Selected Emergency Antidotes With Common Initial Doses*

Antidote	Indication and Dose	Page
N-acetylcysteine	**Acetaminophen:** *Adults IV:* 150 mg/kg in 200 mL D5W infused over 60 min, followed by 50 mg/kg in 500 mL D5W over 4 hours, then 100 mg/kg in 1000 mL D5W over 16 hours. *Oral*: 140 mg/kg, followed by 70 mg/kg every 4 hours for 17 doses. **NOTE:** Special IV dilution required for children.	500
Atropine	**Cholinesterase inhibitors:** *Adults:* 1–5 mg IV, doubled every 3–5 min until bronchorrhea resolves. *Children*: 50 μg/kg (min 0.1 mg; max 0.5 mg) IV, doubled as for adults. **NOTE:** Use 3–5 mg starting dose for adults with severe poisoning. Also for other cholinergics in similar dosing.	1473
L-Carnitine	**Valproic acid–induced hyperammonemia or valproic acid–induced elevated AST/ALT:** *Clinically ill:* 100 mg/kg (up to 6 g) infused IV over 30 min, followed by 15 mg/kg infused over 30 min every 4 hours. *Clinically well:* 100 mg/kg/day oral divided every 6 hours up to 3 grams/day.	711
Deferoxamine	**Iron:** Begin continuous IV infusion at 5 mg/kg/h, titrate to 15 mg/kg/h as tolerated with a total dose of 6–8 g/day.	604
Digoxin-specific antibody fragments (Fab)	**Digoxin:** Known concentration: # of vials = [wt (kg) × concentration (ng/mL)/100] rounded up to nearest vial. Empiric dosing: Acute: 10-20 vials. Chronic: *Adults*: 3–6 vials; *Children*: 1–2 vials. Usually given as IV infusion over 30 min. An IV bolus is acceptable for cardiac arrest. **NOTE: Non-digoxin cardioactive steroids,** use empiric dose.	946
Dimercaprol (BAL)	**Lead encephalopathy:** 75 mg/m^2 (~4 mg/kg) deep IM every 4 hours. First dose to precede edetate calcium disodium ($CaNa_2$ EDTA) by 4 hours. Contraindicated if peanut allergy.	1229
Edetate calcium disodium ($CaNa_2$EDTA)	**Lead encephalopathy:** 1500 mg/m^2/day (~50-75 mg/kg/day) as a continuous IV infusion; maximum dose 3 g/day **NOTE:** Dimercaprol (BAL) should be administered 4 hours prior to starting this dose.	1290
Fomepizole	**Methanol or ethylene glycol:** 15 mg/kg infused IV over 30 min; next 4 doses at 10 mg/kg every 12 hours; additional doses at 15 mg/kg every 12 hours if needed.	1414
Glucagon	**β-Adrenergic antagonists or calcium channel blockers:** IV infusion over 1–2 minutes. *Adults:* 50 μg/kg. *Children:* 50 μg/kg. Dose may be increased up to 10 mg in an adult, as needed.	910
Hydroxocobalamin (Cyanokit)	**Cyanide:** *Adults:* 5 g (2 × 2.5 g). Each 2.5 g reconstituted with 100 mL 0.9% NaCl and infused IV over 7.5 min. *Children*: 70 mg/kg up to 5 g. Repeat second dose as needed. Sodium thiosulfate expected to be synergistic. Do not administer simultaneously through same IV line or inactivation of hydroxocobalamin might occur.	1695
Insulin (Hyperinsulinemic-euglycemic (HIE) therapy	**Calcium channel blockers or β-adrenergic antagonists:** 1 unit/kg IV bolus regular human insulin. Follow with infusion of 0.5 units/kg/h. Titrate to 2 units/kg/h if no improvement in 30 min. Add 0.5 g/kg dextrose if glucose <400 mg/dL. Monitor glucose every 30 min until stable then every 1-2 hours. Maintain glucose 100-250 mg/dL	893
Leucovorin (Folinic acid)	**Methotrexate:** 100 mg/m^2 infused IV over 15–30 min every 3–6 hours for several days or until methotrexate serum conc < 1×10^{-8} M in the absence of bone marrow toxicity.	783
Lipid 20% (Intralipid)	**Cardiac arrest from lipid soluble xenobiotic (CCB, TCA, local anesthetics):** Intralipid 20% 1.5 mL/kg over 1 minute. Follow with infusion at a rate of 0.25 mL/kg/min. Repeat bolus every 3-5 minutes up to 3 mL/kg total dose until circulation is restored. Continue infusion until hemodynamic stability is restored. Increase the rate to 0.5 mL/kg/min if BP declines. Maximum total dose of 8 mL/kg.	976
Methylene blue	**Methemoglobinemia:** 1–2 mg/kg IV over 5 min followed by a 30 mL fluid flush.	1708
Naloxone	**Opioid-induced respiratory depression:** 40-50 μg (0.04-0.05 mg) IV titrated upward to reversal, while avoiding opioid withdrawal.	579
Nitrites and sodium thiosulfate ("Cyanide Antidote Kit")	**Cyanide:** *Adults:* 1) Sodium nitrite: 300 mg (10 mL of a 3% conc) infused IV over 2–5 min. 2) Sodium thiosulfate: 12.5 g (50 mL of a 25% conc) infused IV over 10–30 min or as a bolus. *Children:* 1) Sodium nitrite: 6–8 mL/m^2 (0.2 mL/kg of a 3% conc) (max 300 mg) infused IV over 2–5 min. 2) Sodium thiosulfate: 7 g/m^2 (0.5 g/kg) (max 12.5 g) infused over 10–30 min or as a bolus. NOTE: In both adults and children, avoid sodium nitrite when carboxyhemoglobin is expected to be elevated.	1689
Octreotide	**Sulfonylurea-induced hypoglycemia:** *Adults:* 50 μg SQ every 6 h. *Children:* 1.25 μg/kg (max 50 μg) SQ every 6 hours.	734
Physostigmine	**Anticholinergic syndrome:** IV infusion over 5 min. *Adults:* 1–2 mg. *Children:* 20 μg/kg (max 0.5 mg). The dose can be repeated in 5-10 minutes if an adequate response is not achieved and cholinergic effects are not noted.	759
Pralidoxime	**Cholinesterase inhibitors:** *Adults:* 30 mg/kg (up to 2 grams) over 30 minutes followed by a maintenance infusion of 8 to 10 mg/kg/h (up to 650 mg/h) for sickest patients. *Children:* 20–50 mg/kg (max 1–2 g) infused IV over 30–60 min and then 10–20 mg/kg/h (max 500 mg/h).	1467
Pyridoxine	**Isoniazid:** 1 g for each gram of isoniazid up to 70 mg/kg (max 5 g) infused IV at 0.5 g/min until seizures stop, with the remainder infused IV over 4–6 hours. Empiric dose: *Adults:* 5 g. *Children:* 70 mg/kg at specific dosing rate. May repeat dose if needed.	845
Succimer	**Lead poisoning:** *Adults:* 10 mg/kg orally every 8 hours for five days followed by every 12 hours for 14 days. *Children:* 350 mg/m^2 orally as for adults.	1284

*Consult pages listed for complete information regarding dose, route, duration of therapy, adverse effects, safety issues, contraindications, and other considerations. For up-to-date information, contact your regional poison center at 800-222-1222 or a medical toxicologist.

Goldfrank's Toxicologic Emergencies

NINTH EDITION

Goldfrank's Toxicologic Emergencies

Lewis S. Nelson, MD, FAACT, FACEP, FACMT
Associate Professor of Emergency Medicine
New York University School of Medicine
Attending Physician, Emergency Medicine
Bellevue Hospital Center and New York University Langone Medical Center
Director, Fellowship in Medical Toxicology
New York City Poison Center and New York University School of Medicine
New York, New York

Robert S. Hoffman, MD, FAACT, FACMT
Associate Professor of Emergency Medicine and Medicine (Clinical Pharmacology)
New York University School of Medicine
Attending Physician, Emergency Medicine and Internal Medicine
Bellevue Hospital Center and New York University Langone Medical Center
Director, New York City Poison Center
New York, New York

Neal A. Lewin, MD, FACEP, FACMT, FACP
The Stanley and Fiona Druckenmiller Clinical Professor of Emergency Medicine and Medicine (Pharmacology)
New York University School of Medicine
Director, Didactic Education
Emergency Medicine Residency
Attending Physician, Emergency Medicine and Internal Medicine
Bellevue Hospital Center and New York University Langone Medical Center
Consultant, New York City Poison Center
New York, New York

Lewis R. Goldfrank, MD, FAAEM, FAACT, FACEP, FACMT, FACP
Herbert W. Adams Professor and Chair
Department of Emergency Medicine
New York University School of Medicine
Director, Emergency Medicine
Bellevue Hospital Center and New York University Langone Medical Center
Medical Director, New York City Poison Center
New York, New York

Mary Ann Howland, PharmD, DABAT, FAACT
Clinical Professor of Pharmacy
St. John's University College of Pharmacy
Adjunct Professor of Emergency Medicine
New York University School of Medicine
Bellevue Hospital Center and New York University Langone Medical Center
Senior Consultant in Residence
New York City Poison Center
New York, New York

Neal E. Flomenbaum, MD, FACEP, FACP
Professor of Clinical Medicine
Weill Cornell Medical College of Cornell University
Emergency Physician-in-Chief
New York-Presbyterian Hospital
Weill Cornell Medical Center
Consultant, New York City Poison Center
New York, New York

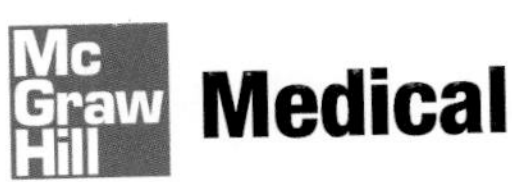

New York Chicago San Francisco Lisbon London Madrid Mexico City
Milan New Delhi San Juan Seoul Singapore Sydney Toronto

Goldfrank's Toxicologic Emergencies, Ninth Edition

The editors' and authors' royalties for this edition, as in the case of the previous editions, are being donated to the department to further the efforts of the New York City Poison Center and to help improve the care of poisoned patients.

2 3 4 5 6 7 8 9 0 CTP/CTP 14 13 12 11

Book ISBN 978-0-07-160593-9
Book MHID 0-07-160593-2
EBook ISBN 978-0-07-160594-6
EBook MHID 0-07-160594-0
OLC ISBN 978-0-07-160595-3
OLC MHID 0-07-160595-9

This book was set in Minion pro by Glyph International.
The editors were Scott Grillo and Christie Naglieri.
The production supervisor was Catherine H. Saggese.
Project management was provided by Gita Raman, Glyph International.
The text designer was Alan Barnett; the cover designer was Pehrsson Design.
China Translation & Printing Services, Ltd was printer and binder.

This book is printed on acid-free paper.

Library of Congress Cataloging-in-Publication Data

Goldfrank's toxicological emergencies.—9th ed./[edited by] Lewis S. Nelson . . . [et al.].
p. ; cm.
Rev. ed. of: Goldfrank's toxicologic emergencies/Neal E. Flomenbaum . . . [et al.]. 8th ed. c2006.
Includes bibliographical references and index.
Summary: "Goldfrank's Toxicological Emergencies is a multi-authored text of approximately 2000 pages prepared by utilizing the education and management principles we apply at the New York City Poison Center and at our clinical sites. In this ninth edition of Goldfrank's Toxicological Emergencies, we proudly offer readers an approach to medical toxicology using evidence based principles viewed through a lens of bedside clinical practice"—Provided by publisher.
ISBN-13: 978-0-07-160593-9 (hardback : alk. paper)
ISBN-10: 0-07-160593-2 (hardback : alk. paper)
1. Toxicological emergencies. 2. Toxicological emergencies—Case studies. I. Nelson, Lewis, 1963- II. Goldfrank, Lewis R., 1941- III. Goldfrank's toxicologic emergencies. IV. Title: Toxicological emergencies.
[DNLM: 1. Emergencies—Case Reports. 2. Emergencies—Examination Questions. 3. Poisoning—Case Reports. 4. Poisoning—Examination Questions. 5. Poisons—Case Reports. 6. Poisons—Examination Questions. QV 600 G618 2011]
RA1224.5.G65 2011
615.9′08—dc22

2009049183

McGraw-Hill books are available at special quantity discounts to use as premiums and sales promotions, or for use in corporate training programs. To contact a representative please e-mail us at bulksales@mcgraw-hill.com.

Digitalis purpurea, the purple foxglove, is a legendary plant that contains the cardiac glycoside digitoxin, closely related to the therapeutically useful but potentially toxic cardiac glycoside digoxin. The electrocardiogram demonstrates high degree atrioventrical nodal blockade in a patient with atrial fibrillation/flutter, an abnormality closely linked to cardioactive steroid poisoning. The vial contains the widely available digoxin-specific Fab antibody fragment that is used to treat poisoning by digoxin and other cardioactive steroids. The 3-dimensional ribbon structure of digoxin specific Fab illustrates its ability engulf and render harmless the active non-glycoside form of the digoxin molecule.

DEDICATION

To the staffs of our hospital emergency departments who have worked with remarkable courage, concern, compassion, and understanding in treating the patients discussed in this text and many thousands more like them

To the staff of the New York City Poison Center who have quietly and conscientiously integrated their skills with ours to serve these patients and to the many others who never needed a hospital visit because of their efforts

To all the faculty, fellows, residents, and students who have studied toxicology with us whose inquisitiveness has helped us continually strive to understand complex and evolving problems and develop methods to teach them to others

To my wife Laura for her unwavering support; to my children Daniel, Adina, and Benjamin for their inquisitiveness and insight; to my parents Dr. Irwin and Myrna Nelson for the foundation they provided; and to my family, friends, and colleagues who keep me focused on what is important in life. (L.N.)

To my wife Gail; to my children Justin and Jesse for their support and patience; and to my parents, who made it possible (N.L.)

To my husband Bob; to my children Robert and Marcy; to my mother and to the loving memory of my father; and to family, friends, colleagues, and students for all their help and continuing inspiration (M.A.H.)

To my wife Ali; my children Casey and Jesse; my parents; and my friends, family, and colleagues for their never-ending patience and forgiveness for the time I have spent away from them (R.H.)

To my children Rebecca, Jennifer, Andrew and Joan, Michelle and James; to my grandchildren Benjamin, Adam, Sarah, Kay, Samantha, and Herbert who have kept me acutely aware of the ready availability of possible poisons; and to my wife, partner, and best friend Susan whose support was and is essential and whose contributions will be found throughout the text (L.G.)

To the memories of my parents Mollie and Lieutenant H. Stanley Flomenbaum whose constant encouragement to help others nonjudgmentally led me to consider toxicologic emergencies many years ago. To my wife Meredith Altman Flomenbaum, RNP, and to my children Adam, David, and Sari who have competed with this text for my attention but who have underscored the importance of these efforts (N.F.)

To the memory of Donald A. Feinfeld, MD. Don was a wonderful collaborator, thoughtful intellectual, nephrologist, and poet who was an active participant at our monthly meetings as well as a critical author for the previous five editions of our text. His warmth, compassion and intellect will be missed.

TABLE OF ANTIDOTES IN DEPTH

Readers of previous editions of Goldfrank's Toxicologic Emergencies *are undoubtedly aware that the editors have always felt that an emphasis on general management of poisoning or overdoses coupled with sound medical management is more important or as important as the selection and use of a specific antidote in the vast majority of cases. Nevertheless, there are some instances where nothing other than the timely use of a specific antidote or therapy will be essential for a patient. For this reason, and also because the use of such strategies may be problematic, controversial, or unfamiliar to the practitioner (as new antidotes continue to emerge), we have included a section (or sections) at the end of each chapter where an in-depth discussion of such antidotes and therapies are relevant. The following Antidotes in Depth are included in this edition.*

TABLE OF CONTENTS

PART A

PART B

SECTION 1

SECTION 2

CONTRIBUTORS

Judith C. Ahronheim, MD
Professor of Medicine
SUNY Downstate
Brooklyn, New York
Adjunct Professor of Medicine and Member
Bioethics Institute, New York Medical College
Valhalla, New York
Chapter 32, "Geriatric Principles"

Kavita M. Babu, MD
Assistant Professor of Emergency Medicine
Brown University Alpert Medical School
Program in Medical Toxicology
Department of Emergency Medicine
Rhode Island Hospital
Providence, Rhode Island
Chapter 25, "Gastrointestinal Principles"
Chapter 82, "Hallucinogens"

Theodore C. Bania, MD, MS
Assistant Professor of Medicine
Columbia University College of Physicians and Surgeons
Director of Research and Toxicology
St. Luke's Roosevelt Hospital Center
New York, New York
Antidote in Depth A21, "Intravenous Fat Emulsions"

Fermin Barrueto, Jr., MD
Clinical Assistant Professor of Emergency Medicine
University of Maryland
Chair, Department of Emergency Medicine
Upper Chesapeake Health Systems
Baltimore, Maryland
Chapter 110, "Sodium Monofluoroacetate and Fluoroacetamide"

James Dave Barry, MD
Program Director, Naval Medical Center
Portsmouth Emergency Medicine Residency
Assistant Adjunct Professor
Uniformed Services University of the Health Sciences
Portsmouth, Virginia
Chapter 58, "Antimalarials"

Joseph M. Betz, PhD
Director, Dietary Supplement Methods and Reference Materials Program
Office of Dietary Supplements
U.S. National Institutes of Health
Bethesda, Maryland
Chapter 118, "Plants"

Michael C. Beuhler, MD, FACMT
Adjunct Assistant Professor of Emergency Medicine
University of North Carolina at Chapel Hill
Medical Director, Carolinas Poison Center
Charlotte, North Carolina
Chapter 111, "Phosphorus"

Steven B. Bird, MD
Assistant Professor of Emergency Medicine
University of Massachusetts Medical School
Worcester, Massachusetts
Chapter 91, "Chromium"

George M. Bosse, MD
Associate Professor of Emergency Medicine
University of Louisville
Medical Director
Kentucky Regional Poison Center
Louisville, Kentucky
Chapter 48, "Antidiabetics and Hypoglycemics"

Nicole C. Bouchard, MD, FRCPC
Assistant Clinical Professor
Columbia University Medical Center
Director of Medical Toxicology
Assistant Site Director
New York-Presbyterian Hospital
New York, New York
Chapter 49, "Thyroid and Antithyroid Medications"

Edward W. Boyer, MD, PhD
Associate Professor of Emergency Medicine
University of Massachusetts Medical School
Chief, Division of Medical Toxicology
UMass-Memorial Medical Center
Worcester, Massachusetts
Chapter 57, "Antituberculous Medications"

Jeffrey R. Brubacher, MD
Assistant Professor
University of British Columbia
Emergency Physician
Vancouver General Hospital
Vancouver, British Columbia, Canada
Chapter 61, "β-Adrenergic Antagonists"

D. Eric Brush, MD
Assistant Professor of Emergency Medicine
Division of Toxicology
University of Massachusetts Medical Center
Worcester, Massachusetts
Chapter 120, "Marine Envenomations"

Keith K. Burkhart, MD
Professor of Clinical Emergency Medicine
Pennsylvania State University College of Medicine
Medical Officer
Center for Drug Evaluation and Research
Food and Drug Administration
Silver Spring, Maryland
Chapter 116, "Methyl Bromide and Other Fumigants"

Michelle Burns Ewald, MD
Assistant Professor of Pediatrics
Harvard Medical School
Fellowship Director, Harvard Medical Toxicology Fellowship
Medical Director, Regional Center for Poison Control and Prevention
Attending Physician, Emergency Medicine
Children's Hospital Boston
Boston, Massachusetts
Chapter 99, "Silver"

Diane P. Calello, MD
Assistant Professor of Pediatrics and Emergency Medicine
Chief, Section of Toxicology
Robert Wood Johnson Medical School
UMDNJ
Staff Toxicologist, New Jersey Poison Information and Education Systems (NJPIES)
New Brunswick, New Jersey
Chapter 98, "Selenium"

Louis R. Cantilena, MD, PhD
Professor of Medicine and Pharmacology
Department of Medicine
Uniformed Services University
Bethesda, Maryland
Chapter 138, "Adverse Drug Events and Postmarketing Surveillance"

Gar Ming Chan, MD
Assistant Clinical Professor of Emergency Medicine
New York University School of Medicine
Attending Physician, North Shore University Hospital
Manhasset, New York
Chapter 92, "Cobalt"

Yiu-cheung Chan, MD, MBBS, FHKAM, FHKCEM, FRCS(Ed)
Associate Consultant, Director of Toxicology Training
Hong Kong Poison Information Centre
Hong Kong SAR, China
Chapter 112, "Strychnine"

Nathan Phillip Charlton, MD
Assistant Professor of Emergency Medicine
University of Virginia
Charlottesville, Virginia
Chapter 128, "Smoke Inhalation"

Alan N. Charney, MD
Clinical Professor of Medicine
New York University School of Medicine
New York, New York
Chapter 16, "Fluid, Electrolyte, and Acid–Base Principles"

William K. Chiang, MD
Associate Professor of Emergency Medicine
New York University School of Medicine
Chief of Emergency Services, Bellevue Hospital Center
Attending Physician
Bellevue Hospital Center and New York University
Langone Medical Center
New York, New York
Chapter 20, "Otolaryngologic Principles"
Chapter 75, "Amphetamines"

Jason Chu, MD
Assistant Professor of Clinical Medicine
Columbia University College of Physicians and Surgeons
Medical Toxicologist
St. Luke's-Roosevelt Hospital Center
New York, New York
Chapter 28, "Genitourinary Principles"
Chapter 51, "Antimigraine Medications"

Richard Church, MD
Fellow in Medical Toxicology
University of Massachusetts Medical Center
Worcester, Massachusetts
Chapter 25, "Gastrointestinal Principles"

Cathleen Clancy, MD
Associate Medical Director
National Capital Poison Center
Associate Professor
Department of Emergency Medicine
George Washington University Medical Center
Attending Physician
Bethesda Naval Emergency Department
Washington, District of Columbia
Chapter 22, "Electrophysiologic and Electrocardiographic Principles"

Richard Franklin Clark, MD
Professor of Medicine
University of California at San Diego
Director, Division of Medical Toxicology
University of California San Diego Medical Center
San Diego, California
Chapter 113, "Insecticides: Organic Phosphorus Compounds and Carbamates"
Antidote in Depth A35, "Antivenom (Scorpion and Spider)"

Steven C. Curry, MD
Director, Department of Medical Toxicology
Banner Good Samaritan Medical Center
Professor of Clinical Medicine
University of Arizona College of Medicine
Phoenix, Arizona
Chapter 13, "Neurotransmitters and Neuromodulators"

John A. Curtis, MD
Assistant Professor of Emergency Medicine
Associate Director, Fellowship in Medical Toxicology
Drexel University College of Medicine
Attending Physician
Hahnemann University Hospital
Philadelphia, Pennsylvania
Chapter 97, "Nickel"

Andrew Dawson, MBBS
Professor, Peradeniya University
Program Director
South Asian Clinical Toxicology Research Collaboration
Peradeniya, Sri Lanka
Chapter 109, "Barium"

Kathleen A. Delaney, MD
Clinical Professor, Division of Emergency Medicine
University of Texas Southwestern Medical School
Dallas, Texas
Chapter 12, "Biochemical and Metabolic Principles"
Chapter 15, "Thermoregulatory Principles"
Chapter 26, "Hepatic Principles"
Antidote in Depth A10, "Dextrose"

Francis Jerome DeRoos, MD
Associate Professor of Emergency Medicine
University of Pennsylvania School of Medicine
Residency Director
Hospital of the University of Pennsylvania
Philadelphia, Pennsylvania
Chapter 60, "Calcium Channel Blockers"
Chapter 62, "Other Antihypertensives"

Suzanne Doyon, MD, FACMT
Medical Director,
Maryland Poison Center
University of Maryland School of Pharmacy
Baltimore, Maryland
Chapter 47, "Anticonvulsants"

Dainius A. Drukteinis, MD, JD
Attending Physician
MetroWest Medical Center
Framingham, Massachusetts
Chapter 140, "Risk Management and Legal Principles"

Michael Eddleston, MD, PhD, MRCP
Clinical Pharmacology Unit
University of Edinburgh
Scottish Poisons Information Bureau
Royal Infirmary of Edinburgh
Edinburgh, United Kingdom
Chapter 113, "Insecticides: Organic Phosphorus Compounds and Carbamates"
Chapter 136, "International Perspectives on Medical Toxicology"

Brenna M. Farmer, MD
Assistant Professor of Medicine
Weill-Cornell Medical College
Attending Physician
New York Presbyterian-Weill-Cornell Medical Center
New York, New York
Chapter 80, "γ-Hydroxybutyric Acid"
Chapter 86, "Aluminum"
Chapter 139, "Medication Safety and Adverse Drug Events"

Donald A. Feinfeld, MD (Deceased)
Nephrology Fellowship Director
Beth Israel Medical Center
Professor of Medicine
Albert Einstein College of Medicine
Consultant in Nephrology
New York City Poison Center
New York, New York
Chapter 27, "Renal Principles"

Kathy Lynn Ferguson, DO
Attending Physician
Emergency Medicine and Medical Toxicology
New York Hospital Queens
Flushing, New York
Chapter 74, "Sedative–Hypnotics"

Jeffrey S. Fine, MD
Assistant Professor of Emergency Medicine and Pediatrics
New York University School of Medicine
Attending Physician
Bellevue Hospital Center and New York University Langone Medical Center New York, New York
Chapter 30, "Reproductive and Perinatal Principles"
Chapter 31, "Pediatric Principles"

Mark A. Flomenbaum, MD, PhD
Associate Professor of Pathology and Laboratory Medicine
Boston University School of Medicine
Director, Autopsy Services
Boston Medical Center
Boston, Massachusetts
Chapter 33, "Postmortem Toxicology"

Neal E. Flomenbaum, MD, FACEP, FACP
Professor of Clinical Medicine
Weill Cornell Medical College of Cornell University
Emergency Physician-in-Chief
New York-Presbyterian Hospital
Weill Cornell Medical Center
Consultant, New York City Poison Center
New York, New York
Chapter 3, "Initial Evaluation of the Patient: Vital Signs and Toxic Syndromes"
Chapter 4, "Principles of Managing the Acutely Poisoned or Overdosed Patient"
Chapter 35, "Salicylates"
Chapter 108, "Pesticides: An Overview of Rodenticides and a Focus on Principles"

Marsha D. Ford, MD
Adjunct Professor of Emergency Medicine
University of North Carolina, Chapel Hill
Director, Carolinas Poison Center
Carolinas Medical Center
Charlotte, North Carolina
Chapter 88, "Arsenic"

Jessica A. Fulton, DO
Attending Physician
Grandview Hospital
Grandview, New Jersey
Chapter 104, "Caustics"

Howard L. Geyer, MD, PhD
Assistant Professor of Neurology
Albert Einstein College of Medicine
Director, Division of Movement Disorders
Montefiore Medical Center
Bronx, New York
Chapter 46, "Botulism"
Antidote in Depth A8, "Botulinum Antitoxin"

Beth Y. Ginsburg, MD
Assistant Professor of Emergency Medicine
Mount Sinai School of Medicine
Attending Physician
Elmhurst Hospital Center
Elmhurst, New York
Chapter 41, "Vitamins"

Jeffrey A. Gold, MD
Associate Professor of Medicine
Oregon Health and Sciences University
Portland, Oregon
Chapter 78, "Ethanol Withdrawal"

David S. Goldfarb, MD
Professor of Medicine and Physiology
New York University School of Medicine
Chief, Nephrology Section
New York Harbor VA Medical Center
New York, New York
Chapter 9, "Principles and Techniques Applied to Enhance Elimination"

Lewis R. Goldfrank, MD, FAACT, FAAEM, FACEP, FACMT, FACP
Herbert W. Adams Professor and Chair
Department of Emergency Medicine
New York University School of Medicine
Director, Emergency Medicine
Bellevue Hospital Center and New York University
Langone Medical Center
Medical Director, New York City Poison Center
New York, New York
Chapter 3, "Initial Evaluation of the Patient: Vital Signs and Toxic Syndromes"
Chapter 4, "Principles of Managing the Acutely Poisoned or Overdosed Patient"
Chapter 117, "Mushrooms"
Antidote in Depth A8, "Botulinum Antitoxin"

Howard A. Greller, MD, FACEP, FACMT
Assistant Professor of Emergency Medicine
New York University School of Medicine
Attending Physician
North Shore University Hospital
Manhasset, New York
Chapter 70, "Lithium"
Workbook Cases and Questions

Martin Griffel, MD
Associate Professor of Anesthesiology
New York University School of Medicine
Director, Cardiovascular ICU
New York University Langone Medical Center
New York, New York
Chapter 67, "Inhalational Anesthetics"

Anne-Bolette Gude, MD
Clinical Pharmacologist
Novo Nordisk
Virum, Denmark
Chapter 7, "Techniques Used to Prevent Gastrointestinal Absorption"

David D. Gummin, MD, FAACT, FACEP, FACMT
Clinical Assistant Professor
Medical College of Wisconsin
Medical Director
Wisconsin Poison Center
Milwaukee, Wisconsin
Chapter 106, "Hydrocarbons"

Jason B. Hack, MD
Associate Professor of Emergency Medicine
Program Director, Medical Toxicology
Brown University, Warren Alpert Medical School
Rhode Island Hospital
Providence, Rhode Island
Chapter 64, "Cardioactive Steroids"

David A. Haggerty, MD
Fellow in Medical Toxicology
Division of Medical Toxicology
Department of Emergency Medicine
Drexel University College of medicine
Philadelphia, Pennsylvania
Chapter 97, "Nickel"

In-Hei Hahn, MD
Assistant Professor of Clinical Medicine
Columbia University College of Physicians and Surgeons
Associate Attending, Emergency Medicine
Assistant Director of Research
St. Luke's-Roosevelt Hospital Center, Danbury Hospital
New York, New York
Chapter 119, "Arthropods"

Sarah Eliza Halcomb, MD
Assistant Professor of Emergency Medicine
Washington University School of Medicine
Section Chief - Medical Toxicology
Washington University-Barnes-Jewish Hospital
St. Louis, Missouri
Chapter 42, "Essential Oils"

Richard J. Hamilton, MD
Professor and Chairman of Emergency Medicine
Drexel University College of Medicine
Philadelphia, Pennsylvania
Chapter 14, "Withdrawal Principles"

Nikolas B. Harbord, MD
Assistant Professor of Medicine
Albert Einstein College of Medicine
Attending Nephrologist
Beth Israel Medical Center
Brooklyn, New York
Chapter 27, "Renal Principles"

Robert G. Hendrickson, MD
Associate Professor of Emergency Medicine
Oregon Health and Science University
Associate Medical Director
Oregon Poison Center
Emergency Physician and Medical Toxicologist
Oregon Health and Science University
Portland, Oregon
Chapter 34, "Acetaminophen"
Antidote in Depth A4, "N-Acetylcysteine"

Fred M. Henretig, MD
Professor of Pediatrics and Emergency Medicine
University of Pennsylvania School of Medicine
Director, Section of Clinical Toxicology
Children's Hospital of Philadelphia
Philadelphia, Pennsylvania
Chapter 94, "Lead"

Christina H. Hernon, MD
Assistant Professor of Emergency Medicine
University of Massachusetts Medical School
Division of Medical Toxicology
University of Massachusetts Memorial Medical Center
Worcester, Massachusetts
Chapter 57, "Antituberculous Medications"

Robert A. Hessler, MD, PhD
Associate Professor of Emergency Medicine
New York University School of Medicine
Attending Physician
Bellevue Hospital Center, New York University Langone Medical Center and Veterans Administration Medical Center, Manhattan
New York, New York
Chapter 23, " Hemodynamic Principles"

Lotte C. G. Hoegberg, MS (Pharm), PhD
Pharmacist, Danish Poison Information Centre
Copenhagen, Denmark
Chapter 7, "Techniques Used to Prevent Gastrointestinal Absorption"

Robert J. Hoffman, MD, MS
Assistant Professor
Albert Einstein College of Medicine
Research Director
Beth Israel Medical Center
New York, New York
Chapter 65, "Methylxanthines and Selective β_2 Adrenergic Agonists"

Robert S. Hoffman, MD, FAACT, FACMT
Associate Professor of Emergency Medicine and Medicine (Pharmacology)
New York University School of Medicine
Attending Physician, Emergency Medicine and Internal Medicine
Bellevue Hospital Center and New York University Langone Medical Center
Director, New York City Poison Center
New York, New York
Chapter 3, "Initial Evaluation of the Patient: Vital Signs and Toxic Syndromes"
Chapter 4, "Principles of Managing the Acutely Poisoned or Overdosed Patient"
Chapter 16, "Fluid, Electrolyte, and Acid-Base Principles"
Chapter 21, "Respiratory Principles"
Chapter 76, "Cocaine"
Chapter 90, "Cadmium"
Chapter 100, "Thallium"
Chapter 135, "Poison Centers and Poison Epidemiology"
Antidote in Depth A24, "Benzodiazepines"
Antidote in Depth A25, "Thiamine Hydrochloride"
Antidote in Depth A29, "Prussian Blue"

Michael G. Holland, MD, FAACT, FACEP, FACMT, FACOEM
Clinical Assistant Professor
SUNY Upstate Medical University
Consultant Medical Toxicologist
Upstate New York Poison Center
Syracuse, New York
Attending Physician
Center for Occupational Health at Glens Falls Hospital
Glens Falls, New York
Chapter 114, "Insecticides: Organic Chlorines, Pyrethrins/Pyrethroids, and Insect Repellents"

Christopher P. Holstege, MD
Associate Professor of Emergency Medicine and Pediatrics
University of Virginia School of Medicine
Director, Division of Medical Toxicology
University of Virginia Health System
Charlottesville, Virginia
Chapter 126, "Cyanide and Hydrogen Sulfide"

William J. Holubek, MD
Attending Physician
Department of Emergency Medicine
New York Methodist Hospital
Brooklyn, New York
Chapter 36, "Nonsteroidal Antiinflammatory Drugs"

Mary Ann Howland, PharmD, DABAT, FAACT
Clinical Professor of Pharmacy
St. John's University
College of Pharmacy
Adjunct Professor of Emergency Medicine
New York University School of Medicine
Bellevue Hospital Center and New York University
Langone Medical Center
Senior Consultant in Residence
New York City Poison Center
New York, New York
Chapter 3, "Initial Evaluation of the Patient: Vital Signs and Toxic Syndromes"
Chapter 4, "Principles of Managing the Acutely Poisoned or Overdosed Patient"
Chapter 8, "Pharmacokinetic and Toxicokinetic Principles"
Chapter 32, "Geriatric Principles"
Antidote in Depth A1, "Syrup of Ipecac"
Antidote in Depth A2, "Activated Charcoal"
Antidote in Depth A3, "Whole-Bowel Irrigation and Other Intestinal Evacuants"
Antidote in Depth A4, "N-Acetylcysteine"
Antidote in Depth A6, "Opioid Antagonists"
Antidote in Depth A7, "Deferoxamine"
Antidote in Depth A9, "L-Carnitine"
Antidote in Depth A11, "Octreotide"
Antidote in Depth A12, "Physostigmine Salicylate"
Antidote in Depth A13, "Leucovorin (Folinic Acid) and Folic Acid"
Antidote in Depth A15, "Pyridoxine"
Antidote in Depth A16, "Vitamin K_1"
Antidote in Depth A17, "Protamine"
Antidote in Depth A19, "Glucagon"
Antidote in Depth A20, "Digoxin-Specific Antibody Fragments (Fab)"
Antidote in Depth A23, "Flumazenil"
Antidote in Depth A24, "Benzodiazepines"
Antidote in Depth A26, "Dimercaprol (British Anti-Lewisite or BAL)"
Antidote in Depth A27, "Succimer (2,3-Dimercaptosuccinic Acid)"
Antidote in Depth A28, "Edetate Calcium Disodium ($CaNa_2EDTA$)"
Antidote in Depth A30, "Calcium"
Antidote in Depth A31, "Fomepizole"
Antidote in Depth A32, "Ethanol"
Antidote in Depth A33, "Pralidoxime"
Antidote in Depth A34, "Atropine"
Antidote in Depth A38, "Sodium and Amyl Nitrite"
Antidote in Depth A39, "Sodium Thiosulfate"
Antidote in Depth A40, "Hydroxocobalamin"
Antidote in Depth A41, "Methylene Blue"

Oliver L. Hung, MD
Attending Physician
Department of Emergency Medicine
Morristown Memorial Hospital
Morristown, New Jersey
Chapter 43, "Herbal Preparations"

Gary E. Isom, PhD
Professor of Toxicology
Purdue University
Clinical Assistant Professor of Pharmacology
Indiana University School of Medicine
West Lafayette, Indiana
Chapter 126, "Cyanide and Hydrogen Sulfide"

David N. Juurlink, BPhm, MD, PhD, FAACT, FACMT, FRCPC
Associate Professor, Faculty of Medicine
University of Toronto
Division Head, Clinical Pharmacology and Toxicology
Sunnybrook Health Sciences Centre
Toronto, Ontario, Canada
Chapter 69, "Antipsychotics"

Bradley J. Kaufman, MD, MPH
Assistant Professor, Department of Emergency Medicine
Albert Einstein College of Medicine
Bronx, New York
Attending Physician
Department of Emergency Medicine
Long Island Jewish Medical Center
New Hyde Park, New York
Division Medical Director
Fire Department of the City of New York
New York, New York
Chapter 130, "Hazmat Incident Response"

Brian Kaufman, MD
Associate Professor of Medicine, Anesthesiology and Neurosurgery
New York University School of Medicine
Co-Director Critical Care
New York University Langone Medical Center
New York, New York
Chapter 66, "Local Anesthetics"
Chapter 67, "Inhalational Anesthetics"

William Kerns, II, MD, FACEP, FACMT
Medical Toxicology Fellowship Director
Division of Medical Toxicology
Department of Emergency Medicine and
Carolinas Poison Center
Attending Toxicologist
Carolinas Medical Center and Carolinas Poison Center
Charlotte, North Carolina
Antidote in Depth A18, "Insulin-Euglycemia Therapy"

Mark A. Kirk, MD
Associate Professor of Emergency Medicine and Pediatrics
University of Virginia
Charlottesville, Virginia
Special Advisor for Chemical Defense and Medical Toxicology
Office of Health Affairs
Department of Homeland Security
Washington, DC
Chapter 10, "Use of the Intensive Care Unit"
Chapter 126, "Cyanide and Hydrogen Sulfide"
Chapter 128, "Smoke Inhalation"

Barbara M. Kirrane, MD
Assistant Professor of Emergency Medicine
Yale University
Attending Physician
New Haven, Connecticut
Chapter 140, "Risk Management and Legal Principles"

Kurt C. Kleinschmidt, MD
Professor of Surgery, Division of Emergency Medicine
University of Texas Southwestern Medical Center
Medical Director, Toxicology
Parkland Memorial Hospital
Dallas, Texas
Chapter 12, "Biochemical and Metabolic Principles"

Edwin K. Kuffner, MD
Senior Director for Medical Affairs
McNeil Pharmaceuticals
Fort Washington, Pennsylvania
Chapter 79, "Disulfiram and Disulfiramlike Reactions"
Chapter 103, "Camphor and Moth Repellents"

Melisa W. Lai Becker, MD
Instructor, Harvard Medical School
Director, Division of Medical Toxicology
Emergency Physician
Department of Emergency Medicine
Cambridge Health Alliance
Cambridge, Massachusetts
Chapter 99, "Silver"

David C. Lee, MD
Clinical Associate Professor of Emergency Medicine
New York University School of Medicine
Director of Research
North Shore University Hospital–Manhasset
Manhasset, New York
Chapter 74, "Sedative–Hypnotics"

Neal A. Lewin, MD, FACEP, FACMT, FACP
The Stanley and Fiona Druckenmiller Clinical Professor of Emergency Medicine and Medicine (Pharmacology)
New York University School of Medicine
Director, Didactic Education
Emergency Medicine Residency
Attending Physician, Emergency Medicine and Internal Medicine
Bellevue Hospital Center and New York University Langone Medical Center
Consultant, New York City Poison Center
New York, New York
Chapter 3, "Initial Evaluation of the Patient: Vital Signs and Toxic Syndromes"
Chapter 4, "Principles of Managing the Acutely Poisoned or Overdosed Patient"
Chapter 29, "Dermatologic Principles"
Chapter 63, "Antidysrhythmics"

Erica L. Liebelt, MD
Professor of Pediatrics and Emergency Medicine
University of Alabama at Birmingham School of Medicine
Director Medical Toxicology Services
Birmingham, Alabama
Chapter 73, "Cyclic Antidepressants"

Heather Long, MD
Assistant Professor of Emergency Medicine
Albany Medical Center
Albany, New York
Chapter 81, "Inhalants"

Nima Majlesi, DO
Research Director
Attending Physician
Staten Island University Hospital
Staten Island, New York
Chapter 101, "Zinc"

Kishor Malavade, MD
Clinical Assistant Professor of Psychiatry
New York University School of Medicine
Director, Comprehensive Psychiatric Emergency Program
Bellevue Hospital Center
New York, New York
Chapter 17, "Psychiatric Principles"

Alex F. Manini, MD, MS
Assistant Professor of Emergency Medicine
Mount Sinai School of Medicine
Co-Director, Toxicology Service and Attending Physician
Elmhurst Hospital Center
New York, New York
Chapter 71, "Monoamine Oxidase Inhibitors"

Jeanna M. Marraffa, PharmD, DABAT
Assistant Professor of Emergency Medicine and Medicine
Section of Clinical Pharmacology
SUNY Upstate Medical University
Clinical Toxicologist
Upstate New York Poison Center
Clinical Toxicologist
Syracuse, New York
Chapter 39, "Dieting Agents and Regimens"

Michael A. McGuigan, MDCM, MBA
Clinical Professor of Emergency Medicine
State University of New York
Stony Brook, New York
Medical Director
Long Island Regional Poison and Drug Information Center
Mineola, New York
Chapter 83, "Cannabinoids"

Charles A. McKay, Jr., MD
Associate Professor of Emergency Medicine
University of Connecticut School of Medicine
Section Chief, Division of Medical Toxicology
Hartford Hospital
Hartford, Connecticut
Chapter 129, "Risk Assessment and Risk Communication"

Maria Mercurio-Zappala, RPh, MS
Associate Director
New York City Poison Control Center
New York, New York
Chapter 100, "Thallium"

Kirk Charles Mills, MD, FACMT
Medical Toxicologist
Wayne State University
Detroit Medical Center
Detroit, Michigan
Chapter 13, "Neurotransmitters and Neuromodulators"

Stephen W. Munday, MD, MPH, MS
Clinical Assistant Professor
University of California, San Diego
Medical Toxicologist
Sharp Rees Stealy Medical Group
San Diego, California
Chapter 88, "Arsenic"

Lewis S. Nelson, MD, FAACT, FACEP, FACMT
Associate Professor of Emergency Medicine
New York University School of Medicine
Attending Physician, Emergency Medicine
Bellevue Hospital Center and New York University
Langone Medical Center
Director, Fellowship in Medical Toxicology
New York City Poison Center and New York University School of Medicine
New York, New York
Chapter 3, "Initial Evaluation of the Patient: Vital Signs and Toxic Syndromes"
Chapter 4, "Principles of Managing the Acutely Poisoned or Overdosed Patient"
Chapter 11, "Chemical Principles"
Chapter 29, "Dermatologic Principles"
Chapter 38, "Opioids"
Chapter 63, "Antidysrhythmics"
Chapter 78, "Ethanol Withdrawal"
Chapter 93, "Copper"
Chapter 124, "Simple Asphyxiants and Pulmonary Irritants"
Antidotes in Depth A6, "Opioid Antagonists"
Antidotes in Depth A24, "Benzodiazepines"

Sean Patrick Nordt, MD, PharmD
Adjunct Assistant Clinical Professor of Medicine
University of California, San Diego
Fellow in Medical Toxicology
Division of Medical Toxicology and
Department of Emergency Medicine
San Diego, California
Chapter 55, "Pharmaceutical Additives"

Ayrn D. O'Connor, MD
Clinical Assistant Professor of Emergency Medicine
Department of Emergency Medicine
University of Arizona College of Medicine
Assistant Fellowship Director
Department of Medical Toxicology
Banner Good Samaritan Medical Center
Phoenix, Arizona
Chapter 13, "Neurotransmitter Principles"

Oladapo A. Odujebe, MD, MT-ACSP
Assistant Professor of Emergency Medicine
Emory University
Medical Toxicologist
Georgia Poison Control Center
Atlanta, Georgia
Chapter 124, "Simple Asphyxiants and Pulmonary Irritants"

Ruben E. Olmedo, MD
Clinical Assistant Professor of Emergency Medicine
Mount Sinai Hospital
Director, Division of Toxicology
Mount Sinai School of Medicine
New York, New York
Chapter 85 "Phencyclidine and Ketamine"

Dean G. Olsen, DO
Attending Staff
New York City Poison Center
Assistant Professor
New York College of Osteopathic Medicine
Old Westbury, New York
Director of Research
Attending Physician
Emergency Medicine, Toxicology
St. Barnabas Hospital
Bronx, New York
Chapter 38, "Opioids"
Work Book: Cases and Questions

Kevin C. Osterhoudt, MD, MS
Associate Professor of Pediatrics and Emergency Medicine
The University of Pennsylvania School of Medicine
Medical Director, The Poison Control Center at The Children's Hospital of Philadelphia
Philadelphia, Pennsylvania
Chapter 137, "Principles of Epidemiology and Research Design"

Mary Emery Palmer, MD
Director, ToxEM LLC
Clinical Assistant Professor of Emergency Medicine
The George Washington University
Washington, District of Columbia
Chapter 118, "Plants"

Jeanmarie Perrone, MD, FACMT
Associate Professor of Emergency Medicine
University of Pennsylvania School of Medicine,
Director, Division of Medical Toxicology
Hospital of the University of Pennsylvania
Philadelphia, Pennsylvania
Chapter 40, "Iron"

Anthony F. Pizon, MD
Assistant Professor
University of Pittsburgh School of Medicine
Medical Director, West Virginia Poison Center
UPMC Presbyterian
Pittsburgh, Pennsylvania
Chapter 121, "Snakes and Other Reptiles"
Antidotes in Depth A36, "Antivenom (Crotaline)"

Dennis P. Price, MD
Assistant Professor of Emergency Medicine
New York University School of Medicine
New York, New York
Attending Physician
Bellevue Hospital Center and New York University
Langone Medical Center
Chapter 127, "Methemoglobin Inducers"

Jane M. Prosser, MD
Assistant Professor
New York Presbyterian Hospital
Weill Cornell Medical College
New York, New York
Chapter 76, "Cocaine"
Special Considerations SC-4, "Internal Concealment of Xenobiotics"

Petrie M. Rainey, MD, PhD
Professor of Laboratory Medicine
University of Washington School of Medicine
Director of Clinical Chemistry
University of Washington Medical Center
Seattle, Washington
Chapter 6, "Laboratory Principles"

Rama B. Rao, MD, FACMT
Assistant Professor
Weill-Cornell Medical College
Emergency Physician and Medical Toxicologist
New York Presbyterian Hospital at the
Weill Cornell Medical Center
New York, New York
Chapter 18, "Neurologic Principles"
Chapter 33, "Postmortem Toxicology"
Chapter 89, "Bismuth"
Special Considerations SC-1, "Organ Procurement from Poisoned Patients"
Special Considerations SC-2, "Intrathecal Administration of Xenobiotics"

Joseph G. Rella, MD
Assistant Professor of Emergency Medicine
School of Medicine and Dentistry of New Jersey
Attending Physician
University Hospital
Newark, New Jersey
Chapter 133, "Radiation"
Antidotes in Depth A42, "Potassium Iodide"
Antidotes in Depth A43, "DTPA [Pentetic Acid or Pentetate (Zinc or Calcium) Trisodium]"

Bradley D. Riley, MD
Assistant Medical Director
Helen DeVos Children's Hospital Regional Poison Center
Attending Physician
Spectrum Health Department of Emergency Medicine
Grand Rapids, Michigan
Chapter 121, "Snakes and Other Reptiles"
Antidotes in Depth A36, "Antivenom (Crotaline)"

Darren M. Roberts, BPharm, MBBS, PhD
Adjunct Associate Professor
University of Canberra
Medical Officer
The Canberra Hospital
Garran, ACT, Australia
Chapter 115, "Herbicides"

Anne-Michelle Ruha, MD
Director, Medical Toxicology Fellowship Program
Banner Good Samaritan Medical Center
Clinical Assistant Professor of Emergency Medicine
University of Arizona College of Medicine
Phoenix, Arizona
Chapter 13, "Neurotransmitters and Neuromodulators"
Chapter 121, "Snakes and Other Reptiles"
Antidotes in Depth A36, "Antivenom (Crotaline)"

Joshua G. Schier, MD, FACMT
Assistant Professor of Emergency Medicine
Section of Toxicology
Emory University School of Medicine
Medical Toxicologist
Centers for Disease Control and Prevention
Chamblee, Georgia
Chapter 37, "Colchicine, Podophyllin, and Vinca Alkaloids"
Special Considerations SC-5, "Diethylene Glycol"

David R. Schwartz, MD
Assistant Professor of Medicine
New York University School of Medicine
Section Chief, Critical Care Medicine
New York University Langone Medical Center
New York, New York
Chapter 66, "Local Anesthetics"

David T. Schwartz, MD
Associate Professor of Emergency Medicine
New York University School of Medicine
Attending Physician
Bellevue Hospital Center and New York University Langone Medical Center
New York, New York
Chapter 5, "Diagnostic Imaging"

Lauren Schwartz, MPH
Public Education Coordinator
New York City Poison Center
New York, New York
Chapter 134, "Poison Prevention and Education"

Mark R. Serper, PhD
Associate Professor of Psychology
Hofstra University
Research Associate Professor of Psychiatry
New York University School of Medicine
New York, New York
Chapter 17, "Psychiatric Principles"

Adhi Sharma, MD
Assistant Professor of Emergency Medicine
Mount Sinai School of Medicine
Chairman, Emergency Medicine
Good Samaritan Hospital Medical Center
West Islip, New York
Chapter 19, "Ophthalmic Principles"

Marco L. A. Sivilotti, MD, MSc
Associate Professor of Emergency Medicine,
Pharmacology and Toxicology
Queen's University
Kingston, Ontario Canada
Consultant, Ontario Poison Centre
Hospital for Sick Children
Toronto, Ontario, Canada
Chapter 24, "Hematologic Principles"

Silas W. Smith, MD
Assistant Professor of Emergency Medicine
Assistant Director of Medical Toxicology Fellowship Program
New York University School of Medicine
Attending Physician
Bellevue Hospital Center and New York University
Langone Medical Center
New York, New York
Chapter 123, "Nanotoxicology"
Antidote in Depth 14, "Glucarpidase (Carboxypeptidase G_2)"

Sari Soghoian, MD
Assistant Professor of Emergency Medicine
New York University School of Medicine
Attending Physician
Bellevue Hospital Center and New York University
Langone Medical Center
New York, New York
Chapter 84, "Nicotine"
Chapter 95, "Manganese"

Andrew Stolbach, MD
Assistant Professor of Emergency Medicine
Johns Hopkins University School of Medicine
Attending Physician
Johns Hopkins Hospital
Baltimore, Maryland
Chapter 21, Respiratory Principles

Christine M. Stork, PharmD, DABAT
Clinical Associate Professor of Emergency Medicine, Medicine and Pharmacology
Upstate Medical University
Clinical Director
Upstate New York Poison Center
Syracuse, New York
Chapter 56, " Antibacterials, Antifungals, and Antivirals"
Chapter 72, "Serotonin Reuptake Inhibitors and Atypical Antidepressants"

Mark Su, MD
Assistant Professor of Emergency Medicine
SUNY Downstate Medical Center
Attending Physician
North Shore University Hospital
Manhasset, New York
Chapter 59, "Anticoagulants"
Chapter 105, "Hydrofluoric Acid and Fluorides"

Jeffrey R. Suchard, MD, FACEP, FACMT
Professor of Clinical Emergency Medicine
Director of Medical Toxicology
University of California, Irvine Medical Center
Orange, California
Chapter 131, "Chemical Weapons"
Chapter 132, "Biological Weapons"

Young-Jin Sue, MD
Clinical Associate Professor of Pediatrics
Division of Pediatric Emergency Medicine
Albert Einstein College of Medicine
Attending Physician
Pediatric Emergency Services
Children's Hospital at Montefiore
Bronx, New York
Chapter 96, "Mercury"

Kenneth M. Sutin, MD
Associate Professor of Anesthesiology and Surgery
New York University School of Medicine
Director of Critical Care and PACU
Department of Anesthesiology
Bellevue Hospital Center
New York, New York
Chapter 68, "Neuromuscular Blockers"
Antidotes in Depth A22, "Dantrolene Sodium"

Asim F. Tarabar, MD, MS
Assistant Professor of Surgery
Section of Emergency Medicine
Department of Surgery
Yale University School of Medicine
Yale New Haven Hospital
New Haven, Connecticut
Chapter 87, "Antimony"

Stephen R. Thom, MD, PhD
Professor of Emergency Medicine
Chief, Hyperbaric Medicine
University of Pennsylvania
Philadelphia, Pennsylvania
Antidotes in Depth A37, "Hyperbaric Oxygen"

Anthony J. Tomassoni, MD, MS
Assistant Professor of Emergency Medicine
Division of Emergency Medical Services
Yale University School of Medicine
Medical Director, Yale New Haven Center for Healthcare Solutions
Yale New Haven Health System
New Haven, Connecticut
Chapter 50,"Antihistamines and Decongestants"

Christian Tomaszewski, MD
Clinical Associate Professor of Emergency Medicine
Department of Emergency Medicine
University of California San Diego
Division of Medical Toxicology
University of California San Diego Medical Center
San Diego, California
Chapter 125, "Carbon Monoxide"

Stephen J. Traub, MD
Assistant Professor of Medicine
Harvard Medical School
Division of Toxicology and Department of Emergency Medicine
Beth Israel Deaconess Medical Center
Boston, Massachusetts
Chapter 11, "Chemical Principles"
Chapter 90, "Cadmium"

Michael G. Tunik, MD
Associate Professor of Emergency Medicine
New York University School of Medicine
Attending Physician
Bellevue Hospital Center
New York, New York
Chapter 45, "Food Poisoning"

Susi U. Vassallo, MD
Associate Professor of Emergency Medicine
New York University School of Medicine
Attending Physician
Bellevue Hospital Center and New York University Langone Medical Center
New York, New York
Chapter 15, "Thermoregulatory Principles"
Chapter 44, "Athletic Performance Enhancers"

Larissa I. Velez, MD
Associate Professor, Associate Program Director
University of Texas Southwestern Medical Center
Staff Toxicologist, North Texas Poison Center
Parkland Health and Hospital System
Dallas, Texas
Antidotes in Depth A10, "Dextrose"

Lisa E. Vivero, PharmD
Manager Drug Information
MedImpact
San Diego, California
Chapter 55, "Pharmaceutical Additives"

Peter H. Wald, MD, MPH
Vice President, Enterprise Medical Director
USAA
San Antonio, Texas
Chapter 122, "Industrial Poisoning: Information and Control"

Richard Y. Wang, DO
Medical Officer
National Center for Environmental Health
Centers for Disease Control and Prevention
Chamblee, Georgia
Chapter 52, "Antineoplastics Overview"
Chapter 53, "Antineoplastics: Methotrexate"
Chapter 54, "Miscellaneous Antineoplastics"
Special Considerations SC-3, "Extravasation of Xenobiotics"

Paul M. Wax, MD, FACMT
Professor, Division of Emergency Medicine
University of Texas Southwestern Medical School
Medical Director, Toxicology Clinic
Dallas, Texas
Executive Director
American College of Medical Toxicology
Phoenix, Arizona
Chapter 1, "Historical Principles and Perspectives"
Chapter 2, "Toxicologic Plagues and Disasters in History"
Chapter 102, "Antiseptics, Disinfectants and Sterilants"
Antidotes in Depth A5, "Sodium Bicarbonate"

Richard S. Weisman, PharmD, DABAT
Associate Dean
University of Miami Miller School of Medicine
Director, Florida Poison Center–Miami
Miami, Florida
Chapter 50,"Antihistamines and Decongestants"

Sage W. Wiener, MD
Assistant Professor of Emergency Medicine
SUNY Downstate Medical Center
Director of Medical Toxicology
SUNY Downstate Medical Center/Kings County Hospital
Brooklyn, New York
Chapter 107, "Toxic Alcohols"

Luke Yip, MD
Assistant Professor
School of Pharmacy, University of Colorado Health Sciences Center
Attending, Rocky Mountain Poison and Drug Center
Attending, Department of Medicine
Denver Health Medical Center
Denver, Colorado
Chapter 77, "Ethanol"

PREFACE

Goldfrank's Toxicologic Emergencies is a multi-authored text of close to 2000 pages prepared by using the education and management principles we apply at the New York City Poison Center and at our clinical sites. In this ninth edition of *Goldfrank's Toxicologic Emergencies*, we proudly offer readers an approach to medical toxicology using evidence-based principles viewed through a lens of bedside clinical practice. The case history is no longer incorporated in the chapter, but these cases and the critical questions appropriate for discussion are available on the website initially established in the eighth edition. We believe that this supplementary use of the cases recreates a learning environment much like the original text published in 1976 and permits us to use additional text space without creating a heavier, less portable text. In this edition, all the chapters have been revised, and several new chapters have been added. The greatest additions are found in the form of both Antidotes in Depth and Special Considerations, which allow us to address major advances in thought in a highly focused fashion.

Our goal is to assist in understanding new intellectual approaches with an emphasis on the ever-expanding role of medical and clinical toxicologists at the beginning of the twenty-first century. We have continued to increase the number of nationally and internationally known authors who have expertise in their respective areas by reassigning many of the chapters to these experts.

The ninth edition expands on our progress in the eighth edition to use the electronic format. The book has been dramatically improved with the use of full-color graphics and a single art style that will expand and enhance the educational value of the imagery of each chapter and of the image section on the website.

The complete "text" now consists of a hard copy component that offers readers the option of holding while consulting, as they have done previously, as well as an electronic workbook component available on our website (goldfrankstoxicology.com).

The workbook, which includes both case studies and annotated multiple-choice questions, is now available on this website and is dramatically enhanced. Many of the cases are relevant classic examples of toxicologic emergencies, and the remainder are new, extensively discussed cases from our regional monthly meetings at the New York City Poison Center. The collective wisdom of many of the current and former text authors continues to guide these sessions as it has for 30 years. Drs. Lewis S. Nelson and Robert S. Hoffman have analyzed these problems, distilled the discussions, and recreated the spirit of these meetings in the printed versions of the cases. Revised annotated multiple-choice questions based on each chapter were developed by the respective chapter authors and edited by Drs. Howard A. Greller and Dean G. Olsen to enhance self-learning and meet the intellectual needs of our readers. Each question has been meticulously meta-tagged by these editors. This allows the learner to sort by a variety of test strategies that are focused on a particular xenobiotic, clinical finding, or therapeutic strategy, to name a few, with the goal of improved individualized learning.

The rewriting and reorganization of this edition of the text has again required an enormous personal effort by each author and the editors as it has in the past, which we hope will facilitate reading, learning, and better patient care. Work on the next edition of this text literally begins the day that the current edition is published because this is such a rapidly evolving field. Although "tearing down" and reconstructing the text between each edition is an extreme exercise, it prevents the editors from accepting and promulgating unfounded treatments and outdated concepts. We hope that you agree that this exercise is worthwhile and that each "new text" continues to serve you well. As always, we encourage your thoughtful comments, and we will do our best, as always, to incorporate your suggestions into future editions.

If this text helps to provide better patient care and stimulates interest in medical toxicology for students of medicine, nursing, and pharmacy and by residents, fellows, and faculty in diverse specialties, our efforts will have indeed been worthwhile.

Lewis S. Nelson
Neal A. Lewin
Mary Ann Howland
Robert S. Hoffman
Lewis R. Goldfrank
Neal E. Flomenbaum

ACKNOWLEDGMENTS

We are grateful to Joan Demas, who worked with authors across the country and the world to ensure that their ideas were effectively expressed. She has assisted all of us in checking the facts, finding essential references, improving the structure and function of our text while dedicating her efforts to ensuring the precision and rigor of the text. The authors' and editors' work is better because of her devotion to excellence, calm demeanor in the face of editorial chaos and consistent presence throughout each stage of the production of this text.

The many letters and verbal communications we have received with the reviews of the previous editions of this book continue to improve our efforts. We are deeply indebted to our friends, associates, and students, who stimulated us to begin this book with their questions and then faithfully criticized our answers.

We thank the many volunteers, students, librarians, and particularly the St. John's University College of Pharmacy students and drug information staff who provide us with vital technical assistance in our daily attempts to deal with toxicologic emergencies.

No words can adequately express our indebtedness to the many authors who worked on earlier editions of many of the chapters in this book. As different authors write and rewrite topics with each new edition, we recognize that without the foundation work of their predecessors this book would not be what it is today.

We appreciate the creative and rigorous advances in design and scientific art that the Mc-Graw Hill team, led by Armen Ovsepyan, Anne Sydor, and John Williams have added to the text. The devotion to the creation of high quality art graphics and tables is greatly appreciated. Anne Sydor's commitment to excellence is most easily recognized in the immense progress in the aesthetics and intellectual rigor of our text.

We appreciate the calm, thoughtful, and cooperative spirit of Karen Edmonson at McGraw-Hill. Her intelligence and ever vigilant commitment to our efforts has been wonderful. We are pleased with the creative developmental editorial efforts of Christie Naglieri. The organized project management by Gita Raman has found errors hiding throughout our pages. Her carefully posed questions have facilitated the process of correcting the text. It has been a pleasure to have her assistance. We greatly appreciate the compulsion and rigor that Kathrin Unger has applied to make this edition's index one of unique value. We appreciate the work of Catherine Saggese in ensuring the quality of production in the finished work.

CHAPTER 1
HISTORICAL PRINCIPLES AND PERSPECTIVES

Paul M. Wax

The term *poison* first appeared in the English literature around the year 1230 A.D. to describe a potion or draught that was prepared with deadly ingredients.[41,140] The history of poisons and poisoning, however, dates back thousands of years. Throughout the millennia, poisons have played an important role in human history—from political assassination in Roman times, to weapons of war, to contemporary environmental concerns, and to weapons of terrorism.

This chapter offers a perspective on the impact of poisons and poisoning on history. It also provides a historic overview of human understanding of poisons and the development of toxicology from antiquity to the present. The development of the modern poison control center, the genesis of the field of medical toxicology, and the recent increasing focus on medication errors and biologic and chemical weapons are examined. Chapter 2 describes poison plagues and unintentional disasters throughout history and examines the societal consequences of these unfortunate events. An appreciation of past failures and mistakes in dealing with poisons and poisoning promotes a keener insight and a more critical evaluation of present-day toxicologic issues and helps in the assessment and management of future toxicologic problems.

POISONS, POISONERS, AND ANTIDOTES OF ANTIQUITY

The earliest poisons consisted of plant extracts, animal venoms, and minerals. They were used for hunting, waging war, and sanctioned and unsanctioned executions. The *Ebers Papyrus*, an ancient Egyptian text written about 1500 B.C. that is considered to be among the earliest medical texts, describes many ancient poisons, including aconite, antimony, arsenic, cyanogenic glycosides, hemlock, lead, mandrake, opium, and wormwood.[91,140] These poisons were thought to have mystical properties, and their use was surrounded by superstition and intrigue. Some agents, such as the Calabar bean (*Physostigma venenosum*) containing physostigmine, were referred to as "ordeal poisons." Ingestion of these substances was believed to be lethal to the guilty and harmless to the innocent.[91] The "penalty of the peach" involved the administration of peach pits, which we now know contain the cyanide precursor amygdalin, as an ordeal poison. Magicians, sorcerers, and religious figures were the toxicologists of antiquity. The Sumerians, in about 4500 B.C., were said to worship the deity Gula, who was known as the "mistress of charms and spells" and the "controller of noxious poisons" (Table 1–1).[140]

ARROW AND DART POISONS

The prehistoric Masai hunters of Kenya, who lived 18,000 years ago, used arrow and dart poisons to increase the lethality of their weapons.[19] One of these poisons appears to have consisted of extracts of *Strophanthus* species, an indigenous plant that contains strophanthin, a digitalis-like substance.[91] Cave paintings of arrowheads and spearheads reveal that these weapons were crafted with small depressions at the end to hold the poison.[141] In fact, the term *toxicology* is derived from the Greek terms *toxikos* ("bow") and *toxikon* ("poison into which arrowheads are dipped").[2,141]

References to arrow poisons are cited in a number of other important literary works. The ancient Indian text *Rig Veda*, written in the 12th century B.C., refers to the use of *Aconitum* species for arrow poisons.[19] In the *Odyssey*, Homer (ca. 850 B.C.) wrote that Ulysses anointed his arrows with a variety of poisons, including extracts of *Helleborus orientalis* (thought to act as a heart poison) and snake venoms.[108] Aristotle (384–322 B.C.) described how the Scythians prepared and used arrow poisons.[143] Finally, reference to weapons poisoned with the blood of serpents can be found in the writings of Ovid (43 B.C.–18 A.D.).[148]

CLASSIFICATION OF POISONS

The first attempts at poison identification and classification and the introduction of the first antidotes took place during Greek and Roman times. An early categorization of poisons divided them into fast poisons, such as strychnine, and slow poisons, such as arsenic. In his treatise, *Materia Medica*, the Greek physician Dioscorides (40–80 A.D.) categorized poisons by their origin—animal, vegetable, or mineral.[141] This categorization remained the standard classification for the next 1500 years.[141]

Animal Poisons Animal poisons usually referred to the venom from poisonous animals. Although the venom from poisonous snakes has always been among the most commonly feared poisons, poisons from toads, salamanders, jellyfish, stingrays, and sea hares are often as lethal. Nicander of Colophon (204–135 B.C.), a Greek poet and physician who is considered to be one of the earliest toxicologists, experimented with animal poisons on condemned criminals.[127] Nicander's poems *Theriaca* and *Alexipharmaca* are considered to be the earliest extant Greek toxicologic texts, describing the presentations and treatment of poisonings from animal toxins.[140] A notable fatality from the effects of an animal toxin was Cleopatra (69–30 B.C.), who reportedly committed suicide by deliberately falling on an asp.[71]

Vegetable Poisons Theophrastus (ca. 370–286 B.C.) described vegetable poisons in his treatise *De Historia Plantarum*.[72] Notorious poisonous plants included *Aconitum* species (aconite, monks-hood), *Conium maculatum* (poison hemlock), *Hyoscyamus niger* (henbane), *Mandragora officinarum* (mandrake), *Papaver somniferum* (opium poppy), and *Veratrum album* (hellebore). Aconite was among the most frequently encountered poisonous plants and was described as the "queen mother of poisons."[140] Hemlock was the official poison used by the Greeks and was used in the execution of Socrates (ca. 470–399 B.C.) and many others.[129] Poisonous plants used in India at this time included *Cannabis indica* (marijuana), *Croton tiglium* (croton oil), and *Strychnos nux vomica* (poison nut, strychnine).[72]

Mineral Poisons The mineral poisons of antiquity consisted of the metals antimony, arsenic, lead, and mercury. Undoubtedly, the most famous of these was lead. Lead was discovered as early as 3500 B.C. Although controversy continues about whether an epidemic of lead poisoning among the Roman aristocracy contributed to the fall of the Roman Empire, lead was certainly used extensively during this period.[53,106] In addition to its considerable use in plumbing, lead was also used in the production of food and drink containers.[60] It was common practice to add lead directly to wine or to intentionally prepare the wine in a lead kettle to improve its taste. Not surprisingly, chronic lead poisoning became widespread. Nicander described the first case of lead poisoning in the 2nd century B.C.[145] Dioscorides, writing in the 1st century A.D., noted that fortified wine was "most hurtful to the nerves."[145] Lead-induced gout ("saturnine gout") may have also been widespread among the Roman elite.[106]

TABLE 1–1. Important Early Figures in the History of Toxicology

Person	Date	Importance
Gula	ca. 4500 B.C.	First deity associated with poisons
Shen Nung	ca. 2000 B.C.	Chinese emperor who experimented with poisons and antidotes and wrote treatise on herbal medicine
Homer	ca. 850 B.C.	Wrote how Ulysses anointed arrows with the venom of serpents
Aristotle	384–322 B.C.	Described the preparation and use of arrow poisons
Theophrastus	ca. 370–286 B.C.	Referred to poisonous plants in *De Historia Plantarum*
Socrates	ca. 470–399 B.C.	Executed by poison hemlock
Nicander	204–135 B.C.	Wrote two poems that are among the earliest works on poisons: *Theriaca* and *Alexipharmaca*
King Mithridates VI	ca. 132–63 B.C.	Fanatical fear of poisons; developed mithradatum, one of the first universal antidotes
Sulla	81 B.C.	Issued *Lex Cornelia*, the first anti-poisoning law
Cleopatra	69–30 B.C.	Committed suicide with deliberate cobra envenomation
Andromachus	37–68 A.D.	Refined mithradatum; known as the Theriac of Andromachus
Dioscorides	40–80 A.D.	Wrote *Materia Medica*, which classified poisons by animal, vegetable, and mineral
Galen	ca. 129–200 A.D.	Prepared "nut theriac" for Roman emperors, a remedy against bites, stings, and poisons; wrote *De Antidotis I* and *II*, which provided recipes for different antidotes, including mithradatum and panacea
Ibn Wahshiya	9th century	Famed Arab toxicologist; wrote toxicology treatise *Book on Poisons*, combining contemporary science, magic, and astrology
Moses Maimonides	1135–1204	Wrote *Treatise on Poisons and Their Antidotes*
Petrus Abbonus	1250–1315	Wrote *De Venenis*, major work on poisoning

Gases Although not animal, vegetable, or mineral in origin, the toxic effects of gases were also appreciated during antiquity. In the 3rd century B.C., Aristotle commented that "coal fumes (carbon monoxide) lead to a heavy head and death"[69] and Cicero (106–43 B.C.) referred to the use of coal fumes in suicides and executions.

POISONERS OF ANTIQUITY

Given the increasing awareness of the toxic properties of some naturally occurring substances and the lack of analytical detection techniques, homicidal poisoning was common during Roman times. In an attempt to curtail this practice, in 81 B.C. the Roman dictator Sulla issued the first law against poisoning, the *Lex Cornelia.* According to its provisions, a perpetrator convicted of poisoning, would be sentenced to either loss of property and exile (if the guilty party was of high social rank) or exposure to wild beasts (if of low social rank). During this period, members of the aristocracy commonly used "tasters" to shield themselves from potential poisoners, a practice also in vogue during the reign of Louis XIV in 16th century France.[148]

One of the most infamous poisoners of ancient Rome was Locusta, who was known to experiment on slaves with poisons that included aconite, arsenic, belladonna, henbane, and poisonous fungi. In 54 A.D., Nero's mother, Agrippina, hired Locusta to poison Emperor Claudius (Agrippina's husband and Nero's stepfather) as part of a scheme to make Nero emperor. As a result of these activities, Claudius, who was a great lover of mushrooms, died from *Amanita phalloides* poisoning,[17] and in the next year, Britannicus (Nero's stepbrother) also became one of Locusta's victims. In his case, Locusta managed to fool the taster by preparing unusually hot soup that required additional cooling after the soup had been officially tasted. At the time of cooling, the poison was surreptitiously slipped into the soup. Almost immediately after drinking the soup, Britannicus collapsed and died. The exact poison remains in doubt, although some authorities suggest that it was a cyanogenic glycoside.[133]

EARLY QUESTS FOR THE UNIVERSAL ANTIDOTE

The recognition, classification, and use of poisons in ancient Greece and Rome were accompanied by an intensive search for a universal antidote. In fact, many of the physicians of this period devoted significant parts of their careers to this endeavor.[140] Mystery and superstition surrounded the origins and sources of these proposed antidotes. One of the earliest specific references to a protective agent can be found in Homer's *Odyssey*, when Ulysses is advised to protect himself by taking the antidote "moli." Recent speculation suggests that moli referred to *Galanthus nivalis*, which contains a cholinesterase inhibitor. This agent could have been used as an antidote against poisonous plants such as *Datura stramonium* (jimsonweed) that contain the anticholinergic alkaloids scopolamine, atropine, and hyoscyamine.[114]

Theriacs and the Mithradatum The Greeks referred to the universal antidote as the *alexipharmaca* or *theriac.*[140] The term alexipharmaca was derived from the words alexipharmakos ("which keeps off poison") and *antipharmakon* ("antidote"). Over the years, alexipharmaca was increasingly used to refer to a method of treatment, such as the induction of emesis by using a feather. Theriac, which originally had referred to poisonous reptiles or wild beasts, was later used to refer to the antidotes. Consumption of the early theriacs (ca. 200 B.C.) was reputed to make people "poison-proof " against bites of all venomous animals except the asp. Their ingredients included aniseed, anmi, apoponax, fennel, meru, parsley, and wild thyme.[140]

The quest for the universal antidote was epitomized by the work of King Mithradates VI of Pontus (132–63 B.C.).[70] After repeatedly being subjected to poisoning attempts by his enemies during his youth, Mithradates sought protection by the development of universal antidotes. To find the best antidote, he performed acute toxicity experiments on criminals and slaves. The theriac he concocted, known as the "mithradatum," contained a minimum of 36 ingredients and was thought to be protective against aconite, scorpions, sea slugs, spiders, vipers, and all other poisonous substances.[69] Mithradates took his concoction every day.

Ironically, when an old man, Mithradates attempted suicide by poison but supposedly was unsuccessful because he had become poison-proof. Having failed at self-poisoning, Mithradates was compelled to have a soldier kill him with a sword. Galen described Mithradates' experiences in a series of three books: *De Antidotis I*, *De Antidotis II*, and *De Theriaca ad Pisonem*.[70,146]

The Theriac of Andromachus, also known as the "Venice treacle" or "galene," is probably the most famous theriac. According to Galen, this preparation, formulated during the 1st century A.D., was considered an improvement over the mithradatum.[146] It was prepared by Andromachus (37–68 A.D.), physician to Emperor Nero. Andromachus added to the mithradatum ingredients such as the flesh of vipers, squills, and generous amounts of opium.[152] Other ingredients were removed. Altogether, 73 ingredients were required. It was advocated to "counteract all poisons and bites of venomous animals," as well as a host of other medical problems, such as colic, dropsy, and jaundice, and it was used both therapeutically and prophylactically.[140,146] As evidence of its efficacy, Galen demonstrated that fowl receiving poison followed by theriac had a higher survival rate than fowl receiving poison alone.[140] It is likely, however, that the scientific rigor and methodology used differed from current scientific practice.

By the Middle Ages, the Theriac of Andromachus contained more than 100 ingredients. Its synthesis was quite elaborate; the initial phase of production lasted months, followed by an aging process that lasted years, somewhat similar to that of vintage wine.[87] The final product was often more solid than liquid in consistency.

Other theriac preparations were named after famous physicians (Damocrates, Nicolaus, Amando, Arnauld, and Abano) who contributed additional ingredients to the original formulation. Over the centuries, certain localities were celebrated for their own peculiar brand of theriac. Notable centers of theriac production included Bologna, Cairo, Florence, Genoa, Istanbul, and Venice. At times, theriac production was accompanied by great fanfare. For example, in Bologna, the mixing of the theriac could take place only under the direction of the medical professors at the university.[140]

Whether these preparations were of actual benefit is uncertain. Some suggest that the theriac may have had an antiseptic effect on the gastrointestinal tract, but others state that the sole benefit of the theriac derived from its formulation with opium.[87] Theriacs remained in vogue throughout the Middle Ages and Renaissance, and it was not until 1745 that their efficacy was finally questioned by William Heberden in *Antitheriaka: An Essay on Mithradatum and Theriaca*.[70] Nonetheless, pharmacopeias in France, Spain, and Germany continued to list these agents until the last quarter of the 19th century, and theriac was still available in Italy and Turkey in the early 20th century.[18,87]

Sacred Earth Beginning in the 5th century B.C., an adsorbent agent called *terra sigillata* was promoted as a universal antidote. This agent, also known as the "sacred sealed earth," consisted of red clay that could be found on only one particular hill on the Greek island of Lemnos. Perhaps somewhat akin to the 20th-century "universal antidote," it was advocated as effective in counteracting all poisons.[140] With great ceremony, once per year, the terra sigillata was retrieved from this hill and prepared for subsequent use. According to Dioscorides, this clay was formulated with goat's blood to make it into a paste. At one time, it was included as part of the Theriac of Andromachus. Demand for terra sigillata continued into the 15th century. Similar antidotal clays were found in Italy, Malta, Silesia, and England.[140]

Charms Charms, such as toadstones, snakestones, unicorn horns, and bezoar stones, were also promoted as universal antidotes. Toadstones, found in the heads of old toads, were reputed to have the capability to extract poison from the site of a venomous bite or sting. In addition, the toadstone was supposedly able to detect the mere presence of poison by producing a sensation of heat upon contact with a poisonous substance.[140]

Similarly, snakestones extracted from the heads of cobras (known as *piedras della cobra de Capelos*) were also reported to have magical qualities.[14] The 17th-century Italian philosopher Athanasius Kircher (1602–1680) became an enthusiastic supporter of snakestone therapy for the treatment of snakebite after conducting experiments, demonstrating the antidotal attributes of these charms "in front of amazed spectators." Kircher attributed the efficacy of the snakestone to the theory of "attraction of like substances." Francesco Redi (1626–1698), a court physician and contemporary of Kircher, debunked this quixotic approach. A harbinger of future experimental toxicologists, Redi was unwilling to accept isolated case reports and field demonstrations as proof of the utility of the snakestone. Using a considerably more rigorous approach, *provando et riprovando* (by testing and retesting), Redi assessed the antidotal efficacy of snakestone on different animal species and different toxins and failed to confirm any benefit.[14]

Much lore has surrounded the antidotal effects of the mythical unicorn horn. Ctesias, writing in 390 B.C., was the first to chronicle the wonders of the unicorn horn, claiming that drinking water or wine from the "horn of the unicorn" would protect against poison.[140] The horns were usually narwhal tusks or rhinoceros horns, and during the Middle Ages, the unicorn horn may have been worth as much as 10 times the price of gold. Similar to the toadstone, the unicorn horn was used both to detect poisons and to neutralize them. Supposedly, a cup made of unicorn horn would sweat if a poisonous substance was placed in it.[85] To give further credence to its use, a 1593 study on arsenic-poisoned dogs reportedly showed that the horn was protective.[85]

Bezoar stones, also touted as universal antidotes, consisted of stomach or intestinal calculi formed by the deposition of calcium phosphate around a hair, fruit pit, or gallstone. They were removed from wild goats, cows, and apes and administered orally to humans. The Persian name for the bezoar stone was *pad zahr* ("expeller of poisons"); the ancient Hebrews referred to the bezoar stone as *bel Zaard* ("every cure for poisons"). Over the years, regional variations of bezoar stones were popularized, including an Asian variety from wild goat of Persia, an Occidental variety from llamas of Peru, and a European variety from chamois of the Swiss mountains.[48,140]

OPIUM, COCA, CANNABIS, AND HALLUCINOGENS IN ANTIQUITY

Although it was not until the mid-19th century that the true perils of opiate addiction were first recognized, juice from the *Papaver somniferum* was known for its medicinal value in Egypt at least as early as the writing of the *Ebers Papyrus* in 1500 B.C. Egyptian pharmacologists of that time reportedly recommended opium poppy extract as a pacifier for children who exhibited incessant crying.[126] In Ancient Greece, Dioscorides and Galen were early advocates of opium as a therapeutic agent. During this time, it was also used as a means of suicide. Mithradates' lack of success in his own attempted suicide by poisoning may have been the result of an opium tolerance that had developed from previous repetitive use.[126] One of the earliest descriptions of the abuse potential of opium is attributed to Epistratos (304–257 B.C.), who criticized the use of opium for earache because it "dulled the sight and is a narcotic."[126]

Cocaine use dates back to at least 300 B.C., when South American Indians reportedly chewed coca leaves during religious ceremonies.[100] Chewing coca to increase work efficacy and to elevate mood has remained commonplace in some South American societies for thousands of years. An Egyptian mummy from about 950 B.C. revealed significant amounts of cocaine in the stomach and liver, suggesting oral use of cocaine during this time period.[104] Large amounts of tetrahydrocannabinol (THC) were also found in the lung and muscle of the same mummy. Another investigation of 11 Egyptian (1079 B.C.–395 A.D.) and 72 Peruvian (200–1500 A.D.) mummies found cocaine, thought to be indigenous only to South America, and hashish, thought to be indigenous only to Asia, in both groups.[113]

Cannabis use in China dates back even further, to around 2700 B.C., when it was known as the "liberator of sin."[100] In India and Iran, cannabis was used as early as 1000 B.C. as an intoxicant known as *bhang*.[103] Other currently abused agents that were known to the ancients include cannabis, hallucinogenic mushrooms, nutmeg, and peyote. As early as 1300 B.C., Peruvian Indian tribal ceremonies included the use of mescaline-containing San Pedro cacti.[100] The hallucinogenic mushroom, *Amanita muscaria*, known as "fly agaric," was used as a ritual drug and may have been known in India as "soma" around 2000 B.C.

EARLY ATTEMPTS AT GASTROINTESTINAL DECONTAMINATION

Nicander's *Alexipharmaca* (*Antidotes for Poisons*) recommended induction of emesis by one of several methods: (a) ingesting warm linseed oil; (b) tickling the hypopharynx with a feather; or (c) "emptying the gullet with a small twisted and curved paper."[87] Nicander also advocated the use of suction to limit envenomation.[141] The Romans referred to the feather as the "vomiting feather" or "pinna." Most commonly, the feather was used after a hearty feast to avoid the gastrointestinal discomfort associated with overeating. At times, the pinna was dipped into a nauseating mixture to increase its efficacy.[90]

TOXICOLOGY DURING THE MEDIEVAL AND RENAISSANCE PERIODS

After Galen (ca. A.D. 129–200), there is relatively little documented attention to the subject of poisons until the works of Ibn Wahshiya in the 9th century. Citing Greek, Persian, and Indian texts, Wahshiya's work, titled *Book of Poisons*, combines contemporary science, magic, and astrology during his discussion of poison mechanisms (as they were understood at that time), symptomatology, antidotes (including his own recommendation for a universal antidote), and prophylaxis. He categorized poisons as lethal by sight, smell, touch, and sound, as well as by drinking and eating. For victims of an aconite-containing dart arrow, Ibn Wahshiya recommended excision, followed by cauterization and topical treatment with onion and salt.[82]

Another significant medieval contribution to toxicology can be found in Moses Maimonides' (1135–1204) *Treatise on Poisons and Their Antidotes* (1198). In part one of this treatise, Maimonides discussed the bites of snakes and mad dogs and the stings of bees, wasps, spiders, and scorpions.[124] He also discussed the use of cupping glasses for bites (a progenitor of the modern suctioning device) and was one of the first to differentiate the hematotoxic (hot) from the neurotoxic (cold) effects of poison. In part two, he discussed mineral and vegetable poisons and their antidotes. He described belladonna poisoning as causing a "redness and a sort of excitation."[124] He suggested that emesis should be induced by hot water, *Anethum graveolens* (dill), and oil, followed by fresh milk, butter, and honey. Although he rejected some of the popular treatments of the day, he advocated the use of the great theriac and the mithradatum as first- and second-line agents in the management of snakebite.[124]

On the subject of oleander poisoning, Petrus Abbonus (1250–1315) wrote that those who drink the juice, spines, or bark of oleander will develop anxiety, palpitations, and syncope.[21] He described the clinical presentation of opium overdose as someone who "will be dull, lazy, and sleepy, without feeling, and he will neither understand nor feel anything, and if he does not receive succor, he will die." Although this "succor" is not defined, he recommended that treatment of opium intoxication include drinking the strongest wine, rubbing the extremities with alkali and soap, and olfactory stimulation with pepper. To treat snakebite, Abbonus suggested the immediate application of a tourniquet, as well as oral suctioning of the bite wound, preferably performed by a servant. Interestingly, from a 21st-century perspective, Abbonus also suggested that St. John's wort had the magical power to free anything from poisons and attributed this virtue to the influence of the stars.[21]

THE SCIENTISTS

Paracelsus' (1493–1541) study on the dose–response relationship is usually considered the beginning of the scientific approach to toxicology (Table 1–2). He was the first to emphasize the chemical nature of toxic agents.[111] Paracelsus stressed the need for proper observation and experimentation regarding the true response to chemicals. He underscored the need to differentiate between the therapeutic and toxic properties of chemicals when he stated in his *Third Defense*, "What is there that is not poison? All things are poison and nothing [is] without poison. Solely, the dose determines that a thing is not a poison."[40]

Although Paracelsus is the best known Renaissance toxicologist, Ambroise Pare (1510–1590) and William Piso (1611–1678) also contributed to the field. Pare argued against the use of the unicorn horn and bezoar stone.[89] He also wrote an early treatise on carbon monoxide poisoning. Piso is credited as one of the first to recognize the emetic properties of ipecacuanha.[121]

MEDIEVAL AND RENAISSANCE POISONERS

Along with these advances in toxicologic knowledge, the Renaissance is mainly remembered as the age of the poisoner, a time when the art of poisoning reached new heights (Table 1–3). In fact, poisoning was so rampant during this time that in 1531, King Henry VIII decreed that convicted poisoners should be boiled alive.[50] From the 15th to 17th centuries, schools of poisoning existed in Venice and Rome. In Venice, poisoning services were provided by a group called the Council of Ten, whose members were hired to perform murder by poison.[148]

Members of the infamous Borgia family were considered to be responsible for many poisonings during this period. They preferred to use a poison called "La Cantarella," a mixture of arsenic and phosphorus.[143] Rodrigo Borgia (1431–1503), who became Pope Alexander VI, and his son, Cesare Borgia, were reportedly responsible for the poisoning of cardinals and kings.

In the late 16th century, Catherine de Medici, wife of Henry II of France, introduced Italian poisoning techniques to France. She experimented on the poor, the sick, and the criminal. By analyzing the subsequent complaints of her victims, she is said to have learned the site of action and time of onset, the clinical signs and symptoms, and the efficacy of poisons.[54]

Murder by poison remained quite popular during the latter half of the 17th and the early part of the 18th centuries in Italy and France.

The Marchioness de Brinvilliers (1630–1676) tested her poison concoctions on hospitalized patients and on her servants and allegedly murdered her husband, father, and two siblings.[52,133] Among the favorite poisons of the Marchioness were arsenic, copper sulfate, corrosive sublimate (mercury bichloride), lead, and tartar emetic (antimony potassium tartrate).[143] Catherine Deshayes (1640–1680), a fortuneteller and sorceress, was one of the last "poisoners for hire" and

TABLE 1–2. Important Figures in Toxicology from Paracelsus to the 1900s

Person	Date	Importance
Paracelsus	1493–1541	Introduced the dose–response concept to toxicology
Ambroise Pare	1510–1590	Spoke out against unicorn horns and bezoars as antidotes
William Piso	1611–1678	First to study emetic qualities of ipecacuanha
Bernardino Ramazzini	1633–1714	Father of occupational medicine; wrote *De Morbis Artificum Diatriba*
Richard Mead	1673–1754	Wrote English-language book about poisoning
Percivall Pott	1714–1788	Wrote the first description of occupational cancer, relating the chimney sweep occupation to scrotal cancer
Felice Fontana	1730–1805	First scientific study of venomous snakes
Philip Physick	1767–1837	Early advocate of orogastric lavage to remove poisons
Baron Guillaume Dupuytren	1777–1835	Early advocate of orogastric lavage to remove poisons
Francois Magendie	1783–1855	Discovered emetine and studied the mechanisms of cyanide and strychnine
Bonaventure Orfila	1787–1853	Father of modern toxicology; wrote *Traite des Poisons*; first to isolate arsenic from humans organs
James Marsh	1794–1846	Developed reduction test for arsenic
Robert Christison	1797–1882	Wrote *Treatise on Poisons*, one of the most influential texts of the early 19th century
Grand Marshall Bertrand	1813	Demonstrated the efficacy of charcoal in arsenic ingestion
Claude Bernard	1813–1878	Studied the mechanisms of toxicity of carbon monoxide and curare
Edward Jukes	1820	Self-experimented with orogastric lavage apparatus known as Jukes' syringe
Theodore Wormley	1826–1897	Wrote *Micro-Chemistry of Poisons*, the first American book devoted exclusively to toxicology
Pierre Touery	1831	Demonstrated the efficacy of charcoal in strychnine ingestion
Hugo Reinsch	1842–1884	Developed qualitative tests for arsenic and mercury
Alfred Garrod	1846	Conducted the first systematic study of charcoal in an animal model
Max Gutzeit	1847–1915	Developed method to quantitate small amounts of arsenic
Benjamin Howard Rand	1848	Conducted the first study of the efficacy of charcoal in humans
O.H. Costill	1848	Wrote the first book on symptoms and treatment of poisoning
Louis Lewin	1850–1929	Studied many toxins, including methanol, chloroform, snake venom, carbon monoxide, lead, opioids, and hallucinogenic plants
Rudolf Kobert	1854–1918	Studied digitalis and ergot alkaloids
Albert Niemann	1860	Isolated cocaine alkaloid
Alice Hamilton	1869–1970	Conducted landmark investigations associating worksite chemical hazards with disease; led reform movement to improve worker safety

was implicated in countless poisonings, including the killing of more than 2000 infants.[54] Better known as "La Voisine," she reportedly sold poisons to women wishing to rid themselves of their husbands. Her particular brand of poison was a concoction of aconite, arsenic, belladonna, and opium known as "la poudre de succession."[143] Ultimately, de Brinvilliers was beheaded, and Deshayes was burned alive for their crimes. In an attempt to curtail these rampant poisonings, Louis XIV issued a decree in 1662 banning the sale of arsenic, mercury, and other poisons to customers not known to apothecaries and requiring poison buyers to sign a register declaring the purpose for their purchase.[133]

A major center for poison practitioners was Naples, the home of the notorious Madame Giulia Toffana. She reportedly poisoned more than 600 people, preferring a particular solution of white arsenic (arsenic trioxide), better known as "aqua toffana," and dispensed under the guise of a cosmetic. Eventually convicted of poisoning, Madame Toffana was executed in 1719.[20]

EIGHTEENTH- AND NINETEENTH-CENTURY DEVELOPMENTS IN TOXICOLOGY

The development of toxicology as a distinct specialty began during the 18th and 19th centuries (see Table 1–2).[112] The mythological and magical mystique of poisoners began to be gradually replaced by an increasingly rational, scientific, and experimental approach to these agents. Much of the poison lore that had survived for almost 2000 years was finally debunked and discarded. The 18th-century Italian Felice Fontana was one of the first to usher in the modern age. He was an early experimental toxicologist who studied the venom of the European viper and wrote the classic text *Traite sur le Venin de la Vipere* in 1781.[75] Through his exacting experimental study on the effects of venom, Fontana brought a scientific insight to toxicology previously lacking and demonstrated that clinical symptoms resulted

TABLE 1–3. Notable Poisoners from Antiquity to the Present

Poisoner	Date	Victim(s)	Poison(s)
Locusta	54–55 A.D.	Claudius and Britannicus	*Amanita phalloides*, cyanide
Cesare Borgia	1400s	Cardinals and kings	La Cantarella (arsenic and phosphorus)
Catherine de Medici	1519–1589	Poor, sick, criminals	Unknown agents
Hieronyma Spara	Died 1659	Taught women how to poison their husbands	Mana of St. Nicholas of Bari (arsenic trioxide)
Marchioness de Brinvilliers	Died 1676	Hospitalized patients, husband, father	Antimony, arsenic, copper, lead, mercury
Catherine Deshayes	Died 1680	>2000 infants, many husbands	La poudre de succession (arsenic mixed with aconite, belladonna, and opium)
Madame Giulia Toffana	Died 1719	>600 people	Aqua toffana (arsenic trioxide)
Mary Blandy	1752	Father	Arsenic
Anna Maria Zwanizer	1807	Random people	Antimony, arsenic
Marie Lefarge	1839	Husband	Arsenic (first use of Marsh test)
John Tawell	1845	Mistress	Cyanide
William Palmer, MD	1855	Fellow gambler	Strychnine
Madeline Smith (acquitted)	1857	Lover	Arsenic
Edmond de la Pommerais, MD	1863	Patient and mistress	Digitalis
Edward William Pritchard, MD	1865	Wife and mother-in-law	Antimony
George Henry Lamson, MD	1881	Brother-in-law	Aconite
Adelaide Bartlett (acquitted)	1886	Husband	Chloroform
Florence Maybrick	1889	Husband	Arsenic
Thomas Neville Cream, MD	1891	Prostitutes	Strychnine
Johann Hoch	1892–1905	Serial wives	Arsenic
Cordelia Botkin	1898	Feminine rival	Arsenic (in chocolate candy)
Roland Molineux	1898	Acquaintance	Cyanide of mercury
Hawley Harvey Crippen, MD	1910	Wife	Hyoscine
Frederick Henry Seddon	1911	Boarder	Arsenic (fly paper)
Henri Girard Landru	1912	Acquaintances	*Amanita phalloides*
Robert Armstrong	1921	Wife	Arsenic (weed killer)
Landru	1922	Many women	Cyanide
Suzanne Fazekas	1929	Supplied poison to 100 wives to kill husbands	Arsenic
Sadamichi Hirasawa	1948	Bank employees	Potassium cyanide
Christa Ambros Lehmann	1954	Friend, husband, father-in-law	E-605 (parathion)
Nannie Doss	1954	11 relatives, including five husbands	Arsenic
Carl Coppolino, MD	1965	Wife	Succinylcholine
Graham Frederick Young	1971	Stepmother, coworkers	Antimony, thallium
Judias V. Buenoano	1971	Husband, son	Arsenic
Ronald Clark O'Bryan	1974	Son and neighborhood children	Cyanide (in Halloween candy)
Unknown	1978	Georgi Markov, Bulgarian dissident	Ricin
Jim Jones	1978	>900 people in mass suicide	Cyanide
Harold Shipman, MD	1974–1998	Patients (100s)	Heroin
Unidentified	1982	Seven people	Extra Strength Tylenol mixed with cyanide
Donald Harvey	1983–1987	Patients	Arsenic
George Trepal	1988	Neighbors	Thallium
Michael Swango, MD	1980s–1990s	Hospitalized patients	Arsenic, potassium chloride, succinylcholine
Charles Cullen, RN	1990s–2003	Hospitalized patients	Digoxin
Unknown	2004	Viktor Yushchenko, Ukrainian presidential candidate	Dioxin
Unknown	2006	Alexander Litvinenko	Polonium-210

from the poison (venom) acting on specific target organs. During the 18th and 19th centuries, attention focused on the detection of poisons and the study of toxic effects of drugs and chemicals in animals.[105] Issues relating to adverse effects of industrialization and unintentional poisoning in the workplace and home environment were raised. Also during this time, early experience and experimentation with methods of gastrointestinal decontamination took place.

DEVELOPMENT OF ANALYTICAL TOXICOLOGY AND THE STUDY OF POISONS

The French physician Bonaventure Orfila (1787–1853) is often called the father of modern toxicology.[105] He emphasized toxicology as a distinct, scientific discipline, separate from clinical medicine and pharmacology.[11] He was also an early medical-legal expert who championed the use of chemical analysis and autopsy material as evidence to prove that a poisoning had occurred. His treatise *Traite des Poisons* (1814)[110] evolved over five editions and was regarded as the foundation of experimental and forensic toxicology.[149] This text classified poisons into six groups: acrids, astringents, corrosives, narcoticoacrids, septics and putrefiants, and stupefacients and narcotics.

A number of other landmark works on poisoning also appeared during this period. In 1829, Robert Christison (1797–1882), a professor of medical jurisprudence and Orfila's student, wrote *A Treatise on Poisons*.[29] This work simplified Orfila's poison classification schema by categorizing poisons into three groups: irritants, narcotics, and narcoticoacrids. Less concerned with jurisprudence than with clinical toxicology, O.H. Costill's *A Practical Treatise on Poisons*, published in 1848, was the first modern clinically oriented text to emphasize the symptoms and treatment of poisoning.[33] In 1867, Theodore Wormley (1826–1897) published the first American book written exclusively on poisons titled the *Micro-Chemistry of Poisons*.[46,151]

During this time, important breakthroughs in the chemical analysis of poisons resulted from the search for a more reliable assay for arsenic. Arsenic was widely available and was the suspected cause of a large number of deaths. In one study, arsenic was used in 31% of 679 homicidal poisonings.[143] A reliable means of detecting arsenic was much needed by the courts.

Until the 19th century, poisoning was mainly diagnosed by its resultant symptoms rather than by analytic tests. The first use of a chemical test as evidence in a poisoning trial occurred in the 1752 trial of Mary Blandy, who was accused of poisoning her father with arsenic.[93] Although Blandy was convicted and hanged publicly, the test used in this case was not very sensitive and depended in part on eliciting a garlic odor upon heating the gruel that the accused had fed to her father.

During the 19th century, James Marsh (1794–1846), Hugo Reinsch, and Max Gutzeit (1847–1915) each worked on this problem. Assays bearing their names are important contributions to the early history of analytic toxicology.[94,105] The "Marsh test" to detect arsenic was first used in a criminal case in 1839 during the trial of Marie Lefarge, who was accused of using arsenic to murder her husband.[133] Orfila's trial testimony that the victim's viscera contained minute amounts of arsenic helped to convict the defendant, although subsequent debate suggested that contamination of the forensic specimen may have also played a role.

In a further attempt to curtail criminal poisoning by arsenic, the British Parliament passed the Arsenic Act in 1851. This bill, which was one of the first modern laws to regulate the sale of poisons, required that the retail sale of arsenic be restricted to chemists, druggists, and apothecaries and that a poison book be maintained to record all arsenic sales.[15]

Homicidal poisonings remained common during the 19th century and early 20th century. Infamous poisoners of that time included William Palmer, Edward Pritchard, Harvey Crippen, and Frederick Seddon.[143] Many of these poisoners were physicians who used their knowledge of medicine and toxicology in an attempt to solve their domestic and financial difficulties by committing the "perfect" murder. Some of the poisons used were aconitine (by Lamson, who was a classmate of Christison), *Amanita phalloides* (Girard), arsenic (by Maybrick, Seddon, and others), antimony (by Pritchard), cyanide (by Molineux and Tawell), digitalis (by Pommerais), hyoscine (by Crippen), and strychnine (by Palmer and Cream) (see Table 1–3).[23,140,143]

In the early 20th century, forensic investigation into suspicious deaths, including poisonings, was significantly advanced with the development of the medical examiner system replacing the much-flawed coroner system that was subject to widespread corruption. In 1918, the first centrally controlled medical examiner system was established in New York City. Alexander Gettler, considered the father of forensic toxicology in the United States, established a toxicology laboratory within the newly created New York City Medical Examiner's Office. Gettler pioneered new techniques for the detection of a variety of substances in biologic fluids, including carbon monoxide, chloroform, cyanide, and heavy metals.[47,105]

Systematic investigation into the underlying mechanisms of toxic substances also commenced during the 19th century. To cite just a few important accomplishments, Francois Magendie (1783–1855) studied the mechanisms of toxicity and sites of action of cyanide, emetine, and strychnine.[45] Claude Bernard (1813–1878), a pioneering physiologist and a student of Magendie, made important contributions to the understanding the toxicity of carbon monoxide and curare.[81] Rudolf Kobert (1854–1918) studied digitalis and ergot alkaloids and authored a textbook on toxicology for physicians and students.[79,108] Louis Lewin (1850–1929) was the first person to intensively study the differences between the pharmacologic and toxicologic actions of drugs. Lewin studied chronic opium intoxication, as well as the toxicity of carbon monoxide, chloroform, lead, methanol, and snake venom. He also developed a classification system for psychoactive drugs, dividing them into euphorics, phantastics, inebriants, hypnotics, and excitants.[88]

THE ORIGIN OF OCCUPATIONAL TOXICOLOGY

The origins of occupational toxicology can be traced to the early 18th century and to the contributions of Bernardino Ramazzini (1633–1714). Considered the father of occupational medicine, Ramazzini wrote *De Morbis Artificum Diatriba* (*Diseases of Workers*) in 1700, which was the first comprehensive text discussing the relationship between disease and workplace hazards.[51] Ramazzini's essential contribution to the care of the patient is epitomized by the addition of a standard question to a patient's medical history: "What occupation does the patient follow?"[49] Altogether Ramazzini described diseases associated with 54 occupations, including hydrocarbon poisoning in painters, mercury poisoning in mirror makers, and pulmonary diseases in miners.

In 1775, Sir Percivall Pott proposed the first association between workplace exposure and cancer when he noticed a high incidence of scrotal cancer in English chimney sweeps. Pott's belief that the scrotal cancer was caused by prolonged exposure to tar and soot was confirmed by further investigation in the 1920s, indicating the carcinogenic nature of the polycyclic aromatic hydrocarbons contained in coal tar (including benzo[*a*]pyrene).[67]

Dr. Alice Hamilton (1869–1970) was another pioneer in occupational toxicology, whose rigorous scientific inquiry had a profound impact on linking chemical toxins with human disease. A physician, scientist, humanitarian, and social reformer, Hamilton became the first female professor at Harvard University and conducted groundbreaking studies of many different occupational exposures and problems, including carbon monoxide poisoning in steelworkers, mercury poisoning in hatters, and wrist drop in lead workers. Hamilton's overriding concerns about these "dangerous trades" and her commitment to improving the health of workers led to extensive voluntary and regulatory reforms in the workplace.[8,58]

ADVANCES IN GASTROINTESTINAL DECONTAMINATION

Using gastric lavage and charcoal to treat poisoned patients was introduced in the late 18th and early 19th century. A stomach pump was first designed by Munro Secundus in 1769 to administer neutralizing substances to sheep and cattle for the treatment of bloat.[24] The American surgeon Philip Physick (1768–1837) and the French surgeon Baron Guillaume Dupuytren (1777–1835) were two of the first physicians to advocate gastric lavage for the removal of poisons.[24] As early as 1805, Physick demonstrated the use of a "stomach tube" for this purpose. Using brandy and water as the irrigation fluid, he performed stomach washings in twins to wash out excessive doses of tincture of opium.[24] Dupuytren performed gastric emptying by first introducing warm water into the stomach via a large syringe attached to a long flexible sound and then withdrawing the "same water charged with poison."[24] Edward Jukes, a British surgeon, was another early advocate of poison removal by gastric lavage. Jukes first experimented on animals, performing gastric lavage after the oral administration of tincture of opium. Attempting to gain human experience, he experimented on himself, by first ingesting 10 drams (600 g) of tincture of opium and then performing gastric lavage using a 25-inch-long, 0.5-inch-diameter tube, which became known as Jukes' syringe.[99] Other than some nausea and a 3-hour sleep, he suffered no ill effects, and the experiment was deemed a success.

The principle of using charcoal to adsorb poisons was first described by Scheele (1773) and Lowitz (1785), but the medicinal use of charcoal dates to ancient times.[32] The earliest reference to the medicinal uses of charcoal is found in Egyptian papyrus from about 1500 B.C.[32] The charcoal used during Greek and Roman times, referred to as "wood charcoal," was used to treat those with anthrax, chlorosis, epilepsy, and vertigo. By the late 18th century, topical application of charcoal was recommended for gangrenous skin ulcers, and internal use of a charcoal-water suspension was recommended for use as a mouthwash and in the treatment of bilious conditions.[32]

The first hint that charcoal might have a role in the treatment of poisoning came from a series of courageous self-experiments in France during the early 19th century. In 1813, the French chemist Bertrand publicly demonstrated the antidotal properties of charcoal by surviving a 5-g ingestion of arsenic trioxide that had been mixed with charcoal.[64] Eighteen years later, before the French Academy of Medicine, the pharmacist Touery survived an ingestion consisting of 10 times the lethal dose of strychnine mixed with 15 g of charcoal.[64] One of the first reports of charcoal used in a poisoned patient was in 1834 by the American Hort, who successfully treated a mercury bichloride–poisoned patient with large amounts of powdered charcoal.[4]

In the 1840s, Garrod performed the first controlled study of charcoal when he examined its utility on a variety of poisons in animal models.[64] Garrod used dogs, cats, guinea pigs, and rabbits to demonstrate the potential benefits of charcoal in the management of strychnine poisoning. He also emphasized the importance of early use of charcoal and the proper ratio of charcoal to poison. Other toxic substances, such as aconite, hemlock, mercury bichloride, and morphine were also studied during this period. The first charcoal efficacy studies in humans were performed by the American physician B. Rand in 1848.[64]

But, it was not until the early 20th century that an activation process was added to the manufacture of charcoal to increase its effectiveness. In 1900, the Russian Ostrejko demonstrated that treating charcoal with superheated steam significantly enhanced its adsorbing power.[32] Despite this improvement and the favorable reports mentioned, charcoal was only occasionally used in gastrointestinal decontamination until the early 1960s, when Holt and Holz repopularized its use.[61]

THE INCREASING RECOGNITION OF THE PERILS OF DRUG ABUSE

Opioids Although the medical use of opium was promoted by Paracelsus in the 16th century, the popularity of this agent was given a significant boost when the distinguished British physician Thomas Sydenham (1624–1689) formulated laudanum, which was a tincture of opium containing cinnamon, cloves, saffron, and sherry. Sydenham also formulated a different opium concoction known as "syrup of poppies."[78] A third opium preparation called Dover's powder was designed by Sydenham's protégé, Thomas Dover; this preparation contained ipecac, licorice, opium, salt-peter, and tartaric acid.

John Jones, the author of the 18th century text *The Mysteries of Opium Reveal'd*, was another enthusiastic advocate of its "medicinal" uses.[78] A well-known opium user himself, Jones provided one of the earliest descriptions of opiate addiction. He insisted that opium offered many benefits if the dose was moderate but that discontinuation or a decrease in dose, particularly after "leaving off after long and lavish use," would result in such symptoms as sweating, itching, diarrhea, and melancholy. His recommendation for the treatment of these withdrawal symptoms included decreasing the dose of opium by 1% each day until the drug was totally withdrawn. During this period, the number of English writers who became well-known opium addicts, included Elizabeth Barrett Browning, Samuel Taylor Coleridge, and Thomas De Quincey. De Quincey, author of *Confessions of an English Opium Eater*, was an early advocate of the recreational use of opiates. The famed Coleridge poem *Kubla Khan* referred to opium as the "milk of paradise," and De Quincey's *Confessions* suggested that opium held the "key to paradise." In many of these cases, the initiation of opium use for medical reasons led to recreational use, tolerance, and dependence.[78]

Although opium was first introduced to Asian societies by Arab physicians some time after the fall of the Roman Empire, the use of opium in Asian countries grew considerably during the 18th and 19th centuries. In one of the more deplorable chapters in world history, China's growing dependence on opium was spurred on by the English desire to establish and profit from a flourishing drug trade.[126] Opium was grown in India and exported east. Despite Chinese protests and edicts against this practice, the importation of opium persisted throughout the 19th century, with the British going to war twice in order to maintain their right to sell opium. Not surprisingly, by the beginning of the 20th century, opium abuse in China was endemic.

In England, opium use continued to increase during the first half of the 19th century. During this period, opium was legal and freely available from the neighborhood grocer. To many, its use was considered no more problematic than alcohol use.[56] The Chinese usually self-administered opium by smoking, a custom that was brought to the United States by Chinese immigrants in the mid-19th century; the English use of opium was more often by ingestion, that is, "opium eating."

The liberal use of opiates as infant-soothing agents was one of the most unfortunate aspects of this period of unregulated opiate use.[79] Godfrey's Cordial, Mother's Friend, Mrs. Winslow's Soothing Syrup, and Quietness were among the most popular opiates for children.[83] They were advertised as producing a natural sleep and recommended for teething and bowel regulation, as well as for crying. Because of the wide availability of opiates during this period, the number of acute opiate overdoses in children was consequential and would remain problematic until these unsavory remedies were condemned and removed from the market.

With the discovery of morphine in 1805 and Alexander Wood's invention of the hypodermic syringe in 1853, parenteral administration of morphine became the preferred route of opiate administration for therapeutic use and abuse.[66] A legacy of the generous use of opium and morphine during the United States Civil War was "soldiers' disease," referring to a rather large veteran population that returned from the war with a lingering opiate habit.[118] One hundred years later, opiate abuse and addiction would again become common among US military serving during the Vietnam War. Surveys indicated that as many as 20% of American soldiers in Vietnam were addicted to opiates during the war—in part because of its widespread availability and high purity there.[123]

Growing concerns about opiate abuse in England led to the passing of the Pharmacy Act of 1868, which restricted the sale of opium to registered chemists. But in 1898, the Bayer Pharmaceutical Company of Germany synthesized heroin from opium (Bayer also introduced aspirin that same year).[134] Although initially touted as a nonaddictive morphine substitute, problems with heroin use quickly became evident in the United States.

Cocaine Ironically, during the later part of the 19th century, Sigmund Freud and Robert Christison, among others, promoted cocaine as a treatment for opiate addiction. After Albert Niemann's isolation of cocaine alkaloid from coca leaf in 1860, growing enthusiasm for cocaine as a panacea ensued.[74] Some of the most important medical figures of the time, including William Halsted, the famed Johns Hopkins surgeon, also extolled the virtues of cocaine use. Halsted championed the anesthetic properties of this drug, although his own use of cocaine and subsequent morphine use in an attempt to overcome his cocaine dependency would later take a considerable toll.[109] In 1884, Freud wrote *Uber Cocaine*,[142] advocating cocaine as a cure for opium and morphine addiction and as a treatment for fatigue and hysteria.

During the last third of the 19th century, cocaine was added to many popular over-the-counter tonics. In 1863, Angelo Mariani, a Frenchman, introduced a new wine, "Vin Mariani," that consisted of a mixture of cocaine and wine (6 mg of cocaine alkaloid per ounce) and was sold as a digestive aid and restorative.[100] In direct competition with the French tonic was the American-made Coca-Cola, developed by J.S. Pemberton. It was originally formulated with coca and caffeine and marketed as a headache remedy and invigorator. With the public demand for cocaine increasing, patent medication manufacturers were adding cocaine to thousands of products. One such asthma remedy was "Dr. Tucker's Asthma Specific," which contained 420 mg of cocaine per ounce and was applied directly to the nasal mucosa.[74] By the end of the 19th century, the first American cocaine epidemic was underway.[102]

Similar to the medical and societal adversities associated with opiate use, the increasing use of cocaine led to a growing concern about comparable adverse effects. In 1886, the first reports of cocaine-related cardiac arrest and stroke were published.[119] Reports of cocaine habituation occurring in patients using cocaine to treat their underlying opiate addiction also began to appear. In 1902, a popular book, *Eight Years in Cocaine Hell*, described some of these problems. *Century Magazine* called cocaine "the most harmful of all habit-forming drugs," and a report in *The New York Times* stated that cocaine was destroying "its victims more swiftly and surely than opium."[39] In 1910, President William Taft proclaimed cocaine to be "public enemy number 1."

In an attempt to curb the increasing problems associated with drug abuse and addiction, the 1914 Harrison Narcotics Act mandated stringent control over the sale and distribution of narcotics (defined as opium, opium derivatives, and cocaine).[39] It was the first federal law in the United States to criminalize the nonmedical use of drugs. The bill required doctors, pharmacists, and others who prescribed narcotics to register and to pay a tax. A similar law, the Dangerous Drugs Act, was passed in the United Kingdom in 1920.[56] To help enforce these drug laws in the United States, the Narcotics Division of the Prohibition Unit of the Internal Revenue Service (a progenitor of the Drug Enforcement Agency) was established in 1920. In 1924, the Harrison Act was further strengthened with the passage of new legislation that banned the importation of opium for the purpose of manufacturing heroin, essentially outlawing the medicinal uses of heroin. With the legal venues to purchase these drugs now eliminated, users were forced to buy from illegal street dealers, creating a burgeoning black market that still exists today.

Sedative-Hypnotics The introduction to medical practice of the anesthetic agents nitrous oxide, ether, and chloroform during the 19th century was accompanied by the recreational use of these agents and the first reports of volatile substance abuse. Chloroform "jags," ether "frolics," and nitrous parties became a new type of entertainment. Humphrey Davies was an early self-experimenter with the exhilarating effects associated with nitrous oxide inhalation. In certain Irish towns, especially where the temperance movement was strong, ether drinking became quite popular.[97] Horace Wells, the American dentist who introduced chloroform as an anesthetic, became dependent on this volatile solvent and later committed suicide.

Until the last half of the 19th century aconite, alcohol, hemlock, opium, and prussic acid (cyanide) were the primary agents used for sedation.[30] During the 1860s, new, more specific sedative-hypnotics, such as chloral hydrate and potassium bromide, were introduced into medical practice. In particular, chloral hydrate was hailed as a wonder drug that was relatively safe compared with opium, and was recommended for insomnia, anxiety, and delirium tremens, as well as for scarlet fever, asthma, and cancer. But within a few years, problems with acute toxicity of chloral hydrate, as well as its potential to produce tolerance and physical dependence, became apparent.[30] Mixing chloral hydrate with ethanol was noted to produce a rather powerful "knockout" combination that would become known as a "Mickey Finn." Abuse of chloral hydrate, as well as other new sedatives such as potassium bromide, would prove to be a harbinger of 20th-century sedative-hypnotic abuse.

Hallucinogens American Indians used peyote in religious ceremonies since at least the 17th century. Hallucinogenic mushrooms, particularly *Psilocybe* mushrooms, were also used in the religious life of Native Americans. These were called "teonanacatl," which means "God's sacred mushrooms" or "God's flesh."[115] Interest in the recreational use of cannabis also accelerated during the 19th century after Napoleon's troops brought the drug back from Egypt, where its use among the lower classes was widespread. In 1843, several French Romantics, including Balzac, Baudelaire, Gautier, and Hugo, formed a hashish club called "Le Club des Hachichins" in the Parisian apartment of a young French painter. Fitz Hugh Ludlow's *The Hasheesh Eater*, published in 1857, was an early American text espousing the virtues of marijuana.[86]

Absinthe, an ethanol-containing beverage that was manufactured with an extract from wormwood (*Artemisia absinthium*), was very popular during the last half of the 19th century.[80] This emerald-colored, very bitter drink was memorialized in the paintings of Degas, Toulouse-Lautrec, and Van Gogh and was a staple of French society during this period.[12] α-Thujone, a psychoactive component of wormwood and a noncompetitive γ-aminobutyric acid type A $GABA_A$ blocker, is thought to be responsible for the pleasant feelings, as well as for the hallucinogenic effects, hyperexcitability, and significant neurotoxicity associated with this drink.[63] Van Gogh's debilitating episodes of psychosis were likely exacerbated by absinthe drinking.[137] Because of the medical problems associated with its use, absinthe was banned throughout most of Europe by the early 20th century.

A more recent event that had significant impact on modern-day hallucinogen use was the synthesis of lysergic acid diethylamide (LSD) by Albert Hofmann in 1938.[62] Working for Sandoz Pharmaceutical Company, Hofmann synthesized LSD while investigating the pharmacologic properties of ergot alkaloids. Subsequent self-experimentation by Hofmann led to the first description of its hallucinogenic effects and stimulated research into the use of LSD as a therapeutic agent. Hofmann is also credited with isolating psilocybin as the active ingredient in *Psilocybe mexicana* mushrooms in 1958.[100]

TWENTIETH-CENTURY EVENTS

EARLY REGULATORY INITIATIVES

The development of medical toxicology as a medical subspecialty and the important role of poison control centers began shortly after World War II. Before then, serious attention to the problem of household poisonings in the United States had been limited to a few federal legislative antipoisoning initiatives (Table 1–4). The 1906 Pure Food and Drug Act was the first federal legislation that sought to protect the public from problematic and potentially unsafe drugs and food. The driving force behind this reform was Harvey Wiley, the chief chemist at the Department of Agriculture. Beginning in the 1880s, Wiley investigated the problems of contaminated food. In 1902, he organized the "poison squad," which consisted of a group of volunteers who did self-experiments with food preservatives.[5] Revelations from the "poison squad," as well as the publication of Upton Sinclair's muckraking novel *The Jungle*[132] in 1906, exposed unhygienic practices of the meatpacking industry and led to growing support for legislative intervention. Samuel Hopkins Adams' reports about the patent medicine industry revealed that some drug manufacturers added opiates to soothing syrups for infants and led to the call for reform.[120] Although the 1906 regulations were mostly concerned with protecting the public from adulterated food, regulations protecting against misbranded patent medications were also included.

The Federal Caustic Poison Act of 1927 was the first federal legislation to specifically address household poisoning. As early as 1859, bottles clearly demarcated "poison" were manufactured in response to a rash of unfortunate dispensing errors that occurred when oxalic acid was unintentionally substituted for a similarly appearing Epsom salts solution.[26] Before 1927, however, "poison" warning labels were not required on chemical containers, regardless of toxicity or availability. The 1927 Caustic Act was spearheaded by the efforts of Chevalier Jackson, an otolaryngologist, who showed that unintentional exposures to household caustic agents were an increasingly frequent cause of severe oropharyngeal and gastrointestinal burns. Under this statute, for the first time, alkali- and acid-containing products had to clearly display a "poison" warning label.[139]

The most pivotal regulatory initiative in the United States before World War II—and perhaps the most significant American toxicologic regulation of the 20th century—was the Federal Food, Drug, and Cosmetic Act of 1938. Although the Food and Drug Administration (FDA) had been established in 1930 and legislation to strengthen the 1906 Pure Food and Drug Act was considered by Congress in 1933, the proposed revisions still had not been passed by 1938. Then the elixir of sulfanilamide tragedy in 1938 (see Chap. 2) claimed the lives of 105 people who had ingested a prescribed liquid preparation of the antibiotic sulfanilamide inappropriately dissolved in diethylene glycol. This event finally provided the catalyst for legislative intervention.[98,147]

Before the elixir disaster, proposed legislation called only for the banning of false and misleading drug labeling and for the outlawing of dangerous drugs without mandatory drug safety testing. After the tragedy, the proposal was strengthened to require assessment of drug safety before marketing, and the legislation was ultimately passed.

THE DEVELOPMENT OF POISON CONTROL CENTERS

World War II led to the rapid proliferation of new drugs and chemicals in the marketplace and in the household.[36] At the same time, suicide was recognized as a leading cause of death from these agents.[9] Both of these factors led the medical community to develop a response to the serious problems of unintentional and intentional poisonings. In Europe during the late 1940s, special toxicology wards were organized in Copenhagen and Budapest,[57] and a poison information service was begun in the Netherlands (Table 1–5).[144] A 1952 American Academy of Pediatrics study revealed that more than 50% of childhood "accidents" in the United States were the result of unintentional poisonings.[60] This study led Edward Press to open the first US poison control center in Chicago in 1953.[116] Press believed that it had become extremely difficult for individual physicians to keep abreast of product information, toxicity, and treatment for the rapidly increasing number of potentially poisonous household products. His initial center was organized as a cooperative effort among the departments of pediatrics at several Chicago medical schools, with the goal of collecting and disseminating product information to inquiring physicians, mainly pediatricians.[117]

By 1957, 17 poison control centers were operating in the United States.[36] With the Chicago center serving as a model, these early centers responded to physician callers by providing ingredient and toxicity information about drug and household products and making treatment recommendations. Records were kept of the calls, and preventive strategies were introduced into the community. As more poison control centers opened, a second important function, providing information to calls from the general public, became increasingly common. The physician pioneers in poison prevention and poison treatment were predominantly pediatricians who focused on unintentional childhood ingestions.[122]

During these early years in the development of poison control centers, each center had to collect its own product information, which was a laborious and often redundant task.[35] In an effort to coordinate poison control center operations and to avoid unnecessary duplication, Surgeon General James Goddard responded to the recommendation of the American Public Health Service and established the National Clearinghouse for Poison Control Centers in 1957.[96] This organization, placed under the Bureau of Product Safety of the Food and Drug Administration, disseminated 5-inch by 8-inch index cards containing poison information to each center to help standardize poison center information resources. The Clearinghouse also collected and tabulated poison data from each of the centers.

Between 1953 and 1972, a rapid, uncoordinated proliferation of poison control centers occurred in the United States.[92] In 1962, there were 462 poison control centers.[1] By 1970, this number had risen to 590,[84] and by 1978, there were 661 poison control centers in the United States, including 100 centers in the state of Illinois alone.[128] The nature of calls to centers changed as lay public–generated calls began to outnumber physician-generated calls. Recognizing the public relations value and strong popular support associated with poison centers, some hospitals started poison control centers without adequately recognizing or providing for the associated responsibilities. Unfortunately, many of these centers offered no more than a part-time telephone service located in the back of the emergency department or pharmacy, staffed by poorly trained personnel.[128]

TABLE 1–4. Protecting Our Health: Important US Regulatory Initiatives Pertaining to Xenobiotics Since 1900

Date	Federal Legislation	Intent
1906	Pure Food and Drug Act	Early regulatory initiative. Prohibits interstate commerce of misbranded and adulterated foods and drugs.
1914	Harrison Narcotics Act	First federal law to criminalize the nonmedical use of drugs. Taxed and regulated distribution and sale of narcotics (opium, opium derivatives, and cocaine).
1927	Federal Caustic Poison Act	Mandated labeling of concentrated caustics.
1930	Food and Drug Administration (FDA)	Established successor to the Bureau of Chemistry; promulgation of food and drug regulations.
1937	Marijuana Tax Act	Applied controls to marijuana similar to those applied to narcotics.
1938	Federal Food, Drug, and Cosmetic Act	Required toxicity testing of pharmaceuticals before marketing.
1948	Federal Insecticide, Fungicide, and Rodenticide Act	Provided federal control for pesticide sale, distribution, and use.
1951	Durham-Humphrey Amendment	Restricted many therapeutic drugs to sale by prescription only
1960	Federal Hazardous Substances Labeling Act	Mandated prominent labeling warnings on hazardous household chemical products.
1962	Kefauver-Harris Drug Amendments	Required drug manufacturer to demonstrate efficacy before marketing
1963	Clean Air Act	Regulated air emissions by setting maximum pollutant standards.
1966	Child Protection Act	Banned hazardous toys when adequate label warnings could not be written.
1970	Comprehensive Drug Abuse and Control Act	Replaced and updated all previous laws concerning narcotics and other dangerous drugs.
1970	Environmental Protection Agency (EPA)	Established and enforced environmental protection standards.
1970	Occupational Safety and Health Act (OSHA)	Enacted to improve worker and workplace safety. Created National Institute for Occupational Safety and Health (NIOSH) as research institution for OSHA.
1970	Poison Prevention Packaging Act	Mandated child-resistant safety caps on certain pharmaceutical preparations to decrease unintentional childhood poisoning.
1972	Clean Water Act	Regulated discharge of pollutants into US waters.
1972	Consumer Product Safety Act	Established Consumer Product Safety Commission to reduce injuries and deaths from consumer products.
1972	Hazardous Material Transportation Act	Authorized the Department of Transportation to develop, promulgate, and enforce regulations for the safe transportation of hazardous materials.
1973	Drug Enforcement Administration (DEA)	Successor to the Bureau of Narcotics and Dangerous Drugs; charged with enforcing federal drug laws.
1973	Lead-based Paint Poison Prevention Act	Regulated the use of lead in residential paint. Lead in some paints was banned by Congress in 1978.
1974	Safe Drinking Water Act	Set safe standards for water purity.
1976	Resource Conservation and Recovery Act (RCRA)	Authorized EPA to control hazardous waste from the "cradle-to-grave," including the generation, transportation, treatment, storage, and disposal of hazardous waste.
1976	Toxic Substance Control Act	Emphasis on law enforcement. Authorized EPA to track 75,000 industrial chemicals produced or imported into the United States. Required testing of chemicals that pose environmental or human health risk.
1980	Comprehensive Environmental Response Compensation and Liability act (CERCLA)	Set controls for hazardous waste sites. Established trust fund (Superfund) to provide cleanup for these sites. Agency for Toxic Substances and Disease Registry (ATSDR) created.
1983	Federal Anti-Tampering Act	Response to cyanide laced Tylenol deaths. Outlawed tampering with packaged consumer products.
1986	Controlled Substance Analogue Enforcement Act	Instituted legal controls on analog (designer) drugs with chemical structures similar to controlled substances.
1986	Drug-Free Federal Workplace Program	Executive order mandating drug testing of federal employees in sensitive positions.
1986	Superfund Amendments and Reauthorization Act (SARA)	Amendment to CERCLA. Increased funding for the research and cleanup of hazardous waste (SARA) sites.
1988	Labeling of Hazardous Art Materials Act	Required review of all art materials to determine hazard potential and mandated warning labels for hazardous materials.
1994	Dietary Supplement Health and Education Act	Permitted dietary supplements including many herbal preparations to bypass FDA scrutiny.
1997	FDA Modernization Act	Accelerated FDA reviews, regulated advertising of unapproved uses of approved drugs
2002	The Public Health Security and Bioterrorism Preparedness and Response Act	Tightened control on biologic agents and toxins; increased safety of the US food and drug supply, and drinking water; and strengthened the Strategic National Stockpile.
2005	Combat Methamphetamine Epidemic Act	Part of the Patriot Act, this legislation restricted nonprescription sale of the methamphetamine precursor drugs ephedrine and pseudoephedrine used in the home production of methamphetamine
2009	Family Smoking Prevention and Tobacco Control Act	Empowered FDA to set standards for tobacco products

TABLE 1-5. Twentieth Century Milestones in the Development of Medical Toxicology

Year	Milestone
1949	First toxicology wards open in Budapest and Copenhagen
1949	First poison information service begins in the Netherlands
1952	American Academy of Pediatrics study shows that 51% of children's "accidents" are the result of the ingestion of potential poisons
1953	First US poison control center opens in Chicago
1957	National Clearinghouse for Poison Control Centers established
1958	American Association of Poison Control Centers (AAPCC) founded
1961	First Poison Prevention Week
1963	Initial call for development of regional Poison Control Centers (PCCs)
1964	Creation of European Association for PCCs
1968	American Academy of Clinical Toxicology (AACT) established
1972	Introduction of microfiche technology to poison information
1974	American Board of Medical Toxicology (ABMT) established
1978	AAPCC introduces standards of regional designation
1983	First examination given for Specialist in Poison Information (SPI)
1985	American Board of Applied Toxicology (ABAT) established
1992	Medical Toxicology recognized by American Board of Medical Specialties (ABMS)
1994	First ABMS examination in Medical Toxicology
2000	Accreditation Council for Graduate Medical Education (ACGME) approval of residency training programs in Medical Toxicology
2000	Poison Control Center Enhancement and Awareness Act
2004	Institute of Medicine (IOM) Report on the future of poison centers is released, calling for a greater integration between public health sector and poison control services

Despite the "growing pains" of these poison control services during this period, there were many significant achievements were made. A dedicated group of physicians and other healthcare professionals began devoting an increasing proportion of their time to poison related matters. In 1958, the American Association of Poison Control Centers (AAPCC) was founded to promote closer cooperation between poison centers, to establish uniform standards, and to develop educational programs for the general public and healthcare professionals.[59] Annual research meetings were held, and important legislative initiatives were stimulated by the organization's efforts.[96] Examples of such legislation include the Federal Hazardous Substances Labeling Act of 1960, which improved product labeling; the Child Protection Act of 1966, which extended labeling statutes to pesticides and other hazardous substances; and the Poison Prevention Packaging Act of 1970, which mandated safety packaging. In 1961, in an attempt to heighten public awareness of the dangers of unintentional poisoning, the third week of March was designated as the Annual National Poison Prevention Week.

Another organization that would become important, the American Academy of Clinical Toxicology (AACT), was founded in 1968 by a diverse group of toxicologists.[31] This group was "interested in applying principles of rational toxicology to patient treatment" and in improving the standards of care on a national basis.[125] The first modern textbooks of clinical toxicology began to appear in the mid-1950s with the publication of Dreisbach's *Handbook of Poisoning* (1955)[43]; Gleason, Gosselin, and Hodge's *Clinical Toxicology of Commercial Products* (1957)[55]; and Arena's *Poisoning* (1963).[10] Major advancements in the storage and retrieval of poison information were also instituted during these years. Information as noted above on consumer products initially appeared on index cards distributed regularly to poison centers by the National Clearinghouse, and by 1978, more than 16,000 individual product cards had been issued.[129] The introduction of microfiche technology in 1972 enabled the storage of much larger amounts of data in much smaller spaces at the individual poison centers. Toxifile and POISINDEX, two large drug and poison databases using microfiche technology, were introduced and gradually replaced the much more limited index card system.[128] During the 1980s, POISINDEX, which had become the standard database, was made more accessible by using CD-ROM technology. Sophisticated information about the most obscure toxins was now instantaneously available by computer at every poison center.

In 1978, the poison control center movement entered an important new stage in its development when the AAPCC introduced standards for regional poison center designation.[92] By defining strict criteria, the AAPCC sought to upgrade poison center operations significantly and to offer a national standard of service. These criteria included using poison specialists dedicated exclusively to operating the poison control center 24 hours per day and serving a catchment area of between 1 and 10 million people. Not surprisingly, this professionalization of the poison center movement led to a rapid consolidation of services. An AAPCC credentialing examination for poison information specialists was inaugurated in 1983 to help ensure the quality and standards of poison center staff.[7]

In 2000, the Poison Control Center Enhancement and Awareness Act was passed by Congress and signed into law by President Clinton. For the first time, federal funding became available to provide assistance for poison prevention and to stabilize the funding of regional poison control centers. This federal assistance permitted the establishment of a single nationwide toll-free phone number (800-222-1222) to access poison centers. At present, 59 centers contribute data to a National Poison Database System (NPDS) which from 1983 to 2006 was known as Toxic Exposure Surveillance System (TESS). Recently, the Centers for Disease Control and Prevention (CDC) has been collaborating with the AAPCC to conduct real-time surveillance of this data to help facilitate the early detection of chemical exposures of public health importance.[150]

A poison control center movement has also grown and evolved in Europe over the past 35 years, but unlike the movement in the United States, it focused from the beginning on establishing strong centralized toxicology treatment centers. In the late 1950s, Gaultier in Paris developed an inpatient unit dedicated to the care of poisoned patients.[57] In the United Kingdom, the National Poison Information Service developed at Guys Hospital in 1963 under Roy Goulding[57] and Henry Matthew initiated a regional poisoning treatment center in Edinburgh about the same time.[117] In 1964, the European Association for Poison Control Centers was formed at Tours, France.[57]

THE RISE OF ENVIRONMENTAL TOXICOLOGY AND FURTHER REGULATORY PROTECTION FROM TOXIC SUBSTANCES

The rise of the environmental movement during the 1960s can be traced, in part, to the publication of Rachel Carson's *Silent Spring* in 1962, which revealed the perils of an increasingly toxic environment.[27] The movement also benefited from the new awareness by those involved with the poison control movement of the growing menace of toxins in the home environment.[25] Battery casing fume poisoning, resulting from the burning of discarded lead battery cases, and acrodynia, resulting from exposure to a variety of mercury-containing products,[38] both demonstrated that young children are particularly vulnerable to low-dose exposures from certain toxins. Worries about the persistence of pesticides in the ecosystem and the increasing number of chemicals introduced into the environment added to concerns of the environment as a potential source of illness, heralding a drive for additional regulatory protection.

Starting with the Clean Air Act in 1963, laws were passed to help reduce the toxic burden on our environment (see Table 1–4). The establishment of the Environmental Protection Agency in 1970 spearheaded this attempt at protecting our environment, and during the next 10 years, numerous protective regulations were introduced. Among the most important initiatives was the Occupational Safety and Health Act of 1970, which established the Occupational Safety and Health Administration (OSHA). This act mandates that employers provide safe work conditions for their employees. Specific exposure limits to toxic chemicals in the workplace were promulgated. The Consumer Product Safety Commission was created in 1972 to protect the public from consumer products that posed an unreasonable risk of illness or injury. Cancer-producing substances, such as asbestos, benzene, and vinyl chloride, were banned from consumer products as a result of these new regulations. Toxic waste disasters such as those at Love Canal, New York, and Times Beach, Missouri, led to the passing of the Comprehensive Environmental Response, Compensation, and Liability Act (CERCLA, also known as the Superfund) in 1980. This fund is designed to help pay for cleanup of hazardous substance releases posing a potential threat to public health. The Superfund legislation also led to the creation of the Agency for Toxic Substances and Disease Registry (ATSDR), a federal public health agency charged with determining the nature and extent of health problems at Superfund sites and advising the US Environmental Protection Agency and state health and environmental agencies on the need for cleanup and other actions to protect the public's health. In 2003, the ATSDR became part of the National Center for Environmental Health of the CDC.

MEDICAL TOXICOLOGY COMES OF AGE

Over the past 25 years, the primary specialties of medical toxicologists have changed. The development of emergency medicine and preventive medicine as medical specialties led to the training of more physicians with a dedicated interest in toxicology. By the early 1990s, emergency physicians accounted for more than half the number of practicing medical toxicologists.[43] The increased diversity of medical toxicologists with primary training in emergency medicine, pediatrics, preventive medicine, or internal medicine has helped broaden the goals of poison control centers and medical toxicologists beyond the treatment of acute unintentional childhood ingestions. The scope of medical toxicology now includes a much wider array of toxic exposures, including acute and chronic, adult and pediatric, unintentional and intentional, and occupational and environmental exposures.

The development of medical toxicology as a medical subspecialty began in 1974, when the AACT created the American Board of Medical Toxicology (ABMT) to recognize physician practitioners of medical toxicology.[6] From 1974 to 1992, 209 physicians obtained board certification, and formal subspecialty recognition of medical toxicology by the American Board of Medical Specialties (ABMS) was granted in 1992. In that year, a conjoint subboard with representatives from the American Board of Emergency Medicine, American Board of Pediatrics, and American Board of Preventive Medicine was established, and the first ABMS-sanctioned examination in medical toxicology was offered in 1994. By 2009, a total of more than 400 physicians were board certified in medical toxicology. The American College of Medical Toxicology (ACMT) was founded in 1994 as a physician-based organization designed to advance clinical, educational, and research goals in medical toxicology. In 1999, the Accreditation Council of Graduate Medical Education (ACGME) in the United States formally recognized postgraduate education in medical toxicology, and by 2009, 25 fellowship training programs had been approved.

During the 1990s in the United States, some medical toxicologists began to work on establishing regional toxicology treatment centers. Adapting the European model, such toxicology treatment centers could serve as referral centers for patients requiring advanced toxicologic evaluation and treatment. Goals of such inpatient regional centers included enhancing care of poisoned patients, strengthening toxicology training, and facilitating research. The evaluation of the clinical efficacy and fiscal viability of such programs is ongoing.

The professional maturation of advanced practice pharmacists and nurses with primary interests in clinical toxicology has also taken place over the past two decades. In 1985, the AACT established the American Board of Applied Toxicology (ABAT) to administer certifying examinations for nonphysician practitioners of medical toxicology who meet their rigorous standards.[5] By 2009, more than 85 toxicologists, who mostly held either a PharmD or a PhD in pharmacology or toxicology, were certified by this board.

RECENT POISONINGS AND POISONERS

Although accounting for just a tiny fraction of all homicidal deaths (0.16% in the United States), notorious lethal poisonings continued throughout the 20th century (Table 1–3).[1]

In England, Graham Frederick Young developed a macabre fascination with poisons.[73] In 1971, at age 14 years, he killed his stepmother and other family members with arsenic and antimony. Sent away to a psychiatric hospital, he was released at age 24 years, when he was no longer considered to be a threat to society. Within months of his release, he again engaged in lethal poisonings, killing several of his coworkers with thallium. Ultimately, he died in prison in 1990.

In 1978, Georgi Markov, a Bulgarian defector living in London, developed multisystem failure and died 4 days after having been stabbed by an umbrella carried by an unknown assailant. The postmortem examination revealed a pinhead-sized metal sphere embedded in his thigh where he had been stabbed. Investigators hypothesized that this sphere had most likely carried a lethal dose of ricin into the victim.[34] This theory was greatly supported when ricin was isolated from the pellet of a second victim who was stabbed under similar circumstances.

In 1982, deliberate tampering with nonprescription tylenol preparations with potassium cyanide caused 7 deaths in Chicago.[44] Because of this tragedy, packaging of nonprescription medications was changed to decrease the possibility of future product tampering.[101] The perpetrator(s) were never apprehended, and other deaths from nonprescription product tampering were reported in 1991.[28]

In 1998, Judias Buenoano, known as the "black widow," was executed for murdering her husband with arsenic in 1971 to collect insurance money. She was the first female executed in Florida in 150 years. The fatal poisoning had remained undetected until 1983, when Buenoano was accused of trying to murder her fiancé with arsenic and by car bombing. Exhumation of the husband's body, 12 years after he died, revealed substantial amounts of arsenic in the remains.[3]

Healthcare providers have been implicated in several poisoning homicides as well. An epidemic of mysterious cardiopulmonary arrests at the Ann Arbor Veterans Administration Hospital in Michigan in July and August 1975 was attributed to the homicidal use of pancuronium by two nurses.[138] Intentional digoxin poisoning by hospital personnel may have explained some of the increased number of deaths on a cardiology ward of a Toronto pediatric hospital in 1981, but the cause of the high mortality rate remained unclear.[22] In 2000, an English general practitioner Harold Shipman was convicted of murdering 15 female patients with heroin and may have murdered as many as 297 patients during his 24-year career. These recent revelations prompted calls for strengthening the death certification process, improving preservation of case records, and developing better procedures to monitor controlled drugs.[65]

Also in 2000, Michael Swango, an American physician, pleaded guilty to the charge of poisoning a number of patients under his care during his residency training. Succinylcholine, potassium chloride, and arsenic were some of the agents he used to kill his patients.[136] Attention to more careful physician credentialing and to maintenance of a national physician database arose from this case because the poisonings occurred at several different hospitals across the country. Continuing concerns about healthcare providers acting as serial killers is highlighted by a recent case in New Jersey in which a nurse, Charles Cullen, was found responsible for killing patients with digoxin.[16]

By the end of the 20th century, 24 centuries after Socrates was executed by poison hemlock, the means of implementing capital punishment had come full circle. Government-sanctioned execution in the United States again favored the use of a "state" poison—this time, the combination of sodium thiopental, pancuronium, and potassium chloride.

The use of a poison to achieve political ends has again resurfaced in several incidents from the former Soviet Union. In December 2004, it was announced that the Ukrainian presidential candidate Viktor Yushchenko was poisoned with 2,3,7,8-tetrachlorodibenzo-*p*-dioxin (TCDD), a potent dioxin.[130] The dramatic development of chloracne over the face of this public person during the previous several months suggested dioxin as a possibly culprit. Given the paucity of reports of acute dioxin poisoning, however, it wasn't until laboratory tests confirmed that Yushenko's dioxin levels were more than 6000 times normal that this diagnosis was confirmed. In another case, a former KGB agent and Russian dissident Alexander Litvinenko was murdered with polonium-210. Initially thought to be a possible case of heavy metal poisoning, Litvinenko developed acute radiation syndrome manifested by acute gastrointestinal symptoms followed by alopecia and pancytopenia before he died.[95]

RECENT DEVELOPMENTS

Medical Errors Beginning in the 1980s, several highly publicized medication errors received considerable public attention and provided a stimulus for the initiation of change in policies and systems. Ironically, all of the cases occurred at nationally preeminent university teaching hospitals. In 1984, 18-year-old Libby Zion died from severe hyperthermia soon after hospital admission. Although the cause of her death was likely multifactorial, drug–drug interactions and the failure to recognize and appropriately treat her agitated delirium also contributed to her death.[13] State and national guidelines for closer house staff supervision, improved working conditions, and a heightened awareness of consequential drug–drug interactions resulted from the medical, legislative, and legal issues of this case. In 1994, a prominent health journalist for the *Boston Globe*, Betsy Lehman, was the unfortunate victim of another preventable dosing error when she inadvertently received four times the dose of the chemotherapeutic agent cyclophosphamide as part of an experimental protocol.[76] Despite treatment at a world-renowned cancer center, multiple physicians, nurses, and pharmacists failed to notice this erroneous medication order. An overhaul of the medication-ordering system was implemented at that institution after this tragic event.

Another highly publicized death occurred in 1999, when 18-year-old Jesse Gelsinger died after enrolling in an experimental gene-therapy study. Gelsinger, who had ornithine transcarbamylase deficiency, died from multiorgan failure 4 days after receiving, by hepatic infusion, the first dose of an engineered adenovirus containing the normal gene. Although this unexpected death was not the direct result of a dosing or drug–drug interaction error, the FDA review concluded that major research violations had occurred, including failure to report adverse effects with this therapy in animals and earlier clinical trials and to properly obtain informed consent.[131] In 2001, Ellen Roche, a 24-year-old healthy volunteer in an asthma study at John Hopkins University, developed a progressive pulmonary illness and died 1 month after receiving 1 g of hexamethonium by inhalation as part of the study protocol.[135] Hexamethonium, a ganglionic blocker, was once used to treat hypertension but was removed from the market in 1972. The investigators were cited for failing to indicate on the consent form that hexamethonium was experimental and not FDA approved. Calls for additional safeguards to protect patients in research studies resulted from these cases.

In late 1999, the problems of medical errors finally received the high visibility and attention that it deserved in the United States with the publication and subsequent reaction to an Institute of Medicine (IOM) report suggesting that 44,000 to 98,000 fatalities each year were the result of medical errors.[77] Many of these errors were attributed to preventable medication errors. The IOM report focused on its findings that errors usually resulted from system faults and not solely from the carelessness of individuals.

Chemical Terrorism and Preparedness The terrorist attacks on the World Trade Center and the Pentagon on September 11, 2001, with the subsequent release of a multitude of toxic substances followed within days by the mailing of letters containing lethal amounts of anthrax in October 2001, resulted in profound changes in preparedness strategies against future terrorist strikes. Defending against biologic and chemical terrorism suddenly took on a much heightened sense of urgency. The asymmetric nature of the terrorism menace has led to increasing concerns that traditional industrial chemicals—so-called "chemical agents of opportunity"—may pose a more likely threat than a military chemical warfare agent attack. Responding to these events, poison centers and medical toxicologists from both emergency response and public health backgrounds are playing an increasingly visible role in terrorism preparedness training and leadership.

These events have led to a new realization that poison control centers serve an essential public health function that extends significantly beyond the traditional prevention of childhood poisonings. Responding to these new challenges, an IOM report released in 2004 calls for a more formal integration of poison center services into local, state, and federal public health preparedness and response.[68]

TOXICOLOGY IN THE TWENTY-FIRST CENTURY

As new challenges and opportunities arise in the 21st century, two new toxicologic disciplines have emerged: toxicogenomics and nanotoxicology.[37,42,107] These nascent fields constitute the toxicologic responses to rapid advances in genetics and material sciences. Toxicogenomics combines toxicology with genomics dealing with how genes and proteins respond to toxic substances. The study of toxicogenomics attempts to better decipher the molecular events underlying toxicologic mechanisms, develop predictors of toxicity through the establishment of better molecular biomarkers, and better understand genetic susceptibilities that pertain to toxic substances such as unanticipated idiosyncratic drug reactions.

Nanotoxicology refers to the toxicology of engineered tiny particles, usually smaller than 100 nm. Given the extremely small size of nanoparticles, typical barriers at portals of entry may not prevent absorption or may themselves be adversely affected by the nanoparticles. Ongoing studies focus on the translocation of these particles to sensitive target sites such as the central nervous system or bone marrow.[107]

SUMMARY

Since the dawn of recorded history, toxicology has impacted greatly on human events, and although over the millennia the important poisons of the day have changed to some degree, toxic substances continue to challenge our safety. The era of poisoners for hire may have long ago reached its pinnacle, but problems with drug abuse, intentional self-poisoning, exposure to environmental chemicals, and the potential for biologic and chemical terrorism continues to challenge us. Unfortunately, knowledge acquired by one generation is often forgotten or discarded inappropriately by the next generation, leading to a cyclical historic course. This historic review is meant to describe the past and to better prepare toxicologists and society for the future.

REFERENCES

1. Adelson L: Homicidal poisoning: A dying modality of lethal violence? *Am J Forensic Med Pathol.* 1987;8:245-251.
2. *American Heritage Dictionary.* Toxicology Boston: Houghton Mifflin; 1991.
3. Anderson C, McGehee S: *Bodies of Evidence: The True Story of Judias Buenoano: Florida's Serial Murderess.* New York: St. Martins; 1993.
4. Anderson H: Experimental studies on the pharmacology of activated charcoal. *Acta Pharmacol.* 1946;2:69-78.
5. Anonymous: American Board of Applied Toxicology. *AACTion.* 1992;1:3.
6. Anonymous: American Board of Medical Toxicology. *Vet Hum Toxicol.* 1987;29:510.
7. Anonymous: Certification examination for poison information specialists. *Vet Human Toxicol.* 1983;25:54-55.
8. Anonymous: Landmark article in occupational medicine. Forty years in the poisonous trades. American Industrial Hygiene Association Quarterly, April 1948. By Alice Hamilton. *Am J Ind Med.* 1985;7:3-18.
9. Anonymous: Suicide: A leading cause of death. *JAMA.* 1952;150:696-697.
10. Arena J: *Poisoning: Chemistry, Symptoms, Treatments.* Springfield, IL: Charles C. Thomas; 1963.
11. Arena JM: The pediatrician's role in the poison control movement and poison prevention. *Am J Dis Child.* 1983;137:870-873.
12. Arnold WN: Vincent van Gogh and the thujone connection. *JAMA.* 1988;260:3042-3044.
13. Asch DA, Parker RM: The Libby Zion case. One step forward or two steps backward? *N Engl J Med.* 1988;318:771-775.
14. Baldwin M: The snakestone experiments. An early modern medical debate. *Isis.* 1995;86:394-418.
15. Bartrip P: A "pennurth of arsenic for rat poison": the Arsenic Act, 1851 and the prevention of secret poisoning. *Med Hist.* 1992;36:53-69.
16. Becker C: Killer credential. In wake of nurse accused of killing patient, the health system wrestles with balancing shortage, ineffectual reference process. *Mod Healthc.* 2003;33:6-7.
17. Benjamin DR: *Mushrooms: Poisons and Panaceas.* New York: WH Freeman; 1995.
18. Berman A: The persistence of theriac in France. *Pharmacy in History.* 1970;12:5-12.
19. Bisset NG: Arrow and dart poisons. *J Ethnopharmacol.* 1989;25:1-41.
20. Bond RT: *Handbook for Poisoners: A Collection of Great Poison Stories.* New York: Collier Books; 1951.
21. Brown HM: De Venenis of Petrus Abbonus: A translation of the Latin. *Ann Med Hist.* 1924;6:25-53.
22. Buehler JW, Smith LF, Wallace EM, et al: Unexplained deaths in a children's hospital. An epidemiologic assessment. *N Engl J Med.* 1985;313:211-216.
23. Burchell HB: Digitalis poisoning: historical and forensic aspects. *J Am Coll Cardiol.* 1983;1:506-516.
24. Burke M: Gastric lavage and emesis in the treatment of ingested poisons: a review and a clinical study of lavage in ten adults. *Resuscitation.* 1972;1:91-105.
25. Burnham JC: How the discovery of accidental childhood poisoning contributed to the development of environmentalism in the United States. *Environ Hist Rev.* 1995;19:57-81.
26. Campbell WA: Oxalic acid, epsom salt and the poison bottle. *Hum Toxicol* 1982;1:187-193.
27. Carson RL: *Silent Spring.* Boston: Houghton Mifflin; 1962.
28. CDC: Cyanide poisonings associated with over-the-counter medication—Washington State, 1991. *MMWR Morb Mortal Wkly Rep.* 1991;40:161,7-8.
29. Christison R: *A Treatise on Poisons.* London: Adam Black; 1829.
30. Clarke MJ: Chloral hydrate: medicine and poison? *Pharm Hist.* 1988;18:2-4.
31. Comstock EG: Roots and circles in medical toxicology: a personal reminiscence. *J Toxicol Clin Toxicol.* 1998;36:401-407.
32. Cooney DO: *Activated Charcoal in Medical Applications.* New York: Marcel Dekker; 1995.
33. Costill OH: *A Practical Treatise on Poisons.* Philadelphia: Grigg, Elliot; 1848.
34. Crompton R, Gall D: Georgi Markov—death in a pellet. *Med Leg J.* 1980;48:51-62.
35. Crotty J, Armstrong G: National Clearinghouse for Poison Control Centers. *Clin Toxicol.* 1978;12:303-307.
36. Crotty JJ, Verhulst HL: Organization and delivery of poison information in the United States. *Pediatr Clin North Am.* 1970;17:741-746.
37. Curtis J, Greenberg M, Kester J, et al: Nanotechnology and nanotoxicology: a primer for clinicians. *Toxicol Rev.* 2006;25:245-260.
38. Dally A: The rise and fall of pink disease. *Soc Hist Med.* 1997;10:291-304.
39. Das G: Cocaine abuse in North America: a milestone in history. *J Clin Pharmacol.* 1993;33:296-310.
40. Deichmann WB, Henschler D, Holmsted B, Keil G: What is there that is not poison? A study of the Third Defense by Paracelsus. *Arch Toxicol Suppl.* 1986;58:207-13.
41. *Dictionary OE*, 2nd ed. Oxford: Clarendon Press; 1989:328.
42. Donaldson K, Stone V, Tran CL, et al: Nanotoxicology. *Occup Environ Med.* 2004;61:727-728.
43. Dreisbach RH. *Handbook of Poisoning: Diagnosis and Treatment.* Los Altos, CA: Lange; 1955.
44. Dunea G: Death over the counter. *Br Med J (Clin Res Ed).* 1983;286:211-212.
45. Earles MP: Early theories of mode of action of drugs and poisons. *Ann Sci.* 1961;17:97-110.
46. Eckert WG: Historical aspects of poisoning and toxicology. *Am J Forensic Med Pathol.* 1981;2:261-264.
47. Eckert WG: Medicolegal investigation in New York City. History and activities 1918-1978. *Am J Forensic Med Pathol.* 1983;4:33-54.
48. Elgood C: A treatise on the bezoar stone. *Ann Med Hist.* 1935;7:73-80.
49. Felton JS: The heritage of Bernardino Ramazzini. *Occup Med (Oxf).* 1997;47:167-179.
50. Ferner RE. *Forensic Pharmacology: Medicine, Mayhem, and Malpractice.* Oxford: Oxford University Press; 1996.
51. Franco G: Ramazzini and workers' health. *Lancet.* 1999;354:858-861.
52. Funck-Brentano F: *Princes and Poisoners: Studies of the Court of Louis IV.* London: Duckworth & Co.; 1901.
53. Gaebel RE: Saturnine gout among Roman aristocrats. *N Engl J Med.* 1983;309:431.
54. Gallo MA: History and scope of toxicology. In: Klassen CD, ed. *Casarett and Doull's Toxicology: The Basic Science of Poisons*, 5th ed. New York: McGraw-Hill; 1996:3-11.
55. Gleason MN, Gosselin RE, Hodge HC: *Clinical Toxicology of Commercial Products: Acute Poisoning (Home and Farm).* Baltimore: Williams & Wilkins; 1957.
56. Golding AM: Two hundred years of drug abuse. *J R Soc Med.* 1993;86:282-286.
57. Govaerts M: Poison control in Europe. *Pediatr Clin North Am.* 1970;17:729-739.
58. Grant MP: *Alice Hamilton: Pioneer Doctor in Industrial Medicine.* London: Abelard-Schuman; 1967.
59. Grayson R: The poison control movement in the United States. *Indust Med Surg.* 1962;31:296-297.

60. Green DW: The saturnine curse: a history of lead poisoning. *South Med J.* 1985;78:48-51.
61. Greensher J, Mofenson HC, Caraccio TR: Ascendency of the black bottle (activated charcoal). *Pediatrics.* 1987;80:949-951.
62. Hofmann A: How LSD originated. *J Psychedelic Drugs.* 1979;11:53-60.
63. Hold KM, Sirisoma NS, Ikeda T, et al: Alpha-thujone (the active component of absinthe): gamma-aminobutyric acid type A receptor modulation and metabolic detoxification. *Proc Natl Acad Sci U S A.* 2000;97:3826-3831.
64. Holt LE, Holz PH: The black bottle: a consideration of the role of charcoal in the treatment of poisoning in children. *J Pediatr.* 1963;63:306-314.
65. Horton R: The real lessons from Harold Frederick Shipman. *Lancet.* 2001;357:82-83.
66. Howard-Jones N: The origins of hypodermic medication. *Sci Am.* 1971;224:96-102.
67. Hunter D: *The Diseases of Occupations*, 6th ed. London: Hodder & Stoughton; 1978.
68. Institute of Medicine: *Forging a Poison Prevention and Control System.* Washington, DC: National Academies Press; 2004.
69. Jain KK: *Carbon Monoxide Poisoning.* St. Louis: Warren H. Green; 1990.
70. Jarcho S: Medical numismatic notes. VII. Mithridates IV. *Bull N Y Acad Med.* 1972;48:1059-1064.
71. Jarcho S: The correspondence of Morgagni and Lancisi on the death of Cleopatra. *Bull Hist Med.* 1969;43:299-325.
72. Jensen LB. *Poisoning Misadventures.* Springfield, IL: Charles C. Thomas; 1970.
73. Johnson H: R v Young—murder by thallium. *Med Leg J.* 1974;42:76-90.
74. Karch SB: The history of cocaine toxicity. *Hum Pathol.* 1989;20:1037-1039.
75. Knoefel PK: Felice Fontana on poisons. *Clio Med.* 1980;15:35-66.
76. Knox RA: Doctor's orders killed cancer patient: Dana Farber admits drug overdose caused death of *Globe* columnist, damage to second woman. *Boston Globe.* March 23, 1995;Sect. 1.
77. Kohn LT, Corrigan J, Donaldson MS, eds: *To Err Is Human: Building a Safer Health System.* Washington, DC: National Academy Press; 2000.
78. Kramer JC: Opium rampant: medical use, misuse and abuse in Britain and the West in the 17th and 18th centuries. *Br J Addict Alcohol Other Drugs.* 1979;74:377-389.
79. Kramer JC: The opiates: two centuries of scientific study. *J Psychedelic Drugs.* 1980;12:89-103.
80. Lanier D. Absinthe: *The Cocaine of the Nineteenth Century.* Jefferson, NC: McFarland; 1995.
81. Lee JA: Claude Bernard (1813-1878). *Anaesthesia.* 1978;33:741-747.
82. Levey M: Medieval Arabic toxicology: The book on poison of Ibn Wahshiya and its relation to early Indian and Greek texts. *Trans Am Philosph Soc.* 1966;56:5-130.
83. Lomax E: The uses and abuses of opiates in nineteenth-century England. *Bull Hist Med.* 1973;47:167-176.
84. Lovejoy FH, Jr., Alpert JJ: A future direction for poison centers. A critique. *Pediatr Clin North Am.* 1970;17:747-753.
85. Lucanie R: Unicorn horn and its use as a poison antidote. *Vet Hum Toxicol.* 1992;34:563.
86. Ludlow FH: *The Hasheesh Eater Microform: Being Passages from the Life of a Pythagorean.* New York: Harper; 1857.
87. Lyon AS: *Medicine: An Illustrated History.* New York: Abradale; 1978.
88. Macht DI: Louis Lewin: pharmacologist, toxicologist, medical historian. *Ann Med Hist.* 1931;3:179-194.
89. Magner LN: *A History of Medicine.* New York: Marcel Dekker; 1992.
90. Major RH: History of the stomach tube. *Ann Med Hist.* 1934;6:500-509.
91. Mann RH: *Murder, Magic, and Medicine.* New York: Oxford University Press; 1992.
92. Manoguerra AS, Temple AR: Observations on the current status of poison control centers in the United States. *Emerg Med Clin North Am.* 1984;2:185-197.
93. Mant AK: Forensic medicine in Great Britain. II. The origins of the British medicolegal system and some historic cases. *Am J Forensic Med Pathol.* 1987;8:354-361.
94. Marsh J: Account of a method of separating small quantities of arsenic from substances with which it may be mixed. *Edinb New Phil J.* 1836;21:229-236.
95. McFee R, Leikin, JB: Death by Polonium-210: Lessons learned from the murder of former Soviet spy Alexander Litvinenko. *JEMS.* 2008;33:18-23.
96. McIntire M: On the occasion of the twenty-fifth anniversary of the American Association of Poison Control Centers. *Vet Hum Toxicol.* 1983;25:35-37.
97. Mead GO: Ether drinking in Ireland. *JAMA.* 1891;16:391-392.
98. Modell W: Mass drug catastrophes and the roles of science and technology. *Science.* 1967;156:346-351.
99. Moore SW: A case of poisoning by laudanum, successfully treated by means of Juke's syringe. *NY Med Phys J.* 1825;4:91-92.
100. Moriarty KM, Alagna SW, Lake CR: Psychopharmacology. An historical perspective. *Psychiatr Clin North Am.* 1984;7:411-433.
101. Murphy DH: Cyanide-tainted Tylenol: what pharmacists can learn. *Am Pharm.* 1986;NS26:19-23.
102. Musto DF: America's first cocaine epidemic. *Wilson Q.* 1989;13:59-64.
103. Nahas GG: Hashish in Islam 9th to 18th century. *Bull N Y Acad Med.* 1982;58:814-831.
104. Nerlich AG, Parsche F, Wiest I, et al: Extensive pulmonary haemorrhage in an Egyptian mummy. *Virchows Arch.* 1995;427:423-429.
105. Niyogi SK: Historic development of forensic toxicology in America up to 1978. *Am J Forensic Med Pathol.* 1980;1:249-264.
106. Nriagu JO: Saturnine gout among Roman aristocrats. Did lead poisoning contribute to the fall of the Empire? *N Engl J Med.* 1983;308:660-663.
107. Oberdorster G, Oberdorster E, Oberdorster J, et al: Nanotoxicology: an emerging discipline evolving from studies of ultrafine particles. *Environ Health Perspect.* 2005;113:823-839.
108. Oehme FW: The development of toxicology as a veterinary discipline in the United States. *Clin Toxicol.* 1970;3:211-220.
109. Olch PD: William S. Halsted and local anesthesia: contributions and complications. *Anesthesiology.* 1975;42:479-486.
110. Orfila MP. *Traites des Poisons.* Paris: Ches Crochard; 1814.
111. Pachter HM: Paracelsus: *Magic into Science.* New York: Collier; 1961.
112. Pappas AA, Massoll NA, Cannon DJ: Toxicology: past, present, and future. *Ann Clin Lab Sci.* 1999;29:253-262.
113. Parsche F, Balabanova S, Pirsig W: Drugs in ancient populations. *Lancet.* 1993;341:503.
114. Plaitakis A, Duvoisin RC: Homer's moly identified as Galanthus nivalis L.: physiologic antidote to stramonium poisoning. *Clin Neuropharmacol.* 1983;6:1-5.
115. Pollack SH: The psilocybin mushroom pandemic. *J Psychedelic Drugs.* 1975;7:73-84.
116. Press E, Mellins RB: A poisoning control program. *Am J Public Health.* 1954;44:1515-1525.
117. Proudfoot AT: Clinical toxicology—past, present and future. *Hum Toxicol.* 1988;7:481-487.
118. Quinones MA: Drug abuse during the Civil War (1861-1865). *Int J Addict.* 1975;10:1007-1020.
119. Randall T: Cocaine deaths reported for century or more. *JAMA.* 1992;267:1045-1046.
120. Regier CC: The struggle for federal food and drugs legislation. *Law Contemp Prob.* 1933;1:3-15.
121. Reid DH: Treatment of the poisoned child. *Arch Dis Child.* 1970;45:428-433.
122. Robertson WO: National organizations and agencies in poison control programs: a commentary. *Clin Toxicol.* 1978;12:297-302.
123. Robins LN, Helzer JE, Davis DH: Narcotic use in southeast Asia and afterward. An interview study of 898 Vietnam returnees. *Arch Gen Psychiatry.* 1975;32:955-961.
124. Rosner F: Moses Maimonides' treatise on poisons. *JAMA.* 1968;205:914-916.
125. Rumack BH, Ford P, Sbarbaro J, et al: Regionalization of poison centers–a rational role model. *Clin Toxicol.* 1978;12:367-375.
126. Sapira JD: Speculations concerning opium abuse and world history. *Perspect Biol Med.* 1975;18:379-398.
127. Scarborough J: Nicander's toxicology II: spiders, scorpions, insects and myriapods. *Pharmacy in History.* 1979;21:73-92.
128. Scherz RG, Robertson WO: The history of poison control centers in the United States. *Clin Toxicol.* 1978;12:291-296.
129. Scutchfield FD, Genovese EN: Terrible death of Socrates: some medical and classical reflections. *Pharos.* 1997;60:30-33.
130. Shane S. Poison's use as political tool: Ukraine is not exceptional. *NY Times.* December 15, 2004;Sect. NY.
131. Silberner J: A gene therapy death. *Hastings Cent Rep.* 2000;30:36.
132. Sinclair U: *The Jungle.* New York: Doubleday; 1906.

133. Smith S: Poisons and poisoners through the ages. *Med Leg J.* 1952;20:153-167.
134. Sneader W: The discovery of heroin. Lancet 1998;352:1697-1699.
135. Steinbrook R: Protecting research subjects—the crisis at Johns Hopkins. *N Engl J Med.* 2002;346:716-720.
136. Stewart JB. Blind Eye: *The Terrifying Story of a Doctor Who Got Away with Murder.* New York: Touchstone; 1999.
137. Strang J, Arnold WN, Peters T: Absinthe: what's your poison? Though absinthe is intriguing, it is alcohol in general we should worry about. *Br Med J.* 1999;319:1590-1592.
138. Stross JK, Shasby M, Harlan WR: An epidemic of mysterious cardiopulmonary arrests. *N Engl J Med.* 1976;295:1107-1110.
139. Taylor HM: A preliminary survey of the effect which lye legislations had had on the incident of esophageal stricture. *Ann Otol Rhinol Laryngol.* 1935;44:1157-1158.
140. Thompson CJ: *Poison and Poisoners.* London: Harold Shaylor; 1931.
141. Timbrell JA: *Introduction to Toxicology.* London: Taylor & Francis; 1989.
142. Freud S: Über Coca, Secundararzt im k.k. Allgemeinen Krandenhause in Wien. Centralblatt für die Gesellschaft Therapie, 2, 289-314; reprinted in English (1984), *J Subst Abuse Treat* 1984;1:206-217.
143. Trestrail JH: *Criminal Poisoning: Investigational Guide for Law Enforcement, Toxicologists, Forensic Scientists, and Attorneys.* Totowa, NJ: Humana Press; 2000.
144. Vale JA, Meredith TJ. Poison information services. In: Vale JA, Meredith TJ, eds. *Poisoning, Diagnosis and Treatment.* London: Update Books; 1981:9-12.
145. Waldron HA: Lead poisoning in the ancient world. *Med Hist.* 1973;17: 391-399.
146. Watson G. *Theriac and Mithradatum: A Study in Therapeutics.* London: Wellcome Historical Medical Library; 1966.
147. Wax PM: Elixirs, diluents, and the passage of the 1938 Federal Food, Drug and Cosmetic Act. *Ann Intern Med.* 1995;122:456-461.
148. Witthaus RA: *Manual of Toxicology.* New York: William Wood; 1911.
149. Witthaus RA, Becker TC: *Medical Jurisprudence: Forensic Medicine and Toxicology.* New York: William Wood; 1894.
150. Wolkin AF, Patel M, Watson W, et al: Early detection of illness associated with poisonings of public health significance. *Ann Emerg Med.* 2006;47:170-176.
151. Wormley TG: *Micro-Chemistry of Poisons.* New York: William Wood; 1869.
152. Wright-St Clair RE: Poison or medicine? *N Z Med J.* 1970;71:224-229.

CHAPTER 2
TOXICOLOGIC PLAGUES AND DISASTERS IN HISTORY

Paul M. Wax

Throughout history, mass poisonings have caused suffering and misfortune. From the ergot epidemics of the Middle Ages to contemporary industrial disasters, these plagues have had great political, economic, social, and environmental ramifications. Particularly within the past 100 years, as the number of toxins and potential toxins has risen dramatically, toxic disasters have become an increasingly common event. The sites of some of these events—Bhopal (India), Chernobyl (Ukraine), Jonestown (Guyana), Love Canal (New York), Minamata Bay (Japan), Seveso (Italy), West Bengal (India)—have come to symbolize our increasingly toxic habitat. Globalization has led to the proliferation of toxic chemicals throughout the world and their rapid distribution. Many chemical factories that store large amounts of potentially lethal chemicals are not secure. Given the increasing attention to terrorism preparedness, an appreciation of chemicals as agents of opportunity for terrorists has suddenly assumed great importance. This chapter provides an overview of some of the most consequential and historically important toxin-associated disasters.

GAS DISASTERS

Inhalation of toxic gases and oral ingestions resulting in food poisoning tend to subject the greatest number of people to adverse consequences of a toxic exposure. Toxic gas exposures may be the result of a natural disaster (volcanic eruption), industrial mishap (fire, chemical release), chemical warfare, or an intentional homicidal or genocidal endeavor (concentration camp gas chamber). Depending on the toxin, the clinical presentation may be acute, with a rapid onset of toxicity (cyanide), or subacute or chronic, with a gradual onset of toxicity (air pollution).

One of the earliest recorded toxic gas disasters resulted from the eruption of Mount Vesuvius near Pompeii, Italy, in 79 A.D. (Table 2–1). Poisonous gases generated from the volcanic activity reportedly killed thousands.[37] A much more recent natural disaster occurred in 1986 in Cameroon, when excessive amounts of carbon dioxide spontaneously erupted from Lake Nyos, a volcanic crater lake.[20] Approximately 1700 human and countless animal fatalities resulted from exposure to this asphyxiant.

A toxic gas leak at the Union Carbide pesticide plant in Bhopal, India in 1984 resulted in one of the greatest civilian toxic disasters in modern history.[136] An unintended exothermic reaction at this carbaryl-producing plant caused the release of more than 24,000 kg of methyl isocyanate. This gas was quickly dispersed through the air over the densely populated area surrounding the factory where many of the workers lived, resulting in at least 2500 deaths and 200,000 injuries.[87] The initial response to this disaster was greatly limited by a lack of pertinent information about the toxicity of this chemical as well as the poverty of the residents. A follow-up study 10 years later showed persistence of small-airway obstruction among survivors.[32] Chronic eye problems were also reported.[2] Calls for improvement in disaster preparedness and strengthened right-to-know laws regarding potential toxic exposures resulted from this tragedy.[53,136]

The release into the atmosphere of 26 tons of hydrofluoric acid at a petrochemical plant in Texas in October 1987 resulted in 939 people seeking medical attention at nearby hospitals. Ninety-four people were hospitalized, but there were no deaths.[144]

More than any other single toxin, carbon monoxide has been involved with the largest number of toxic disasters. Catastrophic fires, such as the Cocoanut Grove Nightclub fire in 1943, have caused hundreds of deaths at a time, many of them from carbon monoxide poisoning.[39] A 1990 fire deliberately started at the Happy Land Social Club in the Bronx, New York, claimed 87 victims, including a large number of nonburn deaths,[80] and the 2003 fire at the Station nightclub in West Warwick, Rhode Island, killed 98 people.[122] Carbon monoxide poisoning was a major determinant in many of these deaths, although hydrogen cyanide gas and simple asphyxiation may have also contributed to the overall mortality.

Another notable toxic gas disaster involving a fire occurred at the Cleveland Clinic in Cleveland, Ohio in 1929, where a fire in the radiology department resulted in 125 deaths.[36] The burning of nitrocellulose radiographs produced nitrogen dioxide, cyanide, and carbon monoxide gases held responsible for many of the fatalities. In 2003, at least 243 people died and 10,000 people became ill after a drilling well exploded in Gaogiao, China, releasing hydrogen sulfide and natural gas into the air.[149] A toxic gas cloud covered 25 square kilometers. Ninety percent of the villagers who lived in the village adjoining the gas well died.

The release of a dioxin-containing chemical cloud into the atmosphere from an explosion at a hexachlorophene production factory in Seveso, Italy in 1976, resulted in one of the most serious exposures to dioxin (2,3,7,8-tetrachlorodibenzo-*p*-dioxin).[52] The lethality of this agent in animals has caused considerable concern for acute and latent injury from human exposure. Despite this apprehension, chloracne was the only significant clinical finding related to the dioxin exposure at 5-year follow-up.[10]

Air pollution is another source of toxic gases that causes significant disease and death. Complaints about smoky air date back to at least 1272, when King Edward I banned the burning of sea-coal.[134] By the 19th century—the era of rapid industrialization in England—winter "fogs" became increasingly problematic. An 1873 London fog was responsible for 268 deaths from bronchitis. Excessive smog in the Meuse Valley of Belgium in 1930, and in Donora, Pennsylvania, in 1948, was also blamed for excess morbidity and mortality. In 1952, another dense sulfur dioxide–laden smog in London was responsible for 4000 deaths.[78] Both the initiation of long-overdue air-pollution reform in England and Parliament's passing of the 1956 Clean Air Act resulted from this latter "fog."

WARFARE AND TERRORISM

Exposure to xenobiotics with the deliberate intent to inflict harm claimed an extraordinary number of victims during the 20th century (Table 2–2). During World War I, chlorine and phosgene gases and the liquid vesicant mustard were used as battlefield weapons, with mustard causing approximately 80% of the chemical casualties.[112] Reportedly, 100,000 deaths and 1.2 million casualties were attributable to these chemical attacks.[37] The toxic exposures resulted in severe airway irritation, acute lung injury, hemorrhagic pneumonitis, skin blistering, and ocular damage. Chemical weapons were used again in the 1980s during the Iran—Iraq war.

TABLE 2–1. Gas Disasters

Xenobiotic	Location	Date	Significance
Poisonous gas	Pompeii, Italy	79 A.D.	>2000 deaths from eruption of Mt. Vesuvius
Smog (SO_2)	London	1873	268 deaths from bronchitis
NO_2, CO, CN	Cleveland Clinic, Cleveland, OH	1929	Fire in radiology department; 125 deaths
Smog (SO_2)	Meuse Valley, Belgium	1930	64 deaths
CO, CN	Cocoanut Grove Night Club, Boston	1942	498 deaths from fire
CO	Salerno, Italy	1944	>500 deaths on a train stalled in a tunnel
Smog (SO_2)	Donora, PA	1948	20 deaths; thousands ill
Smog (SO_2)	London	1952	4000 deaths attributed to the fog/smog
Dioxin	Seveso, Italy	1976	Unintentional industrial release of dioxin into environment; chloracne
Methyl isocyanate	Bhopal, India	1984	>2000 deaths; 200,000 injuries
Carbon dioxide	Cameroon	1986	>1700 deaths from release of gas from Lake Nyos
Hydrofluoric acid	Texas City, TX	1987	Atmospheric release; 94 hospitalized
CO, ?CN	Happy Land Social Club, Bronx, NY	1990	87 deaths in fire from toxic smoke
Hydrogen sulfide	Xiaoying, China	2003	243 deaths and 10,000 became ill from gas poisoning after a gas well exploded
CO, ?CN	West Warwick, RI	2003	98 deaths in fire

The Nazis used poisonous gases during World War II to commit mass murder and genocide. Initially, the Nazis used carbon monoxide to kill. To expedite the killing process, Nazi scientists developed Zyklon-B gas (hydrogen cyanide gas). As many as 10,000 people per day were killed by the rapidly acting cyanide, and millions of deaths were attributable to the use of these gases.

Agent Orange was widely used as a defoliant during the Vietnam War. This herbicide consisted of a mixture of 2,4,5-trichlorophenoxyacetic acid (2,4,5-T) and 2,4-dichlorophenoxyacetic acid (2,4-D), as well as small amounts of a contaminant, 2,3,7,8-tetrachlorodibenzo-*p*-dioxin (TCDD), better known as dioxin. Over the years, a large number of adverse health effects have been attributed to Agent Orange exposure. A 2002 Institute of Medicine study concluded that among Vietnam veterans, there is sufficient evidence to demonstrate an association between this herbicide exposure and chronic lymphocytic leukemia, soft tissue sarcomas, non-Hodgkin lymphomas, Hodgkin disease, and chloracne.[59]

Mass exposure to the very potent organic phosphorus compound sarin occurred in March 1995, when terrorists released this chemical warfare agent in three separate Tokyo subway lines.[102] Eleven people were killed, and 5510 people sought emergency medical evaluation at more than 200 hospitals and clinics in the area.[124] This mass disaster introduced the spectra of terrorism to the modern emergency medical services system, resulting in a greater emphasis on hospital preparedness, including planning for the psychological consequences of such events. Sarin exposure also resulted in several deaths and hundreds of casualties in Matsumoto, Japan in June 1994.[92,99]

During recent wars and terrorism events, a variety of physical and neuropsychologic ailments have been attributed to possible exposure to toxic agents.[27,57] Gulf War syndrome is a constellation of chronic

TABLE 2–2. Warfare and Terrorism Disasters

Toxin	Location	Date	Significance
Chlorine	Iraq	2007	Used against US troops and Iraqi civilians
Chlorine, mustard gas, phosgene	Ypres, Belgium	1915–1918	100,000 dead and 1.2 million casualties from chemicals during World War I
CN, CO	Europe	1939–1945	Millions murdered by Zyklon-B (HCN) gas
Agent Orange	Vietnam	1960s	Contains dioxin; excess skin cancer
Mustard gas	Iraq–Iran	1982	New cycle of war gas casualties
Possible toxin	Persian Gulf	1991	Gulf War syndrome
Sarin	Matsumoto, Japan	1994	First terrorist attack in Japan using sarin
Sarin	Tokyo	1995	Subway exposure; 5510 people sought medical attention
Dust and other particulates	New York City	2001	World Trade Center collapse from terrorist air strike
Fentanyl derivative	Moscow	2002	Used by the Russian military to subdue terrorists in Moscow theatre
Ricin	Washington, DC	2004	Detected in Dirksen Senate Office Building; no illness reported

symptoms, including fatigue, headache, muscle and joint pains, ataxia, paresthesias, diarrhea, skin rashes, sleep disturbances, impaired concentration, memory loss, and irritability, noted in thousands of Persian Gulf War veterans without a clearly identifiable cause. A number of etiologies have been advanced to explain these varied symptoms, including exposure to the smoke from burning oil wells; chemical and biologic warfare agents, including nerve agents; and medical prophylaxis, such as the use of pyridostigmine bromide or anthrax and botulinum toxin vaccines, although the actual etiology remains unclear. An agreed upon toxicologic mechanism remains elusive.[41,57,60,61,62,71,113,133]

After the terrorist attacks on New York City in September 11, 2001, that resulted in the collapse of World Trade Center, persistent cough and increased bronchial responsiveness was noted among 8% of New York City Fire Department workers who were exposed to large amounts of dust and other particulates during the clean-up.[108,109] This condition, known as World Trade Center cough syndrome, is characterized by upper airway (chronic rhinosinusitis) and lower airway findings (bronchitis, asthma, or both) as well as, at times, gastroesophageal reflux dysfunction (GERD).[108] The risk of development of hyperreactivity and reactive airways dysfunction was clearly associated with the intensity of exposure.[17]

The Russian military used a mysterious "gas" to incapacitate Chechen rebels at a Moscow theatre in 2002, resulting in the deaths of more than 120 hostages. Although never publically indentified, the gas may have consisted of a highly potent aerosolized fentanyl derivative such as carfentanil and an inhalational anesthetic such as halothane. Better preparation of the rescuers with suitable amounts of naloxone may have help prevent many of these seemingly unanticipated casualties.[140]

Ricin was found in several government buildings, including a mail processing plant in Greenville, South Carolina in 2003 and the Dirksen Senate Office Building in Washington, DC in 2004. Although no cases of ricin-associated illness ensued, increased concern was generated because the method of delivery was thought to be the mail, and irradiation procedures designed to kill microbials such as anthrax would not inactivate chemical toxins such as ricin.[15,118]

FOOD DISASTERS

Unintentional contamination of food and drink has led to numerous toxic disasters (Table 2–3). Ergot, produced by the fungus *Claviceps purpurea*, caused epidemic ergotism as the result of eating breads and cereals made from rye contaminated by *C. purpurea*. In some epidemics, convulsive manifestations predominated, and in others, gangrenous manifestations predominated.[89] Ergot-induced severe vasospasm was thought to be responsible for both presentations.[88] In 994 A.D.,

TABLE 2–3. Food Disasters

Xenobiotic	Location	Date	Significance
Ergot	Aquitania, France	994 A.D.	40,000 died in the epidemic
Ergot	Salem, Massachusetts	1692	Neuropsychiatric symptoms may be attributable to ergot
Lead	Devonshire, England	1700s	Colic from cider contaminated during production
Arsenious acid	France	1828	40,000 cases of polyneuropathy from contaminated wine and bread
Lead	Canada	1846	134 men died during the Franklin expedition, possibly because of contamination of food stored in lead cans
Arsenic	Staffordshire, England	1900	Arsenic-contaminated sugar used in beer production
Cadmium	Japan	1939–1954	Itai-Itai ("ouch-ouch") disease
Hexachlorobenzene	Turkey	1956	4000 cases of porphyria cutanea tarda
Methyl mercury	Minamata Bay, Japan	1950s	Consumption of organic mercury poisoned fish
Triorthocresyl phosphate	Meknes, Morocco	1959	Cooking oil adulterated with turbojet lubricant
Cobalt	Quebec City, Canada and others	1960s	Cobalt beer cardiomyopathy
Methylenedianiline	Epping, England	1965	Jaundice
Polychlorinated biphenyls	Japan	1968	Yusho ("rice oil disease")
Methyl mercury	Iraq	1971	>400 deaths from contaminated grain
Polybrominated biphenyls	Michigan	1973	97% of state contaminated through food chain
Polychlorinated biphenyls	Taiwan	1979	Yu-Cheng ("oil disease")
Rapeseed oil (denatured)	Spain	1981	Toxic oil syndrome affected 19,000 people
Arsenic	Buenos Aires	1987	Malicious contamination of meat; 61 people underwent chelation
Arsenic	Bangladesh and West Bengal, India	1990s–present	Ground water contaminated with arsenic; millions exposed; 100,000s with symptoms; greatest mass poisoning in history
Tetramine	China	2002	Snacks deliberated contaminated, resulting in 42 deaths and 300 people with symptoms
Arsenic	Maine	2003	Intentional contamination of coffee; one death and 16 cases of illness
Nicotine	Michigan	2003	Deliberate contamination of ground beef; 92 people became ill
Melamine	China	2008	50,000 hospitalized from tainted infant formula

40,000 people died in Aquitania, France, in one such epidemic.[76] Convulsive ergotism was initially described as a "fire which twisted the people," and the term "St. Anthony's fire" (*ignis sacer*) was used to refer to the excruciating burning pain experienced in the extremities that is an early manifestation of gangrenous ergotism. The events surrounding the Salem, Massachusetts witchcraft trials have also been attributed to the ingestion of contaminated rye. The bizarre neuropsychiatric manifestations exhibited by some of the individuals associated with this event may have been caused by the hallucinogenic properties of ergotamine, a lysergic acid diethylamide (LSD) precursor.[23,85]

During the last half of the 20th century, unintentional mass poisoning from food and drink contaminated with toxic chemicals became all too common. One of the more unusual poisonings occurred in Turkey in 1956, when wheat seed intended for planting was treated with the fungicide hexachlorobenzene and then inadvertently used for human consumption. Approximately 4000 cases of porphyria cutanea tarda were attributed to the ingestion of this toxic wheat seed.[119]

Another example of chemical food poisoning took place in Epping, England in 1965. In this incident, a sack of flour became contaminated with methylenedianiline when the chemical unintentionally spilled onto the flour during transport to a bakery. Subsequent ingestion of bread baked with the contaminated flour produced hepatitis in 84 people. This outbreak of toxic hepatitis became known as Epping jaundice.[67]

The manufacture of polybromated biphenyls (PBBs) in a factory that also produced food supplements for livestock resulted in the unintentional contamination of a large amount of livestock feed in Michigan in 1973.[24] Significant morbidity and mortality among the livestock population resulted, and increased human tissue concentrations of PBBs were reported,[145] although human toxicity seemed limited to vague constitutional symptoms and abnormal liver function tests.[22]

The chemical contamination of rice oil in Japan in 1968 caused a syndrome called Yusho ("rice oil disease"). This occurred when heat-exchange fluid containing polychlorinated biphenyls (PCBs) and polychlorinated dibenzofurans (PCDFs) leaked from a heating pipe into the rice oil. More than 1600 people developed chloracne, hyperpigmentation, an increased incidence of liver cancer, or adverse reproductive effects. In 1979 in Taiwan, 2000 people developed similar clinical manifestations after ingesting another batch of PCB-contaminated rice oil. This latter epidemic was referred to as Yu-Cheng ("oil disease").[63]

In another oil contamination epidemic, consumption of illegally marketed cooking oil in Spain in 1981 was responsible for a mysterious poisoning epidemic that affected more than 19,000 people and resulted in at least 340 deaths. Exposed patients developed a multisystem disorder referred to as toxic oil syndrome (or toxic epidemic syndrome), characterized by pneumonitis, eosinophilia, pulmonary hypertension, scleroderma-like features, and neuromuscular changes. Although this syndrome was associated with the consumption of rapeseed oil denatured with 2% aniline, the exact etiologic agent was not definitively identified at the time. Subsequent investigations suggest that the fatty acid oleyl anilide may have been the putative agent.[35,64,65]

In 1999, an outbreak of health complaints related to consuming Coca Cola occurred in Belgium, when 943 people, mostly children, complained of gastrointestinal symptoms, malaise, headaches, and palpitations after drinking Coca Cola.[100] Many of those affected complained of an "off taste" or bad odor to the soft drink. Millions of cans and bottles were removed from the market at a cost of \$103 million.[100] In some of the bottles, the carbon dioxide was contaminated with small amounts of carbonyl sulfide, which hydrolyzes to hydrogen sulfide, and may have been responsible for odor-triggered reactions. Mass psychogenic illness may have contributed to the large number of medical complaints because the concentrations of the carbonyl sulfide (5–14 g/L) and hydrogen sulfide (8–17 g/L) were very low and unlikely to cause systemic toxicity.[42]

Epidemics of heavy metal poisoning from contaminated food and drink have also occurred throughout history. Epidemic lead poisoning is associated with many different vehicles of transmission, including leaden bowls, kettles, and pipes. A famous 18th-century epidemic was known as the Devonshire colic. Although the exact etiology of this disorder was unknown for many years, later evidence suggested that the ingestion of lead-contaminated cider was responsible.[137]

Intentional chemical contamination of food may also occur. Multiple cases of metal poisoning occurred in Buenos Aires in 1987, when vandals broke into a butcher's shop and poured an unknown amount of acaricide (45% sodium arsenite solution) over 200 kg of partly minced meat.[115] The contaminated meat was purchased by 718 people. Of 307 meat purchasers who submitted to urine sampling, 49 had urine arsenic concentrations of 76 to 500 μg/dL, and 12 had urine arsenic concentrations above 500 μg/dL (normal urine arsenic is <50–100 g/dL).

Recent cases of deliberate mass poisoning have heightened concerns about food safety and security. In China in 2002, a jealous food vendor adulterated fried dough sticks, sesame cakes, and rice prepared in a rival's snack bar by surreptitiously putting a large amount of tetramine (tetramethylene disulfotetramine) into the raw pastry material. More than 300 people who consumed these adulterated snacks became ill, and 42 died.[31] In Maine in 2003, a disillusioned parishioner contaminated the communal coffee pot at a church bake sale with arsenic. One victim died within 12 hours, and five others developed hypotension.[146] Also in 2003 in Michigan, 92 people became ill after ingesting contaminated ground beef deliberately contaminated with a nicotine pesticide by a supermarket employee.[6]

At the end of the 20th century and beginning the 21st century, what may be the greatest mass poisoning in history is occurring in Bangladesh and India's West Bengal State.[34,94,110,127] In Bangladesh alone, 60 million people are routinely drinking arsenic-contaminated ground water and at least 220,000 inhabitants of India's West Bengal have been diagnosed with arsenic poisoning.[93] Symptoms reported include melanosis, depigmentation, hyperkeratosis, hepatomegaly, splenomegaly, squamous cell carcinoma, intraepidermal carcinoma, and gangrene.[34] In a country long plagued by dysentery, attempts to purify the water supply led to the drilling of millions of wells into the superficial water table. Unknown to the engineers, this water was naturally contaminated with arsenic, creating several thousand tube wells with extremely high concentrations of arsenic—up to 40 times the acceptable concentration. Although toxicity from arsenic-contaminated groundwater was previously reported from other areas of the world, including Argentina, China, Mexico, Taiwan (black foot disease), and Thailand, the number of people at risk in Bangladesh and West Bengal is by far the largest.

Methyl mercury is responsible for several poisoning epidemics in the past half century. During the 1950s, a Japanese chemical factory that manufactured vinyl chloride and acetaldehyde routinely discharged mercury into Minamata Bay, resulting in contamination of the aquatic food chain. An epidemic of methyl mercury poisoning ensued as the local people ate the poisoned fish.[107,132] Chronic brain damage, tunnel vision, deafness, and severe congenital defects were associated with this outbreak.[107]

Another mass epidemic of methyl mercury poisoning occurred in Iraq in 1971, when the local population consumed homemade bread prepared from wheat seed treated with a methyl mercury fungicide.[16] Six thousand hospital admissions and more than 400 deaths were associated with this disaster. As was the case of the hexachlorobenzene exposure in Turkey 15 years previously, the treated grain, intended for use as seed, was instead used as food.

From 1939 to 1954, contamination of the local water supply with the wastewater runoff from a zinc–lead–cadmium mine in Japan was believed responsible for causing Itai-Itai ("ouch-ouch") disease, an unusual chronic syndrome manifested by extreme bone pain and osteomalacia. The local water was used for drinking and irrigation of the rice fields. Approximately 200 people who lived along the banks of the Jintsu River developed these peculiar symptoms, which were thought most likely to be caused by the cadmium.[3]

More than 50,000 infants were hospitalized in China in 2008 from the ill effects of melamine-contaminated powdered infant formulae.[58] Melamine (1,3,5-triazine–2,4,6-triamine) is a component in many adhesives, glues, plastics, and laminated products (e.g., plywood, cleaners, cement, cleansers, fire-retardant paint). More than 20 Chinese companies produced the tainted formula. Analysis of these formulas found melamine concentrations as high as 2500 ppm. Clinically, exposure to high doses of melamine has been associated with the development of nephrolithiasis, obstructive uropathy, and in some cases acute renal failure. Melamine contamination of pet food resulting in deaths in dogs and cats had previously been reported.[22] The melamine disaster also demonstrates that globalization and international agribusiness may facilitate worldwide distribution of contaminated foodstuffs. After the initial reports of melamine contamination in China, investigation in the United States revealed that certain brands of cookies, biscuits, candies, and milk sold in this country were also tainted with melamine, some of which was traced to an origin in China.[58]

MEDICINAL DRUG DISASTERS

Illness and death as a consequence of therapeutic drug use occur as sporadic events, usually affecting individual patients, or as mass disasters, affecting multiple (sometimes hundreds or thousands) patients. Sporadic single-patient medication-induced tragedies usually result from errors (Chap. 1) or unforeseen idiosyncratic reactions. Mass therapeutic drug disasters have generally occurred secondary to poor safety testing, a lack of understanding of diluents and excipients, drug contamination, or problems with unanticipated drug–drug interactions or drug toxicity (Table 2–4).

In September and October 1937, more than 105 deaths were associated with the use of one of the early sulfa preparations—elixir of sulfanilamide-Massengill—that contained 72% diethylene glycol as the vehicle for drug delivery. Little was known about diethylene glycol toxicity at the time, and many cases of renal failure and death occurred.[44] To avoid similar tragedies in the future, animal drug testing was mandated by the Food, Drug, and Cosmetic Act of 1938.[138] Unfortunately, diethylene glycol continues to be sporadically used in other countries as a medicinal diluent, resulting in deaths in South Africa (1969), India (1986), Nigeria (1990), Bangladesh (1990–1992), and Haiti (1995–1996).[139] In 1996 in Haiti, at least 88 Haitian children died (case fatality rate of 98% for those who remained in Haiti) after ingesting an acetaminophen elixir formulated with diethylene glycol–contaminated glycerin.[101,117] More recently, in Panama in 2006, glycerin contaminated with diethylene glycol found in prescription liquid cough syrup resulted in at least 121 cases of poisoning and 78 deaths (case fatality rate, 65.5%).[19,112] Investigators of this last outbreak discovered that the contaminated glycerin was imported to Panama from China via a European broker, demonstrating that improprieties in pharmaceutical manufacturing may have worldwide implications. In Nigeria in 2009, a tainted teething formula was responsible for 84 deaths in children.[7] The pharmaceutical manufacturers intended to purchase propylene glycol, a component of the teething formula but had bought the diluent in a jerrycan instead of the original container, and the chemical contained diethylene glycol.

A lesser-known drug manufacturing event, also involving an early sulfa antimicrobial, occurred in 1940 to 1941, when at least 82 people died from the therapeutic use of sulfathiazole that was contaminated with phenobarbital (Luminal).[129] The responsible pharmaceutical company, Winthrop Chemical, produced both sulfathiazole and phenobarbital, and the contamination likely occurred during the tableting process because the tableting machines for the two medications were adjacent to each other and were used interchangeably. Each contaminated sulfathiazole tablet contained about 350 mg of phenobarbital (and no

TABLE 2–4. Medicinal Disasters

Xenobiotic	Location	Date	Significance
Thallium	US	1920s–1930s	Treatment of ringworm; 31 deaths
Diethylene glycol	US	1937	Elixir of sulfanilamide; renal failure
Thorotrast	US	1930s–1950s	Hepatic angiosarcoma
Phenobarbital	US	1940–1941	Sulfathiazole contaminated with phenobarbital; 82 deaths
Diethylstilbestrol (DES)	US, Europe	1940s–1970s	Vaginal adenocarcinoma in daughters
Stalinon	France	1954	Severe neurotoxicity from triethyltin
Clioquinol	Japan	1955–1970	Subacute myelooptic neuropathy (SMON); 10,000 symptomatic
Thalidomide	Europe	1960s	5000 cases of phocomelia
Isoproterenol 30%	Great Britain	1961–1967	3000 excess asthma deaths
Pentachlorophenol	US	1967	Used in hospital laundry; nine neonates ill, two deaths
Benzyl alcohol	US	1981	Neonatal gasping syndrome
Tylenol-cyanide	Chicago	1982	Tampering incident resulted in seven homicides
L-Tryptophan	US	1989	Eosinophilia myalgia syndrome
Diethylene glycol	Haiti	1996	Acetaminophen elixir contaminated; renal failure; >88 pediatric deaths
Diethylene glycol	Panama	2006	Cough preparation contaminated with DEG, causing 78 deaths
Diethylene glycol	Nigeria	2009	Teething formula contaminated with DEG, causing 84 deaths

sulfathiazole), and the typical sulfathiazole dosing regimen was several tablets within the first few hours of therapy. Twenty-nine percent of the production lot was contaminated. Food and Drug Administration (FDA) intervention was required to assist with the recovery of the tablets, although 22,000 contaminated tablets were never found.[129]

In the early 1960s, one of the worst drug related modern-day events occurred with the release of thalidomide as an antiemetic and sedative–hypnotic.[33] Its use as a sedative–hypnotic by pregnant women caused about 5000 babies to be born with severe congenital limb anomalies.[89] This tragedy was largely confined to Europe, Australia, and Canada, where the drug was initially marketed. The United States was spared because of the length of time required for review and the rigorous scrutiny of new drug applications by the FDA.[86]

A major therapeutic drug event that did occur in the United States involved the recommended and subsequent widespread use of diethylstilbestrol (DES) for the treatment of threatened and habitual abortions. Despite the lack of convincing efficacy data, as many as 10 million Americans received DES during pregnancy or in utero during a 30-year period, until the drug was prohibited for use during pregnancy in 1971. Adverse health effects associated with DES use include increased risk for breast cancer in "DES mothers" and increased risk of a rare form of vaginal cancer, reproductive tract anomalies, and premature births in "DES daughters."[47,51]

Thorotrast (thorium dioxide 25%) is an intravenous radiologic contrast medium that was widely used between 1928 and 1955. Its use was associated with the delayed development of hepatic angiosarcomas, as well as skeletal sarcomas, leukemia, and "thorotrastomas" (malignancies at the site of extravasated thorotrast).[126,141]

The use of thallium to treat ringworm infections in the 1920s and 1930s also led to needless morbidity and mortality.[48] Understanding that thallium caused alopecia, dermatologists and other physicians prescribed thallium acetate, both as pills and as a topical ointment (Koremlu), to remove the infected hair. A 1934 study found 692 cases of thallium toxicity after oral and topical application and 31 deaths after oral use.[96] "Medicinal" thallium was subsequently removed from the market.

The "Stalinon affair" in France in 1954 involved the unintentional contamination of a proprietary oral medication that was marketed for the treatment of staphylococcal skin infections, osteomyelitis, and anthrax. Although it was supposed to contain diethyltin diiodide and linoleic acid, triethyltin, a potent neurotoxin and the most toxic of organotin compounds, and trimethyltin were present as impurities. Of the approximately 1000 people who received this medication, 217 patients developed symptoms, and 102 patients died.[11,18]

An unusual syndrome, featuring a constellation of abdominal symptoms (pain and diarrhea) followed by neurologic symptoms (peripheral neuropathy and visual disturbances, including blindness) was experienced by approximately 10,000 Japanese people between 1955 and 1970, resulting in several hundred deaths.[70] This presentation, subsequently labeled subacute myelooptic neuropathy (SMON), was associated with the use of the gastrointestinal disinfectant clioquinol, known in the West as Entero-Vioform and most often used for the prevention of travelers' diarrhea.[98] In Japan, this drug was referred to as "sei-cho-zai" ("active in normalizing intestinal function"). It was incorporated into more than 100 nonprescription proprietary medications and was used by millions of people, often for weeks or months. The exact mechanism of toxicity has not been determined, but recent investigators theorize that clioquinol may enhance the cellular uptake of certain metals, particularly zinc, and that the clioquinol–zinc chelate may act as a mitochondrial toxin, causing this syndrome.[14] New cases declined rapidly when clioquinol was banned in Japan.

In 1981, a number of premature neonates died with a "gasping syndrome," manifested by severe metabolic acidosis, respiratory depression with gasping, and encephalopathy.[46] Before the development of these findings, the infants had all received multiple injections of heparinized bacteriostatic sodium chloride solution (to flush their indwelling catheters) and bacteriostatic water (to mix medications), both of which contained 0.9% benzyl alcohol. Accumulation of large amounts of benzyl alcohol and its metabolite benzoic acid in the blood was thought to be responsible for this syndrome.[46]

A nursery mass poisoning occurred in 1967, when nine neonates developed extreme diaphoresis, fever, and tachypnea without rash or cyanosis. Two fatalities resulted, although the other infants responded dramatically to exchange transfusions. The illness was traced to sodium pentachlorophenate used as an antimildew agent in the hospital laundry.[8]

In 1989 and 1990, eosinophilia-myalgia syndrome, a debilitating syndrome somewhat similar to toxic oil syndrome, developed in more than 1500 people who had used the dietary supplement L-tryptophan.[64,135] These patients presented with disabling myalgias and eosinophilia, often accompanied by extremity edema, dyspnea, and arthralgias. Skin changes, neuropathy, and weight loss sometimes developed. Intensive investigation revealed that all affected patients had ingested L-tryptophan produced by a single manufacturer that had recently introduced a new process involving genetically altered bacteria to improve L-tryptophan production. A contaminant produced by this process probably was responsible for this syndrome.[21] The banning of L-tryptophan by the FDA set in motion the passage of the Dietary Supplement Health and Education Act of 1994. This legislation, which attempted to regulate an uncontrolled industry, inadvertently facilitated industry marketing of dietary supplements bypassing FDA scrutiny.

In recent years, a number of therapeutic drugs previously approved by the FDA have been withdrawn from the market because of concerns about health risks.[148] Many more drugs have been given "black box warnings" by the FDA because of their propensity to cause serious or life-threatening adverse effects. In 2009, more than 400 drugs had such black box warnings.[45] Some of the withdrawn drugs had been responsible for causing serious drug–drug interactions (astemizole, cisapride, mibefradil, terfenadine).[95] Other drugs were withdrawn because of a propensity to cause hepatotoxicity (troglitazone), anaphylaxis (bromfenac sodium), valvular heart disease (fenfluramine, dexfenfluramine), rhabdomyolysis (cerivastatin), hemorrhagic stroke (phenylpropanolamine), and other adverse cardiac and neurologic effects (ephedra, rofecoxib). One of the more disconcerting drug problems to arise was the development of cardiac valvulopathy and pulmonary hypertension in patients taking the weight-loss drug combination fenfluramine and phentermine (fen-phen) or dexfenfluramine.[29,123] The histopathologic features observed with this condition were similar to the valvular lesions associated with ergotamine and carcinoid. Interestingly, appetite suppressant medications, as well as ergotamine and carcinoid, all increase available serotonin.

ALCOHOL AND ILLICIT DRUG DISASTERS

Unintended toxic disasters have also involved the use of alcohol and other drugs of abuse (Table 2-5). Arsenical neuropathy developed in an estimated 40,000 people in France in 1828, when wine and bread were unintentionally contaminated by arsenious acid.[84] The use of arsenic-contaminated sugar in the production of beer in England in 1900 resulted in at least 6000 cases of peripheral neuropathy and 70 deaths (Staffordshire beer epidemic).[105]

During the early 20th century, particularly during Prohibition, the ethanolic extract of Jamaican ginger (sold as "the Jake") was a popular ethanol substitute in the southern and midwestern United States.[90] It was sold legally because it was considered a medical supplement to

TABLE 2–5. Alcohol and Illicit Drug Disasters

Xenobiotic	Location	Date	Significance
Triorthocresyl phosphate	US	1930–1931	Ginger Jake paralysis
Methanol	Atlanta, GA	1951	Epidemic from ingesting bootleg whiskey
Methanol	Jackson, MI	1979	Occurred in a prison
MPTP	San Jose, CA	1982	Illicit meperidine manufacturing resulting in drug-induced parkinsonism
Heroin heated on aluminum foil	Netherlands	1982	Spongiform leukoencephalopathy
3-Methyl fentanyl	Pittsburgh, PA	1988	"China-white" epidemic
Methanol	Baroda, India	1989	Moonshine contamination; 100 deaths
Fentanyl	New York City	1990	"Tango and Cash" epidemic
Methanol	New Delhi, India	1991	Antidiarrheal medication contaminated with methanol; >200 deaths
Methanol	Cuttack, India	1992	Methanol-tainted liquor; 162 deaths
Scopolamine	US East Coast	1995–1996	325 cases of anticholinergic poisoning in heroin users
Methanol	Cambodia	1998	>60 deaths
Methanol	Nicaragua	2006	800 became ill, 15 blind, 45 deaths

MPTP, 1-methyl-4-phenyl-1,2,3,6-tetrahydropyridine.

treat headaches and aid digestion and was not subject to Prohibition. For years, the Jake was sold adulterated with castor oil, but in 1930, as the price of castor oil rose, the Jake was reformulated with an alternative adulterant, triorthocresyl phosphate (TOCP). Little was previously known about the toxicity of this compound, and TOCP proved to be a potent neurotoxin. From 1930 to 1931, at least 50,000 people who drank the Jake developed TOCP poisoning, manifested by upper and lower extremity weakness ("ginger Jake paralysis") and gait impairment ("Jake walk" or "Jake leg").[90] A quarter century later, in Morocco, the dilution of cooking oil with a turbojet lubricant containing TOCP caused an additional 10,000 cases of TOCP-induced paralysis.[125]

In the 1960s, cobalt was added to several brands of beer as a foam stabilizer. Certain local breweries in Quebec City, Canada; Minneapolis, Minnesota; Omaha, Nebraska; and Louvain, Belgium added 0.5–5.5 ppm cobalt to their beer. This resulted in epidemics of fulminant heart failure among heavy beer drinkers (cobalt-beer cardiomyopathy).[1,91]

Epidemic methanol poisoning among those seeking ethanol and other inebriants is well described. In one such incident in Atlanta, Georgia in 1951, the ingestion of methanol-contaminated bootleg whiskey caused 323 cases of methanol poisoning, including 41 deaths. In another epidemic in 1979, 46 prisoners became ill after ingesting a methanol-containing diluent used in copy machines.[130]

In recent years, major mass methanol poisonings have continued to occur in developing countries, where store-bought alcohol is often prohibitively expensive. In Baroda, India in 1989, at least 100 people died and another 200 became ill after drinking a homemade liquor that was contaminated with methanol.[5] In New Delhi, India in 1991, an inexpensive antidiarrheal medicine, advertised to contain large amounts of ethanol, was instead contaminated with methanol, causing more than 200 deaths.[28] The following year, in Cuttack, India, 162 people died and an additional 448 were hospitalized after drinking methanol-tainted liquor.[12] A major epidemic of methanol poisoning occurred in 1998 in Cambodia, when rice wine was contaminated with methanol.[4] At least 60 deaths and 400 cases of illness were attributed to the methanol. Most recently, in Nicaragua in 2006, more than 800 people became ill and 45 died after drinking "aguardiente," an alcoholic beverage made with methanol instead of the more expensive ethanol. Fifteen people became blind.[128]

So-called "designer drugs" are responsible for several toxicologic disasters. In 1982, several injection drug users living in San Jose, California who were attempting to use a meperidine analog MPPP (1-methyl-4-phenyl-4-propionoxy-piperidine) developed a peculiar, irreversible neurologic disease closely resembling parkinsonism.[73] Investigation revealed that these patients had unknowingly injected trace amounts of MPTP (1-methyl-4-phenyl-1,2,3,6-tetrahydropyridine), which was present as an inadvertent product of the clandestine MPPP synthesis. The subsequent metabolism of MPTP to MPP^+ resulted in a toxic compound that selectively destroyed cells in the substantia nigra, causing severe and irreversible parkinsonism. The vigorous pursuit of the cause of this disaster led to a better understanding of the pathophysiology of parkinsonism and the development of possible future treatments.

Another example of a "designer drug" mass poisoning occurred in the New York City metropolitan area in 1991, when a sudden epidemic of opioid overdoses occurred among heroin users who bought envelopes labeled "Tango and Cash."[40] Expecting to receive a new brand of heroin, the drug users instead purchased the much more potent fentanyl. Increased and unpredictable toxicity resulted from the inability of the dealer to adjust ("cut") the fentanyl dose properly. Some purchasers presumably received little or no fentanyl, while others received potentially lethal doses. A similar epidemic involving 3-methylfentanyl occurred in 1988 in Pittsburgh, Pennsylvania.[82]

At least 325 cases of anticholinergic poisoning occurred among heroin users in New York City; Newark, New Jersey; Philadelphia, Pennsylvania; and Baltimore, Maryland from 1995 to 1996.[9] The "street drug" used in these cases was adulterated with scopolamine. Whereas naloxone treatment was associated with increased agitation and hallucinations, physostigmine administration resulted in resolution of symptoms. Why the heroin was adulterated was unknown, although the use of an opiate–scopolamine mixture was reminiscent of the morphine–scopolamine combination therapy known as "twilight sleep" that was extensively used in obstetric anesthesia during the early 20th century.[104]

Another unexpected complication of heroin use was observed in the Netherlands in the 1980s, when 47 heroin users developed mutism and spastic quadriparesis that was pathologically documented to be spongiform leukoencephalopathy.[147] In these and subsequent cases in Europe and the United States, the users inhaled heroin vapors after the heroin powder had been heated on aluminum foil, a drug administration technique known as "chasing the dragon."[68,147] The exact toxic mechanism has not been elucidated.

OCCUPATION-RELATED CHEMICAL DISASTERS

Unfortunately, occupation-related toxic epidemics have become increasingly common (Table 2-6). Such poisoning syndromes tend to have an insidious onset and may not be recognized clinically until years after the exposure. A specific toxin may cause myriad problems, among the most worrisome being the carcinogenic and mutagenic potentials.

Although the 18th-century observations of Ramazzini and Pott introduced the concept of certain diseases as a direct result of toxic exposures in the workplace, it was not until the height of the 19th-century industrial revolution that the problems associated with the increasingly hazardous workplace became apparent.[56] During the 1860s, a peculiar disorder, attributed to the effects of inhaling mercury vapor, was described among manufacturers of felt hats in New Jersey.[142] Mercury nitrate was used as an essential part of the felting process at the time. "Hatter's shakes" refers to the tremor that developed in an estimated 10% to 60% of hatters surveyed.[142] Extreme shyness, another manifestation of mercurialism, also developed in many hatters in later studies. Five percent of hatters during this period died from renal failure.

Other notable 19th-century and early 20th-century occupational tragedies included an increased incidence of mandibular necrosis (phossy jaw) among workers in the matchmaking industry who were exposed to white phosphorus,[54] an increased incidence of bladder tumors among synthetic dye makers who used β–Naphthylamine,[49] and an increased incidence of aplastic anemia among artificial leather manufacturers who used benzene.[121] The epidemic of phossy jaw among matchmakers had a latency period of 5 years and a mortality rate of 20% and has been called the "greatest tragedy in the whole story of occupational disease."[25] The problem continued in the United States until Congress passed the White Phosphorus Match Act in 1912, which established a prohibitive tax on white phosphorus matches.[85]

Since antiquity, occupational lead poisoning has been a constant threat. Workplace exposure to lead was particularly problematic during the 19th century and early 20th century because of the large number of industries that relied heavily on lead. One of the most notorious of the "lead trades" was the actual production of white lead and lead oxides. Palsies, encephalopathy, and death from severe poisoning were reported.[50] Other occupations that resulted in dangerous lead exposures included pottery glazing, rubber manufacturing, pigment manufacturing, painting, printing, and plumbing.[81] Given the increasing awareness of harm suffered in the workplace, the British Factory and Workshop Act of 1895 required governmental notification of occupational diseases caused by lead, mercury, and phosphorus poisoning, as well as of occupational diseases caused by anthrax.[75]

Exposures to asbestos during the 20th century have resulted in continuing extremely consequential occupational and environmental disasters.[30,97] Despite the fact that the first case of asbestosis was reported in 1907, asbestos was heavily used in the shipbuilding industries in the 1940s as an insulating and fireproofing material. Since the early 1940s, 8 to 11 million individuals were occupationally exposed to asbestos,[77] including 4.5 million individuals who worked in the shipyards. Asbestos-related diseases include mesothelioma, lung cancer, and pulmonary fibrosis (asbestosis). A threefold excess of cancer deaths, primarily of excess lung cancer deaths, has been observed in asbestos-exposed insulation workers.[120]

The manufacture and use of a variety of newly synthesized chemicals has also resulted in mass occupational poisonings. In Louisville, Kentucky in 1974, an increased incidence of angiosarcoma of the liver was first noticed among polyvinyl chloride polymerization workers who were exposed to vinyl chloride monomer.[38] In 1975, chemical factory workers exposed to the organochlorine insecticide chlordecone (Kepone) experienced a high incidence of neurologic abnormalities, including tremor and chaotic eye movements.[131] An increased incidence of infertility among male Californian pesticide workers exposed to 1,2-dibromochloropropane (DBCP) was noted in 1977.[143]

RADIATION DISASTERS

A discussion of mass poisonings is incomplete without mention of the large number of radiation disasters that have characterized the 20th century (Table 2-7). The first significant mass exposure to radiation occurred among several thousand teenage girls and young women employed in the dial-painting industry.[26] These workers painted luminous numbers on watch and instrument dials with paint that contained radium. Exposure occurred by licking the paint brushes and inhaling radium-laden dust. Studies showed an increase in bone-related cancers, as well as aplastic anemia and leukemia, in exposed workers.[83,106]

TABLE 2–6. Occupational Disasters

Xenobiotic	Location	Date	Significance
Polycyclic aromatic hydrocarbons	England	1700s	Scrotal cancer among chimney sweeps; first description of occupational cancer
Mercury	New Jersey	Mid to late 1800s	Outbreak of mercurialism in hatters
White phosphorus	Europe	Mid to late 1800s	Phossy jaw in matchmakers
β-Naphthylamine	Worldwide	Early 1900s	Bladder cancer in dye makers
Benzene	Newark, NJ	1916–1928	Aplastic anemia among artificial leather manufacturers
Asbestos	Worldwide	20th century	Millions at risk for asbestos-related disease
Vinyl chloride	Louisville, KY	1960s–1970s	Hepatic angiosarcoma among polyvinyl chloride polymerization workers
Chlordecone	James River, VA	1973–1975	Neurologic abnormalities among insecticide workers
1, 2-Dibromochloropropane	California	1974	Infertility among pesticide makers

TABLE 2–7. Radiation Disasters

Xenobiotic	Location	Date	Significance
Radium	Orange, NJ	1910s–1920s	Increase in bone cancer in dial-painting workers
Radium	US	1920s	"Radithor" (radioactive water) sold as radium-containing patent medication
Radiation	Hiroshima and Nagasaki, Japan	1945	First atomic bombs dropped at end of World War II; clinical effects still evident today
Radiation	Chernobyl, Ukraine	1986	Unintentional radioactive release; acute radiation sickness
Cesium	Goiania, Brazil	1987	Acute radiation sickness and radiation burns

At the time of the "watch" disaster, radium was also being sold as a nostrum touted to cure all sorts of ailments, including rheumatism, syphilis, multiple sclerosis, and sexual dysfunction. Referred to as "mild radium therapy" to differentiate it from the higher-dose radium that was used in the treatment of cancer at that time, such particle-emitting isotopes were hailed as powerful natural elixirs that acted as metabolic catalysts to deliver direct energy transfusions.[79]

During the 1920s, dozens of patent medications containing small doses of radium were sold as radioactive tablets, liniments, or liquids. One of the most infamous preparations was Radithor. Each half-ounce bottle contained slightly more than 1 Ci of radium-228 and radium-226. This radioactive water was sold all over the world "as harmless in every respect" and was heavily promoted as a sexual stimulant and aphrodisiac, taking on the glamour of a recreational drug for the wealthy.[79] More than 400,000 bottles were sold. The 1932 death of Eben Byers a Radithor connoisseur from chronic radiation poisoning drew increased public and governmental scrutiny to this unregulated radium industry and helped end the era of radioactive patent medications.[79]

Concerns about the health effects of radiation have continued to escalate since the dawn of the nuclear age in 1945. Long-term follow-up studies 50 years after the atomic bombings at Hiroshima and Nagasaki demonstrate an increased incidence of leukemia, other cancers, radiation cataracts, hyperparathyroidism, delayed growth and development, and chromosomal anomalies in exposed individuals.[66]

The unintentional nuclear disaster at Chernobyl, Ukraine in April 1986 again forced the world to confront the medical consequences of 20th-century scientific advances that created the atomic age.[43] The release of radioactive material resulted in 31 deaths and the hospitalization of more than 200 people for acute radiation sickness. By 2003, the predominant long-term effects of the event appeared to be childhood thyroid cancer and psychological consequences.[111] In some areas of heavy contamination, the increase in childhood thyroid cancer has increased 100-fold.[116]

Another serious radiation event occurred in Goiania, Brazil in 1987 when an abandoned radiotherapy unit was opened in a junkyard and 244 people were exposed to cesium-137. Of those exposed, 104 showed evidence of internal contamination, 28 had local radiation injuries, and eight developed acute radiation syndrome. There were at least four deaths.[103,114]

In September 1999, a nuclear event at a uranium-processing plant in Japan set off an uncontrolled chain reaction, exposing 49 people to radiation.[69] Radiation measured outside the facility reached 4000 times the normal ambient level. Two workers died from the effects of the radiation.

MASS SUICIDE BY POISON

Toxic disasters have also manifested themselves as events of mass suicide. In 1978 in Jonestown, Guyana, 911 members of the Peoples Temple died after drinking a beverage containing cyanide.[13] Although the majority of those deaths may have been by suicide, some appear to have been involuntary.[74]

In 1997, phenobarbital and ethanol (sometimes assisted by physical asphyxiation) was the suicidal method favored by 39 members of the Heavens Gate cult in Rancho Santa Fe, California, a means of suicide recommended in the book *Final Exit*.[55] Apparently, the cult members committed suicide to shed their bodies in hopes of hopping aboard an alien spaceship they believed was in the wake of the Hale-Bopp comet.[72]

SUMMARY

Unfortunately, toxicologic plagues and disasters have had all-too-prominent roles in history. An understanding of the pathogenesis of these toxic plagues pertaining to drug, food, and occupational safety is critically important to prevent future disasters. Such events make us aware that many of the toxic agents involved are potential agents of opportunity for terrorists and nonterrorists who seek to harm others. Given the practical and ethical limitations in studying the effects of many specific toxins in humans, lessons from these unfortunate tragedies must be fully mastered and retained for future generations.

REFERENCES

1. Alexander CS: Cobalt-beer cardiomyopathy. A clinical and pathologic study of twenty-eight cases. *Am J Med.* 1972;53:395-417.
2. Anderson HA, Wolff MS, Lilis R, et al: Symptoms and clinical abnormalities following ingestion of polybrominated-biphenyl-contaminated food products. *Ann N Y Acad Sci.* 1979;320:684-702.
3. Anonymous: Cadmium pollution and Itai-itai disease. *Lancet.* 1971;1:382-383.
4. Anonymous: Cambodian mob kills two Vietnamese in poisoning hysteria. *Deutsche Presse-Agentur.* 1998;September 4.
5. Anonymous: Fatal moonshine in India. *Newsday.* 1989;March 6.
6. Anonymous: Nicotine poisoning after ingestion of contaminated ground beef—Michigan, 2003. *MMWR Morb Mortal Wkly Rep.*. 2003;52:413-416.
7. Anonymous: Nigeria: 12 held over tainted syrup. *The New York Times.* 2009; February 12.
8. Anonymous: Pentachlorophenol poisoning in newborn infants—St. Louis Missouri, April–August 1967. *MMWR Morb Mortal Wkly Rep.* 1996;45:545-549.
9. Anonymous: Scopolamine poisoning among heroin users—New York City, Newark, Philadelphia, and Baltimore, 1995 and 1996. *MMWR Morb Mortal Wkly Rep.* 1996;45:457-460.
10. Anonymous: Seveso after five years. *Lancet.* 1981;2:731-732.
11. Anonymous: Stalinon: A therapeutic disaster. *Br Med J.* 1958;1:515.
12. Anonymous. Tainted liquor kills 162, sickens 228. *Los Angeles Times.* 1992; May 10.
13. Anonymous: The Guyana tragedy—an international forensic problem. *Forensic Sci Int.* 1979;13:167-172.

14. Arbiser JL, Kraeft SK, van Leeuwen R, et al: Clioquinol-zinc chelate: a candidate causative agent of subacute myelo-optic neuropathy. *Mol Med.* 1998;4:665-670.
15. Audi J, Belson M, Patel M, et al: Ricin poisoning: a comprehensive review. *JAMA.* 2005;294:2342-351.
16. Bakir F, Damluji SF, Amin-Zaki L, et al: Methylmercury poisoning in Iraq. *Science.* 1973;181:230-241.
17. Banauch GI, Alleyne D, Sanchez R, et al: Persistent hyperreactivity and reactive airway dysfunction in firefighters at the World Trade Center. *Am J Respir Crit Care Med.* 2003;168:54-62.
18. Barnes JM, Stoner HB: The toxicology of tin compounds. *Pharmacol Rev.* 1959;11:211-232.
19. Barr DB, Barr JR, Weerasekera G, et al: Identification and quantification of diethylene glycol in pharmaceuticals implicated in poisoning epidemics: an historical laboratory perspective. *J Anal Toxicol.* 2007;31:295-303.
20. Baxter PJ, Kapila M, Mfonfu D: Lake Nyos disaster, Cameroon, 1986: the medical effects of large scale emission of carbon dioxide? *Br Med J.* 1989;298:1437-1441.
21. Belongia EA, Hedberg CW, Gleich GJ, et al: An investigation of the cause of the eosinophilia-myalgia syndrome associated with tryptophan use. *N Engl J Med.* 1990;323:357-365.
22. Brown CA, Jeong K-S, Poppenga RH, et al: Outbreaks of renal failure associated with melamine and cyanuric acid in dogs and cats in 2004 and 2007. *J Vet Diagn Invest.* 2007;19:525-531.
23. Caporael LR: Ergotism: The Satan loosed in Salem? *Science.* 1976;192:21-26.
24. Carter LJ: Michigan PBB incident: Chemical mix-up leads to disaster. *Science.* 1976;192:240-243.
25. Cherniack MG: Diseases of unusual occupations: an historical perspective. *Occup Med.* 1992;7:369-384.
26. Clark C: *Radium Girls: Women and Industrial Health Reform, 1910–1935.* Chapel Hill, NC: University of North Carolina Press; 1997.
27. Clauw DJ, Engel CC, Jr., Aronowitz R, et al: Unexplained symptoms after terrorism and war: An expert consensus statement. *J Occup Environ Med.* 2003;45:1040-1048.
28. Coll S: Tainted foods, medicine make mass poisoning rife in India: Critics press for tougher inspections, more accurate labels. *Washington Post.* 1991;December 8:Sect. A36.
29. Connolly HM, Crary JL, McGoon MD, et al: Valvular heart disease associated with fenfluramine-phentermine. *N Engl J Med.* 1997;337:581-588.
30. Corn JK, Starr J: Historical perspective on asbestos: policies and protective measures in World War II shipbuilding. *Am J Indust Med.* 1987;11: 359-373.
31. Croddy E, Croddy E: Rat poison and food security in the People's Republic of China: Focus on tetramethylene disulfotetramine (tetramine). *Arch Toxicol.* 2004;78:1-6.
32. Cullinan P, Acquilla S, Dhara VR: Respiratory morbidity 10 years after the Union Carbide gas leak at Bhopal: A cross sectional survey. The International Medical Commission on Bhopal. *Br Med J.* 1997;314: 338-342.
33. Dally A: Thalidomide: Was the tragedy preventable? *Lancet.* 1998;351: 1197-1199.
34. Das D, Chatterjee A, Mandal BK, et al: Arsenic in ground water in six districts of West Bengal, India: the biggest arsenic calamity in the world. Part 2. Arsenic concentration in drinking water, hair, nails, urine, skin-scale and liver tissue (biopsy) of the affected people. *Analyst.* 1995;120:917-924.
35. de la Paz MP, Philen RM, Borda IA: Toxic oil syndrome: The perspective after 20 years. *Epidemiol Rev.* 2001;23:231-247.
36. Easton WH: Smoke and fire gases. *Ind Med.* 1942;11:466-468.
37. Eckert WG: Mass deaths by gas or chemical poisoning. A historical perspective. *Am J Forensic Med Pathol.* 1991;12:119-125.
38. Falk H, Creech JL Jr, Heath CW Jr, et al: Hepatic disease among workers at a vinyl chloride polymerization plant. *JAMA.* 1974;230:59-63.
39. Faxon NW, Churchill ED: The Coconut Grove disaster in Boston. *JAMA.* 1942;120:1385-1388.
40. Fernando D: Fentanyl-laced heroin. *JAMA.* 1991;265:2962.
41. Ficarra BJ: Medical mystery: Gulf war syndrome. *J Med.* 1995;26:87-94.
42. Gallay A, Van Loock F, Demarest S, et al: Belgian Coca-Cola-related outbreak: Intoxication, mass sociogenic illness, or both? *Am J Epidemiol.* 2002;155:140-147.
43. Geiger HJ: The accident at Chernobyl and the medical response. *JAMA.* 1986;256:609-612.
44. Geiling EHK, Cannon PR: Pathological effects of elixir of sulfanilamide (Diethylene glycol) poisoning: A clinical and experimental correlation—Final report. *JAMA.* 1938;111:919-926.
45. Generali J: *Black Box Warnings, 2008.* Available at http://www.formularyproductions.com/master/showpage.php?dir=blackbox&whichpage=9. Accessed August 17, 2009.
46. Gershanik J, Boecler B, Ensley H, et al: The gasping syndrome and benzyl alcohol poisoning. *N Engl J Med.* 1982;307:1384-1388.
47. Giusti RM, Iwamoto K, Hatch EE: Diethylstilbestrol revisited: a review of the long-term health effects. *Ann Intern Med.* 1995;122:778-788.
48. Gleich M: Thallium acetate poisoning in the treatment of ringworm of the scalp. *JAMA.* 1931;97:851.
49. Goldblatt MW: Vesical tumours induced by chemical compounds. *Br J Indust Med.* 1949;6:65-81.
50. Hamilton A: Landmark article in occupational medicine. "Forty years in the poisonous trades." *Am J Indust Med.* 1985;7:3-18.
51. Herbst AL, Ulfelder H, Poskanzer DC: Adenocarcinoma of the vagina. Association of maternal stilbestrol therapy with tumor appearance in young women. *N Engl J Med.* 1971;284:878-881.
52. Holmstedt B: Prolegomena to Seveso. Ecclesiastes I 18. *Arch Toxicol.* 1980;44:211-230.
53. Hood E: Lessons learned? Chemical plant safety since Bhopal. *Environ Health Perspect.* 2004;112:A352-359.
54. Hughes JP, Baron R, Buckland DH, et al: Phosphorus necrosis of the jaw: A present day study. *Br J Indust Med.* 1962;19:83-99.
55. Humphry D: *Final Exit.* New York: Dell; 1991.
56. Hunter D: *The Diseases of Occupations*, 6th ed. London: Hodder & Stoughton; 1978.
57. Hyams KC, Wignall FS, Roswell R: War syndromes and their evaluation: From the U.S. Civil War to the Persian Gulf War. *Ann Intern Med.* 1996;125:398-405.
58. Ingelfinger JR: Melamine and the global implications of food contamination. *N Engl J Med.* 2008;359:2745-2748.
59. Institute of Medicine: *Veterans and Agent Orange: Update 2002.* Washington, DC: National Academies Press; 2002.
60. Iowa Persian Gulf Study Group: Self-reported illness and health status among Gulf War veterans. A population-based study. *JAMA.* 1997;277:238-245.
61. Ismail K, Everitt B, Blatchley N, et al: Is there a Gulf War syndrome? *Lancet.* 1999;353:179-182.
62. Iversen A, Chalder T, Wessely S, et al: Gulf War Illness: lessons from medically unexplained symptoms. *Clin Psychol Rev.* 2007;27:842-854.
63. Jones GR: Polychlorinated biphenyls: where do we stand now? *Lancet.* 1989;2:791-794.
64. Kilbourne EM, Posada de la Paz M, Abaitua Borda I, et al: Toxic oil syndrome: A current clinical and epidemiologic summary, including comparisons with the eosinophilia-myalgia syndrome. *J Am Coll Cardiol.* 1991;18:711-717.
65. Kilbourne EM, Rigau-Perez JG, Heath CW, Jr., et al: Clinical epidemiology of toxic-oil syndrome. Manifestations of a new illness. *N Engl J Med.* 1983;309:1408-1414.
66. Kodama K, Mabuchi K, Shigematsu I: A long-term cohort study of the atomic-bomb survivors. *J Epidemiol.* 1996;6:S95-S105.
67. Kopelman H, Robertson MH, Sanders PG, Ash I: The Epping jaundice. *Br Med J.* 1966;5486:514-516.
68. Kriegstein AR, Shungu DC, Millar WS, et al: Leukoencephalopathy and raised brain lactate from heroin vapor inhalation ("chasing the dragon"). *Neurology.* 1999;53:1765-1773.
69. Lamar J: Japan's worst nuclear accident leaves two fighting for life. *Br Med J.* 1999;319:937.
70. Lambert ED: *Modern Medical Mistakes.* Bloomington, IN: Indiana University Press; 1978.
71. Landrigan PJ: Illness in Gulf War veterans. Causes and consequences. *JAMA.* 1997;277:259-261.
72. Lang J: Heavens's Gate suicide still a mystery 1 year later. *Arizona Republic.* 1998; March 26:Sect. A11.
73. Langston JW, Ballard P, Tetrud JW, Irwin I: Chronic Parkinsonism in humans due to a product of meperidine-analog synthesis. *Science.* 1983;219:979-980.
74. Layton D: *Seductive Poison: A Jonestown Survivor's story of Life and Death in the Peoples Temple.* New York: Anchor; 1998.
75. Lee WR: The history of the statutory control of mercury poisoning in Great Britain. *Br J Ind Med.* 1968;25:52-62.

76. Leschke E: *Clinical Toxicology: Modern Methods in the Diagnosis and Treatment of Poisoning*. Baltimore: William Wood; 1934.
77. Levin SM, Kann PE, Lax MB: Medical examination for asbestos-related disease. *Am J Indust Med.* 2000;37:6-22.
78. Logan WPD: Mortality in the London fog incident. *Lancet.* 1953;1:336-338.
79. Macklis RM: Radithor and the era of mild radium therapy. *JAMA.* 1990;264:614-618.
80. Magnuson E: The devil made him do it. *Time.* 1990; April 9:38.
81. Markowitz G, Rosner D: "Cater to the children": The role of the lead industry in a public health tragedy, 1900–1955. *Am J Public Health.* 2000;90:36-46.
82. Martin M, Hecker J, Clark R, et al: China White epidemic: An eastern United States emergency department experience. *Ann Emerg Med.* 1991;20:158-164.
83. Martland HS: Occupational poisoning in manufacture of luminous watch dials. *JAMA.* 1929;92:466-73, 552-559.
84. Massey EW, Wold D, Heyman A: Arsenic: Homicidal intoxication. *South Med J.* 1984;77:848-851.
85. Matossian MK: Ergot and the Salem witchcraft affair. *Am Sci.* 1982;70: 355-357.
86. McFadyen RE: Thalidomide in America: A brush with tragedy. *Clio Med.* 1976;11:79-93.
87. Mehta PS, Mehta AS, Mehta SJ, Makhijani AB: Bhopal tragedy's health effects. A review of methyl isocyanate toxicity. *JAMA.* 1990;264:2781-2787.
88. Merhoff GC, Porter JM: Ergot intoxication: historical review and description of unusual clinical manifestations. *Ann Surg.* 1974;180:773-779.
89. Modell W: Mass drug catastrophes and the roles of science and technology. *Science.* 1967;156:346-351.
90. Morgan JP: The Jamaica ginger paralysis. *JAMA.* 1982;248:1864-1867.
91. Morin YL, Foley AR, Martineau G, Roussel J: Quebec beer-drinkers' cardiomyopathy: Forty-eight cases. *Can Med Assoc J.* 1967;97:881-883.
92. Morita H, Yanagisawa N, Nakajima T, et al: Sarin poisoning in Matsumoto, Japan. *Lancet.* 1995;346:290-293.
93. Mudur G: Arsenic poisons 220,000 in India. *Br Med J.* 1996;313:319.
94. Mudur G: Half of Bangladesh population at risk of arsenic poisoning. *Br Med J.* 2000;320:822.
95. Mullins ME, Horowitz BZ, Linden DH, et al: Life-threatening interaction of mibefradil and beta-blockers with dihydropyridine calcium channel blockers. *JAMA.* 1998;280:157-158.
96. Munch JC: Human thallotoxicosis. *JAMA.* 1934;102:1929-1934.
97. Murray R: Asbestos: A chronology of its origins and health effects. *Br J Ind Med.* 1990;47:361-365.
98. Nakae K, Yamamoto S, Shigematsu I, Kono R: Relation between subacute myelo-optic neuropathy (S.M.O.N.) and clioquinol: Nationwide survey. *Lancet.* 1973;1:171-173.
99. Nakajima T, Ohta S, Morita H, et al: Epidemiological study of sarin poisoning in Matsumoto City, Japan. *J Epidemiol.* 1998;8:33-41.
100. Nemery B, Fischler B, Boogaerts M, et al: The Coca-Cola incident in Belgium, June 1999. *Food Chem Toxicol.* 2002;40:1657-1667.
101. O'Brien KL, Selanikio JD, Hecdivert C, et al: Epidemic of pediatric deaths from acute renal failure caused by diethylene glycol poisoning. Acute Renal Failure Investigation Team. *JAMA.* 1998;279:1175-1180.
102. Okumura T, Takasu N, Ishimatsu S, et al: Report on 640 victims of the Tokyo subway sarin attack. *Ann Emerg Med.* 1996;28:129-135.
103. Oliveira AR, Hunt JG, Valverde NJ, et al: Medical and related aspects of the Goiania accident: An overview. *Health Phys.* 1991;60:17-24.
104. Pitcock CD, Clark RB: From Fanny to Fernand: The development of consumerism in pain control during the birth process. *Am J Obstet Gynecol.* 1992;167:581-587.
105. Poisoning FrotRCoA. *Lancet.* 1903;2:1674-1676.
106. Polednak AP, Stehney AF, Rowland RE: Mortality among women first employed before 1930 in the U.S. radium dial-painting industry. A group ascertained from employment lists. *Am J Epidemiol.* 1978;107:179-195.
107. Powell PP: Minamata disease: A story of mercury's malevolence. *South Med J.* 1991;84:1352-1358.
108. Prezant DJ, Prezant DJ: World Trade Center cough syndrome and its treatment. *Lung.* 2008;186(suppl 1):S94-S102.
109. Prezant DJ, Weiden M, Banauch GI, et al: Cough and bronchial responsiveness in firefighters at the World Trade Center site. *N Engl J Med.* 2002;347:806-815.
110. Rahman MM, Chowdhury UK, Mukherjee SC, et al: Chronic arsenic toxicity in Bangladesh and West Bengal, India—a review and commentary. *J Toxicol Clin Toxicol.* 2001;39:683-700.
111. Rahu M: Health effects of the Chernobyl accident: Fears, rumours and the truth. *Eur J Cancer.* 2003;39:295-299.
112. Rentz EL, Lewis L, Mujica, OJ, et al: Outbreak of acute renal failure in Panama in 2006: A case-control study. *Bull World Health Organ.* 2008;86:749-756.
113. Research Advisory Committee on Gulf War Veterans' Illnesses: *Gulf War Illness and the Health of Gulf War Veterans: Scientific Findings and Recommendations 2008.* Available at http://www1.va.gov/RAC-GWVI/. Accessed August 18, 2009.
114. Roberts L: Radiation accident grips Goiania. *Science.* 1987;238:1028-1031.
115. Roses OE, Garcia Fernandez JC, Villaamil EC, et al: Mass poisoning by sodium arsenite. *J Toxicol Clin Toxicol.* 1991;29:209-213.
116. Rytomaa T: Ten years after Chernobyl. *Ann Med.* 1996;28:83-87.
117. Scalzo AJ: Diethylene glycol toxicity revisited: the 1996 Haitian epidemic. *J Toxicol Clin Toxicol.* 1996;34:513-516.
118. Schier JG, Patel MM, Belson MG, et al: Public health investigation after the discovery of ricin in a South Carolina postal facility. *Am J Public Health.* 2007;97(suppl 1):S152-S157.
119. Schmid R: Cutaneous porphyria in Turkey. *N Engl J Med.* 1960;263:397-398.
120. Selikoff IJ, Hammond EC, Seidman H: Mortality experience of insulation workers in the United States and Canada, 1943–1976. *Ann N Y Acad Sci.* 1979;330:91-116.
121. Sharpe WD: Benzene, artificial leather and aplastic anemia: Newark, 1916–1928. *Bull N Y Acad Med.* 1993;69:47-60.
122. Sheridan RL, Schulz JT, Ryan CM, McGinnis PJ: Case records of the Massachusetts General Hospital. Weekly clinicopathological exercises. Case 6-2004. A 35-year-old woman with extensive, deep burns from a nightclub fire. *N Engl J Med.* 2004;350:810-821.
123. Shively BK, Roldan CA, Gill EA, et al: Prevalence and determinants of valvulopathy in patients treated with dexfenfluramine. *Circulation.* 1999;100:2161-2167.
124. Sidell FR: Chemical agent terrorism. *Ann Emerg Med.* 1996;28:223-224.
125. Smith HV, Spalding JM: Outbreak of paralysis in Morocco due to ortho-cresyl phosphate poisoning. *Lancet.* 1959;2:1019-1021.
126. Stover BJ: Effects of Thorotrast in humans. *Health Phys.* 1983;44(suppl 1):253-257.
127. Subramanian KS, Kosnett MJ: Human exposures to arsenic from consumption of well water in West Bengal, India. *Int J Occup Environ Health.* 1998;4:217-230.
128. Surburban Emergency Management Project: *Largest Mass Methanol Poisoning in History Sickens 800 and Kills 45, Nicaragua, September, 2006.* Available at http://www.semp.us/publications/biot_reader.php?BiotID=412. Accessed August 18, 2009.
129. Swann JP: The 1941 sulfathiazole disaster and the birth of good manufacturing practices. *PDA J Pharm Sci Technol.* 1999;53:148-153.
130. Swartz RD, Millman RP, Billi JE, et al: Epidemic methanol poisoning: Clinical and biochemical analysis of a recent episode. *Medicine.* 1981;60:373-382.
131. Taylor JR, Selhorst JB, Houff SA, Martinez AJ: Chlordecone intoxication in man. I. Clinical observations. *Neurology.* 1978;28:626-630.
132. Tsuchiya K: The discovery of the causal agent of Minamata disease. *Am J Indust Med.* 1992;21:275-280.
133. Unwin C, Blatchley N, Coker W, et al: Health of UK servicemen who served in Persian Gulf War. *Lancet.* 1999;353:169-178.
134. Urbinato D: London's historic "pea-soupers." *EPA J.* 1994:59.
135. Varga J, Uitto J, Jimenez SA: The cause and pathogenesis of the eosinophilia-myalgia syndrome. *Ann Intern Med.* 1992;116:140-147.
136. Varma DR, Guest I: The Bhopal accident and methyl isocyanate toxicity. *J Toxicol Environ Health.* 1993;40:513-529.
137. Waldron HA: The Devonshire colic. *J Hist Med Allied. Sci* 1970;25:383-413.
138. Wax PM: Elixirs, diluents, and the passage of the 1938 Federal Food, Drug and Cosmetic Act. *Ann Intern Med.* 1995;122:456-461.
139. Wax PM: It's happening again—another diethylene glycol mass poisoning. *J Toxicol Clin Toxicol.* 1996;34:517-520.
140. Wax PM, Becker CE, Curry SC: Unexpected "gas" casualties in Moscow: A medical toxicology perspective. *Ann Emerg Med.* 2003;41:700-705.
141. Weber E, Laarbaui F, Michel L, Donckier J: Abdominal pain: Do not forget Thorotrast! *Postgrad Med J.* 1995;71:367-368.
142. Wedeen RP: Were the hatters of New Jersey "mad"? *Am J Indust Med.* 1989;16:225-233.

143. Whorton D, Krauss RM, Marshall S, Milby TH: Infertility in male pesticide workers. *Lancet.* 1977;2:1259-1261.
144. Wing JS, Brender JD, Sanderson LM, et al: Acute health effects in a community after a release of hydrofluoric acid. *Arch Environ Health.* 1991;46:155-160.
145. Wolff MS, Anderson HA, Selikoff IJ: Human tissue burdens of halogenated aromatic chemicals in Michigan. *JAMA.* 1982;247:2112-2116.
146. Wolkin AF, Patel M, Watson W, et al: Early detection of illness associated with poisonings of public health significance. *Ann Emerg Med.* 2006;47:170-176.
147. Wolters EC, van Wijngaarden GK, Stam FC, et al: Leucoencephalopathy after inhaling "heroin" pyrolysate. *Lancet.* 1982;2:1233-1237.
148. Wysowski DK, Swartz L, Wysowski DK, Swartz L: Adverse drug event surveillance and drug withdrawals in the United States, 1969–2002: the importance of reporting suspected reactions. *Arch Intern Med.* 2005;165:1363-1369.
149. Yardley J: 40,000 Chinese evacuated from explosion "death zone." *The New York Times.* 2003;December 27:Sect. A3.

PART A

THE GENERAL APPROACH TO MEDICAL TOXICOLOGY

CHAPTER 3
INITIAL EVALUATION OF THE PATIENT: VITAL SIGNS AND TOXIC SYNDROMES

Lewis S. Nelson, Neal A. Lewin, Mary Ann Howland, Robert S. Hoffman, Lewis R. Goldfrank, and Neal E. Flomenbaum

For more than 200 years, American physicians and nurses have attempted to standardize their approach to the assessment of patients. At the New York Hospital in 1865, pulse rate, respiratory rate, and temperature were incorporated into the bedside chart and called "vital signs."[6] It was not until the early part of the 20th century, however, that blood pressure determination also became routine. Additional components of the standard emergency assessment, such as oxygen saturation by pulse oximetry, capillary blood glucose, and pain severity, are now also beginning to be considered vital signs. Although assessment of oxygen saturation, capillary glucose, and pain severity are essential components of the clinical assessment and are important considerations throughout this text, they are not discussed in this chapter.

In the practice of medical toxicology, vital signs play an important role beyond assessing and monitoring the overall status of a patient, as they frequently provide valuable physiologic clues to the toxicologic etiology and severity of an illness. The vital signs also are a valuable parameter, which are used to assess and monitor a patient's response to supportive treatment and antidotal therapy.

Table 3–1 presents the normal vital signs for various age groups. However, this broad range of values considered normal should serve merely as a guide. Only a complete assessment of a patient can determine whether or not a particular vital sign is truly clinically normal. This table of normal vital signs is useful in assessing children because normal values for children vary considerably with age, and knowing the range of normal variation is essential. Normal temperature is defined as 95° to 100.4°F (35° to 38°C).

The difficulty in defining what constitutes "normal" vital signs in an emergency setting has been inadequately addressed and may prove to be an impossible undertaking. Published normal values may have little relevance to an acutely ill or anxious patient in the emergency setting, yet that is precisely the environment in which we must define abnormal vital signs and address them accordingly. Even in nonemergent situations, "normalcy" of vital signs depends on the clinical condition of the patient. A sleeping or comatose patient may have physiologic bradycardia; a slow heart rate appropriate for his or her low energy requiring state. For these reasons, descriptions of vital signs as "normal" or "stable" are too nonspecific to be meaningful and therefore should never be accepted as defining normalcy in an individual patient. Conversely, no patient should be considered too agitated, too young, or too gravely ill for the practitioner to obtain a complete set of vital signs; indeed, these patients urgently need a thorough evaluation that includes all of the vital signs. Also, the vital signs must be recorded as accurately as possible first in the prehospital setting, again with precision and accuracy as soon as a patient arrives in the emergency department, and serially thereafter as clinically indicated.

Many xenobiotics affect the autonomic nervous system, which, in turn, affects the vital signs via the sympathetic pathway, the parasympathetic pathway, or both. Meticulous attention to both the initial and repeated determinations of vital signs is of extreme importance in identifying a pattern of changes suggesting a particular xenobiotic or group of xenobiotics. The value of serial monitoring of the vital signs is demonstrated by the patient who presents with an anticholinergic overdose who is then given the antidote, physostigmine. In this situation, it is important to recognize when tachycardia becomes bradycardia (i.e., anticholinergic syndrome followed by physostigmine excess). Meticulous attention to these changes ensures that the therapeutic interventions can be modified or adjusted accordingly.

Similarly, consider the course of a patient who has opioid-induced bradypnea (a decreased rate of breathing) and then develops tachypnea (an increased rate of breathing) after the administration of the opioid antagonist naloxone. The analysis becomes exceedingly complicated when that patient may have been exposed to two or more substances, such as an opioid combined with cocaine. In this situation, the effects of cocaine may be "unmasked" by the naloxone used to counteract the opioid, and the clinician must then be forced to differentiate naloxone-induced opioid withdrawal from cocaine toxicity. The assessment starts by analyzing diverse information, including vital signs, history, and physical examination.

Table 3–2 describes the most typical toxic syndromes. This table includes only vital signs that are thought to be characteristically abnormal or pathognomonic and directly related to the toxicologic effect of the xenobiotic. The primary purpose of the table, however, is to include many findings, in addition to the vital signs, that together constitute a toxic syndrome. Mofenson and Greensher[5] coined the term *toxidromes* from the words *toxic syndromes* to describe the groups of signs and symptoms that consistently result from particular toxins. These syndromes are usually best described by a combination of the vital signs and clinically apparent end-organ manifestations. The signs that prove most clinically useful are those involving the central nervous system (CNS; mental status), ophthalmic system (pupil size), gastrointestinal system (peristalsis), dermatologic system (skin dryness versus diaphoresis), mucous membranes (moistness versus dryness), and genitourinary system (urinary retention versus incontinence). Table 3–2 includes some of the most important signs and symptoms and the xenobiotics most commonly responsible for these manifestations. A detailed analysis of each sign, symptom, and toxic syndrome can be found in the pertinent chapters throughout the text. In this chapter, the most typical toxic syndromes (see Table 3–2) are considered to enable the appropriate assessment and differential diagnosis of a poisoned patient.

In considering a toxic syndrome, the reader should always remember that the actual clinical manifestations of a poisoning are far more variable than the syndromes described in Table 3–2. The concept of the toxic syndrome is most useful when thinking about a clinical presentation and formulating a framework for assessment. Although some patients may present as "classic" cases, others manifest partial toxic syndromes or formes frustes. These incomplete syndromes may still provide at least a clue to the correct diagnosis. It is important to understand that partial presentations (particularly in the presence of multiple xenobiotics) do not necessarily imply less severe disease and, therefore, are comparably important to appreciate.

In some instances, an unexpected combination of findings may be particularly helpful in identifying a xenobiotic or a combination of xenobiotics. For example, a dissociation between such typically paired changes as an increase in pulse with a decrease in blood pressure (cyclic antidepressants or phenothiazines), or the presentation of a decrease

TABLE 3–1. Normal Vital Signs by Age[a]

Age	Systolic BP (mm Hg)	Diastolic BP (mm Hg)	Pulse (beats/min)	Respirations (breaths/min)[b]
Adult	≤120	<80	60–100	16–24
16 years	≤120	<80	80	16–30
12 years	119	76	85	16–30
10 years	115	74	90	16–30
6 years	107	69	100	20–30
4 years	104	65	110	20–30
4 months	90	50	145	30–35
2 months	85	50	145	30–35
Newborn	65	50	145	35–40

[a] The normal rectal temperature is defined as 95°F to 100.4°F (35°C–38°C) for all ages. For children 1 year of age or younger, these values are the mean values for the 50th percentile. For older children, these values represent the 90th percentile at a specific age for the 50th percentile of weight in that age group.

[b] These values were determined in the emergency department and may be environment and situation dependent.

in pulse with an increase in blood pressure (ergot alkaloids) may be extremely helpful in diagnosing a toxic etiology. The use of these unexpected or atypical clinical findings is demonstrated in Chap. 23 .

BLOOD PRESSURE

Xenobiotics cause hypotension by four major mechanisms: decreased peripheral vascular resistance, decreased myocardial contractility, dysrhythmias, and depletion of intravascular volume. Many xenobiotics can initially cause orthostatic hypotension without marked supine hypotension, and any xenobiotic that affects autonomic control of the heart or peripheral capacitance vessels may lead to orthostatic hypotension (Table 3–3). Hypertension from xenobiotics may be caused by CNS sympathetic overactivity, increased myocardial contractility or increased peripheral vascular resistance, or a combination of these.

Blood pressure and pulse rate may vary significantly as a result of changes in receptor responsiveness, degree of physical fitness, and degree of atherosclerosis. Changing patterns of blood pressure often assist in the diagnostic evaluation: overdose with a monoamine oxidase inhibitor (MAOI) characteristically causes an initial normal blood pressure, to be followed by hypertension, which, in turn, may be followed abruptly by severe hypotension (Chap. 71).

PULSE RATE

Extremely useful clinical information can be obtained by evaluating the pulse rate (Table 3–4 and Chap. 23). Although the carotid artery is usually easily palpable, for reasons of both safety and reliability, the brachial artery is preferred in infants and in adults older than 60 years. The normal heart rate for adults was defined by consensus more than 50 years ago as a regular rate greater than 60 beats/min and less than 100 beats/min. More recent studies[7,8] suggest that 95% of the population have bradycardia and tachycardia thresholds of 50 beats/min and 90 beats/min, respectively. In our text, we have chosen to retain the consensus values.

Because pulse rate is the net result of a balance between sympathetic (adrenergic) and parasympathetic (muscarinic and nicotinic) tone, many xenobiotics that exert therapeutic or toxic effects or cause pain syndromes, hyperthermia, or volume depletion also affect the pulse rate. With respect to temperature, there is a direct correlation between pulse rate and temperature in that pulse rate increases approximately 8 beats/min for each 1.8°F (1°C) elevation in temperature.[4]

The inability to differentiate easily between sympathomimetic and anticholinergic xenobiotic effects by vital signs alone illustrates the

TABLE 3–2. Toxic Syndromes

Group	Vital Signs: BP	P	R	T	Mental Status	Pupil Size	Peristalsis	Diaphoresis	Other
Anticholinergics	–/↑	↑	±	↑	Delirium	↑	↓	↓	Dry mucous membranes, flush, urinary retention
Cholinergics	±	±	–/↑	–	Normal to depressed	±	↑	↑	Salivation, lacrimation, urination, diarrhea, bronchorrhea, fasciculations, paralysis
Ethanol or sedative–hypnotics	↓	↓	↓	–/↓	Depressed, agitated	±	↓	–	Hyporeflexia, ataxia
Opioids	↓	↓	↓	↓	Depressed	↓	↓	–	Hyporeflexia
Sympathomimetics	↑	↑	↑	↑	Agitated	↑	–/↑	↑	Tremor, seizures
Withdrawal from ethanol or sedative–hypnotics	↑	↑	↑	↑	Agitated, disoriented hallucinations	↑	↑	↑	Tremor, seizures
Withdrawal from opioids	↑	↑	–	–	Normal, anxious	↑	↑	↑	Vomiting, rhinorrhea, piloerection, diarrhea, yawning

↑ = increases; ↓ = decreases; ± = variable; – = change unlikely; BP, blood pressure; P, pulse; R, respirations; T, temperature.

TABLE 3–3. Common Xenobiotics That Affect the Blood Pressure[a]

Hypotension	Hypertension
α_1-Adrenergic antagonists	α_1-Adrenergic agonists
α_2-Adrenergic agonists	α_2-Adrenergic antagonists
β-Adrenergic antagonists	Ergot alkaloids
Angiotensin-converting enzyme inhibitors and angiotensin receptor blockers	Lead (chronic)
Antidysrhythmics	Monoamine oxidase inhibitors (overdose early and drug–food interaction)
Calcium channel blockers	Nicotine (early)
Cyanide	Phencyclidine
Cyclic antidepressants	Sympathomimetics
Ethanol and other alcohols	
Iron	
Methylxanthines	
Nitrates and nitrites	
Nitroprusside	
Opioids	
Phenothiazines	
Phosphodiesterase-5 inhibitors	
Sedative-hypnotics	

[a]Chap. 23 lists additional xenobiotics that affect hemodynamic function.

principle that no single vital sign abnormality can definitively establish a toxicologic diagnosis. In trying to differentiate between a sympathomimetic and anticholinergic toxic syndrome, it should be understood that although tachycardia commonly results from both sympathomimetic and anticholinergic xenobiotics, when tachycardia is accompanied by diaphoresis or increased bowel sounds, adrenergic toxicity is suggested, but when tachycardia is accompanied by decreased sweating, absent bowel sounds, and urinary retention, anticholinergic toxicity is likely.

TABLE 3–4. Common Xenobiotics That Affect the Pulse[a]

Bradycardia	Tachycardia
α_2-Adrenergic agonists	Anticholinergics
β-Adrenergic antagonists	Antipsychotics
Baclofen	Cyclic antidepressants
Calcium channel blockers	Disulfiram/ethanol interaction
Cardioactive steroids	Ethanol and sedative–hypnotic withdrawal
Ciguatoxin	Iron
Ergot alkaloids	Methylxanthines
γ-Hydroxybutyric acid	Phencyclidine
Opioids	Sympathomimetics
Organic phosphorus compounds	Thyroid hormone
	Yohimbine

[a]Chap. 23 lists additional xenobiotics that affect the heart rate.

RESPIRATIONS

Establishment of an airway and evaluation of respiratory status are the initial priorities in patient stabilization. Although respirations are typically assessed initially for rate alone, careful observation of the depth and pattern is essential (Table 3–5) for establishing the etiology of a systemic illness or toxicity.[1] Unfortunately, very few investigators have actually measured the respiratory rate in large populations of normal people, let alone in emergency department patients. Two papers[2,3] investigating respiratory rates in emergency department patients differ substantially in their determinations of normal ranges from the remainder of the literature. The combined results of these investigations suggest "normal" respiratory rates are 16 to 24 breaths/min in adults with more rapid rates that are inversely related to age in children.

The term *hyperventilation* may mean tachypnea (an increase in ventilatory rate), hyperpnea (an increase in tidal volume), or both. When hyperventilation results solely or predominantly from hyperpnea, the clinicians may miss this important finding entirely, instead erroneously describing such a hyperventilating patient as normally ventilating or even *hypoventilating* if bradypnea is also present. The ventilatory status of the patient must be viewed in the context of the patient's physiologic condition.

Hyperventilation may result from the direct effect of a CNS stimulant, such as the direct effect of salicylates, on the brainstem. However, salicylate poisoning characteristically produces hyperventilation by tachypnea, but it also produces hyperpnea, with or without tachypnea. Pulmonary injury from any source, including aspiration of gastric contents, may lead to hypoxemia with a resultant tachypnea. Later, tachypnea may change to bradypnea, hypopnea (shallow breathing), or both. Bradypnea may occur when a CNS depressant acts on the brainstem. A progression from fast to slow breathing may also occur in a patient exposed to increasing concentrations of cyanide or carbon monoxide.

TEMPERATURE

Temperature evaluation and control are critical. However, temperature assessment can be done only if safe and reliable equipment is used. The

TABLE 3–5. Common Xenobiotics That Affect Respiration[a]

Bradypnea	Tachypnea
α_2-Adrenergic agonists	Cyanide
Botulinum toxin	Dinitrophenol and congeners
Elapidae venom	Epinephrine
Ethanol and other alcohols	Ethylene glycol
γ-Hydroxybutyric acid	Hydrogen sulfide
Neuromuscular blockers	Methanol
Opioids	Methemoglobin producers
Organic phosphorus compounds	Methylxanthines
Sedative-hypnotics	Nicotine (early)
	Pulmonary irritants
	Salicylates
	Sympathomimetics

[a]Chap. 21 lists additional xenobiotics affecting respiratory rate.

risks of inaccuracy are substantial when an oral temperature is taken in a tachypneic patient, an axillary temperature or a temporal artery temperature is taken in any patient (especially those found outdoors), or a tympanic temperature is taken in a patient with cerumen impaction. Obtaining rectal temperatures using a nonglass probe is essential for safe and accurate temperature determinations in agitated individuals and is considered the standard method of temperature determination in this text.

The core temperature or deep internal temperature (T) is relatively stable (98.6° ± 1.08°F; 37° ± 0.6°C) under normal physiologic circumstances. Hypothermia (T <95°F; <35°C) and hyperthermia (T >100.4°F; >38°C) are common manifestations of toxicity. Severe or significant hypothermia and hyperthermia, unless immediately recognized and managed appropriately, may result in grave complications and inappropriate or inadequate resuscitative efforts. Life-threatening hyperthermia (T >106°F; >41.1°C) from any cause may lead to extensive rhabdomyolysis, myoglobinuric renal failure, and direct liver and brain injury and must therefore be identified and corrected immediately.

Hyperthermia may result from a distinct neurologic response to a signal demanding thermal "upregulation." This signal can be from internal generation of heat beyond the capacity of the body to cool, such as occurs in association with agitation or mitochondrial uncoupling, or from an externally imposed physical or environmental factor, such as the environmental conditions causing heat stroke or the excessive swaddling in clothing causing hyperthermia in infants. Fever, or pyrexia, is hyperthermia due to an elevation in the hypothalamic thermoregulatory set-point.

Regardless of etiology, core temperatures higher than 106°F (41.1°C) are extremely rare unless normal feedback mechanisms are overwhelmed. Hyperthermia of this extreme nature is usually attributed to environmental heat stroke; extreme psychomotor agitation; or xenobiotic-related temperature disturbances such as malignant hyperthermia, the serotonin syndrome, or the neuroleptic malignant syndrome.

A common xenobiotic-related hyperthermia pattern that frequently occurs in the emergency department is defervescence after an acute temperature elevation resulting from agitation or a grand mal seizure. Table 3–6 is a representative list of xenobiotics that affect body temperature. (Chap. 15 provides greater detail.)

Hypothermia is probably less of an immediate threat to life than hyperthermia, but it requires rapid appreciation, accurate diagnosis, and skilled management. Hypothermia impairs the metabolism of many xenobiotics, leading to unpredictable delayed toxicologic effects when the patient is warmed. Many xenobiotics that lead to an alteration of metal status place patients at great risk for becoming hypothermic from exposure to cold climates. Most importantly, a hypothermic patient should never be declared dead without both an extensive assessment and a full resuscitative effort of adequate duration, taking into consideration the difficulties in resuscitating cold but living patients. This is true whenever the body temperature remains less than 95°F (35°C) (Chap. 15).

TABLE 3–6. Common Xenobiotics[a] That Affect Temperature[b]

Hyperthermia	Hypothermia
Anticholinergics	α_2-Adrenergic agonists
Chlorphenoxy herbicides	Carbon monoxide
Dinitrophenol and congeners	Ethanol
Malignant hyperthermia[a]	γ Hydroxybutyric Acid
Monoamine oxidase inhibitors	Hypoglycemics
Neuroleptic malignant syndrome[a]	Opioids
Phencyclidine	Sedative-hypnotics
Salicylates	Thiamine deficiency
Sedative-hypnotic or ethanol withdrawal	
Serotonin syndrome[a]	
Sympathomimetics	
Thyroid hormone	

[a]Three common xenobiotic-induced syndromes are also included.

[b]Chap. 15 lists additional xenobiotics that affect temperature.

SUMMARY

Early, accurate determinations followed by serial monitoring of the vital signs are as essential in medical toxicology as in any other type of emergency or critical care medicine. For this reason, the vital signs are an essential part of the initial evaluation of every case, and serial vital signs are always necessary throughout the patient's clinical evaluation. Careful observation of the vital signs helps to determine appropriate therapeutic interventions and guide the clinician in making necessary adjustments to initial and subsequent therapeutic interventions. When pathognomonic clinical and laboratory findings are combined with accurate initial and sometimes changing vital signs, a toxic syndrome may become evident, which will aid in both general supportive and specific antidotal treatment. Toxic syndromes will also guide further diagnostic testing.

REFERENCES

1. Gravelyn TR, Weg JG: Respiratory rate as an indicator of acute respiratory dysfunction. *JAMA.* 1980;244:1123-1125.
2. Hooker EA, Danzl DF, Brueggmeyer M, Harper E: Respiratory rates in pediatric emergency patients. *J Emerg Med.* 1992;10:407-412.
3. Hooker EA, O'Brien DJ, Danzl DF, et al: Respiratory rates in emergency department patients. *J Emerg Med.* 1989;7:129-132.
4. Karajalainen J, Vitassalo M: Fever and cardiac rhythm. *Arch Intern Med.* 1986;146:1169-1171.
5. Mofenson HC, Greensher J: The unknown poison. *Pediatrics.* 1974;54:336-342.
6. Musher DM, Dominguez EA, Bar-Sela A: Edouard Seguin and the social power of thermometry. *N Engl J Med.* 1987;316:115-117.
7. Opthof T: The normal range and determinants of the intrinsic heart rate in man. *Cardiovasc Res.* 2000;45:177-184.
8. Spodick DH: Normal sinus heart rate: Appropriate rate thresholds for sinus tachycardia and bradycardia. *South Med J.* 1996;89:666-667.

CHAPTER 4
PRINCIPLES OF MANAGING THE ACUTELY POISONED OR OVERDOSED PATIENT

Lewis S. Nelson, Neal A. Lewin, Mary Ann Howland, Robert S. Hoffman, Lewis R. Goldfrank, and Neal E. Flomenbaum

OVERVIEW

For almost 5 decades, medical toxicologists and information specialists have used a clinical approach to poisoned or overdosed patients that emphasizes treating the patient rather than treating the poison. Too often in the past, patients were initially all but neglected while attention was focused on the ingredients listed on the containers of the product(s) to which they presumably were exposed. Although the astute clinician must always be prepared to administer a specific antidote immediately in instances when nothing else will save a patient, all poisoned or overdosed patients will benefit from an organized, rapid clinical management plan (Fig. 4-1).

Over the past 2 decades, some basic tenets and long-held beliefs regarding the initial therapeutic interventions in toxicologic management have been questioned and subjected to an "evidence-based" analysis. For example, in the mid-1970s, most medical toxicologists began to advocate a standardized approach to a comatose and possibly overdosed adult patient, typically calling for the intravenous (IV) administration of 50 mL of $D_{50}W$, 100 mg of thiamine and 2 mg of naloxone along with 100% oxygen at high flow rates. The rationale for this approach was to compensate for the previously idiosyncratic style of overdose management encountered in different healthcare settings and for the unfortunate likelihood that omitting any one of these measures at the time that care was initiated in the emergency department (ED) would result in omitting it altogether. It was not unusual then to discover from a laboratory chemistry report more than 1 hour after a supposedly overdosed comatose patient had arrived in the ED that the initial blood glucose was 30 or 40 mg/dL—a critical delay in the management of unsuspected and consequently untreated hypoglycemic coma. Today, however, with the widespread availability of accurate rapid bedside testing for capillary glucose and pulse oximetry for oxygen saturation, coupled with a much greater appreciation by all physicians of what needs to be done for each suspected overdose patient, clinicians can safely provide a more rational, individualized approach to determine the need for, and in some instances more precise amounts of, dextrose, thiamine, naloxone, and oxygen.

A second major approach to providing more rational individualized early treatment for toxicologic emergencies involves a closer examination of the actual risks and benefits of various gastrointestinal (GI) emptying interventions. Appreciation of the potential for significant adverse effects associated with all types of GI emptying interventions and recognition of the absence of clear evidence-based support of efficacy have led to a significant reduction in the routine use of activated charcoal (AC) and almost complete elimination of syrup of ipecac–induced emesis or orogastric lavage and cathartic-induced intestinal evacuation. In 2004, the American Academy of Pediatricians (AAP) all but entirely abandoned its recommendations for the use of syrup of ipecac in the home. The efficacy of orogastric lavage, even when indicated by the nature or type of ingestion, is limited by the amount of time elapsed since the ingestion. The value of whole-bowel irrigation (WBI) with polyethylene glycol electrolyte solution (PEG-ELS) appears to be much more specific and limited than originally thought, and some of the limitations and (uncommon) adverse effects of AC are now more widely recognized.

Similarly, interventions to eliminate absorbed xenobiotics from the body are now much more narrowly defined or, in some cases, abandoned. Multiple-dose activated charcoal (MDAC) is useful for select but not all xenobiotics. Ion trapping in the urine is only beneficial, achievable, and relatively safe when the urine can be maximally alkalinized after a significant salicylate, phenobarbital, or chlorpropamide poisoning. Finally, the roles of hemodialysis, hemoperfusion, and other extracorporeal techniques are now much more specifically defined. With the foregoing in mind, this chapter represents our current efforts to formulate a logical and effective approach to managing a patient with probable or actual toxic exposure.

Table 4-1 provides a recommended stock list of antidotes and therapeutics for the treatment of poisoned or overdosed patients.

MANAGING ACUTELY POISONED OR OVERDOSED PATIENTS

Rarely, if ever, are all of the circumstances involving a poisoned patient known. The history may be incomplete, unreliable, or unobtainable; multiple xenobiotics may be involved; and even when a xenobiotic etiology is identified, it may not be easy to determine whether the problem is an overdose, an allergic or idiosyncratic reaction, or a drug–drug interaction. Similarly, it is sometimes difficult or impossible to differentiate between adverse effects of a correct dose of medication and the consequences of a deliberate or unintentional overdose. The patient's presenting signs and symptoms may force an intervention at a time when there is almost no information available about the etiology of the patient's condition (Table 4-2), and as a result, therapeutics must be thoughtfully chosen empirically to treat or diagnose a condition without exacerbating the situation.

INITIAL MANAGEMENT OF PATIENTS WITH A SUSPECTED EXPOSURE

Similar to the management of any seriously compromised patient, the clinical approach to the patient potentially exposed to a xenobiotic begins with the recognition and treatment of life-threatening conditions, including airway compromise, breathing difficulties, and circulatory problems such as hemodynamic instability and serious dysrhythmias. After the "ABCs" (airway, breathing, and circulation) have been addressed, the patient's level of consciousness should be assessed because this helps determine the techniques to be used for further management of the exposure.

MANAGEMENT OF PATIENTS WITH ALTERED MENTAL STATUS

Altered mental status (AMS) is defined as the deviation of a patient's sensorium from normal. Although it is commonly construed as a depression in the patient's level of consciousness, a patient with agitation, delirium, psychosis, and other deviations from normal is also

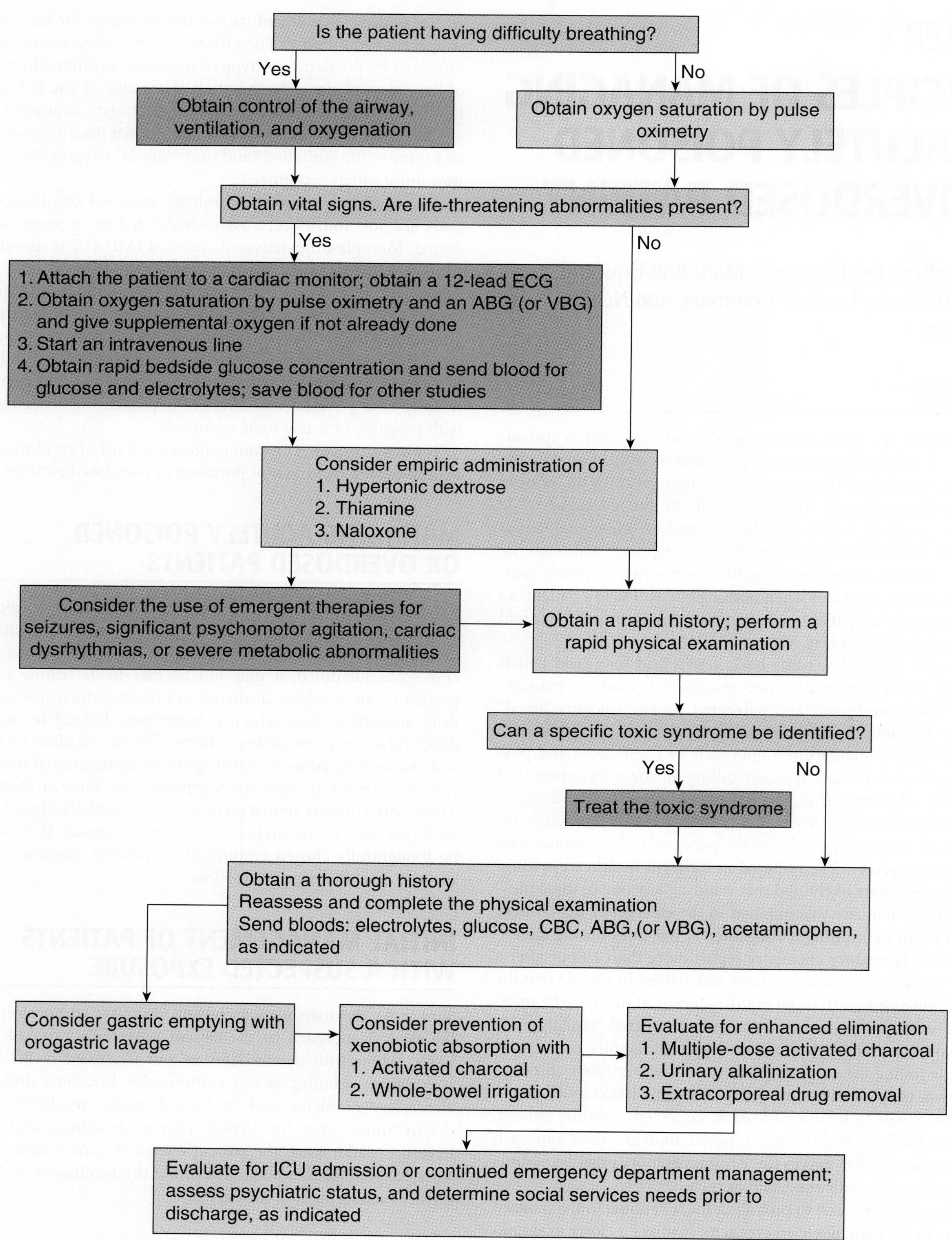

FIGURE 4-1 This algorithm is a basic guide to the management of poisoned patients. A more detailed description of the steps in management may be found in the accompanying text. This algorithm is only a guide to actual management, which must, of course, consider the patient's clinical status.

TABLE 4–1. Antidotes and Therapeutics for the Treatment of Poisonings and Overdoses[a]

Therapeutics[b]	Uses
Activated charcoal (p. 108)	Adsorbs xenobiotics in the GI tract
Antivenom (*Crotalinae*) (p. 1608)	Crotaline snake envenomations
Antivenom (*Elapidae*) (p. 1308)	Coral snake envenomations
Antivenom (*Latrodectus mactans*) (p. 1582)	Black widow spider envenomations
Atropine (p. 1473)	Bradydysrhythmias, cholinesterase inhibitors (organic phosphorus compounds, physostigmine) muscarinic mushrooms (*Clitocybe, Inocybe*) ingestions
Benzodiazepines (p1109)	Seizures, agitation, stimulants, ethanol and sedative–hypnotic withdrawal, cocaine, chloroquine, organic phosphorus compounds
Botulinum antitoxin (ABE-trivalent) (p. 695)	Botulism
Calcium chloride, calcium gluconate (p. 1381)	Fluoride, hydrofluoric acid, ethylene glycol, CCBs, hypomagnesemia, β-adrenergic antagonists
L-Carnitine (p. 711)	Valproic acid
Cyanide kit (nitrites, p. 1689; sodium thiosulfate, p. 1692)	Cyanide
Dantrolene (p. 1001)	Malignant hyperthermia
Deferoxamine mesylate (Desferal) (p. 604)	Iron
Dextrose in water (50% adults; 20% pediatrics; 10% neonates) (p. 728)	Hypoglycemia
Digoxin-specific antibody fragments (Digibind and Digifab) (p. 946)	Cardioactive steroids
Dimercaprol (BAL, British anti-Lewisite) (p. 1229)	Arsenic, mercury, gold, lead
Diphenhydramine	Dystonic reactions, allergic reactions
DTPA (p. 1779)	Radioactive isotopes
Edetate calcium disodium (calcium disodium versenate, $CaNa_2$ EDTA) (p. 1290)	Lead, other selected metals
Ethanol (oral and parenteral dosage forms) (p. 1419)	Methanol, ethylene glycol
Fat emulsion (Intralipid 20% (p. 976)	Cardiac arrest, local anesthetics
Flumazenil (Romazicon) (p. 1072)	Benzodiazepines
Folinic acid (Leucovorin) (p. 783)	Methotrexate, methanol
Fomepizole (Antizole) (p. 1414)	Ethylene glycol, methanol
Glucagon (p. 910)	β-Adrenergic antagonists, CCBs
Glucarpidase (p. 787)	Methotrexate
Hydroxocobalamin (Cyanokit) (p. 1695)	Cyanide
Insulin (p. 893)	β-Adrenergic antagonists, CCBs, hyperglycemia
Iodide, potassium (SSKI) (p. 1775)	Radioactive iodine (I^{131})
Ipecac, syrup of (p. 104)	Induces emesis
Magnesium sulfate or magnesium citrate (p. 114)	Induces catharsis
Magnesium sulfate injection	Cardioactive steroids, hydrofluoric acid, hypomagnesemia, ethanol withdrawal, torsades de pointes
Methylene blue (1% solution) (p. 1708)	Methemoglobinemia
N-acetylcysteine (Acetadote) (p. 500)	Acetaminophen and other causes of hepatotoxicity
Naloxone hydrochloride (Narcan) (p. 579)	Opioids, clonidine
Norepinephrine (Levophed)	Hypotension (preferred for cyclic antidepressants)
Octreotide (Sandostatin) (p. 734)	Oral hypoglycemic induced hypoglycemia
Oxygen (Hyperbaric) (p. 1671)	Carbon monoxide, cyanide, hydrogen sulfide
D-Penicillamine (Cuprimine) (p. 1261)	Copper
Phenobarbital	Seizures, agitation, stimulants, ethanol and sedative–hypnotic withdrawal
Phentolamine (p. 1096)	Cocaine, MAOI interactions, epinephrine, and ergot alkaloids
Physostigmine salicylate (Antilirium) (p. 759)	Anticholinergics
Polyethylene glycol electrolyte solution (p. 114)	Decontaminates GI tract
Pralidoxime chloride, (2-PAM-chloride; Protopam) (p. 1467)	Acetylcholinesterase inhibitors (organic phosphorus agents and carbamates)
Protamine sulfate (p. 880)	Heparin anticoagulation
Prussian blue (Radiogardase) (p. 1334)	Thallium, cesium
Pyridoxine hydrochloride (Vitamin B_6) (p. 845)	Isoniazid, ethylene glycol, gyromitrin-containing mushrooms
Sodium bicarbonate (p. 520)	Ethylene glycol, methanol, salicylates, cyclic antidepressants, methotrexate, phenobarbital, quinidine, chlorpropamide, type 1 antidysrhythmics, chlorphenoxy herbicides
Sorbitol (p. 114)	Induces catharsis
Starch (p. 1349)	Iodine
Succimer (Chemet) (p. 1284)	Lead, mercury, arsenic
Thiamine hydrochloride (Vitamin B_1.) (p. 1129)	Thiamine deficiency, ethylene glycol, chronic ethanol consumption ("alcoholism")
Vitamin K_1 (Aquamephyton) (p. 876)	Warfarin or rodenticide anticoagulants

[a] Each emergency department should have the vast majority of these antidotes immediately available, some of these antidotes may be stored in the pharmacy, and others may be available from the Centers for Disease Control and Prevention, but the precise mechanism for locating each one must be known by each staff member.

[b] A detailed analysis of each of these agents is found in the text in the Antidotes in Depth section on the page cited to the right of each antidote or therapeutic listed.

CCB, calcium channel blocker; DTPA, diethylenetriaminepentaacetic acid; EDTA, ethylenediamine tetraacetic acid; GI, gastrointestinal; MAOI, monoamine oxidase inhibitor; SSKI, saturated solution of potassium iodide.

TABLE 4–2. Clinical and Laboratory Findings in Poisoning and Overdose

Agitation	Anticholinergics,[a] hypoglycemia, phencyclidine, sympathomimetics,[b] withdrawal from ethanol and sedative–hypnotics
Alopecia	Alkylating agents, radiation, selenium, thallium
Ataxia	Benzodiazepines, carbamazepine, carbon monoxide, ethanol, hypoglycemia, lithium, mercury, nitrous oxide, phenytoin
Blindness or decreased visual acuity	Caustics (direct), cocaine, cisplatin, mercury, methanol, quinine, thallium
Blue skin	Amiodarone, FD&C #1 dye, methemoglobinemia, silver
Constipation	Anticholinergics,[a] botulism, lead, opioids, thallium (severe)
Deafness, tinnitus	Aminoglycosides, cisplatin, metals, loop diuretics, quinine, salicylates
Diaphoresis	Amphetamines, cholinergics,[c] hypoglycemia, opioid withdrawal, salicylates, serotonin syndrome, sympathomimetics,[b] withdrawal from ethanol and sedative–hypnotics
Diarrhea	Arsenic and other metals, boric acid (blue-green), botanical irritants, cathartics, cholinergics,[c] colchicine, iron, lithium, opioid withdrawal, radiation
Dysesthesias, paresthesias	Acrylamide, arsenic, ciguatera, cocaine, colchicine, thallium
Gum discoloration	Arsenic, bismuth, hypervitaminosis A, lead, mercury
Hallucinations	Anticholinergics,[a] dopamine agonists, ergot alkaloids, ethanol, ethanol and sedative–hypnotic withdrawal, LSD, phencyclidine, sympathomimetics,[b] tryptamines
Headache	Carbon monoxide, hypoglycemia, monoamine oxidase inhibitor–food interaction (hypertensive crisis), serotonin syndrome
Metabolic acidosis (elevated anion gap)	Methanol, uremia, ketoacidosis (diabetic, starvation, alcoholic), paraldehyde, phenformin, metformin, iron, isoniazid, lactic acidosis, cyanide, protease inhibitors, ethylene glycol, salicylates, toluene
Miosis	Cholinergics,[c] clonidine, opioids, phencyclidine, phenothiazines
Mydriasis	Anticholinergics,[a] botulism, opioid withdrawal, sympathomimetics[b]
Nystagmus	Barbiturates, carbamazepine, carbon monoxide, ethanol, lithium, monoamine oxidase inhibitors, phencyclidine, phenytoin, quinine
Purpura	Anticoagulant rodenticides, clopidogrel, corticosteroids, heparin, pit viper venom, quinine, salicylates, warfarin
Radiopaque ingestions	Arsenic, enteric-coated tablets, halogenated hydrocarbons, metals (e.g., iron, lead)
Red skin	Anticholinergics,[a] boric acid, disulfiram, hydroxocobalamin, scombroid, vancomycin
Rhabdomyolysis	Carbon monoxide, doxylamine, HMG-CoA reductase inhibitors, sympathomimetics,[b] *Tricholoma equestre*
Salivation	Arsenic, caustics, cholinergics,[c] ketamine, mercury, phencyclidine, strychnine
Seizures	Bupropion, camphor, carbon monoxide, cyclic antidepressants, *Gyromitra* mushrooms, hypoglycemia, isoniazid, methylxanthines, ethanol and sedative–hypnotic withdrawal
Tremor	Antipsychotics, arsenic, carbon monoxide, cholinergics,[c] ethanol, lithium, mercury, methyl bromide, sympathomimetics,[b] thyroid replacement
Weakness	Botulism, diuretics, magnesium, paralytic shellfish, steroids, toluene
Yellow skin	Acetaminophen (late), pyrrolizidine alkaloids, β carotene, amatoxin mushrooms, dinitrophenol

[a] Anticholinergics, including antihistamines, atropine, cyclic antidepressants, and scopolamine.

[b] Sympathomimetics, including adrenergic agonists, amphetamines, cocaine, and ephedrine.

[c] Cholinergics, including muscarinic mushrooms; organic phosphorus compounds and carbamates, including select Alzheimer's disease drugs and physostigmine; and pilocarpine and other direct-acting xenobiotics.

HMG-CoA, 3-hydroxy-3-methyl-glutaryl-CoA); LSD, lysergic acid diethylamide; MAOI, monoamine oxidase inhibitor.

considered to have an AMS. After airway patency is established or secured, an initial bedside assessment should be made regarding the adequacy of breathing. If it is not possible to assess the depth and rate of ventilation, then at least the presence or absence of regular breathing should be determined. In this setting, any irregular or slow breathing pattern should be considered a possible sign of the incipient apnea, requiring ventilation with 100% oxygen by bag–valve–mask followed as soon as possible by endotracheal intubation and mechanical ventilation. Endotracheal intubation may be indicated for some cases of coma resulting from a toxic exposure to ensure and maintain control of the airway and to enable safe performance of procedures to prevent GI absorption or eliminate previously absorbed xenobiotics.

Although in many instances, the widespread availability of pulse oximetry to determine O_2 saturation has made arterial blood gas (ABG) analysis less of an immediate priority, pulse oximetry has not eliminated the importance of blood gas analysis entirely. An ABG determination will more accurately define the adequacy not only of oxygenation (PO_2, O_2 saturation) and ventilation (PCO_2) but may also alert the physician to possible toxic-metabolic etiologies of coma characterized by acid–base disturbances (pH, PCO_2) (Chap. 16).

In addition, carboxyhemoglobin determinations are now available by point of care testing and both carboxyhemoglobin and methemoglobin may be determined on venous or arterial blood specimens (Chaps. 125 and 127). In every patient with an AMS, a bedside rapid capillary glucose concentration should be obtained as soon as possible.

After the patient's respiratory status has been assessed and managed appropriately, the strength, rate, and regularity of the pulse should be evaluated, the blood pressure determined, and a rectal temperature obtained. Both a 12-lead electrocardiogram (ECG) and continuous rhythm monitoring are essential. Monitoring will alert the clinician to dysrhythmias that are related to toxic exposures either directly or indirectly via hypoxemia or electrolyte imbalance. For example, a 12-lead ECG demonstrating QRS widening and a right axis deviation might indicate a life-threatening exposure to a cyclic antidepressant or another xenobiotic with sodium channel–blocking properties. In these cases, the physician can anticipate such serious sequelae as ventricular tachydysrhythmias, seizures, and cardiac arrest and consider both the early use of specific treatment (antidotes), such as IV sodium bicarbonate, and avoidance of medications, such as procainamide and other class IA and IC antidysrhythmics, which could exacerbate the situation.

Extremes of core body temperature must be addressed early in the evaluation and treatment of a comatose patient. Life-threatening hyperthermia (temperature >105°F; >40.5°C) is usually appreciated when the patient is touched (although the widespread use of gloves as part of universal precautions has made this less apparent than previously). Most individuals with severe hyperthermia, regardless of the etiology, should have their temperatures immediately reduced to about 101.5°F (38.7°C) by sedation if they are agitated or displaying muscle rigidity and by ice water immersion (Chap. 15). Hypothermia is probably easier to miss than hyperthermia, especially in northern regions during the winter months, when most arriving patients feel cold to the touch. Early recognition of hypothermia, however, helps to avoid administering a variety of medications that may be ineffective until the patient becomes relatively euthermic, which may cause iatrogenic toxicity as a result of a sudden response to xenobiotics previously administered.

For a hypotensive patient with clear lungs and an unknown overdose, a fluid challenge with IV 0.9% sodium chloride or lactated Ringer's solution may be started. If the patient remains hypotensive or cannot tolerate fluids, a vasopressor or an inotropic agent may be indicated, as may more invasive monitoring.

At the time that the IV catheter is inserted, blood samples for glucose, electrolytes, blood urea nitrogen (BUN), a complete blood count (CBC), and any indicated toxicologic analysis can be obtained. A pregnancy test should be obtained in any woman with childbearing potential. If the patient has an AMS, there may be a temptation to send blood and urine specimens to identify any central nervous system (CNS) depressants or so-called drugs of abuse along with other medications. But the indiscriminate ordering of these tests rarely provides clinically useful information. For the potentially suicidal patient, an acetaminophen concentration should be routinely requested, along with tests affecting the management of any specific xenobiotic, such as carbon monoxide, lithium, theophylline, iron, salicylates, and digoxin (or other cardioactive steroids), as suggested by the patient's history, physical examination, or bedside diagnostic tests. In the vast majority of cases, the blood tests that are most useful in diagnosing toxicologic emergencies are not the toxicologic assays but rather the "nontoxicologic" routine metabolic profile tests such as BUN, glucose, electrolytes, and blood gas analysis.

Xenobiotic-related seizures may broadly be divided into three categories: (1) those that respond to standard anticonvulsant treatment (typically using a benzodiazepine); (2) those that either require specific antidotes to control seizure activity or that do not respond consistently to standard anticonvulsant treatment, such as isoniazid-induced seizures requiring pyridoxine administration; and (3) those that may *appear* to respond to initial treatment with cessation of tonic–clonic activity but that leave the patient exposed to the underlying, unidentified toxin or to continued electrical seizure activity in the brain, as is the case with carbon monoxide poisoning and hypoglycemia.

Within the first 5 minutes of managing a patient with an AMS, four therapeutic interventions should be *considered*, and if indicated, administered:

1. High-flow oxygen (8–10 L/min) to treat a variety of xenobiotic-induced hypoxic conditions
2. Hypertonic dextrose: 0.5–1.0 g/kg of $D_{50}W$ for an adult or a more dilute dextrose solution ($D_{10}W$ or $D_{25}W$) for a child; the dextrose is administered as an IV bolus to diagnose and treat or exclude hypoglycemia
3. Thiamine (100 mg IV for an adult; usually unnecessary for a child) to prevent or treat Wernicke encephalopathy
4. Naloxone (0.05 mg IV with upward titration) for an adult or child with opioid-induced respiratory compromise

The clinician must consider that hypoglycemia may be the sole or contributing cause of coma even when the patient manifests focal neurologic findings; therefore, dextrose administration should only be omitted when hypoglycemia can be definitely excluded by accurate rapid bedside testing. Also, while examining a patient for clues to the etiology of a presumably toxic-metabolic form of AMS, it is important to search for any indication that trauma may have caused, contributed to, or resulted from the patient's condition. Conversely, the possibility of a concomitant drug ingestion or toxic metabolic disorder in a patient with obvious head trauma should also be considered.

The remainder of the physical examination should be performed rapidly but thoroughly. In addition to evaluating the patient's level of consciousness, the physician should note abnormal posturing (decorticate or decerebrate), abnormal or unilateral withdrawal responses, and pupil size and reactivity. Pinpoint pupils suggest exposure to opioids or organic phosphorus insecticides, and widely dilated pupils suggest anticholinergic or sympathomimetic poisoning. The presence or absence of nystagmus, abnormal reflexes, and any other focal neurologic findings may provide important clues to a structural cause of AMS. For clinicians accustomed to applying the Glasgow Coma Score (GCS) to all patients with AMS, assigning a score to the overdosed or poisoned patient may provide a useful measure for assessing changes in neurologic status. However, in this situation, the GCS should never be used for prognostic purposes because despite a low GCS, complete recovery from properly managed toxic-metabolic coma is the rule rather than the exception (Chap. 18).

Characteristic breath or skin odors may identify the etiology of coma. The fruity odor of ketones on the breath suggests diabetic or alcoholic ketoacidosis but also the possible ingestion of acetone or isopropyl alcohol, which is metabolized to acetone. The pungent, minty odor of oil of wintergreen on the breath or skin suggests methyl salicylate poisoning. The odors of other substances such as cyanide ("bitter almonds"), hydrogen sulfide ("rotten eggs"), and organic phosphorus compounds ("garlic") are described in detail in Chap. 20 and summarized in Table 20-1.

FURTHER EVALUATION OF ALL PATIENTS WITH SUSPECTED XENOBIOTIC EXPOSURES

Auscultation of breath sounds, particularly after a fluid challenge, helps to diagnose pulmonary edema, acute lung injury, or aspiration pneumonitis when present. Coupled with an abnormal breath odor of hydrocarbons or organic phosphorus compounds, for example, crackles and rhonchi may point to a toxic pulmonary etiology instead of a cardiac etiology; this is important because the administration of certain cardioactive medications may be inappropriate or dangerous in the former circumstances.

Heart murmurs in an injection drug user, especially when accompanied by fever, may indicate bacterial endocarditis. Dysrhythmias may suggest overdoses or inappropriate use of cardioactive xenobiotics, such as digoxin and other cardioactive steroids, β-adrenergic antagonists, calcium channel blockers, and cyclic antidepressants.

The abdominal examination may reveal signs of trauma or alcohol-related hepatic disease. The presence or absence of bowel sounds helps to exclude or to diagnose anticholinergic toxicity and is important in considering whether to manipulate the GI tract in an attempt to remove the toxin.

Examination of the extremities might reveal clues to current or former drug use (track marks, skin-popping scars); metal poisoning (Mees lines, arsenical dermatitis); and the presence of cyanosis or edema suggesting preexisting cardiac, pulmonary, or renal disease (Chap. 29).

Repeated evaluation of the patient suspected of an overdose is essential for identifying new or developing findings or toxic syndromes and for early identification and treatment of a deteriorating condition. Until the patient is completely recovered or considered no longer at risk for the consequences of a xenobiotic exposure, frequent reassessment must be provided, even as the procedures described below are carried out. Toxicologic etiologies of abnormal vital signs and physical findings are summarized in Tables 3–1 to 3–6. Toxic syndromes, sometimes called "toxidromes," are summarized in Table 3-1.

Typically in the management of patients with toxicologic emergencies, there is both a necessity and an opportunity to obtain various diagnostic studies and ancillary tests interspersed with stabilizing the patient's condition, obtaining the history, and performing the physical examination. Chapters 5, 6, and 22 discuss the timing and indications for diagnostic imaging procedures, qualitative and quantitative diagnostic laboratory studies, and the use and interpretation of the ECG in evaluating and managing poisoned or overdosed patients.

THE ROLE OF GASTROINTESTINAL EVACUATION

A series of highly individualized treatment decisions must now be made. As noted previously and as discussed in detail in Chapter 7, the decision to evacuate the GI tract or administer AC can no longer be considered standard or routine toxicologic care for most patients. Instead, the decision should be based on the type of ingestion, estimated quantity and size of pill or tablet, time since ingestion, concurrent ingestions, ancillary medical conditions, and age and size of the patient. The indications, contraindications, and procedures for performing orogastric lavage and for administering WBI, AC, MDAC, and cathartics are listed in Tables 7–1 through 7–4 and are discussed both in Chapter 7 and in the specific Antidotes in Depth sections immediately following Chapter 7.

ELIMINATING ABSORBED XENOBIOTICS FROM THE BODY

After deciding whether or not an intervention to try to *prevent* absorption of a xenobiotic is indicated, the clinician must next consider the applicability of techniques available to eliminate xenobiotics already absorbed. Detailed discussions of the indications for and techniques of manipulating urinary pH (ion trapping), diuresis, hemodialysis, hemoperfusion, hemofiltration, and exchange transfusion are found in Chapter 9. Briefly, patients who may benefit from these procedures are those who have systemically absorbed xenobiotics amenable to one of these techniques and whose clinical condition is both serious (or potentially serious) and unresponsive to supportive care or whose physiologic route of elimination (liver–feces, kidney–urine) is impaired.

Alkalinization of the urinary pH for acidic xenobiotics has only limited applicability. Commonly, sodium bicarbonate can be used to alkalinize the urine (as well as the blood) and enhance salicylate elimination (phenobarbital and chlorpropamide are less common indications), and sodium bicarbonate also prevents toxicity from methotrexate (see Antidotes in Depth: Sodium Bicarbonate). Acidifying the urine to hasten the elimination of alkaline substances is difficult to accomplish, probably useless, and possibly dangerous and therefore has no role in poison management. Forced diuresis also has no indication and may endanger the patient by causing pulmonary or cerebral edema.

If extracorporeal elimination is contemplated, hemodialysis should be considered for overdoses of salicylates, methanol, ethylene glycol, lithium, and xenobiotics that are both dialyzable and cause fluid and electrolyte problems. If available, hemoperfusion or high-flux hemodialysis should be considered for overdoses of theophylline, phenobarbital, and carbamazepine (although rarely, if ever, for the last two). When hemoperfusion is the method of choice (as for a theophylline overdose) but not available, hemodialysis is a logical, effective alternative and certainly preferable to delaying treatment until HP becomes available. Peritoneal dialysis is too ineffective to be of practical utility, and hemodiafiltration is not as efficacious as hemodialysis or hemoperfusion, although it may play a role between multiple runs of dialysis or in hemodynamically compromised patients who cannot tolerate hemodialysis. In theory, both hemodialysis and hemoperfusion *in series* may be useful for a very few life-threatening overdoses such as salicylates. Plasmapheresis and exchange transfusion are used to eliminate xenobiotics with large molecular weights that are not dialyzable (Chap. 9).

AVOIDING PITFALLS

The history alone may not be a reliable indicator of which patients require naloxone, hypertonic dextrose, thiamine, and oxygen. Instead, these therapies should be *considered* (unless specifically contraindicated) only after a clinical assessment for all patients with AMS. The physical examination should be used to guide the use of naloxone. If dextrose or naloxone is indicated, sufficient amounts should be administered to exclude or treat hypoglycemia or opioid toxicity, respectively.

In a patient with a suspected but unknown overdose, the use of vasopressors should be avoided in the initial management of hypotension before administering fluids or assessing filling pressures.

Attributing an AMS to alcohol because of its odor on a patient's breath is potentially dangerous and misleading. Small amounts of alcohol and its congeners generally produce the same breath odor as do intoxicating amounts. Conversely, even when an extremely high blood ethanol concentration is *confirmed* by the laboratory, it is dangerous to ignore other possible causes of an AMS. Because chronic alcoholics may be awake and seemingly alert with ethanol concentrations in excess of 500 mg/dL, a concentration that would result in coma and possibly apnea and death in a nontolerant person, finding a high ethanol concentration does not eliminate the need for further search into the cause of a depressed level of consciousness.

The metabolism of ethanol is fairly constant at 15 to 30 mg/dL/h. Therefore, as a general rule, regardless of the initial blood alcohol concentration, a presumably "inebriated" comatose patient who is still unarousable 3 to 4 hours after initial assessment should be considered to have head trauma, a cerebrovascular accident, CNS infection, or other toxic-metabolic etiology for the alteration in consciousness, until proven otherwise. Careful neurologic evaluation of the completely undressed patient supplemented by a head computed tomography scan or a lumbar puncture is frequently indicated in such cases. This is especially important in dealing with a seemingly "intoxicated" patient who appears to have only a minor bruise because the early treatment of a subdural or epidural hematoma or subarachnoid hemorrhage is critical to a successful outcome.

ADDITIONAL CONSIDERATIONS IN MANAGING PATIENTS WITH A NORMAL MENTAL STATUS

As in the case of the patient with AMS, vital signs must be obtained and recorded. Initially, an assumption may have been made that the patient was breathing adequately, and if the patient is alert, talking, and in no respiratory distress, all that remains to document is the respiratory rate and rhythm. Because the patient is alert, additional history should be obtained, keeping in mind that information regarding the number and types of xenobiotics ingested, time elapsed, prior vomiting, and other critical information may be unreliable, depending in part on whether the ingestion was intentional or unintentional.

When indicated for the potential benefit of the patient, another history should be privately and independently obtained from a friend or relative after the patient has been initially stabilized. Recent emphasis on compliance with the federal Health Insurance Portability and Accountability Act (HIPAA) may inappropriately discourage clinicians from attempting to obtain information necessary to evaluate and treat patients. Obtaining such information from a friend or relative without unnecessarily giving that person information about the patient may be the key to successfully helping such a patient without violating confidentiality.

Speaking to a friend or relative of the patient may provide an opportunity to learn useful and reliable information regarding the ingestion, the patient's frame of mind, a history of previous ingestions, and the type of support that is available if the patient is discharged from the ED. At times, it may be essential to initially separate the patient from any relatives or friends to obtain greater cooperation from the patient and avoid violating confidentiality and because their anxiety may interfere with therapy. Even if the history obtained from a patient with an overdose proves to be unreliable, it may nevertheless provide clues to an overlooked possibility of a second ingestant or reveal the patient's mental and emotional condition. As is often true of the history, physical examination, or laboratory assessment in other clinical situations, the information obtained may confirm but never exclude possible causes.

At this point in the management of a conscious patient, a focused physical examination should be performed, concentrating on the pulmonary, cardiac, and abdominal examinations. A neurologic survey should emphasize reflexes and any focal findings.

APPROACHING PATIENTS WITH INTENTIONAL EXPOSURES

Initial efforts at establishing rapport with the patient by indicating to the patient concern about the problems that led to the ingestion and the availability of help after the xenobiotic is removed (if such procedures are planned) may help make management easier. If GI decontamination is deemed necessary, the reason for and nature of the procedure should be clearly explained to the patient together with reassurance that after the procedure is completed, there will be ample time to discuss related problems and provide additional care. These considerations are especially important in managing the patient with an intentional overdose who may be seeking psychiatric help or emotional support. In deciding on the necessity of GI decontamination, it is important to consider that a resistant patient may transform a procedure of only potential value into one with predictable adverse consequences.

SPECIAL CONSIDERATIONS FOR MANAGING PREGNANT PATIENTS

In general, a successful outcome for both the mother and fetus depends on optimum management of the mother, and proven effective treatment for a potentially serious toxic exposure to the mother should never be withheld based on theoretical concerns regarding the fetus.

PHYSIOLOGIC FACTORS

A pregnant woman's total blood volume and cardiac output are elevated through the second trimester and into the later stages of the third trimester. This means that signs of hypoperfusion and hypotension manifest later than they would in a woman who is not pregnant, and when they do, uterine blood flow may already be compromised. For these reasons, the possibility of hypotension in a pregnant woman must be more aggressively sought and, if found, more rapidly treated. Maintaining the patient in the left-lateral decubitus position helps prevent supine hypotension resulting from impairment of systemic venous return by compression of the inferior vena cava. The left lateral decubitus position is also the preferred position for orogastric lavage, if this procedure is deemed necessary.

Because the tidal volume is increased in pregnancy, the baseline PCO_2 will normally be lower by approximately 10 mm Hg. Appropriate adjustment for this effect should be made when interpreting ABG results.

USE OF ANTIDOTES

Limited data is available on the use of antidotes in pregnancy. In general, antidotes should not be used if the indications for use are equivocal. On the other hand, antidotes should not be withheld if their use may reduce potential morbidity and mortality. Risks and benefits of either decision must be considered. For example, reversal of opioid-induced respiratory depression calls for the use of naloxone, but in an opioid-dependent woman, the naloxone can precipitate acute opioid withdrawal, including uterine contractions and possible induction of labor. Very slow, careful, IV titration starting with 0.05 mg naloxone may be indicated unless apnea is present, cessation of breathing appears imminent, or the PO_2 or O_2 saturation is already compromised. In these instances, naloxone may have to be administered in higher doses (i.e., 0.4–2.0 mg) or assisted ventilation provided or a combination of assisted ventilation and small doses of naloxone used.

An acetaminophen overdose is a serious maternal problem when it occurs throughout pregnancy, but the fetus is at greatest risk in the third trimester. Although acetaminophen crosses the placenta easily, *N*-acetylcysteine has somewhat diminished transplacental passage. During the third trimester, when both the mother and the fetus may be at substantial risk from a significant acetaminophen overdose with manifest hepatoxicity, immediate delivery of a mature or viable fetus may need to be considered.

In contrast to the situation with acetaminophen, the fetal risk from iron poisoning is less than the maternal risk. Because deferoxamine is a large charged molecule with little transplacental transport, deferoxamine should never be withheld out of unwarranted concern for fetal toxicity when indicated to treat the mother.

Carbon monoxide (CO) poisoning is particularly threatening to fetal survival. The normal PO_2 of the fetal blood is approximately 15 to

20 mm Hg. Oxygen delivery to fetal tissues is impaired by the presence of carboxyhemoglobin, which shifts the oxyhemoglobin dissociation curve to the left, potentially compromising an already tenuous balance. For this reason, hyperbaric oxygen is recommended for much lower carboxyhemoglobin concentrations in the pregnant compared with the nonpregnant woman (Chap. 125 and Antidotes in Depth: Hyperbaric Oxygen). Early notification of the obstetrician and close cooperation among involved physicians are essential for best results in all of these instances.

MANAGEMENT OF PATIENTS WITH CUTANEOUS EXPOSURE

The xenobiotics that people are commonly exposed to externally include household cleaning materials; organic phosphorus or carbamate insecticides from crop dusting, gardening, or pest extermination; acids from leaking or exploding batteries; alkalis, such as lye; and lacrimating agents that are used in crowd control. In all of these cases, the principles of management are as follows:

1. Avoid secondary exposures by wearing protective (rubber or plastic) gowns, gloves, and shoe covers. Cases of serious secondary poisoning have occurred in emergency personnel after contact with xenobiotics such as organic phosphorus compounds on the victim's skin or clothing.
2. Remove the patient's clothing, place it in plastic bags, and then seal the bags.
3. Wash the patient with soap and copious amounts of water *twice* regardless of how much time has elapsed since the exposure.
4. Make no attempt to neutralize an acid with a base or a base with an acid. Further tissue damage may result from the heat generated by this reaction.
5. Avoid using any greases or creams because they will only keep the xenobiotic in close contact with the skin and ultimately make removal more difficult.

Chapter 29 discusses the principles of managing cutaneous exposures.

MANAGEMENT OF PATIENTS WITH OPHTHALMIC EXPOSURES

Although the vast majority of toxicologic emergencies result from ingestion, injection, or inhalation, the eyes are occasionally the routes of systemic absorption or are the organs at risk. The eyes should be irrigated with the eyelids fully retracted for no less than 20 minutes. To facilitate irrigation, a drop of an anesthetic (e.g., proparacaine) in each eye should be used, and the eyelids should be kept open with an eyelid retractor. An adequate irrigation stream may be obtained by running 1 L of normal saline through regular IV tubing held a few inches from the eye or by using an irrigating lens. Checking the eyelid fornices with pH paper strips is important to ensure adequate irrigation; the pH should normally be 6.5 to 7.6 if accurately tested, although when using paper test strips, the measurement will often be near 8.0. Chapter 19 describes the management of toxic ophthalmic exposures in more detail.

IDENTIFYING PATIENTS WITH NONTOXIC EXPOSURES

There is a risk of needlessly subjecting a patient to potential harm when a patient with a nontoxic exposure is treated aggressively with GI evacuation techniques and other forms of management indicated for serious exposures. More than 40% of exposures reported to poison centers annually are judged to be nontoxic or minimally toxic. The following general guidelines[1,2] for considering an exposure nontoxic or minimally toxic will assist clinical decision making:

1. Identification of the product and its ingredients is possible.
2. None of the US Consumer Product Safety Commission "signal words" (CAUTION, WARNING, or DANGER) appear on the product label.
3. The history permits the route(s) of exposure to be determined.
4. The history permits a reliable approximation of the maximum quantity involved with the exposure.
5. Based on the available medical literature and clinical experience, the potential effects related to the exposure are expected to be at most benign and self-limited and do not require referral to a clinician.[1,2]
6. The patient is asymptomatic or has developed the expected benign self-limited toxicity.

ENSURING OPTIMAL OUTCOME

The best way to ensure an optimal outcome for the patient with a suspected toxic exposure is to apply the principles of basic and advanced life support in conjunction with a planned and staged approach, always bearing in mind that a toxicologic etiology or coetiology for any abnormal conditions necessitates modifying whatever standard approach is brought to the bedside of a severely ill patient. For example, it is extremely important to recognize that xenobiotic-induced dysrhythmias or cardiac instability require alterations in standard protocols that assume a primary cardiac or nontoxicologic etiology (Chaps. 22 and 23).

Typically, only some of the xenobiotics to which a patient is exposed will ever be confirmed by laboratory analysis. The thoughtful combination of stabilization, general management principles, and specific treatment when indicated will result in successful outcomes in the vast majority of patients with actual or suspected exposures.

SUMMARY

Patients with a suspected overdose or poisoning and an AMS present some of the most serious initial challenges. Conscious patients, asymptomatic patients, and pregnant patients with possible xenobiotic exposures raise additional management issues, as do the victims of toxic cutaneous or ophthalmic exposures. One of the most frequent toxicologic emergencies that clinicians must deal with is a patient with a suspected toxic exposure to an unidentified xenobiotic (medication or substance), sometimes referred to as an *unknown overdose*. Considering not only those patients who have an AMS but also those who are suicidal, those who use illicit drugs, or those who are exposed to xenobiotics of which they are unaware, many toxicologic emergencies at least partly involve an unknown component.

REFERENCES

1. McGuigan MA, Guideline Consensus Panel: Guideline for the out-of-hospital management of human exposures to minimally toxic substances. *J Toxicol Clin Toxicol.* 2003;41:907-917.
2. Mofenson HC, Greensher J: The unknown poison. *Pediatrics* 1974;54:336-342.

CHAPTER 5
DIAGNOSTIC IMAGING

David T. Schwartz

Diagnostic imaging can play a significant role in the management of many toxicologic emergencies. Radiographic studies can directly visualize the xenobiotic in some cases, but in others, they reveal the effects of the xenobiotic on various organ systems (Table 5–1). Radiography can confirm a diagnosis (e.g., by visualizing the xenobiotic), assist in therapeutic interventions such as monitoring gastrointestinal (GI) decontamination, and detect complications of the xenobiotic exposure.[180]

Conventional radiography is readily available in the emergency department (ED) and is the imaging modality most frequently used in acute patient management. However, other imaging modalities can be used in toxicologic emergencies, including computed tomography (CT); enteric and intravascular contrast studies; ultrasonography; transesophageal echocardiography (TEE); magnetic resonance imaging (MRI/MRA); and nuclear scintigraphy, including positron emission tomography (PET) and single-photon emission tomography (SPECT).

VISUALIZING THE XENOBIOTIC

A number of xenobiotics are radiopaque and can potentially be detected by conventional radiography. Radiography is most useful when a substance that is known to be radiopaque has been ingested or injected. When the identity of the xenobiotic is unknown, the usefulness of radiography is very limited. When ingested, a radiopaque xenobiotic may be seen on an abdominal radiograph. Injected radiopaque xenobiotics are also amenable to radiographic detection. If the toxic material itself is available for examination, it can be radiographed outside of the body to detect any radiopaque contents (Fig. 103-1).[76]

RADIOPACITY

The radiopacity of a xenobiotic is determined by several factors. First, the intrinsic radiopacity of a substance depends on its physical density (g/cm^3) and the atomic numbers of its constituent atoms. Biologic tissues are composed mostly of carbon, hydrogen, and oxygen and have an average atomic number of approximately 6. Substances that are more radiopaque than soft tissues include bone, which contains calcium (atomic number 20); radiocontrast agents containing iodine (atomic number 53) and barium (atomic number 56); iron (atomic number 26); and lead (atomic number 82). Some xenobiotics have constituent atoms of high atomic number, such as chlorine (atomic number 17), potassium (atomic number 19), and sulfur (atomic number 16), that contribute to their radiopacity.

The thickness of an object also affects its radiopacity. Small particles of a moderately radiopaque xenobiotic are often not visible on a radiograph. Finally, the radiographic appearance of the surrounding area also affects the detectability of an object. A moderately radiopaque tablet is easily seen against a uniform background, but in a patient, overlying bone or bowel gas often obscures the tablet.

ULTRASONOGRAPHY

Compared with conventional radiography, ultrasonography theoretically is a useful tool for detecting ingested xenobiotics because it depends on echogenicity rather than radiopacity for visualization. Solid pills within the fluid-filled stomach may have an appearance similar to gallstones within the gallbladder. In one in vitro study using a water-bath model, virtually all intact pills could be visualized.[7] The authors were also successful at detecting pills within the stomachs of human volunteers who ingested pills. Nonetheless, reliably finding pills scattered throughout the GI tract, which often contains air and feces that block the ultrasound beam, is a formidable task. Ultrasonography, therefore, has limited clinical practicality.

INGESTION OF AN UNKNOWN XENOBIOTIC

Although a clinical policy issued by the American College of Emergency Physicians in 1995 suggested that an abdominal radiograph should be obtained in unresponsive overdosed patients in an attempt to identify the involved xenobiotic, the role of abdominal radiography in screening a patient who has ingested an unknown xenobiotic is questionable.[6] The number of potentially ingested xenobiotics that are radiopaque is limited. In addition, the radiographic appearance of an ingested xenobiotic is not sufficiently distinctive to determine its identity (Fig. 5–1).[202] However, when ingestion of a radiopaque xenobiotic such as ferrous sulfate tablets or another metal with a high atomic number is suspected, abdominal radiographs are helpful.[5] In addition, knowledge of potentially radiopaque xenobiotics is useful in suggesting diagnostic possibilities when a radiopaque xenobiotic is discovered on an abdominal radiograph that was obtained for reasons other than suspected xenobiotic ingestion, such as in a patient with abdominal pain (Fig. 5–2).[179,186]

Several investigators have studied the radiopacity of various medications.[52,59,81,87,97,147,176,189,197] These investigators used an in vitro water-bath model to simulate the radiopacity of abdominal soft tissues.[176] The studies found that only a small number of medications exhibit some degree of radiopacity. A short list of the more consistently radiopaque xenobiotics is summarized in the mnemonic CHIPES—chloral hydrate, "heavy metals," iron, phenothiazines, and enteric-coated and sustained-release preparations.

The CHIPES mnemonic has several limitations.[176] It does not include all of the pills that are radiopaque in vitro such as acetazolamide and busulfan. Most radiopaque medications are only moderately radiopaque, and when ingested, they dissolve rapidly, becoming difficult or impossible to detect. "Psychotropic medications" include a wide variety of compounds of varying radiopacity.[147,176] For example, whereas trifluoperazine (containing fluorine; atomic number 9) is radiopaque in vitro, chlorpromazine (containing chlorine; atomic number 17) is not.[176]

Finally, sustained-release preparations and those with enteric coatings have variable composition and radiopacity. Pill formulations of fillers, binders, and coatings vary between manufacturers, and even a specific product can change depending on the date of manufacture. Furthermore, the insoluble matrix of some sustained-release preparations is radiopaque, and when seen on a radiograph, these tablets may no longer contain active medication. Some sustained-release cardiac medications such as verapamil and nifedipine have inconsistent radiopacity.[119,188,199]

EXPOSURE TO A KNOWN XENOBIOTIC

When a xenobiotic that is known to be radiopaque is involved in an exposure, radiography plays an important role in patient care.[5] Radiography can confirm the diagnosis of a radiopaque xenobiotic exposure, quantify the approximate amount of xenobiotic involved,

TABLE 5–1. Xenobiotics with Diagnostic Imaging Findings

Xenobiotic	Imaging Study[a]	Finding
Amiodarone	Chest	Phospholipidosis (interstitial and alveolar filling), pulmonary fibrosis
Asbestos	Chest	Interstitial fibrosis (asbestosis), calcified pleural plaques, mesothelioma
Beryllium	Chest	Acute: Airspace filling; chronic: hilar adenopathy
Body packer	Upper GI series or abdominal CT	Ingested packets, ileus, bowel obstruction
Carbon monoxide	Head CT, MRI SPECT, PET	Bilateral basal ganglia lucencies, white matter demyelinization, cerebral dysfunction
Caustic ingestion	Enteric contrast	Esophageal perforation or stricture
Chemotherapeutics (busulfan, bleomycin)	Chest	Interstitial pneumonitis
Cholinergics	Chest	Diffuse airspace filling (bronchorrhea)
Cocaine	Chest, abdominal	Diffuse airspace filling, pneumomediastinum, pneumothorax, aortic dissection, perforation
	Noncontrast Head CT, MRI, TEE, SPECT, PET	SAH, intracerebral hemorrhage, infarction, cerebral dysfunction, dopamine receptor downregulation
Corticosteroids	Skeletal	Avascular necrosis (femoral head)
Ethanol	Chest Head CT, MRI, SPECT, PET	Dilated cardiomyopathy, aspiration pneumonitis, rib fractures, cortical Cortical atrophy, cerebellar atrophy, SDH (head trauma), cerebellar and cortical dysfunction
Fluorosis	Skeletal	Osteosclerosis, osteophytosis, ligament calcification
Hydrocarbons (low viscosity)	Chest	Aspiration pneumonitis
Inhaled allergens	Chest	Hypersensitivity pneumonitis
Iron	Abdominal	Radiopaque tablets
Irritant gases	Chest	Diffuse airspace filling thorax
Lead	Skeletal, abdominal	Metaphyseal bands in children (proximal tibia, distal radius), bullets (dissolution near joints) Ingested leaded paint chips or other leaded compounds
Manganese	Brain MRI	Basal ganglia and midbrain hyperintensity
Mercury (elemental)	Abdominal, skeletal, or chest	Ingested, injected, or embolic deposits
Metals (Pb, Hg, Tl, As)	Abdominal	Ingested xenobiotic
Nitrofurantoin	Chest	Hypersensitivity pneumonitis
Opioids	Chest	Acute lung injury
	Abdominal	Ileus
Phenytoin	Chest	Hilar lymphadenopathy
Procainamide, INH, hydralazine	Chest	Pleural and pericardial effusions (xenobiotic-induced lupus syndrome)
Salicylates	Chest	Acute lung injury
Silica, coal dust	Chest	Interstitial fibrosis, hilar adenopathy (egg-shell calcification)
Thorium dioxide	Abdominal	Hepatic and splenic deposition

[a] Conventional radiography unless otherwise stated.

CT, computed tomography; INH, isoniazid; MRI, magnetic resonance imaging; PET, positron emission tomography; SAH, subarachnoid hemorrhage; SDH, subdural hematoma; SPECT, single-photon emission tomography.

and monitor its removal from the body. Examples include ferrous sulfate, sustained-release potassium chloride,[193] and heavy metals.

IRON TABLET INGESTION

Adult-strength ferrous sulfate tablets are readily detected radiographically because they are highly radiopaque and disintegrate slowly when ingested. Aside from confirming an iron tablet ingestion and quantifying the amount ingested, radiographs repeated after whole-bowel irrigation help to determine whether further GI decontamination is needed (Fig. 5–3).[51,61,101,146,151,153,205] Nonetheless, caution must be exercised in using radiography to exclude an iron ingestion. Some iron preparations are not radiographically detectable. Liquid, chewable, or encapsulated ("Spansule") iron preparations rapidly fragment and disperse after ingestion. Even when intact, these preparations are less radiopaque than ferrous sulfate tablets.[52]

HEAVY METALS

Heavy metals, such as arsenic, cesium, lead, manganese, mercury, potassium, and thallium, can be detected radiographically. Examples of metal exposure include leaded ceramic glaze (Fig. 5–4),[168] paint chips

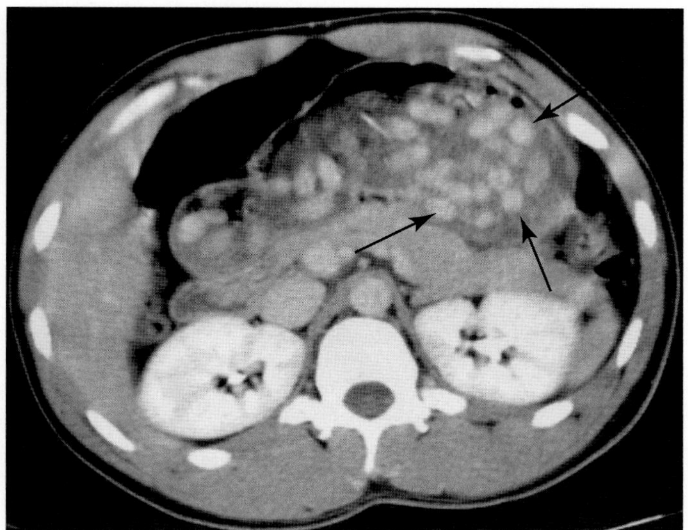

FIGURE 5–1. Ingestion of an unknown substance. A 46-year-old man presented to the emergency department with a depressed level of consciousness. Because he also complained of abdominal pain and mild diffuse abdominal tenderness, a computed tomography (CT) scan of the abdomen was obtained. The CT revealed innumerable tablet-shaped densities within the stomach (*arrows*). The CT finding was suspicious for an overdose of an unknown xenobiotic. Orogastric lavage was attempted, and the patient vomited a large amount of whole navy beans. CT is able to detect small, nearly isodense structures such as these that cannot be seen using conventional radiography. *(Image contributed by Dr. Earl J. Reisdorff, MD, Michigan State University, Lansing, Michigan.)*

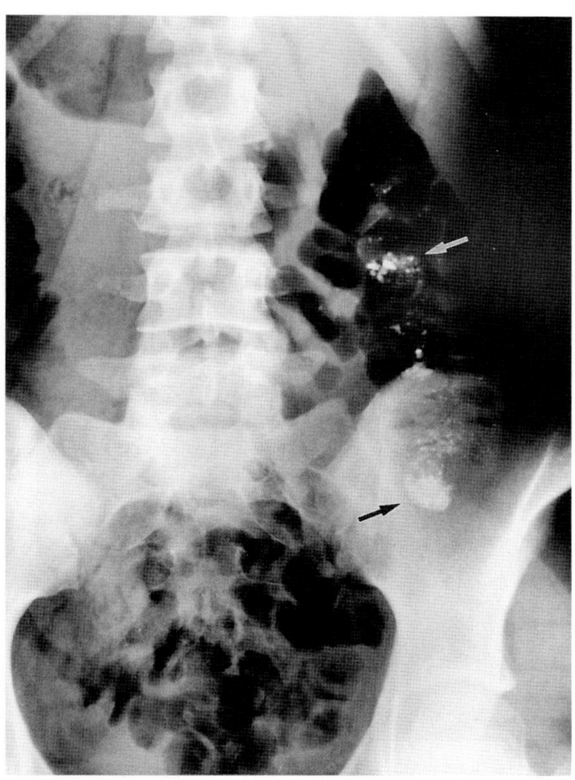

FIGURE 5–2. Detection of a radiopaque substance on an abdominal radiograph. An abdominal radiograph obtained on a patient with upper abdominal pain revealed radiopaque material throughout the intestinal tract (*arrows*). Further questioning of the patient revealed that he had been consuming bismuth subsalicylate (Pepto-Bismol) tablets to treat his peptic ulcer (bismuth, atomic number 83). The identification of radiopaque material does not allow determination of the nature of the substance.

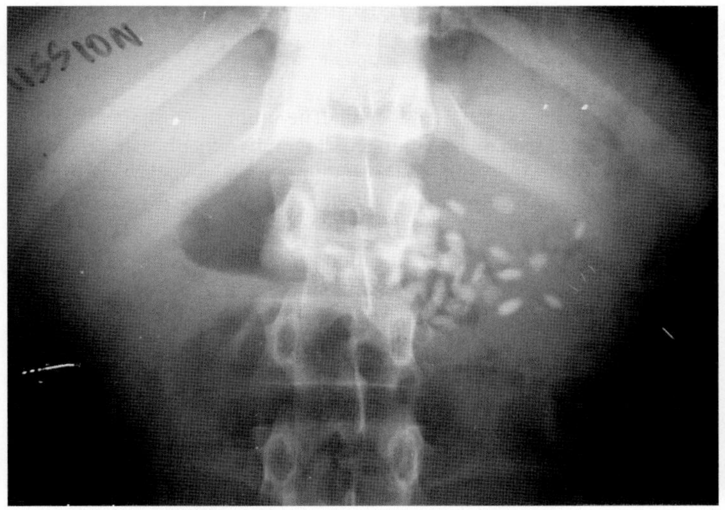

A

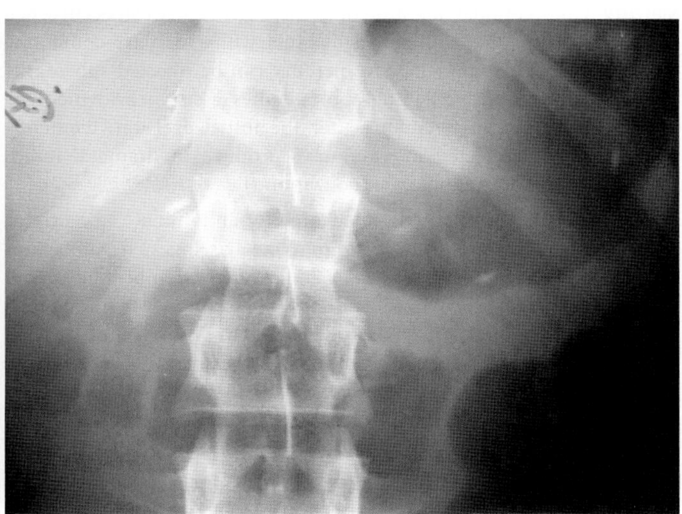

B

FIGURE 5–3. Iron tablet overdose. (**A**) The identification of the large amount of radiopaque tablets confirms the diagnosis in a patient with a suspected iron overdose and permits rough quantification of the amount ingested. (**B**) After emesis and whole-bowel irrigation, a second radiograph revealed some remaining tablets and indicated the need for further intestinal decontamination. A third radiograph after additional bowel irrigation demonstrated clearing of the intestinal tract. *(Images contributed by the Toxicology Fellowship of the New York City Poison Center.)*

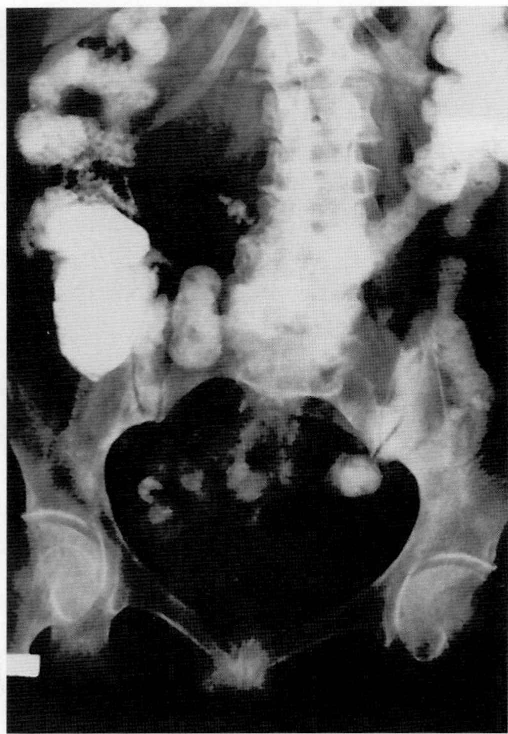

FIGURE 5–4. An abdominal radiograph of a patient who intentionally ingested ceramic glaze containing 40% lead. *(Image contributed by the Toxicology Fellowship of the New York City Poison Center.)*

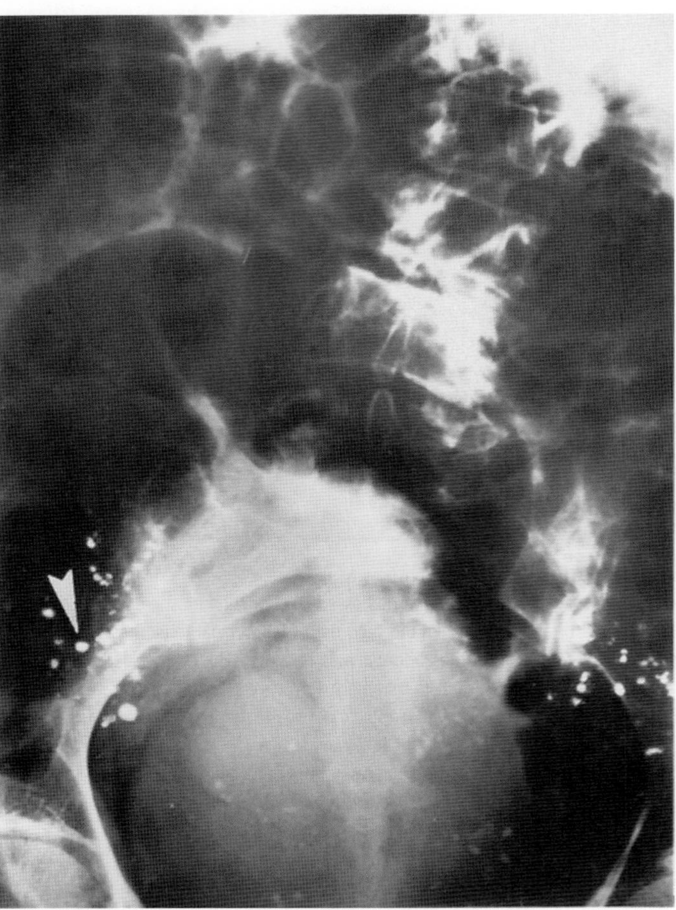

FIGURE 5–5. An abdominal radiograph in an elderly woman incidentally revealed radiopaque material in the pelvic region. This was residual from gluteal injection of antisyphilis therapy she had received 35 to 40 years earlier. The injections may have contained an arsenical. *(Image contributed by Dr. Emil J. Balthazar, Department of Radiology, Bellevue Hospital Center.)*

containing lead (Fig. 94–5),[112,133]mercuric oxide (Fig. 96–1),[122] thallium salts (atomic number 81),[44,134] and zinc (atomic number 30).[23] Arsenic (atomic number 33; Fig. 5–5)[77,116,203] with lower atomic numbers is also radiopaque.

Mercury Unintentional ingestion of elemental mercury can occur when a glass thermometer or a long intestinal tube with a mercury-containing balloon breaks. Liquid elemental mercury can be injected subcutaneously or intravenously. Radiographic studies assist débridement by detecting mercury that remains after the initial excision. Elemental mercury that is injected intravenously produces a dramatic radiographic picture of pulmonary embolization (Fig. 5–6).[23,26,112,126,130,143]

Lead Ingested lead can be detected only by abdominal radiography, such as in a child with lead poisoning who has ingested paint chips (see Fig. 91-5). Metallic lead (e.g., a bullet) that is embedded in soft tissues is not usually systemically absorbed. However, when the bullet is in contact with an acidic environment such as synovial fluid or cerebrospinal fluid (CSF), there may be significant absorption. Over many years, mechanical and chemical action within the joint causes the bullet to fragment and gradually dissolve.[43,45,53,192,196] Radiography can confirm the source of lead poisoning by revealing metallic material in the joint or CSF (Fig. 5–7).

XENOBIOTICS IN CONTAINERS

In some circumstances, ingested xenobiotics can be seen even though they are of similar radiopacity to surrounding soft tissues. If a xenobiotic is ingested in a container, the container itself may be visible.

Body Packers "Body packers" are individuals who smuggle large quantities of illicit drugs across international borders in securely sealed packets.[3,15,16,25,36,56,95,109,125,132,156,181,183,201] The uniformly shaped, oblong packets can be seen on abdominal radiographs either because there is a thin layer of air or metallic foil within the container wall or because the packets are outlined by bowel gas (Fig. 5–8). In some cases, a "rosette" representing the knot at the end of the packet is seen.[183] Intraabdominal calcifications (pancreatic calcifications and bladder stones) have occasionally been misinterpreted as drug-containing packets.[201,217]

The sensitivity of abdominal radiography for such packets is high, in the range of 85% to 90%. The major role of radiography is as a rapid screening test to confirm the diagnosis in individuals suspected of smuggling drugs, such as persons being held by airport customs agents. However, because packets are occasionally not visualized and the rupture of even a single packet can be fatal, abdominal radiography should not be relied on to exclude the diagnosis of body packing. Ultrasonography has also been used to rapidly detect packets, although it also should not be relied on to exclude such a life-threatening ingestion.[33,78,136] After intestinal decontamination, an upper GI series with oral contrast or CT with enteric contrast can reveal any remaining packets.[80,91,148]

Body stuffers A "body stuffer" is an individual who, in an attempt to avoid imminent arrest, hurriedly ingests contraband in insecure packaging.[170] The risk of leakage from such haphazardly constructed

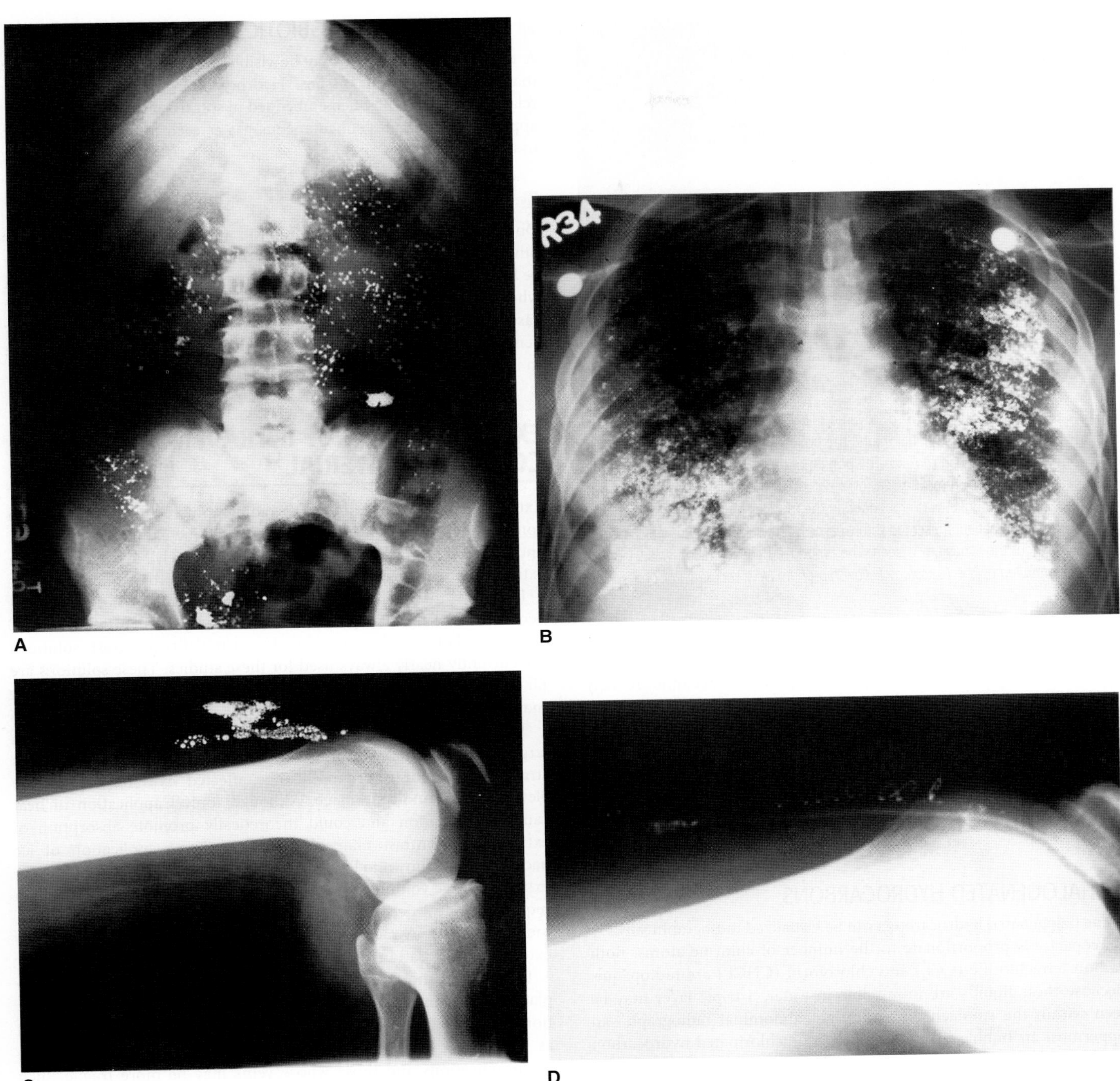

FIGURE 5–6. Elemental mercury exposures. (**A**) Unintentional rupture of a Cantor intestinal tube distributed mercury throughout the bowel. (**B**) The chest radiograph in a patient after intravenous injection of elemental mercury showing metallic pulmonary embolism. The patient developed respiratory failure, pleural effusions, and uremia and expired despite aggressive therapeutic interventions. (**C**) Subcutaneous injection of liquid elemental mercury is readily detected radiographically. Because mercury is systemically absorbed from subcutaneous tissues, it must be removed by surgical excision. (**D**) A radiograph after surgical débridement reveals nearly complete removal of the mercury deposit. Surgical staples and a radiopaque drain are visible. *(Image A contributed by Dr. Richard Lefleur, Department of Radiology, Bellevue Hospital Center; image B contributed by Dr. N. John Stewart, Department of Emergency Medicine, Palmetto Health, University of South Carolina School of Medicine and images C and D contributed by the Toxicology Fellowship of the New York City Poison Center.)*

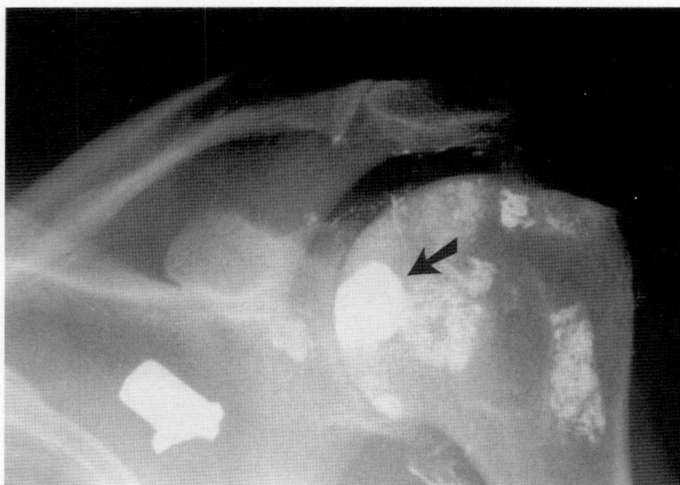

FIGURE 5–7. A "lead arthrogram" discovered many years after a bullet wound to the shoulder. At the time of the initial injury, the bullet was embedded in the articular surface of the humeral head (*arrow*). The portion of the bullet that protruded into the joint space was surgically removed, leaving a portion of the bullet exposed to the synovial space. A second bullet was embedded in the muscles of the scapula. Eight years after the injury, the patient presented with weakness and anemia. Extensive lead deposition throughout the synovium is seen. The blood lead concentration was 91 μg/dL. *(Image contributed by the Toxicology Fellowship of the New York City Poison Center.)*

containers is high. Unfortunately, radiographic studies cannot reliably confirm or exclude such ingestions.[187]

Occasionally, a radiograph will demonstrate the ingested container (Fig. 5–9). If the drug is in a glass or in a hard-plastic crack vial, the container may be seen.[90] If the body stuffer swallows soft plastic bags containing the drug, the containers are not usually visible. However, in three reported cases, "baggies" were visualized by abdominal CT.[37,48,83,105,85,157,180]

HALOGENATED HYDROCARBONS

Some halogenated hydrocarbons can be visualized radiographically.[31,38] Radiopacity is proportionate to the number of chlorine atoms. Both carbon tetrachloride (CCl_4) and chloroform ($CHCl_3$) are radiopaque. Because these liquids are immiscible in water, a triple layer may be seen within the stomach on an upright abdominal radiograph—an uppermost air bubble, a middle radiopaque chlorinated hydrocarbon layer, and a lower gastric fluid layer. However, these ingestions are rare, and the quantity ingested is usually too small to show this effect. Other halogenated hydrocarbons such as methylene iodide are highly radiopaque.[216]

MOTHBALLS

Some types of mothballs can be visualized by radiography. Whereas relatively nontoxic paradichlorobenzene mothballs (containing chlorine; atomic number 17) are moderately radiopaque, more toxic naphthalene mothballs are radiolucent.[194] If the patient is known to have swallowed mothballs, the difference in radiopacity may help determine the type. However, if a mothball ingestion is not already suspected, the more toxic naphthalene type may not be detected. Radiographs of mothballs outside of the patient can help distinguish these two types (see Fig. 103–1).

RADIOLUCENT XENOBIOTICS

A radiolucent xenobiotic may be visible because it is less radiopaque than surrounding soft tissues. Hydrocarbons such as gasoline are relatively radiolucent when embedded in soft tissues. The radiographic appearance resembles subcutaneous gas as seen in a necrotizing soft tissue infection (Fig. 5–10).

SUMMARY

Obtaining an abdominal radiograph in an attempt to identify pills or other xenobiotics in a patient with an unknown ingestion is unlikely to be helpful and is, in general, not warranted. Radiography is most useful when the suspected xenobiotic is known to be radiopaque, as is the case with iron tablets and heavy metals. If the material is available, the xenobiotic can be radiographed within the patient's abdomen, elsewhere in the patient's body, or outside of the patient.

EXTRAVASATION OF INTRAVENOUS CONTRAST MATERIAL

Extravasation of intravenous (IV) radiographic contrast material is a common occurrence. In most cases, the volume extravasated is small, and there are no clinical sequelae.[17,35,54,169] Rarely, a patient has an extravasation large enough to cause cutaneous necrosis and ulceration.

Recently, the incidence of sizable extravasations has increased because of the use of rapid-bolus automated power injectors for CT studies.[208] Fortunately, nonionic low-osmolality contrast solutions are currently nearly always used for these studies. These solutions are far less toxic to soft tissues than older ionic high-osmolality contrast materials.

The treatment of contrast extravasation has not been studied in a large series of human subjects and is therefore controversial. Various strategies have been proposed. The affected extremity should be elevated to promote drainage. Although topical application of heat causes vasodilation and could theoretically promote absorption of extravasated contrast material, the intermittent application of ice packs has been shown to lower the incidence of ulceration.[35] Rarely, an extremely large volume of liquid is injected into the soft tissues, which requires surgical decompression when there are signs of a compartment syndrome. A radiograph of the extremity will demonstrate the extent of extravasation.[35]

Precautions should be taken to prevent extravasation. A recently placed, well-running IV catheter should be used. The distal portions of the extremities (hands, wrist, and feet) should not be used as IV sites for injecting contrast. Patients who are more vulnerable to complications and those whose veins may be more fragile, such as infants, debilitated patients, and those with an impaired ability to communicate, must be closely monitored to prevent or determine if extravasation occurs.

VISUALIZING THE EFFECTS OF A XENOBIOTIC ON THE BODY

The lungs, central nervous system (CNS), GI tract, and skeleton are the organ systems that are most amenable to diagnostic imaging. Disorders of the lungs and skeletal system are seen by plain radiography. For abdominal pathology, contrast studies and CT are more useful, although plain radiographs can diagnose intestinal obstruction, perforation, and radiopaque foreign bodies. Imaging of the CNS uses CT, MRI, and nuclear scintigraphy (PET and SPECT).

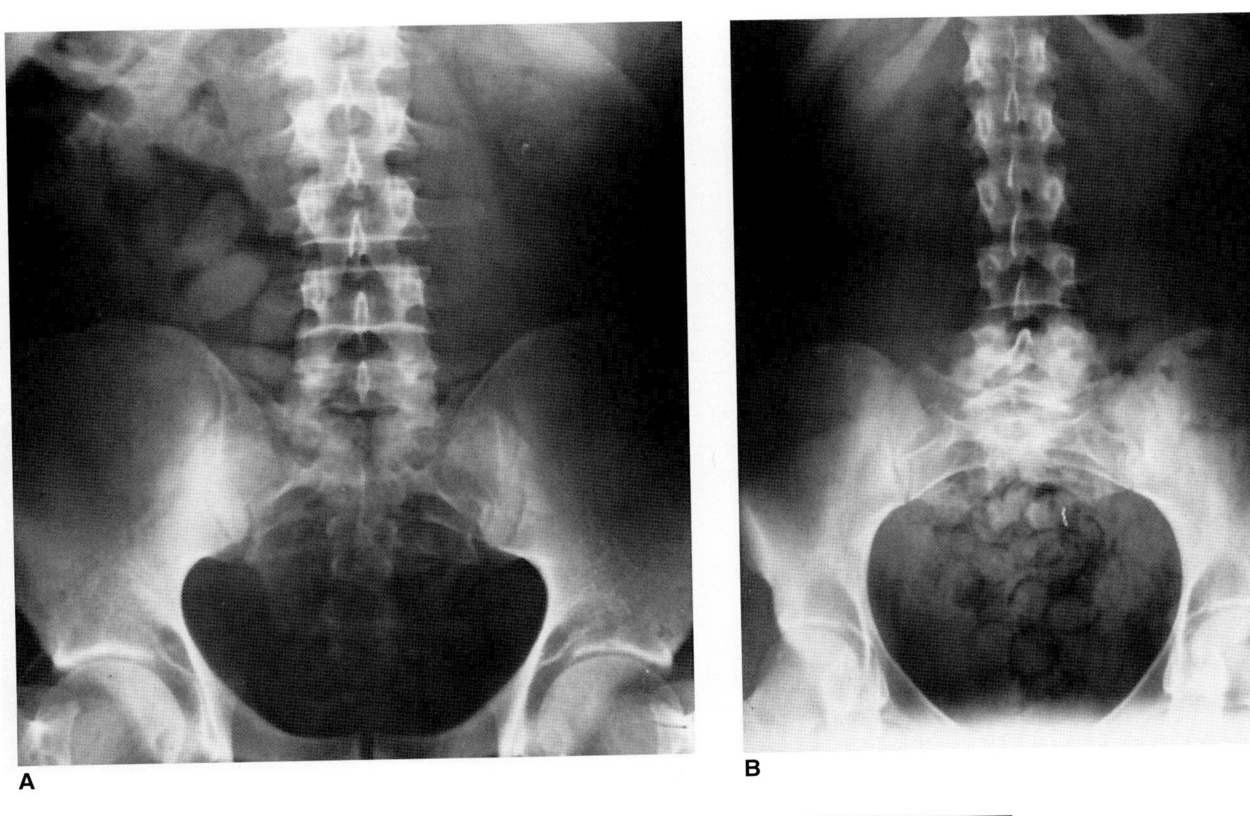

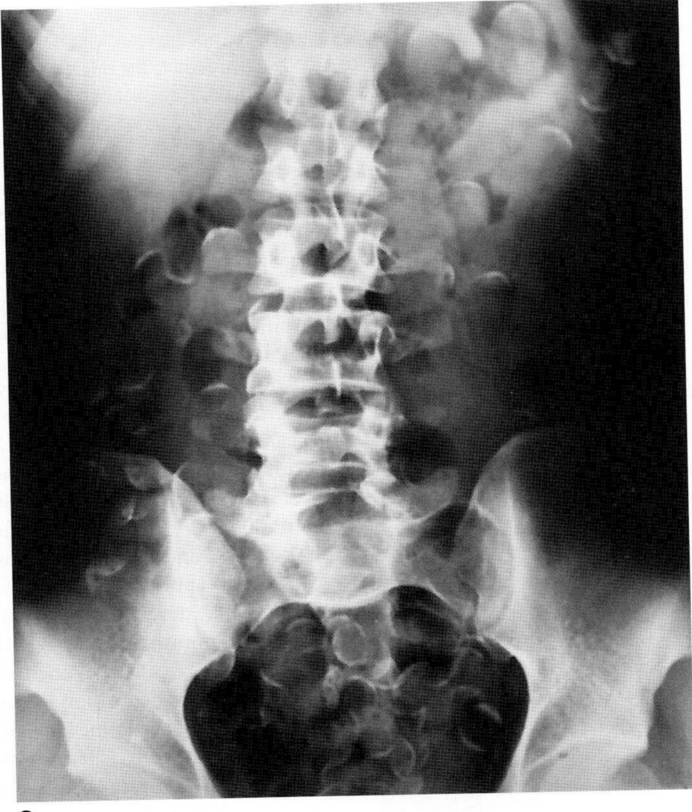

FIGURE 5–8. Radiographs of three "body packers" showing the various appearances of drug packets. Drug smuggling is accomplished by packing the gastrointestinal tract with large numbers of manufactured, well-sealed containers. (**A**) Multiple oblong packages of uniform size and shape are seen throughout the bowel. (**B**) The packets are visible in this patient because they are surrounded by a thin layer of air within the wall of the packet. (**C**) Metallic foil is part of the packet's container wall in this patient. *(Images contributed by Dr. Emil J. Balthazar, Department of Radiology, Bellevue Hospital Center.)*

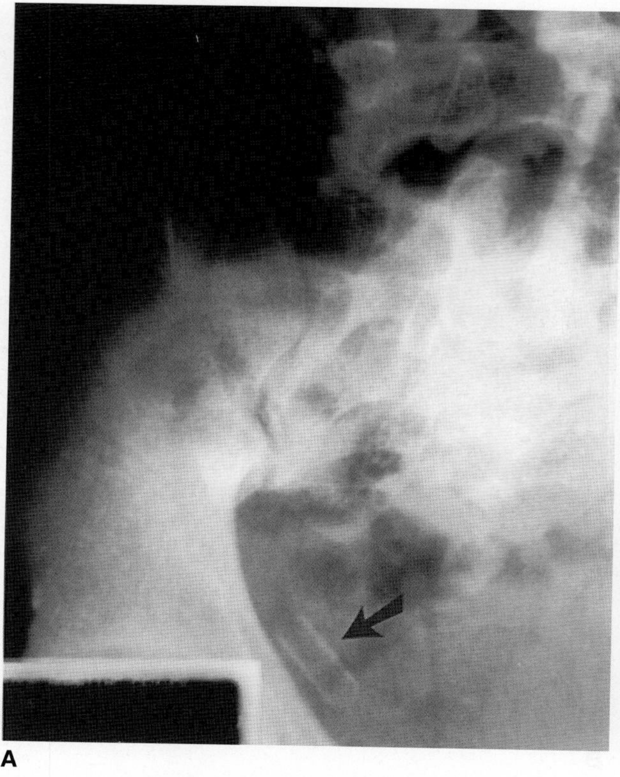

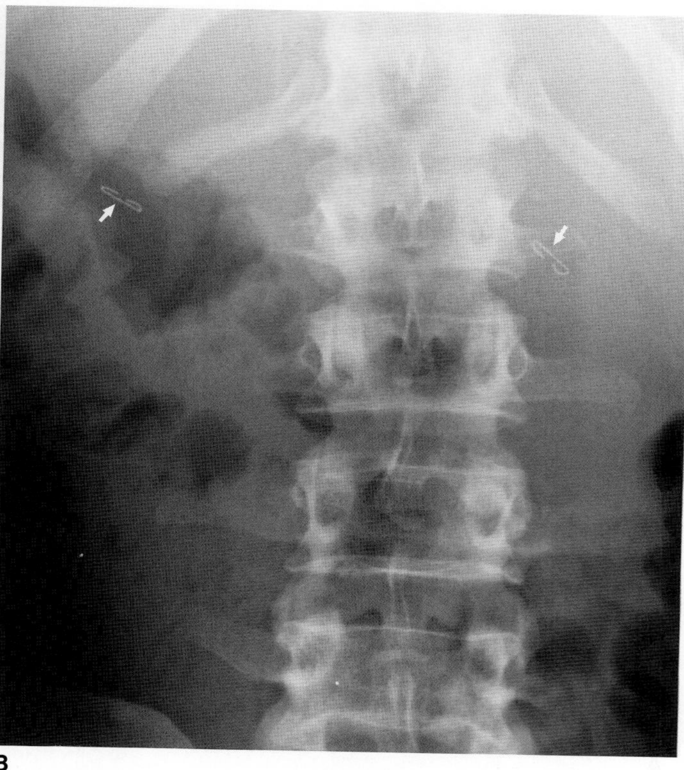

FIGURE 5–9. Two "body stuffers." Radiography infrequently helps with the diagnosis. (**A**) An ingested glass crack vial is seen in the distal bowel (*arrow*). The patient had ingested his contraband several hours earlier at the time of a police raid. Only the tubular-shaped container, and not the xenobiotic, is visible radiographically. The patient did not develop signs of cocaine intoxication during 24 hours of observation. (**B**) Another patient in police custody was brought to the emergency department for allegedly ingesting his drugs. The patient repeatedly denied this. The radiographs revealed "nonsurgical" staples in his abdomen (*arrows*). When questioned again, the patient admitted that he had swallowed several plastic bags that were stapled closed. *(Images contributed by the Toxicology Fellowship of the New York City Poison Center.)*

SKELETAL CHANGES CAUSED BY XENOBIOTICS

A number of xenobiotics affect bone mineralization. Toxicologic effects on bone result in either increased or decreased density (Table 5–2). Some xenobiotics produce characteristic radiographic pictures, although exact diagnoses usually depend on correlation with the clinical scenario.[10,145] Furthermore, alterations in skeletal structure develop gradually and are usually not visible unless the exposure continues for at least 2 weeks.

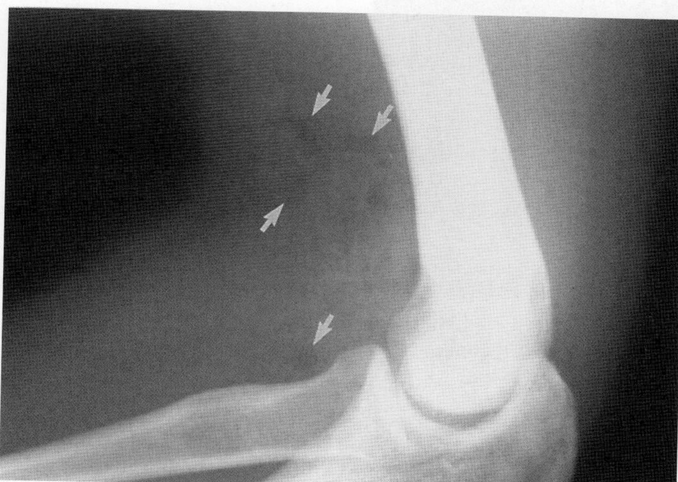

FIGURE 5–10. Subcutaneous injection of gasoline into the antecubital fossa. The radiolucent hydrocarbon mimics gas in the soft tissues that is seen with a necrotizing soft tissue infection such as necrotizing fasciitis or gas gangrene (*arrows*). *(Image contributed by the Toxicology Fellowship of the New York City Poison Center.)*

Lead Poisoning Skeletal radiography may suggest the diagnosis of chronic lead poisoning even before the blood lead concentration is obtained. With lead poisoning, the metaphyseal regions of rapidly growing long bones develop transverse bands of increased density along the growth plate (Fig. 5–11).[21,160,163,174] Characteristic locations are the distal femur and proximal tibia. Flaring of the distal metaphysis also occurs. Such lead lines are also seen in the vertebral bodies and iliac crest. Detected in approximately 80% of children with a mean lead concentration of 49 ± 17 μg/dL, lead lines usually occur in children between the ages of 2 and 9 years.[21] In most children, it takes several weeks for lead lines to appear, although in very young infants (2–4 months old), lead lines may develop within days of exposure.[221] After exposure ceases, lead lines diminish and may eventually disappear.

Lead lines are caused by the toxic effect of lead on bone growth and do not represent deposition of lead in bone. Lead impedes resorption of calcified cartilage in the zone of provisional calcification adjacent to the growth plate. This is termed *chondrosclerosis*.[21,47] Other xenobiotics that cause metaphyseal bands are yellow phosphorus, bismuth, and vitamin D (Chap. 41).

Fluorosis Fluoride poisoning causes a diffuse increase in bone mineralization. Endemic fluorosis occurs where drinking water contains very high levels of fluoride (≥2 or more parts per million), or as an occupational exposure among aluminum workers handling cryolite (sodium–aluminum fluoride). The skeletal changes associated with fluorosis are osteosclerosis (hyperostosis

TABLE 5–2. Xenobiotic Causes of Skeletal Abnormalities

Increased Bone Density	Diminished Bone Density (Either Diffuse Osteoporosis or Focal Lesions)
Metaphyseal bands (children) Lead, bismuth, phosphorus: Chondrosclerosis caused by toxic effect on bone growth **Diffuse increased bone density** Fluorosis: Osteosclerosis (hyperostosis deformans), osteophytosis, ligament calcification; usually involves the axial skeleton (vertebrae and pelvis) and may cause compression of the spinal cord and nerve roots Hypervitaminosis A (pediatric): Cortical hyperostosis and subperiosteal new bone formation; diaphyses of long bones have an undulating appearance Hypervitaminosis D (pediatric): Generalized osteosclerosis, cortical thickening, and metaphyseal bands	Corticosteroids: Osteoporosis: Diffuse Osteonecrosis: Focal lesions, e.g. avascular necrosis of the femoral head; loss of volume with both increased and decreased bone density; osteonecrosis also occurs in alcoholism, bismuth arthropathy, Caisson disease (dysbarism), trauma Hypervitaminosis D (adult): Focal or generalized osteoporosis. Injection drug use: Osteomyelitis (focal lytic lesions) caused by septic emboli; usually affects vertebral bodies and sternomanubrial joint. Vinyl chloride monomer: Acroosteolysis (distal phalanges)

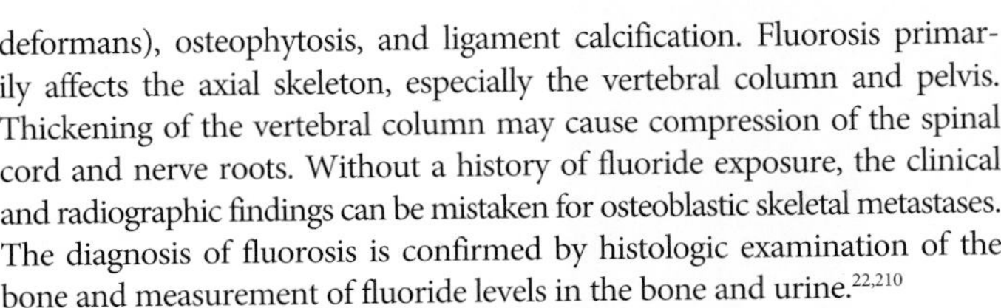

deformans), osteophytosis, and ligament calcification. Fluorosis primarily affects the axial skeleton, especially the vertebral column and pelvis. Thickening of the vertebral column may cause compression of the spinal cord and nerve roots. Without a history of fluoride exposure, the clinical and radiographic findings can be mistaken for osteoblastic skeletal metastases. The diagnosis of fluorosis is confirmed by histologic examination of the bone and measurement of fluoride levels in the bone and urine.[22,210]

Focal Loss of Bone Density Skeletal disorders associated with focal diminished bone density (or mixed rarefaction and sclerosis) include osteonecrosis, osteomyelitis, and osteolysis. Osteonecrosis, also known as avascular necrosis, most often affects the femoral head, humeral head, and proximal tibia.[127] There are many causes of osteonecrosis. Xenobiotic causes include long-term corticosteroid use and alcoholism. Radiographically, focal skeletal lucencies and sclerosis are seen, ultimately with loss of bone volume and collapse (Fig. 5–12A).

Acroosteolysis is bone resorption of the distal phalanges and is associated with occupational exposure to vinyl chloride monomer. Protective measures have reduced its incidence since it was first described in the early 1960s.[164]

Osteomyelitis is a serious complication of injection drug use. It usually affects the axial skeleton, especially the vertebral bodies, as well as the sternomanubrial and sternoclavicular joints (Fig. 5–12B).[74,79] Back pain or neck pain in IV drug users warrants careful consideration. A spinal epidural abscess causing spinal cord compression may accompany vertebral osteomyelitis.[92,125] Radiographs are negative early in the disease course before skeletal changes are visible and the diagnosis is confirmed by MRI or CT (Fig. 5–12C).

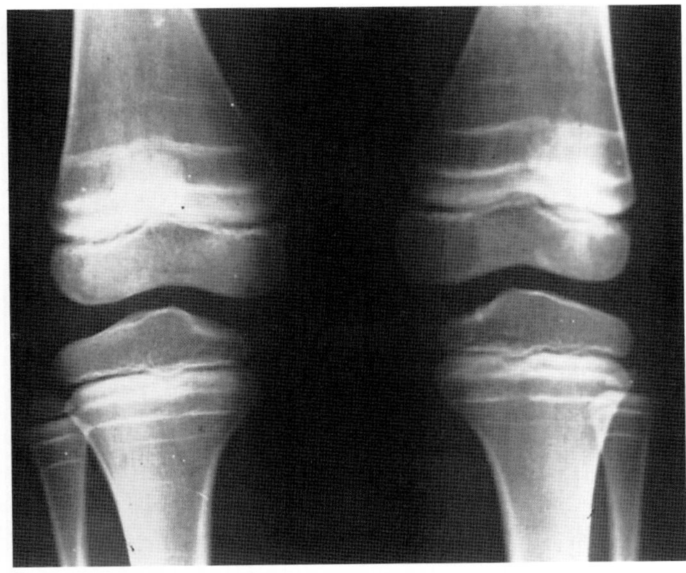

A

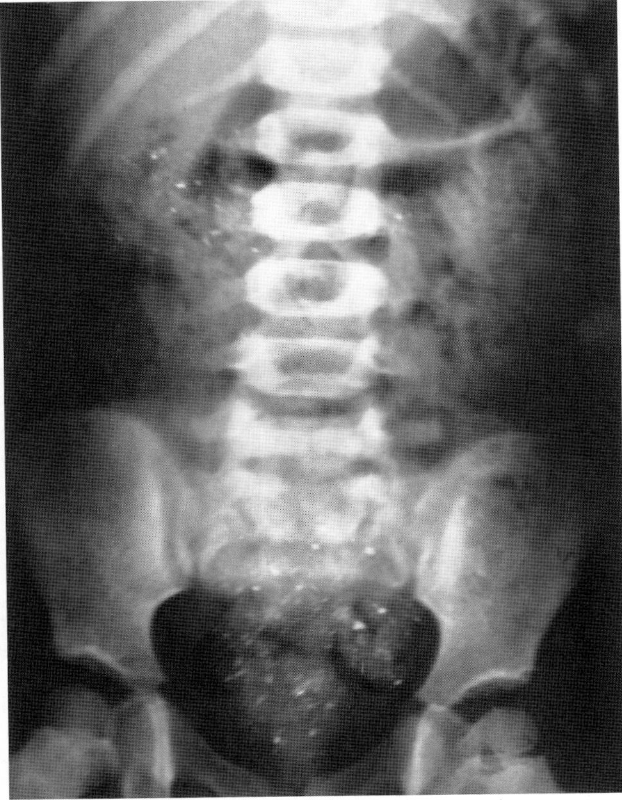

B

FIGURE 5–11. (**A**) A radiograph of the knees of a child with lead poisoning. The metaphyseal regions of the distal femur and proximal tibia have developed transverse bands representing bone growth abnormalities caused by lead toxicity. The multiplicity of lines implies repeated exposures to lead. (**B**) The abdominal radiograph of the child shows many radiopaque flakes of ingested leaded paint chips. Lead poisoning also caused abnormally increased cortical mineralization of the vertebral bodies, which gives them a boxlike appearance. *(Images contributed by Dr. Nancy Genieser, Department of Radiology, Bellevue Hospital Center.)*

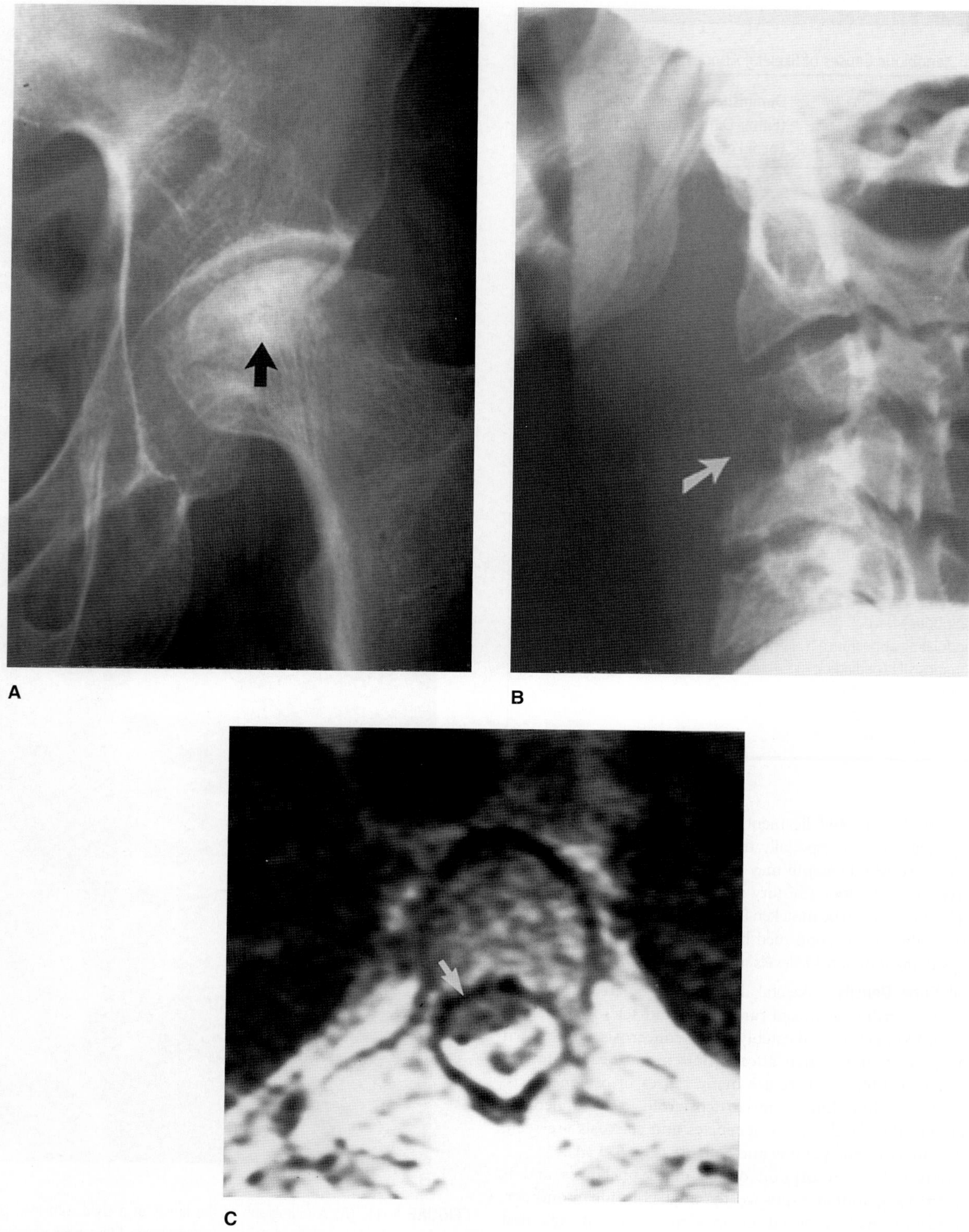

FIGURE 5–12. (A) Avascular necrosis causing collapse of the femoral head in a patient with long-standing steroid-dependent asthma (*arrow*). (B) A patient with vertebral body osteomyelitis complicating injection drug use. Destruction of the intervertebral disk and endplates of C3 and C4 are seen (*arrow*). Operative culture of the bone grew *Staphylococcus aureus*. (C) An injection drug user with thoracic back pain, leg weakness, and low-grade fever. Radiographs of the spine were negative. Magnetic resonance image showing an epidural abscess (*arrow*) compressing the spinal cord. The cerebral spinal fluid in the compressed thecal sac is bright white on this T2-weighted image. *(From Levitan R: Thoracolumbar spine. In: Schwartz DT, Reisdorff EJ, eds:* Emergency Radiology. *New York, McGraw-Hill; 2000:343, with permission.)*

SOFT TISSUE CHANGES

Certain abnormalities in soft tissues, predominantly as a consequence of infectious complications of injection drug use, are amenable to radiographic diagnosis.[74,75,79,99,198] In an injection drug user who presents with signs of local soft tissue infections, radiography is indicated to detect a retained metallic foreign body, such as a needle fragment, or subcutaneous gas, as may be seen in a necrotizing soft tissue infection such as necrotizing fasciitis. CT is more sensitive at detecting soft tissue gas than is conventional radiography. CT and ultrasonography can also detect subcutaneous or deeper abscesses that require surgical or percutaneous drainage.

PULMONARY AND OTHER THORACIC PROBLEMS

Many xenobiotics that affect intrathoracic organs produce pathologic changes that can be detected on chest radiographs.[9,12,24,49,63,75,140,172,219] The lungs are most often affected, resulting in dyspnea or cough, but the pleura, hilum, heart, and great vessels may also be involved.[6] Patients with chest pain may have a pneumothorax, pneumomediastinum, or aortic dissection. Patients with fever, with or without respiratory symptoms, may have a focal infiltrate, pleural effusion, or hilar lymphadenopathy.

Chest radiographic findings may suggest certain diseases, although the diagnosis ultimately depends on a thorough clinical history. When a specific xenobiotic exposure is known or suspected, the chest radiograph can confirm the diagnosis and help in assessment. If a history of xenobiotic exposure is not obtained, a patient with an abnormal chest radiograph may initially be misdiagnosed as having pneumonia or another disorder that is more common than xenobiotic-mediated lung disease.[166] Therefore, all patients with chest radiographic abnormalities must be carefully questioned regarding possible xenobiotic exposures at work or at home, as well as the use of medications or other drugs.

Many pulmonary disorders are radiographically detectable because they result in fluid accumulation within the normally air-filled lung. Fluid may accumulate within the alveolar spaces or interstitial tissues of the lung, producing the two major radiographic patterns of pulmonary disease: airspace filling and interstitial lung disease (Table 5–3). Most xenobiotics are widely distributed throughout the lungs and produce a diffuse rather than a focal radiographic abnormality.

Diffuse Airspace Filling. Overdose with various xenobiotics, including salicylates, opioids, and paraquat, may cause acute lung injury (formerly known as noncardiogenic pulmonary edema) with or without

TABLE 5–3. Chest Radiographic Findings in Toxicologic Emergencies

Radiographic Finding	Responsible Xenobiotic	Disease Processes
Diffuse airspace filling	Salicylates Opioids Paraquat Irritant gases: NO_2 (silo filler's disease), phosgene ($COCl_2$), Cl_2, H_2S	Acute lung injury
	Organic phosphorus compounds, carbamates	Cholinergic stimulation (bronchorrhea)
	Alcoholic cardiomyopathy, cocaine, doxorubicin, cobalt	Congestive heart failure
Focal airspace filling	Low-viscosity hydrocarbons Gastric contents aspiration: CNS depressants, alcohol, seizures	Aspiration pneumonitis
Multifocal airspace filling	Injection drug user	Septic emboli
Interstitial patterns	Inhaled organic allergens: Farmer's lung, pigeon breeder's lung	Hypersensitivity pneumonitis
Fine or coarse reticular or reticulonodular pattern	Nitrofurantoin, penicillamine	
Patchy airspace filling is seen in some cases	Antineoplastics: Busulfan, bleomycin, carmustine, cyclophosphamide, methotrexate	Cytotoxic lung damage
	Amiodarone	Phospholipidosis
	Talcosis (illicit drug contaminant)	Injected particulates
	Pneumoconiosis: Asbestosis, silicosis, coal dust, berylliosis (chronic)	Inhaled inorganic particulates
Pleural effusion	Procainamide, hydralazine, INH, methyldopa	Drug-induced systemic lupus erythematosus
Pneumomediastinum, Pneumothorax	"Crack" cocaine and marijuana (forceful inhalation), ipecac and alcoholism (forceful vomiting), subclavian vein injection puncture	Barotrauma
Pleural plaques (calcified)	Asbestos exposure	Fibrosis or asbestosis
Lymphadenopathy	Phenytoin, methotrexate (rare)	Pseudolymphoma
	Silicosis (eggshell calcification), berylliosis	Pneumoconiosis
Cardiomegaly (chronic exposure)	Ethanol, doxorubicin, cocaine, cobalt amphetamine, ipecac syrup	Dilated cardiomyopathy
	Drug-induced systemic lupus erythematosus (procainamide, hydralazine, INH)	Pericardial effusion
Aortic enlargement	Cocaine	Aortic dissection.

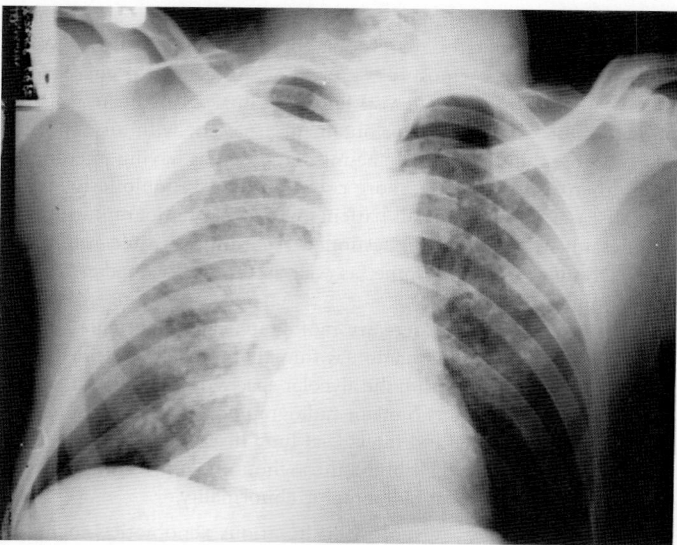

FIGURE 5–13. Diffuse airspace filling. The chest radiograph of a patient who had recently injected heroin intravenously presented with respiratory distress and acute lung injury. The heart size is normal.

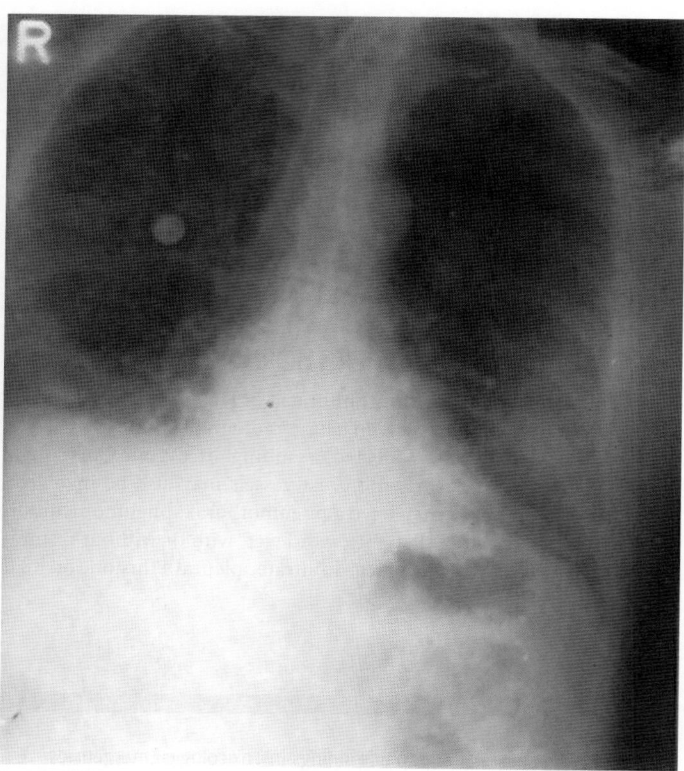

FIGURE 5–14. Focal airspace filling as a result of hydrocarbon aspiration. A 34-year-old man aspirated gasoline. The chest radiograph shows bilateral lower lobe infiltrates.

diffuse alveolar damage and characterized by leaky capillaries (Fig. 5–13).[75,85,89,123,184,191,218] There are, of course, many other causes of acute lung injury, including sepsis, anaphylaxis, and major trauma.[213] Other xenobiotic exposures that may result in diffuse airspace filling include inhalation of irritant gases that are of low water solubility such as phosgene ($COC1_2$), nitrogen dioxide (silo filler's disease), chlorine, hydrogen sulfide, and sulfur dioxide (Chaps. 124, 128).[79,102] Organic phosphorus insecticide poisoning causes cholinergic hyperstimulation, resulting in bronchorrhea (Chap. 113). Smoking "crack" cocaine is associated with diffuse alveolar hemorrhage.[60,75,79,165,219]

Focal Airspace Filling. Focal infiltrates are usually caused by bacterial pneumonia, although aspiration of gastric contents also causes localized airspace disease.[75,195] Aspiration may occur during sedative–hypnotic or alcohol intoxication or during a seizure. During ingestion, low-viscosity hydrocarbons often enter the lungs while they are being swallowed (Figs. 5–14 and 105–2). There may be a delay in the development of radiographic abnormalities, and the chest radiograph may not appear to be abnormal until 6 hours after the ingestion.[8] During aspiration, the most dependent portions of the lung are affected. When the patient is upright at the time of aspiration, the lower lung segments are involved. When the patient is supine, the posterior segments of the upper and lower lobes are affected.[62]

Multifocal Airspace Filling. Multifocal airspace filling occurs with septic pulmonary emboli, which is a complication of injection drug use and right-sided bacterial endocarditis. The foci of pulmonary infection often undergo necrosis and cavitation (Fig. 5–15).[75,79]

Interstitial Lung Diseases. Toxicologic causes of interstitial lung disease include hypersensitivity pneumonitis, use of medications with direct pulmonary toxicity, and inhalation or injection of inorganic particulates.[75] Interstitial lung diseases may have an acute, subacute, or chronic course. On the chest radiograph, acute and subacute disorders cause a fine reticular or reticulonodular pattern (Fig. 5–16). Chronic interstitial disorders cause a coarse reticular "honeycomb" pattern.

Hypersensitivity pneumonitis. Hypersensitivity pneumonitis is a delayed-type hypersensitivity reaction to an inhaled or ingested allergen.[40,96,166] Inhaled organic allergens such as those in moldy hay (farmer's lung) and bird droppings (pigeon breeder's lung) cause hypersensitivity pneumonitis in sensitized individuals. There are two clinical syndromes: an acute, recurrent illness and a chronic, progressive disease. The acute illness presents with fever and dyspnea. In these cases, the

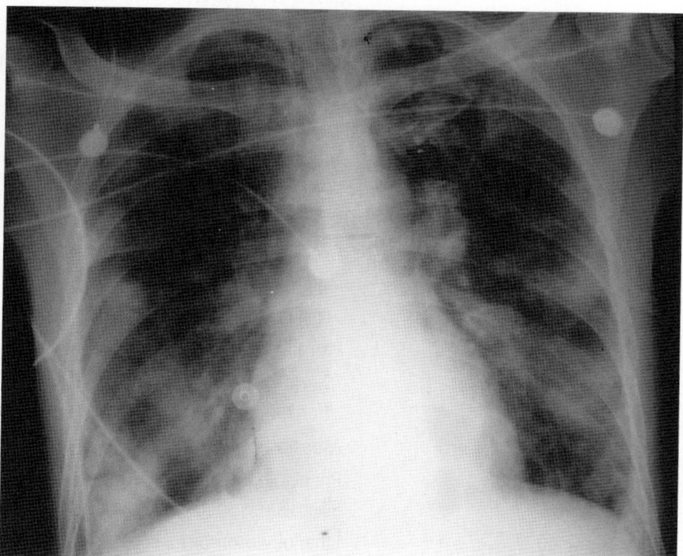

FIGURE 5–15. Multifocal airspace filling. The chest radiograph in an injection drug user who presented with high fever but without pulmonary symptoms. Multiple ill-defined pulmonary opacities are seen throughout both lungs, which are characteristic of septic pulmonary emboli. His blood cultures grew *Staphylococcus aureus.*

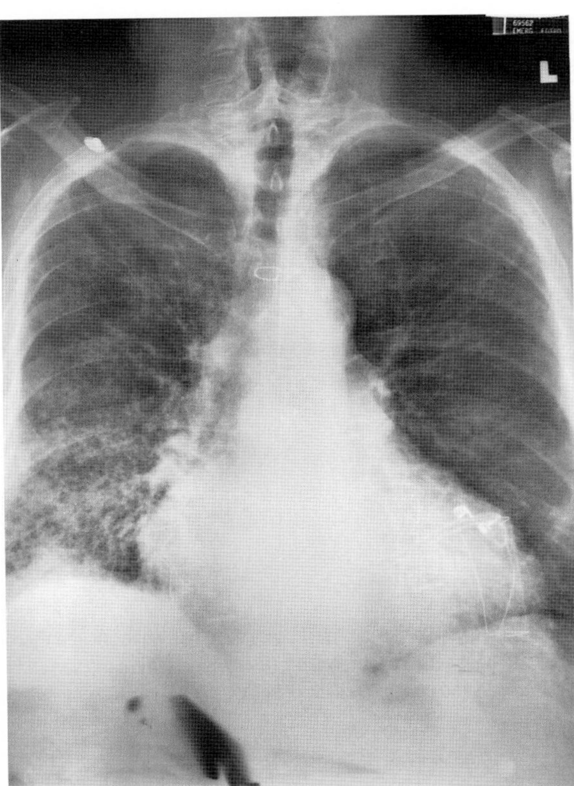

FIGURE 5–16. Reticular interstitial pattern. The chest radiograph of a patient with cardiac disease who presented to the emergency department with progressive dyspnea. The initial diagnostic impression was interstitial pulmonary edema. The patient was taking amiodarone for malignant ventricular dysrhythmias (note the implanted automatic defibrillator). The lack of response to diuretics and the high-resolution CT pattern suggested that this was toxicity to amiodarone. The medication was stopped, and there was partial clearing over several weeks. *(Image contributed by Dr. Georgeann McGuinness, Department of Radiology, New York University.)*

chest radiograph is normal or may show fine interstitial or alveolar infiltrates. Chronic hypersensitivity pneumonitis causes progressive dyspnea, and the radiograph shows interstitial fibrosis.

The most common medication causing hypersensitivity pneumonitis is nitrofurantoin. Respiratory symptoms occur after taking the medication for 1 to 2 weeks. Other medications that may cause hypersensitivity pneumonitis include sulfonamides and penicillins.

Antineoplastics. Various chemotherapeutic agents, such as busulfan, bleomycin, cyclophosphamide, and methotrexate, cause pulmonary injury by their direct cytotoxic effect on alveolar cells.[39,65] The radiographic pattern is usually interstitial (reticular or nodular) but may include airspace filling or mixed patterns. The patient presents with dyspnea, fever, and pulmonary infiltrates that begin after several weeks of therapy. Other causes of these clinical and radiographic findings must be considered, including opportunistic infection, pulmonary carcinomatosis, pulmonary edema, and intraparenchymal hemorrhage. Symptoms usually resolve with discontinuation of the offending medication.

Amiodarone. Amiodarone toxicity causes phospholipid accumulation within alveolar cells and may result in pulmonary fibrosis. An interstitial radiographic pattern is seen, although airspace filling may also occur (see Fig. 5–16) (Chap. 63).

Particulates. Inhaled inorganic particulates, such as asbestos, silica, and coal dust, cause pneumoconiosis. This is a chronic interstitial lung disease characterized by interstitial fibrosis and loss of lung volume.[32,138,167,215] IV injection of illicit xenobiotics that have particulate contaminants, such as talc, causes a chronic interstitial lung disease known as talcosis.[1,55,212]

Pleural Disorders Asbestos-related calcified pleural plaques develop many years after asbestos exposure (Fig. 5–17). These lesions do not cause clinical symptoms and have only a minor association with malignancy and interstitial lung disease. Asbestos-related pleural plaques should not be called *asbestosis* because that term refers specifically to the interstitial lung disease caused by asbestos. Pleural plaques must be distinguished from mesotheliomas, which are not calcified, enlarge at a rapid rate, and erode into nearby structures such as the ribs.

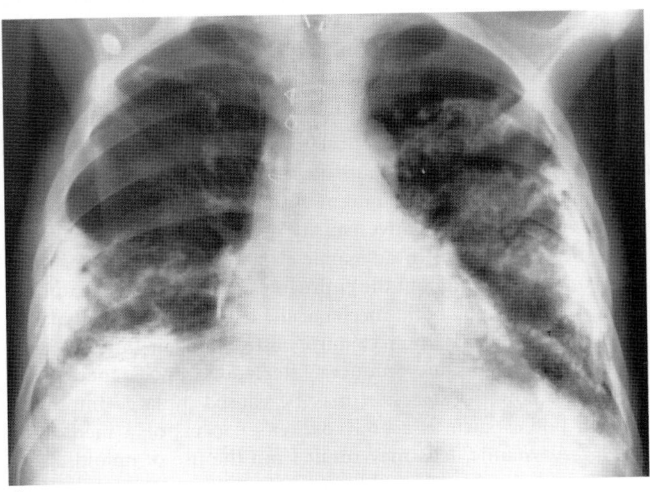

A

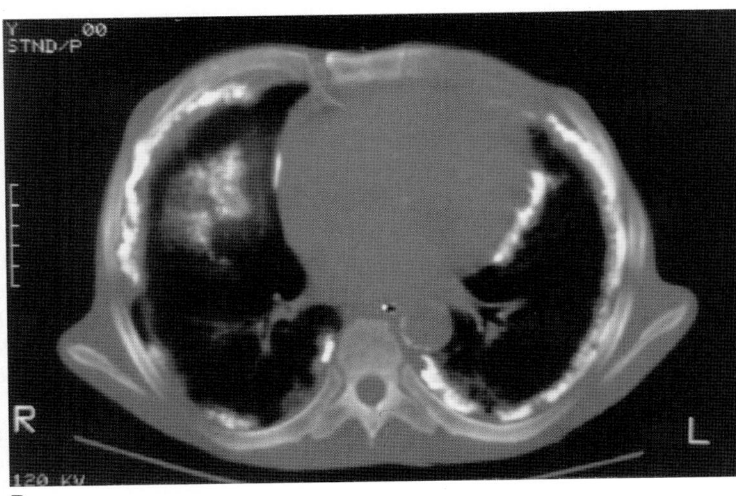

B

FIGURE 5–17. (A) Calcified plaques typical of asbestos exposure are seen on the pleural surfaces of the lungs, diaphragm, and heart. The patient was asymptomatic; this was an incidental radiographic finding. (B) The computed tomography (CT) scan demonstrates that the opacities seen on the chest radiograph do not involve the lung itself. A lower thoracic image shows calcified pleural plaques (the diaphragmatic plaque is seen on the *right*). The CT confirms that there is no interstitial lung disease ("asbestosis").

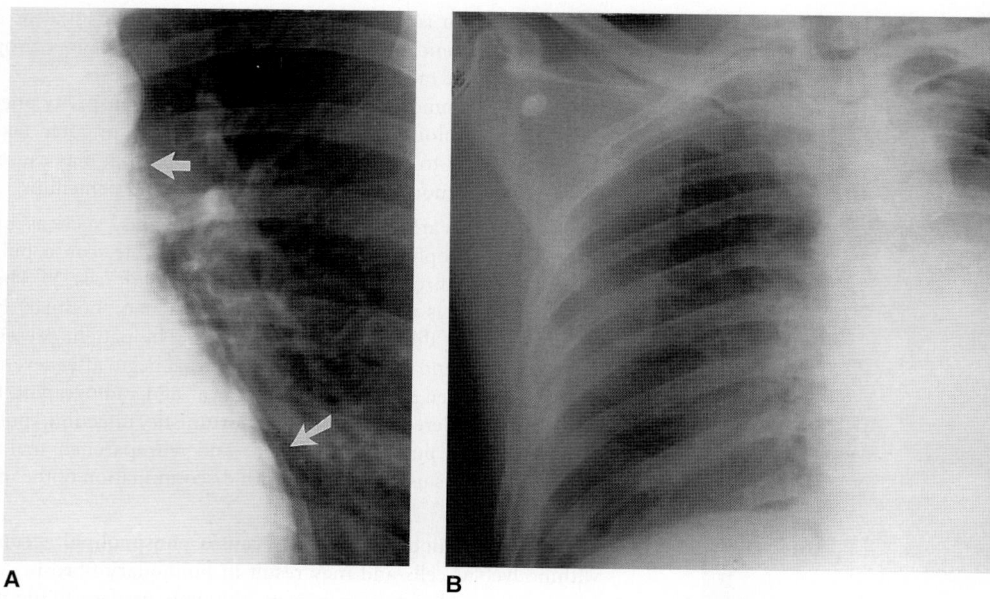

FIGURE 5–18. Two patients with chest pain after cocaine use. (A) Pneumomediastinum after forceful inhalation while smoking "crack" cocaine. A fine white line representing the pleura elevated from the mediastinal structures is seen *(arrows)*. The patient's chest pain resolved during a 24-hour period of observation. (B) Thoracic aortic dissection and rupture after cocaine use. The patient presented with chest pain radiating to the back. Chest radiography reveals a wide and indistinct aortic contour *(arrow)*. *(Images contributed by the Toxicology Fellowship of the New York City Poison Center.)*

Pleural effusions occur with drug-induced systemic lupus erythematosus.[140] The medications most frequently implicated are procainamide, hydralazine, isoniazid, and methyldopa. The patient presents with fever as well as other symptoms of systemic lupus erythematosus.

Pneumothorax and pneumomediastinum are associated with illicit drug use. These complications are related to the route of administration rather than to the particular drug. Barotrauma associated with Valsalva maneuver or intense inhalation with breath holding during the smoking of "crack" cocaine or marijuana results in pneumomediastinum (Fig. 5–18A).[20,50,75,150] Pneumomediastinum is one cause of cocaine-related chest pain that can be diagnosed by chest radiography. Forceful vomiting after ingestion of syrup of ipecac or alcohol may produce a Mallory-Weiss syndrome, pneumomediastinum, and mediastinitis (Boerhaave syndrome).[220] Intravenous drug users who attempt to inject into the subclavian and internal jugular veins may cause a pneumothorax.[46]

Lymphadenopathy Phenytoin may cause drug-induced lymphoid hyperplasia with hilar lymphadenopathy.[140] Chronic beryllium exposure results in hilar lymphadenopathy that mimics sarcoidosis, with granulomatous changes in the lung parenchyma. Silicosis is associated with "eggshell" calcification of hilar lymph nodes.

Cardiovascular Abnormalities Dilated cardiomyopathy occurs in chronic alcoholism and exposure to cardiotoxic medications such as doxorubicin (Adriamycin). Enlargement of the cardiac silhouette may also be caused by a pericardial effusion, which may accompany drug-induced systemic lupus erythematosus. Aortic dissection is associated with use of cocaine and amphetamines.[66,75,114,152,162] The chest radiograph may show an enlarged or indistinct aortic knob and an ascending or descending aorta (Fig. 5–18B).

ABDOMINAL PROBLEMS

Abdominal imaging modalities include conventional radiography, CT, GI contrast studies, and angiography.[68] Conventional radiography is limited in its ability to detect most intraabdominal pathology because most pathologic processes involve soft tissue structures that are not well seen. Plain radiography readily visualizes gas in the abdomen and is therefore usable to diagnose pneumoperitoneum (free intraperitoneal air) and bowel distension caused by mechanical obstruction or diminished gut motility (adynamic ileus). Other abnormal gas collections, such as intramural gas associated with intestinal infarction, are seen infrequently (Table 5–4).[73,120,128,137,186]

Pneumoperitoneum GI perforation is diagnosed by seeing free intraperitoneal air under the diaphragm on an upright chest radiograph. Peptic ulcer perforation is associated with crack cocaine use.[2,29,107] Esophageal or gastric perforation (or tear) can be a complication of forceful emesis induced by syrup of ipecac or alcohol intoxication or attempted placement of a large-bore orogastric tube (Fig. 5–19).[220] Esophageal and gastric perforation may also occur after the ingestion of caustics such as iron, alkali, or acid.[103] Esophageal perforation causes pneumomediastinum and mediastinitis.

Obstruction and Ileus Both mechanical bowel obstruction and adynamic ileus (diminished gut motility) cause bowel distension. With mechanical obstruction, there is a greater amount of intestinal distension proximal to the obstruction and a relative paucity of gas and intestinal collapse distal to the obstruction. In adynamic ileus, the bowel distension is relatively uniform throughout the entire intestinal tract. On the upright abdominal radiograph, both mechanical obstruction and adynamic ileus show air-fluid levels. In mechanical obstruction, air-fluid levels are seen at different heights and produce a "stepladder" appearance.

Mechanical bowel obstruction may be caused by large intraluminal foreign bodies such as a body packer's packets or a medication bezoar.[64,197] Adynamic ileus may result from the use of opioids, anticholinergics, and tricyclic antidepressants (Fig. 5–20).[15,68] Because adynamic ileus is seen in many diseases, the radiographic finding of an ileus is not helpful diagnostically. When the distinction between obstruction and adynamic ileus cannot be made based on the abdominal radiographs, abdominal CT can clarify the diagnosis.[135]

TABLE 5–4. Plain Abdominal Radiography in Toxicologic Emergencies

Radiographic Finding	Xenobiotic
Pneumoperitoneum (hollow viscus perforation)	Caustics: Iron, alkali, acids Cocaine GI decontamination (ipecac, lavage tube)
Mechanical obstruction (intraluminal foreign body) Intestinal gastric outlet } Upper GI esophageal } series	Foreign-body ingestion: Body packer, enteric-coated pills (bezoar)
Ileus (diminished gut motility)	Opioids Anticholinergics Cyclic antidepressants Mesenteric ischemia caused by cocaine, oral contraceptives, cardioactive steroids, hypokalemia, hypomagnesemia
Intramural gas (intestinal infarction) Bowel wall thickening Hepatic portal venous gas (CT is more sensitive)	Cocaine Ergot alkaloids Oral contraceptives Calcium channel blockers Hypotension
Foreign-body ingestion	Iron pills Metals (As, Cs, Hg, K, Pb, Tl) Body packers and stuffers Bismuth subsalicylate Calcium carbonate Enteric-coated and sustained-release tablets Pica (calcareous clay).

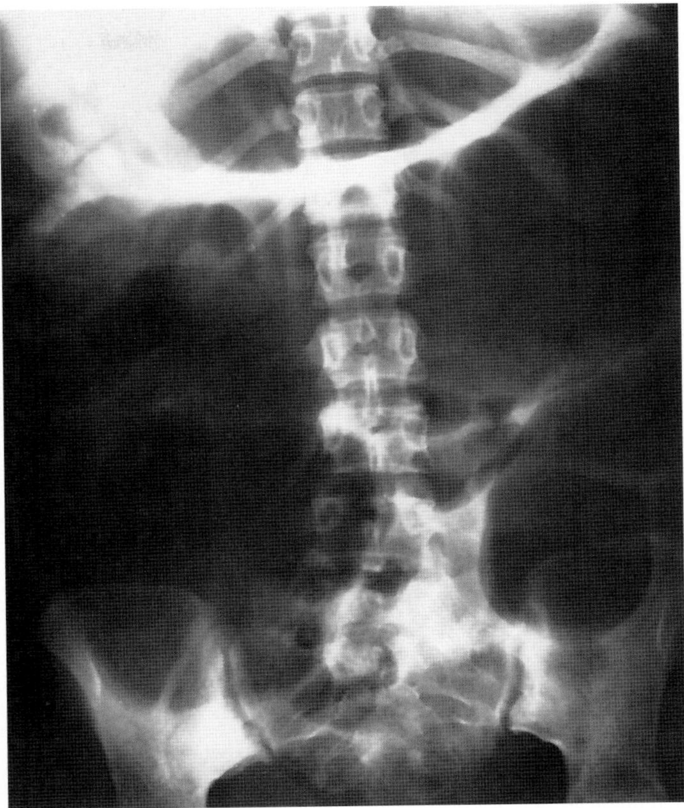

FIGURE 5–20. Methadone maintenance therapy causing marked abdominal distension. The radiograph reveals striking large bowel dilatation, termed *colonic ileus*, caused by chronic opioid use. A similar radiographic picture is seen with anticholinergic poisoning. A contrast enema can clarify the diagnosis. *(Image contributed by Dr. Emil J. Balthazar, Department of Radiology, Bellevue Hospital Center.)*

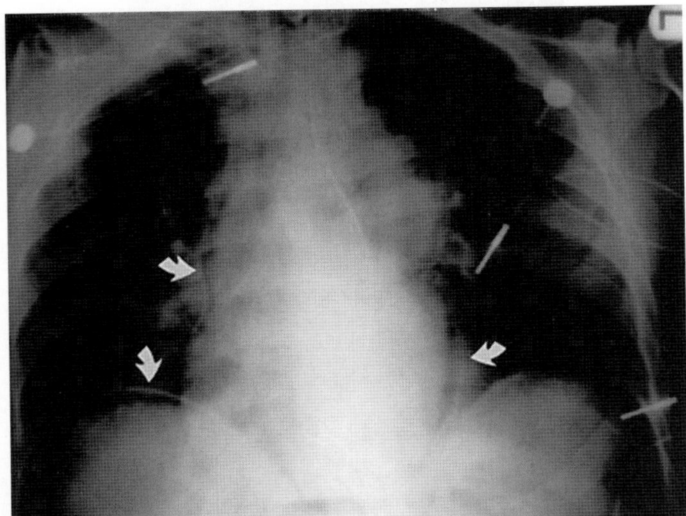

FIGURE 5–19. Gastrointestinal perforation after gastric lavage with a large-bore orogastric tube. The upright chest radiograph shows air under the right hemidiaphragm and pneumomediastinum (*arrows*). An esophagram with water-soluble contrast did not demonstrate the perforation. Laparotomy revealed perforation of the anterior wall of the stomach.

Mesenteric Ischemia In most patients with intestinal ischemia, plain abdominal radiographs show only a nonspecific or adynamic ileus pattern. In a small proportion of patients with ischemic bowel (5%), intramural gas is seen.[15] Rarely, gas is also seen in the hepatic portal venous system. CT is better able to detect signs of mesenteric ischemia, particularly bowel wall thickening.[14]

Intestinal ischemia and infarction may be caused by use of cocaine, other sympathomimetics, and the ergot alkaloids, which induce mesenteric vasoconstriction.[79,110,130] Calcium channel blocker overdoses cause splanchnic vasodilation and hypotension that may result in intestinal ischemia. Superior mesenteric vein thrombosis may be caused by hypercoagulability associated with chronic oral contraceptive use.

Gastrointestinal Hemorrhage and Hepatotoxicity Radiography is not usually helpful in the diagnosis of such common abdominal complications as GI bleeding and hepatotoxicity.

The now obsolete radiocontrast agent thorium dioxide (Thorotrast; thorium, atomic number 90) provides a unique example of pharmaceutical-induced hepatotoxicity. It was used as an angiographic contrast agent until 1947, when it was found to cause hepatic malignancies. The radioactive isotope of thorium has a half-life of 400 years. It accumulates within the reticuloendothelial system and remains there for the life of the patient. It had a characteristic radiographic appearance, with multiple punctate opacities in the liver,

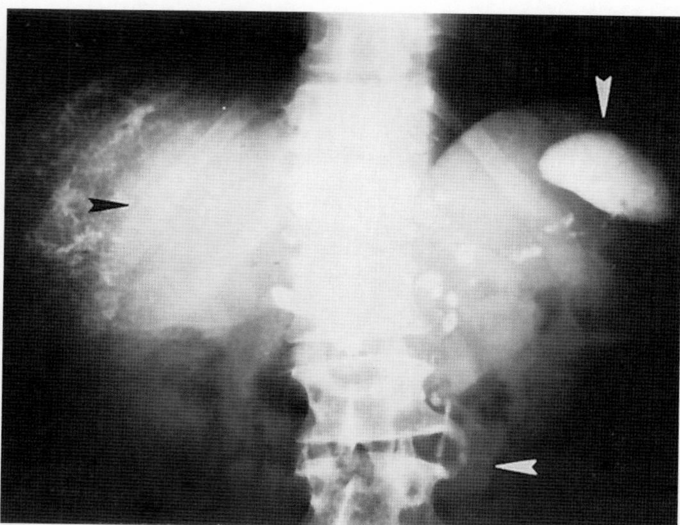

FIGURE 5–21. An abdominal radiograph of a patient who had received thorium dioxide (Thorotrast) for a radiocontrast study many years previously. The spleen (*vertical white arrow*), liver (*horizontal black arrow*), and lymph nodes (*horizontal white arrow*) are demarcated by thorium retained in the reticuloendothelial system. (*Image contributed by Dr. Emil J. Balthazar, Department of Radiology, Bellevue Hospital Center.*)

spleen, and lymph nodes (Fig. 5–21). Patients who received thorium before its removal from the market may still present with hepatic malignancies.[18,204]

Contrast Esophagram and Upper Gastrointestinal Series Ingestion of a caustic may cause severe damage to the mucosal lining of the esophagus. This can be demonstrated by a contrast esophagram. However, in the acute setting, upper endoscopy should be performed rather than an esophagram because it provides more information about the extent of injury and prognosis.[111] In addition, administration of barium will coat the mucosa, making endoscopy difficult. For later evaluation, a contrast esophagram identifies mucosal defects, scarring, and stricture formation (Figs. 5–22 and 104–3).[129]

The choice of radiographic contrast agent (barium or water-soluble material) depends on the clinical situation. If the esophagus is severely strictured and there is risk of aspiration, barium should be used because water-soluble contrast material is damaging to the pulmonary parenchyma. If, on the other hand, esophageal or gastric perforation is suspected, water-soluble contrast is safer because extravasated barium is highly irritating to mediastinal and peritoneal tissues, but extravasated water-soluble contrast is gradually absorbed into the circulation.

Ingested foreign bodies may cause esophageal and gastric outlet obstruction. Esophageal obstruction because of a drug packet can be demonstrated by a contrast esophagram. Concretions of ingested material in the stomach may cause gastric outlet obstruction. This has been reported with potassium chloride tablets and enteric-coated aspirin.[11,185]

Abdominal Computed Tomography CT provides great anatomic definition of intraabdominal organs and plays an important role in the diagnosis of a wide variety of abdominal disorders. In most cases, both oral and IV contrast are administered. Oral contrast delineates the intestinal lumen. IV contrast is needed to reliably detect lesions in hepatic and splenic parenchyma, the kidneys, and the bowel wall.

Certain abdominal complications of poisonings are amenable to CT diagnosis. Intestinal ischemia causes bowel wall thickening; intramural hemorrhage; and at a later stage, intramural gas and hepatic portal venous gas.[14] Splenic infarction and splenic and psoas abscesses

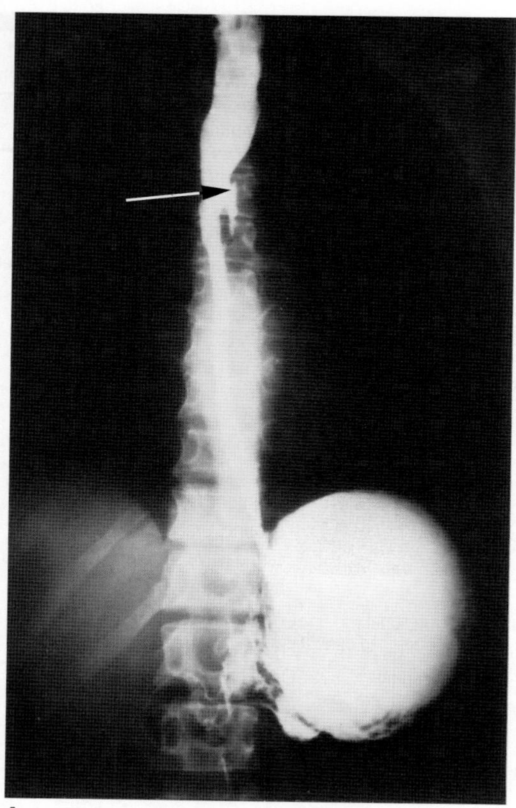

A

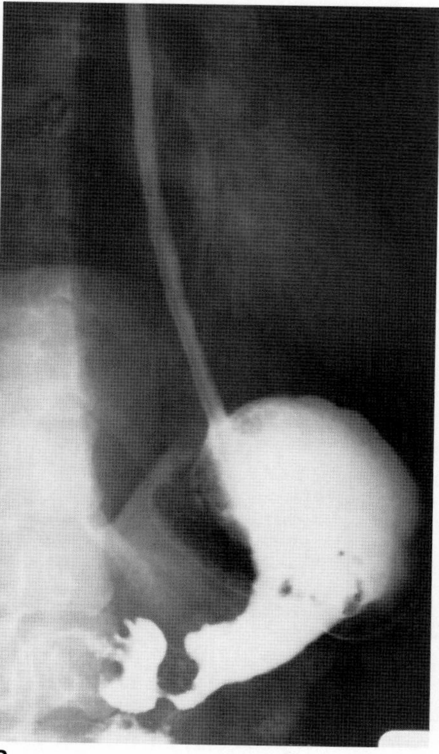

B

FIGURE 5–22. (A) A barium swallow performed several days after ingestion of liquid lye shows intramural dissection and extravasation of barium with early stricture formation. (B) At 3 weeks postingestion, there is an absence of peristalsis, diffuse narrowing of the esophagus, and reduction in size of the fundus and antrum of the stomach as a result of scarring. (*Images contributed by Dr. Emil J. Balthazar, Department of Radiology, Bellevue Hospital Center.*)

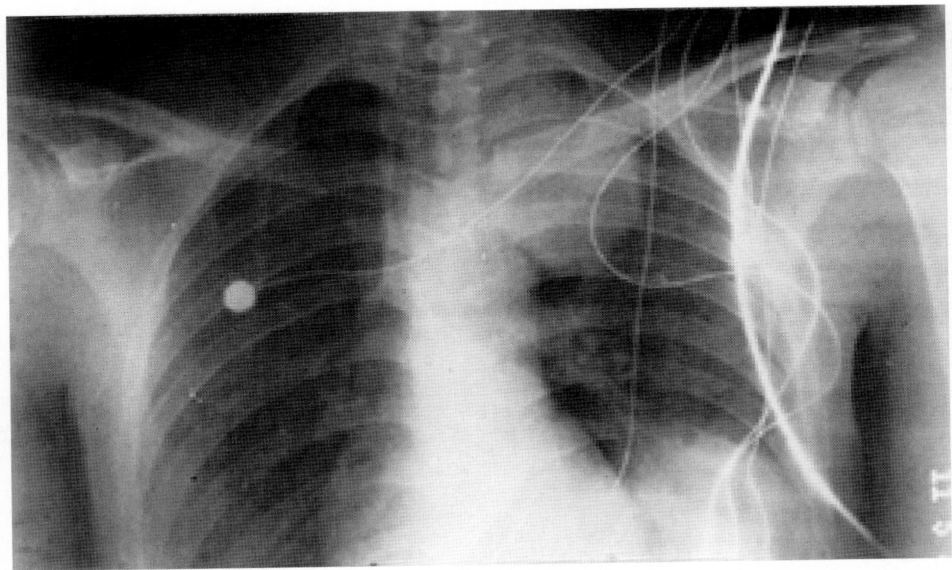
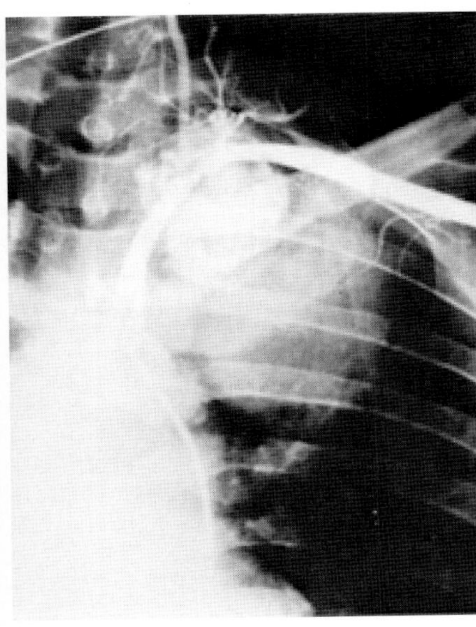

FIGURE 5–23. (**A**) Chest radiograph of a young drug abuser who used the supraclavicular approach for heroin injection. The large mass in the left chest was suspicious for a pseudoaneurysm. (**B**) An arch aortogram performed on the patient revealed a large pseudoaneurysm and hematoma subsequent to an arterial tear during attempted injection. Surgical repair was performed. *(Images contributed by Dr. Richard Lefleur, Department of Radiology, Bellevue Hospital.)*

are complications of IV drug use that may be diagnosed on CT.[15] Radiopaque foreign substances such as intravenously injected elemental mercury may be detected and accurately localized by CT.[126] Radiolucent foreign bodies, such as a body packer's packets, may be detected by using enteric contrast.[83,85]

Vascular Lesions Angiography may detect such complications of injection drug use as venous thrombosis and arterial laceration causing pseudoaneurysm formation (Figs. 5–23 and 5–24). IV injection of amphetamine, cocaine, or ergotamine causes necrotizing angiitis that is associated with microaneurysms, segmental stenosis, and arterial thrombosis. These lesions are seen in the kidneys, small bowel, liver, pancreas, and cerebral circulation (Fig. 5–25).[34,161] Complications include aneurysm rupture and visceral infarction. Renal lesions cause severe hypertension and renal failure.[175]

NEUROLOGIC PROBLEMS

Diagnostic imaging studies have revolutionized the management of CNS disorders.[57,71] Both acute brain lesions and chronic degenerative changes can be detected (Table 5–5).[118] Some xenobiotics have a direct toxic effect on the CNS; others indirectly cause neurologic injury by causing hypoxia, hypotension, hypertension, cerebral vasoconstriction, head trauma, or infection.

Imaging Modalities CT can directly visualize brain tissue and many intracranial lesions.[70] CT is the imaging study of choice in the emergency setting because it readily detects acute intracranial hemorrhage as well as parenchymal lesions that are causing mass effect. CT is fast, widely available on an emergency basis, and can accommodate critical support and monitoring devices. Infusion of IV contrast further delineates intracerebral mass lesions such as tumors and abscesses.

MRI has largely supplanted CT in nonemergency neurodiagnosis. It offers better anatomic discrimination of brain tissues and areas of cerebral edema and demyelination. However, MRI is no better than CT

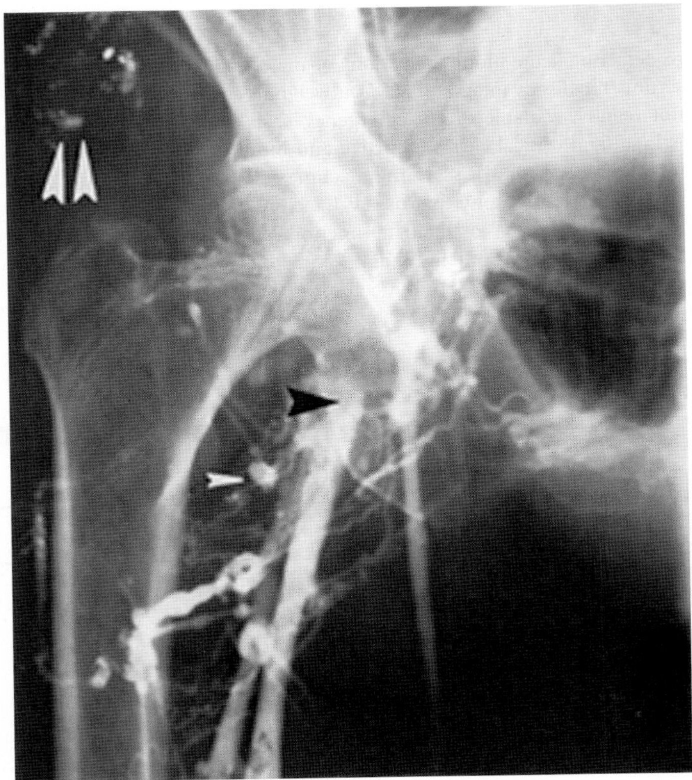

FIGURE 5–24. Venogram of a 50-year-old patient who routinely injected heroin into his groin. Occlusion of the femoral vein (*black arrow*) with diffuse aneurysmal dilation (*small arrow*) and extensive collaterals are shown. Incidental radiopaque materials are noted in the right buttock (*double arrow*). By history, this represents either bismuth or arsenicals he received as antisyphilitic therapy. (*Image contributed by Dr. Richard Lefleur, Department of Radiology, Bellevue Hospital.*)

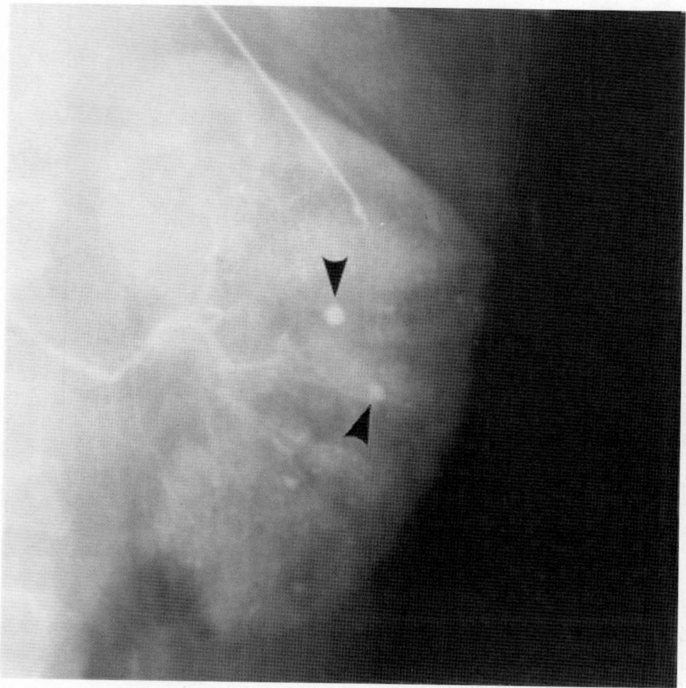

FIGURE 5–25. A selective renal angiogram in an injection methamphetamine user demonstrating multiple small and large aneurysms (*arrows*). *(Image contributed by Dr. Richard Lefleur, Department of Radiology, Bellevue Hospital Center.)*

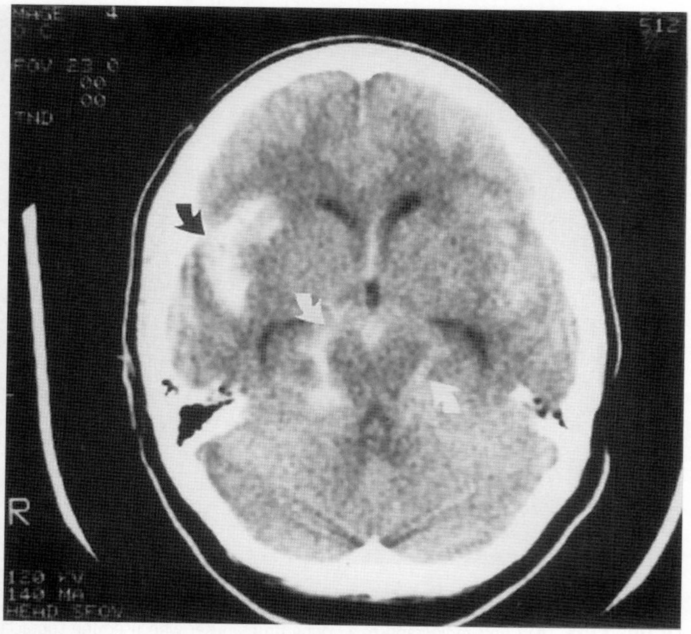

FIGURE 5–26. Subarachnoid hemorrhage after intravenous cocaine use. The patient had sudden severe headache followed by a generalized seizure. Extensive hemorrhage is seen surrounding the midbrain (*white arrows*) and in the right Sylvian fissure (*black arrow*). Angiography revealed an aneurysm at the origin of the right middle cerebral artery.

in detecting acute blood collections or mass lesions. In the emergency setting, the disadvantages of MRI outweigh its strengths. MRI is usually not readily available on an emergency basis, image acquisition time is long, and critical care supportive and monitoring devices are often incompatible with MR scanning machines.[121]

Nuclear scintigraphy that uses CT technology (SPECT and PET) is being used as a tool to elucidate functional characteristics of the CNS. Examples include both immediate and long-term effects of various xenobiotics on regional brain metabolism, blood flow, and neurotransmitter function.[115,154,207]

Emergency Head CT Scanning An emergency noncontrast head CT scan is obtained to detect acute intracranial hemorrhage and focal brain lesions causing cerebral edema and mass effect. Patients with these lesions present with focal neurologic deficits, seizures, headache, or altered mental status. Toxicologic causes of intraparenchymal and subarachnoid hemorrhage include cocaine and other sympathomimetics (Fig. 5–26).[113,117] Cocaine-induced vasospasm may cause ischemic infarction, although this is not well seen by CT until 6 to 24 or more hours after onset of the neurologic deficit (Fig. 5–27). Drug-induced CNS depression, most commonly ethanol intoxication, predisposes the patient to head

TABLE 5–5. Head CT (Noncontrast) in Toxicologic Emergencies

CT Finding	Brain Lesion	Xenobiotic Etiology
Hemorrhage	Intraparenchymal hemorrhage Subarachnoid hemorrhage	Sympathomimetics: cocaine ("crack"), amphetamine, phenylpropanolamine, phencyclidine, ephedrine, pseudoephedrine
		Mycotic aneurysm rupture (IDU)
	Subdural hematoma	Trauma secondary to ethanol, sedative-hypnotics, seizures
		Anticoagulants
Brain lucencies	Basal ganglia focal necrosis (also subcortical white matter lucencies)	Carbon monoxide, cyanide, hydrogen sulfide, methanol, manganese
	Stroke: Vasoconstriction	Sympathomimetics: cocaine ("crack"), amphetamine, phenylpropanolamine, phencyclidine, ephedrine, pseudoephedrine, ergotamine
	Mass lesion: tumor, abscess	Septic emboli, AIDS-related CNS toxoplasmosis or lymphoma
Loss of brain tissue	Atrophy: Cerebral, cerebellar	Alcoholism, toluene

CNS, central nervous system; IDU, injection drug use.

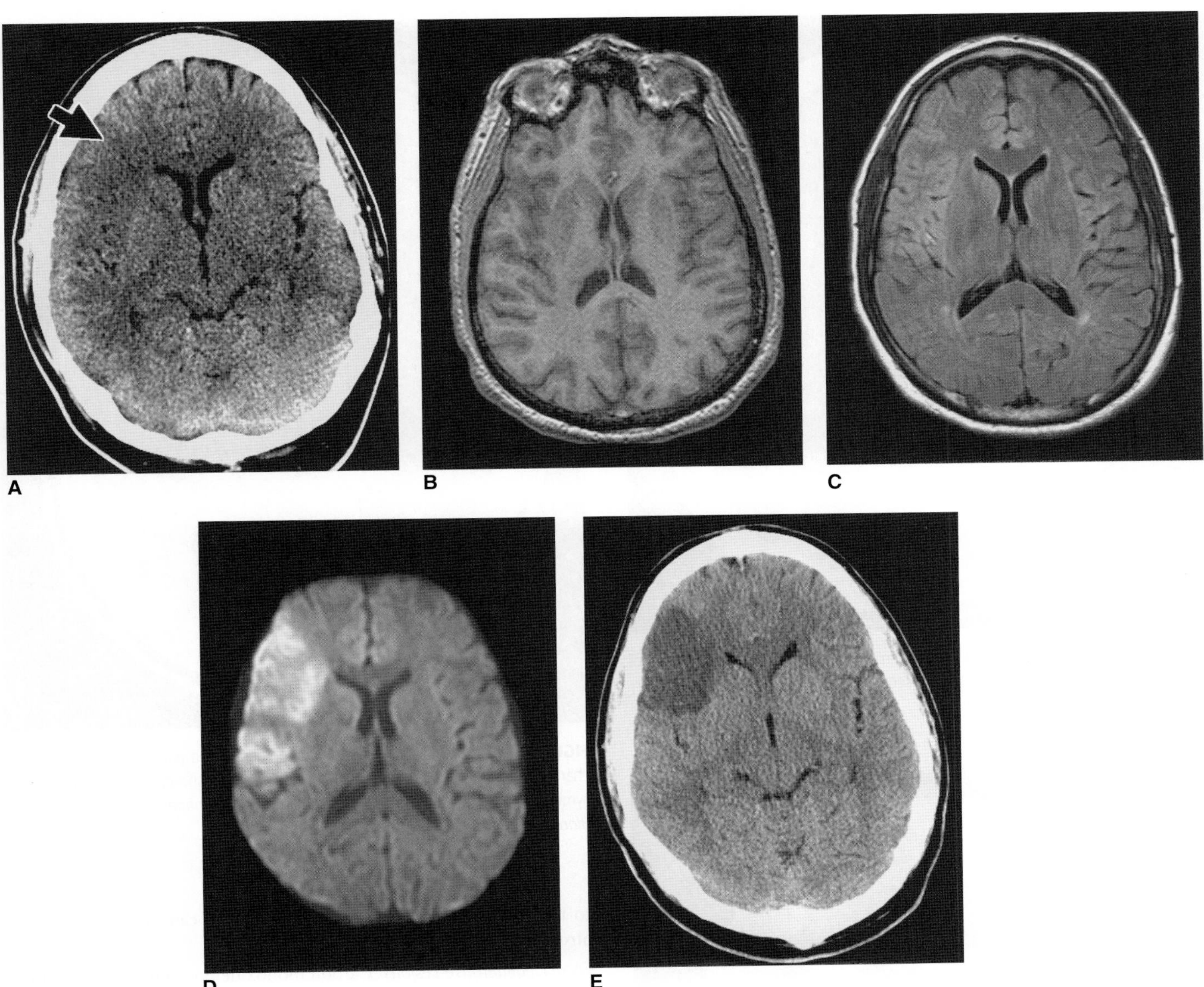

FIGURE 5–27. Acute stroke confirmed by diffusion-weighted magnetic resonance image (MRI). A 39-year-old man presented with left facial weakness that began 3 hours earlier after smoking crack cocaine. He also complained of left arm "tingling" but had a normal examination. A stat noncontrast computed tomography (CT) scan was obtained that was interpreted as normal (**A**), although in retrospect there was subtle loss of the normal gray/white differentiation (*arrow*). MRI was obtained to confirm that the facial palsy was a stroke and not a peripheral seventh cranial nerve palsy. Standard MRI sequence (T1-weighted, T2 weighted, and FLAIR) were normal in this early ischemic lesion (**B** and **C**). Diffusion-weighed imaging (DWI) is able to show such early ischemic change—cytotoxic (intracellular) edema (**D**). The patient's facial paresis improved but did not entirely resolve. A repeat CT scan 2 days later showed an evolving (subacute) infarction with vasogenic edema (**E**). Infarction was presumably due to vasospasm because no carotid artery lesion or cardiac source of embolism was found. *(From Schwartz DT:* Emergency Radiology: Case Studies*, New York, McGraw-Hill; 2008:517, with permission.)*

trauma, which may result in a subdural hematoma or cerebral contusion (Fig. 5-28). Toxicologic causes of intracerebral mass lesions include septic emboli complicating injection drug use and HIV-associated CNS toxoplasmosis and lymphoma (Fig. 5-29).[19,74,79,149] On a contrast CT, such tumors and focal infections exhibit a pattern of "ring enhancement."

Xenobiotic-Mediated Neurodegenerative Disorders A number of xenobiotics directly damage brain tissue, producing morphologic changes that may be detectable using CT and MRI. Such changes include generalized atrophy, focal areas of neuronal loss, demyelinization, and cerebral edema. Imaging abnormalities may help establish a diagnosis or predict prognosis in a patient with neurologic dysfunction after a xenobiotic exposure. In some cases, the imaging abnormality will suggest a toxicologic diagnosis in a patient with a neurologic disorder in whom a xenobiotic exposure was not suspected clinically.[4,13,57,100,104,155,165,214]

Atrophy Ethanol is the most widely used neurotoxin. With long-term ethanol use, there is a widespread loss of neurons and resultant atrophy. In some alcoholics, the loss of brain tissue is especially prominent in the cerebellum. However, the amount of cerebral or cerebellar atrophy does not always correlate with the extent of cognitive impairment or gait disturbance.[42,67,84,86,106,209,211] Chronic solvent exposure, such as

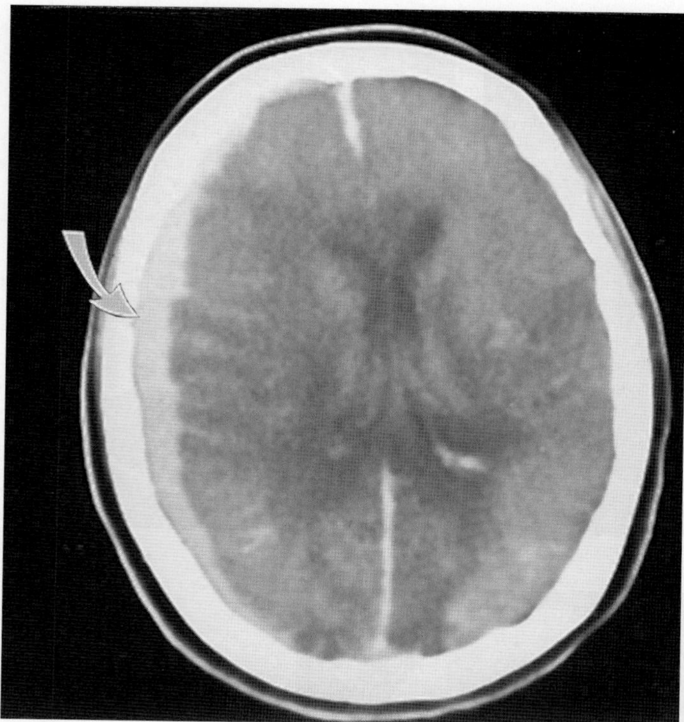

FIGURE 5–28. An acute subdural hematoma in an alcoholic patient after an alcohol binge. A crescent-shaped blood collection is seen between the right cerebral convexity and the inner table of the skull (*arrow*).

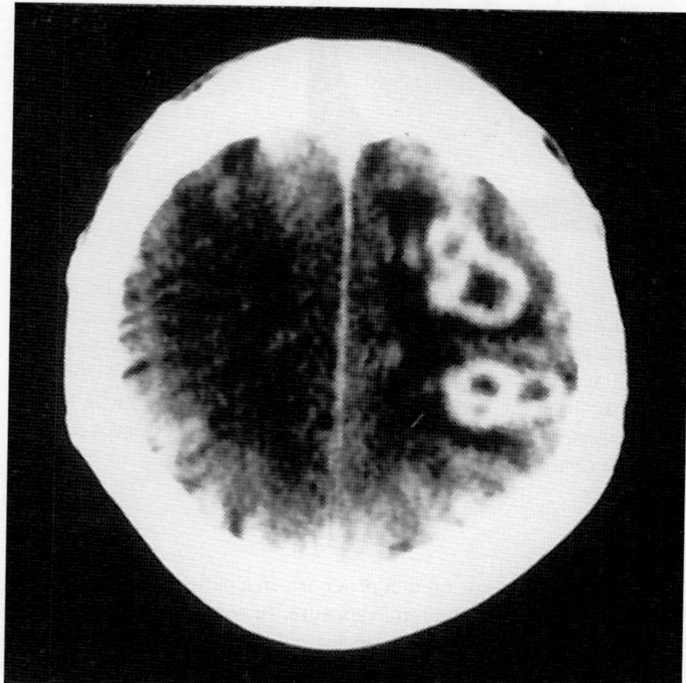

FIGURE 5–29. An injection drug user with ring-enhancing intracerebral lesions. The patient presented with fever and altered mental status. In this patient, the lesions represent multiple septic emboli complicating acute *Staphylococcus aureus* bacterial endocarditis. A similar ring-enhancing appearance is seen with lesions caused by toxoplasmosis or primary central nervous system lymphoma in patients with AIDS. This patient was HIV negative.

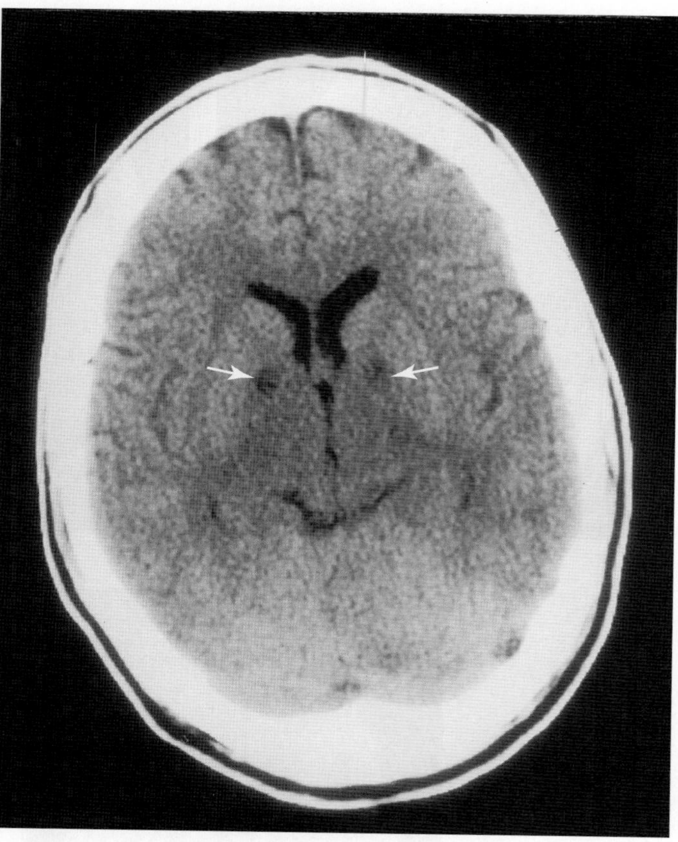

FIGURE 5–30. A head computed tomography scan of a patient with mental status changes after carbon monoxide poisoning. The scan shows characteristic bilateral symmetrical lucencies of the globus pallidus (*arrows*). ***(Image contributed by Dr. Paul Blackburn, Maricopa Medical Center, Arizona.)***

to toluene (occupational and illicit use), also causes diffuse cerebral atrophy.[93,171]

Focal Degenerative Lesions Carbon monoxide poisoning produces focal degenerative lesions in the brain. In about half of patients with severe neurologic dysfunction after carbon monoxide poisoning, CT scans show bilateral symmetric lucencies in the basal ganglia, particularly the globus pallidus (Figs. 5-30 and 125–1).[27,94,100,141,155,158,159,177,178,182,200,206] The basal ganglia are especially sensitive to hypoxic damage because of their limited blood supply and high metabolic requirements. Subcortical white matter lesions also occur after carbon monoxide poisoning. Although less frequent than lesions of the basal ganglia, white matter lesions are more clearly associated with a poor neurologic outcome. MRI is more sensitive than CT at detecting these white matter abnormalities.[27,57,104,159,200]

Basal ganglion lucencies, white matter lesions, and atrophy are caused by other xenobiotics such as methanol,[12,41,69,82,142,173] ethylene glycol, cyanide,[58,139] hydrogen sulfide, inorganic and organic mercury,[131] manganese,[13,190] heroin,[104,108] barbiturates, chemotherapeutic agents, solvents such as toluene,[57,93,17150,83,156] and podophyllin.[28,144] Nontoxicologic disorders may cause similar imaging abnormalities, including hypoxia, hypoglycemia, and infectious encephalitis.[82,88]

Nuclear Scintigraphy Whereas both CT and MRI display cerebral anatomy, nuclear medicine studies provide functional information about the brain. Nuclear scintigraphy uses radioactive isotopes that are bound to carrier molecules (ligands). The choice of ligand depends on the biologic function being studied. Brain cells take up the radiolabeled ligand in proportion to their physiologic activity or the regional blood flow. The radioactive emission from the isotope is detected by a scintigraphic camera, which produces an image showing the quantity and distribution of tracer. Better anatomic detail is provided by using CT techniques to generate cross-sectional images. There are two such technologies: SPECT and PET. These imaging modalities have been used in the research and clinical settings to study the neurologic effects of particular xenobiotics and the mechanisms of xenobiotic-induced neurologic dysfunction.

SPECT uses conventional isotopes such as technetium-99m and iodine-123.[115] These isotopes are bound to ligands that are taken up in the brain in proportion to regional blood flow, reflecting the local metabolic rate.

PET uses radioactive isotopes of biologic elements such as carbon-11, oxygen-15, nitrogen-13, and fluoride-18 (a substitute for hydrogen).[154] These radioisotopes have very short half-lives so that PET scanning requires an onsite cyclotron to produce the isotope. The isotopes are incorporated into molecules such as glucose, oxygen, water, various neurotransmitters, and drugs. Labeled glucose is taken up in proportion to the local metabolic rate for glucose. Uptake of labeled oxygen demonstrates the local metabolic rate for oxygen. Labeled neurotransmitters generate images reflecting their concentration and distribution within the brain.

Both PET and SPECT have been used to study the effects of various xenobiotics on cerebral function. For example, although both CT and MRI can detect cerebellar atrophy in chronic alcoholics, there is a poor correlation between the magnitude of cerebellar atrophy and the clinical signs of cerebellar dysfunction. PET scans may demonstrate diminished cerebellar metabolic rate for glucose, which correlates more accurately with the patient's clinical status.[72,209]

In patients with severe neurologic dysfunction after carbon monoxide poisoning, SPECT regional blood flow measurements show diffuse hypometabolism in the frontal cortex.[30] In one patient, severe perfusion abnormalities improved slightly over several months in proportion to the patient's gradual clinical improvement.[98] In another patient treated with hyperbaric oxygen, a SPECT scan revealed increased blood flow in the frontal lobes, although the blood flow still remained significantly less than normal.[124]

In patients who chronically use cocaine, SPECT blood flow scintigraphy demonstrates focal cortical perfusion defects. The extent of these perfusion defects correlates with the frequency of drug use. Focal perfusion defects probably represent local vasculitis or small areas of infarction.[92,202] PET scanning has been used to demonstrate the effects of cocaine on cerebral blood flow and regional glucose metabolism. PET neurotransmitter studies show promise in elucidating potential mechanisms of action of cocaine. Using radiolabeled dopamine analogs, downregulation of dopamine (D_2) receptors has been noted after a cocaine binge. This finding may be responsible for cocaine craving that occurs during cocaine withdrawal. Using ^{11}C-labeled cocaine, uptake of cocaine can be demonstrated in the basal ganglia, a region rich in dopamine receptors.[207]

Much has been learned about these imaging modalities, and initial applications can be applied to patient care. These imaging modalities are capable of demonstrating abnormalities in many patients with xenobiotic exposures, although other patients with significant cerebral dysfunction have normal studies.

SUMMARY

This chapter has highlighted a variety of situations in which diagnostic imaging studies are useful in toxicologic emergencies. Imaging can be an important tool in establishing a diagnosis, assisting in the treatment of patients, and detecting complications of a toxicologic emergency. The imaging modalities include plain radiography, CT, enteric and intravascular contrast studies, nuclear scintigraphy, and ultrasonography. However, effective use of a diagnostic test requires a firm understanding of the clinical situations in which each test can be useful, knowledge of the capabilities and limitations of the tests, and how the results should be applied to the care of an individual patient.

REFERENCES

1. Akira M, Kozuka T, Yamamoto S, Sakatani M, Morinaga K: Inhalational talc pneumoconiosis: radiographic and CT findings in 14 patients. *AJR Am J Roentgenol.* 2007;188:326-333.
2. Albert P, Sadler MA: Duodenal perforation in a crack cocaine abuser. *Emerg Radiol.* 2000;7:248-249.
3. Algra PR, Brogdon BG, Marugg RC: Role of radiology in a national initiative to interdict drug smuggling: the Dutch experience. *AJR Am J Roentgenol.* 2007;189:331-336.
4. Alphs HH, Schwartz BS, Stewart WF, Yousem DM: Findings on brain MRI from research studies of occupational exposure to known neurotoxicants. *AJR Am J Roentgenol.* 2006;187:1043-1047.
5. American College of Emergency Physicians: Clinical policy for the initial approach to patients presenting with acute toxic ingestion or dermal or inhalation exposure. *Ann Emerg Med.* 1999;33:735-761.
6. American College of Emergency Physicians: Clinical policy for the initial approach to patients presenting with acute toxic ingestion or dermal or inhalation exposure. American College of Emergency Physicians. *Ann Emerg Med.* 1995;25:570-585.
7. Amitai Y, Silver B, Leikin JB, Frischer H: Visualization of ingested medications in the stomach by ultrasound. *Am J Emerg Med.* 1992;10:18-23.
8. Anas N, Namasonthi V, Ginsburg CM: Criteria for hospitalizing children who have ingested products containing hydrocarbons. *JAMA.* 1981;246:840-843.
9. Ansell G: The chest. In: Ansell G, ed. *Radiology of Adverse Reactions to Drugs and Toxic Hazards.* Rockville, MD: Aspen Systems Corp; 1985:1-99.
10. Ansell G: Skeletal system and soft tissues. In: Ansell G, ed. *Radiology of Adverse Reactions to Drugs and Toxic Hazards.* Rockville, MD: Aspen Systems Corp; 1985:254-326.
11. Antonescu CG, Barritt AS 3rd: Potassium chloride and gastric outlet obstruction. *Ann Intern Med.* 1989;111:855-856.
12. Aquilonius SM, Bergstrom K, Enoksson P, et al: Cerebral computed tomography in methanol intoxication. *J Comput Assist Tomogr.* 1980;4:425-428.
13. Arjona A, Mata M, Bonet M: Diagnosis of chronic manganese intoxication by magnetic resonance imaging. *N Engl J Med.* 1997;336:964-965.
14. Balthazar EJ, Hulnick D, Megibow AJ, Opulencia JF: Computed tomography of intramural intestinal hemorrhage and bowel ischemia. *J Comput Assist Tomogr.* 1987;11:67-72.
15. Balthazar EJ, Lefleur R: Abdominal complications of drug addiction: radiologic features. *Semin Roentgenol.* 1983;18:213-220.
16. Beerman R, Nunez D Jr, Wetli CV: Radiographic evaluation of the cocaine smuggler. *Gastrointest Radiol.* 1986;11:351-354.
17. Bellin MF, Jakobsen JA, Tomassin I, et al: Contrast medium extravasation injury: guidelines for prevention and management. *Eur Radiol.* 2002;12:2807-2812.
18. Bensinger TA, Keller AR, Merrell LF, O'Leary DS. Thorotrast-induced reticuloendothelial blockade in man. Clinical equivalent of the experimental model associated with patent pneumococcal septicemia. *Am J Med.* 1971;51:663-668.
19. Berger JR, Donovan-Post MJ, Levy RM: The acquired immunodeficiency syndrome. In: Greenberg JO, Adams RD, eds. *Neuroimaging: A Companion to Adams and Victor's Principles of Neurology.* New York: McGraw-Hill; 1995:413-434.
20. Bernaerts A, Verniest T, Vanhoenacker F, et al: Pneumomediastinum and epidural pneumatosis after inhalation of "Ecstasy." *Eur Radiol.* 2003;13:642-643.
21. Blickman JG, Wilkinson RH, Graef JW: The radiologic "lead band" revisited. *AJR Am J Roentgenol.* 1986;146:245-247.
22. Bruns BR, Tytle T: Skeletal fluorosis. A report of two cases. *Orthopedics.* 1988;11:1083-1087.

23. Burkhart KK, Kulig KW, Rumack B: Whole-bowel irrigation as treatment for zinc sulfate overdose. *Ann Emerg Med.* 1990;19:1167-1170.
24. Camus P, Rosenow EC 3rd: Iatrogenic lung disease. *Clin Chest Med.* 2004;25:XIII-XIX.
25. Caruana DS, Weinbach B, Goerg D, Gardner LB: Cocaine-packet ingestion. Diagnosis, management, and natural history. *Ann Intern Med.* 1984;100:73-74.
26. Celli B, Khan MA: Mercury embolization of the lung. *N Engl J Med.* 1976;295:883-885.
27. Chang KH, Han MH, Kim HS, Wie BA, Han MC. Delayed encephalopathy after acute carbon monoxide intoxication: MR imaging features and distribution of cerebral white matter lesions. *Radiology.* 1992;184:117-122.
28. Chan YW: Magnetic resonance imaging in toxic encephalopathy due to podophyllin poisoning. *Neuroradiology.* 1991;33:372-373.
29. Cheng CL, Svesko V: Acute pyloric perforation after prolonged crack smoking. *Ann Emerg Med.* 1994;23:126-128.
30. Choi IS, Kim SK, Lee SS, Choi YC: Evaluation of outcome of delayed neurologic sequelae after carbon monoxide poisoning by technetium-99m hexamethylpropylene amine oxime brain single photon emission computed tomography. *Eur Neurol.* 1995;35:137-142.
31. Choi SH, Lee SW, Hong YS, et al: Diagnostic radiopacity and hepatotoxicity following chloroform ingestion: a case report. *Emerg Med J.* 2006;23:394-395.
32. Chong S, Lee KS, Chung MJ, et al: Pneumoconiosis: comparison of imaging and pathologic findings. *Radiographics.* 2006;26:59-77.
33. Chung CH, Fung WT: Detection of gastric drug packet by ultrasound scanning. Europ *J Emerg Med.* 2006;13:302-303.
34. Citron BP, Halpern M, McCarron M, et al: Necrotizing angiitis associated with drug abuse. *N Engl J Med.* 1970;283:1003-1011.
35. Cohan RH, Ellis JH, Garner WL: Extravasation of radiographic contrast material: recognition, prevention, and treatment. *Radiology.* 1996;200:593-604.
36. Costello J, Townend W: Best evidence topic report. Abdominal radiography in "body packers." *Emerg Med J.* 2004;21:498.
37. Cranston PE, Pollack CV Jr, Harrison RB: CT of crack cocaine ingestion. *J Comp Assist Tomogr.* 1992;16:560-593.
38. Dally S, Garnier R, Bismuth C: Diagnosis of chlorinated hydrocarbon poisoning by x ray examination. *Br J Indust Med.* 1987;44:424-425.
39. Dee P, Armstrong P: Drug- and radiation-induced lung disease. In: Armstrong P, Wilson AG, Dee P, Hansell DM, eds. *Imaging of Diseases of the Chest*, 2nd ed. St. Louis: Mosby; 1995:461-483.
40. Dee P, Armstrong P: Inhalational lung diseases. In: Armstrong P, Wilson AG, Dee P, Hansell DM, eds. *Imaging of Diseases of the Chest*, 2nd ed. St. Louis: Mosby; 1995:426-460.
41. Degirmencia B, Elab Y, Haktanira A, et al: Methanol intoxication: diffusion MR imaging findings. *Eur J Radiol Extra.* 2007;61:41-44.
42. Demaerel P, Van Paesschen W: Images in clinical medicine. Marchiafava-Bignami disease. *N Engl J Med.* 2004;351:e10.
43. DeMartini J, Wilson A, Powell JS, Powell CS: Lead arthropathy and systemic lead poisoning from an intraarticular bullet. *AJR Am J Roentgenol.* 2001;176:1144.
44. Desenclos JC, Wilder MH, Coppenger GW, Sherin K, Tiller R, VanHook RM: Thallium poisoning: an outbreak in Florida, 1988. *South Med J.* 1992;85:1203-1206.
45. Dillman RO, Crumb CK, Lidsky MJ: Lead poisoning from a gunshot wound. Report of a case and review of the literature. *Am J Med.* 1979;66:509-514.
46. Douglass RE, Levison MA: Pneumothorax in drug abusers. An urban epidemic? *Am Surg.* 1986;52:377-380.
47. Edeiken J, Dalinka M, Karasick D: *Edeiken's Roentgen Diagnosis of Diseases of Bone*, 4th ed. Baltimore, MD. Williams and Wilkins. 1990:1401-1406.
48. Eng JG, Aks SE, Waldron R, Marcus C, Issleib S: False-negative abdominal CT scan in a cocaine body stuffer. *Am J Emerg Med.* 1999;17:702-704.
49. Erasmus JJ, McAdams HP, Rossi SE: High-resolution CT of drug-induced lung disease. *Radiol Clin North Am.* 2002;40:61-72.
50. Eurman DW, Potash HI, Eyler WR, Paganussi PJ, Beute GH: Chest pain and dyspnea related to "crack" cocaine smoking: value of chest radiography. *Radiology.* 1989;172:459-462.
51. Everson GW, Bertaccini EJ, O'Leary J: Use of whole bowel irrigation in an infant following iron overdose. *Am J Emerg Med.* 1991;9:366-369.
52. Everson GW, Oudjhane K, Young LW, Krenzelok EP: Effectiveness of abdominal radiographs in visualizing chewable iron supplements following overdose. *Am J Emerg Med.* 1989;7:459-463.
53. Farber JM, Rafii M, Schwartz D: Lead arthropathy and elevated serum levels of lead after a gunshot wound of the shoulder. *AJR Am J Roentgenol.* 1994;162:385-386.
54. Federle MP, Chang PJ, Confer S, Ozgun B: Frequency and effects of extravasation of ionic and nonionic CT contrast media during rapid bolus injection. *Radiology.* 1998;206:637-640.
55. Feigin DS: Talc: understanding its manifestations in the chest. *AJR Am J Roentgenol.* 1986;146:295-301.
56. Felson B, Spitz HB. Pelvic mass in a 12-year-old girl. *JAMA.* 1977;237:1255-1256.
57. Filley CM, Kleinschmidt-DeMasters BK: Toxic leukoencephalopathy. *N Engl J Med.* 2001;345:425-432.
58. Finelli PF: Case report. Changes in the basal ganglia following cyanide poisoning. *J Comp Assist Tomogr.* 1981;5:755-756.
59. Florez MV, Evans JM, Daly TR: The radiodensity of medications seen on x-ray films. *Mayo Clin Proc.* 1998;73:516-519.
60. Forrester JM, Steele AW, Waldron JA, Parsons PE: Crack lung: an acute pulmonary syndrome with a spectrum of clinical and histopathologic findings. *Am Rev Respir Dis.* 1990;142:462-467.
61. Foxford R, Goldfrank L: Gastrotomy—a surgical approach to iron overdose. *Ann Emerg Med.* 1985;14:1223-1226.
62. Franquet T, Giménez A, Rosón N, et al: Aspiration diseases: findings, pitfalls, and differential diagnosis. *Radiographics.* 2000;20:673-685.
63. Fraser RO, Pare JAP, Pare PD, Fraser RS, Genereux GP: Drug- and poison-induced pulmonary disease. In: Fraser RG, Paré JAP, ed. *Diagnosis of Diseases of the Chest*, 3rd ed. Philadelphia: W.B. Saunders; 1991:2417-2479.
64. Freed TA, Sweet LN, Gauder PJ: Case reports balloon obturation bowel obstruction: a hazard of drug smuggling. *AJR Am J Roengenol.* 1976;127:1033-1034.
65. Fulkerson WJ, Gockerman JP: Pulmonary disease induced by drugs. In: Fishman AP, ed. *Pulmonary Diseases and Disorders*, 2nd ed. New York: McGraw-Hill; 1988:793-811.
66. Gadaleta D, Hall MH, Nelson RL: Cocaine-induced acute aortic dissection. *Chest.* 1989;96:1203-1205.
67. Gallucci M, Amicarelli I, Rossi A, et al: MR imaging of white matter lesions in uncomplicated chronic alcoholism. *J Comp Assist Tomogr.* 1989;13:395-398.
68. Gatenby RA. The radiology of drug-induced disorders in the gastrointestinal tract. *Semin Roentgenol.* 1995;30:62-76.
69. Gaul HP, Wallace CJ, Auer RN, Fong TC: MR findings in methanol intoxication. *AJNR. Am J Neuroradiol.* 1995;16:1783-1786.
70. Gibby WA, Zimmerman RA: X-ray computed tomography. In: Mazziotta JG, Gilman S, eds. *Clinical Brain Imaging: Principles and Applications.* Philadelphia: FA Davis; 1992:3-34.
71. Gilman S: Advances in neurology (1). *N Engl J Med.* 1992;326:1608-1616.
72. Gilman S, Adams K, Koeppe RA, et al: Cerebellar and frontal hypometabolism in alcoholic cerebellar degeneration studied with positron emission tomography. *Ann Neurol.* 1990;28:775-785.
73. Ginaldi S: Geophagia: An uncommon cause of acute abdomen. *Ann Emerg Med.* 1988;17:979-981.
74. Gordon RJ, Lowy FD: Bacterial infections in drug users. *N Engl J Med.* 2005;353:1945-1954.
75. Gotway MB, Marder SR, Hanks DK, et al: Thoracic complications of illicit drug use: An organ system approach. *Radiographics.* 2002;22(suppl):S119-S135.
76. Grabherr S, Ross S, Regenscheit P, et al: Detection of smuggled cocaine in cargos by MDCT. *AJR Am J Roentgenol.* 2008;190:1390-1395.
77. Gray JR, Khalil A, Prior JC: Acute arsenic toxicity—an opaque poison. *Can Assoc Radiol J.* 1989;40:226-227.
78. Greller HA, McDonagh J, Hoffman RS, Nelson LS: Use of ultrasound in the detection of intestinal drug smuggling. *Eur Radiol.* 2005;15:193; author reply 194.
79. Hagan IG, Burney K: Radiology of recreational drug abuse. *Radiographics.* 2007;27:919-940.
80. Hahn IH, Hoffman RS, Nelson LS: Contrast CT scan fails to detect the last heroin packet. *J Emerg Med.* 2004;27:279-283.
81. Handy CA: Radiopacity of oral nonliquid medications. *Radiology.* 1971;98:525-33.
82. Hantson P, Duprez T, Mahieu P: Neurotoxicity to the basal ganglia shown by magnetic resonance imaging (MRI) following poisoning by methanol and other substances. *J Toxicol Clin Toxicol.* 1997;35:151-161.
83. Harchelroad F: Identification of orally ingested cocaine by CT scan. *Vet Hum Toxicol.* 1992;34:350.

84. Haubek A, Lee K: Computed tomography in alcoholic cerebellar atrophy. *Neuroradiology.* 1979;18:77-79.
85. Hibbard R, Wahl M, Kirshenbaum M: Spiral CT imaging of ingested foreign bodies wrapped in plastic: a pilot study designed to mimic cocaine body stuffers [abstract]. *J Toxicol Clin Toxicol.* 1999;37:644.
86. Hillbom M, Muuronen A, Holm L, Hindmarsh T: The clinical versus radiological diagnosis of alcoholic cerebellar degeneration. *J Neurol Sci.* 1986;73:45-53.
87. Hinkel CL: The significance of opaque medications in the gastrointestinal tract, with special reference to enteric coated pills. *Am J Roentgenol Radium Ther Nucl Med.* 1951;65:575-581.
88. Ho VB, Fitz CR, Chuang SH, Geyer CA: Bilateral basal ganglia lesions: pediatric differential considerations. *Radiographics.* 1993;13:269-292.
89. Hoffman CK, Goodman PC: Pulmonary edema in cocaine smokers. *Radiology.* 1989;172:463-465.
90. Hoffman RS, Chiang WK, Weisman RS, Goldfrank LR: Prospective evaluation of "crack-vial" ingestions. *Vet Hum Toxicol.* 1990;32:164-167.
91. Hoffman RS, Smilkstein MJ, Goldfrank LR: Whole bowel irrigation and the cocaine body-packer: a new approach to a common problem. *Am J Emerg Med.* 1990;8:523-527.
92. Holman BL, Mendelson J, Garada B, et al: Regional cerebral blood flow improves with treatment in chronic cocaine polydrug users. *J Nucl Med.* 1993;34:723-727.
93. Hormes JT, Filley CM, Rosenberg NL: Neurologic sequelae of chronic solvent vapor abuse. *Neurology.* 1986;36:698-702.
94. Horowitz AL, Kaplan R, Sarpel G: Carbon monoxide toxicity: MR imaging in the brain. *Radiology.* 1987;162:787-788.
95. Horrocks AW: Abdominal radiography in suspected "body packers." *Clin Radiol.* 1992;45:322-325.
96. Isabela C, Silva S, Churg A, Müller NL: Hypersensitivity pneumonitis: spectrum of high-resolution CT and pathologic findings. *AJR Am J Roentgenol.* 2007;188:334-344.
97. Jaeger RW, Decastro FJ, Barry RC, Gerren LJ, Brodeur AE: Radiopacity of drugs and plants in vivo-limited usefulness. *Vet Hum Toxicol.* 1981;23:2-4.
98. Jibiki I, Kurokawa K, Yamaguchi N: 123I-IMP brain SPECT imaging in a patient with the interval form of CO poisoning. *Eur Neurol.* 1991;31: 149-151.
99. Johnston C, Keogan MT: Imaging features of soft-tissue infections and other complications in drug users after direct subcutaneous injection ("skin popping"). *AJR Am J Roentgenol.* 2004;182:1195-1202.
100. Jones JS, Lagasse J, Zimmerman G: Computed tomographic findings after acute carbon monoxide poisoning. *Am J Emerg Med.* 1994;12:448-451.
101. Kaczorowski JM, Wax PM: Five days of whole-bowel irrigation in a case of pediatric iron ingestion. *Ann Emerg Med.* 1996;27:258-263.
102. Kanne JP, Thoongsuwan N, Parimon T, Stern EJ: Airway injury after acute chlorine exposure. *AJR Am J Roentgenol.* 2006;186:232-233.
103. Kanne JP, Gunn M, Blackmore CC: Delayed gastric perforation resulting from hydrochloric acid ingestion. *AJR Am J Roentgenol.* 2005;185:682-683.
104. Keogh CF, Andrews GT, Spacey SD, Forkheim KE, Graeb DA: Neuroimaging features of heroin inhalation toxicity: "Chasing the dragon." *AJR Am J Roentgenol.* 2003;180:847-850.
105. Keys N, Wahl M, Aks S, et al: Cocaine body stuffers: a case series. *J Toxicol Clin Toxicol.* 1995;33:517.
106. Koller WC, Glatt SL, Perlik S, Huckman MS, Fox JH: Cerebellar atrophy demonstrated by computed tomography. *Neurology.* 1981;31:405-412.
107. Kram HB, Hardin E, Clark SR, Shoemaker WC: Perforated ulcers related to smoking "crack" cocaine. *Am Surg.* 1992;58:293-294.
108. Kriegstein AR, Armitage BA, Kim PY: Heroin inhalation and progressive spongiform leukoencephalopathy. *N Engl J Med.* 1997;336:589-590.
109. Krishnan A, Brown R: Plain abdominal radiography in the diagnosis of the "body packer." *J Accid Emerg Med.* 1999;16:381.
110. Krupski WC, Selzman CH, Whitehill TA: Unusual causes of mesenteric ischemia. *Surg Clin North Am.* 1997;77:471-502.
111. Kuhn JR, Tunell WP: The role of initial cineesophagography in caustic esophageal injury. *Am J Surg.* 1983;146:804-806.
112. Kulshrestha MK: Lead poisoning diagnosed by abdominal X-rays. *J Toxicol Clin Toxicol.* 1996;34:107-108.
113. Landi JL, Spickler EM: Imaging of intracranial hemorrhage associated with drug abuse. *Neuroimag Clin North Am.* 1992;2:187-194.
114. Lange RA, Hillis LD: Cocaine associated cardiovascular events. *N Engl J Med.* 2001;345:351-358.
115. Lassen NA, Holm S: Single photon emission computerized tomography. In: Mazzotta JG, Gilman S, eds. *Clinical Brain Imaging: Principles and Applications.* Philadelphia: FA Davis; 1992:108-134.
116. Lee DC, Roberts JR, Kelly JJ, Fishman SM: Whole-bowel irrigation as an adjunct in the treatment of radiopaque arsenic. *Am J Emerg Med.* 1995;13:244-245.
117. Levine SR, Brust JC, Futrell N, et al: Cerebrovascular complications of the use of the "crack" form of alkaloidal cocaine. *N Engl J Med.* 1990;323:699-704.
118. Lexa FJ: Drug-induced disorders of the central nervous system. *Semin Roentgenol.* 1995;30:7-17.
119. Linowiecki KA, Tillman DJ, Ruggles D, et al: Radiopacity of modified release cardiac medications: a case report and in vitro analysis [abstract]. *Vet Hum Toxicol.* 1992;34:350.
120. Litovitz TL: Button battery ingestions. A review of 56 cases. *JAMA.* 1983;249:2495-2500.
121. Lufkin RB: Magnetic resonance imaging. In: Mazzotti JG, Gilman S, eds. *Clinical Brain Imaging: Principles and Applications.* Philadelphia: FA Davis; 1992:36-69.
122. Ly BT, Williams SR, Clark RF: Mercuric oxide poisoning treated with whole-bowel irrigation and chelation therapy. *Ann Emerg Med.* 2002;39:312-315.
123. Mabry B, Greller HA, Nelson LS: Patterns of heroin overdose-induced pulmonary edema. *Am J Emerg Med.* 2004;22:316.
124. Maeda Y, Kawasaki Y, Jibiki I, Yamaguchi N, Matsuda H, Hisada K: Effect of therapy with oxygen under high pressure on regional cerebral blood flow in the interval form of carbon monoxide poisoning: observation from subtraction of technetium-99m HMPAO SPECT brain imaging. *Eur Neurol.* 1991;31:380-383.
125. Mahoney MS, Kahn M: A medical mystery. *N Engl J Med.* 1998;339:745.
126. Maniatis V, Zois G, Stringaris K: I.V. mercury self-injection: CT imaging. *AJR Am J Roentgenol.* 997;169:1197-1198.
127. Mankin HJ: Nontraumatic necrosis of bone (osteonecrosis). *N Engl J Med.* 1992;326:1473-1479.
128. Maravilla AM, Berk RN: The radiology corner. The radiographic diagnosis of pica. *Am J Gastroenterol.* 1978;70:94-99.
129. Martel W: Radiologic features of esophagogastritis secondary to extremely caustic agents. *Radiology.* 1972;103:31-36.
130. Martin TJ: Cocaine-induced mesenteric ischemia. *N C Med J.* 1991;52:429-430.
131. Matsumoto SC, Okajima T, Inayoshi S, Ueno H: Minamata disease demonstrated by computed tomography. *Neuroradiology.* 1988;30:42-46.
132. McCarron MM, Wood JD: The cocaine "body packer" syndrome. Diagnosis and treatment. *JAMA.* 1983;250:1417-1420.
133. McElvaine MD, DeUngria EG, Matte TD, Copley CG, Binder S: Prevalence of radiographic evidence of paint chip ingestion among children with moderate to severe lead poisoning, St Louis, Missouri, 1989 through 1990. *Pediatrics.* 1992;89:740-742.
134. Meggs WJ, Hoffman RS, Shih RD, Weisman RS, Goldfrank LR: Thallium poisoning from maliciously contaminated food. *J Toxicol Clin Toxicol.* 1994;32:723-730.
135. Megibow AJ, Balthazar EJ, Cho KC, Medwid SW, Birnbaum BA, Noz ME: Bowel obstruction: evaluation with CT. *Radiology.* 1991;180:313-318.
136. Meijer R, Bots ML: Detection of intestinal drug containers by ultrasound scanning: an airport screening tool? *Eur Radiol.* 2003;13:1312-1315.
137. Mengel CE, Carter WA: Geophagia diagnosed by roentgenograms. *JAMA.* 1964;187:955-956.
138. Merchant JA, Schwartz DA: Chest radiography for assessment of the pneumoconioses. In: Rom WN, ed. *Environmental and Occupational Medicine,* 2nd ed. Boston: Little Brown; 1992:215-225.
139. Messing B, Storch B: Computer tomography and magnetic resonance imaging in cyanide poisoning. *Eur Arch Psychiatry Neurol Sci.* 1988;237:139-143.
140. Miller WTJ: Pleural and mediastinal disorders related to drug use. *Semin Roentgenol.* 1995;30:35-48.
141. Miura T, Mitomo M, Kawai R, Harada K: CT of the brain in acute carbon monoxide intoxication: characteristic features and prognosis. *AJNR Am J Neuroradiol.* 1985;6:739-742.
142. Moral AR, Ayanoglu HO, Erhan E: Putaminal necrosis after methanol intoxication. *Intensive Care Med.* 1997;23:234-235.
143. Naidich TP, Bartelt D, Wheeler PS, Stern WZ: Metallic mercury emboli. *Am J Roentgenol Radium Ther Nucl Med.* 1973;117:886-891.
144. Nelson DL, Batnitzky S, McMillan JH, et al: The CT and MRI features of acute toxic encephalopathies. *AJNR Am J Neuroradiol.* 1987;8:951.

145. Neustadter LM, Weiss M: Medication-induced changes of bone. *Semin Roentgenol.* 1995;30:88-95.
146. Ng RC, Perry K, Martin DJ: Iron poisoning: assessment of radiography in diagnosis and management. *Clin Pediatr (Phila).* 1979;18:614-616.
147. O'Brien RP, McGeehan PA, Helmeczi AW, Dula DJ: Detectability of drug tablets and capsules by plain radiography. *Am J Emerg Med.* 1986;4:302-312.
148. Olmedo RE, Hoffman RS, Nelson LS: Limitations of whole bowel irrigation and laparotomy in a cocaine "body packer" [abstract]. *J Toxicol Clin Toxicol.* 1999;37:645.
149. Olsen WL, Cohen W: Neuroradiology of AIDS. In: Federle MP, Megibow AJ, Naidich DP, eds. *Radiology of Acquired Immune Deficiency Syndrome.* New York: Raven Press; 1988:21-45.
150. Palat D, Denson M, Sherman M, Matz R: Pneumomediastinum induced by inhalation of alkaloidal cocaine. *N Y State J Med.* 1988;88:438-439.
151. Palatnick W, Tenenbein M: Leukocytosis, hyperglycemia, vomiting, and positive X-rays are not indicators of severity of iron overdose in adults. *Am J Emerg Med.* 1996;14:454-455.
152. Perron AD, Gibbs M: Thoracic aortic dissection secondary to crack cocaine ingestion. *Am J Emerg Med.* 1997;15:507-509.
153. Peterson CD, Fifield GC: Emergency gastrotomy for acute iron poisoning. *Ann Emerg Med.* 1980;9:262-264.
154. Phelps ME: Positron emission tomography. In: Mazzotta JG, Gilman S, ed. *Clinical Brain Imaging: Principles and Applications.* Philadelphia: FA Davis; 1992:71-106.
155. Piatt JP, Kaplan AM, Bond GR, Berg RA: Occult carbon monoxide poisoning in an infant. *Pediatr Emerg Care.* 1990;6:21-23.
156. Pidoto RR, Agliata AM, Bertolini R, et al: A new method of packaging cocaine for international traffic and implications for the management of cocaine body packers. *J Emerg Med.* 2002;23:149-153.
157. Pollack CV, Biggers DW, Carlton FB: Two crack cocaine body stuffers. *Ann Emerg Med.* 1992;21:1370-1380.
158. Pracyk JB, Stolp BW, Fife CE, Gray L, Piantadosi CA: Brain computerized tomography after hyperbaric oxygen therapy for carbon monoxide poisoning. *Undersea Hyperb Med.* 1995;22:1-7.
159. Prockop LD, Naidu KA: Brain CT and MRI findings after carbon monoxide toxicity. *J Neuroimaging.* 1999;9:175-181.
160. Raber SA: The dense metaphyseal band sign. *Radiology.* 1999;211:773-774.
161. Ramchandani P, Pollack HM: Radiology of drug-related genitourinary disease. *Semin Roentgenol.* 1995;30:77-87.
162. Rashid J, Eisenberg MJ, Topol EJ: Cocaine-induced aortic dissection. *Am Heart J.* 1996;132:1301-1304.
163. Resnick D: Heavy metal poisoning and deficiency. In: Resnick D, ed. *Diagnosis of Bone and Joint Disorders.* Philadelphia: W.B. Saunders; 1995:3353-3364.
164. Resnick D, Niwayama G: Osteolysis and chondrolysis. In: Resnick D, ed. *Diagnosis of Bone and Joint Disorders.* Philadelphia: W.B. Saunders; 1995:4467-4469.
165. Restrepo CS, Carrillo JA, Mart??nez S, et al: Pulmonary complications from cocaine and cocaine-based substances: imaging manifestations. *Radiographics.* 2007;27:941-956.
166. Richerson HB: Hypersensitivity pneumonitis (extrinsic allergic alveolitis). In: Fishman AP, eds. *Pulmonary Diseases and Disorders,* 2nd ed. New York: McGraw-Hill; 1988:667-674.
167. Roach HD, Davies GJ, Attanoos R, Crane M, Adams H, Phillips S: Asbestos: when the dust settles an imaging review of asbestos-related disease. *Radiographics.* 2002;22(suppl):S167-S184.
168. Roberge RJ, Martin TG: Whole bowel irrigation in an acute oral lead intoxication. *Am J Emerg Med.* 1992;10:577-583.
169. Roberts JR: Complications of radiographic contrast material. *Emerg Med News.* 2004;31-34.
170. Roberts JR, Price D, Goldfrank L, Hartnett L: The bodystuffer syndrome: a clandestine form of drug overdose. *Am J Emerg Med.* 1986;4:24-27.
171. Rosenberg NL, Kleinschmidt-DeMasters BK, Davis KA, Dreisbach JN, Hormes JT, Filley CM: Toluene abuse causes diffuse central nervous system white matter changes. *Ann Neurol.* 1988;23:611-614.
172. Rossi SE, Erasmus JJ, McAdams HP, Sporn TA, Goodman PC: Pulmonary drug toxicity: radiologic and pathologic manifestations. *Radiographics.* 2000;20:1245-1259.
173. Rubinstein D, Escott E, Kelly JP: Methanol intoxication with putaminal and white matter necrosis: MR and CT findings. *AJNR Am J Neuroradiol.* 1995;16:1492-1494.
174. Sachs HK: The evolution of the radiologic lead line. *Radiology.* 1981;139:81-85.
175. Saleem TM, Singh M, Murtaza M, Singh A, Kasubhai M, Gnanasekaran I: Renal infarction: a rare complication of cocaine abuse. *Am J Emerg Med.* 2001;19:528-529.
176. Savitt DL, Hawkins HH, Roberts JR: The radiopacity of ingested medications. *Ann Emerg Med.* 1987;16:331-339.
177. Sawada Y, Sakamoto T, Nishide K, et al: Correlation of pathological findings with computed tomographic findings after acute carbon monoxide poisoning. *N Engl J Med.* 1983;308:1296.
178. Sawada Y, Takahashi M, Ohashi N, et al: Computerised tomography as an indication of long-term outcome after acute carbon monoxide poisoning. *Lancet.* 1980;1:783-784.
179. Schabel SI, Rogers CI: Opaque artifacts in a health food faddist simulating ovarian neoplasm. *AJR Am J Roentgenol.* 1978;130:789-790.
180. Schwartz DT: Toxicologic emergencies. In: Schwartz DT, Reisdorff EJ, eds. *Emergency Radiology.* New York: McGraw-Hill; 2000:627-648.
181. Sengupta A, Page P: Window manipulation in diagnosis of body packing using computed tomography. *Emerg Radiol.* 2008;15:203-205.
182. Silver DA, Cross M, Fox B, Paxton RM: Computed tomography of the brain in acute carbon monoxide poisoning. *Clin Radiol.* 1996;51:480-483.
183. Sinner WN: The gastrointestinal tract as a vehicle for drug smuggling. *Gastrointest Radiol.* 1981;6:319-323.
184. Smith DA, Leake L, Loflin JR, Yealy DM: Is admission after intravenous heroin overdose necessary? *Ann Emerg Med.* 1992;21:1326-1330.
185. Sogge MR, Griffith JL, Sinar DR, Mayes GR: Lavage to remove enteric-coated aspirin and gastric outlet obstruction. *Ann Intern Med.* 1977;87:721-722.
186. Spitzer A, Caruthers SB, Stables DP: Radiopaque suppositories. *Radiology.* 1976;121:71-73.
187. Sporer KA, Firestone J: Clinical course of crack cocaine body stuffers. *Ann Emerg Med.* 1997;29:596-601.
188. Sporer KA, Manning JJ: Massive ingestion of sustained-release verapamil with a concretion and bowel infarction. *Ann Emerg Med.* 1993;22:603-605.
189. Staple TW, McAlister WH: Roentgenographic visualization of iron preparations in the gastrointestinal tract. *Radiology.* 1964;83:1051-1056.
190. Stepens A, Logina I, Liguts V, Aldins P, Eksteina I, Platkajis A: A parkinsonian syndrome in methcathinone users and the role of manganese. *N Engl J Med.* 2008;358:1009-1017.
191. Stern WZ, Spear PW, Jacobson HG: The roentgen findings in acute heroin intoxication. *Am J Roentgenol Radium Ther Nucl Med.* 1968;103:522-532.
192. Stromberg BV: Symptomatic lead toxicity secondary to retained shotgun pellets: case report. *J Trauma.* 1990;30:356-357.
193. Su M, Stork C, Ravuri S, et al: Sustained-release potassium chloride overdose. *J Toxicol Clin Toxicol.* 2001;39:641-648.
194. Sue YJ, Saperstein A, Zawin J, et al: Radiopacity of paradichlorobenzene-containing household products. *Vet Hum Toxicol.* 1992;34:350.
195. Swartz MN: Approach to the patient with pulmonary infections. In: Fishman AP, ed. *Pulmonary Diseases and Disorders,* 2nd ed. New York: McGraw-Hill; 1988:1375-1750.
196. Switz DM, Elmorshidy ME, Deyerle WM: Bullets, joints, And lead intoxication. A remarkable and instructive case. *Arch Intern Med.* 1976;136:939-941.
197. Tatekawa Y, Nakatani K, Ishii H, et al: Small bowel obstruction caused by a medication bezoar: report of a case. *Surg Today.* 1996;26:68-70.
198. Theodorou SJ, Theodorou DJ, Resnick D: Imaging findings of complications affecting the upper extremity in intravenous drug users. *Emerg Radiol.* 2008;15:227-239.
199. Tillman DJ, Ruggles DL, Leikin JB: Radiopacity study of extended-release formulations using digitalized radiography. *Am J Emerg Med.* 1994;12:310-314.
200. Tom T, Abedon S, Clark RI, Wong W: Neuroimaging characteristics in carbon monoxide toxicity. *J Neuroimaging.* 1996;6:161-166.
201. Traub SJ, Hoffman RS, Nelson LS: False-positive abdominal radiography in a body packer resulting from intraabdominal calcifications. *Am J Emerg Med.* 2003;21:607-608.
202. Tumeh SS, Nagel JS, English RJ, Moore M, Holman BL: Cerebral abnormalities in cocaine abusers: demonstration by SPECT perfusion brain scintigraphy. Work in progress. *Radiology.* 1990;176:821-824.
203. Vantroyen B, Heilier JF, Meulemans A, et al: Survival after a lethal dose of arsenic trioxide. *J Toxicol Clin Toxicol.* 2004;42:889-895.
204. Velasquez G, Ward CF, Bohrer SP: Thorium dioxide: still around. *South Med J.* 1985;78:743-745.
205. Vernace MA, Bellucci AG, Wilkes BM: Chronic salicylate toxicity due to consumption of over-the-counter bismuth subsalicylate. *Am J Med.* 1994;97:308-309.

206. Vieregge P, Klostermann W, Blumm RG, Borgis KJ: Carbon monoxide poisoning: clinical, neurophysiological, and brain imaging observations in acute disease and follow-up. *J Neurol.* 1989;236:478-481.
207. Volkow ND, Fowler JS, Wolf AP: Use of positron emission tomography to investigate cocaine. In: Nahas GG, Latour C, eds. *Physiopathology of Illicit Drugs: Cannabis, Cocaine, Opiates.* Oxford: Pergamon Press; 1991:129-141.
208. Wang CL, Cohan RH, Ellis JH, Adusumilli S, Dunnick NR: Frequency, management, and outcome of extravasation of nonionic iodinated contrast medium in 69,657 intravenous injections. *Radiology.* 2007;243:80-87.
209. Wang GJ, Volkow ND, Roque CT, et al: Functional importance of ventricular enlargement and cortical atrophy in healthy subjects and alcoholics as assessed with PET, MR imaging, and neuropsychologic testing. *Radiology.* 1993;186:59-65.
210. Wang Y, Yin Y, Gilula LA, Wilson AJ: Endemic fluorosis of the skeleton: radiographic features in 127 patients. *AJR Am J Roentgenol.* 1994;162:93-98.
211. Warach SJ, Charness ME: Imaging the brain lesions of alcoholics. In: Greenberg JO, Adams RD, eds. *Neuroimaging: A companion to Adams and Victor's Principles of Neurology.* New York: McGraw-Hill; 1995:503-515.
212. Ward S, Heyneman LE, Reittner P, Kazerooni EA, Godwin JD, Muller NL: Talcosis associated with IV abuse of oral medications: CT findings. *AJR Am J Roentgenol.* 2000;174:789-793.
213. Ware LB, Matthay MA: The acute respiratory distress syndrome. *N Engl J Med.* 2000;342:1334-1349.
214. Weidauer S, Nichtweiss M, Lanfermann H, Zanella FE: Wernicke encephalopathy: MR findings and clinical presentation. *Eur Radiol.* 2003;13:1001-1009.
215. Weill H, Jones RN: Occupational pulmonary diseases. In: Fishman AP, ed. *Pulmonary Diseases and Disorders*, 2nd ed. New York: McGraw-Hill; 1988:1465-1474.
216. Weimerskirch PJ, Burkhart KK, Bono MJ, Finch AB, Montes JE: Methylene iodide poisoning. *Ann Emerg Med.* 1990;19:1171-1176.
217. Wilgoren J: Misdiagnosis led to man's handcuffing, suit claims. *The New York Times.* December 8, 1998;62.
218. Williams MH: Pulmonary complications of drug abuse. In: Fishman AP, ed. *Pulmonary Diseases and Disorders*, 2nd ed. New York: McGraw-Hill; 1988:819-860.
219. Wolff AJ, O'Donnell AE: Pulmonary effects of illicit drug use. *Clin Chest Med.* 2004;25:203-216.
220. Wolowodiuk OJ, McMicken DB, O'Brien P: Pneumomediastinum and retropneumoperitoneum: an unusual complication of syrup-of-ipecac-induced emesis. *Ann Emerg Med.* 1984;13:1148-1151.
221. Woolf DA, Riach IC, Derweesh A, Vyas H: Lead lines in young infants with acute lead encephalopathy: A reliable diagnostic test. *J Trop Pediatr.* 1990;36:90-93.

CHAPTER 6
LABORATORY PRINCIPLES

Petrie M. Rainey

Medical toxicology addresses harm caused by acute and chronic exposures to excessive amounts of a xenobiotic. The management of toxicologic emergencies is a major component of medical toxicology. Detecting the presence or measuring the concentration of xenobiotics and other acutely toxic xenobiotics is the primary activity of the analytical toxicology laboratory. Such testing is closely intertwined with therapeutic drug monitoring, in which drug concentrations are measured as an aid to optimizing drug dosing regimens. In addition to drugs, measurements may be made of a variety of xenobiotics such as pesticides, herbicides, and poisons found in plants, animals, or the environment. The toxicology laboratory is frequently viewed in much the same way as other clinical laboratories often are—as a "black box" that converts orders into test results. Because toxicology testing volumes are relatively low and menus are extensive, testing is not as highly automated as in other clinical laboratories. Many results may be "hand-made the old-fashioned way." The downside of this may be somewhat longer turnaround times. But the upside is that toxicology laboratory personnel have the incentive and flexibility to develop substantial expertise. Medical toxicologists who understand how toxicology testing is done will be able to apply the results more effectively.

RECOMMENDATIONS FOR ROUTINELY AVAILABLE TOXICOLOGY TESTS

Despite a common focus, there is remarkable variability in the range of tests offered by analytical toxicology laboratories. Test menus may range from once-daily testing for routinely monitored drugs and common drugs of abuse to around-the-clock availability of a broad array of assays with the theoretical potential to identify several thousand compounds. Recently, consensus documents have been developed that recommend tests that should be available to support management of poisoned patients presenting to emergency departments.[22,37] Although they make specific recommendations, these guidelines recognize that no set of recommendations will be universally appropriate and note that it is impossible for a clinical laboratory to offer a full spectrum of toxicology testing in real time.

Decisions on the menu of tests to be offered by any specific laboratory should be decided by the laboratory director in consultation with the medical toxicologists and other clinicians who will use the service and should take into account regional patterns of use of licit and illicit drugs and environmental toxins, as well as resources available and competing priorities.

The recommendations in Table 6–1 were developed by the National Academy of Clinical Biochemists (NACB) from a consensus process that involved clinical biochemists, medical toxicologists, forensic toxicologists, and emergency physicians.[37] Although these tests should be readily available in the clinical laboratory, they should not be considered as a test panel for possibly poisoned patients. As with all laboratory tests, they should be selectively ordered based on the patient's clinical presentation or other relevant factors. Suggested turnaround time for reporting serum concentrations of the drugs listed in Table 6-1 was 1 hour or less. Quantitative tests for serum methanol and ethylene glycol were also recommended, with the reservations that these tests are not needed in all settings and that a realistic turnaround time is 2 to 4 hours. Serum cholinesterase testing with a turnaround time of less than 4 hours was proposed by some participants but did not achieve a general consensus. In the United Kingdom, the National Poisons Information Service and the Association of Clinical Biochemists have recommended a nearly identical list of tests, omitting the anticonvulsants.[22]

Although the consensus for the menu of serum assays was generally excellent, there was less agreement as to the need for qualitative urine assays. This was largely a result of issues of poor sensitivity and specificity, poor correlation with clinical effects, and infrequent alteration of patient management. Although these were potential issues for all of the urine drug tests, they led to explicit omission of tests for tetrahydrocannabinol (THC) and benzodiazepines from the recommended list despite their widespread use. THC results were thought to have little value in managing patients with acute problems, and tests for benzodiazepines were believed to have an inadequate spectrum of detection. Testing for amphetamines, propoxyphene, and phencyclidine were only recommended in areas where use was prevalent. It was also suggested that diagnosis of tricyclic antidepressant (TCA) toxicity not be based solely on the results of a urine screening immunoassay because a number of other drugs may cross-react. The significance of TCA results should always be correlated with electrocardiographic and clinical findings. The only urine test included in the United Kingdom guidelines was a spot test for paraquat.[22] Paraquat testing was omitted in the NACB guidelines because of a very low incidence of paraquat exposure in North America.[37]

The NACB guidelines also recommend the availability of broad-spectrum toxicology testing with the tests in Table 6–1 to be used for selected patients with presentations compatible with poisoning but who remain undiagnosed and who are not improving. In general, such testing should not be ordered until the patient is stabilized and input has been obtained from a medical toxicologist or poison center. This second level of testing may be provided directly by the local laboratory or by referral to a reference laboratory or a regional toxicology center.

Many physicians order a broad-spectrum toxicology screen on a poisoned patient if one is readily available, but only approximately 2% of clinical laboratories provide relatively comprehensive toxicology services (as estimated from proficiency testing data[3]). Although broad-spectrum toxicology screens can identify most drugs present in overdosed patients,[12] the results of broad-spectrum screens infrequently alter management or outcomes.[11,12,15,21,24,25]

The extent to which the NACB recommendations are being followed may be estimated from the numbers of laboratories participating in various types of proficiency testing. Result summaries from the 2007 series of proficiency surveys administered by the College of American Pathologists suggest that quantitative assays for acetaminophen, carbamazepine, carboxyhemoglobin, digoxin, ethanol, iron, lithium, methemoglobin, phenobarbital, salicylate, theophylline, and valproic acid are available in 50% to 60% of laboratories that offer routine clinical testing, as are screening tests for drugs of abuse in urine. About one in four laboratories offers measurement of transferrin or iron-binding capacity.[3]

About 2% of laboratories participated in proficiency testing for a full range of toxicology services. These full-service laboratories typically offer quantitative assays for additional therapeutic drugs, particularly TCAs, as well as assays that are designated as broad-spectrum or comprehensive toxicology screens. About two-thirds of these full-service toxicology laboratories offer testing for volatile alcohols other than ethanol.[3]

Although relatively few laboratories offer a wide range of in-house testing, most laboratories send out specimens to reference laboratories that offer large toxicology menus. The turnaround time for such

TABLE 6–1. Toxicology Assays Recommended by the National Academy of Clinical Biochemists

Quantitative Serum Assays	Qualitative Urine Assays
Acetaminophen	Amphetamines
Carbamazepine	Barbiturates
Cooximetry (carboxyhemoglobin, methemoglobin, oxygen saturation)	Cocaine Opiates
Digoxin	Propoxyphene
Ethanol	Phencyclidine
Iron (plus transferrin or iron-binding capacity)	Tricyclic antidepressants
Lithium	
Phenobarbital	
Salicylate	
Theophylline	
Valproic acid	

"send-out" tests ranges from a few hours to several days, depending on the proximity of the reference laboratory and the type of test requested.

Even in full-service toxicology laboratories, the test menu may vary substantially from institution to institution. Larger laboratories typically offer one or more broad-spectrum testing choices, often referred to as "tox screens." There is as much variety in the range of xenobiotics detected by various toxicologic screens as there is in the total menu of toxicologic tests. Routinely available tests are usually listed in a printed or online laboratory manual. Laboratories with comprehensive services may be able to offer ad hoc chromatographic assays for additional xenobiotics that are not listed. Testing that is sent to a reference laboratory is often not listed in the laboratory manual. The best way to determine if a particular xenobiotic can be detected or quantitated is to ask the director or supervisor of the toxicology or clinical chemistry section because laboratory clerical staff may only be aware of tests listed in the manual.

USING THE TOXICOLOGY LABORATORY

There are many reasons for toxicologic testing. The most common function is to confirm or exclude toxic exposures suspected from a patient's history and physical examination results. A laboratory result provides a level of confidence not readily obtained otherwise and may avert other unproductive diagnostic investigations driven by the desire for completeness and medical certainty. Testing increased diagnostic certainty in more than half of cases,[2,11,15] and in some instances, a diagnosis may be based primarily on the results of testing. This can be particularly important in poisonings with xenobiotics having delayed onset of clinical toxicity, such as acetaminophen, or in patients with ingestion of multiple xenobiotics. In these instances, characteristic clinical findings may not have developed at the time of presentation or may be obscured or altered by the effects of coingestants.

Testing can provide two key parameters that will have a major impact on the clinical course, namely, the xenobiotic involved and the intensity of the exposure. This information can assist in triage decisions, such as whether to admit a patient or to observe the individual for expectant discharge. Serum concentrations can facilitate decisions to use specific antidotes or specific interventions to hasten elimination. Well-defined exposure information can also facilitate provision of optimum advice by poison centers, whose personnel do not have the ability to make decisions based on direct observation of the patient. Serum concentrations can be used to determine when to institute and when to terminate interventions such as hemodialysis or antidote administration and can support the decision to transfer the patient from intensive care or discharge him or her from the hospital. Finally, positive findings for ethanol or drugs of abuse in trauma patients may serve as an indication for substance use intervention as well as a risk marker for the likelihood of future trauma.[11]

The confirmation of a clinical diagnosis of poisoning provides an important feedback function, whereby the physician may evaluate the diagnosis against a "gold standard." Another important benefit is reassurance (e.g., reassurance that an unintentional ingestion did not result in absorption of a toxic amount of xenobiotic). Such reassurance may allow a physician to avoid spending excessive time with patients who are relatively stable. It may also allow admissions to be made and interventions undertaken more confidently and efficiently than would be likely based solely on a clinical diagnosis. Testing may also be indicated for medicolegal reasons. Diagnoses with legal implications should be established "beyond a reasonable doubt." Although testing for illicit drugs is often done for medical purposes, it is almost impossible to dissociate such testing from legal considerations. Documentation is also important in malevolent poisonings, intentional or unintentional child abuse or neglect involving therapeutic or illicit drugs, and pharmacologic elder abuse. When test results may be used to document criminal activity, consideration should be given to having testing done in a forensic laboratory maintaining a full chain of custody. This is usually done in conjunction with a law enforcement request or protocol (e.g., drug-facilitated sexual assault) and not usually for medical purposes.

The documentation function is also important outside the medicolegal arena. Results of testing in a central laboratory are almost invariably entered into the patient's medical record and may often provide definitive confirmation of a problem. Documentation also has an additional importance that goes beyond the individual cases. Medical toxicology does not lend itself readily to experimental human investigation. Much of toxicologic knowledge has been derived from experiments of nature recorded in case reports and case series. Hard data, such as xenobiotic concentrations, may serve as key quantitative variables in summarizing and correlating data. That laboratory results can be reliably and generally easily found in the medical record makes them particularly valuable in retrospective reviews. A related service that the toxicology laboratory may provide is testing in support of experimental investigations.

The key to optimum use of the toxicology laboratory is communication. This begins with learning the laboratory's capabilities, including what xenobiotics are on its menus, which ones can be measured and which merely detected, and what are anticipated turnaround times. For screening assays, one should know which xenobiotics are routinely detected; which ones can be detected if specifically requested; and which ones cannot be detected, even when present at concentrations that result in toxicity.

A key item is learning which specimens are appropriate for the test requested. A general rule is that quantitative tests require serum (red stopper) or heparinized plasma (green stopper) but not ethylenediamine tetraacetic acid (EDTA) plasma (lavender stopper) or citrate plasma (light-blue stopper). EDTA and citrate bind divalent cations that may serve as cofactors for enzymes used as reagents or labels in various assays. Additionally, liquid EDTA and citrate anticoagulants dilute the specimen. Serum or plasma separator tubes (identifiable by the separator gel in the tube) are also acceptable, provided that prolonged gel contact before testing is avoided. Some hydrophobic drugs may diffuse slowly into the gel, leading to falsely low results after several hours. A random, clean urine specimen is generally preferred for toxicology screens because the higher drug concentrations usually found in urine can compensate for the lower sensitivity of the broadly focused screening techniques. A urine specimen of 20 mL is usually optimal. Requirements for all specimens may vary from laboratory to laboratory.

When making a request for a screening test, an important—and often overlooked—item of communication is specifying any xenobiotics that are particularly suspected. This knowledge allows the laboratory to set up the tests for those drugs first and possibly adjust the protocols to increase sensitivity or specificity. This may save an hour or more in the time needed to receive the critical information.

Consultation with the laboratory regarding puzzling cases or unusual needs may allow consensus on an effective and feasible testing strategy. The full capabilities of a toxicology laboratory are often not apparent from published lists of tests available. Most full-service laboratories devote substantial efforts to meeting reasonable requests and often provide consultations at no charge.

The laboratory should also be contacted whenever results appear inconsistent or discrepant with the clinical presentation. The most common causes for this are interferences and preanalytical errors. Analytical interference is caused by materials in the specimen that interfere with the measurement process, leading to falsely high or low results. For example, hemoglobin may interfere with a variety of spectrophotometric tests by absorbing the light used to make the measurement. Preanalytical errors are events that occur before laboratory analysis and produce incorrect or misleading results, such as mislabeling, specimen contamination by intravenous solutions, and incorrect collection time or technique. The laboratory will be familiar with the common sources of discrepant results. If a discrepancy is the result of laboratory error, it is critical that the laboratory be informed so that steps can be taken to understand the source of the error and avoid a recurrence.

METHODS USED IN THE TOXICOLOGY LABORATORY

Most tests in the toxicology laboratory are directed toward the identification or quantitation of xenobiotics. The primary techniques used include spot tests, spectrochemical tests, immunoassays, and chromatographic techniques. Mass spectrometry may also be used, usually in conjunction with gas chromatography (GS) or liquid chromatography. Table 6–2 compares the basic features of these methodologies. Other methodologies include ion-selective electrode measurements of lithium, atomic absorption spectroscopy or inductively coupled plasma mass spectroscopy for lithium and heavy metals, and anodic stripping methods for heavy metals. Many adjunctive tests, including glucose, creatinine, electrolytes, osmolality, metabolic products, and enzyme activities, may also be useful in the management of poisoned patients. The focus here is on the major methods used for directly measuring xenobiotics.

SPOT TESTS

The simplest tests are spot tests. These rely on the rapid reaction of a xenobiotic with a chemical reagent to produce a colored product (e.g., the formation of a colored complex between salicylate and ferric ions). Because the reagents may cause precipitation of serum proteins, spot tests are more commonly performed on urine specimens or gastric aspirates. Such tests were once a mainstay of toxicologic testing. Because of the poor selectivity of chemical reagents, as well as substantial variability in visual interpretation, these assays suffer from fairly frequent false-positive results and occasional false-negative results. As more sensitive and more specific methods have become available, spot tests have waned in popularity. Only a few are still in use, largely to fill gaps in testing menus or to rapidly exclude some common poisonings. The introduction of point-of-care testing devices that have better sensitivity and specificity and are designed to facilitate compliance with regulations is likely to further reduce the use of spot tests.

SPECTROCHEMICAL TESTS

Spectrochemical tests are sophisticated versions of spot tests. They also rely on a chemical reaction to form a light-absorbing substance. They differ in that the reaction conditions and reagent concentrations are carefully controlled and the amount of light absorbed is quantitatively measured at one or more specific wavelengths. The use of specific wavelengths enhances the sensitivity and, particularly, the specificity of the detection, and the measurement of the amount of light absorbed under controlled conditions allows quantitation of the substance.

When an analyte is intrinsically light absorbing, no reaction may be necessary. Cooximetry (also known as hemoximetry) represents

TABLE 6–2. Relative Comparison of Toxicology Methods

Method	Sensitivity	Specificity	Quantitation	Analyte Range	Speed	Cost
Spot test	+	±	No	Few	Fast	$
Spectrochemical	+	+	Yes	Few	Medium	$
Immunoassay	++	++	Yes	Moderate	Medium	$$
TLC	+	++	No	Broad	Slow	$$
HPLC	++	++	Yes	Broad	Medium	$$
GC	++	++	Yes	Broad	Medium	$$
GC/MS	+++	+++	Yes	Broad	Slow	$$$
LC/MS/MS	+++	+++	Yes	Broad	Medium	$$$$

GC, gas chromatography; GC/MS, gas chromatography/mass spectroscopy; HPLC, high-performance liquid chromatography; LC/MS/MS, liquid chromatography/tandem mass spectroscopy; TLC, thin-layer chromatography.
$ = very low
$$$$ = very high cost

a sophisticated application of spectrophotometry to the measurement of various forms of hemoglobin in a hemolyzed blood sample. Measurement of light absorbance at multiple wavelengths allows several hemoglobin species to be simultaneously quantitated. For mathematical reasons, the number of wavelengths used must be greater than the number of different types of hemoglobin present. This is why classic pulse oximetry, which uses only two wavelengths, yields spurious results in the presence of significant amounts of methemoglobin or carboxyhemoglobin (Chaps. 21, 125, and 127).

Most analytes are neither as deeply colored nor as highly concentrated as hemoglobin species. Their detection requires the generation of an intensely light-absorbing product, as is done in spot tests. The difference between a spot test and a spectrochemical one lies in whether the colored product is visually observed or quantitatively measured in a spectrophotometer. Because spectrophotometers can also measure ultraviolet and infrared light, it is not necessary for the product to have a visible color. Early spectrochemical assays typically measured the absorbance after conversion of all of the analyte to the light-absorbing product. Modern assays usually use rate spectrophotometry, taking multiple absorbance measurements over time to determine the rate of change in light absorbance as the reaction proceeds. During the initial phase of the reaction, this rate is constant and proportional to the initial concentration of the analyte. This significantly reduces the time needed to obtain a result because it is not necessary for the reaction to go to completion first, and it allows the averaging of multiple measurements, improving precision. Furthermore, it is unaffected by nonreacting substances that absorb light at the test wavelength because the absorbance of the nonreacting substances is constant and does not contribute to the rate of change in the absorbance.

Rate spectrophotometry remains subject to interference by substances that react to produce a light-absorbing product, thereby falsely increasing the apparent concentration. Substances that inhibit the assay reaction or that consume reagents without producing a light-absorbing product give falsely low results. For example, ascorbic acid produces negative interference in many spectrophotometric assays that use oxidation reactions to generate colored products.

Cooximetry is relatively free of interferences because the concentrations of the hemoglobins are so much higher than other substances in the blood. However, the presence of intensely colored substances (e.g., methylene blue) may cause spurious increases or decreases in the apparent percentages of the hemoglobins. Modern instruments are often able to recognize a significantly atypical pattern of absorbance and generate an error message in addition to or instead of a result.

One way to improve the selectivity of a spectrochemical assay is to increase the selectivity of the reaction that generates the light-absorbing product. Enzymes, which can catalyze highly selective reactions, are often used for this purpose. For example, many assays for ethanol use alcohol dehydrogenase to catalyze the oxidation of ethanol to acetaldehyde, with concomitant reduction of the cofactor NAD^+ (oxidized form of nicotinamide adenine dinucleotide) to NADH (reduced form of nicotinamide adenine dinucleotide). The initial rate of increase in light absorption produced by the conversion of NAD^+ to NADH is proportional to the concentration of ethanol. Although other alcohols, such as isopropanol and methanol, can also be oxidized by alcohol dehydrogenase, they are much poorer substrates with low rates of reaction and correspondingly low levels of interference.

Many other enzymatic assays also rely on measuring the change in light absorption at 340 nm when NAD^+ is converted to NADH or vice versa. These include enzymatic assays for ethylene glycol, as well as some enzyme-linked immunoassays, such as EMIT (enzyme-multiplied immunoassay technique) assays. All such assays are potentially subject to interference by specimens with high concentrations of lactate. Lactate dehydrogenase, which is naturally present in serum, will oxidize this lactate to pyruvate if NAD^+ becomes available for simultaneous reduction to NADH. When a serum specimen with high lactate is mixed with assay reagents that contain NAD^+, oxidation of the lactate contributes to the total rate of NADH production. The increased rate of NADH production results in a false increase in the measured concentration of the target analyte.

IMMUNOASSAYS

The need to measure very low concentrations of an analyte with a high degree of specificity led to the development of immunoassays. The combination of high affinity and high selectivity makes antibodies excellent assay reagents. There are two common types of immunoassays: noncompetitive and competitive. In noncompetitive immunoassays, the analyte is sandwiched between two antibodies, each of which recognizes a different epitope on the analyte. In competitive immunoassays, analyte from the patient's specimen competes for a limited number of antibody binding sites with a labeled version of the analyte provided in the reaction mixture. Because most drugs are too small to have two distinct antibody binding sites, drug immunoassays are usually competitive.

In competitive immunoassays, increasing the concentration of xenobiotic in the specimen results in increased displacement of labeled xenobiotic from the antibodies. The amount of xenobiotic in the specimen can be determined by measuring either the amount of label remaining bound to the assay antibodies or the amount of label free in solution. In the earliest immunoassays, the label was a radioisotope, typically iodine-125, tritium, or carbon-14. The bound and free radioactivity were physically separated, for example, by using a second antibody to cross-link and precipitate the assay antibody, along with its bound radioactivity (Fig. 6–1) or by adsorbing the free label with activated charcoal. Today, radioimmunoassays are relatively uncommon because of problems associated with handling and disposal of radioactivity. They are primarily used for xenobiotics with insufficient demand to justify the development costs of more sophisticated nonisotopic assays.

Nonisotopic immunoassays are currently the most widely used methodologies for the measurement of drugs. They offer high selectivity and good precision and are readily adapted to automated analyzers, thereby decreasing both the cost and the turnaround time of the assays. The effort involved in developing these assays is substantial. Accordingly, the xenobiotics for which immunoassays are available are limited to those for which there is a high demand, such as widely monitored therapeutic drugs and the drugs of abuse included in workplace drug screening. However, after assay development is completed, production costs are relatively low, allowing the tests to be widely distributed at reasonable prices.

The most widely used nonisotopic drug immunoassays are in the category of homogenous immunoassays. Homogenous immunoassays measure differences in the properties of bound and free labels, rather than directly measuring one or the other after their physical separation. Avoiding a separation step allows homogenous immunoassays to be readily adapted to automated analysis. Homogenous techniques that are in wide use include EMIT (Fig. 6–2), kinetic inhibition of microparticles in solution (KIMS), cloned enzyme donor immunoassay (CEDIA), and fluorescence polarization immunoassay (FPIA).

Many of the newest automated immunoassays are again using physical separation techniques. In these assays, the detection antibody is physically attached to a solid support, and separation occurs by a simple wash step. This wash step removes the patient's serum along with many potentially interfering substances. Newer solid supports

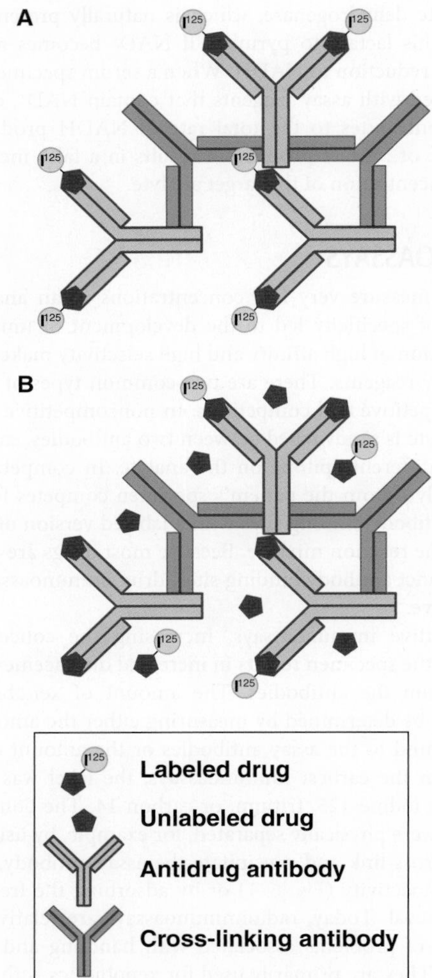

FIGURE 6–1. Competitive radioimmunoassay. (A) No drug from the specimen is present to displace the I^{125} -labeled drug. Adding the cross-linking antibody precipitates the assay antibody, along with high amounts of bound radioactivity. (B) Unlabeled drug in the specimen displaces some of the labeled drug. The displaced label is left in solution when the cross-linking antibody is added, resulting in less radioactivity in the precipitate.

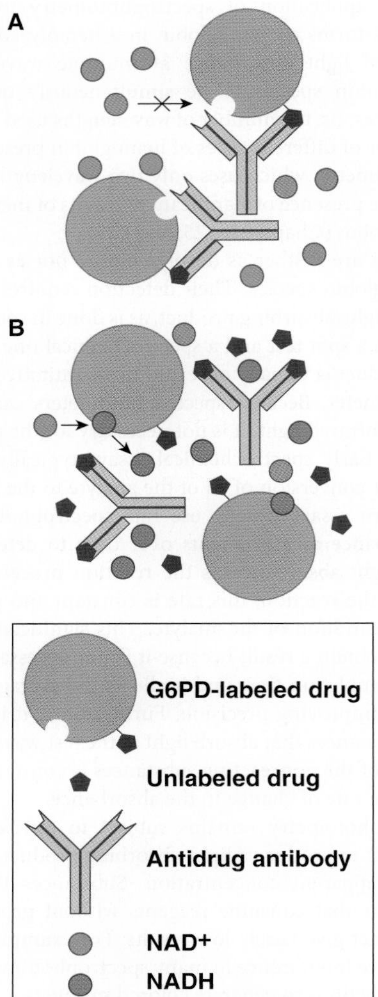

FIGURE 6–2. Enzyme-multiplied immunoassay technique (EMIT) immunoassay. The drug to be measured is labeled by being attached to the enzyme glucose-6-phosphate dehydrogenase (G6PD) near the active site. (A) Binding of the enzyme-labeled drug to the assay antibody blocks the active site, inhibiting conversion of NAD^+ (oxidized form of nicotinamide adenine dinucleotide) to NADH (reduced form of nicotinamide adenine dinucleotide). (B) Unlabeled drug from the specimen can displace the drug-enzyme conjugate from the antibody, thereby unblocking the active site and increasing the rate of reaction.

consist of fine glass fibers or latex microparticles. These have very high total surface areas that allow for rapid equilibration and short assay times. Older assays of this type used antibodies bound to large plastic beads or wells of microtiter plates and required long incubation steps because of substantial times required for diffusion of the reactants to the antibodies.

Fig. 6–3 shows a schematic magnetic microparticle enzyme-labeled chemiluminescent competitive immunoassay. A single enzyme label can generate many photons, allowing high signal amplification. Coupled with a background luminescence that is essentially zero, such assays can measure concentrations below the nanomolar level. Many variations of this approach are in use. Enzyme substrates may be used that result in fluorescent or colored products. Enzymes other than alkaline phosphatase may be used as labels, or non-enzymatic fluorescent, chemiluminescent, or electroluminescent labels may be used. Non-magnetic microparticles may be captured in glass fiber filters during the washing and signal generation steps. These new techniques are readily automated and have higher sensitivities than homogenous immunoassays.

Microparticle capture assays are a type of competitive immunoassays that have become very popular, especially for urine drug-screening tests. The use of either latex or colloidal gold colored microparticles because the label enables the result to be read visually as the presence or absence of a colored band, with no special instrumentation required. Competitive binding occurs as the assay mixture is drawn by capillary action through a porous membrane. This design feature is responsible for alternate names for the technique: lateral flow immunoassay or immunochromatography.

The simplest design uses an antidrug antibody bound to colored microparticles and a capture zone consisting of immobilized drug

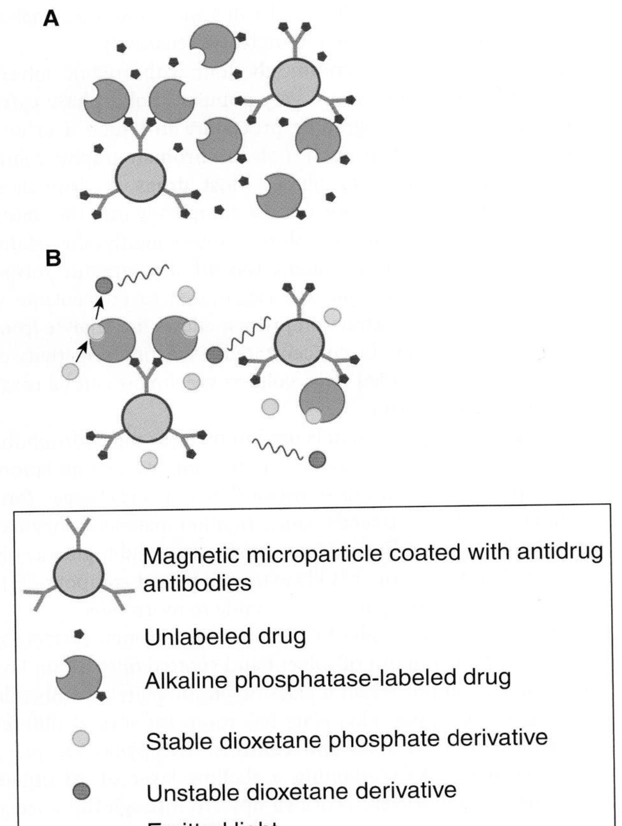

FIGURE 6–3. Magnetic microparticle chemiluminescent competitive immunoassay. (**A**) Unlabeled drug from the specimen competes with alkaline phosphatase-labeled drug for binding to antibody-coated magnetic microparticles. The microparticles are then held by a magnetic field while unbound material is washed away. (**B**) A dioxetane phosphate derivative is added and is dephosphorylated by microparticle-bound alkaline phosphatase to give an unstable dioxetane product that spontaneously decomposes with emission of light. The rate of light production is directly proportional to the amount of alkaline phosphatase bound to the microparticles and inversely proportional to the concentration of competing unlabeled drug from the specimen.

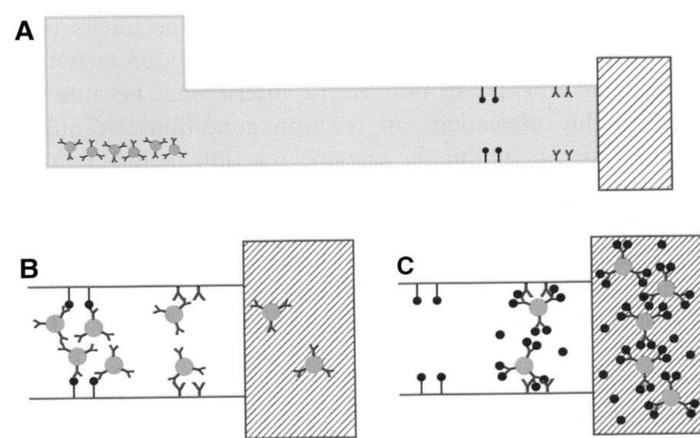

FIGURE 6–4. Microparticle capture immunoassay. (**A**) Diagram of a device before specimen addition. Colored microbeads (about the size of red blood cells) coated with antidrug antibodies (Y) are in the specimen well. At the far end of a porous strip are capture zones with immobilized drug molecules (•) and a control zone with antibodies recognizing the antibodies that coat the microbeads. (**B**) Adding the urine specimen suspends the microbeads, which are drawn by capillary action through the porous strip and into an absorbent reservoir (*hatched area*) at the far end of the strip. In the absence of drug in the urine, the antibodies will bind the beads to the capture zone containing the immobilized drug and form a colored band. Excess beads will be bound by antibody–antibody interactions in the control zone, forming a second colored band that verifies the integrity of the antibodies in the device. (**C**) If the urine contains the drug (•) in concentrations exceeding the detection limit, all of the antibodies on the microbeads will be occupied by drug from the specimen, and the microbeads will not be retained by the immobilized drug in the capture zone. No colored band will form. However, the beads will be bound and form a band in the control zone.

(Fig. 6–4). If the specimen is xenobiotic free, the beads will bind to the immobilized analyte, forming a colored band. When the amount of drug in the patient specimen exceeds the detection limit, all of the antibody sites will be occupied by drug from the specimen, and no labeled antibody will be retained in the capture zone. The use of multiple antibodies and discrete capture zones with different immobilized analytes can allow several xenobiotics to be detected with a single device.

A disadvantage of this design is the potential for causing confusion because a positive test result is indicated by the absence of a band. More complex (and more expensive) variations have been developed in which a colored band denotes a positive test result.

Although immunoassays have a high degree of sensitivity and selectivity, they are also subject to interferences and problems with cross-reactivity. Cross-reactivity refers to the ability of the assay antibody to bind to xenobiotics other than the target analyte. Xenobiotics with similar chemical structures may be efficiently bound, which can lead to falsely elevated results. In some situations, cross-reactivity can be beneficially exploited. For example, some immunoassays effectively detect classes of drugs rather than one specific drug. Immunoassays for opiates use antibodies that recognize various xenobiotics that are structurally related to morphine, including codeine, hydrocodone, and hydromorphone. Oxycodone typically has less cross-reactivity, and higher concentrations are required to give a positive result. However, structurally unrelated synthetic opioids, such as meperidine and methadone, have little or no cross-reactivity and are not detected by opiate immunoassays. Immunoassays for the benzodiazepine class react with a wide variety of benzodiazepines but with varying degrees of sensitivity.[10,17]

Class specificity can be a two-edged sword. Assays for the TCA family have similar reactivity with amitriptyline, nortriptyline, imipramine, and desipramine and can be used to provide a semiquantitative estimate of the total concentration of any combination of these drugs. However, a large number of other drugs with tricyclic structures, including carbamazepine, many phenothiazines, and diphenhydramine, also cross-react and generate a signal, particularly at concentrations found in patients who overdose. Qualitative tests, such as microparticle capture assays, may then yield false-positive results if the signal generated by the cross-reacting drug (e.g., carbamazepine) exceeds the detection limit of the immunoassay. With quantitative or semiquantitative assays, however, the apparent concentration produced by a cross-reacting drug is generally well below TCA concentrations associated with toxicity.

Even when an antibody is selected to be specific to a single drug, it is common that metabolites of the target drug show some cross-reactivity. This, too, may be beneficial. When the metabolite is an active one (e.g., carbamazepine epoxide), the contribution of its cross-reactivity may yield results that correlate better with the drug effect than the true concentration of the parent drug alone.

Immunoassays are also subject to interference by substances that impair detection of the label. Elevated lactate concentrations may lead to spuriously increased drug concentrations in specimens tested by EMIT, as described above. Immunoassays that rely on enzyme labels are particularly sensitive to nonspecific interference because enzyme activity is highly dependent on reaction conditions. A number of substances that can inhibit the enzyme reaction in EMIT assays are used to adulterate urine submitted for drug abuse testing with the intent of producing false-negative results (see the discussion of drug-abuse screening tests under "Special Considerations for Drug Abuse Screening Tests" below). Such adulteration may be detected when the rate of reaction is lower than the rate observed with a drug-free control.

CHROMATOGRAPHY

Chromatography encompasses several related techniques in which analyte specificity is achieved by physical separation. The unifying mechanism for separation is the partition of the analytes between a stationary phase and a moving phase (mobile phase). In most instances, the stationary phase consists of very fine particles arranged in a thin layer or enclosed within a column. The mobile phase flows through the spaces between the particles. Analytes are in a rapid equilibrium between solution in the mobile phase and adsorption to the surfaces of the particles. They move when in the mobile phase and stop when adsorbed to the stationary phase. The average velocity of the analyte xenobiotics depends on the relative time spent in the moving versus stationary phase. Xenobiotics that partition primarily into the mobile phase have average velocities slightly lower than the mobile phase velocity. Average velocity decreases as the proportion of time adsorbed to the stationary phase increases. Under controlled conditions, these average velocities are highly reproducible. Xenobiotics may be provisionally identified based on their characteristic velocity. This is measured as the distance traveled relative to the solvent migration distance in thin-layer chromatography, or the amount of time required to traverse the length of a chromatography column. These characteristic parameters are referred to as the *R_F value* and *retention time*, respectively.

Chromatography is a separation method and must be combined with a detection method to allow identification and measurement of the separated substances. Chromatographic behavior is sufficiently reproducible that the failure to detect a signal at an R_F value or retention time characteristic of a compound effectively excludes the presence of that compound in amounts greater than the detection limit. On the other hand, a number of different substances may have migration velocities that are identical or nearly so. A positive finding is therefore not completely specific. Definitive identification depends on having additional information, which may be obtained through selective detection techniques or by confirmatory testing using a second method. The sensitivity of chromatographic methods depends on both the amount of specimen available and the sensitivity of the detection method. The detection limit may range from less than 10 pg with mass spectrometric detection to more than 10 μg when detection is achieved by forming a colored product using a postchromatographic chemical reaction.

A major advantage of chromatographic techniques is that multiple xenobiotics may be detected and measured in a single procedure. It is not always necessary to know in advance the specific xenobiotic to be looked for. For this reason, chromatographic techniques have a major role in screening for multiple xenobiotics.

Most chromatographic procedures require extraction and concentration of the xenobiotics to be analyzed before the chromatography is done. Extraction results in removal of salts, proteins, and other materials that may exhibit unfavorable interactions with either of the chromatographic phases. Concentration allows the substances to be introduced in a narrow "band," so that compounds with slightly different relative mobilities become completely resolved, or separated from one another, rather than overlapping. This also results in a more intense signal as a band passes through the detector and increases sensitivity.

Extraction of drugs is most commonly done with organic solvents, but "solid-phase extraction" is also very popular.[9] Solid-phase extraction is a modified chromatographic procedure in which a urine or serum specimen is passed through a short chromatography column with a hydrophobic stationary phase. Most drugs are sufficiently hydrophobic so that they partition almost completely into the stationary phase and are retained on the column. Subsequently, the retained xenobiotics are eluted with an organic solvent. The organic solvents from either extraction technique are evaporated to concentrate the extracted xenobiotics. The extraction process allows the analyte from a large volume of specimen to be concentrated. Detection sensitivity can thereby be increased, provided large volume specimens can be readily obtained, as is true with urine.

Often a preextraction treatment is used to increase the hydrophobicity of the substances to be extracted. The most common manipulation is pH adjustment, either upward or downward, to convert charged forms of drugs into uncharged, extractable ones. In other instances, enzymatic or chemical hydrolysis may be used to convert water-soluble glucuronide metabolites back to their more readily extracted parent compounds; for example, conversion of morphine glucuronide to morphine.

In thin-layer chromatography (TLC), the concentrated extracts are redissolved in a small amount of solvent and spotted onto a thin layer of silica gel that is supported on a glass or plastic plate or embedded in a fiber matrix. A typical TLC plate has room for several different spots of extracts from samples and controls. The plates are placed vertically in closed tanks containing a shallow layer of an organic solvent mixture. As the solvent is drawn upward through the silica gel by capillary action, various xenobiotics are carried along at characteristic velocities determined by their partition between the moving organic solvent and the stationary silica gel (Fig. 6–5). Silica gel is

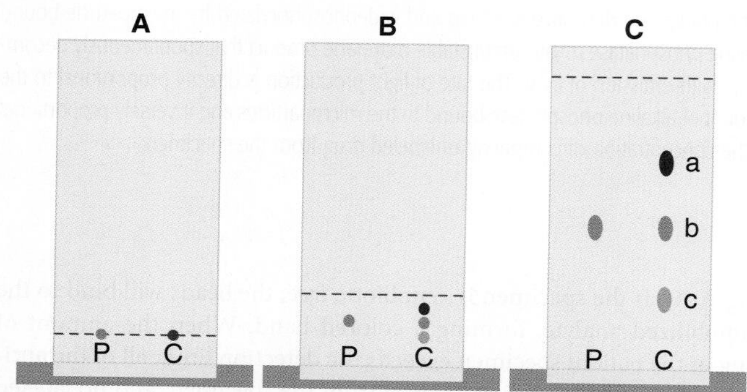

FIGURE 6–5. Thin-layer chromatography. (**A**) Concentrated extracts from patient (*P*) and control (*C*) specimens are dried in small spots on a plate coated with a thin layer of silica gel particles. The plate is placed vertically into an organic solvent mixture, which is being drawn up the plate by capillary action. The leading edge (or solvent front, shown by the *dotted line*) reaches the extracts and begins to dissolve them. (**B**) Various substances are moving at different rates, depending on the relative proportion of time spent in the moving solvent (mobile phase) and adsorbed to the silica gel (stationary phase). (**C**) The development of the chromatogram is stopped when the solvent front nears the top. Various substances are seen at characteristic positions relative to the solvent front. The patient specimen contains a substance that can be tentatively identified as compound *b* in the control mixture based on its relative mobility. Although shown as *shaded spots* here for clarity, most drugs are colorless and are visualized at the end of the chromatography by being dipped or sprayed with reagents that form colored products. The tentative identification of the unknown drug as compound *b* requires that it show the predicted behavior with the visualizing reagents.

polar, so hydrophobic xenobiotics migrate rapidly and hydrophilic ones more slowly. Adjusting the composition of the solvent mixture allows optimization of the migration rates. After sufficient solvent migration, the plates are removed from the tanks, dried, and sprayed with a series of reagents that convert the xenobiotics to be detected into various colored derivatives. The xenobiotics are thereby visualized as colored spots and identified by their migration distance (R_F value), as well as by the various colors produced after each spray. Those that are metabolized can be further confirmed by the finding of additional spots corresponding to characteristic metabolites. Identifications can be most confidently made when an authentic sample of the xenobiotic has been included as a control on the plate.

TLC has the ability to identify the presence of a large number of xenobiotics and is widely used in "drug screens." Visualization as colored spots generally requires fairly large amounts of material. For this reason, TLC is usually used with urine and gastric aspirate specimens because they typically have higher concentrations of many drugs than do corresponding serum specimens and because they are readily available in large volumes.

Drawbacks to TLC include the need for multiple steps—extraction, concentration, chromatography, and a series of detection reactions. This makes TLC a relatively slow and labor-intensive procedure. Interpretation of the spots requires a skilled technologist who knows the TLC behavior of commonly encountered xenobiotics. Quantitation is difficult and rarely attempted. Therefore, TLC is primarily used to demonstrate the presence of a drug. It is of limited value in identifying a drug not previously seen by the chromatographer unless a possible candidate is suggested to the laboratory and an authentic sample (i.e., a standard) can be obtained to verify its behavior in the TLC system. Also, drugs that have limited excretion in the urine might not be readily detected.

In the past, full-service toxicology laboratories used classical TLC procedures to screen urine for a variety of drugs. The development of a commercial kit for TLC of drugs in urine (Toxilab, Varian, Inc., Palo Alto, CA) has reduced the time, labor, and expertise required and has extended its practicability to a broader range of laboratories.[13] The use of a standardized procedure also allows tentative identification of a drug not previously encountered by comparing its characteristics with those of a broad range of drugs provided in a compendium by the manufacturer. Identifications made solely on the basis of agreement with characteristics described in the compendium should be considered provisional until confirmed by additional testing.

In the related technique of high-performance liquid chromatography (HPLC), the stationary phase is packed into a column and the mobile phase is pumped through under high pressure (Fig. 6–6). This allows good flow rates to be achieved, even when solid phases with very small particle sizes are used. Smaller particle size increases surface area, decreases diffusion distances, and improves resolution, but the spaces between the particles are also smaller, increasing the resistance to flow. The use of high pressure and small particles allows better separations in a fraction of the time required for TLC.

Another way that HPLC often differs from TLC is that HPLC typically uses "reverse-phase" chromatography. Reverse-phase chromatography uses stationary phases in which the silica gel particles have had hydrocarbon molecules covalently linked to the outer surface. This reduces the surface charge on the silica, thereby reducing its hydrophilicity, and simultaneously coats the particles with a permanently bonded oil-like layer. At the same time, solvent polarity is increased by using a primarily aqueous mobile phase with varying amounts of organic solvent. Because of these modifications, whereas hydrophobic xenobiotics are more strongly adsorbed by the stationary phase, hydrophilic ones tend to remain in the mobile phase. This results in

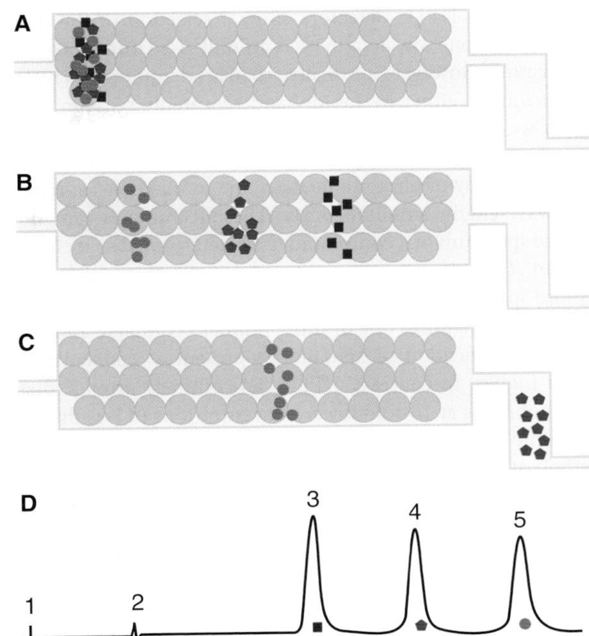

FIGURE 6–6. High-performance liquid chromatography (HPLC). HPLC is schematically shown. **(A)** A mixture of three compounds (■) (●) (⬟) is injected into a column filled with a spherical reversed-phase packing. **(B)** The compounds move through the column at characteristic speeds. The most hydrophilic compound (■) moves most quickly, and the most hydrophobic compound (●) moves most slowly. **(C)** The compound of intermediate polarity (⬟) has reached the detection cell, where it absorbs light directed through the cell and generates a signal proportional to its concentration. **(D)** Illustration of the HPLC tracing that might result: *1* indicates the time of injection. The artifact at *2* results when the injection solvent reaches the detector and indicates the retention time of a completely unretained compound. The peaks at *3*, *4*, and *5* correspond to the separated compounds. For example, peak *4* might be amitriptyline, peak *3* might be the more polar metabolite, nortriptyline, and peak *5* could be the more hydrophobic internal standard *N*-ethylnortriptyline. Later-emerging peaks are typically wider and shorter because of more time for diffusive forces to spread out the molecules.

an order of elution from the column that is approximately the reverse of that seen with organic solvents and unmodified silica gel. Thus, the term *reverse-phase chromatography* is used. Both TLC and HPLC can be done using either "normal-phase" or "reverse-phase" conditions. However, TLC is more commonly done in normal phase and HPLC more commonly in reverse phase. A variety of hydrocarbons can be used to derivatize the silica gel. By far, the most common reverse phase columns use an octadecyl hydrocarbon as the outer coating and are often referred to as C-18 columns.

In HPLC, the xenobiotics are detected after they exit the chromatographic column. In this case, they are identified by their retention time (the characteristic time required to traverse the column). Because most xenobiotics absorb ultraviolet light, detection is commonly by ultraviolet spectroscopy using specially designed flow-through cuvettes. Measuring light absorbance at a selected wavelength allows the amount of the xenobiotic to be determined. Accuracy is often enhanced by comparing the absorbance of the target analyte with absorbance of an internal standard (i.e., a compound with a different retention time that is added in a fixed amount to all specimens). The ratio of the drug absorbance to the internal standard absorbance is proportional to the drug concentration in the specimen.

Although most HPLC detectors allow a selection of the detection wavelength, only one wavelength is commonly used during a given run. Some detectors, however, allow absorbance at multiple wavelengths to be determined, either by rapidly and repeatedly scanning through a range of wavelengths or by breaking white light into its component wavelengths only after it has passed through the detection cuvette and then using an array of photodiode detectors to make measurements at multiple wavelengths simultaneously. These techniques can allow the absorbance spectrum of a compound to be determined as it elutes from the column. This information can supplement the retention time and allow more specific identifications to be made.

TLC generally requires one or more hours to complete and provides qualitative identification of xenobiotics present at concentrations of 1 mg/L or higher. In contrast, HPLC can routinely provide quantitation of xenobiotics at 10-fold lower concentrations in less than 1 hour (provided the calibration was done in advance). Thus, HPLC is often the method of choice for measuring serum concentrations of xenobiotics for which no immunoassay is available. Relative disadvantages of HPLC in comparison with TLC are the much higher costs of the equipment, the inability to analyze multiple samples simultaneously, and a relative inability to analyze drugs with a wide range of polarities with a single assay. The latter limitation inhibits the use of HPLC as a broad drug-screening technique.

GC is similar in principle to HPLC, except that the moving phase is a gas, usually the inert gas helium but occasionally nitrogen. The schematic illustration of HPLC in Figure 6–6 is also applicable to GC. The low flow resistance of gas allows high flow rates that make possible substantially longer columns than are used in HPLC. This offers the dual advantages of high resolution and fast analysis. As was true in HPLC, most GC assays incorporate an internal standard to increase precision.

Because the inert carrier gas does not engage in intermolecular interactions, partition of the analytes into the moving gas phase depends primarily on their natural volatility. Elevated column temperatures are required to achieve sufficient volatility for analysis of most xenobiotics. The use of a temperature gradient (the column temperature is programmed to increase throughout the course of the analysis) can allow xenobiotics with a wide range of volatility to be analyzed in a single run. This feature makes GC suitable for screening assays encompassing a broad range of drugs.

GC is limited to xenobiotics that are reasonably volatile at temperatures below 572°F (300°C), above which the stationary phase may begin to break down. Two principal attributes of a xenobiotic limit its volatility: its size and its ability to form hydrogen bonds. Xenobiotics that form hydrogen bonds via amino, hydroxyl, and carboxylate moieties can be made more volatile by replacing hydrogens on oxygen and nitrogen atoms with a non-bonding, preferably large, substituent. (Large substituents sterically hinder access to the acceptor electron pairs on the nitrogen and oxygen atoms.) A number of derivatizing agents can be used to add appropriate substituents. The most common derivatives involve the trimethylsilyl (TMS) group. Although derivatization with TMS substantially increases the molecular weight, the resulting derivative is much more volatile as a consequence of the loss of hydrogen bonding.

In traditional packed-column GC, the packing may consist of inert support particles with a thin coating of nonvolatile, high-molecular-weight oil that comprises the stationary phase. It is increasingly common for the stationary phase to be covalently bonded to the support particles. A highly useful variant of GC is capillary chromatography. A long, thin capillary tube of fused silica is coated on the inside with a covalently bonded stationary phase. The mobile gas phase flows through the tiny channel in the middle. These capillaries are flexible, allowing very long columns (≥10 m) to be coiled into a small space. The long column length, coupled with highly uniform conditions throughout the column, results in extremely high resolution. The small diameter of the column allows rapid thermal equilibration and the use of steep temperature gradients that can speed analysis. The major drawback to capillary chromatography is a very limited column capacity. Special techniques are needed to restrict the amount of material introduced into the column and thereby to avoid overloading it. High-sensitivity detectors are required to measure the small quantities that can be chromatographed.

A number of detectors are available for GC. The most common detector, particularly for packed columns, is the flame ionization detector. This involves directing the outflow of the column into a hydrogen flame. Organic molecules emerging from the column are burned, creating charged combustion intermediates that can be measured as a current. The amount of current flow is largely determined by the mass of carbon that is being burned. Nitrogen–phosphorus detectors are also widely used in drug analysis. In this modification of a flame ionization detector, a heated bead coated with an alkali metal salt is used to selectively generate ions from xenobiotics containing nitrogen or phosphorus. These devices detect broad ranges of substances but do not identify them. The identity of the compounds detected must be inferred from the retention time.

The mass spectrometer can serve as a highly sensitive GC detector and also possesses the ability to generate highly characteristic mass spectra from the compounds it is detecting. A special requirement of the mass spectrometer is that it requires a high vacuum to prevent the ionic particles that it creates from interacting with other molecules or ions. This requires removal of the inert carrier gas and is easiest when there is a low total gas flow, such as occurs with capillary GC. The mass spectrometer, in turn, provides good sensitivity for the small amounts of analyte that can be accommodated in capillary GC.

This detection process also begins by generating ions from the analyte. This is usually done using electron impact ionization. The gas phase analyte is separated from the bulk of the carrier gas and introduced into an ionization chamber, where it is bombarded by a stream of electrons. Electron impact can dislodge an electron from the analyte, creating a positively charged ion and frequently imparting sufficient energy to the ion to break it into pieces. If fragmentation occurs, conservation of charge requires that one of the resulting fragments be a positively charged ion. The fragments into which a molecular ion can break are characteristic of the xenobiotics because is the relative probability that a given fragment will carry the positive charge.

The mass spectrometer then uses electromagnetic filtering to direct only ions of a specified mass-to-charge (m/z) ratio to a detector. Because most of the ions produced have a single positive charge, the observed peaks generally correspond to the mass of the ions. The detector has sufficient electronic amplification that a single ion could theoretically be detected, accounting for the high sensitivity of mass spectrometric detection. By rapidly scanning through a range of masses that are sequentially allowed to reach the detector, a mass spectrum may be generated. The mass spectrum records the masses of the pieces produced by fragmentation of the parent ion, as well as the relative frequency with which these fragments are produced and detected. The highest mass observed in the spectrum usually corresponds to the mass of intact parent ions generated from collisions that were not energetic enough to cause fragmentation.

Figure 6–7 shows the mass spectrum obtained from a gas chromatograph at a time when the TMS derivative of the cocaine metabolite benzoylecgonine was emerging from the capillary column. The mass spectrum of any compound is highly distinctive and usually unique. The primary exception involves optical enantiomers, both of which have the same mass spectrum. Toxicologically significant examples of

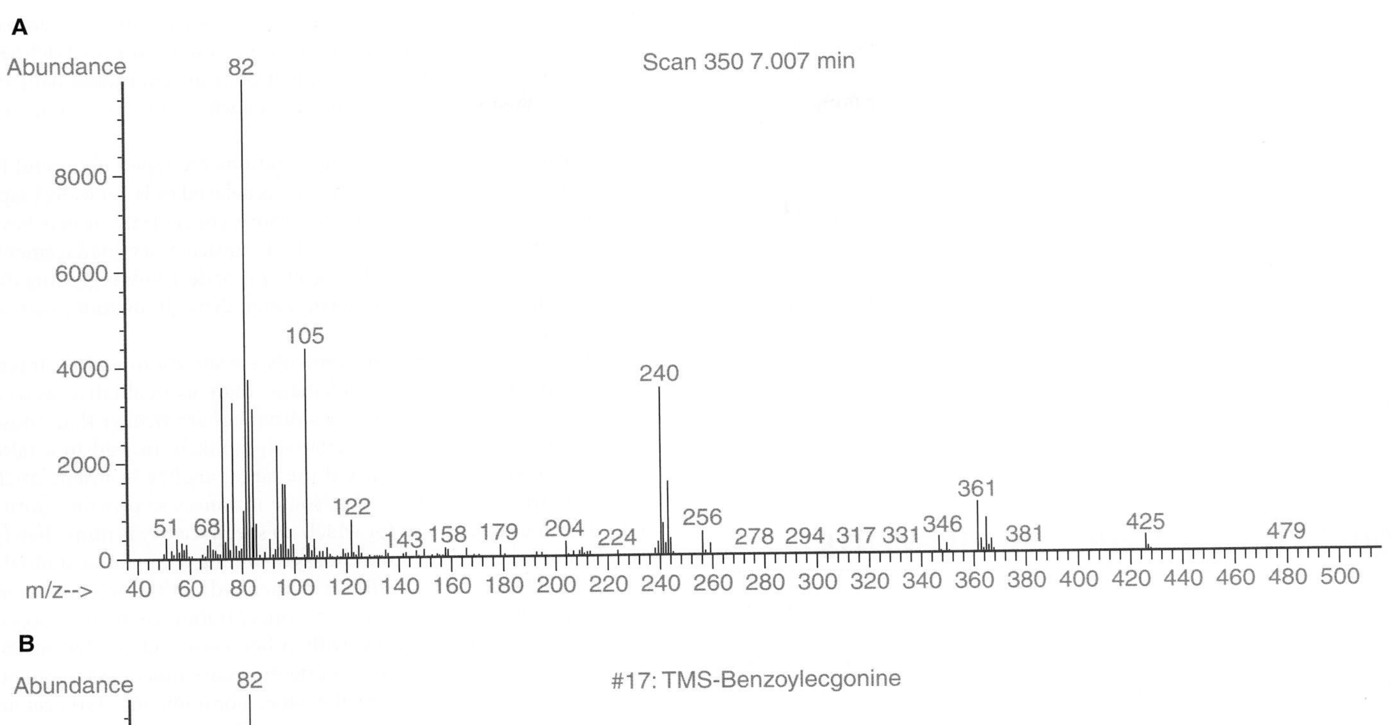

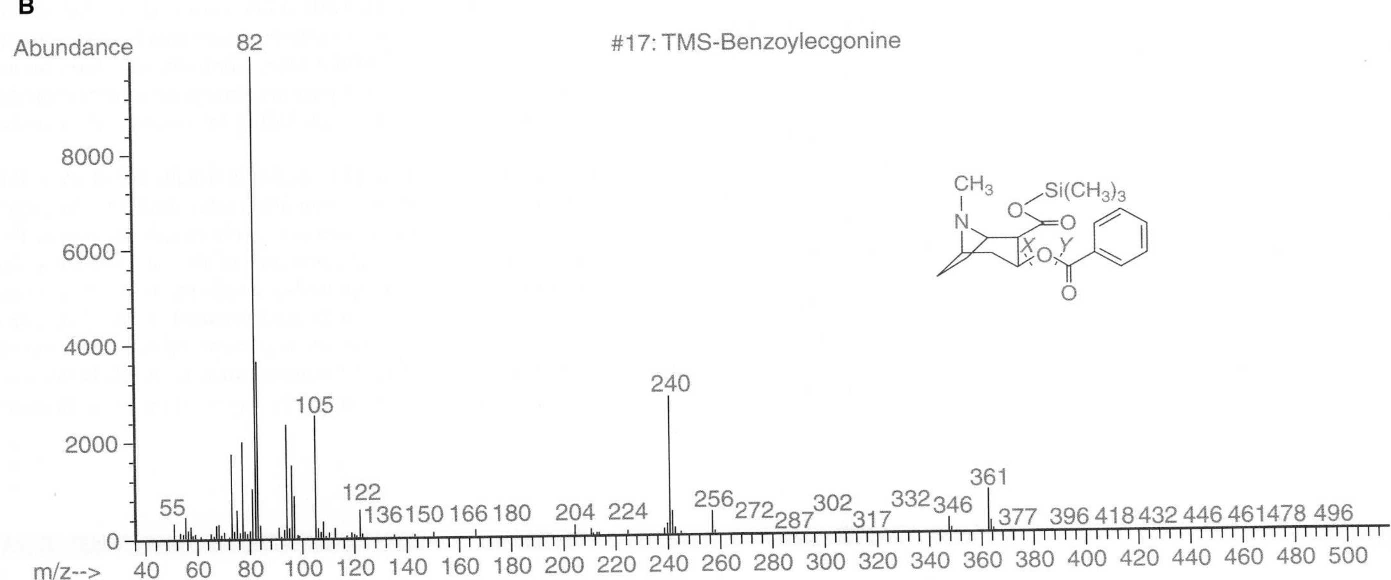

FIGURE 6–7. Mass spectrum of the trimethylsilyl derivative of benzoylecgonine (TMS-BE). (**A**) Mass spectrum of effluent from a gas chromatography (GC) column at the retention time of TMS-BE. The unfragmented parent ion of TMS-BE is at a mass-to-charge (*m/z*) ratio of 361. The two fragment peaks at *m/z* 243 and 259 result from fracture of the bonds at *X* and *Y*, respectively, in structure of TMS-BE (inset in **B**). Additional peaks at *m/z* 243, 259, and 364 are derived from trideuterated TMS-BZE (d_3-TMS-BE) added as an internal standard. The mass spectrometer can identify and quantify TMS-BE and d_3-TMS-BE independently of one another by measuring the heights of the peaks unique for each compound. The peak at *m/z* 425 is from a coeluting contaminant. (**B**) Mass spectrum of pure TMS-BE.

enantiomers include *d*-methamphetamine, a drug of abuse; *l*-methamphetamine, which is found in decongestant inhalers; and dextrorphan, the major metabolite of the cough suppressant dextromethorphan, and levorphan (levorphanol), a controlled substance.

To avoid the need to scan the full range of masses in a typical mass spectrum, selected ion monitoring is often used. Here, the mass spectrometer is typically programmed to filter and detect only three of the larger and more characteristic peaks in the spectrum. In the case of TMS benzoylecgonine (TMS-BE), the peaks at *m/z* 240, 256, and 361 are used. The concentration of TMS-BE in the specimen is determined from the ratio of the peak height at *m/z* 240 to a peak height at *m/z* 243 that results from a corresponding fragment of a triply deuterium-labeled internal standard, d_3-TMS-BE (see Fig. 6-7). The specificity of the identification is verified by finding peaks at *m/z* 256 and *m/z* 361, with peak height ratios to the peak at *m/z* 240 comparable to the ratios seen with authentic TMS-BE. The detection at the correct retention time of a xenobiotic producing all three peaks in the correct ratios produces an extremely specific identification.

The high sensitivity and specificity afforded by GS/mass spectrometry is being further extended by the related hybrid technique of liquid chromatography/tandem mass spectrometry, often abbreviated as LC/MS/MS. Initially restricted to research settings, the technique is now becoming available in a few toxicology laboratories.[19] In LC/MS/MS, a tandem mass spectrometer is used as the detector for liquid chromatography system. The initial ionization is done under conditions that do not promote fragmentation and is commonly achieved by adding or removing a proton rather than forcefully dislodging an electron. The resulting ions have a mass that differs from that of the parent molecule by 1 mass unit ($[M+H]^+$ or $[M-H]^-$) The first mass spectrometer is used to selectively filter only unfragmented ions with the expected molecular mass. As the selected ions exit the first mass spectrometer at high speed, they are allowed to collide with molecules of an inert gas. These collisions cause the ions to break apart to create the fragment mass spectrum that is detected by the second mass spectrometer. The additional selection step provided by the first mass spectrometer greatly enhances specificity and reduces background signal, enhancing sensitivity.

QUANTITATIVE DRUG MEASUREMENTS

When properly used to guide dosing adjustments, drug concentration measurements improve medical outcomes.[6] However, many therapeutic drug measurements are drawn at inappropriate times or are made without an appropriate therapeutic question in mind. An essential requirement for interpretation of xenobiotic concentrations is that the relationship between concentrations and effects must be known. Such knowledge is available for routinely monitored xenobiotics and is often encapsulated in published ranges of therapeutic concentrations and toxic concentrations. Concentrations designated as "toxic" are usually higher than the upper end of the therapeutic range and typically represent concentrations at which toxicity is acute and potentially serious (see back cover).

For most xenobiotics, the relationships between toxic concentrations and effects cannot be systematically studied in humans and consequently are often incompletely defined. These relationships are largely inferred from data provided in overdose case reports and case series. The measurement of xenobiotic concentrations in overdose cases in which concentration–effect relationships are not well defined may contribute more to the management of future overdosed patients than to the management of the patient in whom the measurements were made.

For toxicologists, xenobiotic concentrations are especially useful in two ways. For xenobiotics whose toxicity is delayed or is clinically inapparent during the early phases of an overdose, concentrations may have substantial prognostic value and facilitate anticipatory management. These concentrations may also be used to make decisions regarding the use of antidotes or of interventions to hasten drug elimination, such as hemodialysis.

Quantitative xenobiotic measurements are subject to various interferences, but these are less problematic than in qualitative assays. Signals generated by cross-reacting substances are weaker than those from the target analyte and are relatively unlikely to lead to a false diagnosis of toxicity, particularly if the target analyte is absent. Such cross-reactivity can be exploited in some instances to provide confirmatory evidence of a poison for which no specific assay is immediately available. For example, the immunoassay finding of apparent subtoxic levels of TCAs can help confirm a diphenhydramine overdose, and the finding of a measurable digoxin concentration in an unexposed patient may suggest poisoning with other cardioactive steroids of plant or animal origin. Negative interferences are much less frequent. Table 6–3 summarizes some of the more common interferences in quantitative assays for drugs and poisons. Extensive information on interferences with laboratory tests, including toxicology tests, may be found online.

Interferences in chromatographic methods usually result from the presence of other compounds with migration rates similar to the target analyte. Because the migration rates are rarely exactly the same, the laboratory can often recognize the presence of the interference as an overlapping peak when both compounds are present. In such instances, the interference may impair accurate measurement of the drug concentration. When no target xenobiotic is present, misidentification of the interfering peak as the target becomes much more likely because a single peak is seen at approximately the expected position. Because

TABLE 6–3. Interferences in Quantitative Assays for Xenobiotics

Analyte	Technique	Potential Interferences
Acetaminophen	Spectrochemical	Bilirubin, phenacetin, renal failure, salicylates
	Immunoassay	Phenacetin (clinically a true-positive test result)
Carboxyhemoglobin	Spectrochemical	Fetal hemoglobin, hydroxocobalamin
Digoxin	Immunoassay	Other cardioactive steroids (found in oleander, red squill, Chan Su), endogenous digoxin-like substances (found in hepatic and renal failure, neonates, pregnancy), digoxin metabolites in renal failure, spironolactone, canrenone (spironolactone metabolite), human anti-mouse antibodies, digoxin immune Fab
Iron	Spectrochemical	Citrate, deferoxamine, EDTA, gadolinium contrast agents, hemolysis, oxalate
Lithium	Electrochemical	Hemolysis, lithium heparin (clinically a true positive result) abnormal serum sodium
Methemoglobin	Spectrochemical	Lipemia, methylene blue, sulfhemoglobin
Salicylate	Spectrochemical	Bilirubin, diflunisal, ketosis, salicylamide, salicylsalicylate
	Immunoassay	Diflunisal
Theophylline	Immunoassay	Caffeine, lipemia

EDTA, ethylenediamine tetraacetic acid.

interferences in chromatographic methods are generally unique to a specific method, information about these interferences should be obtained by asking the laboratory.

Xenobiotic measurements are unlike most other laboratory measurements in that the concentrations are highly dependent on the timing of the measurement. Knowledge of the pharmacokinetics of a xenobiotic can substantially enhance the ability to draw meaningful conclusions from a measured concentration. Some xenobiotics alter their pharmacokinetic behavior at very high concentrations. These changes in pharmacokinetics may be predictable from the mechanisms of drug clearance and the extent of binding to plasma proteins and to tissues (Chap. 8).

Knowledge of the relationship between xenobiotic concentrations and effects, or pharmacodynamics, is also important. Effects depend on local concentrations at the site of action, typically at cell membrane receptors or intracellular locations. Serum or plasma concentrations can be correlated with effects only when these concentrations are in equilibrium with concentrations at the site of action. Table 6–4 lists several circumstances that may alter the normal ratio of xenobiotic concentrations measured in serum or plasma to concentrations found at the site of action, thereby altering the usual concentration–effect relationships. During the absorption and distribution phases, the concentration ratio will be higher than its equilibrium value, yet often the only xenobiotic concentration measured after an acute overdose is one obtained while absorption and distribution are still ongoing. This effect may explain some observations of apparent poor correlation between measured concentrations and toxic effects.

For xenobiotics that bind significantly to plasma proteins, it is the concentration of xenobiotic that is not bound to proteins (the free-xenobiotic concentration) that is in equilibrium with concentrations at the site of action. For most drugs at therapeutic concentrations, the free-drug concentration is an approximately constant percentage of the total drug concentration. The total concentration is what is usually measured in the laboratory. Under these conditions, the ratio of total concentration to active site concentration is approximately constant, and a reasonable correlation between total concentration and effects can be expected.

A major change in the free fraction occurs after treatment of digoxin toxicity with digoxin immune Fab, when the free digoxin concentration falls from approximately 75% of the total concentration to less than 1% as a consequence of digoxin binding by the antidigoxin antibody fragments. At the same time, there is extensive redistribution of digoxin from tissues to plasma, leading to substantial increases in total digoxin concentration. This situation may be further complicated by complex digoxin immune Fab interference in many digoxin immunoassays.

Measurement of free-drug concentrations can clarify such situations.[16] Assays for free phenytoin are available in many laboratories. Assays for other free-drug concentrations may require special arrangements. The availability and expected turnaround time can be provided by the laboratory. For example, for patients treated with digoxin immune Fab, newer immunoassays that use antibodies attached to microparticles or glass fibers give results that can be used to set an upper bound on free-digoxin concentrations and thereby verify adequacy of treatment.[26]

TOXICOLOGY SCREENING

A test unique to the toxicology laboratory is the toxicology screen, or "tox screen." Depending on the laboratory, this term may refer to a single testing methodology with the ability to detect multiple xenobiotics, such as a thin-layer or GS, it may refer to a panel of individual tests, such as a drug-abuse screen; or it may be a combination of broad-spectrum and individual tests. The widespread use of the term "tox screen" is unfortunate because this inappropriately implies for many physicians the availability of a test that can confirm or exclude poisoning as a diagnosis. There are many more toxic xenobiotics in the world than there are named diseases. However, a relatively limited number of xenobiotics account for most serious poisonings. As a result, in one study, a comprehensive toxicology screening protocol using multiple detection methods applied to both serum and urine specimens was able to identify more than 98% of implicated xenobiotics.[12] This suggests that a comprehensive "tox screen" can exclude poisoning with a substantial degree of reliability. However, this study was done some time ago, when the rate of introduction of new drugs was much slower than is currently the case. Many newer therapeutic drugs may not be identified even by "comprehensive" screens currently in use.[36] Moreover, comprehensive toxicology screens typically do not detect elemental ions, including bromide, lithium, iron, lead, and other heavy metals, nor do they necessarily detect drugs that are toxic at extremely low concentrations, such as digoxin or fentanyl. Table 6–5 lists a number of xenobiotics encountered in emergency toxicology that may not be detected by routine toxicology screening.

It should therefore be apparent that a negative toxicology screen result cannot exclude poisoning. It is equally true that a positive finding does not necessarily confirm a diagnosis of poisoning. For assays that detect only the presence of a xenobiotic, it is not possible to distinguish

TABLE 6–4. Factors that May Alter Concentration–Effect Relationships

Factor	Effect	Examples
Measurement during absorption phase	Underestimation of eventual effects	Sustained-release preparations; large ingestions of poorly soluble xenobiotics (e.g., salicylates); xenobiotics that slow gastric emptying (e.g., TCAs)
Measurement during distribution phase	Overestimation of effects	Lithium, digoxin, TCAs
Decreased binding to proteins	Underestimation of effects	Phenytoin
Saturation of binding proteins	Underestimation of effects	Salicylate, valproic acid
Binding by antidote	Variable	Digoxin/digoxin immune Fab

TCA, tricyclic antidepressant.

TABLE 6–5. Xenobiotics of Concern that are Often not Detected by Toxicology Screens

Antidysrhythmics	γ-Hydroxybutyrate
Anticholinergics	Herbal preparations
Anticoagulants	Hypoglycemics
Anticonvulsants	Iron
Antipsychotics	Isopropanol
β-Adrenergic agonists and antagonists	Ketamine
	Lithium
Calcium channel blockers	Lysergic acid diethylamide
Carbon monoxide	Methylene dioxyamphetamine
Clonidine	Methylene dioxymethamphetamine
Cyanide	Metals
"Designer drugs"	Methanol
Digoxin	Methemoglobin
Diphenhydramine	Solvents
Ethylene glycol	Serotonin reuptake inhibitors
Fentanyl	Strychnine

TABLE 6–6. Positive and Negative Predictive Values of Toxicology Screens

Sensitivity/ Specificity (%/%)	Prior Probability 10%	50%	95%
98/98 (excellent)	84%/99.8%	98%/98%	99.9%/72%
80/95 (mediocre)	64%/98%	94%/83%	99.7%/20%

benign or therapeutic levels from toxic ones. Quantitative tests may falsely suggest toxicity when drug concentrations are measured during the drug's distribution phase, which may extend for several hours with drugs such as digoxin and lithium. Moreover, the phenomenon of tolerance may allow chronic drug users to be relatively unaffected by concentrations that would be quite toxic to a non-using individual. Because comprehensive drug screens may differ widely between institutions and patterns of exposure also show substantial regional variation, there is limited ability to draw meaningful conclusions from any study of the sensitivity and specificity of such screens for detecting or excluding poisoning.

The predictive power of the result of a toxicology screen depends on a number of factors, including the likelihood of poisoning before receiving the test results (the prior probability or the prevalence), the range of xenobiotics effectively detected, and the frequency of false-positive results. It should be noted that false-positive and false-negative results may be either analytical or clinical in origin. A clinical false-positive result occurs when a xenobiotic is detected that is not contributing to the medical problem (e.g., a therapeutic amount of acetaminophen). A clinical false-negative result may occur when the wrong test is ordered (e.g., a screen for drugs of abuse for a patient with acetaminophen poisoning).

Table 6–6 explores the positive and negative predictive values of two hypothetical toxicology screens. The sensitivity of 98% and specificity of 98% in one scenario reflect the sensitivity of a broadly comprehensive toxicology screen[12] and an achievable false-positive rate of 2%. The second scenario has a sensitivity of only 80% and a specificity of 95% and represents plausible but mediocre performance. Three sets of prior probabilities are considered: 10%, 50%, and 95%. A prior probability of 10% might be seen if screening were indiscriminately applied to all patients in an emergency department or in a scenario in which xenobiotics were being excluded as a secondary cause of lethargy in an older patient who fell and struck his head. Both screens do well at excluding xenobiotics when their presence is already unlikely. However, a positive finding from either does not yield a fully convincing diagnosis of the presence of a xenobiotic. A prior probability of 50% falls into the range of prevalence actually observed in patients for whom toxicology screens were ordered (see below). In this scenario of maximum uncertainty, both screens do a good job of diagnosing poisoning, but xenobiotic exclusion by the mediocre screen will be incorrect in one of six instances.

A prior probability of 95% represents testing in which the clinical presentation strongly suggests poisoning, as in the investigation of lethargy in a known regular drug user. Although positive findings in either screen raise the probability to almost complete certainty, negative findings from the excellent screen are incorrect one time out of four, whereas negative results from the mediocre screen are wrong four times out of five. Overall, toxicology screens have better positive predictive value than negative predictive value. This observation should give pause to those who primarily order toxicology screens "to rule out poisoning."

Although only approximately 2% of laboratories offer comprehensive toxicology screening,[3] most laboratories offer some sort of testing in response to a request for a toxicology screen. This may consist of a panel of immunoassays for drugs of abuse or a urine TLC screen, or it may result in a comprehensive screening test performed at a reference laboratory. Other laboratories may offer a focused, rather than a comprehensive, screening panel. Larger laboratories may have several types of "tox screens" available for use in different situations. Among laboratories that do not limit their tests exclusively to commercially available methods, it is likely that no two will have exactly the same menu of drugs that can be reliably detected. Some laboratories address the issue of providing useful information in a timely fashion through the use of focused, rather than comprehensive, screening protocols.[34] These screens include xenobiotics locally prevalent in overdose cases or drugs for which there are specific interventions. Table 6–7 suggests the possible composition of a focused screen.

Given the trends toward increasing automation and decreasing personnel in clinical laboratories, it is relevant to ask what benefits may be derived from such testing. Studies show that comprehensive toxicologic screening has the potential to provide significant information, with utility varying with the indication for testing. The prevalence of positive results has ranged from 34% to 86% of specimens submitted for testing. When drug exposure, as predicted from the patient's history and physical examination, was compared with screening results, clinically unsuspected substances were found in 7% to 48% of the cases, and clinically suspected xenobiotics were not found in 9% to 25%.[11,12,15,24,25] However, limited utility is suggested by studies showing that the results of comprehensive screening affect management in fewer than 15% of cases,[24] and in many instances, in fewer than 5% of cases.[11,15,21,25,32] A survey of emergency physicians found that more than 75% were not fully aware of the range of drugs detected and not detected by their laboratory's toxicology screen. The majority believed that the screen was more comprehensive than it actually was.[7]

TABLE 6–7. Components of a Focused Toxicology Screen

Serum Tests	Urine Tests
Acetaminophen	Cocaine metabolite
Ethanol	Opiates
Salicylates	TCAs[a]
Tricyclic antidepressants (semiquantitative immunoassay)	
Consider including:	
Barbiturates	Amphetamines
Cooximetry[b]	Barbiturates[a]
Iron	Benzodiazepines
Lithium	Methadone
Theophylline	Phencyclidine
Valproic acid	Propoxyphene
Volatile alcohols[c]	
Other locally prevalent drugs	

[a] If not included in serum tests.

[b] Requires whole-blood specimen.

[c] Methanol, isopropanol (+ acetone).

TCA, tricyclic antidepressant.

One reason for a limited effect on management is the substantial time delay before results of comprehensive screening are available. Generally, more than 3 hours is required for the report of a negative result, and an even longer time is required for confirmation of a positive finding. By this time, most consequential management decisions have been implemented. Another possible explanation for the limited utility of screening is that comprehensive screening is largely available only in major medical centers, where consultation from a medical or clinical toxicologist is more likely to be available. Such experts may be more able to make correct diagnoses and initiate appropriate management relying on clinical findings alone.

Several recently introduced point-of-care devices are capable of rapidly screening urine for the presence of drugs of abuse, as well as TCAs. Results are typically available in 20 to 30 minutes. In a small study of one such device, diagnosis was believed to have been aided in 82% of cases, and clinical management was changed in 25%.[2] Additional studies are needed to ascertain the utility of point-of-care drug screening in emergency toxicology.[35]

A useful alternative to the toxicology screen is the toxicology hold. This is a set of serum and urine specimens drawn at the time of presentation, when xenobiotic concentrations are likely to be near maximum concentrations, and initially held refrigerated or frozen without testing. This allows a specimen to remain available for subsequent testing if needed. Most laboratories hold such specimens for several days.

BEDSIDE TOXICOLOGY TESTS

Testing at the bedside is attractive for emergency toxicology. When a specific diagnosis is being considered, a bedside test can provide confirmation or exclusion quickly and often inexpensively,[18] enabling appropriate management to be initiated. This benefit must be balanced against the generally poorer sensitivity and specificity of bedside tests in comparison with testing in the clinical laboratory, the lack of quantitative information for most tests, the lack of laboratory support, the need to perform testing in accord with regulatory requirements (see below), record-keeping issues, and the erosion of the time advantage when multiple bedside tests are done on the same patient.

Table 6–8 lists some tests that can be conveniently performed at the bedside. Spot tests can also be done at the bedside, although many spot tests use hazardous reagents that may not be suitable for use in many bedside settings. A major problem with bedside tests that are not done with commercial devices is that these are considered "highly complex" tests under federal regulations, although they may be very simple to perform. This classification results from the fact that they are not subject

TABLE 6–8. Bedside Toxicology Tests

Test	Substrate	Drug or Poison	Comments
Alcohol dehydrogenase	Saliva	Ethanol	Other alcohols may interfere. Some tests only give concentration ranges.
Breath analysis	Breath	Carbon monoxide	Ethanol may interfere.
Breath analysis	Breath	Ethanol	Good cooperation is required. Ethanol in the oral cavity interferes. Calibrated to give whole-blood rather than serum concentration.
Ferric chloride	Urine	Salicylate	Acetaminophen and phenothiazines interfere (limited utilization).
Meixner	Mushroom	Amatoxins	Paper must contain lignin (filter paper, which is lignin-free, must be used as a negative control). Requires strong acid. Some false-positives and false-negative test results have been seen
Microparticle agglutination	Urine	Drugs of abuse	KIMS variant with visual endpoint. Separate test for each drug.
Microparticle capture	Urine	Drugs of abuse	Single device detects one or more of the drugs listed in Table 6-10 in a variety of menus available from multiple manufacturers. Some multitest devices include TCAs. Higher false-positive and false-negative rates than for clinical laboratory testing.
Oxalate crystals	Urine	Ethylene glycol	Metabolic end product. Not detected during early stages. Nonspecific.

KIMS, kinetic interaction of microparticles in solution; TCA, tricyclic antidepressant.

to the validation processes required for Food and Drug Administration (FDA)–approved commercial devices. Meeting the regulations requires significant initial and ongoing investment of time. The Meixner test[1] (for amatoxins in mushrooms) and breath analysis (for ethanol or carbon monoxide from human breath) are exempted from these regulations because they are not considered to involve human specimens (see Regulatory Issues Affecting Toxicology Testing below).

In testing in overdose situations, most specimens will have either zero or very high concentrations of target analytes, and correct identification of the presence or absence of a substance is likely even with imprecise methods. Unfortunately, when point-of-care drug-screening devices have been compared with laboratory testing at concentrations near cutoff limits, performance has been variable.[33,35] An extensive study using a more representative range of urine drug concentrations observed higher rates of correct results, but performance remained inferior to that of immunoassays conducted with laboratory instrumentation.[8]

A clinical and methodologic issue with bedside drug-screening assays is whether positive results will subsequently be subjected to confirmatory testing. The extra investment of labor needed to submit a specimen tends to discourage laboratory confirmation. The argument in favor of routine confirmation is that this is an accepted standard of practice, even for screening assays that have lower false-positive rates than the point-of-care devices (see Special Considerations for Drug Abuse Screening Tests below). The counterargument is that if testing is limited to populations with a high prior probability of drug exposure, the predictive value of a positive test result is high. The NACB guidelines actually recommend against routine confirmation of positive results of drug-screening immunoassays done solely for medical reasons but suggest that all such unconfirmed positive results be reported as being "presumptive."[37]

TABLE 6–9. Major Clinical Laboratory Improvement Amendments (CLIA) Requirements for Laboratory Testing

Waived Tests
Certificate of waiver
Follow manufacturer's instructions exactly
Moderate-Complexity Tests
CLIA certificate
Record keeping
Test method verification
Written procedures
Qualified laboratory director
Personnel educational requirements
Documented training of all testing personnel
Annual competency testing of all personnel
Two levels of controls daily
Participate in proficiency testing every 4 months
Verify calibration and reportable range at least every 6 months
Quality assessment program
Biennial inspection and certification
High-Complexity Tests
All moderate-complexity requirements *plus*
Qualified onsite supervisor *or*
Daily review of all results by qualified supervisor

This table lists only the most significant requirements of the regulations implementing CLIA. These regulations continue to evolve. Accrediting agencies such as the Joint Commission may have additional requirements. Consultation with the clinical laboratory or with an institutional point-of-care coordinator is recommended before implementing any testing.

REGULATORY ISSUES AFFECTING TOXICOLOGY TESTING

Since 1992, medical laboratory testing has been governed by federal regulations (42 CFR part 405 et seq) issued under the authority of the Clinical Laboratory Improvement Amendments of 1988 (often referred to as CLIA-88 or simply CLIA). These regulations apply to all laboratory testing of human specimens for medical purposes, regardless of site. They include the universal requirement for possession of an appropriate certificate to perform even the simplest of tests. The remaining requirements depend on the complexity of the test. These regulations become important to the clinician whenever testing is done at the bedside, whether using spot tests or commercial point-of-care devices such as dipsticks, glucose meters, or urine drug-screening devices.

The regulations divide testing into three categories: waived, moderate complexity, and high complexity. Waived tests include a number of specifically designated simple tests, including urine dipsticks, urine pregnancy tests, urine drug-screening immunoassay devices, and blood glucose measurements with a hand-held monitor. The only legal requirement for performing waived testing are the possession of an appropriate CLIA certificate (certificate of waiver or higher) and performance of the test in accordance with the manufacturer's instructions.

There are substantial additional requirements for both moderate and highly complex testing, most of which simply represent good laboratory practice. Table 6–9 lists the most significant of these requirements. Most assays performed with commercial kits or devices are classified as belonging to the moderately complex category. All tests not specifically classified as waived or moderately complex are considered highly complex. This includes essentially all noncommercial tests, including spot tests, because the testing materials have not been subject to review and approval by the FDA.

These regulations have had a substantial impact in all areas of laboratory testing. Some of the most significant effects have been on bedside testing, including spot tests and point-of-care devices. Although clinical laboratories had been following most required practices before the implementation of the regulations, this was usually not the case for testing done at other sites. Most institutions have now established point-of-care testing programs to facilitate compliance with the regulations, as well as with additional requirements of accrediting agencies, such as the Joint Commission. Any toxicologic or other testing done at the point of care should be set up in consultation with the institutional program. Often, all point-of-care testing is done under a CLIA certificate held by the program. There is frequently a point-of-care testing coordinator who may make recommendations or personally assist in efficiently addressing the assorted requirements.

However, such testing may be covered by state laws or by institutional or accrediting agency policies. The NACB guidelines recommend that breath testing be overseen by the clinical laboratory and meet the same standards as other point-of-care testing.[37]

Personnel unaccustomed to quality control and assessment practices may find the CLIA requirements initially burdensome. Nonetheless, compliance is important. Following these practices may lead to a threefold reduction in incorrect results,[31] thereby greatly improving the quality of care provided to the patient. Moreover, noncompliant testing is illegal under federal law and may also be illegal under state law. Any untoward outcome associated with illegal testing creates a major risk management liability for both the institution and the individual. Additionally, billing for any testing that is not CLIA compliant may be considered fraudulent.

Another area in which the CLIA regulations have impacted toxicology testing is in the provision of infrequently requested tests. Meeting regulatory requirements involves a substantial labor investment even when few patient specimens are being tested. Mounting pressures to reduce laboratory costs make it less likely that laboratories will continue to maintain such assays.

Another important regulation, although not part of CLIA regulations, requires that the medical reason for ordering a test be provided with the order. Federal regulations require that the ordering physician provide the diagnosis that establishes the medical necessity for the test, either by name or by diagnostic code (CPT code). Laboratories may not use a "best guess" to assign codes to undocumented test requests.

SPECIAL CONSIDERATIONS FOR DRUG ABUSE SCREENING TESTS

Testing for drugs of abuse is a significant component of medical toxicology testing. These tests are widely used in the evaluation of potential poisonings and are assuming an increasing role is assuring the appropriate use of pain medications.[28] Initial testing is usually done with a screening immunoassay. Although drug-screening immunoassays were initially developed for use in workplace drug-screening programs and are not always optimal for medical purposes, their wide availability low cost and ease of use formats led to their nearly universal adoption in clinical laboratories. Growth of the market for medical drug screening has led to the development of point-of-care tests specifically for medical use, but these devices largely retain the deficiencies of their predecessors. Drug abuse testing for nonmedical reasons is generally considered to be forensic testing, and confirmation of immunoassay results is considered mandatory in such circumstances. Confirmatory testing can compensate for some immunoassay shortcomings but is frequently not performed when screening tests are done for medical purposes. Despite the widespread use of drug-screening immunoassays in medical practice, studies suggest that many physicians do not fully understand the capabilities and limitations of these tests.[28]

The most commonly tested-for drugs are amphetamines, cannabinoids, cocaine, opiates, and phencyclidine. These are often referred to as the NIDA 5, because they are the five drugs that were recommended in 1988 by the National Institute on Drug Abuse (NIDA) for drug screening of federal employees. (Responsibility for recommendations for federal drug testing now lies with the Substance Abuse and Mental Health Services Administration [SAMHSA].) Drug-screening immunoassays are also frequently done for barbiturates and benzodiazepines and less frequently for meperidine, methadone, and propoxyphene. Drug-screening devices intended primarily for medical use may also include tests for acetaminophen or TCAs. Table 6–10 lists some of the general characteristics of these tests. Commercial urine immunoassays are also available for buprenorphine, lysergic acid diethylamide, methaqualone, methylenedioxymethamphetamine (MDMA), and oxycodone. Drug-screening immunoassays are available in a number of formats, which may differ in performance. Almost all of them are designed to be used with urine specimens because these can be obtained noninvasively and generally have higher concentrations than serum, enhancing the sensitivity of the test.

The drug-screening tests for cannabinoids and cocaine are directed toward inactive drug metabolites rather than the active parent compound. The parent drugs, cocaine and tetrahydrocannabinol, are both short lived and persist for no more than a few hours after use. The metabolites remain present substantially longer. Detection of the metabolites increases the ability to detect any recent drug use. However, this limits the utility of the assays for determining whether a patient is currently under the influence of the drug. Because the metabolites are rapidly formed, a negative test result generally excludes toxicity, but a positive test result indicates only use in the recent past, not current toxicity.

To increase sensitivity for detection of less-recent drug use, substrates other than urine can be used for drug screening, including hair and meconium. The latter is used to document intrauterine drug exposure (Chap. 30). SAMHSA is planning to develop regulations governing the use of hair, saliva, and sweat specimens for federal workplace testing after their performance characteristics have been adequately studies. This can be expected to increase the availability of clinical testing using these substrates. However, testing performed on hair and sweat are unlikely to offer advantages over testing of serum and urine for the management of toxicologic emergencies.

The stigma attached to a positive test result for an abused drug requires that special care be exercised in performing and reporting the test results. To protect citizens' rights, many states have legislated specific requirements for workplace drug screening. In some states, the requirements apply only to screening in the workplace, exempting testing for medical purposes. Laws in other states might apply to all drug screening. Although they are not always legally required, some workplace drug-screening practices have been widely applied to all drug screening.

The use of specific cutoff concentrations is nearly universal. Test results are considered positive only when the concentration of drugs in the specimen exceeds a predetermined threshold. This threshold should be set sufficiently high that false-positive results as a consequence of analytic variability or cross-reactivity are extremely infrequent. They should also be low enough to consistently give a positive result in persons who are using drugs. Cutoff concentrations used vary with the drug or drug class under investigation. In some drug-screening immunoassays, the laboratory has the option of selecting from several cutoff values.

The use of cutoff values sometimes creates confusion when a patient who is known to have recently used a drug has a negative result reported on a drug screen. In such instances, the drug is usually present but at a concentration below the cutoff value. Another potential problem occurs when a patient's drug-screening test result is positive after previously having become negative. This is usually interpreted as indicating renewed drug use, but it may actually be an artifact. Urine drug concentrations are directly proportional to the serum drug concentrations but inversely proportional to the rate of urine production. The rate of the urine flow may vary up to 100-fold, with a resulting possible 100-fold change in the urine drug concentration. This effect is often exploited by individuals who drink large quantities of water before taking a urine drug test to increase urine flow and decrease urine drug concentrations. In contrast, a decrease in the rate of urine production may result in a positive test result following a negative one despite no new drug exposure. A similar effect may be produced by changes in urine pH. Drugs containing a basic nitrogen may demonstrate ionic trapping, with increasing concentrations as urine pH decreases. Similarly, excretion of the phenobarbital anion may increase with increasing urine pH. This phenomenon is medically exploited by alkalinizing the urine to increase phenobarbital excretion.

TABLE 6–10. Performance Characteristics of Common Drug Abuse Screening Immunoassays[a]

Drug/Class	Detection Limits[b]	Confirmation Limits[b]	Detection Interval[c]	Comments
Amphetamines	1000 ng/mL	500 ng/mL amphetamine or MDMA	1–2 d (2–4 d)	Decongestants, ephedrine, *l*-methamphetamine, selegilene and bupropion metabolites may give false-positives test results; MDA and MDMA are variably detected. Confirmation of methamphetamine requires detection of >500 ng/mL with >200 ng/mL of metabolite, amphetamine.
Barbiturates	200 ng/mL Secobarbital		2–4 d	Phenobarbital may be detected for up to 4 weeks.
Benzodiazepines	100–300 ng/mL		1–30 d	Benzodiazepines vary in reactivity and potency. Hydrolysis of glucuronides increases sensitivity. False-positive test results maybe be seen with oxaprozin.
Cannabinoids	50 ng/mL; 20ng/mL; 25 ng/mL; 100ng/mL THCA	15 ng/mL THCA	1–3 d (>1 mo)	Screening assays detect inactive and active cannabinoids; confirmatory assay detects inactive metabolite THCA. Duration of positivity is highly dependent on screening assay detection limits.
Cocaine	300 ng/mL BE	150 ng/mL BE	2 d (1 wk)	Screening and confirmatory assays detect inactive metabolite BE. False-positive test results are unlikely.
Opiates	2000 ng/mL; 300 ng/mL	2000 ng/mL; morphine or codeine	1–2 d; 2–4 d (<1 wk)	>10 ng/mL of heroin metabolite 6-monoacetyl morphine is also confirmatory. Semisynthetic opiates derived from morphine show variable cross-reactivity. Fully synthetic opioids (e.g., fentanyl, meperidine, methadone, propoxyphene, tramadol) have minimal cross-reactivity. Quinolones may cross-react.
Methadone	300 ng/mL		1–4 d	Doxylamine may cross-react.
Phencyclidine	25 ng/mL	25 ng/mL	4–7 d (>1 mo)	Dextromethorphan, diphenhydramine, ketamine, and venlafaxine may cross-react.
Propoxyphene	300 ng/mL		3–10 d	Duration of positivity depends on cross-reactivity of metabolite norpropoxyphene.

[a] Performance characteristics vary with manufacturer and may change over time. for the most accurate information, consult the package insert of the current lot or contact the manufacturer.

[b] Substance Abuse and Mental Health Services Administration recommendations[5] are shown as the first value for amphetamines, cannabinoids, cocaine, opiates, and phencyclidine immunoassays and as only values for confirmatory assays. Other commercial immunoassay cutoffs are also listed. Other gas spectrometry cutoffs are set by the laboratory.

[c] Values are after typical use; values in parentheses are after heavy or prolonged use.

BE, benzoylecgonine; MDA, methylenedioxyamphetamine; MDMA, methylenedioxymethamphetamine; THCA, tetrahydrocannabinoic acid.

Another widely used practice is the confirmation of positive screening results using an analytical methodology different from that used in the screen, such as an immunoassay screen followed by chromatographic confirmation. The possibility of simultaneous false-positive results by two distinct methods is quite low. Clinical laboratories may differ in their policies with regard to confirmatory testing. Some may confirm all positive results from screening immunoassays, but others may not provide any confirmatory testing unless it is explicitly requested.

The most common confirmatory method is gas chromatography/mass spectrometry (GS/MS). The high specificity afforded by the combination of the retention time and the mass spectrum makes false-positive results extremely unlikely. GC/MS also has greater sensitivity than the screening immunoassays, minimizing failed confirmations because of drug concentrations below the sensitivity of the confirmatory assay. Some states require GC/MS confirmation for workplace drug screening, and it may be legally required for all drug screening.

Immunoassay results can generally be obtained within 1 hour. Confirmatory testing usually requires at least several hours. This can create a problem when confirmation of initial immunoassay results is considered mandatory. Most laboratories provide a verbal report of a presumptive positive result to facilitate medical management but may not enter the result into a permanent record, such as the laboratory computer, until after confirmation has been completed.

The importance of confirmatory testing in workplace drug screening follows from the relatively low prevalence of positive results. A screening test with both sensitivity and specificity of 98% will produce two false-positive results per 100 subjects tested. A workforce with a 2% prevalence of illicit drug use will yield two true-positive results per 100 subjects. The predictive value of a positive test will only be 50% (two of four). This is an unacceptable level of certainty for results that might be used to terminate employment. Although the prevalence of recent drug use in the workforce is low, rates of positivity of 34% to 86% have been reported for selective drug screening of emergency department populations. Given a 50% prevalence of recent drug use, the positive predictive value of same screening test increases to 98% (see Table 6–6).

A high prior probability of drug positivity for patients tested in medical settings results in a very high posterior probability after a positive test result. Confirmatory testing is much less critical in such a setting, particularly because a positive finding infrequently has consequences that extend beyond the medical management of the patient. An exception may occur when results of testing performed on motor vehicle crash victims can be subsequently subpoenaed as evidence in legal proceedings. Confirmatory testing also becomes more important in drug abuse testing associated with chronic pain management programs, in which unexpected findings may result in termination of care. Chromatographic tests that identify individual opiates can distinguish between prescribed and nonprescribed drugs.

One workplace drug-screening practice that is not widely followed in medical toxicology is maintenance of a chain of custody. Employers generally insist on chain of custody for workplace testing because actions taken in response to a positive result may be contested in court. A chain of custody provides results that are readily defended in court. Laboratories providing testing for medical purposes rarely keep a chain of custody because it is quite expensive and does not benefit the patient. Additionally, the medical personnel responsible for obtaining the specimens are rarely trained in collection requirements for a chain of custody.

The lack of chain of custody may create problems when persons with no medical complaints present at an emergency department or other medical facility requesting the performance of a drug-screening test. Unless the facility is prepared to initiate the chain of custody at the time of specimen collection and the laboratory is prepared to maintain it, such persons should be redirected to a site maintained by a commercial laboratory that routinely performs workplace drug testing and has appropriate procedures in place. Many laboratories have had the experience of unwittingly performing drug abuse testing for nonmedical purposes because the reason for the testing is not always included on the test requisition. To avoid liability issues, the laboratory may choose to include a disclaimer with every drug-screening report indicating that the results are for purposes of medical management only.

Another practice common in workplace testing but rare in medical laboratories is testing for specimen validity. It is common for individuals to try to "beat" a workplace drug test through a variety of means, including diluting the specimen (either physiologically by water ingestion or by direct addition of water to the specimen), substituting "clean" urine obtained from another individual, or adding various substances that will either destroy drugs in the specimen or inactivate the enzymes or antibodies used in the screening immunoassays. Such substances include acids, bases, oxidizing agents (bleach, nitrite, peroxide, peroxidase, iodine, chromate), glutaraldehyde, pyridine, niacin detergents, and soap. SAMHSA requires validity testing for all specimens in federal workplace testing, including measurement of urinary pH, specific gravity, and creatinine concentration, as well as tests for the presence of adulterants.[5] Dipsticks are available that detect the most common adulterants. However, manipulation or adulteration is rarely a problem in medical specimens, and clinical laboratories infrequently provide validity testing.

PERFORMANCE CHARACTERISTICS OF COMMON DRUG-SCREENING ASSAYS

Medical toxicologists, toxicology laboratory directors, and practicing physicians may frequently get questions about the significance of drug-screening assays, particularly about the causes of false-positive results. Often these questions come from an individual who recently had a positive test result. Table 6–10 summarizes drug-screening test performance characteristics, which are discussed in more detail below.

Immunoassays for opiates are directed toward morphine but have good cross-reactivity with many (but not all) structurally similar natural and semisynthetic opiates. The extent of cross-reactivity may vary between manufacturers. For example, oxycodone exhibits approximately 30% cross-reactivity relative to morphine in a fluorescence polarization immunoassay but less than 5% cross-reactivity in a number of other screening assays.[17,28] A failure to appreciate the poor detection of oxycodone can create problems when opiate-screening immunoassays are used to confirm that patients receiving prescription oxycodone for chronic pain are indeed taking it rather than diverting it for illicit sale. If a low cross-reactivity assay is used, a patient taking oxycodone as prescribed might have a negative result, but another patient who is selling the oxycodone and using the proceeds to buy heroin would have a positive result. To address this problem, assays specific for oxycodone have been introduced. These assays are sensitive to therapeutic amounts of oxycodone but relatively insensitive to other opiates.

Synthetic opioids, such as dextromethorphan, fentanyl, meperidine, methadone, propoxyphene, and tramadol, show little or no cross-reactivity in opiate immunoassays. Urine immunoassays specific for meperidine, methadone, and propoxyphene are available. Given the increasing importance of buprenorphine as maintenance therapy for opiate dependency, it is worth noting that the combination of high potency and low cross-reactivity means that buprenorphine will generally not be detected by opiate immunoassays. Immunoassays for detection of buprenorphine have therefore been developed.

A positive immunoassay result may reflect multiple contributions from various opiates and opiate metabolites. Concentrations of morphine glucuronide in the urine may be up to 10-fold higher than the concentrations of unchanged morphine and can contribute substantially to positive results. A positive opiate result after the use of heroin (diacetylmorphine) is primarily a result of the morphine and morphine glucuronide that result from heroin metabolism. Distinguishing heroin from other opiates requires detection of 6-monoacetylmorphine, the heroin-specific metabolite. Small amounts of the metabolite may be detected by GC/MS for up to 24 hours after use. A half-life of 5 minutes means that unchanged heroin can only be found in the urine if sampling is done immediately after use.

The duration of positivity of an opiate immunoassay after last use depends on the identity and amount of the opiate used, the specific immunoassay, the cutoff value, and the pharmacokinetics of the individual. Currently, SAMHSA recommends a cutoff equivalent to 2000 ng/mL of morphine for workplace screening because poppy seeds can rarely produce transient positive results with the previously recommended cutoff of 300 ng/mL. However, most toxicology laboratories continue to use a 300 ng/mL cutoff.

Drug-screening assays for "cocaine" are actually assays for the inactive cocaine metabolite benzoylecgonine, which is eliminated more slowly than cocaine. This extends the duration of positivity after last use from a few hours to 2 days and sometimes to a week or longer after prolonged heavy use. Because the assay is directed toward an inactive metabolite, positive results do not equate with toxicity but merely indicate recent exposure. The assay is highly specific for benzoylecgonine, and false-positive results are extremely uncommon (Chap. 76).

Immunoassays for cannabinoids are also directed toward an inactive metabolite, in this case tetrahydrocannabinoic acid. These immunoassays exhibit cross-reactivity with other cannabinoids but little else. Because cannabinoids are structurally unique and occur only in plants of the genus *Cannabis*, false–positive results are quite uncommon (Chap. 83) It is unusual, although possible, to become exposed to sufficient "second-hand" or sidestream marijuana smoke to develop a positive urine test result.[4] Legal hemp products include fiber, oil, and seedcake derived from *Cannabis* varieties with low concentrations of cannabinoids. Hemp food products contain insufficient amounts of tetrahydrocannabinol to produce psychoactive effects and usually will not increase urinary cannabinoid concentrations above a 50 ng/mL screening threshold.[10,28]

Interpretation of a positive result for cannabinoids can be problematic. Urine may be positive for up to 3 days after occasional recreational use. However, with heavy or prolonged use, there may be significant accumulation of cannabinoids in adipose tissue. These stored cannabinoids are slowly released into the bloodstream and can produce positive findings for 1 month or more. Consequently, little can be concluded from a positive finding in terms of current toxicity. Because positive results in the absence of toxicity are very common and because tetrahydrocannabinol is rarely responsible for serious acute toxicity, NACB guidelines recommend against its routine inclusion in drug screening for patients with acute symptoms.[37]

Amphetamine-screening tests have the greatest problems with false-positive results. A number of structurally related compounds may have significant cross-reactivity, including bupropion metabolites and nonprescription decongestants such as pseudoephedrine, as well as *l*-ephedrine, which is found in a variety of herbal preparations. Some over-the counter nasal inhalers contain *l*-methamphetamine, the less potent levorotary isomer of *d*-methamphetamine. It is particularly problematic because it not only cross-reacts in immunoassays but also cannot be distinguished from the *d*-isomer by mass spectrometry.[10] This cross-reactivity is beneficial from the point of view of the medical toxicologist because all of these compounds may produce serious stimulant toxicity. But it is problematic in drug abuse screening because of the widespread legitimate use of cold medications. Assays with greater selectivity for amphetamine or methamphetamine have been developed. Although these assays produce fewer false-positive results caused by decongestant cross-reactivity, they are also less sensitive for the detection of other abused amphetamine-like compounds, including methylenedioxyamphetamine (MDA), MDMA, and phentermine. Cross-reactivity patterns vary from assay to assay.[17] The manufacturer's literature should be consulted for specific details.

Testing for benzodiazepines is complicated by the wide array of benzodiazepines that differ substantially in their potency, cross-reactivity, and half-lives. There are also substantial differences in the detection patterns of the various immunoassays.[10,17] This heterogeneity complicates the interpretation of benzodiazepine-screening assays. Screening results may be positive in persons using low therapeutic doses of diazepam but negative after an overdose of a highly potent benzodiazepine such as clonazepam. To improve the scope of detection, some assays use antibodies to oxazepam, which is a metabolite of a number of different benzodiazepines. These assays may have poor sensitivity to benzodiazepines that are not metabolized to oxazepam. False-negative results may occur for benzodiazepines that are excreted in the urine almost entirely as glucuronides that have poor cross-reactivity with antibodies directed toward an unmodified benzodiazepine. This is one reason for the poor detectability of lorazepam in some screening assays. The latter situation has led to the recommendation that specimens be treated with β-glucuronidase before analysis.[20] Some assays now include β-glucuronidase in the reagent mixture or use antibodies directed toward glucuronidated metabolites. The frequency of false-negative results, as well as the fact that benzodiazepines are relatively benign in overdose, have led the NACB guidelines to withhold recommendation for routine screening of urine for benzodiazepines until these problems with the immunoassays are addressed.[37]

Barbiturates are comparable to benzodiazepines in their heterogeneity of potency, cross-reactivity, and half-lives, although the differences are less substantial. Specific assays for serum phenobarbital can often help to clarify the significance of a positive barbiturate screen.

Some phencyclidine screening assays may give positive results with dextromethorphan, ketamine, or diphenhydramine but only when these are used in amounts above usual therapeutic quantities. A positive result may serve as a clue to a possible overdose with any of these substances. Furthermore, much of the illicit phencyclidine (PCP) actually consists of a mixture of various congers and byproducts of synthesis. The cross-reactivity of these xenobiotics with the assay varies significantly and may result in false-negative assay results in patients who use PCP.

MEASUREMENT OF ETHANOL CONCENTRATIONS

Measuring ethanol may have ramifications beyond guiding medical management, particularly when performed on crash victims. Although testing for ethanol in urine is common in workplace drug screening, most testing in clinical laboratories is done using serum or plasma. Concentrations are most commonly measured enzymatically using alcohol dehydrogenase. In larger toxicology laboratories, ethanol measurements are often done using a GC assay that can also distinguish and measure isopropanol and methanol, as well as the isopropanol metabolite acetone. Alcohols with lower volatility, including ethylene and propylene glycol, are usually not detected by this assay. Because both enzymatic and chromatographic assays have substantial specificity for ethanol, confirmatory testing with a second method is uncommon.

Breath alcohol analyzers may also be used in assessing ethanol intoxication, as may point-of-care devices that measure salivary ethanol. These measurements are less precise than laboratory assays[14,30] and are more subject to interference by other alcohols and other organic solvents. Breath-alcohol analyzers require good cooperation from the patient to obtain an appropriate breath sample and are typically calibrated to give results approximating whole-blood alcohol concentrations. For the above reasons, confirmation of positive findings with a laboratory measurement may sometimes be desirable.

Blood alcohol concentrations used legally to define driving under the influence have no particular clinical significance but may have risk management implications for patient discharge. Whereas legal standards are written in terms of whole-blood alcohol concentrations, clinical laboratories usually measure alcohol in serum or plasma. Serum and plasma alcohol concentrations are essentially identical, but both will be higher than the alcohol concentration measured in a whole-blood specimen obtained at the same time. This is a result of the lower concentration of alcohol in the red blood cells. The ratio of serum alcohol to whole-blood alcohol varies from individual to individual, with a median value of 1.15.[27] It is more likely than not that an individual with a serum alcohol concentration of less than 92 mg/dL will have a whole-blood alcohol concentration of less than 80 mg/dL (<0.10%, w/v) (Chap. 77).

FOR MORE INFORMATION

For additional information about clinical toxicology laboratories, including topics not covered in this chapter, a recommended reference is *The Clinical Toxicology Laboratory: Contemporary Practice of Poisoning Evaluation*.[29]

REFERENCES

1. Beutler JA, Vergeer PP: Amatoxins in American mushrooms: Evaluation of the Meixner test. *Mycologia.* 1980;72:1142-1149.
2. Buck C, Brunner D, Otten E, et al: Evaluation of rapid urine toxicological testing in patients with altered mental status in the emergency department [abstract]. *J Toxicol Clin Toxicol.* 1999;37:597-598.

3. College of American Pathologists Participant Summaries: *Chemistry Survey Set C-A; Serum Alcohol/Volatiles Survey Set AL2-A; Therapeutic Drug Monitoring (General) Survey Set Z-A; Toxicology Survey Set T-A; Urine Drug Testing (Screening) Set UDS-A; Urine Toxicology Survey Set UT-A.* Northfield, Illinois: College of American Pathologists; 2004.
4. Cone EJ, Johnson RE, Darwin WD, et al: Passive inhalation of marijuana smoke: Urinalysis and room air levels of delta-9-tetrahydrocannabinol. *J Anal Toxicol.* 1987;11:9-96.
5. Department of Health and Human Services, Substance Abuse and Mental Health Services Administration: Mandatory guidelines and proposed revisions to mandatory guidelines for federal workplace drug testing programs. *Fed Reg.* 2004;69:19644-19673.
6. Destache CJ, Meyer SK, Rowley KM: Does accepting pharmacokinetic recommendations impact hospitalization? A cost-benefit analysis. *Thera Drug Monit.* 1990;12:427-433.
7. Durback LF, Scharman EJ, Brown BS: Emergency physicians' perceptions of drug screens at their own hospitals. *Vet Hum Toxicol.* 1998;40:234-237.
8. Ferrara SD, Tedeschi L, Frison G, et al: Drugs-of-abuse testing in urine: Statistical approach and experimental comparison of immunochemical and chromatographic techniques. *J Anal Toxicol.* 1994;18:278-291.
9. Franke JP, de Zeeuw RA: Solid-phase extraction procedures in systematic toxicological analysis. *J Chromatogr B.* 1998;713:51-59.
10. Gourlay DL, Caplan YH, Heit HA: *Urine Drug Testing in Clinical Practice*, 3rd ed. http://www.familydocs.org/files/UDTmonograph.pdf. Accessed August 12, 2008.
11. Hammett-Stabler CA, Pesce AJ, Cannon DJ: Urine drug screening in the medical setting. *Clin Chim Acta.* 2002;315:125-135.
12. Hepler BR, Sutheimer CA, Sunshine I: The role of the toxicology laboratory in emergency medicine. II. Study of an integrated approach. *J Toxicol Clin Toxicol.* 1984–85;22:503-528.
13. Jarvie DR, Simpson D: Drug screening: Evaluation of the Toxi-Lab TLC system. *Ann Clin Biochem.* 1986;23:76-84.
14. Keim ME, Bartfield JM, Raccio-Robak N, et al: Accuracy of an enzymatic assay device for serum ethanol measurement. *J Toxicol Clin Toxicol.* 1999;37:75-81.
15. Kellermann AL, Fihn SD, Logerfro JP, et al: Impact of drug screening in suspected overdose. *Ann Emerg Med.* 1987;16:1206-1216.
16. Kwong TC: Free drug measurements: Methodology and clinical significance. *Clin Chim Acta.* 1985;151:193-216.
17. Magnani B: Concentrations of compounds that produce positive results. In: Shaw LM, Kwong TC, Rosano TG, et al., eds. *The Clinical Toxicology Laboratory: Contemporary Practice of Poisoning Evaluation.* Washington, DC: AACC Press:, 2001:481-497.
18. Mastrovitch TA, Bithoney WG, DeBari VA, Gold NA: Point-of-care testing for drugs of abuse in an urban emergency department. *Ann Clin Lab Sci.* 2002;32:383-386.
19. Maurer HH: Current role of liquid chromatography-mass spectrometry in clinical and forensic toxicology. *Anal Bioanal Chem.* 2007;388:1315–1325.
20. Meatherall R: Benzodiazepine screening using EMIT II and TDx: Urine hydrolysis pretreatment required. *J Anal Toxicol.* 1994;18:385-390.
21. Montague RE, Grace RF, Lewis JH, Shenfield GM: Urine drug screens in overdose patients do not contribute to immediate clinical management. *Ther Drug Monit.* 2001;23:47-50.
22. National Poisons Information Service, Association of Clinical Biochemists: Laboratory analyses for poisoned patients: Joint position paper. *Ann Clin Biochem.* 2002;39:328-339.
23. Nixon AL, Long WH, Puopolo PR, Flood JG. Bupropion metabolites produce false-positive urine amphetamine results: *Clin Chem.* 1995;41:955-956.
24. Osterloh JD: Utility and reliability of emergency toxicologic testing. *Emerg Med Clin North Am.* 1990;8:693-723.
25. Pohjola-Sintonen S, Kivisto KT, Vuori E, et al: Identification of drugs ingested in acute poisoning: Correlation of patient history with drug analyses. *Ther Drug Monit.* 2000;22:749-752.
26. Rainey PM: Digibind and free digoxin. *Clin Chem.* 1999;45:719-720.
27. Rainey PM: Relationship between serum and whole-blood ethanol concentrations. *Clin Chem.* 1993;39:2288-2292.
28. Reisfeld GM, Salazar E, Bertholf RL: Rational use and interpretation of urine drug testing in chronic opioid therapy. *Ann Clin Lab Sci.* 2007; 4:301-314.
29. Shaw LM, Kwong TC, Rosano TG, et al, eds: *The Clinical Toxicology Laboratory: Contemporary Practice of Poisoning Evaluation.* Washington, DC: AACC Press; 2001.
30. Simpson G: Accuracy and precision of breath-alcohol measurements for a random subject in the postabsorptive state. *Clin Chem.* 1987;33:261-268.
31. Stull TM, Hearn TL, Hancock JS, et al: Variation in proficiency testing performance by testing site. *JAMA.* 1998;279:463-467.
32. Sugarman JM, Rodgers GC, Paul RI: Utility of toxicology screening in a pediatric emergency department. *Pediatr Emerg Care.* 1997;13:194-197.
33. von Mach MA, Weber C, Meyer MR, et al: Comparison of urinary on-site immunoassay screening and gas chromatography-mass spectrometry results of 111 patients with suspected poisoning presenting at an emergency department. *Ther Drug Monit.* 2007;29:27-39.
34. Warner A: Setting standards of practice in therapeutic drug monitoring and clinical toxicology: A North American view. *Ther Drug Monit.* 2000;22:93-97.
35. Watson ID, Bertholf R, Hammett-Stabler C, et al: Drugs and ethanol. In Nichols JH, ed. *Evidence-Based Practice for Point-of-Care Testing.* http://www.aacc.org/members/nacb/LMPG/OnlineGuide/PublishedGuidelines/poct/Pages/poctpdf.aspx. Accessed June 2, 2008.
36. Wiley JF II: Difficult diagnoses in toxicology. Poisons not detected by the comprehensive drug screen. *Pediatr Clin North Am.* 1991;38:725-737.
37. Wu AH, McKay C, Broussard LA, et al: National Academy of Clinical Biochemistry laboratory medicine practice guidelines: Recommendations for the use of laboratory tests to support poisoned patients who present to the emergency department. *Clin Chem.* 2003;49:357-379.

CHAPTER 7
TECHNIQUES USED TO PREVENT GASTROINTESTINAL ABSORPTION

Anne-Bolette Gude and Lotte C. G. Hoegberg

Gastrointestinal (GI) decontamination is a controversial issue in medical toxicology. It plays a central role in the initial management of orally poisoned patients and frequently is the only treatment available other than routine supportive care. Unfortunately, as is true in most areas of medical toxicology, valid studies that demonstrate the effects of GI decontamination on clinically meaningful endpoints are difficult to find. The heterogeneity of poisoned patients demands that very large randomized studies be performed because most patients who present to an emergency department (ED) have an unreliable history and a low-risk exposure. These factors, as well as other significant sources of bias, are often hidden in inclusion and exclusion criteria of the available studies. The numerous consequential determinants contribute to the difficulties in designing and completing studies that provide sound evidence for or against a particular therapeutic option. Incontrovertible endpoints, such as complication-specific mortality, also demand exceptionally large studies because the overall morbidity and mortality of poisoned patients is quite low. Whereas other endpoints, such as the length of stay in the hospital or intensive care unit (ICU), change in xenobiotic concentration, the rate of secondary complications, and the need for specific treatments such as expensive antidotes, must be considered, these surrogate markers are not adequately rigorous and are inadequately precise measures of morbidity. In the science of GI decontamination, we are also faced with the dilemma that randomizing half of a group of potentially ill patients to no decontamination is a significant ethical concern—we rarely omit decontamination unless a minimally toxic exposure has occurred or an effective, safe, readily available, and inexpensive antidote exists. Because acetaminophen meets many of these parameters, it has been used both as the xenobiotic of choice in volunteer overdose studies[28,59,67,159] and in a recent Australian evaluation of actually poisoned patients.[37] However, despite its widespread use as a model, the applicability of the management approach for acetaminophen poisoning to other ingestions is limited.

As might be suspected, no available study provides adequate guidance for the management of a patient who has definitely ingested an unknown xenobiotic at an unknown time. Fortunately, in most cases, there is some component of the history or clinical presentation, such as vital signs, physical examination, and focused diagnostic studies such as an ECG and anion gap, that might offer insight into the nature of the ingested xenobiotic (Chap. 3).

For many, the ongoing controversy or debate on GI decontamination culminated in 1997 with the publication of the position statements on activated charcoal, orogastric lavage, syrup of ipecac induced emesis, and whole-bowel irrigation (WBI) from the American Academy of Clinical Toxicology (AACT) and the European Association of Poisons Centres and Clinical Toxicologists (EAPCCT).[29,86,124,125,142,151-153] Contrary to initial expectations, these excellent reviews failed to end the debate; they simply highlighted many shortcomings and ambiguities within this field. A 2000 study concluded that despite having the evidence reviewed and consensus recommendations made, poison specialists at North American poison centers still offered a wide variety of recommendations for GI decontamination.[79] The study evaluated decontamination options for a theoretical patient with a difficult scenario of an overdose of enteric-coated aspirin. The recommendations made were often inconsistent with the published position statements, and in some cases, were frankly dangerous. Even toxicologists who made substantial contributions to the development of these consensus statements disagreed on certain aspects of the treatment, although to a lesser extent. In a similar study, when an interactive questionnaire was sent to 14 European Poison Centers, significant differences in the protocols for the recommended method of GI decontamination, timing, and intervention doses were found.[58] These differences suggest that there is inadequate evidence available to produce a proper evidence-based answer for many of the decisions in question. In most of the clinical studies that provide evidence to form the basis for the consensus statements, either there are very few patients with consequential ingestions included, or these specific patients were excluded from the study. Similarly, there are no studies for most drugs with modified release kinetics or for newly marketed drugs. Thus, the clinician must often make decisions based on a philosophical approach and an understanding of specific principles rather than evidence.

More recent studies investigating the trends in GI decontamination in both the advice given by poison centers and the clinical setting show a considerable decline in the use of all methods of decontamination.[29,88,95] One study specifically evaluating orogastric lavage found that during the years 1993 to 1997, an average of 18.7% of all poisoned patients received orogastric lavage compared with an average of 10.3% of poisoned patients during the years 1998 to 2003. The decline in the use of GI decontamination after the publication of the position statements is also probably a result of the epidemiologic shift in the developed world away from overdoses of more lethal substances, such as barbiturates and tricyclic antidepressants, to benzodiazepines and serotonergic reuptake inhibitors, with a natural resultant decrease in morbidity and mortality. Although true, for the Western world, studies in developing countries indicate a different pattern of poisonings with patients ingesting xenobiotics such as organic phosphorus compounds and other pesticides and herbicides with a more lethal toxicologic profile.[45]

This chapter does not discuss details with regard to the evaluation of the amount and type of xenobiotic ingested or other strategies for managing a patient with an unknown overdose; these issues are discussed in Chapter 4. Rather, the focus is on determining which decontamination technique or combination of techniques is preferred after an indication for GI decontamination has been established. The literature published since the previously mentioned position statements is emphasized, existing evidence is summarized, and areas necessitating further investigation are identified. Detailed discussions of emesis, catharsis, and activated charcoal can be found in the corresponding Antidotes in Depth sections, Syrup of Ipecac, Whole-Bowel Irrigation and Other Intestinal Evacuants, and Activated Charcoal. In addition, when the ingested xenobiotic is known, readers should refer to the decontamination sections found in Chapters 34 through 127, which will offer insight into xenobiotic-specific issues that may alter decontamination strategies.

GASTRIC EMPTYING

The principle theory governing gastric emptying is very simple: If a portion of xenobiotic can be removed before absorption, its potentially toxic effect should either be prevented or minimized. From 1982 to 1995, several important clinical trials attempted to define the role of gastric emptying in poisoned patients.[3,19,32,73,86,104,123,150] Although all of these studies were flawed because of the inclusion of a large number of low-risk patients, numerous restrictive exclusion criteria, and a variety of other biases, they clearly demonstrated that many patients can be successfully managed without aggressive gastric emptying. The clinical parameters listed in Table 7–1 help to identify individuals for whom gastric emptying is usually not indicated based on a risk-to-benefit analysis. In contrast, for a small subset of patients (see Table 7–1), gastric emptying may be indicated. A thorough understanding of this risk analysis is essential when deciding whether gastric emptying is appropriate for a patient who has ingested a xenobiotic.

Time is an important consideration, in that for gastric emptying to be beneficial, a consequential amount of xenobiotic must still be present in the stomach. Demographic studies have found that very few poisoned patients arrive at the ED within 1 to 2 hours after ingestion. In most studies, the average time from ingestion to presentation was approximately 3 to 4 hours, with significant variations.[80,87,124,144] This delay diminishes the likelihood of recovering a large percentage of the xenobiotic from the stomach unless the patient has ingested a xenobiotic that slows gastric emptying rates.

As is discussed in more depth in the Orogastric Lavage section later in this chapter, many authors advise against interventions beyond 1 hour after ingestion. Recent data highlight the arbitrary nature of this limitation. One human volunteer study evaluated the pharmacokinetic effects of diphenhydramine and oxycodone in a simulated acetaminophen overdose.[63] This model is relevant because of the rapid absorption of acetaminophen and the presence of many such combination products in the marketplace. Whereas diphenhydramine did not delay gastric emptying significantly, oxycodone delayed the time to peak acetaminophen concentration by approximately 1 hour. Although GI decontamination was not part of the study protocol, it can be inferred that acetaminophen was available for GI decontamination for a longer time than the 1-hour guideline suggests. Case reports have also reported poisoned patients with the xenobiotic still in the stomach (as confirmed by computed tomography or gastroscopy) as residuals or pharmacobezoars, from 5 hours up to several days after ingestion.[43,84]

In fact, markedly prolonged gastric emptying half-lives and gastric hypomotility were demonstrated using gastric scintigraphy in a prospective study on 85 poisoned patients.[1] Remarkably, these findings occurred with ingestions such as acetaminophen, which are not typically expected to prolong gastric emptying. Patients who underwent orogastric lavage did not have significantly different gastric emptying half-lives, suggesting that the procedure itself was not the cause of the gastroparesis. There was also no evidence that activated charcoal affected gastric emptying rates. The authors speculated that stress in an overdosed patient might be part of the etiology of the hypomotility observed and that the management of patients should not be based on the assumption that GI motility is normal.

Assessment of whether or not gastric emptying is appropriate for a patient continues with an evaluation for potential contraindications (Table 7–2). Regardless of the severity of the ingestion and other contributing factors, such as time, there must be no contraindication to gastric emptying procedures. Because the demonstrable benefit of emptying after ingestion of an unidentified xenobiotic is marginal at best, even relative contraindications usually dictate that the procedure should not be attempted.

After the decision to perform gastric emptying has been made, the clinician must choose between the two available methods. Either emesis can be induced with the administration of syrup of ipecac or orogastric lavage can be performed by cautious aspiration of gastric contents using a large-bore tube and small amounts of water. Although the numerical benefit of either method of gastric emptying has, in several studies, rarely averaged more than a 50% reduction in the absorption of a xenobiotic when performed under optimal research conditions,[86,151] this clinical benefit could be sizable if the ingested dose places the patient on the steep portion of the dose–response curve (Chap. 8). Under these circumstances a small reduction in dose might translate into a significant reduction in toxicity.

TABLE 7–1. Risk Assessment: When to Consider Gastric Emptying

Gastric Emptying Is Usually Not Indicated If[a]	Gastric Emptying May Be Indicated If[b]
The xenobiotic has limited toxicity at almost any dose	There is reason to believe that, given the time of ingestion, a significant amount of the ingested xenobiotic is still present in the stomach.
Although the xenobiotic ingested is potentially toxic, the dose likely ingested is less than that expected to produce significant illness.	The ingested xenobiotic is known to produce serious toxicity *or* the patient has obvious signs or symptoms of life-threatening toxicity.
The ingested xenobiotic is well adsorbed by activated charcoal, and the amount ingested is not expected to exceed the adsorptive capacity of activated charcoal.	The ingested xenobiotic is not adsorbed by activated charcoal or activated charcoal is unavailable.
Significant spontaneous emesis has occurred.	Although the ingested xenobiotic is adsorbed by activated charcoal, the amount ingested exceeds the activated charcoal-to-xenobiotic ratio of 10:1 even when using a dose of activated charcoal that is twice the standard dose recommended.
The patient presents many hours postingestion and has minimal signs or symptoms of poisoning.	The patient has not had spontaneous emesis.
The ingested xenobiotic has a highly efficient antidote (e.g., acetaminophen and NAC).	No highly effective specific antidote exists or alternative therapies (e.g., hemodialysis) pose a significant risk to the patient.

[a] Patients who fulfill these criteria can be decontaminated safely with activated charcoal alone or may require no decontamination at all.

[b] Patients who fulfill these criteria should be considered candidates for gastric emptying *if* there are no contraindications. For individuals who meet some of these criteria but who are judged not to be candidates for gastric emptying, single- or multiple-dose activated charcoal and/or whole-bowel irrigation should be considered.

NAC, *N*-acetylcysteine.

TABLE 7–2. Indications and Contraindications to Orogastric Lavage

Indications	Contraindications
The patient meets criteria for gastric emptying (see Table 7-1). The benefits of gastric emptying outweigh the risks.	The patient does not meet criteria for gastric emptying (see Table 7-1). The patient has lost or will likely lose his or her airway protective reflexes and has not been intubated. (After the patient has been intubated, orogastric lavage can be performed if otherwise indicated.).
	Ingestion of an alkaline caustic
	Ingestion of a foreign body (e.g., a drug packet)
	Ingestion of a xenobiotic with a high aspiration potential (e.g., a hydrocarbon) in the absence of endotracheal intubation
	The patient is at risk of hemorrhage or gastrointestinal perforation because of underlying pathology, recent surgery, or other medical condition that could be further compromised by the use of orogastric lavage.
	Ingestion of a xenobiotic in a form known to be too large to fit into the lumen of the lavage tube (e.g., many modified-release preparations)

OROGASTRIC LAVAGE

Many authors have adopted the consensus approach that orogastric lavage should not be considered unless a patient has ingested a potentially life-threatening amount of a xenobiotic and the procedure can be undertaken within 60 minutes of ingestion.[86,151] Since the publication of the clinical studies cited above,[3,19,32,73,86,104,123,150] studies of orogastric lavage have been scarce. One crossover study used 4 g of an acetaminophen solution as a marker and randomized the subjects to either control or orogastric lavage performed at 30 minutes postingestion. Although the study found a mean 20% reduction in the AUC (area under the plasma drug concentration versus time curve) of acetaminophen with orogastric lavage compared with controls, the confidence interval of ±28% suggests a rather modest and very unreliable effect.[60]

Two other prospective, randomized, crossover studies in volunteers measured the effect of activated charcoal versus orogastric lavage, with interventions at either 5 or 30 minutes postingestion.[90,91] Both studies used therapeutic doses of moclobemide, temazepam, and verapamil. Interestingly, when orogastric lavage was performed 5 minutes after ingestion, there was no significant pharmacokinetic effect on any of the drugs ingested. However, when orogastric lavage was performed 30 minutes after ingestion of moclobemide, the AUC was reduced by 44% compared with controls; there were no effects on the pharmacokinetic profiles of the other two drugs. These results most likely illustrate the very varied and unreliable effect of orogastric lavage even when performed by the same experienced professionals under controlled experimental conditions.

Another study evaluated the effect of activated charcoal compared with activated charcoal followed by orogastric lavage at 30 minutes postingestion.[90] Therapeutic doses of temazepam, ibuprofen, and citalopram were studied. In this model, the combination of activated charcoal and orogastric lavage was not superior to activated charcoal alone. A retrospective case study of 17 patients ingesting *Datura stramonium* seeds found that seeds were recovered in only 57% (eight of 14) of patients subjected to orogastric lavage. There was no significant effect of the removal of the seeds on clinical endpoints such as length of stay in hospital, use of the ICU, or use of the antidote physostigmine.[133]

It is important to highlight the differences between volunteer studies using therapeutic doses of drugs and actual patients with clinically significant overdoses. The most important aspect of this comparison is a bias against gastric emptying and toward a benefit of activated charcoal. The drugs used in these volunteer studies are all well-adsorbed by activated charcoal and the doses of activated charcoal are significantly in excess of its binding capacity for the drug. Larger doses, as might occur in clinically important ingestions are likely to saturate activated charcoal. An additional bias is introduced against gastric emptying because the small amounts of drugs used are unlikely to alter gastric motility and thus the drugs may pass through the pylorus before orogastric lavage can occur. A synthesis of available data can be used to develop indications for orogastric lavage (see Table 7–2). When deciding whether or not to actually perform orogastric lavage on a poisoned patient, these indications, contraindications, and potential adverse effects must be considered. Table 7–3 summarizes the technique of orogastric lavage.

Reported adverse effects of orogastric lavage include injury to the airway, esophagus,[22] and stomach,[40] as well as severe hypernatremia.[105]

TABLE 7–3. The Technique of Performing Orogastric Lavage

Select the correct tube size

Adults and adolescents: 36–40 French

Children: 22–28 French

Procedure

1. If there is potential airway compromise, endotracheal or nasotracheal intubation should precede orogastric lavage.
2. The patient should be kept in the left lateral decubitus position. Because the pylorus points upward in this orientation, this positioning theoretically helps prevent the xenobiotic from passing through the pylorus during the procedure.
3. Before insertion, the proper length of tubing to be passed should be measured and marked on the tube. The length should allow the most proximal tube opening to be passed beyond the lower esophageal sphincter.
4. After the tube is inserted, it is essential to confirm that the distal end of the tube is in the stomach.
5. Any material present in the stomach should be withdrawn and immediate instillation of activated charcoal should be considered for large ingestions of xenobiotics known to be adsorbed by activated charcoal.
6. In adults, 250 mL aliquots of a room-temperature saline lavage solution is instilled via a funnel or lavage syringe. In children, aliquots should be 10 to 15 mL/kg to a maximum of 250 mL.
7. Orogastric lavage should continue for at least several liters in an adult and for at least 0.5 to 1.0 L in a child or until no particulate matter returns and the effluent lavage solution is clear.
8. After orogastric lavage, the same tube should be used to instill activated charcoal if indicated.

A case of hypernatremia resulted from a lavage that was performed using 12 L of hypertonic saline.[105] An observational case series studying 14 consecutive gastric lavages performed in a resource-poor location found three deaths directly related to the procedure, all of which seemed to have resulted from inadequate airway protection.[46] These cases, as well as other well-known complications such as aspiration pneumonitis,[151,153] demonstrate that orogastric lavage is not risk free and should only be considered based on the rigorous indications for gastric emptying listed in Table 7–1.

SYRUP OF IPECAC

A comprehensive summary of the pharmacology and the evidence for induced emesis is available in the Antidotes in Depth: Syrup of Ipecac. Since 1997, very little original work has been published other than reviews and the position statement recommendations.[86] Additionally, a revision of the position paper found no new evidence to support any modification in recommendations.[124] At the time of this writing, no additionally useful materials were found.

Although many animal and human studies show a reduction in drug concentrations with induced emesis, no clinical benefit for this technique has been proven. Furthermore, as the benefits of activated charcoal are recognized and the time to its administration evaluated, it has become evident that the administration of syrup of ipecac delays the administration of activated charcoal, as well as any other oral treatment (symptomatic or specific antidotes).

Syrup of ipecac is absolutely contraindicated when the patient has ingested a caustic or a xenobiotic with a high aspiration potential, such as a hydrocarbon. Because vomiting in the setting of altered consciousness increases the likelihood of pulmonary aspiration, syrup of ipecac can only be used when the patient has a normal mental status *and* can be predicted to have a normal mental status at 1 hour after administration, when emesis may still occur. In the clinical setting, it is rare to identify patients with consequential ingestions who present early enough to require gastric emptying and who are expected to retain their airway protective reflexes for a minimum of 1 hour. Therefore, most consensus statements correctly conclude that, given the lack of evidence demonstrating a clinically meaningful benefit of induced emesis *and* the significant contraindications, the routine administration of syrup of ipecac in the ED should be abandoned.[85,124] Although other emetics and methods to induce emesis exist, data are insufficient to support their routine use.

Gastric decontamination of children in the home has always been an attractive concept because both the xenobiotic and time of ingestion are known and there is a high likelihood that the xenobiotic is still in the stomach. A prospective observational study evaluated 75 cases of probably poisoned children (of 14,603 human exposures) in which home administration of syrup of ipecac had been recommended by a poison specialist.[57] Cases in which syrup of ipecac was indicated but not available in the home were included in this group if the parents stated that syrup of ipecac could be obtained within 15 minutes. The administration of syrup of ipecac occurred in less than 30 minutes in only 20% of cases, and the reported overall mean time to emesis was 58 minutes from ingestion. Initial emesis occurred in less than 60 minutes in only 36% of cases. Numerous studies illustrate that the time to performing GI decontamination is critical. Clearly, the problem with syrup of ipecac is the time delay from administration to onset of emesis. Additionally, the uncertainty of the effect of the administered dose serves as a further delaying factor. A study in 12 adult volunteers showed that with a 20-mL dose, two of six volunteers had not vomited within 4 hours, but all volunteers (six of six) had vomited within 60 minutes after receiving a 30-mL dose.[157]

TABLE 7–4. Indications and Contraindications for Syrup of Ipecac

Indications	Contraindications
The patient meets criteria for gastric emptying (see Table 7-1). Orogastric lavage cannot be performed or is contraindicated because of the size of the xenobiotic formulation. The history and/or physical examination suggest that there is likely to be a clinically significant amount of xenobiotic remaining in the stomach. The benefits of gastric emptying outweigh the risks from the contraindications.	The patient does not meet criteria for gastric emptying (see Table 7–1). Either activated charcoal or another oral therapy is expected to be necessary in the next several hours. Airway protective reflexes might be lost within the next hour Ingestion of a caustic Ingestion of a foreign body such as a drug packet or sharp item Ingestion of a xenobiotic with a high aspiration potential such as a hydrocarbon. The patient is younger than 6 months of age, elderly, or debilitated. The patient has a premorbid condition that would be compromised by vomiting.

A four-limb randomized study using 10 healthy volunteers studied the effect of 30 mL of syrup of ipecac administered at 5, 30, and 60 minutes after the ingestion of 3.9 g of acetaminophen. The fourth limb served as a control. Only the 5-minute intervention was significantly different from control and showed a decrease in bioavailability of approximately 67%.[132] This study also noted that sedation was a significant adverse effect of syrup of ipecac, which makes this therapy difficult to recommend in patients who have ingested any potentially sedating xenobiotic.

A study using the 2003 Toxic Exposure Surveillance System (TESS) database (Chap. 135) evaluated the effect of home use of syrup of ipecac on the rate of referral to EDs across the United States. The study found that there was no reduction in ED use nor any improvement in patient outcome from home administration of syrup of ipecac.[18] Based on these findings and other data, the American Academy of Pediatrics published its policy statement on poison treatment in the home, concluding that syrup of ipecac should no longer be used as a standard home treatment in cases of poisoning.[6] Despite this, some authors still believe that there is a limited role for ipecac-induced emesis.[94] Table 7–4 summarizes the indications and contraindications for administration of syrup of ipecac. The only reasonable conclusion is that induction of emesis has an extremely limited role in the contemporary management of poisoned patients.

PREVENTION OF XENOBIOTIC ABSORPTION

ACTIVATED CHARCOAL

Activated charcoal has long been recognized as an effective method for reducing the systemic absorption of many xenobiotics. For certain xenobiotics, it also enhances elimination through interruption of either the enterohepatic or enteroenteric cycle.[17,33,81] Its superb adsorptive properties theoretically make it the single most useful management strategy for diverse patients with acute oral overdoses.[7-9,18,28,34,72,120,121]

But overall, as is true for the other methods of GI decontamination, there is a lack of sound evidence of its benefits as defined by clinically meaningful endpoints. This opinion is reflected both in the consensus statements and in the overall trend toward no decontamination as shown in AAPCC data (Chap. 135).[29,103,104] The consensus opinion concluded that a single dose of activated charcoal should not be administered routinely in the management of poisoned patients and, based on volunteer studies, the effectiveness of activated charcoal decreased with time, providing the greatest benefit within 1 hour of ingestion. There was no evidence that the administration of a single dose of activated charcoal improved clinical outcome. Additionally, it is generally accepted that unless either airway protective reflexes are intact (and expected to remain so) or the patient's airway has been protected, the administration of activated charcoal is contraindicated.[29]

Only a few studies have used valid clinical endpoints in an attempt to demonstrate a benefit of GI decontamination. A 2-year study concluded that activated charcoal was associated with a higher incidence of vomiting, a more prolonged ED stay, and a failure to improve clinical outcome compared with supportive care.[103] However, despite randomizing 1479 patients to either activated charcoal on even days and of no decontamination on odd days, only 399 patients were placed in the activated charcoal group, and 1080 patients were placed in the control group. This very uneven patient distribution suggest a selection bias that is inadequately described in the study. The authors concluded that there appeared to be no benefit to decontamination procedures, although they admitted that length of stay (one of their endpoints) was more dependent on the wait for psychiatric evaluation and the availability of a mental health bed for patient transfer than the resolution of clinical poisoning. The inclusion of a significant number of low-risk patients in this study introduced a clear bias against determining any benefit of decontamination. Furthermore, the validity of the study is questionable because patients with significant acetaminophen overdoses were excluded given that there are sound data to support improved clinical outcomes or laboratory parameters of diminished hepatotoxicity in acetaminophen-poisoned patients treated with activated charcoal.[21,140]

Theoretically, the early administration of activated charcoal to patients presenting with a significant oral overdose of a potentially toxic xenobiotic would lower systemic exposure to that xenobiotic and thus be of benefit to the patient. Surprisingly, this intuitive result has been difficult to demonstrate using clinically relevant endpoints in large unselected populations of poisoned patients.

A randomized, controlled clinical trial of all oral overdose patients (n = 327) presenting to the ED of a large hospital in an urban setting during 16 consecutive months found no difference in clinical endpoints such as length of stay or other outcomes between patients treated with a single dose of activated charcoal compared with no decontamination. The study excluded seven severely poisoned patients who all arrived within 1 hour of ingestion; the majority of the patients in the trial (nearly 60%) arrived within 2 hours postingestion. The most common xenobiotics ingested were acetaminophen, benzodiazepines, and newer antidepressants with low case-fatality rates.[38]

A large trial (n = 4629) from a rural and resource-poor location (Sri Lanka) studying patients self-poisoned primarily with pesticides and yellow oleander (*Thevetia*) seeds found no difference in mortality rates between no activated charcoal, single-dose activated charcoal, or a regimen of multiple-dose activated charcoal (MDAC). It is important to note that the first 1904 patients in the control group actually received orogastric lavage, as was the case for all patients presenting within 2 hours of ingestion of substantial amounts of pesticides or potentially toxic xenobiotics because of pressure from the national doctors' union. Although the authors claim that logistic regression analysis found no influence of lavage on their results, the data are not presented.[47] Furthermore, in an article on compliance related to activated charcoal, nested within this randomized, controlled trial, it is stated that a large number of patients included in the trial had undergone gastric emptying in some form before being transferred from peripheral hospitals.[106] The results of this trial are probably valid for their particular setting and patient profiles but cannot be generalized to developed nations. In contrast with the lack of effect on clinical endpoints such as death, a pharmacokinetic analysis from another subset of patients (n = 104) from this large trial found a significant increase in plasma clearance of the *Thevetia* cardenolides in patients administered both single-dose activated charcoal and MDAC. There was no difference between groups in mortality, but given the absolute numbers of two to three deaths per group, this could be related to a lack of power in the study design.[127]

Time Factors Many authors state that administration of a single dose of activated charcoal should be considered if a patient has ingested a potentially toxic amount of a xenobiotic (that is known to be adsorbed to activated charcoal) within the previous hour. This position was chosen because there are insufficient data to support or exclude the use of single-dose activated charcoal therapy more than 1 hour beyond xenobiotic ingestion.[29] The efficacy of activated charcoal administered more than 1 hour after xenobiotic ingestion is continuously debated and has been evaluated in several studies. Recent studies support the use of activated charcoal even late after the drug overdose.[55,74,78,140]

In volunteers, the effect of activated charcoal administered 2 and 4 hours after ingestion of acetaminophen demonstrated no significant difference in plasma acetaminophen concentration compared with controls. In contrast, when administered 1 hour after a simulated acetaminophen ingestion, activated charcoal reduced plasma acetaminophen concentrations significantly.[159] Likewise, when the effectiveness of activated charcoal administered 1, 2, and 3 hours after xenobiotic ingestion was determined, only the 1-hour group had a different pharmacokinetic profile from the control group.[59] Although these data do not support the administration of activated charcoal as a GI decontamination strategy more than 1 hour after an overdose, the applicability of these results to actual overdosed patients has not been adequately evaluated. The method in this volunteer study was an 8-hour fast followed by a small meal 1 hour before the administration of 3 to 4 g of acetaminophen.[59,159] Considering the rapid absorption of acetaminophen and the small 3- to 4-g doses used, it is highly probable that little or no acetaminophen would be left in the GI tract to be adsorbed by activated charcoal, limiting the potential time to benefit from activated charcoal to approximately 1 hour.

In contrast, activated charcoal given 3 hours after a xenobiotic overdose was investigated in vivo, again using acetaminophen and a larger-than-standard dose (i.e., 75 g) of activated charcoal. The results demonstrated some benefit in administering activated charcoal 3 hours after an overdose because there were significantly lower serum acetaminophen concentrations in the activated charcoal group than in the control group.[135] In a similar study, activated charcoal was effective in reducing the systemic absorption of a xenobiotic (acetaminophen) when administered 1 and 2 hours after ingestion, although the effect of the 2-hour intervention was substantially less than at 1 hour, reemphasizing the importance of early intervention.[28]

Activated charcoal administered between 0.5 and 4 hours to 17 patients who had ingested potentially toxic doses of citalopram demonstrated a pronounced effect on clearance and bioavailability. The result was a 72% increase in clearance and a 22% decrease in bioavailability when activated charcoal was administered. The data set included concentration–time data from 53 patients studied after 63 citalopram overdose events.[55]

Despite a delay to activated charcoal of 0.5 to 6.0 hours after a quetiapine overdose, a significant benefit for a single dose of activated charcoal was demonstrated. Activated charcoal decreased the fraction absorbed of quetiapine by 35%. No apparent effect on clearance was demonstrated.[75]

A meta-analysis was performed to evaluate the effect of activated charcoal on xenobiotic absorption during the first 6 hours after ingestion. Data were obtained from 64 controlled studies in which activated charcoal was compared with placebo up to 6 hours after drug ingestion in volunteers. Additional considerations were given to the influence of physical and pharmacologic properties, and the activated charcoal-to-drug ratio was evaluated. The authors concluded that activated charcoal was most effective when administered immediately after xenobiotic ingestion. Even with a delay of 4 hours after ingestion, 25% of the participants achieved at least a 32% reduction in absorption, especially when activated charcoal was given with large charcoal-to-drug ratios. Activated charcoal was most effective for xenobiotics with large molecular weights and volumes of distribution (V*d*) where other treatment options, including dialysis, are limited.[78] Activated charcoal should therefore be considered in poisoned patients even when they present late to medical care.

Similarly, when aminotransferase elevations were measured in patients with acetaminophen overdose who presented more than 4 hours after ingestion, patients who received activated charcoal along with *N*-acetylcysteine (NAC) had better outcomes than those who received NAC alone. This study had certain limitations, though, because its observations methodology was neither randomized nor blinded.[140]

Thus, it should be clear that the use of a 1-hour time frame is meant more as a guideline than an absolute cutoff. It is only logical that if an intervention is effective at 59 minutes, it will also be beneficial at 61 minutes. Although it is logical that efficacy decreases as time from ingestion increases, in certain cases, some benefit may be derived many hours postingestion. As discussed above, good data from patients with actual ingestions demonstrate that a significant amount of xenobiotic can be found in the stomach beyond this arbitrary 1-hour time frame. Additional benefits on enhanced elimination are discussed below.

The recommendation that activated charcoal should be administered within 1 hour of ingestion limits the potential to treat most poisoned patients. A study over a 6-month period identifying 63 patients who had taken potentially serious overdoses demonstrated a median time of arrival to healthcare of 136 minutes after the overdose. Only 15 patients presented within 1 hour, and only four of 10 patients who qualified received activated charcoal within 1 hour. The results demonstrate not only the difficulty in clinically assessing patients before 1 hour but also the difficulty in adhering to the principle of treating patients with activated charcoal when they arrive within 1 hour unless activated charcoal could be safely administered to appropriate patients before hospitalization.[80]

Prehospital use of activated charcoal has not gained wide acceptance because of the concern that it would not be administered properly by the untrained lay public and that many children would refuse to drink the charcoal slurry. An 18-month consecutive case series demonstrated that activated charcoal can be administered successfully in the home by the lay public. Home use of activated charcoal significantly reduced the time to activated charcoal administration after xenobiotic ingestion from a mean of 73 ± 18.1 minutes for ED treatment to a mean of 38 ± 18.3 minutes for home treatment.[139] However, many still consider this evidence insufficient to recommend that activated charcoal be stored in the home.

A prospective follow-up study from Finland evaluated the adherence to a new protocol of administering activated charcoal in the prehospital setting. The protocol was implemented by either the first-response unit or paramedics. Activated charcoal was indicated in 722 of 2047 patients. Of these patients, 555 actually received activated charcoal at a mean of 88 minutes after ingestion. There were no adverse effects noted, although 72 patients refused to drink the charcoal. This study shows that it is feasible to administer activated charcoal in the prehospital setting, but its clinical implications are unknown.[2]

In reality, many factors, such as the presence of food in the stomach, sustained-release formulations, and co-ingestions with anticholinergic or opioid properties, which delay gastric emptying can slow the rate of absorption of a xenobiotic. These factors increase the time frame for possible adsorption to activated charcoal. An increased effect of activated charcoal was shown in a randomized, crossover study in which volunteers were administered acetaminophen in either the presence or absence of the anticholinergic drug atropine and subsequently given a single dose of activated charcoal 1 hour later. Activated charcoal was more effective in reducing acetaminophen bioavailability in the presence of an anticholinergic agent.[60]

Dosing The optimal dose of oral activated charcoal has never been fully established. Since the beginning of its clinical use as a GI decontaminant, various factors have been recommended for determining the optimal dose of activated charcoal. Two factors commonly discussed are the patient's weight and the quantity of the xenobiotic ingested. The problem in using the quantity of the xenobiotic as a basis for activated charcoal dosing is that the amount is usually unknown, and there is an implication that nothing else in the GI tract will occupy binding sites on activated charcoal. Additionally, the xenobiotic is often unknown, and xenobiotics vary enormously in their toxicities, rate of absorption, and the clinical effects they produce (e.g., respiratory depression, convulsions, and effect on gastric emptying rate). Some xenobiotics are well adsorbed to activated charcoal, but others are not.[33] Because of variables such as the physical properties of the formulation ingested (liquid, solid, or sustained-release pill), the volume and pH of gastric and intestinal fluids, and the presence of other xenobiotics adsorbed by activated charcoal,[9,13,65,66,94,112,114] the optimal dose cannot be known with certainty in any given patient.

Information concerning the maximum adsorptive capacity of activated charcoal for the particular xenobiotic ingested permits a theoretical calculation of an adequate dose,[4,7,12,14,26,34,109,110,112,113,128,129,131,137,146,149] assuming that the amount of xenobiotic ingested is known. However, clinicians must remain cognizant of the risk of approaching or exceeding the adsorptive capacity of the standard dose of approximately 1 g/kg of body-weight of activated charcoal. This possibility has been investigated in only a few studies.[4,14,24,131]

Thus, the idea that a fixed activated charcoal-to-xenobiotic ratio is appropriate for all xenobiotics is clearly imperfect. It is possible, however, to develop a logical approach to dosing based on available data. The optimal activated charcoal dose is theoretically the minimum dose that completely adsorbs the ingested xenobiotic and, if relevant, that maximizes enhanced elimination. The results of in vitro studies show that the ideal activated charcoal-to-xenobiotic ratio varies widely, but a common recommendation is to deliver an activated charcoal-to-xenobiotic ratio of 10:1 or 50 to 100 g of activated charcoal to adult patients, whichever is greater. From a theoretical perspective, this amount will adsorb 5 to 10 g of a xenobiotic, which should be adequate for most poisonings.[7,8,29,33,96,113] Based on available data from in vivo and in vitro studies, the actual recommended dosing regimen for activated charcoal is 25 to 100 g in adults (1 g/kg of body weight) and 0.5 to 2.0 g/kg of body weight in children.[29,33] These recommendations are generally based more on activated charcoal tolerance than on efficacy. When calculation of a 10:1 ratio exceeds these recommendations, either gastric emptying or MDAC therapy should be considered.

For example, consider a patient who intentionally overdosed by ingesting thirty 0.25-mg digoxin pills (total dose, 7.5 mg). Achieving a 10:1 ratio is quite easy, and a standard dose of 1 g/kg might exceed a 10,000:1 ratio. In comparison, consider a patient who intentionally ingests thirty 325-mg aspirin pills (total dose, 9.75 g). In this case, obtaining a 10:1 activated charcoal-to-xenobiotic ratio is quite difficult and is even less likely if a patient ingests 60 or 100 of the aspirin pills. Poisoning with a combination of xenobiotics may also approach or exceed the maximum adsorption capacity for the standard dose of activated charcoal.

Methods to Increase the Palatability of Activated Charcoal Activated charcoal has a pronounced gritty texture, and it immediately sticks in the throat because it adheres to the mucosal surfaces and begins to cake.[33] In addition, the black appearance and insipid taste of activated charcoal make it less attractive.

There have been numerous attempts at making activated charcoal more appealing by providing flavors, including jam,[41] chocolate syrup,[76,108] cherry extract or syrup,[117,158] juice,[117] sorbitol,[35,39,102] saccharin,[36] strawberry flavor,[116] orange or peppermint oil,[33] melted milk chocolate,[48,49] chocolate milk,[26,117] soda,[26,117,126] yogurt,[67] and ice cream.[26,97,143] Because activated charcoal adsorbs the flavoring agents, the palatable taste often disappears within minutes after mixing.[33,35,36,41] But in cases in which the activated charcoal does not completely adsorb the flavoring agents, they provided a pleasant taste without significantly reducing the adsorptive properties of the activated charcoal.[33,35,36] The general recommendation, however, remains that activated charcoal should be mixed with water.[6,77]

Contraindications and Complications Vomiting frequently complicates the administration of activated charcoal. A prospective cohort study estimating the incidence of vomiting subsequent to the therapeutic administration of activated charcoal to poisoned children younger than 18 years of age showed that one of five of these children vomited. Children with previous vomiting or nasogastric tube administration were at highest risk.[118] This incidence of vomiting appears to be greater when activated charcoal is administered with sorbitol.[152] Also, although rare, inadvertent direct instillation of activated charcoal into the lungs has resulted from a misplaced nasogastric tube, leading to severe pulmonary complications and death. Administration of activated charcoal to already intubated patients is associated with a low incidence of aspiration pneumonia.[107] Another study found that pulmonary complications associated with activated charcoal aspiration might be primarily related to the aspiration of acidic gastric content and not directly related to aspiration of activated charcoal.[130] A retrospective study found that only 1.6% of unselected overdose patients aspirated and that administration of activated charcoal was not found to be an associated risk factor.[74] Pulmonary aspiration in overdose patients who have received activated charcoal is more easily documented because activated charcoal is a very identifiable marker.

Although relatively few reports of clinically significant emesis and pulmonary aspiration resulting from the administration of activated charcoal exist, the severity of these complications is clear. Consequently, it is important to evaluate, particularly in patients determined to be at limited risk from their exposures, whether single-dose activated charcoal therapy is likely to be beneficial based on the indications and contraindications listed in Table 7–5. This is especially true in small children, in whom the risks of a nasogastric tube might outweigh the benefits of activated charcoal.

TABLE 7–5. Indications and Contraindications for Single-Dose Activated Charcoal Therapy without Gastric Emptying

Indications	Contraindications
The patient does not meet criteria for gastric emptying (see Table 7–1) or gastric emptying is likely to be harmful.	Activated charcoal is known not to adsorb a clinically meaningful amount of the ingested xenobiotic.
The patient has ingested a potentially toxic amount of a xenobiotic that is known to be adsorbed by activated charcoal.	Airway protective reflexes are absent or expected to be lost, and the patient is not intubated.
The ingestion has occurred within a time frame amenable to adsorption by activated charcoal or clinical factors are present that suggest that not all of the xenobiotic has already been systemically absorbed.	Gastrointestinal perforation is likely as in cases of caustic ingestions.
	Therapy may increase the risk and severity of aspiration, such as in the presence of hydrocarbons with a high aspiration potential.
	Endoscopy will be an essential diagnostic modality (caustics)

MULTIPLE-DOSE ACTIVATED CHARCOAL

MDAC is typically defined as more than two sequential doses of activated charcoal.[152] In many cases, the actual number of doses administered is substantially greater. This technique serves two purposes: (1) to prevent ongoing absorption of a xenobiotic that persists in the GI tract (usually in the form of a modified-release preparation) and (2) to enhance elimination by either disrupting enterohepatic recirculation or by "gut dialysis" (enteroenteric recirculation).

The 1999 position statement of the AACT and the EAPCCT concluded that based on clinical studies, MDAC should be considered only if a patient has ingested a life-threatening amount of carbamazepine, dapsone, phenobarbital, quinine, or theophylline. Data have confirmed enhanced elimination of these drugs, although no controlled studies have demonstrated clinical benefit. Volunteer studies have demonstrated that MDAC increases the elimination of amitriptyline, dextropropoxyphene, digitoxin, digoxin, disopyramide, nadolol, phenylbutazone, phenytoin, piroxicam, and sotalol, but there are insufficient clinical data to support or exclude the use of this therapy.[152]

Although technically correct, the preceding statements suffer from a lack of evidence. Because the clinical studies used to formulate this opinion all lack sufficient numbers of significantly poisoned patients, they induce a bias against any benefit of MDAC. Additionally, none of the studies included a detailed analysis of sustained- or extended-release formulations, which are widely used today. Three recent studies with clinical endpoints are discussed below. Unfortunately, their results are discordant, which highlights the difficulties within this field of study.

A single-blind, randomized, placebo-controlled trial was designed to assess the efficacy of MDAC in the treatment of patients with yellow oleander (cardioactive steroid) poisoning. This clinical study demonstrated that MDAC (defined as 50 g of activated charcoal every 6 hours for 3 days) effectively reduced life-threatening cardiac dysrhythmias, deaths, and the need for ICU admission.[42] In this dataset, to save one life, only 18 patients needed to receive MDAC. This study demonstrates that consequential benefits of GI decontamination may become evident when investigations are performed in significantly poisoned patients. It further highlights that general recommendations only apply to patients in general and that severely ill patients deserve individualized care.

In contrast with the above-mentioned study are the results from a large (n = 4629) randomized, controlled trial from Sri Lanka in which patients self-poisoned with primarily pesticides and yellow oleander seeds were randomized to no decontamination, single-dose activated charcoal, and MDAC. There was no difference between groups regarding the ultimate clinical endpoint, mortality. As mentioned previously, the "no decontamination group" was not ideal because a large and relatively unaccounted for number of patients had received some form of gastric emptying either before entering the trial (at primary hospital setting) or later on in the trial after pressure from the national doctors' union.[47] In a small study ($n = 12$) of patients poisoned by carbamazepine, individuals were randomized to either single-dose activated charcoal or MDAC. The duration of coma, mechanical ventilation, and length of stay were significantly decreased in the group receiving multiple doses of activated charcoal, corresponding with a measured significantly shorter half-life of carbamazepine.[20]

Similar to single-dose activated charcoal, MDAC can produce emesis, with subsequent pulmonary aspiration of gastric contents containing activated charcoal. It is intuitive that these risks are greater with multiple- than with single-dose therapy. One retrospective study attempted to determine the frequency of complications associated with the use of MDAC.[44] The authors identified nearly 900 patients who had received MDAC and found that only 0.6% of patients had clinically significant pulmonary aspiration. Although no patients developed GI obstruction, 9% had hypernatremia or hypermagnesemia without any clinical consequences noted. The authors did not specify whether the multiple-dose regimens administered included the use of cathartics, but the profile of the adverse reactions listed above suggests that this is probably the case. Despite the obvious limitations, this study demonstrates a reasonably low rate of complications associated with MDAC.

Table 7–6 summarizes the indications and contraindications for MDAC therapy. Because the optimal doses and intervals for repeated doses of activated charcoal have not been established, recommendations are based more on amounts that can be tolerated than on amounts that might be considered pharmacologically appropriate. Table 7–7 lists typical dosing regimens. Larger doses and shorter intervals should be used for patients with more severe toxicity. It is reasonable to base endpoints either on the patient's clinical condition or on xenobiotic concentrations when they are easily measured.

In rats with bile duct externalization, intestinal perfusion with activated charcoal increased the elimination of intravenous acetaminophen and carbamazepine by 7% and 3% within 3.5 hours, respectively. The lack of effect of activated charcoal on the elimination of acetaminophen, carbamazepine, and their metabolites was suggested to be because of the small amounts of the xenobiotics diffusing into the intestine or by inadequate luminal stirring.[51,52]

TABLE 7–6. Indications and Contraindications for Multiple-Dose Activated Charcoal Therapy

Indications	Contraindications
Ingestion of a life-threatening amount of carbamazepine, dapsone, phenobarbital, quinine, or theophylline Ingestion of a life-threatening amount of another xenobiotic that undergoes enterohepatic or enteroenteric recirculation and that is adsorbed to activated charcoal Ingestion of a significant amount of any slowly released xenobiotic or of a xenobiotic known to form concretions or bezoars	Any contraindication to single-dose activated charcoal The presence of an ileus or other causes of diminished peristalsis

TABLE 7–7. Technique of Administering Multiple-Dose Activated Charcoal Therapy

Initial dose orally or via orogastric or nasogastric tube

Adults and children: 1 g/kg of body weight or a 10:1 ratio of activated charcoal to xenobiotic, whichever is greater. After massive ingestions, 2 g/kg of body weight might be indicated if such a large dose can be easily administered and tolerated.

Repeat doses orally or via orogastric or nasogastric tube

Adults and children: 0.5 g/kg of body weight every 4–6 hours for 12–24 hours in accordance with the dose and dosage form of xenobiotic ingested (larger doses or shorter dosing intervals may occasionally be indicated).

Procedure

1. Add 8 parts of water to the selected amount of powdered form. All formulations, including prepacked slurries, should be shaken well for at least 1 minute to form a transiently stable suspension before the patient drinks it or it is instilled via orogastric or nasogastric tube.
2. Activated charcoal can be administered with a cathartic *for the first dose only* when indicated, but cathartics should never be administered routinely and never be repeated with subsequent doses of activated charcoal.
3. If the patient vomits the dose of activated charcoal, it should be repeated. Smaller, more frequent doses or continuous nasogastric administration may be better tolerated. An antiemetic may be needed.
4. If a nasogastric or orogastric tube is used for MDAC administration, time should be allowed for the last dose to pass through the stomach before the tube is removed. Suctioning the tube itself before removal may prevent subsequent activated charcoal aspiration.

MDAC, multiple-dose activated charcoal.

Further clinical and toxicokinetic studies concerning MDAC are needed to establish an optimal dosing regimen and to confirm an effect on relevant endpoints. Readers are referred to Antidotes in Depth: Activated Charcoal for a more detailed discussion of single-dose activated charcoal and MDAC therapy.

WHOLE-BOWEL IRRIGATION

WBI represents a method of purging the GI tract in an attempt to prevent further absorption of xenobiotics. This is achieved through the oral or nasogastric administration of large amounts of an osmotically balanced polyethylene glycol electrolyte lavage solution (PEG-ELS). This decontamination technique was subjected to a thorough literature review, which was published as a position statement in 1997 and revised in 2004.[125,142] The position statement was unable to establish a clear set of evidence-based indications for the use of WBI because no clinical outcome studies have been performed. When experimental, theoretical, and anecdotal human experience is considered, the use of WBI with PEG-ELS can be supported for patients with potentially toxic ingestions of sustained-release pharmaceuticals. Other theoretical indications include the ingestion of large amounts of a xenobiotic with a slow absorptive phase in which morbidity is expected to be high, the ingested xenobiotic is not adsorbed by activated charcoal, and when other methods of GI decontamination are unlikely to be either safe or beneficial. The removal of packets of xenobiotics from body packers can be considered a unique indication for WBI. Similarly, patients who have ingested large amounts of plant or mushroom material might be highly amenable to treatment with WBI.

WBI cannot be applied safely if the GI tract is not intact, there are signs of ileus or obstruction, or there is significant GI hemorrhage or in patients with inadequate airway protection, uncontrolled vomiting, or consequential hemodynamic instability that compromises GI function or integrity. Additionally, the combination of WBI and activated charcoal results in an in vitro decrease in the adsorption of xenobiotics by activated charcoal, especially when the WBI solution is premixed with activated charcoal. Activated charcoal seems to be most efficacious if administered before initiating WBI.[11,70,85,93] Since the publication of the position statement, only three studies of varying degrees of evidence and some case reports have been published, as discussed below.

The effect of WBI on the pharmacokinetics of a modified-release formulation of acetaminophen and the progression of radiopaque markers through the GI tract was studied using a prospective randomized, crossover design.[101] Ten volunteers ingested the acetaminophen in supratherapeutic doses of 75 mg/kg together with a capsule containing 24 small markers. One study day served as control during which no interventions were undertaken. On the intervention day, the volunteers were subjected to WBI beginning 30 minutes after ingestion and continued until rectal effluent was determined to be clear. The average duration of WBI was 6 hours. No tablets or markers were recovered in the effluent. Only two of 10 patients had adverse effects such as nausea and abdominal cramping, and one volunteer vomited. The authors found a nonsignificant 11.5% reduction in the AUC of acetaminophen. The study had an 80% power to detect a 25% difference in AUC, which was arbitrarily set because there is no clinically established minimal relevant difference for a reduction in the AUC of a xenobiotic. The significance of this reduction would also vary in relation to the toxic properties of a xenobiotic (e.g., small versus large therapeutic index, availability of an effective antidote). In theory, for some xenobiotics, an 11% reduction in absorption might mean the difference between serious and life-threatening toxicity. The authors also found that in eight of 10 subjects, whereas the radiopaque markers were all located in the cecum after WBI, the markers were scattered throughout the small intestine in the control group. This observation indicates that WBI has the capability to move objects in the GI tract, at least to some degree. Although the authors stated that they would discontinue WBI when the rectal effluent was clear, this did not occur, and they chose an endpoint in which the final effluent was straw-colored to yellowish-brown, which might have been too short a time. Nevertheless, during the 6-hour mean duration of therapy, they managed to move the markers out of the small intestine more rapidly with WBI, which might limit absorption. Of note, the entire model has limited applicability because WBI would never be considered for a patient with an acetaminophen overdose.

A randomized, three-phase, crossover study using nine volunteers studied the use of activated charcoal alone compared with activated charcoal followed by WBI in preventing the absorption of three different sustained-release drugs (carbamazepine, theophylline, and verapamil), all of which were administered in therapeutic doses. This study also found that WBI seemed to decrease the efficacy of activated charcoal, but that the pharmacokinetic profile was still better than no intervention, although these results were probably largely an effect of activated charcoal.[90] As mentioned above, study designs using activated charcoal and small doses of xenobiotics tend to bias the study toward a benefit of activated charcoal. In an overdose scenario, when activated charcoal adsorptive capacity may be exceeded, it is intuitive that the benefits of other modalities would be more evident.

The third study evaluating the combined use of activated charcoal and WBI found that there were significant decreases in the adsorption of fluoxetine to activated charcoal and an increase in the desorption of the xenobiotic from activated charcoal.[12] Although these data support the findings of the studies previously cited in the position statement, they may have limited applicability as WBI would rarely, if ever, be indicated for fluoxetine overdose. However, they do highlight the potential risk of WBI causing desorption of xenobiotics that have been already adsorbed to activated charcoal.

A small, retrospective, descriptive case series of 16 body packers treated with WBI supports the safety of WBI for body packers. Although the complication rate was reported as 12.5% (two of 16), these complications were not serious. One case of mild cocaine toxicity resulted from leakage, and one heroin body packer had to undergo surgery because of retained packages. There was no correlation between the dose of PEG-ELS, drug type, or packet quantity and length of hospital stay. Because there was no control group, it is not possible to evaluate whether WBI influenced any clinical outcome.[53]

WBI has also been used to treat xenobiotic overdoses in pregnant women and children. One such case involved an iron overdose in a woman during the third trimester of pregnancy; she was treated successfully and without complications.[154] A pediatric case report describes combined WBI with succimer therapy and eventually colonoscopic removal of ingested lead pellets. Abdominal radiographs showed two small lead pellets, which WBI failed to remove, therefore requiring endoscopic removal.[31] Several reports support the use of WBI in children, including an intentional ingestion of mercury,[134] two pediatric body packers,[148] and a 16-month-old boy who had ingested a significant amount of iron.[155] In the latter case, despite WBI, the iron bezoar was not removed, treatment was eventually stopped, and the bezoar was expelled after a normal diet was resumed.[155]

Thus, there is no new convincing evidence of the clinical efficacy of WBI. Additional case reports and series demonstrate the overall safety of this procedure as well as some beneficial effect on secondary endpoints, but the benefits remain generally theoretical. There is some evidence against the simultaneous administration of activated charcoal with WBI, and there is little doubt that PEG-ELS reduces the adsorptive capacity of activated charcoal in vitro.

The indications for WBI must, at the present time, remain theoretical because the only support for the efficacy of this procedure comes from surrogate markers and anecdotal experience. Table 7–8 summarizes the indications and contraindications for WBI.

TABLE 7–8. Indications and Contraindications for Whole-Bowel Irrigation

Indications	Contraindications
Potentially toxic ingestions of sustained-release drugs	Airway protective reflexes are absent or expected to become so in a patient who has not been intubated
Ingestion of a toxic amount of a xenobiotic that is not adsorbed to activated charcoal when other methods of GI decontamination are not possible or not efficacious	GI tract is not intact. Signs of ileus, obstruction, significant GI hemorrhage, or hemodynamic instability that might compromise GI motility
Removal of illicit drug packets from body packers	Persistent vomiting
	Signs of leakage from cocaine packets (indication for surgical removal)

GI, gastrointestinal.

CATHARTICS

At present, there is no indication for the routine use of cathartics as a method of either limiting absorption or enhancing elimination. A single dose can be given as an adjunct to activated charcoal therapy when there are no contraindications and constipation or an increased GI transit time is expected. Multiple-dose cathartics should never be used, and magnesium-containing cathartics should be avoided in patients with renal insufficiency. (See Antidotes in Depth A3: Whole-Bowel Irrigation and Other Intestinal Evacuants for more information on cathartics and WBI.)

SURGERY AND ENDOSCOPY

Surgery and endoscopy are occasionally indicated for decontamination of poisoned patients. As might be expected, no controlled studies have been conducted, and potential indications are based largely on case reports and case series. A prospective, uncontrolled series of 50 patients with cocaine packet ingestion was published more than 20 years ago.[23] The patients were conservatively managed and only underwent surgery if there were signs of leakage or mechanical bowel obstruction. Bowel obstruction occurred in three patients, who promptly underwent successful emergency laparotomy; another six patients chose elective surgery. The authors concluded that body packers should be treated conservatively and only operated on for xenobiotic leakage or bowel obstruction.[23]

Similarly, another study performed a 16-year retrospective analysis of all body packers treated in a single center.[136] Of the 2880 body packers who were identified, 2.2% developed symptoms of severe cocaine toxicity after rupture of a package; 43 (68%) of the symptomatic patients died before surgery could be initiated, and 20 (32%) underwent emergency laparotomy to remove the drug packets and survived.

A recent report described two cases of body packers who successfully underwent surgery to remove drug packets. In one case, the indications were rupture and signs of cocaine toxicity. In the other cases, the indication for surgery was bowel obstruction.[115] Because most packages do not spontaneously rupture, mechanical obstruction is probably the most common reason for surgery on a body packer.[147] Leakage from heroin-containing packages can usually be managed by naloxone infusion, but the lack of antidote when cocaine packages rupture necessitates surgery (Chaps. 38, 76 and SC-4: Internal Concealment of Xenobiotic).[147]

Over the years, a few case reports have presented mixed results for the endoscopic removal of drug packets or pharmacobezoars from the stomach.[27,43,138,141,147] At present, this method is not generally recommended because of concerns about packet rupture. However, under exceptional circumstances, there is certainly a precedent for attempting this procedure in a highly controlled setting such as an ICU or operating room.

In rare cases of massive iron overdoses when emesis, orogastric lavage, and gastroscopy failed, gastrotomy was performed. The significant clinical improvement and postoperative recovery indicated that surgery in these particular cases was the correct approach.[54,76]

OTHER ADJUNCTIVE METHODS USED FOR GASTROINTESTINAL DECONTAMINATION

Other agents, such as cholecystokinin, have been considered as adjuncts to standard measures for GI decontamination.[50,68] Pharmaceuticals that either speed up GI passage or slow down gastric emptying have been administered in an attempt to minimize the absorption of a xenobiotic. In all cases, the results have been negligible, and the potential risks of administering additional pharmacologically active agents to an already poisoned patient seem to outweigh any benefit.[5,156] Agents other than activated charcoal that reduce the absorption of xenobiotics from the GI tract have also been studied, including sodium polystyrene for lithium[16,98-100,145] or thallium overdose.[71] There have also been case reports of the use of the lipid-lowering resins cholestyramine and colestipol to interrupt the enterohepatic circulation of digoxin, digitoxin, and chlordane to increase elimination.[15,56,83,122] With the increased use of activated charcoal and availability of digoxin specific Fab fragments, indications for lipid-lowering resins for cardioactive steroid ingestions seem obsolete.

COMBINATION TREATMENTS

The combination of several different methods of GI decontamination has been studied and, more importantly, is extensively practiced clinically. The combination of gastric emptying (mainly orogastric lavage) followed by activated charcoal is the subject of many investigations, both in volunteers[28] and in two often-discussed clinical studies.[86,123] Only the small subset of significantly ill patients seemed to benefit from combined therapy. On closer examination, this group was comprised of only three patients compared with 17 patients who received activated charcoal alone.[86] This comparison of small, uneven, and unpaired numbers, together with a retrospective stratification, poses consequential statistical problems and limits the potential for generalization of the authors' results.

A volunteer study, although also small in numbers ($n = 12$), used a controlled, randomized, paired design.[28] The subjects received approximately 4 g of acetaminophen (as 30 to 40 tablets of 125-mg strength) 1 hour after a standardized breakfast meal. The interventions (orogastric lavage plus activated charcoal versus activated charcoal alone) were carried out 1 hour after ingestion. There were no significant differences in the AUC of acetaminophen between the two arms (power of 80% to detect a minimum relevant difference of 15%), but there was a 50% reduction for both arms compared with controls. It must be emphasized, however, this was not a clinical endpoint.

Similarly, a clinical study of 981 consecutive acetaminophen poisonings over a 10-year period found that patients who had ingested more than 10 g of acetaminophen by history and had received activated charcoal were significantly less likely to have a concentration of acetaminophen requiring antidotal therapy compared with patients who received no decontamination. Patients who received both orogastric lavage and activated charcoal did not have a further benefit.[21] Thus, the combination of orogastric lavage followed by activated charcoal only seems appropriate in cases in which orogastric lavage is indicated and the xenobiotic is adsorbed to activated charcoal. In cases in which activated charcoal alone is usually beneficial, there is little rationale to expose the patient to the additional risks of orogastric lavage. Although acetaminophen is a reasonable drug to study, the universal availability of a benign and inexpensive antidote contraindicates aggressive gastric emptying in acetaminophen overdose even if some benefit could be demonstrated.

The combination of activated charcoal and WBI would seem to make sense in that it might hasten GI passage and at the same time have the protective adsorptive effect of activated charcoal. However, based on the studies cited previously, it seems that if activated charcoal is administered with WBI, the adsorptive capacity of activated charcoal is reduced. Thus, we recommend administering activated charcoal before PEG-ELS if both are indicated and using WBI with great caution in patients who have already received MDAC. There is concern about the practice of treating asymptomatic cocaine body packers with WBI combined with activated charcoal because severe peritonitis may result if activated charcoal spills into the peritoneum after surgical intervention. The administration of activated charcoal is not expected to prevent routine surgery, and because the use of activated charcoal may increase the risk of surgical complications, activated charcoal should not be used under these circumstances.

GENERAL ASPECTS

Only a few GI decontamination studies provide guidance based on meaningful clinical endpoints. One of the few studies addressing meaningful clinical parameters was a retrospective analysis reviewing the management of all patients presenting to an ED with a diagnosis of deliberate self-poisoning.[64] The study evaluated 561 patients who were treated in 1999, comparing them with patients treated in 1989, 1992, and 1996.[64] The authors found that despite dramatically changing trends of GI decontamination, there were no significant changes in the proportion of patients admitted to the hospital, although there was a reduction in the rate of admission to the ICU. The patient populations did not change significantly over the years with regard to the female-to-male ratio, the age distribution, and the types of xenobiotics ingested. The authors mention that there might be unmeasured differences between the populations and unrecognized differences in practice that might have been influential. However, in 1989, most of the patients were treated with orogastric lavage, almost no patients received activated charcoal, and approximately 33% did not receive any gastric decontamination at all. In comparison, in 1996, more than 50% of patients received activated charcoal alone and fewer than 25% had no GI decontamination at all. In 1999, only 13% of patients received activated charcoal, 0.7% received a combination of orogastric lavage followed by activated charcoal, 0.5% were given WBI, and nearly 86% received no decontamination at all. There were no changes in overall mortality from poisonings over the years, although the number of fatalities was very low. Thus, although the trends in GI decontamination dramatically shifted toward less intervention over the years studied, there was no measurable worsening in outcome when large groups of patients were studied. It must be emphasized that this was a retrospective analysis with fairly nonspecific outcome measures, and possible improvements in other aspects of clinical treatment of poisoned patients were not considered.

The trends in practice noted in the above study reflect the overall combined philosophy of the position statements, which are applicable to the vast majority of poisoned patients. They highlight the benign nature of many exposures and the benefits of good supportive care. In contrast, the previously mentioned survey of recommendations for a theoretical patient with a serious enteric-coated aspirin overdose reveal less consensus in that 36 different courses of action were proposed for the same patient. Most of the poison centers and toxicologists did, however, recommend at least one dose of activated charcoal.[79] This distinction serves as a reminder that the existing studies and consensus statements cannot be applied to all cases and that a lack of data produce significant uncertainty in choices for GI decontamination in either atypical or severely poisoned patients.[69]

It is essential to note that only one study has ever demonstrated a survival advantage for any form of GI decontamination of poisoned patients.[42] Its unique design, involving a cohort of patients with life-threatening toxicity, forces a reassessment of all previous literature and confirms that the principles of decontamination are sound. It also suggests that the failure of most studies to demonstrate a benefit result not from a failure of the techniques used but from applying decontamination techniques to subsets of patients who were likely to have good outcomes regardless of intervention.

SUMMARY

The approach to GI decontamination needs to be more individualized than previously thought. No decontamination method is completely free of risks. The indications and contraindications for GI decontamination must be well defined for each patient, and the method of choice must depend largely on what was ingested, how much was ingested, and when it was ingested. It is important to be aware of the differences in the patterns of ingested xenobiotics when it comes to rural and urban settings as well as industrialized and developing worlds. In some areas, there is a shift towards less toxic pharmaceutical ingestions but also a possible increase in potentially more toxic recreational drug overdoses. Decontamination thus probably must be even more individualized than previously thought. Evidence now points away from the routine GI decontamination of most patients presenting to an ED with an oral drug overdose. A single dose of activated charcoal alone will be sufficient in moderate-risk patients, and only in a small subset of exceptionally high-risk patients will the benefit of orogastric lavage outweigh the risks. This approach is of course dependent on adequate medical assessment of patient history being undertaken promptly at admission without significant delays.

The absolute time frame for when decontamination is indicated depends on many factors, such as the rate of gastric emptying, the rate of xenobiotic absorption, and the possibility of enterohepatic recirculation. The commonly stated short time frame of up to 1 hour postingestion for intervention is most likely an underestimation of the time frame during which a benefit is likely to be realized, although this has not yet been fully investigated.

Judging from the evidence available today, activated charcoal must be the first choice, only accompanied by orogastric lavage when the desirable ratio of activated charcoal to xenobiotic cannot be achieved and the xenobiotic is still thought to be accessible in the stomach. Orogastric lavage as a single intervention is reserved for cases in which the ingested xenobiotic is not adsorbed by activated charcoal and there is reason to believe that the ingested xenobiotic is both life threatening *and* still in the stomach. Syrup of ipecac–induced emesis has a very limited therapeutic role but might be reserved for situations with an absolute need for GI decontamination; when activated charcoal is not expected to be effective; and when orogastric lavage and WBI are, for practical purposes, impossible. Multiple-dose activated charcoal and WBI have narrowly defined indications, which may broaden in the future as more studies focus on subsets of significantly poisoned patients.

The advancement of medical toxicology depends on well-designed clinical studies that concentrate on measuring the effect of GI decontamination using precise, reproducible, and relevant clinical endpoints. For each approach, it must be determined if the benefits of decontamination outweigh the potential risks. If proven beneficial, firm criteria need to be set for the future selection of patients for whom these treatments are beneficial and therefore indicated. One goal must be to reduce complications by identifying patients who can be safely managed without decontamination. At the same time, we must be ever vigilant for patients with ingestions of unstudied highly lethal xenobiotics and massive amounts of studied xenobiotics, as well as those who present early in their clinical course with life-threatening signs and symptoms. This uncommon subset is most likely to benefit from more aggressive GI decontamination. Thus, it is recommended that some form of GI decontamination be considered in *every* patient with potentially life-threatening toxicity regardless of the time since ingestion as long as no absolute contraindications exist.

REFERENCES

1. Adams BK, Mann MD, Aboo A, et al: Prolonged gastric emptying half-time and gastric hypomotility after drug overdose. *Am J Emerg Med.* 2004;22:548-554.
2. Alaspää AO, Kuisma MJ, Hoppu K, Neuvonen PJ: Out-of-hospital administration of activated charcoal by emergency medical services. *Ann Emerg Med.* 2005;45:207-212.

3. Albertson TE, Derlet RW, Foulke GE, et al: Superiority of activated charcoal alone compared with ipecac and activated charcoal in the treatment of acute toxic ingestions. *Ann Emerg Med.* 1989;18:56-59.
4. al-Shareef AH, Buss DC, Routledge PA: Drug adsorption to charcoals and anionic binding resins. *Hum Exp Toxicol.* 1990;9:95-97.
5. Amato CS, Wang RY, Wright RO, Linakis JG: Evaluation of promotility agents to limit the gut bioavailability of extended-release acetaminophen. *J Toxicol Clin Toxicol.* 2004;42:73-77.
6. American Academy of Pediatrics Committee on Injury, Violence, and Poison Prevention: poison treatment in the home. American Academy of Pediatrics Committee on Injury, Violence, and Poison Prevention. *Pediatrics.* 2003;112:1182-1185.
7. Andersen AH: Experimental studies on the pharmacology of activated charcoal. I. Adsorption power of charcoal in aqueous solution. *Acta Pharmacol.* 1946;2:69-78.
8. Andersen AH: Experimental studies on the pharmacology of activated charcoal. II. The effect of pH on the adsorption by charcoal from aqueous solution. *Acta Pharmacol.* 1947;3:199-218.
9. Andersen AH: Experimental studies on the pharmacology of activated charcoal. III. Adsorption from gastrointestinal contents. *Acta Pharmacol.* 1948;4:275-284.
10. Arena JM: Gastric lavage, ipecac, or activated charcoal? *JAMA.* 1970;212:328.
11. Arimori K, Deshimaru M, Furukawa E, Nakano M: Adsorption of mexiletine onto activated charcoal in macrogol-electrolyte solution. *Chem Pharm Bull.* 1993;41:766-768.
12. Atta-Politou J, Kolioliou M, Havariotou M, et al: An in vitro evaluation of fluoxetine adsorption by activated charcoal and desorption upon addition of polyethylene glycol-electrolyte lavage solution. *J Toxicol Clin Toxicol.* 1998;36:117-124.
13. Bailey DN, Briggs JR: The effect of ethanol and pH on the adsorption of drugs from simulated gastric fluid onto activated charcoal. *Ther Drug Monit.* 2003;25:310-313.
14. Bainbridge CA, Kelly EL, Walking WD: In vitro adsorption of acetaminophen onto activated charcoal. *J Pharm Sci.* 1977;66:480-483.
15. Bazzano G, Bazzano GS: Digitalis intoxication. Treatment with a new steroid-binding resin. *JAMA.* 1972;220:828-830.
16. Belanger DR, Tierney MG, Dickinson G: Effect of sodium polystyrene sulfonate on lithium bioavailability. *Ann Emerg Med.* 1992;21:1312-1315.
17. Berlinger WG, Spector R, Goldberg MJ, et al: Enhancement of theophylline clearance by oral activated charcoal. *Clin Pharmacol Ther.* 1983;33:351-354.
18. Bond GR: The role of activated charcoal and gastric emptying in gastrointestinal decontamination: a state-of-the-art review. *Ann Emerg Med.* 2002;39:273-286.
19. Bosse GM, Barefoot JA, Pfeifer MP, Rodgers GC: Comparison of three methods of gut decontamination in tricyclic antidepressant overdose. *J Emerg Med.* 1995;13:203-209.
20. Brahmi N, Kouraichi N, Thabet H, Amamou M: Influence of activated charcoal on the pharmacokinetics and the clinical features of carbamazepine poisoning. *Am J Emerg Med.* 2006;24:440-443.
21. Buckley NA, Whyte IM, O'Connell DL, Dawson AH: Activated charcoal reduces the need for N-acetylcysteine treatment after acetaminophen (paracetamol) overdose. *J Toxicol Clin Toxicol.* 1999;37:753-757.
22. Caravati EM, Knight HH, Linscott MS Jr, Stringham JC: Esophageal laceration and charcoal mediastinum complicating gastric lavage. *J Emerg Med.* 2001;20:273-276.
23. Caruana DS, Weinbach B, Goerg D, Gardner LB: Cocaine-packet ingestion. Diagnosis, management, and natural history. *Ann Intern Med.* 1984;100:73-74.
24. Cassidy SL, Hale A, Buss DC, Routledge PA: In vitro drug adsorption to charcoal, silicas, acrylate copolymer and silicone oil with charcoal and with acrylate copolymer. *Hum Exp Toxicol.* 1997;16:25-27.
25. Cheng A, Ratnapalan S: Improving the palatability of activated charcoal in pediatric patients. *Pediatr Emerg Care.* 2007;23:384-386.
26. Cheng M, Robertson WO: Charcoal "flavored" ice cream. *Vet Hum Toxicol.* 1989;31:332.
27. Choudhary AM, Taubin H, Gupta T, Roberts I: Endoscopic removal of a cocaine packet from the stomach. *J Clin Gastroenterol.* 1998;27:155-156.
28. Christophersen AB, Levin D, Hoegberg LC, et al: Activated charcoal alone or after gastric lavage: a simulated large paracetamol intoxication. *Br J Clin Pharmacol.* 2002;53:312-317.
29. Chyka PA, Seger D: Position statement: single-dose activated charcoal. American Academy of Clinical Toxicology; European Association of Poisons Centres and Clinical Toxicologists. *J Toxicol Clin Toxicol.* 1997;35:721-741.
30. Chyka PA, Winbery SL: Quality improvement process in the adherence to gastric decontamination guidelines for poison exposures as recommended by a poison control center. *Q Manage Health Care.* 2006;15:263-267.
31. Clifton JC, Sigg T, Burda AM, et al: Acute pediatric lead poisoning: combined whole bowel irrigation, succimer therapy, and endoscopic removal of ingested lead pellets. *Pediatr Emerg Care.* 2002;18:200-202.
32. Comstock EG, Boisaubin EV, Comstock BS, Faulkner TP: Assessment of the efficacy of activated charcoal following gastric lavage in acute drug emergencies. *J Toxicol Clin Toxicol.* 1982;19:149-165.
33. Cooney DO: *Activated Charcoal in Medical Applications.* New York: Marcel Dekker; 1995.
34. Cooney DO: In vitro adsorption of phenobarbital, chlorpheniramine maleate, and theophylline by four commercially available activated charcoal suspensions. *J Toxicol Clin Toxicol.* 1995;33:213-217.
35. Cooney DO: Palatability of sucrose-, sorbitol-, and saccharin-sweetened activated charcoal formulations. *Am J Hosp Pharm.* 1980;37:237-239.
36. Cooney DO: Saccharin sodium as a potential sweetener for antidotal charcoal. *Am J Hosp Pharm.* 1977;34:1342-1344.
37. Cooper GM, Buckley NA: Activated charcoal RCT. *Am J Ther.* 2003;10:235-236.
38. Cooper GM, Le Couteur DG, Richardson D, Buckley NA: A randomized clinical trial of activated charcoal for the routine management of oral drug overdose. *Q J Med.* 2005;98:655-660.
39. Cordonnier JA, Van den Heede MA, Heyndrickx AM: In vitro adsorption of tilidine HCl by activated charcoal. *J Toxicol Clin Toxicol.* 1986;24:503-517.
40. Cuperus BK, van der Werf TS, Zijlstra JG: Diagnostic image (65). Unintentional biopsies of the gastric mucosa, obtained by withdrawal of a stomach tube. *Ned Tijdschr Geneeskd.* 2001;145:2271.
41. de-Neve R: Antidotal efficacy of activated charcoal in presence of jam, starch and milk. *Am J Hosp Pharm.* 1976;33:965-966.
42. de Silva HA, Fonseka MM, Pathmeswaran A, et al: Multiple-dose activated charcoal for treatment of yellow oleander poisoning: a single-blind, randomised, placebo-controlled trial. *Lancet.* 2003;361:1935-1938.
43. Djogovic D, Hudson D, Jacka M: Gastric bezoar following venlafaxne overdose. *Clin Toxicol.* 2007;45:735.
44. Dorrington CL, Johnson DW, Brant R: The frequency of complications associated with the use of multiple-dose activated charcoal. *Ann Emerg Med.* 2003;41:370-377.
45. Eddleston M: Patterns and problems of deliberate self-poisoning in the developing world. *QJM.* 2000;93:715-731.
46. Eddleston M, Hagalla S, Reginald K, et al: The hazards of gastric lavage for intentional self-poisoning in a resource poor location. *Clin Toxicol.* 2007;45:136-143.
47. Eddleston M, Juszczak E, Buckley NA, et al: Multiple-dose activated charcoal in acute self-poisoning: a randomised controlled trial. *Lancet.* 2008;371:579-587.
48. Eisen TF, Grbcich PA, Lacouture PG, et al: The adsorption of salicylates by a milk chocolate-charcoal mixture. *Ann Emerg Med.* 1991;20:143-146.
49. Eisen TF, Lacouture PG and Woolf A: The palatability of a new milk chocolate-charcoal mixture in children. *Vet Hum Toxicol.* 1988;30:351-352.
50. el-Bahie N, Allen EM, Williams J, Routledge PA: The effect of activated charcoal and hyoscine butylbromide alone and in combination on the absorption of mefenamic acid. *Br J Clin Pharmacol.* 1985;19:836-838.
51. Eyer F, Jung N, Neuberger H, et al: Enteral exsorption of acetaminophen after intravenous injection in rats: influence of activated charcoal on this clearance path. Basic *Clin Pharmacol Toxicol.* 2007;101:163-171.
52. Eyer F, Jung N, Neuberger H, et al: Seromucosal transport of intravenously administered carbamazepine is not enhanced by oral doses of activated charcoal in rats. *Basic Clin Pharmacol Toxicol.* 2008;102:337-346.
53. Farmer JW, Chan SB: Whole body irrigation for contraband body-packers. *J Clin Gastroenterol.* 2003;37:147-150.
54. Foxford R, Goldfrank L: Gastrotomy—a surgical approach to iron overdose. *Ann Emerg Med.* 1985;14:1223-1226.
55. Friberg LE, Isbister GK, Hackett LP, Duffull SB: The population pharmacokinetics of citalopram after deliberate self-poisoning: a Bayesian approach. *J Pharmacokinet Pharmacodyn.* 2005;32:571-605.
56. Garrettson LK, Guzelian PS, Blanke RV: Subacute chlordane poisoning. *J Toxicol Clin Toxicol.* 1984;22:565-571.

57. Garrison J, Shepherd G, Huddleston WL, Watson WA: Evaluation of the time frame for home ipecac syrup use when not kept in the home. *J Toxicol Clin Toxicol.* 2003;41:217-221.
58. Good AM, Kelly CA, Bateman DN: Differences in treatment advice for common poisons by poison centres—an international comparison. *Clin Toxicol.* 2007;45:234-239.
59. Green R, Grierson R, Sitar DS, Tenenbein M: How long after drug ingestion is activated charcoal still effective? *J Toxicol Clin Toxicol.* 2001;39:601-605.
60. Green R, Sitar DS, Tenenbein M: Effect of anticholinergic drugs on the efficacy of activated charcoal. *J Toxicol Clin Toxicol.* 2004;42:267-272.
61. Grierson R, Green R, Sitar DS, Tenenbein M: Gastric lavage for liquid poisons. *Ann Emerg Med.* 2000;35:435-439.
62. Guenther SE, Junkins EP Jr, Corneli HM, Schunk JE: Taste test: children rate flavoring agents used with activated charcoal. *Arch Pediatr Adolesc Med.* 2001;155:683-686.
63. Halcomb SE, Sivilotti MLA, Goklaney A, Mullins ME: Pharmacokinetic effects of diphenhydramine or oxycodone in simulated acetaminophen overdose. *Acad Emerg Med.* 2005;12:169-172.
64. Hider P, Helliwell P, Ardagh M, Kirk R: The epidemiology of emergency department attendances in Christchurch. *N Z Med J.* 2001;114:157-159.
65. Hoegberg LCG, Angelo HR, Christophersen AB, Christensen HR: Effect of ethanol and pH on the adsorption of acetaminophen (paracetamol) to high surface activated charcoal, in vitro studies. *J Toxicol Clin Toxicol.* 2002;40:59-67.
66. Hoegberg LCG, Angelo HR, Christophersen AJ, Christensen HR: The effect of food and ice cream on the adsorption capacity of paracetamol to high surface activated charcoal, in vitro studies. *Pharmacol Toxicol.* 2003;93:233-237.
67. Hoegberg LC, Christophersen AB, Christensen HR, Angelo HR: Comparison of the adsorption capacities of an activated-charcoal–yogurt mixture versus activated-charcoal–water slurry in vivo and in vitro. *Clin Toxicol.* 2005;43:269-275.
68. Hofbauer RD, Holger JS: The use of cholecystokinin as an adjunctive treatment for toxin ingestion. *J Toxicol Clin Toxicol.* 2004;42:61-66.
69. Hoffman RS: Does consensus equal correctness? *J Toxicol Clin Toxicol.* 2000;38:689-690.
70. Hoffman RS, Chiang WK, Howland MA, et al: Theophylline desorption from activated charcoal caused by whole bowel irrigation solution. *J Toxicol Clin Toxicol.* 1991;29:191-201.
71. Hoffman RS, Stringer JA, Feinberg RS, Goldfrank LR: Comparative efficacy of thallium adsorption by activated charcoal, Prussian blue, and sodium polystyrene sulfonate. *J Toxicol Clin Toxicol.* 1999;37:833-837.
72. Holt LM, Holz PH: The black bottle. A consideration of the role of charcoal in the treatment of poisoning in children. *J Pediatr.* 1963;63:306-314.
73. Hulten BA, Adams R, Askenasi R, et al: Activated charcoal in tri-cyclic antidepressant poisoning. *Hum Toxicol.* 1988;7:307-310.
74. Isbister GK, Downes F, Sibbritt D, et al: Aspiration pneumonitis in an overdose population: frequency, predictors, and outcomes. *Crit Care Med.* 2004;32:88-93.
75. Isbister GK, Friberg LE, Hackett LP, Duffull SB: Pharmacokinetics of quetiapine in overdose and the effect of activated charcoal. *Clin Pharmacol Ther.* 2007;81:821-827.
76. Jaffe JM, Colaizzi JL, Moriarty RW: Activated charcoal-carboxymethylcellulose gel formulation as an antidotal agent for orally ingested aspirin. *Am J Hosp Pharm.* 1976;33:717-719.
77. Jones A, Dargan P: *Churchill's Pocketbook of Toxicology*. London: Churchill Livingstone; 2001.
78. Jürgens G, Hoegberg LCG, Graudal NA: The effect of activated charcoal on drug exposure in healthy volunteers: a meta-analysis. *Clin Pharmacol Ther.* 2009;85:501-505.
79. Juurlink DN, McGuigan MA: Gastrointestinal decontamination for enteric-coated aspirin overdose: what to do depends on who you ask. *J Toxicol Clin Toxicol.* 2000;38:465-470.
80. Karim A, Ivatts S, Dargan P, Jones A: How feasible is it to conform to the European guidelines on administration of activated charcoal within one hour of an overdose? *Emerg Med J.* 2001;18:390-392.
81. Karkkainen S, Neuvonen PJ: Effect of oral charcoal and urine pH on dextropropoxyphene pharmacokinetics. *Int J Clin Pharmacol.* Ther Toxicol 1985;23:219-225.
82. Karkkainen S, Neuvonen PJ: Pharmacokinetics of amitriptyline influenced by oral charcoal and urine pH. *Int J Clin Pharmacol Ther Toxicol.* 1986;24:326-332.
83. Kilgore TL, Lehmann CR: Treatment of digoxin intoxication with colestipol. *South Med J.* 1982;75:1259-1260.
84. Kimura Y, Kamada Y, Kimura S: Case report: a patient with numerous tablets remaining in the stomach even 5 hours after ingestion. *Am J Emerg Med.* 2008;26:118.e1-118.e2.
85. Kirshenbaum LA, Sitar DS, Tenenbein M: Interaction between whole-bowel irrigation solution and activated charcoal: Implications for the treatment of toxic ingestions. *Ann Emerg Med.* 1990;19:1129-1132.
86. Krenzelok EP, McGuigan M, Lheur P: Position statement: ipecac syrup. American Academy of Clinical Toxicology; European Association of Poisons Centres and Clinical Toxicologists. *J Toxicol Clin Toxicol.* 1997;35:699-709.
87. Kulig K, Bar-Or D, Cantrill SV, et al: Management of acutely poisoned patients without gastric emptying. *Ann Emerg Med.* 1985;14:562-567.
88. Lai MW, Klein-Schwartz W, Rodgers GC, et al: 2005 Annual report of the American Association of Poison Control Centers Toxic Exposure Surveillance System. *Clin Toxicol.* 2006;44:803-932.
89. Lamminpaa A, Vilska J, Hoppu K: Medical charcoal for a child's poisoning at home: availability and success of administration in Finland. *Hum Exp Toxicol.* 1993;12:29-32.
90. Lapatto-Reiniluoto O, Kivisto KT, Neuvonen PJ: Activated charcoal alone and followed by whole-bowel irrigation in preventing the absorption of sustained-release drugs. *Clin Pharmacol Ther.* 2001;70:255-260.
91. Lapatto-Reiniluoto O, Kivisto KT, Neuvonen PJ: Efficacy of activated charcoal versus gastric lavage half an hour after ingestion of moclobemide, temazepam, and verapamil. *Eur J Clin Pharmacol.* 2000;56:285-288.
92. Lapatto Levy G, Soda DM, Lampman TA: Inhibition by ice cream of the antidotal efficacy of activated charcoal. *Am J Hosp Pharm.* 1975;32:289-291.
93. Larkin GL, Claassen C: Trends in emergency department use of gastric lavage for poisoning events in the United States, 1993–2003. *Clin Toxicol.* 2007;45:164-168.
94. Levy G, Houston JB: Effect of activated charcoal on acetaminophen absorption. *Pediatrics.* 1976;58:432-435.
95. Linakis JG, Hull KM, Lacouture PG, et al: Enhancement of lithium elimination by multiple-dose sodium polystyrene sulfonate. *Acad Emerg Med.* 1997;4:175-178.
96. Linakis JG, Savitt DL, Trainor BJ, et al: Potassium repletion fails to interfere with reduction of serum lithium by sodium polystyrene sulfonate in mice. *Acad Emerg Med.* 2001;8:956-960.
97. Linakis JG, Savitt DL, Wu TY, et al: Use of sodium polystyrene sulfonate for reduction of plasma lithium concentrations after chronic lithium dosing in mice. *J Toxicol Clin Toxicol.* 1998;36:309-313.
98. Ly BT, Schneir AB, Clark RF: Effect of whole bowel irrigation on the pharmacokinetics of an acetaminophen formulation and progression of radiopaque markers through the gastrointestinal tract. *Ann Emerg Med.* 2004;43:189-195.
99. Makosiej FJ, Hoffman RS, Howland MA, Goldfrank LR: An in vitro evaluation of cocaine hydrochloride adsorption by activated charcoal and desorption upon addition of polyethylene glycol electrolyte lavage solution. *J Toxicol Clin Toxicol.* 1993;31:381-395.
100. Manoguerra AS, Cobaugh DC: Guideline on the use of ipecac syrup in the out-of-hospital management of ingested poisons. *J Toxicol Clin Toxicol.* 2005;43:1-10.
101. Mathur LK, Reiniluoto O, Kivisto KT, Neuvonen PJ: Gastric decontamination performed 5 min after the ingestion of temazepam, verapamil and moclobemide: charcoal is superior to lavage. *Br J Clin Pharmacol.* 2000;49:274-278.
102. Mayersohn M, Perrier D, Picchioni AL: Evaluation of a charcoal-sorbitol mixture as an antidote for oral aspirin overdose. *Clin Toxicol.* 1977;11:561-567.
103. Merigian KS, Blaho KE: Single-dose oral activated charcoal in the treatment of the self-poisoned patient: a prospective, randomized, controlled trial. *Am J Ther.* 2002;9:301-308.
104. Merigian KS, Woodard M, Hedges JR, et al: Prospective evaluation of gastric emptying in the self-poisoned patient. *Am J Emerg Med.* 1990;8:479-483.
105. Mofredj A, Rakotondreantoanina JR, Farouj N: Severe hypernatremia secondary to gastric lavage. *Ann Fr Anesth Reanim.* 2000;19:219-220.
106. Mohamed F, Sooriyarachchi MR, Senarathna L et al: Compliance for single and multiple dose regimens of superactivated charcoal: a prospective study of patients in a clinical trial. *Clin Toxicol.* 2007;45:132-135.
107. Moll J, Kerns W 2nd, Tomaszewski C, Rose R: Incidence of aspiration pneumonia in intubated patients receiving activated charcoal. *J Emerg Med.* 1999;17:279-283.

108. Navarro RP, Navarro KR, Krenzelok EP: Relative efficacy and palatability of three activated charcoal mixtures. *Vet Hum Toxicol.* 1980;22:6-9.
109. Neuvonen PJ, Kannisto H, Lankinen S: Capacity of two forms of activated charcoal to adsorb nefopam in vitro and to reduce its toxicity in vivo. *J Toxicol Clin Toxicol.* 1983;21:333-342.
110. Neuvonen PJ, Olkkola KT, Alanen T: Effect of ethanol and pH on the adsorption of drugs to activated charcoal: studies in vitro and in man. *Acta Pharmacol Toxicol.* 1984;54:1-7.
111. Oderda GM: Letter: activated charcoal and ice cream. *Am J Hosp Pharm.* 1975;32:562.
112. Olkkola KT: Does ethanol modify antidotal efficacy of oral activated charcoal studies in vitro and in experimental animals. *J Toxicol Clin Toxicol.* 1984;22:425-432.
113. Olkkola KT: Effect of charcoal-drug ratio on antidotal efficacy of oral activated charcoal in man. *Br J Clin Pharmacol.* 1985;19:767-773.
114. Olkkola KT, Neuvonen PJ: Effect of gastric pH on antidotal efficacy of activated charcoal in man. *Int J Clin Pharmacol.* Ther Toxicol 1984;22:565-569.
115. Olmedo R, Nelson L, Chu J, Hoffman RS: Is surgical decontamination definitive treatment of "body-packers"? *Am J Emerg Med.* 2001;19:593-596.
116. Oppenheim RC: Strawberry-flavoured activated charcoal. *Med J Aust.* 1980;1:39.
117. Osterhoudt KC, Alpern ER, Durbin D, et al: Activated charcoal administration in a pediatric emergency department. *Pediatr Emerg Care.* 2004;20:493-498.
118. Osterhoudt KC, Durbin D, Alpern ER, Henretig FM: Risk factors for emesis after therapeutic use of activated charcoal in acutely poisoned children. *Pediatrics.* 2004;113:806-810.
119. Peterson CD, Fifield GC: Emergency gastrotomy for acute iron poisoning. *Ann Emerg Med.* 1980;9:262-264.
120. Picchioni AL: Activated charcoal as an antidote for poisons. *Am J Hosp Pharm.* 1967;24:38-39.
121. Picchioni AL: Management of acute poisonings with activated charcoal. *Am J Hosp Pharm.* 1971;28:62-64.
122. Pieroni RE, Fisher JG: Use of cholestyramine resin in digitoxin toxi-city. *JAMA.* 1981;245:1939-1940.
123. Pond SM, Lewis-Driver DJ, Williams GM, et al: Gastric emptying in acute overdose: a prospective randomised controlled trial. *Med J Aust.* 1995;163:345-349.
124. Position paper: ipecac syrup. *J Toxicol Clin Toxicol.* 2004;42:133-143.
125. Position paper: whole bowel irrigation. *J Toxicol Clin Toxicol.* 2004;42:843-854.
126. Rangan C, Nordt SP, Hamilton R, et al: Treatment of acetaminophen ingestion with a superactivated charcoal-cola mixture. *Ann Emerg Med.* 2001;37:55-58.
127. Roberts DM, Southcott E, Potter JM, et al: Pharmacokinetics of digoxin cross-reacting substances in patients with acute yellow oleander (*Thevetia peruviana*) poisoning, including the effect of activated charcoal. *Ther Drug Monit.* 2006;28:784-792.
128. Roivas L, Neuvonen PJ: Drug adsorption onto activated charcoal as a means of formulation. *Methods Find Exp Clin Pharmacol.* 1994;16:367-372.
129. Roivas L, Ojala-Karlsson P, Neuvonen PJ: The bioavailability of two beta-blockers preadsorbed onto charcoal. *Methods Find Exp Clin Pharmacol.* 1994;16:125-132.
130. Roy TM, Ossorio MA, Cipolla LM, et al: Pulmonary complications after tricyclic antidepressant overdose. *Chest.* 1989;96:852-856.
131. Rybolt TR, Burrell DE, Shults JM, Kelley AK: In vitro coadsorption of acetaminophen and N-acetylcysteine onto activated carbon powder. *J Pharm Sci.* 1986;75:904-906.
132. Saincher A, Sitar DS, Tenenbein M: Efficacy of ipecac during the first hour after drug ingestion in human volunteers. *J Toxicol Clin Toxicol.* 1997;35:609-615.
133. Salen P, Shih R, Sierzenski P, Reed J: Effect of physostigmine and gastric lavage in a *Datura stramonium*-induced anticholinergic poisoning epidemic. *Am J Emerg Med.* 2003;21:316-317.
134. Satar S, Toprak N, Gokel Y, Sebe A: Intoxication with 100 grams of mercury: a case report and importance of supportive therapy. *Eur J Emerg Med.* 2001;8:245-248.
135. Sato RL, Wong JJ, Sumida SM, et al: Efficacy of superactivated charcoal administered late (3 hours) after acetaminophen overdose. *Am J Emerg Med.* 2003;21:189-191.
136. Schaper A, Hofmann R, Ebbecke M, et al: Cocaine-body-packing: infrequent indication for laparotomy. *Chirurg.* 2003;74:626-631.
137. Sellers EM, Khouw V, Dolman L: Comparative drug adsorption by activated charcoal. *J Pharm Sci.* 1977;66:1640-1641.
138. Sherman A, Zingler BM: Successful endoscopic retrieval of a cocaine packet from the stomach. *Gastrointest Endosc.* 1990;36:152-154.
139. Spiller HA, Rodgers GC Jr: Evaluation of administration of activated charcoal in the home. *Pediatrics.* 2001;108:E100.
140. Spiller HA, Winter ML, Klein-Schwartz W, Bangh SA: Efficacy of activated charcoal administered more than four hours after acetaminophen overdose. *J Emerg Med.* 2006;30:1-5.
141. Suarez CA, Arango A, Lester JL 3rd: Cocaine-condom ingestion. Surgical treatment. *JAMA.* 1977;238:1391-1392.
142. Tenenbein M: Position statement: whole bowel irrigation. American Academy of Clinical Toxicology; European Association of Poisons Centres and Clinical Toxicologists. *J Toxicol Clin Toxicol.* 1997;35:753-762.
143. Teubner DJO: Absence of ice-cream interference with the adsorption of paracetamol onto activated charcoal. *Emerg Med.* 2000;12:326-328.
144. Thomas SH, Bevan L, Bhattacharyya S, et al: Presentation of poisoned patients to accident and emergency departments in the north of England. *Hum Exp Toxicol.* 1996;15:466-470.
145. Tomaszewski C, Musso C, Pearson JR, et al: Lithium absorption prevented by sodium polystyrene sulfonate in volunteers. *Ann Emerg Med.* 1992;21:1308-1311.
146. Tomaszewski C, Voorhees S, Wathen J, et al: Cocaine adsorption to activated charcoal in vitro. *J Emerg Med.* 1992;10:59-62.
147. Traub SJ, Hoffman RS, Nelson LS: Body packing—the internal concealment of illicit drugs. *N Engl J Med.* 2003;349:2519-2526.
148. Traub SJ, Kohn GL, Hoffman RS, Nelson LS: Pediatric "body packing." *Arch Pediatr Adolesc Med.* 2003;157:174-177.
149. Tsitoura A, Atta-Politou J, Koupparis MA: In vitro adsorption study of fluoxetine onto activated charcoal at gastric and intestinal pH using high performance liquid chromatography with fluorescence detector. *J Toxicol Clin Toxicol.* 1997;35:269-276.
150. Underhill TJ, Greene MK, Dove AF: A comparison of the efficacy of gastric lavage, ipecacuanha and activated charcoal in the emergency management of paracetamol overdose. *Arch Emerg Med.* 1990;7:148-154.
151. Vale JA: Position statement: gastric lavage. American Academy of Clinical Toxicology; European Association of Poisons Centres and Clinical Toxicologists. *J Toxicol Clin Toxicol.* 1997;35:711-719.
152. Vale JA, Krenzelok EP, Barceloux GD: Position statement and practice guidelines on the use of multi-dose activated charcoal in the treatment of acute poisoning. American Academy of Clinical Toxicology; European Association of Poisons Centres and Clinical Toxicologists. *J Toxicol Clin Toxicol.* 1999;37:731-751.
153. Vale JA, Kulig K: Position paper: gastric lavage. American Academy of Clinical Toxicology, European Association of Poisons Centres and Clinical Toxicologists. *J Toxicol Clin Toxicol.* 2004;42:933-943.
154. Van Ameyde KJ, Tenenbein M: Whole bowel irrigation during pregnancy. *Am J Obstet Gynecol.* 1989;160:646-647.
155. Velez LI, Gracia R, Mills LD, et al: Iron bezoar retained in colon despite 3 days of whole bowel irrigation. *J Toxicol Clin Toxicol.* 2004;42:653-656.
156. Visser L, Stricker B, Hoogendoorn M, Vinks A: Do not give paraffin to packers. *Lancet.* 1998;352:1352.
157. Yamashita M, Yamashita M, Azuma J: Urinary excretion of ipecac alkaloids in human volunteers. *Vet Hum Toxicol.* 2002;44:257-259.
158. Yancy RE, O'Barr TP, Corby DG: In vitro and in vivo evaluation of the effect of cherry flavoring on the adsorptive capacity of activated charcoal for salicylic acid. *Vet Hum Toxicol.* 1977;19:163-165.
159. Yeates PJ, Thomas SH: Effectiveness of delayed activated charcoal administration in simulated paracetamol (acetaminophen) overdose. *Br J Clin Pharmacol.* 2000;49:11-14.

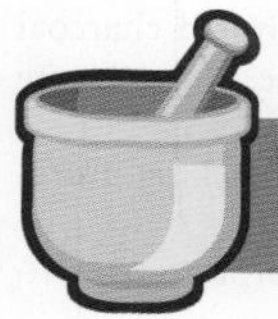

ANTIDOTES IN DEPTH (A1)

SYRUP OF IPECAC

Mary Ann Howland

Emetine

The role of syrup of ipecac has changed dramatically over the past decade. Once the mainstay of poison management, a critical evaluation of animal, volunteer, and a limited number of clinical studies suggests that ipecac administration should be reserved for a very few rare circumstances, if any, rather than administered on a routine basis.[3,5,32] The rationale for this change is based on the facts that (1) most poisonings in children are benign; (2) many adults overdose with xenobiotics that rapidly cause an altered mental status, which constitutes a contraindication to the administration of ipecac; (3) ipecac-induced vomiting may be delayed or persistent, thereby resulting in a delay in the administration of activated charcoal; and (4) the abuse of ipecac by bulimics is substantial.[54]

Syrup of ipecac is an emetic that has been used for the management of poisonings since the 1950s and has been available without prescription since the late 1960s. Pediatricians were encouraged to advise parents to keep syrup of ipecac in their homes. Many physicians currently believe that there is no role for syrup of ipecac in the prehospital or hospital setting and that the abuse of syrup of ipecac by patients with bulimia outweighs any benefit originating from keeping syrup of ipecac as a nonprescription drug. The Food and Drug Administration (FDA) is still reviewing whether to make syrup of ipecac available only by prescription. Advocates for maintaining the nonprescription status of syrup of ipecac support home stocking of ipecac for use in remote areas and limiting use in healthcare facilities to those rare instances when activated charcoal, orogastric lavage, or whole-bowel irrigation with polyethylene glycol electrolyte lavage solution may be inappropriate or inadequate. Changing the availability of syrup of ipecac to prescription status only could result in the complete disappearance of syrup of ipecac from the pharmaceutical market if the FDA requires a new drug application.[51] Under these circumstances, it might not be profitable for any drug company to invest in a new drug application.

COMPOSITION

Ipecac is derived from the dried rhizome and roots of plants found in Brazil belonging to the family Rubiaceae, such as *Cephaelis acuminata* and *Cephaelis ipecacuanha*.[59,60] Cephaeline and emetine are the two alkaloids largely responsible for the production of nausea and vomiting, with cephaeline being the more potent.[31] Each 15-mL dose of syrup of ipecac contains 16 to 21 mg of cephaeline and 6.4 to 21 mg of emetine, resulting in variable cephaeline-to-emetine ratios. Syrup of ipecac also contains a small amount of psychotrine, which does not contribute to emesis but is currently under investigation for its potential anti-HIV effects.

PHARMACOKINETICS OF IPECAC ALKALOIDS

After 20 or 30 mL of syrup of ipecac was administered to human volunteers plasma, vomitus, and urine concentrations of emetine and cephaeline were determined by the use of high-performance liquid chromatography (HPLC).[50,65] Peak plasma concentrations of the alkaloids were reached by 20 minutes to 1 hour and were undetectable at 2 to 6 hours. Only 2% of the total amount of alkaloids in the ipecac were excreted in the urine within 48 hours but remained detectable in the urine for 2 weeks in all 12 volunteers and for 12 weeks in one of two subjects who were tested subsequently.

MECHANISM OF ACTION

Syrup of ipecac induces vomiting by local activation of peripheral emetic sensory receptors in the proximal small intestine and by central stimulation of the chemoreceptor trigger zone that serves as a sensory area, resulting in subsequent activation of the central vomiting center.[55] $5HT_3$ receptors mediate the nausea and vomiting produced by syrup of ipecac by both mechanisms. This was demonstrated in 40 volunteers by administering a specific $5HT_3$ antagonist 30 minutes before administration of syrup of ipecac; the $5HT_3$ antagonist prevented or attenuated the nausea and vomiting in a dose-dependent fashion.[21] In fact, syrup of ipecac is used to assess the efficacy of $5HT_3$ antagonists such as ondansetron and other antiemetics.[8,16,52]

TIME TO ONSET OF VOMITING AND NUMBER OF VOMITING EPISODES

In one of the earliest studies evaluating the delay in onset to vomiting after syrup of ipecac administration, 88% of 214 children who were given 20 mL of syrup of ipecac and copious amounts of water vomited within 30 minutes (mean, 18.7 minutes).[45] Adverse events secondary to syrup of ipecac were not noted. Subsequent studies demonstrated similar findings.[7,14,17,19,23,30,33,57,58]

The onset of emesis after syrup of ipecac administration does not appear to be affected by fluid administration before or after administration of syrup of ipecac, by the temperature of the fluids, or by gentle patient motion or walking.[19,20,23,53] Consequently, it is inadvisable to force fluids and safer to maintain the patient in an appropriate stationary setting (e.g., chair or stretcher). Milk should not be given with the syrup of ipecac because the onset of emesis may be delayed, although the success of inducing vomiting does not appear to be affected.[20] This delay is consistent with the ability of milk to delay gastric emptying and thereby retard contact between ipecac and the peripheral emetic sensory receptors.[61]

The average number of episodes of vomiting after syrup of ipecac administration is three, with a range of one to eight episodes.[30] The duration of syrup of ipecac–induced vomiting averages 23 to 60 minutes.[30,44] Although some investigators have suggested durations lasting up to 3 to 4 hours,[36,39] it is probably reasonable to assume that vomiting that persists for more than 2 hours is unrelated to syrup of ipecac administration, and another cause should be sought. This warning is of particular importance when syrup of ipecac is used at home.

VOLUNTEER STUDIES

Many studies have assessed the effectiveness of syrup of ipecac–induced emesis in decreasing absorption of a xenobiotic and then compared the results with other methods of gastric decontamination, such as gastric lavage or activated charcoal.[39,40,48] These same studies support the concept that the sooner syrup of ipecac is administered after ingestion, the greater the amount of the ingested xenobiotic that will be recovered. The decrease in the amount of xenobiotic absorbed varies from study to study as a result of differences in study design, including time to initiation of the various techniques and the particular xenobiotic used to assess efficacy. Volunteer studies using small lavage tubes were further limited because of both the quantity of the xenobiotic that was administered and the limited potential of the tube to recover the xenobiotic. In a small, well-quantified study, when six adult volunteers were given 20 mL of syrup of ipecac at 5 or 30 minutes after acetaminophen ingestion, absorption was inhibited by 65% and 0%, respectively.[40] In this same volunteer model, absorption was inhibited by 80% and 40% when 50 g of activated charcoal was given at 5 and 30 minutes postingestion.[41]

A subsequent investigation demonstrated that the reduction in the area under the plasma drug concentration versus time curve was equivalent for patients treated with syrup of ipecac–induced emesis and patients treated with activated charcoal plus a cathartic.[58] Comparison of orogastric lavage, syrup of ipecac–induced emesis, and activated charcoal, all given at 60 minutes to adult volunteers, after ingestion of ampicillin showed reductions of 32%, 38%, and 57%, respectively.[58] Adult volunteers given syrup of ipecac 5 minutes after administration of 30 capsules containing a radionucleotide marker demonstrated a mean 54% removal (range, 21%–89%) compared with a mean removal of 35.5% (range, 1%–71%) with orogastric lavage.[66] Other researchers demonstrated recoveries from 0% to 85%.[7,17,18,57] Children given a magnesium hydroxide marker before administration of syrup of ipecac demonstrated a mean recovery of 28%, although the range was 0% to 78%.[17]

OVERDOSED PATIENTS

In one study of self-poisoned adults, they were randomized to receive either syrup of ipecac or orogastric lavage with a 33-French lavage tube. All patients had subsequent gastric endoscopy.[47] Thirteen patients were given syrup of ipecac and vomited within 23 minutes (range, 11–25 minutes). Two of these patients had tablets in the vomitus and on endoscopy, only those two had residual tablets in the stomach. Ten of 17 patients who were lavaged had tablets in the lavage fluid, all of whom had tablets in the stomach at the time of endoscopy. Two additional patients also had residual tablets in the stomach,[47] suggesting a potential additional benefit of activated charcoal after emesis and lavage.

This same group of investigators used barium-marked 3-mm^3 pellets to evaluate the effectiveness of gastric emptying.[48] Forty self-poisoned patients were given 20 pellets on admission and randomized immediately to therapy with either orogastric lavage or syrup of ipecac–induced emesis. Approximately 45% of the pellets were removed in both the orogastric lavage and the syrup of ipecac groups. Two patients in the lavage group and one in the syrup of ipecac group had 100% removal of pellets, and two patients in the lavage group had no removal.[48]

OUTCOME STUDIES

A large emergency department (ED) study addressed whether gastric emptying with either syrup of ipecac followed by activated charcoal or orogastric lavage followed by activated charcoal was more effective than activated charcoal alone in overdosed patients.[28] Syrup of ipecac did not affect the outcome in treated patients.

A study using the Toxic Exposure Surveillance System (TESS) database determined that home use of syrup of ipecac did not reduce the rate of ED referrals.[13] It could have been predicted that this study would not identify an improvement in patient outcome because most children have no clinical sequelae from exposure. Group statistics cannot identify a potentially beneficial effect that occurs rarely.

CONTRAINDICATIONS

Syrup of ipecac should not be administered to patients who have ingested acids or alkalis, are younger than 6 months of age, are expected to deteriorate rapidly, have a depressed mental status, have a compromised gag reflex, have ingested objects such as batteries or sharps, or have a need for rapid gastrointestinal evacuation to prevent absorption. Syrup of ipecac should not be administered to those for whom the hazards of vomiting and aspiration of the ingested substance outweigh the risks associated with systemic absorption (e.g., hydrocarbons), those who have significant prior vomiting, those for whom vomiting will delay administration of an oral antidote, and those with a hemorrhagic diathesis or a nontoxic ingestion, or when toxin is no longer expected to be in the stomach.

ADVERSE EFFECTS

Considering the number of times it has been administered without incident in this country, syrup of ipecac should be considered a relatively safe drug when given in therapeutic doses to patients for whom there are no contraindications. Sedation, especially in children, pulmonary aspiration (most likely from vomiting), and diarrhea are often reported.[32] When ipecac contacts the lower gastrointestinal tract, irritation leads to diarrhea, as was demonstrated in a recent volunteer study.[8] Uncommon problems that have occurred after therapeutic doses of syrup of ipecac include a Mallory-Weiss esophageal tear in an adult given 30 mL of syrup of ipecac for a multidrug overdose,[56] herniation of the stomach into the left chest in a child who had a previously unrecognized underlying congenital defect of the diaphragm,[46] intracerebral hemorrhage,[25] and pneumomediastinum.[63] Additional problems associated with syrup of ipecac administration include pulmonary aspiration of stomach contents, volatile hydrocarbons or foreign bodies, and the associated time delay before it is possible to perform a necessary therapeutic intervention such as administration of activated charcoal or an oral antidote. Another reported problem is the emesis-induced vagal response of bradycardia.[37]

The surreptitious self-administration of frequent doses of syrup of ipecac by patients with bulimia and other related eating disorders results in substantial morbidity, such as extreme muscle weakness, congestive cardiomyopathy, and mortality.[1,10,31,34,42,49,64] Myofibril analysis of ipecac-abusing patients reveals degeneration and a "moth-eaten" appearance, and electron microscopy reveals Z-band streaming and disorganization.[29] When emetine was routinely used for the treatment of amebiasis in the early 1900s, cardiovascular and neuromuscular toxicity occurred. Similarly, inadvertent administration of the fluid extract of ipecac, which is 14 times more potent than syrup of ipecac, produces violent and protracted vomiting, diarrhea, seizures, cardiac toxicity, including PR interval prolongation, T-wave abnormalities, QRS complex abnormalities, atrial dysrhythmias, premature ventricular beats, and ventricular fibrillation, neuromuscular toxicity, including weakness and neuropathy, shock, and death.[31] Surreptitious chronic intentional ipecac poisoning of children, a form of Munchausen Syndrome by Proxy, has also been reported.[11,15,35,62] Self-administration by a child for the purpose of seeking attention and family distraction has also been reported.[43] The findings in these children included vomiting, diarrhea, lethargy, irritability, hypothermia, and hypotonia. The children described had been brought to healthcare providers by their parents for atypical patterns of vomiting and had multiple unsuccessful clinical evaluations.

LABORATORY DETECTION OF SYRUP OF IPECAC

When surreptitious use of syrup of ipecac is suspected as the cause of chronic vomiting, screening the urine, plasma, and vomitus for emetine (thin-layer chromatography screen—Toxi-Lab or HPLC) may be useful.[6,35,65]

CURRENT ROLE OF SYRUP OF IPECAC IN POISON MANAGEMENT

Most authorities agree with the American Academy of Pediatrics' statement that syrup of ipecac should no longer be used routinely.[3,4,32] Instead of promoting the concept of the maintenance of syrup of ipecac in the home, the Academy of Pediatrics currently states that "the first action for a caregiver of a child who may have ingested a toxic substance is to consult with the local poison center."[4] Logically, the sooner that syrup of ipecac is administered after ingestion, the more effective it may be in reducing absorption of the xenobiotic. For this reason, rather than completely abandoning syrup of ipecac, perhaps a targeted approach should be developed. This would mean continuing to promote the stocking of syrup of ipecac in the home setting in remote areas.

Only a few groups of patients are considered appropriate candidates for the use of syrup of ipecac. Patients who are candidates for syrup of ipecac are those who (1) ingest a xenobiotic with considerable risk of toxicity that does not cause a rapid change in mental status, such as acetaminophen or salicylates; (2) consume massive amounts of a toxin that may exceed the binding capacity of activated charcoal, such as salicylates; or (3) ingest a toxin not bound to activated charcoal, such as lithium. Under these circumstances, if the presence of unabsorbed xenobiotic in the stomach remains a potential problem, then the use of syrup of ipecac may be appropriate in rare instances when weighed against the utility of activated charcoal or whole-bowel irrigation with polyethylene glycol electrolyte lavage solution. The time frame for this decision is usually within 1 to 2 hours after ingestion.

ADMINISTRATION

The dose of syrup of ipecac is 15 mL in children 1 to 12 years old and 30 mL in older children and adults. If vomiting does not ensue after the first dose, the same dose may be repeated once 20 to 30 minutes after administration of the first dose. For children 6 to 12 months of age, the dose of syrup of ipecac is 5 to 10 mL, and its use should be limited to a maximum single 10-mL dose.[12,27] Water can be offered but is not essential for success. Vomiting will occur in most patients. Home users should be warned that persistent vomiting for more than 2 hours may indicate toxicity from the primary xenobiotics ingested not the antidote, necessitating medical evaluation.

CONCLUSION

There are very few cases in which syrup of ipecac is indicated in the home setting because typically most ingestions are either nontoxic or, conversely, of such consequence that an imminent deterioration in mental status may occur making syrup of ipecac administration dangerous. Parents in areas with poor access to a healthcare facility should still be encouraged to keep syrup of ipecac and activated charcoal at home as potential first aid measures, but caregivers should be cautioned to use them only on the advice of a regional poison center or physician.

In the ED, the role of syrup of ipecac is extremely limited. One of the only possible candidates for syrup of ipecac in the overdose setting is a child or adult who arrives in the ED shortly after the ingestion of a large number of poorly soluble tablets of a size unlikely to be removed by lavage and also unlikely to cause a rapid change in mental status. One other candidate is a child or adult who has taken such a large amount of a highly toxic substance that a favorable activated charcoal-to-drug ratio cannot be attained with certainty, and an antidote is not available. Whole-bowel irrigation should be considered as a suitable alternative when the xenobiotic has a prolonged absorptive phase.

REFERENCES

1. Adler AG, Walinsky P, Krall RA, Cho SY: Death resulting from ipecac syrup poisoning. *JAMA.* 1980;243:1927-1928.
2. Albertson TE, Derlet RW, Foulke GE, et al: Superiority of activated charcoal alone compared with ipecac and activated charcoal in the treatment of acute toxic ingestions. *Ann Emerg Med.* 1989;18:56-59.
3. American Academy of Clinical Toxicology, European Association of Poison Center and Clinical Toxicologists: Position statement: Ipecac syrup. *J Toxicol Clin Toxicol.* 1997;35:699-709.
4. American Academy of Pediatrics Committee on Injury, Violence and Poison Prevention. Poison treatment in the home. *Pediatrics.* 2003;112:1182-1185.
5. American Academy of Clinical Toxicology and European Association of Poison Centres and Clinical Toxicologists: Position Paper: Ipecac syrup. *J Toxicol Clin Toxicol.* 2004;42:133-144.
6. Asano T, Sadakane C, Ishihara K et al: High performance liquid chromatographic assay with fluorescence detection for the determination of cephaeline and emetine in human plasma and urine. *J Chromatogr B Biomed Sci Appl.* 2001;757:197-206.
7. Auerbach P, Osterloh J, Braun O, et al: Efficacy of gastric emptying: Gastric lavage versus emesis induced with ipecac. *Ann Emerg Med.* 1986;15:692-698.

8. Axelsson P, ThSE, Wattwil M: Betamethasone does not prevent nausea and vomiting induced by ipecacuanha. *Acta Anaesthesiol Scand.* 2004;48:1283-1286.
9. Banner W, Veltri J: The case of ipecac syrup [editorial]. *Am J Dis Child.* 1988;142:596.
10. Bennett H, Spiro A, Pollack M, et al: Ipecac-induced myopathy simulating dermatomyositis. *Neurology.* 1982;32:91-94.
11. Berkner P, Kaster T, Skolnick L: Chronic ipecac poisoning in infancy: A case report. *Pediatrics.* 1988;82:384-386.
12. Boehnert M, Lewander W, Gaudreault P, et al: Advances in clinical toxicology. *Pediatr Clin North Am.* 1985;32:193-211.
13. Bond GR: Home syrup of ipecac does not reduce emergency department use or improve outcome. *Pediatrics.* 2003;112:1061-1064.
14. Boxer L, Anderson F, Rowe D: Comparison of ipecac-induced emesis with gastric lavage in the treatment of acute salicylate ingestion. *J Pediatr.* 1969;74:800-803.
15. Carter KE, Izsak E, Marlow J: Munchhausen syndrome by proxy caused by ipecac poisoning. *Pediatr Emerg Care.* 2006;22:655-666.
16. Cooper M, Sologuren A, Valiente R, Smith J: Effects of lerisetron, a new 5-HT3 receptor antagonist, on ipecacuanha-induced emesis in healthy volunteers. *Arzneimittelforschung.* 2002;52:689-694.
17. Corby D, Decker W, Moran M, et al: Clinical comparison of pharmacologic emetics in children. *Pediatrics.* 1968;42:361-364.
18. Curtis R, Barone J, Giacona N: Efficacy of ipecac and activated charcoal and cathartic: Prevention of salicylate absorption in a simulated overdose. *Arch Intern Med.* 1984;144:48-52.
19. Dean B, Krenzelok E: Syrup of ipecac: 15 mL versus 30 mL in pediatric poisonings. *J Toxicol Clin Toxicol.* 1985;23:165-170.
20. Eisenga B, Meester W: Evaluation of the effect of motility on syrup of ipecac-induced emesis [abstract]. *Vet Hum Toxicol.* 1978;20:462.
21. Forster ER, Palmer JL, Bedding AW, Smith JTL: Syrup of ipecacuanha-induced nausea and emesis is medicated by 5HT3 receptors in man. *J Physiol (London).* 1994;477:72.
22. Freedman G, Pasternak S, Krenzelok E: A clinical trial using syrup of ipecac and activated charcoal concurrently. *Ann Emerg Med.* 1987;16: 164-166.
23. Grande G, Ling L: The effect of fluid volume on syrup of ipecac emesis time. *J Toxicol Clin Toxicol.* 1987;25:473-481.
24. Isner JM: Effects of ipecac on the heart. *N Engl J Med.* 1986;314:1253.
25. Klein-Schwartz W, Gorman R, Oderda G, et al: Ipecac use in the elderly: The unanswered question. *Ann Emerg Med.* 1984;13:1152-1154.
26. Kornberg AE, Dolgen J: Pediatric ingestions: Charcoal alone versus ipecac and charcoal. *Ann Emerg Med.* 1991;20:648-651.
27. Krenzelok K, Dean B: syrup of ipecac in children less than one year of age. *J Toxicol Clin Toxicol.* 1985;23:171-176.
28. Kulig K, Bar-Or D, Cantrill SV, et al: Management of acutely poisoned patients without gastric emptying. *Ann Emerg Med.* 1985;14: 562-567.
29. Lancomis D: Case of the month. Anorexia nervosa. *Brain Pathol.* 1996;6:535-536.
30. MacLean W: A comparison of ipecac syrup and apomorphine in the immediate treatment of ingestion of poisons. *J Pediatr.* 1973;82:121-124.
31. Manno B, Manno J: Toxicology of ipecac. *Clin Toxicol.* 1977;10: 221-242.
32. Manoguerra A, Cobaugh D and the Members of the Guidelines for the Management of Poisonings Consensus Panel: Guideline on the use of ipecac syrup in the out-of-hospital management of ingested poisons. *Clin Toxicol.* 2005;1:1-10.
33. Manoguerra A, Krenzelok E: Rapid emesis from high dose ipecac syrup in adults and children intoxicated with antiemetics and other drugs. *Am J Hosp Pharm.* 1978;35:1360-1362.
34. Mateer J, Farrell B, Chou SM, Gutman L: Reversible ipecac myopathy. *Arch Neurol.* 1985;42:188-190.
35. McClung H, Murray R, Braden N, et al: Intentional ipecac poisoning in children. *Am J Dis Child.* 1988;142:637-639.
36. McNamara R, Aaron C, Gemborys M, Davidheiser S: Efficacy of charcoal versus ipecac in reducing serum acetaminophen in a simulated overdose. *Ann Emerg Med.* 1988;17:243-246.
37. Meester W: Emesis and lavage. *Vet Hum Toxicol.* 1981;22:225-234.
38. Merigian KS, Woodard M, Hedges JR, et al: Prospective evaluation of gastric emptying in the self-poisoned patient. *Am J Emerg Med.* 1990;8:479-483.
39. Neuvonen P: Clinical pharmacokinetics of oral activated charcoal in acute intoxications. *Clin Pharmacokinet.* 1982;7:465-489.
40. Neuvonen P, Olkkola K: Activated charcoal and syrup of ipecac in the prevention of cimetidine and pindolol absorption in man after administration of metoclopramide as an antiemetic. *J Toxicol Clin Toxicol.* 1984;22: 103-114.
41. Neuvonen P, Vartiainen M, Tokola O: Comparison of activated charcoal and ipecac syrup in prevention of drug absorption. *Eur J Clin Pharmacol.* 1983;24:557-562.
42. Palmer E, Guay A: Reversible myopathy secondary to abuse of ipecac in patients with major eating disorders. *N Engl J Med.* 1985;313:1457-1459.
43. Rashid N: Medically unexplained myopathy due to ipecac abuse. *Psychosomatics.* 2006;47:167-169.
44. Rauber A, Maroncelli R: The duration of emetic effect of ipecac: Duration and frequency of vomiting [abstract]. *Vet Hum Toxicol.* 1982;24:281.
45. Robertson WO: Syrup of ipecac: A slow or fast emetic? *Am J Dis Child.* 1962;103:136-139.
46. Robertson WO: Syrup of ipecac associated fatality: A case report. *Vet Hum Toxicol.* 1979;21:87-89.
47. Saetta JP, March S, Gaunt ME, Quinton DN: Gastric emptying procedures in the self-poisoned patient: Are we forcing gastric content beyond the pylorus? *J R Soc Med.* 1991;84:274-277.
48. Saetta JP, Quinton DN: Residual gastric content after gastric lavage and ipecacuanha induced emesis in self-poisoned patients: An endoscopic study. *J R Soc Med.* 1991;84:35-38.
49. Schiff R, Wurzel C, Brunson S, et al: Death due to chronic syrup of ipecac use in a patient with bulimia. *Pediatrics.* 1986;78:412-416.
50. Scharman EJ, Hutzler JM, Rosencrance JG, Tracy TS: Single dose pharmacokinetics of syrup of ipecac. *Ther Drug Monit.* 2000;22:566-573.
51. Shannon M: The demise of ipecac. *Pediatrics.* 2003;112:1180-1181.
52. Soderpalm AH, Schuster A, de Wit H: Antiemetic efficacy of smoked marijuana. Subjective and behavioral effects on nausea induced by syrup of ipecac. *Pharmacol Biochem Behav.* 2001;69:343-350.
53. Spiegel R, Addouch I, Munn D: The effect of temperature on concurrently administered fluid on the onset of ipecac-induced emesis. *Clin Toxicol.* 1979;14:281-284.
54. Steffen KJ, Mitchell JE, Roerig JL, Lancaster KL: The eating disorders medicine cabinet revisited. A clinician's guide to ipecac and laxatives. *Int J of Eat Disord.* 2007:40:360-368.
55. Stewart J: Effects of emetic and cathartic agents on the gastrointestinal tract and the treatment of toxic ingestion. *J Toxicol Clin Toxicol.* 1983;20:199-253.
56. Tandberg D, Liechty E, Fishbein D: Mallory-Weiss syndrome: An unusual complication of ipecac-induced emesis. *Ann Emerg Med.* 1981;10: 521-523.
57. Tandberg D, Diven B, McLeod J: Ipecac-induced emesis versus gastric lavage: A controlled study in normal adults. *Am J Emerg Med.* 1986;4:205-209.
58. Tenenbein M, Cohen, Sitar D: Efficacy of ipecac-induced emesis, orogastric lavage, and activated charcoal for acute drug overdose. *Ann Emerg Med.* 1987;16:838-841.
59. *United States Pharmacopeia 21 and National Formulary 16*(suppl 2). Rockville, MD: US Pharmacopeia Convention; 1985.
60. Vandaveer C: How ipecac was discovered. Available at http://www. killer-plants.com/what's-in-a-name/20030110.asp. Accessed April 25, 2005.
61. Varipapa RJ, Oderda GM: Effect of milk on ipecac-induced emesis. *J Am Pharm Assoc.* 1977;17:510.
62. Wagner C, Bowers W: Cardiomyopathy in a child induced by intentional ipecac abuse. *Air Med J.* 2006;25:236-237.
63. Wolowodiuk O, McMicken D, O'Brien P: Pneumomediastinum and pneumoretroperitoneum: An unusual complication of syrup of ipecac induced emesis. *Ann Emerg Med.* 1984;13:1148-1151.
64. Woolf AD, Grew JM: Acute poisonings among adolescents and young adults with anorexia nervosa. *Am J Dis Child.* 1990;144:785-788.
65. Yamashita M, Yamashita M, Azuma J: Urinary excretion ipecac alkaloids in human volunteers. *Vet Hum Toxicol.* 2002;44:257-259.
66. Young WF, Bruin SMG: Evaluation of gastric emptying using radionucleotides: Gastric lavage versus ipecac-induced emesis. *Ann Emerg Med.* 1993;22:1423-1427.

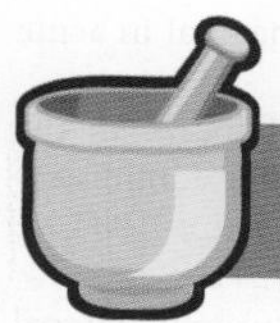

ANTIDOTES IN DEPTH (A2)

ACTIVATED CHARCOAL

Mary Ann Howland

Activated charcoal (AC) is an excellent nonspecific adsorbent. The current debate regarding the role of AC in poison management relies on reconciling evidence-based studies in volunteers and heterogeneous poisoned and overdosed patients with clinical experience.[4] AC should be considered for administration to a poisoned or overdosed patient after a risk-to-benefit assessment for the substance presumably ingested and ideally also for the circumstances of the exposure for a particular patient.[13] The benefits include inactivating a potentially toxic xenobiotic; the risks include vomiting and subsequent aspiration pneumonia. The merits of AC as a decontamination strategy are discussed in detail in Chap. 7.

HISTORY

Activated charcoal, a fine, black, odorless powder, has been recognized for almost two centuries as an effective adsorbent of many substances. In 1930, the French pharmacist Touery demonstrated the powerful adsorbent qualities of AC by ingesting several lethal doses of strychnine mixed with AC in front of colleagues; he suffered no ill effects.[6] An American physician, Holt, first used AC to save a patient from mercury bichloride poisoning in 1934.[6] However, it was not until the 1940s that Anderson began to systematically investigate the adsorbency of AC and unquestionably demonstrated that AC is an excellent broad-spectrum gastrointestinal (GI) adsorbent.[6-8]

ADSORPTION: MECHANISMS AND CONSIDERATIONS

AC is produced in a two-step process, beginning with the pyrolysis of various carbonaceous materials such as wood, coconut, petroleum, or peat. This processing is followed by treatment at high temperatures with a variety of oxidizing (activating) agents such as steam or carbon dioxide to increase adsorptive capacity through formation of an internal maze of pores with a huge surface area.[31,58,109,134] The rate of adsorption depends on external surface area, and the adsorptive capacity depends on the far larger internal surface area.[31,102,108] The adsorptive capacity may be modified by altering the size of the pores. Current AC products have pore sizes that range from 10 to 1000 angstroms (Å), with most of the internal surface area created by 10- to 20-Å-sized pores.[27,29,31] Most xenobiotics are of moderate molecular weight (100–800 daltons) and adsorb well to pores in the range of 10 to 20 Å. Mesoporous charcoals with a pore size of 20 to 200 Å have a greater capacity to adsorb larger xenobiotics as well as those in their larger hydrated forms.[82]

The relationship between AC surface area and adsorptive capacity was studied in vitro and in vivo in animals and in humans. When the surface area is large, the adsorptive capacity is increased, but affinity is decreased because van der Waals forces and hydrophobic forces are diminished.[136] The actual adsorption of a xenobiotic by AC is believed to rely on hydrogen bonding, ion–ion, dipole, and van der Waals forces, suggesting that most xenobiotics are best adsorbed by AC in their dissolved, nonionized form.[31] A superactivated charcoal with a surface area approximately double the current AC formulations demonstrated in both in vitro and in vivo studies a greater maximum adsorptive capacity.[32,121]

Thus, according to the Henderson-Hasselbalch equation, weak bases are best adsorbed at basic pHs, and weak acids are best adsorbed at acidic pHs. For example, cocaine, a weak base, binds to AC with a maximum adsorptive capacity of 273 mg of cocaine per gram of AC at a pH of 7.0; this capacity is reduced to 212 mg of cocaine per gram of AC at a pH of 1.2.[81] Desorption (drug dissociation from AC) may occur, especially for weak acids, as the AC-drug complex passes from the stomach through the intestine and as the pH changes from acidic to basic.[12,46,103,108,133] Whereas strongly ionized and dissociated salts, such as sodium chloride and potassium chloride, are poorly adsorbed, nonionized or weakly dissociated salts, such as iodine and mercuric chloride, respectively, are adsorbed. The adsorption to AC of a weakly dissociated metallic salt such as mercuric chloride ($HgCl_2$) decreases with decreasing pH because the number of complex ions of the type $HgCl_3$ and $HgCl_4$ increases and the number of electroneutral molecules ($HgCl_2$) is reduced.[7] Nonpolar, poorly water-soluble organic substances are more likely to be adsorbed from an aqueous solution than polar, water-soluble substances.[31] Among the organic molecules, aromatics are better adsorbed than aliphatics; molecules with branched chains are better adsorbed than those with straight chains; and molecules containing nitro groups are better adsorbed than those containing hydroxyl, amino, or sulfonic groups.[31]

Desorption may lead to systemic absorption of larger total amounts of xenobiotic over several days; in this case, the elimination half-life of the xenobiotic appears to increase, but peak concentrations remain unaffected.[103] The clinical effects of desorption can be minimized by giving a sufficiently large dose of AC to overcome the decreased affinity of the xenobiotic secondary to pH change such as by using multiple-dose AC.[67,90,101,112,126] Although ethanol and other solvents such as polyethylene glycol are minimally adsorbed by AC, they nonetheless may decrease the adsorptive capacity of AC for a coingested xenobiotic by competing for AC binding with that xenobiotic.[14,103,106]

In vitro studies demonstrate that adsorption begins within about 1 minute of administration of AC but may not reach equilibrium for 10 to 25 minutes.[32,97] AC decreases the systemic absorption of most xenobiotics, including acetaminophen, aspirin, barbiturates, cyclic antidepressants, glutethimide, phenytoin, theophylline, and most inorganic and organic materials.[45,97,111] Notable xenobiotics *not* amenable to AC are the alcohols, acids and alkalis, iron,[49] lithium, magnesium, potassium, and sodium salts. Although the binding of AC to cyanide is less than 4%, the toxic dose is small and 50 g of AC would theoretically be able to bind more than 10 lethal doses of potassium cyanide.

Efficacy of AC is directly related to the quantity administered. The effect of the AC-to-drug ratio on adsorption was demonstrated both in vitro and in vivo with *para*-aminosalicylate (PAS). In vitro, the fraction of unadsorbed PAS decreased from 55% to 3% as the AC-to-PAS ratio increased from 1:1 to 10:1 at a pH of 1.2.[107] This study provides the best scientific basis for the 10:1 AC-to-drug ratio dose typically recommended. In human volunteers, as the AC-to-PAS ratio increased from 2.5:1 to 50:1, the total 48-hour urinary excretion decreased from 37% to 4%.[108] Presumably this occurred because more of the PAS was adsorbed by AC in the lumen of the GI tract rather than being absorbed systemically. These same studies demonstrate AC saturation at low ratios of AC to drug and argue for a 10:1 ratio of AC to xenobiotic.

The clinical efficacy of administered AC is inversely related to the time elapsed after ingestion and depends largely on the rate of absorption of the xenobiotic. For example, early administration of AC is much more important with rapidly absorbed xenobiotics. In this situation, AC functions to prevent the absorption of xenobiotic into the body by achieving rapid adsorption in the GI tract. After a xenobiotic is systemically absorbed or parenterally administered, AC may still enhance elimination through a mechanism referred to as *gastrointestinal dialysis*. This is accomplished with multiple doses of AC.

PALATABILITY

The black and gritty nature of AC has led to the development of many formulations to increase palatability and patient acceptance. Bentonite, carboxymethyl cellulose, and starch[53,96,124] are used as thickening agents, and cherry syrup, chocolate syrup, sorbitol, sucrose, saccharin, ice cream, and sherbet[32,76,83,140] are used as flavoring agents. Most of these additives do not decrease the adsorptive capacity; however, improvement in palatability and acceptance is minimal or nonexistent with all of these formulations.[30] Although a milk chocolate formulation of AC evaluated by children was rated superior in palatability to standard AC preparations,[41] it was never marketed in the United States. A marketed AC product with cherry flavoring was rated by adult volunteers as preferable over plain AC, and a statistically significant larger quantity of the flavored AC was ingested.[26] However, in adult overdosed patients, this was not the case because most patients consumed the entire bottle of AC with or without cherry flavoring. Many of the subjects did not like the taste and actually preferred the plain AC.[63] Two studies in adult overdosed patients compared different brands of AC without additives or flavoring to determine the quantity of AC typically ingested.[18,47] In one study, approximately half of the 50 g of AC offered was ingested, and 7% of the patients vomited.[18] In the other study, 60 g of AC as Liqui-Char or CharcoAid G was offered, and approximately 95% of each formulation was consumed in 20 minutes. There was no difference in the amount consumed even though the palatability of the granular form of AC (CharcoAid G) was rated higher.[47]

Cold cola was used to enhance palatability in volunteer children and adults. Children preferred regular cola over diet cola. The adults rated the cola charcoal combination preferable to the plain charcoal.[118,123]

ADVERSE EFFECTS

The use of AC is relatively safe, although emesis, which especially occurs after rapid administration; constipation; and diarrhea frequently occur after AC administration.[102] Constipation and diarrhea are more likely to result from the ingestion itself than from the AC. However, black stools that are negative for occult blood, black tongues, and mucous membranes are frequently observed. Serious adverse effects of AC include pulmonary aspiration of AC with or without gastric contents[9,43,51,54,55,56,64,91,97,113,125]; peritonitis from spillage of enteric contents, including AC, into the peritoneum after GI perforation caused by orogastric lavage;[84] and intestinal obstruction and pseudo-obstruction, especially after repeated doses of AC in the presence of either dehydration[20,78,93,119,137] or prior bowel adhesions.[52]

Although a significant number of patients aspirate gastric contents before endotracheal intubation and administration of AC,[95,122] the incidence of AC aspiration after endotracheal intubation was reported to vary from 4% to 25%, depending on the nature of the study. A retrospective investigation demonstrated a 1.6% incidence of aspiration pneumonitis in unselected overdosed patients. Altered mental status, spontaneous emesis, and tricyclic antidepressant overdose were associated risk factors; AC was not in itself a risk factor.[62]

HOME AND PREHOSPITAL ADMINISTRATION

Prehospital administration of AC by emergency medical technicians and paramedics may expedite the administration of AC after overdose.[2,138] However, the cost of implementation of such a program would have to be weighed against the small number of patients who would actually benefit.[61]

In a study intended to simulate home administration, the acceptance of a dose of AC given as a water slurry in a paper cup was studied in 50 young children.[22] The children were told to drink the substance, which did not taste bad, and that it would make them feel better and not ill. Eighty-six percent of the children readily drank the AC slurry, and 76% of them consumed 95% to 100% of the total dose. Of seven children in a simulated home environment administered AC in regular cola, three drank 1 g/kg, two drank about half this therapeutic dose, and the other two drank very little.[123] A prospective poison center case series demonstrated successful administration of AC in the home. In this series, the median age of the patients was 3 years, and the median dose of AC ingested was 12 g.[129] However, other attempts at getting children to ingest AC were not as successful; in one study, difficulty was noted in 70% of attempts to administer a standard dose of AC to children in the home setting.[37] A recent review of AC in the home suggested variable success depending on the parent and child.[42]

ADMINISTRATION AND DOSING

AC should not be routinely administered to all poisoned or overdosed patients. Single-dose AC should be administered when a xenobiotic is still expected to be available for adsorption in the GI tract and the benefit of preventing absorption outweighs the risk. The optimal dose of AC is unknown.[4] However, most authorities recommend a minimum dose of AC of 1 g/kg of body weight or a 10:1 ratio of AC to xenobiotic, up to an amount that can be tolerated by the patient and safely administered if the dose is known, which usually represents 50 to 100 g in adults. AC that is not premixed is best administered as a slurry in a 1:8 ratio of AC to suitable liquid, such as water or cola.

Administration may be facilitated by offering children an opaque, decorated, covered cup and a straw.[139] Contraindications to AC include presumed GI perforation and the need for endoscopic visualization, as may occur after caustic ingestion. To prevent aspiration pneumonitis from oral AC administration, it is imperative that the patient's airway be assessed. When the potential for airway compromise is substantial, oral AC should be withheld until airway assessment is accomplished. Subsequently, a risk-to-benefit assessment with regard to the need for airway protection and the need for AC should be made.

Other considerations that must be made before the administration of AC are the determination of normal GI motility, normal bowel sounds, and a normal abdominal examination without distension or signs of an acute abdomen. If bowel function is compromised, AC should be withheld or delayed until the stomach can be decompressed to decrease the risk of subsequent vomiting and aspiration.

THE USE OF ACTIVATED CHARCOAL WITH CATHARTICS OR WHOLE-BOWEL IRRIGATION WITH POLYETHYLENE GLYCOL ELECTROLYTE LAVAGE SOLUTION

Cathartics are often used with AC; however, evidence suggests that AC alone is comparably effective to AC plus a single dose of cathartic (sorbitol or magnesium citrate).[3,67,85,86,90,96,102,110] If a cathartic is used, it should be used only once because repeated doses of magnesium-containing cathartics are associated with hypermagnesemia,[94,128] and repeated doses of any cathartic can be associated with severe and even fatal fluid and electrolyte problems.[44]

Whole-bowel irrigation with polyethylene glycol electrolyte lavage solution may significantly decrease the in vitro and in vivo adsorptive capacity of AC,[57] depending on the individual xenobiotic and its formulation.[10,73] The most likely explanation is competition for the surface of the AC for solute adsorption.

MULTIPLE-DOSE ACTIVATED CHARCOAL

Multiple-dose AC (MDAC) functions to prevent the absorption of xenobiotics that are slowly absorbed from the GI tract and to enhance the elimination of suitable xenobiotics that have already been absorbed.

MDAC decreases xenobiotic absorption when large amounts of xenobiotics are ingested and dissolution is delayed (e.g., masses, bezoars), when xenobiotic formulations exhibit a delayed or prolonged release phase (e.g., enteric coated, extended release), or when reabsorption can be prevented (e.g., enterohepatic circulation of active xenobiotic, active metabolites, or conjugated xenobiotic hydrolyzed by gut bacteria to active xenobiotic).

The ability of MDAC to enhance elimination after absorption had already occurred was first reported in 1982.[15] This report concluded that orally administered MDAC enhanced the total body clearance (nonrenal clearance) of six healthy volunteers given 2.85 mg/kg of body weight of intravenous (IV) phenobarbital.[15] The serum half-life of phenobarbital decreased from 110 ± 8 to 45 ± 6 hours. An accompanying editorial suggested that MDAC enhanced the diffusion of phenobarbital from the blood into the GI tract and trapped it there, to be excreted later in the stool. In this manner, AC was said to perform as an "infinite sink," allowing for "gastrointestinal dialysis" to occur.[75]

These findings were subsequently confirmed by studies in dogs and rats using IV aminophylline.[36,88] Using an isolated perfused rat small intestine, the concept of gastrointestinal dialysis[88] was elegantly demonstrated because AC dramatically affected the pharmacokinetics of theophylline and produced a constant intestinal clearance that was approximately equivalent to intestinal blood flow.[88] The toxicokinetic considerations underlying the ability of MDAC to enhance elimination are similar to those involved in deciding whether hemodialysis would be appropriate for a given xenobiotic and requires the xenobiotic to be in the blood compartment (low volume of distribution), have limited protein binding, and have prolonged endogenous clearance. Although MDAC increases the elimination of digitoxin,[114] phenobarbital,[116] carbamazepine,[17,19], phenylbutazone,[98] dapsone,[99] nadolol,[39] theophylline,[16,80,132] salicylate,[117] quinine,[5] cyclosporine,[59] propoxyphene,[65] nortriptyline, and amitriptyline, its clinical utility remains to be defined.[5,24,66,130]

EXPERIMENTAL STUDIES

An analysis of 28 volunteer studies involving 17 xenobiotics was unable to correlate the physiochemical properties of a particular xenobiotic with the ability of MDAC to decrease the plasma half-life of that xenobiotic.[23] Although the half-life was not thought to be the best marker of enhanced elimination, it was the only parameter consistently evaluated in these exceptionally diverse studies. The xenobiotics with the longest intrinsic plasma half-lives seemed to demonstrate the largest percent reduction in plasma half-life when MDAC was used. A subsequent animal model with therapeutic doses of four simultaneously administered IV xenobiotics (acetaminophen, digoxin, theophylline, and valproic acid) clarified the role of pharmacokinetics on the effectiveness of AC.[25] Theophylline, acetaminophen, and valproic acid all have small volumes of distribution. However, of the three, only valproic acid is highly protein bound at the doses used, which probably accounted for the inability of AC to increase its clearance. An increased clearance with MDAC was demonstrated for the three other xenobiotics. The most rapid and dramatic effect of MDAC was demonstrated on the clearance of theophylline. Large volumes of distribution alone may not exclude benefit from MDAC. Although digoxin has a large volume of distribution, it requires several hours to distribute from the blood to the tissues. MDAC is beneficial as long as the digoxin remains in the blood compartment and distribution is incomplete.

The benefits of MDAC undoubtedly depend on a number of patient variables and xenobiotic exposure characteristics. Most important to remember, however, is that volunteer studies do not accurately reflect the overdose situation[89] in which saturation of plasma protein binding, saturation of first-pass metabolism, and acid–base disturbances may make more free xenobiotic available for an enteroenteric effect and therefore more amenable to MDAC use.

OVERDOSE STUDIES

In a randomized clinical study, patients who overdosed with phenobarbital were given a single dose of AC, and others were given multiple doses.[116] Although the half-life of phenobarbital was significantly decreased in the MDAC group (36 vs. 93 hours), the length of intubation time required by each group did not differ from one another. This study has been criticized as being too small, having unevenly matched groups, and focusing on a single end point (extubation) that may be dependent on factors other than patient condition (e.g., the time of day) to determine the potential clinical benefit.

The most compelling demonstration of the benefits of MDAC in the overdose setting to date comes from a study done in Sri Lanka of patients with severe cardiac toxicity caused by intentional overdose with yellow oleander seeds.[35] An initial dose of 50 g of AC was administered to all patients, who were then randomized to 50 g of AC every 6 hours for 3 days or placebo. There were statistically fewer deaths and fewer life-threatening dysrhythmias in the MDAC group. A more recent randomized, controlled trial compared MDAC, single-dose AC, and no AC in self-poisoned patients.[40] About one-third of the patients ingested yellow oleander seeds, and a little less than one-third ingested organic phosphorous or carbamate pesticides. In contrast to the former study, this trial found no difference in mortality between the groups. It is unclear how these trials done in Sri Lanka apply to management in developed countries such as the United States, where the use of antidotes such as digoxin-specific antibody fragments for cardioactive steroid poisoning and atropine and pralidoxime for organic phosphorous pesticide poisoning routinely complement GI decontamination.

ADMINISTRATION OF MDAC

An initial loading dose of AC should be administered to adults and children in an AC-to-xenobiotic ratio of 10:1 or 1 g/kg of body weight (if xenobiotic exposure amount is unknown). The correct dose and interval of AC for multiple dosing, when it is indicated, is best tailored to the amount and dosage form of the xenobiotic ingested, the severity of the overdose, the potential lethality of the xenobiotic, and the patient's ability to tolerate AC. Benefit should always be weighed against risk. Doses of AC for multiple dosing have varied considerably in the past, ranging from 0.25 to 0.5 g/kg of body weight every 1 to 6 hours to 20 to 60 g for adults every 1, 2, 4, or 6 hours. Some evidence suggests that the total dose administered may be more important than the frequency of administration.[60,135] In some cases, continuous nasogastric administration of AC can be used, especially when vomiting is a problem.[46,105,135] The editors of this text consider a dose of 0.5 g/kg of body weight (~25–50 g in adults) every 4 to 6 hours for up to 12 to 24 hours to be an appropriate regimen in most circumstances.

ADVERSE EFFECTS OF MDAC

The adverse effects of MDAC include diarrhea only when sorbitol-containing charcoal preparations are used, constipation, vomiting with a subsequent risk of aspiration, intestinal obstruction, and reduction of serum concentrations of therapeutically used xenobiotics.[38,93,97,113] Any complication observed with single-dose AC is a possibility with MDAC.

SUMMARY

When benefit exceeds risk and administration is timely, AC is a very effective nonspecific adsorbent. AC should be of benefit to a patient with a potentially life-threatening ingestion involving a xenobiotic expected to be present in the GI tract and that is adsorbable by AC and for whom there are no contraindications. MDAC is useful to prevent systemic absorption of a xenobiotic with a prolonged absorptive phase such as an extended-release formulation. In the postabsorptive phase of managing an exposure, MDAC may decrease the elimination half-lives of a variety of xenobiotics through diverse mechanisms, including GI dialysis, thereby providing potential treatment to some xenobiotic overdoses occurring by any routes. For this postabsorptive effect to be of clinical importance, the xenobiotic or an active metabolite must first be characterized by a lengthy elimination phase because MDAC is given every 4 to 6 hours. In addition, xenobiotics with a small volume of distribution, or that fit a two-compartment model with a prolonged initial distribution phase and low or saturable plasma protein binding, are theoretically most accessible to MDAC. In both the use of AC and MDAC, care must be taken to avoid pulmonary aspiration and intestinal obstruction.

With respect to the use of AC before the patient's arrival at the hospital, home availability of AC should be encouraged in remote locations where healthcare is not immediately available. As more palatable forms of AC are developed, children may accept this therapy more readily, but even without such forms, the benefits are substantial and the risks lower than often suggested.[72,74]

REFERENCES

1. Albertson TE, Derlet RW, Foulke GE, et al: Superiority of activated charcoal alone compared with ipecac and activated charcoal in the treatment of acute toxic ingestions. *Ann Emerg Med.* 1989;18:56-59.
2. Allison T, Gough J, Brown L, Thoms S: Potential time savings by prehospital administration of activated charcoal. *Prehosp Emerg Care.* 1997;1:73-75.
3. Al-Shareef AM, Buss DC, Allen EM, Routledge PA: The effects of charcoal and sorbitol (alone and in combination) on plasma theophylline concentration after a sustained release formulation. *Hum Exp Toxicol.* 1990;9:179-182.
4. American Academy of Clinical Toxicology and European Association of Poison Centers and Clinical Toxicologists: Position statement: Single- dose activated charcoal. *Clin Toxicol.* 2005;43:61-87.
5. American Academy of Clinical Toxicology and European Association of Poison Centers and Clinical Toxicologists: Position statement and practice guidelines on the use of multi-dose activated charcoal in the treatment of acute poisoning. *J Toxicol Clin Toxicol.* 1999;37:731-751.
6. Anderson H: Experimental studies on the pharmacology of activated charcoal. I. Adsorption power of charcoal in aqueous solutions. *Acta Pharmacol.* 1946;2:69-78.
7. Anderson H: Experimental studies on the pharmacology of activated charcoal. II. The effect of pH on the adsorption by charcoal from aqueous solutions. *Acta Pharmacol.* 1947;3:199-218.
8. Anderson H: Experimental studies on the pharmacology of activated charcoal. *Acta Pharmacol.* 1948;4:275-284.
9. Anderson I, Ware C: Syrup of ipecacuanha [letter]. *Br Med J.* 1987;294:578.
10. Atta-Politou J, Kolioliou M, Havariotou M et al: An in vitro evaluation of fluoxetine adsorption by activated charcoal and desorption upon addition of polyethylene glycol-electrolyte lavage solution. *J Toxicol Clin Toxicol.* 1998;36:117-124.
11. Auerbach PS, Osterloh J, Braun O, et al: Efficacy of gastric emptying: Gastric lavage versus emesis induced with ipecac. *Ann Emerg Med.* 1986;15:692-698.
12. Augenstein WL, Kulig KW, Rumack BH: Delayed rise in serum drug levels in overdose patients despite multiple dose charcoal and after charcoal stools [abstract]. *Vet Hum Toxicol.* 1987;29:491.
13. Bailey B: To decontaminate or not to decontaminate? The balance between potential risks and foreseeable benefits. *Clin Ped Emerg Med.* 2008;9:17-23.
14. Bailey D, Briggs J: The effect of ethanol and pH on the adsorption of drugs from simulated gastric fluid onto activated charcoal. *Ther Drug Monit.* 2003;25:310-313.
15. Berg M, Berlinger W, Goldberg M, et al: Acceleration of the body clearance of phenobarbital by oral activated charcoal. *N Engl J Med.* 1982;307:642-644.
16. Berlinger WG, Spector R, Goldberg MJ, et al: Enhancement of theophylline clearance by oral activated charcoal. *Clin Pharmacol Ther.* 1983;33:351-354.
17. Boldy DAR, Heath A, Ruddock C, et al: Activated charcoal for carbamazepine poisoning [letter]. *Lancet.* 1987;1:1027.
18. Boyd R, Hanson J: Prospective single-blinded randomized controlled trial of two orally administered activated charcoal preparations. *J Accid Emerg Med.* 1999;16:24-25.
19. Brahmi N, Kouraichi N, Thabet H, Amamou M: Influence of activated charcoal on the pharmacokinetics and the clinical features of carbamazepine poisoning. *Am J Emerg Med.* 2006;24:440-443.
20. Brubacher JR, Levine B, Hoffman RS: Intestinal pseudo-obstruction (Ogilvie's syndrome) in the theophylline overdose. *Vet Hum Toxicol.* 1996;38:368-370.
21. Burton BT, Bayer MJ, Barron L, Aitchison JP: Comparison of activated charcoal and gastric lavage in the prevention of aspirin absorption. *J Emerg Med.* 1984;1:411-416.
22. Calvert W, Corby D, Herbertson L, Decker W: Orally administered activated charcoal: Acceptance by children. *JAMA.* 1971;215:641.
23. Campbell J, Chyka P: Physiochemical characteristics of drugs and response to repeat dose activated charcoal. *Am J Emerg Med.* 1992;10:208-210.
24. Chyka PA: Multiple dose activated charcoal and enhancement of systemic drug clearance: Summary of studies in animals and human volunteers. *J Toxicol Clin Toxicol.* 1995;33:399-405.
25. Chyka PA, Holley JE, Mandrell TD, Sugathan P: Correlation of drug pharmacokinetics and effectiveness of multiple-dose activated charcoal therapy. *Ann Emerg Med.* 1995;25:356-362.
26. Cohen V, Howland MA, Hoffman RS: Palatability of Insta-Char with cherry flavoring: A human volunteer study [abstract]. *J Toxicol Clin Toxicol.* 1996;34:635.
27. Cooney D: A "superactive" charcoal for antidotal use in poisonings. *Clin Toxicol.* 1977;11:387-390.
28. Cooney D: Palatability of sucrose-sorbitol and saccharin sweetened activated charcoal formulations. *Am J Hosp Pharm.* 1980;37:237-239.

29. Cooney D: "Superactive" charcoal adsorbs drugs as fast as standard antidotal charcoal. *Clin Toxicol.* 1980;16:123-125.
30. Cooney D: Effect of type and amount of carboxymethyl-cellulose on in vitro salicylate adsorption by activated charcoal. *Clin Toxicol.* 1982;19:367-376.
31. Cooney D, ed: *Activated Charcoal in Medical Applications.* New York, Marcel Dekker, 1995.
32. Cooney D: In vitro adsorption of phenobarbital, chlorpheniramine maleate, and theophylline by four commercially available activated charcoal suspensions. *J Toxicol Clin Toxicol.* 1995;33:213-217.
33. Curd-Sneed C, Parks K, Bordelon J, et al: In vitro adsorption of sodium phenobarbital by Superchar, USP, and Darco G-60 ACs. *J Toxicol Clin Toxicol.* 1987;25:1-11.
34. Curtis RA, Barone J, Giacona N: Efficacy of ipecac and activated charcoal/cathartic: Prevention of salicylate absorption in a simulated overdose. *Arch Intern Med.* 1984;144:48-52.
35. de Silva HA, Fonseka M, Pathmeswaran A, et al: Multiple-dose activated charcoal for treatment of yellow oleander poisoning: a single-blind, randomized, placebo controlled trial. *Lancet.* 2003;361:1935-1938.
36. DeVries MH, Rademaker C, Geerlings C, et al: Pharmacokinetic modelling of the effect of activated charcoal on the intestinal secretion of theophylline, using the isolated vascularly perfused rat small intestine. *J Pharm Pharmacol.* 1989;41:528-533.
37. Docksteder LL, Lawrence RA, Bresnick HL: Home administration of activated charcoal: Feasibility and acceptance [abstract]. *Vet Hum Toxicol.* 1986;28:471.
38. Dorrington C, Johnson D, Brant R, et al: The frequency of complications associated with the use of multiple-dose activated charcoal. *Ann Emerg Med.* 2003;41:370-377.
39. DuSoeuch P, Caille G, Larochelle P: Reduction of nadolol plasma half-life by activated charcoal and antibiotics in man [letter]. *Clin Pharmacol Ther.* 1982;31:222.
40. Eddleston M, Juszczak E, Buckley N et al: Multiple-dose activated charcoal in acute self-poisoning: a randomised controlled trial. *Lancet.* 2008;371:579-587.
41. Eisen TF, Grbcich PA, Lacouture PG, Woolf A: The adsorption of salicylates by a milk chocolate-charcoal mixture. *Ann Emerg Med.* 1991;20:143-146.
42. Eldridge DL, Van Eyk J, Kornegay J: Pediatric toxicology. *Emerg Med Clin North Am.* 2007;25:283-308.
43. Elliot CG, Colby TV, Kelly TM, et al: Charcoal lung: Bronchiolitis obliterans after aspiration of activated charcoal. *Chest.* 1989;96:672-674.
44. Farley T: Severe hypernatremic dehydration after use of an AC sorbitol suspension. *J Pediatr.* 1986;109:719-722.
45. Farrar HC, Herold DA, Reed M: Acute valproic acid intoxication enhanced drug clearance with oral activated charcoal. *Crit Care Med.* 1993;21:299-301.
46. Fillippone G, Fish S, Lacouture P, et al: Reversible adsorption (desorption) of aspirin from activated charcoal. *Arch Intern Med.* 1987;147:1390-1392.
47. Fisher T, Singer A: Comparison of the palatabilities of standard and superactivated charcoal in toxic ingestions: A randomized trial. *Acad Emerg Med.* 1999;6:895-899.
48. Freedman G, Pasternak S, Krenzelok E: A clinical trial using syrup of ipecac and activated charcoal concurrently. *Ann Emerg Med.* 1987;16:164-166.
49. Gades NM, Chyka PA, Butler AY, et al: Activated charcoal and the absorption of ferrous sulfate in rats. *Vet Hum Toxicol.* 2003;45:183-187.
50. Gadgil SD, Damle SR, Advani SH, Vaidya AB: Effect of activated charcoal on the pharmacokinetics of high dose methotrexate. *Cancer Treat Rep.* 1982;66:1169-1171.
51. Givens T, Holloway M, Watson S: Pulmonary aspiration of activated charcoal: A complication of its misuse in overdose management. *Pediatr Emerg Care.* 1992;8:137-140.
52. Goulbourne KB, Cisek JE: Small bowel obstruction secondary to activated charcoal and adhesions. *Ann Emerg Med.* 1994;24:108-110.
53. Gwelt P, Perrier D: Influence of thickening agents on the antidotal efficacy of activated charcoal. *Clin Toxicol.* 1976;9:89-92.
54. Hack JB, Gilliland MG, Meggs WJ: Images in emergency medicine. Activated charcoal aspiration. *Ann Emerg Med.* 2006;48:522, 531.
55. Harris CR, Filandrinos D: Accidental administration of activated charcoal into the lung: Aspiration by proxy. *Ann Emerg Med.* 1993;22:143-146.
56. Harsch H: Aspiration of activated charcoal [letter]. *N Engl J Med.* 1986;314:318.
57. Hoffman RS, Chiang WK, Howland MA, et al: Theophylline desorption from activated charcoal caused by whole-bowel irrigation. *J Toxicol Clin Toxicol.* 1991;29:191-202.
58. Holt E, Holz P: The black bottle. *J Pediatr.* 1963;63:306-314.
59. Honcharik N, Anthone S: Activated charcoal in acute cyclosporine overdose. *Lancet.* 1985;1:1051.
60. Ilkhanipour K, Yealy D, Krenzelok E: The comparative efficacy of various multiple dose activated charcoal regimens. *Am J Emerg Med.* 1992;10:298-300.
61. Isbister GK, Dawson AH, Whyte IM: Feasibility of prehospital treatment with activated charcoal: Who could we treat, who should we treat? *J Emerg Med.* 2003;20:375-378.
62. Isbister G, Downes F, Sibbritt D et al: Aspiration pneumonitis in an overdose population. Frequency, predictors and outcome. *Crit Care Med.* 2004;32:88-93.
63. Jaggi M, Cohen V, Howland M, Hoffman R: Activated charcoal versus Insta-Char with cherry flavoring in adult overdose patients [abstract]. *J Toxicol Clin Toxicol.* 1997;35:544.
64. Justiniani F, Hippalgaonkar R, Martinez L: Charcoal-containing empyema complicating treatment for overdose. *Chest.* 1985;87:404-405.
65. Karkkainen S, Neuvonen PJ: Effect of oral charcoal and urine pH on dextropropoxyphene pharmacokinetics. *Int J Clin Pharmacol Ther Toxicol.* 1985;23:219-225.
66. Karkkainen S, Neuvonen P: Pharmacokinetics of amitriptyline influenced by oral charcoal and urine pH. *Int J Clin Pharmacol Ther.* 1986;24:326-332.
67. Keller R, Schwab R, Krenzelok E: Contribution of sorbitol combined with activated charcoal in prevention of salicylate absorption. *Ann Emerg Med.* 1990;19:654-656.
68. Kirshenbaum LA, Sitar DS, Tenenbein M: Interaction between whole-bowel irrigation solution and activated charcoal: Implications for the treatment of toxic ingestions. *Ann Emerg Med.* 1990;19:1129-1132.
69. Kornberg AE, Dolgin J: Pediatric ingestions: Charcoal alone versus ipecac and charcoal. *Ann Emerg Med.* 1991;20:648-651.
70. Krenzelok E, Heller M: Effectiveness of commercially available aqueous activated charcoal products. *Ann Emerg Med.* 1987;16;1340-1343.
71. Kulig KW, Bar-Or D, Cantrill SV, et al: Management of acutely poisoned patients without gastric emptying. *Ann Emerg Med.* 1985;14:562-567.
72. Lamminpaa A, Vilska J, Hoppu K: Medical activated charcoal for a child's poisoning at home: Availability and success of administration in Finland. *Hum Exp Toxicol.* 1993;12:29-32.
73. Lapatto-Reiniluoto O, Kivisto KT, Neuvonen PJ: Activated charcoal alone and followed by whole-bowel irrigation in preventing the absorption of sustained-release drugs. *Clin Pharmacol Ther.* 2001;70:255-260.
74. Lee RJ: Ancient antidote ignored. Activated charcoal is an under-used antidote to a variety of drugs and chemicals, says this author. *Am Pharm.* 1992;32:34-35.
75. Levy G: Gastrointestinal clearance of drugs with activated charcoal [editorial]. *N Engl J Med.* 1982;307:676-678.
76. Levy G, Soda GM, Lampman TA: Inhibition by ice cream of the antidotal efficacy of activated charcoal. *Am J Hosp Pharm.* 1975;32:289-291.
77. Levy G, Tsuchiya T: Effect of activated charcoal on aspirin absorption in man. *Clin Pharmacol Ther.* 1972;13:317-322.
78. Longdson P, Henderson A: Intestinal pseudo-obstruction following the use of enteral charcoal and sorbitol with mechanical ventilation with papaverum sedation for theophylline poisoning. *Drug Saf.* 1992;7:74-77.
79. Lopes de Freitas J, Ferreira MG, Brito MJ: Charcoal deposits in the esophageal and gastric mucosa. *Am J Gastroenterol.* 1997;92:1359-1360.
80. Mahutte CK, True RJ, Michiels TN, et al: Increased serum theophylline clearance with orally administered activated charcoal. *Am Rev Resp Dis.* 1983;128:820-822.
81. Makosiej F, Hoffman RS, Howland MA, et al: An in vitro evaluation of cocaine hydrochloride adsorption by activated charcoal and desorption upon addition of polyethylene glycol electrolyte solution. *J Toxicol Clin Toxicol.* 1993;31:381-386.
82. Malik DJ, Reilly CD, Inman S, et al: The characterization and development of microstructured carbons for the treatment of drug overdose. *J Toxicol Clin Toxicol.* 2003;41:694.
83. Manes M, Mann JF: Easily swallowed formulations of antidote charcoals. *Clin Toxicol.* 1974;7:355-364.
84. Mariani PJ, Poole N: Gastrointestinal tract perforation with charcoal peritoneum complicating orogastric intubation and lavage. *Ann Emerg Med.* 1993;22:606-609.
85. Mathur LK, Jaffe JM, Colaizzi JL, Moriarity RW: Activated charcoal-carboxymethylcellulose gel formulation as an antidotal agent for orally ingested aspirin. *Am J Hosp Pharm.* 1976;33:717-729.

86. Mayersohn M, Perrier D, Picchioni A: Evaluation of a charcoal-sorbitol mixture as an antidote for oral aspirin overdose. *Clin Toxicol.* 1977;11:561-567.
87. McFarland A, Chyka P: Selection of activated charcoal products for the treatment of poisonings. *Ann Pharmacother.* 1993;27:358-361.
88. McKinnon RS, Desmond PV, Harmon PJ, et al: Studies on the mechanisms of action of activated charcoal on theophylline pharmacokinetics. *J Pharm Pharmacol.* 1987;39:522-525.
89. McLuckie A, Forbes AM, Ilett KF: Role of repeated doses of oral activated charcoal in the treatment of acute intoxications. *Anaesth Intensive Care.* 1990;18:375-384.
90. McNamara R, Aaron C, Gemborys M: Sorbitol catharsis does not enhance efficacy of charcoal in simulated acetaminophen overdose. *Ann Emerg Med.* 1988;17:243-246.
91. Menzies DG, Busuttel A, Prescott LF: Fatal pulmonary aspiration of oral activated charcoal. *Br Med J.* 1988;297:459-466.
92. Merigian KS, Woodard M, Hedges JR, et al: Prospective evaluation of gastric emptying in the self-poisoned patient. *Am J Emerg Med.* 1990;8:479-483.
93. Mezutani T, Waits H, Oohashi W: Rectal ulcer with massive hemorrhage due to activated charcoal treatment in oral organophosphate poisoning. *Hum Exp Toxicol.* 1991;10:385-386.
94. Mofenson H, Caraccio T: Magnesium intoxication in a neonate from oral magnesium hydroxide laxative. *J Toxicol Clin Toxicol.* 1991;29:215-222.
95. Moll J, Kerns W, Tomaszewski C: Incidence of aspiration pneumonia in intubated patients receiving activated charcoal. *J Emerg Med.* 1999;17:279-283.
96. Navarro R, Navarro K, Krenzelok E: Relative efficacy and palatability of three activated charcoal mixtures. *Vet Hum Toxicol.* 1980;22:6-9.
97. Neuvonen PJ: Clinical pharmacokinetics of oral activated charcoal in acute intoxications. *Clin Pharmacokinet.* 1982;7:465-489.
98. Neuvonen PJ, Elonen E: Effect of activated charcoal on absorption and elimination of phenobarbitone, carbamazepine, and phenylbuta-zone in man. *Eur J Clin Pharmacol.* 1980;17:51-57.
99. Neuvonen PJ, Elonen E, Mattila MJ: Oral activated charcoal and dapsone elimination. *Clin Pharmacol Ther.* 1980;6:823-827.
100. Neuvonen PJ, Olkkola K: Activated charcoal and syrup of ipecac in prevention of cimetidine and pindolol absorption in man after administration of metoclopramide as an antiemetic agent. *J Toxicol Clin Toxicol.* 1984;22:103-114.
101. Neuvonen PJ, Olkkola K: Effect of purgatives on antidotal efficacy of oral activated charcoal. *Hum Toxicol.* 1986;5:255-263.
102. Neuvonen PJ, Olkkola K: Oral activated charcoal in the treatment of intoxications. *Med Toxicol.* 1988;3:33-58.
103. Neuvonen PJ, Olkkola K, Alanen T: Effect of ethanol and pH on the adsorption of drugs to activated charcoal: Studies in vitro and in man. *Acta Pharmacol Toxicol.* 1984;54:1-7.
104. Neuvonen PJ, Vartiainen M, Tokola O: Comparison of activated charcoal and ipecac syrup in the prevention of drug absorption. *Eur J Clin Pharmacol.* 1983;24:557-562.
105. Ohning B, Reed M, Blumer J: Continuous nasogastric administration of activated charcoal for the treatment of theophylline intoxication. *Pediatr Pharmacol.* 1986;5:241-245.
106. Olkkola K, Neuvonen P: Do gastric contents modify antidotal efficacy of oral activated charcoal? *Br J Clin Pharmacol.* 1984;18:663-669.
107. Olkkola K: Effect of charcoal-drug ratio on antidotal efficacy of oral activated charcoal in man. *Br J Clin Pharmacol.* 1985;19:767-773.
108. Olkkola K: *Factors Affecting the Antidotal Efficacy of Oral Activated Charcoal.* Dissertation. University of Helsinki; 1985.
109. Osol A, ed: *Remington's Practice of Pharmacy*, 16th ed. Easton, PA: Mack Publishing; 1980.
110. Park G, Spector R, Goldberg M, et al: Effect of the surface area of activated charcoal on theophylline clearance. *J Clin Pharmacol.* 1984;24:289-292.
111. Picchioni A: Activated charcoal: A neglected antidote. *Pediatr Clin North Am.* 1970;17:535-543.
112. Picchioni A, Chin L, Gillespie T: Evaluation of activated charcoal-sorbitol suspension as an antidote. *Clin Toxicol.* 1982;19:435-444.
113. Pollack M, Dunbar B, Holbrook P, Fields A: Aspiration of activated charcoal and gastric contents. *Ann Emerg Med.* 1981;10;528-529.
114. Pond SM, Jacobs M, Marks J, et al: Treatment of digitoxin overdose with oral activated charcoal. *Lancet.* 1982;2:1177-1178.
115. Pond SM, Lewis-Driver DJ, Williams G, et al: Gastric emptying in acute overdose: A prospective randomised controlled trial. *Med J Aust.* 1995;163:345-349.
116. Pond SM, Olson KR, Osterloh JD, Tong TG: Randomized study of the treatment of phenobarbital overdose with repeated doses of activated charcoal. *JAMA.* 1984;251:3104-3108.
117. Prescott L, Hillman R: Treatment of salicylate poisoning with repeated oral charcoal. *Br Med J.* 1985;291:1472.
118. Rangan C, Nordt S, Hamilton R, et al: Treatment of toxic ingestions with a superactivated charcoal-cola mixture. *Acad Emerg Med.* 2000;7:496.
119. Ray MJ, Padin DR, Condie JD, Halls JM: Charcoal bezoar: Small bowel obstruction secondary to amitriptyline overdose therapy. *Dig Dis Sci.* 1988;33:106-107.
120. Reynolds JEF, ed: *Martindale: The Extra Pharmacopoeia*, 29th ed. London: Pharmaceutical Press; 1989:835.
121. Roberts JR, Gracely EJ, Schoffetall J: Advantage of high surface area activated charcoal for GI decontamination in a human acetaminophen ingestion model. *Acad Emerg Med.* 1997;4:167-174.
122. Roy TM, Ossorio MA, Cipolla LM, et al: Pulmonary complications after tricyclic antidepressant overdose. *Chest.* 1989;96:852-856.
123. Scharman E, Cloonan H, Durback-Morris L: Home administration of charcoal: Can mothers administer a therapeutic dose? *J Emerg Med.* 2001;21:357-361.
124. Scholtz E, Jaffe J, Colaizzi J: Evaluation of five activated charcoal formulations for inhibition of aspirin adsorption and palatability in man. *Am J Hosp Pharm.* 1978;35:1355-1359.
125. Siberman H, Davis SM, Lee A: activated charcoal aspiration. *N C Med J.* 1990;51:79-80.
126. Sketris I, Mowry J, Czajka P, et al: Saline catharsis: Effect on aspirin bioavailability in combination with activated charcoal. *J Clin Pharmacol.* 1982;22:59-64.
127. Smilkstein MJ, Knapp GL, Kulig KW, Rumack BH: Efficacy of oral N-acetylcysteine in the treatment of acetaminophen overdose: Analysis of the National Multicenter Study (1976–1985). *N Engl J Med.* 1988;319:1557-1562.
128. Smilkstein MJ, Smolinske S, Kulig KW, et al: Severe hypermagnesemia due to multiple-dose cathartic therapy. *West J Med.* 1988;148:208-211.
129. Spiller H, Rodgers G: Evaluation of administration of activated charcoal in the home. *Pediatrics.* 2001;108:E100.
130. Swartz C, Sherman A: The treatment of tricyclic antidepressant overdose with activated charcoal. *J Clin Psychopharmacol.* 1984;4:336-340.
131. Tenenbein M, Cohen S, Sitar DS: Efficacy of ipecac induced emesis, orogastric lavage and activated charcoal for acute drug overdose. *Ann Emerg Med.* 1987;16:838-841.
132. True RJ, Berman JN, Mahutte CK: Treatment of theophylline toxicity with oral activated charcoal. *Crit Care Med.* 1984;12:113-114.
133. Tsuchiya T, Levy G: Relationship between effect of activated charcoal on drug adsorption characteristics in vitro. *J Pharm Sci.* 1972;61:586-589.
134. United States Pharmacopeial Convention: *The United States Pharmacopoeia, 20th rev. The National Formulary*, 15th ed. Easton, PA: Mack Publishing; 1980.
135. Vale JA, Proudfoot AT: How useful is activated charcoal? *Br Med J.* 1993;306:78-79.
136. Van de Graaf W, Thompson WL, Sunshine I, et al: Adsorbent and cathartic inhibition of enteral drug adsorption. *J Pharmacol Exp Ther.* 1982;221:656-663.
137. Watson WA, Cremes KF, Chapman JA: Gastrointestinal obstruction associated with multiple dose activated charcoal. *J Emerg Med.* 1986;4;401-407.
138. Wax P, Cobaugh D: Prehospital gastrointestinal decontamination of toxic ingestions: A missed opportunity Am *J Emerg Med.* 1998;16:114-116.
139. West L: Innovative approaches to the administration of activated charcoal in pediatric toxic ingestions. *Pediatr Nurs.* 1997;23:616-619.
140. Yancy RE, O'Barr TP, Corby DG: In vitro and in vivo evaluation of the effect of cherry flavoring on the adsorptive capacity of activated charcoal for salicylic acid. *Vet Hum Toxicol.* 1980;22:163-165.

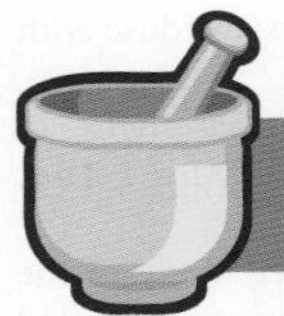

ANTIDOTES IN DEPTH (A3)

WHOLE-BOWEL IRRIGATION AND OTHER INTESTINAL EVACUANTS

Mary Ann Howland

Xenobiotics that promote intestinal evacuation are referred to as *laxatives, cathartics, purgatives, promotility agents*, and *evacuants*. Using different doses, the same xenobiotic may often accomplish any or all of these tasks, but with different side effect profiles. Laxatives promote a soft-formed or semifluid stool within 6 hours to 3 days, depending on the xenobiotic and the dose used. Cathartics promote a rapid, watery evacuation within 1 to 3 hours.[37] The term *purgatives* is used to relate the force associated with bowel evacuation. Promotility agents stimulate gastrointestinal (GI) motor function via the enteric nervous system by affecting acetylcholine, serotonin, motilin, or intestinal chloride channels. Evacuants are commonly used to cleanse the bowel before a procedure, with an onset of action of as little as 30 to 60 minutes, but typically requiring 4 hours for a more complete effect. Although it is far from perfect, the most effective process of evacuating the intestinal tract in poisoned patients is referred to as whole-bowel irrigation (WBI). WBI is typically accomplished using polyethylene glycol 3350 (PEG), which is added to a balanced electrolyte lavage solution (PEG-ELS).

The traditional classification of laxatives into the categories of bulk-forming, softener or emollient, lubricant, stimulant or irritant, saline, hyperosmotic, and evacuant is largely empirical. Bulk-forming agents include high-fiber products such as methylcellulose, polycarbophil, and psyllium; softeners or emollients include docusate calcium. Mineral oil is the sole lubricant. None of these three classes of cathartics is used therapeutically in medical toxicology because their onsets of action are often delayed for several days. In addition, softeners cause an increase in intestinal permeability for a few hours and may therefore increase the absorption of some xenobiotics.[78] Mineral oil may enhance the absorption of lipid-soluble xenobiotics and aspiration could result in a lipoid pneumonia.[102]

Stimulant or irritant laxatives include anthraquinones (sennosides, aloe, and casanthranol), diphenylmethane (bisacodyl), and castor oil. Abdominal discomfort, cramping, and tenesmus are common early manifestations. Long-term use produces bowel habituation and damage to intestinal tissue. Thus, stimulant and irritant laxatives are rarely used today in medical toxicology because of their significant GI side effects.

Saline (meaning salt) cathartics, which include magnesium citrate, magnesium hydroxide, magnesium sulfate, sodium phosphate, and sodium sulfate, are used infrequently and cautiously in medical toxicology. Hyperosmotic agents, including sorbitol and lactulose, are also occasionally considered in poisoned patients.

When different cathartics were compared with respect to time to first stool and number of stools,[38,46,68,69,90] sorbitol produced 10 to 15 watery stools and the most abdominal cramping before catharsis. Sorbitol produced stools in the shortest amount of time but with the highest incidence of nausea, vomiting. generated gas, abdominal cramping, and increased flatus.[42,43,71] The nauseating sweetness of sorbitol resulted in patient preference of magnesium citrate. In comparison, the first bowel movement typically occurs about 1 hour after the start of WBI with PEG-ELS.

Potential adverse effects associated with cathartics and promotility agents include dehydration, absorption of magnesium or other absorbable electrolytes, hypokalemia and metabolic alkalosis from dehydration, activation of the renin–angiotensin–aldosterone system, phosphate-induced renal nephropathy[16,84] and colonic fermentation of digestible sugars. Cathartic-induced rectal prolapse occurred in 2 geriatric patients.[45] The use of repetitive doses of cathartics, either by design or unintentionally, has led to increased risk of hypermagnesemia and death.[40,70,86]

Following the use of hypertonic phosphate enemas and oral sodium phosphate, hypocalcemia, hyperphosphatemia, and hypokalemia were reported.[22,28,31,52,58,79,88] In many of these cases, the recommended dose was used.[22] Frail elderly patients, children, and those with decreased renal function may be most susceptible to adverse effects.[9,11]

Multiple-dose activated charcoal (MDAC) regimens containing 70% sorbitol used to enhance elimination resulted in severe cathartic-related adverse effects in at least four case reports.[1,27,51,62] The potential for sorbitol-related adverse events from the unintentional use of repetitive activated charcoal (AC) dosing was emphasized by a survey revealing that 16% of hospitals surveyed only stocked AC premixed with sorbitol.[103] The retention of sorbitol after repetitive doses in an aperistaltic gut may lead to significant morbidity from gas formation and abdominal distention as a result of the digestive action of gut bacteria.[51]

MECHANISM OF ACTION

The effects of saline cathartics are largely attributed to their relatively nonabsorbable ions that establish an osmotic gradient and draw water into the gut. The increased water leads to increased intestinal pressure and a subsequent increase in intestinal motility.[20] Magnesium ion also leads to the release of cholecystokinin from the duodenal mucosa, which stimulates intestinal motor activity and alters fluid movement, contributing to the cathartic effect.[12,89] The hyperosmotic laxatives, including sorbitol, lactulose, and glycerin, also draw water into the gut, thereby producing diarrhea.

PEG is a nonabsorbable, isoosmotic indigestible molecule that remains in the colon and together with the water diluent is evacuated, resulting in WBI without producing flatus and cramps. A balanced electrolyte solution is added which practically eliminates electrolyte abnormalities and helps prevent fluid shifts across the GI mucosa. Many studies of WBI using PEG-ELS demonstrate patient acceptance, effectiveness, and safety when used for bowel preparation.[3,10,21,23,25,77,94,97]

Promotility agents such as metoclopramide and erythromycin stimulate gut motor function. Metoclopramide mediates GI $5HT_4$ receptor agonist and D_2 receptor antagonist activity which both result in increased acetylcholine release and GI motility. Erythromycin also stimulates gut motor function but via direct stimulation of GI motilin receptors.[75] Lubiprostone is a novel promotility drug that stimulates chloride secretion and enhances the contraction of gastric and colonic musculature.[41] Although lubiprostone has been used with WBI for the treatment of constipation, their combined use has not yet been reported in poisoned patients.

GASTROINTESTINAL EVACUATION AND POISON MANAGEMENT

Although recommended for basic poison management for many years, cathartics should not be used routinely in the management of overdosed patients.[5] Intuitively, the advantages of cathartics appear to result from their ability to decrease the potential for constipation or obstruction from AC and hasten the delivery of AC to the small intestine. However, these theoretical advantages have never been demonstrated clinically.

Studies demonstrate that when administered alone, cathartics such as sorbitol or sodium sulfate may decrease peak or total absorption of some xenobiotics, but no study of cathartics alone has achieved results comparable to that of AC alone.[2,17,61,76,101] When comparing the efficacy of a single dose of AC alone with that of AC plus a single dose of cathartic, studies suggest the combination to be equal to,[2,65,74,76,85] slightly better than,[17,42] or even slightly worse than AC alone.[61,101]

WBI with PEG-ELS is currently advocated to hasten the elimination of poorly absorbed xenobiotics or sustained-release medications before they can be absorbed. This approach is theoretically sound and does not produce the fluid and electrolyte complications associated with cathartics. Unfortunately, evidence of efficacy is limited to anecdotal case reports and volunteer studies.

Animal models suggest that WBI may enhance systemic clearance via GI dialysis, much like MDAC.[50] In actuality, low flow rates, the typical delay in administering WBI in actual clinical situations, and the inconvenience of this procedure make it highly unlikely that enhanced systemic clearance can be achieved in humans.

In human volunteer studies, WBI was more effective than single-dose AC or MDAC for enteric-coated acetylsalicylic acid (ASA),[43] decreased peak lithium [Li], and Li AUC (area under the plasma drug concentration versus time curve) compared with controls[87]; decreased the bioavailability of two sustained-release medications[15,48]; and propelled radiopaque markers through the gut more efficiently than controls.[54]

Not unexpectedly, WBI was inferior to AC with regard to prevention of absorption when administered after 650 mg of immediate-release aspirin.[82] Additionally, after the aspirin was absorbed, WBI was unable to enhance systemic clearance.[60] Likewise, only a small, statistically insignificant effect of WBI could be demonstrated on the absorption of extended-release acetaminophen in a human volunteer study.[54] These findings highlight the limited utility of WBI to assist in the prevention of absorption of relatively rapidly absorbed xenobiotics.

Several reports have shown successful use of WBI in the management of overdoses of iron,[26,57,92,93] sustained-release theophylline,[39] sustained-release verapamil,[13] zinc sulfate,[14] lead,[64,66,72,81] arsenic trioxide,[36] mercuric oxide powder,[55] clonidine patch ingestion,[35] arsenic-containing herbicide,[49] delayed-release fenfluramine[67] and in body packers.[34,95,99] Although some clinicians express enthusiasm for the use of WBI for a variety of ingestions, others question its efficacy.[14,83,91] WBI for 5 hours after ingestion of 10 fluorescent coffee beans by each of seven volunteers removed an average of only four beans (range, 1–8).[83] Similar failures were reported with jequirity beans [91] and button batteries.[92] It can be argued that because of their physical characteristics (density, solubility, size), these xenobiotics might not be representative of xenobiotics amenable to WBI. Additionally, the experience of the editors of this text in caring for body packers demonstrates that WBI may not always evacuate all of the drug packets because of inadequate dosing, partial obstruction, or the nature of the procedure. In a recent case, prolonged WBI failed to clear drug in a methamphetamine body stuffer.[32] As a result of these failures, promotility agents were added to WBI and presumably successfully enhanced bowel evacuation in two body packers suspected of having ingested well-constructed drug packets.[96]

ADVERSE EFFECTS OF WHOLE-BOWEL IRRIGATION

Adverse effects resulting from the use of WBI with PEG-ELS include vomiting, particularly after rapid administration, abdominal bloating, fullness, cramping, flatulence, and pruritus ani. Typically, the patient will need to remain on a commode for 4 to 6 hours to complete the procedure. Slow or low-volume administration of PEG-ELS results in sodium absorption. If a total of 500 mL of PEG-ELS were used instead of multiple liters, potentially 1.5 g of sodium may be absorbed.[24] This adverse effect may have resulted in the exacerbation of congestive heart failure in an unstable patient with cardiac and renal dysfunction.[30]

An unusual complication of WBI is colonic perforation, which occurred in a patient with active diverticulitis.[47] Other adverse effects noted by the manufacturer include isolated reports of upper GI bleeding from a Mallory-Weiss tear, esophageal perforation, aspiration pneumonitis after vomiting, and acute lung injury.

Unintentional administration of PEG-ELS by other than the enteral route has occurred. A 4-year-old child inadvertently received 390 mL of PEG-ELS intravenously with no obvious adverse result.[80] In contrast, acute lung injury developed in an 11-year-old child administered PEG-ELS through a nasogastric tube inadvertently inserted in the trachea.[73] In a similar case, a poorly placed nasogastric tube was responsible for PEG-ELS aspiration in a 3-year old boy, with resultant hypoxia and hemodynamic instability requiring endotracheal intubation.[29]

Finally, a recent report of two cases suggests that vomiting and aspiration may be more frequent than previously recognized in hemodynamically unstable patients.[19] Presumably, the patient's hypotension results in GI hypoperfusion and ileus, which with the continued administration of WBI in the presence of decreased GI motility, produces abdominal distention and vomiting.

INTERACTION OF ACTIVATED CHARCOAL AND WHOLE-BOWEL IRRIGATION

Several in vitro studies demonstrate that the addition of PEG-ELS to AC significantly decreases the adsorptive capacity of AC.[8,33,56] Some interactions were affected by pH and magnified by high ratios of PEG-ELS to AC.[7,44,56] The most likely explanation is competition with the AC surface for solute adsorption. Additionally, in an animal model, WBI appeared to have an adverse effect by washing the AC away from the sustained-release theophylline.[15] One recent case report documents rapid increases in carbamazepine concentrations temporally related to the initiation of WBI.[53] Although the patient had received MDAC and hemoperfusion, xenobiotic concentrations were increasing 58 hours after ingestion. It is possible that PEG-ELS competed for carbamazepine binding to AC, displacing some drug and making it available for absorption.

A similar rapidly increasing drug concentration was noted after the initiation of WBI in a patient with a reported 10-g phenytoin overdose.[18] In this case, AC had not been given before the initiation of WBI. One possible explanation is that the massive dose of phenytoin prevented its own absorption by exceeding its solubility but the administration of WBI provided sufficient diluent to allow phenytoin dissolution before GI emptying with subsequent absorption.

CONTRAINDICATIONS

Contraindications to WBI include prior, current, or anticipated diarrhea; volume depletion; significant GI pathology or dysfunction such as ileus, perforation, colitis, toxic megacolon, hemorrhage, and obstruction; an unprotected or compromised airway; and hemodynamic instability.[4,92]

DOSING

The recommended dose of WBI with PEG-ELS solution is 0.5 L/h or 25 mL/kg/h for small children and 1.5 to 2.0 L/h or 20 to 30 mL/min for adolescents and adults. WBI solution may be administered orally or through a nasogastric tube for 4 to 6 hours or until the rectal effluent becomes clear. An antiemetic such as metoclopramide or a $5HT_3$ serotonin antagonist may be required for the treatment of nausea or vomiting. In select patients, promotility agents may serve as useful adjuncts.[96] If the xenobiotic being removed is radiopaque, a diagnostic imaging technique demonstrating the absence of the xenobiotic may serve as an initial clinical endpoint (Special Considerations: SC4: Internal Concealment of Xenobiotics). WBI with large volumes of fluid was used successfully in two pregnant women at 38 and 26 weeks of gestation.[98,100]

AVAILABLE FORMS OF PEG-ELS FOR WHOLE-BOWEL IRRIGATION

The original WBI solution was GoLYTELY manufactured by Braintree. This solution contained PEG with electrolytes and sodium sulfate as an added laxative. Colyte is manufactured by Schwartz Pharma and is very similar to GoLYTELY. Braintree later introduced NuLYTELY, a PEG formulation with 52% less total salt than GoLYTELY and no added sodium sulfate. These changes in formulation decreased the salty taste and the risk of fluid- or electrolyte-related complications.[63] NuLYTELY is available in flavors. The three available PEG-ELS products are prepared by filling the container to the 4-L mark with water and shaking it vigorously several times to ensure dissolution. Lukewarm water facilitates dissolution, but subsequent chilling improves palatability. Chilled solutions, however, are not recommended for infants because of the risk of hypothermia. The products are stable with refrigeration for 48 hours after reconstitution.

The three available PEG-ELS products differ in the following manner:

1. GoLYTELY contains 236 g (17.6 mmol/L) of PEG, 22.74 g of sodium sulfate (anhydrous) (sulfate, 40 mmol/L), 6.74 g of sodium bicarbonate (bicarbonate, 20 mmol/L), 5.86 g of sodium chloride (total sodium, 125 mmol/L), and 2.97 g of potassium chloride (potassium, 10 mmol/L and total chloride, 35 mmol/L).
2. Colyte contains 240 g (18 mmol/L) of PEG, 22.72 g of sodium sulfate (anhydrous) (40 mmol/L sulfate), 6.72 g of sodium bicarbonate (bicarbonate, 20 mmol/L), 5.84 g of sodium chloride (total sodium, 125 mmol/L), and 2.98 g of potassium chloride (potassium, 10 mmol/L and total chloride, 35 mmol/L).
3. NuLYTELY contains 420 g of PEG 3350, 5.72 g of sodium bicarbonate, 11.2 g of sodium chloride, and 1.48 g of potassium chloride.

MiraLAX (manufactured by Braintree) contains PEG 3350 powder meant for oral administration after dissolution in water, juice, or soda. It is indicated for occasional constipation, with a recommended dose of 1 heaping teaspoon (17 g) in 240 mL liquid per day. For MiraLAX to be useful in WBI, it would need to be administered at a dose of 2 L/h (8 heaping teaspoons in 2 L of water/h) in adults. This is not recommended for WBI because it does not contain any added electrolytes and may result in an electrolyte imbalance.

SUMMARY

Cathartics should never be considered part of routine management of poisoning and overdose in either children or adults. Cathartics should never be used as an AC substitute when xenobiotics known to be adsorbed to AC are involved. Moreover, when total xenobiotic absorption is evaluated, a single dose of a cathartic given with AC appears to be only about as efficacious as AC given alone.

Investigators have studied the rapidity of stool production resulting from the use of various cathartics, promotility agents, and WBI. Administering a cathartic to produce a faster onset of charcoal stools has never been shown to produce a better clinical outcome. In adults, when large amounts of xenobiotics have been ingested or when desorption from charcoal may be an important consideration, as in the case of aspirin ingestion, a single dose of a cathartic, preferably magnesium citrate or sorbitol, may be given with the AC. When MDAC is administered, if a cathartic is used at all, it should only be given with the first dose. Sufficient oral fluids should always be administered with a cathartic to avoid inspissation and dehydration. Unless contraindicated, WBI is preferable to repetitive dose cathartics for evacuation of sustained-release or poorly soluble xenobiotics not adsorbed to AC.

The precise role of WBI and the interactions between AC and PEG-ELS in overdosed patients remain to be defined. No controlled clinical studies have assessed outcome, although theoretically, ingestions of sustained-release xenobiotics (theophylline, glyburide XL, verapamil, and diltiazem), xenobiotics not adsorbed by charcoal (iron, lead, lithium), and drug packets (in body packers) may be amenable to the use of WBI. An added advantage of using PEG-ELS WBI is that if the patient requires endoscopy, diagnostic imaging, or surgery, the GI tract may be more easily visualized, facilitating the intervention or procedure. AC should be given to patients for whom it is indicated, and if WBI is being performed in conjunction, a comparable dose of AC should be given after the WBI, to prevent or overcome the potential xenobiotic desorption and possible further systemic absorption of the xenobiotic.

REFERENCES

1. Allerton J, Strom J: Hypernatremia due to repeated doses of charcoal-sorbitol. *Am J Kidney Dis.* 1991;7:581-584.
2. Al-Shareef AH, Buss DC, Allen EM, Routledge PA: The effects of charcoal and sorbitol (alone and in combination) on plasma theophylline concentration after a sustained release formulation. *Hum Exp Toxicol.* 1990;9:179-182.
3. Ambrose N, Johnson M, Burdon D, et al: A physiologic approach of polyethylene glycol and a balanced electrolyte solution as bowel preparation. *Br J Surg.* 1983;70:428-430.
4. American Academy of Clinical Toxicology and European Association of Poison Centres and Clinical Toxicologists: position statement: whole-bowel irrigation. *J Toxicol Clin Toxicol.* 1997;35:753-762.
5. American Academy of Clinical Toxicology and European Association of Poison Centres and Clinical Toxicologists: position statement: cathartics. *J Toxicol Clin Toxicol.* 1997:35:743-752.
6. American Academy of Clinical Toxicology and the European Association of Poison Centres and Clinical Toxicologists: position paper: whole-bowel irrigation. *J Toxicol Clin Toxicol.* 2004;42:843-854.
7. Atta-Politou J, Macheras P, Koupparis M: The effect of polyethylene glycol on the charcoal adsorption of chlorpromazine studied by ion-selective electrode potentiometry. *J Toxicol Clin Toxicol.* 1996;34:307-316.

8. Atta-Politou J, Kolioliou M, Havariotou M, et al: An in vitro evaluation of fluoxetine adsorption by activated charcoal and desorption upon addition of polyethylene glycol-electrolyte lavage solution. *J Toxicol Clin Toxicol.* 1998;36:117-124.
9. Azzam I, Kovalev Y, Storch S, Elias N: Life threatening hyperphosphataemia after administration of sodium phosphate in preparation for colonoscopy. *Postgrad Med J.* 2004;80:487-488.
10. Beck D, Harford F, diPalma J, et al: Bowel cleansing with polyethylene glycol electrolyte lavage solution. *South Med J.* 1985;78:1414-1416.
11. Beloosesky Y, Grinblat J, Weiss A, et al: Electrolyte disorders following oral sodium phosphate administration for bowel cleansing in elderly patients. *Arch Intern Med.* 2003;163:803-808.
12. Binder H: Pharmacology of laxatives. *Annu Rev Pharmacol Toxicol.* 1977;17:355-367.
13. Buckley N, Dawson A, Howarth D, Whyte I: Slow release verapamil poisoning. *Med J Aust.* 1993;158:202-204.
14. Burkhart KK, Kulig KW, Rumack BH: Whole-bowel irrigation as adjunctive treatment for zinc sulfate overdose. *Ann Emerg Med.* 1990;19:1167-1170.
15. Burkhart KK, Wuerz R, Donovan JW: Whole-bowel irrigation as adjunctive treatment for sustained release theophylline overdose. *Ann Emerg Med.* 1992;21:1316-1320.
16. Carl DE, Sica DA: Acute phosphate nephropathy following colonoscopy preparation. *Am J Med Sci.* 2007;334:151-154.
17. Chin L, Picchioni A, Gillespie T: Saline cathartics and saline cathartics plus activated charcoal as antidotal treatments. *Clin Toxicol.* 1981;18:865-871.
18. Craig S: Phenytoin overdose complicated by prolonged intoxication and residual neurological deficits. *Emerg Med Australas.* 2004;16:361-365.
19. Cumpston KL, Aks SE, Sigg T, Pallasch E: Whole bowel irrigation and the hemodynamically unstable calcium channel blocker overdose: primum non nocere. *J Emerg Med.* 2008 Jul 8. [Epub ahead of print]
20. Darlington RC: Laxatives. In: Griffenhagen GB, Hawkins LL, eds. *Handbook of Nonprescription Drugs*. Washington, DC: American Pharmaceutical Association; 1973:62-76.
21. Davis G, Santa Ana C, Morawsk S, et al: Development of a lavage solution associated with minimal water and electrolyte absorption or secretion. *Gastroenterology.* 1980;78:991-995.
22. Davis R, Eichner J, Bleyer W, et al: Hypocalcemia, hyperphosphatemia, and dehydration following a single hypertonic phosphate enema. *J Pediatr.* 1977;90:484-485.
23. DiPalma J, Brady C, Stewart D, et al: Comparison of colon cleansing methods in preparation for colonoscopy. *Gastroenterology.*1984;86:856-860.
24. DiPalma JA, MacRae DH, Reichelderfer M, et al. Braintree polyethylene glycol (PEG) laxative for ambulatory and long-term care facility constipation patients: report of randomized, cross-over trials. *Online J Dig Health.*1999;1:1-7.
25. Erstoff J, Howard D, Marshall J, et al: A randomized blinded clinical trial of a rapid colonic lavage solution (GoLYTELY) compared with standard preparation for colonoscopy and barium enema. *Gastroenterology.*1983;84:1512-1516.
26. Everson G, Bertaccini E, O'Leary J: Use of whole-bowel irrigation in an infant following iron overdose. *Am J Emerg Med.* 1991;9:366-369.
27. Farley T: Severe hypernatremic dehydration after use of an activated charcoal-sorbitol suspension. *J Pediatr.* 1986;109:719-722.
28. Forman J, Baluarte J, Gruskin A: Hypokalemia after hypertonic phosphate enemas. *J Pediatr.* 1979;94:149-151.
29. Givens ML, Gabrysch J: Cardiotoxicity associated with accidental bupropion ingestion in a child. *Pediatr Emerg Care.* 2007;23:234-237.
30. Granberry MC, White LM, Gardner SF, et al: Exacerbation of congestive heart failure after administration of polyethylene glycol-electrolyte lavage solution. *Ann Pharmacother.* 1995;29:1232-1235.
31. Grissinger M: Bowel preparations might pose problems in renal patients. *P&T.* 2002;27:352.
32. Hendrickson RG, Horowitz BZ, Norton RL, Notenboom H: "Parachuting" meth: a novel delivery method for methamphetamine and delayed-onset toxicity from "body stuffing". *Clin Toxicol.* 2006;44:379-382.
33. Hoffman RS, Chiang WK, Howland MA, et al: Theophylline desorption from activated charcoal caused by whole-bowel irrigation. *J Toxicol Clin Toxicol.* 1991;29:191-202.
34. Hoffman RS, Smilkstein MJ, Goldfrank LR: Whole-bowel irrigation and the cocaine body packer. *Am J Emerg Med.* 1990;8;523-527.
35. Horowitz R, Mazor SS, Aks SE, Leikin JB: Accidental clonidine patch ingestion in a child. *Am J Ther.* 2005;12:272-274.
36. Isbister GK, Dawson AH, Whyte IM: Arsenic trioxide poisoning: a description of two acute overdoses. *Hum Exp Toxicol.* 2004;23:359-364.
37. Jafri S, Pasricha P: Agents for diarrhea, constipation and inflammatory bowel disease. In: Hardman JG, Limbird LE, eds. *Goodman and Gilman's The Pharmacological Basis of Therapeutics*, 10th ed. New York: McGraw-Hill; 2001:1037-1058.
38. James LP, Nichols MH, King WD: A comparison of cathartics in pediatric ingestions. *Pediatrics.* 1995;96:235-238.
39. Janss GJ: Acute theophylline overdose treated with whole bowel irrigation. *S D J Med* 1990;43:7-8.
40. Jones J, Heiselman D, Dougherty J, et al: Cathartic-induced magnesium toxicity during overdose management. *Ann Emerg Med.* 1986;15:1214-1218.
41. Kapoor S: Lubiprostone: clinical applications beyond constipation. *World J Gastroenterol.* 2009;15:1147.
42. Keller R, Schwab R, Krenzelok E: Contribution of sorbitol combined with activated charcoal in prevention of salicylate absorption. *Ann Emerg Med.* 1990;19:654-656.
43. Kirshenbaum L, Mathews SC, Sitar DS, Tenenbein M: Whole-bowel irrigation versus activated charcoal in sorbitol for the ingestion of modified release pharmaceuticals. *Clin Pharmacol Ther.* 1989;46:264-271.
44. Kirshenbaum LA, Sitar DS, Tenenbein M: Interaction between whole-bowel irrigation solution and activated charcoal: implications for the treatment of toxic ingestions. *Ann Emerg Med.* 1990;19:1129-1132.
45. Korkis A, Miskowitz P, Kurt R, Klein H: Rectal prolapse after oral cathartics. *J Clin Gastroenterol.* 1992;14:339-341.
46. Krenzelok EP, Keller R, Stewart RD: Gastrointestinal transit times of cathartics combined with charcoal. *Ann Emerg Med.* 1985;14:1152-1155.
47. Langdon DE: Colonic perforation with volume laxatives. *Am J Gastroenterol.* 1996;91:622-623.
48. Lapatto-Reiniluoto O, Kivisto KT, Neuvonen PJ: Activated charcoal alone and followed by whole bowel irrigation in preventing the absorption of sustained-release drugs. *Clin Pharmacol Ther.* 2001;70: 255-260.
49. Lee DC, Roberts JR, Kelly JJ, Fishman SM: Whole-bowel irrigation as an adjunct in the treatment of radiopaque arsenic. *Am J Emerg Med.* 1995;13:244-245.
50. Lenz K, Oroz R, Kleinberger G, et al: Effect of gut lavage on phenobarbital elimination in rats. *J Toxicol Clin Toxicol.* 1983;20:147-157.
51. Longdon P, Henderson A: Intestinal pseudo-obstruction following the use of enteral charcoal and sorbitol and mechanical ventilation with papaveretum sedation for theophylline poisoning. *Drug Saf.* 1992;7:74-77.
52. Loughnan P, Mullins G: Brain damage following a hypertonic phosphate enema. *Am J Dis Child.* 1977;131:1032.
53. Lurie Y, Bentur Y, Levy Y, Baum E, Krivoy N: Limited efficacy of gastrointestinal decontamination in severe slow-release carbamazepine overdose. *Ann Pharmacother.* 2007;41:1539-1543.
54. Ly BT, Schneir AB, Clark RF: Effect of whole bowel irrigation on the pharmacokinetics of an acetaminophen formulation and progression of radiopaque markers through the gastrointestinal tract. *Ann Emerg Med.* 2004;43:189-195.
55. Ly BT, Williams SR, Clark RF: Mercuric oxide poisoning treated with whole bowel irrigation and chelation therapy. *Ann Emerg Med.* 2002;39:312-315.
56. Makoseij F, Hoffman RS, Howland MA, Goldfrank LR: An in vivo evaluation of cocaine hydrochloride adsorption by activated charcoal and desorption upon addition of polyethylene glycol electrolyte lavage solution. *J Toxicol Clin Toxicol.* 1993;31:381-395.
57. Mann K, Picciotti M, Spevack T, Durban D: Management of acute iron overdose. *Clin Pharm.* 1989;8:428-440.
58. Martin R, Lisehora G, Braxton M, et al: Fatal poisoning from sodium phosphate enema: a case report and experimental study. *JAMA.* 1987;257: 2190-2192.
59. Massanari MJ, Hendeles L, Hill E, et al: The efficacy of sorbitol and activated charcoal in reducing theophylline absorption from a slow release formulation. *Drug Intell Clin Pharm.* 1986;20:471.
60. Mayer L, Sitar DS, Tenenbein M: Multiple-dose charcoal and whole-bowel irrigation do not increase clearance of absorbed salicylate. *Arch Intern Med.* 1992;152:393-396.
61. Mayershohn M, Perrier D, Picchioni A: Evaluation of a charcoal-sorbitol mixture as an antidote for oral aspirin overdose. *Clin Toxicol.* 1977;11:561-567.
62. McCord M: Toxicity of sorbitol-charcoal suspension. *J Pediatr.* 1987;110:307-308.
63. McKee K: A guide to colon preps. *Outpatient Surgery Magazine* February 2002. Available at http://www.outpatientsurgery.net/2002/os02/ f5.shtml. Accessed April 25, 2005.

64. McKinney PE: Acute elevation of blood lead levels within hours of ingestion of quantities of lead shot. *J Toxicol Clin Toxicol.* 2000;38:435-440.
65. McNamara R, Aaron C, Gemborys M: Sorbitol catharsis does not enhance efficacy of charcoal in simulated acetaminophen overdose. *Ann Emerg Med.* 1988;17:243-246.
66. McNutt TK, Chambers-Emerson J, Dethlefsen M, et al: Bite the bullet: lead poisoning after ingestion of 206 lead bullets. *Vet Hum Toxicol.* 2001;43:288-289.
67. Melandri R, Re G, Morigi A, et al: Whole-bowel irrigation after delayed release fenfluramine overdose. *J Toxicol Clin Toxicol.* 1995;33:161-163.
68. Minocha A, Krenzelok EP, Spyker D: Dosage recommendations for activated charcoal-sorbitol treatment. *J Toxicol Clin Toxicol.* 1985;23:579-587.
69. Minocha A, Merold DA, Bruns DE, et al: Effect of activated charcoal in 70% sorbitol in healthy individuals. *J Toxicol Clin Toxicol.* 1984-85;22:529-536.
70. Mofenson HC, Caraccio TR: Magnesium intoxication in a neonate from oral magnesium hydroxide laxative. *J Toxicol Clin Toxicol.* 1991;29:215-222.
71. Muller-Lissner SA: Adverse effects of laxatives: fact and fiction. *Pharmacology* 1993;47(Suppl 1):138-145.
72. Murphy DG, Gerace RV, Peterson RG: The use of whole-bowel irrigation in acute lead ingestion [abstract]. *Vet Hum Toxicol.* 1991;33:353.
73. Narsinghani U, Chadha M, Farrar HC, Anand KS: Life-threatening respiratory failure following accidental infusion of polyethylene glycol electrolyte solution into the lung. *J Toxicol Clin Toxicol.* 2001;39:105-107.
74. Neuvonen P, Olkkola K: Effect of purgatives on antidotal efficacy of oral activated charcoal. *Vet Hum Toxicol.* 1986;5:255-263.
75. Pasricha P: Prokinetic agents, antiemetics, and agents used in irritable bowel syndrome. In: Hardman JG, Limbird LE, eds. *Goodman and Gilman's The Pharmacological Basis of Therapeutics*, 10th ed. New York: McGraw-Hill; 2001:1021-1036.
76. Picchioni A, Chin L, Gillespie T: Evaluation of activated charcoal-sorbitol suspension as an antidote. *Clin Toxicol.* 1982;19:435-444.
77. Postuma R: Whole-bowel irrigation in pediatric patients. *J Pediatr Surg.* 1982;17:350-352.
78. Pray WS: *Nonprescription Product Therapeutics.* Philadelphia, Lippincott Williams & Wilkins; 1999:132-154.
79. Reedy J, Zwiren G: Enema-induced hypocalcemia and hyperphosphatemia leading to cardiac arrest during induction of anesthesia in an outpatient surgery center. *Anesthesiology.* 1983;59:578-579.
80. Rivera W, Velez LI, Guzman DD, Shepherd G: Unintentional intravenous infusion of GoLYTELY in a 4-year-old girl. *Ann Pharmacother.* 2004;38:1183-1185.
81. Roberge RJ, Martin T, Michelson EA, et al: Whole bowel irrigation in acute lead ingestion [abstract]. *Vet Hum Toxicol.* 1991;33:353.
82. Rosenberg PJ, Livingston DJ, McLellan B: Effect of whole bowel irrigation on the antidotal efficacy of oral activated charcoal. *Ann Emerg Med.* 1988;17:681-683.
83. Scharman EJ, Lembersky R, Krenzelok EP: Efficiency of whole-bowel irrigation with and without metoclopramide pretreatment. *Am J Emerg Med.* 1994;12:302-305.
84. Sica DA, Carl D, Zfass AM: Acute phosphate nephropathy—an emerging issue. *Am J Gastroenterol.* 2007;102:1844-1847.
85. Sketris I, Mowry J, Czajka P, et al: Saline catharsis: effect on aspirin bioavailability in combination with activated charcoal. *J Clin Pharmacol.* 1982;22:59-64.
86. Smilkstein MJ, Steedle D, Kulig KW, et al: Magnesium levels after magnesium containing cathartics. *J Toxicol Clin Toxicol.* 1988;26:51-65.
87. Smith S, Ling L, Halstenson C: Whole-bowel irrigation as a treatment for acute lithium overdose. *Ann Emerg Med.* 1991;20:536-539.
88. Sotos J, Cutler E, Finkel M, et al: Hypocalcemic coma following two pediatric phosphate enemas. *Pediatrics.* 1977;60:305-307.
89. Stewart J: Effects of emetic and cathartic agents on the gastrointestinal tract and the treatment of toxic ingestions. *J Toxicol Clin Toxicol.* 1983;20:199-253.
90. Sue YJ, Woolf A, Shannon M: Efficacy of magnesium citrate cathartic pediatric toxic ingestions. *Ann Emerg Med.* 1994;24:709-712.
91. Swanson-Brearman B, Dean BS, Krenzelok EP: Failure of whole-bowel irrigation to decontaminate the GI tract following massive jequirity bean ingestion [abstract]. *Vet Hum Toxicol.* 1992;34:352.
92. Tenenbein M: Whole-bowel irrigation as gastrointestinal decontamination procedure after acute poisoning. *Med Toxicol.* 1988;3:77-84.
93. Tenenbein M, Wiseman N, Yatscoff RW: Gastrotomy and whole-bowel irrigation in iron poisoning. *Pediatr Emerg Care.* 1991;7:286-288.
94. Thomas G, Brozinsky S, Isenberg J: Patient acceptance and effectiveness of a balanced lavage solution (GoLYTELY) versus the standard preparation for colonoscopy. *Gastroenterology.* 1982;82:435-437.
95. Traub SJ, Kohn GL, Hoffman RS, Nelson LS: Pediatric "body packing." *Arch Pediatr Adolesc Med.* 2003;157:174-177.
96. Traub SJ, Su M, Hoffman RS, et al: Use of pharmaceutical promotility agents in the treatment of body packers. *Am J Emerg Med.* 2003;21:511-512.
97. Tuggle D, Hoelzer D, Tunell W, et al: Safety and cost-effectiveness of polyethylene glycol electrolyte solution bowel preparation in infants and children. *J Pediatr Surg.* 1987;22:513-515.
98. Turk J, Aks S, Ampuero F, et al: Successful therapy of iron intoxication in pregnancy with intravenous deferoxamine and whole-bowel irrigation. *Vet Hum Toxicol.* 1993;35:441-444.
99. Utecht M, Stone A, McCarron M: Heroin body packers. *J Emerg Med.* 1990;11:33-40.
100. Van Ameyde K, Tenenbein M: Whole-bowel irrigation during pregnancy. *Am J Obstet Gynecol.* 1989;160:646-647.
101. Van de Graff W, Thompson L, Sunshine I, et al: Absorbent and cathartic inhibition of enteral drug absorption. *J Pharmacol Exp Ther.* 1982;221:656-663.
102. Visser L, Sticker B, Hoogendoorn M, et al: Do not give paraffin to packers. *Lancet.* 1998;352:1352.
103. Wax PM, Wang RY, Hoffman RS, et al: Prevalence of sorbitol in multiple-dose activated charcoal regimens in emergency departments. *Ann Emerg Med.* 1993;22:1807-1812.

CHAPTER 8
PHARMACOKINETIC AND TOXICOKINETIC PRINCIPLES

Mary Ann Howland

Pharmacokinetics is the study of the absorption, distribution, metabolism, and excretion of xenobiotics. *Xenobiotics* are substances that are foreign to the body and include natural or synthetic chemicals, drugs, pesticides, environmental agents, and industrial agents.[49] Mathematical models and equations are used to describe and to predict these phenomena. *Pharmacodynamics* is the term used to describe an investigation of the relationship of xenobiotic concentration to clinical effects. *Toxicokinetics*, which is analogous to pharmacokinetics, is the study of the absorption, distribution, metabolism, and excretion of a xenobiotic under circumstances that produce toxicity. *Toxicodynamics*, which is analogous to pharmacodynamics, is the study of the relationship of toxic concentrations of xenobiotics to clinical effect.

Overdoses provide many challenges to the mathematical precision of toxicokinetics and toxicodynamics because many of the variables, such as dose, time of ingestion, and presence of vomiting, that affect the result are often unknown. In contrast to the therapeutic setting, atypical solubility characteristics are noted, and saturation of enzymatic processes occurs. Intestinal or hepatic enzymatic saturation or alterations in transporters may lead to enhanced absorption through a decrease in first-pass effect. Metabolism before the xenobiotic reaches the blood is referred to as the *first-pass effect*.[2,76] Saturation of plasma protein binding results in more free xenobiotic available in the serum, plasma, and blood. Saturation of hepatic enzymes or active renal tubular secretion leads to prolonged elimination. In addition, age, obesity, gender, genetics, chronopharmacokinetics (diurnal variations), and the effects of illness and compromised organ perfusion all further inhibit attempts to achieve precise analyses.[3,17,40,45,68,72] In addition, various treatments may alter one or more pharmacokinetic and toxicokinetic parameters. There are numerous approaches to recognizing these variables, such as obtaining historical information from the patient's family and friends, performing pill counts, procuring sequential serum concentrations during the phases of toxicity, and occasionally repeating a pharmacokinetic evaluation during therapeutic dosing of that same agent to obtain comparative data.

Despite all of the confounding and individual variability, toxicokinetic principles may nonetheless be applied to facilitate our understanding and to make certain predictions. These principles may be used to help evaluate whether a certain antidote or extracorporeal removal method is appropriate for use, when the serum concentration might be expected to decrease into the therapeutic range (if one exists), what ingested dose might be considered potentially toxic, what the onset and duration of toxicity might be, and what the importance is of a serum concentration. While considering all of these factors, the clinical status of the patient is paramount, and mathematical formulas and equations can never substitute for evaluating the patient. This chapter explains the principles and presents the mathematics in a user-friendly fashion.[79] The application of these principles and mathematical approaches by example and case illustration are found on the website.

ABSORPTION

Absorption is the process by which a xenobiotic enters the body. A xenobiotic must reach the bloodstream and then be distributed to the site or sites of action to cause a systemic effect. Both the rate (k_a) and extent of absorption (F) are measurable and important determinants of toxicity. The rate of absorption often predicts the onset of action and relies on dosage form, and the extent of absorption (*bioavailability*) often predicts the intensity of the effect and depends in part on first-pass effects.[36,37] Figure 8–1 depicts how changes in the rate of absorption may affect toxicity when the bioavailability is held constant versus how toxicity may be affected by changes in bioavailability when the rate of absorption is held constant.

The route by which the xenobiotic enters the body significantly affects both the rate and extent of absorption. As an approximation, the rate of absorption proceeds in the following order from fastest to slowest: intravenous (IV), inhalation > sublingual > intramuscular, subcutaneous, intranasal, oral > cutaneous, rectal. After the oral intake of 200 mg (0.59 mmol) of cocaine hydrochloride, the onset of action is 20 minutes, with an average peak concentration of 200 ng/mL.[71] In marked contrast, smoking 200 mg (0.66 mmol) of cocaine freebase results in an onset of action of 8 seconds and a peak level of 640 ng/mL. When administered IV as 200-mg cocaine hydrochloride, it then has an onset of action of 30 seconds and a peak level of 1000 ng/mL.[71]

A xenobiotic must diffuse through a number of membranes before it can reach its site of action. Figure 8–2 shows the number of membranes through which a xenobiotic typically diffuses. Membranes are predominantly composed of phospholipids and cholesterol in addition to other lipid compounds.[54] A phospholipid is composed of a polar head and a fatty acid tail, which are arranged in membranes so that the fatty acid tails are inside and the polar heads face outward in a mirror image.[58] Proteins are found on both sides of the membranes and may traverse the membrane.[54] These proteins may function as receptors and channels. Pores are found throughout the membranes. The principles relating to diffusion apply to absorption, distribution, certain aspects of elimination, and each instance when a xenobiotic is transported through a membrane.

Transport through membranes occurs via (1) passive diffusion; (2) filtration or bulk flow, which is most important in renal and biliary secretion as the mechanism of transport associated with the movement of molecules with a molecular weight less than 100 daltons, with water directly through aquapores; (3) carrier-mediated active or facilitated transport, which is saturable, and (4) rarely, endocytosis (see Fig. 8–2). Most xenobiotics traverse membranes via simple passive diffusion. The rate of diffusion is determined by the Fick law of diffusion (Eq. 8–1):

$$\text{Rate of diffusion} = \frac{dQ}{dt} = \frac{DAK(C_1 - C_2)}{h} \qquad \text{(Eq. 8–1)}$$

D = diffusion constant
A = surface area of the membrane
h = membrane thickness
K = partition coefficient
$C_1 - C_2$ = difference in concentrations of the xenobiotic at each side of the membrane

The driving force for passive diffusion is the difference in concentration of the xenobiotic on both sides of the membrane. D is

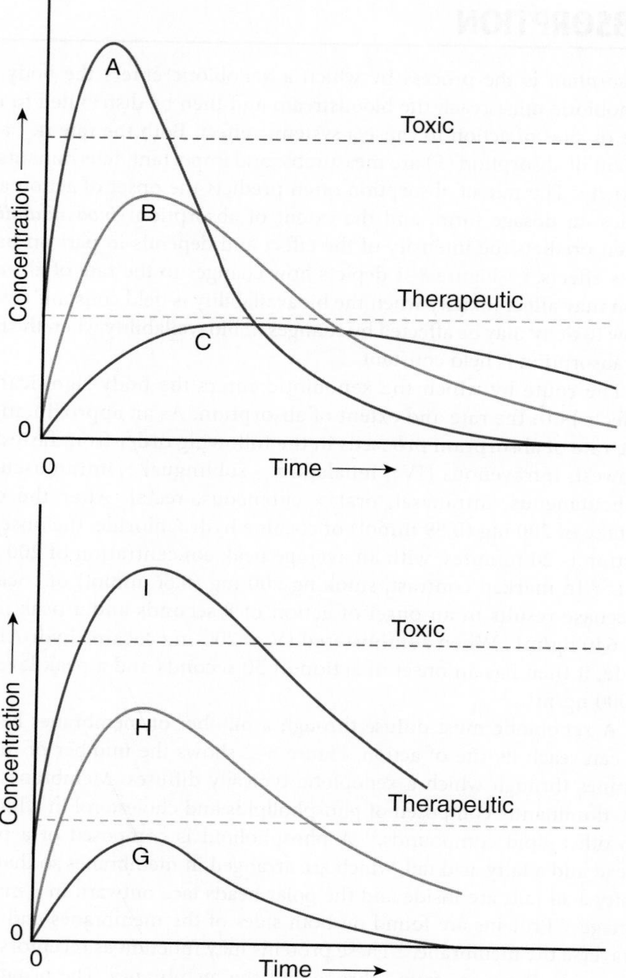

FIGURE 8–1. Effects of changes in k_a (rate of absorption) and F (bioavailability) on the blood concentration time graph and achieving a toxic threshold. In curves A, B, and C, F is constant as k_a decreases. In curves G, H, and I, k_a is constant as F increases from G to I.[48]

a constant for each xenobiotic and is derived when the difference in concentrations between the two sides of the membrane is 1. The larger the surface area A, the higher the rate of diffusion. Most ingested xenobiotics are absorbed more rapidly in the small intestine than in the stomach because of the tremendous increase in surface area created by the presence of microvilli. The partition coefficient K_e represents the lipid-to-water partitioning of the xenobiotic. To a substantial degree, the more lipid soluble a xenobiotic is, the more easily it crosses membranes. Membrane thickness (h) is inversely proportional to the rate at which a xenobiotic diffuses through the membrane. Xenobiotics that are uncharged, nonpolar, of low molecular weight, and of the appropriate lipid solubility have the highest rates of passive diffusion.

The extent of ionization of weak electrolytes (weak acids and weak bases) affects their rate of passive diffusion. Nonpolar and uncharged molecules penetrate faster. The Henderson-Hasselbalch relationship is used to determine the degree of ionization. An acid (HA), by definition, gives up a hydrogen ion, and a base (B) accepts a hydrogen ion. RCOOH (HA) (ie, aspirin, phenobarbital) and RNH_3^+ (BH^+) are acids and $RCOO^-$ (A^-), and RNH_2 (B) (amphetamines, tricyclic antidepressants) are bases. The equilibrium dissociation constant K_a can then be described by Equations 8–2A and 8–2B:

$$\text{For weak acids: } HA = H^+ + A^- \quad K_a = \frac{[H^+][A^-]}{[HA]} \qquad \text{(Eq. 8–2A)}$$

$$\text{For weak bases: } BH^+ = B + H^+ \quad K_a = \frac{[H^+][B]}{[BH^+]} \qquad \text{(Eq. 8–2B)}$$

To work with these numbers in a more comfortable fashion, the negative log of both sides is determined. The results are given in Equations 8–3A and 8–3B.

$$\text{For weak acids:} -\log K_a = -\log[H^+] - \log\frac{[A^-]}{[HA]} \qquad \text{(Eq. 8–3A)}$$

$$\text{For weak bases:} -\log K_a = -\log[H^+] - \log\frac{[B]}{[BH^+]} \qquad \text{(Eq. 8–3B)}$$

By definition, the negative log of $[H^+]$ is expressed as pH, and the negative log of K_a is pK_a. Rearranging the equations gives the familiar forms of the Henderson-Hasselbalch equations, as shown in Equations 8–4A, 8–4B, and 8–4C:

$$pH = pK_a + \log\frac{\text{Unprotonated species}}{\text{Protonated species}} \qquad \text{(Eq. 8–4A)}$$

$$\text{For weak acids: } pH = pK_a + \log\frac{[A^-]}{[HA]} \qquad \text{(Eq. 8–4B)}$$

$$\text{For weak bases: } pH = pK_a + \log\frac{[B]}{[BH^+]} \qquad \text{(Eq. 8–4C)}$$

Because noncharged molecules traverse membranes more rapidly, it is understood that weak acids cross membranes more rapidly in an acidic environment and weak bases move more rapidly in a basic environment. When the pH equals the pK_a, half of the xenobiotic is charged and half is noncharged. An acid with a low pK_a is a strong acid, and a base with a low pK_a is a weak base. For an acid, whereas a pH less than the pK_a favors the protonated or noncharged species facilitating membrane diffusion, for a base, a pH greater than the pK_a achieves the same result. Table 8–1 lists the pH of selected body fluids, and Figure 8–3 illustrates the extent of charged versus noncharged xenobiotic at different pH and pK_a values.

Lipid solubility and ionization each have a distinct influence on absorption. Figure 8–4 demonstrates these characteristics for three different xenobiotics. Although the three xenobiotics have similar pK_a values, their different partition coefficients result in different degrees of absorption from the stomach.

Specialized transport mechanisms are either adenosine triphosphate (ATP) dependent to transport xenobiotics against a concentration gradient (ie, active transport), or ATP independent and lack the ability to transport against a concentration gradient (ie, facilitated transport). These transport mechanisms are of importance in numerous parts of the body, including the intestines, liver, lungs, kidneys, and biliary system. These same principles apply to a small number of lipid-insoluble molecules that resemble essential endogenous agents.[28,64] For example,

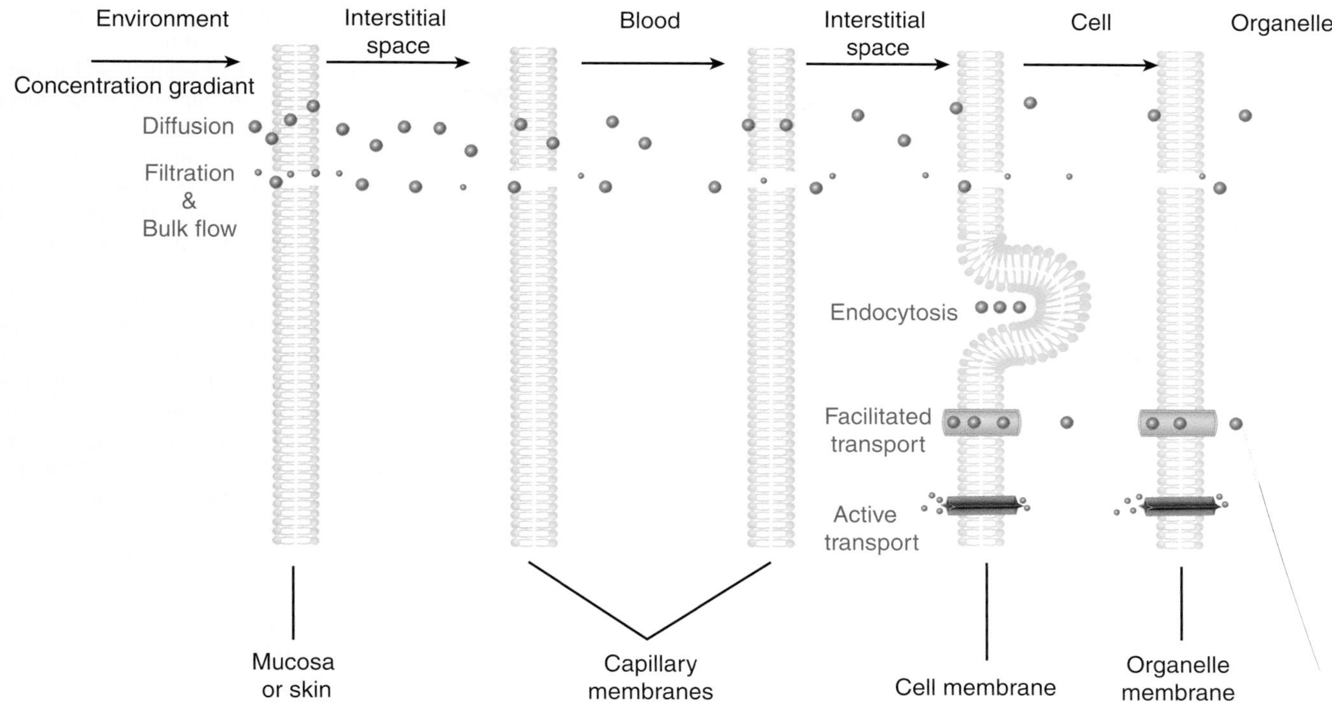

FIGURE 8–2. Illustration of the number of membranes encountered by a xenobiotic in the process of absorption and distribution and the transport mechanisms involved in the passage of xenobiotics across membranes. Examples include diffusion: nonelectrolytes (ethanol) and unionized forms of weak acids (salicylic acid) and bases (amphetamines); endocytosis: Sabin polio virus vaccine; facilitated: 5-fluorouracil, lead, methyldopa, thallium; and active: thiamine and pyridoxine.

5-fluorouracil resembles pyrimidine and is transported by the same system, and thallium and lead are actively absorbed by the endogenous transport mechanisms that absorb and transport potassium and calcium, respectively. Filtration is generally considered to be of limited importance in the absorption of most xenobiotics but is substantially more important with regard to renal and biliary elimination. Endocytosis, which describes the encircling of a xenobiotic by a cellular membrane, is responsible for the absorption of large macromolecules such as the oral Sabin polio vaccine.[64]

TABLE 8–1. pH of Selected Body Fluids

Fluids	pH
Cerebrospinal	7.3
Eye	7–8
Gastric secretions	1–3
Large intestinal secretions	8
Plasma	7.4
Rectal fluid: Infants and children	7.2–12
Saliva	6.4–7.2
Small intestinal secretions: Duodenum	5–6
Small intestinal secretions: Ileum	8
Urine	4–8
Vaginal secretions	3.8–4.5

Gastrointestinal (GI) absorption is affected by xenobiotic-related characteristics such as dosage form, degree of ionization, partition coefficient, and patient factors (eg, GI blood flow; GI motility; and the presence or absence of food, ethanol, or other interfering substances such as calcium) (Fig. 8–5).

The formulation of a xenobiotic is extremely important in predicting GI absorption. Disintegration and dissolution must precede absorption. Disintegration is usually much more rapid than dissolution except for modified-release products. Modified-release products include delayed-release and extended-release formulations. By definition, extended-release formulations decrease the frequency of drug administration by 50% compared with immediate release-formulations, and they include controlled-release, sustained-release, and prolonged-release formulations. These modified-release formulations are designed to release the xenobiotic over a prolonged period of time to simulate the blood concentrations achieved with the use of a constant IV infusion. These formulations minimize blood level fluctuations, reduce peak-related side effects, reduce dosing frequency, and improve patient compliance. A variety of products use different pharmaceutical strategies, including dissolution control (encapsulation or matrix; Feosol), diffusion control (membrane or matrix; Slow K, Plendil ER), erosion (Sinemet CR), osmotic pump systems (Procardia XL, Glucotrol XL), and ion exchange resins (MS Contin suspension). Overdoses with modified-release formulations often result in a prolonged absorption phase, a delay to peak concentrations, and a prolonged duration of effect.[7] Delayed-release preparations are enteric coated and designed to bypass the stomach and to release drug in the small intestine. Enteric-coated (acetylsalicylic acid [ASA], divalproex

pH	Aspirin (pK_a = 3.5)	% Nonionized	Methamphetamine (pK_a = 10)	% Nonionized
1		99.7		
2		97		
3		76		
3.5		50		
4		24		
5		3		0.001
6		0.315		0.01
7		0.032		0.1
10				50
11				90.9
12				99

FIGURE 8–3. Effect of pH on the ionization of aspirin (pK_a = 3.5) and methamphetamine (pKa = 10).

sodium) formulations resist disintegration and delay the time to onset of effect.[6] Dissolution is affected by ionization, solubility, and the partition coefficient, as noted earlier. In the overdose setting, the formation of poorly soluble or adherent masses such as concretions of foreign material termed *bezoars* (verapamil, meprobamate, and bromide) significantly delay the time to onset of toxicity (Table 8–2).[4,11,29,30,60]

Most ingested xenobiotics are primarily absorbed in the small intestine as a result of the large surface area and extensive blood flow of the small intestines.[59] Critically ill patients who are hypotensive, have a reduced cardiac output, or are receiving vasoconstrictors such as norepinephrine have a decreased perfusion of vital organs, including the GI tract, kidneys, and liver.[3] Not only is absorption delayed, but elimination is also diminished.[57] Total GI transit time can be from 0.4 to 5 days, and small intestinal transit time is usually 3 to 4 hours. Extremely short GI transit times reduce absorption. This change in transit time is the unproven rationale for use of whole-bowel irrigation (WBI). Delays in emptying of the stomach impair absorption as a result of the delay in delivery to the small intestine. Delays in gastric emptying occur as a result of the presence of food, especially fatty meals; agents with anticholinergic, opioid, or antiserotonergic properties; ethanol; and any agent that results in pylorospasm (salicylates, iron).

Bioavailability is a measure of the amount of xenobiotic that reaches the systemic circulation unchanged (Eq. 8–5).[38] The fractional absorption (F) of a xenobiotic is defined by the area under the plasma drug concentration versus time curve (AUC) of the designated route of absorption compared with the AUC of the IV route. The AUC for each route represents the amount absorbed.

$$F = \frac{(\mathrm{AUC})_{\text{route under study}}}{(\mathrm{AUC})_{\mathrm{IV}}} \qquad \text{(Eq. 8–5)}$$

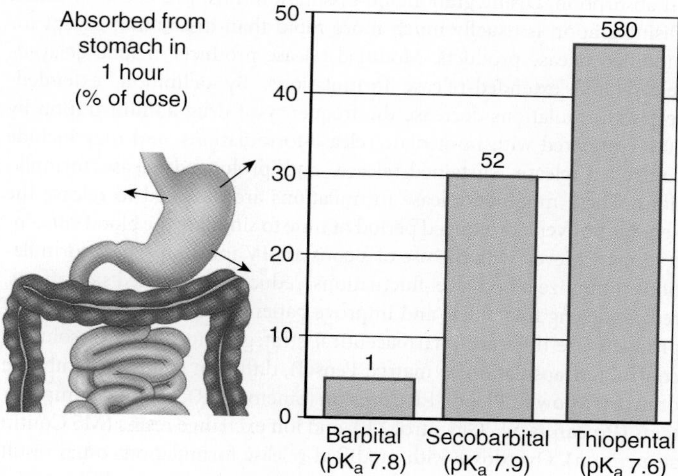

FIGURE 8–4. Influence of increasing lipid solubility on the amount of xenobiotic absorbed from the stomach for three xenobiotics with similar pK_a values. The number above each column is the oil/water equilibrium partition coefficient.

Gastric emptying and activated charcoal are used to decrease the bioavailability of ingested xenobiotics. The oral administration of certain chelators (deferoxamine, D-penicillamine) actually enhances the bioavailability of the complexed xenobiotic. The net effect of some chelators, such as succimer, is a reduction in body burden via enhanced urinary elimination even though absorption is enhanced.[31] Historically, the enteral administration of sodium bicarbonate was used to theoretically reduce the solubility of iron salts; unfortunately, this approach was ineffective and increased toxicity.[15]

Presystemic metabolism may decrease or increase the bioavailability of a xenobiotic or a metabolite.[53] The GI tract contains microbial organisms that can metabolize or degrade xenobiotics such as digoxin and oral contraceptives and enzymes, such as peptidases, that metabolize insulin.[54] However, in rare cases, GI hydrolysis can convert a xenobiotic into a toxic metabolite, as occurs when amygdalin is enzymatically hydrolyzed to produce cyanide, a metabolic step that is not produced after IV amygdalin administration.[27] Xenobiotic metabolizing enzymes and transporters such as P-glycoprotein may also affect bioavailability. Xenobiotic-metabolizing enzymes are found in the lumen of the small intestine and can substantially decrease the absorption of a xenobiotic.[44,73] Some of the xenobiotic that enters the cell can then be removed by the P-glycoprotein transporter out of the cell and back into the lumen to be exposed again to the metabolizing enzymes.[44,73] Venous drainage from the stomach and intestine delivers orally (and intraperitoneally) administered xenobiotics to the liver via the portal vein and avoids direct delivery to the systemic circulation. This venous drainage allows hepatic metabolism to occur before the xenobiotic reaches the blood, and as previously mentioned, is referred to as the *first-pass effect*.[2,76] The hepatic extraction ratio is the percentage of xenobiotic metabolized in one pass of blood through the liver.[47] Xenobiotics that undergo significant first-pass metabolism (eg, propranolol, verapamil) are used at much lower IV doses than oral doses. Some drugs, such as lidocaine and nitroglycerin, are not administered by the oral route because of significant first-pass effect.[4] Instead, sublingual (nitroglycerin), transcutaneous (topical), or rectal administration of drugs is used to bypass the portal circulation and avoid first-pass metabolism.

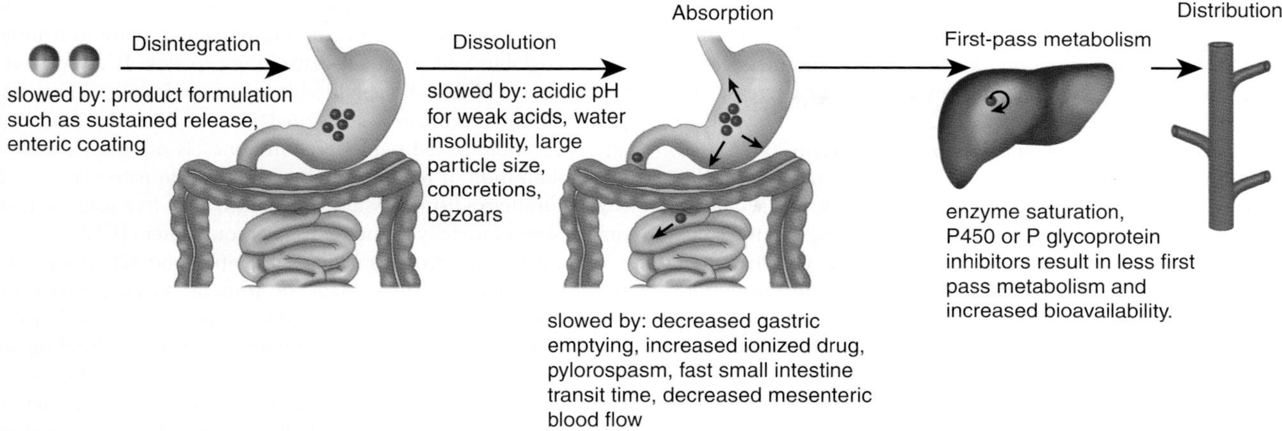

FIGURE 8–5. Determinants of absorption.

In the overdose setting, presystemic metabolism may be saturated, leading to an increased bioavailability of xenobiotics such as cyclic antidepressants, phenothiazines, opioids, and many β-adrenergic antagonists.[56] Hepatic metabolism usually transforms the xenobiotic into a less-active metabolite but occasionally results in the formation of a more toxic agent such as occurs with the transformation of parathion to paraoxon.[51] Biliary excretion into the small intestine usually occurs for these transformed xenobiotics of molecular weights greater than 350 daltons and may result in a xenobiotic appearing in the feces even though it had not been administered orally.[34,54,67] Hepatic conjugated metabolites such as glucuronides may be hydrolyzed in the intestines to the parent form or to another active metabolite that can be reabsorbed by the enterohepatic circulation.[41,49,52,54] The enterohepatic circulation may be responsible for what is termed a *double-peak phenomenon* after the administration of certain xenobiotics.[64] The double-peak phenomenon is characterized as a serum concentration that decreases and then increases again as xenobiotic is reabsorbed from the GI tract. Other causes include variability in stomach emptying, presence of food, or failure of a tablet dosage form.[64]

DISTRIBUTION

After the xenobiotic reaches the systemic circulation, it is available for transport to peripheral tissue compartments and to the liver and kidney for elimination. Both the rate and extent of distribution depend on many of the same principles discussed with regard to diffusion. Additional factors include affinity of the xenobiotic for plasma (plasma protein binding) and tissue proteins, acid–base status of the patient (which affects ionization), drug transporters, and physiologic barriers to distribution (blood–brain barrier, placental transfer, blood–testis barrier).[23,35,58] Blood flow, the percentage of free drug in the plasma, and the activity of transporters account for the initial phase of distribution, and xenobiotic affinities determine the final distribution pattern. Whereas the adrenal glands, kidneys, liver, heart, and brain receive from 55 to 550 mL/min/100 g of tissue of blood flow, the skin, muscle, connective tissue, and fat receive 1 to 5 mL/min/100 g of tissue of blood flow.[62] Hypoperfusion of the various organs in critically ill and injured patients affects absorption, distribution, and elimination.[74]

TABLE 8–2. Xenobiotics that Form Concretions or Bezoars, Delay Gastric Emptying, or Result in Pylorospasm

Anticholinergics	Meprobamate
Barbiturates	Methaqualone
Bromides	Opioids
Enteric-coated tablets	Phenytoin
Glutethimide	Salicylates
Iron	Verapamil

ABC transporters are active ATP-dependent transmembrane protein carriers of which P-glycoprotein was the initial example discovered.[9] Approximately 50 ABC transporters exist, and they are divided into subfamilies based on their similarities. Several members of the ABC superfamily, including P-glycoprotein, are under extensive investigation because of their role in controlling xenobiotic entry into, distribution in, and elimination from the body as well as their contributions to drug interactions.[21,32,73] The discovery of P-glycoprotein resulted from an investigation into why certain tumors exhibit multidrug resistance to many cancer chemotherapy agents. P-glycoprotein (ABCB1) as well as ABCC and ABCG2 are known to be efflux transporters located in the intestines, renal proximal tubules, hepatic bile canaliculi, placenta, and blood–brain barrier and are responsible for the intra- to extracellular transport of various xenobiotics.[16] First-generation transport inhibitors such as amiodarone, ketoconazole, quinidine, and verapamil are responsible for increasing body levels of P-glycoprotein substrates such as digoxin, the protease inhibitors, vinca alkaloids, and paclitaxel. St. John's wort is a transport inducer, and it lowers serum concentrations of these same xenobiotics. Second- and third-generation xenobiotics that will affect transport with a higher affinity and specificity are in development.[18,65] Many of the same xenobiotics that affect cytochrome P450 (CYP) 3A4 also affect P-glycoprotein (Appendix Chapter 12: Cytochrome P450 Substrates Inhibitors and Inducers).

Recently, the organic anion transporting polypeptides (OATPs) have been recognized as another group of transporters found in the liver, kidneys, intestines, brain, and placenta that are also responsible for affecting the absorption, distribution, and elimination of many xenobiotics and contributing to xenobiotic interactions. They include the organic anion transporters (OATs) and the organic cation transporters (OCTs).[18] For example, probenecid increases the serum concentrations of penicillin by inhibiting the OAT responsible for the active secretion of penicillin by the renal tubular cells, and cimetidine inhibits the OCT responsible for the renal elimination of procainamide and metformin. A variety of OAT inhibitors are being investigated to decrease the hepatic uptake of amatoxins[18] (Chap. 117).

Plasma concentration and *serum concentration* are terms often used interchangeably by medical personnel. When a reference or calculation is made with regard to a concentration in the body, it is actually a plasma concentration. When concentrations are measured in the laboratory, a serum concentration (clotted and centrifuged blood) is often determined. In reality, the laboratory measurements of most xenobiotics in serum or plasma are nearly equivalent. Frequently, this is not the case for whole-blood determination if the xenobiotic distributes into the erythrocyte, such as lead and most other heavy metals.

Volume of distribution (Vd) is the proportionality term used to relate the dose of the xenobiotic that the individual receives and the resultant plasma concentration. Vd is an apparent or theoretic volume into which a xenobiotic distributes. It is a measure of how much xenobiotic is located inside and outside of the plasma compartment because only the plasma compartment is routinely assayed. In a 70-kg man, the total body water (TBW) is 60% of total body weight, or 42 L, with two-thirds (28 L) of the fluid accounted for by intracellular fluid. Of the 14 L of extracellular fluid, 8 L is considered interstitial or between the cells; 3 L, or 0.04 L/kg, is plasma; and 6 L, or 0.08 L/kg, is blood. If 42 g of a xenobiotic is administered and remains in the plasma compartment (Vd = 0.04 L/kg), the concentration would be 15 g/L. If the distribution of the 42 g of xenobiotic approximated TBW (methanol; 0.6 L/kg), the concentration would be 100 mg/dL. These calculations can be performed by using Equation 8–6, where S equals the percent pure drug if a salt form is used.

$$V_d = \frac{S \times F \times Dose\ (mg)}{C_0} \quad \text{(Eq. 8–6)}$$

Experimental determination of Vd involves administering an IV dose of the xenobiotic and extrapolating the plasma concentration time curve back to time zero (C_0). If the determination takes place after steady state has been achieved, the volume of distribution is then referred to as the Vdss. For many xenobiotics, the Vd is known and readily available in the literature (Table 8–3). When the Vd and the dose ingested are known, a maximum predicted plasma concentration can be calculated after assuming all of the xenobiotic is absorbed and no elimination occurred. This assumption usually overestimates the plasma concentration. Distribution is complex, and differential affinities for various storage sites, such as plasma proteins, liver, kidney, fat, and bone, in the body determine where a xenobiotic ultimately resides.

For the purposes of determining the utility of extracorporeal removal of a xenobiotic, a low Vd is often considered to be less than 1 L/kg. For some xenobiotics, such as digoxin (Vd = 7 L/kg) and the cyclic antidepressants (Vd = 10–15 L/kg), the Vd is much larger than the actual volume of the body. A large Vd indicates that the xenobiotic resides outside of the plasma compartment, but again, it does not describe the site of distribution.

The site of accumulation of a xenobiotic may or may not be a site of action or toxicity. If the site of accumulation is not a site of toxicity, then the storage depot may be relatively inactive, and the accumulation at that site may be theoretically protective to the animal or person.[58] Selective accumulation of xenobiotics occurs in certain areas of the body because of affinity for certain tissue-binding proteins. For example, the kidney contains metallothionein, which has a high affinity for metals such as cadmium, lead, and mercury.[23] The retina contains the pigment melanin, which binds and accumulates chlorpromazine, thioridazine, and chloroquine.[23] Other examples of xenobiotics accumulating at primary sites of toxicity are carbon monoxide binding to hemoglobin and myoglobin and paraquat distributing to type II alveolar cells in the lungs.[55] Dichlorodiphenyltrichloroethane (DDT), chlordane, and polychlorinated biphenyls are stored in fat, which can be mobilized after starvation.[77] Lead sequestered in bone[33] is not immediately toxic, but mobilization of bone through an increase in osteoclastic activity[58] (hyperparathyroidism, possibly pregnancy) may free lead for distribution to sites of toxicity in the central nervous system (CNS) or blood.

Several plasma proteins bind xenobiotics and act as carriers and storage depots. The percentage of protein binding varies among xenobiotics, as do their affinities and potential for reversibility. After it is bound to plasma protein, a xenobiotic with high binding affinity will remain largely confined to the plasma until elimination occurs. However, dissociation and reassociation may occur if another carrier is available with a higher binding affinity. Most plasma measurements of xenobiotic concentration reflect total drug (bound plus unbound). Only the unbound drug is free to diffuse through membranes for distribution or for elimination. Albumin binds primarily to weakly acidic, poorly water-soluble xenobiotics, which include salicylates, phenytoin, and warfarin, as well as endogenous substances, including free fatty acids, cortisone, aldosterone, thyroxine, and unconjugated bilirubin.[62] α_1-Acid glycoprotein usually binds basic xenobiotics, including lidocaine, imipramine, and propranolol.[62] Transferrin, a β_1-globulin, transports iron, and ceruloplasmin carries copper.

Phenytoin is an example of a xenobiotic whose effects are significantly influenced by changes in concentration of plasma albumin. Only free phenytoin is active. When albumin concentrations are in the normal range, approximately 90% of phenytoin is bound to albumin. As the albumin concentration decreases, more xenobiotic is free for distribution, and a greater clinical response to the same serum phenytoin concentration is often observed. The free plasma phenytoin concentration can be calculated based on the albumin concentration. This achieves an appropriate interpretation (adjusted) of total phenytoin within the conventional therapeutic range of 10 to 20 mg/L of free plus bound phenytoin (Eq. 8–7).

$$\textit{Adjusted phenytoin concentration} = \frac{\textit{Actual phenytoin concentration}}{(0.25 \times [\textit{albumin}]) + 0.1} \quad \text{(Eq. 8–7)}$$

The clinical implications are that a malnourished patient with an albumin of 2 g/dL receiving phenytoin can manifest toxicity with a plasma phenytoin concentration of 14 mg/L. This measurement is total phenytoin (bound + unbound). Because the patient has a reduced albumin concentration, this actually represents a substantially higher proportion and absolute amount of active unbound phenytoin. Substitution into the above equation of 14 mg/L for actual plasma phenytoin concentration and 2 g/dL for albumin gives an adjusted plasma phenytoin concentration of 23.33 mg/L (therapeutic range, 10–20 mg/L).

Although drug interactions are often attributed to the displacement of xenobiotics from plasma protein binding, concurrent metabolic interactions are usually more consequential. Displacement transiently increases the amount of unbound, active drug. This may result in an immediate increase in drug effect. This is followed by enhanced distribution and elimination of unbound drug. Gradually, the unbound plasma concentration returns to predisplacement concentrations.[59]

Saturation of plasma proteins may occur in the therapeutic range for a drug such as valproic acid. Acute saturation of plasma protein binding after an overdose often leads to consequential adverse effects. Saturation of plasma protein binding with salicylates and iron after

TABLE 8–3. Pharmacokinetic Characteristics of Xenobiotics Associated with the Largest Number of Toxicologic Deaths

	Vd (L/kg)	Protein Binding (%)	Renal Elimination (% Unchanged)	Hepatic Metabolism (CYP)	Active Metabolite	Enterohepatic
Analgesics						
Acetaminophen	0.8–1.0	5–20	2	95% 5–10% (2E1)	*N*-acetyl-*p*-benzoquinoneimine	27%–42% excreted in bile
Aspirin	0.15–0.20	50–80 (salicylic acid) saturable	10 (pH dependent)	Majority	Salicylic acid	None
Methadone	3.59	71–87	5–10	Majority (3A4, 2D6)	None?	Yes
Morphine	3–4	35	<10	*n*-Demethylation	15% Morphine 6-glucuronide, 55% morphine 3-glucuronide	Yes
Propoxyphene	12–26	80	<10	>90% (3A4, 2D6)	Norpropoxyphene	Yes?
Antidepressants						
Amitriptyline	8.3 ± 2	96	5	Yes (2C9)	Nortriptyline (2D6)	Yes
Bupropion	18.6	84	0	Yes (2B6)	Hydroxybupropion	No
Citalopram	12	80	0	Yes (3A4, 2C19)	Desmethylcitalopram	Yes
Desipramine	33–42	92	0.3–2.6	Yes (2D6)	None	Yes
Doxepin	20 ± 8	–	0	Yes	Desmethyldoxepin	Yes
Imipramine	15 ± 6	85	0–1.7	Yes (2D6)	Desipramine	Yes
Lithium	0.79	None	89–98	None	None	None
Cardiovascular Drugs						
Digoxin	5.1–7.4	20–25	50–80		Minor amount	Yes
Diltiazem	5.3	70–80	1–3	90% (3A)	Yes, many	No
Nifedipine	0.8–1.4	9–98	?	98% (3A4)	No	No
Propranolol	3.6	93	<0.5	>95% (2C19, 2D6)	No	No
Verapamil	4.7	83–92	3–4%	97% (3A4, 1A2, 2C9)	Norverapamil	No
Stimulants and Drugs of Abuse						
Amphetamine	6.11 (in drug dependent) 3.5–4.6 (in naive)	16	45 (pH dependent)	50%	*p*-Hydroxynorephedrine 0.3%; *p*-hydroxyamphetamine 2%–4%	No
Cocaine	1.96–2.7	8.7	9.5–20 (pH dependent)	5–10%	Norcocaine; (?) others	No
Heroin	25	40	Minor	Yes	Acetylmorphine morphine	No
Methamphetamine	3.2–3.7	pH dependent			Amphetamine 4%–7%; *p*-hydroxymethamphetamine 15%	No
Sedative–Hypnotics						
Alprazolam	1–2	80	100%	None	None	No
Chloral hydrate	0.75	70–80	Minor	Alcohol dehydrogenase	Trichloroethanol	No
Phenobarbital	0.88	40–50	20–50 (pH dependent)	Yes (2C9, 2C19)	None	No
Quetiapine	10	83	0	Yes (3A4)	None	Yes
Alcohols						
Ethanol	0.5–0.6	None	Very little	95% Alcohol dehydrogenase	Acetaldehyde	No
Ethylene glycol	0.6–0.8	None	20	Alcohol dehydrogenase	Oxalic acid	No
Methanol	0.6–0.7	None	3–5	95% alcohol dehydrogenase	Formic acid	No
Miscellaneous						
Cyanide	0.4	60	0		Thiocyanate	None
Theophylline	0.5	50–60	7	90% (1A2, 2 E1 >3A4)	1,3-Dimethyluric acid; caffeine (in neonates)	
Organic Phosphorus Compounds						
Malathion	NA	None		Metabolized by microsomal enzymes	Malaoxon	No
Chlorpyrifos	NA	None		Yes	3,5,6-Trichloro-2 pyridonol	No
Rodenticides						
Brodifacoum	0.985 (rats)	None		Yes		Yes
Strychnine	13	None	10–20 in 24 hr	Yes		No

overdose increase distribution to the CNS (salicylates) or to the liver, heart, and other tissues (iron), increasing toxicity.

Specific therapeutic maneuvers in the overdose setting are designed to alter xenobiotic distribution by inactivating or enhancing elimination to limit toxicity. These therapeutic maneuvers include manipulation of serum or urine pH (salicylates), the use of chelators (lead), and the use of antibodies or antibody fragments (digoxin).

The Vd permits predictions about plasma concentrations and assists in defining whether an extracorporeal method of removal is beneficial for a particular toxin. If the Vd is large (>1 L/ kg), it is unlikely that hemodialysis, hemoperfusion, or exchange transfusion would be effective because most of the xenobiotic is outside of the plasma compartment. Plasma protein binding also influences this decision. If the xenobiotic is more tightly bound to plasma proteins than to activated charcoal, then hemoperfusion is unlikely to be beneficial even if the Vd of the xenobiotic is small. In addition, high plasma protein binding limits the effectiveness of hemodialysis because only unbound xenobiotic will freely cross the dialysis membrane. Exchange transfusion can be effective for a xenobiotic with a small Vd and substantial plasma protein binding because both bound and free xenobiotic are removed simultaneously.

ELIMINATION

Removal of a parent compound from the body (*elimination*) begins as soon as the xenobiotic is delivered to clearance organs such as the liver, kidneys, and lungs. Elimination begins immediately but may not be the predominant kinetic process until absorption and distribution are substantially completed. As expected, the functional integrity of the major organ systems, such as cardiovascular, pulmonary, renal, and hepatic systems, are major determinants of the efficiency of xenobiotic removal and of therapeutically administered antidotes. The xenobiotics themselves (eg, acetaminophen) may cause renal or hepatic failure, subsequently compromising their own elimination. Other factors that influence elimination include age (enzyme maturation), competition or inhibition of elimination processes by interacting xenobiotics, saturation of enzymatic processes, gender, genetics, obesity, and the physicochemical properties of the xenobiotic.[46]

Elimination can be accomplished by biotransformation to one or more metabolites or by *excretion* from the body of unchanged xenobiotic. Excretion may occur via the kidneys, lungs, GI tract, and body secretions (sweat, tears, milk).Because of their water solubility, hydrophilic (polar) or charged xenobiotics and their metabolites are generally excreted via the kidney. The majority of xenobiotic metabolism occurs in the liver, but it also commonly occurs in the blood, skin, GI tract, placenta, or kidneys. Lipophilic (noncharged or nonpolar) xenobiotics are usually metabolized in the liver to hydrophilic metabolites, which are then excreted by the kidneys.[24,51] These metabolites are generally inactive, but if they are active, may contribute to toxicity. Examples of active metabolites include the metabolism of amitriptyline to nortriptyline, procainamide to *N*-acetylprocainamide, and meperidine to normeperidine.

Metabolic reactions catalyzed by enzymes categorized as either phase I or phase II may result in pharmacologically active metabolites; frequently, the latter have different toxicities than the parent compounds. *Phase I* (asynthetic), or preparative metabolism, which may or may not precede phase II, is responsible for introducing polar groups onto nonpolar xenobiotics by oxidation (hydroxylation, dealkylation, deamination), reduction (alcohol dehydrogenase, azo reduction), and hydrolysis (ester hydrolysis). [22,49] *Phase II*, or synthetic reactions, conjugate the polar group with a glucuronide, sulfate, acetate, methyl or glutathione; or amino acids such as glycine, taurine, and glutamic acid, creating less polar metabolites.[14,22,49]

Comparatively, phase II reactions produce a much larger increase in hydrophilicity than phase I reactions. The enzymes involved in these reactions have low substrate specificity, and those in the liver are usually localized to either the endoplasmic reticulum (microsomes) or the soluble fraction of the cytoplasm (cytosol).[49] The location of the enzymes becomes important if they form reactive metabolites, which then concentrate at the site of metabolism and cause toxicity. For example, acetaminophen causes centrilobular necrosis because the CYP 2E1 enzymes, which form *N*-acetyl-*p*-benzoquinoneimine (NAPQI), the toxic metabolite, are located in their highest concentration in that zone of the liver.

The enzymes that metabolize the largest variety of xenobiotics are heme-containing proteins referred to as *CYP monooxygenase enzymes*.[28,49] This group of enzymes, formerly called the *mixed function oxidase system*, is found in abundance in the microsomal endoplasmic reticulum of the liver. These cytochrome P-450 metabolizing enzymes (CYPs) primarily catalyze the oxidation of xenobiotics. Cytochrome P450 in a reduced state (Fe^{2+}) binds carbon monoxide. Its discovery and initial name resulted from spectral identification of the colored CO-bound cytochrome P450, which absorbs light maximally at 450 nm. The cytochrome P450 system is composed of many enzymes grouped according to their respective gene families and subfamilies, of which approximately 57 of these functional human genes have been sequenced. Members of a gene family have more than 40% similarity of their amino acid sequencing, and subfamilies have more than 55% similarity. For example, the *CYP2D6*1a* gene encodes wild-type protein (enzyme) CYP2D6, where 2 represents the family, D the subfamily and 6 the individual gene, and *1a the mutant allele; *CYP2D6.1* represents the most common or wild-type allele.

Toxicity may result from induction or inhibition of CYP enzymes by another xenobiotic, resulting in a consequential drug interaction (Chap. 12) Many of these interactions are predictable based on the known xenobiotic affinities and their capability to induce or inhibit the P450 system.[12,42,49,50,66] However, *polymorphism* (individual genetic expression of enzymes),[1] stereoisomer variability[75](enantiomers with different potencies and isoenzyme affinities), and the capability to metabolize a xenobiotic by alternate pathways contribute to unexpected metabolic outcomes. The pharmaceutical industry is now exploiting the concept of chiral switching (marketing a single enantiomer instead of the racemic mixture) to alter efficacy or side effect profiles. Enantiomers are named either according to the direction in which they rotate polarized light (*l* or – for levorotatory, and *d* or + for dextrorotatory) or according to the absolute spatial orientation of the groups at the chiral center (S or R). *Chiral* means "hand" in Greek, and the latter designations refer to either sinister (left-handed) or rectus (right-handed). There is no direct correlation between levorotatory or dextrorotatory and S and R.[70]

The liver reduces the oral bioavailability of xenobiotics with high extraction ratios. The bioavailabilities of xenobiotics with high extraction ratios are greatly affected by enzyme induction and enzyme inhibition; the reverse is true for xenobiotics with a low extraction ratio. After the xenobiotic is in the blood, the hepatic elimination is affected by blood flow to the liver, the intrinsic hepatic metabolism, and plasma protein binding. If the hepatic metabolism of a xenobiotic is very high, then the only limit to hepatic clearance is blood flow to the liver, and protein binding is not an issue. However, if the intrinsic hepatic metabolism for a xenobiotic is low, then blood flow to the liver is not a consequential factor. Plasma protein binding becomes important because only unbound xenobiotics can be cleared by the liver. Because enzyme inhibition and induction greatly affect intrinsic hepatic metabolism, these factors are also important.

Excretion is primarily accomplished by the kidneys, with biliary, pulmonary, and body fluid secretions contributing to lesser degrees. Urinary excretion occurs through glomerular filtration, tubular secretion, and passive tubular reabsorption. The glomerulus filters unbound xenobiotics of a particular size and shape in a manner that is not saturable (but is subject to renal blood flow and perfusion). Passive tubular reabsorption accounts for the reabsorption of noncharged, lipid-soluble xenobiotics and is therefore influenced by the pH of the urine and the pKa of the xenobiotic. The principles of diffusion discussed earlier permit, for example, the ion trapping of salicylate (pKa = 3.5) in the urine through urinary alkalinization. Tubular secretion is an active process carried out by drug transporters (OATs, OCTs) and subject to saturation and drug interactions (Table 8–4).

Obesity is the accumulation of fat far in excess of that which is considered normal for a person's age and gender. The National Institutes of Health defines obesity as a body mass index (BMI) greater than 30. The BMI is calculated by dividing a person's weight in kilograms by the individual's height in meters squared (m^2). By this criterion, about one-third of the adult US population is obese. Obesity poses problems in determining the correct loading dose and maintenance dose for therapeutic xenobiotics and for the estimation of serum concentrations and elimination times in the overdose setting.[10,26,39,48] A number of formulas have been proposed to classify body size in addition to BMI, but none have been tested adequately in the obese population. Obese patients have not only an increase in adipose tissue but also an increase in lean body mass of 20% to 55% which results in the alteration of the distribution of both lipophilic and hydrophilic xenobiotics. In general, the absorption of xenobiotics in obese patients does not appear to be affected, but distribution is affected. The effect of obesity on hepatic metabolism necessitates additional study, although some studies suggest a nonlinear increase in clearance. Glomerular filtration rate increases in obesity. For example, although aminoglycosides are hydrophilic, because of an increase in fat free mass in obese patients, a dosing weight correction of 40% is used to calculate both the loading dose and the maintenance dose (Dosing body weight = 0.4 × [Actual body weight − Ideal body weight] + Ideal body weight). Preliminary studies with propofol, a very lipophilic drug, suggest that induction and maintenance doses correlate better with actual body weight. These equations are found in Table 8–5. One recent hypothesis suggests using LBW2005 to simplify the calculation of maintenance doses.[26]

TABLE 8–4. Xenobiotics Secreted by Renal Tubules

Organic Anion Transport (OAT)	Organic Cation Transport (OCT)
Acetazolamide	Acetylcholine
Bile salts	Amiodarone
Cephalosporins	Atropine
Indomethacin	Cimetidine
Hydrochlorothiazide	Digoxin
Furosemide	Diltiazem
Methotrexate	Dopamine
Penicillin G	Epinephrine
Probenecid	Morphine
Prostaglandins	Neostigmine
Salicylate	Procainamide
	Quinidine
	Quinine
	Triamterene
	Trimethoprim
	Verapamil

TABLE 8–5. Equations for Determining Body Size

$$\text{BMI} = \frac{\text{Weight (kg)}}{\text{Height (m}^2\text{)}}$$

$$\text{BSA (m}^2\text{)} = \frac{\sqrt{\text{Height (cm)} \times \text{Weight (kg)}}}{\sqrt{3600}}$$

IBW: Males (kg) = 50 + 2.3 (Height > 60 inches)

IBW: Females (kg) = 45.5 + 2.3 (Height > 60 inches)

$$\text{LBW2005: Males (kg)} = \frac{9270 \times \text{Weight (kg)}}{6680 + [(216 \times \text{BMI (kg/m}^2\text{)}]}$$

$$\text{LBW2005: Females (kg)} = \frac{9270 \times \text{Weight (kg)}}{8780 + [(244 \times \text{BMI (kg/m}^2\text{)}]}$$

BMI, body mass index; BSA, body surface area; IBW, ideal body weight; LBW, lean body weight.

CLASSICAL VERSUS PHYSIOLOGIC COMPARTMENT TOXICOKINETICS

Models exist to study and describe the movement of xenobiotics in the body with mathematical equations. Traditional *compartmental* models (one or two compartments) are data based and assume that changes in plasma concentrations represent tissue concentrations (Fig. 8–6).[47] Advances in computer technology facilitate the use of the classic concepts developed in the late 1930s.[69] Physiologic models consider the movement of xenobiotics based on known or theorized biologic processes and are unique for each xenobiotic. This allows the prediction of tissue concentrations while incorporating the effects of changing physiologic parameters and affording better extrapolation from laboratory animals.[79] Unfortunately, physiologic modeling is still in its infancy, and the mathematical modeling it entails is often very complex.[19] Regardless, the most commonly used mathematical equations are based on traditional compartmental modeling.

The *one-compartment model* is the simplest approach for analytic purposes and is applied to xenobiotics that rapidly enter and distribute throughout the body. This model assumes that changes in plasma concentrations will result in and reflect proportional changes in tissue concentrations. Many xenobiotics, such as digoxin, lithium, and lidocaine, do not instantaneously equilibrate with the tissues and are better described by a two-compartment model. In the *two-compartment model*, a xenobiotic is distributed instantaneously to highly perfused tissues (central compartment) and then is secondarily, and more slowly, distributed to a peripheral compartment. Elimination is assumed to take place from the central compartment.

Model 1. One-compartment open model, IV injection.

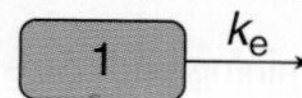

Model 2. One-compartment open model with first-order absorption.

k_a 1 k_e

Model 3. Two-compartment open model, IV injection.

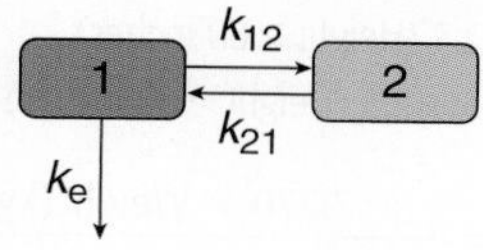

Model 4. Two-compartment open model with first-order absorption.

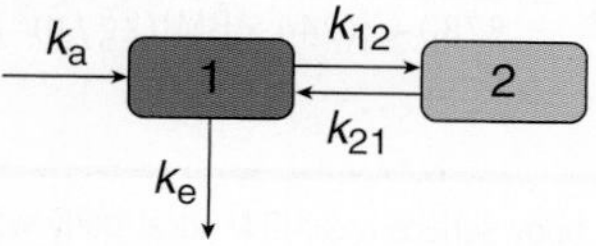

FIGURE 8–6. Various classical compartmental models. k_e = pharmacokinetic rate constants; 1 = plasma or central compartment; 2 = tissue compartment; k_{12} = rate constant into tissue from plasma; k_{21} = rate constant into plasma from tissue; k_a = absorption rate constant.

If the rate of a reaction is directly proportional to the concentration of xenobiotic, it is termed *first order or linear*. Processes that are capacity limited or saturable are termed *nonlinear* (not proportional to the concentration of xenobiotic) and are described by the *Michaelis-Menten* equation, which is derived from enzyme kinetics. Calculus is used to derive the first-order equation, as done by Yang and Andersen.[79] Rate is directly proportional to concentration of xenobiotic, as in Equation 8–8.

$$Rate\ \alpha\ concentration(C) \qquad \text{(Eq. 8–8)}$$

An infinitesimal change in concentration of a xenobiotic (dC) with respect to an infinitesimal change in time (dt) is directly proportional to the concentration (C) of the xenobiotic as in Equation 8–9:

$$\frac{dC}{dt} \propto C \qquad \text{(Eq. 8–9)}$$

The proportionality constant k_e is added to the right side of the expression to mathematically allow the introduction of an equals sign. The constant k_e represents all of the bodily factors, such as metabolism and excretion, that contribute to the determination of concentration (Eq. 8–10).

$$\frac{dC}{dt} = kC \qquad \text{(Eq. 8–10)}$$

Introducing a negative sign to the left-hand side of the equation describes the "decay" or decreasing xenobiotic concentration (Eq. 8–11).

$$-\frac{dC}{dt} = kC \qquad \text{(Eq. 8–11)}$$

This equation is impractical because of the difficulty of measuring infinitesimal changes in C or t. Therefore, the use of calculus allows the integration or summing of all of the changes from one concentration to another beginning at time zero and terminating at time *t*. This relationship is mathematically represented by the integration sign (∫).∫ means to integrate the term from concentration at time zero (C_0) to concentration at a given time *t* (C_t). ∫means the same with respect to time, where t_0 = zero. Prior to this application, the previous equation is first rearranged (Eq. 8–12).

$$-\frac{dC}{C} = kdt$$
$$\int_{C_0}^{C_t} -\frac{dC}{C} = k\int_{t_0}^{t} dt \qquad \text{(Eq. 8–12)}$$

The integration of dC divided by C is the natural logarithm of C (ln C) and the integration of dt is *t* (Eq. 8–13).

$$-In\,C\Big|_{C_0}^{C_t} = kt\Big|_{t_0}^{t}. \qquad \text{(Eq. 8–13)}$$

The vertical straight lines proscribe the evaluation of the terms between those two limits. The following series of manipulations are then performed (Eq. 8–14A–D).

$$-(InC_t - InC_0) = k(t-0) \qquad \text{(Eq. 8–14A)}$$

$$-InC_t + InC_0 = kt \qquad \text{(Eq. 8–14B)}$$

$$-InC_t = -InC_0 + kt \qquad \text{(Eq. 8–14C)}$$

$InC_t =$	$InC_0 -$	kt	
Can be measured	Constant	*Can be selected*	(Eq. 8–14D)

Equation 8–14D can be recognized as taking the form of an equation of a straight line (Eq. 8–15), where the slope is equal to the rate constant k_e and the intercept is C_0.

$$y = b + mx \qquad \text{(Eq. 8–15)}$$

Instead of working with natural logarithms, an exponential form (the antilog) of Equation 8–14D may be used (Eq. 8–16).

$$C_t = C_0 e^{-kt} \qquad \text{(Eq. 8–16)}$$

Graphing the ln (natural logarithm) of the concentration of the xenobiotic at various times for a first-order reaction is a straight line. Equation 8–16 describes the events when only one first-order process occurs. This is appropriate for a one-compartment model (Fig. 8–7).

In this model, regardless of the concentration of the xenobiotic, the rate (percentage) of decline is constant. The absolute amount of xenobiotic eliminated changes continuously while the percent eliminated remains constant. k_e is reported in h^{-1}. A k_e of 0.10 h^{-1} means that the xenobiotic is being processed (eliminated) at a rate of 10% per hour. k_e is often designated as k_e and referred to as the elimination rate constant. The time necessary for the xenobiotic concentration to be reduced by 50% is called the *half-life*. The half-life is determined by

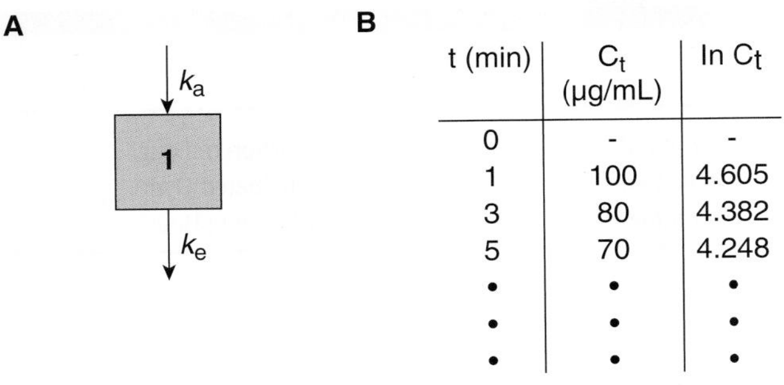

t (min)	C_t (μg/mL)	ln C_t
0	-	-
1	100	4.605
3	80	4.382
5	70	4.248
•	•	•
•	•	•
•	•	•

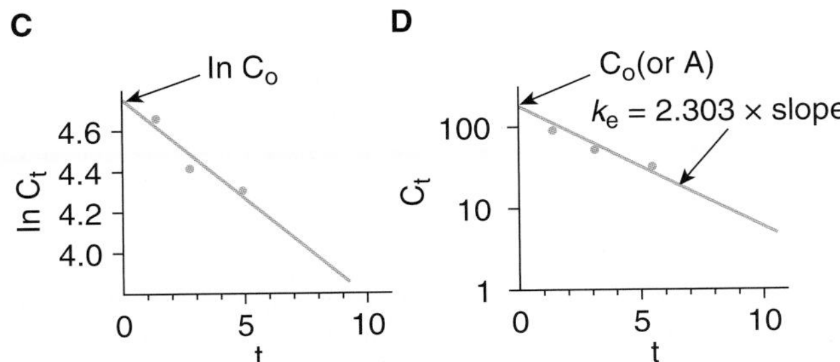

FIGURE 8–7. A one-compartment pharmacokinetic model demonstrating (**A**) graphical illustration, (**B**) hypothetical dataset, (**C**) linear plot, and (**D**) semilogarithmic plot.

a rearrangement of Equation 8–14D whereby C_2 becomes C at time t_2 and C_1 becomes C at t_1 and by rearrangement giving Equation 8–17:

$$(t_1 - t_2) = \frac{(InC_1 - InC_2)}{k_e} \qquad \text{(Eq. 8–17)}$$

Substitution of 2 for C_1 and 1 for C_2 or 100 for C_1 and 50 for C_2 gives Equations 8–18A and 8–18B:

$$t_{1/2} = \frac{(In2 - In1)}{k_e} \qquad \text{(Eq. 8–18A)}$$

$$t_{1/2} = \frac{0.693}{k_e} \qquad \text{(Eq. 8–18B)}$$

The use of semilog paper facilitates graphing the first-order equation. However, because semilog paper plots log (not ln) versus time, to retain appropriate mathematical relationships the rate constant or slope (k) must be divided by 2.303 (see Fig. 8–7).

The mathematical modeling becomes more complex when more than one first-order process contributes to the overall elimination process. The equation that incorporates two first-order rates is used for a two-compartment model and is Equation 8–19.

$$C_t = Ae^{-\alpha t} + Be^{-\beta t} \qquad \text{(Eq. 8–19)}$$

Figure 8–8 demonstrates a two-compartment model where α often represents the distribution phase and β is the elimination phase.

The rate of reaction of a saturable process is not linear (ie, not proportional to the concentration of xenobiotic) when saturation occurs (Fig. 8–9). This model is best described by the Michaelis-Menten

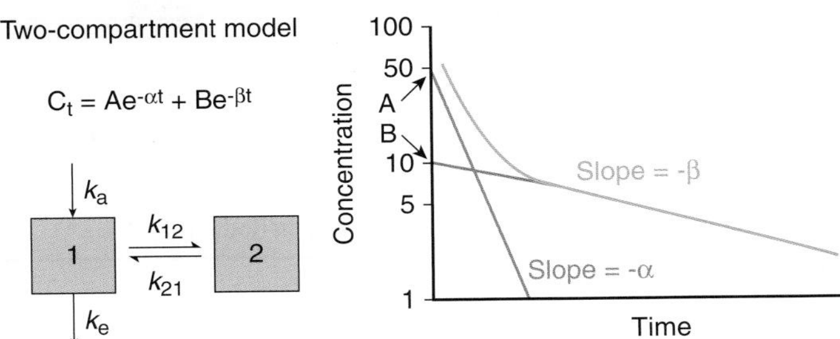

FIGURE 8–8. Mathematical and graphical forms of a two-compartment classical pharmacokinetic model. k_a represents the absorption rate constant, k_e represents the elimination rate constant, α represents the distribution phase, and β represents the elimination phase.

equation used in enzyme kinetics (Eq. 8–20) in which v is the velocity or rate of the enzymatic reaction; C is the concentration of the xenobiotic; V_{max} is the maximum velocity of the reaction between the enzyme and the xenobiotic; and K_m is the affinity constant between the enzyme and the xenobiotic.[79]

$$v = \frac{V_{max} \times C}{K_m + C} \qquad \text{(Eq. 8–20)}$$

Application of this equation to toxicokinetics requires v to become the infinitesimal change in concentration of a xenobiotic (dC) with respect to an infinitesimal change in time (dt) as previously discussed (see Eq. 8–10). V_{max} and K_m both reflect the influences of diverse biologic processes. The Michaelis-Menten equation then becomes Equation 8–21, in which the negative sign again represents decay:

$$\frac{dC}{dt} = \frac{V_{max} \times C}{K_m + C} \qquad \text{(Eq. 8–21)}$$

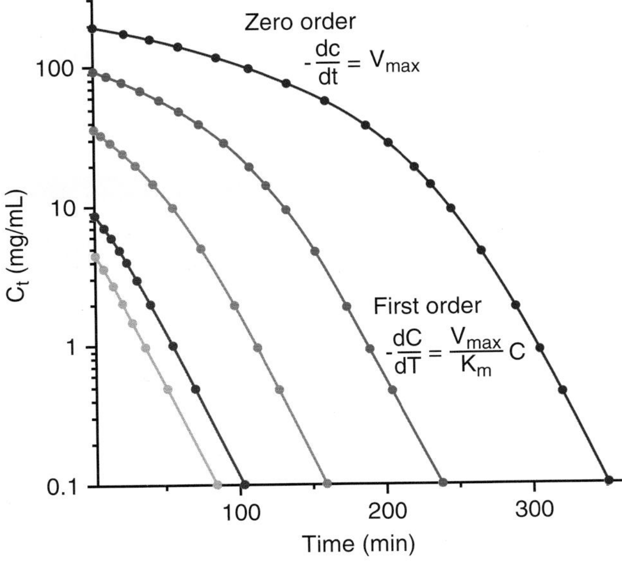

FIGURE 8–9. Concentration versus time curve for a xenobiotic showing nonlinear pharmacokinetics where concentrations below 10 mg/mL represent first-order elimination.

TABLE 8–6A. Illustration of 1000 mg of Xenobiotic in Body After First-Order Elimination

Time After Drug Administration (hour)	Amount of Drug in Body (mg)	Amount of Drug Eliminated Over Preceding Hour (mg)	Fraction of Drug Eliminated Over Preceding Hour
0	1000	–	–
1	850	150	0.15
2	723	127	0.15
3	614	109	0.15
4	522	92	0.15
5	444	78	0.15
6	377	67	0.15

When the concentration of the xenobiotic is very low ($C \lll K_m$), it can be dropped from the bottom right of the equation because its contribution becomes negligible and the resultant equation is described as a first-order process (Eq. 8–22A and 8–22B). Conceptually, this is understandable because at a very low xenobiotic concentration, the process is not saturated.

$$-\frac{dC}{dt} = \frac{V_{max} \times C}{K_m} \qquad \text{(Eq. 8–22A)}$$

Because V_{max} divided by K_m is a constant, K, then:

$$-\frac{dC}{dt} = kC \qquad \text{(Eq. 8–22B)}$$

However, when the concentrations of the xenobiotic are extremely high and exceed the capacity of the system ($C \ggg K_m$), the rate becomes fixed at a constant maximal rate regardless of the exact concentration of the xenobiotic, termed a *zero-order reaction.* Tables 8–6A and 8–6B compare a first-order reaction with a zero-order reaction. In this particular example, zero order is faster, but if the fraction of xenobiotic eliminated in the first-order example were 0.4, then the amount of xenobiotic in the body would decrease below 100 before the xenobiotic in the zero-order example. It is inappropriate to perform half-life calculations on a xenobiotic displaying zero-order behavior because the metabolic rates are continuously changing. After an overdose, enzyme saturation is a common occurrence because the capacity of enzyme systems is overwhelmed.

CLEARANCE

Clearance (Cl) is the relationship between the rate of transfer or elimination of a xenobiotic from a reference fluid (usually plasma) to the plasma concentration of the xenobiotic and is expressed in units of volume per unit time mL/min (Eq. 8–23).[25,47,61]

$$Cl = \frac{\text{Rate of elimination}}{Cp} \qquad \text{(Eq. 8–23)}$$

The determination of creatinine clearance is a well-known example of the concept of clearance. Creatinine clearance (Cl_{CR}) is determined by Equation 8–24:

$$Cl_{creatinine} = \frac{U \times V}{Cp} \qquad \text{(Eq. 8–24)}$$

TABLE 8–6B. Illustration of 1000 mg of Xenobiotic in Body After Zero-Order Elimination

Time After Drug Administration (hour)	Amount of Drug in Body (mg)	Amount of Drug Eliminated Over Preceding Hour (mg)	Fraction of Drug Eliminated Over Preceding Hour
0	1000	–	–
1	850	150	0.15
2	700	150	0.18
3	550	150	0.21
4	400	150	0.27
5	250	150	0.38
6	100	150	0.60

in which U is the concentration of creatinine in urine (mg/mL); V is the volume flow of urine (mL/min); Cp is the plasma concentration of creatinine (mg/mL); and the units for clearance are millimeters per minute. A creatinine clearance of 100 mL/min means that 100 mL of plasma is completely cleared of creatinine every minute. Clearance for a particular eliminating organ or for extracorporeal elimination is calculated with Equation 8–25:

$$Cl = Q_b \times (ER) = Q_b \times \frac{(C_{in} - C_{out})}{C_{in}} \quad \text{(Eq. 8–25)}$$

Cl = clearance for the eliminating organ or extracorporeal device
Q_b = blood flow to the organ or device
ER = extraction ratio
C_{in} = *xenobiotic concentration in fluid (blood or serum) entering the organ or device*
C_{out} = *xenobiotic concentration in fluid (blood or serum) leaving the organ or device*

Clearance can be applied to any elimination process independent of the precise mechanisms (ie, first-order, Michaelis-Menten) and represents the sum total of all of the rate constants for xenobiotic elimination. Total body clearance ($Cl_{total\ body}$) is the sum of the clearances of all of the individual eliminating processes, as seen in Equation 8–26:

$$Cl_{total\ body} = Cl_{renal} + Cl_{hepatic} + Cl_{intestinal} + Cl_{chelation} + \cdots \quad \text{(Eq. 8–26)}$$

For a first-order process (one-compartment model), clearance is given by Equation 8–27:

$$Cl = k_e Vd \quad \text{(Eq. 8–27)}$$

Experimentally, the clearance can be derived by examining the IV dose of xenobiotic in relation to the AUC from time zero to time t (Eq. 8–28). The AUC is calculated using the trapezoidal rule or through integral calculus (units, eg, mg/mL) (Figs. 8–10 and 8–11).

$$Cl = \frac{dose_{IV}}{AUC_{0-t}} \quad \text{(Eq. 8–28)}$$

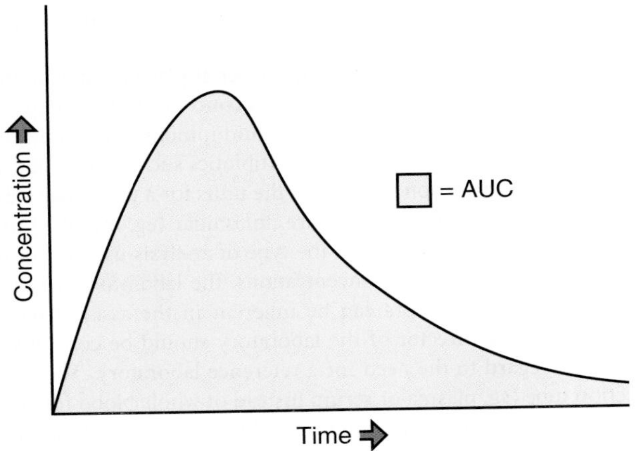

FIGURE 8–10. The AUC profile obtained after extravascular administration of a xenobiotic.

Compartment model

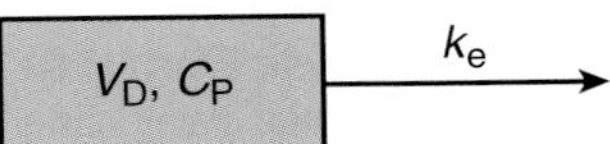

Static volume and first-order elimination is assumed. Plasma flow is not considered. $Cl_T = k_e V_D$.

Physiologic model

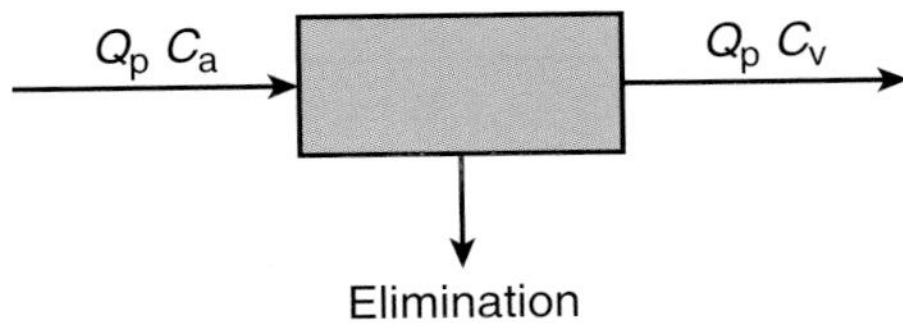

Clearance is the product of the plasma flow (Q_p) and the extraction ratio (ER). Thus, $Cl_T = Q_p$ ER.

Model independent

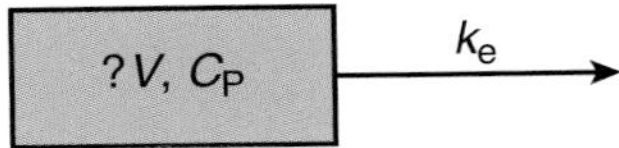

Volume and elimination rate constant not defined. $Cl_T = \text{Dose} \div [\text{AUC}]_0^\infty$.

FIGURE 8–11. General approaches to clearance.

STEADY STATE

When exposure to a xenobiotic occurs at a fixed rate, the plasma concentration of the xenobiotic gradually achieves a plateau level at a concentration at which the rate of absorption equals the rate of elimination and is termed *steady state*. The time to achieve 95% of steady-state concentration for a first-order process is dependent on the half-life and usually necessitates 5 half-lives. The concentration achieved at steady state depends on the Vd, the rate of exposure, and the half-life.

Iatrogenic toxicity may occur in the therapeutic setting when dosing decisions are based on plasma concentrations determined before achieving a steady state. This adverse event is particularly common when using xenobiotics with long half-lives such as digoxin[78] and phenytoin.

PEAK PLASMA CONCENTRATIONS

Peak plasma concentrations (C_{max}) of a xenobiotic occur at the time of peak absorption. At this point in time, the absorption rate is at least equal to the elimination rate. Thereafter, the elimination rate predominates, and plasma concentrations begin to decline. Whereas the C_{max} depends on the dose, the *rate of absorption* (k_a), and *the rate of elimination* (k_e), the *time to peak* (t_{max}) is independent of dose and only depends on the k_a and k_e. For the same dose of xenobiotic, if the k_e remains constant and the rate of absorption decreases, then the t_{max} (see Table 8–7) will occur later and the C_{max} will be slightly lower. Controlled-release dosage forms and xenobiotics that form concretions and have a decreased rate of absorption may not achieve peak concentrations until many hours after an immediate-release preparation with rapid absorption. The AUC will remain the same. However if the k_a remains constant and the k_e is increased, then the tmax occurs sooner, the C_{max} decreases, and the AUC decreases (Table 8–7).[52]

Values are based on a single oral dose (100 mg) that is 100% bioavailable (F = 1) and has an apparent Vd of 10 L. The drug follows a

TABLE 8–7. Pharmacokinetic Effects of the Absorption Rate Constant and Elimination Rate Constant[a]

Absorption Rate Constant k_a (h^{-1})	Elimination Rate Constant k_e (h^{-1})	t_{max} (h)	C_{max} (µg/mL)	AUC (µg·hr/mL)
0.1	0.2	6.93	2.50	50
0.2	0.1	6.93	5.00	100
0.3	0.1	5.49	5.77	100
0.4	0.1	4.62	6.26	100
0.5	0.1	4.02	6.69	100
0.6	0.1	3.58	6.69	100
0.3	0.1	5.49	5.77	100
0.3	0.2	4.05	4.44	50
0.3	0.3	3.33	3.68	33.3
0.3	0.4	2.88	3.16	25
0.3	0.5	2.55	2.79	20

AUC, area under the (plasma drug concentration versus time) curve; C_{max}, peak xenobiotic concentration; t_{max}, time to peak plasma concentration; Reprinted with permission from Shargel L, Yu A: Pharmacokinetics of drug absorption. In: *Applied Biopharmaceutics and Pharmacokinetics*, 3rd ed. Norwalk, CT: Appleton & Lange; 1993:183.

one-compartment open model. The AUC is calculated by the trapezoidal rule from 0 to 24 hours.

In the overdose setting, gastric emptying, single-dose activated charcoal, and WBI decrease k_a. Multiple-dose activated charcoal, manipulation of pH to promote ion trapping to facilitate elimination, and certain chelators (ie, succimer, deferoxamine) increase k_e and are likely to decrease C_{max}, t_{max}, and AUC.

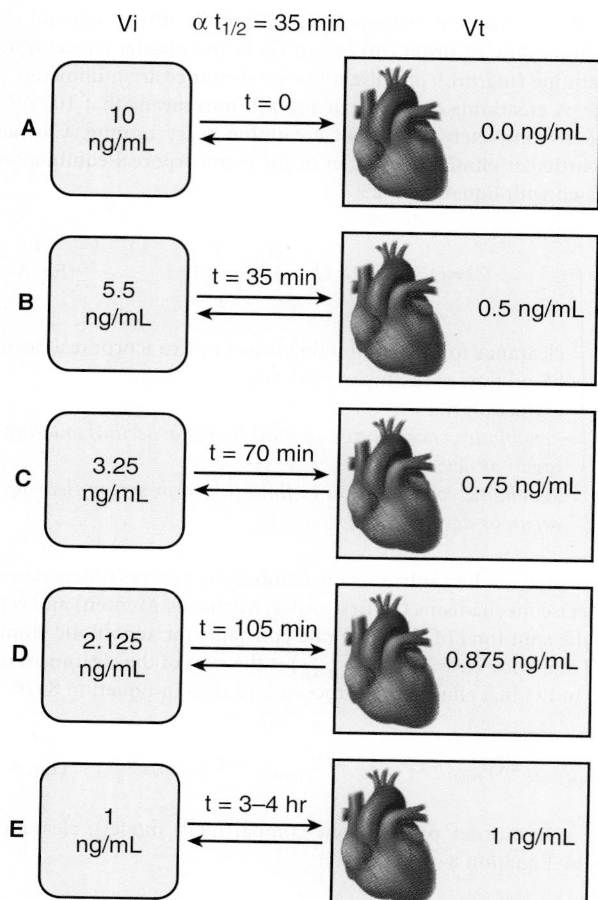

FIGURE 8–12. A theoretical two-compartment model for digoxin. Assume A-E represents the digoxin serum concentration equilibrium at different t (time) intervals between the plasma compartment and the tissue compartment. Vi (initial volume of distribution) is smaller than Vt (tissue volume of distribution). The myocardium sits in Vt. E represents distribution at 5 half lives and it is assumed that the plasma and tissue compartments are now in equilibrium.[78] (Boro MS, Winter ME: Digoxin. In: ME Winter, ed. *Basic Clinical Pharmacokinetics,* 5th ed. Baltimore, MD: Lippincott Williams & Wilkins, 2009:198-239, page 202.)

INTERPRETATION OF PLASMA CONCENTRATIONS

For plasma concentrations to have significance, there must be an established relationship between effect and plasma concentration. Many medications, such as phenytoin, digoxin, carbamazepine, and theophylline, have an established therapeutic range. However, there are also many drugs (eg, diazepam, propranolol, verapamil) for which there is no established therapeutic range. Some xenobiotics (eg, physostigmine) exhibit *hysteresis* in which the effect increases as the plasma concentration decreases. For many xenobiotics, very little information on toxicodynamics is available. Sequential plasma concentrations often are collected for retrospective analysis in an attempt to correlate plasma concentrations and toxicity. Tolerance to drugs, such as ethanol, also influences the interpretation of plasma concentrations. *Tolerance* is an example of a pharmacodynamic or toxicodynamic effect as a result of cellular adaptation, and it occurs when larger doses of a xenobiotic are necessary to achieve the same clinical or pharmacologic result.

Other factors that influence the interpretation of plasma concentrations include chronicity of dosing (a single dose versus multiple doses); whether absorption is still ongoing and therefore concentrations are still increasing; whether distribution is still ongoing and therefore concentrations are uninterpretable (Fig. 8–12); or whether the value is a peak, trough, or steady-state concentration. Clinical examples in which interpretation is dependent on the dosing pattern of a single dose versus multiple doses include theophylline, digoxin, lithium, and acetaminophen. Controlled-release preparations and xenobiotics that delay gastric emptying or form concretions are expected to have prolonged absorptive phases and require serial plasma concentrations to obtain a meaningful analysis of plasma concentrations (Chap. 6). A combination of trough, peak, and minimum inhibitory concentrations is often consequential for monitoring antibiotics such as gentamicin.[8,43]

Pitfalls in interpretation arise when the units for a particular plasma concentration are not obtained or are unfamiliar (eg, mmol/L) to the clinician. In the overdose setting, the type of analysis used is not generally applied to such large concentrations, the laboratory may make errors in dilution, or errors can be inherent in the assay (Chap. 6). In these cases, the director of the laboratory should be consulted for advice with regard to the need for a reference laboratory. The type of collection tube (eg, plasma or serum instead of whole blood for certain metals), or receptacle, or the conditions during delivery of the sample may give rise to inaccurate or inadequate information. When in doubt, the laboratory should be called before sample collection. The laboratory usually measures total xenobiotic (free plus bound), and for agents that are highly plasma protein bound, reductions in albumin increase free concentrations and alter the interpretation of the reported value (see Eq. 8–7). Active metabolites may contribute to toxicity and may not be measured.[37] Collection of accurate data for analysis requires at least 4 data points during 1 elimination half-life. During extracorporeal methods of elimination, ideal criteria for determining the amount removed require assay of the dialysate or charcoal cartridge or multiple simultaneous serum concentrations going into and out of the device rather than random serum concentrations. Clearance calculations for drugs such as lithium that partition significantly into the red cells are more accurate when measurements are taken on whole blood.[13,20] The patient's weight and height and, when indicated, hemoglobin, creatinine, albumin, and other parameters to assess elimination pathways, may be helpful.

REFERENCES

1. Bertilsson L: Geographical/interracial differences in polymorphic drug oxidation. *Clin Pharmacokinet.* 1995;29:192-209.
2. Blaschke TF, Rubin PC: Hepatic first-pass metabolism in liver disease. *Clin Pharmacokinet.* 1979;4:423-432.
3. Bodenham A, Shelly MP, Park GR: The altered pharmacokinetics and pharmacodynamics of drugs commonly used in critically ill patients. *Clin Pharmacokinet.* 1988;14:347-373.
4. Bosse GM, Matyunas NJ: Delayed toxidromes. *J Emerg Med.* 1999;17:679-690.
5. Boyes RN, Scott DB, Jebson PJ, et al: Pharmacokinetics of lidocaine in man. *Clin Pharmacol Ther.* 1971;12:105-116.
6. Brubacher J, Dahghani P, McKnight D: Delayed toxicity following ingestion of enteric-coated divalproex sodium. *J Emerg Med.* 1999;3:463-467.
7. Buckley N, Dawson A, Reith D: Controlled-release drugs in overdose. *Drug Saf.* 1995;12:73-84.
8. Burgess D: Pharmacodynamic principles of antimicrobial therapy in the prevention of resistance. *Chest.* 1999;115:19S-23S.
9. Calcagno A, Kim I, Wu C, et al: ABC drug transporters as molecular targets for the prevention of multidrug resistance and drug-drug interactions. *Curr Drug Deliv.* 2007;4:324-333.
10. Casati A, Putzu M: Anesthesia in the obese patient: pharmacokinetic considerations. *J Clin Anesth.* 2005;17:134-145.
11. Chaikin P, Adir J: Unusual absorption profile of phenytoin in a massive overdose case. *J Clin Pharmacol.* 1987;27:70-73.
12. Ciummo PE, Katz NL: Interactions and drug metabolizing enzymes. *Am Pharm.* 1995;9:41-51.
13. Clendenin N, Pond S, Kaysen G, et al: Potential pitfalls in the evaluation of the usefulness of hemodialysis for the removal of lithium. *J Toxicol Clin Toxicol.* 1982;19:341-352.
14. Dauterman WC: Metabolism of toxicants: phase II reactions. In: Hodgson E, Levi P, eds. *Introduction to Biochemical Toxicology.* Norwalk, CT: Appleton & Lange; 1994:113-132.
15. Dean B, Oehme FW, Krenzelok E: A study of iron complexation in a swine model. *Vet Hum Toxicol.* 1988;30:313-315.
16. de Boer AG, van der Sandt IC, Gaillard PJ: The role of drug transporters at the blood–brain barrier. *Annu Rev Pharmacol Toxicol.* 2003;43:629-656.
17. DeGeorge JJ: Food and drug administration viewpoints on toxicokinetics: the view from review. *Toxicol Pathol.* 1995;23:220-225.
18. Endres CJ, Hsiao P, Chung FS, et al: The role of transporters in drug interactions. *Eur J Pharm Sci.* 2006;27:501-517.
19. Engasser JM, Sarhan F, Falcoz C, et al: Distribution, metabolism and elimination of phenobarbital in rats: Physiologically based pharmacokinetic model. *J Pharm Sci.* 1981;70:1233-1238.
20. Ferron G, Debray M, Buneaux F, et al: Pharmacokinetics of lithium in plasma and red blood cells in acute and chronic intoxicated patients. *Int J Clin Pharmacol Ther.* 1995;33:351-355.
21. Fromm MF: Importance of P-glycoprotein at blood–tissue barriers. *Trends Pharmacol Sci.* 2004;25:423-429.
22. Gillette JR: Factors affecting drug metabolism. *Ann N Y Acad Sci.* 1971;179:43-66.
23. Gram TE: Drug absorption and distribution. In: Craig CR, Stitzel RE, eds. *Modern Pharmacology with Clinical Applications.* Boston: Little, Brown; 1997:13.
24. Guengerich FP, Liebler DC: Enzymatic activation of chemicals to toxic metabolites. *Crit Rev Toxicol.* 1985;14:259-307.
25. Gwilt PR: Pharmacokinetics. In: Craig CR, Stitzel RE, eds. *Modern Pharmacology with Clinical Applications.* Boston: Little, Brown; 1997:49-58.
26. Han PY, Duffull SB, Kirkpatrick CMJ, et al: Dosing in obesity: a simple solution to a big problem. *Clin Pharmacol Ther.* 2007;82:505-508.
27. Hill HZ, Backer R, Hill GJ: Blood cyanide levels in mice after administration of amygdalin. *Biopharm Drug Dispos.* 1980;1:211-220.
28. Hodgson E, Levi PE: Metabolism of toxicants phase I reactions. In: Hodgson E, Levi P, eds. *Introduction to Biochemical Toxicology.* Norwalk, CT: Appleton & Lange; 1994:75-111.
29. Iberti T, Patterson B, Fisher C: Prolonged bromide intoxication resulting from a gastric bezoar. *Arch Intern Med.* 1984;144:402-403.
30. Jenis EH, Payne RJ, Goldbaum LR: Acute meprobamate poisoning: a fatal case following a lucid interval. *JAMA.* 1969;207:361-365.
31. Kapoor SC, Wielopolski L, Graziano JH, LoIacono NJ: Influence of 2,3-dimercaptosuccinic acid on gastrointestinal lead absorption and whole-body lead retention. *Toxicol Appl Pharmacol.* 1989;97:525-529.
32. Kivisto KT, Niemi M, Fromm MF: Functional interaction of intestinal CYP3A4 and P-glycoprotein. *Fundam Clin Pharmacol.* 2004;8:621-626.
33. Klaassen CD, Shoeman DW: Biliary excretion of lead in rats, rabbits and dogs. *Toxicol Appl Pharmacol.* 1974;29:436-446.
34. Klaassen CD, Watkins JB: Mechanisms of bile formation, hepatic uptake, and biliary excretion. *Pharmacol Rev.* 1984;36:1-67.
35. Klotz U: Pathophysiological and disease-induced changes in drug distribution volume: pharmacokinetic implications. *Clin Pharmacokinet.* 1976;1:204-218.
36. Koch-Weser J: Bioavailability of drugs. Part I. *N Engl J Med.* 1974;291:233-237.
37. Koch-Weser J: Bioavailability of drugs. Part II. *N Engl J Med.* 1974;291:503-506.
38. Kwan KC: Oral bioavailability and first-pass effects. *Drug Metab Dispos.* 1997;25:1329-1336.
39. Lee J, Winstead P, Cook A: Pharmacokinetic changes in obesity. *Orthopedics.* 2006;29:984-988.
40. Lemmer B, Bruguerolle B: Chronopharmacokinetics, are they clinically relevant? *Clin Pharmacokinet.* 1994;26:419-427.
41. Levine WG: Biliary excretion of drugs and other xenobiotics. *Ann Rev Pharmacol.* Toxicol 1978;18:81-96.
42. Levy R, Thummel K, Trager W, et al, eds. *Metabolic Drug Interactions.* Philadelphia: Lippincott Williams & Wilkins; 2000.
43. Li R, Zhu M, Shentag J: Achieving optimal outcome in the treatment of infections. *Clin Pharmacokinet.* 1999;37:1-16.
44. Lin JH, Yamazaki M: Role of P-glycoprotein in pharmacokinetics: Clinical implications. *Clin Pharmacokinet.* 2003;42:59-98.
45. Marik P, Varon J: The obese patient in the ICU. *Chest.* 1998;113:492-498.
46. McCarthy J, Gram TE: Drug metabolism and disposition in pediatric and gerontological stages of life. In: Craig CR, Stitzel RE, eds. *Modern Pharmacology with Clinical Applications.* Boston: Little, Brown; 1997:43-48.
47. Medinsky MA, Klaassen CD: Toxicokinetics. In: Klaassen CD, ed. *Casarett & Doull's Toxicology: The Basic Science of Poisons*, 5th ed. New York, McGraw-Hill; 1996:187-198.
48. Pai MP, Bearden DT: Antimicrobial dosing considerations in obese adult patients. *Pharmacotherapy.* 2007;27:1081-1091.
49. Parkinson A: Biotransformation of xenobiotics. In: Klaassen C, ed. *Casarett & Doull's Toxicology: The Basic Science of Poisons*, 5th ed. New York: McGraw-Hill; 1996:113-186.
50. *Pharmacist's Letter.* Stockton, CA: Pharmacy Information Services, University of the Pacific, June 1985.
51. Pirmohamed M, Kitteringham NR, Park BK: The role of active metabolites in drug toxicity. *Drug Saf.* 1994;11:114-144.
52. Plaa OL: The enterohepatic circulation. In: Gillette JR, Mitchell JR, eds. *Handbook of Experimental Pharmacology.* New York: Springer; 1975:28, 130-140, 480.
53. Pond SM, Tozer TN: First-pass elimination: basic concepts and clinical consequences. *Pharmacokinetics.* 1984;9:1-25.
54. Riviere JE: Absorption and distribution. In: Hodgson E, Levi P, eds. *Introduction to Biochemical Toxicology.* Norwalk, CT: Appleton & Lange; 1994:11-48.
55. Rose MS, Lock EA, Smith LL, Wyatt I: Paraquat accumulation: tissue and species specificity. *Biochem Pharmacol.* 1976;25:419-423.
56. Rosenberg J, Benowitz NL, Pond S: Pharmacokinetics of drug overdose. *Clin Pharmacokinet.* 1981;6:161-192.
57. Rowland M, Tozer TN: *Clinical Pharmacokinetics Concepts & Applications*, 2nd ed. Philadelphia, Lea & Febiger; 1989.

58. Rozman KK, Klaassen CD: Absorption, distribution and excretion of toxicants. In: Klaassen CD, ed. *Casarett & Doull's Toxicology: The Basic Science of Poisons*. New York: McGraw-Hill; 1996:91-112.
59. Sansom LN, Evans AM: What is the true clinical significance of plasma protein binding displacement interactions? *Drug Saf.* 1995;12:227-233.
60. Schwartz MD, Morgan BW: Massive verapamil pharmacobezoar resulting in esophageal perforation. *Int J Med Toxicol.* 2004;7:4.
61. Shargel L, Wu-Pong S, Yu A: Drug elimination and clearance. In: *Applied Biopharmaceutics and Pharmacokinetics*, 5th ed. New York: McGraw-Hill; 2005:131-160.
62. Shargel L, Wu-Pong S, Yu A: Physiologic drug distribution and protein binding. In: *Applied Biopharmaceutics and Pharmacokinetics*, 5th ed. New York: McGraw-Hill; 2005:251-301.
63. Shargel L, Wu-Pong S, Yu A: Pharmacokinetics of oral absorption. In: *Applied Biopharmaceutics and Pharmacokinetics*, 5th ed. New York: McGraw-Hill; 2005:pp. 161-184.
64. Shargel L, Wu-Pong S, Yu A: Physiologic factors related to drug absorption. In: *Applied Biopharmaceutics and Pharmacokinetics*, 5th ed. New York: McGraw-Hill; 2005:371-408.
65. Silverman J: P-Glycoprotein. In: Levy R, Thummel K, Trager W, et al, eds. *Metabolic Drug Interactions*. Philadelphia: Lippincott Williams & Wilkins; 2000:135-144.
66. Slaughter RL, Edwards DJ: Recent advances: the cytochrome P450 enzymes. *Ann Pharmacother.* 1995;29:619-623.
67. Stowe CM, Plaa GL: Extrarenal excretion of drugs and chemicals. *Annu Rev Pharmacol.* 1968;8:337-356.
68. Sue Y, Shannon M: Pharmacokinetics of drugs in overdose. *Clin Pharmacokinet.* 1992;23:93-105.
69. Teorell T. Kinetics of distribution of substances administered to the body: I. The extravascular modes of administration. *Arch Intern Pharmacodyn* 1937;57:205–225.
70. Tucker G: Chiral switches. *Lancet.* 2000;355:1085-1087.
71. Verebey K, Gold MS: From coca leaves to crack: the effect of dose and routes of administration in abuse liability. *Psychiatr Ann.* 1988;18:513-520.
72. Vesell ES: The model drug approach in clinical pharmacology. *Clin Pharmacol Ther.* 1991;50:239-248.
73. von Richter O, Burk O, Fromm MF, et al: Cytochrome P450 3A4 and P-glycoprotein expression in human small intestinal enterocytes and hepatocytes: a comparative analysis in paired tissue specimens. *Clin Pharmacol Ther.* 2004;75:172-183.
74. Wagner B, O'Hara D: Pharmacokinetics and pharmacodynamics of sedatives and analgesics in the treatment of agitated critically ill patients. *Clin Pharmacokinet.* 1997;33:426-453.
75. Welling PG: Differences between pharmacokinetics and toxicokinetics. *Toxicol Pathol.* 1995;23:143-147.
76. Wilkinson GR: Influence of hepatic disease on pharmacokinetics. In: Evans WE, Schentag J, Justo W, eds. *Applied Pharmacokinetics: Principles of Therapeutic Drug Monitoring*. Spokane, WA: Applied Therapeutics; 1986:116-138.
77. Wilkinson GR: Plasma and tissue binding considerations in drug disposition. *Drug Metab Rev.* 1983;14:427-465.
78. Winter ME: Digoxin. In: Koda-Kimble MA, Young LY, eds. *Basic Clinical Pharmacokinetics*, 3rd ed. Vancouver, WA: Applied Therapeutics; 1994:198-235.
79. Yang R, Andersen M: Pharmacokinetics. In: Hodgson E, Levi P, eds. *Introduction to Biochemical Toxicology*. Norwalk, CT: Appleton & Lange; 1994:49-73.

CHAPTER 9
PRINCIPLES AND TECHNIQUES APPLIED TO ENHANCE ELIMINATION

David S. Goldfarb

Enhancing the elimination of a xenobiotic from a poisoned patient is a logical step after techniques to inhibit absorption such as orogastric lavage, activated charcoal, or whole-bowel irrigation have been considered. Table 9–1 lists methods that might be used to enhance elimination. Some of these techniques are described in more detail in chapters that deal with specific xenobiotics. In this chapter, hemodialysis, hemoperfusion, and hemofiltration are considered *extracorporeal therapies* because xenobiotic removal occurs in a blood circuit outside the body. Currently these methods are used infrequently as intensive supportive care because most poisonings are not amenable to removal by these methods. Because these elimination techniques have associated adverse effects and complications, they are indicated in only a relatively small proportion of patients.

EPIDEMIOLOGY

Although undoubtedly an underestimate of true use, enhancement of elimination was used relatively infrequently in a cohort of more than 2.4 million patients reported by the American Association of Poison Control Centers (AAPCC) National Poison Data System (NPDS) in 2007 (Chap. 135)[31]. Alkalinization of the urine was reportedly used 9430 times, MDAC 3114 times, hemodialysis 2106 times, hemoperfusion 16 times, and "other extracorporeal procedures" (most likely continuous venovenous hemofiltration [CVVH]) 24 times. As in the past, there continue to be many instances of the use of extracorporeal therapies that are considered inappropriate, such as in the treatment of overdoses of cyclic antidepressants (CAs) or acetaminophen.[31]

Although data reporting remains important in comparing the most recent data with past reports (Table 9–2), there is a continued increase in the reported use of hemodialysis, paralleling a decline in reports of charcoal hemoperfusion (Chap. 135). Lithium and ethylene glycol were the most common xenobiotics for which hemodialysis was used between 1985 and 2005.

Possible reasons for the decline in use of charcoal hemoperfusion are described in the Charcoal Hemoperfusion section below. Various resins and other sorbents once used for hemoperfusion are not currently available in the United States. Peritoneal dialysis (PD), a slower modality that should have little or no role in any poisonings, is no longer separately reported (Chap. 135). "Other extracorporeal procedures" in the AAPCC reports are probably continuous modalities (discussed below in the section Continuous Hemofiltration and Hemodiafiltration) and may include some cases in which PD was used.

Very few prospective, randomized, controlled clinical trials have been conducted to determine which groups of patients actually benefit from enhanced elimination of various xenobiotics and which modalities are most efficacious. For most poisonings, it is unlikely that such studies will ever be performed, given the relative scarcity of appropriate cases of sufficient severity and because of the many variables that would hinder controlled comparisons. Thus, limited evidence predominates. We must therefore rely on an understanding of the principles of these methods to identify the individual patients for whom enhanced elimination is indicated. Isolated case reports in which the kinetics are studied before, during, and after enhanced elimination are also very useful in establishing the efficacy of a method.

GENERAL INDICATIONS FOR ENHANCED ELIMINATION

Enhanced elimination may be indicated for several types of patients:

- *Patients who fail to respond adequately to full supportive care.* Such patients may have intractable hypotension, heart failure, seizures, metabolic acidosis, or dysrhythmias. Hemodialysis or hemoperfusion are much better tolerated than in the past and may represent potentially life-saving opportunities for patients with life-threatening toxicity caused by theophylline, lithium, salicylates, or toxic alcohols.
- *Patients in whom the normal route of elimination of the xenobiotic is impaired.* Such patients may have renal or hepatic dysfunction, either preexisting or caused by the overdose. For example, a patient with chronic renal insufficiency associated with long-term lithium use is more likely to develop lithium toxicity and then require hemodialysis as therapy.
- *Patients in whom the amount of xenobiotic absorbed or its high concentration in serum indicates that serious morbidity or mortality is likely.* Such patients may not appear acutely ill on initial evaluation. Xenobiotics in this group may include ethylene glycol, lithium, methanol, paraquat, salicylate, and theophylline.
- *Patients with concurrent disease or in an age group (very young or old) associated with increased risk of morbidity or mortality from the overdose.* Such patients are intolerant of prolonged coma, immobility, and hemodynamic instability. An example is a patient with both severe underlying respiratory disease and chronic salicylate poisoning.
- *Patients with concomitant electrolyte disorders that could be corrected with hemodialysis.* An example is the lactic acidosis associated with metformin toxicity discussed in the Hemodialysis section of this chapter.

Ideally, these techniques will be applied to poisonings for which studies suggest an improvement in outcome in treated patients compared with patients not treated with extracorporeal removal. As previously mentioned, these data are rarely available.[25]

The need for extracorporeal elimination is less clear for patients who are poisoned with xenobiotics that are known to be removed by the various modalities of treatment but that cause limited morbidity if supportive care is provided. Relatively high rates of endogenous clearance would also make extracorporeal elimination redundant. Examples of such xenobiotics include ethanol and barbiturates. Both are subject to substantial rates of hepatic metabolism, and neither would be expected to lead to significant morbidity after the affected patient has been endotracheally intubated and is mechanically ventilated. There may be instances of severe toxicity from these two xenobiotics for which enhanced elimination will reduce the length of intensive care unit (ICU) stays and the associated nosocomial risks; extracorporeal elimination may then be a reasonable option.[8,50] Dialysis should be avoided if other more effective modalities are available. For example, patients with acetaminophen overdoses should be treated with *N*-acetylcysteine instead of with hemodialysis.

TABLE 9–1. Potential Methods of Enhancing Elimination of Xenobiotics

Cerebrospinal fluid drainage and replacement
Chelation
Cholestyramine
Colestipol
Continuous hemo(dia)filtration
Diuresis
Exchange transfusion
Hemodialysis
Sodium polystyrene sulfonate (Kayexalate)
Manipulation of urinary pH
Multiple-dose activated charcoal
Nasogastric suction
Peritoneal dialysis
Plasmapheresis
Sorbent hemoperfusion (charcoal, others)
Xenobiotic-specific antibody fragments
Whole-bowel irrigation

CHARACTERISTICS OF XENOBIOTICS APPROPRIATE FOR EXTRACORPOREAL THERAPY

The appropriateness of any modality for increasing the elimination of a given xenobiotic depends on various properties of the molecules in question. Effective removal by the extracorporeal procedures and other methods listed in Table 9–1 is limited by a large volume of distribution (Vd). The Vd relates the concentration of the xenobiotic in the blood or serum to the total body burden. The Vd can be envisioned as the apparent volume in which a known total dose of drug is distributed before metabolism and excretion occur:

$$\text{Vd (L/kg)} \times \text{patient weight (kg)} = \text{Dose (mg)/Concentration (mg/L)}$$

The larger the Vd, the less the xenobiotic is available to the blood compartment for elimination. A xenobiotic with a relatively small Vd, considered amenable to extracorporeal elimination, would distribute in an apparent volume not much larger than total body water (TBW). TBW is approximately 60% of total body weight, so a Vd equal to TBW is approximately 0.6 L/kg body weight.

Ethanol is an example of a xenobiotic with a small Vd approximately equal to TBW. A substantial fraction of a dose of ethanol could be removed by hemodialysis. In contrast, an insignificant fraction of digoxin with a large Vd (5–12 L/kg of body weight) would be removed by this therapy. Lipid-soluble xenobiotics and those that are highly protein bound have large volumes of distribution, which can exceed TBW or even total body weight. These high apparent volumes of distribution imply that the xenobiotic is not available to extracorporeal removal because only a small portion would be in the blood and therefore the extracorporeal circuit. In addition to the alcohols, other xenobiotics with a relatively low Vd include phenobarbital, lithium, salicylates, bromide and fluoride ions, and theophylline. Conversely, those with a high Vd (≥1 L/kg of body weight), which would not be removed substantially by hemodialysis, include many β-adrenergic antagonists (with the possible exception of atenolol[59]), diazepam, organic phosphorus compounds, phenothiazines, quinidine, and the cyclic antidepressants.

Pharmacokinetics also influence the ability to enhance elimination of a xenobiotic. Kinetic parameters after an overdose may differ from those after therapeutic or experimental doses. For instance, carrier- or enzyme-mediated elimination processes may be overwhelmed by higher concentrations of the xenobiotic in question, making extracorporeal removal potentially more useful. Similarly, plasma protein- and tissue-binding sites may all be saturated at higher concentrations, making extracorporeal removal feasible in instances in which it would have no role in less significant overdoses. An example is valproic acid, which may be poorly dialyzed at nontoxic concentrations because of high rates of protein binding (although dialysis is rarely indicated). However, higher, potentially toxic concentrations saturate protein-binding sites and lead to a higher proportion of the drug free in the serum, amenable to removal by hemodialysis at a clinically relevant rate.[35] Estimates of the expected endogenous rates of elimination of a xenobiotic in the setting of an overdose should be made, wherever possible, from knowledge of the toxicokinetic characteristics derived from obtained in relevant models of toxicity, not after therapeutic doses.

When assessing the efficacy of any technique of enhanced elimination, a generally accepted principle is that the intervention is worthwhile only if the total body clearance of the xenobiotic is increased by at least 30%.[17] This substantial increase is easier to achieve when the xenobiotic has a low endogenous clearance. Examples of xenobiotics with low endogenous clearances (<4 mL/min/kg) include the toxic alcohols (particularly when their metabolism is blocked), atenolol, sotalol, lithium, paraquat, phenytoin, salicylate, and theophylline. Xenobiotics with high endogenous clearances include many β-adrenergic antagonists, lidocaine, opioids, nicotine, and CAs. Enhancement of elimination is expected to contribute more to overall clearance of the former group than to the latter.

The efficacy of any technique of elimination can be directly assessed by comparing the blood or serum concentrations of the xenobiotic at the beginning and the end of the procedure.[69] For example, a xenobiotic such as theophylline, with one-compartment kinetics, is essentially limited to the extracellular space. The difference between the theophylline concentration before the procedure, minus the concentration at the end of the procedure, divided by the concentration at the beginning, is the fraction of the body burden of the xenobiotic that is eliminated. This calculation would not be appropriate to estimate the effect of treatment on the total body burden of a xenobiotic that distributes in a larger Vd because the changes in blood concentration may not reflect the effect of the treatment on the total amount in other compartments.

TABLE 9–2. Changes in Use of Extracorporeal Therapies[a]

	1986	1990	2001	2004	2007
Hemodialysis	297	584	1280	1726	2106
Charcoal hemoperfusion	99	111	45	20	16
Resin	23	37			
Peritoneal dialysis	62	27			
Other extracorporeal: CVVH, CVVHD, etc			26	33	24

[a] Data derived from American Association of Poison Control Centers annual reports (Chap. 135).

Certain xenobiotics, such as lithium, distribute in part to the intracellular compartment, and equilibrium is established between the intracellular and extracellular compartments. The latter compartment includes the blood from which xenobiotic elimination occurs. An increase in the elimination rate from the extracellular compartment, such as by hemodialysis, alters this equilibrium. The rate of redistribution of the xenobiotic from the intracellular compartment into the now-dialyzed extracellular compartment may be slower than the rate of clearance across the dialysis membrane. In that case, the serum concentration may become relatively low despite a substantial intracellular burden. This low serum concentration reduces the concentration gradient for diffusion from serum to dialysate so that dialysance (the dialysis clearance) is reduced. Thus, although serum concentrations may decrease precipitously during the procedure, the total-body burden of the xenobiotic may not be affected significantly if it does not move from cells to the dialyzable extracellular volume. An example is a 60-kg patient who ingests 100 25-mg amitriptyline tablets, a TCA.[25] Assuming that the drug is fully absorbed, the 2500-mg distributes in an apparent volume of 40 L/kg of body weight to achieve a serum concentration of 1000 ng/mL, a potentially toxic concentration. If charcoal hemoperfusion is performed with a blood flow rate of 350 mL/min (plasma flow rate of 200 mL/min, assuming a hematocrit of approximately 43%) and the extraction ratio is 100% (see Charcoal Hemoperfusion below), the clearance of drug is 200 mL/min or 200 μg/min. In 4 hours (240 minutes) of treatment, only 48 mg (48,000 μg), or less than 2% of the amount ingested, will be removed. The treatment would not have affected toxicity.

Further evidence that a xenobiotic is in a slowly equilibrating compartment is provided by monitoring the concentrations after discontinuation of the procedure and demonstrating rebounding (serum). This rebound indicates postdialysis redistribution (Fig. 9–1). The magnitude of the rebound depends on total-body stores of the xenobiotic. A postdialysis increase in blood concentrations may also result from ongoing absorption from the gastrointestinal (GI) tract.

When assessing overall efficacy, the evidence of enhanced elimination must be considered in the context of the clinical response. In some instances, observed improvement is not predicted by the kinetics of the parent xenobiotic and may not result from the intervention. For example, in severe cases of CA poisoning, unexpected improvement during hemoperfusion could be fortuitous because the toxicity is manifested early and ameliorates rapidly during the initial distribution phase.

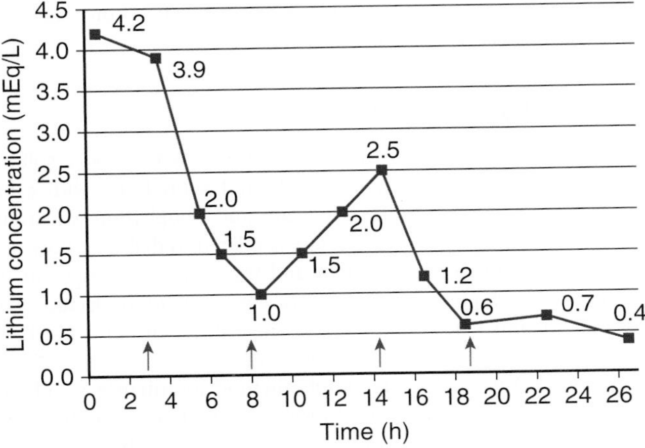

FIGURE 9–1. Repeated serum lithium concentrations after an acute ingestion. *Arrows* indicate beginning (*green arrows*) and end (*red arrows*) of hemodialysis. After a 5-hour hemodialysis treatment, a significant rebound in serum concentration occurred, with recurrence of neurologic impairment. An additional 4-hour hemodialysis treatment was then begun.

Beginning a procedure during the initial distribution phase may increase the fraction of body burden that can be removed. Later, after the xenobiotic has distributed into fat or has been bound by plasma or tissue proteins, administration of extracorporeal treatment may have much lower clearance rates and benefits. Poisonings with paraquat and hepatotoxic mushrooms are other examples in which only early extracorporeal therapy *may* have benefit.[22] An alternative explanation for unanticipated evidence of improvement in some cases is the removal of small amounts of the xenobiotic and active metabolites from a shallow "toxic effect" compartment. This theory has been advanced to explain the response to hemodialysis of patients overdosed with the antipsychotic chlorprothixene[40] or with a combination of diltiazem and metoprolol.[2] Such effects may lead to transient improvements that are not sustained as drug redistributes from one pool to another, leading to early benefit but eventual recurrence of symptoms. Much of the relevant literature fails to provide long-term follow-up to demonstrate prolongation of benefits after extracorporeal therapy is completed and xenobiotics have redistributed.

Other examples also demonstrate that removal of a xenobiotic is a poor surrogate for clinical benefit. Enhanced elimination of phenobarbital[53] or carbamazepine[73] by MDAC did not affect clinical outcomes compared with those of overdosed, untreated control subjects despite a decrease in their serum concentrations. In another study, no difference was observed between patients with lithium poisoning for whom hemodialysis was done and those for whom it was recommended by a poison control center but not done.[9] The conclusion was that hemodialysis should be considered appropriate only for the more severe cases. In acetaminophen toxicity, the efficacy of administration of *N*-acetylcysteine makes extracorporeal removal unnecessary and not part of the recommended treatment strategy.

TECHNIQUES TO ENHANCE REMOVAL OF XENOBIOTICS

Although the efficacy of or need for removal of many xenobiotics remains controversial, consensus regarding the indications for a number of procedures has developed. This consensus has led to consistent application of several techniques of enhanced elimination for some toxic exposures that occur relatively more frequently. The techniques to enhance xenobiotic elimination most commonly applied over the past decade have been alkalinization of the urine for salicylates and hemodialysis for methanol, ethylene glycol, lithium, and salicylates.

FORCED DIURESIS AND MANIPULATION OF URINARY pH

Forced diuresis by volume expansion with isotonic sodium–containing solutions, such as 0.9% NaCl and lactated Ringer solution, may increase renal clearance of some molecules. This therapy would theoretically be most useful for xenobiotics such as lithium for which the glomerular filtration rate (GFR), which is the volume of plasma filtered across the glomerular basement membrane per minute, is an important determinant of excretion. In people with normal extracellular fluid (ECF) volume who have not had loss of sodium via renal, GI, or other routes of excretion, the increase in GFR expected with plasma volume expansion is variable and unpredictable and may not lead to significant increases in xenobiotic elimination. The effect is potentially more important in patients who have had contraction of the ECF volume because of sodium loss. Loss of extracellular volume leads to a reduction of GFR partly as a result of decreased cardiac preload and cardiac output, which, in turn, reduces renal plasma flow. This circumstance is also accompanied by activation of angiotensin II, a small peptide that acts as a pressor and stimulates sodium reabsorption in the proximal tubule. Because small molecules such as lithium are both filtered at the glomerulus and reabsorbed by the proximal tubule, especially when sodium depletion has occurred and angiotensin II has been activated, repletion of ECF volume with isotonic saline will increase GFR and suppress sodium reabsorption. The result is an increase in excretion of low-molecular-weight xenobiotics such as lithium. After the ECF volume is restored, continued infusion of 0.9% NaCl increases urine volume proportionally more than GFR, which may increase excretion of some small molecules such as urea, but which has little efficacy in the case of most poisonings.

The significant risk of this therapy is ECF volume overload, manifested by pulmonary and cerebral edema. This complication may be particularly likely in patients with long-standing lithium use in whom chronic tubulointerstitial disease may lead to renal insufficiency that does not improve with fluid therapy. Other patients with acute kidney injury not mediated by ECF volume depletion are also at risk. Knowing the result of past serum creatinine concentrations may help distinguish acute from chronic renal insufficiency in such cases. Administration of diuretics such as furosemide along with saline may diminish the risk of ECF volume overload but may complicate the therapy, confuse the assessment of ECF volume, and increase the risk of metabolic alkalosis and hypokalemia. The unproven efficacy of forced diuresis in the management of *any* overdose has led most experts to abandon its use. On the other hand, the repletion of ECF volume when it is contracted, as determined by the history and physical examination, is, of course, appropriate.

Many xenobiotics are weak acids or bases that are ionized in aqueous solution to an extent that depends on the pK_a of the compound and the pH of the solution. Knowing these variables, the Henderson-Hasselbalch equation (Chap. 8) may be used to determine the relative proportions of the acids, bases, and buffer pairs. Whereas cell membranes are relatively impermeable to ionized, or polar molecules (eg, an unprotonated salicylate anion), nonionized, nonpolar forms (eg, the protonated, noncharged salicylic acid) may cross more easily. As xenobiotics pass through the kidney, they may be filtered, secreted, and reabsorbed. If the urinary pH is manipulated to favor the formation of the ionized form in the tubular lumen, the xenobiotic is trapped in the tubular fluid and is not passively reabsorbed into the bloodstream. This is referred to as *ion trapping*. Hence, the rate and extent of its elimination can be increased. To make manipulation of urinary pH worthwhile, the renal excretion of the xenobiotic must be a major route of elimination. The 2004 position paper of the American Academy of Clinical Toxicology (AACT) and the European Association of Poisons Centres and Clinical Toxicologists (EAPCCT) emphasizes that, as discussed above for extracorporeal therapies, enhanced removal does not necessarily translate into a clinical benefit with improved outcomes.[55]

Acidification of the urine by systemic administration of HCl or NH_4Cl to enhance elimination of weak bases, such as phencyclidine or the amphetamines, is not useful and is potentially dangerous. The technique has been abandoned because it does not significantly enhance removal of xenobiotics and is complicated by systemic metabolic acidosis.

Alkalinization of the urine to enhance elimination of weak acids has a limited role for xenobiotics such as salicylates,[48] phenobarbital, chlorpropamide, formate, diflunisal, fluoride, methotrexate, and the herbicide 2,4-dichlorophenoxyacetic acid (2,4-D). These weak acids are ionized at alkaline urine pH, and tubular reabsorption is thereby greatly reduced. Alkalinization is achieved by the intravenous (IV) administration of sodium bicarbonate (1 to 2 mEq/kg rapid initial infusion with additional dosing) to increase urinary pH to 7 to 8.

This degree of alkalinization may be difficult, if not impossible, if metabolic acidosis and acidemia are present, as often is the case in patients with salicylate poisoning. In this situation, bicarbonate (administered as the sodium salt) is consumed by titration of plasma protons before it can appear in the urine. On the other hand, salicylate poisoning often causes respiratory alkalosis as well. In that case, when PCO_2 is low, raising serum bicarbonate, equivalent to the induction of metabolic alkalosis, may lead to profound, life-threatening alkalemia. Finally, the risk of ECF volume overload with sodium bicarbonate administration is the same as with the administration of 0.9% NaCl. Hypernatremia may also occur after administration of hypertonic sodium bicarbonate. Bicarbonaturia is also associated with urinary potassium losses, so the patient's serum potassium concentration should be monitored frequently and KCl given liberally as long as GFR is not impaired. A further complication of alkalemia is a decrease of ionized calcium, which becomes bound by albumin as protons are titrated off serum proteins; in this event, tetany may occur.[24] If these complications can be identified and dealt with judiciously and safely, the renal clearance of salicylate may increase fourfold as urine pH increases from 6.5 to 7.5 with alkalinization. Increasing urine pH by decreasing proximal tubular bicarbonate reabsorption via administration of carbonic anhydrase inhibitors such as acetazolamide is not recommended. Although elimination of a xenobiotic may be increased, metabolic acidosis will ensue unless ample sodium bicarbonate is also administered. In the case of salicylates, metabolic acidosis with acidemia may cause increased distribution of drug into the central nervous system. As with $NaHCO_3$ administration, bicarbonaturia is accompanied by urinary potassium losses; hypokalemia may be profound. The role of urinary alkalinization in the management of patients with salicylate poisoning is discussed further in Chapter 35.

Alkalinization is also used to increase the solubility of methotrexate and thereby prevent its precipitation in tubules when patients are given high-dose folinic acid rescue therapy.[15] Precipitation of sulfonamide antibiotics with kidney stones or kidney failure may also be prevented by alkalinization. ECF volume expansion with 0.9% NaCl and $NaHCO_3$ administration also protects the kidneys from the toxic effects of myoglobinuria in patients with extensive rhabdomyolysis. However, because patients with rhabdomyolysis may have acute renal failure, $NaHCO_3$ administration must be used before kidney injury occurs and may lead to ECF volume overload if its administration continues after kidney failure has been established.

PERITONEAL DIALYSIS

Theoretically, PD enhances the elimination of a few water-soluble, low-molecular-weight, poorly protein-bound xenobiotics with a low Vd such as the alcohols, lithium, salicylate, and theophylline. Clearance of xenobiotics in the aqueous dialysate is related to dialysate flow rate, the surface area of the peritoneum, and the molecular weight of the compound. The highest clearances are achieved for molecules with molecular weights below 500 daltons. The efficacy of PD is markedly decreased when the patient has hypotension.

Although PD is a relatively simple method to enhance xenobiotic elimination, it is too slow to be clinically useful. Consequently, PD is never the method of choice unless hemodialysis and hemoperfusion are unavailable and transfer to a center that can offer these techniques is not feasible. Besides exchange transfusion, it may be the only practical option in small children when experience with extracorporeal techniques in younger age groups is lacking or until a child can be transported to an appropriate center.

HEMODIALYSIS

The utility of hemodialysis for the treatment of patients with toxicity caused by lithium, toxic alcohols, salicylates, or theophylline is unquestionable and is not dealt with here in specific detail. Each of these xenobiotics is described in detail in separate chapters that also review in toxicity and indications for extracorporeal therapies. This section describes the hemodialysis procedure in general and its application to some newer situations.

Prompt consultation with a nephrologist is always indicated in the case of any poisoning with a xenobiotic that might benefit from extracorporeal removal. Annual AAPCC data consistently suggest that some salicylate-related deaths, for example, could have been prevented if hemodialysis had been instituted earlier (Chap. 135).[74] To perform hemodialysis, a nephrologist must be available along with a nurse or technician. The dialysis machine requires preparation, and a vascular access catheter has to be inserted into the patient's circulation. A delay of several hours before hemodialysis can be instituted should be anticipated. If indicated, modalities of treatment such as fomepizole or ethanol for poisoning with toxic alcohols should be administered, and other modalities to enhance elimination, such as urinary alkalinization or oral MDAC, should be used when appropriate.

The technical details of performing hemodialysis for treatment of patients with poisonings do not differ markedly from those used in the treatment of patients with acute kidney failure. Vascular access is best attained via the femoral vein. The subclavian and internal jugular veins are also acceptable but have slightly higher rates of complications such as pneumothorax and arterial puncture.[14] Hemostasis after catheter removal is also more easily achieved at the femoral site. Hemodialysis and hemoperfusion (see sections below) are usually performed using a double-lumen catheter manufactured for dialysis that is made of silicon, polyethylene, polyurethane, or Teflon. Blood is pumped through one lumen, passed through the machine, and returned to the venous circulation through the second lumen. Blood flow rates with these catheters can be as high as 450 to 500 mL/min, although 350 mL/min may sometimes be the maximum rate achievable.

The blood lines and artificial kidney (the dialysis membrane) should be primed with an appropriate volume of fluid to reduce or avoid hypotension when the procedure is started. Larger "high-efficiency" or "high-flux" artificial kidneys should be selected. Full anticoagulation with heparin is usually required. A typical adult heparin dose is 4000 to 5000 units as a bolus followed by 400 to 500 units hourly. Alternatively, periodic flushes of the dialysis membrane with heparinized saline expose the patient to very low doses of heparin and little risk of systemic anticoagulation. Regional anticoagulation of the dialysis circuit with citrate or protamine is possible if heparin is absolutely contraindicated, although these agents complicate the procedure. Use of a dialysate that contains citrate may be adequate for anticoagulation and may allow heparin to be avoided.[1]

In poisoned patients, hemodialysis is usually performed for 4 to 8 hours. Assuming that the patient's serum potassium concentration is normal, a standard bicarbonate-based dialysate with a potassium concentration of 3 or 4 mEq/L and a calcium concentration of 3 mEq/L, flowing at 600 to 800 mL/min, is sufficient. If dialysis is performed in a dialysis unit, the dialysate is a mix of a concentrate with $NaHCO_3$ and highly purified water, usually derived by reverse osmosis or deionization. Dialysis procedures done in ICUs should use portable reverse osmosis machines to generate the water for mixing. Although undesirable, tap water can be used if its chlorine content is less than 0.1 ppm.[7]

During conventional hemodialysis, blood flows through hollow fibers, which are semipermeable membranes. The hollow fibers are bathed by a dialysis solution or dialysate. Xenobiotics diffuse across the membrane from blood into the dialysate down their concentration gradients (Fig. 9–2). Table 9–3 lists the characteristics of xenobiotics

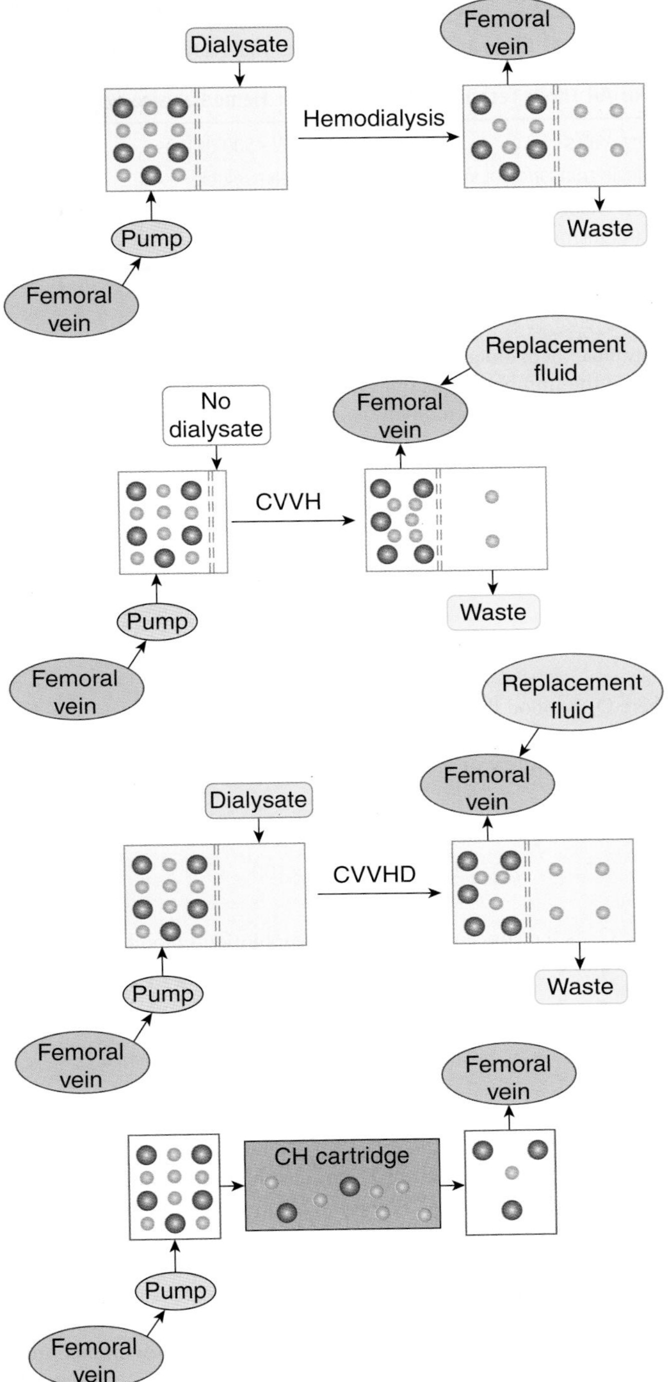

FIGURE 9–2. The comparative schematic layouts of hemodialysis (HD), continuous venovenous hemofiltration (CVVH), continuous venovenous hemofiltration with dialysis (CVHD), and hemoperfusion (HP). *Red circles* are high molecular-weight (MW) xenobiotics, such as methotrexate, whose high MW makes them too large to be removed by HD; *Yellow circles* are low molecular-weight (MW) diffusible solutes such as urea or methanol. In dialysis, solute moves across a semipermeable membrane (*dashed lines*) from a solution in which it is present in a high concentration (blood) to one in which it is at a low concentration (dialysate). In CVVH and CVVHD, plasma moves across a similar membrane in response to hydrostatic pressures; replacement fluid must be provided. The latter also utilizes a dialysate to augment clearance. The availability of blood pumps has made arteriovenous modalities nearly obsolete. Charcoal hemoperfusion (CH) requires movement of blood through a sorbent-containing cartridge and does not include dialysis or hemofiltration.

TABLE 9–3. Characteristics of Xenobiotics That Allow Clearance by Hemodialysis, Hemoperfusion, and Hemofiltration

For All Three Techniques	For Hemodialysis	For Hemoperfusion	For Hemofiltration
Low Vd (<1 L/kg) Single-compartment kinetics Low endogenous clearance (<4 mL/min/kg)	MW <500 daltons Water soluble Not bound to plasma proteins	Adsorption by activated charcoal Binding by plasma proteins does not preclude	MW <10,000 or <40,000 daltons, depending on filter used

MW, molecular weight; Vd, volume of distribution.

that make them amenable to hemodialysis. These requirements greatly reduce the number of xenobiotics that can be expected to be cleared by dialysis. During hemodialysis, clearance of a xenobiotic (Cl_X) can be calculated by:

$$Cl_X = Q_p \times ER$$

where Q_p is the plasma flow rate and ER is the extraction ratio.

$$Q_p = Q_b \times (1 - Hct)$$

where Q_B is blood flow rate and Hct is hematocrit. The extraction ratio (ER) is a measure of the percentage of xenobiotic passing through the artificial kidney or charcoal hemoperfusion cartridge. This can be calculated as:

$$ER = \frac{C_{in} - C_{out}}{C_{in}} \times 100$$

where C_{in} is the concentration of the xenobiotic in blood entering the system and C_{out} is the concentration in blood leaving the system. Then:

$$Cl_X = [Q_p(C_{in} - C_{out})]/C_{in}$$

Several technologic advances now enable patients to tolerate dialysis with better clearances. Although clearance rates reported in the literature of the 1970s and 1980s may significantly underestimate currently achievable clearance rates,[50] these data are still of interest given the relative paucity of more recent reports. Patients undergoing hemodialysis may also experience much less hemodynamic instability than in the past. For instance, the source of base in dialysate is now routinely $NaHCO_3$ rather than sodium acetate; the latter caused hypotension and decreased cardiac output. Computerized machines allow fine control of ultrafiltration rates to limit volume losses; in the past, imprecise calculations and manipulations led to frequent episodes of hypotension. The sodium concentration of the dialysate can be programmed to vary through the course of the procedure, a technique called *sodium modeling*, which may promote hemodynamic stability as well. Better hemodynamic stability and larger dual-lumen catheters allow use of higher blood flows, up to 400 to 500 mL/min. As a result of such innovations, treatment can be delivered in more instances than was previously possible. Hypotension may still occur in critically ill patients. Saline, colloid, vasopressors, or inotropes may also be required in such patients, but if dialysis seems to offer the best chance for the patient's survival, it should usually be attempted.

Dialysis membrane composition has also continually evolved. The hollow-fiber dialyzer, almost universally used today, is composed of thousands of blood-filled capillary tubes held together in a bundle and bathed in the machine-generated dialysate. Older "conventional" dialyzers, much less frequently encountered today, are made of cellulose-derived polymers, most commonly called *cuprophane*. Hemodialysis efficacy for poisonings with low-molecular-weight xenobiotics should improve with the use of larger membranes with larger clearances. The prototypical "middle molecule," the clearance of which is used to express a dialyzer's high-flux dialysance, is β_2-microglobulin (molecular weight, 11,800).

"High-flux," synthetic dialyzers have larger pores that allow more clearance of larger molecules. Because these membranes also have higher water permeability, computerized ultrafiltration control is necessary. These membranes, composed of polysulfone (PS), polyamide, polyacrylonitrile (PAN), and other polymers, have better biocompatibility than older, cellulose-derived membranes. Biocompatibility is measured by the rate of activation or release, after exposure to the membrane, of inflammatory mediators that include white blood cells, platelets, complement, and cytokines. Better biocompatibility means less activation of these potentially damaging mechanisms compared with more bioincompatible membranes.

The influence of biocompatibility on the outcomes of patients receiving long-term hemodialysis for chronic renal failure is still being assessed. Patients with chronic kidney failure are exposed to these membrane materials during at least three treatments a week for many years. It is unlikely that better biocompatibility will affect outcomes for dialysis of poisoned patients who require only one or two treatments.

There are some instances in which high-flux dialyzers might be important in promoting clearance of larger molecules, such as vancomycin, which are not readily removed by conventional low-flux membranes.[26] However, the indications for performing hemodialysis to enhance removal of vancomycin and other xenobiotics with higher molecular weights have not been delineated. Nonetheless, a sound pharmacologic basis for the efficacy of dialysis must still be present; no amount of increased clearance will eliminate a xenobiotic with a large Vd or significant protein or tissue binding.

With that proviso, recent experience suggests a role for high-flux hemodialysis in the clearance of certain xenobiotics that were previously thought to be effectively removed only by charcoal hemoperfusion. The situations in which these modalities are appropriate for these xenobiotics remain exceedingly rare. As valproic acid is increasingly prescribed for neurologic and psychiatric disorders, the incidence of both intentional and unintentional overdoses of this drug will also increase.[68] As discussed previously, valproic acid is largely protein bound at therapeutic serum concentrations. Toxic concentrations saturate protein-binding sites, leading to a higher proportion of unbound drug in the serum and a lower apparent Vd, thereby making the drug more dialyzable. Indeed, several case reports have demonstrated that the clearance of valproic acid with high-flux hemodialysis is at least equivalent to, if not greater than, that of charcoal hemoperfusion.[30,38,39] Although carbamazepine has a low molecular weight and a Vd that would allow for clearance by hemodialysis, its high protein binding and lack of water solubility are expected to impede the efficacy of hemodialysis. Nonetheless, carbamazepine is also effectively cleared with high-flux hemodialysis.[60,70] In a patient who underwent high-flux hemodialysis followed by charcoal hemoperfusion for carbamazepine toxicity, removal rates were similar for the two modalities. Unlike the case for valproic acid, the rationale for these anecdotal reports for enhanced carbamazepine elimination is unclear. Whether the pharmacokinetics of the drug are altered at toxic serum concentrations, as are those of valproic acid, is not known. Because of its potential efficacy and availability and its insignificant effect on cost and adverse events, high-flux hemodialysis should probably replace charcoal hemoperfusion as the treatment modality of choice when extracorporeal elimination of valproic acid or carbamazepine is to be performed. As stated above, however, effective clearance is not necessarily a surrogate for improved outcomes.

In addition to removing xenobiotics, hemodialysis can correct acid–base and electrolyte abnormalities such as metabolic acidosis or alkalosis, hyperkalemia, and ECF volume overload. Consequently, hemodialysis is preferred, if not essential, for poisonings characterized by these disorders, especially when clearance rates resulting from hemoperfusion and hemodialysis are relatively similar. Examples include salicylate poisoning, which is often associated with metabolic acidosis,[33] and propylene glycol toxicity, which is often associated with lactic acidosis, especially in the presence of renal or hepatic impairment.[52]

A more controversial question is the role of dialysis in the treatment of metformin-associated lactic acidosis in patients with diabetes mellitus. If metformin were not primarily responsible for the lactic acidosis, removal of the drug by hemodialysis would then be unlikely to affect the outcome. An inverse relationship exists between serum metformin concentrations and mortality in patients with metformin-associated lactic acidosis.[42] This finding may indicate that many of those patients determined to have metformin-associated lactic acidosis with lower serum metformin concentrations may have another primary cause for lactate production other than metformin. These include sepsis or bowel ischemia, and often these other diagnoses portend worse outcomes. In cases of metformin-associated lactic acidosis in patients with normal renal function, extracorporeal removal is generally not indicated because endogenous clearance of metformin is quite high and prognosis is good without dialysis.[10] Metformin-associated lactic acidosis in the setting of decreased kidney function may constitute an appropriate indication for hemodialysis.

The more important role for hemodialysis is in cases of metformin-associated lactic acidosis involving acute renal failure such as contrast nephropathy without other causes of lactic acidosis in patients with chronic renal failure who are inappropriately treated with metformin, and in patients who overdose on metformin. Here, the small molecular weight and negligible plasma protein binding of metformin may allow for adequate drug removal despite a relatively large Vd. In addition, hemodialysis would correct acidosis via administration of bicarbonate. Clinical improvement with hemodialysis may result as much or more from correction of the acidosis as from removal of the drug.

Complications of acute hemodialysis are relatively rare. Bleeding or thrombosis at the site used for vascular access, usually the femoral vein, is infrequent with normal hemostasis and adequate postprocedure tamponade of the catheter site. Bleeding in the GI tract and elsewhere, caused by systemic anticoagulation with heparin, can be avoided if low doses of heparin are used. Low-dose heparin is an appropriate choice when dialyzing patients for toxic alcohol and salicylate exposures who are at risk for increased intracerebral bleeding. Nosocomial bacteremia may occur if central lines are left in place for prolonged periods; central lines should be removed after 5 days at most. Femoral venous lines should always be removed in patients who are out of bed.

In addition, hemodialysis increases the elimination of some drugs administered therapeutically, such as folic acid and other water-soluble vitamins and xenobiotics. Doses of these drugs should be increased during dialysis or administered immediately afterward. Similarly, the rate of ethanol infusions used in the treatment of patients with toxic alcohol ingestions must be increased. Fomepizole also has a low molecular weight (molecular weight, 82.1 daltons) and a low Vd (0.6–1.0 L/kg), so it can also be dialyzed, but it is not significantly removed by hemofiltration. If necessary, it should be redosed after dialysis (see Antidotes in Depth: Ethanol and Fomepizole). When fomepizole is not available, ethanol removal can be limited in such cases by enriching the dialysate with ethanol to a concentration of 100 mg/dL.[18] Similarly, hypophosphatemia after more prolonged high-flux hemodialysis can be avoided by adding sodium phosphate salts (eg, Fleet Phospho-Soda) to the dialysate or by administering phosphate intravenously. Angiotensin-converting enzyme inhibitors should never be used if dialysis is performed with PAN membranes because the combination is associated with angioedema.[13]

CHARCOAL HEMOPERFUSION

In general, if a xenobiotic is well adsorbed by activated charcoal, charcoal hemoperfusion clearance will exceed that of hemodialysis. During hemoperfusion, blood is pumped through a cartridge containing a very large surface area of sorbent, either activated charcoal or carbon (see Fig. 9–2). The sorbent is coated with a very thin layer of polymer membrane such as cellulose acetate (Adsorba: Gambro, Lakewood, CO), heparin-hydrogel (Biocompatible Hemoperfusion Systems: Clark, New Orleans, LA) or polyHEMA (2-hydroxyl methacrylate or Hemosorba: Asahi, Tokyo, Japan). The membrane prevents direct contact between blood and sorbent, improves biocompatibility, and helps prevent activated charcoal embolization. There may be a further theoretical advantage to the heparin–hydrogel coating to diminish platelet aggregation. The adsorptive capacity of the cartridge is reduced with use because of deposition of cellular debris and blood proteins and saturation of active sites by the xenobiotic in question. Estimation of residual adsorptive capacity by serial serum concentrations is usually not practical because of time delays in obtaining results. The cartridge should therefore be changed after 2 hours of use. As with hemodialysis, patients must be anticoagulated with heparin, and regional heparinization of the cartridge is possible if full anticoagulation is undesirable. The technique can be used in adults[19,74] or children.[16,51] Hemoperfusion is usually performed for 4 to 6 hours at flow rates of 250 to 400 mL/min as tolerated.

The characteristics of xenobiotics that make them amenable to hemoperfusion (summarized in Table 9–3) differ from those for hemodialysis in the important respect that hemoperfusion is not limited by plasma protein binding. This is exemplified in a report in which hemoperfusion but not hemodialysis increased the elimination of the avidly protein-bound oral hypoglycemic agent chlorpropamide.[43] Some xenobiotics are poorly adsorbed by activated charcoal, including the alcohols, lithium, and many metals (see Antidotes in Depth A2: Activated Charcoal), making hemoperfusion inappropriate in their management. Hemoperfusion clearance is calculated in a manner similar to that for hemodialysis. Although hemoperfusion has historically been considered the preferred method to enhance the elimination of carbamazepine, phenobarbital, phenytoin, and theophylline (Table 9–4), recent improvements in hemodialysis technology, such as high-flux membranes, may make older comparisons of hemodialysis and hemoperfusion clearance rates obsolete. Hemodialysis and hemoperfusion have been performed in series for procainamide, thallium, theophylline, and carbamazepine overdoses, with greater apparent clinical efficacy

TABLE 9–4. Properties of Xenobiotics Grouped by Benefit of Extracorporeal Techniques for Elimination

Xenobiotic	MW (daltons)	Water Soluble	Vd (L/Kg)	Protein Binding (%)	Endogenous Clearance (mL/min/kg)	Preferred Method	Comments
Clinically Beneficial							
Bromide	35	Yes	0.7	0	0.1	HD	Falsely elevated chloride measurement
Ethylene glycol	62	Yes	0.6	0	2.0	HD	May have oxaluria
Diethylene glycol	106	Yes	0.5	0	NA	HD	Renal failure
Isopropanol	60	Yes	0.6	0	1.2	HD	No anion gap acidosis
Lithium	7	Yes	0.6–1.0	0	0.4	HD	Cl ↓ in renal failure
Methanol	32	Yes	0.6	0	0.7	HD	Risk CNS hemorrhage
Propylene glycol	76	Yes	0.6	0	1.7	HD	Lactic acidosis, possible acute kidney injury
Salicylate	138	Yes	0.2	50	0.9	HD, HP	Cl and protein binding ↓, with ↑ dose; HD also corrects electrolytes, acid–base disturbance
Theophylline	180	Yes	0.5	56	0.7	HP > HD	HP and HD can also be combined
Valproic acid	144	Yes	0.13–0.22	90	0.1	HD, HP	↑ Concentrations associated with ↓ % protein binding
Possibly Clinically Beneficial							
Amatoxins	373–990	Yes	0.3	0	2.7–6.2	HP	Possibly effective if performed within the first 24 h of exposure
Aminoglycosides	>500	Yes	0.3	1.5	<10	HD, HF	Cl ↓ with renal failure
Atenolol	255	Yes	1.0	2.5	<5	HD, HP	Useful if Cl ↓ caused by renal failure
Carbamazepine	236	No	1.4	74	1.3	HP	Cl ↑ in patients on long-term therapy
Disopyramide	340	No	0.6	1.2	90	HP	Protein binding ↓ as concentration ↑
Fluoride	19	Yes	0.3	50	2.5	HD	Hypocalcemia may be improved by HD; may add little if endogenous renal clearance is preserved
Meprobamate	218	Yes	0.5–0.8	0–30	Low	HP	Most eliminated in 24–36 h
Methotrexate	454	Yes	0.4–0.8	50	1.5	HF	
Paraquat	186	Yes	1.0	6	24.0	HP	Tight tissue binding precludes efficacy unless early in course
Phenobarbital	232	No	0.5	24	0.1	HP	Only for prolonged coma
Phenytoin	252	No	0.6	90	0.3	HP	Cl ↓, as dose ↑
Trichloroethanol	149	Yes	0.6	0.4	0.7	HD	Metabolite of chloral hydrate

Cl, clearance; HD, hemodialysis; HF, hemofiltration; HP, hemoperfusion; MW, molecular weight; NA, not available; Vd, volume of distribution.

than with either procedure alone.[11,21,37] In this technique, blood circulates first through the hemodialysis membrane and then through the charcoal cartridge. If blood traverses the dialysis membrane first, some of the xenobiotic is dialyzed, and the activated charcoal cartridge has less drug to adsorb.[32] The activated charcoal cartridge is exhausted more slowly, and higher extraction ratios are maintained. In a patient who ingested 2 g of propranolol, a hemoperfusion cartridge was inserted into an extracorporeal membrane oxygenation (ECMO) circuit through which the flow rate was less than 3 L/min.[66] The plasma concentrations of propranolol decreased more rapidly during ECMO than after it was discontinued. The high flow rate through the cartridge may have led to substantial clearance of the drug. Hemoperfusion does not correct acid–base and electrolyte disorders, another reason why the combination of the two modalities is attractive for salicylate poisoning.

A practical problem limiting the use of charcoal hemoperfusion is the availability of the cartridges. Many dialysis units do not routinely stock them anymore.[64] The cartridges are expensive ($350–$425 compared with the maximal cost for a high-flux dialysis membrane at about $20–$23). Some have expiration dates, limiting their shelf life. Others, such as the Clark system, have an indefinite shelf life but must be autoclaved before use, which may affect their availability in an emergency. Charcoal cartridges were more available in hemodialysis units when they were more frequently needed for the treatment of patients with chronic aluminum toxicity. The syndromes of aluminum-associated dementia and osteodystrophy were once more prevalent in chronic hemodialysis patients, but aluminum carbonate has been supplanted as a phosphate binder by calcium salts (carbonate and acetate) and sevelamer (Renagel), a phosphate-binding resin. In addition, the most frequent indication for activated charcoal hemoperfusion in the past was theophylline toxicity, and theophylline is rarely used in the treatment of obstructive lung disease and asthma and is consequently less often implicated in acute and chronic poisoning. This accounts for the diminished availability of charcoal cartridges and the relative infrequency with which the procedure is performed. In a survey of New York City hospital dialysis units taking 911 calls, only 10 of 34 units had cartridges. In a recent review of the AAPCC annual data, theophylline was the most common toxin removed by hemoperfusion from 1985 to 2000, but carbamazepine became the most frequent toxin removed by hemoperfusion during 2001 to 2005.[31]

The complications of hemoperfusion are similar to those of hemodialysis. In addition, patients often develop thrombocytopenia, leukopenia, and hypocalcemia. Better membrane encapsulation techniques have made embolization of activated charcoal particles extremely rare. As in the case of hemodialysis, doses of drugs used therapeutically may need to be increased if they are removed by hemoperfusion.

OTHER SORBENTS FOR HEMOPERFUSION

Other adsorptive resins were used for hemoperfusion in the past, such as the synthetic Amberlite XAD-2 and XAD-4 and anion exchange resins such as Dow 1X-2. None of these columns is currently approved or available for use in the United States. The literature regarding their efficacy is scant and relatively anecdotal. Although in vitro evidence suggests that these resins may have greater adsorptive capacities than activated charcoal, there are few, if any, meaningful comparisons in a clinical setting.

A newer concept in sorbents for poisonings is that of albumin dialysis. The procedure is currently available in the United States only for investigational use. The patient's blood flows through a hollow-fiber hemodialyzer. The dialysate bathing the fibers contains human serum albumin that serves as a sorbent to bind the xenobiotic of interest and maintain levels of the free xenobiotic at zero. A steep concentration gradient from blood to dialysate is established so that even highly protein-bound xenobiotics can be removed from the plasma. The membrane is impermeable to albumin, which remains in the dialysate. The albumin is reprocessed by passing through an activated charcoal cartridge as well as an anion exchanger so that it can then be recirculated.

A current proprietary version of this procedure is called Molecular Adsorbents Recirculating System (MARS). The procedure is used in the management of patients with hepatic encephalopathy and liver failure and as a bridge to hepatic transplantation.[67,47] In this setting, the procedure includes a conventional hemodialysis treatment as well as an albumin-bathed dialysis membrane. The mechanism of the significant benefit of the procedure is not completely understood, although it does remove both water-soluble and protein-bound compounds. It is not known which protein-bound molecules are removed from the blood, such as bile salts and aromatic amino acids, to account for the therapeutic advantage in hepatic failure. The MARS system increases the removal of fentanyl and midazolam in an animal model.[62] One case report suggested potential benefit in a patient treated for toxicity with phenytoin, a drug with significant protein binding and therefore one not expected to be removed by hemodialysis or hemoperfusion.[63] Another case report suggests benefit for theophylline toxicity in a patient with hypotension.[41] Whether this relatively expensive, complicated, and nonspecific procedure would offer benefit in a handful of instances in which protein-binding limits removal of xenobiotics is not known. Devices using powdered sorbent may become available in the United States. The report of the initial use of the device in 10 cases of CA overdoses claimed benefit, although the limitations of extracorporeal therapy for this particular class of drugs is discussed above.[5]

MULTIPLE-DOSE ACTIVATED CHARCOAL: "GASTROINTESTINAL DIALYSIS"

Oral administration of multiple doses of activated charcoal increases elimination of some xenobiotics present in the blood. This modality is dealt with in more detail in Antidotes in Depth A2: Activated Charcoal.

CONTINUOUS HEMOFILTRATION AND HEMODIAFILTRATION

Hemofiltration is the movement of plasma across a semipermeable membrane in response to hydrostatic pressure. The addition of dialysate on the other side of the membrane further enhances elimination of toxins, whether xenobiotics or endogenous uremic toxins. A recent review of continuous modalities of dialytic therapy concluded that they are still relatively unproven for the treatment of poisoning.[28] These techniques find relatively widespread usage for the treatment of patients with acute renal failure in the ICU, and in this context, they are referred to collectively as modalities of *continuous renal replacement therapy* (CRRT). The clearances of either urea or xenobiotics that are achieved with these techniques are significantly lower than those achieved with hemodialysis. But as continuous modalities, what they lack in clearance they can make up for in time.

There are several possible advantages of continuous modalities. One is the capability to continue therapy for 24 hours every day, permitting hemofiltration to be instituted after hemodialysis or hemoperfusion to further remove a xenobiotic after it redistributes from tissue to blood.[46] This is an attractive modality for slow, continuous removal of drugs, such as lithium, which distribute slowly from tissue-binding sites or from the intracellular compartment (see Fig. 9–1). Other xenobiotics with volumes of distribution that are large enough to preclude use of dialysis or hemoperfusion might also be eliminated with longer courses.

Hemofiltration, or ultrafiltration, refers to the movement of plasma across a semipermeable membrane in response to hydrostatic pressure gradients. Table 9–3 summarizes the properties of xenobiotics that make them amenable to hemofiltration. However, the rate of removal with this form of therapy may be insufficient to benefit critically ill patients. Patients who can tolerate slower clearance rates may not require this enhanced elimination therapy at all. Whether slow treatment to avoid redistribution of intracellularly distributed lithium, for example, is preferable to repeating conventional hemodialysis is unclear.[45,71] Rebound of serum concentrations indicates that the drug is moving out of the intracellular compartment, where it is toxic, into the extracellular compartment, where it is susceptible to removal by hemodialysis. Therefore, although the continuous modalities are touted as preventing rebound, the importance of this property remains unproven. Despite many case reports demonstrating significant xenobiotic clearance, no data have demonstrated that these continuous techniques affect prognosis or mortality in treatment of patients with xenobiotic toxicity. In most cases, hemodialysis should be considered the preferred initial mode of therapy.

The continuous modalities may be best suited for patients with hypotension who cannot tolerate conventional hemodialysis.[12] These modalities may also have a role after hemodialysis to avoid the need for a repeat session after equilibration of the xenobiotics into plasma. These modalities may have a slight advantage over the use of conventional hemodialysis membranes, but not high-flux membranes, in being able to clear larger molecules such as methotrexate (molecular weight, 454.4).[27] Growing evidence suggests that a significant part of the clearance of many molecules occurs because of adsorption of the molecule to synthetic membranes.[20] However, quantification of the contribution of adsorption to total clearance is difficult and is not usually accomplished in published studies. Adsorption of molecules responsible for adverse effects is being studied as a potential benefit in the management of cytokines and liver failure and could be a property useful in the management of poisoning.[57] At present, this property is difficult to quantify and of uncertain benefit. Another practical advantage of CRRT is that the procedure is usually done now in ICUs by ICU nurses, and when available in such units, might not require dialysis personnel. Familiarity of ICU staff with the procedure is critical to having it available when needed; it is most likely to be used effectively in hospitals with higher incidence rates of acute renal failure.

In pure hemofiltration, sometimes called *slow continuous ultrafiltration* (SCUF), there is no dialysate solution on the other side of the dialysis membrane (see Fig. 9–2). Small solutes, such as urea and sodium, are transported across the membrane with plasma water, a mechanism known as *convective transport* or *bulk flow*. Larger solutes, depending on permeability characteristics of the membrane, are excluded. The ECF volume status of the patient determines whether replacement of all or some of the filtered plasma with physiologic electrolyte solution (lactated Ringer's solution or other commercially available preparations) is indicated. Although this technique can be done intermittently using a hemodialysis machine, it has been adapted for use in ICUs as a continuous form of treatment, particularly when removal of ECF is indicated. The clearance of low-molecular-weight solutes such as urea is relatively low.

Solute clearance may be significantly enhanced by adding dialysis, a diffusive mechanism, by having a dialysate solution bathe the blood-filled capillaries running countercurrent to the blood flow. The combination of hemofiltration with dialysis is known as *hemodiafiltration*. Addition of dialysis also usually suffices to treat supervening acute kidney failure or preexisting chronic kidney failure. Hemodiafiltration, similar to hemodialysis, requires that blood perfuse hollow-fiber dialysis membranes made of synthetic plastics such as polysulfone or polyamide.[23] For all of these procedures, the patient usually must be fully anticoagulated, but some hemofilters are available that may not require anticoagulation. Anticoagulation may be achieved either with heparin or citrate. The hydrostatic pressure required for hemofiltration may be derived either endogenously from the patient's own blood pressure or from a blood pump. In continuous arteriovenous hemofiltration (CAVH), blood is pumped through the filter by the patient's arterial pressure via a single-lumen femoral artery catheter returning to a femoral vein catheter. Arteriovenous modalities are less favored now because they require a large (at least 16-French) catheter in the femoral artery while heparin is administered. CVVH differs from CAVH because a blood pump is required to maintain adequate flow rates, and arterial puncture with large-bore catheters is avoided. However, the need for a blood pump also necessitates an experienced ICU team to be continuously present for more than the 4 to 6 hours needed for acute hemodialysis or hemoperfusion. Both the expense and the complexity of the xenobiotic-removal procedure are thereby increased. One large case series found hemodialysis to be less procedurally complicated than CVVH.[65] The addition of a dialysate bathing solution to the hemofiltration apparatus changes CVVH, or hemofiltration, to the augmented CVVHD, or hemodiafiltration (see Fig. 9–2).

Ultrafiltrate flows of 100 to 6000 mL/h across the membrane can be achieved. Fluid and electrolyte losses must be replaced carefully. Depending on the filter, xenobiotics with a molecular weight of up to 40,000 daltons, as well as water, urea, creatinine, and sodium, pass into the ultrafiltrate. Heparin, myoglobin, insulin, and vancomycin are examples of larger molecules cleared with relative efficiency. CVVH seems to be quite effective in the elimination of theophylline, with clearance rates comparable to those of charcoal hemoperfusion.[29] For protein-bound xenobiotics such as theophylline, continuous removal of the free unbound drug from the plasma may shift the equilibrium so that some drug is always moving from plasma protein to plasma. The cellular components and molecules larger than the pore size of the membrane return to the circulation in the venous line. For instance, a hemofilter with a molecular weight cutoff of 40,000 daltons cannot remove digoxin–antibody complexes (molecular weight, 45,000–50,000).[56] Essential electrolytes lost in the ultrafiltrate are replaced by balanced IV fluids.

Attention must be paid to the undesirable removal of therapeutic drugs such as antimicrobials via these continuous modalities. Drug clearances with different synthetic membranes are available in the literature; the doses necessary to maintain therapeutic drug levels can also be determined.[4]

PLASMAPHERESIS AND EXCHANGE TRANSFUSION

Plasmapheresis and exchange transfusion are intended to eliminate xenobiotics with large molecular weights that are not dialyzable. This includes xenobiotics and endogenous molecules with molecular weights greater than 150,000 daltons, typified by immunoglobulins. The xenobiotic to be eliminated should also have limited endogenous metabolism to make pheresis or exchange worthwhile.[36] By removing plasma proteins, both techniques offer the consequent potential benefit of removal of protein-bound molecules such as *Amanita* toxins,[32] thyroxine, vincristine, or complexes of digoxin and antidigoxin antibodies. However, there is little evidence that either technique affects the clinical course and prognosis of a patient poisoned by any of these or other xenobiotics.

Pheresis is particularly expensive, and both pheresis and exchange transfusion expose the patient to the risks of infection with plasma- or blood-borne diseases. Replacement of the removed plasma during plasmapheresis can be accomplished with fresh-frozen plasma, albumin, or combinations of both. The former is associated with hypersensitivity reactions, such as fever, urticaria, wheezing, and hypotension, in as many as 21% of cases.[36]

A different setting in which exchange transfusion may be an appropriate technique is in the management of small infants or neonates in whom dialysis or hemoperfusion may be technically difficult or impossible. Anticoagulation and MDAC may be hazardous and therefore contraindicated in patients in the neonatal nursery, where the risk of intracerebral bleeding and necrotizing enterocolitis is high. In premature neonates, a single volume exchange appeared to alleviate manifestations of theophylline toxicity.[49] The therapy has been successfully used to treat other pediatric patients with poisonings, including severe salicylism.[44]

TOXICOLOGY OF HEMODIALYSIS

Unlike patients who receive acute hemodialysis once or twice in the management of poisoning, patients with chronic renal failure are repeatedly exposed to large volumes of water derived from municipal reservoirs during the course of their hemodialysis treatments. If an "average" regimen consists of three treatments of 4 hours each week, with dialysate flows of 600 mL/min, patients will be exposed to more than 400 L of water separated from them only by a semipermeable membrane designed to allow solute passage in either direction. Problems with dialysate generation therefore have the potential to be lethal to this population by exposing them to significant quantities of toxins. There are two potential sources of dialysate contamination: the municipality's reservoirs and water treatment plants and the dialysis unit.[54] The quality of water used for dialysate generation is regulated in the United States by the Association for the Advancement of Medical Instrumentation (AAMI).[7] This organization regularly revises its guidelines to incorporate new technology and data.

Contamination of dialysate from the municipal water supply may occur as a result of xenobiotic runoff into reservoirs or as a result of inadvertent or intentional addition of a chemical by the municipality. Chlorine and chloramine are frequently added to municipal water supplies to control bacterial populations. However, chlorine may combine with nitrogenous compounds and form chloramine, which may cause nausea, vomiting, methemoglobinemia, and hemolytic anemia.[72] Recently, chloramine was blamed for decreased bone marrow sensitivity to erythropoietin. Aluminum is present in some municipal water supplies, and before it was recognized as a problem, aluminum led to encephalopathy characterized by seizures, myoclonus, and dementia as well as osteomalacia and microcytic anemia.

Water from the municipal supply entering the dialysis unit is first treated with a water softener to remove calcium and magnesium. It is then run through an activated charcoal bed to adsorb chloramine. The potential toxicity (hemolysis and death) from this compound has caused AAMI to mandate a redundancy in the carbon beds; when the active sites in one carbon bed are exhausted, a second will ensure that no toxicity will occur. Most commonly, water for dialysate is then generated by reverse osmosis, a process that requires that water, in response to applied hydrostatic pressure (and against the osmotic gradient), cross a membrane that is relatively impermeable to solutes, leaving them behind. Alternatively, but less commonly, water can also be purified using deionization, a technique that runs water over an exchange resin, releasing hydroxyl ions in exchange for charged species in the water. Deionization is inferior to reverse osmosis for removal of aluminum and may be associated with release of lethal levels of fluoride when exchange sites are exhausted.[3] General water chemistry testing is mandated annually; testing for chlorine and chloramine must be done daily.

Current requirements are that water be highly purified, but not sterile, because bacteria cannot cross from the dialysate into the blood. However, small quantities of endotoxin (molecular weight, 5–15,000 daltons) can cross, particularly in situations that include the use of high-flux membranes. Endotoxin is suspected of being responsible for activation of circulating cytokines, malnutrition, fever, and other syndromes such as carpal tunnel syndrome, which are associated with chronic inflammation. Recommendations for the frequency of testing for endotoxin and the maximum amounts of endotoxin tolerated are continually debated and have recently become more stringent. Water distribution systems are cleaned at least monthly with bleach, peracetic acid, or other sterilants. Care must be taken that all of these potential toxins are thoroughly flushed from the system before dialysis is restarted. Other products of bacterial metabolism, such as volatile sulfur-containing compounds, generated on the dialysate side of the membrane may be responsible for symptoms in hemodialysis patients.[61]

Unusual microbes have also been associated with serious toxicity. Untreated water at one center in Brazil demonstrated growth of Cyanobacteria (blue-green algae) and production of microcystins, cyclic peptides that cause serious hepatic toxicity; patients dialyzed with the contaminated water had a dramatic rate of death from liver failure.[34] Water contamination should especially be suspected when multiple dialysis patients experience similar symptoms nearly simultaneously. Dialysate distribution systems are always made of polyvinyl chloride (PVC) or other inert plastics, rather than copper, which may also leach into the water and cause hemolytic anemia.

Besides water for dialysate, another potential source of poisoning in hemodialysis units is the process of reusing dialysis membranes. Until recently, up to 70% of dialysis units in the United States reused membranes because of cost considerations. Each dialysis membrane is sterilized with peracetic acid, formaldehyde, or glutaraldehyde. Careful quality assurance programs ensure that there is no significant exposure of the patients to these molecules during the dialysis procedure. Nonetheless, reuse programs are associated with a variety of syndromes such as pyrogenic reactions attributed to patient exposure to germicides or endotoxin caused by inadequate sterilization procedures.[58] Controversial data over the years have suggested, but not proven, higher mortality rates with reuse. Occupational exposure of dialysis personnel to the relevant sterilants has also been monitored closely.

SUMMARY

Further discussions of some of the techniques to enhance elimination that are not discussed here may be found in Chapters 30 (exchange transfusion), SC2 (cerebrospinal fluid drainage and replacement), 64 (toxin-specific antibodies), and 94 (chelation). All of these techniques have limited, very specific indications, and the effect of these interventions on the overall body burden of the intoxicant is usually small.

Urinary alkalinization and many of the other techniques listed in Table 9–1 can be instituted quickly in the emergency department. In contrast, the extracorporeal methods of xenobiotic removal, including hemodialysis, sorbent hemoperfusion, and continuous hemofiltration, all require consultation with a nephrologist or intensivist. Timely use of these techniques requires mobilization of a competent team and preparation of the requisite equipment. Rapid identification of a toxic exposure for which these techniques are appropriate and the presence of more ominous prognostic features should lead to prompt notification of the appropriate consult services so that application of these techniques can proceed in an expeditious manner.

The applicability of these techniques to new xenobiotics should be considered based on the principles discussed here so that these and newer treatment modalities are not used indiscriminately. The relative infrequency of toxicity from specific xenobiotics will continue to hinder accumulation of useful data and limit the numbers of randomized, controlled trials performed. The literature regarding these techniques in general, and for the treatment of specific xenobiotic exposures in particular, should be read critically and with appropriate skepticism.

ACKNOWLEDGMENT

Daniel Matalon contributed to this chapter in a previous edition.

REFERENCES

1. Ahmad S, Callan R, Cole JJ, et al: Dialysate made from dry chemicals using citric acid increases dialysis dose. *Am J Kidney Dis.* 2000;35:493-499.
2. Anthony T, Jastremski M, Elliott W, et al: Charcoal hemoperfusion for the treatment of a combined diltiazem and metoprolol overdose. *Ann Emerg Med.* 1986;15:1344-1348.
3. Arnow PM, Bland LA, Garcia-Houchins S, et al: An outbreak of fatal fluoride intoxication in a long-term hemodialysis unit. *Ann Intern Med.* 1994;121:339-344.
4. Aronoff GR, Bennett Wm, Berns JS, et al: *Drug Prescribing in Renal Failure: Dosing Guidelines for Adults and Children.* Philadelphia: American College of Physicians; 2007.
5. Ash SR, Levy H, Akmal M, et al: Treatment of severe tricyclic antidepressant overdose with extracorporeal sorbent detoxification. *Adv Ren Replace Ther.* 2002;9:31-41.
6. Assael BM, Caccamo ML, Gerna M, et al: Effect of exchange transfusion on elimination of theophylline in premature neonates. *J Pediatr.* 1977;91: 331-332.
7. Association for the Advancement of Medical Instrumentation: *Dialysate for Hemodialysis ANSI/AAMI RD52:2004/A1:2007 and A2:2007.* Arlington, VA: Association for the Advancement of Medical Instrumentation; 2008.
8. Atassi WA, Noghnogh AA, Hariman R, et al: Hemodialysis as a treatment of severe ethanol poisoning. *Int J Artif Organs.* 1999;22:18-20.
9. Bailey B, McGuigan M: Comparison of patients hemodialyzed for lithium poisoning and those for whom dialysis was recommended by PCC but not done: what lesson can we learn? *Clin Nephrol.* 2000;54:388-392.
10. Barrueto F, Meggs WJ, Barchman MJ: Clearance of metformin by hemofiltration in overdose. *J Toxicol Clin Toxicol.* 2002;40:177-180.
11. Bock E, Keller F, Heitz J, et al: Treatment of carbamazepine poisoning by combined hemodialysis/hemoperfusion. *Int J Clin Pharmacol Ther Toxicol.* 1989;27:490-492.
12. Bressolle F, Kinowski JM, de la Coussaye JE, et al: Clinical pharmacokinetics during continuous haemofiltration. *Clin Pharmacokinet.* 1994;26:457-471.
13. Brunet P, Jaber K, Berland Y, et al: Anaphylactoid reactions during hemodialysis and hemofiltration: role of associating AN69 membrane and angiotensin I-converting enzyme inhibitors. *Am J Kidney Dis.* 1992;19: 444-447.
14. Canaud B, Leray-Moragues H, Kamoun K, et al: Temporary vascular access for extracorporeal therapies. *Ther Apher.* 2000;4:249-255.
15. Chan H, Evans WE, Pratt CB: Recovery from toxicity associated with high-dose methotrexate: prognostic factors. *Cancer Treat Rep.* 1977;61:797-804.
16. Chavers BM, Kjellstrand CM, Wiegand C, et al: Techniques for use of charcoal hemoperfusion in infants: experience in two patients. *Kidney Int.* 1980;18:386-389.
17. Cherskov M: Extracorporeal detoxification: still debatable. *JAMA.* 1982;247:3047-3048.
18. Chow MT, DiSilvestro V, Yung CY, et al: Treatment of acute methanol intoxication with hemodialysis using an ethanol-enriched, bicarbonate-based dialysate. *Am J Kidney Dis.* 1997;30:568-570.
19. Cutler RE, Forland SC, Hammond PG, et al: Extracorporeal removal of drugs and poisons by hemodialysis and hemoperfusion. *Annu Rev Pharmacol Toxicol.* 1987;27:169-191.
20. Davies JG, Kingswood JC, Sharpstone P, et al: Drug removal in continuous haemofiltration and haemodialysis. *Br J Hosp Med.* 1995;54:524-528.
21. De BW, Zachee P, Verpooten GA, et al: Thallium intoxication treated with combined hemoperfusion-hemodialysis. *J Toxicol Clin Toxicol.* 1982;19:259-264.
22. Feinfeld DA, Rosenberg JW, Winchester JF: Three controversial issues in extracorporeal toxin removal. *Semin Dial.* 2006;19:358-362.
23. Forni LG, Hilton PJ: Continuous hemofiltration in the treatment of acute renal failure. *N Engl J Med.* 1997;336:1303-1309.
24. Gaiter AM, Bonfant G, Manes M, et al: Relation between blood pH and ionized calcium during acute metabolic alteration of the acid-base balance in vivo. *Scand J Clin Lab Invest.* 1997;57:317-323.
25. Garella S: Extracorporeal techniques in the treatment of exogenous intoxications. *Kidney Int.* 1988;33:735-754.
26. Gatchalian RA, Popli A, Ejaz AA, et al: Management of hypophosphatemia induced by high-flux hemodiafiltration for the treatment of vancomycin toxicity: intravenous phosphorus therapy versus use of a phosphorus-enriched dialysate. *Am J Kidney Dis.* 2000;36:1262-1266.
27. Golper TA, Bennett WM: Drug removal by continuous arteriovenous haemofiltration. A review of the evidence in poisoned patients. *Med Toxicol Adverse Drug Exp.* 1988;3:341-349.
28. Goodman JW, Goldfarb DS: The role of continuous renal replacement therapy in the treatment of poisoning. *Semin Dial.* 2006;19:402-407.
29. Henderson JH, McKenzie CA, Hilton PJ, et al: Continuous venovenous haemofiltration for the treatment of theophylline toxicity. *Thorax.* 2001;56:242-243.
30. Hicks LK, McFarlane PA: Valproic acid overdose and haemodialysis. *Nephrol Dial Transplant.* 2001;16:1483-1486.
31. Holubek WJ, Hoffman RS, Goldfarb DS, et al: Use of hemodialysis and hemoperfusion in poisoned patients. *Kidney Int.* 2008;74:1327-1334.
32. Hootkins R, Sr., Lerman MJ, Thompson JR: Sequential and simultaneous "in series" hemodialysis and hemoperfusion in the management of theophylline intoxication. *J Am Soc Nephrol.* 1990;1:923-926.
33. Jacobsen D, Wiik-Larsen E, Bredesen JE: Haemodialysis or haemoperfusion in severe salicylate poisoning? *Hum Toxicol.* 1988;7:161-163.
34. Jochimsen EM, Carmichael WW, An JS, et al: Liver failure and death after exposure to microcystins at a hemodialysis center in Brazil. *N Engl J Med.* 1998;338:873-878.
35. Johnson LZ, Martinez I, Fernandez MC, et al: Successful treatment of valproic acid overdose with hemodialysis. *Am J Kidney Dis.* 1999;33:786-789.
36. Kale PB, Thomson PA, Provenzano R, et al: Evaluation of plasmapheresis in the treatment of an acute overdose of carbamazepine. *Ann Pharmacother.* 1993;27:866-870.
37. Kar PM, Kellner K, Ing TS, et al: Combined high-efficiency hemodialysis and charcoal hemoperfusion in severe N-acetylprocainamide intoxication. *Am J Kidney Dis.* 1992;20:403-406.
38. Kay TD, Playford HR, Johnson DW: Hemodialysis versus continuous venovenous hemodiafiltration in the management of severe valproate overdose. *Clin Nephrol.* 2003;59:56-58.
39. Kielstein JT, Woywodt A, Schumann G, et al: Efficiency of high-flux hemodialysis in the treatment of valproic acid intoxication. *J Toxicol Clin Toxicol.* 2003;41:873-876.
40. Koppel C, Schirop T, Ibe K, et al: Hemoperfusion in severe chlorprothixene overdose. *Intensive Care Med.* 1987;13:358-360.
41. Korsheed S, Selby NM, Fluck RJ: Treatment of severe theophylline poisoning with the molecular adsorbent recirculating system (MARS). *Nephrol Dial Transplant.* 2007;22:969-970.
42. Lalau JD, Race JM: Lactic acidosis in metformin-treated patients. Prognostic value of arterial lactate levels and plasma metformin concentrations. *Drug Saf.* 1999;20:377-384.
43. Ludwig SM, McKenzie J, Faiman C: Chlorpropamide overdose in renal failure: management with charcoal hemoperfusion. *Am J Kidney Dis.* 1987;10:457-460.
44. Manikian A, Stone S, Hamilton R, et al: Exchange transfusion in severe infant salicylism. *Vet Hum Toxicol.* 2002;44:224-227.
45. Menghini VV, Albright RC, Jr: Treatment of lithium intoxication with continuous venovenous hemodiafiltration. *Am J Kidney Dis.* 2000;36:E21-
46. Meyer RJ, Flynn JT, Brophy PD, et al: Hemodialysis followed by continuous hemofiltration for treatment of lithium intoxication in children. *Am J Kidney Dis.* 2001;37:1044-1047.
47. Mitzner SR, Stange J, Klammt S, et al: Extracorporeal detoxification using the molecular adsorbent recirculating system for critically ill patients with liver failure. *J Am Soc Nephrol* 2001;12(suppl 17):S75-S82.
48. Morgan AG, Polak A: The excretion of salicylate in salicylate poisoning. *Clin Sci.* 1971;41:475-484.
49. Osborn HH, Henry G, Wax P, et al: Theophylline toxicity in a premature neonate—elimination kinetics of exchange transfusion. *J Toxicol Clin Toxicol.* 1993;31:639-644.
50. Palmer BF: Effectiveness of hemodialysis in the extracorporeal therapy of phenobarbital overdose. *Am J Kidney Dis.* 2000;36:640-643.

51. Papadopoulou ZL, Novello AC: The use of hemoperfusion in children. Past, present, and future. *Pediatr Clin North Am.* 1982;29:1039-1052.
52. Parker MG, Fraser GL, Watson DM, et al: Removal of propylene glycol and correction of increased osmolar gap by hemodialysis in a patient on high dose lorazepam infusion therapy. *Intensive Care Med.* 2002;28:81-84.
53. Pond SM, Olson KR, Osterloh JD, et al: Randomized study of the treatment of phenobarbital overdose with repeated doses of activated charcoal. *JAMA.* 1984;251:3104-3108.
54. Pontoriero G, Pozzoni P, Andrulli S, et al: The quality of dialysis water. *Nephrol Dial Transplant.* 2003;18(suppl 7):vii21-vii25; discussion vii56:vii21-vii25.
55. Proudfoot AT, Krenzelok EP, Vale JA: Position paper on urine alkalinization. *J Toxicol Clin Toxicol.* 2004;42:1-26.
56. Quaife EJ, Banner W Jr, Vernon DD, et al: Failure of CAVH to remove digoxin-Fab complex in piglets. *J Toxicol Clin Toxicol.* 1990;28:61-68.
57. Ronco C, Tetta C: Extracorporal blood purification: more than diffusion and convection. Does this help? *Curr Opin Crit Care.* 2007;13:662-667.
58. Rudnick JR, Arduino MJ, Bland LA, et al: An outbreak of pyrogenic reactions in chronic hemodialysis patients associated with hemodialyzer reuse. *Artif Organs.* 1995;19:289-294.
59. Saitz R, Williams BW, Farber HW: Atenolol-induced cardiovascular collapse treated with hemodialysis. *Crit Care Med.* 1991;19:116-118.
60. Schuerer DJ, Brophy PD, Maxvold NJ, et al: High-efficiency dialysis for carbamazepine overdose. *J Toxicol Clin Toxicol.* 2000;38:321-323.
61. Selenic D, varado-Ramy F, Arduino M, et al: Epidemic parenteral exposure to volatile sulfur-containing compounds at a hemodialysis center. *Infect Control Hosp Epidemiol.* 2004;25:256-261.
62. Sen S, Ratnaraj N, Davies NA, et al: Treatment of phenytoin toxicity by the molecular adsorbents recirculating system (MARS). *Epilepsia.* 2003;44:265-267.
63. Sen S, Ytrebo LM, Rose C, et al: Albumin dialysis: a new therapeutic strategy for intoxication from protein-bound drugs. *Intensive Care Med.* 2004;30:496-501.
64. Shalkham AS, Kirrane BM, Hoffman RS, et al: The availability and use of charcoal hemoperfusion in the treatment of poisoned patients. *Am J Kidney Dis.* 2006;48:239-241.
65. Shannon MW: Comparative efficacy of hemodialysis and hemoperfusion in severe theophylline intoxication. *Acad Emerg Med.* 1997;4:674-678.
66. Smith B, Sullivan MJ: Lifesaving use of extracorporeal membrane oxygenation. *Aust J Cardiovasc Perf.* 1990;4:7-11.
67. Stange J, Mitzner SR, Risler T, et al: Molecular adsorbent recycling system (MARS): clinical results of a new membrane-based blood purification system for bioartificial liver support. *Artif Organs.* 1999;23:319-330.
68. Sztajnkrycer MD: Valproic acid toxicity: overview and management. *J Toxicol Clin Toxicol.* 2002;40:789-801.
69. Takki S, Gambertoglio JG, Honda DH, et al: Pharmacokinetic evaluation of hemodialysis in acute drug overdose. *J Pharmacokinet Biopharm.* 1978;6:427-442.
70. Tapolyai M, Campbell M, Dailey K, et al: Hemodialysis is as effective as hemoperfusion for drug removal in carbamazepine poisoning. *Nephron.* 2002;90:213-215.
71. van Bommel EF, Kalmeijer MD, Ponssen HH: Treatment of life-threatening lithium toxicity with high-volume continuous venovenous hemofiltration. *Am J Nephrol.* 2000;20:408-411.
72. Ward DM: Chloramine removal from water used in hemodialysis. *Adv Ren Replace Ther.* 1996;3:337-347.
73. Wason S, Baker RC, Carolan P, et al: Carbamazepine overdose—the effects of multiple dose activated charcoal. *J Toxicol Clin Toxicol.* 1992;30:39-48.
74. Woo OF, Pond SM, Benowitz NL, et al: Benefit of hemoperfusion in acute theophylline intoxication. *J Toxicol Clin Toxicol.* 1984;22:411-424.

CHAPTER 10
USE OF THE INTENSIVE CARE UNIT

Mark A. Kirk

Over the past several decades, the use of the intensive care unit (ICU) and its attendant resources has led to improved patient survival from many serious conditions. This is the direct result of the ability to pay meticulous attention to supportive care, continuously monitor physiologic parameters, and use the most modern medical technology and treatment. Most critically ill poisoned patients have acutely reversible conditions that will clearly benefit from ICU intervention.[55]

Unlike many patients with diseases managed in the ICU, poisoned patients often do not have a well-recognized clinical course or predictable complications. More than almost any other disease managed in the ICU, uncertainties typify toxicologic emergencies. A patient's history is often unreliable with regard to the kind of xenobiotic ingested, time of ingestion, and amount ingested. The xenobiotic may have unknown or unpredictable toxic effects. The therapies, antidotes, and complications of acute poisoning may be unfamiliar to the ICU staff. These uncertainties challenge healthcare providers and influence decisions about admitting patients to the ICU.

Often a patient is admitted to the ICU for observation and monitoring, not for intervention.[71] Of the 12.5 million reported xenobiotic exposures reported in the American Association of Poison Control Centers (AAPCC) National Poison Database System from 2003 to 2007, only 5% were admitted to the hospital (Chap. 135).[7] In addition, fewer than 25% of those hospitalized required specific treatments or antidotes other than gastrointestinal (GI) decontamination.[6,7,71] Many physicians elect to observe poisoned patients in an ICU in anticipation of possible delayed, unrecognized life-threatening toxicity. The ICU provides necessary monitoring and individual nursing care that can help in the early recognition of developing toxicity. ICUs give healthcare providers the best opportunity to minimize morbidity and decrease mortality. However, ICU care is very expensive and has contributed significantly to the escalation of healthcare costs.

The ICU admission guidelines presented in this chapter are intended to encourage effective use of ICU resources without compromising patient care. Effective guidelines must consider the unique characteristics of a xenobiotic, the capabilities of the hospital, and all realistic alternatives for managing and observing poisoned patients without compromising care. Current medical literature allows us to develop only very general guidelines. Future clinical studies addressing the use of healthcare resources for poisoned patients will allow refinement of these guidelines. Although it is impossible to be all-inclusive, this chapter provides a decision-making strategy for most xenobiotics discussed in this text.

CLINICAL OBSERVATIONS AND RISK ASSESSMENT AS THE BASIS FOR ICU ADMISSION

Most critically ill poisoned patients have acutely reversible conditions that will clearly benefit from meticulous supportive care, continuous physiologic monitoring, and the use of the most modern medical technology and treatment. It seems reasonable to assume that a patient's signs and symptoms can be used to decide the need for ICU admission. The presence of certain signs, symptoms, or abnormal diagnostic test results requires ICU observation or intervention, whatever the toxic exposure. This approach is most consistent with the philosophy of "treating the patient and not the poison" and may prove most helpful for patients with polydrug ingestions. Patients with serious central nervous system (CNS), respiratory, cardiovascular, or metabolic manifestations of poisoning need ICU interventions regardless of the exposure. For example, patients with respiratory failure requiring mechanical ventilation, hypotension or cardiac dysrhythmias requiring cardiovascular resuscitation, recurrent seizures requiring airway management and continuous anticonvulsant therapy, or agitation requiring high-dose sedation all require ICU admission.

Beyond managing the obvious end-organ toxicity requiring intervention, the ICU is especially useful for observing for the progression of end-organ effects that may need intervention. Because the natural course of a toxicologic emergency is often unpredictable, consideration must be given to patients at risk of deteriorating to the point that critical care interventions are required.

In acute toxicologic emergencies, the history may be inaccurate or incomplete and the dose uncertain. Therefore, an informal "bedside risk assessment" is a helpful tool for decision making. In this case, "risk assessment" is defined as the process of determining the likelihood of toxicity for an individual after an exposure. This critical care risk assessment takes into account observed clinical effects, estimated dose, pharmacologic and toxicologic characteristics of the suspected xenobiotic, and characteristics of the exposed patient to help determine the need for ICU admission. It is intended to identify patients with conditions requiring meticulous supportive care, physiologic monitoring, or advanced technologic or pharmacologic therapies that can only be provided in the ICU. More importantly, it is needed to predict the likelihood of a patient's deteriorating to the point of needing critical care interventions. This decision-making guide takes into account key clinical observations, current best available evidence from the medical literature, clinical experience, and preferences based on acceptable risks (Table 10–1).

EVIDENCE-BASED CLINICAL CRITERIA FOR ICU ADMISSION

Overcrowded ICUs and escalating healthcare costs have been incentives to develop severity of illness models that predict the benefits of ICU care. The Acute Physiology and Chronic Health Evaluation (APACHE II/III/IV), the Mortality Probability Model (MPM II/III), and the Pediatric Risk of Mortality (PRISM II/III) models are widely studied and generally accepted severity of illness models that score certain physiologic parameters and other factors to estimate risks and predict outcomes in critically ill individuals.[13,61] Additional acute clinical assessment tools, such as the Modified Early Warning Score (MEWS), Simplified Acute Physiology Score (SAPS II), and the Glasgow Coma Score (GCS), are commonly used "bedside" methods of quickly assessing the severity of physiologic derangement and altered neurologic status, respectively.[61,63] These models are most effective for stratifying risks in clinical research trials and comparing quality of care among ICUs. Clinical studies to validate such scoring systems included patients with a variety of medical and surgical conditions, although few trials have validated these scoring systems in large cohorts of poisoned patients. The original APACHE II cohort of 5815 ICU admissions from 13 hospitals included only 153 patients admitted to the ICU with a diagnosis of "drug overdose."[34] APACHE II is limited by its failure

TABLE 10–1. Key Parameters for Informal Risk Assessment

Bedside observations for end-organ toxic effects
Evidence-based clinical criteria and severity of illness models
Need for specific monitoring or therapeutic interventions
Xenobiotic characteristics: Toxicodynamic and toxicokinetic considerations
Patient factors that increase susceptibility to adverse outcomes
At-risk populations
Chronic and other comorbid medical conditions
Risk of life-threatening complications
Anoxic brain injury
Aspiration pneumonitis
Rhabdomyolysis and compartment syndrome

to distinguish between traumatic and nontraumatic causes of altered mental status, a fact of potentially vital import in cases of xenobiotic overdose. The development of APACHE III addressed this shortcoming of its predecessor. However, even this very complicated scoring system with proprietary mathematical modeling has limited value when applied to a wide range of poisoned patients. In fact, when APACHE III was used by its authors to screen a large independent database of almost 40,000 ICU admissions, including 1032 patients admitted with "drug overdose," predicted and actual mortality statistics for these patients were vastly different.[71] Seven deaths (0.7%) were predicted in this cohort, although the actual number turned out to be 25 (2.4%). The difference was highly statistically significant. APACHE IV attempted to further address the shortcomings of its predecessor but it still relies on parameters collected over the first 24 hours in the ICU.[61] Additional articles addressing the usage of severity of illness scoring systems to identify high-risk overdose patients are lacking, although one review of 216 consecutive ICU admissions for intentional overdose found that admission APACHE II and GCS were equally strong predictors of morbidity and mortality.[26] Specifically, a GCS of 12 or less was 88% sensitive and 92% specific in identifying patients at risk of developing morbidity requiring ICU admission.

Results of severity of illness models must be cautiously used.[61] These models lack individual prognostic application, and decisions about individual patients still require clinical judgment. Scores for these models need to be validated for the specific population for which they are to be used. A specific limitation of these models is lead-time bias (ie, pre-ICU care that influences mortality and in which the sole outcome measure is mortality). Therefore, severity of illness models to guide ICU care must be used cautiously when applied specifically to poisoned patients. Few studies have evaluated the use of the ICU for poisoned patients.[6,24,27,29,35,62,65] Prospective studies have focused on mortality rates, use of resources, or types of xenobiotics ingested; other studies, mostly retrospective ones, have focused on patients exposed to a specific xenobiotic. More study is needed before any severity of illness model can be considered reliable in predicting which patients are at the highest risk of developing ICU-requiring morbidity or mortality.

Given the unique characteristics of individual xenobiotics, other authors have attempted to apply severity of illness models in specific instances. APACHE II scores within 24 hours of presentation showed promise as a predictor of mortality when studied prospectively in acetaminophen-induced acute liver failure, revealing similar power to predict a poor outcome when compared against the widely accepted King's College Criteria.[45] Two studies evaluating organic phosphorus compound poisoning used APACHE II and SAPS II scores demonstrated that high scores were predictive of mortality.[38,57] However, some clinical outcome predictors used in these scoring systems, such as neurologic outcome after cardiac arrest, are unreliable in poisoned patients.[17] Patients with severe poisoning may have clinical characteristics that mimic brain death yet have a complete neurologic recovery. Case reports of poisoning from barbiturates, cyclic antidepressants, baclofen, ethylene glycol, botulism, solvents, and sedative–hypnotics provide specific examples of this observation.[3,50,52,66,68,70] In addition, many toxicologic emergencies occur in young patients who are free of underlying disease. This increases the likelihood of surviving significant insults such as prolonged hypotension or hypoxia. Indeed, one prospective trial involving 286 patients admitted to the ICU with nontraumatic coma found that 91% of the 101 xenobiotic-induced coma patients survived, a much higher rate than those patients whose cause of coma was hypoxia (33%), sepsis (28%), focal cerebral (26%), or a general cerebral insult (17%).[23] Despite negative predictors of outcome, aggressive resuscitation efforts may be justified for poisoned patients. Specifically, prolonged cardiac resuscitation should be provided for victims of cardiac arrest resulting from overdoses of cyclic antidepressant, β-adrenergic antagonists, or calcium channel blockers and those with severe hypothermia.[18,30,43,49,58]

A set of criteria was established to determine whether initial clinical assessment could identify poisoned patients who were at risk of developing serious toxicity, thus needing ICU admission.[6] The specific xenobiotic ingested was not considered in defining risks. Criteria defining high-risk patients were need for intubation; unresponsiveness to verbal stimuli; seizures; PCO_2 above 45 mm Hg; systolic blood pressure below 80 mm Hg; QRS duration above 0.12 seconds; or any cardiac rhythm except normal sinus rhythm, sinus tachycardia, or sinus bradycardia. Patients were classified as low risk when none of the above criteria were present in the emergency department (ED). Retrospectively, 209 cases were analyzed using the above parameters. The most commonly ingested xenobiotics in both the high- and low-risk groups were barbiturates, benzodiazepines, cyclic antidepressants, ethanol, opioids, phenothiazines, and salicylates. None of the 151 patients who were considered at low risk developed complications or required ICU interventions after admission. Of the 58 patients deemed high risk, 35 required ICU interventions such as intubation, treatment of dysrhythmias, treatment of seizures, vasopressors, or hemodialysis or hemoperfusion. Seven patients developed high-risk complications such as hypoxia, respiratory failure, hypotension, or seizures after admission, but all of them had other high-risk criteria in the ED. Although the authors concluded that the clinical course of poisoned patients can be predicted during the initial 2 to 3 hours of observation, xenobiotics with delayed or prolonged toxic effects, such as sustained-release products, lithium, and oral hypoglycemics were not prominent in their study population.

In this study population, 70% of the low-risk patients were admitted to the ICU for observation. Because none of these patients developed complications or required ICU intervention, the authors postulated that applying these criteria would have eliminated 50% of the ICU days without compromising care. The limitations of this study are its retrospective design, relatively small study population, and limited variety of xenobiotic exposures. However, it does suggest that with some clinical judgment, many poisoned patients will not require ICU admission.

Ideally, clinical indicators for ICU care should be established for each xenobiotic. Universal criteria cannot be applied to all poisoned patients because of the unique clinical course of some xenobiotics and the uncertainty regarding which xenobiotics were ingested. In one outcome study of elderly poisoned patients, the authors observed that each category of poisoning has its own special risk profile.[46] Until more specific predictors of outcome are developed for individual xenobiotics, nothing will be more useful than experience and good clinical judgment in predicting who may benefit from ICU admission. At present, withholding ICU care from poisoned patients based solely on a nonspecific "score" will not result in significant cost savings in the ICU but may increase the risk of morbidity and mortality.

PHYSIOLOGIC MONITORING AND SPECIALIZED TREATMENT AS REQUIREMENTS FOR ICU ADMISSION

The ICU setting offers the most highly skilled staff and modern technology available to manage complex medical problems. It also provides a nurse-to-patient ratio that allows for frequent or continuous monitoring of basic physiologic parameters. These measurements of vital signs, neurologic status, and fluid intake and output measurements, along with continuous cardiac monitoring, make possible early detection of toxicity, recognition of conditions needing active intervention, and prevention of complications. Medical technologic advances now provide a number of invasive and noninvasive capabilities that can signal or provide trends indicating risk of catastrophic deterioration or provide feedback on response to therapy. For example, monitoring hemodynamic parameters are valuable for managing poisoned patients with hypotension, intravascular volume depletion, or respiratory failure from acute lung injury (ALI). Most importantly, clinicians must recognize that no monitoring device improves clinical outcome unless coupled with a treatment that improves outcome.[25]

Most critically ill poisoned patients have acute reversible conditions requiring supportive care measures (ie, ventilator support, vasopressor support, or both) and close monitoring that only ICUs are equipped to provide. Most often, supportive care measures improve the outcome of critically ill poisoned patients more than antidotes and specialized treatments. Focus on supportive care measures, such as maintaining a patent airway, preventing hypoxia with the administration of oxygen, and treatment of shock, decreased the mortality for patients with barbiturate overdoses from 20% in the 1930s to less than 2% in the 1950s.[12] Both adult and pediatric studies report good outcomes in most critically ill overdosed patients treated with only mechanical ventilation, vasopressor support, and careful monitoring.[17,35]

Many antidotes and specific treatments should be administered in the ED and the ICU settings. Although possibly lifesaving, these treatments may have inherent risks. Because these treatments may be unfamiliar to staff and have their own inherent risks, the ICU is the most appropriate environment to administer or continue such treatments. Whereas some xenobiotics are administered in unconventional doses, other familiar xenobiotics should be avoided in treating patients with toxicologic emergencies. In toxicologic emergencies, a familiar xenobiotic may be an antidotal therapy that requires doses that far exceed conventional regimens or indications that deviate from common treatment protocols. High doses of atropine (ie, hundreds of milligrams) may be necessary for the treatment of patients with organic phosphorus insecticide poisoning.[15,21,37] Direct vasopressors such as norepinephrine or phenylephrine are more appropriate for the treatment of those with xenobiotic-induced hypotension.

A false sense of security can result when an antidote reverses toxicity but has a shorter duration of effect than the xenobiotic. An example is a patient, comatose from an opioid overdose who responds to naloxone, awakens, and refuses further treatment. Toxicity may recur when the short duration of effect of naloxone allows opioid toxicity to recur. These patients must be closely observed for the possible need to readminister the antidote. In a retrospective review of patients presenting with opioid overdosage, 31% of 84 naloxone responders experienced resedation necessitating readministration.[67] Resedation is particularly problematic with long-acting opioids such as methadone and controlled-release preparations of oxycodone and morphine.[28]

Extracorporeal methods of eliminating xenobiotics, such as hemodialysis and continuous venovenous hemofiltration, are ideally performed in the ICU. Invasive procedures, such as extracorporeal membrane oxygenation, cardiopulmonary bypass, and intraaortic balloon pump-assisted perfusion, are used successfully in resuscitating critically ill poisoned patients.[16,30,36]

When the need for surgical intervention or specialized wound care is anticipated, patients with toxicologic emergencies are ideally managed in the ICU. Although transplantation becomes necessary in a minority of critically ill acetaminophen-poisoned patients, this treatment can improve survival to discharge by as much as 75%.[2] Compartment syndrome, from muscle compression after prolonged xenobiotic-induced coma, is a rare but limb-threatening occurrence that sometimes results in the need for fasciotomy.[20] Any poisoned patient with significant rhabdomyolysis, whether localized or more widespread, is at risk for the development of compartment syndrome and acute renal failure. If contemplating fasciotomy, monitoring and specialized postoperative care in an ICU is warranted. Plasmapheresis and specialized wound care in an ICU are necessary in cases of toxic epidermal necrolysis (TEN) secondary to xenobiotics. Mortality and morbidity may be reduced by early referral to a specialized burn center for conditions such as TEN or significant dermal burns from caustics.

ADDITIONAL INFORMATION INFLUENCING ICU ADMISSION OF POISONED PATIENTS

End-organ toxicity and specific monitoring or therapeutic interventions are the most important reasons to admit poisoned patients to the ICU. However, restricting ICU admission to those with only end-organ toxicity is inappropriate. Minimally symptomatic or asymptomatic patients may require ICU admission because other factors must be considered. In addition to end-organ toxicity, the xenobiotic and specific patient characteristics should influence ICU admission decisions.

XENOBIOTIC CHARACTERISTICS AS A BASIS FOR ICU ADMISSION

Both the known and unknown characteristics of a xenobiotic will assist with ICU admission decisions. Some xenobiotics have proven their capability to cause harm or death to humans. Well-described, expected toxic effects assist in early recognition of poisoning. For other xenobiotics, the consequences after human exposure are not yet reported.

ICU admission is warranted for patients with expected serious toxic effects from an ingested xenobiotic. This is especially true for xenobiotics known to be deadly, such as calcium channel blockers, cyanide, cyclic antidepressants, and salicylates. For example, patients with calcium channel blocker poisoning who exhibit hemodynamic compromise require close attention and meticulous continuous treatment available only in the ICU.

Indicators of toxicity should be identified for individual xenobiotics so that high-risk patients may be closely monitored and aggressively treated. Patients who have ingested cyclic antidepressants develop substantial morbidity and mortality and have been studied in great detail to determine indicators of toxicity. These studies demonstrate that a prolonged QRS duration on a 12-lead electrocardiogram (ECG) is predictive of serious complications such as seizures and dysrhythmias.[4,48] Any patient manifesting ECG abnormalities (including QRS ≥0.10 seconds), hypotension, or neurologic signs or symptoms requires ICU monitoring.[9] Unlike cyclic antidepressants, most xenobiotics do not have such an extensive literature to define high-risk patients.

Most acetaminophen-poisoned patients can be safely managed outside of the ICU because they exhibit no end-organ toxicity and their hospital management entails only laboratory monitoring and antidotal therapy with *N*-acetylcysteine. However, acetaminophen poisoning can be lethal, and at some point in the clinical course, manifestations of toxicity require close monitoring and treatments available only in the ICU. Predictors of poor outcome have been studied and can be useful guides for selecting patients who need ICU care. The King's College Criteria are well-established indicators of impending hepatic failure and the need for transplantation. Patients with abnormal clinical and laboratory data approaching these criteria are candidates for ICU admission or transfer to a specialized center with advanced ICU resources and transplantation services.

Decisions can be challenging when the characteristics and clinical course of the xenobiotic are unknown. New pharmaceutical and industrial products are introduced every year with little data on toxic exposure doses or human health effects in overdose. Sometimes animal studies provide the only known toxicologic data, and preclinical trials for new xenobiotics may have excluded the populations at risk, such as infants, children, or the elderly. In these cases, the clinician must often make therapeutic decisions and anticipate potential toxicity with little or no reliable data. Because early recognition of serious toxicity may prevent an adverse outcome, expectant observation may be the only rational approach. For example, intentional and unintentional ingestions followed the introduction of fluoxetine. Because, at that time, clinicians lacked experience treating overdoses of this drug and had no data regarding the natural course and toxic dose, many patients were admitted to the ICU to observe for toxic effects. Now that clinicians have experience with this drug and studies are available demonstrating few severe manifestations, ICU resources are seldom needed to treat such patients.[5,60]

Failure to appreciate the potential for serious, delayed toxic effects is a major pitfall in managing poisoned patients. An asymptomatic patient may be a "time bomb" with the potential to deteriorate rapidly. Delayed or continued absorption, slow tissue distribution, interference with cellular function, production of toxic metabolites, or depletion of target organ reserve capacity are causes of delayed onset of clinical effects.

Certain xenobiotics prolong GI absorption, delaying onset of toxicity.[42] Sustained-release pharmaceutical preparations and those with enteric coatings enhance patient compliance but, in overdose, may delay absorption and, in turn, make the onset of toxicity unpredictable.[44] Published cases of overdoses with sustained-release verapamil, bupropion, and enteric-coated aspirin report delayed onset of toxicity (>6 hours), and peak serum concentrations were measured more than 24 hours after ingestion.[19,59,69]

Serial xenobiotic concentrations measurements are necessary to verify peaks and ensure decreasing concentrations. Serial concentrations may, if available, warn of increasing potential for serious toxic effects. When serum concentrations are unobtainable, extended observation, possibly in the ICU, is required for many patients with overdoses of sustained-release and enteric-coated medications.

Clinical effects may be delayed when toxicity depends on alteration of enzyme functions, cellular reproduction, or metabolic function. For example, toxicity from colchicine may not be apparent for many hours after an overdose but then may progress rapidly to severe toxicity such as cardiovascular collapse. Other xenobiotics may take days to exhibit their toxic effects. For example, methotrexate and other chemotherapeutics may cause life-threatening bone marrow suppression days after exposure. When there is potential for serious delayed toxicity, patients necessitate prolonged close monitoring, typically in an ICU setting.

PATIENT FACTORS AS CRITERIA FOR ICU ADMISSION

Comorbid medical conditions increase a patient's risk for developing toxicity. Many patients who have chronic medical problems do not tolerate major physiologic stressors without significant compromise. For example, a patient with underlying cardiac disease could develop severe myocardial ischemia from a modest carbon monoxide exposure. An elderly or chronically ill or debilitated patient with chronic salicylism is more likely to have major respiratory or CNS complications than a younger or healthier patient. Conditions that alter xenobiotic metabolism or elimination, such as renal or hepatic disease, may prolong toxicity or produce toxicity after lesser amounts are ingested. For many of these reasons, the morbidity and mortality of acute poisoning are higher in elderly patients.[46]

Patients with physical dependency on ethanol, benzodiazepines, or barbiturates may be admitted to the hospital for acute withdrawal or, during hospitalization, go through a period of abstinence that results in an acute withdrawal syndrome. Withdrawal from ethanol and sedative–hypnotics can have serious consequences and complications. ICU management is frequently indicated because large doses of medications with respiratory depressant effects may be required for treatment.

As many as 80% of recognized suicide attempts involve an overdose of medications.[47] Acute complications of poisoning make it difficult to adequately assess suicidal risks. Patients have an increased rate of suicide after discharge from an ICU for drug overdose.[62] Until suicidal risks are adequately assessed, it must be assumed that an overdosed patient needs close observation.

LIFE-THREATENING COMPLICATIONS ASSOCIATED WITH POISONING

Poisoning produces both anticipated and unanticipated complications that can prolong ICU care and decrease survival. Serious complications of poisoning include pulmonary compromise, rhabdomyolysis, compartment syndrome, and anoxic brain injury. Complications such as acute renal or hepatic failure also might prolong an ICU course.

Pulmonary compromise after toxic exposures often develops after several hours or days in the ICU. Pulmonary complications after a toxic exposure include aspiration pneumonitis, ALI, and adult respiratory distress syndrome (ARDS). Aspiration of gastric contents is a common complication after poisoning, especially when a patient's mental status is altered and protective airway reflexes are lost.[11,32] Poisoned patients may aspirate spontaneously while lying unresponsive before being discovered, from stomach dilation secondary to bag-valve-mask ventilation, from GI decontamination procedures such as orogastric lavage, or during insertion of endotracheal or nasogastric tubes.[11,32] In a review of 4562 poisoning admissions, 71 patients clearly has aspiration pneumonitis, giving a rate of 1.6%.[32] In logistic regression analysis older age, a GCS below 15, spontaneous emesis, delayed presentation to the hospital, and ingestion of cyclic antidepressants were associated with aspiration pneumonitis. Not only were the rates of ICU admission and length of stay increased in the patients with aspiration pneumonitis, but mortality was also higher, with a rate of 8.5% compared with 0.4% for those without.

Poisoning may cause global cerebral anoxia from prolonged shock, respiratory failure, or direct toxic metabolic effects. Distinguishing anoxic cerebral injury from reversible encephalopathy can be difficult in poisoned patients. Coma and loss of brainstem reflexes after prolonged, severe cerebral hypoxia indicate a poor prognosis.[39] Although studies are limited in toxicologic patients, newer diagnostic technologies, including diffusion computed tomography, single-photon emission computed tomography, positron emission tomography, cerebral angiography, magnetic resonance imaging, and the use of multimodality evoked potentials, may prove useful in confirming brain death.[1,14,53] Electroencephalography can be particularly misleading in certain overdoses, such as those involving benzodiazepines or barbiturates, in which the lack of brain electrical activity is a direct effect of the ingested xenobiotic. Angiographic imaging via computer tomography or direct arteriography may prove particularly useful in such cases, although such tests can reveal continued blood flow when intracranial hypertension is absent despite severe axonal injury and brain death.[41] Because clinical predictors of outcome may be unreliable when applied to poisoned patients, the diagnosis of brain death should be made cautiously. Cerebral edema is often a secondary effect of global cerebral anoxia, although some xenobiotics have direct cellular effects. Cerebral edema can be a complication of acetaminophen-induced fulminant hepatic failure and the result of direct neuronal injury from salicylate and lead poisoning.[40,54,64] Aggressive ICU care is preferred to treat patients with xenobiotic-induced cerebral injuries.

ALTERNATIVES TO ICU ADMISSION

Placing patients in the ICU solely for observation often is an ineffective use of this expensive resource. Until further clinical studies are available to define patients who are at risk for serious toxicity or life-threatening complications, many poisoned patients will be admitted to the ICU for observation. When information about the xenobiotic, the patient, and the capabilities of the medical unit are all considered, many patients can be safely observed outside the ICU. Table 10–2 presents some items to consider when making disposition decisions.

Alternatives to ICU admission include a medical or pediatric floor bed, an intermediate care unit, a telemetry-monitored bed, a medical psychiatric unit, or an ED observation unit. Capabilities for managing poisoned patients may vary considerably between institutions and in different types of patient care areas. It is essential to understand the capabilities of the unit where a patient is being considered for admission. If the nursing staff is unfamiliar with the potential for rapid deterioration of the patient or the staffing pattern does not allow for close observation, the patient outcome can be severely compromised. For example, it is unrealistic to expect a nurse to manage intravenous fluids, record hourly intake and output measurements, record frequent vital signs, and check hourly urine pH measurements for a salicylate-poisoned patient while caring for eight other patients. ED observation may be an alternative for the care of select poisoned patients.[8,31] These units are capable of frequent monitoring of vital signs, continuous cardiac monitoring, and maintaining a safe environment for suicidal patients.[22] Patients with a low risk of serious toxicity or life-threatening

TABLE 10–2. Considerations for Intensive Care Unit Admission

Xenobiotic Characteristics	**Patient Characteristics**	**Assessing the Capabilities of the Inpatient Unit or Observation Unit**
Are there known serious sequelae (eg, cyclic antidepressant cardiotoxicity)? Can the patient deteriorate rapidly from its toxic effects? Is the onset of toxicity likely to be delayed (eg, sustained-release preparation, slowed GI motility, or delayed toxic effects)? Does the xenobiotic have cardiac effects that will require cardiac monitoring? Is the amount ingested a potentially serious or potentially lethal dose? Is the required or planned therapy unconventional (eg, large doses of atropine for treating overdoses of organic phosphorus insecticides)? Does the therapy have potentially serious adverse effects? Is there insufficient literature to describe the potential human toxic effects? Are potentially serious coingestants likely (must take into account the reliability of the history)?	Does the patient have any signs of serious end-organ toxicity? Is there progression of the end-organ effects? Are laboratory data suggestive of serious toxicity? Are xenobiotic concentrations rising? Is the patient at a high risk for complications requiring ICU intervention? Seizures Unresponsive to verbal stimuli Level of consciousness impaired to the point of potential airway compromise PCO_2 >45 mm Hg Systolic blood pressure <80 mm Hg Cardiac dysrhythmias Abnormal ECG complexes and intervals (QRS duration ≥0.10 seconds; QT prolongation) Does the patient have preexisting medical conditions that could predispose to complications? Chronic alcohol or drug dependence Chronic liver disease Chronic renal failure or insufficiency Heart disease Pregnancy: Is the xenobiotic or the antidote teratogenic? Is the patient suicidal? Is the patient at high risk for complications such as aspiration pneumonitis, anoxic brain injury, rhabdomyolysis, or compartment syndrome?	Does the admitting healthcare team appreciate the potential seriousness of a toxicologic emergency? Is the nursing staff: Familiar with this toxicologic emergency? Familiar with the potential for serious complications? Is the staffing adequate to monitor the patient? What is the ratio of nurses to patients? Are time-consuming nursing activities required and realistic (eg, hourly urine pH assessments or WBI)? Can a safe environment be provided for a suicidal patient? Can a patient have suicide precautions and monitoring with a medical floor bed? Can a one-to-one observer be present in the room with the patient? Can the patient be restrained?

complications who require only observation may be ideal candidates for ED observation units.

Many poisoned patients are placed in the ICU because they are suicide risks. Institutions differ on monitoring policies for suicidal patients not admitted on a psychiatric unit. Other than the ICU, many hospitals cannot provide an alternative for observing high-risk suicidal patients. Less-costly alternatives are available, but they must ensure a safe environment for suicidal patients. An ED observation unit, an intermediate care unit, a medical psychiatric unit, or a one-on-one observer can safely monitor these patients.

Future studies must define prognostic factors for poisoning complications. Patients can then be stratified into high- or low-risk groups. The limitations of current studies prevent generalizing the results to individual patients or certain subgroups. Unfortunately, many current clinical guidelines now being used to ration care may be derived from poorly tested models with no scientific basis and may be motivated by financial concerns. Guidelines should be based on sound evidence so they can provide the best care with less intensive use of health care resources.

CRITERIA FOR SAFE TRANSFER OUT OF THE ICU

After the acute toxic effects have resolved, most patients are safe to transfer out of the ICU. Patients with cyclic antidepressant overdoses were studied to determine when it was safe to discontinue monitoring. Concerns arose from case reports of patients developing sudden death as late as several days after a cyclic antidepressant overdose.[9,42,56] In most cases, delayed complications developed in the setting of continued toxicity evidenced by lethargy or sinus tachycardia. Several subsequent studies demonstrate that dysrhythmias do not occur after signs of toxicity have resolved (ie, CNS and cardiac manifestations).[10,51] The authors of these studies suggested cardiac monitoring for an additional 24 hours after normalization of the ECG and resolution of other signs of continued toxicity such as normalization of the mental status and blood pressure.[10] This additional period of monitoring should occur after discontinuation of all specific forms of therapy, such as serum alkalinization.

Most xenobiotics have not received the level of attention given to cyclic antidepressants, making clinical judgments the only basis for deciding when to discharge a patient from the ICU, pending further research and experience. For example, drug-induced QT interval prolongation may increase the risk of developing torsade de pointes.[33] Cardiac monitoring may be required until other clinical signs of toxicity resolve and the QT interval returns to normal.

The same issues previously mentioned may be pitfalls to a patient's safe discharge from an ICU. Carefully consider discharge decisions about patients exposed to xenobiotics, such as colchicine, with serious delayed clinical effects. Also be mindful that the duration of action of the xenobiotic may be longer than the duration of action of the specific treatment or antidote.

Finally, the patient's suicidal intent must be considered before transfer to a less closely monitored hospital unit. Transfer from the ICU should occur after assessment of suicide risk and other important psychosocial issues. Early involvement of psychiatric services, chemical dependency counseling, and social services can expedite ICU disposition. Disposition and treatment options may be considered at a time when the patient is still medically unstable by interviewing his or her family, friends, and outpatient counselors.

SUMMARY

Acute poisoning challenges medical and nursing staff because of its unpredictable clinical course and unfamiliar therapies. Poisoned patients are especially problematic because their clinical history is incomplete and the medical literature is often limited. These potential unknowns create many uncertainties in management. Because the ICU offers the highest level of skilled staff and modern technology available, most seriously poisoned patients should be admitted there. Whether this is clinically justified or is an effective use of resources for a given patient remains a debated issue because admission of poisoned patients continues to be based mostly on clinical judgment and the best available information.

ACKNOWLEDGEMENT

J. Samuel Pope contributed to this chapter in a previous edition.

REFERENCES

1. Al-Shammri S, Al-Feeli M: Confirmation of brain death using brain radionuclide perfusion imaging technique. *Med Princ Pract.* 2004;13:267-272.
2. Bernal W, Wendon J, Rela M, et al: Use and outcome of liver transplantation in acetaminophen-induced acute liver failure. *Hepatology.* 1998;27:1050-1055.
3. Bird T, Plum F: Recovery from barbiturate overdose coma with a prolonged isoelectric electroencephalogram. *Neurology.* 1968;18:456-460.
4. Boehnert M, Lovejoy F: Value of the QRS duration vs the serum drug level in predicting seizures and ventricular arrhythmias after an acute overdose of tricyclic antidepressants. *N Engl J Med.* 1985;313:474-479.
5. Borys D, Setzer S, Ling L, et al: Acute fluoxetine overdose: a report of 234 cases. *Am J Emerg Med.* 1992;10:115-120.
6. Brett A, Rothchild N, Gray R, Perry M: Predicting the clinical course in intentional drug overdose. *Arch Intern Med.* 1987;147:133-137.
7. Bronstein A, Spyker D, Cantilena J, et al: 2007 Annual Report of the American Association of Poison Control Centers' National Poison Data System (NPDS): 25th Annual Report. *Clin Toxicol.* 2008;46:927-1057.
8. Calello D, Alpern E, McDaniel-Yakscoe M, et al: Observation unit experience for pediatric poison exposures. *J Med Toxicol.* 2009;5:15-19.
9. Callaham M: Admission criteria for tricyclic antidepressant ingestion. *West J Med.* 1982;137:425-429.
10. Callaham M, Kassel D: Epidemiology of fatal tricyclic antidepressant ingestion: implications for management. *Ann Emerg Med.* 1985;14:1-9.
11. Christ A, Arranto CA, Schindler C, et al: Incidence, risk factors, and outcome of aspiration pneumonitis in ICU overdose patients. *Intensive Care Med.* 2006;32:1423-1427.
12. Clemmesen C, Nilsson E: Therapeutic trends in the treatment of barbiturate poisoning: the Scandinavian method. *Clin Pharmacol Ther.* 1961;2:220-229.
13. De Leon AL, Romero-Gutierrez G, Valenzuela CA, Gonzalez-Bravo FE: Simplified PRISM III score and outcome in the pediatric intensive care unit. *Pediatr Int.* 2005;47:80-83.
14. de Tourtchaninoff M, Hantson P, Mahieu P, Guerit J: Brain death diagnosis in misleading conditions. *QJM* 1999;92:407-414.
15. Du Toit P, Muller F, Van Tonder W, Ungerer M: Experience with the intensive care management of organophosphate insecticide poisoning. *S Afr Med J.* 1981;60:227-229.
16. Durward A, Guerguerian A, Lefebvre M, Shemie S: Massive diltiazem overdose treated with extracorporeal membrane oxygenation. *Pediatr Crit Care Med.* 2003;4:372-376.
17. Elk J, Linton D, Potgieter P: Treatment of acute self-poisoning in a respiratory intensive care unit. *S Afr Med J.* 1987;72:532-534.
18. Evans JS, Oram MP: Neurological recovery after prolonged verapamil-induced cardiac arrest. *Anaesth Intensive Care.* 1999;27:653-655.
19. Falkland M, McMorrow J, McKeown R: Bupropion SR in Overdose: subsidized poisoning. *J Toxicol Clin Toxicol.* 2002;40:339-340.
20. Franc-Law J, Rossignol M, Vernec A, et al: Poisoning-induced acute atraumatic compartment syndrome. *Am J Emerg Med.* 2000;18:616-621.
21. Golsousidis H, Kokkas V: Use of 19,590 mg of atropine during 24 days of treatment after a case of unusually severe parathion poisoning. *Hum Toxicol.* 1985;4:339-340.
22. Graff L, Zun L, Leikin J, et al: Emergency department observation beds improve patient care: Society for Academic Emergency Medicine debate. *Ann Emerg Med.* 1992;21:967-975.

23. Grmec S, Gasparovic V: Comparison of APACHE II, MEES and Glasgow Coma Scale in patients with nontraumatic coma for prediction of mortality. Acute Physiology and Chronic Health Evaluation. Mainz Emergency Evaluation System. *Crit Care.* 2001;5:19-23.
24. Gunawardana RH, Abeywarna C: Intensive care utilisation following attempted suicide through self-poisoning. *Ceylon Med J.* 1997;42:18-20.
25. Hadian M, Pinsky M: Functional hemodynamic monitoring. *Curr Opin Crit Care.* 2007;13:318-323.
26. Hamad A, Al-Ghadban A, Carvounis C, et al: Predicting the need for medical intensive care monitoring in drug-overdosed patients. *J Intensive Care Med.* 2000;15:321-328.
27. Henderson A, Wright M, Pond SM: Experience with 732 acute overdose patients admitted to an intensive care unit over six years. *Med J Aust.* 1993;158:28-30.
28. Hendra TJ, Gerrish SP, Forrest ARW: Lesson of the week: fatal methadone overdose. *Br Med J.* 1996;313:481-482.
29. Heyman EN, LoCastro DE, Gouse LH, et al: Intentional drug overdose: predictors of clinical course in the intensive care unit. *Heart Lung.* 1996;25:246-252.
30. Holzer M, Sterz F, Schoerkhuber W, et al: Successful resuscitation of a verapamil-intoxicated patient with percutaneous cardiopulmonary bypass. *Crit Care Med.* 1999;27:2818-2823.
31. Hostetler B, Leikin J, Timmons J, et al: Patterns of use of an emergency department-based observation unit. *Am J Ther.* 2002;9:499-502.
32. Isbister G, Downes F, Sibbritt D, et al: Aspiration pneumonitis in an overdose population: frequency, predictors, and outcomes. *Crit Care Med.* 2004;32:88-93.
33. Kao L, Furbee R: Drug-induced Q-T prolongation. *Med Clin North Am.* 2005;89:1125-1144.
34. Knaus WA, Draper EA, Wagner DP, Zimmerman JE: APACHE II: a severity of disease classification system. *Crit Care Med.* Oct 1985;13:818-829.
35. Lacroix J, Gaudreault P, Gauthier M: Admission to a pediatric intensive care unit for poisoning: a review of 105 cases. *Crit Care Med.* 1989;17:748-750.
36. Lane AS, Woodward AC, Goldman MR: Massive propranolol overdose poorly responsive to pharmacologic therapy: use of the intra-aortic balloon pump. *Ann Emerg Med.* 1987;16:1381-1383.
37. LeBlanc F, Benson B, Gilg A: A severe organophosphate poisoning requiring the use of an atropine drip. *J Toxicol Clin Toxicol.* 1986;24:69-76.
38. Lee P, Tai D: Clinical features of patients with acute organophosphate poisoning requiring intensive care. *Intensive Care Med.* 2001;27:694-699.
39. Levy DE, Bates D, Caronna JJ, et al: Prognosis in nontraumatic coma. *Ann Intern Med.* 1981;94:293-301.
40. Manton WI, Kirkpatrick JB, Cook JP: Does the choroid plexus really protect the brain from lead? *Lancet.* 1984;2:351.
41. Marrache F, Megarbane B, Pirnay S, et al: Difficulties in assessing brain death in a case of benzodiazepine poisoning with persistent cerebral blood flow. *Hum Exp Toxicol.* 2004;23:503-505.
42. McAlpine S, Calabro J, Robinson M, Burkle F: Late death in tricyclic antidepressant overdose revisited. *Ann Emerg Med.* 1986;15:1349-1352.
43. McVey FK, Corke CF: Extracorporeal circulation in the management of massive propranolol overdose. *Anaesthesia.* 1991;46:744-746.
44. Minocha A, Spyker D: Acute overdose with sustained release drug formulations. *Med Toxicol.* 1986;1:300-307.
45. Mitchell I, Bihari D, Chang R, et al: Earlier identification of patients at risk from acetaminophen-induced acute liver failure. *Crit Care Med.* 1998;26:279-284.
46. Muhlberg W, Becher K, Heppner HJ, et al: Acute poisoning in old and very old patients: a longitudinal retrospective study of 5883 patients in a toxicological intensive care unit. *Zeitschrift fur Gerontologie und Geriatrie.* 2005;38:182-189.
47. Murphy G, Wetzel R: Family history of suicidal behavior among suicide attempters. *J Nerv Mental Dis.* 1982;170:86-90.
48. Niemann J, Bessen H, Rothstein R, Laks M: Electrocardiographic criteria for tricyclic antidepressant cardiotoxicity. *Am J Cardiol.* 1986;57:1154-1159.
49. Orr D, Bramble M: Tricyclic antidepressant poisoning and prolonged external cardiac massage during asystole. *Br Med J.* 1981;283:1107-1108.
50. Ostermann ME, Young B, Sibbald WJ, Nicolle MW: Coma mimicking brain death following baclofen overdose. *Intensive Care Med.* 2000;26:1144-1146.
51. Pentel P, Sioris L: Incidence of late arrhythmias following tricyclic antidepressant overdose. *Clin Toxicol.* 1981;18:543-548.
52. Powner D: Drug-associated isoelectric EEGs. A hazard in brain death certification. *JAMA.* 1976;236:1123.
53. Qureshi A, Kirmani J, Xavier A, Siddiqui A: Computed tomographic angiography for diagnosis of brain death. *Neurology.* 2004;62:652-653.
54. Reed JR, Palmisano PA: Central nervous system salicylate. *Clin Toxicol.* 1975;8:623-631.
55. Ron A, Aronne L, Kalb P, et al: The therapeutic efficacy of critical care units. *Arch Intern Med.* 1989;149:338-341.
56. Sedal L, Korman M, Williams P, et al: Overdosage of tricyclic antidepressants: a report of two deaths and a prospective study of 24 patients. *Med J Aust.* 1972;2:74-79.
57. Shadnia S, Darabi D, Pajoumand A, et al: A simplified acute physiology score in the prediction of acute organophosphate poisoning outcome in an intensive care unit. *Hum Exp Toxicol.* 2007;26:623-627.
58. Southall D, Kilpatrick S: Imipramine poisoning: survival of a child after prolonged cardiac massage. *Br Med J.* 1974;4:508.
59. Spiller H, Meyers A, Ziemba T, Riley M: Delayed onset of cardiac arrhythmias from sustained-release verapamil. *Ann Emerg Med.* 1991;20:201-203.
60. Spiller H, Morse S: Fluoxetine ingestion: a one year retrospective study. *Vet Hum Toxicol.* 1990;32:153-155.
61. Strand K, Flaatten H: Severity scoring in the ICU: a review. *Acta Anaesthesiologica Scandinavica.* 2008;52:467-478.
62. Strom J, Thisted B, Krantz T, Bredgaard Sorensen M: Self-poisoning treated in an ICU: drug pattern, acute mortality and short term survival. *Acta Anaesthesiol Scand* 1986;30:148-153.
63. Subbe CP, Kruger M, Rutherford P, Gemmel L: Validation of a modified Early Warning Score in medical admissions [see comment]. *QJM* 2001;94:521-526.
64. Sutherland LR, Muller P, Lewis DR: Massive cerebral edema associated with fulminant hepatic failure in acetaminophen overdose. *Am J Gastroenterol.* 1981;76:446-448.
65. Tay SY, Tai DY, Seow E, Wang YT: Patients admitted to an intensive care unit for poisoning. *Ann Acad Med Singapore.* 1998;27:347-352.
66. van Dijk GW, Vos PE, Eurelings M, et al: [Totally paralyzed or brain dead?]. *Nederlands Tijdschrift voor Geneeskunde.* 2001;145:2513-2516.
67. Watson W, Steele M, Muelleman R, Rush M: Opioid toxicity recurrence after an initial response to naloxone. *J Toxicol Clin Toxicol.* 1998;36:11-17.
68. White A: Overdose of tricyclic antidepressants associated with absent brain-stem reflexes. *Can Med Assoc J.* 1988;139:133-134.
69. Wortzman D, Grunfeld A: Delayed absorption following enteric-coated aspirin overdose. *Ann Emerg Med.* 1987;16:434-436.
70. Yang K, Dantzker D: Reversible brain death: a manifestation of amitriptyline overdose. *Chest.* 1991;99:1037-1038.
71. Zimmerman J, Knaus W, Judson J, et al: Patient selection for intensive care: a comparison of New Zealand and United States hospitals. *Crit Care Med.* 1988;16:318-326.

PART B

THE FUNDAMENTAL PRINCIPLES OF MEDICAL TOXICOLOGY

SECTION 1 BIOCHEMICAL AND MOLECULAR BASIS

CHAPTER 11
CHEMICAL PRINCIPLES

Stephen J. Traub and Lewis S. Nelson

Chemistry is the science of matter; it encompasses the structure, physical properties, and reactivities of atoms and their compounds. In many respects, toxicology is the science of the interactions of matter with physiologic entities. Chemistry and toxicology thereby are intimately linked. The study of the principles of inorganic, organic, and biologic chemistry offer important insight into the mechanisms and clinical manifestations of xenobiotics and poisoning, respectively. This chapter reviews many of these tenets and provides relevance to the current practice of medical toxicology.

THE STRUCTURE OF MATTER

BASIC STRUCTURE

Matter includes the substances of which everything is made. *Elements* are the foundation of matter, and all matter is made from one or more of the known elements. An *atom* is the smallest quantity of a given element that retains the properties of that element. Atoms consist of a nucleus, incorporating protons and neutrons, coupled with its orbiting electrons. The *atomic number* is the number of protons in the nucleus of an atom, and is a whole number that is unique for each element. Thus, elements with 6 protons are always carbon, and all forms of carbon have exactly 6 protons. However, although the vast majority of carbon nuclei have 6 neutrons in addition to the protons, accounting for an *atomic mass* (i.e., protons plus neutrons) of 12 (^{12}C), a small proportion of naturally occurring carbon nuclei, called *isotopes*, have 8 neutrons and a mass number of 14 (^{14}C). This is the reason that the *atomic weight* of carbon displayed on the periodic table is 12.011, and not 12, as it actually represents the average atomic masses of all isotopes found in nature weighted by their frequency of occurrence. Moreover, ^{14}C is actually a *radioisotope*, which is an isotope with an unstable nucleus that emits radiation (particles or rays) until it achieves a stable state (Chap. 133). The atomic weight, measured in grams per mole (g/mol), also indicates the molar mass of the element. That is, in 1 atomic weight (12.011 g for carbon) there is 1 mole of atoms (6.023×10^{23} atoms).

Elements combine chemically to form *compounds*, which generally have physical and chemical properties that differ from those of the constituent elements. The elements in a compound can only be separated by chemical means that destroy the original compound, as occurs during the burning (ie, oxidation) of a hydrocarbon, which releases the carbon as carbon dioxide. This important property differentiates compounds from *mixtures*, which are combinations of elements or compounds that can be separated by physical means. For example, this occurs during the distillation of petroleum into its hydrocarbon components or the evaporation of seawater to leave sodium chloride. With notable exceptions, such as the elemental forms of many metals or halogens (eg, Cl_2), most xenobiotics are compounds or mixtures.

Dimitri Mendeleev, a Russian chemist in the mid-19th century, recognized that when all of the known elements were arranged in order of atomic weight, certain patterns of reactivity became apparent. The result of his work was the Periodic Table of the Elements (Fig. 11–1), which, with some minor alterations, is still an essential tool today. All of the currently recognized elements are represented; those heavier than uranium are not known to occur in nature. Many of the symbols used to identify the elements refer to the Latin name of the element. For example, silver is Ag, for argentum, and mercury is Hg, for hydrargyrum, literally "silver water."

The reason for the periodicity of the table relates to the electrons that circle the nucleus in discrete orbitals. Although the details of quantum mechanics and electronic configuration are complex, it is important to review some aspects in order to predict chemical reactivity. Orbitals, or quantum shells, represent the energy levels in which electrons may exist around the nucleus. The orbitals are identified by various schemes, but the maximum number of electrons each orbital may contain is calculated as $2x^2$, where x represents the numerical rank order of the orbital. Thus, the first orbital may contain 2 electrons, the second orbital may contain 8, the third may contain 18, and so on. However, the outermost shell (designated by s, p, d nomenclature) of each orbital may only contain up to 8 electrons. This is irrelevant through element 20, calcium, because there is no need to fill the third-level or d shells. Even though the third orbital may contain 18 electrons, once 8 are present the 4s electrons dip below the 3d electrons in energy and this shell begins to fill. This occurs at element 21, scandium, and accounts for its chemical properties and those of the other transition elements. Also, because the inert gas elements, which are also known as noble gases, have complete outermost orbitals, they are unreactive under standard conditions. Transition elements are chemically defined as elements that form at least one ion with a partially filled subshell of d electrons.

In general, only electrons in unfilled shells, or *valence shells*, are involved in chemical reactions. This property relates to the fact that the most stable form of an element occurs when the configuration of its valence shell resembles that of the nearest noble gas, found in group 0 on the periodic table. This state can be obtained through the gaining, losing, or sharing of electrons with other elements and is the basis for virtually all chemical reactions.

INORGANIC CHEMISTRY

THE PERIODIC TABLE

Chemical Reactivity Broadly, the periodic table is divided into metals and nonmetals. Metals, in their pure form, are typically malleable solids that conduct electricity, whereas nonmetals are usually dull, fragile,

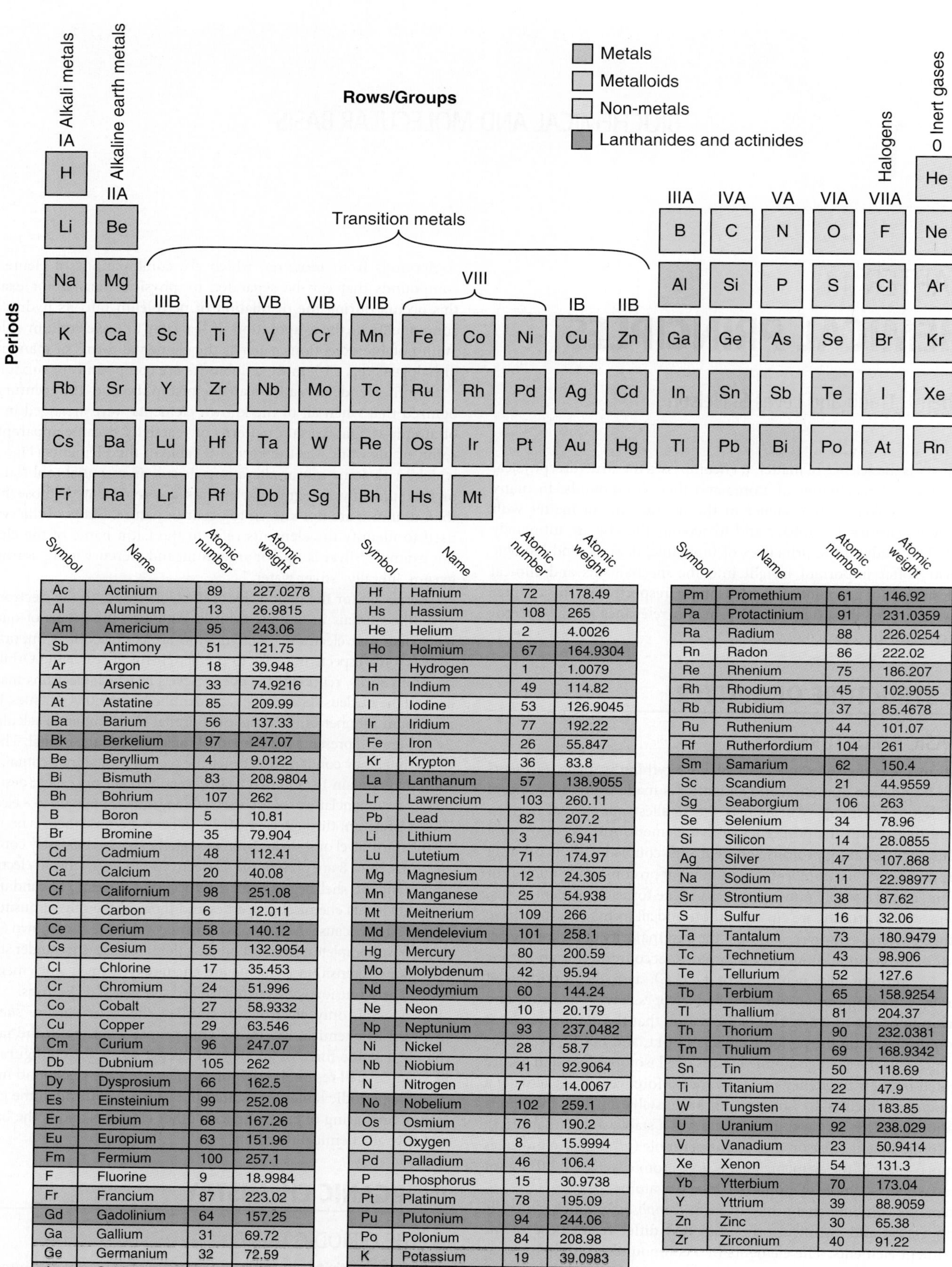

Symbol	Name	Atomic number	Atomic weight
Ac	Actinium	89	227.0278
Al	Aluminum	13	26.9815
Am	Americium	95	243.06
Sb	Antimony	51	121.75
Ar	Argon	18	39.948
As	Arsenic	33	74.9216
At	Astatine	85	209.99
Ba	Barium	56	137.33
Bk	Berkelium	97	247.07
Be	Beryllium	4	9.0122
Bi	Bismuth	83	208.9804
Bh	Bohrium	107	262
B	Boron	5	10.81
Br	Bromine	35	79.904
Cd	Cadmium	48	112.41
Ca	Calcium	20	40.08
Cf	Californium	98	251.08
C	Carbon	6	12.011
Ce	Cerium	58	140.12
Cs	Cesium	55	132.9054
Cl	Chlorine	17	35.453
Cr	Chromium	24	51.996
Co	Cobalt	27	58.9332
Cu	Copper	29	63.546
Cm	Curium	96	247.07
Db	Dubnium	105	262
Dy	Dysprosium	66	162.5
Es	Einsteinium	99	252.08
Er	Erbium	68	167.26
Eu	Europium	63	151.96
Fm	Fermium	100	257.1
F	Fluorine	9	18.9984
Fr	Francium	87	223.02
Gd	Gadolinium	64	157.25
Ga	Gallium	31	69.72
Ge	Germanium	32	72.59
Au	Gold	79	196.9665
Hf	Hafnium	72	178.49
Hs	Hassium	108	265
He	Helium	2	4.0026
Ho	Holmium	67	164.9304
H	Hydrogen	1	1.0079
In	Indium	49	114.82
I	Iodine	53	126.9045
Ir	Iridium	77	192.22
Fe	Iron	26	55.847
Kr	Krypton	36	83.8
La	Lanthanum	57	138.9055
Lr	Lawrencium	103	260.11
Pb	Lead	82	207.2
Li	Lithium	3	6.941
Lu	Lutetium	71	174.97
Mg	Magnesium	12	24.305
Mn	Manganese	25	54.938
Mt	Meitnerium	109	266
Md	Mendelevium	101	258.1
Hg	Mercury	80	200.59
Mo	Molybdenum	42	95.94
Nd	Neodymium	60	144.24
Ne	Neon	10	20.179
Np	Neptunium	93	237.0482
Ni	Nickel	28	58.7
Nb	Niobium	41	92.9064
N	Nitrogen	7	14.0067
No	Nobelium	102	259.1
Os	Osmium	76	190.2
O	Oxygen	8	15.9994
Pd	Palladium	46	106.4
P	Phosphorus	15	30.9738
Pt	Platinum	78	195.09
Pu	Plutonium	94	244.06
Po	Polonium	84	208.98
K	Potassium	19	39.0983
Pr	Praseodymium	59	140.9077
Pm	Promethium	61	146.92
Pa	Protactinium	91	231.0359
Ra	Radium	88	226.0254
Rn	Radon	86	222.02
Re	Rhenium	75	186.207
Rh	Rhodium	45	102.9055
Rb	Rubidium	37	85.4678
Ru	Ruthenium	44	101.07
Rf	Rutherfordium	104	261
Sm	Samarium	62	150.4
Sc	Scandium	21	44.9559
Sg	Seaborgium	106	263
Se	Selenium	34	78.96
Si	Silicon	14	28.0855
Ag	Silver	47	107.868
Na	Sodium	11	22.98977
Sr	Strontium	38	87.62
S	Sulfur	16	32.06
Ta	Tantalum	73	180.9479
Tc	Technetium	43	98.906
Te	Tellurium	52	127.6
Tb	Terbium	65	158.9254
Tl	Thallium	81	204.37
Th	Thorium	90	232.0381
Tm	Thulium	69	168.9342
Sn	Tin	50	118.69
Ti	Titanium	22	47.9
W	Tungsten	74	183.85
U	Uranium	92	238.029
V	Vanadium	23	50.9414
Xe	Xenon	54	131.3
Yb	Ytterbium	70	173.04
Y	Yttrium	39	88.9059
Zn	Zinc	30	65.38
Zr	Zirconium	40	91.22

FIGURE 11–1. The Periodic Table of the Elements.

nonconductive compounds (C, N, P, O, S, Se, halogens). The metals are found on the left side of the periodic table, and account for the majority of the elements, whereas the nonmetals are on the right side. Separating the two groups are the metalloids, which fall on a jagged line starting with boron (B, Si, Ge, As, Sb, Te, At). These elements have chemical properties that are intermediate between the metals and the nonmetals. Each column of elements is termed a family or group, and each row is a period. Although conceived and organized in periods, trends in the chemical reactivity, and therefore toxicity, typically exist within the groups.

The ability of any particular element to produce toxicologic effects relates directly to one or more of its many physicochemical properties, which may, to some extent, be predicted by their location on the periodic table. For example, the substitution of arsenate for phosphate in the mitochondrial production of adenosine triphosphate (ATP) creates adenosine diphosphate monoarsenate (Chap. 12). Because this compound is unstable and not useful as an energy source, energy production by the cell fails; in this manner arsenic interferes with oxidative phosphorylation. Similarly, the existence of an interrelationship between Ca^{2+} and either Mg^{2+} or Ba^{2+} is predictable, although the actual effects are not, that is, under most circumstances Mg^{2+} is a Ca^{2+} antagonist, and patients with hypermagnesemia present with neuromuscular weakness caused by blockade of myocyte calcium channels. Alternatively, Ba^{2+} mimics Ca^{2+} and closes Ca^{2+}-dependent K^+ channels in myocytes, producing life-threatening hypokalemia. Additionally, the physiologic relationship among lithium (Li^+), potassium (K^+), and sodium (Na^+) is consistent with their chemical similarities (all alkali metals in Group IA). However, the clinical similarity between thallium (thallous) ion (Tl^+) and K^+ is not predictable. Other than their monovalent nature (ie, +1 charge), it is difficult to predict the substitution of Tl^+ (Group IIIA, Period 6) for K^+ (Group IA, Period 4) in membrane ion channel functions, until the similarity of their ionic radii is known (Tl^+, 1.47 Å; K^+, 1.33 Å).

Alkali and Alkaline Earth Metals Alkali metals (Group IA: Li, Na, K, Rb, Cs, Fr) and hydrogen (not an alkali metal on earth) have a single outer valence electron and lose this electron easily to form compounds with a valence of 1+. The alkaline earth metals (Group IIA: Be, Mg, Ca, Sr, Ba, Ra) (between the alkali and rare earth, Group IIIB) readily lose 2 electrons, and their cations have a 2+ charge. In their metallic form, members of both of these groups react violently with water to liberate strongly basic solutions accounting for their group names ($2Na^0 + 2H_2O \rightarrow 2NaOH + H_2$). The soluble ionic forms of sodium, potassium, or calcium, which are critical to survival, also produce life-threatening symptoms following excessive intake (Chap. 16). Xenobiotics may interfere with the physiologic role of these key electrolytes. Li^+ may mimic K^+ and enter neurons through K^+ channels, following which it serves as a poor substrate for the repolarizing Na^+-K^+-ATPase. Thus, Li^+ interferes with cellular K^+ homeostasis and alters neuronal repolarization accounting for the neuroexcitability manifesting as tremor. Similarly, as noted previously, the molecular effects of Mg^{2+} and Ba^{2+} may supplant those of Ca^{2+}. More commonly, though, the consequential toxicities ascribed to alkali or alkaline earth salts actually relate to the anionic component. In the case of NaOH or $Ca(OH)_2$, it is a hydroxide anion (not the hydroxyl radical), while it is a CN^- anion in patients poisoned with potassium cyanide (KCN).

Transition Metals Unlike the alkali and alkaline earth metals, most other metallic elements are neither soluble nor reactive. This includes the transition metals (Group IB to VIIIB), a large group that contains several ubiquitous metals such as iron (Fe) and copper (Cu). These elements, in their metallic form, are widely used both in industrial and household applications because of their high tensile strength, density, and melting point, which is partly a result of their ability to delocalize the electrons in the d orbital throughout the metallic lattice. Transition metals also form brightly colored salts that find widespread applications including pigments for paints or fireworks. However, the ionic forms, unlike the metallic form, of these elements are typically highly reactive and toxicologically important. Transition elements are chemically defined as elements which form at least one ion with a partially filled subshell of d electrons. Because the transition metals have partially filled valence shells, they are capable of obtaining several, usually positive, oxidation states. This important mechanism explains the role of transition metals in redox reactions generally as electron acceptors (see Reduction-Oxidation). This reactivity is used by living organisms in various physiologic catalytic and coordination roles, such as at the active sites of enzymes and in hemoglobin, respectively. Expectedly, the substantial reactivity of these transition metal elements is highly associated with cellular injury caused by several mechanisms, including the generation of reactive oxygen species (Fig. 11–2). For example, manganese ion exposure is implicated in the free radical damage of the basal ganglia causing parkinsonism.

Heavy Metals *Heavy metal* is often loosely used to describe all metals of toxicologic significance, but in reality, the term should be reserved to describe only those metals in the lower period of the periodic table, particularly those with atomic masses greater than 200. The chemical properties and toxicologic predilection of this group vary among the elements, but their unifying toxicologic mechanism is electrophilic interference with nucleophilic sulfhydryl-containing enzymes. Some of the heavy metals also participate in the generation of free radicals through Fenton chemistry (Fig. 11–2). The likely determinant of the specific toxicologic effects produced by each metal is the tropism for various physiologic systems, enzymes, or microenvironments; thus the lipophilicity, water solubility, ionic size, and other physicochemical parameters are undoubtedly critical. Also, because the chemistry of metals varies dramatically based on the chemical form (ie, organic, inorganic, or elemental), as well as the charge on the metal ion, prediction of the clinical effects of a particular metal is often difficult.

Mercury. Elemental mercury (Hg^0) is unique in that it is the only metal that exists in liquid form at room temperature, and as such is capable of creating solid solutions, or amalgams, with other metals. Although it is relatively innocuous if ingested as a liquid, it is readily volatilized (ie, high vapor pressure), transforming it into a significant pulmonary mucosal irritant upon inhalation. In addition, this change in the route of exposure raises its systemic bioavailability. Absorbed, or incorporated, Hg^0 undergoes biotransformation in the erythrocyte and brain to the mercuric (Hg^{2+}) form, which has a high affinity for sulfhydryl-containing molecules including proteins. This causes a depletion of glutathione in organs such as the kidney, and also initiates lipid peroxidation. The mercurous form (Hg^+) is considerably less toxic than the mercuric form, perhaps because of its reduced water solubility. Organic

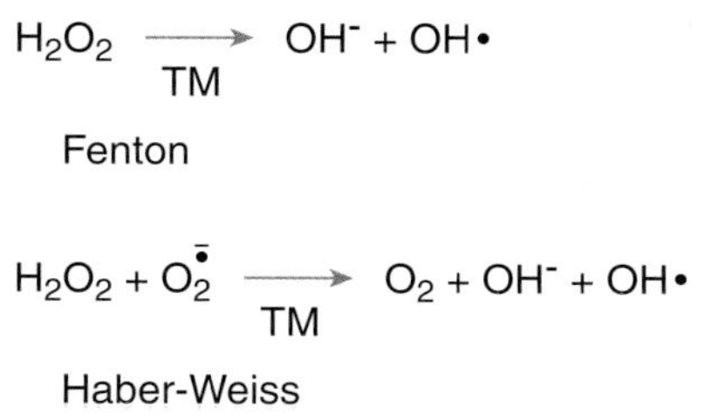

$$H_2O_2 \xrightarrow[TM]{} OH^- + OH\bullet$$

Fenton

$$H_2O_2 + O_2^{\bar{\bullet}} \xrightarrow[TM]{} O_2 + OH^- + OH\bullet$$

Haber-Weiss

FIGURE 11–2. The Fenton and Haber-Weiss reactions, which are the two most important mechanisms to generate hydroxyl radicals, are both mediated by transition metals (TM). Iron (Fe^{2+}) and copper (Cu^+) are typical transition metals.

mercurial compounds, such as methylmercury and dimethylmercury, are environmentally formed by anaerobic bacteria containing the methylating agent methylcobalamin, a vitamin B_{12} analog (Chap. 96).

Thallium. Another toxicologically important member of the heavy metal group is thallium. Metallic thallium is used in the production of electronic equipment and is itself minimally toxic. Thallium ions, however, have physicochemical properties that most closely mimic potassium ions, allowing them to participate in, and potentially alter, the various physiologic activities related to potassium. This property is clinically used during a thallium-stress test to assess for myocardial ischemia or infarction. Because ischemic myocardial cells lack adequate energy for normal Na^+-K^+-ATPase function, they cannot exchange sodium for potassium (or in this scenario radioactive thallium), producing a "cold spot" in the ischemic areas on cardiac scintigraphy (Chap. 100).

Lead. Although lead is not very abundant in the Earth's crust (only 0.002%), exposure may occur during the smelting process or from one of its diverse commercial applications. Most of the useful lead compounds are inorganic plumbous (Pb^{2+}) salts, but plumbic (Pb^{4+}) compounds are also used. The Pb^{2+} compounds are typically ionizable, releasing Pb^{2+} when dissolved in a solvent, such as water. Pb^{2+} ions are absorbed in place of Ca^{2+} ions by the gastrointestinal tract and replace Ca^{2+} in certain physiologic processes. This mechanism is implicated in the neurotoxic effect of lead ions. Pb^{2+} compounds tend to be covalent compounds that do not ionize in water. However, some of the Pb^{4+} compounds are oxidants. Although elemental lead is not itself toxic, it rapidly develops a coating of toxic lead oxide or lead carbonate on exposure to air or water (Chap. 94).

Metalloids Although the metalloids (B, Si, Ge, As, Sb, Te, At) share many physical properties with the metals, they are differentiated because of their propensity to form compounds with both metals and the nonmetals carbon, nitrogen, or oxygen. Thus, metalloids may be either oxidized or reduced in chemical reactions.

Arsenic. Toxicologically important inorganic arsenic compounds exist in either the pentavalent arsenite (As^{5+}) form or the trivalent arsenate (As^{3+}) form. The reduced water solubility of the arsenate compounds, such as arsenic pentoxide, accounts for its limited clinical toxicity when compared to trivalent arsenic trioxide. The trivalent form of arsenic is primarily a nucleophilic toxin, binding sulfhydryl groups and interfering with enzymatic function (Chaps. 12 and 88).

Nonmetals The nonmetals (C, N, P, O, S, Se, halogens) are highly electronegative and, unlike the metals, may be toxic in either their compounded or their elemental form. The nonmetals with large electronegativity, such as O_2 or Cl_2, generally oxidize other elements in chemical reactions. Those with lesser electronegativity, such as C, behave as reducing agents.

Halogens. In their highly reactive elemental form, which contains a covalent dimer of halogen atoms, the halogens (F, Cl, Br, I, At) carry the suffix *-ine* (eg, Cl_2, chlorine). Halogens require the addition of one electron to complete their valence shell; thus, halogens are strong oxidizing agents. Because they are highly electronegative, they form halides (eg, Cl^-, chloride) by abstracting electrons from less electronegative elements. Thus, the halogen ions, in their stable ionic form, generally carry a charge of −1. The halides, although much less reactive than their respective elemental forms, are reducing agents. The hydrogen halides (eg, HCl, hydrogen chloride) are gases under standard conditions, but they ionize when dissolved in aqueous solution to form the hydrohalidic acids (eg, HCl, hydrochloric acid). All hydrogen halides except HF (hydrogen fluoride) ionize nearly completely in water to release H^+ and are considered *strong acids.* Because of its small ionic radius, lack of charge dispersion, and intense electronegativity, HF ionizes poorly and is a *weak acid.* This specific property of HF has important toxicologic implications (Chap. 105).

Group 0: Inert Gases Inert gases (He, Ne, Ar, Kr, Xe, Rn), also known as noble gases, maintain completed valence shells and are thus entirely unreactive except under extreme experimental conditions. However, despite their lack of chemical reactivity, the inert gases are toxicologically important as simple asphyxiants. That is, because they displace ambient oxygen from a confined space, consequential hypoxia may occur, and the expected warning signs may be completely absent (Chap. 124). During high-concentration exposure, inert gases may produce anesthesia, and xenon is used as an anesthetic agent. Radon, although a chemically unreactive gas, is radioactive, and prolonged exposure is associated with the development of lung cancer.

BONDS

Electrons are not generally shared evenly between atoms when they form a compound. Instead, unless the bond is between the same elements, as in Cl_2, one of the elements exerts a larger attraction for the shared electrons. The degree to which an element draws the shared electron is determined by the *electronegativity* of the element (Fig. 11–3). The electronegativity of each element was catalogued by Linus Pauling and relates to the ionic radius, or the distance between the orbiting electron and the nucleus, and the shielding effects of the inner electrons. The electronegativity rises toward the right of the periodic table, corresponding with the expected charge obtained on an element when it forms a bond. Fluoride ion has the highest electronegativity of all elements, which explains many of its serious toxicologic properties.

Several types of bonds exist between elements when they form compounds. When one element gains valence electrons and another loses them, the resulting elements are charged and attract one another in an *ionic,* or *electrovalent,* bond. An example is NaCl, or table salt, in which the electronegativity difference between the elements is 1.9, or greater than the electronegativity of the sodium (see subsequent paragraphs and Fig. 11–3). Thus, the chloride wrests control of the electrons in this bond. In solid form, ionic compounds exist in a crystalline lattice, but when put into solution, as in the serum, the elements may separate and form charged particles, or *ions* (Na^+ and Cl^-). The ions are stable in solution, however, because their valence shells contain 8 electrons and are complete. The properties of ions differ from both the original atom from which the ion is derived and the noble gas with which it shares electronic structure.

It is important to recognize that when a mole of a salt, such as NaCl (molecular weight 58.45 g/mol), is put in aqueous solution, 2 moles of particles result. This is because NaCl essentially ionizes fully in water; that is, it produces 1 mole of Na^+ (23 g/mol) and 1 mole of Cl^- (35.45 g/mol). For salts that do not ionize completely, less than the

IA	IIA		IIIA	IVA	VA	VIA	VIIA	0
H 2.20								He –
Li 0.98	Be 1.57		B 2.04	C 2.55	N 3.04	O 3.44	F 3.98	Ne –
Na 0.93	Mg 1.31		Al 1.61	Si 1.90	P 2.19	S 2.58	Cl 3.16	Ar –
K 0.82	Ca 1.00				As 3.18	Se 2.55	Br 2.96	Kr –

FIGURE 11–3. Electronegativity of the common elements. Note that the inert gases are not reactive and thus do not have electronegativity.

intrinsic number of moles are released and the actual quantity liberated can be predicted based on the defined solubility of the compound, or the solubility product constant (K_{sp}). For ions that carry more than a single charge, the term *equivalent* is often used to denote the number of moles of other particles to which one mole of the substance will bind. Thus, an equivalent of calcium ion will typically bind 2 moles (or equivalents) of chloride ions (which are monovalent) because calcium ions are divalent. Alternatively stated, a 10% calcium chloride ($CaCl_2$) aqueous solution contains approximately 1.4 mEq/mL or 0.7 mmol/mL of Ca^{2+}.

Compounds formed by 2 elements of similar electronegativity have little ionic character because there is little impetus for separation of charge. Instead, these elements share pairs of valence electrons, a process known as *covalence*. The resultant molecule contains a *covalent bond*, which is typically very strong and generally requires a high-energy chemical reaction to disrupt it. There is wide variation in the extent to which the electrons are shared between the participants of a covalent bond, and the physicochemical and toxicologic properties of any particular molecule are in part determined by its nature. Rarely is sharing truly symmetric, as in oxygen (O_2) or chlorine (Cl_2). If sharing is asymmetric and the electrons thus exist to a greater degree around one of the component atoms, the bond is *polar*. However, the presence of a polar bond does not mean that the compound is polar. For example, methane contains a carbon atom that shares its valence electrons with 4 hydrogen atoms, in which there is a small charge separation between the elements (electronegativity [EN] difference = 0.40). Furthermore, because the molecule is configured in a tetrahedral formation, there is no notable polarity to the compound; this compound is *nonpolar*. The lack of polarity suggests that methane molecules have little affinity for other methane molecules and they are held together only by weak intermolecular bonds. This explains why methane is highly volatile under standard conditions.

Because the EN differences between hydrogen (EN = 2.20) and oxygen (EN = 3.44) are greater (EN difference = 1.24), the electrons in the HO bonds in water are drawn toward the oxygen atom, giving it a partial negative charge and the hydrogen a partial positive charge. Furthermore, because H_2O is angular, not linear or symmetric, water is a polar molecule. Water molecules are held together by hydrogen bonds, which are stronger than other intermolecular bonds (for example, van der Waals forces; see later). These hydrogen bonds have sufficient energy to open many ionic bonds and *solvate* the ions. In this process, the polar ends of the water molecule surround the charged particles of the dissolved salt. Thus, because there is little similarity between the nonpolar methane and the polar water molecules, methane is not water soluble. Similarly, salts cannot be solvated by nonpolar compounds, and thus a salt, such as sodium chloride, cannot dissolve in a nonpolar solvent, such as carbon tetrachloride.

Alternatively, the stability and irreversibility of the bond between an organic phosphorus insecticide and the cholinesterase enzyme are a result of covalent phosphorylation of an amino acid at the active site of the enzyme. The resulting bond is essentially irreversible in the absence of another chemical reaction.

Compounds may share multiple pairs of electrons. For example, the two carbon atoms in acetylene (HC≡CH) share three pairs of electrons between them, and each shares one pair with its own hydrogen. Carbon and nitrogen share three pairs of electrons in forming cyanide ($C{\equiv}N^-$), making this bond very stable and accounting for the large number of xenobiotics capable of liberating cyanide. Complex ions are covalently bonded groups of elements that behave as a single element. For example, hydroxide (OH^-) and sulfate (SO_4^{2-}) form sodium salts as if they were simply the ion of a single element (such as chloride).

Noncovalent bonds, such as hydrogen or ionic bonds, are important in the interaction between ligands and receptors, and between ion channels and enzymes. These are low-energy bonds and easily broken. Van der Waals forces, also known as London dispersion forces, are intermolecular forces that arise from induced dipoles as a consequence of nonuniform distribution of the molecular electron cloud. These forces become stronger as the atom (or molecule) becomes larger because of the increased polarizability of the larger, more dispersed electron clouds. This accounts for the fact that under standard temperature and pressure, fluorine and chlorine are gases, whereas bromine is a liquid, and iodine is a solid.

REDUCTION-OXIDATION

Reduction-oxidation (*redox*) reactions involve the movement of electrons from one atom or molecule to another, and actually comprise two dependent reactions: reduction and oxidation. *Reduction* is the gain of electrons by an atom that is thereby *reduced*. The electrons derive from a *reducing agent*, which in the process becomes *oxidized*. *Oxidation* is the loss of electrons from an atom, which is, accordingly, *oxidized*. An *oxidizing agent* accepts electrons and, in the process, is reduced. By definition, these chemical reactions involve a change in the valence of an atom. It is also important to note that acid–base and electrolyte chemical reactions involve electrical charge interactions but no change in valence of any of the involved components. The implications of redox chemistry for medical toxicology are profound. For example, the oxidation of ferrous (Fe^{2+}) to ferric (Fe^{3+}) iron within the hemoglobin molecule creates the dysfunctional methemoglobin molecule.

Also, elemental lead and mercury are both intrinsically harmless metals, but when oxidized to their cationic forms both produce devastating clinical effects. Additionally, the metabolism of ethanol to acetaldehyde involves a change in the oxidation state of the molecule. In this case, an enzyme, alcohol dehydrogenase, acting as a catalyst oxidizes (ie, removes electrons from) the C-O bond and delivers the electrons to oxidized nicotinamide adenine dinucleotide (NAD^+), reducing it to NADH. As in this last example, *oxidation* is occasionally used to signify the gain of oxygen by a substance. That is, when elemental iron (Fe^0) undergoes rusting to iron oxide (Fe_2O_3), it is said to oxidize. The use of this term is consistent because in the process of oxidation, oxygen derives electrons from the atom to which it is binding.

Reactive Oxygen Species Free radicals are reactive molecules that contain one or more unpaired electrons and are typically neutral but may be anionic or cationic. However, because certain toxicologically important reactive molecules do not contain unpaired electrons, such as hydrogen peroxide (H_2O_2) and ozone (O_3), the term *reactive species* is preferred. The reactivity of these molecules directly relates to their attempts to fill their outermost orbitals by receiving an electron; the result is *oxidative stress* on the biologic system. Molecular oxygen is actually a diradical with two unpaired electrons in the outer orbitals. However, its reactivity is less than that of the other radicals because the unpaired electrons have parallel spins, so catalysts (ie, enzymes or metals) are typically involved in the use of oxygen in biologic processes.

Reactive species are continually generated as a consequence of endogenous metabolism and there is an efficient system for their control. Under conditions of either excessive endogenous generation or exposure to exogenous reactive species, the physiologic defense against these toxic products is overwhelmed. When this occurs, reactive species induce direct cellular damage as well as initiate a cascade of oxidative reactions that perpetuate the toxic damage.

Intracellular organelles, particularly the mitochondria, may also be disrupted by various reactive species. This causes further injury to the cell as energy failure occurs. This initial damage is compounded by the activation of the host inflammatory response by chemokines that are released from cells in response to reactive species-induced

TABLE 11–1. Structure of Important Reactive Species

	Structure
Reactive Oxygen Species	
Free radicals	
Hydroxyl radical	OH·
Alcoxyl radical	RO·
Peroxyl radical	ROO·
Superoxide radical	$O_2·^-$ or O_2^-
Nonradicals	
Hydrogen peroxide	H_2O_2
Hypochlorous acid	HOCl
Singlet oxygen	[O] or $^1O_2$
Ozone	O_3
Reactive Nitrogen Species	
Free radicals	
Nitric oxide	NO·
Nitrogen dioxide	$NO_2·$
Nonradicals	
Peroxynitrite anion	$ONOO^-$
Nitronium cation	NO_2^+

damage. This inflammatory response aggravates cellular damage. The resultant membrane dysfunction or damage causes cellular apoptosis or necrosis.

The most important reactive oxygen species in medical toxicology are derived from oxygen, although those derived from nitrogen are also important. Table 11–1 lists some of the important reactive oxygen and nitrogen species.

This biradical nature of oxygen explains both the physiologic and toxicologic importance of oxygen in biologic systems. Physiologically, the majority of oxygen is used by the body to serve as the ultimate electron acceptor in the mitochondrial electron transport chain (Fig. 11–3). In this situation, 4 electrons are added to each molecule of oxygen to form 2 water molecules ($O_2 + 4H^+ + 4e^- \rightarrow 2H_2O$).

Superoxide is generated within neutrophil and macrophage lysosomes as part of the oxidative burst, a method of eliminating infectious agents and damaged cells. Superoxide may subsequently be enzymatically converted, or "dismutated," into hydrogen peroxide by superoxide dismutase (SOD). Hydrogen peroxide may be subsequently converted into hypochlorous acid by the enzymatic addition of chloride by myeloperoxidase. Both hydrogen peroxide and hypochlorite ion are more potent reactive oxygen species than superoxide. However, this lysosomal protective system may also be responsible for tissue damage following poisoning as the innate inflammatory response attacks xenobiotic-damaged cells. Examples include acetaminophen-induced hepatotoxicity (Chap. 34), carbon monoxide neurotoxicity (Chap. 125), and chlorine-induced pulmonary toxicity (Chap. 124), each of which may be altered, at least in experimental systems, by the addition of scavengers of reactive species.

Although superoxide and hydrogen peroxide are reactive species, it is their conversion into the hydroxyl radical (OH·) that accounts for their most consequential effects. The hydroxyl radical is generated by the Fenton reaction (Fig. 11–2), in which hydrogen peroxide is decomposed in the presence of a transition metal. This catalysis typically involves Fe^{2+}, Cu^+, Cd^{2+}, Cr^{5+}, Ni^{2+}, or Mn^{2+}. The Haber-Weiss reaction (Fig. 11–2), in which a transition metal catalyzes the combination of superoxide and hydrogen peroxide, is the other important means of generating the hydroxyl radical. Alternatively, superoxide dismutase, within the erythrocyte, contains an ion of copper (Cu^{2+}) that participates in the catalytic dismutation (reduction) of superoxide to hydrogen peroxide (SOD was originally called erythrocuprein) and the subsequent detoxification of hydrogen peroxide by glutathione peroxidase or catalase.

Transition metal cations may bind to the cellular nucleus where they locally generate reactive oxygen species, most importantly hydroxyl radical. This results in DNA strand breaks and modification, accounting for the promutagenic effects of many transition metals. In addition to the important role that transition metal chemistry plays following iron or copper salt poisoning, the long-term consequences of chronic transition metal poisoning are exemplified by asbestos. The iron contained in asbestos is the origin of the Fenton-generated hydroxyl radicals that are responsible for the pulmonary fibrosis and cancers associated with long-term exposure.

The most consequential toxicologic effects of reactive oxygen species occur on the cell membrane, and are caused by the initiation by hydroxyl radical of the lipid peroxidative cascade. The alteration of these lipid membranes ultimately causes membrane destruction. Identification of released oxidative products such as malondialdehyde is a common method of assessing lipid peroxidation.

Under normal conditions, there is a delicate balance between the formation and immediate endogenous detoxification of reactive oxygen species. For example, the conversion of the superoxide radical to hydrogen peroxide via SOD is rapidly followed by the transformation of hydrogen peroxide to water by glutathione peroxidase or catalase. Furthermore, in order to minimize the formation of hydroxyl radicals, transition metals exist in "free" form in only minute quantities in biologic systems; that is, cells have developed extensive systems by which transition metal ions can be sequestered and rendered harmless. Ferritin (binds iron), ceruloplasmin (binds copper), and metallothionein (binds cadmium) are specialized proteins that safely sequester transition metal ions. Certain proteins and enzymes such as hemoglobin or SOD have critical biological functions associated with the transition metals at their active sites.

Detoxification of certain reactive species is difficult because of their extreme reactivity. Widespread antioxidant systems typically to trap reactive species before tissue damage occurs. An example is the availability of glutathione, a reducing agent and nucleophile, which prevents both exogenous oxidants from producing hemolysis and the acetaminophen metabolite *N*-acetyl-*p*-benzoquinoneimine (NAPQI) from damaging the hepatocyte.

The key reactive nitrogen species is nitric oxide. At typical physiologic concentrations, this radical is responsible for vascular endothelial relaxation through stimulation of guanylate cyclase. However, during oxidative burst, high concentrations of nitric oxide are formed from L-arginine. At these concentrations, nitric oxide has primarily both damaging effects and reacts with the superoxide radical to generate the peroxynitrite anion. This is particularly important because peroxynitrite may spontaneously degrade to form the hydroxyl radical. Peroxynitrite ion is implicated in both the delayed neurologic effects of carbon monoxide poisoning and the hepatic injury from acetaminophen.

Redox Cycling. Although transition metals are an important source of reactive species, certain xenobiotics are also capable of independently generating reactive species. Most do so through a process called *redox cycling*, in which a molecule accepts an electron from a reducing agent and subsequently transfers that electron to oxygen, generating the superoxide radical. At the same time, this second reaction regenerates the parent molecule, which itself can gain another electron and restart the process. The toxicity of paraquat is selectively localized to pulmonary endothelial cells. Its pulmonary toxicity results from redox cycling generation of reactive oxygen species (Fig. 115-3). A similar process, localized to the heart, occurs with anthracycline antineoplastic agents such as doxorubicin.

ACID–BASE CHEMISTRY

Water is *amphoteric*, which means that it can function as either an acid or a base, much the same way as the bicarbonate ion (HCO_3^-). In fact, because of the amphoteric nature of water, H^+, despite the nomenclature, does not ever actually exist in aqueous solution; rather, it is covalently bound to a molecule of water to form the hydronium ion (H_3O^+). However, the term H^+, or proton, is used for convenience.

Even in neutral solution, a tiny proportion of water is always undergoing ionization to form both H^+ and OH^- in exactly equal amounts. It is, however, the quantity of H^+ that is of concern, and this is the basis of using the pH to characterize a solution. In a perfect system at equilibrium, the concentration of H^+ ions in water is precisely 0.0000001, or 10^{-7}, moles per liter and that of OH^- is the same. The number of H^+ ions increases when an acid is added to the solution and falls when an alkali is added. In an attempt to make this quantity more practical, the negative log of the H^+ concentration is calculated, which defines the pH. Thus, the negative log of 10^{-7} is 7, and the pH of a neutral aqueous solution is 7. In actuality, the pH of water is approximately 6 because of dissolution of ambient carbon dioxide to form carbonic acid ($H_2O + CO_2 \rightarrow H_2CO_3$), which ionizes to form H^+ and bicarbonate (HCO_3^-).

There are many definitions of acid and base. The three commonly used definitions are those advanced by (1) Svante Arrhenius, (2) Brønsted and Lowry, and (3) Lewis. Because the focus is on physiologic systems, which are aqueous, the original definition by the Swedish chemist Arrhenius is the most practical. In this view, an acid releases hydrogen ions, or protons (H^+), in water. Similarly, a base produces hydroxyl ions (OH^-) in water. Thus, hydrogen chloride (HCl), a neutral gas under standard conditions, dissolves in water to liberate H^+, and is therefore an acid.

For nonaqueous solutions the Brønsted-Lowry definition is preferable. An acid, in this schema, is a substance that donates a proton and a base is one that accepts a proton. Thus, any molecule that has a hydrogen in the 1+ oxidation state is technically an acid, and any molecule with an unbound pair of valence electrons is a base. Because most of the acids or bases of toxicologic interest have ionizable protons or available electrons, respectively, the Brønsted-Lowry definition is most often considered when discussing acid–base chemistry (ie, $HA + H_2O \rightarrow H_3O^+ + A^-$; $B^- + H_2O \rightarrow HB + OH^-$). However, this is not a defining property of all acids or bases. Thus, Lewis offered the least-restrictive definition of such substances. A Lewis acid is an electron acceptor and a Lewis base is an electron donor. Simplistically, acids are sour and turn litmus paper red, whereas bases are slippery and bitter and turn litmus paper blue.

Because acidity and alkalinity are determined by the number of available H^+ ions, it is useful to classify chemicals by their effect on the H^+ concentration. Strong acids ionize completely in aqueous solution and very little of the parent compound remains. Thus, 0.001 (or 10^{-3}) mole of HCl, a strong acid, added to 1 L of water produces a solution with a pH of 3. Weak acids, on the other hand, obtain an equilibrium between parent and ionized forms, and thus do not alter the pH to the same degree as a similar quantity of a strong acid. This chemical notation defines the strength or weakness of an acid and should not be confused with the concentration of the acid. Thus, the pH of a dilute strong acid solution may be substantially less than that of a concentrated weak acid (Table 11–2).

TABLE 11–2. pH of 0.10 *M* Solutions of Common Acids and Bases Represents the Strength of the Acid or Base

Acid Base	pH
HCl (hydrochloric acid)	1.1
H_2SO_4 (sulfuric acid)	1.2
H_2SO_3 (sulfurous acid)	1.5
H_3PO_4 (phosphoric acid)	1.5
HF (hydrofluoric acid)	2.1
CH_3CO_2H (acetic acid)	2.9
H_2CO_3 (carbonic acid)	3.8
H_2S (hydrogen sulfide)	4.1
HCN (hydrocyanic acid)	5.1
$NaHCO_3$ (sodium bicarbonate)	8.3
NH_4Cl (ammonium chloride)	4.6
$NaCH_3CO_2$ (sodium acetate)	8.9
Na_2HPO_4 (sodium hydrogen phosphate)	9.3
Na_2SO_3 (sodium sulfite)	9.8
NaCN (sodium cyanide)	11.0
NH_4OH (aqueous ammonia)	11.1
Na_2CO_3 (sodium carbonate)	11.6
Na_3PO_4 (sodium phosphate)	12.0
NaOH (sodium hydroxide)	13.0

The degree of ionization of a weak acid is determined by the pK_a, or the negative log of the *ionization constant*, which represents the pH at which an acid is half dissociated in solution. The same relationship applies to the pK_b of an alkali, although by convention the pK_b is expressed as the pK_a ($pK_a = 14 - pK_b$). The lower the pK_a, the stronger the acid; the converse is true for bases. The pK of a strong acid is clinically irrelevant because it is fully ionized under all but the most extreme acid conditions. Knowledge of the pK_a does not itself denote whether a substance is an acid or an alkali. To some extent, this quality may be predicted by its chemical structure or reactivity, or obtained through direct measurement or from a reference source.

Because only uncharged compounds cross lipid membranes spontaneously, the pK_a has clinical relevance. Salicylic acid, a weak acid with a pK_a of 3, is nonionized in the stomach (pH 2) and passive absorption occurs (Fig. 8-3). Because it is predominantly in the ionized form (ie, salicylate) in blood, which has a pH of 7.4, little of the ionized blood-borne salicylate passively enters the tissues. However, because in overdose the serum salicylate rises considerably, enough enters the tissue to have devastating clinical effects. Salicylate, a conjugate base of a weak acid and thus a strong base, equilibrates within the various tissues across the outer mitochondrial membrane. In this intermembrane space (between the inner and outer mitochondrial membrane) abundant protons exist, which are transported there via the electron transport chain of this organelle (Fig. 12-3). Because salicylate is a strong base, it protonates easily in this environment. In this nonionized form, some of the salicylic acid may pass through the inner mitochondrial membrane, into the mitochondrial matrix, and again establish equilibrium by losing a proton. The process just described uncouples oxidative phosphorylation, by dispersing the highly concentrated protons in the intermembrane space that are normally used to generate adenosine triphosphate (Chap. 12). Uncoupling in the skeletal muscle, for example, produces a metabolic acidosis, and this shifts the blood equilibrium of salicylate toward the nonionized, protonated form, enabling salicylic acid to cross the blood–brain barrier. Presumably, once in the brain, the salicylate uncouples the metabolic activity of neurons with the subsequent development of cerebral edema. This is the rationale for serum alkalinization in patients with aspirin overdose (Chap. 35).

In a similar manner, alkalinization of the patient's urine prevents reabsorption by ionization of the urinary salicylate. Conversely, because cyclic antidepressants are organic bases, alkalinization of the urine reduces their ionization and actually decreases the drug's urinary elimination. However, in the management of cyclic antidepressant poisoning, because the other beneficial effects of sodium bicarbonate on the sodium channel outweigh the negative effect on drug elimination, serum alkalinization is recommended (see Chap. 73).

ORGANIC CHEMISTRY

The study of carbon-based chemistry and the interaction of inorganic molecules with carbon-containing compounds is called *organic chemistry*, because the chemistry of living organisms is carbon based. *Biochemistry* (Chap. 12) is a subdivision of organic chemistry; it is the study of organic chemistry within biologic systems. This section reviews many of the salient points of organic chemistry, focusing on those with the most applicability to medicine and the study of toxicology: nomenclature, bonding, nucleophiles and electrophiles, stereochemistry, and functional groups.

CHEMICAL PROPERTIES OF CARBON

Carbon, atomic number 6, has a molecular weight of 12.011 g/mol. With few exceptions (notably cyanide ion and carbon monoxide), carbon forms 4 bonds in stable organic molecules. In organic compounds, carbon is commonly bonded to other carbon atoms, as well as to hydrogen, oxygen, nitrogen, or halide (ie, fluorine, bromine, or iodine) atoms. Under certain circumstances, carbon can be bonded to metals, as is the case with methylmercury.

NOMENCLATURE

The most systematic method to name organic compounds is in accordance with standards adopted by the International Union of Pure and Applied Chemistry (IUPAC); these names are infrequently used, especially for larger molecules, and alternative names are common. The complete details of the IUPAC naming system are beyond the scope of this text and can be reviewed elsewhere (www.iupac.org), but a brief description of the fundamentals of this system is included here.

The carbon backbone serves as the basis of the chemical name. Once the carbon backbone has been identified and named, *substituents* (atoms or groups of atoms that substitute for hydrogen atoms) are identified, named, and numbered. The number refers to the carbon to which the substituent is attached. Some of the common substituents in organic chemistry are –OH (hydroxy), $-NH_2$ (amino), –Br (bromo), –Cl (chloro), and –F (fluoro). Substituents are then alphabetized and placed as prefixes to the carbon chain.

As an example, consider the molecule 2-bromo-2-chloro-1,1,1-trifluoroethane. The molecule has a 2-carbon backbone (ethane), 3 fluoride atoms on the first carbon, a bromine atom on the second carbon, and a chlorine atom on the second carbon (Fig. 11–4A). A basic understanding of a few simple rules of nomenclature thus allows one to quickly generate the molecular structure of a familiar compound, halothane, from what initially appeared to be an intimidating name.

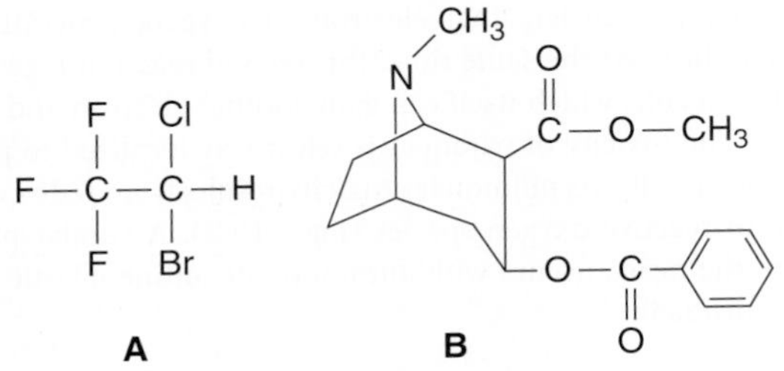

FIGURE 11–4. Nomenclature. (**A**) 2-Bromo-2-chloro-1,1,1-trifluoroethane, or halothane. (**B**) [1R-(exo,exo)]-3-(Benzoyloxy)-8-methyl-8-azabicyclo[3,2,1]-octane-2-carboxylic acid methyl ester, or cocaine.

Although the above-mentioned rules suffice to name simple structures, they are inadequate to describe many others, such as molecules with complex branching or ring structures. The IUPAC rules for naming compounds such as [1R-(exo,exo)]-3-(benzoyloxy)-8-methyl-8-azabicyclo[3,2,1]octane-2-carboxylic acid methyl ester, for example, are too complex to include here. Fortunately, many compounds with complex chemical names have simpler names for day-to-day use; as an example, this molecule is commonly referred to as cocaine (Fig. 11–4B).

Cocaine is an example of a *common* or *trivial* name; one without a systematic basis, but which is generally accepted as an alternative to frequently unwieldy proper chemical names. Common names may refer to the origin of the substance; for example, cocaine is derived from the coca leaf, and wood alcohol (methanol) can be prepared from wood. Alternatively, a common name may refer to the way in which a compound is used; rubbing alcohol is a common name for isopropanol. Common names are often imprecise and may generate some confusion, however, as evidenced by the fact that rubbing alcohol, when commercially marketed, may be ethanol or isopropanol.

An even less precise system of nomenclature is the use of *street* names. A street name is a slang term for a drug of abuse, such as "blow" (cocaine), "weed" (marijuana), or "smack" (heroin). The street name *ecstasy* refers to the stimulant 3,4-methylenedioxymethamphetamine (MDMA), which is most frequently consumed in pill form. It would stand to reason that *liquid ecstasy* might refer to a solution of MDMA, but street names are not necessarily logical. Instead, liquid ecstasy refers to the drug γ-hydroxybutyrate (GHB), a sedative-hypnotic with a completely different pharmacologic and toxicologic profile. Furthermore, there are no standards for the content of ecstasy, and many street pills contain other chemicals or no chemicals at all.

A final consideration must be given to *product names*. Product names are trade names under which a given compound might be marketed, and are frequently different from both the chemical name and common name. Thus, the inhalational anesthetic in Figure 11–4A with the chemical name 2-bromo-2-chloro-1,1,1-trifluoroethane has the common name halothane and the trade name Fluothane.

BONDING IN ORGANIC CHEMISTRY

Whereas much of the bonding in inorganic chemistry is ionic or electrovalent, the vast majority of bonding in organic molecules is *covalent*. Whereas electrons in ionic bonds are described as "belonging" to one atom or another, electrons in covalent bonds are shared between two atoms; this type of bonding occurs when the difference in electronegativity between

2 atoms is insufficient for one atom to wrest control of an electron from another. Single bonds are represented by 1, double bonds by 2, and triple bonds by 3 lines between the atoms.

NUCLEOPHILES AND ELECTROPHILES

Many organic reactions of toxicologic importance can be described as the reactions of *nucleophiles* with *electrophiles*. *Nucleophiles* (literally, nucleus-loving) are species with increased electron density, frequently in the form of a lone pair of electrons (as in the cases of cyanide ion and carbon monoxide). Nucleophiles, by virtue of this increased electron density, have an affinity for atoms or molecules which are electron deficient; such moieties are called *electrophiles* (literally, electron-loving). The electron deficiency of electrophiles can be described as absolute or relative. Absolute electron deficiency occurs when an electrophile is charged, as is the case with cations such as Pb^{2+} and Hg^{2+}. Relative electron deficiency occurs when one atom or group of atoms shifts electrons away from a second atom, making the second atom relatively electron deficient. This is the case for the neurotoxin 2,5-hexanedione (Fig. 11–5); the electronegative oxygen of the carbon-oxygen double bond pulls electron density away from the second and fifth carbon atoms of this molecule, making these carbon atoms electrophilic.

The reaction of a nucleophile with an electrophile involves the movement of electrons, by forming or breaking bonds. This movement of electrons is frequently denoted by the use of curved arrows, which better demonstrates how the nucleophile and electrophile interact. The interaction of acetylcholinesterase with acetylcholine, organic phosphorus pesticides, and pralidoxime hydrochloride provides an excellent example of the way in which nucleophiles and electrophiles interact, and of how the use of curved arrow notation can lead to better understanding of the reactions involved.

Under normal circumstances, the action of acetylcholine is terminated when the serine residue in the active site of acetylcholinesterase attacks this neurotransmitter, forming a transient serine–acetyl complex and liberating choline. This serine–acetyl complex is then rapidly hydrolyzed, producing an acetic acid molecule and regenerating the serine residue for another round of the reaction (Fig. 11–6A). In the presence of an organic phosphorus pesticide, however, this serine residue attacks the electrophilic phosphate atom, forming a stable serine–phosphate bond, which is not hydrolyzed (Fig. 11–6B). The enzyme, thus inactivated, can no longer break down acetylcholine, leading to an increase of this neurotransmitter in the synapse, and possibly to a cholinergic crisis.

The enzyme can be reactivated, however, by the use of another nucleophile. Pralidoxime hydrochloride (2-PAM) is referred to as a *site-directed nucleophile*. Because part of its chemical structure (the charged nitrogen atom) is similar to the choline portion of acetylcholine, this antidote is directed to the active site of acetylcholinesterase. Once in position, the nucleophilic oxime moiety (–NOH) of 2-PAM attacks the electrophilic phosphate atom. This displaces the serine residue, regenerating the enzyme (Fig. 11–6C). For a further discussion of organic phosphorus compound toxicity and the use of 2-PAM, see Chap. 113 and Antidotes in Depth A33: Pralidoxime.

$$CH_3-\overset{\overset{\displaystyle O}{\|}}{C}-CH_2-CH_2-\overset{\overset{\displaystyle O}{\|}}{C}-CH_3$$

FIGURE 11–5. Chemical properties of 2,5-hexanedione. Arrows designate the electrophilic carbon atoms.

A second toxicologically important electrophile is NAPQI (Fig. 11–7). NAPQI is formed when the endogenous detoxification pathways of acetaminophen metabolism (glucuronidation and sulfation) are overwhelmed (Chap. 34). As a result of the electron configuration of NAPQI, the carbon atoms adjacent to the *carbonyl carbon* (a carbonyl carbon is one that is double bonded to an oxygen) are very electrophilic; the sulfur groups of cysteine residues of hepatocyte proteins react with NAPQI to form a characteristic *adduct* (formed when one compound is added to another), 3-(cystein-*S*-yl)acetaminophen, in a multistep process. These adducts are released as hepatocytes die, and can be found in the blood of patients with acetaminophen-related liver toxicity. Figure 11–7 diagrams the mechanism of the protein–NAPQI reaction (Chap. 34).

Nucleophiles can be described by their strength, which by convention is related to the rate at which they react with the reference electrophile CH_3I. Of more use in pharmacology and toxicology, however, are the descriptive terms "hard" and "soft." Although imprecise, the designations hard and soft help to predict, qualitatively, how nucleophiles and electrophiles interact with one another.

Hard species have a charge (or partial charge) that is highly localized; that is, their charge-to-radius ratio is high. Hard nucleophiles are molecules in which the electron density or lone pair is tightly held; fluoride, a small atom that cannot spread its electron density over a large area, is an example. Similarly, hard electrophiles are species in which the positive charge cannot be spread over a large area; ionized calcium, a small ion, is a hard electrophile.

Soft nucleophiles and electrophiles, on the other hand, are capable of delocalizing their charge over a larger area. In this case the charge to mass ratio is low, either because the atom is large or because the charge can be spread over a number of atoms within a given molecule. Sulfur is the prototypical example of a soft nucleophile and the lead ion, Pb^{2+}, is a typical soft electrophile.

The utility of this classification lies in the observation that hard nucleophiles tend to react with hard electrophiles, and soft nucleophiles with soft electrophiles. For example, a principal toxicity of fluoride ion poisoning (Chap. 105) is hypocalcemia; this is because the fluoride ions (hard nucleophiles) readily react with calcium ions (hard electrophiles). On the other hand, the soft nucleophile lead is effectively chelated by soft electrophiles such as the sulfur atoms in the chelating agents dimercaprol (Antidotes in Depth A26: Dimercaprol [British Anti-Lewisite or BAL]) and succimer (Antidotes in depth A27: Succimer [2,3-Dimercaptosuccinic Acid]).

ISOMERISM

Isomerism describes the different ways in which molecules with the same chemical formula (ie, the same number and types of atoms) can be arranged to form different compounds. These different compounds are called *isomers*. Isomers always have the same chemical formula, but differ either in the way that atoms are bonded to each other (*constitutional isomers*) or in the spatial arrangement of these atoms (*geometric isomers* or *stereoisomers*).

Constitutional isomers are conceptually the easiest to understand, because a quick glance shows them to be very different molecules. The chemical formula C_2H_6O, for example, can refer to either dimethyl ether or ethanol (Fig. 11–8). These molecules have very different physical and chemical characteristics, and have little in common other than the number and type of their atomic constituents.

Stereoisomerism, also referred to as *geometric isomerism*, refers to the different ways in which atoms of a given molecule, with the same number and types of bonds, might be arranged. The most important type of stereoisomerism in pharmacology and toxicology is the stereochemistry around a *stereogenic* (sometimes called *chiral*) *carbon*.

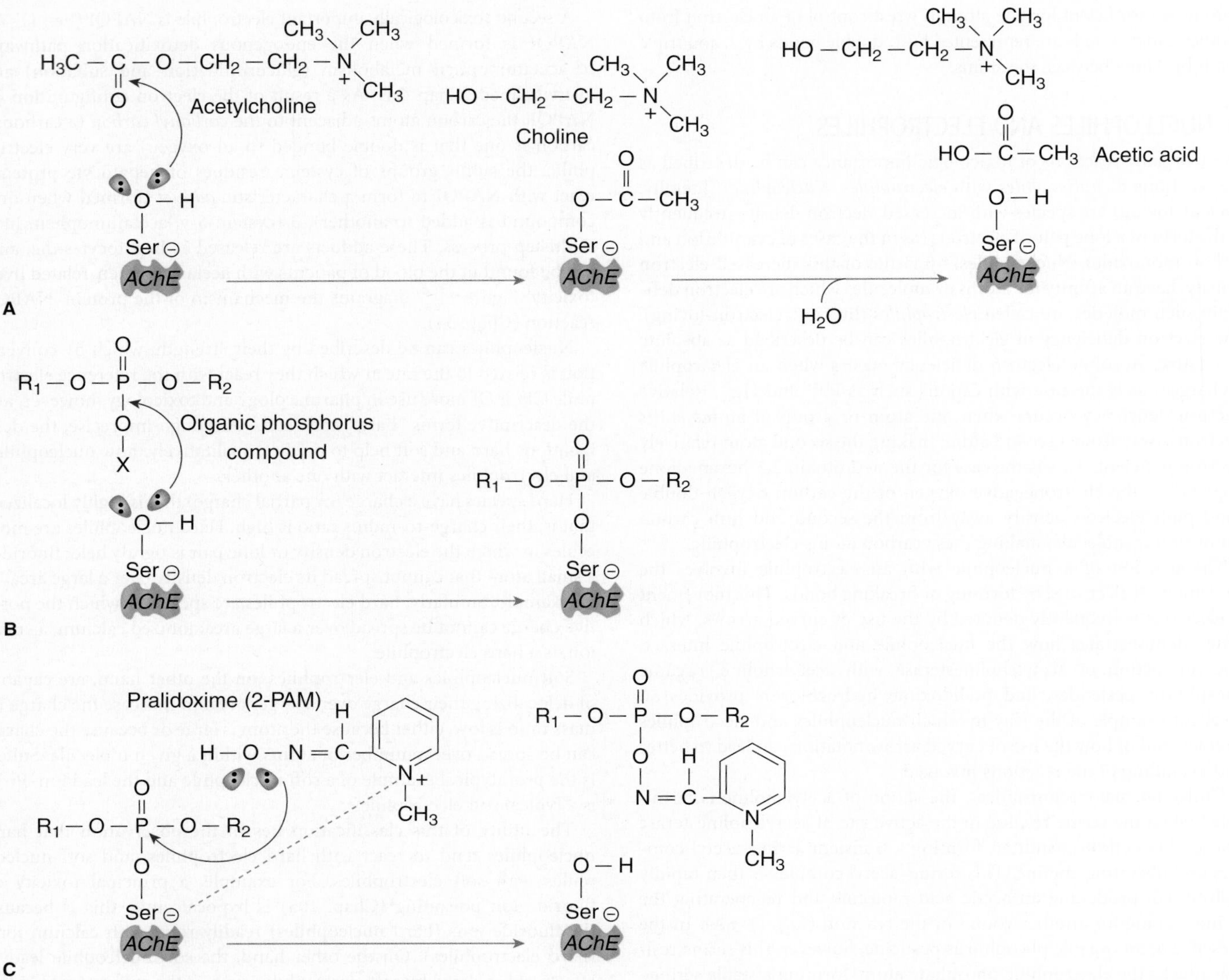

FIGURE 11–6. The reactions of acetylcholinesterase (AChE), organic phosphorus compounds, and pralidoxime hydrochloride (2-PAM). Curved arrows represent the movement of electrons as bonds are formed or broken. (**A**) Normal hydrolysis of acetylcholine by acetylcholinesterase. (**B**) Inactivation (phosphorylation) of acetylcholinesterase by organic phosphorus compound. (**C**) Reactivation by 2-PAM of functional acetylcholinesterase.

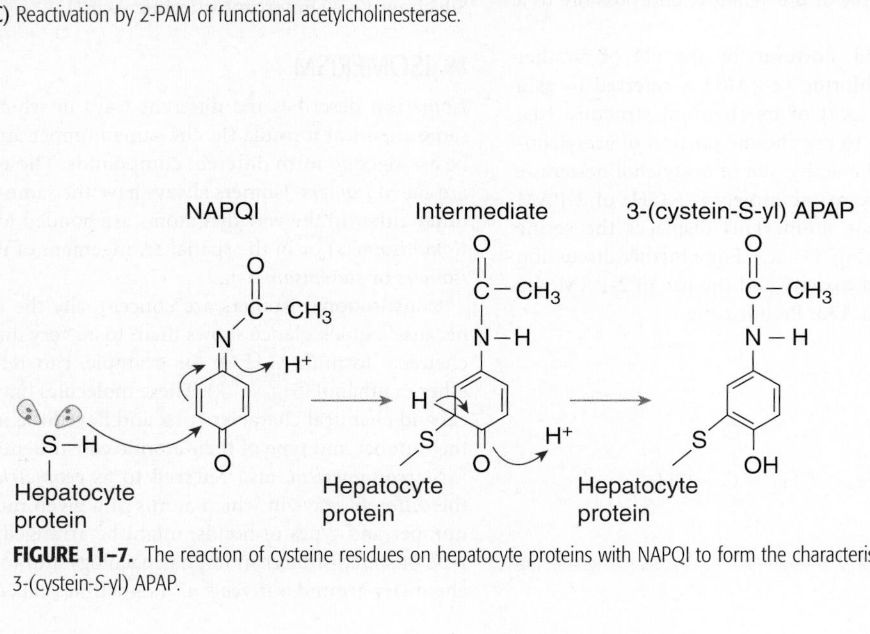

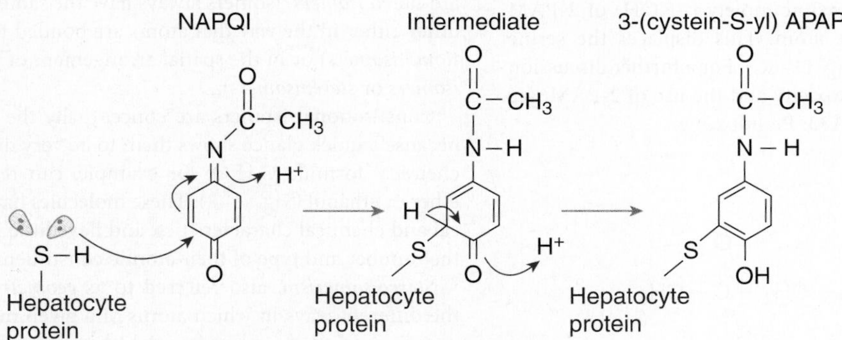

FIGURE 11–7. The reaction of cysteine residues on hepatocyte proteins with NAPQI to form the characteristic adducts 3-(cystein-*S*-yl) APAP.

CH_3-O-CH_3

A

CH_3-CH_2-OH

B

FIGURE 11–8. Two molecules with chemical formula C_2H_6O. (**A**) Dimethylether. (**B**) Ethanol (ethyl alcohol).

Consider the two representations of halothane shown in Figure 11–9. In this figure the straight solid lines and the atoms to which they are bonded exist in the plane of the paper, the solid triangle and the atom to which it is bonded are coming out of the paper, and the dashed triangle and the atom to which it is bonded are receding into the paper. It is clear that, for the molecules in Figure 11–9A and B, no amount of rotation or manipulation will make these molecules superimposable. They are, therefore, different compounds.

The molecules in Figure 11–9A and B are *enantiomers* or *optical isomers*. They differ only in the way in which their atoms are bonded to the chiral carbon. It is important to define the stereochemical configuration of these two molecules, which can be done in one of two ways. In the first classification—the *d*(+)/*l*(−) system—molecules are named empirically based on the direction in which they rotate plane-polarized light. Each enantiomer will rotate plane-polarized light in one direction; the enantiomer that rotates light clockwise (to the right) is referred to as *d*(+), or *dextrorotatory;* the *l*(−), or *levorotatory* enantiomer rotates plane-polarized light in a counterclockwise fashion (to the left).

Alternatively, enantiomers can be named using an elaborate and formal set of rules known as *Cahn-Ingold-Prelog*. These rules establish priority for substituents, based primarily on molecular weight, and then use the arrangement of substituents to assign a configuration. To correctly assign configuration in this system, the molecule is rotated into a projection in which the chiral carbon is in the plane of the page, the lowest priority substituent is directly behind the chiral carbon (and therefore behind the plane of the page), and the other three substituents are arranged around the chiral carbon. Figure 11–10 assigns Cahn-Ingold-Prelog priority to the halothane enantiomers of Figure 11–9, and rearranges the molecules in the appropriate projections.

If the priority of the substituents increases as one moves clockwise (to the right), the enantiomer is *R* (Latin, *rectus* = right); if it increases as one moves counterclockwise, the enantiomer is *S* (Latin, *sinister* = left). Thus, Figure 11–10A is the *R* enantiomer of halothane and Figure 11–10B is the *S* enantiomer.

Enantiomers have identical physical properties, such as boiling point, melting point, and solubility in different solvents; they differ from each other in only two significant ways. The first, as mentioned before, is that enantiomers rotate plane-polarized light in opposite directions; this point has no practical toxicologic importance. The second is that enantiomers may interact in very different ways with other chiral structures (such as proteins and other cell receptors), which is of both pharmacologic and toxicologic significance.

Perhaps the best analogy to explain the toxicologic and pharmacologic importance of stereochemistry is that of the way a hand (analogous to a molecule of drug or toxin) fits into a glove (analogous to the biologic site of activity). Consider the left hand as the *S* enantiomer and the right hand as the *R* enantiomer. There are, qualitatively, three different ways in which the hand can fit into (interact with) a glove.

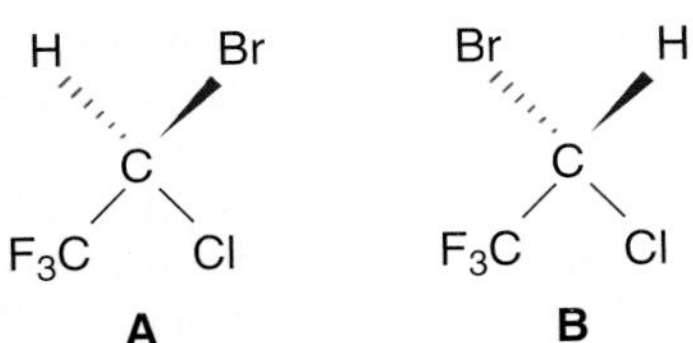

FIGURE 11–9. The graphic representation of the enantiomers of halothane.

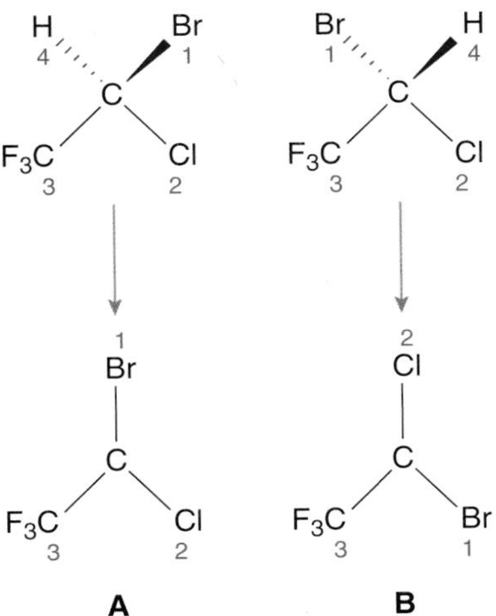

FIGURE 11–10. *R* and *S* enantiomers of halothane. (**A**) The substituents increase in a clockwise fashion, so the configuration is *R*. (**B**) The substituents increase in a counterclockwise fashion, so the configuration is *S*. In this projection, hydrogen atoms are directly behind the carbon atoms.

First, if the glove is very pliable (such as a disposable latex glove), it can accept either the left hand or the right hand without difficulty; this is the case for halothane, whose *R* and *S* enantiomers possess equal activity. Second, if a glove is constructed with greater (but imperfect) specificity, one hand will fit well and the other poorly; this is the case for many substances, such as epinephrine and norepinephrine, whose naturally occurring levorotatory enantiomers are 10-fold more potent than the synthetic dextrorotatory enantiomers. Finally, a glove can be made with exquisite precision, such that one hand fits perfectly, while the other hand does not fit at all. This is the case for physostigmine, in which the (−) enantiomer is biologically active, whereas the (+) enantiomer is inactive.

Even the above analogy is oversimplified, however, as one enantiomer of a drug can be an agonist, while the other enantiomer is an antagonist. Dobutamine, for example, has one stereogenic carbon and thus 2 stereoisomers. At the $\alpha 1$ receptor, *l*-dobutamine is a potent agonist and *d*-dobutamine is a potent antagonist. Because dobutamine is marketed as a *racemic mixture* (a racemic mixture is a 1:1 mixture of enantiomers), however, these effects cancel each other out. Interestingly, at the β_1 receptor, *d*- and *l*-dobutamine have unequal agonist effects, with *d*-dobutamine approximately 10 times more potent than *l*-dobutamine.

FUNCTIONAL GROUPS

There is perhaps no concept in organic chemistry as powerful as that of the *functional group*. Functional groups are atoms or groups of atoms that confer similar reactivity on a molecule; of less importance is the molecule to which it is attached. *Alcohols*, *carboxylic acids*, and *thiols* are functional groups; *hydrocarbons* are generally not considered functional groups per se, but rather are the structural backbone to which functional groups are attached The functional groups discussed below are included because they illustrate important principles, not because this represents an exhaustive list of important functional groups in toxicology.

Hydrocarbons, as their name implies, consist of only carbon and hydrogen. *Alkanes* are hydrocarbons that contain no multiple bonds; they may

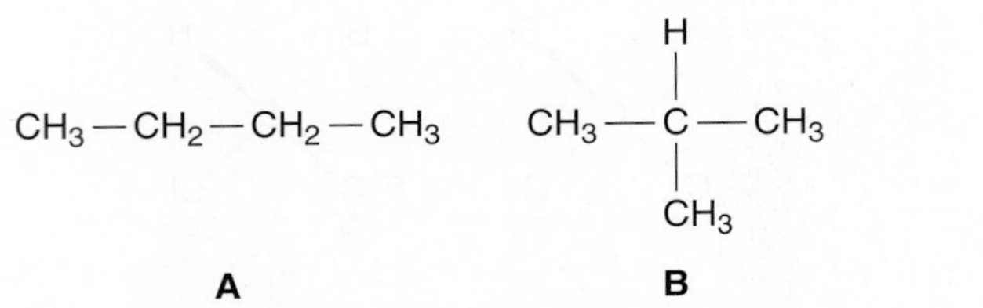

FIGURE 11-11. Two isomers of the 4 carbon alkane, butane. (**A**) *n*-Butane. (**B**) Isobutane.

be straight chain, usually designated by the prefix *n*- (Fig. 11–11A) or, branched (isobutane, Fig. 11–11B); cyclical *Alkenes* contain carbon–carbon double bonds. *Alkynes*, which contain carbon–carbon triple bonds, are of limited toxicologic importance. Butane (lighter fluid) is an alkane, and gasoline is a mixture of alkanes.

Hydrocarbons are of toxicologic importance for two reasons: they are widely abused as inhalational drugs for their CNS depressant effects, and they can cause profound toxicity when aspirated. Although these effects are physiologically disparate, they are readily understood in the context of the chemical characteristics of the hydrocarbon functional group.

Hydrocarbons do not contain *polar groups*, or groups that introduce full or partial charges into the molecule; as such, they interact readily with other nonpolar substances, such as lipids or lipophilic substances. Hydrocarbons readily interact with the myelin of the CNS, disrupting normal ion channel function and causing CNS depression. When aspirated, hydrocarbons interact with the fatty acid tail of surfactant, dissolving this protective substance and contributing to acute lung injury (Chap. 106).

Alcohols possess the hydroxyl (–OH) functional group, which adds polarity to the molecule and makes alcohols highly soluble in other polar substances, such as water. For example, ethane gas (CH_3CH_3) has negligible solubility in water, whereas ethanol (CH_3CH_2OH) is *miscible*, or infinitely soluble, in water. In biologic systems, alcohols are generally CNS depressants, but they can also act as nucleophiles. Ethanol may react with cocaine to form cocaethylene, a longer-acting and more vasoactive substance than cocaine itself (Fig. 11–12; see Chap. 76 for clinical details).

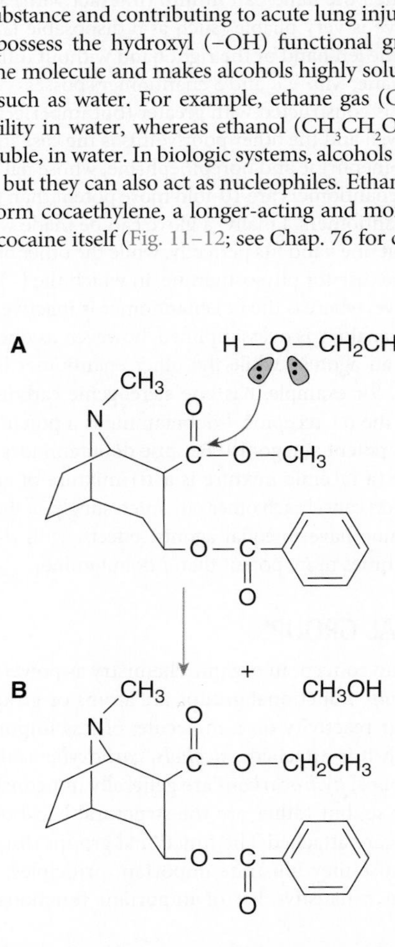

FIGURE 11-12. Reaction of cocaine with ethanol (**A**) to form cocaethylene and methanol (**B**).

Alcohols can be primary, secondary, or tertiary, in which the reference carbon is bonded to 1, 2, or 3 carbons in addition to the hydroxyl group. Methanol, in which the reference carbon is bonded to no other carbons, is not a primary alcohol per se but shares many of the reactivity patterns of primary alcohols. The difference between primary, secondary, and tertiary structures is important, because although the alcohol functional group imparts many qualities to the molecule, the degree of substitution can affect the chemical reactivity. Primary alcohols can undergo multistep oxidation to form carboxylic acids, whereas secondary alcohols generally undergo one-step metabolism to form ketones, and tertiary alcohols do not readily undergo oxidation. This is a point of significant toxicologic importance, and is discussed in more detail later.

Alcohols can be named in many ways; the most common is to add *-ol* or *-yl alcohol* to the appropriate prefix. If the alcohol group is bonded to an interior carbon, the number to which the carbon is bonded precedes the suffix.

Carboxylic acids contain the functional group –COOH. As their name implies, they are weakly acidic, and the pK_a of carboxylic acids are generally 4 or 5, depending on the substitution of the molecule. Carboxylic acids are capable of producing a significant anion gap metabolic acidosis, which is true whether the acids are endogenous or exogenous. Examples of endogenous acids are β-hydroxybutyric acid and lactic acid; examples of exogenous acids are formic acid (produced by the metabolism of methanol) and glycolic, glyoxylic, and oxalic acids (produced by the metabolism of ethylene glycol). Carboxylic acids are named by adding *-oic acid* to the appropriate prefix; the four-carbon straight-chain carboxylic acid is thus butanoic acid.

Thiols contain a sulfur atom, which usually functions as a nucleophile. The sulfur atom of *N*-acetylcysteine can regenerate glutathione reductase, and can also react directly with NAPQI to detoxify this electrophile. The sulfur atoms of many chelators, such as dimercaprol and succimer, are nucleophiles that are very effective at chelating electrophiles such as heavy metal ions. Thiols are generally named by adding the word *thiol* to the appropriate base. Thus, a 2-carbon thiol is ethane thiol.

As noted above, molecules with a given functional group often have more in common with molecules within the same functional group than they have in common with the molecules from which they were derived. The alkanes methane, ethane, and propane are straight-chain hydrocarbons with similar properties. All are gases at room temperature, have almost no solubility in water, and have similar melting and boiling points. When these molecules are substituted with one or more hydroxide functional groups, they become alcohols: examples are methanol, ethanol, ethylene glycol (a *glycol* is a molecule that contains 2 alcohol functional groups), the primary alcohol 1-propanol, and the secondary alcohol 2-propanol (isopropanol). Each of these alcohols is a liquid at room temperature, and all are very water soluble. All have boiling points that are markedly different from the alkane from which they were derived, and quite close to each other.

In addition to conferring different physical properties on the molecule, the addition of the alcohol functional group also confers different chemical properties and reactivities. For example, methane, ethane, and propane are virtually incapable of undergoing oxidation in biologic systems. The alcohols formed by the addition of one or more hydroxyl groups, however, are readily oxidized by alcohol dehydrogenase (Fig. 11–13).

As Figure 11–13 indicates, the oxidation of the primary alcohols methanol and ethanol results in the formation of *aldehydes* (functional groups in which a carbon atom contains a double bond to oxygen and a single bond to hydrogen), whereas the oxidation of the secondary alcohol isopropanol results in the formation of a *ketone* (a functional group in which a carbon is double-bonded to an oxygen atom and

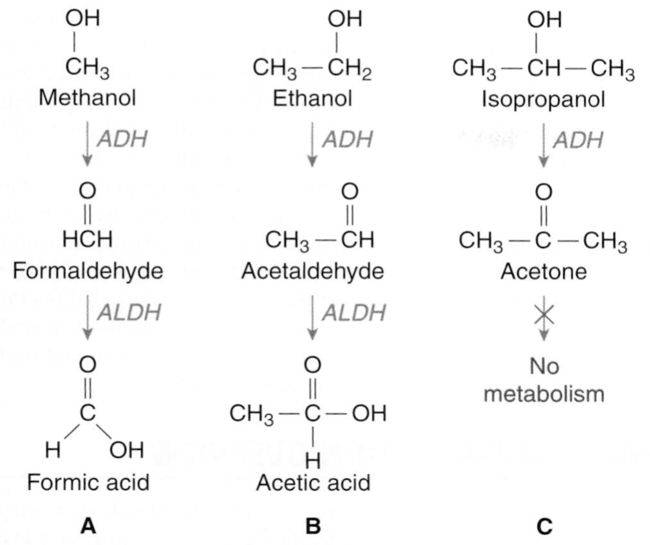

A: Methanol (CH_3OH) —ADH→ Formaldehyde ($HCHO$) —ALDH→ Formic acid ($HCOOH$)

B: Ethanol (CH_3-CH_2OH) —ADH→ Acetaldehyde (CH_3-CHO) —ALDH→ Acetic acid (CH_3-COOH)

C: Isopropanol ($CH_3-CH(OH)-CH_3$) —ADH→ Acetone ($CH_3-CO-CH_3$) ✗→ No metabolism

FIGURE 11–13. Oxidative metabolism of (**A**) methanol, (**B**) ethanol, and (**C**) isopropanol. Note that acetone does not undergo further oxidation in vivo. ADH = alcohol dehydrogenase; ALDH = aldehyde dehydrogenase.

single-bonded to two separate carbon atoms). Although both aldehydes and ketones contain the *carbonyl group* (a carbon-oxygen double bond), aldehydes and ketones are distinctly different functional groups, and have different reactivity patterns. For instance, aldehydes can undergo enzymatic oxidation to carboxylic acids (Figs. 11–13A and B), whereas ketones cannot (Fig. 11–13C).

It is here that recognition of functional groups helps to understand the potential toxicity of an alcohol. Methanol, ethanol, and isopropanol are all alcohols; as such, their toxicity before metabolism is expected to be (and in fact is) quite similar to that of ethanol, producing CNS sedation.

Because these toxins are primary and secondary alcohols, all three can be metabolized to a carbonyl compound, either an aldehyde or a ketone. Here, however, the functional groups on the molecules have changed; whereas aldehydes can be metabolized to carboxylic acids (which can, in turn, cause an anion gap acidosis), ketones cannot. It is for this reason that methanol and ethylene glycol can cause an anion gap acidosis, and isopropanol cannot (Chap. 107).

The concept of functional groups, however useful, has limitations. For example, although both formic acid and oxalic acid are organic acids, they cause different patterns of organ system toxicity. Formic acid is a mitochondrial toxin and exerts effects primarily in areas (such as the retina or basal ganglia) that poorly tolerate an interruption in the energy supplied by oxidative phosphorylation. Conversely, oxalic acid readily precipitates calcium and is toxic to renal tubular cells, which accounts for the hypocalcemia and nephrotoxicity that are characteristic of severe ethylene glycol poisoning. The concept of the functional group is thus an aid to understanding chemical reactivity, but not a substitute for a working knowledge of the toxicokinetic or toxicodynamic effects of xenobiotics in living systems.

SUMMARY

Understanding key principles in inorganic and organic chemistry provides insight into the mechanisms by which xenobiotics act. The periodic table forms the basis for inorganic chemistry and provides insight into the expected reactivity, and to a large extent the clinical effects, of any element. A growing understanding of how reactive species are formed and how they interfere with physiologic processes has led to new insights in the pathogenesis and treatment of toxin-mediated diseases. Organic chemistry forms the basis of life, and is essential to an understanding of biochemistry and pharmacology. Because many xenobiotics are organic compounds there is direct relevance to medical toxicology.

SUGGESTED READINGS

1. Bailey PS, Bailey CA : *Organic Chemistry: A Brief Survey of Concepts and Applications*, 5th ed. Englewood Cliffs, NJ, Prentice Hall, 1995.
2. Bergendi L, Benes L, Durackova Z, Ferencik M: Chemistry, physiology and pathology of free radicals. *Life Sci.* 1999;65:1865–1874.
3. Kasprzak KS: Possible role of oxidative damage in metal-induced carcinogenesis. *Cancer Invest.* 1995;13:411–430.
4. Loudon GM: *Organic Chemistry*, 3rd ed. Redwood City, CA, Benjamin Cummings, 1995.
5. Manahan SE: *Toxicologic Chemistry and Biochemistry*. 3rd ed, Boca Raton, FL, Lewis Publishers, 2003.
6. McMurry J, Castellion ME: *General, Organic, and Biological Chemistry*, 2nd ed. Upper Saddle River, NJ, Prentice Hall, 1996.
7. Oulette RJ, Rawn JD: *Organic Chemistry*. Upper Saddle River, NJ, Prentice Hall, 1996.
8. van der Vliet A, Cross CE: Oxidants, nitrosants, and the lung. *Am J Med.* 2000;109:398–421.

CHAPTER 12
BIOCHEMICAL AND METABOLIC PRINCIPLES

Kurt C. Kleinschmidt and Kathleen A. Delaney

Xenobiotics are compounds that are foreign to a living system. Toxic xenobiotics interfere with critical metabolic processes, causing structural damage to cells or altering the cellular genetic material. The specific biochemical sites of actions that disrupt metabolic processes are well characterized for many xenobiotics although mechanisms of cellular injury are not. This chapter reviews the biochemical principles that are relevant to an understanding of the damaging effects of toxic xenobiotics and the biotransformation enzymes and their clinical implications.

The capacity of a xenobiotic to produce injury is affected by many factors including its absorption, distribution, elimination, site of activation or detoxification, site of action, and capability of cross membranes to access a particular organ. Sites of action include the active sites of enzymes, DNA, and lipid membranes. The route of exposure to a xenobiotic may confine damage primarily to one organ, for example, pulmonary injury that follows inhalation or GI injury that follows a caustic ingestion. Hepatocellular injury results when a toxic xenobiotic is delivered to the liver, either by the portal venous system following ingestion or by the hepatic artery carrying blood with xenobiotics absorbed from other sites of exposure. Various factors affect the ability of a xenobiotic to access a particular organ. For example, many potentially toxic xenobiotics fail to produce CNS injury because they cannot cross the blood–brain barrier. The negligible CNS effects of the mercuric salts when compared with organic mercury compounds are related to their inability to penetrate the CNS. Two potent biologic xenobiotics—ricin (from *Ricinus communis*) and α-amanitin (from *Amanita phalloides*)—block protein synthesis through the inhibition of RNA polymerase. However, they cause different clinical effects because of access to different tissues. Ricin has a special binding protein that enables it to gain access to the endoplasmic reticulum in GI mucosal cells, where it inhibits cellular protein synthesis and causes severe diarrhea.[4] α-Amanitin is transported into hepatocytes by bile salt transport systems, where inhibition of protein synthesis results in cell death.[50,55] The electrical charge on a toxin also affects its ability to enter a cell. Unlike the ionized (charged) form of a xenobiotic, the uncharged form is lipophilic and passes easily through lipid cell membranes to enter the cells. The pK_a of an acidic xenobiotic ($HA \leftrightarrow A^- + H^+$) is the pH at which 50% of the molecules are charged (A^- form) and 50% are uncharged (HA form). A xenobiotic with a low pK_a is more likely to be absorbed in an acidic environment where the uncharged form predominates.

GENERAL ENZYME CONCEPTS

The capability to detoxify and eliminate both endogenous toxins and xenobiotics is crucial to the maintenance of physiologic homeostasis and normal metabolic functions. A simple example is the detoxification of cyanide, a potent cellular poison that is common in the environment and is also a product of normal metabolism. Mammals have evolved the enzyme rhodanese, which combines cyanide with thiosulfate to create the less toxic, renally excreted compound thiocyanate.[6]

Most xenobiotics have lipophilic properties that facilitate absorption across cell membranes in organs that are portals of entry into the body: the skin, GI tract, and lungs. The liver has the highest concentration of enzymes that metabolize xenobiotics. Enzymes found in the liquid matrix of hepatocytes, the cytosol, that are specific for alcohols, aldehydes, esters, or amines act on many different substrates within these broad chemical classes. Enzymes that act on more lipophilic xenobiotics, including the cytochrome P450 (CYP) enzymes, are embedded in the lipid membranes of the cytosol-based endoplasmic reticulum. When cells are mechanically disrupted and centrifuged, these membrane bound enzymes are found in the pellet, or microsomal fraction, hence they are called *microsomal enzymes*. Enzymes located in the liquid matrix of cells are called *cytosolic enzymes* and are found in the supernatant when disrupted cells are centrifuged.[19]

BIOTRANSFORMATION OVERVIEW

The study of xenobiotic metabolism was established as a scientific discipline by the seminal publication of Williams in 1949.[94] Biotransformation is the physiochemical alteration of a xenobiotic, usually as a result of enzyme action. Most definitions also include that this action converts lipophilic substances into more polar, excretable substances.[56,87] The chemical nature of the xenobiotic determines whether it will undergo biotransformation; however, most undergo some degree of biotransformation. The hydrophilic nature of ionized compounds such as carboxylic acids enables the kidneys to rapidly eliminate them. Very volatile compounds, such as enflurane, are expelled promptly via the lungs. Neither of these groups of xenobiotics undergo significant enzymatic metabolism.

Biotransformation usually results in "detoxification," a reduction in the toxicity, by the conversion to hydrophilic metabolites of the xenobiotic that can be renally eliminated.[56] However, this is not always the case. Many parent xenobiotics are inactive and must undergo "metabolic activation," a classic concept introduced in 1947.[59] When metabolites are more toxic than the parent xenobiotic, biotransformation has resulted in "toxification."[87] Biotransformation via acetylation or methylation may enhance the lipophilicity of a xenobiotic. Biotransformation is done by impressively few enzymes, reflecting broad substrate specificity. The predominant pathway for the biotransformation of an individual xenobiotic is determined by many factors including the availability of cofactors, changes in the concentration of the enzyme caused by induction, and the presence of inhibitors. The predominant pathway is also affected by the rate of substrate metabolism, reflected by the K_m (Michaelis-Menten dissociation constant) of the biotransformation enzyme.[87] (Chap. 8)

Biotransformation is often divided into phase I and phase II reactions, terminology first introduced in 1959.[95] Phase I reactions prepare lipophilic xenobiotics for the addition of functional groups or actually add the groups, converting them into more chemically reactive metabolites. This is usually followed by phase II synthetic reactions that conjugate the reactive products of phase I with other molecules that render them more water soluble, further detoxifying the xenobiotics and facilitating their elimination. However, biotransformation often does not follow this stepwise process and it has been suggested that phase I and II terminology be eliminated.[42] Some xenobiotics undergo only a phase I or a phase II reaction prior to elimination. Phase II reactions can precede phase I. While virtually all phase II synthesis reactions cause inactivation, a classic exception is fluoroacetate being metabolized to fluorocitrate, a potent inhibitor of the tricarboxylic acid cycle.[70]

Biotransformed xenobiotics cannot be eliminated until they are moved back across cell membranes, out of the cells. Membrane transporters are proteins that move agents across the membranes without altering their chemical compositions, a process called a phase III reaction because it typically occurs after biotransformation.[42] However, membrane transport does not always occur after phase I or II reactions. Some parent compounds are transported across membranes without any biotransformation at all.

PHASE I BIOTRANSFORMATION REACTIONS

Oxidations are the predominant phase I reactions, adding reactive functional groups suitable for conjugation during phase II. These groups include hydroxyl (–OH), sulfhydryl (–SH), amino (–NH_2), aldehyde (–COH), or carboxyl (–COOH) moieties. Noncarbon elements such as nitrogen, sulfur, and phosphorus are also oxidized in phase I reactions. Other phase I reactions include hydrolysis (the splitting of a large molecule by the addition of water that is divided among the 2 products), hydration (incorporation of water into a complex molecule), hydroxylation (the attachment of –OH groups to carbon atoms), reduction, dehalogenation, dehydrogenation, and dealkylation.[56,87]

The CYP enzymes are the most numerous and important of the phase I enzymes. A common oxidation reaction catalyzed by CYP enzymes is illustrated by the hydroxylation of a xenobiotic R–H to R–OH (Fig. 12–1).[25] Membrane-bound flavin monooxygenase (FMO), an NADPH-dependent oxidase located in the endoplasmic reticulum, is an important oxidizer of amines and other compounds containing nitrogen, sulfur, or phosphorus.[56]

The alcohol, aldehyde, and ketone oxidation systems use predominantly cytosolic enzymes that catalyze these reactions using NADH/NAD^+.[53,87] Two classic phase I oxidation reactions are the metabolism of ethanol to acetaldehyde by alcohol dehydrogenase (ADH) followed by the metabolism of acetaldehyde to acetic acid by aldehyde dehydrogenase (ALDH) (Fig. 12–2). Alcohol dehydrogenase, which oxidizes many different alcohols, is found in the liver, lungs, kidney, and gastric mucosa.[53] Women have less ADH in their gastric mucosa than men. This results in decreased first-pass metabolism of alcohol and increased alcohol absorption. Some populations, particularly Asians, are deficient in ALDH, resulting in increased acetaldehyde concentrations and symptoms of the acetaldehyde syndrome[53] (Chap. 79).

OXIDATION OVERVIEW

Biotransformation often results in the oxidation or reduction of carbon. A substrate is oxidized when it transfers electrons to an electron-seeking (electrophilic or oxidizing) molecule, leading to reduction of the electrophilic molecule. These oxidation-reduction reactions are usually coupled to the cyclical oxidation and reduction of a cofactor, such as the pyridine nucleotides, nicotinamide adenine dinucleotide phosphate (NADPH/$NADP^+$) or nicotinamide adenine dinucleotide (NADH/NAD^+). The nucleotides alternate between their reduced (NADPH, NADH) and oxidized ($NADP^+$, NAD^+) forms. Since xenobiotic oxidation is the most common phase I reaction, the reduced cofactors must have a place to unload their electrons; otherwise, biotransformation ends. The electron transport chain is the major electron recipient.

Electrons resulting from the catabolism of energy sources are extracted primarily by NAD^+, forming NADH. Within the mitochondria,

$$\text{Drug-H} + O_2 \xrightarrow[\text{CYP}]{\text{NADH + H} \;\to\; NAD^+} \text{Drug-OH} + H_2O$$

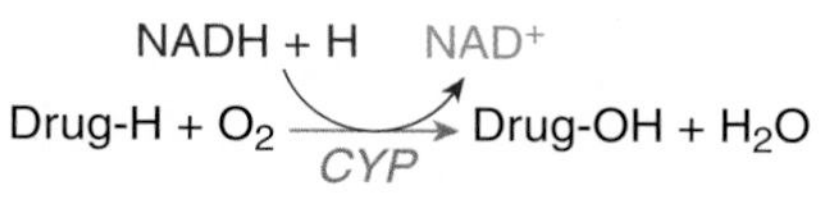

FIGURE 12–1. A common oxidation reaction catalyzed by CYP enzymes: the hydroxylation of Drug-H to Drug-OH.

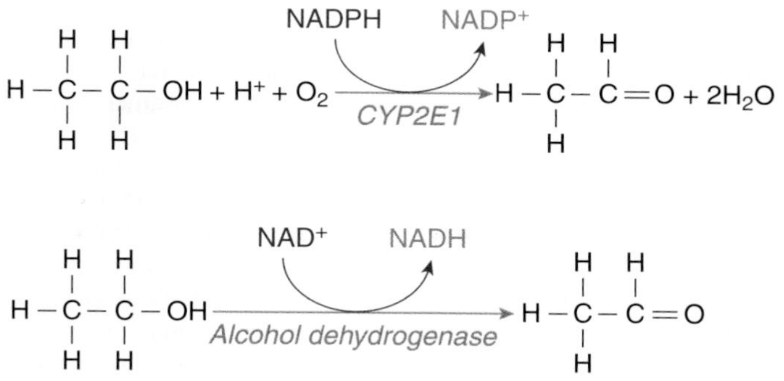

$$\text{H}_3\text{C}-\text{CH}_2-\text{OH} + H^+ + O_2 \xrightarrow[\text{CYP2E1}]{\text{NADPH} \;\to\; NADP^+} \text{H}_3\text{C}-\text{CH}=\text{O} + 2H_2O$$

$$\text{H}_3\text{C}-\text{CH}_2-\text{OH} \xrightarrow[\text{Alcohol dehydrogenase}]{NAD^+ \;\to\; \text{NADH}} \text{H}_3\text{C}-\text{CH}=\text{O}$$

FIGURE 12–2. Conversion of ethanol to acetaldehyde by CYP2E1 that uses NADPH and oxygen and by alcohol dehydrogenase that uses NAD^+. This illustrates how NAD and NADP can function in oxidation reactions in both their oxidized and reduced forms. Alcohol dehydrogenase has a low K_m for ethanol and is the predominant metabolic enzyme in moderate drinkers.

NADH transports its electrons to the cytochrome-mediated electron transport chain. This results in the production of adenosine triphosphate (ATP), the reduction of molecular oxygen, and the regeneration of NAD^+—all parts critical to the maintenance of oxidative metabolism. NADPH, created within the hexose monophosphate shunt, is used in the synthetic (anabolic) reactions of biosynthesis (especially fatty acid synthesis). NADPH is also coupled to the reduction of glutathione, which plays an important role in the protection of cells from oxidative damage.

The oxidation state of a specific carbon atom is determined by counting the number of hydrogen and carbon atoms to which it is connected. The more reduced a carbon, the higher the number of connections. For example, the carbon in methanol (CH_3OH) has three carbon-hydrogen bonds and is more reduced than the carbon in formaldehyde ($H_2C{=}O$), which has two. Carbon–carbon double bonds count as only one connection.

CYTOCHROME ENZYMES—AN OVERVIEW

Cytochromes are a class of hemoprotein enzymes whose function is electron transfer, using a cyclical transfer of electrons between oxidized (Fe^{3+}) or reduced (Fe^{2+}) forms of iron. One type of cytochrome is cytochrome P450 (CYP) whose nomenclature derives from the spectrophotometric characteristics of its associated heme molecule. When bound to carbon monoxide, the maximal absorption spectrum of the reduced CYP (Fe^{2+}) enzyme occurs at 450 nm.[63] CYP enzymes, which incorporate one atom of oxygen into the substrate and one atom into water, were once called *mixed-function oxidases*. This activity is now referred to as a *microsomal monooxygenation reaction*.[63,87]

Cytochrome enzymes perform many functions. The biotransformation CYP enzymes are bound to the lipid membranes of the smooth endoplasmic reticulum. They execute 75% of all xenobiotic metabolisms and most phase I oxidative biotransformations of xenobiotics.[34] A second role for CYP enzymes is synthetic: biotransforming endobiotics (chemicals endogenous to the body) to cholesterol, steroids, bile acids, fatty acids, prostaglandins, and other important lipids. Cytochromes also act as electron transfer xenobiotics within the mitochondrial electron transport chain.[36,63]

While over 6000 CYP genes exist in nature, the human genome project completed in 2003 set the number of human CYP genes at 57.[63] CYP enzymes are categorized according to the similarities of their amino acid sequences. They are in the same "family" if they are more than 40% comparable and same "subfamily" if they are more than 55% similar. Families are designated by an Arabic numeral, subfamilies by a capital letter, and each individual enzyme by another numeral, resulting in the nomenclature CYPnXm for each enzyme. For example, CYP3A4 is enzyme number 4 of the CYP3 family and of the CYP3A subfamily.[32,61] Most xenobiotic metabolism is done by the CYP1, CYP2, and CYP3 families, with a small amount done by the CYP4 family.[12,92] While 15 CYP enzymes metabolize xenobiotics,[69] nearly 90% is done by 6 CYP enzymes: 1A2, 2C9, 2C19, 2D6, 2E1, and 3A4 (Table 12–1).[63]

Most CYP enzymes are found in the liver, where they comprise 2% of total microsomal protein.[69] High concentrations are also in extrahepatic tissues, particularly the gastrointestinal tract and kidney.[21,64] The lungs,[97] heart,[66] and brain[22] have the next highest amounts. Each tissue has a unique profile of CYP enzymes that determines its sensitivity to different xenobiotics.[21] The CYP enzymes in the enterocytes of the small intestine actually contribute significantly to "first-pass" metabolism of some xenobiotics.[44,63] Corrected for tissue mass, the CYP enzyme system in the kidneys is as active as that in the liver. The activity of the renal CYP enzymes is decreased in patients with chronic renal failure, with relative sparing of CYPs 1A2, 2C19, and 2D6 compared with 3A4 and 2C9.[12]

CYTOCHROME P450 ENZYME SPECIFICITY FOR SUBSTRATES

In vitro models have been used to define the specificities of CYP enzymes for their substrates and inhibitors. However, activity in a test tube does not always correlate with that in a cell. These models use substrate and inhibitor concentrations that are much higher than would be encountered in vivo, and the mathematical models that extrapolate to clinically relevant processes yield conflicting results. This has resulted in discrepancies in reported substrates, inhibitors, and inducers of specific CYP enzymes.[93]

The substrate specificity of a CYP enzyme greatly affects its role in biotransformation.[34] CYP enzymes involved in endobiotic biotransformation are highly selective. For example, CYP1A2 specifically catalyzes only the 21-hydroxylation of progesterone, an important step in steroid synthesis.[35] Most CYP enzymes involved in xenobiotic biotransformation have broad substrate specificity and can metabolize many xenobiotics.[34] This is fortunate because the number of xenobiotic substrates may exceed 200,000.[52] Broad substrate specificity often results in multiple CYP enzymes being able to biotransform a xenobiotic. This enables the ongoing biotransformation despite an inhibition or deficiency of an enzyme. When a substrate can be biotransformed by more than one enzyme, the one that has the highest affinity for the substrate usually predominates at low substrate concentrations, while enzymes with lower affinity may be very important at high concentrations. This transition is usually concomitant with, but not dependent on, the saturation of the catalytic capacity of the primary enzyme as it reaches its maximum rate of activity.[34] The K_m, which is defined as the concentration of enzyme that results in 50% of maximal enzyme activity, describes this property of enzymes. For example, ADH in the liver has a very low Km for ethanol, making it the primary metabolic enzyme for ethanol when concentrations are low.[53] Ethanol is also biotransformed by the CYP2E1 enzyme, which has a high K_m for ethanol and only functions when concentrations are high. The CYP2E1 enzyme metabolizes little ethanol in moderate drinkers but accounts for significantly more

TABLE 12–1. Characteristics of Different Cytochrome P450 Enzymes[1,12,21,25,51,63,67]

Enzyme	1A2	2C9	2C19	2D6	2E1	3A4
Percent of liver CYPs	2%	10%–20%	10%–20%	30%	7%	40%–55%
Contribution to enterocyte CYPs	Minor	Minor	Minor	Minor	Minor	70%
Organs other than liver with enzyme	Lung	Small intestine, nasal mucosa, heart	Small intestine, nasal mucosa, heart	Small intestine, kidney, lung, heart	Lung small intestine, kidney	Much in small intestine; some in kidney, nasal mucosa, lung, stomach
Percent of metabolism of typically used drugs	2%–15%	10%–15%		25%–30%		50%–60%
Polymorphism[a]	No	Yes	Yes	Yes	No	No
Poor metabolizer						
African American		1%–2%	20%	2%–8%		
Asian		1%–2%	15%–20%	>1%		
White		1%–3%	3%–5%	5%–10%		
Ultra extensive metabolizer						
Asian				1%		
Ethiopian				30%		
Northern Europeans				1%–2%		
Southern Europeans				10%		

[a] Enzyme variations exist even in those listed as "No" for polymorphism.

biotransformation in alcoholics. As another example, diazepam is metabolized by both CYP2C19 and CYP3A4 enzymes. However, the affinity of CYP3A4 for diazepam is so low (ie, the K_m is high) that most diazepam is metabolized by CYP2C19.[37]

The substrate selectivity of some CYP enzymes is determined by molecular, and physicochemical properties of the substrates. The CYP1A subfamily has greater specificity for planar polyaromatic substrates such as benzo[*a*]pyrene. The CYP2E enzyme subfamily targets low-molecular-weight hydrophilic xenobiotics, whereas the CYP3A4 enzyme has increased affinity for lipophilic compounds. Substrates of CYP2C9 are usually weakly acidic, whereas those of CYP2D6 are more basic.[51] High specificity can also result from key structural considerations such as stereoselectivity. Some xenobiotics are racemic mixtures of stereoisomers. These may be substrates for different CYP enzymes and have distinct affinities for the enzymes, resulting in different rates of metabolism. For example, R-warfarin is biotransformed by CYP3A4 and CYP1A2, whereas S-warfarin is metabolized by CYP2C9.[78,87]

The CYP enzymes that biotransform a specific xenobiotic cannot be predicted by its drug class. Whereas fluoxetine and paroxetine are both major substrates and potent inhibitors of CYP2D6, sertraline is not extensively metabolized and exhibits minimal interaction with other antidepressants.[5] Most β-hydroxy-β-methylglutarylcoenzyme A (HMG-CoA) reductase inhibitors are metabolized by CYP3A4 (lovastatin, simvastatin, and atorvastatin); however, fluvastatin is metabolized by CYP2D6 and pravastatin undergoes virtually no CYP enzyme metabolism at all.[32] Among angiotensin-II receptor blockers, losartan and irbesartan are metabolized by CYP2C9, while valsartan, eprosartan, and candesartan are not substrates for any CYP enzyme. In addition, losartan is a prodrug whose active metabolite provides most of the pharmacologic activity, while irbesartan is the primary active compound. For these two drugs the inhibition of CYP2C9 is predicted to have opposite effects.[28]

CYTOCHROME P450 AND DRUG–DRUG/ DRUG–CHEMICAL INTERACTIONS

Adverse reactions to medications and drug–drug interactions are common causes of morbidity and mortality in hospitalized patients, the risk of which increases with the number of drugs taken (Chaps. 138 and 139). Fifty percent of adverse reactions may be related to pharmacogenetic factors.[30] The most significant interactions are mediated by CYP enzymes.[63] The impact of genetic polymorphism and enzyme induction or inhibition are addressed below.

CYP enzymes are involved in many types of drug interactions. The ability of potential new drugs to induce or inhibit enzymes is an important consideration of industry. Drug development focuses on the potential of new xenobiotics to induce or inhibit during the drug discovery phase. Various in vitro models have been created to enable this early determination.[54]

Many xenobiotics interact with the CYP enzymes. St. John's wort, an herb marketed as a natural antidepressant, induces multiple CYP enzymes including 1A2, 2C9, and 3A4. The induction of CYP3A4 by St. John's wort is associated with a 57% decrease in effective serum concentrations of indinavir when given concomittantly.[71] Xenobiotics contained in grapefruit juice, such as naringin and furanocoumarins, are both substrates and inhibitors of CYP3A4. They inhibit the first-pass metabolism of CYP3A4 substrates by inhibiting CYP3A4 activity in both the gastrointestinal tract and the liver.[18] Polycyclic hydrocarbons found in charbroiled meats and in cigarette smoke induce CYP1A2. For smokers who drink coffee, concentrations of caffeine, a CYP1A2 substrate, will be increased following cessation of smoking.[25]

GENETIC POLYMORPHISM

There is much variation in response to xenobiotics and to coadministration of inhibitory or inducing xenobiotics. The translation of DNA sequences into proteins results in the phenotypic expression of the genes. When a genetic mutation occurs, the changed DNA may continue to exist, be eliminated, or propagate into a polymorphism. A polymorphism is a genetic change that exists in at least 1% of the human population.[30] A polymorphism in a biotransformation enzyme may change its rate of activity. The heterogeneity of CYP enzymes contributes to the differences in metabolic activity between patients.[30] Differences in biotransformation capacity that lead to toxicity, once thought to be "idiosyncratic" drug reactions, are likely caused by these inherited differences in the genetic complement of individuals.

The normal catalytic speed of CYP enzyme activity is called *extensive*. There are 2 major metabolizer phenotypes due to polymorphism: poor (slow) and ultraextensive (rapid).[61,30] The CYP2C19 and CYP2D6 genes are highly polymorphic (Table 12–1).[41] The CYP2D6 gene, which has 76 different alleles, is associated with both ultraextensive and poor metabolism. The CYP2C19 and CYP2C9 genes are both associated with poor metabolizers.[12,63]

The clinical implications of polymorphisms are vast. A prodrug may not be bioactivated because the patient is a poor metabolizer. Conversely, a drug may not reach a therapeutic concentration because the patient is an ultraextensive metabolizer.[30]

Polymorphisms exist for enzymes other than CYP enzymes. A classic one is the inheritance of rapid or slow "acetylator" phenotypes. Acetylation is important for the biotransformation of amines ($R{-}NH_2$) or hydrazines ($NH_2{-}NH_2$). Slow acetylators are at increased risk of toxicity associated with the slower biotransformation of certain nitrogen-containing xenobiotics such as isoniazid, procainamide, hydralazine, and sulfonamides.[24,80]

Polymorphic genes that code for enzymes in important metabolic pathways affect the toxicity of a xenobiotic by altering the response to or the disposition of the xenobiotic. An example occurs in glucose-6-phosphate dehydrogenase (G6PD) deficiency. G6PD is a critical enzyme in the hexose monophosphate shunt, a metabolic pathway located in the red blood cell (RBC) that produces NADPH, which is required to maintain RBC glutathione in a reduced state. In turn, reduced glutathione prevents hemolysis during oxidative stress.[14] In patients deficient in G6PD, oxidative stress produced by electrophilic xenobiotics results in hemolysis.

INDUCTION OF CYP ENZYMES

Biotransformation by induced CYP enzymes results in either increased activity of prodrugs or enhanced elimination of drugs. Stopping an inducing agent may result in the opposite effects. Either way, maintaining therapeutic concentrations of affected drugs is difficult, resulting in either toxicity or subtherapeutic concentrations. Interestingly, not all CYP enzymes are inducible. Inducible ones include CYP2A, CYP2B, CYP2C, CYP2E, and CYP3A.[54]

While varied mechanisms of induction exist, the most common and significant is nuclear receptor (NR)-mediated increase in gene transcription.[54] Nuclear receptors are the largest group of transcription factors, proteins that switch genes on or off.[90] They regulate reproduction, growth, and biotransformation enzymes, including CYP enzymes.[88] Nuclear receptors exist mostly within the cytoplasm of cells. The CYP families 2 and 3 both have gene activation triggered through the nuclear receptors pregnane X receptor (PXR) and constitutive androstane receptor (CAR). The CYP 1A subfamily uses the aryl hydrocarbon receptor (AhR) as its NR. Ligands, molecules that bind to and affect the reactivity of a central molecule, are typically small and lipophilic, enabling them to enter cells. Many xenobiotics are ligands. Ligands bind the NRs, resulting in structural changes that enable the NR-ligand complexes to be translocated into the cell nucleus. Within the nucleus, NR-ligand complexes bind to a heterodimerization partner such as retinoid X receptor (RXR), shared by PXR and CAR, or AhR nuclear translocator (Arnt), by AhR. This new complex then interacts with specific response elements of DNA, initiating the transcription of a segment of DNA, and resulting in the phenotypic expression of the respective CYP enzyme.

The ligand binding domain of the PXR receptor is very hydrophobic and flexible, enabling this pocket to bind many substrates of varied sizes and reflecting why PXR can be activated by such a broad group of ligands.[67,88] For example, xenobiotic ligands that bind the NR PXR that targets the *CYP3A4* gene include rifampin, omeprazole, carbamazepine, and troleandomycin. Phenobarbital, a classic inducing agent, is a ligand that binds CAR.[90] The induction of CYP1A subfamily enzymes is through the interaction with the NR AhR. Exogenous AhR ligands are hydrophobic, cyclic, planar molecules. Classic AhR ligands include polycyclic hydrocarbons such as 2,3,7,8-tetrachlorodibenzo-*p*-dioxin and benzo[*a*]pyrene.[67]

Induction requires time to occur because it involves de novo synthesis of new proteins. Similarly, withdrawal of the inducer results in a slow return to the original enzyme concentration.[54] Polyaromatic hydrocarbons (PAHs) result in CYP1A subfamily induction within 3 to 6 hours with maximum effect within 24 hours.[84] The inducer rifampin does not affect verapamil trough concentrations maximally until 1 week; followed by a 2-week return to baseline steady state after withdrawal of rifampin.[54] Xenobiotics with long half-lives require longer periods to reach steady-state concentrations that maximize induction. Phenobarbital or fluoxetine, which have long half-lives, may fully manifest induction only after weeks of exposure. Conversely, xenobiotics with short half-lives, such as rifampin or venlafaxine, can reach maximum induction within days.[12,32]

Inconsistency in CYP induction exists between individuals. This variability exists for CYP enzymes in all organs.[54,67] In an in vitro study of inducers on 60 livers, differences in enzyme induction ranged from 5-fold for CYP3A4 and CYP2C up to more than 50-fold for CYP2A6 and CYP2D6.[54] The inconsistency likely results from multiple environmental factors including diet, tobacco, and pollutants.[54] There is variation in the extent to which inducers can generate new CYP enzymes. Identical dosing regimens with rifampin have resulted in induction of in vivo hepatic CYP3A4 with up to 18-fold differences between subjects.[54] There is an inverse correlation of the degree of inducibility of an enzyme and the baseline enzyme concentration. Patients with a relatively low baseline concentration of a CYP enzyme will be more inducible than those with a high baseline concentration. Interestingly, the maximum concentrations of CYP enzymes seem to be quantitatively similar among individuals, suggesting a limit to which enzymes can be induced.[54]

While the focus of this section is on CYP enzymes, it appears that all phases of xenobiotic metabolism are regulated by nuclear receptors.[9] Also, just as genetic polymorphisms exist for CYP enzymes, they exist for nuclear receptors including AhR, CAR, and PXR. This results in varied sensitivities to the ligands that complex with the nuclear receptors, ultimately resulting in differences in CYP enzyme induction.[54,90]

INHIBITION OF CYP ENZYMES

CYP enzyme inhibition can result in increased bioavailability of a drug or decreased activity of a prodrug that is no longer able to be metabolically activated.[69] Inhibition of CYP enzymes is the most common cause of harmful drug–drug interactions.[69] Inhibition of CYP enzymes by coadministered xenobiotics has resulted in the removal of many medications from the market in recent years including terfenadine, mibefradil, bromfenac, astemizole, cisapride, cerivastatin, and nefazodone.[93] The appendix at the end of this chapter includes a comprehensive listing of cytochrome P450 substrates, inhibitors, and inducers.

Inhibition mechanisms include irreversible (mechanism-based inhibition) and the more common reversible processes. The most common type of reversible inhibition is competitive, where the substrate and inhibitor both bind the active site of the enzyme.[69,93] Binding is weak and is formed and broken down easily, resulting in the enzyme becoming available again. It occurs rapidly, usually beginning within hours.[12] Because the degree of inhibition varies with the concentration of the inhibitor, the time to reach the maximal effect correlates with the half-life of the xenobiotic in question.[12] A competitive inhibitor can be overcome by increasing the substrate concentration. Each substrate of a CYP enzyme is an inhibitor of the metabolism of all the other substrates of the same enzyme, thereby increasing their concentrations and half life. Noncompetitive inhibition occurs when an inhibitor binds a location on an enzyme that is not the active site, resulting in a structural change that inhibits the active enzyme site. For example, noncompetitive inhibitors of CYP2C9 include nifedipine, tranylcypromine, and medroxyprogesterone acetate.[79] Another reversible mechanism results from competition between one xenobiotic and a metabolite of a second xenobiotic at its CYP enzyme substrate binding site. For example, the metabolites of clarithromycin and erythromycin produced by CYP3A inhibit further CYP3A activity. The effect is reversible and usually increases with repeated dosing.[79] Some reversible inhibitors bind so tightly to the enzyme that they essentially function as irreversible inhibitors.[69]

Irreversible inhibitors have reactive groups that covalently bind the enzyme, permanently. They display time-dependent inhibition because the amount of active enzyme at a given concentration of irreversible inhibitor will be different depending on how long the inhibitor is preincubated with the enzyme. Because the enzyme will never be reactivated, inhibition lasts until new enzyme is synthesized.[69] A relatively rare form of irreversible inhibition occurs when a reactive metabolite of a xenobiotic inhibits further metabolism of the substrate. This so-called suicide inhibition results in the destruction of the bound CYP enzyme.[28,77]

One measure of inhibitor potency is the inhibitory concentration, K_i, the concentration of the inhibitor that produces 50% inhibition of the enzyme. The more potent the inhibitor, the lower the value.[84] Values below 1 μmol/L are regarded as potent.[65] The azole antifungals are very potent with K_i values of 0.02 μmol/L.[84]

The impact of an inhibitor is also affected by the fraction of the substrate that is cleared by the inhibited, target enzyme. The inhibition of a CYP enzyme will have little impact if the enzyme only metabolizes a fraction of the affected drug.[65] Conversely, drugs that are primarily metabolized by a single CYP enzyme are more susceptible to interactions.[69] Astemizole and simvastatin are mainly biotransformed by CYP3A4. The potent and specific CYP3A inhibitor itraconazole prevents their metabolism, resulting in torsade de pointes dysrhythmias or rhabdomyolysis, respectively.[1]

SPECIFIC CYP ENZYMES

CYP1A1 and 1A2 While 1A1 is located primarily in extrahepatic tissue, 1A2 is a hepatic enzyme and is involved in the metabolism of 10 to 15% of all pharmaceuticals used today.[12,54] They both are very inducible by polycyclic aromatic hydrocarbons including those in cigarette smoke and charred food. They bioactivate several procarcinogens including benzo[*a*]pyrene.[45] Xenobiotics activated by the CYP1 enzyme family in the gastrointestinal tract are linked to colon cancer.[63]

CYP2C9 Approximately one-third of human CYP enzymes are in the CYP2 enzyme family, which, with 76 alleles, exhibits the greatest degree of genetic polymorphism.[25] The CYP2C9 enzyme is the most abundant enzyme of the CYP2C enzyme subfamily, which with CYP2C19, comprises approximately 10%–20% of the CYP enzymes in the liver.[25] This enzyme is associated with polymorphisms (Table 12–1).[12,63] This enzyme biotransforms S-warfarin, the more active isomer of warfarin. There is an association between slow metabolism and an increased risk of bleeding in patients on warfarin.[78]

CYP2D6 Twenty-five percent of all drugs used today, including 50% of the commonly used antipsychotics, are substrates for CYP2D6. It is sometimes called debrisoquine hydrolase as it was first identified with studying the metabolism of the antihypertensive agent debrisoquine.[12,41,63]

CYP2E1 This enzyme comprises 7% of the total CYP enzyme content in the human liver.[62] It metabolizes small organic compounds including alcohol, carbon tetrachloride, and halogenated anaesthetic agents.[84] It also biotransforms low-molecular-weight xenobiotics including benzene, acetone, and N-nitrosamines.[84] Some of these substrates are procarcinogens which are bioactivated by CYP2E1. Besides CYP1A2, this is the only other CYP enzyme linked to cancer.[63] The assessment for a relationship to cancer is particularly intense because many of its substrates are environmental xenobiotics. The induction of CYP2E1 is associated with increased liver injury by reactive metabolites of carbon tetrachloride and of bromobenzene[37] (Chap. 26). During the metabolism of substrates that include carbon tetrachloride, ethanol, acetaminophen, aniline, and N-nitrosomethylamine, CYP2E1 actively produces free radicals and other reactive metabolites associated with adduct formation and lipid peroxidation[15] (Chaps. 8 and 34). CYP2E1 is inhibited by acute elevations of ethanol, an effect illustrated by the capacity of acute administration of ethanol to inhibit the metabolism of acetaminophen.[10] The chronic ingestion of ethanol hastens its own metabolism through enzyme induction.

CYP3A4 CYP3A4 is the most abundant CYP in the human liver, comprising 40% to 55% of the mass of hepatic CYP enzymes.[12,25] The CYP3A4 enzyme is the most common one found in the intestinal mucosa and is responsible for much first-pass drug metabolism.[12] Numerous xenobiotics are metabolized by CYP3A4. It is involved in the biotransformation of 50% to 60% of all pharmaceuticals.[62,98] It has such broad substrate specificity because it accommodates especially large lipophilic substrates and can adopt multiple conformations. It can even simultaneously fit two relatively large compounds (ketoconazole, erythromycin) in its active site.[77]

An example of an adverse drug interaction related to this enzyme is the QT interval prolongation and torsades de pointes that occurred in patients taking terfenadine or astemizole in combination with ketoconazole or erythromycin.[68,75] Ketoconazole inhibits CYP3A4, causing a 15-fold to 72-fold increase in serum concentrations of terfenadine.[63] Bioflavonoids in grapefruit juice decrease metabolism of some substrates by 5-fold to 12-fold.[12,63] The CYP3A4 enzyme does not exhibit genetic polymorphism; however, there are large interindividual variations in enzyme concentrations.[98]

PHASE II BIOTRANSFORMATION REACTIONS

Phase II biotransformation reactions are synthetic, catalyzing conjugation of the products of phase I reactions or molecules with sites amenable to conjugation. Conjugation usually terminates the pharmacologic activity of the xenobiotic and greatly increases their water solubility and excretability.[56,87,96] Conjugation occurs most commonly with glucuronic acid, sulfates, and glutathione. Less common phase II reactions include amino acid conjugation, such as glycine, glutamic acid, and taurine; acetylation; and methylation.

Glucuronidation is the most common phase II synthesis reaction.[56] It occurs only within microsomal membranes. Glucuronyl transferase has relatively low substrate affinity but it has high capacity at higher substrate concentrations.[96] The glucuronic acid, donated by uridine diphosphate glucuronic acid (UDPG), is conjugated with the nitrogen, sulfhydryl, hydroxyl, or carboxyl groups of substrates. Smaller conjugates usually undergo renal elimination, whereas larger ones undergo biliary elimination.[51]

Sulfation complements glucuronidation because it is a high affinity but low capacity reaction that occurs primarily in the cytosol. For example, the affinity of sulfate for phenol is very high (the K_m is low), so that when low doses of phenol are administered, the predominant excretion product is the sulfate ester. Because the capacity of this reaction is readily saturated, glucuronidation becomes the main method of detoxification when high doses of phenol are administered.[56,96] Sulfate conjugates are highly ionized and very water soluble. Of note, sulfation is reversible by the action of sulfatases within the liver. The resultant metabolites may be resulfated and the cycle may repeat itself further.[96]

Glutathione *S*-transferases are important because they catalyze the conjugation of the tripeptide glutathione (glycine-glutamate-cysteine, or GSH) with a diverse group of reactive, electrophilic metabolites of phase I CYP enzymes. The reactive compounds initiate an attack on the sulfur group of cysteine, resulting in conjugation with GSH that detoxifies the reactive metabolite. Of the three phase II reactions addressed, hepatic concentrations of glutathione by far account for the greatest amount of cofactors used. While intracellular glutathione is difficult to deplete, when it does occur, severe hepatotoxicity often follows.[96] Some GSH conjugates are directly excreted. More commonly, the glycine and glutamate residues are cleaved and the remaining cysteine is acetylated to form an *N*-acetylcysteine (mercapturic acid) conjugate that is readily excreted in the urine. A familiar example of this detoxification is the avid binding of *N*-acetyl-*p*-benzoquinoneimine (NAPQI), the toxic metabolite of acetaminophen, by glutathione.[5,11]

As with the CYP enzymes, many phase II enzymes are inducible. For example, UDP-glucuronosyltransferase which executes glucuronidation is inducible via PXR, CAR, and AhR nuclear receptors after binding with rifampin, phenobarbital, and PAHs, respectively. Its activity varies 6-fold to 15-fold in liver microsomes.[90]

MEMBRANE TRANSPORTERS

While the focus on drug disposition has traditionally been on biotransformation, membrane transporters also impact drug disposition.[38] Because they usually occur after phase I and II biotransformation, their actions are sometimes called phase III metabolism.[42] Their physiologic role is to transport sugars, lipids, amino acids, and hormones so as to regulate cellular solute and fluid balance. However, they affect drug disposition just as do biotransformation processes by facilitating or preventing the passage of xenobiotics through membranes.[46] Uptake transporters translocate drugs into cells while efflux transporters export xenobiotics, often against concentration gradients, out of cells. Most transporters are in the adenosine triphosphate binding cassette (ABC) family of transmembrane proteins that use energy from ATP hydrolysis.[13,38] This family includes the P-glycoprotein family. Some transporters move substrates both into and out of cells. Organs important for drug disposition have multiple transporters that have overlapping substrate capabilities, a redundancy that enhances protection. In the small intestine, P-glycoprotein is important because it can actively extrude xenobiotics back into the intestinal lumen.[13] The degree of phenotypic expression of P-glycoprotein affects the bioavailability of many xenobiotics including paclitaxel, digoxin, and protease inhibitors. Hepatocyte efflux transporters move biotransformed xenobiotics into bile. Transporters in endothelial cells of the blood–brain barrier prevent

CNS entry of substrate xenobiotics.[13,38] As with biotransformation enzymes and nuclear receptors, membrane transporters may be inhibited or induced. Digoxin, a high affinity substrate for P-glycoprotein, has increased bioavailability when administered with P-glycoprotein inhibitors such as clarithromycin or atorvastatin.[38] Loperamide is a substrate for P-glycoprotein that limits its intestinal absorption or CNS entry. Coadministration with quinidine, a P-glycoprotein inhibitor, results in increased opioid CNS effects of loperamide.[38] As with the biotransformation enzymes, polymorphisms exist for membrane transporters. However, the clinical significance of these is not clear.[17]

MECHANISMS OF CELLULAR INJURY

Ideally and commonly, potentially toxic metabolites produced by phase I reactions are detoxified during phase II reactions. However, detoxification does not always occur. This section reviews mechanisms of cellular injury related to xenobiotic biotransformation.

SYNTHESIS OF TOXINS

Sometimes a xenobiotic is mistaken for a natural substrate by synthetic enzymes that biotransform it into an injurious compound. The incorporation of the rodenticide fluoroacetate into the tricarboxylic acid cycle is an example of this mechanism of toxic injury (Fig. 12–3).[70] Another example is illustrated by analogs of purine or pyrimidine bases that are phosphorylated and inserted into growing DNA or RNA chains, resulting in mutations and disruption of cell division. This mechanism is used therapeutically with 5-fluorouracil (5-FU), an antitumor, pyrimidine base analog. When phosphorylated to 5-fluoro-dUTP and incorporated into growing DNA chains, it causes structural instability of the cellular DNA and inhibits tumor growth.[75]

INJURY BY METABOLITES OF BIOTRANSFORMATION

Many toxic products result from metabolic activation (Table 12–2).[43] The CYP enzymes most associated with bioactivation are 1A1, 1B1, 2A6, and 2E1 while 2C9 and 2D6 yield little toxic activation.[34]

Highly reactive metabolites exert damage at the site where they are synthesized; reacting too quickly with local molecules to be transported elsewhere. This commonly occurs in the liver, the major site of biotransformation of xenobiotics[33,82] (Chap. 26). However, the lungs, skin, kidneys, gastrointestinal tract, and nasal mucosa can also create toxic metabolites that cause local injury.[11,49] Overdoses of acetaminophen lead to excessive hepatic production of the highly reactive electrophile NAPQI, which initiates a damaging covalent bond with hepatocytes[5,10] (Chap. 34). Acute renal tubular necrosis also occurs in patients with overdose of acetaminophen, attributed to its biotransformation by

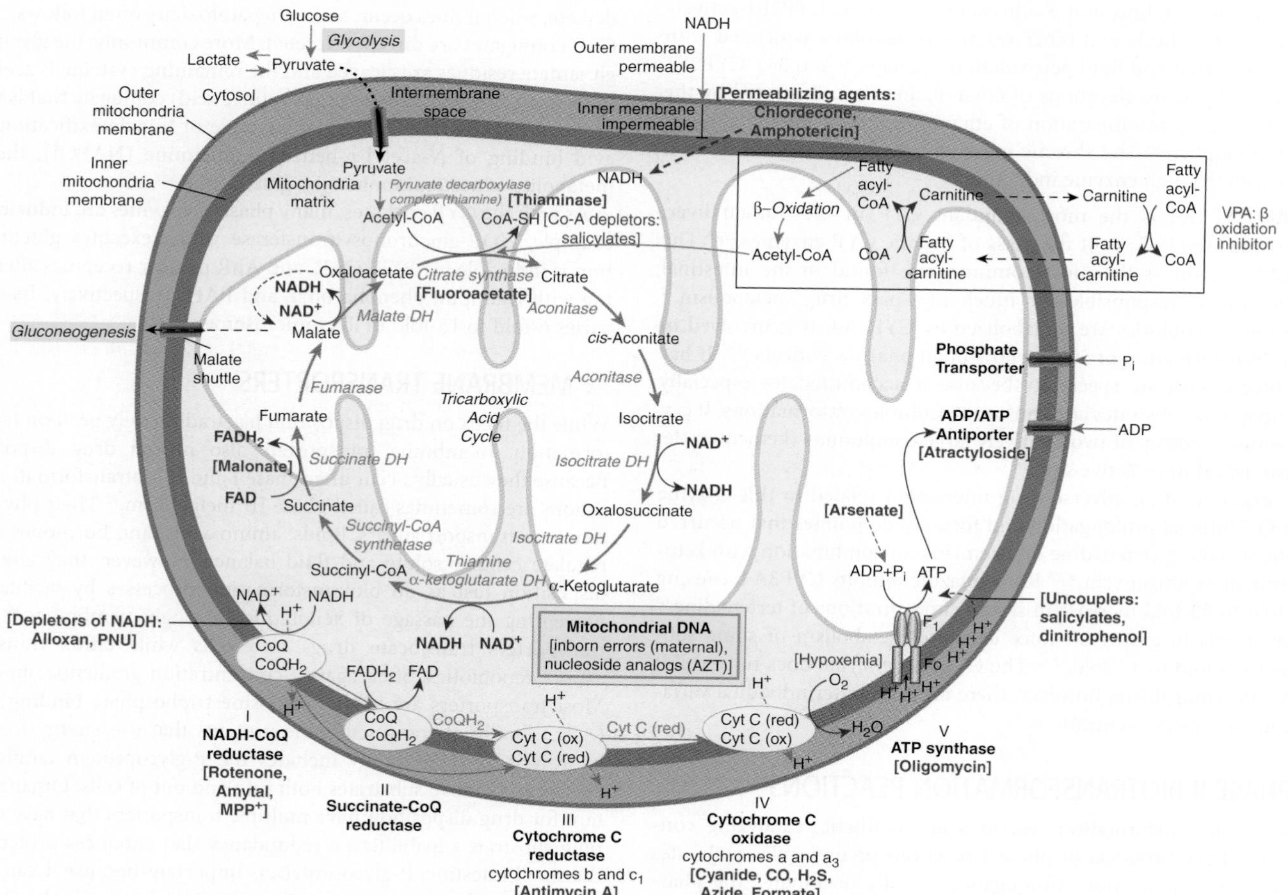

FIGURE 12–3. Pyruvate is converted to acetylcoenzyme A (acetyl-CoA), which enters the Krebs cycle as shown. Reducing equivalents, in the form of NADH, and FADH, donate electrons to a chain of cytochromes beginning with NADH dehydrogenase. These reactions "couple" the energy released during electron transport to the production of ATP. Ultimately, electrons combine with oxygen to form water. The sites of action of xenobiotics that inhibit oxidative metabolism are shown. The sites where thiamine functions as a coenzyme are also illustrated. DH = dehydrogenase.

TABLE 12–2. Examples of Xenobiotics Activated to Toxins by Human Cytochrome P450 Enzymes

CYP Enzyme	Substrate	Toxicity	CYP Enzyme	Substrate	Toxicity
1A1	Benzo[*a*]pyrene (PAH)	IARC Group 1	2E1	Carbon tetrachloride	IARC Group 2B
1A2	Acetaminophen	Hepatotoxicity		Chloroform	IARC Group 2B
	Aflatoxin B (*Aspergillus* mycotoxin)	IARC Group 1		Chloroform	IARC Group 2B
	2-Naphthylamine (azo dye production)	IARC Group 1		Ethylene dibromide (former gas additive and fumigant; still indust. intermediate)	IARC Group 2A
	NNK (nitrosamine in tobacco)	IARC Group 1		Ethyl carbamate (former antineoplastic)	IARC 2A
	NNK (nitrosamine in tobacco)	IARC Group 1		Halothane	Hepatotoxicity
	N-Nitrosodiethylamine (gas and lubricant additive, copolymer softener)	IARC Group 2A		Methylene Chloride	IARC Group 2B
2B6	Chrysene (PAH)	IARC Group 2B		N-Nitrosodimethylamine (formerly in rocket fuel)	IARC Group 2A
	Cyclophosphamide	IARC Group 1		Styrene	IARC Group 2A
2C 8,9	Phenytoin	IARC Group 2B		Trichloroethylene	IARC Group 2A
	Tienilic acid (old diuretic; off market)	Hepatotoxicity		Vinyl chloride	IARC Group 1
	Valproic acid	Hepatotoxicity	3A4	Acetaminophen	Hepatotoxicity
2D6	NNK (nitrosamine in tobacco)	IARC Group 1		Aflatoxin B_1 (*Aspergillus* mycotoxin)	IARC Group 1
2F1	Acetaminophen	Hepatotoxicity		Chrysene (PAH)	IARC Group 2B
	3-Methylindole (in perfumes, cigarettes for flavor)	Pneumotoxicity		Cyclophosphamide	IARC Group 1
	Valproic acid	Hepatotoxicity		1-Nitropyrene (PAH)	IARC Group 2B
2E1	Acetaminophen	Hepatotoxicity		Senecionine (pyrrolizidine alkaloid)	Hepatotoxicity
	Acrylonitrile	IARC Group 2B		Sterigmatocystin (*Aspergillus* mycotoxin)	IARC Group 2B
	Benzene	IARC Group 1			

IARC – International Agency for Research on Cancer of the World Health Organization. Group 1 – known carcinogen; Group 2A – probable carcinogen; Group 2B – possible carcinogen. PAH – polycyclic aromatic hydrocarbon

prostaglandin H synthase within renal tubular cells to a highly reactive semiquinoneimine.[23,48]

Monoamine oxidases (MAOs) are mitochondrial enzymes present in many tissues. They oxidize many amines, including dopamine, epinephrine, and serotonin, and xenobiotics such as primaquine and haloperidol. The metabolic activity of MAOs was responsible for the outbreak of parkinsonism associated with the use of methylphenyltetrahydropyridine (MPTP), an unintended by-product of attempts to synthesize a "designer" analog of meperidine, methylphenylpropionoxypiperidine (MPPP). After crossing the blood–brain barrier, MPTP is biotransformed by MAO in glial cells to methylphenyldihydropyridine ($MPDP^+$), which is nonenzymatically converted to MPP^+. The MPP^+ is subsequently taken up by specific dopamine transport systems into dopaminergic neurons in the substantia nigra, resulting in inhibition of oxidative phosphorylation and subsequent neuronal death.[31]

FREE RADICAL FORMATION

Within an atom, it is energetically favorable for electrons to exist in lone pairs or as a part of a chemical bond. An element or compound with an unpaired electron, called a *radical* or *free radical*, is very reactive and it generally does not exist for long. It rapidly seeks other species in order to obtain another electron. Radicals include the superoxide anion $O_2\bullet^-$, which is produced by adding an electron to O_2, and the highly reactive hydroxyl radical HO•, which is produced by splitting the H_2O_2 molecule into two. The H_2O_2 molecule itself is reactive and is also associated with injury. The superoxide and hydroxyl radicals react with other molecules in order to stabilize; however, by taking an electron in order to do so, they generate new free radical species, potentially initiating a chain reaction. The production of radicals is a normal occurrence and the human body has defense mechanisms. Some xenobiotics promote the formation of reactive oxidizing species to the extent that defensive mechanisms against oxidants are overwhelmed, a condition called *oxidative stress*. Oxidizing species are called such because, by reducing themselves by taking away electrons, they oxidize the species from which they took the electrons.[7]

While oxidative stress may result in oxidative damage to nucleic acids and proteins, other classic targets are polyunsaturated fatty acids (PUFA) in cellular membranes, resulting in lipid peroxidation (the oxidative destruction of lipids). This attack removes the particularly reactive hydrogen atom, with its lone electron, from a methylene carbon of a PUFA; leaving an unpaired electron and causing the formation of a lipid radical. This lipid radical attacks other PUFA, causing a chain reaction that destroys the cellular membrane. Membrane degradation products initiate inflammatory reactions in the cells, resulting in further damage.[82,7]

Molecular oxygen (O_2) has a lone pair of electrons in its orbit. Because oxygen is a relatively weak univalent electron acceptor (and most organic molecules are weak univalent electron donors), oxygen cannot efficiently oxidize amino acids and nucleic acids. However, the unpaired electrons of O_2 readily interact with the unpaired electrons of transition metals and organic radicals. Metals frequently catalyze the creation of oxygen free radicals. The following is an example of hydroxyl radical formation: (1) A first step is the addition of an electron to O_2 to create the superoxide ion. (2) The very reactive superoxide combines with hydrogen and another electron to produce hydrogen peroxide. (3) In the presence of a metal ion catalyst such as iron, hydrogen peroxide undergoes various reactions to produce the hydroxyl radical. The dot in these formulas represents an unpaired electron, the hallmark of a free radical.[40,35,56]

$$(1)\ O_2 + e^- \rightarrow O_2^{\bar{\bullet}}$$

$$(2)\ O_2^{\bar{\bullet}} + 2H^+ + e^- \rightarrow H_2O_2$$

$$(3)\ H_2O_2 \xrightarrow[Fe^{2+}]{} OH^- + OH\bullet \ \text{(Fenton)}$$

$$H_2O_2 + O_2^{\bar{\bullet}} \xrightarrow[Fe^{2+}]{} O_2 + OH^- + OH\bullet \ \text{(Haber-Weiss)}$$

The damaging effects of the free radicals are decreased by reaction with antioxidants such as ascorbate, tocopherols, and glutathione.[56] Deficiencies of antioxidants, especially glutathione, are associated with increased oxidative damage. Free radicals are also neutralized by several enzymes, including peroxidase, superoxide dismutase, and catalase.

The ethanol-inducible CYP2E1 enzyme produces significant amounts of superoxide and peroxide free radicals, and, in the presence of iron, hydroxyl free radicals that readily initiate lipid peroxidation. This has been studied extensively in models of the metabolism of carbon tetrachloride, ethanol, and acetaminophen.[20] The formation of free radicals is implicated in the pulmonary injury caused by paraquat, the myocardial injury caused by doxorubicin, and the liver injury caused by carbon tetrachloride.[60,72] Paraquat reacts with NADPH to form a pyridinyl free radical, which, in turn, reacts with oxygen to generate the superoxide anion radical. Doxorubicin is metabolized to a semiquinone free radical in the cardiac mitochondria, which, in the presence of oxygen, forms a superoxide anion radical that initiates myocardial lipid peroxidation.[60] Carbon tetrachloride (CCl_4) is metabolized to the trichloromethyl radical ($\bullet CCl_3$) that binds covalently to cellular macromolecules. In the presence of oxygen, this is converted to the trichloromethylperoxyl radical ($\bullet CCl_3O_2$) that can initiate lipid peroxidation (Fig. 12–4).[73] See Chap. 106 for a more extensive discussion.

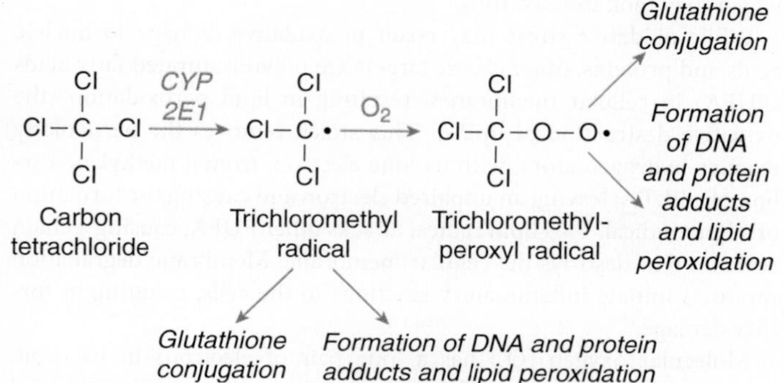

FIGURE 12–4. Carbon tetrachloride metabolism by the hepatocyte. Under hypoxic conditions, the CCl_3 radical is the predominant species formed. At higher oxygen tensions, CCl_3 radical is oxidized to the CCl_3OO radical, which is more readily detoxified by glutathione. Both free radicals bind to hepatocytes and cause cellular injury.

CRITICAL BIOCHEMICAL PATHWAYS AND XENOBIOTICS THAT AFFECT THEM

Energy metabolism is the foundation of cellular function. It provides high-energy fuel, predominantly in the form of ATP, for all energy-dependent cellular processes such as synthesis, active transport, and maintenance of electrolyte balance and membrane integrity. Numerous pathways interconnect glycogen, fat, and protein reserves in many tissues that store and retrieve ATP and glucose. The brain and red blood cells are entirely dependent on glucose for energy production, while other tissues can also use ketone bodies and fatty acids to synthesize ATP. Rapid cell death occurs if the production or use of ATP is inhibited, thus the goal of many metabolic processes is the production and mobilization of cellular energy.

Catabolic pathways that produce cellular energy include glycolysis, the tricarboxylic acid (citric acid, or Krebs) cycle, and oxidative phosphorylation via the electron transport chain. Citric acid occurs in the cytosol while the citric acid cycle and the electron transport chain are located within the mitochondria. Glycolysis produces small amounts of ATP through the anaerobic metabolism of glucose. Pyruvate, the end product of glycolysis, yields far more ATP when it is converted to acetylcoenzyme A (acetyl-CoA) and "processed" in the citric acid cycle (Fig. 12–3). Fat and protein yield their energy through their conversion to acetyl-CoA and other intermediates of the citric acid cycle. The citric acid cycle and oxidative phosphorylation, via the electron transport chain, result in most ATP synthesis. Oxidative phosphorylation disposes of electrons or "reducing equivalents" and converts their energy to ATP. A lack of oxygen stops the electron transport chain and ATP production. Oxidative metabolism is highly energy efficient, producing 36 moles of ATP for each mole of glucose metabolized, compared to the 2 moles of ATP produced by glycolysis. The following sections review the basics of cellular energy metabolism and several important xenobiotics that affect these critical metabolic functions (Table 12–3).[47,25]

GLYCOLYSIS

Glycolysis is the first biochemical pathway in the metabolism of glucose. Other sugars enter the glycolytic pathway after conversion to glycolytic intermediates (Fig. 12–5). The glycolytic process converts 1 molecule of glucose to 2 pyruvate molecules + 2 ATP + 2 NADH. Pyruvate may follow many paths. Under anaerobic conditions, the 2 pyruvates produced from 1 glucose molecule are reduced by lactate dehydrogenase to 2 lactate molecules in an NADH-requiring step that regenerates NAD^+. Thus, anaerobic glycolysis yields 2 molecules of lactate + 2 ATP. When NAD^+ and oxygen are available, pyruvate is converted by pyruvate decarboxylase to acetyl-CoA, which is transported from the cytosol into the mitochondria and condenses with oxaloacetate within the citric acid cycle to form citrate (Fig. 12–3).[47,25] In energy rich conditions, pyruvate is used for fatty acid synthesis.

Arsenate has a toxic effect at the glycolytic step where 3-phosphoglyceraldehyde dehydrogenase (3-PGA) catalyzes the oxidation of glyceraldehyde-3-phosphate to 1,3-diphosphoglycerate; a reaction that preserves a high-energy phosphate bond used to synthesize ATP in the next step of glycolysis (Fig. 12–5).[39] Arsenate acts as an analog of phosphate at this step. While glycolysis continues, the resultant unstable arsenate intermediate is rapidly hydrolyzed, preventing the subsequent synthesis of ATP.[39]

CITRIC ACID CYCLE

The citric acid cycle uses acetyl-CoA derived from glycolysis, fat, or protein to regenerate NADH from NAD^+. The cycle is a major source of

TABLE 12–3. Inhibitors of Glucose Metabolism and ATP Synthesis

Step/Location	Action	Examples
Glycolysis	Inhibits NADH production	Iodoacetate (at GAPDH) NO^+ (at GAPDH)
	Bypasses ATP producing step	Arsenate, As^{5+}
Gluconeogenesis	Inhibits NADH production	4-(Dimethylamino)phenol *p*-benzoquinone Hypoglycin A
Fatty acid metabolism	Inhibits NADH production	Aflatoxin Amiodarone Hypoglycin Perhexiline Protease inhibitors Salicylates Tetracycline Valproic acid
TCA Cycle	Inhibits NADH production	Arsenite, As^{3+} *p*-Benzoquinone Fluoroacetate
Electron-transport chain at complex I	Inhibits electron transport	MPP^+ Paraquat Rotenone
Electron-transport chain at complex III	Inhibits electron transport	Antimycin-A Funiculosin Di- and trivalent metal cations (Zn^{2+}, Hg^{2+}, Cu^{2+}, and Cd^{2+}) Substituted phenols* (are also uncouplers)
Electron-transport chain at complex IV	Inhibits electron transport	Azide Carbon monoxide Cyanide Formate Hydrogen sulfide Nitric oxide Phosphine Protamine
Electron-transport chain at ATP synthase	Inhibits ATP production	Arsenate, As^{5+} Mycotoxins (numerous, including oligomycin) Organic chlorines (DDT and chlordecone) Organotins (cyhexatin) Paraquat
Mitochondria ADP/ATP antiporter	Disrupts the movement of ADP into and ATP out of the mitochondria at the ADP/ATP antiporter	Atractyloside DDT Free fatty acids
Mitochondria inner membrane	Uncouples oxidative phosphorylation by disrupting the proton gradient → stops proton flow at ATP synthase → stops ATP synthesis	Substituted phenols (pentachlorophenol and dinitrophenol) Lipophilic amines (amiodarone, perhexiline, buprenorphine) Benzonitrile Thiadiazole herbicides NSAIDs with ionizable groups (salicylates, diclofenac, indomethacin, piroxicam) Valinomycin Chlordecone
Mitochondria inner membrane	Diverts electrons to alternate pathways (vs. to the electron-transport chain)	Doxorubicin MPP^+ Naphthoquinones (menadione) *N*-nitrosoamines Paraquat

GAPDH = glyceraldehyde 3-phosphate dehydrogenase; MPP^+ = 1-methyl-4-phenylpyridinium; TCA – tricarboxylic acid cycle.

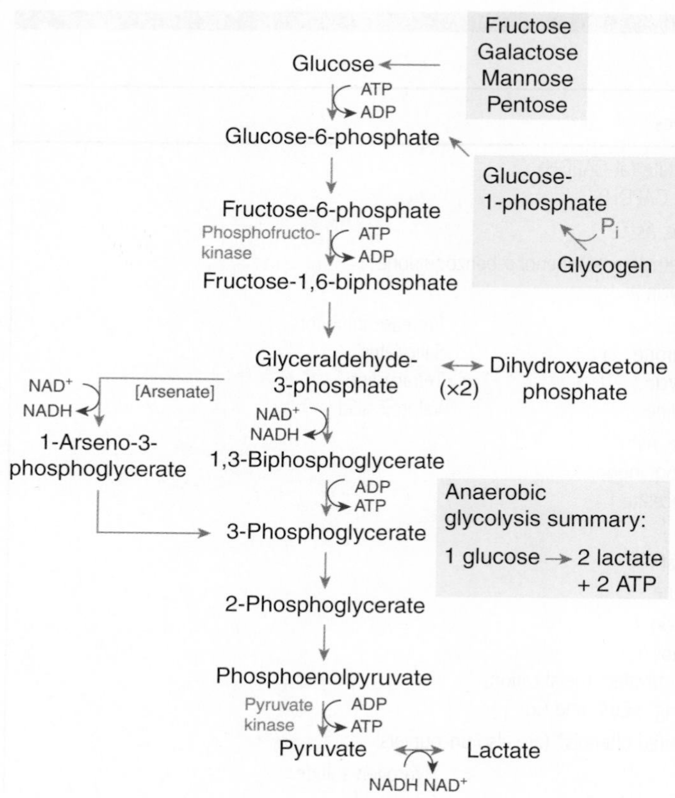

FIGURE 12–5. During glycolysis, the anaerobic metabolism of 1 mole of glucose to 2 moles of pyruvate results in the net production of 2 moles of ATP. Arsenic inhibits 3-phosphoglycerate dehydrogenase, which catalyzes the oxidation of glyceraldehyde-3-phosphate to 1,3-biphosphoglycerate.

electrons (in the form of NADH) and is critical to the aerobic production of ATP (Fig. 12–3). Each acetyl-CoA molecule that is oxidized within the citric acid cycle ultimately forms one molecule each of CO_2 and guanosine triphosphate (GTP), and more importantly, 3 molecules of NADH and one molecule of flavin adenine dinucleotide ($FADH_2$) (reduced form), which enter the electron transport chain, producing a total of 15 molecules of ATP. In addition, the citric acid cycle provides important intermediates for amino acid synthesis and for gluconeogenesis.[47]

Various xenobiotics inhibit the citric acid cycle. The rodenticides, sodium fluoroacetate and fluoroacetamide, are combined with coenzyme A, CoASH, to create fluoroacetyl CoA (FAcCoA). The FAcCoA substitutes for acetyl CoA, entering the TCA cycle by condensation with oxaloacetate to form fluorocitrate, which inhibits citrate metabolism, resulting in inhibition of the cycle and termination of oxidative metabolism (Fig. 12–3) (Chap. 108).[70]

Thiamine is an important cofactor for 2 citric acid cycle enzymes: the conversion of pyruvate to acetyl-CoA by pyruvate decarboxylase and for the conversion of α-ketoglutarate to succinyl-CoA by α-ketoglutarate dehydrogenase (Fig. 12–3).[25] The life-threatening effects of thiamine deficiency are likely related to impairment of these enzyme functions (see Antidotes in Depth: Thiamine Hydrochloride). Arsenite inhibits these thiamine-dependent enzymes within the citric acid cycle.

THE ELECTRON TRANSPORT CHAIN

The electron transport chain is the location where the "phosphorylation" of oxidative phosphorylation occurs. Oxidative phosphorylation is the creation of high energy bonds by phosphorylation of ADP to ATP, "coupled" to the transfer of electrons from reduced coenzymes to molecular oxygen via the electron transport chain. The success of aerobic metabolism requires the disposal of electrons within NADH and FADH, generated by oxidative metabolism within the citric acid cycle. The electron transport chain consists of a series of cytochrome–enzyme complexes within the inner mitochondrial membrane (Fig. 12–3). Within these complexes, NADH is split into $NAD^+ + H^+ +$ 2 electrons at complex I at the beginning of the chain while $FADH_2$ is split into FADH + H^+ + 2 electrons at complex II. These splits have 2 results. First, the regenerated NAD^+ and FADH are recycled back to the citric acid cycle, enabling oxidative metabolism to continue. Second, these actions provide the energy required to pump protons (H^+) from the mitochondrial matrix into the intermembrane space. This action causes the matrix to become relatively alkaline compared to the now acidified intermembrane space, resulting in a proton gradient across the inner mitochondrial membrane. This gradient provides the energy needed to create the high-energy bonds of ATP at complex V. The final step in oxidative phosphorylation is the reduction of molecular oxygen to water by cytochrome a-a_3 (Fig. 12–3).[47,25]

Mitochondria oxidize substrates, consume oxygen, and make ATP. Xenobiotics that interrupt oxidative phosphorylation impair ATP production by either inhibiting specific electron chain complexes or by acting as "uncouplers." Both of these mechanisms result in rapid depletion of cellular energy stores, followed by failure of ATP-dependent active transport pumps, loss of essential electrolyte gradients, and increases in cell volume.[27]

Inhibitors of specific cytochromes block electron transport and cause an accumulation of reduced intermediates proximal to the site of inhibition. This stops the regeneration of oxidized substrates for the citric acid cycle, particularly NAD^+ and FAD, further impairing oxidative metabolism. Cyanide, carbon monoxide, and hydrogen sulfide block the cytochrome a-a_3–mediated reduction of O_2 to H_2O. The very dramatic clinical effects of a significant cyanide exposure illustrate the importance of aerobic metabolism (Chaps. 125, 126). Other xenobiotics are less commonly associated with inhibition of the electron transport chain (Table 12–3).[91]

Severe metabolic acidosis is a clinical manifestation of xenobiotics that inhibits aerobic respiration. This metabolic acidosis is primarily caused by the accumulation of protons in the mitochondrial matrix that are not used in the production of ATP. While lactic acid accumulates, it is only a marker for metabolic acidosis associated with the impairment of oxidative metabolism.[76]

Xenobiotics that uncouple oxidative phosphorylation, like inhibitors of the electron transport chain, stop ATP synthesis. However, protons continue to be pumped into the intermembrane space, electrons continue to flow down the chain to reduce oxygen, and substrate consumption continues. Uncoupling xenobiotics destroy the proton gradient across the mitochondrial inner membrane. They allow the protons to cross back into the mitochondrial matrix, causing the loss of the proton gradient across the inner mitochondria membrane. Since it is the proton gradient that drives the production of ATP at complex V, ATP production is stopped. Thus, oxygen consumption is "uncoupled" from ATP production. The redox energy created by electron transport that cannot be coupled to ATP synthesis is released as heat. Various xenobiotics uncouple ATP synthesis (Table 12–3). A classic one is dinitrophenol, used in the past as an herbicide and as a weight-loss product (Chap. 39). Xenobiotics that are capable of carrying hydrogen ions across membranes are generally lipophilic weak acids. These xenobiotics must have an acid-dissociable group to carry the proton and a bulky lipophilic group to cross a membrane.[91] Dinitrophenol is able to carry its proton from the cytosol into the more alkaline mitochondrial matrix where it dissociates, acidifying the matrix and destroying the proton gradient across the inner mitochondrial membrane. Interestingly, the phenolate anion of dinitrophenol is relatively lipophilic and can cross back out to the cytosol where it gains a new proton and starts the process over again. Long-chain fatty acids uncouple oxidative phosphorylation by a similar mechanism.[91] Fatal exposures to dinitrophenol and to pentachlorophenol, a wood preservative, are associated with severe hyperthermia attributed to heat generation by uncoupled oxidative phosphorylation.[58] Rats develop fatal hyperthermia following oral ingestion of dinitrophenol.[83] The hyperthermia and acidosis associated with severe salicylate poisoning are attributed to its uncoupling of oxidative phosphorylation.[81]

HEXOSE MONOPHOSPHATE SHUNT

The hexose monophosphate (HMP) shunt provides the only source of cellular NADPH. NADPH is used in biosynthetic reactions, particularly fatty acid synthesis, and is an important source of reducing power for the maintenance of sulfhydryl groups that protect the cell from free radical injury.[8,40] As noted earlier, G6PD is a key enzyme in the pathway (Fig. 12–6). Reduced glutathione, which is quantitatively the most important antioxidant in cells, depends on the availability of NADPH. Red blood cells (RBCs) are especially vulnerable to deficiency of NADPH, which results in hemolysis during oxidative stress.

Another manifestation of oxidative stress in RBCs is the oxidation of the iron in hemoglobin from Fe^{2+} to Fe^{3+}, producing methemoglobin that occurs both spontaneously and as a response to xenobiotics such as nitrites and aminophenols. Because most reduction of methemoglobin is done by NADH-dependent methemoglobin reductase, which is not deficient in persons who lack G6PD, such persons do not develop methemoglobinemia under normal circumstances. However, when oxidative stress is severe and methemoglobinemia develops, people who have G6PD deficiency have limited ability to use the alternative NADPH-dependent methemoglobin reductase (Chap. 127).[89]

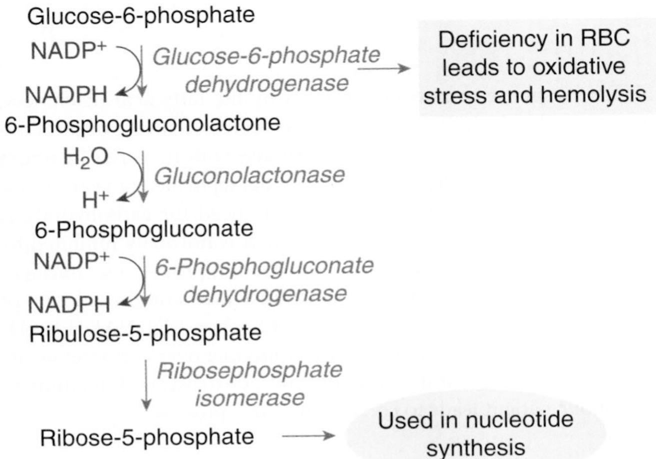

FIGURE 12–6. The oxidation reactions of the hexose monophosphate shunt are an important source of NADPH for reductive biosynthesis and for protection of cells against oxidative stress. Deficiency of G6PD, the first enzyme in the pathway, may result in RBC hemolysis during oxidative stress.

GLUCONEOGENESIS

Gluconeogenesis facilitates the conversion of amino acids and intermediates of the citric acid cycle to glucose. It occurs primarily in the liver but also in the kidney. It is an important source of glucose during fasting and enables maintenance of glycogen stores. Most of the steps in the synthesis of glucose from pyruvate are simply the reverse of glycolysis, with three irreversible exceptions: (1) the conversion of glucose-6-phosphate to glucose; (2) the conversion of fructose-1,6-diphosphate to fructose-6-phosphate; and (3) the synthesis of phosphoenolpyruvate from pyruvate. The synthesis of phosphoenolpyruvate from pyruvate is especially complex. Pyruvate is first converted to oxaloacetate within the mitochondria, then to malate, which is transported out of the mitochondria and converted in the cytosol back to oxaloacetate, and then to phosphoenolpyruvate (Fig. 12–7). Certain amino acids—notably alanine, glutamate, and aspartate—are readily converted to citric acid cycle intermediates and can be used in the synthesis of glucose through this cycle.[47] Glycerol, produced by the breakdown of triglycerides in adipose tissue, is another substrate for gluconeogenesis.

The regulation of gluconeogenesis is opposite to that of glycolysis, stimulated by glucagon and catecholamines but inhibited by insulin. Gluconeogenesis requires the cytosolic NAD^+ and mitochondrial NADH. It is impaired by processes that increase the cytosol-reducing potential as measured by the cytosol NADH/ NAD^+ ratio (see discussion below).

A number of xenobiotics impair gluconeogenesis, resulting in hypoglycemia when glycogen stores are depleted (Table 12–3). Hypoglycin A, an unusual amino acid found in unripe ackee fruit that is the cause of Jamaican vomiting sickness, produces profound hypoglycemia.[26,81,85] Its metabolite methylenecyclopropylacetic acid (MCPA) indirectly inhibits gluconeogenesis by blocking the oxidation of long-chain fatty acids, an important source of NADH in mitochondria. It also inhibits the metabolism of several glycogenic amino acids including leucine, isoleucine, and tryptophan; and blocks their entrance into the citric acid cycle. MCPA may also prevent the transport of malate out of the mitochondria.[74,85,86] Hypoglycemia also occurs in fasting patients with elevated ethanol concentrations.[3,29,49] This is likely a result of the impairment of gluconeogenesis by the increased cytosolic NADH:NAD^+ ratio associated with the metabolism of ethanol. This inhibits the two cytosolic steps that require NAD^+—the conversions of lactate to pyruvate and of malate to oxaloacetate.[2,49,73]

FATTY ACID METABOLISM

Fatty acid metabolism occurs primarily in hepatocytes. Fatty acids mobilized in adipose tissue enter hepatocytes by passive diffusion. Fatty acid synthesis is stimulated by insulin and inhibited by glucagon and epinephrine. Acetyl-CoA is the primary building block of free fatty acids (FFAs). In energy-repleted cells, fatty acids are combined with glycerol phosphate to form triacylglycerol (triglycerides), the first step in the synthesis of fat for storage. Hepatic triglycerides are bound to lipoprotein to form very-low-density lipoprotein (VLDL), then transported and stored in adipocytes. When hepatocytes are energy depleted, triglycerides are broken down to FFA and glycerol. This process is suppressed by insulin but supported by glucagon or epinephrine. FFAs undergo β-oxidation in the mitochondria, a process that breaks the FFA into acetyl-CoA molecules that can then enter the citric acid cycle. FFAs require activation before transport into the mitochondria. This is accomplished by acylcoenzyme A (acyl-CoA) synthetase, which adds a CoA group to the FFA in an energy-dependent synthetic reaction. These are transported into the

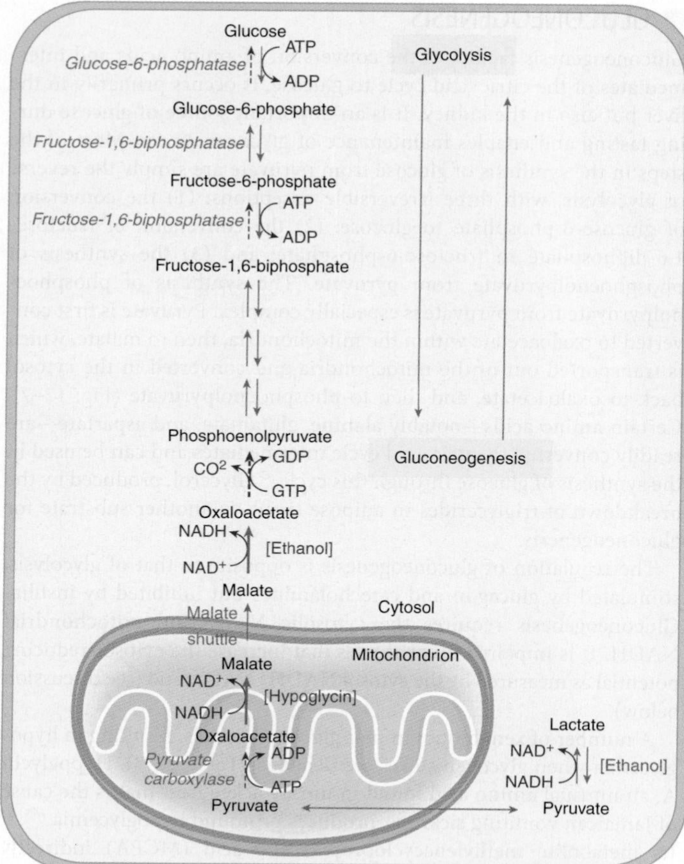

FIGURE 12–7. Gluconeogenesis reverses the steps of glycolysis, with the exception of the bypass of the three irreversible steps shown. The step from pyruvate to phosphoenolpyruvate involves both cytosolic and mitochondrial reactions that use ATP. Hypoglycin A inhibits the intramitochondrial conversion of oxaloacetate to malate by depleting NADH through interference with β-oxidation of fatty acids. Ethanol decreases cytosolic supplies of NAD^+. Pyruvate kinase (PK) and phosphofructokinase (PFK), the enzymes whose activities are regulated by glucagon via cyclic adenosine monophosphate (cAMP)-dependent phosphokinase, are shown.

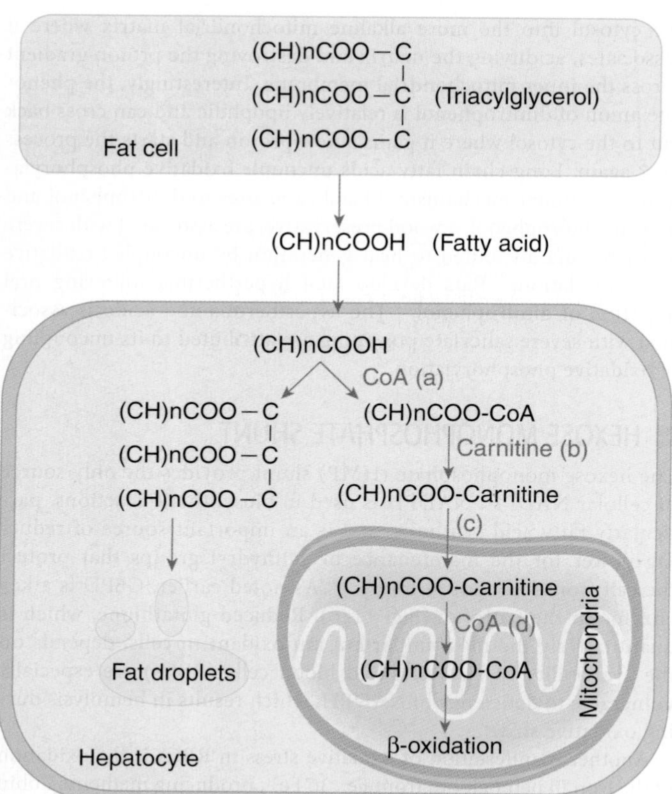

FIGURE 12–8. Steatosis, an accumulation of fat, results when xenobiotics interfere with the oxidation of fatty acids. Other processes that may be associated with intracellular accumulation of fat include: impaired lipoprotein synthesis; impaired lipoprotein release; increased mobilization of free fatty acids; increased uptake of circulating lipids; and increased production of triglycerides. β-Oxidation takes place in the mitochondria after transport of fatty acids from the cellular cytosol across the mitochondrial membrane. The enzymes involved are (a) acyl-CoA synthetase; (b) carnitine palmitoyltransferase I; (c) carnitine acylcarnitine translocase; and (d) carnitine palmitoyltransferase II. Acyl-CoA is the intramitochondrial substrate for β-oxidation. Potential mechanisms of inhibition of β-oxidation include induction of carnitine deficiency, inhibition of the transferase or translocase, and increased $NADH:NAD^+$ ratio via increased use of NAD^+ or by inhibition of NADH use. The specific site of action is not defined for many toxins that cause steatosis.

mitochondria by a process that utilizes cyclical binding to carnitine, a "carnitine shuttle" (Fig. 12–3). Once inside the mitochondria, FFAs are converted to acetyl-CoA by β-oxidation, involving the sequential removal of 2-carbon fragments, each time acting at the second carbon (the β carbon) position of the fatty acid. Each 2-carbon molecule removed from the FFA produces one NADH and one $FADH_2$, which are oxidized in the electron transport chain, and one mole of acetyl-CoA, which enters the TCA cycle. This process produces 1.3 times more ATP per molecule of carbon metabolized than does the oxidative metabolism of glucose or other carbohydrates.[47]

Many xenobiotics interrupt fatty acid metabolism at various steps, resulting in accumulation of triglycerides in the liver (Table 12–3; Fig. 12–8). The mechanisms of disruption of fatty acid metabolism are poorly defined.[16] Some xenobiotics, including ethanol, hypoglycin, and nucleoside analogs (Chap. 56); inhibit β-oxidation, at least indirectly, through effects on NADH concentrations. Protease inhibitors are associated with a syndrome of peripheral fat wasting, central adiposity, hyperlipidemia, and insulin resistance.

The condition of alcoholic ketoacidosis is related in part to inhibition of gluconeogenesis in the alcoholic patient and in part to an exuberant response to nutritional needs by the fatty acid machinery. Vomiting in the alcoholic patient leads to decreased intake of carbohydrate, which stimulates a starvation response with increases in serum glucagon, cortisol, growth hormone, and epinephrine concentrations, and decreases in serum insulin. When the need for carbohydrate is not met by gluconeogenesis, lipolysis, which is normally inhibited by insulin, is intensified and fatty acid mobilization progresses. Glucagon stimulates mitochondrial carnitine acyltransferase, and β-oxidation of fatty acids is increased. The increased mitochondrial $NADH:NAD^+$ ratio favors the production of β-hydroxybutyrate over acetoacetate, its oxidized form. The administration of fluids, dextrose, and thiamine to the alcoholic patient leads to correction of this process.[57]

SUMMARY

Humans are exposed to a wide variety of xenobiotics. Some, including therapeutic drugs, are harmless at low doses and toxic only at high doses. The toxicity of those xenobiotics that interrupt important biologic functions or cause cellular injury is dose related and often rapidly evident. The diverse mechanisms of toxic injury have been discussed in general terms. The capacity of xenobiotics to cause injury is clearly a function of many factors specific to the xenobiotic, the tissue injured, and the individual.

REFERENCES

1. Abernathy D, Flockhart, DA: Molecular basis of cardiovascular drug metabolism implications for predicting clinically important drug interactions. *Circulation*. 2000;101:1749-1753.
2. Albert A: Fundamental aspects of selective toxicity. *Ann N Y Acad Sci.* 1965;123:5-18.
3. Arky RA, Freinkel N: Alcohol hypoglycemia. Effects of ethanol on plasma. 3. Glucose, ketones, and free fatty acids in "juvenile" diabetics: A model for "nonketotic diabetic acidosis"? *Arch Intern Med.* 1964;114:501-507.
4. Audi J, Belson M, Patel M, et al: Ricin poisoning: a comprehensive review. *JAMA*. 2005;294:2342-2351.
5. Badr MZ, Belinsky SA, Kauffman FC, et al: Mechanism of hepatotoxicity to periportal regions of the liver lobule due to allyl alcohol: role of oxygen and lipid peroxidation. *J Pharmacol Exp Ther.* 1986;238:1138-1142.
6. Baud FJ: Cyanide: critical issues in diagnosis and treatment. *Hum Exp Toxicol.* 2007;26:191-201.
7. Bayir H: Reactive oxygen species. *Crit Care Med.* 2005;33:S498-501.
8. Beutler E: Glucose-6-phosphate dehydrogenase deficiency. *N Engl J Med.* 1991;324:169-174.
9. Bock KW, Kohle C: Coordinate regulation of drug metabolism by xenobiotic nuclear receptors: UGTs acting together with CYPs and glucuronide transporters. *Drug Metab Rev.* 2004;36:595-615.
10. Boyland E, Chasseaud LF: The role of glutathione and glutathione S-transferases in mercapturic acid biosynthesis. *Adv Enzymol Relat Areas Mol Biol.* 1969;32:173-219.
11. Brittebo EB: Metabolism of xenobiotics in the nasal olfactory mucosa: implications for local toxicity. *Pharmacol Toxicol.* 1993;72 Suppl 3:50-52.
12. Brown C: Overview of drug interactions modulated by cytochrome P450. *US Pharmacists*. 2001;26:20-35.
13. Callaghan R, Crowley E, Potter S, et al: P-glycoprotein: so many ways to turn it on. *J Clin Pharmacol.* 2008;48:365-378.
14. Cappellini MD, Fiorelli G: Glucose-6-phosphate dehydrogenase deficiency. *Lancet*. 2008;371:64-74.
15. Caro AA, Cederbaum AI: Oxidative stress, toxicology, and pharmacology of CYP2E1. *Annu Rev Pharmacol Toxicol.* 2004;44:27-42.
16. Carr A, Samaras K, Chisholm DJ, et al: Pathogenesis of HIV-1-protease inhibitor-associated peripheral lipodystrophy, hyperlipidaemia, and insulin resistance. *Lancet*. 1998;351:1881-1883.
17. Chinn LW, Kroetz DL: ABCB1 pharmacogenetics: progress, pitfalls, and promise. *Clin Pharmacol Ther.* 2007;81:265-269.
18. Conney AH: Induction of drug-metabolizing enzymes: a path to the discovery of multiple cytochromes P450. *Annu Rev Pharmacol Toxicol.* 2003;43:1-30.
19. Cribb AE, Peyrou M, Muruganandan S, et al: The endoplasmic reticulum in xenobiotic toxicity. *Drug Metab Rev.* 2005;37:405-442.
20. Dai Y, Rashba-Step J, Cederbaum AI: Stable expression of human cytochrome P4502E1 in HepG2 cells: Characterization of catalytic activities and production of reactive oxygen intermediates. *Biochemistry*. 1993;32:6928-6937.
21. Ding X, Kaminsky LS: Human extrahepatic cytochromes P450: Function in xenobiotic metabolism and tissue-selective chemical toxicity in the respiratory and gastrointestinal tracts. *Annu Rev Pharmacol Toxicol.* 2003;43:149-173.
22. Dutheil F, Beaune P, Loriot MA: Xenobiotic metabolizing enzymes in the central nervous system: Contribution of cytochrome P450 enzymes in normal and pathological human brain. *Biochimie*. 2008;90:426-436.
23. Eling TE, Thompson DC, Foureman GL, et al: Prostaglandin H synthase and xenobiotic oxidation. *Annu Rev Pharmacol Toxicol.* 1990;30:1-45.
24. Evans WE: Pharmacogenomics: Marshalling the human genome to individualise drug therapy. *Gut*. 2003;52 Suppl 2:ii10-18.
25. Farabee M. OnLine Biology Book. Vol. 2009; 2009. http://www.emc.maricopa.edu/faculty/farabee/BIOBK/BioBookTOC.html.
26. Feng PC, Patrick SJ: Studies of the action of hypoglycin-A, an hypoglycaemic substance. *Br J Pharmacol.* 1958;13:125-130.
27. Fenteany G. *BioChemWeb*. Vol. 2009; 2009. http://www.biochemweb.org/.
28. Flockhart D, Tanus-Santos, JE: Implications of cytochrome P450 interactions when prescribing medication of hypertension. *Arch Intern Med.* 2002;162:405-412.
29. Freinkel N, Singer, DL, Arky, RA, et al: Alcohol hypoglycemia. I. Carbohydrate metabolism of patients with clinical alcohol hypoglycemia and the experimental reproduction of the syndrome with pure ethanol. *J Clin Invest.* 1963;42:1112-1113.
30. Gardiner SJ, Begg EJ: Pharmacogenetics, drug-metabolizing enzymes, and clinical practice. *Pharmacol Rev.* 2006;58:521-590.
31. Gerlach M, Riederer P, Przuntek H, et al: MPTP mechanisms of neurotoxicity and their implications for Parkinson's disease. *Eur J Pharmacol.* 1991;208:273-286.
32. Goshman L, Fish J, Roller, K.: Clinically significant cytochrome P450 drug interactions. *J Pharm Soc Wisconsin.* 1999:23-38.
33. Guengerich FP: Catalytic selectivity of human cytochrome P450 enzymes: Relevance to drug metabolism and toxicity. *Toxicol Lett.* 1994;70:133-138.
34. Guengerich FP: Cytochrome p450 and chemical toxicology. *Chem Res Toxicol.* 2008;21:70-83.
35. Halpert JR, Guengerich FP, Bend JR, et al: Selective inhibitors of cytochromes P450. *Toxicol Appl Pharmacol.* 1994;125:163-175.
36. Handschin C, Meyer UA: Induction of drug metabolism: The role of nuclear receptors. *Pharmacol Rev.* 2003;55:649-673.
37. Hetu C, Dumont A, Joly JG: Effect of chronic ethanol administration on bromobenzene liver toxicity in the rat. *Toxicol Appl Pharmacol.* 1983;67:166-177.
38. Ho RH, Kim RB: Transporters and drug therapy: Implications for drug disposition and disease. *Clin Pharmacol Ther.* 2005;78:260-277.
39. Hughes MF: Arsenic toxicity and potential mechanisms of action. *Toxicol Lett.* 2002;133:1-16.
40. Imlay JA: Pathways of oxidative damage. *Annu Rev Microbiol.* 2003;57:395-418.
41. Ingleman-Sundberg M: Genetic polymorphisms of cytochrome P450 2D6 (CY2D6): Clinical consequences, evolutionary aspects and functional diversity. *Pharmacogenomics J.* 2005;5:6-13.
42. Josephy D, Guengerich P, Miners JO: "Phase I and Phase II" drug metabolism: Terminology that we should phase out? *Drug Metab Rev.* 2005;37:575-580.
43. Kalgutkar AS, Gardner I, Obach RS, et al: A comprehensive listing of bioactivation pathways of organic functional groups. *Curr Drug Metab.* 2005;6:161-225.
44. Kato M: Intestinal first-pass metabolism of CYP3A4 substrates. *Drug Metab Pharmacokinet.* 2008;23:87-94.
45. Kim D, Guengerich FP: Cytochrome P450 activation of arylamines and heterocyclic amines. *Annu Rev Pharmacol Toxicol.* 2005;45:27-49.
46. Kim RB: Drugs as P-glycoprotein substrates, inhibitors, and inducers. *Drug Metab Rev.* 2002;34:47-54.
47. King M. The Medical Biochemistry Page. Vol. 2009; 2009. http://themedicalbiochemistrypage.org/.
48. Kleinman JG, Breitenfield RV, Roth DA: Acute renal failure associated with acetaminophen ingestion: Report of a case and review of the literature. *Clin Nephrol.* 1980;14:201-205.
49. Krishna DR, Klotz U: Extrahepatic metabolism of drugs in humans. *Clin Pharmacokinet.* 1994;26:144-160.
50. Kroncke KD, Fricker G, Meier PJ, et al: alpha-Amanitin uptake into hepatocytes. Identification of hepatic membrane transport systems used by amatoxins. *J Biol Chem.* 1986;261:12562-12567.
51. Lewis D: On the recognition of mammalian microsomal cytochrome P450 substrates and their characteristics. *Biochem Pharmacol.* 2000;60:293-306.
52. Lewis MS, Youle RJ: Ricin subunit association. Thermodynamics and the role of the disulfide bond in toxicity. *J Biol Chem.* 1986;261:11571-11577.
53. Lieber CS: Metabolism of alcohol. *Clin Liver Dis.* 2005;9:1-35.
54. Lin JH: CYP induction-mediated drug interactions: in vitro assessment and clinical implications. *Pharm Res.* 2006;23:1089-1116.
55. Lindell TJ, Weinberg F, Morris PW, et al: Specific inhibition of nuclear RNA polymerase II by alpha-amanitin. *Science*. 1970;170:447-449.
56. Manahan S: *Toxicological Chemistry and Biochemistry*. 3rd ed. New York: Lewis Publishers; 2003.
57. McGuire LC, Cruickshank AM, Munro PT: Alcoholic ketoacidosis. *Emerg Med J.* 2006;23:417-420.
58. Menon JA: Tropical hazards associated with the use of pentachlorophenol. *Br Med J.* 1958;14:1156-1158.
59. Miller EC, Miller JA: The presence and significance of bound aminoazo dyes in the livers of rats fed p-demethylaminoazobenzene. *Cancer Res.* 1947;7:468-480.

60. Myers CE, McGuire WP, Liss RH, et al: Adriamycin: The role of lipid peroxidation in cardiac toxicity and tumor response. *Science.* 1977;197:165-167.
61. Nagata K: Genetic polymorphism of human cytochrome P450 involved in drug metabolism. *Drug Metabol. Pharmacokin.* 2002;17:167-189.
62. Nelson D: Comparison of cytochrome P450 (CYP) genes from the mouse and human genomes, including nomenclature recommendations for genes, pseudogenes and alternative-splice varients. *Pharmacogenetics.* 2004;14:1-18.
63. Nelson D. Cytochrome P450 homepage. Vol. 2009; 2009. http://drnelson.utmem.edu/CytochromeP450.html.
64. Nolin TD: Altered nonrenal drug clearance in ESRD. *Curr Opin Nephrol Hypertens.* 2008;17:555-559.
65. Obach RS, Walsky RL, Venkatakrishnan K, et al: In vitro cytochrome P450 inhibition data and the prediction of drug-drug interactions: Qualitative relationships, quantitative predictions, and the rank-order approach. *Clin Pharmacol Ther.* 2005;78:582-592.
66. Park B: Cytochrome P450 enzymes in the heart. *Lancet.* 2000;355:945-946.
67. Pavek P, Dvorak Z: Xenobiotic-induced transcriptional regulation of xenobiotic metabolizing enzymes of the cytochrome P450 superfamily in human extrahepatic tissues. *Curr Drug Metab.* 2008;9:129-143.
68. Peck CC, Temple R, Collins JM: Understanding consequences of concurrent therapies. *JAMA.* 1993;269:1550-1552.
69. Pelkonen O, Turpeinen M, Hakkola J, et al: Inhibition and induction of human cytochrome P450 enzymes: Current status. *Arch Toxicol.* 2008;82:667-715.
70. Peters RA, Wakelin RW: The synthesis of fluorocitric acid and its inhibition in acetate. *Biochem J.* 1957;67:280-286.
71. Piscitelli S: Indinavir concentrations and St John's wort. *Lancet.* 2000;355:547-548.
72. Rose MS, Lock EA, Smith LL, et al: Paraquat accumulation: Tissue and species specificity. *Biochem Pharmacol.* 1976;25:419-423.
73. Rosen GM, Rauckman EJ: Carbon tetrachloride-induced lipid peroxidation: A spin trapping study. *Toxicol Lett.* 1982;10:337-344.
74. Ruderman N, Shafrir E, Bressler R: Relation of fatty acid oxidation tgluconeogenesis: Effect of pentenoic acid. *Life Sci.* 1968;7:1083-1089.
75. Santi DV, McHenry CS, Sommer H: Mechanism of interaction of thymidylate synthetase with 5-fluorodeoxyuridylate. *Biochemistry.* 1974;13:471-481.
76. Schafer DF, Sorrell MF: Power failure, liver failure. *N Engl J Med.* 1997;336:1173-1174.
77. Schuster I, Bernhardt R: Inhibition of cytochromes p450: Existing and new promising therapeutic targets. *Drug Metab Rev.* 2007;39:481-499.
78. Schwarz UI, Stein CM: Genetic determinants of dose and clinical outcomes in patients receiving oral anticoagulants. *Clin Pharmacol Ther.* 2006;80:7-12.
79. Si D, Wang Y, Zhou YH, et al: Mechanism of CYP2C9 inhibition by flavones and flavonols. *Drug Metab Dispos.* 2009;37:629-634.
80. Sim E, Lack N, Wang C-J, et al: Arylamine N-acetyltransferases: Structural and functional implications of polymorphisms. *Toxicology.* 2008;254:170-183.
81. Smith MJ, Jeffrey SW: The effects of salicylate on oxygen consumption and carbohydrate metabolism in the isolated rat diaphragm. *Biochem J.* 1956;63:524-528.
82. Southorn PA, Powis G: Free radicals in medicine. I. Chemical nature and biologic reactions. *Mayo Clin Proc.* 1988;63:381-389.
83. Spencer HC RV, Adams EM, Irish DD: Toxicological studies on laboratory animals of certain alkyldinitrophenols used in agriculture. *J Indian Hyg Toxicol.* 1948;30:10-25.
84. Sweeney BP, Bromilow J: Liver enzyme induction and inhibition: Implications for anaesthesia. *Anaesthesia.* 2006;61:159-177.
85. Tanaka K: On the mode of action of hypoglycin A. *J Biol Chem.* 1972;247:7465-7478.
86. Tanaka K, Kean EA, Johnson B: Jamaican vomiting sickness. Biochemical investigation of two cases. *N Engl J Med.* 1976;295:461-467.
87. Timbrell J: *Principles of Biochemical Toxicology.* 3rd ed. Philadelphia: Taylor & Francis; 2000.
88. Timsit YE, Negishi M: CAR and PXR: The xenobiotic-sensing receptors. *Steroids.* 2007;72:231-246.
89. Umbreit J: Methemoglobin—it's not just blue: A concise review. *Am J Hematol.* 2007;82:134-144.
90. Urquhart BL, Tirona RG, Kim RB: Nuclear receptors and the regulation of drug-metabolizing enzymes and drug transporters: Implications for interindividual variability in response to drugs. *J Clin Pharmacol.* 2007;47:566-578.
91. Wallace KB, Starkov AA: Mitochondrial targets of drug toxicity. *Annu Rev Pharmacol Toxicol.* 2000;40:353-388.
92. Waxman D: P450 Gene induction by structurally diverse xenochemicals: Central role of nuclear receptors CAR, P, and PPR. *Arch Biochem Biophys.* 1999;369:11-23.
93. Wienkers LC, Heath TG: Predicting in vivo drug interactions from in vitro drug discovery data. *Nat Rev Drug Discov.* 2005;4:825-833.
94. Williams RT: *Detoxication Mechanisms: The Metabolism of Drugs and Allied Organic Compounds.* 1st ed. London: Chapman and Hall; 1949.
95. Williams RT: *Detoxication Mechanisms: The Metabolism and Detoxication of Drugs, Toxic Substances, and Other Organic Compounds.* 2nd ed. London: Chapman and Hall; 1959.
96. Zamek-Gliszczynski MJ, Hoffmaster KA, Nezasa K, et al: Integration of hepatic drug transporters and phase II metabolizing enzymes: Mechanisms of hepatic excretion of sulfate, glucuronide, and glutathione metabolites. *Eur J Pharm Sci.* 2006;27:447-486.
97. Zhang JY, Wang Y, Prakash C: Xenobiotic-metabolizing enzymes in human lung. *Curr Drug Metab.* 2006;7:939-948.
98. Zhou SF, Xue CC, Yu XQ, et al: Clinically important drug interactions potentially involving mechanism-based inhibition of cytochrome P450 3A4 and the role of therapeutic drug monitoring. *Ther Drug Monit.* 2007;29:687-710.

APPENDIX

Common Cytochrome P450 Substrates, Inhibitors, and Inducers[1]

	SUBSTRATES		INHIBITORS		INDUCERS
1A2	**Analgesics** Acetaminophen Naproxen **Antidepressants** Amitriptyline Clomipramine Duloxetine[2] Fluvoxamine Imipramine Mirtazapine **Antipsychotics** Clozapine Haloperidol Olanzapine Thioridazine	**Cardiovascular** Mexiletine Propranolol Verapamil **Hormones** Estradiol Flutamide **Other Medications** Caffeine Cyclobenzaprine Ondansetron Theophylline[3] Tizanidine[3] Warfarin-R Zolmitriptan	**Antibiotics (Fluoroquinolones)** Ciprofloxacin Norfloxacin **Antibiotics (Macrolides)** Clarithromycin Erythromycin Troleandomycin **Antidepressants** Duloxetine Fluvoxamine	**Cardiovascular** Amiodarone Mexiletine Mibefradil[4] Verapamil **Other Medications** Acyclovir Cimetidine Famotidine Grapefruit juice	**Anticonvulsants** Carbamazepine Phenobarbital Phenytoin **Proton Pump Inhibitors** Lansoprazole Omeprazole **Other** Nafcillin Polycyclic hydrocarbons (chargrilled meat, cigarette smoke) Rifampicin Rifampin Ritonavir[5]
3A4	**Antibiotics** Clarithromycin Dapsone Erythromycin Rifabutin Telithromycin **Antidepressants** (Minor for most) Amitriptyline Buspirone[2] Citalopram Clomipramine Escitalopram Imipramine Mirtazapine Nefazodone Sertraline Trazodone **Antidysrhythmics** Amiodarone Disopyramide Quinidine[3] **Antifungals** Itraconazole Ketoconazole Voriconazole	**Immune Modulators** Cyclosporine[3] Sirolimus[3] Tacrolimus[3] Tamoxifen **Opioids** Alfentanil[3] Buprenorphine Codeine Dextromethorphan Fentanyl[3] Meperidine Methadone Morphine Oxycodone Propoxyphene Sufentanyl Tramadol **Protease Inhibitors** Indinavir Nelfinavir Ritonavir Saquinavir[2]	**Antidepressants** Fluoxetine Fluvoxamine Nefazodone Norfluoxetine Sertraline **Antibiotics (Macrolide)** Clarithromycin Erythromycin Telithromycin **Antibiotics** Chloramphenicol Ciprofloxacin Isoniazid Norfloxacin **Antifungals** Fluconazole Itraconazole Ketoconazole Voriconazole	**Calcium Channel Blockers** Diltiazem Mibefradil[4] Nifedipine Verapamil **Protease Inhibitors** Amprenavir Atazanavir Fosamprenavir Indinavir Nelfinavir[1] Ritonavir[5] Saquinavir **Other** Amiodarone Cimetidine Cisapride Cocaine Cyclosporine Ergotamines Felbamate Grapefruit juice[1]	**Antibiotics** Rifabutin Rifampicin Rifampin Rifapentine **Protease Inhibitors** Amprenavir Efavirenz Nelfinavir[1] Nevirapine Ritonavir[5] **Anticonvulsants** Carbamazepine Felbamate Oxcarbazepine Phenobarbital Phenytoin Topiramate **Steroids** Dexamethasone Methylprednisolone Prednisolone **Other** St. John's wort

	SUBSTRATES		INHIBITORS		INDUCERS
	Antihistamines Astemizole[4] Chlorpheniramine Desloratidine Loratidine Terfenadine[4] **Antipsychotics** (Minor for most) Aripiprazole Clozapine Haloperidol Quetiapine Risperidone Thioridazine Ziprasidone **Benzodiazepines** Alprazolam Clonazepam Diazepam Midazolam[2] Triazolam[2] **Calcium Channel Blockers** Amlodipine Diltiazem Felodipine[2] Nicardipine Nifedipine Nimodipine Nisoldipine Verapamil	**Proton Pump Inhibitors** (Minor for most) Esomeprazole Lansoprazole Omeprazole Pantoprazole Rabeprazole **Statins** Atorvastatin Cerivastatin[4] Lovastatin[2] Simvastatin[2] **Steroids and Hormones** Dexamethasone Estradiol Fluticasone[2] Hydrocortisone Methylprednisolone Prednisone Progesterone **Other Medications** Carbamazepine Cisapride Cyclobenzaprine Diclofenac Ergotamines[3] Losartan Ondansetron Pioglitazone Propranolol Salmeterol Sildenafil[2] Vardenafil[2] Warfarin-R Zaleplon Zolpidem			
2C9	**Angiotensin II Blockers** Irbesartan Losartan **Hypoglycemics** Chlorpropamide Glimepiride Glipizide Glyburide Tolbutamide **NSAIDs** Celecoxib Diclofenac Flurbiprofen Ibuprofen Indomethacin Meloxicam Naproxen Piroxicam	**Other Medications** Amitriptyline Fluoxetine Fluvastatin Phenobarbital Phenytoin[3] Rosiglitazone Tamoxifen Sertraline Rosuvastatin Warfarin-S[3]	**Antibiotics (Macrolide)** Clarithromycin Erythromycin Troleandomycin **Antibiotics** Isoniazid Metronidazole Sulfamethoxazole **Antidepressants** Fluoxetine Fluvoxamine Paroxetine Sertraline	**Antifungals (Azoles)** Fluconazole Itraconazole Ketoconazole Voriconazole **Other** Amiodarone Cimetidine Ritonavir[5] Grapefruit juice Valproic acid	**Anticonvulsants** Carbamazepine Phenobarbital Phenytoin **Other** Nelfinavir Rifampicin Rifampin Rifapentine Ritonavir[5] St. John's wort

	SUBSTRATES		INHIBITORS		INDUCERS
2C19	**Antidepressants** Amitriptyline Citalopram Clomipramine Desipramine Doxepin Escitalopram Fluoxetine Imipramine **Anticonvulsants** Diazepam Phenobarbital Phenytoin	**Proton Pump Inhibitors** (Major for most) Esomeprazole Lansoprazole Omeprazole[2] Pantoprazole Rabeprazole **Other Medications** Atomoxetine Carisoprodol Clopidogrel Cyclophosphamide Indomethacin Nelfinavir Olanzapine Methadone Progesterone Propranolol Voriconazole Warfarin-R	**Antibiotics (Macrolide)** Clarithromycin Erythromycin Troleandomycin **Antidepressants (SSRI)** Citalopram Fluoxetine Fluvoxamine Paroxetine Sertraline **Antifungals (Azoles)** Fluconazole Ketoconazole Voriconazole	**Anticonvulsants** Felbamate Oxcarbazepine Topiramate **Other Medications** Chloramphenicol Cimetidine Grapefruit juice Indomethacin Isoniazid Ritonavir[5] Ticlopidine **Proton Pump Inhibitors** Lansoprazole Omeprazole Pantoprazole Rabeprazole	**Anticonvulsants** Carbamazepine Phenobarbital Phenytoin **Other** Prednisone Rifampicin Rifampin Rifapentine Ritonavir[5] St. John's wort
2D6	**Antidepressants (SSRI)** Escitalopram Fluoxetine Fluvoxamine Paroxetine Sertraline **Antidepressants (Other)** (Major for most) Amitriptyline Clomipramine Desipramine[2] Doxepin Duloxetine Escitalopram Imipramine Maprotiline Mirtazapine Nortriptyline Venlafaxine **Antidysrhythmics** Flecainide Mexiletine Quinidine **Antihistamines** Chlorpheniramine Desloratidine Diphenhydramine Loratadine	**Antipsychotics** (Major for most) Aripiprazole Chlorpromazine Fluphenazine Haloperidol Perphenazine Promethazine Risperidone Thioridazine[3] **β-Adrenergic Antagonists** Metoprolol Pindolol Propranolol Timolol **Opioids** Codeine Dextromethorphan Hydrocodone Oxycodone Tramadol **Other Medications** Amphetamine Atomoxetine Cyclobenzaprine Debrisoquine Metoclopramide Ondansetron Tamoxifen	**Antidepressants** Bupropion Citalopram Duloxetine Escitalopram Fluoxetine Paroxetine Sertraline **Antihistamines** Chlorpheniramine Cimetidine Diphenhydramine Hydroxyzine Ranitidine **Antipsychotics** Chlorpromazine Haloperidol Perphenazine Promethazine Thioridazine	**Other Medications** Amiodarone Celecoxib Chloramphenicol Chloroquine Cocaine Doxorubicin Ticlopidine Methadone Ritonavir[5]	Dexamethasone Rifampicin Rifampin Ritonavir[5] Tramadol

	SUBSTRATES		INHIBITORS	INDUCERS
2E1	Acetaminophen Chlorzoxazone Ethanol Theophylline Isoniazid	**Inhaled Anesthetics** Enflurane Halothane Isoflurane Methoxyflurane	Disulfiram Fomepizole	Ethanol Isoniazid St. John's wort

[1] This list is not complete and may reflect some variation in author opinions as to whether a xenobiotic is a substrate, inhibitor, or inducer. Many drugs are metabolized by several isoenzymes with some representing major pathways and others minor pathways.

[2] The area-under-the-curve of this substrate has been shown to increase 5-fold or more when coadministered with a known CYP3A inhibitor.

[3] This substrate has a narrow therapeutic range and safety concerns occur when coadministered with an inhibitor.

[4] These medications were withdrawn from the market due to complications associated with drug–drug interactions.

[5] Ritonavir has paradoxical dose- and time-dependent inhibitory and induction effects.

NSAID – Non-steroidal anti-inflammatory drugs; PPI – proton pump inhibitors.

REFERENCES

1. Anderson GD: Pharmacogenetics and enzyme induction/inhibition properties of antiepileptic drugs. *Neurology*. 2004;63:S3-8.
2. Armstrong SC, Cozza KL: Antihistamines. *Psychosomatics*. 2003;44:430-434.
3. Bartra J, Valero AL, del Cuvillo A, et al: Interactions of the H1 antihistamines. *J Investig Allergol Clin Immunol*. 2006;16 Suppl 1:29-36.
4. Bertilsson L: Metabolism of antidepressant and neuroleptic drugs by cytochrome p450s: Clinical and interethnic aspects. *Clin Pharmacol Ther*. 2007;82:606-609.
5. Bondy B, Spellmann I: Pharmacogenetics of antipsychotics: Useful for the clinician? *Curr Opin Psychiatry*. 2007;20:126-130.
6. Dixit V, Hariparsad N, Li F, et al: Cytochrome P450 enzymes and transporters induced by anti-human immunodeficiency virus protease inhibitors in human hepatocytes: Implications for predicting clinical drug interactions. *Drug Metab Dispos*. 2007;35:1853-1859.
7. Epocrates: Medication formulary. 2009. Available at: http://www.epocrates.com/
8. FDA: Drug Development and Drug Interactions: Table of Substrates, Inhibitors and Inducers. US Department of Health and Human Services. 2009.
9. Flockhart D: P450 Drug Interaction Table 2009. Available at http://medicine.iupui.edu/clinpharm/ddis/
10. Flockhart D, Tanus-Santos, JE: Implications of cytochrome P450 interactions when prescribing medication of hypertension. *Arch Intern Med*. 2002;162:405-412.
11. Foisy MM, Yakiwchuk EM, Hughes CA: Induction effects of ritonavir: Implications for drug interactions. *Ann Pharmacother*. 2008;42:1048-1059.
12. Furuta T, Sugimoto M, Shirai N, et al: CYP2C19 pharmacogenomics associated with therapy of *Helicobacter pylori* infection and gastro-esophageal reflux diseases with a proton pump inhibitor. *Pharmacogenomics*. 2007;8:1199-1210.
13. Ku HY, Ahn HJ, Seo KA, et al: The contributions of cytochromes P450 3A4 and 3A5 to the metabolism of the phosphodiesterase type 5 inhibitors sildenafil, udenafil, and vardenafil. *Drug Metab Dispos*. 2008;36:986-990.
14. Lotsch J, Skarke C, Liefhold J, et al: Genetic predictors of the clinical response to opioid analgesics: Clinical utility and future perspectives. *Clin Pharmacokinet*. 2004;43:983-1013.
15. Martinez C, Albet C, Agundez JA, et al: Comparative in vitro and in vivo inhibition of cytochrome P450 CYP1A2, CYP2D6, and CYP3A by H2-receptor antagonists. *Clin Pharmacol Ther*. 1999;65:369-376.
16. Mega JL, Close SL, Wiviott SD, et al: Cytochrome p-450 polymorphisms and response to clopidogrel. *N Engl J Med*. 2009;360:354-362.
17. Neuvonen PJ, Niemi M, Backman JT: Drug interactions with lipid-lowering drugs: Mechanisms and clinical relevance. *Clin Pharmacol Ther*. 2006;80:565-581.
18. Nivoix Y, Leveque D, Herbrecht R, et al: The enzymatic basis of drug-drug interactions with systemic triazole antifungals. *Clin Pharmacokinet*. 2008;47:779-792.
19. Nowack R: Review article: Cytochrome P450 enzyme, and transport protein mediated herb-drug interactions in renal transplant patients: Grapefruit juice, St. John's Wort—and beyond! *Nephrology (Carlton)*. 2008;13:337-347.
20. Pai MP, Momary KM, Rodvold KA: Antibiotic drug interactions. *Med Clin N Am*. 2006;90:1223-1255.
21. Pelkonen O, Turpeinen M, Hakkola J, et al: Inhibition and induction of human cytochrome P450 enzymes: current status. *Arch Toxicol*. 2008;82:667-715.
22. Picard N, Cresteil T, Djebli N, et al: In vitro metabolism study of buprenorphine: evidence for new metabolic pathways. *Drug Metab Dispos*. 2005;33:689-695.
23. Ramirez J, Innocenti F, Schuetz EG, et al: CYP2B6, CYP3A4, and CYP2C19 are responsible for the in vitro N-demethylation of meperidine in human liver microsomes. *Drug Metab Dispos*. 2004;32:930-936.
24. Somogyi AA, Menelaou A, Fullston SV: CYP3A4 mediates dextropropoxyphene N-demethylation to nordextropropoxyphene: human in vitro and in vivo studies and lack of CYP2D6 involvement. *Xenobiotica*. 2004;34:875-887.
25. Sweeney BP, Bromilow J: Liver enzyme induction and inhibition: Implications for anaesthesia. *Anaesthesia*. 2006;61:159-177.
26. Wojcikowski J, Maurel P, Daniel WA: Characterization of human cytochrome p450 enzymes involved in the metabolism of the piperidine-type phenothiazine neuroleptic thioridazine. *Drug Metab Dispos*. 2006;34:471-476.
27. Zanger UM, Turpeinen M, Klein K, et al: Functional pharmacogenetics/genomics of human cytochromes P450 involved in drug biotransformation. *Anal Bioanal Chem*. 2008;392:1093-1108.

CHAPTER 13
NEUROTRANSMITTERS AND NEUROMODULATORS

Steven C. Curry, Kirk Charles Mills, Anne-Michelle Ruha, and Ayrn D. O'Connor

This chapter reviews the normal physiology of neurotransmission, the molecular action and biochemistry of several major neurotransmitters and their receptors, and the toxicologic mechanisms by which numerous xenobiotics act at the molecular level. Acetylcholine, norepinephrine, epinephrine, dopamine, serotonin, γ-aminobutyric acid (GABA), γ-hydroxybutyrate (GHB), glycine, glutamate, and adenosine are the neurotransmitters and neuromodulators of toxicologic interest that are discussed in this chapter.

When examining molecular actions of xenobiotics on neurotransmitter systems, it quickly becomes apparent that substances rarely possess single pharmacologic actions. As examples, doxepin, in part, antagonizes voltage-gated sodium channels, histaminic H_1 and H_2 receptors, α-adrenoceptors, muscarinic acetylcholine receptors, dopamine D_2 receptors, and $GABA_A$ receptors; prevents potassium efflux; and inhibits norepinephrine, serotonin, and adenosine uptake. And carbamazepine blocks voltage-gated sodium channels; inhibits uptake of norepinephrine, adenosine, and serotonin; antagonizes adenosine and muscarinic receptors; and activates $GABA_B$ and mitochondrial benzodiazepine receptors. For obvious reasons, then, this chapter cannot include every action of every xenobiotics on the nervous system. Nor is it meant to be a complete discussion of toxic syndromes produced by various xenobiotics, as these are discussed in specific chapters. Rather, it provides a general and basic understanding of the mechanisms of action of various xenobiotics affecting neurotransmitter function and receptors, especially in the central nervous system. With this focus, the clinical effects produced are more easily understood and predicted, and specific treatments can be rationally undertaken. Given the complexity of the nervous system and the numerous actions of a given xenobiotic, it is not always clear which neurotransmitter system is producing an observed effect. Therefore, specific xenobiotics may be found in several sections. An attempt is made to note a xenobiotics main mechanism of action, although other actions are noted when possible.

NEURON PHYSIOLOGY AND NEUROTRANSMISSION

MEMBRANE POTENTIALS, ION CHANNELS, AND NERVE CONDUCTION

Membrane-bound sodium–potassium adenosine triphosphatase (ATPase) moves three sodium ions (Na^+) from inside the cell to the interstitial space while pumping two potassium ions (K^+) into the cell. Because the cell membrane is not freely permeable to large, negatively charged intracellular molecules, such as proteins, an equilibrium results in which the inside of the neuron is negative with respect to the outside. This typical neuronal resting membrane potential is −65 mV.

Sodium, calcium (Ca^{2+}), K^+, and chloride (Cl^-) ions move into and out of neurons through ion channels. Ions always move passively down electrochemical gradients through ion channels, which are long polypeptides comprising several subunits that span the plasma membrane several times. Many different ion channels are structurally comparable, sharing similar amino acid sequences.[15] Channels for a specific ion can also vary in structure, depending on the specific subunits that have combined to form the channel. Because of structural similarity of different channels, it is not surprising that many xenobiotic are able to bind to more than one type of ion channel.

More than 40 different ion channels have been described in various nerve terminals,[102] and it is estimated that a human being contains hundreds of different varieties of ion channels for Na^+, Cl^-, Ca^{2+}, and K^+. Most ion channels fall into two general classes: voltage-gated (voltage-dependent) ion channels and ligand-gated ion channels.[102] Voltage-gated channels open or close in response to changes in membrane potential. Ligand-gated channels open or close when a ligand (eg, neurotransmitter) binds to the channel to change its configuration.

A commonly accepted model describes voltage-gated Na^+ channels and some other voltage-gated ion channels in 3 possible states. Using Na^+ channels as an example, the Na^+ channel is closed at rest and impermeable to Na^+, preventing Na^+ from moving into the cell. When the channel undergoes activation, the channel opens, allowing Na^+ to move intracellularly, down its electrochemical gradient. The channel then undergoes a third conformational change by becoming inactivated, preventing further influx of Na^+. The term *recovery* describes the conversion of inactive channels back to the resting state, a process that requires repolarization of the cell membrane.

Depolarization of a neuron usually results from an initial inward flux of cations (Na^+ or Ca^{2+}), or prevention of K^+ efflux. The fall in membrane potential (movement toward 0 mV) results in further activation of these voltage-dependent Na^+ channels, allowing yet a greater influx of cations. When the membrane potential falls to threshold, Na^+ channels are activated en masse, and there is a large influx of Na^+.

Depolarization of a segment of the neurolemma causes the adjacent neuronal membrane to reach threshold, resulting in the propagation of an action potential down the neuron. Sodium channel activation is quickly followed by inactivation, ending depolarization. Over the short-term, repolarization of the neuron subsequently occurs mainly from efflux of K^+ and some influx of Cl^-.

NEUROTRANSMITTER RELEASE

Neurotransmitters are chemicals that are released from nerve endings into the synapse, where they produce effects by binding to receptors on postsynaptic or presynaptic cell membranes. The receptors may be on either other neurons or effector organs such as smooth muscle. Concentrations of neurotransmitters in cytoplasm are usually low because of rapid enzymatic degradation and diffusion out of the nerve ending. To provide a source of neurotransmitters that is protected from degradation and that can rapidly be released, neurotransmitters are concentrated and stored within vesicles in the axonal nerve terminal. As a wave of depolarization from Na^+ influx reaches the nerve ending, the membrane depolarization causes voltage-gated Ca^{2+} channels to open, allowing Ca^{2+} to move rapidly into the cell. This influx of Ca^{2+} triggers exocytosis of vesicle contents into the synapse. The voltage-gated Ca^{2+} channels responsible for inward Ca^{2+} currents that trigger neurotransmitter release are members of the Ca_v2 subfamily (N, P/Q, and R subtypes).[106,129] Ziconotide is a derivative of a conotoxin that is used for analgesia; it blocks N-type calcium channels on nociceptive neurons in the dorsal root to prevent neurotransmitter release. Cardiovascular calcium channel blockers used in clinical practice do not block these subtypes of voltage-dependent Ca^{2+} channels, but block the L-subtype. However, L-subtype Ca^{2+} channels reside elsewhere on neurons, which explains the ability of traditional Ca^{2+} channel blockers to affect some neurologic functions.

VESICLE TRANSPORT OF NEUROTRANSMITTERS

The pH inside neurotransmitter vesicles is about 5.5, which is lower than that in the cytoplasm. A vacuolar ATPase (V-ATPase) in the vesicular membrane is responsible for movement of protons into the vesicular lumen at the expense of ATP hydrolysis. Vesicular uptake pumps (transporters) that move neurotransmitters or their precursors from the cytoplasm into the vesicle lumen, in turn, are powered by the electrochemical H^+ gradient; that is, the movement of an H^+ out of the vesicle into the cytoplasm is coupled to the movement of a neurotransmitter from the cytoplasm into the vesicle.

Various vesicular transporters for neurotransmitters have been sequenced to date. VGAT transports GABA and glycine. VMAT2 transports all three monoamines, dopamine, norepinephrine, and serotonin (VMAT1 transports monoamines into nonneuronal vesicles). VAChT is responsible for acetylcholine (ACh) transport, and 3 VGluTs (VGluT1-3) move glutamate into vesicles.

Neurotransmitters are confined within the vesicle, to a great extent, by ion trapping, as they are more ionized and less able to diffuse back out of the vesicle at the lower pH. Anything that causes a decrease in the pH gradient across the vesicle membrane results in the movement of neurotransmitters into the cytoplasm.[155] For example, amphetamines move into vesicles, where they buffer protons, causing the movement of monoamine neurotransmitters out of vesicles, and raising cytoplasmic concentrations of neurotransmitters, and ultimately raising the synaptic monoamine concentration.[155,156]

NEUROTRANSMITTER UPTAKE

Although acetylcholine is inactivated in the synapse by enzymatic degradation, other neurotransmitters have their synaptic effects terminated by active uptake into neurons or glial cells. These plasma membrane neurotransmitter transporters are distinct from those transporters responsible for movement of neurotransmitters into vesicles. Cell membrane transporters (uptake pumps) for different neurotransmitters are Na^+-dependent transport proteins, during which the uptake of neurotransmitters is accompanied by the movement of Na^+ across the synaptic membrane.[1]

Neurotransmitter uptake transporters have been subdivided into two main families.[1] One family (SLC6) includes structurally similar uptake pumps for GABA, glycine, norepinephrine, dopamine, and serotonin. They generally comprise 600–700 amino acids and form loops spanning the plasma membrane 12 times. Four GABA uptake transporters (GAT-1 through GAT-4) transport GABA into neurons and glial cells. DAT, SERT, and NET are responsible for uptake of dopamine, serotonin, and norepinephrine, respectively. GLYT-1 and GLYT-2 are responsible for glycine uptake into neurons or astrocytes.

The second family (SLC1) comprises 5 glutamate uptake transporters (excitatory amino acid transporters; EAATs), which appear to traverse the plasma membrane 10 times and move glutamate from the synapse into glial cells and neurons.

Several properties make transporter proteins of particular toxicologic significance. First, they are capable of moving neurotransmitters in either direction; when cytoplasmic neurotransmitter concentrations are significantly elevated, neurotransmitters can be transported back into the synapse. Second, these transporters are not always completely specific. For instance, the uptake transporter for norepinephrine can pump dopamine and other biogenic amines into the neuron. Third, a xenobiotic that acts at the level of the membrane transporter may affect functions of several different neurotransmitters, depending on its specificity for a particular transporter. As an example, fluoxetine is fairly specific at inhibiting uptake of serotonin, whereas cocaine inhibits the uptake of serotonin, norepinephrine, and dopamine.

NEUROTRANSMITTER RECEPTORS

Channel Receptors The first general class of neurotransmitter receptors comprises ligand-gated ion channels (channel receptors or ionotropic receptors), in which the receptor for the neurotransmitter is part of an ion channel. These channels comprise multiple subunits which combine in various combinations to create channels that vary in their response to a given neurotransmitter or other agonist/antagonist. By binding to its receptor, the neurotransmitter allosterically changes the configuration of the ion channel so that ions traverse the channel in greater quantities per unit time. As an example, the acetylcholine nicotinic receptor at the neuromuscular junction is a ligand-gated Na^+ channel. When acetylcholine binds to the nicotinic receptor, the channel's configuration changes, allowing Na^+ to move into the cell and trigger an action potential. (The action potential then propagates down muscle via voltage-gated Na^+ channels.) Table 13–1 lists other examples of channel receptors.

G Protein–Coupled Receptors The second general class of neurotransmitter receptors are linked to G proteins, which are part of a superfamily of proteins with guanosine triphosphatase (GTPase) activity responsible for signal transduction across plasma membranes.[146] G proteins comprise three polypeptide subunits: α, β, and γ chains. These chains span the plasma membrane several times, and they associate with a separately transcribed neurotransmitter receptor that spans the cell membrane 7 times, with an external binding site for neurotransmitters. Some receptors (eg, $GABA_B$ receptor) coupled to G proteins are dimers comprising 2 separate proteins, both of which must be present for activity.

Both the α subunit and the $\beta\gamma$ subunit of a G protein may account for activity resulting from a neurotransmitter binding to its receptor. The α chain normally binds guanosine diphosphate (GDP) in the cytoplasm and is inactive. When a neurotransmitter binds to its receptor on the outside of the cell membrane, GDP dissociates from the α chain and guanosine triphosphate (GTP) binds in its place, activating the α subunit. The activated chain then dissociates from receptor and from the β and γ chains. Both the activated α subunit and $\beta\gamma$ subunits modulate effectors in the plasma membrane.[146] The effector influenced by α or $\beta\gamma$ subunits may be an enzyme that

TABLE 13–1. Types of Neurotransmitter and Neuromodulator Receptors

Ion Channel	G Protein-Coupled Receptor
ACh nicotinic	ACh muscarinic
$GABA_A$, $GABA_C$	$GABA_B$
Glycine (inhibitory)	Dopamine
Glutamate AMPA	Norepinephrine
Glutamate NMDA	$5\text{-HT}_{1,2,4-7}$
Glutamate kainate	Adenosine
5-HT_3	Glutamate metabotropic

ACh = acetylcholine; AMPA = amino-3-hydroxy-5-methyl-4-isoxazole propionate; GABA = γ-aminobutyric acid; 5-HT = 5-hydroxytryptamine (serotonin); NMDA = *N*-methyl-D-aspartate.

the subunits stimulate or inhibit (eg, adenylate cyclase) or an ion channel that is opened or closed directly or through other chemical reactions (eg, channel phosphorylation).[30] Intrinsic GTPase activity in the α chain eventually converts the GTP to GDP, inactivating the α subunit and allowing it to reassociate with the βγ chains and the neurotransmitter receptor, terminating consequences of neurotransmitter binding.[146]

G proteins are mainly categorized by the type of α chain they contain. The three main families of G proteins coupled to neurotransmitter receptors are G_s (containing the α subunit α_s), $G_{i/o}$ (containing α_i or α_o), and G_q (containing α_q). G_s stimulates membrane-bound adenylate cyclase; activation of a neurotransmitter receptor coupled to G_s causes a rise in intracellular 3′,5′-cyclic adenosine monophosphate (cAMP) concentration.[86] Neurotransmitter receptors activating G_i may inhibit adenylate cyclase or modulate K^+ and Ca^{2+} channels. Receptors coupled to G_q act through membrane-bound phospholipase C to increase intracellular calcium concentrations. Table 13–1 lists the neurotransmitter receptors coupled to G proteins. A given neurotransmitter can activate different classes of receptors (eg, ion-channel and G protein) or different types of receptors in the same class. For example, $GABA_A$ receptors are Cl^- channels, whereas $GABA_B$ receptors are coupled to G proteins. Dopamine D_1–like receptors are linked to G_s, whereas D_2–like receptors are linked to G_i or G_o.

Importantly, a single G protein–coupled receptor may activate more than one type of G protein in the same cell, depending on various circumstances, including duration of receptor activation. Receptor downregulation occurs at various levels. For example, prolonged receptor activation results in receptor phosphorylation by G protein kinases (GPKs) which causes receptor binding to a family of proteins, the arrestins, preventing further activation of the G protein by the receptor, and eventually triggers receptor endocytosis.[83,175]

NEURONAL EXCITATION AND INHIBITION

Excitatory neurotransmitters usually act postsynaptically by causing Na^+ or Ca^{2+} influx, or by preventing K^+ efflux, triggering depolarization and an action potential (Fig. 13–1). These effects may be mediated by channel or G protein–coupled receptors.

Postsynaptic inhibition can be mediated by channel receptors or by receptors coupled to G proteins (Fig. 13–1). Inhibition is usually accomplished by neuronal influx of Cl^- or efflux of K^+ to hyperpolarize the neuron and move membrane potential farther away from threshold, making it more difficult for a given stimulus to depolarize the membrane to threshold voltage.

Presynaptic inhibition, the prevention of neurotransmitter release, is usually mediated by receptors coupled to G proteins. When a neurotransmitter released from a neuron binds to a receptor on that same neuron to limit further neurotransmitter release, the receptor is termed an *autoreceptor*.[139] Autoreceptors reside on dendrites, cell bodies, axons, and presynaptic terminals. Autoreceptors on dendrites and cell bodies (somatodendritic autoreceptors) usually inhibit further neurotransmitter release by increasing K^+ efflux, thereby hyperpolarizing the neuron away from threshold (Fig. 13–2). However, activation of autoreceptors found on presynaptic terminals (terminal autoreceptors) usually limits increases in intracellular Ca^{2+} concentration by limiting Ca^{2+} influx or preventing Ca^{2+} release from intracellular stores, impairing exocytosis of neurotransmitter vesicles (Fig. 13–2). Types of neurotransmitter receptors that serve as autoreceptors also usually reside postsynaptically, where they may mediate different physiologic effects.

Presynaptic nerve terminal inhibition of neurotransmitter release is not limited to actions by autoreceptors. Presynaptic terminal inhibitory receptors for various neurotransmitters may be found on a single neuron (heteroreceptors). For example, stimulation of presynaptic α_2 receptors found on postganglionic parasympathetic nerve terminals prevents acetylcholine release.

Finally, stimulation of receptors on presynaptic nerve endings may enhance, rather than inhibit, neurotransmitter release. Such receptors also are usually coupled to G proteins. For example, stimulation of a β_2 receptor on an adrenergic nerve terminal enhances norepinephrine release.

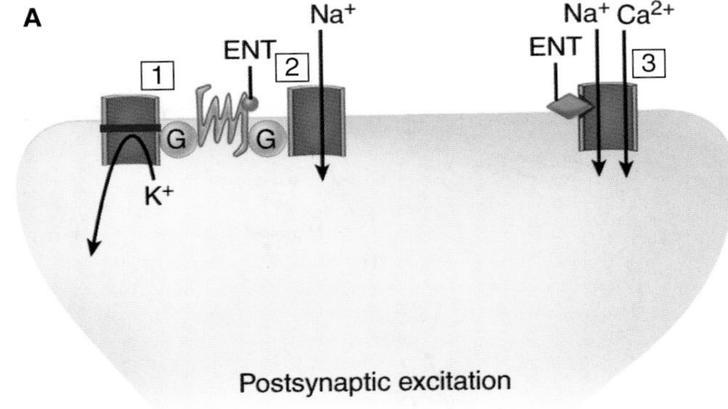

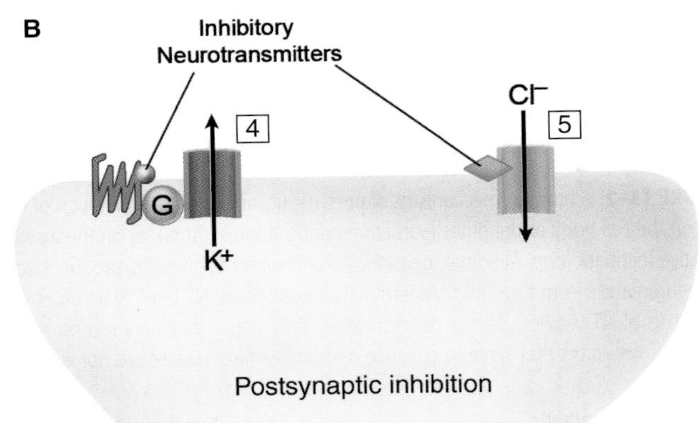

FIGURE 13–1. Common mechanisms of postsynaptic excitation and inhibition. (**A**) An excitatory neurotransmitter (ENT) binds to receptors linked to G proteins to prevent K^+ efflux [1] or to allow Na^+ influx [2], producing membrane depolarization. An ENT may bind to and activate a cation channel [3] to allow Na^+ and/or Ca2+ influx with resultant membrane depolarization. (**B**) An inhibitory neurotransmitter hyperpolarizes the membrane (makes membrane potential more negative) by binding to receptors linked to G proteins to enhance K^+ efflux [4], or to Cl^- channels to allow Cl^- influx [5]. Some Cl^- channels are regulated by G proteins as well. G = G protein.

ACETYLCHOLINE

Acetylcholine (ACh) is a neurotransmitter of the central and peripheral nervous system. Centrally, it is found in both brain and spinal cord; cholinergic fibers project diffusely to the cerebral cortex. Peripherally, ACh serves as a neurotransmitter in autonomic and somatic motor fibers (Fig. 13–3).

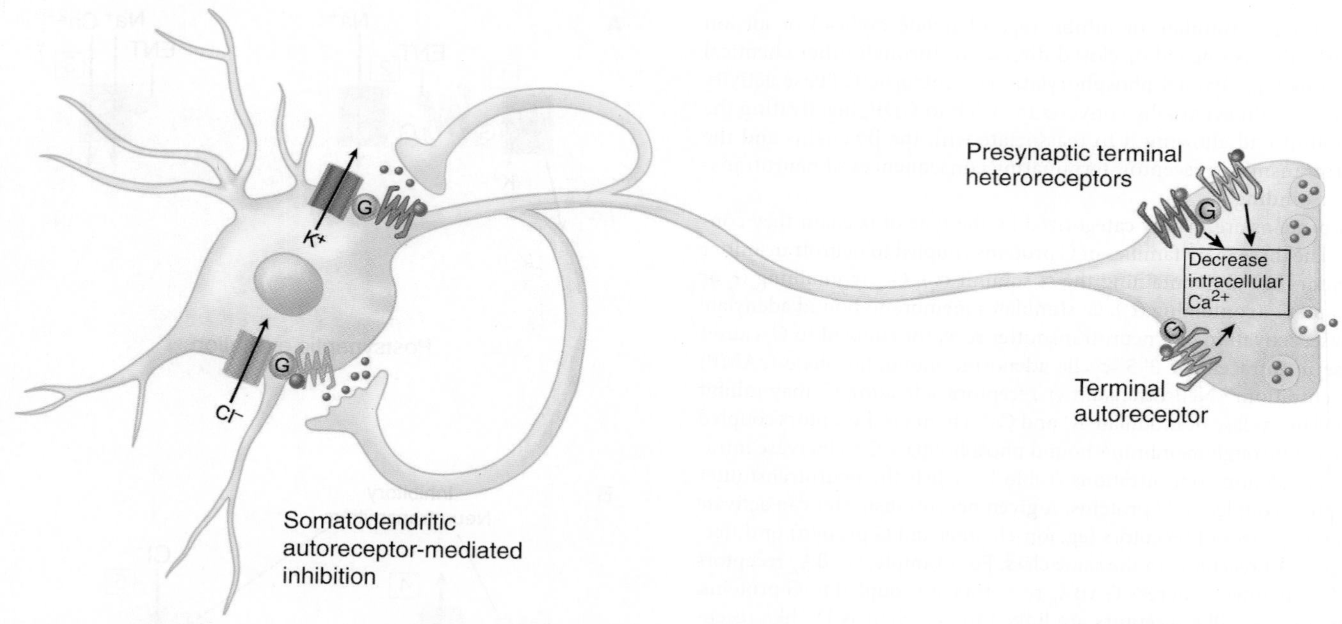

FIGURE 13–2. Common mechanisms of presynaptic inhibition (the inhibition of neurotransmitter [NT] release). A neuron releases NT (green dots), which returns to activate receptors on the cell body or dendrites (somatodendritic autoreceptors), or on the axonal terminal (terminal autoreceptors). Such activation limits further release of NT by completing a negative feedback loop. At somatodendritic autoreceptors, NT binding produces activation of G proteins, which promote either K^+ efflux or Cl^- influx; both processes hyperpolarize the neuron away from threshold. At terminal autoreceptors, NT binding activates G proteins, which, through various mechanisms, lower intracellular Ca^{2+} concentrations to prevent exocytosis of NT vesicles, despite depolarization. Presynaptic inhibitory receptors for other types of NTs (heteroreceptors) are also shown. Excitatory axonal terminal autoreceptors and heteroreceptors that serve to enhance neurotransmitter release are not illustrated. G = G protein.

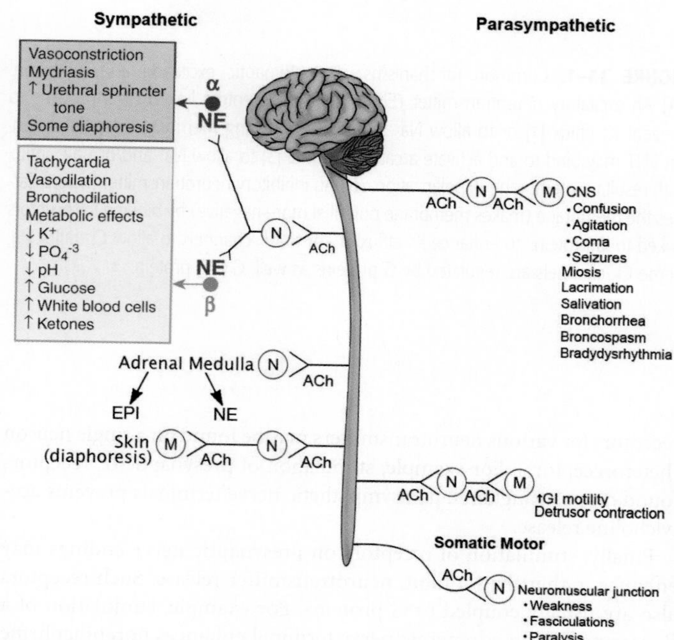

FIGURE 13–3. Diagram of the cholinergic nervous system, including adrenergic involvement in the autonomic nervous system. ACh binds to various nicotinic receptors (N) in CNS, in sympathetic and parasympathetic ganglia, and the adrenal glands. All nicotinic receptors shown are neuronal nicotinic receptors (nnAChRs) except for those at skeletal muscle, which are neuromuscular junction nicotinic receptors (NMJ nAChRs). ACh also binds to various subtypes of muscarinic (M) receptors in the CNS and on effector organs innervated by postsynaptic parasympathetic neurons and to most sweat glands. NE and/or EPI released in response to ACh stimulation of nnAChRs activates α- and β-adrenoceptors. ACh = acetylcholine; CNS = central nervous system; EPI = epinephrine; NE = norepinephrine.

SYNTHESIS, RELEASE, AND INACTIVATION

Acetylcholine is synthesized from acetylcoenzyme A and choline by choline acetyltransferase. Acetylcholine moves into synaptic vesicles via the vesicular membrane transporter, VAChT, where it is stored before release into the synapse by Ca^{2+}-dependent exocytosis. ACh undergoes degradation in the synapse to choline and acetic acid by acetylcholinesterase. A Na^+-dependent transporter in the neuronal membrane (ChT) then pumps choline back into the cytoplasm to be used again as a substrate for ACh synthesis (Fig. 13–4). Pseudocholinesterase (plasma cholinesterase) is made in the liver and plays no role in the degradation of synaptic ACh. However, it does metabolize some xenobiotics, including cocaine and succinylcholine.

ACETYLCHOLINE RECEPTORS

Nicotinic Receptors After release from cholinergic nerve endings, ACh activates two main types of receptors: nicotinic and muscarinic.[84] Nicotinic receptors (nAChRs) reside in the CNS (mainly in spinal cord), on postganglionic autonomic neurons (both sympathetic and parasympathetic), and at skeletal neuromuscular junctions, where they mediate muscle contraction (Fig. 13–3).

Nicotinic receptors at neuromuscular junctions (NMJ nAChRs) are part of a Na^+ channel made of five protein subunits and are thus channel receptors. Stimulation of these receptors by ACh results mainly in Na^+ influx, depolarization of the endplate, and triggering of an action potential that is propagated down the muscle by voltage-gated Na^+ channels.

Nicotinic receptors on central or peripheral neurons or in the adrenal gland are termed neuronal nAChRs. Neuronal nAChRs are also ion channels, although in some cases Ca^{2+} influx through the receptor may be more important than Na^+ influx. Neuronal nAChRs also comprise five subunits.

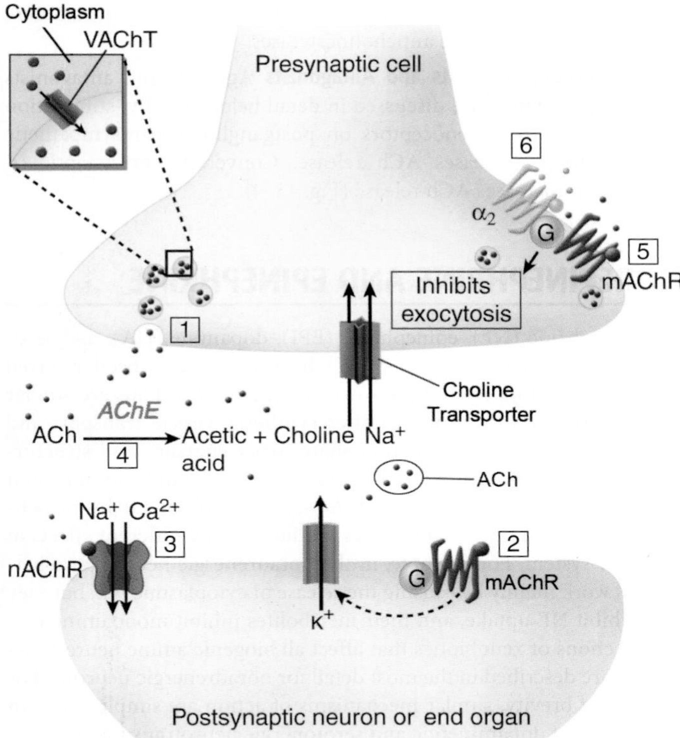

FIGURE 13–4. Cholinergic nerve ending. Activation of postsynaptic muscarinic receptors (mAChR) hyperpolarizes the postsynaptic membrane through G-protein-mediated enhancement of K^+ efflux. Several subtypes of muscarinic receptors coupled to various G proteins exist–a muscarinic receptor coupled to a G protein that opens K^+ channels is shown only as an example [2]. Postsynaptic nicotinic receptor (nAChR) activation causes Na^+ influx and membrane depolarization [3]. Ca^{2+} influx appears to be the main cation involved with some neuronal nicotinic receptors. Presynaptic muscarinic and α_2-adrenoceptor activation prevents ACh release through lowering of intracellular Ca^{2+} concentrations. The agents listed in Table 13-2 may act to enhance or prevent release of ACh [1]; activate or antagonize postsynaptic muscarinic (M) receptors [2]; activate or antagonize nicotinic (N) receptors [3]; inhibit acetylcholinesterase [4]; prevent ACh release by stimulating presynaptic muscarinic autoreceptors [5] or α_2-adrenergic heteroreceptors [6]; or enhance ACh release by antagonizing presynaptic autoreceptors [5] or by antagonizing presynaptic α_2-adrenergic heteroreceptors [6] (on parasympathetic postganglionic terminals). ACh = acetylcholine; AChE = acetylcholinesterase; G = G protein; VAChT = vesicular transporter for ACh. Norepinephrine is shown as light blue dots.

Muscarinic Receptors Muscarinic receptors reside in the CNS (mainly in the brain), on end organs innervated by postganglionic parasympathetic nerve endings, and at most postganglionic sympathetically innervated sweat glands (Fig. 13–4). At least five subtypes of muscarinic receptors, M_{1-5}, are recognized and linked to several G proteins. For example, in the heart, ACh released from the vagus nerve binds to M_2 receptors linked to G_i. G_i opens K^+ channels, allowing efflux of K^+ down its concentration gradient, which makes the inside of the cell more negative and more difficult to depolarize, slowing heart rate. Different subtypes of muscarinic receptors also act as autoreceptors in various locations, M_1 being the most common.

XENOBIOTICS

Table 13–2 provides examples of xenobiotics that affect cholinergic neurotransmission.

Modulators of Acetylcholine Release Figure 13–4 illustrates sites of actions of numerous xenobiotics that influence the cholinergic nervous system. Botulinum toxins, some neurotoxins from pit vipers, and elapid β-neurotoxins prevent release of ACh from peripheral nerve endings.[58] This results in ptosis, other cranial nerve findings, weakness, and respiratory failure. Hypermagnesemia also inhibits ACh release, probably by inhibiting Ca^{2+} influx into the nerve endings.[84]

Guanidine, aminopyridines, and black widow spider venom enhance the release of ACh from nerve endings. Aminopyridines in part block voltage-gated K^+ channels to prevent K^+ efflux; the resultant action potential widening (delayed repolarization) causes prolongation of Ca^{2+} channel activation, enhancing influx of Ca^{2+} and promoting

TABLE 13–2. Examples of Xenobiotics That Affect Cholinergic Neurotransmission

Cholinomimetics	Cholinolytics
Cause ACh release	Direct nicotinic antagonists
α_2-Adrenergic antagonists[a]	α-Bungarotoxin[c]
Aminopyridines	Nondepolarizing neuromuscular blockers
Black widow spider venom	Trimethaphan
Carbachol	Indirect neuronal nicotinic antagonists
Guanidine	Physostigmine
Anticholinesterases	Tacrine
Donepezil	Galantamine
Edrophonium	Direct muscarinic antagonists
N-methylcarbamate insecticides	Antihistamines
Organic phosphorus insecticides	Atropine
Physostigmine	Benztropine
Rivastigmine	Clozapine
Direct nicotinic agonists	Cyclic antidepressants
Carbachol	Cyclobenzaprine
Coniine	Disopyramide
Cytisine	Orphenadrine
Nicotine	Phenothiazines
Succinylcholine[b]	Procainamide
Varenicline	Scopolamine
Indirect neuronal nicotinic agonists	Trihexyphenidyl
Chlorpromazine	Inhibit ACh release
Ethanol	α_2-Adrenergic agonists[d]
Ketamine	Botulinum toxins
Local anesthetics	Crotalinae venoms
Phencyclidine	Elapidae β-neurotoxins
Volatile anesthetics	Hypermagnesemia
Direct muscarinic agonists	
Arecoline	
Bethanechol	
Carbachol	
Cevimeline	
Methacholine	
Muscarine	
Pilocarpine	

ACh = acetylcholine

[a] Antagonism of α_2-adrenoceptors enhances ACh release from parasympathetic nerve endings.

[b] Depolarizing neuromuscular blockers.

[c] α-Bungarotoxin exemplifies many elapid α-neurotoxins that produce paralysis and death from respiratory failure.

[d] Stimulation of presynaptic α_2-adrenoceptors on parasympathetic nerve endings prevents ACh release.

neurotransmitter release. Aminopyridines have been used therapeutically in Lambert–Eaton syndrome, myasthenia gravis, multiple sclerosis, and experimentally in calcium channel blocker overdose.

Black widow spider venom causes ACh release with resultant muscle cramping and diaphoresis.[5]

Nicotinic Receptor Agonists and Antagonists Xenobiotics that bind to and activate nicotinic receptors may stimulate postganglionic sympathetic and parasympathetic neurons, skeletal muscle end-plates, and neurons within the CNS (Fig. 13–3). Prolonged depolarization at the receptor eventually causes diminution of responses to receptor occupancy.[118] For example, poisoning by nicotine, both a neuronal and NMJ nAChR agonist, may produce hypertension, tachycardia, vomiting, diarrhea, muscle fasciculations, and convulsions, followed by hypotension, bradydysrhythmias, paralysis, and coma. Succinylcholine is a neuromuscular blocking agent that initially stimulates and then blocks through prolonged depolarization of NMJ nAChRs.

Xenobiotics that block NMJ nAChRs without stimulation at skeletal neuromuscular junctions produce weakness and paralysis. Examples include curare and atracurium. α-Neurotoxins from elapids (eg, α-bungarotoxin) directly antagonize NMJ nAChRs, producing ptosis, weakness, and respiratory failure from paralysis.[169]

Peripheral neuronal nAChR blockade produces autonomic ganglionic blockade. Trimethaphan was used as a pharmacologic ganglionic blocker; however, it is not entirely specific for neuronal nAChRs. Occasionally, timethaphan may cause weakness and paralysis from NMJ nAChR blockade.

Recent studies demonstrate that the function of neuronal nAChRs can be modulated by a variety of xenobiotics that do not bind to the ACh binding site, but bind instead to a number of distinct allosteric sites on the neuronal nAChR. For example, aside from their ability to inhibit acetylcholinesterase, physostigmine, tacrine, and galantamine bind to a noncompetitive allosteric activator site on neuronal nAChRs to enhance channel opening and ion conductance (there is evidence suggesting that serotonin may bind here as well). Furthermore, a diverse range of xenobiotics, including chlorpromazine, phencyclidine, ketamine, local anesthetics, and ethanol bind to a noncompetitive negative allosteric site(s) to inhibit inward ion fluxes without directly affecting ACh binding. Steroids can desensitize neuronal nAChRs by binding to yet an additional allosteric site.[120]

Muscarinic Receptor Agonists and Antagonists Peripheral muscarinic agonists produce bradycardia, miosis, salivation, lacrimation, vomiting, diarrhea, bronchospasm, bronchorrhea, and micturition. Central muscarinic agonists produce sedation, extrapyramidal dystonias, rigidity, coma, and convulsions. Anticholinergic poisoning syndrome results from blockade of muscarinic receptors and is more appropriately referred to as antimuscarinic poisoning syndrome.[141] Central nervous system muscarinic blockade produces confusion, agitation, myoclonus, tremor, picking movements, abnormal speech, hallucinations, and coma. Peripheral antimuscarinic effects include mydriasis, anhidrosis, tachycardia, and urinary retention. Muscarinic antagonists number in the hundreds; Table 13–2 lists examples.

Acetylcholinesterase Inhibition Xenobiotics inhibiting acetylcholinesterase raise ACh concentrations at both nicotinic and muscarinic receptors, producing a variety of CNS, sympathetic, parasympathetic, and skeletal muscle signs and symptoms.[32] Anticholinesterases include organic phosphorus compounds and *N*-methylcarbamates. Organic phosphorus compounds are usually encountered as insecticides, although topical medicinal organic phosphorus compounds are used for the treatment of glaucoma and lice. *N*-methylcarbamates are found as insecticides and pharmaceuticals. Medicinal *N*-methylcarbamates include physostigmine, pyridostigmine, rivastigmine, and neostigmine. Edrophonium, galantamine, tacrine, donepezil, and metrifonate are noncarbamate, reversible anticholinesterases.

α_2-Adrenoceptor Agonists and Antagonists Agonists and antagonists of α_2-adrenoceptors are discussed in detail below. Briefly, stimulation of presynaptic α_2-adrenoceptors on postganglionic parasympathetic nerve endings decreases ACh release. Conversely, presynaptic α_2 antagonism increases ACh release (Fig. 13–4).

NOREPINEPHRINE AND EPINEPHRINE

Norepinephrine (NE), epinephrine (EPI), dopamine (DA), and serotonin (5-hydroxytryptamine; 5-HT) have historically been referred to as biogenic amines, and their neurotransmitter systems are similar in many respects. Neurotransmitter synthesis, vesicle transport and storage, uptake, and degradation share many enzymes and structurally similar transport proteins. Cocaine, reserpine, amphetamines, and monoamine oxidase inhibitors (MAOIs) affect all four types of neurons. In addition, these xenobiotics produce several different effects in the same system. For example, in the noradrenergic neuron, amphetamines work mainly by causing the release of cytoplasmic NE, but they also inhibit NE uptake, and their metabolites inhibit monoamine oxidase. Actions of xenobiotics that affect all biogenic amine neurotransmitters are described in the most detail for noradrenergic neurons. For the sake of brevity, similar mechanisms of action are simply noted in discussions of dopaminergic and serotonergic neurotransmission.

Norepinephrine is released from postganglionic sympathetic fibers (Fig. 13–3) and is also found in the CNS. The adrenal gland, acting as a modified sympathetic ganglion, releases EPI and lesser amounts of NE in response to stimulation of neuronal nAChRs. Epinephrine-containing neurons also reside in the brainstem.

The locus ceruleus is the main noradrenergic nucleus and resides in the floor of the fourth ventricle on each side of the pons. Axons radiate from this nucleus out to all layers of the cerebral cortex, to the cerebellum, and to other structures. Norepinephrine demonstrates both excitatory and inhibitory actions in the CNS. Norepinephrine released from locus ceruleus projections in the hippocampus increases cortical neuron activity through β-adrenoceptor activation and G protein–mediated inhibition of K^+ efflux. Norepinephrine released in outer cortical areas produces inhibitory effects mediated by α_2-adrenoceptor agonism. Consistent with this, NE demonstrates anticonvulsant actions in animals. Carbamazepine's anticonvulsant action may be partly a result of inhibition of NE uptake.[44] Despite antagonistic actions on different cortical neurons, electrical stimulation of the locus ceruleus produces widespread cortical activation and excitation. This overall effect probably explains a great deal of the hyperattentiveness and lack of fatigue that accompanies use of xenobiotics that mimic or increase noradrenergic activity in the brain. Locus ceruleus neuronal firing increases during waking and dramatically falls during sleep.

SYNTHESIS, RELEASE, AND UPTAKE

Figure 13–5 is a representation of a noradrenergic neuron. Tyrosine hydroxylase is the rate-limiting enzyme in NE synthesis and is sensitive to negative feedback by NE. This enzyme requires Fe^{2+} as a cofactor and exists as a homotetramer and is upregulated by chronic exposure to caffeine and nicotine. Under normal dietary conditions tyrosine hydroxylase is completely saturated by tyrosine, and increasing dietary tyrosine does not appreciably increase dopa synthesis. Dopa undergoes decarboxylation by L-amino acid decarboxylase to DA. L-Amino acid decarboxylase (dopa decarboxylase) is not specific for dopa. For example, it also catalyzes the formation of serotonin from 5-HT.

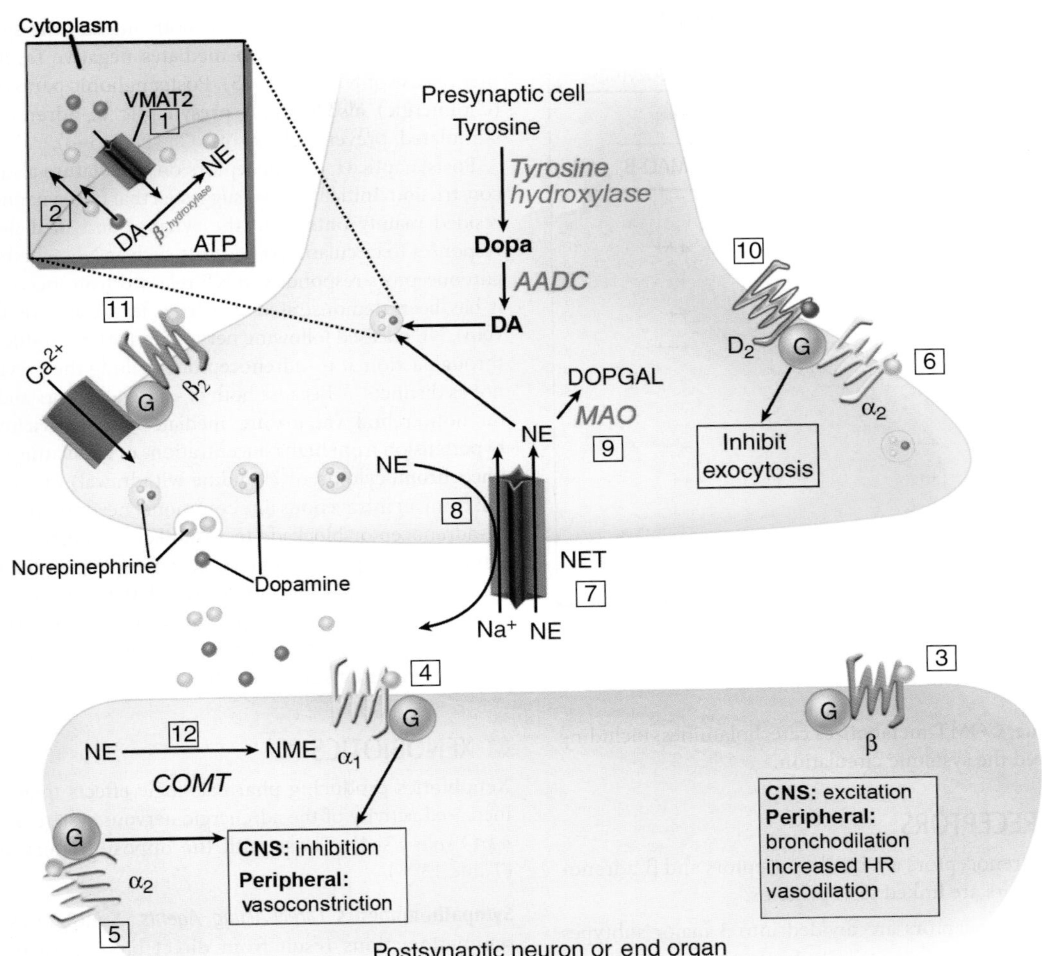

FIGURE 13–5. Noradrenergic nerve ending. The postsynaptic membrane may represent an end organ or another neuron in the CNS. Brief examples of effects resulting from postsynaptic receptor activation are shown. Agents in Tables 13-4 and 13-5 produce effects by inhibiting transport of dopamine (DA) or norepinephrine (NE) into vesicles through VMA2 [1]; causing movement of NE and DA from vesicles into the cytoplasm [2]; activating or antagonizing postsynaptic α- and β-adrenoceptors [3 -5]; modulating NE release by activating or antagonizing presynaptic α_2-autoreceptors [6], dopamine$_2$ (D_2) heteroreceptors [10], or β_2-autoreceptors [11]; blocking uptake of NE (NET inhibition) [7]; causing reverse transport of NE from the cytoplasm into the synapse via NET by raising cytoplasmic NE concentrations [8]; inhibiting monoamine oxidase (MAO) to prevent NE degradation [9]; or inhibiting COMT to prevent NE degradation [12]. AADC = aromatic L-amino acid decarboxylase; β-hydroxylase = dopamine-β-hydroxylase; COMT = catechol-*O*-methyltransferase; CNS = central nervous system; DOPGAL = 3,4-dihydroxyphenylglycoaldehyde; G = G protein; NET = membrane NE uptake transporter; NME = normetanephrine; VMA2 = vesicle uptake transporter for NE.

About one-half of cytoplasmic DA is actively pumped into vesicles by VMAT2. The remaining DA is quickly deaminated.

In the vesicle, DA is converted to NE by dopamine-β-hydroxylase. Vesicles isolated from peripheral nerve endings contain DA, NE, dopamine-β-hydroxylase, and ATP, and all of these substances are released into the synapse during Ca^{2+}-dependent exocytosis triggered by neuronal firing. In neurons containing EPI as a neurotransmitter, NE is released from vesicles into the cytoplasm, where it is converted to EPI by phenylethanolamine-*N*-methyl-transferase. Epinephrine is then transported back into vesicles before synaptic release.[84]

Norepinephrine is removed from the synapse, mainly by uptake into the presynaptic neuron by the NE transporter (NET). Although this transporter has great affinity for NE, it also transports other amines, including DA, tyramine, MAOIs, and amphetamines. Once pumped back into the cytoplasm, NE can either be transported back into vesicles for further storage and release, or can be quickly degraded by monoamine oxidase (MAO), an enzyme expressed on the outer mitochondrial membrane.

MAO is present in all human tissues except red blood cells. It exists as 2 isozymes, MAO-A and MAO-B,[101] each with relatively separate affinities for various substrates (Table 13–3). Neuronal MAO degrades cytoplasmic amines, including neurotransmitters, to prevent elevated cytoplasmic concentrations of biogenic amines. Hepatic and intestinal MAO prevent large quantities of dietary bioactive amines from entering the circulation and producing systemic effects.

Catechol-*O*-methyltransferase (COMT) is an intracellular enzyme widely distributed throughout the body, including the central nervous system, that is responsible for metabolism of DA, L-Dopa, NE, and EPI.

TABLE 13–3. Characteristics of Monoamine Oxidase (MAO) Isozymes

	MAO Isozymes	
	MAO-A	MAO-B
Location		
Brain	+	+++
Intestines	+++	+
Liver	++	++
Platelets	+	++++
Placenta	++++	+
Substrates		
Norepinephrine	++++	+
Epinephrine	++	++
Dopamine	++	++
Serotonin	++++	+
Tyramine	++	++

In extraneuronal tissue, COMT metabolizes catecholamines, including those that have entered the systemic circulation.

ADRENERGIC RECEPTORS

The 2 main types of adrenoceptors are α-adrenoceptors and β-adrenoceptors. All adrenoceptors are linked to G proteins.

β-Adrenoceptors β-Adrenoceptors are divided into 3 major subtypes (β_1, β_2, and β_3), depending on their affinity for various agonists and antagonists.[25,65,68,86] β_1-adrenoceptors and β_2-adrenoceptors are linked to G_s, and their stimulation raises cAMP concentration and/or activates protein kinase A which, in turn, produces several effects, including regulation of ion channels. At least some β_3-adrenoceptors may be coupled not only to G_s, but also to receptors for $G_{i/o}$ proteins. Prolonged activation of β_2 receptors in the heart causes them to become coupled to G_i.[175]

The β-adrenoceptors are polymorphic, with genetic variation in humans.[23] Polymorphism influences response to medications, regulation of receptors, and clinical course of disease.[23,68,86] In general, peripheral β_1-adrenoceptors are found mainly in the heart (along with β_2 receptors), whereas peripheral β_2-adrenoceptors also mediate additional adrenergic effects.[68] Presynaptic β_2-adrenoceptor activation causes release of NE from nerve endings (positive feedback). β_3-Adrenoceptors reside mainly in fat, but they also reside in skeletal muscle, gallbladder, and colon where they regulate metabolic processes. β_3-Adrenoceptors' polymorphism may contribute to clinical expressions of non–insulin-dependent diabetes and obesity.[23,154,171]

α-Adrenoceptors α-Adrenoceptors are linked to G proteins that inhibit adenylate cyclase to lower cAMP levels, affect ion channels, increase intracellular Ca^{2+} through inositol triphosphate and diacylglycerol production, or produce other actions. These receptors are divided into two main types, α_1 and α_2, and at least six subtypes—α_{1A}, α_{1B}, α_{1D}, α_{2A}, α_{2B}, and α_{2C}—are described.[39,65] Most α_1 adrenoceptors are coupled to G_q, whereas most α_2 adrenoceptors are coupled to G_i.

In peripheral tissue, α_1-adrenoceptors reside on the postsynaptic membrane in continuity with the synaptic cleft. Stimulation of these receptors on blood vessels commonly results in vasoconstriction.

α_2-Adrenoceptors reside on both sides of the synapse. Presynaptic α_2-adrenoceptor activation mediates negative feedback, limiting further release of NE (Fig. 13–5). Postganglionic parasympathetic neurons (cholinergic) also contain presynaptic α_2-adrenoceptors that, when stimulated, prevent release of ACh (Fig. 13–4).

Postsynaptic α_2-adrenoceptors on vasculature also can mediate vasoconstriction. Initially, it was suggested that postsynaptic α_2-adrenoceptors resided mainly outside of the synapse and mediated vasoconstrictive responses to circulating α agonists such as NE, whereas postsynaptic α_1-adrenoceptors responded to NE released from nerve endings. However, it has been demonstrated that in at least some tissues (eg, saphenous vein), NE released following nerve stimulation produces vasoconstriction through action at α_2-adrenoceptors, making the previous differentiation not as distinct.[39,76] Because both α_1- adrenoceptors and α_2-adrenoceptors on noncerebral vasculature mediate vasoconstriction, a patient with hypertension from high concentrations of circulating catecholamines (eg, pheochromocytoma or clonidine withdrawal) or from extravasation of NE from an intravenous line commonly needs both α_1-adrenoceptor and α_2-adrenoceptor blockade to vasodilate adequately (eg, phentolamine). Stimulation of postsynaptic α_2-adrenoceptors in the brainstem inhibits sympathetic output and produces sedation (Fig. 13–6). In fact, dexmedetomidine, an imidazole and potent α_{2A}-adrenoceptor agonist, is used for sedation in intensive care patients, although hypotension and bradycardia occur as expected side effects.[13]

XENOBIOTICS

Xenobiotics producing pharmacologic effects that result in or mimic increased activity of the adrenergic nervous system are *sympathomimetics* (Table 13–4). Those with the opposite effect are *sympatholytics* (Table 13–5).

Sympathomimetics ***Direct-Acting Agents.*** Xenobiotics whose sympathomimetic actions result from direct binding to α-adrenoceptors or β-adrenoceptors are called *direct-acting sympathomimetics*. Most do not cross the blood–brain barrier in significant quantities.

Indirect-Acting Agents. Xenobiotics that produce sympathomimetic effects by causing the release of cytoplasmic NE from the nerve ending in the absence of vesicle exocytosis are called *indirect-acting sympathomimetics*. Amphetamine is the prototype of indirect-acting sympathomimetics and is used for the discussion of what is known about their mechanism of action. In general, mechanisms of indirect release of NE

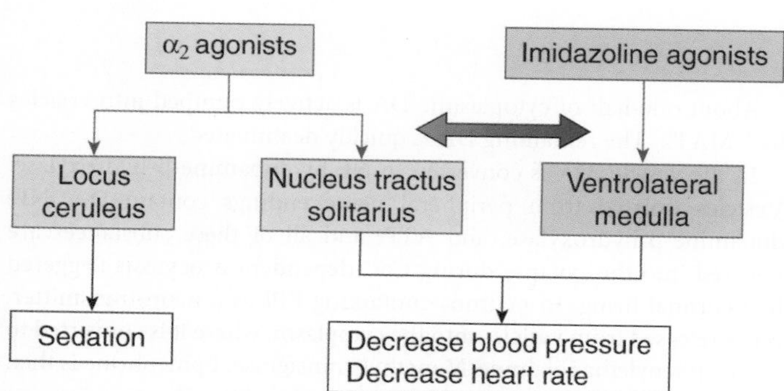

FIGURE 13–6. Central action of agents that activate α_2-adrenoceptors or that bind to type 1 imidazoline binding sites. There are poorly understood interactions between imidazoline binding sites and α_2-adrenoceptors that make delineation of specific effects difficult to attribute to specific receptor activation.

TABLE 13–4. Examples of Sympathomimetics

Direct acting	Selective α_2-adrenoceptor antagonists
α-Adrenoceptor agonists	Idazoxan
Epinephrine	Efaroxan
Ergot alkaloids	Yohimbine
Methoxamine	Imidazoline binding-site antagonists
Midodrine	Idazoxan
Norepinephrine	Efaroxan
Phenylephrine	MAOIs
β-Adrenoceptor agonists	Amphetamine metabolites
Albuterol	Clorgyline
Dobutamine	Isocarboxazid
Epinephrine	Linezolid
Isoproterenol	Moclobemide
Metaproterenol	Pargyline
Norepinephrine	Phenelzine
Terbutaline	Rasagiline
Indirect acting	Selegiline
Amphetamine	Tranylcypromine
Cocaine	Inhibit norepinephrine Uptake
Fenfluramine	Amphetamine
MAOIs	Atomoxetine
Methylphenidate	Benztropine
Pemoline	Bupropion
Phenmetrazine	Carbamazepine
Propylhexedrine	Cocaine
Tyramine	Cyclic antidepressants
Mixed acting	Diphenhydramine
Dopamine	Duloxetine
Ephedrine	Orphenadrine
Mephentermine	Pemoline
Metaraminol	Reboxetine
Phenylpropanolamine	Tramadol
Pseudoephedrine	Trihexyphenidyl
	Venlafaxine

MAOIs = monoamine oxidase inhibitors.

TABLE 13–5. Examples of Sympatholytics

α-Adrenoceptor antagonists	α_2-Adrenoceptor agonists[b]
Clozapine	α-Methyldopa[c]
Cyclic antidepressants	Clonidine
Doxazosin	Dexmedetomidine
Ergot alkaloids	Guanabenz
Olanzapine	Guanfacine
Phenothiazines	Moxonidine
Phenoxybenzamine	Naphazoline
Phentolamine	Oxymetazoline
Prazosin	Rilmenidine
Risperidone	Tetrahydrolozine
Terazosin	Tizanidine
Tolazoline	Xylometazoline
Trazodone	Imidazoline binding-site agonists[b]
Inhibit dopamine-β-hydroxylase	Clonidine
Diethyldithiocarbamate	Guanabenz
Disulfiram	Guanfacine
MAOIs	Moxonidine
β-Adrenoceptor antagonists	Naphazoline
Atenolol	Oxymetazoline
Esmolol	Rilmenidine
Labetalol	Inhibitors of vesicle uptake
Nadolol	Reserpine
Pindolol[a]	Tetrabenazine
Practolol[a]	
Propranolol	
Sotalol	

MAOIs = monoamine oxidase inhibitors.

[a] Partial β-agonist.

[b] Xenobiotics in these categories vary in their relative selectivity for α_2-adrenoceptors or imidazoline binding sites.

[c] Metabolized to α-methylnorepinephrine, which activates α_2-adrenoceptors.

by amphetamines, cocaine, phencyclidine, MAOIs, and mixed-acting xenobiotics noted in Table 13–4 are similar in that their actions depend on their ability to produce elevated cytoplasmic NE concentrations.

Amphetamine and structurally similar indirect-acting sympathomimetics move into the neuron mainly by the membrane transporter that pumps NE into the neuron. (Lipophilic indirect-acting sympathomimetics move into the neuron by diffusion.) From the cytoplasm, amphetamines are transported into neurotransmitter vesicles, where they buffer protons to raise intravesicular pH. As noted earlier, much of the vesicle's ability to concentrate NE (and other neurotransmitters) is a result of ion trapping of NE at the lower pH. The rise in intravesicle pH produced by amphetamines causes NE to leave the vesicle and move into the cytoplasm.[155,156] Such movement may be caused by diffusion or reverse transport of NE by VMAT2. In the cytoplasm, amphetamines also compete with NE and DA for transport into vesicles, which further contributes to elevated cytoplasmic NE concentrations. In the case of amphetamine, the rise in cytoplasmic concentrations of NE may be enhanced by the ability of amphetamine metabolites to inhibit MAO, which impairs NE degradation.

Every time the Na^+-dependent uptake transporter, NET, moves a bioactive amine (eg, tyramine) into the neuron where it is released, a binding site for NE on NET transiently faces inward and becomes available for reverse transport of NE out of the neuron. The normally low concentration of cytoplasmic NE prevents significant reverse transport. In the face of elevated cytoplasmic NE concentrations produced by indirect-acting sympathomimetics, NET moves NE out of the neuron and back into the synapse, where the neurotransmitter stimulates adrenoceptors (indirect action). This process is sometimes referred to as facilitated exchange diffusion, or displacement, of NE from the nerve ending. Evidence supporting reverse transport produced by amphetamines is that inhibitors of the transporter (eg, tricyclic antidepressants) prevent amphetamine-induced NE release.

While all indirect-acting smypathomimetics cause reverse NE transport by increasing cytoplasmic NE concentrations, those that move into the neuron by the membrane transporter (eg, amphetamines, MAOIs, DA, tyramine) further enhance reverse transport because their uptake may cause more NE binding sites on NET to face inward per unit time.

Although cocaine does inhibit NET, it also causes some NE release. In fact, cocaine similarly lessens pH gradients across vesicle membranes[156] to raise cytoplasmic concentrations of NE. That cocaine produces less NE release than amphetamines is partly explained by cocaine-induced inhibition of the membrane transporter and by the fact that cocaine does not move into the neuron by active uptake (ie, does not increase the number of NE binding sites facing inward), but diffuses into the neuron. (Most of cocaine's severe sympathomimetic effects probably result from its action on the brain rather than peripheral nerve endings.[162])

Phencyclidine (PCP) is a hallucinogen that possesses multiple pharmacologic actions. Like toxicity from many hallucinogens, PCP toxicity is accompanied by increased adrenergic activity, which results, in part, from PCP-induced decreases in pH gradients across the vesicle membrane[156] and indirect release of NE. Like cocaine, PCP moves into the neuron by diffusion rather than uptake through the membrane transporter, at least partly explaining less PCP-induced NE release than typically occurs in amphetamine poisoning.

In addition to causing ACh release, black widow spider venom causes vesicle exocytosis of NE, producing hypertension and diaphoresis over the palms, soles, upper lip, and nose. All of the aforementioned indirectly acting sympathomimetics, except black widow spider venom, enter the CNS.

Mixed-Acting Xenobiotics. Mixed-acting sympathomimetics act directly and indirectly. For example, large doses of phenylpropanolamine indirectly cause NE release and act directly as α-adrenoceptor agonists. Intravenously administered DA indirectly causes NE release, explaining most of its vasoconstricting activity, but also directly stimulates dopaminergic and β-adrenoceptors. Direct α-agonism occurs at high doses. Except for DA, these xenobiotics cross the blood–brain barrier to produce central effects.

Uptake Inhibitors. Inhibitors of NE uptake raise concentrations of NE in the synapse to produce excessive stimulation of adrenoceptors.

There are 2 main mechanisms of action for inhibitors of biogenic amine uptake: competitive and noncompetitive. Noncompetitive inhibitors, such as cyclic antidepressants, carbamazepine, venlafaxine, methylphenidate, and cocaine, bind at or near the carrier site on NET to prevent NET from moving NE and similar xenobiotics into or out of the neuron. These inhibitors are not transported into the neuron by this mechanism. Various xenobiotics used for their antimuscarinic effects also block NET noncompetitively. These include benztropine, diphenhydramine, trihexyphenidyl and orphenadrine.[108] Atomexetine also inhibits NET.

The second mechanism, competitive inhibition of NET, characterizes most indirect-acting sympathomimetics, including amphetamines and structurally similar xenobiotics (eg, mixed-acting agents, MAOIs). These xenobiotics prevent NE uptake by competing with synaptic NE for binding to the carrier site on NET, the mechanism by which they move into the neuron. In fact, an additional adrenergic action of amphetamines, mixed-acting agents, MAOIs, and tyramine is to raise synaptic NE concentrations by competing for uptake, thereby compounding their indirect or direct actions.

MAOIs. MAOIs are transported by NET into the neuron, where they act through several mechanisms.[101] Inhibition of MAO, their main pharmacologic effect, results in increased cytoplasmic concentrations of NE and some indirect release of neurotransmitter into the synapse. As a minor effect they also may displace NE from vesicles by raising pH in a manner similar to amphetamines. These actions explain the initial hyperadrenergic findings following MAOI overdose and probably also account for occasional and unpredictable adrenergic crises that occur despite dietary compliance.

Nonspecific MAOIs inhibit both isozymes of MAO, preventing intestinal and hepatic degradation of bioactive amines. A person taking such an MAOI who then is exposed to indirect-acting sympathomimetics (eg, tyramine in cheese, phenylpropanolamine, DA, amphetamines) has a much larger cytoplasmic concentration of NE to transport into the synapse and may, therefore, develop central and peripheral hyperadrenergic findings. MAOIs specific for the MAO-B isozyme are less likely to predispose to food or drug interactions by maintaining significant hepatic and intestinal MAO activity. Furthermore, reversible MAO-A specific inhibitors are also less likely to provoke this reaction because their reversibility allows competition of exogenous amines with the inhibitor, resulting in its displacement from the enzyme and normal metabolism of the bioactive amines.[177] Isozyme specificity is lost as the dose of the MAOI is increased. In fact, selegiline, currently marketed as a selective MAO-B inhibitor, partially inhibits MAO-A activity at therapeutic doses. Specificity might lack importance when indirect-acting agents are administered parenterally (eg, intravenous DA or amphetamines). Linezolid is an antibiotic that produces weak MAO inhibition.

Occasionally, patients suffering from refractory depression respond to a combination of MAOIs and tricyclic antidepressants. This combination therapy is usually unaccompanied by excessive adrenergic activity because the inhibition of the membrane uptake transporter by the tricyclic antidepressant attenuates excessive reverse transport of elevated cytoplasmic NE concentrations produced by MAOIs.

COMT Inhibitors. Inhibitors of COMT are administered in the treatment of Parkinson disease to prevent the catabolism of concomitantly administered L-dopa. Entacapone only acts peripherally, whereas tolcapone also crosses the blood–brain barrier.

α_2-Adrenoceptor Antagonists. Yohimbine blocks α_2-adrenoceptors to produce a mixed clinical picture. Peripheral postsynaptic α_2 blockade produces vasodilation. Blockade of presynaptic α_2-adrenoceptors on cholinergic nerve endings (Fig. 13–4) enhances ACh release, occasionally producing bronchospasm[82] and contributing to diaphoresis. Similar presynaptic actions on peripheral noradrenergic nerves enhance catecholamine release (Fig. 13–5). Antagonism of central α_2-adrenoceptors in the locus ceruleus results in CNS stimulation, whereas blockade of postsynaptic α_2-adrenoceptors in the nucleus tractus solitarius may enhance sympathetic output (Fig. 13–6). The final result includes hypertension, tachycardia, anxiety, fear, agitation, mania, mydriasis, diaphoresis, and bronchospasm.[87]

Sympatholytics ***Direct Antagonists.*** Direct α-adrenoceptor and β-adrenoceptor antagonists are noted in Table 13–5. After overdose, β-adrenoceptor selectivity may be less significant. Some β-adrenoceptor antagonists also are partial agonists.

Xenobiotics That Prevent Norepinephrine Release. Xenobiotics that block the vesicle uptake transporter prevent the movement of NE into vesicles and deplete the nerve ending of this neurotransmitter, also preventing NE release after depolarization. Reserpine and ketanserin inhibit both VMAT1 and VMAT2, whereas tetrabenazine only inhibits VMAT2. Like guanethidine, reserpine causes transient NE release with the initial dose or early in overdose. β-Adrenoceptor antagonists block presynaptic β_2-adrenoceptors to limit catecholamine release from nerve endings, although this does not appear to be their main mechanism of action.

Imidazoline and α_2-Adrenoceptor Agonists. Numerous imidazoline derivatives (eg, clonidine) and structurally similar xenobiotics are used as centrally acting antihypertensives or long-acting topical vasoconstrictors. They are currently divided into first-generation agents (eg, clonidine) that are thought to act at both α_{2A}-adrenoceptor and imidazoline binding sites, and second-generation agents (eg, rilmenidine) that express much greater affinity for imidazoline binding sites than for α_{2A}-adrenergic receptors.

The ventromedial (depressor) and the rostral-ventrolateral (pressor) areas of the ventrolateral medulla (VLM) are responsible for the central regulation of cardiovascular tone and blood pressure. They receive afferent fibers from the carotid and aortic baroreceptors, which form the tractus solitarius via the nucleus tractus solitarius (NTS).[75]

The hypotensive actions of α_2-adrenoceptor agonists were previously attributed entirely to brainstem α_2-adrenoceptor activation, because stimulation of postsynaptic α_2-adrenoceptors in the NTS decreased sympathetic output (Fig. 13–6).[19] The discovery of imidazoline binding sites, however, led to a more complicated analysis. It was discovered that imidazolines and related xenobiotics produced hypotension when applied to the VLM, whereas catecholamines capable of activating α_2-adrenoceptors were claimed to be incapable of producing effects at this site. This led to the hypothesis that receptors specific for imidazolines, different from α_{2A}-adrenoceptors, must exist. Decreased sympathetic output could result from activation of imidazoline binding sites in the VLM and from α_2-adrenoceptor activation in the NTS; sedation and respiratory depression were attributed to α_2-adrenoceptor activation in the locus ceruleus.[46]

Imidazoline binding sites have been characterized and subdivided into I_1, I_2 (with subtypes), and I_3.[41] I_1 binding sites reside on neuronal plasma membranes and are involved in controlling systemic blood pressure. I_2 sites are allosteric sites found on the external membrane of mitochondria and modulate MAO-A and MAO-B.[19,41] The putative I_3 sites are thought to modulate insulin secretion via ATP-sensitive potassium channels in β-islet cells.

The molecular structure of the imidazoline binding sites has not been identified. Endogenous ligands for these binding sites have been discovered: agmatine, imidazole-acetic acid ribotide, harmane, and other β-carbolines.[10,60,132]

Functional evidence suggests that there is significant interaction between the imidazoline sites and α_{2A}-adrenoceptors, and that this interaction is necessary to trigger hypotensive effects.[18,46] As examples, there appears to be a close relationship between "presynaptic" imidazoline sites and "downstream" α_{2A}-adrenoceptors in the VLM mediating hypotension;[59] α_{2A}-adrenoceptors in the VLM appear to be activated as a consequence of imidazoline site activation. Although second-generation agents (rilmenidine and moxonidine) preferentially act via imidazoline binding sites, and although α_{2A}-adrenoceptors are important for the hypotension produced by first-generation agents (clonidine and α-methyldopa), hypotension produced by all of these xenobiotics is dependent on central noradrenergic pathways.[18,59] Some studies report that yohimbine, an α_2-adrenoceptor antagonist, reverses the hypotensive effect of both clonidine and rilmenidine-like drugs when given at high doses. Thus, it appears that there is significant interaction between imidazoline sites and α_{2A}-adrenoceptors, and that centrally acting antihypertensive agents with relatively high affinity for imidazoline binding sites may require both imidazoline specific sites and functional α_{2A}-adrenoceptors to produce their hypotensive actions.

Ingestions of xenobiotics that activate α_{2A}-adrenoceptors and imidazoline binding sites (Table 13–5) produce a mixed clinical picture. Peripheral postsynaptic α_2-adrenoceptor stimulation produces vasoconstriction, pallor, and hypertension, often with reflex bradycardia (Fig. 13–5). Peripheral presynaptic α_2-adrenoceptor stimulation prevents NE release (Fig. 13–5), whereas central α_2-adrenoceptor stimulation in the locus ceruleus accounts for CNS and respiratory depression (Fig. 13–6). Stimulation of postsynaptic α_2-adrenoceptors in the NTS and of central I_1 receptors in the VLM are thought to inhibit sympathetic output and enhance parasympathetic tone, explaining hypotension with bradycardia (Fig. 13–6).[75] Both first-generation and second-generation agents produce dry mouth.[19,41]

Dopamine-β-Hydroxylase Inhibition. Inhibition of dopamine-β-hydroxylase, a copper-containing enzyme (Fig. 13–5), prevents the conversion of DA to NE, resulting in less NE release and less α-adrenoceptor and β-adrenoceptor stimulation with neuronal firing. Disulfiram and diethyldithiocarbamate, copper chelators, produce such inhibition.[43] Because NE release mediates most of DA's ability to cause vasoconstriction, NE is the vasopressor of choice in a hypotensive patient taking disulfiram. MAOIs and α-methyldopa also inhibit dopamine-β-hydroxylase, although this is not their main mechanism of action.[101]

Dopamine is relatively contraindicated in hypotensive patients who have overdosed on MAOIs. First, DA acts indirectly and its administration might produce excessive adrenergic activity and exaggerated rises in blood pressure. Second, even if an adrenergic storm does not occur, most of dopamine's α-mediated vasoconstriction is secondary to NE release. In the presence of MAOIs, NE synthesis may be impaired from concomitant dopamine-β-hydroxylase inhibition, and DA may not reliably raise blood pressure if cytoplasmic and vesicular stores have been depleted. In the presence of impaired NE release or α-adrenoceptor blockade by any cause, unopposed dopamine-induced vasodilatation from action on peripheral DA and β-adrenoceptors may paradoxically lower blood pressure further. Norepinephrine and EPI can be used to support blood pressure relatively safely in patients taking MAOIs, because they have little or no indirect action and are metabolized by COMT when given intravenously.

DOPAMINE

Because DA is the direct precursor of NE, noradrenergic vesicles contain DA. The release of NE from peripheral sympathetic nerves, therefore, always results in release of some DA (Fig. 13–5), as does the release of NE and EPI from the adrenal gland, explaining most of DA in blood. In peripheral tissues, activation of DA receptors causes vasodilatation of renal mesenteric, and coronary vascular beds. Dopamine can also stimulate β-adrenoceptors and, at high doses, can directly stimulate α-adrenoceptors. When DA is administered intravenously, most vasoconstriction is caused by dopamine-induced NE release.

Dopamine accounts for about one-half of all catecholamines in the brain and is present in greater quantities than NE or 5-HT. In contrast to the diffuse projections of noradrenergic neurons, dopaminergic neurons and receptors are highly organized and concentrated in several areas, especially in the basal ganglia and limbic system.[81,140]

Excessive dopaminergic activity in the neostriatum and/or other areas from any cause (eg, increased release, impaired uptake, increased receptor sensitivity) can produce acute choreoathetosis[77] and acute Gilles de la Tourette syndrome, with tics, spitting, and cursing. Excessive dopaminergic activity in the limbic system and, perhaps, in other areas produces paranoid psychosis and is thought responsible for much of the drug craving and addictive behavior in patients abusing sympathomimetics, opioids, alcohol, and nicotine. Diminished dopaminergic tone (eg, impaired release, receptor blockade) in the neostriatum produces various extrapyramidal disorders such as acute dystonias and parkinsonism.[131,151,165]

SYNTHESIS, RELEASE, AND UPTAKE

The steps of DA synthesis and vesicle storage are the same as those for NE, except that DA is not converted to NE after transport into vesicles (Fig. 13–7). Dopamine is removed from the synapse via uptake by DAT, the membrane-bound DA transporter. DAT and NET exhibit 66% homology in their amino acid sequences. Like NET, DAT is not completely specific for DA and transports amphetamines and other structurally similar sympathomimetics. Cytoplasmic DA has a fate similar to NE. It is pumped back into vesicles by VMAT2 (brain) and VMAT1 (neuroendocrine tissue, adrenal glands) or degraded by MAO and COMT.

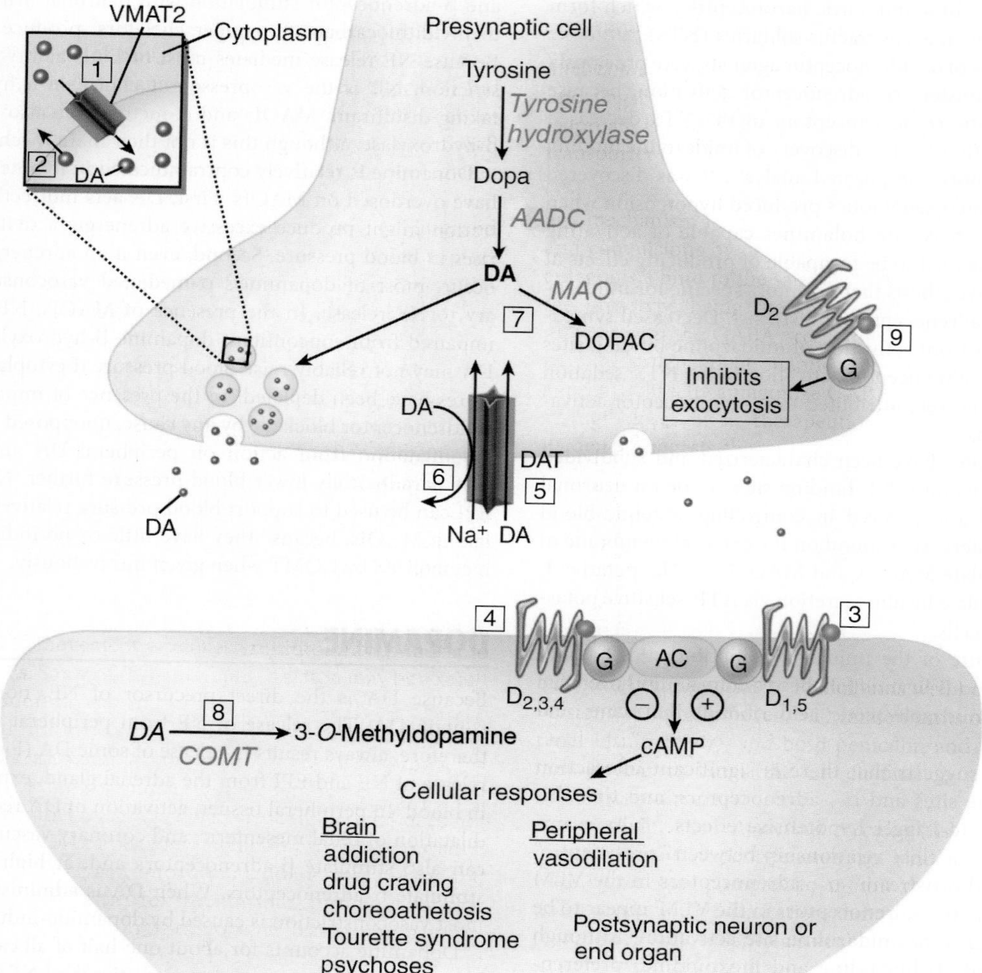

FIGURE 13–7. A dopaminergic nerve ending and postsynaptic membrane. Dopamine (DA) released from nerve endings binds to various postsynaptic DA receptors (D) on neurons or peripheral end organs. Stimulation of presynaptic D_2 receptors [9] lessens DA release. Agents in Table 13-6 may act to inhibit vesicle uptake [1]; cause DA to leave the vesicle and move into the cytoplasm [2]; activate or antagonize DA receptors [3, 4, 9]; inhibit DAT to prevent DA uptake [5]; cause reverse transport of cytoplasmic DA (via DAT) into the synapse by raising cytoplasmic DA concentrations [6]; prevent DA degradation by inhibiting monoamine oxidase (MAO) [7]; or prevent DA degradation by inhibiting catechol-*O*-methyltransferase (COMT) [8]. (Both DA and dopa are substrates for COMT.) AADC = L-aromatic amino acid decarboxylase; DAT = membrane DA uptake transporter; DOPAC = 3,4-dihydroxyphenylacetic acid; VMA2 = vesicle membrane uptake transporter.

DOPAMINE RECEPTORS

All DA receptors are coupled to G proteins and are divided into two main groups, depending on whether they raise or lower cAMP concentrations. Dopamine D_1-like receptors (D_1 and D_5) are expressed as various subtypes and are linked to G_s to stimulate adenylate cyclase and to raise cAMP concentrations.[81] D_1 receptors are found in the basal ganglial nuclei and cerebral cortex, and D_5 receptors are concentrated in the hippocampus and hypothalamus. Dopamine is 5 to 10 times more potent at D_5 receptors than it is at D_1 receptors.

D_2-like receptors (D_2, D_3, D_4) are linked to $G_{i/o}$ to produce several actions, including inhibition of adenylate cyclase and the lowering of cAMP levels. Again, numerous subtypes of receptors exist (eg, D_{2S}, D_{2L}). D_2 receptors are concentrated in the basal ganglia and limbic system. Some D_2 receptors also reside on presynaptic membranes, where their activation limits neurotransmitter release, including the peripheral release of NE (Figs. 13–5 and 13–7). D_3 receptors are concentrated in the hypothalamic and limbic nuclei, whereas D_4 receptors are concentrated in the frontal cortex and limbic nuclei (rather than basal ganglia nuclei). Most agonists bind to the D_3 receptors with higher affinity than to D_2 receptors, whereas most antagonists bind preferentially to D_2 receptors.[81,140] Most agonists and antagonists express a lower affinity for D_4 receptors than they express for D_2 receptors; a notable exception is clozapine.

XENOBIOTICS

Table 13–6 provides examples of xenobiotics that affect dopaminergic neurotransmission.

TABLE 13–6. Examples of Xenobiotics That Affect Dopaminergic Neurotransmission

Dopamine agonism	Increase dopamine receptor sensitivity
Direct stimulation of dopamine receptors	Amphetamine
Apomorphine	Antipsychotics
Bromocriptine	Metoclopramide
Cabergoline[a]	Phenytoin
L-Dopa[b]	Dopamine antagonism
Fenoldopam	Block dopamine receptors
Lisuride	Amoxapine
Pramipexole	Aripiprazole
Ropinirole	Buspirone
Inhibit dopamine metabolism	Butyrophenones
MAOIs	Clozapine
COMTs	Cyclic antidepressants
Indirect acting	Domperidone
Amantadine	Loxapine
Amphetamine	Metoclopramide
Benztropine	Olanzapine
Diphenhydramine	Phenothiazines
MAOIs	Pimozide
Methylphenidate	Quetiapine
Pemoline	Risperidone
Trihexyphenidyl	Thioxanthenes
Inhibit dopamine uptake	Ziprasidone
Amantadine	Destroy dopaminergic neurons
Amphetamine	MPTP/MPP$^+$
Benztropine	Prevent vesicle dopamine uptake
Bupropion	Reserpine
Cocaine	Tetrabenazine
Diphenhydramine	
Methylphenidate	
Orphenadrine	
Trihexyphenidyl	

COMTs = catechol-*o*-methyltransferase inhibitors; MAOIs = monoamine oxidase inhibitors; MPTP = 1-methyl-4-phenyl-1,2,3,6-tetrahydropyridine. MPP$^+$ = 1-methyl-4-phenylpyridinium.

[a] Associated with fibrotic vavlulopathy due to $5HT_{2B}$ agonism.

[b] Metabolized to dopamine, which acts as an agonist.

Dopamine Agonism *Indirect-Acting and Mixed-Acting Xenobiotics.* Most indirect-acting and mixed-acting sympathomimetics cause DA release. The mechanism of action is similar to that causing NE release. These xenobiotics diffuse into the neuron or undergo uptake by DAT before being transported into vesicles by VMAT2 where they buffer protons and displace DA into the cytoplasm for reverse transport by DAT into the synapse. Benztropine, diphenhydramine, trihexyphenidyl, and orphenadrine also cause DA release, perhaps contributing to their abuse potential, which is noted below.[108] Excessive dopaminergic activity following therapeutic doses or overdoses of decongestants (eg, pseudoephedrine), amphetamines, methylphenidate, and pemoline can produce acute choreoathetosis ("crack dancing") and Tourette syndrome.[22,92] Ingestion of excessive doses of L-dopa (which is converted to DA) may present with similar symptoms.

Direct Agonists. Bromocriptine is an ergot derivative that directly activates DA receptors (mainly D_2). Toxic effects include those described above for indirect-acting agents. Apomorphine directly activates D_2 receptors. Such action at the chemoreceptive triggering zone produces vomiting, whereas agonism in the basal ganglia explains the use of apomorphine in the treatment of Parkinson disease. Fenoldopam is a D_1 agonist used as a vasodilator in the treatment of hypertensive emergencies.

D_1-like and D_2-like receptor activation is the predominant mediator of locomotor effects from DA agonists. Activation of either D_1-like or D_2-like receptors produces antiparkinsonian effects.[63,140] Cabergoline, ropinirole, and pramipexole are D_2-like agonists used to treat Parkinson disease.[8,41,57] Dihydrexidine is a D_1-like agonist that has been used for the same purpose.

Uptake Inhibition. Xenobioitics inhibiting DAT prevent DA uptake and include cocaine, amphetamines, methylphenidate, and probably amantadine. Increased dopaminergic activity from cocaine toxicity may produce choreoathetosis and Tourette syndrome. In general, antidepressants are not strong DA uptake blockers. However, bupropion appears to be more active in this regard.[136]

As noted earlier, much of the craving and addiction produced by sympathomimetics probably results from excessive dopaminergic activity in the mesolimbic system.[151] Interestingly, the anticholinergic drugs benztropine, diphenhydramine, trihexyphenidyl, and orphenadrine are also DA uptake inhibitors, possibly explaining their abuse.[108,147] In fact, benztropine is one of the most potent DA uptake inhibitors known. Amantadine, an antiparkinsonian agent that causes DA release and some inhibition of DA uptake (as well as being anticholinergic), is also abused.

Increase of Receptor Sensitivity. Several xenobiotics are thought to increase sensitivity of DA receptors, resulting in choreoathetosis, even with therapeutic doses (eg, phenytoin). Evidence exists that increased DA receptor sensitivity may be responsible for movement disorders resulting from amphetamines.[26] Tardive dyskinesia (discussed below) may also result from increased DA receptor sensitivity and occurs following chronic administration of D_2 receptor antagonists.

MAO Inhibition. MAOIs inhibit the breakdown of cytoplasmic DA. Some of the food and drug interactions with MAOIs results from excessive release of DA from nerve endings.

COMT Inhibition. Peripheral COMT inhibitors (eg, entacapone, tolcapone) are given with levodopa to patients with Parkinson disease to prevent peripheral degradation of levodopa to 3-*O*-methyldopa. This allows more levodopa to traverse the blood–brain barrier and to be converted to DA by neuronal dopa decarboxylase. Tolcapone also inhibits COMT in the brain.[71] Other substrates of COMT include dopa, DA, NE, EPI, and their hydroxylated metabolites. COMT inhibitors might potentiate the effects of these drugs when administered intravenously.[71]

Dopamine Antagonism *Direct Receptor Blockade.* Blockade of DA receptors is the specific aim when using many therapeutic agents. The neuroleptic actions of butyrophenones, phenothiazines, and other antipsychotics mainly correlate with their ability to block D_2-like receptors. Many phenothiazines block both D_1-like and D_2-like receptors, whereas haloperidol mainly blocks D_2-like receptors. Unfortunately, antipsychotics and metoclopramide also block DA receptors in the striatum, producing various extrapyramidal symptoms, including acute parkinsonism and dystonias.

In the last decade, several "atypical" antipsychotics have been marketed that produce fewer extrapyramidal effects and are thought to carry less risk of producing tardive dyskinesia.[134] The relative affinity of an antipsychotic for $5\text{-}HT_{2A}$ receptors over D_2 receptors has predictive value for atypical agents with a lower risk of extrapyramidal symptoms.[124] These include clozapine, olanzapine, quetiapine, risperidone, and ziprasidone.

The ratio of muscarinic (M_1) blockade to D_2-receptor blockade is also important in limiting extrapyramidal symptoms. Antipsychotics exhibiting strong antimuscarinic effects (eg, olanzapine, clozapine, thioridazine) are also less likely to induce extrapyramidal symptoms.[134]

Buspirone, an anxiolytic, antagonizes D_2 receptors, which explains occasional extrapyramidal reactions. Various cyclic antidepressants, especially amoxapine, block D_2 receptors to some extent.

The chronic use of dopamine-blockers causes upregulation of DA receptors. The continued use or, especially, withdrawal of DA antagonists (antipsychotics, metoclopramide, and occasionally antidepressants) can result in excessive dopaminergic activity and tardive dyskinesia, characterized by choreiform movements typical of excessive dopaminergic influence in the neostriatum.

The blockade of DA receptors by numerous xenobiotics, including butyrophenones, phenothiazines, and metoclopramide, can produce a poorly understood disorder called *neuroleptic malignant syndrome.* Neuroleptic malignant syndrome may rarely follow acute withdrawal of DA agonists (eg, stopping L-dopa, bromocriptine, or tolcapone in a patient prior to surgery). Neuroleptic malignant syndrome is characterized, in part, by mental status changes, autonomic instability, rigidity, and hyperthermia.

Indirect Antagonism. Reserpine and tetrabenazine inhibit VMAT to prevent transport of DA into storage vesicles and deplete nerve endings of DA. In fact, reserpine was used as an antipsychotic before the introduction of phenothiazines. 1-Methyl-4-phenyl-1,2,3,6-tetrahydropyridine (MPTP), a meperidine analog, undergoes activation by MAO to a metabolite, 1-methyl-4-phenylpyridinium (MPP^+), that causes death of dopaminergic neurons. Both MPTP and its metabolite undergo uptake not only by DAT, but also by NET and SET, making their way into all biogenic amine neurons. The reasons that dopaminergic neurons are selectively damaged remain unknown. Both MAOIs and inhibitors of DA transporters prevent MPTP-induced destruction of dopaminergic neurons.

SEROTONIN

Serotonin (5-HT, 5-OH-tryptamine) is an indole alkylamine found throughout nature (animals, plants, venoms) and has the most complex receptor family of all known neurotransmitters. In the CNS, several hundred thousand serotonergic neurons lie in or in juxtaposition to numerous midline nuclei in the brainstem (raphe nuclei), from which they project to virtually all areas of the brain, including the basal ganglia. Serotonin is involved with mood, emotion, learning, memory, personality, affect, appetite, aggression, motor function, temperature regulation, sexual activity, pain perception, sleep induction, other basic functions. Serotonin is not essential for any of these processes, but modulates their quality and extent. A number of psychiatric disorders, including depression, anxiety, obsessive-compulsive disorder, dementia, schizophrenia, and eating disorders, are linked to altered serotonin function. Consequently, modification of serotonergic neurotransmission is an integral part of the treatment plan for most of these conditions.

The serotonergic system is extremely diverse, with 14 types of receptors that act to stimulate or inhibit neurons, including those of other neurotransmitter systems. Serotonin is also the precursor for the pineal hormone, melatonin. Despite the important role 5-HT plays in the CNS, less than 5% of the body's 5-HT is found within the CNS, with the great majority of 5-HT being located within enterochromaffin cells of the intestines and a small amount of serotonin sequestered by platelets.[110]

Peripherally, 5-HT is released by enterochromaffin cells in response to intestinal stimulation, which contributes to peristalsis and fluid secretion. Most of this activity is performed automatically at the unconscious level. However, there are two pathways via vagal nerve and spinal cord afferent projections to the CNS that allow for conscious input and feedback between these two systems.[33] Platelets take up 5-HT while passing through the enteric circulation. Serotonin is released from activated platelets to interact with other platelet membranes (promote aggregation) and with vascular smooth muscle.[110]

Experimentally, 5-HT exhibits diverse effects on the cardiovascular and peripheral nervous systems, although the importance of these actions remains uncertain in the normal physiologic state. Serotonin vasoconstricts (stimulation of 5-HT_2, 5-HT_{1B}, and 5-HT_{1D} receptors) most vascular beds, except for coronary arteries and skeletal muscle, where it produces vasodilation in the presence of intact endothelium. 5-HT_{1B} and 5-HT_{1D} agonists (eg, sumatriptan) produce coronary vasoconstriction as an adverse effect to their desired actions on cranial vasculature.[113]

Centrally, it is particularly difficult to ascribe a specific symptom or physical finding to serotonergic neurons because of the diversity of their physiologic actions. However, 5-HT definitely plays an important role in the action of many hallucinogenic or illusionogenic drugs, which act as partial agonists at cortical 5-HT_2 receptors. Proserotonergics are used to treat depression, whereas 5-HT receptors (5-HT_2) antagonists have greater importance in the management of schizophrenia.[51,161]

Generally, in areas where they overlap, 5-HT acts in opposition to DA. For example, 5-HT serves to increase prolactin, adrenocorticotropic hormone (ACTH), and growth hormone secretion, whereas DA decreases prolactin secretion. As another example, activation of basal ganglial 5-HT_{2A} receptors inhibits DA release.[51,161] However, well-known exceptions exist, such as cortical 5-HT_3 receptors[28] and 5-HT_{1A} receptors that are capable of promoting DA release under certain circumstances.[112]

SYNTHESIS, RELEASE, AND UPTAKE

Figure 13–8 illustrates 5-HT synthesis. Tryptophan-5-hydroxylase is the rate-limiting enzyme of 5-HT synthesis. Increases in tryptophan are predictably accompanied by increased 5-HT production. L-Amino acid decarboxylase (dopa decarboxylase) converts 5-hydroxytryptophan to 5-HT. Cytoplasmic 5-HT is transported into vesicles by VMAT2, where it is concentrated by ion trapping before release by Ca^{2+}-dependent exocytosis. In contrast to vesicles containing DA or NE, 5-HT vesicles contain almost no ATP. After release into the synapse, a transporter (SERT) in the neuronal membrane moves 5-HT back into the neuron, where it reenters vesicles or is degraded by MAO.[110]

Serotonin is preferentially metabolized by the MAO-A isozyme. Paradoxically, the serotonergic nerve terminal is almost devoid of MAO-A, but contains abundant amounts of MAO-B. It has been hypothesized that the large amounts of MAO-B metabolize other xenobiotics that might inappropriately promote 5-HT release (eg, dopamine). However, the small amount of MAO-A found in serotonergic neurons provides adequate degradation of 5-HT.[110]

SEROTONIN RECEPTORS

Most authors identify seven major functioning receptors (5-HT_1 through 5-HT_7) and numerous subtypes.

5-HT_1 Receptors Receptors in the 5-HT_1 class are coupled to G proteins and commonly increase K^+ efflux and decrease cAMP concentrations. Members of the 5-HT_1 receptor class express greatest affinity for 5-HT and are thus biologically active under normal physiologic conditions. 5-HT_{1A} receptors reside predominantly on raphe nuclei, where they act as somatodendritic autoreceptors.[104,116] Hippocampal 5-HT_{1A} receptors reside postsynaptically, where they also inhibit through similar mechanisms.[116]

Central 5-HT_{1D} and 5-HT_{1B} receptors primarily act as inhibitory terminal autoreceptors and heteroreceptors. They are found less commonly on postsynaptic membranes.[116] Originally 5-HT_{1B} receptors were not believed to exist in humans. However, most of the actions described in older literature regarding 5-HT_{1D} receptors can now be

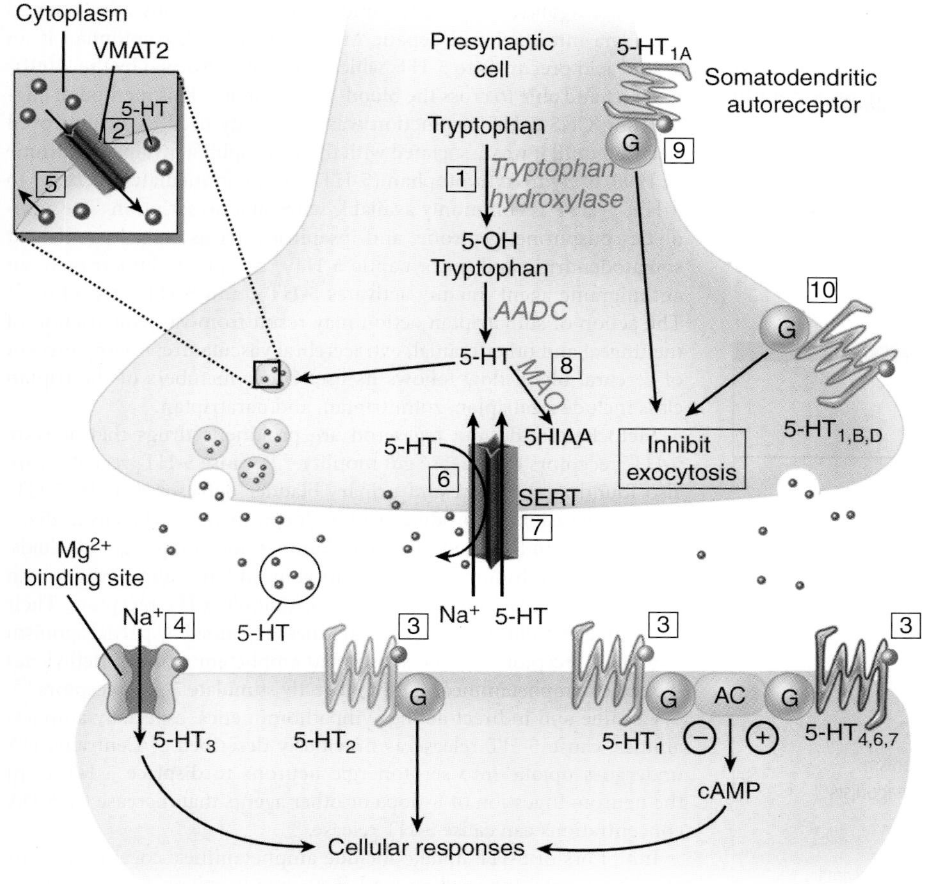

FIGURE 13–8. A serotonergic nerve ending and postsynaptic membrane. Tryptophan hydroxylase [1] converts tryptophan to 5-hydroxytryptophan (5-OH-tryptophan). Aromatic L-amino acid decarboxylase (AADC) then metabolizes 5-OH-tryptophan to serotonin (5-HT). Serotonin is concentrated within vesicles through uptake by VMA2 before exocytosis [2]. After uptake into the neuron by SERT [7], 5-HT is transported back into vesicles or undergoes degradation by monoamine oxidase (MAO) to an intermediate compound, which is converted to 5-hydroxyindoleacetic acid (5-HIAA) [8]. 5-HT$_{1,2,4,6,7}$ receptors [3,9,10] are coupled to G proteins, while 5-HT$_3$ receptors [4] are ligand-gated cation channels that may conduct Na^+ and/or Ca^{2+} (only Na^+ is illustrated). 5-HT$_3$ cation channels also appear to be blocked by Mg^{2+} until the cell is depolarized, allowing Mg^{2+} to dissociate–a mechanism similar to that found at NMDA glutamate receptors. In addition to residing on postsynaptic membranes, 5-HT$_{1A}$, 5-HT$_{1B}$, and 5HT$_{1D}$ receptors serve as presynaptic autoreceptors that, when stimulated, decrease further release of 5-HT [9,10]. Presynaptic 5-HT1A receptors mainly serve as somatodendritic autoreceptors, whereas presynaptic 5-HT1B, and 5-HT1D receptors serve as terminal autoreceptors. Agents in Table 13-7 act to enhance 5-HT synthesis [1]; inhibit VMA2 to prevent vesicle uptake of 5-HT [2]; raise cytoplasmic concentrations of 5-HT, resulting in reverse transport of 5-HT into the synapse by SERT [6]; by displacing 5-HT from vesicles [5] or inhibiting MAO [8]; activate or antagonize 5-HT receptors [3,4,9,10]; or by inhibiting 5-HT uptake [7]. G = G protein; SERT = membrane 5-HT uptake transporter; VMA2 = vesicle membrane uptake transporter.

attributed to 5-HT$_{1B}$ receptors.[116] Cranial blood vessels (eg, meninges) possess 5-HT$_{1D}$ and 5-HT$_{1B}$ receptors, whose activation produces vasoconstriction and decreased inflammation.[113]

5-HT$_{1E}$ and 5-HT$_{1F}$ receptors are more recently discovered members of the 5-HT$_1$ receptor class. Their functional activity is yet to be determined.

5-HT$_2$ Receptors The three subtypes of 5-HT$_2$ receptors are coupled to G proteins, thus serving to decrease K^+ efflux and/or increase intracellular Ca^{2+} concentration by raising concentrations of inositol triphosphate and diacylglycerol.[104] The three subtypes of 5-HT$_2$ receptors are so similar in characterization that investigational probes have great difficulty in distinguishing the subtypes. 5-HT$_{2A}$ receptors are most concentrated in the cerebral cortex, where they serve as excitatory postsynaptic receptors. Their activation increases glutamate release from pyramidal cells, but also can lead to release of GABA.[161] 5-HT$_{2A}$ receptors also reside on platelets, where their activation produces platelet aggregation. 5-HT$_{2C}$ receptors (previously 5-HT$_{1C}$) reside on the choroid plexus, where they regulate cerebrospinal fluid production. Activation of 5-HT$_{2B}$ receptors in the GI tract promotes stomach contraction.[110] At least some xenobiotics that activate 5-HT$_{2B}$ receptors on cardiac valves cause a valvulopathy identical to that of carcinoid syndrome, though both sides of the heart can be involved with drug-induced 5-HT$_{2B}$ agonism.

5-HT$_3$ Receptors 5-HT$_3$ receptors are isopentameric ligand-gated cation channels that are structurally similar to ACh nicotinic receptors, GABA$_A$ Cl^- channels, glycine, and NMDA glutamate receptors.[28] They are localized to both presynaptic and postsynaptic membranes. Upon activation, they stimulate the neuron by opening the channel to cause depolarization through Na^+ and/or Ca^{2+} influx. In addition, these channels are normally blocked by Mg^{2+} in a voltage-dependent manner similar to glutamatergic NMDA receptors (see Glutamate later). Centrally, 5-HT$_3$ receptors are expressed diffusely, but are especially concentrated in the chemoreceptive triggering zone, where their activation induces emesis.[33] In the cerebral cortex, their activation leads to increased release of DA and decreased release of ACh.[28] Cortical 5-HT$_3$ receptors are frequently identified on GABA interneurons where they increase inhibitory, GABAergic tone. In contrast to cerebral actions, activation of peripheral 5-HT$_3$ receptors on cholinergic nerves in the gut enhances ACh release to increase gastrointestinal motility.[33]

5-HT$_4$ Receptors 5-HT$_4$ receptors are coupled to G proteins (G_s). Their activation leads to increased cAMP concentrations. 5-HT$_4$ receptors are scattered diffusely throughout the brain, and their exact role remains undefined, although they are known to increase the release of ACh.[161] Peripheral 5-HT$_4$ receptors reside in the heart, intestines, and adrenal gland where their activation can be demonstrated to produce tachycardia, aldosterone and cortisol release, and contraction of gut and bladder smooth muscle. Whether these actions are important under normal physiologic conditions is not clear, but peripheral 5-HT$_4$ receptors promote the release of ACh and increase gut motility.[33]

5-HT$_5$ Receptors 5-HT$_5$ receptors exist in the form of at least two subtypes, one of which may be coupled to $G_{i/o}$. The 5-HT$_{5a}$ subtype may act as a somatodendritic autoreceptor, but the functionality of this role is unknown, in contrast to the predominant importance of 5-HT$_{1a}$ autoreceptors.[104]

5-HT$_6$ and 5-HT$_7$ Receptors 5-HT$_6$ and 5-HT$_7$ receptors are positively coupled to cAMP formation through G proteins.[104] Their distribution is poorly defined. However, many antidepressants and antipsychotics antagonize these receptors. They are currently a source of great interest because of the possibility of avoiding DA blockade to achieve antipsychotic activity. The 5-HT_7 receptor may be particularly important in regulating circadian rhythms.[161]

XENOBIOTICS

Table 13–7 provides examples of xenobiotics that affect serotonergic neurotransmission.

TABLE 13–7. Examples of Xenobiotics That Affect Serotonergic Neurotransmission

Serotonin agonism
Enhance 5-HT synthesis
L-Tryptophan
5-Hydroxytryptophan
Direct 5-HT agonists
Buspirone
Cisapride
Ergots and indoles
Hallucinogenic substituted amphetamines
mCPP
Lisuride
Mescaline
Metoclopramide
Triptans
Increase 5-HT release
Amphetamine
Cocaine
Dexfenfluramine
Dextromethorphan
L-Dopa
Fenfluramine
MDMA
Mirtazapine
Reserpine (initial)
Increase 5-HT tone by unknown mechanism
Lithium
Inhibit 5-HT breakdown
MAOIs
Inhibit 5-HT uptake
Amoxapine
Amphetamines
Atomoxetine
Carbamazepine
Citalopram
Clomipramine[a]
Cocaine
Cyclic antidepressants
Dextromethorphan
Duloxetine
Escitalopram
Fluoxetine
Fluvoxamine
Lamotrigine
Meperidine
Nefazodone
Sertraline
Tramadol
Trazodone
Venlafaxine
Serotonin Antagonism
Direct 5-HT antagonists
Aripiprazole
Clozapine
Cyclic antidepressants
Cyproheptadine
Ergots and indoles (eg, LSD)
Haloperidol
Ketanserin
Mescaline
Methysergide
Metoclopramide
Mirtazapine
Nefazodone
Olanzapine
Ondansetron
Paliperidone
Phenothiazines
Phentolamine
Propranolol
Quetiapine
Risperidone
Trazodone
Ziprasidone
Enhance 5-HT uptake
Tianeptine
Inhibit vesicle uptake
Reserpine
Ketanserin
Tetrabenazine

5-HT = serotonin; LSD = lysergic acid diethylamide; MAOIs = monoamine oxidase inhibitors; mCPP = *m*-chlorophenylpiperazine (metabolite of trazodone and nefazodone); MDMA methylenedioxymethamphetamine.

[a]Clomipramine is the most potent 5-HT uptake inhibitor of the tricyclic antidepressants.

Serotonin Agonists The body rapidly metabolizes orally administered 5-HT via intestinal and hepatic MAO. However, L-tryptophan is an amino acid precursor to 5-HT, which is readily absorbed by the intestinal tract and able to cross the blood–brain barrier. This method of augmenting CNS 5-HT production was previously used as an unproved sleep aid until it was associated with the eosinophilia myalgia syndrome in 1990. 5-Hydroxytryptophan (5-HTP) is the immediate precursor to 5-HT. 5-HTP is commonly available without a prescription. The anxiolytics buspirone, gepirone, and ipsapirone act as partial agonists at somatodendritic and postsynaptic 5-HT_{1A} receptors. Sumatriptan, an antimigraine agent, mainly activates 5-HT_{1D} and 5-HT_{1B} receptors.[113] The action of sumatriptan action may result from vasoconstriction of meningeal and other cranial, extracerebral vasculature; no impairment of cerebral blood flow follows its use. Other members of the triptan class include rizatriptan, zolmitriptan, and naratriptan.

Metoclopramide and tegaserod are prokinetic drugs that activate 5-HT_4 receptors to increase gut motility.[33] Because 5-HT_4 receptors are also found in the heart and urinary bladder detrusor muscle, 5-HT_4 agonists occasionally produce bladder incontinence and tachycardia.

Numerous indoles and phenylalkylamines, including ergot alkaloids, lysergic acid diethylamide (LSD), psilocybin, and mescaline, exhibit both agonistic and antagonistic properties at multiple 5-HT receptors. Their hallucinogenic/illusionogenic action is best explained by partial agonism at 5-HT_{2A} receptors.[51] Some substituted amphetamines (eg, methylenedioxymethamphetamine, MDMA) directly stimulate 5-HT receptors.[157]

Cocaine and indirect-acting sympathomimetics, especially amphetamines, cause 5-HT release as previously described.[157] Centrally, DA undergoes uptake into serotonergic neurons to displace 5-HT from the neuron. Ingestion of L-dopa or other agents that increase CNS DA concentrations can cause 5-HT release.[104]

Inhibitors of 5-HT uptake include amphetamines, cocaine, various antidepressants, meperidine, and dextromethorphan. Several antidepressants specifically inhibit 5-HT uptake. Examples of selective 5-HT reuptake inhibitors (SSRIs) include fluoxetine, sertraline, paroxetine, and citalopram. The use of SSRIs sometimes produces extrapyramidal side effects for reasons that remain unclear because of the numerous actions of 5-HT in the basal ganglia.[61] Two anticonvulsants, carbamazepine and lamotrigine, appear to inhibit 5-HT uptake.[150] Again, reserpine and tetrabenazine prevent 5-HT uptake into vesicles.

MAO-A accounts for most 5-HT degradation, and nonspecific MAOIs and MAO-A inhibitors (clorgyline, moclobemide) raise 5-HT concentrations and, through indirect action, probably cause 5-HT release.

Serotonin Antagonists Trazodone and nefazodone act mainly as antagonists at 5-HT_2 receptors, but are also weak uptake inhibitors. Both undergo metabolism to *m*-chlorophenylpiperazine (mCPP), which activates most 5-HT receptors, but is especially active at 5-HT_{2C} receptors. Ketanserin and ritanserin specifically antagonize 5-HT_{2C} receptors, while methysergide and cyproheptadine antagonize 5-HT_1 and 5-HT_2 receptors.[110]

Mirtazapine exhibits complex actions, including antagonism of 5-HT_{2A}, 5-HT_{2C}, and 5-HT_3 receptors.[53] It also indirectly increases 5-HT_{1A} activity and enhances release of NE through antagonism of α_2-adrenoceptors. Mirtazapine demonstrates potent antagonism of histaminic and muscarinic receptors.[53]

Most antipsychotics and tricyclic antidepressants antagonize 5-HT_{2A} and, to a lesser extent, 5-HT_{2C} receptors. In fact, investigators are interested in developing antipsychotic agents similar to risperidone that possess potent antagonistic properties at 5-HT_2 receptors, without accompanying DA receptor antagonism, in order to limit extrapyramidal side effects. These investigations have resulted in the introduction of olanzapine, sertindole, ziprasidone, zotepine, quetiapine, and amisulpride.[161]

Ondansetron, granisetron, tropisetron, dolasetron, and alosetron antagonize 5-HT_3 receptors.[33] Their antiemetic action is thought to be explained by several mechanisms. Central antagonism at the chemoreceptor-triggering zone lessens vomiting. Peripheral 5-HT_3 receptor antagonism in the gut prevents ACh release, decreasing gut motility. Finally, antagonism of vagal 5-HT_3 receptors decreases afferent stimulatory signals to the vomiting center in the brainstem. Metoclopramide antagonizes 5-HT_3 and D_2 receptors.[33] Ondansetron and other experimental 5-HT_3 antagonists are being studied in the treatment of schizophrenia because of their ability to prevent DA release.

Tianeptine is an antidepressant that enhances 5-HT uptake, thus lowering synaptic 5-HT concentrations.[128]

Serotonin Syndrome Serotonin syndrome represents an iatrogenic and largely idiosyncratic condition that is most commonly caused by the combination of two or more 5-HT agonists, although it can happen following single 5-HT agonists in overdose or at therapeutic dosages.[107] Animal models indicate that serotonin syndrome can be prevented by the blockade of 5-HT_{1A} receptors and 5-HT_{2A} receptors.[21,110,112] Serotonin syndrome is characterized by alterations in mentation and cognition, autonomic nervous system dysfunction, and neuromuscular abnormalities. Symptoms may include confusion, agitation, convulsions, coma, tachycardia, diaphoresis, hyperthermia, hypertension, shivering, myoclonus, tremor, hyperreflexia, and muscle rigidity (especially of legs).[107] Serotonin syndrome is often confused with neuroleptic malignant syndrome in its more severe presentation due to their similar manifestations. Serotonin syndrome usually responds to supportive care alone but may improve with 5-HT_{1a} and 5-HT_{2a} receptor inhibitors such as cyproheptadine.[21,107] Serotonin syndrome can be caused by xenobiotics that increases CNS 5-HT neurotransmission (Table 13–7). In addition, xenobiotics that act to increase CNS DA concentrations, such as levodopa and bromocriptine, have potential to precipitate serotonin syndrome by indirectly causing 5-HT release (Chap. 72).

γ-AMINOBUTYRIC ACID

GABA is one of two main inhibitory neurotransmitters of the central nervous system (glycine is discussed later; see Glycine as an Inhibitory Neurotransmitter). Xenobiotics that enhance GABA activity are generally used as anticonvulsants, sedative-hypnotics, anxiolytics, and general anesthetics. Xenobiotics that antagonize GABA activity typically produce CNS excitation and convulsions. GABA is synthesized from glutamate, the brain's main excitatory neurotransmitter.

In general, GABA inhibition predominates in the brain. In the spinal cord, through monosynaptic and polysynaptic reflex pathways, GABA mediates a number of physiologically minor peripheral effects outside the CNS (eg, vasodilatation, bladder relaxation). Spinal cord GABA is important in attenuating skeletal muscle reflex arcs.[97]

SYNTHESIS, RELEASE, AND UPTAKE

Figure 13–9 illustrates GABA synthesis. Glutamate is converted to GABA via glutamic acid decarboxylase (GAD) which requires pyridoxal phosphate (PLP) as a cofactor. Pyridoxal phosphate is synthesized from pyridoxine (vitamin B_6) by the enzyme pyridoxine kinase (PK).[105] VGAT, a vesicle-bound transporter, transports GABA into vesicles from where it is released through Ca^{2+}-dependent exocytosis into the synapse.[97] Uptake of GABA from the synapse back into the presynaptic neurons is mediated by the Na^+-dependent transporter, GAT-1, whereas uptake into glial cells and possibly postsynaptic neurons is mediated by GAT-2, GAT-3, and GAT-4. Evidence also suggests that GABA is released into the synapse from cytoplasm by reverse transport under some conditions. In glial cells, cytoplasmic GABA can undergo degradation by GABA-transaminase (GABA-T) to succinic semialdehyde (SSA), part of which then undergoes oxidation to succinate. GABA-T also requires PLP as a cofactor.[115] The transamination of GABA to SSA by GABA-T results in the conversion of α-ketoglutarate to glutamate, which then moves back into neurons to be used for resynthesis of GABA.

GABA RECEPTORS

There are three main types of GABA receptors (Table 13–8).[17] $GABA_A$ receptors are Cl^- channels that mediate inhibition by allowing Cl^- to move into and hyperpolarize the neuron. The majority of $GABA_A$ receptors are located postsynaptically and mediate fast or *phasic* inhibition. About 5% to 10% of $GABA_A$ receptors are located outside the synapse and are responsible for slower *tonic* current that is present at resting membrane potential.[60,91,109,137] Situated at various sites in relation to the GABA recognition site on the Cl^- channel are sites for exogenous and endogenous modulators (Fig. 13–10) where numerous excitatory and depressant xenobiotics bind, and through which $GABA_A$ receptor responsiveness is regulated under normal physiologic conditions. The common denominator for modulation at the $GABA_A$ complex is an increase or decrease in inward Cl^- current.

Throughout the CNS there are regional variations in expressions of multiple subunit genes for the $GABA_A$ complex. $GABA_A$ receptors exist as pentamers, composed most commonly of two α subunits, two β subunits, and either a γ or δ subunit. Multiple isoforms of subunits exist (eg, α_1–α_6), but within a single receptor, the isoforms of individual subunits appear to be identical. While the large numbers of isoforms and different combinations of subunits could theoretically produce more than 2000 different $GABA_A$ Cl^- channels, only a few dozen combinations exist naturally.[35,109] The most common is $\alpha_1\beta_2\gamma_2$.[8,145]

The second type of GABA receptor, $GABA_B$, is found on both presynaptic and postsynaptic membranes. The $GABA_B$ receptors are heterodimers, with companion proteins linked to the receptors, and are coupled to G proteins (probably $G_{i/o}$) that mediate both presynaptic and postsynaptic inhibition.[20] Presynaptic inhibition results from preventing Ca^{2+} influx so as to impair exocytosis of neurotransmitter vesicles, including those containing excitatory amino acids (eg, glutamate). Postsynaptic inhibition is mediated by increasing K^+ efflux through K^+ channels, resulting in hyperpolarization of the membrane away from threshold. Through presynaptic actions, $GABA_B$ receptors also serve as autoreceptors, where their activation in response to synaptic GABA provides feedback inhibition of further neurotransmitter release (Fig. 13–9).

A third GABA receptor, $GABA_C$, is a Cl^- channel that, when activated, allows increased Cl^- influx. The $GABA_C$ receptors are thought to comprise 5 ligand binding sites, whereas $GABA_A$ receptors have 2 ligand binding sites.[17] $GABA_C$ receptors are composed of ρ subunits (ρ_1–ρ_3). ρ_1 subunits are located in the mammalian retina, ρ_2 subunits are present in most brain regions, and ρ_3 subunits are found in the hippocampus. ρ_1 and ρ_2 receptors have also been found outside the CNS.[69] $GABA_C$ receptors are sensitive to *cis*-4-aminocrotonic acid (CACA), are insensitive to baclofen, bicuculline, benzodiazepines, and barbiturates, and are less sensitive to neuroactive steroids and to picrotoxin (Table 13–8).[69] $GABA_C$ receptors are activated at 40-fold lower GABA concentrations than $GABA_A$ receptors, are less liable to desensitization, and remain open longer than $GABA_A$ Cl^- channels.

XENOBIOTICS

Table 13–9 provides examples of xenobiotics that affect GABAergic neurotransmission.

Modulation of GABA Production and Degradation Isoniazid (INH) and other hydrazines (eg, monomethylhydrazine from mushrooms) lower CNS GABA concentrations by several mechanisms. Most important,

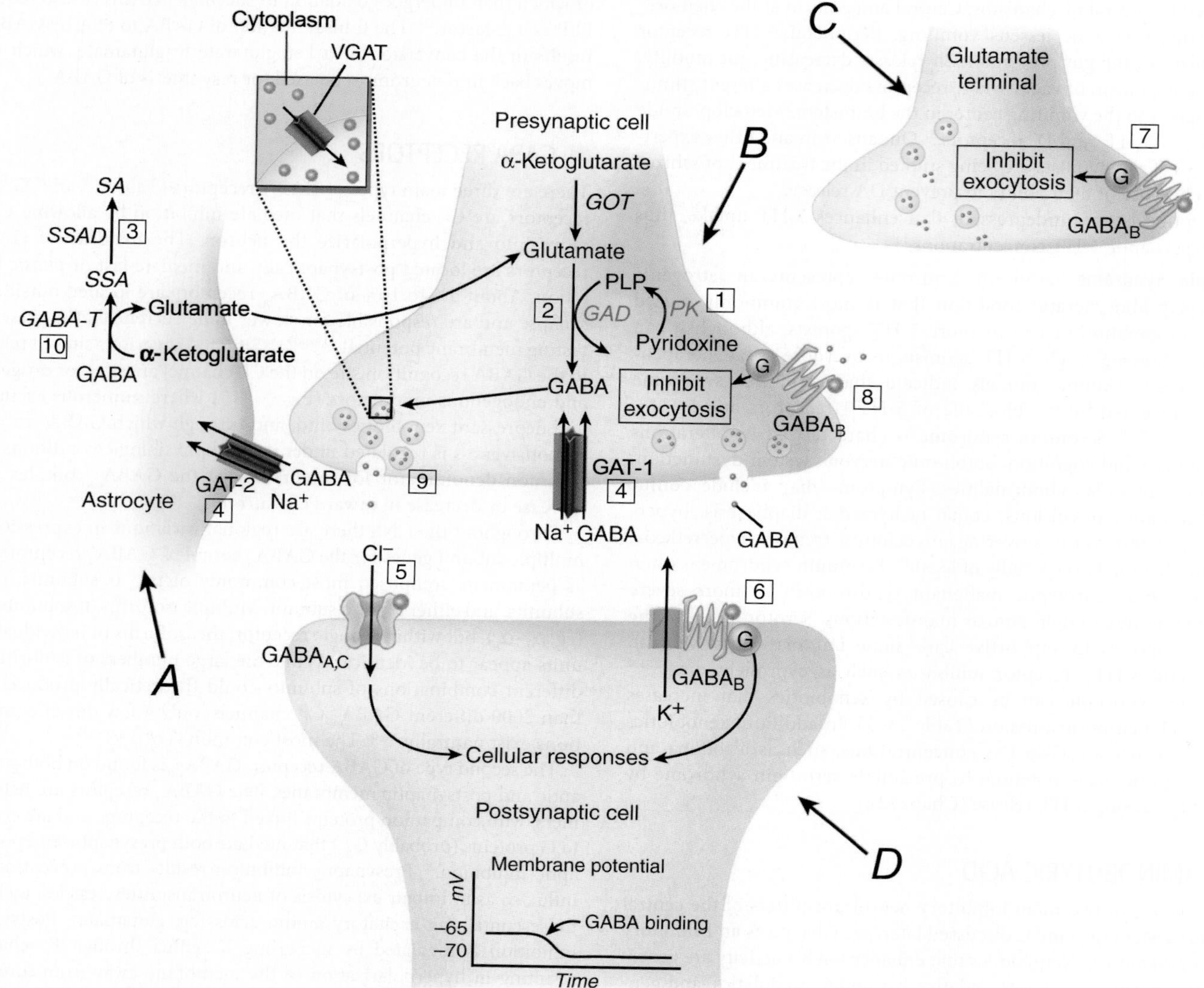

FIGURE 13–9. GABAergic neurotransmission. GABA (γ-aminobutyric acid) released from a presynaptic neuron (B) binds to postsynaptic $GABA_A$, $GABA_B$, or $GABA_C$ receptors to hyperpolarize and inhibit neuron D [5,6] or to presynaptic $GABA_B$ heteroreceptors on neuron C [7] to inhibit neurotransmitter release by blocking Ca^{2+} influx (an excitatory glutamatergic neuron is shown as an example). Stimulation of $GABA_B$ autoreceptors on neuron B [8] also reduces further release of GABA. Synaptic GABA undergoes uptake into the presynaptic neuron by GAT-1, and uptake into glial cells and possibly postsynaptic neurons by GAT-2, GAT-3, and GAT-4 (GAT-2 is shown mediating uptake into glial cell A as an example.) Acute falls in pyridoxal phosphate (PLP) lead to impaired glutamic acid decarboxylase (GAD) activity and low GABA concentrations. Although GABA-transaminase (GABA-T) also requires PLP, acute falls in PLP do not affect this enzyme as dramatically because of tight PLP binding to the GABA-T complex. Agents in Table 13 -9 act to impair PLP formation by inhibiting pyridoxine kinase (PK) [1]; to increase GABA concentrations by either stimulating GAD [2] or inhibiting SSAD [3]; to inhibit GABA uptake [4]; to stimulate or block GABA receptors [5 -8]; to cause GABA release [9]; or to inhibit GABA-T [10]. Glutamic-oxaloacetic transaminase (GOT), GABA-T, and SSAD are mitochondrial enzymes. G = G protein; GAT = membrane GABA uptake transporter; SA = succinic acid; SSA = succinic semialdehyde; SSAD = SSA dehydrogenase; VGAT = vesicle membrane GABA uptake transporter.

they compete with pyridoxine for binding to PK, impairing PLP production.[105] Pyridoxal phosphate binding to the GAD complex is easily reversible.[115] The acute decrease in PLP concentration, then, is rapidly accompanied by impaired GABA synthesis and a decrease in GABA concentration. Lack of normal GABA inhibition produces seizures typical of hydrazine toxicity. Although PLP is also required for GABA degradation by GABA-T, acute decreases in PLP do not affect this enzyme nearly as much, because PLP is more tightly bound to the GABA-T complex and remains associated with the enzyme.[115] To a lesser extent, isoniazid binds to the GAD-PLP complex to prevent GABA formation.

Cyanide inhibits numerous enzymes besides cytochrome oxidase. Inhibition of GAD with a resultant fall in GABA concentration may partly explain seizures that occur in cyanide-poisoned patients. Domoic acid (see Glutamate later) may also inhibit GAD.[36]

In vitro studies demonstrate valproate's ability to increase brain GABA concentrations, either by inhibition of succinic semialdehyde dehydrogenase or by activation of GAD.[70] Gabapentin may increase the rate of GABA synthesis in the brain by stimulating GAD, though gabapentin's main mechanism of action is to bind to calcium channels.[160] Vigabatrin, an anticonvulsant, acts by irreversibly inhibiting GABA-T.[153]

TABLE 13–8. GABA Receptors and Their Characteristics

	$GABA_A$	$GABA_B$	$GABA_C$
Receptor	Cl^- channel	G protein-coupled	Cl^- channel
Bicuculline antagonism	Yes	No	No
Baclofen agonism	No	Yes	No
Benzodiazepine agonism	Yes	No	No
Barbiturate agonism	Yes	No	No
Picrotoxin antagonism	Yes	No	Slight

TABLE 13–9. Examples of Xenobiotics That Affect GABAergic Neurotransmission

GABA agonism	GABA antagonism
Stimulate GAD	Direct $GABA_A$ antagonists
Valproate	Bicuculline
Direct $GABA_A$ agonists	Cephalosporins
Muscimol	Ciprofloxacin
Progabide[a]	Enoxacin
Indirect $GABA_A$ agonists	Imipenem
Avermectin	Nalidixic acid
Barbiturates	Norfloxacin
Benzodiazepines	Ofloxacin
Chloral hydrate	Penicillins
Clomethiazole	Indirect $GABA_A$ antagonists
Ethanol	Aztreonam
Etomidate	Clozapine
Felbamate	Cyclic antidepressants
Ivermectin	Flumazenil
Meprobamate	Lindane
Methaqualone	MAOIs
Propofol	Maprotiline
Steroids	Organic chlorine insecticides
Topiramate	Penicillins
Trichloroethanol	Pentylenetetrazol
Volatile anesthetics	Picrotoxin
Zaleplon	Inhibit GAD
Zolpidem	Cyanide
Zopiclone	Domoic acid
Direct $GABA_B$ agonists	Hydrazines
Baclofen	Isoniazid
GHB	Direct $GABA_B$ antagonists
Inhibit GABA-T	Phaclofen[b]
Vigabatrin	Saclofen[b]
Inhibit GABA uptake	Inhibit PK
Tiagabine	Hydrazines[c]
Valproate	Isoniazid[c]

GABA = γ-aminobutyric acid; GABA-T = GABA transaminase; GAD = glutamic acid decarboxylase; GHB = γ-hydroxybutyric acid; PK = pyridoxine kinase; MAOIs = monoamine oxidase inhibitors.

[a] Directly activates $GABA_A$ and $GABA_B$ receptors as well as being metabolized to GABA.

[b] Thought not to cross blood–brain barrier in meaningful amounts.

[c] Major site of action is PK inhibition, though some direct GAD inhibition occurs.

$GABA_A$ Agonism Figure 13–10 schematically illustrates the $GABA_A$ receptor complex. In general, $GABA_A$ agonists cause CNS depression, ranging from mild sedation and nystagmus to ataxia, stupor, coma, and even general anesthesia. Many indirect agonists that bind to the $GABA_A$ complex have no activity in the absence of GABA. With some exceptions, their pharmacologic actions require the binding of GABA to its receptor and do not result from a direct effect on Cl^- conductance exclusive of GABA binding. Many of these xenobiotics demonstrate additional actions that are not mediated through the $GABA_A$ complex.

Direct GABA Agonists. The main direct GABA agonist of toxicologic interest is muscimol, found in some poisonous mushrooms. Muscimol binds to the GABA receptor on the $GABA_A$ complex to mimic the action of GABA.[117] Ibotenic acid, a direct glutamate agonist found in the same mushrooms, is decarboxylated to muscimol just as glutamate is decarboxylated to GABA.

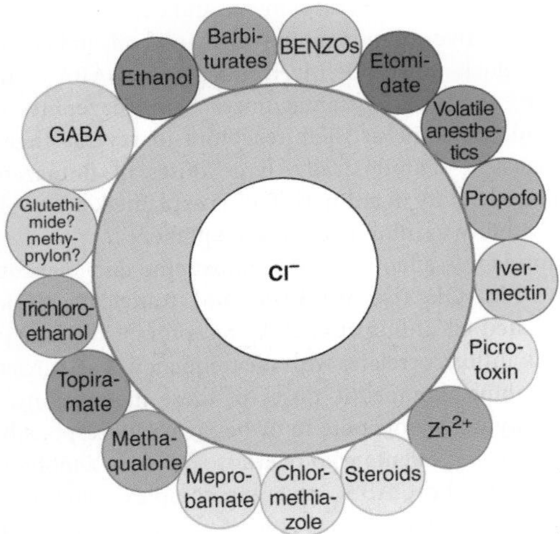

FIGURE 13–10. Representation of the $GABA_A$ Cl^- channel receptor complex. Benzodiazepines (BENZOs), barbiturates, picrotoxin, steroids, and GABA (γ-aminobutyric acid) clearly bind to different sites on the channel. Although separate circles represent different agents capable of binding to and of modulating Cl^- influx through the $GABA_A$ receptor complex, it is not always apparent where these agents bind on the channel. For example, general anesthetics and ethanol may produce their effects by interacting with the steroid binding site. Chloral hydrate undergoes metabolism to trichloroethanol, which interacts with the $GABA_A$ receptor complex. Zolpidem, zopiclone, and zaleplon are nonbenzodiazepines that bind to the benzodiazepine site. Given the structural similarity of glutethimide and methyprylon to barbiturates, it is speculated that their action may be mediated at $GABA_A$ receptors.

Indirect GABA Agonists. Benzodiazepines bind to benzodiazepine receptors on $GABA_A$ complexes to increase the affinity of GABA for its receptor and to increase the frequency of Cl^- channel opening in response to GABA binding.[144] The benzodiazepine binding site on the $GABA_A$ receptor is located in a pocket between an α subunit and a γ_2 subunit.[166] Benzodiazepines also inhibit adenosine uptake apart from $GABA_A$ activity (see Adenosine later).

Various isoforms of $GABA_A$ Cl^- channels differ in their affinity for different benzodiazepines. $GABA_A$ receptors containing γ_2 subunits are more sensitive to benzodiazepines than are $GABA_A$ receptors containing γ_1 and γ_3 subunits. Sensitivity and response to benzodiazepine binding is also highly dependent on the specific α subunit composition of the $GABA_A$ receptor. $GABA_A$ receptors containing an α_4 or α_6 subunit are completely insensitive to and will not bind benzodiazepines, whereas $GABA_A$ receptors containing α_1, α_2, α_3, or α_5 subunits are sensitive to benzodiazepine binding. This has important implications in that the development of tolerance to ethanol confers cross tolerance to benzodiazepines through a change in α subunits (see Chaps. 14 and A24). In addition, specific subunits may mediate different effects of benzodiazepines. For example, sedative effects are mediated through binding to α_1 subunits while anxiolytic effects appear to be mediated by binding to α_2 subunits.[47]

Zolpidem, an imidazopyridine, zaleplon, a pyrazolopyrimidine, and zopiclone are nonbenzodiazepines that act as agonists at the benzodiazepine binding site on the $GABA_A$ receptor. They exhibit a high selectivity for the α_1 subunit and low selectivity for α_2, α_3, and α_5 subunits.[148,166] This selective binding to α_1 subunits is thought to account for their relatively selective sedative properties at therapeutic doses, and lack of anxiolysis, as compared to benzodiazepines.

Numerous steroids, such as alphaxalone and naturally occurring analogs, bind to the $GABA_A$ complex to inhibit or enhance the action of GABA.[50,144] The synthesis of neuroactive steroids is partly regulated by benzodiazepine binding to mitochondrial benzodiazepine receptors (also known as TSPO [translocator proteins]) apart from the $GABA_A$ complex.[79,144] These mitochondrial benzodiazepine binding sites are found both within and outside the CNS and were originally called peripheral benzodiazepine receptors. On binding, benzodiazepines appear to enhance the movement of cholesterol into mitochondria to begin steroid synthesis. Some of carbamazepine's action may be a result of binding at mitochondrial benzodiazepine receptors.[44]

Barbiturates bind to the $GABA_A$ complex to produce several effects.[78,144] All barbiturates enhance the action of GABA by producing more Cl^- influx for a given amount of GABA binding by increasing the duration of Cl^- channel opening. Whereas phenobarbital does not change the affinity of GABA or benzodiazepines for their binding sites, depressant barbiturates, such as pentobarbital, do increase GABA and benzodiazepine receptor affinities for their ligands, further enhancing inward Cl^- currents. At high concentrations, at least some barbiturates directly open Cl^- channels to cause Cl^- influx.[78] Phenobarbital can directly open the Cl^- channel at antiepileptic concentrations. In addition, barbiturates possess other actions that depress all excitable membranes, including cardiac and smooth muscle.

The intravenous anesthetics propofol and etomidate enhance inward $GABA_A$ Cl^- currents, and at high concentrations they directly open chloride channels in the absence of GABA.[7] The respiratory depressant and immobilizing effects of etomidate and propofol are mediated by β_3 subunits, while the sedative effects of these agents are mediated through agonism at β_2 subunits.[149,178] Volatile general anesthetics also directly activate $GABA_A$ Cl^- channels.

Some of ethanol's action is mediated through binding to the $GABA_A$ complex. The degree to which ethanol enhances the effect of GABA on Cl^- influx depends on the $GABA_A$ receptor subunit composition. For example, receptors with an α_4 or α_6 subunit and a δ subunit respond to very low concentrations of ethanol.[158,168]

Methaqualone produces at least part of its pharmacologic effect through indirect $GABA_A$ activity. Little is known of the mechanisms of action of glutethimide and methyprylon. Their structural similarities to barbiturates suggest that they have activity at the $GABA_A$ receptor. Trichloroethanol, a metabolite of chloral hydrate, and clomethiazole interact at the $GABA_A$ complex in a manner similar to barbiturates, although it is not clear whether they are binding to an identical site on the Cl^- channel.[172] Ivermectin, an antihelminthic, activates $GABA_A$ Cl^- channels by increasing GABA binding. Meprobamate displays barbiturate-like action at the $GABA_A$ receptor and, at high concentrations, is able to cause Cl^- influx in the absence of GABA.[133] High concentrations of felbamate also cause inward Cl^- currents in the presence of GABA, although this seems unimportant at therapeutic doses.[133] Part of topiramate's anticonvulsant action may result from enhanced Cl^- influx through binding to $GABA_A$ receptors.[142]

Inhibition of GABA Uptake. Valproate and the anticonvulsants guvacine and tiagabine work, in part, by inhibiting GABA uptake. Although valproate is structurally similar to GABA, its inhibition of the GABA transporter does not appear to be competitive.[114]

$GABA_A$ Antagonism ***Direct $GABA_A$ Antagonists.*** Xenobiotics that act by any mechanism to decrease $GABA_A$ activity can cause CNS excitation and convulsions by decreasing inhibitory inward Cl^- currents. Direct antagonists bind to the same site as GABA to prevent GABA binding, the prototype being the convulsant bicuculline. Various antibiotics interact with the $GABA_A$ receptor to antagonize the action of GABA. In a dose-dependent manner, both imipenem and cephalosporins appear to directly antagonize GABA binding and can produce seizures at high doses or at therapeutic doses in susceptible individuals.[167] Evidence suggests that penicillin may also directly antagonize GABA binding. Electrophysiologic and radioligand binding studies indicate that norfloxacin, ciprofloxacin, ofloxacin, and enoxacin combine with the GABA binding site to prevent GABA binding.[167] Theophylline and at least some NSAIDs markedly enhance GABA antagonism by some fluoroquinolones in vitro.[167] Virol A, from *Cicuta virosa*, appears to directly antagonize binding of GABA to its receptor on the $GABA_A$ complex.[163]

Indirect $GABA_A$ Antagonists. Penicillin is well known for producing convulsions at high doses (eg, >20 million units of penicillin per day with renal insufficiency), and both penicillin and aztreonam, a monobactam, appear to block the Cl^- channel to prevent GABA-mediated inward Cl^- currents.[167]

Picrotoxin, from *Anamirta cocculus* (fish berries), and the experimental convulsant pentylenetetrazol bind to the picrotoxin site of the $GABA_A$ receptor complex to inhibit the action of GABA. Excessive doses produce CNS excitation and convulsions. Some organochlorine insecticides (eg, lindane) also inhibit the action of GABA by binding to what appears to be the picrotoxin site and cause convulsions.[93] Both α-thujone, the active component in wormwood oil, and cicutoxin from the water hemlock noncompetitively antagonize $GABA_A$ activity.[64,164]

Flumazenil competitively antagonizes benzodiazepines, zolpidem, zaleplon, and zopiclone at their receptors to reverse their pharmacologic effects.[17,145] Paradoxically, large doses of flumazenil exhibit anticonvulsant activity in animals. This is explained, at least in part, by flumazenil's ability to inhibit adenosine uptake.[123]

Cyclic antidepressants, including amoxapine and maprotiline, and at least two MAOIs (isocarboxazid and tranylcypromine) inhibit GABA-mediated Cl^- influx at $GABA_A$ receptors.[96,152] Their potency at inhibiting Cl^- influx correlates with the frequency of seizures that occur in patients taking therapeutic doses of these medications. Impaired $GABA_A$ activity may contribute to or be primarily responsible for seizures that occur in patients who overdose on these xenobiotics. Their exact binding on the $GABA_A$ receptor complex remains unknown, although some evidence suggests at least indirect activity at the picrotoxin binding site.

Some subtypes of $GABA_A$ receptors are susceptible to inhibition by zinc ions.[144] What role this plays in normal physiology or toxicology is not established.

$GABA_A$ Withdrawal. Acute withdrawal from all $GABA_A$ direct and indirect agonists appears almost identical except for time course; the common denominator is impaired Cl^- influx. Withdrawal of all $GABA_A$ agonists can cause tremor, hypertension, tachycardia, respiratory alkalosis, diaphoresis, agitation, hallucinations, and convulsions. When $GABA_A$ receptors are chronically exposed to an agonist, changes in gene expression of receptor subunits occur, which lessens

Cl^- influx in response to GABA or drug binding, producing tolerance. Importantly, withdrawal of the agonist produces yet further changes in subunit expression. For example, benzodiazepine-insensitive α_4-subunit expression is increased following withdrawal of many GABA agonists, including benzodiazepines, zolpidem, zopiclone, zaleplon, neurosteroids, and ethanol. (Expression of other subunits, including α_1, γ_2, β_2, and β_1 also change in response to exposure and/or withdrawal of $GABA_A$ agonists.[47]) Alterations in $GABA_A$ receptor subunit composition following chronic exposure to and withdrawal of an agonist can, therefore, affect the ability to successfully treat withdrawal symptoms. While any $GABA_A$ receptor agonist may be used to treat withdrawal from another, some agents work better than others in different clinical settings. For example, patients experiencing severe alcohol withdrawal may have an increased proportion of $GABA_A$ receptors containing benzodiazepine-insensitive α_4 subunits, and contain fewer $GABA_A$ receptors with benzodiazepine-sensitive α_1 subunits.[24] Even extremely high doses of benzodiazepines in these patients may not effectively control severe alcohol withdrawal. A better treatment option in such a setting would be $GABA_A$ agonists such as propofol or phenobarbital that either act on a different site on the $GABA_A$ receptor or directly open the Cl^- channel.[7,24] Phenytoin and carbamazepine do not stop $GABA_A$ withdrawal seizures because their pharmacologic effects are independent of $GABA_A$ agonism.

$GABA_B$ Agonists. The main $GABA_B$ receptor agonist of toxicologic significance is baclofen. Coma, hypothermia, hypotension, bradydysrhythmias, and seizures characterize its toxicity. The convulsions that occur in patients with baclofen overdose are thought to result from disinhibition (inhibition of inhibitory neurons). Carbamazepine's activation of $GABA_B$ receptors has been demonstrated, although this is not thought to explain most of its anticonvulsant action. Some of γ-hydroxybutyrate's actions following pharmacologic doses may be mediated through activation of $GABA_B$ receptors.

$GABA_B$ Withdrawal. Baclofen withdrawal is similar clinically to $GABA_A$ withdrawal. Hallucinations, agitation, tremor, increased sympathetic activity, and convulsions are the main characteristics of baclofen withdrawal. Withdrawal from chronic intrathecal baclofen administration may also be accompanied by large swings in autonomic tone (hypotension, hypertension, tachycardia, bradycardia) and transient cardiomyopathy and shock. Reinstitution of oral baclofen therapy following oral withdrawal, or intrathecal baclofen following intrathecal withdrawal, when possible, is the treatment of choice.[97]

GAMMA-HYDROXYBUTYRATE

γ-Hydroxybutyrate (GHB; γ-hydroxybutyric acid) exists endogenously, but toxicologic interest stems from its use as a drug of abuse and as a treatment for narcolepsy.[11,45,85] GHB is rapidly absorbed and freely crosses the blood–brain barrier. Toxicity resulting from ingestion of GHB is explained by GHB receptor and $GABA_B$ receptor activation, and comprises agitation, tremor, rapid onset of coma, vomiting, bradycardia, hypotension, hypotonia, and apnea that usually resolve within several hours. Although seizure activity has been noted in experimental animals, it is debated whether GHB causes true convulsive activity in human beings. Human experiments with "therapeutic" doses of GHB have not found EEG changes consistent with seizure activity.[85] Some authors have reported "generalized seizures" occurring in patients presenting after GHB overdose. Interestingly, patients with the rare inborn error of metabolism, succinic semialdehyde dehydrogenase (SSAD) deficiency, have elevated GHB concentrations and tend to experience seizures.[52] Valproate similarly elevates endogenous GHB concentrations by inhibiting SSAD.

Controversy exists as to whether GHB should be considered a neurotransmitter or simply a neuromodulator because it is unclear whether this substance is concentrated within vesicles for synaptic release. There is evidence demonstrating a sodium-dependent up-take transporter for GHB.

GHB receptors appear to be heterogeneously distributed throughout the brain, with highest concentrations in the hippocampus, cortex, limbic areas, and thalamus, as well as in regions innervated by dopaminergic terminals and dopaminergic nuclei. GHB receptors exist on neurons, mainly at the synaptic level, but are absent from glial or peripheral cells. At least two general GHB receptors have been described thus far, based on binding affinity for GHB and other ligands. Although γ-butyrolactone (GBL) does not express affinity for GHB binding sites, GBL rapidly undergoes hydrolysis to form GHB by peripheral γ-lactonase.[11,95] 1,4-Butanediol undergoes conversion to GHB via alcohol dehydrogenase and aldehyde dehydrogenase.

Several proposed pathways for endogenous GHB formation exist (Fig. 13–11).[11] Evidence exists for GHB's metabolism back to GABA, although this appears minimal at physiologic GHB concentrations.[45] However, effects resulting from pharmacologic doses of GHB may result, in part, from secondary GABA formation.

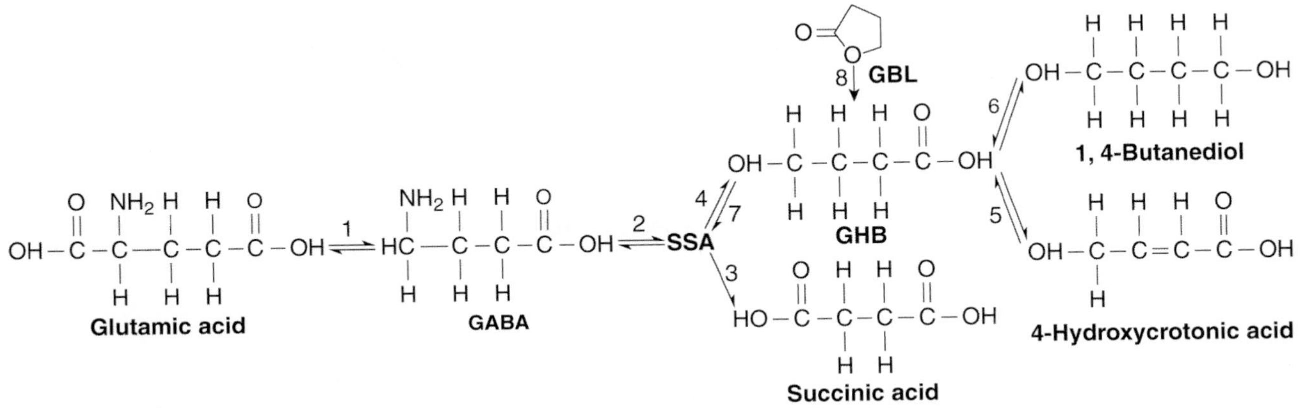

FIGURE 13–11. Potential pathways of GHB (γ-hydroxybutyrate) synthesis and degradation. GABA = γ-aminobutyric acid; GBL = γ-butyrolactone; SSA = succinic semialdehyde; [1] = glutamic acid decarboxylase; [2] = GABA-transaminase; [3] = succinic semialdehyde dehydrogenase; [4] = specific succinic semialdehyde reductase and/or nicotinamide adenine dinucleotide phosphate (NADPH)-dependent aldehyde reductase 2; [5] = mitochondrial β oxidation; [6] = alcohol dehydrogenase and aldehyde dehydrogenase; [7] = GHB dehydrogenase; [8] = γ-lactonase.

Although normal endogenous GHB concentrations are probably not high enough to activate $GABA_B$ receptors, such receptor activation may occur with exogenous administration of GHB. Furthermore, there appears to be functional interplay between GHB and $GABA_B$ receptors.[11]

Specific interactions between GHB and DA are complex and not fully delineated. Treatment with GHB appears to inhibit DA release, probably via stimulation of $GABA_B$ receptors.[173] GHB also affects the firing rates of dopaminergic neurons, DA synthesis, and levels of DA and its major metabolites. GHB is thought to affect sleep cycles, temperature regulation, cerebral glucose metabolism and blood flow, memory, and emotional control, and it may be neuroprotective.

Although GHB can suppress alcohol withdrawal, it is also addictive, and both tolerance and a withdrawal syndrome have been described. Withdrawal is characterized, in part, by insomnia, cramps, paranoia, hallucinations, tremor, and anxiety.

GLYCINE AS AN INHIBITORY NEUROTRANSMITTER

Glycine acts as an inhibitory neurotransmitter in the spinal cord and lower brainstem. In the CNS, serine is converted to glycine by serine hydroxymethyltransferase (SHMT).

RELEASE AND UPTAKE

Glycine is transported into storage vesicles by VGAT and undergoes Ca^{2+}-dependent exocytosis upon neuronal depolarization (Fig. 13–12). Glycine is removed from the synapse through uptake by a Na^+-dependent transporter into presynaptic neurons and into glial cells. Two glycine membrane transporters have been cloned and share homology with GABA uptake transporters. GLYT-1 is found both in astrocytes and neurons, whereas GLYT-2 is localized on axons and terminal boutons of neurons

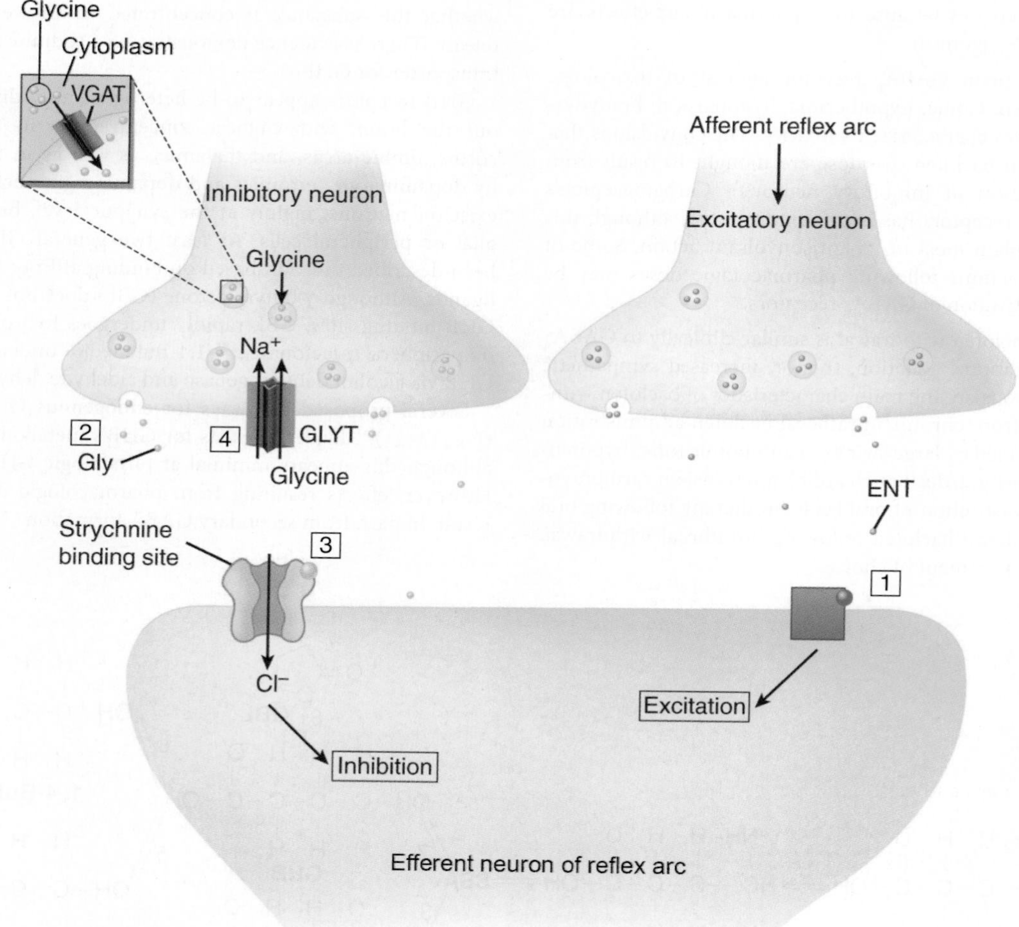

FIGURE 13–12. Inhibitory glycinergic neurotransmission. Glycine is concentrated within vesicles by uptake via VGAT, the vesicle membrane transporter. Signals from the afferent limb of a reflex arc (top right) cause the release of an excitatory neurotransmitter (ENT) that crosses the synapse to bind to a neuron in the efferent limb of the reflex arc [1]. To prevent excessive neuronal firing and motor activity, glycine (Gly) released from a glycinergic inhibitory neuron [2] binds to glycine Cl^- channel receptors [3] and causes inhibition by hyperpolarization through Cl^- influx. Synaptic glycine is transported back into the neuron by at least two subtypes of membrane glycine transporters, GLYT-1 and GLYT-2 [4]. Strychnine binds to the glycinergic Cl^- channel to decrease glycine's binding, which prevents Cl^- influx. Although strychnine is shown to bind to a separate site from glycine, there is evidence that these sites may overlap. GLYT = glycine uptake transporter.

that contain vesicular glycine. Although both transporters are found associated with glycinergic neurons in the brainstem and spinal cord, GLYT-1 is also found in the forebrain in regions devoid of glycinergic neurotransmission. At the latter location, GLYT-1 may regulate extracellular glycine that is available for NMDA receptor activation, and GLYT-1 inhibitors could then enhance NMDA responses (see NMDA Receptor Antagonists). Glycine transporters can also function in reverse, moving glycine out of the cell when the intracellular sodium concentrations rise.[3]

GLYCINE RECEPTORS

The glycine receptor is a Cl^- channel that shares significant amino acid homology with the $GABA_A$ Cl^- channel. Glycine receptors are pentameric proteins made up of α and β subunits. Four isoforms of the α subunit and one isoform of the β subunit have been described.[103] An anchoring protein, gephyrin, binds to the β subunit and allows for clustering of glycine receptors at postsynaptic membranes. Glycine receptors may also be found outside the synapse, although the function of these receptors is not well understood.[170] Glycine receptor activation causes an inward Cl^- current that hyperpolarizes the membrane. Glycine binding is also important for functioning of the NMDA receptor as discussed later.

XENOBIOTICS

Table 13–10 provides examples of xenobiotics that affect inhibitory glycine Cl^- channels. The amino acids D-alanine, taurine, L-alanine, L-serine, and proline can activate glycinergic Cl^- channels. Both ethanol and propofol potentiate glycine-mediated inward Cl^- currents, just as they do at $GABA_A$ Cl^- channels.[99,103] Volatile halogenated anesthetics, ivermectin, Δ-9-tetrahydrocannabinol, and chloromethiazole also potentiate glycinergic transmission.[170] Clozapine inhibits glycine uptake.[67]

Strychnine is the main toxicant affecting glycinergic transmission. Strychnine binds to the α subunit of the glycine receptor to prevent glycine's action on Cl^- influx,[2] at least in part by decreasing glycine's binding to its receptors. This physiologic antagonism of glycine's action produces increased muscle tone, rigidity, opisthotonus, trismus, rhabdomyolysis, and death from respiratory failure. Given the similarity in Cl^- channels, it is not surprising that strychnine binds to the $GABA_A$ complex in vitro. However, strychnine's affinity for this complex is less than that for glycine receptors, and most of its toxicologic action is a result of physiologic antagonism of glycine's inhibitory action.

Picrotoxin binds to the glycine receptor to impair Cl^- influx.[94] Evidence exists for picrotoxin's direct antagonism at the glycine binding site(s), in contrast to $GABA_A$ Cl^- channels, where it acts at a site separate from where GABA binds. Ginkgolide B appears to inhibit the glycine receptor by directly blocking the Cl^- channel.[170] Tetanus toxin produces rigidity and trismus by preventing glycine release from nerve endings in the spinal cord and brainstem.

TABLE 13–10. Examples of Xenobiotics That Affect Inhibitory Glycine Chloride Channels

Glycine agonists	Glycine antagonists
Ethanol	Ginkogolide B
Halogenated anesthetics (volatile)	Picrotoxin
Propofol	Strychnine
D-Serine	Glycine uptake inhibitor
	Clozapine

GLUTAMATE

Glutamate is the main excitatory neurotransmitter in the CNS. It also serves as the immediate precursor to the main inhibitory neurotransmitter, GABA. This exquisite balance between glutamate neuronal stimulation and neuronal inhibition by GABA is essential for the normal functioning and protection of the CNS. Two-thirds of all brain energy expenditure is dedicated to uptake and recycling of glutamate, which insures that glutamate activity is tightly regulated.[67] Glutamate is essential for memory, learning, perception, and locomotion. Although aspartate displays similar actions as glutamate in experimental models, its role as a neurotransmitter in mammalian brains is doubtful, as it is only active at certain types of glutamate receptors and is not a substrate for glutamate neuronal vesicular transporters.[48] Glutamate and aspartate are commonly referred to as excitatory amino acid (EAA) neurotransmitters.

Glutamatergic neurotransmission has been a subject of intense research because of its role in mediating neuronal damage in degenerative neurologic diseases and during trauma, ischemia, hypoglycemia, and status epilepticus.[100] Although glutamate receptor stimulation is necessary for normal brain activity, excessive glutamate receptor activation endogenously or by glutamate agonists can produce convulsions, neuronal damage, and death. Similarly, glutamate antagonists demonstrate anticonvulsant activity and neuroprotective action in animal models of brain and spinal cord injury. A number of psychiatric and neurologic disorders have been identified with altered glutamatergic function, such as schizophrenia, depression, anxiety, posttraumatic stress disorder, and Alzheimer dementia.[67] Glutamate may also play an important role in the development of drug abuse and subsequent withdrawal symptoms. Glutamate antagonists decrease drug craving and withdrawal symptoms in patients addicted to ethanol, benzodiazepines, and opioids.[73]

SYNTHESIS, RELEASE, AND UPTAKE

Glutamate must be synthesized from products of glucose metabolism or other precursors within the CNS because glutamate does not cross the blood–brain barrier. Glutamate is primarily synthesized from glutamine by the enzyme glutaminase located within the mitochondrial compartment.[48] Glutamate is stored within vesicles and then released into the synapse by Ca^{2+}-dependent exocytosis. Synaptic glutamate transported into glial cells undergoes conversion back to glutamine by the enzyme glutamine synthase. Glial cells then release glutamine which is taken up by neurons before conversion back to glutamate and subsequent transport into vesicles (Fig. 13–13). Reverse transport of glutamate from the cytoplasm into the synapse by the membrane transporter may occur under some circumstances.[6] There are five different cell surface excitatory amino acid transporters (EAAT) that differ in their predominant CNS locations. EAAT1 is primarily found on forebrain glial cells. EEAT2 is located on astrocytes and is responsible for 80% of all glutamate update. EAAT3 is located on glutamatergic neurons in the forebrain. EAAT4 serves the same purpose in the cerebellum. EAAT5 is limited to the retina.[74]

GLUTAMATE RECEPTORS

The EAA receptor system is extremely complex, consisting of 11 different receptors. Three of these receptors are ionotropic cation channels, which are responsible for fast excitatory glutamatergic activity. There are eight metabotropic receptors linked to G proteins whose actions are slower, more diverse, and longer lasting than the inotropic receptors.[74] A single neuron may express numerous types of glutamate receptors.

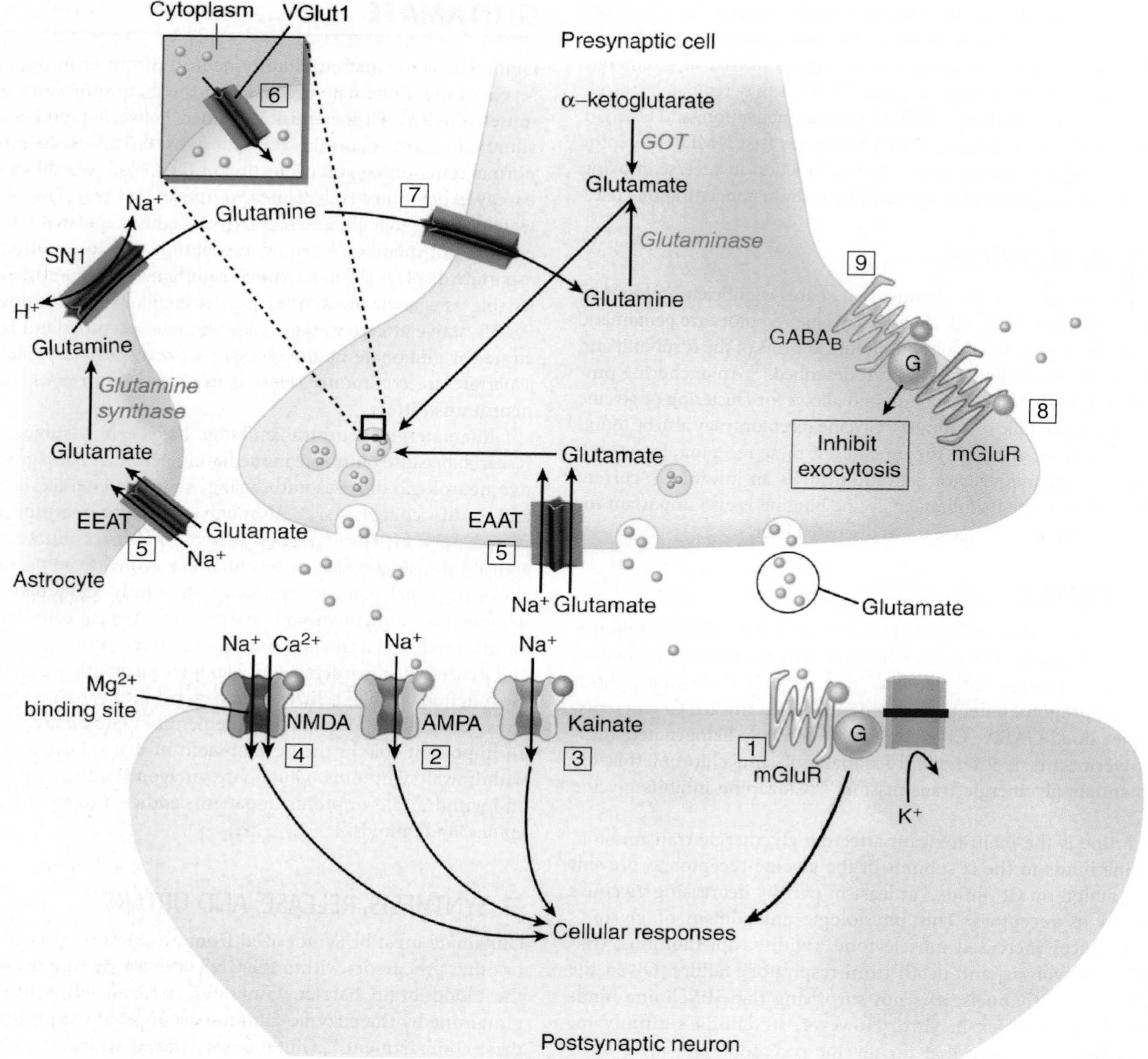

FIGURE 13–13. Glutamatergic neurotransmission. Glutamic oxaloacetic transaminase (GOT) converts α-ketoglutarate to glutamate in mitochondria. Glutamate also forms from glutamine via mitochondrial glutaminase. Glutamate is transported into vesicles [6] by VGlut1 (or possibly other subtypes) for exocytotic release into the synapse. Synaptic glutamate activates four main types of receptors. AMPA [2], kainate [3], and NMDA [4] receptors are cation channels. Membrane depolarization in response to their activation causes neuronal excitation through cation influx. Metabotropic receptors (mGluR) [1,8] are coupled to G proteins and are expressed on pre- and postsynaptic membranes. In addition, some mGluRs reside outside of the synapse. Postsynaptic mGluR excitation in this example [1] results from preventing K^+ efflux, but other mechanisms of excitation exist. Presynaptic mGluRs act to inhibit [8] glutamate (and other neuro-transmitter) release through modulating intracellular Ca^{2+} concentrations, as do presynaptic $GABA_B$ receptors in response to GABA binding [9]. Figure 13 -14 provides a more detailed illustration of the NMDA receptor. Excessive influx of Ca^{2+} through NMDA receptors (and through some AMPA and kainate receptors) causes neuronal damage and cell death. A Mg^{2+} ion normally blocks the NMDA receptor channel to prevent Ca^{2+} influx despite glutamate binding. However, depolarization of the neuronal membrane by cation influx resulting from activation of any of the other receptor types causes Mg^{2+} to dissociate from the NMDA receptor and to allow potentially damaging inward Ca^{2+} currents in response to glutamate binding. Glutamate undergoes uptake by neurons and glial cells by various subtypes of EAAT, the membrane bound glutamate transporter [5]. In glial cells, glutamate is converted to glutamine by glutamine synthase, and glutamine is transported out of glial cells by system N-1 (SN1), a Na^+- and H^+-dependent pump that is structurally similar to VGAT, the vesicle membrane GABA transporter. Glutamine then moves back into neurons [7] where it undergoes conversion back to glutamate. Various agents in Table 13 -11 affect glutamatergic neurotransmission, in part, by stimulating or blocking the various glutamate receptors [1 -4,8] or by preventing glutamate uptake [5]. G = G protein.

Also, every type of glutamate receptor has been identified on both presynaptic and postsynaptic membranes, but many of these receptors are not active under normal physiologic conditions. This complexity is necessary for protection against the devastating effects of uncontrolled excitatory neurotransmission. Presynaptic terminal glutamate receptors modulate the release of various neurotransmitters, including glutamate, while postsynaptic glutamate receptors are usually excitatory, although some inhibitory actions have been demonstrated (Fig. 13–13).[125]

Ionotropic Glutamate Receptors All three types of ionotropic glutamate receptors allow for neuronal excitation through cation influx. These receptors are further categorized and named by their abilities to be activated or antagonized by various substances: kainic acid, α-amino-3-hydroxy-5-methyl-4-isoxazole propionate (AMPA), and *N*-methyl-D-aspartate (NMDA).[74,125]

Kainate receptors are named for their affinity for kainic acid, found in seaweed, and comprise GluR5–7, KA1, and KA2 subunits.[135] Activation allows Na^+ influx and a small amount of K^+ efflux, resulting in neuronal depolarization. Some kainate receptors allow for the passage of Ca^{2+}.[27] Kainate receptors are found both presynaptically and postsynaptically. Their presynaptic behavior is complex in that they initially stimulate neurotramsitter release, but ultimately act more like metabotropic receptors, with the net effect of functioning as autoreceptors, modulating subsequent glutamate release and acting as heteroreceptors via stimulation of presynaptic $GABA_B$ receptors to limit GABA release.[27,135] Postsynaptic kainite receptors contribute to excitability of postsynaptic neurons.

The AMPA receptor is an ion channel structurally similar to the kainate receptor that also mediates Na^+ influx (and lesser amounts of K^+ efflux) on presynaptic and postsynaptic membranes, triggering neuronal depolarization. AMPA receptors comprise GluR1–4 subunits.[27] The AMPA receptor is the most common ionotropic glutamate receptor found in the brain. AMPA receptors appear to be responsible for most glutamatergic excitation under normal conditions.[27]

The NMDA receptor, the most studied of all glutamate receptors, is a Ca^{2+} channel whose activation allows for inward Ca^{2+} and Na^+ currents (and some K^+ efflux), resulting in neuronal depolarization and excitation (Fig. 13–14). NMDA receptors comprise NR1, $NR2_{A-D}$, and $NR3_{A-B}$ subunits.[72] Excessive stimulation of NMDA receptors by glutamate released during ischemia, trauma, hypoglycemia, or convulsions triggers damaging rises in intracellular Ca^{2+} concentrations, activation of numerous enzymes, and free radical formation, all of which incite cell death.[100] Antagonists of NMDA Ca^{2+} channels are anticonvulsants and neuroprotectants.

The NMDA Ca^{2+} channel is normally blocked by Mg^{2+} in a voltage-dependent manner, preventing Ca^{2+} influx despite glutamate binding (Fig. 13–14).[67,72] Only when the neuronal membrane is depolarized by at least 20–30 mV through some other mechanism (eg, activation of another type of glutamate receptor) will Mg^{2+} leave the channel and allow Ca^{2+} influx in response to glutamate binding. Thus, the NMDA glutamate receptor is both a ligand-gated and voltage-gated ion channel. Many neurons express both NMDA and non-NMDA receptors for glutamate. Excessive stimulation of kainate or AMPA receptors by glutamate causes cell damage through Na^+ (and in some instances, Ca^{2+}) influx, because the membrane depolarization they produce causes Mg^{2+} to leave the NMDA receptor and allows for potentially damaging inward Ca^{2+} currents.[38] Calcium ion influx through voltage-gated ion channels (including the L-subtype) on cell bodies that open in response to depolarization also contributes to accumulation of intracellular calcium and cell damage.[72]

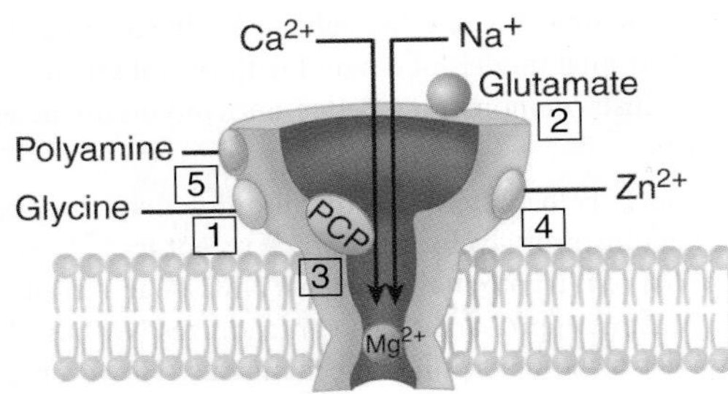

FIGURE 13–14. Representation of the NMDA glutamate receptor. The NMDA receptor is a voltage-gated and ligand-gated Ca^{2+} channel. Glutamate binds to its receptor on the channel [2] to open the Ca^{2+} channel and to allow Ca^{2+} and Na^+ influx and lesser amounts of K^+ efflux. Mg^{2+} normally blocks the Ca^{2+} channel, preventing cation influx in response to glutamate binding. Mg^{2+} leaves the channel when the membrane is depolarized by 20 -30 mV. Glycine must also bind to its site on the NMDA receptor complex for successful glutamate agonism. Polyamines bind on the extracellular surface of the receptor [5]. Zn^{2+} binds [4] to inhibit Ca^{2+} influx. The phencyclidine (PCP) binding site [3] lies within the channel. Agents in Table 13 -11 may antagonize glycine binding [1]; block the Ca^{2+} channel by binding to the PCP binding site [3]; bind to the polyamine binding site [5]; or directly stimulate the glutamate binding site [2].

Glutamate, alone, is incapable of triggering Ca^{2+} influx after binding to NMDA receptors, even after Mg^{2+} has dissociated from the ion channel. Glycine also must bind to its specific receptor on the NMDA receptor complex for successful glutamate agonism (Fig. 13–14), making glycine an indirect agonist of excitatory neurotransmission.[72] Strychnine, a glycine antagonist at neuronal glycine receptors, does not antagonize glycine's excitatory action at NMDA receptors, explaining why glycine NMDA receptors are also known as strychnine-insensitive glycine receptors.

Zinc ions normally bind to the NMDA receptor complex to antagonize the action of glutamate. Binding of spermine or spermidine to a polyamine binding site on the extracellular side of the NMDA receptor results in increased affinity of glycine and glutamate for their binding sites. However, polyamine agonism is not essential for glutamate activation of NMDA receptors.[72]

Metabotropic Glutamate Receptors Metabotropic glutamate receptors (mGluRs) are linked to various G proteins on postsynaptic and presynaptic membranes (Fig. 13–13). Eight different receptors have been isolated. In contrast to ionotropic glutamate receptors, mGluRs may excite or inhibit at postsynaptic membranes, and appear mainly to inhibit at presynaptic locations. Postsynaptic excitation most commonly results from prevention of K^+ efflux or activation of phospholipase C, which serves to raise intracellular Ca^{2+} concentration. Postsynaptic inhibition usually results from enhanced K^+ efflux.[159]

Metabotropic glutamate receptors are commonly subdivided into three main groups based on their sequence homology, intracellular signaling mechanisms, and response to specific experimental agonists.[159] As a general rule, group I receptors (mGlu1, mGlu5) reside postsynaptically; activation produces excitation through blockade of K^+ efflux or by activating phospholipase C, producing rises in intracellular Ca^{2+}. The mGlu5 receptor is the most common and active of the group I receptors. In animal experiments, agonists of group I receptors produce convulsions, while antagonists display anticonvulsant effects.[90]

Groups II (mGlu2, mGlu3) and III (mGlu4, mGlu6, mGlu7, mGlu8) receptors most commonly serve as presynaptic autoreceptors and heteroreceptors and, when activated, inhibit adenylate cyclase activity.[125,159] This, in turn, prevents Ca^{2+} influx and serves to inhibit release of neurotransmitters, including glutamate, GABA, DA, and adenosine. Group II presynaptic autoreceptors may play an especially important role in decreasing further glutamate release during pathologic conditions, when the extracellular concentration of glutamate exceeds normal physiologic levels. They are positioned outside the synaptic active zone and, therefore, only become activated when glutamate spills out of the synapse.[125] The mGlu7 receptor is positioned within the active zone of the synapse, but has a low affinity for glutamate, allowing for a continuous but mild inhibitory effect on glutamate release.[125,159] Agonists of groups II and III metabotropic receptors produce anticonvulsant effects in animals.[98]

XENOBIOTICS

Table 13–11 provides examples of xenobiotics that affect glutamatergic neurotransmission.

Glutamate Agonism Domoic acid produces amnestic shellfish poisoning, partly characterized by confusion, agitation, convulsions, memory disturbance, neuronal damage, and death.[62] The structural similarity

TABLE 13–11. Examples of Xenobiotics That Affect Glutamatergic Neurotransmission

- Glutamate agonism
  - Direct glutamate receptor agonists
    - BMAA
    - BOAA
    - Domoic acid
    - Homoquinolinic acid
    - Ibotenic acid
    - Quisqualate
    - Willardine
  - AMPA receptor modulators
    - BMAA
    - BOAA
    - Cyclothiazide
    - Dysiherbaine
    - Racetams
  - Kainate receptor modulators
    - Concavanalin A
    - Domoic acid
    - Dysiherbaine
  - Glycine NMDA receptor agonists
    - D-Cycloserine
    - Kynerenic acid
    - Milacemide
  - Glutamate uptake inhibitor
    - Clozapine
    - Nitropropionic acid
  - Polyamine aonists
    - Neomycin
- Glutamate antagonism
  - Prevent glutamate release
    - Diazoxide
    - Felbamate
    - Lamotrigine
    - Nimodipine
    - Riluzole
    - Sulfasalazine
  - Increase glutamate reuptake
    - Ceftriaxone
    - Riluzole
  - AMPA receptor antagonists
    - Quinoxalinediones
    - Topiramate
  - NMDA receptor antagonists
    - Amantadine
    - Buprenorphine
    - Dextrorphan
    - Dizocilpine (MK801)
    - Ethanol[a]
    - Ketamine
    - Memantine
    - Meperidine
    - Methadone
    - Orphenadrine
    - Pentamidine
    - Phencyclidine
    - Tramadol
  - NMDA glycine antagonists
    - Felbamate
    - Kynurenic acid
    - Meprobamate
  - Kainate receptor antagonists
    - Quinoxalinediones
    - Topiramate
  - Polyamine antagonists
    - Diethylenetriamine
    - Ifenprodil
    - Eliprodil

BMAA = α-amino-β-methylaminopropionic acid; BOAA = β-*N*-oxalylamino-L-alanine; NMDA = *N*-methyl-D-aspartate.

[a]Ethanol antagonizes glutamate's action at NMDA receptors through an unknown mechanism.

between domoic acid and glutamate is thought to explain excessive activation of kainate receptors with secondary NMDA receptor activation and resultant neuronal dysfunction and damage.

Investigators hypothesize that other naturally occurring glutamate receptor agonists produce additional neurologic diseases. The neurogenic form of lathyrism results from using chickling peas (*Lathyrus sativus*) as a food staple. Chickling peas contain β-*N*-oxalylamino-L-alanine (BOAA), an agonist of AMPA receptors.[80] Neurogenic lathyrism was common in German concentration and prisoner of war camps during World War II and still occurs regularly in some parts of the world. Ibotenic acid, from poisonous mushrooms, activates NMDA and some metabotropic glutamate receptors. It undergoes decarboxylation to muscimol, a direct agonist at $GABA_A$ receptors. Clozapine inhibits glutamate uptake.[67]

Because noncompetitive NMDA receptor antagonism reproduces many signs and symptoms of schizophrenia, investigators are directing efforts at increasing glutamate's activity at NMDA channels in an effort to treat the disease.[143] After crossing the blood–brain barrier, milacemide undergoes conversion to glycine, which is required for NMDA receptor activation.[143] D-Cycloserine also crosses the blood–brain barrier to stimulate glycine receptors on NMDA calcium channels.[72]

Glutamate Antagonism ***Prevention of Glutamate Release.*** Riluzole, used for the treatment of amyotrophic lateral sclerosis, indirectly prevents release of glutamate by blocking Na^+ channels. It also stimulates EAAT activity, thereby facilitating reuptake of glutamate from the synapse.[72] Lamotrigine diminishes glutamate release through blockade of voltage-gated Na^+ channels.[67] Blockade of voltage-gated Ca^{2+} channels by nimodipine also appears to impair glutamate release.[55]

NMDA Receptor Antagonists. Although some experimental xenobiotics antagonize the action of glutamate, most of our knowledge concerns antagonism at NMDA receptors. Phencyclidine and ketamine appear to bind within the ion channel (PCP binding site) to block Ca^{2+} influx following glutamate binding (Fig. 13–14).[67,72] Both possess other pharmacologic actions and can produce convulsions in overdose.

Dextromethorphan and its first-pass metabolite, dextrorphan, exhibit anticonvulsant activity in animals. Dextrorphan's anticonvulsant activity results, in part, from blockade of NMDA receptor Ca^{2+} channels by binding to the PCP binding site. Dextromethorphan does not bind to the NMDA complex but, like dextrorphan, can directly block N-subtype and L-subtype voltage-dependent Ca^{2+} channels.[72]

Dizocilpine (MK-801) is an NMDA receptor antagonist that binds to the PCP binding site in the NMDA Ca^{2+} channel.[40] Human trials of dizocilpine resulted in adverse effects similar to those produced by phencyclidine, preventing further use in humans as a neuroprotective agent. Amantadine, memantine, and orphenadrine act as low-affinity antagonists at the PCP site, but are not associated with insurmountable psychotomimetic adverse effects.[72] Part of amantadine's effectiveness in the treatment of Parkinson disease may be related to NMDA antagonism. Pentamidine also antagonizes glutamate binding at NMDA channels.[40]

Tramadol displays multiple mechanisms of action as an analgesic, including a weak affinity for the opioid receptors, inhibition of monoamine reuptake, and inhibition of NMDA glutamtergic activity at clinically relevant concentrations by an unknown mechanism.[56] Methadone, meperidine, and buprenorphine are opioid analgesics that antagonize NMDA receptors at therapeutic doses, and this mechanism of action may contribute to their analgesic effect.[37]

Ethanol competitively inhibits NMDA receptor activation by an unknown mechanism, resulting in upregulation of this glutamatergic system. It does not appear to act through currently recognized binding sites.[174] In some animal models of ethanol withdrawal seizures, NMDA receptor antagonists demonstrate better anticonvulsant action than $GABA_A$ agonists.

Glycine Antagonists. Felbamate's anticonvulsant activity may result, in part, from antagonism of glycine at NMDA receptors.[122,176] Kynurenic acid, a metabolite of L-tryptophan, prevents NMDA activation through glycine antagonism. Meprobamate also antagonizes NMDA glutamate receptors by a yet-to-be-determined mechanism.[122] However, given the structural similarity to felbamate, meprobamate may act by antagonizing the action of glycine.

Polyamine Antagonism. Ifenprodil and eliprodil antagonize glutamate's action at NMDA channels by preventing polyamine binding.[54]

ADENOSINE

Adenosine is an important modulator of brain activity and body physiology. Adenosine receptors are vastly distributed throughout the body, which emphasizes the pivotal role adenosine plays in neurotransmission and metabolic activity. The overall action of adenosine is to lessen oxygen requirements and to increase oxygen and substrate delivery. Adenosine can be found in small concentrations in most extracellular fluids as a consequence of ATP metabolism. This is in contrast to classical neurotransmitters, which are secreted in discrete quanta upon stimulation of presynaptic neurons. In the brain, adenosine primarily limits glutamate and ACh release, thereby preventing excessive postsynaptic neuronal stimulation. Adenosine also counterbalances the effects of DA stimulation in the basal ganglia.[126] Adenosine contributes to temperature regulation, sleep, anxiety reduction, locomotion, pain perception, and seizure inhibition.[89] Peripheral effects of adenosine include bradycardia, decreased myocardial contractility, vasodilation, bronchoconstriction, decreased glomerular filtration, suppression of overactive immune responses, and anti-inflammatory activity.[66]

SYNTHESIS, RELEASE, AND UPTAKE

Adenosine is derived from the breakdown of ATP, which is commonly co-released with other neurotransmitters (eg, NE, ACh, glutamate) into the synapse before subsequent degradation by ectonucleotidases (Fig. 13–15). During times of adequate oxygen delivery and oxidative phosphorylation, intracellular ATP concentrations are many times greater than those of adenosine, with normal intracellular adenosine concentrations ranging from 50 to 300 n*M*. Intracellular adenosine concentrations increase rapidly during ischemia, hypoxia, or elevated metabolic activity (eg, seizures).[9] A bidirectional Na^+-dependent purine uptake transporter typically moves adenosine from the synapse back into the neuron under normal conditions, but can reverse adenosine transport when intracellular adenosine concentrations become elevated (Fig. 13–15). The overall cellular preference is to convert adenosine back to ATP via adenosine kinase, but adenosine also undergoes conversion to inosine by adenosine deaminase.[89] Synaptic adenosine then activates adenosine receptors on neuronal and non-neuronal tissue (eg, vasculature). Adenosine's actions are terminated by uptake into glial cells and neurons (Fig. 13–15).[9,89] Exogenously administered adenosine used in the treatment of supraventricular tachycardia does not cross the blood–brain barrier and, therefore, is not centrally active. The half-life of adenosine in the blood is less than 10 seconds.

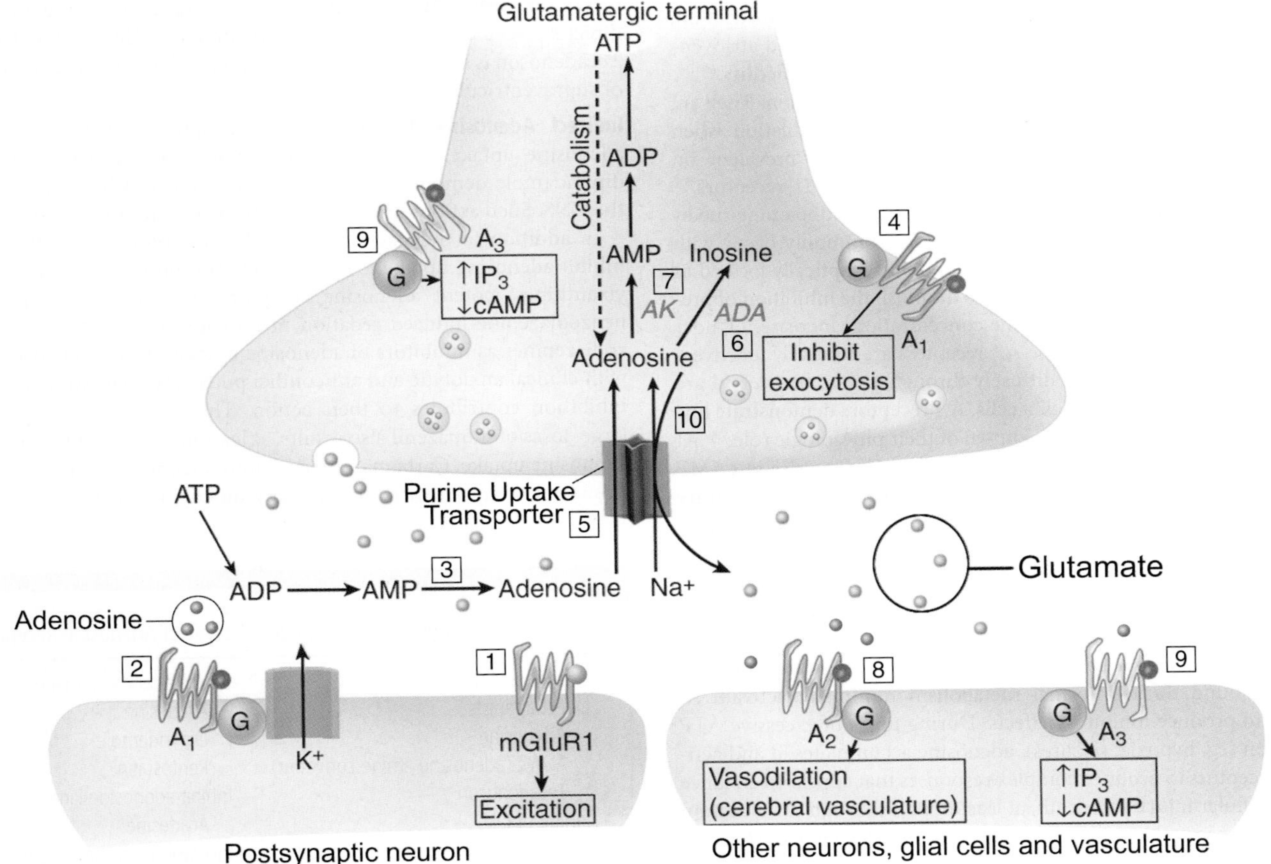

FIGURE 13–15. Adenosine's role in regulating excitatory neurotransmission, using glutamate as an example. In this example, glutamate excites a postsynaptic neuron by activating metabotropic glutamate receptors (mGluR1) [1]. ATP enters the synapse when glutamate is released. Adenosine formed from metabolism of ATP within the synapse [3] binds to postsynaptic A_1 receptors [2], which open K^+ channels to inhibit the neuron through hyperpolarization. Adenosine also activates presynaptic A_1 receptors [4] to lower intracellular Ca^{2+} concentrations, thereby impairing further glutamate release. After uptake [5], adenosine is acted upon either by adenosine kinase (AK) [7] to form AMP, or by adenosine deaminase (ADA) [6] to form inosine. Adenosine also binds to neuronal A_2 receptors (especially in the striatum) and to vascular A_2 receptors to cause vasodilatation [8]. A_3 receptors [9] are not activated by normal concentrations of adenosine. During times of excessive catabolism (e.g., seizures, hypoglycemia, stroke) when intracellular adenosine concentrations rise markedly, adenosine moves into the synapse through reverse transport via the purine uptake transporter [10]. Resultant stimulation of A_1 and A_2 receptors results in inhibitory actions to decrease oxygen requirements and to increase substrate delivery through vasodilatation as described above. However, the resultant stimulation of A_3 receptors [9] may contribute to neuronal damage and death. Agents in Table 13 -12 act to inhibit adenosine uptake [5]; to inhibit ADA [6]; to inhibit AK [7]; to increase adenosine release; and to antagonize A_1 [2,4] and A_2 [8] receptors. ADP = adenosine diphosphate; ATP = adenosine triphosphate; cAMP = cyclic adenosine monophosphate; G = G protein; IP_3 = inositol triphosphate.

ADENOSINE RECEPTORS

The purine P_1 receptor family comprises 4 adenosine receptor subtypes linked to G proteins: A_1, A_{2A}, A_{2B}, and A_3.[9,66,89,138] Postsynaptic A_1 stimulation results in K^+ channel opening and K^+ efflux, with subsequent hyperpolarization of the neuron (Fig. 13–15). Evidence suggests that G protein–mediated Cl^- influx may explain postsynaptic hyperpolarization by A_1 activation in some cases. Presynaptic A_1 stimulation modifies voltage-dependent Ca^{2+} channels, lessening Ca^{2+} influx during depolarization, which limits exocytosis of neurotransmitter. Therefore, activation of A_1 receptors prevents release of neurotransmitters presynaptically and inhibits their responses postsynaptically.[9]

In the central and autonomic nervous systems, A_1 receptors reside on presynaptic and postsynaptic membranes, where they serve as inhibitory modulators for numerous neurotransmitter systems; they are particularly prevalent in association with glutamatergic neurons in the CNS.[126] The A_1 receptor is prevalent throughout the central nervous system, with high levels in the cerebral cortex, hippocampus, cerebellum, thalamus, brain stem, and spinal cord. A_1 receptor stimulation also produces sedation and is important in sleep regulation. Other functions attributed to A_1 receptors include neuroprotection, anxiolysis, temperature reduction, anticonvulsant activity, and spinal analgesia.[9]

Peripheral A_1 receptor activation produces bronchoconstriction, decreased glomerular filtration, decreased heart rate, slowed atrioventricular conduction, and decreased atrial myocardial contractility.[66]

In the CNS, A_{2A} receptors demonstrate limited distribution. They are concentrated on cerebral vasculature and produce vasodilation when stimulated.[66] Additionally, A_{2A} receptors are especially prevalent on neurons in the striatum, where they inhibit the activity of D_2 receptors.[126] Antagonism of A_{2A} receptors in the striatum increases dopamine-mediated motor activity without the dyskinesia that commonly occur with DA agonists.[126] Some A_{2A} receptors are found presynaptically located as heteromers with A_1 receptors. They act to diminish the inhibition of presynaptic A_1 receptors when adenosine concentrations increase.[29] Under normal conditions the presynaptic A_{2A} receptors are relatively inactive.

A_{2B} receptors are expressed diffusely throughout the brain, and are most commonly identified on glial cells. A_{2B} receptors demonstrate low affinity for adenosine, and little is known of their physiologic role.[9,89] At least some A_{2A} and A_{2B} receptors are coupled to G_s. The rise in cAMP concentration resulting from A_{2A} activation on cerebral vasculature and elsewhere explains vasodilatation.[130] For example, peripheral A_2 receptor activation also results in coronary artery vasodilation.[138]

A_3 receptors express low affinity for adenosine. In the CNS, A_3 receptors are expressed primarily in the hippocampus and thalamus. A_3 receptors act through G proteins to decrease adenylate cyclase activity and increase phospholipase C activity.[9] The low concentrations of adenosine found during normal metabolism minimally activate A_3 receptors to produce inhibitory effects. During times of excessive ATP degradation (eg, hypoxia, seizures), adenosine accumulates at and activates A_3 receptors to produce complex responses that appear to enhance ischemic cellular injury and death, at least in part through disinhibition of presynaptic metabotropic glutamate receptor responses. Thus, A_3 receptor antagonists are being examined for neuroprotective actions.[66]

ADENOSINE AND SEIZURE TERMINATION

In humans and in animal models of status epilepticus, including those from xenobiotics, there are two alternating phases of electrical activity noted on electroencephalography. Periods of high-frequency spike activity (ictal) are accompanied by marked increases in cerebral oxygen consumption and metabolic requirements and alternate with interictal periods of isolated spike waves during which metabolic demands are less. The high-frequency phase lasts only a few minutes before suddenly terminating, sometimes with a few seconds of electrocerebral silence. A gradual increase in electrical activity during the interictal phase eventually leads to a recurrence of high-frequency spike activity.[4]

These periodic, spontaneous self-terminations of high-frequency electrical activity initially occur before neurons exhaust oxygen and energy supplies and result from adenosine released from depolarizing neurons (and probably glial cells).[4,16] Adenosine acts on presynaptic receptors to prevent further release of excitatory neurotransmitters and acts on postsynaptic receptors to inhibit their actions.[16]

Any xenobiotic that directly or indirectly enhances adenosine's action at A_1 receptors in the brain will usually exhibit anticonvulsant activity. Conversely, A_1 receptor antagonists lower the seizure threshold and make seizure termination more difficult and less likely to respond to anticonvulsants. Xenobiotics that antagonize A_{2A} receptors produce cerebral vasoconstriction and may limit oxygen delivery during times of increased demand.[4,16]

XENOBIOTICS

Table 13–12 provides examples of xenobiotics that affect adenosine receptors.

Direct Adenosine Agonists ADAC (adenosine amine congener) is a direct A_1 receptor agonist used in the treatment of Huntington disease.[9] Tecadenoson is a selective A_1 receptor agonist that is used for treatment of supraventricular tachycardia.[42]

Indirect Adenosine Agonists Papaverine and dipyridamole inhibit adenosine uptake.[49] Like other adenosine agonists, papaverine and dipyridamole demonstrate anticonvulsant activity when injected into the CNS. Such actions are not achievable with safe systemic doses.

In addition to their actions at $GABA_A$ receptors, benzodiazepines inhibit adenosine uptake.[88] This may explain observations that methylxanthines, potent adenosine receptor antagonists, have reversed benzodiazepine-induced sedation in humans. The potencies of benzodiazepines as inhibitors of adenosine uptake show good correlation with clinical anxiolytic and anticonflict potencies, suggesting that such inhibition contributes to their action. The anticonvulsant effect of large doses of flumazenil also results, at least in part, from inhibition of adenosine uptake. Carbamazepine inhibits adenosine uptake, although this is not thought to account for most anticonvulsive action.

TABLE 13–12. Examples of Xenobiotics That Affect Adenosine Receptors

Adenosine agonism	Inhibit adenosine deaminase
Direct agonists	Acadesine
Adenosine	Dipyridamole
ADAC (adenosine amine congener)	Pentostatin
Tecadenoson	Inhibit adenosine kinase
Inhibit uptake	Acadesine
Acadesine	Increase adenosine release
Acetate[a]	Opioids
Benzodiazepines	Adenosine antagonism
Calcium channel blockers	A_1 blockade
Carbamazepine	Caffeine
Cyclic antidepressants	Carbamazepine
Dipyridamole	Theophylline
Ethanol[a]	A_2 blockade
Indomethacin	Caffeine
Papaverine	Theophylline

[a] Ethanol is metabolized to acetate, which inhibits adenosine uptake.

Adenosine may mediate many of the acute and chronic motor effects of ethanol on the brain. Ethanol, probably through its metabolite, acetate, prevents adenosine uptake, raising synaptic adenosine concentrations.[12] Excessive stimulation of several adenosine receptors in the cerebellum may explain much of the motor impairment from low ethanol concentrations. In fact, animals made tolerant to ethanol develop cross-tolerance to adenosine agonists. In mice, adenosine receptor agonists increase ethanol-induced incoordination, while adenosine antagonists decrease this intoxicating response.[127]

There are numerous inhibitors of adenosine uptake, including propentofylline, nimodipine, cyclic antidepressants, and other calcium channel blockers.[119,121] A_1 receptors located at the spinal cord are important modulators of pain transmission. Cyclic antidepressant-induced inhibition of adenosine uptake may explain some of their effectiveness in treating neuropathic pain.[49] The analgesic effectiveness of opioids can be partially attributed to their ability to increase the release of adenosine within the spinal cord.[9,49]

Dipyridamole inhibits adenosine deaminase, raising adenosine concentrations. During times of elevated adenosine concentrations that occur with cardiac or cerebral ischemia, acadesine further enhances adenosine's beneficial actions by three mechanisms: inhibition of adenosine kinase, inhibition of adenosine deaminase, and inhibition of adenosine uptake.[111]

Adenosine Antagonists The main adenosine antagonists of toxicologic concern are methylxanthines. Theophylline and caffeine are selective P_1 antagonists, blocking both A_1 and A_2 receptors.[9] The response to methylxanthines by A_3 receptors varies widely, depending on the species. Human A_3 receptors demonstrate very low affinity for methylxanthines.[89]

Peripherally, methylxanthines produce excessive release of catecholamines from peripheral nerve endings (and probably the adrenal gland) by blocking presynaptic A_1 receptors. In turn, catecholamine-mediated responses are exaggerated by blockade of inhibitory postsynaptic A_1 receptors on end organs.[4]

Centrally, enhanced release and actions of excitatory neurotransmitters (eg, glutamate) explain methylxanthine-induced convulsions that are frequently refractory to anticonvulsants. The reasons why theophylline convulsions carry such a high mortality stem from lack of A_1-mediated self-termination (continual high-frequency spike activity and large metabolic demands), compounded by vasoconstriction caused by blockade of A_2 receptors. $GABA_A$ receptor agonism, especially by barbiturates, most effectively prevents and terminates methylxanthine-induced seizures. Phenytoin not only is ineffective in treating theophylline-induced seizures, but may actually increase the likelihood of seizures and mortality.[14]

Like phenytoin, carbamazepine's major anticonvulsant effect results from Na^+ channel blockade. Unlike phenytoin, carbamazepine antagonizes A_1 receptors.[31,34] This may explain the higher frequency of seizures after carbamazepine overdose than after phenytoin overdose. The absence of A_2 blockade by carbamazepine theoretically allows for increases in cerebral blood flow to meet metabolic demands of the seizing brain.

SUMMARY

Neurotransmitter systems share common physiologic features, including neurotransmitter uptake, vesicle membrane pumps, ion trapping of neurotransmitters within vesicles, calcium-dependent exocytosis, and receptors coupled to either G proteins or to ion channels. It is not surprising, then, that a single pharmacologic agent frequently produces effects on several different neurotransmitter systems.

As the number of new xenobiotics encountered by man continues to grow, an understanding of their molecular actions in the nervous system helps the physician to anticipate and better understand various pharmacologic and adverse effects resulting from therapeutic or toxic doses.

REFERENCES

1. Albers RW: Membrane transport. In: Seigel GJ, Agranoff BW, Albers RW, Fisher SK, Uhler MD, eds: *Basic Neurochemistry*, 6th ed. Phildelphia: Lippincott Williams & Wilkins; 1999: 95-118.
2. Aprison MH, Galvez-Ruano E, Lipkowitz KB: Identification of a second glycine-like fragment on the strychnine molecule. *J Neurosci Res.* 1995;40:396-400.
3. Aragon C, Lopez-Corcuera B: Structure, function and regulation of glycine neurotransporters. *Eur J Pharmacol.* 2003;479:249-262.
4. Avsar E, Empson RM: Adenosine acting via A1 receptors, controls the transition to status epilepticus-like behaviour in an in vitro model of epilepsy. *Neuropharmacology.* 2004;47:427-437.
5. Baba A, Cooper JR: The action of black widow spider venom on cholinergic mechanisms in synaptosomes. *J Neurochem.* 1980;34:1369-1379.
6. Bak LK, Schousboe A, Waagepetersen HS: The glutamate/GABA-glutamine cycle: Aspects of transport, neurotransmitter homeostasis and ammonia transfer. *J Neurochem.* 2006;98:641-53.
7. Bali M, Akabas MH: Defining the propofol binding site location on the $GABA_A$ receptor. *Mol Pharmacol.* 2004;65:68-76.
8. Barnard EA, Skolnick P, Olsen RW, et al.: International Union of Pharmacology. XV. Subtypes of gamma-aminobutyric acidA receptors: Classification on the basis of subunit structure and receptor function. *Pharmacol Rev.* 1998;50:291-313.
9. Benarroch EE: Adenosine and its receptors: Multiple modulatory functions and potential therapeutic targets for neurologic disease. *Neurology.* 2008;70:231-236.
10. Berkels R, Taubert D, Grundemann D, Schomig E: Agmatine signaling: Odds and threads. *Cardiovasc Drug Rev.* 2004;22:7-16.
11. Bernasconi R, Mathivet P, Bischoff S, Marescaux C: Gamma-hydroxybutyric acid: An endogenous neuromodulator with abuse potential? *Trends Pharmacol Sci.* 1999;20:135-141.
12. Bettler B, Mulle C: Review: Neurotransmitter receptors. II. AMPA and kainate receptors. *Neuropharmacology.* 1995;34:123-139.
13. Bhana N, Goa KL, McClellan KJ: Dexmedetomidine. *Drugs.* 2000;59:263-268; discussion 9-70.
14. Blake KV, Massey KL, Hendeles L, et al.: Relative efficacy of phenytoin and phenobarbital for the prevention of theophylline-induced seizures in mice. *Ann Emerg Med.* 1988;17:1024-1028.
15. Bloom FE: Neurotransmission and the central nervous system. In: Hardman JG, Limbird LE, Molinoff PB, Ruddon RW, Gilman AG, eds.: *The Pharmacological Basis of Therapeutics,* 9th ed. New York: McGraw-Hill; 1995; 267-293.
16. Boison D: Adenosine and epilepsy: From therapeutic rationale to new therapeutic strategies. *Neuroscientist.* 2005;11:25-36.
17. Bormann J: The 'ABC' of GABA receptors. *Trends Pharmacol Sci.* 2000;21:16-19.
18. Bousquet P, Bruban V, Schann S, et al.: Participation of imidazoline receptors and alpha(2-)-adrenoceptors in the central hypotensive effects of imidazoline-like drugs. *Ann N Y Acad Sci.* 1999;881:272-278.
19. Bousquet P, Feldman J: Drugs acting on imidazoline receptors: A review of their pharmacology, their use in blood pressure control and their potential interest in cardioprotection. *Drugs.* 1999;58:799-812.
20. Bowery NG, Enna SJ: γ-Aminobutyric $acid_B$ receptors: First of the functional metabotropic heterodimers. *J Pharmacol Exp Ther.* 2000;292:2-7.
21. Boyer EW, Shannon M: The serotonin syndrome. *N Engl J Med.* 2005;352:1112-1120.
22. Briscoe JG, Curry SC, Gerkin RD, Ruiz RR: Pemoline-induced choreoathetosis and rhabdomyolysis. *Med Toxicol Adverse Drug Exp.* 1988;3:72-76.
23. Buscher R, Herrmann V, Insel PA: Human adrenoceptor polymorphisms: Evolving recognition of clinical importance. *Trends Pharmacol Sci.* 1999;20:94-99.
24. Cagetti E, Liang J, Spigelman I, Olsen RW: Withdrawal from chronic intermittent ethanol treatment changes subunit composition, reduces synaptic function, and decreases behavioral responses to positive allosteric modulators of $GABA_A$ receptors. *Mol Pharmacol.* 2003;63:53-64.

25. Carmichael FJ, Orrego H, Israel Y: Acetate-induced adenosine mediated effects of ethanol. *Alcohol Alcohol Suppl.* 1993;2:411-418.
26. Carpenter CL, Marks SS, Watson DL, Greenberg DA: Dextromethorphan and dextrorphan as calcium channel antagonists. *Brain Res.* 1988;439:372-375.
27. Catarzi D, Colotta V, Varano F: Competitive AMPA receptor antagonists. *Med Res Rev.* 2007;27:239-378.
28. Chameau P, van Hooft JA: Serotonin 5-HT(3) receptors in the central nervous system. *Cell Tissue Res.* 2006;326:573-581.
29. Ciruela F, Casado V, Rodrigues RJ, et al: Presynaptic control of striatal glutamatergic neurotransmission by adenosine A1-A2A receptor heteromers. *J Neurosci.* 2006;26:2080-2087.
30. Clapham DE: Direct G protein activation of ion channels? *Annu Rev Neurosci.* 1994;17:441-464.
31. Clark M, Post RM: Carbamazepine, but not caffeine, is highly selective for adenosine A1 binding sites. *Eur J Pharmacol.* 1989;164:399-401.
32. Clark RF, Curry SC: Organophosphates and carbamates. In: Reisdorff E, Roberts MR, Wiegenstein JG, eds.: *Pediatric Emergency Medicine.* Philadelphia: WB Saunders; 1993: 684-693.
33. Costedio MM, Hyman N, Mawe GM: Serotonin and its role in colonic function and in gastrointestinal disorders. *Dis Colon Rectum.* 2007;50:376-388.
34. Czuczwar SJ, Szczepanik B, Wamil A, et al.: Differential effects of agents enhancing purinergic transmission upon the antielectroshock efficacy of carbamazepine, diphenylhydantoin, diazepam, phenobarbital, and valproate in mice. *J Neural Transm Gen Sect.* 1990;81:153-166.
35. Da Settimo F, Taliani S, Trincavelli ML, et al.: GABA A/Bz receptor subtypes as targets for selective drugs. *Curr Med Chem.* 2007;14:2680-2701.
36. Dakshinamurti K, Sharma SK, Sundaram M: Domoic acid induced seizure activity in rats. *Neurosci Lett.* 1991;127:193-197.
37. De Kock MF, Lavand'homme PM: The clinical role of NMDA receptor antagonists for the treatment of postoperative pain. *Best Prac Res Clin Anaesthesiol.* 2007;21:85-98.
38. Doble A: The role of excitotoxicity in neurodegenerative disease: Implications for therapy. *Pharmacol Ther.* 1999;81:163-221.
39. Docherty JR: Subtypes of functional alpha1- and alpha2-adrenoceptors. *Eur J Pharmacol.* 1998;361:1-15.
40. Dravid SM, Erreger K, Yuan H, et al.: Subunit-specific mechanisms and proton sensitivity of NMDA receptor channel block. *J Physiol.* 2007;581:107-128.
41. Eglen RM, Hudson AL, Kendall DA, et al.: 'Seeing through a glass darkly': Casting light on imidazoline 'I' sites. *Trends Pharmacol Sci.* 1998;19:381-390.
42. Ellenbogen KA, O'Neill G, Prystowsky EN, et al.: Trial to evaluate the management of paroxysmal supraventricular tachycardia during an electrophysiology study with tecadenoson. *Circulation.* 2005;111:3202-3208.
43. Eneanya DI, Bianchine JR, Duran DO, Andresen BD: The actions of metabolic fate of disulfiram. *Annu Rev Pharmacol Toxicol.* 1981;21:575-596.
44. Faingold CL, Browning RA: Mechanisms of anticonvulsant drug action. I. Drugs primarily used for generalized tonic-clonic and partial epilepsies. *Eur J Pediatr.* 1987;146:2-7.
45. Feigenbaum JJ, Howard SG: Gamma hydroxybutyrate is not a GABA agonist. *Prog Neurobiol.* 1996;50:1-7.
46. Feldman J, Greney H, Monassier L, et al.: Does a second generation of centrally acting antihypertensive drugs really exist? *J Auton Nerv Syst.* 1998;72:94-97.
47. Follesa P, Mancuso L, Biggio F, et al.: Changes in GABA(A) receptor gene expression induced by withdrawal of, but not by long-term exposure to, zaleplon or zolpidem. *Neuropharmacology.* 2002;42:191-198.
48. Foster AC, Kemp JA: Glutamate- and GABA-based CNS therapeutics. *Curr Opin Pharmacol.* 2006;6:7-17.
49. Fredholm BB, Chen JF, Masino SA, Vaugeois JM: Actions of adenosine at its receptors in the CNS: Insights from knockouts and drugs. *Ann Rev of Pharmacol Toxicol.* 2005;45:385-412.
50. Gee KW, McCauley LD, Lan NC: A putative receptor for neurosteroids on the $GABA_A$ receptor complex: The pharmacological properties and therapeutic potential of epalons. *Crit Rev Neurobiol.* 1995;9:207-227.
51. Geyer MA, Vollenweider FX: Serotonin research: Contributions to understanding psychoses. *Trends Pharmacol Sci.* 2008;29:445-453.
52. Gibson KM, Hoffmann GF, Hodson AK, et al.: 4-Hydroxybutyric acid and the clinical phenotype of succinic semialdehyde dehydrogenase deficiency, an inborn error of GABA metabolism. *Neuropediatrics.* 1998;29:14-22.
53. Gillman PK: A systematic review of the serotonergic effects of mirtazapine in humans: Implications for its dual action status. *Hum Psychopharmacol.* 2006;21:117-125.
54. Gogas KR: Glutamate-based therapeutic approaches: NR2B receptor antagonists. *Curr Opin Pharmacol.* 2006;6:68-74.
55. Gupta H, Verma D, Ahuja RK, et al,: Intrathecal co-administration of morphine and nimodipine produces higher antinociceptive effect by synergistic interaction as evident by injecting different doses of each drug in rats. *Eur J Pharmacol.* 2007;561:46-53.
56. Hara K, Minami K, Sata T: The effects of tramadol and its metabolite on glycine, γ-aminobutyric $acid_A$, and *N*-methyl-d-aspartate receptors expressed in *Xenopus oocytes. Anesth Analg.* 2005;100:1400-1405.
57. Hasler WL: Serotonin receptor physiology: Relation to emesis. *Dig Dis Sci.* 1999;44:108S-113S.
58. Hawgood B, Bon C: Snake venom presynaptic toxins. In: Tu AT, ed. *Reptile Venoms and Toxins: Handbook of Natural Toxins.* Vol. 5. New York: Marcel Dekker; 1991: 3-52.
59. Head GA, Chan CK, Burke SL: Relationship between imidazoline and alpha2-adrenoceptors involved in the sympatho-inhibitory actions of centrally acting antihypertensive agents. *J Auton Nerv Syst.* 1998;72:163-169.
60. Head GA, Mayorov DN: Imidazoline receptors, novel agents and therapeutic potential. *Cardiovas Hematol Agents Med Chem.* 2006;4:17-32.
61. Hedenmalm K, Guzey C, Dahl ML, et al.: Risk factors for extrapyramidal symptoms during treatment with selective serotonin reuptake inhibitors, including cytochrome P-450 enzyme, and serotonin and dopamine transporter and receptor polymorphisms. *J Clin Psychopharmacol.* 2006;26:192-197.
62. Hesp BR, Clarkson AN, Sawant PM, Kerr DS: Domoic acid preconditioning and seizure induction in young and aged rats. *Epilepsy Res.* 2007;76:103-112.
63. Hobson DE, Pourcher E, Martin WR: Ropinirole and pramipexole, the new agonists. *Can J Neurol Sci.* 1999;26 Suppl 2:S27-33.
64. Hold KM, Sirisoma NS, Ikeda T, et al.: Alpha-thujone (the active component of absinthe): γ-Aminobutyric acid type A receptor modulation and metabolic detoxification. *Proc Natl Acad Sci U S A.* 2000;97:3826-3831.
65. Insel PA: Seminars in medicine of the Beth Israel Hospital, Boston. Adrenergic receptors—evolving concepts and clinical implications. *N Engl J Med.* 1996;334:580-585.
66. Jacobson KA, Gao ZG: Adenosine receptors as therapeutic targets. *Nat Rev Drug Discov.* 2006;5:247-264.
67. Javitt DC: Glutamate as a therapeutic target in psychiatric disorders. *Mol Psychiatry.* 2004;9:984-997.
68. Johnson M: The beta-adrenoceptor. *Am J Respir Crit Care Med.* 1998;158:S146-153.
69. Johnston GA: Medicinal chemistry and molecular pharmacology of GABA(C) receptors. *Curr Top Med Chem.* 2002;2:903-913.
70. Joy RM, Albertson TE: In vivo assessment of the importance of GABA in convulsant and anticonvulsant drug action. *Epilepsy Res Suppl.* 1992;8:63-75.
71. Kaakkola S: Clinical pharmacology, therapeutic use and potential of COMT inhibitors in Parkinson's disease. *Drugs.* 2000;59:1233-1250.
72. Kalia LV, Kalia SK, Salter MW: NMDA receptors in clinical neurology: Excitatory times ahead. *Lancet Neurol.* 2008;7:742-755.
73. Kenny PJ, Markou A: The ups and downs of addiction: Role of metabotropic glutamate receptors. *Trends Pharmacol Sci.* 2004;25:265-272.
74. Kew JN, Kemp JA: Ionotropic and metabotropic glutamate receptor structure and pharmacology. *Psychopharmacology.* 2005;179:4-29.
75. Khan ZP, Ferguson CN, Jones RM: Alpha-2 and imidazoline receptor agonists. Their pharmacology and therapeutic role. *Anaesthesia.* 1999;54:146-165.
76. Kiowski W, Hulthen UL, Ritz R, Buhler FR: Alpha 2 adrenoceptor-mediated vasoconstriction of arteries. *Clin Pharmacol Ther.* 1983;34:565-569.
77. Klawans HL, Weiner WJ: The pharmacology of choreatic movement disorders. *Prog Neurobiol.* 1976;6:49-80.
78. Korpi ER, Mattila MJ, Wisden W, Luddens H: GABA(A)-receptor subtypes: Clinical efficacy and selectivity of benzodiazepine site ligands. *Ann Med.* 1997;29:275-282.
79. Krueger KE, Papadopoulos V: Mitochondrial benzodiazepine receptors and the regulation of steroid biosynthesis. *Annu Rev Pharmacol Toxicol.* 1992;32:211-237.
80. Kuo YH, Defoort B, Getahun H, et al.: Comparison of urinary amino acids and trace elements (copper, zinc and manganese) of recent neurolathyrism patients and healthy controls from Ethiopia. *Clin Biochem.* 2007;40:397-402.
81. Lachowicz JE, Sibley DR: Molecular characteristics of mammalian dopamine receptors. *Pharmacol Toxicol.* 1997;81:105-113.
82. Landis E, Shore E: Yohimbine-induced bronchospasm. *Chest.* 1989;96:1424.
83. Lefkowitz RJ: Historical review: A brief history and personal retrospective of seven-transmembrane receptors. *Trends Pharmacol Sci.* 2004;25:413-422.

84. Lefkowitz RJ, Hoffman BB, Taylor P: The autonomic and somatic motor nervous systems. In: Hardman JG, Limbird LE, Molinoff PB, Ruddon RW, Gilman AG, eds: *The Pharmacological Basis of Therapeutics,* 9 ed. New York: McGraw-Hill; 1995: 105-139.
85. Li J, Stokes SA, Woeckener A: A tale of novel intoxication: A review of the effects of gamma-hydroxybutyric acid with recommendations for management. *Ann Emerg Med.* 1998;31:729-736.
86. Liggett SB: Molecular and genetic basis of beta2-adrenergic receptor function. *J Allergy Clin Immunol.* 1999;104:S42-S46.
87. Linden CH, Vellman WP, Rumack B: Yohimbine: A new street drug. *Ann Emerg Med.* 1985;14:1002-1004.
88. Listos J, Malec D, Fidecka S: Adenosine receptor antagonists intensify the benzodiazepine withdrawal signs in mice. *Pharmacol Rep.* 2006;58:643-651.
89. Livingston M, Heaney LG, Ennis M: Adenosine, inflammation and asthma—a review. *Inflamm Res.* 2004;53:171-178.
90. Loscher W, Dekundy A, Nagel J, et al.: mGlu1 and mGlu5 receptor antagonists lack anticonvulsant efficacy in rodent models of difficult-to-treat partial epilepsy. *Neuropharmacology.* 1006;50:1006-1015.
91. Lovinger DM, Homanics GE: Tonic for what ails us? High-affinity $GABA_A$ receptors and alcohol. *Alcohol.* 2007;41:139-143.
92. Lowe TL, Cohen DJ, Detlor J, et al.: Stimulant medications precipitate Tourette's syndrome. *JAMA.* 1982;247:1168-1169.
93. Lummis SC, Buckingham SD, Rauh JJ, Sattelle DB: Blocking actions of heptachlor at an insect central nervous system GABA receptor. *Proc R Soc Lond B Biol Sci.* 1990;240:97-106.
94. Lynch JW, Rajendra S, Barry PH, Schofield PR: Mutations affecting the glycine receptor agonist transduction mechanism convert the competitive antagonist, picrotoxin, into an allosteric potentiator. *J Biol Chem.* 1995;270:13799-13806.
95. Maitre M: The gamma-hydroxybutyrate signalling system in brain: Organization and functional implications. *Prog Neurobiol.* 1997;51:337-361.
96. Malatynska E, Knapp RJ, Ikeda M, Yamamura HI: Antidepressants and seizure-interactions at the GABA-receptor chloride-ionophore complex. *Life Sci.* 1988;43:303-307.
97. Malcangio M, Bowery NG: GABA and its receptors in the spinal cord. *Trends Pharmacol Sci.* 1996;17:457-462.
98. Marek GJ: Metabotropic glutamate 2/3 receptors as drug targets. *Curr Opin Pharmacol.* 2004;4:18-22.
99. Mascia MP, Mihic SJ, Valenzuela CF, et al.: A single amino acid determines differences in ethanol actions on strychnine-sensitive glycine receptors. *Mol Pharmacol.* 1996;50:402-406.
100. Matute C, Domercq M, Sanchez-Gomez MV: Glutamate-mediated glial injury: Mechanisms and clinical importance. *Glia.* 2006;53:212-224.
101. McDaniel KD: Clinical pharmacology of monoamine oxidase inhibitors. *Clin Neuropharmacol.* 1986;9:207-234.
102. Meir A, Ginsburg S, Butkevich A, et al.: Ion channels in presynaptic nerve terminals and control of transmitter release. *Physiol Rev.* 1999;79:1019-1088.
103. Mihic SJ: Acute effects of ethanol on GABAA and glycine receptor function. *Neurochem Int.* 1999;35:115-123.
104. Millan JM MP, Bockaert J, La Cour CM: Signaling at G-protein-coupled serotonin receptors: Recent advances and future research directions. *Trends Pharmacol Sci.* 2008;29:454-464.
105. Miller J, Robinson A, Percy AK: Acute isoniazid poisoning in childhood. *Am J Dis Child.* 1980;134:290-292.
106. Miller RJ: Presynaptic receptors. *Annu Rev Pharmacol Toxicol.* 1998;38:201-227.
107. Mills KC: Serotonin syndrome. A clinical update. *Crit Care Clin.* 1997;13:763-783.
108. Modell JG, Tandon R, Beresford TP: Dopaminergic activity of the antimuscarinic antiparkinsonian agents. *J Clin Psychopharmacol.* 1989;9:347-351.
109. Mody I, Glykys J, Wei W: A new meaning for "Gin & Tonic": Tonic inhibition as the target for ethanol action in the brain. *Alcohol.* 2007;41:145-153.
110. Mohammad-Zadeh LF, Moses L, Gwaltney-Brant SM: Serotonin: A review. *Vet Pharmacol Ther.* 2008;31:187-199.
111. Muller CE, Scior T: Adenosine receptors and their modulators. *Pharm Acta Helv.* 1993;68:77-111.
112. Muller CP, Carey RJ, Huston JP, De Souza Silva MA: Serotonin and psychostimulant addiction: Focus on 5-HT1A-receptors. *Prog Neurobiol.* 2007;81:133-178.
113. Newman CM, Starkey I, Buller N, et al.: Effects of sumatriptan and eletriptan on diseased epicardial coronary arteries. *Eur J Clin Pharmacol.* 2005;61:733-742.
114. Nilsson M, Hansson E, Ronnback L: Transport of valproate and its effects on GABA uptake in astroglial primary culture. *Neurochem Res.* 1990;15:763-767.
115. Oja SS, Kontro P. Neurochemical aspects of amino acid transmitters and modulators. *Med Biol.* 1987;65:143-152.
116. Olivier B, van Oorschot R: 5-HT1B receptors and aggression: A review. *Eur J Pharmacol.* 2005;526:207-217.
117. Olsen RW: The GABA postsynaptic membrane receptor-ionophore complex. Site of action of convulsant and anticonvulsant drugs. *Mol Cell Biochem.* 1981;39:261-279.
118. Palmer T: Agents acting at the neuromuscular junction and autonomic ganglia. In: Hardman JG, Limbird LE, Molinoff PB, Ruddon RW, Gilman AG, eds: *The Pharmacological Basis of Therapeutics,* 9 ed. New York: McGraw-Hill; 1995:177-197.
119. Parkinson FE, Rudolphi KA, Fredholm BB: Propentofylline: A nucleoside transport inhibitor with neuroprotective effects in cerebral ischemia. *Gen Pharmacol.* 1994;25:1053-1058.
120. Paterson D, Nordberg A: Neuronal nicotinic receptors in the human brain. *Prog Neurobiol.* 2000;61:75-111.
121. Pelleg A, Porter RS: The pharmacology of adenosine. *Pharmacotherapy.* 1990;10:157-174.
122. Pellock JM, Faught E, Leppik IE, et al.: Felbamate: Consensus of current clinical experience. *Epilepsy Res.* 2006;71:89-101.
123. Phillis JW, O'Regan MH: The role of adenosine in the central actions of the benzodiazepines. *Prog Neuropsychopharmacol Biol Psychiatry.* 1988;12:389-404.
124. Pin JP, Bockaert J: Get receptive to metabotropic glutamate receptors. *Curr Opin Neurobiol.* 1995;5:342-349.
125. Pinheiro PS, Mulle C: Presynaptic glutamate receptors: Physiological functions and mechanisms of action. *Nat Rev Neurosci.* 2008;9:423-436.
126. Pinna A, Wardas J, Simola N, Morelli M: New therapies for the treatment of Parkinson's disease: Adenosine A2A receptor antagonists. *Life Sci.* 2005;77:3259-3267.
127. Prediger RD, da Silva GE, Batista LC, et al.: Activation of adenosine A1 receptors reduces anxiety-like behavior during acute ethanol withdrawal (hangover) in mice. *Neuropsychopharmacology.* 2006;31:2210-2220.
128. Proenca P, Teixeira H, Pinheiro J, et al.: Fatal intoxication with tianeptine (Stablon). *Forensic Sci Int.* 2007;170:200-203.
129. Pucilowski O: Psychopharmacological properties of calcium channel inhibitors. *Psychopharmacology (Berl).* 1992;109:12-29.
130. Ralevic V, Burnstock G: Receptors for purines and pyrimidines. *Pharmacol Rev.* 1998;50:413-492.
131. Redgrave P, Prescott TJ, Gurney K: Is the short-latency dopamine response too short to signal reward error? *Trends Neurosci.* 1999;22:146-151.
132. Reis DJ, Regunathan S: Is agmatine a novel neurotransmitter in brain? *Trends Pharmacol Sci.* 2000;21:187-193.
133. Rho JM, Donevan SD, Rogawski MA: Barbiturate-like actions of the propanediol dicarbamates felbamate and meprobamate. *J Pharmacol Exp Ther.* 1997;280:1383-1391.
134. Richelson E: Receptor pharmacology of neuroleptics: Relation to clinical effects. *J Clin Psychiatry.* 1999;60 Suppl 10:5-14.
135. Rodriguez-Moreno A, Sihra TS: Metabotropic actions of kainate receptors in the CNS. *J Neurochem.* 2007;103:2121-2135.
136. Rudorfer MV, Potter WZ: Antidepressants. A comparative review of the clinical pharmacology and therapeutic use of the 'newer' versus the 'older' drugs. *Drugs.* 1989;37:713-738.
137. Santhakumar V, Wallner M, Otis TS: Ethanol acts directly on extrasynaptic subtypes of $GABA_A$ receptors to increase tonic inhibition. *Alcohol.* 2007;41:211-221.
138. Schepp CP, Reutershan J: Bench-to-bedside review: Adenosine receptors—promising targets in acute lung injury? *Crit Care.* 2008;12:226.
139. Scholz KP: Introductory perspective. In: Dunwiddie TV, Lovinger DM, eds: *Presynaptic Receptors in the Mammalian Brain.* Boston: Birkhauser; 1993: 1-11.
140. Sealfon SC: Dopamine receptors and locomotor responses: Molecular aspects. *Ann Neurol.* 2000;47:S12-19; discussion S9-21.
141. Selden BS, Curry SC: Anticholinergics. In: Reisdorff E, Roberts MR, Wiegenstein JG, eds: *Pediatric Emergency Medicine.* Philadelphia: WB Saunders; 1993: 693-700.
142. Shank RP, Gardocki JF, Streeter AJ, Maryanoff BE: An overview of the preclinical aspects of topiramate: Pharmacology, pharmacokinetics, and mechanism of action. *Epilepsia.* 2000;41 Suppl 1:S3-9.

143. Shim SS, Hammonds MD, Kee BS: Potentiation of the NMDA receptor in the treatment of schizophrenia: Focused on the glycine site. *Eur Arch Psy Clin Neurosci.* 2008;258:16-27.
144. Sieghart W: Structure and pharmacology of gamma-aminobutyric acid$_A$ receptor subtypes. *Pharmacol Rev.* 1995;47:181-234.
145. Sigel E, Buhr A: The benzodiazepine binding site of GABA$_A$ receptors. *Trends Pharmacol Sci.* 1997;18:425-429.
146. Simonds WF: G protein-regulated signaling dysfunction in human disease. *J Investig Med.* 2003;51:194-214.
147. Smith JM: Abuse of the antiparkinson drugs: A review of the literature. *J Clin Psychiatry.* 1980;41:351-354.
148. Smith TA: Type A gamma-aminobutyric acid (GABA$_A$) receptor subunits and benzodiazepine binding: Significance to clinical syndromes and their treatment. *Br J Biomed Sci.* 2001;58:111-121.
149. Solt K, Forman SA: Correlating the clinical actions and molecular mechanisms of general anesthetics. *Curr Opin Anaesthesiol.* 2007;20:300-306.
150. Southam E, Kirkby D, Higgins GA, Hagan RM: Lamotrigine inhibits monoamine uptake in vitro and modulates 5-hydroxytryptamine uptake in rats. *Eur J Pharmacol.* 1998;358:19-24.
151. Spanagel R, Weiss F: The dopamine hypothesis of reward: Past and current status. *Trends Neurosci.* 1999;22:521-527.
152. Squires RF, Saederup E: Antidepressants and metabolites that block GABA$_A$ receptors coupled to 35S-t-butylbicyclophosphorothionate binding sites in rat brain. *Brain Res.* 1988;441:15-22.
153. Stahl SM. Anticonvulsants as anxiolytics, part 1: Tiagabine and other anticonvulsants with actions on GABA. *J Clin Psychiatry.* 2004;65:291-292.
154. Strosberg AD. Association of beta 3-adrenoceptor polymorphism with obesity and diabetes: Current status. *Trends Pharmacol Sci.* 1997;18: 449-454.
155. Sulzer D, Maidment NT, Rayport S: Amphetamine and other weak bases act to promote reverse transport of dopamine in ventral midbrain neurons. *J Neurochem.* 1993;60:527-535.
156. Sulzer D, Rayport S: Amphetamine and other psychostimulants reduce pH gradients in midbrain dopaminergic neurons and chromaffin granules: A mechanism of action. *Neuron.* 1990;5:797-808.
157. Sulzer D, Sonders MS, Poulsen NW, Galli A: Mechanisms of neurotransmitter release by amphetamines: A review. *Progr Neurobiol.* 2005;75: 406-433.
158. Sundstrom-Poromaa I, Smith DH, Gong QH, et al.: Hormonally regulated alpha(4)beta(2)delta GABA(A) receptors are a target for alcohol. *Nat Neurosci.* 2002;5:721-722.
159. Swanson CJ, Bures M, Johnson MP, et al.: Metabotropic glutamate receptors as novel targets for anxiety and stress disorders. *Nat Rev Drug Discov.* 2005;4:131-144.
160. Taylor CP: Mechanisms of new antiepileptic drugs. In: Delgado-Escueta AV, Jasper HH, Herbert H, eds: *Jasper's Basic Mechanisms of the Epilepsies,* 3rd ed. Philadelphia: Lippincott Williams & Wilkins; 1999: 1018.
161. Terry AV BJ, Wilson, C: Cognitive dysfunction in neuropsychiatric disorders: Selected serotonin receptor subtypes as therapeutic targets. *Behav Brain Res.* 2008;195:30-38.
162. Tuncel M, Wang Z, Arbique D, et al.: Mechanism of the blood pressure-raising effect of cocaine in humans. *Circulation.* 2002;105:1054-1059.
163. Uwai K, Ohashi K, Takaya Y, et al.: Exploring the structural basis of neurotoxicity in C(17)-polyacetylenes isolated from water hemlock. *J Med Chem.* 2000;43:4508-4515.
164. Uwai K, Ohashi K, Takaya Y, et al.: Virol A, a toxic *trans*-polyacetylenic alcohol of Cicuta virosa, selectively inhibits the GABA-induced Cl^- current in acutely dissociated rat hippocampal CA1 neurons. *Brain Res.* 2001;889:174-180.
165. Vallone D, Picetti R, Borrelli E: Structure and function of dopamine receptors. *Neurosci Biobehav Rev.* 2000;24:125-132.
166. Wafford KA, Macaulay AJ, Fradley R, et al.: Differentiating the role of gamma-aminobutyric acid type A (GABA$_A$) receptor subtypes. *Biochem Soc Trans.* 2004;32:553-556.
167. Wallace KL: Antibiotic-induced convulsions. *Crit Care Clin.* 1997;13:741-762.
168. Wallner M, Hanchar HJ, Olsen RW: Ethanol enhances $\alpha4\beta3\delta$ and $\alpha6\beta3\beta$ γ-aminobutyric acid type A receptors at low concentrations known to affect humans. *Proc Natl Acad Sci U S A.* 2003;100:15218-15223.
169. Watt G, Theakston RD, Hayes CG, et al.: Positive response to edrophonium in patients with neurotoxic envenoming by cobras (Naja naja philippinensis). A placebo-controlled study. *N Engl J Med.* 1986;315:1444-1448.
170. Webb TI, Lynch JW: Molecular pharmacology of the glycine receptor chloride channel. *Curr Pharm Des.* 2007;13:2350-2367.
171. Weyer C, Gautier JF, Danforth E, Jr.: Development of beta 3-adrenoceptor agonists for the treatment of obesity and diabetes—an update. *Diabetes Metab.* 1999;25:11-21.
172. Whiting PJ, McKernan RM, Wafford KA: Structure and pharmacology of vertebrate GABAA receptor subtypes. *Int Rev Neurobiol.* 1995;38:95-138.
173. Wong CG, Gibson KM, Snead OC, 3rd: From the street to the brain: Neurobiology of the recreational drug gamma-hydroxybutyric acid. *Trends Pharmacol Sci.* 2004;25:29-34.
174. Xiao C, Shao X, Olive MF, et al.: Ethanol facilitates glutamatergic transmission to dopamine neurons in the ventral tegmental area. *Neuropsychopharmacology.* 2008.
175. Xiao RP, Zhu W, Zheng M, et al.: Subtype-specific alpha1- and beta-adrenoceptor signaling in the heart. *Trends Pharmacol Sci.* 2006;27:330-337.
176. Yang J, Wetterstrand C, Jones RS: Felbamate but not phenytoin or gabapentin reduces glutamate release by blocking presynaptic NMDA receptors in the entorhinal cortex. *Epilepsy Res.* 2007;77:157-164.
177. Youdim MB, Edmondson D, Tipton KF: The therapeutic potential of monoamine oxidase inhibitors. *Nat Rev Neurosci.* 2006;7:295-309.
178. Zeller A, Arras M, Jurd R, Rudolph U: Identification of a molecular target mediating the general anesthetic actions of pentobarbital. *Mol Pharmacol.* 2007;71:852-859.

CHAPTER 14
WITHDRAWAL PRINCIPLES

Richard J. Hamilton

In the central nervous system (CNS), excitatory neurons fire regularly, and inhibitory neurons inhibit the transmission of these impulses. Whenever action is required, the inhibitory tone diminishes, permitting the excitatory nerve impulses to travel to their end organs. Thus, all action in human neurophysiology can be considered to result from disinhibition.[56,104,108]

Tonic neurological activity of a xenobiotic produces an adaptive change in affected neurons. For example, tonic stimulation of inhibitory neurons reduces their activity so that the baseline level of function is regained. A withdrawal syndrome occurs when the constant presence of this xenobiotic is removed or reduced and the adaptive changes persist. In this example withdrawal produces a dysfunctional condition in which inhibitory neurotransmission is significantly reduced, essentially producing excitation (Fig. 14–1). Every withdrawal syndrome has two characteristics: (1) a pre-existing physiologic adaptation to a xenobiotic, the continuous presence of which prevents withdrawal, and (2) decreasing concentrations of that xenobiotic. In contrast, simple tolerance to a xenobiotic is characterized as a physiologic adaptation that shifts the dose–response curve to the right; that is, greater amounts of a xenobiotic are required to achieve a given effect. Patients with withdrawal syndromes have often developed tolerance, but tolerance does not require the continued presence of the xenobiotic to prevent withdrawal.[41,93]

The *Diagnostic and Statistical Manual of Mental Disorders, Fourth Edition* (DSM-IV) provides a helpful and descriptive set of criteria that mesh with our understanding of the pathophysiology of withdrawal syndromes.[32] According to DSM-IV, withdrawal is manifested by either of the following: (1) a characteristic withdrawal syndrome for the substance or (2) the same (or a closely related) substance is taken to relieve withdrawal symptoms. Note that either criterion fulfills this definition. Logically, all syndromes have the first criterion, so it is the presence of the second criterion that is critical to understanding physiology and therapy.

For the purposes of defining a unifying pathophysiologic pattern of withdrawal syndromes, this chapter considers syndromes in which both features are present. An analysis from this perspective distinguishes xenobiotics that affect the inhibitory neuronal pathways from those that affect the excitatory neuronal pathways, such as cocaine. According to this definition, cocaine does not produce a withdrawal syndrome but rather a postintoxication syndrome that often results in lethargy, hypersomnolence, movement disorders, and irritability. This syndrome does not meet the second of the DSM-IV criteria for a withdrawal syndrome because the same (or a closely related) substance is not taken to relieve or avoid withdrawal symptoms. This postintoxication syndrome, the so-called "crack crash" or "washed-out syndrome," is caused by prolonged use of cocaine, and patients ultimately return to their premorbid function without intervention.[81,94,107] This distinction is important for toxicologists, because (1) withdrawal syndromes that demonstrate both features of the DSM-IV criteria are treated with reinstatement and gradual withdrawal of a xenobiotic that has an effect on the receptor and (2) withdrawal syndromes that do not demonstrate the second feature require only supportive care and resolve spontaneously.

Finally, withdrawal syndromes are best described and treated according to the class of receptors that is primarily affected because this concept also organizes the approach to patient care. For each receptor and its agonists, research has identified genomic and nongenomic effects that produce neuroadaptation and withdrawal syndromes. Six mechanisms appear to be involved: (1) genomic mechanisms via mRNA; (2) second-messenger effects via protein kinases, cyclic adenosine monophosphate (cAMP),[47,49] and calcium ions; (3) receptor endocytosis; (4) expression of various receptor subtypes depending on location within the synapse (synaptic localization); (5) intracellular signaling via effects on other receptors; and (6) neurosteroid modulation. Some or all of these mechanisms are demonstrated in each of the known withdrawal syndromes.[57] These mechanisms develop in a surprisingly rapid fashion and modify the receptor and its function in such complex ways as to depend on the continued presence of the xenobiotic to prevent dysfunction.[55,70,74,76,92,109,112]

GABA$_A$ RECEPTORS (BARBITURATES, BENZODIAZEPINES, ETHANOL, VOLATILE SOLVENTS)

γ-Aminobutyric acid type A (GABA$_A$) receptors have separate binding sites for GABA, barbiturates, benzodiazepines, and picrotoxin, to name only a few xenobiotics (Chap. 13). Barbiturates and benzodiazepines bind to separate receptor sites and enhance the affinity for GABA$_A$ at its receptor site. GABA$_A$ receptors are part of a superfamily of ligand-gated ion channels, including nicotinic acetylcholine receptors and glycine receptors, that exist as pentamers arranged around a central ion channel.[96] When activated, they hyperpolarize the postsynaptic neuron by facilitating an inward chloride current (without a G protein messenger), decreasing the likelihood of the neuron firing an action potential.[56,87]

The GABA receptor is a pentamer comprised of 2 α subunits, 2 β subunits, and 1 additional subunit, most commonly γ, which is a key element in the benzodiazepine binding site. Each receptor has 2 GABA binding sites that are located in a homologous position to the benzodiazepine site between the α and β subunits. Although the mechanism is unclear, benzodiazepines have no direct functional effect without the presence of GABA. Conversely, certain barbiturates (perhaps all, in a dose-dependent manner) can directly increase the duration of channel opening, thereby producing a net increase in current flow without GABA binding.[39,74] This process has therapeutic implications and accounts for why high dose barbiturates are universally successful in stopping status epilepticus and treating severe withdrawal.

Recent evidence demonstrates that this prototypical pentameric GABA$_A$ receptor assembly is derived from permutations and combinations of 2, 3, 4, or even 5 different subunits. The subtypes of GABA receptors can even vary on the same cell.[74] In fact, GABA receptors are heterogeneous receptors with different subunits and distinct regional distribution. Although the preponderance of subtypes $\alpha_1\beta_2\gamma_2$, $\alpha_2\beta_3\gamma_2$, and $\alpha_3\beta_3\gamma_2$ account for 75% of GABA receptors, there are at least 16 others of import.[112] The recognition of additional subunits of GABA$_A$ receptors, has permitted the development of targeted pharmaceuticals.[6] For example, the drug zolpidem achieves its effect of hastened onset of sleep by targeting the BZ$_1$ receptor subunit of GABA$_A$.[91]

Previously, ethanol was thought to have GABA receptor activity, although a clearly identified binding site was not evident. Traditional explanations for this effect included (1) enhanced membrane fluidity and allosteric potentiation (so-called cross-coupling) of the 5 proteins that construct the GABA$_A$ receptor; (2) interaction with a portion of the receptor; and/or (3) enhanced GABA release.[20,56,58,90] Research

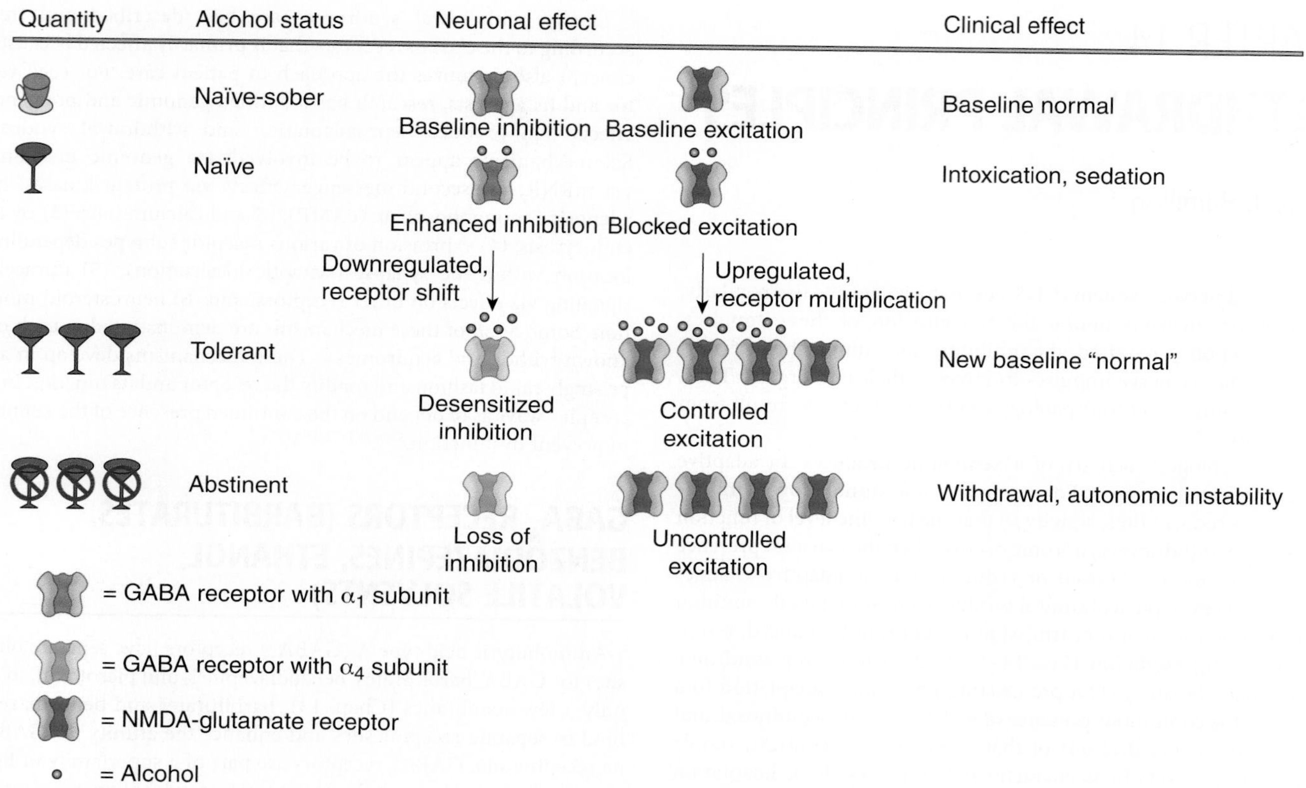

FIGURE 14–1. Alcohol intoxication, tolerance, and withdrawal. Alcohol consumption in alcohol-naive persons produces intoxication and sedation by simultaneous agonism at the γ-aminobutyric acid (GABA) receptor–chloride channel complex and antagonism at the *N*-methyl-D-aspartate (NMDA)-glutamate receptor. Continuous alcohol consumption leads to the development of tolerance through changes in both the GABA receptor–chloride channel complex (a subunit shift from α_1 to α_4 results in reduced sensitivity to the sedating effects of alcohol) and the NMDA subtype of glutamate receptor (upregulation in number, resulting in enhanced wakefulness). There is conceptually a concentration at which the tolerant patient may appear clinically normal despite having an elevated blood alcohol concentration. Tolerant patients who are abstinent lose the tonic effects of alcohol on these receptors, resulting in withdrawal.

with chimeric reconstruction of $GABA_A$ and *N*-methyl-D-aspartate (NMDA) channels demonstrates highly specific binding sites for high doses of ethanol that enhance $GABA_A$ and inhibit NMDA receptor-mediated glutamate neurotransmission.[75] However, research has not clarified whether ethanol at low doses is a direct agonist of $GABA_A$ receptors or a potentiator of $GABA_A$ receptor binding.[59,74,80,83]

Ethanol exhibits all 6 mechanisms of adaptation to chronic exposure and is the prototypical xenobiotic for studying neuroadaptation and withdrawal.[57] These 6 mechanisms appear to apply to benzodiazepines as well.[3,54,80,83] The mechanisms are (1) altered $GABA_A$ receptor gene expression via alterations in mRNA and peptide concentrations of $GABA_A$ receptor subunits in numerous regions of the brain (genomic mechanisms); (2) posttranslational modification through phosphorylation of receptor subunits with protein kinase C (second-messenger effects); (3) subcellular localization by an increased internalization of $GABA_A$ receptor α_1-subunit receptors (receptor endocytosis); (4) modification of receptor subtypes with differing affinities for agonists to the synaptic or nonsynaptic sites (synaptic localization); (5) regulation via intracellular signaling by the NMDA, acetylcholine, serotonin, and β-adrenergic receptors; and (6) neurosteroidal modulation of GABA receptor sensitivity and expression.[12,19,34,37,47,52,58-60,85,110] Furthermore, changes in $GABA_A$ subunit composition and function are evident within 1 hour of administration of a single dose of ethanol.[62]

Intracellular signaling via the NMDA subtype of the glutamate receptor appears to explain the "kindling" hypothesis, in which successive withdrawal events become progressively more severe.[8,11,14,17,36,63,111] The activity of an excitatory neurotransmission increases the more it fires, a phenomenon known as *long-term potentiation*, and is the result of increased activity of mRNA and receptor protein expression, a genomic effect of intracellular signaling.[41,102] As NMDA receptors increase in number and function (upregulation) and $GABA_A$ receptor activity diminishes, withdrawal becomes more severe.[30,46,63,72,85,99] The dizocilpine (MK-801) binding site of the NMDA receptor appears to be the major contributor, and this effect is recognized in neurons that express both NMDA and $GABA_A$ receptors.[4,110,115] Interestingly, animal models suggest that chronic ethanol use induces alterations in the receptor subunit composition of the $GABA_A$ receptor, which may be partly responsible for the development of ethanol tolerance, withdrawal, and kindling.[22,63]

$GABA_A$ agonists induce modulatory changes in the receptors through genomic and nongenomic mechanisms that ultimately alter their function. In this way, withdrawal symptoms represent the clinical manifestation of a change in GABA receptor–complex characteristics.[21,50] When alcohol or any xenobiotic with GABA agonist activity is withdrawn, inhibitory control of excitatory neurotransmission, such as that mediated by the now upregulated NMDA receptors, is lost.[37,70,88]

This loss results in the clinical syndrome of withdrawal: CNS excitation (tremor, hallucinations, seizures), and autonomic stimulation (tachycardia, hypertension, hyperthermia, diaphoresis) (Chap. 78).[42,56,92]

Volatile solvents, such as gasoline, diethyl ether, and toluene, are widely abused xenobiotics whose effects appear to be mediated by the GABA receptor.[84,98] These solvents can produce CNS inhibition and anesthesia at escalating doses via the $GABA_A$ receptor in a fashion similar to that of ethanol.[7,9,48,113]

$GABA_B$ RECEPTORS (GHB AND BACLOFEN)

$GABA_B$ agonists such as γ-hydroxybutyric (GHB) acid and baclofen have similar clinical characteristics with regard to adaptation and withdrawal.[13,24,40,114] The $GABA_B$ receptor is a heterodimer of the $GABA_{B(1)}$ and $GABA_{B(2)}$ receptors. Unlike $GABA_A$, the $GABA_B$ receptor couples to various effector systems through a signal-transducing G protein.[15,69,114] $GABA_B$ receptors mediate presynaptic inhibition (by preventing Ca^{2+} influx) and postsynaptic inhibition (by increasing K^+ efflux). The postsynaptic receptors appear to have an inhibitory effect similar to that of the $GABA_A$ receptors, though the mechanism differs. The presynaptic receptors provide feedback inhibition of GABA release.

GHB is a naturally occurring inhibitory neurotransmitter with its own distinct receptor.[5] Physiologic concentrations of GHB activate at least 2 subtypes of a distinct GHB receptor (antagonist-sensitive and antagonist-insensitive). However, at supraphysiologic concentrations, such as those that occur after overdose and abuse, GHB binds directly to the $GABA_B$ receptor and is metabolized to GABA (which then activates the $GABA_B$ receptor). The GHB withdrawal syndrome clinically resembles the withdrawal syndrome noted from ethanol and benzodiazepines and can be severe.[24] In most cases, distinctive clinical features of GHB withdrawal are the relatively mild and brief autonomic instability and the persistence of psychotic symptoms.[106]

Baclofen is also a $GABA_B$ agonist. The presynaptic and postsynaptic inhibitory properties of baclofen allow it, paradoxically, to cause seizures in cases of both acute overdose (because of decreased release of presynaptic GABA via autoreceptor stimulation) and withdrawal. Withdrawal is probably a result of the loss of the chronic inhibitory effect of baclofen on postsynaptic $GABA_B$ receptors. Discontinuation of baclofen produces hyperactivity of neuronal Ca^{2+} channels (N, P/Q type),[29] leading to seizures, hypertension, hallucinations, psychosis, and coma. However, these manifestations may not differ from the withdrawal symptoms of $GABA_A$ agonists.[86,100]

Typically, the development of a baclofen withdrawal syndrome occurs 24 to 48 hours after discontinuation or a reduction in the dose of baclofen. Case reports highlight the development of seizures, hallucinations, psychosis, dyskinesias, and visual disturbances. The intrathecal baclofen pump has become an effective replacement for oral dosing, but withdrawal can occur following use of this modality as well. Reinstatement of the prior baclofen-dosing schedule appears to resolve these symptoms within 24 to 48 hours. Benzodiazepines and $GABA_A$ agonists (not phenytoin) are the appropriate treatment for seizures induced by baclofen withdrawal.[79]

OPIOID RECEPTORS (OPIOIDS)

Similar to the behavior of ethanol and $GABA_A$ receptors, opioid binding to the opioid receptors results in a series of genomic and nongenomic neuroadaptations, especially via second-messenger effects. When opioids bind to opioid receptors they alleviate pain by inhibiting neurons, while activating G_s proteins and stimulating K^+ efflux currents. The opioid receptors are also linked to the $G_{i/o}$ proteins. They act through adenyl cyclase and activate inward Na^+ current, thus enhancing the intrinsic excitability of a neuron (Chap. 38).[25]

Chronic use of opioids, all xenobiotics with opioid-receptor affinity, results in a decreased efficacy of the receptor to open potassium channels by genomic mechanisms and second-messenger effects. Following chronic opioid use, the expression of adenyl cyclase increases through activation of the transcription factor known as *cAMP response element–binding protein* (*CREB*) (Fig. 14–2).[45,71,77] This situation results in an upregulation of cAMP-mediated responses such as the inward Na^+ channels responsible for intrinsic excitability. The net effect is that only higher concentrations of opioids result in analgesia and other opioid effects. In the dependent patient, when opioid concentrations drop, inward Na^+ flux occurs unchecked, and the patient experiences the opioid withdrawal syndrome. The clinical findings associated with this syndrome are largely a result of uninhibited activity at the locus ceruleus.[23,55,71,73,77]

Furthermore, opioid receptors and central α_2-adrenergic receptors both exert a similar effect on the potassium channel in the locus ceruleus. Clonidine binds to the central α_2-adrenergic receptor and stimulates potassium efflux, as do opioids, and produces similar clinical findings,[2] which explains why clonidine has some efficacy in treating the opioid withdrawal syndrome. In addition, the antagonistic effect of naloxone at the opioid receptor seems to partially reverse the effect of clonidine on this shared potassium efflux channel.[2,38,43]

Rapid opioid detoxification is a form of iatrogenic withdrawal that uses opioid antagonist activity to accelerate a return to premorbid receptor physiology. In theory, inducing opioid withdrawal under general anesthesia with high-dose opioid antagonists permits the transition from drug dependency to naltrexone maintenance without drug withdrawal symptoms.[64-66,95] Naltrexone blocks the euphoric effects of continued opioid use and discourages recidivism by blunting drug craving.[53,65,67,68] Although the mechanism by which naltrexone blocks drug craving is not entirely clear, the speculation is that mere receptor occupancy by an antagonist is sufficient to blunt cravings.[33] However, withdrawal symptoms may still be intense and persist for up to one week after rapid detoxification, suggesting that clinical recovery from the changes induced by chronic opioid use is slow.[26,44,91,97,103]

α_2-ADRENERGIC RECEPTORS (CLONIDINE)

α_2-Adrenergic receptors are located in the central and peripheral nervous systems. Clonidine is a central and peripheral α_2-adrenergic agonist. Stimulation of central presynaptic α_2-adrenergic receptors inhibits sympathomimetic output and results in bradycardia and hypotension.[35] Within 24 hours after the discontinuation of clonidine, norepinephrine concentrations rise as a result of enhanced efferent sympathetic activity.[89] This increase results in hypertension, tachycardia, anxiety, diaphoresis, and hallucinations.[18]

ADENOSINE (A) RECEPTORS (CAFFEINE)

The release of neurotransmitters is accompanied by the passive release of adenosine as a by-product of adenosine triphosphate (ATP) breakdown. The released adenosine binds to postsynaptic A_1 receptors where it typically has inhibitory effects on the postsynaptic neuron. It also binds to presynaptic A_1 autoreceptors to limit further release of neurotransmitters. A_2 receptors are found on the cerebral vasculature and peripheral vasculature where stimulation promotes vasodilation.[28,51] Caffeine and other methylxanthines, such as theophylline, antagonize the inhibitory effect of adenosine, primarily on postsynaptic A_1 receptors.

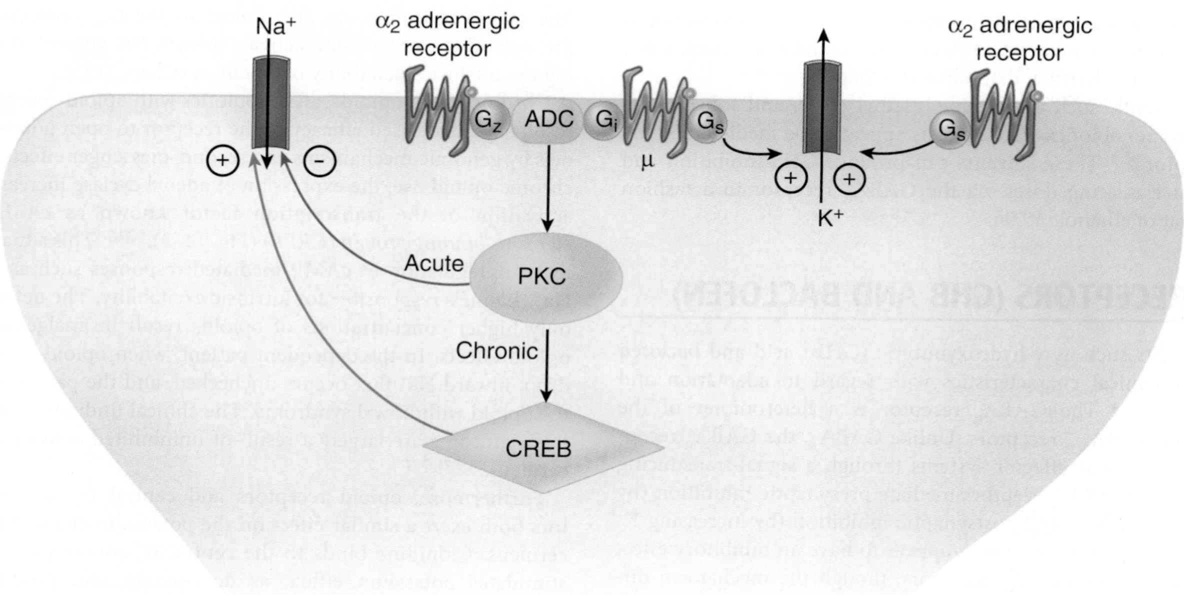

FIGURE 14–2. Immediate and long-term effects of opioids. The immediate effects of both opioids and α_2-adrenergic agonists are to increase inhibition through enhanced potassium efflux and inhibited sodium influx. Long-term effects alter gene expression to enhance sodium influx and restore homeostasis. CREB = cAMP response element-binding protein; AC = adenyl cyclase; PKC = protein kinase C; ( ) = Beta-adrenergic receptor.

As a result, acute use results in increases in heart rate, ventilation, gastrointestinal motility, gastric acid secretion, and motor activity. Chronic caffeine use results in tolerance and the above symptoms diminish.[31] Chronic caffeine use upregulates A_1 receptors by a variety of mechanisms, including increases in receptor number, increases in receptor affinity, enhancement of receptor coupling to the G protein, and increases in G protein–stimulated adenyl cyclase.[61] The results of an animal study demonstrate that the adenosine receptor has a threefold increase in affinity for adenosine at the height of withdrawal symptoms. This model suggests that long-term caffeine administration results in an increase in receptor affinity for adenosine, thus restoring a state of physiologic balance (normal motor inhibitory tone). When caffeine is withdrawn, the enhanced receptor affinity results in a strong adenosine effect and clinical symptoms of withdrawal: headache (cerebral vasodilation), fatigue, and hypersomnia (motor inhibition).[76,101,105]

ACETYLCHOLINE RECEPTORS (NICOTINE)

A nicotinic receptor is a type of acetylcholine receptor located in the autonomic ganglia, adrenal medulla, CNS, spinal cord, neuromuscular junction, and carotid and aortic bodies. Nicotinic receptors are fast-response cation channels that are not coupled to G proteins which distinguishes them from muscarinic receptors, which are coupled to G proteins. Nicotinic acetylcholine receptors have both excitatory and inhibitory effects. As in other withdrawal syndromes, changes brought on by chronic use of nicotinic agonists, such as nicotine in cigarettes, appear to be related to selective upregulation of cAMP.[10,78,109]

SSRI DISCONTINUATION SYNDROME

Upon discontinuation of chronic selective serotonin reuptake inhibitor (SSRI) therapy, patients develop characteristic signs and symptoms. The syndrome complies with the definition of withdrawal syndromes in that symptoms begin when xenobiotic concentrations drop, and the syndrome abates when the xenobiotic is reinstated. Headache, nausea, fatigue, dizziness, and dysphoria are commonly described symptoms. The condition appears to be uncomfortable but not life threatening, rapidly resolves with reinstatement of a xenobiotic of the same class, and slowly resolves when the drug is discontinued after a more gradual taper (Chap. 72).[1,16,24,27,82]

SUMMARY

The understanding of the mechanisms of withdrawal for varied xenobiotics has permitted a more logical approach to these states of altered inhibition of neuronal pathways and those affecting excitatory neuronal pathways. This chapter addresses the related neurophysiologic mechanisms, the characteristics of withdrawal associated with the xenobiotic in question, and the xenobiotic or the types of xenobiotics effective in relieving the withdrawal symptoms.

REFERENCES

1. Agelink MW, Zitzelsberger A, Klieser E: Withdrawal syndrome after discontinuation of venlafaxine [letter]. *Am J Psychiatry.* 1997;154:1473-1474.
2. Aghajanian GK, Wang YY: Common alpha 2- and opiate effector mechanisms in the locus coeruleus: Intracellular studies in brain slices. *Neuropharmacology.* 1987;26:793-799.
3. Allison C, Pratt JA: Neuroadaptive processes in GABAergic and glutamatergic systems in benzodiazepine dependence. *Pharmacol Ther.* 2003;98:171-195.
4. Almiron RS, Perez MF, Ramirez OA: MK-801 prevents the increased NMDA-NR1 and NR2B subunits mRNA expression observed in the hippocampus of rats tolerant to diazepam. *Brain Res.* 2004;1008:54-60.

5. Andriamampandry C, Taleb O, Viry S, et al: Cloning and characterization of a rat brain receptor that binds the endogenous neuromodulator gamma-hydroxybutyrate (GHB). *FASEB J.* 2003;17;1691-1693.
6. Atack JR: Anxioselective compounds acting at the GABA(A) receptor benzodiazepine binding site. *Curr Drug Targets CNS Neurol Disord.* 2003;2:213-232.
7. Bale AS, Tu Y, Carpenter-Hyland EP, et al: Alterations in glutamatergic and gabaergic ion channel activity in hippocampal neurons following exposure to the abused inhalant toluene. *Neuroscience.* 2005;130:197-206.
8. Ballenger JC, Post RM: Kindling as a model for alcohol withdrawal syndromes. *Br J Psychiatry.* 1978;133:1-14.
9. Balster RL: Neural basis of inhalant abuse. *Drug Alcohol Depend.* 1998;51:207-214.
10. Barik J, Wonnacott S: Molecular and cellular mechanisms of action of nicotine in the CNS. *Handb Exp Pharmacol.* 2009;192:173-207.
11. Becker HC, Hale RL: Repeated episodes of ethanol withdrawal potentiate the severity of subsequent withdrawal seizures: An animal model of alcohol withdrawal "kindling." *Alcohol Clin Exp Res.* 1993;17:94-98.
12. Beckley EH, Fretwell AM, Tanchuck MA, et al: Decreased anticonvulsant efficacy of allopregnanolone during ethanol withdrawal in female Withdrawal Seizure-Prone vs. Withdrawal Seizure-Resistant mice. *Neuropharmacology.* 2008;54:365-374.
13. Bernasconi, R, Mathivet P, Bischoff S, Marescaux C: Gamma-hydroxybutyric acid: An endogenous neuromodulator with abuse potential? *Trends Pharmacol Sci.* 1999;20:135-141.
14. Booth BM, Blow FC: The kindling hypothesis: Further evidence from a US national study of alcoholic men. *Alcohol Alcohol.* 1993;28:593-598.
15. Bowery NG, Bettler B, Froestl W, et al: International Union of Pharmacology. XXXIII. Mammalian γ-aminobutyric acid B receptors: Structure and function. *Pharmacol Rev.* 2002;54:247-226.
16. Boyd IW: Venlafaxine withdrawal reactions. *Med J Aust.* 1998;169:91-92.
17. Brown ME, Anton RF, Malcom R, Ballenger JC: Alcohol detoxification and withdrawal seizures: Clinical support for a kindling hypothesis. *Biol Psychiatry.* 1988;23:507-514.
18. Brown M, Salmon D, Rendell M: Clonidine hallucinations. *Ann Intern Med.* 1980;93:456-457.
19. Buck KJ, Hahner L, Sikela J, Harris RA: Chronic ethanol treatment alters brain levels of gamma-aminobutyric acid A receptor subunit mRNAs: Relationship to genetic differences in ethanol withdrawal seizure severity. *J Neurochem.* 1991;57:1452-1455.
20. Buck KJ, Harris RA: Benzodiazepine agonist and inverse agonist actions on $GABA_A$ receptor-operated chloride channels. II. Chronic effects of ethanol. *J Pharmacol Exp Ther.* 1990;253:713-719.
21. Buck KJ, Hood HM: Genetic association of a GABA(A) receptor $gamma_2$ subunit variant with severity of acute physiological dependence on alcohol. *Mamm Genome.* 1998;9:975-978.
22. Cagetti E, Liang J, Spigelman I, Olsen RW: Withdrawal from chronic intermittent ethanol treatment changes subunit composition, reduces synaptic function, and decreases behavioral responses to positive allosteric modulators of $GABA_A$ receptors. *Mol Pharmacol.* 2003;63:53-64.
23. Christie MJ, Williams JT, North RA: Cellular mechanism of opioid tolerance: Studies in single brain neurons. *Mol Pharmacol.* 1987;32:633-638.
24. Craig K, Gomes HF, McManus JL, Bania TC: Severe gamma-hydroxybutyrate withdrawal: A case report and literature review. *J Emerg Med.* 2000;18:65-70.
25. Crain SM, Shen KF: Modulatory effects of G_s-coupled excitatory opioid receptor functions on opioid analgesia, tolerance, and dependence. *Neurochem Res.* 1996;21:1347-1351.
26. Cucchia AT, Monnat M, Spagnoli J, et al: Ultra-rapid opiate detoxification using deep sedation with oral midazolam: short- and long-term results. *Drug Alcohol Depend.* 1998;52:243-250.
27. Dallal A, Chouinard G: Withdrawal and rebound symptoms associated with abrupt discontinuation of venlafaxine. *J Clin Psychopharmacol.* 1998;18:343-344.
28. Daly JW, Fedholm BB: Caffeine—An atypical drug of dependence. *Drug Alcohol Depend.* 1998;51:199-206.
29. Dang K, Bowery NG, Urban L: Interaction of gamma-aminobutyric acid receptor type B receptors and calcium channels in nociceptive transmission studied in the mouse hemisected spinal cord in vitro: Withdrawal symptoms related to baclofen treatment. *Neurosci Lett.* 2004;361:72-75.
30. Davidson M, Shanley B, Wilce P: Increased NMDA-induced excitability during ethanol withdrawal: A behavioural and histological study. *Brain Res.* 1995;674:91-96.
31. Dews PB, Curtis GL, Hanford KJ, O'Brien CP: The frequency of caffeine withdrawal in a population based survey in a controlled, blinded pilot experiment. *J Clin Pharmacol.* 1999;39:1221-1232.
32. *Diagnostic and Statistical Manual of Mental Disorders—Fourth Edition* (DSM-IV). Washington, DC: American Psychiatric Association; 1994.
33. Dijkstra BA, De Jong CA, Bluschke SM, et al: Does naltrexone affect craving in abstinent opioid-dependent patients? *Addict Biol.* 2007;12:176-182.
34. Eckardt MJ, Campbell GA, Marietta CA, et al: Ethanol dependence and withdrawal selectively alter localized cerebral glucose utilization. *Brain Res.* 1992;584:244-250.
35. Farsang C, Kaposci J, Vajda L, et al: Reversal by naloxone of the anti-hypertensive action of clonidine: Involvement of the sympathetic nervous system. *Circulation.* 1984;69:461-467.
36. Ferguson JA, Suelzer CJ, Eckert GJ, et al: Risk factors for delirium tremens development. *J Gen Intern Med.* 1996;11:410-414.
37. Fifkova E, Eason H, Bueltmann K, Lanman J: Changes in GABAergic and non-GABAergic synapses during chronic ethanol exposure and withdrawal in the dentate fascia of LS and SS mice. *Alcohol Clin Exp Res.* 1994;18:989-997.
38. Franz DN, Hare BD, McCloskey KL: Spinal sympathetic neurons: Possible site of opiate-withdrawal suppression by clonidine. *Science.* 1982;215:1643-1645.
39. French-Mullen JMH, Barker JL, Rogawski MA: Calcium current block by pentobarbital, phenobarbital, and CHEB but not (+)pentobarbital in acutely isolated hippocampal CA1 neurons: Comparison with effects on GABA-activated Cl^- current. *J Neurosci.* 1993;13:3211-3221.
40. Galloway GP, Frederick SL, Staggers FE Jr, et al: Gamma-hydroxybutyrate: An emerging drug of abuse that causes physical dependence. *Addiction.* 1997;92:89-96.
41. Glue P, Nutt D: Overexcitement and disinhibition. Dynamic neurotransmitter interactions in alcohol withdrawal. *Br J Psychiatry.* 1990;157:491-499.
42. Golbert TM, Sanz CJ, Rose HD, et al: Comparative evaluation of treatments of alcohol withdrawal syndromes. *JAMA.* 1967;201:99-102.
43. Gold MS, Redmond DE, Kleber HD: Clonidine blocks acute opiate withdrawal symptoms. *Lancet.* 1978;2:599-602.
44. Hamilton RJ, Olmedo RE, Shah S, et al: Complications of ultrarapid opioid detoxification with subcutaneous naltrexone pellets. *Acad Emerg Med.* 2002;9:63-68.
45. Han MH, Bolaños CA, Green TA, et al: Role of cAMP response element-binding protein in the rat locus ceruleus: Regulation of neuronal activity and opiate withdrawal behaviors. *J Neurosci.* 2006;26:4624-4629.
46. Haugbol SR, Ebert B, Ulrichsen J: Upregulation of glutamate receptor subtypes during alcohol withdrawal in rats. *Alcohol Alcohol.* 2005;40:89-95.
47. Hu Y, Lund IV, Gravielle MC, et al: Surface expression of $GABA_A$ receptors is transcriptionally controlled by the interplay of cAMP-response element-binding protein and its binding partner inducible cAMP early repressor. *J Biol Chem.* 2008;283:9328-9340.
48. Jenkins A, Lobo IA, Gong D, et al: General anesthetics have additive actions on three ligand gated ion channels. *Anesth Analg.* 2008;107:486-493.
49. Johnston CA, Watts VJ: Sensitization of adenylate cyclase: A general mechanism of neuroadaptation to persistent activation of $G\alpha_{i/o}$-coupled receptors? *Life Sci.* 2003;73:2913-2925.
50. Kang MH, Spigelman I, Olsen RW: Alteration in the sensitivity of $GABA_A$ receptors to allosteric modulatory drugs in rat hippocampus after chronic intermittent ethanol treatment. *Alcohol Clin Exp Res.* 1998;9;2165-2173.
51. Kaplan GB, Greenblatt DJ, Kent MA, Cotreau-Bibbo MM: Caffeine treatment and withdrawal in mice: Relationships between dosage, concentrations, locomotor activity and A1 adenosine receptor binding. *J Pharmacol Exp Ther.* 1993;266:1563-1571.
52. Keir WJ, Morrow AL: Differential expression of $GABA_A$ receptor subunit mRNAs in ethanol-naive withdrawal seizure resistant (WSR) vs. withdrawal seizure prone (WSP) mouse brain. *Brain Res Mol Brain Res.* 1994;25:2000-2008.
53. Kirchmayer U, Davoli, Vester A: Naltrexone maintenance treatment for opioid dependence. *Cochrane Database Syst Rev.* 2000:CD001333.
54. Klein RL, Whiting PJ, Harris RA: Benzodiazepine treatment causes uncoupling of recombinant $GABA_A$ receptors expressed in stably transfected cells. *J Neurochem.* 1994;63:2349-2352.

55. Koch T, Widera A, Bartzsch K, et al: Receptor endocytosis counteracts the development of opioid tolerance. *Mol Pharmacol.* 2005;67:280-287.
56. Krogsgaard-Larsen P, Scheel-Kruger J, Kofod H, eds: *GABA-Neurotransmitters: Pharmacological, Biochemical, and Pharmacological Aspects.* New York: Academic Press; 1979: 102-103.
57. Kumar S, Fleming RK, Morrow AL: Ethanol regulation of gamma-aminobutyric acid A receptors: Genomic and nongenomic mechanisms. *Pharmacol Ther.* 2004;101:211-226.
58. Kuriyama K, Ueha T: Functional alterations in cerebral $GABA_A$ receptor complex associated with formation of alcohol dependence: Analysis using GABA-dependent $^{36}Cl^-$ influx into neuronal membrane vesicles. *Alcohol Alcohol.* 1992;27:335-343.
59. Kuriyama K, Ueha T, Hirouchi M, et al: Functional alterations in $GABA_A$ receptor complex induced by ethanol. *Alcohol Alcohol.* 1993:2(Suppl);321-325.
60. Läck AK, Diaz MR, Chappell A, et al.: Chronic ethanol and withdrawal differentially modulate pre- and postsynaptic function at glutamatergic synapses in rat basolateral amygdala. *J Neurophysiol.* 2007;98:3185-3196.
61. Leite-Morris KA, Kaplan GB, Smith JG, Sears MT: Regulation of G proteins and adenylyl cyclase in brain regions of caffeine-tolerant and -dependent mice. *Brain Res.* 1998;804:52-62.
62. Liang J, Suryanarayanan A, Abriam A, et al.: Mechanisms of reversible $GABA_A$ receptor plasticity after ethanol intoxication. *J Neurosci.* 2007;27:12367-12377.
63. Little HJ, Stephens DN, Ripley TL, et al: Alcohol withdrawal and conditioning. *Alcohol Clin Exp Res.* 2005;29:453-464.
64. Loimer N, Lenz K, Schmid R, Presslich O: Technique for greatly shortening the transition from methadone to naltrexone maintenance of patients addicted to opiates. *Am J Psychiatry.* 1991;148:933-935.
65. Loimer N, Linzmayer L, Schmid R, Grunberger J: Similar efficacy of abrupt and gradual opiate detoxification. *Am J Drug Alcohol Abuse.* 1991;17:307-312.
66. Loimer N, Schmid R, Lenz K, et al: Acute blocking of naloxone-precipitated opiate withdrawal symptoms by methohexitone. *Br J Psychiatry.* 1990;157:748-752.
67. Loimer N, Schmid W, Presslich O, Lenz K: Continuous naloxone administration suppresses opiate withdrawal symptoms in human opiate addicts during detoxification treatment. *J Psychiatr Res.* 1989;23:81-86.
68. Loimer N, Schmid R, Presslich O, Lenz K: Naloxone treatment for opiate withdrawal syndrome. *Br J Psychiatry.* 1988;153:851-852.
69. Maitre M: The γ-hydroxybutyrate signaling system in brain: Organization and functional implications. *Prog Neurobiol.* 1997;51:337-361.
70. Malcolm RJ: GABA systems, benzodiazepines, and substance dependence. *J Clin Psychiatry.* 2003;64(Suppl 3):36-40.
71. Maldonado R, Blendy JA, Tzavara E, et al: Reduction of morphine abstinence in mice with mutation in the gene encoding CREB. *Science.* 1996;273:657-659.
72. McCown TJ, Breese GR: A potential contribution to ethanol withdrawal kindling: Reduced GABA function in the inferior collicular cortex. *Alcohol Clin Exp Res.* 1993;17:1290-1294.
73. McKim EM: Caffeine and its effects on pregnancy and the neonate. *J Nurse Midwifery.* 1991;36:226-231.
74. Mehta AK, Ticku MK: An update on $GABA_A$ receptors. *Brain Res Brain Res Rev.* 1999;29:196-217.
75. Mihic SJ, Ye Q, Marilee JM: Sites of alcohol and volatile anaesthetic action on $GABA_A$ and glycine receptors. *Nature.* 1997;389:385-389.
76. Nehlig A, Daval JL, Debry G: Caffeine and the central nervous system: Mechanisms of action, biochemical, metabolic and psychostimulant effects. *Brain Res Brain Res Rev.* 1992;17:139-170.
77. Nestler EJ: Molecular mechanisms of drug addiction. *Neuropharmacology.* 2004;47(Suppl 1):24-32.
78. Ochoa EL, Li L, McNamee MG: Desensitization of central cholinergic mechanisms and neuroadaptation to nicotine. *Mol Neurobiol.* 1990;4:251-287.
79. Peng CT, Ger J, Yang CC, et al: Prolonged severe withdrawal symptoms after acute-on-chronic baclofen overdose. *J Toxicol Clin Toxicol.* 1998;36:359-363.
80. Pericic D, Strac DS, Jembrek MJ, Rajcan I: Prolonged exposure to gamma-aminobutyric acid up-regulates stably expressed recombinant $alpha_1$ $beta_2$ $gamma_{2s}$ $GABA_A$ receptors. *Eur J Pharmacol.* 2003;482:117-125.
81. Prakash A, Das G: Cocaine and the nervous system. *Int J Clin Pharmacol Ther Toxicol.* 1993;31:575-581.
82. Precourt A, Dunewicz M, Gregoire G, Williamson DR: Multiple complications and withdrawal syndrome associated with quetiapine/venlafaxine intoxication. *Ann Pharmacother.* 2005;39:153-156.
83. Primus RJ, Yu J, Xu J, et al: Allosteric uncoupling after chronic benzodiazepine exposure of recombinant gamma-aminobutyric acid A receptors expressed in Sf9 cells: Ligand efficacy and subtype selectivity. *J Pharmacol Exp Ther.* 1996;276:882-890.
84. Riegel AC, Ali SF, French ED: Toluene-induced locomotor activity is blocked by 6-hydroxydopamine lesions of the nucleus accumbens and the mGluR2/3 agonist LY379268. *Neuropsychopharmacology.* 2003;28:1440-1447.
85. Ripley TL, Little HJ: Ethanol withdrawal hyperexcitability in vitro is selectively decreased by a competitive NMDA receptor antagonist. *Brain Res.* 1995;699:1-11.
86. Rivas DA, Chancellor MB, Hill K, Freedman MK: Neurological manifestations of baclofen withdrawal. *J Urol.* 1993;150:1903-1905.
87. Rodriguez H, Rhee LM, Ramachandran J, et al: Sequence and functional expression of the $GABA_A$ receptor shows a ligand gated ion channel family. *Nature.* 1987;328:221-227.
88. Rossetti ZL, Carboni S, Brodie BB: Ethanol withdrawal is associated with increased extracellular glutamate in the rat striatum. *Eur J Pharmacol.* 1995;283:177-183.
89. Rupp H, Maisch B, Brilla CG: Drug withdrawal and rebound hypertension: Differential action of the central antihypertensive drugs moxonidine and clonidine. *Cardiovasc Drugs Ther.* 1996;10(Suppl 1):251-262.
90. Saito T, Hashimoto E: Membrane effects of ethanol in the brain. *J Clin Exp Med.* 1990;154:869-873.
91. Sanger DJ, Benavides J, Perrault G, et al: Recent developments in the behavioral pharmacology of benzodiazepine (ω) receptors: Evidence for the functional significance of receptor subtypes. *Neurosci Biobehav Rev.* 1994;18:355-372.
92. Sanna E, Mostallino MC, Busonero F, et al: Changes in GABA(A) receptor gene expression associated with selective alterations in receptor function and pharmacology after ethanol withdrawal. *J Neurosci.* 2003;23:11711-11724.
93. Sanna E, Serra M, Cossu A, et al: Chronic ethanol intoxication induces differential effects on GABAA and NMDA receptor function in the rat brain. *Alcohol Clin Exp Res.* 1993;17:115-123.
94. Satel SL, Price LH, Palumbo JM, et al: Clinical phenomenology and neurobiology of cocaine abstinence: A prospective inpatient study. *Am J Psychiatry.* 1991;148:495-498.
95. Scherbaum N, Klein S, Kaube H, et al: Alternative strategies of opiate detoxification: Evaluation of the so-called ultrarapid detoxification. *Pharmacopsychiatry.* 1998;31:205-209.
96. Schofield PR, Darlison MG, Fujita N, et al: Sequence and functional expression of the $GABA_A$ receptor shows a ligand-gated receptor superfamily. *Nature.* 1987;328:221-227.
97. Seoane A, Carrasco G, Cabre L, et al: Efficacy and safety of two new methods of rapid intravenous detoxification in heroin addicts previously treated without success. *Br J Psychiatry.* 1997;171:340-345.
98. Shar R, Vankar GK, Upadhaya HP: Phenomenology of gasoline intoxication and withdrawal symptoms among adolescents in India: A case series. *Am J Addict.* 1999;8:254-257.
99. Sheela Rani CS, Ticku MK: Comparison of chronic ethanol and chronic intermittent ethanol treatments on the expression of GABA(A) and NMDA receptor subunits. *Alcohol.* 2006;38:89-97.
100. Siegfried RN, Jacobson L, Chobal C: Development of an acute withdrawal syndrome following the cessation of intrathecal baclofen therapy in a patient with spasticity. *Anesthesiology.* 1992;77:1048-1050.
101. Silverman K, Evans SM, Strain EC, et al: Withdrawal syndrome after the double-blind cessation of caffeine consumption. *N Engl J Med.* 1992;327:1109-1114.
102. Smith SS, Shen H, Gong QH, Zhou X: Neurosteroid regulation of GABA(A) receptors: Focus on the alpha4 and delta subunits. *Pharmacol Ther.* 2007;116:58-76.
103. Spangel R, Kirschke C, Tretter F, Holsboer F: Forced opiate withdrawal under anesthesia augments and prolongs the occurrence of withdrawal signs in rats. *Drug Alcohol Depend.* 1998;52:251-256.
104. Spies CD, Nordmann A, Brummer G, et al: Intensive care unit stay is prolonged in chronic alcoholic men following tumor resection of the upper digestive tract. *Acta Anaesthesiol Scand.* 1996;40:649-656.
105. Strain EC, Mumford GK, Silverman K, et al: Caffeine dependence syndrome. *JAMA.* 1994;272:1043-1048.

106. Tarabar AF, Nelson LS: The gamma-hydroxybutyrate withdrawal syndrome. *Toxicol Rev*. 2004;23:45-49.
107. Trabulsy ME: Cocaine washed out syndrome in a patient with acute myocardial infarction. *Am J Emerg Med*. 1995;13:538-539.
108. Tunniclif G, Raess BU: *GABA Mechanism in Epilepsy*. New York: Wiley; 1992: 54-55.
109. Tzavara ET, Monory K, Hanoune J, Nomikos GG: Nicotine withdrawal syndrome: Behavioural distress and selective up-regulation of the cyclic AMP Pathway in the amygdala. *Eur J Neurosci*. 2002;16:149-153.
110. Ulrichsen J, Bech B, Ebert B, et al: Glutamate and benzodiazepine receptor autoradiography in rat brain after repetition of alcohol dependence. *Psychopharmacology (Berl)*. 1996;126:31-41.
111. Veatch LM, Gonzalez LP: Repeated ethanol withdrawal produces site-dependent increases in EEG spiking. *Alcohol Clin Exp Res*. 1996;20:262-267.
112. Wafford KA: $GABA_A$ receptor subtypes: Any clues to the mechanism of benzodiazepine dependence? *Curr Opin Pharmacol*. 2005;5:47-52.
113. Williams JM, Stafford D, Steketee JD: Effects of repeated inhalation of toluene on ionotropic $GABA_A$ and glutamate receptor subunit levels in rat brain. *Neurochem Int*. 2005;46:1-10.
114. Wong C, Guin Ting, Gibson KM, Snead OC: From the street to the brain: Neurobiology of the recreational drug γ-hydroxybutyric acid. *Trends Pharmacol Sci*. 2004;25:29-34.
115. Worner TM: Relative kindling effect of readmissions in alcoholics. *Alcohol Alcohol*. 1996;31:375-380.

SECTION 2 PATHOPHYSIOLOGIC BASIS: ORGAN SYSTEMS

CHAPTER 15

THERMOREGULATORY PRINCIPLES

Susi U. Vassallo and Kathleen A. Delaney

Despite exposure to wide fluctuations of environmental temperatures, human body temperature is maintained within a narrow range.[23,131] Elevation or depression of body temperature occurs when (1) thermoregulatory mechanisms are overwhelmed by exposure to extremes of environmental heat or cold; (2) endogenous heat production is either inadequate, resulting in hypothermia, or exceeds the physiologic capacity for dissipation, resulting in hyperthermia; or (3) disease processes or xenobiotic effects interfere with normal thermoregulatory responses to heat or cold exposure.

METHODS OF HEAT TRANSFER

Heat is transferred to or away from the body through radiation, conduction, convection, and evaporation. *Radiation* involves the transfer of heat from a body to the environment, and from warm objects in the environment, for example, from the sun to a body. *Conduction* involves the transfer of heat to solid or liquid media in direct contact with the body. Water immersion conducts significant amounts of heat away from the body. This effect facilitates cooling in a swimming pool on a hot summer day, or may lead to hypothermia despite moderate ambient temperatures on a rainy day. The amount of heat lost through conduction and radiation depends on the temperature gradient between skin and surroundings, cutaneous blood flow, and insulation such as subcutaneous fat, hair, clothing, or fur in lower animals.[148] In the respiratory tract, heat is lost by conduction to water vapor or gas. In animals unable to sweat, this represents the primary method of heat loss. The amount of heat lost through the respiratory tract depends on the temperature gradient between inspired air and the environment, as well as the rate and depth of breathing.[148] *Convection* is the transfer of heat to the air surrounding the body. Wind velocity and ambient air temperature are the major determinants of convective heat loss. *Evaporation* is the process of vaporization of water, or sweat. Large amounts of heat are dissipated from the skin during this process, resulting in cooling. Ambient temperature, rate of sweating, air velocity, and relative humidity are important factors in determining how much heat is lost through evaporation. On a very humid day, sweat may pour off, rather than evaporate from a person exercising in a hot environment, thereby accomplishing little heat loss. In very warm environments, thermal gradients may be reversed, leading to transfer of heat to the body by radiation, conduction, or convection.[164]

PHYSIOLOGY OF THERMOREGULATION

In the normal human, stimulation of peripheral and hypothalamic temperature-sensitive neurons results in autonomic, somatic, and behavioral responses that lead to the dissipation or conservation of heat. Thermoregulation is the complex physiologic process that serves to maintain hypothalamic temperature within a narrow range of 98.6 ± 0.8°F (37 ± 0.4°C) known as the set point.[131] This hypothalamic set point is influenced by factors including diurnal variation and the menstrual cycle. Maintaining, raising, or lowering the set point results in many outwardly visible physiologic manifestations of thermoregulation such as sweating, shivering, flushing, or panting. In the central nervous system, thermosensitive neurons are located predominantly in the preoptic area of the anterior hypothalamus, although some are found in the posterior hypothalamus. These neurons may be divided into those that are warm sensitive, cold sensitive, or temperature insensitive. Approximately 30% of preoptic neurons are warm sensitive. These increase their firing rate during warming and decrease their firing rate during cooling.[36] Warming of the hypothalamus in conscious animals results in vasodilation, hyperventilation, salivation, and increases in evaporative water loss, as well as a reduction of cold-induced shivering and vasoconstriction.[131] Cooling of the hypothalamus in conscious animals causes shivering, vasoconstriction, and increased metabolic rate, even if the environment is hot.[123] How these temperature-sensitive neurons of the hypothalamus detect temperature changes and effect neuronal transmission is unclear. Altered action potential initiation and propagation caused by temperature-dependent changes in membrane potential, changes in the ratios of Na^+ to Ca^{2+} which alter neuronal excitability and neurotransmitter release, or effects on the Na^+K^+-ATPase (adenosine triphosphatase) pump may be involved.[148] Xenobiotics that increase intracellular cyclic adenosine monophosphate (cAMP) concentrations increase the thermosensitivity of warm-sensitive neurons.[36] In the brainstem, warm-sensitive and cold-sensitive neurons are located in the medullary reticular formation, where information from cutaneous receptors, spinal cord, and preoptic area of the anterior hypothalamus is integrated.[137]

The spinal cord also manifests thermosensitivity. Heat-sensitive and cold-sensitive ascending spinal impulses are conducted in the spinothalamic tract. As in the hypothalamus, local heating or cooling of the spinal cord results in thermoregulatory responses.[131] In addition to the hypothalamus, brainstem, and spinal cord, there is evidence of thermosensitivity in the deep abdominal viscera.[119,131,241] Intra-abdominal heating or cooling results in thermoregulatory responses. Cold-sensitive and warm-sensitive afferent impulses can be recorded from the splanchnic nerves in animals.[119,243] Finally, the skin also contains heat and cold thermosensitive neurons. Cold receptors are free nerve endings that protrude into the basal epidermis, whereas warm-sensitive receptors protrude into the dermis.[130,132] Cutaneous thermoreceptor output is affected by the absolute temperature of the skin, rate of temperature change, and area of stimulation.[131] Cutaneous cold

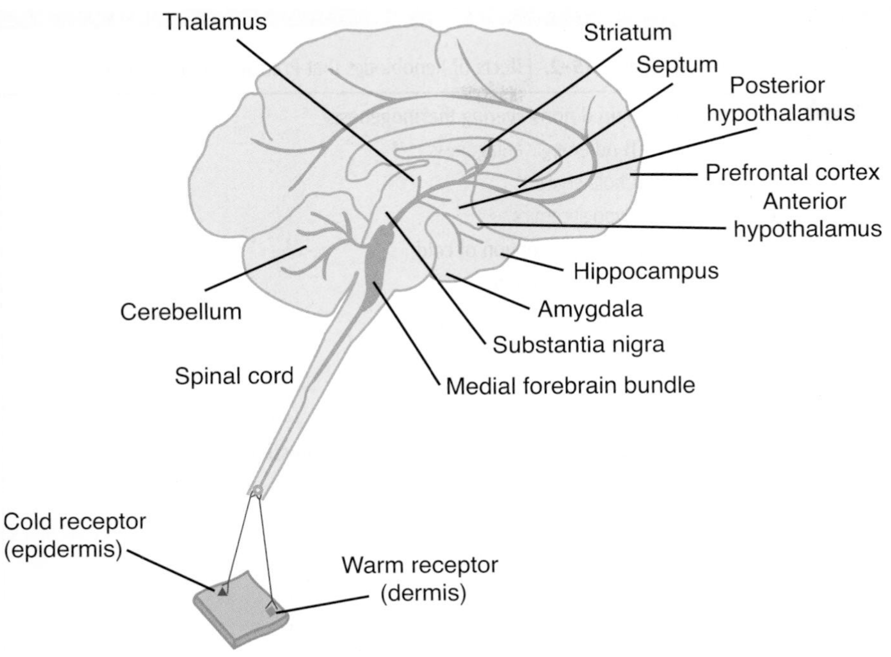

FIGURE 15–1. A representation of the cutaneous thermoreceptive neurons responsive to external temperature change that functions as an early warning to the central nervous system.

receptors are Aδ and C nociceptor afferent fibers. Aδ fibers are small-diameter thinly myelinated fibers that conduct at 5–30 m/sec, and C fibers are small-diameter unmyelinated fibers that conduct at 0.5–2 m/sec.[119] Afferents from heat receptors are primarily C fibers. Cutaneous thermoreceptive neurons respond to external temperature change as well as rate of temperature change, sending early warning to the CNS via afferent impulses. This allows rapid and transient thermoregulatory responses before brain temperature changes (Fig. 15–1).

VASOMOTOR AND SWEAT GLAND FUNCTION

Vasomotor responses to thermoregulatory input differ according to location. The normal thermoregulatory response to heat stress is mediated primarily by heat-sensitive neurons in the hypothalamus. Increased body core temperature results in active vasodilation in the extremities and is under noradrenergic control. Increasing sympathetic stimulation results in vasoconstriction, and decreasing sympathetic stimulation results in vasodilation. Vasodilation in the head, trunk, and proximal limbs is not a result of decreased sympathetic tone; instead, it is a result of an active process that is under the influence of cholinergic sudomotor nerves and local effects of temperature on venomotor tone. Sweat glands release local transmitters, such as vasoactive intestinal polypeptide (VIP) or bradykinins, and vasodilation results. Areas of the body such as the forehead, where sweating is most prominent during heat stress, correspond to areas where active vasodilation is greatest. The neurotransmitters involved in the regulation of relationships between vasodilation and sweating as a response to heat stress are not fully elucidated, but animal evidence suggests the presence of specific vasodilator nerves.[131]

Sweat glands are controlled by sympathetic postganglionic nerve fibers, which are cholinergic, and large amounts of acetylcholinesterase as well as other peptides are involved in neural transmission.[130,131]

NEUROTRANSMITTERS AND THERMOREGULATION

The neurotransmitters involved in thermoregulation include serotonin, norepinephrine, acetylcholine, dopamine, prostaglandins, β-endorphins, and intrinsic hypothalamic peptides such as arginine vasopressin, adrenocorticotropic hormone, thyrotropin-releasing hormone, and melanocyte-stimulating hormone.[56,228] Studies on the effects of individual neurotransmitters in thermoregulation yield contradictory results, depending on the animal species and the route of administration of the exogenous neurotransmitter. Refinements in techniques of microinjection of neurotransmitters into the hypothalamus of animals, rather than intraventricular instillation, have elucidated microanatomic sites where neurotransmitters are active. More research is needed, however, as interspecies variations and theoretical differences in response to exogenous versus endogenous peptides makes this area of study complex.

Apomorphine is a mixed dopamine agonist that causes hypothermia in animals. Studies using selective D_1-receptor and D_2-receptor agonists and antagonists suggest that the hypothermic effect of apomorphine is a result of its effects on D_2 receptors, with some modulation by D_1 receptors in the hypothalamus.[204] Stimulation of D_2 receptors appears to mediate the hypothermia induced by the peptide sauvagine.[40] Stimulation of D_3 by specific agonists caused hypothermia in an animal model.[205,206] There appears to be a link between dopamine D_2 receptors and norepinephrine receptors in the hypothalamus, perhaps leading to vasodilation and hypothermia. The effect of clozapine in producing hypothermia in the rat is caused by D_1 and D_3 stimulation.[206,255] Lesser-known peptides appear to be involved in thermoregulation. For example, neuropeptide Y is an amino acid neurotransmitter that occurs in high concentrations in the preoptic area of the anterior hypothalamus. Administration of neuropeptide Y caused a reduction in core temperature when administered with adrenoceptor antagonists such as prazosin, an α_1-adrenergic antagonist, propranolol, a β-adrenergic antagonist, and clonidine, a central α_2-adrenergic agonist.[90,253] The administration of synthetic cannabinoids induces hypothermia in animals, an effect that is antagonized by adrenergic agonists and enhanced by adrenergic antagonists.[236] Studies on muscarinic receptors suggest the involvement of muscarinic M_2 and M_3 receptors in the production of hypothermia when agonists to these receptors are administered centrally.[256] Blockers of adenosine triphosphate sensitive K^+ channels can reverse the effect of cholinomimetic drugs in producing hypothermia.[238] Finally, studies of the neuroprotective effects of induced hypothermia may better define the role of other neurotransmitters in unintentional hypothermia.[311]

XENOBIOTIC EFFECTS ON THERMOREGULATION

Many xenobiotics have pharmacologic effects that interfere with thermoregulatory responses (Tables 15–1 and 15–2).[188,190,293] α-Adrenergic agonists prevent vasodilation in response to heat stress. Increased endogenous heat production in the setting of increased motor activity also occurs in patients poisoned with cocaine or amphetamines.

TABLE 15–1. Effects of Xenobiotics that Predispose to Hyperthermia

Impaired cutaneous heat loss
Vasoconstriction through α-adrenergic stimulation
Amphetamine and derivatives
Cocaine
Ephedrine
Phenylpropanolamine
Pseudoephedrine
Sweat gland dysfunction
Antihistamines
Belladonna alkaloids
Cyclic antidepressants
Topiramate
Zonisamide
Myocardial depression
Decreased cardiac output
Antidysrhythmics
β-Adrenergic antagonists
Calcium channel blockers
Reduced cardiac filling by salt and winter depletion
Diuretics
Ethanol
Hypothalamic depression
Antipsychotics
Impaired behavioral response
Cocaine
Ethanol
Opioids
Phencyclidine
Sedative-hypnotics
Uncoupling of oxidative phosphorylation
Dinitrophenol
Pentachlorophenol
Salicylates
Increased muscle activity through agitation, seizures, or rigidity
Amphetamines
Caffeine
Cocaine
Isoniazid
Lithium
Monoamine oxidase inhibitors
Phencyclidine
Strychnine
Sympathomimetics
Dystonia
Butyrophenones
Phenothiazines
Withdrawal
Dopamine agonists
Ethanol
Sedative-hypnotics

TABLE 15–2. Effects of Xenobiotics that Predispose to Hypothermia

Impaired nonshivering thermogenesis
β-Adrenergic antagonists
Cholinergics
Hypoglycemics
Impaired perception of cold
Carbon monoxide
Ethanol
Hypoglycemics
Opioids
Sedative-hypnotics
Impaired shivering by hypothalamic depression
Carbon monoxide
Ethanol
General anesthetics
Opioids
Phenothiazines
Sedative-hypnotics
Impaired vasoconstriction
α-Adrenergic antagonists
Ethanol
Phenothiazines

Life-threatening hyperthermia is associated with the use of these xenobiotics. α-Adrenergic antagonists and calcium channel blockers diminish the cardiac reserve available to compensate for heat-induced vasodilation, whereas diuretics decrease cardiac reserve through their effects on intravascular volume.[70] β-Adrenergic antagonists also interfere with the capacity to maintain normothermia under conditions of cold stress, possibly related to their interference with the mobilization of substrates required for thermogenesis.[131,190] Opioids and diverse sedative-hypnotics depress hypothalamic function and predispose to hypothermia in the overdose setting.[92] Carbon monoxide poisoning must also be considered in the hypothermic patient. Organic phosphorous insecticides and other xenobiotics that cause cholinergic stimulation cause hypothermia by stimulation of inappropriate sweating and possibly through depression of the endogenous use of calorigenic substrates.[190] Xenobiotics with anticholinergic effects decrease sweating and predispose to hyperthermia during environmental heat exposure or exercise. Phenothiazines appear to interfere with normal response to both heat and cold. Severe hyperthermia associated with the absence of sweating is frequently described in patients using phenothiazines and may be a consequence of their anticholinergic effects.[257,310] Effects on cold tolerance are attributed to their α-adrenergic antagonist effects, which prevent vasoconstriction in response to cold stress.[189] In addition, hyperthermia associated with severe extrapyramidal rigidity may occur in patients on antipsychotics.[181] This rigidity is attributed to the dopamine-blocking effects of this class of drugs.

ETHANOL

Ethanol is the xenobiotic most commonly related to the occurrence of hypothermia in an urban setting.[68,300,301] The mechanisms by which ethanol predisposes to hypothermia are said to be due to its effects on CNS depression, cutaneous vasodilation, and blunting of behavioral responses to cold. However, thermoregulatory dysfunction associated with ethanol intoxication is undoubtedly more complex.

Ethanol leads to hypothermia in animal models, the extent of which is partly dependent on ambient temperature.[222,244,245] In mice, as the dose of ethanol increased, body temperature decreased. The rate of this decline in body temperature was faster at higher ethanol doses.[217] The decline in body temperature could be reversed by increasing ambient temperature to 96.8°F (36°C) which caused an immediate rise in the body temperature.[217] The poikilothermic effect of ethanol was not a result of hypoglycemia. Poikilothermia is the variation in body temperature greater than ±3.6°F (±2°C) on exposure to environmental temperature changes. Rats treated with equipotent amounts of sodium pentobarbital showed the same effects on body temperature as rats treated with ethanol, suggesting a similar central mechanism of CNS depression resulting in altered thermoregulation.[217]

Numerous mechanisms are involved in the ethanol-induced depression of CNS function.[250] Genetic factors influence the role of ethanol in the production of hypothermia. Mice can be selectively bred for genetic sensitivity or insensitivity to acute ethanol-induced hypothermia, and the differences appear to be mediated by the serotonergic systems.[93,106,209,217] Histidyl-proline–like topiperazine (cyclo His-Pro, or CHP), another neurotransmitter that is found in many animal species, acts at the preoptic-anterior hypothalamus to modulate body temperature.[46,141] Exogenous administration of this neuropeptide produced a dose-dependent decrease in ethanol-induced hypothermia. Attenuation of hypothermia resulted from passive immunization with CHP antibody.[46,141] Ethanol effects may be mediated through modulation of endogenous opioid peptides, as high-dose (10 mg/kg) naloxone reverses ethanol-induced hypothermia in animals.[233]

Pharmacokinetic characteristics of ethanol metabolism change in the presence of hypothermia. Hypothermic piglets infused with ethanol showed slower ethanol metabolism and a smaller volume of distribution and, as a result, higher ethanol concentrations than normothermic controls. Ethanol elimination and metabolism decreased as temperature fell.[169]

Tolerance develops to the ability of ethanol to produce hypothermia in all species.[95,222] The degree of tolerance is proportional to the dose and duration of treatment with ethanol and is not explained by the increased rate of metabolism with chronic exposure.[148] Age is a factor in the development of tolerance; older animals do not display the same degree of tolerance to the hypothermic effects of chronic ethanol administration as do younger animals.[214,231,308] The development of tolerance to ethanol-induced hypothermia is affected by genetic factors. Experimentally, tolerance to ethanol-induced hypothermia increases the incorporation of certain amino acids into proteins in the rat brain. The formation of new proteins in ethanol-tolerant rats suggests stimulation of gene expression related to the tolerant state.[148,296] Deficits in *N*-methyl-D-aspartate (NMDA) receptor systems may also be implicated in the development of ethanol tolerance. In addition, altered nicotinamide adenine dinucleotide (NADH) oxidation to NAD^+, diminished blood flow to the liver, or slowing of metabolism through the microsomal enzyme system may be involved.[250]

Hypothermia alters the breath–ethanol partition in the alveolus, and the temperature of expired breath alters breath–ethanol analysis results. In patients with mild hypothermia, ethanol breath analysis results in lower values by 7.3% per degree centigrade (or 1.8°F) decrease in body temperature.[98] Whether breath–ethanol analysis is also affected by hyperthermia in the test subject remains to be studied.[98]

DISEASE PROCESSES AND THERMOREGULATION

Many disease processes interfere with normal thermoregulation, limiting an individual's capacity to prevent hypothermia or hyperthermia. Extensive dermatologic disease or cutaneous burns impair sweating and vasomotor responses to heat stress.[42] Patients with autonomic disturbances such as diabetes mellitus or peripheral vascular disease also have altered vasomotor responses that impair vasodilation and sweating.[242] Extensive surgical dressings may preclude the evaporation of sweat in an otherwise normal patient. Heat-stressed persons with poor cardiac reserve may not be able to sustain a skin blood flow high enough to maintain normothermia.[82,277] Intense motor activity may lead to excessive endogenous heat production in patients with Parkinson disease or hyperthyroidism. Patients with an agitated delirium or seizures also have significantly elevated rates of endogenous heat production. Hypothalamic injury caused by cerebrovascular accidents, trauma, or infection may disturb thermoregulation.[81,185] Hypothalamic dysfunction can lead to high, unremitting fevers and insufficient stimulation of heat loss mechanisms such as sweating. Hypothalamic damage may predispose to hypothermia by interference with centrally mediated heat conservation.[81,185,258,259] Fever, the normal response to stimulation of the hypothalamus by pyrogens, results in an elevated physiologic temperature set point and is a disadvantage in the heat-stressed individual.[131]

HYPOTHERMIA

Epidemiology Hypothermia is defined as a lowering of the core body temperature to <95°F (<35°C). Between 1999 and 2002, 4607 people had hypothermia-related diagnoses listed on the death certificate as the underlying cause of death.[51] Most of these, 2622, were due to exposure to excessive cold; in the remainder hypothermia resulted from causes other than exposure, such as medical illness[48,49,135,163] (Table 15–3).

Most hypothermic deaths occur in the winter months; however, mildly cool environments and windy wet conditions are also frequently associated with hypothermia. From 1999 to 2002, Alaska, Montana, Wyoming, and New Mexico had the greatest overall death rates from hypothermia.[13] States with milder climates and rapid fluctuations in temperature, such as North Carolina and South Carolina, and western states, such as Arizona, with high elevations and cold nighttime temperatures, report hypothermia-related deaths.[51]

Response to Cold The normal physiologic response to cold is initiated by stimulation of cold-sensitive neurons in the skin, so that the onset of the response to cold occurs prior to cooling of central blood. Cold-sensitive neurons in the skin send afferent impulses to the hypothalamus, resulting in shivering and piloerection. Shivering is the main thermoregulatory response to cold in humans, except in neonates, where nonshivering thermogenesis prevails. Shivering is initiated in the posterior hypothalamus when impulses from cold-sensitive thermoreceptors are integrated in the anterior hypothalamus and communicated to the posterior hypothalamus, or when cold-sensitive neurons in the posterior hypothalamus are activated directly. Efferent stimuli from the posterior hypothalamus travel through the midbrain tegmentum, pons, and lateral medullary reticular formation to the motor pathways of the tectospinal and rubrospinal tracts, resulting in shivering.[28] A mechanism of stimulation of shivering that usually occurs later when core temperature falls is the local cooling of the spinal cord. This leads to shivering by increasing excitability of motor neurons.

Heat produced without muscle contraction is known as *nonshivering thermogenesis*.[41,131] Nonshivering thermogenesis is mediated by the sympathetic nervous system.[62] Catecholamines activate adenylate

TABLE 15–3. Factors Predisposing to Hypothermia

Advanced age
Decreased metabolic rate
Decreased temperature discrimination
Decreased ability to shiver
Reduced peripheral blood flow
Central nervous system depression
Cerebrovascular accident
Ethanol
Hypothalamic dysfunction
Infection
Intracranial hemorrhage
Xenobiotics, diverse
Endocrine
Diabetic ketoacidosis
Hyperosmolar coma
Hypopituitarism
Hypothyroidism
Environmental
Exposure
Hepatic failure
Immobilization
Central nervous system dysfunction
Illness
Spinal cord injury
Trauma
Nutritional
Hypoglycemia
Glycogen depletion
Starvation
Thiamine deficiency
Sepsis
Social
Failure to use indoor heating
Homelessness
Inadequate indoor heating
Poverty
Social isolation
Uremia

cyclase, increasing cAMP, and resulting in mobilization of fat and glucose stores (β-adrenergic receptors).[191,252] Nonshivering thermogenesis is blocked by α-adrenergic receptor antagonism and increased by administration of norepinephrine. Brown adipose tissue is the most important site of nonshivering thermogenesis. In humans, brown fat is found primarily in neonates, although in cold-acclimatized people there may be small amounts found on autopsy.[41] Brown adipose tissue functions as a thermoregulatory effector organ, producing heat by the oxidation of fatty acids when the tissue is stimulated by norepinephrine.[45]

In addition to shivering and nonshivering thermogenesis, efferent sympathetic fibers from the hypothalamus stimulate peripheral vasoconstriction (α-adrenergic receptors). Piloerection and vasoconstriction result in decreased heat loss from the body. Intense vasoconstriction shunts blood away from the periphery to the core and antidiuretic hormone antagonism results in increased urine output and hemoconcentration.

Disease Processes and Hypothermia Several disease processes commonly result in an inability to maintain a normal body temperature in a cool environment (see Table 15–3). Hypothermia may develop in association with sepsis,[183] hypothyroidism, hypoglycemia, uremia, hepatic failure, or poor nutrition.[73,239] Hypothalamic injury may result in chronic poikilothermia.[189] Thiamine deficiency adversely affects the hypothalamus, perhaps because of inefficient glucose metabolism, and leads to hypothermia.[167] Spinal cord transections above the first thoracic segment interrupt hypothalamic-sympathetic outflow pathways, resulting in hypothermia.[242] The frail elderly are at greater risk of hypothermia because of decreased vasomotor responses and decreased capacity to shiver.[62,64] Mentally and physically compromised patients may be unable to make appropriate behavioral responses to hot or cold environments.

Evaluations to determine the presence of underlying diseases are often difficult in the hypothermic patient.[96,183] The mental status may be markedly altered by hypothermia but is not usually abnormal until the temperature falls below 90°F (32.2°C).

Alteration of Pharmacology in Hypothermia The pharmacology of certain xenobiotics is altered in the setting of hypothermia. In hypothermic piglets, the volume of distribution and the clearance of fentanyl are decreased.[169] Similarly, in piglets given gentamycin, the volume of distribution and clearance rate decreased in direct proportion to the decrease in cardiac output and glomerular filtration rate.[168] Hypothermic puppies given intravenous lidocaine showed slower rates of disappearance of the drug than when normothermic.[210] Humans and animals given propranolol showed a reduced volume of distribution and decreased total body clearance, resulting in higher than expected propranolol concentrations.[196,197,220] Decreased hepatic metabolism of propranolol during hypothermia has been shown in vitro.[197] Hypothermia prolongs neuromuscular blockade with *d*-tubocurarine,[121] and increases neuromuscular blockade with suxamethonium.[305] Phenobarbital metabolism and volume of distribution decreased with hypothermia in children.[147] The lethal dose of digoxin was doubled in hypothermic dogs.[24] Digoxin-like substances are present during hypothermia.[102,134]

Reasons for altered metabolism in hypothermia include delayed distribution of the drug and altered enzyme function with temperature and pH changes. Cardiac output decreases, leading to decreased liver perfusion and decreased delivery of drug to hepatic microsomal enzymes.[121,150–152,229] Plasma volume decreases as free water moves intracellularly, causing hemoconcentration and further decreasing organ perfusion.[122] Biliary excretion of atropine, procaine, and sulfanilamide decreases in vitro.[150–152] The glomerular filtration rate decreases in hypothermia.[37] In vitro, the activity of metabolic pathways, including acetylation and hydrolysis, decreases with cooling.[151,152]

Clinical Findings The clinical effects of hypothermia are related to the membrane depressant effects of cold, which result in ionic and electrical conduction disturbances in the brain, heart, peripheral nerves, and other major organs (Table 15–4).[136] Cold tissues are protected by decreases in tissue oxygen requirements. As body temperature decreases, metabolic activity declines at a rate of approximately 7% per 1.8°F (1°C).[307] This effect provides significant protection to

TABLE 15–4. Physiologic and Clinical Manifestations of Hypothermia

Cardiovascular
Variable cardiac output
Normal heart rate or tachycardia, then bradycardia as hypothermia increases
Vasoconstriction and central shunting of blood
ECG
Prolongation of intervals
Atrial fibrillation
Increased ventricular irritability
J-point elevation "Osborn waves"
Central nervous system
Mild: 90°F–95°F (32°C–35°C)
Normal mental status or slightly slowed
Moderate: 80°F–90°F (27°C–32°C)
Lethargic but verbally responsive
Severe: 68°F–80°F (20°C–27°C)
Unlikely to respond verbally, purposefully to noxious stimuli
Profound: <68°F (< 20°C)
Unresponsive, may "appear dead"
Gastrointestinal tract
Decreased motility
Depressed hepatic metabolism
Hematologic
Hemoconcentration
Left shift of oxyhemoglobin dissociation curve
Kidneys
Cold-induced diuresis (Antidiuretic hormone antagonism)
Lungs
Hyperventilation to hypoventilation with increasing hypothermia
Bronchorrhea
Metabolic
Metabolic acidosis
Increased glycogenolysis
Increased serum free fatty acids
Normal thyroid and adrenal function

vital organs despite the potentially deleterious effects of membrane suppression.

Effects on the CNS are temperature dependent and predictable. Mild hypothermia (90°F–95°F; 32.2°C–35°C) usually results in relatively benign clinical manifestations. Ataxia, clumsiness, slowed response to stimuli, and dysarthria are common.[96] As cooling continues, the mental status slowly deteriorates. In moderate hypothermia (80°F–90°F; 27°C–32.2°C), the patient is usually lethargic but still likely to respond verbally. In severe hypothermia (68°F–80°F; 20°C–26.6°C) the patient is unlikely to respond verbally, but will react purposefully to noxious stimuli.[96,127] In profound hypothermia (<68°F; <20°C), the patient is unresponsive to stimuli. Pupils may be fixed and dilated and the patient may appear dead.[127] However, standard criteria of brain death do not apply to hypothermic patients. The hypothermia itself protects against cerebral hypoxic damage.[136] Temperature drop inhibits the release of the excitatory neurotransmitter glutamate and attenuates the release of dopamine in brain ischemia animal models, suggesting a protective effect of hypothermia in brain injury.[44] Ventricular cerebrospinal fluid glutamate concentrations were lower in patients with induced mild hypothermia after brain injury when compared to brain-injured patients kept normothermic.[193] Induced mild hypothermia improves neurological outcomes and survival after return of spontaneous circulation in cardiac arrest.[11,22]

Under controlled circumstances patients have survived with body temperatures as low as 48.2°F (9°C).[99] Vigorous resuscitation is required for these patients. In particular, cardiac resuscitation should not be terminated in the field, where temperatures are seldom taken. The adage that a patient cannot be considered dead until the patient is warm and dead is critical to providing appropriate management. This approach may lead to hours of cardiopulmonary resuscitation of hypothermic patients with ventricular fibrillation, ventricular tachycardia, or asystole, but may be ultimately successful in resuscitating patients initially presumed to be dead.[275]

The cardiac and hemodynamic effects of cold correlate closely with body temperature. As cooling begins there is a transient increase in cardiac output. Tachycardia develops secondary to shivering and sympathetic stimulation. At about 81°F (27.2°C) shivering ceases. Bradycardia develops with maintenance of a normal cardiac stroke volume.[43] This bradycardia is responsible for the decreased myocardial oxygen demand that may be protective in the setting of hypothermia.[43] In profound hypothermia, bradycardia may progress to asystole and death.

Unlike cerebral circulation, where autoregulation is preserved during cooling, coronary autoregulation is disturbed during hypothermia, and myocardial injury may ensue.[43] Attempts to maximize myocardial oxygenation through administration of oxygen and volume replacement to increase diastolic filling pressure are appropriate. Pharmacologic or electrical attempts to increase heart rate may dangerously increase myocardial oxygen demand.

The initial response to cold is hyperventilation; however, as temperature continues to decrease, hypoventilation develops, which may progress to apnea and death. In animal models, this has been attributed to cold-induced failure of phrenic nerve conduction.[159]

The Electrocardiogram The most common ECG abnormality in hypothermia is generalized, progressive depression of myocardial conduction. PR, QRS, and QT intervals are all prolonged, and increasingly profound hypothermia may lead to gradual progression to asystole.[79,289] Ventricular fibrillation occurs in an irritable myocardium most commonly at temperatures less than 86°F (30°C) resulting in a high O_2 consumption dysrhythmia. Atrial fibrillation is the most common dysrhythmia occurring in the presence of hypothermia.[97,230] Shivering may not be clinically evident, but the characteristic fine muscular tremor frequently produces a mechanical artifact in the baseline of the electrocardiogram.[84] A deflection occurring at the junction of the QRS and ST segment is invariably present in patients with temperatures 86°F (<30°C) (Fig. 15–2). First described in a single patient in 1938, the J-point deflection is commonly known as the *Osborn wave*.[85,234,285] The J-point deflection, thought to be a "current of injury" associated with CO_2 retention under hypothermic conditions, was believed to be a poor prognostic sign.[234] Subsequent study does not support any prognostic significance, as the J-point deflection is invariably found in the hypothermic patient when multiple electrocardiographic leads are obtained.[84,85,287,294] The size of the J-point deflection increases as body temperature decreases.[230,294] Atrial dysrhythmias that occur in the

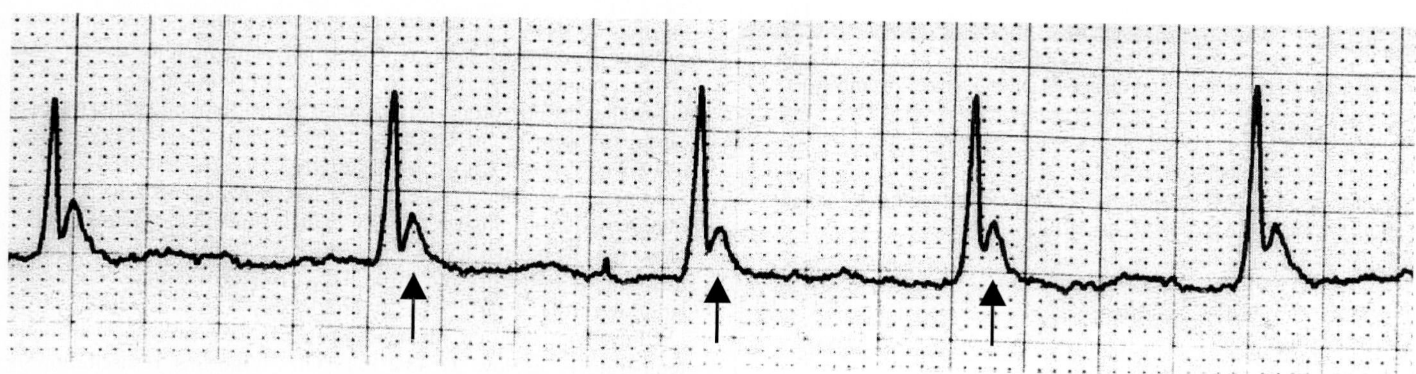

FIGURE 15–2. A characteristic electrocardiographic finding in the patient with profound hypothermia. The arrows (↑) indicate the Osborn wave which appears at terminal phase of the QRS complex.

absence of underlying heart disease invariably disappear solely with rewarming.

Management After blood specimens are drawn, the hypothermic patient in whom hypoglycemia is present should be given 0.5–1.0 g dextrose/kg of body weight as $D_{50}W$ (50% dextrose in water) and 100 mg of thiamine IV. If hypoglycemia is the cause of the hypothermia, the response to dextrose may be dramatic, heralded by the onset of shivering and rapid return to normal body temperature. Wernicke encephalopathy is uncommon, but may be associated with mild hypothermia; thermoregulation and normal ocular motion may return after the initiation of thiamine therapy.[167]

If normal mental status is not regained when the temperature reaches 90°F (32.2°C) during rewarming, underlying CNS structural, toxic, or metabolic problems must be considered.[96,183,239] Failure of the patient to rewarm quickly suggests the presence of underlying disease.[73] (Fig. 15–3). In one study, hypothermic patients without underlying disease are reported to rewarm at a rate of 1.0–3.7°F/h (0.6–2.1°C/h) (average, 2.1°F/h; 1.2°C/h), whereas patients with significant underlying disease (sepsis, gastrointestinal hemorrhage, diabetic ketoacidosis, pulmonary embolus, myocardial infarction) warmed at a rate of 0.25–1.8°F/h (0.1–1.0°C/h) (average, 1°F/h; 0.6°C/h).[300]

Hypothermia shifts the oxygen dissociation curve to the left (Chap. 21), resulting in decreased oxygen unloading to tissues; therefore, oxygen administration may be of benefit.[71] If clinically indicated for airway protection or inadequate ventilation or oxygenation, endotracheal

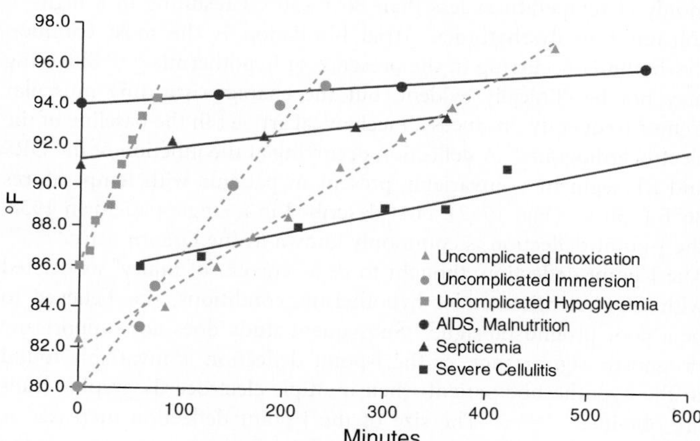

FIGURE 15–3. Relation of rewarming rate to underlying illness.[73]

intubation should be performed and can usually be done without complication.[68,176,207] However, there are case reports of ventricular fibrillation occurring during endotracheal intubation.[20,105,127,235,302] Every effort should be made to limit patient activity and stimulation during the acute rewarming period, as activity may increase myocardial oxygen demand or alter myocardial temperature gradients, increasing the risk of iatrogenic ventricular fibrillation. Although pulmonary artery catheters and central venous lines have been inserted without complications, they should be avoided unless absolutely essential, so as not to precipitate ventricular dysrhythmias.[125,177,286] If a central venous catheter is considered necessary, it should not be allowed to touch the endocardium.[288] Patients who develop ventricular fibrillation or asystole are difficult to manage because they require complex and prolonged resuscitation efforts. In these instances, cardiopulmonary resuscitation (CPR) should be initiated, and the patient intubated and ventilated to maintain a pH of 7.40, **uncorrected** for temperature. Active internal rewarming should be instituted in the patient in cardiac arrest because standard therapy for ventricular fibrillation or asystole may be unsuccessful until rewarming is achieved. There is a risk of toxicity if multiple doses of drugs are administered in the hypothermic patient in whom drug metabolism is altered and circulation is arrested; however, based on current research discussed below, it is reasonable to incorporate pharmacologic agents into the management of hypothermic cardiac arrest. A vasopressor, either epinephrine or vasopressin, may be given to increase the coronary perfusion pressure.[303,304] Amiodarone or lidocaine may then be administered if ventricular fibrillation is present. Defibrillation may not be successful until the temperature exceeds 86°F (30°C); however, it can be successfully accomplished in animals and patients with temperatures of less than 86°F (30°C).[6,20,69,213,303] A reasonable approach is that if defibrillation is unsuccessful, it should not be attempted again until the patient has been warmed several degrees centigrade. Individuals presenting with cardiac arrest and hypothermia may appear dead yet respond to rewarming and resuscitative efforts. The pneumatically powered "thumper" and other devices capable of mechanical chest compression, and cardiopulmonary bypass are used successfully during prolonged hypothermic cardiopulmonary arrests.[20,60,180,276,286]

Arterial Blood Gas Physiochemistry Assessment of the adequacy of ventilation and oxygenation in the hypothermic patient often poses a dilemma to clinicians, as chemical effects of cold on arterial pH and blood gases lead to confusion in the interpretation of arterial blood gas values. Cold inhibits the dissociation of water molecules, causing pH to increase as cooling occurs. In vitro, the pH change of blood as it is cooled increases parallel to the pH change of neutral water. The partial pressures of CO_2 and O_2 decrease as cooling occurs, even as the blood content of those gases remains unchanged. Blood in a syringe taken from a patient whose body temperature is 98.6°F (37°C) yields a pH of 7.40 and a PCO_2 of 40 mm Hg in the blood gas machine at 98.6°F (37°C), but yields a pH of 7.72 and a PCO_2 of 14 mm Hg if the blood is cooled to 61°F (16°C) and the values are measured at that temperature. Specially calibrated laboratory equipment, not routinely available, is required to measure blood gas values directly at other than normal body temperature. A patient whose body temperature is 61°F (16°C) and whose actual in vivo blood gas values are pH 7.72 and PCO_2 14 mm Hg will have values of pH 7.40 and PCO_2 40 mm Hg when the blood is warmed to 98.6°F (37°C) and measured in the standard laboratory blood gas machine. Because the machine measures pH and blood gas pressures only in blood warmed to 98.6°F (37°C) (the uncorrected values), the actual in vivo values in hypothermic patients are approximated using mathematically derived corrected values. Because the pH of neutrality has also increased, it is unclear what clinical meanings these corrected values have. The uncorrected values indicate what the pH and PCO_2 would be if the patient were normothermic. At first glance, the clinician might be content to learn that a hypothermic patient at 61°F (16°C) has a corrected pH of 7.47 and PCO_2 of 40 mm Hg. However, the uncorrected values of pH 7.18 and PCO_2 111 mm Hg indicate that the patient has a significant respiratory acidosis. Attempts to maintain a corrected pH of 7.40 may lead to hypoventilation and risk alveolar collapse and impairment of oxygenation. The preponderance of evidence in the anesthesia and cardiovascular surgery literature suggests that maintenance of ventilation is associated with a decreased incidence of myocardial injury and a decreased incidence of ventricular fibrillation.[71] pH and PCO_2 blood gas values should be left uncorrected after the blood sample is warmed in the blood gas machine and interpreted in the same way as in the normothermic patient.

Hypotension When hypotension occurs in the patient with hypothermia, it may be a result of the presence of bradycardia and volume depletion. However, hypotension may be a predictor of infection, particularly when associated with a slow rewarming rate.[73] Fluid depletion in hypothermia occurs as a result of a variety of mechanisms, including central shunting of blood by vasoconstriction and cold-induced diuresis. Cold diuresis occurs when increases in central blood volume result in inhibition of the release of antidiuretic hormone. Impairment of renal enzyme activity and decreased renal tubular reabsorption contribute to the large quantities of dilute urine known as cold diuresis.[122,126,177,307] Normal saline should be given to expand intravascular volume. Urine output is an important indicator of organ perfusion and the adequacy of intravascular volume in the hypothermic patient, although the initial cold diuresis may lead to underestimation of fluid needs.[307]

Pharmacologic Interventions The best means to affect resuscitation of the hypothermic victim in ventricular fibrillation is controversial. The most recent recommendations of the American Heart Association for the treatment of cardiac arrest when the core body temperature is <86°F (<30°C) do not include the administration of a vasopressor or antidysrhythmic.[1] However, a recent metanalysis of animal studies of antidysrhythmic and vasopressor therapy for ventricular fibrillation in the setting of hypothermia found there was significant improvement in the return of spontaneous circulation (ROSC) in animals that received epinephrine or vasopressin.[304] In this report, the authors could not identify a benefit to the use of amiodarone or bretylium administered without a vasopressor. They postulated that this is most likely due to the improvement in coronary perfusion pressure caused by vasopressors during cardiac arrest.[304]

Epinephrine and Vasopressin The administration of vasopressin to pigs in hypothermic cardiac arrest increased coronary perfusion pressure and improved defibrillation success.[265] However, because of defibrillation, there was no difference in the 1-hour ROSC.[265] In a pig model, when warmed thoracic lavage was utilized, vasopressin increased coronary perfusion pressure and increased the 1-hour survival.[264] In this study the administration of saline resulted in zero episodes of successful defibrillation whereas 8 of 8 vasopressin-treated pigs had restoration of spontaneous circulation after electrical defibrillation and improved short-term survival. The whole body temperature was not increased, but the authors postulated that myocardial warming may have occurred.[264] In another study in which epinephrine was given to one group of pigs and vasopressin to another, increased coronary perfusion pressure and ROSC resulted in both groups.[171,172] In contrast, body temperature significantly increased during CPR with thoracic lavage, and epinephrine increased coronary perfusion pressure, but no improvement in ROSC occurred.[170] The length of time of cardiac arrest, the doses of drug, and the efforts to rewarm differed in these studies. A 19-year-old patient who had a prolonged hypothermic cardiopulmonary arrest showed no improvement following 2 mg of epinephrine but following the administration of vasopressin had immediate restoration of spontaneous circulation.[281] Interactions with epinephrine, vasopressin, and ischemia during CPR are complex and incompletely understood.[173]

Amiodarone Amiodarone is recommended in the current AHA algorithm for ventricular fibrillation in normothermia. In one study comparing the use of amiodarone, bretylium, and placebo in a hypothermic dog model, amiodarone showed no statistical improvement in causing ROSC. There was no significant difference between the groups; only 1 of 10 amiodarone-treated dogs demonstrated ROSC, versus 3 of 10 in the placebo group and 4 of 10 in the bretylium-treated dogs.[280] However, in a study in which hypothermic dogs in ventricular fibrillation were treated with epinephrine before administration of amiodarone 10 mg/kg, there was a significantly higher rate of ROSC.[303]

Bretylium Bretylium tosylate is a benzyl quaternary ammonium compound with a biphasic action, initially causing release of norepinephrine and then blocking its release. This may cause transient hypertension, but hypotension is the most common result.[213,233] Hypothermic dogs given bretylium had significantly lower mean arterial pressures and systemic and pulmonary vascular resistance as compared to controls.[233] The mechanism of the antidysrhythmic effect of bretylium in normothermia may be related to its ability to increase the myocardial refractory period.[233] Bretylium is no longer part of the AHA recommendations and is no longer available in the USA. A single case of successful chemical defibrillation with bretylium is reported in an environmentally exposed patient with a core temperature of 85.1°F (29.5°C).[67]

Dopamine Dopamine increases cardiac output, mean arterial pressure, heart rate, and stroke volume in dogs cooled to 77°F (25°C), and stabilizes pulmonary arterial wedge pressure.[219] In a canine hypothermia model, dopamine infusions provided some protection from ventricular fibrillation. Dopamine lowered the temperature at which ventricular fibrillation occurred and reduced the incidence of ventricular fibrillation, as did infusion of norepinephrine.[10] The added benefit of dopamine in hypothermia may be a result of its renal and splanchnic vasodilating properties, increasing renal perfusion and supporting urine output.[109] Dopamine increases myocardial oxygen demand and decreases peripheral perfusion, potentially detrimental effects in the hypothermic patient.[10] Nevertheless, after the administration of intravenous fluids, dopamine infusion during hypothermia is indicated in the patient requiring blood pressure support.

Rewarming Three types of rewarming modalities are used in the management of hypothermic patients.[63,85] *Passive external rewarming* involves covering the patient with blankets and protecting the patient from further heat loss. Passive external rewarming uses the patient's own endogenous heat production for rewarming and is most successful in healthy patients with mild to moderate hypothermia whose capacity for endogenous heat production is intact.[126] Passive external rewarming is reported to be successful in hypothermic patients with temperatures as low as 69°F (20.6°C).[284,294,301] Advocates of passive external rewarming argue that it allows vasoconstriction to persist and it decreases the afterdrop and shock from vasodilation associated with active skin rewarming.[126,207,284]

Active external rewarming involves the external application of heat to the patient. There is disagreement about the possible detrimental effects of active external rewarming. For example, skin warming may lead to a physiologically detrimental suppression of shivering.[126] Acute vasodilation of peripheral vessels could cause hypotension and an increased peripheral demand on the persistently cold myocardium. The return of cold blood from the extremities to the heart is suggested to exacerbate intramyocardial temperature gradients, which could cause ventricular irritability during hypothermia.[186] However, in pigs, blood returning to the heart was found to be warm before warming of central organs occurred.[110] A new warming method that circulates temperature- controlled water through pads adherent to the skin requires care to prevent skin damage.[115]

Afterdrop is the continuing decrease in temperature once active rewarming begins. The American Heart Association (AHA) Advanced Cardiac Life Support (ACLS) guidelines[1] recommend not in the extremities application of heat to the trunk only, in an attempt to avoid the complications of afterdrop and intramyocardial temperature gradients.[174] In one study of 33 patients with core temperature <82.4°F (< 28°C), no patient experienced afterdrop during peripheral rewarming.[248] There is no scientific evidence to suggest that afterdrop, should it occur, is more dangerous than the very temperature that had existed originally.[187] In addition, there is no evidence of pooling of blood in the periphery, nor of increased flow during surface rewarming.[187,260] Flow studies in the hand, arm, calf, and foot demonstrate that afterdrop has already occurred and is completed before any increase in blood flow occurs in the limbs.[187,298] Initial experiments demonstrating afterdrop were done in inanimate objects and reflected continued cooling of central structures before heat from external sources reached the core.[110,187,298]

Treatment including complete submersion is available in some institutions. Eighteen patients with temperatures of 78.8°F–91.4°F (26°C–33°C) were successfully warmed in a Hubbard tank, although one fatality not associated with rewarming occurred.[309] Submersion must be used with caution, however, because of the inherent difficulties of controlling agitated patients and monitoring and resuscitating patients in water.

Mortality rates for active external rewarming are frequently reported to be higher than for passive external rewarming,[242] but case selection is not controlled in these series. Sicker patients with stable cardiac rhythms who fail to rewarm passively and are then actively rewarmed have a higher mortality rate directly correlated with their underlying disease, rather than the method of therapy.[73] Selection of either passive or active external rewarming in treatment of mild to moderate hypothermic patients with perfusing cardiac rhythms does not appear to influence the prognosis as much as the presence or absence of underlying disease.[73,139,207,300] In our experience, active external rewarming has not resulted in mortality, except in those patients with severe underlying disease.[73,294]

Active internal rewarming involves attempts to increase central core temperature directly, by warming the heart prior to the extremities or periphery. Minimally invasive modalities of active internal rewarming include the administration of heated, humidified oxygen delivered by face mask or endotracheal tube,[128] and gastric lavage with warmed fluids. More invasive modalities, those procedures that are fundamental to the rewarming controversy, include peritoneal lavage with warmed dialysate,[145,224] and the rerouting of blood through external blood rewarming equipment via cardiopulmonary or femoral–femoral bypass and hemodialysis.[47,133,215] Heparin-coated bypass systems are available that avoid systemic anticoagulation, thus decreasing the risk of bleeding complications. It is suggested that extracorporeal venovenous rewarming and continuous arteriovenous rewarming show improved rewarming rates when compared to standard techniques such as saline lavage of the bladder, stomach, or peritoneal cavity.[103] Extracorporeal methods of active internal rewarming should be reserved for severely hypothermic patients (<80°F or <27°C) or those with unstable cardiac rhythms (ventricular fibrillation or tachycardia, or asystole) attributed to hypothermia.[6,72,123] The evidence for the benefit of extracorporeal methods in those patients with stable rhythms is not clear. In patients with stable rhythms, studies are essential to resolve the debate over the merits of passive or active external rewarming versus active internal rewarming. Transcutaneous pacing was successful in improving hemodynamic parameters and speeding rewarming in an animal model.[81]

Unfortunately, current ACLS guidelines for the management of hypothermia make several recommendations that are not supported by the literature. The most glaring is the recommendation of extracorporeal rewarming for stable patients based on a temperature of 86°F (30°C) or less. ACLS guidelines assert that passive rewarming is ineffective in the stable patient with severe hypothermia, which is defined as a temperature below 86°F (30°C). However, many patients with temperatures below 86°F (30°C) have been successfully treated with passive external rewarming with, at most, the addition of warm, humidified oxygen.[73,248,273,294,301] Patient temperature correlates poorly with outcome.[6,69,176,286,289] Treatment recommendations should not be based solely on temperature. Stability of the vital signs and cardiac rhythm and the underlying cause of hypothermia are much more critical considerations in management. It is hard to imagine a patient with a stable cardiac rhythm and core temperature of 80°F–86°F (26.6°C–30°C) in whom extracorporeal rewarming with cardiopulmonary bypass is indicated.

Additionally, ACLS guidelines state that significant hyperkalemia may develop during rewarming, suggesting that this is a complication of rewarming. Hyperkalemia is not described as a consequence of rewarming.[68] In all of the evidence collected with regard to hyperkalemia, this abnormality was present as a consequence of the hypothermia and not the rewarming.[127,191,261]

Prognosis in Hypothermia Except in cases of profound hypothermia,[127] the prognosis is most closely correlated with the presence or absence of underlying disease.[139,207,227,300,301] In patients with hypothermia alone, in the absence of underlying disease, mortality is 0% to 10%. In the presence of a severe underlying disease such as sepsis, mortality is much greater.[73] Morbidity results from associated frostbite and trauma.

Prolonged cardiopulmonary arrest and absolute temperature are not predictive of poor outcome.[6,69,176,286,289] In severely hypothermic patients, profound hyperkalemia ($K^+ > 10$ mEq/L) is associated with unsuccessful resuscitation.[127,191,261]

Frostbite Hypothermia may be accompanied by frostbite when patients are exposed to environmental temperatures that are less than 20°F (6.7°C).[208] Frostbite should be managed by rapid rewarming. The extremity involved may be placed in a large, soft basin of warm water (100°F–108°F; 38°C–43°C) for 30 minutes. The water temperature must be frequently adjusted, as the frozen extremity will cool the water in the basin. Parenteral analgesics may be necessary, as the rewarming process is often painful. Frostbitten areas should never be rubbed, as the tissue is particularly sensitive to trauma. Dextran, alcohol, vasodilators, and anticoagulants have not proven useful. Sympathectomy in this situation is also of unproven benefit and remains highly controversial.[160,175,199]

Prevention Because many patients may not wear (and may not possess) adequate clothing, it is essential that they be assessed for social services support after the acute episode is resolved. In addition, many of these patients live in substandard, inadequately heated (often unheated) housing. Patients should be advised to wear comfortable, warm clothing to prevent future episodes of hypothermia. Adequate clothing is particularly important for patients traveling by automobile during inclement weather conditions. The importance of adequate nutrition should also be stressed.

HYPERTHERMIA

Definition of Heatstroke Heatstroke is defined by a rectal temperature greater than 106°F (41.1°C) in the setting of a neurologic disturbance manifested by mental status changes including confusion, delirium, stupor, coma, and/or convulsions.[164] Temperature criteria cannot be absolute, as information regarding the patient's temperature is rarely available at the time of onset of heatstroke. In some instances the temperature may not be measured for several hours, during which time cooling may have been instituted or occurred spontaneously.[155,156] When appropriate environmental conditions prevail, the diagnosis of heatstroke should be made liberally. Although the absence of sweating was once thought to be an essential component of the definition of heatstroke,[58,226] many patients with heatstroke maintain the ability to sweat.[66,192,270,295]

Epidemiology of Heatstroke Hundreds of people die annually of heatstroke in the United States, and 80% of the victims are older than 50 years of age. When counting heat-related fatalities, the number is underestimated if only death certificates are included in which hyperthermia is listed as the underlying cause of death. Including hyperthermia as a contributing factor to death increased the total number of heat-related deaths by 54% from 1993 to 2003.[12] Several studies show mortality rates from heatstroke to be 5.6% to 80%. Thousands of other victims survive with significant heat-related morbidity.[9,15,33,80,146,157,277] The high morbidity and mortality of heatstroke markedly contrast with those of profound hypothermia, in which the prognosis is related not to the temperature itself, but to the underlying etiology. The overall prognosis in heatstroke depends primarily on how long the temperature has been elevated prior to cooling, the maximum temperature reached, and the affected individual's premorbid health.

Heat-related deaths are preventable, and the public health preparedness of cities, healthcare workers, and the community is essential.[21,50] Mortality during heat waves is increased in urban areas where a heat wave has not occurred for several years.[57,83,146,263] Mortality is decreased when public health interventions improve preparedness. The city of Milwaukee experienced a heat wave in 1995 that resulted in numerous public health and preparedness responses. These efforts may have resulted in a diminution by 49% of the number of heat-related deaths and emergency medical service runs in the heat wave of 1999.[299] After the Chicago heat wave of 1995, public policies targeting the elderly of Chicago may have contributed to a change in the demographics of those who succumbed during a subsequent heat wave in Chicago in 1999. The dead in 1999 were younger; more that 50% of those who died were younger than age 65 years. More than half of the dead were seen or spoken to on either the day of or the day before their death. Psychiatric illness was almost twice as prevalent in the younger victims, compared to those older than 65 years of age.[218]

Heat waves are meteorologic events characterized by air temperatures that are ≥90°F (≥32.2°C) for 3 or more consecutive days.[49] During the summer of 2003, Europe experienced record high temperatures for many consecutive days. The prolonged heat caused extreme increases in mortality across Europe. In France, there were 14,800 excess deaths caused by heat. This is equivalent to a total mortality increase of 60% between August 1 and August 20, 2003.[178,291] In a followup report of 83 of the survivors, the subsequent mortality at 2 years was 71%.[15] Survivors had dramatic decreases in their ability to function.[15] Italy reported 1094 excess deaths from June to August 2003, a 23% increase compared with the average annual number of deaths from 1995 to 2002.[50] Increased mortality was associated with risk factors previously reported, including old age, limited access to care, poor living conditions, and social isolation.[34,266,292]

Socially isolated individuals or those with pre-existing illness, as well as the physically compromised and frail elderly, are at greatest risk of death during heat waves. Confinement to bed was the strongest predictor of death in the Chicago heat wave of 1995, and living alone doubled the risk of death. There were fewer deaths among people with working air conditioners or who had access to an air-conditioned environment.[249,266] Although fans may seem to improve comfort, they do not prevent heat-related illness and may contribute to heat stress when temperatures and humidity exceed approximately 100°F (37.8°C).[153,157,158,218,266,306] In times of heat waves, preventive public health programs should encourage visiting nurses, housekeepers, and community service programs to increase the awareness of the danger of heat and identify those individuals most at risk.[266] A decreased risk of death was found among people with contacts from these agencies during the Chicago heat wave.[266] The media must alert the public and provide information on avoiding heat illness, as well as encourage individuals to help others to stay cool by assuring access to cooling measures.

The number of deaths from exposure-related illness has increased 3-fold in foreign transients attempting to enter the United States from Mexico. Because urban areas are more tightly patrolled, individuals attempting to cross into the United States illegally have turned to the harsh deserts and mountain ranges of the southwestern United States, increasing prolonged exposure and resulting in death from heat, cold, and dehydration. Although many more bodies may remain undiscovered, 99 individuals' deaths were attributed to environmental causes in the year 2000, many of these due to heat.[88]

From 1995 to 2002, 233 children died from heatstroke when left unattended in cars, 75% of whom were either forgotten or left by caretakers who did not expect the temperature to rise dangerously within the automobile. In 25% of the incidents, children were trapped inadvertently while playing. Most of these deaths occurred during the summer months.[117]

Infants may suffer heatstroke under environmental conditions that would not be expected to place the child in danger. Well-meaning parents sometimes overinsulate children with clothing and blankets, inhibiting their cutaneous heat loss and placing them at risk.[19,142,143]

During 2002, the United States military reported 1816 heat-related injuries of active duty soldiers.[7] During Operation Iraqi Freedom, 6 soldiers died from heat-related causes. There were 30 other cases of heatstroke and many other heat-related casualties. During the period 1997–2002, 8084 soldiers were treated as outpatients for heat injuries.[7] The United States military actively promotes heat illness prevention and exhorts its personnel to not repeat history. In comparison, in 1917, 425 British soldiers on active duty in the area on the Persian Gulf formerly known as Mesopotamia, presently known as Iraq, died of heatstroke during 1 month, and 524 died in 1 year.[302] There were 114 heatstroke deaths among football players from 1960 to 2007. From 1995 to 2007, 33 football players died of heatstroke: 25 high school, 5 college, 2 professional, and 1 sandlot.[211,290]

High ambient temperature is associated with an increase in mortality from cocaine overdose. The mean daily number of deaths from cocaine overdose was 33% higher when the ambient temperature exceeded 88°F (31°C).[194]

Thermoregulation and Heat Stress The normal thermoregulatory response to heat stress is mediated primarily by heat-sensitive neurons in the hypothalamus. Increased body core temperature results in active dilation of cutaneous vessels and skin blood flow increases.[131,252] Because increased skin blood flow is attained primarily by an increase in heart rate and stroke volume, the capacity to increase cardiac output is critical to cooling. Compensatory shifting of blood flow from the splanchnic and renal vessels to the skin further increases skin blood flow.[138,252] The combination of vasodilation, increased skin blood flow, and increased sweating results in heat loss through convection and evaporation. Dehydration after profuse sweating increases plasma osmolarity. Heat-sensitive neurons in the preoptic anterior hypothalamus are inhibited by locally increased osmolarity and by input from distal hepatoportal osmoreceptors. The inhibition of heat sensitive neurons results in decreased heat dissipation response.[56,228]

Types of Heatstroke Heatstroke is commonly divided into 2 types: *exertional* and *nonexertional.* Nonexertional, or classic, heatstroke describes heatstroke occurring in the absence of extreme exertion. Nonexertional heatstroke is most commonly described during heat waves, and the victims are predominantly those persons least able to tolerate heat: infants,[19] the aged,[61] those with psychiatric disorders, and the chronically ill.

Exertional heatstroke occurs as a result of increased motor activity. It may occur in young, healthy individuals who are exercising, or in individuals whose increased motor activity results from other causes, such as seizures or agitation. Often a period of significant heat stress in exercising individuals precedes the development of heatstroke. Military recruits who develop heatstroke may sometimes present to the camp infirmary with vague complaints prior to collapse.[270] Published studies of heatstroke in miners, athletes, and military recruits describe several precipitating factors in heatstroke: fatigue associated with a recent deficit in sleep; poor physical conditioning; a recent febrile illness; recent heat-related symptoms such as thirst or weakness; relative volume depletion; failure to allow for acclimatization; and obesity. Symptoms of nausea, weakness, headache, diarrhea, or irritability often precede the development of heatstroke. Although rapid onset of symptoms and acute loss of consciousness are frequently reported in exertional heatstroke, the preceding period of heat stress and insidious symptoms may go unrecognized. Although exertional heatstroke is more likely to occur during intense exertion in a hot, humid environment, it may also occur with moderately intense exercise early in the morning, when environmental conditions do not usually represent a thermoregulatory stress.[16]

Differential Diagnosis of Hyperthermia In addition to exposure and exertion, conditions that predispose to severe hyperthermia include primary hypothalamic lesions; intracranial hemorrhage; agitation; alcohol and sedative-hypnotic withdrawal; seizures; and the use of therapeutic and illicit xenobiotics (Table 15–5).[107,112–114,171,195,282] Included in the differential diagnosis of severe hyperthermia are the serotonin syndrome, malignant hyperthermia, and the neuroleptic malignant syndrome, all of which may result in high temperature, altered mental status, and increased muscle tone.

TABLE 15–5. Differential Diagnosis of Hyperthermia

Increased heat production
Increased muscle activity
Agitation
Catatonia
Ethanol and sedative-hypnotic withdrawal
Exercise
Infectious diseases
Malignant hyperthermia
Monoamine oxidase inhibitor drug interactions
Neuroleptic malignant syndrome
Parkinson disease
Sedative-hypnotic withdrawal
Seizures
Serotonin syndrome
Xenobiotics
Increased metabolic rate
Hyperthyroidism
Pheochromocytoma
Sympathomimetics
Impaired heat loss
Environmental
Heat
Humidity
Lack of acclimatization
Social disadvantage
Isolation
Poverty
Lack of air conditioning
Confinement to bed
Medical illness
Cardiac insufficiency
Diabetes
Hypertension
Pulmonary
CNS dysfunction
Salt and water depletion
Fatigue
Limited behavioral response
Extremes of age
Psychiatric impairment
Mental retardation
Xenobiotics

Serotonin Syndrome The serotonin syndrome results from excess stimulation of the serotonin receptor, primarily the 5-HT_{1A} subtype.[279] Drug interactions are most commonly the cause of the syndrome. Monoamine oxidase inhibitors used in conjunction with tricyclic antidepressants,[21] selective serotonin reuptake inhibitors,[91] L-tryptophan,[91,283] meperidine,[124] dextromethorphan,[246] amphetamines,[171] and sumatriptan are reported to lead to serotonergic hyperstimulation and severe symptoms.[108,279] The clinical condition resulting from excess serotonin includes alterations in consciousness, restlessness, increased muscle tone, tremor, gastrointestinal disturbances, and hyperthermia. Treatment of the syndrome focuses on control of hyperthermia by using aggressive cooling, muscle relaxation primarily by using benzodiazepines, or, in severe cases, endotracheal intubation and paralysis (Chap. 72).

Malignant Hyperthermia Malignant hyperthermia is a very rare disorder that is associated with a congenital disturbance of calcium regulation in striated muscle. Malignant hyperthermia was first reported in 1960. Ten deaths occurred in a single family following general anesthesia.[77] Exposure to anesthetics, depolarizing muscle relaxants, or, rarely, severe exertion precipitates uncontrolled calcium influx into the sarcoplasmic reticulum, leading to severe muscle rigidity and hyperthermia.[116,144] The clinical setting of severe muscle rigidity and hyperthermia following general anesthesia usually is adequate to define the syndrome (Chap. 68).

Neuroleptic Malignant Syndrome Neuroleptic malignant syndrome, a severe extrapyramidal syndrome associated with muscle rigidity, autonomic dysfunction, and altered mental status, was first described in 1968.[74] This disorder develops during the administration of antipsychotics or the withdrawal of dopaminergic xenobiotics. Increased muscle tone, due to dopaminergic blockade of the striatum, as well as central altered hypothalamic thermoregulation lead to hyperthermia.[129] Temperature elevation and alteration of mental status occur after the onset of "lead pipe" muscle rigidity.[27,120] Laboratory findings are not specific and include marked elevation of creatine phosphokinase (CPK) in some patients and leukocytosis with a left shift. Neuroleptic malignant syndrome must be distinguished from the much more common cases of heatstroke in psychiatric patients that are caused by heat intolerance resulting from the anticholinergic effects of antipsychotics or antihistamines prescribed to control extrapyramidal symptoms (Chap. 69).[257,310]

Inflammatory Mediators in Heatstroke The response to heat stress is a coordinated interplay between the mediators of inflammation, including endothelial cells, leukocytes, inflammatory cytokines, and endotoxins. These are important mediators of the systemic immune response. However, in heatstroke they are responsible for systemic inflammation and activation of the coagulation cascade, similar to the sepsis syndrome. Many proinflammatory cytokines are identified in heatstroke, including tumor necrosis factor; interleukin-2, -6, -8, -10, and -12; interferon-α and -β; and granulocyte colony–stimulating factors.[33] In a study of 18 heatstroke patients, circulating cytokine levels correlated with clinical indices of heatstroke severity.[140] Cooling delays the release of interleukin-1B, interleukin-6, and tumor necrosis factor in vitro.[161] Studies in hyperthermic animals focus on the modulation of the mediators of inflammation as possible future adjuncts to cooling. For example, in one report, an interleukin-1 receptor antagonist improved survival.[269] In another, recombinant human activated protein C provided cytoprotection by decreasing release of inflammatory cytokines, but did not improve survival.[35] Whole body cooling restored appropriate levels of cardiac tissue protein associated with loss of structural integrity of the cardiac myocytes, and reversed cardiac dysfunction.[53]

Heat stress causes increased gene transcription of heat shock proteins which render the organism more resistant to heat injury, protecting cells from injury and increasing cell survival. Heat shock protein 72 is protective against injury from heat stress, and the extent of protection correlates with the level of heat shock protein.[188]

During exercise, splanchnic hypoperfusion increases the translocation of bacteria from the gut into the bloodstream, establishing the cascade of inflammation and injury that perpetuate tissue injury after normothermia is established.[89]

Pathophysiologic Characteristics of Heatstroke Hypotension and tachycardia in heatstroke are caused by a number of factors. The patient with heatstroke may have a reduced plasma volume secondary to dehydration. There is peripheral pooling of blood associated with an increase in cutaneous blood flow from 0.5 L/min to 7–8 L/min.[138,252] In addition, patients may manifest primary myocardial insufficiency.[162] Clinically, patients exhibit either a hypodynamic or hyperdynamic circulatory response. The observed circulatory response to heat stress is a function of the patient's cardiac reserve, volume status, and degree of myocardial heat injury. The hyperdynamic condition is characterized by increased cardiac index and decreased systemic vascular resistance.[225] These hemodynamic characteristics occur in patients who are able to maintain a significantly increased cardiac output in response to the circulatory demand of heat stress.

Salt and water depleted patients, or those patients with primary myocardial insufficiency, may exhibit a hypodynamic response. These patients have a decreased cardiac index and increased systemic vascular resistance.[225,278] Whether pulmonary vascular resistance is affected is unclear. High central venous pressures (CVPs) have been found in some patients, with evidence of right heart failure and right heart dilation on autopsy.[192] These findings have led to the suggestion that pulmonary vascular resistance may be elevated.[225] In 22 of 34 patients with heatstroke, CVPs were greater than 3 cm H_2O. Twelve patients had a CVP of 0, and 10 had a CVP that exceeded 10 cm H_2O. These authors cautioned against injudicious infusion of large quantities of intravenous fluids that can result in complications of congestive heart failure and fluid overload. In the study, only 3 patients required more than 2 L of 0.9% sodium chloride solution during cooling. Crystalloid infusion ranged from 500 to 2500 mL, and none of the patients developed problems associated with fluid overload.[267]

A study of compromised elderly patients with heatstroke, using pulmonary artery catheters, showed that pulmonary vascular resistance was low or normal. Pulmonary capillary wedge pressures were not elevated.[277] A study of 13 cases of heatstroke in pilgrims to Mecca, Saudia Arabia, monitored with pulmonary artery catheters, demonstrated a good correlation of CVP with pulmonary capillary wedge pressures.[3] Serial electrocardiograms in 51 of these pilgrims suffering from heatstroke showed normal sinus rhythm in 25%, sinus tachycardia in 52%, atrial fibrillation in 16%, and sinus bradycardia in 6%. ST segment depression and other ST-T wave changes were reported. The QT interval showed no abnormality.[4] ST changes suggestive of acute coronary syndrome may occur and normal coronary arteries are noted upon coronary catherization.[212] In some patients, echocardiography showed pericardial effusions and regional wall motion abnormalities, asymmetric septal hypertrophy, right ventricular dilation, and left ventricular dilation with impaired function.[4]

Autopsy studies of the heart demonstrate right heart dilation, pericardial effusions, interstitial edema, degeneration and necrosis of myocardial fibers, and subendocardial hemorrhages.[156,192] Postmortem examination of the lungs revealed vascular congestion, pleural effusions, and parenchymal hemorrhages.[192,225]

Gastrointestinal hemorrhage, vomiting, and diarrhea occur frequently.[270] At autopsy, edema and hemorrhage of the bowel wall are demonstrated.[52] These changes may be partly a result of the regional ischemia of splanchnic blood vessels and resultant hypoperfusion and hypoxia. Increased bowel wall edema and bleeding predispose to the release of bacteria into the bloodstream from the gut, causing focal microvascular changes in the intestinal villi, leading to bowel wall anoxia and further injury.[86] Liver injury occurs commonly and is not clinically manifest until the second or third day following the temperature increase.[155,270] Centrilobular changes, such as widening of central veins and adjacent sinusoids and pooling of blood, and varying degrees of hepatocellular degeneration are demonstrated on liver biopsy. Repeat biopsies demonstrated that these changes resolve as the patient recovers.[155] In other cases, only congestion and fatty infiltration are reported.[52]

Neuropsychiatric impairment is, by definition, present in all cases of heatstroke. Duration of altered consciousness correlates significantly with mortality.[18,270] Autopsy studies demonstrate a variety of structural and microscopic CNS injuries. Edema and venous congestion are evident. The number of cortical neurons is reduced, with concomitant glial proliferation. Cerebellar Purkinje cell deterioration is marked. The hypothalamus appears to be relatively spared, with limited edema of the neuronal nuclei. Hemorrhages occur throughout the brain.[52,192,270] Carotid artery vasoconstriction occurs in response to heating, in an in vitro model using the carotid arteries of rabbits as a possible mechanism of ischemia and injury in heatstroke.[216] Heatstroke-induced cerebral ischemia is associated with increased glutamate release, activation of cerebral dopaminergic neurons causing dopamine overload, and gliosis. These changes are attenuated by induction of hypothermia in an animal model.[55]

Reports of brain MRIs of patients recovering from heatstroke describe radiographic findings, including hemorrhagic and ischemic abnormalities of the cerebrum and cerebellum, delayed cerebellar atrophy, central pontine myelinolysis, vascular infarcts, and medial thalamic lesions, which correspond anatomically to the paraventricular nucleus.[26,200,201] The paraventricular nucleus is involved with core temperature regulation via the hypothalamic—pituitary—adrenal axis.[25] The clinical symptoms of dysphagia, quadriparesis, wasting extrapyramidal syndrome, and pancerebellar syndrome have corresponding MRI findings.[5] Persistent cerebellar dysfunction occurs, as does lower motor neuron damage, manifested by areflexia and muscle wasting.[75,179] Abnormal nerve conduction studies are documented.[149] Higher cortical functions may be spared in survivors, or may be reversible when they occur.[89,182,203] Permanent neurologic sequelae are correlated with the degree and duration of hyperthermia.

Acute renal failure was the major cause of death in heatstroke victims before the advent of hemodialysis.[262,295] In addition to the direct effects of heat, volume depletion, and hypotension, myoglobinuria secondary to rhabdomyolysis results in further renal tubular injury. This is especially common in the agitated or exercising patient.[59,107,237] The mechanism by which myoglobin contributes to renal failure remains controversial. At autopsy the kidneys are enlarged, with extensive petechial hemorrhage.[192] Acute tubular necrosis is seen on biopsy. In exertional heatstroke with acute renal failure, renal hemodynamics are compromised because of increased vasoconstrictive hormones, such as catecholamines, renin, aldosterone, and endothelin-1, and decreased vasodilatory hormones, such as prostaglandin E_2.[184]

Bleeding is associated with significant morbidity and mortality in many cases of heatstroke. Coagulation disturbances seen in patients with heatstroke appear to be multifactorial. Elevation of the prothrombin time may occur within 30 minutes of temperature elevation and is attributed to direct heat injury of clotting factors.[21] Liver damage may significantly contribute to the coagulation disturbances, although this does not manifest as rapidly.[21,40,217] Two patients with severe liver failure secondary to heatstroke received liver transplantation; both died after chronic rejection.[254] A third patient with extensive liver cell necrosis as a consequence of heatstroke was referred for consideration of liver transplantation, but recovered completely with supportive therapy.[104] Evidence of diffuse capillary basement membrane injury has been demonstrated by electron microscopy and is thought to precipitate consumptive coagulopathy in severe cases of heatstroke.[52,274] Thrombocytopenia is very common and occurs within 30 minutes of onset of heatstroke, frequently in the absence of other evidence of disseminated intravascular coagulation. Direct thermal injury leading to decreased platelet survival and megakaryocyte damage may play a role (Table 15–6).[192,217]

Clinical Evolution in Heatstroke Clinical evaluation of the hyperthermic patient begins with careful assessment of the vital signs. Vital sign abnormalities commonly include tachycardia with heart rates greater than 130 beats per minute, hypotension, and tachypnea with the respiratory

TABLE 15–6. Physiologic and Clinical Manifestations of Heatstroke

Cardiovascular
Hypodynamic states in elderly
Hyperdynamic states in young healthy individuals
Electrocardiogram
Nonspecific
Widening of QRS because of an underlying abnormality (cocaine toxicity, hyperkalemia associated with rhabdomyolysis)
Central nervous system
Altered mental status
Irritability, confusion, ataxia, seizures, coma
Weakness, dizziness, headache
Plantar extension, pupillary abnormalities, decorticate posturing
EEG
Normal or diffuse slowing
CSF
Normal or increased protein
Lymphocytosis
Gastrointestinal
Vomiting, diarrhea, hematemesis
Hematologic
Bleeding diathesis
Prolonged PT and PTT
Disseminated intravascular coagulation
Thrombocytopenia
Petechiae
Purpura
Leukocytosis
Hepatic
Hepatic insufficiency at 12–36 h
Elevated AST, ALT, LDH
Metabolic
Metabolic acidosis and respiratory alkalosis
Electrolyte disturbance
Hypernatremia
Hyponatremia
Hypokalemia
Hypocalcemia
Hypophosphatemia
Muscle
Rhabdomyolysis
Elevated CPK
Renal
Decreased renal perfusion
Myoglobinuria
Proteinuria
Oliguria
Acute tubular necrosis
Interstitial necrosis

rates often above 30 breaths per minute. Most importantly, temperature is elevated. After cooling, there is often a secondary rise in temperature that suggests persistent disturbances of thermoregulation.[192]

Neurologic examination reveals a delirious, comatose, or seizing patient. Pupils may be normal, fixed and dilated, or pinpoint. Decerebrate or decorticate posturing may be evident. Muscle tone is increased, normal, or flaccid. The skin may be hot and dry or diaphoretic. Nasal and oropharyngeal bleeding may be present as a consequence of the acute coagulopathy. Examination of the lungs is often nonspecific, although heatstroke victims are at risk of pulmonary edema as a primary event associated with capillary endothelial damage or following overly aggressive fluid resuscitation. Cardiac auscultation may reveal a flow murmur secondary to high cardiac output or a right ventricular gallop. Neck vein distension indicates increased CVP. Jaundice suggests hepatic injury and occurs on the second or third day following the onset of heatstroke.[54] Nasogastric aspiration or rectal examination may demonstrate gross bleeding. A petechial rash develops, probably secondary to capillary endothelial damage.

Laboratory Findings of Heatstroke Lactic acid dehydrogenase (LDH) rises as a consequence of diffuse tissue injury. Early rises in alanine aminotransferase (ALT) and aspartate aminotransferase (AST), which peak at 48 hours, are indicators of the liver damage that occurs during heatstroke.[155] Muscle enzymes were elevated in all patients in a study of exertional heatstroke,[270] and in 86% of patients in one study of nonexertional heatstroke.[108] Nonspecific ST-wave and T-wave changes on ECG are common. Myocardial enzyme elevation occurs and correlates with ECG changes.[156] Results of lumbar puncture are nonspecific, are often normal, or may demonstrate elevated cerebrospinal fluid (CSF) protein and lymphocytosis.[270]

Other laboratory parameters are affected by heatstroke. Salt and water depletion leads to hemoconcentration in patients exposed to elevated temperatures for a period of time. Hypokalemia is common, with potassium deficits as great as 500 mEq occurring during the early period of heat exposure. Arterial blood gas analysis may show a respiratory alkalosis secondary to direct stimulation of the respiratory center by heat, or a metabolic acidosis with elevated lactate.[66,278] Metabolic acidosis is the most frequent acid–base disturbance, either alone or part of a mixed picture. The prevalence of metabolic acidosis correlates with the degree of hyperthermia; 95% of patients demonstrated metabolic acidosis when the body temperature exceeded 107.6°F (42°C).[33]

Hypophosphatemia is common and is attributed to respiratory alkalosis, which causes intracellular shifts of phosphate. However, 8 of 10 heatstroke patients developed hypophosphatemia and none were alkalemic.[31] The hypophosphatemia in these cases was associated with increased phosphaturia and decreased tubular reabsorption of phosphorus, a finding that reversed after cooling.[165] Renal tubular damage may also lead to phosphate depletion.[118] Phosphate and potassium are elevated when significant muscle injury has occurred. Calcium is normal or low, the latter secondary to binding to damaged muscle tissue. Later, hypercalcemia occurs, possibly as a result of release of this bound calcium.[100,186]

Significant alterations occur in lymphocyte subsets in heatstroke victims. One study reported an increased ratio of T-suppressor to T-cytotoxic cells, as well as increased natural killer cells. There was a significant decrease in the percentages of T and B cells and T-helper cells. These changes correlate with the degree of hyperthermia.[32,35,247] Catecholamines are increased in heatstroke,[2] and may affect the distribution of the lymphocyte subsets.[32] It is possible that the increased susceptibility to infection described in heatstroke and the alterations in lymphocyte populations are related.[32]

Effects of Xenobiotics in Heatstroke Xenobiotics predispose the individual to heatstroke by 2 primary mechanisms: increased production of heat as a result of xenobiotic action and interference with the body's ability to dissipate heat because of pharmacologic or toxicologic effects on thermoregulatory centers (see Table 15–5). Xenobiotic interactions may cause life-threatening increases in temperature, such as the combination of monoamine oxidase inhibitors with meperidine or dextromethorphan resulting in the serotonin syndrome. The uncoupling of oxidative phosphorylation by salicylate, pentachlorophenol, or dinitrophenol leads to the release of metabolic energy as heat, rather than trapping that energy in the form of high energy phosphate bonds in ATP. Sympathomimetics may increase heat production by increasing physical activity.

During heat stress, vasodilation leads to increased cutaneous blood flow, resulting in an increased cardiac output. Parasympathetic stimulation results in increased sweating. Xenobiotics that impair these physiologic mechanisms for heat dissipation predispose the individual to heatstroke. Xenobiotics with anticholinergic effects, such as antihistamines, cyclic antidepressants, and antipsychotics interfere with sweating. Heatstroke as a result of oligohydrosis is reported for zonisamide[166,232] and topiramate.[14,221] The mechanism is postulated to concern the inhibition of carbonic anhydrase, an enzyme associated with eccrine sweat gland function.[38,78] Sympathomimetics stimulate β-adrenergic receptors, impairing vasodilation. Antihypertensives and antianginals (most notably calcium channel blockers and β-adrenergic antagonists) with negative inotropic and chronotropic effects impair the ability of the heart to meet the output requirements of increased skin blood flow. Diuretic-induced volume depletion also limits cardiac output. Antipsychotics cause hypothalamic depression, altering the normal CNS response to heat stress. Finally, xenobiotics such as ethanol, opioids, and sedative-hypnotics impair normal behavioral responses, and heat-related discomfort may go unnoticed.[292]

Heatstroke and Subsequent Heat Intolerance Whether heatstroke victims are subsequently unable to adapt to exercise in a hot environment remains unclear. Is the heatstroke victim genetically predisposed to heat intolerance, or does heatstroke occur as a result of environmental and host factors? Several studies suggest that heatstroke leads to persistent heat intolerance. These studies often use a single heat intolerance test.[87,268,271,272] A study of 10 previous heatstroke victims showed no difference in acclimatization responses, thermoregulation, whole body sodium and potassium balance, sweat gland function, and blood values when compared with controls.[16] The rate of recovery from exertional heatstroke probably differs among individuals. In this study, 1 of 10 patients was found to have recurrent heat intolerance 12 months after the study.[16] Resolution of heat intolerance was delayed for 5 months in an individual who had experienced heatstroke twice.[154]

Treatment of Heatstroke Management must focus on the early recognition of hyperthermia. Body temperatures >106°F (>41.1°C) place the patient at great risk for end organ injury. Rapid cooling is the first priority, and is associated with improved outcomes. Cooling that is delayed allowing body temperatures to remain above 102.2°F (38.9°C) for more than 30 minutes is associated with a high morbidity and mortality. In one report of the Chicago heat wave of 1995, only 1 patient of 58 victims was cooled within 30 minutes, resulting in an in-hospital mortality of 21% and an additional 28% mortality within 1 year.[76] Cooling by covering in ice water was twice as rapid in lowering the core temperature as was cooling by using evaporative spray.[17] Ice water immersion results in faster cooling when compared with all of the evaporative cooling methods in some studies.[65,94,101] A recent report of endovascular cooling using a heat exchange balloon catheter demonstrated dangerously lengthy cooling times and inadequate cooling measures.[202]

Successful treatment requires adequate preparation. Equipment needed for rapid cooling should always be readily available in the emergency department, and includes fans, ice, and tubs for submersion. En route to the hospital, the patient's clothes should be removed and the patient should be covered with ice, if available, and water-soaked sheets. Respiration and cardiovascular status should be stabilized and monitored. Oxygen should be administered. The cause of the heatstroke should be determined and appropriate measures initiated immediately. Xenobiotics, such as antihistamines, butyrophenones, and phenothiazines, and physical restraints that interfere with heat dissipation, such as camisoles and strait jackets, should not be used.[114] Light hand and foot restraints should be used to protect the patient from self-harm. If light restraints are used, the patient should be monitored continuously. The patient who is hyperthermic in the setting of ethanol or sedative-hypnotic withdrawal should be treated with a benzodiazepine.[113] The patient should never be confined to a small, unventilated seclusion room. Adequate cooling, hydration, sedation, and electrolytes and substrate repletion should be ensured.[111]

In the emergency department, appropriate laboratory studies should be performed and an IV line inserted. Administration of 100 mg of thiamine should be considered. A rectal probe should be placed for continuous temperature monitoring. The patient should be immersed in an ice bath with a fan blowing over the patient if possible. In addition to the ice bath, iced gastric lavage may be effective.

Agitation, seizures, and cardiac dysrhythmias must be managed while cooling is accomplished. Benzodiazepines are the treatment of choice for agitation and seizures. Heatstroke patients may have significant volume needs, depending on the amount of fluid lost prior to the onset of heatstroke. Hypotension should be treated with fluids and cooling. Volume repletion should be monitored carefully by parameters such as blood pressure, pulse, CVP, pulmonary wedge pressure, and urine output. As the temperature returns to normal, the hypotension may resolve if significant volume deficits are not present.[58,162,163] In patients with myoglobinuria, an attempt should be made to increase renal blood flow and urine output. The use of sodium bicarbonate and mannitol in the prevention of acute tubular necrosis in these cases is controversial.[29,86,100,251]

Phenothiazines and butyrophenones should not be used as they may depress an already altered mental status, may produce hepatotoxicity in a compromised liver, lower the seizure threshold,[29,113,114] cause acute dystonic reactions, exacerbate hypotension, and interfere with thermoregulation and cooling by affecting the hypothalamus. However, although phenothiazines and butyrophenones may theoretically reduce shivering and the possibility of rebound hyperthermia, their onset of action is slow.[226] When shivering occurs during cooling, we recommend the judicious use of a benzodiazepine. In addition, benzodiazepines treat ethanol and sedative-hypnotic withdrawal and cocaine intoxication, common causes of hyperthermia.

There is no role for antipyretics in the management of heatstroke. Aspirin and acetaminophen lower temperature by reducing the hypothalamic set point, which is only altered in a patient febrile from inflammation or endogenous pyrogens.[77,131] Heatstroke, however, occurs when cooling mechanisms are overwhelmed, and the hypothalamic thermoregulatory set point is not disturbed.[23]

Dantrolene sodium is the preferred drug in the treatment of malignant hyperthermia (see Antidotes in Depth A22: Dantrolene Sodium).[144,297] It acts directly on skeletal muscle and either inhibits the release of calcium or increases calcium uptake through the sarcoplasmic reticulum.[39] Its usefulness has not been demonstrated in other conditions associated with hyperthermia, and there is no evidence to support its administration for other conditions.[8] In a prospective, randomized, double-blind, placebo-controlled study of 52 patients with heatstroke, IV dantrolene sodium at 2 mg/kg of body weight did not alter cooling time.[30] There was no significant difference in the mean number of hospital days necessitated by heatstroke victims who received dantrolene and cooling versus those who received cooling alone. Dantrolene may influence central dopaminergic metabolism in patients with neuroleptic malignant syndrome by affecting calcium-triggered neurotransmitter release in the CNS; however, further study is required.[223] Anecdotal reports of the efficacy of dopamine agonists such as bromocriptine and amantadine have appeared in descriptions of neuroleptic malignant syndrome.[198] No drug therapy should delay the institution of aggressive external cooling (Table 15–7).

TABLE 15–7. Management of Heatstroke

Preparation
Ice and cooling fans available in emergency department
Monitor weather reports
Alert media
On Arrival
Rapid cooling
Clear airway and administer oxygen
Cover with ice and water-soaked sheets
Stabilize respiratory and cardiovascular status
Cool as rapidly as possible
Intravenous access
0.9% NaCl based on CVP or pulmonary artery catheter
Dextrose 0.5–1.0 g/kg, and thiamine 100 mg if indicated
Benzodiazepines for agitation, shivering, seizures
Continous monitoring
Remove from ice bath at 101°F (38.3°C)
Watch for rebound hyperthermia
Cautions
Antipsychotics may have serious adverse effects
Antipyretics do not work
Cooling blankets alone are inadequate

SUMMARY

The thermoregulatory processes responsible for the maintenance of normothermia are complex. Xenobiotics may disturb normal thermoregulation and result in the abnormal conditions of hyperthermia or hypothermia. These disturbances of homeostasis present significant clinical management challenges. Although greater understanding is gained through research and thoughtful analysis, hypothermia and heatstroke are largely preventable conditions and emphasis must be placed on prevention. During heat waves, many socioeconomically disadvantaged and elderly individuals are affected, and it is essential that cities be prepared and that the public be aware of the dangers of heat waves. Similarly, hypothermia is preventable by prudent preparation for harsh environmental conditions, and by policies that provide for shelter for those at greatest risk—the poor, the homeless, and those with underlying medical and psychiatric illnesses.

REFERENCES

1. AHA: 2005 American Heart Association Guidelines for Cardiopulmonary Resuscitation and Emergency Cardiovascular Care. *Circulation.* 2005;112:IV1-203.
2. al-Hadramy MS, Ali F: Catecholamines in heat stroke. *Mil Med.* 1989;154:263-264.
3. al-Harthi SS, El-Deane MS, Akhtar J, et al: Hemodynamic changes and intravascular hydration state in heat stroke. *Ann Saudi Med.* 1989;9: 378-383.
4. al-Harthi SS, Nouh MS, al-Arfaj H, et al: Non-invasive evaluation of cardiac abnormalities in heat stroke pilgrims. *Int J Cardiol.* 1992;37:151-154.
5. Albukrek D, Bakon M, Moran DS, et al: Heat-stroke-induced cerebellar atrophy: Clinical course, CT and MRI findings. *Neuroradiology.* 1997;39:195-197.
6. Althaus U, Aeberhard P, Schupbach P, et al: Management of profound accidental hypothermia with cardiorespiratory arrest. *Ann Surg.* 1982;195:492-495.
7. amsa.army.mil/1Msmr/2003/v09_n04_Article1.htm. Heat-related injuries, US Army, 2002. 2003.
8. Amsterdam JT, Syverud SA, Barker WJ, et al: Dantrolene sodium for treatment of heatstroke victims: Lack of efficacy in a canine model. *Am J Emerg Med.* 1986;4:399-405.
9. Anderson RJ, Reed G, Knochel J: Heatstroke. *Adv Intern Med.* 1983;28: 115-140.
10. Angelakos ET, Daniels JB: Effect of catecholamine infusions on lethal hypothermic temperatures in dogs. *J Appl Physiol.* 1969;26:194-196.
11. Anonymous: Mild therapeutic hypothermia to improve the neurologic outcome after cardiac arrest. *N Engl J Med.* 2002;346:549-556.
12. Anonymous: Heat-related deaths—United States, 1999-2003. *MMWR.* 2006;55:796-798.
13. Anonymous: Hypothermia-related deaths—United States, 1999-2002 and 2005. *MMWR.* 2006;55:282-284.
14. Arcas J, Ferrer T, Roche MC, et al: Hypohidrosis related to the administration of topiramate to children. *Epilepsia.* 2001;42:1363-1365.
15. Argaud L, Ferry T, Le QH, et al: Short- and long-term outcomes of heatstroke following the 2003 heat wave in Lyon, France. *Arch Intern Med.* 2007;167:2177-2183.
16. Armstrong LE, De Luca JP, Hubbard RW: Time course of recovery and heat acclimation ability of prior exertional heatstroke patients. *Med Sci Sports Exerc.* 1990;22:36-48.
17. Armstrong LE, Crago AE, Adams R, et al: Whole-body cooling of hyperthermic runners: Comparison of two field therapies. *Am J Emerg Med.* 1996;14:355-358.
18. Austin MG, Berry JW: Observations on one hundred cases of heatstroke. *J Am Med Assoc.* 1956;161:1525-1529.
19. Bacon C, Scott D, Jones P: Heatstroke in well-wrapped infants. *Lancet.* 1979;1:422-425.
20. Baumgartner FJ, Janusz MT, Jamieson WR, et al: Cardiopulmonary bypass for resuscitation of patients with accidental hypothermia and cardiac arrest. *Can J Surg.* 1992;35:184-187.
21. Beard ME, Hickton CM: Haemostasis in heat stroke. *Br J Haematol.* 1982;52:269-274.
22. Bernard SA, Gray TW, Buist MD, et al: Treatment of comatose survivors of out-of-hospital cardiac arrest with induced hypothermia. *N Engl J Med.* 2002;346:557-563.
23. Bernheim HA, Block LH, Atkins E: Fever: pathogenesis, pathophysiology, and purpose. *Ann Intern Med.* 1979;91:261-270.
24. Beyda EJ, Bellet S, Jung M: Effect of hypothermia on tolerance of dogs to digitalis. *Circ Res.* 1961;9:129-135.
25. Bhatnagar S, Dallman MF: The paraventricular nucleus of the thalamus alters rhythms in core temperature and energy balance in a state-dependent manner. *Brain Res.* 1999;851:66-75.
26. Biary N, Madkour MM, Sharif H: Post-heatstroke parkinsonism and cerebellar dysfunction. *Clin Neurol Neurosurg.* 1995;97:55-57.
27. Birkhimer LJ, DeVane CL: The neuroleptic malignant syndrome: Presentation and treatment. *Drug Intell Clin Pharm.* 1984;18:462-465.
28. Birzis L, Hemingway A: Descending brain stem connections controlling shivering in cat. *J Neurophysiol.* 1956;19:37-43.
29. Bosch X, Poch E, Grau JM: Rhabdomyolysis and acute kidney injury. *N Engl J Med.* 2009;361:62-72.
30. Bouchama A, Cafege A, Devol EB, et al: Ineffectiveness of dantrolene sodium in the treatment of heatstroke. *Crit Care Med.* 1991;19:176-180.
31. Bouchama A, Cafege A, Robertson W, et al: Mechanisms of hypophosphatemia in humans with heatstroke. *J Appl Physiol.* 1991;71:328-332.
32. Bouchama A, al Hussein K, Adra C, et al: Distribution of peripheral blood leukocytes in acute heatstroke. *J Appl Physiol.* 1992;73:405-409.
33. Bouchama A, De Vol EB: Acid-base alterations in heatstroke. *Intensive Care Med.* 2001;27:680-685.
34. Bouchama A, Dehbi M, Mohamed G, et al: Prognostic factors in heat wave related deaths: A meta-analysis. *Arch Intern Med.* 2007;167:2170-2176.
35. Bouchama A, Kunzelmann C, Dehbi M, et al: Recombinant activated protein C attenuates endothelial injury and inhibits procoagulant microparticles release in baboon heatstroke. *Arterioscler Thromb Vasc Biol.* 2008;28:1318-1325.
36. Boulant JA: Hypothalamic neurons. Mechanisms of sensitivity to temperature. *Ann N Y Acad Sci.* 1998;856:108-115.
37. Boylan JW, Hong SK: Regulation of renal function in hypothermia. *Am J Physiol.* 1966;211:1371-1378.
38. Briggman JV, Tashian RE, Spicer SS: Immunohistochemical localization of carbonic anhydrase I and II in eccrine sweat glands from control subjects and patients with cystic fibrosis. *Am J Pathol.* 1983;112:250-257.
39. Britt BA: Dantrolene. *Can Anaesth Soc J.* 1984;31:61-75.
40. Broccardo M, Improta G: Sauvagine-induced hypothermia: Evidence for an interaction with the dopaminergic system. *Eur J Pharmacol.* 1994;258:179-184.
41. Bruck K: Non-shivering thermogenesis and brown adipose tissue in relation to age, and their integration in the thermoregulatory system. In: Lindberg O, ed. *Brown Adipose Tissue.* New York: Elsevier; 1970:117-154.
42. Buchwald I, Davis PJ: Scleroderma with fatal heat stroke. *JAMA.* 1967;201:270-271.
43. Buckberg GD, Brazier JR, Nelson RL, et al: Studies of the effects of hypothermia on regional myocardial blood flow and metabolism during cardiopulmonary bypass. I. The adequately perfused beating, fibrillating, and arrested heart. *J Thorac Cardiovasc Surg.* 1977;73:87-94.
44. Busto R, Globus MY, Dietrich WD, et al: Effect of mild hypothermia on ischemia-induced release of neurotransmitters and free fatty acids in rat brain. *Stroke.* 1989;20:904-910.
45. Cannon B, Houstek J, Nedergaard J: Brown adipose tissue. More than an effector of thermogenesis? *Ann N Y Acad Sci.* 1998;856:171-187.
46. Carlton J, Khan SI, Haq W, et al: Attenuation of alcohol-induced hypothermia by cyclo (His-Pro) and its analogs. *Neuropeptides.* 1995;28: 351-355.
47. Carr ME, Jr., Wolfert AI: Rewarming by hemodialysis for hypothermia: Failure of heparin to prevent DIC. *J Emerg Med.* 1988;6:277-280.
48. Centers for Disease Control: Hypothermia-related deaths—New Mexico, October 1993–March 1994. *MMWR.* 1995;44:933-935.
49. Centers for Disease Control: Heat-related deaths—Chicago, Illinois, 1996–2001, and United States, 1979–1999. *MMWR.* 2003;52:610-613.
50. Centers for Disease Control: Impact of heat waves on mortality—Rome, Italy, June–August 2003. *MMWR.* 2004;53:369-371.
51. Centers for Disease Control: Hypothermia-related deaths—United States, 2003–2004. *MMWR.* 2005;54:173-175.
52. Chao TC, Sinniah R, Pakiam JE: Acute heat stroke deaths. *Pathology.* 1981;13:145-156.
53. Cheng BC, Chang CP, Tsay YG, et al: Body cooling causes normalization of cardiac protein expression and function in a rat heatstroke model. *J Proteome Res.* 2008;7:4935-4945.
54. Chobanian SJ: Jaundice occurring after resolution of heat stroke. *Ann Emerg Med.* 1983;12:102-103.
55. Chou YT, Lin MT, Lee CC, et al: Hypothermia attenuates cerebral dopamine overloading and gliosis in rats with heatstroke. *Neurosci Lett.* 2003;336:5-8.
56. Clark WG, Lipton JM: Brain and pituitary peptides in thermoregulation. *Pharmacol Ther.* 1983;22:249-297.
57. Clarke JF: Some effects of the urban structure on heat mortality. *Environ Res.* 1972;5:93-104.
58. Clowes GH, Jr., O'Donnell TF, Jr.: Heat stroke. *N Engl J Med.* 1974;291: 564-567.
59. Cogen FC, Rigg G, Simmons JL, et al: Phencyclidine-associated acute rhabdomyolysis. *Ann Intern Med.* 1978;88:210-212.
60. Cohen DJ, Cline JR, Lepinski SM, et al: Resuscitation of the hypothermic patient. *Am J Emerg Med.* 1988;6:475-478.

61. Collins KJ, Exton-Smith AN: 1983 Henderson Award Lecture. Thermal homeostasis in old age. *J Am Geriatr Soc.* 1983;31:519-524.
62. Collins KJ. The autonomic nervous system and the regulation of body temperature. In: Bannister R, ed. *Autonmonic Failure: A Textbook of Clinical Disorders of the Autonomic Nervous System*, 3rd ed. New York: Oxford University Press; 1992:212-230.
63. Collis ML, Steinman AM, Chaney RD: Accidental hypothermia: An experimental study of practical rewarming methods. *Aviat Space Environ Med.* 1977;48:625-632.
64. Cooper KE, Ferguson AV: Thermoregulation and hypothermia in the elderly. In: Pozos RS, Wittmers LE, eds. *The Nature and Treatment of Hypothermia.* Minneapolis: University of Minnesota Press; 1983:165-181.
65. Costrini A: Emergency treatment of exertional heatstroke and comparison of whole body cooling techniques. *Med Sci Sports Exerc.* 1990;22:15-18.
66. Costrini AM, Pitt HA, Gustafson AB, et al: Cardiovascular and metabolic manifestations of heat stroke and severe heat exhaustion. *Am J Med.* 1979;66:296-302.
67. Danzl DF, Sowers MB, Vicario SJ, et al: Chemical ventricular defibrillation in severe accidental hypothermia. *Ann Emerg Med* 1982;11:698-699.
68. Danzl DF, Pozos RS, Auerbach PS, et al: Multicenter hypothermia survey. *Ann Emerg Med.* 1987;16:1042-1055.
69. DaVee TS, Reineberg EJ: Extreme hypothermia and ventricular fibrillation. *Ann Emerg Med.* 1980;9:100-102.
70. de Garavilla L, Durkot MJ, Ihley TM, et al: Adverse effects of dietary and furosemide-induced sodium depletion on thermoregulation. *Aviat Space Environ Med.* 1990;61:1012-1017.
71. Delaney KA, Howland MA, Vassallo S, et al: Assessment of acid-base disturbances in hypothermia and their physiologic consequences. *Ann Emerg Med.* 1989;18:72-82.
72. Delaney KA. Hypothermic sudden death. In: Paradis NA, Halaperin HR, Nowak RM, eds. *Cardiac Arrest.* Baltimore: Williams & Wilkins; 1996:745-760.
73. Delaney KA, Vassallo SU, Larkin GL, et al: Rewarming rates in urban patients with hypothermia: Prediction of underlying infection. *Acad Emerg Med.* 2006;13:913-921.
74. Delay J, Deniker P. Drug-induced extrapyramidal syndromes. In: Vinkin PJ, Bruyn GW, eds. *Handbook of Clinical Neurology: Diseases of the Basal Ganglia.* Amsterdam: North Holland; 1969:248-266.
75. Delgado G, Tunon T, Gallego J, et al: Spinal cord lesions in heat stroke. *J Neurol Neurosurg Psychiatry.* 1985;48:1065-1067.
76. Dematte JE, O'Mara K, Buescher J, et al: Near-fatal heat stroke during the 1995 heat wave in Chicago. *Ann Intern Med.* 1998;129:173-181.
77. Dinarello CA, Wolff SM: Pathogenesis of fever in man. *N Engl J Med.* 1978;298:607-612.
78. Dodgson SJ, Shank RP, Maryanoff BE: Topiramate as an inhibitor of carbonic anhydrase isoenzymes. *Epilepsia.* 2000;41 Suppl 1:S35-39.
79. Durakovic Z, Misigoj-Durakovic M, Corovic N, et al: The corrected Q-T interval in the elderly with urban hypothermia. *Coll Antropol.* 1999;23: 683-690.
80. Eichler AC, McFee AS, Root HD: Heat stroke. *Am J Surg.* 1969;118:855-863.
81. el-Gamal N, Frank SM: Perioperative thermoregulatory dysfunction in a patient with a previous traumatic hypothalamic injury. *Anesth Analg.* 1995;80:1245-1247.
82. el-Sherif N, Shahwan L, Sorour AH: The effect of acute thermal stress on general and pulmonary hemodynamics in the cardiac patient. *Am Heart J.* 1970;79:305-317.
83. Ellis FP: Mortality from heat illness and heat-aggravated illness in the United States. *Environ Res.* 1972;5:1-58.
84. Emslie-Smith D: Accidental hypothermia; A common condition with a pathognomic electrocardiogram. *Lancet.* 1958;2:492-495.
85. Emslie-Smith D, Sladden GE, Stirling GR: The significance of changes in the electrocardiogram in hypothermia. *Br Heart J.* 1959;21:343-351.
86. Eneas JF, Schoenfeld PY, Humphreys MH: The effect of infusion of mannitol-sodium bicarbonate on the clinical course of myoglobinuria. *Arch Intern Med.* 1979;139:801-805.
87. Epstein Y, Shapiro Y, Brill S: Role of surface area-to-mass ratio and work efficiency in heat intolerance. *J Appl Physiol.* 1983;54:831-836.
88. Eschbach K, Hagan J, Rodriguez N. Causes and trends in migrant deaths along the U.S.-Mexico border, 1985-1998. Houston, TX: University of Houston Center for Immigration Research Working Paper #01-4; 2001.
89. Eshel GM, Safar P: The role of the central nervous system in heatstroke: Reversible profound depression of cerebral activity in a primate model. *Aviat Space Environ Med.* 2002;73:327-332; discussion 333-324.
90. Esteban J, Chover AJ, Sanchez PA, et al: Central administration of neuropeptide Y induces hypothermia in mice. Possible interaction with central noradrenergic systems. *Life Sci.* 1989;45:2395-2400.
91. Feighner JP, Boyer WF, Tyler DL, et al: Adverse consequences of fluoxetine-MAOI combination therapy. *J Clin Psychiatry.* 1990;51:222-225.
92. Fell RH, Gunning AJ, Bardhan KD, et al: Severe hypothermia as a result of barbiturate overdose complicated by cardiac arrest. *Lancet.*1968;1: 392-394.
93. Feller DJ, Young ER, Riggan JP, et al: Serotonin and genetic differences in sensitivity and tolerance to ethanol hypothermia. *Psychopharmacology (Berl).* 1993;112:331-338.
94. Ferris EB, Blankenhorn MA, Robinson HW, et al: Heat stroke: Clinical and chemical observations on 44 cases. *J Clin Invest.* 1937;17:249-262.
95. Finn DA, Boone DC, Alkana RL: Temperature dependence of ethanol depression in rats. *Psychopharmacology (Berl).* 1986;90:185-189.
96. Fischbeck KH, Simon RP: Neurological manifestations of accidental hypothermia. *Ann Neurol.* 1981;10:384-387.
97. Fleming PR, Muir FH: Electrocardiographic changes in induced hypothermia in man. *Br Heart J.* 1957;19:59-66.
98. Fox GR, Hayward JS: Effect of hypothermia on breath-alcohol analysis. *J Forensic Sci.* 1987;32:320-325.
99. Fruehan AE: Accidental hypothermia. Report of eight cases of subnormal body temperature due to exposure. *Arch Intern Med.* 1960;106:218-229.
100. Gabow PA, Kaehny WD, Kelleher SP: The spectrum of rhabdomyolysis. *Medicine (Baltimore).* 1982;61:141-152.
101. Gaffin SL, Gardner JW, Flinn SD: Cooling methods for heatstroke victims. *Ann Intern Med.* 2000;132:678.
102. Garvie AA, Howland MA, Brubacher JR, Hoffman RS: Endogenous digoxin-like substance in hypothermic patients. *Acad Emerg Med.* 1999;6:377.
103. Gentilello LM, Cobean RA, Offner PJ, et al: Continuous arteriovenous rewarming: Rapid reversal of hypothermia in critically ill patients. *J Trauma.* 1992;32:316-325; discussion 325-317.
104. Giercksky T, Boberg KM, Farstad IN, et al: Severe liver failure in exertional heat stroke. *Scand J Gastroenterol.* 1999;34:824-827.
105. Gillen JP, Vogel MF, Holterman RK, et al: Ventricular fibrillation during orotracheal intubation of hypothermic dogs. *Ann Emerg Med.* 1986;15:412-416.
106. Gilliam DM, Collins AC: Concentration-dependent effects of ethanol in long-sleep and short-sleep mice. *Alcohol Clin Exp Res.* 1983;7:337-342.
107. Ginsberg MD, Hertzman M, Schmidt-Nowara WW: Amphetamine intoxication with coagulopathy, hyperthermia, and reversible renal failure. A syndrome resembling heatstroke. *Ann Intern Med.* 1970;73:81-85.
108. Goldberg LI: Monoamine oxidase inhibitors: Adverse reactions and possible mechanisms. *JAMA.* 1964;190:456.
109. Goldberg LI: Cardiovascular and renal actions of dopamine: potential clinical applications. *Pharmacol Rev.* 1972;24:1-29.
110. Golden FSC, Hervey GR: The "after-drop" and death after rescue from immersion in cold water. In: Adam JM, ed. *Hypothermia Ashore and Afloat.* Abderdeen, TX: Aberdeen University Press; 1981:37-56.
111. Graham BS, Lichtenstein MJ, Hinson JM, et al: Nonexertional heatstroke. Physiologic management and cooling in 14 patients. *Arch Intern Med.* 1986;146:87-90.
112. Granoff AL, Davis JM: Heal illness syndrome and lithium intoxication. *J Clin Psychiatry.* 1978;39:103-107.
113. Greenblatt DJ, Gross PL, Harris J, et al: Fatal hyperthermia following haloperidol therapy of sedative-hypnotic withdrawal. *J Clin Psychiatry.* 1978;39:673-675.
114. Greenland P, Southwick WH: Hyperthermia associated with chlorpromazine and full-sheet restraint. *Am J Psychiatry.* 1978;135:1234-1235.
115. Grocott HP, Mathew JP, Carver EH, et al: A randomized controlled trial of the Arctic Sun Temperature Management System versus conventional methods for preventing hypothermia during off-pump cardiac surgery. *Anesth Analg.* 2004;98:298-302.
116. Gronert GA: Controversies in malignant hyperthermia. *Anesthesiology.* 1983;59:273-274.
117. Guard A, Gallagher SS: Heat related deaths to young children in parked cars: An analysis of 171 fatalities in the United States, 1995-2002. *Inj Prev.* 2005;11:33-37.
118. Guntupalli KK, Sladen A, Selker RG, et al: Effects of induced total-body hyperthermia on phosphorus metabolism in humans. *Am J Med.* 1984;77:250-254.
119. Gupta BN, Nier K, Hensel H: Cold-sensitive afferents from the abdomen. *Pflugers Arch.* 1979;380:203-204.

120. Guze BH, Baxter LR, Jr.: Current concepts. Neuroleptic malignant syndrome. *N Engl J Med.* 1985;313:163-166.
121. Ham J, Miller RD, Benet LZ, et al: Pharmacokinetics and pharmacodynamics of d-tubocurarine during hypothermia in the cat. *Anesthesiology.* 1978;49:324-329.
122. Hamlet MP. Fluid shifts in hypothermia. In: Pozos RS, Wittmers LE, eds. *The Nature and Treatment of Hypothermia.* Minneapolis: University of Minneosta Press; 1983:94-99.
123. Hammel HT: Regulation of internal body temperature. *Annu Rev Physiol.* 1968;30:641-710.
124. Hansen TE, Dieter K, Keepers GA: Interaction of fluoxetine and pentazocine. *Am J Psychiatry.* 1990;147:949-950.
125. Harari A, Regnier B, Rapin M, et al: Haemodynamic study of prolonged deep accidental hypothermia. *Eur J Intensive Care Med.* 1975;1:65-70.
126. Harnett RM, Pruitt JR, Sias FR: A review of the literature concerning resuscitation from hypothermia: Part I—the problem and general approaches. *Aviat Space Environ Med.* 1983;54:425-434.
127. Hauty MG, Esrig BC, Hill JG, et al: Prognostic factors in severe accidental hypothermia: Experience from the Mt. Hood tragedy. *J Trauma.* 1987;27:1107-1112.
128. Hayward JS, Steinman AM: Accidental hypothermia: An experimental study of inhalation rewarming. *Aviat Space Environ Med.* 1975;46:1236-1240.
129. Heiman-Patterson TD: Neuroleptic malignant syndrome and malignant hyperthermia. Important issues for the medical consultant. *Med Clin North Am.* 1993;77:477-492.
130. Hensel H: Cutaneous thermoreceptors. In: Hensel H, ed. *Handbook of Sensory Physiology.* Berlin: Springer-Verlag; 1972:79-110.
131. Hensel H: Neural processes in thermoregulation. *Physiol Rev.* 1973;53:948-1017.
132. Hensel H, Andres KH, von During M: Structure and function of cold receptors. *Pflugers Arch.* 1974;352:1-10.
133. Hernandez E, Praga M, Alcazar JM, et al: Hemodialysis for treatment of accidental hypothermia. *Nephron.* 1993;63:214-216.
134. Hexdall A, Greenblatt B, Garvie AA, et al: Endogenous digoxin-like binding substance in cold cardioplegia. *Acad Emerg Med.* 2000;7:467.
135. Hislop LJ, Wyatt JP, McNaughton GW, et al: Urban hypothermia in the west of Scotland. West of Scotland Accident and Emergency Trainees Research Group. *Brit Med J.* 1995;311:725.
136. Hochachka PW: Defense strategies against hypoxia and hypothermia. *Science.* 1986;231:234-241.
137. Hori T, Harada Y: Responses of midbrain raphe neurons to local temperature. *Pflugers Arch.* 1976;364:205-207.
138. Hubbard RW: The role of exercise in the etiology of exertional heatstroke. *Med Sci Sports Exerc.* 1990;22:2-5.
139. Hudson LD, Conn RD: Accidental hypothermia. Associated diagnoses and prognosis in a common problem. *JAMA.* 1974;227:37-40.
140. Huisse MG, Pease S, Hurtado-Nedelec M, et al: Leukocyte activation: The link between inflammation and coagulation during heatstroke. A study of patients during the 2003 heat wave in Paris. *Crit Care Med.* 2008;36:2288-2295.
141. Jacobs JJ, Prasad C, Wilber JF: Cyclo (His-Pro): Mapping hypothalamic sites for its hypothermic action. *Brain Res.* 1982;250:205-209.
142. Jardine DS: A mathematical model of life-threatening hyperthermia during infancy. *J Appl Physiol.* 1992;73:329-339.
143. Jardine DS, Haschke RH: An animal model of life-threatening hyperthermia during infancy. *J Appl Physiol.* 1992;73:340-345.
144. Jardon OM: Physiologic stress, heat stroke, malignant hyperthermia—a perspective. *Mil Med.* 1982;147:8-14.
145. Jessen K, Hagelsten JO: Peritoneal dialysis in the treatment of profound accidental hypothermia. *Aviat Space Environ Med.* 1978;49:426-429.
146. Jones TS, Liang AP, Kilbourne EM, et al: Morbidity and mortality associated with the July 1980 heat wave in St Louis and Kansas City, Mo. *JAMA.* 1982;247:3327-3331.
147. Kadar D, Tang BK, Conn AW: The fate of phenobarbitone in children in hypothermia and at normal body temperature. *Can Anaesth Soc J.* 1982;29:16-23.
148. Kalant H, Le AD: Effects of ethanol on thermoregulation. *Pharmacol Ther.* 1983;23:313-364.
149. Kalita J, Misra UK: Neurophysiological studies in a patient with heat stroke. *J Neurol.* 2001;248:993-995.
150. Kalser SC, Kelvington EJ, Randolph MM, et al: Drug metabolism in hypothermia. II. C14-Atropine uptake, metabolism and excretion by the isolated, perfused rat liver. *J Pharmacol Exp Ther.* 1965;147:260-269.
151. Kalser SC, Kelvington EJ, Kunig R, et al: Drug metabolism in hypothermia. Uptake, metabolism and excretion of C14-procaine by the isolated, perfused rat liver. *J Pharmacol Exp Ther.* 1968;164:396-404.
152. Kalser SC, Kelvington EJ, Randolph MM: Drug metabolism in hypothermia. Uptake, metabolism and excretion of S35-sulfanilamide by the isolated, perfused rat liver. *J Pharmacol Exp Ther.* 1968;159:389-398.
153. Kellermann AL, Todd KH: Killing heat. *N Engl J Med.* 1996;335:126-127.
154. Keren G, Epstein Y, Magazanik A: Temporary heat intolerance in a heatstroke patient. *Aviat Space Environ Med.* 1981;52:116-117.
155. Kew M, Bersohn I, Seftel H, et al: Liver damage in heatstroke. *Am J Med.* 1970;49:192-202.
156. Kew MC, Tucker RB, Bersohn I, et al: The heart in heatstroke. *Am Heart J.* 1969;77:324-335.
157. Kilbourne EM, Choi K, Jones TS, et al: Risk factors for heatstroke. A case-control study. *JAMA.* 1982;247:3332-3336.
158. Kilbourne EM: Heat-related illness: Current status of prevention efforts. *Am J Prev Med.* 2002;22:328-329.
159. Kiley JP, Eldridge FL, Millhorn DE: The effect of hypothermia on central neural control of respiration. *Respir Physiol.* 1984;58:295-312.
160. Killian H: Cold and frost injuries. In: Frey R, Safer P, eds. *Disaster Medicine.* New York: Springer-Verlag; 1981:9.
161. Kimura A, Sakurada S, Ohkuni H, et al: Moderate hypothermia delays proinflammatory cytokine production of human peripheral blood mononuclear cells. *Crit Care Med.* 2002;30:1499-1502.
162. Knochel JP, Beisel WR, Herndon EG, Jr., et al: The renal, cardiovascular, hematologic and serum electrolyte abnormalities of heat stroke. *Am J Med.* 1961;30:299-309.
163. Knochel JP, Dotin LN, Hamburger RJ: Pathophysiology of intense physical conditioning in a hot climate. I. Mechanisms of potassium depletion. *J Clin Invest.* 1972;51:242-255.
164. Knochel JP: Environmental heat illness. An eclectic review. *Arch Intern Med.* 1974;133:841-864.
165. Knochel JP, Caskey JH: The mechanism of hypophosphatemia in acute heat stroke. *JAMA.* 1977;238:425-426.
166. Knudsen JF, Thambi LR, Kapcala LP, et al: Oligohydrosis and fever in pediatric patients treated with zonisamide. *Pediatr Neurol.* 2003;28:184-189.
167. Koeppen AH, Daniels JC, Barron KD: Subnormal body temperatures in Wernicke's encephalopathy. *Arch Neurol.* 1969;21:493-498.
168. Koren G, Barker C, Bohn D, et al: Influence of hypothermia on the pharmacokinetics of gentamicin and theophylline in piglets. *Crit Care Med.* 1985;13:844-847.
169. Koren G, Barker C, Goresky G, et al: The influence of hypothermia on the disposition of fentanyl—human and animal studies. *Eur J Clin Pharmacol.* 1987;32:373-376.
170. Kornberger E, Lindner KH, Mayr VD, et al: Effects of epinephrine in a pig model of hypothermic cardiac arrest and closed-chest cardiopulmonary resuscitation combined with active rewarming. *Resuscitation.* 2001;50:301-308.
171. Krisko I, Lewis E, Johnson JE, 3rd: Severe hyperpyrexia due to tranylcypromine-amphetamine toxicity. *Ann Intern Med.* 1969;70:559-564.
172. Krismer AC, Lindner KH, Kornberger R, et al: Cardiopulmonary resuscitation during severe hypothermia in pigs: Does epinephrine or vasopressin increase coronary perfusion pressure? *Anesth Analg.* 2000;90:69-73.
173. Krismer AC, Wenzel V, Stadlbauer KH, et al: Vasopressin during cardiopulmonary resuscitation: A progress report. *Crit Care Med.* 2004;32:S432-435.
174. Kuehn LA: Introduction. In: Pozos RS, Wittmers LE, eds. *The Nature and Treatment of Hypothermia.* Minneapolis: University of Minnesota Press; 1983:xi-xxiii.
175. Lapp NL, Jurergens JL: Frostbite. *Mayo Clin Proc.* 1965;40:932.
176. Laufman H: Profound accidental hypothermia. *JAMA.* 1951;147:1201-1212.
177. Ledingham IM, Mone JG: Treatment of accidental hypothermia: a prospective clinical study. *Br Med J.* 1980;280:1102-1105.
178. Ledrans M, Pirard P, Tillaut H, et al: [The heat wave of August 2003: What happened?]. *Rev Prat.* 2004;54:1289-1297.
179. Lefkowitz D, Ford CS, Rich C, et al: Cerebellar syndrome following neuroleptic induced heat stroke. *J Neurol Neurosurg Psychiatry.* 1983;46:183-185.

180. Letsou GV, Kopf GS, Elefteriades JA, et al: Is cardiopulmonary bypass effective for treatment of hypothermic arrest due to drowning or exposure? *Arch Surg.* 1992;127:525-528.
181. Levinson DF, Simpson GM: Neuroleptic-induced extrapyramidal symptoms with fever. Heterogeneity of the 'neuroleptic malignant syndrome'. *Arch Gen Psychiatry.* 1986;43:839-848.
182. Lew HL, Lee EH, Date ES, et al: Rehabilitation of a patient with heat stroke: A case report. *Am J Phys Med Rehabil.* 2002;81:629-632.
183. Lewin S, Brettman LR, Holzman RS: Infections in hypothermic patients. *Arch Intern Med.* 1981;141:920-925.
184. Lin YF, Wang JY, Chou TC, et al: Vasoactive mediators and renal haemodynamics in exertional heat stroke complicated by acute renal failure. *Q J Med.* 2003;96:193-201.
185. Lipton JM, Rosenstein J, Sklar FH: Thermoregulatory disorders after removal of a craniopharyngioma from the third cerebral ventricle. *Brain Res Bull.* 1981;7:369-373.
186. Llach F, Felsenfeld AJ, Haussler MR: The pathophysiology of altered calcium metabolism in rhabdomyolysis-induced acute renal failure. Interactions of parathyroid hormone, 25-hydroxycholecalciferol, and 1,25-dihydroxycholecalciferol. *N Engl J Med.* 1981;305:117-123.
187. Lloyd EL: The cause of death after rescue, *Int J Sports Med.* 1992;13:196-199.
188. Lomax P: Neuropharmacological aspects of thermoregulation. In: Pozos RS, Wittmers LE, eds. *The Nature and Treatment of Hypothermia.* Minneapolis: University of Minnesota Press; 1983:81-94.
189. MacKenzie MA, Hermus AR, Wollersheim HC, et al: Poikilothermia in man: Pathophysiology and clinical implications. *Medicine (Baltimore).* 1991;70:257-268.
190. Maickel RP: Interaction of drugs with autonomic nervous function and thermoregulation. *Fed Proc.* 1970;29:1973-1979.
191. Mair P, Kornberger E, Furtwaengler W, et al: Prognostic markers in patients with severe accidental hypothermia and cardiocirculatory arrest. *Resuscitation.* 1994;27:47-54.
192. Malamud N, Haymaker W, Custer RP: Heatstroke: A clinicopathologic study of 125 fatal cases. *Milit Surg.* 1946;99:397-444.
193. Marion DW, Penrod LE, Kelsey SF, et al: Treatment of traumatic brain injury with moderate hypothermia. *N Engl J Med.* 1997;336:540-546.
194. Marzuk PM, Tardiff K, Leon AC, et al: Ambient temperature and mortality from unintentional cocaine overdose. *JAMA.* 1998;279:1795-1800.
195. McAllister RG, Jr.: Fever, tachycardia, and hypertension with acute catatonic schizophrenia. *Arch Intern Med.* 1978;138:1154-1156.
196. McAllister RG, Jr., Bourne DW, Tan TG, et al: Effects of hypothermia on propranolol kinetics. *Clin Pharmacol Ther.* 1979;25:1-7.
197. McAllister RG, Jr., Tan TG: Effect of hypothermia on drug metabolism. In vitro studies with propranolol and verapamil. *Pharmacology.* 1980;20:95-100.
198. McCarron MM, Boettger ML, Peck JJ: A case of neuroleptic malignant syndrome successfully treated with amantadine. *J Clin Psychiatry.* 1982;43:381-382.
199. McCauley RL, Hing DN, Robson MC, et al: Frostbite injuries: a rational approach based on the pathophysiology. *J Trauma.* 1983;23:143-147.
200. McLaughlin CT, Kane AG, Auber AE: MR imaging of heat stroke: External capsule and thalamic T1 shortening and cerebellar injury. *AJNR Am J Neuroradiol.* 2003;24:1372-1375.
201. McNamee T, Forsythe S, Wollmann R, et al: Central pontine myelinolysis in a patient with classic heat stroke. *Arch Neurol.* 1997;54:935-936.
202. Megarbane B, Resiere D, Delahaye A, et al: Endovascular hypothermia for heat stroke: A case report. *Intensive Care Med.* 2004;30:170.
203. Mehta AC, Baker RN: Persistent neurological deficits in heat stroke. *Neurology.* 1970;20:336-340.
204. Menon MK, Gordon LI, Kodama CK, et al: Influence of D-1 receptor system on the D-2 receptor-mediated hypothermic response in mice. *Life Sci.* 1988;43:871-881.
205. Millan MJ, Audinot V, Rivet JM, et al: S 14297, a novel selective ligand at cloned human dopamine D3 receptors, blocks 7-OH-DPAT-induced hypothermia in rats. *Eur J Pharmacol.* 1994;260:R3-5.
206. Millan MJ, Audinot V, Melon C, et al: Evidence that dopamine D3 receptors participate in clozapine-induced hypothermia. *Eur J Pharmacol.* 1995;280:225-229.
207. Miller JW, Danzl DF, Thomas DM: Urban accidental hypothermia: 135 cases. *Ann Emerg Med.* 1980;9:456-461.
208. Mills W: Accidental hypothermia. In: Pozos RS, Wittmers LE, eds. *The Nature and Treatment of Hypothermia.* Minneapolis: University of Minnesota Press; 1983:182-193.
209. Moore JA, Kakihana R: Ethanol-induced hypothermia in mice: influence of genotype on development of tolerance. *Life Sci.* 1978;23:2331-2337.
210. Morishima HO, Mueller-Heubach E, Shnider SM: Body temperature and disappearance of lidocaine in newborn puppies. *Anesth Analg.* 1971;50:938-942.
211. Mueller F, Colgate B: Annual Survey of Football Injury Research. The American Football Coaches Association 2008:1-28.
212. Muniz A: Ischemic electrocardiographic changes from severe heat stroke. *Southern Med J.* 2004;97:S10-S11.
213. Murphy K, Nowak RM, Tomlanovich MC: Use of bretylium tosylate as prophylaxis and treatment in hypothermic ventricular fibrillation in the canine model. *Ann Emerg Med.* 1986;15:1160-1166.
214. Murphy MT, Lipton JM: Effects of alcohol on thermoregulation in aged monkeys. *Exp Gerontol.* 1983;18:19-27.
215. Murray PT, Fellner SK: Efficacy of hemodialysis in rewarming accidental hypothermia victims. *J Am Soc Nephrol.* 1994;5:422-423.
216. Mustafa S, Thulesius O, Ismael HN: Hyperthermia-induced vasoconstriction of the carotid artery, a possible causative factor of heatstroke. *J Appl Physiol.* 2004;96:1875-1878.
217. Myers RD: Alcohol's effect on body temperature: hypothermia, hyperthermia or poikilothermia? *Brain Res Bull.* 1981;7:209-220.
218. Naughton MP, Henderson A, Mirabelli MC, et al: Heat-related mortality during a 1999 heat wave in Chicago. *Am J Prev Med.* 2002;22:221-227.
219. Nicodemus HF, Chaney RD, Herold R: Hemodynamic effects of inotropes during hypothermia and rapid rewarming. *Crit Care Med.* 1981;9:325-328.
220. Nicodemus HF, Chaney RD, Herold R: Lidocaine/propranolol: hemodynamic effects during hypothermia and rewarming. *J Surg Res.* 1981;30:6-13.
221. Nieto-Barrera M, Nieto-Jimenez M, Candau R, et al: [Anhidrosis and hyperthermia associated with treatment with topiramate]. *Rev Neurol.* 2002;34:114-116.
222. Nikki P, Vapaatalo H, Karppanen H: Effect of ethanol on body temperature, postanaesthetic shivering and tissue monoamines in halothane-anaesthetized rats. *Ann Med Exp Biol Fenn.* 1971;49:157-161.
223. Nisijima K, Ishiguro T: Does dantrolene influence central dopamine and serotonin metabolism in the neuroleptic malignant syndrome? A retrospective study. *Biol Psychiatry.* 1993;33:45-48.
224. O'Connor JP: Use of peritoneal dialysis in severely hypothermic patients. *Ann Emerg Med.* 1986;15:104-105.
225. O'Donnell TF, Jr., Clowes GH, Jr.: The circulatory abnormalities of heat stroke. *N Engl J Med.* 1972;287:734-737.
226. O'Donnell TF, Jr.: Acute heat stroke. Epidemiologic, biochemical, renal, and coagulation studies. *JAMA.* 1975;234:824-828.
227. O'Keeffe K M: Accidental hypothermia: A review of 62 cases. *JACEP.* 1977;6:491-496.
228. Ogawa T, Low PA: Autonomic regulation of temperature and sweating. In: Low PA, ed. *Autonomic Disorders: Evaulation and Management.* Boston: Little, Brown; 1993:79-91.
229. Ohmura A, Wong KC, Westenskow DR, et al: Effects of hypocarbia and normocarbia on cardiovascular dynamics and regional circulation in the hypothermic dog. *Anesthesiology.* 1979;50:293-298.
230. Okada M: The cardiac rhythm in accidental hypothermia. *J Electrocardiol.* 1984;17:123-128.
231. Okuliczkorayn I, Mikolajczak P, Kaminska E: Tolerance to hypothermia and hypnotic action of ethanol in 3 and 14 months old rats. *Pharmacol Res.* 1992;25:63-64.
232. Okumura A, Hayakawa F, Kuno K, et al: [Oligohidrosis caused by zonisamide]. *No To Hattatsu.* 1996;28:44-47.
233. Orts A, Alcaraz C, Goldfrank L, et al: Morphine-ethanol interaction on body temperature. *Gen Pharmacol.* 1991;22:111-116.
234. Osborn JJ: Experimental hypothermia; respiratory and blood pH changes in relation to cardiac function. *Am J Physiol.* 1953;175:389-398.
235. Osborne L, Kamal El-Din AS, Smith JE: Survival after prolonged cardiac arrest and accidental hypothermia. *Br Med J (Clin Res Ed).* 1984;289:881-882.
236. Ovadia H, Wohlman A, Mechoulam R, et al: Characterization of the hypothermic effect of the synthetic cannabinoid HU-210 in the rat. Relation to the adrenergic system and endogenous pyrogens. *Neuropharmacology.* 1995;34:175-180.
237. Patel R, Das M, Palazzolo M, et al: Myoglobinuric acute renal failure in phencyclidine overdose: Report of observations in eight cases. *Ann Emerg Med.* 1980;9:549-553.

238. Patel S, Hutson PH: Hypothermia induced by cholinomimetic drugs is blocked by galanin: Possible involvement of ATP-sensitive K+ channels. *Eur J Pharmacol.* 1994;255:25-32.
239. Paton BC: Accidental hypothermia. *Pharmacol Ther.* 1983;22:331-377.
240. Perchick JS, Winkelstein A, Shadduck RK: Disseminated intravascular coagulation in heat stroke. Response to heparin therapy. *JAMA.* 1975;231:480-483.
241. Rawson RO, Quick KP: Evidence of deep-body thermoreceptor response to intra-abdominal heating of the ewe. *J Appl Physiol.* 1970;28:813-820.
242. Reuler JB: Hypothermia: Pathophysiology, clinical settings, and management. *Ann Intern Med.* 1978;89:519-527.
243. Riedel W: Warm receptors in the dorsal abdominal wall of the rabbit. *Pflugers Arch.* 1976;361:205-206.
244. Ritzmann RF, Tabakoff B: Dissociation of alcohol tolerance and dependence. *Nature.* 1976;263:418-420.
245. Ritzmann RF, Tabakoff B: Body temperature in mice: A quantitative measure of alcohol tolerance and physical dependence. *J Pharmacol Exp Ther.* 1976;199:158-170.
246. Rivers N, Horner B: Possible lethal reaction between Nardil and dextromethorphan. *Can Med Assoc J.* 1970;103:85.
247. Roberts GT, Ghebeh H, Chishti MA, et al: Microvascular injury, thrombosis, inflammation, and apoptosis in the pathogenesis of heatstroke: A study in baboon model. *Arterioscler Thromb Vasc Biol.* 2008;28:1130-1136.
248. Roggla M, Frossard M, Wagner A, et al: Severe accidental hypothermia with or without hemodynamic instability: Rewarming without the use of extracorporeal circulation. *Wien Klin Wochenschr.* 2002;114:315-320.
249. Rogot E, Sorlie PD, Backlund E: Air-conditioning and mortality in hot weather. *Am J Epidemiol.* 1992;136:106-116.
250. Romm E, Collins AC: Body temperature influences on ethanol elimination rate. *Alcohol.* 1987;4:189-198.
251. Ron D, Taitelman U, Michaelson M, et al: Prevention of acute renal failure in traumatic rhabdomyolysis. *Arch Intern Med.* 1984;144:277-280.
252. Rowell LB: Cardiovascular aspects of human thermoregulation. *Circ Res.* 1983;52:367-379.
253. Ruiz de Elvira MC, Coen CW: Centrally administered neuropeptide Y enhances the hypothermia induced by peripheral administration of adrenoceptor antagonists. *Peptides.* 1990;11:963-967.
254. Saissy JM: Liver transplantation in a case of fulminant liver failure after exertion. *Intensive Care Med.* 1996;22:831.
255. Salmi P, Karlsson T, Ahlenius S: Antagonism by SCH 23390 of clozapine-induced hypothermia in the rat. *Eur J Pharmacol.* 1994;253:67-73.
256. Sanchez C, Lembol HL: The involvement of muscarinic receptor subtypes in the mediation of hypothermia, tremor, and salivation in male mice. *Pharmacol Toxicol.* 1994;74:35-39.
257. Sarnquist F, Larson CP, Jr.: Drug-induced heat stroke. *Anesthesiology.* 1973;39:348-350.
258. Satinoff E: Impaired recovery from hypothermia after anterior hypothalamic lesions in hibernators. *Science.* 1965;148:399-400.
259. Satinoff E: Disruption of hibernation caused by hypothalamic lesions. *Science.* 1967;155:1031-1033.
260. Savard GK, Cooper KE, Veale WL, et al: Peripheral blood flow during rewarming from mild hypothermia in humans. *J Appl Physiol.* 1985;58:4-13.
261. Schaller MD, Fischer AP, Perret CH: Hyperkalemia. A prognostic factor during acute severe hypothermia. *JAMA.* 1990;264:1842-1845.
262. Schrier RW, Henderson HS, Tisher CC, et al: Nephropathy associated with heat stress and exercise. *Ann Intern Med.* 1967;67:356-376.
263. Schuman SH: Patterns of urban heat-wave deaths and implications for prevention: Data from New York and St. Louis during July, 1966. *Environ Res.* 1972;5:59-75.
264. Schwarz B, Mair P, Raedler C, et al: Vasopressin improves survival in a pig model of hypothermic cardiopulmonary resuscitation. *Crit Care Med.* 2002;30:1311-1314.
265. Schwarz B, Mair P, Wagner-Berger H, et al: Neither vasopressin nor amiodarone improve CPR outcome in an animal model of hypothermic cardiac arrest. *Acta Anaesthesiol Scand.* 2003;47:1114-1118.
266. Semenza JC, Rubin CH, Falter KH, et al: Heat-related deaths during the July 1995 heat wave in Chicago. *N Engl J Med.* 1996;335:84-90.
267. Seraj MA, Channa AB, al Harthi SS, et al: Are heat stroke patients fluid depleted? Importance of monitoring central venous pressure as a simple guideline for fluid therapy. *Resuscitation.* 1991;21:33-39.
268. Shapiro Y, Magazanik A, Udassin R, et al: Heat intolerance in former heatstroke patients. *Ann Intern Med.* 1979;90:913-916.
269. Shen KH, Chang CK, Lin MT, et al: Interleukin-1 receptor antagonist restores homeostatic function and limits multiorgan damage in heatstroke. *Eur J Appl Physiol.* 2008;103:561-568.
270. Shibolet S, Coll R, Gilat T, et al: Heatstroke: Its clinical picture and mechanism in 36 cases. *Q J Med.* 1967;36:525-548.
271. Shvartz E, Shapiro Y, Magazanik A, et al: Heat acclimation, physical fitness, and responses to exercise in temperate and hot environments. *J Appl Physiol.* 1977;43:678-683.
272. Shvartz E, Shibolet S, Meroz A, et al: Prediction of heat tolerance from heart rate and rectal temperature in a temperate environment. *J Appl Physiol.* 1977;43:684-688.
273. Silfvast T, Pettila V: Outcome from severe accidental hypothermia in Southern Finland—a 10-year review. *Resuscitation.* 2003;59:285-290.
274. Sohal RS, Sun SC, Colcolough HL, et al: Heat stroke. An electron microscopic study of endothelial cell damage and disseminated intravascular coagulation. *Arch Intern Med.* 1968;122:43-47.
275. Southwick FS, Dalglish PH, Jr.: Recovery after prolonged asystolic cardiac arrest in profound hypothermia. A case report and literature review. *JAMA.* 1980;243:1250-1253.
276. Splittgerber FH, Talbert JG, Sweezer WP, et al: Partial cardiopulmonary bypass for core rewarming in profound accidental hypothermia. *Am Surg.* 1986;52:407-412.
277. Sprung CL: Hemodynamic alterations of heat stroke in the elderly. *Chest.* 1979;75:362-366.
278. Sprung CL, Portocarrero CJ, Fernaine AV, et al: The metabolic and respiratory alterations of heat stroke. *Arch Intern Med.* 1980;140:665-669.
279. Sternbach H: The serotonin syndrome. *Am J Psychiatry.* 1991;148:705-713.
280. Stoner J, Martin G, O'Mara K, et al: Amiodarone and bretylium in the treatment of hypothermic ventricular fibrillation in a canine model. *Acad Emerg Med.* 2003;10:187-191.
281. Sumann G, Krismer AC, Wenzel V, et al: Cardiopulmonary resuscitation after near drowning and hypothermia: Restoration of spontaneous circulation after vasopressin. *Acta Anaesthesiol Scand.* 2003;47:363-365.
282. Tavel ME, Davidson W, Batterton TD: A critical analysis of mortality associated with delirium tremens. Review of 39 fatalities in a 9-year period. *Am J Med Sci.* 1961;242:18-29.
283. Thomas JM, Rubin EH: Case report of a toxic reaction from a combination of tryptophan and phenelzine. *Am J Psychiatry.* 1984;141:281-283.
284. Tolman KG, Cohen A: Accidental hypothermia. *Can Med Assoc J.* 1970;103:1357-1361.
285. Tomaszewski W: Changements electrocardiographiques. Ovserves chez un homme mort de froid. *Arch Mal Coeur.* 1938;31:525-528.
286. Towne WD, Geiss WP, Yanes HO, et al: Intractable ventricular fibrillation associated with profound accidental hypothermia—successful treatment with partial cardiopulmonary bypass. *N Engl J Med.* 1972;287:1135-1136.
287. Trevino A, Razi B, Beller BM: The characteristic electrocardiogram of accidental hypothermia. *Arch Intern Med.* 1971;127:470-473.
288. Truscott DG, Firor WB, Clein LJ: Accidental profound hypothermia. Successful resuscitation by core rewarming and assisted circulation. *Arch Surg.* 1973;106:216-218.
289. Tysinger DS, Jr., Grace JT, Gollan F: The electrocardiogram of dogs surviving 1.5 degrees centigrade. *Am Heart J.* 1955;50:816-822.
290. University of North Carolina. www.unc.edu/depts/nccsi/SurveyofFootballInjuries.htm. Vol. 2005.
291. Vandentorren S, Suzan F, Medina S, et al: Mortality in 13 French cities during the August 2003 heat wave. *Am J Public Health.* 2004;94:1518-1520.
292. Vanhems P, Gambotti L, Fabry J: Excess rate of in-hospital death in Lyons, France, during the August 2003 heat wave. *N Engl J Med.* 2003;349:2077-2078.
293. Vassallo SU, Delaney KA: Pharmacologic effects on thermoregulation: Mechanisms of drug-related heatstroke. *J Toxicol Clin Toxicol.* 1989;27:199-224.
294. Vassallo SU, Delaney KA, Hoffman RS, et al: A prospective evaluation of the electrocardiographic manifestations of hypothermia. *Acad Emerg Med.* 1999;6:1121-1126.
295. Vertel RM, Knochel JP: Acute renal failure due to heat injury. An analysis of ten cases associated with a high incidence of myoglobinuria. *Am J Med.* 1967;43:435-451.
296. Walczak DD. Biochemical correlates of alcohol tolerance: Role of cerebral protein synthesis. Phd Thesis 1983. University of Toronto.

297. Ward A, Chaffman MO, Sorkin EM: Dantrolene. A review of its pharmacodynamic and pharmacokinetic properties and therapeutic use in malignant hyperthermia, the neuroleptic malignant syndrome and an update of its use in muscle spasticity. *Drugs*. 1986;32:130-168.
298. Webb P: Afterdrop of body temperature during rewarming: An alternative explanation. *J Appl Physiol*. 1986;60:385-390.
299. Weisskopf MG, Anderson HA, Foldy S, et al: Heat wave morbidity and mortality, Milwaukee, Wis, 1999 vs 1995: An improved response? *Am J Public Health*. 2002;92:830-833.
300. Weyman AE, Greenbaum DM, Grace WJ: Accidental hypothermia in an alcoholic population. *Am J Med*. 1974;56:13-21.
301. White JD: Hypothermia: The Bellevue Experience. *Ann Emerg Med*. 1982;11:417-424.
302. Willcox WH: The nature, prevention, and treatment of heat hyperpyrexia. *BMJ*. 1920:392-397.
303. Wira C, Martin G, Stoner J, et al: Application of normothermic cardiac arrest algorithms to hypothermic cardiac arrest in a canine model. *Resuscitation*. 2006;69:509-516.
304. Wira CR, Becker JU, Martin G, et al: Anti-arrhythmic and vasopressor medications for the treatment of ventricular fibrillation in severe hypothermia: A systematic review of the literature. *Resuscitation*. 2008;78:21-29.
305. Wislicki L: Effects of hypothermia and hyperthermia on the action of neuromuscular blocking agents. I. Suxamethonium. *Arch Int Pharmacodyn Ther*. 1960;126:68-78.
306. Wolfe RM: Death in heat waves: Beware of fans. *Brit Med J*. 2003;327:1228.
307. Wong KC: Physiology and pharmacology of hypothermia. *West J Med*. 1983;138:227-232.
308. York JL, Chan AW: Age effects on chronic tolerance to ethanol hypnosis and hypothermia. *Pharmacol Biochem Behav*. 1994;49:371-376.
309. Zachary L, Kucan JO, Robson MC, et al: Accidental hypothermia treated with rapid rewarming by immersion. *Ann Plast Surg*. 1982;9:238-241.
310. Zelman S, Guillan R: Heat stroke in phenothiazine-treated patients: A report of three fatalities. *Am J Psychiatry*. 1970;126:1787-1790.
311. Zhang H, Zhou M, Zhang J, et al: Therapeutic effect of post-ischemic hypothermia duration on cerebral ischemic injury. *Neurol Res*. 2008;30:332-336.

CHAPTER 16
FLUID, ELECTROLYTE, AND ACID–BASE PRINCIPLES

Alan N. Charney and Robert S. Hoffman

A meaningful analysis of fluid, electrolyte, and acid–base abnormalities must be based on the clinical characteristics of each patient. Although a rigorous appraisal of laboratory parameters often yields the correct differential diagnosis, it is the history and physical examination that provides an understanding of the extracellular fluid volume (ECFV) and pathophysiology, and as well as development of the appropriate treatment strategy. Thus, the evaluation always begins with an overall assessment of the patient's status.

INITIAL PATIENT ASSESSMENT

HISTORY

The history should be directed toward clinical questions associated with fluid and electrolyte abnormalities. Xenobiotic exposure commonly results in fluid losses through the respiratory system (hyperpnea and tachypnea), gastrointestinal tract (vomiting and diarrhea), skin (diaphoresis), and kidneys (polyuria). Patients with ECFV depletion may complain of dizziness, thirst, and weakness. Usually the patients can identify the source of fluid loss.

A history of exposures to nonprescription and prescription medications, alternative or complementary therapies, and other xenobiotics may suggest the most likely electrolyte or acid–base abnormality. In addition, premorbid conditions and the ambient temperature and humidity should always be considered.

PHYSICAL EXAMINATION

The vital signs are invariably affected by significant alterations in ECFV. Whereas hypotension and tachycardia may characterize life-threatening ECFV depletion, an initial finding may be an increase of the heart rate and a narrowing of the pulse pressure. Abnormalities may be recognized through an ongoing dynamic evaluation, realizing that the measurement of a single set of supine vital signs offers useful information only when markedly abnormal. Orthostatic pulse and blood pressure measurements provide a more meaningful determination of functional ECFV status (Chaps. 3 and 23).

The respiratory rate and pattern can give clues to the patient's metabolic status. Hyperventilation (manifested by tachypnea, hyperpnea, or both) may be caused by a primary respiratory stimulus (respiratory alkalosis) or may be a response to the presence of metabolic acidosis. Although hypoventilation (bradypnea or hypopnea or both) is present in patients with metabolic alkalosis, it is rarely clinically significant except in the presence of chronic lung disease. More commonly, hypoventilation is associated with a primary depression of consciousness and respiration, and respiratory acidosis. Unless the clinical scenario (ie, nature of the overdose or poisoning, presence of renal or pulmonary disease, findings on physical examination or laboratory testing) is diagnostic, arterial blood gas analysis is required to determine the acid–base disorder associated with a change in ventilation.

The skin should be evaluated for turgor, moisture, and the presence or absence of edema. The moisture of the mucous membranes can also provide valuable information. These are nonspecific parameters and may not correlate directly with the status of hydration. This dissociation is especially true with xenobiotic exposure, as many xenobiotics alter skin and mucous membrane moisture without necessarily altering ECFV status. For example, antimuscarinics and anticholinergics commonly result in dry mucous membranes and skin without producing ECFV depletion. Conversely, patients exposed to sympathomimetics (eg, cocaine) or cholinergics (eg, organic phosphorus insecticides) may have moist skin and mucous membranes even in the presence of significant fluid losses. This dissociation of ECFV and cutaneous characteristics reinforces the need to assess patients meticulously.

The physical findings associated with electrolyte abnormalities also are nonspecific. Hyponatremia, hypernatremia, hypercalcemia, and hypermagnesemia all may produce a depressed mental status. Neuromuscular excitability such as tremor and hyperreflexia may occur with hypocalcemia, hypomagnesemia, hyponatremia, and hyperkalemia. Weakness may be caused by either hyperkalemia or hypokalemia. Also, multiple, concurrent electrolyte disorders can produce confusing clinical presentations, or patients may appear normal. Rarer diagnostic findings, such as Chvostek and Trousseau signs (primarily found in hypocalcemia), may be useful in assessing patients with potential xenobiotic exposures.

RAPID DIAGNOSTIC TOOLS

The electrocardiogram (ECG) is a useful tool for screening of several common electrolyte abnormalities (Chap. 22). It is easy to perform, rapid, inexpensive, and routinely available. Unfortunately, because poor sensitivity (0.43) and moderate specificity (0.86) were demonstrated when ECGs were used to diagnose hyperkalemia, in actuality, the test is of limited diagnostic value.[168] However, the ECG is valuable for the evaluation of changes in serum potassium and calcium concentrations ($[K^+]$ and $[Ca^{2+}]$) in a single patient.

In many patients, bedside assessment of urine specific gravity by dipstick analysis may provide valuable information about ECFV status. A high urine specific gravity (>1.015) signifies concentrated urine and is often associated with ECFV depletion. However, urine specific gravity may be similarly elevated in states of ECFV excess, such as congestive heart failure or third spacing. Furthermore, when renal impairment is the source of the volume loss, the specific gravity is usually approximately 1.010 (known as isosthenuria). Patients with lithium-induced diabetes insipidus excrete dilute urine (specific gravity <1.010) despite ongoing water losses, and patients with methylenedioxymethamphetamine (MDMA)-induced antidiuretic hormone secretion excrete concentrated urine (specific gravity >1.015) in the presence of a normal to expanded ECFV.

The urine dipstick is particularly useful for rapidly determining the presence of ketones, which are often associated with common causes of metabolic acidosis (eg, diabetic ketoacidosis, salicylate poisoning, alcoholic ketoacidosis). The urine ferric chloride test rapidly detects exposure to salicylates with a high sensitivity and specificity (Chap. 35).

LABORATORY STUDIES

A simultaneous determination of the venous serum electrolytes, blood urea nitrogen (BUN), and glucose, and arterial or venous blood gases is adequate to determine the nature of the most common acid–base, fluid, and electrolyte abnormalities. More complex clinical problems may require determinations of urine and serum osmolalities, urine electrolytes, serum ketones, serum lactate, and other tests. A systematic approach to common problems is discussed in the following sections.

ACID–BASE ABNORMALITIES

DEFINITIONS

The terminology of acid–base disorders often leads to confusion and error. The following definitions provide the appropriate frame of reference for the remainder of the chapter.

The terms *acidosis* and *alkalosis* refer to processes that tend to change pH in a given direction. By definition a patient is said to have:

- A *metabolic acidosis* if the arterial pH is <7.40 and serum bicarbonate concentration ($[HCO_3^-]$) is <24 mEq/L. Because acidemia stimulates ventilation (respiratory compensation), metabolic acidosis is usually accompanied by a PCO_2 <40 mm Hg.
- A *metabolic alkalosis* if the arterial pH is >7.40 and serum $[HCO_3^-]$ is >24 mEq/L. Because alkalemia inhibits ventilation (respiratory compensation), metabolic alkalosis is usually accompanied by a PCO_2 >40 mm Hg.
- A *respiratory acidosis* if the arterial pH is <7.40 and partial pressure of carbon dioxide (PCO_2) is >40 mm Hg. Because an elevated PCO_2 stimulates renal acid excretion and the generation of HCO_3^- (renal compensation), respiratory acidosis is usually accompanied by a serum $[HCO_3^-]$ >24 mEq/L.
- A *respiratory alkalosis* if the arterial pH is >7.40 and PCO_2 is <40 mm Hg. Because a decreased PCO_2 decreases renal net acid excretion and increases the excretion of HCO_3^- (renal compensation), respiratory alkalosis is usually accompanied by a serum $[HCO_3^-]$ <24 mEq/L.

It is important to note that under most circumstances a venous pH permits an approximation of arterial pH (see Chap. 21 for a further discussion of the relationship between arterial and venous pH). Any combination of acidoses and alkaloses can be present in any one patient at any given time. The terms *acidemia* and *alkalemia* refer only to the resultant arterial pH of blood (acidemia referring to a pH <7.40 and alkalemia referring to a pH >7.40). These terms do not describe the processes that led to the alteration in pH. Thus, a patient with acidemia must have a primary metabolic and/or respiratory acidosis, but may have an alkalosis present at the same time. Clues to the presence of more than one acid–base abnormality include the clinical presentation, an apparent excess or insufficient "compensation" for the primary acid–base abnormality, a delta (Δ) anion gap-to-Δ $[HCO_3^-]$ ratio that significantly deviates from 1, and/or an electrolyte abnormality that is uncharacteristic of the primary acid–base disorder.

DETERMINING THE PRIMARY ACID–BASE ABNORMALITY

It is helpful to begin by determining whether the patient is acidemic or alkalemic. This is followed by an assessment of the pH, PCO_2, and the $[HCO_3^-]$. With these three parameters defined, the patient's primary acid–base disorder can be classified using the aforementioned definitions. Next it is important to determine whether the compensation of the primary acid–base disorder is appropriate. It is generally assumed that overcompensation cannot occur.[118] That is, if the primary process is metabolic acidosis, respiratory compensation tends to raise the pH toward normal, but never to >7.40. If the primary process is respiratory alkalosis, compensatory renal excretion of HCO_3^- tends to lower the pH toward normal, but not to <7.40. The same is true for primary metabolic alkalosis and primary respiratory acidosis. As a rule, compensation for a primary acid–base disorder that is inadequate or excessive suggests the presence of a second primary acid–base disorder.

Based on patient data, the Winters equation[7] predicts the degree of the respiratory compensation (the decrease in PCO_2) in metabolic acidosis as follows:

$$PCO_2 = (1.5 \times [HCO_3^-]) + 8 \pm 2 \qquad \text{(Eq. 16–1)}$$

Thus, in a patient with an arterial $[HCO_3^-]$ of 12 mEq/L, the predicted PCO_2 may be calculated as:

$$(1.5 \times 12) + 8 \pm 2$$

or

$$26 \pm 2 \text{ mm Hg}$$

If the actual PCO_2 is substantially lower than is predicted by the Winters equation, it can be concluded that both a primary metabolic acidosis and a primary respiratory alkalosis are present. If the PCO_2 is substantially higher than the predicted value, then both a primary metabolic acidosis and a primary respiratory acidosis are present.

An alternative to the Winters equation is the observation by Narins and Emmett that in compensated metabolic acidosis, the arterial PCO_2 is usually the same as the last two digits of the arterial pH.[117] For example, a pH of 7.26 predicts a PCO_2 of 26 mm Hg.

Guidelines are also available to predict the compensation for metabolic alkalosis,[67] respiratory acidosis, and respiratory alkalosis.[88] Patients with a metabolic alkalosis compensate by hypoventilating, resulting in an increase of their PCO_2 above 40 mm Hg. However, the concomitant development of hypoxemia limits this compensation so that respiratory compensation in the presence of a metabolic alkalosis usually results in a $PCO_2 \leq 55$ mm Hg. It is difficult to be more precise about the expected respiratory compensation for a metabolic alkalosis although the compensation, as in the case of metabolic acidosis, is nearly complete within hours of onset.

By contrast, the degree of compensation in primary respiratory disorders depends on the length of time the disorder has been present. In a matter of minutes, primary respiratory acidosis results in an increase in the serum $[HCO_3^-]$ of 0.1 times the increase (Δ) in the PCO_2. This increase is a result of the production and dissociation of H_2CO_3. Over a period of days, respiratory acidosis causes the compensatory renal excretion of acid. This compensation increases the serum $[HCO_3^-]$ by 0.3 times the ΔPCO_2. Primary respiratory alkalosis acutely decreases the serum $[HCO_3^-]$ by 0.2 times the ΔPCO_2. If a respiratory alkalosis persists for several days, renal compensation, by the urinary excretion of HCO_3, decreases the serum $[HCO_3^-]$ by 0.4 times the ΔPCO_2.

CALCULATING THE ANION GAP

The concept of the anion gap is said to have arisen from the "Gamblegram" originally described in 1939;[50] however, its use was not popularized until the determination of serum electrolytes became routinely available. The law of electroneutrality states that the net positive and negative charges of all fluids must be equal. Thus, all of the negative charges present in the serum must equal all of the positive charges, and the sum of the positive charges minus the sum of the negative charges must equal zero. The problem that immediately arose (and produced an "anion gap") was that all charged species were not routinely measured.

Normally present but not routinely measured cations consist of calcium and magnesium, whereas normally present but not routinely measured anions consist of phosphate, sulfate, albumin, and organic anions (such as lactate or pyruvate).[39,48,120] Sodium and K^+ normally account for 95% of extracellular cations, whereas Cl^- and HCO_3^- account for 85% of extracellular anions.[39] Thus, because more cations than anions are among the electrolytes usually measured, subtracting the anions from the cations normally yields a positive number, known as the anion gap. The anion gap is therefore derived as shown in Equation 16–2:

$$[Na^+] + [K^+] + [\text{Unmeasured Cations } (U_c)] = [Cl^-] + [HCO_3^-] + [\text{Unmeasured Anions } (U_a)]$$

$$\text{Anion Gap} = [U_a] - [U_c]$$

or

$$\text{Anion Gap} = ([Na^+] + [K^+]) - ([Cl^-] + [HCO_3^-]) \quad \text{(Eq. 16–2)}$$

Because the serum $[K^+]$ varies over a limited range of perhaps 1–2 mEq/L above and below normal and therefore rarely significantly alters the anion gap, it is often deleted from the equation for simplicity. Most prefer this approach, yielding Equation 16–3:

$$\text{Anion Gap} = ([Na^+]) - ([Cl^-] + [HCO_3^-]) \quad \text{(Eq. 16–3)}$$

Using Equation 16–3, the normal anion gap was initially determined to be 12 ± 4 mEq/L.[39,166] However, because the normal serum $[Cl^-]$ is higher on modern laboratory instrumentation, the current range for a normal anion gap is 7 ± 4 mEq/L.[165]

A variety of pathologic conditions may result in a rise or fall of the anion gap. High anion gaps result from increased presence of unmeasured anions or decreased presence of unmeasured cations (Table 16–1).[39,48,99,141] Conversely, a low anion gap results from an increase in unmeasured cations or a decrease in unmeasured anions (Table 16–2).[39,48,62,140,150]

ANION GAP RELIABILITY

Several authors have considered the usefulness of the anion gap determination.[20,49,77] When 57 hospitalized patients were studied to determine the cause of elevated anion gaps, in those patients whose anion gap was greater than 30 mEq/L the cause was always lactic acidosis or ketoacidosis.[49] In patients with smaller elevations of the anion gap, the ability to define the cause of the elevation diminished; in only 14% of patients with anion gaps of 17–19 mEq/L could the etiology be determined. Another study determined that although the anion gap is often used as a screening test for hyper-lactatemia (as a sign of poor perfusion), only those patients with the highest serum lactate concentrations had elevated anion gaps.[77] Finally, in a sample of 571 patients, those with higher anion gaps tended to have increased severity of illness. This resulted in higher admission rates, a greater percentage of admissions to intensive care units, and a higher mortality.[20] Thus, although the absence of an increased anion gap does not exclude significant illness, a very elevated anion gap can generally be attributed to a specific cause (typically lactate or ketones) and usually indicates a relatively severe illness.

TABLE 16–1. Xenobiotic and Other Causes of a High Anion Gap

Increase in Unmeasured Anions	Decrease in Unmeasured Cations
Metabolic acidosis (see Table 16–3)	Simultaneous hypomagnesemia, hypocalcemia, and hypokalemia
Dehydration	
Therapy with sodium salts of unmeasured anions	
Sodium citrate	
Sodium lactate	
Sodium acetate	
Therapy with certain antibiotics	
Carbenicillin	
Sodium penicillin	
Alkalosis	

TABLE 16–2. Xenobiotic and Other Causes of a Low Anion Gap

Increase in Unmeasured Cations	Decrease in Unmeasured Anions	Overestimation of Chloride
Hypercalcemia	Hypoalbuminemia	Bromism
Hypermagnesemia	Dilution	Iodism
Hyperkalemia		Nitrate excess
Lithium poisoning		
Multiple myeloma		

METABOLIC ACIDOSIS

Once the diagnosis of metabolic acidosis has been made by finding an arterial pH <7.40, a $[HCO_3^-]$ <24 mEq/L, and a PCO_2 <40 mm Hg, the serum anion gap should be analyzed. Indeed, the popularity of the anion gap is primarily based on its usefulness in categorizing metabolic acidosis as being of the high anion gap or normal anion gap type. This determination should be made after correcting the anion gap for the effect of hypoalbuminemia, a common and important confounding factor in such patients. The anion gap decreases approximately 3 mEq/L per 1 g/dL decrease in the serum [albumin].[45] In general the electrolyte abnormalities that frequently accompany metabolic acidosis usually have only small and insignificant effects on the anion gap.

It should be noted that although many clinicians rely on the mnemonic **MUDPILES** to help remember this differential diagnosis (M, methanol; U, uremia; D, diabetic ketoacidosis; P, paraldehyde; I, iron; L, lactic acidosis; E, ethylene glycol; and S, salicylates), this mnemonic includes rarely used drugs (phenfomin, paraldehyde) and omits important others (such as metformin).

A high anion gap metabolic acidosis results from the absorption or generation of an acid that dissociates into an anion other than Cl^- that is neither excreted nor metabolized. The retention of this "unmeasured" anion (eg, lactate in lactic acidosis) increases the anion gap. Normal anion gap metabolic acidosis results from the absorption or generation of an acid that dissociates into H^+ and Cl^-. In this case, the "measured" Cl^- is retained as HCO_3^- is titrated and reduced during the acidosis, and no increased anion gap is produced. Normal anion gap acidosis, also referred to as hyperchloremic metabolic acidosis, may be caused by intestinal or renal bicarbonate losses as in diarrhea or renal tubular acidosis, respectively. Other causes of high and normal anion gap metabolic acidoses are described elsewhere[1] and shown in Tables 16–3 and 16–4.

TABLE 16–3. Xenobiotic and Other Causes of a High Anion Gap Metabolic Acidosis

Carbon monoxide	Metformin
Cyanide	Methanol
Ethylene glycol	Paraldehyde
Hydrogen sulfide	Phenformin
Isoniazid	Propylene glycol
Iron	Salicylates
Ketoacidoses (diabetic, alcoholic, and starvation)	Sulfur (inorganic)
Lactate	Theophylline
	Toluene
	Uremia (acute or chronic renal failure)

NARROWING THE DIFFERENTIAL DIAGNOSIS OF A HIGH ANION GAP METABOLIC ACIDOSIS

The ability to diagnose the etiology of a high anion gap metabolic acidosis is an essential skill in clinical medicine. The following discussion provides a rapid and cost-effective approach to the problem. As always, the clinical history and physical examination may provide essential clues to the diagnosis. For example, iron poisoning is virtually always associated with significant gastrointestinal symptoms, the absence of which essentially excludes the diagnosis of this poisoning (Chap. 40). Furthermore, when iron overdose is suspected, an abdominal radiograph may show the presence of tablets. The acidosis associated with isoniazid (INH) toxicity results from seizures, the absence of which excludes INH as the cause of a metabolic acidosis (Chap. 57). Methanol toxicity may be associated with visual complaints or an abnormal funduscopic examination (Chap. 107). Methyl salicylate has a characteristic odor (Chap. 20). When these findings are absent, the laboratory analysis must be relied on, as follows:

1. *Begin with the serum electrolytes and glucose:* A rapid blood glucose reagent test should be performed to help confirm or exclude hyperglycemia. While hyperglycemia should raise the possibility of diabetic ketoacidosis, the absence of an elevated serum glucose does not exclude the possibility of euglycemic diabetic ketoacidosis,[79] or alcoholic or starvation ketoacidosis, which are often associated with normal or even low serum glucose concentrations. An elevated BUN and creatinine are essential to diagnose acute or chronic renal failure.
2. *Proceed to the urinalysis:* Do not wait for the laboratory results, as all of these urinary studies are easily performed. In addition, if there is a suspicion of a high anion gap metabolic acidosis, and only the arterial or venous blood gas analysis is completed, the evaluation may begin here, while the electrolyte determination is pending. A urine dipstick for glucose and ketones helps with the diagnosis of diabetic ketoacidosis and other ketoacidoses. However, the absence of urinary ketones does not exclude a diagnosis of alcoholic ketoacidosis (Chap. 77), and ketones are often present in severe salicylism (Chap. 35) and biguanide-associated metabolic acidosis (Chap. 48). The urine of a patient who has ingested fluorescein-containing antifreeze (ethylene glycol) may not fluoresce when exposed to a Wood lamp. Also, because ethylene glycol is metabolized to oxalate, calcium oxalate crystals may be present in the urine of a poisoned patient. Although the presence of a fluorescent urine and calcium oxalate crystals are useful findings, their absence does not exclude ethylene glycol poisoning (Chap. 107). When clinically available, a urine ferric chloride test should be performed. Although highly sensitive and specific for the presence of salicylate, this test is not specific for the diagnosis of salicylism, as small amounts of salicylate will be detected in the urine even days after its last use (Chap. 35). Thus, a serum salicylate concentration must be obtained to quantify the findings of a positive ferric chloride test. A negative ferric chloride test essentially excludes a diagnosis of salicylism.
3. An arterial or venous blood lactate concentration can be helpful. In theory, if the lactate (measured in milliequivalents per liter) can entirely account for the fall in serum $[HCO_3^-]$, then the cause of the increased anion gap can be attributed to lactic acidosis. However, it is important to remember that glycolate (a metabolite of ethylene glycol) can produce a significant false positive elevation of the lactate concentration with many current laboratory techniques.[111,127,167]

When the above analysis of a high anion gap metabolic acidosis is unproductive, the diagnosis is usually toxic alcohol ingestion, starvation, alcoholic ketoacidosis (with minimal urine ketones), or a multifactorial process involving small amounts of lactate and other anions. One approach is to provide the patient with 1–2 hours of intravenous hydration, dextrose, and thiamine. If the acidosis improves, the etiology is either ketoacidosis or lactic acidosis. Alternatively, a more detailed search for the toxic alcohols, involving either the osmol gap or actual methanol and ethylene glycol concentrations, should be initiated (discussed later).

TABLE 16–4. Xenobiotic Causes of a Normal Anion Gap Metabolic Acidosis

Acetazolamide
Acidifying agents
Ammonium chloride
Arginine hydrochloride
Hydrochloric acid
Lysine hydrochloride
Cholestyramine
Mafenide acetate (Sulfamylon)
Toluene
Topiramate

THE Δ ANION GAP-TO-$\Delta[HCO_3^-]$ RATIO

Many patients have mixed acid–base disorders such as metabolic acidosis and respiratory alkalosis. Depending on the relative effects of the acid-base disorders, the patient may have significant acidemia or alkalemia, minor alterations in pH, or even a normal pH. Although the clinical presentation, degree of compensation for the primary acid–base disorder, and the presence of unexpected electrolyte abnormalities may suggest whether more than one primary acid–base disorder is present, comparing the Δ anion gap (ΔAG) with the $\Delta[HCO_3^-]$ gap may be useful.

In the patient with a simple high anion gap metabolic acidosis, each 1 mEq/L decrease in the serum $[HCO_3^-]$ should (at least initially) be associated with a 1 mEq/L rise in the anion gap.[117] This occurs because the unmeasured anion is paired with the acid that is titrating the HCO_3^-. Any deviation from this direct relationship may be an indication of a mixed acid–base disorder.[63,117,123] Thus, the ratio of the change in the anion gap (ΔAG) to the deviation of the serum $[HCO_3^-]$ from normal (Equation 16–4) evolved:

$$\text{Anion Gap Ratio} = \Delta AG/\Delta[HCO_3^-] \qquad \text{(Eq. 16–4)}$$

A ratio close to 1 would suggest a pure high anion gap metabolic acidosis. When the ratio is <1, there is a relative increase in $[HCO_3^-]$ that can result only from a concomitant metabolic alkalosis or renal compensation such as renal generation of HCO_3^- for a respiratory acidosis. Alternatively, when the ratio is >1, the additional presence of either hyperchloremic (normal anion gap) metabolic acidosis or compensated respiratory alkalosis is suggested. Although the usefulness of this relationship has been supported strongly by some authors,[121,123] others suggest that it is often flawed and frequently misleading.[32,136]

After reviewing the arguments, the statements of one author[32] appear to be correct in concluding that "the exact relationship between the ΔAG and $\Delta[HCO_3^-]$ in a high anion gap metabolic acidosis is not readily predictable and deviation of the $\Delta AG/\Delta[HCO_3^-]$ ratio from unity does not necessarily imply the diagnosis of a second acid–base disorder." That being said, very large deviations from a value of 1 usually are associated with the presence of a second acid–base disorder.

THE OSMOL GAP

The osmol gap which is sometimes used to screen for toxic alcohol ingestion, is defined as the difference between the values for the measured osmolality and the calculated osmolarity.[150] Osmolarity is a measure of the total number of particles in 1 L of solution. Osmolality differs from osmolarity in that the number of particles is expressed per kilogram of solution. Thus, osmolarity and osmolality represent molar and molal concentrations of solutes, respectively.[55] In clinical medicine, osmolarity is usually calculated, whereas osmolality is usually measured.

Calculating osmolarity requires a summing of the known particles in solution. Because molarity and milliequivalents are particle-based measurements, unlike weight or concentration, the known constituents of serum have to be converted to molar values. Assumptions are required based on the extent of dissociation of polar compounds (such as NaCl), the water content of serum, and the contributions of various other solutes such as Ca^{2+} and Mg^{2+}. The nature and limitations of these assumptions are beyond the scope of this chapter. The reader is referred to several reviews for more details.[58,71,122] Many equations have been used and evaluated for calculating osmolarity. One investigation that used 13 different methods to evaluate sera from 715 hospitalized patients[34] concluded that Equation 16–5 provided the most accurate calculation:

$$1.86([Na^+] \text{ in mEq/L}) + ([\text{glucose}] \text{ in mg/dL}/18) + ([\text{BUN}] \text{ in mg/dL}/2.8) \qquad \text{(Eq. 16–5)}$$

Obvious sources of potential error in this calculation include laboratory error in determining the measured parameters and the failure to account for a number of osmotically active particles.

The measurement of serum osmolality has the potential for error stemming from the use of different laboratory techniques.[38] It is essential to assure that the freezing point depression technique is used, because when the boiling point elevation method is used xenobiotics with low boiling points (ethanol, isopropanol, methanol) will not be detected.

Conceptual errors may also result. In methanol poisoning, the methanol molecule has osmotic activity that is measured but not calculated, and no increase in the anion gap is present until it is metabolized to formate. Although the metabolite also has osmotic activity, its activity is accounted for by Na^+ in the osmolarity calculation because it is largely dissociated, existing as Na^+ formate. Thus, shortly after a methanol ingestion there will be an elevated osmol gap and a normal anion gap, whereas later, the anion gap will increase and the osmol gap will decrease. This effect is highlighted by several case reports.[9,28,153]

Using Equation 16–5 to calculate osmolarity, it is often stated that the "normal" osmol gap is 10 ± 6 mOsm/L.[34] However, when more than 300 adult samples were studied with a more commonly used equation (Eq. 16–6),

$$2([Na^+] \text{ in mEq/L}) + ([\text{glucose}] \text{ in mg/dL}/18) + ([\text{BUN}] \text{ in mg/dL}/2.8) \qquad \text{(Eq. 16–6)}$$

normal values were −2 ± 6 mOsm.[71] Almost identical results are reported in children.[106]

The largest limitation of the osmol gap calculation is due to the documented large standard deviation around a small "normal" number.[34,71,78,139] An error of 1 mEq/L (<1.0%) in the determination of the serum $[Na^+]$ may result in an error of 2 mOsm in the calculation of the osmol gap. Considering this variability, the molecular weights and relatively modest serum concentrations of the xenobiotics in question (eg, ethylene glycol, MW 62 daltons, at a concentration of 50 mg/dL contributes only 8.1 mOsm/L), and the predicted fall in the osmol gap as metabolism occurs, small or even negative osmol gaps can never be used to exclude toxic alcohol ingestion.[57,71] This overall concept is illustrated by the case of a patient with an osmol gap of 7.2 mOsm (well within the normal range) who ultimately required hemodialysis for severe ethylene glycol poisoning.[153]

Finally, although large osmol gaps may be suggestive of toxic alcohol ingestions, common conditions such as alcoholic ketoacidosis, lactic acidosis, renal failure, and shock are all associated with elevated osmol gaps.[78,139,147] This is surprising because lactate, acetoacetate, and β-hydroxybutyrate should not account for any increase in the osmol gap because they are charged (and accounted for in the osmolarity calculation). Apparently, these conditions are associated with the accumulation of small uncharged molecules in the serum.

Thus although the negative and positive predictive values of the osmol gap are too poor to recommend this test to screen for xenobiotic ingestion, the presence of very high osmol gaps (>50–70 mOsm/L) usually indicate a diagnosis of toxic alcohol ingestion (Chap. 107).

DIFFERENTIAL DIAGNOSIS OF A NORMAL ANION GAP METABOLIC ACIDOSIS

Although the differential diagnosis of a normal anion gap metabolic acidosis is extensive (Table 16–4), most cases result from either urinary or gastrointestinal HCO_3^- losses: renal tubular acidosis (RTA) or diarrhea, respectively. A number of xenobiotics also can cause this disorder, including toluene,[24] which also may cause a high anion gap metabolic acidosis. When the findings of the history and physical examination cannot be used to narrow the differential diagnosis, the use of a urinary anion gap is suggested.[14,131]

The urinary anion gap can be calculated as shown in Equation 16–7:

$$([Na^+] + [K^+]) - [Cl^-] \qquad \text{(Eq. 16–7)}$$

The size of this gap is inversely related to the urinary ammonium (NH_4^+) excretion.[61] As NH_4^+ elimination increases, the urinary anion gap narrows and may become negative, because NH_4^+ serves as an unmeasured urinary cation and is accompanied predominantly by Cl^-.

The normal anion gap metabolic acidosis associated with diarrhea results from HCO_3^- loss. During this process, the kidney's ability to eliminate NH_4^+ is undisturbed; in fact, it increases as a normal response to the acidemia. Thus, with gastrointestinal HCO_3^- losses the urinary anion gap should decrease and may become negative. Alternatively, the patient with RTA has lost the ability to either reabsorb HCO_3^- (type 2 RTA) or increase NH_4^+ excretion (types 1 and 4 RTA) in response to metabolic acidosis, and the urinary anion gap should become more positive. Indeed, when the urinary anion gap was calculated in patients with diarrhea or RTA, it was found that those patients with diarrhea had a mean negative gap (−20 ± 5.7 mEq/L), as compared to a positive gap (23 ± 4.1 mEq/L) in those with RTA.[61] Therefore, when evaluating the patient with a normal anion gap metabolic acidosis, the determination of a urinary anion gap may help to determine the source of the disorder.

ADVERSE EFFECTS OF METABOLIC ACIDOSIS

The acuity of onset and severity of metabolic acidosis determine the consequences of this disorder. Acute metabolic acidosis is usually characterized by obvious hyperventilation (due to respiratory compensation). At arterial pH values <7.20, cardiac and CNS abnormalities also become evident. These may include decreases in blood pressure and cardiac output, cardiac dysrhythmias, and progressive obtundation.[1] Chronic metabolic acidosis is often asymptomatic. The symptoms of anorexia and fatigue may be the only manifestations of chronic acidosis, and compensatory hyperventilation may be undetectable. Because the consequences of even severe metabolic acidosis are not specific, the presence of metabolic acidosis is most often suggested by the clinical evaluation.

MANAGEMENT PRINCIPLES IN PATIENTS WITH METABOLIC ACIDOSIS

The treatment of metabolic acidosis depends on its severity and cause. Most cases of severe poisoning, with a serum [HCO_3^-] concentration <8 mEq/L and an arterial pH value <7.20 should probably be treated with HCO_3^- to increase the pH to >7.20, as described in detail elsewhere.[1] As an example, to raise the serum [HCO_3^-] by 4 mEq/L in a 70-kg person with an estimated HCO_3^- distribution space of 50% of body weight, approximately 140 mEq must be administered. When ECFV overload (caused by heart failure, renal failure, or the sodium bicarbonate therapy itself) cannot be prevented or managed by administering loop diuretics, hemofiltration or hemodialysis may be necessary.

In patients with arterial pH values >7.20, the cause of the acidosis should guide therapy. Metabolic acidosis primarily caused by the overproduction of acid, as in the case of ketoacidosis and lactic acidosis, will require very large quantities of HCO_3^- and may not respond well to sodium bicarbonate therapy. Treatment in these patients should be directed at the cause of acidosis (eg, insulin in diabetic ketoacidosis; fomepizole in methanol and ethylene glycol poisonings [see Antidotes in Depth: Fomepizole]; fluids, glucose, and thiamine in alcoholic ketoacidosis; fluid resuscitation, antibiotics, and vasopressors in sepsis-induced lactic acidosis). Metabolic acidosis primarily caused by underexcretion of acid (eg, acute or chronic renal failure, RTA), should be treated with a low protein diet (if feasible) and oral sodium bicarbonate or substances that generate HCO_3^- during metabolism. Such patients can usually be managed with an oral sodium citrate solution (eg, Shohl's solution yields 1 mEq base/mL). The goal of therapy is to increase the serum [HCO_3^-] to 20 mEq/L, and the pH to 7.30.

METABOLIC ALKALOSIS

ADVERSE EFFECTS OF METABOLIC ALKALOSIS

Life-threatening metabolic alkalosis is rare but can result in tetany (from decreased ionized [Ca^{2+}]),[96] weakness (from decreased serum [K^+]),[107] or altered mental status leading to coma,[91] seizures,[59] and cardiac dysrhythmias.[84] In addition, metabolic alkalosis shifts the oxyhemoglobin dissociation curve to the left, impairing tissue oxygenation (Chap. 21). The expected compensation for a metabolic alkalosis is hypoventilation and increased PCO_2. As discussed before, respiratory compensation is irregular and inadequate at best, invoking the teleologic argument that hypoxia is more undesirable than alkalemia.[117] Several authors, however, have reported that severe hypoventilation and respiratory failure can occur in response to metabolic alkalosis, suggesting an actual, although uncommon, risk.[107,124]

APPROACH TO THE PATIENT WITH METABOLIC ALKALOSIS

Metabolic alkalosis results from gastrointestinal or urinary loss of acid, administration of exogenous base, and/or renal HCO_3^- retention (ie, impaired renal HCO_3^- excretion). Table 16–5 lists the causes of metabolic alkalosis. As compared to metabolic acidosis, metabolic alkalosis is less common and less frequently a consequence of xenobiotic exposure.

The etiologies of metabolic alkalosis can be characterized from a therapeutic standpoint as chloride responsive or chloride resistant. Chloride-responsive etiologies such as diuretic use, vomiting, nasogastric suction, and Cl^- diarrhea are usually associated with a urinary [Cl^-] <10 mEq/L.[67,84] These disorders respond rapidly to infusion of

TABLE 16–5. Xenobiotic and Other Causes of Metabolic Alkalosis

Gastrointestinal acid loss	Urinary acid loss	Base administration	Renal bicarbonate retention
Nasogastric suction (protracted)	Common	Acetate (dialysis or hyperalimentation)	Hypercapnia (chronic)
Vomiting (protracted)	Diuretics	Bicarbonate	Hypochloremia
	Glucocorticoids	Carbonate (antacids)	Hypokalemia
	Rare	Citrate (posttransfusion)	Volume contraction
	Hypercalcemia	Milk alkali syndrome	
	Licorice (containing glycyrrhizic acid)		
	Magnesium deficiency		

0.9% NaCl solution when concomitant therapy addresses the underlying problem.[2] Chloride-resistant disorders exemplified by hyperaldosteronism and severe K^+ depletion are characterized by urinary $[Cl^-]$ >10 mEq/L and tend to be resistant to 0.9% NaCl solution therapy.[52,67] These disorders often require K^+ repletion or drugs that reduce mineralocorticoid effects, such as spironolactone, before correction can occur.[52] When 0.9% NaCl solution repletion is ineffective, or emergent correction of the alkalosis is required, some authors have suggested infusions of lysine or arginine HCl, or dilute HCl.[3,108] However, this technique is rarely necessary.

XENOBIOTIC-INDUCED AND OTHER ALTERATIONS OF WATER BALANCE

Significant fluid abnormalities commonly occur in the setting of xenobiotic exposure. Gastrointestinal losses in the form of vomiting, diarrhea, gastrointestinal hemorrhage, and third spacing such as from gastrointestinal burns result from a variety of xenobiotic toxicities and their management with emetics and cathartics. Renal fluid losses result from the ability of many xenobiotics to increase the glomerular filtration rate (inotropes), impair Na^+ reabsorption (diuretics), or enhance urine volume in response to an obligate solute load (salicylates). Fluid losses also may occur through the skin as a result of sweating (sympathomimetics, cholinergics, and uncouplers of oxidative phosphorylation) or the lung as a result of increased minute ventilation (salicylates and sympathomimetics) or bronchorrhea (cholinergics). To the extent that these lost fluids contain Na^+, various signs, symptoms, and laboratory evidence of ECFV depletion may be present.

The diagnosis and treatment of abnormal serum electrolyte concentrations are usually addressed after repletion of the ECFV deficit with isotonic, Na^+-containing fluids (eg, blood products, 0.9% NaCl solution, lactated Ringer solution). Other fluid balance issues are discussed in Chaps. 25 and 27 and in chapters relating to individual xenobiotics. This section focuses on body water balance (abnormalities of which manifest as hypernatremia and hyponatremia) and specifically on the toxicologically relevant syndromes of diabetes insipidus (DI) and the syndrome of inappropriate secretion of antidiuretic hormone (SIADH).

Sodium concentration in the extracellular space is intrinsically related to and directly reflects total body water balance. This occurs because the sodium cation is largely restricted to the extracellular space, and its serum concentration is primarily, if indirectly, controlled by factors that control water balance. Thus, both the serum $[Na^+]$ and plasma osmolality vary inversely with changes in the quantity of body water.

Plasma osmolality is maintained through a complex interaction between dietary water intake; the hypothalamus, pituitary gland, and kidney; and the effects of hormones such as antidiuretic hormone (ADH) and adrenal mineralocorticoids.[16,19,119,161] Briefly, changes in osmolality are caused by changes in water intake and insensible (dermal, respiratory, and stool) and sensible (urinary, sweat) water losses. Urinary water losses are controlled by the hormone arginine vasopressin (ADH). Increases in the osmolality of the extracellular fluid stimulate anterior hypothalamic osmoreceptors, thereby stimulating thirst and ADH synthesis and release by the posterior pituitary gland. ADH release reaches its maximum level at a plasma osmolality of about 295 mOsm/kg. Antidiuretic hormone is transported to the kidney via the bloodstream, where it stimulates the synthesis of cyclic adenosine monophosphate (cAMP). cAMP increases the water permeability of the distal convoluted tubule and collecting duct (by stimulating the insertion of aquaporin channels in the apical membrane), increasing water reabsorption and urine concentration and minimizing urinary water losses. Conversely, as plasma osmolality falls, thirst and ADH release are diminished. This results in decreased renal cAMP generation, decreased water permeability of the distal convoluted tubule and collecting duct, and the excretion of a relatively dilute urine that ultimately corrects the body water excess. Marked alterations in water intake combined with perturbations of these various processes often lead to hypernatremia or hyponatremia.

HYPERNATREMIA

Table 16–6 summarizes the xenobiotics that cause hypernatremia. Hypernatremia may be caused by the parenteral administration of sodium-containing drugs or rapid and excessive oral Na^+ intake.[3] Oral NaCl and oral sodium citrate have been used as emetics and antiemetics, respectively. As might be expected, both have produced severe hypernatremia.[19] One case of fatal hypernatremia resulted from gargling with a supersaturated salt solution.[110] Similarly, massive ingestion of sodium hypochlorite bleach was associated with hypernatremia.[69,134]

More commonly, hypernatremia results from relatively electrolyte-free (hypotonic) water losses due to xenobiotics or conditions that cause urinary, gastrointestinal, and dermal fluid losses.[3] Indeed, all fluid losses from the body, except hemorrhage and those from fistulas, are hypotonic (and have the potential to cause hypernatremia). The lack of adequate fluid replacement is a key element in the development of hypernatremia because even the large losses caused by DI or cholera-induced diarrhea will not cause hypernatremia if they are adequately replaced. Thus, in patients with hypernatremia caused by fluid losses, the reason why the losses were not replaced by the patient should always be sought.

Xenobiotics that produce significant diarrhea, such as lactulose or cholestyramine, can cause hypernatremia through unreplaced stool water losses. A similar pathogenesis accounts for the hypernatremia caused by the polyethylene-containing solution used for bowel preparation for colonoscopy.[13] Of particular concern is the use of cathartics

TABLE 16–6. Xenobiotic Causes of Hypernatremia

Sodium gain	Water loss	Water loss due to diabetes insipidus
Antacids (baking soda)	Cholestyramine	α-Adrenergic antagonists
Sodium salts (acetate, bicarbonate, chloride, citrate, hypochlorite)	Diuretics	Amphotericin
Seawater	Glycerol	Colchicine
	Lactulose	Demeclocycline
	Mannitol	Ethanol
	Povidone-iodine	Foscarnet
	Sorbitol	Glufosinate
	Urea	Lithium
		Lobenzarit disodium
		Methoxyflurane
		Mesalazine
		Minocycline
		Opioid antagonists
		Propoxyphene
		Rifampin
		Streptozotocin
		Conivaptan and other vasopressin V_2-receptor antagonists

in the management of poisonings, especially when fluid losses are not anticipated. For example, multiple doses of sorbitol can produce severe hypernatremic dehydration and death in both children and adults.[22,41,54,162]

Significant water loss also can occur through the skin. Although diffuse diaphoresis resulting from cocaine or organic phosphorus insecticide toxicity has the potential to produce hypernatremia, this rarely, if ever, occurs. However, application of a remedy containing hyperosmolar povidone-iodine to the skin of burned patients produces significant water losses and hypernatremia.[142]

Diagnosis and Treatment The symptoms of significant hypernatremia consist largely of altered mental status ranging from confusion to coma, and neuromuscular weakness that occasionally results in respiratory paralysis. If hypernatremia is associated with Na^+ losses and marked ECFV depletion, cardiovascular symptoms, tachycardia, and orthostatic hypotension may be present. Treatment consists of first replacing the Na^+ deficit (with isotonic fluids such as 0.9% NaCl solution) if present, and then replacing the water deficit. The water deficit may be estimated by assuming that the fractional increase in serum $[Na^+]$ is equal to the fractional decrease in total body water. Thus, a serum $[Na^+]$ that has increased by 10% (from 144 mEq/L to 158 mEq/L) indicates that the water deficit is 10% (3.6 L in a 60-kg person with 36 L of body water).

When the hypernatremia develops over several hours, for example as occurs after ingestion or administration of a sodium salt, rapid correction is indicated. However, when hypernatremia develops over several days or when the duration is unknown, slow correction of hypernatremia (over several days) is recommended.[3] The adaptation of brain cells to the water deficit (including the gain of intracellular solute) makes cerebral edema a frequent complication of rapid water replacement. Although some sources suggest that 0.9% NaCl solution is an appropriate replacement fluid regardless of the magnitude of the water deficit, recent emphasis has been on the use of hypotonic fluids to correct hypernatremia in the absence of a significant sodium deficit.[3]

DIABETES INSIPIDUS

The greatest water losses and, therefore, the potentially most severe cases of hypernatremia occur during DI, which is always characterized by greater or lesser degrees of hypotonic polyuria. DI may be neurogenic resulting from failure to sense a rising osmolality, or from a failure to release ADH, or nephrogenic resulting from failure of the kidney to respond appropriately to ADH. Although there are many nontoxicologic causes of DI (eg, trauma, tumor, sarcoidosis, vascular and congenital), drug-induced DI is also common, and may be mediated through either central or peripheral mechanisms.

Ethanol, opioid antagonists, and α-adrenergic agonists all suppress ADH release.[9,114] Lithium,[98,146] demeclocycline,[145] methoxyflurane,[102] propoxyphene, foscarnet,[118] mesalazine,[100] streptozotocin, amphotericin,[73] glufosinate,[156] lobenzarit,[135] rifampin,[128] and colchicine[161] are associated with nephrogenic DI (see Table 16-6). In addition, nephrogenic DI may be caused by severe hypokalemia from diuretic use, and hypercalcemia from vitamin D poisoning.[161] Of all these xenobiotics, lithium has been the most extensively evaluated. Although polyuria is a common finding with lithium therapy (occurring in 20%–70% of patients on maintenance therapy), the exact incidence of DI and hypernatremia is unknown. Estimates range from 10%–20% to as high as 80%.

Diagnosis Patients with DI complain of polyuria and polydipsia. Urine volumes typically exceed 30 mL/kg/d[161] and may be as high as 9 L/d with nephrogenic DI[98] and 12–14 L/d with neurogenic (central) DI.[115] Nocturia, fatigue, and decreased work performance are often noted.[161] Neurogenic DI resulting from hypothalamic or pituitary damage is typically associated with other signs of neuroendocrine dysfunction.[115]

Once polyuria is confirmed (eg, in adults, by measuring a urine output >200 mL over 1 hour), the urine osmolality or specific gravity should be measured. The diagnosis of DI is established by the occurrence of dilute urine (urine osmolality <300 mOsm/kg, urine specific gravity <1.010) in the presence of increased serum $[Na^+]$ and an serum osmolality >295 mOsm/kg.[161] Following this determination, a trial of desmopressin (DDAVP), an arginine vasopressin analog, helps to differentiate between neurogenic and nephrogenic DI. If the etiology of the DI is neurogenic, the patient will promptly respond to DDAVP with a decrease in urine output and increase in urine osmolality. In nephrogenic DI, DDAVP will have no significant effect.

Treatment The initial approach to the hypernatremic patient with DI involves the repletion of the water deficit (as described above) and the restoration of electrolyte depletion, if necessary. If a reversible cause for the DI can be established, it should be corrected. Specifically, xenobiotics implicated as the cause of DI should be discontinued or their dose reduced. Patients with neurogenic DI should be maintained on either vasopressin or DDAVP. The latter is preferred because of the lack of vasopressor effects and ease of administration. In the past, patients were occasionally treated with oral medications known to produce SIADH (see later). Patients with nephrogenic DI can be treated with thiazide diuretics,[35] prostaglandin inhibitors,[31,74,93] and/or amiloride, all of which reduce the urine flow rate.[15]

HYPONATREMIA

Hyponatremia may be associated with a high, normal, or low serum osmolality. Patients with myeloma or severe hyperlipidemia may exhibit artifactual hyponatremia whenever the measurement technique requires dilution of the serum sample rather than direct measurement by a sodium electrode. These patients have a normal serum osmolality, no symptoms related to their artifactual hyponatremia, and require no therapy.

Hyperglycemic patients develop hyponatremia because the increase in plasma osmolality caused by hyperglycemia results in a water shift from the intracellular to the extracellular space. The reduction in serum $[Na^+]$, which may cause symptoms, is approximately 1.6 mEq/L for every 100 mg/dL increase in serum glucose concentration. The contribution of hyperglycemia to the hyponatremia should be calculated to determine if other causes of hyponatremia should also be sought. All other causes of hyponatremia are associated with a low plasma osmolality. In fact, in the absence of myeloma, hyperlipidemia, and hyperglycemia, the serum osmolality need not be measured in hyponatremic patients and may be assumed to be low.

Hyponatremia associated with a low plasma osmolality usually results from water intake in excess of the renal capacity to excrete it. When renal water excretion is normal, very large intake is required to cause hyponatremia. Usually such large quantities of water are ingested over a short period of time by people with psychiatric or neurologic disorders such as psychogenic polydypsia.[60,132] Xenobiotic-induced water excess comparable to psychogenic polydipsia is quite uncommon. An example occurs during urologic procedures, such as transurethral resection of the prostate (TURP), where large volumes of irrigation solution are required. Because the wounds are electrically cauterized, these fluids cannot contain conductive electrolytes such as sodium. Sorbitol, dextrose, and mannitol were tried in an attempt to maintain a normal osmolality in these irrigating solutions, but their optical characteristics were undesirable during the surgery. Thus, irrigation during TURP is performed with glycine-containing solutions. When 1.5% glycine (osmolality 220 mOsm/kg) is absorbed through the prostatic venous plexus, a rapid reduction in serum [Na^+] results and will persist until the glycine is metabolized.[70,109] Symptoms in these patients are probably a result of several factors: hyponatremia, the glycine itself, and NH_3, a glycine metabolite. A similar complication has also been described during hysteroscopy.[125,143]

Rarely, hyponatremia results from the loss of a body fluid with a [Na^+] greater than the extracellular fluid (ECF) [Na^+] (of 154 mEq/L). This may occur in patients with adrenal insufficiency through hypertonic urinary losses (although increased ADH secretion as a consequence of ECF sodium depletion is probably a more important mechanism; see later). In burn patients, Na^+ may be lost directly from the ECF. When treated with the topical applications of silver nitrate cream, hyponatremia may develop from the diffusion of sodium through permeable skin into the hypotonic dressing.[26] Ingestion of licorice that contains glycyrrhizic acid produces a syndrome of hyponatremia, hypokalemia, and hypertension that resembles mineralocorticoid excess. Although the exact mechanism of hyponatremia is debated, one report suggested that a glycyrrhizic acid–induced reduction in 11-β-hydroxysteroid dehydrogenase activity could account for the findings.[37,40] Lithium, which is usually associated with DI and hypernatremia, has been reported to cause renal sodium-wasting and hyponatremia that seems to be unrelated to ADH effects.[108]

Most cases of hyponatremia are caused by water intake in excess of a reduced renal excretory capacity. This reduction in urinary water excretion may be physiologic (as during ECF sodium depletion) or pathologic (in association with renal failure, heart failure, or cirrhosis of the liver).[4,13] Because these conditions are accompanied by alterations in renal sodium handling, signs and symptoms of ECFV depletion, such as postural hypotension, or excess, such as edema, usually accompany the hyponatremia. Other patients cannot excrete water normally because malignancy or various brain or pulmonary diseases cause ADH secretion.[4] In fact, in some cases the tumors are associated with paraneoplastic disease and directly secrete ADH. Xenobiotics, such as diuretics, may cause ECFV depletion but most directly stimulate ADH secretion or augment the renal effects of ADH. Drugs such as the thiazide diuretics cause hyponatremia by several mechanisms, including interference with maximal urinary dilution, and by ADH-induced water retention in response to decreased ECFV.[4,44] Patients with excess secretion and/or action of ADH who have near-normal ECFV are said to have SIADH. Table 16–7 summarizes these and other causes of hyponatremia.

TABLE 16–7. Xenobiotic and Other Causes of Hyponatremia

Arginine
Captopril and other angiotensin-converting enzyme inhibitors
Diuretics
Glycine (transurethral prostatectomy syndrome)
Licorice (containing glycyrrhizic acid)
Lithium
Nonsteroidal antiinflammatory drugs
Primary polydipsia
Silver nitrate
SIADH
Amiloride
Amiodarone
Amitriptyline (and other cyclic antidepressants)
Aripiprazole
Atomoxetine
Biguanides (metformin and phenformin)
Bortezomib
Carbamazepine (and oxcarbamazepine)
Cisplatin
Citalopram (and escitalopram)
Clofibrate
Cyclophosphamide
Desmopressin (DDAVP)
Diazoxide
Duloxetine
Indapamide
MDMA (methylenedioxymethamphetamine)
Nicotine
Opioids
Oxytocin
Selective serotonin reuptake inhibitors
Sulfonylureas
Thioridazine
Tramadol
Tranylcypromine
Valproate
Vasopressin
Vincristine and vinblastine

SIADH

SIADH is characterized by hyponatremia and plasma hypotonicity in the absence of abnormalities of ECFV, adrenal, thyroid, or renal function. Early reviews claimed that SIADH was a disorder of volume overload, based largely on evidence of weight gain.[114] The consistent absence of edema, however, and the fact that the decrease in serum [Na^+] cannot be accounted for by the fluid gain (weight gain) suggest that water retention is only part of the mechanism.[87] Urinary Na^+ loss and Na^+ redistribution from the extracellular to the intracellular space are apparently important as well.

There are many nontoxicologic etiologies of SIADH, most of which result from altered pulmonary or intracranial pathophysiology. These causes include infections, malignancies, and surgery.[4,87,114,115] Table 16–7 summarizes xenobiotics known to produce SIADH. The oral hypoglycemics, including drugs from both the sulfonylurea (eg, chlorpropamide) and biguanide (eg, metformin) classes, produce hyponatremia more commonly than other drugs.[113] Their actions are multifactorial and can include both the potentiation of endogenous ADH and the stimulation of ADH release.[113] Many psychiatric medications, including the selective serotonin reuptake inhibitors, cyclic antidepressants, and antipsychotics, are implicated in causing SIADH.[25,85,95,152,159] The effects of these drugs may be mediated by the complex interactions between the dopaminergic and noradrenergic systems that control ADH release.[152] Additional evidence supports a role of serotonin in drug-induced SIADH. Serotonin (specifically 5-HT_2 and/or 5-HT_{1C}) directly stimulates ADH release[10] and water intake.[76] An important role of serotonin is supported by the occurrence of SIADH with methylenedioxymethamphetamine (MDMA) use.[75,164]

Diagnosis The clinical presentation of patients with hyponatremia depends on the cause, the absolute serum [Na^+], and the rate of decline in serum [Na^+]. Patients with associated ECFV excess or depletion will present with evidence of altered ECFV, as well as signs and symptoms of the disease that caused the abnormality in ECFV, such as adrenal insufficiency and heart failure.[5] Rarely, will these patients exhibit symptoms of hyponatremia and hyposmolality of body fluids per se. This may be because of the moderate degree of hyponatremia (>130 mEq/L), the moderate rate of decline in [Na^+], and/or because the loss of Na^+ and water limits the development of cerebral edema.[90] It is important to note that patients with hyponatremia and a low plasma osmolality (excluding those with primary polydipsia) all have a urinary osmolality that is relatively high, regardless of whether they have excess, diminished, or normal ECFV. Consequently, these disorders can only be differentiated by the history, physical examination, and other laboratory tests.

Patients with SIADH, if symptomatic, usually present with signs and symptoms of hyponatremia. As noted above, the clinical manifestations of hyponatremia are dependent on both the absolute serum [Na^+] and its rate of decline.[11,90,115] Chronic, slow depression of the [Na^+] is usually well tolerated, whereas rapid decreases may be associated with symptoms and sometimes catastrophic events. Symptoms include headache, nausea, vomiting, restlessness, disorientation, depression, apathy, irritability, lethargy, weakness, and muscle cramps. In more severe cases, respiratory depression, coma, and seizures may develop.

The diagnosis of SIADH is based on establishing the presence of hyponatremia, a low serum osmolality, and impaired urinary dilution in the absence of edema, hypotension, hypovolemia, and renal, adrenal, or thyroid dysfunction.[87] As discussed above, the presence of any of these clinical findings suggests that another cause of hyponatremia may be present. A serum uric acid concentration may be helpful in differentiating SIADH from other causes of hyponatremia. In the presence of hyponatremia and impaired urinary dilution, patients with SIADH have hypouricemia, whereas patients exhibiting ECFV excess or depletion characteristically have hyperuricemia.[29,151]

Treatment Treatment of patients with demonstrable ECFV excess or depletion should be directed at the abnormal ECFV and its cause, rather than the hyponatremia. In almost all cases, the hyponatremia will improve with correction of the ECFV.[4,90] In a similar way, correction of the serum glucose in hyperglycemic patients and the removal of glycine by hemodialysis in patients with the TURP syndrome will correct the serum [Na^+]. The rate of correction of the serum [Na^+] in these patients is generally not of concern.

In patients with SIADH, treatment begins with fluid restriction. Because the goal of this therapy is to establish a negative fluid balance, careful attention to intake and output is required. If an offending xenobiotic can be identified, it should be discontinued. Although most cases resolve in 1–2 weeks,[87,115] SIADH caused by chronic cerebral or pulmonary conditions or by malignancy often persists. If this occurs, therapy with demeclocycline or lithium may be helpful, because severe fluid restriction is often intolerable. One author suggested that demeclocycline was more efficacious than lithium when the two drugs were compared in a small series of patients with SIADH.[47]

In all asymptomatic or mildly symptomatic patients (usually patients with chronic hyponatremia of more than 2 days duration), correction should proceed slowly, and certainly at a rate less than 0.5 mEq/L/h during the first 24 hours. This is because too rapid correction of hyponatremia may increase the risk of irreversible CNS damage known as central pontine myelinolysis.[4,12,154] Water restriction is usually sufficient, but occasionally demeclocycline may be appropriate in patients in whom a rapid rate of correction represents a greater risk for brain damage than the absolute serum [Na^+]. The use of a vasopressin (V_2) receptor antagonists may make the management of these patients easier.[4,66]

When hyponatremia is associated with life-threatening clinical presentations including respiratory depression, altered mental status, seizures or coma, careful infusion of hypertonic (3%) saline (eg, 1–2 mL/kg/h), with or without furosemide, is indicated.[4,87] Alternatively, conivaptan (a V_2 receptor antagonist) may be administered intravenously as an initial bolus of 20 mg followed by a continuous infusion of 40 mg/d for no more than 4 days.[65,68] In these symptomatic patients, the goal is to increase the serum [Na^+] by 1–2 mEq/L/h, or by 10% over 12–24 hours, or until the symptoms abate.[4,90] After this initial correction and amelioration of symptoms, the serum [Na^+] should be increased at a rate <0.5 mEq/L/h, preferably by water restriction alone. Formulae are available to help calculate the rate of correction of hyponatremia.[4] Equation 16–8 may be helpful.

When 1 L of fluid is infused:

$$\text{Change in serum } [Na^+] = \frac{\text{infusate } [Na^+] - \text{serum } [Na^+]}{\text{Total body water} + 1 \text{ L}} \quad \text{(Eq. 16–8)}$$

where the infusate [Na^+] in mEq/L equals:

3% sodium chloride	513
0.9% sodium chloride	154
Lactated Ringer solution	130
0.45% sodium chloride	77
0.33% sodium chloride	51

XENOBIOTIC-INDUCED ELECTROLYTE ABNORMALITIES

POTASSIUM

Xenobiotic-induced alterations in serum [K^+] are potentially more serious than alterations in other electrolyte concentrations because of the critical role of potassium in a variety of homeostatic processes. Potassium balance is complex.[21,126,138] The total body potassium content of an average adult is about 54 mEq/kg, of which only 2% is located in the intravascular space. The large intracellular store of potassium is maintained by a variety of systems, the most important of which is membrane Na^+-K^+-adenosine triphosphatase (ATPase). The relationship between total body stores and serum [K^+] is not linear, and small changes in the total body potassium may result in dramatic alterations in serum concentrations, and, more importantly, in the ratio of extracellular to intracellular [K^+].

People eating a western diet ingest 50–150 mEq/d of potassium, approximately 90% of which is subsequently eliminated in the urine. The body has two major defenses against a potassium load: acutely, potassium is transferred into cells; chronically, potassium is excreted in the urine by decreased proximal tubular reabsorption and increased distal tubular secretion (to a maximum of 600–700 mEq/d).[21] Following a meal, K^+ transfers into intracellular space through insulin and catecholamine-mediated uptake of potassium in liver and muscle cells.[97,133] Renal potassium excretion is primarily modulated by the renin–angiotensin–aldosterone system. In addition, the gastrointestinal absorption of potassium decreases as the serum [K^+] increases.

Hypokalemia results from decreased oral intake, gastrointestinal losses caused by repeated vomiting or diarrhea, urinary losses through increased K^+ secretion or decreased reabsorption, and processes that shift potassium into the intracellular compartment.[19,21,144,163] Table 16–8 summarizes the xenobiotics commonly associated with hypokalemia.

The neuromuscular manifestations of hypokalemia are reviewed elsewhere.[86] Patients with hypokalemia are often asymptomatic when the decrease in serum [K^+] is mild (serum concentrations of 3.0–3.5 mEq/L). Occasionally, hypokalemia interferes with renal concentrating mechanisms and polyuria is noted. More significant potassium deficits (serum concentrations of 2.0–3.0 mEq/L) cause generalized malaise and weakness. As the [K^+] falls to less than 2 mEq/L, weakness becomes prominent and areflexic paralysis and respiratory failure may occur, often necessitating intubation and mechanical ventilation.[86]

TABLE 16–8. Xenobiotic Causes of Altered Serum Potassium

Hypokalemia	Hyperkalemia
Aminoglycosides	α-Adrenergic agonists (phenylephrine)
Amphotericin	β-Adrenergic antagonists
Barium (soluble salts)	Amiloride
β-Adrenergic agonists	Angiotensin-converting enzyme inhibitors
Bicarbonate	Angiotensin receptor blockers
Caffeine	Arginine hydrochloride
Carbonic anhydrase inhibitors	Cardioactive steroids
Cathartics	Fluoride
Chloroquine	Heparin
Cisplatin	Nonsteroidal antiinflammatory drugs
Dextrose	Penicillin (potassium)
Hydroxychloroquine	Potassium salts
Infliximab	Spironolactone
Insulin	Succinylcholine
Licorice (containing glycyrrhizic acid)	Triamterene
Loop diuretics	Trimethoprim
Metabolic alkalosis	
Osmotic diuretics	
Quinine	
Salicylates	
Sodium penicillin and its analogs	
Sodium polystyrene sulfate	
Sulfonylureas	
Sympathomimetics	
Tenofovir	
Theophylline	
Thiazide diuretics	
Toluene	

Rhabdomyolysis is also likely. These neuromuscular manifestations are so prominent that they may be erroneously attributed to a neuromuscular syndrome such as Guillain-Barré. Other clinical findings associated with hypokalemia include gastrointestinal hypoperistalsis (ileus), manifestations of cardioactive steroid toxicity, worsening hyperglycemia in diabetic patients, and the symptoms and signs of the metabolic abnormalities that often accompany hypokalemia such as hyponatremia, metabolic acidosis, or alkalosis.[163]

Electrocardiographic changes also are common, even with mild potassium depletion, although the absence of ECG changes should never be used to exclude significant hypokalemia. Common ECG findings of hypokalemia include depression of the ST segment, decreased T-wave amplitude, and increased U-wave amplitude (Chap. 22). These findings may herald life-threatening rhythm disturbances.[74,94,163]

Treatment of hypokalemia involves discontinuing or removing the offending xenobiotic and correcting the potassium deficit. Potassium supplementation may be given orally or intravenously. The choice of potassium salt should be based on the associated acid–base abnormality, if present. Thus, potassium chloride should be administered when metabolic alkalosis is present, and another salt of potassium (eg, potassium citrate or potassium bicarbonate[spell out for parallel construction?]) should be administered when metabolic acidosis is present.[163] Potassium phosphate should be part of the K^+ supplement when hypophosphatemia is present, as occurs in diabetic ketoacidosis. Hypomagnesemia, which may cause or accompany hypokalemia (eg, in diuretic-induced hypokalemia), must be corrected because this abnormality may prevent successful potassium replacement.

The debate over the maximum safe infusion rate for intravenous potassium is summarized elsewhere.[89,163] Based on experience with more than 1300 infusions, one group concluded that under intensive care monitoring, intravenous administrations of 20 mEq/h (by central or peripheral vein) were well tolerated. They also found that each 20 mEq of potassium administered resulted in an average increase in serum [K^+] of 0.25 mEq/L. Others have used significantly larger doses (up to 100 mEq/h) in life-threatening circumstances.[30]

Hyperkalemia results from decreased urinary elimination (renal insufficiency, potassium-sparing diuretics, hypoaldosteronism), increased intake (either orally or intravenously), or redistribution from tissue stores.[19,21] The last mechanism is of major toxicologic importance. Overdoses of both cardioactive steroids (Chap. 64) and β-adrenergic antagonists (Chap. 61) cause hyperkalemia by promoting net potassium release from intracellular reservoirs. Presumably because of other protective mechanisms, overdose with a β-adrenergic antagonist produces only a moderate rise in serum [K^+] (usually to 5.0–5.5 mEq/L). By contrast, a similar rise in serum [K^+] as a consequence of blockade of the Na^+-K^+-ATPase pump during cardioactive steroid toxicity may be lethal. This suggests that hyperkalemia per se is not the cause of the lethality of cardioactive steroid toxicity. Thus, the focus of therapy should involve efforts to neutralize or eliminate the cardioactive steroid rather than reduce the serum [K^+].[17] Table 16–8 lists xenobiotics that cause hyperkalemia.

After oral overdoses of potassium salts, patients usually complain of nausea and vomiting. Ileus, and intestinal irritation, bleeding, and perforation may complicate the clinical course.[138] In the absence of potassium ingestion, gastrointestinal symptoms of hyperkalemia are usually very mild. Neuromuscular manifestations include weakness with an ascending flaccid paralysis and respiratory compromise, with intact sensation and cognition.[86,104,126] The similarity of these signs and symptoms to those associated with hypokalemia is striking, suggesting that hyperkalemia may be diagnosed with certainty only by laboratory measurement.

The cardiac manifestations of hyperkalemia are distinct, prominent, and life threatening. Electrocardiographic patterns progress through characteristic changes.[137,138] Although the progression of ECG changes is very reproducible, there is great individual variation with respect to the serum [K^+] at which these ECG findings occur. Initially, the only ECG finding may be the presence of tall, peaked T waves. As the serum [K^+] concentration increases, the QRS complex tends to blend into the T waves, the P-wave amplitude decreases, and the PR interval becomes prolonged. Next, the P wave is lost and ST-segment depression occurs. Finally, the distinction between the S and T waves becomes blurred and the ECG takes on a sine wave configuration (Chap. 22). Hemodynamic instability and cardiac arrest can result. As the patient's serum [K^+] falls with therapy, these ECG changes resolve in a reverse fashion.

The treatment of severe hyperkalemia includes standard airway management and methods to (1) reverse the ECG effects; (2) transfer K^+ to the intracellular space; and (3) enhance K^+ elimination. Pharmacologic interventions, extensively discussed elsewhere,[148] are summarized here. Calcium (eg, $CaCl_2$ 10–20 mEq administered intravenously) works almost immediately to protect the myocardium against the effects of hyperkalemia although it does not reduce the serum [K^+]. However, a potentially life-threatening interaction occurs when the patient with cardioactive steroid toxicity is given calcium salts (Chap. 64); thus, this therapeutic modality is relatively contraindicated in such circumstances.

The administration of insulin (and dextrose to prevent hypoglycemia), sodium bicarbonate, and/or inhalation of a β-adrenergic agonist all stimulate potassium entry into cells.[8] They reduce the serum [K^+] over approximately 30 minutes, but potassium begins to reenter the extracellular space over the next several hours. Cationic exchange resins, such as Na^+ polystyrene sulfonate, take somewhat longer to reduce the serum [K^+] (about 45 minutes), as they enhance gastrointestinal potassium loss. Hemodialysis or peritoneal dialysis may be useful, especially when significant renal impairment is present.

Calcium Calcium is the most abundant mineral in the body and 98%–99% is located in bone. Approximately half of the remaining 1%–2% of calcium in the body is bound to plasma proteins (mostly albumin) and most of the rest is complexed to various anions, with free, ionized calcium representing a very small fraction of extraosseous stores. The serum [Ca^{2+}] is maintained through interactions between dietary intake and renal elimination, modulated by vitamin D activity, parathyroid hormone, and calcitonin. More extensive discussions of calcium physiology are found elsewhere.[6,116]

Xenobiotic-induced hypercalcemia is uncommon and usually caused by an increased dietary calcium as a result of milk or antacid usage, calcium supplements, or a decrease in its renal excretion such as occurs with thiazide use.[6,19] Cholecalciferol, available as a rodenticide, can increase the serum [Ca^{2+}] by increasing its release from bone, increasing gastrointestinal absorption, and decreasing renal elimination (Chap. 108). Vitamin D toxicity from excessive vitamin intake or supplementation of milk also can cause hypercalcemia.[46,81] Table 16–9 lists other causes of hypercalcemia.

TABLE 16–9. Xenobiotic Causes of Altered Serum Calcium

Hypocalcemia	Hypercalcemia
Aminoglycosides	All-trans-retinoic acid (ATRA)
Bicarbonate	Aluminum
Bisphosphonates	Androgens
Calcitonin	Antacids (calcium containing)
Citrate	Antacids (magnesium containing)
Edetate disodium	Cholecalciferol and other vitamin D analogs
Ethanol	Lithium
Ethylene glycol	Milk–alkali syndrome
Fluoride	Tamoxifen
Furosemide	Thiazide diuretics
Mithramycin	Vitamin A
Neomycin	
Phenobarbital	
Phenytoin	
Phosphate	
Theophylline	
Valproate	

Symptoms of hypercalcemia consist of lethargy, muscle weakness, nausea, vomiting, and constipation. Life-threatening manifestations include complications from altered mental status such as aspiration pneumonia and cardiac dysrhythmias (Chap. 22). Treatment of clinically significant hypercalcemia focuses on removing the offending xenobiotic when possible, decreasing gastrointestinal absorption by administering a binding agent, increasing distribution into bone with a bisphosphonate, and enhancing renal excretion through forced diuresis with intravenous 0.9% NaCl solution and furosemide.[6,155] Hemodialysis may be required when significant renal impairment is present.

Xenobiotics more commonly cause hypocalcemia than hypercalcemia. Minor, usually clinically insignificant decreases in serum [Ca^{2+}] can occur in association with anticonvulsant[92] and aminoglycoside therapy.[19] Severe, life-threatening hypocalcemia can occur, however, from ethylene glycol poisoning (Chap. 107) or as a manifestation of fluoride toxicity from either fluoride salts or hydrofluoric acid (Chap. 105).[36,157] Calcium complex formation with fluoride or oxalate ions is responsible for the rapid development of hypocalcemia in these settings. Similar effects occur with excess phosphate[160] or citrate[103,158] intake. This mechanism (calcium complex formation) decreases the ionized [Ca^{2+}], but may or may not reduce the measured total serum [Ca^{2+}]. Other xenobiotics that produce hypocalcemia decrease absorption, enhance renal loss, and/or stimulate calcium entry into cells (Table 16–9).

Symptoms of hypocalcemia consist largely of neuromuscular findings, including paresthesias, cramps, carpopedal spasm, tetany, and seizures. Although ECG abnormalities are common (Chap. 22), life-threatening dysrhythmias are rare. Treatment strategies focus on calcium replacement. When hypomagnesemia or hyperphosphatemia is present, these abnormalities should be corrected or calcium replacement may fail.

MAGNESIUM

Magnesium is the fourth most abundant cation in the body (after Ca^{2+}, Na^+, and K^+), with a normal total body store of about 2000 mEq in a 70-kg person.[129] Approximately 50% of magnesium is stored in bone, with most of the remainder distributed in the soft tissues. Because only approximately 1%–2% of magnesium is located in the extracellular fluid, serum concentrations correlate poorly with total body stores.[130] Magnesium homeostasis is maintained through dietary intake, and renal and gastrointestinal excretion modulated by hormonal effects.[6]

Clinically significant hypermagnesemia is uncommon in the absence of renal failure, except when massive parenteral infusions of magnesium salts overwhelm renal excretory mechanisms. This has been reported with inadvertent intravenous infusion,[18,23,72,112] urologic procedures involving irrigation with magnesium salts,[42,82] and ingestion of large quantities of magnesium-containing antacids[105] and cathartics.[43,51,56] Of concern is iatrogenic overdose from the use of magnesium-containing cathartics used in poison management.[53,83,148] In a series of poisoned patients, a single dose of a magnesium-containing cathartic failed to produce any demonstrable rise in serum [Mg^{2+}].[149] However, patients who received three doses of magnesium sulfate over 8 hours had a significant increase in their serum [Mg^{2+}].[149] Thus the potential for iatrogenic toxicity exists, mandating cautious use of magnesium-containing cathartics, especially in patients with renal insufficiency. Table 16–10 lists xenobiotic causes of hypermagnesemia.

The symptoms of hypermagnesemia correlate with serum concentrations, but depend somewhat on the rate of increase and host factors. At serum [Mg^{2+}] of about 3–10 mEq/L, patients feel weak, nauseated, flushed, and thirsty. Bradycardia, a widened QRS complex on ECG, hypotension, and decreased deep tendon reflexes may be noted. As concentration increases, hypoventilation, muscle paralysis, and

TABLE 16–10. Xenobiotic Causes of Altered Serum Magnesium

Hypomagnesemia	Hypermagnesemia
Aminoglycosides	Antacids (magnesium containing)
Amphotericin	Cathartics (magnesium containing)
Cetuximab	Lithium
Cisplatin	Magnesium sulfate
Citrate	
Cyclosporine	
DDT	
Ethanol	
Fluoride	
Foscarnet	
Insulin	
Laxatives	
Loop diuretics	
Methylxanthines	
Osmotic diuretics	
Phosphates	
Strychnine	
Tacrolimus	
Thiazide diuretics	

ventricular dysrhythmias occur. Serum [Mg^{2+}] greater than 10 mEq/L, and especially those concentrations greater than 15 mEq/L, often cause death.

Hypermagnesemia should be considered a life-threatening disorder. When significant neuromuscular or ECG manifestations are noted, administration of $CaCl_2$ 5–20 mEq intravenously will reverse some of the toxicity.[6,64] Further therapy should focus on enhancing renal excretion by administering fluids and loop diuretics such as furosemide.[64] In the presence of renal failure or inadequate renal excretion, hemodialysis will rapidly correct hypermagnesemia.

Xenobiotic-induced hypomagnesemia is common, but rarely life threatening. Renal losses (caused by diuretics), gastrointestinal losses (caused by ethanol), intracellular shifts due to insulin[101] or β-adrenergic agonists, and complex formation (by fluoride or phosphate) are common.[6] Table 16–10 lists these and other xenobiotic causes of hypomagnesemia. Of note, many causes of hypomagnesemia also cause hypokalemia and hypocalcemia.[5] Therefore, when hypomagnesemia is suspected or discovered, the presence of other electrolyte abnormalities should be sought.

The symptoms of hypomagnesemia are lethargy, weakness, fatigue, neuromuscular excitation (tremor and hyperreflexia), nausea, and vomiting.[27,33] Dysrhythmias may occur, especially in patients treated with cardioactive steroids. Signs and symptoms consistent with hypocalcemia and hypokalemia also may be present.

Treatment involves removing the offending xenobiotic (if it can be identified) and restoring magnesium balance. Although either oral or parenteral supplementation is usually acceptable for mild hypomagnesemia, parenteral therapy is required when significant clinical manifestation is present. When oral therapy is indicated, a normal diet or magnesium oxide, magnesium chloride, or magnesium lactate in divided doses (magnesium 20–100 mEq/d) will often correct the hypomagnesemia.[5,6] When hypomagnesemia is severe or symptomatic, and renal function is normal, magnesium sulfate 16 mEq (2 g) can be given intravenously over several minutes to a maximum of 1 mEq/kg of magnesium in a 24-hour period.[6,27,80] During any substantial magnesium infusion, frequent serum [Mg^{2+}] determinations should be obtained and the presence of reflexes documented. If hyporeflexia occurs, the magnesium infusion should be discontinued.

SUMMARY

The management of poisoned or overdosed patients must include an evaluation of their fluid, electrolyte, and acid–base status. Abnormalities in acid–base and water balance, and alterations in potassium, calcium, and magnesium concentrations are common in such patients,and often are life threatening. Conversely, the possibility of xenobiotic ingestion or administration must always be considered when patients present with abnormalities of water, electrolyte, or acid–base balance. This is because these abnormalities are frequently caused by therapeutic doses of many drugs. Clearly, an appreciation of the pathophysiology of these abnormalities and a rational approach to their correction are essential for reducing morbidity and mortality. Finally, fluid and electrolyte abnormalities may result from the therapy of poisoned or overdosed patients. Thus, these patients must be monitored and reevaluated as treatment progresses to ensure that iatrogenic fluid, electrolyte, or acid–base disorders do not complicate the clinical course.

REFERENCES

1. Adrogue HJ, Madias NE: Management of life-threatening acid–base disorders. First of two parts. *N Engl J Med.* 1998;338:26-34.
2. Adrogue HJ, Madias NE: Management of life-threatening acid–base disorders. Second of two parts. *N Engl J Med.* 1998;338:107-111.
3. Adrogue HJ, Madias NE: Hypernatremia. *N Engl J Med.* 2000;342:1493-1499.
4. Adrogue HJ, Madias NE: Hyponatremia. *N Engl J Med.* 2000;342:1581-1589.
5. Agus ZS: Hypomagnesemia. *J Am Soc Nephrol.* 1999;10:1616-1622.
6. Agus ZS, Wasserstein A, Goldfarb S: Disorders of calcium and magnesium homeostasis. *Am J Med.* 1982;72:473-488.
7. Albert MS, Dell RB, Winters RW: Quantitative displacement of acid–base equilibrium in metabolic acidosis. *Ann Intern Med.* 1967;66:312-322.
8. Allon M, Dunlay R, Copkney C: Nebulized albuterol for acute hyperkalemia in patients on hemodialysis. *Ann Intern Med.* 1989;110:426-429.
9. Ammar KA, Heckerling PS: Ethylene glycol poisoning with a normal anion gap caused by concurrent ethanol ingestion: Importance of the osmolal gap. *Am J Kidney Dis.* 1996;27:130-133.
10. Anderson IK, Martin GR, Ramage AG: Central administration of 5-HT activates 5-HT_{1A} receptors to cause sympathoexcitation and 5-HT_2/5-HT_{1C} receptors to release vasopressin in anaesthetized rats. *Br J Pharmacol.* 1992;107:1020-1028.
11. Auys JC, Arieff AI: Symptomatic hyponatremia: making the diagnosis rapidly. *J Crit Illn.* 1990;5:846-856.
12. Ayus JC, Krothapalli RK, Arieff AI: Treatment of symptomatic hyponatremia and its relation to brain damage. A prospective study. *N Engl J Med.* 1987;317:1190-1195.
13. Ayus JC, Levine R, Arieff AI: Fatal dysnatraemia caused by elective colonoscopy. *BMJ.* 2003;326:382-384.
14. Batlle DC, Hizon M, Cohen E, et al: The use of the urinary anion gap in the diagnosis of hyperchloremic metabolic acidosis. *N Engl J Med.* 1988;318:594-599.
15. Batlle DC, von Riotte AB, Gaviria M, Grupp M: Amelioration of polyuria by amiloride in patients receiving long-term lithium therapy. *N Engl J Med.* 1985;312:408-414.
16. Berl T, Anderson RJ, McDonald KM, Schrier RW: Clinical disorders of water metabolism. *Int Soc Nephrol.* 1976;10:117-132.
17. Bismuth C, Gaultier M, Conso F, Efthymiou ML: Hyperkalemia in acute digitalis poisoning: prognostic significance and therapeutic implications. *Clin Toxicol.* 1973;6:153-162.

18. Bourgeois FJ, Thiagarajah S, Harbert GM Jr, DiFazio C: Profound hypotension complicating magnesium therapy. *Am J Obstet Gynecol.* 1986;154:919-920.
19. Brass EP, Thompson WL: Drug-induced electrolyte abnormalities. *Drugs.* 1982;24:207-228.
20. Brenner BE: Clinical significance of the elevated anion gap. *Am J Med.* 1985;79:289-296.
21. Brown RS: Extrarenal potassium homeostasis. *Kidney Int.* 1986;30:116-127.
22. Caldwell JW, Nava AJ, de Haas DD: Hypernatremia associated with cathartics in overdose management. *West J Med.* 1987;147:593-596.
23. Cao Z, Bideau R, Valdes R Jr, Elin RJ: Acute hypermagnesemia and respiratory arrest following infusion of $MgSO_4$ for tocolysis. *Clin Chim Acta.* 1999;285:191-193.
24. Carlisle EJ, Donnelly SM, Vasuvattakul S, et al: Glue-sniffing and distal renal tubular acidosis: sticking to the facts. *J Am Soc Nephrol.* 1991;1:1019-1027.
25. Catalano G, Kanfer SN, Catalano MC, Alberts VA: The role of sertraline in a patient with recurrent hyponatremia. *Gen Hosp Psychiatry.* 1996;18:278-283.
26. Connelly DM: Silver nitrate. Ideal burn wound therapy? *N Y State J Med.* 1970;70:1642-1644.
27. Cronin RE, Knochel JP: Magnesium deficiency. *Adv Intern Med.* 1983;28:509-533.
28. Darchy B, Abruzzese L, Pitiot O, et al: Delayed admission for ethylene glycol poisoning: lack of elevated serum osmol gap. *Intensive Care Med.* 1999;25:859-861.
29. Decaux G, Schlesser M, Coffernils M, et al: Uric acid, anion gap and urea concentration in the diagnostic approach to hyponatremia. *Clin Nephrol.* 1994;42:102-108.
30. DeFronzo RA, Bia M: Intravenous potassium chloride therapy. *JAMA.* 1981;245:2446.
31. Delaney V, de Pertuz Y, Nixon D, Bourke E: Indomethacin in streptozocin-induced nephrogenic diabetes insipidus. *Am J Kidney Dis.* 1987;9:79-83.
32. DiNubile MJ: The increment in the anion gap: overextension of a concept? *Lancet.* 1988;2:951-953.
33. Dirks JH: The kidney and magnesium regulation. *Kidney Int.* 1983;23:771-777.
34. Dorwart WV, Chalmers L: Comparison of methods for calculating serum osmolality form chemical concentrations, and the prognostic value of such calculations. *Clin Chem.* 1975;21:190-194.
35. Earley LE, Orloff J: The mechanism of antidiuresis associated with the administration of hydrochlorothiazide to patients with vasopressin-resistant diabetes insipidus. *J Clin Invest.* 1963;41:1988-1997.
36. Edelman P: Hydrofluoric acid burns. *Occup Med.* 1986;1:89-103.
37. Edwards CR: Lessons from licorice. *N Engl J Med.* 1991;325:1242-1243.
38. Eisen TF, Lacouture PG, Woolf A: Serum osmolality in alcohol ingestions: differences in availability among laboratories of teaching hospital, nonteaching hospital, and commercial facilities. *Am J Emerg Med.* 1989;7:256-259.
39. Emmett M, Narins RG: Clinical use of the anion gap. *Medicine (Baltimore).* 1977;56:38-54.
40. Farese RV, Biglieri EG, Schackleton CH, et al: Licorice-induced hypermineralocorticoidism. *N Engl J Med.* 1991;325:1223-1227.
41. Farley TA: Severe hypernatremic dehydration after use of an activated charcoal-sorbitol suspension. *J Pediatr.* 1986;109:719-722.
42. Fassler CA, Rodriguez RM, Badesch DB, et al: Magnesium toxicity as a cause of hypotension and hypoventilation. Occurrence in patients with normal renal function. *Arch Intern Med.* 1985;145:1604-1606.
43. Ferdinandus J, Pederson JA, Whang R: Hypermagnesemia as a cause of refractory hypotension, respiratory depression, and coma. *Arch Intern Med.* 1981;141:669-670.
44. Fichman MP, Vorherr H, Kleeman CR, Telfer N: Diuretic-induced hyponatremia. *Ann Intern Med.* 1971;75:853-863.
45. Figge J, Jabor A, Kazda A, Fencl V: Anion gap and hypoalbuminemia. *Crit Care Med.* 1998;26:1807-1810.
46. Fiorino AS: Hypercalcemia and alkalosis due to the milk-alkali syndrome: a case report and review. *Yale J Biol Med.* 1996;69:517-523.
47. Forrest JN Jr, Cox M, Hong C, et al: Superiority of demeclocycline over lithium in the treatment of chronic syndrome of inappropriate secretion of antidiuretic hormone. *N Engl J Med.* 1978;298:173-177.
48. Gabow PA: Disorders associated with an altered anion gap. *Kidney Int.* 1985;27:472-483.
49. Gabow PA, Kaehny WD, Fennessey PV, et al: Diagnostic importance of an increased serum anion gap. *N Engl J Med.* 1980;303:854-858.
50. Gamble JL: *Chemical Anatomy, Physiology, and Pathology of Extra-cellular Fluids: A Lecture Series,* 6th ed. Cambridge, MA: Harvard University Press; 1960.
51. Garcia-Webb P, Bhagat C, Oh T, et al: Hypermagnesaemia and hypophosphataemia after ingestion of magnesium sulphate. *BMJ Clin Res Ed.* 1984;288:759.
52. Garella S, Chazan JA, Cohen JJ: Saline-resistant metabolic alkalosis or "chloride-wasting nephropathy." Report of four patients with severe potassium depletion. *Ann Intern Med.* 1970;73:31-38.
53. Garrelts JC, Watson WA, Holloway KD, Sweet DE: Magnesium toxicity secondary to catharsis during management of theophylline poisoning. *Am J Emerg Med.* 1989;7:34-37.
54. Gazda-Smith E, Synhavsky A: Hypernatremia following treatment of theophylline toxicity with activated charcoal and sorbitol. *Arch Intern Med.* 1990;150:689.
55. Gennari FJ: Current concepts. Serum osmolality. Uses and limitations. *N Engl J Med.* 1984;310:102-105.
56. Gerard SK, Hernandez C, Khayam-Bashi H: Extreme hypermagnesemia caused by an overdose of magnesium-containing cathartics. *Ann Emerg Med.* 1988;17:728-731.
57. Glaser DS: Utility of the serum osmol gap in the diagnosis of methanol or ethylene glycol ingestion. *Ann Emerg Med.* 1996;27:343-346.
58. Glasser L, Sternglanz PD, Combie J, Robinson A: Serum osmolality and its applicability to drug overdose. *Am J Clin Pathol.* 1973;60:695-699.
59. Goldman MA, Lisak R, Matz R, Davidson FZ: Hypochloremic alkalosis with symptoms of seizure disorder. *N Y State J Med.* 1970;70:306-308.
60. Goldman MB, Luchins DJ, Robertson GL: Mechanisms of altered water metabolism in psychotic patients with polydipsia and hyponatremia. *N Engl J Med.* 1988;318:397-403.
61. Goldstein MB, Bear R, Richardson RM, et al: The urine anion gap: a clinically useful index of ammonium excretion. *Am J Med. Sci.* 1986; 292:198-202.
62. Goldstein RJ, Lichtenstein NS, Souder D: The myth of the low anion gap. *JAMA.* 1980;243:1737-1738.
63. Goodkin DA, Krishna GG, Narins RG: The role of the anion gap in detecting and managing mixed metabolic acid–base disorders. *Clin Endocrinol Metab.* 1984;13:333-349.
64. Graber TW, Yee AS, Baker FJ: Magnesium: physiology, clinical disorders, and therapy. *Ann Emerg Med.* 1981;10:49-57.
65. Greenber A, Verbalis JG: Vasopressin receptor antagonists. *Kidney Int.* 2006;69:2124-2130.
66. Gross P, Reimann D, Henschkowski J, Damian M: Treatment of severe hyponatremia: conventional and novel aspects. *J Am Soc Nephrol.* 2001;12:S10-S14.
67. Harrington JT. Metabolic alkalosis. *Kidney Int.* 1984;26:88-97.
68. Hays RM: Vasopressin antagonists—progress and promise. *N Engl J Med.* 2006;355:2146-2148
69. Hilbert G, Bedry R, Cardinaud JP, Benissan GG: Euro bleach: fatal hypernatremia due to 13.3% sodium hypochlorite. *J Toxicol Clin Toxicol.* 1997;35:635-636.
70. Hoekstra PT, Kahnoski R, McCamish MA, et al: Transurethral prostatic resection syndrome—a new perspective: encephalopathy with associated hyperammonemia. *J Urol.* 1983;130:704-707.
71. Hoffman RS, Smilkstein MJ, Howland MA, Goldfrank LR: Osmol gaps revisited: normal values and limitations. *J Toxicol Clin Toxicol.* 1993;31:81-93.
72. Hoffman RS, Smilkstein MJ, Rubenstein F: An "amp" by any other name: the hazards of intravenous magnesium dosing. *JAMA.* 1989;261:557.
73. Hohler T, Teuber G, Wanitschke R, Meyer zum Buschenfeld KH: Indomethacin treatment in amphotericin B induced nephrogenic diabetes insipidus. *Clin Invest.* 1994;72:769-771.
74. Hohnloser SH, Verrier RL, Lown B, Raeder EA: Effect of hypokalemia on susceptibility to ventricular fibrillation in the normal and ischemic canine heart. *Am Heart J.* 1986;112:32-35.
75. Holden R, Jackson MA: Near-fatal hyponatraemic coma due to vasopressin over-secretion after "ecstasy" (3,4-MDMA). *Lancet.* 1996;347:1052.
76. Hubbard JI, Lin N, Sibbald JR: Subfornical organ lesions in rats abolish hyperdipsic effects of isoproterenol and serotonin. *Brain Res Bull.* 1989;23:41-45.
77. Iberti TJ, Leibowitz AB, Papadakos PJ, Fischer EP: Low sensitivity of the anion gap as a screen to detect hyperlactatemia in critically ill patients. *Crit Care Med.* 1990;18:275-277.
78. Inaba H, Hirasawa H, Mizuguchi T: Serum osmolality gap in postoperative patients in intensive care. *Lancet.* 1987;1:1331-1335.

79. Ireland JT, Thomson WS: Euglycemic diabetic ketoacidosis. *BMJ.* 1973;3:107.
80. Iseri LT, Freed J, Bures AR: Magnesium deficiency and cardiac disorders. *Am J Med.* 1975;58:837-846.
81. Jacobus CH, Holick MF, Shao Q, et al: Hypervitaminosis D associated with drinking milk. *N Engl J Med.* 1992;326:1173-1177.
82. Jenny DB, Goris GB, Urwiller RD, Brian BA: Hypermagnesemia following irrigation of renal pelvis. Cause of respiratory depression. *JAMA.* 1978;240:1378-1379.
83. Jones J, Heiselman D, Dougherty J, Eddy A: Cathartic-induced magnesium toxicity during overdose management. *Ann Emerg Med.* 1986;15:1214-1218.
84. Kassirer JP, Berkman PM, Lawrenz DR, Schwartz WB: The critical role of chloride in the correction of hypokalemic alkalosis in man. *Am J Med.* 1965;38:172-189.
85. Kessler J, Samuels SC: Sertraline and hyponatremia. *N Engl J Med.* 1996;335:524.
86. Knochel JP: Neuromuscular manifestations of electrolyte disorders. *Am J Med.* 1982;72:521-535.
87. Kovacs L, Robertson GL: Syndrome of inappropriate antidiuresis. *Endocrinol Metab Clin North Am.* 1992;21:859-875.
88. Krapf R, Beeler I, Hertner D, Hulter HN: Chronic respiratory alkalosis. The effect of sustained hyperventilation on renal regulation of acid–base equilibrium. *N Engl J Med.* 1991;324:1394-1401.
89. Kruse JA, Carlson RW: Rapid correction of hypokalemia using concentrated intravenous potassium chloride infusions. *Arch Intern Med.* 1990;150:613-617.
90. Lauriat SM, Berl T: The hyponatremic patient: practical focus on therapy. *J Am Soc Nephrol.* 1997;8:1599-1607.
91. Lavie CJ, Crocker EF Jr, Key KJ, Ferguson TG: Marked hypochloremic metabolic alkalosis with severe compensatory hypoventilation. *South Med J.* 1986;79:1296-1299.
92. Lee WL, Yang CC, Deng JF, et al: A case of severe hyperammonemia and unconsciousness following sodium valproate intoxication. *Vet Hum Toxicol.* 1998;40:346-348.
93. Libber S, Harrison H, Spector D: Treatment of nephrogenic diabetes insipidus with prostaglandin synthesis inhibitors. *J Pediatr.* 1986;108:305-311.
94. Lichstein E, Chadda K, Fenig S: Atrial pacing in the treatment of refractory ventricular tachycardia associated with hypokalemia. *Am J Cardiol.* 1972;30:550-553.
95. Liu BA, Mittmann N, Knowles SR, Shear NH: Hyponatremia and the syndrome of inappropriate secretion of antidiuretic hormone associated with the use of selective serotonin reuptake inhibitors: a review of spontaneous reports. *CMAJ.* 1996;155:519-527.
96. Lubash GD, Cohen BD, Young CW, et al: Severe metabolic alkalosis with neurologic abnormalities; report of a case. *N Engl J Med.* 1958;258:1050-1052.
97. Lundborg P: The effect of adrenergic blockade on potassium concentrations in different conditions. *Acta Med Scand Suppl.* 1983;672:121-126.
98. Lydiard RB, Gelenberg AJ: Hazards and adverse effects of lithium. *Ann Rev Med.* 1982;33:327-344.
99. Madias NE, Ayus JC, Adrogue HJ: Increased anion gap in metabolic alkalosis: the role of plasma-protein equivalency. *N Engl J Med.* 1979;300: 1421-1423.
100. Masson EA, Rhodes JM: Mesalazine associated nephrogenic diabetes insipidus presenting as weight loss. *Gut.* 1992;33:563-564.
101. Matsumura M, Nakashima A, Tofuku Y: Electrolyte disorders following massive insulin overdose in a patient with type 2 diabetes. *Intern Med.* 2000;39:55-57.
102. Mazze RI, Trudell JR, Cousins MJ: Methoxyflurane metabolism and renal dysfunction: clinical correlation in man. *Anesthesiology.* 1971;35:247-252.
103. McCarthy LJ, Danielson CF, Skipworth EM, Thompson CF: Hypocalcemia secondary to citrate toxicity. *Ther Apher.* 1998;2:249.
104. McCarty M, Jagoda A, Fairweather P: Hyperkalemic ascending paralysis. *Ann Emerg Med.* 1998;32:104-107.
105. McGuire JK, Kulkarni MS, Baden HP: Fatal hypermagnesemia in a child treated with megavitamin/megamineral therapy. *Pediatrics.* 2000; 105:E18.
106. McQuillen KK, Anderson AC: Osmol gaps in the pediatric population. *Acad Emerg Med.* 1999;6:27-30.
107. Mennen M, Slovis CM: Severe metabolic alkalosis in the emergency department. *Ann Emerg Med.* 1988;17:354-357.
108. Mercado R, Michelis MF: Severe sodium depletion syndrome during lithium carbonate therapy. *Arch Intern Med.* 1977;137:1731-1733.
109. Mizutani AR, Parker J, Katz J, Schmidt J: Visual disturbances, serum glycine levels and transurethral resection of the prostate. *J Urol.* 1990;144:697-699.
110. Moder KG, Hurley DL: Fatal hypernatremia from exogenous salt in-take: report of a case and review of the literature. *Mayo Clin Proc.* 1990;65:1587-1594.
111. Morgan TJ, Clark C, Clague A: Artifactual elevation of measured plasma L-lactate concentration in the presence of glycolate. *Crit Care Med.* 1999;27:2177-2179.
112. Morisaki H, Yamamoto S, Morita Y, et al: Hypermagnesemia-induced cardiopulmonary arrest before induction of anesthesia for emergency cesarean section. *J Clin Anesth.* 2000;12:224-226.
113. Moses AM, Miller M: Drug-induced dilutional hyponatremia. *N Engl J Med.* 1974;291:1234-1239.
114. Moses AM, Miller M, Streeten DH: Pathophysiologic and pharmacologic alterations in the release and action of ADH. *Metab Clin Exp.* 1976;25:697-721.
115. Moses AM, Notman DD: Diabetes insipidus and syndrome of inappropriate antidiuretic hormone secretion (SIADH). *Adv Intern Med.* 1982;27:73-100.
116. Mundy GR: The hypercalcemia of malignancy. *Kidney Int.* 1987;31:142-155.
117. Narins RG, Emmett M: Simple and mixed acid-base disorders: a practical approach. *Medicine.* 1980;59:161-187.
118. Navarro JF, Quereda C, Quereda C, et al: Nephrogenic diabetes insipidus and renal tubular acidosis secondary to foscarnet therapy. *Am J Kidney Dis.* 1996;27:431-434.
119. Nielsen S, Frokiaer J, Marples D, et al: Aquaporins in the kidney: from molecules to medicine. *Physiol Rev.* 2002;82:205-244.
120. Oh MS, Carroll HJ: The anion gap. *N Engl J Med.* 1977;297:814-817.
121. Oster JR, Perez GO, Materson BJ: Use of the anion gap in clinical medicine. *South Med J.* 1988;81:229-237.
122. Osterloh JD, Kelly TJ, Khayam-Bashi H, Romeo R: Discrepancies in osmolal gaps and calculated alcohol concentrations. *Arch Pathol Lab Med.* 1996;120:637-641.
123. Perez GO, Oster JR: Acid–base disorders: II. Use of AG/ HCO3 in evaluating mixed acid–base disorders—a patient management problem. *South Med J.* 1986;79:882-886.
124. Perrone J, Hoffman RS: Compensatory hypoventilation in severe metabolic alkalosis. *Acad Emerg Med.* 1996;3:981-982.
125. Phillips DR, Milim SJ, Nathanson HG, et al: Preventing hyponatremic encephalopathy: comparison of serum sodium and osmolality during operative hysteroscopy with 5.0% mannitol and 1.5% glycine distention media. *J Am Assoc Gynecol Laparosc.* 1997;4:567-576.
126. Ponce SP, Jennings AE, Madias NE, Harrington JT: Drug-induced hyperkalemia. *Medicine (Baltimore).* 1985;64:357-370.
127. Porter WH, Crellin M, Rutter PW, Oeltgen P: Interference by glycolic acid in the Beckman synchron method for lactate: A useful clue for unsuspected ethylene glycol intoxication. *Clin Chem.* 2000;46:874-875.
128. Quinn BP, Wall BM: Nephrogenic diabetes insipidus and tubulointerstitial nephritis during continuous therapy with rifampin. *Am J Kidney Dis.* 1989;14:217-220.
129. Randall RE Jr, Cohen MD, Spray CC Jr, Rossmeisl EC: Hypermagnesemia in renal failure. Etiology and toxic manifestations. *Ann Intern Med.* 1964;61:73-88.
130. Reinhart RA: Magnesium metabolism. A review with special reference to the relationship between intracellular content and serum levels. *Arch Intern Med.* 1988;148:2415-2420.
131. Richardson RM, Halperin ML: The urine pH: a potentially misleading diagnostic test in patients with hyperchloremic metabolic acidosis. *Am J Kidney Dis.* 1987;10:140-143.
132. Riggs AT, Dysken MW, Kim SW, Opsahl JA: A review of disorders of water homeostasis in psychiatric patients. *Psychosomatics.* 1991;32:133-148.
133. Rosa RM, Silva P, Young JB, et al: Adrenergic modulation of extrarenal potassium disposal. *N Engl J Med.* 1980;302:431-434.
134. Ross MP, Spiller HA: Fatal ingestion of sodium hypochlorite bleach with associated hypernatremia and hyperchloremic metabolic acidosis. *Vet Hum Toxicol.* 1999;41:82-86.
135. Sakane N, Yoshida T, Umekawa T, et al: Nephrogenic diabetes insipidus induced by lobenzarit disodium treatment in patients with rheumatoid arthritis. *Intern Med.* 1996;35:119-122.
136. Salem MM, Mujais SK: Gaps in the anion gap. *Arch Intern Med.* 1992;152:1625-1629.

137. Saxena K: Death from potassium chloride overdose. *Postgrad Med.* 1988;84:97-98.
138. Saxena K: Clinical features and management of poisoning due to potassium chloride. *Med Toxicol Adverse Drug Exp.* 1989;4:429-443.
139. Schelling JR, Howard RL, Winter SD, Linas SL: Increased osmolal gap in alcoholic ketoacidosis and lactic acidosis. *Ann Intern Med.* 1990;113:580-582.
140. Schnur MJ, Appel GB, Karp G, Osserman EP: The anion gap in asymptomatic plasma cell dyscrasias. *Ann Intern Med.* 1977;86:304-305.
141. Schwartz SM, Carroll HM, Scharschmidt LA: SubliMed (inorganic) sulfur ingestion. A cause of life-threatening metabolic acidosis with a high anion gap. *Arch Intern Med.* 1986;146:1437-1438.
142. Scoggin C, McClellan JR, Cary JM: Hypernatraemia and acidosis in association with topical treatment of burns. *Lancet.* 1977;1:959.
143. Scott SM: Pulmonary edema and hyponatremia during hysteroscopic resection of uterine fibroids: Case report. *CRNA.* 1998;9:113-117.
144. Sigue G, Gamble L, Pelitere M, et al: From profound hypokalemia to life-threatening hyperkalemia: A case of barium sulfide poisoning. *Arch Intern Med.* 2000;160:548-551.
145. Singer I, Rotenberg D: Demeclocycline-induced nephrogenic diabetes insipidus. In vivo and in vitro studies. *Ann Intern Med.* 1973;79:679-683.
146. Singer I, Rotenberg D: Mechanisms of lithium action. *N Engl J Med.* 1973;289:254-260.
147. Sklar AH, Linas SL: The osmolal gap in renal failure. *Ann Intern Med.* 1983;98:481-482.
148. Smilkstein MJ, Smolinske SC, Kulig KW, Rumack BH: Severe hypermagnesemia due to multiple-dose cathartic therapy. *West J Med.* 1988;148:208-211.
149. Smilkstein MJ, Steedle D, Kulig KW, et al: Magnesium levels after magnesium-containing cathartics. *J Toxicol Clin Toxicol.* 1988;26:51-65.
150. Smithline N, Gardner KD, Jr: Gaps—Anionic and osmolal. *JAMA.* 1976;236:1594-1597.
151. Sonnenblick M, Rosin A: Increased uric acid clearance in the syndrome of inappropriate secretion of antidiuretic hormone. *Isr J Med Sci.* 1988;24:20-23.
152. Spigset O, Hedenmalm K: Hyponatraemia and the syndrome of inappropriate antidiuretic hormone secretion (SIADH) induced by psychotropic drugs. *Drug Saf.* 1995;12:209-225.
153. Steinhart B: Case report: Severe ethylene glycol intoxication with normal osmolal gap—"A chilling thought." *J Emerg Med.* 1990;8: 583-585.
154. Sterns RH, Riggs JE, Schochet SS Jr: Osmotic demyelination syndrome following correction of hyponatremia. *N Engl J Med.* 1986; 314: 1535-1542.
155. Suki WN, Yium JJ, Von Minden M, et al: Acute treatment of hypercalcemia with furosemide. *N Engl J Med.* 1970;283:836-840.
156. Takahashi H, Toya T, Matsumiya N, Koyama K: A case of transient diabetes insipidus associated with poisoning by a herbicide containing glufosinate. *J Toxicol Clin Toxicol.* 2000;38:153-156.
157. Tepperman PB: Fatality due to acute systemic fluoride poisoning following a hydrofluoric acid skin burn. *J Occup Med.* 1980;22:691-692.
158. Uhl L, Maillet S, King S, Kruskall MS: Unexpected citrate toxicity and severe hypocalcemia during apheresis. *Transfusion.* 1997;37: 1063-1065.
159. Van Amelsvoort T, Bakshi R, Devaux CB, Schwabe S: Hyponatremia associated with carbamazepine and oxcarbazepine therapy: a review. *Epilepsia.* 1994;35:181-188.
160. Vincent JC, Sheikh A: Phosphate poisoning by ingestion of clothes washing liquid and fabric conditioner. *Anaesthesia.* 1998;53:1004-1006.
161. Vokes TJ, Robertson GL: Disorders of antidiuretic hormone. *Endocrinol Metab Clin North Am.* 1988;17:281-299.
162. Wax PM, Wang RY, Hoffman RS, et al: Prevalence of sorbitol in multiple-dose activated charcoal regimens in emergency departments. *Ann Emerg Med.* 1993;22:1807-1812.
163. Weiner ID, Wingo CS: Hypokalemia—consequences, causes, and correction. *J Am Soc Nephrol.* 1997;8:1179-1188.
164. Wilkins B: Cerebral oedema after MDMA ("ecstasy") and unrestricted water intake. Hyponatraemia must be treated with low water input. *BMJ.* 1996;313:689-690.
165. Winter SD, Pearson JR, Gabow PA, et al: The fall of the serum anion gap. *Arch Intern Med.* 1990;150:311-313.
166. Witte DL, Rodgers JL, Barrett DA: The anion gap: its use in quality control. *Clin Chem.* 1976;22:643-646.
167. Woo MY, Greenway DC, Nadler SP, Cardinal P: Artifactual elevation of lactate in ethylene glycol poisoning. *J Emerg Med.* 2003;25:289-293.
168. Wrenn KD, Slovis CM, Slovis BS: The ability of physicians to predict hyperkalemia from the ECG. *Ann Emerg Med.* 1991;20:1229-1232.

CHAPTER 17
PSYCHIATRIC PRINCIPLES

Kishor Malavade and Mark R. Serper

Psychiatric problems may be the cause or the effect of many toxicologic presentations. Suicide attempts and aggressive behaviors are commonly associated with toxicity and can be uniquely difficult to assess and manage. Patient behaviors are often viewed as either totally intentional and deliberate or totally "out of control" and irrational. The truth is usually more complex, with some aspects occurring within the awareness and control of the patient and other aspects either unknown or overwhelming to the patient. This chapter addresses suicide and violence to enable the physician to adopt the appropriate role of both diagnostician and medical decision maker.

SUICIDE AND SELF-INJURIOUS BEHAVIOR

Although suicide may be attempted or accomplished in a variety of settings and by a variety of means it is most typically associated with psychiatric disorders and/or substance abuse, especially ethanol, and is typically accomplished with psychoactive xenobiotics alone or in combination.[37,39]

Suicide is a leading cause of death and injury in the United States and throughout the world. Suicide was the 11th leading cause of death in 2005, with the 32,637 known cases representing 1.3% of the total deaths in the United States that year. The age-adjusted death rate in 2005 was 10.9 deaths by suicide for every 100,000 persons, or 0.0109%.[13] Suicidal ideation and attempts are far more frequent than actual suicide. Recent studies published since 1999 have demonstrated that among individuals age 18 and above, lifetime prevalence rates for suicidal ideation are 5.6%–14.3%. The lifetime prevalence rate for suicidal plans is 3.9% and the lifetime prevalence rates for suicide attempts are 1.9%–8.7%.[13,14]

Although the prevalence of suicide and suicidal behaviors shows significant overlap, one notable area of difference is the consistent pattern of higher rates of suicide attempts among women and of completed suicides among men.[13,14] For adolescents aged 12–17, lifetime prevalence rates for suicidal ideation are 19.8%–24.0%. Lifetime prevalence rates for suicide attempts are 3.1%–8.8%. Twelve-month prevalence rates for suicidal ideation are 15.0%–29.0%. Twelve-month prevalence rates for suicide attempts are 7.3%–10.6%. Twelve-month prevalence rates for suicide plans are 12.6%–19.0%. There are no lifetime data on suicide plans.[14,15,46]

Given that the act of suicide is a statistically rare event in the overall population, it is virtually impossible to predict who will actually commit suicide. It is therefore critical to identify risk factors that increase the likelihood that any individual might attempt suicide, and to identify risk factors that are modifiable. The identification of modifiable risk factors provides opportunities for interventions that may decrease suicide risk. Additionally, there are protective factors that mitigate the risk for suicide, and it is important to assess for the presence or absence of these factors in determining the overall risk for suicide in a patient.

TERMINOLOGY OF SUICIDE

The terms and definitions of suicide and suicidal behaviors used in this chapter have been outlined in several reports on the subject.[24,32,54] The term *suicide* refers to self-inflicted death with evidence (either explicit or implicit) that the person intended to die. The term *suicidal ideation* refers to thoughts of serving as the agent of one's own death. Suicidal ideation may vary in seriousness depending on the specificity of suicide plans and the degree of suicidal intent. The term *suicidal intent* refers to the subjective expectation and desire for a self-destructive act to end in death. The term suicidal plan refers to the formulation of a specific method through which one intends to die. The term *suicide attempt* refers to self-injurious behavior with a nonfatal outcome accompanied by evidence (either explicit or implicit) that the person intended to die. The term *self-harm* refers to self-inflicting of painful, destructive, or injurious acts without intent to die. Lethality of suicidal behavior is the objective danger to life associated with a suicide method or action. Note that lethality is distinct from and may not always coincide with an individual's expectation of what is medically dangerous.

PSYCHIATRIC MANAGEMENT OF SELF-POISONING

Table 17–1 depicts a case of suspected self-poisoning from the starting point of prehospital care through the completion of a comprehensive assessment and treatment planning.

FOCUSED PSYCHIATRIC ASSESSMENT

At a relatively early point in the patient's course, when the patient can be cooperative, a focused psychiatric assessment is critical to address specific clinical concerns. A thorough psychiatric consultation is warranted, once the patient is medically stable. The determination that the patient is stable is not solely established on the basis of blood concentrations of a xenobiotic or ancillary medical tests, but rather when the emergency physician or medical toxicologist with an understanding of pharmacokinetics deems it appropriate.[36] Psychiatric examination is not warranted until an altered mental status has cleared. There are several reasons for this approach.

The physician should not unequivocally attribute altered mental status to poisoning or toxicity until the signs of altered consciousness have resolved and cognitive functions have returned to normal. Until that time, other toxic metabolic and structural conditions that might coexist with, or masquerade as, toxicity cannot be excluded. If the patient's cognitive functioning is impaired by xenobiotics critical historical details may be unreliable.[19] It should be understood that much of what the patient reports may be ephemeral, caused by the predictable temporary and reversible effects on mood of these xenobiotics.[9]

A focused assessment is necessary to ascertain elopement risk or decisional capacity. Subacute residual CNS effects of ingestions such as confusion, fatigue, and fear can dispose patients to wander or elope. Additionally, the patient's intentions remain unclear at this point, and the question of unintentional versus intentional exposure to a xenobiotic cannot be completely resolved. For these reasons, a high level of supervision should be maintained, and a patient should not be allowed to leave until an adequate assessment of the patient's mental status is completed. Depending on the architecture and organization of the emergency department (ED) and personnel, it may be sufficient to place the patient in an open area in the direct line of sight of the medical staff. If such an arrangement is not possible, or if the patient is agitated and disruptive, it may be necessary to separate the patient from the general population. Under these circumstances, an individual aide should be assigned to observe the patient on a one-to-one basis. Safe physical and/or chemical restraints may be necessary to prevent further injury to both the patient and the staff.

TABLE 17–1. Case Presentation: Suspected Self-Poisoning

	Case		Evolution		Disposition
Patient course	Patient found in the community unresponsive	Patient monitored in the ED; vital signs stable; still unresponsive	Patient lethargic but cooperative; answers simple questions	Patient fully awake and alert	Evaluation complete
Treatment course	Prehospital	Triage medical assessment	Observation and monitoring	Formal psychiatric evaluation	Treatment planning
Physician course	Patient identification Search for prescription drugs, drug paraphernalia Assessment of cardiac and respiratory function	Orogastric lavage(?) Activated charcoal(?) Diagnostic testing (blood studies, ECG, urine toxicology) Contact collateral sources for history Prior records	Focused psychiatric assessment: elopement, aggressive behavior, decisional capacity, addressing confidentiality, and immediate suicide risk	Comprehensive psychiatric assessment: diagnostic interviewing, risk factors, future risk	Treatments: medication, hospitalization, substance abuse, crisis intervention or family therapy

In general, patients are presumed competent and must consent to treatment, but the issue of decisional capacity frequently arises. Patients may request their discharge, refuse care, or become aggressive. Aggression may arise from lingering effects of ingestion or a xenobiotic-withdrawal, severe anxiety, fear, anger at the loss of autonomy, or the discomfort associated with unpleasant procedures.[52] Although patients may respond to verbal limit setting and repeated explanations of their care, they may also require pharmacologic or physical restraint and involuntary treatment. Patients are not allowed to make poor health-care decisions if their ability to weigh the risks and benefits of the proposed care is limited by cognitive deficits or mental illness. In the setting of toxicity, appropriate care may be provided under the doctrine of implied consent.

The emergency exception to the doctrine of informed consent may also apply in circumstances where self-injury is suspected. The emergency exception permits forcible detention, restraint, medication over objection, and necessary medical care until psychiatric assessment can be accomplished. After the management of the immediate medical emergency and resolution of toxicity, suspected self-injury is sufficient evidence of impaired decisional capacity for the emergency physician to hold a patient for further psychiatric assessment. The emergency physician should document the patient's objections in the patient's medical record and indicate the basis for the determination of diminished capacity.

After the intentionally self-poisoned patient is stabilized, there may be a need for a more thorough assessment of decisional capacity. Psychiatric consultation is appropriate at this stage to help document the degree of impairment, determine the etiology, and predict the likely course.

Immediate Risk After these safety considerations are addressed, the aim of the focused psychiatric assessment moves toward a determination of immediate suicide risk. This examination should answer the following questions: What is the patient's attitude toward lifesaving care? What are the patient's current wishes with regard to living or dying? What are the patient's thoughts about his or her rescue and likely recovery?

These questions can only be answered in the course of a frank discussion between the patient and the emergency physician. The physician should not be concerned about "provoking" further self-injurious impulses by having this vital discussion; many patients will be relieved that the healthcare provider is speaking directly about their distress.

Reliability and Confidentiality Mention should be made here about the difficult issues of reliability and confidentiality with regard to gathering history. Evasiveness, lack of detail, inconsistency, and improbability may lead to an unreliable history. It is appropriate to confront the patient with the implausible aspects of this history and offer an opportunity for the patient to rethink his or her history. This is often successful, although subsequent reports are, of course, equally suspect.

The most important step from the standpoint of both clinical care and risk management is to locate other sources of information to clarify the patient's situation. A careful review of any previous medical and psychiatric records is critical. Any pattern to a patient's presentations such as increasing frequency, more aggravated behavior, or disheveled appearance should be noted.

Collateral contacts are another important source of information, although the level of involvement, sophistication, and reliability of the collaterals must also be taken into account. In the interest of providing necessary medical and psychiatric care for a patient, the ED staff may make contacts that are limited to soliciting information without specific consent. An effort should be made to obtain consent for any broader discussion with family, friends, or other physicians. The patient may express concern about the ED staff contacting a family member or counselor. Any information to be imparted to third parties can be discussed in advance with the patient. The patient may restrict consent to receiving information only and may withhold consent to impart certain information. More caution is indicated in contacting an employer. Although disclosing information about the patient without the patient's consent is a breach of confidentiality, a physician may do so in the interest of protecting the patient.[4]

COMPREHENSIVE PSYCHIATRIC ASSESSMENT

The comprehensive psychiatric assessment includes a characterization of the suicidal ideation present, exploration of risk factors, and the formulation of a diagnostic impression. These three elements help to determine the attendant risk and guide treatment planning.[70]

Stress Vulnerability Model The best understanding of suicide at this time is that it results from intrinsic vulnerability factors interacting with extrinsic circumstances. Intrinsic vulnerability may be conferred by a variety of traits such as impulsivity or conditions such as depression, anxiety, and hopelessness. Extrinsic factors include stressful life events, access to lethal means, and a host of other factors, positive and negative.

Characterization of Suicidal Ideation The core of the suicide risk assessment is a detailed discussion of the patient's suicidal thoughts and urges. This must be included in every mental status examination. It is important to establish rapport and introduce the topic in an appropriate context in order to improve the patient's candor. This evaluation requires significant time and skillful interviewing, for which there is no substitute. This approach will enhance the therapeutic quality of the interview as well as its reliability. For example, almost everyone has had some period in life when he or she was discouraged. The clinician may spend a few moments talking with the patient about the point in life when the patient was most disheartened. This is done by asking the patient if he or she has been feeling "down" lately; and if the patient has, by asking if this is the worst the patient has ever felt. If the patient denies recent depression altogether, or indicates that this is not the worst, it is helpful, for several reasons, to ask the patient to describe the point in his or her life when he or she felt worst. Depression may fluctuate markedly, and characterizing the worst period assures that a prior history of major depression will not be overlooked.

At some point, the physician should ask if, during that worst period in the patient's life, he or she ever felt that perhaps things would never get better (hopelessness), that he or she could not go on (helplessness), or perhaps that he or she would be better off dead (passive suicidal ideation). If failing others was involved in the patient's demoralization (guilt), the physician should ask if the patient had ever felt that others would be better off without him or her. These are common thoughts that most people can endorse without much difficulty and lay the groundwork for discussing more troublesome ideas in the suicidal spectrum. Ultimately, the patient must be asked directly if he or she has ever felt like killing himself or herself (active suicidal ideation). Nothing else will do. The more generic form, "hurting" himself or herself, which might seem to cover more, is in fact confusing to patients—even those who wish to die do not usually consciously intend to be hurt in the process. The latter is more typical of multiple suicide attempters than suicide completers.

For those patients who have felt like killing themselves at some point, the next step in this scenario might be to establish how the patient is currently and to compare this to a prior episode(s). One dimension to assess is the progression from passive to active suicidal ideation. Suicidal feelings may take the form of a relatively inchoate wish to die, perhaps from a fatal disease or injury, and then proceed to consideration of various active means of hastening death. Planning might range from fleeting thoughts or images of a variety of methods from which the patient recoils, to a more detailed consideration of a particular, realistic method of choice, to serious planning concerning acquisition of the means, and so-called last acts. At some point the patient goes beyond thinking to acting by hoarding pills or completing his or her will. An astute family member may observe a series of odd conversations including phone calls to distant friends and family members as the suicidal individual begins to implement the plan with a series of vague farewells. In psychological autopsy studies, approximately 50%–70% of those who completed suicides gave some warning of their intention, and 30%–40% of individuals who completed suicides disclosed a direct and specific intent to kill themselves.[6,57]

Other dimensions of suicidal ideation to assess include frequency, urgency, chronicity, reactivity to positive and negative external events, and subjective distress. Table 17–2 presents a schema for the detailed characterization of suicidal ideation.

The communication of suicidal ideas either directly or indirectly should not be misconstrued as a "cry for help" and hence evidence of lower risk. Communication is probably related to the degree of preoccupation with morbid thoughts and to personality characteristics that dispose individuals to revealing their thoughts to various degrees.[40]

RISK FACTORS FOR SUICIDE

The goal of the suicide risk assessment is to identify factors that may increase or decrease the level of suicide risk in a particular patient and develop a plan that addresses the modifiable factors that contribute to suicide risk and the overall safety of the patient. The clinical determination of suicide risk, at the culmination of the suicide assessment, ultimately is a clinical judgment, since no study has identified one specific risk factor or set of risk factors as specifically predictive of suicide or other suicidal behavior. Despite the lack of such predictive factors for suicide, there is a large body of evidence on the multiple risk factors that contribute to suicide risk, and a growing body of evidence on protective factors. Knowledge of this evidence is critical to informing the clinical determination of suicide risk.

TABLE 17–2. Characterization of Suicidal Ideation

Dimension	Benign	Intermediate	Malignant
Onset	None, acute	Chronic, stable	New or fluctuating
Frequency	Occasional	Daily	Constant
Persistence	Fleeting thoughts	Persistent thoughts	Preoccupation
Urgency	Disinterested	Engaged	Intense
Complexity	Simple	Some detail	Elaborate
Activity	Passive ideas	Plans without action	Action
Emotional response	Death repellent	Ambivalent	Death desirable
Circumstances	Victim identifies one clear precipitant	Several complex contributory stressors	Either noncontributory or overwhelming stressors
Alternatives	Some, realistic	Few, problematic	Seems hopeless
Insight	Recognizes remediable psychological problem	Overvalued ideas present, temporarily reassured	Morbid delusions present, reassurance impossible
Intent	Opposed to suicide	Suicide acceptable but prefers to live	Resolutely suicidal

The risk of suicide increases 50 to 100 times within the first 12 months after an episode of self-harm compared to the general population risk. About half of all people who commit suicide have a history of self-harm, and this ratio increases by 60% in juveniles.[5]

While much is known about the risk of suicide for various groups over time, little can be said with certainty about an individual patient at a particular point in time. There is no one type of "typical" suicidal patient or clinically useful test or rating scale at this time. Albeit, while one investigator was able to prospectively identify almost all of those who ultimately died by suicide (97% sensitivity), the investigator overpredicted suicide by almost half (56% specificity).[54] However, there is also no patient in distress for whom the risk of suicide is so remote that it need not be considered. Assessment of the potentially suicidal patient begins with a screen for psychiatric illness, substance abuse, and history of self-harm.

Psychiatric Illness and Suicide One major consideration in suicide risk assessment is the occurrence of severe mental illness. Suicide risk for individuals with severe mental illness is 20–40 times higher than it is for the general population.[41] Psychological autopsy studies in the United States and Europe over the years have consistently revealed major psychiatric illness to be a factor in suicide, present in 93% of adult suicides.[38,41,55,58] This is also true of those who make medically serious suicide attempts.[8,38] In particular, prospective cohort studies and retrospective case control investigations have revealed clinical depression and bipolar disorder to dramatically increase suicide risk.[33,40,69] For mood disorders, factors correlated with acute suicidality include current depression, severe anxiety, anhedonia, panic, insomnia, ambivalence, and acute alcohol abuse.[40] After mood disorders, chronic alcoholism is the most commonly reported disorder; it is present in approximately 20% of cases. Moreover, alcoholic patients who also suffer from periodic episodes of depression are at more risk for suicide than patients who present with either disorder separately. As a result, any assessment conducted on a patient with a substance abuse history must include an examination of symptoms of major depression or bipolar illness.[25,71]

Schizophrenic patients are at risk for suicide at rates comparable to major depression and are 20 times more likely to attempt suicide than the general population.[68] Approximately 50% of schizophrenic patients will attempt suicide and 13% of schizophrenic patients will complete suicide.[10,68] Additionally, between 5% and 18% of patients with severe borderline personality disorder (especially those patients with comorbid depression) ultimately kill themselves.[27,38,63]

The ability to treat psychiatric disorders such as mood disorders, schizophrenia, and alcoholism suggests that most suicides are preventable. Indeed, a suicide prevention program directed at general practitioners in Sweden was able to demonstrate prevention based on the detection and treatment of depression.[56] The Centers for Disease Control and Prevention (CDC) reported that psychiatric problems in US emergency departments represented approximately 3% of the visits, which is significantly lower than the national psychiatric rate of 20%–28%.[12] This suggests significant psychiatric underdiagnosis is occurring in the ED. Emergency physicians, consequently, must enhance the comprehensive nature of their psychiatric screening in order to identify suicidality and concomitant mental disorders in presenting self-injurious patients.

Demographic Risk Factors Factors have been identified empirically that place groups of individuals at high risk for suicide; although this level of prediction is actuarial and reflective of groups rather than individuals, knowledge of these risk factors is important.

Table 17–3 presents risk factors that are associated with increased suicide risk. Table 17–4 presents protective factors that are associated with mitigating suicide risk. Risk factors are additive, with suicide risk increasing with the number of risk factors that are present, but certain risk factors interact synergistically to increase suicide risk. The combined risk of concomitant depression and alcohol intoxication may be greater than the sum of the risk associated with each in isolation. Certain risk factors, such as a recent suicide attempt associated with a high degree of lethality, or the presence of a suicide note, should be considered serious on its own, regardless of whether other risk factors are present.[20]

Although not specifically predictive, suicide is statistically more common in men than women and in whites than in nonwhites. Younger black men, however, have approximately the same suicide rate as white men of the same age. Suicide rates for both black and white adolescents (15 to 19 years of age) are increasing. In contrast, suicide rates in the those over 65 years of age have decreased 3-fold since 1940, but still occur in disproportionately high numbers.[41,69]

Previous suicide attempts are a significant risk factor. However, those who attempt suicide appear to be a somewhat different group demographically and diagnostically. Parasuicidal behavior is more common in 25- to 44-year-olds than in the elderly, and more common in women than men. Existing data also indicate that those who unsuccessfully attempt suicide are equally prevalent across racial and ethnic groups.[24,49] Many individuals who kill themselves seem to do so on the first attempt. Although that suicide attempt is still the strongest predictor of suicidal outcome, only about 1 in 10 attempters is ultimately successful.[34,54] Multiple attempters also appear to have higher risk than those who make a single attempt.[32,64] Medically serious attempts may be a better marker of risk. Those who make serious attempts tend to share with completers a higher rate of serious mental illness.[7]

A number of avenues of inquiry suggest that violent suicide attempts are associated with a persistent deficiency in brain serotonin levels. Impulsive types of aggression and impulsive suicidal behavior have been linked to serotonergic dysfunction in prefrontal cortical regions of the brain.[21] This deficiency has been measured in postmortem brains and spinal fluid of suicide victims and survivors of violent attempts compared to nonviolent attempts and to other patients. Hopelessness has also received a significant amount of study as a potential predictor of suicide. However, hopelessness appears to have high sensitivity but low specificity.[8] Identifying hopelessness as a problem also suggests possible interventions.

Ultimately, most persons belonging to a high-risk group do not commit suicide, and some individuals with no apparent risk factors do. Many risk factors are not modifiable. This type of information, then, weighs most heavily in the assessment in the absence of other more specific data, early in the hospital course, or in the case of the uncooperative or hostile patient. The best foundation for treatment planning and clinical decision making is direct examination and clinical diagnosis.[30]

TREATMENT

Following the comprehensive psychiatric assessment, the next step is deciding on treatment alternatives. Any patient who has made a suicide attempt must be considered to be at risk, and some further intervention is warranted. The risk of a subsequent lethal attempt is approximately 1% per year over the first 10 years. The risk is highest in the first month to 1 year.

The treatment alternatives available will depend on the psychiatric sophistication of the staff available to the ED at any given time. This section describes the commonly used interventions in the ED; they can be used singly or in combination.

TABLE 17–3. Factors Associated with an Increased Risk for Suicide

Psychiatric Risk Factors	Neurological and Medical Factors	Sociodemographic Factors	Genetic and Familial Factors
Major depressive disorder	Diseases of the nervous system	Male gender (suicide)	Family history of suicide (particularly in first-degree relatives)
Bipolar disorder	Multiple sclerosis	Female gender (suicide attempts)	Family history of mental illness, including substance use disorders
Schizophrenia	Huntington disease	Widowed, divorced, or single marital status, particularly for men	
Alcohol use disorder	Brain and spinal cord injury	Elderly age group	
Other substance use disorders	Seizure disorders	Adolescent and young adult age groups	
Alcohol intoxication	Malignant neoplasms	White race	
Personality disorders	HIV/AIDS	Gay, lesbian, or bisexual orientation	
Concomitant disorders	Pain syndromes	Recent lack of social support (including living alone)	
Helplessness	Functional impairment	Unemployment	
Hopelessness		Drop in socioeconomic status	
Impulsiveness		Domestic partner violence	
Aggression, including violence against others		Recent stressful life event	
Agitation		Childhood sexual abuse	
Factors related to current or past suicidal behavior		Childhood physical abuse	
Suicide attempts		Access to firearms	
Suicidal ideation			
Suicidal plans			
Suicidal intent and lethality			

Medications can be used acutely in the treatment of severe anxiety or psychosis; however, in the case of antidepressants, a period of weeks is required for therapeutic effect, so their immediate use is not indicated in the ED. In fact, there are concerns about prescribing medications with relatively high potential for lethality in overdose, such as the cyclic antidepressants and nonselective monoamine oxidase inhibitors, to persons who have recently attempted suicide. However, newer antidepressants, particularly the selective serotonin reuptake inhibitors (SSRIs), can be used as first-line drugs for treatment of most depressions and are relatively safe in overdose. Nonetheless, the initiation of antidepressant therapy by the nonpsychiatric physician is not recommended unless a tight linkage can be made between discharge and immediate (within days) aftercare by either a community outreach team or a crisis clinic.

TABLE 17–4. Factors Associated with Protective Effects for Suicide

Children in the home
Effective clinical care for mental, physical, and substance abuse disorders
Pregnancy
Family and community support (connectedness)
Religious beliefs and cultural practices
Positive social support
Skills in problem solving and conflict resolution

Patients with depressive disorders may suffer from significant anxiety, as may patients with overwhelming situational stressors such as job loss, new financial hardship, bereavement, or divorce. The prescription of a short course of a benzodiazepine may provide significant relief to the patient in crisis.

After the patient's immediate symptoms have been treated in the ED, the next treatment decision is determining the setting in which further treatment may safely be provided. Not all patients with suicidal ideation or even significant attempts necessarily require hospitalization, and there is still a substantial stigma attached to psychiatric hospitalization. In general, hospitalization should be used if less restrictive measures cannot insure the patient's safety. If significant doubt exists about the safety of outpatient treatment, the patient should be held in the ED for further evaluation, admitted to a general hospital with close nursing supervision, or admitted to a psychiatric unit. "Holding beds" now available in some larger psychiatric EDs are ideal for this purpose. Some localities may also have crisis outreach services that follow the patient after discharge from the ED and improve appropriate monitoring and continuity of care.

Patients most likely to respond to interventions in the ED are individuals who, until recently have been stable but who, as a result of some external event, find their way of life threatened. This acute change results in a painful state of anxiety and the mobilization of some combination of adaptive and maladaptive coping strategies. Finally, a second event, the precipitant, intensifies the anxiety to the point that the patient cannot tolerate the instability and is thrown into crisis.

The patient then feels desperate and may be completely immobilized or vulnerable to various strong impulses including the impulse to run away, strike out at someone else, or kill himself or herself. Reality testing is preserved, and no major psychiatric syndrome is present. The patient accurately perceives his or her situation, understands that the current reaction is a psychological problem, and is highly motivated to obtain help. The crisis may last for a matter of hours or weeks prior to the ED presentation and will ultimately resolve. Such patients respond well to crisis intervention and may actually undergo some positive development in the course of treatment.

By contrast, patients whose condition has been deteriorating for some time in the absence of significant stressors, and who appear on examination to be suffering from severe depressive symptoms, are unlikely to benefit rapidly from supportive techniques. If such patients present with suicidal ideation or attempts, it will be difficult, though not impossible, to manage them outside the hospital.

Outpatient settings have the advantage of maintaining the patient's functioning as much as possible. Work and childcare responsibilities, financial obligations, and social relationships are not disrupted. Unnecessary regression is halted. The patient is able to assume more responsibility for his or her outcome, and independence helps preserve self-esteem. These individuals remain closer to and more engaged with the people and situations with whom and with which they must learn to cope. Their morale may be rapidly improved by the combination of support, planning, and modest early treatment successes.

In some cases, though, these same factors may be disadvantageous. Routine tasks may seem overwhelming. High levels of conflict may render major relationships at least temporarily unworkable. Inpatient settings offer the advantage of respite, high levels of structure, more intensive professional and peer support, constant supervision, and, usually, more rapid pharmacologic and psychosocial intervention.

The choice of inpatient or outpatient setting will depend on the balance of strengths and weaknesses of the patient, the involvement and competence of family or friends, the availability of a therapist in the community, and the ongoing stresses in the patient's life, and this decision is best made by a psychiatrist. Because a psychiatrist is not always present in many facilities, a trained mental health professional should be on call to every ED. This may be a psychiatric social worker, nurse clinician, or psychologist. When such services are not available, it is appropriate to detain patients in the ED until a practitioner with specific competence is available or to transfer the patient to another facility for evaluation. Every state has laws that provide for the involuntary commitment of the mentally ill under circumstances that vary from state to state. Any acute, deliberately self-injurious behavior would generally qualify. Chronic, repetitive dangerous behavior that is not deliberate, such as frequent unintentional opioid, alcohol, sedative-hypnotic, or illicit "recreational" psychoactive drug overdoses, warrants careful evaluation. In the absence of psychiatric illness, involuntary treatment is usually not necessary. The practitioner should be familiar with the criteria for commitment and the classes of healthcare providers so empowered under state law.

There are other treatment interventions that can be provided in the emergency setting, including crisis intervention, substance abuse counseling, and family therapy. A single session in the ED may be sufficient to defuse a crisis or to spur the drug-abusing patient to seek help. Alternatively, the intervention may be initiated in the ED and continued as an outpatient.

Crisis intervention is a brief, highly focused therapy that seeks to deconstruct how a crisis occurred, with the intent of examining the patient's role. Often, patients have distorted perceptions of the crisis, and a gentle "correction" of catastrophic thinking can be extremely helpful.

The crisis is presented to the patient as an unfortunate and perhaps tragic experience that the patient can overcome. Ideally, the patient should have a relief of symptoms and learn how crises may be avoided in the future. This insight intervention will likely fail for patients with severe depression because of the presence of profound hopelessness. It is most successful for patients who give a history of high functioning just prior to the crisis.

Substance abuse treatment is ultimately an intermediate (weeks to months) to long-term (months to years) intervention. However, there are powerful initial steps that the emergency physician can take. Central among these is confronting the patient about the medical consequences of substance use. This can take the form of discussion only, or the physician can invite the patient to examine clinical laboratory results or view remarkable clinician/diagnostic findings (hepatomegaly, repeated fractures from falls, increased liver enzymes, or evidence of "silent" past myocardial infarction). There is little to be lost from a respectful but blunt confrontation of the patient's deterioration, and he or she may listen to a physician rather than family or friends. Peer counseling is particularly useful in addictive disorders; if possible, patients should be referred to community 12-step programs such as Narcotics Anonymous and Alcoholics Anonymous. Family therapy can occur as a series of sessions over the long term or can be useful in the emergency setting to defuse a crisis, reinstate social supports for the patient, or educate families about mental illness. It is most important to respect a patient's request as to the level of family involvement, because in the emergency setting a patient may be either too angry or ashamed to confront his or her family. It is prudent to defer to the patient's wishes, and to assure the family that the patient is safe and that you will keep them as informed as confidentiality and discretion allow at a later date.

VIOLENCE

Aggression also presents unique challenges to the emergency physician. Moreover, aggression is intimately related to suicidal behavior. Chronic aggression and impulsivity are risk factors for suicidal behavior. Like suicidal patients, aggressive patients are difficult to treat and they tend to elicit strong negative reactions in ED personnel.[60] In one study of violence in the ED, directors of emergency medicine residency programs were surveyed as to the frequency of verbal threats, physical attacks, and the presence of weaponry in the area. Of the 127 institutions surveyed, 74.7% of the residency directors responded; 41 (32%) reported receiving at least one verbal threat each day; moreover, 23 (18%) reported that weapons were displayed as a threat at least once each month. Fifty-five program directors (43%) noted that a physical attack on medical staff occurred at least once a month.[43] Another study involved a retrospective review of university police log records and ED staff incident reports to examine the problem of violence in the ED setting. Almost 75% of the incidents occurred during the evening or night. Of the 686 episodes of violence in this study, more than 25% required physical restraint or removal from the premises. In addition, it was found that the police responded to the ED nearly twice daily.[53] These studies underscore the need for timely identification of the violent patient, as well as appropriate management for this diagnostically heterogeneous group.[22] The assessment and management of the violent patient should include provisions for patient and staff safety as well as a thorough search for the cause of violent behavior.[60] This section addresses the differential diagnosis of violent behavior, the pharmacotherapy of aggressive and/or agitated behavior, and the use of seclusion and restraint. It also provides an overview of potential risk factors for violent behavior.

STRESS-VULNERABILITY MODEL OF AGGRESSION

As in the case of suicide, there are many and varied causes of violent behavior, some more social and some more medical in nature. The stress-vulnerability model suggests that violence should be considered as the outcome of a dynamic interaction among numerous factors both intrinsic and extrinsic to the individual, some of which promote and some of which ameliorate the potential for violent behavior at any given moment. This is the stress-vulnerability model. Education may provide alternatives to violence, but xenobiotic-induced delirium may cause an otherwise nonviolent person to misinterpret healthcare efforts, in which case education is of no benefit at that time. Hence, the individual becomes violent under circumstances that would not normally be sufficient to provoke a violent outburst. Some patients, on the other hand, come from cultures in which aggressive behavior is more acceptable, and these patients require little stress or provocation before responding in what can be perceived as aggression by western cultural standards.

In the ED, likely medical sources of vulnerability include metabolic derangements, exposure to xenobiotics—both licit and illicit, withdrawal syndromes, seizure disorders, head trauma, psychotic states, and personality disorders. Additionally, patients with severe pain, delirium, or extreme anxiety can respond to the efforts of emergency personnel with resistance, hostility, or frank aggression.

PREDICTION

Research on risk factors for community violence may not apply to the prediction of inpatient violence. Some researchers have postulated that violence committed outside the hospital may not be predictive of inpatient violence and that hospital violence may result from the interaction of patients with specific factors found in the hospital environment.[35,60] Other studies are contradictory.[62] Consequently, prior violence is not a perfect predictor of future violence. Other factors, such as mental illness and substance abuse, need to be examined in order to make meaningful predictions of inpatient violence for each individual case.[60] One study found that the most common types of hospital violence were incidents of aggression against objects in the hospital (56.7%), violence directed against the hospital staff (27.8%), and violence directed against other patients (14.4%).[61] In this study, men were not found to be committing significantly greater incidents of violence than women. Other studies concur that men are not necessarily more of a risk for inpatient violence than women inpatients. For example, researchers examining inpatient violence found that close to half of the violent incidents were committed by women patients,[42,55] and the number of violence-related injuries committed by men and women inpatients were almost proportional to the ratio of men and women inpatients on the unit. The conclusion was that gender should not be considered a risk factor for inpatient violence. Long hospitalization was not considered a factor predictive of violence for the majority of inpatients. As with outpatient violence, the correlation of violence with younger age appears to hold true in the inpatient setting.[48,55,56]

SUBSTANCE USE

The association between substance use and violence is well established. Alcohol is found in the offender, the victim, or both in one-half to two-thirds of homicides and serious assaults.[16,55] Substance abuse is seldom the sole cause, but it may contribute to violence in a number of ways. The direct pharmacologic effects include disinhibition and misinterpretation, suspiciousness, or paranoia. Psychological effects of substance use include cultural expectations of appropriate behavior under the influence and the ability to excuse or disavow inappropriate behavior that occurs while intoxicated. Substance use then interacts with other physiologic, cognitive, psychological, situational, and cultural factors including any underlying mental illness. A tripartite model has been described: (1) systemic violence related to drug distribution, (2) economic compulsive violence associated with the criminal activity necessary to sustain a drug habit, and (3) psychopharmacologic violence resulting from the direct effects of the particular xenobiotic.[29,31]

MENTAL ILLNESS

The relationship between mental illness and violence is also complex. Efforts made to destigmatize mental illness have confused the issue, but it seems clear that mental illness is associated with an increased risk for violence.[55] In one large epidemiologic study, the prevalence of violence for those with no disorder was 2%. Schizophrenia was associated with an 8% rate of violent behavior, and other mental disorders all had similar prevalences of approximately 12%. But of all respondents reporting violent behaviors, 42% had a substance use disorder. Substance use more than tripled the rate of violence for individuals with schizophrenia. Mental illness appears to reduce the threshold for aggression, and the more comorbid conditions present, the greater the risk.[51,65,66]

Researchers consistently find a greater prevalence of personality disorders among violent inpatients than among nonviolent inpatients.[50,52] However, antisocial personality is the condition most strongly associated with both substance use and aggression. In one study, when the history of juvenile deviance was controlled for alcohol, the drug most commonly associated with violence, accounted for only 2% of the violent behavior.

In conclusion, some aggressive behavior is attributable to the direct pharmacologic effects of xenobiotics, but probably represents only a modest fraction. Substance use is also a part of the setting of violent behavior in the community, a coincidental part of the lifestyle of violent individuals, and both substance use and violence are related to common underlying characteristics such as a character disorder.

MEDICATION NONCOMPLIANCE

Many research studies currently list medication noncompliance as a risk factor for violence that is as serious as substance use or mental illness. One such study associated medication noncompliance and substance use with increased violence risk in the mentally ill.[67] It suggested that medication noncompliance may lead to self-medicating through the use of illicit xenobiotics, and substance use may lead to further medication noncompliance. These two factors together may then have the effect of increasing violence for the mentally ill. This study also suggested that low insight into their illness can be associated with greater violence. However, they found that poor insight was correlated with substance use and medication noncompliance, so it is unclear if poor insight is truly predictive. These findings have been replicated.[66]

Patients entering the ED who did not adhere to their medications as outpatients may be more of a risk for inpatient violence. Furthermore, inpatients who refuse to adhere to medication prescribed in the hospital also are more of a risk for violence, especially when comorbid with substance abuse disorders.

ADDITIONAL FACTORS IN AGGRESSIVE BEHAVIOR

Many of the factors correlated with aggression are easy to observe and monitor in the hospital. However, some additional factors that influence violent behavior may not be as easy to detect. For example, one study examining violent behavior found that most violent incidents in the hospital occur on Mondays and Fridays, with very few incidents on weekends. These violence research investigators suggested that the analysis was comparable in the general population as Mondays and Fridays have special significance in that the work-week and weekends are usually less stressful. This finding illustrates the point that seemingly minor social stressors can be as conducive to violent behavior as any other factor.

Furthermore, researchers have postulated a seasonal variation of violence.[18] There is an increase in the frequency of assaults by inpatients during the winter months, and it has been hypothesized that increased population density, cold temperature, and less sunlight during the day could account for the increased violence. This finding is in contrast to the literature on outpatient violence, which has reported greater incidence of violence during the warmer months.[5] However, this same review conceded that any extreme temperature could evoke aggressive feelings and frustration. Yet another study examined the relationship between temperature and violence and found that more aggressive acts occur during the summer months, both in the hospital and in the community.[26] They cited several explanations, one of which was that the high rate of staff turnover, as vacations are taken, disrupts the social networks that the patients have established, evoking aggressive feelings.

Although it is unclear whether the cold can provoke aggression as much as it has been established that heat can, it does seem clear that overcrowding and social stressors can lead to violent behavior. If the effects of temperature and social stressors (eg, holidays) correlate so drastically with violence in the community, it is likely that such effects would have even more impact when comorbid with severe mental illness, substance use, or any of the other risk factors of aggression.

ASSESSMENT

The comprehensive evaluation of the violent patient should include a complete physical examination. The examination may reveal the underlying cause of the violent behavior as well as insuring the treatment of any secondary patient injuries. Laboratory analysis may include blood chemistries (thyroid-stimulating hormone, glucose, electrolytes including calcium and liver enzymes), a complete blood count, lumbar puncture, and neuroimaging as guided by the examination and clinical history.

Illicit xenobiotic and alcohol use often present with symptoms of violence. Acute cocaine toxicity can produce extreme psychomotor agitation, delirium, and transient psychosis characterized by paranoia and hallucinations; a clinically indistinguishable syndrome can occur following the use of amphetamines. Phencyclidine toxicity is manifested by assaultiveness, muscle rigidity, dysarthria, nystagmus, autonomic instability, and ataxia. Alcohol intoxication is characterized by typical signs of cerebellar dysfunction such as slurred speech, gait ataxia, and incoordination; however, patients who are intoxicated are also at risk for violent behavior. Cannabis does not typically produce violent or aggressive behavior but paranoia can occur with intoxication and can secondarily promote reactions of extreme fear associated with distorted perception, as can occur with lysergic acid diethylamide (LSD) and psilocybin, particularly in the naive user (see Chaps. 77–85)

Withdrawal syndromes from specific xenobiotics can also promote aggressive behavior as a consequence of physical discomfort or anticipatory anxiety. Opioid withdrawal is characterized by myalgias, rhinorrhea, and piloerection with a clear sensorium, whereas alcohol, benzodiazepines, and barbiturates share a common syndrome of autonomic hyperreactivity, seizures, and subsequent delirium. Patients suffering from any of these signs and symptoms may become aggressive, verbally abusive, or threatening. Prompt recognition of these syndromes and immediate treatment can prevent some aggressive outbursts. Because drug use is often concealed, is difficult to ascertain on clinical grounds, and frequently contributes to violent behavior, urine and blood toxicologic studies may be useful to enhance the understanding and long-range treatment of some patients[55] (see Chaps. 14, 28, and 78).

Delirium can be a cause of aggression. Patients are often suddenly confused, frightened, or frankly psychotic as a result of impaired perception. Patients may require sedation or physical restraint in order to prevent injury to themselves as well as staff.

Although persons suffering from psychotic disorders are not generally aggressive, there are aspects of the psychosis state that place patients at risk for aggressive behavior. Paranoid ideation can serve to promote misperceptions of impending bodily harm ("They're trying to kill me"), sexual victimization ("Men and women are raping me"), and humiliation ("Everyone is laughing at me"). It follows that these fearful perceptions might provoke violent reactions in a patient. Hallucinations can cause aggression, either as a result of command hallucinations or in reaction to the anxiety and irritation that patients experience with loud or persistent auditory hallucinations ("hearing voices"). Patients with either borderline or antisocial personality disorder are at risk for violent acting out as a result of poor impulse control.

Violence risk is also associated with cognitive dysfunction. Both acute mental illness and chronic substance use can result in neurologic impairment. Psychiatric patients with compromised cognitive abilities such as impaired attention, memory, or executive functioning such as reasoning and planning are found to be at increased risk for violence.[55] Patients presenting with cognitive impairment may also be at increased risk for committing acts of violence in the ED.

TREATMENT

The acute pharmacotherapy of violent behavior is directed simply at reducing the level of arousal. A recent review of this issue proposed a model for the efficient use of medication for the control of episodic, as opposed to chronic, agitation and aggression.[2] In this model, agitation and violent outbursts are viewed as transient disturbances of the usual treatment relationship between the physician and patient. Pharmacotherapy and seclusion or restraint are to be used only as needed to restore that relationship, for the benefit of the patient as well as other members in the environment. The restoration of the treatment relationship is necessary in order to take measures to understand and address the cause of the agitation, with the input and consent of the patient, thus preventing future incidents. For this reason, sleep is considered an undesirable use of medication. Sleep delays, rather than promotes, assessment, may further frighten or anger the patient, and does not even guarantee elimination of the agitated state on awakening.

As aggression derives from varied and multiple etiologies, it follows that there is much debate about the specific sedative that should be used, the route of administration, and the dosing interval. Studies examining the treatment of aggression and/or agitation have included such diverse populations as schizophrenics, acutely intoxicated patients (alcohol), trauma patients, postoperative patients, patients in alcohol withdrawal, and patients with presumed personality disorders. Treatment settings for these studies included psychiatric inpatient units and intensive care units, and the ED found that both benzodiazepines and antipsychotics resulted in rapid control of agitation and aggression.[11,23,40,42]

It seems, however, that there are specific clinical situations when benzodiazepines and antipsychotics might be preferentially used. Haloperidol has been safely used in the treatment of agitation and aggression in patients with psychoses, acute alcohol intoxication, and delirium.[1,11,40,42] The drug can be administered orally, intravenously, or intramuscularly. Dosing intervals range from 30 minutes to 2 hours, with a usual regimen of haloperidol 5 mg given every 30–60 minutes; most patients respond after 1–3 doses. The dose of haloperidol needed to achieve sedation rarely exceeds a total of 50 mg in acute management.[44,45]

Benzodiazepines are also quite effective for sedation; their use has been examined in patients with psychoses, stimulant intoxication, sedative-hypnotic and alcohol withdrawal, and postoperative agitation.[28,47]

Diazepam may be given as 5 to 10 mg IV, with rapid repeat dosing titrated to desired effect. Because diazepam is poorly absorbed from intramuscular sites, its route of administration is either intravenous or oral. Lorazepam 1 to 2 mg may be given orally or parenterally and repeated at 15- or 30-minute intervals, respectively, until the patient is calm (see Antidotes in Depth A24: Benzodiazepines). Benzodiazepines may have a unique role in the treatment of agitation secondary to cocaine intoxication (Chap. 76). Antipsychotics, particularly low-potency antipsychotics, are known to lower the seizure threshold in animals, so their use for patients with cocaine or amphetamine toxicity, or alcohol or sedative hypnotic withdrawal should be avoided. Although some studies suggest that the combined use of lorazepam with antipsychotics in patients with known psychiatric illness and delirium afforded relief of psychotic symptoms while allowing for a reduced dose of antipsychotic medications,[1,17,59] the authors generally discourage the combined use of these drugs in cases of unclear etiology and favor the predictable pharmacodynamics of intravenous diazepam or midazolam. Concerns regarding respiratory depression mandate careful observation of patients receiving sedation with any xenobiotic.

PHYSICAL RESTRAINT

Isolation and restraint are also used in the treatment of violent behavior. Isolation or seclusion can help to diminish environmental stimuli and thereby reduce hyperreactivity. However, a few aspects are worth mentioning: Because seclusion is defined by a condition of very limited interactive and environmental cues, it is not indicated for patients with unstable medical conditions, delirium, dementia, self-injurious behavior (cutting, head banging), or who are suffering extrapyramidal reactions as a consequence of antipsychotic medication.[3] Restraint is used to prevent patient and staff injury. All facilities should have clear, written policy guidelines for restraint that address monitoring, provisions for patient comfort, and documentation.

TRAINING

Finally, training in the management of aggression helps to reduce violence and injuries through the early identification of impending episodes of violence, use of verbal techniques to defuse incidents, and appropriate physical techniques to minimize injuries in those that occur. It is necessary for healthcare providers to maintain their skills through training and to advocate for continuing medical education on this topic at the workplace.[10]

SUMMARY

Both violent and suicidal behavior in the ED may be the cause or the effect of many toxicologic presentations. Patients presenting with suicidal or aggressive behavior pose unique problems for the clinician who must make appropriate assessment and management decisions. It is incumbent on all emergency physicians to screen patients for psychiatric emergency presentations as part of a comprehensive screening for self-harm.

Identifying risk factors for suicide and aggression can aid the clinician in employing preventive or early intervention strategies in the ED. Important risk factors for both suicidal and violent behavior include past history of the behavior, comorbid mental illness, drug and alcohol intoxication, and young age. Mental status examination for suicidality should focus on extrinsic factors such as current ideation, intent, lethality of plan, current life stressors, as well as intrinsic vulnerability factors such as comorbid mental illness, feelings of hopelessness, and impulsivity. In terms of violence risk assessment, drug and alcohol intoxication, mental illness, and psychiatric medication noncompliance (alone or in combination) are robust predictors of aggressive behavior in the ED and other inpatient settings. Early detection and rapid intervention for patients at risk for suicide or violence is, to date, the best means for preventing injury or death.

ACKNOWLEDGMENT

Michael H. Allen, Wendy Rives (deceased), Brett R. Goldberg, and Cherie Elfenbein contributed to this chapter in previous editions.

REFERENCES

1. Adams F: Neuropsychiatric evaluation and treatment of delirium in the critically ill cancer patient. *Cancer Bull.* 1984;36:156-160.
2. Allen MH: Managing the agitated psychotic patient: a reappraisal of the evidence. *J Clin Psychiatry.* 2000;61(Suppl 14):11-20.
3. American Psychiatric Association: Clinician Safety. Task Force Report No. 33. Washington, DC: American Psychiatric Association; 1992;266.
4. American Psychiatric Association: The Principles of Medical Ethics with Annotations Especially Applicable to Psychiatry. Washington, DC: American Psychiatric Association' 1989.
5. Anderson CA: Temperature and aggression: ubiquitous effects of heat on occurrence of human violence. *Psychol Bull.* 1989;106:74-96.
6. Barraclough B, Bunch J, Nelson B, Sainsbury P: A hundred cases of suicide: clinical aspects. *Br J Psychiatry.* 1974;125:355-373.
7. Beautrais AL, Joyce PR, Mulder RT, et al: Prevalence and comorbidity of mental disorders in persons making serious suicide attempts: a case control study. *Am J Psychiatry.* 1996;153:1009-1014.
8. Beck A, Steer R, Kovacs M, Garrison B: Hopelessness and eventual suicide: a 10-year prospective study of patients hospitalized with suicidal ideation. *Am J Psychiatry.* 1985;142:559-563.
9. Bentur Y, Raikhlin-Eisenkraft B, Lavee M: Toxicological features of deliberate self-poisonings. *Hum Exp Toxicol.* 2005;23:331-337.
10. Carmel H, Hunter M: Compliance with training in managing assaultive behavior and injuries from inpatient violence. *Hosp Commun Psychiatry.* 1990;41:558-560.
11. Carter G, Reith DM, Whyte I, Mcpherson M: Repeated self-poisoning: increasing severity of self-harm as a predictor of subsequent suicide. *Br J Psychiatry.* 2005;186:253-257.
12. Centers for Disease Control and Prevention, National Center for Injury Prevention and Control (producer): Web-based Injury Statistics Query and Reporting System (WISQARS) [online]. 2005. Available online at: http://www.cdc.gov/ncipc/wisqars/default.htm. Last accessed May 4, 2009.
13. Centers for Disease Control and Prevention: Homicides and suicides – national violent death reporting system, United States, 2004-2004. *Morb Mortal Wkly Rep.* 2006;55:721-724.
14. Centers for Disease Control and Prevention: Toxicology testing and results for suicide victims – 13 States, 2004. *MMWR Morb Mortal Wkly Rep.* 2006;55:1245-1248.
15. Centers for Disease Control and Prevention: Youth risk behavior surveillance – United States, 2007. *MMWR Morb Mortal Wkly Rep.* 2008;57:SS-4.
16. Clinton JE, Sterner S, Steimachers Z, Ruiz E: Haloperidol for sedation of disruptive emergency patients. *Ann Emerg Med.* 1987;16:319-322.
17. Cohen S, Khan A, Johnson S: Pharmacological management of manic psychosis in an unlocked setting. *J Clin Psychopharmacol.* 1987;7:261-264.
18. Coldwell JB, Naismith LJ: Violent incidents in special hospitals. *Br J Psychiatry.* 1989;154:270.
19. Crome P: The toxicity of drugs used for suicide. *Acta Psychiatr Scand.* 1993;371(Suppl):33-37.
20. CrosbyAE, Cheltenham MP, Sacks, JJ: Incidence of suicidal ideation and behavior in the United States. *Suicide Life Threat Behav.* 1999;29:131-140.
21. Davidson RJ, Putnam, KM, Larson CL: Dysfunction in the neural circuitry of emotion regulation: a possible prelude to violence. *Science.* 2000;289:591-594.
22. DeLeo D, Bertolote J, Lester D: Self-directed violence. In: Krug EG, Dahlberg LL, Mercy JA, et al, eds. *World Report on Violence and Health.* Geneva: World Health Organization; 2002:183-212.

23. Dubin W: Rapid tranquilization: antipsychotics or benzodiazepines? *J Clin Psychiatry*. 1988;49(Suppl 12):5-12.
24. Fawcett J, Clark DC, Busch KA: Assessing and treating the patient at risk for suicide. *Psychiatr Ann*. 1993;23:244-255.
25. Fawcett J, Scheftner WA, Fogg L, et al: Time-related predictors of suicide in major affective disorder. *Am J Psychiatry*. 1990;144:923-926.
26. Flannery RB, Penk WE: Cyclical variations in psychiatric patient-to-staff assaults: preliminary inquiry. *Psychol Rep*. 1993;72:642.
27. Frances A, Blumenthal S: Personality as a predictor of youthful suicide. In: *Risk Factors for Youth Suicide*. Report of the Secretary's Task Force on Youth Suicide, Vol. 2. U.S. Department of Human Services Alcohol, Drug Abuse, and Mental Health Administration. DHHS pub. no. (ADM) 89-1624. Washington, DC: US Government Printing Office; 1989: 160-171.
28. Garza-Trevino E, Hollister LE, Overall JE, Alexander WF: Efficacy of combinations of intramuscular antipsychotics and sedative-hypnotics for control of psychotic agitation. *Am J Psychiatry*. 1989;146:1598-1601.
29. Goldfrank LR, Hoffman RS: The cardiovascular effects of cocaine. *Ann Emerg Med*. 1991;20:165-175.
30. Goldsmith SK, Pellmar TC, Kleinman AM, Bunney WE, eds. *Reducing Suicide: A National Imperative*. Washington, DC: National Academy Press; 2007.
31. Goldstein PJ: The drugs-violence nexus: a tripartite conceptual framework. *J Drug Issues*. 1986;15:493-506.
32. Goldstein R., Black D, Nasrallah A, Winokur G: The prediction of suicide: sensitivity, specificity, and predictive value of a multivariate model applied to suicide among 1906 patients with affective disorders. *Arch Gen Psychiatry*. 1991;48:418-422.
33. Hagnell O, Lanke J, Rorsman B: Suicide rates in the Lundby study: mental illness as a risk factor for suicide. *Neuropsychobiology*. 1981;7:248-253.
34. Harris EC, Barraclough B: Suicide as an outcome for mental disorders: a meta-analysis. *Br J Psychiatry*. 1997;170:205-227.
35. Hassan SD, Sobel RN: Violence in the community as a predictor of violence in the hospital. *Psychiatr Serv*. 2001;52:240-241.
36. Henry JA: A fatal toxicity index for antidepressant poisoning. *Acta Psychiatr Scand*. 1989;354:37-45.
37. Hoffman RS, Wipfler MG, Maddaloni MA, Weisman RS: The effect of the triplicate benzodiazepine prescription regulation on sedative-hypnotic overdoses. *N Y State J Med*. 1991;91:436-439.
38. Inskip HM, Harris EC, Barraclough B: Lifetime risk of suicide for affective disorder, alcoholism and schizophrenia. *Br J Psychiatry*. 1998; 172:35-37.
39. Kapur S, Mieczkowski T, Mann JJ: Antidepressant medications and the relative risk of suicide attempt and suicide. *JAMA*. 1992;268:3441-3445.
40. Kessler RC, Borges G, Walters EE: Prevalence of and risk factors for lifetime suicide attempts in the National Comorbidity Survey. *Arch Gen Psychiatry*. 1999;56:617-633.
41. Kochanek KD, Murphy SL, Anderson RN, Scott C: Deaths: final data for 2002. *Natl Vital Stat Rep*. 2004;53:55.
42. Lam JN, McNiel DE, Binder RL: The relationship between patients' gender and violence leading to injuries. *Psychiatr Serv*. 2000;51:1167-1170.
43. Lavoie F, Carter G, Danzi D, Berg R: Emergency department violence in United States teaching hospitals. *Ann Emerg Med*. 1988;17:1227-1233.
44. Lenehan G, Gastfriend DR, Stetler C: Use of haloperidol in the management of agitated or violent, alcohol-intoxicated patients in the emergency department: a pilot study. *J Emerg Nurs*. 1985;11:72-79.
45. Lerner Y, Lwow E, Levitin A, Belmaker R: Acute high-dose parenteral haloperidol treatment of psychosis. *Am J Psychiatry*. 1979;136:1061-1064.
46. McCaig LF, Nawar EN: National Hospital Ambulatory Medical Care Survey: 2004 Emergency Department Summary. Advance Data from Vital and Health Statistics Hyattsville, MD, National Center for Health Statistics, 2006 Report No. 3702.
47. Modell JG, Lenox RH, Weiner S: Inpatient clinical trial of lorazepam for the management of manic agitation. *J Clin Psychopharmacol*. 1985;5:109-113.
48. Monk M: Epidemiology of suicide. *Epidemiol Rev*. 1987;9:51-69.
49. Moscicki EK, O'Carroll P, Rae DS, et al: Suicide attempts in the epidemiologic catchment area study. *Yale J Biol Med*. 1988;61:259-268.
50. National Center for Injury Prevention and Control: Suicide in the United States. Available at: http://www.cdc.gov/ViolencePrevention/suicide/index.html. Last accessed May 4, 2009.
51. Nolan KA, Volavka J, Mohr P, et al: Psychopathy and violent behavior among patients with schizophrenia or schizoaffective disorder. *Psychiatr Serv*. 1999;50:787-792.
52. Owen C, Tarantello C, Jones M, et al: Violence and aggression in psychiatric units. *Psychiatr Serv*. 1998;49:1452-1457.
53. Pane G, Winiarski A, Salness K: Aggression directed toward emergency department staff at a university teaching hospital. *Ann Emerg Med*. 1991;20:283-286.
54. Pokorny AD: Prediction of suicide in psychiatric patients. *Arch Gen Psychiatry*. 1983;40:249-257.
55. Rich CL, Young D, Fowler RC: San Diego suicide study, I: Young vs. old subjects. *Arch Gen Psychiatry*. 1986;43:577-582.
56. Rihmer Z, Rutz W, Pihlgren H: Depression and suicide on Gotland: an intensive study of all suicides before and after a depression-training programme for general practitioners. *J Affect Disord*. 1995;35:147-152.
57. Robins E, Gassner S, Kayes J, et al: The communication of suicidal intent: a study of 134 consecutive cases of successful (completed) suicide. *Am J Psychiatry*. 1959;115:724-733.
58. Robins E, Murphy GE, Wilkinson RH, et al: Some clinical considerations in the prevention of suicide based on a study of 134 successful suicides. *Am J Public Health*. 1959;49:888-889.
59. Salzman C, Green A, Rodriguez-Villa F, et al: Benzodiazepines combined with neuroleptics for management of severe disruptive behavior. *Psychosomatics*. 1986;27(Suppl):17-21.
60. Serper M, Bergman AJ: *Psychotic Violence: Methods, Motives, Madness*. New York: International University Press Inc; 2003.
61. Soliman AE-D, Reza H: Risk factors and correlates of violence among acutely ill adult psychiatric inpatients. *Psychiatr Serv*. 2001;52:75-80.
62. Spiessl H, Krischker S, Cording C: Aggression in the psychiatric hospital. A psychiatric basic documentation based 6-year study of 17,943 inpatient admissions. *Psychiatr Prax*. 1998;25:227-230.
63. Stone MH: The course of borderline personality disorder. In: Tasman A, Hales RE, Frances AJ, eds: *Review of Psychiatry*, Vol. 8. Washington, DC: American Psychiatric Press; 1987: 103-122.
64. Suominen K, Isometsä E, Suokas J, Haukka J, Achte K, Lönnqvist J: Completed suicide after a suicide attempt: a 37-year follow-up study. *Am J Psychiatry*. 2004;161:562-563.
65. Swanson J, Holzer C, Ganju V, Jono R: Violence and psychiatric disorder in the community: evidence from the Epidemiologic Catchment Area Survey. *Hosp Commun Psychiatry*. 1990;41:761-770.
66. Swanson JW, Swartz MS, Borum R, et al: Involuntary out-patient commitment and reduction of violent behavior in persons with severe mental illness. *Br J Psychiatry*. 2000;176:324-331.
67 Swartz MS, Swanson JW, Hiday VA, et al: Violence and severe mental illness: the effects of substance abuse and nonadherence to medication. *Am J Psychiatry*. 1998;155:226-231.
68. Tandon R, Jibson MD: Suicidal behavior in schizophrenia: diagnosis, neurobiology, and treatment implications. *Curr Opin Psychiatry*. 2003;16:193-197.
69. US Department of Commerce: Statistical Abstracts of the United States, 116th ed. Washington, DC: US Government Printing Office; 1996.
70. US Public Health Service: The surgeon general's call to action to prevent suicide. Washington, DC: US Department of Health and Human Services; 1999. Available at http://www.surgeongeneral.gov/library/calltoaction/. Last accessed May 12, 2009.
71. Vijayakumar L, Rajkumar S: Are risk factors for suicide universal? A case-control study in India. *Acta Psychiatr Scand*. 1999;99:407-411.

CHAPTER 18
NEUROLOGIC PRINCIPLES

Rama B. Rao

INTRODUCTION

The central nervous system (CNS) coordinates responses to the fluctuating metabolic requirements of the body and modulates behavior, memory, and higher levels of thinking. These functions require a diversity of cells: astrocytes, neurons, ependymal cells, and vascular endothelial cells. Disruption or death of any one cell type can cause critical changes in the function or viability of another. This cellular interdependence, along with the high metabolic demands of the CNS, make neurons especially vulnerable to injury from both endogenous neurotoxins and xenobiotics. Endogenous neurotoxins like the metals iron, copper, and manganese, are substances that may be critical to CNS function, but are harmful when their penetration into the CNS is poorly controlled.

The understanding of the normal chemical and molecular functions of the CNS is limited at best. Interestingly, cellular mechanisms have sometimes been revealed by investigating xenobiotic-induced neuronal injuries.[38,66] For example, the pathophysiology of Parkinson disease, which affects movement and motor tone, was elucidated by the inadvertent exposure of individuals to 1-methyl-4-phenyl-1,2,3,6-tetrahydropyridine (MPTP). The mechanisms of axonal transport were elucidated by investigations of the effects of acrylamide exposures in human and animal models.[57] The neurodegenerative changes of amyotrophic lateral sclerosis have a promising xenobiotic model in β-methylamino-L-alanine (BMAA), a neurotoxin found in the cyanobacteria associated with cycad plants ingested by the Chamorro people of Guam.[67]

There are few minimally invasive methods available to investigate xenobiotic-induced CNS injury. Biomarkers are usually nonspecific and not readily available. Xenobiotic concentrations of blood and urine rarely reflect tissue concentrations of the CNS.[58] Cerebrospinal fluid may be useful in excluding CNS injury from infection, hemorrhage and inflammatory processes, but is, with few exceptions, poorly reflective of the mechanisms of neuronal injuries.[88] Similarly, electroencephalograms and electromyelograms are useful in only a few types of xenobiotic exposures, and neuroimaging, while progressively evolving,[54] is a poor substitute for neuroanatomical evaluations which are usually only available on autopsy. Much of the current study to elucidate the mechanisms of CNS injury uses animal models, cultured astrocytes, and other tissue, or postmortem investigations. Less commonly, occupational evaluations, such as the enzyme activity of cholinesterases in pesticide workers, are employed.

This chapter reviews some basic anatomic and physiological principles of the nervous system and the common mechanisms by which xenobiotics exploit the functional and protective components of the CNS with a few relevant examples. The multiple factors determining the clinical expression of neurotoxicity are reviewed.

CELLS OF THE NERVOUS SYSTEM: AN OVERVIEW

NEURONS

Neurons are the major route of cellular communication in the CNS. Having one of the highest metabolic rates in the body, these cells are especially sensitive to changes in the microenvironment and are dependent on astrocytes, choroidal epithelium, and capillary endothelium to confer protection and deliver glucose and other sources of energy.

While each neuron is capable of receiving information through different neurotransmitters and receptor subtypes at the dendrite, neurons typically produce and release a single type of neurotransmitter at the axonal terminal. This specificity allows for cellular classification of neurons based on the neurotransmitter released, for example, serotonergic, cholinergic, and dopaminergic neurons (see Chap. 13). Other substances such as adenosine may be produced and released that are less specific to the neuron type.

The anatomic structure of neurons facilitates their function. Dendrites located on the cell body are lined with receptors that bind neurotransmitters and affect cellular changes via several mechanisms (see Chap. 13). The soma, or cell body is responsible for coordination and production of multiple proteins required to carry out normal physiological functions. This synthesis occurs at a rate several times greater than the liver or kidney. These proteins, organelles, and substrates must then be transported across long distances to the terminal axon. This energy-dependent function is supported by a cytoskeleton comprised of neurofilaments, microfilaments, microtubules, and complex transport proteins. Fast anterograde transport of membrane-bound organelles occurs through *kinesin,* a transport protein, at a rate of 200–400 mm/d. Channel proteins, synaptic vesicles, mitochondria, Na^+, K^+-ATPase, glycolipids, and other substances are transported by kinesin. Slow anterograde transport also occurs at a substantially slower rate (0.5–4 mm/d). The retrograde transport protein, *dyenin,* is produced in the soma and delivered to the nerve terminal for the movement of larger vesicles and reusable proteins back to the cell body.

In the CNS, groups of neurons are organized into complex functional pathways, with a single class of neuron regulating different functions and clinical effects depending on the brain region affected. As an example, dopaminergic neurons regulate cravings, movement, and resting muscle tone, each of which is determined not only by dopaminergic neurons and receptor subtype, but the part of the cortex or basal ganglia specifically affected (see Chap. 13).

Neurons must be able to respond to changes in the local environment and alter the expression of different receptors in response to signaling from neurotrophic factors, variations in metabolic requirements, and xenobiotic interactions. This "neuroplasticity" accounts for the diversity of clinical responses to substances that induce tolerance to xenobiotics like ethanol (see Chap. 14).

GLIAL CELLS

Glial cells are comprised of *astrocytes, oligodendrocytes, Schwann cells,* and *microglia.* These cells serve to support the neurons both structurally and functionally.

Astrocytes comprise between 25% and 50% of the brain volume.[1-3,11] In addition to the anatomic contribution to the blood–brain barrier (BBB), astrocytes play a critical role in maintaining neuronal function.[3,4,91] They contribute to three major areas: homeostasis of the extraneuronal environment, provision of energy substrates, and limitation of oxidative stress. In addition astrocytes contribute to the "plasticity" of cells and receptor expression in the CNS (see later).

In order for cells of all types to function in the CNS, membrane potentials must be adequately maintained. Astrocytes contribute to this by closely regulating the extracellular pH, free water, and, like brain capillaries, the extracellular potassium concentration. Metallothioneins, which control the entry of heavy metals necessary for CNS function, are produced by astrocytes.[28,91] Astrocytes also release energy substrates such as lactate, citrate, alanine, glutathione, and α-ketoglutarate for utilization by neurons.[11]

Astrocytes metabolize glutamate, the main excitatory amino acid (EAA) neurotransmitter in the CNS, as well as ammonia. These cells also produce superoxide dismutase and gluthathione peroxidase to reduce free radical propagation. Glutathione, the major antioxidant for the brain, is predominantly located in the astrocytes. It can be released into the extracellular space or cleaved for neuronal uptake and intracellular reformulation.[11]

Through the release of complex trophic factors, astrocytes control the expression of endothelial transporters of the BBB and the production of tight junctions in both the blood–cerebrospinal fluid barrier (B-CSFB) and BBB. Angiogenesis is similarly astrocyte regulated, as is detection of neuronal injury, immune mediation, and neurotransmitter production. The growth of neurites, the branches of neuronal cell bodies that eventually become dendrites or axons, are similarly modulated by astrocytes.

Oligodendrocytes are a type of glial cell that provide anatomical support, protective insulation, and facilitate rapid neuronal depolarization by the production of myelin. Myelin is the primary constituent of white matter in the CNS. The production of myelin in the peripheral nervous system (PNS) is performed by the Schwann cells. While oligodendrocytes support several axons, each Schwann cell is anatomically dedicated to a single axon.

Finally, microglial cells modulate immune response, inflammation, and tissue repair from a variety of CNS injuries. Like neurons, microglia are dependent on signaling from astrocytes.

MECHANISMS OF NEUROPROTECTION

The nervous system has multiple protective mechanisms. Xenobiotics are prevented from accessing the CNS by the blood–brain and blood–CSF barriers. For xenobiotics that enter the CNS, there are multiple cellular specializations to limit oxidant stress. These protective mechanisms are reviewed.

BLOOD–BRAIN BARRIER

The BBB confers an anatomic and enzymatic barrier to xenobiotic entry into the CNS. Brain capillaries are surrounded by the foot processes of adjacent astrocytes. The potential spaces between endothelial cells are limited by tight junctions, or zonulae occludentes, which are between 50 and 100 times tighter than those found on peripheral capillaries.[2-4,52,61] This anatomic barrier prevents movement of substances between cells, also known as the paracellular aqueous pathway, due to osmotic and oncotic forces.[2-4,52,61]

Transendothelial movement of critical substrates and, potentially, xenobiotics occurs through three major mechanisms: diffusion, transport proteins, and endocytosis.[2,3] These routes allow carefully controlled entry of critical substrates and cofactors while limiting the potential for injury from either endogenous or exogenous neurotoxins.

Lipophilic substances may move directly across the luminal and abluminal endothelial membranes abutting the CNS. Other substances may enter the endothelium through bidirectional transport proteins on the luminal surface. These proteins may be specific, such as the GLUT-1 protein for uptake of glucose, or less specific large neutral amino acid transporters (LNAA) that move amino acids and xenobiotics, such as baclofen, intracellularly. These transporters also line the abluminal surface of the endothelial cell for movement of substrates and xenobiotics into the CNS. The third line of entry for larger proteins is via endocytosis. This can be adsorptive, or mediated through specific receptors such as insulin or transferrin.[2-4,52,61,91]

Endothelial cells have other protective properties, including intracellular enzymes, to metabolize xenobiotics and efflux proteins to transport certain xenobiotics back into the capillary lumen. These efflux proteins include energy-dependent P-glycoproteins which are ATP-binding cassette transporters and are sometimes referred to as multidrug-resistant (MDR) proteins. Several hydrophobic xenobiotics are prevented from accumulating in the CNS through these transporters including vinca alkaloids, digoxin, cyclosporine A, and protease inhibitors. Nonsedating antihistamines may have limited sedative properties due, in part, to efflux through P-glyproteins.[25] Another type of saturable transporter, known as organic acid transport (OAT) protein, facilitates the efflux of hydrophilic xenobiotics such as valproic acid or baclofen. The expression of each of these transporters may be upregulated under certain conditions such as intermittent disruptions in the BBB from seizures. This expression upregulation is theorized to account for the resistance of anticonvulsant medications in patients with epilepsy. Comprehensive lists of xenobiotics that are substrates for these transporters are available elsewhere.[2,52,53]

BLOOD–CSF BARRIER

The ventricles of the brain are lined by the epithelial cells of the choroid. These cells also have tight junctions, but not as extensive as those of the BBB. They are, however, rich in glutathione peroxidase and other xenobiotic-metabolizing enzymes in concentrations approximating those of the liver. Similar to brain capillary cells, the choroid contains efflux transporters for organic anions and cations, as well as MDR efflux proteins (P-glycoproteins) to limit entry of xenobiotics into the CSF.[2,3,52,91]

NEUROTOXIC PRINICPLES

EXCITOTOXICITY

Neuronal function is strictly dependent on aerobic metabolism with the adequate supply of substrates and functioning mitochondria for the production of ATP. When energy expenditure exceeds production, cellular dysfunction and ultimately cell death, or apoptosis, results. The specific cascade of molecular events relating to this process is termed *excitoxicity*.[10,71]

The initial event is traced to an oxidant stress and excessive stimulation of NMDA receptors by glutamate, an EAA neurotransmitter. An influx of intracellular calcium changes membrane potentials across the cellular and mitochondrial membranes. The mitochondria become progressively more inefficient at ATP production and handling the resulting reactive oxygen species. As membrane damage is propagated, calcium further depolarizes the mitochondria, activating a permeability transition pore across the mitochondrial membrane. Gradients are further disrupted, precipitating more injury, energy failure, and ultimately cell death.

Excitotoxicity is considered a common mechanism of cell death due to xenobiotic, ischemic, traumatic, infectious, neoplastic, or neurodegenerative injury. It is the subject of study for many therapeutic interventions in CNS injury.

DETERMINANTS OF NEUROTOXICITY

The clinical expression of neurotoxicity is related to many factors. These include the chemical properties of the xenobiotic, the dose and route of administration, xenobiotic interactions, and underlying patient characteristics including age, gender, and comorbid conditions.

CHEMICAL PROPERTIES OF XENOBIOTICS

One of the most important determinants of neurotoxicity is the ability of a xenobiotic to penetrate the BBB. Water-soluble molecules larger than M_r 200 to 400 (molecular weight ratio, or mass of a molecule relative to the mass of an atom) are unable to bypass the tight junctions.[2] Xenobiotics with a high octanol/water partition coefficient are more likely to passively penetrate the capillary endothelium, and potentially the BBB, while those with a low partition coefficient may require energy-dependent facilitated transport.[61] Xenobiotics that are substrates for capillary endothelial efflux mechanisms will have limited penetration regardless of the coefficient.[2,3,52,61]

ROUTE OF ADMINISTRATION

The route of xenobiotic administration may also be consequential. While most xenobiotics gain access to the nervous system through the circulatory system, aerosolized solvent and heavy metals in industrial and occupational exposures gain CNS access through inhalation, traveling via olfactory and circulatory routes. Alternatively, some agents may move from the PNS via retrograde axonal transport to the CNS. Naturally occurring proteins such as tetanospasmin, and rabies, polio, and herpes use this mechanism to access the PNS and CNS.[13,16,47] The toxalbumins ricin and abrin as well as bismuth salts may also use this mechanism to a limited extent.[83,89] This understanding may prove beneficial from a therapeutic perspective. For example, in one small series of patients experiencing severe pain, doxorubicin was injected into the involved peripheral nerves. Therapeutically, a chemical ganglionectomy occurred through retrograde "suicide" transport of doxorubicin, providing substantial relief in these patients in this experimental therapy.[50]

Some xenobiotics may be delivered directly into the CSF (intrathecally), the consequences of which are variable (see Special Considerations SC-2: Intrathecal Xenobiotic Administration).

XENOBIOTIC INTERACTIONS

Coadministration of xenobiotics may precipitate neurotoxicity by several mechanisms.[45] Extra-axially (outside of the CNS), xenobiotic interactions that increase the blood concentration of one or both agents may overwhelm the protective mechanisms of the BBB.[20] Similar effects may occur in the PNS where elevated blood concentrations may have enhanced clinical effects resulting in peripheral neuropathies.[91]

Xenobiotic interactions can be synergistic, acting on the same neuroreceptor with additive effects. Benzodiazepines and ethanol, for example, both stimulate the $GABA_A$ receptor.[14] The excessive neuroinhibition can result in deep coma and even respiratory depression when these agents are administered together.

In some circumstances, xenobiotic interactions result in excessive neurotransmitter availability.[9] This is demonstrated in patients with the serotonin syndrome, the result, for example, of coadministration of a monoamine oxidase inhibitor and a serotonin reuptake inhibitor or other serotonergics (see Chap. 72).

Access to the CNS may be altered by one of the xenobiotics, allowing the other to bypass the BBB. For example, mannitol causes transient opening of the BBB; as a result, therapeutic use of mannitol is under investigation for the delivery of antineoplastic agents which might otherwise be unable to access the nervous system.[53] Similarly, some xenobiotics, such as verapamil, cyclosporine, and probenicid, are blockers of capillary endothelium efflux.[2,91] These theoretically limit efflux of other substrates of P-glycoprotein or OAT. The clinical utility of employing such efflux blockers is under investigation as was done in a study in which primates received intrathecal methotrexate. The CSF clearance of methotrexate was reduced in animals administered intrathecal probenecid.[12,74]

PATIENT CHARACTERISTICS

Patient-specific variables may affect the ability of a xenobiotic to penetrate the BBB and/or the clinical effects of a given exposure. For example, age of the patient at the time of exposure is critical, especially in the fetus and neonates.[76] The structural and enzymatic development of the BBB is incomplete, and synaptogenesis, or formation of intercellular relationships, is especially sensitive to impaired protein synthesis or other excitotoxic events. This is demonstrated classically by maternal exposure to methylmercury. The mother may be minimally affected, but the developing fetus suffers profound neurological and developmental consequences (see Chaps. 30 and 96).

In neonates, immature liver function may lead to the accumulation of circulating bilirubin. Due to incomplete formation of the BBB, the bilirubin may access the CNS and produce a form of encephalopathy known as *kernicterus*.

Elderly patients may also have increased susceptibility to neurotoxins as a result of relatively impaired circulation or age-related changes in mitochondrial function that predispose to excitotoxicity.[79] Xenobiotic-induced parkinsonism, or the unmasking of subclinical idiopathic Parkinson disease, may occur more readily than in younger patients. Animal models also suggest age-related sensitivity with one study noting increased manganese toxicity with advanced age.[36]

The role of gender in expression of xenobiotic-induced neurological injury is potentially contributory. In animal models, the presence of estrogen-related and progesterone-related compounds may be neuroprotective for some xenobiotic injuries.[62,69] In humans women are more susceptible to some movement disorders such as xenobiotic-induced parkinsonism and tardive dyskinesia, whereas dystonias and bruxism are more prevalent in young male patients.[72] The etiologies of these gender-related differences are incompletely understood.

NEUROLOGIC COMORBIDITIES

Conditions affecting the integrity of the BBB can affect CNS penetration of xenobiotics and endogenous neurotoxins. For example, glutamate concentrations are normally higher in the circulatory system than the CNS.[56] Patients with trauma, ischemia, or lupus vasculitis[1] may experience neuropsychiatric disorders as a result of increased penetration of glutamate or sensitivity to additional xenobiotics. Similarly, meningitis and encephalitis cause openings in the BBB and this may be exploited therapeutically. Intravenous penicillin achieves a higher CSF concentration in animals with meningeal inflammation than in those without meningitis.[75]

In some patients previously undiagnosed diseases become evident on exposure to xenobiotics. This is especially true in patients with peripheral neuropathies. For example, patients being treated with therapeutic doses of vincristine suffered a severe polyneuropathy due to unmasking of a previously undiagnosed Charcot-Marie-Tooth disease.[9,22] Similarly, patients with diabetes mellitus, which is the most common cause of peripheral neuropathy, or HIV disease may have exacerbation of symptoms in the presence antiretroviral agents.[24,70] Patients with myasthenia gravis may have exacerbation of weakness with aminoglycoside administration which can affect transmission at the neuromuscular junction (NMJ).[90]

Chronic exposures to some neuroinhibitory xenobiotics such as ethanol may alter neuronal receptor expression and upregulate or increase the amount of receptors for EAAs. In addition to receptor augmentation, neurotransmitter concentrations of the excitatory neurotransmitters glutamate and aspartate are increased, as is homocysteine. These changes induce a tolerance to neuroinhibitory xenobiotics acting on the same receptor, and patients require escalating doses to achieve the same clinical effect. In such patients cessation of ethanol intake results in a relative deficiency of exogenous inhibitory tone. The patient experiences neuroexcitability and the clinical syndrome of withdrawal[17,18] (see Chap. 14).

Adequate nutritional status is important for the maintenance of normal neurological function. The BBB may not be adequately maintained in patients with malnutrition. Deficiencies of heavy metal cofactors such as manganese, copper, zinc, and iron can affect neurological function. In some cases the deficiencies enhance absorption of other xenobiotics. For example, iron deficiency enhances lead and manganese absorption in the gastrointestinal tract which can ultimately overwhelm neuroprotective mechanisms. Vitamins serve as enzymatic cofactors in modulating the production of glutamate, homocysteine, and other amino acids. Specific vitamin deficiencies can precipitate neurological syndromes such as Wernicke encephalopathy in thiamine-depleted patients (see Antidotes in Depth A25: Thiamine Hydrochloride, and Chap. 41). The toxicity of xenobiotics may also be enhanced. For example, a relative pyridoxine deficiency in patients with acute isoniazid overdose may result in seizures as a result of a relative excess of EAAs (see Antidote in Depth: Pyridoxine, and Chap. 57). Glucose is a critical energy substrate that can cause profound neurological impairment when delivery is inadequate (see Antidotes in Depth A10: Dextrose, and Chap. 48).

Interestingly, certain conditions such as temperature may affect the toxicity of xenobiotics. For example, cooling may limit the impedance of ACh neurotransmission caused by botulinum toxin.[41]

EXTRA-AXIAL ORGAN DYSFUNCTION

Renal failure may impair metabolism of xenobiotics or endogenous neurotoxins such as urea rendering it more available to the CNS. Hyperglycemia in patients with diabetes mellitus may also increase formation of CNS reactive oxygen species. Similarly, patients with liver failure may have elevations in CNS manganese. These patients may suffer Parkinson syndrome[51,77] (see Parkinson Syndrome later).

Hepatic encephalopathy illustrates the concept of excitotoxicity from endogenous neurotoxins. Hyperammonemia increases oxidative stress and free radical formation in astrocytes. Ammonia potentially decreases critical metabolic enzymes such as catalases, superoxide dismutase, and glutathione peroxidase. Nitric oxide production is increased due to elevations in NO synthetase. Under these conditions, astrocytes upregulate the expression of the peripheral benzodiazepine receptor (PBR) on the outer mitochondrial membrane. The PBR modulates the production of neurosteroids and, in turn, the $GABA_A$ receptor. Continued CNS exposure to ammonia and other endogenous solutes propagates this oxidative and nitrosative stress to the mitochondrial membrane, potentially opening a channel named the mitochondrial permeability transition pore. Osmotic swelling of the mitochondrial membrane followed by excitotoxicity results in cerebral edema and hepatic encephalopathy.[63,64]

SPECIFIC MECHANISMS OF NEUROTOXICTY

ALTERATION OF ENDOGENOUS NEUROTRANSMISSION

Xenobiotics can induce neurotoxicity by triggering changes in neurotransmission in either the CNS or PNS. In some cases xenobiotics enhance neurotransmission through a specific receptor subtype. This enhanced transmission can occur through inhibition of presynaptic metabolism (monoamine oxidase inhibitors), stimulation of neurotransmitter release (amphetamines), impairment of neurotransmitter reuptake (cocaine), or inhibition of synaptic degradation (acetylcholinesterase inhibitors).

Alternatively, synaptic neurotransmission may be impaired.[78] Xenobiotics may inhibit the presynaptic release of neurotransmitters (botulinum toxin), block receptors (antimuscarinics), or alter membrane potentials at the postsynaptic membrane (tetrodotoxin).[32,33] Patients may present with a clinical syndrome of toxicity associated with altered neurotransmission of the specific receptor (see Chap. 3).

DIRECT RECEPTOR INTERACTION

Some xenobiotics are able to directly stimulate receptors. Both kainate and α-amino-3-hydroxy-5methyl-4-isoxazole propionate (AMPA) are subclasses of the glutamate receptor, which are targeted by some naturally occurring xenobiotics.[42] An example is β-*N*-oxalylamino-L-alanine (BOAA) found in the grass pea, *Lathyrus sativus*. BOAA stimulates the AMPA and inhibits specific mitochondrial enzymes resulting in the spastic paraparesis of lathyrism.[67] Domoic acid stimulates the kainate receptor and causes the neuroexcitation associated with neurotoxic shellfish poisoning.

Direct inhibition is also possible, as exemplified by phencyclidine, an NMDA (*N*-methyl-D-aspartate) receptor antagonist.

ENZYME AND TRANSPORTER EXPLOITATION

The classic example of xenobiotics that exploit endogenous enzymes and/or transporters is MPTP.[38] Once MPTP crosses the BBB, it is converted by monoamine oxidase to the neurotoxic compound MPP^+ (1-methyl-4-phenylpyridine) in astrocytes. MPP^+ is taken up by dopamine transporters into the neurons of the substantia nigra pars compacta. MPP^+ inhibits complex I of the mitochondrial electron transport chain resulting in dopaminergic excitotoxicity and the clinical syndrome similar to Parkinson disease (see Disorders of Movement and Tone, and Chap. 38).

ALTERED CONDUCTION ALONG MEMBRANES: DEMYELINATING NEUROTOXINS

Aside from xenobiotics that affect neurotransmission at the postsynaptic membrane, some affect the production or maintenance of myelin by oligodendrocytes and Schwann cells.[23,34,37,48] In the CNS these are often associated with white matter abnormalities and a leukoencephalopathy.[34] Agents such as hexachlorophene, arsenic, inhibitors of tumor necrosis factor α, neural tissue–derived rabies vaccine, and the act of "chasing the dragon" or inhaling volatilized heroin are associated with a demyelinating neurotoxicity.[23] In the PNS, nitrous oxide, suramin, and tacrolimus are associated with peripheral demyelination.[46]

INHIBITION OF INTRACELLULAR FUNCTIONS

Some xenobiotics are nonspecific inhibitors of cellular function.[29] The neurotoxicity of substances such as carbon monoxide (CO) or cyanide can result in diffuse dysfunction or, depending on the dose and specific vulnerabilities of an exposed patient, be more focal. For example, patients surviving CO exposure may experience delayed neurological sequelae that is a diffuse impairment of neuropsychiatric function, or more focally, present with a xenobiotic-induced Parkinson syndrome (see later and Chap. 125).

Antineoplastics can affect the production of critical proteins required for cellular maintenance. These can be very specific such as the ability of vincristine to impair cytoskeletal transport in the peripheral nervous system (see Chap. 37).

CLINICALLY RELEVANT XENOBIOTIC-MEDIATED CONDITIONS

ALTERATIONS IN CONSCIOUSNESS

The toxicological differential of xenobiotics that induce alterations in mental status or consciousness is expansive. These xenobiotics can be broadly divided into those agents that produce some form of neuroexcitation, and those that produce neuroinhibition. While some agents such as phencyclidine have elements of both depending on dose, this categorization facilitates a general clinical understanding of neurotoxic alterations in mental status.

Xenobiotics resulting in neuroexcitation are agents that enhance neurotransmission of EAA, or diminish inhibitory input from GABAergic neurons. The clinical presentation of the patient can vary; some patients may be alert and confused, or suffering from an agitated delirium, hallucinations, or a seizure.

Neuroinhibitory xenobiotics typically enhance GABA-mediated neurotransmission. These patients may be somnolent or in deep coma. Benzodiazepines hyperpolarize cells by increasing inward movement of Cl^- ions through the chloride channel of the $GABA_A$ receptor. This hyperpolarization limits subsequent neurotransmission (see Chap. 13). Less commonly, neuroinhibition is a result of diminution of EAA. Patients presenting the day after binging on cocaine may be sleepy but arousable and oriented in what is termed cocaine "washout," theoretically related to depletion of EAA and dopamine. Xenobiotics that cause diffuse cortical dysfunction through impairment in the delivery or utilization of oxygen or glucose can also present with depressed or altered consciousness.

Clinical evaluation of patients with altered consciousness includes obtaining complete history including medications, comorbid conditions, occupation, and suicidal intent when relevant or available. Patients should have a complete physical examination, with particular attention paid to vital sign abnormalities or findings that may indicate a toxic syndrome. Assessment and correction of hypoxia or hypoglycemia should be performed. An electrocardiogram may be useful in some circumstances (see Chaps. 22 and 23).

TABLE 18–1. Xenobiotics that Commonly Induce Seizures

Concentration-Related	Idiosyncratic	Withdrawal Related	Tonic-Clonic Seizure-like
Antihistamines			
Baclofen	Bupropion	Baclofen	Strychnine
Camphor*	Carbamazepine	Barbiturates	Tetanus toxin
Carbon monoxide	Ergotamines	Benzodiazepines	
Chloroquine*	GHB	Ethanol	
Cicutoxin*	Mefenamic acid	GHB	
CNS stimulants	Phenylbutazone		
Cyanide	Tramadol		
Diphenhydramine			
Domoic acid			
Isoniazid*			
Hypoglycemics			
Gyromitrin*			
Lidocaine			
Meperidine			
Organic chlorines			
Organic phosphorous compounds			
Propoxyphene			
Strychnine			
Tetramethylenedisulfotetramine (TETS)*			
Thallium			
Theophylline*			
Zinc phosphide			

* High concentrations may result in status epilepticus.

XENOBIOTIC-INDUCED SEIZURES

Seizures are the most extreme form of neuroexcitation. As with alterations of consciousness, this may be due to enhanced EAA neurotransmission (domoic acid, sympathomimetics) or inhibition of GABAergic tone (isoniazid). Unlike patients with traumatic or idiopathic seizure disorders who have an identifiable seizure focus, the initiation and propagation of xenobiotic-induced seizures is diffuse. It is for this reason that most non-sedative-hypnotic anticonvulsants such as phenytoin are unlikely to be effective in terminating seizures.

Seizures may be idiopathic as described with tramadol and bupropion, or they may be concentration-dependent events as described with theophylline and isoniazid toxicity. Alternatively, seizures may be a result of withdrawal from GABAergic substances.

Status epilepticus is variably defined, but involves two or more seizures without a lucid interval, or continuous seizure activity for greater than 15 minutes. True xenobiotic-induced status epilepticus is rare. Cicutoxin, the toxin in water hemlock, *Cicuta maculata*, is a potent inhibitor of $GABA_A$ neurotransmission and may cause status epilepticus.

Theophylline toxicity precipitates seizures and status epilepticus through a different mechanism. Normally, endogenous termination of seizures is mediated through presynaptic release of adenosine during the release of the primary neurotransmitter at the terminal axon. Adenosine functions as a feedback inhibitor of the presynaptic neuron, disrupting propagation of excitatory neurotransmission. Theophylline is an adenosine antagonist. However, adenosine administration is not a useful therapy for theophylline-induced seizures as adenosine is unable to cross the BBB. Generally high-dose sedative-hypnotics, affecting $GABA_A$ receptors are required for seizure control.

Some clinical conditions appear to be centrally mediated tonic–clonic movements, but are due to glycine inhibition in the spinal cord. Glycine is the major inhibitory neurotransmitter of motor neurons of the spinal cord. Under normal conditions glycine contributes to termination of reflex arcs. Glycine inhibition results in myoclonus, hyperreflexia, and opisthotonos often without alteration in consciousness. Presynaptic glycine release inhibition is caused by tetanospasmin, the major neurotoxin from *Clostridium tetani*. Postsynaptic glycine inhibition is caused by strychnine, the toxin in *Strychnos nux-vomica*. Patients with exposures to these agents are often treated in quiet environments where the stimuli to initiate hyperreflexia are minimized (see Chap. 112 and Table 18–1.)

XENOBIOTIC-INDUCED MOOD DISORDERS

Certain xenobiotics are inconsistently associated with alterations in mood.[5,19] What predisposes individuals to xenobiotic-induced mood alterations is unclear. In some circumstances patients with previously undiagnosed bipolar disorder are given a xenobiotic that unmasks their disease. Interestingly antibiotic-induced mania is found in some patients without a previous psychiatric history. The symptoms of mania are usually evident within the first week of therapy and, unlike the mania of purely psychiatric origin, readily abate within 48–72 hours of the last antibiotic dose. Some patients with clarithomycin-induced mania have documented recurrence on rechallenge of the antibiotic.[5] In general xenobiotic-induced manias are idiopathic and very rare.

TABLE 18–2. Xenobiotics Commonly Inducing Mood and Neuropsychiatric Disorders

Mania	Depression	Psychosis
Acyclovir	β-adrenergic antagonists	Amantadine
Amantadine	Amiodarone	Corticosteroids
Caffeine	Interferon	CNS stimulants
Chloroquine	Isoretinoic acid	
Clarithromycin	Ribavirin	
CNS stimulants		
Corticosteroids		
Dextromethorphan		
Dehydroepiandrosterone		
Efavirenz		
Flenfluramine		
Floroquinolones		
Gabapentin		
Ginseng		
Interferon-α		
Isophosphamide		
Isoniazid		
L-dopa		
Mefloquine		
Phentermine		
Phenylpropanolamine		
Pseudoephedrine		
Quetiapine		
St. John's wort		
Testosterone		
Tramadol		

More common are either psychosis from chronic CNS stimulant use or depression from ethanol or the agents listed in Table 18–2.

DISORDERS OF MOVEMENT AND TONE

CNS-Mediated Disorders Most movement disorders, including akathisia, bradykinesia, tics, chorea, and dystonias are mediated by the complex dopaminergic pathways of the basal ganglia. Different dopamine receptor subtypes, modulated by GABAergic, glutaminergic, and cholinergic neurons are involved (see Chap. 13). Chorea occurs in some cases of carbamazepine overdose, therapeutic oral contraceptive use,[31] and after cocaine use when the stimulant effects have subsided.[72]

Dopamine receptor antagonists can precipitate acute dystonic reactions. The D_2 receptor antagonists, in conjunction with alterations in muscarinic cholinergic tone, are usually implicated. Animal models suggest possible mediation through σ receptors, the craniofacial distribution of which corresponds to the common clinical manifestations of acute dystonias.[49]

Diffusely increased motor tone may be seen with glycine antagonists such as tetanospasmin and strychnine, and in adrenergic states such as acute intoxication with CNS stimulants, or withdrawal from sedative-hypnotics.

Other centrally mediated disorders of tone include serotonin syndrome and neuroleptic malignant syndrome (NMS). Both of these potentially life-threatening syndromes consist of altered consciousness, hyperthermia, rigidity, and autonomic insufficiency. NMS may occur in patients on dopamine receptor antagonists such as antipsychotic medications, or in patients with idiopathic Parkinson disease who abruptly stop their dopaminergic therapy. Dopamine receptor agonists such as bromocriptine or restoration of antiparkinson medications are used therapeutically in these circumstances (see Chaps. 15 and 69).

Parkinsonism Xenobiotic-induced parkinsonism is a syndrome of unstable posture, rigidity, gait disturbance, loss of facial expression, hypokinesis, and variable presence of tremor.[7] The common neuroanatomic target involves the dopaminergic neurons of the basal ganglia, specifically the substantia nigra.[26,84] In some circumstances the toxicity is transient and the mechanism inadequately understood.

Some xenobiotics such as carbon monoxide and heroin produce tissue hypoxia and ischemia in the basal ganglia which occasionally results in xenobiotic-induced Parkinson syndrome.

Other xenobiotics such as MPTP, carbon disulfide, manganese, and the endogenous neurotoxin copper in patients with Wilson disease produce predictable mitochondrial impairment of the basal ganglia neurons. Viscose rayon workers exposed to carbon disulfide may present with a Parkinson syndrome refractory to L-dopa administration[43,44] (see Enzyme and Transporter Exploitation later).

Manganese is a critical substrate for production and metabolism of several neurotransmitters including glutamate. Excessive manganese interferes with normal uptake of glutamate and is critical to the function of superoxide dismutase and glutamine synthetase.[30,35] In patients with liver failure who accumulate manganese from occupational exposure, reversal or treatment of liver disease may result in resolution of parkinsonism.[36,77]

A recent review of patients who intravenously injected the illicit agent metcathinone described a Parkinson syndrome thought to be secondary to contamination with manganese from a precursor, potassium permanganate, which is used in metcathinone production. Unlike patients with idiopathic parkinsonism, these patients did not suffer from a resting tremor, and they had a specific gait abnormality in which they walked on the balls of their feet.[82] Like those with occupational manganese exposures and normal liver function, these patients did not respond to L-dopa (see Table 18–3).

Tremors Tremors may be observed in adrenergic states, with specific xenobiotics such as lithium, or as a result of sedative-hypnotic withdrawal. These are well reviewed elsewhere.[60]

The Neuromuscular Junction Flaccid paralysis usually occurs as a result of impaired transmission at the NMJ[14,15,78] or from xenobiotics causing demyelination. Mechanisms of NMJ transmission impairment include

TABLE 18–3. Xenobiotics Commonly Inducing Parkinsonism

Reversible*	Irreversible
Amlodipine	Carbon disulfide
Antineoplastics	Carbon monoxide
Cyclosporine	Copper
Calcium channel blockers	Cyanide
Dopaminergic agents (withdrawal)	Heroin
Kava Kava	Manganese
Progesterone	MPTP
Sertraline	
Valproate	
Trazadone	

* May improve with removal of xenobiotic, sometimes requiring persistent administration of dopaminergic therapy.

impeded propagation of the action potential on the terminal neuron, impaired release of acetylcholine, depression of motor end-plate potential with failure of depolarization, and impedance of myofibril excitation[78] (see also Chap. 68).

Rarely toxins can enhance transmission at the NMJ. Latrotoxin, the toxic compound in the black widow spider (*Latrodectus* spp), causes enhanced release of acetylcholine at the NMJ with severe, painful muscle contractions (see Chap. 119).

NEUROPATHIES AND MYOPATHIES

CRANIAL NERVES

Xenobiotics are a relatively rare cause of cranial nerve impairment. Some neuropathies are a result of direct delivery of the xenobiotic to the affected cranial nerve. For example, some patients may have optic nerve impairment from intraorbital installation of silicone

TABLE 18–4. Cranial Neuropathies

Cranial Nerve	Sign	Symptom	Toxin
I[a]		Failure to detect odor	Hydrogen sulfide: olfactory fatigue
II	Pupil unresponsive to light	Blindness	Amiodarone, ammonia, cisplatin, clioquinol, deferoxamine, diethylene glycol (DEG), dimethyl mercury, α_2-interferon, holocyclotoxin, methanol, methotrexate, methyl iodide, oxaliplatin, quinine, solvents
III	In paralysis : Ptosis, pupil unresponsive to light In excess: stimulation	Photophobia Dim vision Muscarinic cholinergics	Amiodarone, antimuscarinics, botulinum toxin, DEG, holocyclotoxin, hypoglycemics, α_2-interferon, methyl iodide, thallium, Venoms: Elapidae, scorpion
IV	Paralysis of the superior oblique muscle of eye with weakness of downward gaze, slight upward gaze of affected eye	Vertical and torsional diplopia which worsens on adduction, and may improve with tilt of head	Barbiturates, botulinum toxin, DEG, holocyclotoxin, thallium, venoms
V	Diminished facial sensation, weakness in chewing and swallowing Excessive contraction: trismus	Parasthesias face, weakness in chewing Difficulty opening mouth/jaw Tetanus and strychnine[b]	Botulinum toxin, ethylene glycol, holocylotoxin, oxaliplatin, vincristine. Tetanus toxin and strychnine[b]
VI	Failure to abduct eye on lateral gaze	Diplopia	DEG, holocyclotoxin, intrathecal water soluble contrast agents, lithium, local anesthetics, MDMA, nitroglycerin, ornithine-ketoacid transaminase, oxaliplatin, thallium, thiamine deficiency, Elapid venom, vitamin A
VII[a]	Weakness of facial muscles, impaired expression	Facial droop, impaired taste	DEG, ethylene glycol, holocyclotoxin
VIII[a]	Impaired hearing on auditory testing, nystagmus	Alterations in hearing, potential alterations in balance	Cisplatin, DEG, ethylene glycol, oxalosis, quinine, salicylates, solvents
IX[c]	Impaired gag reflex	Impaired taste	Botulinum toxin, ethylene glycol, stibanate, cholinergic compounds[c]
X[c,d]	Decreased gag reflex when paralyzed May be enhanced with cholinergic or impaired with anticholinergic: Autonomic instability, altered bowel sounds	Choking, change in voice	Botulinum toxin, ethyleme glycol, stibanate, cholinergic compounds[c]
XI[c]	Weakness shoulder shrug	Weakness neck/shoulders	Botulinum toxin, cholinergic compounds[c]
XII[c]	Impaired speech, tongue deviation	Dysarthria	Botulinum toxin, cholinergic compounds[c]

[a] See also Chap. 20.

[b] Tetanus causes indirect effects on masseter muscles; see section on xenobiotic-induced seizures or Chap. 111.

[c] Weakness of cranial nerves IX–XII is often referred to as bulbar palsy and can be seen in the intermediate syndrome after acute cholinesterase poisoning. This syndrome is often accompanied by paralysis of extraocular muscles (see Chap. 112).

[d] See Chap. 3.

oil,[6] or inadvertent deep space injection of a local anesthetic during dental anesthesia with a resultant abducens palsy.[59] In some cases, a xenobiotic is converted into a toxic substance such as formic acid in the retina.

The neuromuscular junction of the cranial nerves is sensitive to disruptions in neurotransmission. In xenobiotics affecting the occulomotor nerves (CN III, IV, VI) patients may describe diplopia or have gaze palsies on examination. Botulinum toxin, diethylene glycol toxicity, elapid snake venom, and the cranial neuropathy associated with the organic phosphorus insecticide-induced intermediate syndrome are some examples.

Absence of critical substrates such as glucose or thiamine can result in an ophthalmoplegia. In most cases, however, the mechanisms underlying the cranial neuropathy are poorly understood, such as is the case with chemotherapeutic agents. Similarly, some patients who survive ethylene glycol poisoning experience transient ophthalmoplegia days after the initial exposure[55,81] (see Table 18–4 and Chap. 19).

PERIPHERAL NERVES

Complaints of pain, paresthesias, numbness, or weakness of extremities are clinically termed *neuropathies*. The mechanisms of evolution are variable. Common to most xenobiotic-induced neuropathies is early bilateral involvement of the lower extremities. This may be due in part to the patient's rapid recognition of impairment during an attempt to ambulate. Additionally, the axons serving the lower extremities are longer. Maintenance and transportation of substrates is more energy dependent and sensitive to xenobiotic-induced disruptions.

In some cases the anatomic structure of the nerve is maintained, but the xenobiotic affects neurotransmission. This may be due to direct impairment of specific enzymes at the NMJ, such as cholinesterase inhibitors.[27] Tri-ortho-cresyl phosphate (TOCP) is an inhibitor of neuropathic target esterase. Contamination of food and the beverage Ginger Jake with TOCP resulted in irreversible lower extremity paralysis in several epidemic exposures.[68,86] Indirectly, the extracellular environment may be altered as in the case of hypermagnesemia, or hypokalemia which can be induced by multiple agents (see Chap. 16) Ciguatoxin, a sodium channel opener, affects neurotransmission causing paresthesias and the unusual symptom of sensory reversal in which the perception of temperature is reversed to the stimulus.

Xenobiotics such as amiodarone and tacrolimus induce peripheral demyelination. Patients present with weakness and flaccidity. Nitrous oxide impairs the production of *S*-adenosyl methionine essential to the production of myelin and is additive to the nitrous oxide disruptions of vitamin B_{12} which further impair axonal function.[87]

Other xenobiotics affect the structure or intracellular function of the peripheral nerves. Those that induce death of the cell body are termed *neuronopathies* and they may be clinically indistinguishable from those that affect the axon, or *axonopathies*.

Peripheral nerve cell death is usually linked to injury at the spinal cord as was described above by the doxorubicin injection of the peripheral nerves.[50] Pyridoxine overdose is another cause of neuronopathy. However, neuronopathies are an unusual mechanism of peripheral nerve toxicity.

Unlike neuronopathies, axonopathies are potentially reversible and are the most common mechanism of xenobiotic-induced peripheral neuropathy. Xenobiotic-induced axonal injuries to the peripheral nerves are usually diffuse and bilateral, with preservation of the proximal cell body. These often target the cytoskeleton and impair the capacity for the microtubule system to deliver functional substrates.[21,40] Patients with occupational exposure to 2,5-hexanedione, a γ-diketone metabolite of n-hexane present in certain glues, suffer from a sensorimotor axonopathy due to cross-linking of neurofilaments and impaired substrate transport.[65] Progressive neuropathy may occur long after the initial exposure. Vincristine similarly effects axonal transport. Acrylamide impairs fast anterograde and retrograde transport with animal models suggesting effects on both kinesin and dyenin.

Nucleoside reverse transcriptase inhibitors cause peripheral neuropathy by decreasing the production of mitochondrial DNA.

TABLE 18–5. Xenobiotics Associated with Muscle Toxicity

Amiodarone	HMG-CoA reductase inhibitors
Azidothymine	Hydroxychloroquine
Bothrops spp, and Agkistrodon spp venoms	Ipecac
Chloroquine	*Loxosceles* spp venom
Cimetidine	Niacin
Clofibrate	Organic phosphorous compounds
Clostridium toxins	D-Penicillamine
Cocaine	Phencyclidine
Colchine	Procainamide
Crotaline and other tissue-toxic snake venoms	Propylthiouracil
Cyclosporine	Rifampin
Doxylamine	Sulfonamides
Epsilon aminocaproic acid	Suxamethonium
Ethanol	Toxic oil syndrome
Ethchlorvynol	L-Tryptophan
Glucocorticoids	Vincristine
Heroin	Zidovudine

MYOPATHIES

Some patients experience local muscle damage as a result of direct injury from extravasation of tissue toxic substances or enzymatic degradation associated with crotalid snake envenomations.

Most xenobiotic-induced muscle injuries or myopathies are more diffuse.[39,73,80,85] HMG Co-A reductase inhibitors can cause myalgias, cramping, myositis, or rhabdomyolysis. The incidence appears to be higher in patients taking other medications which share the same liver metabolic enzymes. The mechanism underlying the myopathy may be related to impaired cholesterol synthesis in myocytes, or diminished production of regulatory proteins such as ubiquinone and GTP-binding proteins required for mitochondrial function.

Another myopathy that presents predominantly with weakness is the acute quadriplegic myopathy of intensive care patients. This syndrome was originally described in ventilated patients with asthma who received glucocorticoids and nondepolarizing neuromuscular blockers, but is also reported in other critically ill patients[8] (see Chap. 68). The mechanisms underlying quadriplegic myopathy, eosinophilia myalgia syndrome, and toxic oil syndrome are poorly described. Xenobiotics associated with muscle injury can be found in Table 18–5.

CONCLUSIONS

The principles involving xenobiotic-induced neurological injury are an area of intensive and evolving investigation. With improved understanding of these neurotoxic principles, therapeutic medications can be better delivered to the CNS while limiting the entry of potentially toxic substances. Toxicological models for the investigation of neurodegenerative disorders can be further developed as can new and creative therapies for mood disorders, hepatic encephalopathy, and injuries from infections, trauma, and ischemia. Elucidation of neurotoxicologic principles shows promise for the treatment of many nervous system disorders. The chemical properties of the xenobiotic and the characteristics of the patient exposed are critical to the clinical expression of neurotoxicity.

ACKNOWLEDGMENT

E. John Gallagher contributed to this chapter in previous editions.

REFERENCES

1. Abbott NJ, Mendonca LL, Dolman DE: The blood-brain barrier in systemic lupus erythematosus. *Lupus*. 2003;12:908-915.
2. Abbott NJ, Romero IA: Transporting therapeutics across the blood-brain barrier. *Mol Med Today*. 1996;2:106-113.
3. Abbott NJ: Astrocyte-endothelial interactions and blood-brain barrier permeability. *J Anat*. 2002;200:629-638.
4. Abbott NJ: Inflammatory mediators and modulation of blood-brain barrier permeability. *Cell Mol Neurobiol*. 2000;20:131-147.
5. Abouesh A, Stone C, Hobbs WR: Antimicrobial-induced mania (antibiomania): a review of spontaneous reports. *J Clin Psychopharmacol*. 2002;22:71-81.
6. Agrawal R, Soni M, Biswas J, Sharma T, Gopal L: Silicone oil-associated optic nerve degeneration. *Am J Ophthalmol*. 2002;133:429-430.
7. Anonymous. Parkinsonian syndrome and calcium channel blockers. *Prescrire Int*. 2003;12:62.
8. Argov Z: Drug-induced myopathies. *Curr Opin Neurol*. 2000;13:541-545.
9. Ariffin H, Omar KZ, Ang EL, Shekhar K: Severe vincristine neurotoxicity with concomitant use of itraconazole. *J Paediatr Child Health*. 2003;39:638-639.
10. Arundine M, Tymianski M: Molecular mechanisms of calcium-dependent neurodegeneration in excitotoxicity. *Cell Calcium*. 2003;34:325-337.
11. Aschner M, Sonnewald U, Tan KH: Astrocyte modulation of neurotoxic injury. *Brain Pathol*. 2002;12:475-481.
12. Balis FM, Blaney SM, McCully CL, et al: Methotrexate distribution within the subarachnoid space after intraventricular and intravenous administration. *Cancer Chemother Pharmacol*. 2000;45:259-264.
13. Bearer EL, Schlief ML, Breakefield XO, et al: Squid axoplasm supports the retrograde axonal transport of herpes simplex virus. *Biol Bull*. 1999;197:257-258.
14. Ben-Ami M, Giladi Y, Shalev E: The combination of magnesium sulphate and nifedipine: a cause of neuromuscular blockade. *Br J Obstet Gynaecol*. 1994;101:262-263.
15. Best JA, Marashi AH, Pollan LD: Neuromuscular blockade after clindamycin administration: a case report. *J Oral Maxillofac Surg*. 1999;57:600-603.
16. Bhatia R, Prabhakar S, Grover VK: Tetanus. *Neurol India*. 2002;50:398-407.
17. Bleich S, Degner D, Bandelow B, et al: Plasma homocysteine is a predictor of alcohol withdrawal seizures. *Neuroreport*. 2000;11:2749-2752.
18. Bleich S, Degner D, Sperling W, et al: Homocysteine as a neurotoxin in chronic alcoholism. *Prog Neuropsychopharmacol Biol Psychiatry*. 2004;28:453-464.
19. Boffi BV, Klerman GL: Manic psychosis associated with appetite suppressant medication, phenylpropanolamine. *J Clin Psychopharmacol*. 1989;9:308-309.
20. Burneo JG, Limdi N, Kuzniecky RI, et al: Neurotoxicity following addition of intravenous valproate to lamotrigine therapy. *Neurology*. 2003;60:1991-1992.
21. Chang MH, Liao KK, Wu ZA, Lin KP: Reversible myeloneuropathy resulting from podophyllin intoxication: an electrophysiological follow up. *J Neurol Neurosurg Psychiatry*. 1992;55:235-236.
22. Chauvenet AR, Shashi V, Selsky C, et al: Vincristine-induced neuropathy as the initial presentation of Charcot-Marie-Tooth disease in acute lymphoblastic leukemia: a Pediatric Oncology Group study. *J Pediatr Hematol Oncol*. 2003;25:316-320.
23. Chen CY, Lee KW, Lee CC, et al: Heroin-induced spongiform leukoencephalopathy: value of diffusion MR imaging. *J Comput Assist Tomogr*. 2000;24:735-737.
24. Cherry CL, McArthur JC, Hoy JF, et al: Nucleoside analogues and neuropathy in the era of HAART. *J Clin Virol*. 2003;26:195-207.
25. Chishty M, Reichel A, Siva J, et al: Affinity for the P-glycoprotein efflux pump at the blood-brain barrier may explain the lack of CNS side-effects of modern antihistamines. *J Drug Target*. 2001;9:223-228.
26. Chuang C, Constantino A, Balmaceda C, et al: Chemotherapy-induced parkinsonism responsive to levodopa: an underrecognized entity. *Mov Disord*. 2003;18:328-331.
27. Chuang CC, Lin TS, Tsai MC: Delayed neuropathy and myelopathy after organophosphate intoxication. *N Engl J Med*. 2002;347:1119-1121.
28. Chung RS, West AK: A role for extracellular metallothioneins in CNS injury and repair. *Neuroscience*. 2004;123:595-599.
29. Cliff J, Lundqvist P, Martensson J, et al: Association of high cyanide and low sulphur intake in cassava-induced spastic paraparesis. *Lancet*. 1985;2:1211-1213.
30. Dobson AW, Erikson KM, Aschner M: Manganese neurotoxicity. *Ann N Y Acad Sci*. 2004;1012:115-128.
31. Driesen JJ, Wolters EC: Bilateral ballism induced by oral contraceptives. A case report. *J Neurol*. 1986;233:379.
32. Dutta D, Fischler M, McClung A: Angiotensin converting enzyme inhibitor induced hyperkalaemic paralysis. *Postgrad Med J*. 2001;77:114-115.
33. Elinav E, Chajek-Shaul T: Licorice consumption causing severe hypokalemic paralysis. *Mayo Clin Proc*. 2003;78:767-768.
34. Ellis WG, Sobel RA, Nielsen SL: Leukoencephalopathy in patients treated with amphotericin B methyl ester. *J Infect Dis*. 1982;146:125-137.
35. Erikson KM, Aschner M: Manganese neurotoxicity and glutamate-GABA interaction. *Neurochem Int*. 2003;43:475-480.
36. Erikson KM, Dorman DC, Lash LH, et al: Airborne manganese exposure differentially affects end points of oxidative stress in an age- and sex-dependent manner. *Biol Trace Elem Res*. 2004;100:49-62.
37. Freimer ML, Glass JD, Chaudhry V, et al: Chronic demyelinating polyneuropathy associated with eosinophilia-myalgia syndrome. *J Neurol Neurosurg Psychiatry*. 1992;55:352-358.
38. Fukuda T: Neurotoxicity of MPTP. *Neuropathology*. 2001;21:323-332.
39. George KK, Pourmand R: Toxic myopathies. *Neurol Clin*. 1997;15:711-730.
40. Graham DG: Neurotoxicants and the cytoskeleton. *Curr Opin Neurol*. 1999;12:733-737.
41. Grattan-Smith PJ, et al. Clinical and neurophysiological features of tick paralysis. *Brain*. 1997;120:1975-1987.
42. Hampson DR, Manalo JL: The activation of glutamate receptors by kainic acid and domoic acid. *Nat Toxins*. 1998;6:153-158.
43. Huang CC, Chu CC, Wu TN, et al: Clinical course in patients with chronic carbon disulfide polyneuropathy. *Clin Neurol Neurosurg*. 2002;104:115-120.
44. Huang CC, Yen TC, Shih TS, et al: Dopamine transporter binding study in differentiating carbon disulfide induced parkinsonism from idiopathic parkinsonism. *Neurotoxicology*. 2004;25:341-347.
45. Israel ZH, Lossos A, Barak V, et al: Multifocal demyelinative leukoencephalopathy associated with 5-fluorouracil and levamisole. *Acta Oncol*. 2000;39:117-120.
46. Iwata K, O'Keefe GB, Karanas A: Neurologic problems associated with chronic nitrous oxide abuse in a non-healthcare worker. *Am J Med Sci*. 2001;322:173-174.
47. Jackson AC: Rabies virus infection: an update. *J Neurovirol*. 2003;9:253-258.
48. Jarosz JM, Howlett DC, Cox TC, Bingham JB: Cyclosporine-related reversible posterior leukoencephalopathy: MRI. *Neuroradiology*. 1997;39:711-715.
49. Jeanjean AP, Laterre EC, Maloteaux JM: Neuroleptic binding to sigma receptors: possible involvement in neuroleptic-induced acute dystonia. *Biol Psychiatry*. 1997;41:1010-1019.
50. Kato S, Otsuki T, Yamamoto T, et al: Retrograde adriamycin sensory ganglionectomy: novel approach for the treatment of intractable pain. *Stereotact Funct Neurosurg*. 1990;54-55:86-89.
51. Klos KJ, Ahlskog E, Josephs KA, et al. Neurologic spectrum of chronic liver failure and basal ganglia T1 hyperintensity on magnetic resonance imaging. *Arch Neurol*. 2005;62:1385-1390
52. Kroll RA, Neuwelt EA: Outwitting the blood-brain barrier for therapeutic purposes: osmotic opening and other means. *Neurosurgery*. 1998;42:1083-1099.
53. Kroll RA, Pagel MA, Muldoon LL, et al: Improving drug delivery to intracerebral tumor and surrounding brain in a rodent model: A comparison of osmotic versus bradykinin modification of the blood-brain and/or blood-tumor barriers. *Neurosurgery*. 1998;43:879-886.

54. Lang CJ: The use of neuroimaging techniques for clinical detection of neurotoxicity: a review. *Neurotoxicology*. 2000;21:847-855.
55. Lewis LD, Smith BW, Mamourian AC: Delayed sequelae after acute overdoses or poisonings: cranial neuropathy related to ethylene glycol ingestion. *Clin Pharmacol Therap*. 1997;61:692-699.
56. Lo EH, Singhal AB, Torchilin VP, Abbott NJ: Drug delivery to damaged brain. *Brain Res Brain Res Rev*. 2001;38:140-148.
57. LoPachin RM: The changing view of acrylamide neurotoxicity. *Neurotoxicology*. 2004;25:617-630.
58. Manzo L, Castoldi AF, Coccini T, Prockop LD: Assessing effects of neurotoxic pollutants by biochemical markers. *Environ Res*. 2001;85:31-36.
59. Marinho RO: Abducent nerve palsy following dental local analgesia. *Br Dent J*. 1995;179:69-70.
60. Morgan JC, Sethi KD. Drug-induced tremors. *Lancet Neurol*. 2005;4:866-876.
61. Neuwelt EA: Mechanisms of disease: the blood-brain barrier. *Neurosurgery*. 2004;54:131-140.
62. Nilsen J, Diaz Brinton R: Mechanism of estrogen-mediated neuroprotection: regulation of mitochondrial calcium and Bcl-2 expression. *Proc Natl Acad Sci U S A*. 2003;100:2842-2847.
63. Norenberg MD, Jayakumar AR, Rama Rao KV: Oxidative stress in the pathogenesis of hepatic encephalopathy. *Metab Brain Dis*. 2004;19:313-329.
64. Norenberg MD: Oxidative and nitrosative stress in ammonia neurotoxicity. [comment]. *Hepatology*. 2003;37:245-248.
65. Oge AM, Yazici J, Boyaciyan A, et al: Peripheral and central conduction in n-hexane polyneuropathy. *Muscle Nerve*. 1994;17:1416-1430.
66. Orth M, Tabrizi SJ: Models of Parkinson's disease. *Mov Disord*. 2003;18:729-737.
67. Pai KS, Ravindranath V: L-BOAA induces selective inhibition of brain mitochondrial enzyme, NADH-dehydrogenase. *Brain Res*. 1993;621:215-221.
68. Parascandola J: The Public Health Service and Jamaica ginger paralysis in the 1930s. *Public Health Rep*. 1995;110:361-363.
69. Picazo O, Azcoitia I, Garcia-Segura LM: Neuroprotective and neurotoxic effects of estrogens. *Brain Res*. 2003;990:20-27.
70. Pourmand R: Diabetic neuropathy. *Neurol Clin*. 1997;15:569-576.
71. Reynolds IJ: Mitochondrial membrane potential and the permeability transition in excitotoxicity. *Ann N Y Acad Sci*. 1999;893:33-41.
72. Rodnitzky RL: Drug-induced movement disorders in children. *Semin Pediatr Neurol*. 2003;10:80-87.
73. Rosenson RS: Current overview of statin-induced myopathy. *Am J Med*. 2004;116:408-416.
74. Salzer W, Widemann B, McCully C, et al: Effect of probenecid on ventricular cerebrospinal fluid methotrexate pharmacokinetics after intralumbar administration in nonhuman primates. *Cancer Chemother Pharmacol*. 2001;48:235-240.
75. Sande MA, Sherertz RJ, Zak O, et al: Factors influencing the penetration of antimicrobial agents into the cerebrospinal fluid of experimental animals. *Scand J Infect Dis Suppl*. 1978;160-163.
76. Saunders NR, Knott GW, Dziegielewska KM: Barriers in the immature brain. *Cell Mol Neurobiol*. 2000;20:29-40.
77. Schaumberg HH, Herskovitz S, Cassano VA. Occupational manganese neurotoxicity provoked by hepatitis C. *Neurology*. 2006;67:322-323.
78. Senanayake N, Roman GC: Disorders of neuromuscular transmission due to natural environmental toxins. *J Neurol Sci*. 1992;107:1-13.
79. Shigenaga MK, Hagen TM, Ames BN: Oxidative damage and mitochondrial decay in aging. *Proc Natl Acad Sci U S A*. 1994;91:10771-10778.
80. Sieb JP, Gillessen T: Iatrogenic and toxic myopathies. *Muscle Nerve*. 2003;27:142-156.
81. Spillane L, Roberts JR, Meyer AE: Multiple cranial nerve deficits after ethylene glycol poisoning. *Ann Emerg Med*. 1991;20:208-210.
82. Stepens A, Logina I, Liguts V, et al. A Parkinsonian syndrome in methcathione users and the role of manganese. *New Engl J Med*. 2008;358:1009-1017.
83. Stoltenberg M, Schionning JD, Danscher G: Retrograde axonal transport of bismuth: an autometallographic study. *Acta Neuropathol*. 2001;101:123-128.
84. Teive HA, Germiniani FM, Werneck LC: Parkinsonian syndrome induced by amlodipine: case report. *Mov Disord*. 2002;17:833-835.
85. Thompson PD, Clarkson P, Karas RH: Statin-associated myopathy. *JAMA*. 2003;289:1681-1690.
86. Tosi L, Righetti C, Adami L, Zanette G: October 1942: a strange epidemic paralysis in Saval, Verona, Italy. Revision and diagnosis 50 years later of tri-ortho-cresyl phosphate poisoning. *J Neurol Neurosurg Psychiatry*. 1994;57:810-813.
87. Waclawik AJ, Luzzio CC, Juhasz-Pocsine K, Hamilton V: Myeloneuropathy from nitrous oxide abuse: Unusually high methylmalonic acid and homocysteine levels.[erratum appears in *WMJ* 2003;102:5]. *WMJ*. 2003;102:43-45.
88. Wagner AK, Bayir H, Ren D, et al: Relationships between cerebrospinal fluid markers of excitotoxicity, ischemia, and oxidative damage after severe TBI: the impact of gender, age, and hypothermia. *J Neurotrauma*. 2004;21:125-136.
89. Wiley RG, Blessing WW, Reis DJ: Suicide transport: destruction of neurons by retrograde transport of ricin, abrin, and modeccin. *Science*. 1982;216:889-890.
90. Yamada S, Kuno Y, Iwanaga H: Effects of aminoglycoside antibiotics on the neuromuscular junction: Part I. *Int J Clin Pharmacol Ther Toxicol*. 1986;24:130-138.
91. Zheng W, Aschner M, Ghersi-Egea JF: Brain barrier systems: a new frontier in metal neurotoxicological research. *Toxicol Appl Pharmacol*. 2003;192:1-11.

CHAPTER 19
OPHTHALMIC PRINCIPLES

Adhi Sharma

While it is arguable that the eyes are the mirror to the soul, it is certain that the eyes can reveal a great deal of information with regard to toxicology. In addition to exhibiting findings of systemic toxicity, they are also subject to the direct effects of xenobiotics and can serve as a portal of entry for systemic absorption. An understanding of ophthalmic principles will allow the clinician to make timely and more accurate diagnoses that can be sight-saving or lifesaving and is essential to efficient, organized patient care.

OPHTHALMIC EXAMINATION

As a matter of convention, the routine eye examination is performed in the following sequence: visual acuity, pupillary response, extraocular muscle function, funduscopy, and, when indicated, a slit-lamp examination. Examination of the pupillary size and response to light can help determine the presence of a toxic syndrome. For example, opioids and cholinergics may produce miosis, whereas anticholinergics and sympathomimetics may produce mydriasis. Assessment of the extraocular muscles can reveal xenobiotic-induced nystagmus. Funduscopy can reveal pink discs characteristic of poisoning by methanol or carbon monoxide. The slit-lamp examination allows for evaluation of toxic exposure to the lids, lacrimal systems, conjunctiva, sclera, cornea, and anterior chamber. However, before considering specific xenobiotic exposures in detail, it is important to review the anatomy and physiology of the visual pathways and how alteration of the normal physiology and anatomy correlate with clinical signs and symptoms.

OCULAR ANATOMY AND PHYSIOLOGY

The eye is a roughly spherical structure referred to as a globe. The globe is divided into anterior and posterior structures (Fig. 19–1). The most anterior structures are the cornea, conjunctiva, and sclera. Posterior to the cornea are the iris, the lens, and the ciliary body. The space between the cornea and the iris is the anterior chamber, and the space between the iris and the retina is the posterior chamber. The anterior chamber contains *aqueous humor,* which is produced by the ciliary processes; this fluid nourishes the cornea, iris, and lens. The iris, the ciliary processes, and the choroid compose the uvea. The posterior chamber is filled with a transparent gelatinous mass termed the *vitreous humor*. The vitreous humor is an important body fluid in forensic toxicology as it is less susceptible to postmortem redistribution (Chap. 33). The fundus is the most posterior structure and includes the retina, retinal vessels, and the head of the optic nerve or disc.

VISUAL ACUITY AND COLOR PERCEPTION

Normal vision is dependent on light transmission to intact neural elements. Appropriate light transmission requires a clear cornea and aqueous humor, proper pupil size, an unclouded lens, and clear vitreous. The neural elements include the retina, optic nerve, and the optic cortex; all of these structures require intact blood circulation for proper function. Decreased acuity can result from abnormalities anywhere in the visual system that affect either light transmission or neural elements.[4,12,21] Corneal injury or edema may result in blurring of vision, characteristically described as "halos" around lights. Toxicologic causes of corneal abnormalities include direct exposure to chemicals, failure of corneal protective reflexes because of local anesthetic effects or a profoundly decreased level of consciousness, and incomplete eyelid closure during coma. Mydriasis, secondary to various xenobiotics (Table 19–1), may interfere with the pupillary constriction necessary for accommodation, thereby resulting in decreased acuity for near objects. Lens clouding or cataract formation causes blurred vision and decreased light perception, as does blood (hyphema) or other deposits in the aqueous humor or vitreous humors. Xenobiotic-induced lens abnormalities caused by chronic exposures are well described (Table 19–2),[17,21,27] but are unimportant in the evaluation of an acute toxicologic emergency. Even if light reaches the retina without distortion, abnormal reception or transmission can result from ischemia or injury to any neural element from the retina to the optic cortex. Direct, acute, visual neurotoxic injury is rare and is caused almost exclusively by methanol or quinine. Indirect injury following xenobiotic-induced CNS ischemia or hypoxia is far more common. Alterations in color perception generally result from abnormalities in retinal or optic nerve function. Color-vision abnormalities are attributed to hundreds of xenobiotics, but unlike those caused by chronic xenobiotic exposure such abnormalities are rare and inconsistent features of acute toxicity.[17,21]

PUPIL SIZE AND REACTIVITY

Generally, pupils are round and symmetric with an average diameter of 3–4 mm under typical light conditions. Physiologic anisocoria (unequal pupils) is a normal variant and is defined as a difference in pupil size of 1 mm or less. However, in the absence of a history of physiologic anisocoria, any asymmetry in pupil size should be considered an abnormal finding. Pupils react directly and consensually to light intensity by either constricting or dilating. Constriction is also a component of the near reflex (accommodation) that occurs when the eye focuses on near objects. The iris controls pupil size through a balance of cholinergic innervation of the sphincter (constrictor) muscle by cranial nerve III and sympathetic innervation of the radial (dilator) muscle.[12]

Pupillary dilation (mydriasis) can result from increased sympathetic stimulation of the radial muscle by endogenous catecholamines, or from xenobiotics such as cocaine, amphetamines, and other sympathomimetics as well as ophthalmic instillation of sympathomimetic agents such as phenylephrine. Mydriasis can also result from inhibition of muscarinic cholinergic-mediated innvervation of the sphincter secondary to systemic or ophthalmic exposure to anticholinergic agents (Chap. 50). Because pupillary constriction in response to light is a major determinant of normal pupil size, blindness from ocular, retinal, or optic nerve disorders also leads to mydriasis as exemplified by methanol and quinine toxicity. As such, the reactivity of mydriatic pupils to light varies with the etiology of the mydriasis.[21] Although often difficult to appreciate, constriction to light can usually be elicited after sympathomimetic exposures because constrictor function is preserved, whereas this is often not the case when mydriasis results from anticholinergic excess since constrictor function is potently antagonized. Light reactivity is absent in cases of complete blindness, but may be preserved if there is some remaining light perception.

Miosis can result from increased cholinergic stimulation such as opioids, pilocarpine, and cholinesterase inhibitors such as organic phosphorus compounds, or inhibition of sympathetic dilation caused by clonidine. Miosis was the most common finding in victims of the Tokyo subway sarin attack of 1995 and was used to distinguish between mild and moderate exposure.[33]

There are conflicting reports regarding the pupillary reactions to many xenobiotics. Depending on the stage and severity of toxicity,

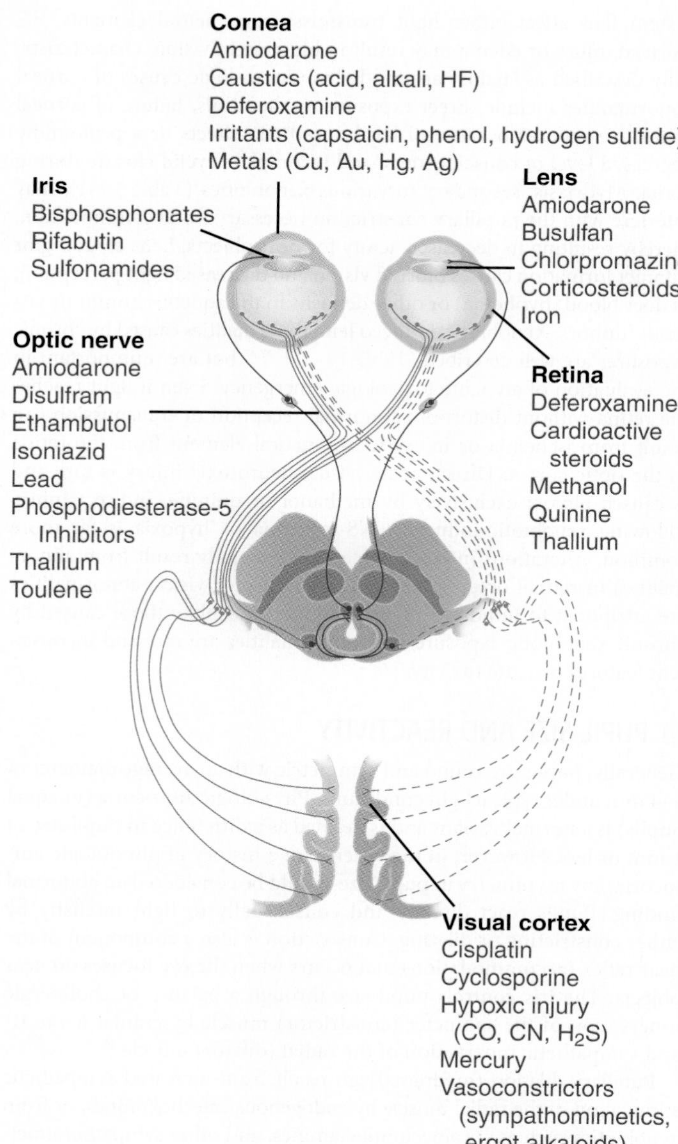

FIGURE 19–1. The major xenobiotics and their areas of ophthalmic injury.

TABLE 19–1. Ophthalmic Findings Caused by Acute Xenobiotic Exposures

Disconjugate gaze
Botulism
Elapid envenomation
Neuromuscular blockers
Paralytic shellfish poisoning
Secondary to decreased level of consciousness (many causes)
Tetrodotoxin
Thiamine deficiency
Funduscopic abnormalities
Carbon monoxide (red)
Cocaine (vasoconstriction)
Cyanide (retinal vein arteriolization)
Ergot alkaloids (vasoconstriction; disc pallor)
Intravenous drug use (attenuation or loss of small vessels due to emboli)
Methanol (disc and retinal pallor or hyperemia)
Methemoglobin (cyanosis)
Miosis
Cholinesterase inhibitors (carbamates, organic phosphorus compounds)
Coma from sedative-hypnotics (barbiturates, benzodiazepines, ethanol)
Decreased sympathetic tone (clonidine, opioids)
Increased cholinergic tone
Mydriasis
Decreased cholinergic tone
Nicotine
Increased sympathetic tone (cocaine, sedative-hypnotic withdrawal)
Nystagmus
Carbamazepine
Dextromethorphan
Ethanol
Ketamine
Lithium
Monoamine oxidase inhibitors (oscillopsia or ping-pong nystagmus)
Phencyclidine (usually rotary nystagmus)
Phenytoin
Sedative-hypnotics
Thiamine deficiency
Papilledema (see causes of idiopathic intracranial hypertension (Table 41–2) for a more detailed list)
Amiodarone
Lead
Phenytoin
Vitamin A

the presence of co-ingestants or coexistent hypoxemia, and numerous other factors, many individual xenobiotics (eg, phencyclidine and barbiturates) are reported to cause either mydriasis, miosis, or hippus, the fluctuation between miosis and mydriasis.[21,28] For some xenobiotics, the pupillary examination provides consistent information (Table 19–1), but many factors are involved and the significance of the pupil size and reactivity must always be considered in the context of the remainder of the patient evaluation.

EXTRAOCULAR MOVEMENT, DIPLOPIA, AND NYSTAGMUS

Maintenance of normal eye position and movement requires a coordinated function of a complex circuit involving bilateral frontal and occipital cortices, multiple brainstem nuclei, cranial nerves, and extraocular muscles.[2,12] Because of the many elements necessary for normal function, abnormalities of eye movement can result from several causes and are extremely common.[21] Probably the most common abnormality is reversible nystagmus or rhythmic oscillations of the globes (Table 19–1). Nystagmus is divided into two types: jerk nystagmus has a slow phase and a fast phase, while pendular nystagmus is a rhythmic oscillation. Either type can be torsional (rotary) or in a horizontal or vertical direction. Xenobiotic-induced nystagmus can take many forms, but is most commonly jerk nystagmus, as opposed to pendular. The nystagmus may be evident at rest but is accentuated by visual pursuit and extreme lateral gaze. Although nystagmus with extreme lateral gaze is a normal finding, it extinguishes within 2–5 beats; if nystagmus

TABLE 19–2. Examples of Ocular Abnormalities Caused by Chronic Systemic Xenobiotic Exposures[a]

Category	Examples
Alteration of color vision	Sildenafil Citrate (cyanopsia); Styrene (color blindness); Tertiary amines (glaucopsia)
Cataracts	Busulfan[c]; Corticosteroids[b]; Deferoxamine; Dinitrophenol (internal use)[d]; Trinitrotoluene[d]
Corneal deposits	Amiodarone[b]; Chloroquine; Chlorpromazine; Copper[d]; Gold; Mercury[d]; Retinoids; Silver (argyria)[d]; Vitamin D
Corneal/Conjunctival inflammation	Cytosine arabinoside (Ara-C); Isotretinoin[b]; Mercury (acrodynia); Practolol[c]
Cortical blindness	Cisplatin; Cyclosporine; Glycine; Interleukin[c]; Methylmercury compounds[d]; Tacrolimus
Lens deposits	Amiodarone[b]; Chlorpromazine; Copper[d]; Iron; Mercury[d]; Silver[d]
Myopia[c]	Acetazolamide; Diuretics (chlorthalidone, thiazides, spironolactone); Retinoids; Sulfonamides
Retinal injury	Carbon disulfide[d]; Carmustine[c]; Chloramphenicol[c]; Chloroquine; Cinchona alkaloids (quinine); Deferoxamine[c]; Ethambutol; Methanol; Thallium; Vigabatrin; Vincristine[c]
Retrobulbar and optic neuropathy	Carbon disulfide[d]; Chloramphenicol[d]; Dinitrobenzene[d]; Dinitrochlorobenzene[d]; Dinitrotoluene[d]; Disulfiram; Ethambutol[b]; Isoniazid[c]; Lead[c]; Thallium; Vincristine[c]
Uveitis	Bisphosphonates; Pamidronate; Rifabutin; Sulfonamides

[a] This list includes only selected examples and is not intended to be comprehensive.

[b] Particularly important example.

[c] Reported, but extremely rare from this exposure.

[d] Mostly of historical interest; associated with patterns of use that are no longer common.

persists, it is evidence of underlying pathology. Vertical nystagmus in other settings is usually associated with a structural lesion of the CNS. However, xenobiotic-induced vertical nystagmus occurs with phencyclidine, ketamine, dextromethorphan, or phenytoin toxicity. Loss of conjugate gaze commonly results from CNS depression of any etiology, typically after sedative-hypnotic or ethanol poisoning. Except after extremely rare exposures to neurotoxins (Table 19–1), diplopia without a decreased level of consciousness should not be attributed to an acute toxicologic etiology. In addition to the transient effects of some xenobiotics, thallium, carbon disulfide, and carbon monoxide may cause sustained gaze disorders as a consequence of residual cranial nerve and CNS injury.[21] Nystagmus and ophthalmoplegia caused by thiamine deficiency (Wernicke) usually improves after therapy, but the nystagmus may not completely resolve.[43]

DIRECT OCULAR TOXINS

CAUSTICS

The initial approach to all patients with ocular caustic exposures should be immediate decontamination by irrigating with copious amounts of fluids.[9,44] Water, normal saline, lactated Ringer solution, and balanced salt solution (BSS) are all appropriate choices.[37] In theory, BSS is ideal, because it is both isotonic and buffered to physiologic pH. Lactated Ringer solution (pH 6–7.5) and 0.9% sodium chloride solution (pH 4.5–7) are also isotonic and therefore theoretically preferable to water.[22] The use of an ocular anesthetic is usually required to perform irrigation properly. Irrigation is intended to accomplish at least four objectives: immediate dilution of the offending agent; removal of the agent; removal of any foreign body; and, in some cases, normalization of anterior chamber pH. As delays of even seconds can dramatically affect outcome,[21] there is no justification for waiting for any specific solution if water is the first available agent. Irrigation must include the external and internal palpebral surfaces, as well as the cornea and bulbar conjunctiva and its recesses. Effective irrigation includes lid retraction and eversion or use of a scleral shell or other irrigating device. After irrigation, visual acuity testing, inspection of the eye, and slit-lamp examination should be performed. The immediacy with which an ophthalmologic consultation must be obtained will depend on the degree of injury.

SULFUR MUSTARD

The alkylating agent reacts with ocular tissues resulting in early and late toxic effects. Of note, there is a latency of 30 minutes to 8 hours during which time victims are asymptomatic. Immediate effects include pain, foreign body sensation (grittiness), lacrimation, photophobia, blepharospasm, corneal ulceration, and blindness.[24] Generally, injury is limited to the anterior chamber. More than 90% of exposed victims will experience late complications associated with conjunctival sensitivity to irritants with resultant recurrent blepharoconjunctivitis. Less than 1% of severely intoxicated victims will suffer delayed keratopathy, resulting in thinning, neovascularization, and epithelial defects of the cornea.[24]

Management is directed at removal from the exposure and aggressive decontamination of the skin and eyes. Any of the irrigation solutions mentioned above will suffice. The goal is to provide irrigation as soon as possible; to this end, even tap water is an acceptable solution. Animal studies have suggested that topical anti-inflammatory agents are helpful; as such, a short course of ocular steroids may be beneficial.[5] Steroid treatment should only be rendered in consultation with an ophthalmologist. Late complications are best managed by referral to an ophthalmologist.

EXPOSURE-SPECIFIC IRRIGATING SOLUTIONS

Despite theoretical concern, there is probably no toxic exposure for which standard aqueous solutions are contraindicated. Of greatest concern are

TABLE 19–3. Irrigation Solutions for Various Xenobiotics

Xenobiotic	Irrigation Solution	Duration of Irrigation[a]
Caustics (acids/alkalis)	NS, LR, BSS	1–2 h
HF (hydrofluoric acid)	NS	1–2 h[a]
Phenol	NS, LR, BSS	15–20 min
Cyanoacrylate adhesives	Typically none needed	N/A
Capsaicin (pepper spray)	NS, LR, BSS	15–20 min

NS = 0.9% sodium chloride (pH ~5.5), LR = lactated Ringer's solution (pH ~6.5), BSS = balanced saline solution (pH ~7.0).

[a] Duration of irrigation can also be determined by other endpoints, including symptoms or conjunctival pH. See text for further discussion.

agents such as white or yellow phosphorus, metallic sodium, metallic potassium, and calcium oxide (cement) that may react violently in the presence of water, leading to heat or mechanical injury, or resulting in the generation of sodium hydroxide, potassium hydroxide, and calcium hydroxide.[21] Although not well studied, irrigation with large amounts of water probably dissipates the heat of the initial hydration reaction with conjunctival moisture more than it initiates a thermochemical reaction. In addition to removing the offending material, irrigation serves to dilute and remove the alkaline by-products formed by reaction with conjunctival water. Table 19–3 summarizes irrigation solutions for various xenobiotics.

The use of special irrigating solutions for more uncommon exposures, including hydrofluoric acid and phenols, is also debated. Recent animal models of alkaline injury suggest irrigation with amphoteric or buffered solutions rapidly restores anterior chamber pH.[38] The authors have gone further to conclude that normal saline should be avoided as an irrigation solution.[35] These were all ex vivo models, and the majority of the published human data have been case reports. Therefore, at this time these solutions are probably best suited for first aid treatment at worksite eyewash stations and are neither practical nor proven in the emergency department setting for prolonged irrigation.

Hydrofluoric Acid For hydrofluoric acid exposures (Chap. 105), experimental irrigation with calcium salt solutions was too irritating to the eye, but isotonic magnesium chloride solutions appear effective and not irritating.[29,30] From a practical standpoint, however, 0.9% sodium chloride solution remains readily available, well studied, and effective. In one animal model, it was suggested that irrigation beyond the initial liter yielded worse outcomes; however, this has not been demonstrated in a human model.[29]

Phenol For phenol exposure, topical low-molecular-weight polyethylene glycol (PEG) solutions are effective for treatment of experimental skin exposure; for eyes, copious water irrigation appears to be as effective as PEG.[7] There is, however, a report of superior efficacy of PEG-400 over water in treatment of actual phenol eye burns.[26] Although PEG-400 may be readily available at worksites where phenols are used, it is not a realistic option in the emergency department, and there should be no hesitation to use water, 0.9% sodium chloride solution, lactated Ringer solution, or BSS as lavage solutions.

Cyanoacrylate Adhesives Ocular exposures to cyanoacrylate adhesives such as Dermabond and Krazy Glue occasionally result in rapid adherence between upper and lower eyelids that may persist for days. Such occurrences may be associated with corneal abrasions,[13] but are otherwise relatively harmless. In fact, cyanoacrylate has been safely used for decades to treat corneal perforations.[46] Solvents, such as acetone or ethanol, which are often effective treatment for dermal-to-dermal adhesions caused by cyanoacrylates, should never be used in or around the eyes as they can result in a severe keratitis. Expectant management is the safest approach as spontaneous rejection of the glue will occur over time. Application of gauze pads coated with antibiotic ophthalmic ointment may speed recovery.[25] A thorough eye examination should be performed once the eyelids can be fully opened.

Other xenobiotic-specific treatments have been tried experimentally or clinically,[22] but none should be considered prior to or instead of copious irrigation, most are not advocated, and consideration of such agents should be vanishingly rare.

Duration of Irrigation To accomplish the desired goals of irrigation, the appropriate duration varies with the exposure. Most solvents, for example, do not penetrate deeper than the superficial cornea, and brief (10–20 minutes) irrigation is generally sufficient.[21] After exposure to acids or alkalis, normalization of the conjunctival pH is often suggested as a useful end point. Testing of pH should be done in every case of acid or alkali exposure, but the limitations of testing must be understood. When measured by sensitive experimental methods, normal pH of the conjunctival surface is 6.5–7.6.[1] This is highly method dependent, however, and normal values in the literature range from 5.2 to 8.6.[10] When measured by touching pH-sensitive paper to the moist surface of the conjunctival cul-de-sac, normal pH is most often near 8.[3] Therefore, after irrigation following alkali burns, pH should not be expected to reach 7 and is more likely to stabilize near 8.[21] In this setting, lower pH values may indicate the pH of the irrigant rather than of the ocular surface. Waiting for an interval of several minutes between irrigation and pH testing allows washout of any residual irrigant.[11] Choice of testing paper is important, as some are intended for use at extremes of pH and lack sensitivity in the clinically useful range.

Despite these limitations, a logical role for pH assessment can be described: Probably a minimum of 500–1000 mL of irrigant should be used for each affected eye before any assessment of pH, and after 7–10 minutes, the pH of the lower fornix conjunctiva should be checked. Thereafter, cycles of 10–15 minutes of irrigation followed by rechecks should be continued until the pH is 7.5–8. This is certainly adequate for exposures to weak acids, which do not penetrate well, and for alkaline exposures where the pH is less than 12.

For strong or concentrated acid or alkali exposures normal surface pH is not an adequate end point (see Alkalis later). After these burns, irrigation should be continued for at least 2–3 hours, regardless of surface pH, in an attempt to correct anterior chamber pH;[21,36,44] in addition, immediate ophthalmologic consultation is mandatory. Following this lengthy irrigation, it is important to verify that conjunctival pH has normalized. If not, irrigation must be continued, sometimes for 24–48 hours.

OTHERS

Most solvents cause immediate pain and superficial injury because of dissolution of corneal epithelial lipid membranes, but do not penetrate or react significantly with deeper tissue.[21] The epithelial defect may be large or complete, but the limited depth of injury usually allows rapid regeneration of normal epithelium. Detergents and surfactants cause variable injury, ranging from minor irritation from soaps to extensive injury from cationic agents such as concentrated benzalkonium chloride.[21] Ocular exposure to A-200 Pyrinate pediculicide shampoo causes typical detergent-surfactant injury, leading to extensive loss of corneal epithelium but with normal underlying stroma, and therefore complete healing within days. Lacrimators (tear gases), such as chloroacetophenone, stimulate corneal nerve endings and cause pain, burning, and tearing, but produce no structural injury at low concentrations. At high concentrations, these agents can produce significant corneal injury.

Pepper spray, often used for self-protection by civilians or law enforcement agents, contains the active ingredient oleoresin capsicum (OC). OC results in rapid depolarization of nociceptors containing substance P, resulting in immediate pain, blepharospasm, tearing, and blurred vision. In general, ocular injury is uncommon, although corneal erosions can occur. The solvent used for the spray can be more injurious to the eye than the OC itself. Although most sprays use a water-based or oil-based solvent, some use alcohol, which can result in significant corneal damage.[47] Management of pepper spray exposure consists of rapid irrigation and pain control. Corneal erosions can be treated with artificial tears but corneal abrasions should be treated with topical antistaphylococcal antibiotics. Specific information on thousands of agents is readily available if needed.[21]

GENERAL MEASURES

There is a wide array of options for adjunctive therapy of chemical burns of the eye. In all cases in which serious injury is evident, the treatment plan must include consultation with an ophthalmologist. Generally, patients with corneal injury should be treated with an ocular topical antibiotic providing antistaphylococcal and antipseudomonal coverage. Cycloplegics not only reduce pain from ciliary spasm, but also decrease the likelihood of posterior synechiae (scar) formation. Topical NSAIDs and systemic analgesics also improve patient comfort. It is never appropriate to dispense topical ophthalmic anesthetics, because repeated use leads to further corneal disruption both by direct chemical effects and by eliminating corneal protective reflex sensation.

DISPOSITION

Disposition of patients with chemical burns of the cornea can be challenging. Patients with extensive burns to other parts of the body should be evaluated for transfer to a burn center. Grading the degree of injury in patients with isolated ocular injury can guide disposition. The most commonly used grading system is the Roper-Hall modification of the Ballen classification system. Injury is graded on a four-tier scale: Patients with mild conjunctival injection with corneal epithelial loss and minimal corneal haziness are classified as grades 1 and 2 (mild to moderate). These patients can be safely discharged from the emergency department with ophthalmology followup within 24–48 hours. Patients with severe corneal haziness or opacification with significant limbal ischemia are classified as grades 3 or 4 (moderate to severe) and should receive immediate consultation with an ophthalmologist; transfer to a burn unit should be considered.

SYSTEMIC ABSORPTION AND TOXICITY FROM OCULAR EXPOSURES

Systemic absorption from ocular exposure has caused serious toxicity, morbidity, and even death.[14,23] Although the patterns of toxicity are characteristic of the xenobiotics involved, recognition may be delayed as a result of a failure to appreciate the eye as a significant route of absorption. Although transcorneal diffusion of xenobiotics is limited, there is substantial nasal mucosal absorption after nasolacrimal drainage, and absorption via conjunctival capillaries and lymphatics, which is markedly increased during conjunctival inflammation. Unlike the gastrointestinal route of absorption, there is no significant first-pass hepatic removal after ocular absorption; consequently, bioavailability is much greater.[20,23,39] If nasolacrimal outflow is normal, up to 80% of instilled drug may be absorbed systemically.[14] Unfortunately, by the time toxicity is apparent, there is no role for ocular decontamination to prevent further absorption. After instillation of eye drops, absorption is generally complete within 7 minutes.

Children appear to be at greatest risk, possibly because of the higher relative drug dose they experience when systemic absorption does occur.[14,34,39] Diligent attempts to comply with prescribed dosing in a struggling, crying infant may also result in excessive dosing. As eyedrop size (40–50 μL) exceeds ocular cul-de-sac capacity (30 μL), overflow often occurs and is assumed to represent a failed instillation, which leads to unnecessary reinstillation. Also, as doses of ocular medications are typically not adjusted based on patient weight, the consequences of equivalent degrees of systemic absorption are much greater for an infant than for an adult. Toxicity from eye drops is also a problem among the immunocompromised, probably because of the combination of greater use of potentially toxic ophthalmic medications and the presence of comorbid conditions.

Prevention of systemic toxicity from topical ophthalmic medications requires recognition of the risk, a careful history, use of the lowest effective concentration and dose, and patient education including proper administration instructions. To minimize inadvertent absorption, no more than one drop of any eyedrop solution should be instilled at one time in the superolateral corner of the eye while using gentle finger compression of the medial canthus to limit nasolacrimal drainage.[14,23]

MYDRIATICS

Mydriatics are used almost exclusively to dilate the pupils prior to diagnostic evaluation of the eyes. This common practice is not generally considered to be potentially dangerous; however, the risk may be substantial if the precautions outlined are not considered. Anticholinergic poisoning (Chap. 50), including substantial morbidity and mortality, is well described after ocular use of atropine, cyclopentolate, or scopolamine eyedrops, especially in infants.

The use of the α-adrenergic agonist phenylephrine eyedrops in a 10% solution may cause severe hypertension, subarachnoid hemorrhage, ventricular dysrhythmias, and myocardial infarction.[16] Fortunately, these effects are rare if the 2.5% ocular phenylephrine is used. Mydriatics can also precipitate acute angle closure glaucoma in susceptible individuals.

MIOTICS AND OTHER ANTIGLAUCOMA DRUGS

Miosis can be induced by the cholinesterase inhibitor echothiphate (sometimes used to treat glaucoma or accommodative esotropia) which can exacerbate asthma, parkinsonism, cardiac disease, and prolong the metabolism of certain medications such as succinylcholine.[23] Miosis can also be produced by use of direct cholinergic agonists, such as pilocarpine. Although absorption is limited, nausea and abdominal cramps can occur at recommended doses. After excessive dosing, salivation, diaphoresis, bradycardia, and hypotension may occur.

β-Adrenergic antagonists, such as timolol, levobunolol, metipranolol, carteolol, and betaxolol, are used to lower intraocular pressure but may cause a variety of adverse effects, including bradycardia, hypotension, myocardial infarction, syncope, transient ischemic attacks, congestive heart failure, exacerbation of asthma, and respiratory arrest. Timolol has exacerbated symptoms in patients with myasthenia gravis and is implicated in both causing and masking symptoms of hypoglycemia in diabetics.[41,42] Nonspecific complaints of anorexia, anxiety, depression, fatigue, hallucinations, headache, and nausea are also described after use of timolol eye drops. Despite the cardioselectivity of betaxolol, respiratory toxicity has occurred.[14]

Dipivefrin, an esterified epinephrine derivative sometimes used to treat glaucoma, can cause adrenergic systemic effects, although much fewer than those caused by epinephrine. Ophthalmic formulations of highly selective α_2-adrenergic agonists, brimonidine (Alphagan) and apraclonidine (Iopidine), were introduced to treat glaucoma.[14,45] Apraclonidine is expected to have a lower potential for toxicity because of limited CNS penetration. Systemic absorption of brimonidine eye drops in a child has led to bradycardia, hypotension, and a decreased level of consciousness, similar to the central effects of other α_2-adrenoceptor agonists (eg, clonidine),[6] apparently mediated through both α_2-adrenoceptors and imidazoline receptors[8] (see Chap. 62).

ANTIMICROBIALS

Life-threatening reactions to ophthalmic antimicrobials are unusual. Aplastic anemia has occurred after prolonged use of chloramphenicol eye preparations,[15] and Stevens-Johnson syndrome was reported after short-term use of ophthalmic sulfacetamide in a patient with a history of allergy to sulfa drugs.[20]

TOXICITY TO OCULAR STRUCTURES FROM NONOCULAR EXPOSURES

Ocular toxicity from systemic xenobiotics is almost always the result of chronic exposure, and the manifestations develop over a prolonged period of time. Thousands of xenobiotics are implicated, affecting every element of the visual system from the cornea to the optic cortex. Thorough discussion of this topic is beyond the scope of this text, but Table 19–2 lists examples of causative xenobiotics.[17,21] Many topical and systemic medications are associated with inflammation of the eye, ie, uveitis (inflammation of the iris, ciliary process, or choroids membrane).[18] Unlike many other ocular abnormalities caused by xenobiotics, uveitis should prompt immediate ophthalmologic consultation. Because in many cases the etiology is related to commonly prescribed medications, adverse drug effects should always be considered when patients present with visual abnormalities or unusual ocular findings.

In the setting of emergency care, xenobiotic-induced disturbances of normal vision from systemic exposures take many forms. Impaired near-vision from mydriasis, and diplopia or nystagmus from interference with normal control of extraocular movements, are examples of common, usually harmless visual effects. Serious effects generally result from injury or dysfunction of the neural elements from the retina to the cortex. Such toxicity can be direct (neurotoxic) or indirect (hypoxia, ischemia). Many xenobiotics historically reported to cause acute visual loss directly are no longer available.[21] Methanol and quinine are currently the most important xenobiotics that cause direct visual toxicity after acute oral poisoning. Many xenobiotics capable of causing vasospasm, hypotension, or embolization also cause acute visual loss (Table 19–4).[40] Blindness and other visual defects are described following recovery from severe toxicity with barbiturates and other sedative-hypnotics, opioids, carbon monoxide, and many others.[21]

TABLE 19–4. Xenobiotics Reported to Cause Visual Loss After Acute Exposures

Direct causes	Indirect causes[b]
Caustics	Vasoactive agents
Methanol	Amphetamines
Quinine	Cocaine
Lead[a]	Ergot alkaloids
Mercuric chloride[a]	Hypotension (eg, calcium channel blockers)
	Cisplatin
	Combined endocrine agents (thyrotropin-releasing hormone with gonadotropin-releasing hormone and glucagon)
	Embolization of foreign material (intravenous injection)

[a] Distinctly rare with these poisonings.

[b] Distinctly rare with use of these agents; visual loss often instantaneous, secondary to sudden hypotension, vascular spasm, or embolization.

OCULAR COMPLICATIONS OF DRUG ABUSE

In addition to the well-known ocular pupillary signs of opioid, cocaine, amphetamine, and phencyclidine toxicity, a number of complications may result from short-term or long-term use of these and other agents.[31] Quinine amblyopia (see Quinine earlier) caused by intravenous use of quinine-containing heroin is one of many ocular complications caused by injection of contaminants. Talc contaminants have resulted in talc retinopathy, which was first described after prolonged intravenous use of adulterated methylphenidate,[19] but was also noted after intravenous use of heroin, methadone,[32] codeine, meperidine, and pentazocine. Talc retinopathy develops only after extensive intravenous drug use. In one study of intravenous methadone abusers, only patients who had injected more than 9000 tablets developed this complication.[32] Infectious complications, such as fungal (*Candida, Aspergillus*) or bacterial (*Staphylococcus* spp, *Bacillus cereus*) endophthalmitis, are well known as both direct effects of intravenous drug use and secondary complications of AIDS. In addition to AIDS-related ophthalmic infections such as cytomegalovirus, cryptococcus, toxoplasmosis retinitis, and choroidal *Mycobacterium avium-intracellulare* complex (MAC), other disorders include retinal cotton-wool spots, conjunctival Kaposi sarcoma, and ocular motility disorders caused by infectious or neoplastic meningitis. Corneal defects have been noted after smoking cocaine alkaloid ("crack eye").[37] Cocaine that is either volatilized or inadvertently introduced by direct contact probably results in corneal anesthesia and loss of corneal protective reflex sensation. Minor trauma, such as eye rubbing, then leads to corneal epithelial defects. In addition, there appears to be an increased incidence of infectious keratitis and corneal ulceration in these patients. The ability of local anesthetics to interfere with corneal epithelial adhesion may also play a role.

SUMMARY

Both systemic and local toxicologic emergencies occur in the ophthalmic system. This discussion has focused on research in the treatment of damage to the eye caused by xenobiotics. Although the obvious physical injuries are apparent to the clinician, the more subtle clues to toxicologic mechanisms that involve the ophthalmic and neurologic systems are made only by a meticulous examination of the eye. A careful ophthalmic examination often leads to early recognition of a toxicologic emergency.

ACKNOWLEDGMENT

Martin J. Smilkstein and Frederick W. Fraunfelder contributed to this chapter in previous editions.

REFERENCES

1. Abelson MB, Udell IJ, Weston JH: Normal human tear pH by direct measurement. *Arch Ophthalmol.* 1981;99:301.
2. Adams RD, Victor M: Disorders of ocular movement and pupillary function. In: Adams RD, Victor M, eds: *Principles of Neurology*, 5th ed. New York: McGraw-Hill; 1993: 225-246.
3. Adler IN, Wlodyga RJ, Rope SJ: The effects of pH on contact lens wearing. *J Am Optom Assoc.* 1968;39:1000-1001.
4. Albert DM, Jakobiec FA, eds: *Principles and Practice of Ophthalmology*, 2nd ed. Philadelphia: WB Saunders; 2000.
5. Amir A, Turetz J, Chapman S, et al.: Beneficial effects of topical anti-inflammatory drugs against sulfur mustard-induced ocular lesions in rabbits. *J Appl Toxicol.* 2000;20(Suppl 1):S109-14.
6. Berlin R, Sing K, Lee U, Steiner R: Toxicity from the use of brimonidine ophthalmic solution in an infant and reversal with naloxone [abstract]. *J Toxicol Clin Toxicol.* 1997;35:506.
7. Brown VKH, Box VL, Simpson BJ: Decontamination procedures for skin exposed to phenolic substances. *Arch Environ Health.* 1975;30:1-6.
8. Burke J, Kharlamb A, Shan T, et al: Adrenergic and imidazoline receptor-mediated responses to UK-14,304-18 (brimonidine) in rabbits and monkeys. A species difference. *Ann N Y Acad Sci.* 1995;763:78-95.
9. Burns FR, Paterson CA: Prompt irrigation of chemical eye injuries may avert severe damage. *Occup Health Saf.* 1989;58:33-36.
10. Carney LG, Hill RM: Human tear pH: diurnal variations. *Arch Ophthalmol.* 1976;94:821-824.
11. Chen FS, Maurice DM: The pH in the precorneal tear film and under a contact lens measured with a fluorescent probe. *Exp Eye Res.* 1990;50: 251-259.
12. Davson H: *Physiology of the Eye*, 5th ed. New York: Pergamon Press; 1990.
13. Dean BS, Krenzelok EP: Cyanoacrylates and corneal abrasions. *J Toxicol Clin Toxicol.* 1989;27:169-172.
14. Flach AJ: Systemic toxicity associated with topical ophthalmic medications. *J Fla Med Assoc.* 1994;81:256-260.
15. Fraunfelder FT, Bagby GC, Kelly DJ: Fatal aplastic anemia following topical administration of ophthalmic chloramphenicol. *Am J Ophthalmol.* 1982;93:356-360.
16. Fraunfelder FT, Fraunfelder FW, Jensvold B: Adverse systemic effects from pledgets of topical ocular phenylephrine 10%. *Am J Ophthalmol.* 2002;134:624-625.
17. Fraunfelder FT, Fraunfelder FW, eds: *Drug-Induced Ocular Side Effects*, 5th ed. Boston: Butterworth Heinemann; 2001.
18. Fraunfelder FW, Rosenbaum JT: Drug-induced uveitis incidence, prevention and treatment. *Drug Saf.* 1997;17:197-207.
19. Friberg TR, Gragoudas ES, Regan CDJ: Talc emboli and macular ischemia in intravenous drug abuse. *Arch Ophthalmol.* 1979;97: 1089-1091.
20. Gottschalk HR, Stone Orville J: Stevens-Johnson syndrome from ophthalmic sulfonamides. *Arch Dermatol.* 1976;112:513-514.
21. Grant WM, Schuman JS: *Toxicology of the Eye*, 4th ed. Springfield, IL: Charles C Thomas; 1993: 1531.
22. Herr RD, White GL, Bernhisel K, et al: Clinical comparison of ocular irrigation fluids following chemical injury. *Am J Emerg Med.* 1991;9:228-231.
23. Hugues FC, Le Jeunne C: Systemic and local tolerability of ophthalmic drug formulations. An update. *Drug Saf.* 1993;8:365-380.
24. Javadi MA, Yazdani S, Sajjadi H, et al.: *Chronic and delayed-onset mustard gas keratitis: report of 48 patients and review of literature. Ophthalmology.* 2005;112:617-25.
25. Kimbrough RL, Okereke PC, Stewart RH: Conservative management of cyanoacrylate ankyloblepharon: a case report. *Ophthalmic Surg.* 1986;17:176-177.
26. Lang K: Treatment of phenol burns of the eye with polyethyleneglycol-400. *Z Arztl Fortbild (Jena).* 1969;63:705-708.
27. Mattox C: Table of toxicology. In: Albert DM, Jakobiec FA, eds: *Principles and Practice of Ophthalmology*, 2nd ed. Philadelphia: WB Saunders; 2000: 496-507.
28. McCarron MM, Schulze BW, Thompson GA, et al: Acute phencyclidine toxicity: incidence of clinical findings in 1,000 cases. *Ann Emerg Med.* 1981;10:237-242.
29. McCulley JP: Ocular hydrofluoric acid burns: animal model, mechanism of injury and therapy. *Trans Am Ophthalmol Soc.* 1990;88:649-684.
30. McCulley JP, Whiting DW, Petitt MG, Lauber SE: Hydrofluoric acid burns of the eye. *J Occup Med.* 1983;25:447-450.
31. McLane NJ, Carroll DM: Ocular manifestations of drug abuse. *Surv Ophthalmol.* 1986;30:298-311.
32. Murphy SB, Jackson WB, Dare JA: Talc retinopathy. *Can J Ophthalmol.* 1977;95:861-868.
33. Okumura T, Takasu N, Ishimatsu S, et al.: *Report on 640 victims of the Tokyo subway sarin attack. Ann Emerg Med.* 1996 Aug;28:129-35.
34. Palmer EA: How safe are ocular drugs in pediatrics? *Ophthalmology.* 1986;93:1038-1040.
35. Rihawi S, Frentz M, Reim M, Schrage NF: *Rinsing with isotonic saline solution for eye burns should be avoided. Burns.* 2008;34:1027-32. Epub 2008.
36. Saari KM, Leinonen J, Aine E: Management of chemical eye injuries with prolonged irrigation. *Acta Ophthalmol.* 1984;161(Suppl 16):52–59.
37. Sachs R, Zagelbaum BM, Hersh PS: Corneal complications associated with the use of crack cocaine. *Ophthalmology.* 1993;100:181-191.
38. Schrage NF, Kompa S, Haller W, Langefeld S: Use of an amphoteric lavage solution for emergency treatment of eye burns. First animal type experimental clinical considerations. *Burns.* 2002;28:782-786.
39. Shell JW: Pharmacokinetics of topically applied ophthalmic drugs. *Surv Ophthalmol.* 1982;26:207-217.
40. Smilkstein MJ, Kulig KW, Rumack BH: Acute toxic blindness: unrecognized quinine poisoning. *Ann Emerg Med.* 1987;16:98-101.
41. Velde TM, Kaiser FE: Ophthalmic timolol treatment causing altered hypoglycemic response in a diabetic patient. *Arch Intern Med.* 1983;143:1627.
42. Verkijk A: Worsening of myasthenia gravis with timolol maleate eye-drops. *Ann Neurol.* 1985;17:211-212.
43. Victor M, Adams RD: The effect of alcohol on the nervous system. *Res Publ Assoc Res Nerv Ment Dis.* 1953;32:526-573.
44. Wagoner MD: Chemical injuries of the eye: current concepts in pathophysiology and therapy. *Surv Ophthalmol.* 1997;41:275-312.
45. Walters TR: Development and use of brimonidine in treating acute and chronic elevations of intraocular pressure: a review of safety, efficacy, dose response, and dosing studies. *Surv Ophthalmol.* 1996;41(Suppl 1):S19-S26.
46. Webster RG, Slansky HH, Refojo MF, et al: The use of adhesive for the closure of corneal perforations: report of two cases. *Arch Ophthalmol.* 1968;80:705-709.
47. Zollman TM, Bragg RM, Harrison DA: Clinical effects of oleoresin capsicum (pepper spray) on the human cornea and conjunctiva. *Ophthalmology.* 2000;107:2186-2189.

CHAPTER 20

OTOLARYNGOLOGIC PRINCIPLES

William K. Chiang

Many xenobiotics adversely affect the senses of olfaction, gustation, and cochlear-vestibular functions. These toxic effects are not life threatening and frequently considered less important than they actually are to the patient. Because of the lack of standardized diagnostic techniques and normal parameters, such adverse effects may be overlooked and dismissed by healthcare providers, despite significant patient distress and dysfunction. This is particularly true for disorders of olfaction and gustation. This chapter reviews the anatomy and physiology of these senses; describes the effects of xenobiotics on these senses and examines the significant diagnostic information these senses contribute to identifying the presence of xenobiotics. Understanding the effects of xenobiotics on the senses may allow for early detection, which occasionally can be lifesaving.

OLFACTION

ANATOMY AND PHYSIOLOGY

Olfactory receptors are bipolar neurons located in the superior nasal turbinates and the adjacent septum. There are 10 to 20 million receptor cells per nasal chamber, and the receptor portion of the cell undergoes continuous renewal from the olfactory epithelium.[106,110] Renewed olfactory receptors regenerate neural connections to the olfactory bulb. These olfactory receptor neurons are distinctive in their ability to regenerate.[22] The axons of these cells form small bundles that traverse the fenestrations of the cribriform plate of the ethmoid bone to the dura. Within the dura, these bundles form connections with the olfactory bulb from which neural projections then connect to the olfactory cortex. There are extensive interconnections to other parts of the brain, such as the hippocampus, thalamus, hypothalamus, and frontal lobe, suggesting effects on other biologic functions.[106] Although primary odor detection is a function of the olfactory nerve (I), some irritant odors, such as ammonia and acetone, are transmitted through the trigeminal nerve (V) and its receptors.[40,144]

The actual olfactory receptor sites are structurally similar to the taste receptors of the mouth and the photoreceptors of the retina. The receptor is a single polypeptide chain consisting of approximately 350 amino acids, which folds back and forth on itself to traverse the cellular membrane seven times. The outer end of the polypeptide contains an amine group (N-terminal) and the cytosol end contains a carboxyl group (C-terminal). The transmembranous portions determine the receptor shape and characteristics of the binding site. When a molecule binds to a specific receptor site, the resultant conformational change leads to the activation of the G protein system and calcium and/or sodium channel activation and neurotransmission.[72]

Smelling is an extremely sensitive mechanism of detecting xenobiotics. Olfactory receptors can detect the presence of a few molecules of certain xenobiotics with a sensitivity that is superior to some of the most sophisticated laboratory detection instruments.[65]

LIMITATIONS OF THE OLFACTORY SENSES

The sense of smell can be extremely useful as a toxicologic warning system. Human olfaction is a variable trait.[5,117,174] For example, 40%–45% of people have specific anosmia (inability or loss of smell) for the bitter almond odor of cyanide.[41,86,117] There are limited data on the inheritance characteristics or genetic basis of these specific forms of anosmia. While some studies suggest that the ability to detect the odor of cyanide is a sex-linked recessive trait,[55] other studies yield conflicting results.[5,17,88] Women have a greater ability to detect androsterone, which is prominent in human underarm secretion.[65] Human olfaction usually can distinguish a mixture of no more than four xenobiotics,[92] and therefore specific odors may be masked by other stimuli.

Olfactory fatigue is the process of olfactory adaptation following exposure to a stimulus for a variable period of time. This leads to a temporal diminution of the smell. Unfortunately, this adaptation may lead to a false sense of security with continued exposure to a xenobiotic. For example, hydrogen sulfide, which inhibits cytochrome oxidase, is readily detectable as distinct and offensive at the very low concentration of 0.025 ppm. At the higher and potentially toxic concentration of 50 ppm, the odor is less offensive, and recognition may disappear after 2–15 minutes of exposure.[8,149] At higher concentration still when toxicity is likely, the onset of olfactory fatigue is even more rapid. The combination of the rapid onset of olfactory fatigue and systemic toxicity at high concentrations of hydrogen sulfide exposure has contributed to numerous fatalities (Chap. 126).[1,23,161]

In industrial settings, it is important to be aware of impaired olfactory function in any worker who may be exposed to chemical vapors or gases.[70,154] Such workers are at increased risk for toxic injury. The National Institute for Occupational Safety and Health (NIOSH) requires that an individual using an air-purifying respirator be capable of detecting the odor of a xenobiotic at concentrations below those producing toxicity.[6,154] Sensory perception at this concentration ensures that the individual can detect filter cartridge "breakthrough" or failure at a safe concentration.[154] The odor safety factor refers to the ratio of the time-weighted average (TWA) threshold limit value (TLV) to the odor threshold for a given xenobiotic. A xenobiotic with a high odor safety factor can be detected despite prolonged exposure.[6] Nontoxic xenobiotics, such as ethyl mercaptan, with a very high odor safety factor, can be added to xenobiotics that are odorless with lower safety factors, so that olfactory detection is predictable. This enhanced sensory awareness is the basis for the addition of mercaptans to the odorless natural gases used in the home so as to limit the potential for unrecognized hazardous exposure.

CLINICAL USE OF ODOR RECOGNITION

The recognition of odors has traditionally been considered an important diagnostic skill in clinical medicine. Some diseases can be diagnosed accurately by recognizable associated odors of various affected parts of the body such as the breath, sweat, urine, and wounds: diabetic ketoacidosis as a characteristically fruity odor; diphtheria as sweet; scurvy as putrid; typhoid fever as fresh-baked brown bread; and scrofula as stale beer.[35] Odors are also described for disorders of amino acid and fatty acid metabolism, such as phenylketonuria, maple syrup urine disease, hypermethioninemia, and isovaleric acidemia.[35]

The recognition of odors continues to be an important diagnostic skill for the rapid detection of some xenobiotics (Table 20–1). To increase awareness of odors of toxic xenobiotics, a "sniffing bar" of commonly available odors may be prepared.[60] Nontoxic xenobiotics that simulate the odors of toxic xenobiotics are placed in test tubes, numbered, and inserted in a test tube rack for circulation among staff. The sniffing bar, brief descriptions of clinical presentations, and a table of diagnostic odors (Table 20–1) may be used to teach the recognition of odors in medical toxicology.[60]

TABLE 20–1. Odors Suggestive of a Xenobiotic

Odor	Xenobiotic
Bitter almond	Cyanide
Carrots	Cicutoxin (water hemlock)
Disinfectants	Creosote, phenol
Eggs (rotten)	Carbon disulfide, disulfiram, hydrogen sulfide, mercaptans, *N*-acetylcysteine
Fish or raw liver (musty)	Aluminum phosphide, zinc phosphide
Fruit	Nitrites (amyl, butyl)
Garlic	Arsenic, dimethyl sulfoxide (DMSO), organic phosphorus compounds, phosphorus, selenium, tellurium, thallium,
Hay	Phosgene
Mothballs	Camphor, naphthalene, *p*-dichlorobenzene,
Pepper	*O*-chlorobenzylidene malonitrile
Rope (burnt)	Marijuana, opium
Shoe polish	Nitrobenzene
Sweet fruity	Acetone, chloral hydrate, chloroform, ethanol, isopropanol, lacquer, methylbromide, paraldehyde, trichloroethane
Tobacco	Nicotine
Vinegar	Acetic acid
Violets	Turpentine (metabolites excreted in urine)
Wintergreen	Methyl salicylate

TABLE 20–2. Xenobiotics Responsible for Disorders of Smell

Hyposmia/Anosmia	Dysosmia/Cacosmia/Phantosmia
Acrylic acid	Amebicides/antihelminthics: metronidazole
Antihyperlipidemics: cholestyramine, clofibrate, gemfibrozil, HMG-CoA reductase inhibitors	Anesthetics, local
Cadmium	Anticonvulsants: carbamazepine, phenytoin
Chlorhexidine	Antihistamines
Cocaine	Antihypertensives: ACE inhibitors, diazoxide
Formaldehyde	Antimicrobials
Gentamicin nose drops	Antiinflammatory
Hydrocyanic acid	Antirheumatics: allopurinol, colchicine, gold, D-penicillamine
Hydrocarbons (volatile)	Antiparkinson drugs: levodopa, bromocriptine
Hydrogen sulfide	Antithyroid drugs: methimazole, methylthiouracil, propylthiouracil
Methylbromide	β-Adrenergic antagonists
Nutritional	Calcium channel blockers
Vitamin B_{12} deficiency	DMSO (dimethylsulfoxide)
Zinc deficiency	Ethacrynic acid
Pentamidine	Insecticides
Sulfur dioxide	Lithium
	Nicotine
	Opioids
	Sympathomimetics
	Toothpastes
	Vitamin D

Anosmia = the loss of smell; cacosmia = sensation of a foul smell; dysosmia = a distorted perception of smell; hyposmia = a decreased perception of smell; phantosmia = sensation of smell without stimulus.

CLASSIFICATION OF OLFACTORY IMPAIRMENT

There are different types of olfactory dysfunction. Anosmia, the inability to detect odors, and hyposmia, a decrease in the perception of certain odors, are the most common forms of olfactory impairment. The etiology of olfactory impairment may be classified as conductive, from anatomic obstruction of inspired air, or perceptive, from dysfunction of the olfactory receptors or signal transmission. Most conductive olfactory dysfunction results in hyposmia, because the obstruction is usually incomplete.[106,141]

The most common causes of anosmia and hyposmia are viral infections, trauma, xenobiotics, tumors, and congenital and psychiatric disorders (Table 20–2).[40,127,133,141,144] Viral infections may result in olfactory impairment either by obstructing nasal airflow or by causing damage to the olfactory epithelium.[73] Trauma to the head or nose can shear fragile olfactory nerves crossing the cribriform plate.[144,163]

Chronic exposures to numerous xenobiotics are associated with olfactory dysfunction (Table 20–2). The most common toxic mechanism related is perceptive olfactory dysfunction. This may be a result of a direct injury, or of a structural alteration of the receptor or its components such as G proteins, adenylate cyclase, or receptor kinase.[71,72] Anosmia or hyposmia from hydrocarbons, formaldehyde, cadmium, and antineoplastics such as cytarabine results from direct effects on the receptor sites.[44,72,77] Local effects on the epithelium and the receptors from antibiotic nose drops may lead to temporary anosmia and hyposmia.[83,173] Inhaled corticosteroids may have local effects on the epithelium, as well as direct effects on both G proteins and adenylate cyclase.[74] Cocaine insufflation causes direct local effects, as well as effects on receptor functions.[61,63,69] Because of local effects of most xenobiotics and the regenerative ability of the olfactory receptor neurons, most xenobiotic-induced olfactory dysfunction is reversible.

Many individuals determined to have anosmia actually have congenital anosmia for select molecules, such as hydrogen cyanide, *N*-butyl mercaptan, trimethylamine, and isovaleric acid.[7,40] Some extreme forms of congenital anosmia are associated with other abnormalities, such as Kallmann syndrome, a hereditary form of anosmia associated with hypogonadotropic hypogonadism where agenesis of the olfactory bulbs and incomplete development of the hypothalamus are responsible for the anosmia.[40,144]

Dysosmia or parosmia is the distorted perception of smell (Table 20–2). Subclassifications of dysosmia include the perception of foul smell or cacosmia, the sensation of smell without a stimulus, or phantosmia, and the sensation of the smell of a burnt or metallic material, torqosmia.[141] The etiologies are classified as peripheral or central. Peripheral etiologies include abnormalities of the nose, sinuses, and upper respiratory tract. Central etiologies may be related to disorders such as Addison disease, hypothyroidism, temporal lobe epilepsy, psychosis, or pregnancy.[40,106,142] How these conditions actually alter the perception of smell is unclear. A number of xenobiotics with similar effects are listed in Table 20–2. Bromocriptine alters dopaminergic transmission and inhibits adenylate cyclase. Levodopa affects the dopaminergic transmission as well as chelating zinc, which is important in the maintenance of normal receptor functions.[72,74]

EVALUATION OF OLFACTORY IMPAIRMENT

General evaluation of olfactory function should include a detailed history, focusing on types, duration, and progression of symptoms, recent illnesses, head and nose trauma, sinus problems, family history, occupational history, hobbies, and xenobiotic history.[36,64] A physical examination with a detailed examination of the nasopharynx and sinuses should be performed to assess the potential for inflammation or structural abnormality. A simple set of olfactory stimulants, such as ground coffee, almond extract, peppermint extract, and musk, should be used to test each nostril individually with the patient's eyes closed.[64,144] Standardized smell tests such as the UPSIT (University of Pennsylvania Smell Identification Test) and the CCCRC (Connecticut Chemosensory Clinical Research Center) tests are commercially available, and a composite score based on a panel of tests can determine the degree of olfactory dysfunction.[98] Pungent odors or stimulation associated with ammonia, capsaicin, acetone, and menthol are dependent on the trigeminal nerve (V) olfactory function, which is mainly responsible for tactile pressure, pain, and temperature sensation in the mouth and nasal cavity. A patient who has olfactory nerve damage should be able to detect these substances; conversely, a person with hysteria may deny detection of these substances that should physiologically be recognized.[64,144,173] If a xenobiotic-mediated mechanism is suspected, the offending xenobiotic should be discontinued. A coronal CT of the sinuses and nose or an MRI of the brain should be obtained if structural abnormalities are suspected.[144,173] Gas chromatographic analysis of the urine may be useful in patients with fish odor syndrome associated with trimethylaminuria.[93,151] Complicated cases and patients with significant impairment should be referred to an otolaryngologist or neurologist.

GUSTATION

ANATOMY AND PHYSIOLOGY

Taste, the sensory interpretation of orally ingested materials, is determined by taste buds on the tongue, palate, throat, and upper third of the esophagus. The cells in the taste buds have a life span of 10 days and are constantly renewed.[11,141] The taste buds on the anterior two-thirds of the tongue and the palate are innervated by the facial (VII) nerve, those on the posterior one-third of the tongue by the glossopharyngeal (IX) nerve, and those on the laryngeal and epiglottal regions by the vagus (X) nerve. There are at least 13 known chemical taste receptors responsible for the five primary taste sensations—sweet, sour, bitter, brothy, and salty: two sodium receptor types; two potassium receptor types; one chloride receptor; one adenosine receptor; two inosine receptor; two sweet receptor types; two bitter receptor types; one glutamate receptor; and one hydrogen ion receptor.[66] One substrate will typically activate multiple taste receptors; the combined effects of these stimulated receptors determine the taste of the substance.[53]

The structure of the taste receptors is similar to that of the olfactory receptors, in that they are coupled to G proteins and sodium and calcium channels permitting neural stimulation. Each receptor is capable of interacting with various classes of xenobiotics, of varying sizes. The pH of the xenobiotic determines sour or acid taste, whereas sodium or potassium concentrations determine salty taste. Many xenobiotics such as sugars, glycols, aldehydes, ketones, amides, amino acids, inorganic salts of lead, and bretylium activate the sweet receptors. Bitter taste may be the result of long-chain organic substances containing nitrogen, or alkaloids, including quinine, strychnine, caffeine, and nicotine.[66] Umami taste is a more recently accepted primary taste, associated with a brothy flavor. The primary xenobiotic that stimulates umami receptor is glutamate, such as monosodium-L-glutamate. Umami receptor stimulation can be enhanced by such 5′-ribonucleotide monophosphates as IMP and GMP.[177] Salivary proteins, such as zinc-containing gustin and ebnerin, are important in the regulation of taste sensation.[72,76,95,150] These molecules may serve as binding proteins and growth factors for the regeneration of taste receptors. Taste is also affected significantly by the appreciation of aromas or odors and, to a lesser extent, by visual perception.[142]

CLASSIFICATION OF GUSTATORY DYSFUNCTION

Types of gustatory dysfunction include ageusia, the inability to perceive taste; hypogeusia, the diminished sensitivity of taste; and dysgeusia, the distortion of normal taste. There are several variations of dysgeusia, such as cacogeusia, which is a perceived foul, perverted, or metallic taste.[64,103] Taste impairment is commonly related to direct damage to the taste receptors, adverse effects on their regeneration, or effects on receptor mechanisms.[73] These effects can result from a xenobiotic, disease, aging, and nutritional disorder (Table 20–3).[59,66,132,159] Any abnormality that interferes with either the direct contact of a xenobiotic with the gustatory cells of the tongue or cranial nerves VII, IX, or X dramatically affects taste.[141] Most common forms of xenobiotic-induced dysgeusia are related to direct effects on the

TABLE 20–3. Xenobiotics Responsible for Alterations of Taste

Hypogeusia/Ageusia	Dysgeusia	Metallic Taste
Local	*Local*	ACE inhibitors
Chemical and thermal burns	Chemical burn	Acetaldehyde
	Radiation therapy	Allopurinol
Radiation therapy	*Systemic*	Arsenicals
Systemic	ACE inhibitors	Cadmium
ACE inhibitors	Adriamycin	Ciguatoxin
Amiloride	Amphotericin B	Copper
Amrinone	Botulism (in recovery)	*Coprinus* spp
Carbon monoxide	Bretylium	Dipyridamole
Cocaine	Carbamazepine	Disulfiram
DMSO (dimethylsulfoxide)	DMSO (dimethylsulfoxide)	Ethambutol
	5-Fluorouracil	Ferrous salts
Gasoline	Griseofulvin	Flurazepam
Hydrochlorothiazide	Isotretinoin	Iodine
Methylthiouracil	Levodopa	Lead
Nitroglycerin	NSAIDs	Levamisole
NSAIDs	Nicotine	Lithium
Penicillamine	Nifedipine	Mercury
Propranolol	Phenylthiourea (hereditary)	Methotrexate
Pyrethrins	Quinine	Metformin
Smoking	Zinc deficiency	*Metoclopramide*
Spironolactone		Metronidazole
Triazolam		Pentamidine
		Procaine penicillin
		Propafenone
		Snake envenomation
		Tetracycline

taste receptor site or effects related to receptor mechanisms such as G proteins, adenylate cyclase, and calcium channels.[91] Other forms of dysgeusia may result from direct stimulation of chemical receptors by xenobiotics.[66,72]

Angiotensin-converting enzyme (ACE) inhibitors commonly cause gustatory impairment, usually hypogeusia and dysgeusia.[16,61,105,175] ACE inhibitors work by inhibiting zinc-dependent ACE, and chelating zinc from taste receptors and salivary proteins results in gustatory dysfunction. Calcium channel blockers act by inhibiting calcium channels of the taste receptor mechanisms.[66] Many diuretics cause zinc depletion by enhancing zinc elimination in the urine,[72] whereas furosemide and spironolactone may also chelate zinc. Numerous xenobiotics also cause gustatory dysfunction through variable degrees of zinc chelation, among them amrinone, ethambutol, hydralazine, methyldopa, the nonsteroidal antiinflammatory drugs (NSAIDs), the antithyroid agents, penicillamine, and phenytoin.[66,72,176] Metals such as arsenic, mercury, chromium, and lead may either chelate zinc or replace zinc in salivary proteins because of a higher level of affinity. Antineoplastics and the antimicrotubular colchicine inhibit cellular division and taste-receptor regeneration. The oral antiseptic chlorhexidine directly alters taste-receptor function.[52] Acetazolamide causes cacogeusia when carbonated beverages are consumed. The exact mechanism is unclear, but is postulated to be a result of the inhibition of carbonic anhydrase causing carbon dioxide accumulation and an increased tissue bicarbonate.[72,84,107]

HEARING

ANATOMY AND PHYSIOLOGY

Normal hearing begins when sound waves are captured by the external auricle, traverse the external auditory canal, and are conducted to the tympanic membrane, the three auditory ossicles of the middle ear, and through the oval window to the perilymph in the scala vestibuli of the cochlea (Figs. 20–1 and 20–2). The sound wave is then transferred through the Reissner membrane at the roof of the cochlear duct, to the endolymph and the organ of Corti.[48,155] The specialized hair cells of the organ of Corti convert mechanical waves into neurologic signals. The hair cells contain cross-linked stereocilia projections that detect transmitted shear forces, which lead to the influx of potassium from the endolymph through opened potassium channels.[38,96] Depolarization of the hair cells results in calcium influx and neurotransmitter release to the cochlear nerve. Neurologic signals from the cochlear nerve are conducted to the cochlear nucleus of the pons; bilateral projections are then sent to the superior olivary nucleus of the midbrain, nuclei of lateral lemnisci, inferior colliculus, medial geniculate body of the thalamus, and then to the auditory cortex of the temporal lobe.[155] Interruption or damage to any part of the hearing mechanism may lead to auditory impairment.

The anatomy and physiology of the cochlea and its importance in the biomechanics of hearing are reviewed in order to better understand the potential for xenobiotic injury. The word *cochlea* is derived from the Greek word *kochlias*, meaning snail, and describes its general structure—a 2.5-turn, spirally wound tube. The cochlea is further divided into three inner tubular structures: the upper tube or scala vestibuli, the middle tube or cochlear duct, and the lower tube or scala tympani. The scala vestibuli and the scala tympani contain the perilymph fluid. The cochlear duct contains endolymph fluid, the Reissner membrane at the roof, and the organ of Corti.[155] The cochlear fluids serve multiple functions: to conduct sound waves to the hair cells; to provide nutrients for and remove waste from the cells lining the cochlear duct; to control pressure distribution in the cochlea; and to maintain an electrochemical gradient for the function of the hair cells. The sodium concentration of the perilymph is similar to that of the extracellular fluid, and the potassium concentration of the endolymph is similar to that of the

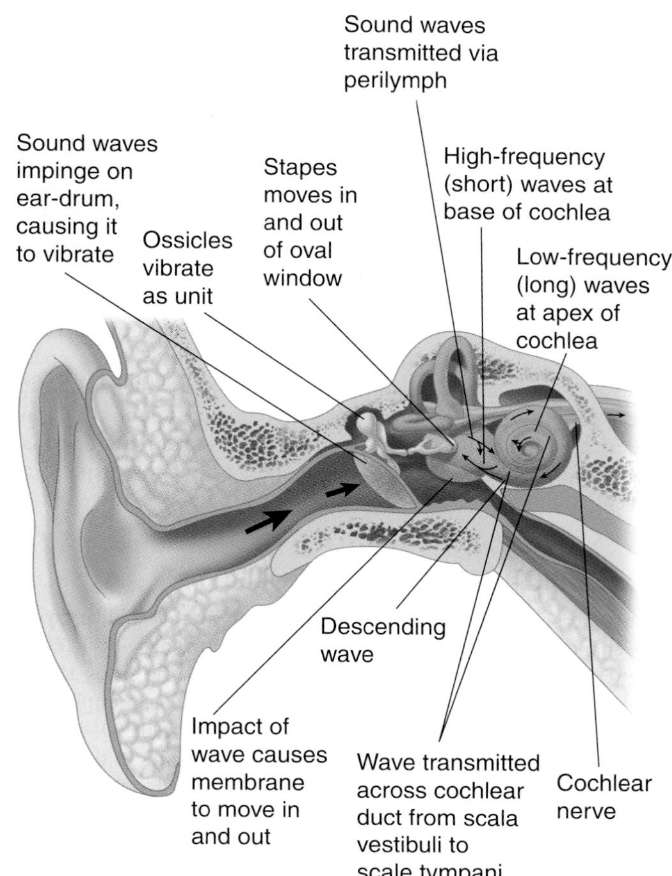

FIGURE 20–1. Pathways of sound conduction in the ear.

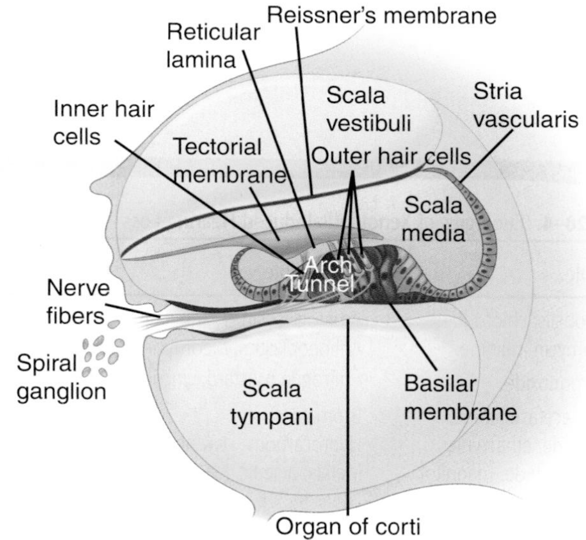

FIGURE 20–2. Cross-section of the organ of Corti.

intracellular fluid.[50] Any significant alterations of the sodium or potassium concentrations will depress the cochlear potential and function. The stria vascularis controls the production of the cochlear fluids and the repolarization of the hair cells, and maintains the electrochemical gradient between the endolymph and the perilymph. The stria vascularis contains a high concentration of the oxidative enzymes, Na^+-K^+-adenosine triphosphatase (ATPase), adenylate cyclase, and carbonic anhydrase, which are all highly susceptible to xenobiotics.[18,77,139]

Although human speech is composed of sounds in the frequency of 250–3000 Hz, humans can normally detect sounds in the frequency range of 20–20,000 Hz.[116] The cochlea is a "tuned" structure with varying width and stiffness, such that different regions can receive different sound waves. The stiffer and wider base of the cochlea serves as a receptacle for higher-frequency sounds, whereas the apex is responsible for receiving the lower-frequency sounds.[48] Because various regions of the cochlea are susceptible to different forms of injury, appropriate audiologic testing should be tailored specifically to each patient.[25]

XENOBIOTIC-INDUCED OTOTOXICITY

Ototoxicity includes effects on the cochlear and vestibular system. This chapter focuses on cochlear toxicity. Quinine and salicylates were widely recognized in the 1800s and streptomycin in the 1940s as causes of ototoxicity.[78,134] Several hundred xenobiotics have been implicated as causes of other reversible or irreversible ototoxicity (Table 20–4).[21,82,89,113] Ototoxic xenobiotics primarily affect two different sites in the cochlea: the organ of Corti—specifically the outer hair cells—and the stria vascularis. Because of the limited regenerative capacity of the sensory hair cells and other supporting cells, when significant cellular damage occurs, the loss is often permanent.[42,48,78,153] Although cell death of the outer hair cells from inflammation and necrosis is expected when sufficient insults occur, apoptotic cell death is now postulated to be a major mechanism of ototoxicity from certain xenobiotics such as cisplatin and aminoglycosides.[18,21,39,78,82,131] Inhibition of caspases and calpain associated with apoptosis of the hair cells is demonstrated to decrease ototoxicity from cisplatin and aminoglycosides in animals.[131,152] Evidence supports the concept that otic injury can be potentiated by loud noises. Although the actual cellular mechanisms for many forms of ototoxicity remain unclear,[172] some of the mechanisms are known.[56] Loop diuretics, such as furosemide, bumetanide, and ethacrynic acid, cause physiologic dysfunction and edema at the stria vascularis, resulting in reversible hearing loss.[78,101,168] The underlying mechanisms appear to be the inhibition of potassium pumps and G proteins associated with adenyl cyclase.[9] Studies of loop diuretics demonstrate decreased potassium activity in the endolymph and a decreased endocochlear potential.[136] Permanent hearing loss associated with furosemide and ethacrynic acid is also reported, and may be related to direct interference with oxidative metabolism in the outer hair cells.[90,101,136]

Salicylates are a well-known cause of ototoxicity. Aspirin (acetylsalicylic acid)-induced hearing impairment was first reported in 1877.[85] Salicylate-induced hearing loss is generally mild to moderate (a 20–40 dB loss) and reversible.[15,80] Animal studies demonstrate immediate hearing impairment with the use of high doses of salicylates.[14,102,103,123] The mechanism of salicylate-induced ototoxicity is unclear, although multiple factors are postulated. Salicylates and other NSAIDs inhibit cyclooxygenase, which converts arachidonic acid to prostaglandin G_2 and prostaglandin H_2. These effects may interfere with Na^+-K^+-ATPase pump function at the stria vascularis, and also decrease cochlear blood flow.[27,45,85] A reversible decrease in outer hair cell turgor secondary to membrane permeability changes may impair otoacoustic emissions.[122,126] In support of these theories, pretreatment of animals with leukotriene antagonists and α-adrenergic receptor antagonists attenuates or prevents salicylate-induced ototoxicity.[85]

NSAIDs and quinine also cause reversible hearing loss, particularly at the higher frequencies.[29,78] Occasionally, quinine-induced hearing loss may be permanent.[78,140] The primary mechanism is related to prostaglandin inhibition.[85] Quinine inhibits phospholipase A_2 enzyme, which converts phospholipids to arachidonic acid. Quinine also inhibits calcium channels that interact with prostaglandins.[85]

Certain antineoplastics, such as cisplatin, vinblastine, and vincristine, can cause permanent ototoxicity.[78] Cisplatin is the most toxic of the group, with clinically apparent hearing loss noted in 30%–70% of the patients receiving doses of 50–100 mg/m^2. These antineoplastics typically damage the outer hair cells but may also affect the stria vascularis.[78] The underlying mechanisms may be related to the inhibition of adenyl cyclase in the stria vascularis, the inhibition of protein synthesis, and the formation of oxygen free radicals.[9,78,145] The generation of oxygen free radicals and the depletion of antioxidants result in the irreversible damage to the hair cells.[47] Furthermore, cranial radiation will cause synergistic toxicity if radiation precedes cisplatin therapy. Various antioxidants and free radical scavengers prevent cisplatin-induced ototoxicity in animals.[94,108,111,128,135,157,171] Newer xenobiotics also prevent cisplatin-induced toxicity in animals, perhaps preventing oxidative injury–induced apoptosis to hair cells.[131] Amifostine, a precursor to a thiol free radical scavenger, is available to prevent cisplatin-induced nephrotoxicity. However, amifostine does not appear to prevent cisplatin-induced ototoxicity.[138]

The aminoglycosides are best known for their association with irreversible ototoxicity,[121] but they are not concentrated in the cochlea. It is postulated that toxicity is related to the metabolites of aminoglycosides and not the parent compounds because toxicity can be reproduced in vivo, but not in vitro.[139] The endolymph concentration of gentamicin is approximately 10% of that in the serum. Neomycin and kanamycin are the most ototoxic, although all aminoglycosides are potentially toxic.[90] With the development of the newer aminoglycosides and therapeutic drug monitoring, the incidence of aminoglycoside-related ototoxicity appears to be decreasing. The reported rates of ototoxicity for the more commonly used aminoglycosides gentamicin and tobramycin are between 5% and 8%.[100] In China, where aminoglycosides are readily available as nonprescription medications, as much as 66% of deaf-mutism may be directly related to aminoglycoside toxicity.[54,97] A genetic predisposition to aminoglycoside-induced ototoxicity has been identified.[68] The genetic transmission appears to be maternal via mitochondrial DNA.[51] Chinese patients with this genetic defect may

TABLE 20–4. Etiologies of Xenobiotic-Induced Hearing Loss

Reversible	Irreversible
Antimicrobials: chloroquine, erythromycin, quinine	Aminoglycosides
Carbon monoxide	Antineoplastics: bleomycin, cisplatin, nitrogen mustard, vincristine, vinblastine
Diuretics: acetazolamide, bumetanide, ethacrynic acid, furosemide, mannitol	Bromates
NSAIDs	Hydrocarbons: styrene, toluene, xylene
Salicylates	Metals: arsenic, lead, mercury

suffer rapid and severe hearing loss compared to whites with a similar aminoglycoside exposure.[131]

Several mechanisms of ototoxicity have been postulated including antagonism of calcium channels of the outer hair cells of the cochlea, blocking transduction of the hair cells and resulting in acute, reversible hearing deficits as well as binding to polyphosphoinositides of cell membranes to alter their functions. Polyphosphoinositides are essential for the generation of the second messengers diacylglycerol and inositol triphosphate and their ultimate cellular function, for the maintenance of lipid membrane structure and permeability, and as a source for arachidonic acid.[165] Aminoglycosides interact with iron and copper to generate free radicals, damaging the hair cells. Aminoglycosides also inhibit ornithine decarboxylase which is important for cellular recovery following an injury and makes the cell more susceptible to toxicity.[139] The outer hair cells of the cochlea are increasingly susceptible to aminoglycosides and damage progresses from the inner row of the outer hair cells to the basal turn of the cochlea, and, ultimately, to the apex.[4,7,90,130]

The risks of ototoxicity are increased with a duration of therapy of greater than 10 days, concomitant use of other ototoxic xenobiotics, and the development of elevated serum concentrations.[7,49,137] There is no evidence that single daily dosing of aminoglycosides alters the risk of ototoxicity.[118,166] Loop diuretics increase aminoglycoside toxicity by increasing aminoglycoside penetration into the endolymph. In animal models, certain free radical scavengers, such as glutathione, amifostine, and deferoxamine, decrease aminoglycoside-induced ototoxicity.[57,140,158,164,167] Fosfomycin, a phosphonic antibiotic, has limited efficacy in reducing aminoglycoside-induced ototoxicity, and salicylates are also suggested to reduce ototoxicity.[115,149] Salicylates may act as free radical scavengers in low doses. Leupeptin and Z-DEVD-FNK, a calpain and caspase inhibitor, respectively, that affects the apoptotic pathway, is demonstrated in animal models to decrease ototoxicity.[30,56,148,152] Further studies are required to determine their applicability to humans.

Erythromycin, vancomycin, and their respective analogs are ototoxic. There are a number of reports of hearing loss following erythromycin therapy in humans and an animal study supporting the ototoxic potential. Most deficits in humans are transient, although several cases of permanent hearing loss are reported.[19,20] The mechanisms of toxicity remain unclear, although the proposed effects are on the central auditory pathways. Erythromycin-induced hearing loss occurs at both lower and higher frequencies for speech, allowing for recognition in the early stages of ototoxicity.[19] Ototoxicity from the newer macrolide antibiotics clarithromycin and azithromycin is also reported.

The evidence for vancomycin-induced ototoxicity is less convincing. Although numerous cases of presumed vancomycin-related ototoxicity are reported, concomitant use of other ototoxic antibiotics was common or audiometric studies were not performed. In limited animal studies, vancomycin alone does not induce ototoxicity, but the xenobiotic increases ototoxicity when administered concomitantly with an aminoglycoside. Vancomycin analogs such as teicoplanin and daptomycin probably have similar ototoxic potentials.

Bromates are among the most extensively studied ototoxic xenobiotics.[31,33,99,124] Bromates are used in hair "neutralizers," bread preservatives, and as fuses in explosive devices.[79,124,160] The stria vascularis and hair cells of the organ of Corti are irreversibly damaged.[124] Substantial exposure to bromates may also cause renal failure which in turn increases its ototoxic potential.[79,124]

It is intriguing that xenobiotics such as the bromates, loop diuretics, and aminoglycosides primarily affect both the cochlea and the kidneys. One possible explanation is that the stria vascularis and the renal tubules have similar functions in maintaining electrochemical gradients.[124,125] However, renal tubules may regenerate while damage to the hair cells and the stria vascularis of the cochlea is more likely to be permanent.

Other xenobiotics implicated as ototoxins are carbon monoxide, lead, arsenic, mercury, toluene, xylene, and styrene.[75,154] However, both human and animal data are quite limited. Carbon disulfide, carbon tetrachloride, and trichloroethylene are also suspected of being ototoxic, but toxicity has not been demonstrated in humans.[75,154] Because exposures to xenobiotics are frequently occupational, they are of great concern as they may potentiate or be additive to other types of occupational hearing impairments.[87,129]

High-frequency hearing is most vulnerable, and early or limited impairment may not be noticeable unless audiometry, especially at 8000 kHz and above, is performed.[165] These hearing tests can be performed in infants using the measurement of auditory brainstem response.[12]

NOISE-INDUCED HEARING IMPAIRMENT

Noise-induced hearing impairment has been recognized for hundreds of years, but became a great concern and increasingly prevalent with the industrial revolution and the discovery of gunpowder.[48] Some of the anatomic changes in the organ of Corti and the audiometric features of noise-induced hearing impairment were well described by 1900.[2,3,104] Unfortunately, few longitudinal studies on noise-induced hearing impairment have been performed.

Although noises of sufficient magnitude may cause hearing impairment with limited exposure, most noise-induced hearing losses result from preventable prolonged cumulative occupational exposure. NIOSH has estimated that up to 1.7 million workers in the United States between 50 and 59 years of age have significant occupation-related hearing loss.[116] Noise can be defined as any unwanted sound, which can be further characterized by duration, time pattern (continuous, intermittent, or impulsive), frequency, and intensity. The intensity is measured in sound pressure levels (SPLs) and expressed in a logarithmic scale in decibels (dB). The intensity of a normal conversation is approximately 65 dB (Table 20–5).[116] The risk of noise-induced hearing loss

TABLE 20–5. Typical Sound Levels on the Decibel Scale

Sound	Decibels
Weakest sound that humans can detect	10
Quiet bedroom, soft whisper	20
Broadcast studio	25–30
Insulated lounge	50
Normal conversation	65
Television-audio	70
Vacuum cleaner	80
Machine press, subway car (35 mph)	95
Spray painting, snowmobile	105
Power saw	110
Car horn	115
Armored personnel carrier; ear pain begins	120
Jet plane engine, gunshot	145
Highest sound level that can occur	194

TABLE 20–6. OSHA Standard for Permissible Noise Exposure

dBA[a]	Duration of Exposure Per Day in Hours
85	16
90	8
92	6
95	4
97	3
100	2
102	1.5
105	1
110	0.5
115	≤0.25

[a] Decibels using the A-scale filter.

is related to cumulative duration of exposure, intensity, and individual susceptibility.[114,119,170] Much of the risk assessment of noise-induced hearing loss is inexact. Most authorities agree that sounds with maximal intensity below 75–80 dB will not cause hearing impairment, regardless of the duration of exposure.[114] At higher intensity, the risk of hearing impairment increases with increased duration of exposure. Continued occupational exposure at 90–94 dB typically causes some high-frequency hearing loss in approximately 10 years.[2,119] Further exposure results in hearing loss in the lower-frequency range. The Occupational Safety and Health Administration (OSHA) established guidelines for permissible occupational noise exposure based on an analysis of the average intensity and duration of exposure (Table 20–6).[2,170]

The pathophysiology of noise-induced hearing impairment is related to an excessive energy impact on the cochlea, but the exact biochemical changes are unclear. Apoptotic death of the hair cells has now been demonstrated and inhibition of apoptosis pathways mitigates noise-induced toxicity in animal models. A limited exposure to excessive noise results in a temporary hearing impairment or temporary threshold shift with a duration of hours to weeks. However, prolonged exposure results in a permanent threshold shift or hearing impairment.[3,48,170] Initially, outer hair cells are lost, but more significant exposures result in damage to both inner and outer hair cells and all supporting structures in the organ of Corti. Cochlear nerve fibers degenerate after hair cell damage.[48,170] The section of the cochlea most at risk from loud noises is at the 9–13 mm region (the total length is 32 mm).[104] This region is responsible for hearing at the 3000–6000 kHz range, corresponding to the typical noise-induced hearing loss pattern.

Much of the clinical assessment and monitoring of noise-induced hearing loss is based on pure tone hearing loss, demonstrating an audiometric deficit at 3000–6000 kHz.[116,119,170] Although human speech is composed mainly of low frequency sounds, the ability to perceive the higher frequency sounds is extremely important in speech recognition. For this reason, the major impairment in patients with noise-induced hearing loss is an inability to discriminate speech, particularly from background noise.[2,37] Currently, the science of the investigation of speech discrimination is limited with extensive areas for research.

Blast injury to the ear results from exposure of extremely short duration, but very high-intensity sound waves, usually greater than 140 dB. Military personnel are particularly at risk.[28,120,162,165] Hearing loss from blast injury may be related to rupture of the tympanic membrane, disruption of the ossicles, temporary cochlear dysfunction, and permanent cochlear dysfunction from labyrinthine fistulae and basilar membrane rupture.[26] When a large tympanic membrane rupture or disruption of the ossicles occurs, surgical intervention may be required to treat hearing impairment.[26]

Prevention of any type of noise-induced hearing loss remains the best solution. Various hearing-protection devices are available if the noise exposure cannot be reduced. Better monitoring and more longitudinal studies are required on noise-induced hearing loss. Exposure to xenobiotics that can impair hearing may have synergistic effects with noise-induced hearing loss.[87,89] These factors should be considered when noise exposure is evaluated. Furthermore, noise exposure is not limited to the workplace. Significant noise exposure may occur at home or from leisure activities, such as power tools, stereo, and ambient exposure.[13,34,67,119] The impact of noise exposure outside of the workplace has only recently attracted the attention of investigators.

TINNITUS

Tinnitus is the sensation of sound not resulting from mechano-acoustic or electric signals. Virtually all humans experience tinnitus during their lives. The exact mechanism or mechanisms resulting in tinnitus are largely unknown.[143] Tinnitus may or may not be associated with hearing loss. Several theories are proposed, but none is completely satisfactory. Tinnitus may result from spontaneous neurologic discharges when the hair cells or cochlear nerve is injured. Altered sound perception may result from local or central effects when feedback mechanisms are interrupted.[43,46,81,103] Severing the cochlear nerve terminates tinnitus in less than half of affected patients, suggesting important central mechanisms.[10] Furthermore, certain etiologies of tinnitus, such as migraine headache and temporal lobe seizures, do not affect hearing directly. *N*-methyl-D-aspartate (NMDA) glutamate receptor activation (and enhanced cochlear signal transmission) has been implicated as a mechanism for tinnitus in animal models; NMDA receptor activation may result from cyclooxygenase inhibition or neurologic injuries.[69] Xenobiotics, including salicylate, may cause hair cell dysfunction and may modify neurotransmission centrally in both the cochlear nucleus and the inferior colliculis.[58,169] Although the probable sites involved in tinnitus may be classified as peripheral (external ear, middle ear, or cochlear [VIII]), central, or extra-auditory (vascular, nasopharyngeal), some etiologies may affect peripheral and central sites, and many etiologies remain unknown.[32,46,103]

Numerous xenobiotics are associated with tinnitus (Table 20–7), but the incidence is probably low and the implied relationships have usually been supported only by case reports.[31,146,147] Tinnitus may or may not be associated with transient or permanent hearing loss. It is probable that the xenobiotics associated with hearing loss affect cochlear function, while those that produce tinnitus without hearing loss probably act on signal transmission at the cochlear and the CNS. Xenobiotics that frequently produce tinnitus are streptomycin, neomycin, indomethacin, doxycycline, ethacrynic acid, furosemide, heavy metals, and high doses of caffeine.[62,146,147] Only a few xenobiotics, such as quinine and salicylates, consistently cause tinnitus at toxic doses.[14,46] These two xenobiotics also serve as examples of how the presence of tinnitus may be an indicator of drug toxicity.

Tinnitus associated with salicylates usually begins when serum concentrations are in the high therapeutic or low toxic range of approximately 20–40 mg/dL.[109] Membrane permeability changes cause a loss of outer hair cell turgor in the organ of Corti which may impair acoustic emissions, explaining tinnitus to some extent[122,123,126] (see Xenobiotic-Induced Ototoxicity earlier). Before the wide availability of serum salicylate measurements , physicians treating gout or rheumatoid arthritis often titrated the salicylate dosage until tinnitus developed.[34] Tinnitus

TABLE 20–7. Xenobiotics That Cause Tinnitus
β-Adrenergic antagonists
Anticonvulsants: carbamazepine
Antidepressants: cyclic antidepressants, amoxapine, lithium, trancylcypromine
Antifungals: amphotericin B
Antihistamines
Antimicrobials: Aminoglycosides, vancomycin, dapsone, tetracyclines, sulpha drugs, metronidazole, thiabendazole, clindamycin
Antineoplastics: cisplatin, nitrogen mustard, 6-aminonicotinamide, methotrexate, vinblastine
Antiparasitics: chloroquine, hydroxychloroquine
Antipsychotics: haloperidol, molindone
Bromates
Cinchona alkaloids: quinine, quinidine
Diuretics: furosemide, ethacrynic acid, bumetanide
Hydrocarbons: benzene
Local anesthetics: mepivacaine, bupivacaine, lidocaine
Nonsteroidal antiinflammatory drugs
Oral contraceptives
Salicylates
Sympathomimetics: caffeine, theophylline, metaproterenol, albuterol, methylphenidate

and other signs and symptoms of salicylism (Chap. 35) should be sufficient for physicians to diagnose salicylate toxicity before serum salicylate concentrations are available. However, tinnitus may not be evident in patients with hearing impairment despite significantly elevated salicylate concentrations.[109] The classic constellation of symptoms of quinine and salicylate toxicity, called cinchonism, includes nausea, vomiting, tinnitus, and visual disturbances.[4,24,112] Because serum quinine concentrations are not readily available, symptoms of quinine toxicity define the clinical diagnosis (Chap. 58).[156]

SUMMARY

Numerous xenobiotics commonly affect the sense of smell, taste, and hearing. They may cause significant patient morbidity. Some of the events may be predictable, whereas others will require monitoring and appropriate testing. Significant patient risk and discomfort may be avoided by an understanding of the basic pathophysiology of the otolaryngologic organs and by a heightened suspicion on the part of healthcare providers. Current knowledge about the pathophysiology of xenobiotics and these special organs at the molecular level is expanding rapidly. It is particularly encouraging and exciting to understand and witness the development of potential therapeutic xenobiotics.

REFERENCES

1. Adelson L, Sunshine I: Fatal hydrogen sulfide poisoning. Report of three cases occurring in a sewer. *Arch Pathol.* 1966;81:375-380.
2. Alberti PW: Noise-induced hearing loss. *BMJ.* 1992;304:522.
3. Alberti PW: Occupational hearing loss. In: Ballenger JJ, ed: *Diseases of the Nose, Throat, Ear, Head, and Neck,* 14th ed. Philadelphia: Lea & Febiger; 1991:1053-1068.
4. Alvan G, Karlsson KK, Villen T: Reversible hearing impairment related to quinine blood concentration in guinea pigs. *Life Sci.* 1989;45:751-755.
5. Amoore JE, Hautala E: Odor as an aid to chemical safety: odor thresholds compared with threshold limit values and volatilities for 214 industrial chemicals in air and water diluted. *J Appl Toxicol.* 1983;3:272-290.
6. Amoore JE: Olfactory genetics and anosmia. In: Beidler LM, ed: *Handbook of Sensory Physiology,* Vol 4. Chemical Senses, Part I. Berlin: Springer-Verlag; 1971: 145-156.
7. Assael BM, Parini R, Rusconi F: Ototoxicity of aminoglycoside antibiotics in infants and children. *Pediatr Infect Dis.* 1982;1:357-365.
8. Audeau FM, Gnanaharan C, Davey K: Hydrogen sulfide poisoning: associated with pelt processing. *N Z Med J.* 1985;98:145-147.
9. Bagger-Sjoback D, Filipek CS, Schacht J: Characteristics and drug responses of cochlear and vestibular adenylate cyclase. *Arch Otorhinolaryngol.* 1980;228:217-222.
10. Barrs DM, Brackmann DE: Translabyrinthine nerve section: effect on tinnitus. *J Laryngol Otolaryngol.* 1984;98(S9):287-293.
11. Beidler LM: Renewal of cells within taste buds. *J Cell Biol.* 1965;27:263-272.
12. Bergstorm L, Thompson PL: Ototoxicity. In: Brown RD, Daigneault EA, eds: *Pharmacology of Hearing: Experimental and Clinical Basis.* New York: Wiley; 1981:119-134.
13. Bess FH, Poynor RE: Noise-induced hearing loss and snowmobiles. *Arch Otolaryngol.* 1974;99:45-51.
14. Boettcher FA, Bancroft BR, Salvi RJ, et al: Effects of sodium salicylate on evoked-response measures of hearing. *Hear Res.* 1989;42:129-142.
15. Boettcher FA, Salvi RJ: Salicylate ototoxicity: review and synthesis. *Am J Otolaryngol.* 1991;12:33-47.
16. Boyd O: Captopril-induced taste disturbance. *Lancet.* 1993;342:304.
17. Brown KS, Robinette RR: No simple pattern of inheritance in ability to smell solutions of cyanide. *Nature.* 1967;215:406-408.
18. Brown RD, Penny JE, Henley CM, et al: Ototoxicity drugs and noise. In: Evered D, Lawrenson G, eds: *Tinnitus.* Ciba Foundation Symposium 85. London: Pitman; 1981: 151-171.
19. Brummett RE, Traynor J, Brown R, et al: Cochlear damage resulting from kanamycin and furosemide. *Acta Otolaryngol.* 1975;80:86-92.
20. Brummett RE: Ototoxicity of erythromycin and analogues. *Otolaryngol Clin North Am.* 1993;26:811-819.
21. Brummett RE: Ototoxicity of vancomycin and analogues. *Otolaryngol Clin North Am.* 1993;26:821-827.
22. Buckland ME, Cunninghamb AM: Alterations in the neurotrophic factors BDNE, GDNF and CNTF in the regenerating olfactory system. *Ann N Y Acad Sci.* 1998;855:260-265.
23. Burnett WW, King EG, Grace M, et al: Hydrogen sulfide poisoning: review of 5 years' experience. *Can Med Assoc J.* 1977;117:1277-1280.
24. Burst JCM, Richter RW: Quinine amblyopia related to heroin addiction. *Ann Intern Med.* 1971;74:84-86.
25. Campbell KCM, Durrant J: Audiologic monitoring for ototoxicity. *Otolaryngol Clin North Am.* 1993;26:903-914.
26. Casler JD, Chait RH, Zajtchuk JT: Treatment of blast injury to the ear. *Ann Otol Rhinol Laryngol.* 1989;98:13-22.
27. Cazals Y, Li XQ, Aurousseau C, et al: Acute effects of noradrenaline related vasoactive agents on the ototoxicity of aspirin: an experimental study in guinea pigs. *Hear Res.* 1988;36:89-96.
28. Chait R, Casler J, Zajtchuk JT: Blast injury of the ear: historical perspective. *Ann Otol Rhinol Laryngol.* 1989;98:9-12.
29. Chapman P: Naproxen and sudden hearing loss. *J Laryngol Otol.* 1982;96:163-166.
30. Chen Y, Huang WG, Zha DJ, et al: Aspirin attenuates gentamicin ototoxicity: from the laboratory to the clinic. *Hear Res.* 2007;226:178-182.
31. Chiu JJ, Hsu CJ, Lin-Shiau SY: The detrimental effects of potassium bromate and thioglycolate on auditory brainstem response of guinea pig. *Chin J Physiol.* 2000;30:91-96.
32. Ciba Foundation Symposium 85: A central or peripheral source of tinnitus. In: Evered D, Lawrenson G, eds: *Tinnitus.* London: Putnam; 1981: 279-294.
33. Ciba Foundation Symposium 85: Appendix I: Definition and classification of tinnitus. In: Evered D, Lawrenson G, eds: *Tinnitus.* London: Pitman' 1981: 300-302.
34. Clark WW: Noise exposure from leisure activities. *J Acoust Soc Am.* 1991;90:175-181.
35. Cone TE Jr: Diagnosis and treatment: some diseases, syndromes, and conditions associated with an unusual odor. *Pediatrics.* 1968;41:993-995.

36. Davidson TM: The loss of smell. *Emerg Med.* 1988;20:104-116.
37. Davignon DD, Leshowitz BH: The speech-in-noise test: a new approach to the assessment of communication capability of elderly persons. *Int J Aging Hum Dev.* 1986;23:149-160.
38. Davis H: Advances in the neurophysiology and neuroanatomy of the cochlea. *J Acoust Soc Am.* 1962;34:1377-1385.
39. Devarajan P, Savoca M, Castaneda M, et al: Cisplatin-induced apoptosis in auditory cells: role of death receptor and mitochondrial pathways. *Hear Res.* 2002;174:45-54.
40. Doty RL: A review of olfactory dysfunctions in man. *Am J Otolaryngol.* 1979;1:57-79.
41. Drewnowski A: Genetics of taste and smell. *World Rev Nutr Diet.* 1990;63:194-208.
42. Duckert LG, Rubel EW: Current concepts in hair regeneration. *Otolaryngol Clin North Am.* 1993;26:873-901.
43. Eggermont JJ: On the pathophysiology of tinnitus: a review and a peripheral model. *Hear Res.* 1990;48:111-123.
44. Emmett EA: Parosmia and hyposmia induced by solvent exposure. *Br J Ind Med.* 1976;3:196-198.
45. Escoubet B, Amsallem P, Ferrary E, et al: Prostaglandin synthesis by the cochlea or the guinea pig. Influence of aspirin, gentamicin, and acoustic stimulation. *Prostaglandins.* 1985;29:589-599.
46. Evans EF: Chairman's closing remarks. In: Evered D, Lawrenson G, eds: *Tinnitus.* Ciba Foundation Symposium 85. London: Putman; 1981: 295-302.
47. Evans P, Halliwel B: Free radicals and hearing. Cause, consequence, and criteria. *Ann N Y Acad Sci.* 1999;884:19-40.
48. Falk SA: Pathophysiological responses of the auditory organ to excessive noise. In: Lee DHK, Falk HL, Geiger SR, eds: *Handbook of Physiology: Reactions to Environmental Agents.* Bethesda, MD: American Physiological Society; 1977: 17-30.
49. Fee WE Jr: Aminoglycoside ototoxicity in the human. *Laryngoscope.* 1980;90(Suppl 24):1-19.
50. Feldman AM: Cochlear fluids: physiology, biochemistry, and pharmacology. In: Brown RD, Daigneault EA, eds: *Pharmacology of Hearing. Experimental and Clinical Basis.* New York: Wiley; 1981: 81-97.
51. Fischel-Ghodsian N: Genetic factors in aminoglycoside toxicity. *Ann N Y Acad Sci.* 1999;884:99-109.
52. Flotra L, Gjermo P, Rolla G, et al: Side effects of chlorhexidine mouth washes. *J Dent Res.* 1971;79:119-125.
53. Froloff N, Faurion A, MacLeod P: Multiple human taste receptor sites: a molecular modeling approach. *Chem Senses.* 1996;21:425-445.
54. Fu DM: Survey of 1583 deaf mutes. *Qinghai Med J.* 1985;1:105-112.
55. Fukumoto Y, Nakajima H, Uetake M, et al: Smell ability to solution of potassium cyanide and its inheritance. *Jpn J Hum Genet.* 1957;2: 7-16.
56. Gao W: Role of neurotrophins and lectins in prevention of ototoxicity. *Ann N Y Acad Sci.* 1999;884:312-327.
57. Garetz SL, Altschuler RA, Schacht J: Attenuation of gentamicin ototoxicity by glutathione in the guinea pig in vivo. *Hear Res.* 1994;77:81-87.
58. Gerken GM: Central tinnitus and lateral inhibition: An auditory brainstem model. *Hear Res.* 1996;97:75-83.
59. Glover J, Dibble S, Miaskoski C, et al: Changes in taste associated with intravenous administration pentamidine. *J Assoc Nurses AIDS Care.* 1995;6:43-48.
60. Goldfrank LR, Weisman R, Flomenbaum N: Teaching the recognition of odors. *Ann Emerg Med.* 1982;11:684-686.
61. Gomez HJ, Cirillo VJ, Irvin JD: Enalapril: a review of human pharmacology. 1985;30S:13-24.
62. Goodey RJ: Drugs in the treatment of tinnitus. In: Evered D, Lawrenson G, eds: *Tinnitus.* Ciba Foundation Symposium 85. London: Putnam; 1981: 263-278.
63. Gordon AS, Moran DT, Jafek BW, et al: The effect of chronic cocaine abuse on human olfaction. *Arch Otolaryngol Head Neck Surg.* 1990;116:1415-1418.
64. Gordon CB: Practical approach to the loss of smell. *Am Fam Physician.* 1982;26:191-193.
65. Gorman W: The sense of smell. *Eye Ear Nose Throat.* 1964;43:54-58.
66. Griffin JP: Drug-induced disorder of taste. *Adv Drug React Rev.* 1992;11:229-239.
67. Grumet GW: Pandemonium in the modern hospital. *N Engl J Med.* 1993;322:433-437.
68. Guan MX, Fischel-Ghodsian N, Attardi G: A biochemical basis for the inherited susceptibility to aminoglycoside ototoxicity. *Hum Mol Genet.* 2000;9:1787-1793.
69. Guitton MJ, Caston J, Ruel J, et al: Salicylate induces tinnitus through activation of cochlear NMDA receptors. *J Neurosci.* 2003;23:3944-3952.
70. Hastings L: Sensory neurotoxicology: use of the olfactory system in the assessment of toxicity. *Neurotoxicol Teratol.* 1990;12:455-459.
71. Henkin RI, Larson AL, Powell RD: Hypogeusia, dysgeusia, hyposmia, and dysosmia following influenza-like infection. *Ann Otol Rhinol Laryngol.* 1975;84:672-682.
72. Henkin RI, Lippoldt RE, Bilstad J, et al: A zinc protein isolated from human parotid saliva. *Proc Natl Acad Sci U S A.* 1975;72:488-492.
73. Henkin RI: Concepts of therapy in taste and smell dysfunction: repair of sensory receptor functions as primary treatment. In: Kurihara K, Suzuki N, Ogawa H, eds: *Olfaction and Taste.* Tokyo: Springer-Verlag; 1994: 568-570.
74. Henkin RI: Drug-induced taste and smell disorders. Incidence, mechanisms and management related primarily to treatment of sensory receptor dysfunction. *Drug Saf.* 1994;11:318-377.
75. Hetu R, Phaneuf R, Marien C: Non-acoustic environmental factor influences on occupational hearing impairment: a preliminary discussion. Paper presented at the second international conference on the combined effects of environmental factors, Kanazama, Japan, 1986, pp. 17-31.
76. Heyneman CA: Zinc deficiency and taste disorders. *Ann Pharmacother.* 1996;30:186-187.
77. Hotz P, Tshchopp A, Soderstrom D, et al: Smell or taste disturbances, neurological symptoms, and hydrocarbon exposure. *Int Arch Occup Environ Health.* 1992;63:525-530.
78. Huang MY, Shacht J: Drug-induced ototoxicity: pathogenesis and prevention. *Med Toxicol.* 1989;4:452-467.
79. Hymes LC, Bruner BS, Rauber AP: Bromate poisoning from hair permanent preparations. *Pediatrics.* 1985;76:975-978.
80. Jardini L, Findlay R, Burgi E, et al: Auditory changes associated with moderate blood salicylate levels. *Rheumatol Rehab.* 1978;14:233-236.
81. Jastreboff PJ: Phantom auditory perception (tinnitus): mechanisms of generation and perception. *Neurosci Res.* 1990;8:221-254.
82. Jobe PC, Brown RD: Auditory pharmacology. *Trends Pharmacol Sci.* 1980;1:202-206.
83. Jojart G: Sense of smell after gentamicin nose-drops. *Lancet.* 1992; 339:313.
84. Joyce PW: Taste disturbance with acetazolamide [letter]. *Lancet.* 1990; 336:1446.
85. Jung TTK, Rhee CK, Lee CS, et al: Ototoxicity of salicylate, nonsteroidal anti-inflammatory drugs, and quinine. *Otolaryngol Clin North Am.* 1993;26:791-810.
86. Kare MR, Mattes RD: A selective overview of the chemical senses. *Nutr Rev.* 1990;48:39-48.
87. Keeve JP: Ototoxic drugs and the workplace. *Am Fam Physician.* 1988;38:177-181.
88. Kirk RL, Stenhouse NS: Ability to smell solutions of potassium cyanide. *Nature.* 1953;171:698-699.
89. Kisiel DL, Bobbin RP: Miscellaneous ototoxic agents. In: Brown RD, Daigneault EA, eds: *Pharmacology of Hearing: Experimental and Clinical Basis.* New York: Wiley; 1981: 231-269.
90. Koegel L: Ototoxicity: a contemporary review of aminoglycosides, loop diuretics, acetylsalicylic acid, quinine, erythromycin, and cis-platinum. *Am J Otolaryngol.* 1985;6:190-199.
91. Kusakabe Y, Abe K, Tanemura K, et al: GUST27 and closely related G-protein-coupled receptors are localized in taste buds together with G_i-protein alpha-subunit. *Chem Senses.* 1996;21:335-340.
92. Laing DG, Francis GW: The capacity of humans to identify odors in mixtures. *Physiol Behav.* 1989;46:809-814.
93. Leopold DA, Preti G, Mozell MM, et al: Fish-odor syndrome presenting as dysosmia. *Arch Otolaryngol Head Neck Surg.* 1990;116: 354-355.
94. Li G, Sha SH, Zotova E, et al: Salicylate protects hearing and kidney function from cisplatin toxicity without compromising its oncolytic action. *Lab Invest.* 2002;82:585-96.
95. Li XJ, Snyder SH: Molecular cloning of ebnerin, a von Ebner's gland protein associated with taste buds. *J Biol Chem.* 1995;270:17674-17679.
96. Lim DJ: Functional structure of the organ of Corti: a review. *Hear Res.* 1986;22:117-146.
97. Lu YF: Cause of 611 deaf mutes in schools for deaf children in Shanghai. *Shanghai Med J.* 1987;10:159.
98. Mann NM: Management of smell and taste problems. *Cleve Clin J Med.* 2002;69:329-336.

99. Matsumoto I, Morizona T, Paparella MM: Hearing loss following potassium bromate: two case reports. *Otolaryngol Head Neck Surg*. 1980;88:625-629.
100. Matz GJ: Aminoglycoside cochlear ototoxicity. *Otolaryngol Clin North Am*. 1993;26:705-736.
101. Matz GJ: The ototoxic effects of ethacrynic acid in man and animals. *Laryngoscope*. 1976;86:1065-1086.
102. McFadden D, Plattsmier HS: Aspirin abolishes spontaneous otoacoustic emissions. *J Acoust Soc Am*. 1984;76:443-448.
103. McFadden D: *Tinnitus: Facts, Theories, and Treatment*. Washington, DC, National Academy Press, 1982, pp. 10-24.
104. McGill TJ, Schuknecht HF: Human cochlear changes in noise induced hearing loss. *Laryngoscope*. 1976;86:1293-1302.
105. McNeil JJ, Anderson A, Christophidis N, et al: Taste loss associated with oral captopril treatment. *Br Med J*. 1979;15:1555-1556.
106. Meyerhoff WL: Physiology of the nose and paranasal sinuses. In: Paparella MM, Schumrick DA, eds: *Otolaryngology: Basic Sciences and Related Disciplines*, Vol. 1. Philadelphia: WB Saunders; 1980: 308-311.
107. Miller LG, Miller SM: Altered taste secondary to acetazolamide. *J Fam Pract*. 1990;31:199-200.
108. Minami SB, Sha SH, Schacht J: Antioxidant protection in a new animal model of cisplatin-induced ototoxicity. *Hear Res*. 2004;137-143.
109. Mongan E, Kelly P, Nies K, et al: Tinnitus as an indication of therapeutic serum salicylate levels. *JAMA*. 1973;226:142-145.
110. Mott AE, Leopold DA: Disorders of taste and smell. *Med Clin North Am*. 1991;75:1321-1353.
111. Muldoon LL, Pagel MA, Kroll RA, et al: Delayed administration of sodium thiosulfate in animal models reduces platinum ototoxicity without reduction of antitumor activity. *Clin Cancer Res*. 2000;6:309-315.
112. Myers EN, Bernstein JM: Salicylate ototoxicity. *Arch Otolaryngol*. 1965;82:483-493.
113. Nadol JB Jr: Hearing loss. *N Engl J Med*. 1993;329;1092-1102.
114. National Institutes of Health: Noise and hearing loss. Consensus Development Conference statement. *JAMA*. 1990;263:3185-3190.
115. Ohtani I, Ohtsuki K, Aikawa T, et al: Mechanism of protective effect of fosfomycin against aminoglycoside ototoxicity. *Auris Nasus Larynx*. 1984;11: 119-124.
116. Olishifski JB: Occupational hearing loss, noise, and hearing conservation. In: Zenz C, ed: *Occupational Medicine: Principles and Practical Applications*. Chicago: Year Book; 1988: 274-323.
117. Patterson PM, Lauder BA: The incidence and probable inheritance of "smell blindness." *J Hered*. 1948;39:295-297.
118. Peloquin CA, Berning SE, Nitta AT, et al: Aminoglycoside toxicity: daily versus thrice-weekly dosing for treatment of mycobacterial diseases. *Clin Infect Dis*. 2004;38:1538-1544.
119. Phaneur R, Hetu R: An epidemiological perspective of the causes of hearing loss among industrial workers. *J Otolaryngol*. 1990;19:31-40.
120. Phillips YY, Zajtchuk JT: Blast injuries of the ear in military operations. *Ann Otol Rhinol Laryngol*. 1989;98:3-4.
121. Prazma J: Ototoxicity of aminoglycoside antibiotics. In: Brown RD, Daigneault EA, eds: *Pharmacology of Hearing: Experimental and Clinical Basis*. New York: Wiley; 1981: 155-193.
122. Puel JL: Cochlear NMDA receptor blockade prevents salicylate-induced tinnitus. *B-ENT*. 2007;3(Suppl 7):19-22.
123. Puel JL, Guitton MJ. Salicylate-induced tinnitus: molecular mechanisms and modulation by anxiety. *Prog Brain Res*. 2007;166:141-146.
124. Quick CA, Chole RA, Mauer SM: Deafness and renal failure due to potassium bromate poisoning. *Arch Otolaryngol*. 1975;101:494-495.
125. Quick CA, Fish A, Brown C: The relationship between cochlea and kidney. *Laryngoscope*. 1973;83:1469-1482.
126. Ramsden RT, Latif A, O'Malley S: Electrocochleographic changes in acute salicylate overdosage. *J Laryngol Otol*. 1985;99:1269-1273.
127. Razani J, Murphy C, Davidson TM, et al: Odor sensitivity is impaired in HIV-positive cognitively impaired patients. *Physiol Behav*. 1996;59:877-881.
128. Reser D, Rho M, Dewan D, et al: L- and D-methionine provide equivalent long-term protection against CDDP-induced ototoxicity in vivo, with partial in vitro and in vivo retention of antineoplastic activity. *Neurotoxicology*. 1999;20:731-748.
129. Riggs LC, Brummett RE, Guitjens SK, et al: Ototoxicity resulting from combined administration of cisplatin and gentamicin. *Laryngoscope*. 1996;106:401-406.
130. Roche RJ, Silamut K, Pukrittayakamee S, et al: Quinine induces reversible high-tone hearing loss. *Br J Clin Pharmacol*. 1990;29:780-782.
131. Roland PS: New developments in our understanding of ototoxicity. *Ear Nose Throat J*. 2004;83:15-17.
132. Rollin H: Drug-related gustatory disorders. *Ann Otolaryngol*. 1978;87:37-42.
133. Rose CS, Heywood PG, Costanzo RM: Olfactory impairment after chronic occupational cadmium exposure. *J Occup Med*. 1992;34:600-605.
134. Rutka J, Alberti PW: Toxic and drug-induced disorders in otolaryngology. *Otolaryngol Clin North Am*. 1984;17:761-774.
135. Rybak LP, Husain K, Whitworth C, et al: Dose dependent protection by lipoic acid against cisplatin-induced ototoxicity in rats: antioxidant defense system. *Toxicol Sci*. 1999;47:195-202.
136. Rybak LP: Ototoxicity of loop diuretics. *Otolaryngol Clin North Am*. 1993;26:829-844.
137. Rybak MJ, Abate BJ, Kang SL, et al: Prospective evaluation of the effect of an aminoglycoside dosing regimen on rates of observed nephrotoxicity and ototoxicity. *Antimicrob Agents Chemother*. 1999;43:1549-1555.
138. Santini V, Giles FJ: The potential of amifostine: from cytoprotective to therapeutic agent. *Hematologia*. 1999;84:1035-1042.
139. Schacht J: Biochemical basis of aminoglycoside ototoxicity. *Otolaryngol Clin North Am*. 1993;26:845-856.
140. Schacht J: Molecular mechanisms of drug-induced hearing loss. *Hear Res*. 1986;22:297-304.
141. Schiffman SS: Taste and smell in disease (Part 1). *N Engl J Med*. 1983;308: 1275-1279.
142. Schiffman SS: Taste and smell in disease (Part 2). *N Engl J Med*. 1983;308: 1337-1343.
143. Schleuning AJ: Management of the patient with tinnitus. *Med Clin North Am*. 1991;75:1225-1237.
144. Schneider BA: Anosmia: verification and etiologies. *Ann Otolaryngnol*. 1972;81:272-277.
145. Schweitzer VG: Ototoxicity of chemotherapeutic agents. *Otolaryngol Clin North Am*. 1993;26:759-789.
146. Seidman MD, Jacobson GP: Update on tinnitus. *Otolaryngol Clin North Am*. 1996;29:455-465.
147. Seligmann H, Podoshin L, Ben-David J, et al: Drug-induced tinnitus and other hearing disorders. *Drug Saf*. 1996;14:198-212.
148. Sha SH, Qiu JA, Schacht J: Aspirin to prevent gentamicin-induced hearing loss. *N Engl J Med*. 2006;354:1856-1857.
149. Sha SH, Schacht J: Salicylate attenuates gentamicin-induced ototoxicity. *Lab Invest*. 1999;79:807-13.
150. Shatzman AR, Henkin RI: Metal-binding characteristics of the parotid salivary protein gustin. *Biochim Biophys Acta*. 1980;623:107-118.
151. Shelley WB: A diagnosis you can smell. *Emerg Med*. 1992;24:232-235.
152. Shimizu A, Takumida M, Anniko M, Suzuki M: Cisplatin and caspase inhibitors protect vestibular sensory cells from gentamicin ototoxicity. *Acta Otolaryngol*. 2003;123:4549-465.
153. Shulman A: The cochleovestibular system/ototoxicity/clinical issues. *Ann N Y Acad Sci*. 1999;884:433-436.
154. Shusterman DJ, Sheedy JE: Occupational and environmental disorders of the special senses. *Occup Med*. 1992;7:515-542.
155. Silverstein H, Wolfson RJ, Rosenberg S: Diagnosis and management of hearing loss. *Clin Symp*. 1994;44:1-32.
156. Smilkstein MJ, Kulig KW, Rumack BH: Acute toxic blindness: unrecognized quinine poisoning. *Ann Emerg Med*. 1987;16:98-101.
157. Smoorenburg GF, De Groot JC, Hamers FP, et al: Protection and spontaneous recovery from cisplatin-induced hearing loss. *Ann N Y Acad Sci*. 1999;884:192-210.
158. Song BB, Schacht J: Variable efficacy of radical scavengers and iron chelators to attenuate gentamicin ototoxicity in guinea pig in vivo. *Hear Res*. 1996;94:87-93.
159. Stevens JC, Cruz LA, Hoffman JM, et al: Taste sensitivity and aging: high incidence of decline revealed by repeated threshold. *Chem Senses*. 1995;20:451-459.
160. Stewart TH, Sherman Y, Politzer WM: An outbreak of food-poisoning due to a flour improver, potassium bromate. *South Afr Med J*. 1969; 200-202.
161. Stine R, Slosberg B, Beacham BE: Hydrogen sulfide intoxication. *Ann Intern Med*. 1976;85:756-758.
162. Sullivan P: MD launches study to determine amount of job-related hearing loss in military. *CMAJ*. 1992;146:2061-2062.
163. Sumner D: Post-traumatic anosmia. *Brain*. 1964;87:107-120.
164. Takumida M, Anniko M: Brain-derived neurotrophic factor and nitric oxide synthase inhibitor protect the vestibular organ gentamicin ototoxicity. *Acta Otolaryngol*. 2002;122:10-15.

165. Tange RA, Dreschler WA, van der Hulst RJ: The importance of high-tone audiometry in monitoring for ototoxicity. *Arch Otorhinolaryngol.* 1985;242:77-81.
166. Turnidge MB: Pharmacodynamics and dosing of aminoglycosides. *Infect Dis Clin North Am.* 2003;17:503-528.
167. Unal OF, Ghoreishi SM, Atas A, et al: Prevention of gentamicin induced ototoxicity by trimetazidine in animal model. *Int J Pediatr Otorhinolaryngol.* 2005;69:193-199.
168. Verdel BM, van Puijenbroek EP, Souverein PC: Drug-related nephrotoxic and ototoxic reactions—a link through a predictive mechanistic commonality. *Drug Saf.* 2008;31:877-884.
169. Wallhauser-Frank E, Braun S, Langner G: Salicylate alters 2-DG uptake in the auditory system: a model for tinnitus? *Neuroreport.* 1996;7:1585-1588.
170. Ward WD: Noise-induced hearing loss. In: Northern JL, ed: *Hearing Disorder,* 2nd ed. Boston: Little, Brown; 1984:143-152.
171. Watanabe KI, Hess A, Bloch W, et al: Nitric oxide synthase inhibitor suppresses the ototoxic side effects of cisplatin in guinea pig. *Anti-cancer Drugs.* 2000;11:401-406.
172. Willems PJ: Genetic causes of hearing loss. *N Engl J Med.* 2000;342:1101-1109.
173. Wright HN: Characterization of olfactory dysfunction. *Arch Otolaryngol Head Neck Surg.* 1987;113:163-168.
174. Wysocki CJ, Gilbert AN: The National Geographic Smell Survey: the effects of age are heterogenous. *Ann N Y Acad Sci.* 1989;561:12-28.
175. Zazgornick J, Kaiser W, Biesenbach G: Captopril induced dysgeusia [letter]. *Lancet.* 1993;341:1542.
176. Zeller JA, Machetanz J, Kessler C: Ageusia as an adverse effect of phenytoin. *Lancet.* 1998;351:1101.
177. Zhang F, Klebansky B, Fine RM, et al: Molecular mechanism for the umami taste synergism. *Proc Natl Acad Sci U S A.* 2008;105:20930-20934.

CHAPTER 21
RESPIRATORY PRINCIPLES

Andrew Stolbach and Robert S. Hoffman

The primary function of the lungs is to exchange gases. Specifically, this involves the transport of oxygen (O_2) into the blood, and the elimination of carbon dioxide (CO_2) from the blood. In addition, the lungs serve as minor organs of metabolism and elimination for a number of xenobiotics, a source of insensible water loss, and a means of temperature regulation.

Cellular oxygen use is dependent on many factors, including respiratory drive; percent of oxygen in inspired air; airway patency; chest wall and pulmonary compliance; diffusing capacity; ventilation–perfusion mismatch; hemoglobin content; hemoglobin oxygen loading and unloading; cellular oxygen uptake; and cardiac output. Xenobiotics have the unique ability to inhibit or impair each of these factors necessary for oxygen use and result in respiratory dysfunction. This chapter illustrates how xenobiotics interact acutely with the mechanisms of gas exchange and oxygen use. Discussion of chronic occupational lung injury is beyond the scope of this text; the reader is referred to a number of reviews for further information.[5,14,18,91]

PULMONARY MANIFESTATIONS OF XENOBIOTIC EXPOSURES

RESPIRATORY DRIVE

Respiratory rate and depth are regulated by the need to maintain a normal PCO_2 and pH. Most of the control for ventilation occurs at the level of the medulla, although it is modulated both by involuntary input from the pons and voluntary input from the higher cortices. Changes in PCO_2 are measured primarily by a central chemoreceptor which measures cerebral spinal fluid (CSF) pH, and secondarily by peripheral chemoreceptors in the carotid and aortic bodies, which measure PCO_2. Input with regard to PO_2 is obtained from carotid and aortic chemoreceptors. Stretch receptors in the chest relay information about pulmonary dynamics, such as the volume and pressure.

Xenobiotics can affect respiratory drive in one of several ways: direct suppression of the respiratory center; alteration in the response of chemoreceptors to changes in PCO_2; direct stimulation of the respiratory center; increase in metabolic demands such as result from agitation or fever, which, in turn, increases total body oxygen consumption; or indirectly, as a result of the creation of acid–base disorders. For example, opioids (Chap. 38) depress respiration by decreasing the responsiveness of chemoreceptors to CO_2 and by direct suppression of the pontine and medullary respiratory centers.[34,78,104] Any xenobiotic that causes a decreased respiratory drive or a decreased level of consciousness can produce bradypnea (a decreased respiratory rate), hypopnea (a decreased tidal volume), or both, resulting in hypoventilation (Chap. 3).

Methylxanthines, cocaine, and other sympathomimetics may cause an increase in respiratory drive as well as an increase in oxygen consumption. Salicylates produce hyperventilation by both central and peripheral effects via respiratory alkalosis and metabolic acidosis. The net consequence of increased respiratory drive, increased oxygen consumption, or metabolic acidosis is the generation of either tachypnea (an elevated respiratory rate), hyperpnea (an increased tidal volume), or both. Either alone or in combination, tachypnea and hyperpnea produce hyperventilation. Tables 21–1 and 21–2 list xenobiotics that commonly produce hypo- and hyperventilation.

DECREASED INSPIRED FIO_2

Barometric pressure at sea level ranges near 760 mm Hg. At this pressure, 21% of ambient air is comprised of oxygen (FIO_2 21%), and after subtracting for the water vapor normally present in the lungs, PAO_2 (the alveolar partial pressure of oxygen) is about 150 mm Hg. Any reduction in FIO_2 decreases the PAO_2, thereby producing signs and symptoms of hypoxemia (a low PaO_2 [the arterial partial pressure of oxygen]). At an FIO_2 of 12%–16%, patients experience tachypnea, tachycardia, headache, mild confusion, and impaired coordination. A further decrease to an FIO_2 of 10%–14% produces severe fatigue and cognitive impairment and when the FIO_2 decreases to between 6% and 10%, nausea, vomiting, and lethargy develop. An $FIO_2 < 6\%$ is incompatible with life.[63]

This effect on PAO_2 is typically observed as elevation increases above sea level, because while FIO_2 remains 21%, barometric pressure falls. At 18,000 feet, barometric pressure is only 380 mm Hg, and the PAO_2 falls to below 70 mm Hg. At 63,000 feet, the barometric pressure falls to 47 mm Hg, a level where the PAO_2 equals 0 mm Hg. Although it is important to remember this relationship, altitude-induced decreases in PAO_2 are rarely important in clinical medicine, even in commercial airline flights, where the cabins are pressurized to a maximum of several thousand feet above sea level. However, in closed or low-lying spaces, oxygen may be replaced or displaced by other gases that have no intrinsic toxicity. Common examples of these gases, referred to as simple asphyxiants (Table 21–3), are found alone or in combination with more toxic gases. Because they have little or no toxicity other than their ability to replace oxygen, removal of the victim from exposure and administration of supplemental oxygen are curative if permanent injury as a consequence of hypoxia has not already developed (Chap. 124).

The potential magnitude of toxicity from simple asphyxiants was best exemplified by the disasters in Cameroon near the Lakes of Monoun and Nyos, in 1984 and 1986, respectively. For unclear reasons, Lake Nyos, a volcanic lake, released a cloud of carbon dioxide (CO_2) gas of approximately a quarter million tons. Because CO_2 is 1.5 times heavier than air, the gas cloud flowed into the surrounding low-lying valleys, killing by asphyxia more than 1700 people, and affecting countless more people because of hypoxia. Most survivors recovered without complications.[9,38] Smaller scale, but equally serious, toxicity from CO_2 results from improper handling of dry ice or release into a closed space.[39,44]

CHEST WALL

Hypoventilation can result from a decrease in either respiratory rate or tidal volume. Thus, even when the stimulus to breathe is normal, adequate ventilation is dependent on the coordination and function of the muscles of the diaphragm and chest wall. Changes in this function can result in hypoventilation by two separate mechanisms; both muscle weakness and muscle rigidity may impair the patient's ability to expand the chest wall. Toxicologic causes of muscle weakness include botulinum toxin,[86] electrolyte abnormalities such as hypokalemia,[57,105] or hypermagnesemia,[232] organic phosphorus compounds,[68,87] and neuromuscular blockers.[13,50] Patients with hypoventilation caused by muscle weakness respond well to assisted ventilation and correction of the underlying problem (Chaps. 16, 46, 68, and 113). Chest-wall rigidity impairing ventilation can occur in strychnine poisoning,[15,55,62] tetanus,[23,55,93] and fentanyl use[22,24] (Chaps. 38 and 112). Often these patients are difficult to ventilate despite tracheal intubation and may require muscle relaxants, neuromuscular blocking agents, or naloxone (for fentanyl).

TABLE 21–1. Xenobiotics that Produce Hypoventilation

Baclofen	γ-Hydroxybutyrate and analogs
Barbiturates	Isopropanol
Botulinum toxin	Methanol
Carbamates	Neuromuscular blockers
Clonidine	Nicotine
Conium maculatum (*Poison Hemlock*)	Opioids
Colchicine	Organic phosphorus compounds
Cyclic antidepressants	Sedative-hypnotics
Elapid envenomation	Strychnine
Electrolyte abnormalities	Tetanus toxin
Ethanol	Tetrodotoxin
Ethylene glycol	

AIRWAY PATENCY

The airway may be compromised in several ways. As a patient's mental status becomes impaired, the airway is often obstructed by the tongue.[41] Alternatively, vomitus, or aspiration of activated charcoal or a foreign body, can directly obstruct the trachea or major bronchi with resultant hypoxia[41,52,65,69,81,97] Obstruction may also result from increased secretions produced during organic phosphorus compound poisoning. Laryngospasm may occur either as a manifestation of systemic reactions, such as anaphylaxis, as a result of edema from thermal or caustic injury (Chaps. 104 and 128), or as a direct response to an irritant gas (Chap. 124). Similarly, the tongue can become swollen in response to thermal or caustic injury or toxic exposure to plants such as *Dieffenbachia* spp, or as a result of angioedema from drugs such as angiotensin-converting enzyme inhibitors (Chaps. 62, 104, 118, and 128).[34] Regardless of the mechanism, upper airway obstruction results in hypoventilation, hypoxemia, and hypercapnia (hypercarbia) with the persistence of a normal A-a gradient (see discussion of A-a gradients). Upper airway obstruction is often acute and severe and requires immediate therapy to prevent further clinical compromise. Bronchospasm may be a manifestation of anaphylaxis, as well as exposure to pyrolyzed cocaine,[84,95,96] smoke, irritant gases[43,48, 76] (Table 21–4), or dust (eg, cotton in byssinosis), or as a result of work-related asthma[61,91] and hypersensitivity pneumonitis[96,109] (Chaps. 124 and 128).

Airway collapse may result from pneumothorax caused by barotrauma, which more commonly results from the manner of administration of illicit xenobiotics than from actual drug overdose. Barotrauma may also result from nasal insufflation or inhalation of drugs. This form of barotrauma occurs most often in cocaine (particularly in the form of "crack") and marijuana users, who either smoke or insufflate these xenobiotics and then perform prolonged Valsalva maneuvers in an attempt to enhance the effects of these xenobiotics. (Chaps. 76 and 83).[11,20,74,89,106] The increased airway pressure leads to rupture of an alveolar bleb, and free air dissects along the peribronchial paths into the mediastinum and pleural cavities. Nitrous oxide abuse also causes barotrauma.[53] Siphoning of nitrous oxide from low-pressure tanks meant for inhalation is not typically associated with barotrauma. In contrast, inhalation of nitrous oxide, used as a propellant in whipped cream cans, generates tremendous pressure that sometimes results in severe barotrauma (Chap. 81).

TABLE 21–2. Xenobiotics that Produce Hyperventilation

Amphetamines	Isopropanol
Anticholinergics	Methanol
Camphor	Metformin
Carbon monoxide	Methemoglobin inducers
Cocaine	Methylxanthines
Cyanide	Nucleoside reverse transcriptase inhibitors
Dinitrophenol	Paraldehyde
Ethanol (ketoacidosis)	Pentachlorophenol
Ethylene glycol	Phenformin
Gyromitra spp.	Progesterone
Hydrogen sulfide	Salicylates
Iron	Sodium monofluoroacetate
Isoniazid	

TABLE 21–3. Simple Asphyxiants

Argon	Hydrogen
Carbon dioxide	Methane
Ethane	Nitrogen
Helium	Propane

VENTILATION–PERFUSION MISMATCH

Ventilation–perfusion (V/Q) mismatch is manifested at the extremes by aeration of the lung without arterial blood supply (as in pulmonary embolism from injected contaminants), and by a normal blood supply to the lung without any ventilation. Impaired blood supply to a normal lung and normal blood supply to an inadequately ventilated lung constitute an infinite number of gradations that exist between the extremes. The normal response to regional variations in ventilation is to shunt blood away from an area of lung that is poorly ventilated, thereby preferentially delivering blood to an area of the lung where gas exchange is more efficient. An hypoxia-induced reduction in local nitric oxide pro-

TABLE 21–4. Irritant Gases

Ammonia	Isocyanates
Chloramine	Nitrogen dioxide
Chlorine	Ozone
Chlorocetophenone (CN)	Phosgene
Chlorobenzylidene-malonitrile (CS)	Phosphine
Fluorine	Sulfur dioxide
Hydrogen chloride	

duction appears to be responsible for the regional vasoconstriction that occurs.[1] This effect, commonly known as hypoxic pulmonary vasoconstriction, is best described in patients with chronic obstructive lung disease and facilitates compensation for the V/Q mismatch associated with that disorder. It is unclear whether xenobiotic-induced alterations in pulmonary nitric oxide production are significant determinants in the V/Q mismatch that occurs in poisoning.

In toxicology, V/Q mismatch most commonly results from perfusion of an abnormally ventilated lung, as may occur following aspiration of gastric contents, a frequent complication of many types of poisoning.[52,69] Although alterations in consciousness and loss of protective airway reflexes are predisposing factors, certain xenobiotics, such as hydrocarbons, directly result in aspiration pneumonitis because of their specific characteristics of high volatility, low viscosity, and low surface tension (Chap. 106).

The diagnosis of aspiration pneumonitis often relies on the chest radiograph for confirmation. The location of the infiltrate depends significantly on the patient's position when the aspiration occurred. Most commonly, aspiration occurs in the right mainstem bronchus, because the angle with the carina is not as acute as it is for entry into the left mainstem bronchus. When aspiration occurs in the supine position, the subsequent infiltrate is usually manifest in the posterior segments of the upper lobe and superior segments of the lower lobe. Aspiration typically involves vomitus; but secretions, activated charcoal, teeth, dentures, food, and other foreign bodies are also frequently aspirated.

DIFFUSING CAPACITY ABNORMALITIES

Severe impairment in diffusing capacity commonly results from local injury to the lungs in disorders such as interstitial pneumonia, aspiration, toxic inhalations, and near drowning, and from systemic effects of sepsis, trauma, and various other medical disorders.[8] When this process is acute and associated with clinical criteria including crackles, hypoxemia, and bilateral infiltrates on a chest radiograph demonstrating a normal heart size, it has been traditionally referred to as *noncardiogenic pulmonary edema*; throughout this chapter and text, however, the term *acute lung injury* (ALI) is used, which reflects current nomenclature.[8] ALI is the presence of increased intraalveolar fluid in the lungs with a normal cardiac output. More rigid criteria, such as a Pao_2/Fio_2 ratio < 300 mm Hg (regardless of positive end-expiratory pressure [PEEP]), bilateral infiltrates on the chest radiograph, and either a pulmonary artery wedge pressure that is ≤ 18 mm Hg or no clinical evidence of left atrial hypertension, are used to further define the ALI.[8] When these same criteria are met, but the patient's Pao_2/Fio_2 ratio is < 200 mm Hg (regardless of PEEP), the term *acute respiratory distress syndrome* (ARDS) is used.[8,59] Approximately 150,000 Americans develop ARDS annually, many as a result of xenobiotics; ARDS has a fatality rate near 50%.[4]

Commonly, patients are chronically exposed to xenobiotics associated with reduced diffusing capacity by smoking tobacco and other xenobiotics or working with asbestos, silica, and coal, which slowly causes pulmonary fibrosis or promotes emphysema. More recent work also emphasizes the ability of chronically smoked cocaine to alter pulmonary function.[96] Acutely, ALI from opioids, salicylates, or phosgene and delayed severe fibrosis from paraquat can cause profound alterations in diffusion (Chaps. 35, 38, 115, and 124).[72,82,111] Associated parenchymal damage is almost always present and causes both reduction in lung volumes and V/Q mismatch. Intravenous injection of talc, a common contaminant found in drugs of abuse,[75] and septic emboli from right-sided endocarditis[73,92] may result in isolated vascular defects with reduction in diffusion capacity. Similarly, cocaine-induced pulmonary spasm can obstruct vascular channels and alter pulmonary function, creating V/Q mismatch.[27]

Acute lung injury with or without progression to ARDS is a common occurrence from poisoning. The edema fluid (and the resulting hypoxia, pulmonary crackles, and radiographic abnormalities) may develop in part because of increased permeability of the alveolar and capillary basement membrane.[21,25,64,82] Proteinaceous fluid leaks from the capillaries into the alveoli and interstitium of the lung. Several mechanisms are proposed as the cause for ALI, although there is no single unifying mechanism for all of the xenobiotics that have been implicated. Acute lung injury may result from exposure to xenobiotics that produce hypoventilation by at least three different mechanisms: hypoxia may injure the vascular endothelial cells; autoregulatory vascular redistribution may cause localized capillary hypertension; or alveolar microtrauma may occur as alveolar units collapse, only to be reopened suddenly during reventilation.[82] These and other events may activate neutrophils and release inflammatory cytokines.[3,103] Other xenobiotics may be directly toxic to the capillary epithelial cells or may be partly responsible for the release of vasoactive substances.[3] The effects of salicylates and other NSAIDs may be mediated via effects on prostaglandin synthesis. Finally, sympathomimetic stimulants may cause "neurogenic" pulmonary edema, which is thought to be mediated by massive catecholamine discharge. Elevated catecholamine concentrations are also noted in experimental opioid overdose, possibly representing support for a link between hypoxia, hypercarbia, and the catecholamine hypothesis of ALI.[67]

In the 1880s, William Osler described "oedema of left lung" in a morphine user. The opioids are still among the most common causes of ALI (Chap. 38), but it is now recognized that there are many types of xenobiotics that can cause or are associated with ALI, such as the sedative-hypnotics, salicylates, cocaine, carbon monoxide, diuretics, and calcium channel blockers (Table 21–5).[29,31,33,36,37,42,45,49,56,77,79,90,92,111] The route of xenobiotic administration is not usually the determining factor; ALI can result from oral, intravenous, and inhalational exposure. Because the source of the problem is increased pulmonary capillary permeability, patients with ALI have a normal pulmonary-capillary wedge pressure, unlike patients with cardiogenic pulmonary edema.

Cardiogenic pulmonary edema may also occur as the result of poisoning. Etiologies for this phenomenon include the ingestion of large amounts of a xenobiotic with negative inotropy (eg, β-adrenergic antagonists, type IA antidysrhythmics) or myocardial infarction (from cocaine). Because many overdoses are mixed overdoses, the distinction between cardiogenic pulmonary edema and ALI is often difficult to establish by physical examination and requires invasive monitoring techniques.

Although the treatments for cardiogenic pulmonary edema and ALI have many similarities, critical aspects of the therapy differ, and therefore

TABLE 21–5. Common Xenobiotic Causes of Acute Lung Injury

Amiodarone	Ethchlorvynol
Amphetamines	Irritant gases
Amphotericin	Lidocaine
Bleomycin	Opioids
Calcium channel blockers	Protamine
Carbon monoxide	Salicylates
Cocaine	Sedative-hypnotics
Colchicine	Smoke inhalation
Cyclic antidepressants	Streptokinase
Cytosine arabinoside	Vinca alkaloids

an accurate diagnosis must be established. Most diagnostic tests are not helpful in differentiating between the two diseases. Physical examination reveals the presence of crackles with both entities. An S_3 gallop, if present, suggests a cardiac cause of pulmonary edema, but its absence does not establish the diagnosis of ALI. In both entities, the arterial blood-gas analysis demonstrates hypoxia and the chest radiograph shows perihilar, basilar, or diffuse alveolar infiltrates. The presence of "vascular redistribution" on the chest radiograph, however, is suggestive of a cardiogenic etiology; a normal-sized heart is more commonly associated with ALI, whereas an enlarged heart is more typical of cardiogenic pulmonary edema. The diagnostic tests that may be useful in establishing the correct diagnosis include echocardiography, transcutaneous bioimpedance, pulmonary artery catheter pressure measurements, and radionuclide ventriculography ("gated-pool" scan). Although the radionuclide scan accurately measures cardiac output, it is not routinely available in the emergency department (ED) or ICU and usually requires the transport of a critically ill patient to the nuclear medicine suite. Although echocardiography can be performed as a portable "bedside" technique, it is less sensitive and less specific for determinations of cardiac output. Therefore, the most definitive diagnostic procedure in the emergency setting is the insertion of a pulmonary artery catheter for hemodynamic monitoring. Cardiogenic pulmonary edema results from an elevated left-atrial filling pressure (elevated pulmonary-capillary wedge pressure) and a decreased cardiac output. In patients with ALI, the pulmonary artery wedge pressure and the cardiac output are normal. Although not specifically well-investigated in poisoning, recent experiences with transcutaneous bioimpedance measurements of cardiac output show promise for this portable noninvasive technique.[8,26,70]

The basic treatment for ALI and ARDS is supportive care while the xenobiotic is eliminated and healing occurs in the pulmonary capillaries.[3,59] The most important specific therapeutic maneuver in patients with ALI/ARDS involves the use of low tidal-volume ventilation (≤ 6 mL/kg predicted body weight).[1,40,103]

This results in reduced airway pressures which seem to "rest" the lung and allow healing to occur. The efficacy of jet ventilators or membrane oxygenators is inadequately studied. Some studies suggested a potential role for extracorporeal membrane oxygenation in the treatment of ALI and ARDS.[54] PEEP, which may derive its benefit from keeping alveoli open, has traditionally been considered an essential component in the management of ARDS.[30,40]

The PEEP should be maintained in the range of 5–12 cm H_2O, to maintain a Po_2 of at least 55 mm Hg, or an oxygen saturation of 88%, with an inspired oxygen concentration of ≤ 40%. Higher PEEP settings are not always beneficial and can cause an increased incidence of pneumothorax or hypotension. An increase in PEEP may result in a modest increase in Po_2, but a larger decrease in venous return and decreased cardiac output. Therefore, with each change in PEEP, the resulting increase (or perhaps decrease) in oxygen delivery to the body should be determined.[4]

A conservative fluid strategy has been shown to improve oxygenation and decrease ICU stay without increasing the incidence of shock or the need for dialysis. A conservative fluid management strategy is recommended for patients with ARDS who are not in shock, have not been in shock for at least 12 hours and do not have other reasons to require liberal fluid administration.[71]

HEMOGLOBIN AND THE CHEMICAL ASPHYXIANTS

Disorders of hemoglobin oxygen content, as well as of hemoglobin loading and unloading, result in cellular hypoxia, which, in turn, results in hyperventilation. Anemia is a common complication of the infectious diseases associated with injection drug use. In addition, many xenobiotics result in hemolysis or direct bone marrow suppression. Among the latter group are the heavy metals, lead, benzene, and ethanol. Hemolysis may occur in individuals exposed to lead, copper, or arsine gas, and in patients with glucose-6-phosphate dehydrogenase (G6PD) deficiency exposed to oxidants (Chap. 24).

The oxygen-carrying capacity of blood declines in almost direct proportion to hemoglobin content,[97] as seen in Figure 21–1. As shown in Figure 21–1A, under most normal conditions the dissolved oxygen content of the blood contributes little, and thus the last portion of the equation can be eliminated. Anemia resulting in a decrease of the hemoglobin content to 7.5 g/dL (a hematocrit of ~ 22%) decreases the oxygen content of the blood to about 10.2 mL O_2/dL (Fig. 21–1B). Because central cyanosis is only visible with a concentration of reduced deoxyhemoglobin of at least 5 g/dL, unless an abnormal hemoglobin is present, anemia can significantly impair oxygen-carrying capacity without the development of this common physical manifestation (Chap. 127).

In contrast, as the Po_2 reaches higher values (as in hyperbaric oxygen [HBO] chambers), the dissolved oxygen content becomes significant and may be of therapeutic value, particularly when the oxygen-carrying content of hemoglobin is compromised. The Po_2 corresponding to an Fio_2 of 100% is approximately 575 mm Hg. In HBO at 3 atm and 100% oxygen, Po_2 values in excess of 1500 mm Hg can be achieved.[63] Under these conditions, the dissolved oxygen content of the blood rises dramatically (to as much as 4.5 mL O_2/dL) and may be adequate to sustain life, even in the absence of any contribution from hemoglobin (Fig. 21–1C).

The chemical asphyxiants that produce methemoglobin, carboxyhemoglobin, and sulfhemoglobin interfere with oxygen loading and/or unloading to various degrees. Methemoglobin inhibits oxygen loading, producing cyanosis that is unresponsive to supplemental oxygen

Oxygen content (O_2 content) = hemoglobin bound oxygen + dissolved oxygen

A. Normal conditions: hemoglobin (Hb) = 15 g/dL; PO_2 = 100 mm Hg, oxygen saturation (O_2 Sat) = 95%

O_2 content = [(Hb)(O_2 sat) (constant) + (another constant)(PO_2)]
= [(Hb)(O_2 sat)(1.39 mL O_2/g%)
+ (0.003 mL O_2 /dL/mm Hg)(PO_2)]
= [(15 g/dL)(95%)(1.39 mL O_2/g%)
+ (0.003 mL O_2/dL/mm Hg)(100 mm Hg)]
= [(19.8 mL O_2/dL) + (0.3 mL O_2/dL)]
= 20.1 mL O_2/dL = 20.1 vol%

B. Anemia: Hb = 7.5 g/dL; PO_2 = 100 mm Hg, O_2 Sat = 95%

O_2 content = [(Hb)(O_2 sat)(1.39 mL O_2/g%)
+ (0.003 mL O_2/dL/mm Hg)(PO_2)]
= [(7.5 g/dL)(95%)(1.39 mL O_2/g%)
+ (0.003 mL O_2/dL/mm Hg)(100 mm Hg)]
= [(9.9 mL O_2/dL) + (0.3 mL O_2/dL)]
= 10.2 mL O_2/dL = 10.2 vol%

C. Hyperbaric oxygen: Hb = 15 g/dL; PO_2 = 1500 mm Hg, O_2 Sat = 100%

O_2 content = [(Hb)(O_2 sat)(1.39 mL O_2/g%)
+ (0.003 mL O_2dL/mm Hg)(PO_2)]
= [(15 g/dL)(100%)(1.39 mL O_2/g%)
+ (0.003 mL O_2/dL/mm Hg)(1500 mm Hg)]
= [(20.9 mL O_2/dL) + (4.5 mL O_2/dL)]
= 25.4 mL O_2/dL = 25.4 vol%

FIGURE 21–1. Examples of calculations of the oxygen content of the blood under various conditions.

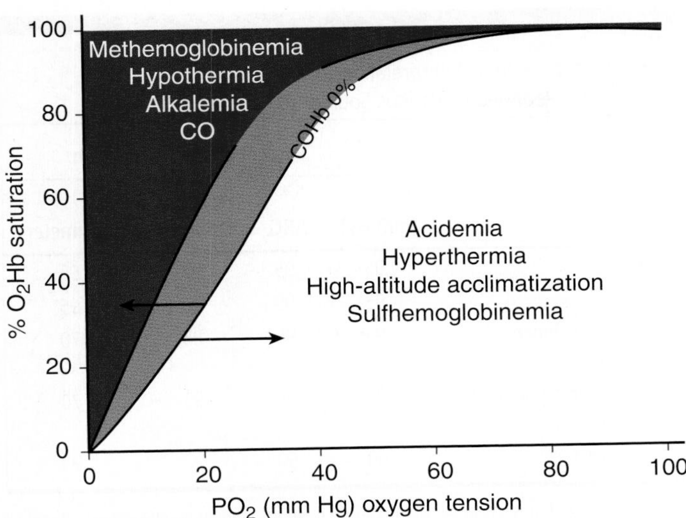

FIGURE 21–2. Oxyhemoglobin dissociation curve at 98.6°F (37°C) and pH 7.40. Hematocrit does not alter this relationship.

(Chaps. 125, and A37). In addition, the oxyhemoglobin saturation curve is shifted to the left, interfering with unloading (Fig. 21–2). Carboxyhemoglobin has similar effects on oxygen loading and unloading, but carboxyhemoglobin is not associated with cyanosis (Chap. 125). Sulfhemoglobin has similar effects on oxygen loading, but shifts the oxyhemoglobin saturation curve to the right, favoring unloading. Cyanide, hydrogen sulfide, and sodium azide primarily affect oxygen use by interfering with the cytochrome oxidase system (Chap. 126).

CARDIAC OUTPUT

Any xenobiotic that causes a decreased cardiac output or hypotension may result in tissue hypoxia and tachypnea. This occurs most frequently with overdoses of β-adrenergic antagonists and calcium channel blockers, antidysrhythmics, cyclic antidepressants, and phenothiazines (Chap. 23).

ASTHMA AND OCCUPATIONAL EXPOSURES

Usually considered a cause of morbidity more than mortality, work-related asthma is frequently encountered by the practitioner. The pathophysiology of these illnesses is still being elucidated, and appears to result from both IgE and non–IgE-related mechanisms.[14]

Work-related asthma can be divided into three distinct clinical entities:

1. Work-aggravated asthma: Preexisting asthma worsened by allergens in the workplace.
2. Occupational asthma: Asthma caused by workplace exposure and not factors outside the workplace. There is a latency period between the symptoms and the first exposure, possibly as long as several years.
3. Reactive airway dysfunction syndrome (RADS): Asthma caused by nonimmunogenic stimuli in the workplace, occurring for the first time within 24 hours of exposure to an inhaled irritant xenobiotic.[5,19,102]

Occupational exposures are thought to be responsible for a substantial proportion of adult-onset asthma, estimated at 10%–25% in one international prospective study.[18]

A large number of xenobiotics and occupations are associated with the development of work-aggravated and work-related asthma. Because researchers rely on surveys and interviews, the latency period between exposure and symptoms makes identification of these associations a challenge.

Many high molecular weight xenobiotics, usually plant or animal derived, have been identified, such as arthropod and mite related materials, latex, flour, molds, endotoxins, and biological enzymes. Lower molecular weight xenobiotics associated with work-related asthma include isocyanates (used in spray paints and foam manufacturing), cleaning agents, anhydrides, amines, dyes and glues. For more information on specific xenobiotics see Chapters 124 and 127.

In one study, the following occupations were found, in decreasing order, to be associated with the development of occupational asthma: printing, woodworking, nursing, agriculture and forestry, cleaning and caretaking and electrical processors.[58]

In contrast to the occupational asthma and work-related asthma, the latency period between exposure and symptoms in RADS is short or absent, so the clinician may more easily identify the precipitant from history. Xenobiotics frequently associated with RADS include cleaning materials (including chlorine, hypochlorite, ammonia, and chloramines), solvents, toluene diiosocyanate, acids, alkali, nitrogen oxides, smoke, and diesel exhaust.[46,88]

APPROACH TO THE POISONED PATIENT

The initial assessment of each patient must involve the evaluation of upper airway patency. Adequacy of ventilation should then be determined. If concomitant injury is suspected, care must be taken to protect the cervical spine. When airway patency is in question, maneuvers to establish and protect the airway are of prime importance. Often this may simply involve repositioning the chin, jaw, or head, or suctioning secretions or vomitus from the airway. However, insertion of an oral or nasopharyngeal airway, or nasopharyngeal or endotracheal intubation, or surgical cricothyroidotomy may be required as clinically indicated. After the airway is secured, high-flow supplemental oxygen should be provided and the depth, rate, and rhythm of respirations evaluated. An acceptable tidal breath is one that transports 10–15 mL of air/kg of body weight.[4]

Hypoventilation that results from an inadequate respiratory rate or tidal volume is arbitrarily defined as P_{CO_2} > 44 mm Hg and leads to hypoxia and ventilatory failure if uncorrected.[107] The symptoms of hypoxia and or hypercarbia are nonspecific and resemble toxicity from many xenobiotics. Initially, patients appear restless and confused. Signs of sympathetic discharge, such as tachycardia and diaphoresis, may be noted. Later, patients may complain of headache, only to become sedated and subsequently comatose, as further deterioration occurs. Because these signs and symptoms are nonspecific, arterial blood-gas analysis must be used early in the assessment of patients who present with xenobiotic overdose and possible ventilatory failure.

A trial of naloxone, hypertonic dextrose, and thiamine may be indicated for the patient with an altered mental status and or respiratory compromise (Chap. 4). Because opioid overdose and hypoglycemia are rapidly reversible, potential causes of respiratory failure, these diagnoses should be addressed before most other interventions are considered. Failure to identify and reverse these conditions may result in unnecessary diagnostic and therapeutic interventions in addition to irreversible neurologic sequelae.

Having assured an acceptable airway, the remainder of the evaluation can proceed. A rapid assessment of the remainder of the vital signs (Chap. 3) should then occur. Obtaining a history and physical examination, pulse oximetry, arterial blood-gas analysis, measured oxygen saturation, and a chest radiograph are sufficient to determine the diagnosis of pulmonary pathology in most cases. However, adjuncts, such as measurement of negative inspiratory force (NIF), invasive hemodynamic monitoring, evaluation of the arterial–venous oxygen difference, xenon ventilation and technetium scanning, and CT scanning may be required.

HISTORY

A directed history must include questions on the nature, onset, and duration of symptoms; substance use and abuse; home and occupational exposures; and underlying pulmonary pathology. If the patient is suffering from a significant degree of respiratory compromise, most or all of the history may have to be obtained from friends, relatives, paramedics, coworkers, or others.

PHYSICAL EXAMINATION

The physical evaluation must include a detailed assessment of depth, rate, and rhythm of respirations, use of accessory muscles, direct evaluation of the oropharynx, position of the trachea, and presence and quality of breath sounds. Skin, nail bed, and conjunctival color must be observed for pallor or cyanosis. Funduscopic examination is a useful adjunct to the examination. Papilledema may be noted in the presence of acute hypercapnia. Additionally, because cyanide poisoning interferes with oxygen delivery to tissue, the venous oxygen saturation remains high. During the funduscopic examination, this may appear as arteriolization of the retinal veins, where the veins take on a color more characteristic of arteries (Chap. 126). A general assessment of muscle tone, with a specific emphasis on ocular and neck muscles may give clues to flaccidity or rigidity syndromes that interfere with respiration. When in doubt, a determination of the NIF will provide a rapid, objective, quantifiable bedside assessment of respiratory strength.

PULSE OXIMETRY

Pulse oximeters have gained widespread acceptance as rapid, noninvasive indicators of hemoglobin oxygen saturation. As defined, hemoglobin oxygen saturation is the ratio of oxyhemoglobin to total hemoglobin. By using two light-emitting diodes, the pulse oximeter is able to measure absorbance at the peak wavelengths for oxy- and deoxyhemoglobin (typically at 940 and 660 nm). Thus, the ratio of oxyhemoglobin to oxyhemoglobin plus deoxyhemoglobin (total hemoglobin) can be calculated. The clinician may then estimate the Po_2 from the oxygen saturation.

Limitations of this approach require elaboration. Because the oxyhemoglobin saturation curve becomes quite flat above 90% saturation (see Fig. 21–2), small changes in saturation greater than 90% may represent very large changes in Po_2. Thus, a decrease from 97% saturation to 95% saturation may represent a substantial decrease in Po_2. Although a low saturation is an early indicator of hypoxic hypoxia, this is only one of many causes of tissue hypoxia. If total hemoglobin is low, oxygen-carrying capacity is inadequate even with excellent saturation (see Fig. 21–1). Dyshemoglobinemias, such as carboxyhemoglobin, methemoglobin, and possibly sulfhemoglobin, interfere with the accuracy of pulse oximeter determinations and are of particular concern in the poisoned patient. Specifically, using a standard pulse oximeter, the presence of elevated concentrations of methemoglobin will tend to make the saturation approach 84%–86% (Chap. 127).[7,73] Carboxyhemoglobin is falsely interpreted by the pulse oximeter as mostly oxyhemoglobin, thus readings tend to appear normal even with significant carbon monoxide poisoning,[98] as Table 21–6 illustrates.

Accurate response by the pulse oximeter also requires adequate blood pressure, lack of strong venous pulsations (as might occur in a patient with tricuspid regurgitation), translucent nails (some shades of nail polish may interfere), absence of circulating dyes (methylene blue), and a near-normal temperature. Finally, we are often more interested in Pco_2 than Po_2 because it is a better measure of ventilation. The pulse oximeter gives no information with regard to Pco_2. Although the pulse oximeter may give early clues to the presence of hypoxic hypoxia, extrapolation of oxygen saturation to standard arterial blood-gas values may be difficult because of the many possible sources of error. Pulse oximetry is therefore best used as an initial screening tool for hypoxic hypoxia and later in combination with the initial arterial blood-gas measurement, as a determination of the patient's response to therapy. Although not widely used in clinical practice, a new pulse-cooximeter (noninvasive spectral analysis cooximeter), designed to measure carboxyhemoglobin and methemoglobin in addition to hemoglobin oxygen saturation, is available.

TABLE 21–6. Sample Interpretations of Oxygen Saturations Reported by Various Sources of Measurement

	Percent Oxygen Saturation			
Condition	Po_2 (mm Hg)	ABG	Pulse Oximeter	Cooximeter
Normal	95	95	95	95
Anemia	95	95	95	95*
Methemoglobinemia (30%)	95	95	85	70
Carboxyhemoglobinemia (30%)	95	95	95	70
Hypoxemia	60	90	90	90

The table demonstrates limitations of the various methods for determining oxygen saturation (O_2 saturation). The arterial blood gas (ABG) calculates the O_2 saturation from the dissolved oxygen content (Po_2) and becomes abnormal only when the Po_2 falls. The pulse oximeter uses only two wavelengths of light and produces substantial errors in the presence of a dyshemoglobinemia. Because the cooximeter uses more wavelengths of light than the pulse oximeter, it can correctly identify the presence of carboxyhemoglobin and methemoglobin. The cooximeter has the additional advantage (*) of calculating the total hemoglobin and oxygen content, so that it is useful in the setting of anemia. All techniques are acceptable for the assessment of hypoxemia.

Use of this device could potentially facilitate early, noninvasive diagnosis of carbon monoxide poisoning and methemoglobinemia, as well as minimize erroneous interpretations of standard pulse oximetry caused by the presence of these abnormal hemoglobins. A volunteer study, sponsored by the manufacturer of the device, demonstrated the ability to measure carboxyhemoglobin with an uncertainty of ± 2% within the range of 0%–15% and methemoglobin with an uncertainty of 0.5% within the range of 0%–12%.[6]

The device has already been used to identify carbon monoxide poisoning at emergency department triage, although another author found the device to have a large number of false positives for carboxyhemoglobin when used for this purpose.[51,94]

BLOOD-GAS ANALYSIS

Arterial blood-gas analysis is an easy and rapid means of evaluating both acid–base status and gas exchange. Attention must be paid to the method for determining oxygen saturation, specifically whether it is measured or calculated from Po_2. If the measured O_2 saturation is lower than would be predicted from the Po_2 (the calculated O_2 saturation), the presence of an abnormal hemoglobin (such as carboxyhemoglobin or methemoglobin) must be suspected. A normal calculated O_2 saturation does not exclude these disorders ("Use of the Cooximeter").

Because it is easier to obtain, venous blood-gas analysis is often used as a substitute for arterial blood-gas analysis.[16] In comparison with arterial values, venous pH and Po_2 are lower, whereas Pco_2 is higher. Errors can be introduced by increased muscle activity of the extremity being tested (eg, seizures) or the prolonged placement of a tourniquet while attempting phlebotomy. Although a venous blood gas is generally acceptable for assessment of the blood pH, it cannot provide a good evaluation of gas exchange.

Mixed venous blood (defined as right-heart blood), however, is required for accurate determination of the arterial–venous oxygen extraction and is an excellent indicator of acid–base status, cardiovascular function, and oxygen use. Unfortunately, a central venous catheter is required for sampling. When performing a peripheral venous blood-gas analysis, it is usually assumed that this is only an approximation of mixed venous blood.

The arterial Po_2 is generally considered adequate only if it lies within the flat portion at the upper right of the sigmoidal-shaped oxyhemoglobin dissociation curve (see Fig. 21–2). That portion of the curve includes the Po_2 range from 60 to 100 mm Hg, which corresponds to oxygen saturations > 90%. As mentioned earlier, within this flat portion there can be discernible changes in Po_2 with little change in oxygen saturation. For instance, an arterial Po_2 of 80 mm Hg corresponds roughly to an oxygen saturation of 95%. If the Po_2 falls to 60 mm Hg, the oxygen saturation falls to 90%. This insignificant decrease in the oxygen-carrying capacity of the blood is of minimal clinical concern. If the Po_2 falls another 20 mm Hg, however, there is a more significant reduction in oxygen saturation, to ~ 70%. Thus, changes in Po_2 > 60 mm Hg are usually not of acute therapeutic significance, because the O_2 saturation is > 90%. These changes are, however, frequently of diagnostic significance.

An exception to this concept applies to the patient who is under metabolic stress, as might result from low cardiac output, impaired vascular flow, anemia, or dyshemoglobinemia. Under these circumstances even the modest gain achieved by increasing both dissolved oxygen content and hemoglobin saturation > 90% may be desirable, as discussed earlier ("Hemoglobin and Chemical Asphyxiants"). Also, even if a Po_2 > 60 mm Hg or an O_2 saturation > 90% is considered acceptable in most acute settings, it is still desirable to achieve greater values, when feasible, to create a safety zone in case of clinical deterioration.

SIGNIFICANCE OF A DECREASED Po_2

In a patient with a diminished Po_2, five clinically relevant mechanisms for the hypoxemia should be considered: (a) alveolar hypoventilation; (b) V/Q mismatch; (c) shunting; (d) diffusion abnormality; and, rarely, (e) a decrease in Fio_2. In most clinical circumstances, diffusion defects cannot be distinguished from V/Q mismatch. Usually, the responsible mechanism can be identified by calculating the alveolar-arterial (A-a) oxygen gradient. In patients with alveolar hypoventilation, the A-a gradient is completely normal (≤ 15 mm Hg when breathing room air). Patients with V/Q mismatch have an A-a gradient that is increased but which normalizes when 100% oxygen is administered for at least 20 minutes. A normal A-a gradient is defined as < 100 mm Hg on 100% oxygen. The arterial Po_2 on 100% oxygen reaches approximately 575 mm Hg. In contrast, a patient with a shunt will also have an increased A-a gradient while breathing room air, but when 100% oxygen is administered, the arterial Po_2 falls to substantially less than 575 mm Hg and the A-a gradient does not normalize. Finally, in the case of a patient with hypoxia resulting from breathing in an environment in which the Fio_2 is < 21%, the Po_2 should correct rapidly when the patient is removed from the environment or supplemental oxygen is delivered.

In general, a low Po_2 can be improved by supplying supplemental oxygen. Although in this instance the patient's laboratory values may be corrected, the underlying process persists. It is important to remember that the laboratory correlate of hypoventilation is hypercapnia on the arterial blood-gas analysis. If hypercapnia is associated with a low arterial pH (< 7.35), assisted ventilation should be considered, regardless of whether the Po_2 corrects with supplemental oxygen.

USE OF THE COOXIMETER

Routine analysis of an arterial blood-gas yields a measured pH, measured Po_2, and measured Pco_2. Ordinarily, the serum bicarbonate, base excess, and percent oxygen saturation of hemoglobin are all calculated values. The oxygen saturation is of clinical significance because it usually correlates with the oxygen content of the blood, and thus the oxygen available to the tissues. However, implied in this relationship is a normal amount of functional hemoglobin. Because the oxygen saturation is calculated from the measured Po_2 using the oxyhemoglobin dissociation curve, it represents only the saturation of normal hemoglobin. Thus, in the presence of even a small percentage of abnormal hemoglobin, the calculated oxygen saturation overestimates the total oxygen content of the blood. For example, a patient with Po_2 of 95 mm Hg has a calculated oxygen saturation of 95%. If the patient also has a 30% methemoglobinemia, only 70% of the total hemoglobin is saturated to 95% and the actual saturation is only 67%. This gap is clinically important because hemoglobin saturations of < 90% do not provide adequate oxygen delivery to the tissues.

Despite the development of bedside noninvasive pulse-cooximetry, most clinicians still depend on laboratory cooximeters for measurement of carboxyhemoglobin and methemoglobin. Most cooximeters spectrophotometrically measure total hemoglobin, oxyhemoglobin, deoxyhemoglobin, carboxyhemoglobin, and methemoglobin (Fig. 21–3). The resultant saturation is a measured oxygen saturation of the total hemoglobin by including four common hemoglobin variants, and thus correlates with the total oxygen content of the blood.

The difference between measured and calculated oxygen saturation represents the percentage of abnormal hemoglobin present. This gap is helpful in the diagnosis of methemoglobin and carboxyhemoglobin, and is useful in assessing the adequacy of therapy for these disorders.

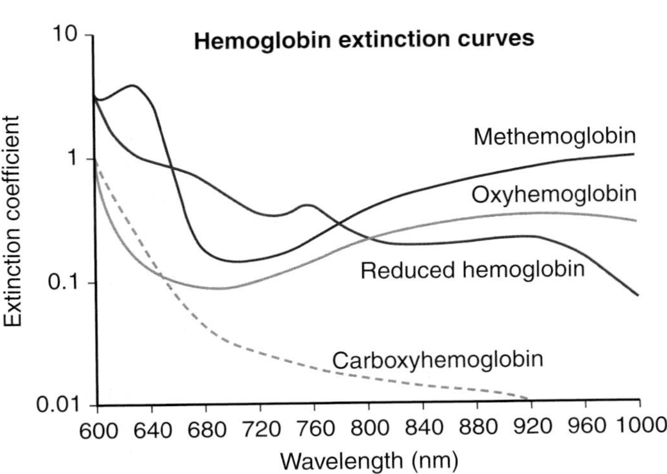

FIGURE 21–3. Cooximetry curves for normal and abnormal hemoglobin variants. Transmitted light absorbance spectra are shown for four hemoglobin species: oxyhemoglobin, reduced (deoxy) hemoglobin, carboxyhemoglobin, and methemoglobin.

Common indications for cooximetry include cyanosis that is unresponsive to oxygen (methemoglobin and sulfhemoglobin), known use of methemoglobin-forming xenobiotics (such as dapsone), smoke inhalation (carboxyhemoglobin and possibly methemoglobin), and evaluation of therapy for cyanide toxicity (methemoglobin).

Like so many other tools, the cooximeter is not perfect. Its biggest limitation occurs when dealing with uncommon hemoglobins. Because only four wavelengths of light are used by most cooximeters, they have the ability to define only four hemoglobin variants. Consequently, rare dyshemoglobinemias, such as sulfhemoglobin, are interpreted as one or a combination of the four common hemoglobin variants, giving erroneous results. This phenomenon is commonly noted in neonates, where fetal hemoglobin may be interpreted as carboxyhemoglobin.[100,108] Although this error rarely adds greater than 10% to the true carboxyhemoglobin value, this amount can be significant because of the difficulties in assessing the neuropsychiatric status of infants possibly exposed to carbon monoxide. Some newer cooximeters are unaffected by fetal hemoglobin, and should be used in neonatal cases of suspected carbon monoxide poisoning.[101,112] Similarly, these newer models are now beginning to provide measurements of sulfhemoglobin as well.[28,110,112] Additionally, cooximeters tend to interpret low levels (< 2.5%) of carboxyhemoglobin inconsistently.[66] Fortunately, this rarely has clinical implications.

CHEST RADIOGRAPHY

Radiographic detection of a pneumothorax or pneumomediastinum, cardiogenic pulmonary edema, ALI and ARDS, aspiration pneumonitis, or the presence of a foreign body is crucial, but can usually be delayed until the initial evaluation is completed. Confirmation of endotracheal tube placement is necessary but initially can be ascertained by auscultating bilateral breath sounds following compression of a bag valve mask, or using a variety of marketed devices such as end tidal CO_2 detectors designed to help confirm tube placement. For patients with occupational disorders, the chest radiograph is essential to confirm and stage exposures to asbestos, silica, coal, and other causes of pneumoconiosis.

THERAPEUTIC OPTIONS

SUPPLEMENTAL OXYGEN

Supplemental oxygen is indicated for all patients with suspected or confirmed respiratory insufficiency. Although it is generally advisable to begin with high flow (12 L/min) via a nonrebreather mask, lower concentrations of oxygen can be used in more stable patients. It is important to remember that a normal saturation on pulse oximetry does not imply that there is no need for supplemental oxygen. This can be determined only after a more complete assessment. Initially, there should be limited concern over worsening hypercapnia in patients with chronic obstructive pulmonary disease (COPD) and respiratory failure. This concern should not deter one from providing needed oxygen as many of these patients will require intubation for their hypoventilation. If time and the patient's clinical condition permit, an arterial blood-gas analysis should be obtained prior to administering supplemental oxygen or mechanical ventilation so that the patient's intrinsic respiratory status can be adequately defined. In many situations, the patient's condition will not permit delay, and subsequent arterial blood-gas analyses will be needed to determine the ability to decrease the Fio_2 or the need for intubation. Hyperbaric oxygen is indicated for carbon monoxide poisoning and rarely other exposures (Antidotes in Depth A37: Hyperbaric Oxygen).

Additional respiratory support can be offered from bilevel positive airway pressure (BiPAP). Some experimental evidence supports the use of BiPAP for patients with acute respiratory dysfunction in the emergency department.[80] Although this technique may be useful in overdosed patients, it should be considered only as a temporizing measure for patients who are expected to recover rapidly, or while preparing for intubation.

INTUBATION

After the decision for mechanical ventilation has been made, the route needs to be selected. The editors of this text prefer oral intubation because it permits the use of a larger endotracheal tube—usually 8 mm or larger in adults—than does nasal intubation. If the patient later needs bronchoscopy, it can be done through the endotracheal tube. Some data suggest that bronchoscopy with bronchoalveolar lavage may be of both diagnostic[99] and therapeutic[60] benefit for selected poisoned patients. However, in an awake patient, nasotracheal intubation done blindly or with the aid of a flexible fiberoptic laryngoscope may be more easily performed. An advantage of nasotracheal intubation over oral intubation is that orogastric lavage can be performed more easily when the oral cavity is unimpeded. After the trachea is intubated, the tube should be checked to ensure that it is correctly positioned.

All patients who sustain overdoses and show signs or symptoms of respiratory insufficiency should have chest radiographs performed. Unfortunately, intubated patients usually have portable radiographs performed and the carina may be difficult to visualize because of the poor quality of the study. When seen, the carina is visualized between T-5 and T-7 in most patients. Thus, the tip of the endotracheal tube should be above T-5 for proper (safe) placement. When a portable chest radiograph is obtained, the patient's neck may be extended or flexed, altering the location of the endotracheal tube tip. For this reason it is essential to note the position of the neck during the radiograph, because the tip of the endotracheal tube may move up (with flexion) or down (with extension) by almost 2 cm.[12]

MECHANICAL VENTILATION

After a patient is intubated for ventilatory support, the respirator mode—assist, control, or intermittent mandatory ventilation (IMV)—is selected. Patients with pure hypoventilation usually require a controlled fixed rate that can be easily adjusted based on serial arterial blood-gas analyses. Patients with pulmonary parenchymal processes, such as ALI, ARDS, or pneumonia, usually do well when placed on either assist or IMV mode. With the IMV mode, a given number of mandatory breaths is administered at the set tidal volume. The patient may take additional breaths without assistance, permitting lower mean airway pressure, which theoretically may reduce the risk of barotrauma and hemodynamic compromise. Although the lower airway pressures associated with IMV are desirable, many authorities recommend the use of the assist mode because it eliminates the patient's work of breathing.[59]

The next step is to determine the appropriate Fio_2 to be delivered to the patient. A number of formulas have been devised. One simple approach is to intubate a patient, control breathing, administer 100% oxygen, and decrease to an Fio_2 of < 50% as quickly as possible in an attempt to prevent oxygen toxicity.[3] Although the toxic effects of oxygen are well known for paraquat (Chap. 115), evidence suggests that oxygen may be an important mediator of other xenobiotic-induced pulmonary injuries such as with iron.[47] A Po_2 of 55 mm Hg or a measured oxygen saturation > 88% is generally acceptable; thus, there is little reason to expose patients to much higher concentrations of oxygen once these conditions are met.[1,103] Many clinicians feel more comfortable establishing a "buffer" against deterioration by increasing the Po_2 to somewhat greater than 55 mm Hg, but prolonged exposure to higher values is rarely indicated. In patients with pure alveolar hypoventilation, the tidal volume should be set at 10–15 mL/kg/breath. If oxygenation

Two 30-year-old patients who overdosed were brought to the ED. Each had ingested substantial amounts of barbiturates and diazepam. An arterial blood gas drawn from patient 1 while he was breathing room air revealed a pH of 7.18, PCO_2 of 70 mm Hg, PO_2 of 50 mm Hg, and a calculated bicarbonate of 24 mEq/L. An arterial blood gas drawn from patient 2, also breathing room air, revealed a pH of 7.31, PCO_2 of 50 mm Hg, PO_2 of 50 mm Hg, and a calculated bicarbonate of 25 mEq/L. Quick analysis showed that patient 1 was hypercapnic with a significant respiratory acidosis. Patient 2 did not appear as ill; his PCO_2 was not very elevated and his pH was not significantly reduced. The A-a gradients were calculated to be 12.5 mm Hg for patient 1 and 37.5 mm Hg for patient 2 (Fig. 21–4A and B).

A. Arterial PCO_2 approximates alveolar PCO_2 and is substituted as:

$$PAO_2 = PiO_2 - \frac{PCO_2}{R}$$

$$PiO_2 = (FiO_2)\,(PB - PH_2O)$$

where PAO_2 is alveolar PO_2, PiO_2 is partial pressure of inspired O_2, $PaCO_2$ is arterial PCO_2, and R is the respiratory exchange ratio. Therefore:

$$PAO_2 = [(FiO_2)(PB - PH_2O)] - \frac{PCO_2}{R}$$

where FiO_2 is the inspired O_2 fraction, PH_2O is water vapor pressure, and PB is barometric pressure. On room air at sea level, FiO_2 – 21%. At steady state, R = 0.8. At sea level, PB = 760 mm Hg, and PH_2O = 47 mm Hg.
Therefore:

$$PAO_2 = [(FiO_2)(PB - PH_2O)] - \frac{PCO_2}{R}$$

$$= [(0.21)(760 - 47)] - \frac{PCO_2}{R}$$

$$= 150 - [(1.25)(PCO_2)]$$

Because the A-a gradient is equal to $PAO_2 - PaO_2$ it can be expressed as:

$150 - [(1.25)(PCO_2)] - PaO_2$ or $150 - [(1.25)(PCO_2) + PaO_2]$

A normal A-a gradient is 10–15 mm Hg, but this increases with age. A rough estimate of the normal A-a gradient is one-third the patient's age.

B. Referring to the two overdosed patients above, the A-a gradient for patient 1 is:

$$150 - [(1.25)(70) + 50] = 12.5 \text{ mm Hg}$$

This calculation reveals a normal gradient, indicating that the etiology for hypoxemia and hypoventilation is extrinsic to the lung itself. In patient 2 the A-a gradient is:

$$150 - [(1.25)(50) + 50] = 37.5 \text{ mm Hg}$$

This abnormally high A-a gradient is consistent with the aspiration which was pneumonia seen on the patient's chest radiograph.

FIGURE 21–4. (A) Derivation of the definition of alveolar-arterial (A-a) oxygen gradients. (B) Using the A-a gradients.

cannot be maintained with $Fio_2 \leq 50\%$, PEEP may be used, with careful reassessment of serial arterial blood-gas analyses, changes in effective compliance, and hemodynamic data with each increment in PEEP. In patients with ALI or ARDS, however, lower tidal volumes (on the order of 6 mL/kg/breath) decrease both mortality and the total number of days on the ventilator.[1]

PHARMACOLOGIC ADJUNCTS

Only a few pharmacologic agents have a significant role in reversing xenobiotic-induced respiratory dysfunction. Naloxone may have the greatest role. Atropine and pralidoxime may be useful for respiratory dysfunction from cholinesterase inhibitors (Antidotes in Depth A33: Pralidoxime and Chap. 113). Elapid antivenom and botulinum antitoxin are rarely used but may be lifesaving. Neostigmine can reverse muscle weakness from nondepolarizing neuromuscular blockers (Chap. 68). More commonly, clinicians are required to treat bronchospasm from exposure to pulmonary irritants. The use of β_2-selective adrenergic-agonist bronchodilators is effective in these patients.[35] The role of corticosteroids remains controversial.[3]

When treating patients with bronchospasm from one of the work-related asthma syndromes, it is reasonable that management should be similar to that of any patient with pulmonary bronchospasm: emphasizing inhaled bronchodilators and corticosteroids (Fig. 21–4).

An inhaled solution of 2% sodium bicarbonate may provide symptomatic relief for patients with pulmonary exposure to hydrogen chloride or to chlorine (Antidotes in Depth A5: Sodium Bicarbonate).

Exogenous nitric oxide has been considered for a variety of pulmonary conditions. Specifically, nitric oxide may be useful as a bronchodilator,[17] a means to reverse hypoxic pulmonary vasoconstriction,[3] and as a treatment for ARDS.[2] Unfortunately, controlled studies fail to demonstrate a benefit for nitric oxide in ALI/ARDS patients.[3,103] Similarly, the results are disappointing for glucocorticoids, surfactants, and a variety of antiinflammatory agents.[4,103]

SUMMARY

Xenobiotics affect tissue oxygenation adversely at every step required for oxygen delivery. This process begins with lowering the partial pressure of inspired oxygen (simple asphyxiants) and ends with inhibition or blockade of cytochrome oxidase (carbon monoxide, cyanide, hydrogen sulfide). Although the clinical manifestations of hypoxia are constant regardless of the etiology, the history, physical examination, and some simple laboratory testing will often allow the clinician to determine the specific mechanism of hypoxia. Once the specific mechanism for hypoxia is identified, potential etiologies can be appreciated, and specific treatments begun. While the diagnosis is being determined, the first responses to tissue hypoxia always involve administration of supplemental oxygen, assisted ventilation if necessary, and assuring the adequacy of circulation.

REFERENCES

1. Acute Respiratory Distress Syndrome Network. Ventilation with lower tidal volumes as compared with traditional tidal volumes for acute lung injury and the acute respiratory distress syndrome. *N Engl J Med.* 2000;342:1301-1308.
2. Adnot S, Raffestin B, Eddahibi S. NO in the lung. *Respir Physiol.* 1995;101:109-120.
3. Albertson TE, Walby WF, Allen RP, Tharratt RS. The pharmacology and toxicology of three new biologic agents used in pulmonary medicine. *J Toxicol Clin Toxicol.* 1995;33:427-438.
4. Artigas A, Bernard GR, Carlet J, et al. The American-European Consensus Conference on ARDS, part 2. Ventilatory, pharmacologic, supportive therapy, study design strategies and issues related to recovery and remodeling. *Intensive Care Med.* 1998;24:378-398.
5. Banks DE, Jalloul A. Occupational asthma, work-related asthma, and reactive airways dysfunction syndrome. *Curr Opin Pulm Med.* 2007;13:131-136.
6. Barker SJ, Curry J, Redford D, Morgan S. Measurement of carboxyhemoglobin and methemoglobin by pulse oximetry: a human volunteer study. *Anesthesiology.* 2006;105:892-897.
7. Barker SJ, Tremper KK, Hyatt J. Effects of methemoglobinemia on pulse oximetry and mixed venous oximetry. *Anesthesiology.* 1989;70:112-117.
8. Baumann BM, Perrone J, Hornig SE, et al. Cardiac and hemodynamic assessment of patients with cocaine-associated chest pain syndromes. *J Toxicol Clin Toxicol.* 2000;38:283-290.

9. Baxter PJ, Kapila M, Mfonfu D. Lake Nyos disaster, Cameroon, 1986: The medical effects of large scale emission of carbon dioxide? *BMJ.* 1989;298:1437-1441.
10. Bernard GR, Artigas A, Brigham KL, et al. The American-European Consensus Conference on ARDS. Definitions, mechanisms, relevant outcomes, and clinical trial coordination. *Am J Resp Crit Care Med.* 1994;149:818-824.
11. Birrer RB, Calderon J. Pneumothorax, pneumomediastinum, and pneumopericardium following Valsalva's maneuver during marijuana smoking. *N Y State J Med.* 1984;84:619-620.
12. Blanc VF, Tremblay NA. The complications of tracheal intubation: A new classification with a review of the literature. *Anesth Analg.* 1974;53: 202-213.
13. Book WJ, Abel M, Eisenkraft JB. Adverse effects of depolarizing neuromuscular blocking agents. Incidence, prevention and management. *Drug Saf.* 1994;10:331-349.
14. Boulet LP, Lemière C, Gautrin D, Cartier A. New insights into occupational asthma. *Curr Opin Allergy Clin Immunol.* 2007;7:96-101.
15. Boyd RE, Brennan PT, Deng JF, et al. Strychnine poisoning. Recovery from profound lactic acidosis, hyperthermia, and rhabdomyolysis. *Am J Med.* 1983;74:507-512.
16. Brandenburg MA, Dire DJ. Comparison of arterial and venous blood gas values in the initial emergency department evaluation of patients with diabetic ketoacidosis. *Ann Emerg Med.* 1998;31:459-465.
17. Brett SJ, Evans TW. Nitric oxide: Physiological roles and therapeutic implications in the lung. *Br J Hosp Med.* 1996;55:487-490.
18. Brooks SM. An approach to patients suspected of having an occupational pulmonary disease. *Clin Chest Med.* 1981;2:171-178.
19. Brooks SM, Weiss MA, Bernstein IL. Reactive airways dysfunction syndrome (RADS). Persistent asthma syndrome after high level irritant exposures. *Chest.* 1985;88:376-384.
20. Bush MN, Rubenstein R, Hoffman I, Bruno MS. Spontaneous pneumomediastinum as a consequence of cocaine use. *N Y State J Med.* 1984;84: 618-619.
21. Byrne K, Sugerman HJ. Experimental and clinical assessment of lung injury by measurement of extravascular lung water and transcapillary protein flux in ARDS: A review of current techniques. *J Surg Res.* 1988;44: 185-203.
22. Caspi J, Klausner JM, Safadi T, et al. Delayed respiratory depression following fentanyl anesthesia for cardiac surgery. *Crit Care Med.* 1988;16: 238-240.
23. Cherubin CE. Epidemiology of tetanus in narcotic addicts. *N Y State J Med.* 1970;70:267-271.
24. Christian CM 2nd, Waller JL, Moldenhauer CC. Postoperative rigidity following fentanyl anesthesia. *Anesthesiology.* 1983;58:275-277.
25. Cope DK, Grimbert F, Downey JM, Taylor AE. Pulmonary capillary pressure: A review. *Crit Care Med.* 1992;20:1043-1056.
26. Cotter G, Moshkovitz Y, Kaluski E, et al. Accurate, noninvasive continuous monitoring of cardiac output by whole-body electrical bioimpedance. *Chest.* 2004;125:1431-1440.
27. Delaney K, Hoffman RS. Pulmonary infarction associated with crack cocaine use in a previously healthy 23-year-old woman. *Am J Med.* 1991;91: 92-94.
28. Demedts P, Wauters A, Watelle M, Neels H. Pitfalls in discriminating sulfhemoglobin from methemoglobin. *Clin Chem.* 1997;43: 1098-1099.
29. Duberstein JL, Kaufman DM. A clinical study of an epidemic of heroin intoxication and heroin-induced pulmonary edema. *Am J Med.* 1971;51:704-714.
30. Esteban A, Anzueto A, Frutos F, et al. Characteristics and outcomes in adult patients receiving mechanical ventilation: a 28-day international study. *JAMA.* 2002;287:345-355.
31. Ettinger NA, Albin RJ. A review of the respiratory effects of smoking cocaine. *Am J Med.* 1989;87:664-668.
32. Fassler CA, Rodriguez RM, Badesch DB, et al. Magnesium toxicity as a cause of hypotension and hypoventilation. Occurrence in patients with normal renal function. *Arch Intern Med.* 1985;145:1604-1606.
33. Fein A, Grossman RF, Jones JG, et al. Carbon monoxide effect on alveolar epithelial permeability. *Chest.* 1980;78:726-731.
34. Finley CJ, Silverman MA, Nunez AE. Angiotensin-converting enzyme inhibitor-induced angioedema: Still unrecognized. *Am J Emerg Med* 1992;10:550-552.
35. Flury KE, Dines DE, Rodarte JR, Rodgers R. Airway obstruction due to inhalation of ammonia. *Mayo Clin Proc.* 1983;58:389-393.
36. Frand UI, Shim CS, Williams MH Jr. Heroin-induced pulmonary edema. Sequential studies of pulmonary function. *Ann Intern Med.* 1972;77: 29-35.
37. Frand UI, Shim CS, Williams MH Jr. Methadone-induced pulmonary edema. *Ann Intern Med.* 1972;76:975-979.
38. Freeth SJ: Lake Nyos disaster. *BMJ.* 1989;299:513.
39. Gill JR, Ely SF, Hua Z. Environmental gas displacement: Three accidental deaths in the workplace. *Am J Forensic Med Pathol.* 2002;23:26-30.
40. Girard TD, Bernard GR. Mechanical ventilation in ARDS: a state of the art review. *Chest.* 2007;131:921-929.
41. Glassroth J, Adams GD, Schnoll S. The impact of substance abuse on the respiratory system. *Chest.* 1987;91:596-602.
42. Glauser FL, Smith WR, Caldwell A, et al. Ethchlorvynol (Placidyl)-induced pulmonary edema. *Ann Intern Med.* 1976;84:46-48.
43. Griffith DE, Levin JL. Respiratory effects of outdoor air pollution. *Postgrad Med.* 1989;86:111-116.
44. Halpern P, Raskin Y, Sorkine P, Oganezov A. Exposure to extremely high concentrations of carbon dioxide: A clinical description of a mass casualty incident. *Ann Emerg Med.* 2004;43:196-199.
45. Heffner JE, Sahn SA. Salicylate-induced pulmonary edema. Clinical features and prognosis. *Ann Intern Med.* 1981;95:405-409.
46. Henneberger PK, Derk SJ, Davis L, et al. Work-Related Reactive Airways Dysfunction Syndrome Cases from Surveillance in Selected US States. *J Occup Environ Med.* 2003;45:360-368).
47. Howland MA. Risks of parenteral deferoxamine for acute iron poisoning. *J Toxicol Clin Toxicol.* 1996;34:491-497.
48. Hu H, Fine J, Epstein P, et al. Tear gas—Harassing agent or toxic chemical weapon? *JAMA.* 1989;262:660-663.
49. Humbert VH Jr, Munn NJ, Hawkins RF. Noncardiogenic pulmonary edema complicating massive diltiazem overdose. *Chest.* 1991;99:258-259.
50. Hunter JM. New neuromuscular blocking drugs. *N Engl J Med.* 1995;332:1691-1699.
51. O'Malley GF. Non-invasive carbon monoxide measurement is not accurate. *Ann Emerg Med.* 2006;48:477-478.
52. Isbister GK, Downes F, Sibbritt D, et al. Aspiration pneumonitis in an overdose population: Frequency, predictors, and outcomes. *Crit Care Med.* 2004;32:88-93.
53. Joseph WL, Fletcher HS, Giordano JM, Adkins PC. Pulmonary and cardiovascular implications of drug addiction. *Ann Thorac Surg.* 1973;15:263-274.
54. Katz NM, Buchholz BJ, Howard E, et al. Venovenous extracorporeal membrane oxygenation for noncardiogenic pulmonary edema after coronary bypass surgery. *Ann Thorac Surg.* 1988;46:462-464.
55. King WW, Cave DR. Use of esmolol to control autonomic instability of tetanus. *Am J Med.* 1991;91:425-428.
56. Klein MD. Noncardiogenic pulmonary edema following hydrochlorothiazide ingestion. *Ann Emerg Med.* 1987;16:901-903.
57. Knochel JP. Neuromuscular manifestations of electrolyte disorders. *Am J Med.* 1982;72:521-535.
58. Kogevinas M, Zock J, Jarvis D, et al. Exposure to substances in the workplace and new-onset asthma: an international prospective population-based study (ECRHS-II). *Lancet.* 2007;370:336-341.
59. Kollef MH, Schuster DP. The acute respiratory distress syndrome. *N Engl J Med.* 1995;332:27-37.
60. Kulling P. Hospital treatment of victims exposed to combustion products. *Toxicol Lett.* 1992;64-65:283-289.
61. Lam S, Chan-Yeung M. Occupational asthma: Natural history, evaluation and management. *Occup Med.* 1987;2:373-381.
62. Lambert JR, Byrick RJ, Hammeke MD. Management of acute strychnine poisoning. *CMAJ.* 1981;124:1268-1270.
63. Leach RM, Rees PJ, Wilmshurst P. Hyperbaric oxygen therapy. *BMJ.* 1998;317:1140-1143.
64. Leeman M. The pulmonary circulation in acute lung injury: A review of some recent advances. *Intensive Care Med.* 1991;17:254-260.
65. Little JW, Smith LH. Pulmonary aspiration. *West J Med.* 1979;131: 122-129.
66. Mahoney JJ, Vreman HJ, Stevenson DK, Van Kessel AL. Measurement of carboxyhemoglobin and total hemoglobin by five specialized spectrophotometers (CO-oximeters) in comparison with reference methods. *Clin Chem.* 1993;39:1693-1700.
67. Mills CA, Flacke JW, Miller JD, et al. Cardiovascular effects of fentanyl reversal by naloxone at varying arterial carbon dioxide tensions in dogs. *Anesth Analg.* 1988;67:730-736.

68. Minton NA, Murray VS. A review of organophosphate poisoning. *Med Toxicol Adverse Drug Exp.* 1988;3:350-375.
69. Moll J, Kerns W 2nd, Tomaszewski C, Rose R. Incidence of aspiration pneumonia in intubated patients receiving activated charcoal. *J Emerg Med.* 1999;17:279-283.
70. Moshkovitz Y, Kaluski E, Milo O, et al. Recent developments in cardiac output determination by bioimpedance: Comparison with invasive cardiac output and potential cardiovascular applications. *Curr Opin Cardiol.* 2004;19:229-237.
71. National Heart, Lung, and Blood Institute Acute Respiratory Distress Syndrome (ARDS) Clinical Trials Network. Wiedemann HP, Wheeler AP, Bernard GR, et al. Comparison of two fluid-management strategies in acute lung injury. *N Engl J Med.* 2006 Jun 15;354(24):2564-2575.
72. Onyeama HP, Oehme FW. A literature review of paraquat toxicity. *Vet Hum Toxicol.* 1984;26:494-502.
73. Osei C, Berger HW, Nicholas P. Septic pulmonary infarction: Clinical and radiographic manifestations in 11 patients. *Mt Sinai J Med.* 1979;46: 145-148.
74. Palat D, Denson M, Sherman M,.Matz R. Pneumomediastinum induced by inhalation of alkaloidal cocaine. *N Y State J Med.* 1988;88: 438-439.
75. Pare JA, Fraser RG, Hogg JC, et al. Pulmonary 'mainline' granulomatosis: Talcosis of intravenous methadone abuse. *Medicine (Baltimore).* 1979;58:229-239.
76. Park S, Giammona ST. Toxic effects of tear gas on an infant following prolonged exposure. *Am J Dis Child.* 1972;123:245-246.
77. Parsons PE. Respiratory failure as a result of drugs, overdoses, and poisonings. *Clin Chest Med.* 1994;15:93-102.
78. Pentiah P, Reilly F, Borison HL. Interactions of morphine sulfate and sodium salicylate on respiration in cats. *J Pharmacol Exp Ther.* 1966;154: 110-118.
79. Persky VW, Goldfrank LR. Methadone overdoses in a New York City hospital. *JACEP.* 1976;5:111-113.
80. Pollack C Jr, Torres MT, Alexander L. Feasibility study of the use of bilevel positive airway pressure for respiratory support in the emergency department. *Ann Emerg Med.* 1996;27:189-192.
81. Pollack MM, Dunbar BS, Holbrook PR, Fields AI. Aspiration of activated charcoal and gastric contents. *Ann Emerg Med.* 1981;10:528-529.
82. Reed CR, Glauser FL. Drug-induced noncardiogenic pulmonary edema. *Chest.* 1991;100:1120-1124.
83. Reynolds KJ, Palayiwa E, Moyle JT, et al. The effect of dyshemoglobins on pulse oximetry: Part I, theoretical approach and part II, experimental results using an in vitro test system. *J Clin Monit.* 1993;9:81-90.
84. Rubin RB, Neugarten J. Cocaine-associated asthma. *Am J Med.* 1990;88: 438-439.
85. Saba GP 2nd, James AE Jr, Johnson BA, et al. Pulmonary complications of narcotic abuse. *Am J Roentgenol Radium Ther Nucl Med.* 1974;122:733-739.
86. Schmidt-Nowara WW, Samet JM, Rosario PA. Early and late pulmonary complications of botulism. *Arch Intern Med.* 1983;143:451-456.
87. Senanayake N, Karalliedde L. Neurotoxic effects of organophosphorus insecticides. An intermediate syndrome. *N Engl J Med.* 1987;316: 761-763.
88. Shakeri MS, Dick FD, Ayres JG. Which agents cause reactive airways dysfunction syndrome (RADS)? A systematic review. *Occup Med (Lond).* 2008;58:205-211. [Epub ahead of print]
89. Shesser R, Davis C, Edelstein S. Pneumomediastinum and pneumothorax after inhaling alkaloidal cocaine. *Ann Emerg Med.* 1981;10:213-215.
90. Sklar J, Timms RM. Codeine-induced pulmonary edema. *Chest.* 1977;72: 230-231.
91. Smith DD. Top ten list in occupational pulmonary disease. *Chest.* 2004;126:1360-1363.
92. Stern WZ. Roentgenographic aspects of narcotic addiction. *JAMA.* 1976;236:963-965.
93. Sun KO, Chan YW, Cheung RT, et al. Management of tetanus: A review of 18 cases. *J R Soc Med.* 1994;87:135-137.
94. Suner S, Partridge R, Sucov A, et al. Non-invasive pulse co-oximetry screening in the emergency department identifies occult carbon monoxide toxicity. *J Emerg Med.* 2008;34:441-450.
95. Tashkin DP. Airway effects of marijuana, cocaine, and other inhaled illicit agents. *Curr Opin Pulm Med.* 2001;7:43-61.
96. Thadani PV. NIDA conference report on cardiopulmonary complications of "crack" cocaine use. Clinical manifestations and pathophysiology. *Chest.* 1996;110:1072-1076.
97. Treacher DF, Leach RM. Oxygen transport-1. Basic principles. *BMJ.* 1998;317:1302-1306.
98. Vegfors M, Lennmarken C. Carboxyhaemoglobinaemia and pulse oximetry. *Br J Anaesth.* 1991;66:625-626.
99. Vijayan VK, Pandey VP, Sankaran K, et al. Bronchoalveolar lavage study in victims of toxic gas leak at Bhopal. *Indian J Med Res.* 1989;90: 407-414.
100. Vreman HJ, Ronquillo RB, Ariagno RL, et al. Interference of fetal hemoglobin with the spectrophotometric measurement of carboxyhemoglobin. *Clin Chem.* 1988;34:975-977.
101. Vreman HJ, Stevenson DK. Carboxyhemoglobin determined in neonatal blood with a CO-oximeter unaffected by fetal oxyhemoglobin. *Clin Chem.* 1994;40:1522-1527.
102. Wagner GR, Wegman DH: Occupational asthma: prevention by definition. *Am J Ind Med.* 1998;33:427-429.
103. Ware LB, Matthay MA. The acute respiratory distress syndrome. *N Engl J Med.* 2000;342:1334-1349.
104. Weil JV, McCullough RE, Kline JS, Sodal IE. Diminished ventilatory response to hypoxia and hypercapnia after morphine in normal man. *N Engl J Med.* 1975;292:1103-1106.
105. Wetherill SF, Guarino MJ, Cox RW. Acute renal failure associated with barium chloride poisoning. *Ann Intern Med.* 1981;95:187-188.
106. Wiener MD, Putman CE. Pain in the chest in a user of cocaine. *JAMA.* 1987;258:2087–2088.
107. Williams AJ. ABC of oxygen: Assessing and interpreting arterial blood gases and acid-base balance. *BMJ.* 1998;317:1213-1216.
108. Wimberley PD, Siggaard-Andersen O, Fogh-Andersen N. Accurate measurements of hemoglobin oxygen saturation, and fractions of carboxyhemoglobin and methemoglobin in fetal blood using radiometer OSM3: Corrections for fetal hemoglobin fraction and pH. *Scand J Clin Lab Invest Suppl.* 1990;203:235-239.
109. Woodard ED, Friedlander B, Lesher RJ, et al. Outbreak of hypersensitivity pneumonitis in an industrial setting. *JAMA.* 1988;259:1965-1969.
110. Wu C, Kenny MA. A case of sulfhemoglobinemia and emergency measurement of sulfhemoglobin with an OSM3 CO-oximeter. *Clin Chem.* 1997;43:162-166.
111. Zimmerman GA, Clemmer TP. Acute respiratory failure during therapy for salicylate intoxication. *Ann Emerg Med.* 1981;10:104-106.
112. Zwart A, Buursma A, Zijlstra WG. A new trend in blood gas chemistry: The measurement of clinically relevant hemoglobin derivatives. performance of the OSM3 hemoximeter. *Scand J Clin Lab Invest Suppl.* 1987;188:57-60.

CHAPTER 22
ELECTROPHYSIOLOGIC AND ELECTROCARDIOGRAPHIC PRINCIPLES

Cathleen Clancy

ELECTROPHYSIOLOGIC PRINCIPLES

The clinical tool most commonly used to assess cardiac function is the surface electrocardiogram (ECG). The ECG records the sum of the electrical changes occurring within the myocardium. The electrophysiologic basis of cardiac function and of the ECG, are complex and are subject to functional alternation by numerous xenobiotics. Ion currents flowing through various ion channels are responsible for cardiac function. Electrophysiologic studies have identified the functional types of membrane receptors and ion channels. Molecular genetic studies have identified the gene coding for the key cardiac ion channels and have elucidated the structural and physiologic relationships that lead to the toxic effects of many xenobiotics. These channels are critical for maintenance of the intracellular ion concentrations necessary for action potential development, impulse conduction throughout the heart, and myocyte contraction. This chapter will first review the individual ion channels and their currents, and then review them in summary through the perspective of their contribution and effects on the ECG.

ION CHANNELS OF THE MYOCARDIAL CELL MEMBRANE

SODIUM CHANNELS

The voltage-sensitive sodium channels are responsible for the initiation of depolarization of the myocardial membrane. All currently identified voltage-sensitive channels, including the sodium and calcium channel, have structures similar to the functional potassium channel assembly. The sodium channel gene encodes a single protein that contains four functional domains (D I—D IV). Each of these domains has the 6 membrane-spanning regions characteristic of the voltage-gated potassium channel and is structurally similar to an α subunit of the potassium channel (Fig. 22–1A). The single, large α subunit of the sodium channel assembles with regulatory β subunits to form the functional unit of the sodium channel. The best characterized of the sodium channels, the SCN5A gene-encoded α channel, is inactivated by xenobiotic interactions between the D III and the D IV domains to physically block the inner mouth of the sodium channel pore.[26]

POTASSIUM CHANNELS

Ion channels that change their conductance of current with changes in the transmembrane voltage potential are called *rectifying channels*. The voltage sensitive potassium channels are categorized based upon their speed of activation and their voltage response. They include the "delayed rectifier" potassium currents, particularly the I_{Kr} (rapidly activating) and the I_{Ks} (slowly activating) channels.[40]

The various voltage gated potassium channels share an underlying structural similarity. The α subunit is a protein molecule with 6 membrane-spanning α-helical domains, termed S1–S6 (Fig. 22–1B). The pore domain is located between the S5 and S6 regions of the α subunit, and the S4 region is the voltage sensor region.[26,49] Four of the α subunits encoded by the KvLQT1 gene assemble with β units encoded by the minK gene (originally thought to be the minimal potassium channel subunit) to form the I_{Ks} potassium channel.[26] Human ether a-go-go related gene (HERG) encodes the α subunit that assembles with β subunit proteins encoded by the minK related protein 1 (MiRPI) gene to form the I_{Kr} potassium channel. The C-terminus region of the α subunit encoded by HERG has a cyclic nucleotide binding domain and an N-terminus region similar to domains involved in signal transduction in cells.[26]

Many xenobiotics interact with the HERG-encoded subunit of the potassium channel to reduce the current through the I_{Kr} channel and prolong the action potential duration. The HERG α subunit of the channel is particularly susceptible to xenobiotic-induced interactions due to two important differences from the other channels. First, the S6 domain of the HERG channel has aromatic domains on the inner cavity pore that can bind to aromatic xenobiotics. Additionally, the inner cavity and entrance of the HERG channel is larger than the other voltage-gated potassium channels.[26] This larger pore can accommodate larger xenobiotics that are then trapped within the pore when the channel closes.[26,48,49,54]

CALCIUM CHANNELS

Calcium channel conductivity across the myocardial cell membrane is critical for maintaining the appropriate duration of cell membrane depolarization and for initiation of cellular contraction. The best characterized of the calcium channels are the slow (L-type), the fast (T-type), and the ryanodine receptor calcium channel. They are more prominently involved in cardiac contractility and discussed in Chap. 23.

ION CHANNELS AND THE MYOCARDIAL CELL ACTION POTENTIAL

An understanding of the basic electrophysiology of the myocardial cell is essential to understand the toxicity of xenobiotics and to plan appropriate therapy. Figure 22–2 shows the typical action potential of myocardial cell depolarization, the electrolyte fluxes responsible for the action potential, and the resulting ECG complex. The action potentials of the contractile and the conductive cells are depicted.

The action potential is divided into 5 phases: phase 0, depolarization; phase 1, overshoot; phase 2, plateau; phase 3, repolarization; and phase 4, resting. Phase 0 begins when the cell is excited either by a stimulus from an adjoining cell or by spontaneous depolarization of a pacemaker cell. Selective voltage-gated fast sodium channels (I_{Na^+}) open, resulting in rapid depolarization of the membrane. At the end of phase 0, the voltage-sensitive sodium channels close and a transient outward potassium current (I_{To}) occurs, resulting in a partial repolarization of the membrane—this constitutes phase 1.

During phase 2 (plateau phase), the inward depolarizing calcium currents are largely balanced by the outward repolarizing potassium currents. Voltage-sensitive calcium channels open that allow Ca^{2+} movement down the concentration gradient into the cell. The intracellular Ca^{2+} concentration is 5000–10,000 times lower than the extracellular concentration. The voltage-gated calcium channels that allow movement of Ca^{2+} down its concentration gradient into the cell are categorized based on their conductance (fast or slow) and their

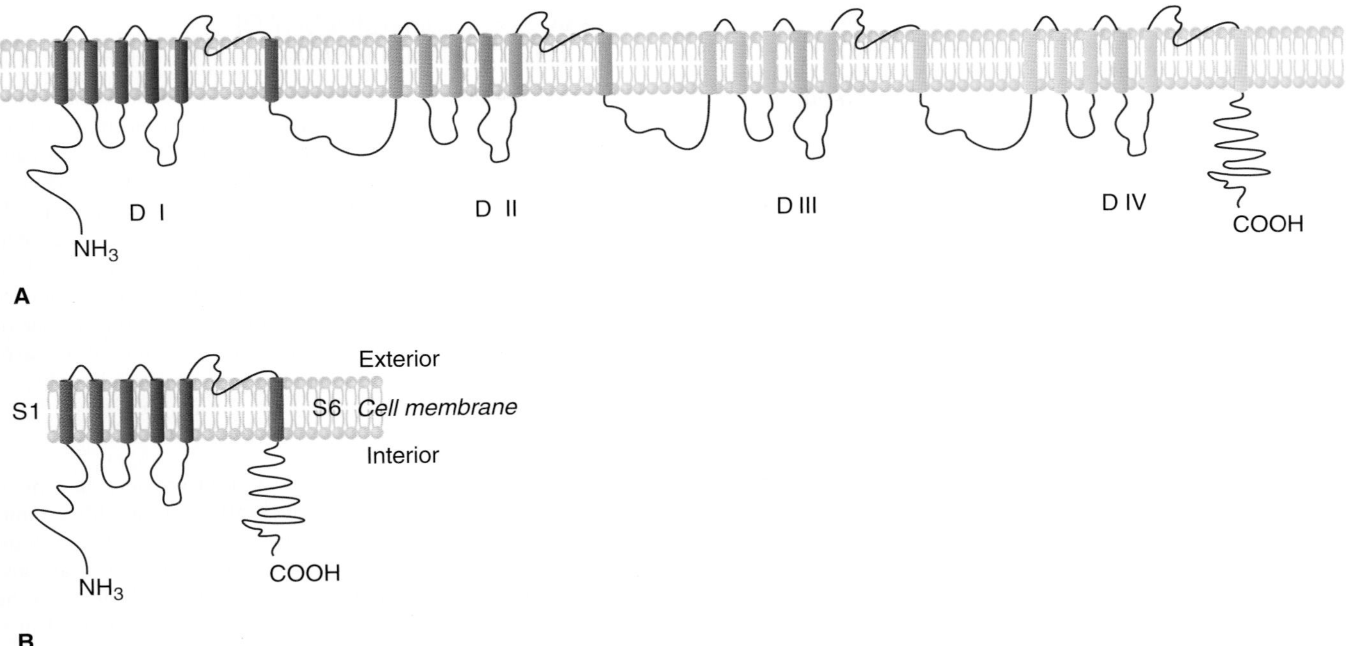

FIGURE 22–1. Structure of the potassium and sodium ion channels. (**A**) The structure of the α subunit of the sodium channel. The protein molecule has 4 domains (D I–D IV) each analagous to one of the potassium channel α subunits. One of these molecules assembles with β subunits to form the membrane sodium channel. (**B**) The structure of the α subunit of the voltage gated potassium channel. The protein molecule has 6 membrane spanning regions (S1–S6); the voltage sensitive region is S4 and the actual ion channel is located between S5 and S6. Four of these α subunits assemble with 4 β subunits to form the potassium channel complex.

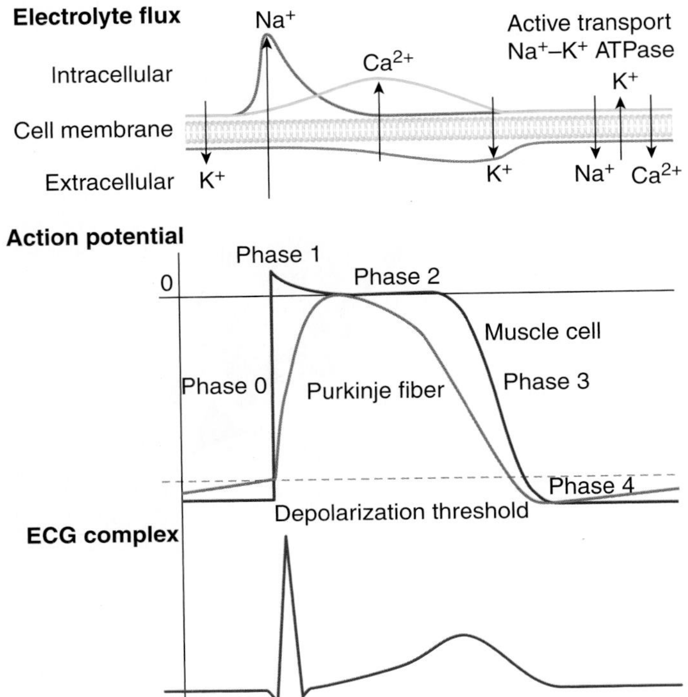

FIGURE 22–2. Relationship of electrolyte movement across the cell membrane to the action potential and the surface ECG recording.

sensitivity to voltage changes.[14,45] The calcium currents (mostly the "long-lasting" current) gradually decrease as the channels inactivate. Simultaneously, the outward potassium "delayed rectifier" currents, particularly the I_{Kr} (rapidly activating) and the I_{Ks} (slowly activating) currents, increase terminating the plateau phase of the action potential and initiating cellular repolarization (phase 3). Other, smaller, outward potassium currents (not shown in Fig. 22–2) play a lesser role in the duration of the action potential and development of phase 3, including I_{Kur} (ultrarapid), I_{Kp} (plateau), $I_{K\text{-}Ach}$ (acetylcholine-dependent), and $I_{K\text{-}ATP}$ (adenosine triphosphate-dependent) currents.

Phase 4 is the resting state for much of the myocardium, except the pacemaker cells, and corresponds to diastole in the cardiac cycle. During phases 3 and 4, active transport of Na^+, K^+, and Ca^{2+} against their electrochemical gradients return the myocyte to the baseline resting state. The transmembrane electrochemical gradient is maintained during the resting state by a Ca^{2+}-Na^+ exchange mechanism and by ATP-dependent pumps in the membrane that together move Ca^{2+} out of the cells.[45] In the pacemaker cells, during phase 4 of the action potential, gradual electrical depolarization of the membrane occurs due to potassium currents (called the I_f for "funny" or the I_h for "hyperpolarization-activated" current).[16] The membrane potential gradually increases in these pacemaker cells until the threshold potential is reached, the fast inward sodium channels open, and the I_{Na} current initiates the next phase 0. This electrical impulse is then propagated via the His-Purkinje conducting system of the heart.

During phases 0–2, the cell cannot be depolarized again with another stimulus; the cell is absolutely refractory. During the latter half of phase 3, as the calcium channels convert from their inactivated to their resting state, an electrical stimulus of sufficient magnitude may cause another depolarization; the cell is relatively refractory. During phase 4, the cell is no longer refractory and any appropriate stimulus that reaches the threshold level may cause depolarization.

In addition to its role in myocardial contractility, Ca^{2+} influx is also important in pacemaker function. Although spontaneous pacemaker cell depolarization has traditionally been ascribed to inward cation current through "pacemaker channels"[1,16] recent research suggests that it may actually be driven by rhythmic release of calcium from the sarcoplasmic reticulum.[33,34] Regardless, Ca^{2+} fluxes play an important role in the spontaneous depolarization (phase 4) of the action potential in the sinoatrial (SA) node.[35] The rate of pacemaker cell depolarization is enhanced by β-adrenergic stimulation through phosphorylation of proteins on the sarcoplasmic reticulum and by a phosphorylation-independent action of cAMP at the pacemaker channels.[1,33] Depolarization of cells in the SA node spreads to surrounding atrial cells where it triggers the opening of fast sodium channels and impulse propagation. Calcium flux also allows normal propagation of electrical impulses via the specialized myocardial conduction tissues in the atrioventricular (AV) node.

ELECTROCARDIOGRAPHY

The ECG measures the sum of all electrical activity in the heart. It is used extensively in medicine and its interpretation is widely understood by physicians of nearly all disciplines. It is an invaluable diagnostic tool for patients with cardiovascular complaints. However, it is also a valuable source of information in poisoned patients and has the potential to enhance and direct their care. Although it seems obvious that an ECG would be required following exposure to a medication used for cardiovascular indications, many medications with no overt cardiovascular effects at therapeutic doses, are cardiotoxic in overdose. Furthermore, in patients with unknown exposures, the ECG can suggest specific xenobiotics or demonstrate electrolyte abnormalities, long before blood is drawn. For example, oropharyngeal or dermal burns in a patient whose ECG has evidence of hyperkalemia or hypocalcemia suggests exposure to hydrofluoric acid[58] (Chap. 105). Alternatively, a patient manifesting signs of the opioid toxidrome with runs of torsades de pointes might have been exposed to methadone(Chap. 38).[20] QT prolongation may be a clue to the etiology of an overdose with an atypical antipsychotic such as quetiapine (Chap. 69). The ECG can also be used to predict complications of poisoning, such as seizures following a cyclic antidepressant overdose (Chap. 73). Therefore, an ECG should be examined early in the initial evaluation of most poisoned patients.

HISTORY OF THE ECG

In the 1900s, Willem Einthoven graphically displayed the electrical activity of the heart and named the different waves—P, QRS, and T. He called this tracing an "elektrokardiogramme," and was awarded a Nobel Prize in 1924 for his efforts. The acronym *EKG*, still employed by some authors, was derived from Einthoven's spelling. The acronym *ECG*, which is consistent with our current spelling of electrocardiogram, is used throughout this text.

Since this initial description, both the normal electrophysiology of the heart and the pharmacologic effects of various xenobiotics on the ECG have been described. Despite the large number, diversity, and complexity of the various cardiac toxins, there are only a limited number of electrocardiographic manifestations.

BASIC ELECTROPHYSIOLOGY OF AN ELECTROCARDIOGRAM

Simplistically, a positive or upward deflection on the oscilloscope is generated when an electrical force moves toward an electrical sensor or electrode, and a downward deflection occurs if the force moves away. An ECG represents the sum of movement of all electrical forces in the heart in relation to the surface electrode, and the height above baseline represents the magnitude of the force (Fig. 22–3). Only during depolarization or repolarization does the ECG tracing leave the isoelectric baseline, because it is only during these periods that measurable currents are flowing in the heart. During the other periods, mechanical effects are occurring in the myocardium, but large amounts of current are not flowing.

LEADS

Although the reading from a single ECG lead provides an immense amount of information, to visualize the heart in a nearly three-dimensional perspective, multiple leads must be assessed simultaneously. Given the cylindrical nature of both the heart and thorax, at any given moment some of these leads will record positive voltage and others negative. The lead placement that was described and refined in the early 1900s by Einthoven forms the basis for the bipolar or limb leads, described as I, II, and III (Fig. 22–4). The Einthoven triangle is an equilateral triangle formed by the sum of these leads. Unipolar limb leads and precordial leads were subsequently added to the standard ECG. Unipolar leads were created when the limb leads were connected to a common point where the sum of the potentials from leads I, II, and III was zero. The currently used unipolar augmented (a) leads (aV_R, aV_L, and aV_F) are based on these unipolar leads (see Fig. 22–3). The voltage potential of these unipolar, "augmented leads" is small, thus it is amplified by incorporating the voltage change of the other two augmented leads. Together, leads I, II, III, aV_R, aV_F, and aV_L form the hexaxial reference system that is used to calculate the electrical axis of

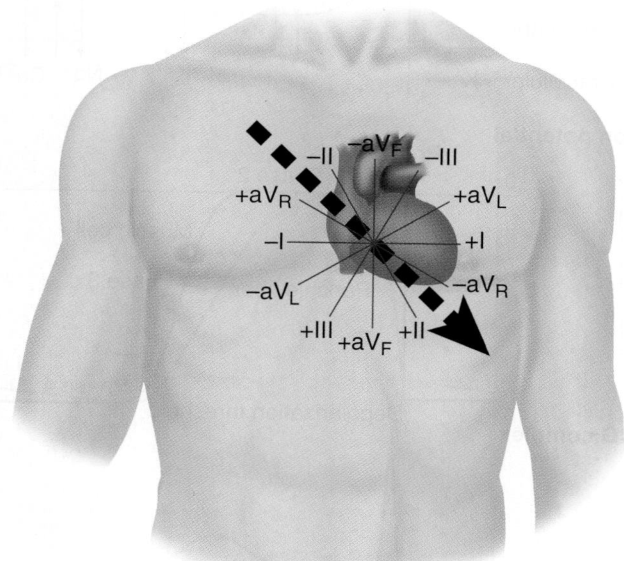

FIGURE 22–3. The hexaxial reference system derived from the Einthoven equilateral triangle defining the electrical potential vectors of electrocardiography showing the relationship between cardiac anatomy and electrocardiographic leads.

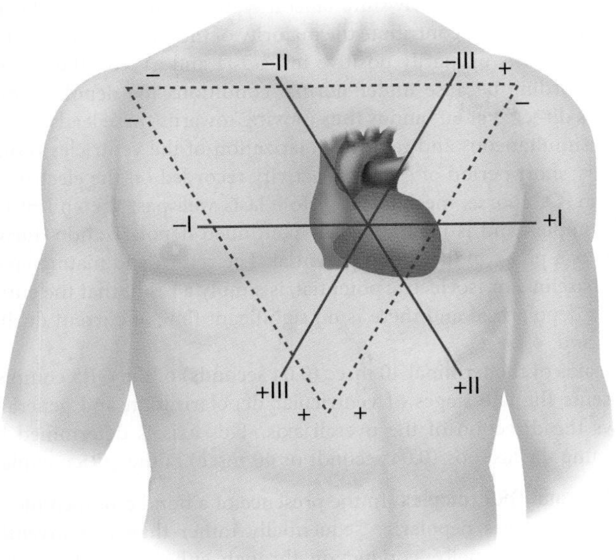

FIGURE 22–4. The hexaxial reference system derived from the Einthoven equilateral triangle defining the electrical potential vectors of electrocardiography. The relationships of the original three limb leads are illustrated. The equiangular (60°) Einthoven triangle formed by leads I, II, and III is shown (*dotted lines*) with positive and negative poles of each of the leads indicated. Leads I, II, and III are also presented as a triaxial reference system that intersects in the center of the ventricles.

the heart in the frontal plane. The precordial leads, called V_1 through V_6, are also unipolar measurements of the change in electric potential measured from a central point to the 6 anterior and left lateral chest positions (Fig. 22–5). If V_2 is placed over the right ventricle, part of the initial positive ventricular deflection (QRS complex) reflects right ventricular activation, with electrical forces moving toward the electrode.

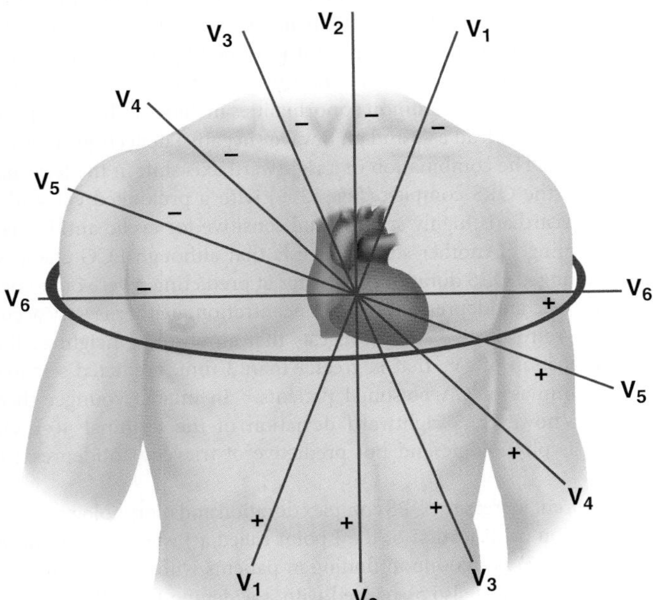

FIGURE 22–5. Visualized as a cross-section, each of the chest leads is oriented through the atrioventricular (AV) node and exits through the patient's back, which is negative.

The majority of the subsequent terminal negative deflection reflects activation of other muscle tissue (septum, left ventricular wall) when the electrical forces are moving away from the electrode. Recordings from each of these 12 leads (I, II, III, aV_R, aV_L, aV_F, V_{1-6}) evaluate the heart from two different planes in 12 different positions, yielding a three-dimensional electrical "picture" of the heart, with respect to time and voltage.

A continuous cardiac monitor often relies on recordings from one of two bipolar leads: a modified left chest lead (MCL_1) or a lead II. The recording from an MCL_1, in which the positive electrode is in the V_1 position, is similar in appearance to a V_1 recording on a 12-lead ECG. This lead visualizes ventricular activity well; however, lead II shows atrial activity (ie, the P wave) much more clearly.

THE VARIOUS INTERVALS AND WAVES

The ECG tracing has specific nomenclature to define the characteristic patterns. Waves refer to positive or negative deflections from baseline, such as the P, T, or U wave. A segment is defined as the distance between two waves, such as the ST segment, and an interval measures the duration of a wave plus a segment, such as QT or PR interval. Complexes are a group of waves without intervals or segments between them (QRS). Electrophysiologically, the P wave and PR interval on the ECG tracing represent the depolarization of the atria. The QRS complex represents the depolarization of the ventricles. The plateau is depicted by the ST segment and repolarization is visualized as the T wave and the QT interval (QT). The U wave, when present, generally represents an afterdepolarization (Fig. 22–6).

THE P WAVE

The P wave is the initial deflection on the ECG that occurs with the initiation of each new cardiac cycle.

Electrophysiology The early, middle, and late portions of the P wave are represented sequentially by the electrical potential initiated by the sinus node. The impulse is propagated directly through the right atrial muscle, producing contraction. The impulse is also propagated by specialized conduction tissue across the interatrial septum, to produce contraction of the left atrium. Additionally, internodal pathways rapidly conduct the impulse to the AV node. The electrical excitation of the sinus node differs from that of the ventricular myocardium in that current is mediated primarily by calcium ion influx via slow T-type calcium channels, not by Na^+ entering through fast sodium channels. Furthermore, the vagus nerve exerts a profound suppressive influence on the nodal tissues.

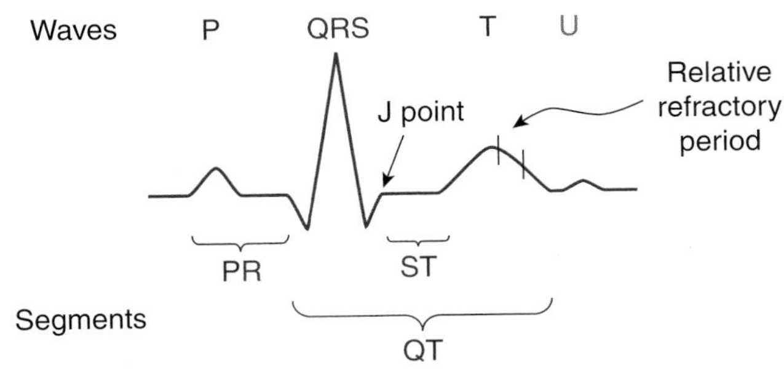

FIGURE 22–6. The normal ECG: P wave, atrial depolarization; QRS, ventricular depolarization; ST segment, T wave, QT interval, and U wave, ventricular repolarization. The U wave is the small, positive deflection following the T wave.

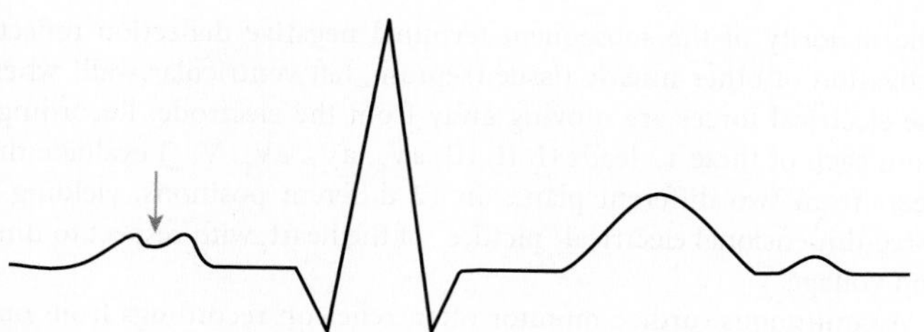

FIGURE 22–7. A notched p wave (arrow) suggests delayed conduction across the atrial septum and is characteristic of quinidine poisoning.

The Abnormal P Wave Clinically, abnormalities of the P wave occur with xenobiotics that depress automaticity of the sinus node, causing sinus arrest and nodal or ventricular escape rhythms (β-adrenergic antagonists, calcium channel blockers). The P wave is absent in rhythms with sinus arrest, such as occurs with xenobiotics that produce vagotonia such as cardioactive steroids and cholinergics. A notched P wave suggests delayed conduction across the atrial septum and is characteristic of quinidine poisoning or atrial enlargement (Fig. 22–7). P waves decrease in amplitude as hyperkalemia becomes more severe until they become indistinguishable from the baseline (Chap. 16).

THE PR INTERVAL

The PR interval is measured from the beginning of the P wave to the beginning of the QRS complex (normal is 120–200 msec).

Electrophysiology Despite rapid conduction by specialized conduction tissue from the SA to the AV node, the AV node delays transmission of the impulse into the ventricles, ostensibly to allow for complete atrial emptying. Thus, the PR interval represents the interval between the onset of atrial depolarization and the onset of ventricular depolarization. Children usually have more rapid conduction and a shorter PR interval, and older adults generally have a longer PR interval. The segment between the end of the P wave and the beginning of the QRS complex (the PQ segment) reflects atrial contraction and is usually isoelectric. Atrial repolarization coincides with the Q wave, but its ECG findings, or atrial T waves, are obscured by the QRS complex.

The abnormal PR interval Xenobiotics that decrease interatrial or AV nodal conduction cause marked lengthening of the PR segment until such conduction completely ceases. At this point, the P wave no longer relates to the QRS complex; this is AV dissociation, or complete heart block. Some xenobiotics suppress AV nodal conduction by blocking calcium channels in nodal cells, as does magnesium, β-adrenergic receptor antagonists, or cholinergics through enhanced vagal tone. Although the therapeutic concentrations of digoxin, as well as early cardioactive steroid poisoning, cause PR prolongation through vagotonic effects, direct electrophysiologic effects account for the bradycardia of poisoning ("Bradydysrhythmias," Chap. 64, and Antidotes in Depth A20: Digoxin-Specific Antibody Fragments [DSFab]).

THE QRS COMPLEX

The QRS complex is the second and typically largest deflection on the ECG. The normal QRS duration in adults varies between 60 and 120 msec. The normal QRS complex axis in the frontal plane lies between −30° and 90°, although most individuals will have axes between 30° and 75°. This axis will vary with the weight and age of the patient. Alterations in myocardial function may also alter the electrical axis of the heart.

Electrophysiology The QRS complex reflects the electrical forces generated by ventricular depolarization mediated primarily by Na^+ influx into the myocardial cells. Although under normal conditions both ventricles depolarize nearly simultaneously, the greater mass of the left ventricle causes it to contribute the majority of the electrical forces. The QRS complex is primarily positive in leads I and aV_L on the surface ECG recording because under normal conditions the depolarization vector is directed at 60° and is thus moving towards these leads.

The simultaneous and rapid depolarization of the ventricles results in a very short period of electrical activity recorded on the electrocardiogram. Of course, mechanical systole lasts well past the end of the QRS complex and is maintained by continued depolarization during the plateau phase of the action potential. The return and maintenance of the baseline, or isoelectric potential, is simply a result that the entire heart is depolarized and there is no significant flow of current during this period.

The axis of the terminal 40 msec (0.04 seconds) of the QRS complex represents the late stages of ventricular depolarization and generally follows the direction of the overall axis. This axis is determined by examining the last box (0.04 seconds or 40 msec) of the QRS complex.

The abnormal QRS complex In the presence of a bundle-branch block, the two ventricles depolarize sequentially rather than concurrently. Although, conceptually, conduction through either the left or right bundle may be affected (Fig. 22–8) many xenobiotics preferentially affect the right bundle. The specific reasons for this effect are unclear, but it may be related to differing refractory periods of the tissues. This effect typically results in the left ventricle depolarizing slightly more rapidly than the right. The consequence on the ECG is both a widening of the QRS complex and the appearance of the right ventricular electrical forces that were previously obscured by those of the left ventricle. These changes are typically the result of the effects of a xenobiotic that blocks fast sodium channels. Implicated xenobiotics include cyclic antidepressants,[9,11] quinidine and other type IA and IC antidysrhythmics[17] phenothiazines, amantadine,[51] diphenhydramine,[52]carbamazepine,[27] and cocaine.[2] In the setting of cyclic antidepressant poisoning, an increased QRS duration has both prognostic and therapeutic value (Chap. 73).[6,11,23] In one prospective analysis of ECGs, the maximal limb lead QRS duration was prognostic of seizures (0% if < 100 msec; 30% if greater) and ventricular dysrhythmias (0% if < 160 msec; 50% if greater).[11]

The terminal 40-msec axis of the QRS complex also contains information regarding the likelihood, but not the extent, of poisoning by sodium channel blockers. In a patient poisoned by a sodium channel blocker, the terminal portion of the QRS has a rightward deviation greater than 120°. The common abnormalities include, an R wave (positive deflection) in lead aV_R and an S wave (negative deflection) in leads I and aV_L.[10,30] The combination of a rightward axis shift in the terminal 40 msec of the QRS complex (Fig. 22–9) with a prolonged QT and a sinus tachycardia is highly specific and sensitive for cyclic antidepressant poisoning.[41] Another study suggests that although ECG changes, like a prolonged QRS duration, are better at predicting severe outcomes than the cyclic antidepressant (CA) concentration, neither is very accurate.[6] One retrospective study suggests that an absolute height of the terminal portion of aV_R that is greater than 3 mm, predicted seizures or dysrhythmias in CA-poisoned patients.[29] In infants younger than 6 months, however, a rightward deviation of the terminal 40-msec QRS axis is physiologic and not predictive of tricyclic antidepressant toxicity.[9]

An apparent increase in QRS complex duration and morphology, which is an elevation or distortion of the J point called a J wave or an Osborn wave (Fig. 15–3) is a common finding in patients with hypothermia.[43,57] Hypermagnesemia is also associated with a widening the QRS complex duration and a slight narrowing of the QRS complex may occur with hypomagnesemia. Significant elevation in the serum concentration K^+ may also cause widening and distortion of the QRS complex.

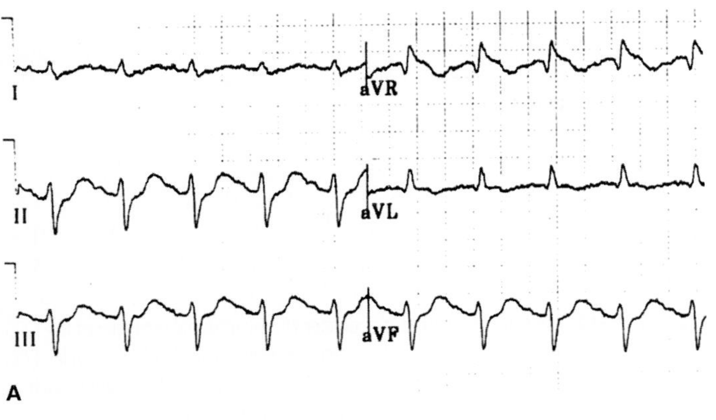

A

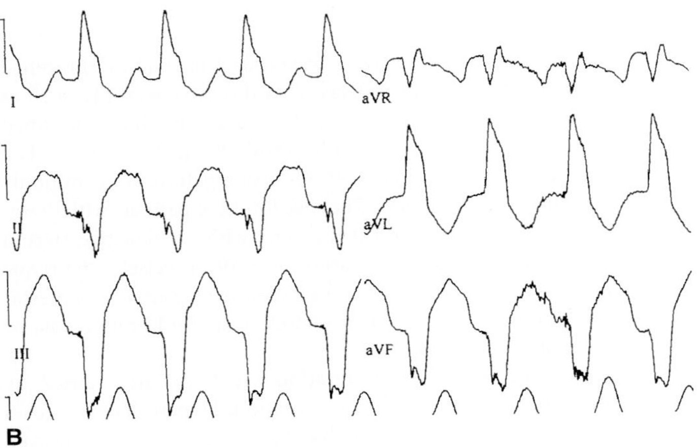

B

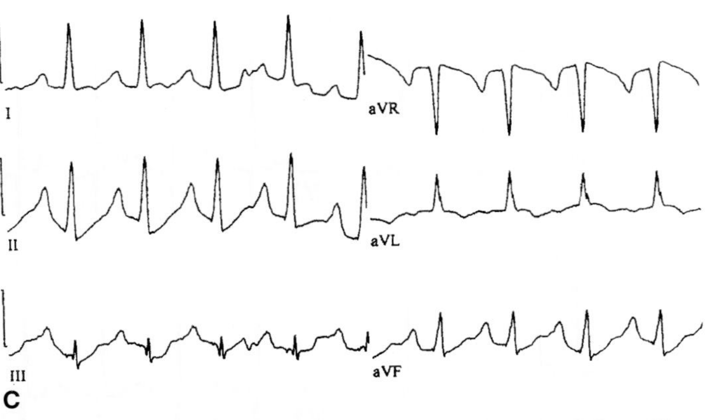

C

FIGURE 22–8. A 35-year-old woman was found unresponsive in a hallway with an empty bottle of doxepin. Note the progression from (**A**) a wide QRS interval (108 msec, axis +10), to (**B**) At over 35 minutes: a RBBB with an axis of -50 and a rightward shift of the terminal 40 msec of the QRS axis, and (C) In the next hour: marked improvement after hypertonic sodium bicarbonate therapy.

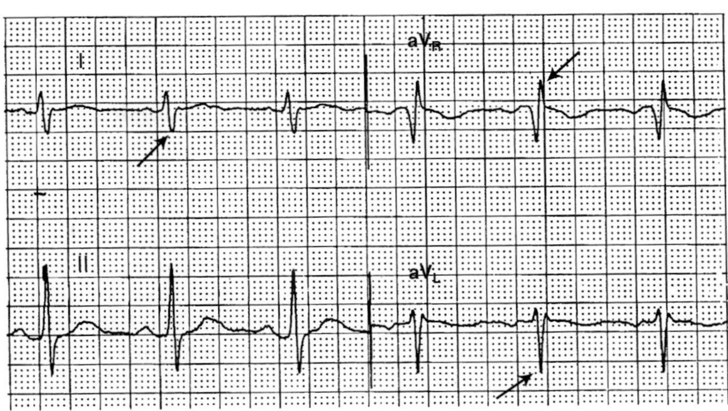

FIGURE 22–9. ECG of a patient with a tricyclic antidepressant overdose. The arrows highlight prominent S wave in leads I and aV_L and R wave in aV_R demonstrate the terminal 40-msec rightward axis shift.

THE ST SEGMENT

The ST segment is defined as the distance between the end of the QRS complex and the beginning of the T wave.

Electrophysiology The ST segment reflects the period of time between depolarization and the start of repolarization, or the plateau phase of the action potential. During this period, no major currents flow within the myocardium, which explains why under normal circumstances the ST segment is isoelectric. Although both the degree of displacement from the baseline and the length of this segment are important, the ST segment duration is usually measured by its effects on the QT duration (see "The QT Interval").

The abnormal ST segment Displacement of the ST segment from its baseline typically characterizes myocardial ischemia or infarction (Fig. 22–10). The subsequent appearance of a Q wave is diagnostic of myocardial infarction. The ECG patterns of these entities reflect the different underlying electrophysiologic states of the heart. Ischemic regions are highly unstable and produce currents of injury because of

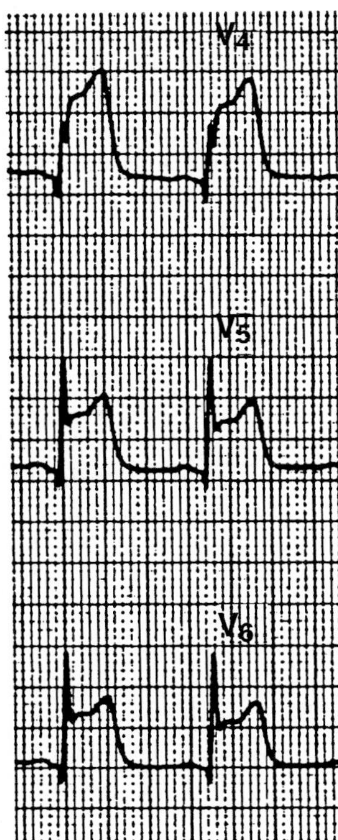

FIGURE 22–10. Leads V_4–V_6 suggestive of a lateral STEMI are shown from the ECG of a 27-year-old man with substernal chest pain after using crack cocaine.

inadequate repolarization, which is related to lack of energy substrate to power the Na^+-K^+ ATPase. Myocardial infarction represents the loss of electrical activity from the necrotic, inactive ventricular tissue, allowing the contralateral ventricular forces to be predominant on the ECG. Patients who are poisoned by xenobiotics that cause vasoconstriction, such as cocaine (Chap. 76), other α-adrenergic agonists, or the ergot alkaloids, are particularly prone to develop focal myocardial ischemia and infarction. The specific ECG manifestations help to identify the region of injury and may, to some extent, be correlated with an arterial flow pattern: inferior (leads II, III, aV_F; right coronary artery); anterior (leads I, aV_L; left anterior descending artery); or lateral (leads aV_L, V_{5-6}; circumflex branch). However, any poisoning that results in profound hypotension or hypoxia may also result in ECG changes of ischemia and injury. In this patient, the injury may be more global, involving more than one arterial distribution. Diffuse myocardial damage may not be identifiable on the ECG because of global, symmetric electrical abnormalities. In this patient, the diagnosis is established by other noninvasive testing, such as by echocardiogram or by finding elevated concentrations of serum markers for myocardial injury such as troponin.

Many young, healthy patients have ST segment abnormalities that mimic those of myocardial infarction. The most common normal variant is termed "early repolarization" or "J-point elevation," and is identified as diffusely elevated, upwardly concave ST segments, located in the precordial leads and typically with corresponding T waves of large amplitude (Fig. 22–11).[12] The J point is located at the beginning of the ST segment just after the QRS complex. Because this ECG variant is common in patients with cocaine-associated chest pain (Chap. 76),[22] its recognition is critical to instituting appropriate therapy.

The Brugada electrocardiographic pattern (Fig. 22–12) is characterized by terminal positivity of the QRS complex and ST-segment elevation in the right precordial leads. The Brugada pattern is found in some patients with mutations of the gene that codes for the α subunit of the sodium channel. These patients are at risk for sudden death, but a similar ECG pattern often occurs in patients who are poisoned by sodium channel blocking xenobiotics, including CAs, cocaine, class IA (procainamide), and class IC (flecainide, encainide) antidysrhythmic.[31] In CA-poisoned patients this pattern is associated with an increased risk of hypotension, but not sudden death or dysrhythmias.[8] This pattern is also associated with lithium toxicity.

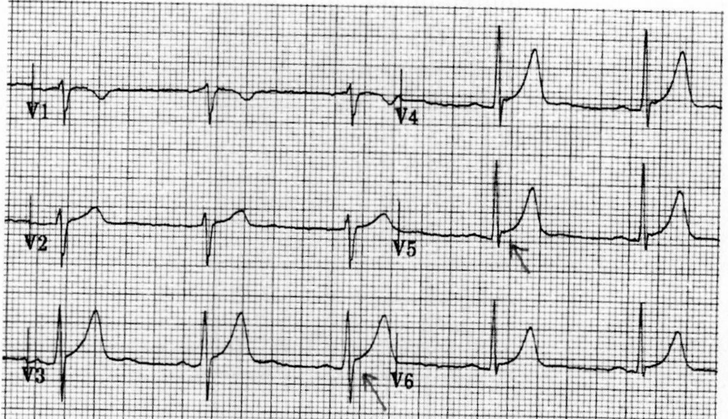

FIGURE 22–11. Healthy 34-year-old male whose ECG demonstrates diffusely elevated, upwardly concave ST segments in leads V3–V5, and T waves of large amplitude suggestive of an "early repolarization" abnormality.

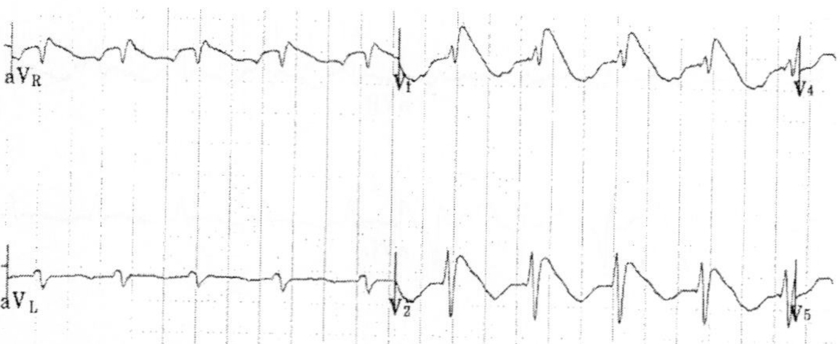

FIGURE 22–12. The Brugada pattern is characterized by terminal positivity of the QRS complex and ST-segment elevation in the right precordial leads and is a similar ECG pattern to that noted in patients poisoned by sodium channel blocking agents such as cyclic antidepressants.[4] (Image contributed by Vikhyat Bebarta, MD.)

Sagging ST segments, inverted T waves, and normal or shortened QT intervals are characteristic effects of cardioactive steroids, such as digoxin. These repolarization abnormalities are sometimes identified by their similar appearance to "Salvador Dali's mustache" (Fig. 22–13). As a group, these findings, along with PR prolongation, are commonly described as the "digitalis effect." They are found in patients with therapeutic drug concentrations and in patients with cardioactive steroid poisoning. As the serum concentration or, more precisely, the tissue concentration increases, clinical and electrocardiographic manifestations of toxicity will appear, which include profound bradycardia or ventricular dysrhythmias.

Changes in the ST segment duration are frequently caused by abnormalities in the serum Ca^{2+} concentration. Hypercalcemia causes shortening of the ST segment through enhanced calcium influx during

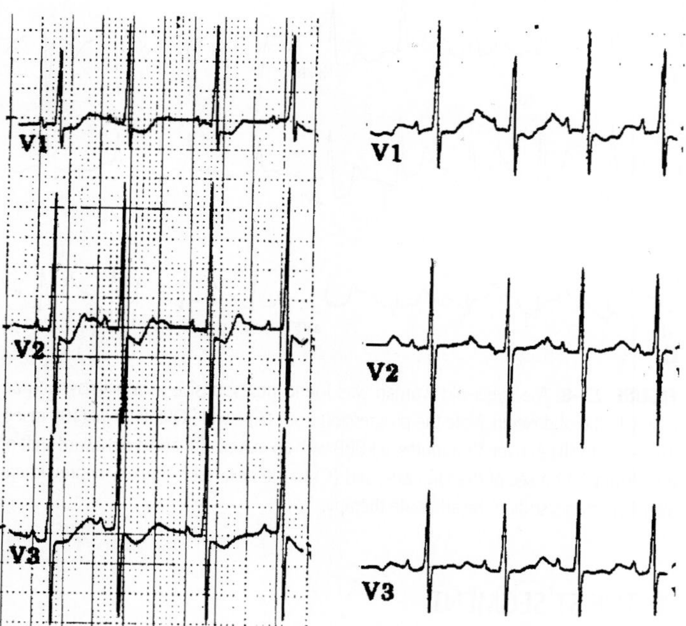

FIGURE 22–13. Two-day-old boy erroneously given 50 mcg/kg of digoxin, presented with heart rate 60 bpm, given digibind. (**A**) ECG from hospital day #2, after digoxin-specific Fab, and shows "digitalis effect" of the ST segment in leads V1–V3 (*free* digoxin concentration 4 ng/mL). (**B**) This finding resolves after the child was switched to amiodarone; notice the mild QT prolongation. The scooping of the ST segment has been likened to the scooping of Salvador Dali's mustache.

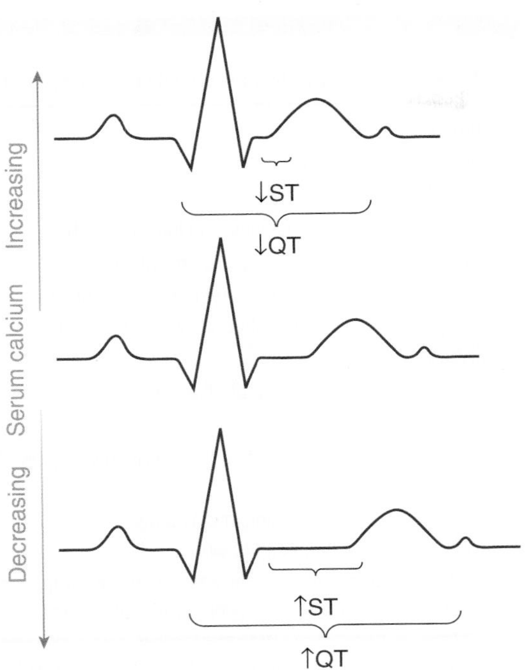

FIGURE 22–14. Electrocardiographic findings associated with changes in serum calcium concentration.

the plateau phase of the cardiac cycle speeding the onset of repolarization. For practical purposes this effect is more commonly identified by reduction of the QT duration (Fig. 22–14). In patients with hypercalcemia, the morphology and duration of the QRS complex and T and P waves remain unchanged. Xenobiotic-induced hypercalcemia may result from exposure to antacids (milk alkali syndrome), diuretics (eg, hydrochlorothiazide), cholecalciferol (vitamin D), vitamin A, and other retinoids. Hypocalcemia causes prolongation of the ST segment and QT interval (see Fig. 22–14).

THE T WAVE

The T wave is the third deflection that occurs on the ECG.

Electrophysiology The T wave represents ventricular repolarization, during which time current is again flowing, although at a cellular level in the opposite direction from that during depolarization. Cardiac repolarization on the larger level generally follows the same pattern as depolarization and thus the deflection is usually in the same direction as the QRS complex. During repolarization, the intracellular potential of the cardiac myocyte becomes more negative as a result of a net loss of positive charge because of the increasing outward flow of potassium ions. As repolarization progresses, the voltage-dependent ion channels "reset" themselves as the intracellular potential falls past their set points. Thus, the initial part of the T wave represents the absolute refractory period of the heart, because at this time there are an insufficient number of reset voltage-dependent calcium channels to allow an impulse to cause a contraction. The latter part of the T wave represents the relative refractory period of the heart, during which time a sufficient number of these calcium channels are available to open with an aberrant depolarization and initiate a contraction.

The abnormal T wave Isolated peaked T waves are usually evidence of early hyperkalemia.[36] Hyperkalemia initially causes tall, tented T waves with normal QRS and QT interval, and a normal P wave (Fig. 22–15).

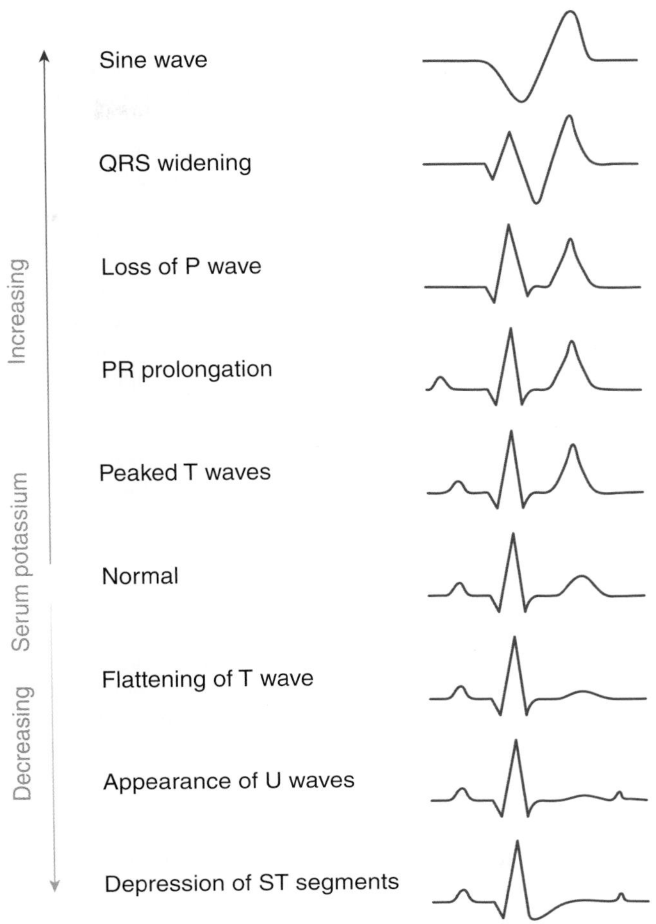

FIGURE 22–15. Electrocardiographic manifestations associated with changes in serum potassium concentration.

As the serum potassium concentration rises to 6.5–8 mEq/L, the P wave diminishes in amplitude and the PR and QRS intervals prolong. Progressive widening of the QRS complex causes it to merge with the ST segment and T wave, forming a "sine wave." ECG manifestations of hyperkalemia may occur following chronic exposure to numerous xenobiotics, including potassium-sparing diuretics, angiotensin-converting enzyme inhibitors, angiotensin receptor blockers, (Chap. 16), or potassium supplements. Either fluoride, arsine or cardioactive steroid poisoning produces acute hyperkalemia, but the latter rarely produces hyperkalemic ECG changes. Peaked T waves also occur following myocardial ischemia and may also be confused with early repolarization effects ("The ST Segment"). Consequently, the ability to properly identify electrolyte abnormalities by electrocardiography is often limited.

Hypokalemia typically reduces the amplitude of the T wave and, ultimately, causes the appearance of prominent U waves (see Fig. 22–15). Its effects on the ECG are manifestations of altered myocardial repolarization. Lithium similarly affects myocardial ion fluxes and causes reversible changes on the ECG that may mimic mild hypokalemia, although documentation of low cellular potassium concentrations is lacking. Patients chronically poisoned with lithium have more T-wave abnormalities (typically flattening) than do those who are poisoned acutely, but these abnormalities are rarely of clinical significance.[55]

THE QT INTERVAL

The QT is measured from the beginning of the QRS complex to the end of the T wave. The QT interval normally varies because of biologic diurnal effects and autonomic tone; technical issues with the environment or with processing and acquiring the ECG; and intra- and inter-observer variability.[3,37,38] The bipolar limb lead with the largest T wave should therefore be used for this measurement.

The QT interval is normally prolonged at slower heart rates and shortens as the heart rate increases. This is especially important since many of the xenobiotics that affect the QT interval also affect the heart rate. As the normal QT varies also with the heart rate, numerous formulas and tables are available to obtain the corrected QT, known as the QTc. [21] Using the QTc allows the determination of the appropriateness of the QT independent of the heart rate.

With a rate of 50–90 beats/min, the commonly used Bazett formula (QTc (msec) = QT (msec)/$\sqrt{\text{RR interval (sec)}}$is adequate for determining a rate corrected QT interval (QTc). The RR interval is calculated as 60/heart rate per minute. In this heart rate range, 99% of men have a QTc < 450 msec and 99% of women have a QTc < 460 msec.[39] A QTc interval > 500 msec weakly correlates with an increased risk of developing ventricular dysrhythmias. However, at higher heart rates, a normal patient will have an inaccurately calculated "prolonged" QTc interval using the Bazett formula. Studies suggest that medications such as bupropion prolong the QT interval when the "increase" in the QTc may be only a result of the increased heart rate.[24] A variety of formulas and corrections are proposed to attempt to identify normal QT intervals on ECGs at higher heart rates,[5, 15, 32] including the Friderician formula (QTc = QT/$\sqrt[3]{\text{RR interval (sec)}}$) and the Framingham linear regression analysis (QTLC = QT + 0.154 (1-RR)).[50] Which correction formula is optimal remains unknown, and the FDA requests that sponsors use multiple calculations when performing a "thorough QT study" for any drug with prodysrhythmic potential.[19]

With slow heart rates, a prominent U wave can obscure the terminal portion of the T wave and with fast heart rates the subsequent P wave can obscure the terminal portion of the T wave. In these patients the QTc should be estimated by following the downslope of the T wave. The QTc is often measured to approximate repolarization, although this is not fully appropriate because alterations in depolarization, such as excess Na^+ entry, may affect it.

QT interval measurements from the computerized ECG algorithms are less accurate than careful manual determinations of the interval.[25] In August 2000, a panel of experts convened to address these issues and suggested that the QT interval should be measured manually in one of the limb leads that best shows the end T wave; the QT interval should be measured and averaged over 3 to 5 beats; and large U waves should be included in the QT interval measurement if they merge into the T wave and obscure the end of the T wave.[4] However, a subsequent study of 334 healthcare practitioners found that only 60% of the physicians were able to correctly measure a sample QT interval on the survey, although nearly all indicated correctly the measurement should be from the beginning of the QRS to the end of the T wave.[28]

Electrophysiology The QT represents the entire duration of ventricular systole and thus is made up of several electrophysiologic periods. Prolongation of the QT interval generally corresponds to an increase in the duration of phase 2 or phase 3 of the action potential. Although as noted above depolarization abnormalities can affect the QT, these are uncommon, and the plateau phase and repolarization are primarily reflected by the QT. Variations in the speed of the paper, [18] T-wave morphology, irregular baseline, and the presence of U waves may make this determination difficult.[4]

The abnormal QT interval A prolonged QT reflects an increase in the time period that the heart is "vulnerable" to the initiation of ventricular dysrhythmias (Table 22–1, Fig. 22–16). This occurs because although some myocardial fibers are refractory during this time period, others are not (ie, relative refractory period). Early afterdepolarizations (EADs) may occur in patients with lengthened repolarization time (Table 22–2). An EAD occurs when a myocardial cell spontaneously depolarizes before its repolarization is complete (Fig. 22–17). If this depolarization is of sufficient magnitude, it may capture and initiate a premature ventricular contraction, which itself may initiate ventricular tachycardia, ventricular fibrillation, or torsades de pointes. There are two types of EADs based on whether they occur during phase 2 (type 1) or phase 3 (type 2) of the cardiac action potential. The ionic basis of EADs is unclear, but may be via the L-type calcium channel; EADs are suppressed by magnesium.[7]

Xenobiotics that cause sodium channel blockade (Chap. 63) prolong the QT duration by slowing cellular depolarization during phase 0. Thus, the QT duration increases because of a prolongation of the QRS complex duration, and the ST segment duration remains near normal. Xenobiotics that cause potassium channel blockade similarly prolong the QT, but through prolongation of the plateau and repolarization phases. This specifically prolongs the ST segment duration. Although at a cellular level these xenobiotics are antidysrhythmic, the multicellular effects may be prodysrhythmic. The highly selective serotonin reuptake inhibitor citalopram, causes QT prolongation due

TABLE 22–1. Xenobiotic Causes of an Acquired Long QT Syndrome*

Antidysrhythmics
Class IA, IC, and III antidysrhythmics
Antifungals: itraconazole, ketoconazole
Antihistamines: astemizole and terfenadine (no longer available)
Antihypertensives: angiotensin converting enzyme inhibitors
Antimicrobials: amantadine, chloroquine, erythromycin, halofantrin, fluoroquinolones, pentamidine, trimethoprim-sulfamethoxazole,
Electrolyte disturbances
Hypocalcemia: oxalate (eg, ethylene glycol), fluoride
Hypokalemia: barium
Hypomagnesemia: (eg, diuretics, digoxin, amphotericin, phosphates [IV], ethanol)
Other: arsenic trioxide, cisapride, cocaine, methadone, organic phosphorus insecticides, vasopressin
Psychotropics: atypical antipsychotics, cyclic antidepressants, droperidol, haloperidol, pimozide, phenothiazines, zisprasidone, citalopram

*Additional information can be found at www.qtdrugs.org, hosted by the Arizona CERT

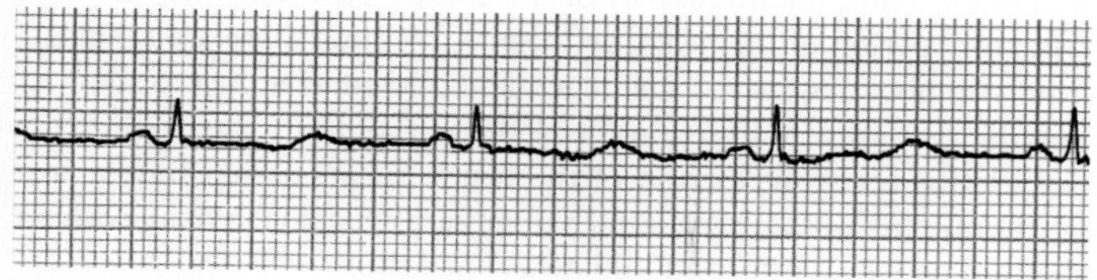

FIGURE 22–16. 33-year-old woman who ingested excessive methadone along with ethanol 3 hours before admission. Her ECG shows a sinus bradycardia and QT prolongation.

TABLE 22–2. The Electrophysiologic Basis for Delayed Afterdepolarization and Early Afterdepolarization

	Phase of Action Potential Affected by Depolarization	Clinical Effect	Mechanism
Delayed after depolarization (DAD)	Phase 4	Cardioactive steroid–induced dysrhythmias	↑ Intracellular Ca^{2+} → Activation of a nonselective cation channel or Na^+-Ca^{2+} exchanger → Transient inward current carried mostly by Na^+ ions
Early after depolarization (EAD)	Phase 2 Phase 3	↑ Repolarization time Long QT syndrome (hereditary and acquired)	Possibly via L-type calcium channels
		Drug-induced torsades de pointes, ventricular tachycardia	Suppressed by magnesium

to the sodium and calcium channel blocking effects of its metabolite didemethyl-citalopram. In a recent large retrospective cohort study, users of both typical antipsychotics (thioridazine and haloperidol) and atypical antipsychotics (clozapine, quetiapine, olanzapine, risperidone) had a risk of sudden cardiac death that was twice that of non users of antipsychotics. Xenobiotic induced QT prolongation and the subsequent risk of dysrhythmias is the postulated etiology.[46] Hypocalcemia may produce a prolonged QT interval, and is caused by a number of xenobiotics, including fluoride, calcitonin, ethylene glycol, phosphates, and mithramycin (Table 16-9). Hypokalemia alone does not usually prolong the QT. Arsenic poisoning may cause prolongation of the QT and result in torsades de pointes. The mechanism is unknown, although either a direct dysrhythmogenic effect or an autoimmune myocarditis are postulated.

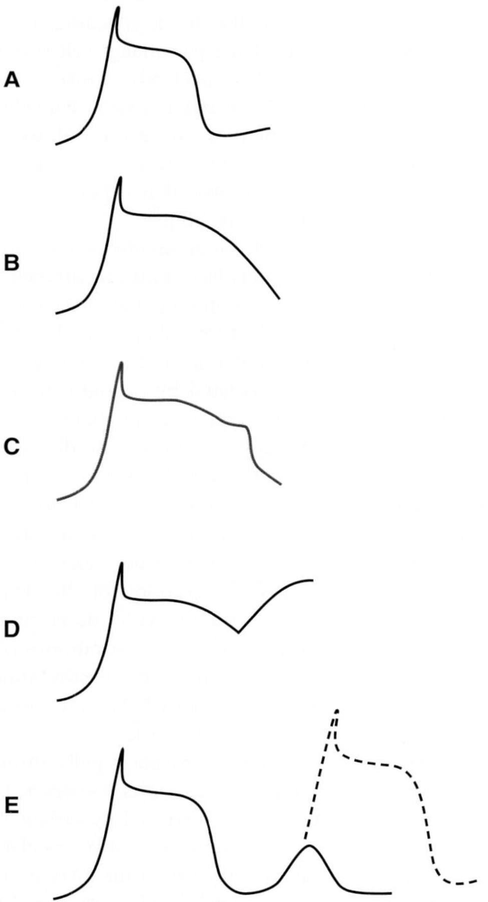

FIGURE 22–17. Afterdepolarization. (**A**) The normal action potential. (**B**) Prolonged duration action potential. (**C**) Prolonged duration action potential with an early afterdepolarization (EAD) (↓) occurring during the downslope of phase 3 of the action potential. (**D**) Early afterdepolarization that reaches the depolarization threshold and initiates another depolarization, or a triggered beat. (**E**) Delayed afterdepolarization (↓) which occurs after repolarization is complete.

QT dispersion The QT interval may vary in duration from lead to lead, reflecting a dispersion or variability in regional myocardial repolarization. The normal QT interval dispersion is around 30 to 70 msec. The conduction characteristics vary regionally throughout the heart. For example, the subendocardial cells have a longer action potential duration than do epicardial cells; this is called dispersion of repolarization and is normal. This is important to allow the heart to contract and relax in an appropriate manner even though the impulse takes time to travel through the full thickness of the myocardial wall, from endocardium to epicardium. The subpopulations of the various ion channels (primarily potassium channels in the setting of repolarization) differ in character and density and account for this variation.[40] Ischemia and drugs preferentially affect certain layers of the myocardium and alter, generally increase, the regional heterogeneity of repolarization. This is reflected on the ECG as an increase in QT dispersion. This prolonged vulnerable phase is associated with occurrences of ventricular dysrhythmias. A measured QT dispersion greater than 80 msec after myocardial infarction was associated with VT with a sensitivity of 73% and a specificity of 86%.[44] This heterogeneity is also correlated with both the efficacy and prodysrhythmic potential of therapy.[53] Overall however, assessment of QT dispersion (from a standard 12-lead ECG) has not gained popularity as a useful clinical tool in part due to technologic limitations.

THE U WAVE

The U wave is a small deflection that occurs after the T wave and usually with a similar orientation. Distinguishing a U wave from a notched T wave is difficult. The apices of a notched T wave are usually < 150 msec apart, and the peaks of a TU complex are > 150 msec apart.

Electrophysiology U waves occur when there is fluctuation in the membrane potential following myocardial repolarization. Prominent U waves are generally representative of an underlying electrophysiologic abnormality, although they may be physiologic. Physiologic U waves may be caused by repolarization of the Purkinje fibers, or they may correspond to late repolarization of myocardial cells in the mid-myocardium, and are implicated in the initiation of cardiac dysrhythmias.[4]

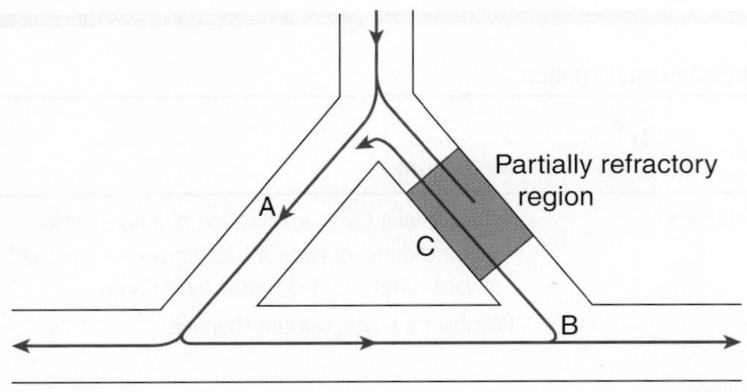

FIGURE 22–18. Mechanism of reentry dysrhythmias. An impulse traveling down a conduction pathway reaches a branch point with one branch refractory (*C*). The impulse is conducted down branch *A* and spreads through the myocardium eventually to reach *B*, the distal end of the originally refractory branch. However, branch *C* is no longer refractory, and the impulse is conducted retrograde up through branch *C*, again to be conducted down branch *A*. The myocardium is depolarized during each loop around the circuit as the impulse spreads from the distal end of branch *A* to the rest of the heart.

The abnormal U wave Abnormal U waves are typically caused by spontaneous afterdepolarization of membrane potential that occurs in situations where repolarization is prolonged (see Fig. 22–17). EAD occurs in situations where the prolonged repolarization period allows calcium channels (which are both time and voltage dependent) to close and spontaneously reopen because they may close at a membrane potential that is above their threshold potential for opening. In this situation, the opening of the calcium channels produces a slight membrane depolarization that is identified as a U wave. Delayed afterdepolarization (DAD) occurs when the myocyte is overloaded with Ca^{2+}, as in the setting of cardioactive steroid toxicity. The excess intracellular Ca^{2+} can trigger the ryanodine receptors on the myocyte sarcoplasmic reticulum to release Ca^{2+}, causing slight depolarization that is recognized as a U wave. If the U waves are of sufficient magnitude to reach threshold, the cell may depolarize and initiate a premature ventricular contraction. Transient U-wave inversion can also be caused by myocardial ischemia or systemic hypertension.

The abnormal QU interval The QU interval is the distance between the end of the Q wave and the end of the U wave. Differentiation between the QU and the QT intervals is difficult if the T and U waves are superimposed. When hypomagnesemia coexists with hypokalemia, as is usually the case, QU prolongation and torsades de pointes may occur.[56]

CARDIAC DYSRHYTHMIAS AND CONDUCTION ABNORMALITIES

Xenobiotics may produce adverse effects on the electrical activity of the heart, often by acting directly on the myocardial cells. Because metabolic abnormalities (especially acidemia, hypotension, hypoxia, and electrolyte abnormalities) can further exacerbate the toxicity, or can actually be the sole cause of the cardiovascular abnormalities, correction of metabolic abnormalities must be a high priority in the treatment of patients with cardiovascular manifestations of poisoning. The terminal phase of any serious poisoning may include nonspecific hemodynamic abnormalities and cardiac dysrhythmias. However, many xenobiotics directly or primarily affect cardiac rhythm or conduction, often through effects on the cardiac ion channels.

The distinction between xenobiotics that cause a rapid rate and those that cause a slow rate on the ECG is somewhat artificial, because many can do both. For example, patients poisoned by CAs almost always develop sinus tachycardia, but most die with a wide complex bradycardia. In either case, abnormalities in the pattern or rate on the ECG can provide the clinician with immediate information about a patient's cardiovascular status. ECG disturbances in many poisoned patients may be categorized in more than one manner (abnormal pattern, fast rate, slow rate). In any case, when electrocardiographic abnormalities are detected, appropriate interpretation, evaluation, and therapy must be rapidly performed.

Xenobiotics that directly cause dysrhythmias or cardiac conduction abnormalities usually affect the myocardial cell membrane. Other xenobiotics that modify ion channels may alter the transmembrane potentials within myocytes and may result in the spontaneous generation of an abnormal rhythm.

MECHANISMS OF DYSRHYTHMIA INITIATION AND PROPAGATION

Dysrhythmias can be related to one or more of 3 mechanisms: abnormal spontaneous depolarization (enhanced automaticity), afterdepolarization (triggered automaticity), and reentry.[40] In normal myocardium, spontaneous, phase 4 depolarization occurs most rapidly in the sinus node, the normal pacemaker for the heart. Speeding or slowing the rate of phase 4 depolarization of the pacemaker cell results in sinus tachycardia or sinus bradycardia, respectively. However, xenobiotics can also speed the depolarization of other myocardial cells that have pacemaker potential allowing them to overtake the sinus node as the primary pacemaker. This mechanism, called increased automaticity, accounts for many of the dysrhythmias that occur with cardioactive steroid and β-adrenergic agonist poisoning.

Dysrhythmias can also result from spontaneous oscillations in the membrane potential, called afterdepolarizations, mentioned above, that occur during phase 3 or 4 of the action potential. If the oscillations are of sufficient magnitude to reach the threshold potential, the fast sodium channels open and an action potential occurs. These spontaneous oscillating depolarizations are mediated by depolarizing inward Ca^{2+} currents, primarily through the L-type calcium channels. EADs occur during the plateau phase (phase 2) or during the downslope (phase 3) of the action potential. Oscillations in the membrane potential that occur after repolarization is complete, during phase 4, are called DADs. EADs most commonly occur in situations in which the action potential is prolonged, typically as a consequence of the blockade of I_{Kr} (such as by antidysrhythmic agents). EADs account for the "trigger beats" that initiate episodes of VT, commonly torsades de pointes (TdP), as discussed below. DADs occur primarily under conditions of increased intracellular Ca^{2+}, and account for many of the dysrhythmias that are associated with cardioactive steroid toxicity.[40] The increased Ca^{2+} may also come from extensive sympathetic stimulation.

Most afterdepolarizations do not propagate rapidly throughout the myocardium and do not generate ectopic beats. However, because the normal dispersion of repolarization is increased by certain xenobiotics, ectopic beats (eg, an atrial premature contraction or ventricular premature contraction) may propagate abnormally within the myocardium. Ectopy is the ECG manifestation of myocardial depolarization initiated from a site other than the sinus node. Ectopy may be lifesaving under circumstances in which the atrial rhythm cannot be conducted to the ventricles (ie,"escape rhythm"), as during high-degree AV blockade induced by cardioactive steroids. (Chap. 64). Alternatively, ectopy may lead to dramatic alterations in the physiologic function of the heart or deteriorate into lethal ventricular dysrhythmias.

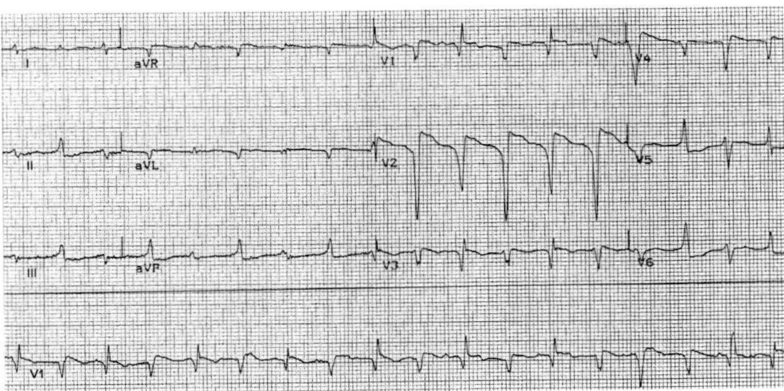

FIGURE 22–19. Digoxin-induced bidirectional ventricular tachycardia. The ECG demonstrates the alternating QRS axis characteristic of bidirectional ventricular tachycardia and is nearly pathognomonic for cardioactive steroid poisoning. The 89-year-old patient's serum digoxin concentration was 4.0 ng/mL. (Image contributed by Ruben Olmedo, MD, Mount Sinai School of Medicine.)

Occasionally, because of the altered regional repolarization, an impulse may reach a branch point with a partial block (ie, relatively refractory) to conduction in one of the branches (Fig. 22–18). The impulse is carried through only one of the branches and then spreads through the myocardial cells. After a short delay, the impulse reaches the distal end of the previously blocked pathway. By this time, the region is no longer refractory and conducts the impulse in a retrograde fashion. The impulse may continue in a continuous loop circuit, depolarizing the heart with each passage; this process is called reentry. Reentry mechanisms appear to be responsible for the majority of the malignant tachydysrhythmias attributable to poisoning.

TACHYDYSRHYTHMIAS

Both supraventricular and ventricular tachydysrhythmias can occur in poisoned patients (Table 22–3). Sinus tachycardia is the most common rhythm disturbance that occurs in poisoned patients. Parasympatholytic xenobiotics, such as atropine, raise the heart rate to its innate rate by eliminating the inhibitory tonic vagal influence. However, more rapid rates require direct myocardial stimulatory effects, generally mediated by β-adrenergic agonism. For example, catecholamine excess, as occurs in patients with cocaine use, psychomotor agitation, or fever, may cause sinus tachycardia with rates faster than 150 beats/min. Ventricular dysrhythmias frequently accompany hypotension, hypoxia, acidemia, electrolyte abnormalities, and other metabolic derangements that may be present in poisoned patients or may be a direct effect of the xenobiotic.

The intrinsic pacemaker cells of the heart undergo spontaneous depolarization and reach threshold at a predictable rate. Under normal circumstances the sinus node is the most rapidly firing pacemaker cell of the heart; and as a result it controls the heart rate. Spontaneous depolarization occurs via ion entry through potassium, sodium, and calcium channels via phase 4 of the action potential. Other potential pacemakers exist in the heart, but their rate of spontaneous depolarization is considerably slower than that of the sinus node. Thus, they are reset during depolarization of the myocardium and they never spontaneously reach threshold. Xenobiotics, such as sympathomimetics, which speed the rate of rise of phase 4, or diastolic depolarization, speed the rate of firing of the pacemaker cells. As long as the sinus node is preferentially affected, it maintains the pacemaker activity of the heart. If the firing rate of another intrinsic pacemaker exceeds that of the sinus node, ectopic rhythms may develop. This effect may be either pathologic or lifesaving, depending on the clinical circumstances.

TABLE 22–3. Xenobiotics that Cause Ventricular and Supraventricular Tachydysrhythmias

Amantadine
Antidysrhythmics
Anticholinergics
Antihistamines
Botanicals and plants
Carbamazepine
Cardioactive steroids
Chloroquine and quinine
Cyclic antidepressants
Cyclobenzaprine
Hydrocarbons and solvents
Halogenated hydrocarbons
Inhalational anesthetics
Jellyfish venom
Metal salts
Arsenic
Iron
Lithium
Magnesium
Potassium
Pentamidine
Phenothiazines
Phosphodiesterase inhibitors (eg, Methylxanthines)
Propoxyphene
Sedative-hypnotics
Chloral Hydrate
Ethanol
Sympathomimetics (eg, cocaine)
Thyroid hormone

Certain xenobiotics are highly associated with ventricular tachydysrhythmias following poisoning. Those that increase the adrenergic tone on the heart, either directly, or indirectly, may cause ventricular dysrhythmias. Whether a result of excessive circulating catecholamines observed with cocaine and sympathomimetics, myocardial sensitization secondary to halogenated hydrocarbons or thyroid hormone, or increased second messenger activity secondary to theophylline, the extreme inotropic and chronotropic effects cause dysrhythmias. Altered repolarization, increased intracellular Ca^{2+} concentrations, or myocardial ischemia can cause the dysrhythmia. Additionally, xenobiotics that produce focal myocardial ischemia, such as cocaine, ephedrine, or ergots can lead to malignant ventricular dysrhythmias. Finally, an uncommon cause of xenobiotic-induced ventricular dysrhythmias is persistent activation of sodium channels, such as following aconitine poisoning. Although not all wide QRS complex tachydysrhythmias are ventricular in origin, making this assumption is generally considered to be prudent. For example, in a patient known to be poisoned with cyclic antidepressants, cocaine, or similar agents ("The QRS Complex"),

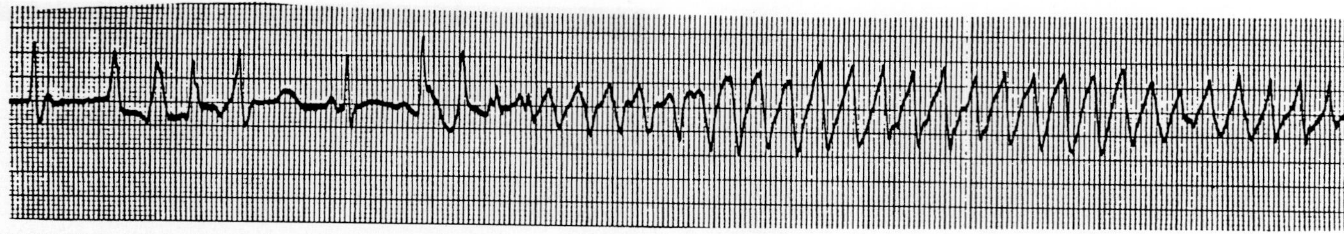

FIGURE 22–20. Torsades de pointes in a patient who ingested an unknown amount of thioridazine.

the differentiation of aberrantly conducted sinus tachycardia (common) from ventricular tachycardia (rare) is important, but difficult. Although guidelines for determining the origin of a wide complex tachydysrhythmia exist,[13] they are imperfect, difficult to apply, and unstudied in poisoned patients.

TABLE 22–4. Xenobiotics That Cause Conduction Abnormalities and/or Heart Block

α_1-Adrenergic agonists
α_2-Adrenergic agonists
β-Adrenergic antagonists
Amantadine
Anesthetics (local)
Antidepressants
Antidysrhythmics (class I and III)
Antihistamines
Antimicrobials
Chloroquine and quinine
Macrolides
Quinolones
Antipsychotics
Atypical antipsychotics (quetiapine, olanzapine, risperidone)
Droperidol
Haloperidol
Phenothiazines
Calcium channel blockers
Carbamazepine
Cardioactive steroids
Cholinergics
Cocaine
Cyclic antidepressants
Cyclobenzaprine
Electrolytes
Potassium
Magnesium
Metal salts
Arsenic
Methadone
Pentamidine
Propoxyphene

Bidirectional ventricular tachycardia is associated with severe cardioactive steroid toxicity and results from alterations of intraventricular conduction, junctional tachycardia with aberrant intraventricular conduction, or, on rare occasions, alternating ventricular pacemakers (see Figure 22–19). Aconitine, usually obtained from traditional Chinese or other alternative therapies that contain plants of the Aconitum spp (such as *Aconitum napellus* (monkshood)), may cause bidirectional ventricular tachycardia (Chaps. 43 and 118).

TACHYDYSRHYTHMIA ASSOCIATED WITH A PROLONGED QT INTERVAL: TORSADES DE POINTES

Xenobiotics that alter myocardial repolarization and prolong the QT interval predispose to the development of afterdepolarization-induced contractions during the relative refractory period (R on T phenomena), which may initiate ventricular tachycardia. If torsades de pointes (TdP) is noted this is undoubtedly the mechanism, and the QT interval should be carefully assessed and appropriate treatment initiated (Fig. 22–20).

Ventricular tachycardia, including TdP, is usually a reentrant-type rhythm. The presence of a prolonged QT interval on the ECG may indicate the possible existence of conditions within the myocardium that favor occurrence of reentry dysrhythmias, as discussed above. The long action potential duration resulting from prolongation in the duration of phase 2 or phase 3 increases the occurrence of EADs. These, in combination with an increased dispersion of repolarization, increase the risk for reentrant dysrhythmias, particularly TdP.

Many xenobiotics may also interact with cardiac membrane ion channels and increase the risk of TdP. Most of these xenobiotics interact with the HERG-encoded subunit of the potassium channel to reduce the current through the I_{Kr} channel and prolong the action potential duration. The HERG subunit of the channel is particularly susceptible to xenobiotic interactions because of the larger inner cavity with aromatic binding domains.[48,47,54] Acquired QT interval prolongation and TdP from xenobiotics occur most often with class Ia and Ic antidysrhythmics, the cyclic antidepressants, and the antipsychotics. Although the class Ic antidysrhythmics (such as encainide and flecainide) cause greater QT prolongation, the class Ia agents (such as quinidine and procainamide) are responsible for more reported cases. This is probably a result of the relatively infrequent use of the class Ic antidysrhythmics, due paradoxically, to concerns about the higher risk of prodysrhythmic effects. Class Ib agents, such as lidocaine, have no significant effect on potassium channels and the QT interval, and do not cause TdP. Acquired QT interval prolongation and TdP also commonly result from metabolic and electrolyte abnormalities, particularly hypocalcemia, hypomagnesemia, and hypokalemia (Chapters 16 and 63).

BRADYDYSRHYTHMIAS

Bradycardia, heart block, and asystole are the terminal events following fatal ingestions of many xenobiotics, but some xenobiotics tend to cause sinus bradycardia (see Table 23–2) and conduction abnormalities (see Table 23–3) early in the course of toxicity. Sinus bradycardia with an otherwise normal electrocardiogram is characteristic of xenobiotics that reduce central nervous system outflow (Chap. 23). Xenobiotics that cause CNS sedation, such as the sedative-hypnotics, most opioids, and α_2-adrenergic receptor agonist ("centrally acting") antihypertensive drugs, will usually decrease sympathetic outflow to the heart and produce a heart rate in the range of 40–60 beats/min. Differentiating among these xenobiotics is not possible based on ECG criteria alone. Xenobiotics that directly affect ion flux across myocardial cell membranes cause abnormalities in AV nodal conduction. Calcium channel blockers, β-adrenergic receptor antagonists, and cardioactive steroids (Chaps. 60, 61, and 64) are the leading causes of sinus bradycardia and conduction disturbances. Indirect metabolic effects may also be contributory; such as severe hyperkalemia (which may accompany any acidosis) that results in a wide complex, sinusoidal bradycardic rhythm.

Xenobiotics that have direct depressant effects on the cardiac pacemaker are most likely to produce bradycardia. The ECG manifestations of calcium channel blocker and β-adrenergic antagonist overdoses are difficult to distinguish. In general, both drug classes cause decreased dromotropy (conduction), although the specific pharmacologic actions of the drugs differ even within the class. For example, most members of the dihydropyridine subclass of calcium channel blockers do not have any antidromotropic effect, whereas verapamil and diltiazem routinely produce PR prolongation. Similarly, while most β-adrenergic antagonists produce sinus bradycardia and first-degree heart block, certain members of this group, such as propranolol, may prolong the QRS complex through their sodium channel blocking abilities (Chap. 61). Others, such as sotalol, which have properties of the class III antidysrhythmics, block myocardial potassium channels and prolong the QT interval duration. The bradycardia produced by cardioactive steroids is typically accompanied by electrocardiographic signs of "digitalis effect," including PR prolongation and ST segment depression (Chap. 64).

TABLE 22–5. Classes of Antidysrhythmics

Class	Pharmacologic Blockade: Sodium Channels	Pharmacologic Blockade: Potassium Channels	Pharmacologic Blockade: Calcium Channels	Prolongation of ECG Intervals: PR	Prolongation of ECG Intervals: QRS	Prolongation of ECG Intervals: QT	Examples
Sodium channel blockers							
IA	++/+++	++	0	±	↑	↑	Disopyramide Procainamide Quinidine
IB	+/++	±	0	±	±	±	Lidocaine Phenytoin Mexiletine Tocainide
IC	+++	++/+++	0	↑	↑	↑↑	Encainide Flecainide Propafenone Moricizine
β-Adrenergic antagonists							
II	0	0	+(indirect)	↑	±	±	Propranolol Atenolol Esmolol Metoprolol Timolol
Potassium channel blockers							
III	+	++	0	↑	±	↑	Amiodarone Bretylium Sotalol Ibutilide[a]
Calcium channel blockers							
IV	0	0	+++	↑	±	±	Verapamil Diltiazem

+ = Mild blockade; + + = moderate blockade; + + + = marked blockade; ↑ = increases; ± = no significant effect

[a] Ibutilide activates a slow inward sodium channel rather than blocking outward potassium currents, but is classified as class III because of its increased action potential duration and atrial and ventricular refractoriness, which are typical of class III Antidysrhythmics. ∗ = Vaughan-Williams classification.

CONDUCTION ABNORMALITIES AND ATRIOVENTRICULAR NODAL BLOCK

The cardiac toxicity of some xenobiotics results from their effects on the propagation of the electrical impulse through the conduction system of the heart. The ECG abnormalities produced may be a result of effects on the AV node, producing first-, second-, or third-degree (complete) heart block, or on the His-Purkinje system, producing intraventricular conduction delays such as bundle-branch blocks. The effects of xenobiotics on myocardial conduction are often mediated through interactions with the sodium or potassium membrane channels. For example, xenobiotics that affect the fast inward I_{Na} currents (such as the type I antidysrhythmics and cyclic antidepressants) prolong the action potential duration, slow ventricular myocyte depolarization, and slow intraventricular conduction. This produces widening of the QRS complex and prolongation of the QT interval on the ECG. Table 22–4 lists some of the xenobiotics that cause conduction abnormalities. Many of the antidysrhythmics derive their clinical benefit from their ability to alter sodium and potassium channel function and slow conduction through the myocardium. Xenobiotics that depress phase 0 (the inward I_{Na} currents) produce slowing of conduction and widening of the QRS complex. Xenobiotics that prolong depolarization and repolarization (phase 2 or phase 3 of the action potential) produce prolongation of the QT interval on the ECG. The classes of the antidysrhythmics, their effects on the ion channels and on the action potential, and the resulting ECG abnormalities, are shown in Table 22–5 and discussed in detail in Chap. 63.

THE PEDIATRIC ELECTROCARDIOGRAM

THE NORMAL PEDIATRIC ECG

The normal pediatric ECG differs in many ways from the normal adult ECG. The resting heart rate of infants and children is substantially faster than that of adults and, in general, conduction is faster. In a term infant, the right ventricle is substantially larger than the left, and the ECG demonstrates prominent R waves in the right precordium and deep S waves in the left lateral precordium.[42] This may be misinterpreted as cyclic antidepressant toxicity.[9] An adult ratio of left to right ventricular size is usually reached by the age of 6 months. In infants, Q waves commonly exist in the inferior and lateral precordial leads, but are abnormal in leads I and aV_L. The T waves are the most notable difference between pediatric and adult ECGs. The T waves in the right precordial leads in children are deeply inverted until 7 years and sometimes older, in which case it is called a persistent juvenile T-wave pattern.

THE ABNORMAL PEDIATRIC ECG

Although congenital heart disease is the most common cause of ECG abnormalities in children, electrolyte disorders and xenobiotics may also cause changes in electrophysiology that are reflected on the ECG. Abnormalities that are useful markers on the adult ECG may not always be as useful in children. For example, in older children, a retrospective chart review of 37 children diagnosed with tricyclic antidepressant overdose and 35 controls (all younger than 11 years) found interpatient variability, unrelated to age, so great that a rightward deviation of the terminal 40-msec QRS axis could not distinguish between poisoned and healthy children.[9]

SUMMARY

The ECG is one of the few widely available diagnostic procedures that reveals immediate, useful clinical information. This has far-reaching implications in toxicology, where other diagnostic test results often return too late to effectively impact the care of an acutely poisoned patient.

REFERENCES

1. Accili EA, Proenza C, Baruscotti M, et al. From funny current to HCN channels: 20 years of excitation. *News Physiol Sci.* 2002;17:32-37.
2. Afonso L, Mohammad T, Thatai D. Crack whips the heart: a review of the cardiovascular toxicity of cocaine. *Am J Cardiol.* 2007;100:1040-1043.
3. Al-Khatib SM, LaPointe NM, Kramer JM, et al. What clinicians should know about the QT interval. *JAMA.* 2003;289:2120-2127.
4. Anderson ME, Al-Khatib SM, Roden DM, et al. Cardiac repolarization: current knowledge, critical gaps, and new approaches to drug development and patient management. *Am Heart J.* 2002;144:769-781.
5. Aytemir K, Maarouf N, Gallagher MM, et al. Comparison of formulae for heart rate correction of QT interval in exercise electrocardiograms. *Pacing Clin Electrophysiol.* 1999;22:1397-1401.
6. Bailey B, Buckley NA, Amre DK. A meta-analysis of prognostic indicators to predict seizures, arrhythmias or death after tricyclic antidepressant overdose. *J Toxicol Clin Toxicol.* 2004;42:877-888.
7. Bailie DS, Inoue H, Kaseda S, et al. Magnesium suppression of early afterdepolarizations and ventricular tachyarrhythmias induced by cesium in dogs. *Circulation.* 1988;77:1395-1402.
8. Bebarta VS, Phillips S, Eberhardt A, et al. Incidence of Brugada electrocardiographic pattern and outcomes of these patients after intentional tricyclic antidepressant ingestion. *Am J Cardiol.* 2007;100:656-660.
9. Berkovitch M, Matsui D, Fogelman R, et al. Assessment of the terminal 40-millisecond QRS vector in children with a history of tricyclic antidepressant ingestion. *Pediatr Emerg Care.* 1995;11:75-77.
10. Bessen HA, Niemann JT. Improvement of cardiac conduction after hyperventilation in tricyclic antidepressant overdose. *J Toxicol Clin Toxicol.* 1985;23:537-546.
11. Boehnert MT, Lovejoy FH Jr. Value of the QRS duration versus the serum drug level in predicting seizures and ventricular arrhythmias after an acute overdose of tricyclic antidepressants. *N Engl J Med.* 1985;313:474-479.
12. Brady WJ. Benign early repolarization: electrocardiographic manifestations and differentiation from other ST segment elevation syndromes. *Am J Emerg Med.* 1998;16:592-597.
13. Brugada P, Brugada J, Mont L, et al. A new approach to the differential diagnosis of a regular tachycardia with a wide QRS complex. *Circulation.* 1991;83:1649-1659.
14. Catterall WA, Perez-Reyes E, Snutch TP, et al. International Union of Pharmacology. XLVIII. Nomenclature and structure-function relationships of voltage-gated calcium channels. *Pharmacol Rev.* 2005;57:411-425.
15. Desai M, Li L, Desta Z, et al. Variability of heart rate correction methods for the QT interval. *Br J Clin Pharmacol.* 2003;55:511-517.
16. DiFrancesco D, Borer JS. The funny current: cellular basis for the control of heart rate. *Drugs.* 2007;67Suppl 2:15-24.
17. Ducroq J, Printemps R, Guilbot S, et al. Action potential experiments complete hERG assay and QT-interval measurements in cardiac preclinical studies. *J Pharmacol Toxicol Methods.* 2007;56:159-170.
18. Faber TS, Kautzner J, Zehender M, et al. Impact of electrocardiogram recording format on QT interval measurement and QT dispersion assessment. *Pacing Clin Electrophysiol.* 2001;24:1739-1747.
19. Food and Drug Administration. Guidance for Industry E14 Clinical Evaluation of QT/QTc Interval Prolongation and Proarrhythmic Potential for Non-Antiarrhythmic Drugs. http://www.fda.gov/CDER/GUIDANCE/6922fnl.htm. Accessed April 27, 2009.
20. Food and Drug Administration. Methodone hydrochloride (marketed as Dolophine) information: Death, narcotic overdose, and serious cardiac arrhythmias. [FDA Alert]. http://www.fda.gov/cder/drug/infopage/methadone/default.htm. Accessed April 24, 2009.
21. Funck-Brentano C, Jaillon P. Rate-corrected QT interval: techniques and limitations. *Am J Cardiol.* 1993;72:17B-22B.
22. Hollander JE, Lozano M, Fairweather P, et al. "Abnormal" electrocardiograms in patients with cocaine-associated chest pain are due to "normal" variants. *J Emerg Med.* 1994;12:199-205.
23. Hulten BA, Adams R, Askenasi R, et al. Predicting severity of tricyclic antidepressant overdose. *J Toxicol Clin Toxicol.* 1992;30:161-170.

24. Isbister GK, Balit CR. Bupropion overdose: QTc prolongation and its clinical significance. *Ann Pharmacother.* 2003;37:999-1002.
25. Kautzner J. QT interval measurements. *Card Electrophysiol Rev.* 2002;6:273-277.
26. Keating MT, Sanguinetti MC. Molecular and cellular mechanisms of cardiac arrhythmias. *Cell.* 2001;104:569-580.
27. Kenneback G, Bergfeldt L, Vallin H, et al. Electrophysiologic effects and clinical hazards of carbamazepine treatment for neurologic disorders in patients with abnormalities of the cardiac conduction system. *Am Heart J.* 1991;121:1421-1429.
28. LaPointe NM, Al-Khatib SM, Kramer JM, et al. Knowledge deficits related to the QT interval could affect patient safety. *Ann Noninvasive Electrocardiol.* 2003;8:157-160.
29. Liebelt EL, Francis PD, Woolf AD. ECG lead aVR versus QRS interval in predicting seizures and arrhythmias in acute tricyclic antidepressant toxicity. *Ann Emerg Med.* 1995;26:195-201.
30. Liebelt EL, Ulrich A, Francis PD, et al. Serial electrocardiogram changes in acute tricyclic antidepressant overdoses. *Crit Care Med.* 1997;25:1721-1726.
31. Littmann L, Monroe MH, Kerns WP 2nd, et al. Brugada syndrome and "Brugada sign": clinical spectrum with a guide for the clinician. *Am Heart J.* 2003;145:768-778.
32. Malik M, Hnatkova K, Batchvarov V. Differences between study-specific and subject-specific heart rate corrections of the QT interval in investigations of drug induced QTc prolongation. *Pacing Clin Electrophysiol.* 2004;27:791-800.
33. Maltsev VA, Lakatta EG. Normal heart rhythm is initiated and regulated by an intracellular calcium clock within pacemaker cells. *Heart Lung Circ.* 2007;16:335-348.
34. Maltsev VA, Vinogradova TM, Lakatta EG. The emergence of a general theory of the initiation and strength of the heartbeat. *J Pharmacol Sci.* 2006;100:338-369.
35. Mangoni ME, Nargeot J. Genesis and regulation of the heart automaticity. *Physiol Rev.* 2008;88:919-982.
36. Mattu A, Brady WJ, Robinson DA. Electrocardiographic manifestations of hyperkalemia. *Am J Emerg Med.* 2000;18:721-729.
37. Molnar J, Zhang F, Weiss J, et al. Diurnal pattern of QTc interval: how long is prolonged? Possible relation to circadian triggers of cardiovascular events. *J Am Coll Cardiol.* 1996;27:76-83.
38. Morganroth J, Brozovich FV, McDonald JT, et al. Variability of the QT measurement in healthy men, with implications for selection of an abnormal QT value to predict drug toxicity and proarrhythmia. *Am J Cardiol.* 1991;67:774-776.
39. Moss AJ: Long QT Syndrome. *JAMA* .2003;289:2041-2044.
40. Nelson LS. Toxicologic myocardial sensitization. *J Toxicol Clin Toxicol.* 2002;40:867-879.
41. Niemann JT, Bessen HA, Rothstein RJ, et al. Electrocardiographic criteria for tricyclic antidepressant cardiotoxicity. *Am J Cardiol.* 1986;57:1154-1159.
42. O'Connor M, McDaniel N, Brady WJ. The pediatric electrocardiogram: part I: Age-related interpretation. *Am J Emerg Med.* 2008;26:506-512.
43. Osborn JJ. Experimental hypothermia; respiratory and blood pH changes in relation to cardiac function. *Am J Physiol.* 1953;175:389-398.
44. Puljevic D, Smalcelj A, Durakovic Z, et al. QT dispersion, daily variations, QT interval adaptation and late potentials as risk markers for ventricular tachycardia. *Eur Heart J.* 1997;18:1343-1349.
45. Ravens U, Wettwer E, Hala O. Pharmacological modulation of ion channels and transporters. *Cell Calcium.* 2004;35:575-582.
46. Ray WA, Chung CP, Murray KT, et al. Atypical antipsychotic drugs and the risk of sudden cardiac death. *N Engl J Med.* 2009;360:225-235.
47. Roden DM. Role of the electrocardiogram in determining electrophysiologic end points of drug therapy. *Am J Cardiol.* 1988;62:34H-38H.
48. Roden DM. Drug-induced prolongation of the QT interval. *N Engl J Med.* 2004;350:1013-1022.
49. Roden DM, Balser JR, George AL Jr., et al. Cardiac ion channels. *Annu Rev Physiol.* 2002;64:431-475.
50. Sagie A, Larson MG, Goldberg RJ, et al. An improved method for adjusting the QT interval for heart rate (the Framingham Heart Study). *Am J Cardiol.* 1992;70:797-801.
51. Schwartz M, Patel M, Kazzi Z, et al. Cardiotoxicity after massive amantadine overdose. *J Med Toxicol.* 2008;4:173-179.
52. Sharma AN, Hexdall AH, Chang EK, et al. Diphenhydramine-induced wide complex dysrhythmia responds to treatment with sodium bicarbonate. *Am J Emerg Med.* 2003;21:212-215.
53. Stone PH. Ranolazine: new paradigm for management of myocardial ischemia, myocardial dysfunction, and arrhythmias. *Cardiol Clin.* 2008;26:603-614.
54. Teschemacher AG, Seward EP, Hancox JC, et al. Inhibition of the current of heterologously expressed HERG potassium channels by imipramine and amitriptyline. *Br J Pharmacol.* 1999;128:479-485.
55. Tilkian AG, Schroeder JS, Kao JJ, et al. The cardiovascular effects of lithium in man. A review of the literature. *Am J Med.* 1976;61:665-670.
56. Tzivoni D, Keren A, Cohen AM, et al. Magnesium therapy for torsades de pointes. *Am J Cardiol.* 1984;53:528-530.
57. Vassallo SU, Delaney KA, Hoffman RS, et al. A prospective evaluation of the electrocardiographic manifestations of hypothermia. *Acad Emerg Med.* 1999;6:1121-1126.
58. Wrenn KD, Slovis BS, Slovis CM. The ability of physicians to predict electrolyte deficiency from the ECG. *Ann Emerg Med.* 1990;19:580-583.

CHAPTER 23
HEMODYNAMIC PRINCIPLES

Robert A. Hessler

Adequate tissue perfusion depends on maintenance of volume status, vascular resistance, cardiac contractility, and cardiac rhythm. The components of the hemodynamic system are vulnerable to the effects of xenobiotics. Cardiovascular toxicity may therefore be manifested by the development of hemodynamic instability, heart failure, cardiac conduction abnormalities, or dysrhythmias. The presence of a specific pattern of cardiovascular anomalies (toxicologic syndrome or "toxidrome") may suggest a particular class or type of xenobiotic. Conduction and rhythm disturbances are discussed in detail in Chapter 22.

An alteration in hemodynamic functioning may be a result of indirect metabolic effects. Poisoning with a xenobiotic may lead to hemodynamic changes secondary to the development of acid base disturbances, hypoxia, or electrolyte abnormalities. In these patients, supportive care with ventilation, oxygenation, and fluid and electrolyte repletion will usually improve the cardiovascular status

PHYSIOLOGY OF THE HEMODYNAMIC SYSTEM

Maintaining cardiac contractility, heart rate and rhythm, and vascular resistance requires complex modulation of the cardiac and vascular systems. Xenobiotics can cause hemodynamic abnormalities as a result of direct effects on the myocardial cells, on the cardiac conduction system, or on the arteriolar smooth muscle cells. These effects are frequently mediated by interactions with cellular ion channels or cell membrane neurohormonal receptors. Ion channels are discussed in detail in Chapter 22.

THE AUTONOMIC NERVOUS SYSTEM AND HEMODYNAMICS

In addition to the voltage dependent ion channels, the cell membrane contains channels that open in response to receptor binding of neurotransmitters or neurohormones.[42,43,44] The hemodynamic effects of many xenobiotics are mediated by interactions with membrane receptors and by changes in the autonomic nervous system. The autonomic nervous system is functionally divided into the sympathetic (ie, adrenergic) and parasympathetic (ie, cholinergic) systems. The two systems, which share certain common features, function semi-independently of each other. Through complex feedback, the two systems provide the balance needed for existence under changing external conditions.

The sympathetic nervous system is primarily responsible for the maintenance of arteriolar tone and cardiac function. Although the ganglionic neurotransmitter of the sympathetic nervous system is acetylcholine, norepinephrine is its primary postganglionic neurotransmitter. On release into the synapse, norepinephrine binds to the postsynaptic adrenergic receptors to elicit an effect by the postsynaptic cell.

ADRENERGIC RECEPTORS

CELLULAR PHYSIOLOGY OF ADRENERGIC RECEPTORS

The effects of adrenergic xenobiotics on the cell are primarily mediated through a secondary messenger system of cyclic adenosine monophosphate (cAMP). The intracellular cAMP concentration is regulated by the membrane interaction of three components: the adrenergic receptor, a "G-protein" complex, and adenyl cyclase, the enzyme that synthesizes cAMP in the cell.[7,19,59,60] These receptors are described in detail in Chap. 13.

The G protein serves as a "signal transducer" between the receptor molecule in the cell membrane and the effector enzyme, adenyl cyclase, in the cytosol. The G proteins consist of 3 subunits: α, β, and γ.[11,37,38] The α subunit of the G protein complex binds to the adrenergic receptor in the cell membrane and to the adenyl cyclase enzyme. The G protein complex exists in several isomeric forms, depending on their interactions with the adenyl cyclase enzyme. G_s proteins contain α_s subunits that stimulate adenyl cyclase when "activated" by adrenergic receptor interaction. β_1- and β_2-adrenergic receptors interact primarily with β_s subunits in stimulatory G_s protein complexes. The α_i subunits of G_i proteins inhibit the activity of adenyl cyclase. β_2-adrenergic receptors and α_2-adrenergic receptors interact with inhibitory G_i proteins. A third form, G_q, interacts with the α_1-adrenergic receptors, but does not interact directly with adenyl cyclase. Instead, the G_q interacts with phospholipase C to mediate the cell response to α_1-adrenergic stimulation.

In the absence of a catecholamine at the receptor site, the receptor protein is bound to the β and βγ dimers of the G protein, and guanosine diphosphate (GDP) is bound to the α subunit. Catecholamine binding to the receptor causes a conformational change in the α subunit; GDP dissociates and guanosine triphosphate (GTP) binds to the α subunit. The α subunit (with GTP bound) then dissociates from the receptor and from the βγ dimer. This "activated" α subunit can now interact with adenyl cyclase or other effector enzymes. Interaction of the α_s subunit with adenyl cyclase increases the activity of the enzyme resulting in a rapid increase in the intracellular cAMP (Fig. 23–1).[7,11,32,37,50]

cAMP acts as a secondary messenger in the cell. cAMP interacts with protein kinase A (PKA) and other cAMP-dependent protein kinases to increase their protein phosphorylating activity.[31] In the absence of cAMP, PKA is a tetramer of two regulatory and two catalytic subunits. cAMP binds to the regulatory subunits to release the active enzymatic units from the tetramer (see Fig. 23–1). The activated protein kinases then transfer phosphate groups from ATP to serine (as well as to threonine and tyrosine amino acid groups) on enzymes that are involved in intracellular regulation and activities. Phosphorylation may increase or decrease the activity of specific enzymes, and specific protein kinases are highly selective in the proteins that they phosphorylate.[56,57]

PKA phosphorylates a variety of cellular proteins involved in Ca^{2+} regulation, including the voltage-sensitive calcium channel, phospholamban, and troponin.[23,24,55] Phosphorylation of the L-type calcium channel increases the entry of calcium ions during membrane depolarization.[41] Phosphorylation of phospholamban decreases its activity to inhibit the calcium ATPase pump on the SR. This decreased inhibition of the calcium ATPase pump increases the efficiency of Ca^{2+} storage in the SR, which enhances both cellular contractility as the Ca^{2+} is released into the cell cytosol and the relaxation of muscle fibers as the Ca^{2+} is pumped back into the SR.[41]

Intracellular calcium, calcium channels, and myocyte contractility The contraction and relaxation cycle of the myocyte is controlled by the

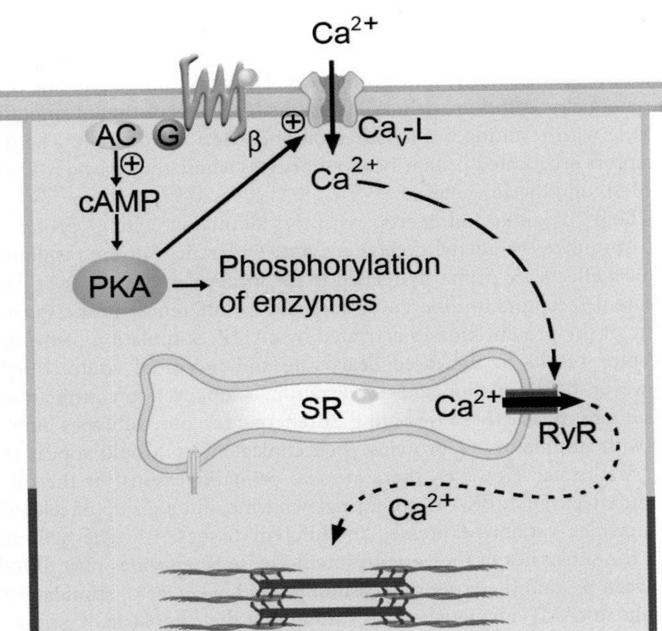

FIGURE 23–1. Binding of the β-adrenergic agonist to the β receptor of a myocardial cell causes the Gs protein to activate adenyl cyclase (AC) to produce cyclic adenosine monophosphate (cAMP). The cAMP interacts with and activates protein kinase A (PKA). Subsequent phosphorylation by PKA changes the activity of multiple other various cellular proteins including phospholambam, calcium channels, and troponin, all of which increase the activity of the myocardial cell. (see text). Ca_V-L = L type voltage dependent calcium channel; SR = sarcoplasmic reticulum; RyR = ryanodyne receptor.

flux of Ca^{2+} into and out of the SR into the cytoplasm.[12,30,47] Only a small proportion of the Ca^{2+} involved in myofibril contraction actually enters the cell through the exterior cell membrane during the action potential and membrane depolarization. Invaginations of the myocyte membrane known as T-tubules place L-type calcium channels in close approximation to calcium release channels (ryanodine receptors [RyR]) on the sarcoplasmic reticulum (SR). The local increase in Ca^{2+} concentration that follows the opening of a single L-type calcium channel triggers the opening of the associated RyR channels resulting in a large release of Ca^{2+} from the SR.[9] Myocytes contain tens of thousands of *couplons*, clusters of L-type calcium channels and RyR channels. The Ca^{2+} released from one couplon is not sufficient to trigger firing of neighboring couplons. Myocyte contraction requires synchronized release of Ca^{2+} from numerous couplons throughout the myocyte. This process depends on membrane depolarization to synchronize opening of L-type channels and subsequent Ca^{2+} release.[13,41] This phenomenon of calcium-induced calcium release results in a rapid increase in the intracellular Ca^{2+} concentration, and initiates a rapid myosin and actin interaction.[12]

At the conclusion of cellular contraction, an SR-associated Ca^{2+} ATPase adenosine triphosphatase pump returns the cytosolic Ca^{2+} into the SR. This SR associated Ca^{2+} ATPase pump is regulated by phospholamban, a cellular protein. Phosphorylation of phospholamban decreases its affinity for binding to the Ca^{2+} pump; dissociation of the phosphorylated phospholamban increases the activity of the Ca^{2+} ATPase pump. β-Adrenergic stimulation leads to phosphorylation of phospholamban, dissociation of the phosphorylated phospholamban from the pump, and increase in the total SR Ca^{2+} stores.[16,17] The increased activity of the SR associated Ca^{2+} pump enhances the contractility and increases the rate of relaxation of the myocytes.

Cellular contraction occurs when myosin filaments interact with the actin-tropomyosin helix. A complex of troponin T, troponin I, and troponin C binds to the actin helix near the myosin binding site and act as regulators of the interaction. Troponin T binds the regulatory complex to the actin helix, troponin I prevents myosin from accessing its binding site on the actin helix, and troponin C acts as a Ca^{2+} trigger to initiate contraction. When the intracellular Ca^{2+} concentration increases, 4 molecules of Ca^{2+} bind to troponin C and a conformational shift occurs in the troponin complex. Troponin I shifts and the myosin-binding site is exposed; myosin binds to the exposed site and myofibril contraction occurs (Figure 23–2).[26,27,48,49]

Calcium transport through the cellular membrane ion channels is critical for normal cardiac muscle function and contractility and for maintenance of vascular smooth muscle tone. The physiologic response to calcium channel blockers and to xenobiotics that interact with the α- or β-adrenergic receptors is mediated through changes in the intracellular Ca^{2+}. Calcium channel blockers in current clinical use primarily block the L-type calcium channel, although their specificity differs for the calcium channels on the vascular smooth muscle cells versus myocardial cells. This results in variable effects of different calcium channel blockers on the vascular tone and peripheral vascular resistance, and on the contractility and electrical activity of the myocardial cells. Certain calcium channel blockers block neuronal calcium channels, such as the P/Q type, and are used to treat neurologic disorders such as migraine headache.

Patients poisoned by calcium channel blockers have less Ca^{2+} entry into the cell during cardiac membrane depolarization. Administration of exogenous Ca^{2+} increases the concentration gradient across the cell membrane, enhances flow through available Ca^{2+} channels and restores the triggered response of the RyR-2 channels to release Ca^{2+} from the sarcoplasmic reticulum (see Antidotes in Depth A30: Calcium). Because β-adrenergic antagonists have negative effects on Ca^{2+} handling by the SR, similar effects occur in the myocyte affected by these xenobiotics.

In the vascular smooth muscle, the cytosolic Ca^{2+} concentration maintains basal tone and any decrease of Ca^{2+} influx results in relaxation and arterial vasodilation.[39] The rapid influx of calcium binds

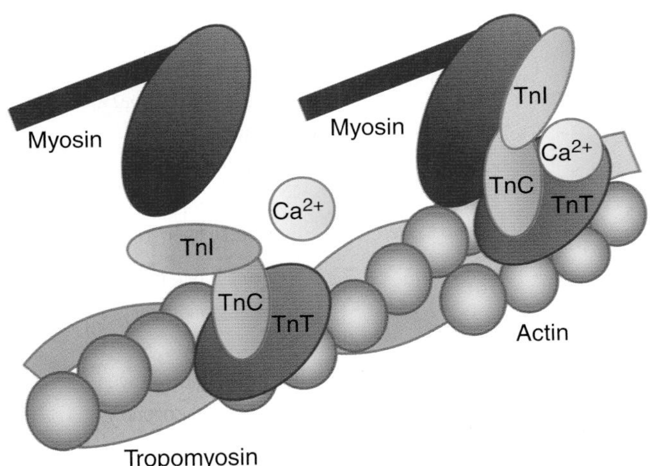

FIGURE 23–2. Troponin regulation of actin and myosin interaction. On the left, Troponin I (TnI) blocks the binding site for myosin on the tropomyosin-actin helix. On the right, calcium binding to troponin C (TnC) causes a conformational shift in the troponin molecules, and myosin is able to bind to the actin helix and initiate myofibril contraction. TnT is Troponin T.

calmodulin, and the resulting complex stimulates myosin light-chain kinase activity.[35] The myosin light-chain kinase phosphorylates, and thus activates, myosin, which subsequently binds actin, causing a contraction to occur (Fig. 60–1).[4,27]

PHYSIOLOGIC EFFECTS OF ADRENERGIC RECEPTORS

The existence of two types of adrenergic receptors, α and β, was first proposed in 1948 to explain both the excitatory and the inhibitory effects of catecholamines on different smooth muscle tissue.[1] The α receptor was subsequently further subdivided into α_1 and α_2 when norepinephrine and other α-adrenergic agonists were found to inhibit the release of additional norepinephrine from neurons into the synapse. The α_1-adrenergic receptors are located on postsynaptic cells outside the central nervous system, primarily on blood vessels, and mediate arteriole constriction. The "autoregulatory" α_2 receptors are primarily located on the presynaptic neuronal membrane and, when stimulated, decrease release of additional norepinephrine into the synapse. Some α_2-adrenergic receptors are also found on the postsynaptic membrane. Activation of these postsynaptic α_2-receptors in the cardiovascular control centers in the medulla and elsewhere in the central nervous system decreases sympathetic outflow from the brain. Therefore, α_2-adrenergic agonists generally cause decreased peripheral vascular resistance, decreased heart rate, and decreased blood pressure. The α_1 and α_2 adrenergic receptors also interact with circulating catecholamines and other sympathomimetics. The effects of sympathomimetics vary in the different organ systems due to differences in the adrenergic receptors and in the cellular responses to the receptor interactions.

The β-adrenergic receptors have been subclassified into 3 subtypes: β_1, β_2, and β_3 (Table 23–1). The most prevalent β-adrenergic subtype in the heart is β_1 (80%), although β_2 (20%) and β_3 (few) receptors are also present.[6,14,18,43] Stimulation of the β_1-adrenergic receptors increases heart rate, contractility, conduction velocity, and automaticity. The β_2-adrenergic receptors are primarily responsible for relaxation of smooth muscle with resulting bronchodilation and arteriolar dilation. The β_3 receptors are located primarily on adipocytes where they play a role in lipolysis and thermogenesis.[8]

The β_1, β_2, and α_2 adrenergic receptors all interact with G_s proteins and stimulate the adenyl cyclase enzyme. Differences in the resultant clinical effects are primarily related to the location and number of the different receptors in different tissues and to differences in the specificity of the protein kinases activated by cAMP. Stimulation of the β_1 receptor results in increased heart rate and increased contractility. However, β_2 stimulation causes relaxation, as opposed to contraction, of smooth muscle. Because both β-adrenergic receptor subtypes interact with stimulatory G_s proteins, their clinical effects would appear to be paradoxical. However, there are two primary reasons for the different effect. First, PKA is not a single enzyme, but a group of related isoenzymes variably expressed in different tissues.[5,25,40] The actions and the substrates of the varied protein kinase isoenzymes may differ between β_1- and β_2-responsive tissues. Second, whereas β_1 stimulation results in cAMP-mediated effects throughout the cytoplasm, β_2 stimulation is compartmentalized within the cell. The effect of β_2 stimulation of G_s type receptors is localized phosphorylation of the L-type calcium channels, increasing their activity.[10,28,64,65] β_2 receptors are also coupled to G_i-type receptors that inhibit adenyl cyclase and prevent the diffuse cytoplasmic increases in cAMP.[52,53,64] Additionally, β_2-receptor stimulation does not result in phosphorylation of phospholamban[29] or troponins.[10]

The α_2-adrenergic receptor interacts with a G_i protein that has an inhibitory interaction with adenyl cyclase. Binding of α_2-adrenergics to the receptor results in inhibition (not stimulation) of adenyl cyclase and to a decrease in the intracellular cAMP.

The α_1-adrenergic receptors also are associated with G proteins. However, rather than being associated with G_s proteins and adenyl cyclase, the α_1-adrenergic receptors are associated with G_q proteins that are linked to phospholipase C.[58] Binding to the receptor activates the hydrolysis of phosphatidyl inositol 4,5-bisphosphate (PIP_2) to 1,2-diacylglycerol (DAG) and inositol triphosphate (IP_3).[22] The IP_3, acting as an intracellular messenger, binds to receptors on the SR and initiates the release of calcium ion.[3] DAG activates protein kinase C, which phosphorylates slow calcium channels and other intracellular proteins, and increases the influx of calcium ion into the cell (Figure 23–3).[45,51,67]

Many xenobiotics interact with G-protein membrane receptors and alter the intracellular cAMP or Ca^{2+} concentration. β-Adrenergic antagonist overdose results in decreased stimulation of adenyl cyclase by G_s proteins, decreased production of cAMP, decreased activation of the cAMP-dependent kinases, and decreased Ca^{2+} release (Chap. 61). Similarly, by different mechanisms, calcium channel blocker overdose results in decreased cytoplasmic calcium concentration (Chap. 60).

Glucagon receptors, which are similar to the β-adrenergic receptors, are coupled to G_s proteins and stimulate adenyl cyclase activity.[2,20,29,62,66] The ability of glucagon to increase cAMP is further enhanced by its inhibitory activity on phosphodiesterase (preventing cAMP breakdown).[15,36] Phosphodiesterase inhibitors, such as amrinone, milrinone, and enoximone, exert at least some of their inotropic activity by preventing the degradation of cAMP and enhancing calcium cycling.[33,61,63] In a canine model of propranolol poisoning, amrinone significantly increased inotropy, stroke volume, and cardiac output.[33]

TABLE 23–1. Types and Function of the Beta-Adrenergic Receptor

Type	Location	Function
β_1	Heart	Increase rate
		Increase inotropy
		Increase SA and AV node conduction
	Kidney	Increase renin
	Eye	Increase aqueous humor
	Adipose tissue	increase lipolysis
β_2	Heart	Increase rate (?)
		Increase inotropy
	Liver	Increase glycogenolysis
		Increase gluconeogenesis
	Skeletal muscle	Increase glycogenolysis
	Smooth muscle (bronchi, arterioles, GI tract, uterus)	Relaxation
β_3	Adipose tissue	Increase lipolysis
		Increase thermogenesis
	Heart	Decrease inotropy (?)

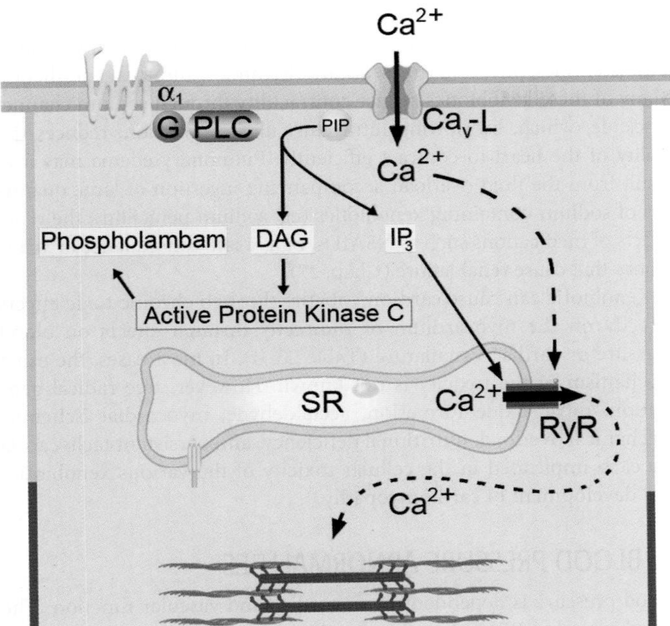

FIGURE 23–3. Binding of the α-adrenergic agonist to the α-1 adrenergic receptor causes the G protein to activate phospholipase C (PLC). PLC catalyzes the hydrolysis of 4,5-bisphosphate (PIP) to produce 1,2-diacylglycerol (DAG) and inositol triphosphate (IP_3). IP_3 interacts with the ryanodyne receptor (RyR) on the sarcoplasmic reticulum to enhance release of calcium from this cellular store. The calcium and DAG activate protein kinase C, which phosphorylates and changes the activity of various cellular proteins including phospholambam (see text) Ca_V-L = L type voltage dependent calcium channel.

TABLE 23–2. Xenobiotics that Cause Bradycardia

α_1-Adrenergic agonists (reflex bradycardia)
Phenylephrine
Phenylpropanolamine
α_2-Adrenergic agonists (centrally acting)
Clonidine
Methyldopa
β-Adrenergic antagonists
Antidysrhythmics
Amiodarone
Sotalol
Calcium channel blockers
Cardioactive steroids
Cholinergics
Carbamates or organic phosphorus compounds
Edrophonium
Neostigmine
Physostigmine
Opioids
Sedative hypnotics
Sodium channel openers
Aconitine
Andromedotoxin
Ciguatoxin
Veratridine

CARDIOVASCULAR EFFECTS OF XENOBIOTICS

Xenobiotics may produce adverse effects on the cardiovascular system by acting on the myocardial cells or the autonomic nervous system to affect the heart rate, blood pressure or cardiac contractility, directly. Because metabolic abnormalities (especially acidemia, hypotension, hypoxia, and electrolyte abnormalities) can further exacerbate the toxicity, or can be the sole cause of the cardiovascular abnormalities, correction of metabolic abnormalities must be a high priority in the treatment of patients with cardiovascular manifestations of poisoning. The terminal phase of any serious poisoning may include nonspecific hemodynamic abnormalities and cardiac dysrhythmias.

HEART RATE ABNORMALITIES

Xenobiotics that directly cause dysrhythmias or cardiac conduction abnormalities usually affect the myocardial cell membrane. These abnormal rhythms, cardiac conduction abnormalities, and heart blocks are discussed in Chapter 22.

Bradycardia Sinus bradycardia is probably the most common xenobiotic-induced bradycardia. Xenobiotics (Table 23–2) produce bradycardia through different mechanisms. The xenobiotic may affect the central or peripheral nervous system, or may affect rhythm generation or conduction in the heart. Most xenobiotics that cause CNS sedation, such as the sedative-hypnotics, opioids, and α_2 adrenergic receptor agonist ("centrally acting") antihypertensives, will usually decrease sympathetic outflow to the heart and produce sinus bradycardia in the range of 40–60 beats/min. Digoxin, certain cholinergics, and α_1 agonists may produce bradycardia and heart block through the enhancement of vagal tone. Sodium channel activators, such as aconitine, cause bradycardia due to intracellular Na^+ overload with a resultant alteration in calcium Ca^{2+} handling. The most profound bradycardia results from overdoses of xenobiotics that have direct depressant effects on the cardiac pacemakers.[54] The ultimate manifestation of pacemaker failure is asystole. Similarly, the inability to propagate an impulse within the cardiac conducting system may produce bradycardia. Examples of xenobiotics that can produce pacemaker or conduction effects include calcium channel blockers and β-adrenergic antagonists.

Bradycardia, heart block, and asystole are frequently the terminal events in patients with massive overdose of many noncardiotoxic xenobiotics. These dysrhythmias may occur as a result of direct effects on the myocardial system or of indirect metabolic effects. For instance, severe hyperkalemia or metabolic acidosis results in a wide complex, sinusoidal bradycardic rhythm.

Tachycardia Sinus tachycardia is the most common rhythm disturbance that occurs in poisoned patients. Parasympatholytic drugs, such as atropine, raise the heart rate by elimination of the inhibitory tonic vagal influence. However, more rapid rates require direct myocardial stimulatory effects, generally mediated by β-adrenergic agonism. For example, catecholamine excess (eg, cocaine, psychomotor agitation, methylxanthines, sedative-hypnotic withdrawal) may cause sinus tachycardia with rates faster than 150 beats/min. Tachycardia may also

TABLE 23–3. Xenobiotics that Cause Sinus Tachycardia and Tachydysrhythmias

Amantadine
Antidysrhythmics
Anticholinergics
Antihistamines
Botanicals and plants (Chap. 118)
Carbamazepine
Cardioactive steroids
Chloroquine and quinine
Cyclic antidepressants
Cyclobenzaprine
Flumazenil
Hydrocarbons and solvents
Halogenated hydrocarbons
Inhalational anesthetics
Jellyfish venom
Metal salts
Arsenic
Iron
Lithium
Magnesium
Potassium
Pentamidine
Phenothiazines
Phosphodiesterase inhibitors
Amrinone
Methylxanthines
Propoxyphene
Sedative-hypnotics
Chloral Hydrate
Ethanol
Sympathomimetics
Catecholamines
Cocaine
Thyroid hormone preparations

be an indirect effect as occurs in response to hypotension, hypoxia, acidemia, fever electrolyte abnormalities, and other metabolic derangements that may be present in poisoned patients (Table 23–3).

DECREASED CARDIAC CONTRACTILITY AND CONGESTIVE HEART FAILURE

Xenobiotics can reduce cardiac contractility with a resulting decrease in cardiac ejection fraction and cardiac output, a decrease in blood pressure, and development of congestive heart failure (CHF). Cardiogenic pulmonary edema generally occurs as a result of the direct effects of the xenobiotic on the contractility, or inotropy, of the heart, or through increases in the preload or afterload. Acute cardiogenic pulmonary edema, resulting from impaired left heart filling (which may be due to decreased cardiac output), occurs in patients poisoned by a non-dihydropyridine calcium channel blocker or β-adrenergic receptor antagonist. Other xenobiotics that can exert direct depressant effects on cardiac contractility include antihistamines, phenothiazines, antidysrhythmics, and local anesthetics. Many of these xenobiotics reduce contractility through sodium channel blockade, which, by slowing intraventricular conduction, reduces the ability of the heart to contract efficiently. Pulmonary edema may also result from the fluid overload accompanying ingestion of large quantities of sodium-containing xenobiotics (eg, sodium penicillin), the renal effects of medications such as NSAIDs, or as a late consequence of xenobiotics that cause renal failure (Chap. 27).

Xenobiotic can cause cardiomyopathy through chronic toxic effects directly on the myocardium or indirectly through effects on blood pressure or cardiac vasculature (Table 23–4). In most cases, the exact mechanism of the toxicity is not known. However, free radical generation, nitric oxide formation, acetaldehyde, myocardial ischemia, mechanical overload, nutritional deficiency, and persistent tachycardia are each implicated in the cellular toxicity of the various xenobiotics and development of cardiomyopathy.

BLOOD PRESSURE ABNORMALITIES

Blood pressure is dependent upon cardiac and vascular function. The blood pressure (BP) is directly related to the heart rate (HR), the stroke volume (SV), and the systemic vascular resistance (SVR): $BP = HR \times SV \times SVR$. The systolic component of the blood pressure measurement is a reflection of the inotropic state of the myocardium, whereas the diastolic component reflects the vascular tone. It is important to consider both components of the blood pressure. Blood pressure may be expressed also the mean arterial pressure (MAP) during a single cardiac cycle. Since at normal heart rates the duration of diastole is approximately twice that of systole, the MAP is calculated as $[(2 \times \text{diastolic}) + \text{systolic}]/3$. Xenobiotics may affect either component and compensatory mechanisms within the cardiovascular system may produce recognizable patterns of blood pressure alterations.

Many xenobiotics affect blood pressure by modulation of normal neurotransmission at the postganglionic sympathetic neurons. Through these effects they may cause, for example, vasoconstriction (α agonism) or inotropy (β_1 agonism). Because of the functional similarity of most sympathomimetics, physical examination alone seldom identifies the specific causative xenobiotic in any patient. However, often a clinical constellation of signs and symptoms can be identified that is associated with this general class. For example, patients who ingest sympathomimetic amines such as cocaine or amphetamines typically have central nervous system stimulation, hypertension, and tachycardia (Chap. 3).

Hypertension caused by xenobiotics Hypertension may be the result of an increase in either inotropy or vascular resistance or both. For example, stimulation of the α_1-adrenergic receptor causes hypertension

TABLE 23–4. Xenobiotics Commonly Associated with Cardiomyopathy

Anthracyclines (dactinomycin, daunorubicin, idarubicin, and doxorubicin),
Antimony
Cobalt
Cocaine
Ethanol
Emetine from syrup of ipecac
HMG Co-A reductase inhibitors

through vasoconstriction, and stimulation of the β_1-receptor causes hypertension through enhanced myocardial contractility (Table 23–5).

The hemodynamic results of a xenobiotic overdose depend on the specific xenobiotic ingested and the relative action on the various types of receptors (see Table 23–1). This suggests that, among β-adrenergic agonists, only those with a predominant β_1 adrenergic effect cause hypertension. Nonselective β-adrenergic agonists (those that agonize at both β_1 and β_2) produce β_1-mediated systolic hypertension (through inotropic effects) with β_2-mediated vascular vasodilation and diastolic hypotension. This may result in a widened pulse pressure, which is the numerical difference between the systolic and diastolic pressures. Thus after exposure to selective β agonist (eg, albuterol), tachycardia and enhanced inotropy may occur, resulting in a widened pulse pressure in a manner analagous to a nonselective beta agonist. The resulting blood pressure depends on the relative physiologic balance between inotropy and vasodilation.

Xenobiotics that interact only with the α_1-adrenergic receptor (such as phenylephrine) cause vasoconstriction and hypertension. Barorecptors detect the increased blood pressure and signal the parasympathetic nervous system neurons of the vagus nerve to fire and slow the heart rate. In the absence of β-adrenergic stimulation, a "reflex" bradycardia results. Norepinephrine is an α_1- adrenergic agonist with additional β-adrenergic activity. Profound hypertension is the primary hemodynamic toxic effect due to the activity of norepinephrine as both a positive inotrope (β_1) and a vasoconstrictor (α_1). Reflex bradycardia does not occur as a result of stimulation of the cardiac β-adrenergic receptors.

TABLE 23–5. Xenobiotics that Commonly Cause Hypertension

Hypertensive effects mediated by α-adrenergic receptor interaction	Hypertensive effects not mediated by α-adrenergic receptor interaction
Direct α-receptor agonists	β-Adrenergic receptor agonists[b]
Clonidine[a]	Nonselective
Epinephrine	Isoproterenol
Ergotamines	Cholinergics[a]
Methoxamine	Corticosteroids
Norepinephrine	Nicotine[a]
Phenylephrine	Thromboxane A_2
Tetrahydrozoline	Vasopressin
Indirect-acting agonists	
Amphetamines	
Cocaine	
Dexfenfluramine	
Monoamine oxidase inhibitors	
Phencyclidine	
Yohimbine	
Direct- and indirect-acting agonists	
Dopamine	
Ephedrine	
Metaraminol	
Naphazoline	
Oxymetazoline	
Phenylpropanolamine	
Pseudoephedrine	

[a] These may cause transient hypertension followed by hypotension.

[b] These can also cause hypotension.

Hypotension caused by xenobiotics Typically, hypotension in adults is arbitrarily defined as a systolic blood pressure of less than 90 mm Hg or a MAP of less than 70 mm Hg. However, this is not an adequate clinical parameter. Young children and adults with a small body habitus may have a normal systolic pressure less than 90 mm Hg (Chap. 3). Patients with hypothermia have decreased metabolic demands, and a lower blood pressure may be considered "normal" for these patients. Most importantly, patients with long-standing hypertension may have inadequate tissue perfusion even with a MAP of more than 70 mm Hg. The cerebral arterioles normally constrict or dilate to maintain a relatively constant cerebrovascular blood flow despite changes in the peripheral blood pressure. Chronically hypertensive patients lose this autoregulatory response as a consequence of atherosclerotic disease, arteriolar hypertrophy, or arteriolar smooth muscle constriction. These narrowed arterioles may require a higher peripheral blood pressure to properly perfuse the brain.

Hypotension is clinically defined as a blood pressure that is inadequate to perfuse tissues. The clinical assessment of tissue perfusion is based on the vital signs, skin color, capillary refill, mental status, urine output and concentration, and acid—base balance (eg, serum lactate concentration). However, if a xenobiotic directly affects one or more of these clinical parameters, the clinical assessment of volume and hemodynamic status may be difficult. Measurement of central venous pressure is beneficial in the early treatment of the sepsis syndrome, and most likely would be beneficial in the treatment of other causes of hypotension, including those occurring in poisoned patients. Invasive measurement of cardiac filling pressure, cardiac output, systemic vascular resistance, and arterial pressures may be necessary in critically ill patients with severe poisoning.[46]

Poor tissue perfusion may result from hypovolemia, decreased peripheral vascular resistance, myocardial depression, or a dysrhythmia that reduces the cardiac output. A single xenobiotic may exert several effects on the hemodynamic system, such as diltiazem, a calcium channel blocker that causes negative inotropy and vasodilation. Appropriate treatment of the hypotension requires an understanding of the pathophysiologic consequences of the xenobiotic and the resultant hemodynamic derangement (Table 23–6).

A common etiology of hypotension in a poisoned patient is intravascular volume depletion. Intravascular volume may decrease due to gastrointestinal, urinary, or insensible losses; or fluid may redistribute from the intravascular space into the intracellular, interstitial, pleural, or peritoneal spaces. Xenobiotics can cause significant intravascular volume depletion through all of these mechanisms.

Hypotension may also be caused by xenobiotics that affect the venous tone. These xenobiotics increase venous capacitance, decrease the central venous pressure, and result in a relative hypovolemia. The effects may be mediated via central effects on the sympathetic nervous system or direct effects on the peripheral vasculature. Sedative hypnotics and central α_2-adrenergic agonists (eg, clonidine) decrease the central sympathetic outflow and may result in hypotension. Other xenobiotics directly block peripheral α_1-adrenergic receptors or stimulate β_2-adrenergic receptors on the blood vessels to produce vascular smooth muscle relaxation, venodilation, and hypotension. A large number of xenobiotics are reported to cause hypotension. However, the hypotension often is not a direct action of the xenobiotic. Rather, the cause of hypotension is coexisting hypoxia, acidosis, anaphylaxis, volume depletion, or dysrhythmias.

Identification of the specific xenobiotic causing hypotension requires the integration of a detailed history, complete physical examination, and laboratory studies. Often the identification of the specific xenobiotic responsible for hypotension is based on other physical findings associated with the xenobiotic or recognition of a specific toxic syndrome.

TABLE 23–6. Heart Rate and ECG Abnormalities of Xenobiotics that Cause Hypotension

	Characteristic ECG Abnormalities		
Heart Rate	**Sinus Rhythm**	**Heart Block or Prolonged Intervals**	**Dysrhythmia**
Bradycardia	α_2-Adrenergic agonists Opioids Sedative-hypnotics	β-Adrenergic antagonists Calcium channel blockers Cholinergics Cardioactive steroids Magnesium (severe) Methadone Propafenone Sotalol	Cardioactive steroids Plant toxins Aconitine Andromedotoxin Veratrine Propafenone Propoxyphene Sotalol
Tachycardia	Angiotensin-converting enzyme inhibitors Anticholinergics Arterial vasodilators Bupropion Cocaine Disulfiram Diuretics Iron Yohimbine	Anticholinergics Antidysrhythmics Antihistamines Arsenic Bupropion Cocaine Cyclic antidepressants Phenothiazines Quinine/chloroquine	Anticholinergics Antidysrhythmics Antihistamines Arsenic Chloral hydrate Cocaine Cyclic antidepressants Methylxanthines Noncyclic antidepressants Phenothiazines Sympathomimetics

ASSESSMENT OF VOLUME STATUS IN THE POISONED PATIENT

Assessment of volume status may be particularly difficult in the poisoned patient because of functional alterations in the patient's autonomic nervous system and the pharmacologic effects of the xenobiotic. For example, the usual signs of salt and water depletion, such as dry mucous membranes, dry skin, low blood pressure, tachycardia, narrowed pulse pressure, clouded sensorium, and decreased urine output, can be mimicked by a number of xenobiotics, including tricyclic antidepressants. Additionally, hypovolemic patients may present with diaphoresis, flushed skin, hypertension, bradycardia, or increased urine output after the exposure to a cholinergic xenobiotic such as an organic phosphorus compound. In most cases, clinical assessment of central venous pressures and neck vein distension or the hemodynamic response to a fluid bolus can assist in the determination of the patient's volume status. A central venous or pulmonary artery pressure catheter may be required in some critically ill patients.

Additional information about the adequacy of the patient's volume status may be obtained by orthostatic vital sign testing (Table 23–7).[21] Normally, the cardiovascular system responds to sitting or standing with vasoconstriction and a slight increase in heart rate. Even with a 30% or greater volume loss, the supine blood pressure may remain normal in young, previously healthy patients. However, patients with hypovolemia are unable to maintain adequate intravascular pressure when upright and have either an exaggerated reflex increase in heart rate or a drop in blood pressure (ie, orthostasis).

A variety of xenobiotics can produce orthostatic blood pressure changes (Table 23–8).[21,34] Volume depletion is the most common cause of xenobiotic-induced orthostatic vital sign changes. However, xenobiotics may produce orthostatic vital sign changes even with a normal volume status. For instance, α_1-adrenergic antagonists or direct acting vasodilators may prevent an adequate vasoconstrictor response or β adrenergic antagonists may block the normal slight heart rate increase, and result in positive orthostatic vital sign testing. In these cases, cardiac output and blood pressure decrease when the patient is upright.

TABLE 23–7. Orthostatic Vital Signs ("Tilt" Testing)

1. After the patient is supine for 2 minutes, determine the blood pressure and pulse rate.
2. Stand the patient for at least 1 minute and determine the blood pressure and pulse rate again, and observe for any orthostatic symptoms such as dizziness or light-headedness. If it is impossible for the patient to stand, have the patient sit up with feet dangling for at least 2 minutes before determining vital signs.

The test is positive if *any one* of the following is true:
- Systolic blood pressure decreases > 20 mm Hg
- Diastolic blood pressure decreases > 10 mm Hg
- Pulse increases > 10 beats/min
- Development of clinical symptoms of hypovolemia (dizziness, syncope, light-headedness)

Significance of a positive test: 10-15 mL|Kg volume loss.

TABLE 23–8. Xenobiotics that Cause Orthostatic Hypotension

Antianginals
β-Adrenergic antagonists
Calcium channel blockers
Nitrates
Antidepressants
Cyclic antidepressant
MAO inhibitors
Antihypertensives
Angiotensin-converting enzyme inhibitors
Angiotensin receptor antagonists
Central α_2-adrenergic agonists
Clonidine
Guanabenz
Guanfacine
Methyldopa
Antiparkinsons
Bromocriptine
L-Dopa
Pergolide mesylate
Antipsychotics
Butyrophenones
Phenothiazines
CNS depressants
Ethanol
Opioids
Sedative-hypnotics
Diuretics
Loop diuretics
Thiazides
Ganglionic blockers
Trimethaphan
Miscellaneous
Reserpine
Peripheral α-adrenergic antagonists
Phenoxybenzamine
Prazosin
Vasodilators
Hydralazine

TABLE 23–9. Clues that an Unanticipated Xenobiotic Might be the Cause of Hemodynamic Compromise or Dysrhythmia

History
New-onset, concomitant seizure
Gastrointestinal disturbances (colicky pain, nausea, vomiting, diarrhea)
Prior ingestion of medications (consider possibility that the container is mislabeled or misidentified)
Depression (even if patient denies ingestion)
Suspected myocardial ischemia in patient younger than 35 years old
Past medical history
Treatment with *any* cardiac medications (especially antidysrhythmics or digoxin)
History of psychiatric illness, asthma, or hypertension
History of drug use or abuse
Physical examination and vital signs
Heart rate
Sinus tachycardia with rate >130 beat/min
Sinus tachycardia without apparent identified cause
Sinus bradycardia
Respiratory rate
Any unexplained depression or elevation in rate
Temperature
Elevation especially if > 106°F (> 41.1°C)
Hypothermia
Dissociation between typically paired changes, for example:
Hypotension and bradycardia (tachycardia expected)
Fever and dry skin (diaphoresis expected)
Hypertension and tachycardia (reflex bradycardia anticipated)
Depressed mental status and tachypnea (decreased respirations common)
Relatively rapid changes in vital signs
Initial hypertension becomes hypotension
Increasing sinus tachycardia or hypertension
General
Alteration in consciousness, such as depressed mental status, confusion, or agitation
Findings usually not associated with cardiovascular diseases
Ataxia, bullae, dry mucous membranes, lacrimation, miosis or mydriasis, nystagmus, unusual odor, flushed skin, salivation, tinnitus, tremor, visual disturbances
Findings consistent with a toxic syndrome
Especially findings consistent with anticholinergics, sympathomimetics, or sedative hypnotics
Laboratory tests
Any unexpected or unexplained laboratory result, especially:
Metabolic acidosis
Respiratory alkalosis
Hypokalemia or hyperkalemia

SUMMARY

Xenobiotics can interact with the heart or blood vessels to produce hypotension or hypertension, congestive heart failure, dysrhythmias (including bradycardias and tachycardias), or cardiac conduction delays. These toxic effects often occur through interactions with specific receptors or with the ion channels in the cell membrane. Disruption of the normal cellular regulation of metabolic processes or of the cellular ionic status leads to the cardiovascular and hemodynamic compromise.

The occurrence of these abnormalities, individually or in combination, might suggest a particular xenobiotic or class of xenobiotics as the etiologic (toxic syndrome) and might dictate initial treatment. Often, however, significant abnormalities in vital signs must be corrected before the xenobiotic is identified. By understanding both the pharmacology of the xenobiotic and the physiology of the heart and vasculature, appropriately tailored treatment can be delivered.

Definitive care of the poisoned patient with hemodynamic compromise or a dysrhythmia begins with recognition that a xenobiotic may be present. Infectious, cardiovascular disease, and other metabolic disorders must always be considered; however, the toxic effects of xenobiotics must be included in the differential diagnosis. A variety of clinical clues, when present, should heighten the clinician's suspicion that a xenobiotic effect may be responsible for the hemodynamic or dysrhythmic problem (Table 23–9).

REFERENCES

1. Ahlquist RP. A study of the adrenotropic receptors. *Am J Physiol.* 1948;153:586-600.
2. Bailey B. Glucagon in beta-blocker and calcium channel blocker overdoses: a systematic review. *J Toxicol Clin Toxicol.* 2003;41:595-602.
3. Berridge MJ. Inositol trisphosphate and calcium signalling. *Nature.* 1993;361:315-325.
4. Berridge MJ. Smooth muscle cell calcium activation mechanisms. *J Physiol.* 2008; 586(Pt 21):5047-5061.
5. Blackshear PJ, Nairn AC, Kuo JF. Protein kinases 1988: a current perspective. *FASEB J.* 1988;2:2957-2969.
6. Brodde OE. The functional importance of beta 1 and beta 2 adrenoceptors in the human heart. *Am J Cardiol.* 1988;62:24C-29C.
7. Casey PJ, Gilman AG. G protein involvement in receptor-effector coupling. *J Biol Chem.* 1988;263:2577-2580.
8. Celi FS. Brown adipose tissue—when it pays to be inefficient. *N Engl J Med.* 2009;360:1553-1556.
9. Chakraborti S, Das S, Kar P, et al. Calcium signaling phenomena in heart diseases: a perspective. *Mol Cell Biochem.* 2007;298:1-40.
10. Chen-Izu Y, Xiao RP, Izu LT, et al. G(i)-dependent localization of beta(2)-adrenergic receptor signaling to L-type Ca(2+) channels. *Biophys J.* 2000;79:2547-2556.
11. Clapham DE, Neer EJ. G protein beta gamma subunits. *Annu Rev Pharmacol Toxicol.* 1997;37:167-203.
12. Dibb KM, Graham HK, Venetucci LA, Eisner DA, Trafford AW. Analysis of cellular calcium fluxes in cardiac muscle to understand calcium homeostasis in the heart. *Cell Calcium.* 2007;42:503-512.
13. Eisner DA, Choi HS, Díaz ME, O'Neill SC, Trafford AW. Integrative analysis of calcium cycling in cardiac muscle. *Circ Res.* 2000;87:1087-1094.
14. Enocksson S, Shimizu M, Lonnqvist F, et al. Demonstration of an in vivo functional beta 3-adrenoceptor in man. *J Clin Invest.* 1995;95:2239-2245.
15. Fant JS, James LP, Fiser RT, Kearns G. The use of glucagon in nifedipine poisoning complicated by clonidine ingestion. *Pediatr Emerg Care.* 1997;13:417-419.
16. Frank K, Kranias EG. Phospholamban and cardiac contractility. *Ann Med.* 2000;32:572-578.
17. Frank KF, Bolck B, Erdmann E, Schwinger RH. Sarcoplasmic reticulum Ca2+-ATPase modulates cardiac contraction and relaxation. *Cardiovasc Res.* 2003;57:20-27.
18. Gauthier C, Tavernier G, Charpentier F, Langin D, Le Marec H. Functional beta3-adrenoceptor in the human heart. *J Clin Invest.* 1996;98:556-562.
19. Gilman AG. The Albert Lasker Medical Awards. G proteins and regulation of adenylyl cyclase. *JAMA.* 1989;262:1819-1825.
20. Glick G, Parmley WW, Wechsler AS, Sonnenblick EH. Glucagon. Its enhancement of cardiac performance in the cat and dog and persistence of its inotropic action despite beta-receptor blockade with propranolol. *Circ Res.* 1968;22:789-799.
21. Gorgas DL. Vital sign measurement. In: Roberts JR, Hedges JR, eds. *Clinical Procedures in Emergency Medicine.* 4th ed. Philadelphia: WB Saunders; 2004.
22. Graham RM, Perez DM, Hwa J, Piascik MT. Alpha 1-adrenergic receptor subtypes. Molecular structure, function, and signaling. *Circ Res.* 1996;78:737-749.
23. Hartzell HC, Hirayama Y, Petit-Jacques J. Effects of protein phosphatase and kinase inhibitors on the cardiac L-type Ca current suggest two sites are phosphorylated by protein kinase A and another protein kinase. *J Gen Physiol.* 1995;106:393-414.
24. Hirayama Y, Hartzell HC. Effects of protein phosphatase and kinase inhibitors on Ca2+ and Cl- currents in guinea pig ventricular myocytes. *Mol Pharmacol.* 1997;52:725-734.
25. Jaken S. Protein kinase C isozymes and substrates. *Curr Opin Cell Biol.* 1996;8:168-173.
26. Katz AM. A growth of ideas: role of calcium as activator of cardiac contraction. *Cardiovasc Res.* 2001;52:8-13.
27. Katz AM, Lorell BH. Regulation of cardiac contraction and relaxation. *Circulation.* 2000;102:IV69-74.
28. Kuschel M, Zhou YY, Cheng H, Zhang SJ, Chen Y, Lakatta EG, Xiao RP. G(i) protein-mediated functional compartmentalization of cardiac beta(2)-adrenergic signaling. *J Biol Chem.* 1999;274:22048-22052.
29. Lee J. Glucagon use in symptomatic beta blocker overdose. *Emerg Med J.* 2004;21:755.
30. Lennon NJ, Ohlendieck K. Impaired Ca2+-sequestration in dilated cardiomyopathy. *Int J Mol Med.* 2001;7:131-141.
31. Levitzki A, Marbach I, Bar-Sinai A. The signal transduction between beta-receptors and adenylyl cyclase. *Life Sci.* 1993;52:2093-2100.
32. Limbird LE. Receptors linked to inhibition of adenylate cyclase: additional signaling mechanisms. *FASEB J.* 1988;2:2686-2695.
33. Love JN, Leasure JA, Mundt DJ, Janz TG. A comparison of amrinone and glucagon therapy for cardiovascular depression associated with propranolol toxicity in a canine model. *J Toxicol Clin Toxicol.* 1992;30:399-412.
34. Mader SL. Orthostatic hypotension. *Med Clin North Am.* 1989;73:1337-1349.
35. Marston S, El-Mezgueldi M. Role of tropomyosin in the regulation of contraction in smooth muscle. *Adv Exp Med Biol.* 2008;644:110-123.
36. Mery PF, Brechler V, Pavoine C, Pecker F, Fischmeister R. Glucagon stimulates the cardiac Ca^{2+} current by activation of adenylyl cyclase and inhibition of phosphodiesterase. *Nature.* 1990;345:158-161.
37. Neer EJ. Heterotrimeric G proteins: organizers of transmembrane signals. *Cell.* 1995;80:249-257.
38. Neer EJ, Clapham DE. Roles of G protein subunits in transmembrane signalling. *Nature.* 1988;333:129-134.
39. Oloizia B, Paul RJ. Ca^{2+} clearance and contractility in vascular smooth muscle: evidence from gene-altered murine models. *J Mol Cell Cardiol.* 2008;45:347-362.
40. Paakkari P, Paakkari I, Feuerstein G, Siren AL. Evidence for differential opioid mu 1- and mu 2-receptor-mediated regulation of heart rate in the conscious rat. *Neuropharmacology.* 1992;31:777-782.
41. Petrovic MM, Vales K, Putnikovic B, et al. Ryanodine receptors, voltage-gated calcium channels and their relationship with protein kinase A in the myocardium. *Physiol Res.* 2008;57:141-149.
42. Rasmussen H. The calcium messenger system (1). *N Engl J Med.* 1986;314:1094-1101.
43. Rasmussen H. The calcium messenger system (2). *N Engl J Med.* 1986;314:1164-1170.
44. Rasmussen H, Barrett P, Smallwood J, Bollag W, Isales C. Calcium ion as intracellular messenger and cellular toxin. *Environ Health Perspect.* 1990;84:17-25.
45. Reuter H. Calcium channel modulation by beta-adrenergic neurotransmitters in the heart. *Experientia.* 1987;43:1173-1175.
46. Rivers EP, Coba V, Whitmill M. Early goal-directed therapy in severe sepsis and septic shock: a contemporary review of the literature. *Curr Opin Anaesthesiol.* 2008;21:128-140.

47. Roden DM, Balser JR, George AL Jr, Anderson ME. Cardiac ion channels. *Annu Rev Physiol.* 2002;64:431-475.
48. Ruegg JC. Cardiac contractility: how calcium activates the myofilaments. *Naturwissenschaften.* 1998;85:575-582.
49. Ruegg JC. Pharmacological calcium sensitivity modulation of cardiac myofilaments. *Adv Exp Med Biol.* 2003;538:403-410.
50. Saunders C, Limbird LE. Localization and trafficking of alpha2-adrenergic receptor subtypes in cells and tissues. *Pharmacol Ther.* 1999;84:193-205.
51. Sperelakis N, Xiong Z, Haddad G, Masuda H. Regulation of slow calcium channels of myocardial cells and vascular smooth muscle cells by cyclic nucleotides and phosphorylation. *Mol Cell Biochem.* 1994;140:103-117.
52. Steinberg SF. The cellular actions of beta-adrenergic receptor agonists: looking beyond cAMP. *Circ Res.* 2000;87:1079-1082.
53. Steinberg SF. The molecular basis for distinct beta-adrenergic receptor subtype actions in cardiomyocytes. *Circ Res.* 1999;85:1101-1111.
54. Stinson J, Walsh M, Feely J. Ventricular asystole and overdose with atenolol. *BMJ.* 1992;305:693.
55. Sulakhe PV, Vo XT. Regulation of phospholamban and troponin-I phosphorylation in the intact rat cardiomyocytes by adrenergic and cholinergic stimuli: roles of cyclic nucleotides, calcium, protein kinases and phosphatases and depolarization. *Mol Cell Biochem.* 1995;149-150:103-126.
56. Sunahara RK, Beuve A, Tesmer JJ, Sprang SR, Garbers DL, Gilman AG. Exchange of substrate and inhibitor specificities between adenylyl and guanylyl cyclases. *J Biol Chem.* 1998;273:16332-16338.
57. Sunahara RK, Dessauer CW, Gilman AG. Complexity and diversity of mammalian adenylyl cyclases. *Annu Rev Pharmacol Toxicol.* 1996;36:461-480.
58. Talosi L, Kranias EG. Effect of alpha-adrenergic stimulation on activation of protein kinase C and phosphorylation of proteins in intact rabbit hearts. *Circ Res.* 1992;70:670-678.
59. Tang WJ, Gilman AG. Type-specific regulation of adenylyl cyclase by G protein beta gamma subunits. *Science.* 1991;254:1500-1503.
60. Taussig R, Tang WJ, Hepler JR, Gilman AG. Distinct patterns of bidirectional regulation of mammalian adenylyl cyclases. *J Biol Chem.* 1994;269:6093-6100.
61. Travill CM, Pugh S, Noble MI. The inotropic and hemodynamic effects of intravenous milrinone when reflex adrenergic stimulation is suppressed by beta-adrenergic blockade. *Clin Ther.* 1994;16:783-792.
62. Walter FG, Frye G, Mullen JT, et al. Amelioration of nifedipine poisoning associated with glucagon therapy. *Ann Emerg Med.* 1993;22:1234-1237.
63. Whitehurst VE, Vick JA, Alleva FR, et al. Reversal of propranolol blockade of adrenergic receptors and related toxicity with drugs that increase cyclic AMP. *Proc Soc Exp Biol Med.* 1999;221:382-385.
64. Xiao RP. Cell logic for dual coupling of a single class of receptors to G(s) and G(i) proteins. *Circ Res.* 2000;87:635-637.
65. Xiao RP, Cheng H, Zhou YY, Kuschel M, Lakatta EG. Recent advances in cardiac beta(2)-adrenergic signal transduction. *Circ Res.* 1999;85:1092-1100.
66. Yagami T. Differential coupling of glucagon and beta-adrenergic receptors with the small and large forms of the stimulatory G protein. *Mol Pharmacol.* 1995;48:849-854.
67. Zaugg M, Schaub MC. Cellular mechanisms in sympatho-modulation of the heart. *Br J Anaesth.* 2004;93:34-52.

CHAPTER 24
HEMATOLOGIC PRINCIPLES

Marco L.A. Sivilotti

Blood is rightfully considered the vital fluid, as every organ system depends on the normal function of blood. Blood delivers oxygen and other essential substances throughout the body, removes waste products of metabolism, transports hormones from their origin to site of action, signals and defends against threatened infection, promotes healing via the inflammatory response and maintains the vascular integrity of the circulatory system. It also contains the central compartment of classical pharmacokinetics, and thereby comes into direct contact with virtually every systemic toxin that acts on the organism.[162] The ease and frequency with which blood is assayed, its central role in functions vital to the organism, and the ability to analyze its characteristics, at first by light microscopy and more recently with molecular techniques, have enabled a detailed understanding of blood that has advanced the frontier of molecular medicine.

In addition to transporting xenobiotics throughout the body, blood and the blood-forming organs can at times be directly affected by these same xenobiotics. For example, decreased blood cell production, increased blood cell destruction, alteration of hemoglobin, and impairment of coagulation can all result from exposure to many xenobiotics. The response in many cases depends on the nature and quantity of the xenobiotic, and the capacity of the system to respond to the insult. In other cases, no clear and predictable dose–response relationship can be determined, especially when the interaction involves the immune system. These latter reactions are often termed idiosyncratic, reflecting an incomplete understanding of their causative mechanism. In general, such reactions can often be reclassified when advancing knowledge identifies the characteristics which render the individual vulnerable.

HEMATOPOIESIS

Hematopoiesis is the development of the cellular elements of blood. The majority of the cells of the blood system may be classified as either lymphoid (B, T, and natural-killer lymphocytes) or myeloid (erythrocytes, megakaryocytes, granulocytes, and macrophages). All of these cells are descended from a small common pool of totipotent cells called hematopoietic stem cells.[182] Indeed, the study of this process and its regulation has provided fundamental insight into embryogenesis, stem cell pluripotency, and complex cell-to-cell signaling and interaction.

BONE MARROW

Marrow spaces within bone begin to form in humans at about the 5th fetal month and become the sole site of granulocyte and megakaryocyte proliferation. Erythropoiesis moves from the liver to the marrow by the end of the last trimester. At birth, all marrow contributes to blood cell formation and is red, containing very few fat cells. By adulthood, the same volume of hematopoietic marrow is normally restricted to the sternum, ribs, pelvis, upper sacrum, proximal femora and humeri, skull, vertebrae, clavicles and scapulae. So-called extramedullary hematopoiesis in the liver and spleen may reemerge as a compensatory mechanism under severe stimulation.

Progenitor cells must interact with a supportive microenvironment to sustain hematopoiesis. The hematopoietic stroma consists of macrophages, fibroblasts, adipocytes, and endothelial cells. The extracellular matrix is produced by the stromal cells and is composed of various fibrous proteins, glycoproteins, and proteoglycans, such as collagen, fibronectin, laminin, hemonectin, and thrombospondin. Hematopoietic progenitor cells have receptors to particular matrix molecules. The extracellular matrix provides a structural network to which the progenitors are anchored. As the cells approach maturity, they lose their surface receptors, allowing them to leave the hematopoietic space and enter the venous sinuses. Blood cell release depends upon the development of a pressure gradient that drives mature cells through channels in endothelial cell cytoplasm.[191] Pressure within the marrow is increased by erythropoietin and by granulocyte colony-stimulating factor (G-CSF).[83,84]

STEM CELLS

A stem cell is capable of self-renewal, as well as differentiating into a specific cell type. The pluripotent hematopoietic stem cells can therefore continuously replicate while awaiting the appropriate signal to differentiate into either a myeloid stem cell (for myelo-, erythro-, mono-, or megakaryopoiesis) or a lymphoid stem cell (for lymphopoiesis of T, B, null, and natural-killer cells) (Fig. 24–1). The stem cell pool represents approximately 1 in 100,000 of the nucleated cells of the bone marrow, and the majority of these stem cells are usually quiescent. Nevertheless, these relatively few cells are directly responsible for the estimated 3 billion red cells, 2.5 billion platelets, and 1.5 billion granulocytes per kilogram of body weight produced each day. In response to hemolysis or infection, substantially larger numbers of blood cells can be produced.[130]

Hematopoietic stem cells are found in umbilical cord blood, bone marrow, and peripheral blood.[108] With subsequent division and maturation, these cells progressively display the antigenic, biochemical, and morphologic features characteristic of mature cells of the appropriate lineages, and lose their capacity for self-renewal. Multiple steps are involved in the commitment of less-differentiated cells to more mature cell lines. The final steps in the maturation of erythrocytes alone, for example, involve extensive remodeling, the restructuring of cellular membranes, the accumulation of hemoglobin, and the loss of nuclei and organelles. In the case of granulocytes, granules containing proteolytic enzymes are formed in cell cytoplasm, and the nucleus condenses to form the multilobulated nucleus of the mature cell. Megakaryocyte cytoplasm demarcates into units that are split off eventually as platelets.

Multipotent mesenchymal stem cells capable of differentiating into other tissue lines including hepatic, renal, muscle and perhaps nerves are also found in the bone marrow.[64] Furthermore, tissue-specific stem cells capable of self-renewal are believed to reside in numerous other organs and to play a fundamental role in repair and regeneration.[35] A variety of strategies have likely evolved to protect the stem cell from injury due to xenobiotics and radiation, and a better understanding of these effects promises to improve our understanding of toxicity and treatment. The hematopoietic stem cell has provided fundamental insights into regenerative biology, and remains a focus of intense research given the profound implications for organ homeostasis, tissue repair and gene therapy.[99,105]

CYTOKINES

Cytokines are soluble mediators secreted by cells for cell-to-cell communication. Initially termed growth factors, it is now recognized that not all cytokines are growth factors. Cytokines promote or inhibit the differentiation, proliferation, and trafficking of blood cells and their precursors. Importantly, they can also inhibit apoptosis, and their

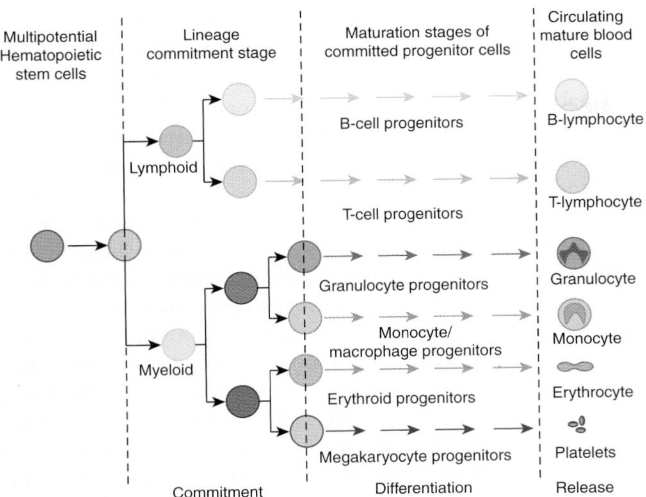

FIGURE 24–1. Principles of hematopoiesis. Commitment refers to the apparent inability of progenitor cells to generate hematopoietic stem cells. Following differentiation, the various mature blood cells are released into the circulation.

absence therefore results in the self-destruction of unwanted cells. They include growth factors or colony-stimulating factors (CSFs), interleukins, monokines, interferons, and chemokines. At baseline, these act in concert to maintain normal blood counts. In response to antigens or other stimuli, cytokines are released to combat perceived infection. Recombinant cytokines are being developed for therapeutic use in immunocompromised patients, transplant recipients, sepsis, and cancer. They have also been used in clinical toxicology for the treatment of colchicine and podophyllum toxicity.[45,69]

The growth factors are glycoproteins necessary for the differentiation and maturation of individual or multiple cell lines.[83,93,94,123] They fall into two families based on their target receptors. The ligands of the cytokine receptor family include growth hormone, interleukin-2 (IL-2), macrophage colony-stimulating factor-1 (CSF-1), granulocyte-macrophage colony-stimulating factor (GM-CSF), γ-interferon, and granulocyte colony-stimulating factor (G-CSF), to name a few. The second group, the tyrosine kinase family, includes Kit ligand and insulinlike growth factor-I receptor (IGF-1R), a member of the insulin family. The complete development of all of the mature blood cells from stem cells or multilineage progenitors requires the action of growth factors, either alone or in combination, for successful differentiation and final maturation.

CELL SURFACE ANTIGENS

Using monoclonal antibody technology, cell surface antigens are used to characterize cell types. The cluster designation (CD) nomenclature was introduced by immunologists to ensure a common language when confronted with multiple antibodies to the same leukocyte cell-surface molecule, and hundreds of such unique molecules have been classified.[198] For example, the CD34 antigen is a 115-kilodalton (kDa) highly glycosylated transmembrane protein that is selectively expressed by primitive multipotent hematopoietic stem cells shortly after activation, but is absent from mature T and B lymphocytes.[108] Advances in genomics and proteomics now complement the immunologic designation, but the ability to subtype blood cells phenotypically has transformed the approach to the leukemias, autoimmune disease, transplantation medicine and thromboembolic disease.

APLASTIC ANEMIA

Aplastic anemia is characterized by pancytopenia on peripheral smear, a hypocellular marrow, and delayed plasma iron clearance. Severe aplastic anemia denotes a granulocyte count of less than 500 cells/mm^3, a platelet count of less than 20,000/mm^3, and a reticulocyte count of less than 1% after correction for anemia. Following acute insult and depletion of extracirculatory reserves, cell line counts fall at a rate inversely proportional to their life span: granulocytes (half-life 6–12 hours in the circulation) disappear within days, platelets (life span of 7–10 days) decline by half in about one week, while erythrocytes (normal life span 120 days) decline over weeks in the absence of bleeding or hemolysis. Approximately 1000 new cases of aplastic anemia are diagnosed yearly in the United States. The incidence is two to three times higher in Asia, perhaps due to a combination of genetic, environmental and infectious factors.[195] Aplastic anemia may be inborn (as in Fanconi anemia) or acquired. A variety of xenobiotics have been associated with acquired aplastic anemia, such as benzene, environmental pesticides and chloramphenicol (Table 24–1).[32,196] However, much of this older literature is suspect given uncertain case ascertainment and other biases. More recent epidemiologic studies have shown that specific causes are identified in relatively few cases.[82]

Generally speaking, the majority of cases of so-called idiosyncratic aplastic anemia are caused by autoimmune attack on CD34+

TABLE 24–1. Xenobiotics Associated with Aplastic Anemia

Analgesics	Antirheumatics
Acetaminophen	Gold salts
Acetylsalicylic acid	Methotrexate
Diclofenac	D-Penicillamine
Dipyrone	Antithyroids
Indomethacin	Propylthiouracil
Phenylbutazone	Antineoplastics[a]
Antibiotics	Adriamycin[a]
Azidothymidine	Antimetabolites
Chloramphenicol	Colchicine
Mefloquine	Daunorubicin[a]
Penicillin	Mustards
Anticonvulsants	Vinblastine
Carbamazepine	Vincristine
Felbamate	Diuretics
Antidysrhythmics	Acetazolamide
Tocainide	Metolazone
Antihistamines	Occupational
Cimetidine	Arsenic[a]
Antiplatelets	Benzene[a]
Ticlopidine	Cadmium
Antipsychotics	Copper
Chlorpromazine	Pesticides
Clozapine	Pesticides
	Radiation[a]

[a]Denotes agents that predictably result in bone marrow aplasia following a sufficiently large exposure.

hematopoietic stem cells. Following an exposure to an inciting antigen, cytotoxic T cells secrete interferon-γ and tumor necrosis factor α which destroy progenitor cells, causing loss of circulating mature leukocytes, erythrocytes and platelets.[196] As with other autoimmune diseases, certain histocompatibility antigen patterns are associated with the condition, namely the human leukocyte antigen (HLA) DR2, indicating a genetic predisposition. Clozapine-induced agranulocytosis is associated with the HLA B38, DR4, and DQ3 haplotypes.[132] Immunosuppressive therapy or allogenic stem cell transplantation allow recovery of hematopoiesis, and survival is now expected.[195]

It is important to distinguish immunologic xenobiotic-induced aplastic anemia from the direct myelotoxic effects of radiation and chemotherapy. Following exposure to ionizing radiation, a pancytopenia ensues due to injury to both stem and progenitor cells. Nevertheless, atom bomb survivors rarely develop aplastic anemia.[79] Vacuolated pronormoblasts can be found in the bone marrow when aplasia is due to a myelotoxic drug, and treatment consists of stopping the offending agent. Other nonimmunologic mechanisms of aplasia have also been identified in specific cases. For example, the severe pancytopenia seen following 5-fluorouracil therapy is caused by a deficiency of dihydropyrimidine dehydrogenase present in 3% to 5% of whites.[187]

THE ERYTHRON

The erythron can be considered to be a single yet dispersed tissue, defined as the entire mass of erythroid cells from the first committed progenitor cell to the mature circulating erythrocyte. This functional definition emphasizes the integrated regulation of the erythron, both in health and disease. Homeostasis of the erythron is primarily maintained by the equilibrium between stimulation via the hormone erythropoietin, and apoptosis controlled by two receptors, Fas and FasL, expressed on the membranes of erythroid precursors. At the other extreme, erythrocytes are culled from the circulation at the end of their life span, primarily by the action of the spleen. Senescent erythrocytes less able to negotiate the narrow red pulp passages are phagocytosed by macrophages, thereby minimizing both entrapment in the microvasculature of other organs, and spillage of intracellular contents into the intravascular circulation.

The primary function of the erythron is to transport molecular oxygen throughout the organism. To accomplish this, adequate number of circulating erythrocytes must be maintained. These erythrocytes must be able to preserve their structure and flexibility to circuit repeatedly through the microcirculation and to resist oxidant stress accumulated during their life span.[150] The erythrocyte also plays a key role in modulating vascular tone. Interactions between oxyhemoglobin and nitric oxide help match vasomotor tone to local tissue oxygen demands.[46,62,68,119,160]

ERYTHROPOIETIN

Erythropoietin (EPO) is a glycoprotein hormone of molecular weight 34,000 Da that is produced in the epithelial cells lining the peritubular capillaries in the normal kidney. Anemia and hypoxemia stimulate its synthesis.[2,3] EPO receptors are found in human erythroid cells, megakaryocytes, and fetal liver. EPO promotes erythroid differentiation, the mobilization of marrow progenitor cells, and the premature release of marrow reticulocytes.[2] The cell most sensitive to EPO is a cell between the erythroid colony-forming unit (CFU-E) and the proerythroblast.[3] The absence of EPO results in DNA cleavage and erythroid cell death.

THE MATURE ERYTHROCYTE

The mature erythrocyte (red blood cell) is a highly specialized cell, designed primarily for oxygen transport. Accordingly, it is densely packed with hemoglobin, which constitutes approximately 90% of the dry weight of the erythrocyte. During maturation, the erythrocyte loses its nucleus, mitochondria and other organelles, rendering it incapable of synthesizing new protein, replicating, or using the oxygen being transported for oxidative phosphorylation. Its metabolic repertoire is also severely limited, and largely restricted to a few pathways described below under Metabolism. In general, the enzymatic pathways are those required for optimizing oxygen and carbon dioxide exchange, transiting the microcirculation while maintaining cellular integrity and flexibility, and resisting oxidant stress on the iron and protein of the cell. The characteristic biconcave discocyte shape is dynamically maintained, increasing membrane surface to cell volume.[117] This shape both decreases intracellular diffusion distances to the extracellular membrane[104] and allows plastic deformation when squeezing through the microcirculation.[36,161] The shape is the net sum of elastic and electrostatic forces within the membrane, surface tension, and osmotic and hydrostatic pressures. The cell membrane contains globular proteins floating within the phospholipid bilayer. The major blood group antigens are carried on membrane ceramide glycolipids and proteins, particularly glycophorin A and the Rh proteins.[40] Membrane proteins generally serve to maintain the structure of the cell, to transport ions and other substances across the membrane, or to catalyze a limited number of specific chemical reactions for the cell.

Structural proteins The cell membrane is coupled to, and interacts dynamically with the cytoskeleton, allowing changes in cell shape such as tank treading or rotation of the membrane relative to the cytoplasm. This cytoskeleton consists of a hexagonal lattice of proteins, especially spectrin, actin, and protein 4.1, which interact with ankyrin and band 3 in the membrane to provide a strong but flexible structure to the membrane.[21,101,159] Other essential structural proteins include tropomyosin, tropomodulin, and adducin. Absence or abnormalities of these proteins can result in abnormal erythrocyte shapes such as spherocytes and elliptocytes.

Transport proteins Many specialized transport proteins are embedded in the erythrocyte membrane. These include anion and cation transporters, glucose and urea transporters, and water channels.[177] The erythrocyte membrane is relatively impermeable to ion flux. Band 3 anion-exchange protein plays an important role in the chloride-bicarbonate exchanges that occur as the erythrocyte moves between the lung and tissues. Glucose, the sole source of energy of the erythrocyte, crosses the membrane by facilitated diffusion mediated by a transmembrane glucose transporter. Sodium-potassium adenosine triphosphatase (Na^+,K^+-ATPase) maintains the primary cation gradient by pumping sodium out of the erythrocyte in exchange for potassium.

Membrane-associated enzymes At least 50 membrane-bound or membrane-associated enzymes are known to exist in the human erythrocyte. Acetylcholinesterase is an externally oriented enzyme whose role in the function of the erythrocyte remains obscure.[178] Its function is inhibited by certain xenobiotics, most notably the organic phosphorus insecticides, and it can be conveniently assayed as a marker for such exposures (Chap. 113).

Metabolism Lacking mitochondria and the ability to generate adenosine triphosphate (ATP) using molecular oxygen, the mature erythrocyte has a severely limited repertoire of intermediary metabolism compared to most mammalian cells. Its metabolic capacity is also limited once its nucleus, ribosomes, and translational apparatus are lost. Unable to synthesize new enzymes, the capacity declines over the lifetime of the cell because of declining enzyme function with time. Fortunately, the metabolic demands of the erythrocyte are usually modest, but under conditions of stress the capacity can be overwhelmed, especially among senescent cells. The greatest expenditure of energy under physiologic conditions is for the maintenance of transmembrane gradients and for the contraction of cytoskeletal elements. However, oxidant stress can put severe strain on the metabolic reserves of the erythrocyte, and lead ultimately to the premature destruction of the cell, a process termed hemolysis.

Figure 24–2 illustrates the main metabolic pathways and their purpose. The Embden-Meyerhof glycolysis is the only source of ATP for the erythrocyte, and consumes approximately 90% of the glucose imported by the cell. The reduced nicotinamide adenine dinucleotide (NADH) generated during glycolysis, which would ordinarily be used for oxidative phosphorylation in cells containing mitochondria, is directed toward the reduction of either methemoglobin to hemoglobin by cytochrome b5 reductase, or pyruvate to lactate. Both pyruvate and lactate are exported from the cell. During glycolysis, metabolism can be diverted into the Rapoport-Luebering shunt, generating 2,3-bisphosphoglycerate (2,3-BPG, formerly known as 2,3-diphosphoglycerate or 2,3-DPG) in lieu of ATP. 2,3-BPG binds to deoxyhemoglobin to modulate oxygen affinity and allow unloading of oxygen at the capillaries. In response to anemia, altitude, or changes in cellular pH, the activity of the shunt increases, thereby favoring synthesis of 2,3-BPG and increasing oxygen delivery considerably.[42,113] Reduced levels of 2,3-BPG in stored blood are believed to result in impaired oxygen delivery for approximately 12 hours following massive transfusion.[183]

As an alternative to glycolysis, glucose can be directed toward the hexose monophosphate shunt during times of oxidant stress. This pathway results in the generation of reduced nicotinamide adenine dinucleotide phosphate (NADPH), which the erythrocyte uses to maintain reduced glutathione which, in turn, inactivates oxidants and protects the sulfhydryl groups of hemoglobin and other proteins. The initial, rate-limiting step of this pathway is controlled by glucose-6-phosphate dehydrogenase (G6PD). Accordingly, cells deficient in this enzyme are less able to maintain glutathione in a reduced state, and

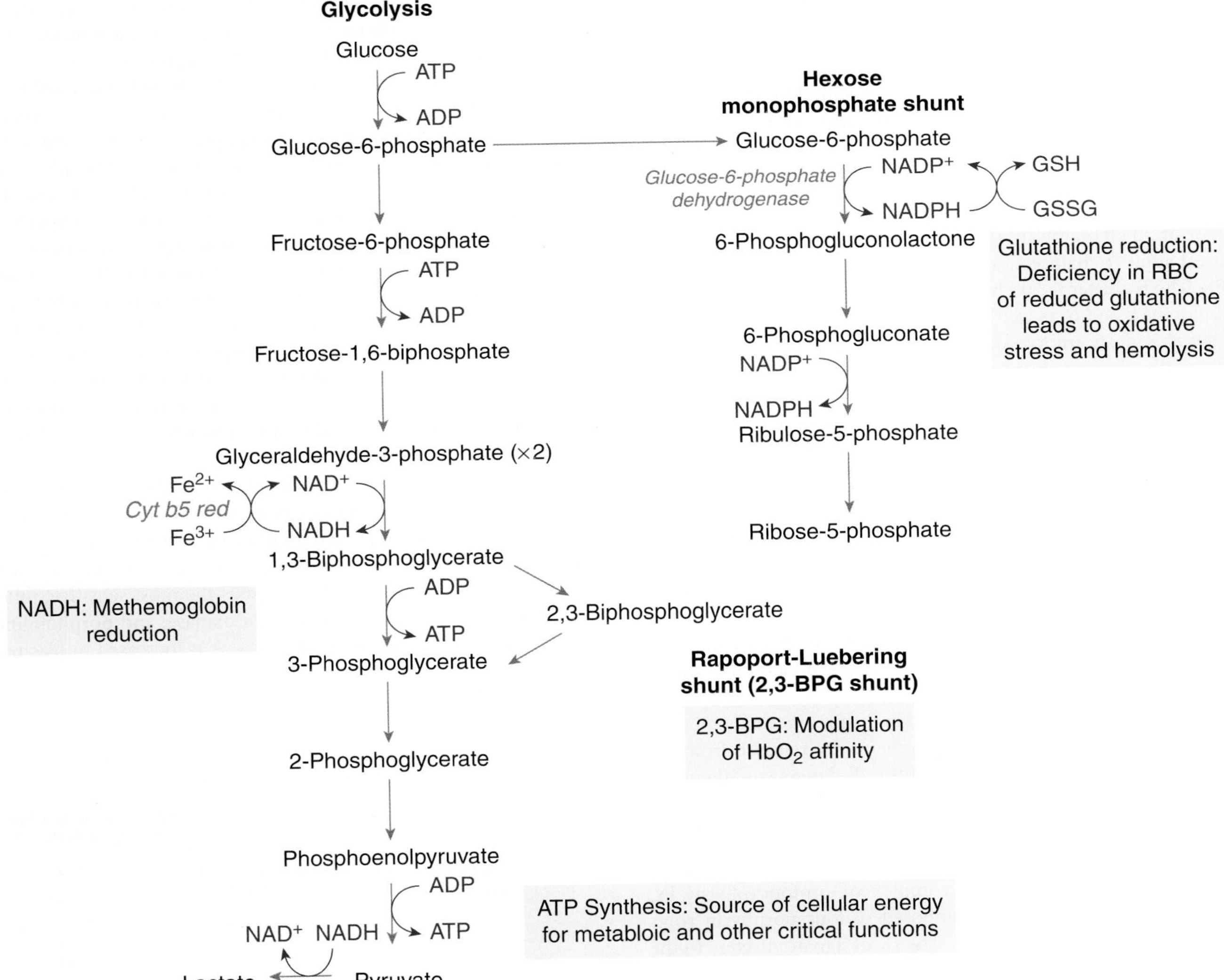

FIGURE 24–2. Metabolic pathways of the erythrocyte. The main metabolic pathways available to the mature erythrocyte are shown (rectangles). Glucose is imported into the cell, while pyruvate, lactate, and oxidized glutathione (GSSG) are exported. 2,3-BPG = 2,3-Biphosphoglycerate; ADP = adenosine diphosphate; ATP = adenosine triphosphate; cyt b5 red = cytochrome b5 reductase; G6PD = glucose-6-phosphate dehydrogenase; GSH = reduced glutathione; Hb = hemoglobin; NADH reduced form of nicotinamide adenine dinucleotide (NAD^+); NADPH = reduced form of nicotinamide adenine dinucleotide phosphate ($NADP^+$); RBC = red blood cell (erythrocyte).

are vulnerable to irreversible damage under oxidant stress. The consequences of this deficiency are discussed in greater detail below under Glucose-6-Phosphate Dehydrogenase Deficiencies.

The erythrocyte also contains enzymes to synthesize glutathione (γ-glutamyl-cysteine synthetase and glutathione synthetase), to convert CO_2 to bicarbonate ion (carbonic anhydrase I), to remove pyrimidines resulting from the degradation of RNA (pyrimidine 5′-nucleotidase), to protect against free radicals (catalase, superoxide dismutase, glutathione peroxidase), and to conjugate glutathione to electrophiles (ρ glutathione-*S*-transferase).

HEMOGLOBIN

Hemoglobin, the major constituent of the cytoplasm of the erythrocyte, is a conjugated protein with a molecular weight of 64,500 Da. One molecule is composed of 4 protein or globin chains, each attached to a prosthetic group called heme. Heme contains an iron molecule complexed at the center of a porphyrin ring. The globin chains are held together by noncovalent electrostatic attraction into a tetrahedral array. Hemoglobin is so efficient at binding and carrying oxygen that it enables blood to transport 100 times as much oxygen as could be carried by plasma alone (Chap. 21). In addition, the capacity of hemoglobin to modulate oxygen binding under different conditions allows adaptation to a wide variety of environments and demands. Three complex and integrated pathways are required for the formation of hemoglobin: globin synthesis, protoporphyrin synthesis, and iron metabolism.

Globin synthesis The protein chains of hemoglobin are produced with information from two different genetic loci. The α-globin gene cluster spans 30 kb on the short arm of chromosome 16, and codes for 2 identical adult α-chain genes, as well as the ζ -chain, an embryonic globulin. The β cluster is 50 kb on chromosome 11, and codes for the 2 adult globins β and δ, as well as 2 nearly identical γ chains expressed in the fetus and an embryonic globulin ε. The expression of genes in each family changes during embryonic, fetal, neonatal, and adult development. Until 8 weeks of intrauterine life, ε, ζ, γ, and α chains are produced and assembled in various combinations in yolk sac-derived erythrocytes. With the shift in erythropoiesis from yolk sac to fetal liver and spleen, embryonic hemoglobin is no longer detectable, and the α and γ globin chains are paired into fetal hemoglobin (HbF = $\alpha_2\gamma_2$). Erythrocytes containing HbF have a higher O_2 affinity than those containing adult hemoglobin, which is important for oxygen transfer across the placenta into the relatively hypoxic uterine environment. Beginning shortly before birth, expression shifts to the α and β globins, which constitute the predominant adult hemoglobin termed hemoglobin A ($\alpha_2\beta_2$). Approximately 2.5% of normal adult hemoglobin is in the form of hemoglobin A_2 ($\alpha_2\,\delta_2$).

The rate of globin synthesis is increased in the presence of heme, and inhibited in its absence.[116] As the globin chains are released from the ribosomes, they spontaneously assemble into αβ dimers, and then into $\alpha_2\beta_2$ tetramers. The thalassemias, a group of inherited disorders, result from defective synthesis of one or more of the globin chains. Clinically this results in a hypochromic, microcytic anemia.[65,116]

Heme synthesis Heme is the iron complex of protoporphyrin IX. Protoporphyrin IX is a tetramer composed of four porphyrin rings joined in a closed, flat-ring structure. The IX designation refers to the order in which it was first synthesized in Hans Fischer's laboratory. Of the 15 possible isomers, only protoporphyrin IX occurs in living organisms. Technically, only iron complexes with the iron in the Fe^{2+} state can be called heme, but the term is commonly used to refer to the prosthetic group of metalloproteins such as peroxidase (ferric) and cytochrome c (both ferric and ferrous), whether the iron is in the Fe^{2+} or Fe^{3+} state. The terms "hemiglobin" and "ferrihemoglobin" are synonymous with methemoglobin but rarely used. All animal cells can synthesize heme, with the notable exception of mature erythrocytes.[143] Hemoproteins are involved in a multitude of biologic functions, including oxygen binding (hemoglobin, myoglobin), oxygen metabolism (oxidases, peroxidases, catalases, and hydroxylases), and electron transport (cytochromes), as well as metabolism of xenobiotics (cytochrome P450 family).[144] Erythroid cells synthesize 85% of total body heme, with the liver synthesizing most of the balance. Hemoglobin is the most abundant hemoprotein, containing 70% of total body iron.[143]

The first step in the synthesis of heme takes place in the mitochondrion and is the condensation of glycine- and succinylcoenzyme A (CoA) to form 5-aminolevulinic acid (ALA) (Fig. 24–3).[116] The formation of 5-ALA is catalyzed by aminolevulinic acid synthase (ALAS), the rate-limiting step of the pathway. The rate of heme synthesis is closely controlled, given that free intracellular heme is toxic and that this first step is essentially irreversible.

Of the two isoforms of ALAS known to exist in mammals, erythroid cells express the ALAS 2 isoform which resides on the X chromosome. Comparatively more is known about ALAS 1 (chromosome 3), a housekeeping gene with a short half-life expressed ubiquitously allowing the synthesis of cellular and mitochondrial hemoproteins. ALAS 1 activity is induced by many factors, which can increase its expression by two orders of magnitude. Moreover, it is strongly inhibited by heme in a classical negative feedback fashion.[143] ALAS 2 is constitutively expressed at very high levels in erythroid precursors, allowing sustained synthesis of heme during erythropoiesis. Pyridoxal phosphate (active vitamin B_6) serves as a cofactor to both isoforms of ALAS. The clinical consequences of pyridoxine deficiency may include a hypochromic, microcytic anemia, iron overload, and neurologic impairment.

The next step in the synthesis of hemoglobin is the formation of the monopyrrole porphobilinogen via the condensation of two molecules of ALA. The subsequent steps in heme synthesis involve the condensation of four molecules of porphobilinogen into a flat ring, which is transported back into the mitochondrion by an unknown mechanism. The final step is the insertion of iron into protoporphyrin IX, a reaction that is catalyzed by ferrochelatase (also known as heme synthase) to form heme.

Understanding this carefully regulated synthetic pathway is relevant to understanding the laboratory evidence of lead exposure, and predicting the response of porphyric patients to a range of xenobiotics. Most steps in the heme biosynthetic pathway are inhibited by lead (see Fig. 24–3; Chap. 94). ALA dehydratase is the most sensitive, followed by ferrochelatase, coproporphyrinogen oxidase, and porphobilinogen (PBG) deaminase. As a consequence, ALA is increased in plasma and

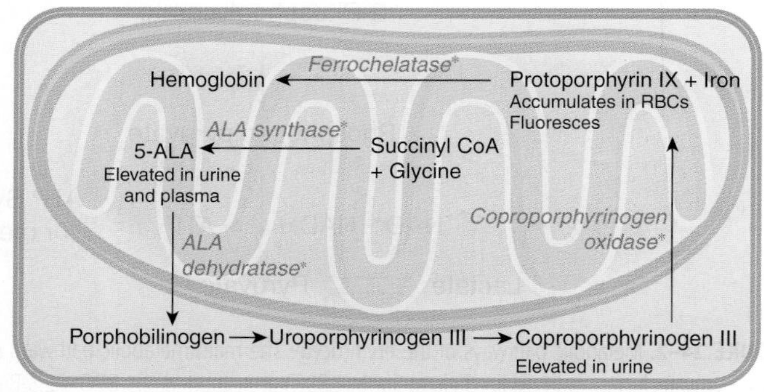

FIGURE 24–3. The heme synthesis pathway. The enzymatic steps inhibited by lead are marked with an asterisk (*) RBCs red blood cells; 5-ALA = 5-aminolevulinic acid.

especially urine. With increasing exposure, ferrochelatase inhibition coupled with iron deficiency causes zinc protoporphyrin to accumulate in erythrocytes, which can easily be detected by fluorescence. Coproporphyrinogen III also appears in the urine. These effects have served as the basis for a number of tests of lead exposure.

The porphyrias are a group of disorders resulting from an inherited deficiency of any given enzyme which follows ALAS on the heme biosynthetic pathway. As such, when ALAS activity outpaces the activity of this enzyme, the rate-limiting step shifts downstream, and intermediate metabolites accumulate. These metabolites can cause characteristic neuropsychiatric symptoms and palsies (due to 5-ALA and porphobilinogen), and cutaneous reactions including photosensitivity (caused by the fluorescence of the porphyrins). For example, porphobilinogen is excreted in large quantities by patients with acute intermittent porphyria (porphobilinogen deaminase deficiency), and the urine darkens with exposure to air and light due to oxidation to porphobilin and to non-enzymatic assembly into porphyrin rings. A variety of xenobiotics can precipitate a crisis in susceptible individuals, by inducing ALAS 1 and overloading the deficient enzyme.[181] The molecular mechanisms which allow xenobiotics to induce the ALAS 1 gene closely resemble those accounting for induction of the cytochrome P450 (CYP) genes, not surprisingly since both components are required to form the hemoprotein. The xenobiotic typically interacts with either the constitutive androstane receptor (CAR) or the pregnane X receptor (PXR), the two main so-called orphan nuclear receptors.[194] These transcriptional factors are DNA-binding proteins which induce the expression of a range of drug metabolizing and transporting genes in response to the presence of a xenobiotic, and have been termed "xenosensors." When activated, they associate with the 9-*cis* retinoic acid xenobiotic receptor (RXR), and then attach to enhancer sequences near the apoCYP or ALAS1 genes to enhance transcription.[142] The multifunctional inducers capable of activating a wide range of hepatic enzymes are therefore extremely porphyrogenic, and include phenobarbital, phenytoin, carbamazepine, and primidone. Furthermore, because CYP 3A4 and 2C9 represent nearly half of the hepatic CYP pool, inducers of these isoforms can also stimulate heme synthesis and induce a porphyric crisis. Examples of these agents included the anticonvulsants, nifedipine, sulfamethoxazole, rifampicin, ketoconazole, and the reproductive steroids progesterone, medroxyprogesterone and testosterone. Glucocorticoids, on the other hand, despite binding to PXR, suppress ALAS1 induction and translation, and are not porphyrogenic.[181]

Iron metabolism Unless appropriately chelated, free iron not bound by transport or storage proteins can generate harmful oxygen free radicals that damage cellular structures and metabolism (Chaps. 11 and 40).[145] For this reason, serum iron circulates bound to a transfer protein, transferrin, and is stored in the tissues using ferritin. Although each molecule of transferrin can bind two iron atoms, ferritin has a large internal cavity, approximately 80 Å in diameter, that can hold up to 4500 iron atoms per molecule. The amount of iron transported through plasma depends on total-body iron stores and the rate of erythropoiesis. Only about one-third of the iron-binding sites of circulating transferrin are normally saturated, as demonstrated by the usual serum iron content of 60–170 μg/dL (10–30 μmol/L) as compared to the total iron-binding capacity of 280–390 μg/dL (50–70 μmol/L).

Only transferrin can directly supply iron for hemoglobin synthesis.[143] The iron–transferrin complex binds to transferrin receptors on the surface of developing erythroid cells in bone marrow. Iron in the erythroid cell is used for hemoglobin synthesis or is stored in the form of ferritin.

The absorption of non-heme, free ferrous iron from the diet occurs via the divalent metal transporter of the duodenal enterocyte, which then passes it into the circulation via ferroportin. Oxidized to the ferric form, iron then circulates bound to transferrin.[71] Dietary iron complexed with heme can also be absorbed via the recently discovered heme carrier protein 1, which transports either iron or zinc protoporphyrin into the erythrocyte.[164] The iron may then be freed by microsomal heme oxygenase, and follow the transport of atomic iron, or perhaps heme itself can be transferred to the circulation via specific export proteins, and circulate bound to its carrier protein, hemopexin.[9]

The senescent erythrocyte is usually removed from the circulation by splenic macrophages. Heme is degraded by heme oxygenase to carbon monoxide and biliverdin, and the iron extracted.[145] Some iron may remain in macrophages in the form of ferritin or hemosiderin. Most is delivered again by ferroportin back to the plasma, and bound to transferrin.

Iron homeostasis is largely regulated at the level of absorption, with little physiologic control over its rate of loss. Excess absorption relative to body stores is the hallmark of hereditary hemochromatosis. The iron regulatory hormone hepcidin produced by the liver is now believed to play a central role in iron control, including the anemia of chronic disease caused by inflammatory signals.[71] Hepcidin is a 25-amino acid peptide that senses iron stores, and controls the ferroportin-mediated release of iron from enterocytes, macrophages and hepatocytes. The liver is an important reservoir of iron as it can store considerable amounts of iron taken from portal blood, and release it when needed.

OXYGEN-CARBON DIOXIDE EXCHANGE

The evolutionary transition of organisms from anaerobic to aerobic life allowed the liberation of 18 times more energy from glucose. Vertebrates have developed 2 important systems to overcome the relatively small quantities of oxygen dissolved in aqueous solutions under atmospheric conditions: the circulatory system and hemoglobin. The circulatory system allows delivery of oxygen and removal of carbon dioxide throughout the organism. Hemoglobin also plays an essential role in the transport and exchange of both gases.[74] Moreover, the interactions between these gases and hemoglobin are directly linked in a remarkable story of molecular evolution. Understanding this interplay has allowed fundamental insight into protein conformation and the importance of allosteric interactions between molecules.

The binding of oxygen to each of the 4 iron molecules in heme results in conformational changes that affect binding of oxygen at the remaining sites. This phenomenon is known as cooperativity, and is a fundamental property to allow both the transport of relatively large quantities of oxygen and the unloading of most of this oxygen at tissue sites. Cooperativity results from the intramolecular interactions of the tetrameric hemoglobin, and is expressed in the sigmoidal shape of the oxyhemoglobin dissociation curve (Chap. 21). Conversely, the monomeric myoglobin has a hyperbolic oxygen binding curve. The partial pressure of oxygen at which 50% of the oxygen bindings sites of hemoglobin are occupied is about 26 mm Hg, in contrast with about 1 mm Hg for myoglobin. Moreover, hemoglobin is nearly 100% saturated at partial oxygen pressures of about 100 mm Hg in the pulmonary capillaries, transporting 1.34 mL of oxygen per gram of hemoglobin A. About one-third of this oxygen can be unloaded under normal conditions at tissue capillaries with partial oxygen pressures around 35 mm Hg. The proportion rises during exercise and sepsis, and with poisons that uncouple oxidative phosphorylation. Elite athletes can extract up to 80% of the available oxygen under conditions of maximal aerobic effort.

The oxygen reserve, however, is only one of the reasons for the large quantity of hemoglobin in circulation. The ability of hemoglobin to buffer the acid equivalent of CO_2 in solution is equally vital to respiratory physiology, as it allows the removal of large quantities of CO_2 from metabolically active tissues with minimal changes in blood pH. To put things in perspective, the typical adult male has approximately 75 mL/kg of blood containing 15 g/100 mL of hemoglobin, or nearly 1 kg of hemoglobin. His 0.3-kg heart must pump this entire mass of hemoglobin every minute at rest, a substantial work expenditure. This expenditure may be explained in part by the observation that hemoglobin is by far the largest buffer in circulation, accounting for nearly seven times the buffer capacity of the serum proteins combined (28 vs. 4 mEq H^+/L of whole blood). For every 1 mol of oxygen unloaded in the tissue, about 0.5 mol of H^+ is loaded onto hemoglobin.

The linked interaction between oxygen and carbon dioxide transport can be first considered from the perspective of oxygen binding to hemoglobin. The affinity of oxygen for hemoglobin is directly affected by pH, which is a function of the CO_2 content of the blood. The oxyhemoglobin dissociation curve shifts to the left in lungs, where the level of carbon dioxide, and thus carbonic acid, are kept relatively low as a result of ventilation, an effect that promotes oxygen binding. The curve shifts to the right in tissues where cellular respiration increases CO_2 concentrations. This phenomenon, known as the *Bohr effect*, promotes the uptake of oxygen in the lungs and the release of oxygen at tissue sites.

From the perspective of carbon dioxide transport, hemoglobin also plays an essential albeit indirect role. Carbon dioxide dissolves into serum, and is slowly hydrated to carbonic acid which dissociates to H+ and HCO_3^-(pK_a 6.35). The hydration reaction is accelerated from about 40 seconds to 10 msec by the abundant enzyme carbonic anhydrase located within the erythrocyte. Most carbon dioxide collected at the tissues diffuses into erythrocytes where it becomes H^+ and HCO_3^-. This HCO_3^- is then rapidly transported back to the serum in exchange for chloride ion via the band 3 anion exchange transporter located in the erythrocyte membrane, thereby shifting serum Cl^- into the erythrocyte (the *chloride shift*).[177] The hydrogen ion is accepted by hemoglobin, largely at the imidazole ring of histidine residues which have a pK_a of about 7.0. A small amount of CO_2 reacts directly with the amino terminal of the globin chains to form carbamino residues ($HbNHCOO^-$). Thus, most of the transported carbon dioxide is transformed by the erythrocyte into bicarbonate ion that is returned to the serum, and hydrogen ion that is buffered by hemoglobin. Each liter of venous blood typically carries 0.8 mEq dissolved CO_2 and 16 mEq HCO_3^- in the serum, and 0.4 mEq dissolved CO_2, 4.6 mEq HCO_3^-, and 1.2 mEq $HbNHCOO^-$ in the erythrocyte (a total of 23 mEq CO_2, equivalent to 510 mL CO_2/L blood). Although two-thirds of the total CO_2 content appears to be carried in the serum, all of the serum bicarbonate is originally generated within erythrocytes. In the capillaries of the lungs, the reverse reactions occur to eliminate CO_2. Because deoxyhemoglobin is better able to buffer hydrogen ions, the release of oxygen from hemoglobin at the tissues facilitates the uptake of carbon dioxide into venous blood. This effect is known as the *Haldane effect.* In fact, 1 L of venous blood at 70% oxygen saturation can transport an additional 20 mL of CO_2 compared to arterial blood. Both the Bohr and Haldane effects can have important consequences, either at the extremes of acid–base perturbations or because of interference with oxygen metabolism, as can occur in a number of poisonings.

Finally, in addition to inactivating nitric oxide, hemoglobin can also reversibly bind it as *S*-nitrosohemoglobin, thereby playing an important role in the regulation of microvascular circulation and oxygen delivery. The ability of hemoglobin to vasodilate the surrounding microvasculature in response to oxygen desaturation using nitric oxide provides new insight into oxygen delivery, and may be pivotal in such disorders as septic shock, pulmonary hypertension, and senescence of stored red blood cells.[167]

ABNORMAL HEMOGLOBINS

Several alterations of the hemoglobin molecule are encountered in clinical toxicology. A detailed understanding of their molecular basis, clinical manifestations, and effects on gas exchange are essential. Unfortunately, the nomenclature can be ambiguous and overlap with distinct clinical entities such as oxidant injury and hemolysis. Therefore, although a detailed discussion of these abnormal hemoglobins appears elsewhere (Chaps. 125 and 127), an overview of the subject is presented here. It is helpful to recall that the iron atom has six binding positions. Four of these positions are attached in a single plane to the protoporphyrin ring to form heme. The remaining 2 binding positions lie on opposite sides of this plane. Iron is ordinarily bonded on one side to the F8 proximal histidine residue of the globin chain. The remaining site is available for binding molecular oxygen, but can also bind carbon monoxide, nitric oxide, cyanide, hydroxide ion, or water. The E7 distal histidine residue facilitates the binding of oxygen, while stearically hindering carbon monoxide binding.

Methemoglobin Methemoglobin (ferrihemoglobin or hemiglobin) is the oxidized form of deoxyhemoglobin in which at least one heme iron is in the oxidized (Fe^{3+}) valence state. A number of valency hybrids can occur depending on the number of ferric versus ferrous heme units within the tetramer. Methemoglobin therefore represents oxidation (loss of electrons) of the hemoglobin molecule at the iron atom. It occurs spontaneously as a consequence of interactions between the iron and oxygen. Normally, in deoxygenated hemoglobin, the heme iron is in the ferrous (Fe^{2+}) valence state. In this state, there are 6 electrons in the outer shell, 4 of which are unpaired. When oxygen is bound, one of these electrons is partially transferred to it and the iron is reversibly oxidized. When O_2 is released, the electron is usually transferred back to heme iron, yielding the normal reduced state. Sometimes, the electron remains with the O_2 yielding a superoxide anion radical O_2^- rather than molecular oxygen. In this case, heme iron is left in the Fe^{3+}, or oxidized, state and is unable to release another electron to bind oxygen. This oxidation is primarily reversed via the action of cytochrome b5 reductase, also known as NADH methemoglobin reductase, which uses the electron carrier NADH generated by glycolysis ("Metabolism" and Chap. 12).[77,112] Minor pathways are also involved in methemoglobin reduction, including NADPH methemoglobin reductase, which normally reduces only approximately 5% of the methemoglobin, and vitamin C, a nonenzymatic reducing agent. The activity of NADPH methemoglobin reductase may be significantly accelerated by the presence of the electron donor methylene blue (Antidotes in Depth: Methylene Blue and Chap. 127) or riboflavin.[91] Equilibrium is maintained with methemoglobin concentrations of 1% of total hemoglobin. Many xenobiotics are capable of increasing the rate of methemoglobin formation as much as 1000-fold. Nitrites, nitrates, chlorates, and quinones are capable of directly oxidizing hemoglobin.[30] Certain individuals may be especially vulnerable because of deficient methemoglobin reduction.[44] The fetus and neonate are more susceptible to methemoglobinemia than the adult, as HbF is more susceptible to oxidation of the heme iron than adult hemoglobin. The newborn also has a limited capacity to reduce methemoglobin, because levels of cytochrome b5 reductase only reach adult levels around 6 months of age.

Carboxyhemoglobin Carbon monoxide (CO) can reversibly bind to heme iron in lieu of molecular oxygen. The affinity of CO for hemoglobin is 200–300 times that of oxygen, despite the stearic hindrance of the E7 distal histidine. The presence of CO thereby precludes the binding of oxygen. In addition, CO binding within any one heme subunit degrades the cooperative binding of oxygen at the remaining heme groups of the same hemoglobin molecule. The oxyhemoglobin dissociation curve is therefore shifted to the left, reflecting the fact that oxygen is more tightly bound by hemoglobin and less able to be unloaded to the tissues. In addition, CO binds to the heme group of myoglobin and the cytochromes, interfering with cellular respiration, exacerbating the clinical symptoms of hypoxia (Chap. 125).[66]

Sulfhemoglobin Sulfhemoglobin is a bright green molecule in which the hydrosulfide anion HS^- irreversibly binds to ferrous hemoglobin. The sulfur atom is probably attached to a β carbon in the porphyrin ring, and not at the normal oxygen-binding site.[125] It has a spectrophotometric absorption band at approximately 618 nm,[23] is ineffective in oxygen transport, and clinically resembles cyanosis. The oxygen affinity of sulfhemoglobin is approximately 100 times less than that of oxyhemoglobin, shifting the oxyhemoglobin dissociation curve to the right, in favor of O_2 unbinding. Thus, the symptoms of hypoxia are not as severe with sulfhemoglobinemia as with carboxy- or methemoglobinemia.[136]

Oxidation of the globin chain Oxidation can also occur at the amino acid side chains of the globin protein. In particular, sulfhydryl groups can oxidize to form disulfide links between cysteine residues, which leads to the unfolding of the protein chain, exposure of other side chains and further oxidation. When these disulfide links join adjacent hemoglobin molecules, they cause the precipitation of the concentrated hemoglobin molecules out of solution. Covalent links can also form between hemoglobin and other cytoskeletal and membrane proteins.[39] Eventually, aggregates of denatured and insoluble protein are visible on light microscopy as Heinz bodies. The distortion of the cellular architecture, and the loss of fluidity in particular, is a signal to reticuloendothelial macrophages to excise sections of erythrocyte membrane ("bite cells") or to remove the entire erythrocyte from the circulation ("Hemolysis"). To guard against these oxidation reactions, the erythrocyte maintains a pool of reduced glutathione via the actions of the NADPH generated in the hexose monophosphate shunt (assuming adequate G6PD activity to initiate this pathway). This glutathione transfers electrons to break open disulfide links and to preserve sulfhydryl groups in their reduced state.

HEMOLYSIS

Hemolysis is merely the acceleration of the normal process by which senescent or compromised erythrocytes are removed from the circulation.[168] The normal life span of a circulating erythrocyte is approximately 120 days, and any reduction in this life span represents some degree of hemolysis. If sufficiently rapid, hemolysis can overwhelm the regenerative capacity of the erythron, resulting in anemia. Intravascular hemolysis occurs when the rate of hemolysis exceeds the capacity of the reticuloendothelial macrophages to remove damaged erythrocytes, and free hemoglobin and other intracellular contents of the erythrocyte appear in the circulation.

Reticulocytosis, polychromasia, unconjugated hyperbilirubinemia, increased serum lactate dehydrogenase, and decreased serum haptoglobin are characteristic of hemolysis. A normal or elevated RBC distribution width and thrombocytosis are usually present on the automated complete blood count. The presence of spherocytes on peripheral blood smear suggests an autoimmune or hereditary process, and can be pursued with a Coombs' test. Schistocytes suggest thrombotic thrombocytopenic purpura (TTP) or hemolytic uremic syndrome, disseminated intravascular coagulation, or valvular hemolysis. TTP and hemolytic uremic syndrome are characterized by a microangiopathic anemia, thrombocytopenia and normal coagulation parameters (unlike disseminated intravascular coagulation). TTP is discussed under platelet disorders below. Hemoglobinemia, hemoglobinuria, and hemosiderinuria can occur with intravascular hemolysis. Specialized tests to measure hemolysis detect shortened erythrocyte survival, increased endogenous carbon monoxide generation from heme oxygenase, and increased fecal urobilinogen.[175]

Table 24–2 presents a brief classification of acquired causes of hemolysis relevant to toxicology. Oxidant injury following xenobiotic exposure is one of the triggers of hemolysis, as it may cause irreversible changes in the erythrocyte. Xenobiotics can also interact with the immune system to cause hemolysis. Finally, erythrocytes deficient in G6PD by virtue of cell age or enzyme mutations are particularly vulnerable to hemolysis following oxidant stress due to limited capacity to generate NADPH and reduced glutathione.[168]

TABLE 24–2. Xenobiotics Causing Acquired Hemolysis

Immune-mediated
Type I: IgG against drug tightly bound to red cell
Type II: Complement activated by antibodies against drug-membrane complex
Type III: True autoimmune response to red cell membrane
Nonimmune-mediated
Oxidants
Aniline[107]
Benzocaine[52;103]
Chlorates[47;85]
Dapsone[88]
Hydrogen peroxide
Hydroxylamine[174]
Methylene blue[166]
Naphthalene[184]
Nitrites[16;28;31;154]
Nitrofurantoin
Oxygen[102;121]
Phenacetin[122]
Phenazopyridine[53;131]
Phenol
Platin salts[109]
Sulfonamides[190]
Nonoxidants
Arsine (AsH_3)
Copper
Lead
Pyrogallic acid
Stibine (SbH_3)
Microangiopathic (eg, ticlopidine, clopidogrel, cyclosporine, tacrolimus)[(17;19;49;73;165;186)]
Venoms (snake, spider)[(60;78;127;189)]
Osmotic agents (eg, water)[(76;98)]
Hypophosphatemia[(5;90;120)]

NONIMMUNE-MEDIATED CAUSES OF XENOBIOTIC-INDUCED HEMOLYSIS

A number of xenobiotics or their reactive metabolites can cause hemolysis via oxidant injury; Table 24–2 provides a partial list. A Heinz-body hemolytic anemia can result, which typically resolves within a few weeks of drug discontinuation. Some xenobiotics cause hemolysis in the absence of overt oxidant injury (see Table 24–2). Copper sulfate hemolysis is described in Chap. 93, and the delayed hemolysis following exposure to arsine or stibine is described below.

Arsine Arsine (AsH_3) is a colorless, odorless, nonirritating gas that is 2.5 times denser than air (Chap. 88). Clinical signs and symptoms appear after a latent period of up to 24 hours after exposure to concentrations above 30 ppm, and may include headache, malaise, dyspnea, abdominal pain with nausea and vomiting, hepatomegaly, hemolysis with hemoglobinuric renal failure, and death.[38,54,87,97,141] The mechanism of hemolysis is believed to involve the fixation of arsine by sulfhydryl groups of hemoglobin and other essential proteins.[63,192] Interestingly, hemolysis is prevented in vitro by conversion to carboxy- or methemoglobin.[70] Impairment of membrane proteins including Na^+-K^+-ATPase is another potential mechanism for arsine-induced hemolysis.[148] Chronic exposure to low levels of arsine can produce clinically significant disease.[38] Stibine (SbH_3) an antimony derivative likely causes hemolysis via similar mechanisms.

IMMUNE-MEDIATED HEMOLYTIC ANEMIA

The immune-mediated hemolytic anemias occur when ingested xenobiotics trigger an antigen antibody reaction (see Table 24–2).[138] In general, these molecules are too small to be sensitizing agents, but antigenicity can be acquired after binding to carrier proteins in blood. The particulars of the xenobiotic-carrier immune activation sequence form the basis for the classification of this group of hemolytic anemias.[13]

The first class of reaction (hapten model, or drug adsorption) occurs when the xenobiotic acts as a hapten and binds tightly to cell membrane glycoproteins on the surface of the erythrocyte. IgG antibodies develop against the bound drug, leading to removal of the erythrocyte by splenic macrophages. The prototype of this reaction is the hemolytic anemia observed following high dose penicillin therapy.[55] Historically, approximately 3% of patients treated with megadose penicillin over weeks for infectious endocarditis developed a positive direct Coombs test, demonstrating erythrocytes become coated with IgG or complement. The positive direct Coombs test is a necessary, but insufficient, condition for the hemolytic reaction. The hemolysis is usually subacute, and requires at least a week to develop, but can become life threatening if the cause is not recognized. Discontinuation of the xenobiotic results in cessation of hemolysis, because its presence is needed for antibody binding.

The second class of reaction (immune complex, or neoantigen) occurs with drugs that have low affinity for cellular membrane glycoproteins. Examples are quinine, quinidine, stibophen and newer-generation cephalosporins, such as cefotetan, cefotaxime, and ceftriaxone. Antibodies are formed against the joint drug-membrane complex (neoantigen), and erythrocyte injury is primarily mediated by complement. Unlike the hapten model, small doses of xenobiotics are sufficient to trigger sudden intravascular hemolysis and hemoglobinuria, leading to renal failure. The direct Coombs test is positive only for complement, but the presence of drug is again necessary.

The third class of reaction (true autoimmune) occurs when the xenobiotic alters the natural suppressor system, allowing the formation of antibody to cellular components. This is a true autoantibody reaction directed against erythrocyte surface antigen rather than the drug.[15] The classic example is α-methyldopa, but chlorpromazine, cladribine, cyclosporine, fludarabine, levodopa, and procainamide can also trigger autoimmune hemolysis.[15,128,153] An indirect Coombs test that is positive in the absence of drug demonstrates the presence of IgG autoantibodies in the patient's serum when incubated with normal erythrocytes. The severity of hemolysis is variable, and its onset insidious, but hemolysis can continue for weeks to months despite removal of the inciting agent.

Glucose-6-phosphate dehydrogenase deficiencies (G6PD) G6PD is the enzyme that catalyzes the first step of the hexose monophosphate shunt: the conversion of glucose-6-phosphate to phosphogluconolactone (see Fig. 12-5). In the process, $NADP^+$ is reduced to NADPH, which the erythrocyte uses to maintain a supply of reduced glutathione and to defend against oxidation. It follows that erythrocytes deficient in G6PD activity are less able to resist oxidant attack and, in particular, to maintain sulfhydryl groups of hemoglobin in their reduced state, resulting in hemolysis. It is important to recognize that the term G6PD deficiency encompasses a wide range of differences in enzyme activities among individuals. These differences may result from decreased enzyme synthesis, altered catalytic activity, or reduced stability of the enzyme. Approximately 7.5% of the world population is affected to some degree, with more than 400 variants having been identified. Most cases involve relatively mild deficiency and minimal morbidity.[25,37,114] Ethnic populations from tropical and subtropical countries (the so-called malaria belt) have a much higher prevalence of G6PD deficiency, possibly because that phenotype protects against malaria.[129]

The gene that encodes for G6PD resides near the end of the long arm of the X-chromosome. Most mutations consist of a single amino acid substitution, as complete absence of this enzyme is lethal. Although males hemizygous for a deficient gene are more severely affected, females randomly inactivate one X-chromosome during cellular differentiation according to the Lyon hypothesis. Thus, female carriers heterozygous for a deficient G6PD gene have a mosaic of erythrocytes, some proportion of which expresses the deficient gene during maturation. Accordingly, approximately 10% of carrier females may be nearly as severely affected as a male hemizygous for the same deficient gene. Because of the high gene frequency in certain ethnic groups, another approximately 10% of females may be homozygous for the deficient gene.

Normal G6PD has a half-life of about 60 days. Because the erythrocyte cannot synthesize new protein, the activity of G6PD normally declines by approximately 75% over its 120-day life span. Consequently, even in unaffected individuals, susceptibility to oxidant stress varies based on the age mix of circulating erythrocytes. In all cases, older erythrocytes are less likely to recover following exposure to an oxidant and will hemolyze first. Moreover, after an episode of hemolysis following acute exposure to an oxidant stress, the higher G6PD activity of surviving erythrocytes will confer some resistance against further hemolysis in most individuals with relatively mild deficiency, even if the offending xenobiotic is continued. Phenotypic testing for G6PD deficiency is best done 2 to 3 months after a hemolytic crisis, after the reticulocyte count has normalized.

The World Health Organization classification of G6PD is based on the degree of enzyme deficiency and severity of hemolysis.[27] Both class I and class II patients are severely deficient, with less than 10% of normal G6PD activity. Class I individuals are prone to chronic hemolytic anemia, whereas class II patients experience intermittent hemolytic crises. Class III patients have only moderate (10%–60%) enzyme deficiency, and experience self-limiting hemolysis in response to certain drugs and infections. Approximately 11% of African Americans have a class III deficiency, traditionally termed type A^-, and experience a decline of no more than 30% of the red blood cell mass during any single hemolytic episode. Another 20% of African Americans have type A^+ G6PD enzyme, which is functionally normal, and therefore of no consequence despite a 1-base substitution compared to wild-type B. The Mediterranean type found in Sardinia, Corsica, Greece, the Middle East, and India is a class II deficiency, and hemolysis can occur spontaneously or in response to ingestion of oxidants, such as the β-glycosides found in fava (*Vicia fava)* beans.

The most common clinical presentation of previously unrecognized G6PD deficiency is the acute hemolytic crisis. Typically, hemolysis begins 1 to 4 days following the exposure to an offending xenobiotic or infection (Table 24–3). Jaundice, pallor, and dark urine may occur

TABLE 24–3. Representative Xenobiotics That Can Cause Hemolysis in Patients with Class I, II, or III G6PD Deficiency

Doxorubicin	Phenylhydrazine
Furazolidone	Primaquine
Isobutyl nitrite	Sulfacetamide
Methylene blue	Sulfamethoxazole
Nalidixic acid	Sulfanilamide
Naphthalene	Sulfapyridine
Nitrofurantoin	Toluidine blue
Phenazopyridine	Trinitrotoluene

Data adapted from Beutler E: Glucose-6-phosphate dehydrogenase deficiency. N Engl J Med 1991;324:169–174, and Beutler E: G6PD deficiency. Blood 1994;84:3613–3636.

with abdominal and back pain. A decrease in the concentration of hemoglobin occurs. The peripheral smear demonstrates cell fragments and cells that have had Heinz bodies excised. Bone marrow stimulation results in a reticulocytosis by day 5 and an increased erythrocyte mass. In general, a normal bone marrow can compensate for ongoing hemolysis, and can return the hemoglobin concentration to normal. Most crises are self-limiting because of the higher G6PD activity of younger erythrocytes. Historically, the anemia observed when primaquine was administered to type A^- military recruits for malaria prophylaxis resolved within 3 to 6 weeks in most patients.[26] Some xenobiotics, including acetaminophen, vitamin C, and sulfisoxazole, are safe at therapeutic doses but can cause hemolysis in G6PD-deficient patients following overdose.[24,170,193]

Other presentations of more severe variants of G6PD include neonatal jaundice and kernicterus, chronic hemolysis with splenomegaly and black pigment gallstones, megaloblastic crisis caused by folate deficiency, and aplastic crisis after parvovirus B19 infection.

MEGALOBLASTIC ANEMIA

Vitamin B_{12} and folate are essential for one-carbon metabolism in mammals. One-carbon fragments are necessary for the biosynthesis of thymidine, purines, serotonin and methionine, as well as the methylation of DNA, histones and other proteins, and the complete catabolism of branched chain fatty acids and histidine. Unable to synthesize vitamin B_{12} or folate, mammals are dependent on dietary sources and microorganisms for these cofactors. The hematologic manifestation of vitamin B_{12} or folate deficiency is a characteristic panmyelosis termed megaloblastic anemia. The hallmark nuclear-cytoplasmic asynchrony is due to disrupted DNA synthesis, halted interphase and ineffective erythropoiesis.[146] The hyperplastic bone marrow contains precursor cells with abnormal nuclei filled with incompletely condensed chromatin. Among circulating blood cells, macrocytic anemia (macro-ovalocytes) without reticulocytosis is followed by the appearance of granulocytes with an abnormally large, distorted nucleus (hypersegmented neutrophils with six or more lobes). Lymphocytes and platelets may appear normal but are also functionally impaired.

In addition to dietary deficiencies which have become less common, macrocytic anemia with or without megaloblastosis in adults is usually caused by chronic ethanol abuse, chemotherapy or antiretroviral agents, especially when mean corpuscular volumes are only moderately elevated (100–120 fL).[158] The folate antagonists aminopterin, methotrexate, hydantoins, pyrimethamine, proguanil, sulfasalazine, trimethoprim-sulfamethoxazole and valproate can interfere with DNA synthesis. Ethanol affects folate metabolism and transport. Vitamin B_{12} deficiency can be induced by chronic exposure to nitrous oxide, biguanides, colchicine, neomycin, and the proton pump inhibitors. Purine analogs (eg, azathioprine, 6-mercaptopurine, 6-thioguanine, acyclovir) and pyrimidine analogs (eg, 5-fluorouracil, floxuridine, 5-azacitidine, and zidovudine) also disrupt nucleic acid synthesis. Hydroxyurea and cytarabine, which inhibit ribonucleotide reductase, also delay nuclear maturation and function and frequently cause megaloblastosis.

PURE RED CELL APLASIA

Pure red cell aplasia is an uncommon condition in which erythrocyte precursors are absent from an otherwise normal bone marrow. It results in a normocytic anemia with inappropriately low reticulocyte count. The other blood cell lines are unaffected, unlike aplastic anemia. Drugs cause less than 5% of cases of this uncommon condition, having been implicated in fewer than 100 human reports.[180] Only phenytoin, azathioprine, and isoniazid meet criteria for definite causality; chlorpropamide and valproic acid can only be considered as possible causes.[180] Most other xenobiotics are cited only in single case reports, and drug rechallenge was not used, making the association uncertain.

In part because of its rarity, a cluster of 13 cases in France of pure red cell aplasia in hemodialysis patients receiving subcutaneous recombinant erythropoietin ultimately led to an international effort by researchers, regulatory authorities and industry to identify the etiology.[20,41] To reduce theoretical concerns regarding transmission of variant Creutzfeldt-Jakob disease, human serum albumin was replaced with polysorbate 80 as the stabilizer in a formulation used in Europe and Canada. It is suspected that this change allowed rubber to leach from the uncoated stopper of prefilled syringes, triggering an immune response against both recombinant and endogenous erythropoietin in some patients.[118] This episode not only serves as a recent example of successful pharmacovigilence for rare adverse drug effects, but has also influenced safety assessments for an emerging class of biological therapies which include simple peptides, monoclonal antibodies and recombinant DNA proteins.[18,118]

ERYTHROCYTOSIS

Erythrocytosis denotes an increase in the red cell mass, either in absolute terms or relative to a reduced plasma volume. An increasingly recognized cause of drug-induced absolute erythrocytosis is the abuse of recombinant human erythropoietin by athletes to enhance aerobic capacity.[34,57,61,173] Autologous blood transfusions (doping) are also used in this population, and both can cause dangerous increases in blood viscosity. Cobalt was once considered for the treatment of chronic anemia[50] because of its ability to cause a secondary erythrocytosis. The mechanism may involve impaired degradation of the transcription factor Hypoxia Inducible Factor 1α, thereby prolonging erythropeitin transcription. This effect is more pronounced in high altitude dwellers, in whom elevated serum erythropoietin concentrations despite hematocrits in excess of 75% and chronic mountain sickness have been associated with increased serum cobalt concentrations.[86]

THE LEUKON

The leukon represents all leukocytes (white blood cells), including precursor cells, cells in the circulation, and the large number of extravascular cells. It includes the granulocytes (neutrophils, eosinophils, and basophils), lymphocytes, and monocytes. Neutrophils (polymorphonuclear leukocytes) are highly specialized mediators of the inflammatory response, and are a primary focus of concern regarding hematologic toxicity of xenobiotics. B and T lymphocytes are involved in antibody production and cell-mediated immunity. Monocytes migrate out of the vascular compartment to become tissue macrophages and to regulate immune system function.

Immunity is generally divided into the *innate* and the *adaptive* responses. Innate immunity is an immediate but less specific defenses that is highly conserved in evolutionary terms. It is centered on the neutrophil response, and involves monocytes and macrophages as well as complement, cytokines and acute phase proteins. The innate system responds primarily to extracellular pathogens, especially bacteria, by recognizing structures commonly found on pathogens, namely lipopolysaccharide (Gram negative cell walls), lipotechoic acid (Gram positive) and mannans (yeast). Adaptive immunity is demonstrated only in higher animals, and is an antigen-specific response via T- and B-lympocytes after antigen presentation and recognition. While this reaction is more specific, it requires several days to develop, unless that antigen has previously triggered a response (so-called immune memory). This response can also at times be directed against self antigens, resulting in autoimmune disorders.

The recruitment and activation of neutrophils provide the primary defense against the invasion of bacterial and fungal pathogens. They emerge from the bone marrow with the biochemical and metabolic machinery needed for the efficient killing of microorganisms. Activated macrophages release granulocyte and granulocyte-macrophage colony stimulating factors, which stimulate myeloid differentiation and can be recognized on blood testing as the classic neutrophil leucocytosis. Neutrophils are activated when circulating cells detect chemokines released from sites of inflammation. On activation, they undergo conformational and biochemical changes that transform them into powerful host defenders.[115] These changes allow rolling along the endothelial lining of postcapillary venules, migration toward the site of inflammation, adherence to the endothelium, migration through the endothelium to tissue sites, ingestion, killing, and digestion of invading organisms.[115]

Neutrophils migrate to sites of infection along gradients of chemoattractant mediators. An acute inflammatory stimulus leads to the accumulation of neutrophils along the endothelium of postcapillary venules.[33] The major molecules involved in this process are adhesion molecules, chemoattractants, and chemokines. Loose adhesions between neutrophils and endothelium are made and broken, resulting in the slow movement of leukocytes along endothelium and a more intense exposure of neutrophils to activating factors. Chemotaxis requires responses involving actin polymerization–depolymerization adhesion events mediated by integrins and involving microfilament–membrane interactions.[29] All leukocytes including lymphocytes localize infection using these same mediators. Colchicine depolymerizes microfilaments, causing the dissolution of the fibrillar microtubules in granulocytes and other motile cells, impairing this response.

Opsonized particles, immune complexes, and chemotactic factors activate neutrophils in tissues by binding to cell surface receptors. The neutrophil makes tight contact with its target, and the plasma membrane surrounds the organism completely enclosing it. Two mechanisms are then responsible for the destruction of the organism: the oxygen-dependent respiratory burst and the oxygen-independent response involving cationic enzymes found in cytoplasmic granules. The respiratory burst is caused by an NADPH oxidase complex that assembles at the phagosomal membrane. Electrons are transferred from cytoplasmic NADPH to oxygen on the phagosomal side of the membrane, generating superoxide, hydrogen peroxide, hydroxyl radical, singlet oxygen, hypochlorous acid, chloramines, nitric oxide, and peroxynitrite.[67] Cytoplasmic granules within the neutrophil fuse with the phagosome and empty their contents into it. There are at least four different classes of granules.[67] The components of these granules include myeloperoxidase (MPO), elastase, lipases, metalloproteinases, and a pool of CD11b/CD18 proteins required for adhesion and migration.[149] Finally, the phagocytized organism is digested and eliminated by the neutrophil. Overstimulation of this complex and highly regulated but somewhat non-specific system can at times become deleterious, as is postulated to occur with reperfusion injury or carbon monoxide poisoning, to cite two examples.[179,188] Vasculitis and the systemic inflammatory response syndrome are further examples of excessive activation of the innate response.

NEUTROPENIA AND AGRANULOCYTOSIS

Neutropenia is a reduction in circulating neutrophils at least two standard deviations below the norm, but the threshold of $1500/mm^3$ ($1.5 \times 10^9/L$) is often used instead.[75] Severe neutropenia is termed *agranulocytosis,* and is generally defined to be an absolute neutrophil count of less than $500/mm^3$ ($0.5 \times 10^9/L$). Neutropenia can result from decreased production, increased destruction or retention of neutrophils in the various storage pools. Their high rate of turnover renders neutrophils vulnerable to any xenobiotic that inhibits cellular reproduction. As such, the various antineoplastic xenobiotics including antimetabolites, alkylating agents and antimitotics will predictably cause neutropenia. This predictable, dose-dependent reaction represents an important dose-limiting adverse effect of therapy. On the other hand, a number of xenobiotics are implicated in idiosyncratic neutropenia.[7,8] The parent drug or a metabolite usually act as a hapten to trigger antineutrophil antibodies. Table 24–4 provides an abbreviated list.[139,176] A recent

TABLE 24–4. Selected Causes of Idiosyncratic Drug-Induced Agranulocytosis

Anticonvulsants	Antipsychotics
Carbamazepine	Clozapine*
Phenytoin	Phenothiazines
Antiinflammatory agents	Antithyroid agents
Aminopyrine	Methimazole*
Ibuprofen	Propylthiouracil*
Indomethacin	Cardiovascular agents
Phenylbutazone	Hydralazine
Antimicrobials	Lidocaine
β-Lactams, including penicillin G*	Procainamide*
Cephalosporins	Quinidine
Chloramphenicol	Ticlopidine*
Dapsone*	Vesnarinone
Ganciclovir	Diuretics
Isoniazid	Acetazolamide
Rifampicin	Hydrochlorothiazide
Sulfonamides	Hypoglycemics
Vancomycin	Chlorpropamide
Antirheumatics	Tolbutamide
Gold salts	Sedative-hypnotics
Levamisole[197]	Barbiturates
Penicillamine	Flurazepam
Sulfasalazine*	Other
	Deferiprone

*denotes at least 10 cases reported[6]

systematic review of published case reports identified a small subset of xenobiotics (denoted by an asterisk in the table) which were implicated in at least 10 cases and which account for the majority of reports deemed definitely or probably drug-induced. [6]

EOSINOPHILIA

Eosinophils are primarily responsible for protecting against parasitic infection. Allergic reactions and malignancies such as lymphoma are also common causes of eosinophilia, especially where nematode infection is rare.[155] Eosinophils bind to antigen-specific IgE, and discharge their large granules which contain major basic protein, peroxidase, and eosinophil-derived neurotoxin onto the surface of the antibody-coated organism. Two unusual toxicologic outbreaks were characterized by eosinophilia, acute cough, fever, and pulmonary infiltrates, followed by severe myalgia, neuropathy, and eosinophilia. The first outbreak, called the toxic oil syndrome, took place in central Spain in 1981, when industrial-use rapeseed oil denatured with 2% aniline was fraudulently sold as olive oil by door-to-door salesmen.[58] The precise causative agent remains uncertain, but may include fatty acid esters of 3-(*N*-phenylamino)-1,2-propanediol.[58] The second outbreak, called the eosinophilia-myalgia syndrome, occurred during 1988 and 1989 in users of L-tryptophan supplements traced back to a single wholesaler in Japan.[10] The causative contaminant has not been identified, but is believed to have been present in only trace quantities in the L-tryptophan purified from microbial culture. Both syndromes appear to be mediated by immunologic mechanisms.

LEUKEMIA

The leukemias represent the malignant, unregulated proliferation of hematopoietic cells. Although monoclonal in origin, they affect all cell lines derived from the progenitor cell. Acute myeloid leukemia (AML) and the myelodysplastic syndromes are the most common leukemias associated with xenobiotics. The long-recognized association between AML and occupational benzene exposure, radiation, or treatment with alkylating antineoplastic agents has helped to advance understanding of the molecular mechanisms underlying leukemogenesis.[22] The necessary events are believed to involve several sequential genetic and epigenetic alterations, as evidenced by a distinct pattern of chromosomal deletions preceding the development of AML.[80,81] Other recognized xenobiotics that can cause leukemia include topoisomerase II inhibitors, 1,3-butanediol, styrol, ethylene oxide, and vinyl chloride.[92] In many cases, the latency period between exposure and illness is prolonged. For example, leukemia linked to benzene is preceded by several months of anemia, neutropenia, and thrombocytopenia. Benzene or other petroleum products are not believed to cause multiple myeloma.[22]

HEMOSTASIS

In the absence of pathology, blood remains in a fluid form with cells in suspension. Injury triggers coagulation and thrombosis. The resulting clot formation, retraction, and dissolution involve an interaction between the vessel endothelium, soluble constituents of the coagulation system, and proteins located on and within platelets. Platelets respond to signals within their immediate environment and from injured components of the distant microcirculation. A dynamic balance must be maintained between coagulation and fibrinolysis to maintain the integrity of the circulatory system (Fig. 24–4).

COAGULATION

Two basic pathways termed *intrinsic* and *extrinsic* are involved in the initiation of coagulation. Activation of the intrinsic system occurs when blood is exposed to tissue factor in damaged blood vessels or on the surface of activated leukocytes. Tissue factor binds factor VIIa, forming the intrinsic tenase complex, which activates factors IX and X. Factor IXa binds to the surface of activated platelets together with VIIIa and calcium, forming the extrinsic tenase complex. Factor X, which is activated by extrinsic and intrinsic tenase, binds to factor Va on the surface of activated platelets, forming the prothrombinase complex. The prothrombinase complex activates prothrombin, which results in the generation of thrombin activity. Thrombin activates platelets, promotes its own generation by activation of factors V, VIII, and XI, and converts fibrinogen to fibrin (Chap. 59).[72]

XENOBIOTIC-INDUCED DEFECTS IN COAGULATION

Warfarin The recognition of a hemorrhagic disease in cattle in the 1920s and the isolation of the causative agent dicoumarol from spoiled sweet clover in the 1940s resulted in the development of the warfarin-type anticoagulants (Chap. 59). This group of anticoagulants indirectly

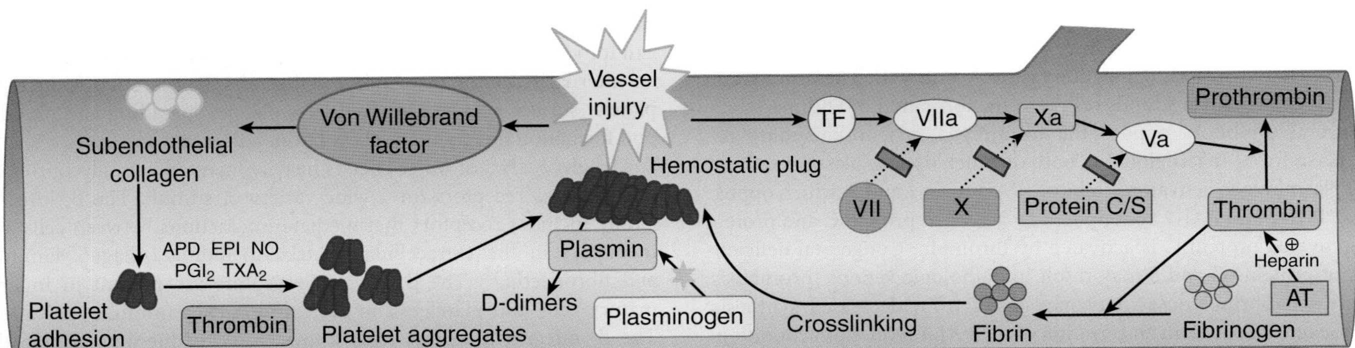

FIGURE 24–4. The general relationships between thrombosis, coagulation, and fibrinolysis. Although these pathways are shown independently, they are intricately linked as outlined in the text. Von Willebrand factor stabilizes factor VIII and platelets on the surface of exposed endothelium. The star indicates that plasminogen is activated by t-PA, which itself is inhibited by plasminogen activator inhibitor (PAI; not shown). Recombinant t-PA (rt-PA) is commercially available. (▬) indicate inhibition; ⊕ denotes activation of catalytic activity. For a more detailed version, see Figure 59–1. AT = antithrombin; t-PA = tissue plasminogen activator.

inhibits hepatic synthesis of coagulation factors II, VII, IX, X, and proteins C and S.[140] Hepatic γ-carboxylation of glutamic acid residues by vitamin K-dependent carboxylase results in the formation of the vitamin K-dependent clotting factors. Vitamin K must be available in its reduced form, vitamin K quinol, to effectively catalyze this reaction. The carboxylation reaction oxidizes vitamin K quinol to vitamin $K^{2,3}$ epoxide, which must be reduced to vitamin K by reductase enzymes. The warfarin anticoagulants inhibit the reductase that is responsible for the regeneration of vitamin K quinone from vitamin K epoxide, impairing the synthesis of the vitamin K-dependent proteins.[95,171]

Heparin Heparin is a highly sulfated glycosaminoglycan that is normally present in tissues. Commercial unfractionated heparin is either bovine or porcine in origin, and consists of a mixture of polysaccharides with molecular weights ranging from 4000–30,000 Da. It is used extensively for the prophylaxis and treatment of venous thrombosis and thromboembolism. It is ineffective orally. This same property makes it safe for use during pregnancy because heparin cannot cross the placenta.[157] The anticoagulant activity of heparin is through its catalytic activation of antithrombin III. Antithrombin III acts as a suicide inhibitor of the serine proteases thrombin and factors IXa, Xa, XIa and XIIa.[126]

The low-molecular-weight heparins (LMWHs) have a mean molecular weight of 4000–6000 Da.[72] The pharmacokinetics and bioavailability of the LMWHs are more predictable, eliminating the need for close monitoring. They exhibit lower protein binding and a longer half-life than unfractionated heparin, making them more convenient to use.[126]

Other anticoagulants Heparinoids are glycosaminoglycans not derived from heparin with anticoagulant effects. This class includes dermatan sulfate, which activates the thrombin inhibitor heparin cofactor II, and danaparoid sodium, which inhibits factor Xa. Fondaparinux is a synthetic pentasaccharide that also inhibits factor Xa, and therefore acts upstream of thrombin. Several direct thrombin inhibitors are also in clinical use, including lepirudin, argatroban, bivalirudin, and dabigatran. These agents prolong the activated partial thromboplastin time and whole-blood activated clotting time, but also affect the INR.

FIBRINOLYSIS

The coagulation system is opposed by three major inhibitory systems. Components of the fibrinolytic system circulate as zymogens, activators, inhibitors, and cofactors.[51] Plasminogen can be activated to plasmin by an intrinsic pathway involving factor XII, prekallikrein, and high-molecular-weight kininogen. This produces the degradation products and fibrin monomers that are found in disseminated intravascular coagulation. The extrinsic pathway involves the release of tissue plasminogen activator (t-PA) from tissues and urokinase plasminogen activator (u-PA) from secretions.[51] Once activated, plasmin can degrade fibrinogen, fibrin, and coagulation factors V and VIII. The degradation of cross-linked fibrin strands results in the formation of D-dimers.

Several inhibitors oppose the fibrinolytic system, including α_2-antiplasmin, α_2-macroglobulin, both of which oppose plasmin activity, and plasminogen activator inhibitor (PAI) types 1 and 2, which oppose t-PA. PAI-1 and PAI-2 are opposed by activated protein C and protein S. Activated protein C is activated by thrombin. Congenital deficiencies of proteins C and S may result in pathologic venous thrombosis. Decreased fibrinolytic activity may result from decreased synthesis, release of t-PA, or from an elevation of the PAI-1 level. Both conditions have been observed postoperatively, with the use of oral contraceptives, in the third trimester of pregnancy, and in obesity. The activity of α_2-antiplasmin and α_2-macroglobulin are increased in pulmonary fibrosis, malignancy, infection, and myocardial infarction, and in thromboembolic disease.[51]

TABLE 24–5. Xenobiotics which impair Fibrinolysis

Antineoplastics
Anthracyclines
L-Asparaginase
Methotrexate
Mithramycin
Antifibrinolytics
Aminocaproic acid
Aprotinin
Desmopressin
Tranexamic acid
Coagulation factors
Cytokines
Erythropoietin
Thrombopoietin
Hormones, including conjugated estrogens

XENOBIOTIC-INDUCED DEFECTS IN FIBRINOLYSIS.

Table 24–5 lists xenobiotics associated with an acquired defect of fibrinolysis. The antitumor agents may result in a reduction in serine protease inhibitors such as antithrombin. L-Asparaginase is associated with a reduction in circulating t-PA levels. Methotrexate can damage vascular endothelium, which may trigger thrombosis (Chap. 53).[51] Hemostatic drugs used therapeutically include the synthetic lysine derivatives aminocaproic acid and tranexamic acid, which bind reversibly to plasminogen; the bovine protease inhibitor aprotinin, which inhibits kallikrein; the vasopressin analog desmopressin, which increases plasma concentrations of factor VIII and vWF; and conjugated estrogens, which normalize bleeding times in uremia.[111]

PLATELETS

In the resting state, platelets maintain a discoid shape. The platelet membrane is a typical trilaminal membrane with glycoproteins, glycolipids, and cholesterol embedded in a phospholipid bilayer. The plasma membrane is in direct continuity with a series of channels, the surface-connected canalicular system (SCCS), which is sometimes referred to as the open canalicular system. The SCCS provides a route of entry and exit for various molecules, a storage pool for platelet glycoproteins, and an internal reservoir of membrane that may be recruited to increase platelet surface area.[133] This facilitates platelet spreading and pseudopod formation during the process of cell adhesion.

The glycocalyx, or outer coat, is heavily invested with glycoproteins that serve as receptors for a wide variety of stimuli. The β_1-integrin family includes receptors that mediate interactions between cells and mediators in the extracellular matrix, including collagen, laminin, and fibronectin.[169] The β_2-integrin receptors are present in inflammatory cells and platelets and are important in immune activation. The β_3-integrin receptors (also known as cytoadhesins) include the glycoprotein (GP) IIb-IIIa fibrinogen receptor, as well as vitronectin.[72] Vitronectin has binding sites for other integrins, collagen, heparin, and components of complement. All of the integrins are active in the process of platelet adhesion to surfaces. Platelet aggregation is mediated by the GP IIb-IIIa receptors.[72]

The submembrane region contains actin filaments that stabilize the platelets' discoid shape and are involved in the formation and stabilization of pseudopods. They also generate the force needed for the movement of receptor-ligand complexes from the outer plasma membrane to the SCCS. These mobile receptors are important in the spreading of platelets on surfaces, and for binding fibrin strands and other platelets. Platelet cytoplasm contains three types of membrane bound secretory granules.[72] The α granules contain β-thromboglobulin, which mediates inflammation, binds and inactivates heparin, and blocks the endothelial release of prostacyclin. In addition, platelet factor-4, which inactivates heparin, and fibrinogen are contained within the α granules. Dense granules store adenine nucleotides, serotonin, and calcium, which are secreted during the release reaction. Platelet lysosomes contain hydrolytic enzymes. Stimulation by platelet agonists causes the granules to fuse with the channels of the SCCS, driving the contents out of the platelets and into the surrounding media.

Platelet adhesion In the vessel wall, collagen, von Willebrand factor (vWF), and fibronectin are the adhesive proteins that play the most prominent role in the adhesion of platelets to vascular subendothelium.[169] On the exposure of collagen (eg, following a laceration or the rupture of an atherosclerotic plaque), platelet adhesion is triggered. Under conditions of high shear (flowing blood), platelet adhesion is mediated by the binding of GP Ib-V-IX receptors on platelet membranes to vWF in the vascular subendothelium.[72,169] Following adherence of platelets to subendothelial vWF, a conformational change in GP IIb-IIIa on platelet membrane occurs, activating this receptor complex to ligate vWF and fibrinogen. The result is the amplification of platelet adhesion and aggregation. An important interaction occurs between thrombosis and inflammation. Platelet-activating factor is synthesized and coexpressed with P-selectin on the surface of the endothelium in response to mediators such as hista-mine or thrombin. Platelet-activating factor interacts with a receptor on the surface of neutrophils that activates the CD11/CD18 adhesion complex, and results in adhesion of neutrophils to endothelium and to platelets. This results in the synthesis of leukotrienes and other mediators of inflammation.

Platelet activation Thrombin, collagen, and epinephrine can activate platelets. In response to thrombin, granules fuse with each other and with elements of the SCCS to form secretory vesicles.[133] These vesicles are believed to fuse with the surface membrane, releasing their contents into the surrounding medium. The membranes of the secretory granules become incorporated into the platelet surface membrane.

Platelet aggregation Following activation, GP IIb-IIIa is expressed in active form on platelet surface, serving as the final common pathway for platelet aggregation regardless of inciting stimulus. This receptor binds exogenous calcium and fibrinogen. GP IIb-IIIa ligates fibrinogen along with fibronectin, vitronectin, and vWF, resulting in the binding of platelets to other platelets, and ultimately the formation of the platelet plug. Collagen-induced platelet aggregation is mediated by adenosine diphosphate (ADP) and thromboxane A_2. ADP binds to the metabotropic purine receptors P2Y1 and P2Y12, leading to transient and sustained aggregation, respectively.[56] Thromboxane A_2 is formed from arachidonic acid by the action of cyclooxygenase 1. It is a potent vasoconstrictor and inducer of platelet aggregation and release reactions.[72] Platelets participate in triggering the coagulation cascade by binding coagulation factors II, VII, IX, and X to membrane phospholipid, a calcium-dependent process.

ANTIPLATELET AGENTS

Aspirin Aspirin inhibits prostaglandin H synthase (cyclooxygenase [COX]) by irreversibly acetylating a serine residue at the active site of the enzyme. Aspirin inhibition of the COX-1 isoform of this enzyme is 100–150 times more potent than its inhibition of the COX-2 isoform. The inhibition of COX-1 results in the irreversible inhibition of thromboxane A_2 formation. Because platelets can be activated by other mechanisms including thrombin, thrombosis can develop despite aspirin therapy (Chap. 35).[163]

Selective COX-2 inhibitors Platelets express primarily COX-1 and use it to produce mostly thromboxane A_2, which leads to platelet aggregation and vasoconstriction. Endothelial cells express COX-2 and use it to produce prostaglandin I_2, an inhibitor of platelet aggregation and a vasodilator. Whereas aspirin and traditional (nonselective) nonsteroidal antiinflammatory medications inhibit the production of thromboxane A_2 and prostaglandin I_2 at both sites, the selective COX-2 inhibitors do not affect platelet derived thromboxane A_2, perhaps accounting for the increase in cardiovascular events associated with long-term use of some of these xenobiotics.[43,89,100,110,172,185]

GP IIb-IIIa antagonists The GP IIb-IIIa antagonist abciximab is a chimeric human-murine monoclonal antibody that binds the GP IIb-IIIa receptor of platelets and megakaryocytes. Two synthetic ligand-mimetic antagonists have also been developed: eptifibatide and tirofiban. These parenteral agents are used primarily in patients undergoing percutaneous coronary interventions.[72] By blocking the fibrogen binding site of IIb-IIIa, platelet aggregation is blocked and even reversed regardless of the inciting activation. Reversible thrombocytopenia can occur within hours of initiation of these xenobiotics.[156]

Thienopyridines The prodrugs clopidogrel and ticlopidine antagonize ADP-mediated platelet aggregation by noncompetitive inhibition of ADP binding to the P2Y12 receptor.[137,147] Both prodrugs are associated with thrombotic thrombocytopenic purpura, as well as neutropenia and aplastic anemia.[17,19,134,135,147]

Dipyridamole The pyrimidopyrimidine derivative dipyridamole inhibits cyclic nucleotide phosphodiesterase in platelets, resulting in the accumulation of cyclic adenosine monophosphate and perhaps cyclic guanine monophosphate.

XENOBIOTIC-INDUCED THROMBOCYTOPENIA

Multiple drugs are reported to cause thrombocytopenia, either via the formation of drug-dependent antiplatelet antibodies or as thrombotic thrombocytopenic purpura. Drug-induced platelet antibodies are estimated to occur in 1 in 100,000 drug exposures. Reversible drug binding to platelet epitopes such as GP Ib-V-IX, GP IIb-IIIa, and platelet–endothelial cell adhesion molecule-1, lead to a structural change that can form or expose a neoepitope target for antibody formation.[11,152] The presence of the drug is required for antibody binding and increased platelet destruction, but there is no covalent bond (as occurs in the hapten model of penicillin binding to the erythrocyte membrane).

Thrombocytopenia can also occur as a result of spurious clumping, pregnancy, hypersplenism with cirrhosis, idiopathic thrombocytopenic purpura, heparin-induced thrombocytopenia (Chap. 59), bone marrow toxicity, and thrombotic thrombocytopenic purpura. After excluding these conditions and nontherapeutic exposures, a systematic literature search updated annually lists more than 1000 cases reported in English involving more than 150 xenobiotics.[1] Table 24–6 lists the xenobiotics appearing in multiple cases satisfying criteria for probable to definite causality including drug rechallenge. Nevertheless, a common clinical problem is to distinguish drug-induced thrombocytopenia from idiopathic thrombocytopenic purpura in a patient on multiple medications who develops thrombocytopenia. In the absence of validated laboratory assays for drug-dependent platelet antibodies other than heparin, diagnosis still depends on the clinical course following drug discontinuation and perhaps rechallenge. Large databases provide

TABLE 24–6. Xenobiotics Reported to Cause Thrombocytopenia as a Result of Antiplatelet Antibodies[a]

Abciximab	Indinavir
Acetaminophen	Levamisole
Aminoglutethimide	Linezolid
Aminosalicylic acid	Meclofenamic acid
Amiodarone	Nalidixic acid
Amphotericin B	Orbofiban
Carbamazepine	Oxprenolol
Cimetidine	Phenytoin
Danazol	Piperacillin
Diclofenac	Procainamide
Digoxin	Quinidine
Dipyridamole	Quinine
Eptifibatide	Rifampin
Famotidine	Tirofiban
Furosemide	Trimethoprim-sulfamethoxazole
Gold salts	Valproate
Heparin	Vancomycin
Imipenem-cilastatin	

[a]Xenobiotics reported in at least 2 cases to have definitely caused immune thrombocytopenia, or in at least 5 cases to have probably caused immune thrombocytopenia following therapeutic use.

Data adapted from George JN, Raskob GE, Shah SR, et al: Drug-induced thrombocytopenia: A systematic review of published case reports. Ann Intern Med 1998;129:886–890; Li X, Swisher KK, Vesely SK, George JN: Drug-induced thrombocytopenia: an updated systematic review. Drug Safety 2007;30:185–186 and http://w3.ouhsc.edu/platelets. Accessed January 12, 2009.

some guidance regarding past reported experience.[1,59,106,151] Severe (< 20,000 platelets/mm^3), or acute transient thrombocytopenia are more likely to be drug-induced.[14]

In patients administered the sensitizing agent de novo, 5 to 7 days are typically required for the development of the immune response. During rechallenge, thrombocytopenia can develop within 12 hours.[14] Interestingly, the unique ability of GP IIb/IIIa inhibitors such as abciximab to cause thrombocytopenia within hours of first use suggests the presence of preformed antibodies directed against platelet epitopes, perhaps accounting for ex vivo clumping of platelets observed in each of approximately 500 normal patients.[152] Clinically, fever, chills, pruritus, and lethargy may occur. The onset of life-threatening bleeding may be abrupt. Hemorrhagic vesicles may be seen in the oral mucosa. Laboratory investigations will demonstrate an absence of platelets on peripheral smear, prolongation of the bleeding time, deficient clot retraction, and an abnormal prothrombin consumption test. Bone marrow aspiration will demonstrate normal or increased numbers of megakaryocytes and immature forms. Treatment includes the transfusion of blood products, glucocorticoids, and the withdrawal of the offending agent.[14]

Thrombotic thrombocytopenic purpura Thrombotic thrombocytopenic purpura (TTP) is characterized by the triad of microangiopathic hemolytic anemia, severe thrombocytopenia, and fluctuating neurologic abnormalities.[124] Fever and renal dysfunction are also common, although overt renal failure is rare. The hallmark is the presence of platelet aggregates throughout the microvasculature, without fibrin clot, unlike the fibrin-rich thrombi seen in disseminated intravascular coagulation or the hemolytic uremic syndrome. In the acquired form, drug-induced autoantibodies inactivate a circulating zinc metalloprotease ADAMTS13, thereby blocking its ability to depolymerize large multimers of vWF and leading to platelet clumping.[11,12,17,186] Plasma exchange with fresh frozen plasma replensishes ADAMTS13 and removes the inhibitory antibodies. Prior to understanding of the molecular mechanism, other causes of microvascular hemolysis with thrombocytopenia were often confused with TTP. These causes included hemolytic uremic syndrome due to shiga toxin, the HELLP syndrome of pregnancy, Rocky Mountain spotted fever, and paroxysmal nocturnal hemoglobinuria. Also included were cases secondary to xenobiotics such as cyclosporine, cocaine, gemcitabine, mitomycin C and cisplatin, in which ADAMTS13 antibodies are not present.[48,186]

Heparin-induced thrombocytopenia An immune response to heparin, manifested clinically by the development of thrombocytopenia and, at times, venous thrombosis, is now recognized to result from antibodies to a complex of heparin and platelet factor 4.[4] The diagnosis is confirmed by testing for these antibodies. The heparin–platelet factor 4 antibody complex can directly activate platelets, and is believed to be the mechanism for the paradoxical thrombosis associated with this condition, which can be limb- or life-threatening[96] (Chap. 59).

SUMMARY

The mechanisms of toxic injury to the blood are extremely varied, reflecting the complexity of this vital fluid. The response to injury may be idiosyncratic, as in many xenobiotic-related causes of agranulocytosis and aplastic anemia, or predictable, as in the case of significant exposures to ionizing radiation or to benzene. Injury may depend on the presence of certain host factors, such as G6PD deficiency. Xenobiotics may directly injure mature cells, or prohibit their development by injuring the stem cell pool. Toxicity may result from the amplification of a potentially therapeutic intervention, such as occurs with many chemotherapeutic agents and anticoagulants. A common theme in hematologic toxicity is the perturbation of homeostatic equilibria that exist between cell proliferation and apoptosis, between immune activation and suppression, or between thrombophilia and thrombolysis. An improved awareness of these complex pathways allows the toxicologist to better understand, diagnose, and treat toxic injury to the blood.

ACKNOWLEDGMENT

Dr. Diane Sauter contributed to this chapter in previous editions.

REFERENCES

1. Glucose-6-phosphate dehydrogenase deficiency. WHO Working Group. *Bull World Health Organ.* 1989; 67(6):601-611.
2. Adamson J. Erythropoietin, iron metabolism, and red blood cell production. *Semin Hematol.* 1996; 33:5-9.
3. Adamson JW. Regulation of red blood cell production. *Am J Med.* 1996;101(Suppl:2A):4S-6S.
4. Alberio L. Heparin-induced thrombocytopenia: some working hypotheses on pathogenesis, diagnostic strategies and treatment. *Curr Opin Hematol.* 2008;15(5):456-464.

5. Altuntas Y, Innice M, Basturk T, et al. Rhabdomyolysis and severe haemolytic anaemia, hepatic dysfunction and intestinal osteopathy due to hypophosphataemia in a patient after Billroth II gastrectomy. *Eur J Gastroenterol Hepatol.* 2002;14(5):555-557.
6. Andersohn F, Konzen C, Garbe E. Systematic review: agranulocytosis induced by nonchemotherapy drugs. *Ann Intern Med.* 2007;146(9):657-665.
7. Andres E, Maloisel F. Idiosyncratic drug-induced agranulocytosis or acute neutropenia. *Curr Opin Hematol.* 2008;15(1):15-21.
8. Andres E, Noel E, Kurtz JE, et al. Life-threatening idiosyncratic drug-induced agranulocytosis in elderly patients. *Drugs & Aging.* 2004;21(7):427-435.
9. Andrews NC. Understanding heme transport. *N Engl J Med.* 2005;353(23):2508-2509.
10. Armstrong C, Lewis T, D'Esposito M, Freundlich B. Eosinophilia-myalgia syndrome: selective cognitive impairment, longitudinal effects, and neuroimaging findings. *J Neurol Neurosurg Psychiatry.* 1997;63(5):633-641.
11. Aster RH. Drug-induced immune thrombocytopenia: an overview of pathogenesis. *Semin Hematol.* 1999;36(1 Suppl 1):2-6.
12. Aster RH. Thrombotic thrombocytopenic purpura (TTP)–an enigmatic disease finally resolved? *Trends Mol Med.* 2002;8(1):1-3.
13. Aster RH. Drug-induced immune cytopenias. *Toxicology* 2005; 209(2):149-153.
14. Aster RH, Bougie DW. Drug-induced immune thrombocytopenia. *N Engl J Med.* 2007; 357(6):580-587.
15. Bakemeier RF, Leddy JD. Erythrocyte autoantibody associated with alpha-methyldopa: Heterogeneity of structure and specificity. *Blood.* 1968;32:1-14.
16. Beaupre SR, Schiffman FJ. Rush hemolysis. A 'bite-cell' hemolytic anemia associated with volatile liquid nitrite use. *Arch Fam Med.* 1994; 3(6):545-548.
17. Bennett CL, Connors JM, Carwile JM, et al. Thrombotic thrombocytopenic purpura associated with clopidogrel. *N Engl J Med.* 2000; 342(24):1773-1777.
18. Bennett CL, Cournoyer D, Carson KR, et al. Long-term outcome of individuals with pure red cell aplasia and antierythropoietin antibodies in patients treated with recombinant epoetin: a follow-up report from the Research on Adverse Drug Events and Reports (RADAR) Project. *Blood.* 2005;106(10):3343-3347.
19. Bennett CL, Weinberg PD, Rozenberg-Ben-Dror K, et al. Thrombotic thrombocytopenic purpura associated with ticlopidine. A review of 60 cases. *Ann Intern Med.* 1998;128(7):541-544.
20. Bennett CL, Luminari S, Nissenson AR, et al. Pure Red-Cell Aplasia and Epoetin Therapy. *N Engl J Med.* 2004;351(14):1403-1408.
21. Bennett V. Spectrin-based membrane skeleton: a multipotential adaptor between plasma membrane and cytoplasm. *Physiol Rev.* 1990;70(4):1029-1065.
22. Bergsagel DE, Wong O, Bergsagel PL, et al. Benzene and multiple myeloma: appraisal of the scientific evidence. *Blood.* 1999;94(4):1174-1182.
23. Berzofsky JA, Peisach J, Blumberg WE. Sulfheme proteins. I. Optical and magnetic properties of sulfmyoglobin and its derivatives. *J Biol Chem.* 1971;246(10):3367-3377.
24. Beutler E. Glucose-6-phosphate dehydrogenase deficiency. *N Engl J Med.* 1991;324(3):169-174.
25. Beutler E. G6PD deficiency. *Blood.* 1994;84(11):3613-3636.
26. Beutler E, Dern RJ, Alving AS. The hemolytic effect of primaquine. IV. The relationship of cell age to hemolysis. *J Lab Clin Med.* 1954;44(3):439-442.
27. Beutler E, Vulliamy TJ. Hematologically important mutations: glucose-6-phosphate dehydrogenase. *Blood Cells Mol Dis.* 2002;28(2):93-103.
28. Bogart L, Bonsignore J, Carvalho A. Massive hemolysis following inhalation of volatile nitrites. *Am J Hematol.* 1986;22(3):327-329.
29. Bokoch GM. Chemoattractant signaling and leukocyte activation. *Blood.* 1995;86:1649-1660.
30. Bradberry SM. Occupational methaemoglobinaemia. Mechanisms of production, features, diagnosis and management including the use of methylene blue. *Tox Rvws.* 2003;22(1):13-27.
31. Brandes JC, Bufill JA, Pisciotta AV. Amyl nitrite-induced hemolytic anemia. *Am J Med.* 1989;86(2):252-254.
32. Brodsky RA. Biology and management of acquired severe aplastic anemia. *Curr Opin Oncol.* 1998;10:95-99.
33. Brown E. Neutrophil adhesion and the therapy of inflammation. *Semin Hematol.* 1997;34:319-326.
34. Brown KR, Carter W, Jr., Lombardi GE. Recombinant erythropoietin overdose. *Am J Emerg Med.* 1993;11(6):619-621.
35. Bryder D, Rossi DJ, Weissman IL. Hematopoietic stem cells: the paradigmatic tissue-specific stem cell. *Am J Pathol.* 2006;169(2):338-346.
36. Bull BS. The biconcavity of the red cell: An analysis of several hypotheses. *Blood.* 1973;41:833-844.
37. Bulliamy T, Luzzatto L, Hirono A, Beutler E. Hematologically important mutations: glucose-6-phosphate dehydrogenase. *Blood Cells Mol Dis.* 1997;23(2):302-313.
38. Bulmer FMR, Rothwell HE, Polack SS, et al. Chronic arsine poisoning among workers employed in the cyanide extraction of gold: A report of fourteen cases. *J Ind Hygiene Tox.* 1940;22:111-124.
39. Cappellini MD, Tavazzi D, Duca L, et al. Metabolic indicators of oxidative stress correlate with haemichrome attachment to membrane, band 3 aggregation and erythrophagocytosis in beta-thalassaemia intermedia. *Br J Haematol.* 1999;104(3):504-512.
40. Cartron JP. Defining the Rh blood group antigens. *Biochem Mol Gen.* 1994;8:199-212.
41. Casadevall N, Nataf J, Viron B et al. Pure red-cell aplasia and antierythropoietin antibodies in patients treated with recombinant erythropoietin. *N Engl J Med.* 2002;346(7):469-475.
42. Chanutin A, Curnish RR. Effect of organic and inorganic phosphates on the oxygen equilibrium of human erythrocytes. *Arch Biochem Biophys.* 1967;121:96-102.
43. Clark DW, Layton D, Shakir SA. Do some inhibitors of COX-2 increase the risk of thromboembolic events? Linking pharmacology with pharmacoepidemiology. *Drug Safety.* 2004;27(7):427-456.
44. Coleman MD, Coleman NA. Drug-induced methaemoglobinaemia. Treatment issues. *Drug Safety.* 1996;14(6):394-405.
45. Critchley JA, Critchley LA, Yeung EA, et al. Granulocyte-colony stimulating factor in the treatment of colchicine poisoning. *Hum Exp Toxicol.* 1997;16(4):229-232.
46. Datta B, Tufnell-Barrett T, Bleasdale RA, et al. Red blood cell nitric oxide as an endocrine vasoregulator: a potential role in congestive heart failure. *Circulation.* 2004;109(11):1339-1342.
47. Davies P. Potassium-chlorate poisoning with oliguria treated by the Bull regime. *Lancet.* 1956;270(6923):612-613.
48. Dlott JS, Danielson CF, Blue-Hnidy DE, McCarthy LJ. Drug-induced thrombotic thrombocytopenic purpura/hemolytic uremic syndrome: a concise review. *Ther Apher.* 2004;8(2):102-111.
49. Dzik WH, Georgi BA, Khettry U, Jenkins RL. Cyclosporine-associated thrombotic thrombocytopenic purpura following liver transplantation—successful treatment with plasma exchange. *Transplantation.* 1987;44(4):570-572.
50. Edwards MS, Curtis JR. Use of cobaltous chloride in anaemia of maintenance hemodialysis patients. *Lancet.* 1971;2(7724):582-583.
51. Fareed J, Hoppensteadt DA, Jeske WP, et al. Acquired defects of fibrinolysis associated with thrombosis. *Semin Thromb Hemost.* 1999;25:367-374.
52. Ferraro-Borgida MJ, Mulhern SA, DeMeo MO, Bayer MJ. Methemoglobinemia from perineal application of an anesthetic cream. *Ann Emerg Med.* 1996; 27(6):785-788.
53. Fincher ME, Campbell HT. Methemoglobinemia and hemolytic anemia after phenazopyridine hydrochloride (Pyridium) administration in end-stage renal disease. *South J Med.* 1989;82(3):372-374.
54. Fowler BA, Weissberg JB. Arsine poisoning. *N Engl J Med.* 1974;291(22): 1171-1174.
55. Funicella T, Weinger RS, Moake JL, et al. Penicillin-induced immunohemolytic anemia associated with circulating immune complexes. *Am J Hematol.* 1977;3:219-223.
56. Gachet C. ADP receptors of platelets and their inhibition. *Thromb Haemost.* 2001;86(1):222-232.
57. Gareau R, Audran M, Baynes RD, et al. Erythropoietin abuse in athletes. *Nature.* 1996;380(6570):113.
58. Gelpi E, de la Paz MP, Terracini B, et al. The Spanish toxic oil syndrome 20 years after its onset: a multidisciplinary review of scientific knowledge. *Environ Health Perspect.* 2002;110(5):457-464.
59. George JN, Raskob GE, Shah SR, et al. Drug-induced thrombocytopenia: a systematic review of published case reports. *Ann Intern Med.* 1998;129(11):886-890.
60. Gibly RL, Walter FG, Nowlin SW, Berg RA. Intravascular hemolysis associated with North American crotalid envenomation. *J Toxicol Clin Toxicol.* 1998;36(4):337-343.
61. Gore CJ, Parisotto R, Ashenden MJ, et al. Second-generation blood tests to detect erythropoietin abuse by athletes. *Haematologica.* 2003;88(3):333-344.

62. Gow AJ, Luchsinger BP, Pawloski JR, et al. The oxyhemoglobin reaction of nitric oxide. *Proc Natl Acad Sci (USA).* 1999;96(16):9027-9032.
63. Graham AF, Crawford TBB, Marian GF. The action of arsine on blood: Observations on the nature of the fixed arsenic. *Biochem J.* 1946;40:256-260.
64. Gregory CA, Prockop DJ, Spees JL. Non-hematopoietic bone marrow stem cells: Molecular control of expansion and differentiation. *Exp Cell Res.* 2005;306(2):330-335.
65. Grosveld F, DeBoer E, Dillon N, et al. The dynamics of globin gene expression and gene therapy vectors. *Ann N Y Acad Sci.* 1998;850:18-27.
66. Haab P. The effect of carbon monoxide on respiration. *Experientia.* 1990;46:1202-1203.
67. Hampton MB, Kettle AJ, Winterbourne CC. Inside the neutrophil phagosome: oxidants, myeloperoxidase, and bacterial killing. *Blood.* 1998;92:3007-3017.
68. Hare JM. Nitroso-redox balance in the cardiovascular system. *N Engl J Med.* 2004;351(20):2112-2114.
69. Harris R, Marx G, Gillett M, et al. Colchicine-induced bone marrow suppression: treatment with granulocyte colony-stimulating factor. *J Emerg Med.* 2000;18(4):435-440.
70. Hatlelid KM, Brailsford C, Carter DE. Reactions of arsine with hemoglobin. *J Toxicol Environ Health.* 1996;47(2):145-157.
71. Hentze MW, Muckenthaler MU, Andrews NC. Balancing acts: molecular control of mammalian iron metabolism. *Cell.* 2004;117(3):285-297.
72. Hirsh J, Weitz I. Thrombosis and anticoagulation. *Semin Hematol.* 1999;36:118-132.
73. Holman MJ, Gonwa TA, Cooper B, et al. FK506-associated thrombotic thrombocytopenic purpura. *Transplantation.* 1993;55(1):205-206.
74. Hsia CC. Respiratory function of hemoglobin. *N Engl J Med.* 1998;338(4):239-247.
75. Hsieh MM, Everhart JE, Byrd-Holt DD, et al. Prevalence of neutropenia in the U.S. population: age, sex, smoking status, and ethnic differences. *Ann Intern Med.* 2007;146(7):486-492.
76. Hulten JO, Tran VT, Pettersson G. The control of haemolysis during transurethral resection of the prostate when water is used for irrigation: monitoring absorption by the ethanol method. *BJU International.* 2000;86(9):989-992.
77. Hultquist DE, Passon PG. Catalysis of methaemoglobinemia reduction by erythrocyte cytochrome B5 and cytochrome B5 reductase. *Nat New Biol.* 1971;229:252-254.
78. Hung DZ, Wu ML, Deng JF, Lin-Shiau SY. Russell's viper snakebite in Taiwan: differences from other Asian countries. *Toxicon.* 2002;40(9):1291-1298.
79. Ichimaru M, Ishimaru T, Tsuchimoto T, Kirshbaum JD. Incidence of aplastic anemia in A-bomb survivors. Hiroshima and Nagasaki, 1946-1967. *Radiat Res.* 1972;49(2):461-72.
80. Irons RD. Molecular models of benzene leukemogenesis. *J Toxicol Environ Health A.* 2000;61(5-6):391-397.
81. Irons RD, Stillman WS. The process of leukemogenesis. *Environ Health Perspect.* 1996;104Suppl6:1239-1246.
82. Issaragrisil S, Kaufman DW, Anderson T, et al. The epidemiology of aplastic anemia in Thailand. *Blood.* 2006;107(4):1299-1307.
83. Iversen PO, Nicolaysen G, Benestad HB. Blood flow to bone marrow during development of anemia or polycythemia in the rat. *Blood.* 1992;79(3):594-601.
84. Iversen PO, Nicolaysen G, Benestad HB. The leukopoietic cytokine granulocyte colony-stimulating factor increases blood flow to rat bone marrow. *Exp Hematol.* 1993;21(2):231-235.
85. Jackson RC, Elder WJ, McDonnell H. Sodium-chlorate poisoning complicated by acute renal failure. *Lancet.* 1961;2:1381-1383.
86. Jefferson JA, Escudero E, Hurtado ME, et al. Excessive erythrocytosis, chronic mountain sickness, and serum cobalt levels. *Lancet.* 2002;359(9304):407-408.
87. Jenkins GC, Ind JE, Kazantzis G, Owen R. Arsine poisoning: Massive haemolysis with minimal impairment of renal function. *BMJ.* 1965;5453:78-80.
88. Jollow DJ, Bradshaw TP, McMillan DC. Dapsone-induced hemolytic anemia. *Drug Metab Rev.* 1995;27(1-2):107-124.
89. Juni P, Nartey L, Reichenbach S, et al. Risk of cardiovascular events and rofecoxib: cumulative meta-analysis. *Lancet.* 2004;364(9450):2021-2029.
90. Kaiser U, Barth N. Haemolytic anaemia in a patient with anorexia nervosa. *Acta Haematologica.* 2001;106(3):133-135.
91. Kaplan JC, Chirouze M. Therapy of recessive congenital methaemoglobinaemia by oral riboflavin. *Lancet.* 1978;2:1043-1044.
92. Karp JE, Smith MA. The molecular pathogenesis of treatment-induced (secondary) leukemias: foundations for treatment and prevention. *Semin Oncol.* 1997;24(1):103-113.
93. Kaushansky K. Thrombopoietin. *N Engl J Med.* 1998;339:746-754.
94. Kaushansky K. Thrombopoietin and hematopoietic stem cell development. *Ann N Y Acad Sci.*1999;872:314-319.
95. Keller C, Matzdorff AC, Kemkes-Matthes B. Pharmacology of warfarin and clinical implications. *Semin Thromb Hemost.* 1999;25:13-16.
96. Kelton JG, Warkentin TE. Heparin-induced thrombocytopenia: a historical perspective. *Blood.* 2008;112(7):2607-2616.
97. Kleinfeld MJ. Arsine poisoning. *J Occup Med.* 1980;22(12):820-821.
98. Knutsen OH, Jansson U. [Hemolysis and pulmonary edema after a near-drowning accident in chlorated water]. *Lakartidningen.* 1988;85(52):4646-4647.
99. Korbling M, Estrov Z. Adult stem cells for tissue repair—a new therapeutic concept? *N Engl J Med.* 2003;349(6):570-582.
100. Krum H, Liew D, Aw J, Haas S. Cardiovascular effects of selective cyclooxygenase-2 inhibitors. *Exp Rev Cardiovasc Ther* 2004;2(2):265-270.
101. Lambert S, Bennett V. From anemia to cerebellar dysfunction. A review of the Ankyrin gene family. *Eur J Biochem.* 1993;211:1-6.
102. Larkin EC, Williams WT, Ulvedal F. Human hematologic responses to 4 hr of isobaric hyperoxic exposure (100 per cent oxygen at 760 mm Hg). *J Appl Physiol.* 1973;34(4):417-421.
103. Lee E, Boorse R, Marcinczyk M. Methemoglobinemia secondary to benzocaine topical anesthetic. *Surg Laparosc Endosc.* 1996;6(6):492-493.
104. Lenard JG. A note on the shape of the erythrocyte. *Bull Math Biol.* 1974;36(1):55-58.
105. Lennard AL, Jackson GH. Stem cell transplantation. *BMJ.* 2000;321(7258):433-437.
106. Li X, Swisher KK, Vesely SK, George JN. Drug-induced thrombocytopenia: an updated systematic review, 2006. *Drug Safety.* 2007;30(2):185-186.
107. Lubash GD, Phillips RE, Shields JD, III, Bonsnes RW. Acute aniline poisoning treated by hemodialysis. Report of a case. *Arch Intern Med.* 1964;114:530-532.
108. Majeti R, Park CY, Weissman IL. Identification of a Hierarchy of Multipotent Hematopoietic Progenitors in Human Cord Blood. *Cell Stem Cell.* 2007;1(6):635-645.
109. Maloisel F, Kurtz JE, Andres E, et al. Platin salts-induced hemolytic anemia: cisplatin- and the first case of carboplatin-induced hemolysis. *Anti-Cancer Drugs.* 1995;6(2):324-326.
110. Mamdani M, Juurlink DN, Lee DS, et al. Cyclo-oxygenase-2 inhibitors versus non-selective non-steroidal anti-inflammatory drugs and congestive heart failure outcomes in elderly patients: a population-based cohort study. *Lancet.* 2004;363(9423):1751-1756.
111. Mannucci PM. Hemostatic drugs. *N Engl J Med.* 1998;339(4):245-253.
112. Mansouri A. Methemoglobin reduction under near physiological conditions. *Biochem Med Metab Biol.* 1989;42(1):43-51.
113. Marschner JP, Seidlitz T, Rietbrock N. Effect of 2,3-diphosphoglycerate on O2-dissociation kinetics of hemoglobin and glycosylated hemoglobin using the stopped flow technique and an improved in vitro method for hemoglobin glycosylation. *Int J Clin Pharmacol Ther.* 1994;32(3):116-121.
114. Mason PJ. New insights into G6PD deficiency. *Br J Haematol.* 1996;94(4):585-591.
115. Matzner Y. Acquired neutrophil dysfunction and diseases with an inflammatory component. *Semin Hematol.* 1997;34:291-302.
116. May BK, Bawden MJ. Control of heme biosynthesis in animals. *Semin Hematol.* 1989;26:150-156.
117. Mayhew TM, Mwamengele GL, Self TJ, Travers JP. Stereological studies on red corpuscle size produce values different from those obtained using haematocrit- and model-based methods. *Br J Haematol.* 1994;86(2):355-360.
118. McKoy JM, Stonecash RE, Cournoyer D, et al. Epoetin-associated pure red cell aplasia: past, present, and future considerations. *Transfusion.* 2008;48(8):1754-1762.
119. McMahon TJ, Moon RE, Luschinger BP, et al. Nitric oxide in the human respiratory cycle. *Nat Med.* 2002;8(7):711-717.
120. Melvin JD, Watts RG. Severe hypophosphatemia: a rare cause of intravascular hemolysis. *Am J Hematol.* 2002;69(3):223-224.
121. Mengel CE, Kann HE, Jr., Heyman A, Metz E. Effects of in vivo hyperoxia on erythrocytes. Ii. Hemolysis in a human after exposure to oxygen under high pressure. *Blood.* 1965;25:822-829.
122. Millar J, Peloquin R, De Leeuw NK. Phenacetin-induced hemolytic anemia. *CMAJ.* 1972; 106(7):770-775.

123. Miyazaki H, Kato T. Thrombopoietin: biology and clinical potentials. *Int J Hematol.* 1999;70:216-225.
124. Moake JL. Thrombotic microangiopathies. *N Engl J Med.* 2002;347(8):589-600.
125. Morell DB, Chang Y. The structure of the chromophore of sulphmyoglobin. *Biochim Biophys Acta.* 1967;136(1):121-130.
126. Mousa SA. Comparative efficacy of different low-molecular-weight heparins (LMWHs) and drug interactions with LMWH: Interactions for management of vascular disorders. *Semin Thromb Hemost.* 2000;26(Suppl1):1-46.
127. Mukherje AK, Ghosal SK, Maity CR. Some biochemical properties of Russell's viper (Daboia russelli) venom from Eastern India: correlation with clinico-pathological manifestation in Russell's viper bite. *Toxicon.* 2000;38(2):163-175.
128. Myint H, Copplestone JA, Orchard J, et al. Fludarabine-related autoimmune haemolytic anaemia in patients with chronic lymphocytic leukaemia. *Br J Haematol.* 1995; 91(2):341-344.
129. Nagel RL, Roth EF Jr. Malaria and red cell genetic defects. *Blood.* 1989;74(4):1213-1221.
130. Nardi NB, Alfonso ZZC. The hematopoietic stroma. *Braz J Med Biol Res.* 1999;32:601-609.
131. Nathan DM, Siegel AJ, Bunn HF. Acute methemoglobinemia and hemolytic anemia with phenazopyridine: possible relation to acute renal failure. *Arch Intern Med.* 1977;137(11):1636-1638.
132. Nimer SD, Ireland P, Meshkinpour A, Frane M. An increased HLA DTR2 frequency is seen in aplastic anemia patients. *Blood.* 1994;84:923-927.
133. Nurden P, Heilman E, Paponneau A, Nurden A. Two-way trafficking of membrane glycoproteins on thrombin-activated human platelets. *Semin Hematol.* 1994;31:240-250.
134. Paradiso-Hardy FL, Angelo CM, Lanctot KL, Cohen EA. Hematologic dyscrasia associated with ticlopidine therapy: evidence for causality. *CMAJ.* 2000;163(11):1441-1448.
135. Paradiso-Hardy FL, Papastergiou J, Lanctot KL, Cohen EA. Thrombotic thrombocytopenic purpura associated with clopidogrel: further evaluation. *Can J Cardiol.* 2002;18(7):771-773.
136. Park CM, Nagel RL. Sulfhemoglobinemia: Clinical and molecular aspects. *N Engl J Med.* 1984;310:1579-1584.
137. Patrono C, Coller B, Dalen JE, et al. Platelet-active drugs : the relationships among dose, effectiveness, and side effects. *Chest.* 2001;119(1Suppl):39S-63S.
138. Petz LD. Drug-induced autoimmune hemolytic anemia. *Transfus Med Rev.* 1993;7(4):242-254.
139. Piga A, Roggero S, Vinciguerra T, et al. Deferiprone: new insight. *Ann NY Acad Sci.* 2005;1054:169-174.
140. Pindur G, Morsdorf S, Schenk JF, et al. The overdosed patient and bleedings with oral anticoagulation. *Semin Thromb Hemost.* 1999;25:85-88.
141. Pinto SS. Arsine poisoning: Evaluation of the acute phase. *J Occup Med.* 1976;18:633-635.
142. Podvinec M, Handschin C, Looser R, Meyer UA. Identification of the xenosensors regulating human 5-aminolevulinate synthase. *Proc Natl Acad Sc U S A.* 2004;101(24):9127-32.
143. Ponka P. Tissue-specific regulation of iron metabolism and heme synthesis: Distinct control mechanisms in erythroid cells. *Blood.* 1997;89:1-25.
144. Ponka P. Cell biology of heme. *Am J Med Sci.* 1999;318:241-256.
145. Ponka P, Beaumont C, Richardson DR. Function and regulation of transferrin and ferritin. *Semin Hematol.* 1998;35:35-54.
146. Provan D, Weatherall D. Red cells II: acquired anaemias and polycythaemia. *Lancet.* 2000;355(9211):1260-1268.
147. Quinn MJ, Fitzgerald DJ. Ticlopidine and clopidogrel. *Circulation.* 1999;100(15):1667-1672.
148. Rael LT, Ayala-Fierro F, Carter DE. The effects of sulfur, thiol, and thiol inhibitor compounds on arsine-induced toxicity in the human erythrocyte membrane. *Toxicol Sci.* 2000;55(2):468-477.
149. Rainger GE, Rowley AF, Nash GB. Adhesion-dependent release from human neutrophils in a novel flow-based model: specificity of different chemotactic agents. *Blood.* 1998;92:4819-4827.
150. Reiter CD, Wang X, Tanus-Santos JE, et al. Cell-free hemoglobin limits nitric oxide bioavailability in sickle-cell disease. *Nat Med.* 2002;8(12):1383-1389.
151. Rizvi MA, Kojouri K, George JN. Drug-induced thrombocytopenia: an updated systematic review. *Ann Intern Med.* 2001;134(4):346.
152. Rizvi MA, Shah SR, Raskob GE, George JN. Drug-induced thrombocytopenia. *Curr Opin Hematol.* 1999;6(5):349-353.
153. Robak T, Blasinska-Morawiec M, Krykowski E, et al. Autoimmune haemolytic anaemia in patients with chronic lymphocytic leukaemia treated with 2-chlorodeoxyadenosine (cladribine). *Eur J Haematol.* 1997;58(2):109-113.
154. Romeril KR, Concannon AJ. Heinz body haemolytic anaemia after sniffing volatile nitrites. *Med J Austral.* 1981;1(6):302-303.
155. Rothenberg ME. Eosinophilia. *N Engl J Med.* 1998;338(22):1592-1600.
156. Said SM, Hahn J, Schleyer E, et al. Glycoprotein IIb/IIIa inhibitor-induced thrombocytopenia: diagnosis and treatment. *Clin Res Cardiol.* 2007;96(2):61-69.
157. Samama MM, Gerotziafas GT. Comparative pharmacokinetics of LMWHs. *Semin Thromb Hemost.* 2000;26(Suppl1):1-38.
158. Savage DG, Ogundipe A, Allen RH, et al. Etiology and diagnostic evaluation of macrocytosis. *Am J Med Sci.* 2000;319(6):343-352.
159. Schafer DA, Cooper JA. Control of actin assembly at filament ends. *Annual Rev Cell Dev Biol.* 1995;11:497-518.
160. Schechter AN, Gladwin MT. Hemoglobin and the paracrine and endocrine functions of nitric oxide. *N Engl J Med.* 2003;348(15):1483-1485.
161. Schmid-Schonbein H, Wells RE Jr. Rheological properties of human erythrocytes and their influence upon the "anomalous" viscosity of blood. *Ergebnisse der Physiologie, Biologischen Chemie und Experimentellen Pharmakologie.* 1971;63:146-219.
162. Schrijvers D. Role of red blood cells in pharmacokinetics of chemotherapeutic agents. *Clin Pharmacokinet.* 2003;42(9):779-791.
163. Schror K. Aspirin and platelets: the antiplatelet action of aspirin and its role in thrombosis and treatment prophylaxis. *Semin Thromb Hemost.* 1997;23:349-356.
164. Shayeghi M, Latunde-Dada GO, Oakhill JS, et al. Identification of an intestinal heme transporter. *Cell.* 2005;122(5):789-801.
165. Shitrit D, Starobin D, Aravot D, et al. Tacrolimus-induced hemolytic uremic syndrome case presentation in a lung transplant recipient. *Trans Pros.* 2003;35(2):627-628.
166. Sills MR, Zinkham WH. Methylene blue-induced Heinz body hemolytic anemia. *Arch Pediatr Adolesc Med.* 1994;148(3):306-310.
167. Singel DJ, Stamler JS. Chemical physiology of blood flow regulation by red blood cells: the role of nitric oxide and S-nitrosohemoglobin. *Annual Rev Physiol.* 2005;67:99-145.
168. Sivilotti MLA. Oxidant stress and hemolysis of the human erythrocyte. *Toxicol Rev.* 2004;23(3):169-188.
169. Sixma J, van Zanten H, Banga JD, et al. Platelet adhesion. *Semin Hematol.* 1995;32:89-98.
170. Sklar GE. Hemolysis as a potential complication of acetaminophen overdose in a patient with glucose-6-phosphate dehydrogenase deficiency. *Pharmacotherapy.* 2002;22(5):656-658.
171. Smith RE. The INR: a perspective. *Semin Thromb Hemost.* 1997;23:547-549.
172. Solomon DH, Schneeweiss S, Glynn RJ, et al. Relationship between selective cyclooxygenase-2 inhibitors and acute myocardial infarction in older adults. *Circulation.* 2004;109(17):2068-2073.
173. Spivak JL. Erythropoietin use and abuse: when physiology and pharmacology collide. *Adv Exp Med Biol.* 2001;502:207-224.
174. Spooren AA, Evelo CT. Hydroxylamine treatment increases glutathione-protein and protein-protein binding in human erythrocytes. *Blood Cells Mol Dis.* 1997;23(3):323-336.
175. Stevenson DK, Vreman HJ. Carbon monoxide and bilirubin production in neonates. *Pediatrics.* 1997;100(2:Pt 1):t-4.
176. Stock W, Hoffman R. White blood cells 1: non-malignant disorders. *Lancet.* 2000;355(9212):1351-1357.
177. Tanner MLA. Molecular and cellular biology of the erythrocyte anion exchanger (AE1). *Semin Hematol.* 1993;30:34-57.
178. Telen MJ. Erythrocyte blood group antigens: polymorphisms of functionally important molecules. *Semin Hematol.* 1996;33(4):302-314.
179. Thom SR. Leukocytes in carbon monoxide-mediated brain oxidative injury. *Toxicol Applied Pharmacol.* 1993;123:234-247.
180. Thompson DF, Gales MA. Drug-induced pure red cell aplasia. *Pharmacotherapy.* 1996;16(6):1002-1008
181. Thunell S, Pomp E, Brun A. Guide to drug porphyrogenicity prediction and drug prescription in the acute porphyrias. *Br J Clin Pharmacol.* 2007;64(5):668-679.
182. Till JE, McCulloch EA. A direct measurement of the radiation sensitivity of normal mouse bone marrow cells. *Radiat Res.* 1961;14:213-222.
183. Tinmouth A, Chin-Yee I. The clinical consequences of the red cell storage lesion. *Transfus Med Rev.* 2001;15(2):91-107.

184. Todisco V, Lamour J, Finberg L. Hemolysis from exposure to naphthalene mothballs. *N Engl J Med.* 1991;325(23):1660-1661.
185. Topol EJ. Arthritis medicines and cardiovascular events—"house of coxibs". *JAMA.* 2005;293(3):366-368.
186. Tsai HM. Current concepts in thrombotic thrombocytopenic purpura. *Annual Rev Med.* 2006;57:419-436.
187. Vandendries ER, Drews RE. Drug-associated disease: hematologic dysfunction. *Crit Care Clin.* 2006;22(2):347-355,viii.
188. VanUffelen BE, de Koster BM, VanStevenink J, et al. Carbon monoxide enhances human neutrophil migration in a cyclic GMP-dependent way. *Biochem Biophys Res Commun.* 1996;226:21-26.
189. Vetter RS, Visscher PK, Camazine S. Mass envenomations by honey bees and wasps. *West J Med.* 1999;170(4):223-227.
190. Ward PC, Schwartz BS, White JG. Heinz-body anemia: "bite cell" variant—a light and electron microscopic study. *Am J Hematol.* 1983;15(2):135-146.
191. Waugh RE, Sassi M. An in vitro model of erythroid egress in bone marrow. *Blood.* 1986;68:250-257.
192. Winski SL, Barber DS, Rael LT, Carter DE. Sequence of toxic events in arsine-induced hemolysis in vitro: implications for the mechanism of toxicity in human erythrocytes. *Fundam Appl Toxicol.* 1997;38(2):123-128.
193. Wright RO, Perry HE, Woolf AD, Shannon MW. Hemolysis after acetaminophen overdose in a patient with glucose-6-phosphate dehydrogenase deficiency. *J Toxicol Clin Toxicol.* 1996;34(6):731-734.
194. Xie W, Uppal H, Saini SP, et al. Orphan nuclear receptor-mediated xenobiotic regulation in drug metabolism. *Drug Discovery Today.* 2004;9(10):442-449.
195. Young NS, Kaufman DW. The epidemiology of acquired aplastic anemia. *Haematologica.* 2008;93(4):489-492.
196. Young NS, Scheinberg P, Calado RT. Aplastic anemia. *Curr Opin Hematol.* 2008;15(3):162-168.
197. Zhu NY, LeGatt DF, Turner AR. Agranulocytosis after consumption of cocaine adulterated with levamisole. *Ann Intern Med.* 2009;0000605-200902170.
198. Zola H, Swart B, Nicholson I, et al. CD molecules 2005: human cell differentiation molecules. *Blood.* 2005;106(9):3123-3126.

CHAPTER 25
GASTROINTESTINAL PRINCIPLES

Richard G. Church and Kavita M. Babu

Humans are constantly in contact with a variety of xenobiotics. The gastrointestinal (GI) tract forms an important initial functional barrier, in addition to its critical role in absorbing nutrients. An understanding of the structure, physiology, and enteric autonomic system is critical to toxicologic concepts of absorption, gastric motility and appreciating the unique vulnerabilities of the GI tract to xenobiotics. This chapter discusses the role of the GI tract and its relation to toxicology. Anatomic, pathologic, and microbiologic principles are discussed, including the role of the GI tract in the metabolism of xenobiotics. Examples of GI pathologies and their clinical manifestations are discussed.

STRUCTURE AND INNERVATION OF THE GASTROINTESTINAL TRACT

The luminal gastrointestinal tract can be divided into five distinct structures: oral cavity and hypopharynx, esophagus, stomach, small intestine, and colon. These environments differ in luminal pH, specific epithelial cell receptors, and endogenous flora. The transitional areas between these distinct organs have specialized epithelia and muscular sphincters with specific functions and vulnerabilities. Knowledge of the anatomy of these transition zones is particularly important to the localization and management of foreign bodies. The functions of the pancreas and liver are closely integrated with those of the luminal organs, although they are not within the nutrient stream. The pancreas is discussed here; the liver and its metabolic functions are discussed in Chapters 12 and 26.

The visceral structures of the GI tract are composed of several layers, including the epithelium, lamina propria, submucosa, muscle layers and serosa (the last only in intraperitoneal organs). As the transition is made throughout the GI tract differences in luminal pH, epithelial cell receptors, muscularity and endogenous flora are encountered, affecting absorption and metabolism of individual xenobiotics.

The epithelium, the innermost layer of the GI tract, is the most specialized cell type in the intestine and is composed of epithelial, endocrine and receptor cells. Epithelial cells have polarity, with the basal surface facing the lamina propria and the apical surface facing the lumen. They are further specialized for specific functions of secretion or absorption. Additionally, the epithelial cell forms part of the mucosal immune defense, to detect the presence of microbial pathogens and down-regulate the immune system in the presence of nonpathogenic or probiotic microbes. The major barrier to penetration of xenobiotics and microbes is the GI epithelium, a single cell thick membrane.[13] The cell membrane is a lipid bilayer that contains proteins, which act as aqueous pores through which certain materials can pass, dependent on size or molecular structure, providing the basis for semi-permeability. The membrane is not continuous as it consists of individual epithelial cells; however, these cells are joined to each other by structures known as tight junctions, which are located on the lateral surfaces of the cells, near the apical membranes. The tight junctions have a gap of about 8 angstroms, which allows passage only of water, ions, and low-molecular weight substances.

The muscle layer found beneath the lamina propria is made up of the muscularis mucosa, the circular muscles and the longitudinal muscles. Contraction of the muscularis mucosa causes a change in the surface area of the gut lumen that alters secretion or absorption of nutrients. Depolarization of circular muscle leads to contraction of a ring of smooth muscle and a decrease in the diameter of that segment of the GI tract whereas depolarization of longitudinal muscle leads to contraction in the longitudinal direction and a decrease in the length of that segment. The function of the muscle layers is integrated with the enteric nervous system to provide for a coordinated movement of luminal contents through the GI tract so as to maximize absorption and minimize bacterial growth. This integration facilitates the flow of chyme (undigested food) via a coordinated sequence of muscular contractions and relaxations, leading to segmentation of luminal contents, peristaltic movements, and unidirectional flow through the intestine.

The GI tract is innervated by the autonomic nervous system via both extrinsic and intrinsic pathways. The extrinsic innervation permits communication between the brain, spinal cord, and chemoreceptors and mechanoreceptors located in the gut. Parasympathetic stimulation in the extrinsic pathway tends to be excitatory ("rest and digest"), and is carried via the vagus, splanchnic and pelvic nerves to the myenteric and submucosal plexuses. In contrast, increased sympathetic tone ("fight or flight") inhibits digestive and peristaltic activity via fibers that originate in the thoracolumbar cord and terminate in the myenteric and submucosal plexuses. The intrinsic innervation of the GI tract, or enteric nervous system, is responsible for the determination of parasympathetic and sympathetic tone to the GI tract. The intrinsic innervation provides local control of peristalsis and endocrine secretions, via the myenteric (Auerbach) and submucosal (Meissner) plexuses, respectively.

THE IMMUNE SYSTEM AND MICROBIOLOGY OF THE GI TRACT

An elaborate mucosal immune system has evolved to protect the GI tract from pathogens.[38] Mucosal immunity can be divided into an afferent limb, which recognizes a pathogen and induces the proliferation and differentiation of immunocompetent cells, and an efferent limb, which coordinates and affects the immune response. The afferent system includes the lymphoid follicles, and specialized M-cells found therein, that promote transit of antigens to antigen-presenting cells.[26] Once sensitized, immune cells undergo a complicated process of clonal expansion and differentiation, which occurs in mucosal and mesenteric lymphoid follicles, as well as in extraintestinal sites. Immunocompetent cells then return to the intestine and other mucous membranes, and are scattered diffusely within the epithelial and lamina propria compartments.

The normal endogenous flora in the GI tract includes more than 400 species of bacteria; the intestinal mucosa is normally colonized by nonpathogenic strains of *Esterichia coli, Proteus spp., Enterobacter spp., Serratia spp., and Klebsiella spp*. En masse, these bacteria are more metabolically active than the liver. The concentration of luminal bacteria varies by site, from lowest in the proximal small intestine to highest in the large intestine. Endogenous bacteria occupy unique niches related to host physiology, environmental pressures, and microbial interactions, which result in long-term stability.[17] The flora may be altered by various insults (particularly antibiotics), but usually returns to baseline once the insult is removed.

The endogenous flora has multiple metabolic functions. A primary function in the colon is the salvage of malabsorbed carbohydrates by fermentation and production of short-chain fatty acids, which is a preferred substrate for colonic epithelial cells. Hydrolysis of urea occurs following its passive diffusion into the intestinal lumen, producing NH_3

and a carbon skeleton. Elevated concentrations of nitrogenous compounds, including ammonia, may result from increased dietary load, or from gastrointestinal hemorrhage, or by decreased clearance, as occurs in patients with end-stage liver disease and hepatic encephalopathy.

Bacterial metabolism can significantly affect the disposition of enteral compounds. For example, the bacterial metabolism of digoxin contributes to its steady state concentrations, and antibiotic treatment may reduce or eradicate the intestinal flora, predisposing to digoxin toxicity.[7] Bacterial contribution to vitamin K metabolism is also demonstrated, necessitating dose adjustments of warfarin during and after antibiotic therapy. The metabolic activity of intraluminal bacteria has been exploited in treatment strategies. For example, sulfasalazine, used in the treatment of ulcerative colitis is created through the linkage of 5-aminosalicylic acid to sulfapyridine. The azo bonds of the nonabsorbable sulfasalazine are broken by bacterial azoreductases, permitting the absorption of active metabolites in the colon at the site of inflammation.[30]

The normal flora of the gut consists of probiotics—live, nonpathogenic bacteria and fungi that can also be used as prophylactic or therapeutic agents. These bacteria compete for and displace pathogenic bacteria, directly modulate intestinal immune function and exert a trophic effect on the gastrointestinal tract. They are used to decrease traveler's diarrhea, suppress antibiotic-induced diarrhea, and reduce inflammation in ileal pouches after colectomy in patients with ulcerative colitis.[10,15]

REGULATORY SUBSTANCES OF THE GASTROINTESTINAL TRACT

There are three groups of regulatory materials that act on target cells within the GI tract. These gastrointestinal hormones are released from endocrine cells in the GI mucosa into the portal circulation, enter the systemic circulation with resultant physiologic actions on target cells. Gastrin, cholecystokinin (CCK), secretin, and gastric inhibitory peptide (GIP) are considered the primary GI hormones. Somatostatin and histamine make up the paracrines, hormones that are released from endocrine cells and diffuse over short distances to act on target cells located in the GI tract. Vasoactive intestinal peptide (VIP), GRP (bombesin) and enkephalins compose the last group known as neurocrines, substances that are synthesized in neurons of the GI tract, move by axonal transport down the axon, and are then released by action potentials in the nerves. Effects on these regulatory substances are in summarized Table 25–1.[8]

ANATOMIC AND PHYSIOLOGIC PRINCIPLES

OROPHARYNX AND HYPOPHARYNX

The main functions of the mouth and oropharynx are chewing, lubrication of food with saliva, and swallowing. Saliva initiates digestion of

TABLE 25–1. Regulatory Substances of the GI Tract[8]

Substance	Site of Secretion/Release	Stimulus for Secretion/Release	Actions
Gastrin	G cells of gastric antrum	Small peptides and amino acids Stomach distention Vagal stimulation (via GRP) Inhibited by H^+ in stomach (negative feedback)	↑ gastric H^+ secretion, ↑ growth of gastric mucosa
Cholecystokinin	I cells of duodenum and jejunum	Small peptides and amino acids Fatty acids and monoglycerides	↑ contraction of gallbladder and relaxation of sphincter of Oddi ↑ pancreatic enzyme and HCO_3^- secretion ↑ growth of exocrine pancreas/gallbladder ↓ gastric emptying (allow more time for digestion and absorption)
Secretin	S cells of duodenum	H^+ in duodenal lumen Fatty acids in duodenal lumen	Coordinated to reduce small intestinal H^+ ↑ pancreatic HCO_3^- secretion ↑ biliary HCO_3^- secretion ↓ gastric H^+ secretion ↑growth of exocrine pancreas
Gastric Inhibitory Peptide	Duodenum and jejunum	Fatty acids, amino acids, oral glucose	↓ H^+ secretion by gastric parietal cells ↑ insulin release
Somatostatin	Throughout GI tract	H^+ in GI tract lumen Inhibited by vagal stimulation	↓ release of all GI hormones ↓ gastric H^+ secretion
Histamine	Mast cells of gastric mucosa	Vagal stimulation gastrin	↑ gastric H^+ secretion
Vasoactive Intestinal Peptide	GI tract mucosa and smooth muscle neurons	H^+ in duodenal lumen	Smooth muscle relaxation ↑ pancreatic HCO_3^- secretion ↓ gastric H^+ secretion
Bombesin	Vagus nerves that innervate G cells	Vagal stimulation	↑ gastrin release from G cells
Enkephalins (met-enkephalin, leu-enkephalin)	GI tract mucosa and smooth muscle neurons		↑ contraction of GI smooth muscle ↓ intestinal secretion of fluid and electrolytes

starch by α-amylase (ptyalin), triglyceride digestion by lingual lipase, lubrication of ingested food by mucus, and protection of the mouth and esophagus by dilution and buffering of ingested foods.

Saliva production is unique in that it is increased by both parasympathetic and sympathetic activity. Parasympathetic stimulation, via cranial nerves VII and IX acts on muscarinic cholinergic receptors on acinar and ductal cells, increases saliva production by causing vasodilation and increasing transport processes in the acinar and ductal cells. Parasympathetic pathways are stimulated by food in the mouth, smells, conditioned reflexes, and nausea, and are inhibited by sleep, dehydration, and fear. Sympathetic stimulation, originating from preganglionic nerves in the thoracic segments T1-3, requires receipt of norepinephrine by β-adrenergic receptors on acinar and ductal cells, leading to increases in the production of saliva, but at a rate less than that of parasympathetic stimulation.[8] Dysfunction of saliva production can lead to dry mouth, or xerostomia.

ESOPHAGUS

The normal esophagus is a distensible muscular tube that extends from the epiglottis to the gastroesophageal junction. The lumen of the esophagus narrows at several points along its course, first at the cricopharyngeus muscle, then midway down alongside the aortic arch and then distally where it crosses the diaphragm. The upper esophageal sphincter (UES) and lower esophageal sphincter (LES) are physiologic high-pressure regions that remain closed except during swallowing, and have no anatomic features to distinguish them from the intervening esophageal musculature.

The wall of the esophagus reflects the general structural organization of the GI tract noted previously, consisting of mucosa, submucosa, muscularis propria, and adventitia. The mucosal layer has three components. The nonkeratinizing stratified squamous epithelial layer faces the lumen, provides protection for underlying tissue, and houses several specialized cell types such as melanocytes, endocrine cells, dendritic cells, and lymphocytes. The lamina propria is the nonepithelialized portion of the mucosa, and the muscularis mucosa, a layer of longitudinally oriented smooth-muscle bundles is the third component.

The submucosa consists of loose connective tissue, and submucosal glands secrete a mucin-containing fluid via squamous epithelium-lined ducts which facilitates lubrication of the esophageal lumen. The muscularis propria consists of an inner circular and outer longitudinal coat of smooth muscle; this layer also contains striated muscle fibers in the proximal esophagus that is responsible for voluntary swallowing.

The esophagus has no serosal lining. Only small segments of the intraabdominal esophagus are covered by adventitia, a sheath-like structure that also surrounds the adjacent great vessels, tracheobronchial tree, and other structures of the mediastinum.

The esophagus provides a conduit for food and fluids from the pharynx to the stomach, and the sphincters generally prevent reflux of gastric contents into the esophagus. Normal transit of food involves coordinated motor activity including a wave of peristaltic contraction, relaxation of the LES (facilitated by nitric oxide and VIP), and subsequent closure of the LES (facilitated by several hormones and neurotransmitters such as gastrin, acetylcholine, serotonin, and motilin). Because of the rapid transit time of swallowed substances through this portion of the GI tract, digestion does not take place and passive diffusion of substances from the food into the bloodstream is prevented.[8,24]

STOMACH

The stomach is a saccular organ covered entirely by peritoneum that has a capacity greater than 3 liters. The stomach is divided into five anatomic regions: the cardia, fundus, corpus or body, antrum, and pyloric sphincter. The gastric wall consists of mucosa, submucosa, muscularis propria, and serosa. The interior surface of the stomach is marked by coarse rugae, or longitudinal folds. The mucosa is made up of a superficial epithelial cell compartment and a deep glandular compartment. The glandular compartment consists of gastric glands, which vary between regions of the stomach. The mucus glands of the cardia, fundus and body secrete mucus and pepsinogen. Oxyntic, or acid-forming glands, found in the fundus and body contain parietal, chief, and endocrine cells. The parietal cells contain vesicles that house hydrochloric acid-secreting proton pumps and also secrete intrinsic factor, a substance necessary for the ileal absorption of vitamin B_{12}. Chief cells secrete the proteolytic proenzyme pepsinogen which is cleaved to its active form, pepsin, upon exposure to the low luminal gastric pH of 3 to 4. Pepsin is subsequently inactivated in the duodenum when the pH increases to 6.0. The endocrine, or enterochromaffin-like (ECL), cells found in the mucosa of the body of the stomach produce histamine, which increases acid production and decreases gastric pH by stimulating H_2 receptors on the parietal cells. Somatostatin and endothelin, both modulators of acid production, are also produced in ECL cells (Fig. 50–3).

Hydrochloric acid is secreted when cephalic, gastric and intestinal signals converge on the gastric parietal cells to activate proton pumps and release hydrochloric acid in an ATP-dependent process. During the cephalic phase, or the preparatory phase of the brain for eating and digestion, acetylcholine is released from vagal afferents in response to sight, smell, taste, and chewing. Acetylcholine stimulates the parietal cells via muscarinic receptors, resulting in an increase in cytosolic calcium and activation of the proton pump. G cells, located in the antrum of the stomach, produce and release gastrin in response to luminal amino acids and peptides. Gastrin activates receptors within parietal cells, leading to a similar increase in cytosolic calcium. Additionally, gastrin and vagal afferents induce the release of histamine from ECL cells, which stimulates parietal cell H_2 receptors. Lastly, the intestinal phase is initiated when food containing digested protein enters the proximal small intestine and involves gastrin as well as a number of other polypeptides in the secretion of hydrochloric acid from the stomach.[24] See Fig 25–1.

The gastric mucosa is protected from the acidic secretions of the stomach by several mechanisms, including a thin layer of surface mucus, and channels that allow acid- and pepsin- containing fluids to exit glands without contact with the surface epithelium. Additionally, the surface epithelium secretes bicarbonate, creating a more neutral pH at the cell surface. Prostaglandins produced in the mucosal cells stimulate production of bicarbonate and mucus, and inhibit parietal cell production of acid; prostaglandin inhibition plays an important role in the pathogenesis of peptic ulcer disease.[24]

In the stomach, ingested products are ground to particle sizes of less than 0.2 mm, which are then further processed and digested in preparation for absorption of nutrients in the small intestine.[25] Many xenobiotics are weak acids that are no longer ionized in the acidic environment of the stomach, facilitating absorption through the lipid bilayer at the level of the stomach. Other factors that affect xenobiotic absorption include particle size, transit time, and type of drug delivery system. Different types of drug formulations, such as time-release, enteric coating, slowly dissolving matrices, dissolution control via osmotic pumps, ion exchange resins, and pH-sensitive mechanisms can affect bioavailability, as well as the site of maximal release within the GI tract.

Following processing, the stomach delivers the products to the small intestine.

The time required for gastric emptying is determined by the complex interplay of GI innervation, muscle action, underlying illness, and xenobiotic exposure. Digestion and absorption are time-dependent

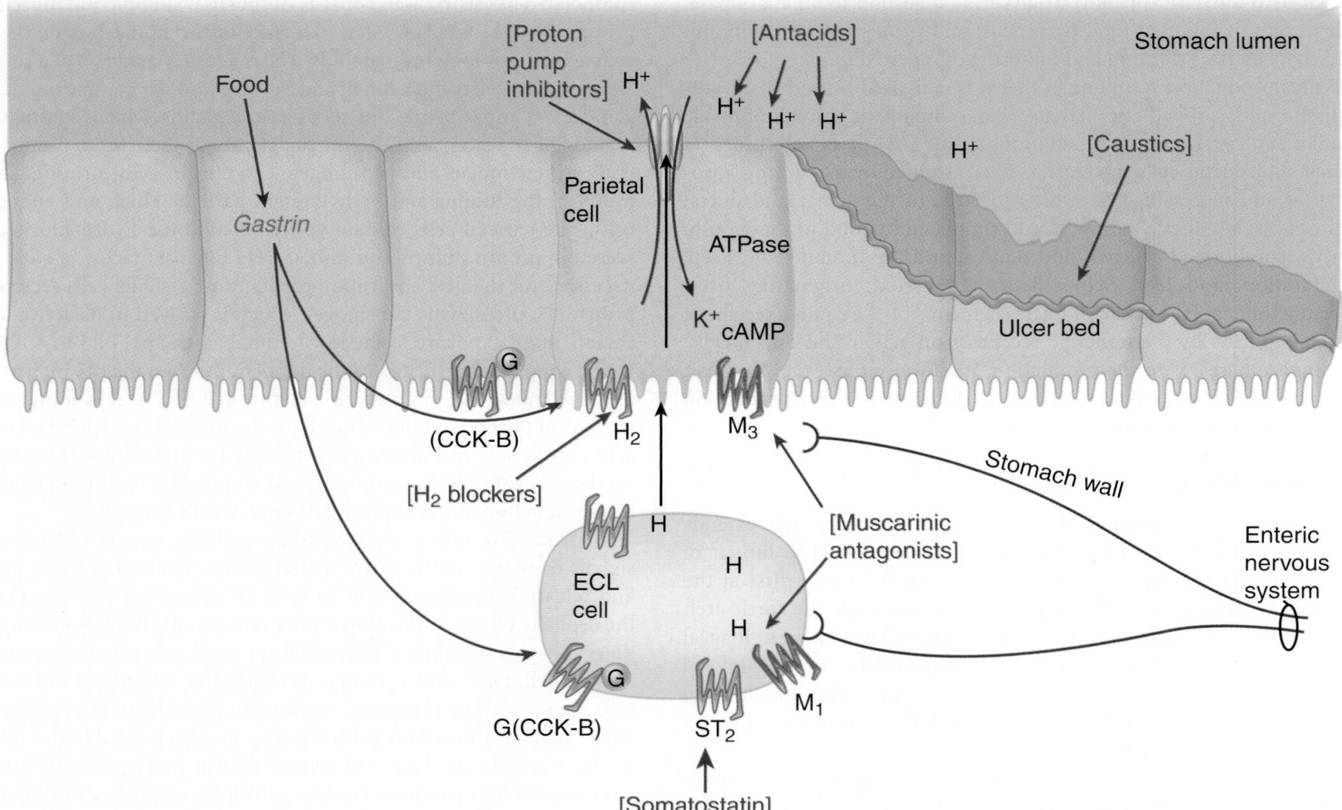

FIGURE 25–1. Effects of various xenobiotics on the gastrointestinal tract. ECL cell, enterochromaffin-like cell; CCK-B, cholecystokinin receptor B; H, histamine; H_2, histamine-2 (H_2) receptor; M_1, M_3; muscarinic receptors; ST2, somatostatin-2 receptor.

processes and optimal absorption requires adjustment of the luminal environment through secretion of ions and water, to accommodate meals that vary considerably in nutrient composition and density. Osmoreceptors and chemoreceptors in the GI tract fine-tune the digestive and absorptive processes by regulating transit and secretion, using a variety of neurocrine, paracrine and endocrine mechanisms. Interference with this integrated response may lead to stasis and bacterial overgrowth, or rapid transit with decreased absorption and development of diarrhea. A large number of mediators affect motility, including common neurotransmitters, such as acetylcholine and norepinephrine, hormones, cytokines, inflammatory compounds, and others. In general, parasympathetic impulses promote motility, whereas sympathetic stimulation inhibits motility. Other transmitters, such as serotonin, promote transit, whereas dopamine and enkephalins can slow motility.

SMALL AND LARGE INTESTINES

In the average adult, the small intestine is approximately 6 meters in length, and begins retroperitoneally as the duodenum, becoming peritoneal at the jejunum and ileum. Small intestine transitions to large intestine at the ileocecal valve, and the large intestine typically measures 1.5 meters in an adult. The large intestine or colon is further divided into cecal, ascending, transverse, descending, and sigmoid segments. The sigmoid colon transitions to the rectum, and terminates at the anus. Anterograde and retrograde peristalsis occurs in the small intestine, whereas anterograde peristalsis predominates in the large intestine. This movement allows for mixing of food, maximizes contact with the mucosa, and is mediated by both the extrinsic and intrinsic nervous systems. The remarkable absorptive capacity of the small intestine is created by innumerable villi of the intestinal wall, which are small epithelial-lined “fingers” that extend into the lumen. The epithelial border of the small intestine also contains mucin-secreting goblet cells, endocrine cells, and specialized absorptive cells; functionally, these cells create an ideal environment for maximal nutrient absorption. The mucosa of the large intestine is devoid of villi. The large intestine functions primarily to absorb electrolytes and water, secrete potassium, salvage any remaining nutrients, and to store and release waste.

Intestinal epithelial cells also have the ability to metabolize xenobiotics, a function typically attributed to the liver. Epithelial cells contain many of the same metabolic enzymes as the liver and are capable of performing multiple types of reactions including hydroxylation, sulfation, acetylation, and glucuronidation. These metabolic processes affect the amount of orally administered xenobiotic that enters the body and contributes to the first-pass effect, or presystemic disposition. Variations in intestinal metabolism also may influence the pharmacokinetics of a xenobiotic.

Regeneration of injured or senescent intestinal epithelial cells begins in the crypts, with differentiation occurring as these cells migrate towards to the intestinal lumen. This process occurs rapidly, with turnover of the small intestinal epithelium occurring every 4 to 6 days, and large intestinal epithelium every 3 to 8 days. This rapid regeneration leaves the intestinal epithelium vulnerable to processes that interfere with cell replication. The sloughing of GI epithelium, typically manifested by hemorrhagic enteritis, is subsequently a valuable marker for xenobiotic insults that lead to mitotic arrest.

PANCREAS

The pancreas is a retroperitoneal organ that serves dual exocrine and endocrine functions. The exocrine portion of the gland produces digestive enzymes and occupies more than 80%–85% of the mass of the pancreas. The exocrine pancreas is comprised of acinar cells, specialized epithelial cells housing zymogen granules that release digestive enzymes and proenzymes on secretion. The digestive enzymes enter the duodenum, while columnar epithelial cells produce mucin and ductal cuboidal epithelial cells secrete a bicarbonate-rich fluid that neutralizes gastric acids. The pancreas secretes 2–2.5 liters per day of this mixed solution. Typically, the digestive enzymes are released as proenzymes, such as trypsinogen, chymotrypsinogen, and procarboxypeptidase, are activated upon contact with the higher pH of the duodenum; this process helps to prevent autodigestion of the pancreas itself. Enzymes on the brush border of the duodenum, including enteropeptidase, cleave proenzymes to their active forms. Only pancreatic amylase and lipase are secreted in their active forms.

Secretion of pancreatic enzymes is regulated by multiple factors, the most important of which are cholecystokinin and secretin, both produced in the duodenum. Cholecystokinin is released from the duodenum in response to fatty acids and the products of protein catabolism such as peptides and amino acids. Cholecystokinin stimulates acinar cells to release digestive enzymes and proenzymes. Secretin is released by the duodenum in the presence of lowered pH caused by gastric acids and luminal fatty acids. Secretin triggers ductal cells to secrete bicarbonate and water. Acetylcholine also plays a role in the regulation of pancreatic exocrine function, by stimulating digestive enzyme secretion from the acinus and potentiating the effects of secretin. Vagal reflexes increase acetylcholinergic tone in the setting of decreased pH, protein breakdown products, and fatty acids in the duodenal lumen.

The endocrine portion of the pancreas is comprised of approximately one million clusters of cells known as the islets of Langerhans which secrete insulin, glucagons, and somatostatin. Other products of the endocrine pancreas include serotonin and VIP. Injury to the endocrine pancreas can result in impaired glucose homeostasis.

XENOBIOTIC METABOLISM

Although the liver is usually identified as the site of xenobiotic metabolism, similar functions occur in the luminal GI tract. Biotransformation is a property both of luminal bacteria and enterocytes. Metabolism by the intestine affects the amount of orally administered xenobiotic that actually enters the body and therefore contributes to the first-pass effect, or presystemic disposition.

One of the most well-described families of export proteins, P-glycoprotein (PGP), is found in the mucosa of the small and large intestines, hepatocytes, the adrenal cortex, renal tubules, and the capillary cells lining the blood-brain barrier.[43] The PGPs are susceptible to induction and inhibition in a manner similar to hepatic cytochrome oxidase enzymes. Many of the substrates of CYP3A have inhibitory effects on PGPs. Inhibitors of PGPs may raise serum concentrations of the parent drug or metabolite, although inducers of PGPs may prevent therapeutic drug concentrations from ever reaching the target cell. The PGP system is important in drug interactions and drug resistance (Chap. 8).

TABLE 25–2. Xenobiotics Causing Discoloration of the Teeth and Gums[1]

Areca catecha leaves	Red
Cadmium	Yellow
Ciprofloxacin	Green
Doxycycline	Yellow
Fluoride	White flecking
Chlorhexidine oral rinse	Brown
Tetracycline	Yellow to brown-grey

PATHOLOGIC CONDITIONS OF THE GI TRACT

Oral Pathology Discoloration of the teeth has been reported with a number of medications, most notably tetracyclines. Medications known to cause dental pigmentation are listed in Table 25–2. Gingival hyperplasia in an uncommon, but reported adverse effect of the chronic use of several xenobiotics, including multiple anticonvulsants. Gingival hyperplasia describes overgrowth of the gums around the teeth which can result in loosening of teeth and severe periodontal disease. Some medications implicated in causing gingival hyperplasia include calcium channel blockers, cyclosporine, lithium, phenobarbital, phenytoin, topiramate, and valproic acid.[1] Xerostomia, or pathologic dryness of the mouth, is an uncomfortable adverse effect of many xenobiotics that can lead to increased dental decay. Xenobiotics that can cause xerostomia is extensive, and the most commonly implicated classes of xenobiotics causing xerostomia are listed in Table 25–3. Chronic methamphetamine use has been linked to characteristic oral pathology known as "meth mouth." This condition is characterized by extensive and severe tooth decay, and has been linked to poor hygiene, bruxism, and xerostomia associated with methamphetamine use.[9]

Esophagitis and Dysphagia Xenobiotic-induced esophageal injury includes esophagitis, ulceration, perforation, and stricture. The most common presenting complaint is a foreign body sensation in the throat.[5,18] Xenobiotics commonly implicated in the causation of esophagitis or esophageal ulcerations are listed in Table 25–4. Patient features that predict likelihood of esophageal pathology include preexisting esophageal motility disorderts. Conditions like Parkinsonism, cerebrovascular accidents, scleroderma, and myasthenia gravis can contribute to dysphagia. Xenobiotics with a gelatin matrix, rapid dissolvability, and large size predispose to esophageal injury. Although most symptoms resolve with withdrawal of the offending xenobiotics, patients with persistent or severe odynophagia should be evaluated with endoscopy to identify pathology and prevent perforation caused by retained pills.[11]

TABLE 25–3. Xenobiotics that Commonly Cause Xerostomia[1,40]

α_1-adrenergic receptor antagonists
α_2-adrenergic receptor agonists
Anticholinergics
Antidepressants (CAs, maprotiline)
Antihistamines
Antipsychotics (phenothiazines)
Protease inhibitors

TABLE 25–4. Xenobiotics Implicated in Esophagitis and Esophageal Ulcerations[28]

Antipsychotics
Bisphosphonates
NSAIDs
Potassium chloride
Quinine
Tetracycline

Webs, strictures, and esophageal malignancy Caustic injury is one of the most common causes of esophageal strictures. Some authors have also postulated the role of pill esophagitis in the evolution of esophageal strictures.[4] Caustic injury is also implicated in the causation of esophageal malignancy. As great as 4% of patients with esophageal cancer report a history of caustic injury and patients with a prior history of caustic ingestion may have more than a 1000-fold higher risk of developing an esophageal malignancy than the general population.[19,20] Other xenobiotics known to cause esophageal strictures include aluminum phosphide and ionizing radiation.[37]

Gastritis/Peptic Ulcer Disease Gastritis, or inflammation of the gastric mucosa, and peptic ulcer disease (PUD) are commonly related to xenobiotic exposure (Table 25–5). Symptoms of gastritis and PUD include epigastric pain, nausea and vomiting, but may include hematemesis and melena.[29] The primary distinction between gastritis and peptic ulcer disease is appearance at endoscopy where gastritis is characterized by diffuse inflammation of the gastric mucosa, whereas an ulcer is a discrete lesion of the mucosa. Nonsteroidal antiinflammatory drugs (NSAIDs) remain an important part of the pathogenesis of gastric and PUD by decreasing prostaglandin secretion and subsequently affecting the integrity of the gastric mucosal barrier to acid. Cyclooxygenase-2 (COX-2) selective inhibitors promised to decrease the incidence of gastric pathology caused by chronic NSAID use; however, the available COX-2 inhibitors now carry a black box warning in the United States that desribe an increased risk of significant adverse cardiovascular events.[14]

Chronic treatment of peptic ulcer disease with antacids, H_2 blockers, or proton pump inhibitors can lead to hypochlorhydria or achlorhydria, the reduction or absence of gastric acid, respectively. These conditions increase risk of bacterial overgrowth, atrophic gastritis, hip fracture (possibly caused by impaired calcium absorption), *Salmonella* and *Vibrio cholerae* infection, and gastric carcinoma.[32,42]

TABLE 25–5. Xenobiotics Commonly Implicated in Gastritis and Peptic Ulcer Disease

Aspirin
Corticosteroids
Ethanol
Isopropyl alcohol
Nicotine
NSAIDs
Radiation (Ionizing)

TABLE 25–6. Xenobiotic-induced Enteritis

Mechanism	Xenobiotic
Mechanical irritation	Aloe Bacterial food poisoning Laxatives Mushrooms
Cholinergic stimulation	Carbamates Neostigmine, physostigmine Nicotine Organic Phosphorous compounds
Inhibitors of mucosal regeneration (Hemorrhagic enteritis)	Arsenic Colchicine Mercuric salts Iron Monochloroacetic acid Podophyllin Pokeweed (*Phytolacca americana*) Radiation (ionizing) Thallium

Enteritis The symptoms of GI distress are nonspecifically associated with xenobiotic exposure, as well as a myriad of infectious etiologies. However, certain xenobiotics that increase gastric emptying and peristalsis can result in significant diarrhea. Opioid withdrawal and serotonin syndrome are important toxidromes that may feature diarrhea as a prominent symtom. Additionally, the rapid turnover of the GI mucosa makes it uniquely susceptible to xenobiotics that cause cell death and mitotic arrest. Hemorrhagic enteritis, manifested by hematochezia, can be a characteristic finding of certain xenobiotic exposures (Table 25–6).

Pancreatitis Pancreatitis is an acute inflammatory process that results in autolysis of the pancreas from digestive enzymes.[41] Cases range from mild to severe, with mortality of 5%.[16] The most common causes of pancreatitis are alcohol abuse and gallbladder disease; however, xenobiotic-induced pancreatitis accounts for 0.1%–2% of cases of acute pancreatitis.[2] Populations at higher risk of drug-induced pancreatitis include children, women, the elderly, and patients with HIV and inflammatory bowel disease.[2] In acute pancreatitis, the most common diagnostic criterion is elevation of serum pancreatic enzymes, amylase or lipase, to more than three times the upper limit of the reference range. The diagnosis of xenobiotic-induced pancreatitis can be impossible to confirm, as no diagnostic test or pattern of injury distinguishes xenobiotic-induced pancreatitis from other etiologies. However, the symptoms and laboratory abnormalities associated with xenobiotic-induced pancreatitis tend to resolve shortly after withdrawal of the offending xenobiotic; again, this can be challenging to differentiate from the natural course of mild to moderate disease. It is unclear whether rechallenge with a culprit xenobiotic will cause pancreatitis again; however, any xenobiotic suspected of causing pancreatitis should be withheld unless the benefits outweigh this risk. The management of xenobiotic-induced pancreatitis does not differ from other causes, and hinges on aggressive volume resuscitation, bowel rest, and careful monitoring. Patients at the extremes of age, manifesting end organ dysfunction, acute lung injury, or signs of shock are at greatest risk of death.

There are numerous xenobiotics associated with pancreatitis, and the strength of that association has been described as definite, likely, or possible; representative xenobiotics are listed in Table 25–7. The pathogenic mechanism varies with the specific xenobiotic. The nucleoside reverse transcriptase inhibitor, didanosine, and exposure to dioxin,

TABLE 25–7. Xenobiotics Commonly Associated with Pancreatitis[2]

Alcohols: Ethanol and methanol
Analgesics: Acetaminophen, NSAIDs
Antibiotics: Clarithromycin, isoniazid, metronidazole, sulfonamides, tetracycline
Anticonvulsants: Valproic acid
Antihyperlipidemics: HMG-CoA reductase inhibitors
Cardiovascular: ACE inhibitors
Diuretics: Furosemide, thiazides
HIV medications: Didanosine, lamivudine, nelfinavir
Hormones: Corticosteroids, estrogens
Immunosuppressants: Azathioprine, corticosteroids
Pesticides: Organic Phosphorous compounds
Sitagliptin
Venoms: *Buthus quiquestriatus, Tityus discrepans*

may promote pancreatitis as a result of mitochondrial injury.[27,33,34] Cholinergic xenobiotics, like parathion and certain scorpion venoms, may result in pancreatitis caused by overstimulation.[21,31] Vasospasm and ischemia are also purported as a mechanism, as in cases of pancreatitis secondary to ergot alkaloids.[12]

The endocrine pancreas is also susceptible to injury from pancreatitis or toxic insult. Typically, dysfunction of the endocrine pancreas results from injury to pancreatic beta cells and impaired glucose homeostasis, similar to diabetes. There are rare xenobiotics that can cause damage to alpha cells in animal models; however, they do not consistently cause hypoglycemia (Table 25–8).

TABLE 25–8. Xenobiotics Associated with Endocrine Pancreatic Dysfunction

Alpha cells
Cobalt salts
Decamethylene diguanidine
Phenylethylbiguanide
Beta cells
Alloxan
Androgens
Cyclizine
Cyproheptadine
Diazoxide
Dihydromorphanthridine
Epinephrine
Glucagon
Glucorticoids
Growth hormone
Pentamidine
Streptozocin
Sulfonamides
Vacor

FOREIGN BODIES

The esophagus is the most common site of symptomatic foreign bodies. They tend to be found in the cervical esophagus, at the level of the aortic notch, just above the gastroesophageal junction, or just proximal to an esophageal narrowing.[6] The likelihood that a foreign object will lodge in the esophagus is related to its size and shape. The major complications of foreign bodies in the esophagus include pain, bleeding, obstruction or perforation, which may lead to subsequent mediastinitis or fistula. The general rule is that conservative means can be employed for up to 12 hours after ingestion of the esophageal foreign body. If serial radiographs demonstrate no movement after 12 hours, endoscopic retrieval or surgery should be considered, as the risk of perforation increases after that time; some authors will extend this observation period to 24 hours.[3,35] Ingestion of button batteries proves an important exception to this rule. Esophageal button batteries can cause significant mucosal injury in four hours, with perforation in as little as 6 hours.[22] Proposed mechanisms for the rapid development of esophageal injury include alkaline burn, local current and pressure necrosis.[23,36] As a result, all suspected esophageal button batteries should undergo immediate endoscopic removal, and success rates with this modality have been reported as excellent.[23]

Foreign bodies are also commonly found in the stomach. Many small foreign bodies will pass through the stomach and the remainder of the GI tract without difficulty. Objects greater than 5 cm in length or 2 cm in diameter may be unable to traverse the duodenum, and may require endoscopic or surgical removal. Foreign bodies beyond the duodenum may not require any intervention except observation; however, some objects may become stuck at the ileocecal valve. Serial examinations and radiographs can be appropriate for asymptomatic patients; however, increasing abdominal pain or tenderness may mandate further imaging and surgical consultation. Body packers represent an unusual exception to these rules. Patients who are discovered to be internally concealing large quantities of illicit drugs may require whole bowel irrigation to facilitate transit of colonic packets, and even emergency laparotomy for obstruction or suspected packet rupture in cases of cocaine or methamphetamine smuggling.[39]

SUMMARY

The GI tract is vulnerable to a wide variety of pathogenic agents with diverse physical, chemical, and biologic forms. Understanding the effects of such xenobiotics on the GI tract requires an appreciation of its normal anatomy and physiology. Because of its potential as a site of severe local or systemic effects, and the role that GI signs and symptoms play in various toxic syndromes, the GI tract is an important consideration in many toxicologic emergencies.

ACKNOWLEDGMENT

Donald P. Kotler and Neal E. Flomenbaum contributed to this chapter in previous editions.

REFERENCES

1. Abdollahi M, Rahimi R, Radfar M. Current opinion on drug-induced oral reactions: a comprehensive review. *J Contemp Dent Pract.* 2008;9:1-15.
2. Balani AR, Grendell JH. Drug-induced pancreatitis: incidence, management and prevention. *Drug Saf.* 2008;31:823-837.
3. Bloom RR, Nakano PH, Gray SW, Skandalakis JE. Foreign bodies of the gastrointestinal tract. *Am Surg.* 1986;52:618-621.

4. Bonavina L, DeMeester TR, McChesney L, Schwizer W, Albertucci M, Bailey RT. Drug-induced esophageal strictures. *Ann Surg.* 1987;206:173-183.
5. Carlborg B, Densert O, Lindqvist C. Tetracycline induced esophageal ulcers. a clinical and experimental study. *Laryngoscope.* 1983;93:184-187.
6. Chaikhouni A, Kratz JM, Crawford FA. Foreign bodies of the esophagus. *Am Surg.* 1985;51:173-179.
7. Constantine PA. Antibiotic therapy and serum digoxin toxicity. *Am Fam Physician.* 1998;57:1239-1240.
8. Costanzo L. *Physiology.* Philadelphia: Saunders; 2002.
9. Curtis EK. Meth mouth: a review of methamphetamine abuse and its oral manifestations. *Gen Dent.* 2006;54:125-129; quiz 130.
10. D'Souza AL, Rajkumar C, Cooke J, Bulpitt CJ. Probiotics in prevention of antibiotic associated diarrhoea: meta-analysis. *BMJ.* 2002;324:1361.
11. de Groen PC, Lubbe DF, Hirsch LJ, et al. Esophagitis associated with the use of alendronate. *N Engl J Med.* 1996;335:1016-1021.
12. Deviere J, Reuse C, Askenasi R. Ischemic pancreatitis and hepatitis secondary to ergotamine poisoning. *J Clin Gastroenterol.* 1987;9:350-352.
13. Diamond JM. Channels in epithelial cell membranes and junctions. *Fed Proc.* 1978;37:2639-2643.
14. Flower RJ. The development of COX2 inhibitors. *Nat Rev Drug Discov.* 2003;2:179-191.
15. Gionchetti P, Rizzello F, Helwig U, et al. Prophylaxis of pouchitis onset with probiotic therapy: a double-blind, placebo-controlled trial. *Gastroenterology.* 2003;124:1202-1209.
16. Granger J, Remick D. Acute pancreatitis: models, markers, and mediators. *Shock.* 2005;24 Suppl 1:45-51.
17. Hooper LV, Gordon JI. Commensal host-bacterial relationships in the gut. *Science.* 2001;292:1115-1118.
18. Kikendall JW. Pill esophagitis. *J Clin Gastroenterol.* 1999;28:298-305.
19. Kiviranta. U. Corrosion carcinoma of the esophagus. *Cancer.* 1953;6:1159-1164.
20. Kochhar R, Sethy PK, Kochhar S, Nagi B, Gupta NM. Corrosive induced carcinoma of esophagus: report of three patients and review of literature. *J Gastroenterol Hepatol.* 2006;21:777-780.
21. Lankisch PG, Muller CH, Niederstadt H, Brand A. Painless acute pancreatitis subsequent to anticholinesterase insecticide (parathion) intoxication. *Am J Gastroenterol.* 1990;85:872-875.
22. Litovitz T, Schmitz BF. Ingestion of cylindrical and button batteries: an analysis of 2382 cases. *Pediatrics.* 1992;89:747-757.
23. Litovitz TL. Button battery ingestions. A review of 56 cases. *JAMA.* 1983;249:2495-2500.
24. Liu C, Crawford J., The gastrointestinal tract. In: Kumar V, Abbas AK, Fausto N, editors. *In*: Robbins and Cotran, *Pathologic Basis of Disease.* 7th ed. . Philadelphia: Elsevier Saunders; 2005:799-875.
25. Meyer J, ed. *Motility of the Stomach and Gastroduodenal Junction.* 2nd ed. New York: Raven; 1987:613.
26. Neutra MR. M cells in antigen sampling in mucosal tissues. *Curr Top Microbiol Immunol.* 1999;236:17-32.
27. Nyska A, Jokinen MP, Brix AE, et al. Exocrine pancreatic pathology in female Harlan Sprague-Dawley rats after chronic treatment with 2,3,7,8-tetrachlorodibenzo-p-dioxin and dioxin-like compounds. *Environ Health Perspect.* 2004;112:903-909.
28. O'Neill JL, Remington TL. Drug-induced esophageal injuries and dysphagia. *Ann Pharmacother.* 2003;37:1675-1684.
29. Parfitt JR, Driman DK. Pathological effects of drugs on the gastrointestinal tract: a review. *Hum Pathol.* 2007;38:527-536.
30. Peppercorn MA. Sulfasalazine. Pharmacology, clinical use, toxicity, and related new drug development. *Ann Intern Med.* 1984;101:377-386.
31. Possani LD, Martin BM, Fletcher MD, Fletcher PL Jr. Discharge effect on pancreatic exocrine secretion produced by toxins purified from Tityus serrulatus scorpion venom. *J Biol Chem.* 1991;266:3178-3185.
32. Recker RR. Calcium absorption and achlorhydria. *N Engl J Med.* 1985;313:70-73.
33. Rozman K, Pereira D, Iatropoulos MJ. Histopathology of interscapular brown adipose tissue, thyroid, and pancreas in 2,3,7,8-tetrachlorodibenzo-p-dioxin (TCDD)-treated rats. *Toxicol Appl Pharmacol.* 1986;82:551-559.
34. Seidlin M, Lambert JS, Dolin R, Valentine FT. Pancreatitis and pancreatic dysfunction in patients taking dideoxyinosine. *Aids.* 1992;6:831-835.
35. Silverberg M, Tillotson R. Case report: esophageal foreign body mistaken for impacted button battery. *Pediatr Emerg Care.* 2006;22:262-265.
36. Studley JG, Linehan IP, Ogilvie AL, Dowling BL. Swallowed button batteries: is there a consensus on management? *Gut.* 1990;31:867-870.
37. Talukdar R, Singal DK, Tandon RK. Aluminium phosphide-induced esophageal stricture. *Indian J Gastroenterol.* 2006;25:98-99.
38. Tomasi TB Jr, Tan EM, Solomon A, Prendergast RA. Characteristics of an immune system common to certain external secretions. *J Exp Med.* 1965;121:101-124.
39. Traub SJ, Hoffman RS, Nelson LS. Body packing—the internal concealment of illicit drugs. *N Engl J Med.* 2003;349:2519-2526.
40. Tredwin CJ, Scully C, Bagan-Sebastian JV:. Drug-induced disorders of teeth. *J Dent Res.* 2005;84:596-602.
41. Whitcomb DC. Clinical practice. Acute pancreatitis. *N Engl J Med.* 2006;354:2142-2150.
42. Yang YX, Lewis JD, Epstein S, Metz DC. Long-term proton pump inhibitor therapy and risk of hip fracture. *JAMA.* 2006;296:2947-2953.
43. Yu DK. The contribution of P-glycoprotein to pharmacokinetic drug-drug interactions. *J Clin Pharmacol.* 1999;39:1203-1211.

CHAPTER 26
HEPATIC PRINCIPLES

Kathleen A. Delaney

The liver plays an essential role in the maintenance of metabolic homeostasis. Hepatic functions include the synthesis, storage, and breakdown of glycogen. In addition, the liver is important in the metabolism of lipids; the synthesis of albumin, clotting factors, and other important proteins; the synthesis of the bile acids necessary for absorption of lipids and fat-soluble vitamins; and the metabolism of cholesterol.[20,54] Hepatocytes facilitate the excretion of metals, most importantly iron, copper, zinc, manganese, mercury, and aluminum; and the detoxification of products of metabolism, such as bilirubin and ammonia.[29,62] Generalized disruption of these important functions results in manifestations of liver failure: hyperbilirubinemia, coagulopathy, hypoalbuminemia, hyperammonemia, and hypoglycemia.[41,74] The hepatic functions can also be selectively altered by exposure to hepatotoxins.[54] Disturbances of more specific functions result in accumulation of fat, metals, and bilirubin, and the development of fat-soluble vitamin deficiencies.[20,54]

The liver is also the primary site of biotransformation and detoxification of xenobiotics.[46,133] Its interposition between the gut and systemic circulation makes it the first-pass recipient of xenobiotics absorbed from the gastrointestinal tract into the portal vein. The liver also receives blood from the systemic circulation and participates in the detoxification and elimination of xenobiotics that reach the bloodstream through other routes, such as inhalation or cutaneous absorption.[20,118]

Many xenobiotics are lipophilic inert substances that require chemical activation followed by conjugation to make them sufficiently soluble to be eliminated. The liver contains the highest concentration of enzymes involved in phase I oxidation-reduction reactions, the first stage of detoxification for many lipophilic xenobiotics.[46,133] Conjugation of the reactive products of phase I biotransformation with molecules such as glucuronide facilitates excretion.[133] (Chap. 12) Although many xenobiotics that are detoxified in the liver are subsequently excreted in the urine, the biliary tract provides a second essential route for the elimination of detoxified xenobiotics and products of metabolism.[20,29]

MORPHOLOGY AND FUNCTION OF THE LIVER

Two pathologic concepts are used to describe the appearance and function of the liver; a structural one represented by the hepatic lobule, and a functional one represented by the acinus. The basic structural unit of the liver characterized by light microscopy is the hepatic lobule, a hexagon with the central hepatic vein at the center and the portal triads at the angles. The portal triad consists of the portal vein, the common bile duct, and the hepatic artery. Cords of hepatocytes are oriented radially around the central hepatic vein, forming sinusoids. The acinus, or "metabolic lobule" is a functional unit of the liver. Located between two central hepatic veins, it is bisected by terminal branches of the hepatic artery and portal vein that extend from the bases of the acini toward hepatic venules at the apices. The acinus is subdivided into three metabolically distinct zones. Zone 1 lies near the portal triad, zone 3 near the central hepatic vein, and zone 2 is intermediate.[20,54] Figure 26–1 illustrates the relationship of the structural and functional concepts of the liver.

Approximately 75% of the blood supply to the liver is derived from the portal vein, which drains the alimentary tract, spleen, and pancreas. The blood is enriched with nutrients and other absorbed xenobiotics and is poor in oxygen. The remainder of the hepatic blood flow comes from the hepatic artery, which delivers well-oxygenated blood from the systemic circulation.[20] Blood from the hepatic artery and portal vein mixes in the sinusoids, coming in close contact with cords of hepatocytes before it exits through small holes in the wall of the vein. Oxygen content diminishes several fold as blood flows from the portal area to the central hepatic vein.[54,118]

There are six types of cells in the liver. Hepatocytes and bile duct epithelia make up the parenchyma. Cells found in the vicinity of the sinusoids include endothelial cells, fixed macrophages (Kupffer cells), hepatic stellate cells (Ito cells) that store fat, and large lymphocytic "pit cells" that roam the sinusoids.[118] The sinusoidal lining formed by endothelial cells is thin and fenestrated, allowing transfer of fluid, chylomicrons, and proteins across the space of Disse, an extrasinusoidal space filled with microvilli.[20,54,118] Kupffer cells scavenge particulate materials and cell debris within the sinusoids. When immunologically activated by xenobiotics, Kupffer cells contribute to the generation of oxygen free radicals[115,144] and may also participate in the production of autoimmune injury to hepatocytes.[33,61,115] Hepatic stellate cells (Ito cells) are primary sites for the storage of fat and vitamin A.[43] In a quiescent state they spread out between the sinusoidal endothelium and hepatic parenchymal cells. Filled with microtubules and microfilaments, they project cytoplasmic extensions that contact several cell types.[54,118] Activated stellate cells produce collagen, proteoglycans, and adhesive glycoproteins, which are crucial to the development of hepatic fibrosis.[118] Kupffer cells also contribute to the activation of hepatic stellate cells.[118] "Pit cells" are antigenically related to circulating natural killer cells. They actively lyse tumor cells and cells infected by virus[118] (Fig. 26–2).

Bile acids, organic anions, bilirubin, phospholipids, xenobiotics, and other molecules excreted in bile are actively transported across the hepatocyte plasma membrane into the bile canaliculi at sites that have specificity for acids, bases, and neutral compounds.[20,54] Tight junctions separate the contents of the bile canaliculi from the sinusoids and hepatocytes, maintaining a rigid and functionally necessary compartmentalization. Bile acids use three active transport systems: a sodium-dependent bile salt transporter in the sinusoidal membrane; an adenosine triphosphate (ATP)-dependent bile salt carrier in the canalicular membrane; and a canalicular membrane transport site driven by the membrane voltage potential.[54,67,118] Glucuronidated xenobiotics are substrates for the bile acid transport systems and are actively secreted into bile. Xenobiotics with molecular weights greater than 350 daltons are also preferentially secreted into bile. Like the transport and concentration of constituents from the sinusoids and hepatocytes, the flow of bile through the canaliculi is also an active process facilitated by ATP-dependent contractions of actin filaments that encircle the canaliculi.[67,139]

The enterohepatic circulation of bile acids and some vitamins plays a crucial role in their conservation. Unfortunately, this physiologically important process impedes the fecal elimination of some xenobiotics by reabsorbing and returning them back into the systemic circulation, prolonging their half lives and toxicity. Xenobiotics that have low molecular weights and are not ionized at intestinal pH, such as methyl mercury, phencyclidine, and nortriptyline, are most likely to be reabsorbed.[29,114]

The liver is especially vulnerable to toxic injury, due to its location at the end of the portal system and its substantial complement of biotransformation enzymes. Although phase I activation of xenobiotics is usually followed by phase II conjugation that results in detoxification, it can also lead to the production of xenobiotics with increased toxicity, which is often manifest at the site of their synthesis.[46,82,133]

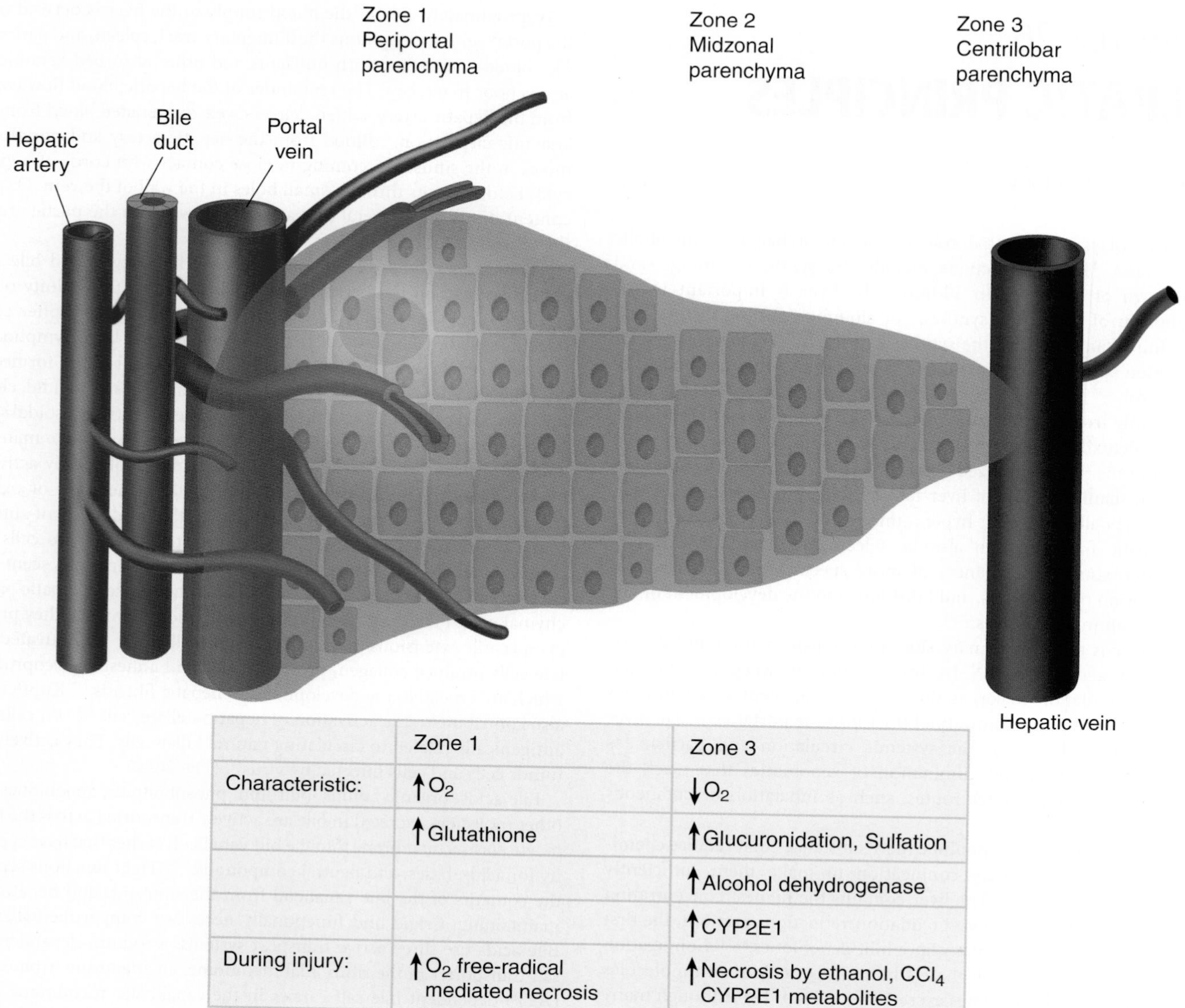

	Zone 1	Zone 3
Characteristic:	↑O_2	↓O_2
	↑Glutathione	↑Glucuronidation, Sulfation
		↑Alcohol dehydrogenase
		↑CYP2E1
During injury:	↑O_2 free-radical mediated necrosis	↑Necrosis by ethanol, CCl_4 CYP2E1 metabolites

FIGURE 26–1. The acinus is defined by three functional zones. Specific contributions of each zone to the biotransformation of xenobiotics reflect various metabolic factors that include differences in oxygen content of blood as it flows from the oxygen-rich portal area to the central hepatic vein; differences in glutathione content; different capacities for glucuronidation and sulfation; and variations in content of metabolic enzymes such as CYP2E1.The hepatic lobule (not shown) is a structural concept, a hexagon with the central vein at the center surrounded by 6 portal areas that contain branches of the hepatic artery, bile duct, and portal vein. Injury to hepatocytes that is confined to zone 3 is called "centrilobular" because in the structure of the lobule, zone 3 encircles the central vein, which is the center of the hepatic lobule.

FACTORS THAT AFFECT THE ANATOMIC LOCALIZATION OF HEPATIC INJURY

Hepatocellular injury that occurs near the portal vein is called *periportal,* or *zone 1* necrosis. The terms *centrilobular* or *zone 3* necrosis refer to injury that surrounds the central hepatic vein.[20] Figure 26–3 shows centrilobular necrosis caused by exposure to bromobenzene. Metabolic characteristics of the zones of the acinus have important relevance to the anatomic distribution of toxic liver injury. Because of its location in the periportal area, zone 1 has a two-fold higher oxygen content than zone 3. Hepatic injury that results from the metabolic production of oxygen free radicals predominates in zone 1. Allyl alcohol, an industrial chemical that is metabolized to a highly reactive aldehyde, is associated with oxygen dependent lipid peroxidation injury to hepatocytes in zone 1.[8] The tendency for centrilobular or zone 3 accumulation of fat in patients with alcoholic steatosis is attributed to the effect of relative hypoxia in the central vein area on the oxidation potential of the hepatocyte.[80] The availability of substrates for detoxification and the localization of enzymes involved in biotransformation also affect the site of injury. Zone 1 has a higher concentration of glutathione, whereas zone 3 has a greater capacity for glucuronidation and sulfation.[134] Zone 3 has higher concentrations of alcohol dehydrogenase, which may lead to increased production of toxic acetaldehyde at centrilobular sites.[28,54,80,84] Zone 3 also has high concentrations of cytochrome oxidase CYP2E1, which converts many xenobiotics including acetaminophen, nitrosamines, benzene, and carbon tetrachloride (CCl_4) to reactive intermediates that may cause centrilobular injury. Although CCl_4 can be metabolized to a

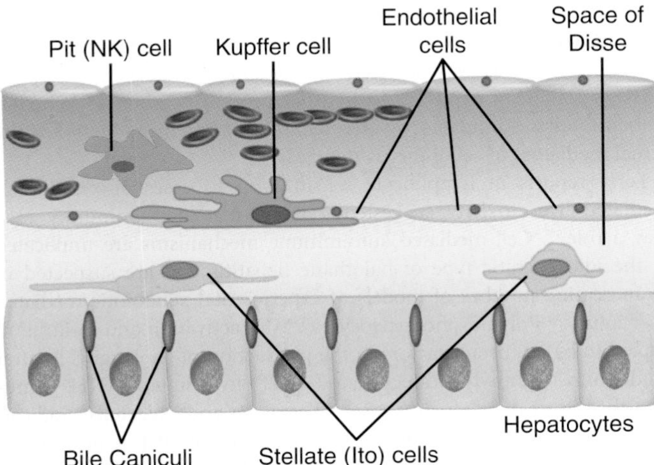

FIGURE 26–2. Blood flowing through the hepatic sinusoids is separated from hepatocytes by fenestrated endothelium that allows passage of many substances across the Space of Disse. This figure shows 6 types of cells found in the liver and their localization in relation to the sinusoid. Stellate cells are fat storage cells that promote fibrosis when activated. Kupffer cells are fixed macrophages that participate in immune surveillance and are a source of free radicals when activated. Pit cells float freely in the sinusoids and have activities similar to natural killer (NK) cells. Hepatocytes and bile epithelial cells form the hepatic parenchyma.

highly reactive oxygen free radical in zone 1, it primarily injures zone 3 for the following reasons:[16] CCl_4 is metabolized by CYP2E1 in zone 3 to a trichloromethyl free radical ($\cdot CCl_3$) that can form covalent bonds with cellular proteins, cause lipid peroxidation, or spontaneously react with oxygen to form the more highly reactive trichloromethyl peroxy radical ($CCl_3OO\cdot$).[16,33,81] Higher oxygen tension in zone 1 fosters the formation of $CCl_3OO\cdot$ which is rapidly detoxified by glutathione. Since the less reactive $\cdot CCl_3$ that predominates in zone 3 is not readily detoxified by glutathione, zone 3 incurs the greater amount of injury. Hyperbaric oxygen increases the oxygen tension throughout the liver and decreases liver injury caused by CCl_4, possibly by increasing the formation of $CCl_3OO\cdot$ in zone 3, which is then efficiently detoxified by glutathione.[16,133] The observed effects of isoniazid (an inhibitor of the enzyme CYP2E1) and chronic ethanol intake (an inducer of the CYP2E1 gene) on injury in cell cultures from periportal and centrilobular areas exposed to CCl_4 support the association of CCl_4 injury with the localization of CYP2E1 activity. Acute exposure to isoniazid significantly decreases the injury associated with exposure of zone 3 cells to CCl_4, whereas chronic treatment with ethanol significantly enhances it.[81]

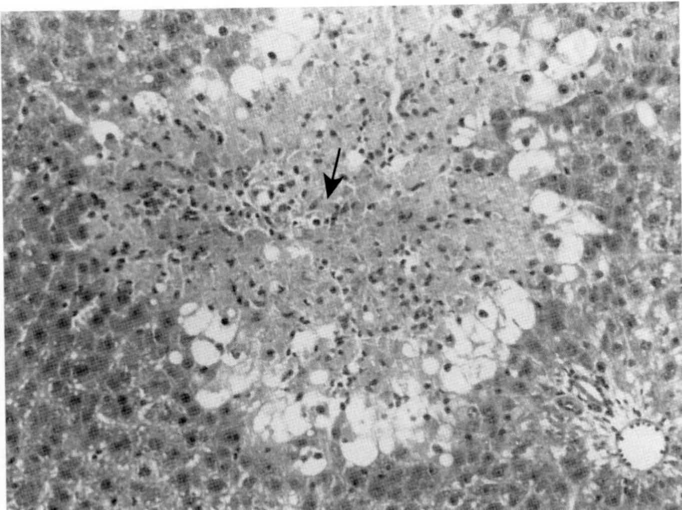

FIGURE 26–3. Centrilobular necrosis in a rat liver caused by bromobenzene administration. Note the polymorphonuclear leukocyte infiltration surrounded by vacuolated hepatocytes in the necrotic area. (Reprinted, with permission, from Hetu C, Dumont A, Joly JG, et al. Effect of chronic ethanol administration on bromobenzene liver toxicity in the rat. *Toxicol Appl Pharm.* 1983;676:166.)

HOST FACTORS THAT AFFECT THE DEVELOPMENT OF HEPATOTOXICITY

Xenobiotics that produce liver damage in all humans in a predictable and dose-dependent manner are called *intrinsic* hepatotoxins. They include acetaminophen, CCl_4, and yellow phosphorous. Those that cause liver damage in a small number of individuals and whose effect is not apparently dose dependent or predictable are called *idiosyncratic* hepatotoxins. Some idiosyncratic hepatotoxins cause hepatotoxicity very rarely, whereas others produce it commonly. The majority of hepatotoxins fall into the category of idiosyncratic xenobiotics.[75,82] The inhaled anesthetic halothane is both an intrinsic and an idiosyncratic hepatotoxin. A mild degree of hepatitis occurs in as great as 20% of patients exposed to halothane.[32] This form of halothane hepatitis, which can be reliably induced in animals, is likely caused by direct toxicity.[117] A more severe idiosyncratic form appears to be caused by an autoimmune response induced by halothane that targets liver proteins[13,127] (Chap. 67).

Sporadic unpredicted hepatotoxicity is not idiosyncratic, but is more likely a result of the combined effects of genetic and other factors that result in the overproduction or decreased clearance of toxic metabolites. Idiosyncratic toxicity may be related to individual variability in the capacity to metabolize a specific xenobiotic and would most likely be predictable, rather than "idiosyncratic," if the exposed individual's metabolic capabilities could be prospectively defined (Chap. 12). An individual's susceptibility to a hepatotoxin depends on numerous factors, including the activity of biotransformation enzymes, the availability of substrates such as glutathione, and the immune competence of the individual. In turn, these are affected by age, sex, diet, underlying diseases, concurrent exposure to other xenobiotics, and genetic factors. Many enzymes involved in biotransformation show genetic polymorphism.[46,51,75,82] The susceptibility to toxic effects of a xenobiotic may be determined by inherited variations in CYP enzymes. For example, approximately 8% of whites are deficient in CYP2D6, which is responsible for the metabolism of a number of xenobiotics, including debrisoquine (an antihypertensive first identified as the substrate of this enzyme), several antidepressants and antidysrhythmics, some opioids, and phenformin.[75,125] Perhexiline, an antianginal agent marketed in Europe in the 1980s, caused severe liver disease and peripheral neuropathy in persons with a demonstrated inability to metabolize debrisoquine.[125] The congenital disorder that results in Gilbert syndrome is characterized by impaired glucuronyltransferase. Patients demonstrate decreased glucuronidation and increased bioactivation of acetaminophen during chronic therapeutic dosing, suggesting an increased risk of hepatic injury following ingestions of acetaminophen.[25]

EFFECTS OF XENOBIOTICS ON ENZYME FUNCTION

Changes in the activities of biotransformation enzymes that result in increased formation of hepatotoxic metabolites increase susceptibility to hepatic injury. Chronic administration of isoniazid (INH) induces CYP2E1 activity.[145] During chronic ethanol exposure proliferation of the smooth endoplasmic reticulum in the centrilobular areas is associated with increased activity of CYP2E1.[23,65,81,83,99] In one rat study, the administration of an average of 9.2 gm/kg of ethanol in increasing doses for 4 weeks resulted in a significant increase in the extent of injury to cultured zone 3 hepatocytes when exposed to CCl_4. This was associated with a higher expression of CYP 2E1 in the livers of ethanol treated rats.[81] Bromobenzene is a xenobiotic whose metabolism and hepatotoxicity are similar to that of acetaminophen. When administered to rats chronically exposed to ethanol, the onset of hepatotoxicity occurs more rapidly in study animals, with only a small increase in the extent of hepatic necrosis. The dose of bromobenzene required for hepatic injury to occur is not altered by pretreatment with ethanol.[48] Chronic administration of phenobarbital to rats results in a very significant increase in the hepatotoxic effects of bromobenzene.[98,109] Hepatic toxicity caused by solvents such as CCl_4, dimethylformamide, and bromobenzene may be exacerbated by chronic exposure to ethanol.[48,81,86,107] Whether ethanol increases the clinical risk of acetaminophen hepatotoxicity in humans is debated.[68,103,120,124,148] There is no evidence that the chronic use of ethanol increases the risk of liver injury due to therapeutic doses of acetaminophen.[54]

Some xenobiotic combinations increase the possibility of hepatotoxic reactions because one xenobiotic alters the metabolism of the other, leading to the production of toxic metabolites.[102] This is the case with combinations of rifampin and isoniazid;[55] amoxicillin and clavulanic acid;[72,106] and trimethoprim and sulfamethoxazole.[3]

Immune Mediated Hepatic Injury Immune-mediated liver injury is an idiosyncratic and host-dependent hypersensitivity response to exposure to xenobiotics.[9,82] It is differentiated from liver injury caused by other autoimmune disorders by the absence of self-perpetuation, that is, there is a need for continuous exposure to the xenobiotic to perpetuate the injury.[82] Hypersensitivity reactions result in forms of liver injury that include hepatitis, cholestasis, and mixed disorders. Drugs with hypersensitivity reactions that typically present with hepatitis include halothane,[13,59,127] trimethoprim-sulfamethoxazole,[3,98] anticonvulsants,[77] and allopurinol.[4,126] Drugs that typically present with cholestatic signs and symptoms (pruritus, jaundice, insignificant elevations of aspartate aminotransferase [AST] and alanine aminotransferase [ALT]) include chlorpromazine, erythromycin, penicillins, rifampin, and sulfonamides.[67,137] Signs of injury typically begin 1 to 8 weeks following the initiation of the drug, although they may begin as late as 20 weeks for drugs such as isoniazid or dantrolene. The onset of signs of injury associated with the oxypenicillins may occur as great as 2 weeks after the drug is stopped.[82] In all cases, the onset is earlier when the patient is rechallenged with the drug. Although eosinophilia, atypical lymphocytosis, fever, and rash are common clinical manifestations of hypersensitivity, their absence does not exclude an autoimmune mechanism of drug-associated liver injury.[64,82]

How the immune response ultimately leads to cell injury is not well defined. Damage to the hepatocyte may be mediated by complement- or antibody-directed lysis; by specific cell-mediated cytotoxicity; or by an inflammatory response stimulated by immune complexes and complement.[10,14,31,59,61,92] The covalent binding of a reactive electrophilic metabolite with a hepatocellular protein resulting in the formation of a neoantigen is a well-defined first step in the development of xenobiotic-related autoimmune liver injury. This covalent binding creates an "adduct" that is perceived as foreign by the immune system and induces an immune response. In cases where the metabolite is highly unstable, the electrophilic attack may be directed against the CYP enzyme at the site of formation of the metabolite.[13,77,82] Adducts and associated autoantibodies have been demonstrated for acetaminophen,[18] minocycline,[10] halothane,[13,31,127] dihydralazine,[14] phenytoin,[77] and germander.[71] The most severe form of idiosyncratic halothane liver injury is manifest as fulminant hepatic failure associated with formation of adducts of its trifluoroacetyl chloride (TFA) metabolite with numerous hepatoproteins that include CYP2E1 and pyruvate dehydrogenase.[9,31,59,127] Autoantibodies against the CYP2E1 enzyme have been demonstrated in halothane liver injury (Chap. 67).[13,59] Autoantibodies specifically directed against CYP enzymes have also been demonstrated for dihydralazine,[14] and phenytoin.[77] A trifluoroacetyl protein adduct similar to that associated with halothane hepatitis was detected in workers who developed hepatic necrosis following exposure to hydrochlorofluorocarbons.[49] Whether autoantibodies stimulated by the xenobiotic-protein adducts are the actual mediators of cell injury is not clear.

Early reports of lymphocyte sensitization in cases of xenobiotic-mediated liver toxicity suggested that cell-mediated immunity may play a role.[137] Cell-mediated autoimmune mechanisms are implicated in the idiosyncratic type of halothane hepatitis and are suspected in an increasing number of models of experimental xenobiotic-mediated liver injury.[32] Polymorphonucleocyte (PMN) activation and infiltration appear to be important factors in the production of cholangitis in a rat model of α-naphthyl-isothiocyanate (ANIT) liver injury. ANIT stimulates the release of cytotoxic lysosomal enzymes and oxygen free radicals by activated PMNs.[92] Antibodies directed against circulating neutrophils to decrease the extent of liver damage caused by ANIT.[22] Natural killer T cells are ubiquitous in the liver and their possible role in the facilitation of cell-mediated autoimmune liver injury is being investigated.[21,45]

Availability of Substrates The availability of substrates for detoxification may significantly affect both the likelihood and localization of hepatic injury.[73] The metabolism of acetaminophen illustrates the effect of glutathione concentration on the delicate balance between detoxification and the production of injurious metabolites. In healthy adults taking therapeutic amounts of acetaminophen, approximately 90% of hepatic metabolism results in formation of glucuronidated or sulfated metabolites.[25,133] Most of the remainder undergoes oxidative metabolism to the toxic electrophile *N*-acetyl-*p*-benzoquinoneimine (NAPQI) and is rapidly detoxified by conjugation with glutathione.[18,54] Glutathione may be depleted during the course of metabolism of acetaminophen by otherwise normal livers, or it may be decreased by inadequate nutrition or liver disease.[73,75] Excessive amounts of acetaminophen result in increased synthesis of NAPQI, which, in the absence of glutathione, reacts avidly with hepatocellular macromolecules. The cellular concentration of glutathione correlates inversely with the demonstrable covalent binding of NAPQI to liver cells.[18] Centrilobular (zone 3) necrosis predominates in acetaminophen induced hepatic injury, possibly related to the centrilobular localization of CYP2E1 and the relatively low glutathione concentrations compared to the periportal areas (zone 1).[54]

MORPHOLOGIC AND BIOCHEMICAL MANIFESTATIONS OF HEPATIC INJURY

The liver responds to injury in a limited number of ways.[57] Cells may swell (ballooning degeneration) and accumulate fat (steatosis) or biliary material. They may necrose and lyse or undergo the slower process of apoptosis, forming shrunken, nonfunctioning, eosinophilic bodies. Necrosis may be focal or bridging, linking the periportal or centrilobular areas; zonal or panacinar; or it may be massive. An inflammatory cell response may precede or follow necrosis.[20,75] Injury to the bile ducts results in cholestasis. Vascular injuries may cause obstruction to venous flow.[69,143] The vascular effects of cocaine may cause ischemic liver injury.[75,135] The variety and spectrum of injury caused by NSAIDS illustrates the difficulty in categorizing and characterizing all of the forms and causes of xenobiotic hepatic injury. These xenobiotics are associated with most forms of injury including asymptomatic aminotransferase elevations, simple cholestasis, hepatitis, bile duct injury, fulminant necrosis, and steatosis.[57] Both azathioprine[27] and ethanol[54,80,84] are associated with a multitude of histopathologic manifestations of hepatocellular injury. Table 26–1 lists characteristic morphologies of hepatic injury and associated xenobiotics.

Table 26–1. Morphology of Liver Injury by Selected Xenobiotics

Acute Hepatocellular Necrosis
Acetaminophen[a]
Allopurinol
Amatoxin[a]
Arsenic
Carbamazepine
Carbon tetrachloride[a]
Chlordecone (less severe)
Hydralazine
Iron
Isoniazid
Methotrexate[a]
Methyldopa
Nitrofurantoin
Phenytoin
Phosphorus (yellow)[a]
Procainamide
Propythiouracil
Quinine
Propythiouracil
Quinine
Sulfonamides
Tetrachlorethane
Tetracycline
Trinitrotoluene
Troglitazone
Vinyl Chloride

Steatohepatitis
Amiodarone
Dimethyl formamide

Microvesicular Steatosis
Aflatoxin
Cerulide
Fialuridine
Hypoglycin
Margosa oil
Nucleoside analogs (Antiretrovirals)
Tetracycline
Valproic acid

Granulomatous Hepatitis
Allopurinol
Aspirin
Beryllium
Carbamazepine
Copper Salts
Diltiazem
Halothane
Hydralazine
Isoniazid
Metolazone
Methyldopa
Nitrofurantoin
Penicillins
Phenytoin
Procainamide
Quinidine
Quinine
Sulfonamides
Sulfonylureas

Cholestasis
Allopurinol
Amoxacillin/clavulanic acid
Androgens
Chlorpromazine
Chlorpropamide
Erythromycin estolate
Hydralazine
Nitrofurantoin
Oral contraceptives
Rifampin
Tetracycline
Trimethaprim-sulfamethoxazole

Fibrosis and Cirrhosis
Ethanol
Methotrexate
Vitamin A

Neoplasms
Androgens
Contraceptive steroids
Vinyl chloride

Venoocclusive Disease
Cyclophosphamide
Pyrrozolidine alkaloids

Cannicular Cholestasis
Chlorpromazine
Cyclosporine
Estrogens
Methylene dianiline

Bile Duct Damage
α-napthylisothiocyanate
Amoxicillin
Carbamazepine
Nitrofurantoin
Oral contraceptives

Autoimmune Hepatitis
Dantrolene
Diclofenac
Methyldopa
Methyldopa
Nafcillin
Nitrofurantoin
Methyldopa
Nafcillin
Nitrofurantoin
Propylthiouracil

[a] Intrinsic hepatotoxin.

ACUTE HEPATOCELLULAR NECROSIS

Numerous xenobiotics have been associated with hepatocellular necrosis (see Table 26–1). Acetaminophen is a common cause, as are herbal remedies, whose risks are increasingly recognized.[34,50,52,71,97] Many halogenated hydrocarbons that include carbon tetrachloride,[16,81] bromobenzene,[48,109] hydrochlorofluorocarbons,[49] halothane[13,59,127] and antituberculous drugs[93,94,101] also produce hepatocellular necrosis. A study of greater than 11,000 patients exposed to isoniazid during preventive treatment showed that hepatocellular necrosis occurred in 0.10% of those starting treatment, and in 0.15% of those completing treatment.[94] Risk factors for the development of hepatotoxicity from isoniazid exposure are female sex, increasing age, coadministration with rifampin, and alcoholism[101] (Chap. 57). The thiazolidinedione agents troglitazone and rosiglitazone, marketed for the treatment of type 2 diabetes, are associated with acute hepatocellular necrosis.[5,44] The much greater incidence of liver injury attributed to troglitazone led to its withdrawal from the market in March 2000.[79] Occupational exposure to solvents that include dimethylformamide and CCl_4 cause dose-related hepatocellular necrosis.[86,107,108]

Acute necrosis of a hepatocyte disrupts all aspects of its function. Because there is a great deal of functional reserve in the liver, hepatic function may be preserved despite the development of focal necrosis. Extensive necrosis results in functional liver failure. The processes that lead to cell necrosis are not well known. Cell lysis is preceded by the formation of blebs in the lipid membrane and leakage of cytosolic enzymes, primarily aminotransferases and lactate dehydrogenase. Coalescence of blebs leads to rupture of the cellular membrane and acute irreversible cell death, with disintegration of the nucleus and termination of all cellular function. Prior to membrane rupture, this injury is reversible by membrane repair processes.[92] The release of intracellular constituents attracts circulating leukocytes and results in an inflammatory response in the hepatic parenchyma. A proposed mechanism of rapid injury to the cell membrane is the initiation of a cascading lipid peroxidation reaction following attack by a free radical. The CYP2E1 enzyme has a significant potential to produce oxygen free radicals, as do activated PMNs and Kupffer cells.[23,33,92,115,144] Oxidant stress is an important cause of liver injury during the metabolism of ethanol by CYP2E1.[28] This results in cell death and the stimulation of stellate cells, which promotes fibrosis.[28] In addition to peroxidation of membrane lipids, the oxidation of proteins, phospholipid fatty acyl side chains, and nucleosides appear to be widespread. Mitochondrial injury and resultant ATP depletion may also be associated with necrosis.[58,85] Acetaminophen is the commonest xenobiotic cause of fulminant hepatic failure and NAPQI, its reactive metabolite of acetaminophen, may target mitochondrial enzymes.[79] Other xenobiotics known to cause mitochondrial injury include antiviral drugs,[19,24,79,88,90] tetracycline,[122] valproic acid,[11] hypoglycin, margosa oil, and cerulide.[85,119]

STEATOSIS

Steatosis is the abnormal accumulation of fat in hepatocytes. It reflects abnormal cellular metabolism in conditions that include responses to xenobiotics. Cell injury depends on the severity of the underlying metabolic disturbance, steatosis per se is normally well tolerated and reversible in many cases although approximately one-third of patients with nonalcoholic steatosis may develop steatohepatitis.[37,54,70] Nonalcoholic steatosis associated with obesity, insulin resistance, and the metabolic syndrome may account for many cases of cryptogenic cirrhosis.[37] Intracellular fat accumulation may occur as a result of any one or more of the following mechanisms: impaired synthesis of lipoproteins; increased mobilization of peripheral adipose stores; increased uptake of circulating lipids; increased triglyceride production; decreased binding of triglycerides to lipoprotein; and decreased release of very-low-density lipoproteins from the hepatocytes.[7,54,70,80] There are two light microscopic manifestations of steatosis: macrovesicular steatosis, in which the nucleus is displaced by large droplets of intracellular fat, and microvesicular steatosis, which is characterized by tiny cytoplasmic fat droplets that do not displace the nucleus. Xenobiotics associated with macrovesicular steatosis include ethanol and amiodarone. Ethanol increases the uptake of fatty acids into hepatocytes and decreases lipoprotein secretion. In addition, the increased ratio of the reduced form of nicotinamide adenine dinucleotide (NADH) to the oxidized form of nicotinamide adenine dinucleotide (NAD^+), associated with hepatic metabolism of ethanol, decreases oxidation of fatty acids and promotes fatty acid synthesis.[54,80] An early pathologic lesion that occurs in alcoholic liver disease is reversible macrovesicular steatosis. Mallory bodies, eosinophilic cytoplasmic deposits of keratin filaments in degenerating hepatocytes, are also common microscopic findings in alcoholic liver disease.[20,54,80,84] Amiodarone hepatic toxicity resembles that of alcoholic hepatitis, with steatosis, Mallory bodies, and potential for progression to cirrhosis.[75] Lamellated intralysosomal phospholipid inclusion bodies are specific for amiodarone toxicity.[112] Figure 26–4 shows macrovesicular steatosis with Mallory bodies caused by amiodarone.

Steatosis Associated with Mitochondrial Dysfunction Microvesicular steatosis is caused by severe impairment of β-oxidation of fatty acids. The β-oxidation of fatty acids depends on a steady synthesis of cellular energy in the form of ATP and takes place in the mitochondia. Mechanisms of impaired β-oxidation of fatty acids include direct inhibition or sequestration of critical cofactors such as coenzyme-A and L-carnitine.[70] An association between deficiency of carnitine, microsteatosis, and the development of hyperammonemia is observed in children treated with valproic acid.[11,104,136] Valproic acid causes mild elevations of aminotransferases in approximately 11% of patients, usually during the first few months of therapy. The earliest pathologic

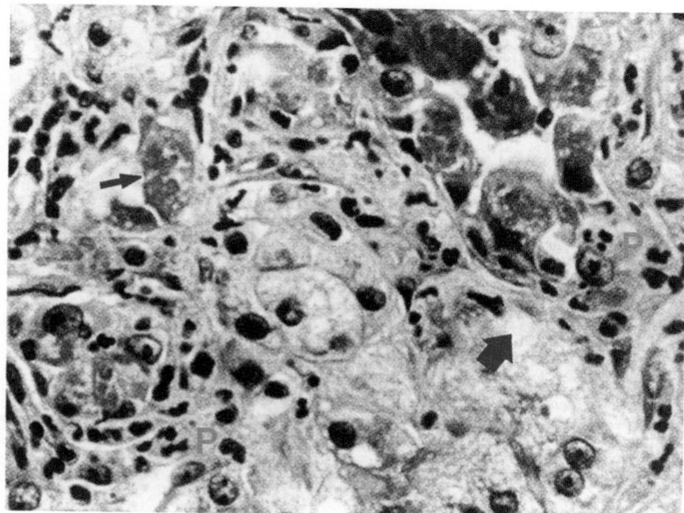

FIGURE 26–4. Macrovesicular steatosis associated with administration of amiodarone. The *small arrow* indicates the presence of Mallory bodies. The *large arrow* points to accumulated intracellular fat. (Note that the nuclei are displaced.) Polymorphonuclear leukocytes (*P*) are also present. (Reprinted, with permission, from Lee WM. Drug-induced hepatotoxicity. *N Engl J Med.* 1995;333:1118.)

lesion that signals progression of liver injury is microvesicular steatosis, which occurs in the absence of necrosis. A small percentage of patients progress to fulminant hepatic failure characterized by centrilobular necrosis.[146] The incidence of fatal hepatocellular injury is highest in children, approaching 1 in 800 children younger than age 2 years.[104] Other mechanisms of impairment of β-oxidation of fatty acids include processes that disrupt cellular ATP production, either directly by xenobiotics such as sodium azide or cyanide that inhibit electron transport in the respiratory chain; by xenobiotics that increase permeability of mitochondrial membranes and degrade the proton gradient that is critical to ATP synthesis; or by xenobiotics that uncouple oxidative ph osphorylation.[7,42,78,90,119,122] Nucleoside analogs that inhibit viral reverse transcriptase also inhibit mitochondrial DNA synthesis, leading to depletion of mitochondria.[19,70,90,119] Microvesicular steatosis is described in patients taking antiretrovirals such as zidovudine, zalcitabine, and didanosine.[24,88,128,131] Failure of the mitochondrial power supply may or may not be associated with hepatocyte necrosis and elevation of hepatocellular enzymes.[85,90,119] In all cases, metabolic acidosis with elevated lactate is a prominent biochemical feature.[24,42,119] The nucleoside analog fialuridine caused severe hepatotoxicity during a study of its use in the treatment of chronic hepatitis B infection. Microscopic examinations of liver specimens in these cases showed marked accumulation of fat with minimal necrosis or structural injury. Severe acidosis and failure of hepatic synthetic function suggested failure of cellular energy production. Mitochondria examined under the electron microscope were demonstrably abnormal.[90] Figure 26–5 demonstrates microvesicular steatosis in a patient with fialuridine hepatotoxicity. High doses of tetracycline produce microvesicular steatosis associated with moderate elevations of aminotransferases, markedly prolonged prothrombin time, and progression to fulminant hepatic failure.[122] Microvesicular steatosis attributed to failure of mitochondrial energy production was reported in a fatal case of *Bacillus cereus* food poisoning, where high concentrations of the bacterial emetic toxin cereulide were found in the bile and liver. In this case, microvesicular steatosis was associated with extensive hepatocellular necrosis.[85] Other xenobiotics that cause mitochondrial failure are hypoglycin, the cause of Jamaican vomiting sickness, aflatoxin, and margosa oil.[119] Steatosis is also observed following exposure to the industrial solvent dimethylformamide. Liver biopsies in patients with acute illness show focal hepatocellular necrosis and microvesicular steatosis. More prolonged, less symptomatic exposures result in significant macrovesicular steatosis with mild aminotransferase elevations.[107,108]

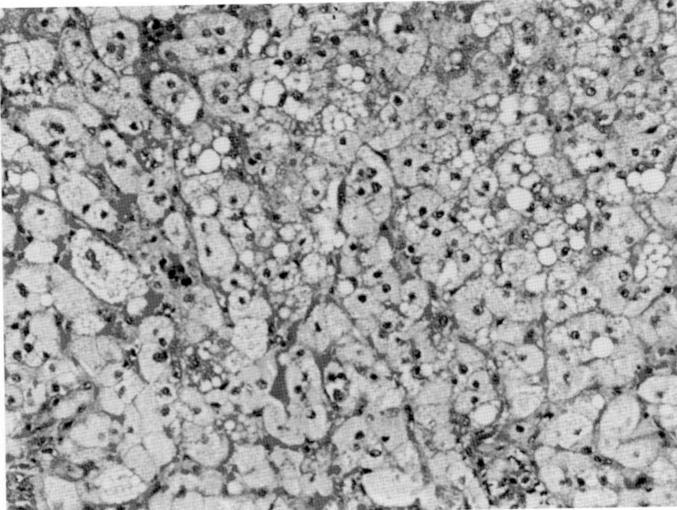

FIGURE 26–5. This figure shows severe microvesicular steatosis in a patient treated with fialuridine. Note the central location of the nuclei. (Reprinted, with permission, from McKenzie R, Fried MW, Sallie R, et al. Hepatic failure and lactic acidosis due to fialuridine, an investigational nucleoside analogue for chronic hepatitis B. *N Engl J Med.* 1995;333:1099.)

CHOLESTASIS

Xenobiotics induce cholestasis by targeting specific mechanisms of bile synthesis and flow or by damaging canicular cells.[54,67] Cholestasis may occur with or without associated hepatitis. The development of jaundice following hepatic necrosis is a manifestation of general failure of liver function. More discrete mechanisms that result in intrahepatic cholestasis include (a) impairment of the integrity of tight membrane junctions that functionally isolate the canaliculus from the hepatocyte and sinusoids; (b) failure of transport of bile components across the hepatocytes; (c) blockade of specific membrane active transport sites; (d) decreased membrane fluidity resulting in altered transport; and (e) decreased canalicular contractility resulting in decreased bile flow.[12,54,67,121] Estrogens cause intrahepatic cholestasis by altering the composition of the lipid membrane and inhibiting the rate of secretion of bile into the canaliculi.[67,79,121] Rifampin impedes the uptake of bilirubin into hepatocytes. Methyltestosterone and C-17 alkylated anabolic steroids impair the secretion of bilirubin into canaliculi.[79] Exposure to chlorpromazine is associated with cholestasis and periductal inflammation. This may be caused by inhibition of Na^+, K^+-adenosine triphosphatase (ATPase), which results in decreased canalicular contractility.[116] Cyclosporine inhibits sodium-dependent uptake of bile salts across the sinusoidal membrane and blocks ATP-dependent bile salt transport across the canalicular membrane.[12] Floxacillin causes cholestasis with minimal inflammation or evidence of hepatocellular injury.[137] Exposure of rats to ANIT causes a specific injury localized to the tight junctions that separate the hepatocyte from the canaliculi. This results in reflux of bile constituents into the sinusoidal space and increased access of sinusoidal molecules to the biliary tree.[22,67,92]

VENOOCCLUSIVE DISEASE

Hepatic venoocclusive disease is caused by toxins that injure the endothelium of terminal hepatic venules, resulting in intimal thickening, edema, and nonthrombotic obstruction. Central and sublobular hepatic veins may also become edematous and fibrosed. There is intense sinusoidal dilation in the centrilobular areas that is associated with liver cell atrophy and necrosis.[142] The gross pathologic appearance is that of a "nutmeg" liver.[69,143] Massive hepatic congestion and ascites ensue.[69,111] Hepatic venoocclusive disease is rapidly fatal in 15% to 20% of cases. It is associated with exposure to pyrrolizidine alkaloids found in many plant species including *Symphytum* (comfrey tea),[140,143] *Heliotrope, Senecio,* and *Crotalaria.*[69] It has occurred in epidemic proportions; in South Africa after the ingestion of flour contaminated with ragwort (*Senecio*); in Jamaica after the ingestion of "bush teas" (*Crotalaria spp*); and in India and Afghanistan when food was contaminated with *Heliotropium lasiocarpine* and *Crotalaria.*[15,95,132] A rapidly progressive form has been reported in bone marrow transplant patients following high-dose treatment with cyclophosphamide.[89]

CHRONIC HEPATITIS

A form of hepatitis that clinically resembles nontoxic autoimmune hepatitis occurs with the chronic administration of drugs such as methyldopa, nitrofurantoin, propylthiouracil, nafcillin, dantrolene, and diclofenac.[4,60,76,88,110,123,130] Many cases are associated with positive antinuclear antibody (ANA), smooth muscle antibody (SMA), and hyperglobulinemia. Jaundice is prominent and hepatocellular enzymes are elevated 5- to 60-fold. Liver biopsy commonly reveals intrahepatic cholestasis, as well as centrilobular inflammation.[82]

Granulomatous hepatitis is characterized by infiltration of the hepatic parenchyma with caseating granulomata. As great as 60 drugs are associated with this disorder. Fever and systemic symptoms are common, 25% have splenomegaly. Liver enzymes are mixed, reflecting variable degrees of cholestasis and hepatocellular injury. Eosinophilia occurs in 30% as an extrahepatic manifestation of drug hypersensitivity. Continued exposure may result in a more severe form of liver disease. Small vessel vasculitis, which may involve the skin, lungs, and kidney, is a disturbing sign associated with increased mortality.[75,91,147] Table 26–1 lists a number of the xenobiotics that have been implicated in this disorder.

CIRRHOSIS

Cirrhosis is caused by progressive fibrosis and scarring of the liver, which results in irreversible hepatic dysfunction and portal hypertension. This causes shunting of blood away from hepatocytes and subsequent hepatocellular dysfunction. Activated stellate cells produce collagen, proteoglycans, and adhesive glycoproteins, which are deposited in the space of Disse and are crucial to the development of hepatic fibrosis.[118] Kupffer cells contribute to the activation of hepatic stellate cells.[118] In alcoholic cirrhosis, acetaldehyde also stimulates collagen production by hepatic stellate cells, as do other aldehydes that are products of lipid peroxidation.[54,80] Alcoholic hepatitis generally precedes cirrhosis, although cirrhosis may develop in its absence.[84] Chronic ingestion of excessive amounts of vitamin A (25,000 U/d for 6 years or 100,000 U/d for 2.5 years) results in cirrhosis. An increase in the fat content of the sinusoidal stellate cells with increasing degrees of collagen formation are characteristic lesions that occur early in vitamin A toxicity (Chap. 41). Portal hypertension may be early and striking.[43] Like vitamin A, methyldopa and methotrexate also cause a slow progressive development of cirrhosis with few clinical symptoms.[76,141] Methotrexate-induced hepatic fibrosis is dose dependent. Risk factors include associated alcohol intake and preexisting liver disease. Reduced dosing has largely eliminated the risk of the development of cirrhosis in patients receiving methotrexate.[58,141]

HEPATIC TUMORS

There is persuasive evidence that the use of oral contraceptive steroids increases the risk of hepatic adenomas.[63] There is also evidence that oral contraceptives increase the overall risk of hepatocellular carcinoma; however, the number of cases associated with estrogen therapy is low.[53] Anabolic steroids are rarely associated with the development of both benign and malignant hepatic tumors.[38] Angiosarcoma is strongly associated with exposure to vinyl chloride, in addition to arsenic, thorium dioxide, and steroid hormones.[36]

HEPATIC INJURY ASSOCIATED WITH PLANTS AND HERBS

In addition to the venoocclusive disease associated with pyrrolizidine alkaloids described above, herbal remedies are increasingly recognized as a cause of acute hepatocellular injury. Numerous plants or plant products are known or suspected to cause hepatic injury (Chaps. 43 and 118).[30,34,50,52,71,97]

CLINICAL PRESENTATION OF TOXIC LIVER INJURY

Clinical presentations of toxic liver injury range from indolent, often asymptomatic progression of impairment of hepatic function to rapid development of hepatic failure. Jaundice and pruritis are due to increased concentrations of bile acids and bilirubin in the blood. Failure of hepatocellular synthetic function results in bleeding due to coagulopathy and edema due to hypoalbuminemia. Encephalopathy may be due to hypoglycemia, impaired neurotransmission, or accumulation of toxic products of metabolism such as ammonia. Fever may occur with autoimmune mediated liver injury. Impaired hepatic blood flow results in familiar manifestations of portal hypertension such as caput medusa, splenomegaly, ascites and varices. Spider angiomata and gynecomastia also occur due to altered estrogen metabolism.[20]

FULMINANT HEPATIC FAILURE

Fulminant hepatic failure (FHF) is defined as liver injury that progresses to coagulopathy and encephalopathy within 8 weeks of the onset of illness in a patient without preexisting liver disease.[41,74] Complications from FHF include encephalopathy, cerebral edema, coagulopathy, renal dysfunction, hypoglycemia, hypotension, acute lung injury, sepsis, and death. In some cases, a patient may progress from health to death in as little as 2-10 days.[17,39,40,41,74,85,100] Table 26–2 shows the clinical progression of encephalopathy as hepatic failure develops. The prognosis of FHF is related to the time that passes between the onset of jaundice and the onset of encephalopathy. Perhaps surprisingly, a better prognosis is associated with shorter (2-4 weeks) jaundice-to-encephalopathy intervals.[113] Most cases of FHF are caused by xenobiotics or viral hepatitis. FHF is usually associated with extensive necrosis,

TABLE 26–2. Stages of Hepatic Encephalopathy

Clinical Stage	Mental Status	Neuromotor Function
Subclinical	Normal physical examination	Subtle impairment of neuromotor function → driving or work injury hazard
I	Euphoric, irritable, depressed, fluctuating mild confusion, poor attention, sleep disturbance	Poor coordination; may have asterixis alone
II	Impaired memory, cognition, or simple mathematical tasks	Slurred speech, tremor, ataxia
III	Difficult to arouse, persistent confusion, incoherent	Hyperactive reflexes, clonus, nystagmus
IV	Coma; may respond to noxious stimuli	May have decerebrate posturing; Cheyne-Stokes respirations; pupils are reactive and the oculocephalic reflex is intact; may have signs of ↑ intracranial pressure

although it may occur in the absence of demonstrable necrosis following exposures to xenobiotics that injure mitochondria.[85,90,131] Some xenobiotics that are associated with fulminant hepatic necrosis are clove oil, amanitin cyclopeptides, acetaminophen, tetracycline, yellow phosphorus, halogenated hydrocarbons, isoniazid, methyldopa, and valproic acid.[30,74,96,107,108,113,122]

HEPATIC ENCEPHALOPATHY

Hepatic encephalopathy (HE) is a severe manifestation of liver failure that is potentially fully reversible, even in cases of deep coma.[39,40,41] HE is associated with a fluctuating sensorium that ranges from barely discernible confusion to coma. Neuromotor signs such as asterixis and rigidity are common.[17] Table 26–2 lists the clinical stages of acute HE. Ammonia is produced in the colon by bacterial breakdown of ingested proteins then transported to the liver via the portal circulation where it is detoxified to glutamine and urea.[40] Ammonia concentrations are elevated in 60% to 80% of patients with HE.[40] Processes that raise CNS ammonia concentrations include infection, hypokalemia, alkalosis, increased muscle wasting, volume depletion, azotemia, or gastrointestinal bleeding.[40] Alkalosis and hypokalemia facilitate conversion of NH_4^+ to NH_3, which moves more easily across the blood–brain barrier. The demonstration that ammonia is not elevated in many cases suggests that there are other pathogenic etiologies and the etiology is multifactorial. Disruption of central neurotransmitter regulation including dopamine receptor binding may contribute.[138] There is evidence that liver failure is associated with the accumulation of substances that stimulate central benzodiazepine receptors, leading to inhibition of γ-aminobutyric acid (GABA) transmission.[6] Nonnitrogenous HE is precipitated by sedatives, especially benzodiazepines, hypoxia, hypoglycemia, hypothyroidism, and anemia.[40] Although it is clear that sedatives that depress GABAergic transmission can make encephalopathy worse, studies of the use of flumazenil to reverse encephalopathy show conflicting results.[6] Significant short-term improvement was demonstrated in some patients who already have a highly favorable prognosis. Although there is no clear evidence that all patients will benefit from flumazenil, some individuals may benefit for a short time. Certainly, the administration of benzodiazepines should be avoided.[6]

EVALUATION OF THE PATIENT WITH LIVER DISEASE

The history is critical in establishing the diagnosis of the patient with liver disease. A medication history should include careful investigation of nonprescription xenobiotics, especially acetaminophen and the possible use of alternative or complementary therapies including herbal therapies. Nearly all chronically used medications should be suspect. An occupational history may indicate exposure to vinyl chloride (plastics industry), dimethylformamide (leather industry), or other industrial solvents. Table 26–3 lists occupational exposures that result in liver injury. Alcohol abuse is a common cause of acute hepatitis and the most common cause of cirrhosis in this country.[80,84] A history of male homosexual contacts, healthcare occupation, or intravenous drug use indicates the possibility of hepatitis B and C. Recent travel to an underdeveloped country suggests the possibility of hepatitis A. In patients with significant pain, the possibility of cholelithiasis should be considered.

TABLE 26–3. Occupational Exposures Associated with Liver Injury

Xenobiotic	Type of Injury
Arsenic	Cirrhosis, angiosarcoma
Beryllium	Granulomatous hepatitis
Carbon tetrachloride	Acute necrosis
Chlordecone	Minor hepatocellular injury
Copper salts	Granulomatous hepatitis, angiosarcoma
Dimethylformamide	Steatohepatitis
Methylenedianiline	Acute cholestasis
Phosphorus	Acute necrosis
Tetrachloroethane	Acute, subacute necrosis
Tetrachloroethylene	Acute necrosis
Toluene	Steatosis, minor hepatocellular injury
Trichloroethane	Steatosis, minor hepatocellular injury
Trinitrotoluene	Acute necrosis
Vinyl chloride	Acute necrosis, fibrosis, angiosarcoma
Xylene	Steatosis, minor hepatocellular injury

BIOCHEMICAL PATTERNS OF LIVER INJURY

There are two basic biochemical patterns associated with liver injury induced by xenobiotics. The hepatocellular pattern is characterized by elevation of liver transaminases due to the injury of hepatocytes by apoptosis or necrosis. The cholestatic pattern is characterized by elevation of the serum alkaline phosphatase concentration and usually results from injury or functional impairment of the bile ductules.[1] Processes associated with intrahepatic cholestasis in the absence of hepatitis may not lead to significant aminotransferase elevation.[98,106,147]

Aminotransferases Laboratory tests are helpful and certain patterns may be suggestive of specific etiologies (Table 26–4). Elevation of hepatocellular enzymes, especially the AST and ALT, indicates hepatocellular injury, and within a given clinical context, has useful diagnostic significance. Aminotransferases may be increased up to 500 times normal when hepatic necrosis is extensive, such as in severe acute viral or toxic hepatitis.[2,74] The degree of elevation does not always reflect the severity of injury as concentrations may decline as FHF progresses. Only moderately elevated, or occasionally normal aminotransferase concentrations occur in some patients with hepatic failure caused by mitochondrial failure, cirrhosis, or venoocclusive disease.[43,69,90,146] Aminotransferase concentrations may be normal or only slightly elevated in processes associated with intrahepatic cholestasis in the absence of hepatitis.[98,106,147] In alcoholic liver disease, in contrast to other forms of hepatitis, the AST concentration is typically two to three times greater than the ALT. This is attributed to impairment of ALT synthesis because of pyridine-5′-phosphate deficiency in alcoholics. This effect is reversed by pyridoxine supplementation. Elevation of either of these enzymes greater than 300 IU/L is inconsistent with injury caused by ethanol.[2] During acute extrahepatic obstruction of the biliary tract, the AST or ALT may be as high as 1000 IU/L, indicating inflammation caused by reflux of bile acids into the biliary tree.[2] The measurement of γ-glutamyl transpeptidase (GGTP) is not very useful as it is present throughout the liver and its elevation is often nonspecific.[2]

Alkaline Phosphatase In patients with cholestasis, bile acids stimulate the synthesis of alkaline phosphatase by hepatocytes and biliary epithelium in response to a number of pathologic processes in the liver. Elevations of the alkaline phosphatase as great as 10-fold may occur with infiltrative liver diseases, but are most commonly associated with extrahepatic obstruction.[2] Although the alkaline phosphatase may be normal or elevated only minimally in hepatocellular injury, it is

TABLE 26–4. Laboratory Tests that Evaluate the Liver

Disorder	Alkaline Phosphatase	AST, ALT	Albumin	Prothrombin Time	Bilirubin	Ammonia	Anion Gap
Hepatocellular necrosis, acute focal (hepatitis)	N or ↑	↑↑↑	N	N or ↑	↑↑	N	N
Hepatocellular necrosis, acute massive	N or ↑	↑↑↑	N	↑↑	↑↑↑	↑↑	↑
Chronic infiltrative disease (tumor, fatty liver)	↑↑↑	↑	N	N	N	N	N
Acute mitochondrial failure	N or ↑	N or ↑	N	↑↑	↑	↑↑	↑↑↑
Cholelithiasis	↑	N or ↑	N	N	N or ↑	N	N
Cholestasis	↑↑	N or ↑	N	N	↑	N	N
Chronic hepatitis	N or ↑	↑	N or ↓	N	N or ↑	N or ↑	N
Cirrhosis	N or ↑	↑	↓	N or ↑	N or ↑	N or ↑	N

↑ = increase; ↓ = decrease; N = normal.

unusual for obstruction to occur without some elevation of the alkaline phosphatase. Elevations of alkaline phosphatase and GGTP parallel each other in disease of the biliary tract.[2]

Bilirubin Elevation of conjugated, or direct, bilirubin implies impairment of secretion into bile while elevation of unconjugated, or indirect, bilirubin implies impairment of conjugation. Unconjugated hyperbilirubinemia also occurs during hemolysis and in rare disorders of hepatic conjugation such as Gilbert or Crigler-Najjar syndromes. Except in cases of pure unconjugated hyperbilirubinemia, the fractionation of bilirubin in the case of hepatobiliary disorders does not have any important diagnostic utility, and will not distinguish patients with parenchymal disorders of the liver from intrinsic or extrinsic cholestasis. The presence of bilirubin in the urine implies elevation of conjugated (direct) bilirubin which is water soluble and filtered by the glomerulus obviating the need for laboratory fractionation.[2]

Urobilinogen is produced by the bacterial metabolism of bilirubin in the bowel lumen. It is absorbed and excreted in the urine. Its presence in the urine indicates the normal excretion of bilirubin in bile, while its absence is associated with complete biliary obstruction. As a result of more modern methods of detection of complete obstruction of the biliary tract, this test is mainly of historical interest.

Serum Albumin Quantitatively, albumin is the most important protein that is made in the liver. With a half-life as great as 20 days, the albumin is usually normal in the previously healthy patient with acute liver injury. In the absence of disorders that affect albumin, such as nephrotic syndrome, protein-losing enteropathy, or starvation, a low serum albumin is a useful marker for the severity of chronic liver disease.[2]

Coagulation Factors Impairment of coagulation is a marker of the severity of hepatic dysfunction in both acute and chronic liver disease. Unlike the case with serum albumin, with its half-life of 20 days, the onset of coagulopathy as a consequence of impaired synthesis of the short-lived vitamin K-dependent clotting factors II, VII, IX, and X is rapid. Very acute changes in coagulation reflect the concentration of factor VII, which has the shortest half life.[56] The extrinsic coagulation pathway, as measured by the prothrombin time (PT) or the international normalized ratio (INR), is affected by reductions in factors II, VII, and X. Elevation of the INR or PT in acute hepatitis is associated with a higher risk of FHF.[47,74,90] In addition to failure of hepatic synthesis, inadequate levels of factors II, VII, IX, and X may also result from ingestion of warfarin anticoagulants or malabsorption of vitamin K (Chap. 59).[2]

Because different thromboplastin reagents give different PT values on the same sample, the INR was developed to normalize PT measurements in patients treated with warfarin, allowing comparisons of therapeutic outcomes across different care settings and across the literature. The INR uses the International Sensitivity Index (ISI) that is derived from a cohort of patients on stable anticoagulant therapy. It normalizes the responsiveness of a given thromboplastin reagent in comparison to a WHO reference standard that is assigned a value of 1.0.[66] There is little controversy regarding the value of the INR in comparison with the PT ratio for measuring the extent of warfarin-induced anticoagulation. Because factor deficiencies in patients with liver disease are different from those in patients on warfarin, there is considerable controversy regarding which measurement is best for patients with liver disease.[2,26,66] Although comparison of factor levels in warfarin-treated patients with those with liver disease showed no difference in factor VII, there are significant differences in factors II, V, X, and fibrinogen. Comparison of the PT with INR in the evaluation of test results with three different thromboplastin reagents showed consistency among the control groups of warfarin-treated patients, but no consistency among PT or INR measurements using the same thromboplastin reagents in patients with liver disease.[66] Because of a failure to demonstrate an advantage, liver specialists who have expressed an opinion support the continued use of the PT to describe the degree of liver injury, lacking the availability of a single reliable standard that would help predict operative risk.[2,26,66] In patients with liver disease, use of the INR implies a normalized correlation that does not exist and is therefore potentially misleading. The implication for toxicologists is that caution should be exercised in relying too heavily on published

INR values that purportedly predict the severity of illness in patients with acute liver failure.

Ammonia Severe generalized impairment of hepatic function leads to a rise in the serum ammonia concentration as a result of impairment of detoxification of ammonia produced during catabolism of proteins. The absolute concentration is not clearly associated with mental status alteration. Elevations of serum ammonia concentrations occur in 60% to 80% of patients with hepatic encephalopathy, suggesting that hyperammonemia is not the only cause of hepatic encephalopathy.[40]

Some patients treated with valproic acid have developed alterations in mental status associated with elevated ammonia concentrations, sometimes in the absence of other laboratory indicators of hepatic injury, and without demonstrable toxic concentrations of valproic acid. This has been attributed to selective impairment of urea cycle enzymes ornithine transcarbamylase or carbamyl phosphate synthetase by pentanoic acid metabolites (Chap. 47).[35,105] As noted above, an association between deficiency of carnitine, microsteatosis, and the development of hyperammonemia is observed in children treated with valproic acid. This is attributed to impairment of carnitine-dependent beta-oxidation of sodium valproate and free fatty acids in the mitochondria.[11,104,136]

OTHER LABORATORY TESTS

Serologic Studies for the Presence of Markers of Hepatitis A, B, and C Should be Done Routinely in Patients with Hepatitis. In the patient with severe liver injury, hypoglycemia is a major concern because of impairment of glycogen storage and gluconeogenesis. Hyperglycemia also occurs as a result of the liver's inability to handle a large glucose load. The arterial blood-gas value commonly shows a respiratory alkalosis. Severe metabolic acidosis with elevated lactate occurs in patients with hepatic failure caused by mitochondrial injury. Measurements of serum lactate concentration may be useful in identifying the cause of acidosis in a patient with suspected toxic liver injury.[85,90,119]

The CT and MRI scans are useful tests for evaluation of parenchymal disease of the liver. An ultrasound examination reliably demonstrates dilation of the extrahepatic bile ducts. Liver biopsy may be helpful but is not specifically diagnostic of xenobiotic-induced hepatic injury.

MANAGEMENT

In many patients, toxic liver injury resolves with simple withdrawal of the offending xenobiotic. In patients with severe injury, significant improvement in survival is associated with good supportive care in an intensive care environment.[74] Early referral to a transplant center for patients with evidence of severe or rapidly progressive toxic injury is indicated. For discussion of indications for the use of *N*-acetylcysteine and discussion of indications for transplantation, see Antidotes in Depth A4: *N*-Acetylcysteine.

SUMMARY

The primary role of the liver in the biotransformation of xenobiotics results in an increased risk of hepatotoxicity. Xenobiotic-induced liver injury can be dose-dependent and predictable or idiosyncratic and unpredictable. Idiosyncratic injury is affected by host characteristics that include genetic makeup, concomitant or previous exposure to drugs and toxins, and the underlying condition of the liver. The spectrum of liver injury includes combinations of cholestasis, steatosis, hepatocellular necrosis, apoptosis, and fibrosis. Injury may be a result of cellular or antibody-mediated immune mechanisms; free radical initiation of lipid peroxidation; mitochondrial injury; formation of adducts with critical cellular enzymes; and other, less-well-defined mechanisms.

ACKNOWLEDGMENT

Charles Maltz and Todd Bania contributed to this chapter in a previous edition.

REFERENCES

1. Abboud G, Kaplowitz N. Drug-induced liver injury. *Drug Safety*. 2007: 277-294.
2. Ahmed A, Keeffe EB. Liver chemistry and function tests. In: Feldman M, Friedman L, Sleisenger M, et al., eds. *Sleisenger & Fordtran's Gastrointestinal and Liver Disease: Pathophysiology, Diagnosis, Management*. 8th ed. Philadelphia: Saunders; 2006:1575-1579 .
3. Alberti-Flor JJ, Hernandez ME, Ferrer JP, et al. Fulminant liver failure and pancreatitis associated with the use of sulfamethoxazoletrimethoprim. *Am J Gastroenterol*. 1989;84:1577-1579.
4. Al-Kawas FH, Seeff LB, Berendson RA, et al. Allopurinol hepatotoxicity. Report of two cases and review of the literature. *Ann Intern Med*. 1981;95:588-590.
5. Al-Salman J, Arjomand H, Kemp DG, Mittal M. Hepatocellular injury in a patient receiving rosiglitazone: a case report. *Ann Intern Med*. 2000;132:121-124.
6. Als-Nielsen B, Gluud LL, Gluud C. Benzodiazepine receptor antagonists for hepatic encephalopathy. *Cochrane Database of Systematic Reviews*. 2004, Issue2.Art.No. CD002798. DOI:10.1002/14651858.CD002798.pub2.
7. Amacher DE. Drug-associated mitochondrial toxicity and its detection. *Curr Med Chem*. 2005;12:1829-1839.
8. Badr MZ, Belinsky SA, Kauffman FC, et al. Mechanism of hepatotoxicity to periportal regions of the liver lobule due to allyl alcohol: role of oxygen and lipid peroxidation. *J Pharmacol Exp Ther*. 1986;238:1138-1142.
9. Beaune PH, Lecoeur S. Immunotoxicology of the liver: adverse reactions to drugs. *J Hepatol*. 1997;26(Suppl2):37-42.
10. Bhat G, Jordan J Jr., Sokalski S, et al. Minocycline-induced hepatitis with autoimmune features and neutropenia. *J Clin Gastroenterol*. 1998;27:74-75.
11. Bohan TP, Helton E, McDonald I, et al. Effect of L-carnitine treatment for valproate-induced hepatotoxicity. *Neurology*. 2001;56:1405-1409.
12. Bohme M, Muller M, Leier I, et al. Cholestasis caused by inhibition of the adenosine triphosphate-dependent bile salt transport in rat liver. *Gastroenterology*. 1994;107:255-265.
13. Bourdi M, Chen W, Peter RM, et al. Human cytochrome P450 2E1 is a major autoantigen associated with halothane hepatitis. *Chem Res Toxicol*. 1996;9:1159-1166.
14. Bourdi M, Gautier JC, Mircheva J, et al. Anti-liver microsomes autoantibodies and dihydralazine-induced hepatitis: specificity of autoantibodies and inductive capacity of the drug. *Mol Pharmacol*. 1992;42:280-285.
15. Bras G, Jelliffe DB, Stuart KL. Veno-occlusive disease of liver with nonportal type of cirrhosis, occurring in Jamaica. *Arch Pathol*. 1954;57:285-300.
16. Burk RF, Reiter R, Lane JM. Hyperbaric oxygen protection against carbon tetrachloride hepatotoxicity in the rat. Association with altered metabolism. *Gastroenterology*. 1986;90:812–818.
17. Butterworth RF. Complications of cirrhosis. III: hepatic encephalopathy. *J Hepatol*. 2000;32(Suppl1):171-180.
18. Corcoran GB, Racz WJ, Smith CV, et al. Effects of *N*-acetylcysteine on acetaminophen covalent binding and hepatic necrosis in mice. *J Pharmacol Exp Ther*. 1985;232:864-872.
19. Cote HC, Brumme ZL, Craib KJ, et al. Changes in mitochondrial DNA as a marker of nucleoside toxicity in HIV-infected patients. *N Engl J Med*. 2002;346:811-820.
20. Crawford JM. The liver and the biliary tract. In: Kumar V, Fausto N, Abbas A, eds. *Robbins and Cotran's Pathologic Basis of Disease*. 7th ed. Philadelphia: Elsevier; 2005:877-938.
21. Crispe IN, Mehal WZ. Strange brew: T cells in the liver. *Immunol Today*. 1996;17:522-525.

22. Dahm LJ, Schultze AE, Roth RA. An antibody to neutrophils attenuates alpha-naphthylisothiocyanate–induced liver injury. *J Pharmacol Exp Ther.* 1991;256:412-420.
23. Dai Y, Rashba-Step J, Cederbaum AI. Stable expression of human cytochrome P450 2E1 in HepG2 cells: characterization of catalytic activities and production of reactive oxygen intermediates. *Biochemistry.* 1993;32:6928-6937.
24. Day L, Shikuma C, Gerschenson M. Mitochondrial injury in the pathogenesis of antiretroviral-induced hepatic steatosis and lactic acidemia. *Mitochondrion.* 2004;4:95-109.
25. de Morais SM, Uetrecht JP, Wells PG. Decreased glucuronidation and increased bioactivation of acetaminophen in Gilbert's syndrome. *Gastroenterology.* 1992;102:577-586.
26. Denson KW, Reed SV, Haddon ME. Validity of the INR system for patients with liver impairment. *Thromb Haemost.* 1995;73:162.
27. DePinho RA, Goldberg CS, Lefkowitch JH. Azathioprine and the liver. Evidence favoring idiosyncratic, mixed cholestatic-hepatocellular injury in humans. *Gastroenterology.* 1984;86:162-165.
28. Dey A, Cederbaum AI. Alcohol and oxidative liver injury. *Hepatology.* 2006;43:S63-S74.
29. Dutczak WJ, Clarkson TW, Ballatori N. Biliary-hepatic recycling of a xenobiotic: gallbladder absorption of methyl mercury. *Am J Physiol.* 1991;260:G873-G880.
30. Eisen JS, Koren G, Juurlink DN, et al. *N*-Acetylcysteine for the treatment of clove oil-induced fulminant hepatic failure. *J Toxicol Clin Toxicol.* 2004;42:89-92.
31. Eliasson E, Kenna JG. Cytochrome P450 2E1 is a cell surface autoantigen in halothane hepatitis. *Mol Pharmacol.* 1996;50:573-582.
32. Elliott RH, Strunin L. Hepatotoxicity of volatile anaesthetics. *Br J Anaesth.* 1993;70:339-348.
33. El-Sisi AE, Earnest DL, Sipes IG. Vitamin A potentiation of carbon tetrachloride hepatotoxicity: role of liver macrophages and active oxygen species. *Toxicol Appl Pharmacol.* 1993;119:295-301.
34. Estes JD, Stolpman D, Olyaei A, et al. High prevalence of potentially hepatotoxic herbal supplement use in patients with fulminant hepatic failure. *Arch Surg.* 2003;138:852-858.
35. Eze E, Workman M, Donley B. Hyperammonemia and coma developed by a woman treated with valproic acid for affective disorder. *Psychiatr Serv.* 1998;49:1358-1359.
36. Falk H, Thomas LB, Popper H, et al. Hepatic angiosarcoma associated with androgenic-anabolic steroids. *Lancet.* 1979;2:1120-1123.
37. Farrell GC, Larter CZ. Non-alcoholic fatty liver disease. *Hepatology.* 2006;43:S99-S112.
38. Farrell GC, Joshua DE, Uren RF, et al. Androgen-induced hepatoma. *Lancet.* 1975;1:430-432.
39. Ferenci P. Brain dysfunction in fulminant hepatic failure. *J Hepatol.* 1994;21:487-490.
40. Fitz JG. Hepatic encephalopathy. In: Feldman M, Friedman L, Sleisenger M, et al., eds. *Sleisenger & Fordtran's Gastrointestinal and Liver Disease: Pathophysiology, Diagnosis, Management.* 8th ed. Philadelphia: Saunders; 2006:1966-1971.
41. Fontana RJ. Acute liver failure. In: Feldman M, Friedman L, Sleisenger M, et al., eds. *Sleisenger & Fordtran's Gastrointestinal and Liver Disease: Pathophysiology, Diagnosis, Management.* 8th ed. Philadelphia: Saunders; 2006:1993-2003 .
42. Fromenty B, Pessayre D. Inhibition of mitochondrial β-oxidation as a mechanism of hepatotoxicity. *Pharmacol Ther.* 1995;67:101-154.
43. Geubel AP, de Galoscy C, Alves N, et al. Liver damage caused by therapeutic vitamin A administration: estimate of dose-related toxicity in 41 cases. *Gastroenterology.* 1991;100:1701-1709.
44. Gitlin N, Julie NL, Spurr CL, et al. Two cases of severe clinical and histologic hepatotoxicity associated with troglitazone. *Ann Intern Med.* 1998;129:36-38.
45. Godfrey DI, Hammond KJ, Poulton LD, et al. NKT cells: facts, functions and fallacies. *Immunol Today.* 2000;21:573-583.
46. Guegenrich F. Catalytic selectivity of human cytochrome P450 enzymes: relevance to drug metabolism and toxicity. *Toxicol Lett.* 1994;70:133-138.
47. Harrison PM, O'Grady JG, Keays RT, et al. Serial prothrombin time as prognostic indicator in paracetamol induced fulminant hepatic failure. *BMJ.* 1990;301:964-966.
48. Hetu C, Dumont A, Joly JG. Effect of chronic ethanol administration on bromobenzene liver toxicity in the rat. *Toxicol Appl Pharmacol.* 1983;67:166-177.
49. Hoet P, Graf ML, Bourdi M, et al. Epidemic of liver disease caused by hydrochlorofluorocarbons used as ozone-sparing substitutes of chlorofluorocarbons. *Lancet.* 1997;350:556-559.
50. Horowitz RS, Feldhaus K, Dart RC, et al. The clinical spectrum of Jin Bu Huan toxicity. *Arch Intern Med.* 1996;156:899-903.
51. Huang YS, Chern HD, Su WJ, et al. Cytochrome P450 2E1 genotype and the susceptibility to antituberculous drug-induced hepatitis. *Hepatology.* 2003;37:924-930.
52. Humberston CL, Akhtar J, Krenzelok EP. Acute hepatitis induced by kava kava. *J Toxicol Clin Toxicol.* 2003;41:109-113.
53. Ishak KG. Hepatic lesions caused by anabolic and contraceptive steroids. *Semin Liver Dis.* 1981;1:116-128.
54. Jaeschke H. Toxic responses of the liver. In: Klaassen CD, ed. *Casarett and Doull's Toxicology The Basic Science of Poisons.* 7th ed. New York: McGraw Hill Medical; 2007:557-582.
55. Jenner PJ, Ellard GA. Isoniazid-related hepatotoxicity: a study of the effect of rifampicin administration on the metabolism of acetyl isoniazid in man. *Tubercle.* 1989;7093-101.
56. Johnston M, Harrison L, Moffat K, et al. Reliability of the international normalized ratio for monitoring the induction phase of warfarin: comparison with the prothrombin time ratio. *J Lab Clin Med.* 1996;128:214-217.
57. Kanel GC. Histopathology of drug-induced liver disease. In: Kaplowitz N, DeLeve LD, eds. *Drug-Induced Liver Disease.* 2nd ed. Informa Health Care; New York, NY. 2007:237.
58. Kaplowitz N. Mechanisms of liver cell injury. *J Hepatol.* 2000;32:39-47.
59. Kenna JG: Immunoallergic drug-induced hepatitis: lessons from halothane. *J Hepatol.* 1997;26(Suppl1):5-12.
60. Kim HJ, Kim BH, Han YS, et al. The incidence and clinical characteristics of symptomatic propylthiouracil-induced hepatic injury in patients with hyperthyroidism: a single-center retrospective study. *Am J Gastroenterol.* 2001;96:165-169.
61. Kita H, Mackay IR, Van De Water J, et al. The lymphoid liver: considerations on pathways to autoimmune injury. *Gastroenterology.* 2001;120:1485-1501.
62. Klaassen CD. Biliary excretion of metals. *Drug Metab Rev.* 1976;5:165-193.
63. Knowles DM 2nd, Casarella WJ, Johnson PM, et al. The clinical, radiologic, and pathologic characterization of benign hepatic neoplasms. Alleged association with oral contraceptives. *Medicine.*1978;57:223-237.
64. Knudtson E, Para M, Boswell H, et al. Drug rash with eosinophilia and systemic symptoms syndrome and renal toxicity with a nevirapine-containing regimen in a pregnant patient with human immunodeficiency virus. *Obstet Gynecol.* 2003;101:1094-1097.
65. Konishi M. Ishii H. Role of microsomal enzymes in development of alcoholic liver diseases. *J Gastroenterol Hepatol.* 2007;22(Suppl1):S7-S10.
66. Kovacs MJ, Wong A, MacKinnon K, et al. Assessment of the validity of the INR system for patients with liver impairment. *Thromb Haemost.* 1994;71:727-730.
67. Krell H, Metz J, Jaeschke H, et al. Drug-induced intrahepatic cholestasis: characterization of different pathomechanisms. *Arch Toxicol.* 1987;60:124-130.
68. Kuffner EK, Dart RC, Bogdan GM, et al. Effect of maximal daily doses of acetaminophen on the liver of alcoholic patients: a randomized, double-blind, placebo-controlled trial. *Arch Intern Med.* 2001;161:2247-2252.
69. Kumana CR, Ng M, Lin HJ, et al. Herbal tea induced hepatic venoocclusive disease: quantification of toxic alkaloid exposure in adults. *Gut.* 1985;26:101-104.
70. Labbe G, Pessayre D, Fromenty B. Drug-induced liver injury through mitochondrial dysfunction: mechanisms and detection during preclinical safety studies. *Fundam Clin Pharmacol.* 2008;22:335-53.
71. Laliberte L, Villeneuve JP. Hepatitis after the use of germander, a herbal remedy. *CMAJ.* 1996;154:1689-1692.
72. Larrey D, Vial T, Micaleff A, et al. Hepatitis associated with amoxicillin-clavulanic acid combination. Report of 15 cases. *Gut.* 1992;33:368-371.
73. Lauterburg BH, Velez ME. Glutathione deficiency in alcoholics: risk factor for paracetamol hepatotoxicity. *Gut.* 1988;29:1153-1157.
74. Lee WM. Acute liver failure. *N Engl J Med.* 1993;329:1862-1872.
75. Lee WM. Drug-induced hepatotoxicity. *N Engl J Med.* 1995;333:1118-1127.
76. Lee WM, Denton WT. Chronic hepatitis and indolent cirrhosis due to methyldopa: the bottom of the iceberg? *J S C Med Assoc.* 1989;85:75-79.
77. Leeder JS, Lu X, Timsit Y, et al. Non-monooxygenase cytochromes P450 as potential human autoantigens in anticonvulsant hypersensitivity reactions. *Pharmacogenetics.* 1998;8:211-225.

78. Leverve XM. Mitochondrial function and substrate availability. *Crit Care Med.* 2007;35(Suppl):S454-S460.
79. Lewis JH. Drug-induced liver disease. *Med Clin North Am.* 2000;84:1275-1311.
80. Lieber CS. Alcohol and the liver: 1994 update. *Gastroenterology.* 1994;106:1085-1105.
81. Lindros KO, Cai YA, Penttila KE. Role of ethanol-inducible cytochrome P-450 IIE1 in carbon tetrachloride-induced damage to centrilobular hepatocytes from ethanol-treated rats. *Hepatology.* 1990;12:1092-1097.
82. Liu ZX, Kaplowitz N. Immune-mediated drug-induced liver disease. *Clin Liver Dis.* 2002;6:467-486.
83. Lu Y, Cederbaum AI. CYP2E1 and oxidative liver injury by alcohol. *Free Radical Biol Med.* 2008;44:723-738.
84. Maddrey WC. Alcohol-induced liver disease. *Clin Liver Dis.* 2000;4:116-130.
85. Mahler H, Pasi A, Kramer JM, et al. Fulminant liver failure in association with the emetic toxin of *Bacillus cereus. N Engl J Med.* 1997;336:1142-1148.
86. Manno M, Rezzadore M, Grossi M, et al. Potentiation of occupational carbon tetrachloride toxicity by ethanol abuse. *Hum Exp Toxicol.* 1996;15:294-300.
87. Mazuryk H, Kastenberg D, Rubin R, et al. Cholestatic hepatitis associated with the use of nafcillin. *Am J Gastroenterol.* 1993;88:1960-1962.
88. McComsey GA, Libutti DE, O'Riordan M, et al. Mitochondrial RNA and DNA alterations in HIV lipoatrophy are linked to antiretroviral therapy and not to HIV infection. *Antiviral Therapy.* 2008;13:715.
89. McDonald GB, Hinds MS, Fisher LD, et al. Venoocclusive disease of the liver and multiorgan failure after bone marrow transplantation: a cohort study of 355 patients. *Ann Intern Med.* 1993;118:255-267.
90. McKenzie R, Fried MW, Sallie R, et al. Hepatic failure and lactic acidosis due to fialuridine (FIAU), an investigational nucleoside analogue for chronic hepatitis B. *N Engl J Med.* 1995;333:1099-1105.
91. McMaster KR 3rd, Hennigar GR. Drug-induced granulomatous hepatitis. *Lab Invest.* 1981;44:61-73.
92. Mehendale HM, Roth RA, Gandolfi AJ, et al. Novel mechanisms in chemically induced hepatotoxicity. *FASEB J.* 1994;8:1285-1295.
93. Mitchell I, Wendon J, Fitt S, et al. Anti-tuberculous therapy and acute liver failure. *Lancet.* 1995;345:555-556.
94. MMWR. Centers for Disease Control and Prevention: severe isoniazid-associated hepatitis—New York, 1991–1993. *Morb Mortal Wkly Rep.* 1993;42:545-547.
95. Mohabbat O, Younos MS, Merzad AA, et al. An outbreak of hepatic venoocclusive disease in north-western Afghanistan. *Lancet.* 1976;2:269-271.
96. Moses PL, Schroeder B, Alkhatib O, et al. Severe hepatotoxicity associated with bromfenac sodium. *Am J Gastroenterol.* 1999;94:1393-1396.
97. Nadir A, Agrawal S, King PD, et al. Acute hepatitis associated with the use of a Chinese herbal product, ma-huang. *Am J Gastroenterol.* 1996;91:1436-1438.
98. Nair SS, Kaplan JM, Levine LH, et al. Trimethoprim-sulfamethoxazole-induced intrahepatic cholestasis. *Ann Intern Med.* 1980;92:511-512.
99. Nakajima T, Okino T, Sato A. Kinetic studies on benzene metabolism in rat liver—Possible presence of three forms of benzene metabolizing enzymes in the liver. *Biochem Pharmacol.* 1987;36:2799-2804.
100. Nicolas F, Rodineau P, Rouzioux JM, et al. Fulminant hepatic failure in poisoning due to ingestion of T 61, a veterinary euthanasia drug. *Crit Care Med.* 1990;18:573-575.
101. Nolan CM, Goldberg SV, Buskin SE. Hepatotoxicity associated with isoniazid preventive therapy: a 7-year survey from a public health tuberculosis clinic. *JAMA.* 1999;281:1014-1018.
102. Peck CC, Temple R, Collins JM. Understanding consequences of concurrent therapies. *JAMA.* 1993;269:1550-1552.
103. Prescott LF. Paracetamol, alcohol and the liver. *Br J Clin Pharmacol.* 2000;49:291-301.
104. Raskind JY, El-Chaar GM. The role of carnitine supplementation during valproic acid therapy. *Ann Pharmacother.* 2000;34:630-638.
105. Rawat S, Borkowski WJ, Jr., Swick HM. Valproic acid and secondary hyperammonemia. *Neurology.* 1981;31:1173-1174.
106. Reddy KR, Brillant P, Schiff ER. Amoxicillin-clavulanate potassium-associated cholestasis. *Gastroenterology.* 1989;96:1135-1141.
107. Redlich CA, Beckett WS, Sparer J, et al. Liver disease associated with occupational exposure to the solvent dimethylformamide. *Ann Intern Med.* 1988;108:680-686.
108. Redlich CA, West AB, Fleming L, et al. Clinical and pathological characteristics of hepatotoxicity associated with occupational exposure to dimethylformamide. *Gastroenterology.* 1990;99:748-757.
109. Reid WD, Christie B, Krishna G, et al. Bromobenzene metabolism and hepatic necrosis. *Pharmacology.* 1971;6:41-55.
110. Reinhart HH, Reinhart E, Korlipara P, et al. Combined nitrofurantoin toxicity to liver and lung. *Gastroenterology.* 1992;102:1396-1399.
111. Ridker PM, Ohkuma S, McDermott WV, et al. Hepatic venoocclusive disease associated with the consumption of pyrrolizidine-containing dietary supplements. *Gastroenterology.* 1985;88:1050-1054.
112. Rigas B, Rosenfeld LE, Barwick KW, et al. Amiodarone hepatotoxicity. A clinicopathologic study of five patients. *Ann Intern Med.* 1986;104:348-351.
113. Riordan SM, Williams R. Fulminant hepatic failure. *Clin Liver Dis.* 2000;4:25-45.
114. Roberts MS, Magnusson BM, Burczynski FJ, et al. Enterohepatic circulation: physiological, pharmacokinetic and clinical implications. *Clin Pharmacokinet.* 2002;41:751-790.
115. Roberts RA, Ganey PE ,Ju C, et al. Role of the Kupffer cell in mediating hepatic toxicity and carcinogenesis. *Toxicol Sci.* 2007;96:2-15.
116. Ros E, Small DM, Carey MC. Effects of chlorpromazine hydrochloride on bile salt synthesis, bile formation and biliary lipid secretion in the rhesus monkey: a model for chlorpromazine-induced cholestasis. *Eur J Clin Invest.* 1979;9:29-41.
117. Ross WT Jr, Daggy BP, Cardell RR Jr. Hepatic necrosis caused by halothane and hypoxia in phenobarbital-treated rats. *Anesthesiology.* 1979;51:321-326.
118. Roy-Chowdhury N, Roy-Chowdhury J. Liver physiology and energy metabolism. In: Feldman M, Friedman L, Sleisenger M, et al., eds. *Sleisenger & Fordtran's Gastrointestinal and Liver Disease: Pathophysiology, Diagnosis, Management.* 7th ed. Philadelphia: Saunders; 2006:1551-1565.
119. Schafer DF, Sorrell MF. Power failure, liver failure. *N Engl J Med.* 1997;336:1173-1174.
120. Schiodt FV, Rochling FA, Casey DL, Lee WM. Acetaminophen toxicity in an urban county hospital. *N Engl J Med.* 1997;330:1907.
121. Schreiber AH, Simon FR. Estrogen-induced cholestasis. Clues to pathogenesis and treatment. *Hepatology.* 1983;3:607-613.
122. Schultz JC, Adamson JS Jr, Workman WW, et al. Fatal liver disease after intravenous administration of tetracycline in high dosage. *N Engl J Med.* 1963;269:999-1004.
123. Scully LJ, Clarke D, Barr RJ. Diclofenac induced hepatitis. 3 cases with features of autoimmune chronic active hepatitis. *Dig Dis Sci.* 1993;38:744-751.
124. Seeff LB, Cuccherini BA, Zimmerman HJ, et al. Acetaminophen hepatotoxicity in alcoholics. *Ann Intern Med.* 1986;104:399-404.
125. Shah RR, Oates NS, Idle JR, et al. Impaired oxidation of debrisoquine in patients with perhexiline neuropathy. *Br Med J (Clin Res Ed).* 1982;284:295-299.
126. Simmons F, Feldman B, Gerety D. Granulomatous hepatitis in a patient receiving allopurinol. *Gastroenterology.* 1972;62:101-104.
127. Smith GC, Kenna JG, Harrison DJ, et al. Autoantibodies to hepatic microsomal carboxylesterase in halothane hepatitis. *Lancet.* 1993;342:963-964.
128. Soriano V, Puoti M, Garcia-Gasco P, et al. Antiretroviral drugs and liver injury. *AIDS.* 2008;22:1-13.
130. Stricker BH, Blok AP, Claas FH, et al. Hepatic injury associated with the use of nitrofurans: a clinicopathological study of 52 reported cases. *Hepatology.* 1988;8:599-606.
131. Sundar K, Suarez M, Banogon PE, et al. Zidovudine-induced fatal lactic acidosis and hepatic failure in patients with acquired immunodeficiency syndrome: report of two patients and review of the literature. *Crit Care Med.* 1997;25:1425-1430.
132. Tandon BN, Tandon HD, Tandon RK, et al. An epidemic of venoocclusive disease of liver in central India. *Lancet.* 1976;2:271-272.
133. Timbrell J. Factors affecting toxic responses: metabolism. In: *Principles of Biochemical Toxicology.* 3rd ed. London: Taylor and Francis Ltd; 2000:65-110.
134. Tsutsumi M, Lasker JM, Shimizu M, et al. The intralobular distribution of ethanol-inducible P450IIE1 in rat and human liver. *Hepatology.* 1989;10:437-446.
135. Van Thiel DH, Perper JA. Hepatotoxicity associated with cocaine abuse. *Recent Dev Alcohol.* 1992;10:335-341.
136. Verrotti A, Greco R, Morgese G, et al. Carnitine deficiency and hyperammonemia in children receiving valproic acid with and without other anticonvulsant drugs. *Int J Clin Lab Res.* 1999;29:36-40.
137. Victorino RM, Maria VA, Correia AP, et al. Floxacillin-induced cholestatic hepatitis with evidence of lymphocyte sensitization. *Arch Intern Med.* 1987;147:987-989.

138. Watanabe Y, Kato A, Sawara K, et al. Selective alterations of brain dopamine D(2) receptor binding in cirrhotic patients: results of a (11)C-N-methylspiperone PET study. *Metabol Br Dis.* 2008;23:265-74.
139. Watanabe N, Tsukada N, Smith CR, et al. Permeabilized hepatocyte couplets. Adenosine triphosphate-dependent bile canalicular contractions and a circumferential pericanalicular microfilament belt demonstrated. *Lab Invest.* 1991;65:203-213.
140. Weston CF, Cooper BT, Davies JD, et al. Veno-occlusive disease of the liver secondary to ingestion of comfrey. *Br Med J (Clin Res Ed).* 1987;295:183.
141. Whiting-O'Keefe QE, Fye KH, Sack KD. Methotrexate and histologic hepatic abnormalities: a meta-analysis. *Am J Med.* 1991;90:711-716.
142. Williams DE, Reed RL, Kedzierski B, et al. Bioactivation and detoxication of the pyrrolizidine alkaloid senecionine by cytochrome P-450 enzymes in rat liver. *Drug Metab Dispos.* 1989;17:387-392.
143. Yeong ML, Swinburn B, Kennedy M, et al. Hepatic venoocclusive diseaseassociated with comfrey ingestion. *J Gastroenterol Hepatol.* 1990;5:211-214,144.
144. Younis HS, Parrish AR, Sypes IG, et al. The role of hepatocellular oxidative stress in Kuppfer cell activation during 1-2 dichlorobenzene-induced hepatocellular toxicity. *Toxicol Sci.* 2003;76:201-211.
145. Zand R, Nelson SD, Slattery JT, et al. Inhibition and induction of cytochrome P4502E1-catalyzed oxidation by isoniazid in humans. *Clin Pharmacol Ther.* 1993;54:142-149.
146. Zimmerman HJ, Ishak KG. Valproate-induced hepatic injury: analyses of 23 fatal cases. *Hepatology.* 1982;2:591-597.
147. Zimmerman HJ, Lewis JH. Chemical- and toxin-induced hepatotoxicity. *Gastroenterol Clin North Am.* 1995;24:1027-1045.
148. Zimmerman HJ, Maddrey WC. Acetaminophen (paracetamol) hepatotoxicity with regular intake of alcohol: analysis of instances of therapeutic misadventure. *Hepatology.* 1995;22:767-773.

CHAPTER 27
RENAL PRINCIPLES

Donald A. Feinfeld and Nikolas B. Harbord

OVERVIEW OF RENAL FUNCTION

ANATOMIC CONSIDERATIONS

The kidneys lie in the paravertebral grooves at the level of the T12-L3 vertebrae. The medial margin of each is concave whereas the lateral margins are convex, giving the organ a bean-shaped appearance. In the adult, each kidney measures 10 to 12 cm in length, 5 to 7.5 cm in width, and 2.5 to 3.0 cm in thickness. In an adult man, each kidney weighs 125 to 170 g; in an adult woman, each kidney weighs 115 to155 g.

On the concave surface of the kidney is the hilum, through which the renal artery, vein, renal pelvis, a nerve plexus, and numerous lymphatics pass. On the convex surface, the kidney is surrounded by a fibrous capsule, which protects it, and a fatty capsule with a fibroareolar capsule called the *renal fascia*, which offers further protection and serves to anchor it in place.

The arterial supply begins with the renal artery, which is a direct branch of the aorta. On entering the hilum, this artery subdivides into branches supplying the five major segments of each kidney: the apical pole, the anterosuperior segment, the anteroinferior segment, the posterior segment, and the inferior pole. These arteries subsequently divide within each segment to become lobar arteries. In turn, these vessels give rise to arcuate arteries that diverge into the sharply branching interlobular arteries, which directly supply the glomerular tufts.

The cut surface of the kidney reveals a pale outer rim and a dark inner region corresponding to the cortex and medulla, respectively. The cortex is 1 cm thick and surrounds the base of each medullary pyramid. The medulla consists of between 8 and 18 cone-shaped areas called *medullary pyramids;* the apex of each area forms a papilla containing the ends of the collecting ducts. Urine empties from these ducts into the renal pelvis, flows into the ureters, and, subsequently, into the urinary bladder.

The kidneys maintain the constancy of the extracellular fluid by creating an ultrafiltrate of the plasma that is virtually free of cells and larger macromolecules, and then processing that filtrate, reclaiming what the body needs and letting the rest escape as urine. Every 24 hours, an adult's kidneys filter nearly 180 L of water (total body water is ~ 25–60 L), and 25,000 mEq of sodium (total body Na^+ is 1200–2800 mEq). Under normal circumstances, the kidneys regulate these two substances independent of each other, depending on the body's needs. Approximately 1% of the filtered water and 0.5% to 1% of the filtered Na^+ are excreted.

Renal function begins with filtration at the glomerulus, a highly permeable capillary network stretched between two arterioles in series. The relative constriction or dilation of these vessels normally controls the glomerular filtration rate (GFR). Under normal circumstances, approximately 20% of the plasma water in the blood entering the glomeruli goes through the filter, carrying with it electrolytes, small metabolites such as glucose, amino acids, lactate, and urea, and leaving behind the blood cells and nearly all the larger proteins, including albumin and globulins. The filtrate then enters a series of tubules that reabsorb and secrete certain substances, such as organic acids and bases, into the urinary space. The proximal tubule performs bulk reabsorption, isotonically reclaiming 65% to 70% of the filtrate. Distal to the proximal tubule is the loop of Henle, which controls concentration and dilution of the urine, and the distal nephron, which does the fine-tuning in the balance between excretion and reclamation. Reabsorption of sodium is controlled proximally by hydrostatic and oncotic pressures in the peritubular capillaries, and distally by hormones such as aldosterone. Control of water reclamation depends first on function of the ascending limb of the loop of Henle, which absorbs solute without water. This produces a dilute tubular fluid and at the same time makes the medullary interstitium hypertonic. Final regulation of water reabsorption is related to the concentration of antidiuretic hormone (ADH), which opens water-reabsorbing channels (aquaporins) into the membranes of the final nephron segments (collecting ducts). The kidneys also regulate balance for potassium and hydrogen ion (both of which are influenced by the effect of aldosterone on the distal nephron), and calcium and phosphate (both of which are influenced by the blood concentration of parathormone).

Injury to the vasculature, glomeruli, tubules, or interstitium can lead to renal dysfunction; that is, to a decrease in glomerular filtration. As the kidneys fail, serum concentrations of the marker substances urea and creatinine increase. However, the relationship between these concentrations and the level of GFR is hyperbolic, not linear, therefore a small initial elevation in serum concentrations of these substances denotes a large decrease in renal function. By the time blood urea nitrogen (BUN) or serum creatinine exceeds the upper limit of normal, GFR is reduced by more than 50%.

Many xenobiotics cause or aggravate renal dysfunction. The kidneys are particularly susceptible to toxic injury for four reasons:[151] (a) they receive 20% to 25% of cardiac output yet make up less than 1% of total body mass implying a relatively large renal exposure in almost all circumstances; (b) they are metabolically active, and thus vulnerable to xenobiotics that disrupt metabolism or are activated by metabolism such as acetaminophen; (c) they remove water from the filtrate and may build up a high concentration of xenobiotics; and (d) the glomeruli and interstitium are susceptible to attack by the immune system. Many factors, such as renal perfusion, can affect an individual's reaction to a particular nephrotoxin.[10] The clinician should be aware of these factors and, when possible, alter them to minimize the adverse effect after a toxic exposure.

FUNCTIONAL TOXIC RENAL DISORDERS

Although most toxic renal injury results in decreased renal function, there are three functional disorders that upset body balance despite normal GFR in anatomically normal kidneys: renal tubular acidosis, syndrome of inappropriate secretion of ADH, and nephrogenic diabetes insipidus.

Renal tubular acidosis (RTA) is a loss of ability to reclaim the filtered bicarbonate (proximal RTA) or a decreased ability to generate new bicarbonate to replace that lost in buffering the daily acid load (distal RTA). In either case, there is a nonaniongap metabolic acidosis, usually accompanied by hypokalemia.

The primary defect in distal RTA involves the decreased secretion of hydrogen (H^+) from the intercalated cells of the distal tubule. This most often denotes a defect in the H^+-translocating adenosine triphosphatase (ATPase) on the luminal surface of these cells. Less frequently occurring mechanisms include abnormalities of the chloride-bicarbonate exchanger, which is responsible for returning bicarbonate generated within the cell to the systemic circulation. Also, given the voltage dependence of hydrogen secretion, if there is a decrease in the degree of luminal electronegative charge, there will be a decrease in this secretion. Most of this voltage is created by the activity of the Na^+-K^+-ATPase on the peritubular capillary side of the adjacent cell. (*Note:* Cells adjacent to the intercalated cells are called principal cells and primarily control K^+ secretion.) As this pump malfunctions, less sodium is returned to the capillaries, creating a decreased gradient from the lumen to the cell. Thus, the lumen becomes more electropositive, diminishing the transmembrane potential. Amphotericin causes distal RTA by allowing secreted H^+ to leak back into the tubular cells.[38]

The primary defect in proximal RTA is incompletely understood. Normally, the Na^+-H^+ exchanger in the luminal membrane, the Na^+-K^+-ATPase in the basolateral membrane, and the enzyme carbonic anhydrase, are the key systems necessary for proximal tubular bicarbonate reabsorption. If one or more of these mechanisms becomes disordered, the resorptive capacity of the proximal tubule is diminished. Proximal RTA often occurs as part of the Fanconi syndrome, a generalized failure of proximal tubular transport (proximal RTA plus aminoaciduria, renal glycosuria, and hyperphosphaturia), which may occur during treatment with some chemotherapy agents or antiretroviral drugs.

Syndrome of inappropriate secretion of antidiuretic hormone (SIADH) occurs when the body produces ADH despite a fall in plasma osmolality, which normally inhibits ADH secretion. ADH primarily affects the collecting tubule and causes increased water reabsorption by increasing the aquaporin channels in this segment. There are three common patterns of altered physiology: altered secretion of ADH; a resetting of the osmostat (ie, the threshold for ADH secretion); and the inability to decrease ADH secretion in the face of a water load. The increased hormonal effect of ADH serves to augment normal free water retention, which subsequently leads to the main clinical manifestations of SIADH: concentrated urine (as reflected in a relative increase in urine osmolality) and hyponatremia in the setting of euvolemia. Although this manifestation most often occurs as a complication of intracranial lesions or from ectopic ADH production by a tumor or in a diseased lung, many xenobiotics (eg, chlorpropamide, antidepressants, vincristine, opioids, and methylenedioxymethamphetamine [MDMA or Ecstasy]) can also cause inappropriate ADH release (Chap. 16).

Nephrogenic diabetes insipidus (NDI) is the reverse of SIADH and is the inability of the kidneys to respond to ADH stimulation despite severe losses of body water in urine. NDI will typically present with polyuria, or hypernatremia if water intake is limited or insufficient. Although genetic disorders, disease states, or electrolyte perturbations are usually implicated, several xenobiotics also cause NDI. Lithium, demeclocycline, foscarnet and clozapine are drugs that can cause this syndrome (Chap. 16). NDI from lithium toxicity is thought to result from impaired aquaporin-2 channel synthesis and transport despite normal ADH binding to vasopressin type-2 receptors at the collecting tubule.[199]

MAJOR TOXIC SYNDROMES OF THE KIDNEY

Most nephrotoxicity involves histologic renal injury. Although xenobiotics can affect any part of the nephron (Fig. 27–1), there are three major syndromes of toxic renal injury: (a) chronic kidney disease; (b) nephrotic syndrome; and, especially, (c) acute kidney injury (Table 27–1). For purposes of continuity, acute kidney injury is discussed last. Because nephrotoxins usually affect the tubules, the most metabolically active segment of the nephron, most nephrotoxicity involves either acute or chronic tubular injury, although glomerular injury sometimes results from xenobiotics. The processes are not mutually exclusive, and toxic nephropathy may impinge on more than one part of the nephron (eg, nonsteroidal antiinflammatory drug [NSAID]-induced acute kidney injury and nephrotic syndrome). When one of these patterns of renal injury occurs, the clinician should consider possible toxic etiologies.

Chronic kidney disease refers to a disease process that causes progressive decline of renal function over a period of months to years. There is usually a gradual rise in BUN and serum creatinine concentration as glomerular filtration falls; often there are no symptoms other than nocturia (indicating loss of urinary concentrating ability).

The most common lesion of nephrotoxic chronic kidney disease is chronic interstitial nephritis (Fig. 27–2), which involves destruction of tubules over a prolonged period,[75] with tubular atrophy, fibrosis, and a variable cellular infiltrate (see Fig. 27–2), sometimes accompanied by papillary necrosis. Acute interstitial nephritis may progress to chronic interstitial nephritis, if exposure to xenobiotics is prolonged.[217] The onset is usually insidious and relatively asymptomatic, often presenting as secondary hypertension or unexplained chronic azotemia. The major symptom is nonspecific nocturia. Papillary necrosis may lead to ureteral colic via papillary sloughing. There is mild to moderate proteinuria that remains well under the nephrotic range. Unlike other chronic renal disorders, interstitial nephritis is characterized by failure of the diseased tubules to adapt to the renal impairment, resulting in metabolic imbalances such as hyperchloremic metabolic acidosis, sodium wasting, and hyperkalemia early in the disease course.[71] Injury to erythropoietin-secreting cells may produce a disproportionate anemia.

Nephrotic syndrome is characterized by massive proteinuria (>3 g/d, in the adult), hypoalbuminemia, hyperlipidemia, and the edema that usually prompts the patient to seek medical attention. Although the relationships among these findings are not completely understood, the underlying event is injury to the glomerular barrier that normally prevents macromolecules from passing from the capillary lumen into the urinary space. Xenobiotics induce nephrotic syndrome (Table 27–2) in two ways. First, they may release hidden antigens into the blood, which leads to antigen–antibody complex formation after the immune response is elicited. These complexes subsequently deposit in the

TABLE 27–1. Major Nephrotoxic Syndromes

Chronic Renal Disease (slowly increasing azotemia)	Nephrotic Syndrome (proteinuria, hypoalbuminemia, edema)	Acute Renal Injury (rapidly increasing azotemia)
Chronic interstitial nephritis	Minimal glomerular change	Acute prerenal failure
Papillary necrosis	Membranous nephropathy	Acute urinary obstruction
Chronic glomerulosclerosis	Focal segmental glomerulosclerosis	Acute tubular necrosis
		Acute interstitial nephritis
		Acute vasculitis or glomerular injury (rare)

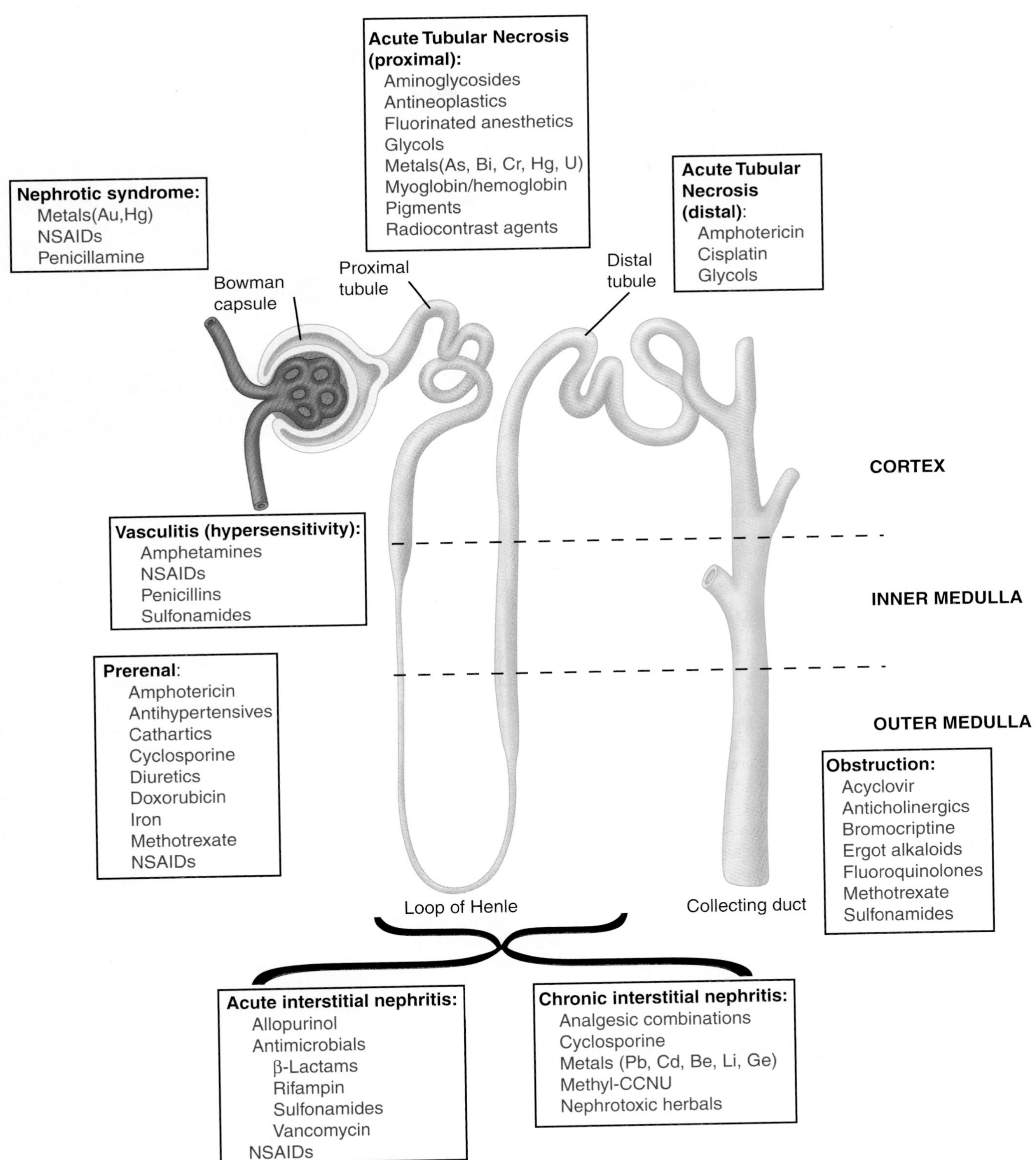

FIGURE 27–1. Schematic showing the major nephrotoxic processes and the sites on the nephron that they chiefly affect.

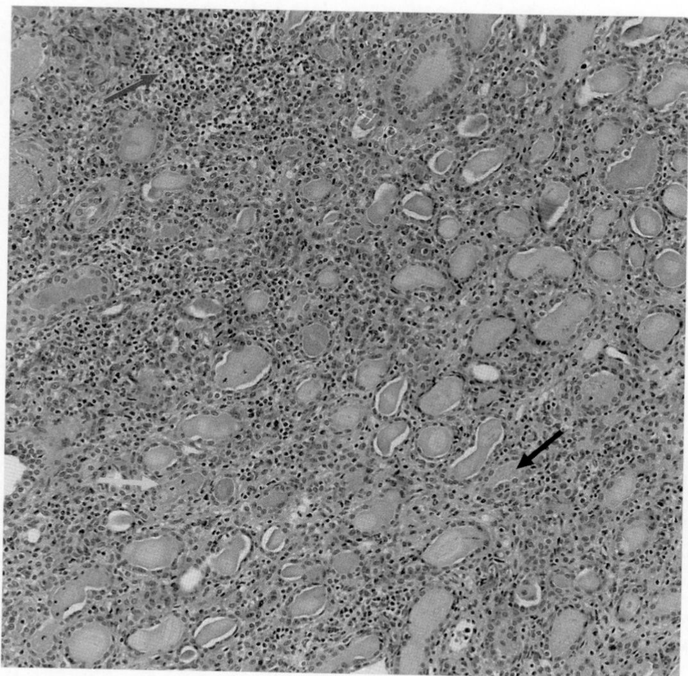

FIGURE 27–2. Chronic interstitial nephritis (secondary to NSAIDs). Interstitial fibrosis (⟶), lymphocytic infiltration (↗), and tubular atrophy (↙). H&E × 225. (Image contributed by Dr. Rabia Mir.)

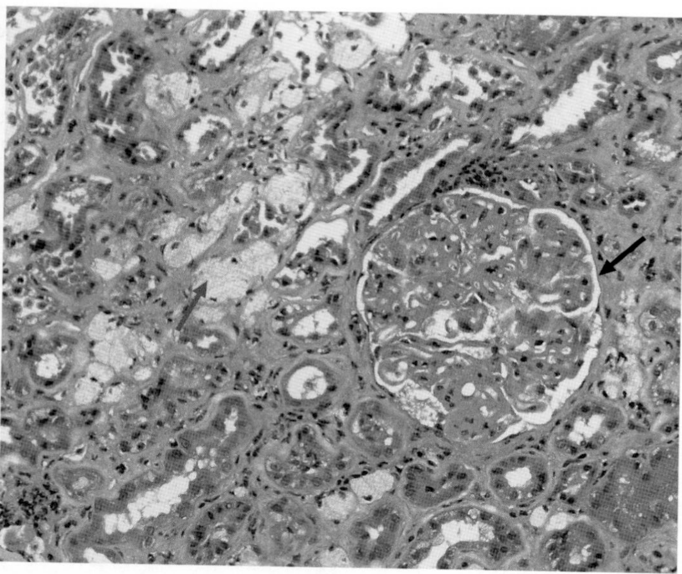

FIGURE 27–3. Membranous glomerulonephropathy (secondary to gold), a cause of nephrotic syndrome. Globally thickened glomerular capillaries (↙) and interstitial foam cells (↗) are seen. H&E × 450. (Image contributed by Dr. Rabia Mir.)

glomerular basement membrane, thereby changing its consistency (eg, gold) (Fig. 27–3). Second, they can upset the immunoregulatory balance (eg, NSAIDs). A less-common glomerular lesion is hypersensitivity vasculitis. The pathologic appearance of the glomeruli may be described as secondary minimal glomerular change, membranous glomerulopathy, or focal segmental glomerulosclerosis. Albumin loss usually exceeds urinary excretion as a result of renal tubular catabolism of filtered protein. The tubules also retain sodium, causing expansion of the extracellular space and edema. The glomerular lesion may progress to renal failure if the pathologic process continues.

Acute kidney injury (formerly called "acute renal failure") is defined as an abrupt decline in renal function that impairs the capacity of the kidney to maintain metabolic balance. The three main categories of acute kidney injury are prerenal, postrenal, and intrinsic renal failure.

TABLE 27–2. Xenobiotics that Cause Nephrotic Syndrome

Antimicrobials (rifampicin, cefixime)
Captopril
Drugs of abuse (heroin, cocaine)
Insect venom
Interferon α
Metals (gold, mercury, lithium)
NSAIDs
Penicillamine

Prerenal failure involves impaired renal perfusion, which can occur with volume depletion, systemic vasodilatation, heart failure, or preglomerular vasoconstriction. Hence, toxic events that cause bleeding (overdose of anticoagulants), volume depletion (diuretics, cathartics, or emetics), cardiac dysfunction (β-adrenergic antagonists), or hypotension from any cause can lead to acute prerenal failure.[67]

An example of vascular constriction is the hepatorenal syndrome, or renal hypoperfusion caused by liver failure. This syndrome is characterized by impaired renal function and marked constriction of the renal arterial vasculature associated with severe chronic or acute hepatic failure. Many neurohumoral disturbances lead to the renal and systemic hemodynamic changes that occur in the syndrome. Splanchnic and systemic vasodilation- likely secondary to portal hypertension decrease mean arterial pressure and compromise renal blood flow. Circulating mediators of vasoconstriction are subsequently increased, resulting in hepatorenal syndrome. Angiotensin, norepinephrine, vasopressin, endothelin, and isoprostane F_2 all contribute to an extreme cortical vasoconstriction. That this renal insufficiency is extrarenal is best illustrated by the fact that when a kidney from a patient with hepatorenal syndrome is transplanted into a uremic patient, the function of the graft promptly returns to normal.

Postrenal failure, such as urinary tract obstruction, may result from crystalluria (eg, oxalosis in ethylene glycol poisoning) or blocked urinary flow (eg, retroperitoneal fibrosis from methysergide; bladder dysfunction from anticholinergic drugs). Regardless of the cause of urinary tract obstruction, there are characteristic histologic and pathophysiologic alterations in the kidney. Microscopically, tubular dilation, predominantly in the distal nephron segments (ie, the collecting ducts and distal tubules), occurs initially and glomerular structure is preserved, subsequently dilation of the Bowman space occurs, and finally periglomerular fibrosis develops.

Pathophysiologically, GFR falls as tubule pressure counteracts the capillary hydraulic pressure gradient. Subsequently there is a fall in

TABLE 27–3. Xenobiotics that Cause Acute Tubular Necrosis

Acetaminophen	**Halogenated hydrocarbons**
Antimicrobials	**Metals**
Aminoglycosides	Arsenic
Amphotericin	Bismuth
Pentamidine	Chromium
Tenofovir, cidofovir, adefovir	Mercury
Polymyxins	Uranium
Antineoplastics	**Mushrooms**
Cisplatin	*Cortinarius spp*
Ifofamide	*Amanita smithiana*
Methotrexate	**Pigments**
Mithramycin	Myoglobin
Streptozotocin	Hemoglobin
Fluorinated anesthetics	**Radiocontrast agents**
Foscarnet	Those that cause hypotension or hypovolemia
Glycols	
Ethylene glycol	
Diethylene glycol	

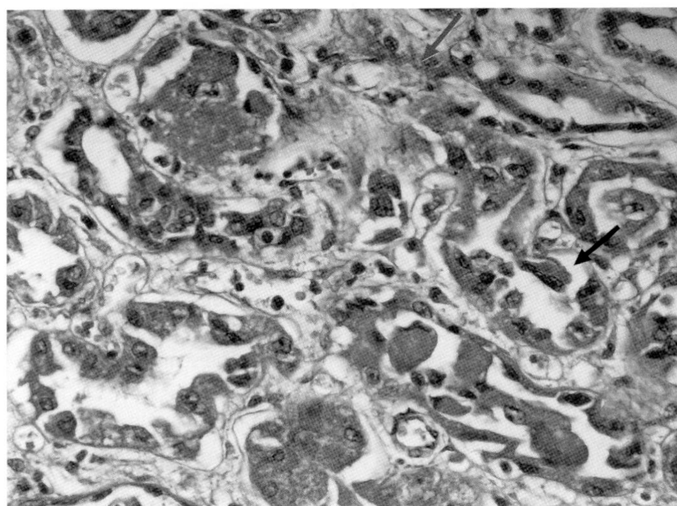

FIGURE 27–4. Acute tubular necrosis (secondary to mercury). Proximal tubular epithelial necrosis (↙) and sloughing are associated with interstitial edema (↗). H&E × 450. (Photo contributed by Dr. Rabia Mir.)

renal perfusion leading to ischemic damage to nephrons. Tubular function is impaired such that concentrating ability, potassium secretory function, and urinary acidification mechanisms are all altered.

Acute tubular necrosis (Table 27–3), the most common nephrotoxic event,[4] is characterized pathologically by patchy necrosis of tubules, usually the proximal segments (Fig. 27–4). The lesion is associated with three different processes: direct toxic injury, ischemic injury from renal hypoperfusion, and pigmenturia.[181]

Direct toxicity accounts for approximately 35% of all cases of acute tubular necrosis.[130,235] Direct acting xenobiotics affect different segments of the renal tubules; for example, uranium attacks the proximal tubule and amphotericin the distal tubule (see Fig. 27–1). However, the clinical pattern of rapidly declining renal function, often accompanied by oliguria, is identical in all forms of tubular necrosis. Poisoning may also lead to ischemic tubular necrosis if hypotension or cardiac failure causes ischemia of nephron segments (proximal straight tubule and inner medullary collecting duct) that are particularly vulnerable to hypoxia.

Pigmenturia refers either to myoglobinuria from rhabdomyolysis (skeletal muscle necrosis) or to hemoglobinuria from massive hemolysis.[61] Either pigment may cause tubular injury and necrosis by precipitating in the tubular lumen.[73,181] Myoglobinuria follows necrosis of striated muscle. Alcohol and cocaine can be directly myotoxic in some individuals,[190] as can the β-hydroxy-β-methylglutaryl-coenzyme A (HMG-CoA) reductase inhibitors (statins) used to lower blood cholesterol.[107] Rhabdomyolysis causing myoglobinuric acute tubular necrosis can occur after extensive bee or wasp stings[128] or fire ant bites.[134] Xenobiotics that produce hypokalemia (eg, diuretics and laxatives) or predispose to hyperthermia (antipsychotics) can cause muscle necrosis on this basis. Most often, poisoning leads to muscle breakdown from pressure necrosis following prolonged unconsciousness (opioids and sedative-hypnotics), excessive muscle contraction (cocaine), or grand mal seizures (alcohol withdrawal, theophylline).[82] Pigmenturic acute renal failure may also complicate poisoning with carbon monoxide, copper sulfate, and zinc phosphate.[34,130,259]

Myoglobin is normally excreted without causing toxicity. A study of patients with rhabdomyolysis suggests that the concentration of myoglobin in the urine may affect the development of renal failure.[73] If myoglobin inspissates in the tubular lumen because of renal hypoperfusion and high water absorption, it dissociates in the relatively acidic environment as H^+ is secreted, releasing tubulotoxic hematin.[61] This toxicity may stem from the iron-catalyzing production of oxygen free radicals.

Myoglobinuric acute tubular necrosis is diagnosed when acute kidney injury occurs following muscle breakdown. There is a simultaneous elevation of concentration of serum muscle enzymes such as creatinine kinase and aldolase. A positive urine orthotolidine test, with no erythrocytes in the sediment, and urine myoglobin may be measured. However, because primary renal failure may cause detectable myoglobinuria that does not worsen renal function,[71] finding myoglobin in the urine does not prove the diagnosis.

Myoglobinuric acute tubular necrosis can be prevented by early volume expansion if renal injury has not yet occurred.[200] Alkalinizing the urine may prevent dissociation of myoglobin and minimize tubular necrosis. However, massive rhabdomyolysis can lead to severe hypocalcemia resulting from the release of large amounts of phosphate into the blood. Alkalemia in this setting can cause tetany or seizures, worsening muscle injury.[130] Hence, the risk of alkalinization must be weighed against the benefit.

Hemoglobinuria follows hemolysis, which can be caused by a number of xenobiotics, including snake and spider venoms, cresol, phenol, aniline, arsine, stibine, naphthalene, dichromate, and methylene chloride. Sensitivity reactions to drugs (hydralazine, quinine) can also cause hemolysis.[61] The pathophysiology of hemoglobinuric acute tubular necrosis resembles that of myoglobinuria. The pigment deposits in the tubules and dissociates, causing necrosis to occur.[181] Volume depletion and acidosis precipitate the disorder, so volume expansion and alkalinization may help prevent kidney injury.

Although there is controversy about how a tubular lesion leads to glomerular shutdown, it is generally felt that tubular obstruction,

TABLE 27–4. Xenobiotics that Cause Acute Interstitial Nephritis

More Common	Less Common
Allopurinol	Anticonvulsants
Antimicrobials	Carbamazepine
β-Lactams, especially ampicillin, methicillin, penicillin	Phenobarbital
	Phenytoin
Moxifloxacin	Captopril
Rifampin	Diuretics
Sulfonamides (including mesalamine)	Furosemide
Vancomycin	Thiazides
Proton-pump inhibitors	Zoledronate
Azathioprine	
NSAIDs	

back-leak of filtrate across injured epithelium, renal hypoperfusion, and decreased glomerular filtering surface combine to impair glomerular filtration.[232] Additionally, filtration pressure is diminished by neutrophil infiltration and status in the vasa recta.[239] Recent evidence suggests that prolonged medullary ischemia, perhaps caused by an imbalance in the production of vasoconstrictors such as endothelin and vasodilators such as nitric oxide, is important in prolonging the renal dysfunction after the tubular injury develops.[142]

Clinically, acute tubular necrosis presents as a rapid deterioration of renal function, usually first noted as azotemia. Muddy brown casts or renal tubular cells may be seen in the urinary sediment, but hematuria and leukocyturia are unusual. Disorders of metabolic balance, such as hyperkalemia and metabolic acidosis, are also common. Although tubular sodium reabsorption is decreased, the fall in glomerular filtration usually leads to positive sodium and water balance, as renal output of these substances is fixed.[159]

Acute interstitial nephritis (Table 27–4) is clinically similar to acute tubular necrosis and often must be diagnosed by renal biopsy, which shows a cellular infiltrate separating tubular structures (Fig. 27–5). Nearly all acute interstitial nephritis is caused by hypersensitivity.[238] In many patients, the renal failure is accompanied by manifestations of systemic allergy such as fever, rash, or eosinophilia. Finding eosinophils in the urine is consistent with this disorder.[177] However, approximately 25% of patients with xenobiotic-induced interstitial nephritis have no signs of hypersensitivity. Unlike those with tubular necrosis, most patients with acute interstitial nephritis have hematuria and leukocyturia,[9] particularly eosinophiluria.[10] Secondary fever at the onset of azotemia is common, and flank pain or arthralgia may be present. The lesion usually improves after the xenobiotic is removed. Corticosteroids may hasten recovery;[89,147] many physicians use this treatment only if the renal failure does not improve promptly when the xenobiotic exposure is stopped.

DIFFERENTIAL DIAGNOSIS OF ACUTE KIDNEY INJURY

Patients who present with acutely deteriorating renal function often represent a difficult diagnostic challenge. Not only are there three major etiologic categories, but each category has several subdivisions; and more than one factor may be present. For example, a patient with an opioid overdose may have neurogenic hypotension (prerenal), together with muscle necrosis causing myoglobinuric renal failure (intrinsic renal), and opioid-induced urinary retention (postrenal). Because renal, prerenal, and postrenal processes are not mutually exclusive and require different interventions, all three should always be considered, even when one appears to be the most obvious cause of the renal failure.

Prerenal failure (renal hypoperfusion) initiates a sequence of events leading to renal salt and water retention.[12] Renin is released, causing

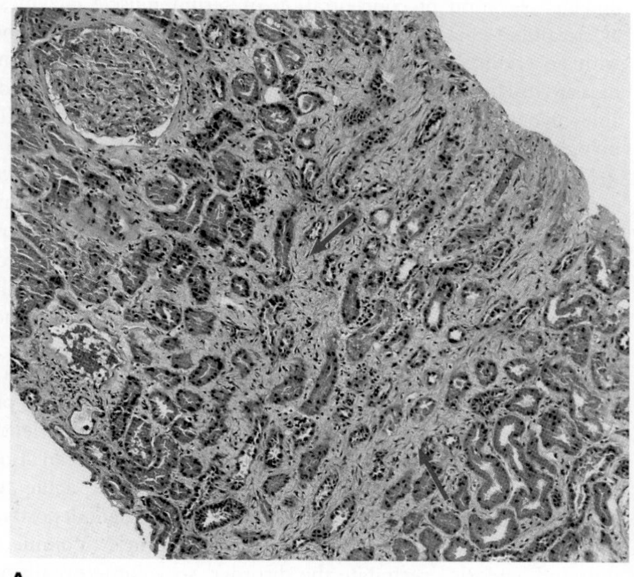

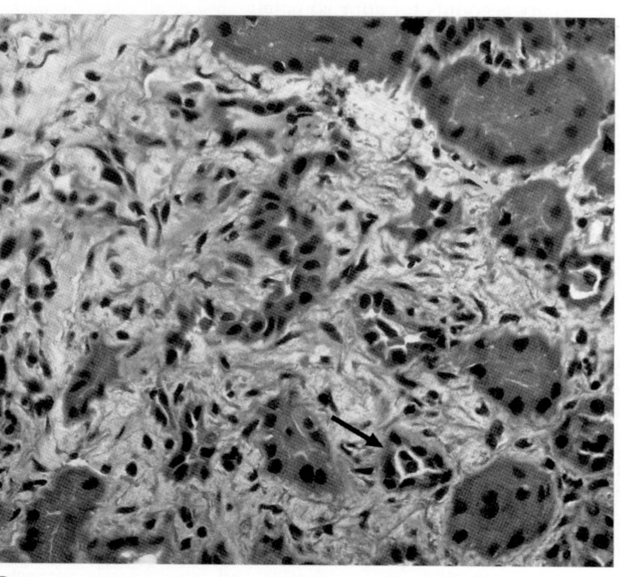

FIGURE 27–5. Acute interstitial nephritis (secondary to rifampin). Interstitial edema and patchy lymphocyte, plasma cell, and eosinophil infiltration occurs without fibrosis (↗). Tubular epithelium shows degenerative and regenerative changes (↙) and mononuclear cell infiltration (tubulitis) (→)(**A**) H&E × 112; (**B**) H&E × 450. (Images contributed by Dr. Rabia Mir.)

TABLE 27–5. Tests of Renal Function

Acute	Chronic
To differentiate prerenal failure from acute tubular necrosis: 1. BUN-to-creatinine ratio; usually > 20:1 in prerenal failure 2. Urine Na^+ usually < 20 mEq/L in prerenal failure; usually > 40 mEq/L in acute tubular necrosis 3. Fractional Na^+ excretion (FE_{Na}) is most reliable test: $FE_{Na} = \frac{\text{Urine[Na]/Plasma [Na}^+]}{\text{Urine[Creatinine]/Plasma [Creatinine]}} \times 100$ FE_{Na} < 1% (ie, normal) in prerenal failure, if the patient has not received diuretics or large infusions of sodium, which increase Na^+ excretion despite normal tubular function. In tubular necrosis or interstitial nephritis, renal Na^+ absorption is decreased, and FE_{Na} > 1%. This is useful except in pigmenturic or iodinated radiocontrast-associated renal failure, when the test is of no benefit.	Creatinine clearance (C_{cr}) = U × V/P (normal range 90–130 mL/min), where U is urine creatinine concentration, V is urine flow in mL/min, and P is plasma creatinine concentration. Urine collection must be complete (not necessarily 24 hours), and U and P must be in the same units. In steady states, C_{cr} in adults can be approximated by dividing the patient's weight in kilograms by the serum creatinine in mg/dL (multiply by 0.8 in women);[3] from the Cockroft-Gault equation,[44] $C_{cr} = \frac{(140-\text{age})\times \text{ideal body weight (kg)}}{72\times \text{serum creatinine}} (\times 0.85 \text{ for women})$ or more formally, GFR can be estimated from the MDRD formula, 186 × serum creatinine$^{-1.154}$ × age$^{-0.203}$ (× 0.742 if female); × (1.21 if African-American).[140]

Go to website http://www.nephron.com/MDRD_GFR.cgi

N.B. If renal function is unstable, these formulae are meaningless.

production of angiotensin, which enhances proximal tubular sodium reabsorption and stimulates adrenal aldosterone release, thus increasing distal sodium reabsorption. Prerenal failure is, therefore, accompanied by low urinary sodium excretion (Table 27–5). Release of ADH increases water and urea retention. Unresolving renal hypoperfusion may cause ischemic tubular necrosis.

Xenobiotics may decrease renal blood flow without causing intrinsic renal injury (see Fig. 27–1). Diuretics or cathartics can decrease blood volume and antihypertensive agents can excessively reduce blood pressure. Some xenobiotics (eg, cyclosporine, tacrolimus, amphotericin, methotrexate) cause prerenal vasoconstriction. NSAIDs lower filtration rate by inhibiting production of vasodilatory prostaglandins in the afferent arteriole. Finally, cardiotoxins, such as doxorubicin, can cause severe heart failure. Some xenobiotics cause a hypersensitivity vasculitis (see Fig. 27–1).

Although it is not a renal injury, the clinician should bear in mind that an estimated creatinine clearance (C_{cr}) or GFR < 40 carries the risk of nephrogenic systemic fibrosis in patients exposed to gadolinium for contrast MRI studies.[236]

Urinary tract obstruction should always be considered when the kidneys fail rapidly. Although complete obstruction leads to anuria, partial obstruction, which is more common, is usually associated with alternating oliguria and polyuria. Continued production of urine in the presence of obstruction leads to distension of the urinary tract above the blockage. Calyceal dilatation is common. Obstruction of the bladder outlet or urethra may distend the bladder.

Obstruction may be caused by xenobiotics (Table 27–6).[75] Most do so by impairing contraction of the bladder through anticholinergic action (atropine, antidepressants). Rarely, certain xenobiotics, particularly methysergide,[230] cause retroperitoneal fibrosis and ureteral constriction. Finally, a few xenobiotics lead to crystalluria and intratubular obstruction. Sometimes the xenobiotic itself forms precipitates (sulfonamides,[48] indinavir, or methotrexate) or causes excretion of a precipitating chemical such as oxalate (ethylene glycol and fluorinated anesthetics).

PATIENT EVALUATION

Evaluation of a patient with suspected toxic renal injury should include extrarenal as well as renal factors. The kidney's response to xenobiotics is affected by previous renal function, renal blood flow, and the presence of urinary tract obstruction that can exert back-pressure on the nephrons, all of which must be considered.

HISTORY

A past history of renal disease or conditions that can affect the kidney (eg, diabetes, hypertension, cardiovascular disease) should be noted. Flank pain, hematuria, or an abnormal pattern of urine output are important findings. The patient's intravascular volume status affects renal perfusion. Thus, a history of heart disease or a disorder that

TABLE 27–6. Xenobiotics that Cause Urinary Obstruction

Bladder Dysfunction	Crystal Deposition
Anticholinergics	Acyclovir (intravenous)
Antihistamines	Ethylene glycol
Atropine	Fluorinated anesthetics
Cyclic Antidepressants	Fluoroquinolones
Scopolamine	Heme pigments
Antipsychotics	Indinavir
Butyrophenones	Methotrexate
Phenothiazines	Phenylbutazone
Atypicals	Sulfonamides
Bromocriptine	**Retroperitoneal Fibrosis**
CNS depressants	Ergotamines (Methysergide, LSD)
	Chinese herbs (*Stephania spp, Aristolochia spp*)

TABLE 27–7. Nephrotoxic Effects of Metals

	Toxic Acute Tubular Necrosis	Shock Acute Tubular Necrosis	Hemolysis	Acute Interstitial Nephritis	Chronic Interstitial Nephritis	Tubular Dysfunction	Nephrotic Syndrome	Glomerulo-nephritis
Antimony[35]	+							
Arsenic[137,167,243,245]	+++	+++	++	+	+			
Barium[204,255]	+							
Beryllium[16]					++			
Bismuth[20,21,211]	++			+		+	+	
Cadmium[124,254,121]					+++	+++		
Chromium[181,250]	+++							
Copper[210,180]		+	+					
Gadolinium[87,106,216]	+							
Germanium[149,179]					+			
Gold[7,56,173,241]	+						+++	
Iron[41,153,240]		++			+			
Lead[6,19,34,39,45,50,113,145,14,6,178,253]	+		+		+++	+++		
Lithium[30,53,78,104,221,156]	+				++	++	+	
Mercury[25,83,166,diamond, stachiatti]	+++	+				+	+	
Platinum (cisplatin)[90,95,206,224,258]	++				++	++		
Silicon[122]								+
Silver[150,153]	+							
Thallium[215]	+			+				
Uranium[181,186]	+							

+++ = common; + = uncommon.

lowers plasma volume such as vomiting or diarrhea is important. Prior cancer chemotherapy with drugs such as cisplatin or methyl-CCNU (methyl-1-[2-chloroethyl]-3-cyclohexyl-1-nitrosourea) should be noted. All current xenobiotics should be evaluated for potential renal effects, both those with direct and indirect nephrotoxic effects.[92] The patient's intake of alcohol and drugs of abuse should be explored. A careful occupational history and assessment of hobbies and lifestyle are crucial, with emphasis on exposure to nephrotoxic xenobiotics.

TABLE 27–8. Nephrotoxic Hydrocarbons and Mechanisms of Toxicity

Solvents	Glycols
Carbon tetrachloride[153,181,222,223] Hepatic failure leading to hepatorenal syndrome Occasional acute nephrotoxic renal failure Tetrachloroethylene[215] Hepatic failure leading to hepatorenal syndrome Occasional acute nephrotoxic renal failure Trichloroethylene[13] Acute tubular necrosis Toluene[198] Hippuric acidosis	Ethylene glycol[37,135] Metabolized to glycolic acid (metabolic acidosis) Further metabolized to oxalic acid (acute tubular necrosis) Diethylene glycol[96,181] Direct tubular toxin (acute tubular necrosis) Hyperoxaluria may add to renal injury Propylene glycol[261,262] Metabolic acidosis and acute kidney injury May cause hemolysis and hemoglobinuric renal failure

PHYSICAL EXAMINATION

The patient's hemodynamic status should be carefully assessed. Postural changes in pulse and blood pressure, and either engorgement or decreased filling of the neck veins, give important information about the intravascular volume. The skin should be examined for lesions. Funduscopy may reveal evidence of chronic hypertension or diabetes. All aspects of cardiac function should be noted, including presence or absence of edema. Injuries or scars in the suprapubic area or evidence of past urologic or retroperitoneal surgery may suggest obstruction, as may a palpable or percussible bladder.

LABORATORY EVALUATION

Nephrotoxic injury is not always apparent clinically, so the laboratory is exceedingly important. Acute loss of renal function may be suspected if urine output decreases, but oliguria is not universal. The most important parameter of renal function is glomerular filtration. Because urea and creatinine are largely excreted by this route, serum concentrations of these substances are used as markers of renal function. However, the concentration of any substance depends on both production and excretion. Azotemia—elevation of BUN or creatinine—is a standard

TABLE 27–9. Nephrotoxic Antimicrobials

Acute glomerular Injury	Acute Tubular Necrosis	Acute Interstitial Nephritis	Hypersensitivity Vasculitis	Obstruction (Crystalluria)	Tubular Dysfunction
Crystalline deposits	Aminoglycosides[27,54,184,205,220]	β-Lactams (penicillins,[9,169] cephalosporins[10,129])	Penicillins[169]	Acyclovir (IV)[22]	Aminoglycosides (K^+ and Mg^{2+} wasting)[111]
Foscarnet[260]	Gentamicin,[111] tobramycin,[226] amikacin[138]	Sulfonamides[162] (including cotrimoxazole[147])	Sulfonamides[169]	Indinavir[120]	Amphotericin
Nephrotic syndrome	Amphotericin[5,17,38,98,244]	Vancomycin[8,64]		Sulfonamides[162]	Renal tubular acidosis[100]
Cefixime[114]	Fluoroquinolones (ciprofloxacin, levofloxacin)[88,227]	Rifampin and Rifampicin[174,197,47]			K^+ and Mg^{2+} wasting[18]
Rifampicin[237]	Polymyxins B and E[131]	Nitrofurantoin[168]			Nephrogenic diabetes insipidus[81]
	Pentamidine[229]	Aminoglycosides (rare)[164,207]			Tetracyclines (Fanconi syndrome,[80] hypercatabolism[192])
	Acyclovir[22]	Tetracyclines (rare)[251]			
	Foscarnet[32]	Polymyxins[24]			
	Ritonavir[55]				
	Phenazopyridine[77]				
	Tenofovir, cidofovir, adefovir[154]				

indication of renal insufficiency. However, BUN or creatinine in the normal range does not exclude a substantial degree of renal impairment because of the previously discussed hyperbolic relationship between these parameters and GFR. In addition, decreased production of urea (starvation or liver failure) or creatinine (amputation, muscle wasting) may result in a normal BUN or creatinine in the presence of significant renal impairment. Conversely, decreased renal perfusion (prerenal failure) is often associated with a disproportionate rise in BUN in comparison with the rise in creatinine, because urea is partially reabsorbed along with salt and water, whose reabsorption is increased when the kidneys are underperfused. Thus, a BUN-to-creatinine ratio > 20 is suggestive of prerenal failure (see Table 27–5). Because many nephrotoxic xenobiotics are associated with nonoliguric acute renal failure (urine volume > 400 mL/d), progressive azotemia without oliguria should always raise suspicion of a drug-related cause. Tubular injury, especially in lead poisoning and myoglobinuria, can cause hyperuricemia from decreased tubular secretion of uric acid.

TABLE 27–10. Nephrotoxic Effects of Antiarthritic Drugs[40,43,62,188,213]

Acute tubular necrosis
Colchicine[231]
Acetaminophen[33,52]

Acute interstitial nephritis
Allopurinol[85]
Sulfinpyrazone[109,147]

Acute worsening of kidney function (prerenal)[84]
Indomethacin and other NSAIDS

Chronic interstitial nephritis[31]
5-Aminosalicylate[2]
Aspirin/phenacetin or aspirin/acetaminophen "analgesic nephropathy"[66,101,153,209,213]

Hyperkalemia[213]

Hyponatremia[43]

Nephrotic syndrome[31,76,252]
Penicillamine[202]
Probenecid[103]

Certain xenobiotics alter measured concentrations of urea and creatinine in the absence of any change in renal function.[171] The most obvious is exogenous creatine taken to build muscle mass. Cefoxitin, nitromethane, and ketones absorb light at the same frequency as the creatinine reaction product, thus artifactually increasing the measured level. Drugs that block renal creatinine secretion, such as cimetidine and trimethoprim, may also increase serum creatinine. BUN may be raised independently of renal function by tetracycline or corticosteroids, which increase protein catabolism.

In patients with chronic kidney disease it is necessary to assess the remaining renal function to manage the patient properly. Clearance measurements are generally used to determine glomerular filtration rate. The most common is endogenous Ccr (see Table 27–5).

Determining Ccr in acute kidney injury is not helpful, as the accuracy of a clearance implies a steady state. Changing GFR during a clearance time period distorts the resulting estimation. There is also a lag period between changes in kidney function and changes in BUN or creatinine concentrations. In general, a patient with acute kidney injury should be treated as if glomerular filtration were < 10 mL/min. In patients with acute kidney injury, a random sample of urine may be sent promptly to the laboratory for sodium and creatinine measurements to determine fractional sodium excretion, which may help discriminate prerenal azotemia from tubular necrosis (see Table 27–5).

Examination of the urine is essential in cases of poisoning. Although urine is sent to the laboratory, it can also be examined carefully by the physician. Standard dipsticks will detect albumin and glucose. The dipstick test for blood is useful for confirming the presence of small amounts of blood or myoglobin, but is not a substitute for careful microscopic examination of the sediment. Clinicians should look not only for red or white cells but also for crystals, tubular elements, casts, and bacteria. If acute interstitial nephritis is a consideration, a fresh urine sample should be stained for eosinophils.[164]

TABLE 27–11. Nephrotoxic Medications

Diuretics
- Prerenal failure (volume depletion)
- Acute interstitial nephritis[147,151,152]
- Acute renal failure (mannitol)[28,93]
- Hyperkalemia (K⁺-sparing diuretics)[72]
- Hyponatremia

Antihypertensives
- Prerenal failure (excessive dosage)
- Acute interstitial nephritis
  - Methyldopa[256]
  - Captopril[233]
- Nephrotic syndrome
  - Captopril[196]
- Obstruction (retroperitoneal fibrosis)
  - Methyldopa[141]

Anticonvulsants
- Acute interstitial nephritis
- Carbamazepine[108]
- Phenobarbital[182]
- Phenytoin[9,112]
- Nephrotic syndrome
  - Trimethadione[15]
  - Paramethadione

Anesthetics
- Acute tubular necrosis
- Methoxyflurane[185]
- Halothane[86]
- Enflurane[63]

Antineoplastics
- Acute tubular necrosis
- Cisplatin[90,206]
- Methotrexate[46,99,193,116]
- Mithramycin[126]
- Ifosfamide[219]
- Streptozotocin[214]
- Chronic interstitial nephritis
  - Cisplatin[95]
  - Nitrosoureas[64,217]
- Thrombotic microangiopathy
  - Mitomycin C[139,187]

Immunosuppressants
- Acute tubular necrosis and/or chronic interstitial nephritis
- Cyclosporine[74,110,158,172,189]
- Tacrolimus[173,235]
- Acute interstitial nephritis
  - Azathioprine[225]
- Renal tubular acidosis
  - Tacrolimus[97]

Radiocontrast agents
- Acute renal failure, especially the high osmolal and ionic agents[11,28,68,123,165,166,179,195,249]
- Osmotic nephropathy and renal vasoconstriction [gadolinium]

TABLE 27–12. Nephrotoxicity of Miscellaneous Xenobiotics

Acute glomerular injury
Focal segmental glomerulosclerosis
- Pamidronate (collapsing type)[155]
- Interferon alpha[176,257]

Acute tubular necrosis
- Aluminum phosphide[127]
- Deferoxamine[41]
- Epinephrine (in neonate)[141]
- Etidronate[183]
- Mycotoxins[57]
- Paraquat, diquat[248]

Acute interstitial nephritis
- Cimetidine[147,157]
- Clofibrate[51]
- Phenylpropanolamine[26]
- Proton-pump inhibitors[84A]
- Ranitidine[79]
- Ticlopidine[201]

Acute renal failure
- Mushrooms
  - *Amanita* (especially *A. smithiana*)[172]
  - *Cortinarius* spp[136]
- Pigments[67]
  - Hemoglobin
  - Myoglobin

Obstruction (retroperitoneal fibrosis)
- Bromocriptine[29]

Renal stones and aminoaciduria
- Worcestershire sauce[170]

Thrombotic microangiopathy
- Clopidogrel[25]
- Cyclosporine[246]
- Mitomycin C[139]
- *Possible* (IL-2, Interferon alpha, imatinib, gemcitabine)
- Quinine[132]
- Tacrolimus[144]
- Ticlopidine[36]

TABLE 27–13. Nephrotoxicity of Drugs of Abuse

Nephrotic Syndrome	Amyloidosis	Obstruction (Retroperitoneal Fibrosis)	Acute Renal Failure (Myoglobinuria)	Chronic Renal Failure (Vasculitis)
Adulterated heroin[119,60,148,161] Adulterated cocaine[119]	Adulterated heroin (injection use)[49,117]	Lysergic acid diethylamide (LSD)[230]	Amphetamines[102,125] Cocaine[203]	Amphetamines[42]

TABLE 27–14. Nephrotoxicity of "Complementary" Medical Treatments

Acute Interstitial Nephritis	Acute Tubular Necrosis	Obstruction (Retroperitoneal Fibrosis)
Stephania tetrandra, Magnolia officinalis[69,247] (Chinese herbs, often irreversible) *Hypericum*[69] *Ledum*[69]	Grass carp gallbladder[143] Disodium edetate[45,183]	*Stephania tetrandra, Magnolia officinalis*[69,247]

Further evaluation of the patient with acute renal failure should include tests for obstruction, which can be caused by a number of substances (see Table 27–6). Renal ultrasonography should be performed to look for hydronephrosis. Postvoiding residual urine volume may be measured as appropriate by catheterization; if the volume is in excess of 75 to 100 mL, suspect bladder dysfunction or obstruction.

Nephrotoxic complications of specific xenobiotics are found in Tables 27–7 through 27–14.

SUMMARY

The kidneys are exposed to exogenous or endogenous xenobiotics in their role as primary defenders against harmful xenobiotics entering the bloodstream. The environment, the workplace, and, especially, the administration of medications, represent potential sources of nephrotoxicity. Consequently, it is important to determine, by history and observation, to which xenobiotics a patient may have been exposed and to be aware of their potential to harm the kidneys. It is equally crucial to work the other way when a patient presents with renal dysfunction: review all xenobiotics, both conventional and complementary, all xenobiotic exposures, and any conditions that can adversely affect the kidneys.

ACKNOWLEDGMENT

Vincent L. Anthony contributed to this chapter in a previous edition.

REFERENCES

1. Agharazii M, Marcotte J, Boucher D, et al. Chronic interstitial nephritis due to 5-aminosalicylic acid. *Am J Nephrol.* 1999;19:373-376.
2. Albini B, Glurich I, Andres GA. Mercuric chloride-induced immunologically mediated diseases in experimental animals. In: Porter GA, ed. *Nephrotoxic Mechanisms of Drugs and Environmental Toxins.* New York: Plenum; 1982:413-423.
3. Ali F, Boldur A, Winchester JF, Feinfeld DA. A simplified, reliable estimate of creatinine clearance. *J Am Soc Nephrol.* 2006;17:893A-894A.
4. Anderson HL Jr, Feinfeld DA. Mechanisms of drug-induced renal failure. *Hosp Physician.* 1987;23:27-40.
5. Andreoli T. On the anatomy of amphotericin B-cholesterol pores in lipid bilayer membranes. *Kidney Int.* 1973;4:337-345.
6. Angevine JM, Kappas A, DeGowin RL, et al. Renal tubular nuclear inclusions of lead poisoning: a clinical and experimental study. *Arch Pathol.* 1962;73:486-494.
7. Antonovych TT. Gold nephropathy. *Ann Clin Lab Sci.* 1981;11:386-391.
8. Appel GB, Given DB, Levine LR, et al. Vancomycin and the kidney. *Am J Kidney Dis.* 1986;8:75-80.
9. Appel GB, Kunis CL. Acute tubulointerstitial nephritis. *Contemp Issues Nephrol.* 1983;10:151-185.
10. Appel GB, Neu HC. Acute interstitial nephritis induced by beta-lactam antibiotics. In: Fillastre JH, Whelton A, Tulkens P, eds. *Antibiotic Nephrotoxicity.* Paris: INSERM; 1982:195-212.
11. Aron NB, Feinfeld DA, Peters AT, et al. Acute renal failure associated with ioxaglate, a low-osmolality radiocontrast agent. *Am J Kidney Dis.* 1989;13:189-193.
12. Badr KF, Ichikawa I: Prerenal failure. A deleterious shift from renal compensation to decompensation. *N Engl J Med.* 1988;319:623-629.
13. Baerg RD, Kimberg DV. Centrilobular hepatic necrosis and acute renal failure in "solvent sniffers." *Ann Intern Med.* 1970;73:713-720.
14. Ball BU, Sorensen LB. Pathogenesis of hyperuricemia in saturnine gout. *N Engl J Med.* 1969;280:1199-1202.
15. Bar-Khayim Y, Teplitz C, Garella S, et al. Trimethadione (Tridione)-induced nephrotic syndrome. *Am J Med.* 1973;54:272-280.
16. Barnett RN, Brown DS, Cadorna CB, et al. Beryllium disease with death from renal failure. *Conn Med.* 1961;25:142-147.
17. Barquist E, Fein E, Shadick D, et al. A randomized prospective trial of amphotericin B lipid emulsion versus dextrose colloidal solution in critically ill patients. *J Trauma.* 1999;47:336-340.
18. Barton CH, Pahl M, Vaziri N, et al. Renal magnesium wasting associated with amphotericin B therapy. *Am J Med.* 1984;77:471-474.
19. Batuman V, Maesaka JK, Haddad B, et al. The role of lead in gouty nephropathy. *N Engl J Med.* 1981;304:520-523.
20. Beattie JW. Nephrotic syndrome following sodium bismuth tartrate therapy in rheumatoid arthritis. *Ann Rheum Dis.* 1953;12:144-146.
21. Beaver DL, Burr RE. Bismuth inclusions in the human kidney: a long-term autopsy study. *Arch Pathol.* 1963;76:89-94.
22. Becker BN, Fall P, Hall C, et al. Rapidly progressive acute renal failure due to acyclovir: case report and review of the literature. *Am J Kidney Dis.* 1993;22:611-615.
23. Becker CG, Becker EF, Maher JF, et al. Nephrotic syndrome after contact with mercury: a report of five cases, three after the use of ammoniated mercury ointment. *Arch Intern Med.* 1962;110:178-186.
24. Beirne GJ, Hansing CE, Octaviano GW, et al. Acute renal failure caused by hypersensitivity to polymyxin B sulfate. *JAMA.* 1967;202:156-158.
25. Bennett CL, Connors JM, Carwile JM, et al. Thrombotic thrombocytopenic purpura associated with clopidogrel. *N Engl J Med.* 2000;342:1773-1777.
26. Bennett WM. Hazards of the appetite suppressant phenylpropanolamine. *Lancet.* 1979;2:42-43.
27. Bennett WM, Gilbert DN, Houghton D, et al. Gentamicin nephrotoxicity: morphologic and pharmacologic features. *West J Med.* 1977;126:65-68.
28. Better OS, Winaver JM, Knochel JP. Mannitol therapy revisited (1940–1997). *Kidney Int.* 1997;51:886-894.
29. Bowler JV, Ormerod IE, Legg NJ. Retroperitoneal fibrosis and bromocriptine. *Lancet.* 1986;2:466.
30. Bosquet S, Descombes E, Gauthier T, et al. Nephrotic syndrome during lithium therapy. *Nephrol Dial Transplant.* 1997;12:2728-2731.
31. Brezin JH, Katz SM, Schwartz AB, et al. Reversible renal failure and nephrotic syndrome associated with non-steroidal anti-inflammatory drugs. *N Engl J Med.* 1979;301:1271-1273.
32. Cacoub P, Deray G, Baumelou A, et al. Acute renal failure induced by foscarnet. *Clin Nephrol.* 1988;29:315-318.
33. Campbell NR, Baylis B. Renal impairment associated with an acute paracetamol overdose in the absence of hepatotoxicity. *Postgrad Med J.* 1992;68:116-118.
34. Catsch A, Harmuth-Hoene AE. The chelation of heavy metals. In: Levine WG, ed. *International Encyclopedia of Pharmacology and Therapeutics.* New York: Pergamon; 1979:107-224.
35. Charlas R, Benabadji A. Néphrite azotémique au cours du traitement par l'antimoine d'un cas de leishmaniase viscérale infantile. *Maroc Med.* 1962;41:1180-1182.
36. Chen DK, Kim JS, Sutton DM. Thrombotic thrombocytopenic purpura associated with ticlopidine use: a report of 3 cases and review of the literature. *Arch Intern Med.* 1999;159:311-314.
37. Cheng JT, Beysolow TD, Kaul B, et al. Clearance of ethylene glycol by kidneys and hemodialysis. *J Toxicol Clin Toxicol.* 1987;25:95-108.
38. Cheng JT, Feinfeld DA. Amphotericin B and the kidney. *Hosp Physician.* 1988;24:68-72.
39. Chisolm JJ Jr, Harrison HC, Eberlein WR, et al. Aminoaciduria, hypophosphatemia, and rickets in lead poisoning. *Am J Dis Child.* 1955;89:159-168.
40. Ciabbatoni G, Cinotti GA, Pierucci A, et al. Effects of sulindac and ibuprofen in patients with chronic glomerular disease. *N Engl J Med.* 1984;310:279-283.
41. Cianciulli P, Sorrentino F, Forte L, et al. Acute renal failure occurring during intravenous desferrioxamine therapy: recovery after hemodialysis. *Haematologica.* 1992;77:514-515.
42. Citron BP, Halpern M, McCarron M, et al. Necrotizing angiitis associated with drug abuse. *N Engl J Med.* 1970;283:1003-1011.
43. Clive DM, Stoff J. Renal syndromes associated with non-steroidal anti-inflammatory drugs. *N Engl J Med.* 1984;310:563-572.
44. Cockroft DW, Gault MH. Prediction of creatinine clearance from serum creatinine. *Nephron.* 1976;16:31-41.
45. Collet JT. EDTA-chelation therapy. *Ned Tijdschr Geneeskd.* 1992;136:191-192.
46. Condit PT, Chanes PE, Joel W. Renal toxicity of methotrexate. *Cancer.* 1969;23:126-131.
47. Covic A, Golea O, Segall L, et al. A clinical description of rifampicin-induced acute renal failure in 170 consecutive cases. *J Indian Med Assoc.* 2004;102:20,22-25.

48. Crespo M, Quereda C, Pascual J, et al. Patterns of sulfadiazine acute nephropathy. *Clin Nephrol.* 2000;54:68-72.
49. Crowley S, Feinfeld DA, Janis R. Resolution of nephrotic syndrome and lack of progression of heroin-associated renal amyloidosis. *Am J Kidney Dis.* 1989;13:333-335.
50. Crutcher JC. Clinical manifestations and therapy of acute lead intoxication due to the ingestion of illicitly distilled alcohol. *Ann Intern Med.* 1963;59:707-715.
51. Cumming A. Acute renal failure and interstitial nephritis after clofibrate treatment. *Br Med J.* 1980;281:1529-1530.
52. Davenport A, Finn R. Paracetamol (acetaminophen) poisoning resulting in acute renal failure. *Nephron.* 1988;50:55-56.
53. Davies B, Kincaid-Smith P. Renal biopsy studies of lithium and prelithium patients and comparison with cadaver transplant kidneys. *Neuropharmacology.* 1979;18:1001-1002.
54. DeBroe ME, Giuliano R, Verpooten G. Choice of drug and dosage regimen: two important risk factors for aminoglycoside nephrotoxicity. *Am J Med.* 1986;80:115-118.
55. Deray G, Bochet M, Katlama C, et al. Nephrotoxicity of ritonavir. *Presse Med.* 1998;27:1801-1803.
56. Derot M, Kahn J, Mazalton A, et al. Néphrite anurique aigue mortelle après traitement aurique, chrysocyanose associée. *Bull Mem Soc Med Hop Paris.* 1954;70:234-239.
57. Di Paolo N, Guarnieri A, Loi F, et al. Acute renal failure from inhalation of mycotoxins. *Nephron.* 1993;64:621-625.
58. Diamond GL, Zalups RK. Understanding renal toxicity of heavy metals. *Toxicol Pathol.* 1998;26:92-103.
59. Dorfman LE, Smith JP. Sulfonamide crystalluria: a forgotten disease. *J Urol.* 1970;104:482-483.
60. do Sameiro Faria M, Sampaio S, Faria V, et al. Nephropathy associated with heroin abuse in Caucasian patients. *Nephrol Dial Transplant.* 2003;18:2308-2313.
61. Dubrow A, Flamenbaum W. Acute renal failure associated with myoglobinuria and hemoglobinuria. In: Brenner BM, Lazarus JM, eds. *Acute Renal Failure.* 2nd ed. New York: Churchill Livingstone; 1988:279-293.
62. Dunn MJ. Are Cox-2 selective inhibitors nephrotoxic? *Am J Kidney Dis.* 2000;35;976-977.
63. Eichhorn JH, Hedley-White J, Steinman TI, et al. Renal failure following enflurane anesthesia. *Anesthesiology.* 1976;45:557-560.
64. Eisenberg ES, Robbins N, Lenci M. Vancomycin and interstitial nephritis. *Ann Intern Med.* 1981;95:658.
65. Ellis ME, Weiss RB, Kuperminc M. Nephrotoxicity of lomustine. *Cancer Chemother Pharmacol.* 1985;15:174-175.
66. Elseviers MM, De Broe ME. Analgesic nephropathy: is it caused by multi-analgesic abuse of single substance use? *Drug Saf.* 1999;20:15-24.
67. Espinel CH, Gregory AW. Differential diagnosis of acute renal failure. *Clin Nephrol.* 1980;13:73-77.
68. Fang LS, Sirota RA, Ebert TH, et al. Low fractional excretion of sodium with contrast media-induced acute renal failure. *Arch Intern Med.* 1980;140:531-533.
69. Farrell J, Campbell E, Walshe JJ. Renal failure associated with alternative medical therapies. *Ren Fail.* 1995;17:659-664.
70. Feinfeld DA, Ansari N, Nuovo M, et al. Tubulointerstitial nephritis associated with minimal self reexposure to rifampin. *Am J Kidney Dis.* 1999;33:E3.
71. Feinfeld DA, Briscoe AM, Nurse HM, et al. Myoglobinuria in chronic renal failure. *Am J Kidney Dis.* 1986;8:111-114.
72. Feinfeld DA, Carvounis CP. Fatal hyperkalemia and hyperchloremic acidosis: association with spironolactone in the absence of renal impairment. *JAMA.* 1978;240:1516.
73. Feinfeld DA, Cheng JT, Beysolow TD, et al. A prospective study of urine and serum myoglobin levels in patients with acute rhabdomyolysis. *Clin Nephrol.* 1992;38:193-195.
74. Feinfeld DA, D'Agati V, Benvenisty A, et al. Cyclosporin A and urine glutathione-*S*-transferase. *Proc Eur Dial Transplant Assoc Eur Ren Assoc.* 1985;22:561-565.
75. Feinfeld DA, Nurse HM, Hotchkiss JL, et al. The clinical spectrum of chronic interstitial nephritis. *Hosp Physician.* 1985;21:102-104.
76. Feinfeld DA, Olesnicky L, Pirani CL, et al. Nephrotic syndrome associated with the use of non-steroidal anti-inflammatory drugs. *Nephron.* 1984;37:174-179.
77. Feinfeld DA, Ranieri R, Lipner HI, Avram MM. Renal failure in phenazopyridine overdose. *JAMA.* 1978;240:2661.
78. Forrest JN Jr, Marcy TW, Biemesderfer D, et al. Cytoskeletal defect in cortical collecting duct cells in lithium-induced polyuria [abstract]. *Kidney Int.* 1981;19:200.
79. Freeman HJ. Ranitidine-associated interstitial nephritis in a patient with celiac sprue. *Can J Gastroenterol.* 1988;2:35.
80. Frimpter GW, Timpanelli AE, Eisenmenger WJ, et al. Reversible "Fanconi syndrome" caused by degraded tetracycline. *JAMA.* 1963;184:111-113.
81. Fujita Y, Kasahara K, Uno K, et al. Amphotericin B-induced nephrogenic diabetes insipidus in a case of cryptococcemia. *Intern Med.* 2005;44:458-461.
82. Gabow PA, Kaehny WD, Kelleher SP. The spectrum of rhabdomyolysis. *Medicine (Baltimore).* 1982;61:141-152.
83. Gade R, Feinfeld DA, Gade MF. A microradiographic study of nephrons in mercuric chloride-induced acute renal failure in the rabbit. *Invest Radiol.* 1983;18:183-188.
84. Galler M, Folkert VW, Schlondorff D. Reversible acute renal insufficiency and hyperkalemia following indomethacin therapy. *JAMA.* 1981;246:154-155.

84A. Geevasinga N, Coleman PL, Webster AC, Roger SD. Proton pump inhibitors and acute interstitial nephritis. *Clin Gastroenterol Hepatol.* 2006;4:597-604.

85. Gelbart DR, Weinstein AB, Fajardo LF. Allopurinol-induced interstitial nephritis. *Ann Intern Med.* 1977;86:196-198.
86. Gelman ML, Lichtenstein N. Halothane-induced nephrotoxicity. *Urology.* 1981;17:323-327.
87. Gemery J, Idelson B, Reid S, et al. Acute renal failure after arteriography with gadolinium-based contrast agent. *AJR Am J Roentgenol.* 1998;171:1277-1278.
88. Gerritsen WR, Peters A, Henny FC, et al. Ciprofloxacin-induced nephrotoxicity. *Nephrol Dial Transplant.* 1987;2:382-383.
89. Gilbert DN, Gourley R, d'Agostino A, et al. Interstitial nephritis due to methicillin, penicillin, and ampicillin. *Ann Allergy.* 1970;28:378-385.
90. Goldstein RS, Mayor GH. The nephrotoxicity of cisplatin. *Life Sci.* 1983;32:685-690.
91. Gradus D, Rhoads M, Bergstrom LB, et al. Acute bromate poisoning associated with renal failure and deafness presenting as hemolyticuremic syndrome. *Am J Nephrol.* 1984;4:188-191.
92. Greven J, Klein H. Renal effects of furosemide in glycerol-induced acute renal failure of the rat. *Pflugers Arch.* 1976;365:81-87.
93. Gudallah MF, Lynn M, Work J. Case report: mannitol nephrotoxicity syndrome. *Am J Med Sci.* 1995;309:219-222.
94. Halpren BA, Kempson RC, Coplon NS. Interstitial fibrosis and chronic renal failure following methoxyflurane anesthesia. *JAMA.* 1973;233:1239-1242.
95. Hayes DM, Cvitkovic E, Golbey RB, et al. High dose cisplatinum diamine dichloride: amelioration of renal toxicity by mannitol diuresis. *Cancer.* 1977;39:1372-1381.
96. Hébert JL, Auzépy P, Durand A. Acute human and experimental poisoning with diethylene glycol. *Sem Hop Paris.* 1983;59:344-349.
97. Heering P, Ivens K, Aker S, et al. Distal renal tubular acidosis induced by FK-506. *Clin Transplant.* 1998;12:465-471.
98. Heidemann HT, Gerkens JF, Spickard WA, et al. Amphotericin B nephrotoxicity in humans decreased by salt repletion. *Am J Med.* 1983;75:476-481.
99. Hempel L, Misselwitz J, Fleck C, et al. Influence of high-dose methotrexate therapy (HD-MTX) on glomerular and tubular kidney function. *Med Pediatr Oncol.* 2003;40:348-354.
100. Hemstreet BA. Antimicrobial-associated renal tubular acidosis. *Ann Pharmacother.* 2004;38:1031-1038.
101. Henrich WL, Agodoa LE, Barrett B, et al. Analgesics and the kidney: summary and recommendations to the scientific advisory board of the National Kidney Foundation from an ad hoc committee of the National Kidney Foundation. *Am J Kidney Dis.* 1996;27:162-165.
102. Henry JA, Jeffreys KJ, Dawling S. Toxicity and deaths from 3,4-methylenedioxyamphetamine ("ecstasy"). *Lancet.* 1992;340:384-387.
103. Hertz P, Yager H, Richardson JB. Probenecid-induced nephrotic syndrome. *Arch Pathol.* 1972;94:241-243.
104. Hestbech J, Aurell M. Lithium-induced uremia. *Lancet.* 1979;1:212-213.
105. Hestbech J, Hansen HE, Amdisen A, et al. Chronic renal lesions following long-term treatment with lithium. *Kidney Int.* 1977;12:205-213.
106. Heuck A, Reiser M. Nephrotoxicity of contrast medium in magnetic resonance tomography. *Internist (Berl).* 1997;38:1234-1235.

107. Hill MD, Bilbao JM. Case of the month: February 1999—54-year-old man with severe muscle weakness. *Brain Pathol.* 1999;9:607-608.
108. Hogg RJ, Sawyer M, Hecox K, et al. Carbamazepine-induced acute tubulointerstitial nephritis. *J Pediatr.* 1981;98:830-832.
109. Howard T, Hoy RH, Warren S, et al. Acute renal dysfunction due to sulfinpyrazone therapy in post-myocardial infarction: cardiomegaly, reversible hypersensitivity, interstitial nephritis. *Am Heart J.* 1981;102:294-295.
110. Humes HD, Jackson NM, O'Connor RP, et al. Pathogenetic mechanisms of nephrotoxicity: insights into cyclosporine nephrotoxicity. *Transplant Proc.* 1985;17(Suppl 1):51-62.
111. Humes HD, Weinberg JM, Knauss TC. Clinical and pathophysiologic aspects of aminoglycoside toxicity. *Am J Kidney Dis.* 1982;2:5-29.
112. Hyman LR, Ballow M, Knieser MR. Diphenylhydantoin interstitial nephritis: roles of cellular and humoral immunologic injury. *J Pediatr.* 1978;92:915-920.
113. Inglis JA, Henderson DA, Emmerson BT. The pathology and pathogenesis of chronic lead nephropathy occurring in Queensland. *J Pathol.* 1978;124:65-76.
114. Işlek I, Gök F, Albayrak D, et al. Nephrotic syndrome following cefixime therapy in a 10-month-old girl: spontaneous resolution without corticosteroid treatment. *Nephrol Dial Transplant.* 1999;14:25-27.
115. Iversen BM, Nordahl E, Thunold S, et al. Retroperitoneal fibrosis during treatment with methyldopa. *Lancet.* 1975;2:302-304.
116. Izzedine H, Launay-Vacher V, Karie S, et al. Is low-dose methotrexate nephrotoxic? Case report and review of the literature. *Clin Nephrol.* 2005;64:315-319.
117. Jacob H, Charytan C, Rascoff JH, et al. Amyloidosis secondary to drug abuse and chronic skin suppuration. *Arch Intern Med.* 1978;138:1150-1151.
118. Jadoul M, de Plaen JF, Cosyns JP, et al. Adverse effects from traditional Chinese medicines. *Lancet.* 1993;341:892-893.
119. Jaffe JA, Kimmel PL. Chronic nephropathies of cocaine and heroin abuse: a critical review. *Clin J Am Soc Nephrol.* 2006;1:655-667.
120. Jaradat M, Phillips C, Yum MN, et al. Acute tubulointerstitial nephritis attributable to indinavir therapy. *Am J Kidney Dis.* 2000;35:E16.
121. Järup L. Cadmium overload and toxicity. *Nephrol Dial Transplant.* 2002;17S2:35-39.
122. Kallenberg CGM. Renal disease—another effect of silica exposure. *Nephrol Dial Transplant.* 1995;10:1117-1119.
123. Katholi RE, Woods WT Jr, Taylor GJ, et al. Oxygen free radicals and contrast nephropathy. *Am J Kidney Dis.* 1998;32:64-71.
124. Kazantzis G. Renal tubular dysfunction and abnormalities of calcium metabolism in cadmium workers. *Environ Health Perspect.* 1979;28:155-159.
125. Kendrick WC, Hull, AR, Knochel JP. Rhabdomyolysis and shock after intravenous amphetamine administration. *Ann Intern Med.* 1977;86:381-387.
126. Kennedy BJ. Metabolic and toxic effects of mithramycin during tumor therapy. *Am J Med.* 1970;49:494-503.
127. Khosla SN, Nand N, Khosla P. Aluminium phosphide poisoning. *J Tropic Med Hyg.* 1988;91:196-198.
128. Kim YO, Yoon SA, Kim KJ, et al. Severe rhabdomyolysis and acute renal failure due to multiple wasp stings. *Nephrol Dial Transplant.* 2003;18:1235.
129. Kleinknecht D, Vanhille P, Morel-Maroger L. Acute interstitial nephritis due to drug hypersensitivity: an up-to-date review with a report of 19 cases. *Adv Nephrol.* 1983;12:277-308.
130. Knochel JP. Rhabdomyolysis and myoglobinuria. In: Suki WN, Kknoyan G, eds. *The Kidney in Systemic Disease.* 2nd ed. New York: Wiley; 1981:263-284.
131. Koch-Weser J, Sidel V, Federman ER, et al. Adverse effects of sodium colistimethate: manifestations and specific reaction rates during courses of therapy. *Ann Intern Med.* 1970;72:857-868.
132. Kojouri K, Vesely SK, George JN. Quinine-associated thrombotic thrombocytopenic purpura-hemolytic uremic syndrome: frequency, clinical features, and long-term outcomes. *Ann Intern Med.* 2001;135:1047-1051.
133. Koren G. The nephrotoxic potential of drugs and chemicals: pharmacologic basis and clinical relevance. *Med Toxicol.* 1989;4:59-72.
134. Koya S, Crenshaw D, Agarwal A. Rhabdomyolysis and acute renal failure after fire ant bites. *J Gen Intern Med.* 2007;22:145-147.
135. Kraut JA, Kurtz I. Toxic alcohol ingestions: clinical features, diagnosis, and management. *Clin J Am Soc Nephrol.* 2008;3:208-225.
136. Lampe KF. Toxic effects of plant toxins. In: Klaassen CD, Amdur MO, Doull J, eds. *Casarett and Doull's Toxicology.* 3rd ed. New York: Macmillan; 1986:757-770.
137. Landrigan PJ. Arsenic. In: Rom WN, ed. *Environmental and Occupational Medicine.* Boston: Little, Brown; 1983:473-480.
138. Lerner SA, Schmitt B, Seligsohn R, et al. Comparative study of ototoxicity and nephrotoxicity in patients randomly assigned to treatment with amikacin or gentamicin. *Am J Med.* 1986;80:90-104.
139. Lesesne JB, Rothschild N, Erickson B, et al. Cancer-associated hemolytic-uremic syndrome: analysis of 85 cases from a national registry. *J Clin Oncol.* 1989;7:781-789.
140. Levey AS, Bosch JP, Lewis JB, Greene T, Rogers N, Roth D. A more accurate method to estimate glomerular filtration rate from serum creatinine: a new prediction equation. Modification of Diet in Renal Disease Study Group. *Ann Intern Med.* 1999;130:461-470.
141. Levine DH, Levkoff AH, Pappu LD, et al. Renal failure and other serious sequelae of epinephrine toxicity in neonates. *South Med J.* 1985;78:874-877.
142. Lieberthal W. Biology of acute renal failure: therapeutic implications. *Kidney Int.* 1997;52:1102-1115.
143. Lim PS, Lin JL, Hu SA, et al. Acute renal failure due to ingestion of the gallbladder of grass carp: report of 3 cases with review of literature. *Ren Fail.* 1993;15:639-644.
144. Lin CC, King KL, Chao YW, et al. Tacrolimus-associated hemolytic uremic syndrome: a case analysis. *J Nephrol.* 2003;16:580-585.
145. Lin JL, Tan DT, Ho HH, et al. Environmental lead exposure and urate excretion in the general population. *Am J Med.* 2002;113:563-568.
146. Lin JL, Yu CC, Lin-Tan DT, et al. Lead chelation therapy and urate excretion in patients with chronic renal diseases and gout. *Kidney Int.* 2001;60:266-271.
147. Linton AL, Clark WF, Drieger AA, et al. Acute interstitial nephritis due to drugs: review of the literature with a report of nine cases. *Ann Intern Med.* 1980;93:735-741.
148. Llach F, Descoeudres C, Massry SG. Heroin-associated nephropathy: clinical and histological studies in 19 patients. *Clin Nephrol.* 1979;11:7-12
149. Luck BE, Mann H, Melzer H, Dunemann L, Begerow J. Renal and other organ failure caused by germanium intoxication. *Nephrol Dial Transplant.* 1999;14:2464-2468.
150. Lucké B. Lower nephron nephrosis: the renal lesions of crush syndrome of burns, transfusions and other conditions affecting the lower segment of the nephrons. *Mil Surg.* 1946;99:371-396.
151. Lyons H, Pinn VW, Cortell S, et al. Allergic interstitial nephritis causing reversible renal failure in four patients with idiopathic nephrotic syndrome. *N Engl J Med.* 1973;288:124-128.
152. Magil AB, Ballon HS, Cameron ECC, et al. Acute interstitial nephritis associated with thiazide diuretics: clinical and pathological observations in three cases. *Am J Med.* 1980;69:939-943.
153. Maher JF. Toxic nephropathy. In: Brenner BM, Rector FC Jr, eds. *The Kidney.* Philadelphia: WB Saunders; 1976:1355-1395.
154. Malik A, Abraham P, Malik N. Acute renal failure and Fanconi syndrome in an AIDS patient on tenofovir treatment: case report and review of literature. *J Infect.* 2005;51:E61-E65.
155. Markowitz GS, Appel GB, Fine PL, et al. Collapsing focal segmental glomerulosclerosis following treatment with high-dose pamidronate. *J Am Soc Nephrol.* 2001;12:1164-1172.
156. Markowitz GS, Radhakrishnan J, Kambham N, et al. Lithium nephrotoxicity: a progressive combined glomerular and tubulointerstitial nephropathy. *J Am Soc Nephrol.* 2000;11:1439-1448.
157. McGowan WR, Vermillion SE. Acute interstitial nephritis related to cimetidine therapy. *Gastroenterology.* 1980;79:746-749.
158. Mihatsch MJ, Thiel G, Spichtin HD, et al. Morphological findings in kidney transplants after treatment with cyclosporine. *Transplant Proc.* 1983;15:2821-2835.
159. Miller TJ, Anderson RJ, Linas SL, et al. Urinary diagnostic indices in acute renal failure: A prospective study. *Ann Intern Med.* 1978;89:47-50.
160. Mitchel DH Amanita mushroom poisoning. *Annu Rev Med.* 1980; 31:51-57.
161. Moody C, Kaufman R, McGuire D, et al. The role of adulterants in heroin nephropathy (abstract). *Natl Kidney Found.* 1985;15:A12.
162. More RH, McMillan GC, Duff GL. The pathology of sulfonamide allergy in man. *Am J Pathol.* 1946;22:703-705.
163. Moreau JF, Droz D, Noel LH. Tubular nephrotoxicity of water soluble iodinated contrast media. *Invest Radiol.* 1980;15(Suppl 6):S54-S60.

164. Morin JP, Viotte G, Vandewalle A, et al. Gentamicin-induced nephrotoxicity: A cell biology approach. *Kidney Int.* 1980;18:583-590.
165. Mudge GH, Meier FA, Ward KK. Pathogenesis of renal impairment induced by radiocontrast drugs. In: Solez K, Whelton A, eds. *Acute Renal Failure.* New York: Marcel Dekker; 1984:361-388.
166. Mudge GH. Nephrotoxicity of urographic radiocontrast drugs. *Kidney Int.* 1980;18:540-552.
167. Muehrcke RC, Pirani CL. Arsine induced anuria: a correlative clinicopathologic study with electron microscopic observations. *Ann Intern Med.* 1968;68:853-866.
168. Muehrcke RC, Pirani CL, Kark RM. Interstitial nephritis: a clinico-pathological renal biopsy study. *Ann Intern Med.* 1967;66:1052.
169. Mullick FG, McAllister HA Jr, Wagner BM, et al. Drug-related vasculitis: clinicopathologic correlations in 30 patients. *Hum Pathol.* 1979;10:313-325.
170. Murphy KJ. Bilateral renal calculi and aminoaciduria after excessive intake of Worcestershire sauce. *Lancet.* 1967;2:401-403.
171. Muther RS. Drug interference with renal function tests. *Am J Kidney Dis.* 1983;3:118-120.
172. Myers BD, Ross J, Newton L, et al. Cyclosporine-associated chronic nephropathy. *N Engl J Med.* 1984;311:699-705.
173. Nagi AH, Alexander F, Barbas AZ. Gold nephropathy in rats: light and electron microscopic studies. *Exp Mol Pathol.* 1971;15:354-362.
174. Nessi R, Bonoldi GL, Redaelli B, et al. Acute renal failure after rifampicin: a case report and survey of the literature. *Nephron.* 1976;16:148-159.
175. Neylan J, Whelchel J, Laskow D, et al. Adverse events in the comparative dose finding trial of FK-506 in primary renal transplantation. *Am Soc Transplant Phys.* 1993;12:154.
176. Nishimura S, Miura H, Yamada H, et al. Acute onset of nephrotic syndrome during interferon-alpha retreatment for chronic active hepatitis C. *J Gastroenterol.* 2002;37:854-858.
177. Nolan CR, Anger MS, Kelleher SP. Eosinophiluria: a new method of detection and definition of the clinical spectrum. *N Engl J Med.* 1986;315:1516-1519.
178. Nolan CV, Shaikh ZA. Lead nephrotoxicity and associated disorders: biochemical mechanisms. *Toxicology.* 1992;73:127-146.
179. Obara K, Saito T, Sato H, et al. Germanium poisoning: clinical symptoms and renal damage caused by long-term intake of germanium. *Jpn J Med.* 1991;30:67-72.
180. Oldenquist G, Salem M. Parenteral copper sulfate poisoning causing acute renal failure. *Nephrol Dial Transplant.* 1999;14:441-443.
181. Oliver J, MacDowell M, Tracy A. The pathogenesis of acute renal failure associated with traumatic and toxic injury: renal ischemia, nephrotoxic damage and the ischemuric episode. *J Clin Invest.* 1951;30:1307-1351.
182. Ooi BS, First MR, Pesce AJ, et al. IgE levels in interstitial nephritis. *Lancet.* 1974;1:1254-1256.
183. O'Sullivan TL, Akbari A, Cadnapaphornchai P. Acute renal failure associated with the administration of parenteral etidronate. *Ren Fail.* 1994;16:767-773.
184. Paller MS. Drug-induced nephropathies. *Med Clin North Am.* 1990;74:909-916.
185. Panner BJ, Freeman, RB, Roth-Mayo VA, et al. Toxicity following methoxyflurane anesthesia. *JAMA.* 1970;214:86-90.
186. Pavlakis N, Pollack CA, McLean G, et al. Deliberate overdose of uranium: toxicity and treatment. *Nephron.* 1996;72:313-317.
187. Pavy MD, Wiley EL, Abeloff MD. Hemolytic-uremic syndrome associated with mitomycin therapy. *Cancer Treat Rep.* 1982;66:457-461.
188. Perazella MA, Eras J. Are selective COX-2 inhibitors nephrotoxic? *Am J Kidney.* Dis 2000;35:937-940.
189. Perico N, Ruggenenti P, Gaspari P, et al. Daily renal hypoperfusion induced by cyclosporine in patients with renal transplantation. *Transplantation.* 1992;54:56-60.
190. Perkoff GT, Dioso MM, Bleisch V, et al. A spectrum of myopathy associated with alcoholism. I. Clinical and laboratory features. *Ann Intern Med.* 1967;67:493-510.
191. Peterson BA, Collins AJ, Vogelzang NJ, et al. 5-Azacytidine and renal tubular dysfunction. *Blood.* 1981;57:182-185.
192. Phillips ME, Eastwood JB, Curtis JR, et al. Tetracycline poisoning in renal failure. *Br Med J.* 1974;2:149-151.
193. Pitman SW, Parker LM, Tattersall MHN, et al. Clinical trials of high-dose methotrexate with citrovorum factor: toxicologic and therapeutic observations. *Cancer Chemother Rep.* 1975;6:43-49.
194. Poole G, Stradling P, Worlledge S. Potentially serious side effects of high-dose twice-weekly rifampicin. *Br Med J.* 1971;3:343-347.
195. Porter GA. Radiocontrast-induced nephropathy. *Nephrol Dial Transplant.* 1994;9(Suppl 4):146-156.
196. Prins EJL, Hoorntje SJ, Weening JJ, et al. Nephrotic syndrome in patients on captopril. *Lancet.* 1979;2:306-307.
197. Qunibi WY, Godwin J, Eknoyan G. Toxic nephropathy during continuous rifampin therapy. *South Med J.* 1980;73:791-792.
198. Reisin E, Teicher A, Jaffe R, et al. Myoglobinuria and renal failure in toluene poisoning. *Br J Ind Med.* 1975;32:163-164.
199. Robben JH, Knoers NV, Deen PM. Cell biological aspects of the vasopressin type-2 receptor and aquaporin 2 water channel in nephrogenic diabetes insipidus. *Am J Physiol Renal Physiol.* 2006;291:F257-F270
200. Ron D, Taitelman MD, Michaelson MD, et al. Prevention of acute renal failure in traumatic rhabdomyolysis. *Arch Intern Med.* 1984;144:277-280.
201. Rosen H, El-Hennawy AS, Greenberg S, et al. Acute interstitial nephritis associated with ticlopidine. *Am J Kidney Dis.* 1995;25:934-936.
202. Ross JH, McGinty F, Brewer DG. Penicillamine nephropathy. *Nephron.* 1980;26:184-186.
203. Roth D, Alarcon FJ, Fernandez JA, et al. Acute rhabdomyolysis associated with cocaine intoxication. *N Engl J Med.* 1988;319:673-677.
204. Roza O, Berman LB. The pathophysiology of barium: hypokalemic and cardiovascular effects. *J Pharmacol Exp Ther.* 1971;177:433-439.
205. Rybak MJ, Abate BJ, Kang SL, et al. Prospective evaluation of the effect of an aminoglycoside-dosing regimen on rates of observed nephrotoxicity and ototoxicity. *Antimicrob Agents Chemother.* 1999;43:1549-1555.
206. Safirstein R, Winston J, Goldstein M, et al. Cisplatin nephrotoxicity. *Am J Kidney Dis.* 1986;8:356-367.
207. Saltissi D, Pulsey CD, Rainford DJ. Recurrent acute renal failure due to antibiotic-induced interstitial nephritis. *Br Med J.* 1979;1:1182-1183.
208. Sandhu JS, Sood A, Midha V, et al. Non-traumatic rhabdomyolysis with acute renal failure. *Ren Fail.* 2000;22:81-86.
209. Sandler DP, Smith JC, Weinberg CR, et al. Analgesic use and chronic renal disease. *N Engl J Med.* 1989;320:1238-1243.
210. Sanghvi LM, Sharma R, Mirsa SN, et al. Sulfhemoglobinemia and acute renal failure after copper sulfate poisoning: report of two fatal cases. *Arch Pathol.* 1957;63:172-175.
211. Sarikaya M, Sevinc A, Ulu R, et al. Bismuth subcitrate nephrotoxicity. a reversible cause of acute oliguric renal failure. *Nephron.* 2002;90:501-502.
212. Schacht RG, Feiner HD, Gallo GR, et al. Nephrotoxicity of nitrosoureas. *Cancer.* 1981;38:1328-1334.
213. Scharschmidt LA, Feinfeld DA. Renal effects of nonsteroidal antiinflammatory drugs. *Hosp Physician.* 1989;25:29-33.
214. Schein PS, O'Connell MJ, Blom J, et al. Clinical antitumor activity and toxicity of streptozotocin. *Cancer.* 1974;34:993-1000.
215. Schreiner GE, Maher JF. Toxic nephropathy. *Am J Med.* 1965;38:409-449.
216. Schuhmann-Giamperi G, Krestin G. Pharmacokinetics of Gd-DTPA in patients with chronic renal insufficiency. *Invest Radiol.* 1991;26:975-979.
217. Schwarz A, Krause PH, Kunzendorf U, et al. The outcome of acute interstitial nephritis: risk factors for the transition from acute to chronic interstitial nephritis. *Clin Nephrol.* 2000;54:179-190.
218. Shils ME. Renal disease and the metabolic effects of tetracycline. *Ann Intern Med.* 1963;58:389-408.
219. Shore R, Greenberg M, Geary D, et al. Iphosphamide-induced nephrotoxicity in children. *Pediatr Nephrol.* 1992;6:162-165.
220. Simmons CF, Bogusky RT, Humes HD. Inhibitory effects of gentamicin on renal mitochondrial oxidative phosphorylation. *J Pharmacol Exp Ther.* 1980;214:709-715.
221. Singer I. Lithium and the kidney. *Kidney Int.* 1981;19:374-387.
222. Sinicrope RA, Gordon JA, Little JR, et al. Carbon tetrachloride nephrotoxicity: a reassessment of pathophysiology based upon the urinary diagnostic indices. *Am J Kidney Dis.* 1984;3:362-365.
223. Sipes IG, Krishna G, Gillette JR. Bioactivation of carbon tetrachlo-ride, chloroform, and bromotrichloromethane: role of cytochrome. *Life Sci.* 1977;20:1541-1548.
224. Sleijfer DTH, Smit EF, Meijer S, et al. Acute and cumulative effects of carboplatin on renal function. *Br J Cancer.* 1989;60:116-120.
225. Sloth K, Thomsen AC. Acute renal insufficiency during treatment with azathioprine. *Act Med Scand.* 1971;189:145-148.
226. Smith CR, Lipsky JJ, Laskin OL, et al. Double-blind comparison of the nephrotoxicity and auditory toxicity of gentamicin and tobramycin. *N Engl J Med.* 1980;302:1106-1109.

227. Solomon NM, Mokrzycki MH. Levofloxacin-induced allergic interstitial nephritis. *Clin Nephrol.* 2000;54:356.
228. Stacchiotti A, Borsani E, Rodella L, et al. Dose-dependent mercuric chloride tubular injury in rat kidney. *Ultrastruct Pathol.* 2003;27:253-259.
229. Stahl-Bayliss CM, Kalman CM, Laskin OL. Pentamidine-induced hypoglycemia in patients with the acquired immune deficiency syndrome. *Clin Pharmacol Ther.* 1986;39:271-275.
230. Stecker JF Jr, Rawls HP, Devine CJ, et al. Retroperitoneal fibrosis and ergot derivatives. *J Urol.* 1974;112:30-32.
231. Stefanidis I, Bohm R, Hagel J, et al. Toxic myopathy with kidney failure as a colchicine side effect in familial Mediterranean fever. *Dtsch Med Wochenschr.* 1992;117:1237-1240.
232. Stein JH, Lifschitz MD, Barnes LD. Current concepts of the pathophysiology of acute renal failure. *Am J Physiol.* 1978;234:F171-F181.
233. Steinman TI, Silva P. Acute renal failure, skin rash, and eosinophilia associated with captopril therapy. *Am J Med.* 1983;75:154-156.
234. Sterne TL, Whitaker C, Webb CH. Fatal cases of bismuth intoxication. *J La State Med Soc.* 1955;107:332-335.
235. Su Q, Weber L, Lettir M, et al. Nephrotoxicity of cyclosporin A and FK-506: inhibition of calcineurin phosphatase. *Ren Physiol Biochem.* 1995;18:128-139.
236. Swaminathan S, Shah SV. New insights into nephrogenic systemic fibrosis. *J Am Soc Nephrol.* 2007;18:2636-2643.
237. Tada T, Ohara A, Nagai Y, et al. A case report of nephrotic syndrome associated with rifampicin therapy. *Nippon Jinzo Gakkai Shi.* 1995;37:145-150.
238. Ten RM, Torres VE, Milliner DS, et al. Acute interstitial nephritis: immunologic and clinical aspects. *Mayo Clin Proc.* 1988;63:921-930.
239. Thadhani R, Pascual M, Bonventre J. Medical progress: Acute renal failure. *N Engl J Med.* 1996;334:1448-1460.
240. Thompson J. Ferrous sulfate poisoning: its incidence, symptomatology, treatment, and prevention. *Br Med J.* 1950;1:645-646.
241. Tornroth T, Skrifvars B. Gold nephropathy prototype of membranous glomerulonephritis. *Am J Pathol.* 1974;75:573-590.
242. Tubbs RR, Gephardt GN, McMahon JT, et al. Membranous glomerulonephritis associated with industrial mercury exposure. *Am J Clin Pathol.* 1982;77:409-413.
243. Uldall PR, Khan HA, Ennis JE, et al. Renal damage from industrial arsine poisoning. *Br J Ind Med.* 1970;27:372-377.
244. Ullmann AJ, Sanz MA, Tramarin A, et al. Prospective study of amphotericin B formulations in immunocompromised patients in 4 European countries. *Clin Infect Dis.* 2006;43:e29-e38.
245. Vallee BL, Ulmer DD, Wacker WEC. Arsenic toxicology and biochemistry. *Arch Ind Health.* 1960;21:132-151.
246. Van Buren D, Van Buren CT, Flechner SM, et al. De novo hemolytic uremic syndrome in renal transplant recipients immunosuppressed with cyclosporine. *Surgery.* 1985;98:54-62.
247. Vanherweghem JL, Depierreux M, Tielemans C, et al. Rapidly progressive interstitial renal fibrosis in young women: association with slimming regimen including Chinese herbs. *Lancet.* 1993;341:387-391.
248. Vanholder R, Colardyn F, De Reuck J, et al. Diquat intoxication: report of two cases and review of the literature. *Am J Med.* 1981;70:1267-1271.
249. VanZee BE, Hoy WE, Talley TE, et al. Renal injury associated with intravenous pyelography in nondiabetic and diabetic patients. *Ann Intern Med.* 1978;89:51-54.
250. Varma A, Jha V, Ghosh AK, et al. Acute renal failure in a case of fatal chromic acid poisoning. *Ren Fail.* 1994;16:653-657.
251. Walker RG, Thomson NM, Dowling JP, Ogg CS. Minocycline-induced acute interstitial nephritis. *Br Med J.* 1979;1:524.
252. Warren GV, Korbet SM, Schwartz MM, et al. Minimal change glomerulopathy associated with nonsteroidal anti-inflammatory drugs. *Am J Kidney Dis.* 1989;13:127-130.
253. Weaver VM, Jaar BG, Schwartz BS, et al. Associations among lead dose biomarkers, uric acid, and renal function in Korean lead workers. *Environ Health Perspect.* 2005;113:36-42.
254. Wedeen RP, Batuman V. Tubulo-interstitial nephritis induced by heavy metals and metabolic disturbances. *Contemp Issues Nephrol.* 1983;10:211-241.
255. Wetherill SF, Guarine MJ, Cox RW. Acute renal failure associated with barium chloride poisoning. *Ann Intern Med.* 1981;95:187-188.
256. Wilson M, Brown DJ, Brown RW, et al. Renal failure from alpha-methyldopa therapy. *Aust N Z J Med.* 1974;4:415-416.
257. Willson RA. Nephrotoxicity of interferon alfa-ribavirin therapy for chronic hepatitis C. *J Clin Gastroenterol.* 2002;35:89-92.
258. Woolf AD, Ebert TH. Toxicity after self-poisoning by ingestion of potassium chloroplatinite. *J Toxicol Clin Toxicol.* 1991;29:467-472.
259. Wolff E. Carbon monoxide poisoning with severe myonecrosis and acute renal failure. *Am J Emerg Med.* 1994;12:347-349.
260. Zanetta G, Maurice-Estepa L, Mousson C, et al. Foscarnet-induced crystalline glomerulonephritis with nephrotic syndrome and acute renal failure after kidney transplantation.*Transplantation.* 1999;67:1376-1378.
261. Zar T, Graeber C, Perazella MA. Recognition, treatment, and prevention of propylene glycol toxicity. *Semin Dial.* 2007;20:217-219.
262. Zar T, Yusufzai I, Sullivan A, et al. Acute kidney injury, hyperosmolality and metabolic acidosis associated with lorazepam. *Nat Clin Pract Nephrol.* 2007;3:515-520.

CHAPTER 28
GENITOURINARY PRINCIPLES

Jason Chu

The genitourinary system encompasses two major organ systems: the reproductive and the urinary systems. Successful reproduction requires interaction between two sexually mature individuals. Xenobiotic exposures to either individual can have an adverse impact on fertility, which is the successful production of children, and fecundity, which is an individual's or a couple's capacity to produce children. The role of occupational and environmental exposures in the development of infertility is difficult to define.[10,37,89,93] Well-designed and conclusive epidemiologic studies are lacking due to the following factors: laboratory tests used to evaluate fertility are relatively unreliable; clinical endpoints are unclear; xenobiotic exposure is difficult to monitor; and indicators of biologic effects are imprecise. The negative impact on fertility as an adverse effect of xenobiotics is often ignored, but the evaluation of infertility is incomplete without a thorough xenobiotics and occupational history. Differences in the toxicity of xenobiotics in individuals may be sex- and/or age-related. Xenobiotic-related, primary infertility may be the result of effects on the hypothalamic-pituitary-gonadal axis or of a direct toxic effect on the gonads.[78] Fertility is also affected by exposures that cause abnormal sexual performance. Table 28–1 lists xenobiotics associated with infertility.

Aphrodisiacs are used to heighten sexual desire and to counteract sexual dysfunction. Historically, humans have continued to search for the perfect aphrodisiac. Efficacy is variable, and toxic consequences occur commonly. Various treatments have been available for male sexual dysfunction, or erectile dysfunction.

Although many people search for a cure for impotence or infertility, others explore xenobiotics that can be used as abortifacients. Routes of administration used include oral, parenteral, and intravaginal, with an end result of pregnancy termination. Toxicity results not only in the termination of pregnancy but also from the systemic effects of the various xenobiotics.

This chapter examines these issues, as well as the impact of xenobiotics on the urinary system, specifically, urinary retention and incontinence, and abnormalities detected in urine specimens. Renal (Chap. 27), teratogenic, (Chap. 30), and carcinogenic principles are discussed elsewhere in this text.

MALE FERTILITY

Male fertility is dependent on a normal reproductive system and normal sexual function. The male reproductive system is comprised of the central nervous system (CNS) endocrine organs and the male gonads. The hypothalamus and the anterior pituitary gland form the CNS portion of the male reproductive system. Both organs begin low-level hormone secretion as early as in utero gestation. At puberty, the hypothalamus begins pulsatile secretion of gonadotropin-releasing hormone (GnRH). This stimulates the anterior pituitary gland to release follicle-stimulating hormone (FSH) and luteinizing hormone (LH) in a pulsatile fashion. The hormones exert their effects on the male target organs, inducing spermatogenesis and secondary body sexual characteristics (Fig. 28–1).

Disruption of normal function at any part of the system affects fertility. There are a number of xenobiotics that can adversely affect the male reproductive system and sexual function.

SPERMATOGENESIS

Central to the male reproductive system is the process of spermatogenesis, which occurs in the testes. The bulk of the testes consist of seminiferous tubules with germinal spermatogonia and Sertoli cells. The remainder of the gonadal tissue is interstitium with blood vessels, lymphatics, supporting cells, and Leydig cells. Spermatogenesis begins with the maturation and differentiation of the germinal spermatogonia. The process is controlled by the secretion of gonadotropin-releasing hormone (GnRH) from the hypothalamus, which stimulates the pituitary to release follicle-stimulating hormone (FSH) and luteinizing hormone (LH). Follicle-stimulating hormone stimulates the development of Sertoli cells in the testes, which are responsible for the maturation of spermatids to spermatozoa. Luteinizing hormone promotes production of testosterone by Leydig cells. Testosterone concentrations must be maintained to ensure the formation of spermatids.[19] Both FSH and testosterone are required for initiation of spermatogenesis, but testosterone alone is sufficient to maintain the process.

Testicular Xenobiotics Xenobiotics can affect any part of the male reproductive tract, but, invariably, the end result is decreased sperm production defined as oligospermia, or absent sperm production, azoospermia. In contrast to oogenesis in women, spermatogenesis is an ongoing process throughout life but can be inhibited by decreases in FSH and/or LH or Sertoli cell toxicity. Spermatogenic capacity is evaluated by semen analysis, including sperm count, motility, sperm morphology, and penetrating ability. Normal sperm count is greater than 40 million sperm/mL semen, and a count less than 20 million/mL is indicative of infertility.[19] Decreased motility (asthenospermia) less than 40% of normal or abnormal morphology (teratospermia) of greater than 40% of the total number of sperm also indicates infertility.[19,101]

Physiology of Erection The penis is composed of two corpus cavernosa and a central corpus spongiosum. The internal pudendal arteries supply blood to the penis via four branches. Blood outflow is via multiple emissary veins draining into the dorsal vein of the penis and plexus of Santorini. Within the penis, the corpora cavernosa share vascular supply and drainage due to extensive arteriolar, arteriovenous, and sinusoidal anastomoses.[120] When penile blood flow is greater than 20–50 mL/min, erection occurs. Maintenance of tumescence occurs with flow rates of 12 mL/min. The tunica albuginea limits the absolute size of erection.

In the flaccid state, sympathetic efferent nerves maintain helicine resistance arteriole constriction primarily through norepinephrine induced α-adrenergic agonism. α-Adrenergic receptor agonism in the erectile tissues decreases cAMP to produce flaccidity, while α-Adrenergic antagonism can result in pathologic erection (priapism) as a consequence of parasympathetic dominance.[120] Other vasoconstrictors, such as endothelin, prostaglandin F_{2a}, and thromboxane A_2 play a role in maintaining corpus cavernosal smooth muscle tone in contraction, which results in a flaccid state.[84]

Normal penile erection is a result of both neural and vascular effects. Psychogenic neural stimulation arising from the cerebral cortex inhibits norepinephrine release from thoracolumbar sympathetic pathways, stimulates nitric oxide (NO) and acetylcholine release from sacral parasympathetic tracts, and stimulates acetylcholine release from somatic pathways. In animals, dopamine and NO play a role in erection.[84] Reflex stimulation can also occur from the sacral spinal cord. The

TABLE 28–1. Xenobiotics Associated with Infertility

Men	
Xenobiotic	**Effects**
Anabolic steroids	↓ LH, oligospermia
Androgens	↓ testosterone production
Antineoplastics	Gonadal toxicity
Cyclophosphamide	Oligospermia
Chlorambucil	Oligospermia
Methotrexate	Oligospermia
Combination chemotherapy (COP, CVP, MOPP, MVPP)	Oligospermia
Carbon disulfide	↓ FSH, ↓ LH, ↓ spermatogenesis
Cimetidine	Oligospermia
Chlordecone	Asthenospermia, oligospermia
Dibromochloropropane (DBCP)	Azoospermia, oligospermia
Diethylstilbestrol	Testicular hypoplasia
Ethanol	↓ Testosterone production, Leydig cell damage, asthenospermia, oligospermia, teratospermia
Ethylene oxide	Asthenospermia (in monkeys), oligospermia
Glycol ethers	Azoospermia, oligospermia, testicular atrophy
Ionizing radiation	↓ Spermatogenesis
Opioids	↓ LH,, ↓ testosterone
Lead	↓ Spermatogenesis, asthenospermia, teratospermia
Nitrofurantoin	↓ Spermatogenesis
Sulfasalazine	↓ Spermatogenesis
Tobacco	↓ Testosterone
Women	
Xenobiotic	**Effects**
Antineoplastics	Gonadal toxicity
Cyclophosphamide	Ovarian failure
Busulphan	Amenorrhea
Combination chemotherapy (MOPP, MVPP)	Amenorrhea
Diethylstilbestrol	Spontaneous abortions
Ethylene oxide	Spontaneous abortions
Lead	Spontaneous abortions, still births
Oral contraceptives	Affect hypothalamic-pituitary axis, end-organ resistance to hormones, amenorrhea
Thyroid hormone	↓ Ovulation

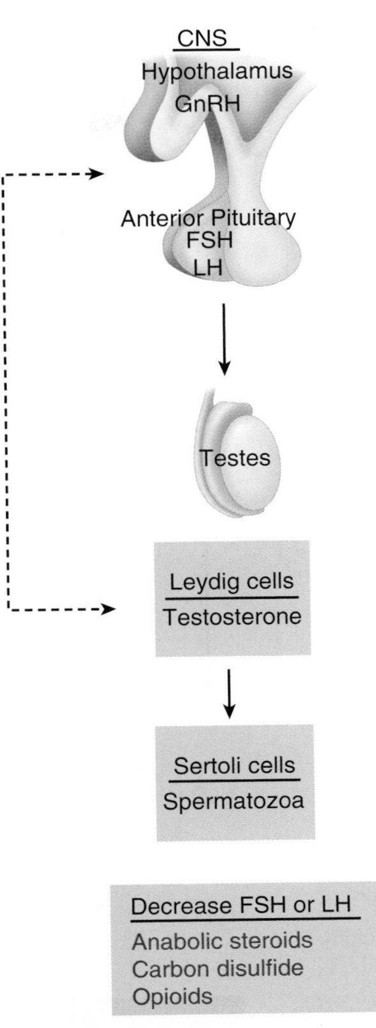

FIGURE 28–1. A schematic of the male reproductive axis and sites of xenobiotic effects. FSH = follicle stimulating hormone; GnRH = Gonadotropin releasing hormone; LH = Luteinizing hormone.

afferent limb of the reflex arc is supplied by the pudendal nerves and the efferent limb by the nervi erigentes (pelvic splanchnic nerves).

The central impulses stimulate various neurotransmitters to be released by peripheral nerves in the penis. Nonadrenergic-noncholinergic nerves and endothelial cells produce NO, which is the principal neurotransmitter mediating erection. Nitric oxide activates guanylate cyclase conversion of guanosine triphosphate (GTP) to cyclic guanosine monophosphate (cGMP). Increasing concentrations of cGMP act as a second messenger, mediating arteriolar and trabecular smooth-muscle relaxation to enable increased cavernosal blood flow and penile erection.[84] Both cGMP and cyclic adenosine

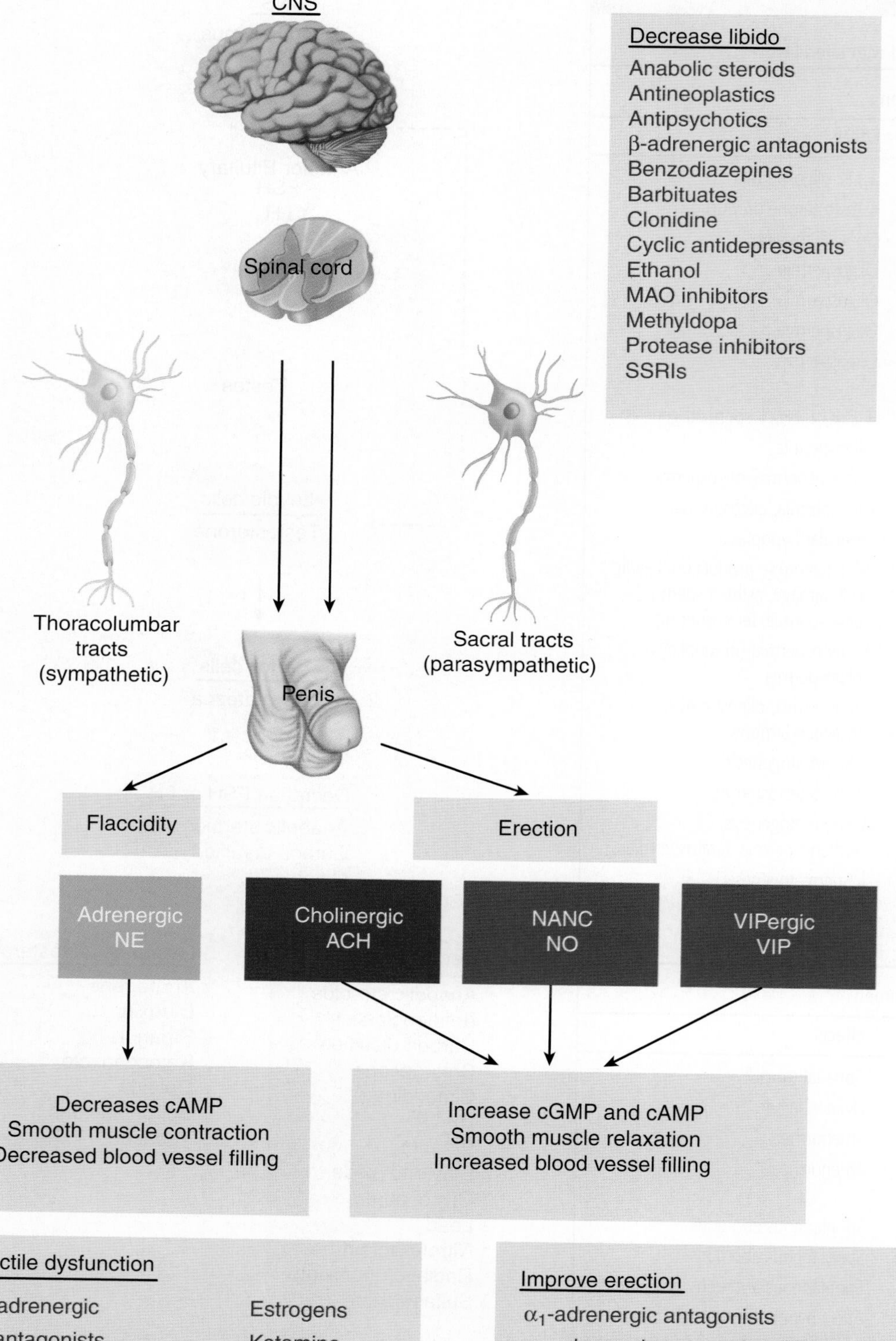

FIGURE 28–2. A schematic of the erection and xenobiotics that cause sexual dysfunction. NE = norepinephrine; ACH = acetylcholine; NANC = nonadrenergic-noncholinergic; NO = nitric oxide; VIP = vasoactive intestinal peptide.

monophosphate (cAMP) pathways mediate smooth-muscle relaxation. Cholinergic nerves release acetylcholine, which stimulates endothelial cells via M_3 receptors to produce NO and prostaglandin E_2 (PGE). Prostaglandin E_2 and nerves containing vasoactive intestinal peptide (VIP) and calcitonin gene-related peptide (CGRP) increase cellular cAMP to potentiate smooth-muscle relaxation.

Penile corpus cavernosal smooth muscle relaxation allows increased blood flow into the corpus cavernosal sinusoids. Expansion of the sinusoids compresses the venous outflow and enables penile erection (Fig. 28–2).

SEXUAL DYSFUNCTION

Sexual dysfunction can result from decreased libido (sexual desire), impotence, diminished ejaculation, and erectile dysfunction. Dopamine, norepinephrine, oxytocin, and adrenocorticotrophic hormone (ACTH) are central neurotransmitters and hormones which facilitate sexual function. Serotonin, prolactin, endogenous opioids and GABA inhibit sexual function centrally.[6] Libido can be decreased by xenobiotics that block central dopaminergic or adrenergic pathways or by xenobiotics that increase serotonin or prolactin levels. Conversely, xenobiotics that increase dopamine can improve sexual function. Sexual dysfunction can also be caused by xenobiotics that decrease testosterone production and by xenobiotics that produce dysphoria. Xenobiotics that affect spinal reflexes can cause diminished ejaculation and erectile dysfunction.[118]

Approximately 30 million men in the United States suffer from erectile dysfunction, with an increased prevalence in older men.[53] Erectile dysfunction is defined as the inability to achieve and/or maintain an erection for a sufficiently long period of time to permit satisfactory sexual intercourse[3] and is divided into the following classifications: psychogenic, vasculogenic, neurologic, endocrinologic, and xenobiotic-induced. Xenobiotic-induced erectile dysfunction is associated with the following categories of xenobiotics: antidepressants, antipsychotics, centrally and peripherally-acting antihypertensives, CNS depressants, anticholinergics, exogenous hormones, antibiotics, and antineoplastics.[74,100,118] Treatment of this disorder is varied and includes vacuum-constriction devices, penile prostheses, vascular surgery, and medications (intracavernosal, transdermal, and oral agents).

Antihypertensives Erectile dysfunction is reported as an adverse effect with all antihypertensives and may be caused, in part, by a decrease in hypogastric artery pressure, which impairs blood flow to the pelvis.[117] Methyldopa and clonidine both are centrally acting α_2-adrenergic agonists that inhibit sympathetic outflow from the brain. Sexual dysfunction is reported in 26% of patients receiving methyldopa and in 24% of patients receiving clonidine.[14,87] Erectile dysfunction associated with thiazide diuretics may be related to decreased vascular resistance, diverting blood from the penis.[20] Spironolactone acts as an antiandrogen by inhibiting the binding of dihydrotestosterone to its receptors. Impotence related to use of β-adrenergic antagonists, is well documented[1,57,114] and may be caused by unopposed α-mediated vasoconstriction resulting in reduced penile blood flow.

Ethanol Ethanol is directly toxic to Leydig cells. Chronic alcohol abuse causes decreased libido, erectile dysfunction, and is associated with testicular atrophy. In alcoholics liver disease contributes to sexual dysfunction resulting from decreased testosterone and increased estrogen production. Alcoholics can have autonomic neuropathies affecting penile nerves and subsequent erection. Heavy drinkers suffer more from erectile dysfunction than episodic drinkers.[116]

Antipsychotics Individuals who take antipsychotics therapeutically have varying degrees of sexual dysfunction related to their underlying disease and their medications. All psychoactive medications are associated with sexual dysfunction to some degree. Monoamine oxidase inhibitors (MAOIs), cyclic antidepressants (CAs), antipsychotics, and selective serotonin reuptake inhibitors (SSRIs) are associated with decreased libido and erectile dysfunction in men.[31] Thioridazine is associated with significantly lower LH and testosterone levels in men in comparison with other antipsychotics.[19] Antidepressants such as bupropion, nefazodone, mirtazapine, and duloxetine have lower incidences of sexual dysfunction in comparison with other antidepressants.[102] Table 28–2 lists xenobiotics associated with sexual dysfunction.

TABLE 28–2. Xenobiotics Associated with Sexual Dysfunction (Particularly Diminished Libido and Impotence)

α_1-Adrenergic antagonists	Diuretics
α_2-Adrenergic agonists	Ethanol
β-Adrenergic antagonists*	Lead
Anabolic Steroids	Lithium
Anticholinergics*	Methyldopa
Anticonvulsants	Monamine oxidase inhibitors*
Antiestrogens	Opioids
Benzodiazepines	Oral contraceptives
Calcium channel blockers	Phenothiazines
Cimetidine	Selective serotonin reuptake inhibitors
Clonidine	Spironolactone
Cyclic Antidepressants	

*Associated with erectile dysfunction

XENOBIOTICS USED IN THE TREATMENT OF ERECTILE DYSFUNCTION

Intracavernosal Agents. The three most commonly used intracavernosal agents used for erectile dysfunction are papaverine, prostaglandin E_1, and phentolamine. Papaverine is a benzylisoquinoline alkaloid derived from the poppy plant *Papaver somniferum*. It exerts its effects through nonselective inhibition of phosphodiesterase, leading to increased cAMP and cGMP levels and subsequent cavernosal vasodilation. Papaverine was used for the treatment of cardiac and cerebral ischemia but had limited efficacy. Presently, it is used as intracavernosal therapy for erectile dysfunction alone or in conjunction with phentolamine. Systemic side effects include dizziness, nausea, vomiting, hepatotoxicity, lactic acidosis with oral administration, and cardiac dysrhythmias with intravenous use. Intracavernosal administration is associated with penile fibrosis which is usually dose-related phenomenon, although fibrosis can also occur with limited use.[33] More concerning is the development of priapism with papaverine use.

Prostaglandin E_1 (Alprostadil) is a nonspecific agonist of prostaglandin receptors resulting in increased concentrations of intracavernosal cAMP, cavernosal smooth muscle relaxation and penile erection. It is effective via intracavernosal administration as a single agent. Other preparations include an intraurethral preparation, which is less effective, and a topical gel formulation.[54] Penile fibrosis can occur but the incidence is lower compared to papaverine. Other adverse effects include penile pain, secondary to its effects as a nonspecific prostaglandin receptor agonist, and priapism.

Phentolamine is a competitive α-adrenergic antagonist at α_1 and α_2 receptors. It effects erection by inhibiting the normal resting adrenergic tone in cavernosal smooth muscle, thus allowing increased arterial blood flow and erection. Intracavernosal use can cause systemic hypotension, reflex tachycardia, nasal congestion, and gastrointestinal upset. Penile fibrosis and priapism are also reported.

Oral Agents Since the development of the phosphodiesterase 5 inhibitors, oral therapy has replaced intracavernosal injections as the mainstay for treatment of erectile dysfunction. Sildenafil was the first agent developed, followed by vardenafil and tadalafil. These medications are pharmacodynamically similar but differ in their pharmacokinetics. Phosphodiesterase 5 inhibitors increase NO-induced cGMP concentrations by preventing phosphodiesterase breakdown of cGMP, enhancing NO-induced vasodilation to promote penile vascular relaxation and erection.[18]

After oral administration, sildenafil is rapidly absorbed with a bioavailability of 40% and a median peak serum concentration of 60 minutes. Its mean volume of distribution is 105 L, and its elimination half-life is 3 to 5 hours. Metabolism is primarily by the CYP3A4 pathway with some minor metabolic activity via the CYP2C9 pathway. Serum concentrations of sildenafil are increased in patients older than 65 years as well as those with hepatic dysfunction, severe renal dysfunction (creatinine clearance <30 mL/min), and when used with CYP3A4 inhibitors (macrolide antibiotics, cimetidine, antifungal agents, protease inhibitors).[26]

Vardenafil has more selective inhibition of phosphodiesterase 5 enzymes and less inhibition of phosphodiesterase 6 enzymes compared to sildenafil. After oral administration, it has a 14% bioavailability, a volume of distribution of 208 L, a median peak serum concentration of 60 minutes and an elimination half-life of 4 to 5 hours. The CYP3A4 pathway is the primary hepatic metabolic pathway with minor contributions from CYP3A5 and CYP2C9 enzymes.[13,15] The primary metabolite, M1, has phosphodiesterase 5 inhibitory activity but is four times less potent than vardenafil.[15] As with sildenafil, vardenafil concentrations are increased in patients older than 65 years, and those with hepatic dysfunction, severe renal dysfunction (creatinine clearance <30 mL/min), and when used with CYP3A4 inhibitors (macrolide antibiotics, cimetidine, antifungal agents, protease inhibitors).[62]

Tadalafil has a median peak serum concentration of 2 hours and a mean elimination half-life of 17.5 hours. It is predominantly metabolized by CYP3A4 enzymes. Unlike sildenafil and vardenafil, serum concentrations are not affected by age, hepatic dysfunction, renal dysfunction or CYP3A4 inhibitors. However, the FDA has issued recommendations to decrease the dosage of all phosphodiesterase 5 inhibitors if used in conjunction with atazanavir.[2]

The most common adverse effects of the phosphodiesterase 5 inhibitors are headache, flushing, dyspepsia, and rhinitis, which are related to phosphodiesterase 5 inhibitory effects on extracavernosal tissue.[53] Blurred vision, increased light perception and transient blue-green tinged vision are also reported and are related to the weak phosphodiesterase 6 inhibition of sildenafil in the retina.[53] Vardenafil and tadalafil are associated with infrequent abnormal vision, including blurred and abnormal color vision.[55]

More serious adverse effects of sildenafil include myocardial infarction, when used alone or with nitrates, subaortic obstruction, stroke, transient ischemic attack, priapism, and anterior optic ischemia.[9,41,61,103,106] Tadalafil use is associated with anterior ischemic optic neuropathy.[16]

When taken alone, the vasodilatory effects of phosphodiesterase 5 inhibitors cause a modest decrease in systemic blood pressure. However, because of their mechanism of action via cGMP inhibition and vascular vasodilation, phosphodiesterase 5 inhibitors can have synergistic interactions with the vasodilatory effects of nitrates resulting in profound hypotension.[18,63] A study of healthy male volunteers taking sildenafil demonstrated significantly less tolerance to a glyceryl trinitrate infusion in comparison with placebo.[115] Because of this interaction, patients with acute myocardial ischemic syndromes using phosphodiesterase 5 inhibitors should avoid taking organic nitrates as well.[26] α_1-Adrenergic antagonists are also contraindicated with concomitant phosphodiesterase 5 inhibitor use because of increased hypotensive effects.[63] Hypotension occurred in patients using vardenafil with terazosin and tamsulosin,[63] and in patients using tadalafil with doxazosin.[64] However, patients using tadalafil with tamsulosin did not develop hypotension.[64]

Yohimbine, an indole alkylamine alkaloid from the West African yohimbe tree (*Corynanthe yohimbe*), is an α_2-adrenergic antagonist with cholinergic activity used to treat erectile dysfunction and postural hypotension associated with anticholinergic drugs.[71] It is structurally similar to reserpine. Other names for yohimbine include Aphrodyne, corynine, hydroaergotocin, quebrachine, and the street name "yo-yo."[72] Its use in the treatment of impotence is based on the theory that erection is linked to cholinergic stimulation and α_2 antagonism, resulting in an increase inflow and decrease outflow of blood to the penis. Although the agent Aphrodex, which contained 5 mg yohimbine, 5 mg methyltestosterone, and 5 mg strychnine, improved performance in males with erectile failure,[75] its distribution was halted in 1973 because of safety concerns.[98]

Yohimbine can be obtained by prescription, but extracts are also available in "health food" products marketed as "vitalizing agents for men and women."[35] Yohimbine can also be extracted from the Rauwolfia root.[46] The "therapeutic" dose is 2 to 6 mg 3 times daily. The drug is rapidly absorbed, with peak serum concentrations occurring in 45 to 60 minutes. The half-life is 36 minutes, and clearance is by hepatic metabolism without renal excretion.[90] Maximum pharmacologic effects occur 1 to 2 hours after ingestion and effects persist for 3 to 4 hours.[72]

Because the erectile process involves various neurotransmitters, a single agent would be expected to only have a partial effect. In a double-blind study of 100 males with erectile failure treated with 18 mg/d of yohimbine, 42.6% of the treatment group and 27.6% of the placebo group reported some improvement in erectile function, which was not statistically significant.[83] Another study that compared a higher dose of yohimbine and placebo in 82 elderly males showed a statistically significant improvement with treatment.[108]

Adverse effects can occur with relatively low doses of yohimbine. Tachycardia, hypertension, mydriasis, diaphoresis, lacrimation, salivation, nausea, vomiting, and flushing can occur following intravenous administration.[58] Ten milligrams of yohimbine can elicit manic symptoms in patients with bipolar disorder,[95] and 15 mg/d is associated with bronchospasm[66] and a lupuslike syndrome.[99] A 16-year-old woman who ingested 250 mg of yohimbine powder, purchased for its purported aphrodisiac activity, developed an acute dissociative reaction with weakness, paresthesias, headache, nausea, palpitations, and chest pain. She also developed tachycardia, tachypnea, diaphoresis, tremors, and a rash. Her symptoms resolved after 36 hours without treatment.[72] Another report describes a 62-year-old man who ingested 200 mg of yohimbine and developed tachycardia, hypertension, and a brief period of anxiety that resolved without treatment.[46] Symptomatic patients who ingest yohimbine should receive activated charcoal and should be observed until asymptomatic. Clonidine has been recommended for treatment of yohimbine's central and peripheral effects.[72] β-Adrenergic antagonists may attenuate some of the peripheral toxicity, but may also result in unopposed α_1-adrenergic activity and worsening of hypertension, and should be avoided. Benzodiazepine administration may be sufficient for the treatment of agitation and sympathomimetic effects related to yohimbine.

Sublingual apomorphine effects erection through activation of central dopaminergic pathways; most likely D_2 receptors in the paraventricular nucleus of the hypothalamus.[56] It reaches maximum serum concentrations within 40 to 60 minutes after sublingual administration and is metabolized hepatically with a half-life of 2 to 3 hours.[8] Common adverse effects are nausea, vomiting, headache, dizziness and syncope. Unlike the phosphodiesterase 5 inhibitors, apomorphine is not associated with hypotension when used with antihypertensive, such as nitrates.

Priapism Priapism is defined as prolonged involuntary erection, which is painful, unassociated with sexual stimulation, and can result in impotence. It most commonly occurs during the third and fourth decades of life and is caused by inflow of blood to the penis in excess of outflow. The corpora cavernosa become firm and the corpus spongiosum flaccid. Intracavernosal pressures can exceed arterial systolic pressure, resulting in cell death. Priapism can occur from an imbalance in neural stimuli, interference with venous outflow, or as a result of xenobiotic-induced inhibition of penile detumescence. α-Adrenergic antagonists prevent constriction of blood vessels supplying erectile tissue, resulting in priapism.[120] One out of 10,000 patients taking trazodone develop priapism, which is thought to be related to its α-adrenergic antagonist effects.[98] A common cause of priapism is iatrogenic, resulting from the injection of papaverine for the treatment of impotence.[109] Other xenobiotics associated with xenobiotic-induced priapism include prazosin, labetalol, guanethidine, hydralazine, phenothiazines, androgens, anticoagulants, ethanol, marijuana, and cantharidin[60,120] (Table 28–3).

The goal in the treatment of priapism is detumescence with retention of potency. Initial therapy includes sedation with benzodiazepines, analgesia with opioids, and ice packs, and early urologic consultation. Oral terbutaline (5–10 mg) was effective for prostaglandin E_1-induced priapism and may be effective for other xenobiotic-induced priapism.[73,96] Aspiration and normal saline irrigation of the corpora cavernosa may be effective. If priapism occurs secondary to α_1-adrenergic antagonism, an α_1-adrenergic agonist (0.02 mg norepinephrine or 0.2 mg phenylephrine) diluted with normal saline to 10 mL volume can be instilled by placing a 19-gauge butterfly needle into the corpora cavernosa. If the above measures fail, operative venous shunt placement may be required.[109,120]

TABLE 28–3. Xenobiotics Associated with Priapism

Androgens	**Antipsychotics**
Anticoagulants	Butyrophenones
Dalteparin	Clozapine
Heparin	Neuroleptics
Warfarin	Olanzapine
Antidepressants	Quetiapine
Buproprion	Risperidone
Phenelzine	Ziprasidone
SSRIs	**Cantharidin**
Trazodone	**Cocaine**
Antihypertensives	**Diazepam**
α Adrenergic antagonists	**Papaverine**
Guanethidine	**Phosphodiesterase 5 inhibitors**
Hydralazine	
Labetalol	
Phentolamine	

FEMALE FERTILITY

The female reproductive system consists of the female gonadal organs and the respective hormonal system (Fig. 28–3). Fertility encompasses the reproductive system, the process of oocyte fertilization and gestation. Female infertility may result from changes in hormone concentrations, direct toxicity to the ovum, interference with the transport of the ovum, or inhibition of implantation of the ovum in the uterus. Women usually notice reproductive abnormalities more quickly than men, because menses may be affected; although infertility may occur while normal menses persists. Evaluation of female fertility is more difficult because of the complexity of the systems involved and the inaccessibility of the female germ cell, but it is feasible and involves investigations of the anatomy and hormonal concentrations. The following is a discussion of oogenesis, agents that disrupt oogenesis, and xenobiotics that affect early embryo gestation.

OOGENESIS

In contrast to men, women have a limited number of reproductive cells (ovarian follicles). Follicles are most numerous while the fetus is in utero, with the number decreasing to approximately 2 million at birth. By the time a woman reaches puberty, the majority of follicles have degenerated, leaving 300,000 to 400,000 ova, of which approximately 400 will eventually produce mature ova during a woman's reproductive years. In contrast, men produce millions of spermatozoa each day. The process of oogenesis requires secretion of GnRH from the hypothalamus, resulting in production of LH and FSH from the pituitary, which are required for ovarian follicle maturation.[19] FSH induces early maturation by stimulating granulosa and thecal cell proliferation and estrogen

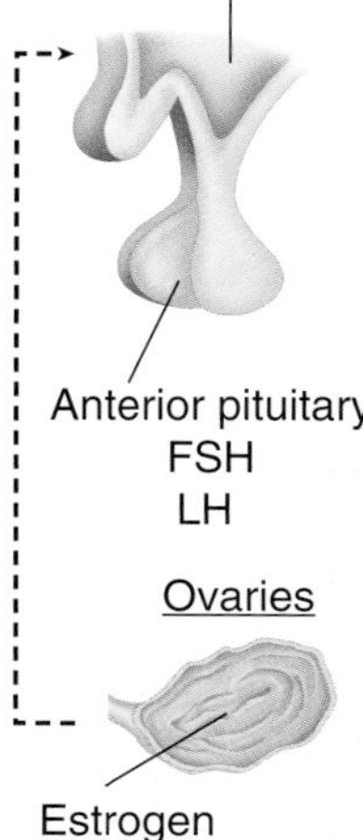
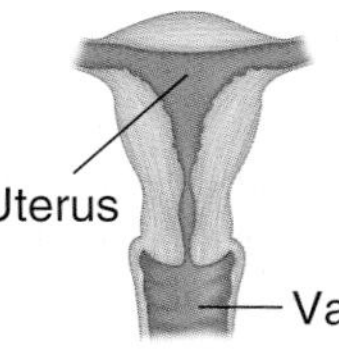

FIGURE 28–3. A schematic of female reproductive axis and sites of xenobiotic action. FSH = follicle stimulating hormone; GnRH = gonadotropin releasing hormone; LH = Luteinizing hormone.

TABLE 28–4. Xenobiotics Used as Abortifacients

Source	Common Name	Xenobiotic	Miscellaneous/Toxicity
		Inhibit implantation	
Abrus precatorius	Jequirity pea	Abrin	Cytotoxic toxalbumin
Acanthospermum hispidum	Bristly starbur	*Acanthospermum hispidum*	Preimplantation effects
Aristolochia sp.	Birthwort	Aristolochic acid	Nephrotoxicity
Momordica charantia	Bitter melon	α-Momorcharin	Similar to trichosanthin
Cajanus cajan	Pigeon pea	*Cajanus cajan*	Preimplantation effects
Lagenaria breviflora	Wild colocynth	*Lagenaria breviflora*	Preimplantation effects
–	–	Mifepristone	Nausea, vomiting, abdominal pain, vaginal bleeding
Juniperus sabina	Savin	Oil of savin	Hepatotoxicity in mice
Ruta graveolens	Rue	Chalepesin	Hepatotoxicity, nephrotoxicity, photodermatitis
		Abortive	
Ranunculus spp.	Buttercup	Devil's claw	Similar to pennyroyal oil
Angelica sinesis	Dong quai	Furanocoumarin, phytoestrogen	Anticoagulant effects, gynecomastia, photodermatitis
Daphne genkwa	Lilac daphne	Yuanhuacine	
–	–	Lysol disinfectant	Death after intrauterine administration
Mentha pulegium	Pennyroyal	Pulegone	Hepatotoxicity
–	–	Methotrexate	Cytotoxic effects
–	–	Mifepristone	Nausea, vomiting, abdominal pain, vaginal bleeding
Momordica charantia	Bitter melon	α-momorcharin	Similar to trichosanthin
Moringa oleifera	Horseradish tree	*Moringa oleifera*	100% abortifacient in rats
Podophyllum peltatum	Mayapple	Podophyllin	Podophyllum toxicity
Trichosanthes kirilowii	Snake gourd	Tricosanthin (compound Q)	Inhibits protein synthesis, ↓HCG, ↓progesterone
		Oxytocic	
Aristolochia sp.	Birthwort	Aristolochic acid	Nephrotoxicity
Caulophyllum thalictroides	Blue cohosh	Methylcytisine	Toxicity similar to nicotine
Cimicifuga racemosa	Black cohosh	unknown	Nausea, vomiting, headache, rare hepatotoxicity
Cinchona spp.	Quinine bark	Quinine	Cinchonism
Claviceps purpurea	Ergot	Ergotamines	Vasospasm
Lagenaria breviflora Robert	Wild colocynth	*Lagenaria breviflora* Robert	Antiimplantation, oxytocic
Misoprostol		Prostaglandin E analogue	Marketed as Cytotec for gastric ulcers and arthrotec

production. LH is required for ovulation and for the formation of the corpus luteum. The corpus luteum continues estrogen production and produces progesterone, which stimulates the uterus to develop an endometrium receptive to any fertilized ovum. Successful ovulation requires not only hormone secretion but also appropriate cyclic secretion.

FEMALE SEXUAL DYSFUNCTION

The National Health and Social Life Survey found that 43% of women in the United States (in comparison with 31% of men) reported having sexual dysfunction.[67] In 1999, a consensus panel of the American Foundation for Urologic Disease revised the classification of female sexual dysfunction into the following four categories: a) sexual desire disorders, which include hypoactive sexual desire disorder and sexual aversion disorder; b) sexual arousal disorder; c) orgasmic disorder; and d) sexual pain disorders, which include dyspareunia, vaginismus, and noncoital sexual pain disorder.[11] The organic etiologies of female sexual dysfunction parallel those of male sexual and erectile dysfunction: vasculogenic, neurogenic, muscuologenic, psychogenic, endocrinologic, and xenobiotic-induced causes. The medications implicated in female sexual dysfunction are similar to the above-mentioned agents that decrease female fertility with antihypertensives, antidepressants and antipsychotics as the most frequent causes.[42]

Treatments for xenobiotic-induced female sexual dysfunction include decreasing medication dosages, switching to alternate medications with less adverse effects on sexual function (ie, bupropion and nefazodone), temporary cessation of the medication (drug holiday), or adding another medication to stimulate sexual function. Bupropion alone was as effective as fluoxetine for the treatment of depression but with less sexual dysfunction, [32] and when used in conjunction with SSRIs, bupropion improved sexual function compared to SSRIs alone.[30] Sildenafil was successful for treating spinal cord-induced[105] and antidepressant-induced sexual dysfunction[88] whereas larger trials had mixed results with sildenafil for sexual arousal disorder.[12,22] Sublingual apomorphine improved sexual function in women with hypoactive sexual disorder.[21]

The majority of medical therapy for female sexual dysfunction is centered on hormonal agents; both estrogen and androgen supplementation. Estrogen replacement therapy is available in oral, dermal, vaginal ring, and topical cream formulations alone or in combination with progesterone.[113] Estrogen therapy is associated with a higher incidence of coronary disease, breast cancer, stroke, and venous thromboembolism. Androgen therapy includes testosterone, which is available in oral, dermal and topical preparations, and dehydroepiandrosterone.[4] Adverse effects are weight gain, increased cholesterol, and androgenization.

Abortifacients An abortifacient is defined as a xenobiotic that affects early embryonic gestation to induce abortion. Xenobiotics may act by flushing the zygote from the fallopian tube, blocking the uterine horn, inhibiting implantation, inducing fetal resorption, or by producing oxytocin like activity that results in uterine irritation and contraction. Abortifacients may also indirectly affect pregnancy by altering hormonal concentrations through placental inhibition of HCG or progesterone production or through interference with progesterone receptors.

The toxic effects of abortifacients are varied. Many produce gastrointestinal symptoms such as abdominal pain, nausea, and vomiting. Abdominal pain may be related to the oxytocic effects of the xenobiotic (eg, misoprostol and mifepristone) on the uterus, cytotoxic effects of the xenobiotic (eg, methotrexate) on the gastrointestinal lining leading to stomatitis and ulcers, or hepatoxicity (eg, pennyroyal).[27] Abortifacients that inhibit implantation or have abortive effects can have severe vaginal bleeding (eg, mifepristone). Other toxic effects are not necessarily related to their abortive mechanisms but due to the specific xenobiotic. Plant derived abortifacients can cause nephrotoxicity (eg, aristolochia), photosensitivity (eg, dong quai), seizures (eg, blue cohosh), or cardiac dysrhythmias (eg, quinine).[86] Congenital abnormalities (scalp and skull defects, cranial nerve palsies, limb defects such as talipes equinovarus) are also reported with misoprostol use that did not terminate pregnancy[28] (Table 28–4).

In a US poison center study, 5 of 43 pregnant women who intentionally overdosed used known abortifacients, including quinine, misoprostol, methylergonovine, and oral contraceptives. Four of these patients developed vaginal bleeding and cramping, but no short-term (1–3 days) fetal demise was reported.[94] The use of abortifacients is more common in underdeveloped countries and in people without access to safer methods for termination or prevention of pregnancy.

TOXICITY OF APHRODISIACS

Aphrodisiacs heighten sexual desire, pleasure, and/or performance and include xenobiotics from the plant, animal, and mineral kingdoms.[34] The search for an effective aphrodisiac has continued for thousands of years. Ancient fertility cults used *Datura,* belladonna, and henbane as aphrodisiacs. Yohimbine has been used by African cultures to enhance sexual prowess, and mandrake was used in medieval Europe. Other xenobiotics recommended include oysters, vitamin E, and ginseng. Because there are no measurable objective parameters, research in this area is lacking. Most published studies evaluating aphrodisiacs have been conducted in male rodents, and little information is available in humans. Toxicity can result from the aphrodisiac or adulterants[39] (Table 28–5).

Dopamine, NO, oxytocin, and ACTH facilitate sexual behavior. Dopamine stimulates the forebrain and midbrain and leads to an increase in sexual response and arousal. In animals, dopamine agonists, such as apomorphine and quinpirole, have proerectile effects through stimulation of dopamine pathways, increasing NO in the paraventricular nucleus in the hypothalamus, and releasing oxytocin.[84] Other preparations tested for the treatment of impotence include bromocriptine,[5,17] glyceryl trinitrate,[85] zinc,[7] oxytocin,[70] and LH.[69] Endogenous opioids, GABA, and norepinephrine are associated with decreased sexual behavior. Serotonin is generally inhibitory to sexual function but the effects are dependent on the receptor subclass. $5\text{-}HT_{1A}$ receptor stimulation inhibits erection but facilitates ejaculation in rats, whereas $5\text{-}HT_{2C}$ receptors facilitate male sexual behavior.[84] Various serotonergic drugs, including trazodone, nefazodone, bupropion, and clomipramine, are reported to improve sexual dysfunction.[98,119]

TABLE 28–5. Xenobiotics Used as Aphrodisiacs

Xenobiotic	Toxicity
Oral	
Cantharidin	Vesicant actions–GI mucositis & hemorrhage, hematuria
Cathinone (hagigot)	Hypertension, tachycardia
Dapsone	Methemoglobinemia, hemolysis
Ginseng	Ginseng abuse syndrome, vaginal bleeding
Lead	Anemia, GI upset, abdominal pain
Nutmeg (myristicin)	Hallucinogen, GI upset
Tribulus terrestris (Puncturevine)	Gynecomastia
Yohimbine	Paresthesias
Topical	
Cantharidin	Vesicant actions–GI mucositis & hemorrhage, hematuria
Bufotoxin	Cardioactive steroid
Inhalation	
Alkyl nitrites (amyl, butyl, isobutyl nitrites)	Hemolytic anemia, methemoglobinemia

URINARY SYSTEM

The urinary system is composed of the kidneys, ureters, bladder, and urethra. Many xenobiotics are concentrated by the kidneys and eliminated in the urine. The following discusses the effect of xenobiotics on the bladder and urine (Chapter 27).

Bladder Anatomy and Physiology The bladder is a hollow, muscular reservoir composed of two parts— the body and the neck—and normally stores up to 350 to 450 mL of urine in adults. A smooth muscle, the detrusor muscle, makes up the bulk of the body and contracts during urination. Urine from the ureters enters the bladder at the uppermost part of the trigone, an area in the posterior wall of the bladder, and leaves via the neck and the posterior urethra. Surrounding the neck and posterior urethra is smooth muscle interlaced with elastic tissue to form the internal sphincter. Sympathetic innervation from the lumbar

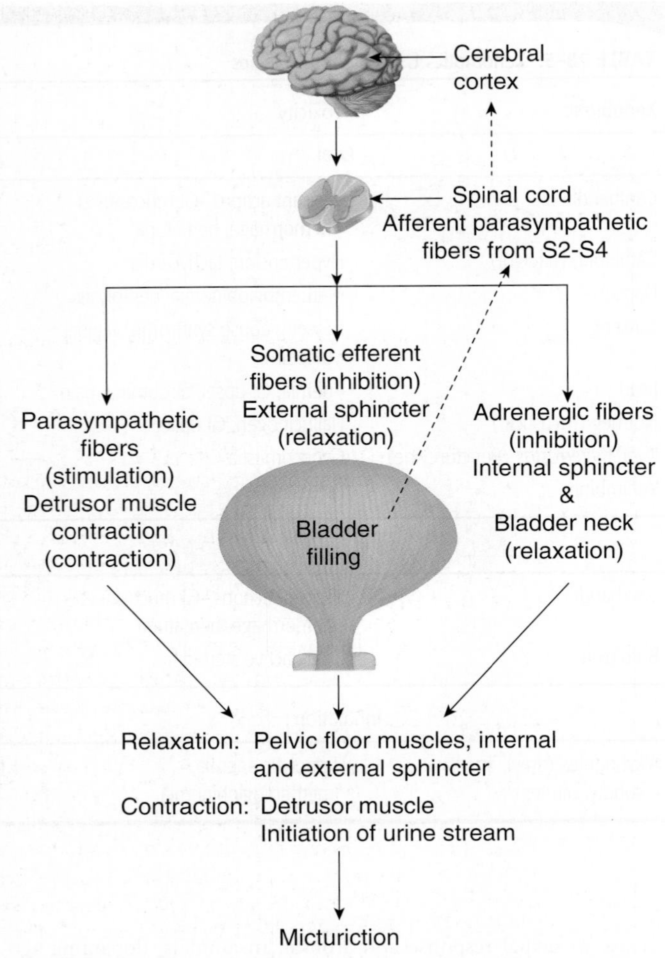

FIGURE 28–4. A schematic description of the physiology of micturition. (The dotted lines show efferent pathway.)

spinal cord to the internal sphincter maintains smooth muscle contraction. Distal to the internal sphincter is an area with voluntary skeletal muscle that forms the external sphincter and is innervated by somatic pudendal nerves.

The nerve supply and neurophysiology of urination involves interplay between lumbar sympathetic nerves, sacral parasympathetic nerves and sacral somatic nerves. Figure 28–4 illustrates the physiology of micturition. With bladder filling, norepinephrine is released by sympathetic postganglionic fibers. α-adrenergic receptors predominate in the internal sphincter and the bladder neck while β-adrenergic receptors supply the detrusor wall of the bladder. Stimulation of α-adrenergic receptors results in internal sphincter contraction and increased bladder outlet resistance, and stimulation of β-adrenergic receptors leads to detrusor relaxation and bladder filling.[111] In micturition, parasympathetic pre- and post-ganglionic fibers release acetylcholine to M_2 and M_3 muscarinic receptors in the detrusor muscle. Stimulation of M_3 receptors is responsible for detrusor muscle contraction and bladder emptying.[25] Conversely, anticholinergics prevent bladder emptying and result in urinary retention.[23,24,29,45,50,82]

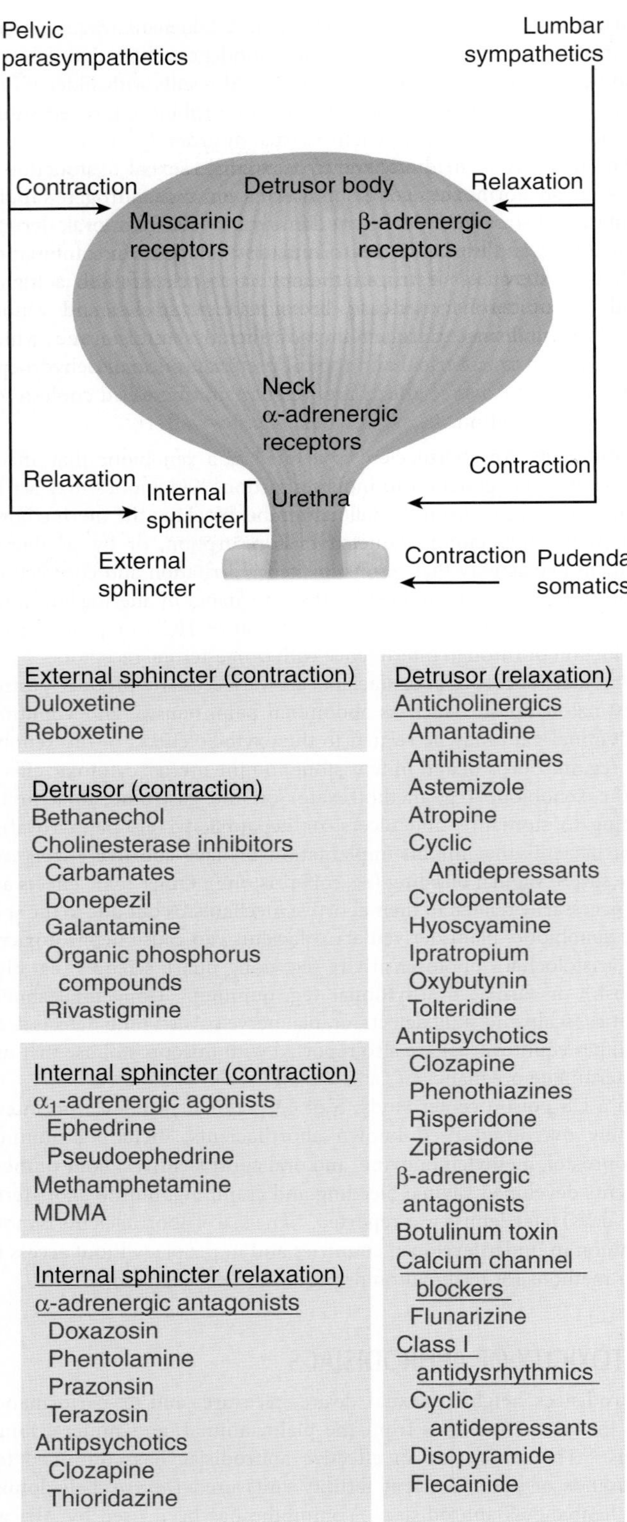

FIGURE 28–5. A graphic of the bladder and sites of xenobiotic effects.

Urinary Abnormalities Urinary incontinence is common in the elderly. As age increases, bladder size decreases, resulting in more frequent emptying. Early detrusor contraction, even with low bladder volumes, occurs more commonly in the elderly causing a sense of urgency. There are many etiologies for urinary incontinence, including various xenobiotic exposures (Fig. 28–5). General or regional anesthesia, bladder instrumentation, and medications may produce bladder atony leading to incontinence.[29] Functional incontinence can also result from use of any medication that causes impaired cognition or decreased mobility (sedative/hypnotics, opioids, etc).[29] Pharmacologic agents used in the treatment of urinary incontinence include anticholinergics (tolterodine, oxybutynin, trospium chloride), imipramine, botulinum toxin A, and duloxetine. Duloxetine is a serotonin and norepinephrine reuptake inhibitor that acts centrally at the sacral cord pudendal motor nucleus to stimulate urethral rhabdosphincter contraction.[38] Urinary retention can be obstructive, neurogenic, psychogenic or pharmacologic in origin. Medications associated with urinary retention include sympathomimetics, anticholinergics, antidysrhythmics (quinidine, procainamide, disopyramide), antidepressants, antipsychotics, hormonal agents (progesterone, estrogen, testosterone), and muscle relaxants.[29,45] In men older than 50 years, benign prostatic hyperplasia is the most common cause of bladder outlet obstruction, leading to decreased urinary output and urinary retention. Treatment of benign prostatic hyperplasia consists of 5α-reductase inhibitors and α-adrenergic antagonists. 5α-reductase inhibitors (finasteride, dutasteride) block the conversion of testosterone to dihydrotestosterone in order to decrease prostate volume.[79] α_1-adrenergic antagonists (doxazosin, terazosin, alfuzosin, tamsulosin) decrease urethral α-adrenergic contraction.[47] Table 28–6 lists xenobiotics associated with urinary retention and incontinence.

TABLE 28–6. Xenobiotics that Cause Urinary Retention and Incontinence

Retention	Incontinence
α_1-Adrenergic agonists	**α_1-Adrenergic antagonists**
Amantadine	**Antipsychotics**
Antihistamines	Clozapine
Anticholinergics	Chlorpromazine
Atropine	Haloperidol
Dicyclomine	Thioridazine
Hyoscyamine	**Cholinesterase inhibitors**
Oxybutynin	**Diuretics**
Tolterodine	**Naloxone** (for opiate-induced retention)
Antipsychotics	
Aripiprazole	
Phenothiazines	
Risperidone	
Quetiapine	
Benzodiazepines	
Botulinum toxin	
Calcium channel blockers	
Cyclic antidepressants	
Cyclopentolate	
NSAIDs	
Opioids	
SSRIs	
Citalopram	
Duloxetine	
Fluoxetine	
Fluvoxamine	
Reboxetine	

TABLE 28–7. Xenobiotics that Cause Crystalluria

Acyclovir	Indinavir
Ampicillin	Nitrofurantoin
Amoxicillin	Primidone
Ascorbic acid	Sulfadiazine
Ciprofloxacin	Sulfamethoxazole
Ethylene glycol	Thiabendazole
Flucytosine	Triamterene

Abnormalities in Urinalysis Abnormalities of the urinalysis are often useful in identifying xenobiotic exposures. Crystalluria is a common finding and may be normal but the presence of crystals may aid in diagnosis. Crystal formation is dependent on supersaturation of the urine and changes in the urine temperature or pH. The most common crystals are calcium oxalate, uric acid, and phosphate. However, crystals of various xenobiotics alone or in combination with other crystals may be seen in ingestions.[43] The urinalysis in patients who ingest ethylene glycol often (but not always) reveals calcium oxalate or hippurate crystals. Calcium oxalate crystals are monohydrates (prism or needlelike) or dihydrates (envelope shaped). Hippurate crystals are needle shaped.[91] Crystalluria is present in 50% of cases of ethylene glycol poisoning. B irefringent single or conglomerates of hexagonal crystals are noted after massive primidone poisoning and result from precipitation of primidone in the urine.[110] Crystalluria is also described after therapeutic doses of salicylate, phenacetin, sulfonamide, and quinolones. After large ingestions, crystals can be seen with methotrexate, amoxicillin, cephalexin, ampicillin, and indinavir. (Table 28–7)

Urine color is dependent on several factors, including pH, concentration, natural pigments, and length of time exposed to air.[52] Normal urine specimens should be clear and yellow in coloration. Dilute urine secondary to diuretic use, diabetes mellitus, diabetes insipidus, or overhydration can appear colorless, whereas concentrated urine is usually orange. The presence of fluorescein, detected by illumination of the urine with a Wood lamp, suggests ethylene glycol (commercial antifreeze) ingestion, but this diagnostic test has poor sensitivity and specificity.[112] One study utilized urine samples from a group of unpoisoned children and three urine samples with added sodium fluorescein to examine physicians ability to detect urinary fluorescence with a Wood lamp against a fluorometer. The fluorometer reported fluorescence in 100% of the urine samples whereas the physicians reported fluorescence in 70% to 80% of the samples.[92] Urinary fluorescence, even when present, is not useful as a diagnostic test. Table 28–8 lists other causes of colored urine.

There are multiple causes of hematuria.[76] (Table 28–9). It can occur with xenobiotic interstitial nephritis, a condition distinguished by fever, rash, eosinophilia, azotemia, and oliguria.[36] Hemorrhagic cystitis is a more frequent cause of hematuria, and is associated with a number of xenobiotics. The clinical presentation of hemorrhagic cystitis includes hematuria, dysuria, and urinary frequency. Criteria for diagnosis include a history of gross hematuria, laboratory findings of gross hematuria (>5 RBC/HPF), platelet count above 50,000/mm,[7] and a negative urine culture.[97] When in doubt, the diagnosis may be confirmed by cystoscopy, which reveals an inflamed, hyperemic, and sometimes ulcerated bladder mucosa.

Cyclophosphamide-related hemorrhagic cystitis was first described in 1959,[81] and is the best-documented type of drug-induced hemorrhagic

TABLE 28–8. Xenobiotics that Cause Colored Urine

Milky white	Chloroquine
Chyle	Fava beans
Lipids	Nitrofurantoin
Neutrophils	Primaquine
Reddish-brown	Rhubarb
Anthraquinone	Sulfamethoxazole
Bilirubin	**Yellow**
Chloroquine	Fluorescein
Ibuprofen	Phenacetin
Levodopa	Quinacrine
Methyldopa	Riboflavin
Phenacetin	Santonin
Phenazopyridine	**Yellow-orange**
Phenothiazines	Aminopyrine
Phenytoin	Anisindione
Porphyrins	Carrots
Trinitrophenol	Sulfasalazine
Reddish-orange	Vitamin A
Aminopyrine	Warfarin
Aniline dyes	**Black**
Antipyrine	Alcaptonuria
Chlorzoxazone	Homogentisic acid
Doxorubicin	Melanin
Ibuprofen	*p*-Hydroxyphenylpyruvic acid
Mannose	**Brown-black**
Phenacetin	Cascara
Phenazopyridine	Iron
Phenothiazines	Methyldopa
Phenytoin	Phenylhydrazine
Rifampin	Senna
Salicylazosulfapyridine	**Greenish-blue**
Red	Amitriptyline
Anthraquinones	Anthraquinones
Beets	Biliverdin
Blackberries	Chlorophyll breath mints
Eosin	Flavin derivatives
Erythrocytes	Food dye & Color Blue No. 1
Hemoglobin	Indicans
Myoglobin	Indigo blue
Porphyrins	Magnesium salicylate
Rhubarb	Methylene blue
Yellow-brown	Phenol
Aloe	Thymol
Anthraquinones	

TABLE 28–9. Xenobiotics that Cause Hematuria

Acyclovir	**Isoniazid**
Amitraz	**Ketamine**
Anticoagulants	**Mesalamine**
Brodifacoum	**NSAIDs**
Clopidogrel	Indomethacin
Heparin	Phenacetin
Warfarin	Tiaprofenic acid
Antineoplastics	**Orthotoluidine**
Busulfan	**Penicillamine**
Cyclophosphamide	**Penicillins**
Dacarbazine	Carbenicillin
Ifosfamide	Methicillin
Methotrexate	Nafcillin
Pentostatin	Penicillin G
Aspirin	Piperacillin
Baclofen	**Protease inhibitors**
BCG (intravesicular)	**Radiation**
Cantharidin	**Solvents**
Colchicine	Cyclohexane
COX-2 inhibitors	Toluene
Celecoxib	Xylene
Rofecoxib	**Statins**
Crotaline envenomation	Atorvastatin
Danazol	Rosuvastatin
Fibrinolytics	
Fluoroquinolones	
Ciprofloxacin	
Gatifloxacin	

cystitis.[48] As many as 46% of patients receiving cyclophosphamide will develop hemorrhagic cystitis.[40,59,65,68] Acrolein, the causative xenobiotic, is a metabolite of cyclophosphamide that damages the urothelium when excreted. (Chap. 54).[94,107]

An outbreak of hemorrhagic cystitis occurred in workers in a packaging plant after exposure to chlordimeform, a formamidine insecticide used to control mites and insects on cotton. Nine workers developed abdominal pain, dysuria, urgency, and hematuria, with biopsy-proven hemorrhagic cystitis.[44] Eight young adults developed painful hematuria after consuming "bootleg" methaqualone. The cause was orthotoluidine, a compound utilized in the synthesis of methaqualone, and the symptoms occurred within 6 hours of ingestion.[51] Cases of hemorrhagic cystitis have also been described with ticarcillin,[77] nafcillin, penicillin G, carbenicillin, piperacillin, isoniazid, indomethacin, tiaprofenic acid, and busulphan.[49,80,104]

SUMMARY

Toxicologic evaluation of the reproductive system is challenging because reproduction is an intermittent phenomenon. Adverse effects from xenobiotic exposures to both the male and female reproductive systems may not be noticed until fertility is desired. Xenobiotics can affect the hormonal controls, the organs of gametogenesis or cause sexual dysfunction. Alternatively, patients with sexual dysfunction may take xenobiotics to treat their condition but can result in toxicity. Once pregnant, some patients may opt for abortifacients that also can have unexpected toxicity.

Xenobiotic effects on the urinary system can result in disorders of urination, either urinary retention or incontinence, and abnormalities of urine in terms of color, crystals, and hematuria. A thorough history including past and present medications, illicit drug use, occupational and environmental exposures, or the use of herbal or alternative therapies is mandatory in the evaluation of patients with genitourinary complaints.

REFERENCES

1. Anonymous: Adverse reactions to bendrofluazide and propranolol for the treatment of mild hypertension. Report of Medical Research Council Working Party on Mild to Moderate Hypertension. *Lancet.* 1981;2:539-543.
2. Atazanavir (Reyataz): New recommendations if combined with tenofovir (Viread)—and warning on Viagra, Cialis, and Levitra. *AIDS Treat News.* 2004:5.
3. NIH Consensus Conference. Impotence. NIH Consensus Development Panel on Impotence. *JAMA.* 1993;270:83-90.
4. Sexual dysfunction: *Obstet Gynecol.* 2004;104:85S-91S.
5. Ambrosi B, Bara R, Travaglini P, et al. Study of the effects of bromocriptine on sexual impotence. *Clin Endocrinol (Oxf).* 1977;7:417-421.
6. Andersson KE, Wagner G. Physiology of penile erection. *Physiol Rev.* 1995;75:191-236.
7. Antoniou LD, Shalhoub RJ, Sudhakar T, et al. Reversal of uraemic impotence by zinc. *Lancet.* 1977;2:895-898.
8. Argiolas A, Hedlund H. The pharmacology and clinical pharmacokinetics of apomorphine SL. *BJU Int.* 2001;88Suppl3:18-21.
9. Arora RR, Timoney M, Melilli L. Acute myocardial infarction after the use of sildenafil. *N Engl J Med.* 1999;341:700.
10. Baranski B. Effects of the workplace on fertility and related reproductive outcomes. *Environ Health Perspect.* 1993;101(Suppl2):81-90.
11. Basson R, Berman J, Burnett A, et al. Report of the international consensus development conference on female sexual dysfunction: definitions and classifications. *J Urol.* 2000;163:888-893.
12. Basson R, McInnes R, Smith MD, et al. Efficacy and safety of sildenafil citrate in women with sexual dysfunction associated with female sexual arousal disorder. J *Womens Health Gend Based Med.* 2002;11:367-377.
13. Basu A, Ryder RE. New treatment options for erectile dysfunction in patients with diabetes mellitus. *Drugs.* 2004;64:2667-2688.
14. Beeley L. Drug-induced sexual dysfunction and infertility. *Adverse Drug React Acute Poisoning Rev.* 1984;3:23-42.
15. Bischoff: Vardenafil preclinical trial data: potency, pharmacodynamics, pharmacokinetics, and adverse events. *Int J Impot Res.* 2004;16Suppl1:S34-S37.
16. Bollinger K, Lee MS. Recurrent visual field defect and ischemic optic neuropathy associated with tadalafil rechallenge. *Arch Ophthalmol.* 2005;123:400-401.
17. Bommer J, Ritz E, del Pozo E, et al. Improved sexual function in male haemodialysis patients on bromocriptine. *Lancet.* 1979;2:496-497.
18. Boolell M, Allen MJ, Ballard SA, et al. Sildenafil: an orally active type 5 cyclic GMP-specific phosphodiesterase inhibitor for the treatment of penile erectile dysfunction. *Int J Impot Res.* 1996;8:47-52.
19. Buchanan JF, Davis LJ. Drug-induced infertility. *Drug Intell Clin Pharm.* 1984;18:122-132.
20. Buffum J. Pharmacosexology update: prescription drugs and sexual function. *J Psychoactive Drugs.* 1986;18:97-106.
21. Caruso S, Agnello C, Intelisano G, et al. Placebo-controlled study on efficacy and safety of daily apomorphine SL intake in premenopausal women affected by hypoactive sexual desire disorder and sexual arousal disorder. *Urology.* 2004;63:955-959.
22. Caruso S, Intelisano G, Lupo L, et al. Premenopausal women affected by sexual arousal disorder treated with sildenafil: a double-blind, cross-over, placebo-controlled study. *Bjog.* 2001;108:623-628.
23. Castleden CM, Duffin HM, Gulati RS. Double-blind study of imipramine and placebo for incontinence due to bladder instability. *Age Ageing.* 1986;15:299-303.
24. Chapple CR, Parkhouse H, Gardener C, et al. Double-blind, placebo-controlled, cross-over study of flavoxate in the treatment of idiopathic detrusor instability. *Br J Urol.* 1990;66:491-494.
25. Chapple CR, Yamanishi T, Chess-Williams R. Muscarinic receptor subtypes and management of the overactive bladder. *Urology.* 2002;60:82-88; discuss88-89.
26. Cheitlin MD, Hutter AM, Brindis RG, et al. ACC/AHA expert consensus document. Use of sildenafil (Viagra) in patients with cardiovascular disease. American College of Cardiology/American Heart Association. *J Am Coll Cardiol.* 1999;33:273-282.
27. Christin-Maitre S, Bouchard P, Spitz IM. Medical termination of pregnancy: *N Engl J Med.* 2000;342:946-956.
28. Christin-Maitre S, Bouchard P, Spitz IM. Medical termination of pregnancy. *N Engl J Med.* 2000;342:946-956.
29. Chutka DS, Fleming KC, Evans MP, et al. Urinary incontinence in the elderly population. *Mayo Clin Proc.* 1996;71:93-101.
30. Clayton AH, Warnock JK, Kornstein SG, et al. A placebo-controlled trial of bupropion SR as an antidote for selective serotonin reuptake inhibitor-induced sexual dysfunction. *J Clin Psychiatry.* 2004;65:62-67.
31. Clayton DO, Shen WW. Psychotropic drug-induced sexual function disorders: diagnosis, incidence and management. *Drug Saf.* 1998;19:299-312.
32. Coleman CC, King BR, Bolden-Watson C, et al. A placebo-controlled comparison of the effects on sexual functioning of bupropion sustained release and fluoxetine. *Clin Ther.* 2001;23:1040-1058.
33. Corriere JN, Fishman IJ, Benson GS, et al. Development of fibrotic penile lesions secondary to the intracorporeal injection of vasoactive agents. *J Urol.* 1988;140:615-617.
34. Czajka P, Field J, Novak P, et al. Case report: accidental aphrodisiac ingestion. *J Tenn Med Assoc.* 1978;71:747-750.
35. De Smet PA, Smeets OS. Potential risks of health food products containing yohimbe extracts. *BMJ.* 1994;309:958.
36. Ditlove J, Weidmann P, Bernstein M, et al. Methicillin nephritis. *Medicine.* 1977;56:483-491.
37. Dlugosz L, Bracken MB. Reproductive effects of caffeine: a review and theoretical analysis. *Epidemiol Rev.* 1992;14:83-100.
38. Dmochowski RR, Miklos JR, Norton PA, et al. Duloxetine versus placebo for the treatment of North American women with stress urinary incontinence. *J Urol.* 2003;170:1259-1263.
39. Dolan G, Jones AP, Blumsohn A, et al. Lead poisoning due to Asian ethnic treatment for impotence. *J R Soc Med.* 1991;84:630-631.
40. Droller MJ, Saral R, Santos G. Prevention of cyclophosphamide-induced hemorrhagic cystitis. *Urology.* 1982;20:256-258.
41. Egan R, Pomeranz H. Sildenafil (Viagra) associated anterior ischemic optic neuropathy. *Arch Ophthalmol.* 2000;118:291-292.
42. Finger WW, Lund M, Slagle MA. Medications that may contribute to sexual disorders. A guide to assessment and treatment in family practice. *J Fam Pract.* 1997;44:33-43.
43. Fogazzi GB. Crystalluria: a neglected aspect of urinary sediment analysis. *Nephrol Dial Transplant.* 1996;11:379-387.
44. Folland DS, Kimbrough RD, Cline RE, et al. Acute hemorrhagic cystitis. Industrial exposure to the pesticide chlordimeform. *JAMA.* 1978;239:1052-1055.
45. Fontanarosa PB, Roush WR. Acute urinary retention. *Emerg Med Clin North Am.* 1988;6:419-437.
46. Friesen K, Palatnick W, Tenenbein M. Benign course after massive ingestion of yohimbine. *J Emerg Med.* 1993;11:287-288.
47. Furuya S, Kumamoto Y, Yokoyama E, et al. Alpha-adrenergic activity and urethral pressure in prostatic zone in benign prostatic hypertrophy. *J Urol.* 1982;128:836-839.
48. Gellman E, Kissane J, Frech R, et al. Cyclophosphamide cystitis. *J Can Assoc Radiol.* 1969;20:99-101.
49. Ghose K. Cystitis and nonsteroidal antiinflammatory drugs: an incidental association or an adverse effect? *N Z Med J.* 1993;106:501-503.
50. Gilja I, Radej M, Kovacic M, et al. Conservative treatment of female stress incontinence with imipramine. *J Urol.* 1984;132:909-911.
51. Goldfarb M, Finelli R. Necrotizing cystitis. Secondary to "bootleg" methaqualone. *Urology.* 1974;3:54-55.
52. Goldfrank L, Osborn H. Rainbow urine. *Hosp Phys.* 1978;3:22-26.

53. Goldstein I, Lue TF, Padma-Nathan H, et al. Oral sildenafil in the treatment of erectile dysfunction. Sildenafil Study Group. *N Engl J Med.* 1998;338:1397-1404.
54. Goldstein I, Payton TR, Schechter PJ. A double-blind, placebo-controlled, efficacy and safety study of topical gel formulation of 1% alprostadil (Topiglan) for the in-office treatment of erectile dysfunction. *Urology.* 2001;57:301-305.
55. Goldstein I, Young JM, Fischer J, et al. Vardenafil, a new phosphodiesterase type 5 inhibitor, in the treatment of erectile dysfunction in men with diabetes: a multicenter double-blind placebo-controlled fixed-dose study. *Diabetes Care.* 2003;26:777-783.
56. Heaton JP. Central neuropharmacological agents and mechanisms in erectile dysfunction: the role of dopamine. *Neurosci Biobehav Rev.* 2000;24:561-569.
57. Hogan MJ, Wallin JD, Baer RM. Antihypertensive therapy and male sexual dysfunction. *Psychosomatics.* 1980;21:234-237.
58. Holmberg G, Gershon S. Autonomic and psychic effects of yohimbine hydrochloride. *Psychopharmacologia.* 1961;2:93-106.
59. Jayalakshmamma B, Pinkel D. Urinary-bladder toxicity following pelvic irradiation and simultaneous cyclophosphamide therapy. *Cancer.* 1976;38:701-707.
60. Karras DJ, Farrell SE, Harrigan RA, et al. Poisoning from "Spanish fly" (cantharidin). *Am J Emerg Med.* 1996;14:478-483.
61. Kassim AA, Fabry ME, Nagel RL. Acute priapism associated with the use of sildenafil in a patient with sickle cell trait. *Blood.* 2000;95:1878-1879.
62. Keating GM, Scott LJ. Vardenafil: a review of its use in erectile dysfunction. *Drugs.* 2003;63:2673-2703.
63. Kloner RA. Novel phosphodiesterase type 5 inhibitors: assessing hemodynamic effects and safety parameters. *Clin Cardiol.* 2004;27:I20-I25.
64. Kloner RA, Jackson G, Emmick JT, et al. Interaction between the phosphodiesterase 5 inhibitor, tadalafil and 2 alpha-blockers, doxazosin and tamsulosin in healthy normotensive men. *J Urol.* 2004;172:1935-1940.
65. Kotsonis FN, Dodd DC, Regnier B, et al. Preclinical toxicology profile of misoprostol. *Dig Dis Sci.* 1985;30:142S-146S.
66. Landis E, Shore E. Yohimbine-induced bronchospasm. *Chest.* 1989;96:1424.
67. Laumann EO, Paik A, Rosen RC. Sexual dysfunction in the United States: prevalence and predictors. *JAMA.* 1999;281:537-544.
68. Lawrence HJ, Simone J, Aur RJ. Cyclophosphamide-induced hemorrhagic cystitis in children with leukemia. *Cancer.* 1975;36:1572-1576.
69. Levitt NS, Vinik AI, Sive AA, et al. Synthetic luteinizing hormone-releasing hormone in impotent male diabetics. *S Afr Med J.* 1980;57:701-704.
70. Lidberg L, Sternthal V. A new approach to the hormonal treatment of impotentia erectionis. *Pharmakopsychiatr Neuropsychopharmakol.* 1977;10:21-25.
71. Lin SC, Hsu T, Fredrickson PA, et al. Yohimbine- and tranylcypromine-induced postural hypotension. *Am J Psychiatry.* 1987;144:119.
72. Linden CH, Vellman WP, Rumack B. Yohimbine: a new street drug. *Ann Emerg Med.* 1985;14:1002-1004.
73. Lowe FC, Jarow JP. Placebo-controlled study of oral terbutaline and pseudoephedrine in management of prostaglandin E1-induced prolonged erections. *Urology.* 1993;42:51-53;discuss53-54.
74. Lue TF. Erectile dysfunction. *N Engl J Med.* 2000;342:1802-1813.
75. Margolis R, Prieto P, Stein L, et al. Statistical summary of 10,000 male cases using Afrodex in treatment of impotence. *Curr Ther Res Clin Exp.* 1971;13:616-622.
76. Marks LB, Carroll PR, Dugan TC, et al. The response of the urinary bladder, urethra, and ureter to radiation and chemotherapy. *Int J Radiat Oncol Biol Phys.* 1995;31:1257-1280.
77. Marx CM, Alpert SE. Ticarcillin-induced cystitis. Cross-reactivity with related penicillins. *Am J Dis Child.* 1984;138:670-672.
78. Mattison DR, Plowchalk DR, Meadows MJ, et al. Reproductive toxicity: male and female reproductive systems as targets for chemical injury. *Med Clin North Am.* 1990;74:391-411.
79. McConnell JD. Benign prostatic hyperplasia. Hormonal treatment. *Urol Clin North Am.* 1995;22:387-400.
80. Millard RJ. Busulphan haemorrhagic cystitis. *Br J Urol.* 1978;50:210.
81. Miller LJ, Chandler SW, Ippoliti CM. Treatment of cyclophosphamide-induced hemorrhagic cystitis with prostaglandins. *Ann Pharmacother.* 1994;28:590-594.
82. Moore KH, Hay DM, Imrie AE, et al. Oxybutynin hydrochloride (3 mg) in the treatment of women with idiopathic detrusor instability. *Br J Urol.* 1990;66:479-485.
83. Morales A, Condra M, Owen JA, et al. Is yohimbine effective in the treatment of organic impotence? Results of a controlled trial. *J Urol.* 1987;137:1168-1172.
84. Moreland RB, Hsieh G, Nakane M, et al. The biochemical and neurologic basis for the treatment of male erectile dysfunction. *J Pharmacol Exp Ther.* 2001;296:225-234.
85. Mudd JW. Impotence responsive to glyceryl trinitrate. *Am J Psychiatry.* 1977;134:922-925.
86. Netland KE, Martinez J. Abortifacients: toxidromes, ancient to modern—a case series and review of the literature. *Acad Emerg Med.* 2000;7:824-829.
87. Newman RJ, Salerno HR. Letter: sexual dysfunction due to methyldopa. *Br Med J.* 1974;4:106.
88. Nurnberg HG, Hensley PL, Lauriello J, et al. Sildenafil for women patients with antidepressant-induced sexual dysfunction. *Psychiatr Serv.* 1999;50:1076-1078.
89. Olsen J. Is human fecundity declining—and does occupational exposures play a role in such a decline if it exists? *Scand J Work Environ Health.* 1994;20:72-77.
90. Owen JA, Nakatsu SL, Fenemore J, et al. The pharmacokinetics of yohimbine in man. *Eur J Clin Pharmacol.* 1987;32:577-582.
91. Parry MF, Wallach R. Ethylene glycol poisoning. *Am J Med.* 1974;57:143-150.
92. Parsa T, Cunningham SJ, Wall SP, et al. The usefulness of urine fluorescence for suspected antifreeze ingestion in children. *Am J Emerg Med.* 2005;23:787-792.
93. Paumgartten FJ, Castilla EE, Monteleone-Neto R. Risk assessment in reproductive toxicology as practiced in South America. In: Neubert D, Kavlock R, Merker H, et al., eds. *Risk Assessment of Prenatally Induced Adverse Health Effects.* Berlin: Springer-Verlag; 1992:163-179.
94. Perrone J, Hoffman RS. Toxic ingestions in pregnancy: abortifacient use in a case series of pregnant overdose patients. *Acad Emerg Med.* 1997;4:206-209.
95. Price LH, Charney DS, Heninger GR. Three cases of manic symptoms following yohimbine administration. *Am J Psychiatry.* 1984;141:1267-1268.
96. Priyadarshi S. Oral terbutaline in the management of pharmacologically induced prolonged erection. *Int J Impot Res.* 2004;16:424-426.
97. Relling MV, Schunk JE. Drug-induced hemorrhagic cystitis. *Clin Pharm.* 1986;5:590-597.
98. Rosen RC, Ashton AK. Prosexual drugs: empirical status of the "new aphrodisiacs." *Arch Sex Behav.* 1993;22:521-543.
99. Sandler B, Aronson P. Yohimbine-induced cutaneous drug eruption, progressive renal failure, and lupus-like syndrome. *Urology.* 1993;41:343-345.
100. Schlegel PN, Chang TS, Marshall FF. Antibiotics: potential hazards to male fertility. *Fertil Steril.* 1991;55:235-242.
101. Schrag SD, Dixon RL. Occupational exposures associated with male reproductive dysfunction. *Annu Rev Pharmacol Toxicol.* 1985;25:567-592.
102. Segraves RT. Sexual dysfunction associated with antidepressant therapy. *Urol Clin North Am.* 2007;34:575-579,vii.
103. Shah PK. Sildenafil in the treatment of erectile dysfunction. *N Engl J Med.* 1998;339:699.
104. Shieh CC, Chen BW, Lin KH. Late onset hemorrhagic cystitis after allogeneic bone marrow transplantation. *Taiwan Yi Xue Hui Za Zhi.* 1989;88:508-511.
105. Sipski ML, Rosen RC, Alexander CJ, et al. Sildenafil effects on sexual and cardiovascular responses in women with spinal cord injury. *Urology.* 2000;55:812-815.
106. Stauffer JC, Ruiz V, Morard JD. Subaortic obstruction after sildenafil in a patient with hypertrophic cardiomyopathy. *N Engl J Med.* 1999;341:700-701.
107. Stillwell TJ, Benson RC Jr. Cyclophosphamide-induced hemorrhagic cystitis. A review of 100 patients. *Cancer.* 1988;61:451-457.
108. Susset JG, Tessier CD, Wincze J, et al. Effect of yohimbine hydrochloride on erectile impotence: a double-blind study. *J Urol.* 1989;141:1360-1363.
109. Tackett RE. Priapism. In: Stine R, Chudnofsky C, eds. *A Practical Approach to Emergency Medicine.* Boston: Little, Brown; 1994:710-711.
110. van Heijst AN, de Jong W, Seldenrijk R, et al. Coma and crystalluria: a massive primidone intoxication treated with haemoperfusion. *J Toxicol Clin Toxicol.* 1983;20:307-318.
111. Verhamme KM, Sturkenboom MC, Stricker BH, et al. Drug-induced urinary retention: incidence, management and prevention. *Drug Saf.* 2008;31:373-388.

112. Wallace KL, Suchard JR, Curry SC, et al. Diagnostic use of physicians' detection of urine fluorescence in a simulated ingestion of sodium fluorescein-containing antifreeze. *Ann Emerg Med.* 2001;38:49-54.
113. Walsh KE, Berman JR. Sexual dysfunction in the older woman: an overview of the current understanding and management. *Drugs Aging.* 2004;21:655-675.
114. Warren SC, Warren SG. Propranolol and sexual impotence. *Ann Intern Med.* 1977;86:112.
115. Webb DJ, Freestone S, Allen MJ, et al. Sildenafil citrate and blood-pressure-lowering drugs: results of drug interaction studies with an organic nitrate and a calcium antagonist. *Am J Cardiol.* 1999;83:21C-28C.
116. Wetterling T, Veltrup C, Driessen M, et al. Drinking pattern and alcohol-related medical disorders. *Alcohol Alcohol.* 1999;34:330-336.
117. Whorton MD, Foliart DE. Mutagenicity, carcinogenicity and reproductive effects of dibromochloropropane (DBCP). *Mutat Res.* 1983;123:13-30.
118. Wilson B. The effect of drugs on male sexual function and fertility. *Nurse Pract.* 1991;16:12-17, 21-24.
119. Woodrum ST, Brown CS. Management of SSRI-induced sexual dysfunction. *Ann Pharmacother.* 1998;32:1209-1215.
120. Yealy DM, Hogya PT. Priapism. *Emerg Med Clin North Am.* 1988;6:509-520.

CHAPTER 29
DERMATOLOGIC PRINCIPLES

Neal A. Lewin and Lewis S. Nelson

The skin shields the internal organs from harmful xenobiotics in the environment and maintains internal organ integrity. The adult skin covers an average surface area of 2 meters^2. Despite its outwardly simple structure and function, the skin is extraordinarily complex. The skin can be affected by xenobiotic exposures that occur through any route. Dermal exposures account for a few percent of the cases and for approximately 1% of the fatalities reported to the American Association of Poison Control Centers (AAPCC) (Chap. 135). The principles of an adverse cutaneous reaction can be used to make relevant predictions, such as the physical and chemical properties of the xenobiotic and whether the effect of a response will be local or systemic. The clinician must obtain essential information as to the dose, timing, route, and location of exposure. The location of xenobiotic injury determines the histologic morphology, the severity of the reaction pattern, and the overall clinical findings. It should be noted, however, that different xenobiotics may produce clinically similar skin changes and conversely that many xenobiotics may produce diverse dermal lesions. The classical dermatologic lesions are defined in Table 29–1. The dermatology lexicon to assist the clinician is available at www.dermatologylexicon.org.

SKIN ANATOMY AND PHYSIOLOGY

The skin has three main components that interconnect anatomically and interact functionally: the epidermis, the dermis, and the subcutis or hypodermis (Figure 29–1). The three reactive units are the superficial reactive unit; the reticular layer of the dermis; and the subcutaneous tissue.[24] The primary physiologic role of the epidermis, the most external layer of the skin, is to maintain water homeostasis and to establish immunologic surveillance. It is composed of five layers: the horny, transitional, granular, spinous, and basal layers. The keratinocyte, which is an ectodermal derivative, represents the majority of the epidermis. The thin stratum corneum, or horny layer, is predominantly responsible for the protective function of the skin. Disruption or inadequate formation of the stratum corneum leads to a breakdown of this barrier function and many disease processes. The cells of the stratum corneum serve as a buffer to acidic and alkaline substances. Barrier function is also partly maintained by the granular layer. In this layer, there are Odland bodies, also known as membrane-coating granules, lamellar granules, and keratinosomes. The contents of these organelles provide a barrier to water loss while mediating stratum corneum cell cohesion.[10]

The stratum corneum is covered by a surface film composed of sebum emulsified with sweat and breakdown products from the horny layer.[22] The surface film functions as an external barrier to protect the entry of bacteria, viruses, and fungi. The role of the surface film, however, is limited with regard to percutaneous absorption. The major barrier molecules to percutaneous absorption in the skin are lipids called *ceramides*.[22] Diseases characterized by dry skin, such as eczema, atopic dermatitis, and psoriasis, are caused by decreased concentrations of ceramide in the stratum corneum, which allows increased xenobiotic penetration because of barrier degradation.[22] Similarly, hydrocarbon solvents, such as gasoline or methanol, or detergents, commonly produce a "defatting dermatitis" by keratolysis or the dissolution of these surface lipids.

The degree of barrier function of the epidermis varies with its thickness as well. Differences in thickness are observed on different regions of the body. The epidermis varies from 1.5 mm on the glabrous surfaces (palms and soles) to 0.1 mm on the eyelids. The cells of the basal layer control the renewal of the epidermis. The basal layer contains stem cells and transient amplifying cells, which are the proliferative cells resulting in new epidermal formation that occurs every 59 to 75 days. As the basal cells migrate toward the skin surface they flatten, lose their nuclei, develop keratohyalin granules, and eventually develop into the horny layer. Patients with primary cutaneous diseases, such as psoriasis, have a significantly shortened epidermal renewal or turnover time resulting in a thicker epidermis (hyperkeratosis) and potentially less direct penetration of xenobiotics.[2] The basal layer is adjacent to the basement membrane zone and is also populated by melanocytes and Langerhans cells. Melanocytes contain melanin, which is the major chromophore in the skin that is responsible for absorbing ultraviolet and other light energies. Melanocytes are primarily responsible for producing skin pigmentation. The *Langerhans cells* are bone marrow–derived cells with a primary role in immunosurveillance. Langerhans cells function in the recognition, uptake, processing, and presentation of antigens to previously sensitized T lymphocytes. Langerhans cells may also carry antigens via dermal lymphatics to regional lymph nodes. The cells express chemokine CCR6 which allows tracking of peripatetic leukocytes to migrate from the dermis to the epidermis, and without CCR7 migration to lymph nodes is not possible.

The basement membrane zone, which consists of three layers—the lamina lucida, the lamina densa, and the sublamina densa—separates the epidermis from the dermis. It provides a site of attachment for keratinocytes and permits epidermal–dermal interaction.

The dermal-epidermal junction (DEJ) functions as a basement membrane to provide resistance against trauma, give support to the overlying structures, organize the cytoskeleton in the basal cells, and serve as a semipermeable barrier. The dermis, the second reactive unit, is deep to the epidermis and contains the adnexal structures, blood vessels, and nerves. It is arranged into two major regions, the upper papillary dermis and the deeper reticular dermis, which comprise the bulk of dermis. The dermis provides structural integrity and contains many important appendageal structures. The structural support is provided by both collagen and elastin fibers embedded in glycosaminoglycans, such as chondroitin A and hyaluronic acid. Mature dermis is predominantly composed of type I collagen (80%–90%); type III (8%–12%), type V (<5%); types VI, VII and IV collagen maintain a less important role. Collagen accounts for 70% of the dry weight of the skin, whereas elastic fibers are equivalent to 1% to 2% of the skin's dry weight. Several important cells, including fibroblasts, macrophages and mast cells, are transient circulating cells of the immune system present in the dermis. Traversing the dermis are venules, capillaries, arterioles, nerves, and glandular structures.

The arteriovenous framework of the skin consists of a deep plexus in the region of the subcutaneous dermal junction. From this deep plexus, smaller arterioles transverse upward to the junction of the reticular and papillary dermis, where they form the superficial plexus. Capillary-venules form superficial vascular loops that ascend into and descend from the dermal papillae. The communicating blood vessels provide channels in which xenobiotics exposed to the skin can be transported internally. In addition, they transport internally absorbed xenobiotics and cells of the immune system to the skin.

Parallel to the vasculature are cutaneous nerves, which serve the dual function of receiving sensory input and carrying sympathetically mediated autonomic stimuli that induce piloerection and sweating.[12]

TABLE 29–1. Dermatologic Diagnostic Descriptions of Lesions of the Skin

Primary Cutaneous Lesions	Secondary Cutaneous Lesions
Bulla: a circumscribed collection of free fluid > 0.5 cm in diameter Comedone: open and closed dilated pores (blackheads and whiteheads) Macule: a circumscribed flat variation of color that may be brown, blue, yellow, red, or hypopigmented (no thickness) Nodule: a circumscribed elevation of ≥ 0.5 cm in diameter Papule: an elevation of < 0.5 cm in diameter Plaque: a circumscribed elevation of > 0.5 cm in diameter Pustule: a circumscribed collection of leukocytes and free fluid that vary in size Tumor: an elevation of > 0.5 cm in diameter Vesicle: a circumscribed collection of free fluid ≥ 0.5 cm in diameter Wheal: a firm edematous plaque resulting from infiltration of the dermis with fluid	Erosion: a loss of the epidermis up to the full thickness of the epidermis but not through the basement membrane Hypertrophy: a thickening of the skin Lichenification: a secondary process with noted accentuation of skin surface markings Scale: flaking that is separate from the original surface of a lesion Scar: a thickened, often discolored, surface Ulcer: a loss of full-thickness epidermis and papillary dermis, reticular dermis, or subcutis

The apocrine glands consist of secretory coils and intradermal ducts ending in the follicular canal. The secretory coil is located in the subcutis and consists of a large lumen surrounded by columnar to cuboidal cells with eosinophilic cytoplasm.[12] Apocrine glands, which are located in select areas of the body such as the axilla, produce secretions that are rendered odoriferous by cutaneous bacterial flora.

The eccrine glands, in contrast, produce an isotonic to hypotonic secretion that is modified by the ducts and emerges on the skin surface as sweat. The eccrine unit consists of a secretory gland as well as intradermal and intraepidermal ducts. The coiled secretory gland is located in the area of the deep dermis and subcutis. Xenobiotics can be concentrated in the sweat and increase the intensity of the local skin reactions.

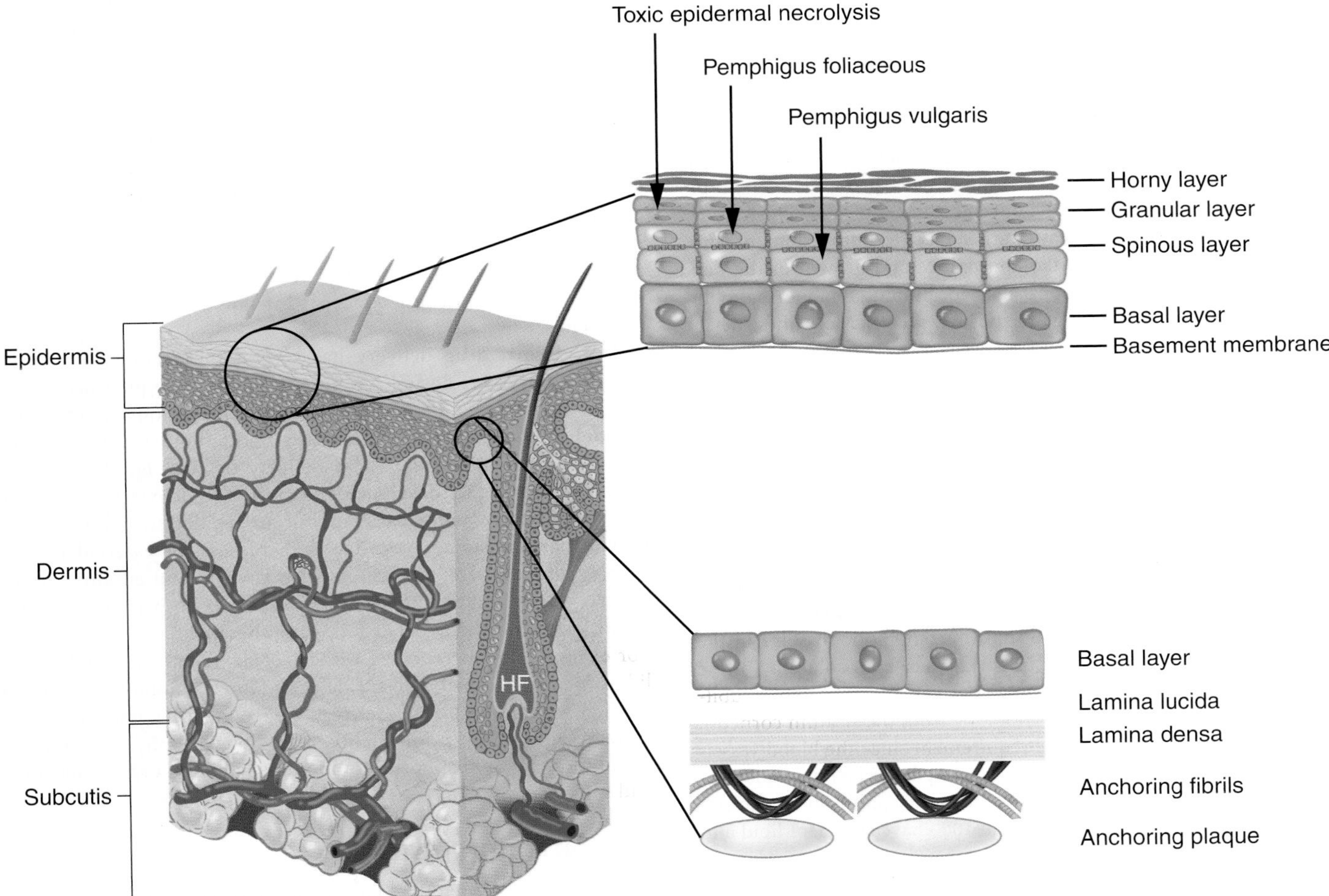

FIGURE 29–1. Skin histology and pathology. Intraepidermal cleavage sites in various xenobiotic-induced blistering diseases. In pemphigus foliaceous, the cleavage is below or within the granular layer, whereas in pemphigus vulgaris, it is suprabasilar. This accounts for the differing types of blisters found in the two diseases. HF = Hair Follicle

Certain antineoplastics, such as cytarabine or bleomycin, directly damage the eccrine sweat glands, resulting in anhidrosis.

Sebaceous glands also reside in the dermis. They produce an oily, lipid-rich secretion that functions as an emollient for the hair and skin, and can be a reservoir of noxious environmental xenobiotics. Pilosebaceous follicles, which are present all over the body, consist of a hair shaft, hair follicle, sebaceous gland, sensory end organ, and erector pili. Certain halogenated aromatic chemicals, such as polychlorinated biphenyls (PCBs), dioxin, and 2,4-dichlorophenoxyacetic acid, are excreted in the sebum and cause hyperkeratosis of the follicular canal. This produces a syndrome, chloracne, that looks like acne vulgaris, because of plugging of the ducts. Similar syndromes result from exposure to brominated and iodinated compounds, and are known as bromoderma and ioderma, respectively.[40]

The tissues of the hypodermis or subcutaneous tissue, serves to insulate, cushion, and allow for mobility of the overlying skin structures. Adipocytes represent the majority of cells found in this layer. Leptin, an adipose-derived hormone responsible for long-term feedback of appetite and satiety signaling, is synthesized and regulates fat mass (adiposity) in this layer.

The hair follicle is divided into three portions.[34] The deepest portion of the hair follicle contains the bulb with matrix cells. The matrix cells are highly mitotically active and often are the target of cytotoxic xenobiotics. The rate of growth and the type of hair are unique for different body sites. Hair growth proceeds through three distinct phases: the active prolonged growth phase (anagen phase) during which matrix cell mitotic activity is high; a short involutional phase (catagen phase); and a resting phase (telogen phase). Understanding the phases and biochemical structure of hair growth is important because hair growth can be used to identify clues regarding the timing and mechanism of action of a xenobiotic.

The nail, which is often considered analogous to the hair, is also a continuously growing structure. Fingernails grow at average of 0.1 mm/d and toenails grow at about one-third that rate. The mitotically active cells of the nail matrix are subject to both traumatic and xenobiotic injury that affects the appearance and growth of the nail plate. Because nail growth is consistent, location of an abnormality in the plate can predict the timing of exposure, such as Mees lines.

TOPICAL TOXICITY

TRANSDERMAL XENOBIOTIC ABSORPTION

Although there is no active uptake mechanism for xenobiotics by the skin, many undergo percutaneous absorption by passive diffusion. Lipid solubility, concentration gradient, molecular weight, and certain specific skin characteristics are important determinants of dermal absorption. Absorption is generally considered to occur though intercellular movement, requiring that the xenobiotic dissolve in the ceramides. This accounts for the importance of lipid solubility of the xenobiotic in transdermal absorption. However, excessive lipid solubility limits the partitioning of the xenobiotic from the stratum corneum into the aqueous dermis, a critical requirement since the blood vessels are in this deeper layer.[13,14,31,32] The relationship between lipid and water solubility is often described by the octanol-water partition coefficient. Xenobiotics with values between 10 and 1000 have sufficient lipid and water solubility to permit skin permeation.

For example, morphine sulfate, with an octanol water partition coefficient of approximately 1, is not absorbed when applied topically, whereas fentanyl, with a coefficient of approximately 700, is widely used as a transdermally delivered medication. The dermal toxicity of the various organic phosphorus compounds may be predicted based on this coefficient.[9] Although metal ions such as Hg^+ have limited skin penetration, the addition of a methyl group, to form methylmercury, increases its lipophilicity and its systemic absorption. Dimethylmercury, has even better absorption and may produce life-threatening systemic effects with a minute amount applied to the skin (Chap. 96). Similarly, the nonionized component of the weakly acidic hydrofluoric (HF) acid is able to penetrate deeply through skin and even bone. The proton (H^+) and fluoride ion (F^-) are unable to penetrate the lipids of the skin individually because of their charged nature; however, once in the dermis, the HF acid may ionize and cause both acid-induced tissue necrosis and fluoride-induced toxicity (Chap. 105).[4]

Children appear particularly at risk for toxicity from percutaneous absorption because their skin is more penetrable than an adult's and specific anatomic sites, such as the face, often represent larger percentage of body surface areas than in the adult.[37] Furthermore, there is enhanced absorption on anatomic parts of the body with thinner skin, such as the mucous membranes, eyelids, and intertriginous areas (axillae, groin, inframammary, and intergluteal). Under certain circumstances, such as with more highly lipophilic xenobiotics, the stratum corneum may serve a depot function leading to slow onset and continued systemic exposure despite apparent removal of the xenobiotic. For example, applied topically in the form of a transdermal device, fentanyl does not result in peak concentration for 24 to 72 hours after initial application. When removed, the serum fentanyl concentrations fall with an average half-life of 17 hours, which is substantially longer than when administered intravenously.[18] The vehicle of a xenobiotic may also influence absorption; indeed, transdermal drug-delivery systems are based on their ability to alter the skin partition coefficient through the use of an optimized vehicle. Similarly, through localized dermal occlusion, transdermal systems hydrate the skin and raise its temperature to increase absorption. Despite these techniques to enhance drug delivery, transdermal systems require that large amounts of drug be present externally to maximize the transcutaneous gradient. Much of the drug typically remains in the patch when it is removed following its intended course of therapy, raising concerns for safe disposal, especially for children.[13,14,31,32]

Transdermal drug delivery has several therapeutic advantages, such as continuous dosing resulting in more stable pharmacokinetics, prolonged drug delivery resulting in a more convenient dosing schedule (eg, weekly device changes), and the avoidance of first pass hepatic metabolism. These delivery devices, familiarly called "patches," are highly developed and crafted to deliver their content at a specified rate. Some variability occurs related to skin thickness, dermal barrier damage (eg, dry skin, rashes), or external factors, such as ambient temperature. As with any route of administration, adverse effects and toxicity caused by excessive absorption following patch application may occur following therapeutic use and misuse. For example, this is reported with nicotine, fentanyl, NSAIDS, and lidocaine transdermal delivery devices. Other xenobiotics, topically applied without a specific delivery device, may be associated with systemic morbidity and mortality, including podophyllin, camphor, phenol, organic phosphorus compounds, ethanol, organochlorines, and nitrates.

CONTACT DERMATITIS

Allergic contact dermatitis from plants and dyes such as fragrances and paraphenylenediamine (henna) is increasing in frequency. Miconidin and miconidin methyl ester were isolated from *Primula obconica* (primrose). Parthenolide is an ingredient in feverfew and can cause an airborne contact dermatitis. Triethanolamine polyethylene glycol-3

(TEA-PEG-3) cocamide sulfate was identified recently to cause allergic reactions in coconut oil.

DIRECT DERMAL TOXICITY

Exposure to any of a myriad of industrial and environmental xenobiotics can result in dermal "burns." Although the majority of these xenobiotics injure the skin through chemical reactivity rather than thermal damage, the clinical appearances of the two are often identical. Injurious xenobiotics may act as oxidizing or reducing agents, corrosives, protoplasmic poisons, desiccants, or vesicants. Often an injury may initially appear to be mild or superficial with only faint erythema, blanching, or discoloration of the skin. Over the subsequent 24 to 36 hours there may be progression to extensive necrosis of the skin and its underlying tissues.

Acids are water soluble and many readily penetrate into the subcutaneous tissue. The damaged tissue coagulates and forms a thick leathery eschar that limits the spread of the xenobiotic. The histopathologic finding following acid injury is termed *coagulative necrosis*. Alkali exposures characteristically produce *a liquefactive necrosis*, which allows continued penetration of the corrosive xenobiotic; consequently, dermal injury following alkali exposure is typically more severe than after an acid exposure of an equivalent magnitude.[7]

Thermal damage can also be the result of a toxicologic exposure. For example, the exothermic reaction generated by the wetting of elemental phosphorus or sodium may result in a thermal burn. In these circumstances, the products of reactivity, phosphoric acid and sodium hydroxide respectively, may produce secondary chemical injury. Alternatively, skin exposure to a rapidly expanding gas, such as nitrous oxide from a whipped cream cartridge or compressed liquefied nitrogen, or to frozen substances, such as dry ice, can produce a freezing injury, or frostbite.

Hydrocarbon-based solvents are typically liquids that are capable of dissolving non–water-soluble solutes.[7] Although the most prominent effect is a dermatitis due to loss of ceramides from the stratum corneum, prolonged exposure can result in deeper dermal irritation and destruction.

PRINCIPLES OF DERMAL DECONTAMINATION

On contact with xenobiotics, the skin should be thoroughly cleansed to prevent direct effects and systemic absorption. In general, a copious amount of water is the decontamination agent of choice for skin irrigation. Soap should be used when adherent xenobiotics are involved. Following exposures to airborne xenobiotics, the mouth, nasal cavities, eyes, and ear canals should be irrigated with appropriate solutions such as water or a 0.9% NaCl solution. For nonambulatory patients, the decontamination process may need to be conducted using special collection stretchers if available.[6]

There are a few situations in which water should not be used for skin decontamination. The situations include contamination involving the reactive metallic forms of the alkali metals, sodium, potassium, lithium, cesium, and rubidium, which react with water to form strong bases. The dusts of pure magnesium, sulfur, strontium, titanium, uranium, yttrium, zinc, and zirconium will ignite or explode on contact with water. Following exposure to these metals, any residual metal should be removed mechanically with forceps, gauze, or towels and stored in mineral oil. Additionally, phenol has a tendency to thicken and become difficult to remove following exposure to water. Suggestions for phenol decontamination include high-flow water or low-molecular-weight polyethylene glycol solution. Lime, or CaO, thickens and forms $Ca(OH)_2$ following wetting, suggesting that mechanical removal is appropriate.[6]

DERMATOLOGIC SIGNS OF SYSTEMIC DISEASES

CYANOSIS

Normal cutaneous and mucosal pigmentation is caused by several factors, one of which is the visualization of the capillary beds through the translucent dermis and epidermis. Cyanosis manifests as a blue or violaceous appearance of the skin, mucous membranes, and nailbeds. It occurs when excessive concentrations of reduced hemoglobin (>5g/dL) are present, as in hypoxia or polycythemia, or when oxidation of the iron moiety of heme to the ferric state forms methemoglobin, which is deeply pigmented (Chap. 127). The presence of the more deeply colored hemoglobin moiety within the dermal plexus results in cyanosis that is most pronounced on the skin surfaces with the least overlying tissue, such as the mucous membranes or fingernails.

XANTHODERMA

Xanthoderma is a yellow to yellow-orange macular discoloration of skin.[16] Xanthoderma can be caused by xenobiotics such as carotenoids, which deposit in the stratum corneum, and causes carotenoderma. Carotenoids are lipid soluble and consist of α-carotene, β-carotene, β-cryptoxanthin, lycopene, lutein, and zeaxanthan, and serve as precursors of vitamin A (retinol). The carotenoids are excreted via sweat, sebum, urine, and GI secretions.

Jaundice is typically a sign of hepatocellular failure or hemolysis and is caused by hyperbilirubinemia either conjugated or unconjugated, a condition in which the yellow pigment deposits in the subcutaneous fat. True hyperbilirubinemia is differentiated from hypercarotenemia by the presence of scleral icterus in patients with the former which is absent in patients with the latter. In addition, the cutaneous discoloration seen in hypercarotenemia can be removed by wiping the skin with an alcohol swab. Lycopenemia, an entity similar to carotenemia, is caused by the excessive consumption of tomatoes. Additionally, topical exposure to dinitrophenol or picric acid or stains from cigarette use produces localized yellow discoloration of the skin.

URTICARIAL DRUG REACTIONS

Urticarial drug reactions are characterized by transient, pruritic, edematous, pink papules, or wheals that arise in the dermis, which blanch on palpation and are frequently associated with central clearing. Approximately 40% of patients with urticaria experience angioedema and anaphylactoid reactions as well.[1] The reaction pattern is representative of a type I, or IgE-dependent, immune reaction and commonly occurs as part of clinical anaphylaxis or anaphylactoid (non–IgE-mediated) reactions. Widespread urticaria may occur following systemic absorption of an allergen or following a minimal localized exposure in patients highly sensitized to the allergen. Following limited exposure, a localized form of urticaria also may occur. Regardless of the specific clinical presentation, the reaction occurs when immunologic recognition occurs between IgE molecules and a putative antigen triggering the immediate degranulation of mast cells, which are distributed along the dermal blood vessels, nerves, and appendages. The release of histamine, complements C3a and C5a, and other vasoactive mediators result in leakage of fluid from dermal capillaries as their endothelial cells contract. This produces the characteristic urticarial lesions described above. Activation of the nearby sensory neurons produces pruritus. Nonimmunologically mediated mast cell degranulation producing an identical urticarial syndrome may also occur, following exposure to any xenobiotic.[8]

Pruritus is a common manifestation of urticarial reactions, but it may also be of nonimmunologic origin. Patients with hepatocellular disease frequently suffer from pruritus, which is mediated by the release of bile acids. In addition, in patients with chronic liver disease and obstructive jaundice, pruritus can be caused by central mechanisms, as suggested by elevated central nervous system (CNS) endogenous opioid concentrations. Pruritus can also be caused by topical exposure to the urticating hairs of Tarantula spiders, spines of the stinging nettle plant (*Urtica spp*), or via stimulation of substance P by certain xenobiotics such as capsaicin.[15]

Xenobiotics can also evoke a type III immune reaction that causes mast cells to degranulate. The cellular inflammatory response to released chemotactic factors leads to increased vascular permeability.

FLUSHING

Vasodilation of the dermal arterioles leads to flushing. Flushing can occur following autonomically-mediated vasodilation, as occurs with stress, anger, or exposure to heat, or it can be chemically induced by vasoactive xenobiotics. Those xenobiotics that cause histamine release through a type I hypersensitivity reaction are the most frequent cause of xenobiotic-induced flush. Histamine and saurine poisoning can result from the consumption of scombrotoxic fish, and can produce flushing. Flushing after the consumption of ethanol is common in patients of Asian and Inuit descent and is similar to the reaction following ethanol consumption in patients exposed to disulfiram or similar agents (Chap. 79). The increased production of and inability to efficiently metabolize acetaldehyde, the initial metabolite of ethanol, results in the characteristic syndrome of vomiting, headache, and flushing. Niacin causes flushing through an arachidonic acid–mediated pathway that is generally prevented by aspirin.[5,38] Vancomycin if too rapidly infused causes a transient bright red flushing, mediated by histamine. This reaction typically occurs during and immediately after the infusion, and is termed "red man syndrome." Other nontoxicologic causes of flushing including carcinoid syndrome, pheochromocytoma, mastocytosis, anaphylaxis, medullary carcinoma of the thyroid, pancreatic cancer, and renal carcinoma must be entertained in the flushed patient.[17]

SKIN MOISTURE

Xenobiotic-induced diaphoresis may be part of a physiologic response to heat generation or may be pharmacologically mediated following parasympathetic or sympathomimetic xenobiotic use. Because the postsynaptic receptor on the eccrine glands is muscarinic, most muscarinic agonists stimulate sweat production. Sweat most commonly occurs following exposure to cholinesterase inhibitors, such as organic phosphorus compounds, but it may also occur with direct-acting muscarinic agonists such as pilocarpine. Alternatively, antimuscarinic agents, such as belladonna alkaloids or antihistamines, reduce sweating and produce dry skin.

METALLIC PIGMENTATION

Pigmentary changes can result from the deposition of fine metallic particles. The particles can be ingested and carried to the skin by the blood, or may permeate the skin from topical applications. Argyria, a slate-colored pigmentation of the skin resulting from the systemic deposition of silver particles in the skin, can be localized or widespread. The discoloration tends to be most prominent in areas exposed to sunlight, probably secondary to the fact that silver stimulates melanocyte proliferation. Histologically, fine black granules are found in the basement membrane zone of the sweat glands, blood vessel walls, the dermoepidermal junction, and along the erector pili muscles (Chap. 99). Gold, which was historically used parenterally in the treatment of rheumatoid arthritis, caused a blue or slate-gray pigmentation known as *chrysiasis*. The pigmentation is also accentuated in light-exposed areas but, unlike in argyria, sun-protected areas do not histologically demonstrate gold. Also, melanin is not increased in the areas of hyperpigmentation. The hyperpigmentation is probably secondary to the gold itself, but the cause of its distribution pattern remains unknown. Histologically, the gold is distributed in a perivascular pattern in the dermis with granules accentuated at the basement membrane zone of sweat glands.

Bismuth produces a characteristic oral finding of the metallic deposition in the gums and tongue known as bismuth lines. Arsenic, which is found in certain pesticides and in contaminated well water, causes cutaneous hyperpigmentation with areas of scattered hypopigmentation. Chronic lead poisoning can produce a characteristic "lead hue" with pallor. Lead also deposits in the gums, causing the characteristic "lead line." Intramuscular injection of iron can cause staining of the skin, resulting in pigmentation similar to that seen in tattoos, and iron storage problems, known as *hemochromatosis*, can result in a bronze appearance of the skin.[11]

SPECIFIC SYNDROMES

Dermatology is a specialty whereby visual inspection may allow a rapid diagnosis. Some authors suggest a brief examination prior to a lengthy history due to some of the classic skin conditions with such obvious morphologies that a "doorway diagnosis" can be made. Irrespective of the initial complaint a total body examination with proper lighting needs to be accomplished on all patients. The tools the physician needs are readily available: magnifying glass, glass slide (diascopy), flashlight, alcohol pad to remove scale or makeup, scalpel, and at times a Wood lamp. Universal precautions should always be used.

The ability to describe lesions accurately is an important skill, as is the ability to recognize specific patterns. Such abilities help clinicians in their approach to the patient with a rash. Several cutaneous reaction patterns account for the majority of clinical presentations occurring in patients with xenobiotic-induced dermatotoxicity (Table 29–2).

Toxic epidermal necrolysis (TEN) and Stevens-Johnson syndrome (SJS) (Fig. 29–2) are considered to be related disorders that belong to a spectrum of increasingly severe skin failure.[27] Toxic epidermal necrosis is often considered to be the most severe manifestation of the spectrum of syndromes represented by erythema multiforme. Erythema multiforme is characterized by target-shaped, erythematous macules and patches on the palms and soles, as well as the trunk and extremities. The Nikolsky sign, consisting of sloughing of the epidermis when direct pressure is exerted on the skin lesion, is absent. Contact sensitization to sulfonamides, phenytoin, antihistamines, many antibiotics, dinitrochlorobenzene (DNCB), diphenylcyclopropenone (DPCP), isopropyl-*p*-phenylenediamine (IPPD), rosewood, and urushiol can elicit erythema multiforme. The Stevens-Johnson syndrome is considered to be an overlap reaction with erythema multiforme major when greater than 30% of body surface area is involved. However, although erythema multiforme shares many clinical characteristics with SJS/TEN, many now consider it as a distinct disease. It should also be noted that SJS occurs predominantly in children and TEN occurs in all age groups.

Toxic epidermal necrolysis is a rare, life-threatening dermatologic emergency with a 30% mortality. Its incidence is estimated at 0.4 to 1.2 cases per 1 million population, and xenobiotics are causally implicated in 80% to 95% of the cases. The cutaneous reaction pattern is characterized by tenderness and erythema of the skin and mucosa, followed by

TABLE 29–2. Xenobiotics Commonly Associated with Various Cutaneous Reaction Patterns

Acneiform
- ACTH
- Amoxapine
- Androgens
- Azathioprine
- Bromides
- Corticosteroids
- Danazol
- Dantrolene
- Halogenated hydrocarbons
- Iodides
- Isoniazid
- Lithium
- Oral contraceptives
- Phenytoin

Alopecia
- Anticoagulants
- Antineoplastics
- Hormones
- NSAIDs
- Phenytoin
- Radiation
- Retinoids
- Selenium
- Thallium

Contact dermatitis
- Bacitracin
- Balsam of Peru
- Benzocaine
- Carba mix
- Catechol
- Cobalt
- Diazolidinyl urea
- Ethylenediamine dihydrochloride
- Formaldehyde
- Fragrance mix
- Imidazolidinyl urea
- Lanolin
- Methylchloroisothiazolinone/methylisothiazolinone
- Neomycin sulfate
- Nickel
- *p*-Tert-butylphenol formaldehyde resin
- *p*-Phenylenediamine
- Quaternium-15
- Rosin (colophony)
- Sesquiterpene lactones
- Thimerosal

Erythema multiforme
- Antimicrobials
- Allopurinol
- Barbiturates
- Carbamazepine
- Cimetidine
- Codeine
- Gold
- Glutethimide
- Ethinyl estradiol
- Furosemide
- Ketoconazole
- Methaqualone
- NSAIDs
- Nitrogen mustard
- Phenolphthalein
- Phenothiazines
- Phenytoin
- Sulfonamides
- Thiazides

Exfoliative Dermatitis
- Allopurinol
- Anticonvulsants
- Calcium channel blockers
- Cimetidine
- Dapsone
- Gold
- Lithium
- Penicillins
- Quinidine
- Sulfonamides
- Vancomycin

Fixed drug eruptions
- Acetaminophen
- Allopurinol
- Barbiturates
- Captopril
- Carbamazepine
- Chloral hydrate
- Chlordiazepoxide
- Chlorpromazine
- Erythromycin
- D-Penicillamine
- Fiorinal
- Gold
- Griseofulvin
- Lithium
- Phenacetin
- Phenolphthalein
- Methaqualone
- Metronidazole
- Minocycline
- Naproxen
- NSAIDs
- Oral contraceptives
- Salicylates
- Sulindac

Maculopapular reactions
- Antimicrobials
- Anticonvulsants
- Antihypertensive agents
- Antiinflammatory agents

Photosensitivity reactions
- Amiodarone
- Benoxaprofen
- Chlorpromazine
- Ciprofloxacin
- Dacarbazine
- 5-Fluorouracil
- Furosemide
- Griseofulvin
- Hydrochlorothiazide
- Hematoporphyrin (Porphyria)
- Levofloxacin
- Nalidixic acid
- Naproxen
- Piroxicam
- Psoralen
- Sulfanilamide
- Tetracyclines
- Tolbutamide
- Vinblastine

Photoirritant contact dermatitis
- Celery
- Dispense blue 35
- Eosin
- Fig
- Fragrance materials
- Lime
- Parsnip
- Pitch

Toxic epidermal necrolysis
- Allopurinol
- L-Asparaginase
- Amoxapine
- Bactrim
- Mithramycin
- Nitrofurantoin
- NSAIDs
- Penicillin
- Phenytoin
- Prazosin
- Pyrimethamine–sulfadoxine
- Streptomycin
- Sulfonamides
- Sulfasalazine

Vasculitis
- Allopurinol
- Cefaclor
- Cimetidine
- Gold
- Hydralazine
- Levamisole
- Minocycline
- NSAIDs
- Penicillamine
- Penicillin
- Phenytoin
- Propylthiouracil

Vesiculobullous
- Amoxapine
- Barbiturates
- Captopril
- Carbon monoxide
- Chemotherapeutics
- Dipyridamole
- Furosemide
- Griseofulvin
- Penicillamine
- Penicillin
- Rifampin
- Sulfonamides

Xanthoderma
- Generalized
  - Hepatic jaundice (Acetominophen, isoniazid)
  - Hemolytic jaundice
  - Carotenoderma
    - Canthaxanthin (tanning pills)
  - Dipyridamole (yellow compound)
  - Quinacrine
- Localized
  - Dihydroxyacetone (spray tanning)
  - Picric acid
  - Methylenedianiline
  - Phenol, topical

Nail changes
Beau lines (Onychodystrophy) & Mees lines (Leukonychia)
- Cyclophosphamide
- Doxorubicin
- Hydroxyurea
- Paclitaxel

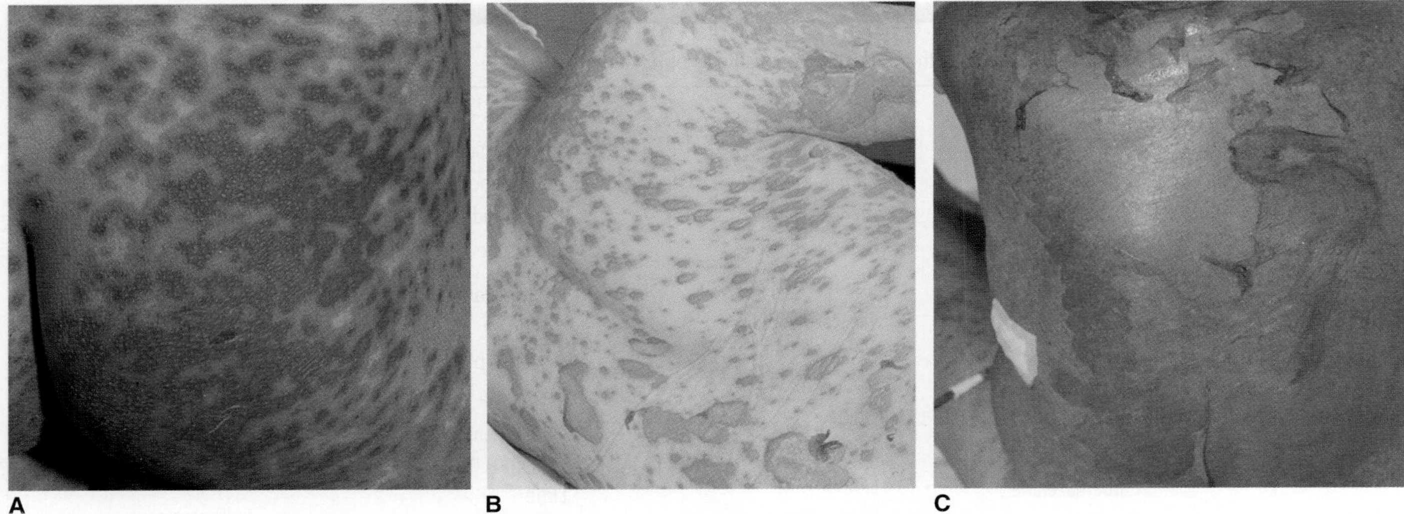

FIGURE 29–2. Toxic Epidermal Necrolysis **(A)** Early eruption. Erythematous dusky red macules (flat atypical target lesions) that progressively coalesce and show epidermal detachment. **(B)** Advanced eruption. Blisters and epidermal detachment have led to large confluent erosions. **(C)** Full-blown epidermal necrolysis characterized by large erosive areas reminiscent of scalding. (Reproduced, with permission, from Wolff K, Goldsmith LA, Katz SI, Gilchrest BA, Paller AS, Lefferell DJ. *Fitzpatrick's Dermatology in General Medicine.*, 7th ed. McGraw-Hill, 2008.)

extensive cutaneous and mucosal exfoliation. The incidence is higher in HIV-infected patients with advanced disease. [27,36] There is general agreement that the keratinocyte cell death in TEN is the result of *apoptosis* not *necrosis*. Furthermore, apoptosis is suggested based on electronic microscopic studies with DNA fragmentation analysis.[27]

Greater than 220 xenobiotics are implicated in causing TEN. Classically, the eruption is painful and occurs within days of the exposure to the implicated xenobiotic(s). The eruption is preceded by malaise, headache, abrupt onset of fever, myalgia, arthralgia, nausea, vomiting, diarrhea, chest pain, or cough. Initially, a macular erythema develops that subsequently becomes raised and morbilliform ("measles-like"). The face, neck, and central trunk are usually the initial areas affected. The disease generally progresses to involve the extremities and with the remainder of the body the lesions progress over a period of 2 to 15 days. Individual lesions are reminiscent of target lesions because of their dusky centers. The entire thickness of the epidermis, including the nails, becomes necrotic and may slough off. The mucosal surfaces of the lips, oropharynx, conjunctivae, vagina, urethra, and anus may show erythema and sloughing. This mucositis precedes the skin lesions by a few days.[30] A Nikolsky sign may occur,[3] and although suggestive, is not pathognomonic of TEN as it occurs in a variety of other dermatoses, including pemphigus vulgaris. If the diagnosis is suspected, a biopsy should be performed and treatment initiated immediately. The histopathology typically shows partial- or full-thickness epidermal necrosis, with subepidermal bullae with a sparse infiltrate, and vacuolization with numerous dyskeratotic keratinocytes along the dermoepidermal junction adjacent to the necrotic epidermis. Cytotoxic T lymphocytes are the main effector cells and experimental evidence points to involvement of both the Fas-Fas ligand and perforin/granzyme pathways. Anemia and lymphopenia are common, neutropenia portends a poor prognosis. Early stages consist mainly of CD8 lymphocytes in the epidermis and blisters containing CD4 lymphocytes in dermis.

Removal of the inciting xenobiotic as soon as possible is critical to survival. Patients with TEN related to a xenobiotic with a long half-life have poorer prognosis, and should be transferred to a burn or other specialized center for sterile wound care. The use of porcine xenografts or human skin allografts including amniotic membrane transplantation has been utilized and is a widely accepted therapy.[29] Although glucocorticoids are not generally recommended, there is emerging support for the use of immunosuppressive or immunomodulatory agents, such as intravenous immunoglobulins, cyclophosphamide, and cyclosporine.[29] Reported mortality is as great as 30%, particularly in patients with gastrointestinal and tracheobronchial involvement.[36] The "acute skin failure" patients have metabolic abnormalities, sepsis, multiorgan failure, pulmonary emboli and gastrointestinal hemorrhages. The major causes of sepsis is *S. aureus* and *P. aerogenosa*. In a patient with SJS/TEN with ophthalmologic complications early ophthalmologic consultation is necessary because blindness is a potential complication.

Simulators of TEN include staphylococcal scalded skin syndrome; linear IgA dermatosis: paraneoplastic pemphigus; acute graft versus host disease; drug-induced pemphigoid and pemphigus vulgaris and acute generalized exanthematous pustulosis; discussion of these entities is beyond the scope of the chapter.

BLISTERING REACTIONS

Xenobiotic-related cutaneous blistering reactions may be clinically indistinguishable from autoimmune blistering reactions, such as pemphigus vulgaris or bullous pemphigoid (Fig. 29–3). Certain topically-applied xenobiotics cause blistering by disrupting the anchoring filaments of basal cell desmosomes at the dermal–epidermal junction. In high concentrations, the xenobiotics can lead to necrosis of both skin and mucous membranes. Other xenobiotics cause a similar reaction pattern mediated by the production of antibody directed against the cells at the dermal–epidermal junction (Table 29–3).

A number of medications, many of which contain a "thiol group" such as penicillamine and captopril, can induce either pemphigus, a superficial blistering disorder in which the blister is at the level of the stratum corneum, or pemphigus vulgaris, in which blistering occurs at the suprabasilar level (see Fig. 29–1). Other xenobiotics, such as diuretics, produce the tense bullae that resemble pemphigoid. Immunofluorescence studies might show epidermal intracellular immunoglobulin deposits at the dermal–epidermal junction. Treatment options include immunosuppressants. The reaction may persist for up to 6 months after the offending xenobiotic is withdrawn.

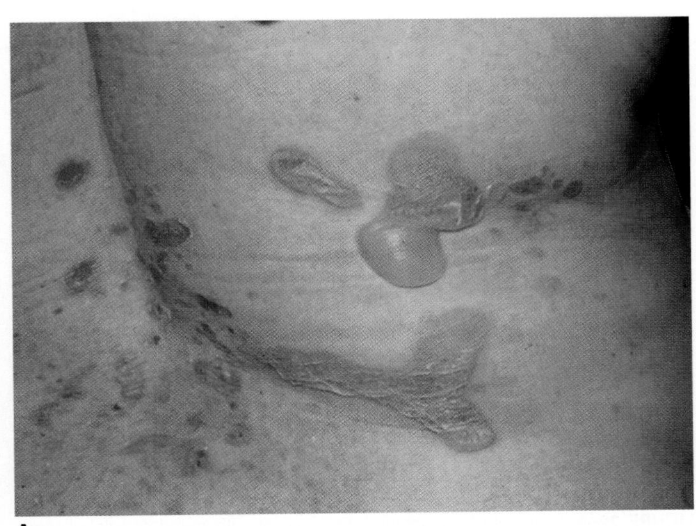
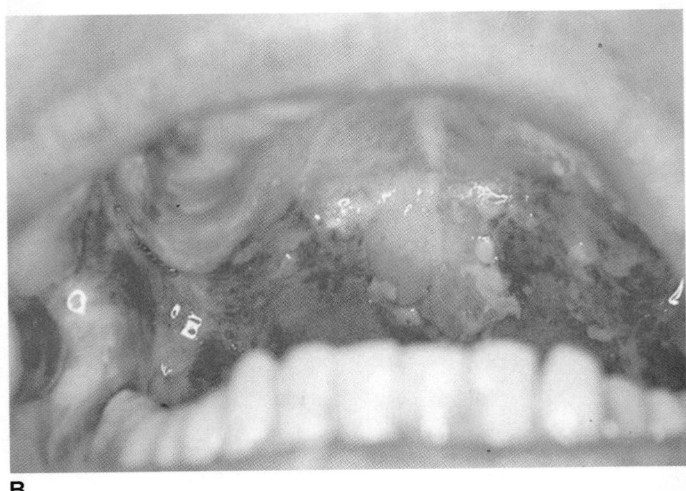

A B

FIGURE 29–3. Pemphigus vulgaris. **(A)** Flaccid blisters. **(B)** Oral erosions. (Part **A,** contributed by Lawrence Lieblich, MD. Part **B,** reproduced, with permission, from Wolff K, Goldsmith LA, Katz SI, Gilchrest BA, Paller AS, Lefferell D. *Fitzpatrick's Dermatology in General Medicine,* 7th ed. McGraw-Hill, 2008.)

"Coma bullae" are flaccid bullae that occur occasionally in patients with sedative-hypnotic overdoses, particularly phenobarbital, or carbon monoxide poisoning. Although these blisters are thought to result predominantly from pressure-induced epidermal necrosis, they occasionally occur in non–pressure-dependent areas, suggesting a systemic mechanism. An intraepidermal or subepidermal blister may occur. There is accompanying eccrine duct and gland necrosis.

BULLOUS DRUG ERUPTIONS

Multiple, large, ill-defined, dull, purplish-livid patches sometimes accompanied by large flaccid blisters characterize these eruptions. Typical locations include acral extremities, genitals, and intertriginous sites, and this process may be confused with TEN if widely confluent. However, bullous drug eruptions spare the mucous membranes. This reaction pattern is generally not life-threatening. Bullous fixed-drug reactions result from exposure to diverse medications such as angiotensin converting enzyme inhibitors and a multitude of antibiotics.

The drug hypersensitivity syndrome known as drug rash with eosinophilia and systemic symptoms (DRESS) can be severe and potentially life threatening. The skin may be involved with systemic xenobiotic-induced immunologic diseases. The hypersensitivity syndromes are characterized by the triad of fever, skin eruption, and internal organ involvement.[20] The frequency has been estimated between 1 in 1000 to 1 in 10,000 with anticonvulsants or sulfonamide antibiotic exposures and usually begins within 2 to 6 weeks after the initial exposure.

TABLE 29–3. Differential Diagnosis of Xenobiotic-induced Blistering Disorders

Disease	Fever	Mucositis	Morphology	Onset	Miscellaneous
Xenobiotic-induced pemphigoid	No	Rare	Tense bullae (sometimes hemorrhagic)	Acute	Diuretics a common cause, especially spironolactone; often pruritic
Staphylococcal scalded skin syndrome	Yes	Absent	Erythema, skin tenderness, periorificial crusting	Acute	Affects children < 5 years, adults on dialysis, and those on immunosuppressive therapy
Xenobiotic-induced pemphigus	No	Usually absent	Erosions, crusts, patchy erythema (resembles pemphigus foliaceous)	Gradual	Commonly caused by penicillamine and other "thiol" drugs; resolves after inciting inciting agent is discontinued
Xenobiotic-triggered pemphigus	No	Present	Mucosal erosions, flaccid bullae	Gradual	Caused by "non-thiol" drugs; persists after discontinuation of drug; may require long-term immunosuppressive therapy
Paraneoplastic pemphigus	No	Present (usually severe)	Polymorphous skin lesions, flaccid bullae	Gradual	Resistant to treatment; associated with malignancy, especially lymphoma
Acute graft-versus host disease	Yes	Present	Morbilliform rash, bullae and erosions	Acute	Closely resembles TEN
Acute generalized exanthematous	Yes	Rare	Superficial pustules	Acute	Self-limiting on discontinuation of drug
Xenobiotic-induced linear IgA bullous dermatosis	No	Rare	Tense, subepidermal bullae	Acute	Vancomycin is most commonly implicated

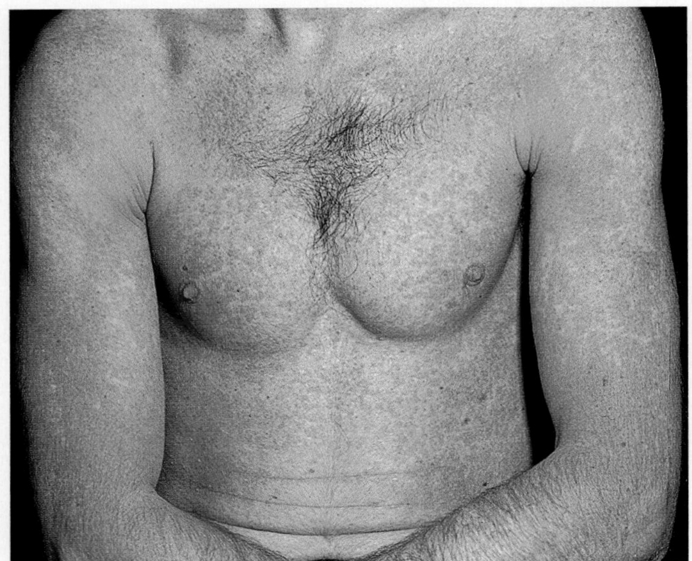

FIGURE 29–4. A patient with a hypersensitivity syndrome associated with phenytoin. He has a symmetric, bright red, and exanthematous eruption, confluent in some sites. The patient had associated lymphadenopathy. (Reproduced with permission from Klaus Wolff; Richard Allen Johnson. *Fitzpatrick's Color Atlas and Synopsis of Clinical Dermatology,* 6e, p. 22-10. McGraw-Hill, 2009.)

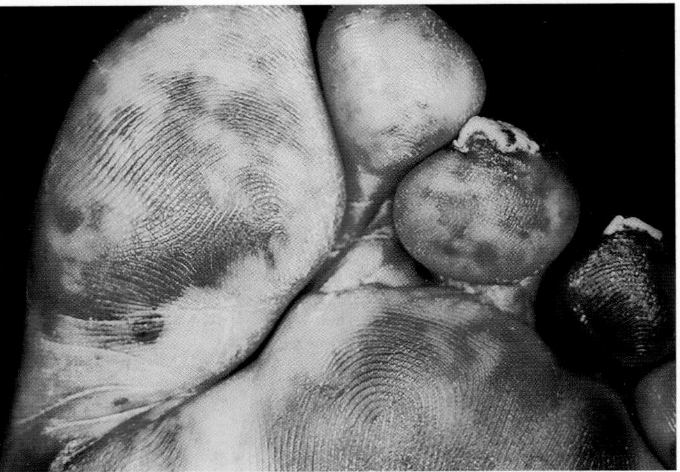

FIGURE 29–5. Leukocytoclastic vasculitis in a patient with mixed cryoglobulinemia manifested as palpable purpura and acrocyanosis. Patient with tuberculosis, positive antinuclear antibody, and hepatitis.(Reproduced, with permission, from Wolff K, Goldsmith LA, Katz SI, Gilchrest BA, Paller AS, Lefferell DJ. *Fitzpatrick's Dermatology in General Medicine,* 7th ed. McGraw-Hill, 2008.)

Fever, malaise, pharyngitis and cervical lymphodenpathy are the usual presenting clinical findings. Atypical lymphocytes and eosinophilia, occur initially. The exanthem is generalized and conjunctivitis and angioedema may occur. One-half of these patients have hepatitis, interstitial nephritis, vasculitis, CNS manifestations (including encephalitis, aseptic meningitis), interstitial pneumonitis, ARDS, and autoimmune hypothyroidism. Colitis with bloody diarrhea and abdominal pain may occur. The aromatic anticonvulsants, allopurinol, sulfonamide antibiotics, and dapsone are the common xenobiotics that induce this syndrome. Treatment is supportive.[26,39] Although the role of systemic corticosteroids is controversial; most clinicians start prednisone at a dose of 1–2 mg/kg/d if symptoms are severe.

EXFOLIATIVE ERYTHRODERMAS

Exfoliative erythrodermic eruptions (Fig. 29–4) can result from any xenobiotic and are characterized by widespread erythema and scale with the potential for multisystem organ failure. The process may persist for months. Such patients require aggressive fluid and electrolyte repletion and nutritional support. Boric acid toxicity causes a bright red eruption ("lobster skin"), followed usually within 1 to 3 days by a generalized exfoliation.

VASCULITIS

Xenobiotic-induced vasculitis (Fig. 29–5) comprises 10% of acute cutaneous vasculitides. It generally occurs from 7 to 21 days after exposure to the xenobiotic and is a small vessel disease. Hypersensitivity vasculitis is characterized by purpuric, nonblanching macules that usually become raised and palpable. The purpura tends to occur predominantly on gravity-dependent areas, including the lower extremities, feet, and buttocks. Sometimes the reaction pattern can have edematous purpuric wheals (urticarial vasculitis), hemorrhagic bullae, or ulcerations. The underlying cytopathology consistently shows a leukocytoclastic vasculitis, which is characterized by fibrin deposition in the vessel walls. There is a perivascular infiltrate with intact and fragmented neutrophils that appear as black dots, known as "nuclear dust," visible only by electron microscopy. This reaction pattern may be limited to the skin, or may be more serious and involve other organ systems, particularly the kidneys, joints, liver, lungs, and brain. The purpura results from circulating immune complexes, which form as a result of a hypersensitivity to a xenobiotic. Treatment consists of withdrawing the putative agent and systemic corticosteroid therapy.

Purpura Purpura is the multifocal extravasation of blood into the skin or mucous membranes (Fig. 29–6). Ecchymoses are, therefore, considered to be purpuric lesions. Cytotoxic medications that either diffusely suppress the bone marrow or specifically depress platelet counts below 30,000/mm^3, predispose to purpuric macules. Xenobiotics that interfere with platelet aggregation, such as, aspirin, clopidogrel, ticlopidine, and valproic acid, may cause purpura, as may thrombolytics. Anticoagulants, such as heparin and warfarin, may also result in purpura (Chaps. 24 and 59).

Anticoagulant Skin Necrosis Skin necrosis from warfarin, low molecular weight heparin, or unfractionated heparin usually begins 3 to 5 days after the initiation of treatment (Fig. 29–7). The estimated risk is 1 in 10,000 persons. It is four times higher in women especially if obese with peaks in sixth to seventh decades. The necrosis is secondary to thrombus formation in vessels of the dermis and subcutaneous fat. There may be blisters, ecchymosis, ulcers, and massive subcutaneous necrosis, usually in areas of abundant subcutaneous fat, such as the breasts, buttocks, abdomen, thighs, and calves. It may be associated with protein C or S deficiency, anticardiolipin antibody syndrome, as well as Factor V Leiden mutations.[28] Of note is acute generalized exanthematous pustulosis from dalteparin is reported.[21]

Treatment involves stopping the medication, administration of vitamin K and, if coumarin induced, changing to heparin. Treatment may include fresh frozen plasma and Protein C. Skin grafting may be necessary if full thickness necrosis occurs.

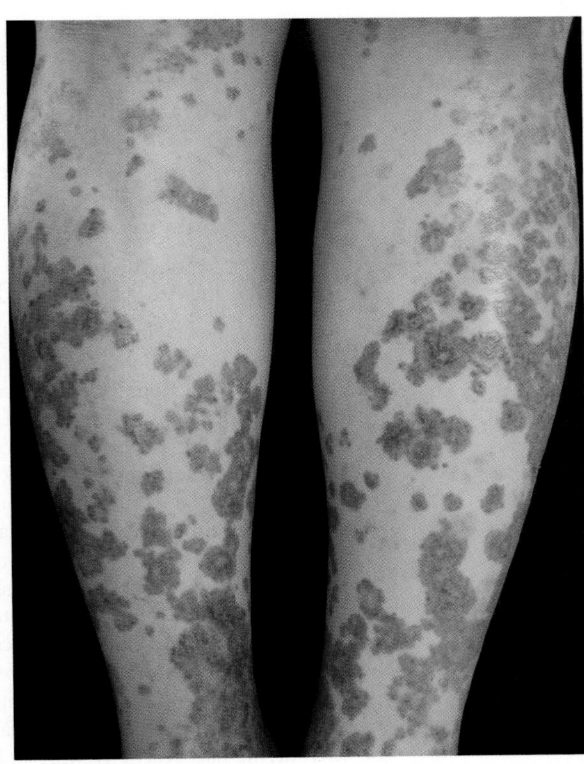

FIGURE 29–6. Purpura. Non-blanching red erythematous papules and plaques (palpable purpura) on the legs, representing leukocytoclastic vasculitis. (Reproduced, with permission, from Wolff K, Goldsmith LA, Katz SI, Gilchrest BA, Paller AS, Lefferell DJ. *Fitzpatrick's Dermatology in General Medicine,* 7th ed. McGraw-Hill, 2008.)

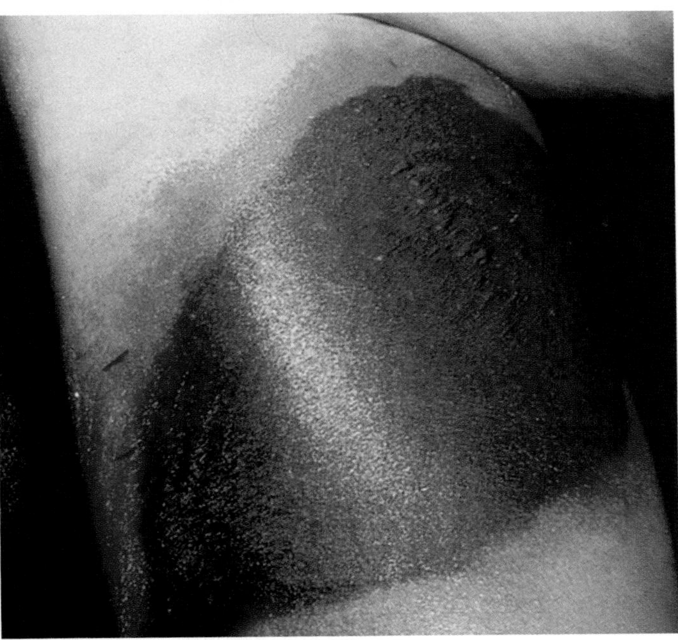

FIGURE 29–7. Skin necrosis in a patient after 4 days of warfarin therapy. (Reproduced, with permission, from Wolff K, Goldsmith LA, Katz SI, Gilchrest BA, Paller AS, Lefferell DJ. *Fitzpatrick's Dermatology in General Medicine,* 7th ed. McGraw-Hill, 2008.)

CONTACT DERMATITIS

When a xenobiotic comes in contact with the skin, it can result in either an allergic contact dermatitis or an irritant dermatitis. Contact dermatitis is characterized by inflammation of the skin with spongiosis (intercellular edema) of the epidermis that results from the interaction of a xenobiotic with the skin. Erythema, induration, pruritus, or blistering may be noted on areas in direct contact with the xenobiotic, while the remaining areas are spared.

Allergic contact dermatitis fits into the classic delayed hypersensitivity, or type IV, immunologic reaction. The development of this reaction requires prior sensitization to an allergen, which, in most cases, acts as a hapten by binding with an endogenous molecule that is then presented to an appropriate immunologic T cell. Upon reexposure, the hapten diffuses to the Langerhans cell, is chemically altered, bound to an HLA-DR, and the complex is expressed on the Langerhans cell surface. This complex interacts with primed T cells either in the skin or lymph nodes, causing the Langerhans cells to make interleukin-1 and the activated T cells to make interleukin-2 and interferon. This subsequently activates the keratinocytes to produce cytokines and eicosanoids that activate mast cells and macrophages, leading to an inflammatory response (Fig. 29–8).[19]

Many allergens are associated with contact dermatitis; a complete list is beyond the scope of this chapter. Among the most common plant-derived sensitizers are urushiol (poison ivy), sesquiterpene lactone (ragweed), and tuliposide A (tulip bulbs). Metals, particularly nickel, are commonly implicated in contact dermatitis. Several industrial chemicals, such as the thiurams (rubber) and urea formaldehyde resins (plastics), account for the majority of occupational contact dermatitis. Medications, particularly topical medications such as neomycin, commonly cause contact dermatitis. Management strategies commonly employed are outlined in Table 29–4.

Irritant dermatitis, although clinically indistinguishable, results from direct damage to the skin and does not require prior antigen sensitization. Still, the inflammatory response to the initial mild insult is the cause of the majority of the damage. Irritant xenobiotics include acids, bases, solvents, and detergents, many of which, in their concentrated form or following prolonged exposure, can cause direct cellular injury. The specific site of damage varies with the chemical nature of the xenobiotic. Many xenobiotics can affect the lipid membrane of the keratinocyte, whereas others can diffuse through the membrane, injuring the lysosomes, mitochondria, or nuclear components. When the cell membrane is injured, phospholipases are activated and affect the release of arachidonic acid and the synthesis of eicosanoids. The second-messenger system is then activated, leading to the expression of genes and the synthesis of various cell surface molecules and cytokines. Interleukin-1 is secreted, which can activate T cells directly and indirectly by stimulation of granulocyte-macrophage colony-stimulating factor production. Treatment is similar to contact dermatitis.

PHOTOSENSITIVITY REACTIONS

Photosensitivity may be caused by topical or systemic xenobiotics. Nonionizing radiation, particularly to ultraviolet A (320–400 nm) and less often to ultraviolet B (280–320 nm) are the wavelengths that commonly cause the photosensitivity diagnosis. There are generally two types of xenobiotic related reaction patterns: phototoxic and photoallergic.[25] *Phototoxic* drug reactions occur within 24 hours of the first dose and are dose-related. These reactions result from direct tissue injury caused by the absorption by the xenobiotics of activating

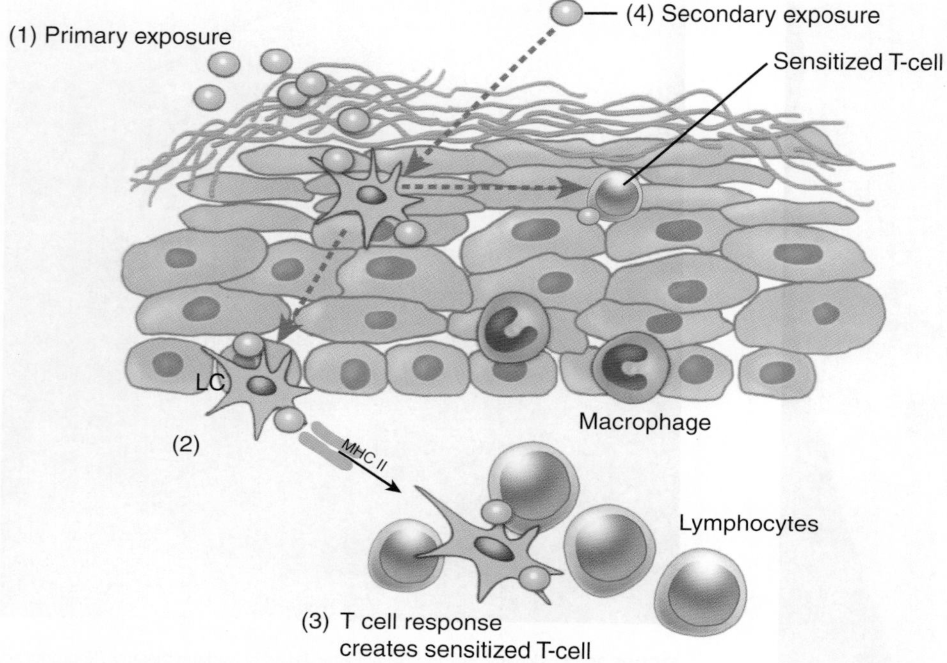

FIGURE 29–8. Contact dermatitis. **(1)** Causative xenobiotic, typically a hapten of < 500 daltons, diffuses through stratum corneum and binds to receptor on Langerhans cell (LC). **(2)** The antigen is processed with major histocompatibility complex II (MHC II) receptor site, presented to T-helper lymphocytes, and carried through the lymphatics to regional lymph nodes. **(3)** There it undergoes the sensitization phase by producing memory, effector, and suppressor T lymphocytes. **(4)** On reexposure to the same, or to a cross-reactive antigen, the LC represents the antigen to T lymphocytes (··········➤), which are now sensitized. This initiates an inflammatory process that appears as indurated, scaly patches. NK, Natural Killer.

wavelengths of nonionizing radiation. The clinical findings include erythema, edema, and vesicles in a light-exposed distribution, and resemble an exaggerated sunburn that can last for days to weeks (Fig. 29–9). *Photoallergic reactions* occur less commonly, may occur following even small exposures, and are characterized by lichenoid papules or eczematous changes on exposed areas. These are type IV hypersensitivity reactions that develop in response to a xenobiotic that has been altered by absorption of nonionizing radiation, acting as a hapten and eliciting an immune response on first exposure. Only on recurrent exposure do to the lesions typically develop. Photoallergic reactions can be diagnosed by the use of patch tests. Both phototoxic and photoallergic reactions are managed with symptomatic therapy, including topical or, if needed, systemic corticosteroids. The patient should be advised to avoid sun exposure or wear a sunscreen that blocks both ultraviolet A and ultraviolet B with a sun protection factor (SPF) of 15 or greater and is devoid of para-aminobenzoic acid (PABA), a sensitizing agent to many patients.

TABLE 29–4. Overview of Treatment of Acute Contact Dermatitis

Avoidance
Drying agents, such as topical aluminum sulfate/calcium acetate: if weeping
Emollients: lichenified lesions
Corticosteroids, topical, rarely systemic: for severe reactions
Calcineurin inhibitors
Cyclosporin (oral)
Tacrolimus or picrolimus
Phototherapy, UVA or UVB

SCLERODERMA-LIKE REACTIONS

A number of environmental xenobiotics are associated with a localized or diffuse scleroderma-like reactions. Sclerodermatous changes refer to a tightened indurated surface change of the skin. These typically occur on the face, hands, forearms, and trunk and are three times more common in women. This may be accompanied by facial telangiectasias and Raynaud syndrome. Raynaud syndrome consists of skin color changes of white, blue, and red accompanied by intense pain with exposure to cold, and can cause acral ulcerations, if untreated. The fibrotic process usually does not remit with removal of the external stimulus. The association of scleroderma-like reactions with polyvinyl chloride manufacture is likely related to exposure to vinyl chloride monomer. Similar reports of this syndrome are associated with exposure to trichloroethylene and perchlorethylene, which are structurally similar to vinyl chloride. Epoxy resins, silica, and organic solvents have been implicated as environmental causes. The xenobiotics bleomycin, carbidopa, pentazocine are causative.

In Spain, patients exposed to imported rapeseed oil mixed with an aniline denaturant developed widespread cutaneous sclerosis. This became known as the "toxic oil syndrome." A similar syndrome, following ingestion of impure L-tryptophan as a dietary supplement, used as a sleeping aid resulted in the eosinophilia myalgia syndrome, which is characterized by myalgia, paralysis, edema, arthralgias, alopecia, urticaria, mucinous yellow papules, and erythematous plaques.[33]

HAIR LOSS

Anagen effluvium, hair loss during the anagen stage of the growth cycle, is caused by interruption of the rapidly dividing cells of the hair matrix producing rapid hair loss. *Telogen effluvium*, or toxicity during the resting stage of the cycle, might not produce hair loss for 2 to 4 weeks. Anagen toxicity is the most common mechanism and occurs with chemotherapeutics such as doxorubicin, cyclophosphamide, vincristine, and thallium exposures.[35] Many antineoplastics reduce the mitotic activity of the rapidly dividing hair matrix cells, leading to the formation of a thin shaft that breaks easily topical minoxidil may hasten resolution of the alopecia. Thallium, a toxin classically associated with hair loss, causes alopecia by two mechanisms. Thallium distributes intracellularly, like potassium, altering potassium-mediated processes and thereby disrupting protein synthesis. By binding sulfhydryl groups, thallium also inhibits the normal incorporation of cysteine into keratin. Selenium may produce alopecia by similar mechanisms. Thallium toxicity results in alopecia 1 to 4 weeks after exposure. Within 4 days of exposure a hair mount observed using light microscopy will demonstrate tapered or bayonet anagen hair with a characteristic

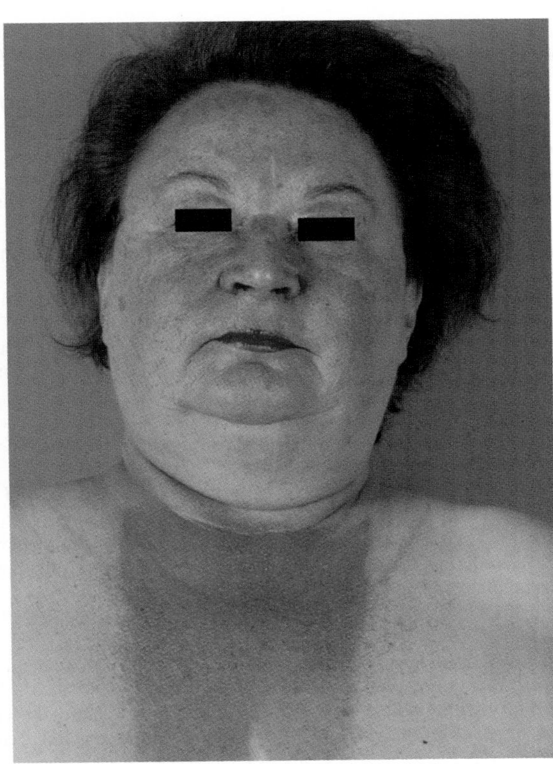

FIGURE 29–9. Phototoxicity associated with a heterocyclic antidepressant. Note erythema and edema on sun-exposed areas and sparing of sun-protected chest and shaded upper lip and neck. (Photo contributed by Dr. Adrian Tanew. Reproduced, with permission, from Wolff K, Goldsmith LA, Katz SI, Gilchrest BA, Paller AS, Lefferell DJ. *Fitzpatrick's Dermatology in General Medicine,* 7th ed. McGraw-Hill, 2008.)

bandlike black pigmentation at the base. Seeing this anagen effect can reveal the timing of exposure (Chap. 100).

Soluble barium salts, such as barium sulfide, are applied topically as a depilatory to produce localized hair loss. The mechanism of hair loss is undefined.

NAILS

The nail consists of a horny layer the "nail plate" and four specialized epithelia: proximal nail fold, nail matrix, nail bed and hyponychium. The nail matrix consists of keratinocytes, melanocytes, Langerhans cells and Merkel cells.

Nail hyperpigmentation occurs for unclear reasons, but may be caused by focal stimulation of melanocytes in the nail matrix. The pigment deposition can be longitudinal, diffuse, or perilunar in orientation, and typically develop several weeks after chemotherapy.[35] Black dark-skinned patients are more commonly affected due to a higher concentration of melanocytes. Cyclophosphamide, doxorubicin, hydroxyurea, and bleomycin are most often implicated in nail hyperpigmentation, and the pigmentation generally resolves with cessation of therapy.

Nail findings may serve as important clues to xenobiotic exposures that have occurred in the recent past. Matrix keratinization in a programmed and scheduled pattern, leads to the formation of the nail plate. Certain changes in nails, such as Mees lines and Beau lines, result from a temporary arrest of the proximal nail matrix proliferation. These lines can be used to predict the timing of a toxic exposure because of the reliability of rate of growth of the nails at approximately 0.1 mm per day. Mees lines, first described in 1919 in the setting of arsenic poisoning, can be used to approximate the date of the insult by the position of growth of the Mees line a patterned leukonychia (not indentation) causing transverse white lines.[23] Multiple Mees lines suggests multiple exposures. Arsenic, thallium, doxorubicin, vincristine, cyclophosphamide, methotrexate, and 5 fluorouracil are examples of xenobiotics that cause Mees lines, but Mees lines may be noted after any period of critical illness such as sepsis or trauma. Beau lines, or onychodystrophy, are transverse grooves or indentations that are similar to Mees lines in origin and etiology (Fig. 29–10).

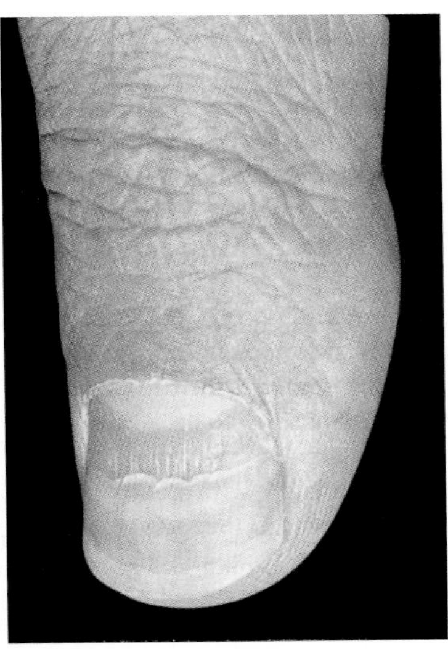

FIGURE 29–10. Presence of proximal indented Beau line and distal band of leukonychia due to cyclophosphamide 3 months after bone marrow transplantation. (Reproduced, with permission, from Wolff K, Goldsmith LA, Katz SI, Gilchrest BA, Paller AS, Lefferell DJ. *Fitzpatrick's Dermatology in General Medicine,* 7th ed. McGraw-Hill, 2008.)

SUMMARY

The integument is constantly exposed to both topical and systemic xenobiotics and the exposure may result in reactive dermatoses. Prompt attention and diagnosis is imperative in treating such exposures. The skin, hair, and nails may provide invaluable clues about the route and nature of the xenobiotic. With a careful history, clinical examination, and appropriate biopsy when indicated the etiology and nature of the reaction can be ascertained and treatment initiated in a timely and an effective manner.

ACKNOWLEDGMENT

Dr. Dina Began contributed to this chapter in previous editions.

REFERENCES

1. Amar SM, Dreskin SC. Urticaria. *Prim Care.* 2008;35:141-57, vii–viii.
2. Baden HP. Biology of the epidermis and pathophysiology of psoriasis and certain ichthyosiform dermatoses. In: Soter, Nicholas A and Baden, Howard P. eds. *Pathophysiology of Dermatologic Diseases.* 2nd ed. New York: McGraw-Hill; 1991:131-158.
3. Bastuji-Garin S, Rzany B, Stern RS, Shear NH, Naldi L, Roujeau JC. Clinical classification of cases of toxic epidermal necrolysis, Stevens-Johnson syndrome, and erythema multiforme. *Arch Dermatol.* 1993;129:92-96.
4. Bertolini JC. Hydrofluoric acid: a review of toxicity. *J Emerg Med.* 1992;10:163-168.

5. Brown BG. Expert commentary: niacin safety. *Am J Cardiol.* 2007;99:32C-34C.
6. Burgess JL, Kirk M, Borron SW, Cisek J. Emergency department hazardous materials protocol for contaminated patients. *Ann Emerg Med.* 1999;34:205-212.
7. Cartotto RC, Peters WJ, Neligan PC, Douglas LG, Beeston J. Chemical burns. *Can J Surg.* 1996;39:205-211.
8. Clark S, Camargo CA Jr. Epidemiology of anaphylaxis. *Immunol Allergy Clin North Am.* 2007;27:145-63,v.
9. Czerwinski SE, Skvorak JP, Maxwell DM, Lenz DE, Baskin SI. Effect of octanol: water partition coefficients of organophosphorus compounds on biodistribution and percutaneous toxicity. *J Biochem Mol Toxicol.* 2006;20:241-246.
10. Fartasch M, Diepgen TL: The barrier function in atopic dry skin. Disturbance of membrane-coating granule exocytosis and formation of epidermal lipids? *Acta Derm Venereol Suppl (Stockh).* 1992;176:26-31.
11. Granstein RD, Sober AJ. Drug- and heavy metal-induced hyperpigmentation. *J Am Acad Dermatol.* 1981;5:1-18.
12. Groscurth P. Anatomy of sweat glands. *Curr Probl Dermatol.* 2002;30:1-9.
13. Guy RH, Hadgraft J. Physicochemical aspects of percutaneous penetration and its enhancement. *Pharm Res.* 1988;5:753-758.
14. Hadgraft J, Lane ME. Skin permeation: the years of enlightenment. *Int J Pharm.* 2005;305:2-12.
15. Harvell J, Bason M, Maibach H. Contact urticaria and its mechanisms. *Food Chem Toxicol.* 1994;32:103-112.
16. Haught JM, Patel S, English JC 3rd. Xanthoderma: a clinical review. *J Am Acad Dermatol.* 2007;57:1051-1058.
17. Izikson L, English JC 3rd, Zirwas MJ. The flushing patient: differential diagnosis, workup, and treatment. *J Am Acad Dermatol.* 2006;55:193-208.
18. Duragesic [package insert]. Janssen, division of Ortho-McNeil-Janssen Pharmaceuticals. Titusville, New Jersey. 2008.
19. Kligman AM. The spectrum of contact urticaria. Wheals, erythema, and pruritus. *Dermatol Clin.* 1990;8:57-60.
20. Knowles SR, Shear NH. Recognition and management of severe cutaneous drug reactions. *Dermatol Clin.* 2007;25:245-53,viii.
21. Komericki P, Grims R, Kranke B, Aberer W. Acute generalized exanthematous pustulosis from dalteparin. *J Am Acad Dermatol.* 2007;57:718-721.
22. Lebwohl M, Herrmann LG. Impaired skin barrier function in dermatologic disease and repair with moisturization. *Cutis.* 2005;76:7-12.
23. Mees RA. Een verschijnsel bij polyneuritis arsenicosa. *Ned Tijdsch Geneeskd.* 1919;1:391-396.
24. Mihm MC, Kibbi AG, Wolff K. Basic Pathologic Reactions of the Skin. In: Fitzpatrick TB, Wolff K, eds. *Fitzpatrick's Dermatology in General Medicine.* 7th ed. New York: McGraw-Hill Medical; 2008.
25. Morison WL. Clinical practice. Photosensitivity. *N Engl J Med.* 2004;350:1111-1117.
26. Morkunas AR, Miller MB. Anticonvulsant hypersensitivity syndrome. *Crit Care Clin.* 1997;13:727-739.
27. Pereira FA, Mudgil AV, Rosmarin DM. Toxic epidermal necrolysis. *J Am Acad Dermatol.* 2007;56:181-200.
28. Peterson CE, Kwaan HC. Current concepts of warfarin therapy. *Arch Intern Med.* 1986;146:581-584.
29. Prasad JK, Feller I, Thomson PD. Use of amnion for the treatment of Stevens-Johnson syndrome. *J Trauma.* 1986;26:945-946.
30. Revuz J, Roujeau JC, Guillaume JC, Penso D, Touraine R. Treatment of toxic epidermal necrolysis. Creteil's experience. *Arch Dermatol.* 1987;123:1156-1158.
31. Riviere JE, Brooks JD. Prediction of dermal absorption from complex chemical mixtures: incorporation of vehicle effects and interactions into a QSPR framework. *SAR QSAR Environ Res.* 2007;18:31-44.
32. Scheindlin S. Transdermal drug delivery: past, present, future. *Mol Interv.* 2004;4:308-312.
33. Silver RM, Heyes MP, Maize JC, Quearry B, Vionnet-Fuasset M, Sternberg EM. Scleroderma, fasciitis, and eosinophilia associated with the ingestion of tryptophan. *N Engl J Med.* 1990;322:874-881.
34. Stenn KS, Paus R. Controls of hair follicle cycling. *Physiol Rev.* 2001;81:449-494.
35. Susser WS, Whitaker-Worth DL, Grant-Kels JM. Mucocutaneous reactions to chemotherapy. *J Am Acad Dermatol.* 1999;40:367-98.
36. Viard I, Wehrli P, Bullani R, et al. Inhibition of toxic epidermal necrolysis by blockade of CD95 with human intravenous immunoglobulin. *Science.* 1998;282:490-493.
37. Wester RC, Maibach HI. Percutaneous absorption of drugs. *Clin Pharmacokinet.* 1992;23:253-266.
38. Wilkin JK. The red face: flushing disorders. *Clin Dermatol.* 1993;11:211-223.
39. Wolverton SE. Update on cutaneous drug reactions. *Adv Dermatol.* 1997;13:65-84.
40. Zugerman C. Chloracne. Clinical manifestations and etiology. *Dermatol Clin.* 1990;8:209-213.

SECTION

3 SPECIAL POPULATIONS

CHAPTER 30

REPRODUCTIVE AND PERINATAL PRINCIPLES

Jeffrey S. Fine

Reproductive and perinatal principles in toxicology are derived from many areas of basic science and are applied to many aspects of clinical practice. This chapter reviews several principles of reproductive medicine that have implications for toxicology: the physiology of pregnancy and placental xenobiotic transfer, the effects of xenobiotics on the developing fetus and the neonate, and the management of overdose in the pregnant woman.

One of the most dramatic effects of exposure to a xenobiotic during pregnancy is the birth of a child with congenital malformations. Teratology, the study of birth defects, has principally been concerned with the study of physical malformations. A broader view of teratology includes "developmental" teratoge ns—agents that induce structural malformations, metabolic or physiologic dysfunction, or psychological or behavioral alterations or deficits in the offspring, either at or after birth.[245] Only 4% to 6% of birth defects are related to known pharmaceuticals or occupational and environmental exposures.[41,245]

Reproductive effects of xenobiotics may occur before conception. Female germ cells are formed in utero; adverse effects from xenobiotic exposure can theoretically occur from the time of a woman's own intrauterine development to the end of her reproductive years. An example of a xenobiotic that had both teratogenic and reproductive effects is diethylstilbestrol (DES), which caused vaginal and/or cervical adenocarcinoma in some women who had been exposed to DES in utero and also had effects on fertility and pregnancy outcome.[23,31]

Men generally receive less attention with respect to reproductive risks. Male gametes are formed after puberty; only from that time on are they susceptible to xenobiotic injury. An example of a toxin affecting male reproduction is dibromochloropropane, which reduces spermatogenesis and, consequently, fertility. In general, much less is known about the paternal contribution to teratogenesis.[301]

Occupational exposures to xenobiotics are potentially important but are often poorly defined. In 2004, it was estimated that there were 41 million women of reproductive age in the workforce.[281] Although approximately 90,000 chemicals are used commercially in the United States, only a few thousand industrial and pharmaceutic agents have been specifically evaluated for reproductive toxicity. Many xenobiotics have teratogenic effects when tested in animal models, but relatively few well-defined human teratogens have been identified (Table 30–1).[256] Thus, most tested xenobiotics do not appear to present a human teratogenic risk, but most xenobiotics have not been tested. Some of the presumed safe xenobiotics may have other reproductive, nonteratogenic toxicities. Several excellent reviews and online resources are available.[93,209,218,219,245,256]

Another type of xenobiotic exposure for a pregnant woman is intentional overdose. Although a xenobiotic taken in overdose may have direct toxicity to the fetus, fetal toxicity frequently results from maternal pulmonary and/or hemodynamic compromise, such as hypoxia or shock, further emphasizing the critical nature of the maternal–fetal dyad.

Xenobiotic exposures before and during pregnancy can have effects throughout gestation and may extend into and beyond the newborn period. In addition, the effects of xenobiotic administration in the perinatal period and the special case of delivering xenobiotics to an infant via breast milk deserve special consideration.

PHYSIOLOGIC CHANGES DURING PREGNANCY THAT AFFECT DRUG PHARMACOKINETICS

Many physical and physiologic changes that occur during pregnancy affect both absorption and distribution of xenobiotics in the pregnant woman and consequently affect the amount of xenobiotics delivered to the fetus.[278]

During pregnancy there is delayed gastric emptying, decreased gastrointestinal (GI) motility, and increased transit time through the GI tract. These changes result in delayed but more complete GI absorption of xenobiotics and, consequently, lower peak plasma concentrations. Because blood flow to the skin and mucous membranes is increased, absorption from dermal exposure may be increased. Similarly, absorption of inhaled xenobiotics may be increased because of increased tidal volume and decreased residual lung volume.

An increased free xenobiotic concentration in the pregnant woman can be caused by several factors, including decreased plasma albumin, increased binding competition, and decreased hepatic biotransformation, during the later stages of pregnancy. Fat stores increase during the early stages of pregnancy; free fatty acids are released during the later stages and, with them, xenobiotics that are lipophilic and may have accumulated in the lipid compartment. The increased concentration of free fatty acids can compete with circulating free xenobiotic for binding sites on albumin.

Other factors may lead to decreased free xenobiotic concentrations. Early in pregnancy, increased fat stores, as well as the increased plasma and extracellular fluid volume, lead to a greater volume of distribution. Increased renal blood flow and glomerular filtration may result in increased renal elimination.

Cardiac output increases throughout pregnancy, with the placenta receiving a gradually increasing proportion of total blood volume. Xenobiotic delivery to the placenta may therefore increase over the course of pregnancy.

These processes interact dynamically, and it is difficult to predict their net effect. The concentrations of many xenobiotics, such as

Table 30–1. Known and Probable Human Teratogens

Xenobiotic	Reported Effects	Comments
Amiodarone	Transient neonatal hypothyroidism, with or without goiter; hyperthyroidism	Amiodarone contains 39% iodine by weight. Small to moderate risk from 10 weeks to term for thyroid dysfunction.
Androgens (eg, methyltestosterone, danazol)	Virilization of the female external genitalia: clitoromegaly, labioscrotal fusion	Effects are dose dependent. Stimulates growth of sex-steroid-receptor–containing tissue.
Alkylating agents (eg, busulfan, chlorambucil, cyclophosphamide, mechlorethamine, nitrogen mustard)	Growth retardation, cleft palate, microphthalmia, hypoplastic ovaries, cloudy corneas, renal agenesis, malformations of digits, cardiac defects, other anomalies	A 10%–50% malformation rate, depending on the agent. Cyclophosphamide-induced damage requires cytochrome P450 oxidation.
Angiotensin converting enzyme inhibitors/angiotensin II type 1 receptor inhibitors (sartans)	Fetal/neonatal death, prematurity, oligohydramnios, neonatal anuria, IUGR, secondary skull hypoplasia, limb contractures, pulmonary hypoplasia	Do not interfere with organogenesis. Significant risk of effects related to chronic fetal hypotension during second/third trimester. If used during early pregnancy, can be switched during first trimester.[9,10,41]
Carbamazepine	Upslanting palpebral fissures, epicanthal folds, short nose with long philtrum, fingernail hypoplasia, developmental delay, NTD[128]	1% risk for NTD. Risk of other malformations is unquantified, but may be significant for minor anomalies. Risk is increased in setting of therapy with multiple anticonvulsants, particularly valproic acid. Mechanism may involve an epoxide intermediate. High-dose folate is recommended to prevent NTD.
Carbon monoxide	Cerebral atrophy, mental retardation, microcephaly, convulsions, spastic disorders, intrauterine/death	With severe maternal poisoning, high risk for neurologic sequelae; no increased risk in mild exposures.
Cocaine	IUGR, microcephaly, neurobehavioral abnormalities, vascular disruptive phenomenon (limb amputation, cerebral infarction, visceral/urinary tract abnormalities)	Vascular disruptive effects because of decreased uterine blood flow and fetal vascular effects from first trimester through the end of pregnancy. Risk for major disruptive effects is low (see text).
Corticosteroids	Cleft palate, decreased birth weight (up to 9%) and head circumference (up to 4%)	Low risk. Most information related to prednisone or methylprednisolone.
Coumadin (Warfarin)	Fetal warfarin syndrome: nasal hypoplasia, chondrodysplasia punctata, brachydactyly, skull defects, abnormal ears, malformed eyes, CNS malformations, microcephaly, hydrocephalus, skeletal deformities, mental retardation, spasticity	A 10%–25% risk of malformation for first-trimester exposure, 3% risk of hemorrhage, 8% risk of stillbirth. Bleeding is an unlikely explanation for effects produced in the first trimester. CNS defects may occur during second/third trimesters and may be related to bleeding.[128,289]
Diazepam	Cleft palate, other anomalies	Controversial association, probably low risk.[42,77,93] Risk may extend to other benzodiazepines. Also risk for neonatal sedation or withdrawal following maternal use near delivery.
Diethylstilbestrol (DES)	*Female offspring:* vaginal adenosis, clear cell carcinoma, irregular menses, reduced pregnancy rates, increased rate of preterm deliveries, increased perinatal mortality and spontaneous abortion *Male offspring:* epididymal cysts, cryptorchidism, hypogonadism, diminished spermatogenesis	A synthetic nonsteroidal estrogen that stimulates estrogen receptor–containing tissue and may cause misplaced genital tissue with propensity to develop cancer. A 40%–70% risk of morphologic changes in vaginal epithelium. Risk of carcinoma approximately 1/1000 for exposure before the 18th week. Most patients exposed to DES in utero can conceive and deliver normal children.
Ethanol	Fetal alcohol syndrome (FAS): pre-/postnatal growth retardation, mental retardation, fine motor dysfunction, hyperactivity, microcephaly, maxillary hypoplasia, short palpebral fissures, hypoplastic philtrum, thinned upper lips, joint, digit anomalies	FAS in 4% of offspring of alcoholic women consuming ethanol above 2 g/kg/d (6 oz/d) over the first trimester. There may be a threshold for effects, but a safe dose has not been identified. Can see partial expression or other congenital anomalies (see text). Other effects: increased incidence of spontaneous abortion, premature delivery, and stillbirth; neonatal withdrawal.
Fluconazole	Brachycephaly, abnormal facies, abnormal calvarial development, cleft palate, femoral bowing, thin ribs and long bones, arthrogryposis, and congenital heart disease	Risk related to high dose (400–800 mg/d), chronic, parenteral use. Single 150-mg oral dose probably safe.

Table 30–1. Known and Probable Human Teratogens (*Continued*)

Xenobiotic	Reported Effects	Comments
Indomethacin	Premature closure of the ductus arteriosus; in premature infants, oligohydramnios, anuria, intestinal ischemia	NSAIDs generally labeled as category B. However, there is concern when used after 34 weeks' gestation and for more than 48 hours and/or immediately prior to delivery. Risk may extend to other NSAIDs.
Iodine and iodine-containing products	Thyroid hypoplasia after the 8th week of development	High doses of radioiodine isotopes can additionally produce cell death and mitotic delay. Tissue and organ-specific damage is dependent on the specific radioisotope, dose, distribution, metabolism, and localization.
Lead	Lower scores on developmental tests	Higher risk when maternal lead is >10 μg/dL.
Lithium carbonate	Ebstein anomaly	Low risk.
Methimazole	Aplasia cutis, skull hypoplasia, dystrophic nails, nipple abnormalities, hypo- or hyperthyroidism	Small risk of anomalies or goiter with first-trimester exposure. Hypothyroidism risk after 10 weeks' gestation.
Methotrexate, Aminopterin (amethopterin)	Hydro-/microcephaly; meningoencephalocele; anencephaly; abnormal cranial ossification; cerebral hypoplasia; growth retardation; eye, ear, and nose malformations; cleft palate; malformed extremities/fingers; reduction in derivatives of first branchial arch; developmental delay[288]	These folate antagonists inhibit dihydrofolate reductase. High rate of malformations. Methotrexate is used to terminate ectopic pregnancies.
Methyl mercury, mercuric sulfide	Normal appearance at birth; cerebral palsy–like syndrome after several months; microcephaly, mental retardation, cerebellar symptoms, eye/dental anomalies	Inhibits enzymes, particularly those with sulfhydryl groups. Of 220 babies born following the Minamata Bay exposure, 13 had severe disease. Mothers of affected babies ingested 9–27 ppm mercury; greater risk with ingestion at 6–8 months' gestation. In acute poisoning, the fetus is 4–10 times more sensitive than an adult. Pathologically, there is atrophy and hypoplasia of the brain cortex and abnormalities in cytoarchitecture.[110,294]
Methylene blue (intraamniotic injection)	Intestinal atresia, hemolytic anemia, neonatal jaundice	This xenobiotic was used to identify twin amniotic sacs during amniocentesis.[63]
Misoprostol	Vascular disruptive phenomena (eg, limb reduction defects); Moebius syndrome (paralysis of 6th and 7th facial nerves)	Synthetic prostaglandin E_1 analog. Effects mostly observed in women after unsuccessful attempts to induce abortion.
Oxazolidine-2,4-diones (trimethadione, paramethadione)	Fetal trimethadione syndrome: V-shaped eyebrows; low-set ears with anteriorly folded helix; high-arched palate; irregular teeth; CNS anomalies; severe developmental delay; cardiovascular, genitourinary, and other anomalies	An 83% risk of at least one major malformation with any exposure; 32% die. Characteristic facial features are associated with chronic exposure.
Penicillamine	Cutis laxa, hyperflexibility of joints	Copper chelator—copper deficiency inhibits collagen synthesis/maturation. Few case reports; low risk.
Phenytoin	Fetal hydantoin syndrome: microcephaly, mental retardation, cleft lip/palate, hypoplastic nails/phalanges, characteristic facies—low nasal bridge, inner epicanthal folds, ptosis, strabismus, hypertelorism, low-set ears, wide mouth	Phenytoin has a direct effect on cell membranes and on folate and vitamin K metabolism. May reduce the availability of retinoic acid derivatives or alter the genetic expression of retinoic acid. Epoxide intermediate may play a role in teratogenesis. Effects seen with chronic exposure. A 5%–10% risk of typical syndrome, 30% risk of partial syndrome. Risks confounded by those associated with epilepsy itself and use of other anticonvulsants. Possible increased risk of developing tumors, in particular, neuroblastoma, although absolute risk is very low.
Polychlorinated biphenyls	Cola-colored children; pigmentation of gums, nails, and groin; hypoplastic, deformed nails; IUGR; abnormal skull calcifications	Cytotoxic agent. Body residue can affect subsequent offspring for up to 4 years after exposure. Most cases followed high consumption of PCB-contaminated rice oil; 4%–20% of offspring were affected.[125]

(*Continued*)

Table 30–1. Known and Probable Human Teratogens (*Continued*)

Xenobiotic	Reported Effects	Comments
Progestins (eg, ethisterone, norethindrone)	Masculinization of female external genitalia	Progestogens are converted into androgens or may have weak androgenic activity. Stimulates or interferes with sex-steroid receptors. Effects occur only after exposure to high doses of some testosterone-derived progestins and may be at the rate of <1% of those exposed. Oral contraceptives containing these agents are not thought to present teratogenic risk, despite their category X designation.
Quinine	Hypoplasia of 8th nerve, deafness, abortion	Effects related to high doses used as abortifacients.
Radiation, ionizing	Microcephaly, mental retardation, eye anomalies, growth retardation, visceral malformations	Significant doses of radiation from diagnostic or therapeutic sources produce cell death and mitotic delay. There is no measurable risk with X-ray exposures of 5 rads or less at any stage of pregnancy.[29,39]
Retinoids (isotretinoin, etretinate, high-dose vitamin A)	Spontaneous abortions; micro-/hydrocephalus; deformities of cranium, ears, face, heart, limbs, liver	Retinoids can cause direct cytotoxicity and alter apoptosis. Neural crest cells are particularly sensitive. For isotretinoin, 38% risk of malformations; 80% are CNS malformations. Effects are associated with vitamin A doses of 25,000–100,000 international units (IU)/day. Exposures below 10,000 IU/day present no risk to fetus. Topical retinoids are not considered a reproductive risk.[273]
Smoking	Placental lesions, IUGR, increased perinatal mortality, increased risk of SIDS, neurobehavioral effects such as learning deficits and hyperactivity.[121,230]	Possible mechanisms include vasoconstriction (nicotine effect); hypoxia secondary to hypoperfusion, CO, and CN; and altered development of neurons and neural pathways via stimulation of nicotinic acetylcholine receptors.[260,261]
Streptomycin	Hearing loss	Rare reports. A low-risk phenomenon that could be associated with long-duration maternal therapy during pregnancy.
Tetracycline	Yellow, gray-brown, or brown staining of deciduous teeth, hypoplastic tooth enamel	Effects seen after 4 months of gestation, because tetracyclines must interact with calcified tissue. Effects occur in 50% of fetuses exposed to tetracycline and in 12.5% of fetuses exposed to oxytetracycline.
Thalidomide	Limb phocomelia, amelia, hypoplasia, congenital heart defects, renal malformations, cryptorchidism, abducens paralysis, deafness, microtia, anotia	Approximately 20% risk for exposure during days 34–50 of gestation.
Trimethoprim	NTD, oral clefts, hypospadias, and cardiovascular defects	Approximately 1% risk of NTD for first-trimester exposure. Mechanism is folic acid inhibition.
Valproic acid	Lumbosacral spina bifida with meningomyelocele; CNS defects, microcephaly, cardiac defects; narrow face with high forehead, epicanthal folds, broad, low nasal bridge with short nose, long philtrum with a thin vermilion border; long, thin fingers and toes	Risk for spina bifida is approximately 1%, but the risk for dysmorphic facies may be greater. The mechanism of teratogenicity is unknown. Possible explanations include interference with glutathione, folate, or zinc metabolism, or regulation of intracellular pH. Risk is confounded by those risks associated with epilepsy itself or use of other anticonvulsants.
Vitamin D	Possible association with supravalvular aortic stenosis, elfin facies, and mental retardation	Large doses of vitamin D may disrupt cellular calcium regulation. Genetic susceptibility may play a role.

IUGR, intrauterine growth retardation; NSAID, nonsteroidal antiinflammatory drug; NTD, neural tube defect; SIDS, sudden infant death syndrome Data adapted from Brent RL: Environmental causes of human congenital malformations: The pediatrician's role in dealing with these complex clinical problems caused by a multiplicity of environmental and genetic factors. *Pediatrics*. 2004;113:957-968; Nulman I, Izmaylov Y, Staroselsky A, Koren G: Teratogenic drugs and chemicals in humans. In: Koren G, ed: *Medication Safety in Pregnancy and Breastfeeding*. New York, McGraw-Hill, 2007, pp. 21-30; and Polifka JE, Friedman JM: Medical genetics: 1. Clinical teratology in the age of genomics. *CMAJ*. 2002;167:265–273. .

lithium, gentamicin, and carbamazepine, decrease during pregnancy, even if the administered dose is not changed.[97]

Although not specifically related to the physiologic changes occurring during pregnancy, the fetus may be exposed to xenobiotics that accumulated in adipose tissue before pregnancy. For example, malformations typically ascribed to retinoid use were seen in a baby born to a woman whose pregnancy began 1 year after she discontinued use of the xenobiotic etretinate (retinoic acid).[148]

XENOBIOTIC EXPOSURE IN PREGNANT WOMEN

Exposure to xenobiotics during pregnancy is common. Between 30% and 80% of pregnant women take xenobiotics sometime during pregnancy—primarily analgesics, antipyretics, antimicrobials, and antiemetics, as well as vitamins, caffeine, ethanol, and nicotine.[34,47,60,71,179,236,237] Some pregnant women use xenobiotics to treat chronic disease; others unknowingly use various prescription and nonprescription xenobiotics prior to recognizing that they are pregnant.

Pharmaceutical manufacturers are required by law to label their products with respect to use in pregnancy, according to standards promulgated by the US Food and Drug Administration (FDA) (Table 30–2).[282] Similar classification systems have been developed in Sweden and Australia.[7,225,243] The original intent of the US regulations was to inform practitioners about the nature of the available evidence regarding risk in pregnancy. However, the general impression is that the categories refer to teratogenic risk—a hierarchy of harmful effects according to the letter categories and an equivalence of risk within each letter category.[76,146,225,249,250] For example, in the US system, a category C medication is generally considered more dangerous than a category B medication in pregnancy, even though category C is the default category for medications about which there is little or no specific information available, and for which the risk is unknown. Approximately 90% of medications are classified as category C.[160]

There is significant discordance between the use-in-pregnancy labeling and the teratogenic risk, as determined by clinical teratologists,[160] and the FDA system has been criticized for being too conservative.[92] Manufacturers may label certain medications as category X even when there is only limited information associating the medication with any adverse fetal or neonatal effects. For example, oral contraceptives generally carry a category X classification, even though they are not considered teratogenic; category X is assigned because there is no indication for use of oral contraceptives in pregnancy.[146] Certain agents with a category D classification may cause problems only at certain times during pregnancy. Even medications that are classified as category D or X may only have a very low risk of teratogenicity or other adverse effect, and exposure to these xenobiotics, even during the first trimester, may not be a sufficient indication to terminate a pregnancy.

The difficulty regarding appropriate drug labeling reflects many complex questions regarding the use of medications during pregnancy. How should animal data in general be evaluated? How should animal data be extrapolated to humans? How should the teratogenic risk be defined and quantified for any particular xenobiotic? How should the risk of not treating a particular disease be compared with the risk of using a particular medication to treat that disease? Finally, how should the answers to these questions be communicated to practitioners and the public?[250] In an attempt to address many of these problems, the FDA has proposed changes to the labeling of medications for use in pregnancy and lactation.[146,283]

Specific current information on individual xenobiotics can be obtained from local and regional teratogen information services[6] and published books,[42,93,245,255] some of which also have online versions.[191,218,219,276] Motherisk is a Canadian program that uses accumulated evidence and experience to advise women about the actual risk to them of using a particular medication or being exposed to a particular xenobiotic in a current or planned pregnancy.[190,191]

Although most women are concerned about the teratogenic effects of medications, in utero exposure to therapeutic medications can have

Table 30–2. FDA Use-in-Pregnancy Ratings

Category	Risk to Human Fetus	Example(s)	Basis
A	No known risk	Multiple vitamins	*Controlled studies show no risk.* Adequate, well-controlled studies in pregnant women do not demonstrate a risk to the fetus and if animal studies exist, they do not demonstrate a risk.
B	Unlikely risk	Acetaminophen, penicillin	*No evidence of risk in humans.* Either animal studies show risk but human studies do not, or if no adequate human studies have been done, animal studies show no risk.
C	Unknown risk	Albuterol	*Risk cannot be excluded.* Animal studies may or may not show risk, but human studies do not exist. However, benefits may justify the potential or unknown risk.
D	Known risk, but benefit may outweigh risk	Tetracycline	*Positive evidence of risk.* Investigational or postmarketing data or human studies show risk to the fetus. Nevertheless, potential benefits may outweigh the potential risk; for example, if the drug is needed in a life-threatening situation or serious disease for which safer drugs cannot be used or are ineffective.
X	Known risk but risk significantly outweighs benefit	Isotretinoin	*Contraindicated in pregnancy.* Studies in animals or humans or investigational or postmarketing reports have shown fetal risk that clearly outweighs any possible benefit to the patient.

other pharmacologic effects on the newborn infant, such as hyperbilirubinemia or withdrawal reactions.[42,73]

Estimates of substance use in pregnancy vary tremendously, depending on the geographic location, practice environment, patient population, and screening method.[54,150] Among a large national sample screened for xenobiotic use during pregnancy, 20% of pregnant women smoked, 20% drank ethanol, 3% used marijuana, 0.5% used cocaine, 0.1% used methadone, and fewer than 0.1% used heroin. Women tend to decrease their exposure to xenobiotics once they know they are pregnant.[35,124,127]

PLACENTAL REGULATION OF XENOBIOTIC TRANSFER TO THE FETUS

With respect to the transfer of xenobiotics from mother to fetus, the placenta functions in a manner similar to other lipoprotein membranes. Most xenobiotics enter the fetal circulation by passive diffusion down a concentration gradient across the placental membranes. The characteristics of a substance that favor this passive diffusion are low molecular weight (MW), lipid solubility, neutral polarity, and low protein binding.[212] Polar molecules and ions may be transported through interstitial pores.[279]

Xenobiotics with an MW greater than 1000 Da do not diffuse passively across the placenta, and this characteristic is used to therapeutic advantage. For example, warfarin (MW 1000 Da) easily crosses the placenta and causes specific fetal malformations.[289] However, heparin (MW 20,000 Da), which is too large to cross the placenta, is not teratogenic and, consequently, is the preferred anticoagulant during pregnancy. Most therapeutic medications have molecular weights between 250 and 400 Da and easily cross the placenta. For example, thiopental is highly lipid soluble and crosses the placenta rapidly. Fetal plasma concentrations reach maternal concentrations within a few minutes. Neuromuscular blockers such as vecuronium are more polar and cross the placenta slowly.[79]

Although the state of ionization is a limiting factor for diffusion, some highly charged compounds can still diffuse across the placenta. Valproic acid (pK_a 4.7) is nearly completely ionized at physiologic pH, yet there is rapid equilibration across the placental membrane. The small amount of xenobiotic that exists in the nonionized form rapidly crosses the placenta; as equilibrium is reestablished, a new, small amount of nonionized xenobiotic becomes available for diffusion.[195]

Fetal blood pH changes during gestation. Embryonic intracellular pH is high relative to the intracellular pH of the pregnant woman. During this developmental stage, weak acids will diffuse across the placenta to the embryo and remain there because of "ion trapping." Many teratogens, such as valproic acid, trimethadione, phenytoin, thalidomide, warfarin, and isotretinoin, are weak acids. Although ion trapping does not explain the mechanism of teratogenesis, it may explain how xenobiotics accumulate in an embryo. Late in gestation the fetal blood is 0.10 to 0.15 pH units more acidic than the mother's blood; this pH differential may permit weakly basic xenobiotics to concentrate in the fetus during this period.[212]

The relative concentrations of protein binding sites in the pregnant woman and fetus also have an impact on the extent of xenobiotic transfer to the fetus.[212] As maternal free fatty acid concentrations increase near term, these fatty acids can displace xenobiotics such as valproic acid or diazepam from maternal protein binding sites and make more free xenobiotic available for transfer to the fetus. Fetal albumin concentrations increase during gestation and exceed maternal albumin concentrations by term. Because the fetus does not have high concentrations of free fatty acids to compete for protein binding sites, these sites are available for binding the xenobiotics. At birth, when neonatal free fatty acid concentrations increase two- to threefold, they displace stored xenobiotic from the binding protein. In the cases of valproic acid and diazepam, the elevated concentrations of free xenobiotic have adverse effects on the newborn infant.[100,126,195,217]

The placenta may also affect xenobiotic presentation to the fetus by ion trapping and xenobiotic metabolism. The placenta blocks the transfer of some positively charged ions such as cadmium and mercury[110] and may even accumulate them. This barrier does not necessarily protect the fetus, however, because these heavy metal ions interfere with normal placental function and may lead to placental necrosis and subsequent fetal death.[189]

The placenta contains xenobiotic-metabolizing enzymes capable of performing both phase I and phase II reactions (Chaps. 12 and 26). However, the concentration of biotransforming enzymes in the placenta is significantly lower than that in the liver, and it is unlikely that the level of enzymatic activity is protective for the fetus. Moreover, the fetus may be exposed to reactive intermediates that form during these processes. On the other hand, glutathione may also be present in the placenta and detoxify some of these reactive intermediates.[130]

Placental transfer of xenobiotics can have a positive effect when it provides fetal therapy. For example, if a fetus is found to have a supraventricular tachycardia or atrial flutter, digoxin can be given to the mother in order to treat the tachydysrhythmia in the fetus.[142,233]

EFFECTS OF XENOBIOTICS ON THE DEVELOPING ORGANISM

A basic premise of teratogenicity is that the particular toxic effects of a xenobiotic are determined by the organism's stage of development.[40,251] Although the fertilized ovum is generally thought to be resistant to toxic insult before implantation,[40] xenobiotics in the fallopian or uterine secretions may prevent implantation of the embryo. Xenobiotic exposure leading to cell loss or chromosomal abnormalities may also lead to a spontaneous abortion, possibly even before pregnancy has been detected. If the preimplantation embryo survives a xenobiotic exposure, the functional cells usually proceed to normal development.[251] Teratogens that act in such a manner elicit an "all-or-none response"; that is, the exposed embryo will either die or go on to normal development.

Teratogens generally behave according to a dose–response curve; there is a threshold dose below which no effects occur and as the dose of the teratogen increases above the threshold, the magnitude of the effect increases. The effects might be the number of offspring that die or suffer malformations, or the extent or severity of malformations. A strict definition is teratogenic effects are those that occur at doses that do not cause maternal toxicity because maternal toxicity itself might be responsible for an observed adverse or teratogenic effect on the developing organism.[40]

Organogenesis occurs during the embryonic stage of development between days 18 and 60 of gestation. Most gross malformations are determined before day 36, although genitourinary and craniofacial anomalies occur later.[40] The period of susceptibility to teratogenic effects varies for each organ system (Fig. 30–1). For instance, the palate has a very short period of sensitivity, lasting approximately 3 weeks, whereas the central nervous system (CNS) remains susceptible throughout gestation.

Theoretically, knowing the exact time of teratogen exposure during gestation would allow prediction of a teratogenic effect; this is true in animal models, where dose and time can be strictly controlled. It is also

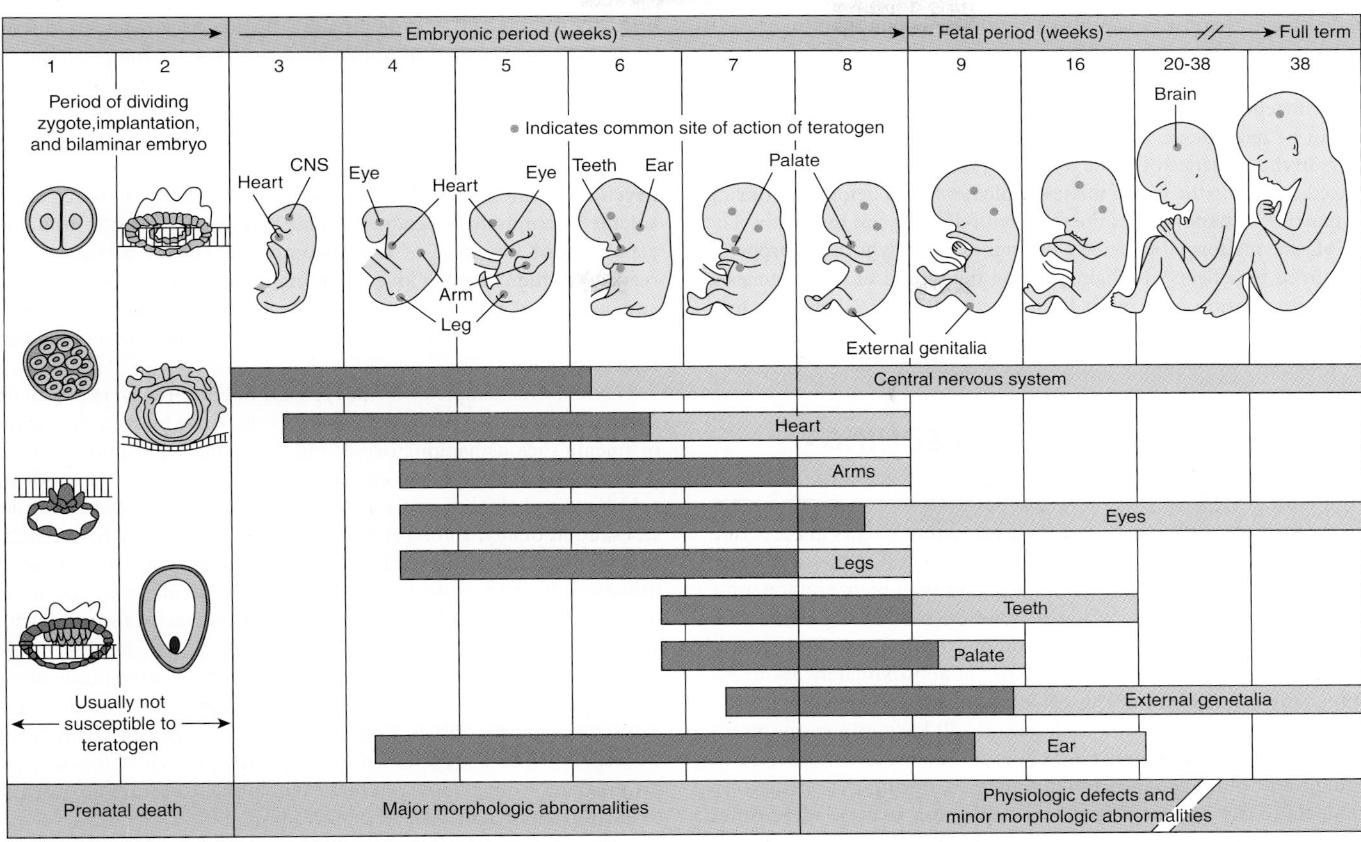

FIGURE 30–1. Critical periods of fetal development. (Modified with permission from Moore KL, Persaud TVN: *The Developing Human: Clinically Oriented Embryology*, 7th ed. Philadelphia, WB Saunders, 2003, p. 520.)

true for thalidomide, where different limb anomalies are specifically related to exposures on particular days of gestation.[251] In many clinical situations, for xenobiotics administered either for a short course or chronically, relating teratogenicity to a particular xenobiotic exposure is difficult because the exact time of conception is unknown and the exact time of exposure is unknown. This is particularly true when the primary exposure precedes the pregnancy but there is secondary or ongoing exposure during pregnancy as xenobiotic is redistributed from tissue storage sites.[148]

During the fetal period, formed organs continue their cellular differentiation and grow to functional maturity. Exposure to xenobiotics such as cigarettes and their toxic constituents (for example, nicotine) during this period generally lead to growth retardation. Teratogenic malformations or death may still occur as a result of disruption or destruction of growing organs, as has been the result of exposure to angiotensin-converting enzyme inhibitors during the second and third trimesters.[27]

Another concern during the fetal period is the initiation of carcinogenesis. Significant cellular replication and proliferation lead to a dramatic growth in size of the organism. At the same time, when the fetus is exposed to xenobiotics, development of biotransformation systems may expose the organism to reactive metabolites that might initiate tumor formation. Some tumors, such as neuroblastoma, appear early in postnatal life, suggesting a prenatal origin. In pregnant rats given ethylnitrosourea during the embryonic period, lethal or teratogenic effects occur.[220] If ethylnitrosourea is administered during the fetal period, there is an increased incidence of tumors in the offspring. Clear cell vaginal and cervical adenocarcinomas are seen in the female offspring of women exposed to DES during pregnancy.[31]

MECHANISMS OF TERATOGENESIS

Cytotoxicity is one mechanism of teratogenesis and is the characteristic result of exposure to alkylating or antineoplastic xenobiotics. Aminopterin, for example, inhibits dihydrofolate reductase activity and leads to suppression of mitosis and cell death. If exposure to a cytotoxic xenobiotic occurs very early in development, the conceptus may die, whereas sublethal exposure during organogenesis may result in maldevelopment of particular structures. There is evidence that following cell death, the remaining cells in an affected region may try to repair the damage caused by the missing cellular elements. This "restorative growth" may lead to uncoordinated growth and exacerbate the original malformation.

In the case of the cytotoxic xenobiotics, the mechanism of action is understood, although it is not always clear why particular xenobiotics affect particular structures. With other xenobiotics, the structural effects have a clearer relationship to the site of action. For instance, when glucocorticoids are administered in large doses to some experimental animals during the period of organogenesis, malformations of the palate occur. Glucocorticoid receptors are found in high concentrations in the palate of the developing mouse embryo.[213]

Corticosteroid exposure can also cause cleft palate in humans at a low frequency.[207,255]

Caloric deficiency is not considered teratogenic during the period of organogenesis. However, specific nutritional or vitamin deficiencies can be teratogenic; an increased incidence of neural tube defects occurs in the presence of folate deficiency, and the incidence has been reduced following the use of folate supplementation before and during pregnancy.[201] Ethanol affects the fetus both directly and indirectly. The craniofacial malformations seen in fetal alcohol syndrome probably result from the effects of ethanol during the period of organogenesis. Growth retardation may result from direct effects of ethanol on fetal growth, or from indirect effects resulting from ethanol-induced maternal nutritional deficiencies.

MANAGEMENT OF ACUTE POISONING IN THE PREGNANT WOMAN

For most women, pregnancy and the postpartum period are a period of emotional happiness. However, women have a lifetime prevalence of depression that is two to three times higher than men, and for some women psychiatric illness during pregnancy, particularly depression and anxiety, represents a significant complication. A new first episode or recurrence of major depression occurs in approximately 3% to 5% of pregnant women and 1% to 6% of postpartum women; an additional 5% to 6% of women in each period will have minor symptoms of depression.[96] Overall, these rates of depression are about the same in pregnant and nonpregnant women; however, during the postpartum period, the onset of new episodes of depression may be three times higher than for nonpregnant women. Pregnant teenagers may also be at higher risk of depression in pregnancy.[159]

Postpartum blues are common; typically involve relatively mild symptoms including mood swings, irritability, anxiety, and crying spells; and generally resolve by 2 weeks postpartum.[164] Postpartum blues do not include suicidal ideation. True depression is manifested by feelings of hopelessness or helplessness and may include suicidal ideation.[164] Postpartum psychosis, typically associated with bipolar disorder, is uncommon but it represents a true psychiatric emergency because there is a high risk of suicide and/or infanticide.[164]

Risk factors for perinatal depression include an unplanned pregnancy, ambivalence about the pregnancy, poor social support, marital difficulties, adverse life events, and chronic stressors such as financial problems.[164] Of particular importance is a personal or family history of depression, particularly previous perinatal depression. Discontinuation of antidepressant medications represents a significant risk for relapse of disease, although relapse is possible even while a woman is on antidepressant medication. Additional risk factors for depression include miscarriage, stillbirth, and preterm delivery.

Depression in pregnancy has adverse effects on both the mother and the fetus.[33] For the pregnant woman, adverse effects include noncompliance with prenatal care; self-medication with tobacco, alcohol, and drugs; poor sleep; poor appetite; and poor weight gain. In addition there may be increased risk of spontaneous abortion, preeclampsia, preterm delivery, and growth retardation. For many of these outcomes, it is difficult to separate out the contributions from multiple confounding and interacting factors including psychopathology, socioeconomic status, acute and chronic stressors, smoking, and the use of alcohol and other substances. Infants born to women being treated with antidepressant medications are also at risk for neonatal withdrawal symptoms.[139]

One of the most extreme outcomes of depression is suicide. Suicidal ideation occurs in about 5% of pregnant women in community samples and up to 20% in women with underlying psychiatric illness.[159,198] Even so, suicide and suicide attempts during pregnancy are uncommon. Each year a small number of women die during pregnancy or the postpartum period; 1% to 5% of these pregnancy-related deaths may be the result of suicide.[52,69,202] Between 2% and 12% of women who attempt or commit suicide may be pregnant.[138,210,297] Overall, completed suicide occurs less frequently during pregnancy.[16,159,178] Psychiatric illness including previous suicide attempts predisposes to suicide attempts in pregnancy. Acute stressors leading to impulsive acts account for most of the uncompleted suicide attempts; these reasons include loss of a lover, economic crisis, prior loss of children, and unwanted pregnancy and desire for an abortion.[66,156,297] Fewer than half the suicide attempts are specifically related to a pregnancy-related problem.

Women who complete suicide typically have more severe psychiatric illness. In particular, these women are likely to use more violent means of suicide such as hanging or self-inflicted gunshot wounds, although poisonings are a significant contributor to these deaths.[202] In addition, substance and alcohol use is a significant contributing factor in many cases; additionally, some pregnancy-related deaths may be secondary to complications of substance use, such as overdose.[202] In one series, initiation of child-protection proceedings, particularly in the setting of maternal substance use, was a significant risk factor for postpartum suicide.[202]

Medication ingestion is a common method of attempting suicide during pregnancy. Analgesics, vitamins, iron, antibiotics, and antipsychotics account for 50% to 79% of the reported ingestions by pregnant women.[210,214] These xenobiotics are frequently prescribed for, and used by, pregnant women. Some of these xenobiotic exposures are attempts to terminate pregnancy (see Chap. 28).[210]

Although the focus of this section is on medical management, it goes without saying that any woman who attempts suicide during pregnancy should have a psychiatric evaluation after she is medically stabilized. In particular, there are a growing number of specialized units or teams that focus on pregnant or postpartum women and attempt to keep women and infants together in the postpartum period.[164,202]

Managing any acute overdose during pregnancy provokes discussion of several questions. Is the general management different? Do altered metabolism and pharmacokinetics increase or decrease the woman's risk of morbidity or mortality from a xenobiotic overdose? Is the fetus at risk of poisoning from a maternal overdose? Is there a teratogenic risk to the fetus from an acute overdose or poisoning? Is the use of an antidote contraindicated, or should use be modified? When should a potentially viable fetus be emergently delivered to prevent toxicity? When should termination of a pregnancy be recommended?

As described above, physiologic changes during pregnancy affect pharmacokinetics; xenobiotics taken in overdose also have unpredictable toxicokinetics. In any significant overdose during pregnancy, pregnancy-related alterations in pharmacokinetics are unlikely to protect the woman from significant morbidity or mortality.

Although a single high-dose exposure to a xenobiotic during the period of organogenesis might seem analogous to an experimental model to induce teratogenesis, most xenobiotics ingested as a single, acute overdose do not induce physical deformities.[67] Anticonvulsants are teratogenic and may be ingested in toxic doses, but their teratogenicity is probably related more to chronic exposure. Acute acetaminophen intoxication in the first trimester may lead to an increased risk of spontaneous abortion,[223] suggesting a teratogenic effect similar to the all-or-none response described earlier. In general, however, it is extremely difficult to ascribe teratogenicity to a particular xenobiotic exposure based on a single case report. There is, for example, a report of multiple severe congenital malformations in the stillborn fetus of a woman who overdosed on isoniazid during the 12th week of pregnancy.[154] However, because the background incidence of congenital malformations is 3% to 6%, it is almost impossible to determine for a single individual whether a particular xenobiotic exposure is the etiology of any observed malformations.[68] Considering the successful outcome of most pregnancies that progressed following an acute overdose, it is very unlikely that the small risk of possible teratogenesis would ever lead to a recommendation for termination of pregnancy after an acute overdose of most xenobiotics.

In general, any condition that leads to a severe metabolic derangement in the pregnant woman is likely to have an adverse impact on the developing fetus. Therefore, the management of overdose in a pregnant woman usually follows the principles outlined in Chapter 4, with close attention paid to the airway, oxygenation, and hemodynamic stability. The use of naloxone or dextrose has not been specifically assessed in pregnancy, but should be guided by the same considerations raised in managing the nonpregnant patient with alterations in respiratory or neurologic function. Opioid-induced respiratory failure in the pregnant patient will lead to fetal hypoxia and adverse effects; opioid withdrawal in a pregnant woman, whether induced by abstinence or the use of naloxone, may adversely affect the fetus or the pregnancy. Consideration of the benefits and risks of the use of naloxone for an opioid-poisoned woman in respiratory distress or coma suggests that reduced morbidity, for both mother and fetus, may be achieved by the use of carefully titrated doses of naloxone to minimize the likelihood of maternal withdrawal (see Chap. 38 and Antidotes in Depth A–6: Opioid Antagonists).

Gastrointestinal decontamination is frequently a part of the early management of acute poisoning in the nonpregnant patient. Gastric lavage is not specifically contraindicated for the pregnant patient and the usual concerns about protecting the airway apply. Even though syrup of ipecac is no longer recommended as a standard therapy for the management of typical pediatric and adult ingestions, pregnancy was previously considered a relative contraindication to its use because vomiting increases both intrathoracic and intraabdominal pressure.

There is no specific contraindication to the use of activated charcoal in a pregnant woman. There may be a specific role for whole-bowel irrigation in the management of several xenobiotic exposures, particularly in the treatment of iron overdose in pregnancy.[284] The use of oral polyethylene glycol is safe in pregnant women.[196]

Almost all antidotes are designated as FDA pregnancy-risk category C; that is, there is little specific information to guide their use. Ethanol is labeled as category D (positive evidence of risk), although this is presumably related to chronic use throughout pregnancy. Fomepizole, which has replaced ethanol as the preferred antidote for toxic alcohol poisoning, is labeled as category C. Pyridoxine and thiamine are category A xenobiotics; *N*-acetylcysteine (NAC), magnesium, glucagon, and naloxone are category B xenobiotics.

Thus far, there are no reports of adverse effects on the fetus from antidotal treatment of a poisoned pregnant woman. Conversely, in at least one case, withholding deferoxamine therapy may have contributed to the death of both a woman and her fetus.[174,271]

ACETAMINOPHEN

Acetaminophen is the most common analgesic and antipyretic used during pregnancy and is one of the most common xenobiotics ingested in overdose during pregnancy.[185,223] There are two published series, as well as a number of individual reports, totaling more than 100 cases of acute acetaminophen overdose during all trimesters of pregnancy. In the two large series representing 112 acute and chronic overdoses, 33 patients had serum acetaminophen concentrations in the toxic range.[185,223] These studies, in addition to the case reports described below, demonstrate that most pregnant women recover from an acetaminophen ingestion without adverse effects to themselves or their babies.

In the two large series of acetaminophen overdose during pregnancy,[185,223] eight of 28 women who overdosed in the first trimester and continued their pregnancy experienced spontaneous abortions, most within 2 weeks of the ingestion. Of the eight women, five had toxic serum acetaminophen concentrations; one woman received NAC within 8 hours, and four received NAC between 12 and 17 hours after ingestion. In one of these cases both maternal and fetal death occurred. Five patients with toxic serum acetaminophen concentrations and 14 with nontoxic serum concentrations delivered healthy term newborns. Ten women had elective terminations of pregnancy.

The two large series included 32 second-trimester acute overdoses.[185,223] Two women who had nontoxic serum acetaminophen concentrations had spontaneous abortions—one had symptoms of a threatened abortion several days prior to the overdose, and the second was assaulted the day before the overdose and aborted the next day. Six women with toxic serum acetaminophen concentrations delivered full-term healthy infants; 19 women with nontoxic serum concentrations delivered full-term babies, and one woman with a nontoxic serum concentration delivered a premature infant 2 months after the overdose. Four women had elective terminations of pregnancy.

There are three case reports of women with acute overdoses in the second trimester. One woman who overdosed at 15.5 weeks of gestation had a toxic serum acetaminophen concentration, was treated with intravenous NAC beginning 20 hours after the ingestion, and developed hepatotoxicity. She had a spontaneous rupture of membranes at 31 weeks and delivered a male infant at 32 weeks.[163] One woman who overdosed at 16 weeks had a toxic serum acetaminophen concentration, was treated with NAC within 8 hours, and did not develop hepatotoxicity.[228] She delivered a normal female infant at term. One woman overdosed at 20 weeks, received intravenous NAC starting some time between 8 and 18 hours after ingestion, and developed hepatotoxicity. She had labor induced at 41 weeks because of weight loss and delivered a male infant.[268] The infant was irritable and developed hyperbilirubinemia, both of which resolved after phototherapy.

The two large series described above included 39 third-trimester overdoses.[185,223] Twelve women had toxic serum acetaminophen concentrations: eight delivered healthy term infants; two women who had no evidence of hepatotoxicity delivered premature infants 2 days after the overdose; one woman with hepatotoxicity delivered a moderately ill premature infant at 32 weeks of gestation; and one woman with severe hepatotoxicity delivered a stillborn infant with hepatic necrosis at 33 weeks of gestation (Table 30–3). Twenty-seven women had nontoxic serum acetaminophen concentrations: two delivered premature infants (one of whom had respiratory distress), and 25 delivered full-term infants. Of these full-term infants, one developed a withdrawal syndrome, one developed pyloric stenosis, and three had physical anomalies. Altogether, in these two series, six of 39 women with third-trimester overdoses had premature delivery, usually within 2 to 3 days of the overdose.

In addition to the large series described, there are 11 case reports of third-trimester acetaminophen overdoses (Table 30–3). Three additional third-trimester cases are briefly described: two women had an acute overdose and one had a chronic overdose. All three women had toxic serum acetaminophen concentrations, were treated with NAC, and delivered healthy infants while receiving NAC.[120] There are also several case reports of adverse pregnancy outcome in the setting of chronic use of acetaminophen, or acute overdose associated with chronic substance use.[53,120,145,165,223] It is difficult to interpret these

Table 30–3. Reported Cases of Third-Trimester Acetaminophen Overdose

Gestational Age (Weeks)	Maternal: APAP Concentration (μg/mL) (Time[a])	Maternal: AST Peak (IUnits/L) (Time[a])	Infant: APAP Concentration (μg/mL) (Time[a])	Infant: Hepatotoxicity (Yes/No)	Comment	Ref
27	0 (36 h)	1226 (36 h)	ND	No	C/S for fetal distress. Infant: mild respiratory distress syndrome	94
27–28	56 (16 h)	6226 (96 h)	ND	Yes	Ingestion over 24 h. No fetal movements at presentation. PO NAC started at 20 h. Induced labor at 4 d. Infant: stillborn with diffuse hepatic necrosis. Hepatic APAP 250 μg/g.	107
29	160 (10 h)	4300 (50 h)	76 (16 h, cord)	No	Ingestion of aspirin, caffeine, and quinine, followed 17 h later by APAP. Presented in labor. Treated with oral methionine. Spontaneous delivery at 16 h. Infant: moderate hyaline membrane disease. Peak AST 86 (cord). Four whole-blood exchange transfusions. Discharged home at 54 d of life. Died at 106 d, no apparent cause.	153
31	40 (26)	13320 (60 h)	41 (27)	Yes	APAP only, C/S for fetal distress 1 h after initial maternal evaluation. Infant's birth weight was 1620 g. Apgars 0, 0, 1.[b] Infant died at 34 h of life. Mother died at 34 h post ingestion. No autopsy of mother or child.	286
32	448 (12 h)	5269 (48 h)	0 (84 h, cord)	No	IV NAC started at 12 h. Induced delivery at 84 h. Infant: transient hypoglycemia, mild respiratory distress, mild jaundice. Peak AST 56 (day 1 of life).	185,235
33	135 (28 h)	6237 (66 h)	330 (3 d, cord)	Yes	Oral NAC at 12 h. Fetal death at 2 d, spontaneous delivery at 3 d. Infant: stillborn with diffuse hepatic necrosis.	223
36	280 (3–4 h)	Normal	217 (6–7 h, cord)	No	Ingestion of APAP, ethanol, barbiturates. Elective C/S at 6–7 h. Infant: double volume exchange transfusion at 18 h. Discharge at 40 d, "cot death" at 157 d.	227
36	200 (5 h)	25 (24 h)	ND	No	Oral NAC (? time). Infant: spontaneous delivery 6 weeks after ingestion. Normal neonatal course.	48
38	216 (4 h)	Normal	13 (17 h, cord)	No	NAC (? route). Infant: normal neonatal course.	144,239
"Term"	147 (9 h)	28 (9 h)	133 (9 h, 4 h of life)	No	Infant PT 44 at 4 h of life. IV NAC. No problems. AST 86 at 4 h of life.	21
Term?	89 (11 h)	326 (35 h)	144 (11 h, 4 h of life)	No	Mother presented in labor at 6 h. Infant received IV NAC at 4 h of life. AST 55 at 4 h of life.	241

APAP, acetaminophen; AST, aspartate aminotransferase; C/S, cesarean section; IV, intravenous; NAC, *N*-acetylcysteine; ND, not done or not reported; PO, oral; PT, prothrombin time.

[a] Time after maternal ingestion.

[b] Apgars are at 1, 5, and 10 minutes.

reports with respect to specific acetaminophen effect because of the confounders of chronic disease, chronic use, or use of additional medications or substances.

Acetaminophen is an FDA use-in-pregnancy category B medication; at recommended doses, it is considered safe for use during pregnancy. However, in overdose, it may put the developing fetus at risk. As the third-trimester cases described above demonstrate, acetaminophen crosses the placenta to reach the developing fetus. The clinical series[185,223] suggest that there may be some increased risk of spontaneous abortion after overdose during the first trimester, but not with therapeutic use.[157] There is also a question about whether overdose during the first trimester can lead to late sequelae, for instance, premature labor.

Some experimental work may help to explain early pregnancy loss after overdose. Acetaminophen prevented the development of preimplantation (two-cell stage) mouse embryos in culture, an effect that was not associated with alterations in glutathione concentrations,[151] and also led to abnormal neuropore development in cultured rat embryos.[267] These data suggest that acetaminophen may be directly toxic to the immature organism. However, other work reported that similar embryotoxic effects were associated with reductions in glutathione concentrations[293] and that *N*-acetyl-*p*-benzoquinoneimine (NAPQI) produced nonspecific toxicity when added to the rat embryo culture medium.[267]

The fetal liver has some ability to metabolize acetaminophen to a reactive intermediate in vitro. Cytochrome P450 (CYP) activity was detected in intact hepatocytes, as well as in microsomal fractions isolated from the livers of fetuses aborted between 18 and 23 weeks of gestation, although fetal CYP activity was only 10% of the activity of hepatocytes isolated from adults following brain death; fetal CYP activity increased with increasing gestational age.[231] In two clinical cases, cysteine and mercapturate conjugates were identified in newborns exposed to acetaminophen in utero, suggesting that the fetus and neonate can metabolize acetaminophen through the CYP system.[153,227] These data suggest that the fetus in utero and the neonate can generate a toxic metabolite; the clinical cases suggest that the fetal liver is susceptible to injury.

This CYP activity has not been further characterized. However, CYP2E1, one of the cytochromes responsible for acetaminophen metabolism, is present in human fetal tissues as early as 16 weeks of gestation.[187] CYP3A4 and CYP1A2 are also involved in acetaminophen metabolism, but are not present in fetal liver. CYP3A7 is a functional fetal form of the CYP3 family, but its metabolic activity with respect to acetaminophen has not been studied.[108]

The most difficult questions relate to management of overdose during the third trimester. Can acetaminophen overdose lead to premature labor even if a pregnant woman does not have a toxic serum concentration or develop hepatotoxicity? Should a woman be emergently delivered following overdose? Does NAC treatment of the mother help the fetus? What is the appropriate treatment of a neonate exposed to acetaminophen in utero?

The clinical cases may help address the last two questions (see Table 30–3). Six women, all less than 36 weeks of gestation, developed hepatotoxicity. Two infants died in utero with evidence of severe hepatotoxicity, although what effect in utero postmortem changes may have had on serum acetaminophen concentrations or liver pathology is unclear. One infant died on the second day of life with hepatotoxicity. The other three infants experienced problems associated with prematurity but did not develop obvious hepatotoxicity. One of these three had an exchange transfusion and an unexplained death at 3 months of age. Five women, all at 36 or more weeks of gestation, did not develop hepatotoxicity. One infant had an exchange transfusion and did not develop hepatotoxicity but died a "cot death" at 5 months of age. One infant received IV NAC and had a transient elevation of aspartate aminotransferase (AST) and prothrombin time. Two infants were not treated; both did well, although one had a transient elevation of AST. One infant was born 6 weeks after the overdose and was normal.

Severe maternal hepatotoxicity that is associated with any sign of fetal distress is an indication for urgent delivery. Although a fetus with prolonged exposure to acetaminophen in utero is at risk of developing severe hepatotoxicity, not all at-risk infants are affected. What role gestational age, maternal disease state, or other maternal factors may play is unknown. Although there are insufficient case data to suggest that acetaminophen overdose per se is an indication for urgent delivery, there may be an indication for urgent delivery when the maternal serum acetaminophen concentration is in the toxic range but hepatotoxicity has not yet developed.[275] Significant acetaminophen overdose with or without hepatotoxicity can precipitate premature spontaneous labor, and even women with nontoxic serum concentrations may be at a slightly increased risk.

In two cases, exchange transfusion was employed to treat the exposed neonate. In both cases, the acetaminophen half-life was prolonged, and in neither case was this affected by the transfusion. Disturbingly, these two infants had unexplained deaths at several months of age. There is insufficient information on which to base a recommendation regarding exchange transfusion as therapy for prenatal exposure.

The pregnant woman with acute toxic acetaminophen ingestion should be treated with *N*-acetylcysteine (see Chap. 34 and Antidotes in Depth A–4: *N*-Acetylcysteine). This is therapy to treat the mother. Although maternal hepatoxicity or delayed NAC therapy may be associated with fetal toxicity,[223] there is insufficient information to indicate that prevention of maternal toxicity will prevent fetal toxicity in either the first or the third trimester. NAC was found in cord blood after administration to four mothers before delivery,[120] although NAC did not cross the sheep placenta in vivo[252] or the perfused human placenta in vitro.[124] Even if NAC does cross the placenta, whether it prevents fetal hepatotoxicity is unknown because not all exposed fetuses develop hepatotoxicity.

In four third-trimester cases where the mothers overdosed at or after 36 weeks of gestation and did not develop hepatotoxicity, the infants did well. One infant received NAC. There are anecdotal reports of infants who received NAC soon after delivery and did well. Current theory suggests that infants and young children are less likely than teenagers or adults to develop hepatotoxicity after acetaminophen overdose because of immature CYP activity and increased sulfation activity. It is intriguing to consider that this metabolic protection might extend to the newborn exposed to acetaminophen in utero. It also makes it difficult to know to what extent postnatal NAC therapy for the prenatally exposed newborn might prevent toxicity. Although there are no reported cases, it would seem that the premature newborn exposed in utero might be the best candidate for postnatal NAC therapy.

IRON

Iron is another common ingestant during pregnancy; maternal toxicity is generally greater than fetal toxicity. In two reported cases, normal babies were delivered although the mothers died.[206,221] In another case, the mother had severe iron toxicity with acidosis, shock, renal failure, and disseminated intravascular coagulation but was not treated with deferoxamine because of concerns about its teratogenic risks. Instead, the mother received an exchange transfusion followed 45 minutes later by a spontaneous abortion of the 16-week fetus.[174,271] Neonatal and cord blood iron concentrations were not elevated. In several cases, pregnant women who had signs and symptoms of iron poisoning and elevated serum iron concentrations were treated with deferoxamine and subsequently delivered normal babies.[32,136,147,215,246,280]

Although the placenta transports iron to the fetus efficiently,[20] it also blocks the transfer of large quantities of iron. In a sheep model of iron poisoning, only a small amount of iron was transferred across the placenta despite significantly elevated serum iron concentrations.[65]

Deferoxamine is an effective antidote for iron poisoning (see Chap. 40 and Antidotes in Depth A–7: Deferoxamine), but it is reported to be an animal teratogen that causes skeletal deformities and abnormalities of ossification (FDA class C pregnancy risk). An animal model observed similar effects, but only with doses of deferoxamine that caused maternal toxicity.[36] Experimentally, in sheep, little transfer of deferoxamine across the placenta was demonstrated[65]; therefore, the reported fetal effects may be secondary to chelation of essential nutrients (such as trace metals) on the maternal side of the placenta.[275]

In clinical case reports of iron overdose for which deferoxamine was used, there have been no adverse effects on the fetus, although most have been either second- or third-trimester poisonings.[32,136,147,206,215,246,280] In a case series of 49 patients with iron poisoning during pregnancy, few of the patients exhibited any clinical toxicity other than vomiting and diarrhea; 25 received deferoxamine, most by the oral route.[184] One woman with a first-trimester overdose, eight women with second-trimester overdoses, and 12 women with third-trimester overdoses were treated with deferoxamine and subsequently delivered full-term infants. One infant whose mother overdosed at 30 weeks of gestation had webbed fingers on one hand. One woman overdosed at 20 weeks, had minimal clinical toxicity, received deferoxamine, and delivered a 2.5-kg male infant at 34 weeks. One woman with a first-trimester overdose and two women with second-trimester overdoses elected to terminate their pregnancies.

Further support for the safe use of deferoxamine in pregnancy is the experience with its use for pregnant women with thalassemia. For many years deferoxamine has been administered as part of the therapy for posttransfusion iron overload without adverse effects.[259]

Deferoxamine is probably safe for use in pregnant women. Considering the potentially fatal nature of severe iron poisoning, deferoxamine should be administered when signs and symptoms indicate significant poisoning.

Iron overdose may be one of the few specific indications for whole-bowel irrigation because iron is not adsorbed to activated charcoal (see Antidotes in Depth A–2: Activated Charcoal). A case report demonstrated elimination of pill fragments following treatment of a pregnant woman with whole-bowel irrigation.[284]

CARBON MONOXIDE

Carbon monoxide is the leading cause of poisoning fatalities in the United States. In contrast to iron and most other xenobiotics, when pregnant women are exposed to carbon monoxide, the fetus may be at greater risk of toxicity than the woman herself. There are reports of both the mother and fetus dying, the mother surviving but the fetus dying, and both the mother and fetus surviving but with adverse neonatal outcome, primarily brain damage resembling that seen following severe cerebral ischemia.[49,64,143,161,175,200,284,300] Similar clinical effects have also been observed in animal models.[78,101,162]

The case literature suggests increased risk of poor fetal outcome with clinically severe maternal poisoning or significantly elevated carboxyhemoglobin concentrations.[143,200] Women with minimal symptoms and/or low concentrations of carboxyhemoglobin have a low risk of fetal toxicity, but a lower limit of exposure without effect has not been specifically defined.[143]

In animal models, under physiologic conditions, the fetus has a carboxyhemoglobin concentration 10% to 15% higher than the mother. After exposure to carbon monoxide, the fetus achieves peak carboxyhemoglobin concentrations 58% higher than those achieved by the mother at steady state, and the time to peak concentration is also delayed compared to the mother. Similarly, the elimination of carbon monoxide occurs more slowly in the fetus than in the mother.[115,161,162] One case report describes such a phenomenon: after 1 hour of supplemental oxygen, the maternal carboxyhemoglobin was 7% and the fetal carboxyhemoglobin was 61% at the time of death in utero.[83]

Carbon monoxide leads to fetal hypoxia by several mechanisms: (1) maternal carboxyhemoglobin leads to a decrease in the oxygen content of maternal blood, and therefore less oxygen is delivered across the placenta to the fetus, which normally has an arterial PO_2 of only 20 to 30 mm Hg; (2) fetal carboxyhemoglobin causes a decrease in fetal PO_2; (3) carbon monoxide shifts the oxyhemoglobin dissociation curve to the left and decreases the release of oxygen to the fetal tissues (an exacerbation of the physiologic left shift found with normal fetal hemoglobin); and (4) carbon monoxide may inhibit cytochrome oxidase or other mitochondrial functions (Chap. 125).

The treatment for severe carbon monoxide poisoning is hyperbaric oxygen therapy (HBO) (see Chap. 125 and Antidotes in Depth A–37: Hyperbaric Oxygen). There are questions about the use of HBO in pregnant women because animal models suggest HBO adversely effects the embryo or fetus.[88,188,244,274] The applicability of the animal models to humans is difficult to assess; many of the animal models used hyperbaric conditions of greater pressures and duration than those clinically used for humans.

HBO has been used therapeutically for carbon monoxide poisoning in pregnancy with good results reported, although there are limited data on the long-term follow-up of the children.[44,87,95,105,116,143,285] One large series reported 44 women who were exposed to carbon monoxide during pregnancy and were treated with HBO, regardless of clinical severity or gestational age: 33 had term births; one had a premature delivery 22 weeks after HBO, during an episode of maternal fever; two had spontaneous miscarriages (one 12 hours after severe poisoning and one 15 days after mild poisoning); one delivered a child with Down syndrome; one had an elective abortion; and six were lost to follow-up.[83] Unfortunately, details regarding trimester of exposure, maternal carboxyhemoglobin level, and severity of symptoms are not available, making it difficult to interpret the reported outcomes. Although HBO appears safe for pregnant women and seems to present little risk to the fetus, it is not clear whether HBO prevents carbon monoxide–related fetal toxicity for those at risk. Carbon monoxide can have a severe impact on fetal health and development and, as noted above, the maternal carboxyhemoglobin concentration may not accurately reflect the fetal carboxyhemoglobin concentration.

HBO should be considered for any pregnant woman exposed to carbon monoxide, especially for a woman with an elevated serum carboxyhemoglobin concentration or any evidence of fetal distress. In order to allow the fetal carboxyhemoglobin to be eliminated, if HBO therapy is not available, 100% oxygen should be administered to a pregnant woman for five times as long as the time needed for her carboxyhemoglobin to return to the normal range. Thus if a pregnant woman's carboxyhemoglobin level returns to normal in 30 minutes she should continue to receive 100% oxygen for a total of 150 minutes.

SUBSTANCE USE DURING PREGNANCY

One of the most complex areas of toxicology deals with issues of substance use during pregnancy and its effects on the woman, on the pregnancy itself, and on fetal and postnatal development. This section reviews of some of the important aspects of this topic.

Clinical research in the area of substance use during pregnancy is very difficult to perform. With the increased use of cocaine during the latter half of the 1980s and 1990s, there was great interest in determining the effects of cocaine use during pregnancy. As research in this area progressed, many of the critical methodologic issues related to substance use research were highlighted.[89,123,155,197,303]

Substance-using women often have multiple risk factors for adverse pregnancy outcomes, such as low socioeconomic status, polysubstance use, ethanol and cigarette use, sexually transmitted diseases, AIDS, malnutrition, and lack of prenatal care. Lack of prenatal care is highly correlated with premature birth, and smoking is associated with spontaneous abortion, growth retardation, and sudden infant death syndrome (SIDS).[133,295] Other factors not specifically related to substance use such as age, race, gravidity, and prior pregnancies also affect pregnancy outcome. Each of these factors represents a significant potential confounding variable when the effects of a particular xenobiotic such as cocaine or marijuana are evaluated during pregnancy and must be controlled for in research design. Many of these factors are also significant confounders in evaluation of postnatal growth and development.

There may be bias in the selection of study subjects. For example, if all the patients are selected from an inner-city hospital obstetrics service, there is potential for overestimating the effects of the xenobiotic being studied. If cohorts are followed over a long time, study subjects are frequently lost to follow-up. Are the ones who continue more motivated, or do they have more problems that need attention?

Categorizing patients into substance-use groups is difficult. Self-reporting of substance use is frequently unreliable or inaccurate, and making determinations about the nature, frequency, quantity (dose), or timing (with respect to gestation) of xenobiotic exposure is difficult. Because substance users frequently use multiple xenobiotics, it may be difficult to categorize subjects into particular xenobiotic-use groups, and patients using different xenobiotics may be grouped together. In fact, there may be no actual xenobiotic-free control groups.

When urine drug screens are used to identify substance users, there is a high probability of false negatives because drug screens reflect only recent use. This factor is particularly important because substance use tends to decrease later in pregnancy, and a negative urine drug screen in the third trimester or at delivery may fail to identify a woman who was using xenobiotics early in pregnancy. Testing for xenobiotics in hair or meconium may improve the accuracy of the analysis with regard to the entire pregnancy.[37,140]

Another bias involves selection of infants who are exposed to xenobiotics. Evaluating newborns who are "at risk," show signs of withdrawal, or have positive urine drug screens will miss some exposed infants. When research concerns the neurobehavioral development of children exposed in utero to substances, it is important that the examiners performing the evaluation be blinded to the infants' xenobiotic exposure category.

Finally, there may be a bias against publishing research that shows a negative or no significant effect.[141]

ETHANOL

Chronic ethanol use during pregnancy produces a constellation of fetal effects. The most severe effects are seen in the fetal alcohol syndrome (FAS), which is characterized by (1) intrauterine or postnatal growth retardation, (2) mental retardation or behavioral abnormalities, and (3) facial dysmorphogenesis, particularly microcephaly, short palpebral fissures, epicanthal folds, maxillary hypoplasia, cleft palate, hypoplastic philtrum, and micrognathia.[30,173] A child can be diagnosed with FAS even when a history of regular gestational alcohol use cannot be confirmed.

In an attempt to formalize diagnostic criteria for FAS and other gestational-alcohol-related effects, the Institute of Medicine proposed some additional descriptors which are in common use.[269] *Partial FAS* is applied to a child with some of the characteristic facial features and with either growth retardation, neurodevelopmental abnormalities, or other behavioral problems. *Alcohol-related birth defects* are congenital anomalies other than the characteristic facial features described above, for example, cleft palate, which are sometimes seen with regular gestational alcohol use. *Alcohol-related neurodevelopmental disorder* describes neurodevelopmental abnormalities or other behavioral problems, which are sometimes seen with regular gestational alcohol use. Fetal alcohol spectrum disorders (FASD) is an umbrella term describing the range of effects that can occur in an individual whose mother drank alcohol during pregnancy.[30,263]

Differential expression of the syndrome may reflect the effects of varying quantities of ethanol ingested at critical periods specific for particular effects. The craniofacial anomalies probably represent teratogenic effects during organogenesis, whereas some central nervous system abnormalities and growth retardation may result from adverse effects later in gestation.

There is considerable controversy about what level of alcohol consumption can cause fetal alcohol spectrum disorder.[193,203] Approximately 10% of women consume some alcohol during pregnancy, 2% are frequent users and 2% binge. Of women who might become pregnant, about 50% drink some alcohol, 13% drink frequently, and 12% binge.[50] Some researchers believe that the fetal alcohol spectrum disorder is a result of alcoholism—chronic regular use or frequent binging—rather than to low levels of gestational ethanol exposure, no matter how little or how infrequent.[4,104] A high level of consumption would be in the range of 50 to 100 mL of 100% ethanol (four to six "standard" drinks of hard liquor) regularly throughout pregnancy[269] or binge drinking (at least five standard drinks per occasion), with a significantly elevated peak blood ethanol concentration.[3,170] On the other hand, some behavioral abnormalities have been associated with the reported consumption of as little as one drink per week.[264] In this regard, neither a no-effect amount nor a safe amount of ethanol use in pregnancy has been determined[129] and therefore the US Surgeon General recommends no alcohol consumption during pregnancy.[205]

The incidence of FAS is 0.5 to 3 per 1000 live births; 4% of women who drink heavily may give birth to children with FAS.[2,181] This means that several hundred children with FAS and several thousand with fetal alcohol effects will be born each year; ethanol use is considered the leading preventable cause of mental retardation in this country.[269] Although the primary determinant of FAS and its effects is the level of maternal ethanol consumption, there is some evidence that paternal ethanol exposure may play a contributing role.[1]

Ethanol use during pregnancy may lead to an increased incidence of spontaneous abortion, premature deliveries, stillbirths,[171] neonatal ethanol withdrawal,[25,199] and possibly carcinogenesis.[137] Infants may be irritable or hypertonic and may have problems with habituation and arousal. Long-term behavioral and intellectual effects include decreased IQ, learning disability, memory deficits, speech and language disorders, hyperactivity, and dysfunctional behavior in school.[180,264,270]

Brain autopsies of children with FAS demonstrate malformations of gray and white matter, a failure of certain regions such as the corpus callosum to develop, a failure of certain cells such as the cerebellar astrocytes to migrate, and a tendency for tissue in certain regions to die.[86] The mechanisms of ethanol-induced teratogenesis are not fully elucidated.[26,109] Much of the work in animals has focused on the developing nervous system, where ethanol adversely affects nerve cell growth, differentiation, and migration, particularly in areas of the neocortex, hippocampus, sensory nucleus, and cerebellum.[106,272]

Several mechanisms are potential contributors to the effects of ethanol.[103] Ethanol interferes with a number of different growth factors, which may affect neuronal migration and development.[296] In addition, ethanol interferes with the development and function of both serotonin and *N*-methyl-D-aspartate (NMDA) receptors. Ethanol, or its metabolite acetaldehyde, may also cause necrosis of certain cells directly or through the generation of free radicals and excessive apoptosis.[59,86,113] In particular, craniofacial abnormalities may be related to apoptosis of neural crest cells through the formation of free radicals, a deficiency of retinoic acid, or the altered expression of homeobox genes which regulate growth and development.[272]

One integrative model of ethanol-induced teratogenesis proposes that sociobehavioral risk factors, such as drinking behavior, smoking behavior, low socioeconomic status, and cultural/ethnic influences, create provocative biologic conditions, such as high peak blood ethanol concentrations, circulating tobacco constituents, and undernutrition. These provocative factors exacerbate fetal vulnerability to potential teratogenic mechanisms, such as ethanol-related hypoxia or free radical–induced cell damage.[5]

Table 30–4. Signs and Symptoms of Neonatal Opioid Withdrawal

Neurologic Excitability	Gastrointestinal Dysfunction	Autonomic Signs
Exaggerated Moro reflex	Dehydration	Fever
Frequent yawning and sneezing	Diarrhea	Increased sweating
High-pitched crying	Poor feeding	Mottling
Hyperactive deep tendon reflexes	Poor weight gain	Nasal stuffiness
Increased muscle tone	Uncoordinated and constant sucking	Temperature instability
Increased wakefulness		
Irritability	Vomiting	
Seizures		
Tremors		

Reproduced with permission from the Committee on Drugs. Neonatal drug withdrawal. *Pediatrics*. 1998;101:1079–1088.

OPIOIDS

Opioid use in pregnancy remains a significant cause of both maternal and neonatal morbidity. In past month surveys, heroin use is reported by approximately 0.1% of pregnant women,[204] and up to 75,000 babies per year may be exposed to methadone or heroin in utero.[194] Almost all clinical research regarding opioid toxicity during pregnancy relates to the use of heroin or methadone, although recent surveys indicate that approximately 0.1% of women use oxycodone (OxyContin) during pregnancy and the lay press has begun to report on fetal OxyContin exposure.[204,234]

Pregnant opioid users are at increased risk for many medical complications of pregnancy, such as hepatitis, sepsis, endocarditis, sexually transmitted diseases, and AIDS, and may be at increased risk for obstetric complications, such as miscarriage, premature delivery, or stillbirth.[89,102] Some of the obstetric complications may be related to associated risk factors in addition to the opioid use.

Maternal opioid use most commonly affects fetal growth.[89,102,303] There is an increased incidence of low birth weight in babies born to opioid-using mothers, compared to controls, and the effect is greater for heroin than for methadone. Women who receive low-dose methadone and good prenatal care have birth outcomes similar to nonusers, but they are at increased risk for pregnancy-related complications.[89]

The most significant acute neonatal complication of opioid use during pregnancy is the neonatal withdrawal syndrome (NWS), characterized by hyperirritability, gastrointestinal dysfunction, respiratory distress, and vague autonomic symptoms, including yawning, sneezing, mottling, and fever (Table 30–4).[13] Myoclonic jerks or seizures may also signify neurologic irritability. Withdrawing infants are recognizable by their extreme jitteriness, despite efforts at consolation; ecchymoses and contusions may be found on the tips of their fingers or toes, as a result of trauma from striking the sides of the bassinet. From 60% to 90% of methadone, heroin, and probably other chronic opioid-exposed offspring will show some signs of withdrawal.[89]

Some of the manifestations of the neonatal withdrawal syndrome may be caused by enhanced α-adrenergic activity in the locus coeruleus. Firing of neurons in this region of the brain leads to such NWS-like behaviors as wakefulness and tremors—effects that are inhibited by opioid agonists. Chronic opioid administration leads to tolerance, as well as an increased number of α_2-adrenergic receptors. Presumably, withdrawal of opioids causes increased stimulation of a large number of receptors in this region, leading to clinical signs of withdrawal.

Opioid withdrawal symptoms typically occur within 2 weeks of birth. Heroin withdrawal usually occurs within the first 24 hours; however, methadone withdrawal may be delayed because it has a larger volume of distribution and slower metabolism in the neonate, and therefore an increased half-life. In one study, methadone withdrawal occurred when the plasma concentration fell below 0.06 mg/mL.[232] The onset and severity of symptoms may be related to whether heroin, methadone, or both were used; how much was used chronically; how much was used near the time of delivery; the character of the labor; whether analgesics or anesthetics were used; and the maturity, nutrition, and medical condition of the neonate.[72] Acute neonatal withdrawal symptoms generally last from days to weeks, but some symptoms may persist for months.[13]

From 5% to 7% of babies showing signs of withdrawal experience seizures, generally by 10 days after birth.[114] Seizures may be more likely after methadone withdrawal than after heroin withdrawal.[302] These seizures do not necessarily predispose to idiopathic epilepsy; in one small study, children who had withdrawal seizures were normal at 1-year follow-up.[75]

Treatment of withdrawal begins by providing a comforting environment: swaddling or tightly wrapping the infant, minimal handling or stimulation, and demand feeding. More severe symptoms may require pharmacologic therapy. One way of determining the need for therapy is the application of a severity-scoring scale. In general, babies who are extremely irritable; have feeding difficulties, diarrhea, or significant tremors; or are crying continuously are candidates for pharmacologic therapy.[11,131]

Opioid agonists such as morphine, methadone, tincture of opium and paregoric, and sedative-hypnotic agents such as diazepam and phenobarbital have been used to treat withdrawal symptoms.[11,131] Tincture of opium, diluted to a final dose of 0.4 mg/mL of morphine equivalent, may be preferred because it is a pure opioid agonist, and the formulation has no additives. However, there are few well-controlled trials evaluating the relative efficacy of the different agents.[89]

Opioid agonists may be more effective at preventing withdrawal seizures from heroin or methadone than from phenobarbital or diazepam.[114,132] However, sedative-hypnotics are commonly used by heroin users or adults maintained on methadone, and sedative-hypnotic withdrawal seizures may contribute to the overall neonatal abstinence symptomatology. In this setting there may be a role for phenobarbital. Because oral administration of phenobarbital may delay achieving a therapeutic concentration, parenteral administration may be required.

Infants of opioid-using mothers have a two to three times increased risk for SIDS compared to controls.[133,134] The mechanism may be related to a decreased medullary responsiveness to CO_2, or the effect may be related to some condition of the postnatal environment.[89]

Although young children born to opioid users do not seem to have significant differences in behavior compared to controls, older children have increased learning problems and school dysfunction particularly related to behavior difficulties.[303]

COCAINE

Approximately 1% of pregnant women in the United States use cocaine at some time during their pregnancy.[194] The rate may be as high as 15% in certain populations,[70] and it is estimated that more than 100,000 infants born in the United States each year may be exposed to cocaine in utero.[54] The consequences of cocaine use during pregnancy have been extensively reviewed.[118,211,253]

The incidence of abruptio placentae may be significant when related to acute cocaine use.[257] Some uncommon perinatal problems include seizures, cerebral infarctions, and other CNS effects.[57,211]

Cocaine use is significantly related to decreases in gestational age, birth weight, length, and head circumference, although these growth parameters generally correct by several years of age.[253] In addition, these growth effects are exacerbated by concomitant alcohol, tobacco, and opiate use.[253] Good prenatal care can mitigate many of these adverse effects of cocaine.[166,222,303]

Significant congenital malformations were reported among some infants who were exposed to cocaine in utero, specifically genitourinary malformations, cardiovascular malformations, and limb-reduction defects.[46,93] However, in one large population-based study, there was no increase in the incidence of malformations.[176]

Teratogenic effects have been observed in animal models of in utero cocaine exposure. Decreased maternal and fetal weight gain and an increased frequency of fetal resorption were demonstrated in rats[85]; sporadic physical anomalies have also been observed.[58] Teratogenic effects similar to those observed in humans were reported in mice: bony defects of the skull, cryptorchidism, hydronephrosis, ileal atresia, cardiac defects, limb deformities, and eye abnormalities.[90,167,168,186] Cocaine caused hemorrhage and edema of the extremities and, subsequently, limb-reduction defects in rats when administered during midgestation in the postorganogenic period.[290]

The perinatal effects of cocaine are probably mediated through a vascular mechanism. Cocaine administration in the pregnant ovine model causes increased uterine vascular resistance, decreased uterine blood flow, increased fetal heart rate and arterial blood pressure, and decreased fetal PO_2 and O_2 content.[19,298] Similar effects have been seen in rats.[208] Fetal hypoxia may cause rupture of fetal blood vessels and infarction in developing organ systems such as the genitourinary system[56,186,262] or the CNS.[55,74,291] Hyperthermia or direct effects of cocaine in the fetus may exacerbate these effects.[38] Limb-reduction defects similar to those attributed to cocaine have been produced after mechanical clamping of the uterine vessels.[38,292] A developing concept is that following vasospasm and ischemia, reperfusion occurs with the generation of oxygen free radicals and subsequent injury.[298,299]

Despite the reported malformations and a possible mechanism, neither the human epidemiology nor the effects observed in animal models suggest a specific teratogenic syndrome. The risk of a significant malformation from prenatal cocaine exposure is low, but the effect, if one occurs, may be severe.[40,80,93]

One of the greatest concerns about prenatal cocaine exposure is the potential adverse effect on the developing child, and this is an intensive area of epidemiologic research. The most common findings in early infancy are lability of behavior and autonomic regulation, decreased alertness and orientation, and abnormal reflexes, tone, and motor maturity; however, many studies show no effect especially after controlling for confounding variables.[84,253] For some children, effects may manifest in later infancy as difficulty with information processing and learning. For school-age children, observed cognitive deficits may also be related to the home environment, even for those children who showed some of the typical neonatal behaviors.[91,253] Nonetheless, there is evidence of impairment in modulating attention and impulsivity, which makes handling unfamiliar, complex, and stressful tasks more difficult,[183,253] and these effects are also observed in animal models of prenatal cocaine exposure.[80,111,158,265]

The mechanism of neurotoxicity has not been specifically elucidated. As described above, for many of the maternal and fetal physical defects, cocaine may have direct toxicity or, alternatively, effects may be mediated through hypoxia or oxygen free radicals. Because cocaine interferes with neurotransmitter reuptake, it is likely that cocaine also disrupts normal neural ontogeny by interfering with the trophic functions of neurotransmitters on the developing brain, in particular dysfunction of signal transduction via the dopamine D1 receptor.[111,158,172,182] These mechanisms may be more important in the etiology of neurobehavioral effects.

BREAST-FEEDING

In the United States, breast-feeding is the recommended method of infant nutrition because it offers nutritional, immunologic, and psychological benefits. Many women use prescription and nonprescription xenobiotics while breast-feeding, and are concerned about the possible ill effects on the infant of these xenobiotics in the breast milk. This concern extends to the possible exposure of the infant to occupational and environmental xenobiotics via breast milk.[229,248] The response to many of these concerns can be determined by the answer to the following question: Does the risk to an infant from a xenobiotic exposure via breast milk exceed the benefit of being breast-fed?[152]

Pharmacokinetic factors determine the amount of xenobiotic available for transfer from maternal plasma into breast milk; only free xenobiotic can traverse the mammary alveolar membrane. Most xenobiotics are transported by passive diffusion. A few xenobiotics, such as ethanol and lithium, are transported through aqueous-filled pores. The factors that determine how well a xenobiotic diffuses across the membrane are similar to those for other biologic membranes such as the placenta: molecular weight, lipid solubility, and degree of ionization.

Large-molecular-weight xenobiotics, such as heparin or insulin, will not pass into breast milk. Lipid solubility is important not only for diffusion but also for xenobiotic accumulation in breast milk, because breast milk is rich in fat, especially breast milk that is produced in the postcolostral period (approximately 3 to 4 days postpartum). With a pH near 7.0, breast milk is slightly more acidic than plasma. Consequently, xenobiotics that are weak acids in plasma exist largely as ionized molecules and cannot be easily transported into milk. Conversely, xenobiotics that are weak bases exist in plasma largely as nonionized molecules and are available for transport into breast milk. Once in the breast milk, ionization of the weak base xenobiotics occurs, and the xenobiotic is concentrated as a result of ion trapping. In other words, xenobiotics that are weak bases may concentrate in breast milk.

Sulfacetamide (pK_a 5.4, a weak acid) has a concentration in plasma 10 times its concentration in breast milk, whereas sulfanilamide (pK_a 10.4, a weak base) is found in equal concentrations in both plasma and breast milk.[152]

The net effect of these physiologic processes is expressed in the milk-to-plasma (M/P) ratio. Xenobiotics with higher M/P ratios have relatively greater concentrations in breast milk. The M/P ratio does not, however, reflect the absolute concentration of a xenobiotic in the breast milk, and a xenobiotic with a high M/P *ratio* is not necessarily found at a high *concentration* in the breast milk. For example, morphine has an M/P ratio of 2.46 (is concentrated in breast milk), but only 0.4% of a maternal dose is excreted into the breast milk.[18] In general, for most pharmaceuticals, approximately 1% to 2% of the maternally administered dose is presented to the infant in breast milk.[152]

The M/P ratio has several limitations. It does not account for differences in xenobiotic concentration that may result from (1) repeat or chronic dosing, (2) breast-feeding at different times relative to maternal xenobiotic dosing, (3) differences in milk production during the day or even during a particular breast-feeding session, (4) the time postpartum (days, weeks, or months) when the measurement is made, and (5) maternal disease.

While being cognizant of the limitations, a spot breast milk xenobiotic concentration or a concentration estimate based on the M/P ratio allows a simplistic estimation of the quantity of xenobiotic to which an infant is exposed, assuming a constant breast-milk concentration:

$$\text{Infant dose} = \text{Breast-milk concentration} \times \text{amount consumed}$$

The effect of this dose on the infant depends on the bioavailability of the xenobiotic in breast milk, the pharmacokinetic parameters that determine xenobiotic concentrations in the infant, and the infant's receptor sensitivity to the xenobiotic. These parameters are often different in neonates than in adults and may lead to xenobiotic accumulation; generally, absorption is greater, but metabolism and clearance are reduced.[17] These effects are exaggerated in premature infants.[216,226] The amount of most xenobiotics delivered to infants in breast milk is usually adequately metabolized and eliminated.[152]

Many of the considerations above are theoretical, and the number of specifically contraindicated xenobiotics is quite small.[14] Published guidelines on the advisability of breast-feeding during periods of maternal therapy are generally based on the expected effects of full doses in the infant or on case reports of adverse occurrences. Interestingly, when the reports of adverse effects were reviewed, 37% of cases were in infants younger than 2 weeks old, 63% were in infants younger than 1 month old, and 78% were in infants younger than 2 months old; 18% were in infants 2 to 6 months old; and only 4% were in infants older than 6 months.[15] It seems, therefore, that adverse effects are most likely to be observed in the first few weeks of life, when an infant's metabolic capacity is only 20% to 40% that of an adult.[8]

Every few years the American Academy of Pediatrics (AAP) publishes recommendations regarding breast-feeding in the setting of xenobiotic exposure. In the latest revision, the AAP continues to discourage the use of xenobiotics such as cocaine or heroin during the breast-feeding period because of direct effects on the baby, as well as detrimental effects on the physical and emotional health of the mother and on the caregiving environment.[14] Although ethanol is not specifically contraindicated for the breast-feeding mother, decreased milk production and adverse effects in the infant are noted with maternal consumption of large amounts of ethanol.[152]

The AAP recommends the temporary cessation of breast-feeding when the mother is exposed to metronidazole, an in vitro mutagen, or to certain radiopharmaceuticals, specifically isotopes of copper, gallium, indium, iodine, sodium, and technetium. In these cases, breast milk can be collected and stored before medication use for later feeding to the baby. Breast-feeding is resumed when the milk is no longer radioactive, generally 1 to 3 days for most of the isotopes mentioned except gallium, after which radioactivity may be present for 2 weeks. Metronidazole can be administered as a single 2-g dose, allowing breast-feeding to be discontinued for only 12 to 24 hours.[152]

Although there are few data demonstrating specific effects, the AAP suggests caution with regard to breast-feeding while using sedative-hypnotics, antidepressants, and antipsychotics. These medications modulate neurotransmitters in the CNS, which can adversely affect the developing nervous system.

For most xenobiotics, a risk-to-benefit analysis must be made. For example, lithium is transferred in breast milk and may lead to measurable, although subtherapeutic, serum concentrations in the breast-fed infant. Although the effects of such exposure to lithium are unknown, many practitioners believe that the benefit of treating a mother's bipolar illness outweighs the potential risk to the infant.[152,247]

Similarly, the breast-fed infant of a woman who smokes is exposed to nicotine and other tobacco constituents, both by inhalation and via breast milk. Although this child may be at increased risk for respiratory illness as a result of exposure to tobacco smoke, some of the risk may be reduced by breast feeding.[14,224]

Many xenobiotics, including pharmaceuticals, foods, and environmental xenobiotics, have been found in breast milk, and Table 30–5 lists some of their effects. In addition to the effects listed, there may be a small increased risk of carcinogenicity associated with exposure to some environmental xenobiotics through breast milk.[229]

In most cases, women do not need to stop breast-feeding while using pharmaceuticals, such as most common antibiotics. However, "compatibility" with breast-feeding is generally based on a lack of reported adverse effects, which may reflect limited clinical experience with a particular xenobiotic in breast-feeding patients. Therefore, in the setting of limited information, exposure to a xenobiotic through breast milk should be regarded as a small potential risk, and the infant should receive appropriate medical follow-up. Not all "compatible" medications are safe in all situations. For instance, phenobarbital can produce CNS depression in an infant if the mother's serum concentration is in the high therapeutic or supratherapeutic range, which often occurs while dosage adjustments are being made. Such a concentration may or may not produce CNS depression in the mother. Nalidixic acid, nitrofurantoin, sulfapyridine, and sulfisoxazole, although generally safe, can cause hemolysis in a breast-fed infant with glucose-6-phosphate dehydrogenase deficiency.

Decisions on breast-feeding should be made with the informed involvement of the woman, her physicians and, when necessary, a consultant with special expertise in this field. Guidelines are available from several sources.[28,42,152,190]

TOXICOLOGIC PROBLEMS IN THE NEONATE

Physiologic differences between adults and newborn infants affect xenobiotic absorption, distribution, and metabolism.[17,135,287] Appropriate administration of xenobiotics to newborn infants therefore requires an understanding of the appropriate developmental state for medication dosing and pharmacokinetics. Even so, approximately 8% of all medication doses administered in neonatal intensive care units (NICUs) may be up to 10 times greater or lesser than the dose ordered,[62] and as many as 30% of newborns in NICUs may sustain adverse drug effects, some of which may be life threatening or fatal.[18] Pharmacokinetic differences between adults and newborns may account for some cases of unanticipated xenobiotic toxicity seen in the newborn infant.

Table 30–5. Xenobiotics Associated With Effects on Some Nursing Infants

Xenobiotic	Effect
Use With Caution	
5-Aminosalicylic acid	Diarrhea
Acebutolol, atenolol, nadolol, sotalol, timolol	Hypotension, bradycardia, tachypnea, cyanosis
Amiodarone	Possible hypothyroidism
Antineoplastics: Cyclophosphamide, cyclosporine, doxorubicin, methotrexate	Neutropenia, thrombocytopenia, ? immune suppression; ? effect on growth or carcinogenesis
Aspirin	Metabolic acidosis; may affect platelet function; rash
Bromocriptine	Suppresses lactation
Chloramphenicol	Potential risk for aplastic anemia or gray-baby syndrome[131]
Chlorpromazine	Galactorrhea in mother; drowsiness and lethargy in infant; decline in developmental scores
Cimetidine	Possible antiandrogenic effects[152]
Clemastine	Drowsiness, irritability, refusal to feed, high-pitched cry, meningismus
Clofazimine	Possible increased skin pigmentation
Codeine	CNS and respiratory depression
Ergotamine	Vomiting, diarrhea, seizures; may inhibit prolactin secretion and lactation
Fluoxetine	Colic, irritability, feeding and sleeping disorders, slow weight gain
Haloperidol	Decline in developmental scores
Lamotrigine	Potential therapeutic serum concentrations in infant
Lithium	Subtherapeutic concentrations in infant
Metronidazole, tinidazole	In vitro mutagen
Phenindione	Risk of hemorrhage
Phenobarbital	Sedation, withdrawal after weaning from phenobarbital-containing milk; methemoglobinemia
Primidone	Sedation, feeding problems
Propylthiouracil, methimazole	May cause thyroid suppression and goiter[152]
Salicylates	Metabolic acidosis; may affect platelet function; rash
Sulfapyridine, sulfisoxazole	Caution in infant with jaundice or G6PD deficiency and in ill, stressed, or premature infant
Sulfasalazine	Bloody diarrhea
Tetracycline	May cause staining of infant teeth after prolonged maternal use[131]
Use Is Compatible With Breast-Feeding Despite Known Effect	
Ethanol	Large doses: ↓ milk ejection reflex. Infant: drowsiness, diaphoresis, ↓ growth and weight gain
Bendroflumethiazide	Suppresses lactation
Caffeine	Irritability, poor sleeping pattern (no effect with usual amount of caffeinated beverages)
Carbimazole	Goiter
Chloral hydrate	Sleepiness
Chlorthalidone	Excreted slowly
Contraceptive pills with estrogen/progesterone	Rare breast enlargement; decrease in milk production and protein content (unconfirmed)
Danthron	Increased bowel activity
Dexbrompheniramine maleate with *d*-isoephedrine	Crying, irritability, poor sleeping pattern
Estradiol	Withdrawal vaginal bleeding
Indomethacin	Seizure
Iodine topical	Odor of iodine on infant's skin
Iodine, iodides	Goiter
Methyprylon	Drowsiness
Nalidixic acid	Hemolysis in infant with G6PD deficiency
Nitrofurantoin	Hemolysis in infant with G6PD deficiency
Phenytoin	Methemoglobinemia
Theophylline	Irritability
Specific Risk Categories	
Aspartame	Caution if mother has phenylketonuria
Chocolate (theobromine)	Irritability or increased bowel activity if mother consumes large amounts
Fava beans	Hemolysis in infant with G6PD deficiency
Hexachlorobenzene	Skin rash, diarrhea, vomiting, dark urine, neurotoxicity, death
Lead	Possible neurotoxicity
Methylmercury, mercury	Possible neurodevelopmental toxicity
Polyhalogenated biphenyls	Lack of endurance, hypotonia, sullen expressionless facies
Silicone	Esophageal dysmotility
Tetrachloroethylene	Obstructive jaundice, dark urine
Vegetarian diet	Vitamin B_{12} deficiency

GI absorption of xenobiotics in the neonate is generally slower than in adults.[17,135,287] This delay may be related to decreased gastric acid secretion, decreased gastric emptying and transit time, and decreased pancreatic enzyme activity. The GI environment of the newborn and young infant may allow the growth of *Clostridium botulinum* and the subsequent development of infantile botulism (see Chap. 46). Infantile botulism has been reported in infants several weeks of age.[122,277]

Although it is uncommon, cutaneous absorption of xenobiotics may be a route of toxic exposure in the newborn.[82,240] Aniline dyes used for marking diapers are absorbed, causing methemoglobinemia,[240] and contaminated diapers were responsible for one epidemic of mercury poisoning.[22] The absorption of hexachlorophene antiseptic wash has led to neurotoxicity with marked vacuolization of myelin seen microscopically.[149,177,258] The dermal application of antiseptic ethanol has caused hemorrhagic necrosis of the skin of some premature infants. Iodine antiseptics have led to hypothyroidism in mature newborns.[51] Increased potential for absorption and toxicity has followed the application of corticosteroids[98,238] and boric acid[81] to the skin of children with cutaneous disorders.

Other routes of exposure have led to clinical poisoning. Several children aspirated talcum powder and died.[43,192] Inhalation of mercury from incubator thermometers may be a potential risk.[12] One child died following the ophthalmic instillation of cyclopentolate hydrochloride.[24]

Because of differences in total body water and fat compared to the adult, the distribution of absorbed xenobiotics may differ in neonates.[17,135,287] Water represents 80% of body weight in a full-term baby, compared to 60% in an adult. Approximately 20% of a term baby's body weight is fat, compared to only 3% in a premature baby. The increased volume of water means that the volume of distribution for some water-soluble xenobiotics, such as theophylline or phenobarbital, is increased.

Protein binding of xenobiotics is reduced in newborns compared to adults: the serum concentration of proteins is lower, there are fewer receptor sites that become saturated at lower xenobiotic concentrations, and binding sites have decreased binding affinity.[17,135,287] Protein binding has potential relevance with respect to bilirubin, an endogenous metabolite that at very high concentrations can cause kernicterus; bilirubin competes with exogenously administered xenobiotics for protein binding sites. In vitro, certain xenobiotics, such as sulfonamides and ceftriaxone, displace bilirubin from protein receptor sites, which might increase the risk of kernicterus, although this has not been clinically demonstrated. Conversely, bilirubin may itself displace other xenobiotics, such as phenobarbital or phenytoin, leading to increased plasma xenobiotic concentrations.

Newborn infants have decreased hepatic metabolic capacity compared with adults, which may lead to xenobiotic toxicity.[17,135] For example, caffeine, used in the treatment of neonatal apnea, has an extremely prolonged half-life in newborns because CYP1A2 has only 5% of the normal adult activity.[17] Except for CYP1A2, most of the CYP enzymes reach approximately 25% of adult activity in newborns by about 1 month of age.

Two syndromes related to immature metabolic function have been described. The "gasping baby syndrome," characterized by gasping respirations, metabolic acidosis, hypotension, central nervous system depression, convulsions, renal failure, and occasionally death, is attributed to high concentrations of benzyl alcohol and benzoic acid in the plasma of affected infants.[11,45,99] Benzyl alcohol, a bacteriostatic agent, was added to intravenous flush solutions and accumulated in newborns after repetitive doses. The high concentrations of benzoic acid could not be further metabolized to hippuric acid by the immature liver. Immature glucuronidation in the neonate is responsible for the "gray-baby syndrome" following high doses of chloramphenicol (Chaps. 31 and 55).[117]

The umbilical vessels are a common site of vascular access in sick neonates. Because blood drains into the portal vein, it is possible that IV medications experience a "first-pass" effect, although whether this route of xenobiotic administration affects metabolism or clearance has not been well studied. Most renal functions, including glomerular filtration rate and tubular secretion, are relatively immature at birth[17]; the glomerular filtration rate of the newborn is approximately 30% of that of an adult. Xenobiotics such as aminoglycosides and digoxin are excreted unchanged by the kidney and, therefore, depend on glomerular filtration for clearance. Dosing of these xenobiotics in the newborn must account for these differences.

An interesting association has been made periodically over the years between the use of erythromycin, particularly in the first 2 weeks of life, and idiopathic hypertrophic pyloric stenosis.[61,119,169,242,266] Although erythromycin is known to interact with motilin receptors in the antrum of the stomach, no specific etiology has been defined.[112]

Very little information is available to guide the clinician in the management of xenobiotic poisoning in the newborn infant. Cutaneous absorption is probably already complete by the time toxicity is noted, although further exposure may be prevented. Gastrointestinal decontamination is not generally performed in neonates, and the neonate may be at increased risk of fluid, electrolyte, and thermoregulatory problems following gastric lavage or the use of cathartic agents. Multiple-dose activated charcoal was used in a 1.4-kg 2-week-old premature infant to treat theophylline poisoning.[254] Hemodialysis, hemoperfusion, and exchange transfusion are used in neonates to treat xenobiotic toxicity (Chaps. 9 and 31).

SUMMARY

The use of xenobiotics in the pregnant or breast-feeding woman is a complex area of medical practice and presents the clinician with potentially difficult management decisions. This chapter highlights some of the important principles of xenobiotic effects in both the pregnant woman and the fetus. Appropriate management of many of the potential problems will be facilitated by the coordinated efforts of obstetricians, perinatologists, neonatologists, pediatricians, and toxicologists.

REFERENCES

1. Abel E. Paternal contribution to fetal alcohol syndrome. *Addict Biol.* 2004;9:127-133; discussion 135-126.
2. Abel EL. An update on incidence of FAS: FAS is not an equal opportunity birth defect. *Neurotoxicol Teratol.* 1995;17:437-443.
3. Abel EL. *Fetal Alcohol Abuse Syndrome.* New York: Plenum Press; 1998.
4. Abel EL. Fetal alcohol syndrome: a cautionary note. *Curr Pharm Des.* 2006;12:1521-1529.
5. Abel EL, Hannigan JH. Maternal risk factors in fetal alcohol syndrome: provocative and permissive influences. *Neurotoxicol Teratol.* 1995;17:445-462.
6. Addis A, Moretti ME, Schuller-Faccini L. Teratogen information services around the world. In: Koren G, ed. *Medication Safety in Pregnancy and Breastfeeding.* New York: McGraw-Hill; 2007:289-294.
7. Addis A, Sharabi S, Bonati M. Risk classification systems for drug use during pregnancy: are they a reliable source of information? *Drug Saf.* 2000;23:245-253.
8. Alcorn J, McNamara PJ. Pharmacokinetics in the newborn. *Adv Drug Deliv Rev.* 2003;55:667-686.
9. Alwan S, Polifka JE, Friedman JM. Addendum: sartan treatment during pregnancy. *Birth Defects Res A Clin Mol Teratol.* 2005;73:904-905.
10. Alwan S, Polifka JE, Friedman JM. Angiotensin II receptor antagonist treatment during pregnancy. *Birth Defects Res A Clin Mol Teratol.* 2005;73:123-130.

11. American Academy of Pediatrics. Benzyl alcohol: toxic agent in neonatal units. *Pediatrics.* 1983;72:356-358.
12. American Academy of Pediatrics. Mercury vapor contamination of infant incubators: a potential hazard. *Pediatrics.* 1984;67:637.
13. American Academy of Pediatrics. Neonatal drug withdrawal. *Pediatrics.* 1998;101:1079-1088.
14. American Academy of Pediatrics. Transfer of drugs and other chemicals into human milk. *Pediatrics.* 2001;108:776-789.
15. Anderson PO, Pochop SL, Manoguerra AS. Adverse drug reactions in breastfed infants: less than imagined. *Clin Pediatr.* 2003;42:325-340.
16. Appleby L. Suicide during pregnancy and in the first postnatal year. *BMJ.* 1991;302:137-140.
17. Aranda JV, Edwards DJ, Hales BF, Rieder MJ. Developmental pharmacology. In: Fanaroff AA, Martin RJ, eds. *Neonatal-Perinatal Medicine, Vol. 1.* St. Louis: Mosby; 2002:144-166.
18. Aranda JV, Portuguez-Malavasi A, Collinge JM, Germanson T, Outerbridge EW. Epidemiology of adverse drug reactions in the newborn. *Dev Pharmacol Ther.* 1982;5:173-184.
19. Arbeille P, Maulik D, Salihagic A, et al. Effect of long-term cocaine administration to pregnant ewes on fetal hemodynamics, oxygenation, and growth. *Obstet Gynecol.* 1997;90:795-802.
20. Atkinson DE, Boyd RDH, Sibley CP. Placental transfer. In: Neill JD, ed. *Knobil and Neill's Physiology of Reproduction, Vol. 2.* Amsterdam: Elsevier; 2006:2787-2827.
21. Aw MM, Dhawan A, Baker AJ, Mieli-Vergani G. Neonatal paracetamol poisoning. *Arch Dis Child Fetal Neonatal Ed.* 1999;81:F78.
22. Banzaw TM. Mercury poisoning in Argentine babies linked to diapers. *Pediatrics.* 1981;67:637.
23. Barnes AB, Colton T, Gundersen J, et al. Fertility and outcome of pregnancy in women exposed in utero to diethylstilbestrol. *N Engl J Med.* 1980;302:609-613.
24. Bauser CR, Trottier MCT, Stern L. Systemic cyclopentolate (Cyclogyl) toxicity in the newborn infant. *J Pediatr.* 1973;82:501.
25. Beattie JO. Transplacental alcohol intoxication. *Alcohol Alcohol.* 1986;21:163-166.
26. Becker HC, Diaz-Granados JL, Randall CL. Teratogenic actions of ethanol in the mouse: a minireview. *Pharmacol Biochem Behav.* 1996;55: 501-513.
27. Beckman DA, Brent RL. Teratogenesis: alcohol, angiotensin-converting-enzyme inhibitors, and cocaine. *Curr Opin Obstet Gynecol.* 1990;2: 236-245.
28. Bennett PN, Jensen AA. *Drugs and Human Lactation: A Comprehensive Guide to the Content and Consequences of Drugs, Micronutrients, Radiopharmaceuticals, and Environmental and Occupational Chemicals in Human Milk.* 2nd ed. Amsterdam: New York; 1996.
29. Bentur Y. Ionizing and nonionizing radiation in pregnancy. In: Koren G, ed. *Medication Safety in Pregnancy and Breastfeeding.* New York: McGraw-Hill; 2007:221-248.
30. Bertrand J, Floyd RL, Weber MK, et al. *Fetal Alcohol Syndrome: Guidelines for Referral and Diagnosis.* Atlanta, GA: Centers for Disease Control and Prevention; 2004.
31. Bibbo M, Gill WB, Azizi F, et al. Follow-up study of male and female offspring of DES-exposed mothers. *Obstet Gynecol.* 1977;49:1-8.
32. Blanc P, Hryhorczuk D, Danel I. Deferoxamine treatment of acute iron intoxication in pregnancy. *Obstet Gynecol.* 1984;64:12S-14S.
33. Bonari L, Pinto N, Ahn E, et al. Perinatal risks of untreated depression during pregnancy. *Can J Psychiatry.* 2004;49:726-735.
34. Bonati M, Bortolus R, Marchetti F, Romero M, Tognoni G. Drug use in pregnancy: an overview of epidemiological (drug utilization) studies. *Eur J Clin Pharmacol.* 1990;38:325-328.
35. Bonati M, Fellin G. Changes in smoking and drinking behaviour before and during pregnancy in Italian mothers: implications for public health intervention. ICGDUP (Italian Collaborative Group on Drug Use in Pregnancy). *Int J Epidemiol.* 1991;20:927-932.
36. Bosque MA, Domingo JL, Corbella J. Assessment of the developmental toxicity of deferoxamine in mice. *Arch Toxicol.* 1995;69:467-471.
37. Boumba VA, Ziavrou KS, Vougiouklakis T. Hair as a biological indicator of drug use, drug abuse or chronic exposure to environmental toxicants. *Int J Toxicol.* 2006;25:143-163.
38. Brent RL. Relationship between uterine vascular clamping, vascular disruption syndrome, and cocaine teratogenicity. *Teratology.* 1990;41: 757-760.
39. Brent RL. Saving lives and changing family histories: appropriate counseling of pregnant women and men and women of reproductive age, concerning the risk of diagnostic radiation exposures during and before pregnancy. *Am J Obstet Gynecol.* 2009;200:4-24.
40. Brent RL. The application of the principles of toxicology and teratology in evaluating the risks of new drugs for treatment of drug addiction in women of reproductive age. *NIDA Res Monogr.* 1995;149:130-184.
41. Brent RL, Beckman DA. Angiotensin-converting enzyme inhibitors, an embryopathic class of drugs with unique properties: information for clinical teratology counselors. *Teratology.* 1991;43:543-546.
42. Briggs GG, Freeman RK, Yaffe SJ. *Drugs in Pregnancy and Lactation.* 8th ed. Phildelphia: Lippincott Williams & Williams; 2008.
43. Brouillette F, Weber ML. Massive aspiration of talcum powder by an infant. *Can Med Assoc J.* 1978;119:354-355.
44. Brown DB, Mueller GL, Golich FC. Hyperbaric oxygen treatment for carbon monoxide poisoning in pregnancy: a case report. *Aviat Space Environ Med.* 1992;63:1011-1014.
45. Brown WJ, Buist NR, Gipson HT, Huston RK, Kennaway NG. Fatal benzyl alcohol poisoning in a neonatal intensive care unit. *Lancet.* 1982;1:1250.
46. Buehler BA, Conover B, Andres RL. Teratogenic potential of cocaine. *Semin Perinatol.* 1996;20:93-98.
47. Buitendijk S, Bracken MB. Medication in early pregnancy: prevalence of use and relationship to maternal characteristics. *Am J Obstet Gynecol.* 1991;165:33-40.
48. Byer AJ, Traylor TR, Semmer JR. Acetaminophen overdose in the third trimester of pregnancy. *JAMA.* 1982;247:3114-3115.
49. Caravati EM, Adams CJ, Joyce SM, Schafer NC. Fetal toxicity associated with maternal carbon monoxide poisoning. *Ann Emerg Med.* 1988;17: 714-717.
50. Centers for Disease Control and Prevention. Alcohol consumption among women who are pregnant or who might become pregnant—United States, 2002. *MMWR Morb Mortal Wkly Rep.* 2004;53:1178-1181.
51. Chabrolle JP, Rossier A. Goitre and hypothyroidism in the newborn after cutaneous absorption of iodine. *Arch Dis Child.* 1978;53:495-498.
52. Chang J, Berg CJ, Saltzman LE, Herndon J. Homicide: a leading cause of injury deaths among pregnant and postpartum women in the United States, 1991-1999. *Am J Public Health.* 2005;95:471-477.
53. Char VC, Chandra R, Fletcher AB, Avery GB. Letter: Polyhydramnios and neonatal renal failure–a possible association with maternal acetaminophen ingestion. *J Pediatr.* 1975;86:638-639.
54. Chasnoff IJ. Drug use and women: establishing a standard of care. *Ann N Y Acad Sci.* 1989;562:208-210.
55. Chasnoff IJ, Bussey ME, Savich R, Stack CM. Perinatal cerebral infarction and maternal cocaine use. *J Pediatr.* 1986;108:456-459.
56. Chavez GF, Mulinare J, Cordero JF. Maternal cocaine use during early pregnancy as a risk factor for congenital urogenital anomalies. *JAMA.* 1989;262:795-798.
57. Chiriboga CA. Neurological correlates of fetal cocaine exposure. *Ann N Y Acad Sci.* 1998;846:109-125.
58. Church MW, Dintcheff BA, Gessner PK. Dose-dependent consequences of cocaine on pregnancy outcome in the Long-Evans rat. *Neurotoxicol Teratol.* 1988;10:51-58.
59. Cohen-Kerem R, Koren G. Antioxidants and fetal protection against ethanol teratogenicity. I. Review of the experimental data and implications to humans. *Neurotoxicol Teratol.* 2003;25:1-9.
60. Collaborative Group on Drug Use in Pregnancy. Medication during pregnancy: an intercontinental cooperative study. *Int J Gynaecol Obstet.* 1992;39:185-196.
61. Cooper WO, Griffin MR, Arbogast P, et al. Very early exposure to erythromycin and infantile hypertrophic pyloric stenosis. *Arch Pediatr Adolesc Med.* 2002;156:647-650.
62. Cotten CM, Turner BS, Miller-Bell M. Pharmacology in neonatal care. In: Merenstein GB, Gardner SL, eds. *Handbook of Neonatal Intensive Care.* St. Louis: Mosby Elsevier; 2006:184.
63. Cragan JD. Teratogen update: methylene blue. *Teratology.* 1999;60:42-48.
64. Cramer CR. Fetal death due to accidental maternal carbon monoxide poisoning. *J Toxicol Clin Toxicol.* 1982;19:297-301.
65. Curry SC, Bond GR, Raschke R, Tellez D, Wiggins D. An ovine model of maternal iron poisoning in pregnancy. *Ann Emerg Med.* 1990;19: 632-638.
66. Czeizel A, Lendvay A. Attempted suicide and pregnancy. *Am J Obstet Gynecol.* 1989;161:497.

67. Czeizel AE, Gidai J, Petik D, Timmerman G, Puhó EH. Self-poisoning during pregnancy as a model for teratogenic risk estimation of drugs. *Toxicol Ind Health.* 2008;24:11-28.
68. Czeizel AE, Tomcsik M, Timar L. Teratologic evaluation of 178 infants born to mothers who attempted suicide by drugs during pregnancy. *Obstet Gynecol.* 1997;90:195-201.
69. Dannenberg AL, Carter DM, Lawson HW, et al. Homicide and other injuries as causes of maternal death in New York City, 1987 through 1991. *Am J Obstet Gynecol.* 1995;172:1557-1564.
70. Day NL, Cottreau CM, Richardson GA. The epidemiology of alcohol, marijuana, and cocaine use among women of childbearing age and pregnant women. *Clin Obstet Gynecol.* 1993;36:232-245.
71. De Vigan C, De Walle HE, Cordier S, et al. Therapeutic drug use during pregnancy: a comparison in four European countries. OECM Working Group. Occupational Exposures and Congenital Anomalies. *J Clin Epidemiol.* 1999;52:977-982.
72. Desmond MM, Wilson GS. Neonatal abstinence syndrome: recognition and diagnosis. *Addict Dis.* 1975;2:113-121.
73. Diav-Citrin O, Koren G. Direct drug toxicity to the fetus. In: Koren G, ed. *Medication Safety in Pregnancy and Breastfeeding.* New York: McGraw-Hill; 2007:85-119.
74. Dixon SD, Bejar R. Echoencephalographic findings in neonates associated with maternal cocaine and methamphetamine use: incidence and clinical correlates. *J Pediatr.* 1989;115:770-778.
75. Doberczak TM, Shanzer S, Cutler R, et al. One-year follow-up of infants with abstinence-associated seizures. *Arch Neurol.* 1988;45:649-653.
76. Doering PL, Boothby LA, Cheok M. Review of pregnancy labeling of prescription drugs: is the current system adequate to inform of risks? *Am J Obstet Gynecol.* 2002;187:333-339.
77. Dolovich LR, Addis A, Vaillancourt JM, et al. Benzodiazepine use in pregnancy and major malformations or oral cleft: meta-analysis of cohort and case-control studies. *BMJ.* 1998;317:839-843.
78. Dominick MA, Carson TL. Effects of carbon monoxide exposure on pregnant sows and their fetuses. *Am J Vet Res.* 1983;44:35-40.
79. Douglas MJ. Perinatal physiology and pharmacology. In: Norris MC, ed. *Obstetric Anesthesia.* Philadelphia: Lippincott Williams & Wilkins; 1999:113-134.
80. Dow-Edwards D. Comparability of human and animal studies of developmental cocaine exposure. *NIDA Res Monogr.* 1996;164:146-174.
81. Ducey J, Williams DB. Transcutaneous absorption of boric acid. *J Pediatr.* 1953;43:644-651.
82. Elhassani SB. Neonatal poisoning: causes, manifestations, prevention, and management. *South Med J.* 1986;79:1535-1543.
83. Elkharrat D, Raphael JC, Korach JM, et al. Acute carbon monoxide intoxication and hyperbaric oxygen in pregnancy. *Intensive Care Med.* 1991;17:289-292.
84. Eyler FD, Behnke M. Early development of infants exposed to drugs prenatally. *Clin Perinatol.* 1999;26:107-150, vii.
85. Fantel AG, Macphail BJ. The teratogenicity of cocaine. *Teratology.* 1982;26:17-19.
86. Farber NB, Olney JW. Drugs of abuse that cause developing neurons to commit suicide. *Brain Res Dev Brain Res.* 2003;147:37-45.
87. Farrow JR, Davis GJ, Roy TM, McCloud LC, Nichols GR 2nd. Fetal death due to nonlethal maternal carbon monoxide poisoning. *J Forensic Sci.* 1990;35:1448-1452.
88. Ferm VH. Teratogenic effects of hyperbaric oxygen. *Proc Soc Exp Biol Med.* 1964;116:975-976.
89. Finnegan LP, Kandall SR. Maternal and neonatal effects of alcohol and drugs. In: Lowinson JH, Ruiz P, Millman RB, Langrod JG, eds. *Substance Abuse: A Comprehensive Textbook.* Philadelphia: Lippincott Williams & Wilkins; 2005:805-839.
90. Finnell RH, Toloyan S, van Waes M, Kalivas PW. Preliminary evidence for a cocaine-induced embryopathy in mice. *Toxicol Appl Pharmacol.* 1990;103:228-237.
91. Frank DA, Augustyn M, Knight WG, Pell T, Zuckerman B. Growth, development, and behavior in early childhood following prenatal cocaine exposure: a systematic review. *JAMA.* 2001;285:1613-1625.
92. Friedman JM. Report of the Teratology Society Public Affairs Committee symposium on FDA classification of drugs. *Teratology.* 1993;48:5-6.
93. Friedman JM, Polifka JE. *Teratogenic Effects of Drugs: A Resource for Clinicians (TERIS).* Baltimore: The Johns Hopkins University Press; 2000.
94. Friedman S, Gatti M, Baker T. Cesarean section after maternal acetaminophen overdose. *Anesth Analg.* 1993;77:632-634.
95. Gabrielli A, Layon AJ. Carbon monoxide intoxication during pregnancy: a case presentation and pathophysiologic discussion, with emphasis on molecular mechanisms. *J Clin Anesth.* 1995;7:82-87.
96. Gaynes BN, Gavin N, Meltzer-Brody S, et al. *Perinatal Depression: Prevalence, Screening Accuracy, and Screening Outcomes. Evidence Report/Technology Assessment No. 119. AHRQ Publication No. 05-E006-2.* Rockville, MD: Agency for Healthcare Research and Quality; 2005.
97. Gedeon C, Koren G. Gestational changes in drug disposition in the maternal-fetal unit. In: Koren G, ed. *Medication Safety in Pregnancy and Breastfeeding.* New York: McGraw-Hill; 2007:5-11.
98. Gemme G, Ruffa G, Bonioli E, Lagorio V, Feingold M. Picture of the month. Cushing's syndrome due to topical corticosteroids. *Am J Dis Child.* 1984;138:987-988.
99. Gershanik J, Boecler B, Ensley H, McCloskey S, George W. The gasping syndrome and benzyl alcohol poisoning. *N Engl J Med.* 1982;307:1384-1388.
100. Gillberg C. "Floppy infant syndrome" and maternal diazepam. *Lancet.* 1977;2:244.
101. Ginsberg MD, Myers RE. Fetal brain injury after maternal carbon monoxide intoxication. Clinical and neuropathologic aspects. *Neurology.* 1976;26:15-23.
102. Glantz JC, Woods JR. Cocaine, heroin, and phencyclidine: obstetric perspectives. *Clin Obstet Gynecol.* 1993;36:279-301.
103. Goodlett CR, Horn KH. Mechanisms of alcohol-induced damage to the developing nervous system. *Alcohol Res Health.* 2001;25:175-184.
104. Gray R, Henderson J. *Review of the Fetal Effects of Prenatal Alcohol Exposure: National Perinatal Epidemiology Unit.* Oxford: University of Oxford; 2006.
105. Greingor JL, Tosi JM, Ruhlmann S, Aussedat M. Acute carbon monoxide intoxication during pregnancy. One case report and review of the literature. *Emerg Med J.* 2001;18:399-401.
106. Guerri C. Neuroanatomical and neurophysiological mechanisms involved in central nervous system dysfunctions induced by prenatal alcohol exposure. *Alcohol Clin Exp Res.* 1998;22:304-312.
107. Haibach H, Akhter JE, Muscato MS, Cary PL, Hoffman MF. Acetaminophen overdose with fetal demise. *Am J Clin Pathol.* 1984;82:240-242.
108. Hakkola J, Tanaka E, Pelkonen O. Developmental expression of cytochrome P450 enzymes in human liver. *Pharmacol Toxicol.* 1998;82:209-217.
109. Hannigan JH. What research with animals is telling us about alcohol-related neurodevelopmental disorder. *Pharmacol Biochem Behav.* 1996;55:489-499.
110. Harada M. Congenital Minamata disease: intrauterine methylmercury poisoning. *Teratology.* 1978;18:285-288.
111. Harvey JA. Cocaine effects on the developing brain: current status. *Neurosci Biobehav Rev.* 2004;27:751-764.
112. Hauben M, Amsden GW. The association of erythromycin and infantile hypertrophic pyloric stenosis: causal or coincidental? *Drug Saf.* 2002;25:929-942.
113. Henderson GI, Chen JJ, Schenker S. Ethanol, oxidative stress, reactive aldehydes, and the fetus. *Front Biosci.* 1999;4:D541-550.
114. Herzlinger RA, Kandall SR, Vaughan HG Jr. Neonatal seizures associated with narcotic withdrawal. *J Pediatr.* 1977;91:638-641.
115. Hill EP, Hill JR, Power GG, Longo LD. Carbon monoxide exchanges between the human fetus and mother: a mathematical model. *Am J Physiol.* 1977;232:H311-323.
116. Hollander DI, Nagey DA, Welch R, Pupkin M. Hyperbaric oxygen therapy for the treatment of acute carbon monoxide poisoning in pregnancy. A case report. *J Reprod Med.* 1987;32:615-617.
117. Holt D, Harvey D, Hurley R. Chloramphenicol toxicity. *Adverse Drug React Toxicol Rev.* 1993;12:83-95.
118. Holzman C, Paneth N. Maternal cocaine use during pregnancy and perinatal outcomes. *Epidemiol Rev.* 1994;16:315-334.
119. Honein MA, Paulozzi LJ, Himelright IM, et al. Infantile hypertrophic pyloric stenosis after pertussis prophylaxis with erythromcyin: a case review and cohort study. *Lancet.* 1999;354:2101-2105.
120. Horowitz RS, Dart RC, Jarvie DR, Bearer CF, Gupta U. Placental transfer of *N*-acetylcysteine following human maternal acetaminophen toxicity. *J Toxicol Clin Toxicol.* 1997;35:447-451.
121. Huizink AC, Mulder EJ. Maternal smoking, drinking or cannabis use during pregnancy and neurobehavioral and cognitive functioning in human offspring. *Neurosci Biobehav Rev.* 2006;30:24-41.
122. Hurst DL, Marsh WW. Early severe infantile botulism. *J Pediatr.* 1993;122:909-911.

123. Hutchings DE. The puzzle of cocaine's effects following maternal use during pregnancy: are there reconcilable differences? *Neurotoxicol Teratol.* 1993;15:281-286.
124. Ihlen BM, Amundsen A, Sande HA, Daae L. Changes in the use of intoxicants after onset of pregnancy. *Br J Addict.* 1990;85:1627-1631.
125. Jacobson JL, Jacobson SW. Teratogen update: polychlorinated biphenyls. *Teratology.* 1997;55:338-347.
126. Jager-Roman E, Deichl A, Jakob S, et al. Fetal growth, major malformations, and minor anomalies in infants born to women receiving valproic acid. *J Pediatr.* 1986;108:997-1004.
127. Johnson SF, McCarter RJ, Ferencz C. Changes in alcohol, cigarette, and recreational drug use during pregnancy: implications for intervention. *Am J Epidemiol.* 1987;126:695-702.
128. Jones KL. *Smith's Recognizable Patterns of Human Malformation.* 6th ed. Philadelphia: WB Saunders; 2005.
129. Jones KL, Chambers CD. What really causes FAS? A different perspective. *Teratology.* 1999;60:249-250.
130. Juchau MR, Rettie AE. The metabolic role of the placenta. In: Fabro S, Scialli AR, eds. *Drug and Chemical Action in Pregnancy.* New York: Marcel Dekker, Inc.; 1986:153-169.
131. Kandall SR. Treatment strategies for drug-exposed neonates. *Clin Perinatol.* 1999;26:231-243.
132. Kandall SR, Doberczak TM, Mauer KR, Strashun RH, Korts DC. Opiate v CNS depressant therapy in neonatal drug abstinence syndrome. *Am J Dis Child.* 1983;137:378-382.
133. Kandall SR, Gaines J. Maternal substance use and subsequent sudden infant death syndrome (SIDS) in offspring. *Neurotoxicol Teratol.* 1991;13:235-240.
134. Kandall SR, Gaines J, Habel L, Davidson G, Jessop D. Relationship of maternal substance abuse to subsequent sudden infant death syndrome in offspring. *J Pediatr.* 1993;123:120-126.
135. Kearns GL, Abdel-Rahman SM, Alander SW, et al. Developmental pharmacology—drug disposition, action, and therapy in infants and children. *N Engl J Med.* 2003;349:1157-1167.
136. Khoury S, Odeh M, Oettinger M. Deferoxamine treatment for acute iron intoxication in pregnancy. *Acta Obstet Gynecol Scand.* 1995;74:756-757.
137. Kiess W, Linderkamp O, Hadorn HB, Haas R. Fetal alcohol syndrome and malignant disease. *Eur J Pediatr.* 1984;143:160-161.
138. Kleiner GJ, Greston WM. Suicide during pregnancy. In: Cherry SH, Merkatz IR, eds. *Complications of Pregnancy: Medical, Surgical, Gynecologic, Psychosocial, and Perinatal.* Baltimore: William & Wilkins; 1991.
139. Klinger G, Merlob P. Selective serotonin reuptake inhibitor induced neonatal abstinence syndrome. *Isr J Psychiatry Relat Sci.* 2008;45:107-113.
140. Koren G, Chan D, Klein J, Karaskov T. Estimation of fetal exposure to drugs of abuse, environmental tobacco smoke, and ethanol. *Ther Drug Monit.* 2002;24:23-25.
141. Koren G, Graham K, Shear H, Einarson T. Bias against the null hypothesis: the reproductive hazards of cocaine. *Lancet.* 1989;2:1440-1442.
142. Koren G, Klinger G, Ohlsson A. Fetal pharmacotherapy. *Drugs.* 2002;62:757-773.
143. Koren G, Sharav T, Pastuszak A, et al. A multicenter, prospective study of fetal outcome following accidental carbon monoxide poisoning in pregnancy. *Reprod Toxicol.* 1991;5:397-403.
144. Kumar A, Goel KM, Rae MD. Paracetamol overdose in children. *Scott Med J.* 1990;35:106-107.
145. Kurzel RB. Can acetaminophen excess result in maternal and fetal toxicity? *South Med J.* 1990;83:953-955.
146. Kweder SL. Drugs and biologics in pregnancy and breastfeeding: FDA in the 21st century. *Birth Defects Res A Clin Mol Teratol.* 2008;82:605-609.
147. Lacoste H, Goyert GL, Goldman LS, Wright DJ, Schwartz DB. Acute iron intoxication in pregnancy: case report and review of the literature. *Obstet Gynecol.* 1992;80:500-501.
148. Lammer EJ. A phenocopy of the retinoic acid embropathy following maternal use of etretinate that ended one year before conception. *Teratology.* 1988;37:42.
149. Lampert P, O'Brien J, Garrett R. Hexachlorophene encephalopathy. *Acta Neuropathol (Berl).* 1973;23:326-333.
150. Land DB, Kushner R. Drug abuse during pregnancy in an inner-city hospital: prevalence and patterns. *J Am Osteopath Assoc.* 1990;90:421-426.
151. Laub DN, Elmagbari NO, Elmagbari NM, Hausburg MA, Gardiner CS. Effects of acetaminophen on preimplantation embryo glutathione concentration and development in vivo and in vitro. *Toxicol Sci.* 2000;56:150-155.
152. Lawrence RA, Lawrence RM. *Breastfeeding: A Guide for the Medical Professional.* 6th ed. St. Louis: Mosby, Inc.; 2005.
153. Lederman S, Fysh WJ, Tredger M, Gamsu HR. Neonatal paracetamol poisoning: treatment by exchange transfusion. *Arch Dis Child.* 1983;58:631-633.
154. Lenke RR, Turkel SB, Monsen R. Severe fetal deformities associated with ingestion of excessive isoniazid in early pregnancy. *Acta Obstet Gynecol Scand.* 1985;64:281-282.
155. Lester BM, LaGasse L, Freier K, Brunner S. Studies of cocaine-exposed human infants. *NIDA Res Monogr.* 1996;164:175-210.
156. Lester D, Beck AT. Attempted suicide and pregnancy. *Am J Obstet Gynecol.* 1988;158:1084-1085.
157. Li DK, Liu L, Odouli R. Exposure to non-steroidal anti-inflammatory drugs during pregnancy and risk of miscarriage: population based cohort study. *BMJ.* 2003;327:368.
158. Lidow MS. Consequences of prenatal cocaine exposure in nonhuman primates. *Brain Res Dev Brain Res.* 2003;147:23-36.
159. Lindahl V, Pearson JL, Colpe L. Prevalence of suicidality during pregnancy and the postpartum. *Arch Womens Ment Health.* 2005;8:77-87.
160. Lo WY, Friedman JM. Teratogenicity of recently introduced medications in human pregnancy. *Obstet Gynecol.* 2002;100:465-473.
161. Longo LD. The biological effects of carbon monoxide on the pregnant woman, fetus, and newborn infant. *Am J Obstet Gynecol.* 1977;129:69-103.
162. Longo LD, Hill EP. Carbon monoxide uptake and elimination in fetal and maternal sheep. *Am J Physiol.* 1977;232:H324-330.
163. Ludmir J, Main DM, Landon MB, Gabbe SG. Maternal acetaminophen overdose at 15 weeks of gestation. *Obstet Gynecol.* 1986;67:750-751.
164. Lusskin SI, Pundiak TM, Habib SM. Perinatal depression: hiding in plain sight. *Can J Psychiatry.* 2007;52:479-488.
165. Maalouf EF, Battin M, Counsell SJ, Rutherford MA, Manzur AY. Arthrogryposis multiplex congenita and bilateral mid-brain infarction following maternal overdose of co-proxamol. *Eur J Paediatr Neurol.* 1997;1:183-186.
166. MacGregor SN, Keith LG, Bachicha JA, Chasnoff IJ. Cocaine abuse during pregnancy: correlation between prenatal care and perinatal outcome. *Obstet Gynecol.* 1989;74:882-885.
167. Mahalik MP, Gautieri RF, Mann DE Jr. Teratogenic potential of cocaine hydrochloride in CF-1 mice. *J Pharm Sci.* 1980;69:703-706.
168. Mahalik MP, Hitner HW. Antagonism of cocaine-induced fetal anomalies by prazosin and diltiazem in mice. *Reprod Toxicol.* 1992;6:161-169.
169. Mahon BE, Rosenman MB, Kleiman MB. Maternal and infant use of erythromycin and other macrolide antibiotics as risk factors for infantile hypertrophic pyloric stenosis. *J Pediatr.* 2001;139:380-384.
170. Maier SE, West JR. Drinking patterns and alcohol-related birth defects. *Alcohol Res Health.* 2001;25:168-174.
171. Makarechian N, Agro K, Devlin J, et al. Association between moderate alcohol consumption during pregnancy and spontaneous abortion, stillbirth and premature birth: a meta-analysis. In: Koren G, ed. *Medication Safety in Pregnancy and Breastfeeding.* New York: McGraw-Hill; 2007.
172. Malanga CJ, Kosofsky BE. Mechanisms of action of drugs of abuse on the developing fetal brain. *Clin Perinatol.* 1999;26:17-37, v-vi.
173. Manning MA, Eugene Hoyme H. Fetal alcohol spectrum disorders: a practical clinical approach to diagnosis. *Neurosci Biobehav Rev.* 2007;31:230-238.
174. Manoguerra AS. Iron poisoning: report of a fatal case in an adult. *Am J Hosp Pharm.* 1976;33:1088-1090.
175. Margulies JL. Acute carbon monoxide poisoning during pregnancy. *Am J Emerg Med.* 1986;4:516-519.
176. Martin ML, Khoury MJ, Cordero JF, Waters GD. Trends in rates of multiple vascular disruption defects, Atlanta, 1968-1989: is there evidence of a cocaine teratogenic epidemic? *Teratology.* 1992;45:647-653.
177. Martin-Bouyer G, Lebreton R, Toga M, Stolley PD, Lockhard J. Outbreak of accidental hexachlorophene poisoning in France. *Lancet.* 1982;1:91-95.
178. Marzuk PM, Tardiff K, Leon AC, et al. Lower risk of suicide during pregnancy. *Am J Psychiatry.* 1997;154:122-123.
179. Matsui D, Knoppert D. Drugs and chemicals most commonly used by pregnant women. In: Koren G, ed. *Medication Safety in Pregnancy and Breastfeeding.* New York: McGraw-Hill; 2007:75-83.
180. Mattson SN, Riley EP. A review of the neurobehavioral deficits in children with fetal alcohol syndrome or prenatal exposure to alcohol. *Alcohol Clin Exp Res.* 1998;22:279-294.

181. May PA, Gossage JP. Estimating the prevalence of fetal alcohol syndrome. A summary. *Alcohol Res Health.* 2001;25:159-167.
182. Mayes LC. Developing brain and in utero cocaine exposure: effects on neural ontogeny. *Dev Psychopathol.* 1999;11:685-714.
183. Mayes LC, Grillon C, Granger R, Schottenfeld R. Regulation of arousal and attention in preschool children exposed to cocaine prenatally. *Ann N Y Acad Sci.* 1998;846:126-143.
184. McElhatton PR, Roberts JC, Sullivan FM. The consequences of iron overdose and its treatment with desferrioxamine in pregnancy. *Hum Exp Toxicol.* 1991;10:251-259.
185. McElhatton PR, Sullivan FM, Volans GN, Fitzpatrick R. Paracetamol poisoning in pregnancy: an analysis of the outcomes of cases referred to the Teratology Information Service of the National Poisons Information Service. *Hum Exp Toxicol.* 1990;9:147-153.
186. Mehanny SZ, Abdel-Rahman MS, Ahmed YY. Teratogenic effect of cocaine and diazepam in CF1 mice. *Teratology.* 1991;43:11-17.
187. Miller MS, Juchau MR, Guengerich FP, Nebert DW, Raucy JL. Drug metabolic enzymes in developmental toxicology. *Fundam Appl Toxicol.* 1996;34:165-175.
188. Miller PD, Telford IR, Haas GR. Effect of hyperbaric oxygen on cardiogenesis in the rat. *Biol Neonate.* 1971;17:44-52.
189. Miller RK. Placental transfer and function: the interface for drugs and chemicals in the conceptus. In: Fabro S, Scialli AR, eds. *Drug and Chemical Action in Pregnancy.* New York: Marcel Dekker, Inc.; 1986:123-152.
190. Moretti ME. Motherisk: the Toronto model for counseling in reproductive toxicology. In: Koren G, ed. *Medication Safety in Pregnancy and Breastfeeding.* New York: McGraw-Hill; 2007:295-307.
191. Motherisk. http://www.motherisk.org. Accessed May 19, 2009.
192. Motomatsu K, Adachi H, Uno T. Two infant deaths after inhaling baby powder. *Chest.* 1979;75:448-450.
193. Nathanson V, Jayesinghe N, Roycroft G. Is it all right for women to drink small amounts of alcohol in pregnancy? No. *BMJ.* 2007;335:857.
194. National Institute of Drug Abuse. *National Pregnancy & Health Survey: Drug Use among Women Delivering Livebirths: 1992.* Rockville, MD: National Institutes of Health; 1996.
195. Nau H, Helge H, Luck W. Valproic acid in the perinatal period: decreased maternal serum protein binding results in fetal accumulation and neonatal displacement of the drug and some metabolites. *J Pediatr.* 1984;104:627-634.
196. Neri I, Blasi I, Castro P, et al. Polyethylene glycol electrolyte solution (Isocolan) for constipation during pregnancy: an observational open-label study. *J Midwifery Womens Health.* 2004;49:355-358.
197. Neuspiel DR. Behavior in cocaine-exposed infants and children: association versus causality. *Drug Alcohol Depend.* 1994;36:101-107.
198. Newport DJ, Levey LC, Pennell PB, Ragan K, Stowe ZN. Suicidal ideation in pregnancy: assessment and clinical implications. *Arch Womens Ment Health.* 2007;10:181-187.
199. Nichols MM. Acute alcohol withdrawal syndrome in a newborn. *Am J Dis Child.* 1967;113:714-715.
200. Norman CA, Halton DM. Is carbon monoxide a workplace teratogen? A review and evaluation of the literature. *Ann Occup Hyg.* 1990;34:335-347.
201. Oakley GP. Preventing all folic acid-preventable spina bifida. In: Wyszynski DF, ed. *Neural Tube Defects: From Origin to Treatment.* Oxford: Oxford University Press; 2006:335-341.
202. Oates M. Deaths from psychiatric causes. In: Lewis G, ed. *Saving Mothers' Lives: Reviewing Maternal Deaths to Make Motherhood Safer-2003-2005. The Seventh Report on Confidential Enquiries into Maternal Deaths in the United Kingdom.* London: CEMACH; 2007:152-172.
203. O'Brien P. Is it all right for women to drink small amounts of alcohol in pregnancy? Yes. *BMJ.* 2007;335:856.
204. Office of Applied Studies. *Results from the 2005 National Survey on Drug Use and Health: National Findings (DHHS Publication No. SMA 06-4194, NSDUH Series H-30).* Rockville, MD: Substance Abuse and Mental Health Services Administration (SAMHSA); 2006.
205. Office of the Surgeon General. *U.S. Surgeon General Releases Advisory on Alcohol Use in Pregnancy.* Washington, DC: US Department of Health and Human Services; 2005.
206. Olenmark M, Biber B, Dottori O, Rybo G. Fatal iron intoxication in late pregnancy. *J Toxicol Clin Toxicol.* 1987;25:347-359.
207. Park-Wyelie L, Mazzotta P, Moretti M, et al. Birth defects after maternal exposure to corticosteroids: prospective controlled cohort study and a meta-analysis of epidemiological studies. In: Koren G, ed. *Medication Safety in Pregnancy and Breastfeeding.* New York: McGraw-Hill; 2007:541-548.
208. Patel TG, Laungani RG, Grose EA, Dow-Edwards DL. Cocaine decreases uteroplacental blood flow in the rat. *Neurotoxicol Teratol.* 1999;21:559-565.
209. Paul M. *Occupational and Environmental Reproductive Hazards: A Guide for Clinicians.* Baltimore: Williams & Wilkins; 1993.
210. Perrone J, Hoffman RS. Toxic ingestions in pregnancy: abortifacient use in a case series of pregnant overdose patients. *Acad Emerg Med.* 1997;4:206-209.
211. Plessinger MA, Woods JR. Cocaine in pregnancy. Recent data on maternal and fetal risks. *Obstet Gynecol Clin North Am.* 1998;25:99-118.
212. Plonait SL, Nau H. Physicochemical and structural properties regulating placental drug transfer. In: Polin RA, Fox WW, eds. *Fetal and Neonatal Physiology, Vol. 1.* Philadelphia: Saunders; 2004:197-211.
213. Pratt R, Salomon DS. Biochemical basis for the teratogenic effects of glucocorticoids. In: Juchau MR, ed. *The Biochemical Basis of Chemical Teratogenesis.* New York: Elsevier/North Holland; 1981:179-199.
214. Rayburn W, Aronow R, DeLancey B, Hogan MJ. Drug overdose during pregnancy: an overview from a metropolitan poison control center. *Obstet Gynecol.* 1984;64:611-614.
215. Rayburn WF, Donn SM, Wulf ME. Iron overdose during pregnancy: successful therapy with deferoxamine. *Am J Obstet Gynecol.* 1983;147:717-718.
216. Reed MD, Besunder JB. Developmental pharmacology: ontogenic basis of drug disposition. *Pediatr Clin North Am.* 1989;36:1053-1074.
217. Rementeria JL, Bhatt K. Withdrawal symptoms in neonates from intrauterine exposure to diazepam. *J Pediatr.* 1977;90:123-126.
218. Reprorisk System. http://www.micromedex.com/products/reprorisk/. Accessed May 19, 2009.
219. Reprotox. http://www.reprotox.org/. Accessed May 19, 2009.
220. Rice JM, Donovan PJ. Mutagenesis and carcinogenesis. In: Fabro S, Scialli AR, eds. *Drug and Chemical Action in Pregnancy.* New York: Marcel Dekker, Inc.; 1986:205-236.
221. Richards R, Brooks SE. Ferrous sulphate poisoning in pregnancy (with afibrinogenaemia as a complication). *West Indian Med J.* 1966;15:134-140.
222. Richardson GA, Day NL. Maternal and neonatal effects of moderate cocaine use during pregnancy. *Neurotoxicol Teratol.* 1991;13:455-460.
223. Riggs BS, Bronstein AC, Kulig K, Archer PG, Rumback BH. Acute acetaminophen overdose during pregnancy. *Obstet Gynecol.* 1989;74:247-253.
224. Riordan J. Drugs and breastfeeding. In: Riordan J, Auerbach KG, eds. *Breastfeeding and Human Lactation.* Sudbury: Jones and Bartlett; 1999:163-219.
225. Ritchie H, Bolton P. The Australian categorisation of risk of drug use in pregnancy. *Aust Fam Physician.* 2000;29:237-241.
226. Rivera-Calimlim L. The significance of drugs in breast milk. Pharmacokinetic considerations. *Clin Perinatol.* 1987;14:51-70.
227. Roberts I, Robinson MJ, Mughal MZ, Ratcliffe JG, Prescott LF. Paracetamol metabolites in the neonate following maternal overdose. *Br J Clin Pharmacol.* 1984;18:201-206.
228. Robertson RG, Van Cleave BL, Collins JJ Jr. Acetaminophen overdose in the second trimester of pregnancy. *J Fam Pract.* 1986;23:267-268.
229. Rogan WJ. Breastfeeding in the workplace. *Occup Med.* 1986;1:411-413.
230. Rogers JM. Tobacco and pregnancy: overview of exposures and effects. *Birth Defects Res C Embryo Today.* 2008;84:1-15.
231. Rollins DE, von Bahr C, Glaumann H, Moldéus P, Rane A. Acetaminophen: potentially toxic metabolite formed by human fetal and adult liver microsomes and isolated fetal liver cells. *Science.* 1979;205:1414-1416.
232. Rosen TS, Pippenger CE. Pharmacologic observations on the neonatal withdrawal syndrome. *J Pediatr.* 1976;88:1044-1048.
233. Rosenberg AA, Galan HL. Fetal drug therapy. *Pediatr Clin North Am.* 1997;44:113-135.
234. Rosenberg D. Oxy's offspring. *Newsweek.* 2002;139:37.
235. Rosevear SK, Hope PL. Favourable neonatal outcome following maternal paracetamol overdose and severe fetal distress. Case report. *Br J Obstet Gynaecol.* 1989;96:491-493.
236. Rubin JD, Ferencz C, Loffredo C. Use of prescription and non-prescription drugs in pregnancy. The Baltimore-Washington Infant Study Group. *J Clin Epidemiol.* 1993;46:581-589.
237. Rubin PC, Craig GF, Gavin K, Sumner D. Prospective survey of use of therapeutic drugs, alcohol, and cigarettes during pregnancy. *Br Med J (Clin Res Ed).* 1986;292:81-83.

238. Ruiz-Maldonado R, Zapata G, Lourdes T, Robles C. Cushing's syndrome after topical application of corticosteroids. *Am J Dis Child.* 1982;136:274-275.
239. Ruthnum P, Goel KM. ABC of poisoning: paracetamol. *Br Med J (Clin Res Ed).* 1984;289:1538-1539.
240. Rutter N. Percutaneous drug absorption in the newborn: hazards and uses. *Clin Perinatol.* 1987;14:911-930.
241. Sancewicz-Pach K, Chmiest W, Lichota E. Suicidal paracetamol poisoning of a pregnant woman just before a delivery. *Przegl Lek.* 1999;56:459-462.
242. SanFilippo JA. Infantile hypertrophic pyloric stenosis related to ingestion of erythromycine estolate: a report of five cases. *J Pediatr Surg.* 1976;11:177-180.
243. Sannerstedt R, Lundborg P, Danielsson BR, et al. Drugs during pregnancy: an issue of risk classification and information to prescribers. *Drug Saf.* 1996;14:69-77.
244. Sapunar D, Saraga-Babic M, Peruzovic M, Marusic M. Effects of hyperbaric oxygen on rat embryos. *Biol Neonate.* 1993;63:360-369.
245. Schardein JL. *Chemically Induced Birth Defects.* 3rd ed. New York: Marcel Dekker, Inc.; 2000.
246. Schauben JL, Augenstein WL, Cox J, Sato R. Iron poisoning: report of three cases and a review of therapeutic intervention. *J Emerg Med.* 1990;8:309-319.
247. Schou M. Lithium treatment during pregnancy, delivery, and lactation: an update. *J Clin Psychiatry.* 1990;51:410-413.
248. Schreiber JS. Parents worried about breast milk contamination. What is best for baby? *Pediatr Clin North Am.* 2001;48:1113-1127, viii.
249. Scialli AR. Identifying teratogens: the tyranny of lists. *Reprod Toxicol.* 1997;11:555-559.
250. Scialli AR, Buelke-Sam JL, Chambers CD, et al. Communicating risks during pregnancy: a workshop on the use of data from animal developmental toxicity studies in pregnancy labels for drugs. *Birth Defects Res A Clin Mol Teratol.* 2004;70:7-12.
251. Scialli AR, Fabro S. The stage dependence of reproductive toxicology. In: Fabro S, Scialli AR, eds. *Drug and Chemical Action in Pregnancy.* New York: Marcel Dekker, Inc.; 1986:191-204.
252. Selden BS, Curry SC, Clark RF, et al. Transplacental transport of *N*-acetylcysteine in an ovine model. *Ann Emerg Med.* 1991;20:1069-1072.
253. Shankaran S, Lester BM, Das A, et al. Impact of maternal substance use during pregnancy on childhood outcome. *Semin Fetal Neonatal Med.* 2007;12:143-150.
254. Shannon M, Amitai Y, Lovejoy FH Jr. Multiple dose activated charcoal for theophylline poisoning in young infants. *Pediatrics.* 1987;80:368-370.
255. Shepard TH, Brent RL, Friedman JM, et al. Update on new developments in the study of human teratogens. *Teratology.* 2002;65:153-161.
256. Shepard TH, Lemire RJ. *Catalog of Teratogenic Agents.* 12th ed. Baltimore: The Johns Hopkins University Press; 2007.
257. Shiono PH, Klebanoff MA, Nugent RP, et al. The impact of cocaine and marijuana use on low birth weight and preterm birth: a multicenter study. *Am J Obstet Gynecol.* 1995;172:19-27.
258. Shuman RM, Leech RW, Alvord EC Jr. Neurotoxicity of hexachlorophene in humans. II. A clinicopathological study of 46 premature infants. *Arch Neurol.* 1975;32:320-325.
259. Singer ST, Vichinsky EP. Deferoxamine treatment during pregnancy: is it harmful? *Am J Hematol.* 1999;60:24-26.
260. Slotkin TA. Fetal nicotine or cocaine exposure: which one is worse? *J Pharmacol Exp Ther.* 1998;285:931-945.
261. Slotkin TA. If nicotine is a developmental neurotoxicant in animal studies, dare we recommend nicotine replacement therapy in pregnant women and adolescents? *Neurotoxicol Teratol.* 2008;30:1-19.
262. Slutsker L. Risks associated with cocaine use during pregnancy. *Obstet Gynecol.* 1992;79:778-789.
263. Sokol RJ, Delaney-Black V, Nordstrom B. Fetal alcohol spectrum disorder. *JAMA.* 2003;290:2996-2999.
264. Sood B, Delaney-Black V, Covington C, et al. Prenatal alcohol exposure and childhood behavior at age 6 to 7 years: I. dose-response effect. *Pediatrics.* 2001;108:E34.
265. Spear LP, Campbell J, Snyder K, Silveri M, Katovic N. Animal behavior models. Increased sensitivity to stressors and other environmental experiences after prenatal cocaine exposure. *Ann N Y Acad Sci.* 1998;846:76-88.
266. Stang H. Pyloric stenosis associated with erythromycin ingested through breastmilk. *Minn Med.* 1986;69:669-670, 682.
267. Stark KL, Lee QP, Namkung MJ, Harris C, Juchau MR. Dysmorphogenesis elicited by microinjected acetaminophen analogs and metabolites in rat embryos cultured in vitro. *J Pharmacol Exp Ther.* 1990;255:74-82.
268. Stokes IM. Paracetamol overdose in the second trimester of pregnancy. Case report. *Br J Obstet Gynaecol.* 1984;91:286-288.
269. Stratton K, Howe C, Battaglia FC. *Fetal Alcohol Syndrome: Diagnosis, Epidemiology, Prevention, and Treatment.* Washington, DC: Committee to Study Fetal Alcohol Syndrome, Institute of Medicine, National Academy Press; 1996.
270. Streissguth AP, O'Malley K. Neuropsychiatric implications and long-term consequences of fetal alcohol spectrum disorders. *Semin Clin Neuropsychiatry.* 2000;5:177-190.
271. Strom RL, Schiller P, Seeds AE, Bensel RT. Fatal iron poisoning in a pregnant female. *Minn Med.* 1976;59:483-489.
272. Sulik KK. Genesis of alcohol-induced craniofacial dysmorphism. *Exp Biol Med.* 2005;230:366-375.
273. Teelmann K. Retinoids: toxicology and teratogenicity to date. *Pharmacol Ther.* 1989;40:29-43.
274. Telford IR, Miller PD, Haas GF. Hyperbaric oxygen causes fetal wastage in rats. *Lancet.* 1969;2:220-221.
275. Tenenbein M. Poisoning in pregnancy. In: Koren G, ed. *Maternal-Fetal Toxicology: A Clinician's Guide.* New York: Marcel Dekker, Inc.; 2001.
276. TERIS (Teratogen Information System). http://depts.washington.edu/~terisweb/teris/. Accessed May 19, 2009.
277. Thilo EH, Townsend SF, Deacon J. Infant botulism at 1 week of age: report of two cases. *Pediatrics.* 1993;92:151-153.
278. Thornburg KL, Bagby SP, Giraud GD. Maternal adaptation to pregnancy. In: Neill JD, ed. *Knobil and Neill's Physiology of Reproduction, Vol. 2.* Amsterdam: Elsevier; 2006:2899-2919.
279. Thornburg KL, Faber JJ. Transfer of hydrophilic molecules by placenta and yolk sac of the guinea pig. *Am J Physiol.* 1977;233:C111-124.
280. Turk J, Aks S, Ampuero F, Hryhorczuk DO. Successful therapy of iron intoxication in pregnancy with intravenous deferoxamine and whole bowel irrigation. *Vet Hum Toxicol.* 1993;35:441-444.
281. US Census Bureau American FactFinder. 2004 American Community Survey: Detailed Table B23001. Sex by age by employment status for the population 16 years and over. http://factfinder.census.gov. Accessed May 19, 2009.
282. US Food and Drug Administration. Labeling and prescription drug advertising: content and format for labeling for human prescription drugs. *Fed Register.* 1979;44.
283. US Food and Drug Administration. Pregnancy and lactation labeling. http://www.fda.gov/cber/safety/preglac.htm. Accessed May 19, 2009.
284. Van Ameyde KJ, Tenenbein M. Whole bowel irrigation during pregnancy. *Am J Obstet Gynecol.* 1989;160:646-647.
285. Van Hoesen KB, Camporesi EM, Moon RE, Hage ML, Piantadosi CA. Should hyperbaric oxygen be used to treat the pregnant patient for acute carbon monoxide poisoning? A case report and literature review. *JAMA.* 1989;261:1039-1043.
286. Wang PH, Yang MJ, Lee WL, et al. Acetaminophen poisoning in late pregnancy. A case report. *J Reprod Med.* 1997;42:367-371.
287. Ward RM, Lugo RA. Drug therapy in the newborn. In: MacDonald MG, Seshia MMK, Mullet MD, eds. *Avery's Neonatology: Pathophysiology & Management of the Newborn.* Philadelphia: Lippincott Williams & Wilkins; 2005:1507-1556.
288. Warkany J. Aminopterin and methotrexate: folic acid deficiency. *Teratology.* 1978;17:353-357.
289. Warkany J. Warfarin embryopathy. *Teratology.* 1976;14:205-209.
290. Webster WS, Brown-Woodman PD. Cocaine as a cause of congenital malformations of vascular origin: experimental evidence in the rat. *Teratology.* 1990;41:689-697.
291. Webster WS, Brown-Woodman PD, Lipson AH, Ritchie HE. Fetal brain damage in the rat following prenatal exposure to cocaine. *Neurotoxicol Teratol.* 1991;13:621-626.
292. Webster WS, Lipson AH, Brown-Woodman PD. Uterine trauma and limb defects. *Teratology.* 1987;35:253-260.
293. Weeks BS, Gamache P, Klein NW, et al. Acetaminophen toxicity to cultured rat embryos. *Teratog Carcinog Mutagen.* 1990;10:361-371.
294. Weiss B, Doherty RA. Methylmercury poisoning. *Teratology.* 1975;12:311-313.
295. Werler MM. Teratogen update: smoking and reproductive outcomes. *Teratology.* 1997;55:382-388.

296. West JR, Chen WJ, Pantazis NJ. Fetal alcohol syndrome: the vulnerability of the developing brain and possible mechanisms of damage. *Metab Brain Dis.* 1994;9:291-322.
297. Whitlock FA, Edwards JE. Pregnancy and attempted suicide. *Compr Psychiatry.* 1968;9:1-12.
298. Woods JR. Maternal and transplacental effects of cocaine. *Ann N Y Acad Sci.* 1998;846:1-11.
299. Woods JR, Plessinger MA, Fantel A. An introduction to reactive oxygen species and their possible roles in substance abuse. *Obstet Gynecol Clin North Am.* 1998;25:219-236.
300. Woody RC, Brewster MA. Telencephalic dysgenesis associated with presumptive maternal carbon monoxide intoxication in the first trimester of pregnancy. *J Toxicol Clin Toxicol.* 1990;28:467-475.
301. Working PK. *Toxicology of the Male and Female Reproductive Systems.* New York: Hemisphere; 1989.
302. Zelson C, Rubio E, Wasserman E. Neonatal narcotic addiction: 10 year observation. *Pediatrics.* 1971;48:178-189.
303. Zuckerman B, Frank D, Brown E. Overview of the effects of abuse and drugs on pregnancy and offspring. *NIDA Res Monogr.* 1995;149:16-38.

CHAPTER 31
PEDIATRIC PRINCIPLES

Jeffrey S. Fine

Phone calls to poison centers regarding childhood exposures to potential xenobiotics are more frequent than those regarding any other age group. Because of this and the frequent role of poisoning as a cause of pediatric injury, pediatricians have been active for many years in helping to establish and promote the study of medical toxicology, as well as in establishing and supporting the use of regional poison centers. Although the basic approaches to the medical management of toxicologic problems outlined in Chapters 3 and 4 are generally applicable to both children and adults, issues, such as abuse by poisoning, are of particular concern in children. This chapter provides a pediatric perspective to the application of generally accepted toxicologic principles.

EPIDEMIOLOGY

To analyze the problem of pediatric poisoning, it is necessary to understand the magnitude of the problem. When assessing the impact of a particular type of injury such as poisoning, epidemiologists examine multiple parameters, such as exposure, morbidity, mortality, and cost, to measure the effect of the injury; however, these parameters are difficult to measure accurately. An important source for information on the extent and effects of poisoning exposures in the United States is the American Association of Poison Control Centers (AAPCC). Every year, the AAPCC compiles standardized data collected from poison centers throughout the United States; the 2007 annual review includes information submitted by 61 poison centers. In the following discussion, comments on AAPCC data refer to cumulative information from the previous five published reports covering the years 2003 to 2007 (see Chap. 135)

Each year, the AAPCC reports approximately 1.6 million potentially toxic exposures in children and adolescents ages 0 to 19 years, which account for 65% of all reported exposures. In fact, children younger than age 6 years account for 52% of all reported exposures. Of the reported exposures in children and adolescents, children younger than age 6 years account for 79%, children between 6 and 12 years of age account for 10%, and adolescents between 13 and 19 years of age account for 11%. Girls represent 47% of the reported poisoning exposures in young children and 55% of the reported exposures among adolescents.

Among the AAPCC-reported xenobiotic exposures in children younger than age 6 years, 99% are labeled unintentional. In contrast, only 48% of the reported adolescent exposures are unintentional; 47% exposures in adolescents are labeled intentional, mostly resulting from substance use or suicide attempts. The high frequency of intentional poisoning in adolescents has been reported by others.[35,150,199] The remaining 5% of adolescent exposures include adverse drug events and other miscellaneous or unknown causes. Differences in the reasons for exposure between young children and adolescents account for differences in the outcomes of these exposures.

Approximately 118,000 xenobiotic exposures each year are classified by the AAPCC as therapeutic errors, accounting for approximately 6% of exposures in children younger than 6 years of age, 21% in children 6 to 12 years of age, and 9% in adolescents. An additional 13,000 exposures each year are classified as adverse drug reactions, which account for approximately 0.4% of exposures in children younger than 6 years of age, 2% in children 6 to 12 years of age, and 3% in adolescents.

Table 31–1 shows the leading causes of reported exposures in children and adolescents. According to the AAPCC, approximately 55% of childhood exposures are to xenobiotics that are commonly found around the house, such as cleaning products, cosmetics, plants, hydrocarbons, and insecticides; approximately 45% are to pharmaceuticals. In older children and adolescents, approximately 47% of exposures are to nonpharmaceutical xenobiotics, and approximately 53% are to pharmaceuticals. Most hospitalizations and deaths in both groups are caused by pharmaceuticals.

Table 31–1 lists the most common reported *exposures*, but not all of these xenobiotics lead to serious morbidity and mortality (Table 31–2). For example, children frequently ingest cosmetic products, so the number of reported exposures is large, but most cosmetics manufactured in the United States are nontoxic. Poisoning is unusual in children younger than age 6 months but may result from the inadvertent administration of an incorrect drug or drug dose by a parent,[38,61] intentional administration of a drug by a parent or sibling,[46,79]or passive exposure (eg, to the smoke of "crack" cocaine or phencyclidine).[16,78,133,173,208] Any poisoning in a child younger than 1 year of age should be carefully evaluated for possible child abuse or neglect (see below).[79]

Several typical characteristics associated with ingestions by toddlers differentiate them from ingestions by adolescents or adults: (1) they are without suicidal intent; (2) there is usually only one xenobiotic involved; (3) the xenobiotics are usually nontoxic; (4) the amount is usually small; and (5) toddlers usually present for evaluation relatively soon after the ingestion is discovered, generally within 1 to 2 hours. As many as 30% of children who experience one ingestion will experience a repeat ingestion; adolescents may be particularly prone to recidivism.[62,89] Children who ingest poisons may also be at a greater risk for other types of injuries.[14,52]

The peak age for childhood poisoning is between 1 and 3 years.[30] Unintentional ingestion is unusual after age 5 years, although when it occurs it can be the result of mistaken consumption of a xenobiotic from a mislabeled container.[26] Between the ages of 5 and 9 years, poisoning may result from intrafamilial stress or suicidal intent. After age 9 years and through adolescence overdose or poisoning frequently results from either suicidal gestures and attempts, or from the adverse effects of alcohol or substance use. Unintentional poisonings are largely preventable. (see Chap. 135)

Because many children are exposed to nontoxic xenobiotics or to only small amounts of potentially toxic xenobiotics, the proportion of children and adolescents who suffer significant morbidity is small (Table 31–3). However, because there are millions of such exposures each year, the number of children and adolescents who experience at least moderate effects is large.

Another source of data related to poisoning morbidity is the National Injury Surveillance database maintained by the United States Centers for Disease Control and Prevention (CDC), which provides information on emergency department (ED) visits and hospitalizations.[31] For the period 2001 to 2007, the CDC estimates approximately 66,000 ED visits (274 per 100,000) and 6300 hospitalizations (10%) per year for children 0 to 5 years who were exposed to a xenobiotic. Children 6 to 12 years accounted for 12,000 ED visits (38 per 100,000) and 1900 hospitalizations (16%), and adolescents 13 to 19 years old account for 103,000 ED visits (198 per 100,000) and 36,000 hospitalizations (35%). Approximately 80% of the patients hospitalized were adolescents, and approximately 75% of those cases were intentional poisonings.

These numbers are consistent with estimates of 100,000 to 170,000 ED visits for poisoning and overdose per year, or approximately 300 to 840

TABLE 31–1. Average Annual Xenobiotic Exposures Reported to the American Association of Poison Control Centers (2003–2007)[a]

Age <6 Years		Age 6–19 Years	
Category	Number of Exposures	Category	Number of Exposures
Cosmetics and personal care items	165,637	Analgesics	46,047
Cleaning substances	119,500	Cough and cold preparations	20,510
Analgesics	98,743	Cosmetics and personal care items	17,412
Topicals	88,555	Bites and envenomations	17,252
Cough and cold preparations	65,044	Cleaning substances	16,512
Plants	49,058	Antidepressants	15,423
Insecticides, pesticides, and rodenticides	48,096	Sedative–hypnotics	15,050
Vitamins	46,519	Stimulants and street drugs	12,943
Antihistamines	33,845	Antihistamines	12,138
Antimicrobials	33,495	Food products and poisoning	10,856

[a] See Chap. 135 for references and discussion.

[b] Does not include the American Association of Poison Control Centers' category "foreign bodies."

TABLE 31–2. Xenobiotics Responsible for Significant Pediatric Poisoning Morbidity and Mortality

	<6 Years Old						13–19 Years Old	
	Reported Major Effects[a,b]		Reported Deaths[a]		Reported Deaths 2003–2007[c,d]		Reported Deaths 2003–2007[c,d]	
Category	Number	%	Number	%	Number	%	Number	%
Alcohols	53	2	9	7	1	1	17	5
Analgesics	119	5	8	7	39	27	125	37
Anticonvulsants	106	5	4	3	4	3	4	1
Antidepressants and antipsychotics	182	8	9	7	7	5	39	12
Antihistamines and cough and cold medications	92	4	8	7	19	13	15	4
Bites and envenomations	100	4	0	0	3	2	0	0
Carbon monoxide	42	2	18	15	27	18	22	7
Cardiovascular agents	182	8	7	6	4	3	4	1
Cleaning agents and chemicals	297	13	10	8	4	3	3	1
Hydrocarbons	168	7	5	4	7	5	16	5
Insecticides, pesticides, rodenticides	123	5	7	6	4	3	2	1
Iron	52	2	7	6	0	0	0	0
Sedative–hypnotics	151	7	0	0	2	1	9	3
Stimulants and street drugs	84	4	1	1	1	1	52	15
Theophylline	38	2	3	2	0	0	0	0
Other or unknown	481	21	26	21	25	17	28	8
Totals	2270		122		147		336	

[a] Data from Litovitz T, Manoguerra A: Comparison of pediatric poisoning hazards: an analysis of 3.8 million exposure incidents. *Pediatrics.* 1992;89:999–1106.

[b] Major effect is defined as life-threatening signs and symptoms or significant residual disability or disfigurement.

[c] Data from American Association of Poison Control Centers (AAPCC),2003–2007.

[d] The AAPCC does not report specific outcomes other than death, by age, for individual xenobiotics; consequently, the number of major effects cannot be calculated from annual reports.

TABLE 31–3. Outcome of Reported Pediatric Xenobiotic Exposures (2003–2007)[a]

	Effects (% of Reported Exposures)[b]			
Age (years)	Minor or None	Moderate	Major	Death
0–5	99	1	0.05	0.003
6–12	97	3	0.15	0.008
13–19	88	11	1	0.04
All children and adolescents 0–19	97	2	0.19	0.008

[a] See Chap. 135 for references and discussion.

[b] Minor = minimal signs and symptoms often not requiring therapy; moderate = more pronounced, prolonged, or systemic signs and symptoms often requiring therapy; major = life-threatening signs and symptoms.

visits per 100,000 for children younger than 5 years of age and 290 to 360 per 100,000 visits for adolescents. Hospitalization rates are 10% to 20%.[29,30,53,60,125,196]

As mentioned, adolescents are more frequently hospitalized than children after exposure to xenobiotics.[62] However, it is unclear whether this reflects medical hospitalization for management of the xenobiotic exposure or for patients' psychiatric problems. The peak age for hospitalizing young children exposed to xenobiotics is between 1 and 3 years, reflecting the peak age of exposure. Whereas among hospitalized children younger than age 2 years, exposure to nonpharmaceutical xenobiotics is more common; children older than age 2 years and adolescents are more commonly exposed to pharmaceuticals.[53,62,199]

Although the AAPCC reports overall outcome related to age, it does not generally stratify outcome of exposure to individual xenobiotics by age. In a multiyear review published in 1992, the AAPCC reported the xenobiotics that caused the greatest number of major and fatal effects in children younger than 6 years old.[116] Table 31–2 lists the xenobiotics that caused significant morbidity and mortality. Other reports of hospitalized patients include a similar distribution of xenobiotics that cause significant morbidity.[8,32,85,213] However, in rural areas of many developing countries, kerosene and pesticides are the leading causes of poison-related hospitalizations, and the spectrum of pharmaceutical exposures is often different[2,72,74,140,142] (see Chap. 136).

Poisoning accounts for approximately 2% of childhood and 6% of adolescent injury-related deaths in the United States.[31] Based on information from death certificates filed in state vital statistics offices as well as demographic information provided by funeral directors, the CDC reports 593 deaths in children younger than 6 years of age from 1999 to 2005 for an average of about 85 per year. These deaths represent 10% of the reported poisoning fatalities for all age groups for those years and an 81% decrease from the 456 deaths reported by the CDC in 1959.[30] This dramatic decrease in childhood poisoning mortality may be the result of improved poisoning prevention such as child-resistant closures and improved medical care or may reflect a decrease in reporting (see Chap. 135).

Thirty-seven percent of the AAPCC-reported childhood fatalities result from unintentional ingestions; 20% are from environmental exposures, mostly carbon monoxide poisoning; 16% are caused by therapeutic errors and adverse reactions; and 11% are malicious or related to abuse. The remaining 16% have miscellaneous causes or are unknown. In contrast, 42% of AAPCC-reported adolescent fatalities are the result of suicide and 37% follow abuse or misuse of substances; only 5% are related to environmental exposures, and only 3% are caused by medication errors and adverse reactions; the remaining 13% have miscellaneous or unknown causes.

Although the AAPCC data provide a remarkable amount of epidemiologic information, there are questions about the accuracy of the data.[75,77,206] For example, as mentioned above, whereas the CDC reported 593 poisoning-related deaths in children younger than 6 years of age from 1999 to 2005, the AAPCC reported 184 for those same years based on voluntary calls. Thus, there is a recognition that many significant poisonings are not reported to poison centers. Physicians managing "common" toxicologic problems may not feel the need for the assistance of a local or regional poison center and may not feel compelled to participate in the reporting process. Therapeutic misadventures may also go unreported. In Rhode Island, only 45 of 369 poisoning deaths were reported to the regional poison center[114] (see Chap. 135).

The most notable difference between the xenobiotics listed in Table 31–2 and studies from the 1960s and 1970s is that salicylates are no longer a leading cause of reported poisoning morbidity and mortality.[40,45] This change may be related to federal regulations requiring child-resistant closures as well as to the decreased availability of aspirin at home for use in children after the recognition of its association with Reye syndrome (see Chap. 35).[19,37,86,134,160]

There are some significant etiologic differences between children and adolescents (see Table 31–1), particularly with regard to the lethality of xenobiotics. For 2003 to 2007, the xenobiotics causing the greatest number of childhood deaths were analgesics, carbon monoxide, and antihistamines and cough and cold preparations, which together account for 58% of all reported poisoning deaths. The xenobiotics causing the greatest number of adolescent deaths were analgesics, antidepressants, and stimulants and street drugs, which together account for 64% of reported poisoning deaths.

With respect to AAPCC-reported analgesic-related deaths, there are significant differences between children and adolescents for this population of possibly exposed individuals. For children younger than 6 years, opioids are suggested to account for 69% of the deaths (methadone, 39%; oxycodone or hydrocodone, 23%), and acetaminophen-containing products accounted for 28%. The high frequency of childhood exposures to these xenobiotics has been identified as a significant consequence of both the therapeutic and illicit use of prescription opioid analgesics.[11] These fatalities were related to unintentional exposures in 43% of the children (mostly opioids), malicious exposures in 18% (all opioids), and therapeutic errors in 13% (mostly acetaminophen); the reasons in the rest of the cases were unknown. In adolescents, opioids accounted for 60% of the deaths (methadone, 31%; oxycodone or hydrocodone,15%), and acetaminophen-containing products accounted for 38%. Forty-four percent of the fatalities were the result of abuse or misuse, and 40% were suicides.

Hydrocarbon-related fatalities occur in both children and adolescents; whereas the hydrocarbon deaths of young children generally result from unintentional aspiration, almost all of the hydrocarbon-related deaths in adolescents are related to inhalational abuse of hydrocarbons such as trichloroethanes or chlorofluorocarbons.

Poisoning also has an economic cost. Charges for hospitalized patients range from $2000 to $10,000, depending on the length of stay and outcome.[98,192,213] In a large-scale economic analysis of the cost of injury in the United States in 1985, the estimated average lifetime cost was $495 per child and $10,839 per adolescent or young adult injured or killed by poisoning for a total lifetime cost of approximately $140 million for children and $1.5 billion for adolescents and young adults.[152]

BEHAVIORAL, ENVIRONMENTAL, AND PHYSICAL ISSUES

An oversimplification of the etiology of childhood poisonings would be the formulation that unobserved toddlers exploring their environment inadvertently ingest xenobiotics. However, this approach ignores the complex interplay of factors that may contribute to some ingestions in children.

One approach to understanding injury causation that can be applied to poisoning uses an infectious disease–like model.[73] According to this model, there are three interacting factors: host, agent, and environment. These factors interact during three phases: preinjury, injury, and postinjury. The factors themselves contribute to the likelihood, nature, magnitude of, and host response to an injury.

During the preinjury phase, there is an interaction of the host, agent, and environment. Under the proper circumstances, an injury may occur. Modification of these factors may help to prevent an injury. For example, if a 2-year-old child finds two pills on a bedside table, there is a fair chance the child will ingest the tablets. However, storing the pills out of reach of the child can prevent the ingestion.

The injury phase covers both the ingestion and the initial pathophysiologic host response. Again particular factors determine the nature and extent of injury. Continuing the above example, if the two pills are 325-mg acetaminophen tablets, the ingestion will not lead to injury. However, if the pills are 0.2-mg clonidine tablets, there is a high likelihood of toxicity.

The postinjury phase is concerned both with the ongoing host response and the medical management of the patient who has been poisoned. In this phase, it would be determined whether the 2-year-old child with a clonidine ingestion manifests signs of toxicity, such as coma or hypotension; whether the child requires treatment with activated charcoal (AC), intravenous fluid, or naloxone; and whether the child requires hospital admission.

This paradigm is only a model; in reality, it is often difficult to examine any individual factor independently, and the relative contributions of these factors are not well defined. Nonetheless, consideration of the individual factors of host, agent, and environment allows us to focus on several relevant aspects of poisoning in children.

Childhood and adolescence are times of tremendous growth and development.[215] Some of these physical and social changes place children and teenagers at increased risk for poisonings. By 7 months of age, an infant sitting up can pivot in order to grab an object; by 9 to 10 months of age, most infants can creep and crawl; by 15 months of age, most toddlers are walking quite competently and eagerly exploring. Between 9 and 12 months of age, a skillful pincer grasp with the thumb and forefinger develops that allows the child to pick up small objects. Throughout this period, one of the child's primary sensory experiences is sucking on or gumming objects that are placed in the mouth. Thus, the combination of three developmental skills—the ability to move around the home and go beyond the immediate view of a guardian, the ability to pick up and manipulate small objects, and the tendency of children to put things in their mouths—places them at risk for poisoning.

As children develop socially, they desire to become more like their parents, and they tend to imitate behaviors, such as taking medicine or using mouthwash. Children are taught that medicine is good for them when they are sick. Many children's medicines are sweetened and flavored to make them more palatable, and many parents inappropriately encourage their children to take medicines by telling them "it tastes like candy." Children have been observed "making tea" from plants or "making pizza" with mushrooms from the yard.[26]

As children become more mobile, agile, and curious, xenobiotics that were previously outside their reach become accessible, even when stored in some difficult-to-reach places. There is some evidence suggesting that parents underestimate the developmental skills of their children.[52] The meaning of the term *unintentional* with respect to childhood poisoning should also be reconsidered—the toddler quite purposefully intends to get to a pill and eat it, but the child does *not* intend to injure him- or herself.

Some of the reasons why a child wants to ingest a pill are because it is there, it looks and maybe tastes like candy or food, or that the child is mimicking the behavior of a parent who ingests medicines or vitamins to cure illness and improve health. However, these reasons may not be sufficient to explain why xenobiotic exposures occur. Another aspect of poisoning that must be considered is the interaction between the child's temperament and the social environment.

Many authors have tried to identify psychosocial predictors for childhood poisoning in general and for repeat poisoning in particular.[22,54,91,94,186] As many as 30% of children repeatedly ingest xenobiotics, frequently the same xenobiotic. Certain risk factors have been identified for single and repeat episodes of childhood poisoning, such as hyperactivity, impulsive risk-taking behavior, rebelliousness, and negativistic attitude. Other factors seem to be associated more with the quality of supervision by parents or guardians, who themselves are experiencing medical illnesses, depression, or social isolation.[94] Finally, a stressful environment or a major social problem may also contribute.[181,187] It is not difficult to imagine a situation of a parent who is depressed, uses antidepressant medication that is kept at the bedside, and cannot give adequate attention to a demanding child. In a bid for attention, or as an expression of anger or frustration, the child ingests some of the parent's medication.

With regard to the agent, a number of issues affect the preinjury and injury phases, and modification of any one of the interacting factors of host, agent, or environment may potentially prevent or reduce the severity of injury. When household products of lower toxicity are available around the house, the likelihood of injury is reduced if one of these products is ingested. For example, less-toxic rodenticides such as warfarin have replaced more toxic ones such as thallium or sodium monofluoroacetate, and relatively nontoxic paradichlorobenzene mothballs have largely replaced the relatively more toxic camphor-containing mothballs.

It may also be possible to reduce the likelihood of ingestion by making a xenobiotic unpalatable. Denatonium benzoate is an aversive bittering xenobiotic that is added to some liquids such as windshield washer fluid and antifreeze to prevent unintentional poisoning.[87] However, some trials show that whereas older children may respond negatively to these xenobiotics with the first taste, younger children may ingest 1 to 2 teaspoonfuls before being deterred by the bitter flavor.[20,180] This is an important consideration because even a small amount of a xenobiotic such as methanol can be toxic (see below). The actual usefulness of denatonium benzoate in poison prevention is largely unstudied.[161]

The problem of unintentional ingestions is compounded by poison "look-alikes," that is, xenobiotics that resemble candy or food products.[55] Some common examples are ferrous sulfate tablets and vitamins that look like common candies and fuel oils that come in cans resembling soft drink containers. Many shampoos and dishwashing detergents are given lemon or strawberry scents and have pictures of fruits on the labels. Children are not always able to distinguish poison "look-alikes" from real candies, fruits, and sodas, and they may be attracted to bright colors, pleasant smells, and appealing packages. Eliminating these "look-alikes" might prevent some unintentional ingestions.

Probably the most significant changes have occurred in the physical characteristics with regard to packaging and dispensing of pharmaceuticals and some other xenobiotics with child-resistant closures mandated by the Poison Prevention Packaging Act of 1972 (see Chap. 134). This legislation is credited with causing a significant reduction in morbidity and mortality due to poisoning from aspirin and other regulated products, although this analysis has been challenged.[37,159,201] Child-resistant closures have also been credited with reducing the number of toxic exposures to kerosene.[107]

Nonetheless, problems with child-resistant closures include the dispensing of pharmaceuticals in nonresistant containers, not properly closing child-resistant containers, and leaving pharmaceuticals out of the child-resistant container.[29,184] Seventy percent of potentially toxic pharmaceuticals may be in non–child-resistant or in improperly functioning child-resistant containers. Several studies have identified poor functioning of the closures when there is sticky liquid or pill residue around the top or in the screw threads of the child-resistant container.[89,98,212]

Although child-resistant containers are a significant deterrent to unintentional ingestions in toddlers, they are not completely effective, and even without the problems noted, some children can open them. A false sense of security associated with these closures may lead some parents to be less compulsive regarding safe storage of the containers. A double barrier, such as a unit-dose dispenser within a child-resistant container or a blister pack, has been recommended for a few pharmaceuticals associated with a large number of significant poisonings such as iron and antidepressants.[98]

In fact, in 1997, the Food and Drug Administration (FDA) issued a regulation to package products with 30 mg or more of elemental iron per tablet in unit-dose packages such as blister packs.[66] The intent of this regulation was to reduce the likelihood of iron poisoning in children. Even before this regulation was instituted, the number of fatal childhood iron ingestions had declined significantly; therefore, it is not known how much if any of the decrease is related to the mandated packaging changes. In any case, the rule was overturned in 2003, when it was determined that the FDA did not have the statutory authority to regulate a drug for the purpose of poison prevention.[139] As yet there is no evidence of an resurgence of iron-related fatalities.

A discussion of containers and storage naturally leads to a consideration of the third factor in the injury-causation model discussed above, the environment, which is particularly important in the preinjury and the injury phases. Approximately 80% of childhood pharmaceutical ingestions occur at home; the remainder occurs at the homes of grandparents, other relatives, and friends. At home, the medicine usually belongs either to the child or to a parent, although a significant number of medications, both at home and away from home, belong to a grandparent.[89,115] Grandparents, other relatives, and family friends without children at home may not obtain or retain medications in child-resistant containers and may not be as attentive to safe storage practices. Poison prevention education directed to these groups may be particularly helpful.[128]

Medications are frequently kept in the kitchen or bedroom while they are being used.[89,212] In the kitchen, medications are stored in the refrigerator, on the table, or on the counter, and in the bedroom, medications are left on a dresser or bedside table. A mother's or grandmother's purse is another location where medications are commonly found. Interestingly, there are no significant differences in the storage practices in the homes of children who ingest and those who do not ingest medicines, so storage practices alone cannot predict the likelihood of childhood poisoning.[186,212]

One important caveat relates to the storage of nonpharmaceutical xenobiotics, particularly those in liquid form. These types of xenobiotics should never be transferred for storage to familiar household containers, such as food jars or wine or soda bottles, stored in areas low to the ground such as beneath sinks, or kept in cabinets that do not have child-resistant locks. Both children and adults have been unintentionally exposed to xenobiotics, such as sodium hydroxide, pesticides, hydrocarbons, and potassium cyanide that was stored in bottles in the refrigerator.[197] Many of the kerosene exposures reported from developing countries occur because the kerosene is stored in water bottles, jugs, or other containers in easily accessible locations. When the weather is hot, children may mistake the clear liquid kerosene for water.[1,2,179]

HISTORY OF THE INGESTION

The appropriate management of any poisoned patient is influenced by the history of the exposure. Except in rare cases of child abuse–related poisoning, parents or guardians will generally provide information to the fullest extent possible. As a rule, in the case of children, the xenobiotic and time of ingestion are known. However, the reported number of pills or volume of liquid ingested may not be as accurate. Clues to the amount ingested are the number of pills or volume of liquid in a bottle before and after an ingestion, the number of pills set out on the night table, or the area of a spot of liquid after a spill. When symptoms are suggestive of poisoning but the history is inadequate, information about possible exposure outside of the home, such as with a babysitter, grandparent, friend, or other relative, should be obtained because approximately 15% of childhood poisonings occur outside the home.[89,145]

In contrast, adolescents may not be forthcoming when relating the history of an intentional ingestion, especially when they are depressed, suicidal, or concerned about the response of their guardian or parent. When caring for these patients, the clinician must use the history provided but should remain skeptical about the reported type and number of xenobiotics ingested, as well as the time of ingestion.

When a child may be the victim of abuse or intentionally poisoned by a parent or guardian, the healthcare provider must ensure that (1) the history of the poisoning remains consistent over time and among people providing the details of the event, (2) the child's clinical presentation is consistent with the history of the poisoning, and (3) the reported actions are consistent with the child's developmental level.

GASTROINTESTINAL DECONTAMINATION

Chapter 7 is devoted to a complete discussion of gastrointestinal (GI) decontamination. This section reiterates and emphasizes only a few important points.

As described above, children generally ingest small quantities of single xenobiotics. For most of these ingestions, gastric emptying is unnecessary. Some examples of nontoxic ingestions are eating a crayon or the leaf of a jade plant, licking the cap of a household bleach container, or swallowing two adult-strength acetaminophen tablets.

Orogastric lavage is the preferred method of gastric emptying when indicated for most serious ingestions. Small children can generally tolerate orogastric lavage with a large-bore 28- or 34-French tube; however, the smaller "large-bore" tubes may not be effective for removing large pills or fragments from the stomach of a small child. Placement of an orogastric tube is an unpleasant and frightening procedure for an infant or small child to undergo. Some local trauma may result from tube placement and, rarely, there may be more serious injury, such as esophageal perforation. Also, many children vomit during placement of an orogastric tube. Therefore, the use of orogastric lavage should be limited to cases in which the risk of significant morbidity or mortality is high, the likelihood of benefit is at least moderate, and the likely risk of injury to the child from the procedure is small. Orogastric lavage should never be used as a form of punishment. The patient should be intubated to protect the airway before orogastric lavage is used in a child with a diminished gag reflex or a depressed level of consciousness.

Previously, administration of syrup of ipecac to poisoned patients was considered a primary emergency intervention, and the availability of ipecac in the home was a primary tenet of pediatric anticipatory guidance. The AAPCC reports that the use of syrup of ipecac for case management declined from 13% in 1983 to 0.1% by 2005. This is not surprising because syrup of ipecac is contraindicated in cases associated with hemodynamic instability, seizures, or a depressed level of consciousness. Although syrup of ipecac is highly effective at making children vomit, the efficacy of preventing morbidity after an ingestion is questionable.

Even before the use of syrup of ipecac was abandoned, it had been used only infrequently in the ED management of poisonings, with lavage favored when evacuation of the stomach was considered important. However, it was, until recently, still advocated for use at home at the direction of a poison center to avoid an unnecessary evaluation in an ED. However, in 2003, the American Academy of Pediatrics recommended against the use of ipecac at home, and in 2004, the American Academy of Clinical Toxicology and the European Association of Poison Control Centres and Clinical Toxicologists recommended against the general use of syrup of ipecac for the management of poisoning.[4,6] The reasons for the new recommendations include its unproven benefit, its adverse effects, its interference with and complication of subsequent ED evaluation, its abuse potential, and its administration in cases in which there is no indication or there is a contraindication because of lack of consultation with a poison center.

Notwithstanding these position statements, some toxicologists believe there may still be a role for home use of ipecac syrup in very specific limited circumstances.[158] Thus, there may still be a very limited role for the use of syrup of ipecac in the management of some cases (see Chap. 7 and Antidotes in Depth A1: Syrup of Ipecac).

AC is a current mainstay of poison treatment in the ED.[3,36] Children generally will not drink AC willingly, although some children can be coaxed to do so if the AC is disguised in a baby bottle or soft drink container or sweetened with juice or sorbitol.[209] A nasogastric or orogastric tube may have to be inserted to administer AC. This can be a small-bore tube because it is not intended for lavage, although the smaller the bore, the more difficult it is to administer the thick slurry of AC. Placement of the tube, the presence of AC in the stomach, the effects of the xenobiotic, or the previous use of an emetic all may make the child vomit, making aspiration of AC or stomach contents a risk. For AC to be used safely in a patient who is comatose and who does not have a gag reflex, the patient should be intubated and the airway protected. Because of this risk, AC alone is unnecessary for a nontoxic or minimally toxic ingestion.

AC is available for home use.[108,190] Administration of AC at home or by prehospital personnel allows for administration significantly earlier than can be achieved after arrival and evaluation in the ED.[41,190] Although it would seem to have potential benefit as home therapy, AC is unpalatable, quite messy, and not always available; as a result, it has not achieved widespread use in the home.[138,158] It is also unclear how well parents can administer AC at home.[169,170,191] Whether the earlier administration of AC would affect outcome is unknown. If AC is to replace syrup of ipecac for home therapy, it will require a substantial reeducation effort on the part of pediatricians, toxicologists, and pharmacists.

METHODS OF ENHANCED ELIMINATION

For consequential poisoning with xenobiotics such as methanol, ethylene glycol, salicylates, lithium, and theophylline, either hemodialysis or charcoal hemoperfusion is the optimal technique to enhance elimination, depending on the particular xenobiotic. These extracorporeal techniques can be performed on newborns or small infants in specially equipped centers with dedicated personnel. The primary limiting factor is the ability to obtain vascular access.[18,49,51,198] However, even large centers that routinely do hemodialysis in children may not be able to manage very small infants. There has been a report of the use of peritoneal dialysis for the treatment of alcohol intoxication in a child,[71] but this technique is not generally recommended.

Exchange transfusion is occasionally used to enhance xenobiotic elimination. This technique might be useful when multiple-dose AC cannot be administered, the xenobiotic is poorly adsorbed to charcoal, or access to specialized hemodialysis or hemoperfusion is not readily available. Exchange transfusion has been used successfully for poisoning by salicylates[50,124] and theophylline.[15,141,176] Another xenobiotic for which exchange transfusion may be a therapeutic alternative is chloral hydrate.[9]

XENOBIOTICS THAT MAY BE TOXIC OR FATAL IN SMALL QUANTITIES

When children ingest even small quantities of toxic xenobiotics, they are potentially ingesting large relative doses because of their small size. There are a number of xenobiotics that may cause significant toxicity or even death with as little as one pill or one teaspoonful.[13,113] Table 31–4 lists these xenobiotics.

XENOBIOTICS THAT MAY CAUSE DELAYED TOXICITY IN CHILDREN

Several xenobiotics warrant particular concern because their effects may be significantly delayed. Classic examples are atropine-diphenoxylate (Lomotil)[23,43,126] and sulfonylureas such as glipizide.[69,148,194] Both of these xenobiotics may cause serious morbidity with initial symptoms or recurrence of symptoms delayed by as much as 24 hours after ingestion.

TABLE 31–4. Xenobiotics that May Cause Severe Toxicity to an Infant After a Small Adult Dose, a Single pill or a Small Volume

Benzocaine
β-Adrenergic antagonists (sustained release)
Calcium channel blockers (sustained release)
Camphor
Clonidine
Cyclic antidepressants
Diphenoxylate and atropine (Lomotil)
Methanol or ethylene glycol
Methylsalicylate
Monoamine oxidase inhibitors
Opioids (methadone, codeine, OxyContin)
Phenothiazines
Quinine or chloroquine
Sulfonylureas
Theophylline

Children with real or possible ingestions of Lomotil or a sulfonylurea should be admitted for observation and monitoring, even if they are asymptomatic, because effects may not become apparent for 24 hours (see Chaps. 38 and 48).

With the advent of new modified-release formulations of calcium channel blockers and β-adrenergic antagonists, concern for delayed toxicity and possibly death has become even greater and has been extended to other xenobiotics.

XENOBIOTICS THAT CAUSE UNUSUAL OR IDIOSYNCRATIC REACTIONS IN CHILDREN

BENZYL ALCOHOL: GASPING SYNDROME

Benzyl alcohol is a preservative added to liquid pharmaceutical preparations; for small-volume medications administered to adults, the benzyl alcohol additive is quite safe (Chap. 55). At toxic doses, benzyl alcohol may cause respiratory failure, vasodilation, hypotension, convulsions, and paralysis. Intravenous flush solutions containing benzyl alcohol were implicated as the cause of the "gasping syndrome" in sick newborns; the syndrome includes severe metabolic acidosis, encephalopathy, respiratory depression, and gasping.[5] The association was made when infants with this syndrome were found to have elevated concentrations of benzoic acid and hippuric acid, metabolites of benzyl alcohol.[28,63] Benzyl alcohol is metabolized by the conjugation of benzoic acid with glycine to form hippuric acid; this pathway may not be functional in premature infants. Benzyl alcohol administration has also been associated with kernicterus and intraventricular hemorrhage in premature infants.[81,90] Although benzyl alcohol has been removed from many of the medications used for neonates, some preparations may still contain this agent.[207]

IMIDAZOLINES AND CLONIDINE: CENTRAL NERVOUS SYSTEM EFFECTS

Imidazolines such as tetrahydrozoline, oxymetazoline, xylometazoline, and naphazoline are nonprescription sympathomimetics used as nasal decongestants and conjunctival vasoconstrictors (see Chap. 50). Clonidine is an imidazoline derivative used as an antihypertensive (see Chap. 62). In small children, these xenobiotics can cause central nervous system (CNS) depression, respiratory depression, bradycardia, miosis, and hypotension.[12,123,210] The presumed mechanism of action is by stimulation of central $alpha_2$-adrenergic and imidazole receptors. Although naloxone has been reported to reverse some of the CNS effects of clonidine, there have been no reports of its successful use with the other imidazolines (see Chap. 62).

ETHANOL: HYPOGLYCEMIA

Ethanol is the primary component of alcoholic beverages, as well as a major constituent of many liquid preparations, such as mouthwash, vanilla flavoring, and perfume. Besides its well-known sedative–hypnotic effects, ethanol poisoning in children is associated with hypoglycemia because of reduced hepatic glycogen stores in children.[42,112,121,202] Ethanol-induced hypoglycemia may cause seizures and may exacerbate the other CNS effects induced by ethanol poisoning. Hypoglycemia results from the inhibition of gluconeogenesis in the setting of alcohol poisoning. There does not seem to be a blood alcohol concentration threshold for the development of hypoglycemia, which has been reported with blood alcohol concentrations as low as 20 mg/dL[42] (see Chap. 77).

CHLORAMPHENICOL: GRAY BABY SYNDROME

Chloramphenicol is a broad-spectrum antibiotic that has been used in pediatrics because of its activity against *Haemophilus influenzae*. It has largely been replaced by other antibiotics in the United States because of its association with aplastic anemia. When administered at high doses, chloramphenicol can produce the "gray baby syndrome," which includes abdominal distension, vomiting, metabolic acidosis, progressive pallid cyanosis, irregular respirations, hypothermia, hypotension, and vasomotor collapse. Although these effects occur primarily in premature newborn infants, they may also occur in older children and adults (see Chap. 56).

Gray baby syndrome is associated with serum concentrations greater than 100 mg/L. Increased chloramphenicol concentrations may result from (1) inadequate conjugation of chloramphenicol with glucuronic acid because of inadequate activity of glucuronyl transferase in the newborn liver and (2) decreased renal elimination of unconjugated chloramphenicol. The exact mechanism of toxicity is unknown; there is speculation that free radicals produced during the metabolism of chloramphenicol may interfere with mitochondrial function.[84]

MEDICATION ERRORS

Ever since the publication of the Institute of Medicine's report titled *To Err is Human* in 1999, increasing attention has been paid to the issue of medical errors in medicine.[100] Although most of the research regarding medication errors has focused on adults (see Chap. 139), this problem also affects children. Remarks in this section are generally limited to the pediatric literature.

Approximately 113,000 exposures each year are classified as therapeutic errors, accounting for approximately 6% of exposures in children younger than 6 years of age, 21% in children 6 to 12 years of age, and 9% in adolescents. For 2003 to 2007, there were a total of 26 deaths attributed to therapeutic errors, representing 5% of all reported deaths in children and adolescents. Although only 6% of the AAPCC-reported exposures in young children were related to therapeutic errors, approximately 12% of the reported deaths were related to therapeutic errors. This is in contrast to adolescents, for whom 9% of the calls but only 2% of the reported deaths were related to therapeutic errors.

Medication errors may occur at any phase of a process that includes ordering, order transcription, pharmacy dispensing, preparation and administration of the medication, and monitoring of medication effects. In fact, the same types of errors can usually occur at different points in the process. Table 31–5 lists the types of errors that can occur, and Table 31–6 provides some examples of errors.

Most of the analyses of medication errors have occurred in inpatient settings. The reported frequencies of medication errors vary widely—from 0.47% to 5.7% of written orders and from 0.51 to 157 per 1000 patient-days.[56,82,92,96,167] The variance largely depends on whether the definition of "error" does or does not include prescribing errors, regardless of whether or not they are corrected, and whether potential, or only actual, adverse drug events are included. The reported frequencies also vary depending on whether there is active case finding or whether there is only voluntary reporting.

In a 2001 study of pediatric inpatients in which orders were actively monitored for a 6-week period, 5.7% of 10,778 prescriptions had errors in the order for the medication, transcription of the order, dispensing or administration of the medication, or monitoring of medication effects (56 per 100 admissions, 157 per 1000 patient-days);[96] 1.1% could have *potentially* caused an adverse effect (10 per 100 admissions, 29 per 1000 patient-days). Eighty-four percent of the errors occurred during the ordering or transcription phase, so most of the errors were intercepted

TABLE 31–5. Types of Medication Errors

1. Wrong patient—someone else's drug
2. Wrong drug
   a. Wrong individual drug
   b. Wrong formulation
   c. Known allergy
   d. Known drug–drug interactions
   e. Wrong indication
   f. Contraindication
   g. Expired
   h. Deteriorated
3. Wrong dose
   a. Miscalculation
      i. Decimal point error
      ii. Wrong formula
      iii. Right formula using wrong dose, frequency, units, weight
      iv. Pound/kilogram confusion
      v. Mg/g units confusion
      vi. Dilution error
   b. Appropriate individual dose divided into multiple doses
   c. Total daily dose for an individual dose
   d. Wrong IV infusion rate
   e. Measuring error
4. Wrong route
5. Wrong frequency
   a. Increased or decreased dosing interval
   b. Omitted, delayed, or added dose
   c. Delay or failure to supply
6. Transcription errors
7. Documentation (order, prescription, transcription, logs)
   a. Illegible
   b. Incomplete or missing information (weight, signature, maximum daily dose, stop date)
8. Monitoring
9. Miscellaneous
   a. Wrong label
   b. Wrong information or advice
   c. Failure to detect error
   d. Breast milk exposure

Data based on Kaushal R, Bates DW, Landrigan C, et al: Medication errors and adverse drug events in pediatric inpatients. *JAMA.* 2001;285:2114–2120; Lesar TS: Errors in the use of medication dosage equations. *Arch Pediatr Adolesc Med.* 1998;152:340–344; and Wilson DG, McArtney RG, Newcombe RG, et al: Medication errors in paediatric practice: Insights from a continuous quality improvement approach. *Eur J Pediatr.* 1998;157:769–774.

and corrected before drug administration. There were 26 true adverse drug events, but only five were considered preventable errors (0.05%, 0.52 per 100 admissions, 1.8 per 1000 patient-days). Although the overall error rate was similar to that reported by the same group in a study of adults, the rate of errors that could *potentially* have caused harm was three times greater; 41% of the potentially harmful errors were not intercepted.

Generally, error rates are higher in intensive care units, where the sickest patients are cared for; such patients often receive multiple medications with complex administration regimens[56,82,96,149,167,200,211] Results similar to those from inpatient settings have been reported in pediatric EDs.[105,109,135,156,174]

TABLE 31–6. Examples of Medication Errors

1. **Wrong drug.** In one nursery, an epidemic mimicking neonatal sepsis was caused when racemic epinephrine was inadvertently administered instead of vitamin E because both drugs were manufactured by the same company, distributed in nearly identical bottles, and stored near each other inside the nursery refrigerator.[189]
2. **Wrong drug formulation.** Acetaminophen suppositories (120 mg) were ordered for a toddler, but adult-strength suppositories (650 mg) were distributed and administered every 4 hours. The child developed hepatotoxicity requiring hospitalization and therapy (see Chap. 34).
3. **Wrong dose.** A 1-kg premature infant required sedation for a diagnostic study. A high dose of chloral hydrate, 100 mg/kg, was miscalculated to be 1 g (1000 mg) instead of 100 mg. The child had a cardiopulmonary arrest and died. When drugs require milligram per kilogram dosing, it is easy to make decimal mistakes in the calculation or in the transcription.
4. **Wrong dose/wrong route.** A recommendation was made to treat a baby with penicillin G benzathine, 50,000 U/kg intramuscularly (IM). The recommendation was transcribed as "penicillin G 50,000 units/kg." The order was handwritten as "Benzathine Pen G 150,000 U IM" but was misread or misinterpreted as 1,500,000 U intravenously. The patient had a cardiopulmonary arrest and died.[185]
5. **Wrong dose.** A patient had the dose of cyclosporine changed from 10 mg to 7 mg twice daily. The child received 70 mg (0.7 mL of solution) instead of 7 mg (0.07 mL). When the prescription was refilled, the parents received a 5-mL syringe to use instead of a 1-mL syringe they had used previously.[47]

The studies cited above suggest that the frequency of significant errors leading to significant adverse drug events is low; however, even a low frequency applied to a large population of patients could result in a large number of patients being harmed. The most important outcome of the analysis would be to try to reduce the overall number of errors to reduce the number of potential and actual adverse drug events.

The causes of medication errors are numerous, varied, and complex; they are organizational, environmental, and personal, which includes factors such as the level of training, knowledge and competence, the time of day, workload, staff interactions, communications, number of distractions or interruptions, ambient noise, and drug formulation and drug packaging[44,58,65,100,205] (see Chap. 139).

Children may be placed at increased risk of a medication error for several reasons: (1) someone other than the child administers the medication, so there is little opportunity to prevent or limit drug administration; (2) a young child cannot warn practitioners about possible problems such as allergies; (3) a young child cannot inform practitioners when he or she is experiencing an adverse event; (4) medication ordering and administration in children frequently requires dose calculations; (5) inexperienced practitioners may be uncomfortable with pediatric dosing or related calculations; and (6) incorrect measurement or dilution of concentrated stock solutions may yield a small volume, which is not perceived as containing a relatively large dose of medication.[33,47,65]

The most common error attributed to physicians is prescription of an incorrect dose, particularly in children, in whom almost every prescription requires a determination of weight and calculation of the dose.[96,106,111] In addition, even the milligram per kilogram dose may vary depending on the age of the patient or the diagnosis. Although pediatric doses are generally determined on a milligram per kilogram basis, if the weight is recorded in pounds and this weight is used in the calculation, there will be a built-in twofold error. Calculation errors also occur when drug preparation requires dilution of a concentrated stock solution or special compounding. Further confusion can arise when *mg* is written or interpreted as *mL* or *mcg* in a calculation.

When an extra zero is added or a required zero is omitted from calculations, written or verbal prescriptions, or in dispensed and administered medications, a 10-fold error occurs. These large errors are common and result in significant under- or overdosing; 10-fold errors have been reported in testing scenarios, case series, and case reports.[27,47,68,102,103,106,136,149,154,163,167,183,185] These errors are of particular concern because the risk of toxicity generally increases with significant overdose.

Because the causes of medication error are numerous and complex, the solutions must be multifaceted and interdisciplinary. The approach to the problem is contained within the field of human factors research and potentially requires changes in individual factors such as knowledge; environmental factors such as interruptions; and system problems such as how medications are ordered, stocked, and dispensed[100,193,205] (see Chap. 139).

The most commonly recommended solutions to reduce the frequency of medication errors are computerized physician order entry (CPOE) with clinical decision support systems; ward-based clinical pharmacists; and improved communication among physicians, nurses, and pharmacists.[95,110,157,193] In one of the studies cited above, it was estimated that these three solutions together could have prevented more than 90% of the potential errors,[57] although the effect of interventions other than CPOE have generally not been studied.

In its simplest form, CPOE eliminates errors related to legibility. Decision support adds the ability to check a prescription against age, weight, dose, allergies, and drug–drug interactions, but it may not prevent ordering the wrong drug or dose, so there is still a need for education and human oversight in additional to other safeguards. The implementation of CPOE is generally associated with at least some reduction in errors related to medication ordering,[39,83,99,146,204] although in one controversial study, CPOE was associated with an increase in mortality,[76] and this may have been related to the method of implementation.[88,117,166] Occasionally, other problems are associated with computerized systems.[101,127,203]

Some years from now, all inpatient medication orders and outpatient prescriptions may be transmitted electronically, but until that time, it will be necessary to ensure that prescriptions are written legibly and correctly. The Joint Commission and many other groups have issued a number of recommendations to reduce errors in medication ordering (see chapter 139).

Standardized tests of the math skills necessary to calculate doses and administer medications have demonstrated deficiencies in both nursing and physician groups.[17,21,137,143,147,162,168] These kinds of tests may be a way to identify practitioners at risk for making calculation errors, highlight areas in need of remediation, and serve as an ongoing educational tool.

As described above, there may be an increased risk of medication errors in critical care areas because of severity of illness and intensity of medication therapy. In many cases, such as during resuscitations, critically ill patients require immediate therapy, verbal orders are common, and there is often insufficient time to carefully review all of the particulars related to medication ordering and administration.[106,109,119,144]

Critical care areas, including the ED, benefit from having precalculated dosing charts available for resuscitation medications and for other commonly prescribed medications; this is a recommendation of the American Heart Association.[7] Many clinical units have developed their own dosing schemes. Commercial products, such as the Broselow-Luten system, are also available and have been shown to reduce the number of medication errors in simulated [118,120,175] and real resuscitations.[93]

The previous discussion has been almost exclusively related to hospital-based medication use, but significant errors also may occur in outpatient settings.

Antipyretics are among the most frequently recommended medications for children. Although significant toxicity after unintentional ingestions in toddlers is now rare, administration of multiple supratherapeutic doses of acetaminophen is common and may cause significant hepatotoxicity.[104]

In fact, many parents have difficulty calculating the appropriate dose of acetaminophen and measuring out the appropriate amount after it is calculated despite having received appropriate instructions and graduated cups or oral-dosing syringes.[70,122,130,182,188] The most commonly used measuring device is also the most inaccurate; the household teaspoon is not standardized for volume and can easily be confused with a household tablespoon.[122] Although graduated syringes are considered the most accurate of the measuring instruments available and are recommended by the American Academy of Pediatrics for young children, acetaminophen and ibuprofen elixirs are typically packaged with a graduated cup for administration. Visual cues using pictograms in the discharge instructions or color-coded or premarked syringes may be one way to improve the accuracy of parental medication dosing.[59,214]

INTENTIONAL POISONING AND CHILD ABUSE

Intentional poisoning of children is an unusual, though significant, form of child abuse. There are several types of intentional poisoning, some of which define pathologic characteristics of the parent or guardian: (1) undifferentiated child abuse, neglect, or impulsive acts under stress; (2) factitious illness (Munchausen syndrome by proxy [MSBP]); (3) overt parental psychosis; (4) altruistic motivation or bizarre childrearing practices; and (5) the Medea complex, or the vengeful killing of a child out of spite for one's spouse.[79,165,195]

Intentional poisoning is rarely suspected unless the patient dies and an autopsy is performed, a wide-ranging drug screen is ordered, or the history is bizarre enough to raise suspicions. In many cases in which children are later found to be poisoned, the initial diagnoses were sepsis, meningitis, seizures, intracranial hemorrhage, gastroenteritis, apnea, apparent life-threatening events, or metabolic derangements.[79] In addition to many pharmaceuticals, salt, pepper, water, caffeine, ethylene glycol, herbs, plants, and traditional remedies have been used to poison children.[48,79]Although the death rate from unintentional poisoning in children is much less than 1%, the death rate from inflicted poisoning may be as high as 20% to 30%.[48,79,195]

Intentional poisoning may be associated with other forms of abuse; approximately 20% of poisoned children may have evidence of physical abuse.[48,79] Of children presenting to the ED after presumed unintentional poisoning, 36% had previous ED visits for trauma, 7% for poisoning, 6% for both trauma and poisoning, and 1.4% for failure to thrive. At the time of the visit, only 7% were evaluated for possible abuse, and 2.7% were considered neglected.[79] These data do not prove an association between poisoning and physical trauma; however, in some children, repeat episodes of trauma or poisoning may be a manifestation of significant intrafamilial stress. Healthcare providers must remain vigilant to the possibility that a presumed unintentional poisoning may have been inflicted, especially in the setting of a repeat ingestion or when there have been previous evaluations for trauma.

Substance abuse by a parent or guardian may play a role in unintentional or intentional poisoning of children. Children have been intoxicated with cocaine or phencyclidine by passive inhalation,[16,78,133,172,208] unintentional ingestion,[97,155] and rectal adminstration,[151] as well as through breast milk.[34] Children have been given doses of alcohol, methadone, and other xenobiotics to quiet them or to prevent withdrawal.[45,80,153] There have also been reports of babysitters blowing marijuana smoke into babies' faces to "get them high" or to quiet them.[173]

In 1977, the term *Munchausen syndrome by proxy* was used to describe a condition in which a parent or guardian, typically the mother, fabricates a history of nonexistent disease(s) in a child or creates the signs and symptoms of disease in a child (factitious illness).[131,132,165] This is usually a manifestation of the parent's complex psychiatric illness, which may include Munchausen syndrome itself.[24,67,171] There may be only a fine line separating MSBP from an intentional poisoning with intent to harm or kill a child. However, regardless of the specific intent, this condition is considered a form of child abuse.

Over the years, child protection experts have tried to develop more specific terminology than MSBP. In light of the fact that this entity involves two individuals—the child victim and the adult perpetrator—the American Professional Society on the Abuse of Children recommends that the child victim be diagnosed with "pediatric condition falsification" and that the psychiatric diagnosis of "factitious disorder by proxy" be applied to the adult perpetrator. The diagnosis of MSBP requires that both criteria be met.[10,171]

A child's fabricated illness may lead to multiple medical evaluations by several different physicians, frequent hospitalizations, unnecessary surgeries and diagnostic testing, unneeded prescribing and administration of medication, and at times even the death of the child. Administration of medications to the child by the adult perpetrator is frequently how a particular set of signs and symptoms is created. Xenobiotics used to create factitious illness have included analgesics, antidepressants, insulin, syrup of ipecac, Lomotil, phenothiazines, sedative–hypnotics, warfarin, phenolphthalein, and hydrocarbons.[164] Several warning signals may suggest a diagnosis of MSBP (Table 31–7).

In one illustrative case of MSBP, a 29-month-old boy who had undergone a previous appendectomy was hospitalized multiple times for vomiting, diarrhea, and dehydration.[64] Evaluation included multiple blood and stool analyses, a gastric pH probe, computed tomography, magnetic resonance imaging, endoscopy, and upper GI series. On the fourth admission, a small bowel obstruction was identified, and the child had lysis of adhesions. Nonetheless, symptoms recurred every 2 to 4 months, necessitating hospitalization. The child failed to thrive and required a nasoduodenal tube for feeding, which frequently became dislodged. The child went on to have a jejunostomy tube and a permanent central venous catheter placed. Eighteen months after his initial presentation, the child presented in congestive heart failure with evidence of cardiomyopathy. A urine screen identified emetine and cephaline, components of syrup of ipecac. The child was removed from his home to protective custody after which he recovered and remained asymptomatic on a regular diet.

Siblings of children evaluated and treated for poisoning may also have suffered from factitious illness. In addition, significant psychiatric problems may be manifested by the victim, parents, and siblings.[25,129,171,177]

Child abuse or neglect must be part of the differential diagnosis of any case of childhood poisoning. Intentional poisoning should be considered for

1. An "ingestion" in a child younger than 1 year of age
2. A case with a confusing history or presentation
3. A child with a previous poisoning or a child whose siblings have previously been evaluated for poisoning
4. A child with a previous presentation for a rare or unexplained medical condition
5. A child with apnea, unexplained seizures, or an apparent life-threatening event
6. A massive ingestion by a small child
7. An ingestion of multiple xenobiotics by a small child
8. An exposure to substances of abuse
9. An intoxication with a xenobiotic to which a child could or would not typically have access
10. "Accidental ingestions" in a school-age child
11. A history of previous trauma, child abuse, or neglect
12. Sudden infant death syndrome or an unexplained death[79,80]

TABLE 31–7. Factitious Illness (Munchausen Syndrome by Proxy): Suggestive Characteristics in Clinical Situations

1. The child has a persistent or recurrent illness that cannot be explained.
2. The history of disease or results of diagnostic tests are inconsistent with the general health and appearance of the child.
3. The signs and symptoms cause the clinician to remark, "I've never seen anything like this before!"
4. The signs and symptoms do not occur when the child is separated from the parent.
5. The parent is particularly attentive and refuses to leave the child's bedside, even for a few minutes.
6. The parent develops particularly close relations with hospital staff.
7. The parent seems less worried than the physician about the child's condition.
8. Treatments are not tolerated (eg, intravenous lines fall out frequently, prescribed medications lead to vomiting).
9. The proposed diagnosis is a rare disease.
10. "Seizures" are unwitnessed by medical staff and reportedly do not respond to any treatment.
11. The parent has a complicated medical or psychiatric history.
12. The parent is or was associated with the healthcare field.

These considerations of child abuse notwithstanding, rare diseases do occur. One child's rare, inherited metabolic disorder, methyl malonic acidemia, was misdiagnosed as ethylene glycol poisoning because of the chromatographic appearance of the metabolite propionic acid, which was similar to that of ethylene glycol.[178]

SUMMARY

Children are frequently exposed to potentially toxic xenobiotics; fortunately, most childhood exposures are ingestions of nonpoisonous xenobiotics or small nontoxic quantities of potentially toxic xenobiotics. When a child sustains a significant toxic exposure, management follows general toxicologic principles. Although most childhood exposures are unintentional, the clinician should be alert to the possibility of intentional poisoning of a child with pharmaceutical or household products.

The normal development of children places them at risk for unintentional ingestions. A chaotic home environment or a disorganized social structure may compound these risks. Small size puts children at increased risk for medication dosing and dispensing errors, and their immature metabolic processes may lead to unexpected toxicity from pharmaceutical agents.

Toxicologists should encourage parents to provide as safe a home environment as possible to prevent unintentional ingestions and must encourage practitioners to exercise special vigilance when administering medications to children.

REFERENCES

1. Abu-Ekteish F: Kerosene poisoning in children: a report from northern Jordan. *Trop Doct.* 2002;32:27-29.
2. Adejuyigbe EA, Onayade AA, Senbanjo IO, Oseni SE: Childhood poisoning at the Obafemi Awolowo University Teaching Hospital, Ile-Ife, Nigeria. *Niger J Med.* 2002;11:183-186.
3. American Academy of Clinical Toxicology; European Association of Poisons Centres and Clinical Toxicologists: position statement and practice guidelines on the use of multi-dose activated charcoal in the treatment of acute poisoning. *J Toxicol Clin Toxicol.* 1999;37:731-751.
4. American Academy of Clinical Toxicology; European Association of Poisons Centres and Clinical Toxicologists: position paper: ipecac syrup. *J Toxicol Clin Toxicol.* 2004;42:133-143.
5. American Academy of Pediatrics: Benzyl alcohol: toxic agent in neonatal units. *Pediatrics.* 1983;72:356-358.
6. American Academy of Pediatrics: Poison treatment in the home. American Academy of Pediatrics Committee on Injury, Violence, and Poison Prevention. *Pediatrics.* 2003;112:1182-1185.
7. American Heart Association. *PALS Provider Manual*; Dallas, TX. 2002.
8. Andiran N, Sarikayalar F: Pattern of acute poisonings in childhood in Ankara: what has changed in twenty years? *Turk J Pediatr.* 2004;46:147-152.
9. Anyebuno MA, Rosenfeld CR: Chloral hydrate toxicity in a term infant. *Dev Pharmacol Ther.* 1991;17:116-120.
10. Ayoub CC, Alexander R, Beck D, et al: Position paper: definitional issues in Munchausen by proxy. *Child Maltreat.* 2002;7:105-111.
11. Bailey JE, Campagna E, Dart RC: The underrecognized toll of prescription opioid abuse on young children. *Ann Emerg Med.* 2009;53:419-424.
12. Bamshad MJ, Wasserman GS: Pediatric clonidine intoxications. *Vet Hum Toxicol.* 1990;32:220-223.
13. Bar-Oz B, Levichek Z, Koren G: Medications that can be fatal for a toddler with one tablet or teaspoonful: a 2004 update. *Paediatr Drugs.* 2004;6:123-126.
14. Baraff LJ, Guterman JJ, Bayer MJ: The relationship of poison center contact and injury in children 2 to 6 years old. *Ann Emerg Med.* 1992;21:153-157.
15. Barazarte V, Rodriguez Z, Ceballos S, et al: Exchange transfusion in a case of severe theophylline poisoning. *Vet Hum Toxicol.* 1992;34:524.
16. Bateman DA, Heagarty MC: Passive freebase cocaine ("crack") inhalation by infants and toddlers. *Am J Dis Child.* 1989;143:25-27.
17. Bayne T, Bindler R: Medication calculation skills of registered nurses. *J Contin Educ Nurs.* 1988;19:258-262.
18. Bebeukelear MM, Batisky DL, Melber SL. Acute hemodialysis in children. In Henrich WL, ed. *Principles and Practice of Dialysis.* Philadelphia: Williams & Wilkins; 1999:534-548.
19. Belay ED, Bresee JS, Holman RC, et al: Reye's syndrome in the United States from 1981 through 1997. *N Engl J Med.* 1999;340:1377-1382.
20. Berning CK, Griffith JF, Wild JE: Research on the effectiveness of denatonium benzoate as a deterrent to liquid detergent ingestion by children. *Fundam Appl Toxicol.* 1982;2:44-48.
21. Bindler R, Bayne T: Do baccalaureate students possess basic mathematics proficiency? *J Nurs Educ.* 1984;23:192-197.
22. Bithoney WG, Snyder J, Michalek J, Newberger EH: Childhood ingestions as symptoms of family distress. *Am J Dis Child.* 1985;139:456-459.
23. Block SM, Dansky R, Davis MD: Lomotil poisoning in children: two case reports. *S Afr Med J.* 1977;51:553-554.
24. Bools C, Neale B, Meadow R: Munchausen syndrome by proxy: a study of psychopathology. *Child Abuse Negl.* 1994;18:773-788.
25. Bools CN, Neale BA, Meadow SR: Co-morbidity associated with fabricated illness (Munchausen syndrome by proxy). *Arch Dis Child.* 1992;67:77-79.
26. Brayden RM, MacLean WE, Jr., Bonfiglio JF, Altemeier W: Behavioral antecedents of pediatric poisonings. *Clin Pediatr.* 1993;32:30-35.
27. Brown ET, Corbett SW, Green SM: Iatrogenic cardiopulmonary arrest during pediatric sedation with meperidine, promethazine, and chlorpromazine. *Pediatr Emerg Care.* 2001;17:351-353.
28. Brown WJ, Buist NR, Gipson HT, et al: Fatal benzyl alcohol poisoning in a neonatal intensive care unit. *Lancet.* 1982;1:1250.
29. Centers for Disease Control: Unintentional poisoning among young children—United States. *MMWR Morb Mortal Wkly Rep.* 1983;32:117-118.
30. Centers for Disease Control: Update: childhood poisonings—United States. *MMWR Morb Mortal Wkly Rep.* 1985;34:117-118.
31. Centers for Disease Control and Prevention: Web-based Injury Statistics Query and Reporting System (WISQUARS). Washington, DC: National Center for Injury Control and Prevention; 2009.
32. Chan TY, Chan AY, Pang CW: Epidemiology of poisoning in the New Territories south of Hong Kong. *Hum Exp Toxicol.* 1997;16:204-207.
33. Chappell K, Newman C: Potential tenfold drug overdoses on a neonatal unit. *Arch Dis Child Fetal Neonatal Ed.* 2004;89:F483-484.
34. Chasnoff IJ, Lewis DE, Squires L: Cocaine intoxication in a breast-fed infant. *Pediatrics.* 1987;80:836-838.
35. Cheng TL, Wright JL, Pearson-Fields AS, Brenner RA: The spectrum of intoxication and poisonings among adolescents: surveillance in an urban population. *Inj Prev* 2006;12:129-132.
36. Chyka PA, Seger D: Position statement: single-dose activated charcoal. American Academy of Clinical Toxicology; European Association of Poisons Centres and Clinical Toxicologists. *J Toxicol Clin Toxicol.* 1997;35:721-741.
37. Clarke A, Walton WW: Effect of safety packaging on aspirin ingestion by children. *Pediatrics.* 1979;63:687-693.
38. Coco TJ, King WD, Slattery AP: Descriptive epidemiology of infant ingestion calls to a regional poison control center. *South Med J.* 2005;98:779-783.
39. Conroy S, Sweis D, Planner C, et al: Interventions to reduce dosing errors in children: a systematic review of the literature. *Drug Saf.* 2007;30:1111-1125.
40. Craft AW: Circumstances surrounding deaths from accidental poisoning 1974–80. *Arch Dis Child.* 1983;58:544-546.
41. Crockett R, Krishel SJ, Manoguerra A, et al: Prehospital use of activated charcoal: a pilot study. *J Emerg Med.* 1996;14:335-338.
42. Cummins LH: Hypoglycemia and convulsions in children following alcohol ingestion. *J Pediatr.* 1961;58:23-26.
43. Cutler EA, Barrett GA, Craven PW, Cramblett HG: Delayed cardiopulmonary arrest after Lomotil ingestion. *Pediatrics.* 1980;65:157-158.
44. Dean B, Schachter M, Vincent C, Barber N: Causes of prescribing errors in hospital inpatients: a prospective study. *Lancet.* 2002;359:1373-1378.
45. Deeths TM, Breeden JT: Poisoning in children—a statistical study of 1,057 cases. *J Pediatr.* 1971;78:299-305.
46. Densen-Gerber J: The forensic pathology of drug-related child abuse. *Leg Med Annu.* 1978:135-147.
47. Diav-Citrin O, Ratnapalan S, Grouhi M, et al: Medication errors in paediatrics: a case report and systematic review of risk factors. *Paediatr Drugs.* 2000;2:239-242.
48. Dine MS, McGovern ME: Intentional poisoning of children—an overlooked category of child abuse: report of seven cases and review of the literature. *Pediatrics.* 1982;70:32-35.
49. Donckerwolcke RA, Bunchman TE: Hemodialysis in infants and small children. *Pediatr Nephrol.* 1994;8:103-106.
50. Done AK, Otterness LJ: Exchange transfusion in the treatment of oil of wintergreen (methyl salicylate) poisoning. *J Pediatrics.* 1956;18:80-85.
51. Ellis EN. Infant hemodialysis. In: Nissenson AR, Fine RN, eds. *Dialysis Therapy.* Philadelphia: Hanley & Belfus; 2002:459-461.
52. Eriksson M, Larsson G, Winbladh B, Zetterstrom R: Accidental poisoning in pre-school children in the Stockholm area. Medical, psychosocial and preventive aspects. *Acta Paediatr Scand.* 1979;275(suppl):96-101.
53. Ferguson JA, Sellar C, Goldacre MJ: Some epidemiological observations on medicinal and non-medicinal poisoning in preschool children. *J Epidemiol Community Health.* 1992;46:207-210.
54. Flagler SL, Wright L: Recurrent poisoning in children: a review. *J Pediatr Psychol.* 1987;12:631-641.
55. Flomenbaum NE, Howland MA: Pretty poison. *Emerg Med.* 1986;4:69-84.
56. Folli HL, Poole RL, Benitz WE, Russo JC: Medication error prevention by clinical pharmacists in two children's hospitals. *Pediatrics.* 1987;79:718-722.

57. Fortescue EB, Kaushal R, Landrigan CP, et al: Prioritizing strategies for preventing medication errors and adverse drug events in pediatric inpatients. *Pediatrics.* 2003;111:722-729.
58. Fox GN: Minimizing prescribing errors in infants and children. *Am Fam Phys.* 1996;53:1319-1325.
59. Frush KS, Luo X, Hutchinson P, Higgins JN: Evaluation of a method to reduce over-the-counter medication dosing error. *Arch Pediatr Adolesc Med.* 2004;158:620-624.
60. Gallagher SS, Finison K, Guyer B, Goodenough S: The incidence of injuries among 87,000 Massachusetts children and adolescents: results of the 1980–81 Statewide Childhood Injury Prevention Program Surveillance System. *Am J Public Health.* 1984;74:1340-1347.
61. Gaudreault P, McCormick MA, Lacouture PG, Lovejoy FH Jr: Poison exposures and use of ipecac in children less than 1 year old. *Ann Emerg Med.* 1986;15:808-810.
62. Gauvin F, Bailey B, Bratton SL: Hospitalizations for pediatric intoxication in Washington State, 1987–1997. *Arch Pediatr Adolesc Med.* 2001;155:1105-1110.
63. Gershanik J, Boecler B, Ensley H, et al: The gasping syndrome and benzyl alcohol poisoning. *N Engl J Med.* 1982;307:1384-1388.
64. Goebel J, Gremse DA, Artman M: Cardiomyopathy from ipecac administration in Munchausen syndrome by proxy. *Pediatrics.* 1993;92:601-603.
65. Goldmann D, Kaushal R: Time to tackle the tough issues in patient safety. *Pediatrics.* 2002;110:823-826.
66. *Good Manufacturing Practice for Dietary Supplements.* 1997;21 CFR 111.50.
67. Gray J, Bentovim A: Illness induction syndrome: paper I—a series of 41 children from 37 families identified at The Great Ormond Street Hospital for Children NHS Trust. *Child Abuse Negl.* 1996;20:655-673.
68. Green SM, Clark R, Hostetler MA, et al: Inadvertent ketamine overdose in children: clinical manifestations and outcome. *Ann Emerg Med.* 1999;34:492-497.
69. Greenberg B, Weihl C, Hug G: Chlorpropamide poisoning. *Pediatrics.* 1968;41:145-147.
70. Gribetz B, Cronley SA: Underdosing of acetaminophen by parents. *Pediatrics.* 1987;80:630-633.
71. Grubbauer HM, Schwarz R: Peritoneal dialysis in alcohol intoxication in a child. *Arch Toxicol.* 1980;43:317-320.
72. Gupta SK, Peshin SS, Srivastava A, Kaleekal T: A study of childhood poisoning at National Poisons Information Centre, All India Institute of Medical Sciences, New Delhi. *J Occup Health.* 2003;45:191-196.
73. Haddon W Jr: Advances in the epidemiology of injuries as a basis for public policy. *Public Health Rep.* 1980;95:411-421.
74. Hamid MH, Butt T, Baloch GR, Maqbool S: Acute poisoning in children. *J Coll Physicians Surg Pak.* 2005;15:805-808.
75. Hamilton RJ, Goldfrank LR: Poison center data and the Pollyanna phenomenon. *J Toxicol Clin Toxicol.* 1997;35:21-23.
76. Han YY, Carcillo JA, Venkataraman ST, et al: Unexpected increased mortality after implementation of a commercially sold computerized physician order entry system. *Pediatrics.* 2005;116:1506-1512.
77. Harchelroad F, Clark RF, Dean B, Krenzelok EP: Treated vs reported toxic exposures: discrepancies between a poison control center and a member hospital. *Vet Hum Toxicol.* 1990;32:156-159.
78. Heidemann SM, Goetting MG: Passive inhalation of cocaine by infants. *Henry Ford Hosp Med J.* 1990;38:252-254.
79. Henretig FM, Paschall RT, Donaruma-Kwoh MM. Child abuse by poisoning. In: Reece RM, Christian CW, eds. *Child Abuse: Medical Diagnosis and Management.* American Academy of Pediatrics; Farmington Hills, Michigan. 2009:549-599.
80. Hickson GB, Altemeier WA, Martin ED, Campbell PW: Parental administration of chemical agents: a cause of apparent life-threatening events. *Pediatrics.* 1989;83:772-776.
81. Hiller JL, Benda GI, Rahatzad M, et al: Benzyl alcohol toxicity: impact on mortality and intraventricular hemorrhage among very low birth weight infants. *Pediatrics.* 1986;77:500-506.
82. Holdsworth MT, Fichtl RE, Behta M, et al: Incidence and impact of adverse drug events in pediatric inpatients. *Arch Pediatr Adolesc Med.* 2003;157:60-65.
83. Holdsworth MT, Fichtl RE, Raisch DW, et al: Impact of computerized prescriber order entry on the incidence of adverse drug events in pediatric inpatients. *Pediatrics.* 2007;120:1058-1066.
84. Holt D, Harvey D, Hurley R: Chloramphenicol toxicity. *Adverse Drug React Toxicol Rev.* 1993;12:83-95.
85. Hon KL, Ho JK, Leung TF, et al: Review of children hospitalised for ingestion and poisoning at a tertiary centre. *Ann Acad Med Singapore.* 2005;34:356-361.
86. Hurwitz ES: Reye's syndrome. *Epidemiol Rev.* 1989;11:249-253.
87. Jackson MH, Payne HA: Bittering agents: their potential application in reducing ingestions of engine coolants and windshield wash. *Vet Hum Toxicol.* 1995;37:323-326.
88. Jacobs BR, Brilli RJ, Hart KW: Perceived increase in mortality after process and policy changes implemented with computerized physician order entry. *Pediatrics.* 2006;117:1451-1452; author reply 1455-1456.
89. Jacobson BJ, Rock AR, Cohn MS, Litovitz T: Accidental ingestions of oral prescription drugs: a multicenter survey. *Am J Public Health.* 1989;79:853-856.
90. Jardine DS, Rogers K: Relationship of benzyl alcohol to kernicterus, intraventricular hemorrhage, and mortality in preterm infants. *Pediatrics.* 1989;83:153-160.
91. Jones JG: The child accident repeater: a review. *Clin Pediatr.* 1980;19:284-288.
92. Juntti-Patinen L, Neuvonen PJ: Drug-related deaths in a university central hospital. *Eur J Clin Pharmacol.* 2002;58:479-482.
93. Kaji AH, Gausche-Hill M, Conrad H, et al: Emergency medical services system changes reduce pediatric epinephrine dosing errors in the prehospital setting. *Pediatrics.* 2006;118:1493-1500.
94. Katrivanou A, Lekka NP, Beratis S: Psychopathology and behavioural trends of children with accidental poisoning. *J Psychosom Res.* 2004;57:95-101.
95. Kaushal R, Barker KN, Bates DW: How can information technology improve patient safety and reduce medication errors in children's health care? *Arch Pediatr Adolesc Med.* 2001;155:1002-1007.
96. Kaushal R, Bates DW, Landrigan C, et al: Medication errors and adverse drug events in pediatric inpatients. *JAMA.* 2001;285:2114-2120.
97. Kharasch S, Vinci R, Reece R: Esophagitis, epiglottitis, and cocaine alkaloid ("crack"): "accidental" poisoning or child abuse? *Pediatrics.* 1990;86:117-119.
98. King WD, Palmisano PA: Ingestion of prescription drugs by children: an epidemiologic study. *South Med J.* 1989;82:1468-1471, 1478.
99. King WJ, Paice N, Rangrej J, et al: The effect of computerized physician order entry on medication errors and adverse drug events in pediatric inpatients. *Pediatrics.* 2003;112:506-509.
100. Kohn LT, Corrigan JM, Donaldson MS. *To Err Is Human: Building a Safer Health System.* Washington, DC: Committee on Quality of Health Care in America, Institute of Medicine, National Academy Press; 1999.
101. Koppel R, Metlay JP, Cohen A, et al: Role of computerized physician order entry systems in facilitating medication errors. *JAMA.* 2005;293:1197-1203.
102. Koren G, Barzilay Z, Modan M: Errors in computing drug doses. *Can Med Assoc J.* 1983;129:721-723.
103. Koren G, Haslam RH: Pediatric medication errors: predicting and preventing tenfold disasters. *J Clin Pharmacol.* 1994;34:1043-1045.
104. Kozer E, Barr J, Bulkowstein M, et al: A prospective study of multiple supratherapeutic acetaminophen doses in febrile children. *Vet Hum Toxicol.* 2002;44:106-109.
105. Kozer E, Scolnik D, Macpherson A, et al: Variables associated with medication errors in pediatric emergency medicine. *Pediatrics.* 2002;110:737-742.
106. Kozer E, Seto W, Verjee Z, et al: Prospective observational study on the incidence of medication errors during simulated resuscitation in a paediatric emergency department. *Br Med J.* 2004;329:1321.
107. Krug A, Ellis JB, Hay IT, et al: The impact of child-resistant containers on the incidence of paraffin (kerosene) ingestion in children. *S Afr Med J.* 1994;84:730-734.
108. Lamminpaa A, Vilska J, Hoppu K: Medical charcoal for a child's poisoning at home: availability and success of administration in Finland. *Hum Exp Toxicol.* 1993;12:29-32.
109. Larose G, Bailey B, Lebel D: Quality of orders for medication in the resuscitation room of a pediatric emergency department. *Pediatr Emerg Care.* 2008;24:609-614.
110. Leape LL, Berwick DM, Bates DW: What practices will most improve safety? Evidence-based medicine meets patient safety. *JAMA.* 2002;288:501-507.
111. Lesar TS: Errors in the use of medication dosage equations. Ar*ch Pediatr Adolesc Med.* 1998;152:340-344.
112. Leung AK: Ethyl alcohol ingestion in children. A 15-year review. *Clin Pediatr.* 1986;25:617-619.
113. Liebelt EL, Shannon MW: Small doses, big problems: a selected review of highly toxic common medications. *Pediatr Emerg Care.* 1993;9:292-297.

114. Linakis JG, Frederick KA: Poisoning deaths not reported to the regional poison control center. *Ann Emerg Med.* 1993;22:1822-1828.
115. Litovitz T, Klein-Schwartz W, Veltri J, Manoguerra A: Prescription drug ingestions in children: whose drug? *Vet Hum Toxicol.* 1986;28:14-15.
116. Litovitz T, Manoguerra A: Comparison of pediatric poisoning hazards: an analysis of 3.8 million exposure incidents. A report from the American Association of Poison Control Centers. *Pediatrics.* 1992;89:999-1006.
117. Longhurst C, Sharek P, Hahn J, et al: Perceived increase in mortality after process and policy changes implemented with computerized physician order entry. *Pediatrics.* 2006;117:1450-1451; author reply 1455-1456.
118. Lubitz DS, Seidel JS, Chameides L, et al: A rapid method for estimating weight and resuscitation drug dosages from length in the pediatric age group. *Ann Emerg Med.* 1988;17:576-581.
119. Luten R, Wears RL, Broselow J, et al: Managing the unique size-related issues of pediatric resuscitation: reducing cognitive load with resuscitation aids. *Acad Emerg Med.* 2002;9:840-847.
120. Luten RC, Wears RL, Broselow J, et al: Length-based endotracheal tube and emergency equipment in pediatrics. *Ann Emerg Med.* 1992;21:900-904.
121. MacLaren NK, Valman HB, Levin B: Alcohol-induced hypoglycaemia in childhood. *Br Med J.* 1970;1:278-280.
122. Madlon-Kay DJ, Mosch FS: Liquid medication dosing errors. *J Fam Pract.* 2000;49:741-744.
123. Mahieu LM, Rooman RP, Goossens E: Imidazoline intoxication in children. *Eur J Pediatr.* 1993;152:944-946.
124. Manikian A, Stone S, Hamilton R, et al: Exchange transfusion in severe infant salicylism. *Vet Hum Toxicol.* 2002;44:224-227.
125. McCaig LF, Burt CW: Poisoning-related visits to emergency departments in the United States, 1993–1996. *J Toxicol Clin Toxicol.* 1999;37:817-826.
126. McCarron MM, Challoner KR, Thompson GA: Diphenoxylate-atropine (Lomotil) overdose in children: an update (report of eight cases and review of the literature). *Pediatrics.* 1991;87:694-700.
127. McDonald CJ: Computerization can create safety hazards: a bar-coding near miss. *Ann Intern Med.* 2006;144:510-516.
128. McFee RB, Caraccio TR: "Hang up your pocketbook"—an easy intervention for the granny syndrome: grandparents as a risk factor in unintentional pediatric exposures to pharmaceuticals. *J Am Osteopath Assoc.* 2006;106:405-411.
129. McGuire TL, Feldman KW: Psychologic morbidity of children subjected to Munchausen syndrome by proxy. *Pediatrics.* 1989;83:289-292.
130. McMahon SR, Rimsza ME, Bay RC: Parents can dose liquid medication accurately. *Pediatrics.* 1997;100:330-333.
131. Meadow R: Munchausen syndrome by proxy. The hinterland of child abuse. *Lancet.* 1977;2:343-345.
132. Meadow R: Munchausen syndrome by proxy. *Arch Dis Child.* 1982;57:92-98.
133. Mirchandani HG, Mirchandani IH, Hellman F, et al: Passive inhalation of free-base cocaine ('crack') smoke by infants. *Arch Pathol Lab Med.* 1991;115:494-498.
134. Monto AS: The disappearance of Reye's syndrome—a public health triumph. *N Engl J Med.* 1999;340:1423-1424.
135. Morgan N, Luo X, Fortner C, Frush K: Opportunities for performance improvement in relation to medication administration during pediatric stabilization. *Qual Saf Health Care.* 2006;15:179-183.
136. Narayanan M, Schlueter M, Clyman RI: Incidence and outcome of a 10-fold indomethacin overdose in premature infants. *J Pediatr.* 1999;135:105-107.
137. Nelson LS, Gordon PE, Simmons MD, et al: The benefit of house officer education on proper medication dose calculation and ordering. *Acad Emerg Med.* 2000;7:1311-1316.
138. Nordt SP, Manoguerra A, Williams SR, Clark RF: The availability of activated charcoal and ipecac for home use. *Vet Hum Toxicol.* 1999;41:247-248.
139. *Nutritional Health Alliance v. FDA.* 318 F.3d 2003:92.
140. Oguche S, Bukbuk DN, Watila IM: Pattern of hospital admissions of children with poisoning in the Sudano-Sahelian North eastern Nigeria. *Niger J Clin Pract.* 2007;10:111-115.
141. Osborn HH, Henry G, Wax P, et al: Theophylline toxicity in a premature neonate—elimination kinetics of exchange transfusion. *J Toxicol Clin Toxicol.* 1993;31:639-644.
142. Paudyal BP: Poisoning: pattern and profile of admitted cases in a hospital in central Nepal. *JNMA J Nepal Med Assoc.* 2005;44:92-96.
143. Perlstein PH, Callison C, White M, et al: Errors in drug computations during newborn intensive care. *Am J Dis Child.* 1979;133:376-379.
144. Peth HA Jr: Medication errors in the emergency department: a systems approach to minimizing risk. *Emerg Med Clin North Am.* 2003;21:141-158.
145. Polakoff JM, Lacouture PG, Lovejoy FH Jr: The environment away from home as a source of potential poisoning. *Am J Dis Child.* 1984;138:1014-1017.
146. Potts AL, Barr FE, Gregory DF, et al: Computerized physician order entry and medication errors in a pediatric critical care unit. *Pediatrics.* 2004;113:59-63.
147. Potts MJ, Phelan KW: Deficiencies in calculation and applied mathematics skills in pediatrics among primary care interns. *Arch Pediatr Adolesc Med.* 1996;150:748-752.
148. Quadrani DA, Spiller HA, Widder P: Five year retrospective evaluation of sulfonylurea ingestion in children. *J Toxicol Clin Toxicol.* 1996;34:267-270.
149. Raju TN, Kecskes S, Thornton JP, et al: Medication errors in neonatal and paediatric intensive-care units. *Lancet.* 1989;2:374-376.
150. Ramisetty-Mikler S, Mains D, Rene A: Poisoning hospitalizations among Texas adolescents: age and gender differences in intentional and unintentional injury. *Tex Med.* 2005;101:64-71.
151. Reinhart MA: Child abuse: cocaine absorption by rectal administration. *Clin Pediatr.* 1990;29:357..
152. Rice DP, MacKenzie EJ, AS ASJ, et al *Cost of Injury in the United States: A Report to Congress.* San Francisco: Institute for Health and Aging, University of California Injury Prevention Center, Johns Hopkins University; 1989.
153. Richards RG, Cravey RH: Infanticide due to ethanolism. *J Analyt Toxicol.* 1978;2:60-61.
154. Rieder MJ, Goldstein D, Zinman H, Koren G: Tenfold errors in drug dosage. *CMAJ.* 1988;139:12-13.
155. Riggs D, Weibley RE: Acute hemorrhagic diarrhea and cardiovascular collapse in a young child owing to environmentally acquired cocaine. *Pediatr Emerg Care.* 1991;7:154-155.
156. Rinke ML, Moon M, Clark JS, et al: Prescribing errors in a pediatric emergency department. *Pediatr Emerg Care.* 2008;24:1-8.
157. Risser DT, Rice MM, Salisbury ML, et al: The potential for improved teamwork to reduce medical errors in the emergency department. The MedTeams Research Consortium. *Ann Emerg Med.* 1999;34:373-383.
158. Robertson WO: Conflicting views in poison treatment. *Pediatrics.* 2002;110:199-200; author reply 199-200.
159. Rodgers GB: The safety effects of child-resistant packaging for oral prescription drugs. Two decades of experience. *JAMA.* 1996;275:1661-1665.
160. Rodgers GB: The effectiveness of child-resistant packaging for aspirin. *Arch Pediatr Adolesc Med.* 2002;156:929-933.
161. Rodgers GC Jr, Tenenbein M: The role of aversive bittering agents in the prevention of pediatric poisonings. *Pediatrics.* 1994;93:68-69.
162. Rolfe S, Harper NJ: Ability of hospital doctors to calculate drug doses. *Br Med J.* 1995;310:1173-1174.
163. Romano MJ, Dinh A: A 1000-fold overdose of clonidine caused by a compounding error in a 5-year-old child with attention-deficit/hyperactivity disorder. *Pediatrics.* 2001;108:471-472.
164. Rosenberg DA: Web of deceit: a literature review of Munchausen syndrome by proxy. *Child Abuse Negl.* 1987;11:547-563.
165. Rosenberg DA. Munchausen syndrome by proxy. In: Reece RM, Christian CW, eds. *Child Abuse: Medical Diagnosis and Management.* American Academy of Pediatrics; Farmington Hills, Michigan. 2009:513-547.
166. Rosenbloom ST, Harrell FE, Jr., Lehmann CU, et al: Perceived increase in mortality after process and policy changes implemented with computerized physician order entry. *Pediatrics.* 2006;117:1452-1455; author reply 1455-1456.
167. Ross LM, Wallace J, Paton JY: Medication errors in a paediatric teaching hospital in the UK: five years operational experience. *Arch Dis Child.* 2000;83:492-497.
168. Rowe C, Koren T, Koren G: Errors by paediatric residents in calculating drug doses. *Arch Dis Child.* 1998;79:56-58.
169. Scharman EJ: Home administration of charcoal: can mothers administer a therapeutic dose? *J Emerg Med.* 2002;22:421-422.
170. Scharman EJ, Cloonan HA, Durback-Morris LF: Home administration of charcoal: can mothers administer a therapeutic dose? *J Emerg Med.* 2001;21:357-361.
171. Schreier H: Munchausen by proxy. *Curr Probl Pediatr Adolesc Health Care.* 2004;34:126-143.
172. Schwartz RH, Einhorn A: PCP intoxication in seven young children. *Pediatr Emerg Care.* 1986;2:238-241.
173. Schwartz RH, Peary P, Mistretta D: Intoxication of young children with marijuana: a form of amusement for 'pot'-smoking teenage girls. *Am J Dis Child.* 1986;140:326.

174. Selbst SM, Levine S, Mull C, et al: Preventing medical errors in pediatric emergency medicine. *Pediatr Emerg Care.* 2004;20:702-709.
175. Shah AN, Frush K, Luo X, Wears RL: Effect of an intervention standardization system on pediatric dosing and equipment size determination: a crossover trial involving simulated resuscitation events. *Arch Pediatr Adolesc Med.* 2003;157:229-236.
176. Shannon M, Wernovsky G, Morris C: Exchange transfusion in the treatment of severe theophylline poisoning. *Pediatrics.* 1992;89:145-147.
177. Shaw RJ, Dayal S, Hartman JK, DeMaso DR: Factitious disorder by proxy: pediatric condition falsification. *Harv Rev Psychiatry.* 2008;16:215-224.
178. Shoemaker JD, Lynch RE, Hoffmann JW, Sly WS: Misidentification of propionic acid as ethylene glycol in a patient with methylmalonic acidemia. *J Pediatr.* 1992;120:417-421.
179. Shotar AM: Kerosene poisoning in childhood: a 6-year prospective study at the Princess Rahmat Teaching Hospital. *Neuro Endocrinol Lett.* 2005;26:835-838.
180. Sibert JR, Frude N: Bittering agents in the prevention of accidental poisoning: children's reactions to denatonium benzoate (Bitrex). *Arch Emerg Med.* 1991;8:1-7.
181. Sibert R: Stress in families of children who have ingested poisons. *Br Med J.* 1975;3:87-89.
182. Simon HK, Weinkle DA: Over-the-counter medications. Do parents give what they intend to give? *Arch Pediatr Adolesc Med.* 1997;151:654-656.
183. Simpson JH, Lynch R, Grant J, Alroomi L: Reducing medication errors in the neonatal intensive care unit. *Arch Dis Child Fetal Neonatal Ed.* 2004;89:F480-482.
184. Slagle MA, Chyka PA, Holley JE: Pharmacists' use of safety caps on refilled prescriptions. *Am Pharm.* 1994;NS34:37-40.
185. Smetzer JL: Lesson from Colorado. Beyond blaming individuals. *Nurs Manage.* 1998;29:49-51.
186. Sobel R: Traditional safety measures and accidental poisoning in childhood. *Pediatrics.* 1969;44(suppl):811-816.
187. Sobel R: The psychiatric implications of accidental poisoning in childhood. *Pediatr Clin North Am.* 1970;17:653-685.
188. Sobhani P, Christopherson J, Ambrose PJ, Corelli RL: Accuracy of oral liquid measuring devices: comparison of dosing cup and oral dosing syringe. *Ann Pharmacother.* 2008;42:46-52.
189. Solomon SL, Wallace EM, Ford-Jones EL, et al: Medication errors with inhalant epinephrine mimicking an epidemic of neonatal sepsis. *N Engl J Med.* 1984;310:166-170.
190. Spiller HA, Rodgers GC, Jr.: Evaluation of administration of activated charcoal in the home. *Pediatrics.* 2001;108:E100.
191. Spiller HA: Home administration of charcoal. *J Emerg Med.* 2003;25:106-107; author reply 107.
192. Stremski ES: Accidental pediatric ingestion, hospital charges and failure to utilize a poison control center. *WMJ.* 1999;98:29-33.
193. Stucky ER: Prevention of medication errors in the pediatric inpatient setting. *Pediatrics.* 2003;112:431-436.
194. Szlatenyi CS, Capes KF, Wang RY: Delayed hypoglycemia in a child after ingestion of a single glipizide tablet. *Ann Emerg Med.* 1998;31:773-776.
195. Tenenbein M: Pediatric toxicology: current controversies and recent advances. *Curr Probl Pediatr.* 1986;16:185-233.
196. Thomas SH, Bevan L, Bhattacharyya S, et al: Presentation of poisoned patients to accident and emergency departments in the north of England. *Hum Exp Toxicol.* 1996;15:466-470.
197. Thompson JN: Corrosive esophageal injuries. I. A study of nine cases of concurrent accidental caustic ingestion. *Laryngoscope.* 1987;97:1060-1068.
198. Tolman IJ, Done GA: Hemodialysis of the neonate weighing less than 4 kg. *ANNA J.* 1989;16:421-424.
199. Trinkoff AM, Baker SP: Poisoning hospitalizations and deaths from solids and liquids among children and teenagers. *Am J Public Health.* 1986;76:657-660.
200. Vincer MJ, Murray JM, Yuill A, et al: Drug errors and incidents in a neonatal intensive care unit. A quality assurance activity. *Am J Dis Child.* 1989;143:737-740.
201. Viscusi WK: Consumer behavior and the safety effects of product safety regulation. *J Law Econom.* 1985;28:527-554.
202. Vogel C, Caraccio T, Mofenson H, Hart S: Alcohol intoxication in young children. *J Toxicol Clin Toxicol.* 1995;33:25-33.
203. Walsh KE, Adams WG, Bauchner H, et al: Medication errors related to computerized order entry for children. *Pediatrics.* 2006;118:1872-1879.
204. Walsh KE, Landrigan CP, Adams WG, et al: Effect of computer order entry on prevention of serious medication errors in hospitalized children. *Pediatrics.* 2008;121:e421-427.
205. Wears R, Leape LL: Human error in emergency medicine. *Ann Emerg Med.* 1999;34:370-372.
206. Weisman RS, Goldfrank L: Poison center numbers. *J Toxicol Clin Toxicol.* 1991;29:553-557.
207. Weissman DB, Jackson SH, Heicher DA, Rockoff MA: Benzyl alcohol administration in neonates. *Anesth Analg.* 1990;70:673-674.
208. Welch MJ, Correa GA: PCP intoxication in young children and infants. *Clin Pediatr.* 1980;19:510-514.
209. West L: Innovative approaches to the administration of activated charcoal in pediatric toxic ingestions. *Pediatr Nurs.* 1997;23:616-619.
210. Wiley JF 2nd, Wiley CC, Torrey SB, Henretig FM: Clonidine poisoning in young children. *J Pediatr.* 1990;116:654-658.
211. Wilson DG, McArtney RG, Newcombe RG, et al: Medication errors in paediatric practice: insights from a continuous quality improvement approach. *Eur J Pediatr.* 1998;157:769-774.
212. Wiseman HM, Guest K, Murray VS, Volans GN: Accidental poisoning in childhood: a multicentre survey. 2. The role of packaging in accidents involving medications. *Hum Toxicol.* 1987;6:303-314.
213. Woolf A, Wieler J, Greenes D: Costs of poison-related hospitalizations at an urban teaching hospital for children. *Arch Pediatr Adolesc Med.* 1997;151:719-723.
214. Yin HS, Dreyer BP, van Schaick L, et al: Randomized controlled trial of a pictogram-based intervention to reduce liquid medication dosing errors and improve adherence among caregivers of young children. *Arch Pediatr Adolesc Med.* 2008;162:814-822.
215. Zuckerman BS, Duby JC: Developmental approach to injury prevention. *Pediatr Clin North Am.* 1985;32:17-29.

CHAPTER 32
GERIATRIC PRINCIPLES

Judith C. Ahronheim and Mary Ann Howland

PREVALENCE, LETHALITY, AND UNDERRECOGNITION OF TOXIC EXPOSURE

In developed countries, the population is aging steadily. In the United States, those older than 65 years of age comprise not only an increasing proportion of the population at large (12%) but also an increasing proportion of patients seen in medical practices. Compared with all other age groups, patients older than 65 years of age account for one-third of emergency department (ED) ambulance arrivals and the highest proportion of patients in EDs triaged as emergent.[80]

Although the elderly account for only a small minority of toxicologic exposures, after they have been exposed, they have a high mortality rate. Among exposures reported to the American Association of Poison Control Centers (AAPCC) in 2006, the fatality ratio (ie, number of cases divided by number of deaths) increased with age in a bimodal pattern, with peaks in the middle and latest decades of life (see Chap. 135). Previous AAPCC surveys had shown a steady increase in fatality ratio. In addition to possible methodologic changes and smaller numbers of exposures in the latest decades of life, potential explanations for the current change to a bimodal pattern may include an increase in intentional exposures in midlife and physiologic vulnerability in the later decades. However, this only accounts for part of the difference because suicide fatality ratios increase steadily with age (see Suicide and Intentional Poisonings below). In a separate study, seven specific pharmaceuticals were selected from the AAPCC database for analysis based on their prevalent use and potential toxicity from 1995 through 2002. These pharmaceuticals were theophylline, digoxin, benzodiazepines, tricyclic antidepressants (TCAs), calcium channel blockers, acetaminophen, and salicylate.[97] The death rate from intentional or unintentional exposure to these pharmaceuticals was found to increase by 35% for each decade of life after age 19 years.[97]

Toxic exposures reported to the AAPCC may underestimate the serious consequences for elderly people exposed to toxic substances. Data from the National Electronic Injury Surveillance System—Cooperative Adverse Drug Event Surveillance Project (NEISS-CADES) indicate that patients aged 65 years and older accounted for 25% of estimated visits related to adverse drug events (ADEs) and almost 50% of such visits requiring hospitalization or prolonged monitoring in the ED.[10] The problem may be even greater because the NEISS-CADES study did not capture recognized or unrecognized ADEs in patients treated or dying outside of EDs.

Underrecognition of toxic exposures in the elderly may occur for several reasons. First, because of pharmacokinetic and pharmacodynamic changes that occur as one ages,[31] a "standard" therapeutic dose may produce an unexpected serious effect. Second, the presentation of disease, including drug toxicity, is often atypical in the elderly.[59] For example, falls in the elderly may be a presenting sign of xenobiotic toxicity and are commonly due to prescribed xenobiotics, with sedative–hypnotics, antipsychotics, antidepressants, and class Ia antidysrhythmics (quinidine and procainamide) most often associated with an increased risk of falling.[108] If the patient is cognitively impaired and the fall is unwitnessed, the immediate consequences of the fall may be adequately addressed, but the xenobiotic causing it may not.[67] Likewise, the toxicologic etiology of neurologic deficits may not be recognized. For example, severe hypoglycemia can produce signs of classic stroke,[116] which could be attributed to other etiologies, particularly in someone who is elderly and otherwise predisposed (see Chap. 48). Another important syndrome in older patients is delirium, which may be caused by many factors but is a common presentation of xenobiotic toxicity[87] (see Chap. 18).[87] A large variety of xenobiotics may cause mental status changes, which may mistakenly be attributed to for nonxenobiotic-related causes in the elderly.[104] Conversely, altered mental status may be unrecognized[75] and, even when obvious, misdiagnosed—for example, as Alzheimer's disease.

A striking case of drug-induced mental status changes is represented by a previously normal 66-year-old man who developed psychosis and attempted suicide after taking increasing doses of dextromethorphan-containing cough syrup for a respiratory infection. The patient was treated with psychiatric medications, and several months elapsed before providers realized that his behavior had been xenobiotic induced rather than due to a primary psychiatric condition.[79]

Finally, the presentation of drug toxicity may be delayed in elderly individuals. Drugs with long half-lives may not reach a steady state and hence not achieve peak action until days after the drug therapy is initiated. In some older patients, the active metabolite of flurazepam, desalkylflurazepam, has a half-life of up to 100 hours or longer, which requires days to achieve a steady state.[47] When peak effects are delayed in this way, drug toxicities may easily be mistaken for nondrug-related illnesses.

Table 32–1 lists xenobiotics commonly responsible for toxicity in the elderly.

SUICIDE AND INTENTIONAL POISONINGS

The risk of suicide by all methods increases steadily with age, particularly among men. Although data for individual ethnic groups are limited, white men have a substantially higher risk of suicide than age-matched cohorts among the African American population.[20] Another high-risk group appears to be Native American and Alaskan Native men,[61] although the number of deaths from all causes among elderly men in those groups is too low to make meaningful comparisons.[20] Although less likely than men to complete suicide, women are more likely to attempt it.[20] The male-to-female ratio of suicide attempts narrows with increasing age, and in the oldest age groups, men attempt suicide slightly more often than women, when all methods of attempted suicide are considered (Chap. 17).[20,102]

Data published in 2000 from eight states reveal that for all attempted and successful suicides combined, the case fatality rate increases with age and is highest for those aged 65 years and older compared with all other age groups (30.7% compared with 14.8% in the next highest group, which is those between 45 and 64 years old).[102] Although the elderly are more likely to select a highly lethal method, the fatality rate is highest among the elderly regardless of method used. In the United States, firearms are the most frequent means of death by suicide. Among men older than age 65 years, xenobiotic overdose accounts for only 3% of completed suicides, and firearms account for 73%. In contrast, xenobiotic overdose and firearms each account for approximately 25% of successful suicides in women. When death by toxic inhalation is included, poison exposure may surpass gunshot wounds as a cause of death among elderly women.[82] Xenobiotic overdose is an important factor in suicide *attempts* by the elderly of both genders.[41]

Geographic and cultural factors also determine the method of suicide. In countries other than the United States, firearms are only

TABLE 32–1. Xenobiotics that Pose an Increased Risk of Toxicity in the Elderly[a]

Anticholinergics
Anticoagulants
Antidepressants
Antipsychotics
Cardiovascular medications
β-Adrenergic antagonists
Calcium channel blockers
Digoxin
Insulin and oral hypoglycemics
Magnesium-containing laxatives
Nonsteroidal antiinflammatory drugs
Opioids
Salicylates
Sedative–hypnotics
Sodium phosphate laxatives
Warfarin

[a] In addition, polypharmacy may lead to toxicity as a result of diverse drug–drug interactions.

rarely used to commit suicide at any age; suicide by oral overdose and toxic inhalation consequently comprise a much greater proportion.[106] A study of medical examiner–certified suicides in New York City between 1990 and 1998 revealed that falls from a height was the most common method used by people 65 years of age and older and accounted for 33.6% of suicides by people 85 years and older.[2] These data likely represent a local phenomenon because they are inconsistent with national statistics.[20] Falls from a substantial height in Manhattan, with its skyscrapers, landmarks, and bridges, accounts for 34% of suicides among residents and 43% of suicides among visitors.[61]

Among the elderly, the pattern of medications responsible for suicidal deaths may be changing because selective serotonin reuptake inhibitors (SSRIs) are increasingly prescribed for depression instead of TCAs.[15] In the United States, higher suicide rates have been associated with greater use of TCAs than non-TCA antidepressants,[45] which could be related to greater lethality of TCAs in overdose or poorer tolerability of TCAs, leading to nonadherence and enhanced suicide risk. In a Swedish study examining autopsy-confirmed suicides that included analysis of legal xenobiotics, the incidence of suicidal fatalities attributed to benzodiazepines was reported to be increasing despite a marked decrease in benzodiazepine prescriptions.[15] Overdose of benzodiazepines is rarely fatal unless it is accompanied by alcohol or another toxic ingestion or occurs in the presence of serious medical conditions.[35] However, the likelihood of fatality from an overdose of benzodiazepine taken alone increases markedly with each decade of life,[97] perhaps because benzodiazepines in frail elderly people commonly lead to secondary morbidity and mortality from aspiration pneumonia, falls including hip fracture, and other medical complications that may be only the proximate cause of death in the case of overdose.

Notably, flunitrazepam and nitrazepam, the two most frequently implicated in single benzodiazepine suicides in Sweden,[16] are not available in the United States. However, single-drug suicides have been reported with other benzodiazepines that are available, such as flurazepam, triazolam, diazepam, and oxazepam.[16,28,81]

UNINTENTIONAL POISONING, ADVERSE DRUG EVENTS, AND THERAPEUTIC ERRORS

Although poisoning exposures are much less frequent in the elderly than in other age groups, the incidence of ADEs among adults increases steadily with age and increases steeply from age 65 years through the tenth decade of life (Fig. 32–1).[10] An ADE is defined as "one that occurs with normal, prescribed, labeled or recommended use of the [drug]."[9] ADEs are more likely to be serious in the elderly than in younger adults. Serious ADEs are those resulting in death, hospitalization, life-threatening outcome, disability, or other serious outcome[18] and are most prevalent among people 85 years of age and older.[13]

It may be challenging for a clinician to distinguish an intentional or unintentional overdose from an ADE in an elderly patient. The history, if available, must be explored carefully to identify and prevent recurrent problems. However, exposures in persons older than age 60 years are more likely the result of therapeutic errors and "misuse" than in younger adults.[24,29] A therapeutic error is defined as "an unintentional deviation from a proper therapeutic regimen that results in the wrong dose, incorrect route of administration, administration to the wrong person, or administration of the wrong substance" and includes "unintentional administration of xenobiotics or foods which are known to interact." [9] These age-related differences may be because of physiologic changes that affect xenobiotic disposition or effect, patient errors caused by cognitive or visual impairment, or lack of provider proficiency in geriatric prescribing principles.

In contrast to serious consequences of therapeutic errors, reactions such as the serotonin syndrome and neuroleptic malignant syndrome (NMS), which are potentially life threatening, may occur with correctly prescribed therapeutic doses or drug interactions.[5] Although abnormalities in thermoregulation are more common in late life,[8] the risk of developing NMS has not been linked to advanced age per se.[17] However, these syndromes can be overlooked in a patient with comorbidities that could obscure a precise diagnosis. For example, NMS must be distinguished from such geriatric syndromes as cerebrovascular events, heat stroke, or neuroleptic sensitivity syndrome seen in Lewy body dementia.[17]

Both serotonin syndrome and NMS, which are relatively unpredictable, and can occur at any age, are relatively rare. Among elderly

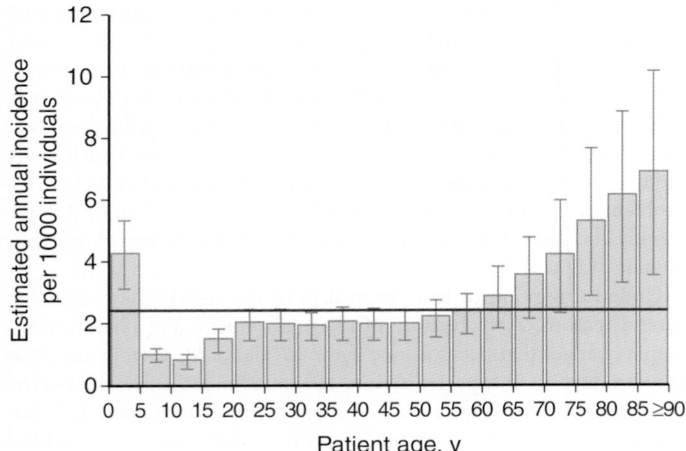

FIGURE 32–1. Estimated annual incidence of adverse drug events treated in 63 US emergency departments: based on 21,298 cases. (Reprinted with permission from Budnitz DS, Pollock DA, Weidenbach KN, et al: National surveillance of emergency department visits for outpatient adverse drug events. *JAMA*. 2006;296:1858-1866.)

TABLE 32–2. Pharmacokinetic Considerations in the Elderly

	Young	Elderly	Effect on Kinetics
Fat (% of body weight)	15	↑30	↑Vd for xenobiotics distributing to fat (amitriptyline, diazepam)
Intracellular water (% of body weight)	42	↓30	↓Vd for water-soluble xenobiotics
Muscle (% of body weight)	17	↓12	↓Vd for xenobiotics distributing into lean tissue (acetaminophen, caffeine, digoxin, ethanol)
Albumin (g/dL)	4	↓With acute or chronic illness	↑Free concentrations of xenobiotics if > 90% bound to albumin, especially in overdose; interpretation of serum concentration altered
Liver	Normal	↓Size ↓Hepatic blood flow	Liver enzymes not predictive of compromise; concentrations of xenobiotics with high extraction (propranolol, triazolam) may increase; ↓hepatic oxidation (diazepam, chlordiazepoxide)
Kidney	Normal	↓Renal blood flow ↓GFR ↓Tubular secretion	↑Accumulation (lithium, aminoglycosides, *N*-acetyl procainamide, ACE inhibitors, cimetidine, digoxin, opioid metabolites

ACE, angiotensin-converting enzyme; GFR, glomerular filtration rate; Vd, volume of distribution.

patients, serious or life-threatening ADEs are more typically caused by commonly prescribed drugs, such as anticoagulants; insulin and oral hypoglycemics; and drugs that cause delirium, such as sedative–hypnotics, opioids, and anticholinergic agents (see Table 32–1).

As many as 42% of serious ADEs reported in elderly patients are potentially preventable.[4,51] National data from the NEISS-CADES study revealed that drugs requiring careful outpatient monitoring were disproportionately represented among ED visits attributed to unintentional drug overdose. Data gathered as recently as 2004 and 2005 show that hypoglycemics, warfarin, certain anticonvulsants, lithium, digitalis glycosides, and perhaps surprisingly, theophylline account for more than 50% of unintentional overdoses among all age groups and 42% of all estimated hospitalizations.[10] These xenobiotics pose a particular problem for patients 65 years of age and older, being implicated in 85% of visits attributed to unintentional overdose, 87% of overdoses requiring hospitalizations, and 54% of hospitalizations overall.[10] Insulin, warfarin, and digoxin were the most common specific xenobiotics implicated in such events.

The above-mentioned xenobiotics are generally monitored with routine blood testing. Other drugs that commonly cause ADEs in the elderly must be monitored clinically, and these ADEs are often best prevented by not prescribing these xenobiotics to vulnerable patients or by cautioning against their use when they are available without prescription. Criteria have been developed to guide clinicians regarding "inappropriate" medications in elderly patients.[38] Xenobiotics deemed inappropriate in the elderly cause numerically fewer ADEs than more frequently prescribed xenobiotics.[11] However, there is consensus as well as evidence that these xenobiotics pose great risk to older adults, especially those who are frail.[42,72] For example, the elderly are at enhanced risk of severe upper gastrointestinal (GI) bleeding from nonsteroidal antiinflammatory drugs (NSAIDS).[119] Although this could be partly explained by increased exposure to and regular use of these drugs, for chronic conditions, older adults are more vulnerable to their effects because of underlying atrophic gastritis. There is controversy as to cause of age-related gastric mucosal changes, but they may partly be caused by underlying *Helicobacter pylori* infection, which appears to increase with age.[3,33] The elderly are also at greater risk of prolonged hypoglycemia from certain sulfonylureas, particularly glyburide.[100] Age-related mechanisms to explain this vulnerability to glyburide may include a decreased counterregulatory hormonal response to xenobiotic-induced hypoglycemia,[84] inappropriate stimulation of insulin in response to hypoglycemia,[105] or reduced excretion of a renally eliminated active metabolite of glyburide.[60] Other age-related factors involved in enhanced susceptibility to ADEs are given in Tables 32–2 and 32–3.

SUBSTANCE ABUSE IN THE ELDERLY

Substance abuse declines with age[39] but is important to consider in older adults under relevant clinical circumstances. Alcohol is the most common substance of abuse in people older than age 65 years. Abuse of alcohol or other xenobiotics may be a continuation of long-term habits, but some individuals may first begin to use and abuse xenobiotics late in life.[63]

Substance abuse in late life is probably underrecognized and underreported.[96] In one Illinois study of patients presenting to a trauma facility, only 5% of those aged 65 years and older were tested for alcohol or other substances, but among those younger than age 65 years, 22% were tested for alcohol and 29% for other xenobiotics.[122] However, almost half of the elderly patients tested for alcohol were positive and 72% of those had a blood alcohol level of 80 mg/dL (the legal limit in Illinois) or above, results that were comparable to those of younger patients who were studied, 75% of whom tested positive. For a comparable amount of alcohol ingested, the blood alcohol concentration of an elderly person will be higher than that of a younger adult because changes in body composition reduce the volume of distribution (Vd) of ethanol.[109,113] Moreover, because of an age-associated diminished tolerance to alcohol, the impact on cognitive or motor function tends to be greater.

In the Illinois study noted above, 11% of elderly patients who were tested had positive urine toxicology screening results compared with 43% of tested younger adults.[122] The most common xenobiotics detected in the elderly were benzodiazepines, opioids, and barbiturates, which, like alcohol, are more likely to impair older than younger adults. The failure to consider use of these xenobiotics, whether illicit or by prescription, may have serious consequences. When admitted to hospitals, if a careful history is not elicited, withdrawal from these xenobiotics may be missed, be misdiagnosed, and as a result be inappropriately managed.

TABLE 32–3. Pathophysiologic Disorders Exacerbated or Unmasked by Xenobiotics in the Elderly[a]

Disorder or Alteration	Drug	Possible Outcome
ADH secretion (increased)	Antipsychotics, SSRIs	Hyponatremia
Androgenic hormones (decreased in men)	Digoxin, spironolactone	Gynecomastia
Baroreceptor dysfunction, venous insufficiency	Antipsychotics, diuretics, CAs, α_1-adrenergic antagonists	Orthostatic hypotension
Bladder dysfunction	Diuretics	Incontinence
Cardiac disease	Thiazolidinediones	Congestive heart failure
Dementia	Sedatives, anticholinergics, many others	Confusion
Gastritis (atrophic)	NSAIDs, salicylates	Gastric hemorrhage
Immobility, cathartic bowel	Anticholinergics, opioids, CCBs	Constipation; fecal impaction
Nodal disease (sinus or AV)	β-Adrenergic antagonists, digoxin, CCBs	Bradycardia
Parkinson's disease; Lewy body dementia	Antipsychotics, metoclopramide	Parkinsonism
Prostatic hyperplasia	Anticholinergics, CAs, disopyramide	Urinary retention
Thermoregulation, disordered	Antipsychotics	Hypo- or hyperthermia
Venous insufficiency	CCBs, gabapentin, others	Edema

[a] Disorder may be preclinical.

ADH, antidiuretic hormone; AV, atrioventricular; CCB, calcium channel blocker; SSRI, serotonin reuptake inhibitor; CA, cyclic antidepressant.

PHARMACOKINETICS

Age-related pharmacokinetic changes have important clinical implications for elderly patients. The most consistent pharmacokinetic change that occurs with aging is a decrease in renal function. Glomerular filtration rate (GFR) declines, on the average, by 50% between the ages of 30 and 80 years[32,98] and cannot be accurately predicted by serum creatinine, which does not increase significantly with age,[98] because muscle mass, the source of serum creatinine, declines with age.[68,89]

Because it is impractical and often difficult to measure 24-hour creatinine clearance before instituting therapy with a renally excreted xenobiotic, clinicians commonly estimate creatinine clearance using age-adjusted formulas or nomograms. Frequently applied formulas are fairly predictive of renal function when renal function is stable.[88] However, age-related declines in GFR are not universal, and limited data from longitudinal studies suggest that as many as 33% of elderly individuals do not experience this age-related decline.[77] Conversely, predictive formulas could significantly overestimate actual creatinine clearance in chronically ill, debilitated elderly people, especially those with renal insufficiency.[71] Modifications to the Cockcroft-Gault equation to correct for body surface area[58,99] have been proposed to better reflect renal function (see Table 27–5 for details). However, anthropomorphic measurements are unreliable in the elderly,[66,101] and physiologic variability is great. Alternative measurements, such as the Modification of Diet in Renal Disease(MDRD) Study Group equation, serum cystatin C, and others have also been proposed, but no current method of estimating renal function in the elderly appears to be superior for use in the clinical setting.[111] For all of these reasons, it is difficult to accurately predict the renal elimination of xenobiotics or their metabolites in the elderly. A practical solution is to assume that renal function has declined significantly and to exercise caution when prescribing maintenance doses of drugs with a narrow therapeutic-to-toxic ratio (Table 32–4). Failure to do so is an important cause of toxicity.[74]

The nature and degree of impact of age-related hepatic changes on drug elimination is controversial. Liver mass decreases with an associated decrease in hepatic blood flow,[120] which results in decreased efficiency of hepatic extraction. Enzymatic processes are often unpredictable,[65] and although hepatic oxidation appears to decline with age,[31] this change is difficult to demonstrate. There is substantial genetic variability among cytochrome P450 isoenzymes, making it difficult to interpret studies of age-related alterations in oxidative metabolism. Some studies that consider cofactors that could affect hepatic enzymes, such as concurrent

TABLE 32–4. Xenobiotics with Narrow Therapeutic-to-Toxic Ratios and Potential for Accumulation in the Presence of Diminished Renal Function

- Antimicrobials
  - Aminoglycosides
  - Imipenem
  - Pyrazinamide
  - Vancomycin
- Opioids with active metabolites that may cause toxicity
  - Morphine (morphine 6-glucuronide): respiratory depression; (morphine 3 glucuronide): neuroexcitation
  - Codeine (morphine)
  - Hydromorphone (hydromorphone 3-glucuronide): potential for neuroexcitation
  - Meperidine (normeperidine: neuroexcitation, seizures)
- Digoxin
- Heparins (Low-molecular-weight)
- Lithium
- Metformin
- NSAIDs
- Procainamide (*N*-acetyl procainamide)
- Salicylates.

medications or cigarette smoking, or that determine isoenzyme genotype may demonstrate that there is no age-related change in hepatic oxidative enzyme function.[7]

Hepatic conjugation does not decline significantly with age, so xenobiotics such as temazepam and oxazepam that are metabolized by these processes do not have prolonged elimination half-lives. In contrast, xenobiotics such as diazepam and flurazepam, which are metabolized by hepatic oxidative enzymes, are eliminated more slowly with age.[47] Similar to many oxidized xenobiotics, metabolites of diazepam and flurazepam are active, undergo further metabolism, and remain in circulation after the parent xenobiotic has been metabolized. The active metabolites of some drugs, such as opioids, are renally eliminated, and excretion may be prolonged because of an age-related decline in renal function (see Table 32–4).

Other changes in enzyme systems may occur late in life. For example, a decline in gastric alcohol dehydrogenase level increases the bioavailability of ingested ethanol in the elderly.[93] The decline in this enzyme is attributed to the increased incidence of gastric atrophy with age (see below). Whether age-related changes occur in metabolic enzymes that are present in the intestines, brain, kidneys, and other organ systems and what impact such changes have on drug disposition and drug interactions are likely to become active areas of research. Studies to date have not demonstrated a substantial effect of age on P-glycoprotein, a transmembrane transport protein involved in xenobiotic interactions in the kidneys, intestines, and other organs.[7]

Age-related alterations in body composition may affect xenobiotic disposition in later life (see Table 32–2). For example, lean muscle mass and total body water decline, and the fat-to-lean ratio increases with advancing age.[68,89] Thus, highly lipid-soluble xenobiotics tend to have an increased volume of distribution. As a result, there may be a delay before steady state is reached, and peak effect and toxicity may occur later than expected. This mechanism may be an additional reason xenobiotics such as diazepam and flurazepam have prolonged half-lives in otherwise healthy elderly patients. In contrast, xenobiotics that distribute in water, such as ethanol, have a smaller Vd, leading to higher peak concentrations, accounting at least in part for the more pronounced peak effect of ethanol in the elderly. This may also account for the increased blood alcohol concentration attained in an older adult drinking an equivalent amount of alcohol as a younger person, as noted above.[109,113]

Protein reserve diminishes with age as a consequence of decreased muscle mass and decreased protein synthesis.[95] Although serum albumin concentration remains in the normal range in healthy elderly individuals,[14] people in this age group are more likely to experience a rapid decrease in albumin concentrations when experiencing acute or chronic illness or when their protein intake diminishes.[27,121] A decline in serum protein level increases the free or active fraction of xenobiotics that are otherwise highly protein bound. Free xenobiotic is able to travel more readily to the liver and kidney for metabolism or excretion, so a gradual change in the serum protein concentration is unlikely to lead to a change in the patient's response to the xenobiotic. However, these changes may be clinically important for interpreting serum concentrations of highly protein bound xenobiotics. Clinical laboratories typically measure total xenobiotic concentrations, which include both free and bound xenobiotic. Because most xenobiotic is bound, the reported value reflects mostly bound xenobiotic; therefore, the total xenobiotic concentration may be in the therapeutic range even though the active unbound fraction is actually elevated. Phenytoin, which is highly bound to albumin, serves as an illustrative example. If the serum concentration of phenytoin is reported as subtherapeutic, the physician might order a dose increase even though the free fraction of phenytoin actually is in the therapeutic range. With a dose increase, the free or active fraction may increase to toxic concentrations. Basic xenobiotics are not bound to albumin but to α-1-acid glycoprotein (AAG), an acute-phase reactant that tends to increase, rather than decrease, with age.[1] However, the increase attributed to age is most likely related to underlying disease. These unpredictable changes would be expected to have the reverse effect on the ratio of bound to unbound xenobiotic in any laboratory report. However, the correlation between clinical effect and free xenobiotic concentrations requires further study because there may be complex factors involved, for example, alterations in Vd, tissue-specific xenobiotic concentrations, and the contribution of other serum proteins to xenobiotic binding.

The precise contributions of gastric and intestinal tract mechanisms to toxicity have not been adequately determined. Changes in gastric absorption with age are not substantial enough to have an important clinical impact, and if anything, there is a modest decline, partly because of delayed gastric emptying, which could cause a delay in absorption of certain xenobiotics. However, age-associated changes in the gastric mucosa may account for enzymatic changes, as demonstrated in the case of alcohol dehydrogenase, noted above.

PHARMACODYNAMICS

Pharmacodynamic factors may also affect a patient's response to a particular xenobiotic. In general, age-related physiologic changes in target or nontarget organs lead to increased sensitivity to most xenobiotics, although sensitivity to some xenobiotics may also be decreased. For example, there is evidence that β-adrenergic receptor sensitivity declines with aging, leading to a diminished response to both β-adrenergic agonists and antagonists, although this is not necessarily demonstrated clinically.[26,40,114]

The observation of enhanced sensitivity to xenobiotics is probably due to altered pharmacokinetics in many, if not most, cases.[50] Proving that enhanced sensitivity is related to altered pharmacodynamics would require demonstrating that the concentration of drug at the tissue site was not increased as the result of diminished elimination. Regardless of the mechanism, it is important to recognize that the response to a given xenobiotic might be altered in specific ways among the elderly. These altered responses are probably caused less by chronologic aging and more by an increased prevalence of disease.[23,50] Table 32–3 provides examples of pathologic or physiologic changes that frequently occur in the elderly and disorders that are worsened or unmasked by xenobiotics.

ADVERSE DRUG EVENTS: RECOGNIZING RISK AND AVOIDING PITFALLS

A complicated xenobiotic regimen reduces adherence,[86] increases medication errors, and increases the risk of clinically important drug interactions. The likelihood of experiencing an ADE increases with the increasing number of xenobiotics taken.[55] Geriatric patients take more prescription and nonprescription xenobiotics than any other patient group.[62] ADEs may occur as a consequence of xenobiotic–xenobiotic interactions, but the exact relationship between the two phenomena is sometimes difficult to quantitate.[55]

Concurrent disease in target or nontarget organs may also alter the patient's sensitivity to a xenobiotic,[87] resulting in a serious ADE even when the patient is given a standard or previously used xenobiotic dose. Coexistent disease is often subclinical, and the patient's enhanced sensitivity may not be anticipated. A patient with subclinical Alzheimer's disease whose cognitive function is overtly normal may acutely develop delirium or symptoms of dementia when given standard doses of drugs such as sedative–hypnotics and CAs. Delirium is a medical emergency and an important cause of ED visits by the elderly.[57]

Another contributing factor to an ADE is physician lack of knowledge with regard to the principles of geriatric prescribing.[37,52,91] New xenobiotics are sometimes promoted as being safer than older ones, but problems often become apparent after marketing and use by large numbers of patients. For example, the hypnotic agent zolpidem was marketed as a safe alternative to benzodiazepines for the elderly. However, similar to benzodiazepines, zolpidem may also cause confusion, global amnesia, memory loss, and falls.[115,117] Low-molecular-weight heparins (LMWHs), such as enoxaparin and dalteparin, are other examples. LMWHs have more predictable pharmacokinetics than unfractionated heparin and are associated with a lower rate of overall bleeding. However, because therapeutic monitoring requires measurement of antifactor Xa activity, which is not as readily available as standard tests such as activated partial thromboplastin time (aPTT), they have not been recommended for routine use.[54] LMWHs such as enoxaparin and dalteparin are eliminated by the kidneys, and repeated doses lead to progressive increases in antifactor Xa activity when creatinine clearance is 30 mL/min or below,[21,76] a degree of renal insufficiency that is common in frail elderly patients. Less severe levels of renal impairment may also result in reduced enoxaparin clearance that might be avoided with lowered doses.[56] Most reported cases of serious, unexpected enoxaparin-induced bleeding, occur in elderly patients who are receiving "standard," not age-appropriate, dosing.[83,110,112]

In addition to dosing incautiously, clinicians often prescribe drugs considered inappropriate for the elderly at any dose,[30] drugs such as CAs, long-acting benzodiazepines, and anticholinergics.[22] In all of these cases, attention to geriatric risk factors might prevent ADEs.

Compounding the problem of lack of knowledge is the common practice of not adequately studying the effects of new xenobiotics in the elderly (see Chap. 138 for further details).[12,73] Reactions occurring in a small percentage of patients in a special subgroup can easily be missed during the initial drug evaluations. Even when a substantial number of subjects older than age 60 years are studied, a much smaller proportion of patients older than age 70 years may be included in clinical trials.[73] Thus, the adults at highest risk for many forms of xenobiotic toxicity are in a population that is often the least studied. Xenobiotic testing is typically carried out in subjects who are young adults and disease free, so pharmacokinetic profiles do not reflect patterns of xenobiotic disposition characteristic of geriatric patients. Pharmacokinetic testing may be limited to a one-time dose, and frequently the evaluation takes place over a short period of time. On average, approximately 5 half-lives of a xenobiotic are necessary to achieve steady-state xenobiotic concentrations. Thus, a xenobiotic with a half-life of 24 hours might not reach a steady state for 5 days, and in the presence of prolonged elimination associated with age-related factors, a steady state might not be reached for substantially longer. As a result, even if elderly subjects are included in a xenobiotic trial, the ultimate effect of that xenobiotic might not be appreciated during testing intervals designed for younger patients.

Morbidity and mortality in elderly patients as a result of specific xenobiotics might be avoided if the responsible xenobiotics were studied under the predictably high-risk conditions typically present in the elderly. For example, xenobiotics eliminated by the kidney need to be evaluated after repeated dosing in elderly subjects. Gatifloxacin was removed from the market only after several years of use when it was finally linked to both hypoglycemia and hyperglycemia in large numbers of elderly subjects.[49,92] Adverse events from xenobiotics that are studied in the elderly or others with chronic illness may be less obvious in the presence of comorbidity in the population at risk. The cyclooxygenase-2 (COX-2) inhibitor rofecoxib (Vioxx) was withdrawn from the market in 2004 after it was shown to increase the risk of myocardial infarction and stroke, especially in older adults.[34] Based on the complex actions of COX-1 and COX-2 in many tissues, the possibility existed that COX-2 inhibition might increase cardiovascular morbidity, for example, by leaving COX-1–mediated platelet aggregation unopposed while inhibiting prostacyclin-induced vasodilation or by leading to fluid retention and increased blood pressure via renal mechanisms.[53,94] Because elderly individuals typically have one or more chronic illnesses[23] as well as occult disease, extra vigilance is required when new xenobiotics are given, and clinicians and clinical investigators must be very mindful of the theoretical possibilities of adverse outcomes. In view of the vulnerability of older patients to many medications, the Food and Drug Administration (FDA) now requires that sponsors of new drug applications present effectiveness and safety data for important demographic subgroups, including the elderly, in their FDA submission data.[19] However, exceptions to the rule are allowed, for example, when studies have included insufficient numbers of subjects older than age 65 years to determine whether the elderly respond differently to the drug, the labeling must state this, but the statement is a poor substitute for providing actual efficacy and safety data.[25] Also, unfortunately, geriatric recommendations in the package insert may thus be insufficiently specific to provide guidance for drugs commonly used in this population.[103]

Xenobiotics, such as digoxin, warfarin, and diuretics, commonly prescribed in the elderly population are frequently involved in serious drug interactions. This situation is complicated by the frequency with which elderly patients who often have multisystem disease visit multiple physicians, who prescribe medications without specific knowledge of, or attention to, the remainder of the patient's xenobiotic regimen, thereby increasing the risk of inappropriate xenobiotic combinations.[46,107] Problems can also arise when patients obtain prescriptions from more than one pharmacy or mail order service.

Herbal preparations used by the elderly also may interact with prescription medications.[43,85] The use of herbal preparations has increased substantially in recent years, particularly among patients with illnesses such as cancer, dementia, and depression that commonly affect the elderly. Very few patients voluntarily report use of these or other nonprescribed therapies to their physicians, and too often the physician fails to inquire specifically about such "alternative" or "complementary" therapies. Poisonings, herb–drug interactions, and other problems related to herbal preparations are discussed further in Chap. 43.

The use of nonprescription pharmaceuticals may also cause serious adverse effects. For example, excessive use of magnesium-containing preparations frequently causes severe toxicity in older individuals. Impaired renal clearance, decreased GI motility, and other medical comorbidities are just three risk factors that potentiate magnesium toxicity in the elderly. The source of magnesium in these cases may include the cathartics that contain magnesium hydroxide (Milk of Magnesia) and magnesium citrate, antacid preparations, and magnesium sulfate (Epsom salts).[44] Magnesium-containing laxatives are still sometimes used in hospital settings with serious outcomes.[90] Likewise, oral sodium phosphate formulations, frequently used to cleanse the large intestine before endoscopy, may harm renal function in certain elderly patients despite normal baseline creatinine.[64] Virtually all of the most popular nonprescription medications [62] are more likely to produce problems in the elderly than in younger patients, including GI bleeding (aspirin and other NSAIDs), enhanced warfarin sensitivity (cimetidine), confusion and urinary retention (anticholinergic antihistamines), and cardiovascular symptoms (pseudoephedrine).

Outdated and discontinued xenobiotics are an additional problem for the elderly, who often retain unused or partially used products in their homes for decades or may continue to request prescription renewals when safer or more effective alternatives are available. Patients may be unwilling to change or physicians may continue to renew the prescription without sufficiently reevaluating the patient. Potential examples include digoxin and theophylline, which are still responsible for large numbers of adverse events diagnosed in EDs,[10] as well as diazepam, propoxyphene, and sedating antihistamines and other anticholinergics.

Other age-related factors may increase the risk of unintentional poisonings in geriatric patients; impaired vision, hearing, and memory may lead to misunderstanding or an inability to follow directions concerning the use of prescription and nonprescription drugs. Dementia is another important risk factor in unintentional poisonings. In addition to cognitive impairment, patients with dementia sometimes exhibit abnormal feeding behaviors, which may lead to ingestion of toxic substances.[118]

MANAGEMENT

Management decisions must be made with the foregoing principles in mind. GI decontamination should proceed as in younger patients. Because constipation is a more frequent problem in the elderly, when multiple-dose activated charcoal is used, particular attention must be paid to GI function and motility. The specific precautions and contraindications in the basic management and GI decontamination detailed in Chapter 7 are particularly pertinent for the geriatric population.

The presence of clinical or subclinical heart failure or renal failure may increase the risk of fluid overload when sodium bicarbonate is used. In the elderly, hemodialysis or hemoperfusion may be indicated earlier in cases of aspirin, lithium, or theophylline poisoning, in which elimination may be hampered by a decreased creatinine clearance or reduced endogenous clearance.

A problem that may go unrecognized in geriatric patients is the development of alcohol or xenobiotic withdrawal symptoms. Because elderly patients are typically not perceived as xenobiotic users, a physician evaluating an unfamiliar patient may not be aware of the patient's chronic use of prescribed benzodiazepines or opioids and consequently might fail to consider the possibility of substance withdrawal when unanticipated complications occur during hospitalization.

Strategies to limit unintentional toxic exposures in elderly patients with cognitive or sensory impairment should be similar to those used in young children, who are also at high risk of ingesting toxic substances or pharmaceuticals prescribed for others in the household. The strategies should include the removal of potentially dangerous substances and unnecessary xenobiotics from the patient's environment. The physician should request that the patient or caregiver bring all medications to the office in the original bottles and then make an effort to limit the number of medications prescribed or to seek alternative medications with a safer therapeutic index or appropriate geriatric safety profile. Administration and control of the medications by directly observed therapy may, of necessity, become the responsibility of the caregiver rather than the patient.

ADMISSION CRITERIA

When geriatric patients are evaluated in the ED for poisonings or serious ADEs, the need for hospital admission should be guided by concerns about the patient's frailty weighed carefully against the known hazards of hospitalization for the elderly.[28] The physician should be particularly alert to certain situations that might mandate admission, including elder abuse or neglect, unexplained mental status changes, inadequate home care manifested by unexplained falls, and overdose of xenobiotics with prolonged durations of action.

When there is concern that the established caregivers at home may be abusing or neglecting the patient, the patient requires further observation, removal from the environment, and possibly hospitalization. Signs of actual physical abuse may be more obvious than signs of neglect.[69] Vulnerable elderly who are physically disabled or cognitively impaired may be brought to the hospital because of presumed illness, but the source of the problem may actually be the caregiver. The caregiver, frequently a family member, may be depleting the patient's funds for personal use. Patients may become ill because funds were diverted from the purchase of food or because the patient's prescription drugs were sold on the street. More direct abuse may take the form of intentional poisoning of the patient by overdose of the patient's own prescription drugs. Provision for follow-up care, such as an alternative place to live and guardian appointment, is essential because abuse and neglect are associated with serious outcomes.[70]

Unresolved mental status changes may require close observation and hospitalization. Elderly patients who are confused or unable to walk are sometimes mistakenly assumed to be chronically impaired. However, incomplete explanation of an altered mental status or physical impairment should prompt careful inquiry into the patient's baseline functional status. Functional deterioration should never be assumed to be age related. Many very elderly patients are cognitively normal, physically robust, and independent in all activities of daily living.

Patients with overdoses with long-acting medications require careful monitoring. Because the durations of action of certain xenobiotics may be markedly prolonged among geriatric patients, a higher degree of vigilance is required. A classic example is associated with the use of the long-acting benzodiazepine flurazepam, mentioned above. Although this drug has been less often used in the United States in recent years, other long-acting benzodiazepines, such as flunitrazepam and nitrazepam, are still widely used in other countries.[36] The ultra-long-acting sulfonylurea chlorpropamide is rarely used today, but glyburide may cause relatively prolonged hypoglycemia compared with other hypoglycemics, as noted above.

SUMMARY

Older patients may account for only a small fraction of total poisoning victims, but when poisoned, they have a high mortality rate. More importantly, the elderly are much more likely to experience serious ADEs as a consequence of both appropriate and inappropriate use of medications. Attention to risk factors is essential in this vulnerable population. Important risk factors include pharmacokinetic and pharmacodynamic changes; the presence of overt or subclinical disease, including dementia; patient and provider error; suicide risk; complex therapeutic drug regimens; and a general lack of knowledge about the principles of prescribing for the geriatric population.

REFERENCES

1. Abernethy DR, Kerzner L: Age effects on alpha-1-acid glycoprotein concentration and imipramine plasma protein binding. *J Am Geriatr Soc.* 1984;32:705-708.
2. Abrams RC, Marzuk PM, Tardiff K, et al: Preference for fall from height as a method of suicide by elderly residents of New York City. *Am J Public Health.* 2005;95:1000-1002.
3. Banatvala N, Mayo K, Megraud F, et al: The cohort effect and *Helicobacter pylori. J Infect Dis.* 1993;168:219-221.
4. Bates DW, Cullen DJ, Laird N, et al: Incidence of adverse drug events and potential adverse drug events. Implications for prevention. ADE Prevention Study Group. *JAMA.* 1995;274(1):29-34.

5. Boyer EW, Shannon M: The serotonin syndrome. *N Engl J Med.* 2005;352:1112-1120.
6. Brenner SS, Herrlinger C, Dilger K, et al: Influence of age and cytochrome P450 2C9 genotype on the steady-state disposition of diclofenac and celecoxib. *Clin Pharmacokinet.* 2003;42:283-292.
7. Brenner SS, Klotz U: P-glycoprotein function in the elderly. *Eur J Clin Pharmacol.* 2004;60:97-102.
8. Brody GM: Hyperthermia and hypothermia in the elderly. *Clin Geriatr Med.* 1994;10:213-229.
9. Bronstein AC, Spyker DA, Cantilena LR, et al: 2006 Annual Report of the American Association of Poison Control Centers' National Poison Data System (NPDS). *Clin Toxicol.* 2007;45:815-917. Available at http://www.aapcc.org/archive/Annual%20Reports/06Report/2006%20Annual%20Report%20Final.pdf. Accessed June 9, 2008.
10. Budnitz DS, Pollock DA, Weidenbach KN, et al: National surveillance of emergency department visits for outpatient adverse drug events. *JAMA.* 2006;296:1858-1866.
11. Budnitz DS, Shehab N, Kegler SR, et al: Medication use leading to emergency department visits for adverse drug events in older adults. *Ann Intern Med.* 2007;147:755-765.
12. Bugeja G, Kumar A, Banerjee AK: Exclusion of elderly people from clinical research: a descriptive study of published reports. *Br Med J.* 1997;315:1059.
13. Burke LB, Jolson H. Goetsch R, et al: Geriatric drug use and adverse drug event reporting in 1990: a descriptive analysis of the two national data bases. *Annu Rev Gerontol Geriatr.* 1992;12:1-28.
14. Campion EW, deLabry LO, Glynn RJ: The effect of age on serum albumin in healthy males: report from the normative aging study. *J Gerontol.* 1988;43:M18-M20.
15. Carlsten A, Waern M, Allebeck P: Suicides by drug poisoning among the elderly in Sweden 1969–1996. *Soc Psychiatry Psychiatr Epidemiol.* 1999;34:609-614.
16. Carlsten A, Waern M, Holmgren P, et al: The role of benzodiazepines in elderly suicides. *Scand J Public Health.* 2003;31:224-228.
17. Caroff SN, Campbell EC, Sullivan KA: Neuroleptic malignant syndrome in elderly patients. *Expert Rev Neurother.* 2007;7:423-431.
18. Center for Drug Evaluation and Research: *Adverse Event Reporting System.* Available at http://www.fda.gov/Cder/aers/statistics/aers_patient_outcome.htm. Accessed June 14, 2008.
19. Center for Drug Evaluation and Research: *Guidance for Industry: Content and Format for Geriatric Labeling, October 2001.* Available at http://www.fda.gov/cder/guidance/3636fnl.PDF. Accessed June 6, 2008.
20. Centers for Disease Control and Prevention: *Web-Based Injury Statistics Query and Reporting System.* Available at http://www.cdc.gov/ncipc/wisqars/. Accessed June 29, 2008.
21. Chow SL, Zammit K, West K, et al: Correlation of antifactor Xa concentrations with renal function in patients on enoxaparin. *J Clin Pharmacol.* 2003;43:586-590.
22. Chutka DS, Takahashi PY, Hoel RW: Inappropriate medications for elderly patients. *Mayo Clin Proc.* 2004;79:122-139.
23. Cigolle CT, Langa KM, Kabeto MU, et al: Geriatric conditions and disability: the Health and Retirement Study. *Ann Intern Med.* 2007;147:156-64.
24. Cobaugh DJ, Krenzelok EP: Adverse drug reactions and therapeutic errors in older adults: a hazard factor analysis of poison center data. *Am J Health Syst Pharm.* 2006;63:2228-2234.
25. Code of Federal Regulations: 21 CFR 201.57(c)(9)(v)(B)(1).
26. Connolly MJ, Crowley JJ, Charan NB, et al: Impaired bronchodilator response to albuterol in healthy elderly men and women. *Chest.* 1995;108:401-406.
27. Covinsky KE, Covinsky MH, Palmer RM, et al: Serum albumin concentration and clinical assessments of nutritional status in hospitalized older people: different sides of different coins? *J Am Geriatr Soc.* 2002;50:631-637.
28. Creditor MC: Hazards of hospitalization of the elderly. *Ann Intern Med.* 1993;118:219-223.
29. Crouch BI, Caravati EM: Poisoning in older adults: a 5-year experience of US poison control centers. *Ann Pharmacother.* 2004;38:2005-2011.
30. Curtis LH, Ostbye T, Sendersky V, et al: Inappropriate prescribing for elderly Americans in a large outpatient population. *Arch Intern Med.* 2004;164:1621-1625.
31. Cusack BJ. Pharmacokinetics in older persons. *Am J Geriatr Psychother.* 2004;2:274-302.
32. Davies DF, Shock NW: Age changes in glomerular filtration rate: effective renal plasma flow and tubular excretory capacity in adult males. *J Clin Invest.* 1950;29:496-507.
33. Dooley CP, Cohen H, Fitzgibbons PL, et al: Prevalence of *Helicobacter pylori* infection and histologic gastritis in asymptomatic persons. *N Engl J Med.* 1989;321:1562-1566.
34. Drazen J: Cox-2 Inhibitors—a lesson in unexpected problems. *N Engl J Med.* 2005;352:1131-1132.
35. Drummer OH, Ranson DL: Sudden death and benzodiazepines. *Am J Forensic Med Pathol.* 1996;17:336-342.
36. Engeland A, Skurtveit S, Morland J: Risk of road traffic accidents associated with the prescription of drugs: a registry-based cohort study. *Ann Epidemiol.* 2007;17:597-602.
37. Ferry ME, Lamy PP, Becker LA: Physicians' lack of knowledge of prescribing for the elderly: a study in primary care physicians in Pennsylvania. *J Am Geriatr Soc.* 1985;33:616-625.
38. Fick DM, Cooper JW, Wade WE et al: Updating the Beers criteria for potentially inappropriate medication use in older adults: results of a US consensus panel of experts. *Arch Intern Med.* 2003;163:2716-2724.
39. Fink A, Hays RD, Moore AA, et al: Alcohol-related problems in older persons: determinants, consequences and screening. *Arch Intern Med.* 1996;156:1150-1156.
40. Fitzergald JD: Age-related effects of beta blockers and hypertension. *J Cardiovasc Pharmacol.* 1988;12(suppl):S83-S92.
41. Frierson RL: Suicide attempts by the old and the very old. *Arch Intern Med.* 1991;151:141-144.
42. Fu AZ, Liu GG, Christensen DB: Inappropriate medication use and health outcomes in the elderly. *J Am Geriatr Soc.* 2004;52:1934-1939.
43. Fugh-Berman A: Herb–drug interactions. *Lancet.* 2000;355:134-138.
44. Fung MC, Weintraub M, Bowel DL: Hypermagnesemia. Elderly over-the-counter drug users at risk. *Arch Fam Med.* 1995;4:718-723.
45. Gibbons RD, Hur K, Bhaumik DK, et al: The relationship between antidepressant medication use and rate of suicide. *Arch Gen Psychiatry.* 2005;62:165-72.
46. Green JL, Hawley JN, Rask KJ: Is the number of prescribing physicians an independent risk factor for adverse drug events in an elderly outpatient population? *Am J Geriatr Pharmacother.* 2007;5:31-39.
47. Greenblatt DJ, Divoll M, Harmatz JS, et al: Kinetics and clinical effects of flurazepam in young and elderly noninsomniacs. *Clin Pharmacol Ther.* 1981;30:475-486.
48. Gross C, Piper TM, Bucciarelli A, et al: Suicide tourism in Manhattan, New York City, 1990–2004. *J Urban Health.* 2007;84:755-765.
49. Gurwitz JH: Serious adverse drug effects—seeing the trees through the forest. *N Engl J Med.* 2006;354:1413-1415.
50. Gurwitz JH, Avorn J: The ambiguous relation between aging and adverse drug reactions. *Ann Intern Med.* 1991;114:956-966.
51. Gurwitz JH, Field TS, Harrold LR, et al: Incidence and preventability of adverse drug events among older persons in the ambulatory setting. *JAMA.* 2003;289(9):1107-1116.
52. Hastings S, Schmader KE, Sloane RJ, et al: Quality of pharmacotherapy and outcomes for older veterans discharged from the emergency department. *J Am Geriatr Soc.* 2008;56:875-880.
53. Hawkey CJ: COX-2 inhibitors. *Lancet.* 1999;353:307-314.
54. Hirsh J, Bauer KA, Donati MB, et al: Parenteral anticoagulants. *Chest.* 2008;133(6 suppl):141S-159S.
55. Hohl CM, Dankoff J, Colacone A, et al: Polypharmacy, adverse drug-related events, and potential adverse drug interactions in elderly patients presenting to an emergency department. *Ann Emerg Med.* 2001;38:666-671.
56. Hulot JS, Montalescot G, Lechat P, et al: Dosing strategy in patients with renal failure receiving enoxaparin for the treatment of non-ST-segment elevation in acute coronary syndrome. *Clin Pharmacol Ther.* 2005;77:542-552.
57. Hustey FM, Meldon SW: The prevalence and documentation of impaired mental status in elderly emergency department patients. *Ann Emerg Med.* 2002;39:248-253.
58. Ibrahim H, Mondress M, Tello A, et al: An Alternative formula to the Cockcroft-Gault and the modification of diet in renal diseases formulas in predicting GFR in individuals with type 1 diabetes. *J Am Soc Nephrol.* 2005;16:1051-1060.
59. Jarrett PG, Rockwood K, Carver D: Illness presentation in elderly patients. *Arch Intern Med.* 1995;155:1060-1064.

60. Jonsson A, Hallengren B, Rydberg T, et al: Effects and serum levels of glibenclamide and its active effects and serum levels of glibenclamide and its active metabolites in patients with type 2 diabetes. *Diabetes Obes Metab.* 2001;3:403-409.
61. Karch DL, Lubell KM, Friday J, et al: Surveillance for violent deaths—National Violent Death Reporting System, 16 states, 2005. *MMWR Surveill Summ.* 2008;57(3):1-45. Available at http://www.cdc.gov/MMWR/preview/mmwrhtml/ss5703a1.htm#tab14. Accessed June 16, 2008.
62. Kaufman DW, Kelly JP, Rosenberg L, et al: Recent patterns of medication use in the ambulatory adult population in the United States. The Slone Survey. *JAMA.* 2002;287:337-344.
63. Kausch O: Cocaine abuse in the elderly: a series of three case reports. *J Nerv Ment Dis.* 2002;190:562-565.
64. Khurana A, McLean L, Atkinson S, et al: The effect of oral sodium phosphate drug products on renal function in adults undergloing bowel endoscopy. *Arch Intern Med.* 2008;168:593-597.
65. Kinirons MT, Crome P: Clinical pharmacokinetics considerations in the elderly. An update. *Clin Pharmacokinet.* 1997;33:302-312.
66. Kirk SFL, Hawke T, Sanford S, et al: Are the measures used to calculate BMI accurate and valid for the use in older people? *J Human Nutr Dietetics.* 2003;16:365-370.
67. Kruse W: Problems and pitfalls in the use of benzodiazepines in the elderly. *Drug Saf.* 1990;5:328-344.
68. Kyle UG, Genton L, Hans D, et al: Total body mass, fat mass, fat-free mass, and skeletal muscle in older people: cross-sectional differences in 60 year-old persons. *J Am Geriatr Soc.* 2001;49:1633-1640.
69. Lachs M, Pillemer K: Abuse and neglect of elderly persons. *N Engl J Med.* 1995;332:437-443.
70. Lachs MS, Williams CS, O'Brien S, et al: The mortality of elder mistreatment. *JAMA.* 1998;280:428-432.
71. Lamb EJ, Webb MC, Simpson DE, et al: Estimation of glomerular filtration rate in older patients with chronic renal insufficiency: is the modification of diet in renal disease formula an improvement? *J Am Geriatr Soc.* 2003;51:1012-1017.
72. Lau DT, Kasper JD, Potter DE, et al: Hospitalization and death associated with potentially inappropriate medication prescriptions among elderly nursing home residents. *Arch Intern Med.* 2005;165:68-74.
73. Lee PY, Alexander KP, Hammill BG, et al: Representation of elderly persons and women in published randomized trials of acute coronary syndromes. *JAMA.* 2001;286:708-713.
74. Lesar TS, Briceland L, Stein DS: Factors related to errors in medication prescribing. *JAMA.* 1997;277:312-317.
75. Lewis LM, Miller DK, Morley JE, et al: Unrecognized delirium in ED geriatric patients. *Am J Emerg Med.* 1995;13:142-145.
76. Lim W, Dentali F, Eikelboom JW, et al: Meta-analysis: Low-molecular-weight heparin and bleeding in patients with severe renal insufficiency. *Ann Intern Med.* 2006;144:673-684.
77. Lindeman R, Tobin J, Shock NW: Longitudinal studies on the rate of decline in renal function with age. *J Am Geriatr Soc.* 1985;33:278-285.
78. Martello S, Oliva A, De Giorgio F, et al: Acute flurazepam intoxication: a case report. *Am J Forensic Med Pathol.* 2006;27:55-57.
79. Matin N, Kurani A, Kennedy CA: Dextromethorphan-induced near-fatal suicide attempt in a slow metabolizer at cytochrome P450 2D6. *Am J Geriatr Pharmacother.* 2007;5:162-165.
80. McCaig LF, Nawar EW: National Hospital Ambulatory Medical Care Survey: 2004 Emergency Department Summary. *Adv Data.* 2006;Jun 23(372):1-29 Available at: http://www.cdc.gov/nchs/data/ad/ad372.pdf. Accessed May 31, 2008.
81. McIntyre IM, Syrjanen ML, Lawrence KL, et al: A fatality due to flurazepam. *J Forensic Sci.* 1994;39:1571-1574.
82. Meehan PJ, Saltzman LE, Sattini RW: Suicides among older United States residents: epidemiologic characteristics and trends. *Am J Public Health.* 1991;81:1198-1200.
83. Melde SL: Enoxaparin-induced retroperitoneal hematoma. *Ann Pharmacother.* 2003;37:822-824.
84. Meneilly GS, Cheung E, Tuokko H: Counterregulatory hormone responses to hypoglycemia in the elderly patient with diabetes. *Diabetes.* 1994;43:403-410.
85. Miller LG. Herbal medicinals. Selected clinical considerations focusing on known or potential drug–herb interactions. *Arch Intern Med.* 1998;158:2200-2211.
86. Monane M, Bohn RL, Gurwitz JH, et al: The effects of initial drug choice and comorbidity on antihypertensive therapy compliance: results from a population-based study in the elderly. *Am J Hypertens.* 1997;10 (7 Pt 1): 697-704.
87. Moore AR, O'Keeffe ST: Drug-induced cognitive impairment in the elderly. *Drugs Aging.* 1999;15:15-28.
88. National Kidney Foundation: K/DOQI clinical practice guidelines for chronic kidney disease: evaluation, classification and stratification. Kidney Disease Outcome Quality Initiative. *Am J Kidney Dis.* 2002;39(suppl 1):S1-S266.
89. Novak LP: Aging, total body potassium, fat-free mass, and cell mass in males and females between ages 18 and 85 years. *J Gerontol.* 1972;27:428-443.
90. Onishi S, Yoshino S: Cathartic-induced fatal hypermagnesemia in the elderly. *Intern Med.* 2006;45:207-210.
91. Papaioannou A, Clarke JA, Campbell G, et al: Assessment of adherence to renal dosing guidelines in long-term care facilities. *J Am Geriatr Soc.* 2000;48:1470-1473.
92. Park-Wyllie LY, Juurlink DN, Kopp A, et al: Outpatient gatifloxacin therapy and dysglycemia in older adults. *N Engl J Med.* 2006;354:1352-1361.
93. Pozzato G, Moretti M, Franzin F, et al: Ethanol metabolism and aging: the role of "first pass metabolism" and gastric alcohol dehydrogenase activity. *J Gerontol.* 1995;50:B135-B141.
94. Psaty BM, Furberg CD: COX-2 inhibitors—lessons in drug safety. *N Engl J Med.* 2005;352:1133-1135.
95. Rattan SI, Derventzi A, Clark BFC: Protein synthesis, posttranslational modifications, and aging. *Ann N Y Acad Sci.* 1992;663:48-62.
96. Reid MC, Tinetti ME, Brown CJ, et al: Physician awareness of alcohol use disorders among older patients. *J Gen Intern Med.* 1998;13:729-734.
97. Rogers JJ, Heard K: Does age matter? Comparing case fatality rates for selected poisonings reported to U.S. poison centers. *Clin Toxicol.* 2007;45:705-708.
98. Rowe J, Andres R, Tobin J, et al: The effect of age on creatinine clearance in men: a cross-sectional and longitudinal study. *J Gerontol.* 1976;31:155-163.
99. Shoker A, Hossain MA, Koru-Sengul T, Raju DL, Cockcroft D: Performance of creatinine clearance equations on the original Cockcroft-Gault population. *Clin Nephrol.* 2006;66(2):89-97.
100. Shorr RI, Ray WA, Daugherty JR, et al: Individual sulfonylureas and serious hypoglycemia in older people. *J Am Geriatr Soc.* 1996;44:751-755.
101. Sorkin JD, Muller DC, Andres R: Longitudinal change in height of men and women: implications for interpretation of the body mass index. *Am J Epidemiol.* 1999;150:969-976.
102. Spicer RS, Miller TR: Suicide acts in 8 states: incidence and case fatality rates by demographics and method. *Am J Public Health.* 2000;90:1885-1891.
103. Steinmetz KL, Coley KC, Pollock BG: Assessment of geriatric information on the drug label for commonly prescribed drugs in older people. *J Am Geriatr Soc.* 2005;53:891-894.
104. Svenson J: Obtundation in the elderly patient. *Am J Emerg Med.* 1987;5:524-527.
105. Szoke E, Gosmanov NR, Sinkin JC et al: Effects of glimepiride and glyburide on glucose counterregulation and recovery from hypoglycemia. *Metabolism.* 2006;55:78-83.
106. Tadros G, Salib E: Age and methods of fatal self harm (FSH). Is there a link? *Int J Geriatr Psychiatry.* 2000;15:848-852.
107. Tamblyn RM, McLeod PJ, Abramowitz M, Laprise R: Do too many cooks spoil the broth? Multiple physician involvement in medical management of elderly patients and potentially inappropriate drug combinations. *CMAJ.* 1996;154:1177-1184.
108. Tinetti ME: Preventing falls in older persons. *N Engl J Med.* 2003;348:42-49.
109. Tupler LA, Hege S, Ellinwood EH: Alcohol pharmacodynamics in young-elderly adults contrasted with you and middle-aged subjects. *Psychopharmacology (Berlin).* 1995;118:460-470.
110. Vadnerkar A, Brensilver JM: Enoxaparin-associated spontaneous retroperitoneal hematoma in elderly patients with impaired creatinine clearance: a report of two cases. *J Am Geriatr Soc.* 2004;52:477-479.
111. Van Den Noortgate NJ, Janssens WH, Delanghe JR, et al: Serum cystatin C concentration compared with other markers of glomerular filtration rate in the old old. *J Am Geriatr Soc.* 2002;50:1278-1282.
112. Vaya A, Mira Y, Aznar J, et al: Enoxaparin-related fatal spontaneous retroperitoneal hematoma in the elderly. *Thromb Res.* 2003;110:69-71.

113. Vestal RE, McGuire EA, Tobin JD, et al: Aging and ethanol metabolism. *Clin Pharm Ther.* 1977;21:343-354.
114. Vestal RE, Wood AJJ, Shand DG: Reduced beta-adrenoceptor sensitivity in the elderly. *Clin Pharmacol Ther.* 1979;26:181-186.
115. Wagner AK, Zhang F, Soumerai SB, et al: Benzodiazepine use and hip fractures in the elderly. Who is at greatest risk? *Arch Intern Med.* 2004;164:1567-1572.
116. Wallis WE, Donaldson I, Scott RS, et al: Hypoglycemia masquerading as cerebrovascular disease (hypoglycemic hemiplegia). *Ann Neurol.* 1985;18:510-512.
117. Wang PS, Bohn RL, Glynn RJ: Zolpidem use and hip fractures in older people. *J Am Geriatr Soc.* 2001;49:1685-1690.
118. Welker JA, Zaloga GP: Pine oil ingestion. A common cause of poisoning. *Chest.* 1999;116:1822-1826.
119. Wolfe MM, Lichtenstein DR, Singh G: Gastrointestinal toxicity of nonsteroidal anti-inflammatory agents. *N Engl J Med.* 1999;340:1888-1899.
120. Woodhouse KW, Wynne HA: Age-related changes in liver size and hepatic blood flow: the influence on drug metabolism in the elderly. *Clin Pharmacokinet.* 1988;15:287-294.
121. Young VR: Amino acids and proteins in relation to the nutrition of elderly people. *Age Ageing.* 1990;19:S10-S24.
122. Zautcke JL, Coker SB, Morris RW, et al: Geriatric trauma in the state of Illinois: Substance use and injury patterns. *Am J Emerg Med.* 2002;20:14-17.

CHAPTER 33

POSTMORTEM TOXICOLOGY

Rama B. Rao and Mark A. Flomenbaum

Postmortem toxicology is the study of the presence, distribution, and quantification of a xenobiotic after death. This information is used to account for physiologic effects of a xenobiotic at the time of death through its quantification and distribution in the body at the time of autopsy. Several variables may cause changes in xenobiotic concentrations during the interval between the time of death and subsequent autopsy and the storage interval between the time of sampling and the time of testing. Toxicologists and forensic pathologists are frequently asked to interpret postmortem xenobiotic concentrations and decide whether the reported values are meaningful and, if so, whether these substances were incidental or contributory to the cause of death.

The development of the field of forensic toxicology and the improvement of laboratory technology now permit more refined identification and quantification of xenobiotics. The interpretation of postmortem xenobiotic concentrations and their significance, however, continues to evolve.

This chapter reviews factors that affect xenobiotic concentrations identified at autopsy and discusses an approach for interpreting postmortem toxicologic reports as they relate to the cause and manner of death.[37,40,42,48,49,50,58,68,78,96]

HISTORY AND ROLE OF MEDICAL EXAMINERS

The relationship between antemortem xenobiotic exposures and death has been a subject of investigation for centuries. In 12th-century England, an appointee of the royal court, eventually named the *coroner*, was designated to record and identify causes of death.[72] In suspicious circumstances, coroners investigated poisonings, but scientific methods were primitive, and conclusions regarding such deaths were conjecture at best.

By the mid-19th century however, techniques for detecting certain compounds in postmortem tissue were developed and focused generally on identifying heavy metals as a cause of death in homicides.[43,72,76,93,98] At that time, coroners were still elected or appointed individuals with little or no medical training. However, with better laboratory techniques and autopsies performed by trained pathologists, the specialty of forensic medicine continued to develop. In late 19th-century Massachusetts, trained pathologists, referred to as *medical examiners*, ultimately replaced the coroner system and were eventually empowered by the state to investigate deaths (medicolegal autopsies).[72] Currently in the United States, legal jurisdiction of death investigations is the responsibility of either a coroner or a medical examiner depending upon the state or county, with 19 states using medical examiner systems almost exclusively.[47]

The medicolegal autopsy is performed by a forensic pathologist who attempts to establish the cause and manner of death (Table 33–1). The *cause of death* is the physiologic agent or event necessary for death to occur. For example, the presence of cyanide in the toxicologic evaluation may be sufficient to establish cardiorespiratory arrest from cyanide poisoning. The *manner of death* is an explanation of how the death occurred and broadly distinguishes natural from nonnatural (or violent) deaths. Nonnatural deaths, depending on the jurisdiction, may be divided into several categories (Table 33–2). With the identification of cyanide, the manner of death cannot be considered natural because a poisoning is a "chemically traumatic" (violent) event. The medical examiner must make the best determination of the manner of death based on the available evidence.[98,105] An unintentional exposure may be classified as an *accident* (a legal term for some unintentional nonnatural deaths), and intentional self-exposure may be classified as a *suicide*. If the circumstances indicate an exposure due to the acts of another person, the manner of death is classified as a *homicide*.

Determination of the manner of death has important consequences. Homicide necessitates involvement of law enforcement officials for further investigation. Cases deemed suicide not only impact survivors psychologically but also may nullify life insurance payments. Conversely, a case deemed an "accident" may have a double-indemnity insurance clause. Assignment of financial responsibility for workplace disasters may be similarly affected when illicit drugs are identified in the postmortem specimens of involved workers.

Recognition of xenobiotic-related deaths also has significant public health consequences. The forensic pathologist may be the first to identify and report critical information regarding fatal drug reactions, medication errors, or rapidly fatal epidemics associated with illicit drug use or malicious intent activities. In cases of occupational and environmental xenobiotic-related fatalities, interventions can be implemented to prevent subsequent morbidity and mortality. In addition, the pathologist describes gross and microscopic autopsy findings that may elucidate mechanisms of xenobiotic toxicity.

Postmortem toxicologic techniques may be used in other types of investigations as well. For example, when carboxyhemoglobin is identified in the burned human remains from an airplane crash, a cabin fire before descent is more probable than a fire on impact. This type of postmortem analysis is useful in the reconstruction of events leading to the crash.[8,54,63,97]

THE TOXICOLOGIC INVESTIGATION

Ordinarily, toxicologic samples are collected as part of a complete autopsy. In the hospital, when a death is assumed to be from natural causes, the hospital pathologist may perform an autopsy with the consent of the family. In a medicolegal investigation, however, the forensic pathologist determines the need for a complete or partial autopsy and has statutory authority to act on that determination independent of familial consent. Occasionally, only fluid samples may need to be obtained along with an external inspection of the body if a complete autopsy is either unnecessary or the family has legal or religious grounds for objection. The precise list of xenobiotics screened in postmortem samples varies greatly by jurisdiction. Large cities may routinely screen for hundreds of illicit, therapeutic, and environmental xenobiotics. Occasionally, the suspicions of the medical examiner or death scene investigator warrant special assays that are performed only upon request.

The sampling of fluid and tissue may be obtained minutes to years after death. The *postmortem interval*, defined by the degree of bodily decomposition, varies depending on environmental conditions such as ambient temperature, humidity, and immersion under water.[64] Samples may be collected from a body during advanced stages of decomposition, after exhumation from graves, or even after embalming.[8,36,37,44,61,77] Knowing the condition of the body at the time of sampling assists in interpreting the toxicologic findings. These postmortem changes are reviewed below.

TABLE 33–1. Information Used by Forensic Pathologists

Autopsy
Evidence from the crime scene
Laboratory investigations
Medical consultants
Available history
Medical records
Police reports
Interviews with contacts

DECOMPOSITION AND POSTMORTEM BIOCHEMICAL CHANGES

The first stage of decomposition is autolysis during which endogenous enzymes are released and normal mechanisms maintaining cellular integrity fail.[57] Chemicals move across leaky cellular membranes down relative concentration gradients. Glycolysis continues in the red blood cells until intracellular glucose is depleted, and then lactate is produced. Ultimately, intracellular ions and proteins are released into the blood, and tissue and blood acidemia develops (Table 33–3).[98]

The next stage of decomposition is putrefaction. This stage involves digestion of tissue by bacterial organisms, which typically colonize the bowel or respiratory system. Later, other organisms may be introduced by insects or other external sources. As the putrefactive process advances, the colors of the skin and organ change; epithelial blebs may form and separate from the underlying dermis; and gases may accumulate, forming foul odors and bloating.[98]

If death occurs in a very warm, dry climate, such as a desert or comparably arid environment, the body may desiccate so rapidly that putrefactive changes may not occur. This results in mummification and produces a lightweight cadaver with a tight, dry skin enveloping a prominent bony skeleton.[98]

If the environment is very cold and devoid of oxygen, such as at great depths under water, putrefaction will be slowed. Anoxic decomposition of fatty tissues occurs, forming a white, cheesy material known as adipocere.

Another phase of decomposition, anthropophagia, occurs in unprotected environments where insects or other animals feed on the remains.[98]

Because most postmortem changes are driven by chemical reactions, they are temperature dependent, with increased temperatures accelerating the process and cooler temperatures retarding it. In general, morgue refrigerators achieve low enough temperatures (40°F; 4°C) to prevent further gross decomposition and many associated postmortem changes.

Another process that alters natural decomposition is embalming, a process of chemically preserving tissues that may be performed in a variety of ways.[45,46] Typically, blood is drained through large vessel pumps, and an embalming fluid is injected intravascularly to perfuse and preserve the face or other tissues. Intracavitary spaces may be injected with the preserving substances, and solid organs may or may not be removed.

TABLE 33–2. Categories of Manner of Death

Natural
Nonnatural
Homicide
Suicide
Accident
Therapeutic complication[a]
Undetermined

[a] Not all jurisdictions recognize therapeutic complication as a manner of death.

TABLE 33–3. Postmortem Biochemical Changes Over the First 3 Days[a]

Increased	Decreased	Stable	Variable
Amino acids	Cl^-	BUN/Cr (vitreous)	Lipids
Ammonia	Glucose	Cholinesterases	T_3
Ca^{2+}	Na^+	Cortisol (serum)	
Epinephrine	pH	Proteins (serum)	
Hepatic enzymes	T_4	Sulfates	
Insulin (especially right heart blood)			
K^+			
Mg^{2+}			

[a] In refrigerated bodies.

BUN, blood urea nitrogen; Cr, creatinine; T_3, triiodothyronine; T_4, thyroxine.

SAMPLES USED FOR TOXICOLOGIC ANALYSIS

Unless the medical examiner is suspicious about a death, only standard autopsy samples will be available in an otherwise intact body.[23,37,52,59,81,96] These typically include samples of blood, gastric contents, bile, urine, and occasionally solid organs such as the liver or brain. Less commonly, vitreous humor is obtained for analysis (Table 33–4). If the decedent was hospitalized before death, antemortem specimens may also be available for evaluation and comparison. These specimen analyses are reviewed in greater detail below.

BLOOD

Postmortem cell lysis prevents the reporting of plasma concentrations, and "blood" concentrations are reported instead. Intravascular blood

TABLE 33–4. Sampling Sites[16,20,24,36,50,91]

Routine	Infrequent	Uncommon
Bile	Antemortem blood	Extravasated blood
Blood	CSF	Extravasated fluid
Brain	Fat	Casket fluid
Liver	Hair	Insect larvae
Gastric contents	Kidneys	Pupae casings
Vitreous humor	Muscle	
	Nails	
	Skin	

CSF, cerebrospinal fluid.

from the subclavian or femoral vessels is a common source for toxicologic examination. In patients with a prolonged postmortem interval and in cases where intravascular blood is coagulated, right heart blood may serve as a sample site. Just one site is usually sampled unless an unusual xenobiotic with nonuniform distribution is suspected of causing the death. Ideally, femoral blood is obtained.

Other sources of blood may sometimes be available to the forensic pathologist. These frequently include antemortem samples and occasionally extravasated blood, which is unlikely to undergo extensive metabolism. Intracranial clots, in particular, serve as useful comparative samples in patients with a prolonged survival period after exposure to a xenobiotic.[65]

In advanced states of decomposition, blood from the abdominal or thoracic cavities is less useful because it may be contaminated by bacteria or other substances that may affect xenobiotic recovery or analysis.

VITREOUS HUMOR

Because of the relatively avascular and acellular nature of the fluid, the vitreous humor is well protected from the early decompositional changes that typically occur in blood.[16,18,19,20,24] When bodies are immediately refrigerated, creatinine, blood urea nitrogen, and sodium can be reliably approximated from vitreous humor samples for up to 3 or 4 days. Potassium concentrations are less reliable as cell lysis causes intracellular release. When vitreous glucose is elevated, hyperglycemia at the time of death can be assumed. A low vitreous glucose level, however, is inconclusive with regard to the antemortem serum glucose concentration. A low vitreous glucose level may be attributable to either antemortem hypoglycemia or postmortem glycolysis (even in the relatively avascular vitreous).

The aqueous content of the vitreous is normally higher than that of blood and may affect the partitioning of certain water-soluble xenobiotics.

URINE

Urine may be available during the autopsy and may reveal renally eliminated substances or their metabolites. Because the bladder serves as a reservoir in which metabolism is unlikely to occur, the concentrations of xenobiotics obtained during the autopsy reflect antemortem urine concentrations. An isolated urine sample is of limited quantitative value but may be useful when compared with other sample sites.

GASTRIC CONTENTS

The gross contents of the stomach are inspected for color; odor; and the presence or absence of pill fragments, food particles, activated charcoal, and other foreign materials.[96] Typically, gastric concentrations of xenobiotics are reported as milligrams of substance per gram of total gastric contents. Xenobiotic-induced pylorospasm, diminished intestinal motility, or decreased splanchnic blood flow may all decrease gastric emptying and affect the quantitive values obtained from sampling different parts of the gastrointestinal tract.

SOLID ORGANS AND OTHER SOURCES

Xenobiotic concentrations in solid organs, such as the liver and brain, are usually reported as milligrams of substance per kilogram of tissue. Other tissue samples, including hair and nails, are used for thiol-avid agents such as metals. Rarely, tracheal aspirates of gases may be analyzed to confirm inhalational exposures. Pleural fluid analysis of postmortem xenobiotics typically yields qualitative results in decomposed bodies because redistribution of xenobiotics from the stomach and intestines may occur.[31,88]

OTHER SAMPLING SOURCES

In an embalmed body, either the organs or tissues that remain relatively unembalmed, such as deep leg muscle,[67] or the embalming fluid itself may be used for analysis. Some authorities regulate the contents of embalming fluid to specifically avoid confounding postmortem analysis. Most embalming fluid in the United States consists of formaldehyde, sodium borate, sodium nitrate, glycerin and water. When a body is disinterred, soil samples are usually obtained from above and below the coffin to permit identification of chemicals that may have leeched into or out from the body.[77]

On rare occasions, cremated remains, often referred to as *cremains*, are the only source of sampling available. Most metallic implants, such as pacemakers, are removed before cremation, and only dental remains, particulate matter, and occasionally calcified blood vessels are available for analysis.[4,104] In most cremations performed in the United States, the incineration process is followed by mechanical grinding to yield a fine particulate matter.[104] The ability to extract xenobiotics from such samples is markedly limited at best, and little published data are available on the subject. A new technique to identify heavy metals such as lead from cremains has been described but is not routinely used at present.[4,104]

ENTOMOTOXICOLOGY

In putrefied bodies or bodies that have undergone anthropophagy, fluids and even insect parts can be analyzed. Forensic entomologists can collect samples of these insects from the remains. After taking into account the stage of insect life, environmental conditions, and the season, the approximate time of death can be extrapolated. The species *Calliphoridae*, or the bluebottle fly, is attracted to unprotected remains by a very fine scent that develops in the cadaver within hours of death. The adult fly lays eggs on mucosal surfaces or in open wounds. After the eggs hatch, the larvae feed on the decomposing tissue. Larval samples can then be examined for the presence of xenobiotics. To achieve accurate analysis, these samples must be preserved immediately after collection because living larvae can continue to metabolize certain xenobiotics. In another phase of their life cycle, the larvae undergo pupation, secreting a substance that encloses them into pupal casings until they hatch as adults. These pupal casings are often found in the soil beneath the body. Some xenobiotics have been identified in the casings long after the adult fly has emerged[86] (Table 33–5). A variety of other anthropophagic insect species may also demonstrate the presence

TABLE 33–5. Xenobiotics Reported From Larvae and Pupae Casings

Benzoylecgonine
Cocaine
Heroin
Malathion
Mercury
Methamphetamine
Morphine
Nortriptyline
Oxazepam
Phenobarbital
Triazolam

of toxicological substances.[1,41,61,62] This process of analysis is termed *entomotoxicology*.

INTERPRETATION OF POSTMORTEM TOXICOLOGY RESULTS

After fluid and tissue samples have been collected and analyzed for the presence of xenobiotics, the process of interpreting these results begins. This complex task attempts to account for the clinical effects of a xenobiotic at the time of death by integrating medical history, autopsy and crime scene findings, and toxicologic reports. Multiple confounding variables may affect the sample concentrations of xenobiotics from the time of death to the time of testing after the autopsy. Variables include the nature, metabolism, and distribution of the xenobiotic; the state of health of the decedent; physical and environmental variables during the postmortem interval; the techniques of analysis; and other findings of the autopsy (Tables 33–6, 33–7).

VARIABLES RELATING TO THE XENOBIOTIC

Postmortem Redistribution The xenobiotic blood concentration may be higher during the autopsy than at the time of death if the agent undergoes significant postmortem redistribution.[53,80,103–110] Redistribution occurs most often with substances that have large volumes of distribution and when decomposition results in release of intracellular xenobiotic into the extracellular compartment.[84] For example, amitriptyline may be released from tissue stores into the blood as autolysis progresses, resulting in a higher blood concentration during the autopsy than at the time of death. If postmortem redistribution is not considered, xenobiotic concentrations obtained during the autopsy may be misinterpreted as being supratherapeutic or even toxic, and the cause of death may be inappropriately attributed to this agent.

Postmortem Metabolism Less commonly, xenobiotic concentration may decrease secondary to postmortem metabolism. For example, cocaine continues to be degraded after death by endogenous enzymes such as cholinesterases in the blood, which are stable in postmortem tissue and in vitro. Unless blood is collected immediately after death and placed in tubes containing enzyme inhibitors such as sodium fluoride, the concentration of cocaine will continue to decrease, and the analysis will not accurately reflect the concentration of the drug at the time of death.[58,70,97,101] All available information regarding postmortem redistribution or metabolism of a specific xenobiotic must be considered for the proper interpretation of the toxicologic results.

State of Absorption and Distribution Both in the living and deceased, the state of absorption, distribution, and other toxicokinetic principles affect the apparent concentration of a sampled xenobiotic. For a xenobiotic with minimal postmortem metabolism or redistribution, the phase of absorption is suggested by the relative quantity of the agent in different fluids and solid organs. For example, a high concentration of xenobiotic pill fragments in the gastric contents, with progressively lower concentrations in the liver, blood, vitreous, and brain, suggests an early phase of absorption at the time of death. When an agent is orally administered and the tissue concentration is highest in the liver, the relationship suggests a postabsorption phase but a predistribution concentration. A concentration found to be highest in the urine suggests that the xenobiotic was in an elimination phase at the time of death. Although this approach has limitations, it may be important for correlating the state of absorption and the expected clinical course of the xenobiotic. Unfortunately, multiple samples may not always be available at the time of autopsy or the interpretation of reports, and opportunities for subsequent sampling are often limited.

Xenobiotic Stability Xenobiotic stability refers to the ability of an agent to maintain its molecular integrity despite postmortem changes such as decomposition of the body, adverse storage conditions, or the lack of preservatives.[5,13,15,55,56,61,91,99,106,108,109] Postmortem xenobiotic stability was assessed in homogenized liver tissue infused with various concentrations of xenobiotics.[99] The samples were allowed to putrefy outdoors, and sequential sampling of xenobiotic concentrations was performed. The xenobiotics that decreased in concentration as putrefaction progressed were considered labile, but samples with a constant concentration were considered stable. The authors proposed that the chemical moieties of a xenobiotic determine its stability. For example, labile agents share the molecular configuration of an oxygen–nitrogen bond, thiono groups, or aminophenols. Conversely, chemical structures that enhance stability include single-bonded sulfur groups, carbon–oxygen and carbon–nitrogen bonds, and sulfur–oxygen and hydrogen–nitrogen bonds. Although not explicitly studied in otherwise intact but putrefying bodies, logically, a less stable xenobiotic may be recovered in a lower concentration than the actual concentration at the time of death. This must be considered when information regarding stability is available and the body of a decedent is in an advanced stage of decomposition.

TABLE 33–6. Considerations in Interpreting Postmortem Xenobiotic Concentrations

Xenobiotic Dependent	Decedent Dependent	Autopsy Dependent	Other
Pharmacokinetic considerations State of absorption or distribution at time of death Postmortem redistribution Postmortem metabolism Pharmacodynamic considerations Expected clinical effects Synergistic interactions Postmortem xenobiotic stability during Putrefaction Preservation	Comorbid conditions Tolerance Pharmacogenetic variability	Postmortem interval: State of preservation or decomposition Previously undiagnosed conditions Specimens sampled Sample sites Handling and preservation	Laboratory techniques Evidence at scene Previously published tissue concentrations

TABLE 33–7. Xenobiotic Stability and Laboratory Recovery[10,12,22,27,73,79,80,87]

Quantitative recovery affected by preservatives	
As, Pb, Hg, Cu, Ag	
Cyanide	
Carbon monoxide	
Ethchlorvynol	
Nortriptyline (converted to amitriptyline in fixatives)	
Chemical stability in formalin	
Stable	**Labile**
Succinylcholine	Desipramine
Phenobarbital	
Diazepam	
Phenytoin (30 days)	
Chemical stability in putrefying liver	
Stable	**Labile**
Acetaminophen	*o,p*-Aminophenols
Amitriptyline	Chlordiazepoxide
Barbiturates	Chlorpromazine
Chloroform	Clonazepam
Clemastine	Malathion
Dextropropoxyphene	Metronidazole
Diazepam	Nitrofurazone
Doxepin	Nitrazepam
Flurazepam	*p*-Nitrophenol
Glutethimide	Obidoxime
Hydrochlorothiazide	Perphenazine
Imipramine	Trifluoperazine
Lorazepam	
Methaqualone	
Morphine	
Nicotine	
Paraquat	
Pentachlorophenol	
Quinine	
Plant alkaloids	
Strychnine	

Xenobiotic Chemical Interactions An artifact may result from a chemical interaction with a xenobiotic added during the postmortem interval, such as embalming fluid.[38] In a study of xenobiotic-spiked blood and formalin in test tubes, amitriptyline was formed by the methylation of nortriptyline.[26,109] Identification of amitriptyline, which was not present at the time of death, could confuse the interpretation of toxicologic analyses.

Expected Clinical Effects of the Xenobiotic For a fatality to be attributed to a xenobiotic, the expected clinical course from the exposure should be consistent with the autopsy findings. For example, what are the implications of a person found dead[90] minutes after having been seen ingesting pills, if a large concentration of acetaminophen is identified in both the gastric contents and blood but not in other tissues of at autopsy? Although suicidal intent may be supported by this finding, the onset of death within minutes is inconsistent with a fatality due to an acetaminophen overdose. Thus, another cause of death must be sought. Interpretation of postmortem toxicology must also incorporate clinically relevant consequences of xenobiotic interactions. For example, the combined ingestion of phenobarbital and ethanol can cause fatal respiratory depression. Although neither may be fatal alone, their clinical synergy must be acknowledged during toxicological interpretation.

VARIABLES RELATED TO THE DECEDENT

Comorbid Conditions The clinical response to a xenobiotic may be affected by acquired and inherited physiologic conditions that are not always identified or identifiable on autopsy. A thorough medical history is important, and may assist in interpreting the clinical effects of a xenobiotic exposure. Similarly, certain clinical conditions may produce substances that interfere with postmortem laboratory assays. For example, an individual with a critical illness may produce digoxin-like immunoreactive substances (DLIS), which may cross-react with the postmortem digoxin assay.[6] Without knowledge of DLIS production, the results may confound toxicologic analysis.

Tolerance Tolerance is an acquired condition in which increasingly higher xenobiotic concentrations are required to produce a given clinical effect. It is an important consideration for deaths in the presence of opioids, ethanol, and sedative–hypnotic agents. For example, respiratory depression and death from methadone may be easily diagnosed in an opioid-naive individual with a history of methadone exposure and methadone-positive postmortem samples. However, the same methadone concentrations in a patient on chronic methadone maintenance therapy will not produce the same outcome. Unfortunately, no autopsy markers are available to indicate tolerance, and no biochemical or histologic markers are available during autopsy that may be used to predict clinically dangerous xenobiotic concentrations in tolerant individual.[27] Complex postmortem assays analyzing opioid receptors are not routinely used.[35] Postmortem assessment of tolerance ultimately depends on knowledge of the patient, pharmacokinetics of the agent, and the best judgment of the investigator.

Pharmacogenetics There is genetic variability in the expression of certain metabolic enzymes. For example, pharmacogenetic differences in metabolic enzymes, such as CYP2D6, predispose some individuals to fatal hypotension from an inability to metabolize debrisoquine. Such distinctions are not routinely identifiable on autopsy.[28]

VARIABLES RELATING TO THE AUTOPSY

State of Decomposition In decedents in advanced stages of decomposition, xenobiotics may diffuse from depot compartments such as the stomach or bladder into adjacent tissues and blood vessels or secondarily affecting their sample concentrations.[22,37,65,75–77,83–85]

During putrefaction, bacteria cause fermentation of endogenous carbohydrates, resulting in ethanol formation. In decedents without gross evidence of putrefaction, especially those in cool, dry environments, endogenous ethanol production is minimal.[17,21] With a longer postmortem interval or in an environment that is more conducive to ethanol production, the distinction between endogenous and exogenous sources of ethanol becomes more difficult. Sampling from multiple sites is often useful in making the distinction.[100] A comprehensive review of interpreting postmortem ethanol concentrations is available elsewhere.[65]

Handling of the Body or Samples Inappropriate handling of the body may result in artifacts.[90,92] In one reported case, methanol was detected in the vitreous humor of a decedent after embalming.[12] The methanol was subsequently traced to a spray cleanser that likely settled on the surface of open eyes during washing of the body.

In addition, inappropriate handling of samples may affect xenobiotic concentrations. In one study, autopsy blood was obtained from a diabetic man who died of bronchopneumonia. The samples were stored at 4°C and tested at 2 and 5 days postmortem. The blood ethanol increased from 0.4g/L to 3.5 g/L because of an inadequate addition of fluoride preservative to the samples. The combination of inadequate preservation, hyperglycemia (vitreous glucose of 996 mg/dL), and bacterial sepsis created an ideal environment for ethanol production.[65]

In the United States, preservatives containing metals are currently banned for use in embalming because they may contaminate subsequent evaluation for metal poisoning. Formalin may also affect stability or quantitative identification of some xenobiotics. When necessary, an analysis of embalming fluid used by the mortician or soil sampling around disinterred bodies may facilitate the toxicologic investigation.[19,33]

Autopsy Findings In many xenobiotic-related deaths, the anatomic findings are nonspecific.[107] In some cases, the autopsy reveals confirmatory or supportive findings. A large quantity of undigested pills in the stomach is consistent with an intentional overdose, and suicide should be considered. Centrilobular hepatic necrosis may be found in decedents with a history of acetaminophen overdose. The autopsy may also reveal other findings such as coronary artery narrowing, chronic hypertension, renal abnormalities, or a clinically silent myocardial injury. Such information may be useful to assess the potential effects of a xenobiotic in a patient with previously undiagnosed conditions. In other cases, the absence of a chronic condition may be strongly suggestive of a xenobiotic-related death. For example, a decedent with an autopsy finding of aortic dissection in the absence of chronic hypertensive findings or other predisposing conditions may suggest a xenobiotic-induced hypertensive crisis as may occur from use of cocaine or other sympathomimetics.

Artifacts Related to Sampling Sites Site-specific differences in postmortem xenobiotic blood concentrations are common.[34] For example, blood drawn from femoral vessels may have low glucose levels because of postmortem glycolysis, but the blood glucose concentration removed from the right heart chambers may be high as a result of perimortem release of liver glycogen stores. Hyperglycemic states are more reliably assessed from sampling the vitreous humor. An elevated vitreous glucose concentration suggests antemortem hyperglycemia. The individual interpreting the toxicologic report must know the exact site from which the sample was taken.[19,59]

Ideally, samples from more than one site would be available for comparison; unfortunately, multiple blood samples are not often routinely obtained. Comparison of concentrations from different sites may reveal important information regarding the state of xenobiotic absorption at the time of death and acute versus chronic exposure.[9–11,19,25,29,51,66,71,79,81,83,87–89,94,95,100,102]

Other Considerations Published therapeutic, toxic, and fatal postmortem xenobiotic concentrations are available to aid in the interpretation of postmortem specimens.[3,69] However, the conditions associated with reported concentrations do not necessarily permit comparisons with the concentrations of the particular case under investigation. Thus, these resources are valuable but should be used mainly as guidelines and not accepted as absolute values that define either toxic or therapeutic concentrations. Similarly, formulas available for assessing xenobiotic doses or concentrations in the living are not usually applicable when analyzing postmortem samples.

OTHER LIMITATIONS

Although there are generalized standards of practice in forensic investigations, specimen collection and laboratory methodology may vary.[2,3] Some xenobiotic concentrations may be falsely elevated or depressed depending on the chosen methodology.[31,71] Descriptions of specific toxicology laboratory techniques are beyond the scope of this chapter, but these variables must also be given consideration in the interpretations of results. Other limitations may include a lack of information relating to the circumstances of death and possible compromises in specimen handling because of the required protocols for the maintenance of proper chain of custody (often of paramount importance in forensic autopsies).[36,37]

SUMMARY

To accurately interpret postmortem toxicologic reports, it is essential to understand potential biochemical changes and other artifacts that affect postmortem testing. Unfortunately, because of the complexity and variety of all possible circumstances, no single resource can absolutely correlate postmortem xenobiotic blood and tissue concentrations to those at the actual time of death. Postmortem toxicology is an evolving discipline that may permit only the most likely truths associated with the xenobiotic identified and the circumstances in question.[14,32,73] Progress in this field will depend on the continued collaboration between the treating physicians, medical and forensic toxicologists, and forensic pathologists.

REFERENCES

1. Amendt J, Krettek R, Zehner R: Forensic entomology. *Naturwissenschaften.* 2004;91:51-56.
2. Andollo W: Quality assurance in postmortem toxicology. In: Karch SB, ed. *Drug Abuse Handbook.* Boca Raton, FL: CRC Press; 1998:953-969.
3. Baselt RC, ed: *Disposition of Toxic Drugs and Chemicals in Man,* 5th ed. Foster City, CA: Chemical Toxicology Institute; 2000.
4. Barry M: Metal residues after cremation. *Br Med J.* 1994;308:390.
5. Battah AH, Hadidi KA: Stability of trihexyphenidyl in stored blood and urine specimens. *Int J Legal Med.* 1998;111:111-114.
6. Bentur Y, Tsipiniuk A, Taitelman U: Postmortem digoxin-like immunoreactive substance (DLIS) in patients not treated with digoxin. *Hum Exp Toxicol.* 1999;18:67-70.
7. Berryman HE, Bass WM, Symes SA, Smith OC: Recognition of cemetery remains in the forensic setting. *J Forensic Sci.* 1991;36:230-237.
8. Blackmore DJ: Aircraft accident toxicology: UK experience 1967–1972. *Aerospace Med.* 1974;45:987-994.
9. Bonnichsen R, Gerrtinger P, Maehly AC: Toxicological data on phenothiazine drugs in autopsy cases. *J Legal Med.* 1970;67:158-169.
10. Briglia EJ, Bidanset JH, Dal Cortivo LA: The distribution of ethanol in postmortem blood specimens. *J Forensic Sci.* 1993;38:1019-1021.
11. Caplan YH, Levine B: Vitreous humor in the evaluation of postmortem blood ethanol concentrations. *J Anal Toxicol.* 1990;14:305-307.
12. Caughlin J: An unusual source for postmortem findings of methyl ethyl ketone and methanol in two homicide victims. *Forensic Sci Int.* 1994;67:27-31.
13. Chace DH, Goldbaum LR, Lappas NT: Factors affecting the loss of carbon monoxide from stored blood samples. *J Anal Toxicol.* 1986;10:181-189.
14. Chamberlain RT: Role of the clinical toxicologist in court. *Clin Chem.* 1996;42:1337-1341.
15. Chikasue F, Yashiki T, Kojima T: Cyanide distribution in five fatal cyanide poisonings and the effect of storage conditions on cyanide concentration in tissue. *Forensic Sci Int.* 1988;38:173-183.
16. Choo-Kang E, McKoy C, Escoffery C: Vitreous humor analytes in assessing the postmortem interval and the antemortem clinical status. *West Med J.* 1983;32:23-26.

17. Clark MA, Jones JW: Studies on putrefactive ethanol production. I: lack of spontaneous ethanol production in intact human bodies. *J Anal Toxicol.* 1982;27:366-371.
18. Coe JI: Comparative postmortem chemistries of vitreous humor before and after embalming. *J Forensic Sci.* 1976;21:583-586.
19. Coe JI: Postmortem chemistry of blood, cerebrospinal fluid, and vitreous humor. *Legal Med Ann.* 1977;76:55-92.
20. Coe JI: Use of chemical determinations on vitreous humor in forensic pathology. *J Forensic Sci.* 1972;17:541-546.
21. Coe JI, Sherman RE: Comparative study of postmortem vitreous humor and blood alcohol. *J Forensic Sci.* 1970;15:185-190.
22. Cook DS, Braithwaite RA, Hale KA: Estimating the antemortem drug concentrations from postmortem drug samples: the influence from postmortem redistribution. *J Clin Pathol.* 2000;53:282-285.
23. Craig PH: Standard procedures for sampling—a pathologist's prospective view. *Clin Toxicol.* 1979;15:597-603.
24. Daae LN, Teige B, Svaar H: Determination of glucose in human vitreous humor. *J Legal Med.* 1978;80:287-290.
25. Davis GL: Postmortem alcohol analyses of general aviation pilot fatalities, Armed Forces Institute of Pathology 1962–1967. *Aerospace Med.* 1973;44:80-83.
26. Dettling RJ, Briglia EJ, Dal Cortivo LA, Bidanset JH: The production of amitriptyline from nortriptyline in formaldehyde-containing solutions. *J Anal Toxicol.* 1990;14:325-326.
27. Devgun MS, Dunbar JA: Post-mortem estimation of gamma-glutamyl transferase in vitreous humor and its association with chronic abuse of alcohol and road-traffic deaths. *Forensic Sci Int.* 1985;28:179-180.
28. Druid H, Holmgren P: A compilation of fatal and control concentrations of drugs in postmortem femoral blood. *J Forensic Sci.* 1997;42:79-87.
29. Druid H, Holmgren P, Carlsson B, Ahlner J: Cytochrome P450 2D6 (CYP2D6) genotyping on postmortem blood as a supplementary tool for interpretation of forensic toxicological results. *Forensic Sci Int.* 1999;99:25-34.
30. Drummer OH: Postmortem toxicology of drugs of abuse. *Forensic Sci Int.* 2004;142:101-113.
31. Drummer OH, Gerostamoulos J: Postmortem drug analysis: analytical and toxicological aspects. *Ther Drug Monit.* 2002;24:199-209.
32. Ernst MF, Poklis A, Gantner GE: Evaluation of medicolegal investigators' suspicions and positive toxicology findings in 100 drug deaths. *J Anal Toxicol.* 1982;27:61-65.
33. Falconer B, Moller M: The determination of carbon monoxide in blood treated with formaldehyde. *J Legal Med.* 1971;68:17-19.
34. Felby S, Olsen J: Comparative studies of postmortem barbiturate and meprobamate in vitreous humor, blood and liver. *J Forensic Sci.* 1969;14:507-514.
35. Ferrer-Alcon M, La Harpe R, Garcia-Sevilla JA: Decreased immunodensities of μ opioid receptors, receptor kinases, GRK 2/6 and β-arrestin-2 in postmortem brains of opioid addicts. *Molec Brain Res.* 2004;121:114-122.
36. Flanagan RJ, Connally G. Interpretation of analytical toxicology results in life and at postmortem. *Toxicol Rev.* 2005;24:51-62.
37. Flanagan RJ, Connally G, Evans JM: Analytical toxicology: guidelines for sample collection postmortem. *Toxicol Rev.* 2005;24:63-71.
38. Fomey RB, Carroll FT, Nordgren IK, et al: Extraction, identification and quantitation of succinylcholine in embalmed tissue. *J Anal Toxicol.* 1982:6:115-119.
39. Forrest AR: Obtaining samples at post mortem examination for toxicological and biochemical analyses. *J Clin Pathol.* 1993;46:292-296.
40. Garriott JC: Interpretive toxicology. *Clin Lab Med.* 1983;3:367-384.
41. Goff ML, Lord WD: Entomotoxicology. A new area for forensic investigation. *Am J Forensic Med Pathol.* 1994;15:51-57.
42. Goldman P, Ingelfinger JA: Completeness of toxicological analyses. *JAMA.* 1980;243:2030-2031.
43. Goulding R: Poisoning as a fine art. *Med Legal J.* 1978;46:6-17.
44. Grellner W, Glenewinkel F: Exhumations: synopsis of morphologic findings in relation to the postmortem interval. Survey on a 20-year the literature. *Forensic Sci Int.* 1997;90:139-159.
45. Halmai J: Common thyme (*Thymus vulgaris*) as employed for the embalming. *Ther Hungarica.* 1972;20:162-165.
46. Hanzlick R: Embalming, body preparation, burial, and disinterment. *Pathology.* 1994;15:122-131.
47. Hanzlick R: Medical examiner and coroner systems: history and trends. *JAMA.* 1998;279:870-874
48. Hearn WL, Keran EE, Wei H, Hime G: Site dependent postmortem changes in blood cocaine concentrations. *J Forensic Sci.* 1991;36:673-684.
49. Hearn WL, Walls HC: Common methods in postmortem toxicology In: Karch SB, ed. *Drug Abuse Handbook.* Boca Raton, FL: CRC Press; 1998:890-926.
50. Hearn WL, Walls HC: Introduction to postmortem toxicology. In: Karch SB, ed. *Drug Abuse Handbook.* Boca Raton, FL: CRC Press; 1998:863-873.
51. Hearn WL, Walls HC: Strategies for postmortem toxicological investigation. In: Karch SB, ed. *Drug Abuse Handbook.* Boca Raton, FL: CRC Press; 1998:926-953.
52. Helper BR, Isenschmid DS: Specimen selection, collection, preservation, and security In: Karch SB, ed. *Drug Abuse Handbook.* Boca Raton, FL: CRC Press; 1998:873-889.
53. Hilberg T, Rogde S, Morland J: Postmortem drug redistribution—human cases related to results in experimental animals. *J Forensic Sci.* 1999;44:3-9.
54. Hill IR: Toxicological findings in fatal aircraft accidents in the United Kingdom. *Am J Forensic Med Pathol.* 1986;7:322-326.
55. Høiseth G, Karinen R, Johnsen L, Normann PT, Christophersen AS, Mørland J: Disappearance of ethyl glucuronide during heavy putrefaction. *Forensic Sci Int.* 2008;176:147-151.
56. Høiseth G, Kristoffersen L, Larssen B, Arnestad M, Hermansen NO, Mørland J: In vitro formation of ethanol in autopsy samples containing fluoride ions. *Int J Legal Med.* 2008;122:63-66.
57. Iwasa Y, Onaya T: Postmortem changes in the level of calcium pump triphosphatase in rat heart sarcoplasmic reticulum. *Forensic Sci Int.* 1988;39:13-22.
58. Jones GR: Interpretation of postmortem drug levels. In: Karch SB, ed. *Drug Abuse Handbook.* Boca Raton, FL: CRC Press; 1998:970-985.
59. Jones GR, Pounder DJ: Site dependence of drug concentrations in postmortem blood—a case study. *J Anal Toxicol.* 1987;11:186-190.
60. Karch SB: Introduction to the forensic pathology of cocaine. *Am J Forensic Med Pathol.* 1991;12:126-131.
61. Karger B, Lorin de la Grandmaison G, Bajanowski T, Brinkmann B: Analysis of 155 consecutive forensic exhumations with emphasis on undetected homicides. *Int J Legal Med.* 2004;118:90-94.
62. Kintz P, Tracqui A, Ludes B, et al: Fly larvae and their relevance in forensic toxicology. *Am J Forensic Med Pathol.* 1990;11:63-65.
63. Klette K, Levine B, Springate C, Smith ML: Toxicological findings in military aircraft fatalities from 1986–1990. *Forensic Sci Int.* 1992;53:143-148.
64. Krompecher T: Experimental evaluation of rigor mortis. v. effect of various temperatures on the evolution of rigor. *Forensic Sci Int.* 1981;17:19-26.
65. Kugelberg FC, Jones AW: Interpreting results of ethanol analysis in postmortem specimens: a review of the literature. *Forensic Sci Int.* 2007;165:10-29.
66. Kunsman GW, Rodriguez R, Rodriguez P: Fluvoxamine distribution in postmortem cases. *Am J Forensic Med Pathol.* 1999;20:78-83.
67. Langford AM, Taylor KK, Pounder DJ: Drug concentration in selected skeletal muscles. *J Forensic Sci.* 1998;43:22-27.
68. Levine BS, Smith ML, Froede RC: Postmortem forensic toxicology. *Clin Lab Med.* 1990;10:571-589.
69. Lewin JF, Pannell LK, Wilkinson LF: Computer storage of toxicology methods and postmortem drug determinations. *Forensic Sci Int.* 1983;23:225-232.
70. Logan BK, Smirnow D, Gullberg RG: Lack of predictable site-dependent differences and time-dependent changes in postmortem concentrations of cocaine, benzoylecgonine, and cocaethylene in humans. *J Anal Toxicol.* 1997;20:23-31.
71. Long C, Crifasi J, Maginn D, et al: Comparison of analytical methods in the determination of two venlafaxne fatalities. *J Anal Toxicol.* 1997;21:166-169.
72. Mellen PF, Bouvieer EC: Nineteenth-century Massachusetts coroner inquests. *Am J Forensic Med Pathol.* 1996;17:207-210.
73. Messite J, Stellman SD: Accuracy of death certificate completion. *JAMA.* 1996;275:794-796.
74. Moriya F. Hashimoto Y: Postmortem diffusion of drugs from the bladder into femoral blood. *Forensic Sci Int.* 2001;123;248-253.
75. Moriya F. Hashimoto Y: Redistribution of basic drugs into cardiac blood from surrounding tissues during early stages postmortem. *J Forensic Sci.* 1999;44:10-16.
76. Niyogi SK: Historic development of forensic toxicology in America up to 1978. *Am J Forensic Med Pathol.* 1980;1:249-264.
77. Oxley DW: Examination of the exhumed body and embalming artifacts. *Med Legal Bull.* 1984;33:1-7.

78. Peat MA: Advances in forensic toxicology. *Clin Lab Med.* 1998;18:263-278.
79. Peclet C, Picotte P, Iobin F: The use of vitreous humor levels of glucose, lactic acid and blood levels of acetone to establish antemortem hyperglycemia in diabetics. *Forensic Sci Int.* 1994:65:1-6.
80. Pelissier-Alicot AL, Gaulier JM, Champsaur P, Marquet P: Mechanisms underlying postmortem redistribution of drugs: a review. *J Anal Toxicol.* 2003;27:533-544.
81. Pla A, Hernandez AF, Gil F, et al: A fatal case of oral ingestion of methanol. Distribution in postmortem tissues and fluids including pericardial fluid and vitreous humor. *Forensic Sci Int.* 1991;49:193-196.
82. Polson CJ, Gee DJ, Knight B: *The Essentials of Forensic Medicine*, 4th ed. Oxford: Pergamon Press; 1985:3-39.
83. Pounder DJ, Carson DO, Johnston K, Orihara Y: Electrolyte concentration differences between left and right vitreous humor samples. *J Forensic Sci.* 1998;43:604-607.
84. Pounder DJ, Davies JI: Zopiclone poisoning: tissue distribution and potential for postmortem diffusion. *Forensic Sci Int.* 1994;65:177-183.
85. Pounder DJ, Fuke C, Cox DE, et al: Postmortem diffusion of drugs from gastric residue: an experimental study. *Am J Forensic Med Pathol.* 1996;17:1-7.
86. Pounder DJ: Forensic entomo-toxicology. *Forensic Sci Soc.* 1991;31:469-472.
87. Prouty RW, Anderson WH: A comparison of postmortem heart blood and femoral blood ethyl alcohol concentrations. *J Anal Toxicol.* 1987;11:191-197.
88. Prouty RW, Anderson WH: The forensic science implications of site and temporal influences on postmortem blood-drug concentrations. *J Forensic Sci.* 1990;35:243-270.
89. Ritz S, Harding P, Martz W: Measurement of digitalis-glycoside levels in ocular tissues. *Int J Legal Med.* 1992;105:155-159.
90. Rivers RL: Embalming artifacts. *J Forensic Sci.* 1978;23:531-535.
91. Robertson MD, Drummer OR: Stability of nitrobenzodiazepines in postmortem blood. *J Forensic Sci.* 1998;43:5-8.
92. Rohrig TP: Comparison of fentanyl concentrations in unembalmed and embalmed liver samples. *J Anal Toxicol.* 1998;22:253.
93. Rosenfeld L: Alfred Swaine Taylor (1806–1880), pioneer toxicologist—and a slight case of murder. *Clin Chem.* 1985;31:1235-1236.
94. Schonheyder RC, Renriques U: Postmortem blood cultures. Evaluation of separate sampling of blood from the right and left cardiac ventricle. *APMIS.* 1997;105:76-78.
95. Schoning P, Strafuss AC: Analysis of postmortem canine blood, cerebrospinal fluid, and vitreous humor. *Am J Vet Res.* 1981;42:1447-1449.
96. Skopp G: Preanalytic aspects in postmortem toxicology. *Forensic Sci Int.* 2004;142:75-100.
97. Smith PW, Lacefield DJ, Crane CR: Toxicological findings in aircraft accident investigation. *Aerospace Med.* 1970;41:760-762.
98. Spitz WU, ed: *Spitz's and Fischers Medicolegal Investigation of Death.* Springfield, IL: Charles C Thomas; 1993.
99. Stevens HM: The stability of some drugs and poisons in putrefying human liver tissues. *J Forensic Sci.* Soc 1984;24:577-589.
100. Stone BE, Rooney PA: A study using body fluids to determine blood alcohol. *J Anal Toxicol.* 1984;8:95-96.
101. Tardiff K, Gross E, Wu J, et al: Analysis of cocaine positive fatalities. *J Forensic Sci.* 1989;34:53-63.
102. Vermeulen T: Distribution of paroxetine in three postmortem cases. *J Anal Toxicol.* 1998;22:541-544.
103. Vorpahl TE, Coe JI: Correlation of antemortem and postmortem digoxin levels. *J Forensic Sci.* 1978;23:329-334.
104. Warren MW, Falsetti AB, Hamilton WF, Levine LJ: Evidence of arteriosclerosis in cremated remains. *Am J Forensic Med Pathol.* 1999;20:277-280.
105. Wetli CV: Investigation of drug-related deaths—an overview. *Am J Forensic Med Pathol.* 1984;5:111-120.
106. Winek CL, Esposito FM, Cinicola DP: The stability of several compounds in formalin fixed tissues and formalin-blood solutions. *Forensic Sci Int.* 1990;44:159-168.
107. Winek CL, Wahba WW: The role of trauma in postmortem blood alcohol determination. *Forensic Sci Int.* 1995;74:213-214.
108. Winek CL, Wahba WW, Rozin L, Winek CL Jr: Determination of ethchlorvinyl in body tissues and fluids after embalmment. *Forensic Sci Int.* 1988;37:161-166.
109. Winek CL, Zaveri NR, Wahba WW: The study of tricyclic antidepressants in formalin fixed human liver and formalin solutions. *Forensic Sci Int.* 1993;61:175-183.
110. Worm K, Dragsholt C, Simonsen K, Kringsholm B: Citalopram concentrations in samples from autopsies and living persons. *Int J Legal Med.* 1998;111:188-190.

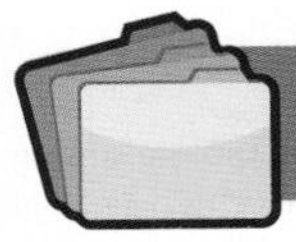

SPECIAL CONSIDERATIONS (SC1)

ORGAN PROCUREMENT FROM POISONED PATIENTS

Rama B. Rao

Xenobiotics can cause brain death due to the unique vulnerabilities of the central nervous system. With supportive care however, such patients may be suitable candidates for organ donation.[7,8,11,27,33] Early identification of donors is critical as the viability of transplantable tissue diminishes as duration of brain death progresses.[24,33] Timely identification may be further complicated by the presence of xenobiotics that mimic brain death.[3,8,31]

A variety of protocols to establish brain death are reviewed elsewhere.[3,8,31] Once brain death is established, organ procurement personnel assist in: obtaining familial consent, deciding which organs are most suitable for transplant, and maximizing physiological support and perfusion until organ procurement occurs.[33]

Successful transplantation of organs is reported from poisoned donors associated with a multitude of xenobiotics[1,2,4,6-8,10,14,23,25-30] (Tables SC1-1, SC1-2). Although some xenobiotics are highly toxic, such as cyanide and carbon monoxide (CO), transfer of clinical poisoning to the organ recipient is not reported. This is likely caused by several factors including xenobiotic metabolism, tissue redistribution or binding prior to procurement, as well as the means of handling organs during the transplantation process. For example, some xenobiotic clearance may occur in the myocardium during organ rinsing and cardiopulmonary bypass.[25] Furthermore, individual organs may not uniformly manifest toxicity in response to xenobiotic insults. For example, the heart of a CO poisoned donor was examined after a transplantation failed for technical reasons. The myocardium did not demonstrate histological signs of CO poisoning.[30]

Probably more critical to transplantation success is adequate tissue perfusion and well maintained cellular morphology. For example, patients suffering brain death from acetaminophen poisoning are not suitable liver donors given the hepatoxicity. Alternatively, xenobiotics considered toxic to organ function by impairing enzymes have resulted in successful transplantation if the cellular structure is otherwise maintained. For example, a death from cardioactive steroid poisoning did not preclude successful heart transplantation even when the donor had a bradydysrhythmia, an elevated serum digoxin concentration,

Table SC–1. Organs Transplanted After Donor Poisonings

Organ	Poisons Identified in Donors
Cornea*[1,23,25,26,29]	brodifacoum, cyanide
Heart[8,14,25,28,30]	acetaminophen, alkylphosphate, benzodiazepine, beta-adrenergic antagonists, brodifacoum, carbamazepine, carbon monoxide, chlormethiazole, cyanide, digitalis, digoxin, ethanol, flurazepam, glibenclamide, insulin, meprobamate, methanol, propoxyphene, thiocyanide
Kidney*[2,4,6,10,25,26,29]	acetaminophen, brodifacoum, carbon monoxide, *Conium maculatum*, cyanide, ethylene glycol, Insulin, malathion, methanol, tricyclic antidepressants
Liver[4,6,7,10,14]	brodifacoum, carbon monoxide, *Conium maculatum*, cyanide, ethylene glycol, insulin, malathion, methanol, Methaqualone, tricylic antidepressants
Lung[5,7,14,25,27,29]	brodifacoum, carbon monoxide, methanol
Pancreas[6,7,10,25]	acetaminophen, brodifacoum, carbon monoxide, *Conium maculatum*, cyanide, ethylene glycol, methanol, tricyclic antidepressants
Skin[7,27]	cyanide, methanol

*Can be cadaveric procurement.

Table SC–2. Xenobiotic Related Deaths Resulting in Successful Organ Donation

Alkylphosphate
Barbiturates
Benzodiazepines
Beta-adrenergic antagonists
Brodifacoum
Carbamazepine
Carbon monoxide
Cardioactive steroids
Chlormethiazole
Conium maculatum
Cyanide
Ethanol
Ethylene glycol
Glibenclamide
Ibuprofen
Insulin
Malathion
Methaqualone
Meprobamate
Methanol
Propoxyphene
Tricyclic antidepressants

and required cardiopulmonary resuscitation.[30] Similarly, the liver of a patient poisoned with brodifacoum was transplanted after administration of fresh frozen plasma and vitamin K_1. The recipient's INR post-transplant was 2 and corrected rapidly with supportive care. Recipient concentrations of brodifacoum were not reported and not clearly causative of the elevated INR.[25] In both examples the target of toxicity was enzymatic and the tissue morphology was otherwise minimally affected. Organs from a patient who suffered hypoxic brain death after malathion poisoning were procured 2 weeks after the exposure at which time which no further evidence of acute cholinergic toxicity was present and[4] successfully transplanted. Most transplant failures from poisoned donors, are due to rejection, sepsis, or technical reasons. The 1-year survival in recipients from poisoned donors approximates that from nonpoisoned donors, one series reported at 75% survival.[10] In another review 5-year survival was between 33% and 100% with heart transplant recipients the lowest.[7]

Ideally, a comprehensive international registry of transplants from poisoned donors will be established to improve understanding of transplants from such patients. It appears that patients who suffer brain death from poisoning are potentially suitable donors when cellular infrastructure is preserved.[20,22,24,33] Consideration for organ procurement should not be limited by the xenobiotic.

REFERENCES

1. Basu PK. Experimental and clinical studies on corneal grafts from donors dying of drug overdose: a review. *Cornea.* 1984–85;3:262-267.
2. Brown PW, Buckels JA, Jain AB, McMaster P. Successful cadaveric transplantation from a donor who died of cyanide poisoning. *Br Med J Clin Res.* 1987;294:1325.
3. de Tourtchaninoff M, Hantson P, Mahieu P, Geurit JM. Brain-death diagnosis in misleading conditions. *QJM.* 1999;92:404-414.
4. Dribben WH, Kirk MA. Organ procurement and successful transplantation after malathion poisoning. *J Toxicol Clin Toxicol.* 2001;39:633-636.
5. Evrard P, Hantson P, Ferrant E, et al. Successful double lung transplantation with a graft obtained from a methanol-poisoned donor. *Chest.* 1999;115:1458-1459.
6. Foster PF, McFadden R, Trevino R. Successful transplantation of donor organs from a hemlock poisoning victim. *Transplantation.* 2003;76:874-876.
7. Hantson P. Organ donation after fatal poisoning: an update and recent literature data. *Adv in Exper Med Biol.* 2004;550:207-213.
8. Hantson P, de Tourtchaninoff M, Guerit JM, et al. Multimodality evoked potentials as a valuable technique for brain death diagnosis in poisoned patients. *Transpl Proc.* 1997;29:3345-3346.
9. Hantson P, Kremer Y, Lerut J, et al. Successful liver transplantation with a graft from a methanol-poisoned donor. *Transpl Int.* 1996;9:437.
10. Hantson P, Mahieu P, Hassoun A, Otte JB. Outcome following organ removal from poisoned donors in brain death status: a report of 12 cases and review of the literature. *J Toxicol Clin Toxicol.* 1995;33:709-712.
11. Hantson P, Mahieu P. Organ donation after fatal poisoning. *QJM.* 1999;92:415-418.
12. Hantson P, Squifflet JP, Vanormelingen P, Mahieu P. Organ transplantation after fatal cyanide poisoning. *Clin Transpl.* 1999;13:72-73.
13. Hantson P, Wittbole X, Liolios A. Strategies to increase the lung donors' pool. *Eur Respir J.* 2004;24:889-890.
14. Hantson P, Vanormelingen P, Lecomte C, et al. Fatal methanol poisoning and organ donation: experience with seven cases in a single center. *Transpl Proc.* 2000;32:491-492.
15. Hantson P, Vanormelingen P, Squifflet JP, et al. Methanol poisoning and organ transplantation. *Transplantation.* 1999;68:165-166.
16. Hantson P, Vekemans MC, Laterre PF, et al. Heart donation after fatal acetaminophen poisoning. *J Toxicol Clin Toxicol.* 1997;35:325-326.
17. Hantson P, Vekemans MC, Squifflet JP, Mahieu P. Organ transplantation from victims of carbon monoxide poisoning. *Ann Emerg Med.* 1996;27:673-674.
18. Hantson P, Vekemans MC, Squifflet JP, Mahieu P. Outcome following organ removal from poisoned donors: experience with 12 cases and a review of the literature. *Transpl Int.* 1995;8:185-189.
19. Hantson P, Vekemans MC, Vanormelingen P, De Meester J, et al. Organ procurement after evidence of brain death in victims of acute poisoning. *Transpl Proc.* 1997;29:3341-3342.
20. Jones AL, Simpson KJ. Drug abusers and poisoned patients: a potential source of organs for transplantation? *QJM.* 1998;91:589-592.
21. Koerner MM, Tenderich G. Minami K, et al. Extended donor criteria: use of cardiac allografts after carbon monoxide poisoning. *Transplantation.* 1997;63:1358-1360.
22. Leikin JB, Heyn-Lamb R, Aks S, et al. The toxic patient as a potential organ donor. *Am J Emerg Med.* 1994;12:151-154.
23. Lindquist TD, Oiland D, Weber K. Cyanide poisoning victims as corneal transplant donors. *Am J Opthalmol.* 1988;106:354-355.
24. Lopez-Navidad A, Caballero F. Extended criteria for organ acceptance: Strategies for achieving organ safety and for increasing organ pool. *Clin Transpl.* 2003;17:308-324.
25. Ornstein DL, Lord KE, Yanofsky NN, et al. Successful donation and transplantation of multiple organs after fatal poisoning with brodifacoum, a long-acting anticoagulant rodenticide: case report. *Transplantation.* 1999;67:475-478.
26. Ravishankar DK, Kashi SH, Lam FT. Organ transplant from a donor who died of cyanide poisoning. *Clin Transpl.* 1998;12:142-143.
27. Shennib H, Adoumie R, Fraser R. Successful transplantation of a lung allograft from a carbon monoxide poisoning victim. *J Heart Lung Transpl.* 1992;11:68-71.
28. Smith JA, et al. Successful heart transplantation with cardiac allografts exposed to carbon monoxide poisoning. *J Heart Lung Transpl.* 1992;11:698-700.
29. Swanson-Bieraman B, Krenzelok EP, Snyder JW, et al. Successful donation and transplantation of multiple organs from a victim of cyanide poisoning. *J Toxicol Clin Toxicol.* 1993;31:95-99.
30. Tenderich G, Koerner MM, Posival H, et al. Hemodynamic follow-up of cardiac allografts from poisoned donors. *Transplantation.* 1998;66:1163-1167.
31. Wijdicks EF. The diagnosis of brain death: *N Engl J Med.* 2001;3444:1215-1221.
32. Wood DM, Dargan PI, Jones AL. Poisoned patients as potential organ donors: postal survey of transplant centres and intensive care units. *Crit Care (London).* 2003;7:147-154.
33. Wood KE, Becker BN, McCartney JG, et al. Care of the potential organ donor. *N Engl J Med.* 2004;351:2730-2739.

PART C

THE CLINICAL BASIS OF MEDICAL TOXICOLOGY

SECTION

1 A. ANALGESICS AND ANTIINFLAMMATORY MEDICATIONS

CHAPTER 34

ACETAMINOPHEN

Robert G. Hendrickson

Structure			
H—N—C(=O)—CH_3 on benzene ring with OH	MW	=	151 daltons
	Therapeutic serum concentration	=	10–30 μg/mL
		=	66–199 μmol/L

HISTORY AND EPIDEMIOLOGY

Acetaminophen (*N*-acetyl-*p*-aminophenol [APAP]), a metabolite of phenacetin, was first used clinically in the United States in 1955.[137,154,161] The well-known toxicity of phenacetin led to unfounded concerns about acetaminophen safety that delayed widespread acceptance of acetaminophen until the 1970s. Acetaminophen has since proved to be a remarkably safe drug at appropriate dosage, which has led to its popularity, as evidenced by sales of more than 90 million tablets per year.[70] Acetaminophen is available alone in myriad single-agent dose formulations and delivery systems, and in a variety of combinations with opioids, other analgesics, sedatives, decongestants, expectorants, and antihistamines.[161]

The diversity and wide availability of acetaminophen products dictate that acetaminophen toxicity be considered not only after identified ingestions but also after exposure to unknown or multiple drugs in settings of intentional drug overdose, drug abuse, and therapeutic misadventures.

Despite enormous experience with acetaminophen toxicity, many controversies and challenges are unresolved. New formulations and new analogs will be introduced in the future, which will require reassessments of the knowledge in this area.[303] To best understand the continuing evolution in approach to acetaminophen toxicity, it is critical to start with an analysis of certain fundamental principles and then to apply these principles to both typical and atypical presentations in which acetaminophen toxicity must be considered.

PHARMACOLOGY

Acetaminophen (APAP) is an analgesic and antipyretic with weak peripheral antiinflammatory and antiplatelet properties. Analgesic activity is reported at a serum acetaminophen concentration of 10 μg/mL and antipyretic activity at 4 to 18 μg/mL.[323]

APAP has a unique mechanism of action among the analgesic antipyretics. Most of the nonsteroidal antiinflammatory drugs (NSAIDs) occupy the cyclooxygenase (COX) binding site on the enzyme prostaglandin H_2 synthase (PGH_2) and prevent arachidonic acid from physically entering the site and being converted to prostaglandin H_2. APAP also inhibits prostaglandin H_2 production but does so indirectly by reducing a heme on the peroxidase (POX) portion of the PGH_2,[177] and indirectly inhibiting COX activation.[9,138,173] In this way, APAP function is highly dependent on cellular location and intracellular conditions.[8,102,211] APAP strongly inhibits prostaglandin synthesis where concentrations of POX and arachidonic acid ("peroxide tone") are low, such as the brain.[92] In conditions of high peroxide tone, such as inflammatory cells (macrophages) and platelets, prostaglandin synthesis is less affected by APAP.[9,34,102,110,173,203,211] This explains APAP's strong central antipyretic and analgesic effect but weak peripheral antiinflammatory and antiplatelet effects. Functionally, APAP predominantly acts as a central indirect inhibitor of COX-2 enzymes,[121,201,203] with some mild peripheral COX-2 inhibition[164] and minimal COX-1 inhibition (see chap. 36).[53]

Antipyresis and analgesia are predominantly mediated by this central indirect COX-2 inhibition and the resulting decrease in prostaglandin E_2 (PGE_2) synthesis.[89,102,150,168,203] Additional analgesic effects may be mediated by APAP's centrally mediated indirect stimulation of serotonergic and opioid descending pathways or activation of the cannabinoid system. Stimulation of descending serotonergic pathways has been demonstrated in rats[32] and humans,[102,216] and the analgesic effect of APAP may be inhibited by several serotonin antagonists or serotonin depletion.[2,216,218,219,252] In rats, the analgesic effect of APAP is attenuated by opioid receptor antagonists.[47,253] However, APAP poorly binds to opioid receptors,[230,231,232] and the exact mechanism of opioid stimulation remains unexplained.[254] Finally, activation of the central or peripheral endogenous cannabinoid system, potentially from an APAP metabolite,[123] has been theorized but remains controversial.[22,67,109,210]

PHARMACOKINETICS

After oral (PO) ingestion of a therapeutic dose immediate-release acetaminophen is rapidly absorbed from the small intestine with a time to peak [APAP] of approximately 30 minutes for liquids and 45 minutes for tablets.[4,77,95] Extended-release acetaminophen has a time to peak of 1 to 2 hours but is almost entirely absorbed by 4 hours.[79] The time to peak may be delayed by food[77] and coingestion of opioids or anticholinergics.[108,200] The oral bioavailability is 60% to 98%,[234] and the volume of distribution is 1 L/kg.[4,95] Peak [APAP] after recommended doses typically ranges from 8 to 20 μg/mL.[4,7,163] After administration of 20 to 25 mg/kg rectal suppositories, the peak [APAP] ranges from 4.1 to 13.6 μg/mL, the time to peak [APAP] is 2 to 4 hours (range, 0.4–8 hours), and the bioavailability is 30% to 40%.[15,28,107] Acetaminophen is available in several countries in the intravenous (IV) form as an acetaminophen solution and as a pro-drug (eg, propacetamol) and is currently in Phase lll trials in the United States. The time to peak of the

IV formulations are immediate (<15 min), and peak [APAP] after a 2-g infusion of IV APAP is approximately 75 μg/mL with a large range of 31 to 161 μg/mL.[93,104,215] Acetaminophen has total protein binding of 10% to 30% that does not change in overdose.[186] APAP crosses the placenta; the blood–brain barrier; and in small amounts (<2% of ingested dose), into breast milk.[100,167,207]

After it has been absorbed, approximately 90% of acetaminophen normally undergoes hepatic conjugation with glucuronide (40%–67%) and sulfate (20%–46%) to form inactive metabolites, which are eliminated in the urine.[256] A small fraction of unchanged acetaminophen (<5%) and other minor metabolites reach the urine.[192,253] The remaining fraction, which usually ranges from 5% to 15%, is oxidized by CYP2E1 (and, to a lesser extent, CYP3A4, CYP2A6 and CYP1A2),[116,176] resulting in the formation *N*-acetyl-*p*-benzoquinoneimine (NAPQI).[62] Glutathione quickly combines with NAPQI,[191] and the resulting complex is converted to nontoxic cysteine or mercaptate conjugates, which are eliminated in the urine (Fig. 34–1).[185,192] The elimination half-life of acetaminophen is approximately 2 to 3 hours after a nontoxic dose[4,228] but may become prolonged in patients who develop hepatotoxicity.[227]

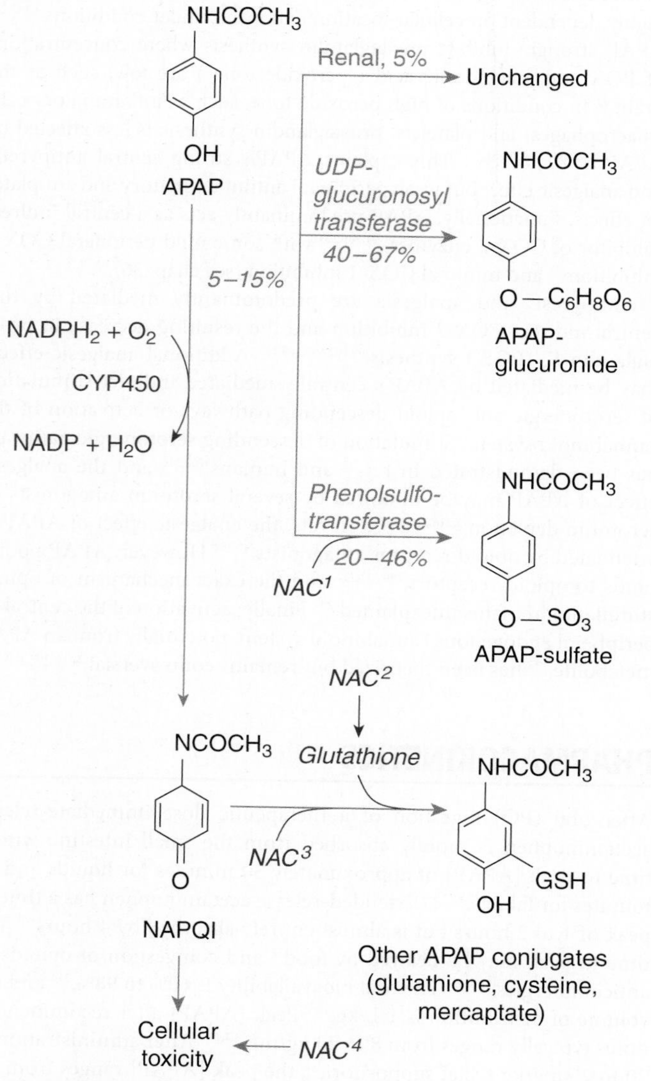

FIGURE 34–1. Important routes of acetaminophen metabolism in humans and mechanisms of *N*-acetylcysteine (NAC) hepatoprotection. NAC^1 augments sulfation, NAC^2 is a glutathione (GSH) precursor, NAC^3 is a GSH substitute, and NAC^4 improves multiorgan function during hepatic failure and possibly limits the extent of hepatocyte injury. APAP = *N*-acetyl-*p*-aminophenol = acetaminophen.

TOXICOKINETICS

Even after overdose, the majority of acetaminophen absorption occurs within 2 hours. Peak plasma concentrations generally occur within 4 hours, although later peaks or double peaks are rarely documented in overdoses.[298] Evidence suggests that NAPQI production is largely the result of activity of the CYP2E1 enzyme after both therapeutic and supratherapeutic doses of APAP.[116] Contributions of CYP1A2, CYP3A4, and CYP2A6 to the production of NAPQI in humans are small and insignificant in most cases, but they may be variable, depending on individual host factors and dosage.[116,213,233,295] After clinically significant overdose, nontoxic sulfation metabolism of APAP may become saturated,[147] and the amount of NAPQI formed is increased out of proportion to the acetaminophen dose. Glucuronidation rates are likely not saturatable in humans (see Fig. 34–1).[73,147,224]

PATHOPHYSIOLOGY

The safety of appropriate acetaminophen dosing results from the availability of electron donors such as reduced glutathione (GSH) and other thiol (S-H)-containing compounds. After therapeutic acetaminophen dosing, GSH supply and turnover far exceed that required to detoxify NAPQI, and no toxicity occurs. After overdose, the rate and quantity of NAPQI formation outstrip supply and turnover of GSH, resulting in free NAPQI rapidly binding to hepatocyte constituents. In animal experiments of acetaminophen overdose, hepatotoxicity becomes evident only when hepatic [GSH] decreases to 30% of baseline or below.[190] This affords acetaminophen a remarkably safe therapeutic index. Whereas a therapeutic acetaminophen dose is 10 to 15 mg/kg, significant toxicity after a single acute overdose generally involves doses that are higher than 150 mg/kg.[225]

When NAPQI formation overwhelms the supply of thiol-containing compounds, it covalently binds[86,221] and arylates proteins throughout the cell,[61,133,137] inducing a series of events that result in cell death.[135] Covalent binding and arylation occur rapidly after glutathione depletion and within hours of ingestion.[27,133,135,236] Both covalent binding and glutathione deficiency are necessary for hepatotoxicity; however, the selective arylation of specific cellular proteins is more predictive of toxicity than total covalent binding.[61,128]

After covalent protein binding and glutathione depletion occur, a cascade of events follows that alters normal cell function and impairs cell defenses against endogenous reactive oxygen species.[137,236,299] This cascade can be ameliorated with *N*-acetylcysteine (NAC) even after covalent binding occurs.[43,75,98,133,236] These events include mitochondrial dysfunction,[48,78] an increase in mitochondrial permeability,[236] mitochondrial oxidant stress or peroxynitrite formation,[63,120,144] hepatocellular hypoxia,[249] DNA fragmentation[63] resulting from interactions with topoisomerase 2-α,[18,267] calcium dyshomeostasis,[196,300] lipid peroxidation,[105,318] nitric oxide release,[250] inflammatory cell mobilization and activation,[125,156,169] inflammatory cytokine release,[132,133,156,169] and up- or downregulation of protein expression.[25,128,129,249] Which specific event is critical and irreversibly commits the cell to death is not known and is an active area of research.

The final pathway of hepatic cell death is predominantly cellular necrosis,[106] although evidence suggests that apoptosis may occur early in APAP toxicity.[175,235] Macrophages, neutrophils, and inflammatory cells infiltrate after necrosis[125,159,169] followed by a cascade of inflammatory cytokines such as IL-6, IL-8, and MCP-1.[125,132,133,169]

Hepatocellular destruction caused by secondary inflammation, impairment of microcirculation,[188] and hepatic nitric oxide release[133,250] are all demonstrated, although none appear to be necessary for hepatic injury.[63,129,130,159] The exact mechanism and sequence of events involved in hepatocellular damage remains controversial.[127,128,133]

Hepatotoxicity initially and most profoundly occurs in hepatic zone III (centrilobular) because this zone is the area with the largest concentration of oxidative metabolism (CYP2E1)[23] (see Fig. 26-1). In more severe hepatotoxicity, necrosis may extend into zones I and II, destroying the entire liver parenchyma.

Renal injury after acute overdose is typically acute tubular necrosis (ATN) that may be caused by local production of NAPQI by renal CYP2E1 enzymes.[40,84,124] However, several other nephrotoxic mechanisms have been proposed.[113] Conversion of acetaminophen and hepatically derived acetaminophen–glutathione[195] to nephrotoxic *p*-aminophenol[52] are both demonstrated in selected animal models.[80,85,182] NAPQI formation via renal prostaglandin synthetase[308] and prostaglandin-mediated renal medullary ischemia[227] are also suspected of contributing to chronic analgesic nephropathy from acetaminophen alone or in combination with other analgesics.[94,165,251] In patients with hepatic failure, volume depletion and hepatorenal syndrome may be the most important contributory cofactors because the rate of renal failure is similar regardless of the cause of hepatic failure.[322] Dose-related renal potassium wasting[212,315] after acute APAP overdose may be related to APAP-induced renal vasoconstriction due to COX inhibition or a NAC effect, or both.[99,212]

Direct injury to organs other than the liver and kidney is rarely reported. The mechanism of early central nervous system (CNS) depression after APAP ingestion is undefined, but theoretical mechanisms include serotonin and opioid effects as well as CNS glutathione depletion.[26,54] Acidosis and hyperlactatemia early after massive APAP ingestion may be the result of alterations in mitochondrial respiratory function, but the exact mechanism is unknown.[46,88,287] Rare cases of metabolic acidosis with 5-oxoprolinemia and 5-oxoprolinuria are reported and appear to be more likely in women with chronic APAP use and renal insufficiency.[42,90,122] In this rare condition, it is theorized that chronic APAP use combined with acute oxidative stress and inflammatory mediators may lead to an alteration of the γ-glutamyl cycle and elevations of γ-glutamylcysteine and 5-oxoproline.[42,90,122]

The remaining sequelae of severe toxicity are secondary effects of fulminant hepatic failure rather than direct acetaminophen effects, and the pathophysiology of these complex multisystem problems is well described.[162] For example, myocardial injury and pancreatitis have both been reported in patients with acetaminophen-induced fulminant hepatic failure. The ability of NAC to ameliorate secondary multiorgan failure via extrahepatic mechanisms suggests that the oxidation of vital thiols and the loss of normal microvascular function are important components of secondary organ failure.[89,112]

CLINICAL MANIFESTATIONS

Early recognition and treatment of patients with acetaminophen poisoning are essential to minimize morbidity and mortality. This task is made difficult by the lack of early predictive clinical findings, and clinicians should not be reassured by the absence of clinical symptoms shortly after ingestion. The first symptoms after acetaminophen overdose may be those of hepatic injury, which develop many hours after the ingestion, when antidotal therapy will have diminished efficacy.

The clinical course of acute acetaminophen toxicity can be divided into four stages.[247] During stage I, hepatic injury has not yet occurred, and even patients who ultimately develop severe hepatotoxicity may be asymptomatic. Clinical findings, when present, are nonspecific and may include nausea, vomiting, malaise, pallor, and diaphoresis. Laboratory indices of liver function are normal. In rare cases of massive overdose, a decreased level of consciousness,[91,103,149,242,285] metabolic acidosis,[103,149,184,242] and even death[33,296] may occur during this stage in the absence of signs or symptoms of hepatotoxicity.[33,91,149,242,285,328] These clinical findings should never be attributed to acetaminophen alone without thorough evaluation of other possible causes.

Stage II represents the onset of liver injury, which occurs in fewer than 5% of those who overdose.[276] Aspartate aminotransferase (AST) is the most sensitive, widely available measure to detect the onset of hepatotoxicity, and AST abnormalities always precede evidence of actual liver dysfunction (prolonged prothrombin time (PT), international normalized ratio (INR), elevated bilirubin concentration, hypoglycemia, and metabolic acidosis). When stage II occurs, onset of AST elevation is most common within 24 hours after ingestion but is nearly universal by 36 hours.[268] In the most severely poisoned patients, AST concentrations may increase as early as 12 hours after ingestion.[268] Symptoms and signs during stage II vary with the severity of liver injury. By convention, acetaminophen-induced *hepatotoxicity* is defined as a peak AST concentration above 1000 IU/L. Although lower peak concentrations of AST represent some injury to hepatic tissue, they rarely have any clinical relevance.

Stage III, defined as the time of maximal hepatotoxicity, most commonly occurs between 72 and 96 hours after ingestion. The clinical manifestations of stage III include fulminant hepatic failure with encephalopathy, coma, or rarely exsanguinating hemorrhage. Results of laboratory studies are variable; AST and alanine aminotransferase (ALT) concentrations above 10,000 IU/L are common, even in patients without other evidence of liver failure. Much more important than the degree of aminotransferase concentration elevation, abnormalities of PT and INR, glucose, lactate, creatinine and pH are essential determinants of prognosis and treatment.

Renal function abnormalities are rare overall[225] but occur in as many as 25% of patients with significant hepatotoxicity[225] and in more than 50% of those with hepatic failure.[155,322] Renal abnormalities may be more common after sustained, repeated excessive dosing[155] and in adolescents and young adults.[35,180,197] After acute ingestions, elevations of serum creatinine typically occur between 2 and 5 days after ingestion, peak on day 7 (range, 3–16 days), and normalize over a month.[180] When overt renal failure necessitating hemodialysis occurs, it nearly always does so among patients with marked hepatic injury.[50] Infrequently, mild renal insufficiency occurs without elevations in aminotransferase concentrations.[1,35,60]

Fatalities from fulminant hepatic failure generally occur between 3 and 5 days after an acute overdose. Death results from either single or combined complications of multiorgan failure, including hemorrhage, acute respiratory distress syndrome, sepsis, and cerebral edema. Patients who survive this period reach stage IV, defined as the recovery phase. Survivors have complete hepatic regeneration, and no cases of chronic hepatic dysfunction have been reported. The rate of recovery varies; in most cases, AST, pH, PT and INR, and lactate are normal by 7 days in survivors of acute overdoses. ALT may remain elevated longer than AST, and creatinine may be elevated for more than 1 month. The recovery time is much longer in severely poisoned patients, and histologic abnormalities may persist for months.[166,178,220]

DIAGNOSTIC TESTING

ASSESSING THE RISK OF TOXICITY

Principles That Guide the Diagnostic Approach The majority of acetaminophen exposures result in no toxicity, and the overall mortality rate after acute APAP ingestion is less 0.5%.[276] However, APAP is commonly ingested and is now the leading cause of acute liver failure in the United States, United Kingdom, and much of Europe.[155,161] To maintain the seemingly divergent goals of avoiding the enormous cost of overtreatment while eliminating patient risk, clinicians must understand the basis for and sensitivity of current toxicity screening methods. A discussion of the diagnostic approach follows.

When considering risk determination, it is useful to separate different categories of acetaminophen exposure. There is an extensive body of experience and literature on acute overdose in typical circumstances, permitting a more systematic approach with demonstrated efficacy. For issues related to repeated excessive acetaminophen dosing, uncertain circumstances, patients with possible predispositions to toxicity, new acetaminophen formulations, and many other permutations, there is an important conceptual framework for decision making but little in the way of validated strategies. For these challenges, the central concepts and one approach are presented here, with the understanding that they are dynamic and that more than one approach may have validity.

The clinician must rely solely on the often unreliable ingestion history and measurement of [APAP] in the patient to assess the risk for subsequent toxicity and thus the need for treatment. The ideal model for determining risk after acetaminophen overdose would assess the individual's metabolic enzyme activity (CYP2E1, UDP-glucuronosyl transferase, and sulfotransferase activity), the amount and rate of NAPQI formation, the availability of hepatic GSH, and the balance of NAPQI formation and hepatic GSH turnover.[189,243] At present, none of these measures is available to clinicians.

Protein adducts, which indicate binding of NAPQI to hepatocyte proteins[71,131,199,229,317] and the profile of urinary APAP metabolism[73] can be determined but have been inadequately studied to be useful in risk assessment. Plasma GSH concentration can be measured or approximated using the plasma γ-glutamyl transferase (GGT) concentration but have an uncertain relationship to hepatic GSH availability.[265,279]

Risk Determination After Acute Overdose Determining risk in a patient with acute overdose consists of determining the initial risk based on dosing history and then potentially further risk stratifying with serum [APAP].

Acute overdose usually is considered a single ingestion, although many patients actually overdose incrementally over a brief period of time. For purposes of this discussion, an *acute overdose* is arbitrarily defined as one in which the entire ingestion occurs within a single 8-hour period.[69] Figures of 7.5 g in an adult or 150 mg/kg in a child are widely disseminated as the lowest acute dose capable of causing toxicity.[226] These standards are likely quite conservative but have stood the test of time as sensitive markers and have been corroborated with some data in humans.[313] However, it is more likely that doses of at least 12 g in an adult or 200 mg/kg in a child are necessary to cause hepatotoxicity in most patients.[193,313]

Higher dose cutoffs for consideration of risk would improve specificity; however, the value of improving specificity has not been weighed against the current sensitive lower cutoff. In the face of an enormous variety of potential outliers, the near absence of screening failures almost certainly results from the use of these standards and of a very sensitive screening nomogram. The adult standard may be considered less controversial than that for children because massive ingestions, unreliable histories, and factors that might predispose to toxicity occur primarily in adults, justifying continued use of 7.5 g as a screening amount to avoid missing serious toxicity. In patients younger than 6 years old, with unintentional ingestions, use of a higher 200-mg/kg cutoff has been suggested[51,193,290] and may be appropriate but has been incompletely studied.

The dose history should be used in the assessment of risk only if there is reliable corroboration or direct evidence of validity. Although the amount ingested by history roughly correlates with risk of toxicity and an [APAP] over the treatment line,[313] historical information is not sufficiently reliable in all patients to exclude significant ingestion, particularly in patients with self-harm or drug abuse. In fact, patients with suicidal ingestions who do not confirm an ingestion of acetaminophen may have a measurable concentration of it in 1.4% to 8.4% of cases[10,172] and a concentration over the treatment line in up to 0.2% to 2.2%.[10,172] Therefore, when the history suggests possible risk, the patient should be further assessed using determination of [APAP].

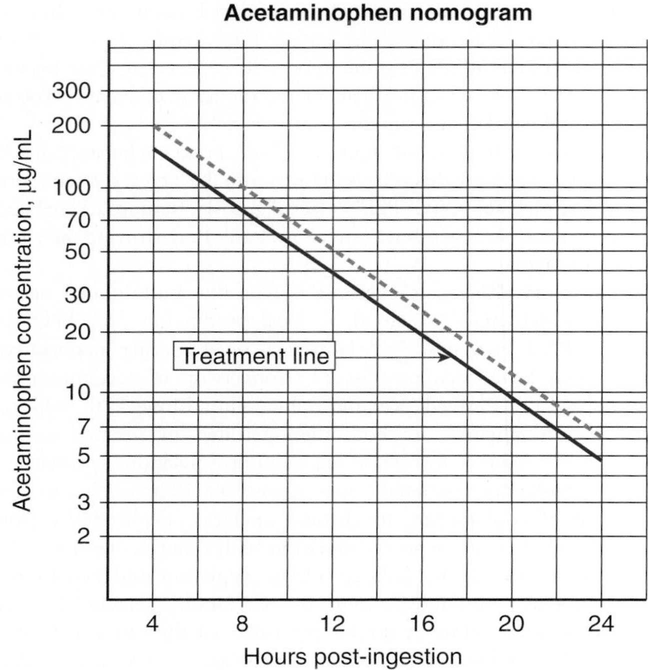

FIGURE 34–2. The Rumack-Matthew nomogram (reconstructed) for determining the risk of acetaminophen-induced hepatoxicity after a single acute ingestion. Serum concentrations above the treatment line on the nomogram indicate the need for *N*-acetylcysteine therapy.

Interpretation of [APAP] after acute exposures is based on adaptation of the Rumack-Matthew nomogram (Fig. 34–2).[243] The original nomogram was based on the observation that untreated patients who subsequently developed AST or ALT concentrations above 1000 IU/L could be separated from those who did not on the basis of the initial [APAP]. A nomogram was constructed that plotted the initial concentration versus time since ingestion, and a discriminatory line was drawn to separate patients who developed hepatotoxicity from those who did not. The initial discriminatory line stretched from [APAP] of 300 μg/mL at 4 hours to 50 μg/mL at 12 hours but was lowered to between 200 μg/mL at 4 hours and 50 μg/mL at 12 hours after evaluation of additional patients.[243] The half-life of acetaminophen was not a factor in the development of the nomogram, and the slope of the treatment line does not reflect any discriminatory APAP half-life or acetaminophen kinetics.[243] The nomogram is designed and validated using a single value obtained at or greater than 4 hours after ingestion to allow for complete APAP absorption. Although patients who develop hepatotoxicity may have acetaminophen half-lives greater than 4 hours,[228] plotting multiple points on the nomogram or using an APAP half-life to determine risk has not been adequately studied and has significant limitations.[145,278] The nomogram was later extrapolated to 24 hours using the same slope of the original nomogram line.[243]

It is important to realize that the line was based on aminotransferase concentration elevation rather than on hepatic failure or death, and it was chosen to be very sensitive, with little regard to specificity. Without antidotal therapy, only 60% of those with an initial [APAP] above this original line will develop hepatotoxicity as defined by aminotransferase concentrations above 1000 IU/L, but the risk of hepatotoxicity is not the same for all such patients. Elevated aminotransferase concentration develops in virtually all untreated patients with [APAP] far above the line, and serious hepatic dysfunction occurs frequently; the incidence of hepatotoxicity among untreated people with [APAP] immediately above the line is very low, and the risk of hepatic failure or death is far less.[225,270]

The original line ("200-line") is used in the United Kingdom, Canada, Europe, Australia, and other locations throughout the world. The line used in the United States runs parallel to the original but was arbitrarily lowered by 25% to add even greater sensitivity.[243,247] The lower line, subsequently referred to as the *treatment line* or *150-line,* starts at a concentration of 150 μg/mL at 4 hours after ingestion; declines with a 4-hour half-life, and ends at 4.7 μg/mL 24 hours after the overdose. The treatment line is one of the most sensitive screening tools used in medicine. The incidence of nomogram failures in the United States using this line is only 1% to 3% (depending on time to treatment) and most likely results predominately from inaccurate ingestion histories.[243] A vanishingly small number of anecdotal cases of nomogram failure involve special circumstances of increased risk,[56,181,202] questionable facts, or both.[274]

The higher line ("200-line") has had reported nomogram failures, although they are likely rare. Several authors have recommended that the 200-line is not sensitive enough for patients with comorbid factors that potentially predispose them to hepatotoxicity, and a lower line starting at 100 μg/mL ("100-line") is used in some countries.[39,41,56,72,274,304] In retrospective series, six patients developed hepatotoxicity with [APAP] between the 150-line and the 200-line, and one died of liver failure.[17,41] It has been estimated that of all patients with [APAP] between the 150-line and 200-line, if untreated 3% to 10% develop hepatotoxicity (AST >1000 IU/L),[243,276] and 0.08% develop hepatic failure.[17]

Based on these observations and more than 20 years of use, the 150-line should be considered adequate in nearly all cases and is reliable when rigorously followed. When using the acetaminophen nomogram, it is essential to precisely define the time window during which acetaminophen exposure occurred and, if the time is unknown, to use the earliest possible time as the time of ingestion. Using this approach, patients with [APAP] below the treatment line, even if only slightly so, do not require further evaluation or treatment for acute acetaminophen overdose. This also applies to most patients with factors that may predispose them to acetaminophen-induced hepatotoxicity. There appears to be adequate experience with acute acetaminophen overdose in the settings of potentially predisposing factors such as chronic alcohol abuse, chronic medication with CYP-inducing drugs, and inadequate nutrition to recommend that no special approach is required in such cases. Further study is needed to determine if rare events, such as acute APAP ingestion in the setting of chronic INH use,[202] may uniquely predispose patients to toxicity[87,327] and require alteration of this approach.

The goal should be to determine [APAP] at the earliest point at which it will be meaningful in decision making. Measurement of [APAP] 4 hours after ingestion or as soon as possible thereafter is used to confirm the patient's risk of toxicity and thus the need to initiate NAC. No established guidelines are available for the use of determinations made less than 4 hours after ingestion, and because of variability in absorption, such values have less predictive value. Although it is optimal to start NAC therapy as soon as possible after confirmation of risk, most patients have excellent outcomes if therapy is started earlier than 6 to 8 hours after the overdose.[270,276] This allows clinicians some leeway to wait for the laboratory results before starting therapy in patients in whom the history of ingestion suggests that the 4 hour concentration will fall below the treatment line. It should be noted, however, that delaying NAC therapy longer than 6 to 8 hours after ingestion may increase the patient's risk. If there is any concern about the availability of an acetaminophen concentration before this time, treatment with NAC should be initiated. Only if the results cannot be obtained within 6 to 8 hours of the overdose should history alone be considered adequate to consider the patient at risk and as an indication to start NAC. In such cases, [APAP] still should be determined as soon as possible. The results, when they become available, should be interpreted according to the treatment line on the acetaminophen nomogram and NAC either continued or discontinued on the basis of this result. In the unusual circumstance in which no determination of [APAP] can ever be obtained, evidence of possible risk by history alone is sufficient to initiate and complete a course of NAC therapy post ingestion.

Early Measurement of [APAP] Measurement of [APAP] between 1 and 4 hours after ingestion may be helpful only to exclude ingestion of APAP. If [APAP] is below 10 μg/mL in this time frame, significant APAP overdose can likely be excluded. However, a concentration that is detectable between 1 and 4 hours cannot be definitively interpreted and mandates repeat testing at 4 hours.

DETERMINATION OF RISK WHEN THE ACETAMINOPHEN NOMOGRAM IS NOT APPLICABLE

Risk Determination When the Time of Ingestion Is Unknown With careful questioning of the patient, family, and others, it is almost always possible to establish a time window during which the APAP ingestion must have occurred. The *earliest possible time* of ingestion ("worst-case scenario") is used for risk-determination purposes. If this time window cannot be established or is so broad that it encompasses a span of more than 24 hours, the following approach is suggested. Determine both [APAP] and AST concentrations. If the AST concentration is elevated, regardless of [APAP], treat the patient with NAC. If the time of ingestion is completely unknown and [APAP] is detectable, it is prudent to assume that the patient is at risk and to initiate treatment with NAC. If [APAP] is below the lower level of detection and the AST concentration is normal, there is little evidence that subsequent consequential hepatic injury is possible; NAC is unnecessary.

Risk Assessment After Extended-Release Acetaminophen An extended-release formulation of acetaminophen (Extended Relief Tylenol, Tylenol 8 Hour, Tylenol Arthritis Pain) was released in the United States in 1994, and others exist worldwide. The pill available in the United States consists of a 325-mg immediate-release acetaminophen dose and an additional 325-mg dose designed for delayed dissolution.[70] This results in the immediate release of acetaminophen with delayed release of an additional dose. Pharmacokinetic analysis of the product reveals that the majority of acetaminophen is absorbed within 4 hours,[79,305] the peak [APAP] is within 4 hours,[55,79,286] and a small number of patients may have an initial [APAP] below the treatment line, but then have a subsequent [APAP] above the treatment line ("nomogram crossing").[55,305] This "nomogram crossing" is not unique to the extended-release product and occurs in up to 10% of acute ingestions of immediate-release APAP.[44] There is little evidence that nomogram crossing effects outcome[70] and no evidence that an alternate approach to extended-release products should be used. In a 9-year review of isolated extended-release acetaminophen overdoses, no deaths were reported from acute overdose.[70] Therefore, a single [APAP] can reliably be plotted on the treatment nomogram after APAP extended-release ingestion. The validity of this approach, of course, is specific to the current product, and any new type of extended-release acetaminophen formulation must be evaluated individually.

Patients with Signs or Symptoms of Hepatic Injury After Acute Ingestion Patients who present with signs or symptoms of hepatic injury after acute acetaminophen ingestion should be immediately started on NAC and measurements of AST and acetaminophen concentrations should be obtained. In patients with elevated AST and acetaminophen concentrations below the treatment line, the history should be reviewed with respect to the timing of ingestion and repeat excessive acetaminophen dosing. The patients should be thoroughly evaluated for causes of hepatic failure and for other causes of elevated AST concentration.

Risk Determination After Chronic Overdose Exposure No well-established guidelines are available for determining risk after chronic exposure to APAP. Conceptually, several factors must be considered before assessing and determining an individual's risk of toxicity. It has been well established that therapeutic dosing of APAP is safe; however, some risk factors may put individual patients at risk for toxicity at supratherapeutic doses.

The chronic ingestion of "maximal therapeutic" doses (4 g/d) in normal adults without special circumstances appears to be safe. Several randomized, controlled trials have used maximal therapeutic doses of APAP (4 g/d) in hundreds of patients over periods from 4 weeks to 2 years with no reported increase in adverse events or hepatic injury.[38,96,152,217] A transient increase in transaminases up to 10 times the normal concentration has been detected in some patients taking therapeutic doses,[316] but these abnormalities resolve spontaneously despite continued use and have not led to hepatic dysfunction.[152,316] Finally, several studies have evaluated abstaining chronic alcoholics administered APAP 4 g/d for up to 10 days with no evidence of hepatic damage, although elevations in transaminases were detected in both APAP and control groups.[66,153]

Although therapeutic dosing appears to be safe, repeated supratherapeutic ingestions (RSTIs) may lead to toxicity. Given the amount of APAP use, the incidence of serious acetaminophen toxicity after repeated doses is small, and hepatotoxicity appears to occur only after massive dosing[66,165,179,312] or prolonged excessive dosing.[36,66] The risk of hepatotoxicity is likely proportional to both the total amount of APAP ingested and the duration of the exposure; however, exact cutoffs for safe dosing are difficult to determine and are likely subject to factors of the individual. In an ideal setting, the interaction of an individual's CYP2E1 activity and therefore NAPQI production with the rate of hepatic glutathione turnover would be determined and considered, but these evaluation tools are currently not available.

Although short-term prospective studies of supratherapeutic dosing (6–8 g/d) have not identified alterations in APAP kinetics or hepatotoxicity,[97] several series and case reports have identified patients with hepatotoxicity who retrospectively report therapeutic or slightly supratherapeutic doses. Retrospective dosage reporting is prone to significant errors, and a substantial portion of these cases involve parental dosing errors, iatrogenic errors, alcoholic patients, or other issues in which those giving the history may be unable or unwilling to report accurately. Furthermore, because APAP is commonly used in patients with alcoholism and viral infections, it is unclear in which cases APAP was causative, contributory, or unrelated to hepatotoxicity.

Conceptually, the groups that are at "high risk" for hepatotoxicity after RSTI of APAP have either potentially increased activity of CYP2E1 and therefore additional NAPQI formation or have decreased glutathione stores and turnover rate. In fact, nearly all reported cases of APAP toxicity from RSTI involve patients who have a factor that influences their glutathione supply or turnover, NAPQI production, or both, including infants with febrile illness who have received excessive dosing,[49,59,74,80,118,206,289,388] chronic alcohol users,[194,264,330] and patients chronically taking CYP-inducing medications.[36,39] The interplay of NAPQI and glutathione may also be an important factor. For example, malnutrition has been theorized to increase the risk of APAP toxicity[320]; however, both CYP2E1 activity[58] and glutathione supply[143] are decreased in malnourished patients, and their relative impact on risk is unknown.

When there is concern about toxicity risk after RSTI dosing, several approaches are suggested. The goal should be to select patients at risk based on dosing history and other risk factors and to then use limited laboratory testing to determine the need for NAC. A logical screening laboratory evaluation consists of determination of [APAP] and AST concentrations, with additional testing as indicated by these results and other clinical features. The objective is to identify the two conditions that warrant NAC therapy—remaining acetaminophen yet to be metabolized and potentially serious liver injury.

Role of History and Physical Examination in Chronic Overdose The first consideration when evaluating a patient with a history of repeated supratherapeutic acetaminophen dosing is the presence or absence of signs or symptoms of hepatotoxicity. Regardless of risk factors or dosing history, such findings should prompt treatment with NAC and laboratory evaluation. This is particularly important because most reported cases of serious toxicity after repeated dosing are symptomatic for more than 24 hours before diagnosis, and earlier diagnosis should improve outcome.

In asymptomatic patients, a reasonable approach is to perform laboratory evaluation for those who have ingested more than 200 mg/kg/d (or 10 g/d, whichever is less) in a 24-hour period or more than 150 mg/kg/d (or 6 g/d, whichever is less) in a 48-hour period.[66,69,174] In children younger than age 6 years, laboratory evaluation should be performed if the reported ingestion is more than 100 mg/kg/d over a 72-hour period or greater.

Several factors or characteristics place patients at higher risk for chronic APAP toxicity. High-risk factors that have been theorized include chronic alcoholism; chronic ingestion of isoniazid; febrile illnesses in infants and young children; and malnutrition, AIDS, or anorexia. In some cases, animal or basic science studies show evidence of increased risk, and in most cases, there have been multiple anecdotal reports of toxicity at therapeutic or slightly supratherapeutic doses. Whether these patients require a lower threshold for laboratory screening is unknown and controversial.

Role of Laboratory Evaluation in Chronic Overdose After a patient is determined to be at risk, an [APAP] and AST concentrations should be determined. These should be interpreted using the concept that a patient may be at risk of hepatotoxicity if there is evidence of hepatic injury (elevation of AST) or there remains enough APAP to produce further hepatic damage.

Using the strategy described here, patients with elevated AST concentrations are considered at risk, regardless of [APAP]. An [APAP] is useful in patients with normal AST concentrations as a tool to determine only whether sufficient acetaminophen remains to lead to subsequent NAPQI formation and delayed hepatotoxicity. In many cases, AST concentration is normal and [APAP] is below 10 μg/mL, obviating the need for NAC. If the AST concentration is normal, the patient should be considered at risk if [APAP] is 10 μg/mL or above.

Patients who develop highly elevated AST after chronic acetaminophen overdose should be treated and further evaluated with laboratory tests to assess hepatotoxicity and prognosis (creatinine, PT and INR, and pH; phosphate; lactate).

The measurement of APAP protein adducts in urine has been described and theoretically could quantify NAPQI production in the liver. Although this test has promise as an early detection tool, it remains largely unavailable and has been insufficiently studied for clinical use.[71,133,199]

Patients who are identified as at risk, with an elevated AST or a normal AST and an elevated [APAP], should be treated with NAC.

RISK DETERMINATION AFTER ACETAMINOPHEN EXPOSURE IN CHILDREN

Serious hepatotoxicity or death after acute acetaminophen overdose is extremely rare in children.[30,245,290] Predominant theories[5] for resistance to toxicity include a relative hepatoprotection in children because of increased sulfation capacity[185] or differences in the characteristics of children's poisonings, including smaller ingested doses, overestimation of liquid doses, and unique formulations.[293] This has led some to suggest higher screening values and a higher nomogram line for children.[6,31,301] However, no significant change in NAPQI production has been demonstrated in children,[307] and a more liberal approach to children's acute APAP ingestions has been inadequately studied and is not recommended. After repeated supratherapeutic acetaminophen dosing, there is no evidence that children are relatively protected. In fact, infants and children with acute febrile illnesses comprise one of the few groups in which toxicity after repeated excessive dosing is well described.[49,59,74,80,119,120,206,239,280,288] Common sources of dosing errors include substitution of adult for pediatric preparations; substitution of drops (100 mg/mL) for elixir (32 mg/mL), overzealous dosing by amount or frequency in attempts to maximize effect, and failure to read the label and dose carefully.[5] Age younger than 2 years is an independent risk factor for development of toxicity.[139] These rare cases of toxicity in febrile children with repeated supratherapeutic dosing may simply reflect that these children constitute the most common setting for pediatric acetaminophen use and that children are at greater relative risk for excessive dosing because of their size. Although logically one can argue that inflammatory oxidant stress and short-term fasting during febrile infectious illnesses affect oxidative drug metabolism and decrease glutathione supply, these relationships are complex and not well defined. Of the reported cases of repeated supratherapeutic APAP dosing in children with hepatic injury, the cause was likely an isolated infectious illness in some, acetaminophen in others, and a combination of the two in still others.

RISK DETERMINATION AFTER ACETAMINOPHEN EXPOSURE IN PREGNANCY

The initial risk of toxicity of a pregnant patient is similar to that of a nonpregnant patient with a few exceptions. Little evidence suggests that any alteration of the treatment line is necessary. In fact, there have been no reported cases of fetal or maternal toxicity in women with [APAP] below the treatment line[183] or in those treated with NAC within 10 hours of an acute ingestion.[238] However, there is controversy in assessing the risk of fetal toxicity after the mother has been determined to be at risk. To better understand the issues, a review of maternal–fetal physiology and pharmacokinetics related to APAP and NAC is necessary.

Acetaminophen is capable of crossing the human placenta,[11,167,205,240] and APAP may be present in concentrations that are similar to maternal serum concentrations within hours after ingestion.[11,205,240] Fetal metabolism of APAP probably is inefficient but is not completely understood. Fetal sulfation and oxidative metabolism of APAP are slower than in adults, and glucuronidation is undetectable until 23 weeks of gestation.[241] CYP450 enzymes that are capable of oxidizing APAP are present in the fetus as early as 18 weeks gestation.[241] However, the activity of these enzymes is less than 10% that of adult enzymes at 18 weeks gestation and increases to only 20% activity at 23 weeks.[241] How the opposing forces of decreased overall metabolism of APAP and decreased NAPQI formation impact fetal risk is unclear.

The mechanism of fetal risk in patients with [APAP] over the treatment line remains controversial. The degree of fetal toxicity that is attributable to fetal metabolism of APAP or to maternal illness is unclear. In clinical case series, the majority of pregnant women who overdose on APAP have uneventful pregnancies.[183,238] Pregnant women who develop APAP toxicity in the first trimester have an increased risk of spontaneous abortion,[238] and those who develop APAP toxicity in the third trimester have a potential risk of fetal hepatotoxicity because of fetal metabolism. However, reports of third-trimester fetal hepatotoxicity are rare[183,238] and are only associated with severe maternal toxicity.[238,310] The factors associated with poor fetal outcome after a large APAP overdose are delayed treatment with NAC and young gestational age.

The decision to treat a pregnant woman with NAC requires consideration of what is known about the efficacy and beneficial effects as well as the adverse effects of NAC for both the fetus and the mother. Every indication suggests that NAC is both safe and effective in treating the mother,[238] but there are inadequate data to evaluate efficacy in the fetus, although fetal outcome has generally been excellent after maternal treatment with NAC.[238] Given that NAC has been safely used in many pregnancies[183,238] and fetal mortality is linked to delays to treatment, NAC should be initiated in pregnant women whose [APAP] is over the treatment line. The necessary length of NAC therapy is difficult to determine. The 20-hour IV protocol probably is the most commonly recommended NAC protocol used for pregnant women worldwide, with *published* experience supporting NAC treatment courses shorter than the PO 72-hour protocol (see chap. 30).[183,238]

ETHANOL AND RISK DETERMINATION

The effects of ethanol on acetaminophen toxicity are complex and are best described by clearly separating experimental animal data from actual human overdose experience, acute from chronic ethanol abuse, and single from repeated supratherapeutic acetaminophen dosing. Although not entirely consistent, both animal and human data suggest that acute ethanol coingestion with APAP may be hepatoprotective. Ethanol coingestion decreases NAPQI formation presumably by inhibiting CYP2E1 in both humans[3,13,296,297] and animals.[255,296,302] In large retrospective evaluations of human overdoses, acute ethanol ingestion independently decreases the risk of severe hepatotoxicity in chronic alcoholics[260] and in nonalcoholics,[270] but does not significantly decrease the risk of hepatotoxicity (ALT >1000 IU/L) in a smaller prospective study.[314]

Chronic ethanol administration however, increases the risk of hepatotoxicity from acetaminophen dosing in animals[302,329] and increases human NAPQI formation[294] on the basis of induced CYP2E1 metabolism or decreased mitochondrial glutathione supply or regeneration.[158,329]

After acute acetaminophen overdose, alcoholics may be at a slightly increased risk; however, this elevated risk appears to be of little clinical importance given the sensitivity of the treatment line.[244,275,297] There is no credible evidence that chronic ethanol use should alter the approach after an APAP acute overdose using the treatment line. Given the paucity of data linking alcoholism to nomogram failures, it appears that the treatment line is adequately sensitive for screening after an acute APAP overdose, regardless of the patient's pattern of ethanol use.

The relationship between chronic ethanol use and chronic APAP use is complex. Hepatotoxicity has been sporadically reported in patients with chronic ethanol abuse after repeated supratherapeutic acetaminophen dosing.[194,264,323] Complicating these reports are the clinical challenges of obtaining accurate histories in alcoholics, failure to exclude non-APAP causes of hepatotoxicity, and other factors. Alcoholics commonly use supratherapeutic doses both chronically and acutely and use combinations of multiple APAP-containing products.[265] In contrast, prospective evidence demonstrates minimal risk of hepatotoxicity in alcoholic patients who ingest therapeutic doses of APAP.[14,117,151,153] In prospective trials of ingestion of 4g/d of APAP in moderate to heavy ethanol drinkers for up to 10 days, no clinically relevant increases in AST versus placebo have been identified.[14,117,151,153] It should be noted, however, that in studies involving alcoholics, mild AST elevations (<120 IU/L) were noted in 40% of both study and control subjects, and more significant increases (>120 IU/L or three times normal) were noted in 4% of 6% of subjects.[151,153] In addition, in all studies, a small group of patients developed significant increases in transaminases, but most were unchanged. Patients who develop elevated transaminases after therapeutic dosing who are then rechallenged with additional APAP develop similar AST increases,[117] implying that individual factors are likely more important than the chronic ethanol use itself.

CYP INDUCERS AND RISK DETERMINATION

Inducers of the CYP enzymes have long been theorized to increase the risk of toxicity from APAP because of a proportionally increased production of NAPQI.[246] It is now clear that APAP is metabolized to NAPQI largely by CYP2E1[116,176] and that only induction of this specific enzyme is likely to increase the risk of hepatotoxicity.

Although ethanol and isoniazid are known inducers of CYP2E1, there is no evidence that the clinical approach to these patients should be altered. Similarly, several other medications, including phenytoin, carbamazepine, and phenobarbital, have been theorized to increase APAP toxicity because of nonspecific CYP induction activity. None of these anticonvulsants induces CYP2E1, although there is some evidence that they increase NAPQI formation in cultured human hepatocyte and animal models, possibly through inhibition of glucuronidation.[29,81,190,222] Clinical experience, however, suggests that there is no need to change the clinical approach to these patients.[301]

ASSESSING ACTUAL TOXICITY: CRITICAL COMPONENTS OF THE DIAGNOSTIC APPROACH

Earlier protocols and guidelines recommended extensive and ongoing laboratory assessment after acetaminophen overdose.[247] Based on the pathophysiology and time course of toxicity, a simplified and far more cost-effective approach is logical.

Initial Testing The acetaminophen concentration should be measured in patients with acute acetaminophen overdose and no evident hepatotoxicity, but no other initial laboratory assessment is required. AST concentration should be measured in patients considered to be at risk for APAP toxicity according to the nomogram or history (in the case of repeated supratherapeutic dosing) or in those suspected of already having mild hepatotoxicity by history and physical examination.

Unless evidence of serious hepatotoxicity is present, AST concentration is sufficient indication of hepatic conditions, and no additional testing is initially needed. Death of hepatocytes, resulting in release of measurable hepatic enzymes, precedes all cases of serious liver dysfunction. Even if abnormalities of other markers precede elevation of AST concentration, there is no evidence that their detection benefits the patient.[16] Mild renal toxicity may rarely occur without hepatotoxicity[35]; however, at least minimal elevation of AST concentration generally precedes evidence of clinically significant nephrotoxicity.[1,50] Exceptions are rare,[35,54,142,] and routine screening of renal function in the absence of elevated AST concentration is probably unnecessary.

Acetaminophen overdose may lead to minor prolongation of PT even without causing hepatotoxicity.[321] This most commonly occurs between 4 and 24 hours after ingestion and may be a result of NAPQI-related inhibition of vitamin K–dependent γ-carboxylation of factors II, VII, IX, and X.[292,321] These minor prolongations (resulting in PT that usually is less than twice control) are rarely clinically relevant, are not evidence of hepatotoxicity, and should not be used as prognostic factors or indications for NAC treatment. In fact, treatment with NAC may prolong PT[134,148] by interfering with the PT assay, by reversing an APAP/NAPQI effect,[292] or by direct NAC effects.[292] Clinical interpretation of these minor prolongations of PT is clouded by preexisting conditions, treatment with NAC, and laboratory error. Even in cases in which PT and INR are prolonged, if consequential liver injury does develop, elevation of AST concentration precedes serious liver dysfunction.

Ongoing Monitoring and Testing If no initial elevation of AST concentration is noted, repeated AST determination alone—without other biochemical testing—is sufficient to exclude the development of hepatotoxicity. AST should be determined at the end of the protocol (eg, at 21 hours if using the 21-hour protocol) or every 24 hours if using a longer protocol. If elevated AST concentration is noted, then PT and INR and creatinine concentration should be measured and repeated every 24 hours or more frequently if clinically indicated. Results of other liver tests, such as γ-glutamyltransferase, alkaline phosphatase, lactate dehydrogenase, and bilirubin, which are useful when determining the cause of liver abnormalities, will be abnormal in cases of serious acetaminophen-induced hepatotoxicity but provide little additional useful information if the cause is certain.

If evidence of actual liver failure is noted, then careful monitoring of blood glucose, pH, PT and INR, creatinine, lactate, and phosphate concentrations are important in assessing extrahepatic organ toxicity and are vital in assessing hepatic function and the patient's potential need for transplant (see Assessing Prognosis). In addition, meticulous bedside evaluation is necessary to detect and document vital signs, neurologic status, and evidence of bleeding. Many additional tests may be useful in the setting of liver failure based on clinical condition and local protocols. Testing for other rare acetaminophen-associated conditions by electrocardiography, lipase determination, or other studies should be performed on a case-by-case basis only.

MANAGEMENT

GASTROINTESTINAL DECONTAMINATION

In cases of very early presentation or coingestion of agents that delay gastrointestinal (GI) absorption, gastric emptying may be appropriate for some patients. In general, however, gastric emptying is not a consideration for patients with isolated acetaminophen overdose because of the very rapid GI absorption of acetaminophen and the availability of an effective antidote.

Administration of activated charcoal (AC) shortly after APAP ingestion may decrease the number of patients who have an [APAP] above the treatment line.[45] Although activated charcoal is most effective when given within the first 1 to 2 hours after APAP ingestion, it may be reasonable to consider AC at later times provided there are no contraindications.[283]

Interactions between AC and PO administered NAC are likely clinically unimportant. In the majority of cases, there should be no interaction because GI absorption of APAP, and therefore the necessity to give AC, is complete by 4 hours after ingestion, and NAC typically is administered between 4 and 8 hours after ingestion. As a result, there is generally no difficulty separating the doses.

If delayed or repeated AC dosing is indicated because of suspected delayed absorption or coingestants, then a strategy using an IV NAC protocol should be considered. Alternatively, PO NAC and AC doses may be separated by 1 to 2 hours, with NAC given the priority for the first dose because time to administration of NAC correlates with risk of hepatotoxicity.[270,276] NAC is absorbed high in the GI tract and is not likely to interact with AC if they are not administered simultaneously.

In unusual cases, as a result of coingestants, timing of presentation, and unavailability of IV NAC, PO NAC and AC may be administered simultaneously. Although there is clear in vitro evidence of binding between AC and NAC[57,248,291] and volunteer data suggest that AC causes statistically significant decreases in NAC absorption,[83] there is no evidence that this interaction is clinically significant or that a dose adjustment is necessary.[282]

SUPPORTIVE CARE

General supportive care consists primarily of controlling nausea and vomiting and managing the hepatic injury, renal dysfunction, and other manifestations. Treatment of these problems is based on general principles and is not acetaminophen dependent. Discussion of the management of liver failure is clearly beyond the scope of this chapter, but certain aspects deserve mention. Monitoring for and treatment of hypoglycemia as a result of liver failure are critical because hypoglycemia is one of the most readily treatable of the life-threatening effects of liver failure. If adequate viable hepatocytes are present, vitamin K may produce some improvement in coagulopathy; thus, trial dosing is logical as liver injury develops and as it resolves. Administration of fresh-frozen plasma (FFP) should be based on specific indications rather than PT and INR alone.

One of the most important advances is use of prolonged NAC for treatment of fulminant hepatic failure. Parenteral NAC, other advances in supportive care, and successful liver transplantation programs appear to have substantially improved survival from APAP-related liver failure.[101,174,259]

Antidotal Therapy with N-acetylcysteine

Mechanism of Action of N-acetylcysteine Conceptually, it is helpful to think of NAC as serving three distinct roles. During the metabolism of acetaminophen to NAPQI, NAC *prevents toxicity* by limiting the formation of NAPQI. More importantly, it *increases the capacity to detoxify* NAPQI that is formed (see Fig. 34–1). In fulminant hepatic failure, NAC *treats toxicity* through nonspecific mechanisms that preserve multiorgan function. A complete discussion of NAC can be found in Antidotes in Depth A4: *N*-Acetylcysteine. A brief review follows.

NAC prevents toxicity by serving as a glutathione precursor[157] and as a glutathione substitute, combining with NAPQI, and being converted to cysteine and mercaptate conjugates.[46] NAC may also lead to increased substrate for nontoxic sulfation, allowing less metabolism by oxidation to NAPQI.[271] Each of these preventive mechanisms must be in place early, and none is of benefit after NAPQI has initiated cell injury. Time is required to saturate nontoxic metabolism from excessive NAPQI, deplete GSH, and overcome GSH production; thus there is a window of opportunity after exposure to an APAP overdose during which NAC can be initiated before the onset of liver injury without any loss of efficacy. Based on large clinical trials, it appears that NAC efficacy is nearly complete as long as it is initiated within 6 to 8 hours of an acute overdose.[141,270,276,277] However, the relationship between the time to administration of NAC and the risk of hepatotoxicity should be considered a continuous variable, with the risk of hepatotoxicity beginning to increase at 6 hours for patients with very high [APAP] and closer to 8 hours for patients with [APAP] just over the treatment line.[270,284] For this reason, NAC therapy should not be unnecessarily delayed past 6 hours if it can be safely administered earlier.

Several observations illustrate the effectiveness of NAC by other mechanisms of action even after NAPQI formation and binding. NAC actually reverses NAPQI oxidation in both a mouse model[62] and an in vitro human hepatocyte model,[175] and even after cell injury is initiated, NAC may diminish hepatocyte injury.[43] Most significantly, a prospective, randomized trial found that even after fulminant hepatic failure was evident, starting IV NAC diminished the need for vasopressors and the incidences of cerebral edema and death.[140] In this study, despite improved organ function and survival in the NAC-treated group, there was no apparent difference in the degree of hepatic injury, implying that much of the benefit of NAC in this setting may not be derived from hepatic effects. Whether based on its nonspecific antioxidant effects, its increase in oxygen delivery and utilization,[76,112,136,281,309,310] its ability to enhance glutathione supply, or its role in mediating microvascular tone, NAC improves function in several organs affected by multisystem failure.[64,76,306] In fact, NAC may preserve cerebral blood flow and perfusion in the setting of cerebral edema[319] more effectively than traditional therapies such as mannitol and hyperventilation, which may actually be detrimental.

Although NAC has a defined role in preventing and treating APAP-induced hepatic injury, its role in treating APAP-induced renal injury is less clear. When used early after ingestion in animals, NAC produces a small reduction in renal injury.[195,272] In retrospective reviews of human data, NAC has had little effect on renal injury[82] but does not appear to be harmful.[197] However, little data is available to recommend NAC therapy in treating isolated renal injury or renal injury after resolution of hepatic injury.

N-acetylcysteine administration NAC may be administered via the PO or IV routes and in protocols that vary in length. The two most common regimens are a 21-hour IV infusion and a 72-hour PO dosing protocol. These are described at length in Antidotes in Depth A4: *N*-Acetylcysteine.

With the exception of established liver failure, for which only the IV route has been investigated,[140] the IV and PO routes of NAC are equally efficacious in preventing or treating acetaminophen toxicity.[44,223] The decision to treat with IV or PO dosing is complex and is described in Antidotes in Depth A4: *N*-Acetylcysteine. In brief, whereas IV NAC has been associated with rare but severe anaphylactoid reactions and medication errors.[115] PO NAC is associated with a greater than 50% risk of vomiting. There are three scenarios in which IV NAC is generally recommended: APAP toxicity in pregnant women, APAP-induced liver failure, and intractable vomiting preventing PO treatment.

Duration of N-acetylcysteine Treatment Known mechanisms of action and the observation that all studied durations of NAC are effective when started within 8 hours[44] suggest that all courses of treatment currently published are effective when NAC is used for its early preventive actions. Results from use of the traditional 20-hour IV NAC protocol, the 48- and 36-hour IV NAC protocols studied in the United States,[273] one 20-hour PO protocol,[325] and other "short-course" dosing protocols[24,324] indicate that all therapies are safe and effective in this scenario.[289,326]

It is important to realize that even in low-risk patients (those treated within 8 hours), regardless of the protocol (20, 36, 48, or 72 hour) or formulation of NAC (IV, PO) initiated, that NAC therapy should be continued until APAP metabolism is complete (the [APAP] is below detection) and there are no signs of hepatotoxicity.[85,180] With this concept in mind, it may seem reasonable to *shorten* a set course of NAC if the patient is low risk and the above criteria are met [APAP] undetectable, AST normal, PT/INR normal, and no encephalopathy).[24,68,270] This approach is conceptually reasonable; however, adequate studies have not definitively confirmed its safety.[266,270] For that reason, shortened courses cannot currently be recommended until additional studies are completed.

However, NAC therapy should be continued *beyond* the prescribed protocol length if there is evidence of significant liver injury (AST concentration above normal or INR elevated or encephalopathy is present) or acetaminophen metabolism is incomplete ([APAP] detectable). This likely will not be an issue in the vast majority of cases because the aminotransferases of approximately half of all NAC-treated patients with [APAP] above the treatment line will remain below 100 IU/L.[277] The IV NAC dosing protocol that has proved beneficial in patients with liver failure is the same initial dosing as the 1-hour IV protocol but with the third IV infusion continued until resolution of liver failure. These observations suggest that rather than a single duration of therapy for all patients, it is appropriate to extend treatment protocols based on the clinical course of the patient.[68]

After NAC therapy is extended beyond a set-length protocol, the decision to discontinue therapy should be entirely based on the patient's condition. For patients who develop liver failure, IV NAC is continued until the PT or INR is near normal and encephalopathy, if present, is resolved.[174] For patients without liver failure but with elevated AST concentration, NAC is often continued until all liver abnormalities resolve (AST concentration is decreasing and <1000 IU/L).

Hepatic Transplantation Liver transplantation may increase survival for a select group of severely ill patients who have acetaminophen-induced fulminant hepatic failure.[174,208] Tremendous improvements in transplantation and supportive hepatic care have increased immediate survival rates after hepatic transplantation to 75% to 78% with 3-year survival rates of 56% to 66%.[21,174] Patients who meet criteria for transplant but do not receive an organ have had survival rates ranging from 5% to 17%,[19,20,155,174,187,209] but survival rates have recently been reported as high as 66%.[259]

Concerns that patients who receive transplants for acetaminophen-induced fulminant hepatic failure will have lower survival rates and be unable to maintain posttransplant medication regimens have resulted in the majority of patients not being listed for transplant.[21] However, those who meet psychosocial criteria for transplantation have high rates of survival,[21,174] and only 12% later die from intentional rejection or suicide attempts.[21] Techniques that allow subtotal hepatectomy with transplantation and eventual weaning of immunosuppressants are promising and may allow for higher rates of transplantation.[171]

Assessing Prognosis Determining a patient's prognosis and predicting patients who require transplantation early in the course of the disease is an important area of current research.

The most commonly used indicator of the need for immediate transplantation is the King's College Criteria (KCC), which was developed and validated on patients with acetaminophen-induced fulminant hepatic failure. The criteria include a serum pH below 7.30 after fluid resuscitation or the combination of creatinine above 3.3 mg/dL, PT above 100 seconds (INR > 5 is commonly used), and grade III or IV encephalopathy. The survival rate of patients who meet the KCC but do not receive an organ remains below 20% in most centers.[12,21,209] Significantly higher survival rates in patients meeting transplant criteria have recently been reported and may be due to improved supportive care for patients with acute liver failure.[101,259]

When determining the KCC, interpretation of PT and INR must include awareness of therapy with vitamin K or FFP and/or NAC. The use of vitamin K, if effective, implies that transplant may be unnecessary because viable liver remains. If vitamin K is ineffective, PT and INR can be used as discussed in the previous paragraph. Transfusion of exogenous clotting factors, such as FFP, alters interpretation because improvement in PT and INR may not indicate improvement in liver function. The prognostic importance of monitoring PT and INR in this setting suggests that FFP should be given only with evidence of bleeding, with risk of bleeding from known concomitant trauma, or before invasive procedures and not based merely on the PT and INR value.

A blood lactate concentration above 3.5 mmol/L at a median of 55 hours after APAP ingestion or blood lactate concentration above 3.0 mmol/L after fluid resuscitation are shown to be both sensitive and a specific predictor of patient death without transplant.[20,65] Additional studies confirmed lactate as an independent predictor of prognosis but suggest that it does not add significantly to the KCC .[263] Others have confirmed a lower specificity than initially reported[101,263] and suggested that a higher cutoff (4 mmol/L) may be more specific.[263]

Unfortunately, patients often meet the KCC and lactate criteria quite late in their course of disease, so these criteria are not useful as early predictors or as standards for transfer to a facility that performs hepatic transplant. Several attempts at determining early predictors of death or the need for transplant have proven to be no more effective than the KCC, including serum phosphate (day 2),[19,261] Model for Endstage Liver Disease score,[170,262] serum Gc-globulin,[160,257] factor V concentration,[126,214] Factor VIII:V ratio,[37,214] worsening day 4 PT and INR,[111] and PT (in seconds) larger than the number of hours since ingestion.[204]

An Acute Physiology and Chronic Health Evaluation (APACHE) II score above 15 in isolated APAP ingestions may be as specific as the above KCC criteria and slightly more sensitive.[187] These criteria may be beneficial in determining whether to transfer a patient to a transplant center because the score is easily calculated, is sensitive, and is available within the first day of admission; however, confounders such as coingestants may decrease its utility. Furthermore, an APACHE III score above 60 may be helpful in identifying additional patients with multiorgan dysfunction who may require transplantation.[21]

Several early factors may be useful in identifying patients at high risk of hepatotoxicity but not necessarily patients who require transplantation or who may die. The time from ingestion to the initiation of NAC and serum APAP concentration are directly proportional to the patient's risk of developing hepatotoxicity and hepatic failure.[258,270,276] Using these principles, a nomogram has been produced that may be used to determine the risk of hepatotoxicity on patient arrival. Unfortunately, this only predicts the risk of a peak aminotransferase above 1000 IU/L and has not been studied to determine the risk of death or transplant.

SUMMARY

Several key concepts will help clinicians effectively manage patients with acetaminophen exposures. For patients with intentional overdoses, measurement of [APAP] should be considered part of the initial evaluation. In cases in which risk assessment for acetaminophen toxicity is merited, treatment with NAC should be initiated as soon as possible and ideally within 6-8 hours from the time of ingestion. IV NAC should be preferentially used in cases of fulminant hepatic failure or intractable vomiting and in pregnant patients. Otherwise, the efficacy of the PO and IV formulations should be considered the same. Patients who present after repeated excessive APAP dosing should be assessed for evidence of hepatic injury and for the possibility of ongoing production of NAPQI. Factors that potentially predispose patients to hepatotoxicity after repeated dosing should be taken into account when deciding which patients to assess further for hepatic injury.

Patients showing evidence of severe hepatotoxicity or hepatic encephalopathy and those at risk for fulminant hepatic failure may require admittance to the ICU. All of these patients require frequent neurologic checks, monitoring of vital signs, and additional and repeated laboratory studies. Consultations with a regional poison center, gastroenterologist (or hepatologist) consultant, and regional transplant center are important to guide treatment strategies and to coordinate transplantation when needed. Early psychiatric consultation may be helpful in assessing transplant eligibility. Absolute indications for transplantation vary and should be discussed early with the appropriate local transplant center, poison control center, medical toxicologist(s) and hepatologist(s).

Although our understanding of acetaminophen toxicity has advanced significantly and additional therapeutic modalities (primarily IV NAC) have become more widely available, many important challenges remain. Development of an entirely new method of toxicity screening to accurately determine the risk of toxicity in atypical patients, high-risk patients, and those who present after repeated excessive dosing of APAP is needed. Ongoing study of antidotal therapy dosing protocols is needed to assess the validity of many assumptions. Most importantly, improved methods to determine the indication for liver transplantation early after APAP ingestion are desperately needed. These and other issues predict that further changes are likely. Hopefully, the principles and current strategies presented in this chapter will serve as a strong foundation for these important future advances.

ACKNOWLEDGMENT

Martin J. Smilkstein and Kenneth Bizovi contributed to this chapter in previous editions.

REFERENCES

1. Akca S, Suleymanlar I, Tuncer M, et al. Isolated acute renal failure due to paracetamol intoxication in an alcoholic patient. *Nephron.* 1999;83:270-271.
2. Alloui A, Chassaing C, Schmidt J, et al. Paracetamol exerts a spinal, tropisetron-reversible, antinociceptive effect in an inflammatory pain model in rats. *Eur J Pharmacol.* 2002;443:71-77.
3. Altomare E, Vendemiale G, Trizio T, Albano O. Does acute ethanol really protect against acetaminophen hepatotoxicity? *Am J Gastroenterol.* 1986;81(1):91-92.
4. Ameer B, Divoll M, Abernethy D, et al. Absolute and relative bioavailability of oral acetaminophen preparations. *J Pharm Sci.* 1983;72:955-958.
5. American Academy of Pediatrics. Acetaminophen toxicity in children. *Pediatrics.* 2001;108:1020-1024.
6. Anderson BJ, Holford NHG, Armishaw JC, et al. Predicting concentrations in children presenting with acetaminophen overdose. *J Pediatr.* 1999;135:290-295.
7. Andreasen PB, Hutter L. Paracetamol (acetaminophen) clearance in patients with cirrhosis of the liver. *Acta Med Scand.* 1979;624:99-105.
8. Aronoff D, Neilson E. Antipyretics: mechanism of action and clinical use in fever suppression. *Am J Med.* 2001;111:304-315.
9. Aronoff DM, Oates JA, Boutaud O. New insights into the mechanism of action of acetaminophen: its clinical pharmacologic characteristics reflect its inhibition of the two prostaglandin H2 synthases. *Clin Pharmacol Ther.* 2006;79:9-19.
10. Ashbourne JF, Olson KR, Khayam-Bashi H. Value of rapid screening for acetaminophen in all patients with intentional drug overdose. *Ann Emerg Med.* 1989;18:1035-1038.
11. Aw MM, Dhawan A, Baker AJ, Mieli-Vergani G. Neonatal paracetamol poisoning. *Arch Dis Child Fetal Neonatal Ed.* 1999;81:F78.
12. Bailey B, Amre DK, Gaudreault P. Fulminant hepatic failure secondary to acetaminophen poisoning: a systematic review and meta-analysis of prognostic criteria determining the need for liver transplantation. *Crit Care Med.* 2003;31:299-305.
13. Banda PW, Quart BD. The effect of mild alcohol consumption on the metabolism of acetaminophen in man. *Res Comm Chem Path Pharm.* 1982;38:57-70.
14. Bartels S, Sivilotti M, Crosby D, Richard J. Are recommended doses of acetaminophen hepatotoxic for recently abstinent alcoholics? A randomized trial. *Clin Toxicol.* 2008;46:243-249.
15. Beck DH, Schenk MR, Hagemann K, Doepfmer UR, Kox WJ. The pharmacokinetics and analgesic efficacy of larger dose rectal acetaminophen (40 mg/kg) in adults: a double-blinded, randomized study. *Anesth Analg.* 2000;90:431-436.
16. Beckett GJ, Donovan JW, Hussey AJ, et al. Intravenous N-acetylcysteine, hepatotoxicity and plasma glutathione S-transferase in patients with paracetamol overdosage. *Hum Exp Toxicol.* 1990;9:183-186.
17. Beer C, Pakravan N, Hudson M, et al. Liver unit admission following paracetamol overdose with concentrations below current UK treatment thresholds. *Q J Med.* 2007:100;93-96.
18. Bender RP, Lindsey RH, Jr, Burden DA, Osheroff N. N-acetyl-benzoquinone imine, the toxic metabolite of acetaminophen, is a topoisomerase poison II. *Biochemistry.* 2004;43:3731-3739.
19. Bernal W, Wendon J. More on serum phosphate and prognosis of acute liver failure. *Hepatology.* 2003;38:533-534.
20. Bernal W, Donaldson N, Wyncoll D, Wendon J. Blood lactate as an early predictor of outcome in paracetamol-induced acute liver failure: a cohort study. *Lancet.* 2002;359:558-563.
21. Bernal W, Wendon J, Rela M, et al. Use and outcome of liver transplantation in acetaminophen-induced acute liver failure. *Hepatology.* 1998;27:1050-1055.
22. Bertolini A, Ferrari A, Ottani A, et al. Paracetamol: new vistas of an old drug. *CNS Drug Rev.* 2006;12:250-275.
23. Bessems JGM, Vermeulen NPE. Paracetamol (acetaminophen-)-induced toxicity: molecular and biochemical mechanisms, analogues and protective approaches. *Crit Rev Toxicol.* 2001;31:55-138.
24. Betten DP, Cantrell FL, Thomas SC, et al. A prospective evaluation of shortened course oral N-acetylcysteine for the treatment of acute acetaminophen poisoning. *Ann Emerg Med.* 2007;50:272-279.
25. Beyer RP, Fry RC, Lasarev MR, et al. Multicenter study of acetaminophen hepatotoxicity reveals the importance of biological endpoints in genomic analyses. *Toxicol Sci.* 2007;99:326-337.
26. Bien E, Vick K, Skorka G. Effects of exogenous factors on the cerebral glutathione in rodents. *Arch Toxicol.* 1992;66:279-285.
27. Birge RB, Bartolone JB, Hart SG, et al. Acetaminophen hepatotoxicity: correspondence of selective protein arylation in human and mouse liver in vitro, in culture, and in vivo. *Toxicol Appl Pharmacol.* 1990;105: 472-482.
28. Birmingham PK, Tobin MJ, Henthorn TK, et al. Twenty-four-hour pharmacokinetics of rectal acetaminophen in children: an old drug with new recommendations. *Anesthesiology.* 1997;87:244-252.
29. Blouin RA, Dickson P, McNamara PJ, et al. Phenobarbital induction and acetaminophen hepatotoxicity: resistance in the obese Zucker rodent. *J Pharmacol Exp Ther.* 1987;243:565-570.
30. Bond G. Reduced toxicity of acetaminophen in children: it's the liver. *J Toxicol Clin Toxicol.* 2004;42:149-152.
31. Bond GR, Krenzelok EP, Normann SA, et al. Acetaminophen ingestion in childhood: cost and relative risk of alternative referral strategies. *J Toxicol Clin Toxicol.* 1994;32:513-525.
32. Bonnefont J, Alloui A, Chapuy E, et al. Orally administered paracetamol does not act locally in the rat formalin test: evidence for a supraspinal, serotonin-dependent antinociceptive mechanism. *Anesthesiology.* 2003;99:976-981.
33. Bourdeaux C, Bewley J. Death from paracetamol overdose despite appropriate treatment with N-acetylcysteine. *Emerg Med J.* 2007;24:e31
34. Boutaud O, Aronoff D, Richardson J, et al. Determinants of the cellular specificity of acetaminophen as an inhibitor of prostaglandin H(2) synthases. *Proc Natl Acad Sci U S A.* 2002;99:7130-7135.
35. Boutis K, Shannon M. Nephrotoxicity after acute severe acetaminophen poisoning in adolescents. *J Toxicol Clin Toxicol.* 2001;39:441-445.
36. Brackett CC, Bloch JD. Phenytoin as a possible cause of acetaminophen hepatotoxicity: case report and review of the literature. *Pharmacotherapy.* 2000;20:229-233.
37. Bradberry SM, Hart M, Bareford D, et al. Factor V and Factor VII:V ratio as prognostic indicators in paracetamol poison. *Lancet.* 1995;1:646-647.
38. Bradley JD, Brandt KD, Katz BP, et al. Comparison of an antiinflammatory dose of ibuprofen, an analgesic dose of ibuprofen, and acetaminophen in the treatment of patients with osteoarthritis of the knee. *N Engl J Med.* 1991;325:87-91.
39. Bray GP, Harrison PM, O'Grady JG, et al. Long-term anticonvulsant therapy worsens outcome in paracetamol-induced fulminant hepatic failure. *Hum Exp Toxicol.* 1992;11:265-270.
40. Breen K, Wandscheer JC, Peignoux M, Pessayre D. In situ formation of the acetaminophen metabolite covalently bound in kidneys and lung: supportive evidence provided by total hepatectomy. *Biochem Pharmacol.* 1982, 31:115-116.
41. Bridger S, Henserson K, Glucksman E, et al. Lesson of the week: deaths from low dose paracetamol poisoning. *Br Med J.* 1998;316:1724-1725.
42. Brooker G, Jeffery J, Nataraj T, et al. High anion gap metabolic acidosis secondary to pyroglutamic aciduria (5-oxoprolinuria): association with prescription drugs and malnutrition. *Ann Clin Biochem.* 2007;44: 406-409.

43. Bruno MK, Cohen S, Khairallah EA. Antidotal effectiveness of N-acetylcysteine in reversing acetaminophen-induced hepatotoxicity: Enhancement of the proteolysis of arylated proteins. *Biochem Pharmacol.* 1988;37:4319-4325.
44. Buckley NA, Whyte IM, O'Connell DL, Dawson AH. Oral or intravenous N-acetylcysteine: which is the treatment of choice for acetaminophen (paracetamol) poisoning. *J Toxicol Clin Toxicol.* 1999;37:759-767.
45. Buckley NA, Whyte IM, O'Connell DL. Activated charcoal reduces the need for N-Acetylcysteine treatment after acetaminophen (paracetamol) overdose. *J Toxicol Clin Toxicol.* 1999;37:753-757.
46. Buckpitt AR, Rollins DE, Mitchell JR. Varying effects of sulfhydryl nucleophiles on acetaminophen oxidation and sulfhydryl adduct formation. *Biochem Pharmacol.* 1979;28:2941-2946.
47. Bujalska M. Effect of nonselective and selective opioid receptors antagonists on antinociceptive action of acetaminophen. *Pol J Pharmacol.* 2004;56:539-545.
48. Burcham PC, Harman AW. Acetaminophen toxicity results in site specific mitochondrial damage in isolated mouse hepatocytes. *J Biol Chem.* 1991;266:5049-5054.
49. Calvert LJ, Linder CW. Acetaminophen poisoning. *J Fam Pract.* 1978;7: 953-956.
50. Campbell NR, Baylis B. Renal impairment associated with an acute paracetamol overdose in the absence of hepatotoxicity. *Postgrad Med J.* 1992;68:116-118.
51. Caravati EM. Unintentional acetaminophen ingestion in children and the potential for hepatotoxicity. *Clin Toxicol.* 2000;38:291-296.
52. Carpenter HM, Mudge GH. Acetaminophen nephrotoxicity: studies on renal acetylation and deacetylation. *J Pharmacol Exp Ther.* 1981;218: 161-167.
53. Catella-Lawson F, Reilly MP, Kapoor SC, et al. Cyclooxygenase inhibitors and the antiplatelet effects of aspirin. *N Engl J Med.* 2001;345:1809-1817.
54. Cerretani D, Micheli L, Fiaschi AI, et al. MK-801 potentiates the glutathione depletion induced by acetaminophen in rat brain. *Curr Ther Res.* 1994;55:707-717.
55. Cetaruk EW, Dart RC, Hurlbut KM, et al. Tylenol Extended Relief overdose. *Ann Emerg Med.* 1997;30:104-108.
56. Cheung L, Potts R, Meyer K. Acetaminophen treatment nomogram. *N Engl J Med.* 1994;330:1907-1908.
57. Chinouth RW, Czajka PA, Peterson RG. N-acetylcysteine absorption by activated charcoal. *Vet Hum Toxicol.* 1980;22:392-394.
58. Cho M, Kim Y, Kim S, Lee MG. Suppression of rat hepatic cytochrome P450s by protein-calorie malnutrition: complete or partial restoration by cysteine or methionine supplementation. *Arch Biochem Biophys.* 1999;372:150-158.
59. Clark JH, Russell GJ, Fitzgerald JF. Fatal acetaminophen toxicity in a 2-year-old. *J Indiana State Med Assoc.* 1983;76:832-835.
60. Cobden I, Record CO, Ward MK, Derr DNS. Paracetamol-induced acute renal failure in the absence of fulminant liver damage. *Br Med J.* 1982;284:21-22.
61. Cohen SD, Khairallah EA. Selective protein arylation and acetaminophen-induced hepatotoxicity. *Drug Metab Rev.* 1997;29:59-77.
62. Corcoran GB, Mitchell JR, Vaishnav YN, Horning EC. Evidence that acetaminophen and N-hydroxyacetaminophen form a common arylating intermediate, N-acetyl-p-benzoquinoneimine. *Mol Pharmacol.* 1980;18:536-542.
63. Cover C, Liu J, Farhood A, et al. Pathophysiological role of the acute inflammatory response during acetaminophen hepatotoxicity. *Toxicol Appl Pharmacol.* 2006;216:98-107.
64. Cuzzocrea S, Constantino G, Mazzon E, Caputi AP. Protective effect of N-acetylcysteine on multiple organ failure induced by zymosan in the rat. *Crit Care Med.* 1999;27:1524-1532.
65. Dabos KJ, Newsome PN, Parkinson JA, et al. A biochemical prognostic model of outcome in paracetamol-induced acute liver injury. *Transplantation.* 2005;80:1712-1717.
66. Daly FF, O'Malley GF, Heard K, et al. Prospective evaluation of repeated supratherapeutic acetaminophen (paracetamol) ingestion. *Ann Emerg Med.* 2004;44:393-398.
67. Dani M, Guindon J, Lambert C, Beaulieu P. The local antinociceptive effects of paracetamol in neuropathic pain are mediated by cannabinoid receptors. *Eur J Pharm.* 2007;573:214-215.
68. Dart RC, Rumack BH. Patient-tailored acetylcysteine administration. *Ann Emerg Med.* 2007;50:280-281.
69. Dart RC, Erdman AR, Olson KR, et al. Acetaminophen poisoning: an evidence-based consensus guideline for out-of-hospital management. *Clin Toxicol.* 2006;44:1-18.
70. Dart RC, Green JL, Bogdan GM. The safety profile of sustained release paracetamol during therapeutic use and following overdose. *Drug Saf.* 2005;28:1045-1056.
71. Davern TJ, James LP, Hinson JA, et al. Measurement of serum acetaminophen-protein adducts in patients with acute liver failure. *Gastroenterology.* 2006;130:687-694.
72. Davie A. Acetaminophen poisoning and liver function [letter]. *N Engl J Med.* 1994;331:1311.
73. Davis M, Simmons CJ, Harrison NG, Williams R. Paracetamol overdose in man: relationship between pattern of urinary metabolites and severity of liver damage. *Q J Med.* 1976;45:181-191.
74. Day A, Abbott GD. Chronic paracetamol poisoning in children: a warning to health professionals. *NZ Med J.* 1994;107:201.
75. Devalia JL, Ogilvie RC, McLean AEM. Dissociation of cell death from covalent binding of paracetamol by flavones in a hepatocyte system. *Biochem Pharmacol.* 1982;31:3745-3749.
76. Devlin J, Ellis AE, McPeake J, et al. N-acetylcysteine improves indocyanine green extraction and oxygen transport during hepatic dysfunction. *Crit Care Med.* 1997;25:236-242.
77. Divoll M, Greenblatt DJ, Ameer B, Abernathy DR. Effect of food on acetaminophen absorption in young and elderly subjects. *J Clin Pharmacol.* 1982;22:571-576.
78. Donnelly PG, Walker RN, Racz WJ. Inhibition of mitochondrial respiration in vivo is an early event in acetaminophen-induced hepatotoxicity. *Arch Toxicol.* 1994;68:110-118.
79. Douglas DR, Sholar JB, Smilkstein MJ: A pharmacokinetic comparison of acetaminophen products (Tylenol Extended Relief vs regular Tylenol). *Acad Emerg Med.* 1996;3:740-744.
80. Douidar SM, Al-Khalil I, Habersang RW. Severe hepatotoxicity, acute renal failure, and pancytopenia in a young child after repeated acetaminophen overdosing. *Clin Pediatr.* 1994;33:42-45.
81. Douidar SM, Ahmed AE. A novel mechanism for the enhancement of acetaminophen hepatotoxicity by phenobarbital. *J Pharmacol Exp Ther.* 1987;240:578-583.
82. Eguia L, Materson BJ. Acetaminophen-related acute renal failure without fulminant liver failure. *Pharmacotherapy.* 21997;17:363-370.
83. Ekins B, Ford DC, Thompson MIB, et al. The effect of activated charcoal on N-acetylcysteine absorption in normal subjects. *Am J Emerg Med.* 1987;5:483-487.
84. Emeigh Hart SG, Beierschmitt WP, Wyand DS, Khairallah EA, Cohen SD. Acetaminophen nephrotoxicity in CD-1 mice. I. Evidence of a role for in situ activation in selective covalent binding and toxicity. *Toxicol Appl Pharmacol.* 1994;126:267-275.
85. Emeigh Hart SG, Beierschmitt WP, Bartolone JB, et al. Evidence against deacetylation and for cytochrome P450-mediated activation in acetaminophen-induced nephrotoxicity in the CD-1 mouse. *Toxicol Appl Pharmacol.* 1991;107:1-15.
86. Emeigh Hart SG, Birge RB, Cartun RW, et al. In vivo and in vitro evidence for situ activation and selective covalent binding of acetaminophen (APAP) in mouse kidney. *Adv Exp Med Biol.* 1991;283:711-716.
87. Epstein MM, Nelson SD, Slatterly JT, et al. Inhibition of the metabolism of paracetamol by isoniazid. *Br J Clin Pharmacol.* 1991;31:139-142.
88. Esterline RL, Ji S. Metabolic alterations resulting from the inhibition of mitochondrial respiration by acetaminophen in vivo. *Biochem Pharmacol.* 1989;38:2390-2392.
89. Feldberg W, Gupta K. Pyrogen fever and prostaglandin-like activity in cerebrospinal fluid. *J Physiol.* 1973;228:41-53.
90. Fenves AZ, Kirkpatrick HM, Patel VV, et al. Increased anion gap metabolic acidosis as a result of 5-oxoproline (pyrogluatamic acid): a role for acetaminophen. *Clin J Am Soc Nephrol.* 2006;1:441-447.
91. Flanagan RJ, Mant TGK. Coma and metabolic acidosis early in severe acute paracetamol poisoning. *Hum Toxicol.* 1986;5:256-259.
92. Flower R, Vane J. Inhibition of prostaglandin synthetase in brain explains the anti-pyretic activity of paracetamol (4-acetamidophenol). *Nature.* 1972;240:410-411.
93. Flouvat B, Leneveu A, Fitoussi S, et al. Bioequivalence study comparing a new paracetamol solution for injection and propacetamol after single intravenous infusion in healthy subjects. *Int J Clin Pharm Ther.* 2004;42(1):50-57.

94. Fored CM, Ejerblad E, Lindblad P, et al. Acetaminophen, aspirin, and chronic renal failure. *N Engl J Med.* 2001;345:1801-1808.
95. Forrest JAH, Clements JA, Prescott LF. Clinical pharmacokinetics of paracetamol. *Clin Pharm.* 1982;7:93-107.
96. Geba GP, Weaver AL, Polis AB, et al. Efficacy of rofecoxib, celecoxib, and acetaminophen in osteoarthritis of the knee: a randomized trial. *JAMA.* 2002;287:64-71.
97. Gelotte CK, Auiler JF, Temple AR, et al. Clinical features of a repeat dose multiple-day pharmacokinetics trial of acetaminophen at 4, 6, and 8g/day. *J Toxicol Clin Toxicol.* 2003;41:726.
98. Gerber JG, MacDonald JS, Harbison RD, et al. Effect of N-acetylcysteine on hepatic covalent binding of paracetamol (acetaminophen). *Lancet.* 1977;1:657-658.
99. Godber IM, Jarvis SJ, Maguire D. Hypokalaemia following paracetamol overdose in two teenage girls. *Ann Clin Biochem.* 2007;44:403-405.
100. Godfrey L, Morselli A, Bennion P, et al. An investigation of binding sites for paracetamol in the mouse brain and spinal cord. *Eur J Pharm.* 2005;508:99-106.
101. Gow PJ, Warrilow S, Lontos S, et al. Time to review the selection criteria for transplantation in paracetamol-induced fulminant hepatic failure? *Liver Transplant.* 2007;13:1762-1763.
102. Graham GG, Kieran FS. Mechanism of action of paracetamol. *Am J Ther.* 2005;12:46-55.
103. Gray TA, Buckley BM, Vale JA. Hyperlactataemia and metabolic acidosis following paracetamol overdose. *Q J Med.* 1987;65:811-821.
104. Gregoire N, Hovsepian L, Gualano V, et al. Safety and pharmacokinetics of paracetamol following intravenous administration of 5g during the first 24 h with a 2-g starting dose. *Clin Pharm Ther.* 2007;81:401-405.
105. Grypioti AD, Kostopanagiotou G, Mykoniatis M. Platelet-activating factor inactivator (rPAF-AH) enhances liver's recovery after paracetamol intoxication. *Dig Dis Sci.* 2007;52:2580-2590.
106. Gujral JS, Knight TR, Farhood A, et al. Mode of cell death after acetaminophen overdose in mice: apoptosis or oncotic necrosis? *Toxicol Sci.* 2002;67:322-328.
107. Hahn TW, Henneberg SW, Holm-Knudsen RJ, et al. Pharmacokinetics of rectal paracetamol after repeated dosing in children. *Br J Anaesth.* 2000;85:512-519.
108. Halcomb S, Sivilotti M, Goklaney A, Mullins ME. Pharmacokinetic effects of diphenhydramine or oxycodone in simulated acetaminophen overdose. *Acad Emerg Med.* 2005;12:169-172.
109. Haller VL, Cichewicz DL, Welch SP. Non-cannabinoid CB1, non-cannabinoid CB2 antinociceptive effects of several novel compounds in the PPQ stretch test in mice. *Eur J Pharm.* 2006:546;60-68.
110. Hanel AM, Lands WE. Modification of anti-inflammatory drug effectiveness by ambient lipid peroxides. *Biochem Pharmacol.* 1982;31:3307-3311.
111. Harrison PM, O'Grady JG, Keays RT, et al. Serial prothrombin time as prognostic indicator in paracetamol induced fulminant hepatic failure. *Br Med J.* 1990;310:964-966.
112. Harrison PM, Wendon JA, Gimson AES, et al. Improvement by acetylcysteine of hemodynamics and oxygen transport in fulminant hepatic failure. *N Engl J Med.* 1991;324:1852-1857.
113. Hart SG, Beierschmitt WP, Wyand DS, et al. Acetaminophen nephrotoxicity in CD-1 mice. Evidence of a role for in situ activation in selective covalent binding and toxicity. *Toxicol Appl Pharmacol.* 1994;126:216-275.
114. Harvison PJ, Egan RW, Gale PH, et al. Acetaminophen and analogs as cosubstrates and inhibitors of prostaglandin H synthase. *Chem Biol Interactions.* 1988;64:251-266.
115. Hayes BD, Klein-Schwartz W, Doyon S. Frequency of medication errors with intravenous acetylcysteine for acetaminophen overdose. *Ann Pharmacother.* 2008;42:766-770.
116. Hazai E, Vereczkey L, Monostory K. Reduction of toxic metabolite formation of acetaminophen. *Biochem Biophys Res Commun.* 2002;291:1089-1094.
117. Heard K, Green JL, Bailey JE, et al. A randomized trial to determine the change in alanine aminotransferase during 10 days of paracetamol (acetaminophen) administration in subjects who consume moderate amounts of alcohol. *Aliment Pharmacol Ther.* 2007;26:283-290.
118. Henretig FM, Selbst SM, Forrect C, et al. Repeated acetaminophen overdosing: causing hepatotoxicity in children. *Clin Pediatr.* 1989;28:267-275.
119. Heubi JE, Barbacci MB, Zimmerman HJ. Therapeutic misadventures with acetaminophen: hepatoxicity after multiple doses in children. *J Pediatr.* 1998;132:22-27.
120. Hinson JA, Pike SL, Pumford NR, Mayeux PR. Nitrotyrosine-protein adducts in hepatic centrilobular areas following toxic doses of acetaminophen in mice. *Chem Res Toxicol.* 1998;11:604-607.
121. Hinz B, Cheremina O, Brune K. Acetaminophen (paracetamol) is a selective cyclooxygenase-2 inhibitor in man. *FASEB J.* 2007;22:383-390.
122. Hodgman MJ, Horn JF, Stork CM, et al. Profound metabolic acidosis and oxoprolinuria in an adult. *J Med Toxicol.* 2007;3:119-124.
123. Hogestatt ED, Jonsson BAG, Ermund A, et al. Conversion of acetaminophen to the bioactive N-acylphenolamine AM404 via fatty acid amide hydrolase-dependent arachidonic acid conjugation in the nervous system. *J Biol Chem.* 2006;280:31405-31412.
124. Hoivik DJ, Manautou JE, Tviet A, et al. Gender-related differences in susceptibility to acetaminophen-induced protein arylation and nephrotoxicity on the CD-1 mouse. *Toxicol Appl Pharmacol.* 1995;130:257-271.
125. Ishida Y, Kondo T, Kimura A, et al. Opposite roles of neutrophils and macrophages in the pathogenesis of acetaminophen-induced acute liver injury. *Eur J Immunol.* 2006;36:1028-1038.
126. Izumi S, Langley PG, Wendon J, et al. Coagulation factor V levels as a prognostic indicator in fulminant hepatic failure. *Hepatology.* 1996;23:1507-1511.
127. Jaeschke H. How relevant are neutrophils for acetaminophen hepatotoxicity? *Hepatology.* 2006;43:1191-1194.
128. Jaeschke H, Bajt ML. Intracellular signaling mechanisms of acetaminophen-induced liver cell death. *Toxicol Sci.* 2006;89:31-41.
129. Jaeschke H, Liu J. Neutrophil depletion protects against murine acetaminophen hepatotoxicity: another perspective. *Hepatology.* 2007;45:1588-1589.
130. Jaeschke H, Smith SW. Role of neutrophils in acetaminophen induced liver injury. *Toxicologist.* 1991;11:32.
131. James LP, Alonso EM, Hynan LS. Detection of acetaminophen protein adducts in children with acute liver failure of indetermined cause. *Pediatrics.* 2006;118:e676-e681.
132. James L, Simpson PM, Farrar HC, et al. Cytokines and toxicity in acetaminophen overdose. *J Clin Pharm.* 2005;45:1165-1171.
133. James LP, McCullough SS, Lamps LW, Hinson JA. Effect of Nacetylcysteine on acetaminophen toxicity in mice: relationship to reactive nitrogen and cytokine formation. *Toxicol Sci.* 2003;75:458-467.
134. Jepsen S, Hansen AB. The influence of N-acetylcysteine on the measurement of prothrombin time and activated partial thromboplastin time in healthy subjects. *Scand J Clin Lab Invest.* 1994;54:543-547.
135. Jollow DJ, Mitchell JR, Potter WZ, et al. Acetaminophen-induced hepatic necrosis. II. Role of covalent binding in vivo. *J Pharmacol Exp Ther.* 1973;187:195-202.
136. Jones AL. Mechanism of action and value of N-acetylcysteine in the treatment of early and late acetaminophen poisoning: a critical review. *J Toxicol Clin Toxicol.* 1998;36:277-285.
137. Josephy PD. The molecular toxicology of acetaminophen. *Drug Metab Rev.* 2005;37:581-594.
138. Karthein R, Dietz R, Nastainczyk W, Ruf HH. Higher oxidation states of prostaglandin H synthase. EPR study of a transient tyrosyl radical in the enzyme during the peroxidase reaction with prostaglandin G2. *Eur J Biochem.* 1988;171:321-328.
139. Kearns GL, Leeder JS, Wasserman GS. Acetaminophen intoxication during treatment: what you don't know can hurt you. *Clin Pediatr.* 2000;39:133-144.
140. Keays R, Harrison PM, Wendon JA, et al. Intravenous acetylcysteine in paracetamol induced fulminant hepatic failure: a prospective controlled trial. *Br Med J.* 1991;303:1026-1029.
141. Kerr F, Dawson A, Whyte I, et al. The Australasian Clinical Toxicology Investigators Collaboration randomized trial of different loading infusion rates of N-acetylcysteine. *Ann Emerg Med.* 2005;45:402-408.
142. Kher K, Makker S. Acute renal failure due to acetaminophen ingestion without concurrent hepatotoxicity. *Am J Med.* 1987;82:1280-1281.
143. Kim Y, Kim S, Kwon J, et al. Effects of cysteine on amino acid concentrations and transsulfuration enzyme activities in rat liver with protein-calorie malnutrition. *Life Sci.* 2003;72:1171-1181.
144. Knight TR, Kurtz A, Bajt ML, Hinson JA, Jaeschke H. Vascular and hepatocellular peroxynitrite formation during acetaminophen-induced liver injury: role of mitochondrial oxidant stress. *Toxicol Sci.* 2001;62:212-220.
145. Kobrinsky NO, Hartfield D, Horner H, et al. Treatment of advanced malignancies with high-dose acetaminophen. *Cancer Invest.* 1996;14:202-210.
146. Kociancic T, Reed M: Acetaminophen intoxication and length of treatment: how long is long enough? *Pharmacotherapy.* 2003;23:1052-1059.

147. Kostrubsky SE, Sinclair JF, Strom SC, et al. Phenobarbital and phenytoin increased acetaminophen hepatotoxicity due to inhibition of UDP-glucuronosyltransferases in cultured human hepatocytes. *Toxicol Sci.* 2005;87:146-155.
148. Koterba AP, Smolen S, Joseph A, et al. Coagulation protein function. II. Influence of thiols upon acetaldehyde effects. *Alcohol.* 1995;12:49-57.
149. Koulouris Z, Tierney MG, Jones G. Metabolic acidosis and coma following a severe acetaminophen overdose. *Ann Pharmacother.* 1999;33:1191-1194.
150. Kozer E, Hahn Y, Berkovitch M, et al. The association between acetaminophen concentration in the cerebrospinal fluids and temperature decline in febrile infants. *Ther Drug Monit.* 2007;29:819-823.
151. Kuffner EK, Green JL, Bogdan GM, et al. The effect of acetaminophen (four grams a day for three consecutive days) on hepatic test in alcoholic patients—a multicenter randomized study. *BMC Med.* 2007;5:13-22.
152. Kuffner EK, Temple AR, Cooper KM, et al. Retrospective analysis of transient elevations in alanine aminotransferase during long-term treatment with acetaminophen in osteoarthritis clinical trials. *Curr Med Res Opin.* 2006;22:2137-2148.
153. Kuffner EK, Dart RC, Bogdan GM, et al. Effect of maximal daily doses of acetaminophen on the liver of alcoholic patients: a randomized, double-blind, placebo-controlled trial. *Arch Intern Med.* 2001;161:2247-2252.
154. Larson AM. Acetaminophen hepatotoxicity. *Clin Liver Dis.* 2007:11;525-548.
155. Larson AM, Polson J, Fontana RJ, et al. Acetaminophen-induced acute liver failure: results of a United States multicenter, prospective study. *Hepatology.* 2005:42;1364-1372.
156. Laskin DL, Gardner CR, Price VF, Jollow DJ. Modulation of macrophage functioning abrogates the acute hepatotoxicity of acetaminophen. *Hepatology.* 1995;21:1045-1050.
157. Lauterburg BH, Corcoran GB, Mitchell JR: Mechanism of action of N-acetylcysteine in the protection against hepatotoxicity of acetaminophen in rats in vivo. *J Clin Invest.* 1983;71:980-991.
158. Lauterburg BH, Velez ME: Glutathione deficiency in alcoholics: risk factor for paracetamol hepatotoxicity. *Gut.* 1988;29:1153-1157.
159. Lawson JA, Farhood A, Hopper RD, et al. The hepatic inflammatory response after acetaminophen overdose: role of neutrophils. *Toxicol Sci.* 2000;54:509-516.
160. Lee WH, Galbraith RM, Watt GH, et al. Predicting survival in fulminant hepatic failure using serum Gc protein concentrations. *Hepatology.* 1995;21:101-105.
161. Lee WM. Acetaminophen toxicity: changing perceptions on a social/medical issue. *Hepatology.* 2007(a);46:966-970
162. Lee WM. Acute liver failure. *N Engl J Med.* 1993;329:135-138.
163. Lee WH, Kramer WG, Granville GE. The effect of obesity on acetaminophen pharmacokinetics in man. *J Clin Pharmacol.* 1981;21:284-287.
164. Lee YS, Kim H, Brahim JS, et al. Acetaminophen selectively suppresses peripheral prostaglandin E2 release and increases COX-2 gene expression in a clinical model of acute inflammation. *Pain.* 2007;129:279-286.
165. Leibowitz J, Huhn JA. Acetaminophen overdosage, a case presentation and review of current therapy. *Del Med J.* 1980;52:135-138.
166. Lesna M, Watson AJ, Douglas AP, et al. Evaluation of paracetamol-induced damage in liver biopsies. *Virchows Arch Pathol.* 1976;370:333-344.
167. Levy G, Garrettson L, Soda D. Evidence of placental transfer of acetaminophen [letter]. *Pediatrics.* 1974;55:895.
168. Li S, Wang Y, Matsumura K, et al. The febrile response to lipopolysaccharide is blocked in cyclooxygenase-2, -/- , but not in cyclooxygenase-1, -/- mice. *Brain Res.* 1999;825:86-94.
169. Liu ZX, Han D, Guanawan B, Kaplowitz N. Neutrophil depletion protects against murine acetaminophen hepatotoxicity. *Hepatology.* 2006;43:1220-1230.
170. Llado L, Figueras J, Memba R, et al. Is MELD really the definitive score for liver allocation? *Liver Transpl.* 2002;8:795-798.
171. Lodge JPA, Dasgupta D, Prasad KR, et al. Emergency subtotal hepatectomy: a new concept for acetaminophen-induced acute liver failure: temporary hepatic support by auxiliary orthotopic liver transplantation enables long-term success. *Ann Surg.* 2008;247:238-249.
172. Lucanie R, Chiange WK, Reilly R. Utility of acetaminophen screening in unsuspected suicidal ingestions. *Vet Hum Toxicol.* 2002;44:171-173.
173. Lucas R, Warner TD, Vojnovic I, Mitchell JA. Cellular mechanisms of acetaminophen: role of cyclooxygenase. *FASEB J.* 2005;19:635-637.
174. Makin AJ, Wendon J, Williams R. A 7-year experience of severe acetaminophen-induced hepatotoxicity (1987–1993). *Gastroenterology.* 1995;109:1907-1916.
175. Manov I, Hirsh M, Iancu TC. N-acetylcysteine does not protect HepG2 cells against acetaminophen-induced apoptosis. *Basic Clin Pharmacol Toxicol.* 2004;94:213-225.
176. Manyike PT, Kharasch ED, Kalhorn TF, Slattery JT. Contribution of CYP2E1 and CYP3A to acetaminophen reactive metabolite formation. *Clin Pharmacol Ther.* 2000;67:275-282.
177. Markey CM, Alward A, Weller PE, Marnett LJ. Quantitative studies of hydroperoxide reduction by prostaglandin H synthase. *J Biol Chem.* 1987;13:6266-6279.
178. Mathew J, Hines JE, James OFW, Burt AD. Non-parenchymal cell responses in paracetamol (acetaminophen)-induced liver injury. *J Hepatol.* 1994;20:537-541.
179. Mathis RD, Walker JS, Kuhns DW. Subacute acetaminophen overdose after incremental dosing. *J Emerg Med.* 1988;6:37-40.
180. Mazer M, Perrone J. Acetaminophen-induced nephrotoxicity: pathophysiology, clinical manifestations, and management. *J Med Toxicol.* 2008;4:2-6.
181. McClements BM, Hyland M, Callender ME, et al. Management of paracetamol poisoning complicated by enzyme induction due to alcohol or drugs. *Lancet.* 1990;335:1526.
182. McCrae TA, Furuhama K, Roberts DW, et al. Evaluation of 3-(cysteine-S-yl) acetaminophen in the nephrotoxicity of acetaminophen in rats. *Toxicologist.* 1989;9:47.
183. McElhatton PR, Sullivan FM, Volans GN. Paracetamol overdose in pregnancy analysis of the outcomes of 300 cases referred to the Teratology Information Service. *Reprod Toxicol.* 1997;11:85-94.
184. Mendoza CD, Heard K, Dart RC. Coma, metabolic acidosis and normal liver function in a child with a large serum acetaminophen level. *Ann Emerg Med.* 2006;48:637.
185. Miller RP, Roberts RJ, Fischer LJ. Acetaminophen elimination kinetics in neonates, children, and adults. *Clin Pharmacol Ther.* 1976;19:676-684.
186. Milligan TP, Morris HC, Hammond PM, Price CP. Studies on paracetamol binding to serum proteins. *Ann Clin Biochem.* 1994;31:492-496.
187. Mitchell I, Bihari D, Chang R, et al. Earlier identification of patients at risk from acetaminophen-induced acute liver failure. *Crit Care Med.* 1998;26:279-284.
188. Mitchell JR. Acetaminophen toxicity. *N Engl J Med.* 1988;319:1601-1602.
189. Mitchell JR. Host susceptibility and acetaminophen liver injury. *Ann Intern Med.* 1977;87:377-378.
190. Mitchell JR, Jollow DJ, Potter WZ, et al. Acetaminophen-induced hepatic necrosis. I. Role of drug metabolism. *J Pharmacol Exp Ther.* 1973;187:185-194.
191. Mitchell JR, Jollow DJ, Potter WZ, et al. Acetaminophen-induced hepatic necrosis. IV. Protective role of glutathione. *J Pharmacol Exp Ther.* 1973;187:211-217.
192. Mitchell JR, Thorgeirsson SS, Potter WZ, et al. Acetaminophen-induced hepatic injury: protective role of glutathione in man and rationale for therapy. *Clin Pharmacol.* Ther 1974;16:676-684.
193. Mohler CR, Nordt SP, Williams SR, et al. Prospective evaluation of mild to moderate pediatric acetaminophen exposures. *Ann Emerg Med.* 2000;35:239-244.
194. Moling O, Cairon E, Rimenti G, et al. Severe hepatotoxicity after therapeutic doses of acetaminophen. *Clin Ther.* 2006;28:755-760.
195. Moller-Hartmann W, Siegers CP. Nephrotoxicity of paracetamol in the rate-mechanistic and therapeutic aspects. *J Appl Toxicol.* 1991;11:141-146.
196. Moore M, Thor H, Moore G, et al. The toxicity of acetaminophen and N-acetyl-p-benzoquinoneimine in isolated hepatocytes is associated with thiol depletion and increased cytosolic Ca2+. *J Biol Chem.* 1985;260:13035-13040.
197. Mour G, Feinfeld DA, Caraccio T, McGuigan M. Acute renal dysfunction in acetaminophen poisoning. *Renal Failure.* 2005;27:381-383.
198. Mroz LS, Krenzelok EP. Angioedema with oral N-acetylcysteine. *Ann Emerg Med.* 1997;30:240-241.
199. Muldrew KL, James LP, Coop L, et al. Determination of acetaminophen-protein adducts in mouse liver and serum and human serum after hepatotoxic doses of acetaminophen using high-performance liquid chromatography with electrochemical detection. *Drug Metab Disp.* 2002;30:446-451.
200. Muller FO, van Achterbergh SM, Hundt HK. Paracetamol overdose: protective effect of concomitantly ingested antimuscarinic drugs and codeine. *Hum Toxicol.* 1983;2:473-477.
201. Murakami M, Naraba H, Tanioka T. Regulation of prostaglandin E2 biosynthesis by membrane-associated prostaglandin E2 synthase that acts in concert with cyclooxygenase-2. *J Biol Chem.* 2000;276:32783-32792.

202. Murphy R, Swartz R, Watkins PB. Severe acetaminophen toxicity in a patient receiving isoniazid. *Ann Intern Med.* 1990;113:799-800.
203. Muth-Selbach U, Tegeder I, Brune K, et al. Acetaminophen inhibits spinal prostaglandin E2 release after peripheral noxious stimulation. *Anesthesiology.* 1999;91:231-239.
204. Mutimer DJ, Ayres RCs, Neuberger JM, et al. Serious paracetamol poisoning and the results of liver transplantation. *Gut.* 1994;35:809-814.
205. Naga Rani MA, Joseph T, Narayanan R. Placental transfer of paracetamol. *J Indian Med Assoc.* 1989;87:182-183.
206. Nogen AG, Bremner JE. Fatal acetaminophen overdosage in a young child. *J Pediatr.* 1978;92:832-833.
207. Notarianni L, Oldham H, Bennett P. Passage of paracetamol into breast milk and its subsequent metabolism by the neonate. *Br J Clin Pharmacol.* 1987;24:63-67.
208. O'Grady JG, Alexander GJM, Hayllar KM, Williams R. Early indicators of prognosis in fulminant hepatic failure. *Gastroenterology.* 1989;97:439-445.
209. O'Grady JG, Wendon J, Tan KC, et al. Liver transplantation after paracetamol overdose. *Br Med J.* 1991;303:221-223.
210. Ottani A, Leone S, Sandrini M, Ferrari A, Bertolini A. The analgesic activity of paracetamol is prevented by the blockade of cannabinoid CB1 receptors. *Eur J Pharm.* 2006;531:280-281.
211. Ouellet M, Percival MD. Mechanism of acetaminophen inhibition of cyclooxygenase isoforms. *Arch Biochem Biophys.* 2001;387:273-280.
212. Pakravan N, Bateman DN, Goddard J. Effect of acute paracetamol overdose on changes in serum and urine electrolytes. *Br J Clin Pharm.* 2007;64:824-832.
213. Patten CJ Thomas PE, Guy RL, et al. Cytochrome P450 enzymes involved in acetaminophen activation by rat and human liver microsomes and their kinetics. *Chem Res Toxicol.* 1993;6:511-518.
214. Pereira LMMB, Langley PG, Hayllar KM, et al. Coagulation factor V and VII/V ratio as predictors of outcome in paracetamol induced fulminant hepatic failure: relation to other prognostic indicators. *Gut.* 1992;33:98-102.
215. Pettersson PH, Owall A, Jakobsson J. Early bioavailability of paracetamol after oral or intravenous administration. *Acta Anaesthesiol Scand.* 2004;48:867-870.
216. Pickering G, Loriot MA, Libert F, et al. Analgesic effect of acetaminophen in humans: first evidence of a central serotonergic mechanism. *Clin Pharmacol Ther.* 2006;79:371-378.
217. Pincus T, Koch GG, Sokka T, et al. A randomized, double-blind, crossover clinical trial of diclofenac plus misoprostol versus acetaminophen in patients with osteoarthritis of the hip or knee. *Arthritis Rheum.* 2001;44:1587-1598.
218. Pini L, Sandrini M, Vitale G. The antinociceptive action of paracetamol is associated with changes in the serotonergic system in the rat brain. *Eur J Pharm.* 1996;308:31-40.
219. Pini L, Vitale G, Ottani A, Sandrini M. Naloxone-reversible antinociception by paracetamol in the rat. *J Pharmacol Exp Ther.* 1997;280:934-940.
220. Portmann B, Talbot IC, Day DW, et al. Histopathological changes in the liver following a paracetamol overdose: correlation with clinical and biochemical parameters. *J Pathol.* 1975;117:169-181.
221. Potter WZ, Davis DC, Mitchell JR, et al. Acetaminophen induced hepatic necrosis III: Cytochrome P450 mediated covalent binding in vitro. *J Pharmacol Exp Ther.* 1973;187:203-210.
222. Poulsen HE, Lerche A, Pedersen NT. Phenobarbital induction does not potentiate hepatotoxicity but accelerates liver cell necrosis from acetaminophen overdose in the rat. *Pharmacology.* 1985;30:100-108.
223. Prescott L. Oral or intravenous N-acetylcysteine for acetaminophen poisoning? *Ann Emerg Med.* 2005;45:409-413.
224. Prescott L: Drug conjugation in clinical toxicology. *Biochem Soc Trans.* 1984;12:96-99.
225. Prescott LF: Paracetamol overdosage: pharmacological considerations and clinical management. *Drugs.* 1983;25:290-314.
226. Prescott LF. Kinetics and metabolism of paracetamol and phenacetin. *Br J Clin Pharmacol.* 1980;10(suppl 2):291S-298S.
227. Prescott LF, Mattison P, Menzies DG, Manson LM. The comparative effects of paracetamol and indomethacin on renal function in health female volunteers. *Br J Clin Pharmacol.* 1990;29:403-412.
228. Prescott LF, Wright N, Roscoe P, Brown SS. Plasma-paracetamol half-life and hepatic necrosis in patients with paracetamol overdosage. *Lancet.* 1971;1:519-522.
229. Pumford NR, Hinson JA, Potter, et al. Immunochemical quantitation of 3-(Cystein-S-yl) acetaminophen adducts in serum and liver proteins of acetaminophen-treated mice. *J Pharmacol Exp Ther.* 1989;248:190-196.
230. Raffa R, Stone D, Tallarida R. Discovery of 'self-synergistic' spinal/supraspinal antinociception produced by acetaminophen (paracetamol). *J Pharmacol Exp Ther.* 2000;295:291-294.
231. Raffa R, Walker E, Sterious S. Opioid receptors and acetaminophen (paracetamol). *Eur J Pharmacol.* 2004;503:209-210.
232. Raffa RB, Codd EE. Lack of binding of acetaminophen to 5-HT receptor or uptake sites (or eleven other binding/uptake assays). *Life Sci.* 1996;59:PL37-40.
233. Raucy JL, Sker JML, Lieber CS, Black M: Acetaminophen activation by human liver cytochromes P-450 IIE1 and P-450 IA2. *Arch Biochem Biophys.* 1989;271:270-283.
234. Rawlins MD, Henderson DB, Hijab AR. Pharmacokinetics of paracetamol after intravenous and oral administration. *Eur J Clin Pharmacol.* 1977;11:283-286.
235. Ray SD, Mumaw VR, Raje RR, Fariss MW. Protection of acetaminophen-induced hepatocellular apoptosis and necrosis by cholesteryl hemisuccinate pretreatment. *J Pharmacol Exp Ther.* 1996;279:1470-1483.
236. Reid AB, Kurten RC, McCullough SS, et al. Mechanisms of acetaminophen-induced hepatotoxicity: role of oxidative stress and mitochondrial permeability transition in freshly isolated mouse hepatocytes. *J Pharmacol Exp Ther.* 2004;311:855-863.
237. Rexrode KM, Buring JE, Glynn RJ, et al. Analgesic use and renal function in men. *JAMA.* 2001;286:315-21.
238. Riggs BS, Bronstein AC, Kulig K, et al. Acute acetaminophen overdose during pregnancy. *Obstet Gynecol.* 1989;74:247-253.
239. Rivera-Penera T, Gugig R, Davis J, et al. Outcome of acetaminophen overdose in pediatric patients and factors contributing to hepatotoxicity. *J Pediatr.* 1997;130:300-304.
240. Roberts I, Robinson MJ, Mughal MZ, et al. Paracetamol metabolites in the neonate following maternal overdose. *Br J Clin Pharmacol.* 1984;18:201-206.
241. Rollins DE, Von Bahr C, Glaumann H, et al. Acetaminophen: potentially toxic metabolite formed by human fetal and adult liver microsomes and isolated fetal liver cells. *Science.* 1979;205:1414-1416.
242. Roth B, Woo O, Blanc P. Early metabolic acidosis and coma after acetaminophen ingestion. *Ann Emerg Med.* 1999;33:452-456.
243. Rumack BH. Acetaminophen hepatotoxicity: the first 35 years. *J Toxicol Clin Toxicol.* 2002;40:3-20.
244. Rumack BH. Acetaminophen overdose. *Am J Med.* 1983;75(suppl 5A):104-112.
245. Rumack BH. Acetaminophen overdose in young children: treatment and effects of alcohol and other additional ingestants in 417 cases. *Am J Dis Child.* 1984;138:428-433.
246. Rumack BH, Matthew H. Acetaminophen poisoning and toxicity. *Pediatrics.* 1975;55:871-876.
247. Rumack BH, Peterson RG, Koch GG, Amara IA. Acetaminophen overdose. 662 cases with evaluation of oral acetylcysteine treatment. *Arch Intern Med.* 1981;141:380-385.
248. Rybolt TR, Burrell DE, Shults JM, Kelly AK. In vitro coadsorption of acetaminophen and N-acetylcysteine onto activated carbon powder. *J Pharm Sci.* 1986;75:904-906.
249. Salhanick SD, Belikoff B, Orlow D, et al. Hyperbaric oxygen reduces acetaminophen toxicity and increases HIF-1alpha expression. *Acad Emerg Med.* 2006;13:707-714.
250. Salhanick SD, Orlow D, Holt DE, et al. Endothelially derived nitric oxide affects the severity of early acetaminophen-induced hepatic injury in mice. *Acad Emerg Med.* 2006;13:479-485.
251. Sandler DP: Analgesic use and chronic renal disease. *N Engl J Med.* 1989;320:399-404.
252. Sandrini M, Pini L, Vitale G. Differential involvement of central 5-HT1B and 5-HT receptor subtypes in the antinociceptive effect of paracetamol. *Inflamm Res.* 2003;52:347-352.
253. Sandrini M, Romualdi P, Capobianco A, et al. The effect of paracetamol on nociception and dynorphin A levels in the rat brain. *Neuropeptides.* 2001;35:110-116.
254. Sandrini M, Vitale G, Ruggieri V, Pini LA. Effect of acute and repeated administration of paracetamol on opioidergic and serotonergic systems in rats. *Inflamm Res.* 2007;56:139-142.
255. Sato C, Lieber CS. Mechanism of the preventive effect of ethanol on acetaminophen-induced hepatotoxicity. *J Pharm Exper Ther.* 1981;218:811-815.
256. Schenker S, Speeg K, Perez A, Finch J. The effects of food restriction in man on hepatic metabolism of acetaminophen. *Clin Nutr.* 2001;20:145-150.

257. Schiodt FV, Bondesen S, Petersen I, et al. Admission levels of serum Gc-globulin: predictive value in fulminant hepatic failure. *Hepatology.* 1996;23:713-718.
258. Schiodt FV, Bondesen S, Tygstrup N, Christensen E. Prediction of hepatic encephalopathy in paracetamol overdose: a prospective and validated study. *Scand J Gastroenterol.* 1999;7:723-728.
259. Schiodt FV, Rossaro L, Stravitz RT, et al. Gc-globulin and prognosis in acute liver failure. *Liver Transpl.* 2005;11:1223-1227.
260. Schmidt LE, Dalhoff K, Poulsen HE. Acute versus chronic alcohol consumption in acetaminophen-induced hepatotoxicity. *Hepatology.* 2002;35:876-882.
261. Schmidt LE, Dalhoff K. Serum phosphate is an early predictor of outcome in severe acetaminophen-induced hepatotoxicity. *Hepatology.* 2002;36:659-665.
262. Schmidt LE, Larsen FS. MELD score as a predictor of liver failure and death in patients with acetaminophen-induced liver failure. *Hepatology.* 2007;45:789-796.
263. Schmidt LE, Larson FS. Prognostic implications of hyperlactatemia, multiple organ failure and systemic inflammatory response syndrome in patients with acetaminophen-induced acute liver failure. *Crit Care Med.* 2006;34:337-343.
264. Seeff LB, Cuccherini BA, Zimmerman HJ, et al. Acetaminophen hepatotoxicity in alcoholics. A therapeutic misadventure. *Ann Intern Med.* 1986;104:309-404.
265. Seifert CF, Anderson DC. Acetaminophen usage patterns and concentrations of glutathione and gamma-glutamyl transferase in alcoholic subjects. *Pharmacotherapy.* 2007;27:1473-1482.
266. Shah NL, Gordon FD. N-acetylcysteine for acetaminophen overdose: when enough is enough. *Hepatology.* 2007;46:939-941.
267. Shen W, Kamendulis LM, Ray SD, Corcoran GB. Acetaminophen-induced cytotoxicity in cultured mouse hepatocytes: effects of CA 2+-endonuclease, repair DNA, and glutathione depletion inhibitors on DNA fragmentation and cell death. *Toxicol Appl Pharmacol.* 1992;112:34-40.
268. Singer AJ, Carracio TR, Mofenson HC: The temporal profile of increased transaminase levels in patients with acetaminophen-induced liver dysfunction. *Ann Emerg Med.* 1995;26:49-53.
269. Singer PP, Jones GR, Bannach BG, Denmark L. Acute fatal acetaminophen overdose without liver necrosis. *J Forensic Sci.* 2007;52(4):992-994.
270. Sivilotti MLA, Yarema MC, Juurlink DN, et al. A risk quantification instrument for acute acetaminophen overdose patients treated with N-acetylcysteine. *Ann Emerg Med.* 2005;46:263-271.
271. Slattery JT, Wilson JM, Kalhorn TF, et al. Dose-dependent pharmacokinetics of acetaminophen: Evidence for glutathione depletion in humans. *Clin Pharmacol Ther.* 1987;41:413-418.
272. Slitt AL, Dominick PK, Roberts JC, Cohen SD. Standard of care may not protect against acetaminophen-induced nephrotoxicity. *Basic Clin Pharm Toxicol.* 2004;95:247-248.
273. Smilkstein MJ, Bronstein AC, Linden C, et al. Acetaminophen overdose: a 48-hour intravenous N-acetylcysteine treatment protocol. *Ann Emerg Med.* 1991;20:1058-1063.
274. Smilkstein MJ, Douglas DR, Daya MR. Acetaminophen poisoning and liver function. *N Engl J Med.* 1994;330:1310-1311.
275. Smilkstein MJ, Knapp GL, Kulig KW, Rumack BH. N-Acetylcysteine in the treatment of acetaminophen overdose. *N Engl J Med.* 1989;320:1418.
276. Smilkstein MJ, Knapp GL, Kulig KW, Rumack BH. Efficacy of oral N-acetylcysteine in the treatment of acetaminophen overdose: analysis of the national multicenter study (1976–1985). *N Engl J Med.* 1988;3190:1557-1562.
277. Smilkstein MJ, Knapp GL, Kulig KW, et al. Acetaminophen overdose: how critical is the delay to N-acetylcysteine [abstract]? *Vet Hum Toxicol.* 1987;29:486.
278. Smilkstein MJ, Rumack BH. Elimination half-life as a predictor of acetaminophen-induced hepatotoxicity [abstract]. *Vet Hum Toxicol.* 1994;36:377.
279. Smith CV, Jones DP, Guenther TM, et al. Compartmentation of glutathione: Implications for the study of toxicity and disease. *Toxicol Appl Pharmacol.* 1996;140:1-12.
280. Smith DW, Isakson G, Frankel LR, Kerner JA. Hepatic failure following ingestion of multiple doses of acetaminophen in a young child. *J Pediatr Gastroenterol Nutr.* 1986;5:822-825.
280a. Smith SW, Howland MA, Hoffman RS, Nelson LS: Acetaminophen overdose with altered acetaminophen pharmacokinetics and hepatotoxicity associated with premature cessation of intravenous *N*-acetylcysteine therapy. *Ann Pharmacother.* 2008;42:1333-1339.
281. Spies CD, Reinhart K, Witt I, et al. Influence of N-acetylcysteine on indirect indicators of tissue oxygenation in septic shock patients. *Crit Care Med.* 1994;22:1738-1746.
282. Spiller HA, Krenzelok EP, Grande GA, et al. A prospective evaluation of the effect of activated charcoal before oral N-acetylcysteine in acetaminophen overdose. *Ann Emerg Med.* 1994;23:519-523.
283. Spiller HA, Winter ML, Klein-Schwartz W, Bangh SA. Efficacy of activated charcoal administered more than four hours after acetaminophen overdose. *J Emerg Med.* 2006;30:1-5
284. Spyker D, Connelly R, Davalloo S, et al. Response surface analysis of acetaminophen (APAP) overdose hepatotoxicity—unmasking the data. *Clin Pharmacol Ther.* 2003;73:27.
285. Steelman R, Goodman A, Biswas S, Zimmerman A. Metabolic acidosis and coma in a child with acetaminophen toxicity. *Clin Pediatr.* 2004;43:201-203.
286. Stork CM, Rees S, Howland MA, et al. Pharmacokinetics of extended relief vs regular release Tylenol in simulated human overdose. *J Toxicol Clin Toxicol.* 1996;34:157-162.
287. Strubelt O, Younes M. The toxicological relevance of paracetamol-induced inhibition of hepatic respiration and ATP depletion. *Biochem Pharmacol.* 1992;44:163-170.
288. Swetnam SM, Florman AL. Probable acetaminophen toxicity in an 18-month-old infant due to repeated overdosing. *Clin Pediatr.* 1984;23:104-105.
289. Taylor SE. Acetaminophen intoxication and length of treatment: how long is long enough? A comment. *Pharmacotherapy.* 2004;24:694-696.
290. Tenenbein M. Acetaminophen: the 150 mg/kg myth. *J Toxicol Clin Toxicol.* 2004;42:145-148.
291. Tenenbein PK, Sitar DS, Tenenbein M: Interaction between Nacetylcysteine and activated charcoal: implications for the treatment of acetaminophen poisoning. *Pharmacotherapy.* 2001;21:1331-1336.
292. Thijssen HH, Soute BA, Vervoort LM, Claessens JG. Paracetamol (acetaminophen) warfarin interaction: NAPQI, the toxic metabolite of paracetamol, is an inhibitor of enzymes in the vitamin K cycle. *Thromb Haemost.* 2004;92:797-802.
293. Thomsen MS, Loft S, Roberts DW, Poulsen HE. Cytochrome P4502E1 inhibition by propylene glycol prevents acetaminophen (paracetamol) hepatotoxicity in mice without cytochrome P4501A2 inhibition. *Pharmacol Toxicol.* 1995;76:395-399.
294. Thummel K, Slattery J, Ro H, et al. Ethanol and production of the hepatotoxic metabolite of acetaminophen in healthy adults. *Clin Pharmacol Ther.* 2000;67:591-599.
295. Thummel KE, Lee CA, Kunze KL, Nelson SD. Oxidation of acetaminophen to N-acetyl-p-benzoquinone imine by human CYP3A4. *Biochem Pharmacol.* 1993;45:1563-1569.
296. Thummel KE, Slattery JT, Nelson SD. Mechanism by which ethanol diminishes the hepatotoxicity of acetaminophen. *J Pharmacol Exp Ther.* 1988;245:129-136.
297. Thummel KE, Slattery JT, Nelson SD, et al. Effect of ethanol on hepatotoxicity of acetaminophen in mice and on reactive metabolite formation by mouse and human liver microsomes. *Toxicol Appl Pharmacol.* 1989;100:391-397.
298. Tighe TV, Walter FG. Delayed toxic acetaminophen level after initial four hour nontoxic level. *J Toxicol Clin Toxicol.* 1994;32:431-434.
299. Tirmenstein MA, Nelson SD. Acetaminophen-induced oxidation of protein thiols: contributions of impaired thiol-metabolizing enzymes and the breakdown of adenosine nucleotides. *J Biol Chem.* 1990;265:3059-3065.
300. Tirmenstein MA, Nelson SD. Subcellular binding and effects on calcium homeostasis produced by acetaminophen and a non-hepatotoxic regioisomer 3-hydroxyacetoanilide in mouse liver. *J Biol Chem.* 1989;264:9814-9819.
301. Tomlinson B, Young RP, Ng MC, et al. Selective liver enzyme induction by carbamazepine and phenytoin in Chinese epileptics. *Eur J Clin Pharm.* 1996;50:411-415.
302. Tredger JM, Smith HM, Read RB, Williams R. Effects of ethanol ingestion on the metabolism of a hepatotoxic dose or paracetamol in mice. *Xenobiotica.* 1986;16:661-670.
303. Vaccarino AL, Paul D, Mukherjee PK, et al. Synthesis and in vivo evaluation of non-hepatotoxic acetaminophen analogs. *Biorg Med Chem.* 2007;15:2206-2215.
304. Vale JA, Proudfoot AT. Paracetamol (acetaminophen) poisoning. *Lancet.* 1996;346:547-552.

305. Vassallo S, Khan AN, Howland MA. Use of the Rumack-Matthew nomogram in cases of extended-release acetaminophen toxicity. *Ann Intern Med.* 1996;125:940.
306. Vaughan D, Yanay O, Zimmerman JJ. Deciphering the oxyradical inflammation Rosetta stone: O2-NO, OONO-, polymorphonuclear neutrophils, poly(ADP-ribose) synthetase, systemic inflammatory response syndrome, and multiple organ dysfunction syndrome. *Crit Care Med.* 1999;27:1666-1669.
307. Volans GN. Antipyretic analgesic overdosage in children. Comparative risks. *Br J Clin Pract.* 1991;70(suppl):26-29.
308. Walker RJ, Fawcett JP. Drug nephrotoxicity: the significance of cellular mechanisms. *Prog Drug Res.* 1993;41:51-94.
309. Walsh TS, Hopton P, Philips BJ, et al. The effect of N-acetylcysteine on oxygen transport and uptake in patients with fulminant hepatic failure. *Hepatology.* 1998;27:1332-1340.
310. Walsh TS, Lee A. N-acetylcysteine administration in the critically ill. *Intensive Care Med* 1999;25:432-434.
311. Wang PH, Yang MJ, Lee WL, et al. Acetaminophen poisoning in late pregnancy. *J Reprod Med.* 1997;42:367-371.
312. Ware AJ, Upchurch KS, Eigenbrodt EH, Norman DA. Acetaminophen and the liver. *Ann Intern Med.* 1978;88:267-268.
313. Waring WS, Robinson ODG, Stephen AFL, et al. Does the patient history predict hepatotoxicity after acute paracetamol overdose? *Q J Med.* 2008;101:121-125.
314. Waring WS, Stephen AF, Malkowska AM, Robinson ODG. Acute ethanol coingestion confers a lower risk of hepatotoxicity after deliberate acetaminophen overdose. *Acad Emerg Med.* 2008;15:54-58.
315. Waring WS, Stephen AFL, Malkowska AM, Robinson ODG. Acute acetaminophen overdose is associated with dose-dependent hypokalemia: a prospective study of 331 patients. *Basic Clin Pharm Toxicol.* 2007;102:325-328.
316. Watkins PB, Kaplowitz N, Slattery JT, et al. Aminotransferase elevations in healthy adults receiving 4 grams of acetaminophen daily. *JAMA.* 2006;296:87-93.
317. Webster PA, Roberts DW, Benson RW, Kearns GL. Acetaminophen toxicity in children: diagnostic confirmation using a specific antigenic biomarker. *J Clin Pharmacol.* 1996;36:397-402.
318. Wendel A, Feuerstein S, Konz KH. Acute paracetamol intoxication of starved mice leads to lipid peroxidation in vivo. *Biochem Pharmacol.* 1979;28:2051-2055.
319. Wendon JA, Harrison PM, Keays R, Williams R. Cerebral blood flow and metabolism in fulminant liver failure. *Hepatology.* 1994;19:1407-1413.
320. Whitcomb DC, Block GD. Association of acetaminophen hepatotoxicity with fasting and ethanol use. *JAMA.* 1994;272:1845-1850.
321. Whyte IM, Buckley NA, Reith DM, et al. Acetaminophen causes an increased international normalized ratio by reducing functional factor VII. *Ther Drug Monit.* 2000;22:742-748.
322. Wilkinson SP, Moodie H, Arroyo VA, Williams R. Frequency of renal impairment in paracetamol overdose compared with other causes of acute liver damage. *J Clin Pharmacol.* 1977;30:220-224.
323. Wilson JT, Brown AD, Bocchini JA, Kearns GL. Efficacy, disposition, and pharmacodynamics of aspirin, acetaminophen and choline salicylate in young febrile children. *Ther Drug Monit.* 1982;4:147-180.
324. Woo OF, Mueller PD, Olson KR, et al. Shorter duration of oral N-acetylcysteine therapy for acute acetaminophen overdose. *Ann Emerg Med.* 2000;35:363-368.
325. Yip L, Dart RC. A 20-hour treatment for acute acetaminophen overdose. *N Engl J Med.* 2003;348:2471-2472.
326. Yip L, Dart R, Hurlbut KM. Intravenous administration of oral N-acetylcysteine. *Crit Care Med.* 1998;26:40-43.
327. Zand R, Nelson SD, Slattery JT, et al. Inhibition and induction of cytochrome P4502E1-catalyzed oxidation by isoniazid in humans. *Clin Pharmacol Ther.* 1993;54:142-149.
328. Zezulka A, Wright N. Severe metabolic acidosis early in paracetamol poisoning. *Br Med J.* 1982;285:851-852.
329. Zhao P, Kalhorn TF, Slattery JT. Selective mitochondrial glutathione depletion by ethanol enhances acetaminophen toxicity in rat liver. *Hepatology.* 2002;36:326-335.
330. Zimmerman HJ, Maddrey WC. Acetaminophen (paracetamol) hepatotoxicity with regular intake of alcohol: analysis of instances of therapeutic misadventure. *Hepatology.* 1995;22:767-773.

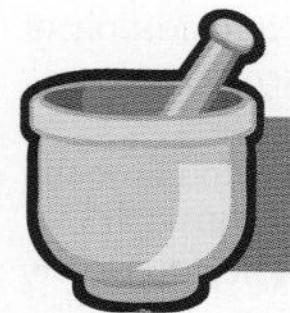

ANTIDOTES IN DEPTH (A4)

N-ACETYLCYSTEINE

Mary Ann Howland and Robert G. Hendrickson

N-acetylcysteine

Glutathione

Methionine

Cysteamine

N-acetylcysteine (NAC) is the cornerstone of therapy for patients with potentially lethal acetaminophen (APAP) overdoses. If administered early in the course of exposure, NAC can prevent APAP-induced hepatotoxicity. Administered after the onset of hepatotoxicity, NAC can improve outcome and decrease mortality. NAC also has a role in limiting hepatotoxicity caused by other xenobiotics that cause glutathione depletion and free radical formation, such as cyclopeptide-containing mushrooms, carbon tetrachloride, chloroform, pennyroyal oil, clove oil, and possibly liver failure from chronic valproic acid use.[27,47,48,145] Finally, NAC is useful in the management of patients with fulminant hepatic failure caused by other nontoxicologic etiologies.[17,70,76,127] Its beneficial effects are also under investigation in critically ill patients with a variety of stress-induced disorders,[79,124,139] in the prevention of further renal impairment in patients with chronic renal insufficiency administered a radiographic contrast agent,[46,55,71,114] and in those with hepatorenal syndrome.[57] Furthermore, NAC may enhance the elimination of boron, cobalt, cadmium, chromium, gold, and methylmercury, although this evidence is limited.[27,78]

HISTORY

Shortly after the first case of APAP hepatotoxicity was reported, Mitchell and coworkers described the protective effect of glutathione.[87,111] Prescott et al.[99] first suggested the use of NAC for APAP poisoning in 1974. Early experiments demonstrated that NAC could prevent APAP-induced hepatotoxicity in mice and that the oral (PO) and intravenous (IV) routes were equally efficacious when treatment was initiated early after ingestion.[94] Mitchell et al.,[87] Prescott et al.,[98,99] and Rumack and Peterson[112] performed human research with PO and IV NAC in the 1970s. The United States Food and Drug Administration (FDA) approved NAC for PO use in 1985 and for IV administration in 2004.

Cysteamine, methionine, and NAC, which are all glutathione precursors or substitutes, have been used successfully to prevent hepatotoxicity, but cysteamine and methionine both produce more adverse effects than NAC, and methionine is less effective than NAC. Therefore, NAC has emerged as the preferred treatment.[96,118,138]

MECHANISM OF ACTION IN ACETAMINOPHEN POISONING

NAC has several distinct roles in the treatment of APAP poisoning. Early after ingestion and during the metabolism of APAP to *N*-acetyl benzoquinoneimine (NAPQI), NAC prevents toxicity by rapidly detoxifying NAPQI that has formed. After hepatotoxicity is evident, NAC decreases toxicity through several nonspecific mechanisms, including free radical scavenging, increasing oxygen delivery, antioxidant effects, and alteration of microvascular tone.

NAC effectively prevents APAP-induced hepatotoxicity if it is administered before glutathione stores are depleted to 30% of normal. This level of depletion occurs approximately 6 to 8 hours after toxic APAP ingestion.[98,107,121] In this preventive role, NAC acts primarily as a precursor for the synthesis of glutathione.[73] NAC is a thiol-containing compound that is deacetylated to cysteine, an amino acid that is used intracellularly. Cysteine is then used with the amino acids glycine and glutamate to synthesize glutathione.[110] The availability of cysteine is the rate-limiting step in the synthesis of glutathione, and NAC is effective in replenishing diminished supplies of both cysteine and glutathione. Additional minor mechanisms of NAC in preventing hepatotoxicity include acting as a substrate for sulfation,[120] as an intracellular glutathione substitute by directly binding to NAPQI,[25] and by enhancing the reduction of NAPQI to *N*-acetyl-*p*-aminophenol (APAP).[73]

After NAPQI covalently binds to hepatocytes and other tissues,[107] NAC modulates the subsequent cascade of inflammatory events in a variety of ways.[51] NAC may act directly as an antioxidant or as a precursor to glutathione. Glutathione protects cells against electrophilic compounds by acting as both a reducing agent and an antioxidant.[110] NAC improves oxygen delivery[34,51,62,126,139,140] and utilization in extrahepatic organs such as the brain, heart, and kidney, probably by improving blood flow in the microvasculature, although the exact mechanism is unclear.[79,114,123] In addition, in vitro studies demonstrate a suppressive action on macrophages, neutrophils, leukocyte endothelial cell adhesion, and cytokines.[70]

CLINICAL USE

In acute overdose, treatment with NAC should be initiated if the serum APAP is plotted on or above the treatment line on the Rumack-Matthew nomogram or the patient's history suggests an acute APAP ingestion of 150 mg/kg or above and the results of blood tests will not be available within 8 hours of ingestion. In chronic APAP ingestions, treatment with NAC should be initiated if either aspartate aminotransferase (AST) is above normal or the APAP concentration is above 10 μg/mL (see Chap. 34 for details).

PHARMACOKINETICS

Administered NAC is present in plasma in the reduced or oxidized state and is either free or bound to plasma proteins or with other thiols and SH groups to form mixed disulfides such as NAC–cysteine.[97] NAC has a relatively small volume of distribution (Vd) (0.5 L/kg), and protein binding is 83%. NAC is metabolized to many sulfur-containing compounds such as cysteine, glutathione, methionine, cystine, and disulfides, as well as conjugates of electrophilic compounds, which are not measured.[42,93,97] Thus, the pharmacodynamic study of NAC is complex. In addition, the pharmacokinetics of NAC are complicated based on whether total or free NAC is being measured.[97]

PHARMACOKINETICS OF ORAL *N*-ACETYLCYSTEINE

PO NAC is rapidly absorbed, but the bioavailability is low (10%–30%) because of significant first-pass metabolism.[42,93,97] The mean time to maximum peak concentration is 1.4 ± 0.7 hours. The mean elimination half-life is 2.5 ± 0.6 hours and is linear with increasing dose up to 3200 mg/m^2/d given as a single daily dose. Intersubject plasma NAC concentrations vary 10-fold.[93] Chronic administration leads to a decrease in plasma concentrations from a C_{max} of 8.9 mg/L (55 μmol/L) at the end of 1 month to 5.1 mg/L (31 μmol/L) at the end of 6 months.[93]

Conflicting in vitro[26,68,113] and in vivo[24,40,90,103] data regarding the concomitant use of PO NAC and activated charcoal suggest that the resultant bioavailability of NAC is either decreased or unchanged. This interaction is likely of limited clinical importance, and either PO or IV NAC can be initiated without concern for charcoal interaction (see Chap. 34).

PHARMACOKINETICS OF INTRAVENOUS *N*-ACETYLCYSTEINE

When only free NAC was measured and analyzed, 600 mg of IV NAC given to healthy volunteers resulted in a peak serum NAC concentration of (300 μmol/L) 49 mg/L with a half-life of 2.27 hours compared with a peak serum concentration of (16 μmol/L) 2.6 mg/L after 600 mg PO.[20] Serum concentrations after IV administration of an initial loading dose of 150 mg/kg over 15 minutes reach approximately 500 mg/L (3075 μmol/L).[97] A steady-state plasma concentration of 35 mg/L (10–90 mg/L) is reached in approximately 12 hours with the standard IV protocol.[97] Approximately 30% is eliminated renally. Although an early study suggested that severe liver damage did not appear to affect NAC elimination,[97] a more recent study suggests that the half-life is increased because of a reduction in clearance, while the Vd did not change.[62]

ORAL VERSUS INTRAVENOUS *N*-ACETYLCYSTEINE

INTRAVENOUS VERSUS ORAL ADMINISTRATION

As with many issues related to APAP toxicity, the choice of PO versus IV NAC is complex. The available information suggests that each has advantages and disadvantages, and each may be more appropriate than the other in certain settings. Because no controlled studies have compared IV with PO NAC, conclusions about the relative benefit of each are largely speculative.

With the exception of fulminant hepatic failure, for which only the IV route has been investigated, IV and PO NAC administration are equally efficacious in treating patients with APAP toxicity.[100] Initial concerns about the apparent superiority of PO NAC over IV NAC when started 16 to 24 hours after overdose have been resolved by data showing equivalent results between the two protocols.[100] Any difference in outcome for these patients almost certainly is related to the *duration* and *dose* of NAC therapy rather than the route itself. The decision of which route to use should depend on the rate of side effects, safety, availability, and ease of use. Efficacy should not be a consideration.

Safety is the best understood of these issues. Nausea and vomiting may occur in more than 50% of patients treated with PO NAC,[86] and diarrhea is prevalent, but there is no credible evidence of more serious complications resulting from PO NAC. Reports of skin rash and unusual complications are rare.[88] In contrast, IV NAC is associated with a 2% to 6% rate of anaphylactoid reactions,[58,63,144,148] although rates of up to 14% to 18% have been reported in prospective trials.[67] Most of these reactions are mild and include rash, flushing, vomiting, and bronchospasm.[9,67,121] Anaphylactoid reactions may be severe in 1% of cases[67,85] and in rare instances may lead to hypotension and death.[5,15,30,63,83,85,121,148] Anaphylactoid reactions are attributed to both the dose and concentration of NAC. Reaction rate may be decreased by using a more dilute NAC solution[63,67,148] and slowing NAC infusions in some studies.[24] In one prospective study, prolongation of the loading infusion from 15 to 60 minutes did not decrease the anaphylactoid rate significantly (from 18% to 14%).[67] Unfortunately, this study lacked blinding; was underpowered; and had insufficient comparisons of coingestions, medical histories, and APAP concentration, so its generalizability is limited.[43,82]

Minor reactions, such as rash, generally do not require treatment, rarely recur, and do not preclude administration of subsequent NAC doses.[9,121,148] Even when urticaria, angioedema, and respiratory symptoms develop, they usually are easily treated, and NAC can be subsequently restarted with a very low incidence of recurrence.[9,95] Although proper dosing of IV NAC is very safe, it nevertheless must be considered less safe than PO NAC because of the possibility of severe anaphylactoid reactions, the risk of dosing errors,[52] and the possibility of nontreatment because of anaphylactoid reactions.[58,95]

Additional safety concerns have involved dosing for both small infants and obese adults. The IV NAC dosing regimen includes a milligrams per kilograms dose in a fixed water volume, leading to variability of IV NAC concentration.[23,58] This leads to a large free water dose for children, with one case of hyponatremic seizures,[128] and high concentration NAC for obese adults, with concern for anaphylactoid reactions. This has led to alternative dosing for both children (constant 3% concentration)[23] and obese adults (ceiling weight of 100 kg) (see Dosing below).[37]

The main disadvantage of the PO formulation of NAC is the high rate of vomiting and the concern that vomiting may delay therapy.[100] Delays in administration of NAC are correlated with an increased risk of hepatotoxicity.[122] The IV route avoids an increased rate of vomiting in patients who typically are already nauseated and avoids the use of high-dose antiemetics that may alter mental status.[86] Another potential disadvantage of PO NAC is that its absorption may be delayed up to 1 hour compared with IV NAC.[56] However, although short delays in delivery of NAC to the liver are probable in some instances, the equivalent rates of hepatotoxicity in patients treated with PO and IV NAC early after APAP ingestion suggest the delays associated with the

PO route may not be clinically relevant. PO NAC doses may be difficult to administer to patients with alterations of mental status because of the risk of aspiration, so IV NAC offers a distinct advantage in these instances.

One theoretical, albeit unproven, advantage of PO NAC early in the course of toxicity is that direct delivery via the portal circulation yields a higher concentration of NAC in the liver. Because of this first-pass clearance, PO NAC results in circulating NAC 20- to 30-fold lower than after IV dosing, suggesting that most PO NAC ended up in the liver.[20,56] However, elevated serum NAC may be an advantage of IV NAC administration when the liver is not the target organ of NAC, as with cerebral edema or in pregnancy. Lower costs of care are emphasized as an advantage of PO NAC, particularly in the United States, where the IV formulation is more expensive than the generic PO formulation.[74] However, the shorter length of stay for most patients treated with IV NAC (21 vs. 72 hours) may negate or reverse this difference. With the increasing use of "patient-tailored" NAC therapy, whether a major cost difference remains is unknown.[16,29]

Historically, before the current IV formulation in the United States, the PO formulation was used intravenously for years with an excellent safety profile[36,63,148] and without published evidence of infectious or febrile consequences.[36,63] This IV use of the PO formulation for this purpose is not generally recommended but is historically effective and may be necessary in cases in which only the PO formulation is available and the patient has intractable vomiting or APAP-induced hepatic failure.[74]

SPECIFIC INDICATIONS FOR IV NAC

In addition to decisions based on cost, duration, safety, and ease of use, three situations exist for which the available information suggests IV NAC is preferable to PO NAC: fulminant hepatic failure, inability to tolerate PO NAC, and APAP poisoning in pregnancy. Each of these requires further study for validation, but all three seem well supported by current information.

Fulminant hepatic failure is an important indication for IV NAC. The choice of IV over PO NAC is based on several observations. Most importantly, IV is the only route that has been studied in liver failure.[66] PO NAC may prove effective but has not yet been demonstrated. Second, evidence that (some or all of) the benefit of NAC in liver failure is extrahepatic suggests that IV NAC is preferable.[51] IV NAC results in higher blood NAC concentrations, which presumably leads to more NAC delivery to critical organs. Finally, concomitant gastrointestinal bleeding, use of lactulose, and other factors make IV NAC more practical.

A more common indication for IV NAC use is for patients with very high APAP concentrations who are approaching or are more than 6 to 8 hours from the time of ingestion and who are unable to tolerate PO NAC after a brief aggressive trial of antiemetic therapy. Use of IV NAC is logical to prevent further delays and resultant loss of NAC efficacy, even without proof that continued vomiting significantly limits NAC absorption.

The most controversial indication for IV NAC use is during pregnancy. Administration of IV NAC to the mother has the theoretical advantage of increased delivery to the fetus over PO NAC use. IV administration circumvents first-pass metabolism, presumably exposing the fetal circulation to higher maternal serum concentrations with IV dosing. Some studies have suggested that placental transfer of NAC to the fetus is limited.[61,116] However, one case series found that the NAC concentration in cord or neonatal blood after PO maternal NAC administration equaled the NAC concentration seen in patients treated with PO NAC.[59] Of course, an equivalent serum NAC concentration does not prove adequacy of therapy. Unlike the neonates studied, patients treated with PO NAC have extensive first-pass hepatic uptake before NAC entry into the serum, where NAC concentration was measured.[20,56] Whether serum NAC concentration in the neonates studied reflects any significant hepatic NAC delivery is uncertain.

SAFETY IN PREGNANCY AND NEONATES

Untreated APAP toxicity is a far greater threat to fetuses than is NAC treatment.[28,105] NAC traverses the human placenta and produces cord blood concentrations comparable to maternal blood concentrations.[59] NAC is FDA Pregnancy Category B.

Limited data exist with regard to the management of neonatal APAP toxicity,[7,75,108,117] although IV and PO NAC have been used safely.[1,7] No adverse effects were observed when preterm newborns were treated with IV NAC[1] (see Chaps. 30 and 34). The elimination half-life of NAC in preterm neonates was 11 hours compared with 5.6 hours in adults.[1] IV administration has the advantage of assuring adequate antidotal delivery. PO administration in general is associated with necrotizing enterocolitis in neonates, although NAC has been orally administered safely in neonates.

OTHER USES (NON-ACETAMINOPHEN)

Diverse investigations of NAC as a treatment for a number of xenobiotics associated with free radical or reactive metabolite toxicity have been reported. Some of these xenobiotics include acrylonitrile, amatoxins, cadmium, chloroform, carbon tetrachloride, cyclophosphamide, 1,2-dichloropropane, doxorubicin, eugenol, pulegone, ricin, and zidovudine.[27,39,42,138,145] NAC has not been adequately studied for any of these xenobiotics in humans to definitively recommend it as a therapeutic intervention. However, the best evidence supports the use of NAC in cases of acute exposures to cyclopeptide-containing mushrooms (see below) and carbon tetrachloride.[27,42,138] NAC has also decreased cisplatin-induced nephrotoxicity in both rats and human cell cultures, but little human data exist.[6,109] NAC may be considered in cases of acute pennyroyal oil (ie, pulegone) or clove oil (eg, eugenol) ingestions based on their similarities to APAP-induced hepatotoxicity in which NAC has been proven beneficial and preventative. Both pulegone and eugenol are converted to reactive metabolites and induce glutathione depletion, leading to centrilobular necrosis.[131-134] NAC may be effective in treating patients with hepatotoxicity from chronic valproate use given the evidence that the 2,4-diene valproic acid metabolite acts as an electrophile and reduces hepatic glutathione.[47,48] However, there is no evidence that NAC is effective in treating patients with acute valproate toxicity and no evidence or theoretical efficacy in treating valproate-induced hyperammonemia. NAC has been demonstrated to increase excretion of several metals and other elements in animal studies, including boron, cadmium, chromium, cobalt, gold, and methylmercury.[11,13,27,53] The clinical usefulness of this effect remains unclear.

NAC has been studied as a chemopreventive agent[32,79,110] against cancer,[2] lung injury,[31,33] cardiac injury,[123,124] multiorgan failure from trauma and sepsis,[49,101,115,125,] traumatic brain injury,[12,130,147] and malnutrition. NAC has extracellular antimutagenic effects, enhances repair of nuclear DNA damaged by carcinogens, and inhibits malignant cell invasion and metastases.[32,92,102] PO NAC added to prednisone and azathioprine preserves vital capacity in patients with idiopathic pulmonary fibrosis.[33] Rescue NAC therapy has been studied with high-dose APAP (>20 g/m^2) in patients with specific advanced malignancies.[69]

NAC has been extensively studied to determine its effect on the risk of contrast-induced nephropathy in procedures requiring IV contrast. Both PO[3,18,21,35,45,65,119] and IV[10,38,84] formulations have been studied before angiography with mixed results, with some small studies showing large reductions in nephropathy rates, but several studies showing no advantage over placebo. Absolute creatinine change in the positive studies remains quite small and are typically below 0.2 mg/dL.[46,71] Studies using higher IV NAC doses[10,84] have shown greater reductions in nephropathy rates and will likely be further studied. One recent study showed a dose-related effect on both nephropathy and in-hospital mortality when comparing 600 mg to 1200 mg IV with placebo.[84] Routes and doses have varied in these studies, and understanding of the appropriate dose continues to evolve. Most studies use 400 to 600 mg PO NAC 2-3 times a day for 1 to 2 days before and 1 to 2 days after cardiac catheterization.[3,18,21,35,45,65,119,129] Other studies have used IV NAC boluses of 600 mg, 1200 mg,[38,84] and 150 mg/kg over 30 minutes.[10]

NAC has been used for decades in cases of cyclopeptide-containing mushroom poisoning, particularly poisoning with amanita phalloides. NAC therapy for amatoxin poisoning is largely based on the similarity of toxicity of amatoxin and APAP, including delayed onset of centrilobular hepatic necrosis. Decreases in intracellular glutathione stores have been identified in isolated rat hepatocytes that were exposed by amanita extracts,[64] leading to the reasonable conclusion that supplying the tissue with thiols may decrease toxicity. In retrospective studies, patients treated with NAC have lower mortality rates than those treated with supportive care[41]; however, in animal studies, NAC has little effect on hepatotoxicity.[135]

ADVERSE EFFECTS AND SAFETY ISSUES

PO NAC may cause nausea, vomiting, flatus, diarrhea, gastroesophageal reflux, and dysgeusia; generalized urticaria occurs rarely. Generalized anaphylactoid reactions described after IV NAC dosing[4,15,19,30,44,54,81,83,97,104,137,141] are not noted after PO therapy and may be related to rate, concentration, or high serum NAC concentrations.[14,97]

The IV route ensures delivery, but rate-related anaphylactoid reactions are possible. The manufacturer of IV NAC categorizes the number of anaphylactoid reactions occurring in 109 patients receiving the previously recommended 15-minute loading dose as mild (6%), moderate (10%), and severe (1%).[1] Of the adverse events occurring in more than 2000 patients who received IV NAC over 15 minutes, vasodilation, rash, and pruritus account for approximately 10%, hypotension 4%, bronchospasm 6%, and angioedema 8%.[1] An interesting yet unexplainable observation demonstrated a 25% incidence of anaphylactoid reactions to IV NAC administered over 15 minutes when the APAP 4-hour plasma concentration was less than 150 μg/mL compared with a 3% incidence when the serum concentration was 300 μg/mL.[142]

If angioedema or an anaphylactoid reaction characterized by hypotension; shortness of breath; or wheezing, flushing, or erythema occurs, NAC should be stopped and standard symptomatic therapy instituted. After the reaction resolves, NAC can be carefully readministered at a slower rate after 1 hour, assuming NAC is still indicated. If the reaction persists or worsens, IV NAC should be discontinued and a switch to PO NAC should be considered. Adverse reactions confined to flushing and erythema are usually transient, and NAC can be continued with meticulous monitoring for systemic symptoms that indicate the need to stop the NAC. Urticaria can be managed with diphenhydramine with the same precautions.[9] Iatrogenic overdoses with IV NAC have resulted in severe reactions and even death in children.[1,9,83]

IV NAC decreases clotting factors and increases the prothrombin time (PT) in healthy volunteers and overdose patients without hepatic damage.[60,80,89,143] This effect occurs within the first hour, stabilizes after 16 hours of continuous IV NAC, and rapidly returns to normal when the infusion is stopped.[60] Because the INR is used as a marker of the severity of toxicity and is one of the criteria for transplantation, this adverse effect of NAC should always be considered when evaluating the patient's condition. An elevated INR without other indicators of hepatic damage is probably related to the NAC.

DOSING

The standard 21-hour IV NAC protocol is a loading dose of 150 mg/kg up to a maximum of 15 g in 200 mL of 5% dextrose in water (D_5W) (for adults) infused over 60 minutes followed by a first maintenance dose of 50 mg/kg up to a maximum of 5 g in 500 mL D_5W (for adults) infused over 4 hours followed by a second maintenance dose of 100 mg/kg up to a maximum of 10 g in 1000 mL D_5W (for adults) infused over 16 hours. The loading dose was changed to a 60-minute infusion rate from a previously recommended 15-minute infusion rate.

When NAC is administered orally, the patient should receive a 140-mg/kg loading dose either orally or by enteral tube. Starting 4 hours after the loading dose, 70 mg/kg should be given every 4 hours for an additional 17 doses, for a total dose of 1330 mg/kg. The solution should be diluted to 5% and can be mixed with a soft drink to enhance palatability. If any dose is vomited within 1 hour of administration, the dose should be repeated[77] or IV delivery used. Antiemetics (eg, metoclopramide or a serotonin receptor antagonist) should be used to ensure absorption.

Several other regimens, including a 48-hour IV, 36-hour IV, 36-hour PO, and 20-hour PO protocols, have been described; however, none of these has been adequately studied for general use[29,121,146,149] (see Chap. 34).

Regardless of the protocol initiated, NAC should be continued beyond the protocol length if the serum APAP concentration is detectable or the AST is elevated. A NAC infusion should be continued until the APAP concentration is undetectable, the serum AST is normal or has significantly improved (eg, two consecutive decreasing values and AST <1000 IU/L), and any evidence of hepatic failure (international normalized ratio [INR] >2, encephalopathy) has resolved.[29]

There are no specific dosing guidelines for obese patients. However, it may be reasonable to limit PO and IV NAC dosing using a maximum weight of 100 kg. This maximum limit is not based on experimental evidence; however, patients who are larger than 100 kg have an equivalent hepatic volume and similar ingestion amounts as patients who weight less than 100 kg. The current NAC dosing is sufficient for a patient of any weight with an APAP dose of 16 g, postulating that 4% is converted to the toxic metabolite, NAPQI. Although dosing with a maximum weight is logical, it has not yet been adequately studied in obese humans.

For the rare patient who ingests exceptionally large doses of APAP, or who has prolonged and significantly elevated APAP concentrations, consideration should be given to treating with greater amounts of NAC once prolonged, massive APAP concentrations are evident.[122a,115a] No data exists to determine which, if any, alternative NAC dosing strategy is superior, however it seems reasonable to increase NAC dosing if the hepatic exposure to APAP is prolonged and massive. Several strategies have been theorized, but none studied, including: 1) increasing the maintenance IV dose to 200 mg/kg over 16 hours (12.5 mg/kg/h) (in 1000 mL D5W for patients >40 kg) possibly preceded by a repeat of the IV loading dose or 2) adding the standard oral protocol (140 mg/kg oral loading dose followed by 70 mg/kg orally every 4 hours) to the standard IV regimen (6.25 mg/kg/h).

Previously dosing information for IV NAC was not available for patients weighing less than 40 kg, and problems with osmolarity, sodium concentrations and fluid requirements became apparent when improper dilutions were used. The package insert now gives specific information for dosing in these patients.

The IV dosing of NAC is complicated because three different preparations must be prepared with each based on weight. A recent

TABLE A4–1. Three-Bag Method Dosage Guide[1] by Weight for Patients Weighing 40 kg or Above [a]

Body Weight		Loading Dose (150 mg/kg in 200 mL D_5W over 60 min)	Second Dose (50 mg/kg in 500 mL D_5W over 4 h)	Third Dose (100 mg/kg in 1000 mL D_5W over 16 h)
(kg)	(lb)	Acetadote (mL)[b]	Acetadote (mL)[b]	Acetadote (mL)[b]
100	220	75	25	50
90	198	67.5	22.5	45
80	176	60	20	40
70	154	52.5	17.5	35
60	132	45	15	30
50	110	37.5	12.5	25
40	88	30	10	20

[a] The total volume administered should be adjusted for patients weighing less than 40 kg and for those requiring fluid restriction.

[b] Acetadote is available in 30 mL 200-mg/mL single-dose glass vials.

D_5W, 5% dextrose in water.

TABLE A4–2. Three-Bag Method Dosage Guide[1] by Weight for Patients Weighing Less Than 40 kg[1a]

Body Weight		Loading Dose (150 mg/kg over 60 min)		Second Dose (50 mg/kg over 4 h)		Third Dose (100 mg/kg over 16 h)	
(kg)	(lb)	Acetadote(mL)	D_5W (mL)[b]	Acetadote(mL)[b]	D_5W (mL)	Acetadote(mL)[b]	D_5W (mL)
30	66	22.5	100	7.5	250	15	500
25	55	18.75	100	6.25	250	12.5	500
20	44	15	60	5	140	10	280
15	33	11.25	45	3.75	105	7.5	210
10	22	7.5	30	2.5	70	5	140

[a] Acetadote is hyperosmolar (2600 mOsm/L) and is compatible with D_5W, ½ normal saline (0.45% sodium chloride injection), and water for injection.

[b] Acetadote is available in 30 mL 200-mg/mL single-dose glass vials.

D_5W, 5% dextrose in water.

retrospective study estimated that there was a 33% medication error rate in the preparation and delivery of IV NAC.[52] To limit these errors, the Tables A4–1 and A4–2 from the package insert give the appropriate doses and dilutions for adults and patients weighing less than 40 kg.[1] In addition, the following web site has a dosage calculator: http://acetadote.net/dosecalc.shtml.

If hepatic failure intervenes, IV NAC should be administered at a dose of 150 mg/kg in D_5W infused over 24 hours and continued until the patient has a normal mental status (or recovers from hepatic encephalopathy)[51] and the patient's INR becomes below 2.0[106] or until the patient receives a liver transplant.[22,50,66]

AVAILABILITY

NAC (Acetadote) is available as a 20% concentration in 30-mL single-dose vials designed for dilution before IV administration. NAC for PO administration is available in 10-mL vials of 10% and 20% for PO administration and should also be diluted before administration.

ACKNOWLEDGMENT

Martin Jay Smilkstein, MD, contributed to this Antidotes in Depth in a previous edition.

REFERENCES

1. Acetadote package insert. Nashville, TN: Cumberland Pharmaceuticals, Inc., February 2006.
2. Agarwal A, Munoz-Najar U, Klueh U, et al. N-acetyl-cysteine promotes angiostatin production and vascular collapse in an orthotopic model of breast cancer. *Am J Pathol.* 2004;164:1683-1696.
3. Allaqaband S, Tumuluri R, Malik AM, et al. Prospective randomized study of N-acetylcysteine, fenoldopam, and saline for prevention of radiocontrast-induced nephropathy. *Cathet Cardiovasc Intervent.* 2002;57:279-283.
4. Anonymous. Death after N-acetylcysteine. *Lancet.* 1984;1:1421.
5. Appelboam AV, Dargan PI, Knighton J. Fatal anaphylactoid reaction to N-acetylcysteine: caution in patients with asthma. *Emerg Med J.* 2002;19:594-595.

6. Appenroth D, Winnefeld K, Heinz S, et al. Beneficial effect of acetylcysteine on cisplatin nephrotoxicity in rats. *J Appl Toxicol.* 1993;13:189-198.
7. Aw MM, Dhawan A, Baker AJ, Mieli-Vergani G. Neonatal paracetamol poisoning. *Arch Dis Child Fetal Neonatal Ed.* 1999;81:F78.
8. Bailey B, Blais R, Letarte A. Status epilepticus after a massive intravenous N-acetylcysteine overdose leading to intracranial hypertension and death. *Ann Emerg Med.* 2004;44:401-406.
9. Bailey B, McGuigan M. Management of anaphylactoid reactions to intravenous N-acetylcysteine. *Ann Emerg Med.* 1998;31:710-715.
10. Baker CSR, Wragg A, Kumar S, et al. A rapid protocol for the prevention of contrast-induced renal dysfunction: the RAPPID study. *J Am Coll Cardiol.* 2003;41:2114-2118.
11. Ballatori N, Lieberman MW, Wang W. N-acetylcysteine as an antidote in methylmercury poisoning. *Environ Health Perspect.* 1998;106:267-271.
12. Baltzer WI, McMichael MA, Hosgood GL, et al. Randomized, blinded, placebo-controlled clinical trials of N-acetylcysteine in dogs with spinal cord trauma from acute intervertebral disc disease. *Spine.* 2008;33:1397-1402.
13. Banner Jr W, Koch M, Capin DM, et al. Experimental chelation therapy in chromium, lead, and boron intoxication with N-acetylcysteine and other compounds. *Toxicol Appl Pharmacol.* 1986;83:142-7.
14. Barrett KE, Minor JR, Metcalfe DD. Histamine secretion induced by N-acetyl cysteine. *Agents Actions.* 1985;16:144-146.
15. Bateman DN, Woodhouse KW, Rawlins MD. Adverse reactions to N-acetylcysteine. *Hum Toxicol.* 1984;3:393-398.
16. Betten DP, Cantrell FL, Thomas SC, et al. A prospective evaluation of shortened course oral N-acetylcysteine for the treatment of acute acetaminophen poisoning. *Ann Emerg Med.* 2007;50:272-279.
17. Bne-Ari Z, Vaknin H, Tur-Kaspa R. N-acetylcysteine in acute hepatic failure (non-paracetamol-induced). *Hepatogastroenterology.* 2000;47:786-789.
18. Boccalandro F, Amhad M, Smalling RW, Sdringola S. Oral acetylcysteine does not protect renal function from moderate to high doses of intravenous radiographic contrast. *Cathet Cardiovasc Intervent.* 2003;58:336-341.
19. Bonfiglio M, Traeger S, Hulisz D, et al. Anaphylactoid reaction to IV acetylcysteine associated with electrocardiographic abnormalities. *Pharmacotherapy.* 1992;26:22-25.
20. Borgstrom L, Kagedal B, Paulsen O. Pharmacokinetics of N-acetylcysteine in man. *Eur J Clin Pharmacol.* 1986;31:217-222.
21. Briguori C, Manganelli F, Scarpato P, et al. Acetylcysteine and contrast agent-associated nephrotoxicity. *J Am Coll Cardiol.* 2002;40:298-303.
22. Bromley PN, Cottam SJ, Hilmi I, et al. Effects of intraoperative N-acetylcysteine in orthotopic liver transplantation. *Br J Anaesth.* 1995;75:352-354.
23. Brush DE, Boyer EW. Intravenous N-acetylcysteine for children. *Pediatr Emerg Care.* 2004;20:649-650.
24. Buckley N, Whyte I, O'Connell DL, Dawson A. Activated charcoal reduces the need for N-acetylcysteine treatment after acetaminophen (paracetamol) overdose. *J Toxicol Clin Toxicol.* 1999;37:753-757.
25. Buckpitt AR, Rollins DE, Mitchell JR. Varying effects of sulfhydryl nucleophiles on acetaminophen oxidation and sulfhydryl adduct formation. *Biochem Pharmacol.* 1979;28:2841-2946.
26. Chinough R, Czajka P. N-Acetylcysteine adsorption by activated charcoal. *Vet Hum Toxicol.* 1980;22:392-394.
27. Chyka P, Butler A, Holliman B, Herman M. Utility of acetylcysteine in treatment poisonings and adverse drug reactions. *Drug Saf.* 2000;2:123-148.
28. Crowell C, Lyew RV, Givens M, et al. Caring for the mother, concentrating on the fetus: intravenous N-acetylcysteine in pregnancy. *Am J Emerg Med.* 2008 6:735-738.
29. Dart R, Rumack B. Patient tailored acetylcysteine administration. *Ann Emerg Med.* 2007;50:280-281.
30. Dawson A, Henry D, McEwen J. Adverse reactions to N-acetylcysteine during treatment for paracetamol poisoning. *Med J Aust.* 1989;150:329-331.
31. De Backer WA, Amsel B, Jorens PG, et al. N-Acetylcysteine pretreatment of cardiac surgery patients influences plasma neutrophil elastase and neutrophil influx in bronchoalveolar lavage fluid. Intensive *Care Med.* 1996;22:900-908.
32. De Flora S, Cesarone CE, Balansky RM, et al. Chemopreventive properties and mechanisms of N-acetylcysteine. The experimental background. *J Cell Biochem.* 1995;22(suppl):33-41.
33. Demedts M, Behr J, Buhl R, et al. High-dose acetylcysteine in idiopathic pulmonary fibrosis. *N Engl J Med.* 2005;353:2229-2242.
34. Devlin J, Ellis AE, McPeake J, et al. N-acetylcysteine improves indocyanine green extraction and oxygen transport during hepatic dysfunction. *Crit Care Med.* 1997;25:236-242.
35. Diaz-Sandoval LJ, Kosowsky BD, Losordo DW. Acetylcysteine to prevent angiography-related renal tissue injury (The APART Trial). *Am J Cardiol.* 2002;89:356-358.
36. Dribben WH, Porto SM, Jeffords BK. Stability and microbiology of inhalant N-acetylcysteine used as an intravenous solution for the treatment of acetaminophen poisoning. *Ann Emerg Med.* 2003;42:9-13.
37. Duncan R, Cantlay G, Paterson B. New recommendation for N-acetylcysteine dosing may reduce incidence of adverse effects. *Emerg Med J.* 2006;23:584-585.
38. Durham JD, Caputo C, Dokko J, et al. A randomized controlled trial of N-acetylcysteine to prevent contrast nephropathy in cardiac angiography. *Kidney Int.* 2002;62:2202-2207.
39. Eisen JS, Koren G, Juurlink DN, et al. N-acetylcysteine for the treatment of clove oil-induced fulminant hepatic failure. *Clin Toxicol.* 2004;42(1):89-92.
40. Ekins B, Ford D, Thompson M, et al. The effect of activated charcoal on N-acetylcysteine absorption in normal subjects. *Am J Emerg Med.* 1987;5:483-487.
41. Enjalbert F, Rapior S, Nouguier-Soule J, et al. Treatment of amatoxin poisoning: 20-year retrospective analysis. *Clin Toxicol.* 2002;40:715-757.
42. Flanagan R, Meredith TJ. Use of N-acetylcysteine in clinical toxicology. *Am J Med.* 1991;91:131S-139S.
43. Gawarammana IB, Greene SL, Dargan PI, Jones AL. Australian Clinical Toxicology Investigators Collaboration randomized trial of different loading infusion rates of N-acetylcysteine. *Ann Emerg Med.* 2006;47:124.
44. Gervais S, Lussier-Labelle F, Beaudet G. Anaphylactoid reaction to acetylcysteine. *Clin Pharm.* 1984;3:586-587.
45. Goldenberg I, Shechter M, Matetzky S, et al. Oral acetylcysteine as an adjunct to saline hydration for the prevention of contrast-induced nephropathy following coronary angiography. *Eur Heart J.* 2004;25:212-218.
46. Gonzales DA, Norsworthy KJ, Kern SJ, et al. A meta-analysis of N-acetylcysteine in contrast-induced nephrotoxicity: unsupervised clustering to resolve heterogeneity. *BMC Med.* 2007;5:32.
47. Gopaul SV, Farrell K, Abbott FS. Identification and characterization of N-acetylcysteine conjugates of valproic acid in humans and animals. *Drug Metab Dispos.* 2000;28:823-832.
48. Gopaul S, Farrell K, Abbott F. Effects of age and polytherapy, risk factors of valproic acid (VPA) hepatotoxicity, on the excretion of thiol conjugates of (E)-2,4-diene VPA in people with epilepsy taking VPA. *Epilepsia.* 2003;44:322-328.
49. Gundersen Y, Vaagenes P, Thrane I, et al. N-acetylcysteine administered as part of the immediate post-traumatic resuscitation regimen does not significantly influence initiation of inflammatory responses or subsequent endotoxin hyporesponsiveness. *Resuscitation.* 2005;64:377-382.
50. Harrison P, Keays R, Bray G, et al. Improved outcome of paracetamol-induced fulminant hepatic failure by late administration of acetylcysteine. *Lancet.* 1990;335:1572-1573.
51. Harrison P, Wendon J, Gimson A, et al. Improvement by acetylcysteine of hemodynamics and oxygen transport in fulminant hepatic failure. *N Engl J Med.* 1991;324:1852-1857.
52. Hayes B, Klein-Schwartz W, Dyon S. Frequency of medication errors with intravenous acetylcysteine for acetaminophen overdose. *Ann Pharmacotherapy.* 2008;42:766-770.
53. Henderson P, Hale TW, Shum S. N-acetylcysteine therapy of acute heavy metal poisoning in mice. *Vet Human Toxicol.* 1985;27:522-5.
54. Ho SW, Beilin JJ. Asthma associated with N-acetylcysteine infusion and paracetamol poisoning: report of two cases. *Br Med J.* 1983;287:876-877.
55. Hoffmann U, Fischereder M, Kruger B. The value of N-acetylcysteine in the prevention of radiocontrast agent-induced nephropathy seems questionable. *J Am Soc Nephrol.* 2004;15:407-410.
56. Holdiness MR. Clinical pharmacokinetics of N-acetylcysteine. *Clin Pharm.* 1991;20:123-134.
57. Holt S, Goodier D, Marley R, et al. Improvement in renal function in hepatorenal syndrome with N-acetylcysteine. *Lancet.* 1999;353:294-295.
58. Horowitz BZ, Hendrickson RG, Pizarro-Osilla. Not so fast! *Ann Emerg Med.* 2006;47:122-123.
59. Horowitz R, Dart R, Jarvie D, et al. Placental transfer of N-acetylcysteine following human maternal acetaminophen toxicity. *J Toxicol Clin Toxicol.* 1997;35:447-451.
60. Jepsen S, Hansen AB. The influence of N-acetylcysteine on the measurement of prothrombin time and activated partial thromboplastin time in healthy subjects. *Scand J Clin Lab Invest.* 1994;54:543-547.
61. Johnson D, Simone C, Koren G. Transfer of N-acetylcysteine by the human placenta. *Vet Hum Toxicol.* 1993;35:365.

62. Jones A, Jarvie D, Simpson D, et al. Pharmacokinetics of N-acetylcysteine are altered in patients with chronic liver disease. *Aliment Pharmacol Ther.* 1997;11:787-791.
63. Kao LW, Kirk MA, Furbee RB. What is the rate of adverse events after oral N-acetylcysteine administered by the intravenous route to patients with suspected acetaminophen poisoning? *Ann Emerg Med.* 2003;42:741-750.
64. Kawaji A, Sone T, Natsuki R, et al. In vitro toxicity test of poisonous mushroom extracts with isolated rat hepatocytes. *J Toxicol Sci.* 1990; 15:145-156.
65. Kay J, Chow WH, Chan TM, et al. Acetylcysteine for prevention of acute deterioration of renal function following elective coronary angiography and intervention: a randomized controlled trial. *JAMA.* 2003;289:553-558.
66. Keays R, Harrison P, Wendon J, et al. Intravenous acetylcysteine in paracetamol-induced fulminant hepatic failure: a prospective controlled trial. *Br Med J.* 1991;303:1026-1029.
67. Kerr F, Dawson A, Whyte I, et al. The Australasian clinical toxicology intervention collaboration randomized trial of different loading infusion rates of N-acetylcysteine. *Ann Emerg Med.* 2005;45:402-409.
68. Klein Schwartz W, Oderda G. Adsorption of oral antidotes for acetaminophen poisoning (methionine and N-acetylcysteine) by activated charcoal. *Clin Toxicol.* 1981;18:283-290.
69. Kobrinsky NL, Hartfield D, Horner H, et al. Treatment of advanced malignancies with high-dose acetaminophen and N-acetylcysteine rescue. *Cancer Invest.* 1996;14:202-210.
70. Kortsalioudaki C, Taylor R, Cheeseman P, et al. Safety and efficacy of N-acetylcysteine in children with non-acetaminophen-induced acute liver failure. *Liver Transplant.* 2008;14:25-30.
71. Kshirsagar AV, Poole C, Mottl A, et al. N-acetylcysteine for the prevention of radiocontrast induced nephropathy: a meta-analysis of prospective controlled trials. *J Am Soc Nephrol.* 2004;15:761-769.
72. Lauterburg BH, Corcoran GB, Mitchell JR. Mechanism of action of N-acetylcysteine in the protection against the hepatotoxicity of acetaminophen in rats. *J Clin Invest.* 1983;71:980-991.
73. Lauterburg BH, Velez M. Glutathione deficiency in alcoholics: risk factor for paracetamol hepatotoxicity. *Gut.* 1988;29:1153-1157.
74. Lavonas EJ, Farhood A, Hopper RD, et al. Intravenous administration of N-acetylcysteine: oral and parenteral formulations are both acceptable. *Ann Emerg Med.* 2005;45:223-224.
75. Lederman S, Fysh WJ, Tredger M, Gamsu HR. Neonatal paracetamol poisoning: treatment by exchange transfusion. *Arch Dis Child.* 1983;58:631-633.
76. Leonis M, Balistreri W. Is there a "Nac" to treating acute liver failure. *Liver Transplant.* 2008;14:7-8.
77. Linden CH, Rumack BH. Acetaminophen overdose. *Emerg Med Clin North Am.* 1984;2:103-119.
78. Llobet JM, Domingo JL, Corbella J. Comparative effects of repeated parenteral administration of several chelators on the distribution and excretion of cobalt. *Res Commun Chem Pathol Pharmacol.* 1988;60:225-233.
79. Lovat R, Preiser JC. Antioxidant therapy in intensive care. *Curr Opin Crit Care.* 2003;9:266-270.
80. Lucena MI, Lopez-Torres E, Verge C. The administration of Nacetylcysteine causes a decrease in prothrombin time in patients with paracetamol overdose but without evidence of liver impairment. *Eur J Gastroenterol Hepatol.* 2005;17:59-63.
81. Lynch RM, Robertson R. Anaphylactoid reactions to intravenous Nacetylcysteine: a prospective case controlled study. *Accid Emerg Nurs.* 2004;12:10-15.
82. Manini AF, Snider C. Intravenous loading infusion rates of N-acetylcysteine. *Ann Emerg Med.* 2006;47:123.
83. Mant TGK, Tompowski JH, Volans GN, Talbot JC. Adverse reactions to acetylcysteine and effects of overdose. *Br Med J.* 1984;289:217-219.
84. Marenzi G, Assanelli E, Marana I, et al. N-acetylcysteine and contrast-induced nephropathy in primary angioplasty. *N Engl J Med.* 2006;354:2773-2882.
85. Merl W, Koutsogiannis Z, Kerr D, Kelly AM. How safe is intravenous N-acetylcysteine for the treatment of paracetamol poisoning. *Hong Kong J Emerg Med.* 2007;14:198-203.
86. Miller MA, Navarro M, Bird SB, Donovan JL. Antiemetic use in acetaminophen poisoning: how does the route of N-acetylcysteine administration affect utilization? *J Med Toxicol.* 2007;3:152-156.
87. Mitchell JR, Thorgeirsson SS, Potter WZ, et al. Acetaminophen-induced hepatic injury: protective role of glutathione in man and rationale for therapy. *Clin Pharmacol Ther.* 1974;16:676-684.
88. Mour G, Feinfeld DA, Caraccio T, McGuigan M. Acute renal dysfunction in acetaminophen poisoning. *Renal Failure.* 2005;27:381-383.
89. Mullins ME, Schmidt RU Jr, Jang TB. What is the rate of adverse events with intravenous versus oral N-acetylcysteine in pediatric patients? *Ann Emerg Med.* 2004;44:547-548.
90. North D, Peterson RG, Krenzelok E. Effect of activated charcoal administration on acetylcysteine serum levels in humans. *Am J Hosp Pharm.* 1981;38:1022-1024.
91. Ozcan EE, Guneri S, Akdeniz B, et al. Sodium bicarbonate, N-acetylcysteine, and saline for prevention of radiocontrast-induced nephropathy. A comparison of 3 regimens for protecting contrast-induced nephropathy in patients undergoing coronary procedures. A single-center prospective controlled trial. *Am Heart J.* 2007;154:539-544.
92. Peake J, Suzuki K. Neutrophil activation, antioxidant supplements and exercise-induced oxidative stress. *Exerc Immunol Rev.* 2004;10:129-141.
93. Pendyala L, Creaven PJ. Pharmacokinetic and pharmacodynamic studies of N-acetylcysteine, a potential chemopreventive agent during a phase 1 trial. *Cancer Epidemiol Biomarkers Prev.* 1995;4:245-251.
94. Piperno E, Berssenbruegge DA. Reversal of experimental paracetamol toxicosis with N-acetylcysteine. *Lancet.* 1976;2:738-739.
95. Pizon AF, LoVecchio F. Adverse reaction from use of intravenous N-acetylcysteine. *J Emerg Med.* 2006;31:434-435.
96. Prescott LF, Sutherland GR, Park J, et al. Cysteamine, methionine, and penicillamine in the treatment of paracetamol poisoning. *Lancet.* 1976;2:109-113.
97. Prescott LF, Donovan JW, Jarvie DR, et al. The disposition and kinetics of intravenous N-acetylcysteine in patients with paracetamol over-dosage. *Eur J Clin Pharmacol.* 1989;37:501-506.
98. Prescott LF, Illingworth RN, Critchley JAJH, et al. Intravenous N-acetylcysteine: the treatment of choice for paracetamol poisoning. *Br Med J.* 1979;2:1097-1100.
99. Prescott LF, Newton RW, Swainson CP, et al. Successful treatment of severe paracetamol overdosage with cysteamine. *Lancet.* 1974;1:588-592.
100. Prescott L. Oral or intravenous N-acetylcysteine for acetaminophen poisoning? *Ann Emerg Med.* 2005;45:409-413.
101. Rank N, Michel C, Haertel C, et al. N-acetylcysteine increases liver blood flow and improves liver function in septic shock patients: results of a prospective, randomized, double-blind study. *Crit Care Med.* 2000;28:3799-3807.
102. Reliene R, Fischer E, Schiestl R. The effect of N-acetylcysteine cysteine on oxidative DNA damage and the frequency of DNA deletions in atm-deficient mice. *Cancer Res.* 2004;64:5148-5153.
103. Renzi F, Donovan J, Morgan L, et al. Concomitant use of activated charcoal and N-acetylcysteine. *Ann Emerg Med.* 1985;14:568-572.
104. Reynard K, Riley A, Walker BE. Respiratory arrest after N-acetylcysteine for a paracetamol overdose. *Lancet.* 1992;340:675.
105. Riggs BS, Bronstein AC, Kulig KW, et al. Acute acetaminophen overdose during pregnancy. *Obstet Gynecol.* 1989;74:247-253.
106. Riordan SM, Williams R. Fulminant hepatic failure. *Clin Liver Dis.* 2000;4:25-45.
107. Roberts DW, Bucci TJ, Benson RW, et al. Immunohistochemical localization and quantification of the 3 (cystein-5-yl) acetaminophen protein adduct in acetaminophen hepatotoxicity. *Am J Pathol.* 1991;138:359-371.
108. Roberts I, Robinson M, Mughal MZ, et al. Paracetamol metabolites in the neonate following maternal overdose. *Br J Clin Pharmacol.* 1984;18:201-201.
109. Roller A, Weller M. Antioxidants specifically inhibit cisplatin cytotoxicity of human malignant glioma cells. *Anticancer Res.* 1998;18:4493-4498.
110. Ruffmann R, Wendel A. GSH rescue by N-acetylcysteine. *Klin Wochenschr.* 1991;69:857-862.
111. Rumack BH. Acetaminophen toxicity: the first 35 years. *J Toxicol Clin Toxicol.* 2002;40:3-20.
112. Rumack BH, Peterson RG. Acetaminophen overdose: incidence, diagnosis and management in 416 patients. *Pediatrics.* 1978;62(suppl):898-903.
113. Rybolt T, Burrell D, Shults J, Kelley A. In vitro coadsorption of acetaminophen and N-acetylcysteine onto activated carbon powder. *J Pharm Sci.* 1986;75:904-905.
114. Safirstein R, Andrade L, Vieira J. Acetylcysteine and nephrotoxic effects of radiographic contrast agents—a new use for an old drug. *N Engl J Med.* 2000;343:210-212.
115. Schaller G, Pleiner J, Mittermayer F, et al. Effects of N-acetylcysteine against systemic and renal hemodynamic effects of endotoxin in healthy humans. *Crit Care Med.* 2007;35:1869-1875.

115a. Schwartz EA, Hayes BD, Sarmiento KF. Development of hepatic failure despite use of intravenous acetylcysteine after a massive ingestion of acetaminophen and diphenhydramine. *Ann Emerg Med.* 2009;54:421-423.

116. Selden BS, Curry SC, Clark RF, et al. Transplacental transport of N-acetylcysteine in an ovine model. *Ann Intern Med.* 1991;20:1069-1072.
117. Sharma A, Howland MA, Hoffman RS, et al. The dilemma of NAC therapy in a premature infant. *J Toxicol Clin Toxicol.* 2000;38:57.
118. Shriner K, Goetz M. Severe hepatotoxicity in a patient receiving both acetaminophen and zidovudine. *Am J Med.* 1992;93:94-96.
119. Shyu KG, Cheng JJ, Kuan P. Acetylcysteine protects against acute renal damage in patients with abnormal renal function undergoing a coronary procedure. *J Am Coll Cardiol.* 2002;40:1383-1388.
120. Slattery JT, Wilson JM, Kalhorn TF, Nelson SD. Dose-dependent pharmacokinetics of acetaminophen: evidence of glutathione depletion in humans. *Clin Pharmacol Ther.* 1987;41:413-418.
121. Smilkstein MJ, Bronstein AC, Linden CH, et al. Acetaminophen overdose: a 48-hour intravenous N-acetylcysteine protocol. *Ann Emerg Med.* 1991;20:1058-1063.
122. Smilkstein MJ, Knapp GL, Kulig KW, et al. Efficacy of oral N-acetylcysteine in the treatment of acetaminophen overdose. Analysis of the national multicenter study (1976–1985). *N Engl J Med.* 1988;319:1557-1562.
122a. Smith SW, Howland MA, Hoffman RS, Nelson LS. Acetaminophen overdose with altered acetaminophen pharmacokinetics and hepatotoxicity associated with premature cessation of intravenous *N*-acetylcysteine therapy. *Ann Pharmacother.* 2008;42:1333-1339.
123. Sochman J. N-acetylcysteine in acute cardiology: 10 years later: what do we know and what would we like to know? *J Am Coll Cardiol.* 2002;39:1422-1428.
124. Sochman J, Vrbska J, Musilova B, et al. Infarct size limitation: acute N-acetylcysteine defense (ISLAND) trial. Start of the study. *Int J Cardiol.* 1995;49:181-182.
125. Spapen HD, Diltoer MW, Nguyen DN, et al. Effects of N-acetylcysteine on microalbuminuria and organ failure in acute severe sepsis: results of a pilot study. *Chest.* 2005;127:1413-1419.
126. Spies CD, Reinhart K, Witt I, et al. Influence of N-acetylcysteine on indirect indicators of tissue oxygenation in septic shock patients. *Crit Care Med.* 1994;22:1738-1746.
127. Stravitz RT, Kramer AH, Davern T, et al. Intensive care of patients with acute liver failure: recommendations of the U.S. Acute Liver Failure Study Group. *Crit Care Med.* 2007;35:2498-2508.
128. Sung L, Simons J, Dayneka N. Dilution of intravenous N-acetylcysteine as a cause of hyponatremia. *Pediatrics.* 1997;100:389-391.
129. Tepel M, VanDer Giet M, Schwarzfeld C, et al. Prevention of radiographic-contrast-agent-induced reductions in renal function by acetylcysteine. *N Engl J Med.* 2000;343:180-184.
130. Thomale UW, Griebenow M, Kroppenstedt SN, et al. The effect of N-acetylcysteine on posttraumatic changes after controlled cortical impact in rats. *Intensive Care Med.* 2006;32:149-155.
131. Thomassen D, Knebel N, Slattery JT, McClanahan RH, Nelson SD. Reactive intermediates in the oxidation of menthofuran by cytochromes P-450. *Chem Res Toxicol.* 1992;5:123-130.
132. Thomassen D, Slattery JT, Nelson SD. Menthofuran-dependent and independent aspects of pulegone hepatotoxicity: roles of glutathione. *J Pharmacol Exp Ther.* 1990;253:567-572.
133. Thompson DC, Barhoumi R, Burghardt RC. Comparative toxicity of eugenol and its quinine methide metabolite in cultured liver cells using kinetic fluorescence bioassays. *Toxicol Appl Pharmacol.* 1998;149:55-63.
134. Thompson DC, Constantin-Teodosiu D, Egestad B, et al. Formation of glutathione conjugates during oxidation of eugenol by microsomal fractions of rat liver and lung. *Biochem Pharmacol.* 1990;39:1587-1595.
135. Tong TC, Hernandez M, Richardson WH 3rd, et al. Comparative treatment of alpha-amanitin poisoning with N-acetylcysteine, benzylpenicillin, cimetidine, thioctic acid, and silybin in a murine model. *Ann Emerg Med.* 2007;50:282-283.
136. Vale JA, Meredith TJ, Goulding R. Treatment of acetaminophen poisoning. The use of oral methionine. *Arch Intern Med.* 1981;141:394-396.
137. Vale JA, Wheeler DC. Anaphylactoid reactions to N-acetylcysteine. *Lancet.* 1982;2:988.
138. Valles EG, de Castro CR, Castro JA. N-acetyl cysteine is an early but also a late preventive agent against carbon tetrachloride-induced liver necrosis. *Toxicol Lett.* 1994;71:87-95.
139. Walsh TS, Lee A. N-Acetylcysteine administration in the critically ill. *Intensive Care Med.* 1999;25:432-434.
140. Walsh TS, Hopton P, Philips BJ, et al. The effect of N-acetylcysteine on oxygen transport and uptake in patients with fulminant hepatic failure. *Hepatology.* 1998;27:1332-1340.
141. Walton NG, Mann TN, Shaw KM. Anaphylactoid reaction to N-acetylcysteine. *Lancet.* 1979;2:1298.
142. Waring WS, Stephen AF, Robinson OD. Lower incidence of anaphylactoid reactions to N-acetylcysteine in patients with high acetaminophen concentrations after overdose. *Clin Toxicol. (Phila).* 2008;46:496-500.
143. Wasserman GS, Garg U. Intravenous administration of N-acetylcysteine: interference with coagulopathy testing. *Ann Emerg Med.* 2004;44:546-547.
144. Whyte IM, Francis B, Dawson AH. Safety and efficacy of intravenous N-acetylcysteine for acetaminophen overdose: analysis of the Hunter Area Toxicology Service (HATS) database. *Curr Med Res Opin.* 2007;23:2359-2368.
145. Wong CK, Ooi VE, Kim C. Protective effects of N-acetylcysteine against carbon tetrachloride and trichloroethylene-induced poisoning in rats. *Environ Toxicol Pharmacol.* 2003;14:109-116.
146. Woo OF, Mueller PD, Olson KR, et al. Shorter duration of oral Nacetylcysteine therapy for acute acetaminophen overdose. *Ann Emerg Med.* 2000;35:363-368.
147. Yi JH, Hoover R, McIntosh TK, Hazell AS. Early, transient increase in complexin I and complexin II in the cerebral cortex following traumatic brain injury is attenuated by N-acetylcysteine. *J Neurotrauma.* 2006;23:86-96.
148. Yip L, Dart R, Hurlbut K. Intravenous administration of oral N-acetylcysteine. *Crit Care Med.* 1998;26:40-43.
149. Yip L, Dart RC. A 20-hour treatment for acute acetaminophen overdose. *N Engl J Med.* 2003;348:2471-2472.

CHAPTER 35
SALICYLATES

Neal E. Flomenbaum

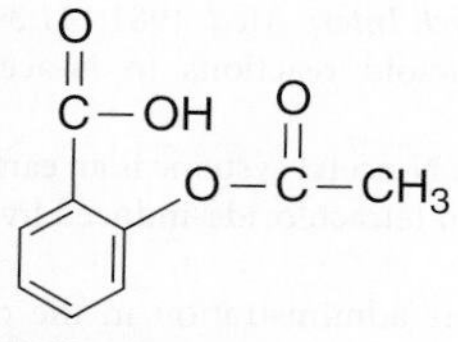

Acetylsalicylic acid

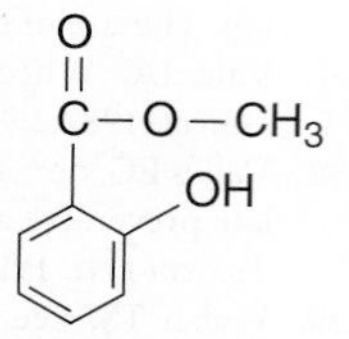

Methylsalicylic acid

Salicylic Acid

MW	=	138 daltons
Therapeutic serum concentration	=	15–30 mg/dL
	=	1.1–2.2 mmol/L

Salicylate overdose remains a consequential concern for clinicians. Unintentional salicylate toxicity may occur in patients who are unaware that fixed-dose cold preparations may contain aspirin and who concomitantly take aspirin, seeking further relief of their symptoms. Serious adolescent and adult salicylate poisonings frequently result from suicide attempts. Even in this setting, rapid diagnosis and appropriate therapy initiated quickly can reduce mortality. Salicylism should be considered in patients who have tachypnea, acid–base disorders, and acute lung injury (ALI), particularly anyone using salicylates. Unexplained neurologic abnormalities should also raise concern, particularly in patients in the aforementioned groups.[4]

HISTORY AND EPIDEMIOLOGY

Hippocrates may have been among the first to use willow bark and leaves to relieve fever, but it was not until 1829 that the glycoside salicin was extracted from the willow bark and used as an antipyretic. Seven years later, salicylic acid was isolated, and by the late 1800s, it was being used to treat gout, rheumatic fever, and elevated temperatures. The less irritating acetylated compound was first synthesized in 1833, and in 1899 acetylsalicylic acid was commercially introduced as aspirin by Bayer.[19] With that, the modern era of aspirin therapy and salicylate toxicity began.

Since 2000, the category of analgesics, which includes both aspirin and acetaminophen, has consistently ranked first among the xenobiotics most frequently reported in human exposures. In 2007, the American Association of Poison Control Centers (AAPCC) National Poison Data System (NPDS) reported 309,431 analgesic exposures in the United States. Of the 1239 deaths judged to be poison-related fatalities, aspirin alone accounted for 63. Isolated aspirin poisoning is the 14th most common cause of death from toxic exposures recorded by AAPCC NPDS (see Chap. 135).

Safety packaging, together with the increased use of nonsteroidal antiinflammatory drugs (NSAIDs), acetaminophen, and other alternatives to aspirin have contributed to the decreased incidence of unintentional salicylate poisoning. On the other hand, the widespread availability of salicylate preparations without prescription and the toxicity caused by small increments in salicylate dosage when used chronically have contributed to its continued implication in poisoning.[79]

Over the past 2 decades, popular brand and product names previously associated exclusively with salicylates or acetaminophen have been applied to other analgesic-containing products. For example, the names Alka-Seltzer, Anacin, and Excedrin, which once were used exclusively for salicylate-containing products, are now used as brand names for products containing aspirin, acetaminophen, or both. Bayer, a company once associated exclusively with aspirin, now also markets a line of products called Bayer Select, which contain ibuprofen or acetaminophen. Clinicians should be vigilant for parents and healthcare providers who, while seeking to give acetaminophen to avoid Reye syndrome,[10,72] may inadvertently give their children a product containing aspirin.[27] Intentional or unintentional overdose of nonprescription brands or products might involve aspirin.[27] Salicylate toxicity may also result from confusion regarding the correct dosage: Terms such as *grains* and *milligrams* and *baby*, *children's*, *junior*, and *adult aspirin* are often misunderstood.

PHARMACOLOGY AND TOXICOLOGY OF SALICYLATES

There are two types of salicylic acid esters: phenolic esters such as aspirin and carboxylic acid esters, including methyl salicylate, phenyl salicylate, and glycosalicylate.[34] Most of the studies of salicylate metabolism involve aspirin.[34] The implicit assumption is that all members of the salicylate class have similar properties after they are converted to salicylic acid.

Aspirin and other salicylates are analgesics, antiinflammatories, and antipyretics, a combination of traits shared by all medications of varying structures known as NSAIDs. Most of the beneficial effects of NSAIDs result from the inhibition of cyclooxygenase (COX). This enzyme enables the synthesis of prostaglandins, which in turn mediate inflammation and fever.[116,136] Contributing to the antiinflammatory effects and independent of the effects on prostaglandins, salicylates and other NSAIDs may also directly inhibit neutrophils.[12]

Salicylates and NSAIDs are purportedly most effective in treating the pain accompanying inflammation and tissue injury. Such pain is elicited by prostaglandins liberated by bradykinin and other cytokines. Fever is also mediated by cytokines such as interleukin (IL)-1β, IL-6, α and β interferons, and tumor necrosis factor-α, all of which increase synthesis of prostaglandin E2.[19] In turn, this inflammatory mediatory increases cyclic AMP, triggering the hypothalamus to elevate the body temperature set point, resulting in increased heat generation and decreased heat loss.[26]

Because platelets cannot regenerate COX-1, a daily dose of as little as 30 mg of aspirin inhibits COX-1 for the 8- to 12-day life of the platelet.[19] Adverse effects of aspirin and some NSAIDs related to alteration of COX include gastrointestinal (GI) ulcerations and bleeding, interference with platelet adherence,[119] and a variety of metabolic and organ-specific effects described below under Gastrointestinal Effects.

To achieve an antiinflammatory effect for patients with chronic conditions such as rheumatoid arthritis, salicylates typically have been prescribed in doses sufficient to achieve serum salicylate concentrations of 15 to 30 mg/dL, which is considered the therapeutic range. Concentrations higher than 30 mg/dL are associated with signs and symptoms of toxicity.

Salicylate is rapidly absorbed from aspirin tablets in the stomach. The pK_a of aspirin is 3.5, and the majority of salicylate is nonionized (ie, salicylic acid) in the acidic stomach (pH, 1–2).[34,67] Although absorption of salicylate may be less efficient in the small bowel because of its higher pH, it is substantial and rapid due to the large surface area and the increase in pH increases the solubility of salicylate.[19,97,98] The dosage form of salicylates (eg, effervescent, enteric coated) influences the absorption rate.[118,121,145] Delayed absorption of aspirin may result from salicylate-induced pylorospasm or pharmacobezoar formation.[14,118]

After ingestion of therapeutic doses of immediate-release salicylate, significant serum concentrations are achieved in 30 minutes, and maximum concentrations are often attained in less than 1 hour.[34] The apparent volume of distribution (Vd) increases from 0.2 L/kg at low concentrations to more than 0.3 L/kg (possibly as high as 0.5 L/kg) at higher concentrations.[87,88,130] There is a decrease in protein (albumin) binding from 90% at therapeutic concentrations to less than 75% at toxic concentrations caused by saturation of protein binding sites.[2,15,41]

Salicylates have substantially longer apparent half-lives at toxic concentrations than at therapeutic concentrations, varying from 2 to 4 hours at therapeutic concentrations to as long as 20 hours at high concentrations.[37,89] Salicylates are conjugated with glycine and glucuronides in the liver and are eliminated by the kidneys. Approximately 10% of salicylates are excreted in the urine as free salicylic acid, 75% as salicyluric acid, 10% as salicylic phenolic glucuronides, 5% as acylglucuronides, and 1% as gentisic acid.[19] As the concentration of salicylates increases, two of the five pathways of elimination—those for salicyluric acid and the salicylic phenolic glucuronide—become saturated and exhibit zero-order kinetics. As a result of this saturation, overall salicylate elimination changes from first-order kinetics to zero-order kinetics.[87] When administered chronically, a small increase in dosage or a small decrease in metabolism or renal function may result in substantial increases in serum salicylate concentrations and toxicity.[79] At very high serum concentrations, first-order elimination may become more prominent because of an increasing fraction of renal clearance. Figure 35–1 illustrates the main features of salicylate metabolism (see Chap. 8).

Free salicylic acid is filtered through the glomerulus and both passively reabsorbed and secreted from the proximal tubules. More than 30% of ingested salicylate may be eliminated in alkaline urine and as little as 2% in acidic urine.[139] Salicylate conjugates (glycine and glucuronides) are filtered and secreted by the proximal tubules; salicylate conjugates are not reabsorbed across renal tubular cells because of poor lipid solubility, and the amount eliminated is dependent on glomerular filtration rate and proximal tubule secretion but not urine pH. Protein-binding abnormalities, urine and plasma pH variations, and delayed absorption all influence the maximum salicylate concentrations and the rates of decline.[98,118]

PATHOPHYSIOLOGY

ACID–BASE DISTURBANCES CAUSED BY SALICYLATE POISONING

Salicylate stimulates the respiratory center in the brainstem, leading to hyperventilation and respiratory alkalosis.[134] In addition, salicylates are weak acids, and in toxic concentrations, they titrate approximately 2 to 3 mEq/L of plasma bicarbonate. Toxic concentrations of salicylate impair renal hemodynamics, leading to the accumulation of inorganic acids. Salicylate interferes with the Krebs cycle, which limits production of adenosine triphosphate (ATP).[77] It also uncouples oxidative phosphorylation, causing accumulation of pyruvic and lactic acids

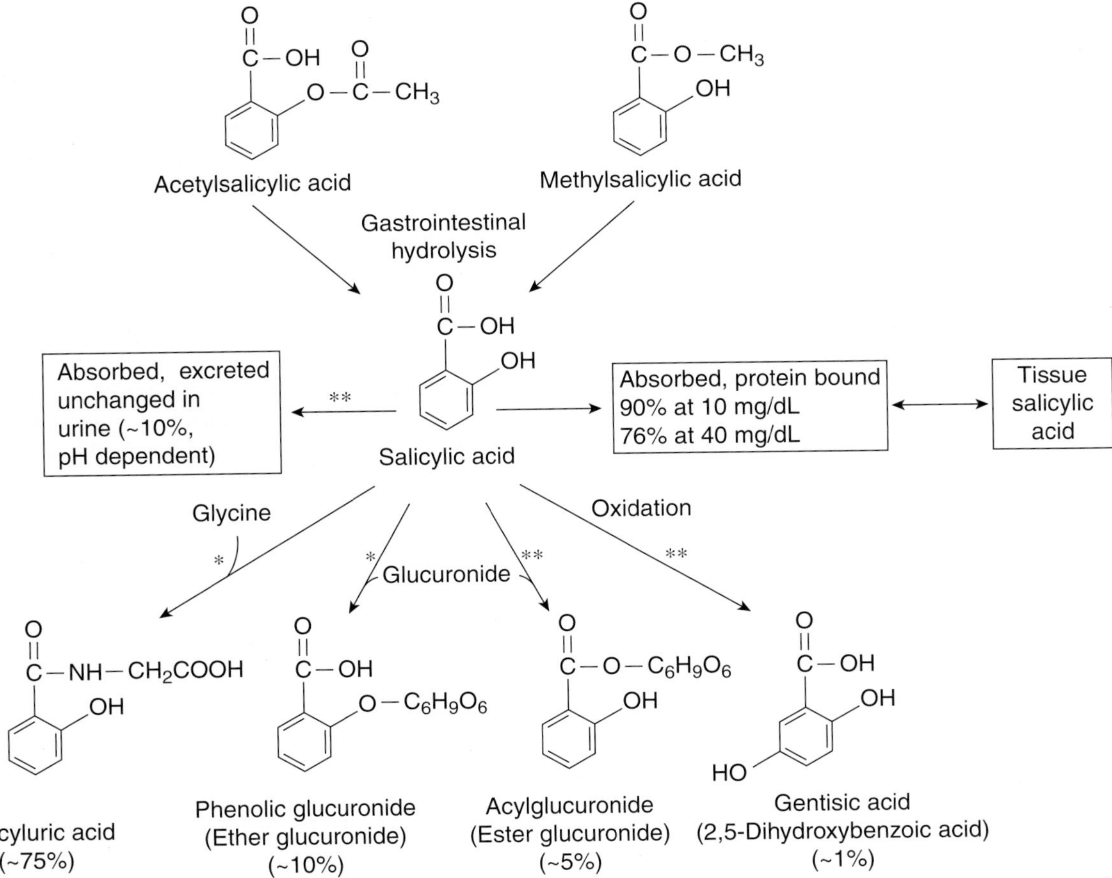

FIGURE 35–1. Salicylic acid metabolism. At excessive doses, the 4 mechanisms of salicylic acid metabolism are overloaded, leading to increased tissue binding, decreased protein binding, and increased excretion of unconjugated salicylic acid.* = Michaelis-Menten kinetics; ** = first-order kinetics.

and releasing energy as heat[83] (see Chap. 12). Salicylate-induced increased fatty acid metabolism generates ketone bodies, including β-hydroxybutyric acid, acetoacetic acid, and acetone. The net result of all of these metabolic processes is an anion gap metabolic acidosis (see Chap. 16), in which the unmeasured anions include salicylate and its metabolites, lactate, ketoacids, and inorganic acids.

Neurologic Effects The central nervous system (CNS) effects are the most visible and most consequential clinical effects in salicylate-poisoned patients. With increasing CNS salicylate concentrations, neuronal energy depletion likely develops as salicylate uncouples neuronal and glial oxidative phosphorylation,[96] resulting in neuronal dysfunction and ultimately cerebral edema.

Correlation Between Cerebrospinal Fluid and Serum Salicylate Concentrations. Salicylate concentrations in the cerebrospinal fluid (CSF) directly correlate with death in primates.[64] Inhalation of carbon dioxide in a dog resulted in a precipitous decrease in serum salicylate concentrations, which returned to baseline rapidly after the discontinuation of CO_2.[65] This suggests that the salicylate redistributed into tissue during the period of induced respiratory acidosis and reequilibrated after its correction. Autoradiographs of cat brain after administration of radiolabeled salicylate visually and objectively document the profound effect that acidosis has on the distribution of salicylate into the brain.[56] However, even if CSF salicylate concentrations in humans are more accurate predictors of toxicity than serum concentrations, their use in clinical management is currently impractical. Furthermore, serum salicylate concentrations in the presence of acidemia may have little or no correlation with the CSF salicylate concentration.

Glucose Metabolism Salicylate poisoning may produce a discordance between serum and CSF glucose concentrations.[117] Despite normal serum glucose concentrations, CSF glucose concentration decreased 33% in salicylate-poisoned mice compared with controls.[135] In other words, the rate of CSF glucose use exceeded the rate of supply, even in the presence of a normal serum glucose concentration. There was also a marked increase in oxygen consumption in mice, even with low salicylate concentrations, highlighting the importance of salicylate-induced uncoupling of oxidative phosphorylation.[64]

Hepatic Effects Salicylate-poisoned mice had a marked decrease in hepatic glycogen and a dramatic increase in serum lactate concentration compared with control subjects.[65] This is likely because of increased glycogenolysis and glycolysis to compensate partly for the energy loss caused by uncoupling of oxidative phosphorylation.[96] Salicylates reduce lipogenesis by blocking the incorporation of acetate into free fatty acids and increase peripheral fatty acid metabolism as an energy source, resulting in ketone formation.

Through the depletion of intrahepatocyte coenzyme A (Co-A), fatty acids entering the hepatocyte cytoplasm cannot be transported into the mitochondria for beta-oxidation. The buildup of fatty acids in the hepatocyte results in microvesicular steatosis, which is characteristic of Reye syndrome.

Otolaryngologic Effects The molecular mechanism of salicylate ototoxicity is not completely understood but appears to be multifactorial. Inhibition of cochlear COX by salicylate increases arachidonate, enabling calcium flux and neural excitatory effects of *N*-methyl-D-aspartic acid (NMDA) on cochlear spinal ganglion neurons.[112,123] Also, the prevention of prostaglandin synthesis interferes with the Na^+-K^+-adenosine triphosphatase (ATPase) pump in the stria vascularis, and the vasoconstriction decreases cochlear blood flow.[16,21,45,74] Membrane permeability changes cause a loss of outer hair cell turgor in the organ of Corti, which may impair otoacoustic emissions.[113,115] See Chapter 20 for a more complete description of the pathophysiology of salicylate-induced ototoxicity and sensorineural alterations as well as comparisons with the patterns of other ototoxic xenobiotics.

Pulmonary Effects ALI results from increased pulmonary capillary permeability and subsequent exudation of high-protein edema fluid into the interstitial or alveolar spaces.[69] Hypothalamic insults from increased intracranial pressure or salicylate CNS poisoning may be the critical factor, with resultant adrenergic overactivity. This "central" ALI shifts blood from the systemic to the pulmonary circulation because of a loss of left ventricular compliance with left atrial and pulmonary capillary hypertension (see Chap. 21). Additionally, the resulting hypoxia results in pulmonary arterial hypertension and a local release of vasoactive substances, worsening ALI.[70]

Gastrointestinal Effects GI manifestations result from local gastric irritation at lower doses and from stimulation of the medullary chemoreceptor trigger zone at higher doses. Hemorrhagic gastritis, decreased gastric motility, and pylorospasm also result from the direct gastric irritant effects of salicylates.[121]

Renal Effects The kidneys clearly play a major role in the handling and excretion of salicylate and its metabolites. Although some believe that salicylates are nephrotoxic, the majority of studies and experimental evidence do not strongly support this notion.[32,43,106] Most of the adverse renal effects historically associated with salicylates occurred with use of combination products such as aspirin–phenacetin–caffeine (APC) tablets and appear to have been mostly caused by the phenacetin.[43] Renal papillary necrosis and chronic interstitial nephritis, initially characterized by reduced tubular function and reduced concentrating ability, rarely occur in adults using salicylates unless they have chronic illnesses that already compromise renal function.

Chronic nephrotoxicity from long-term use of aspirin alone has been demonstrated in humans in only one case-control series. In adults with preexisting glomerulonephritis, cirrhosis, or chronic renal insufficiency and in children with congestive heart failure, short-term therapeutic doses of aspirin may precipitate reversible acute renal failure, possibly because of inhibition of the vasodilatory prostaglandins necessary to maintain renal blood flow in people with these conditions.[32] In healthy adults, however, short-term therapeutic doses of aspirin do not adversely affect creatinine clearance, urine volume, or sodium and potassium clearance. Aspirin doses above 300 mg/kg may cause acute renal failure, and chronic aspirin poisoning may cause reversible or irreversible acute renal failure.[32]

Hematologic Effects The hematologic effects of salicylate poisoning include hypoprothrombinemia and platelet dysfunction.[105] The platelet dysfunction, caused by irreversible acetylation of COX-1 and -2, prevents the formation thromboxane A_2, which is normally responsible for platelet aggregation. The platelets themselves are numerically and morphologically intact but are unresponsive to thrombogenic stimulation. Hypoprothrombinemia is the result of interruption of vitamin K cycling, similar to that of warfarin.[103] Anemia in patients who chronically abuse salicylates may be a result of the effects of both platelet dysfunction and GI bleeding.[105] Hemolysis is unusual, and alterations in leukocyte function are of no apparent clinical significance.[122]

Musculoskeletal Effects Rhabdomyolysis after salicylate overdose probably results from uncoupling of muscular oxidative phosphorylation.[86,96,97] Paratonia, characterized by extreme muscle postmortem rigidity, was present in three of the 51 salicylate deaths reviewed in Ontario between 1983 and 1984.[95] Rapid rigor mortis and paratonia (which are not unique to salicylate poisoning) are probably related to the extreme depletion of myocyte ATP and the inability of the muscle fibers to relax.

CLINICAL MANIFESTATIONS OF SALICYLATE POISONING

ACUTE SALICYLATE TOXICITY

The earliest signs and symptoms of salicylate toxicity, which include nausea, vomiting, diaphoresis, and tinnitus, typically develop within 1 to 2 hours of acute exposure.[16,53,131] As CNS salicylate concentrations increase, tinnitus is rapidly followed by diminished auditory acuity that sometimes leads to deafness.[16] Other early CNS effects may include vertigo and hyperventilation manifested as hyperpnea or tachypnea (see Chap. 3), hyperactivity, agitation, delirium, hallucinations, convulsions, lethargy, and stupor. Coma is rare and generally occurs only with severe acute poisoning or mixed overdoses (Table 35–1).[53] A marked elevation in temperature resulting from the uncoupling of oxidative phosphorylation caused by salicylate poisoning [96] is one indication of severe toxicity and is typically a preterminal condition.

TABLE 35–1. Clinical Manifestations and Diagnostic Testing Results of Salicylate Toxicity

Acid–Base and Electrolyte Disturbances	**Gastrointestinal**
Anion gap increased	Nausea
Respiratory alkalosis (predominates early)	Vomiting
Metabolic acidosis	Hemorrhagic gastritis
Respiratory acidosis (late, grave prognosis)	Decreased motility
Metabolic alkalosis (vomiting)	Pylorospasm
Hyponatremia or hypernatremia	**Hepatic**
Hypokalemia	Abnormal liver enzymes
Central Nervous System	Altered glucose metabolism
Tinnitus	**Metabolic**
Diminished auditory acuity	Diaphoresis
Vertigo	Hyperthermia
Hallucinations	Hypoglycemia
Agitation	Hyperglycemia
Hyperactivity	Hypoglycorrhachia
Delirium	Ketonemia
Stupor	Ketonuria
Coma	**Pulmonary**
Lethargy	Hyperpnea
Convulsions	Tachypnea
Cerebral edema	Respiratory alkalosis
Syndrome of inappropriate antidiuretic hormone	Acute lung injury
Coagulation Abnormalities	**Renal**
Hypoprothrombinemia	Tubular damage
Inhibition of factors V, VII, and X	Proteinuria
Platelet dysfunction	NaCl and water retention
	Hypouricemia

Unfortunately, many of the signs and symptoms of salicylate toxicity are vague and may be mistakenly attributed to another illness with disastrous consequences.[28,131] In the review of all salicylate deaths in Ontario, Canada, in 1983 and 1984, the author noted that in six of the 23 (26%) patients who arrived alert, no salicylate determination appears to have been made and that probably neither the diagnosis nor the severity of the salicylate poisoning was recognized.[95]

Acid–Base Disturbances Caused by Salicylate Poisoning A primary respiratory alkalosis predominates initially, although a metabolic acidosis begins to develop early in the course of consequential salicylate toxicity. By the time a symptomatic adult patient presents to the hospital after a substantial acute or chronic salicylate overdose, a mixed acid–base disturbance is often prominent.[54] This latter finding includes two primary processes, a respiratory alkalosis and a metabolic acidosis, and is discernible by arterial blood gas (ABG) and serum electrolyte analyses. In one study of 66 salicylate-poisoned adults, 22% had respiratory alkalosis and 56% had mixed respiratory alkalosis and metabolic acidosis.[54]

The predominant primary respiratory alkalosis that initially characterizes salicylate poisoning in adults may be missed in young children.[55,131] Possible reasons for this include the limited ventilatory reserve of small children that prevents the same degree of sustained hyperpnea as occurs in adults, the fact that children may present later for healthcare, or the exposure to salicylates per body weight may be much larger. The typical acidemic presentation of a seriously poisoned child led some investigators in the past to incorrectly suggest that pediatric salicylate poisoning produces only metabolic acidosis. Although after a significant salicylate exposure, some children present with a mixed acid–base disturbance and a normal or high pH, most present with acidemia.[55]

The mixed acid–base pattern is so characteristic of adult salicylate poisoning that any salicylate-poisoned adult who presents with respiratory acidosis almost certainly has salicylate-induced ALI, severe fatigue from the strenuous exercise of hyperventilating for a prolonged period, or CNS depression (eg, mixed overdose). Mixed xenobiotic overdoses in adult populations are fairly common, as demonstrated by the findings of one study that one-third of patients with a presumed primary salicylate overdose had taken other xenobiotics.[54] Benzodiazepines, barbiturates, alcohol, and cyclic antidepressants all blunt the centrally induced hyperventilatory response to salicylates, resulting in either actual respiratory acidosis (PCO_2 >40 mm Hg) or metabolic acidosis without an apparently appropriate degree of respiratory compensation (PCO_2 <40 mm Hg but inappropriately high for the concomitant degree of metabolic acidosis). In both adults and children, the development of respiratory acidosis may occur as salicylate poisoning progresses. The combination of metabolic and respiratory acidosis in a salicylate-poisoned adult resulting in severe and worsening acidemia indicates an exceedingly grave situation and almost invariably is a preterminal event.[109]

Neurologic Effects Hyperventilation is centrally mediated, and detection requires an assessment of both the ventilatory rate and depth. Patients may develop a spectrum of CNS abnormalities that includes confusion, agitation, lethargy, and then ultimately seizures and coma. The most severe clinical findings are likely associated with the development of cerebral edema and portend a poor prognosis.

Otolaryngologic Effects The pattern of salicylate-induced auditory sensorineural alterations is different than the pattern characterizing other ototoxic drugs.[20] Tinnitus, which is a subjective sensation of ringing or hissing, with or without hearing loss as well as loss of absolute acoustic sensitivity, and alterations of perceived sounds are the three effects resulting from exposure to large doses of salicylates.[20] Tinnitus and subsequent reversible hearing loss typically occurs with serum salicylate concentrations of 20 to 45 mg/dL or higher.[16,20,100] Occasionally, investigators have questioned whether salicylate ototoxicity may be used as an indicator of serum salicylate concentration, only to note that whereas some patients with therapeutic concentrations of salicylates complained of tinnitus, many with higher or toxic concentrations had no tinnitus. In a study of 94 patients with salicylate concentrations above 30 mg/dL on one or more occasions, tinnitus only correlated with serum salicylate concentrations in 30%; 55% had no tinnitus, although audiologic testing results were usually abnormal regardless of the presence or absence of tinnitus.[59] Thus, symptomatic ototoxicity is too nonspecific and too insensitive to serve as an indicator of serum salicylate concentrations.

Pulmonary Effects When a patient with salicylate poisoning presents with the clinical and radiographic manifestations of pulmonary edema or ALI, major causes that must be considered include aspiration pneumonitis, viral and bacterial infections, neurogenic ALI, and salicylate-induced ALI[70,78] (see Chap. 21). In 111 consecutive patients with peak salicylate concentrations above 30 mg/dL, ALI occurred in 35% of patients older than 30 years of age and none of the 55 patients younger than 16 years of age. Risk factors for developing ALI included cigarette smoking, chronic salicylate ingestion, and the presence of neurologic symptoms on admission. The average arterial blood pH was 7.37 in the six adult patients with ALI and 7.46 in the 30 adults without ALI. There was no significant difference in salicylate concentrations, which were approximately 57 mg/dL in both groups.[141] In a 2-year review of all salicylate deaths in Ontario, Canada, 59% of 39 autopsies revealed pulmonary pathology, mostly "pulmonary edema" (ALI).[95]

Hepatic Effects Salicylate-induced hepatitis occurred in children who were being treated with high (average concentration, 30.9 mg/dL) chronic doses of salicylates for rheumatic fever and juvenile rheumatoid arthritis.[60,93,124] Another form of liver disease associated with salicylates that also occurs primarily in children is Reye syndrome, which is characterized by nausea, vomiting, hypoglycemia, elevated concentrations of liver enzymes (aspartate aminotransferase [AST], alanine aminotransferase [ALT], fatty infiltration of the liver, and coma after a viral illness, usually influenza or varicella.[7,10] Although the link between Reye syndrome and salicylates has never been fully proven, the existence of such a link is fairly mechanistically certain, and the decreasing incidence that has occurred concomitantly with the decreased use of salicylates in children is highly suggestive.[10,22,140] Apart from the few cases still attributable to salicylate use, Reye or "Reye-like" syndromes may occur from other etiologies, including possible biochemical disturbances induced by viral or bacterial infections; microbial toxins; hypoglycin from unripe Ackee fruit; and valproic acid, tetracycline, zidovudine, diclofenac sodium, as well as a variety of antineoplastics.[114]

CHRONIC SALICYLATE TOXICITY

Chronic salicylate poisoning most typically occurs in elderly individuals as a result of unintentional overdosing on salicylates used to treat chronic conditions such as rheumatoid arthritis and osteoarthritis[5,39,79] (Table 35–2). Presenting signs and symptoms of chronic salicylate poisoning include hearing loss and tinnitus; nausea; vomiting; dyspnea and hyperventilation; tachycardia; hyperthermia; and neurologic manifestations such as confusion, delirium, agitation, hyperactivity, slurred speech, hallucinations, seizures, and coma.[4,40,53,85] Although there is considerable overlap with some of the presenting signs and symptoms of acute salicylate poisoning, the slow onset and less severe appearance of some of these signs of chronic poisoning in elderly individuals frequently cause delayed recognition of the true cause of the patient's presentation.[54]

TABLE 35–2. Differential Characteristics of Acute and Chronic Salicylate Poisoning

	Acute	Chronic
Age	Younger	Older
Etiology	Overdose usually intentional	Therapeutic misadventures; iatrogenic
Diagnosis	Easily recognized	Frequently unrecognized
Other diseases	None	Underlying disorders (especially chronic pain conditions)
Suicidal ideation	Typical	Usually absent
Serum concentrations	Marked elevation	Intermediate elevation
Mortality	Uncommon when recognized and properly treated	More common because of missed diagnosis

Typically, ill patients who have chronic salicylate poisoning may be misdiagnosed as having delirium, dementia, encephalopathy of undetermined origin, diseases such as sepsis (fever of unknown origin), alcoholic ketoacidosis, respiratory failure, or cardiopulmonary disease.[4,8,28,44,53] Unfortunately, many of the signs and symptoms of chronic salicylate toxicity may be mistakenly attributed to the illness for which the salicylates were administered, with serious consequences.[28,131] In a study of 73 consecutive adults hospitalized with salicylate poisoning, 27% were not correctly diagnosed for as long as 72 hours after admission.[4] These patients manifested toxicity with standard or excessive therapeutic regimens and had significant associated diseases without a history of previous overdoses. In this group, 60% of the patients had a previous neurologic consultation before the diagnosis of salicylism was established. When diagnosis is delayed in elderly individuals, the morbidity and mortality associated with salicylate poisoning are high. Mortality was reported to be as high as 25% in the 1970s,[4] and there are no data to suggest that survival after delayed diagnosis is substantially better today (see Table 35–2).

Underrecognition or misdiagnosis of chronic salicylate poisoning is not confined to elderly patients and may be a problem at the other end of the age spectrum as well. In one study of all children admitted to a district hospital in Kenya over a 3-month period with the primary diagnosis of severe malaria, 90% had detectable blood salicylate concentrations, and six of 143 had serum concentrations 20 mg/dL or above. All six of the children with serum salicylate concentrations of 20 mg/dL or above had neurologic impairment and metabolic acidosis, and four had hypoglycemia, suggesting that salicylates may be associated with the complications of malaria that have substantial morbidity and mortality.[44]

DIAGNOSTIC TESTING

Careful observation of the patient, correlation of the serum salicylate concentrations with blood pH, and repeat determinations of serum salicylate concentrations every 2 to 4 hours are essential until the patient is clinically improving and has a low serum salicylate concentration in the presence of a normal or high blood pH. In all cases, after

Prior to alkalinization

Tissues pH 6.8	Plasma pH 7.1	Urine pH 6.5
HA ⇄	HA ⇄	HA
↓↑	↓↑	↓↑
$H^+ + A^-$	$H^+ + A^-$ →	$H^+ + A^-$

After alkalinization

Tissues pH 6.8	Plasma pH 7.4	Urine pH 8.0
HA ⇄	HA ⇄	HA
↓↑	↓↑	↓↑
$H^+ + A^-$	$H^+ + A^-$ →	$H^+ + A^-$

FIGURE 35–2. Rationale for alkalinization.[131] Alkalinization of the plasma with respect to the tissues and alkalinization of the urine with respect to plasma shifts the equilibrium to the plasma and urine and away from the tissues, including the brain. This equilibrium shift results in "ion trapping."[131] (From Temple AR. Acute and chronic effects of aspirin toxicity and their treatment. *Arch Intern Med.* 1981;141:364-369.)

a presumed peak serum salicylate concentration has been reached, at least one additional serum concentration should be obtained several hours later. Analyses should be obtained more frequently in managing seriously ill patients to assess the efficacy of treatment and the possible need for hemodialysis (HD).

Serum salicylate concentrations may provide useful clinical correlations at a normal or high blood pH, but they should not be used as the sole determinant of the degree of toxicity. A concurrent arterial or venous blood pH should be determined when a serum salicylate concentration is obtained because in the presence of acidemia, more salicylic acid leaves the blood and enters the CSF and other tissues (Fig. 35–2), increasing the toxicity. In other words, meaningful interpretation of serum salicylate concentrations must take into account the effect of blood pH on salicylate distribution unless the serum salicylate concentration is so high that HD is indicated regardless of the pH. A decreasing serum salicylate concentration may be difficult to interpret because it may reflect either an increased tissue distribution with increasing toxicity or an increased clearance with decreasing toxicity. A decreasing serum salicylate concentration accompanied by a decreasing or low blood pH should be presumed to reflect a serious or worsening situation, not a benign or improving one.

In summary, when the patient's clinical signs and symptoms are given the highest priority and the serum salicylate concentration is interpreted in conjunction with a simultaneously obtained blood pH, the severity of toxicity usually can be predicted and the need for HD most accurately assessed.

RAPID CONFIRMATION OF SALICYLATE EXPOSURE

Rapid "point-of-care" determinations that may suggest salicylate poisoning in the proper clinical setting are (1) a positive urine ketone determination reflecting ketogenesis from increased fatty acid metabolism[66] or (2) a whole-blood electrolyte determination performed on a handheld analyzer, which can quickly demonstrate acid–base disturbance(s) characteristic of salicylate poisoning.

Serum salicylate concentrations are relatively easy to obtain in most hospital laboratories, and with proper attention to the units reported (mg/dL vs. mg/L) and concomitant arterial or venous blood pH values, clinicians can quickly confirm or exclude toxic salicylate concentrations. The historical bedside urine qualitative tests for the presence of salicylate (not for poisoning per se) using either ferric chloride or mercuric chloride (Trinder assay) can no longer be performed outside of a certified laboratory as they are not permissible under the federal Clinical Laboratory Improvement Amendments (CLIA) in the United States.

SERUM SALICYLATE CONCENTRATIONS AND CORRELATION WITH TOXICITY

Serum salicylate concentrations should be requested when clinically significant salicylate exposures are suspected and not as part of a general toxicologic screen. There is often confusion in correctly identifying aspirin and acetaminophen products, and the possibility that either or both may be used in a suicide attempt may suggest the need for determinations of both. Four studies, including one in the United States,[127] one in Hong Kong,[25] and two in the United Kingdom,[57,144] concluded that universal salicylate screening is not indicated for all patients with acute self-poisonings. The lack of initial symptoms after acetaminophen ingestion highlights the importance in routine laboratory screening for acetaminophen. The London, UK study of 596 patients concluded that routine measurements of serum salicylate concentration are not required in the absence of a positive history of salicylate ingestion, an inability to obtain a valid history (because of reduced level of consciousness, for example) and the absence of clinical features of salicylate poisoning. A prospective study in Glasgow, UK, considering routine testing for serum paracetamol and salicylate concentrations in 134 alert overdose patients found that no patient who had denied taking salicylate or paracetamol subsequently tested positive. In the absence of any clinical indications of toxicity, routine ASA testing may not be necessary for fully conscious patients. [57] In current practice, insufficient information is often obtained from patients to identify the clinical features of toxicity, and there is a need for focused clinical investigation for signs and symptoms of salicylate poisoning in at-risk groups.[144]

ERRORS IN THE INTERPRETATION OF SERUM SALICYLATE CONCENTRATIONS

Laboratory reporting errors for serum salicylate concentrations are relatively common due partly to the use of several different units. Analyzing and reporting salicylate concentrations as milligrams per liter when the clinician is accustomed to receiving results as milligrams per deciliter or inadvertently reporting actual milligrams per liter (before internal laboratory conversion) results erroneously because "mg/dL" provides the true salicylate concentration multiplied by 10.[58] These may suggest a toxic salicylate concentration in a patient whose serum salicylate concentration is actually within the therapeutic range (eg, "165 mg/L" instead of "16.5 mg/dL"). Most errors can be eliminated before initiation of aggressive therapy, such as HD, by determining whether the reported salicylate concentration is consistent with the clinical presentation and ABG or venous blood gas results and, when time permits, repeating the salicylate determination with appropriate consideration for methodology and conversion calculations.[58] Using the above example, a patient with a serum salicylate concentration of 165 mg/dL would undoubtedly show clinical signs of salicylate toxicity and have a profound acid–base abnormality.

The Done nomogram for classifying aspirin poisoning,[37] which was first published in 1960, was based on data predominantly from children, intended to be applied at only 6 hours or more after a single acute ingestion of nonenteric-coated, orally ingested aspirin and in patients with a blood pH of approximately 7.4 or higher. Such conditions rarely apply to patients with serious salicylate poisoning, explaining why the Done nomogram showed poor predictive value when applied to a group of 55 predominantly adults with salicylate poisoning.[39]

MANAGEMENT

Evidence-based consensus guidelines were developed to assist poison center staff with appropriate out-of-hospital triage decisions of patients with suspected salicylate exposures.[29] Management recommendations for in-hospital use may contain inadequate, misleading, or dangerous advice for managing patients with salicylate overdoses, as demonstrated by a 2001 report from Canada.[18] Additionally, there is significant discordance among medical directors of poison centers regarding the optimal method of GI decontamination of a patient who ingested a large quantity of enteric-coated aspirin.[75,76]

For a salicylate-poisoned patient who presents severely ill and requires mechanical ventilation for airway stabilization or sedation, maintenance of hyperventilation requires an extremely careful approach if death is to be avoided.[11,128] The complexity of the decision-making process and practical implementation of this common practice is highlighted in patients with salicylate poisoning. Airway protection is the reason often invoked when a patient with altered mental status undergoes endotracheal intubation. Although this is often appropriate, it must be performed efficiently because death has occurred after sedation during initial airway management.[11] Additionally, the postintubation ventilator settings must be properly chosen to avoid the development of hypoventilation relative to the preintubation degree of spontaneous ventilation. This is discussed further below under Alkalemia by Hyperventilation versus Sodium Bicarbonate and Risks Associated with Assisted Ventilation.

Frequent blood gas monitoring is required for all salicylate-poisoned patients. Although maintaining alkalemia clearly is essential for treatment, blood pH probably should not be allowed to increase above 7.55 because alkalemia shifts the oxyhemoglobin dissociation curve to the left and may be otherwise detrimental. Note, however, that even with a blood pH of 7.45 to 7.50 in patients with moderately severe salicylism, boluses of bicarbonate have been given without necessarily further increasing the pH. Frequent reassessment of blood pH, fluid status, and urinary pH almost always allows administration of more sodium bicarbonate than was initially thought possible.

GASTRIC DECONTAMINATION AND USE OF ACTIVATED CHARCOAL

The use of orogastric lavage and activated charcoal (AC) is discussed throughout this text. Their effects on the absorption and elimination of salicylates have been extensively studied. In vitro studies suggest that each gram of AC can adsorb approximately 550 mg of salicylic acid.[90,101] In humans, AC reduces the absorption of therapeutic doses of aspirin by 50% to 80%, effectively adsorbing aspirin from enteric-coated and sustained-release preparations in addition to immediate-release tablets.[90] Presumably, the sooner AC is given after salicylate ingestion, the more effective it will be in reducing absorption. A 10:1 ratio of AC to ingested salicylate appears to result in maximal efficacy. Although peak serum concentrations are markedly decreased from predicted concentrations, aspirin desorption from the aspirin–AC complex may diminish the impact of AC on total absorption.[49,94,101] The addition of a cathartic to the initial dose of AC has been questioned and largely abandoned for most xenobiotics, but a benefit of adding sorbitol to AC in preventing salicylate absorption was demonstrated in one study.[80]

Repetitive or multiple-dose AC (MDAC) probably limits desorption, which may reduce the concentration of initially absorbed salicylate to only 15% to 20%.[49] MDAC appears to increase the elimination of unabsorbed salicylates over that achieved by single-dose AC.[9,66] Thus, the use of MDAC to decrease GI absorption of salicylate overdoses is warranted, particularly if a pharmacobezoar or extended-release preparation is suspected (see Antidotes in Depth A2: Activated Charcoal).

The value of MDAC in enhancing salicylate elimination through GI dialysis is controversial and is not generally warranted.[3,73] In one volunteer study of 2800 mg of aspirin followed by 25 g of AC at 4, 6, 8, and 10 hours after ingestion, the total amount of salicylate excreted from the body increased by 9% to 18% but was not considered statistically significant.[82] The efficacy will likely be greater in the overdose situation, when more unbound salicylate is available because of decreased protein binding. However, in another study of the effects of MDAC on the clearance of high-dose intravenous (IV) aspirin in a porcine model, MDAC did not enhance the clearance of salicylates under alkaline conditions when the venous bicarbonate was kept at ≥15 mEq/L and urine pH kept at ≥7.5.[73] In contrast to the findings of both of these studies, two children with salicylate overdoses were successfully treated with MDAC given every 4 hours for 36 hours.[138] Overall, extensive use of MDAC is currently discouraged, but the administration of two to four properly timed doses is reasonable (see Chap. 7).

Theoretical support may be found for the use of whole-bowel irrigation (WBI) consisting of polyethylene glycol electrolyte lavage solution (PEG-ELS) in addition to AC to reduce systemic absorption, particularly for enteric-coated aspirin preparations.[133] Moreover, WBI alone may be effective in preventing absorption of other xenobiotics. However, the addition of WBI to MDAC does not increase the clearance of absorbed salicylate.[94]

FLUID REPLACEMENT

There is a need to differentiate between restoration of fluid and electrolyte balance in salicylate-poisoned patients as opposed to increasing the fluid load presented to the kidneys in an attempt to achieve "forced diuresis." Fluid losses from salicylate poisoning are prominent, especially in children, and can be attributed to tachypnea, hyperpnea, vomiting, fever, a hypermetabolic state, and insensible perspiration.[132] The kidneys also respond to salicylate poisoning by excreting an increased solute load, including large quantities of bicarbonate, sodium, potassium, and organic acids.[5] For all of these reasons, the patient's volume status must be adequately assessed and corrected if necessary, along with any glucose and electrolyte abnormalities. As in other cases, accurate management of volume status in poisoned patients may require invasive monitoring with a central venous pressure monitor or, preferably, a pulmonary artery catheter, especially in patients with cardiac disease, ALI, or renal compromise.

Increasing fluids beyond restoration of fluid balance to achieve forced diuresis is a practice that was inappropriately promoted in the past. Although forced diuresis theoretically increases renal tubular flow and reduces the urine tubular cell diffusion gradient for reabsorption, renal excretion of salicylate depends much more on urine pH than on flow rate, and use of forced diuresis alone is not effective regardless of whether diuretics, osmotic agents, or fluid volumes are used to achieve the diuresis.[108] Although renal salicylate clearance varies in direct proportion to flow rate, its relation to pH is logarithmic.[84] In summary, although fluid imbalance must be corrected, forced saline diuresis does little more than oral fluids to enhance elimination over a 24-hour period[108] and subjects the patient to the hazards of fluid overload.

ALKALEMIA BY HYPERVENTILATION VERSUS SODIUM BICARBONATE

Alkalinization of the serum by a substance that does not easily cross the blood–brain barrier such as intravenously administered sodium bicarbonate reduces the fraction of salicylate in the nonionized form and increases the pH gradient with the CSF. This both prevents entry and helps remove salicylate from the CNS[56,62,64,65,131] (see Fig. 35–2). Hyperventilation alone should not be relied upon, and $NaHCO_3$ should be used for alkalinization.

Alkalinization with IV sodium bicarbonate should be considered for symptomatic patients whose serum salicylate concentrations exceed the therapeutic range and for clinically suspected cases of salicylism until a salicylate concentration and simultaneously obtained blood pH are available to guide treatment. Patients on therapeutic regimens of salicylates who feel well with salicylate concentrations of 30 to 40 mg/dL and who do not manifest toxicity do not require intervention. Oral bicarbonate administration should never be substituted for IV bicarbonate to achieve alkalinization because the oral route may increase salicylate absorption from the GI tract by enhancing dissolution.

Alkalinization may be achieved with a bolus of 1 to 2 mEq/kg IV followed by an infusion of 3 ampules of sodium bicarbonate (132 mEq) in 1 L of 5% dextrose in water (D_5W), administered at 1.5 to 2.0 times the maintenance fluid range. Urine pH should be maintained at 7.5 to 8.0, and hypokalemia must be corrected (see below) to achieve maximum urinary alkalinization. Calcium concentrations should be monitored because decreases in both ionized[38] and total serum calcium[52] are also complications of bicarbonate therapy. Volume load should remain modest while repleting previous losses. Early HD must be considered when a patient cannot tolerate the increased solute load that results from alkalinization because of ALI, congestive heart failure, renal failure, or cerebral edema. However, even when the decision for HD has been made, alkalinization (when possible) helps to achieve a more rapid initial reduction in blood concentrations.[63]

RISKS ASSOCIATED WITH ASSISTED VENTILATION

Although induced hyperventilation may effectively increase the blood pH in certain patients, endotracheal intubation followed by assisted ventilation of a salicylate-poisoned patient poses particular risks if it is not meticulously performed. Although early endotracheal intubation to maintain hyperventilation may aid in the management of patients whose respiratory efforts are faltering, healthcare providers must maintain appropriate hypocarbia through hyperventilation. Ventilator settings that result in an increase in the patient's PCO_2 relative to pre-mechanical ventilation (p-MV) will produce a relative respiratory acidosis, even if serum pH remains in the alkalemic range.

In a search of a poison center database of patients with salicylate poisoning between 2001 and 2007, seven patients were identified with salicylate concentrations above 50 mg/dL, who had both pre-MV and post-MV data. All seven had a post-MV pH values below 7.4, and five of the six for whom recorded PCO_2 values were available had post-MV PCO_2 above 50 mm Hg, suggesting substantial underventilation. Two of the seven patients died after intubation, and one sustained neurologic injury. Inadequate MV of patients with salicylate poisoning was associated with respiratory acidosis, a decrease in the serum pH, and clinical deterioration.[128] Even when achieved, however, respiratory alkalosis sustained by hyperventilation (assisted or unassisted) alone should never be considered a substitute for use of either sodium bicarbonate (to achieve both alkalemia and alkalinuria) or HD (when indicated).

ENHANCED SALICYLATE ELIMINATION BY URINE ALKALINIZATION

Because salicylic acid is a weak acid (pK_a 3.5), it will be ionized in an alkaline milieu and theoretically can be "trapped" there. This occurs because there is no specific uptake mechanism in the kidney for salicylate, and passive reabsorption of a charged molecule is very limited. Thus, alkalinization of the urine (defined as pH ≥7.5) with sodium bicarbonate results in enhanced excretion of the ionized salicylate ion.

Alkalinization of the urine should be considered as first-line treatment for patients with moderately severe salicylate poisoning who do not meet the criteria for HD.[111] It should also be administered to salicylate-poisoned patients who require HD as long as it is thought clinically safe to do so. Although salicylic acid is almost completely ionized within physiologic pH limits, small changes in pH obtained by alkalinization may have substantial changes in the relative amount of salicylate in the charged form. Regardless of the reason for the change in serum PH, renal excretion of salicylate is very dependent on urinary pH[108,139] (see Fig. 35–2 and Antidotes in Depth A5: Sodium Bicarbonate).

Alkalinization increases free salicylate secretion from the proximal tubule but does not affect renal elimination of salicylate conjugates. The percentage of a single dose of 1.5 g of sodium salicylate administered to volunteers that was excreted unchanged increased from 2.3% ± 1.5% under acidic conditions to 30.5% ± 9.1% under alkaline conditions. When urine acidity was maintained using ammonium chloride, salicylic acid had a terminal $t_{1/2}$ value of 3.29 ± 0.52 hours, which was significantly reduced to 2.50 ± 0.41 hours when an alkaline urine was maintained with sodium bicarbonate treatment. The total body clearance of salicylic acid was significantly less under acidic urine conditions (1.38 ± 0.43 L/h) than under alkaline urine conditions (2.27 ± 0.83 L/h).[139]

Alkalinizing the urine from a pH of 5 to 8 logarithmically increased renal salicylate clearance from 1.3 to 100 mL/min.[99] Assuming an overdose Vd of 0.5 L/kg, this increased clearance would decrease salicylate half-life from 310 to 4 hours. However, alkalinizing the urine from a pH of 5 to 8 has a more modest effect on serum salicylate clearance.[108] The apparent serum half-life decreased from 48 to 6 hours. This difference between serum and renal half-lives reflects the fact that renal clearance only applies to free salicylate, but serum clearance applies to both free and protein-bound salicylate.

Although the administration of acetazolamide, a noncompetitive carbonic anhydrase inhibitor, results in the formation of bicarbonate-rich alkaline urine, it also causes a systemic metabolic acidosis and acidemia.[48,62,65] The effect of acetazolamide is usually self-limited and mild but nevertheless increases the concentration of freely diffusible nonionized molecules of salicylic acid, thereby increasing the Vd and most probably enhancing the penetrance of salicylate into the CNS.[65,89]

HYPOKALEMIA

Hypokalemia is a common complication of salicylate poisoning and prevents urinary alkalinization unless corrected. Hypokalemia results from the movement of potassium into cells in exchange for hydrogen ions in the presence of alkalemia, potassium losses in the urine or feces, and vomiting with subsequent metabolic alkalosis and bicarbonaturia.[53] Furthermore, in the presence of hypokalemia, the renal tubules reabsorb potassium ions in exchange for hydrogen ions, preventing urinary alkalinization. If urinary alkalinization cannot be achieved easily, hypokalemia, excretion of organic acids, and salt and water depletion should be considered possible reasons.

EXTRACORPOREAL REMOVAL

Unfortunately, delays in initiating HD remain a potentially preventable cause of death despite repeated calls over many years for prompt HD for patients with salicylate poisoning.[47] Extracorporeal measures are indicated if the patient has severe signs or symptoms, a very high serum salicylate concentration regardless of clinical findings, severe fluid or electrolyte disturbances, or ALI or is unable to eliminate the salicylates (Table 35–3). In most instances of severe salicylate poisoning, HD is the extracorporeal technique of choice, not only to clear the

TABLE 35–3. Indications for Hemodialysis in Salicylate-Poisoned Patients

Renal failure
Congestive heart failure (relative)
Acute lung injury
Persistent CNS disturbances
Progressive deterioration in vital signs
Severe acid–base or electrolyte imbalance despite appropriate treatment
Hepatic compromise with coagulopathy
Salicylate concentration (acute) >100 mg/dL (in the absence of the above)[a]

[a] Hemodialysis for patients with chronic poisoning is indicated for those with concerning symptoms regardless of salicylate concentrations.

salicylate but also to rapidly correct fluid, electrolyte, and acid–base disorders that will not be corrected by hemoperfusion (HP) alone. The combination of HD and HP in series is feasible and theoretically may be useful for treating patients with severe or mixed overdoses,[35] but it is rarely used. Rapid reduction of serum salicylate concentrations in severely poisoned patients has been described with the use of continuous venovenous hemodiafiltration, a technique that may be especially valuable for patients who are too unstable to undergo HD or when HD is unavailable[146] (see Chap. 9).

A combination of therapies that is both useful and practical is to ensure effective alkalinization with sodium bicarbonate while the patient is waiting for and then while undergoing HD. In one unique case report, a patient who overdosed twice on salicylates within a 2-month period was treated in the first instance with 4 hours of HD but no effective alkalinization and in the second instance with sodium bicarbonate alkalinization but no HD. In both instances, blood concentrations of salicylates were above 65 mg/dL. Although similar decreases in salicylate concentrations were achieved with each technique, the rate of decline during the first 4 hours was faster with alkalinization and HD.[63] Combining the two therapies makes sense even if part of the reason for the increased early effectiveness of sodium bicarbonate treatment is related to the rapidity with which it can be achieved compared with the 2 to 4 hours required to institute HD after a patient presents under even the most favorable circumstances.[63]

Peritoneal dialysis (PD) was sometimes suggested in the past as a simpler extracorporeal procedure for eliminating salicylates in the setting of hemodynamic compromise, coagulopathy, or inability to perform HP or HD. However, PD is only 10% to 25% as efficient as HP or HD and not even as efficient as renal excretion itself. The 24-hour clearance of salicylates with PD is less than the 4-hour clearance of salicylates by HP or HD; therefore, PD is not recommended (see Chap. 9).

In a recent animal model of salicylate poisoning, IV infusion of 1.25 g/kg of albumin was accompanied by a 14% decline in median brain salicylate concentration.[31] If this effect is achievable in humans, it could (along with rapid $NaHCO_3$ infusions) allow additional time for HD to be instituted.

OTHER FORMS OF SALICYLATE

Topical Salicylate Methyl Salicylate (Oil of Wintergreen) and Salicylic Acid Topical salicylates, which are used as keratolytics (salicylic acid) or as rubifacients (≤30% methyl salicylate) are rarely responsible for salicylate poisoning when used in their intended manner because absorption through normal skin is very slow. However, particularly in children, extensive application of topical preparations containing methyl salicylate may result in consequential poisoning.[17,143] After 30 minutes of contact time, only 1.5% to 2.0% of a dose is absorbed, and even after 10 hours of contact with methyl salicylate, only 12% to 20% of the salicylates is systemically absorbed.[18,120] Heat, occlusive dressings, young age, inflammation, and psoriasis all increase topical salicylate absorption.[24]

Ingestion of methyl salicylate may be disastrous, but its highly irritating characteristics probably limit most ingestions. When ingested, 1 mL of 98% oil of wintergreen contains an equivalent quantity of salicylate as 1.4 g of aspirin. In a 10-kg child, the minimum toxic salicylate dose of approximately 150 mg/kg body weight can almost be achieved with 1 mL of oil of wintergreen, which contains 140 mg/kg of salicylates for the child (see Chap. 42). In Hong Kong, medicated oils containing methyl salicylate accounted for 48% of acute salicylate poisoning cases treated in one hospital.[23] Methyl salicylate is rapidly absorbed from the GI tract and much, but not all, of the ester is rapidly hydrolyzed to free salicylates. Despite rapid and complete absorption, serum concentrations of salicylates are much less than predicted after ingestion of methyl salicylate containing liniment compared with oil of wintergreen.[143] Vomiting is common, along with abdominal discomfort. Onset of symptoms usually occurs within 2 hours of ingestion.[24] Patients with methyl salicylate exposure have died in less than 6 hours, emphasizing the need for early determinations of salicylate concentrations in addition to frequent testing after such exposures.

Bismuth Subsalicylate Bismuth subsalicylate, which is found in the popular medication Pepto Bismol, releases the salicylate moiety in the GI tract, which is subsequently absorbed. Each milliliter of bismuth subsalicylate contains 8.7 mg of salicylic acid.[46] After a large therapeutic dose (60 mL), peak salicylate concentrations may reach 4 mg/dL at 1.8 hours after ingestion.[46] Patients with diarrhea and infants with colic using large quantities of this antidiarrheal agent may develop salicylate toxicity.[91,137] Chronic use should raise concerns for bismuth toxicity (see Chap. 89).

PREGNANCY

Considered a rare event, salicylate poisoning during pregnancy poses a particular hazard to the fetus because of the acid–base and hematologic characteristics of the fetus and placental circulation. Salicylates cross the placenta and are present in higher concentrations in the fetus than in the mother. The respiratory stimulation that occurs in the mother after toxic exposures does not occur in the fetus, which has a decreased capacity to buffer acid. The ability of the fetus to metabolize and excrete salicylates is also less than in the mother. In addition to its toxic effects on the mother, including coagulation abnormalities, acid–base disturbances, tachypnea, and hypoglycemia, repeated exposure to salicylates late in gestation displaces bilirubin from protein-binding sites in the fetus, causing kernicterus.

A case report described fetal demise in a woman who claimed to ingest 50 aspirin tablets per day for several weeks during the third trimester of pregnancy. This raises concerns that the fetus is at greater risk from salicylate exposures than is the mother. Emergent delivery of near-term fetuses of salicylate-poisoned mothers should be considered on a case-by-case basis[102] (see Chap. 30).

SUMMARY

The initial assessment of a patient who has ingested excessive amounts of salicylates includes a determination of the vital signs, particularly the depth and frequency of respiration as well as the temperature. The clinical presentation of a patient with a salicylate overdose may be characterized by an early onset of nausea, vomiting, abdominal pain, blood-tinged vomitus or gross hematemesis, tinnitus, and lethargy. The presence of hyperventilation, hyperthermia, confusion, coma, seizures, and any other nonspecific neurologic presentation should heighten suspicion of salicylate poisoning (see Tables 35–1 and 35–2). Using a combination of symptoms, signs, and characteristic ABG findings along with the results of point-of-care testing and laboratory studies, the clinician can rapidly confirm a significant salicylate ingestion and then institute immediate alkalinization with sodium bicarbonate; achieve gastric decontamination by orogastric lavage (if indicated), AC, or MDAC (if indicated); and consider the need for HD (or perhaps hemodiafiltration) early in the course of management.

In patients with pulmonary and CNS manifestations of salicylate toxicity, the protective nature of hyperventilation in maintaining alkalemia may be disastrously compromised by assisted ventilation unless the clinician is extremely skilled at adjusting the ventilator to ensure hyperventilation, decreased PCO_2, and high pH (7.5) at all times. Moreover, any unnecessary delays to HD places the patient at greater risk for morbidity or mortality. Serum and urinary alkalinization with sodium bicarbonate to eliminate salicylates is important even though use of sodium bicarbonate may further complicate electrolyte abnormalities. Maintenance of eukalemia is important to ensure success, and fluid and electrolyte replacement is essential.

ACKNOWLEDGMENT

Eddy A. Bresnitz, MD, Donald Feinfeld, MD and Lorraine Hartnett, MD, contributed to this chapter in a previous edition.

REFERENCES

1. Abdallah HY, Mayersohn M, Conrad KA. The influence of age on salicylate pharmacokinetics in humans. *J Clin Pharmacol.* 1991;31:380-387.
2. Alvan G, Bergman V, Gustafsson L. High unbound fraction of salicylate in plasma during intoxication. *Br J Clin Pharmacol.* 1981;11:625-626.
3. American Academy of Clinical Toxicology and European Association of Poisons Centers and Clinical Toxicologists. Position statement and practice guidelines on the use of multi-dose activated charcoal in the treatment of acute poisoning. *J Toxicol Clin Toxicol.* 1999;37:731-751.
4. Anderson RJ, Potts DE, Gabow PA, et al. Unrecognized adult salicylate intoxication. *Ann Intern Med.* 1976;85:745-748.
5. Arena FP, Dugowson C, Saudek CD. Salicylate-induced hypoglycemia and ketoacidosis in a nondiabetic adult. *Arch Intern Med.* 1978;138:1153-1154.
6. Armstrong CP, Blower AL. Non-steroidal anti-inflammatory drugs and life-threatening complications of peptic ulceration. *Gut.* 1987;28:527-532.
7. Arrowsmith JB, Kennedy DL, Kuritsky JN, et al. National patterns of aspirin use and Reye syndrome reporting. United States 1980 to 1985. *Pediatrics.* 1987;79:858-863.
8. Bailey RB, Jones SR. Chronic salicylate intoxication: a common cause of morbidity in the elderly. *J Am Geriatr Soc.* 1989;37:556-561.
9. Barone J, Raia J, Huang YC. Evaluation of the effects of multiple-dose activated charcoal on the absorption of orally administered salicylate in a simulated toxic ingestion model. *Ann Emerg Med.* 1988;17:34-37.
10. Belay ED, Bresee JJ, Holman RC, et al. Reye's syndrome in the United States from 1981 through 1997. *N Engl J Med.* 1999;340:1377-1382.
11. Berk WA, Anderson JC. Salicylate associated asystole: report of two cases. *Am J Med.* 1989;86:505-506.
12. Bertolini A, Ottani A, Sandrini A. Dual acting anti-inflammatory drugs: a reappraisal. *Pharmacol Res.* 2001;44:437-450.
13. Bhutta AT, Squell VH, Schexnayder SM. Reye's syndrome: down but not out. *South Med J.* 2003;96:43-45.
14. Bogazc K, Caldron P. Enteric-coated aspirin bezoar: elevation of serum salicylate level by barium study. *Am J Med.* 1981;83:783-786.
15. Borga O, Odar-Cederlof I, Ringberger VA, et al. Protein binding of salicylate in uremic and normal plasma. *Clin Pharmacol Ther.* 1976;20:464-475.
16. Brien J. Ototoxicity associated with salicylates. *Drug Saf.* 1993;9:143-148.
17. Brubacher JR, Hoffman RS. Salicylism from topical salicylates: review of the literature. *J Toxicol Clin Toxicol.* 1996;34:431-436.
18. Brubacher JR, Purssell R, Kent DA. Salty broth for salicylate poisoning? Adequacy of overdose management advice in the 2001 compendium of pharmaceuticals and specialties. *CMAJ.* 2002;167:992-996.
19. Burke A, Smyth E, FitzGerald GA. Analgesic-antipyretic agents; pharmacotherapy of gout. In: Brunton LL, Lazo JS, Parker KL, eds. *Goodman & Gilman's The Pharmacological Basis of Therapeutics*, 11th ed. New York: McGraw-Hill; 2006:671-715.
20. Cazals Y. Auditory sensorineural alterations induced by salicylate. *Prog Neurobiol.* 2000;62:583-631.
21. Cazals Y, Li XQ, Aurousseau C, et al. Acute effects of noradrenaline related vasoactive agents on the ototoxicity of aspirin: an experimental study in guinea pigs. *Heart Res.* 1988;36:89-96.
22. Centers for Disease Control and Prevention. Reye's syndrome surveillance—United States 1989. *MMWR Morb Mortal Wkly Rep.* 1991;40:88-89.
23. Chan TYK. Medicated oils and severe salicylate poisoning: quantifying the risk based on methyl salicylate content and bottle size. *Vet Human Toxicol.* 1996;38:133-134.
24. Chan TYK. Potential dangers from topical preparations containing methyl salicylate. *Hum Exp Toxicol.* 1996;15:747-750.
25. Chan TYK, Chan AYW, Ho CS. The clinical value of screening for salicylates in acute poisoning. *Vet Human Toxicol.* 1995;37:37-38.
26. Childs C. Human brain temperature: regulation, measurement and relationship with cerebral trauma: part 1. *Br J Neurosurg.* 2008;22:486-496.
27. Chow EL, Cherry JD. Reassessing Reye syndrome. *Arch Pediatr Adolesc Med.* 2003;157:1241-1242.
28. Chui PT. Anesthesia in a patient with undiagnosed salicylate poisoning presenting as intraabdominal sepsis. *J Clin Anesth.* 1999;11:251-253.
29. Chyka PA, Erdman AR, Christianson G, et al. Salicylate poisoning: an evidence-based consensus guideline for out-of-hospital management. *Clin Toxicol.* 2007;45:95-131.
30. Coggon D, Langman MJS, Spiegelhalter D. Aspirin, paracetamol, hematemesis and melena. *Gut.* 1982;23:340-344.
31. Curry SC, Pizon AF, Riley BD, et al. Effect of intravenous albumin infusion on brain salicylate concentration. *Acad Emerg Med.* 2007;14:508-514.
32. D'Agati V. Does aspirin cause acute or chronic renal failure in experimental animals and in humans? *Am J Kidney Dis.* 1996;28(1 suppl 1):S24-S29.
33. Davis JE: Are one or two dangerous? Methyl salicylate exposure in toddlers. *J Emerg Med.* 2007;32:63-69.
34. Davison C. Salicylate metabolism in man. *Ann N Y Acad Sci.* 1971;179: 249-268.
35. DeBroe ME, Verpooten GA, Christiaens ME, et al. Clinical experience with prolonged combined hemoperfusion-hemodialysis treatment of severe poisoning. *Artif Organs.* 1981;5:59-66.
36. Dinis-Oliveira RJ, de Pinho PG, Ferreira AC, et al. Reactivity of paraquat with sodium salicylate: formation of stable complexes. *Toxicology.* 2008;249:130-139.
37. Done AK: Salicylate intoxication: significance of measurements of salicylate in blood in cases of acute ingestion. *Pediatrics.* 1960;26:800-807.
38. Done AK, Temple AR. Treatment of salicylate poisoning. *Mod Treat.* 1971;8:528-551.
39. Dugandzic RM, Tierney MG, Dickinson GE, et al. Evaluation of the validity of the Done nomogram in the management of acute salicylate intoxication. *Ann Emerg Med.* 1989;18:1186-1190.
40. Durnas C, Cusack BJ. Salicylate intoxication in the elderly. Recognition and recommendations on how to prevent it. *Drugs Aging.* 1992;2:20-34.
41. Ekstrand R, Alvan A, Borga O. Concentration dependent plasma protein binding of salicylate in rheumatoid patients. *Clin Pharmacokinet.* 1979;4:137-143.
42. Elseviers MM, DeBroe ME. Combination analgesic involvement in the pathogenesis of analgesic nephropathy: the European perspective. *Am J Kidney Dis.* 1996;28(suppl 1):S48-S55.
43. Emkey RD. Aspirin and renal disease. *Am J Med.* 1983;74:97-101.
44. English M, Marsh V, Amukoye E, et al. Chronic salicylate poisoning and severe malaria. *Lancet.* 1996;347:1736-1737.
45. Escoubet B, Amsallem P, Ferrary E, et al. Prostaglandin synthesis by the cochlea or the guinea pig. Influence of aspirin, gentamicin, and acoustic stimulation. *Prostaglandins.* 1985;29:589-599.

46. Feldman S, Chen SL, Pickering LK. Salicylate absorption from bismuth subsalicylate preparation. *Clin Pharmacol Ther.* 1981;29:788-792.
47. Fertel BS, Nelson LS, Goldfarb DS. The underutilization of hemodialysis in patients with salicylate poisoning. *Kidney Int.* 2009;75(12):1349-1353.
48. Feuerstein RC, Finberg L, Fleishman BS. The use of acetazolamide in the therapy of salicylate poisoning. *Pediatrics.* 1960;25:215-227.
49. Fillippone G, Fish S, Lacouture P, et al. Reversible adsorption (desorption) of aspirin from activated charcoal. *Arch Intern Med.* 1987;147:1390-1392.
50. Fisher CJ, Albertson TE, Foulke GE. Salicylate induced pulmonary edema. Clinical characteristics in children. *Am J Emerg Med.* 1985;3:33-37.
51. Ford M, Tomaszewski C, Kerns W, et al. Bedside ferric chloride urine test to rule out salicylate intoxication [abstract]. *Vet Hum Toxicol.* 1994;36:364.
52. Fox GN. Hypocalcemia complicating bicarbonate therapy for salicylate poisoning. *West J Med.* 1984;141:108-109.
53. Gabow PA. How to avoid overlooking salicylate intoxication. *J Crit Illness.* 1986;1:77-85.
54. Gabow PA, Anderson RJ, Potts DE, Schrier RW. Acid-base disturbances in the salicylate poisoning in adults. *Arch Intern Med.* 1978;138:1481-1484.
55. Gaudreault P, Temple AR, Lovejoy FH Jr. The relative severity of acute versus chronic salicylate poisoning in children: a clinical comparison. *Pediatrics.* 1982;70:566-569.
56. Goldberg MA, Barlow CF, Roth LJ. The effects of carbon dioxide on the entry and accumulation of drugs in the central nervous system. *J Pharmacol Exp Ther.* 1961;131:308-318.
57. Graham CA, Irons AJ, Munro PT. Paracetamol and salicylate testing: routinely required for all overdose patients? *Eur J Emerg Med.* 2006;13:26-28.
58. Hahn IH, Chu J, Hoffman RS, Nelson LS. Errors in reporting salicylate levels. *Acad Emerg Med.* 2000;7:1336-1337.
59. Halla JT, Atchison SL, Hardin JG. Symptomatic salicylate ototoxicity: a useful indicator of serum salicylate concentration? *Ann Rheum Dis.* 1991;50:682-684.
60. Hamdan JA, Manasra K, Ahmed M. Salicylate-induced hepatitis in rheumatic fever. *Am J Dis Child.* 1985;139:453-455.
61. Harris FC. Pyloric stenosis: holdup of enteric-coated aspirin tablets. *Br J Surg.* 1973;60:979-981.
62. Heller I, Halevy J, Cohen S, et al. Significant metabolic acidosis induced by acetazolamide: not a rare complication. *Arch Intern Med.* 1985;145:1815-1817.
63. Higgins RM, Connolly JO, Hendry BM. Alkalinization and hemodialysis in severe salicylate poisoning: comparison of elimination techniques in the same patient. *Clin Nephrol.* 1998;50:178-183.
64. Hill JB. Salicylate intoxication. *N Engl J Med.* 1973;288:1110-1113.
65. Hill JB. Experimental salicylate poisoning: observations on the effects of altering blood pH on tissue and plasma salicylate concentrations. *Pediatrics.* 1971;47:658-665.
66. Hillman RJ, Prescott LF. Treatment of salicylate poisoning with repeated oral charcoal. *Br Med J.* 1986;291:1472.
67. Hogben CAM, Schanker LS, Jocco DJ, Brodie BB. Absorption of drugs from the stomach. II: the human. *J Pharmacol Exp Ther.* 1957;120:540-545.
68. Hoffman RJ, Nelson LS, Hoffman RS. Use of ferric chloride to identify salicylate-containing poisons. *J Toxicol Clin Toxicol.* 2002;40:547-549.
69. Hormaechea E, Carlson RW, Rogove H, et al. Hypovolemia, pulmonary edema and protein changes in severe salicylate poisoning. *Am J Med.* 1979;66:1046-1050.
70. Hrnicek G, Skelton J, Miller W. Pulmonary edema and salicylate intoxication. *JAMA.* 1974;230:866-867.
71. Huff RW, Fred HL. Postictal pulmonary edema. *Arch Intern Med.* 1966;117:824-828.
72. Hurwitz ES, Barrett MJ, Bregman D, et al. Public Health Service study on Reye's syndrome and medications: report of the pilot phase. *N Engl J Med.* 1985;313:849-857.
73. Johnson D, Eppler J, Giesbrecht E, et al. Effect of multiple-dose activated charcoal on the clearance of high-dose intravenous aspirin in a porcine model. *Ann Emerg Med.* 1995;26:569-574.
74. Jung TTK, Rhee CK, Lee CS, et al. Ototoxicity of salicylate, nonsteroidal anti-inflammatory drugs, and quinine. *Otolaryngol Clin North Am.* 1993;26:791-810.
75. Juurlink DN, McGuigan MA. Gastrointestinal decontamination for enteric-coated aspirin overdose: what to do depends on who you ask. *J Toxicol Clin Toxicol.* 2000;38:465-470.
76. Juurlink DN, Szalai JP, McGuigan MA. Discrepant advice from poison centres and their medical directors. *Can J Clin Pharmacol.* 2002;9:101-105.
77. Kaplan E, Kennedy J, David J. Effects of salicylate and other benzoates on oxidative enzymes of the tricarboxylic acid cycle in rat tissue homogenates. *Arch Biochem Biophys.* 1954;51:47-61.
78. Karliner J. Noncardiogenic forms of pulmonary edema. *Circulation.* 1972;46:212-215.
79. Karsh J. Adverse reactions and interactions with aspirin—considerations in the treatment of the elderly patient. *Drug Saf.* 1990;5:317-327.
80. Keller RE, Schwab RA, Krenzelok EP. Contribution of sorbitol combined with activated charcoal in prevention of salicylate absorption. *Ann Emerg Med.* 1990;19:654-656.
81. King JA, Storrow AB, Finkelstein JA. Urine Trinder spot test: a rapid salicylate screen for the emergency department. *Ann Emerg Med.* 1995;26:330-333.
82. Kirshenbaum LA, Mathews SC, Sitar DS, Tenenbein M. Does multiple-dose charcoal therapy enhance salicylate excretion? *Arch Intern Med.* 1990;150:1281-1283.
83. Krebs HG, Woods HG, Alberti KG. Hyperlactatemia and lactic acidosis. *Essays Med Biochem.* 1975;1:81-103.
84. Lawson AAH, Proudfoot AT, Brown SS, et al. Forced diuresis in the treatment of acute salicylate poisoning in adults. *Q J Med.* 1969;38:31-48.
85. Lemesh RA. Accidental chronic salicylate intoxication in an elderly patient: major morbidity despite early recognition. *Vet Hum Toxicol.* 1993;35:34-36.
86. Leventhal LJ, Kuritsky L, Ginsburg R, et al. Salicylate-induced rhabdomyolysis. *Am J Emerg Med.* 1989;7:409-410.
87. Levy G. Clinical pharmacokinetics of salicylates: a reassessment. *Br J Clin Pharmacol.* 1980;10:285S-290S.
88. Levy G. Clinical pharmacokinetics of aspirin. *Pediatrics.* 1978;62(suppl):867-872.
89. Levy G. Pharmacokinetics of salicylate elimination in man. *J Pharm Sci.* 1965;54:959-967.
90. Levy G, Tsuchiya T. Effect of activated charcoal on aspirin absorption in man. *Clin Pharmacol Ther.* 1972;13:317-322.
91. Lewis TV, Badillo R, Schaeffer S, Hagemann TM, McGoodwin L. Salicylate toxicity associated with administration of Percy medicine in an infant. *Pharmacotherapy.* 2006;26:403-109.
92. Macpherson CR, Milne MD, Evans BM. The excretion of salicylate. *Br J Pharmacol.* 1955;10:484-489.
93. Manso C, Taranta A, Nydick I. Effect of aspirin administration on serum glutamic oxaloacetic and glutamic pyruvic transaminases in children. *Proc Soc Exp Biol Med.* 1956;93:84-88.
94. Mayer AL, Sitar DS, Tenenbein M. Multiple-dose charcoal and whole-bowel irrigation do not increase clearance of absorbed salicylate. *Arch Intern Med.* 1992;152:393-396.
95. McGuigan MA. A two year review of salicylate deaths in Ontario. *Arch Intern Med.* 1987;147:510-512.
96. Miyahara JT, Karler R. Effect of salicylate on oxidative phosphorylation and respiration of mitochondrial fragments. *Biochem J.* 1965;97:194-198.
97. Montgomery H, Porter JC, Bradley RD. Salicylate intoxication causing a severe systemic inflammatory response and rhabdomyolysis. *Am J Emerg Med.* 1994;12:531-532.
98. Montgomery PR, Berger LG, Mitenko PA, Sitar DS. Salicylate metabolism: effects of age and sex in adults. *Clin Pharmacol Ther.* 1986;39:571-576.
99. Morgan AG, Polak A. The excretion of salicylate in salicylate poisoning. *Clin Sci.* 1971;41:475-484.
100. Myers EN, Bernstein JM, Fostiropolous G. Salicylate ototoxicity. *N Engl J Med.* 1965;273:587-590.
101. Neuvonen PJ, Elfving SM, Elonen E. Reduction of absorption of digoxin, phenytoin, and aspirin by activated charcoal in man. *Eur J Clin Pharmacol.* 1978;13:213-218.
102. Palatnick W, Tenenbien M. Aspirin poisoning during pregnancy: increased fetal sensitivity. *Am J Perinatol.* 1998;15:39-41.
103. Park BK, Leck JB. On the mechanism of salicylate-induced hypothrombinaemia. *J Pharm Pharmacol.* 1981;33:25-28.
104. Partin JS, Partin JC, Schubert WK, Hammond JG. Serum salicylate concentration in Reye's disease: a study of 130 biopsy proven cases. *Lancet.* 1982;1:191-194.
105. Patrono C, Baigent C, Hirsh J, Roth G. Antiplatelet drugs: American College of Chest Physicians Evidence-Based Clinical Practice Guidelines (8th edition). *Chest* 2008;133(6 suppl):199S-233S.
106. Phillips BM, Hartnagel RE, Leeling JL, Gurtoo HL. Does aspirin play a role in analgesic nephropathy? *Aust NJ Med.* 1976;6(suppl 1):48-53.
107. Porter GA. Acetaminophen/aspirin mixtures: experimental data. *Am J Kidney Dis.* 1996;28(suppl 1):S30-S33.

108. Prescott LF, Balali-Mood M, Critchley JA, et al. Diuresis or urinary alkalinization for salicylate poisoning? *Br Med J.* 1982;285:1383-1386.
109. Proudfoot AT, Brown SS. Acidaemia and salicylate poisoning in adults. *Br Med J.* 1969;2:547-550.
110. Proudfoot AT, Krenzelok EP, Brent J, Vale JA. Does urine alkalinization increase salicylate elimination? If so, why? *Toxicol Rev.* 2003;22:129-136.
111. Proudfoot AT, Krenzelok EP, Vale JA. Position paper on urine alkalinization. *J Toxicol Clin Toxicol.* 2004;42:1-26.
112. Puel JL. Cochlear NMDA receptor blockade prevents salicylate-induced tinnitus. *B-ENT* 2007;3(suppl 7):19-22.
113. Puel JL, Guitton MJ. Salicylate-induced tinnitus: molecular mechanisms and modulation by anxiety. *Prog Brain Res.* 2007;166:141-146.
114. Pugliese A, Beltramo T, Torre D. Reye's and Reye's-like syndromes. *Cell Biochem Funct.* 2008;26:741-746.
115. Ramsden RT, Latif A, O'Malley S. Electrocochleographic changes in acute salicylate overdosage. *J Laryngol Otol.* 1985;99:1269-1273.
116. Rao P, Knaus EE. Evolution of nonsteroidal anti-inflammatory drugs (NSAIDs): cyclooxygenase (COX) inhibition and beyond. *J Pharm Sci.* 2008;11:81s-110s.
117. Raschke R, Arnold-Capell P, Richeson R, Curry SC. Refractory hypoglycemia secondary to topical salicylate intoxication. *Arch Intern Med.* 1991;151:591-593.
118. Rivera W, Kleinschmidt KC, Velez LI, et al. Delayed salicylate toxicity at 35 hours without early manifestations following a single salicylate ingestion. *Ann Pharmacother.* 2004;38:1186-1188.
119. Roberts MS, Cossum PA, Kilpatrick DO. Implications of hepatic and extrahepatic metabolism of aspirin in selective inhibition of platelet cyclooxygenase. *N Engl J Med.* 1985;312:1388-1389.
120. Roberts MS, Favretto WA, Meyer A, et al. Topical bioavailability of methyl salicylate. *Aust N Z J Med.* 1982;12:303-305.
121. Romankiewicz JA, Reidenberg MM. Factors that modify drug absorption. *Ration Drug Ther.* 1978;12:1-6.
122. Rothschild BM. Hematologic perturbations associated with salicylate. *Clin Pharmacol Ther.* 1979;26:145-150.
123. Ruel J, Chabbert C, Nouvian R, et al. Salicylate enables cochlear arachidonic-acid-sensitive NMDA receptor responses. *J Neurosci.* 2008;28:7313-7323.
124. Schaller JG. Chronic salicylate administration in juvenile rheumatoid arthritis: Aspirin "hepatitis" and its clinical significance. *Pediatrics.* 1978;62(suppl):916-925.
125. Schanker LS, Tocco DJ, Brodie BB, Hogben CAM. Absorption of drugs from the rat's small intestine. *J Pharmacol Exp Ther.* 1958;123:81-88.
126. Sogge MR, Griffith JL, Sinar DR, Mayes GR. Lavage to remove enteric-coated aspirin and gastric outlet obstruction. *Ann Intern Med.* 1977;87:721-722.
127. Sporer KA, Khayam-Bashi H. Acetaminophen and salicylate serum levels in patients with suicidal ingestion or altered mental status. *Am J Emerg Med.* 1996;14:443-447.
128. Stolbach AI, Hoffman RS, Nelson LS. Mechanical ventilation was associated with acidemia in a case series of salicylate-poisoned patients. *Acad Emerg Med.* 2008;15:866-869.
129. Sweeney KR, Chapron DJ, Brandt JL, et al. Toxic interaction between acetazolamide and salicylate: case reports and a pharmacokinetic explanation. *Clin Pharmacol Ther.* 1986;40:518-524.
130. Swintosky JV. Illustrations and pharmaceutical interpretations of first-order drug elimination rate from the bloodstream. *J Am Pharm Assoc.* 1956;45:395-400.
131. Temple AR. Acute and chronic effects of aspirin toxicity and their treatment. *Arch Intern Med.* 1981;141:364-369.
132. Temple AR, George DJ, Done AK, Thompson JA. Salicylate poisoning complicated by fluid retention. *Clin Toxicol.* 1976;9:61-68.
133. Tenenbein M. Whole-bowel irrigation as a gastrointestinal decontamination procedure after acute poisoning. *Med Toxicol.* 1988;3:77-84.
134. Tenney SM, Miller RM. The respiratory and circulatory action of salicylate. *Am J Med.* 1955;19:498-508.
135. Thurston JH, Pollock PG, Warren SK, Jones EM. Reduced brain glucose with normal plasma glucose in salicylate poisoning. *Clin Invest.* 1970;49:2139-2145.
136. Vane JR, Botting RM. The mechanism of action of aspirin. *Thromb Res.* 2003;110:255-258.
137. Vernace MA, Bellucci AG, Wilkes BM. Chronic salicylate toxicity due to consumption of over-the-counter bismuth subsalicylate. *Am J Med.* 1994;97:308-309.
138. Vertrees JE, McWilliams BC, Kelly HW. Repeated oral administration of activated charcoal for treating aspirin overdose in young children. *Pediatrics.* 1990;85:594-597.
139. Vree TB, Van Ewijk-Beneken Kolmer EWJ, Verwey-Van Wissen CPWGM, Hekster YA. Effect of urinary pH on the pharmacokinetics of salicylate acid, with its glycine and glucuronide conjugates in humans. *Int J Clin Pharmacol Ther.* 1994;32:550-558.
140. Waldman RJ, Hall WN, McGee H, Van Amburg G. Aspirin as a risk factor in Reye's syndrome. *JAMA.* 1982;247:3089-3094.
141. Walters JS, Woodring JH, Stelling CB, et al. Salicylate-induced pulmonary edema. *Radiology.* 1983;146:289-293.
142. Weisberg HF. Water and electrolytes. In: Davidsohn I, Wells BB, eds. Clinical *Diagnosis by Laboratory Methods.* Philadelphia: WB Saunders; 1962:500.
143. Wolowich WR, Hadley CM, Kelley MT, et al. Plasma salicylate from methyl salicylate cream compared to oil of wintergreen. *J Toxicol Clin Toxicol.* 2003;41:353-358.
144. Wood DM, Dargan PI, Jones AL. Measuring plasma salicylate concentrations in all patients with drug overdose or altered consciousness: is it necessary? *Emerg Med J.* 2005;22:401-403.
145. Wortzman DJ, Grunfeld A. Delayed absorption following enteric-coated aspirin overdose. *Ann Emerg Med.* 1987;16:434-436.
146. Wrathall G, Sinclair R, Moore A, Pogson D. Three case reports of the use of haemodiafiltration in the treatment of salicylate overdose. *Hum Exp Toxicol.* 2001;20:491-495.
147. Zenser TV, Mattammal MB, Rapp NS, Davis BB. Effect of aspirin on metabolism of acetaminophen and benzidine by renal inner medulla prostaglandin hydroperoxidase. *J Lab Clin Med.* 1983;101:58-65.

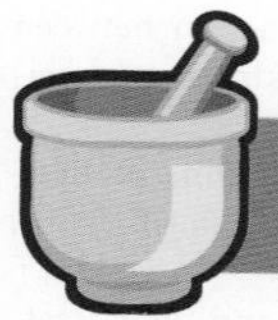

ANTIDOTES IN DEPTH (A5)

SODIUM BICARBONATE

Paul M. Wax

Sodium bicarbonate is a nonspecific antidote effective in the treatment of a variety of poisonings by means of a number of distinct mechanisms (Table A5–1). However, the support for its use in these settings is predominantly based on animal evidence, case reports, and consensus.[9] It is most commonly used in the treatment of patients with cyclic antidepressant (CA) and salicylate poisonings. Sodium bicarbonate also has a role in the treatment of phenobarbital, chlorpropamide, and chlorophenoxy herbicide poisonings and wide-complex tachydysrhythmias induced by type IA and IC antidysrhythmics and cocaine. Correcting the life-threatening acidosis generated by methanol and ethylene glycol poisoning and enhancing formate elimination are other important indications for sodium bicarbonate. Use of sodium bicarbonate in the treatment of rhabdomyolysis, metabolic acidosis with elevated lactate, cardiac resuscitation, and diabetic ketoacidosis is controversial and is not addressed in this Antidote in Depth.[1,4,15,45,91,92]

ALTERED XENOBIOTIC IONIZATION RESULTING IN ALTERED XENOBIOTIC DISTRIBUTION

CYCLIC ANTIDEPRESSANTS

The most important role of sodium bicarbonate in toxicology appears to be its ability to reverse potentially fatal cardiotoxic effects of the CAs and other type IA and IC antidysrhythmics. Use of sodium bicarbonate for CA overdose developed as an extension of sodium bicarbonate use in the treatment of patients with other cardiotoxic exposures. Noting similarities in electrocardiographic (ECG) findings between hyperkalemia and quinidine toxicity (ie, QRS widening), investigators in the 1950s began to use sodium lactate (which is rapidly metabolized in the liver to sodium bicarbonate) for the treatment of quinidine toxicity.[3,8,95] In a canine model, quinidine-induced ECG changes and hypotension were consistently reversed by infusion of sodium lactate.[7] Clinical experience confirmed this benefit.[8] Similar efficacy in the treatment of patients with procainamide cardiotoxicity was also reported.[95]

With the introduction of the CAs during the late 1950s, conduction disturbances, dysrhythmias, and hypotension occurring after overdose were soon reported. Extending the use of sodium lactate from the type I antidysrhythmics to the CAs, uncontrolled observations in the early 1970s showed a decrease in mortality from 15% to less than 3% when sodium lactate was administered to patients with CA poisoning.[29] In 1976, the first report of successful use of sodium bicarbonate in the treatment of a series of CA-induced dysrhythmias in children was reported.[17] In this series, nine of 12 children who had developed multifocal premature ventricular contractions (PVCs), ventricular tachycardia, or heart block reverted to normal sinus rhythm with sodium bicarbonate therapy alone. An early canine experiment of amitriptyline-poisoning demonstrated resolution of dysrhythmias upon alkalinization of the blood to a pH above 7.40.[17] Other methods of alkalinization, including hyperventilation and administration of the nonsodium buffer tris (hydroxymethyl) aminomethane (THAM), were also effective in reversing the dysrhythmias.[18,42]

A better understanding of the mechanism and utility of sodium bicarbonate has come from a series of animal experiments during the 1980s. In amitriptyline-poisoned dogs, sodium bicarbonate reversed conduction slowing and ventricular dysrhythmias and suppressed ventricular ectopy.[62] When comparing sodium bicarbonate, hyperventilation, hypertonic sodium chloride, and lidocaine, sodium bicarbonate and hyperventilation proved most efficacious in reversing ventricular dysrhythmias and narrowing QRS prolongation. Although lidocaine transiently antagonized dysrhythmias, this antagonism was demonstrable only at nearly toxic lidocaine concentrations and was associated with hypotension. Furthermore, prophylactic alkalinization protected against the development of dysrhythmias in a pH-dependent manner.

In desipramine-poisoned rats, the isolated use of either sodium chloride or sodium bicarbonate was effective in decreasing QRS duration.[69] Both sodium bicarbonate and sodium chloride also increased mean arterial pressure, but hyperventilation or direct intravascular volume repletion with mannitol did not. In further studies both in vivo and on isolated cardiac tissue, alkalinization and increased sodium concentration improved CA effects on cardiac conduction.[79,80] Although respiratory alkalosis and sodium chloride each independently improved conduction velocity, this effect was greater when sodium bicarbonate was administered.

Another study on amitriptyline-poisoned rats demonstrated that treatment with sodium bicarbonate was associated with shorter QRS interval, longer duration of sinus rhythm, and increased survival rates.[44] Sodium bicarbonate seems to work independently of initial blood pH. Animal studies show that cardiac conduction improves after treatment with sodium bicarbonate or sodium chloride in both normal pH and acidemic animals.[69] Clinically, TCA-poisoned patients who already were alkalemic also responded to repeat doses of sodium bicarbonate.[59]

Although several authors suggest that the efficacy of sodium bicarbonate is modulated via a pH-dependent change in plasma protein binding that decreases the proportion of free drug,[18,49] further study failed to support this hypothesis.[72] The administration of large doses of a binding protein α_1-acid glycoprotein (AAG) (to which CAs show great affinity) to desipramine-poisoned rats only minimally decreased cardiotoxicity. Although the addition of AAG increased the concentrations of total desipramine and protein-bound desipramine in the serum, the concentration of active free desipramine did not decline significantly. A redistribution of CA from peripheral sites may have prevented lowering of free desipramine concentration. The persistence of other CA-associated toxicity, such as the anticholinergic effects and seizures, also argues against changes in protein-binding modulating toxicity. In vitro studies performed in plasma protein-free bath further support that the efficacy of sodium bicarbonate is independent of plasma protein binding.[79]

Sodium bicarbonate has a crucial antidotal role in CA poisoning by increasing the number of open sodium channels, thereby partially

TABLE A5–1. Sodium Bicarbonate: Mechanisms, Site of Action, and Uses in Toxicology

Mechanism	Site of Action	Uses
Altered interaction between xenobiotic and sodium channel	Heart	Amantadine Carbamazepine Cocaine Diphenhydramine Flecainide Mesoridazine Procainamide Propoxyphene Quinidine Quinine Thioridazine cyclic antidepressants
Altered xenobiotic ionization leads to altered tissue distribution	Brain	Formic acid Phenobarbital Salicylates
Altered xenobiotic ionization leads to enhanced xenobiotic elimination	Kidneys	Chlorophenoxy herbicides Chlorpropamide Formic acid Methotrexate Phenobarbital Salicylates
Correct life-threatening acidosis	Metabolic	Cyanide Ethylene glycol Methanol Metformin
Increase xenobiotic solubility	Kidneys	Methotrexate
Neutralization	Lungs	Chlorine gas, HCl
Maintenance of chelator effect	Kidneys	Dimercaprol (BAL)–metal
Reduce free radical formation	Kidneys	Contrast media

BAL, British anti-Lewisite.

reversing fast sodium channel blockade. This decreases QRS prolongation and reduces life-threatening cardiovascular toxicity such as ventricular dysrhythmias and hypotension.[62,69,79] The animal evidence supports two distinct and additive mechanisms for this effect: a pH-dependent effect and a sodium-dependent effect. The pH-dependent effect increases the fraction of the more freely diffusible nonionized xenobiotic. Both the ionized xenobiotic and the nonionized forms are able to bind to the sodium channel, but assuming CAs act like local anesthetics, it is estimated that 90% of the block results from the ionized form. By increasing the nonionized fraction, less xenobiotic is available to bind to the sodium channel binding site. The sodium-dependent effect increases the availability of sodium ions to pass through the open channels. Decreased ionization should not significantly decrease the rate of CA elimination because of the small contribution of renal pathways to overall CA elimination (<5%).

Although many anecdotal accounts support the efficacy of sodium bicarbonate in treating CA cardiotoxicity in humans,[36] these reports are all uncontrolled observations; controlled studies are not available. In one of the largest retrospective observational studies involving 91 patients who received sodium bicarbonate after CA overdose, QRS prolongation corrected in 39 of 49 patients who had QRS durations above 0.12 seconds, and hypotension corrected within 1 hour in 20 of 21 patients who had systolic blood pressures below 90 mm Hg.[37] Use of sodium bicarbonate was not associated with any complications in this study.

Prospective validation of treatment criteria for use of sodium bicarbonate after CA overdose has not been performed. The most common indications are conduction delays manifested by QRS above 0.10 seconds or right bundle-branch block, wide-complex tachydysrhythmias, and hypotension.[45] Because studies show that there is a critical threshold QRS duration at which ventricular dysrhythmias may occur (≥0.16 seconds),[12] it seems reasonable that narrowing the QRS interval through use of sodium bicarbonate or hyperventilation may prophylactically prevent against development of dysrhythmias. Practice patterns vary considerably with regard to the use of sodium bicarbonate when the QRS interval is below 0.16 seconds.[83] Although sodium bicarbonate has no proven efficacy in either the treatment or prophylaxis of TCA-induced seizures, seizures often cause acidemia, which rapidly increases the risks of conduction disturbances and ventricular dysrhythmias. Administering sodium bicarbonate when the QRS duration is 0.10 seconds or above may establish a theoretical margin of safety in the event the patient suddenly deteriorates, without adding significant demonstrable risk. When the QRS duration is below 0.10 seconds (given the negligible risk of seizures or dysrhythmias), prophylactic use of sodium bicarbonate is not indicated. In patients exhibiting a Brugada ECG pattern (right bundle branch block with downsloping ST segment elevation in V1–V3) and QRS widening after CA ingestion, sodium bicarbonate administration may narrow the QRS without reversing the Brugada pattern[5] (see Chap. 22).

Because cardiotoxicity may worsen during the first few hours after ingestion, we recommend starting sodium bicarbonate immediately if the QRS interval widens to greater than 0.10 seconds. Because CA-induced hypotension also responds to sodium bicarbonate, hypotension is another indication for sodium bicarbonate. However, no evidence supports a role for sodium bicarbonate in CA-poisoned patients who present with altered mental status or seizures without QRS widening or hypotension.

Because the potential benefits of alkalinization in CA overdose usually outweigh the risks, sodium bicarbonate should be administered regardless of whether the patient has an acidemic or normal pH. The most commonly used preparations are an 8.4% solution (1 M) containing 1 mEq each of sodium and bicarbonate ions per milliliter (calculated osmolarity of 2000 mOsm/L) and a 7.5% solution containing 0.892 mEq each of sodium and bicarbonate ions per milliliter (calculated osmolarity of 1786 mOsm/L). Fifty-milliliter ampules of the 8.4% and 7.5% solutions contain 50 and 44.6 mEq of $NaHCO_3$, respectively. One to two milliequivalents of sodium bicarbonate per kilogram body weight should be administered intravenously (IV) as a bolus over a period of 1 to 2 minutes.[70] Greater amounts may be required to treat patients with unstable ventricular dysrhythmias. Sodium bicarbonate can be repeated as needed to achieve a blood pH of 7.50 to 7.55.[71,85] The end point of treatment is narrowing of the QRS interval. Excessive alkalemia (pH >7.55) and hypernatremia should be avoided. Because sodium bicarbonate has a brief duration of effect, a continuous infusion usually is required after the IV bolus. Three 50-mL ampules should be placed in 1 L of 5% dextrose in water (D_5W) and run at twice maintenance with frequent checks of QRS and pH depending on the fluid requirements and blood pressure of the patient. Frequent evaluation of the fluid status should be performed to avoid precipitating pulmonary edema. An optimal duration of therapy has not been established. The time to resolution of conduction abnormalities during continuous bicarbonate infusion varies significantly, ranging from several hours to several days.[50] In a case of prolonged clinical effects from modified-release amitriptyline poisoning, sodium bicarbonate was administered on multiple occasions over 110 hours after the initial ingestion to reverse ongoing sodium channel conduction disturbances.[64] Sodium bicarbonate infusion usually is discontinued as soon as there is improvement in hemodynamics and cardiac conduction and resolution in altered mental status, although controlled data supporting such an approach are lacking.

OTHER SODIUM CHANNEL BLOCKING XENOBIOTICS

Sodium bicarbonate is useful in treating patients with cardiotoxicity from other xenobiotics, with sodium channel blocking effects manifested by widened QRS complexes, dysrhythmias, and hypotension. Isolated case reports provide the bulk of the evidence in these situations. The utility of sodium bicarbonate in treating patients with type IA and IC antidysrhythmics, diphenhydramine, propoxyphene, and quinine has been demonstrated.[7,11,77,84,88,95]

Use of sodium bicarbonate in the treatment of patients with amantadine overdose manifested by prolongation of the QRS and QT intervals was associated with narrowing of the QT but not the QRS interval.[25] Although the usefulness of sodium bicarbonate in reversing QT prolongation occasionally observed during fluoxetine and citalopram overdose has been reported,[19,24,30] sodium channel disturbances are uncommon in most cases of selective serotonin reuptake inhibitor (SSRI) overdose, and routine use of alkalinization therapy in this setting is unwarranted. Sodium bicarbonate may help in the management of patients with other ingestions associated with type IA-like cardiac conduction abnormalities and dysrhythmias, such as carbamazepine and the phenothiazines thioridazine and mesoridazine, but documentation of such benefit is lacking.

The role of sodium bicarbonate as an antidote has been studied in experimental models of calcium channel blocker toxicity and β-adrenergic antagonist toxicity. In the calcium channel blocker study, hypertonic sodium bicarbonate increased mean arterial pressure and cardiac output in verapamil-poisoned swine.[89] Possible explanations for this beneficial effect include the increase in serum pH, reversal of a sodium channel effect, lowering of serum potassium concentration, or volume expansion. In a canine model of propranolol toxicity, sodium bicarbonate failed to increase heart rate or blood pressure.[51]

Cocaine, a local anesthetic with membrane-stabilizing properties resembling other type I antidysrhythmics may cause similar conduction disturbances. In several canine models of cocaine toxicity, 2 mEq/kg of sodium bicarbonate successfully reversed cocaine-induced QRS prolongation[6,68] and improved myocardial function.[97] Of interest, sodium loading by itself (2 mEq/kg of sodium chloride) failed to produce a benefit. Similar findings were demonstrated in cocaine-treated guinea pig hearts.[98] Patients with cocaine-induced cardiotoxicity responded to treatment with sodium bicarbonate.[41,66,94] In many of these cases, simultaneous treatment with sedation, active cooling, and hyperventilation confounds the contribution of the sodium bicarbonate to overall recovery.

ALTERED XENOBIOTIC IONIZATION RESULTING IN ENHANCED ELIMINATION

SALICYLATES

Although there is no known specific antidote for salicylate toxicity, judicious use of sodium bicarbonate is an essential treatment modality of salicylism. Through its ability to change the concentration gradient of the ionized and nonionized fractions of salicylates, sodium bicarbonate is useful in decreasing tissue (eg, brain) concentrations of salicylates and enhancing urinary elimination of salicylates.[74] This therapy may limit the need for more invasive treatment modalities, such as hemodialysis.

Salicylate is a weak acid with a pK_a of 3.0. As pH increases, more of the xenobiotic is in the ionized form. Ionized molecules penetrate lipid-soluble membranes less rapidly than do nonionized molecules because of the presence of polar groups on the ionized form. Consequently, when the ionized forms predominate weak acids, such as salicylates, may accumulate in an alkaline milieu, such as an alkaline urine.[56,86]

Although alkalinizing the urine to increase salicylate elimination is an important intervention in the treatment of patients with salicylate poisoning, increasing the serum pH in patients with severe salicylism may prove even more consequential by protecting the brain from a lethal central nervous system (CNS) salicylate burden. Using sodium bicarbonate to "trap" salicylate in the blood (ie, keeping it out of the brain) may prevent clinical deterioration of salicylate-poisoned patients. Salicylate lethality is directly related to primary CNS dysfunction, which, in turn, corresponds to a "critical brain salicylate level."[35] At physiologic pH, at which a very small proportion of the salicylate is in the nonionized form, a small change in pH is associated with a significant change in amount of nonionized molecules (eg, at a pH of 7.4, 0.004% of the salicylate molecules is in the nonionized form; at a pH of 7.2, 0.008% of the salicylate is in the nonionized form). In experimental models, lowering the blood pH produces a shift of salicylate into the tissues.[20] Hence, acidemia that is observed in significant salicylate poisonings can be devastating. In salicylate-poisoned rats, increasing the blood pH with sodium bicarbonate produced a shift in salicylate out of the tissues and into the blood.[34] This change in salicylate distribution did not result from enhanced urinary excretion because occlusion of the renal pedicles failed to alter these results.

Enhancing the urinary elimination of salicylate by trapping ionized salicylate in the urine also provides great benefit. Salicylate elimination at low therapeutic concentrations consists predominantly of first-order hepatic metabolism. At these low concentrations, without alkalinization, only approximately 10% to 20% of salicylate is eliminated unchanged in the urine. With increasing concentrations, enzyme saturation occurs (Michaelis-Menten kinetics); thus, a larger percentage of elimination occurs as unchanged free salicylate. Under these conditions, in an alkaline urine, urinary excretion of free salicylate becomes even more significant, accounting for 60% to 85% of total elimination.[31,75]

The exact mechanism of pH-dependent salicylate elimination has generated controversy. The pH-dependent increase in urinary elimination initially was ascribed to "ion trapping," which is the filtering of both ionized and nonionized salicylate while reabsorbing only the nonionized salicylate.[82] However, limiting reabsorption of the ionizable fraction of filtered salicylate cannot be the primary mechanism responsible for enhanced elimination produced by sodium bicarbonate.[52] Because the quantitative difference between the percentage of molecules trapped in the ionized form at a pH of 5.0 (99% ionized) and a pH of 8.0 (99.999% ionized) is small, decreases in tubular reabsorption cannot fully explain the rapid increase in urinary elimination seen at a pH above 7.0.

"Diffusion theory" offers a reasonable alternative explanation. Fick's law of diffusion states that the rate of flow of a diffusing substance is proportional to its concentration gradient. A large concentration gradient between the nonionized salicylate in the peritubular fluid (and blood) and the tubular luminal fluid is found in alkaline urine. Because at a higher urinary pH, a greater proportion of secreted nonionized molecules quickly becomes ionized upon entering the alkaline environment, more salicylate (ie, nonionized salicylate) must pass from the peritubular fluid into the urine in an attempt to reach equilibrium with the nonionized fraction. In fact, as long as nonionized molecules are rapidly converted to ionized molecules in the urine, equilibrium in the alkaline milieu will never be achieved. The concentration gradient of peritubular nonionized salicylates to urinary nonionized salicylates continues to increase with increasing urinary pH. Hence, increased tubular diffusion, not decreased reabsorption, probably accounts for most of the increase in salicylate elimination observed in the alkaline urine.[52]

Controversies regarding the indications for alkalinization in the treatment of patients with salicylism persist. Although urinary alkalinization undoubtedly works to lower serum salicylate concentrations and enhance urinary elimination, the risks associated with alkalinization in the management of salicylism are of concern. Concerns regarding excessive alkalemia, hypernatremia, fluid overload, hypokalemia, and hypocalcemia, as well as the potential delay in achieving alkalinization with sodium bicarbonate (as opposed to more rapid response achieved with hyperventilation), have all been raised.[27,48,70,75,82] Early on, patients with pure respiratory alkalosis often have alkaluria, as well as alkalemia, and do not require urinary alkalinization. In the more common scenario in which patients present with a mixed respiratory alkalosis and metabolic acidosis, sodium bicarbonate must be administered cautiously. Young children who rapidly develop metabolic acidosis often require alkalinization but should be at less risk for complications of this therapy.[65]

Sodium bicarbonate is indicated in the treatment of salicylate poisoning for most patients with evidence of significant systemic toxicity. Although some authors have suggested alkali therapy for asymptomatic patients with concentrations above 30 mg/dL,[96] limited data support this approach. For patients with chronic poisoning, concentrations are not as helpful and may be misleading; clinical criteria remain the best indicators for therapy. Patients with contraindications to sodium bicarbonate use, such as renal failure and acute lung injury, should be considered candidates for intubation and subsequent hyperventilation, but extracorporeal removal is often required because of the difficulty and danger of intubation.

Dosing recommendations depend on the acid–base status of the patient. For patients with acidemia, rapid correction is indicated with IV administration of 1 to 2 mEq of sodium bicarbonate per kilogram of body weight.[90] After the blood is alkalinized or if the patient has already presented with an alkalemia, continued titration with sodium bicarbonate over 4 to 8 hours is recommended until the urinary pH reaches 7.5 to 8.0.[87,90] Alkalinization can be maintained with a continuous sodium bicarbonate infusion of 100 to 150 mEq in 1 L of D_5W at 150 to 200 mL/hr (or about twice the maintenance requirements in a child). Obtaining a urinary pH of 8.0 is difficult but is considered to be the goal. Fastidious attention to the patient's changing acid–base status is required. Systemic pH should not go above 7.55 to prevent complications of alkalemia.

Hypokalemia can make urinary alkalinization particularly problematic.[48,81] In hypokalemic patients, the kidneys preferentially reabsorb potassium in exchange for hydrogen ions. Urinary alkalinization will be unsuccessful as long as hydrogen ions are excreted into the urine. Thus, appropriate potassium supplementation to achieve normokalemia may be required to alkalinize the urine.[99]

In the past, proper urinary alkalinization was thought to require forced diuresis to maximize salicylate elimination.[23,48] Suggestions included administering enough fluid (2 L/h) to produce a urine output of 500 mL/h. Because forced alkaline diuresis appears unnecessary and is potentially harmful as a result of its unnecessarily large fluid load, the goal is alkalinization at a rate of approximately twice maintenance requirements to achieve a urine output of 3 to 5 mL/kg/h.

PHENOBARBITAL

Although cardiopulmonary support is the most critical intervention in the treatment of patients with severe phenobarbital overdose, sodium bicarbonate may be a useful adjunct to general supportive care. The utility of sodium bicarbonate is particularly important considering the long plasma half-life (~100 hours) of phenobarbital. Phenobarbital is a weak acid (pK_a, 7.24) that undergoes significant renal elimination. As in the case of salicylates, alkalinization of the blood and urine may reduce the severity and duration of toxicity. In a study of mice, the median anesthetic dose for mice receiving phenobarbital increased by 20% with the addition of 1 g/kg of sodium bicarbonate (increasing the blood pH from 7.23 to 7.41), demonstrating decreased tissue concentrations associated with increased pH.[93] Extrapolating the animal evidence to humans has suggested that phenobarbital-poisoned patients in deep coma might develop a respiratory acidosis secondary to hypoventilation, with the acidemia enhancing the entrance of phenobarbital into the brain, thus worsening CNS and respiratory depression. Alternatively, increasing the pH with bicarbonate, ventilatory support, or both would enhance the passage of phenobarbital out of the brain, thus lessening toxicity. Given the relatively high pK_a of phenobarbital, significant phenobarbital accumulation in the urine is evident only when urinary pH is increased above 7.5.[10] As the pH approaches 8.0, a threefold increase in urinary elimination occurs. The urine-to-serum ratio of phenobarbital, although much higher in alkaline urine than in acidic urine, remains less than unity, thereby suggesting less of a role for tubular secretion than in salicylate poisoning.

Clinical studies examining the role of alkalinization in phenobarbital poisoning have been inadequately designed. Many are poorly controlled and fail to examine the effects of alkalinization, independent of coadministered diuretic therapy. In one uncontrolled study, a 59% to 67% decrease in the duration of unconsciousness in patients with phenobarbital overdoses occurred in patients administered alkali compared with nonrandomized control subjects.[58] In other older studies, treatment with sodium lactate and urea reduced mortality and frequency of tracheotomy to 50% of control subjects, enhanced elimination, and shortened coma.[47,61] In a later human volunteer study, urinary alkalinization with sodium bicarbonate was associated with a decrease in phenobarbital elimination half-life from 148 to 47 hours.[28] However, this beneficial effect was less than the effect achieved by multiple-dose activated charcoal (MDAC), which reduced the half-life to 19 hours.[28] In a nonrandomized study of phenobarbital-poisoned patients comparing urinary alkalinization alone, MDAC alone, and both methods together, both the phenobarbital half-life decreased most rapidly and the clinical course improved most rapidly in the group of patients who received MDAC alone.[57] Interesting, the combination approach proved inferior to MDAC alone but was better than alkalinization alone. The authors speculated that when both treatments were used together, the increased ionization of phenobarbital resulting from sodium bicarbonate infusion may have decreased the efficacy of MDAC. These studies suggest that MDAC is more efficacious than urinary alkalinization in the treatment of phenobarbital-poisoned patients, although both approaches are beneficial and indicated.

Sodium bicarbonate therapy does not appear warranted in the treatment of patients with ingestions of other barbiturates, such as pentobarbital and secobarbital, most of which have a pK_a above 8.0 or are predominantly eliminated by the liver.

CHLORPROPAMIDE

Chlorpropamide is a weak acid (pK_a, 4.8) and has a long half-life (30–50 hours). In a human study using therapeutic doses of chlorpropamide, urinary alkalinization with sodium bicarbonate significantly increased renal clearance of the drug.[63] This study showed that whereas nonrenal clearance was the more significant route of elimination at a urinary pH of 5 to 6 (only slightly above pK_a), at a pH of 8.0, renal clearance was 10 times that of nonrenal clearance. Alkalinization reduced the area under the curve (AUC) almost fourfold and shortened the elimination half-life from 50 to 13 hours. Acidification increased the AUC by 41% and increased the half-life to 69 hours. Although not a study in overdose patients, this report suggests that sodium bicarbonate may be useful in the management of patients with chlorpropamide overdose. The effect of urinary alkalinization on elimination of other sulfonylureas is unnecessary because the benefit presumably is limited as these agents are largely metabolized in the liver.

CHLOROPHENOXY HERBICIDES

Alkalinization is indicated in the treatment of patients with poisonings from weed killers that contain chlorophenoxy compounds, such as 2,4-dichlorophenoxyacetic acid (2,4-D) or 2-(4-chloro-2-methylphenoxy) propionic acid (MCPP).[73] Poisoning results in muscle weakness, peripheral neuropathy, coma, hyperthermia, and acidemia. These compounds are weak acids (pK_a 2.6 and 3.8 for 2,4-D and MCPP, respectively) that are excreted largely unchanged in the urine. In an uncontrolled case series of 41 patients poisoned with a variety of chlorophenoxy herbicides, 19 of whom received sodium bicarbonate, alkaline diuresis significantly reduced the half-life of each by enhancing renal elimination.[26] In one patient, resolution of hyperthermia and metabolic acidosis and improvement in mental status were associated with a transient elevation of serum concentration, perhaps reflecting chlorophenoxy compound redistribution from the tissues into the more alkalemic blood. The limited data suggest that the increased ionized fractions of the weak-acid chlorophenoxy compounds produced by alkalinization is trapped in both the blood and the urine (as demonstrated with salicylates and phenobarbital); thus, its use ameliorates toxicity and shortens the duration of effect.

CORRECTING METABOLIC ACIDOSIS

TOXIC ALCOHOLS

Sodium bicarbonate has two important roles in treating patients with toxic alcohol ingestions. As an immediate temporizing measure, administration of sodium bicarbonate may reverse the life-threatening acidemia associated with methanol and ethylene glycol ingestions. In rats poisoned with ethylene glycol, the administration of sodium bicarbonate alone resulted in a fourfold increase in the median lethal dose.[13] Clinically, titrating the endogenous acid with bicarbonate greatly assists in reversing the consequences of severe acidemia, such as hemodynamic instability and multiorgan dysfunction.

The second role of bicarbonate in the treatment of toxic alcohol poisoning involves its ability to favorably alter the distribution and elimination of certain toxic metabolites.[76] In cases of methanol poisoning, the proportion of ionized formic acid can be increased by administering bicarbonate, thereby trapping formate in the blood compartment.[40,53] Consequently, decreased visual toxicity results from removal of the toxic metabolite from the eyes. In cases of formic acid (pK_a of 3.7) ingestion, sodium bicarbonate decreases tissue penetration of the formic acid and enhances urinary elimination.[60] Further investigation is required to delineate the beneficial effects of sodium bicarbonate in the treatment of patients with toxic alcohol ingestions.

Early treatment of acidemia with sodium bicarbonate is strongly recommended in cases of methanol and ethylene glycol poisoning.[33] Sodium bicarbonate should be administered to toxic alcohol-poisoned patients with an arterial pH below 7.30.[46] More than 400 to 600 mEq of sodium bicarbonate may be required in the first few hours.[39] In cases of ethylene glycol toxicity, sodium bicarbonate administration may worsen hypocalcemia, so the serum calcium concentration should be monitored. Combating the acidemia, however, is not the mainstay of therapy, and concurrent administration of IV fomepizole or ethanol and preparation for possible hemodialysis are almost always indicated.

METFORMIN

Metformin toxicity, either from overdose or therapeutic use in the setting of renal failure, may cause severe, life-threatening lactic acidosis. The use of high-dose sodium bicarbonate to correct the metabolic acidosis, as well as extracorporeal removal of the metformin, has been recommended in these cases.[32]

INCREASING XENOBIOTIC SOLUBILITY: METHOTREXATE

Urinary alkalinization with sodium bicarbonate is routinely used during high-dose methotrexate cancer chemotherapy therapy. Methotrexate is predominantly eliminated unchanged in the urine. Unfortunately, it is poorly water soluble in acidic urine. Under these conditions, tubular precipitation of the methotrexate may occur, leading to nephrotoxicity and decreased elimination, increasing the likelihood of methotrexate toxicity. Administration of sodium bicarbonate (as well as intensive hydration) during high-dose methotrexate infusions increases methotrexate solubility and the elimination of methotrexate.[22,78]

NEUTRALIZATION: CHLORINE GAS

Nebulized sodium bicarbonate serves as a useful adjunct in the treatment of patients with pulmonary injuries resulting from chlorine gas inhalation.[2,21] Inhaled sodium bicarbonate neutralizes the hydrochloric acid that is formed when the chlorine gas reacts with the water in the respiratory tree. Although oral sodium bicarbonate is not recommended for neutralizing acid ingestions because of the problems associated with the exothermic reaction and production of carbon dioxide in the relatively closed gastrointestinal tract, the rapid exchange in the lungs of air with the environment facilitates heat dissipation. In a chlorine-inhalation sheep model, animals treated with 4% nebulized sodium bicarbonate solution demonstrated higher PO_2 and lower PCO_2 than did the normal, saline-treated animals.[21] There was no difference, however, in 24-hour mortality or pulmonary histopathology. In a retrospective review, 86 patients with chlorine gas inhalation were treated with nebulized sodium bicarbonate.[14] Sixty-nine patients were sent home from the emergency department, 53 of whom had clearly improved. In a more recent study, 44 patients who were diagnosed with reactive airway dysfunction syndrome after an acute exposure to chlorine gas were randomized to receive either nebulized sodium bicarbonate (4 mL of 4.2% $NaHCO_3$ solution) or nebulized placebo.[2] Both groups also received IV corticosteroids and inhaled β_2 agonists. Compared with the placebo group, the nebulized sodium bicarbonate group had significantly higher forced expiratory volume in 1 second (FEV_1) values at 120 and 240 minutes and scored significantly higher on a posttreatment quality of life questionnaire.

MAINTENANCE OF CHELATION EFFECT: DIMERCAPROL–METAL CHELATION

Adverse effects and safety concerns may be associated with the dissociation of the dimercaprol (British anti-Lewisite [BAL]) metal binding that occurs in acid urine. Because dissociation of the BAL-metal chelate occurs in acidic urine, the urine of patients receiving BAL should be alkalinized with hypertonic $NaHCO_3$ to a pH of 7.5 to 8.0 to prevent renal liberation of the metal.[43]

REDUCTION IN FREE RADICAL FORMATION: CONTRAST MEDIA

Recent studies have suggested that sodium bicarbonate may be beneficial in preventing contrast-induced nephropathy (CIN).[55] A randomized trial of 119 patients compared an infusion of 154 mEq/L of either sodium bicarbonate or sodium chloride before (3 mL/kg for 1 hour) and after (1 mL/kg/h for 6 hours) iopamidol administration. CIN, defined as a 25% or greater increase in serum creatinine concentration within 2 days of contrast, occurred in eight patients in the sodium chloride group and one patient in the sodium bicarbonate group. In another study comparing sodium bicarbonate with sodium chloride before emergency coronary angiography or intervention, the incidence of CIN was also significantly lower in the sodium bicarbonate group than in the sodium chloride group (7% vs. 35%).[54] It is suggested that increasing medullary pH with sodium bicarbonate infusion might protect the kidneys from oxidant injury by slowing free radical production. The addition of *N*-acetylcysteine to a sodium bicarbonate hydration regimen to prevent CIN does not appear to offer any benefit compared with the use of only sodium bicarbonate hydration.[67] Further study to define the optimal hydration strategy is recommended.[38]

SUMMARY

Despite the increasing tendency to avoid sodium bicarbonate administration in critically ill acidemic patients, sodium bicarbonate remains an important antidote in the treatment of a wide variety of xenobiotic exposures. In fact, its utility in poisoned patients continues to expand. Sodium bicarbonate is effective in the treatment of patients with poisonings by CAs[16] and other sodium channel blockers through its effects on drug ionization and subsequent diffusion from the sodium channel binding site. Sodium bicarbonate is effective for salicylates, phenobarbital, and other weak acids because of its ability to ion trap in the blood or brain and keep toxins away from the target organ.[68] Sodium bicarbonate is effective as a neutralizing agent for inhaled acids such as chlorine gas. In the more common causes of metabolic acidosis with elevated lactate, specific therapy such as antibiotics, volume resuscitation, and inotropic support usually takes precedence over bicarbonate administration.

REFERENCES

1. Aschner JL, Poland RL, Aschner JL, Poland RL. Sodium bicarbonate: basically useless therapy. *Pediatrics.* 2008;122:831-835.
2. Aslan S, Kandis H, Akgun M, et al. The effect of nebulized NaHCO3 treatment on "RADS" due to chlorine gas inhalation. *Inhal Toxicol.* 2006;18:895-900.
3. Bailey D. Cardiotoxic effects of quinidine and their treatment. *Arch Intern Med.* 1960;105:37-46.
4. Bar-Joseph G, Abramson NS, Kelsey SF, et al. Improved resuscitation outcome in emergency medical systems with increased usage of sodium bicarbonate during cardiopulmonary resuscitation. *Acta Anaesthesiol Scand.* 2005;49:6-15.
5. Bebarta VS, Waksman JC, Bebarta VS, Waksman JC. Amitriptyline-induced Brugada pattern fails to respond to sodium bicarbonate. *Clin Toxicol (Phila).* 2007;45:186-188.
6. Beckman KJ, Parker RB, Hariman RJ, et al. Hemodynamic and electrophysiological actions of cocaine. Effects of sodium bicarbonate as an antidote in dogs. *Circulation.* 1991;83:1799-1807.
7. Bellet S, Hamdan G, Somiyo A, Lara R. The reversal of cardiotoxic effects of quinidine by molar sodium lactate: an experimental study. *Am J Med Sci.* 1959;237:165-176.
8. Bellet S, Wasserman F. The effects of molar sodium lactate in reversing the cardiotoxic effect of hyperpotassemia. *Arch Intern Med.* 1957;100:565-581.
9. Blackman K, Brown SG, Wilkes GJ. Plasma alkalinization for tricyclic antidepressant toxicity: a systematic review. *Emerg Med (Fremantle).* 2001;13:204-210.
10. Bloomer HA. A critical evaluation of diuresis in the treatment of barbiturate intoxication. *J Lab Clin Med.* 1966;67:898-905.
11. Bodenhamer JE, Smilkstein MJ. Delayed cardiotoxicity following quinine overdose: a case report. *J Emerg Med.* 1993;11:279-285.
12. Boehnert MT, Lovejoy FH Jr. Value of the QRS duration versus the serum drug level in predicting seizures and ventricular arrhythmias after an acute overdose of tricyclic antidepressants. *N Engl J Med.* 1985;313:474-479.
13. Borden TA, Bidwell CD. Treatment of acute ethylene glycol poisoning in rats. *Invest Urol.* 1968;6:205-210.
14. Bosse GM. Nebulized sodium bicarbonate in the treatment of chlorine gas inhalation. *J Toxicol Clin Toxicol.* 1994;32:233-241.
15. Boyd JH, Walley KR, Boyd JH, Walley KR. Is there a role for sodium bicarbonate in treating lactic acidosis from shock? *Curr Opin Crit Care.* 2008;14:379-383.
16. Bradberry SM, Thanacoody HK, Watt BE, et al. Management of the cardiovascular complications of tricyclic antidepressant poisoning: role of sodium bicarbonate. *Toxicol Rev.* 2005;24:195-204.
17. Brown TC. Sodium bicarbonate treatment for tricyclic antidepressant arrhythmias in children. *Med J Aust.* 1976;2:380-382.
18. Brown TC, Barker GA, Dunlop ME, Loughnan PM. The use of sodium bicarbonate in the treatment of tricyclic antidepressant-induced arrhythmias. *Anaesth Intensive Care.* 1973;1:203-210.
19. Brucculeri M, Kaplan J, Lande L, et al. Reversal of citalopram-induced junctional bradycardia with intravenous sodium bicarbonate. *Pharmacotherapy.* 2005;25:119-122.
20. Buchanan N, Kundig H, Eyberg C. Experimental salicylate intoxication in young baboons. A preliminary report. *J Pediatr.* 1975;86:225-232.
21. Chisholm C, Singletary E, Okerberg C, Langlinais P. Effect of hydration on sodium bicarbonate therapy for chlorine inhalation injuries [abstract]. *Ann Emerg Med.* 1988;18:466.
22. Christensen ML, Rivera GK, Crom WR, et al. Effect of hydration on methotrexate plasma concentrations in children with acute lymphocytic leukemia. *J Clin Oncol.* 1988;6:797-801.
23. Dukes D, Blainey J, Cumming G, Widdowson G. The treatment of severe aspirin poisoning. *Lancet.* 1963;2:329-331.
24. Engebretsen KM, Harris CR, Wood JE. Cardiotoxicity and late onset seizures with citalopram overdose. *J Emerg Med.* 2003;25:163-166.
25. Farrell S, Lee D, McNamara R. Amantadine overdose: considerations for the treatment of cardiac toxicity [abstract]. *J Toxicol Clin Toxicol.* 1995;33:516-517.
26. Flanagan RJ, Meredith TJ, Ruprah M, et al. Alkaline diuresis for acute poisoning with chlorophenoxy herbicides and ioxynil. *Lancet.* 1990;335:454-458.
27. Fox GN. Hypocalcemia complicating bicarbonate therapy for salicylate poisoning. *West J Med.* 1984;141:108-109.
28. Frenia ML, Schauben JL, Wears RL, et al. Multiple-dose activated charcoal compared to urinary alkalinization for the enhancement of phenobarbital elimination. *J Toxicol Clin Toxicol.* 1996;34:169-175.
29. Gaultier M. Sodium bicarbonate and tricyclic-antidepressant poisoning [letter]. *Lancet.* 1976;2:1258.
30. Graudins A, Vossler C, Wang R. Fluoxetine-induced cardiotoxicity with response to bicarbonate therapy. *Am J Emerg Med.* 1997;15:501-503.
31. Gutman A, Sirota J. A study by simultaneous clearance techniques of salicylate excretion in man: effects of alkalinization of the urine by bicarbonate administration: effect of probenecid. *J Clin Invest.* 1955;34:711-722.
32. Harvey B, Hickman C, Hinson G, et al. Severe lactic acidosis complicating metformin overdose successfully treated with high-volume venovenous hemofiltration and aggressive alkalinization. *Pediatr Crit Care Med.* 2005;6:598-601.
33. Herken W, Rietbrock N. The influence of blood-pH on ionization, distribution, and toxicity of formic acid. *Naunyn Schmiedebergs Arch Exp Pathol Pharmakol.* 1968;260:142-143.

34. Hill JB. Experimental salicylate poisoning: observations on the effects of altering blood pH on tissue and plasma salicylate concentrations. *Pediatrics.* 1971;47:658-665.
35. Hill JB. Salicylate intoxication. *N Engl J Med.* 1973;288:1110-1113.
36. Hoffman JR, McElroy CR. Bicarbonate therapy for dysrhythmia and hypotension in tricyclic antidepressant overdose. *West J Med.* 1981;134:60-64.
37. Hoffman JR, Votey SR, Bayer M, Silver L. Effect of hypertonic sodium bicarbonate in the treatment of moderate-to-severe cyclic antidepressant overdose. *Am J Emerg Med.* 1993;11:336-341.
38. Hogan SE, L'Allier P, Chetcuti S, et al. Current role of sodium bicarbonate-based preprocedural hydration for the prevention of contrast-induced acute kidney injury: a meta-analysis. *Am Heart J.* 2008;156:414-421.
39. Jacobsen D, McMartin KE. Methanol and ethylene glycol poisonings. Mechanism of toxicity, clinical course, diagnosis and treatment. *Med Toxicol.* 1986;1:309-334.
40. Jacobsen D, Webb R, Collins TD, McMartin KE. Methanol and formate kinetics in late diagnosed methanol intoxication. *Med Toxicol Adverse Drug Exp.* 1988;3:418-423.
41. Kerns W 2nd, Garvey L, Owens J. Cocaine-induced wide complex dysrhythmia. *J Emerg Med.* 1997;15:321-329.
42. Kingston ME. Hyperventilation in tricyclic antidepressant poisoning. *Crit Care Med.* 1979;7:550-551.
43. Klaassen CD. Heavy metals and heavy metal antagonist. In: Hardman JG, Limbird LE, eds. *The Pharmacological Basis of Therapeutics*, 10th ed. New York: Macmillan; 2001:1851-1875.
44. Knudsen K, Abrahamsson J. Epinephrine and sodium bicarbonate independently and additively increase survival in experimental amitriptyline poisoning. *Crit Care Med.* 1997;25:669-674.
45. Kraut JA, Kurtz I. Use of base in the treatment of severe acidemic states. *Am J Kidney Dis.* 2001;38:703-727.
46. Kulig K, Duffy J, Linden C, Rumack B. Toxic effects of methanol, ethylene glycol, and isopropyl alcohol. *Top Emerg Med.* 1984;6:14-28.
47. Lassen N. Treatment of severe acute barbiturate poisoning by forced diuresis and alkalinization of the urine. *Lancet.* 1960;2:338-342.
48. Lawson AA, Proudfoot AT, Brown SS, et al. Forced diuresis in the treatment of acute salicylate poisoning in adults. *Q J Med.* 1969;38:31-48.
49. Levitt MA, Sullivan JB Jr, Owens SM, et al. Amitriptyline plasma protein binding: effect of plasma pH and relevance to clinical overdose. *Am J Emerg Med.* 1986;4:121-125.
50. Liebelt EL, Ulrich A, Francis PD, Woolf A. Serial electrocardiogram changes in acute tricyclic antidepressant overdoses. *Crit Care Med.* 1997;25:1721-1726.
51. Love JN, Howell JM, Newsome JT, et al. The effect of sodium bicarbonate on propranolol-induced cardiovascular toxicity in a canine model. *J Toxicol Clin Toxicol.* 2000;38:421-428.
52. Macpherson C, Milne MD, Evans B. The excretion of salicylate. *Br J Pharmacol.* 1955;10:484-489.
53. Martin-Amat G, McMartin KE, Hayreh SS, et al. Methanol poisoning: ocular toxicity produced by formate. *Toxicol Appl Pharmacol.* 1978;45:201-208.
54. Masuda M, Yamada T, Mine T, et al. Comparison of usefulness of sodium bicarbonate versus sodium chloride to prevent contrast-induced nephropathy in patients undergoing an emergent coronary procedure. *Am J Cardiol.* 2007;100:781-786.
55. Merten GJ, Burgess WP, Gray LV, et al. Prevention of contrast-induced nephropathy with sodium bicarbonate: a randomized controlled trial. *JAMA.* 2004;291:2328-2334.
56. Milne M, Scribner B, Crawford M. Non-ionic diffusion and the excretion of weak acids and bases. *Am J Med.* 1958;24(5):709-729.
57. Mohammed Ebid AH, Abdel-Rahman HM. Pharmacokinetics of phenobarbital during certain enhanced elimination modalities to evaluate their clinical efficacy in management of drug overdose. *Ther Drug Monit.* 2001;23:209-216.
58. Mollaret P, Rapin M, Pocidalo J, Monsallier J. Treatment of acute barbiturate intoxication through plasmatic and urinary alkalinization. *Presse Med.* 1959;67:1435-1437.
59. Molloy DW, Penner SB, Rabson J, Hall KW. Use of sodium bicarbonate to treat tricyclic antidepressant-induced arrhythmias in a patient with alkalosis. *Can Med Assoc J.* 1984;130:1457-1459.
60. Moore DF, Bentley AM, Dawling S, et al. Folinic acid and enhanced renal elimination in formic acid intoxication. *J Toxicol Clin Toxicol.* 1994;32:199-204.
61. Myschetzky A, Lassen N. Urea-induced, osmotic diuresis and alkalization of urine in acute barbiturate intoxication. *JAMA.* 1963;185:936-942.
62. Nattel S, Mittleman M. Treatment of ventricular tachyarrhythmias resulting from amitriptyline toxicity in dogs. *J Pharmacol Exp Ther.* 1984;231:430-435.
63. Neuvonen PJ, Karkkainen S. Effects of charcoal, sodium bicarbonate, and ammonium chloride on chlorpropamide kinetics. *Clin Pharmacol Ther.* 1983;33:386-393.
64. O'Connor N, Greene S, Dargan P, et al. Prolonged clinical effects in modified-release amitriptyline poisoning. *Clin Toxicol (Phila).* 2006;44:77-80.
65. Oliver T, Dyer M. The prompt treatment of salicylism with sodium bicarbonate. *Am J Dis Child.* 1960;99:553-564.
66. Ortega-Carnicer J, Bertos-Polo J, Gutierrez-Tirado C. Aborted sudden death, transient Brugada pattern, and wide QRS dysrrhythmias after massive cocaine ingestion. *J Electrocardiol.* 2001;34:345-349.
67. Ozcan EE, Guneri S, Akdeniz B, et al. Sodium bicarbonate, N-acetylcysteine, and saline for prevention of radiocontrast-induced nephropathy. A comparison of 3 regimens for protecting contrast-induced nephropathy in patients undergoing coronary procedures. A single-center prospective controlled trial. *Am Heart J.* 2007;154:539-544.
68. Parker RB, Perry GY, Horan LG, Flowers NC. Comparative effects of sodium bicarbonate and sodium chloride on reversing cocaine-induced changes in the electrocardiogram. *J Cardiovasc Pharmacol.* 1999;34:864-869.
69. Pentel P, Benowitz N. Efficacy and mechanism of action of sodium bicarbonate in the treatment of desipramine toxicity in rats. *J Pharmacol Exp Ther.* 1984;230:12-19.
70. Pentel PR, Benowitz NL. Tricyclic antidepressant poisoning. Management of arrhythmias. *Med Toxicol.* 1986;1:101-121.
71. Pentel PR, Goldsmith SR, Salerno DM, et al. Effect of hypertonic sodium bicarbonate on encainide overdose. *Am J Cardiol.* 1986;57:878-880.
72. Pentel PR, Keyler DE. Effects of high dose alpha-1-acid glycoprotein on desipramine toxicity in rats. *J Pharmacol Exp Ther.* 1988;246:1061-1066.
73. Prescott LF, Park J, Darrien I. Treatment of severe 2,4-D and mecoprop intoxication with alkaline diuresis. *Br J Clin Pharmacol.* 1979;7:111-116.
74. Proudfoot AT, Krenzelok EP, Brent J, Vale JA. Does urine alkalinization increase salicylate elimination? If so, why? *Toxicol Rev.* 2003;22:129-136.
75. Reimold EW, Worthen HG, Reilly TP Jr. Salicylate poisoning. Comparison of acetazolamide administration and alkaline diuresis in the treatment of experimental salicylate intoxication in puppies. *Am J Dis Child.* 1973;125:668-674.
76. Roe O. Methanol poisoning: its clinical course, pathogenesis, and treatment. *Acta Med Scand.* 1946;126(suppl 182):1-253.
77. Salerno DM, Murakami MM, Johnston RB, et al. Reversal of flecainide-induced ventricular arrhythmia by hypertonic sodium bicarbonate in dogs. *Am J Emerg Med.* 1995;13:285-293.
78. Sand TE, Jacobsen S. Effect of urine pH and flow on renal clearance of methotrexate. *Eur J Clin Pharmacol.* 1981;19:453-456.
79. Sasyniuk BI, Jhamandas V. Mechanism of reversal of toxic effects of amitriptyline on cardiac Purkinje fibers by sodium bicarbonate. *J Pharmacol Exp Ther.* 1984;231:387-394.
80. Sasyniuk BI, Jhamandas V, Valois M. Experimental amitriptyline intoxication: treatment of cardiac toxicity with sodium bicarbonate. *Ann Emerg Med.* 1986;15:1052-1059.
81. Savege TM, Ward JD, Simpson BR, Cohen RD. Treatment of severe salicylate poisoning by forced alkaline diuresis. *Br Med J.* 1969;1:35-36.
82. Segar WE. The critically ill child: salicylate intoxication. *Pediatrics.* 1969;44:440-444.
83. Seger DL, Hantsch C, Zavoral T, Wrenn K. Variability of recommendations for serum alkalinization in tricyclic antidepressant overdose: a survey of U.S. Poison Center medical directors. *J Toxicol Clin Toxicol.* 2003;41:331-338.
84. Sharma AN, Hexdall AH, Chang EK, et al. Diphenhydramine-induced wide complex dysrhythmia responds to treatment with sodium bicarbonate. *Am J Emerg Med.* 2003;21:212-215.
85. Smilkstein MJ. Reviewing cyclic antidepressant cardiotoxicity: wheat and chaff. *J Emerg Med.* 1990;8:645-648.
86. Smith P, Gleason H, Stoll C. Studies on the pharmacology of salicylates. *J Pharmacol Exp Ther.* 1946;87:237-255.
87. Snodgrass W, Rumack BH, Peterson RG, Holbrook ML. Salicylate toxicity following therapeutic doses in young children. *Clin Toxicol.* 1981;18:247-259.
88. Stork CM, Redd JT, Fine K, Hoffman RS. Propoxyphene-induced wide QRS complex dysrhythmia responsive to sodium bicarbonate—a case report. *J Toxicol Clin Toxicol.* 1995;33:179-183.
89. Tanen DA, Ruha AM, Curry SC, et al. Hypertonic sodium bicarbonate is effective in the acute management of verapamil toxicity in a swine model. *Ann Emerg Med.* 2000;36:547-553.

90. Temple AR. Acute and chronic effects of aspirin toxicity and their treatment. *Arch Intern Med.* 1981;141:364-369.
91. Viallon A, Zeni F, Lafond P, et al. Does bicarbonate therapy improve the management of severe diabetic ketoacidosis? *Crit Care Med.* 1999;27:2690-2693.
92. Vukmir RB, Katz L, Sodium Bicarbonate Study Group. Sodium bicarbonate improves outcome in prolonged prehospital cardiac arrest. *Am J Emerg Med.* 2006;24:156-161.
93. Waddell W, Butler T. The distribution and excretion of phenobarbital. *J Clin Invest.* 1957;36:1217-1226.
94. Wang RY. pH-dependent cocaine-induced cardiotoxicity. *Am J Emerg Med.* 1999;17:364-369.
95. Wasserman F, Brodsky L, Dick M, et al. Successful treatment of quinidine and procainamide intoxication. *N Engl J Med.* 1958;259:797-802.
96. Whitten C, Kesaree N, Goodwin J. Managing salicylate poisoning in children. *Am J Dis Child.* 1961;101:178-194.
97. Wilson LD, Shelat C. Electrophysiologic and hemodynamic effects of sodium bicarbonate in a canine model of severe cocaine intoxication. *J Toxicol Clin Toxicol.* 2003;41:777-788.
98. Winecoff AP, Hariman RJ, Grawe JJ, et al. Reversal of the electrocardiographic effects of cocaine by lidocaine. Part 1. Comparison with sodium bicarbonate and quinidine. *Pharmacotherapy.* 1994;14:698-703.
99. Yip L, Dart RC, Gabow PA. Concepts and controversies in salicylate toxicity. *Emerg Med Clin North Am.* 1994;12:351-364.

CHAPTER 36 NONSTEROIDAL ANTIINFLAMMATORY DRUGS

William J. Holubek

Nonsteroidal antiinflammatory drugs (NSAIDs) comprise a class of xenobiotics with analgesic, antipyretic, and antiinflammatory properties. These desirable clinical effects account for the extensive list of approved clinical uses, including the treatment of pain, inflammation, and fever, as well as the management of connective tissue, immunologic, and rheumatologic diseases.[55] In addition to the countless benefits of NSAIDs, some deleterious and life-threatening effects are associated with both their therapeutic use and overdose. In an attempt to circumvent some of these adverse effects, selective cyclooxygenase-2 (COX-2) inhibitors were introduced to the market but one was withdrawn because of their own toxicity profiles. The term *NSAID* used in this chapter does not refer to salicylates, which are unique members of the NSAID class and are covered in Chapter 35.

HISTORY AND EPIDEMIOLOGY

The discovery of NSAIDs began with the creation of acetyl salicylic acid (aspirin) by Felix Hoffman in 1897.[59] Searching for an antirheumatic xenobiotic with less adverse gastrointestinal (GI) effect than aspirin, Stewart Adams and John Nicholson discovered and developed 2-(4-isobutylphenyl) propionic acid, now known as ibuprofen, in 1961. Ibuprofen was initially marketed under the trade name Brufen in the United Kingdom in 1969 and was introduced to the U.S. market in 1974. Ibuprofen became available without a prescription in the United States by 1984. More than a decade later, in 1999, the first selective COX-2 inhibitor, rofecoxib, was approved by the U.S. Food and Drug Administration (FDA), but it was withdrawn in 2004 after increased myocardial infarctions and cerebrovascular accidents were associated with its use.

The American Association of Poison Control Centers (AAPCC) compiles data from participating poison centers throughout the United States using the National Poison Data System (NPDS), formerly known as the Toxic Exposure Surveillance System (TESS). Approximately 4% of all human exposures reported to the AAPCC from 2003 to 2007 were to NSAIDs (including COX-2 inhibitors, ibuprofen, ibuprofen with hydrocodone, indomethacin, ketoprofen, naproxen, and others), which translates to about 90,000 to 100,000 calls annually. In 2006, the AAPCC introduced a Fatality Review Team, which attempts to determine the relationship between exposure and death. The 2006 and 2007 annual reports assigned five deaths and 107 life-threatening manifestations to NSAID exposure (see Chap. 135).

Ibuprofen, naproxen, and ketoprofen are currently the only nonprescription NSAIDs in the United States. NSAIDs are also contained in cough and cold preparations and in prescription combination drugs (eg, ibuprofen with hydrocodone) and have occasionally been found as adulterants in herbal preparations.[64]

NSAIDs are considered among the most commonly used and prescribed medications in the world.[10,75] An estimated one in seven patients with rheumatologic diseases is given a prescription for NSAIDs, and another one in five U.S. citizens uses NSAIDs for acute common complaints.[99]

PHARMACOLOGY

These chemically heterogeneous compounds can be divided into carboxylic acid and enolic acid derivatives and COX-2 selective inhibition (Table 36–1). They all share the ability to inhibit prostaglandin (PG) synthesis. PG synthesis begins with the activation of phospholipases (commonly, phospholipase A_2 or PLR) that cleave phospholipids in the cell membrane to form arachidonic acid (AA). AA is metabolized by PG endoperoxide G/H synthase, otherwise known as COX, to form many eicosanoids, including PGs and the prostanoids, prostacyclin (PGI_2) and thromboxane (TXA_2). AA can also be metabolized by lipoxygenase (LOX) to form hydroperoxy eicosatetraenoic acid (HPETE), which is converted to many different leukotrienes (LTs) that are involved in creating a proinflammatory environment (Fig. 36–1).

The COX enzyme responsible for PG production exists in two isoforms termed *COX-1* and *COX-2*. COX-1 is constitutively expressed by virtually all cells throughout the body but is the only isoform found within platelets. This enzyme produces eicosanoids that govern "housekeeping" functions, including vascular homeostasis and hemostasis, gastric cytoprotection, and renal blood flow and function.[11,79] COX-2, on the other hand, is rapidly induced (within 1 to 3 hours) in inflammatory tissue by laminar shear (or mechanical) forces and cytokines, producing PGs involved in the inflammatory response. COX-2 is also upregulated by several cytokines, growth factors, and tumor promoters involved with cellular differentiation and mitogenesis, suggesting a role in cancer development.[11,31,85]

Glucocorticoids can both inhibit PLA and downregulate the induced expression of COX-2, which decreases the production of eicosanoids and PGs, respectively. Most NSAIDs nonselectively inhibit the COX enzymes in a competitive or time-dependent, reversible manner, unlike salicylates which irreversibly acetylate COX (see Chap. 35). Inhibiting COX-1 can interrupt tissue homeostasis, leading to deleterious clinical effects. In what may seem advantageous, some NSAIDs (eg, etodolac, meloxicam, and nimesulide) preferentially inhibit COX-2 over COX-1; others were specifically designed to selectively inhibit COX-2 (eg, celecoxib).[97] As will be discussed later in this chapter, many of the selective COX-2 inhibitors (sometimes referred to as *coxibs*) were removed from the market in the United States because of their increased risk of adverse cardiovascular events.

NSAIDs do not directly affect the LOX enzyme and the production of LTs; however, some data suggest that blocking the COX enzymes allows AA to be shunted toward the LOX pathway, increasing the production of proinflammatory and chemotactic-vasoactive LTs.[55,99]

PHARMACOKINETICS AND TOXICOKINETICS

Most NSAIDs are organic acids with extensive protein binding (>90%) and small volumes of distribution of approximately 0.1 to 0.2 L/kg. Oral absorption of most NSAIDs occurs rapidly, resulting in bioavailabilities above 80%. Time to peak plasma concentrations achieved by NSAIDs can differ widely (see Table 36–1).[17]

NSAIDs differ with regard to their sites of both action and accumulation within the body. For example, significant synovial concentrations are attained by indomethacin, tolmetin, diclofenac, ibuprofen, and piroxicam.[17] Some NSAIDs cross the blood–brain barrier, achieving significant cerebrospinal fluid (CSF) concentrations. The mechanism and chemical properties related to these properties are not well defined, but evidence suggests that NSAIDs with either very high or very low lipophilicity do

TABLE 36–1. Classes and Pharmacology of Selected Nonsteroidal Antiinflammatory Drugs[8,17,18,29,56,65]

	Time to Peak Plasma Concentration (h)	Half-Life (h)	Pharmacokinetics	Unique Features
CARBOXYLIC ACIDS				
Acetic Acids				
Diclofenac[a,e]	2–3	1–2	First-pass effect; hepatic metabolism (CYP2C9)	Decreases leukocyte AA concentration; topical activity; hepatotoxic
Etodolac	1	7	Hepatic metabolism	Inhibits PMN motility; coronary vasoconstrictor effect
Indomethacin	1–2	2.5	Demethylation (50%)	Poor antiinflammatory effect; topical activity
Ketorolac	< 1	4–6	Urinary excretion	
Sulindac	1–2	7	Active metabolite with a half-life of 18 hr	Prodrug; hepatotoxic
Tolmetin	< 1	5	Hepatic metabolism	Accumulates in synovia
Fenamates				
Meclofenamate	0.5–2.0	2–3		Seizures; GI inflammation
Mefenamic acid	2–4	3–4	Urinary excretion (50%)	Seizures; PG antagonist
Propionic Acids				
Fenoprofen	2	2–3	Decreased oral absorption (~85%)	Increased C_{CSF}
Flurbiprofen	1–2	6		Increased C_{CSF}
Ibuprofen[b,f]	<0.5	2–4	Hepatic metabolism; urinary excretion	Also formulated as IV caldolor
Indobufen[c]	2	6–7	Urinary excretion (70%–80%)	In Europe, used as prophylaxis for thrombus formation
Ketoprofen[b]	1–2	2	Hepatic metabolism; urinary excretion	Bradykinin antagonist; stabilizes lysosomal membranes
Naproxen[b]	1	14	Increased half-life with renal dysfunction	Inhibitory effect on leukocytes; prolonged platelet inhibition
Oxaprozin	3–6	40–60		Once-daily administration
Salicylates (see Chapter 35)				
ENOLIC ACIDS				
Oxicams				
Meloxicam[a]	5–10	15–20		High COX-2 selectivity
Nabumetone	3–6	24	Hepatic metabolism; active metabolites	Prodrug
Piroxicam	3–5	45–50	Hepatic metabolism (CYP2C9)	Inhibits neutrophil activation
Pyrazolone				
Phenylbutazone[c]	2	54–99	Hepatic metabolism; active metabolites	Irreversible agranulocytosis; aplastic anemia
COX-2 SELECTIVE INHIBITORS[d]				
Celecoxib	2–4	6–12	Hepatic metabolism (CYP2C9)	Inhibits CYP2D6
Nimesulide[c]	1–3	2–5	Urinary excretion (60%); active metabolites	Inhibits neutrophil activation

AA, arachidonic acid; C_{CSF}, cerebrospinal fluid concentration; COX, cyclooxygenase; GI, gastrointestinal; PMN, polymorphonuclear leukocytes; PG, prostaglandin.

[a] COX-2 preferential.

[b] Nonprescription.

[c] Not available in the United States.

[d] Rofecoxib (Vioxx) and valdecoxib (Bextra) are no longer available.

[e] Available in combination with misoprostol.

[f] Available in combination with oxycodone and hydrocodone.

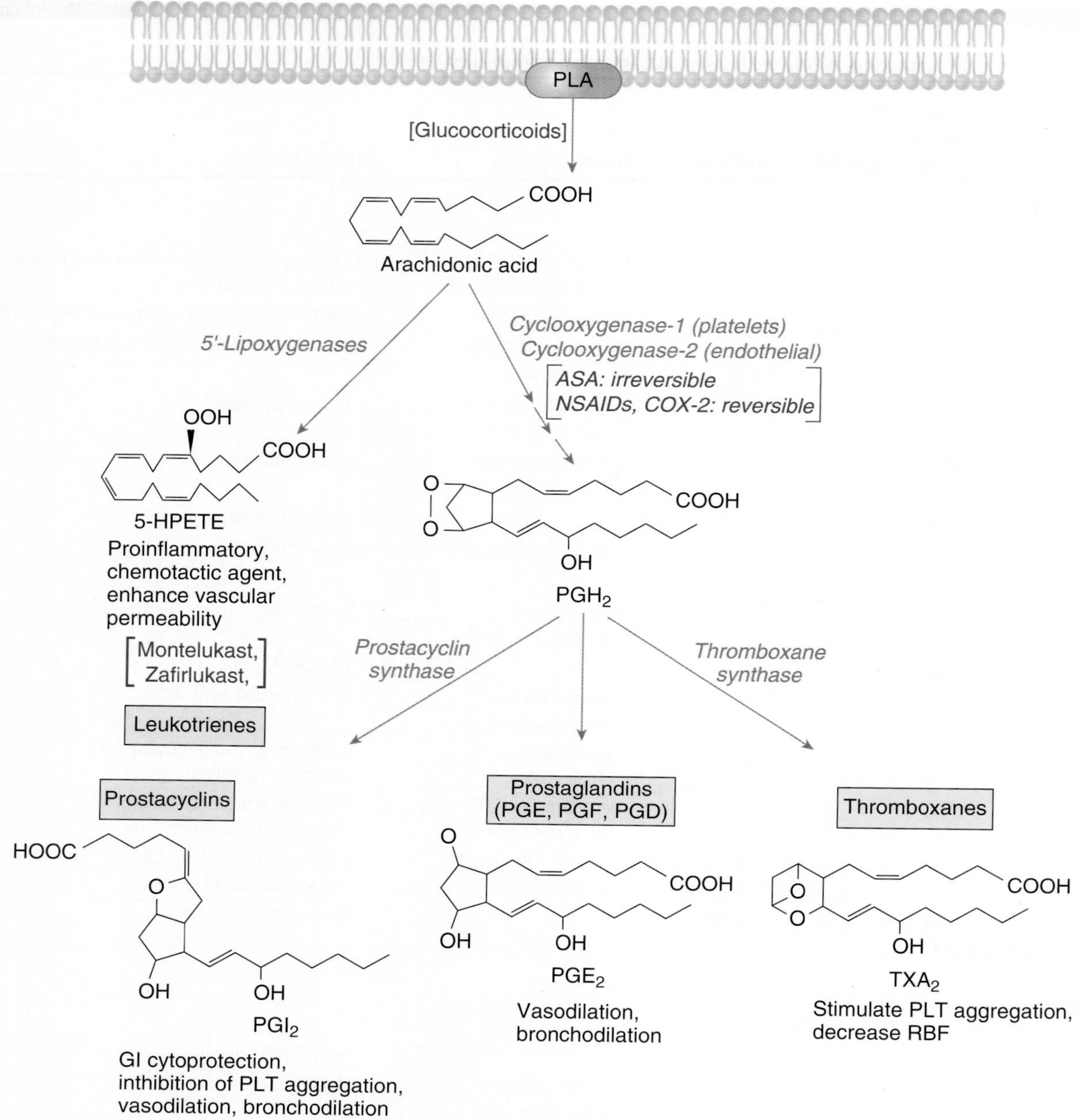

FIGURE 36–1. Arachidonic acid (AA) metabolism. This figure also illustrates some of the major differences between cyclooxygenase-1 (COX-1) and cyclooxygenase-2 (COX-2). Phospholipase A is stimulated by physical, chemical, inflammatory, and mitogenic stimuli and releases AA from cell membranes. The COX-1 enzyme synthesizes prostaglandins (PGs) that maintain cellular and vascular homeostasis. The COX-2 enzyme produces PGs within activated macrophages and endothelial cells that accompany inflammation. Whereas nonsteroidal antiinflammatory drugs reversibly inhibit both COX isoforms, selective COX-2 inhibitors inhibit the COX-2 isoform. Some authors suggest that inhibiting the COX enzymes shunts AA metabolism toward the production of chemotactic-vasoactive leukotrienes. Glucocorticoids inhibit PLA and downregulate induced expression of COX-2. 5-HPETE, hydroperoxy eicosatetraenoic acid; PLA, phospholipase A; PGI_2, prostacyclin; PGE_2, prostaglandin E_2; PLT, platelet; RBF, renal blood flow; TXA_2, thromboxane.

not cross the blood–brain barrier well.[3,56] Ketorolac and diclofenac have topical activity and are used in ophthalmologic solutions.[17]

Serum half-lives with therapeutic dosing vary from as short as 1 to 2 hours for diclofenac and ibuprofen to 50 to 60 hours for oxaprozin and piroxicam (see Table 36–1). Most NSAIDS undergo hepatic metabolism with renal excretion of metabolites. Whereas diclofenac undergoes extensive first-pass metabolism, 10% to 20% of indomethacin and ketorolac are excreted unchanged in the urine. Variable amounts of NSAIDs are recovered in the feces.[17]

The kinetics of NSAIDs may change in overdose, depending on the particular xenobiotic. Therapeutic and supratherapeutic doses of naproxen (250 mg–4 g) result in the same half-life and time to peak plasma concentration, but the clearance and volume of distribution increase proportionately.[67,78] When plasma protein binding of naproxen becomes saturated, the free drug concentration increases more rapidly than the total drug concentration, resulting in increased urinary excretion.[78] Overdoses of ibuprofen do not appear to prolong its elimination half-life.[36,57,101]

PATHOPHYSIOLOGY

GI toxicity is the most common adverse effect from NSAID use (Table 36–2). Normally, the COX-1 enzyme expressed in the gastric epithelial cells leads to the production of PGs (PGE_2 and PGI_2), which are responsible for maintaining GI mucosal integrity by increasing mucous production and decreasing acid production. NSAIDs not only inhibit the production of these cytoprotective PGs and platelet aggregatory TXA_2 but also have a direct cytotoxic effect, increasing the risk of gastric and duodenal ulcers, perforations, and hemorrhage.[24,70,75] Esophageal and small intestinal ulcers and strictures are also associated with NSAID use. Small intestinal diaphragms (or webs) are concentric web-like septa arising from submucosal fibrosis that can eventually cause a small bowel obstruction. These diaphragms rarely occur but are considered pathognomonic for NSAID use.[24]

Selective COX-2 inhibitors to decreased the incidence of significant GI toxicity compared with some nonselective NSAIDs, a benefit that is lost in patients concomitantly taking warfarin or low-dose aspirin.[4,12,31,98] Although *Helicobacter pylori* and NSAID use both individually increase the risk of gastroduodenal ulcers, there are conflicting data regarding the relationship between the two, given the wide array of study designs, individual responses to infection and treatments, and different gastric acid suppressants. Current evidence suggests that eradicating *H. pylori* before initiating NSAID therapy in NSAID-naïve patients may decrease this risk.[10,19,24,75]

Locally, the kidney produces homeostatic PGs largely via COX-1, including PGI_2, PGE_2, and PGD_2, which cause renal vasodilation and maintain renal blood flow and function.[31,99] Patients with volume contraction (dehydration) or poor cardiac output (congestive heart failure) have elevated concentrations of renal vasoconstrictor substances from stimulation of both the renin–angiotensin–aldosterone axis and the sympathetic nervous system. In these patients, NSAIDs inhibit the synthesis of the compensatory vasodilatory PGs, resulting in unopposed renal vasoconstriction and causing decreased renal blood flow and glomerular filtration rate (GFR). This effect may lead to medullary ischemia and possibly acute renal failure, particularly in elderly individuals.[72] This vasoconstrictive effect appears to be reversible upon discontinuation of therapy. This same effect is associated with COX-2 selective inhibitors.[63,72,99]

Some PGs mediate natriuretic and diuretic effects by maintaining adequate GFR by renal vasodilation, inhibiting sodium chloride absorption, and antagonizing the action of antidiuretic hormone (vasopressin). In addition to opposing homeostatic renal vasodilation, NSAIDs also augment sodium reabsorption, blunting the antihypertensive effect of thiazide and loop diuretics. NSAIDs also decrease renin synthesis, a mechanism shared by beta-adrenergic antagonists, rendering this antihypertensive therapy less effective.[99]

Normal platelet function depends partly on endothelial-derived PGI_2 (largely via COX-1), which blocks platelet activation and causes vasodilation, allowing blood to flow freely within vessels. At the site of vascular injury, platelets are activated by binding to collagen-bound von Willebrand factor and synthesize and release TXA_2, a potent platelet stimulator and vasoconstrictor. The antiplatelet activity of NSAIDs stems from their ability to inhibit COX-1 which is necessary for platelet-stimulating TXA_2 synthesis. Some in vitro evidence suggests that PGI_2 synthesis is largely dependent on COX-2.[16] Inhibiting the antiaggregatory PGI_2 may counter the antiplatelet effect, creating a prothrombotic environment. This is the predominant theory of how selective COX-2 inhibitors increase the risk of adverse cardiovascular events (see below for further discussion).[79]

PGs play a major role during the initiation of parturition. Exogenous administration of $PGF_{2\alpha}$ and PGE_2 has been used to induce uterine activity, and indomethacin has been used successfully as a tocolytic agent blunting PG-mediated uterine stimulation. However, a major clinical drawback in using NSAIDs as a tocolytic agent is the potential to cause premature constriction or closure of the ductus arteriosus in utero. Vasodilatory PGs are required to keep the fetal ductus arteriosus open and patent, and inhibiting these PGs has been shown to cause fetal ductal constriction, leading to pulmonary hypertension and persistent fetal circulation after birth.[61]

TABLE 36–2. Selected Adverse Effects of Nonsteroidal Antiinflammatory Drugs

Gastrointestinal
Chronic: dyspepsia, ulceration, perforation, hemorrhage, elevated hepatic aminotransferases, hepatocellular injury (rare)
Acute: same as above
Renal
Chronic: acute renal failure, fluid and electrolyte retention, hyperkalemia, interstitial nephritis, nephrotic syndrome, papillary necrosis, azotemia
Acute: same as above
Hypersensitivity or Pulmonary
Chronic: angioedema, drug-induced lupus
Acute: asthma exacerbation, anaphylactoid and anaphylactic reactions, urticaria, angioedema, acute lung injury, drug-induced lupus
Hematologic
Chronic: increased bleeding time, agranulocytosis, aplastic anemia, thrombocytopenia, neutropenia, hemolytic anemia
Acute: same as above
Central Nervous System
Chronic: headache, dizziness, lethargy, coma, aseptic meningitis, delirium, cognitive dysfunction, hallucinations, psychosis
Acute: same as above
Drug Interactions
Aminoglycosides: increased risk of aminoglycoside toxicity[80]
Anticoagulants (eg, warfarin): increased risk of GI bleeding[11,79]
Antihypertensives (especially diuretics, β-adrenergic antagonists, and ACE inhibitors): reduced antihypertensive effects[99]
Digoxin: increased risk of digoxin toxicity[89]
Ethanol: increased bleeding time[79]
Lithium: increased risk of lithium toxicity[69]
Methotrexate: increased risk of methotrexate toxicity[69]
Sulfonylureas: increased hypoglycemic effect[87]

CARDIOVASCULAR RISK OF SELECTIVE CYCLOOXYGENASE-2 INHIBITORS AND NONSELECTIVE NSAIDs

Atherosclerosis is a dynamic process of thrombus formation and inflammation involving numerous tissue factors and inflammatory mediators.[32] Given the ability to inhibit synthesis of proinflammatory PGs, selective COX-2 inhibitors would be expected to be antithrombotic; however, their ability to inhibit endothelial-derived PGI_2 combined with their relative inability to inhibit platelet-activating TXA_2 (a predominantly COX-1 effect) may shift the balance toward thrombus formation.[62]

In 2000, the Vioxx Gastrointestinal Outcomes Research (VIGOR) study reported a slightly higher incidence of myocardial infarction in patients taking rofecoxib compared with those taking naproxen (0.4% vs. 0.1%). This was thought to be because of a substantial number of patients who were not taking daily aspirin but should have been (based on FDA criteria) and that naproxen may have had a cardioprotective effect.[12,58,62]

In 2004, Merck pharmaceutical company withdrew rofecoxib from the worldwide market given the prepublication results of a study demonstrating an undisputed elevated cardiovascular risk.[14] Results from a meta-analysis[44] spawned controversy within the medical literature regarding the extent of delay before the withdrawal of rofecoxib from the market.[27,42,48,91] Several other studies addressing selective COX-2 inhibitors have shown similar results of increased risk of adverse cardiovascular events, suggesting this to be a class effect.[27,68,86] Valdecoxib has subsequently been removed from the market, leaving celecoxib as the only selective COX-2 inhibitor available; however, it carries a U.S. FDA alert on a possible increased cardiovascular risk.[86]

The data on nonselective NSAID use and cardiovascular risk remain controversial. Many of the currently published studies and meta-analyses use large databases and are unable to exclude significant confounding factors, including smoking, body mass index, chronic disease, concurrent aspirin use, and socioeconomic status.[96] Some of the nonselective NSAIDs that show a trend toward elevated cardiovascular risk include diclofenac, meloxicam, indomethacin, and (to a lesser extent) ibuprofen.[34,58,81,96] In 2005, the U.S. FDA asked manufacturers of all nonprescription NSAIDs to revise their package inserts to provide more information on the potential cardiovascular risks pending further investigation.

CLINICAL MANIFESTATIONS OF TOXICITY

NSAIDs are a heterogeneous class of drugs, some carrying a unique toxicity profile or effect. Fortunately, most nonselective NSAIDs behave similarly in overdose, although much of the medical literature specifically describes ibuprofen. Regardless of the particular NSAID ingested, symptoms, if they develop, typically manifest within 4 hours after ingestion.[36,37,38,53,57,95,100]

Initial clinical manifestations are usually mild and predominantly include GI symptoms such as nausea, vomiting, abdominal pain, or neurologic symptoms such as drowsiness, headache, tinnitus, blurred vision, diplopia, and dizziness. More moderate and severe findings are rare and include coma, seizures, central nervous system (CNS) depression, metabolic acidosis, hypotension, hypothermia, rhabdomyolysis, electrolyte imbalances, cardiac dysrhythmias, and acute oliguric renal failure.[20,36,37,53,57,60,76,95] Massive NSAID ingestions may lead to multisystem organ failure and death.[22,41,84,93,101]

NEUROLOGIC EFFECTS

The neurologic effects of NSAID use vary from the mild drowsiness, headache, and dizziness with therapeutic dosing to the more life-threatening CNS depression, coma, and seizures in overdose. The mechanism associated with the depressed level of consciousness is unknown; however, several animal studies suggest a relationship with opioid receptors, and a human case report documents a dramatic return of consciousness in a child after IV administration of high-dose naloxone.[28] Other miscellaneous neurologic manifestations reported include optic neuritis, toxic amblyopia, color blindness, transient diplopia, other visual disturbances, transient loss of hearing, acute psychosis, and cognitive dysfunction.[39,54,69]

Drug-induced aseptic meningitis has been reported with several NSAIDs, including tolmetin, rofecoxib, naproxen, sulindac, piroxicam, and diclofenac, but ibuprofen is more commonly implicated perhaps because of its widespread use.[66] Clinical findings include fever and chills, headache, meningeal signs, nausea, vomiting, and altered mental status, as well as CSF pleocytosis, elevated protein, and normal glucose.[66] Recent studies suggest an immunologic mechanism because NSAID-induced aseptic meningitis appears to be more common in patients with systemic lupus erythematosus or mixed connective tissue disease.[39,66,69]

Muscle twitching and generalized tonic-clonic seizures are described with mefenamic acid overdose and usually occur within 7 hours after ingestion.[2] Seizures are also associated with ibuprofen overdose.[71] The specific mechanism for NSAID-induced seizures is unknown.

RENAL AND ELECTROLYTE EFFECTS

Both acute overdose and chronic therapeutic dosing of NSAIDs may have deleterious effects of renal function, most of which are reversible but in rare cases permanent. These include sodium retention and edema, hyperkalemia, acute renal failure, membranous nephropathy, nephrotic syndrome, interstitial nephritis, and both acute and chronic renal papillary necrosis.[39,74,99] General risk factors for NSAID-induced renal dysfunction include congestive heart failure, volume depletion, diabetes mellitus, underlying renal disease, systemic lupus erythematosus, cirrhosis, diuretic therapy, and advanced age.[55]

Acute tubulointerstitial nephritis (ATIN) is one of the more common forms of NSAID-induced renal impairment, and it may occur with short-term therapeutic dosing.[25,55] Many cases of ATIN probably go undiagnosed because clinical symptoms usually do not appear until significant renal impairment occurs.[25,77] Significant elevations in blood urea nitrogen (azotemia) may occur in elderly patients within 5 to 7 days of initiating NSAID therapy but return to baseline within 2 weeks of discontinuation.[35]

Analgesic abuse nephropathy is a condition whose pathogenesis is not well defined, but it develops from excessive, chronic therapeutic consumption of NSAIDs. This results in acute renal failure manifested by renal papillary necrosis, often requiring hemodialysis.[82,99] Analgesic abuse nephropathy was originally described with the use of analgesic combinations including phenacetin and aspirin in addition to caffeine and has decreased in prevalence after the removal of phenacetin from many world markets.

Anion gap metabolic acidosis, with and without acute renal failure, complicates many acute, massive ibuprofen ingestions and may be profound.[26,41,52,73,101,102] The cause of the acidosis in this setting is most likely multifactorial, involving elevated lactate concentrations from profound hypotension and tissue hypoperfusion, as well as the accumulation of ibuprofen and its two major metabolites, all weak acids.[53] An elevated anion gap metabolic acidosis with elevated lactate concentrations is also described after naproxen overdose, suggesting this to be a class effect given that all NSAIDs are acid derivatives.[13]

Use of NSAIDs by pregnant women is associated with reversible oligohydramnios and is used therapeutically as a treatment modality for polyhydramnios. Decreased fetal urine output and neonatal acute and chronic renal failure, including transient oligoanuria, have been associated with gestational NSAID use, commonly indomethacin.[5,30,45]

GASTROINTESTINAL EFFECTS

Numerous studies have reported an increased risk in serious, adverse GI effects with therapeutic use of NSAIDs.[33,50,70] The relative risk of developing gastroduodenal perforation, ulcer, or hemorrhage during chronic NSAID therapy ranges from 2.7 to 5.4, with ketorolac posing the greatest risk.[70,92] Acute NSAID overdoses are reported to cause bloody emesis,[100] fecal occult blood,[20]; and severe, life-threatening GI hemorrhage.[52]

NSAID-induced hepatotoxicity is a well known adverse effect that has prompted the removal of several NSAIDs from the market. Hepatotoxicity occurs with an incidence less than 0.1% and can be quite difficult to diagnose because many patients on chronic NSAID therapy have underlying conditions, such as systemic lupus or rheumatoid arthritis, which may cause hepatotoxicity. NSAID-induced hepatotoxicity is an idiosyncratic reaction primarily causing hepatocellular injury and does not depend on the chemical class. Diclofenac and sulindac are most commonly implicated.[90]

IMMUNOLOGIC AND DERMATOLOGIC EFFECTS

The non-immunologic anaphylactoid and IgE-mediated anaphylactic reactions that are reported with the use of NSAIDs are clinically indistinguishable from one another, producing flushing, urticaria, bronchospasm, edema, and hypotension.[7] Evidence for anaphylactic reactions includes the presence of NSAID-specific IgE antibodies, positive wheal-and-flare skin reactions, and lack of cross-reactivity with oral challenges of aspirin and other NSAIDs.[7] The proposed mechanism of NSAID-induced anaphylactoid reactions involves the inhibition of COX-1, which not only inhibits the production of PGE_2 (which causes bronchodilation and inhibits the release of histamine from mast cells and basophils) but also shunts the AA metabolism to increased production of bronchoconstricting LTs.

The term *aspirin-sensitive asthmatic* is a bit of a misnomer because it refers to anaphylactoid reactions that may occur with any COX-1 inhibiting NSAID, not only aspirin.[7,88] Selective COX-2 inhibitors cause similar clinical reactions but with an unclear mechanism. There appears to be very little cross-reactivity between NSAIDs and selective COX-2 inhibitors, and reports of reactions to one COX-2 inhibitor and not another suggest a predominant IgE-mediated mechanism.[7,47,88]

The most common skin reactions include angioedema and facial swelling, urticaria and pruritus, bullous eruptions, and photosensitivity.[39] Although rare, toxic epidermal necrolysis and Stevens-Johnson syndrome have been reported.[39]

HEMATOLOGIC EFFECTS

As a class, NSAIDs are frequently implicated as a cause of thrombocytopenia and are reported to have caused adverse effects on most other cell lines and function, including agranulocytosis, aplastic anemia, hemolytic anemia, methemoglobinemia, neutropenia, and pancytopenia.[23,39,46,65,94] Specifically, phenylbutazone in chronic, therapeutic doses is associated with agranulocytosis and aplastic anemia,[84] prompting its removal from the U.S. market in the 1970s. The inhibitory effect of NSAIDs on granulocyte adherence, activation, and phagocytosis has been suggested as the mechanism responsible for the association between NSAID use and necrotizing fasciitis, causing a delay in the onset of symptoms.[40]

The ability of a particular type of NSAID to inhibit platelet aggregation and affect bleeding time depends on the dose and half-life because NSAIDs reversibly inhibit COX. One dose of ibuprofen prolongs the bleeding time within 2 hours and persists for up to 12 hours; however, this increase in bleeding time usually remains within the upper limit of normal range. This is in contrast to aspirin, which irreversibly inhibits COX, and typically doubles the bleeding time within 12 hours, returning to normal within 24 to 48 hours.[79] Compared with placebo, flurbiprofen and indobufen have been shown to clinically inhibit platelet function, thereby decreasing vascular reocclusion after angioplasty and preventing thromboembolic complications.[9,15] The concern for ketorolac to potentiate postoperative bleeding remains controversial, but many studies support its safety and efficacy.[1,21]

Furthermore, NSAID use may potentiate bleeding risk in patients already at higher risk. These patients include those with thrombocytopenia, coagulation factor deficiencies, or von Willebrand disease and those ingesting alcohol or on warfarin therapy.[79]

CARDIOVASCULAR EFFECTS

Although no evidence supports a direct cardiotoxic effect of NSAIDs or their metabolites, acute and massive NSAID overdoses may be complicated by persistent, severe hypotension; myocardial ischemia; and cardiac conduction abnormalities and dysrhythmias, including bradycardia, ventricular tachycardia or fibrillation, and prolonged QT interval.[26,41,76,83,101] The cause of these findings is yet to be elucidated, although these effects are reported only in severely ill patients with acid–base abnormalities and multisystem organ involvement (see Cardiovascular Risk above).

PULMONARY EFFECTS

Although there is no evidence of direct pulmonary toxicity, some case reports describe the development of acute lung injury with[51,60] and without[26,41] hypoxia. Because this is described with salicylate toxicity, it may be mechanism based. Although chest radiographic findings such as bilateral pulmonary infiltrates appear to resolve rapidly, one study reported persistent clinical abnormalities associated with exertional dyspnea 1 month later (see Immunologic Effects above).[60]

DIAGNOSTIC TESTING

Serum concentrations of most NSAIDs can be determined but usually only by a specialty laboratory requiring several days to report results. Although ibuprofen nomograms were constructed in an attempt to correlate serum concentrations with clinical toxicity,[36,43] the utility of these nomograms proved limited because serum concentrations do not reliably correlate with clinical toxicity.[38,57,83]

Laboratory measurements, including complete blood count, serum electrolytes, blood urea nitrogen, and creatinine should be obtained for all symptomatic patients, patients with intentional ingestion, ibuprofen ingestion of greater than 400 mg/kg in a child, or ibuprofen ingestion of greater than 6 g in an adult.[38] For patients presenting with significant neurologic effects, such as CNS depression, further evaluation of acid–base and ventilatory status by blood gas, hepatic aminotransferases, and prothrombin time should be obtained. Additionally, one must always be cognizant of other potential medical and infectious causes (eg, encephalitis and meningitis) and consider the utility of a lumbar puncture. An acetaminophen concentration should always be determined in patients with intentional ingestions and in patients presenting with an unclear history because many people mistake acetaminophen for NSAIDs because of confusing labeling and packaging or unawareness that they are completely different types of analgesics. For similar reasons, one may also consider obtaining a salicylate concentration.

MANAGEMENT

Management of a patient with an NSAID overdose is largely supportive and guided by the clinical signs and symptoms. Most asymptomatic patients with intentional overdose and those with normal vital signs require observation for 4 to 6 hours and a serum acetaminophen concentration before being medically cleared. Children with ibuprofen ingestions of less than 100 mg/kg can be observed at home, but those who ingest greater than 400 mg/kg are at high risk for toxicity and require medical evaluation.[38] GI decontamination with activated charcoal (AC) should be considered for an asymptomatic patient with the potential for a large ingestion, symptomatic patients, and children with a history of ibuprofen ingestion greater than 400 mg/kg.[38,49] Serum concentrations of ibuprofen have been demonstrated to increase after the time of emergency department arrival,[101] so gastric lavage for massive overdose followed by AC should be considered. Multiple-dose AC may be useful for patients with massive overdoses of sustained-release preparations.[101]

Patients who develop severe, life-threatening manifestations usually present with lethargy or unresponsiveness.[26,41,60,71,83,101] Aggressive, supportive care is indicated in these patients, including stabilization of the airway and intravenous (IV) fluid therapy. An early electrocardiogram is essential to detect any significant electrolyte abnormalities or conduction disturbances. Electrolyte imbalances should be corrected and sodium bicarbonate therapy considered for severe metabolic acidosis. Hypotension should be treated initially with IV fluid therapy followed by direct-acting vasopressors if necessary. Electrocardiograms should be monitored for the development of any life-threatening electrolyte imbalances or cardiac conduction abnormalities.

Given their high protein binding, NSAIDs do not appear to be amenable to extracorporeal removal methods; however, in cases of persistent metabolic acidosis or renal failure, hemodialysis or continuous renal replacement therapies may be useful to correct the acid–base status.[6,51] Patients with seizures, which are characteristic of mefenamic acid overdose,[2] should be treated with IV benzodiazepines. Phenylbutazone overdose, in particular, carries a high morbidity and mortality rate and requires early and aggressive treatment.[22,65]

The most common adverse effect of therapeutic NSAID use is dyspepsia, and the most serious GI effect is ulcer formation, which has the potential for perforation and hemorrhage. Most patients with dyspepsia do not have ulcers.[24] To help prevent the development of ulcers, concomitant use of misoprostol (a PGE_1 analog), an H_2-blocker, or a proton pump inhibitor (PPI) is often used; however, PPIs may be superior for both preventing and healing gastroduodenal ulcers resulting from chronic NSAID therapy.[75]

SUMMARY

NSAIDs are among the most commonly used drugs in the world. Each NSAID is unique in its chemical structure, but they all share the ability, among other properties, of inhibiting COX-1. Most NSAID overdoses produce nonspecific symptoms, including nausea and abdominal discomfort, requiring very little management, if any. Although the management of patients with larger ingestions involves administration of AC and general supportive care, all patients with intentional NSAID overdoses require the exclusion of acetaminophen coingestion. Massive ingestions may cause life-threatening complications, including coma, metabolic acidosis, renal failure, GI hemorrhage, seizures, and cardiovascular collapse. In these rare cases, therapy depends on hemodynamic monitoring, appropriate resuscitation, and supportive care.

ACKNOWLEDGMENT

Martin G. Belson, MD and William A. Watson, PharmD contributed to this chapter in previous editions.

REFERENCES

1. Agrawal A, Gerson CR, Seligman I, Dsida RM. Postoperative hemorrhage after tonsillectomy: use of ketorolac tromethamine. *Otolaryngol Head Neck Surg*. 1999;120:335-339.
2. Balali-Mood M, Proudfoot AT, Critchley J, et al. Mefenamic acid overdosage. *Lancet*. 1981;2:1324-1356.
3. Bannwarth B, Netter P, Pourel J, et al. Clinical pharmacokinetics of nonsteroidal anti-inflammatory drugs in the cerebrospinal fluid. *Biomed Pharmacother*. 1989;43:121-126.
4. Battistella M, Mamdami MM, Juurlink DN, et al. Risk of upper gastrointestinal hemorrhage in warfarin users treated with nonselective NSAIDs or COX-2 inhibitors. *Arch Intern Med*. 2005;165:189-192.
5. Benini D, Fanos V, Cuzzolin L, Tato L. In utero exposure to nonsteroidal anti-inflammatory drugs: neonatal renal failure. *Pediatr Nephrol*. 2004;19:232-234.
6. Bennett RR, Dunkelberg JC, Marks ES. Acute oliguric renal failure due to ibuprofen overdose. *S Med J*. 1985;78:491-492.
7. Berkes EA. Anaphylactic and anaphylactoid reactions to aspirin and other NSAIDs. *Clin Rev Allergy Immunol*. 2003;24:137-148.
8. Bernareggi A. Clinical pharmacokinetics of nimesulide. *Clin Pharmacokinet*. 1998;35:247-274.
9. Bhana N, McClellan. Indobufen: an updated review of its use in the management of atherothrombosis. *Drugs and Aging* 2001;18:369-388.
10. Bjorkman DJ. Current status of nonsteroidal anti-inflammatory drug (NSAID) use in the United States: risk factors and frequency of complications. *Am J Med*. 1999;107:3S-10S.
11. Bjorkman DJ. The effect of aspirin and nonsteroidal anti-inflammatory drugs on prostaglandins. *Am J Med*. 1998;105:8S-12S.
12. Bombardier C, Laine L, Reicin A, et al. Comparison of upper gastrointestinal toxicity of rofecoxib and naproxen in patients with rheumatoid arthritis. *N Engl J Med*. 2000;343:1520-1528.
13. Bortone E, Bettoni L, Buzio S, et al. Triphasic waves associated with acute naproxen overdose: a case report. *Clin Electroencephalogr*. 1998;29:142-145.
14. Bresalier RS, Sandler RS, Quan H. Cardiovascular events associated with rofecoxib in a colorectal adenoma chemoprevention trial. *N Engl J Med*. 2005;352:1092-1102.
15. Brochier ML. Evaluation of flurbiprofen for prevention of reinfarction and reocclusion after successful thrombolysis or angioplasty in acute myocardial infarction. *Eur Heart J*. 1993;14:951-957.
16. Brock TG, McNish RW, Peters-Golden M. Arachidonic acid is preferentially metabolized by cyclooxygenase-2 to prostacyclin and prostaglandin E2. *J Biol Chem*. 1999;274:11660-11666.
17. Burke A, Smyth E, FitzGerald GA. Analgesic-antipyretic agents; pharmacotherapy of gout. In: Brunton LL, Lazo JS, Parker KL, eds. *Goodman and Gilman's the Pharmacologic Basis of Therapeutics*, 11th ed. New York: McGraw-Hill; 2006:671-715.
18. Capone ML, Tacconelli S, Sciulli MG, et al. Clinical pharmacology of platelet, monocyte, and vascular cyclooxygenase inhibition by naproxen and low-dose aspirin in healthy subjects. *Circulation*. 2004;109:1468-1471.
19. Chan FL. NSAID-induced peptic ulcers and Helicobacter pylori infection. *Drug Saf*. 2005;28:287-300.
20. Chelluri L, Jastremski MS. Coma caused by ibuprofen overdose. *Crit Care Med*. 1986;14:1078-1079.
21. Chin KR, Sundram H, Marcotte P. Bleeding risk with ketorolac after lumbar microdiscectomy. *J Spinal Disord Tech*. 2007;20:123-126.
22. Court H, Volans G. Poisoning after overdose with nonsteroidal antiinflammatory drugs. *Adverse Drug React Acute Poisoning Rev*. 1984;3:1-21.
23. Cramer RL, Aboko-Cole VC, Gualtieri RJ. Agranulocytosis associated with etodolac. *Ann Pharmacother*. 1994;28:428-460.
24. Cryer B, Kimmey MB. Gastrointestinal side effects of nonsteroidal anti-inflammatory drugs. *Am J Med*. 1998;105:20S-30S.
25. Dixit MP, Nguyen C, Carson T, et al. Non-steroidal anti-inflammatory drugs-associated acute interstitial nephritis with granular tubular basement membrane deposits. *Pediatr Nephrol*. 2008;23:145-148.
26. Downie A, Ali A, Bell D. Severe metabolic acidosis complicating massive ibuprofen overdose. *Postgrad Med J*. 1993;69:575-577.
27. Drazen JM. COX-2 inhibitors—a lesson in unexpected problems. *N Engl J Med*. 352;11:1131-1132.
28. Easley RB, Altemeier WA. Central nervous system manifestations of an ibuprofen overdose reversed by naloxone. *Ped Emerg Care*. 2000;16:39-41.
29. Edlund A, Berglund B, van Dorne D, et al. Coronary flow regulation in patients with ischemic heart disease: release of purines and prostacyclin and the effect of inhibitors of prostaglandin formation. *Circulation*. 1985;71:1113-1120.
30. Fieni S, Gramellini D, Vadora E. Oligohydramnios and fetal renal sonographic appearances related to prostaglandin synthetase inhibitors. *Fetal Diagn Ther*. 2004;19:224-227.
31. FitzGerald GA, Patrono C. The coxibs, selective inhibitors of cyclooxygenase-2. *N Engl J Med*. 2001;345:433-442.

32. Furie B, Furie BC. Mechanisms of thrombus formation. *N Engl J Med.* 2008;359:938-949.
33. Gabriel SE, Jaakkimainen L, Bombardier C. Risk for serious gastrointestinal complications related to use of nonsteroidal anti-inflammatory drugs. *Ann Intern Med.* 1991;115:787-796.
34. Graham DJ. COX-2 inhibitors, other NSAIDs, and cardiovascular risk: the seduction of common sense. *JAMA.* 2006;296:1653-1656.
35. Gurwitz JH, Avorn J, Ross-Degnan D, Lipsitz LA. Nonsteroidal anti- inflammatory drug-associated azotemia in the very old. *JAMA.* 1990;264:471-475.
36. Hall AH, Smolinske SC, Conrad FL, et al. Ibuprofen overdose: 126 cases. *Ann Emerg Med.* 1986;15:1308-1313.
37. Hall AH, Smolinske SC, Kulig KW, et al. Ibuprofen overdose: a prospective study. *West J Med.* 1988;48:653-656.
38. Hall AH, Smolinske SC, Stover B, et al. Ibuprofen overdose in adults. *J Toxicol Clin Toxicol.* 1992;30:23-37.
39. Halpern SM, Fitzpatrick R, Volans GN. Ibuprofen toxicity. A review of adverse reactions and overdose. *Adverse Drug React Toxicol Rev.* 1993;12:107-128.
40. Holder EP, Moore PT, Brown BA. Nonsteroidal anti-inflammatory drugs and necrotising fasciitis: an update. *Drug Saf.* 1997;17:369-373.
41. Holubek W, Stolbach A, Nurok S, et al. A report of two deaths from massive ibuprofen ingestion. *J Med Toxicol.* 2007;3:52-55.
42. Horton R. Vioxx, the implosion of Merck, and the aftershocks at the FDA. *Lancet.* 2004;364:1995-1996.
43. Jenkinson ML, Fitzpatrick R, Streete PJ, Volans GN. The relationship between plasma ibuprofen concentrations and toxicity in acute ibuprofen overdose. *Hum Toxicol.* 1988;7:319-324.
44. Juni P, Nartey L, Reichenbach S. Risk of cardiovascular events and rofecoxib: cumulative meta-analysis. *Lancet.* 2004;364:2021-2029.
45. Kaplan BS, Restaino I, Raval DS, et al. Renal failure in the neonate associated with in utero exposure to nonsteroidal antiinflammatory agents. *Pediatr Nephrol.* 1994;8:700-704.
46. Kaushik P, Zuckerman SJ, Campo NJ, et al. Celecoxib-induced methemoglobinemia. *Ann Pharmacother.* 2004;38:1635-1638.
47. Kelkar PS, Butterfield JH, Teaford HG. Urticaria and angioedema from cyclooxygenase-2 inhibitors. *J Rheumatol.* 2001;28:2553-2554.
48. Kim PS, Reicin AS, Lievre M, et al. Discontinuation of Vioxx: authors' reply. *Lancet.* 2005;365:23-28.
49. Lapatto-Reiniluoto O, Divisto KT, Neuvonen PJ. Effect of activated charcoal alone or given after gastric lavage in reducing the absorption of diazepam, ibuprofen and citalopram. *Br J Clin Pharmacol.* 1999;48:148-153.
50. Laporte JR, Ibanez L, Vidal X, et al. Upper gastrointestinal bleeding associated with the use of NSAIDs. *Drug Saf.* 2004;27:411-420.
51. Le HT, Bosse GM, Tsai Y. Ibuprofen overdose complicated by renal failure, adult respiratory distress syndrome, and metabolic acidosis. *Clin Toxicol.* 1994;32:315-320.
52. Lee CY, Finkler A. Acute intoxication due to ibuprofen overdose. *Arch Pathol Lab Med.* 1986;110:747-749.
53. Linden CH, Townsend PL. Metabolic acidosis after acute ibuprofen overdosage. *J Pediatr.* 1987;111:922-925.
54. Lund BC, Neiman RF. Visual disturbance associated with celecoxib. *Pharmacotherapy.* 2001;21:114-155.
55. Marasco WA, Gikas PW, Azziz-Baumgartner R, et al. Ibuprofen-associated renal dysfunction. *Arch Intern Med.* 1987;147:2107-2116.
56. Matoga M, Pehourcq F, Lagrange F, et al. Influence of molecular lipophilicity on the diffusion of arylpropionate non-steroidal anti-inflammatory drugs into the cerebrospinal fluid. *Arzneimittelforschung.* 1999;49:477-482.
57. McElwee NE, Veltri JC, Bradford DC, Rollins DE. A prospective, population-based study of acute ibuprofen overdose: complications are rare and routine serum levels not warranted. *Ann Emerg Med.* 1990;19:657-662.
58. McGettigan P, Henry D. Cardiovascular risk and inhibition of cyclooxygenase: a systematic review of the observational studies of selective and nonselective inhibitors of cyclooxygenase 2. *JAMA.* 2006;296:1633-1644.
59. Mehta A. Aspirin. *Chem Engin News.* 2005;83:1-5.
60. Menzies DG, Conn AG, Williamson IJ, Prescott LF. Fulminant hyperkalaemia and multiple complications following ibuprofen overdose. *Med Toxicol Adverse Drug Exp.* 1989;4:468-471.
61. Moise KJ, Huhta JC, Sharif DS, et al. Indomethacin in the treatment of premature labor: effects on the fetal ductus arteriosus. *N Engl J Med.* 1988;319:327-331.
62. Mukherjee D, Nissen SE, Topol EJ. Risk of cardiovascular events associated with selective COX-2 inhibitors. *JAMA.* 2001;286:954-959.
63. Murray MD, Brater DC. Adverse effects of nonsteroidal antiinflammatory drugs on renal function. *Ann Intern Med.* 1990;112:559-560.
64. Nelson L, Shih R, Hoffman R. Aplastic anemia induced by an adulterated herbal medication. *J Toxicol Clin Toxicol.* 1995;33:467-470.
65. Newton T, Rose R. Poisoning with equine phenylbutazone in a racetrack worker. *Ann Emerg Med.* 1991;20:204-207.
66. Nguyen HT, Juurlink DN. Recurrent ibuprofen-induced aseptic meningitis. *Ann Pharmacother.* 2004;38:408-410.
67. Niazi SK, Alam SM, Ahmad SI. Dose-dependent pharmacokinetics of naproxen in man. *Biopharm Drug Dispos.* 1996;17:355-361.
68. Nussmeier NA, Whelton AA, Brown MT, et al. Complications of the COX-2 inhibitors parecoxib and valdecoxib after cardiac surgery. *N Engl J Med.* 2005;352:1081-1091.
69. O'Brien WM, Bagby GF. Rare adverse reaction to nonsteroidal anti-inflammatory drugs. *J Rheumatol.* 1985;12:785-790.
70. Ofman JJ, Maclean CH, Straus WL, et al. A metaanalysis of severe upper gastrointestinal complications of nonsteroidal antiinflammatory drugs. *J Rheumatol.* 2002;29:804-812.
71. Oker EE, Hermann L, Baum CR, et al. Serious toxicity in a young child due to ibuprofen. *Acad Emerg Med.* 2000;7:821-823.
72. Perazella MA, Eras J. Are selective COX-2 inhibitors nephrotoxic? *Am J Kidney Dis.* 2000;35:937-940.
73. Primos W, Bhatnager A, Bishop P, Evans OB. Acute metabolic acidosis due to ibuprofen overdose. *J Miss State Med Assoc.* 1987;28:233-234.
74. Radford MG, Holley KE, Grande JP, et al. Reversible membranous nephropathy associated with the use of nonsteroidal anti-inflammatory drugs. *JAMA.* 1996;276:466-469.
75. Raskin JB. Gastrointestinal effects of nonsteroidal anti-inflammatory therapy. *Am J Med.* 1999;106:3S-12S.
76. Ritter A, Eskin B. Ibuprofen overdose presenting with severe agitation and hypothermia. *Am J Emerg Med.* 1998;16:549-550.
77. Rossert J. Drug-induced acute interstitial nephritis. *Kidney Int.* 2001;60: 804-817.
78. Runkel R, Chaplin M, Savelium H, et al. Pharmacokinetics of naproxen overdoses. *Clin Pharmacol Toxicol.* 1976;20:269-277.
79. Schafer AI. Effects of nonsteroidal anti-inflammatory therapy on platelets. *Am J Med.* 1999;106(5B):25S-36S.
80. Scott CS, Retsch-Bogart GZ, Henry MM. Renal failure and vestibular toxicity in an adolescent with cystic fibrosis receiving gentamicin and standard-dose ibuprofen. *Pediatr Pulmonol.* 2001;31:314-316.
81. Scott PA, Kingsely GH, Smith CM, et al. Non-steroidal anti-inflammatory drugs and myocardial infarctions: comparative systematic review of evidence from observational studies and randomized controlled trials. *Ann Rheum Dis.* 2007;66:1296-1304.
82. Segasothy M, Samad SA, Zulfigar A, Bennett WM. Chronic renal disease and papillary necrosis associated with the long-term use of nonsteroidal anti-inflammatory drugs as the sole or predominant analgesic. *Am J Kidney Dis.* 1994;24:17-24.
83. Seifert SA, Bronstein AC, McGuire T. Massive ibuprofen ingestion with survival. *Clin Toxicol.* 2000;38:55-57.
84. Smolinske S, Hall A, Vandenberg S, et al. Toxic effects of nonsteroidal antiinflammatory drugs in overdose. *Drug Saf.* 1990;5:252-274.
85. Smyth EM, Burke A, Fitzgerald GA. Lipid-derived autacoids: eicosanoids and platelet-activating factor. In: Brunton LL, Lazo JS, Parker KL, eds. *Goodman and Gilman's the Pharmacologic Basis of Therapeutics*, 11th ed. New York: McGraw-Hill; 2006:653-670.
86. Solomon SD, McMurray JV, Pfeffer MA, et al. Cardiovascular risk associated with celecoxib in a clinical trial for colorectal adenoma prevention. *N Engl J Med.* 2005;352:1071-1080.
87. Sone H, Takahashi A, Yamada N. Ibuprofen-related hypoglycemia in a patient receiving sulfonylurea. *Ann Intern Med.* 2001;134:344.
88. Stevenson DD. Anaphylactic and anaphylactoid reactions to aspirin and other nonsteroidal anti-inflammatory drugs. *Immunol Allergy Clin N Am.* 2001;21:745-768.
89. Stollberger C, Finsterer J. Nonsteroidal anti-inflammatory drugs in patients with cardio- or cerebrovascular disorders. *Z Kardiol.* 2003;92:721-729.
90. Tolman KG. Hepatotoxicity of non-narcotic analgesics. *Am J Med.* 1998;105:13S-19S.
91. Topol EJ. Failing the public health: rofecoxib, Merck and the FDA. *N Engl J Med.* 2004;351:1707-1708.
92. Traversa G, Walker AM, Ippolito FM, et al. Gastroduodenal toxicity of different nonsteroidal antiinflammatory drugs. *Epidemiology.* 1995;6:49-54.

93. Vale JA, Meredith TJ. Acute poisoning due to non-steroidal anti-inflammatory drugs: clinical features and management. *Med Toxicol.* 1986;1:12-31.
94. Van den Bemt P, Meyboom R, Egberts A. Drug-induced immune thrombocytopenia. *Drug Saf.* 2004;27:1243-1252.
95. Volans G, Monaghan J, Colbridge M. Ibuprofen overdose. *Int J Clin Pract Suppl.* 2003;135:54-60.
96. Waksman JC, Brody A, Phillips SD. Nonselective nonsteroidal antiinflammatory drugs and cardiovascular risk: are they safe? *Ann Pharmacother.* 2007;41:1163-1173.
97. Warner TD, Giuliano F, Vojnovic I, et al. Nonsteroid drug selectivities for cyclo-oxygenase-1 rather than cyclo-oxygenase-2 are associated with human gastrointestinal toxicity: a full in vitro analysis. *Proc Natl Acad Sci USA.* 1999;96:7563-7568.
98. Weideman RA, Kelly KC, Dazi S, et al. Risks of clinically significant upper gastrointestinal events with etodolac and naproxen: a historical cohort analysis. *Gastroenterology.* 2004;127:1322-1328.
99. Whelton A. Nephrotoxicity of nonsteroidal anti-inflammatory drugs: physiologic foundations and clinical implications. *Am J Med.* 1999;106: 13S-24S.
100. Wolfe TR. Ibuprofen overdose. *Am J Emerg Med.* 1995;13:375.
101. Wood DM, Monaghan J, Streete, et al. Fatality after deliberate ingestion of sustained-release ibuprofen: a case report. *Crit Care.* 2006;10:R44.
102. Zuckerman GB, Uy CC. Shock, metabolic acidosis, and coma following ibuprofen overdose in a child. *Ann Pharmacother.* 1995;29:869-871.

CHAPTER 37
COLCHICINE, PODOPHYLLIN AND THE VINCA ALKALOIDS

Joshua G. Schier

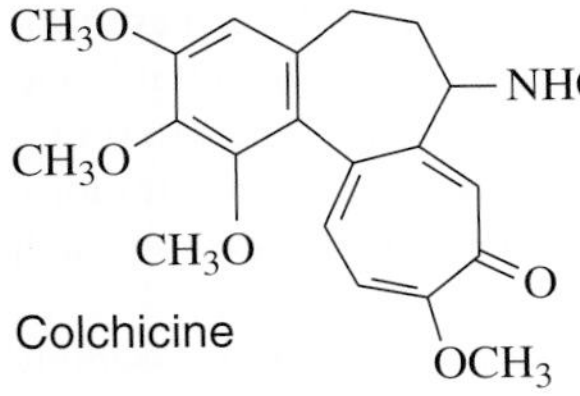

Colchicine

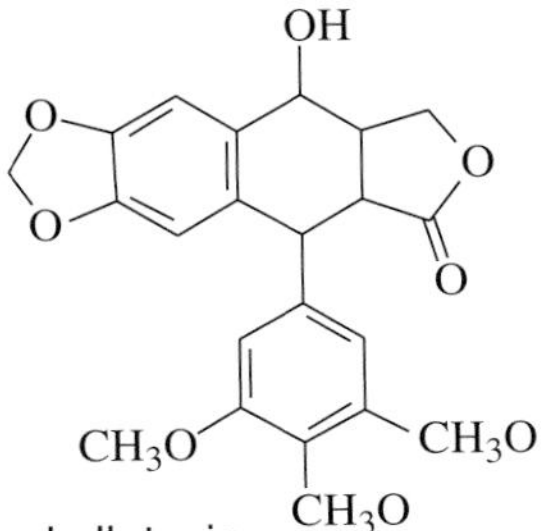

Podophyllotoxin

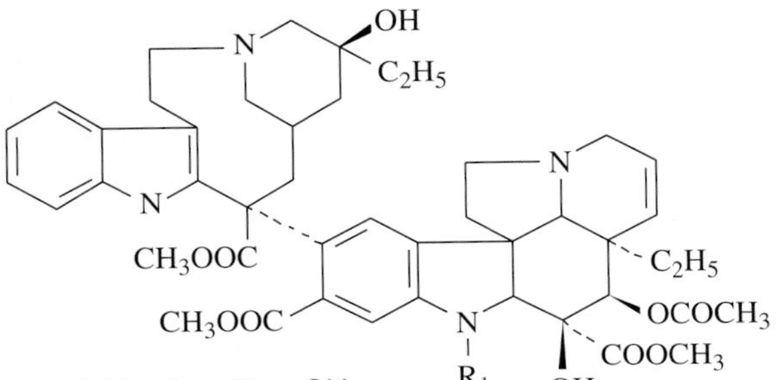

Vinblastine: $R_1 = CH_3$
Vincristine: $R_1 = CHO$

Colchicine, podophyllotoxin, and the vinca alkaloids exert their primary toxicity by binding to tubulin and interfering with microtubule structure and function. The ubiquitous nature of microtubules within human cells and the heavy reliance on them for maintenance of normal cell functions present numerous opportunities for these xenobiotics to cause dysfunction at a cellular, organ, and organ system level in a dose-dependent fashion.

COLCHICINE

HISTORY AND EPIDEMIOLOGY

The origins of colchicine and its history in poisoning can be traced back to Greek mythology. Medea was the evil daughter (and a known poisoner) of the king of Colchis, a country that lay east of the Black Sea in Asia Minor. After being betrayed by her husband Jason (of Jason and the Argonauts), she killed their children and her husband's lover. Medea often used plants of the Liliaceae family, of which *Colchicum autumnale* is a member, to poison her victims.[17,134,176] The use of colchicum for medicinal purposes is also reported in *Pedanius Dioscorides De Materia Medica*, an ancient medical text, written in the first century A.D.[17,134,176] and subsequently in the 6th century A.D. by Alexander of Trallis, who recommended it for arthritic conditions.[17,30,110,176] However, colchicum fell out of favor, perhaps because of its pronounced gastrointestinal (GI) effects, until it was introduced for dropsy and various other nonrheumatic conditions in 1763.[17,176] In the late 18th century, a colchicum-containing product known as *Eau Medicinale* appeared, which reportedly had strong anti-gout effects.[176] Colchicine, the active alkaloidal component in colchicum, was isolated in 1820 and rapidly became popular as an anti-gout medication.[134,176] Benjamin Franklin reportedly had gout and is credited with introducing colchicine in the United States.[134] Colchicine is still used in the treatment of gout and has been used in a multitude of other disorders, including amyloidosis, Behçet 's syndrome, familial Mediterranean fever, pericarditis, arthritis, pulmonary fibrosis, vasculitis, biliary cirrhosis, pseudogout, certain spondyloarthropathies, calcinosis, and scleroderma.[7,17,122,127] Systematic data supporting the efficacy of colchicine therapy in many of these other diseases are lacking.

Colchicine is derived from two plants of the Liliaceae family, *C. autumnale* (autumn crocus, meadow saffron, wild saffron, naked lady, son-before-the-father) and *Gloriosa superba* (glory lily).[176] The autumn crocus may contain different amounts of colchicine by weight, depending on the plant part (bulb, 0.8%; flowers, 0.1%; seeds, 0.8%; and the corm or underground stem, 0.6%).[110,134,159] Colchicine concentrations within the plant peak during the summer months.[134] The leaves of *C. autumnale* closely resemble those of the *Allium ursinum* or wild garlic and have been mistaken for them.[33,34,98] The tubers of *G. superba* may be confused with *Ipomoea batatas* (sweet potatoes).[176]

There is a lack of good epidemiologic data on colchicine poisoning. The American Association of Poison Control Centers records several hundred overall exposures annually. The majority of these exposures are in adults and are categorized as unintentional. Of the cases with a recorded outcome, approximately 10% reportedly to have major toxicity or resulted in death (see Chap. 135). At least 50 adverse events (23 of which were fatalities) have been linked to the use of intravenous (IV) colchicine.[216] The United States Food and Drug Administration recently announced its intent to stop the marketing of injectable compounds containing colchicine,[216] and serious questions remain about the utility of colchicine in light of its extremely narrow therapeutic index.

PHARMACOLOGY

Colchicine is a potent inhibitor of microtubule formation and function, which interferes with cellular mitosis, intracellular transport mechanisms, and maintenance of cell structure and shape.[127,176] The ubiquitous presence of microtubules in cells throughout the body presents a wide variety of targets for colchicine in poisoning.[127,176] Colchicine accumulates in leukocytes and has inhibitory effects on leukocyte adhesiveness, ameboid motility, mobilization, lysosome degranulation, and chemotaxis.[17,40,49,74,81,127,136,137,171-173,177] At doses used clinically, colchicine inhibits neutrophil and synovial cell release of chemotactic glycoproteins.[180,202] Colchicine also inhibits microtubule polymerization, which disrupts inflammatory cell-mediated chemotaxis and phagocytosis.[184] It reduces expression of adhesion molecules on endothelial and white blood cells and affects polymorphonuclear cell cytokine production.[5,18,152] Colchicine also acts as a competitive antagonist at $GABA_A$ receptors.[226]

PHARMACOKINETICS AND TOXICOKINETICS

Colchicine is rapidly absorbed in the jejunum and ileum and has a bioavailability generally between 25% and 50%.[17,123,176,188] It is highly lipid soluble[12,17,176] with a volume of distribution that ranges from 2.2 to 12 L/kg and that may increase to 21 L/kg in overdose.[158,164,176,181,182,214,223] Colchicine binding to plasma proteins approaches 50%.[17,127,153,176] Protein binding is principally to albumin, although some binding to α-1-glycoprotein acid and other lipoproteins is reported.[188] During the first several hours after acute overdose, colchicine is sequestered in white and red blood cells in concentrations 5-10 times higher than serum.[188] Peak serum concentrations after ingestion occur between 1 to 3 hours.[127] Toxic effects usually do not occur with concentrations less than 3 ng/mL.[75,153,222]

Colchicine is primarily metabolized through the liver with up to 20% of the ingested dose excreted unchanged in the urine.[108,176,214] Colchicine undergoes demethylation by the cytochrome P450 3A4.[108,127,164,213] Detoxification mainly occurs through deacetylation, demethylation, biliary secretion, and excretion in the stool.[108,127,150,186,188,213] Enterohepatic recirculation of colchicine occurs.[1,164,176]

Serum elimination half-lives ranging from 9 to 108 minutes have been reported.[10,95,176,188,223] On closer examination, however, these times probably more accurately reflect a rapid initial distribution phase. The drug undergoes a more delayed terminal elimination phase, which ranges from 1.7 to 30 hours, depending on the individual compartment model used to estimate elimination and the amount of colchicine absorbed.[1,79,176,182,186,188,214] These values are on the same order as and probably reflect the tubulin—colchicine complex disassociation time.[164] Individuals with renal failure and liver cirrhosis may have elimination half-lives that are prolonged up to 10-fold.[127] Colchicine can remain in measurable tissue quantities for a long time, as evidenced by its detection in white blood cells after 10 days and in urine 7 to 10 days after exposure.[74,176] Colchicine can cross the placenta and is secreted in breast milk, but it is not dialyzable.[127] Postmortem examination of colchicine-poisoned patients reveals high concentrations within the bone marrow, testicles, spleen, kidney, lung, brain, and heart.[181]

Drug Interactions Colchicine metabolism is susceptible to drug interactions. Because colchicine is detoxified through CYP3A4, blood concentrations are susceptible to xenobiotics that alter the function of this enzyme, such as erythromycin, clarithromycin, and grapefruit juice.[42,67,87,127] In particular, coadministration of clarithromycin and colchicine, especially in patients with renal insufficiency, increases the risk of fatal interaction.[107] P-glycoprotein (PGP) expels and clears colchicine, and drugs that inhibit PGP may directly affect the amount of colchicine eliminated and hence, toxicity.[164] For example, cyclosporine increases colchicine toxicity.[127,200,201]

PATHOPHYSIOLOGY

Microtubules play a vital role in cellular mitosis and possess a high amount of dynamic instability.[14,73,116,194] Microtubules are made up of tubulin protein subunits, of which three are known to exist: α, β, and γ.[116,146,194] These structures are highly dynamic with α-β tubulin heterodimers, constantly being added at one end and removed at the other.[116,117] Microtubules undergo two forms of dynamic behavior: dynamic instability, in which microtubule ends switch between growth and shortening phases, and treadmilling, in which there is a net growth (addition of heterodimers) at one end and a shortening (loss) at the other.[20] Assembly and polymerization dynamics are regulated by additional proteins known as stabilizing microtubule-associated proteins (MAPs) and destabilizing MAPs.[20] These dynamic behaviors and a resultant equilibrium are needed for multiple cell functions, including cell support, transport, and mitotic spindle formation for cell replication.[116] Xenobiotics that bind to specific regions on tubulin can interfere with microtubule structure and function, thereby causing mitotic dysfunction and arrest.[146,194] This leads to cellular dysfunction and death.[194] Xenobiotics that target microtubules can be generally divided into two categories: polymerization inhibitors (ie, vinca alkaloids, colchicine) and polymerization promoters (ie, taxanes, laulimalides).[20]

Colchicine binds to a tubulin dimer at a specific region known as the *colchicine-binding domain*, which is located at the interphase of the α and β subunits of the tubulin heterodimer.[20,99,116,167,194,217] This binding is relatively slow, temperature dependent, and generally irreversible, resulting in an alteration of the protein's secondary structure.[99,116,167,189] Colchicine binds at a second reversible but lower-affinity site on tubulin.[116,133] Current evidence suggests that the colchicine—tubulin complex binds to the microtubule ends and prevents further growth by sterically blocking further addition of dimers.[20] Conformational changes in the tubulin and colchicine complex also result as colchicine concentrations increase, which weakens the lateral bonds at the microtubule end.[20,146,194] Lateral and longitudinal interactions between dimers within a microtubule help stabilize the structure. The number of tubulin—colchicine dimers incorporated into the microtubule determines the stability of the microtubule ends.[20] All of these processes may prevent adequate binding of the next tubulin subunit and result in cessation of microtubule growth.[146,194] At low concentrations, colchicine arrests microtubule growth, where as at high concentrations, colchicine can actually cause microtubule depolymerization through disassociation of tubulin dimers.[20]

These conformational changes ultimately result in disassembly of the microtubule spindle in metaphase of cellular mitosis, cellular dysfunction, and death.[77,99,116,167,189,194] The effects of colchicine are dose dependent, with high concentrations inhibiting further microtubule polymerization, as well as inducing depolymerization of already formed microtubules.[130] Low concentrations can simply affect new microtubule formation and have no effect on preestablished polymer mass.[130] Colchicine also inhibits microtubule-mediated intracellular granule transport.[17,127] Some in vitro animal studies have also shown that colchicine might inhibit DNA synthesis by changing cell regulatory events at a critical time during the mitotic cycle.[72,78,101,130]

TOXIC DOSE

The toxic dose for colchicine is not well established. An early case series suggested that patients with ingestions of greater than 0.8 mg/kg uniformly died and those with ingestions above 0.5 mg/kg but less than 0.8 mg/kg would survive if given supportive care.[23] This information was based on a limited series of patients and is likely not generalizable.[156] More recent literature suggests that severe toxicity and even death may occur with smaller doses, and patients may survive ingestions in excess of 0.8 mg/kg.[63,81,88,94,156,204] This inability to accurately quantify the toxic dose in humans is likely due in great part to difficulty in dose estimation from the patient's history and significant advances in supportive care.

CLINICAL PRESENTATION

The clinical findings in poisoned patients is commonly described as triphasic (Table 37–1).[103,142,158,204] GI irritant effects, such as nausea, vomiting, abdominal distress, and diarrhea, occur initially within several hours after an overdose[3,32,34,59,66,118,142,147,219] and may lead to severe volume depletion.[87,106,137,156,158,160,204,225] This first stage usually persists for the first 12 to 24 hours after ingestion.[106,142] The second stage is characterized by widespread organ system dysfunction, particularly the bone marrow, and lasts for several days.[34,63,156,158,204] The final phase is characterized by recovery or death, and the progression can usually be defined within 1 week.[103,106,142,204]

After overdose, the hematopoietic effects of colchicine are characterized by an initial peripheral leukocytosis, which may be as high as 30,000/mm^3. This is followed by a profound leukopenia, which may be lower than 1000/mm^3. It is commonly accompanied by pancytopenia, usually beginning 48 to 72 hours after overdose.[17,32,79,87,102,142,161] The hematopoietic manifestations occur as a result of colchicine's effects

TABLE 37–1. Colchicine Poisoning: Common Clinical Findings, Timing of Onset, and Treatment

Phase	Time[a]	Signs and Symptoms	Therapy/Followup
I	0–24 hours	Nausea, vomiting, diarrhea	Antiemetics Consider GI decontamination
		Dehydration	IV fluids
		Leukocytosis	Close observation for leukopenia
II	1–7 days	Possible risk of sudden cardiac death (24–36 hours)	ICU admission and appropriate resuscitation
		Pancytopenia	G-CSF
		Renal failure	Hemodialysis
		Sepsis	Antibiotics
		Acute respiratory distress syndrome	Oxygen, mechanical ventilation
		Electrolyte imbalances	Repletion as needed
		Rhabdomyolysis	IV fluids, hemodialysis
III	>7 days	Alopecia	Follow-up within 1–2 months
		Myopathy, neuropathy, or myoneuropathy	EMG testing, biopsy and neurological follow-up as needed

[a] The interval time course is not absolute, and overlap of symptom presentation may occur.
EMG, electromyography; G-CSF, granulocyte-colony stimulating factor.

on bone marrow cell division.[30,106,145,181,225] A rebound leukocytosis and recovery of all cell lines occur if the patient survives.

Colchicine toxicity is associated with the development of dysrhythmias and cardiac arrest.[30,103,106,142,158] Sudden cardiovascular collapse from colchicine typically occurs between 24 to 36 hours after ingestion.[30,41,142,145,156] Profound hypovolemia and shock may contribute to this collapse,[17,87,156,158,204] but colchicine has direct toxic effects on skeletal and cardiac muscle, causing rhabdomyolysis.[26,50,140,148,157,220,225]

Myopathy,[35,36,193,229] neuropathy,[8,130] and a combined myoneuropathy[6,52,61,70,125,126,178,199,233] are described as a result of both long-term therapy and acute poisoning.[130] A combined myoneuropathy is reported more often, with myopathy dominating the clinical picture.[6,52,61,70,125,126,178,199,233] The myoneuropathy is often initially misdiagnosed as polymyositis or uremic neuropathy (caused by coexistent renal insufficiency).[6,126] Myoneuropathy usually develops in the context of chronic, therapeutic dosing in patients with some baseline renal impairment,[6,52,61,70,125,126,178,199,233] although it may also occur in the presence of normal renal function.[175] Patients may present with proximal limb weakness, distal sensory abnormalities, distal areflexia, and nerve conduction problems consistent with an axonal neuropathy.[126,169] A small amount of myelin degeneration is reported on autopsy, which suggests a myelinopathic component.[31] The myopathy is characterized by vacuolar changes on biopsy and accompanied by lysosome accumulation.[6,70,126,233] Elevated serum creatine kinase activity is present concurrently with symptoms.[126,158] Weakness usually resolves within several weeks of drug discontinuation.[126] Myopathy may also occur when concomitant use of hydroxymethylglutaryl—coenzyme A reductase inhibitors are used in patients with renal insufficiency.[2] Myopathy symptoms typically resolve within 4 to 6 weeks, although it may take up to 6 to 8 months in some patients.[229]

Acute respiratory distress syndrome occurs with colchicine toxicity.[11,59,102,150,191,195] The etiology is not well understood but may result from several factors, including respiratory muscle weakness, multisystem organ failure, and possibly direct pulmonary toxicity.[59,142,150,191,212] Other indirect effects of colchicine include renal failure and various electrolyte abnormalities resulting from fluid loss and impaired kidney function.[17,63,87,130,158]

Alopecia, which is usually reversible, is a well-described complication that occurs 2 to 3 weeks after poisoning in survivors.[17,79,87,88,106,133,211] Dermatologic complications range in severity from epithelial cell atypia to toxic epidermal necrolysis.[4,9,77,86,185]

Neurologic effects, including delirium, stupor, coma, and seizures, might be at least partly attributable to the multisystem disease caused by poisoning and not necessarily a direct effect of colchicine.[35,161,176,195] The cause of seizures is unclear but it might be partly attributable to antagonism of $GABA_A$ receptors.[226]

Other reported complications of colchicine poisoning include bilateral adrenal hemorrhage,[54,208] disseminated intravascular coagulation,[106,176,195] pancreatitis,[161] and liver dysfunction.[35,158,176]

DIAGNOSTIC TESTING

Colchicine concentrations in body fluids are not available in a clinically relevant fashion and have no well-established correlation with severity of illness. However, effective steady-state serum concentrations for treatment of patients with various illnesses are reported as 0.5 to 3.0 ng/mL.[153] Concentrations greater than 3.0 ng/mL are generally associated with toxicity.[75,153,222] Serum concentrations do not correlate well with the amount of xenobiotic ingested in massive oral overdose settings.[62] Initial laboratory monitoring should include a complete blood count (CBC), serum electrolytes, renal and liver function tests, creatine kinase, phosphate, calcium, magnesium, prothrombin time, activated partial thromboplastin time, and urinalysis. The need for other laboratory studies, such as a troponin, arterial blood gases, lactate, fibrinogen, and fibrin split products, should be considered, depending on the clinical situation. If cardiac toxicity is present or suspected, serial troponins (every 6–12 hours) should be performed because increasing concentrations may be predictive of cardiovascular collapse.[84,220] An electrocardiogram and chest radiograph should also be obtained. Serial CBCs are indicated (at least every 12 hours) to evaluate for the development of depression in cell lines.

MANAGEMENT

Treatment for patients with colchicine toxicity is mainly supportive, which includes IV fluid replacement, vasopressor use, hemodialysis (for renal failure), antibiotics for suspected secondary infection, colony-stimulating factors and adjunctive respiratory therapy (endotracheal intubation, positive end-expiratory pressure), as indicated. Consultation with nephrology and hematology specialists should be obtained in the case of impaired renal function or evidence of hematotoxicity.

Gastrointestinal Decontamination Because most patients with an acute oral colchicine overdose present several hours after their ingestion, vomiting has already begun, and the utility of GI decontamination is inadequately defined. However, given the extensive morbidity and mortality associated with colchicine overdose, orogastric lavage probably should be performed in patients who present within 1 to 2 hours of ingestion and are not vomiting.[25,218] A dose of activated charcoal (AC) should be administered after lavage, or in its place, and multiple-dose AC (MDAC) should be considered because of enterohepatic recirculation.[1,176] The delay in presentation to a health care facility coupled with the presence of GI symptoms such as vomiting significantly complicates using MDAC. However, antiemetic medications can be given to control emesis and facilitate AC administration.

Antidotal Therapy Experimental colchicine-specific antibodies can restore colchicine-affected tubulin activity in vitro and were successfully used in a single case of severe colchicine poisoning.[13] The administration of Fab fragments was temporally associated with a dramatic improvement in clinical and hemodynamic status. This improvement was also associated with a significant increase in serum colchicine concentrations, which suggests a redistribution of drug into the intravascular space.[13] Unfortunately, this therapy is not commercially available.

Granulocyte-colony stimulating factor (G-CSF) has been useful in the treatment of patients with colchicine-induced leukopenia and thrombocytopenia.[57,97,120,232] The dose of G-CSF, the dosing frequency, and the route of administration were variable in the reported cases.[57,97,120,232] G-CSF should be started if the patient begins to manifest evidence of leukopenia. Dosing should be in accordance with the manufacturer's instructions.

Extracorporeal Elimination Hemodialysis and hemoperfusion are not viable options for patients with colchicine poisoning based on its large volume of distribution, but hemodialysis may be required if renal failure is present.[16,21,22,181,182,214,223]

Disposition Because of the significant morbidity and mortality associated with colchicine toxicity, all symptomatic patients with suspected or known overdoses should be admitted to the hospital for observation. Because these patients have a risk of sudden cardiovascular collapse within the first 24 to 48 hours[156] intensive care unit monitoring is recommended for at least this initial time period. Troponin should be ordered every 6 to 12 hours during this period because increasing results may suggest an increased risk of cardiotoxicity and cardiovascular collapse.[84,220] Poisoned patients manifest GI signs and symptoms within several hours of ingestion and should be observed for at least 8 to 12 hours. Patients who do not manifest GI signs and symptoms within that time period after ingestion are unlikely to be significantly poisoned.

PODOPHYLLUM RESIN OR PODOPHYLLIN

HISTORY AND EPIDEMIOLOGY

Podophyllin is the name often used to refer to a resin extract from the rhizomes and roots of certain plants of the genus *Podophyllum*.[64,91] Examples include the North American perennial *Podophyllum peltatum* (mayapple or mandrake), the related Indian species *Podophyllum emodi*, and the Taiwanese *Podophyllum pleianthum*.[64] It is more descriptive to refer to it as podophyllum resin.[64,91] Podophyllum resin, or podophyllin, contains at least 16 active compounds.[45,64,91] These include a variety of lignins and flavonols, including podophyllotoxin, picropodophyllin, α- and β-pellatins, desoxypodophyllotoxin, and quercetin.[43,45,64,91] Podophyllotoxin, a component of podophyllin, is a potent microtubular poison, similar to colchicine, and causes similar effects in overdose.[64]

The first reported modern era medicinal use of podophyllin preparations was as a laxative in the 19th century.[43,45,173] Its cathartic properties, as well as its potential toxicity, were noted as early as 1890, when the first fatality from podophyllin was recorded.[69,196] Podophyllin was used to treat individuals with a variety of other health issues, including liver disease, scrofula, syphilis, warts, and cancer.[64] Etoposide and teniposide are semisynthetic derivatives of podophyllotoxin used as chemotherapeutics.[64]

Poisoning usually is caused by systemic absorption after topical application, after ingestion of the resin or plant, and after consumption of a commercial preparation of the extract. Systemic toxicity is described after unintentional dispensing of the incorrect herb, as well as after ingestion of herbal preparations containing podophyllin.[46,48,65]

PHARMACOLOGY

Podophyllin is primarily used in modern pharmacopeia as a topical treatment for patients with verruca vulgaris and condyloma acuminatum.[43,76,129] The active ingredient is believed to be podophyllotoxin.[12,64,119,196,210,221,230] Podophyllotoxin exists in the plant as a β-D-glucoside[76,119,196] Numerous synthetic and semisynthetic derivatives of podophyllotoxin exist; however, the most important are probably the chemotherapeutics etoposide and teniopside.[64] The antitumor effect of etoposide and teniposide results from their interaction with topoisomerase II and free radical production, leading to DNA strand breakage, an effect not shared by podophyllin and colchicine.[39,64] Use of etoposide and teniposide may also lead to a cessation of cell growth in the late S or early G2 phase of the cell cycle.[39,64,85] Further discussion of these xenobiotics can be found in the Chapter 52.

PHARMACOKINETICS AND TOXICOKINETICS

Very limited information exists regarding the pharmacokinetics (absorption, distribution, metabolism, and elimination) of podophyllin as a preparation or for its major active ingredient, podophyllotoxin. Podophyllotoxin is highly lipid soluble and can easily cross cell membranes.[76,89,163,196] It can be eliminated through the bile with a half-life of 48 hours.[43,53] However, review of the referenced articles failed to adequately support this elimination and may have been based solely on clinical course.[53]

Absorption of podophyllotoxin was measured in seven men after application of various amounts of a 0.5% ethanol podophyllotoxin preparation for condylomata acuminata.[221] Peak serum concentrations of 1 to 17 ng/mL were achieved within 1 to 2 hours after administration of doses ranging from 0.1 to 1.5 mL (0.5—7.5 mg).[221] Patients treated with less than or equal to 0.05 mL had no detectable podophyllotoxin in their serum. Administration of 0.1 mL yielded peak serum concentrations up to 5 ng/mL within 1 to 2 hours and up to 3 ng/mL at 4 hours. Administration of 1.5 mL yielded peak serum levels ranging from 5 to 9 ng/mL within 1 to 2 hours, levels of 5 to 7 ng/mL at 4 hours, 3 to 4.5 ng/mL at 8 hours, and 3.5 ng/mL at 12 hours.[221]

PATHOPHYSIOLOGY

The components of podophyllin have numerous actions within the cell, including inhibition of purine synthesis, inhibition of purine incorporation into RNA, reduction of cytochrome oxidase and succinoxidase activity, and inhibition of microtubule structure and function.[43,85,224] Podophyllotoxin causes its toxicity similar to colchicine[64,230] because it is able to bind to tubulin subunits and interfere with subsequent microtubule structure and function.[64,230] Interestingly, radiolabeled podophyllotoxin can inhibit colchicine binding to tubulin, suggesting that their binding sites overlap.[64] Podophyllotoxin binds more rapidly than colchicine, and binding is reversible in contrast to colchicine.[64] Podophyllotoxin also inhibits fast axoplasmic transport similar to colchicine by interference with microtubule structure and function.[170] Many other compounds, such as the vinca alkaloids, cryptophycins, and halichondrins, also inhibit microtubule polymerization in a similar manner.[117]

CLINICAL PRESENTATION

Poisoning is described after ingestion,[38,48,65,80,104,143,187,228] as well as after absorption from topical application of podophyllin.[83,144,151,154,168,205,207] Toxicity also is reported after IV administration of podophyllotoxin[192] and ingestion of mandrake root or herbal remedies containing podophyllin.[65,69,80] Nausea, vomiting, abdominal pain, and diarrhea usually begin within several hours after ingestion.[53,69,83,89,104,144,149,151,187,192,196,205,228] Symptoms of poisoning might be delayed for 12 hours or more after topical exposure to podophyllin and are often caused by improper usage (excessive topical exposure, interruption in skin integrity, or failure to remove the preparation after a short time period).[144,149,154,196] Initial clinical findings are not necessarily dictated by the route of exposure.[144]

Alterations in central and peripheral nervous system function tend to predominate in podophyllin toxicity. Patients might present with, or rapidly progress to confusion, obtundation, and coma.[38,53,65,83,143,149,151,154,187,205,207,210,228]

Delirium and both auditory and visual hallucinations occur during the initial presentation.[55,76,207] Patients develop paresthesias, lose deep tendon reflexes, and might develop a Babinski sign.[38,45,48,53,65,83,143,151,154,166,196,207] Cranial nerve involvement, including diploplia,[45] nystagmus,[53] dysmetria,[48] dysconjugate gaze,[207] and facial nerve paralysis,[55] are all reported. Patients who recover from the initial event are at risk of developing a peripheral sensorimotor axonopathy.[48,53,65,76,83,143,151,163,166,196,207] The reported duration for recovery from podophyllin-induced axonopathy is variable but can take several months.[53,65,83,151,163] Dorsal radiculopathy[89] and autonomic neuropathy have also been reported.[129] There may be a mild myelopathic component in the neuropathy.[47]

Hematologic toxicity from podophyllin most likely results from its antimitotic effects. A review of the limited literature suggests that it is similar to colchicine but is not nearly as consistent in its pattern, severity, and frequency. An initial leukocytosis[83,151,154,196] may occur after poisoning, which can be followed by leukopenia, thrombocytopenia, or generalized pancytopenia.[104,129,149,151,196,205] In patients who recover, cell lines tend to reach their nadir within 4 to 7 days after exposure.[76,83,104,151,205]

Other complications of poisoning include fever,[149] ileus,[76,149,207] elevated liver function tests,[65,104,151,205,228] and hyperbilirubinemia,[104] coagulopathy,[104] seizures,[55,187] and renal insufficiency or failure.[149,228] Teratogenic effects resulting from exposure during pregnancy may also occur.[45,119]

DIAGNOSTIC TESTING

Podophyllin or podophyllotoxin concentrations are not readily available. Routine testing for suspected or known podophyllin poisoning should include routine laboratory tests and other targeted testing, as needed. Serial cell blood counts should be obtained in cases of poisoning to evaluate for pancytopenia.

MANAGEMENT

Management primarily consists of supportive and symptomatic care. Orogastric lavage may be considered in patients with serious ingestions if presentation occurs within several hours of ingestion based on its high toxicity profile.[25,218] If the patient presents within the first several hours of ingestion, a dose of AC should be given. Any topically applied podophyllin should be removed and the area thoroughly cleansed. Supportive and symptomatic care should be instituted as needed. Patients either progress to multisystem organ dysfunction and death or recover with supportive care.

A few case reports of treatment with extracorporeal elimination techniques exist. These reports include resin hemoperfusion[100] and charcoal hemperfusion.[151,196] The role these procedures played in the patients' clinical courses is unclear. As a result, firm recommendations regarding the use of these techniques cannot be made at this time.

DISPOSITION

Patients with significant ingestions of podophyllin develop GI symptoms within a few hours,[48,69,80,104,166,228] but patients may also present with primarily neurologic symptoms, such as confusion or obtundation.[38,43,76,144] An isolated number of cases suggest the onset of toxicity can be delayed for as long as 12 hours.[38,43,53,65] Dermal exposure might result in even further delayed toxicity because systemic absorption is delayed and symptom onset is more insidious.[76,83,129,154,196,205,207] Patients probably should be observed for toxicity for at least 12 hours after ingestion and perhaps even longer after a significant dermal exposure.

VINCRISTINE AND VINBLASTINE

PHARMACOLOGY

Vincristine and vinblastine are derived from the periwinkle plant (*Catharanthus roseus*) and used for the treatment of patients with leukemias, lymphomas, and certain solid tumors. Their mechanism of activity is similar to that of colchicine, podophyllotoxin, and the taxoids (eg, paclitaxel, docetaxel).[60,71] These chemotherapeutics disrupt microtubule assembly from tubulin subunits by either preventing their formation or depolymerization, both of which are necessary for routine cell maintenance. Vinblastine binds to the β-subunit of the tubulin heterodimer at a specific region known as the *vinblastine binding site*.[20] Microtubules are responsible for several basic cellular functions, including cell division, axonal transport of nutrients and organelles, and cellular movement. Mitotic metaphase arrest is commonly observed because of the inability to form spindle fibers from the microtubules. Cell death quickly ensues as a result of the interruption of these homeostatic functions, accounting for the clinical manifestations.

PHARMACOKINETICS

After IV administration, vincristine is rapidly distributed to tissue stores and highly bound to proteins and red blood cells.[37] The capacity of vincristine to be bound by plasma proteins ranges from 50% to 80%.[174] In more than 50% of children given IV vincristine, serum concentrations were not detected 4 hours after administration.[155] The vinca alkaloids are primarily eliminated through the liver. Patients with hepatic dysfunction are susceptible to toxicity. Elimination of vincristine occurs via the hepatobiliary system,[37] and it has a terminal plasma half-life of about 24 hours.[162] Vincristine overdose is the most frequently reported antineoplastic overdose in the literature. This is because there are at least four different potential inappropriate ways to dose and administer vincristine, including confusing it with vinblastine, misinterpreting the dose, administering it by the wrong route, and confusing two different-strength vials. The normal dose of vincristine is 0.06 mg/kg, and a single dose is not to exceed 2 mg for either an adult or child.

CLINICAL MANIFESTATIONS

Despite their similarity in structure, vincristine and vinblastine differ in their clinical toxicity. Vincristine produces less bone marrow suppression and more neurotoxicity than does vinblastine. During the therapeutic use of vincristine, myelosuppression occurs in only 5% to 10% of patients.[105] However, this effect is common in the overdose setting, and when it occurs, the need for replacement blood products and concern for overwhelming infection is apparent.[132] The decrease in cell counts begins within the first week and may last for up to 3 weeks. Other manifestations of acute vincristine toxicity are mucositis, central nervous system (CNS) disorders, and the syndrome of inappropriate secretion of antidiuretic hormone (SIADH) (see Chap. 16).

CNS disorders are varied and unusual during therapeutic vincristine therapy because of its poor penetrance of the blood—brain barrier. They are, however, more common when there is delayed elimination, damage to the blood brain—barrier, overdose, or inadvertent intrathecal administration. Generalized seizures from toxicity or secondary effects may occur from 1 to 7 days after exposure.[109,115,121,206] Other manifestations are depression, agitation, insomnia, and hallucinations. Vincristine stimulation of the hypothalamus may be responsible for the fevers and SIADH noted in overdosed patients.[183] The fevers begin 24 hours after exposure and last 6 to 96 hours. Serum electrolytes need to be monitored, typically for 10 days.

Autonomic dysfunction is observed, and it commonly includes ileus, constipation, and abdominal pain. Atony of the bladder, hypertension, and hypotension may also occur.[121]

Ascending peripheral neuropathies occur during vincristine therapy and can be limited by keeping the total for a single dose below 2 mg.[197] Neuropathy may appear after an overdose, starting at about 2 weeks and lasting for 6 to 7 weeks. Paresthesias, neuritic pain, ataxia, bone pain, wrist drop, foot drop, involvement of cranial nerves III to VII and X, and diminished reflexes may be observed.[227] The incidence of paresthesia increases with dose and is reported to be 56% in patients treated at doses between 12.5 and 25 μg/kg.[105] At a dose of 75 μg/kg, the incidence of patients with a sensory disorder increased by sixfold. The loss of reflexes, the earliest and most consistent sign of vincristine neuropathy, is maximal at 17 days after a single massive dose. Muscular weakness is a limiting point in therapy and typically involves the distal dorsiflexors of the extremities, although laryngeal involvement is also reported.[128,190] These severe neurologic symptoms may be reversed by either withholding therapy or reducing dosage upon manifestation of these findings.[128] The mechanism of toxicity is not well understood but appears to be related to inhibition of microtubular synthesis, which leads to axonal degeneration.[90,165] A brain biopsy of a patient suffering a vincristine-related death showed neurotubular dissociation, which is characteristic of vincristine damage in experimental animals.[28,51] Unlike the vinca alkaloids, Taxol-induced peripheral neuropathy is predominantly sensory and resolves faster with discontinuation.[131] This is because of the different effects on microtubule assembly by these agents. Nerve conduction studies and the Achilles tendon reflex are useful in monitoring patients for toxicity after exposure.

Vincristine-induced myocardial infarctions have been reported, but their cause is not understood.[138,198,209,231] They may be related to vinca alkaloid—induced platelet aggregation, coronary artery spasm, or increased sensitivity of myocardium to hypoxia.

MANAGEMENT

Patients receiving an inadvertent amount of an IV dose of vincristine should be admitted to a cardiac-monitored bed and observed for 24 to 72 hours.[135] Treatment of generalized seizures with benzodiazepines or phenobarbital is usually successful, and phenytoin was used successfully in a patient with barbiturate hypersensitivity.[121] Prophylactic phenobarbital and benzodiazepine agents were used to prevent seizures in two patients.[44,124] Dysrhythmias and alterations in blood pressure may also be expectantly managed. Calcium channel blockers (nifedipine and amlodipine) were used to control hypertension in a patient with vincristine overdose.[44] Blood counts must be monitored daily, and G-CSF may be used to treat neutropenia.[44,132,206] However, the red blood cell response from the use of erythropoietin may be limited because of the induction of metaphase arrest in the erythroblasts.[141]

If patients remain asymptomatic during the observation period, they can be discharged with follow-up for bone marrow suppression and SIADH; otherwise, depending on the patient's clinical condition, continual observation for progression of neurologic symptoms is warranted.[19] The symptoms of acute toxicity usually last for 3 to 7 days, and the neurologic sequelae may last for months before some resolution is observed.

In a controlled clinical trial for vincristine-induced peripheral neuropathy, glutamic acid therapy had limited efficacy. Patients receiving vincristine therapy were given glutamic acid as 500 mg orally 3 times a day.[114] There was a decreased incidence in loss of the Achilles tendon reflex and a delayed onset of paresthesias in the glutamic acid—treated group. No reported adverse effects with glutamic acid were observed in this investigation. Animal studies involving the administration of glutamic and aspartic acid to mice poisoned with either vinblastine or vincristine demonstrate increased survival and decreased sensorimotor peripheral neuropathy.[27,58,112] The mechanisms of these observed effects with glutamic acid remain unclear, but several authors have suggested the ability of glutamic acid to competitively inhibit a common cellular transport mechanism for vincristine,[24,56] its ability to assist in the stabilization of tubulin and promote its polymerization into microtubules,[29,96] and the ability of glutamic acid to improve cellular metabolism by overcoming the inhibition in the Krebs cycle.[68,179] Although the role of glutamic acid in acute toxicity needs further study, it is not harmful and should be considered. Glutamic acid may be initiated as 500 mg orally three times a day and continued until the serum vincristine concentration is below toxicity.[114] L-Glutamic acid is the preferred stereoisomer because it is biologically active, and this product is available as a powder from various distributors in the United States.

Leucovorin may shorten the course of vincristine-induced peripheral neuropathy[92] and myelosuppression.[124] The mechanism is attributed to leucovorin's ability to overcome a vincristine-mediated block of dihydrofolate reductase and thymidine synthetase.[92] However, neither leucovorin[15,111,215] nor pyridoxine[113] has been definitely shown to be effective. An initial experimental investigation evaluating the efficacy of antibody therapy to limit vinca alkaloid toxicity shows promise.[93]

One case of vinblastine overdose was reported to be successfully managed with plasma exchange procedures performed at 4 hours and 18 hours after vinblastine administration.[203]

ENHANCED ELIMINATION

Vincristine's rapid distribution and high protein binding characteristics favor early intervention and methods other than hemodialysis. Double-volume exchange transfusion was performed at 6 hours postexposure in 3 children who were overdosed with 7.5 mg/m^2 of IV vincristine.[124] This procedure replaced approximately 90% of the circulating blood volume by exchanging twice the patient's blood volume. Of the two survivors, their respective postexchange serum vincristine concentrations were 57% and 71% lower than their preexchange concentrations. The amount of vincristine removed was not determined. Although these patients developed peripheral neuropathies, myelosuppression, and autonomic instability, the author noted that the duration of illness was shorter than previously reported. Thus, based on the pharmacokinetic profile of vincristine and these two reports, exchange transfusion in children is the preferred method of enhanced elimination when the patient presents soon after the administration of the drug, and plasmapheresis is the preferred method in adults.

Plasmapheresis was attempted with vinca alkaloid overdoses.[132,174] In an 18-year-old patient who received two 8-mg IV doses of vincristine at 12-hour intervals, the procedure was performed 6 hours after the second dose, and 1.5 times the plasma volume was plasmapheresed.[174] Postplasmapheresis serum vincristine concentration was 23% lower than the starting concentration. The patient survived with myelosuppression, neurotoxicity, and SIADH. Additional information on the toxicity of intrathecal administration of the vinca alkaloids can be found in Special Considerations SC2: Intrathecal Administration of xenobiotics.

SUMMARY

Colchicine toxicity may be evident several hours after ingestion and consists of severe nausea, vomiting, diarrhea and abdominal pain followed by pancytopenia several days later. Colchicine-poisoned patients

TABLE 37–2. Comparison of General Antimitotic Xenobiotics in Overdose

	Colchicine	Podophyllum Resin	Vincristine	Vinblastine
Route of exposure	PO	PO and topical	IV	IV
Initial symptoms	GI[a]	GI[a] and/or neurologic effects (obtundation, confusion, delirium)	GI effects,[a] fever, neurologic effects	GI effects,[a] fever, myalgias, neurologic effects
Initial symptom onset	Several hours after ingestion; delayed presentation beyond 12 hours is very unlikely	Several hours after ingestion; delayed presentation (past 12 h) is possible, especially in those with a cutaneous route of exposure	Usually within 24–48 hours	Usually within 24–48 hours
Hematotoxic effects	Leukocytosis (24–48 hours after ingestion); pancytopenia (beginning 48–72 h after ingestion)	Similar to colchicine; however, not well characterized and reported less frequently	Hematotoxicity may occur; *less* toxicity compared with vinblastine	Hematotoxicity may occur; *more* toxicity compared with vincristine
CNS effects	Late (after 48–72 h after ingestion); obtundation, confusion, and lethargy secondary to progression of MSD	Can be early (<12 h after ingestion); CNS toxicity may occur later or secondary to progression of MSD	Variable; cranial neuropathies; seizures; obtundation, confusion, and lethargy may occur because of progression of MSD	Variable; cranial neuropathies; obtundation, confusion, and lethargy may occur because of progression of MSD[b]
Delayed PNS effects	Myoneuropathy most common; reported most often in chronic colchicine users with renal insufficiency	Peripheral sensorimotor axonopathy	Autonomic and ascending peripheral neuropathy; *increased* severity compared with vinblastine	Can see autonomic and peripheral neuropathy; *decreased* severity compared with vincristine
Clinical course	Recovery or MSD and death	Recovery or MSD and death	Recovery or MSD and death; May develop SIADH	Recovery or MSD and death; may develop SIADH
Management	Supportive; GI decontamination; G-CSF for neutropenia	Supportive; consider GI decontamination for oral exposures and skin decontamination for topical exposures	Primarily supportive; G-CSF for neutropenia; see Special Considerations: Intrathecal Administration of Xenobiotics	Primarily supportive; G-CSF[c] for neutropenia; treatment of intrathecal overdoses; Special Considerations SC2: Intrathecal Administration of Xenobiotics

[a] Nausea, vomiting, diarrhea, abdominal discomfort.

MSD, multi-system organ dysfunction; PNS, peripheral nervous system.

may have a higher risk of sudden cardiac death, especially during the period between 24 and 36 hours after ingestion; increasing serial troponin levels in these patients may suggest a higher risk of cardiovascular complications. Podophyllum toxicity may be less pronounced but may occur after dermal application (Table 37–2).

Management of patients with toxicity from colchicine, podophyllotoxin, and the vinca alkaloids is generally similar after oral exposure. Serial blood counts should be done to identify the development of cytopenias. G-CSF may be of benefit in patients with colchicine-induced neutropenia. Early GI decontamination and supportive treatment are the hallmarks of therapy for all colchicine and podophyllin exposure because there are no commercially available and proven antidotes. The particular aspects and complications of unintentional or excessive IV or intrathecal exposure are described in detail in this chapter, and experimental antidotes for vincristine and vinblastine exposure were discussed.

The findings and conclusions in this article are those of the authors and do not necessarily represent the views of the Centers for Disease Control and Prevention or the Agency for Toxic Substances and Disease Registry.

ACKNOWLEDGEMENT

Richard Wang, DO, contributed to this chapter in a previous edition.

The findings and conclusions in this article are those of the authors and do not necessarily represent the views of the Centers for Disease Control and Prevention or the Agency for Toxic Substances and Disease Registry.

REFERENCES

1. Achtert G, Scherrmann JM, Christen MO. Pharmacokinetics/bioavailability of colchicine in healthy male volunteers. *Eur J Drug Metab Pharmacokinet.* 1989;14:317-322.
2. Alayli G, Cengiz K, Canturk F, et al. Acute myopathy in a patient with concomitant use of pravastatin and colchicine. *Ann Pharmacother.* 2005;39:1358-61.
3. Aleem HMA. Gloriosa superba poisoning. *J Assoc Physicians India.* 1992;40:541-542.
4. Alfandari S, Beuscart C, Delaporte E, et al. Toxic epidermal necrolysis in a patient suffering from acquired immune deficiency syndrome. *Infection.* 1994;22:365.

5. Allen JN, Herzyk OJ, Wewers MD. Colchicine has an opposite effect on interleukin 1b and tumor necrosis factor. *Am J Physiol.* 1991;261:315-321.
6. Altiparmak MR, Pamuk ON, Pamuk GE, et al. Colchicine neuromyopathy: a report of six cases. *Clin Exp Rheumatol.* 2002;20(suppl 26):S13-S16.
7. Angulo P, Lindor KD. Management of primary biliary cirrhosis and autoimmune cholangitis. *Clin Liver Dis.* 1998;2:333-351.
8. Angunawela RM, Fernando HA. Acute ascending polyneuropathy and dermatitis following poisoning by tubers of *Gloriosa superba*. *Ceylon Med J.* 1971;233-235.
9. Arroyo MP, Sanders S, Yee H, et al. Toxic epidermal necrolysis-like reaction secondary to colchicine overdose. *Br J Dermatol.* 2004;150:581-588.
10. Back A, Walaszek EJ, Uyeki E. Distribution of radioactive colchicine in some organs of normal and tumor-bearing mice. *Proc Soc Exp Biol Med.* 1951;77:667-669.
11. Baldwin LR, Talbert RL, Samples R. Accidental overdose of insufflated colchicine. *Drug Saf.* 1990;5:305-312.
12. Bargman H. Is podophyllin a safe drug to use and can it be used in pregnancy? *Arch Dermatol.* 1988;124:1718-1719.
13. Baud FJ, Sabouraud A, Vicaut E, et al. Treatment of severe colchicine overdose with colchicine-specific Fab fragments. *N Engl J Med.* 1995;332; 642-645.
14. Bayley PM, Martin SR. Microtubule dynamic instability: basic mechanisms and numerical modeling by computer simulation. *Comments Theor Biol.* 1992;2:403-427.
15. Beer M, Cavalli F, Martz G. Vincristine overdose: treatment with and without leucovorin rescue. *Cancer Treat Rep.* 1983;67:746-747.
16. Ben-Chetrit E, Backenroth R, Levy M. Colchicine clearance by high-flux polysulfone dialyzers. *Arthritis Rheum.* 1998;41:749-750.
17. Ben-Chetrit E, Levy M. Colchicine: 1998 update. *Semin Arthritis Rheum.* 1998;28:48-59.
18. Ben-Chetrit E, Navon P. Colchicine-induced leucopenia in a patient with familiar Mediterranean fever: the cause and a possible approach. *Clin Exp Rheumatol.* 2003;21(suppl 30)S38-S40.
19. Berenson MP. Recovery after inadvertent massive overdosage of vincristine. *Cancer Chemother Rep.* 1971;55:525-526.
20. Bhattacharyya B, Panda D, Gupta S, Banerjee M. Anti-mitotic activity of colchicine and the structural basis for its interaction with tubulin. *Med Res Rev.* 2008;28:155-183.
21. Bismuth C. Biological valuation of extra-corporeal techniques in acute poisoning. *Acta Clin Belg Suppl.* 1990;13:20-28.
22. Bismuth C, Fournier PE, Galliot M. Biological evaluation of hemoperfusion in acute poisoning. *J Toxicol Clin Toxicol.* 1981;18:1213-1223.
23. Bismuth C, Gaultier M, Conso F. Medullary aplasia after acute colchicine poisoning. 20 cases *Nouv Presse Med.* 1977;6:1625-1629 [Article in French].
24. Bleyer WA, Frisby SA, Oliverio VT. Uptake and binding of vincristine by murine leukemia cells. *Biochem Pharmacol.* 1975;24:633-639.
25. Bond GR. The role of activated charcoal and gastric emptying in gastrointestinal decontamination: a state-of-the-art review. *Ann Emerg Med.* 2002;39:273-286.
26. Boomershine KH. Colchicine-induced rhabdomyolysis. *Ann Pharmacother.* 2002;36:824-826.
27. Boyle FM, Wheeler HR, Shenfield GM. Glutamate ameliorates experimental vincristine neuropathy. *J Pharmacol Exp Ther.* 1996;279:410-415.
28. Bradley WG, Lassman LP, Pearce GW, Walton JN. The neuromyopathy of vincristine in man: clinical electrophysiological and pathological studies. *J Neurol Sci.* 1970;10:107-131.
29. Brady ST. Basic properties of fast axonal transport and the role of fast axonal transport in axonal growth. In: Elam JS, ed. *Axonal Transport in Neuronal Growth and Regeneration.* New York: Plenum; 1984:13-27.
30. Brncic N, Viskovic I, Peric R, et al. Accidental plant poisoning with *Colchicum autumnale*: report of two cases. *Croat Med J.* 2001;42:673-675.
31. Brown WO, Seed L. Effects of colchicine on human tissues. *Am J Clin Pathol.* 1945;15:189-195.
32. Bruns BJ. Colchicine toxicity. *Australas Ann Med.* 1968;17:341-344.
33. Brvar M, Kozelj G, Mozina M, Bunc M. Acute poisoning with autumn crocus (*Colchicum autumnale* L.). *Wien Klin Wochenschr* 2004;116:205-208.
34. Brvar M, Ploj T, Kozelj G, et al. Case report. Fatal poisoning with *Colchicum autumnale*. *Crit Care.* 2004;8:R56-R59.
35. Caglar K, Odabasi Z, Safali M, Colchicine-induced myopathy with myotonia in a patient with chronic renal failure. *Clin Neurol Neurosurg.* 2003;105:274-276.
36. Caglar K, Safali M, Yavuz I, et al. Colchicine-induced myopathy with normal creatine phosphokinase level in a renal transplant patient. *Nephron.* 2002;92:922-924.
37. Calabresi P, Chabner BA. Antineoplastic agents. In: Goodman LS, Limbird LE, Milinoff PB, Gilman AG, Rall TW, eds. *The Pharmacological Basis of Therapeutics*, 9th ed. New York: McGraw-Hill; 1996:1224-1287.
38. Campbell A. Accidental poisoning with podophyllin. *Lancet.* 1980;8161:206-207.
39. Canel C, Moraes RM, Dayan FE, Ferreira D. Podophyllotoxin. *Phytochemistry.* 2000;54:115-120.
40. Caner JEZ. Colchicine inhibition of chemotaxis. *Arthritis Rheum.* 1965;8:757-764.
41. Caplan YH, Orloff KG, Thompson BC. A fatal overdose with colchicine. *J Analytical Toxicol.* 1980;4:153-155.
42. Caraco Y, Putterman C, Rahamimov R, Ben-Chetrit E. Acute colchicine intoxication—possible role of erythromycin administration. *J Rheumatol.* 1992;19:491-496.
43. Cassidy DE, Drewry J, Fanning JP. Podophyllum toxicity: a report of a fatal case and a review of the literature. *J Toxicol Clin Toxicol.* 1982;19:35-44.
44. Chae L, Moon HS, Kim SC. Overdose of vincristine: experience with a patient. *J Korean Med Sci.* 1998;13:334-348.
45. Chamberlain MJ, Reynolds AL, Yeoman WB. Toxic effect of podophyllum application in pregnancy. *Br Med J.* 1972;3:391-392.
46. Chan TYK, Critchley AJH. The spectrum of poisonings in Hong Kong: an overview. *Vet Hum Toxicol.* 1994;36:135-137.
47. Chang MH, Liao KK, Wu ZA, Lin KP. Reversible myeloneuropathy resulting from podophyllin intoxication: an electrophysiological follow-up. *J Neurol Neurosurg Psychiatry.* 1992;55:235-236.
48. Chang MH, Lin KP, Wu ZA, Liao KK. Acute ataxic sensory neuronopathy resulting from podophyllin intoxication. *Muscle Nerve.* 1992;15:513.
49. Chappey ON, Niel E, Waitier JL, et al. Colchicine disposition in human leukocytes after single and multiple oral administration. *Clin Pharmacol Ther.* 1993;54:360-362.
50. Chattopadhyay I, Shetty HGM, Routledge PA, Jeffery J. Colchicine induced rhabdomyolysis. *Postgrad Med J.* 2001;77:191-192.
51. Cho ED, Lowndes HE, Goldstein BD. Neurotoxicology of vincristine in the cat. *Arch Toxicol.* 1983;52:83-90.
52. Choi SS, Chan KF, Ng HK, Mak WP. Colchicine-induced myopathy and neuropathy. *Hong Kong Med J.* 1999;5:204-207.
53. Clark ANG, Parsonabe MJ. A case of podophyllum poisoning with involvement of the nervous system. *Br Med J.* 1957;2:1155.
54. Clevenger CV, August TF, Shaw LM. Colchicine poisoning: report of a fatal case with body fluid analysis by GC/MS and histopathologic examination of postmortem tissues. *J Anal Toxicol.* 1991;15:151-154.
55. Coruh M, Argun G. Podophyllin poisoning. A case report. *Turk J Pediatrics.* 1965;7:100-103.
56. Creasey WA, Bensch KB, Malawista SE. Colchicine, vinblastine and griseofulvin pharmacological studies with human leukocytes. *Biochem Pharmacol.* 1971;20:1579-1588.
57. Critchley JAJH, Critchley LAH, Yeung EA, et al. Granulocyte-colony stimulating factor in the treatment of colchicine poisoning. *Hum Exp Toxicol.* 1997;16:229-232.
58. Cutts HJ. Effects of other agents on the biologic responses to vincaleukoblastine. *Biochem Pharmacol.* 1964;13:421-430.
59. Davies HO, Hyland RH, Morgan CD, Laroye GJ. Massive overdose of colchicine. *CMAJ.* 1988;138:335-336.
60. Deconti RC, Creasey WA. Clinical aspects of the dimeric Catharan-thus alkaloids. In: Taylor WI, Farnsworth NR, eds. *The Catharanthus Alkaloids: Botany, Chemistry, Pharmacology and Clinical Use.* New York: Marcel Dekker; 1975:237-278.
61. De Deyn PP, Ceuterick C, Saxena V, et al. Chronic colchicine-induced myopathy and neuropathy. *Acta Neurol Belg.* 1995;95:29-32.
62. Deveaux M, Hubert N, Demarly C. Colchicine poisoning: case report of two suicides. *Forensic Sci Int.* 2004;143:2004:219-22.
63. De Villota ED, Galdos P, Mosquera JM, Tomas MI. Colchicine overdose: an unusual origin of multiorgan failure. *Crit Care Med.* 1979;7:278-279.
64. Desbene S, Giorgi-Renault S. Drugs that inhibit tubulin polymerization: the particular case of podophyllotoxin and analogues. *Curr Med Chem Anti Cancer Agents.* 2002;2:71-90.
65. Dobb GJ, Edis RH. Coma and neuropathy after ingestion of herbal laxative containing podophyllin. *Med J Aust.* 1984;140:495-496.
66. Dodds AJ, Lawrence PJ, Biggs JC. Colchicine overdose. *Med J Aust.* 1978;2:91-92.
67. Dogukan A, Oymak FS, Taskapan H, et al. Acute fatal colchicine intoxication in a patient on continuous ambulatory peritoneal dialysis (CAPD). Possible role of clarithromycin administration. *Clin Nephrol.* 2001;55:181-182.

68. Dorr RT, Fritz WL. *Cancer Chemotherapy Handbook*. New York: Elsevier; 1980:677-684.
69. Dudley WH. Fatal podophyllum poisoning. *Med Rec.* 1890;37:409.
70. Dupont P, Hunt I, Goldberg L, Warrens A. Colchicine myoneuropathy in a renal transplant patient. *Transpl Int.* 2002;15:374-376.
71. Dustin P. Microtubule poisons. In: Justin P, ed. *Microtubules*. Berlin: Springer-Verlag; 1984:167-225.
72. Epstein B, Epstein JH, Fukuyama K. Autoradiographic study of colchicine inhibition of DNA synthesis and cell migration in hairless mouse epidermis in vivo. *Cell Tissue Kinet.* 1983;16:313-319.
73. Erickson H, O'Brien E. Microtubule dynamic instability and GTP hydrolysis. *Annu Rev Biophys Biomol Struct.* 1992;21:145.
74. Ertel NH, Wallace SL. Measurement of colchicine in urine and peripheral leukocytes [abstract]. *Clin Res.* 1971;19:348.
75. Ferron GM, Rochdi M, Jusko WJ, Scherrmann JM. Oral absorption characteristics and pharmacokinetics of colchicine in healthy volunteers after single and multiple doses. *J Clin Pharmacol.* 1996;36:874-883.
76. Filley CM, Graff-Radford NR, Lacy JR, et al. Neurologic manifestations of podophyllin toxicity. *Neurology.* 1982;32:309-311.
77. Finger JE, Headington JT. Colchicine-induced epithelial atypia. *Am J Clin Pathol.* 1963;40:605-609.
78. Fitzgerald PH, Brehaut LA. Depression of DNA synthesis and mitotic index by colchicine in cultured human lymphocytes. *Exp Cell Res.* 1970;59:27-31.
79. Folpini A, Furfori P. Colchicine toxicity—clinical features and treatment. Massive overdose case report. *J Toxicol Clin Toxicol.* 1995;33:71-77.
80. Frasca T, Brett AS, Yoo, SD. Mandrake toxicity: a case of mistaken identity. *Arch Intern Med.* 1997;157:2007-2009.
81. Fruhman GJ. Inhibition of neutrophil mobilization by colchicine. *Proc Soc Exp Biol Med.* 1960;104:284-286.
82. Gabrscek L, Lesnicar G, Krivec B, et al. Accidental poisoning with Autumn crocus. *J Toxicol Clin Toxicol.* 2004;42:85-88.
83. Gate RG, Leche J, Chervenak C. Podophyllin toxicity. *Ann Intern Med.* 1979;90:723.
84. Gaze DC, Collinson PO. Cardiac troponins as biomarkers of drug- and toxin-induced cardiac toxicity and cardioprotection. *Exp Opin Drug Metab Toxicol.* 2005;1:715-725.
85. Georgatsos JG, Karembyllis R. Action of podophyllic acid on malignant tumors. II. Effects of podophyllic acid ethyl hydrazide on the incorporation of precursors into the nucleic acids of mouse mammary tumors and livers in vivo. *Biochem Pharmacol.* 1968;17:1489.
86. Gilbert JD, Byard RW. Epithelial cell mitotic arrest—a useful postmortem histologic marker in cases of possible colchicine toxicity. *Forensic Sci Int.* 2002;126:150-152.
87. Goldbart A, Press J, Sofer S, Kapelushnik J. Near fatal acute colchicine intoxication in a child: a case report. *Eur J Pediatr.* 2000;159:895-897.
88. Gooneratne BWM. Massive generalized alopecia after poisoning by *Gloriosa superba*. *Br Med J.* 1966;1:1023-1024.
89. Gorin F, Kindall D, Seyal M. Dorsal radiculopathy resulting from podophyllin toxicity. *Neurology.* 1989;39:607-608.
90. Green LS, Donoso JA, Heller-Bettinger IE, Samson FE. Axonal transport of disturbances in vincristine-induced peripheral neuropathy. *Ann Neurol.* 1977;12:255-262.
91. Gruber M. Podophyllum versus podophyllin. *J Am Acadf Dermatol.* 1984;10:302-303.
92. Grush OC, Morgan SK. Folinic acid rescue for vincristine toxicity. *Clin Toxicol.* 1979;14:71-78.
93. Gutowski MC, Fix DV, Corvalan JR, Johnson DA. Reduction of toxicity of a vinca alkaloid by an anti-vinca alkaloid antibody. *Cancer Invest.* 1995;13:370-374.
94. Guven AG, Bahat E, Akman S, et al. Late diagnosis of severe colchicine intoxication. *Pediatrics.* 2002;109:971-973.
95. Halkin H, Dany S, Greenwald M, et al. Colchicine kinetics in patients with familial Mediterranean fever. *Clin Pharmacol Ther.* 1980;28:82-87.
96. Hamel E, Lin CM. Glutamate induced polymerization of tubulin: characteristics of the reaction and application to the large-scale purification of tubulin. *Arch Biochem Biophys.* 1981;209:29-40.
97. Harris R, Marx G, Gillett M, et al. Colchicine-induced bone marrow suppression: treatment with granulocyte colony-stimulating factor. *J Emerg Med.* 2000;18:435-440.
98. Hartung EF. History of the use of colchicum and related medicaments in gout with suggestions for further research. *Ann Rheum Dis.* 1954;13: 190-200.
99. Hastie SB. Interactions of colchicine with tubulin. *Pharm Ther.* 1991;51:377-401.
100. Heath A, Mellstrand T, Ahlmen J. Treatment of podophyllin poisoning with resin hemoperfusion. *Hum Toxicol.* 1982;373-378.
101. Hell E, Cox DG. Effects of colchicine and colchemid on synthesis of deoxyribonucleic acid in the skin of the guinea pig's ear in vitro. *Nature.* 1963;197:287-288.
102. Hill RN, Spragg RG, Wedel MK, Moser KM. Adult respiratory distress syndrome associated with colchicine toxicity. *Ann Intern Med.* 1975;83:523-524.
103. Hobson CH, Rankin APN. A fatal colchicine overdose. *Anaesth Intensive Care.* 1986;14:453-464.
104. Holdright DR, Jahangiri M. Accidental poisoning with podophyllin. *Hum Exp Toxicol.* 1990;9:55-56.
105. Holland JF. Vincristine treatment of advanced cancer: a cooperative study of 392 cases. *Cancer Res.* 1973;33:1258-1265.
106. Hood RL. Colchicine poisoning. *J Emerg Med.* 1994;12:171-177.
107. Hung IFN, Wu AKL, Cheng VCC, et al. Fatal interaction between clarithromycin and colchicine in patients with renal insufficiency: a retrospective study. *CID.* 2005;41:291-300.
108. Hunter AL, Klaassen CD. Biliary excretion of colchicine. *J Pharmacol Exp Ther.* 1975;192:605-617.
109. Hurwitz RL, Mahoney DH, Armstrong DL, Browder TM. Reversible encephalopathy and seizures as a result of conventional vincristine administration. *Med Pediatr Oncol.* 1988;16:216-219.
110. Insel PA. Analgesic-antipyretics and antiinflammatory agents: drugs employed in the treatment of rheumatoid arthritis and gout. In: Gilman AG, Goodman LS, Rall TW, et al (eds). *Goodman and Gilman's: The Pharmacological Basis of Therapeutics*, 8th ed. New York: MacMillan; 1990:674-676.
111. Jackson DV, McMahan RA, Pope EK, et al. Clinical trial of folinic acid to reduce vincristine neurotoxicity. *Cancer Chemother Pharmacol.* 1986;17:281-284.
112. Jackson DV, Pope EK, Case LD, et al. Improved tolerance of vincristine by glutamic acid. A preliminary report. *J Neurooncol.* 1984;2:219-222.
113. Jackson DV, Pope EK, McMahan RA, et al. Clinical trial of pyridoxine to reduce vincristine neurotoxicity. *J Neurol.* Oncol 1986;4:37-41.
114. Jackson DV, Wells HB, Atkins JN, et al. Amelioration of vincristine neurotoxicity by glutamic acid. *Am J Med.* 1988;84:1016-1022.
115. Johnson FL, Bernstein ID, Hartman JR. Seizures associated with vincristine sulfate therapy. *J Pediatr.* 1973;82:699-702.
116. Jordan A, Hadfield JA, Lawrence NJ, et al. Tubulin as a target for anticancer drugs: agents which are known to interact with the mitotic spindle. *Med Res Rev.* 1998;18:259-296.
117. Jordan MA. Mechanism of action of anti-tumor drugs that interact with microtubules and tubulin. *Curr Med Chem Anti Cancer Agents.* 2002;2:1-17.
118. Jose J, Ravindran M. A rare case of poisoning by *Gloriosa superba*. *J Assoc Physicians India.* 1988;36:451-452.
119. Karol MD, Conner CS, Watanabe AS, Murphrey KJ. Podophyllum: suspected teratogenicity from topical application. *J Toxicol Clin Toxicol.* 16:283-286.
120. Katz R, Chuang LC, Sutton JD. Use of granulocyte colony-stimulating factor in the treatment of pancytopenia secondary to colchicine overdose. *Ann Pharmacother.* 1992;26:1087-1088.
121. Kaufman IA, Kung FH, Koenig HM, Giammona ST. Overdosage with vincristine. *J Pediatr.* 1976;89:671-674.
122. Kim KY, Schumacher HR, Hunsche E, et al. A literature review of the epidemiology and treatment of acute gout. *Clin Ther.* 2003;25:1593-1617.
123. Klintschar M, Beham-Schmidt C, Radner H, et al. Colchicine poisoning by accidental ingestion of meadow saffron (*Colchicum autumnale*): pathological and medicolegal aspects. *Forensic Sci Int.* 1999;106:191-200.
124. Kosmidos HV, Bouhoutsou DO, Varvoutsi MC, et al. Vincristine overdose: experience with 3 patients. *Pediatr Hematol Oncol.* 1991;8:171-178.
125. Kuncl RW, Cornblath DR, Avila O, Duncan G. Electrodiagnosis of human colchicine myoneuropathy. *Muscle Nerve.* 1989;12:360-364.
126. Kuncl RW, Duncan G, Watson D, et al. Colchicine myopathy and neuropathy. *N Engl J Med.* 1987;316:1562-1568.
127. Lange U, Schumann C, Schmidt KL. Current aspects of colchicine therapy: classical indications and new therapeutic uses. *Eur J Med Res.* 2001;6:150-160.
128. Legha SS. Vincristine neurotoxicity, pathophysiology and management. *Med Toxicol.* 1986;1:421-427.
129. Leslie KO, Shitamoto B. The bone marrow in systemic podophyllin toxicity. *Am J Clin Pathol.* 1982;77:478-480.

130. Levy M, Spino M, Read S. Colchicine: a state of the art review. *Pharmacotherapy.* 1991;11:196-211.
131. Lipton RB, Apfel SC, Dutcher JP, et al. Taxol produces a predominantly sensory neuropathy. *Neurology.* 1989;39:368-373.
132. Lotz JP, Chapiro J, Voinea A, et al. Overdosage of vinorelbine in a woman with metastatic non—small-cell lung carcinoma. *Ann Oncol.* 1997:7:714-715.
133. Ludena RF, Roach MC. Tubulin sulfhydryl groups as probes and targets for antimitotic and antimicrotubule agents. *Pharm Ther.* 1991;49:133-152.
134. Mack RB. Achilles and his evil squeeze. Colchicine poisoning. *North Carolina Med J.* 1991;52:581-583.
135. Maeda K, Ueda M, Ohtaka H, et al. A massive dose of vincristine. *Jpn J Clin Oncol.* 1987;7:247-253.
136. Malawista SE. Sols, gels and colchicine: a common formulation for the effects of colchicine in gouty inflammation and cell division. *Arthritis Rheum.* 1964;7:325-326.
137. Malawista SE. The action of colchicine in acute gout. *Arthritis Rheum.* 1965;8:752-756.
138. Mandel EM, Lewinski U, Djaldetti M. Vincristine-induced myocardial infarction. *Cancer.* 1975;36:1979-1982.
139. Marijuana. Erowid. Available at http://www.erowid.org/plants/cannabis/cannabis_cultivation14.shtml; accessed January 3, 2005.
140. Markland ON, D'Agostino AN. Ultrastructural changes in skeletal muscle induced by colchicine. *Arch Neurol.* 1971;24:72-81.
141. Marmont AM. Selective metaphasic arrest of erythroblasts by vincristine in patients receiving high doses of recombinant human erythropoietin for myelosuppressive anemia. *Leukemia.* 1992;4:167-170.
142. Maxwell MJ, Muthu P, Pritty PE. Accidental colchicine overdose. A case report and literature review. *Emerg Med J.* 2002;19:265-267.
143. McFarland MF, McFarland J. Accidental ingestion of podophyllum. *J Toxicol Clin Toxicol.* 1981;18:973-977.
144. McGuigan M. Toxicology of topical therapy. *Clin Dermatol.* 1989;32-37.
145. McIntyre IM, Ruszkiewicz AR, Crump K, Drummer OH. Death following colchicine poisoning. *J Forensic Sci.* 1994;39:280-286.
146. Melki R, Carlier M, Pantaloni D, Timasheff SN. Cold depolymerization of microtubules to double rings: geometric stabilization of assemblies. *Biochemistry.* 1989;28:9143-9152.
147. Mendis S. Colchicine cardiotoxicity following ingestion of *Gloriosa superba* tubers. *Postgrad Med J.* 1989;65:752-755.
148. Mery P, Riou B, Chemla D, Lecarpentier Y. Cardiotoxicity of colchicine in the rat. *Intensive Care Med.* 1994;20:119-123.
149. Miller RA. Podophyllin. *Int J Dermatol.* 1985;24:491-498.
150. Milne ST, Meek PD. Fatal colchicine overdose: report of a case and review of the literature. *Am J Emerg Med.* 1998;16:603-608.
151. Moher LM, Maurer SA. Podophyllum toxicity: case report and literature review. *J Fam Pract.* 1979;9:237-240.
152. Molad Y, Reibman J, Levin RI, et al. A new mode of action for an old drug: colchicine decreases surface expression of adhesion molecules on both neutrophils (PMNs) and endothelium [abstract]. *Arthritis Rheum.* 1992;35(suppl):S35.
153. Molad Y. Update on colchicine and its mechanism of action. *Curr Rheumatol Rep.* 2002;4:252-256.
154. Montaldi DH, Giambrone JP, Courey NG, Taefi P. Podophyllin poisoning associated with the treatment of condyloma acuminatum: a case report. *Am J Obstet Gynecol.* 1974;119:1130-1131.
155. Morasca L, Rainisio C, Masera G. Duration of cytotoxicity activity of vincristine in the blood of leukemia in children. *Eur J Cancer.* 1969;5:79-84.
156. Mullins ME, Carrico EA, Horowitz BZ. Fatal cardiovascular collapse following acute colchicine ingestion. *J Toxicol Clin Toxicol.* 2000;38:51-54.
157. Mullins ME, Robertson DG, Norton RL. Troponin I as a marker of cardiac toxicity in acute colchicine overdose. *Am J Emerg Med.* 2000;18:743-744.
158. Murray SS, Kramlinger KG, McMichan JC, Mohr DN. Acute toxicity after excessive ingestion of colchicine. *Mayo Clin Proc.* 1983 Aug;58:528-532.
159. Muzaffar A, Brossi A. Chemistry of colchicine. *Pharm Ther.* 1991;49: 105-109.
160. Nagaratnam N, De Silva DPKM, De Silva N. Colchicine poisoning following ingestion of *Gloriosa superba* tubers. *Trop Geogr Med.* 1972;25:15-17.
161. Naidus RM, Rodvien R, Mielke CH. Colchicine toxicity: a multi-system disease. *Arch Intern Med.* 1977;137:394-396.
162. Nelson RL. The comparative clinical pharmacology and pharmacokinetics of vindesine, vincristine, and vinblastine in human patients with cancer. *Med Pediatr Oncol.* 1982;10:115-127.
163. Ng THK, Chan YW, Yu YL, et al. Encephalopathy and neuropathy following ingestion of a Chinese herbal broth containing podophyllin. *J Neurol Sci.* 1991;101:107-113.
164. Niehl E, Scherrmann JM. Colchicine today. *Joint Bone Spine.* 2006;73:672-678.
165. Ochs S, Worth R. Comparison of the block of fast axoplasmic transport in mammalian nerve by vincristine, vinblastine, and desacetyl vinblastine amide sulfate (DVA). *Proc Am Assoc Cancer Res.* 1975;16:70-75.
166. O'Mahony S, Keohane C, Jacobs J, et al. Neuropathy due to podophyllin intoxication. *J Neurol.* 1990;237:110-112.
167. Panda D, Daijo JE, Jordan MA. Kinetic stabilization of microtubule dynamics at steady state in vitro by substoichiometric concentrations of tubulin-colchicine complex. *Biochemistry.* 1995;34:9921-9929.
168. Pascher F. Systemic reactions to topically applied drugs. *Bull NY Acad Med.* 1973;49:613-627.
169. Paulson JC, McClure WO. Inhibition of axoplasmic transport by colchicine, podophyllotoxin and vinblastine: an effect on microtubules. *Ann NY Acad Sci.* 1975;253:517-527.
170. Paulson JC, McClure WO. Microtubules and axoplasmic transport. Inhibition of transport by podophyllotoxin: an interaction with microtubule protein. *J Cell Biol.* 1975;67:461-467.
171. Phelps P. Appearance of chemotactic activity following intracellular injection of monosodium urate crystals: effect of colchicine. *J Lab Clin Med.* 1970;71:622-631.
172. Phelps P. Polymorphonuclear leukocyte activity in vitro. IV. Colchicine inhibition of chemotactic activity formation after phagocytosis of urate crystals. *Arthritis Rheum.* 1970;13:1-9.
173. Phillips RA, Love AHG, Mitchell TG, Neptune EM Jr. Cathartics and the sodium pump. *Nature.* 1965;206:1367-1368.
174. Pierga JY, Beuzeboc P, Dorval T, et al. Favorable outcome after plasmapheresis for vincristine overdose. *Lancet.* 1992;640:185.
175. Pirzada NA, Medell M, Ali I. Colchicine induced neuromyopathy in a patient with normal renal function. *J Clin Rheumatol.* 2001;7:374-376.
176. Putterman C, Ben-Chetrit E, Caraco Y, Levy M. Colchicine intoxication: clinical pharmacology, risk factors, features, and management. *Semin Arthritis Rheum.* 1991;21:143-155.
177. Rajan RT. Lysosomes and gout. *Nature.* 1966;210:959-960.
178. Rana SS, Giuliani MJ, Oddis CV. Acute onset of colchicine myoneuropathy in cardiac transplant recipients: case studies of three patients. *Clin Neurol Neurosurg.* 1997;99:266-270.
179. Reynolds JEF. Vinblastine. In: Reynolds JEF, ed. *Martindale: The Extra Pharmacopoeia.* London: Pharmaceutical Press; 1989:655-657.
180. Roberts W, Liang MH, Stern SH. Colchicine in acute gout. Reassessment of risks and benefits. *JAMA.* 1987;257:1920-1922.
181. Rochdi M, Sabouraud A, Baud FJ, et al. Toxicokinetics of colchicine in humans: analysis of tissue plasma and urine data in ten cases. *Hum Exp Toxicol.* 1992;11:510-516.
182. Rochdi M, Sabouraud A, Girre C, et al. Pharmacokinetics and absolute bioavailability of colchicine after iv and oral administration in healthy human volunteers and elderly subjects. *Eur J Clin Pharmacol.* 1994;46:351-354.
183. Rosenthal S, Kaufman S. Vincristine neuropathy. *Ann Intern Med.* 1974;81:733-737.
184. Rott KT, Agudelo CA. Gout. *JAMA.* 2003;289:2857-2860.
185. Roujeau JC, Guillaume JC, Fabre JP, et al. Toxic epidermal necrolysis (Lyell syndrome). *Arch Dermatol.* 1990;126:37-42.
186. Rudi J, Raedsch R, Gerteis C, et al. Plasma kinetics and biliary excretion of colchicine in patients with chronic liver disease after oral administration of a single dose and after long-term treatment. *Scand J Gastroenterol.* 1994;29:346-351.
187. Rudrappa S, Vijaydeva L. Podophyllin poisoning. *Ind Pediatr.* 2002;39:598-599.
188. Sabouraud A, Rochdi M, Urtizberea M, et al. Pharmacokinetics of colchicine: a review of experimental and clinical data. *Z Gastroenterol* 1992;30(suppl 1):35-39.
189. Sackett D, Varma J. Molecular mechanism of colchicine action: induced local unfolding of beta-tubulin. *Biochemistry.* 1993;32:13560-13565.
190. Sandler SG, Tobin W, Henderson ES. Vincristine induced neuropathy: a clinical study of fifty leukemic patients. *Neurology.* 1969;19:367-374.
191. Sauder P, Kopferschmitt J, Jaeger A, Mantz JM. Haemodynamic studies in eight cases of colchicine poisoning. *Hum Toxicol.* 1983;2:169-173.
192. Savel H. Clinical experience with intravenous podophyllotoxin. *Proc Am Assoc Cancer Res.* 1964;5:56.

193. Sayarlioglu M, Sayarlioglu H, Ozen S, et al. Colchicine-induced myopathy in a teenager with familial Mediterranean fever. *Ann Pharmacother.* 2003;37:1821-1824.
194. Shi Q, Chen K, Morris-Natschke SL, Lee KH. Recent progress in the development of tubulin inhibitors as antitumor agents. *Curr Pharm Design.* 1998;4:219-248.
195. Simons RJ, Kingma DW. Fatal colchicine toxicity. *Am J Med.* 1989;86:356-357.
196. Slater GE, Rumack BH, Peterson RG. Podophyllin poisoning—systemic toxicity following cutaneous application. *Obstet Gynecol.* 1978;52:94.
197. Slimowitz R. Thoughts on a medical disaster. *Am J Health Syst Pharm.* 1995;52:1464-1465.
198. Somers G, Abramow M, Witter M, Naets JP. Myocardial infarction: a complication of vincristine treatment? *Lancet.* 1976;308:690.
199. Soto O, Hedley-Whyte ET. Case 33-2003: a 37-year old man with a history of alcohol and drug abuse and sudden onset of leg weakness. *N Engl J Med.* 2003;349:1656-1663.
200. Speeg AU, Maldonado AL, Liaci J, Muirhead D. Effect of cyclosporine on colchicine secretion by a liver canalicular transporter studied in vivo. *Hepatology.* 1992;15:899-903.
201. Speeg KV, Maldonado AL, Liaci J, Muirhead D. Effect of cyclosporine on colchicine secretion by the kidney multidrug transporter studied in vivo. *J Pharmacol Exp Ther.* 1992;261;50-55.
202. Spilberg I, Gallacher A, Mehta JM, Mandell B. Urate crystal-induced chemotactic factor: isolation and partial characterization. *J Clin Invest.* 1976;58:815-819.
203. Spiller M, Marson P, Perilongo G, et al. A case of vinblastine overdose managed with plasma exchange. *Pediatr Blood Cancer.* 2005;45:344-346.
204. Stapczynski JS, Rothstein RJ, Gaye WA, Niemann JT. Colchicine overdose: report of two cases and review of the literature. *Ann Emerg Med.* 1981;10:364-368.
205. Stoehr GP, Peterson AL, Taylor WJ. Systemic complications of local podophyllin therapy. *Ann Intern Med.* 1978;89:362-363.
206. Stones DK. Vincristine overdosage in paediatric patients. *Med Pediatr Oncol.* 1998;30:193.
207. Stoudemire A, Baker L, Thompson II TL. Delirium induced by topical application of podophyllin. A case report. *Am J Psychiatry.* 1981;138:1505-1506.
208. Stringfellow HF, Howat AJ, Temperley JM, Phillips M. Waterhouse-Friderichsen syndrome resulting from colchicine overdose. *J Royal Soc Med.* 1993;86:680.
209. Subar M, Muggia FM. Apparent myocardial ischemia associated with vinblastine administration. *Cancer Treat Rep.* 1986;70:690-691.
210. Sullivan M, Follis RH, Hilgartner M. Toxicology of podophyllin. *Proc Soc Exp Biol Med.* 1951;77:269.
211. Sullivan TP, King Jr LE, Boyd AS. Colchicine in dermatology. *J Am Acad Dermatol.* 1998;39:993-999.
212. Tanios MA, El Gamal H, Epstein SK, Hassoun PM. Severe respiratory muscle weakness related to long-term colchicine therapy. *Respiratory Care.* 2004;49:189-191.
213. Tateiski T, Soucek S, Caraco Y, et al. Colchicine biotransformation by human liver microsomes: identification of CYP 3A4 as a major isoform responsible for colchicine demethylation. *Biochem Pharmacol.* 1997;10:111-116.
214. Thomas G, Girre C, Scherrmann JM, et al. Zero-order absorption and linear disposition of oral colchicine in healthy volunteers. *Eur J Clin Pharmacol.* 1989;37:79-84.
215. Thomas LL, Brasst PC, Somers R, Goudsmit R. Massive vincristine overdose: failure of leucovorin to reduce toxicity. *Cancer Treat Rep.* 1982;66:1967-1969.
216. United States Food and Drug Administration. *FDA Takes Action to Stop the Marketing of Unapproved Injectable Drugs Containing Colchicine.* Available at http://www. fda. gov/bbs/topics/NEWS/2008/NEW01791. html; accessed on May 28, 2008.
217. Uppuluri S, Knipling L, Sackett D, Wolff J. Localization of the colchicine-binding site of tubulin. *J Proc Nat Acad Sci.* 1993;90:11598-11602.
218. Vale JA, Kulig K. American Academy of Clinical Toxicologists. Position statement: gastric lavage. *J Toxicol Clin Toxicol.* 1997;35:711-719.
219. Valenzuela P, Paris E, Oberpauer B, et al. Overdose of colchicine in a three-year old child. *Vet Hum Toxicol.* 1995;37:366-367.
220. Van Heyningen C. Troponin for prediction of cardiovascular collapse in acute colchicine overdose. *Emerg Med J.* 2005;22:599-600.
221. Von Krogh G. Podophyllotoxin in serum: absorption subsequent to three-day repeated applications of a 0. 5% ethanolic preparation on condylomata acuminate. *Sex Transm Dis.* 1982;9:26-33.
222. Wallace SL, Ertel NH. Plasma levels of colchicine after oral administration of a single dose. *Metabolism.* 1973;22:749-753.
223. Wallace SL, Omokoku B, Ertel NH. Colchicine plasma levels. Implications as to pharmacology and mechanism of action. *Am J Med.* 1970;48:443-448.
224. Waravdekar VS, Paradis AD, Leiter J. Enzyme changes induced in normal and malignant tissues with chemical agents. V. Effect of acetylpodophylo-toxin-ω-pyridinium chloride on uricase, adenosine deaminase, nucleoside phosphorylase, and glutamic dehydrogenase activities. *J Natl Cancer Inst.* 1955;16:99.
225. Weakley-Jones B, Gerber JE, Biggs G. Colchicine poisoning: case report of two homicides. *Am J Forensic Med Pathol.* 2001;22:203-206.
226. Weiner JL, Buhler AV, Whatley VJ, et al. Colchicine is a competitive antagonist at human recombinant γ-aminobutyric $acid_A$ receptors. *J Pharmacol Exp Ther.* 1998;284:95-102.
227. Weiss HD, Walker MD, Wiernick PH. Neurotoxicity of commonly used antineoplastic agents. *N Engl J Med.* 1974;29:75-81.
228. West WM, Ridgeway NA, Morris AJ, Sides PJ. Fatal podophyllin ingestion. *South Med J.* 1982;75:1269-1270.
229. Wilbur K, Makowsky M. Colchicine myotoxicity: case reports and literature review. *Pharmacotherapy.* 2004;24:1784-92.
230. Wisniewski H, Shelanski ML, Terry RD. Effects of mitotic spindle inhibitors on neurotubules and neurofilaments in anterior horn cells. *J Cell Biol.* 1968;38:224-231.
231. Yancey RS, Talpaz M. Vindesine-associated angina and ECG changes. *Cancer Treat Rep.* 1982;66:587-589.
232. Yoon KH. Colchicine induced toxicity and pancytopenia at usual doses and treatment with granulocyte-colony stimulating factor. *J Rheumatol.* 2001;28:1199-1200.
233. Younger DS, Mayer SA, Weimer LH, et al. Colchicine-induced myopathy and neuropathy. *Neurology.* 1991;41:943.

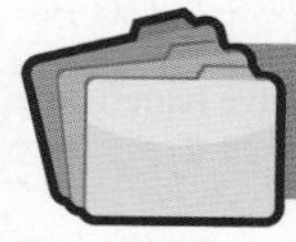

SPECIAL CONSIDERATIONS (SC2)

INTRATHECAL ADMINISTRATION OF XENOBIOTICS

Rama B. Rao

Cerebrospinal fluid (CSF) is produced by the choroid plexus lining the ventricles at a rate of 15–30 mL/h, or approximately 500 mL/d in adults.[46] Cerebrospinal fluid flows in a rostral to caudal direction and is resorbed through the arachnoid villi directly into the venous circulation. The estimated total volume of CSF in a healthy adult is between 130–150 mL, and 35 mL in infants.[46,62,82]

For over 100 years, a variety of experimental and therapeutic xenobiotics have been delivered directly into the CSF.[53,109] The most common current indications for intrathecal xenobiotic administration include analgesia, anesthesia, and treatment of spasticity or CNS neoplasms. The clinical advantages of this route of administration include targeted delivery and lower medication dosages with fewer systemic effects. Medications are usually administered via a spinal needle or an indwelling intrathecal catheter. Catheters may be attached to either an external or subcutaneous pump. Less commonly, substances are administered into a reservoir of an intraventricular shunt (Table SC2–1). The distribution of intrathecal xenobiotics is determined by a variety of factors. Some authors speculate that the xenobiotic movement is often attributed to both diffusion and convection, and that the dilution of xenobiotics administered via a lumbar catheter is attributed to the outflow of CSF from the fourth ventricle.[79] In a radiolabelled tracer study of 5 patients with lumbar catheters, individuals received intrathecally the hydrophilic radiolabeled diethylene triamine pentaacetic acid (^{111}In- DTPA). Neuroimaging revealed a drop in concentration of the tracer as the fluid moved rostrally.[55] The steady state lumbar to cervical concentration for hydrophilic xenobiotics is 4:1 with marked interindividual variability.[79] Depending on the lipophilicity the xenobiotic reaches the brain within a few minutes to 1 hour. Patient position, and interindividual variations in lumbosacral CSF fluid volume may affect xenobiotic distribution and may account for the differences in the level of spinal anesthesia among patients administered the same local anesthetic dosages.[44] Baricity which is the ratio of the specific gravity of the xenobiotic to the specific gravity of CSF at 98.6° F (37° C) is also a consequential variable. Hyperbaric xenobiotics typically distribute in accordance with gravitational forces.[44] In overdose or administration of xenobiotics unintended for intrathecal administration, distribution, resorption, and clinical effects may not follow predictable models.

Complications can occur from preparation and dosing errors or inadvertent penetration of the dura and admixture with the CSF during epidural anesthesia or analgesia.[24,43,44] Medications intended for intrathecal delivery may be administered into the wrong port of a pump delivery system resulting in a massive overdose. Another potentially fatal error involves inadvertent administration of the wrong medication into the CSF.[49] This error occurs with misidentification or mislabeling of medications during pharmacy preparation, or at the bedside. For patients with indwelling devices, medications intended for intravenous delivery may be misconnected to the intrathecal catheter which also operates via Luer lock system.

Several factors affect the clinical toxicity of intrathecal medication errors.[110] The properties of the xenobiotic are important. Ionized xeniobiotics are likely to disrupt normal neurotransmission and cause toxicity, as may hyperosmolar or lipophilic xenobiotics. The site of administration may be important as well. Patients administered the wrong xenobiotic into an Ommaya reservoir may suffer more immediate alterations in mental status depending upon the agent administered. While intrathecal administration of preservatives and excipients are investigated in animal models, the characteristics of these adjuvants in medication errors is not likely to be of value in predicting clinical effect.[45]

Patients may present with exaggerated symptoms typically associated with the xenobiotic. For example, patients with intrathecal morphine overdose may present with symptoms of opioid toxicity.[51] Other manifestations of intrathecal errors, regardless of the xenobiotic, include pain and paresthesias, often ascending in nature, autonomic instability especially with extremes of blood pressure, and hyperreflexic myoclonic spasms similar to those seen in patients with tetanus. Seizures, or a depressed level of consciousness may also occur. The time of onset of these life-threatening symptoms may be determined by the dose and characteristics of the xenobiotic. For example, a woman inadvertently administered intrathecal potassium chloride complained immediately of severe back pain.[67] Myoclonic spasms, seizures, and coma followed and the patient died within 3 hours despite a normal serum potassium concentration. Patients with inadvertent vincristine exposures may be asymptomatic for many hours and die within a few days to a few weeks.

Once a medication delivery error is identified, rapid intervention is mandatory especially for ionic agents, chemotherapeutics, or iodinated water soluble contrast agents as these xenobiotics usually reach the brain within an hour. In cases in which outcome is uncertain or not previously described, the exposure should be treated as potentially fatal. Any existing access to the CSF, ideally in the lumbosacral area, should be maintained.[103] Immediate withdrawal of CSF, in volumes as high as 75 mL in adults is indicated. This can be replaced with isotonic solutions: lactated ringers 0.9% salineplasma-lyte or a combination of these. Some older cases utilized Elliot B solution. Some authors recommend the initial large volume removal be performed in 20–30 mL aliquots. For children, multiple aliquots of between 5–10 mL can be removed and replaced with isotonic fluid. If the patient can tolerate an upright position, this may limit cephalad movement of xenobiotics, but positioning for any critical life support measures should take precedence.

Delays to initial CSF drainage should be minimized as the interval between the exposure and CSF drainage may also affect the total xenobiotic recovered (see below). In the interim, a neurosurgical consultation should be obtained to consider the placement of ventricular access for the performance of continuous CSF lavage. This procedure, also known as ventriculolumbar perfusion, involves continuous ventricular instillation of an isotonic solution with CSF drainage through a lumbar site. Another intervention involves placement of an epidural catheter into the intrathecal space at a space above the lumbar drainage site.

TABLE SC2–1. Xenobiotics Administered Intrathecally*

Analgesics/anesthetics	**Antiinflammatory**
Anesthetics (local)	Corticosteroids
Clonidine[20]	**Antispasmodic**
Ketamine[42]	Baclofen
Midazolam[112]	**Chemotherapeutics**
Morphine[59]	Liposomal cytarabine[15]
Neostigmine[59]	Methotrexate
Octreotide[72,77]	**Vasoactive**
Opioids[65]	Epinephrine
Zinconitide[16]	Papaverine[99]
Antibiotics	Phenylephrine
Amikacin[13,25]	**Other**
Amphotericin B	Bethanecol[76]
Arbekacin[36]	Colistin[105]
Cefotetan	Somatostatin
Ceftriaxone[21]	Tetanus immunoglobulin[2]
Gentamicin[94]	
Levofloxacin[13]	
Penicillin	
Polymixin E[12]	
Vancomycin[1,66]	

*Few of these xenobiotics are FDA approved for intrathecal administration. Most were utilized in clinical trials or as rescue xenobiotics for refractory CNS infections.

An isotonic solution can be perfused through the catheter and drained caudally. This serves as a readily available, rapid intervention for patients awaiting placement of an emergent ventriculostomy.[69,96]

For ventriculolumbar perfusion, lavage flow rates can be as great as 150 mL/h. Fresh frozen plasma can be added to the lavage fluid after several hours to increase the CSF protein content. The ideal lavage fluid, protein components, and infusion rates are not known.[40] Some protocols previously utilized are listed in Table SC2–2. Although artificial CSF formulations exist, their role in the treatment of such medication errors is not evaluated.[70]

Depending on the xenobiotic exposure, specific antidotes or rescue agents can be employed. With most intrathecal exposures, these rescue agents will be administered via oral, intramuscular or intravenous routes. Extreme caution should be under taken to avoid delivery of antidotes directly into the CSF, unless specific data supports their use.

XENOBIOTIC RECOVERY FROM CSF

Immediate, aggressive CSF removal and lavage resulted in nearly 95% recovery of vincristine in the lavage fluid of a patient with inadvertent exposure. Of the published cases in which xenobiotic recovery is reported, percentages relate to both the lavage method and quantity of CSF removed. For example, withdrawal of 10 mL of CSF 45 minutes after a methotrexate overdose in a 4-year-old patient recovered 20% of the initial dose.[3] Withdrawal of 200 mL of CSF in aliquots, 45 minutes after methotrexate overdose in a 9-year-old patient recovered 78% of the initial dose.[30] The specific xenobiotic may affect recovery as well. For example a patient underwent withdrawal of 30 mL of CSF at 18 minutes after an overdose of simultaneously administered lidocaine, epinephrine, and fentanyl. Approximately 39% of lidocaine was recovered, whereas the recovery of fentanyl was only 7%.[95]

SPECIFIC EXPOSURES

IONIC CONTRAST AGENTS

Several xenobiotics have been utilized historically for contrast myelography. Many of these agents were abandoned because of their propensity to cause adhesive arachnoiditis chronic pain syndromes or other complications (Thorotrast). Low osmolar, nonionic contrast media are currently utilized, but unfortunately, other hyperosmolar ionic media are readily available in radiographic suites and sometimes inadvertently administered. Some patients develop cranial neuropathies.[34] Exposed patients become symptomatic within 30 minutes to 6 hours after administration with hyperreflexia and myoclonic spasms following minimal stimulation.[84,86,100] Clinical symptoms typically begin in the lower extremities and move in a cephalad direction, sometimes progressing to opisthotonos. This is likely due to alterations in inhibitory neurotransmission as occur in patients with tetanus, and has been termed ascending tonic-clonic syndrome (ATCS). In one review, nearly one-third of patients died as a result of their exposures.[104] Immediate large volume CSF drainage should be performed in 20 mL aliquots with isotonic fluid replacement. Ventriculolumbar perfusion should be considered in severe cases.

CHEMOTHERAPEUTICS

Methotrexate is administered intrathecally for the prevention and treatment of leukemic meningitis or other CNS neoplasms.[8] Errors are generally dose related.[3,28-30,41,47,58,83,101] In most reported cases, aggressive drainage of CSF as great as 250 mL in aliquots with isotonic fluid replacement was utilized without ventriculolumbar perfusion. Experimental treatment of patients with intrathecal carboxypeptidase G_2 ($CPDG_2$) has been described without obvious adverse events.[71,107] The patients underwent lumbar drainage followed by intrathecal $CPDG_2$. Drainage removed between 32% and 58% of the methotrexte, and the antidote reduced the methotrexte concentrations by 98%. The patients received 2000 U of intrathecal $CPDG_2$ in 12mL of normal saline over 5 minutes (Antidote in Depth A14: Carboxypeptidase).

Intrathecal leucovorin is *absolutely contraindicated* as its use results in fatalities. Following intrathecal methotrexate overdose, the intravenous administration of leucovorin is appropriate[48,102] (Antidote in Depth: Leucovorin).

Vincristine is typically administered intravenously and does not cross the blood brain barrier. There are no therapeutic indications for intrathecal vincristine, and such errors are almost always fatal.[4-6,14,26,33,37,38,56] As soon as the exposure is identified, immediate CSF drainage should be instituted and rapid neurosurgical consultation should be obtained. The few known survivors with cognitive function underwent early neurosurgical intervention for ventriculolumbar perfusion.[6,69,80] One of the patients had an epidural catheter placed intrathecally above the drainage site for lumbolumbar perfusion while awaiting ventriculostomy. This method of intrathecal perfusion should be considered in all patients with intrathecal vincristine exposures until definitive ventriculolumbar perfusion can be established. Ideally tubing systems would be readily available to prevent intrathecal medication errors.[73,98] Other rescue medications are covered in Chap. 53.

TABLE SC2–2. Adverse Intrathecal Exposures

Agent	Age (y) Sex (M,F)	Mechanism	Symptoms	Intervention	Outcome
Baclofen[114]	8/M	Probable pump malfunction	Coma, vomiting, bradycardia	20 mL CSF removed at undetermined time	Survived
Bupivcaine[32]	34/M	Inadvertent dural puncture	Hypotension, ascending paralysis at 10 minutes	Not described	Survived
Cefotetan[17]	66/M	Catheter misconnection	Dyspnea, hypotension, myoclonic spasm, pain at 2 hours	10 mL CSF removed at 20 hours	Rhabdomyolysis Survived
Ceftriaxone[21]	74/F	Overdose	Bilateral lower extremity pain	240 mL CSF removed in 20 mL aliquots, with 0.9% NaCl replacement. Started at unknown time.	Survived
Cytarabine[57]	4	Overdose	Mydriasis, delayed onset, gait impairment, tremor	50 mL CSF removed in 5 mL aliquots, with 0.9% NaCl replacement. Started at 65 minutes. Estimated 27%–36% cytarabine recovery	Died of unknown cause
Dactinomycin[54]	5/F	Medication error	Hypotonia, fasciculations, hyperreflexia at 2 hours	50 mL CSF removed with 0.9% NaCl replacement at 1 hour, then ventriculolumbar perfusion started at 1.5 hours using 0.9% NaCl 100 mL/h with 2.5 mg/mL hydrocortisone for 26 hours Other adjuncts	Ascending paraplegia, obstructive hydrocephalus, Survived
Doxorubicin[7]	12/F	Medication error	Fever, headache, vomiting at 12 hours, seizures, hydrocephalus	No attempt at removal	Survived without sequelae at 56 days
Doxorubicin[50]	31/F	Medication error 14.5 mg	Hypoesthesia, paraparesis, incontinence over 7 days, T8 sensory level, bowel and bladder incontinence, meningismus, adhesive arachnoiditis at 3 weeks	CSF exchange at 20 cm^3/h for 500 cm^3 per publication. Methyl predinsolone 500 mg/d and immunoglobulin 22 g/d initiated at 1 week. Treatment of arachnoiditis with ventriculoperitoneal shunt placement.	Lower extremity weakness 3/5 at 8 months, eventual ambulation with resolution of incontinence at 14 months
Furosemide[19]	36/M	Medication error	None	No attempt at removal	Survived
Gadolinium[8]	64/M	Medication error: gadopentetate dimeglumine	Confusion, nausea, vomiting, ataxia, nystagmus, hallucinations, blurred vision, depressed mental status	Not described	Survived
Gallamine[39]	48/M	Medication error	Hyperreflexic nyoclonic spasm, onset 1 hour 45 minutes; fever, hypertension, tachycardia, miosis, coma at 3 hours	15 mL CSF drainage Started at 6 hours	Survived
Iohexol[34]	–	Medication error	Cranial neuropathy	Not described	Survived
Iohexol[85]	52/M	Dural perforation	ATCS at 30 minutes Coma, hypoxia, fever	Not described	Survived

TABLE SC2–2. Adverse Intrathecal Exposures (*Continued*)

Agent	Age (y) Sex (M,F)	Mechanism	Symptoms	Intervention	Outcome
Ioxitalmate Contrast[104]	48/M	Medication error	ATCS, opisthotonos	Sitting position, intubation 145 mL CSF removal in 10–20 mL aliquots Other adjuncts	Survived
Leucovorin[48]	11/M	Therapeutic error	Seizures	Not described	Died on day 5
Lidocaine, epinephrine, fentanyl[95]					
Patient 1	28/F	Dural perforation	Hypotension, numbness at 5 minutes	20 mL CSF drained within 5 minutes 51% lidocaine recovery, 4% fentanyl recovery	Survived
Patient 2	68/F	Dural perforation	C_5- C_6 sensory impairment at 18 minutes	30 mL CSF drained at 18 minutes 39% lidocaine recovery, 7% fentanyl recovery	Survived
Magnesium sulfate[61]	23/F	Misidentification; 2 mL of 50% magnesium sulfate	Backache, lower extremity motor, weakness sensation intact, normotension	Fowlers position	Recovery within 7 h
Meglumine diatrizoate[86] (ionic contrast)	67/M	Medication error	ATCS at 30 minutes	None	Survived
Mercury antiseptic[97]	69/F	Inadvertent Mercurochrome Injection into CSF fistula	Local pain, nuchal rigidity; coma at 24 hours	Lumbar drain Parenteral chelation	Sensorimotor polyneuropathy Survived
Methotrexate[29]	2/F	Overdose	Headaches	Not specified	Survived
Methotrexate[35]	34/M	Overdose	Confusion, seizures, ARDS; coma at 2 hours	200 mL CSF drained and replaced with 0.9% NaCl. Started at 6 hours in aliquots over 48 hours, then another 150 mL CSF exchange over 36 hours (patient also received intrathecal leucovorin)	Cognitive and motor deficits
Methotrexate[30]	9/M	Overdose	Lower extremity numbness, seizures, flaccid paralysis, cranial neuropathy, posturing	200 mL CSF drained in 30–40 mL aliquots Started at 45 minutes 78% drug recovery	Died
Methotrexate Series I[3]		Overdose			
Patient 1	12/M		Headache, vomiting at 45 minutes	30 mL CSF drained Started at 2 hours. 28% drug recovery	Survived until relapse leukemia
Patient 2	4/M		Not described	10 mL CSF drained at 45 minutes 20% drug recovery	Survived

(*Continued*)

TABLE SC2–2. Adverse Intrathecal Exposures (*Continued*)

Agent	Age (y) Sex (M,F)	Mechanism	Symptoms	Intervention	Outcome
Methotrexate Series II[47]					
Patient 1	4/M	Not described	Not described	250 mL CSF drained in 20 mL aliquots. Replacement with 0.9% NaCl. Started at 5 hours.	Survived
Patient 2	11/M	Not described	Not described	20 mL CSF withdrawn then 210 mL CSF drained in 5 mL aliquots. Replacement with 0.9% NaCl. Started at 3 hours. 31% drug recovery	Survived
Methotrexate[60]	3/F	Medication error: 125 mg	Seizures at 3 hours	No CSF exchange; IV folinic acid rescue and dexamethasone	Survived
Methotrexate[96]	26/M	Medication error: 62 5mg	Immediate pain in leg; coma and flaccid paralysis followed; renal failure	70 mL CSF drained at 2 hours; Ventriculolumbar perfusion with 240 mL 0.9% NaCl over 3 hours; intrathecal administration of 1000 U glucarpidase at 8.5 hours 32% recovery in initial drainage fluid, 58% recovery from perfusion drainage	Survived
Methotrexate[107]	Case series n = 7	Medication errors 155–600 mg	5/7 patients with seizures, some with headache, nausea, vomiting	Various interventions including ventriculolumbar perfusion started within 1 hour with 500 mL 0.9% NaCl over 4 hours	All survived
Methylene blue[31]	Case series n = 14	10–100 mg	Pain headache, paralysis	Not described	11/14 residual paraplegia or weakness
Methylene blue[91]	59/M	6 mL of 1% solution	Vomiting, hypotension day 1; paralysis and urinary retention.	Not described	Paraplegia and death at 5 years
Morphine[87]	45/F	Inadvertent filling wrong port of subcutaneous infusion pump. 450 mg	Seizures, hypertension, subarachnoid hemorrhage	12 mL CSF withdrawn then 550 mL CSF drained at 10 mL/h by gravity over 2–3 days. Other adjuncts.	Survived
Morphine[51]	81/M	5 mg	Coma at 4 hours	50 mL CSF drained over 6 minutes, replacement with 50 mL 0.9% NaCl	Survived
Morphine[115]	47/F	510 mg into wrong port of pump	Myoclonic spasms, coma, seizures, cranial neuropathy, hypertension then hypotension	No CSF interventions	Survived
Neostigmine[63]	26/M	Medication error	Not described	None	Survived
Penicillin[18]	22/M	Dosing error into Ommaya reservoir	Coma, hyporeflexia, tonic-clonic seizures, absence seizures, hypotension at 30 minutes	10 mL CSF withdrawal then ventriculolumbar CSF drainage. Replacement with Ringer lactate over 30 minutes.	Survived

TABLE SC2–2. Adverse Intrathecal Exposures (*Continued*)

Agent	Age (y) Sex (M,F)	Mechanism	Symptoms	Intervention	Outcome
Potassium chloride[67]	42/F	Medication error during labor	Immediate cramps, pain, seizures, normal serum potassium	None	Maternal-fetal death at 3 hours
Rifampin[90]	41/M	Medication error 600 mg	None reported	None	Survived
Tramadol[10]	75/F	Connection error	Diaphoresis, hypotension at 10 minutes. Myoclonic spasms, opisthotonos		Died at 48 hours
Tranexamic acid[113]	49/F	Medication error, wrong route	Immediate back pain, hypertension; seizure at 2 minutes; ventricular fibrillation	None	Died at 1.5 h
Vincristine[64]	5/F	0.9 mg	Headache at 10 hours, opisthotonos, nystagmus, flaccidity	Not described	Died on day 18
Vincristine[88]	2.5/F	3 mg error	Opisthotonos day 2	200 mL CSF drainage in 10 mL aliquots. Replacement with 0.9% NaCl	Died on day 3
Vincristine[58]	27/F	Medication error into Ommaya reservoir	Ascending paralysis	Detail limited- CNS"washout" FFP and "lactate solution" in undefined quantities. Timing not described	Died on day 10
Vincristine[108]	16/M	Mislabeled	Ascending paralysis at 2 hours, fever, coma	None	Died
Vincristine[28]	Adult	Medication error	Ascending paralysis	CSF drainage unreported quantity and replacement with Ringer lactate immediately. Ventriculolumbar perfusion 150 mL/h for > 24 hours then 25 mL FFP in 1L isotonic solution at 75 mL/h for undefined time. 95% recovery of vincristine	Lower extremity neuropathy
Vincristine[33]	4/F	Medication error 1.5 mg	Nystagmus, encephalopathy, ascending paralysis, transient improvement	Immediate drainage 18 mL CSF in 3 mL aliquots. Replacement 0.9% NaCl. An additional 30–40 mL drained over 30 minutes, starting at 10 minutes. Ventriculolumbar perfusion using Plasmalyte to replace 200 mL CSF over at unknown rate. Then 6 mL FFP in 250 mL Plasmalyte at 50 mL/h for 4 hours.	Died on day 13
Vincristine[4]	1.25/M	0.7mg	Febrile and irritable at 10 hours then lower ext pain, nuchal rigidity, opisthotonos, ileus, hypotonia at day 2; ascending paralysis, encephalopathy by day 5; respiratory arrest at day 7	Intrathecal corticosteroids at 10 hours	Died on day 75 (withdrawal of life support)

(*Continued*)

TABLE SC2–2. Adverse Intrathecal Exposures (*Continued*)

Agent	Age (y) Sex (M,F)	Mechanism	Symptoms	Intervention	Outcome
Vincristine[5]	7/F	0.5 mg	Ascending weakness, pain, paraplegia	Upright position; immediate drainage 75 mL CSF within 15 minutes, replaced with Ringer lactate; ventriculolumbar perfusion started within 2 hours with 150 mL/h of Ringer lactate for 10 hours then FFP I15 mL in 1L Ringer lactate as irrigant at 55 mL/h for 24 hours. Other adjuncts	Paraplegia, neurogenic bladder; survived
Vincristine[6]	12/F	Medication error: 2 mg	Asymptomatic for 48 hours, then ascending paralysis, hiccup, cranial neuropathy, coma	35 mL CSF drained at 30 minutes then additional drainage of 15 mL CSF replaced with Ringer lactate; ventriculolumbar perfusion at 3 hours using FFP 15 mL in 1L Ringer lactate for total drainage of 615 mL CSF over 10 h; 0.785 mg recovered	Died on day 83
Vincristine[14]	23/M	Error: 2 mg	Headache day 1; leg weakness at day 2–3; ascending myeloencephalopathy with coma at day 10; seizures	Drainage of 100 mL CSF at 10 minutes, "large volume lumbar punctures" day 2 and 3	Prolonged coma, died at 11 months
Vincristine series[26]		Medication error			
	5/F		Ascending paralysis, opisthotonos, coma	Not described	Died on day 7
	57/M		Ascending paralysis	"Flushing the subarachnoid space"	Died at 4 weeks
Vincristine[56]	3/M	Medication error	Leg pain day 1; headache, nuchal rigidity at day 2; bladder dysfunction, fever, lower extremity paralysis, opisthotonos at day 3, coma	Not described	Died on day 6
Vincristine[68]	59/F	Medication error into ommaya reservoir; 2 mg	Nausea, vomiting day 1; altered mental status, tremor, chills, hiccups, nystagmus, coma over 1 week.	50 mL CSF drainage at 10 minutes followed by 75 mL CSF drainage at 30 mintes; ventriculolumbar perfusion with Ringer lactate and FFP over 24 hours	Died on day 40
Vincristine[69]	10/F	Medication error	Asymptomatic for 6 days, then ascending paralysis with incontinence	Immediate drainage of CSF for 15 minutes; epidural catheter above the lumbar drainage site with lumbolumbar irrigation using 12.5 mL FFP in 500 mL Ringer lactate with 96 mL drained; ventriculolumbar perfusion within 90 minutes for 24 hours	Survived with sensory-motor deficits of the extremities and urinary incontinence

TABLE SC2–2. Adverse Intrathecal Exposures (*Continued*)

Agent	Age (y) Sex (M,F)	Mechanism	Symptoms	Intervention	Outcome
Vindesine[101]	25/F	Medication error	Ascending parethesia, paraplegia, coma	40 mL drainage immediately. Subsequent irrigation delayed by 24 hours	Died at 6 weeks
Vincristine[92]	5.5/	1.2 mg	Headache, vomiting and backache at 3 h, nystagmus, extremity weakness at 72 h, autinoimic instability, hiccups, encephalopathy	Drainage of 20 mL CSF at 30 min, repeated on day 2, intrathecal corticosteroids, 23% recovery of dose	Died on day 12
Vincristine[93]	29/F	2 mg	Headache, ascending paraplegia, cranial neuropathy, coma	Intrathecal infusion 5mL 0.9% NaCl with drainage of 10 mL CSF, positioned upright, additional 60 mL CSF drained at 3 hours	Died on day 14, pulmonary embolus at autopsy
Zinconitide series[78]		Overtitration of therapeutic dosage in each case			
	47/M		Nystagmus, auditory and visual hallucinations, dysmetria, ataxia	Not described	Resolution with discontinuation of medication
	62/M (for pain of multiple sclerosis)		Agitation, disorientation, waxing and waning mental status, hallucinations, allodynia, bradycardia	Not described	Resolution with discontinuation of medication. Worsening MS at 1 year
	45/M		Nausea, lightheadedness, nystagmus, bradycardia, agitation	Not described	Resolution with discontinuation

CSF = cerebrospinal fluid

ARDS = adult respiratory distress syndrome; ATCS = ascending tonic clonic syndrome- myoclonus, hyperreflexia on minimal stimulation, beginning in the lower extremities.

CSF = cerebrospinal fluid; FFP = fresh frozen plasma

PUMP MALFUNCTIONS AND ERRORS

Some implantable pumps contain two access sites, one of which is contiguous with the intrathecal space and allows for CSF withdrawal or injection of nonionic contrast media for imaging. The other pump is a depot port that is intermittently filled with concentrated amounts of drug (usually an opioid analgesic or baclofen) to be delivered through a programmable pump. In some patients a template must be placed on the skin overlying subcutaneous pumps to ascertain the proper medication port. Errors occur when a concentrated bolus is inadvertently injected into the wrong port resulting in a massive, sometimes fatal, overdose.[49,111] Massive intrathecal morphine overdose can have severe rapid symptoms, including hypertensive crises. Either reaccessing the CSF port immediately or placing spinal needle into the intrathecal space at another site is critical for the withdrawal of CSF. Large volume drainage with isotonic fluid replacement is required, as well as other supportive measures such as intravenous naloxone. The patients usually require intubation and care in an intensive care unit. The clinical service that placed the pump should be consulted to assist in further CSF access and perform interrogation of the pump in cases where malfunction is suspected.[27] If the consultant is not readily available, emptying the deport port will automatically cause the pump motor to stop.

The other pump problem encountered is sudden, insufficient delivery of either baclofen or opioid pain medication.[81] This may occur because of pump malfunction. Alternatively the intrathecal catheter may kink, migrate, or become obstructed by an inflammatory mass.[22,23,49,74] Patients with chronic use of baclofen or morphine may suffer severe withdrawal symptoms when intrathecal delivery is disrupted.[106] Intrathecal doses are 100 to 1000 times more potent than the equivalent dose administered intravenously.[52] The patients may therefore require very high oral or intravenous doses to treat withdrawal until intrathecal delivery can be reestablished. The clinical service that implanted the pump should be consulted, and a thorough neurologic examination should be performed to evaluate for spinal cord compression symptoms.[49] An anteroposterior and lateral radiograph can be obtained to assess for kinking or fracture of the catheter.

SUMMARY

Intrathecal medication errors can be life threatening. Rapid intervention with CSF drainage should be considered when a dosing or medication error occurs. More aggressive therapies may be required for chemotherapeutic medications, depending on the administered agent.

REFERENCES

1. Aalfs RL, Connelly JF. Comment: dilution of vancomycin for intrathecal or intraventricular administration. *Ann Pharmacother.* 1996;30:415.
2. Abrutyn E, Berlin JA. Intrathecal therapy in tetanus. A meta-analysis. *JAMA.* 1991;266:2262-2267.
3. Addiego JE, Jr, Ridgway D, Bleyer WA. The acute management of intrathecal methotrexate overdose: pharmacologic rationale and guidelines. *J Pediatr.* 1981;98:825-828.
4. al Fawaz IM. Fatal myeloencephalopathy due to intrathecal vincristine administration. *Ann Trop Paediatr.* 1992;12:339-342.
5. Al Ferayan A, Russell NA, Al Wohaibi M, et al. Cerebrospinal fluid lavage in the treatment of inadvertent intrathecal vincristine injection. *Childs Nervous System.* 1999;15:87-89.
6. Alcaraz A, Rey C, Concha A, Medina A. Intrathecal vincristine: fatal myeloencephalopathy despite cerebrospinal fluid perfusion. *J Toxicol Clin Toxicol.* 2002;40:557-561.
7. Arico M, Nespoli L, Porta F, et al. Severe acute encephalopathy following inadvertent intrathecal doxorubicin administration. *Med Pediatr Oncol.* 1990;18:261-263.
8. Arlt S, Cepek L, Rustenbeck HH, et al. Gadolinium encephalopathy due to accidental intrathecal administration of gadopentetate dimeglumine. *J Neurol.* 2007;254:810-812.
9. Balis FM, Blaney SM, McCully CL, et al. Methotrexate distribution within the subarachnoid space after intraventricular and intravenous administration. *Cancer Chemother Pharmacol.* 2000;45:259-264.
10. Barrett NA, Sundaraj SR. Inadvertent intrathecal injection of tramadol. *Br J Anaesth.* 2003;91:918-920.
11. Bearer EL, Schlief ML, Breakefield XO, et al. Squid axoplasm supports the retrograde axonal transport of herpes simplex virus. *Biol Bull.* 1999;197:257-258.
12. Benifla M, Zucker G, Cohen A, Alkan M. Successful treatment of Acinetobacter meningitis with intrathecal polymyxin E. *J Antimicrob Chemother.* 2004;54:290-292.
13. Berning SE, Cherry TA, Iseman MD. Novel treatment of meningitis caused by multidrug-resistant Mycobacterium tuberculosis with intrathecal levofloxacin and amikacin: case report. *Clin Infect Dis.* 2001;32: 643-646.
14. Bleck TP, Jacobsen J. Prolonged survival following the inadvertent intrathecal administration of vincristine: Clinical and electrophysiologic analyses. *Clin Neuropharmacol.* 1991;14:457-462.
15. Bomgaars L, Geyer JR, Franklin J, et al. Phase I trial of intrathecal liposomal cytarabine in children with neoplastic meningitis. *J Clin Oncol.* 2004;22:3916-3921.
16. Bonicalzi V, Canavero S. Intrathecal ziconotide for chronic pain. *JAMA.* 2004;292:1681-1682.
17. Brossner G, Engelhardt K, Beer R, et al. Accidental intrathecal infusion of cefotiam: clinical presentation and management. *Eur J Clin Pharmacol.* 2004;60:373-375.
18. Callaghan JT, Ausman JI, Clubb R. CSF perfusion to treat intraventricular penicillin toxicity. *Arch Neurol.* 1981;38:390-391.
19. Cardan E. Intrathecal frusemide. *Anaesthesia.* 1985;40:1025.
20. Chiari A, Lorber C, Eisenach JC, et al. Analgesic and hemodynamic effects of intrathecal clonidine as the sole analgesic agent during first stage of labor: a dose-response study. *Anesthesiology.* 1999;91:388-396.
21. Clara N. CSF exchange after the erroneous intrathecal injection of 800 mg ceftriaxone for pneumococcal meningitis. *J Antimicrob Chemother.* 1986;17:263-265.
22. Coffey RJ, Burchiel K. Inflammatory mass lesions associated with intrathecal drug infusion catheters: report and observations on 41 patients. *Neurosurgery.* 2002;50:78-86.
23. Coffey RJ, Edgar TS, Francisco GE, et al. Abrupt withdrawal from intrathecal baclofen: recognition and management of a potentially life-threatening syndrome.[erratum appears in *Arch Phys Med Rehabil.* 2002;83:1479]. *Arch Phys Med Rehabil.* 2002;83:735-741.
24. Collier C. Collapse after epidural injection following inadvertant dural perforation. *Anesthesiology.* 1982;57:427-428.
25. Corpus KA, Weber KB, Zimmerman CR. Intrathecal amikacin for the treatment of pseudomonal meningitis. *Ann Pharmacother.* 2004;38: 992-995.
26. Dettmeyer R, Driever F, Becker A, et al. Fatal myeloencephalopathy due to accidental intrathecal vincristin administration: a report of two cases. *Forensic Sci Int.* 2001;122:60-64.
27. Dressnandt J, Weinzierl FX, Tolle TR, et al. Acute overdose of intrathecal baclofen. *J Neurol.* 1996;243:482-483.
28. Dyke RW. Treatment of inadvertent intrathecal injection of vincristine. *N Engl J Med.* 1989;321:1270-1271.
29. Ettinger LJ, Freeman AI, Creaven PJ. Intrathecal methotrexate overdose without neurotoxicity: case report and literature review. *Cancer.* 1978;41:1270-1273.
30. Ettinger LJ. Pharmacokinetics and biochemical effects of a fatal intrathecal methotrexate overdose. *Cancer.* 1982;50:444-450.
31. Evans JP, Keegan HR. Danger in the use of intrathecal methylene blue. *JAMA.* 1960;174:856-859.
32. Evans PJ, Lloyd JW, Wood GJ. Accidental intrathecal injection of bupivacaine and dextran. *Anaesthesia.* 1981;36:685-687.
33. Fernandez CV, Esau R, Hamilton D, et al. Intrathecal vincristine: an analysis of reasons for recurrent fatal chemotherapeutic error with recommendations for prevention. *J Pediatr Hematol Oncol.* 1998;20: 587-590.
34. Ferrara VL. Post myelographic nerve palsy in association with contrast agent iopanidol. *J Clin Neuroophthalmol.* 1991;11:74.
35. Finkelstein Y, Zevin S, Heyd J, et al. Emergency treatment of life-threatening intrathecal methotrexate overdose. *Neurotoxicology.* 2004;25: 407-410.
36. Fujita T, Kayama T, Sato I, et al. MRSA meningitis and intrathecal injection of arbekacin. *Surg Neurol.* 1997;48:69.
37. Gaidys WG, Dickerman JD, Walters CL, Young PC. Intrathecal vincristine. Report of a fatal case despite CNS washout. *Cancer.* 1983;52:799-801.
38. Gilbar PJ, Carrington CV. Preventing intrathecal administration of vincristine. *Med J Austra* 2004;181:464.
39. Goonewardene TW, Sentheshanmuganathan S, Kamalanathan S, Kanagasunderam R. Accidental subarachnoid injection of gallamine. A case report. *Brit J Anaesth.* 1975;47:889-893.
40. Gopal G. Preliminary studies on cerebrospinal fluid exchange transfusion. *Indian Pediatr.* 1979;16:227-228.
41. Gosselin S, Isbister GK. Re: Treatment of accidental intrathecal methotrexate overdose. *J Natl Cancer Inst.* 2005;97:609-610.
42. Govindan K, Krishnan R, Kaufman MP, et al. Intrathecal ketamine in surgeries for lower abdomen and lower extremities. *Proc West Pharmacol Soc.* 2001;44:197-199.
43. Hew CM, Cyna AM, Simmons SW. Avoiding inadvertent epidural injection of drugs intended for non-epidural use. *Anaesth Intensive Care.* 2003;31: 44-49.
44. Hocking G, Wildsmith JA. Intrathecal drug spread. *Br J Anaesth.* 2004;93:568-578.
45. Hodgson PS, Neal JM, Pollock JE, Liu SS. The neurotoxicity of drugs given intrathecally (spinal). *Anesth Analg.* 1999;88:797-809.
46. Huang TY, Chung HW, Chen MY, et al. Supratentorial cerebrospinal fluid production rate in healthy adults: quantification with two-dimensional cine phase-contrast MR imaging with high temporal and spatial resolution. *Radiology.* 2004;233:603-608.
47. Jakobson AM, Kreuger A, Mortimer O, et al. Cerebrospinal fluid exchange after intrathecal methotrexate overdose. A report of two cases. *Acta Paediatrica.* 1992;81:359-361.

48. Jardine LF, Ingram LC, Bleyer WA. Intrathecal leucovorin after intrathecal methotrexate overdose. *J Pediatr Hematol Oncol.* 1996;18:302-304.
49. Jones TF, Feler CA, Simmons BP, et al. Neurologic complications including paralysis after a medication error involving implanted intrathecal catheters. *Am J Med.* 2002;112:31-36.
50. Jordan B, Pasquier Y, Schnider A. Neurological improvement and rehabilitation potential following toxic myelopathy due to intrathecal injection of doxorubicin. *Spinal Cord.* 2004;42:371-373.
51. Kaiser KG, Bainton CR. Treatment of intrathecal morphine overdose by aspiration of cerebrospinal fluid. *Anesth Analg.* 1987;66:475-477.
52. Kao LW, Amin Y, Kirk MA, Turner MS. Intrathecal baclofen withdrawal mimicking sepsis. *J Emerg Med.* 2003;24:423-427.
53. Kaplan KM, Brose WG. Intrathecal methods. *Neurosurg Clin N Am.* 2004;15:289-296.
54. Kavan P, Valkova J, Koutecky J. Management and sequelae after misapplied intrathecal dactinomycin. *Med Pediatr Oncol.* 2001;36:339-340.
55. Kroin JS, Ali A,York M, Penn RD. The distribution of medication along the spinal canal after chronic intrathecal administration. *Neurosurg* 1993;33;226-230.
56. Kwack EK, Kim DJ, Park TI, et al. Neural toxicity induced by accidental intrathecal vincristine administration. *J Korean Med Sci.* 1999;14: 688-692.
57. Lafolie P, Liliemark J, Bjork O, et al. Exchange of cerebrospinal fluid in accidental intrathecal overdose of cytarabine. *Med Toxicol Adverse Drug Exp.* 1988;3:248-252.
58. Lau G. Accidental intraventricular vincristine administration: an avoidable iatrogenic death. *Med Sci Law.* 1996;36:263-265.
59. Lauretti GR, Reis MP, Prado WA, Klamt JG. Dose-response study of intrathecal morphine versus intrathecal neostigmine, their combination, or placebo for postoperative analgesia in patients undergoing anterior and posterior vaginoplasty. *Anesth Analg.* 1996;82:1182-1187.
60. Lee AC, Wong KW, Fong KW, So KT. Intrathecal methotrexate overdose. [see comment]. *Acta Paediatrica.* 1997;86:434-437.
61. Lejuste MJ. Inadvertant intrathecal administration of magnesium sulfate. *S Afr Med J.* 1985;68:367-368.
62. Mahajan R, Gupta R. Cerebrospinal fluid physiology and cerebrospinal fluid drainage. *Anesthesiology.* 2004;100:1620.
63. Maheshwari S, Sharma K, Chawla R, Bhattyacharya A. Accidental intrathecal injection of a very large dose of neostigmine methylsulphate. *Indian J Anaesth.* 2003;47:299-301.
64. Manelis J, Freudlich E, Ezekiel E, Doron J. Accidental intrathecal vincristine administration. Report of a case. *J Neurol.* 1982;228:209-213.
65. Mason N, Gondret R, Junca A, Bonnet F. Intrathecal sufentanil and morphine for post-thoracotomy pain relief. *Br J Anaesth.* 2001;86:236-240.
66. Matsubara H, Makimoto A, Higa T, et al. Successful treatment of meningoencephalitis caused by methicillin-resistant Staphylococcus aureus with intrathecal vancomycin in an allogeneic peripheral blood stem cell transplant recipient. *Bone Mar Trans.* 2003;31:65-67.
67. Meel B. Inadvertent intrathecal administration of potassium chloride during routine spinal anesthesia: case report. *Am J Forens Med Pathol.* 1998;19:255-257.
68. Meggs WJ, Hoffman RS. Fatality resulting from intraventricular vincristine administration. *J Toxicol Clin Toxicol.* 1998;36:243-246.
69. Michelagnoli MP, Bailey CC, Wilson I, et al. Potential salvage therapy for inadvertent intrathecal administration of vincristine.[erratum appears in *Br J Haematol.* 1998;101:398]. *Br J Haematol.* 1997;99:364-367.
70. Oka K, Yamamoto M, Nonaka T, Tomonaga M. The significance of artificial cerebrospinal fluid as perfusate and endoneurosurgery. *Neurosurgery.* 1996;38:733-736.
71. O'Marcaigh AS, Johnson CM, Smithson WA, et al. Successful treatment of intrathecal methotrexate overdose by using ventriculolumbar perfusion and intrathecal instillation of carboxypeptidase G2. *Mayo Clin Proc.* 1996;71:161-165.
72. Paice JA, Penn RD, Kroin JS. Intrathecal octreotide for relief of intractable nonmalignant pain: 5-year experience with two cases. *Neurosurgery.* 1996;38:203-207.
73. Palmieri C, Barron N, Vigushin DM. The Vincotube System:a design solution to prevent the accidental administration of intrathecal vinca alkaloids. *J Clin Oncol.* 2004;22:965.
74. Peng P, Massicotte EM. Spinal cord compression from intrathecal catheter-tip inflammatory mass: case report and a review of etiology. *Reg Anesth Pain Med.* 2004;29:237-242.
75. Penn RD, Kroin JS. Treatment of intrathecal morphine overdose. *J Neurosurg.* 1995;82:147-148.
76. Penn RD, Martin EM, Wilson RS, et al. Intraventricular bethanechol infusion for Alzheimer's disease: results of double-blind and escalating-dose trials. *Neurology.* 1988;38:219-222.
77. Penn RD, Paice JA, Kroin JS. Octreotide: a potent new non-opiate analgesic for intrathecal infusion. *Pain.* 1992;49:13-19.
78. Penn RD, Paice JA. Adverse effects associated with intrathecal administration of zinconitide. *Pain.* 2000;85:291-296.
79. Penn RD. Intrathecal medication delivery. Neurosurg Clinics of North America 2003;14:381-387.
80. Qweider M, et al. Inadvertant intrathecal vincristine administration: a neurosurgical emergency. *J Neurosurg Spine.* 2007;6:280-283.
81. Reeves RK, Stolp-Smith KA, Christopherson MW. Hyperthermia, rhabdomyolysis, and disseminated intravascular coagulation associated with baclofen pump catheter failure. *Arch Phys Med Rehabil.* 1998;79: 353-356.
82. Reiber H. Flow rate of cerebrospinal fluid (CSF)—a concept common to normal blood-CSF barrier function and to dysfunction in neurological diseases. *J Neurol Sci.* 1994;122:189-203.
83. Root T. Accidental injection of vincristine. *J Oncol Phar Pract.* 2005;11:35.
84. Rosati G, Leto di Priolo S, Tirone P. Serious or fatal complications after inadvertent administration of ionic water-soluble contrast media in myelography. *Eur J Radiol.* 1992;15:95-100.
85. Rosenberg H, Grant M. Ascending tonic-clonic syndrome secondary to intrathecal omnipaque. *J Clin Anesth.* 2004;16:299-300.
86. Salvolini U, Bonetti MG, Ciritella P. Accidental intrathecal injection of ionic water-soluble contrast medium: report of a case, including treatment. *Neuroradiology.* 1996;38:349-351.
87. Sauter K. Correction: treatment of high dose intrathecal morphine overdose. *J Neurosurg.* 1994;81:813.
88. Schochet SS Jr, Lampert PW, Earle KM. Neuronal changes induced by intrathecal vincristine sulfate. *J Neuropathol Exp Neurol.* 1968;27:645-658.
89. Segal-Maurer S, Mariano N, Qavi A, et al. Successful treatment of ceftazidime-resistant Klebsiella pneumoniae ventriculitis with intravenous meropenem and intraventricular polymyxin B: case report and review. *Clin Infect Dis.* 1999;28:1134-1138.
90. Senbaga N, Davies EM. Inadvertent intrathecal administration of rifampicin. *Brit J Clin Pharmacol.* 2005;60:116.
91. Sharr MM, Weller RO, Brice JG. Spinal cord necrosis after intrathecal injection of methylene blue. *J Neurol Neurosurg Psychiatry.* 1978;41: 384-386.
92. Shepherd DA, Steuber CP, Starling KA, Fernbach DJ. Accidental intrathecal administration of vincristine. *Med Pediatr Oncol.* 1978;5:85-88.
93. Slyter H, Liwnicz B, Herrick MK, Mason R. Fatal myeloencephalopathy caused by intrathecal vincristine. *Neurology.* 1980;30:867-871.
94. Smilack J, McCloskey RV. Intrathecal gentamicin. *Ann Intern Med.* 1972;77:1002-1003.
95. Southorn P, Vasdev GM, Chantigian RC, Lawson GM. Reducing the potential morbidity of an unintentional spinal anaesthetic by aspirating cerebrospinal fluid. *Br J Anaesth.* 1996;76:467-469.
96. Spiegel RJ, Cooper PR, Blum RH, et al. Treatment of massive intrathecal methotrexate overdose by ventriculolumbar perfusion. *N Engl J Med.* 1984;311:386-388.
97. Stark AM, Barth H, Grabner JP, Mehdorn HM. Accidental intrathecal mercury application. *Eur Spine J.* 2004;13:241-243.
98. Stefanou A, Dooley M. Simple method to eliminate risk of inadvertent intrathecal vincristine administration. *J Clin Oncol.* 2003:21:2044.
99. Svensson LG, Grum DF, Bednarski M, et al. Appraisal of cerebrospinal fluid alterations during aortic surgery with intrathecal papaverine administration and cerebrospinal fluid drainage. *J Vasc Surg.* 1990;11: 423-429.
100. Tartiere J, Gerard JL, Peny J, et al. Acute treatment after accidental intrathecal injection of hypertonic contrast media. *Anesthesiology.* 1989; 71:169.
101. Tournel G, Bécart-Robert A, Courtin P, et al. Fatal accidental intrathecal injection of vindesine. *J Forensic Sci.* 2006;51:1166-1168.
102. Trinkle R, Wu JK. Intrathecal methotrexate overdoses.[comment]. *Acta Paediatr.* 1998;87:116-117.
103. Tsui BC, Malherbe S, Koller J, Aronyk K. Reversal of an unintentional spinal anesthetic by cerebrospinal lavage. *Anesth Analg.* 2004;98: 434-436.

104. van der Leede H, Jorens PG, Parizel P, Cras P. Inadvertent intrathecal use of ionic contrast agent. *Eur Radiol.* 2002;12:S86-S93.
105. Vasen W, Desmery P, Ilutovich S, Di Martino A. Intrathecal use of colistin. *J Clin Microbiol.* 2000;38:3523.
106. Walker RH, Danisi FO, Swope DM, et al. Intrathecal baclofen for dystonia: benefits and complications during six years of experience. *Mov Disord.* 2000;15:1242-1247.
107. Widemann BC, Balis FM, Shalabi A, et al. Treatment of accidental intrathecal methotrexate overdose with intrathecal carboxypeptidase G2. *J Natl Cancer Inst.* 2004;96:1557-1559.
108. Williams ME, Walker AN, Bracikowski JP, et al. Ascending myeloencephalopathy due to intrathecal vincristine sulfate. A fatal chemotherapeutic error. *Cancer.* 1983;51:2041-2047.
109. Wolman L. The neuropathological effects resulting from the intrathecal injection of chemical substances. *Paraplegia.* 1966;4:97-115.
110. Woods K. The prevention of intrathecal medication errors. A report to the Chief Medical Officer. Department of Health, UK, Crown Copyright. 2001.
111. Wu CL, Patt RB. Accidental overdose of systemic morphine during intended refill of intrathecal infusion device. *Anesth Analg.* 1992;75:130-132.
112. Yegin A, Sanli S, Dosemeci L, et al. The analgesic and sedative effects of intrathecal midazolam in perianal surgery. *Eur J Anaesthesiol.* 2004;21:658-662.
113. Yeh HM, Lau HP, Lin PL, et al. Convulsions and refractory ventricular fibrillation after intrathecal injection of a massive dose of tranexamic acid. *Anesthesiology.* 2003;98:270-272.
114. Yeh RN, Nypaver MM, Deegan TJ, Ayyangar R. Baclofen toxicity in an 8-year-old with an intrathecal baclofen pump. *J Emerg Med.* 2004;26:163-167.
115. Yilmaz A, Sogut A, Kilinc M, Sogut AG. Successful treatment of intrathecal morphine overdose. *Neurol India.* 2003;51:410-411.

CHAPTER 38
OPIOIDS

Lewis S. Nelson and Dean Olsen

Morphine

Opioids are among the oldest therapies in our armamentarium, and clinicians recognize their universal utility to limit human distress from pain. Although opioids enjoy widespread use as potent analgesics, they have the potential for abuse because of their psychoactive properties. Although the therapeutic and toxic doses are difficult to predict because of the development of tolerance with chronic use, the primary adverse event from excessive dosing is respiratory depression.

HISTORY AND EPIDEMIOLOGY

The medicinal value of opium, the dried extract of the poppy plant *Papaver somniferum*, was first recorded around 1500 B.C. in the Ebers papyrus. Raw opium is typically composed of at least 10% morphine, but extensive variability exists depending on the environment in which the poppy is grown.[82] Although reformulated as laudanum (deodorized tincture of opium; 10 mg morphine/mL) by Paracelsus, paregoric (camphorated tincture of opium; 0.4 mg morphine/mL), Dover's powder (pulvis Doveri), and Godfrey's cordial in later centuries, the contents remained largely the same: phenanthrene poppy derivatives, such as morphine and codeine. Over the centuries since the Ebers papyrus, opium and its components have been exploited in two distinct manners: medically to produce profound analgesia and nonmedically to produce psychoactive effects.

Currently, the widest clinical application of opioids is for acute or chronic pain relief. Opioids are available in various formulations that allow administration by virtually any route: epidural, inhalational, intranasal, intrathecal, oral, parenteral (ie, subcutaneous [SC], intravenous [IV], intramuscular [IM]), rectal, transdermal, and transmucosal. Patients also may benefit from several of the nonanalgesic effects engendered by certain opioids. For example, codeine and hydrocodone are widely used as antitussives, and diphenoxylate as an antidiarrheal.

Unfortunately, the history of opium and its derivatives is marred by humankind's endless quest for xenobiotics that produce pleasurable effects. Opium smoking was so problematic in China by the 1830s that the Chinese government attempted to prohibit the importation of opium by the British East India Company. This act led to the Opium Wars between China and Britain. China eventually accepted the importation and sale of the drug and was forced to turn over Hong Kong to British rule. The euphoric and addictive potential of the opioids is immortalized in the works of several famous writers, such as Thomas de Quincey (*Confessions of an English Opium Eater*, 1821), Samuel Coleridge (*The Rime of the Ancient Mariner*, 1798), and Elizabeth Barrett Browning (*Aurora Leigh*, 1856).

Because of mounting concerns of addiction and toxicity in the United States, the Harrison Narcotic Act, enacted in 1914, made nonmedicinal use of opioids illegal. Since that time, recreational and habitual use of heroin and other opioids have remained epidemic in the United States and worldwide despite extensive and diverse attempts to curb their availability.

Morphine was isolated from opium by Armand Séquin in 1804. Charles Alder Wright synthesized heroin from morphine in 1874. Ironically, the development and marketing of heroin as an antitussive agent by Bayer, the German pharmaceutical company, in 1898 legitimized the medicinal role of heroin.[153] Subsequently, various xenobiotics with opioidlike effects were marketed, each promoted for its presumed advantages over morphine. This assertion proved true for fentanyl because of its pharmacokinetic profile. However, in general, the advantages of such medications have fallen short of expectations, particularly with regard to their potential for abuse.

The terminology used in this chapter recognizes the broad range of xenobiotics commonly considered to be opiumlike. The term *opiate* specifically refers to the relevant alkaloids naturally derived directly from the opium poppy: morphine; codeine; and, to some extent, thebaine and noscapine. *Opioids* are a much broader class of xenobiotics that are capable of either producing opiumlike effects or binding to opioid receptors. A *semisynthetic opioid*, such as heroin or oxycodone, is created by chemical modification of an opiate. A *synthetic opioid* is a chemical, not derived from an opiate, that is capable of binding to an opioid receptor and producing opioid effects clinically. Synthetic opioids, such as methadone and meperidine, bear little structural similarity to the opiates. Opioids also include the naturally occurring animal-derived opioid peptides such as endorphin and nociceptin/orphanin FQ. The term *narcotic* refers to sleep-inducing xenobiotics and initially was used to connote the opioids. However, law enforcement and the public currently use the term to indicate any illicit psychoactive substance. The term *opioid* as used hereafter encompasses the opioids and the opiates.

PHARMACOLOGY

OPIOID-RECEPTOR SUBTYPES

Despite nearly a century of opioid studies, the existence of specific opioid receptors was not proposed until the mid-20th century. Beckett and Casy noted a pronounced stereospecificity of existing opioids (only the L-isomer is active) and postulated that the drug needed to "fit" into a receptor.[7] In 1963, after studies on the clinical interactions of nalorphine and morphine, the theory of receptor dualism[155] postulated the existence of two classes of opioid receptors. Such opioid binding sites were not demonstrated experimentally until 1973.[126] Intensive experimental scrutiny using selective agonists and antagonists continues to permit refinement of receptor classification. The current, widely accepted schema postulates the coexistence of three major classes of opioid receptors, each with multiple subtypes, and several poorly defined minor classes.

Initially, the reason such an elaborate system of receptors existed was unclear because no endogenous ligand could be identified. However, evidence for the existence of such endogenous ligands was uncovered in 1975 with the discovery of metenkephalin and leuenkephalin[102] and the subsequent identification of β-endorphin and dynorphin. As a group, these endogenous ligands for the opioid receptors are called *endorphins* (*endo*genous mo*rphine*). Each is a five–amino acid peptide cleaved from a larger precursor peptide: proenkephalin, proopiomelanocortin, and prodynorphin, respectively. More recently, a minor related endogenous opioid (nociceptin/orphanin FQ) and its receptor ORL have been described.

All three major opioid receptors have been cloned and sequenced. Each consists of seven transmembrane segments, an amino terminus, and a carboxy terminus. Significant sequence homology exists between the transmembrane regions of opioid receptors and those of other members of the guanosine triphosphate (GTP)–binding protein (G-protein)–binding receptor superfamily. However, the extracellular and intracellular segments differ from one another. These nonhomologous segments probably represent the ligand-binding and signal transduction regions, respectively, which would be expected to differ among the three classes of receptors. The individual receptors have distinct distribution patterns within the central nervous system (CNS) and peripherally on nerve endings within various tissues, mediating unique but not entirely understood clinical effects. Until recently, researchers used varying combinations of agonists and antagonists to pharmacologically distinguish between the different receptor subtypes. However, knockout mice (ie, mutant mice lacking the genes for an individual opioid receptor) promise new insights into this complex subject.[51]

Because multiple opioid receptors exist and each elicits a different effect, determining the receptor to which an opioid preferentially binds should allow prediction of the clinical effect of the opioid. However, binding typically is not limited to one receptor type, and the relative affinity of an opioid for differing receptors accounts for the clinical effects (Table 38-1). Even the endogenous opioid peptides exhibit substantial crossover among the receptors.

Although the familiar pharmacologic nomenclature derived from the Greek alphabet is used throughout this textbook, the International Union of Pharmacology (IUPHAR) Committee on Receptor Nomenclature has twice recommended a nomenclature change from the original Greek symbol system to make opioid receptor names more consistent with those of other neurotransmitter systems.[173] In the first new schema, the receptors were denoted by their endogenous ligand (*o*pioid *p*eptide [OP]), with a subscript identifying their chronologic order of discovery.[37] The δ receptor was renamed OP_1, the κ receptor was renamed OP_2, and the μ receptor was renamed OP_3. However, adoption of this nomenclature met with significant resistance, presumably because of problems that would arise when merging previously published work that had used the Greek symbol nomenclature. The currently proposed nomenclature suggests the addition of a single letter in front of the OP designation and the elimination of the number. In this schema, the μ receptor is identified as MOP. In addition, the latest iteration formally recognizes the nociceptin/orphanin FQ or NOP receptor as a fourth receptor family.

TABLE 38–1. Clinical Effects Related to Opioid Receptors

1996 Conventional Name	Proposed IUPHAR Name	IUPHAR Name	Important Clinical Effects of Receptor Agonists
μ_1	OP_{3a}	MOP	Supraspinal analgesia
			Peripheral analgesia
			Sedation
			Euphoria
			Prolactin release
μ_2	OP_{3b}		Spinal analgesia
			Respiratory depression
			Physical dependence
			GI dysmotility
			Pruritus
			Bradycardia
			Growth hormone release
κ_1	OP_{2a}	KOP	Spinal analgesia
			Miosis
			Diuresis
κ_2	OP_{2b}		Psychotomimesis
			Dysphoria
κ_3	OP_{2b}		Supraspinal analgesia
δ	OP_1	DOP	Spinal and supraspinal analgesia
			Modulation of μ-receptor function
			Inhibit release of dopamine
Nociceptin/ orphanin FQ	OP_4	NOP	Anxiolysis
			Analgesia

GI, gastrointestinal; IUPHAR, International Union of Pharmacology Committee on Receptor Nomenclature.

Mu Receptor (μ, MOP, OP_3) The early identification of the μ receptor as the *m*orphine binding site gave this receptor its designation.[109] Although many exogenous xenobiotics produce supraspinal analgesia via μ receptors, the endogenous ligand is elusive. Nearly all of the recognized endogenous opioids have some affinity for the μ receptor, although none is selective for the receptor. Endomorphin-1 and -2 are nonpeptide ligands present in brain that may represent the endogenous ligand.

Experimentally, two subtypes (μ_1 and μ_2) are well defined, although currently no xenobiotics have sufficient selectivity to make this dichotomy clinically relevant. Experiments with knockout mice suggest that both subtypes derive from the same gene and that either posttranslational changes or local cellular effects subsequently differentiate them. The μ_1 subtype appears to be responsible for supraspinal (brain) analgesia and for the euphoria sometimes engendered by these xenobiotics. Although stimulation of the μ_2 subtype produces spinal-level analgesia, it also produces respiratory depression. All of the currently available μ agonists have some activity at the μ_2 receptor and therefore produce some degree of respiratory compromise. Localization of μ receptors to regions of the brain involved in analgesia (periaqueductal gray, nucleus raphe magnus, medial thalamus), euphoria and reward (mesolimbic system), and respiratory function (medulla) is not unexpected.[69] Predictably, μ receptors are found in the medullary cough center, peripherally in the gastrointestinal (GI) tract, and on various sensory nerve endings, including the articular surfaces (see analgesia under Clinical Manifestations below).

Kappa Receptor (κ, KOP, OP_2) Although dynorphins now are known to be the endogenous ligands for these receptors, originally they were identified by their ability to bind ketocyclazocine and thus were labeled κ.[109] κ receptors exist predominantly in the spinal cords of higher animals, but they also are found in the antinociceptive regions of the brain and the substantia nigra. Stimulation is responsible for spinal analgesia, miosis, and diuresis (via inhibition of antidiuretic hormone release). Unlike μ-receptor stimulation, κ-receptor stimulation is not associated with significant respiratory depression or constipation. The receptor currently is subclassified into three subtypes. The κ_1 receptor subtype is responsible for spinal analgesia. This analgesia is not reversed by μ-selective antagonists,[116] supporting the role of κ receptors as independent mediators of analgesia. Although the function of the κ_2 receptor subtype is largely unknown, stimulation of cerebral κ_2 receptors by xenobiotics such as pentazocine and salvinorin A produces psychotomimesis in distinction to the euphoria evoked by μ agonists.[144] The κ_3 receptor subtype is found throughout the brain and participates in supraspinal analgesia. This receptor is primarily responsible for the action of nalorphine, an agonist–antagonist opioid. Nalbuphine, another agonist–antagonist, exerts its analgesic effect via both κ_1 and κ_3 agonism, although both nalorphine and nalbuphine are antagonists to morphine at the μ receptor.[128]

Delta Receptor (δ, DOP, OP_1) Little is known about δ receptors, although the enkephalins are known to be their endogenous ligands.

Opioid peptides identified in the skin and brain of *Phyllomedusa* frogs, termed *dermorphin* and *deltorphin*, respectively, are potent agonists at the δ receptor. δ receptors may be important in spinal and supraspinal analgesia (probably via a noncompetitive interaction with the μ receptor) and in cough suppression. δ receptors may mediate dopamine release from the nigrostriatal pathway, where they modulate the motor activity associated with amphetamine.[69] δ receptors do not modulate dopamine in the mesolimbic tracts and have only a slight behavioral reinforcing role. Subpopulations, specifically $\delta_1$and δ_2, are postulated based on in vitro studies but presently are not confirmed in vivo.[173]

Nociceptin/Orphanin FQ Receptor (ORL$_1$, NOP, OP$_4$) The ORL$_1$ receptor was identified in 1994 based on sequence homology during screening for opioid-receptor genes with DNA libraries. It has a similar distribution pattern in the brain and uses similar transduction mechanisms as the other opioid-receptor subtypes. It binds many different opioid agonists and antagonists. Its insensitivity to antagonism by naloxone, often considered the sine qua non of opioid character, delayed its acceptance as an opioid-receptor subtype. Simultaneous identification of an endogenous ligand, called *nociceptin* by the French discoverers and *orphanin* FQ by the Swiss investigators, allowed the designation OP$_4$. A clinical role has not yet been defined, but anxiolytic and analgesic properties are described.[25]

Sigma Receptor (σ) Although originally conceived as an opioid subtype, the σ receptor is no longer considered opioid in character, and it has not been given an IUPHAR OP designation. Investigation of this receptor revealed that it is insensitive to antagonism by naloxone, prefers ligands with a dextrorotatory stereochemistry, and has no endogenous ligand, all features in contradistinction to the other opioid receptors. Nonetheless, the effects of the σ receptor are relevant to opioid pharmacology because certain opioids, such as dextromethorphan and pentazocine, are σ-receptor agonists. Stimulation of the σ receptor is implicated in psychotomimesis and movement disorders, effects that are reported with both dextromethorphan and pentazocine independently.[65] Hallucinogens, such as ibogaine, and antipsychotics, such as haloperidol, are known σ-receptor antagonists.

Other Receptors (Epsilon [ε], Zeta [ζ]) Two other opioid receptor subtypes are largely uncharacterized in humans. The ε receptor is postulated based on in vivo binding assays and has no known clinical role. The ζ receptor has been proposed and may serve as an opioid growth factor receptor.

OPIOID-RECEPTOR SIGNAL TRANSDUCTION MECHANISMS

Figure 38–1 illustrates opioid-receptor signal transduction mechanisms. Continuing research on the mechanisms by which an opioid receptor induces an effect has produced confusing and often contradictory results. Despite the initial theory that each receptor subtype is linked to a specific transduction mechanism, individual receptor subtypes may use one or more mechanisms, depending on several factors, including receptor localization (eg, presynaptic vs postsynaptic). As noted, all opioid-receptor subtypes are members of a superfamily of membrane-bound receptors that are coupled to G proteins.[173] The G proteins are responsible for signaling the cell that the receptor has been activated and for initiating the desired cellular effects. The G proteins are generally of the pertussis toxin-sensitive, inhibitory subtype known as G_i or G_o, although coupling to a cholera toxin-sensitive, excitatory G_s subtype has been described. Regardless of subsequent effect, the G proteins consist of three conjoined subunits, α, β, and γ. The βγ subunit is liberated upon GTP binding to the subunit. When the α subunit dissociates from the βγ subunit, it modifies specific effector systems, such as phospholipase C or adenylate cyclase, or it may directly affect a channel or transport protein. GTP subsequently is hydrolyzed by a GTPase intrinsic to the α subunit, which prompts its reassociation with the βγ subunit and termination of the receptor-mediated effect.

CLINICAL MANIFESTATIONS

Table 38–2 outlines the clinical effects of opioids.

THERAPEUTIC EFFECTS

Analgesia Although classic teaching attributes opioid analgesia solely to the brain, opioids actually appear to modulate cerebral cortical pain perception at supraspinal, spinal, and peripheral levels. The regional distribution of the opioid receptors confirms that μ receptors are responsible for most of the analgesic effects of morphine within the brain. They are found in highest concentration within areas of the brain classically associated with analgesia—the periaqueductal gray, nucleus raphe magnus, locus ceruleus, and medial thalamus. Microelectrode-induced electrical stimulation of these areas[130] or iontophoretic application of agonists into these regions results in profound analgesia.[9] Specifically, enhancement of inhibitory outflow from these supraspinal areas to the sensory nuclei of the spinal cord (dorsal roots) dampens nociceptive neurotransmission. Additionally, inactivation of the μ-opioid–receptor gene in embryonic mouse cells results in offspring that are insensitive to morphine analgesia.[110]

Interestingly, blockade of the *N*-methyl-D-aspartate (NMDA) receptor, a mediator of excitatory neurotransmission, enhances the analgesic effects of μ-opioid agonists and may reduce the development of tolerance (see Dextromethorphan below).[1] Even more intriguing is the finding that low-dose naloxone (0.25 μg/kg/h) actually improves the efficacy of morphine analgesia.[48] Administration of higher-dose, but still low-dose, naloxone (1 μg/kg/h) obliterated its opioid-sparing effect. Although undefined, the mechanism may be related to selective inhibition of G_s-coupled excitatory opioid receptors by extremely low concentrations of opioid-receptor antagonist.[28,27]

δ and κ receptors also are responsible for mediation of analgesia, but they exert their analgesic effect predominantly in the spinal cord. Conceptually, these receptors modulate nociceptive impulses in transit to the thalamus via the spinothalamic tract, reducing the perception of pain by the brain. Xenobiotics with strong binding affinity for δ receptors in humans produce significantly more analgesia than morphine administered intrathecally. Indeed, the use of spinal and epidural opioid analgesia is predicated on the direct administration of opioid near the κ and δ receptors in the spinal cord. Agonist–antagonist opioids, with agonist affinity for the κ receptor and antagonist effects at the μ receptor, maintain analgesic efficacy.

Interestingly, communication between the immune system and the peripheral sensory nerves occurs in areas of tissue inflammation. In response to inflammatory mediators, such as interleukin-1, immune cells locally release opioid peptides, which bind and activate peripheral opioid receptors on sensory nerve terminals.[174] Agonism at these receptors reduces afferent pain neurotransmission and may inhibit the release of other proinflammatory compounds, such as substance P.[157] Of note, intraarticular morphine (1 mg) administered to patients after arthroscopic knee surgery produces significant, long-lasting analgesia that can be prevented with intraarticular naloxone.[156] The clinical analgesic effect of 5 mg of intraarticular morphine is equivalent to 5 mg of morphine given IM.[22] Intraarticular analgesia is locally mediated by μ receptors.[44]

Despite their well-defined analgesic properties and their recommendation by many clinical practice guidelines, opioids continue to be underprescribed for patients with acute and chronic pain. Reluctance often stems from the fear that patients may become addicted or abuse the opioid. However, despite extensive investigation, this is of limited

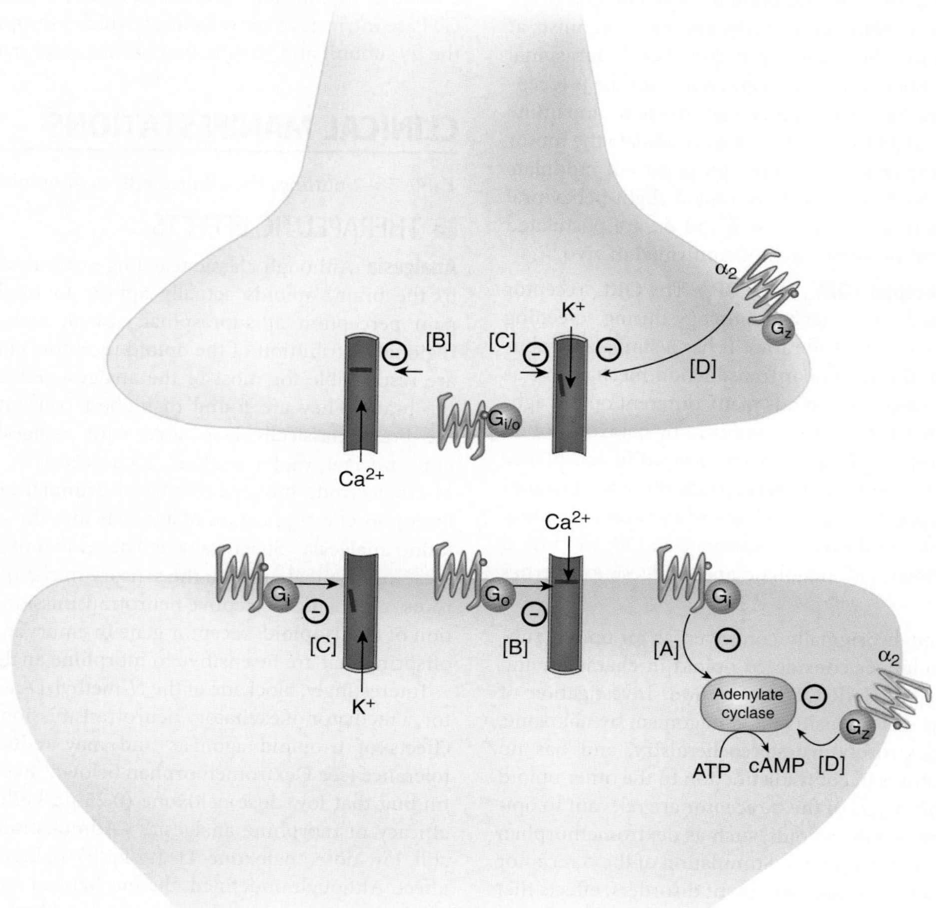

FIGURE 38–1. Opioid-receptor signal transduction mechanisms. Upon binding of an opioid agonist to an opioid receptor, the respective G protein is activated. G proteins may **(A)** reduce the capacity of adenylate cyclase to produce cAMP; **(B)** close calcium channels that reduce the signal to release neurotransmitters; or **(C)** open potassium channels and hyperpolarize the cell, which indirectly reduces cell activity. Each mechanism has been found coupled to each receptor subtype, depending on the location of the receptor (pre- or postsynaptic), and the neuron within the brain (see text). Note that α_2 receptors **(D)** mediate similar effects, using a different G protein (G_z).
***Adenylate cyclase/cAMP* (A).** Inhibition of adenylate cyclase activity by G_i or G_o is the classic mechanism for postsynaptic signal transduction invoked by the inhibitory μ receptors. However, this same mechanism also has been identified in cells bearing either δ or κ receptors. Activation of cAMP production by adenylate cyclase, with subsequent activation of protein kinase A, occurs after exposure to very-low-dose opioid agonists and produces excitatory, antianalgesic effects.[39]
***Calcium (Ca^{2+}) channels* (B).** Presynaptic μ receptors inhibit norepinephrine release from the nerve terminals of cells of the rat cerebral cortex. Adenylate cyclase does not appear to be the modulator for these receptors because inhibition of norepinephrine release is not enhanced by increasing intracellular cAMP levels by various methods.[208] Opioid-induced blockade is, however, prevented by increased intracellular calcium levels that are induced either by calcium ionophores, which increase membrane permeability to calcium, or by increasing the extracellular calcium concentration.[208] This implies a role for opioid-induced closure of N-type calcium channels, presumably via a G_o protein. Reduced intraterminal concentrations of calcium prevent the neurotransmitter-laden vesicles from binding to the terminal membrane and releasing their contents. Nerve terminals containing dopamine appear to have an analogous relationship with inhibitory κ receptors, as do acetylcholine-bearing neurons with opioid receptors.[208]
***Potassium(K^+) channels* (C).** Increased conductance through a potassium channel, generally mediated by G_i or G_o, results in membrane hyperpolarization with reduced neuronal excitability. Alternatively, protein kinase A–mediated reduction in membrane potassium conductance enhances neuronal excitability.

concern.[80,89] Furthermore, opioid analgesics often are better tolerated, safer, and less expensive than the alternatives, such as the nonsteroidal antiinflammatory drugs.

Euphoria The pleasurable effects of many xenobiotics used by humans are mediated by the release of dopamine in the mesolimbic system. This final common pathway is shared by all opioids that activate the μ–δ receptor complex in the ventral tegmental area, which, in turn, indirectly promotes dopamine release in the mesolimbic region. Opioids also may have a direct reinforcing effect on their self-administration through μ receptors within the mesolimbic system.[67]

The sense of well-being and euphoria associated with strenuous exercise appears to be mediated by endogenous opioid peptides and μ receptors. This so-called "runner's high" is reversible with naloxone.[143] Naloxone may also reverse euphoria or even produce dysphoria in nonexercising, highly trained athletes. Even in normal individuals, high-dose naloxone (≤4 mg/kg) may produce dysphoria.[23]

TABLE 38–2. Clinical Effects of Opioids

Cardiovascular	Bradycardia
	Orthostatic hypotension
	Peripheral vasodilation
Dermatologic	Flushing (histamine)
	Pruritus
Endocrinologic	Reduced antidiuretic hormone (ADH) release
	Prolactin release
	Reduced gonadotrophin release
Gastrointestinal	Increased anal sphincter tone
	Increased biliary tract pressure
	Reduced gastric acid secretion
	Reduced motility
Neurologic	Analgesia
	Antitussive
	Euphoria
	Sedation, coma
	Seizures (meperidine, propoxyphene)
Ophthalmic	Miosis
Pulmonary	Acute lung injury
	Bronchospasm (histamine)
	Respiratory depression

Exogenous opioids do not induce uniform psychological effects. Some of the exogenous opioids, particularly those that are highly lipophilic such as heroin, are euphorigenic, but morphine is largely devoid of such pleasurable effects.[150] However, morphine administration results in analgesia, anxiolysis, and sedation. Because heroin has little affinity for opioid receptors and must be deacetylated to morphine for effect, these seemingly incompatible properties likely are related to pharmacokinetic differences in blood–brain barrier penetration.[123] Chronic users note that fentanyl produces effects that are subjectively similar to those of heroin.[94] This effect may explain the higher prevalence of fentanyl, as opposed to other accessible opioids, as an abused drug by anesthesiologists.[11,177] In distinction, certain opioids, such as pentazocine, produce dysphoria, an effect that is related to their affinity for κ or σ receptors.

Antitussive Codeine and dextromethorphan are two opioids with cough-suppressant activity. Cough suppression is not likely mediated via the μ_1 opioid receptor because the ability of other opioids to suppress the medullary cough centers is not correlated with their analgesic effect. Various models suggest that cough suppression occurs via agonism of the μ_2 or κ opioid receptors or antagonism of the δ opioid receptor and that the σ or NMDA receptors also are involved.[163]

TOXIC EFFECTS

When used appropriately for medical purposes, opioids are remarkably safe and effective. However, excessive dosing for any reason may result in serious toxicity. Most adverse or toxic effects are predictable based on "opioid" pharmacodynamics (eg, respiratory depression), although several xenobiotics produce unexpected "nonopioid" or xenobiotic-specific responses. Determining that a patient is suffering from opioid toxicity is generally more important than identifying the specific opioid involved. Notwithstanding some minor variations, patients poisoned by all available opioids predictably develop a constellation of signs, known as the *opioid syndrome* (see Chap. 3). Mental status depression, hypoventilation, miosis, and hypoperistalsis are the classic elements.

Respiratory Depression Experimental use of various opioid agonists and antagonists consistently implicates μ_2 receptors in the respiratory depressant effects of morphine.[144] Through these receptors, opioid agonists reduce ventilation by diminishing the sensitivity of the medullary chemoreceptors to hypercapnea.[180] In addition to loss of hypercarbic stimulation, opioids depress the ventilatory response to hypoxia.[95] The combined loss of hypercarbic and hypoxic drive leaves virtually no stimulus to breathe, and apnea ensues. Equianalgesic doses of the available opioid agonists produce approximately the same degree of respiratory depression.[42,145] This reasoning is supported by experiments in MOR-deficient knockout mice.[134] Patients chronically exposed to opioid agonists, such as those on methadone maintenance, experience chronic hypoventilation, although tolerance to loss of hypercarbic drive may develop over several months.[106] However, such patients never develop complete tolerance to loss of hypoxic stimulation.[136] Although some opioids, notably the agonist–antagonists and partial agonists, demonstrate a ceiling effect on respiratory depression, such sparing generally occurs at the expense of analgesic potency. The different activity profiles likely are a result of differential activities at the opioid-receptor subtypes; that is, agonist–antagonists are predominantly κ-receptor agonists and either partial agonists or antagonists at μ sites.

It is important to recognize that ventilatory depression may be secondary to a reduction in either respiratory rate or tidal volume. Thus, although respiratory rate is more accessible for clinical measurement, it is not an ideal index of ventilatory depression. In fact, morphine-induced respiratory depression in humans initially is related more closely to changes in tidal volume.[145] Large doses of opioids also result in a reduction of respiratory rate.

Acute Lung Injury Reports linking opioids with the development of acute pulmonary abnormalities became common in the 1960s, although the first report was made by William Osler in 1880.[125] Almost all opioids are implicated, and opioid-related acute lung injury (ALI) is reported in diverse clinical situations. Typically, the patient regains normal ventilation after a period of profound respiratory depression, either spontaneously or after the administration of an opioid antagonist, and over the subsequent several minutes to hours develops hypoxemia and pulmonary crackles. Occasionally, classic frothy, pink sputum is present in the patient's airway or in the endotracheal tube of an intubated patient. Acute lung injury was described in 71 (48%) of 149 hospitalized heroin overdose patients in New York City.[40] The outcome generally depends on comorbid conditions and the delay to adequate care. ALI may be an isolated finding or may occur in the setting of multisystem organ damage.

No single mechanism can be consistently invoked in the genesis of opioid-associated ALI. However, several prominent theories are each well supported by experimental data. Although several authors ascribe ALI to naloxone, the majority of affected patients had already experienced respiratory arrest and had been given naloxone to reestablish spontaneous breathing. In these patients, naloxone likely "uncovered" the clinical findings of ALI that were not evident because an adequate examination could not be performed. Other evidentiary cases involve surgical patients given naloxone postoperatively who subsequently awoke with clinical signs of pulmonary edema. In addition to presumably receiving the naloxone for ventilatory compromise or hypoxia, these patients received multiple intraoperative medications, further obscuring the etiology.[129] Although naloxone ordinarily is safe when appropriately administered to nonopioid-tolerant individuals, the production of acute opioid withdrawal may be responsible for "naloxone-induced" ALI. In this situation, as in patients with "neurogenic" pulmonary edema, massive sympathetic discharge from the CNS occurs and produces "cardiogenic" pulmonary edema from the acute effects of catecholamines on the myocardium. In an interesting series of experiments, precipitated opioid withdrawal in nontolerant dogs was associated with dramatic cardiovascular changes and abrupt elevation of serum catecholamine concentrations.[117,118] The effects were more dramatic in dogs with an elevated PCO_2 than in those with a normal or low PCO_2, suggesting the potential benefit of adequately ventilating patients before opioid reversal with naloxone. Similar effects occur in humans undergoing ultrarapid opioid detoxification (UROD; see below).[43]

Even though abrupt precipitation of withdrawal by naloxone may contribute to the development of ALI, it cannot be the sole etiology. Alveolar filling was noted in 50% to 90% of the postmortem examinations performed on heroin overdose patients, many of whom were declared dead before arrival to medical care and thus never received naloxone.[66,70] In addition, neither naloxone nor any other opioid antagonist was available when Osler and others described their initial cases of pulmonary edema. Alternatively, the negative intrathoracic pressure generated by attempted inspiration against a closed glottis creates a large pressure gradient across the alveolar membrane and draws fluid into the alveolar space. This mechanical effect, also known as the *Müller maneuver*, was invoked as the cause of ventilator-associated ALI before the advent of demand ventilators and neuromuscular blockers. In the setting of opioid poisoning, glottic laxity may prevent adequate air entry during inspiration. This effect may be especially prominent at the time of naloxone administration, in which case breathing may be reinstituted before the return of adequate upper airway function.

Cardiovascular Arteriolar and venous dilation secondary to opioid use may result in a mild reduction in blood pressure.[178] This effect is clinically useful for treatment of patients with acute cardiogenic pulmonary edema. However, although patients typically do not develop significant supine hypotension, orthostatic changes in blood pressure and pulse routinely occur. Bradycardia is unusual, although a reduction in heart rate is common as a result of the associated reduction in CNS stimulation. Opioid-induced hypotension appears to be mediated by histamine release, although induction of histamine release does not appear to occur through interaction with an opioid receptor. It may be related to the nonspecific ability of certain xenobiotics to activate mast cell G proteins,[6] which induce degranulation of histamine-containing vesicles. Many opioids share this ability, which seems to be conferred by the presence of a positive charge on a hydrophobic molecule. Accordingly, not all opioids are equivalent in their ability to release histamine.[6] After administration of one of four different opioids to 60 healthy patients, meperidine produced the most hypotension and elevation of serum histamine concentrations; fentanyl produced the least.[47] The combination of H_1 and H_2 antagonists is effective in ameliorating the hemodynamic effects of opioids in humans.[127]

Cardiovascular toxicity may occur with use of propoxyphene, which causes wide-complex dysrhythmias and negative contractility through sodium channel antagonism similar to that of type IA antidysrhythmics (see Propoxyphene below). Adulterants or coingestants may also produce significant cardiovascular toxicity. For example, quinine-adulterated heroin is associated with dysrhythmias. Cocaine, surreptitiously added to heroin, may cause significant myocardial ischemia or infarction. Similarly, concern that naloxone administration may "unmask" cocaine toxicity in patients simultaneously using cocaine and heroin ("speedball") probably is warranted but rarely is demonstrated unequivocally.

Certain opioids at therapeutic concentrations, particularly methadone, may interfere with normal cardiac repolarization and produce QT interval prolongation, an effect that predisposes to the development of torsades de pointes.[92,121] Many patients who receive methadone experience minor increases in QT interval, although a small percentage of patients experience a substantial increase to more than 500 msec.[92] Methadone and levo-α-acetylmethadol (LAAM) both prolong the QT interval via interactions with cardiac K^+ channels.[85] Additionally, certain opioids, primarily propoxyphene, may alter the function of myocardial Na^+ channels in a manner similar to that of the antidysrhythmics (see Chap. 63).

Miosis The mechanisms by which opioids induce miosis remain controversial. Support for each of several mechanisms can be found in the literature. Stimulation of parasympathetic pupilloconstrictor neurons in the Edinger-Westphal nucleus of the oculomotor nerve by morphine produces miosis. Additionally, morphine increases firing of pupilloconstrictor neurons to light,[98] which increases the sensitivity of the light reflex through central reinforcement.[181] Although sectioning of the optic nerve may blunt morphine-induced miosis, the consensual reflex in the denervated eye is enhanced by morphine. Because opioids classically mediate inhibitory neurotransmission, hyperpolarization of sympathetic nerves or of inhibitory neurons to the parasympathetic neurons (removal of inhibition) ultimately may be found to mediate the classic "pinpoint pupil" associated with opioid use.

Not all patients using opioids present with miosis. Meperidine has a lesser miotic effect than other conventional opioids, and propoxyphene use does not result in miosis.[54] Use of opioids with predominantly κ-agonist effects, such as pentazocine, may not result in miosis. Mydriasis may occur in severely poisoned patients secondary to hypoxic brain insult. Additionally, concomitant drug abuse or the presence of adulterants may alter pupillary findings. For example, the combination of heroin and cocaine ("speedball") may produce virtually any size pupil, depending on the relative contribution by each xenobiotic. Similarly, patients ingesting diphenoxylate and atropine (Lomotil) or those using scopolamine-adulterated heroin typically develop mydriasis.[61]

Seizures Seizures are a rare complication of therapeutic use of most opioids. In patients with acute opioid overdose, seizures most likely are caused by hypoxia. However, experimental models demonstrate a proconvulsant effect of morphine in that it potentiates the convulsant effect of other xenobiotics.[185] These effects are variably inhibited by naloxone, suggesting the involvement of a mechanism other than opioid receptor binding. In humans, morphine-induced seizures are reported in neonates and are reversed by naloxone,[30] although opioid withdrawal seizures in neonates are more common.

Seizures should be anticipated in patients with meperidine, propoxyphene, tapentadol or tramadol toxicity. Naloxone antagonizes the convulsant effects of propoxyphene in mice, although it is only moderately effective in preventing seizures resulting from meperidine or its metabolite normeperidine.[55] Interestingly, naloxone potentiates the anticonvulsant effects of benzodiazepines and barbiturates, but in a single study, it antagonized the effects of phenytoin.[78] The ability of fentanyl and its analogs to induce seizures is controversial. They are used to activate epileptiform activity for localization in patients with temporal lobe epilepsy who are undergoing surgical exploration.[113] However, electroencephalography (EEG) performed on patients undergoing fentanyl anesthesia did not identify seizure activity even though the clinical assessment suggested that approximately one-third of them had seizures.[152] It appears likely that the rigidity and myoclonus associated with fentanyl use are readily misinterpreted as a seizure.

Movement Disorders Patients may experience acute muscular rigidity with rapid IV injection of certain high-potency opioids, especially fentanyl and its derivatives.[161] This condition is particularly prominent during induction of anesthesia and in neonates.[46] The rigidity primarily involves the trunk and may impair chest wall movement sufficiently to exacerbate hypoventilation. Chest wall rigidity may have contributed to the lethality associated with epidemics of fentanyl-adulterated or fentanyl-substituted heroin. Although the mechanism of muscle rigidity is unclear, it may be related to blockade of dopamine receptors in the basal ganglia. Other postulated mechanisms include γ-aminobutyric acid (GABA) antagonism and NMDA agonism. Opioid antagonists generally are therapeutic but may produce adverse hemodynamic effects, withdrawal phenomena, or uncontrollable pain, depending on the situation.[46] Although not a problem for patients taking stable doses of methadone, rapid escalation of methadone doses may produce choreoathetoid movements.[10]

Gastrointestinal Effects Historically, the morphine analog apomorphine was used as a rapidly acting emetic whose clinical use was limited by its tendency to depress the patient's level of consciousness. Emesis induced by apomorphine is mediated through agonism at D_2 receptor subtypes within the chemoreceptor trigger zone of the medulla. Many opioids, particularly morphine, produce significant nausea and vomiting when used therapeutically.[20] Whether these effects are inhibited by naloxone is not clearly established, but they likely are not.

Although diphenoxylate and loperamide are widely used therapeutically to manage diarrhea, opioid-induced constipation is most frequently a bothersome side effect of both medical and nonmedical use of opioids. Constipation, mediated by μ_2 receptors within the smooth muscle of the intestinal wall,[73] is ameliorated by oral naloxone. Provided the first pass hepatic glucuronidative capacity is not exceeded (at doses of ~6 mg), enteral naloxone is poorly bioavailable and thus induces few, if any, opioid withdrawal symptoms.[115] Methylnaltrexone and alvimopan are bioavailable, peripherally acting opioids that antagonize the effects of other opioids on the GI tract opioid receptors.[187] Opioid withdrawal does not occur because methylnaltrexone and alvimopan cannot cross the blood–brain barrier.[114] (see Antidote in Depth A6: Opioid Antagonists)

DIAGNOSTIC TESTING

LABORATORY CONSIDERATIONS

Although it is always tempting to seek laboratory confirmation of an ingested xenobiotic in acutely poisoned patients, current laboratory methodology suffers from several important limitations and the potential for many confounding variables. The most apparent impediment to use of laboratory testing in the acute care setting is the lack of timely reporting of results. Patients may experience grave consequences if therapy is withheld pending test results. Opioid poisoned patients are particularly appropriate for a rapid clinical diagnosis because of the unique characteristics of the opioid syndrome. Additionally, even in situations where the assay results are available rapidly, the fact that several distinct classes of opioids and nonopioids can produce similar opioid effects limits the use of laboratory tests, such as immunoassays, that rely on structural features to identify xenobiotics. Furthermore, because opioids may be chemically detectable long after their clinical effects have dissipated, assay results cannot be considered in isolation but rather viewed in the clinical context. Several well-described problems with laboratory testing of opioids are described below and in Chapter 6.

Cross-Reactivity Many opioids share remarkable structural similarities, such as methadone and propoxyphene, but they do not necessarily share the same clinical characteristics (Fig. 38–2). Because most clinical assays depend on structural features for identification, structurally similar xenobiotics may be detected in lieu of the desired one. Whether a similar xenobiotic is noted by the assay depends on the sensitivity and specificity of the assay and the serum concentration of the xenobiotic. Some cross-reactivities are predictable, such as that of codeine with

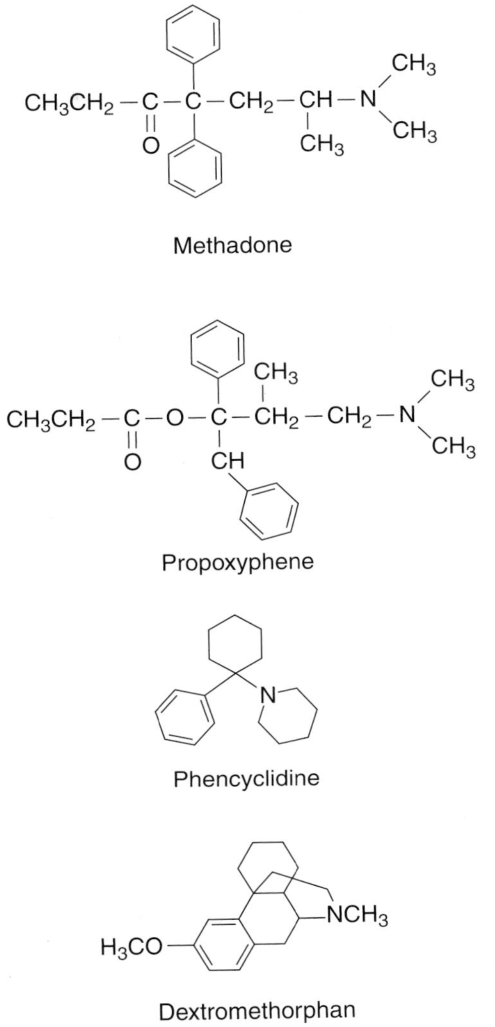

Methadone

Propoxyphene

Phencyclidine

Dextromethorphan

FIGURE 38–2. Structural similarity between methadone and propoxyphene and between phencyclidine and dextromethorphan.

morphine, on a variety of screening tests. Other cross-reactivities are less predictable, as in the case of the cross-reaction of dextromethorphan and the phencyclidine (PCP) component of the fluorescence polarization immunoassay (Abbott TDx),[138] a widely used drug abuse screening test (see Chap. 6).[158]

Congeners and Adulterants Commercial opioid assays, which are specific for morphine, likely will not detect most of the semisynthetic and synthetic opioids. In some cases, epidemic fatalities involving fentanyl derivatives remained unexplained despite obvious opioid toxicity until the ultrapotent fentanyl derivative α-methylfentanyl (although initially misidentified as 3-methylfentanyl) was identified by more sophisticated testing.[91,108] Oxycodone, hydrocodone, and other common morphine derivatives have variable detectability by different opioid screens.[100,151]

Drug Metabolism A fascinating dilemma may arise in patients who ingest moderate to large amounts of poppy seeds.[87] These seeds, which are widely used for culinary purposes, are derived from poppy plants and contain both morphine and codeine. After ingestion of a single poppy seed bagel, patients may develop elevated serum morphine and codeine concentrations and test positive for morphine.[119,133] Because the presence of morphine on a drug abuse screen may suggest illicit heroin use, the implications are substantial. Federal workplace testing regulations thus require corroboration of a positive morphine assay with assessment of another heroin metabolite, 6-monoacetylmorphine, before reporting a positive result.[120,172] Humans cannot acetylate morphine and therefore cannot synthesize 6-monoacetylmorphine, but humans can readily deacetylate heroin, which is diacetylmorphine.

A similar problem may occur in patients taking therapeutic doses of codeine. Because codeine is demethylated to morphine by CYP2D6, a morphine screen may be positive as a result of metabolism and not structural cross-reactivity.[50] Thus, determination of the serum codeine or 6-monoacetylmorphine concentration is necessary in these patients. Determination of the serum codeine concentration is not foolproof, however, because codeine is present in the opium preparation used to synthesize heroin.

Forensic Testing Decision making regarding the cause of death in the presence of systemic opioids often is complex.[32] Variables that often are incompletely defined contribute substantially to the difficulty in attributing or not attributing the cause of death to the opioid. These variables include the specifics regarding the timing of exposure, the preexisting degree of sensitivity or tolerance, the role of cointoxicants (including parent opioid metabolites), and postmortem redistribution and metabolism.[39,84] Interesting techniques to help further elucidate the likely cause of death that have been studied include the application of postmortem pharmacogenetic principles[79] and the use of alternative specimens (see Chap. 33).

MANAGEMENT

The consequential effects of acute opioid poisoning are CNS and respiratory depression. Although early support of ventilation and oxygenation is generally sufficient to prevent death, prolonged use of bag-valve-mask ventilation and endotracheal intubation may be avoided by cautious administration of an opioid antagonist. Opioid antagonists, such as naloxone, competitively inhibit binding of opioid agonists to opioid receptors, allowing the patient to resume spontaneous respiration. Naloxone competes at all receptor subtypes, although not equally, and is effective at reversing almost all adverse effects mediated through opioid receptors. (Antidotes in Depth A6: Opioid Antagonists contains a complete discussion of naloxone and other opioid antagonists.)

Because many clinical findings associated with opioid poisoning are nonspecific, the diagnosis requires clinical acumen. Differentiating acute opioid poisoning from other etiologies with similar clinical presentations may be challenging. Patients manifesting opioid toxicity, those found in an appropriate environment, or those with characteristic physical clues such as fresh needle marks require little corroborating evidence. However, subtle presentations of opioid poisoning may be encountered, and other entities superficially resembling opioid poisoning may occur. Hypoglycemia, hypoxia, and hypothermia may result in clinical manifestations that share features with opioid poisoning and may exist concomitantly. Each can be rapidly diagnosed with routinely available, point-of-care testing, but their existence does not exclude opioid toxicity. Other xenobiotics responsible for similar clinical presentations include clonidine, PCP, phenothiazines, and sedative–hypnotics (primarily benzodiazepines). In such patients, clinical evidence usually is available to assist in diagnosis. For example, nystagmus nearly always is noted in PCP-intoxicated patients, hypotension or electrocardiographic (ECG) abnormalities in phenothiazine-poisoned patients, and coma with virtually normal vital signs in patients poisoned by benzodiazepines. Most difficult to differentiate on clinical grounds may be toxicity produced by the centrally acting antihypertensive agents such as clonidine (see Clonidine below and Chap. 62). Additionally, myriad traumatic, metabolic, and infectious etiologies may occur simultaneously and must always be considered and evaluated appropriately.

ANTIDOTE ADMINISTRATION

The goal of naloxone therapy is not necessarily complete arousal; rather, the goal is reinstitution of adequate spontaneous ventilation. Because precipitation of withdrawal is potentially detrimental and often unpredictable, the lowest practical naloxone dose should be administered initially, with rapid escalation as warranted by the clinical situation. Most patients respond to 0.04 to 0.05 mg of naloxone administered IV, although the requirement for ventilatory assistance may be slightly prolonged because the onset may be slower than with larger doses. Administration in this fashion effectively avoids endotracheal intubation and allows timely identification of patients with nonopioid causes of their clinical condition yet diminishes the risk of precipitation of acute opioid withdrawal. SC administration may allow for smoother arousal than the high-dose IV route but is unpredictable in onset and likely prolonged in offset.[176] Prolonged effectiveness of naloxone by the SC route can be a considerable disadvantage if the therapeutic goal is exceeded and the withdrawal syndrome develops.

In the absence of a confirmatory history or diagnostic clinical findings, the cautious empiric administration of naloxone may be both diagnostic and therapeutic. Naloxone, even at extremely high doses, has an excellent safety profile in opioid-naïve patients receiving the medication for nonopioid-related indications, such as spinal cord injury or acute ischemic stroke. However, administration of naloxone to opioid-dependent patients may result in adverse effects; specifically, precipitation of an acute withdrawal syndrome should be anticipated. The resultant agitation, hypertension, and tachycardia may produce significant distress for the patient and complicate management for the clinical staff and occasionally may be life threatening. Additionally, emesis, a common feature of acute opioid withdrawal, may be particularly hazardous in patients who do not rapidly regain consciousness after naloxone administration. For example, patients with concomitant ethanol or sedative–hypnotic exposure and those with head trauma are at substantial risk for pulmonary aspiration of vomitus if their airways are unprotected.

Identification of patients likely to respond to naloxone conceivably would reduce the unnecessary and potentially dangerous precipitation of withdrawal in opioid-dependent patients. Routine prehospital administration of naloxone to all patients with subjectively assessed altered mental status or respiratory depression was not beneficial in 92% of patients.[186] Alternatively, although not perfectly sensitive, a respiratory rate of 12 breaths/min or less in an unconscious patient presenting via Emergency Medical Services best predicted a response to naloxone.[71] Interestingly, neither respiratory rate below 8 breaths/min nor coma was able to predict a response to naloxone in hospitalized patients.[183] It is unclear whether the discrepancy between the latter two studies is a result of the demographics of the patient groups or whether patients with prehospital opioid overdose present differently than patients with iatrogenic poisoning. Regardless, relying on the respiratory rate to assess the need for ventilatory support or naloxone administration is not ideal because hypoventilation secondary to hypopnea may precede that caused by bradypnea.[131,147]

The decision to discharge a patient who awakens appropriately after naloxone administration is based on practical considerations. Patients presenting with profound hypoventilation or hypoxia are at risk for development of ALI or posthypoxic encephalopathy. Thus, it seems prudent to observe these patients for at least 24 hours in a medical setting. Patients manifesting only moderate signs of poisoning who remain normal for at least several hours after parenteral naloxone likely

TABLE 38–3. How to Use a Naloxone Infusion

1. If a naloxone bolus (start with 0.04 mg IV and titrate) is successful, administer two-thirds of the effective bolus dose per hour by IV infusion; frequently reassess the patient's respiratory status.
2. If respiratory depression is not reversed after the bolus dose:
   Intubate the patient, as clinically indicated.
   Administer up to 10 mg of naloxone as an IV bolus. If the patient does not respond, do not initiate an infusion.
3. If the patient develops withdrawal after the bolus dose:
   Allow the effects of the bolus to abate.
   If respiratory depression recurs, administer half of this new bolus dose and begin an IV infusion at two-thirds of the initial bolus dose per hour. Frequently reassess the patient's respiratory status.
4. If the patient develops withdrawal signs or symptoms during the infusion:
   Stop the infusion until the withdrawal symptoms abate.
   Restart the infusion at half the initial rate; frequently reassess the patient's respiratory status.
   Exclude withdrawal from other xenobiotics.
5. If the patient develops respiratory depression during the infusion:
   Readminister half of the initial bolus and repeat until reversal occurs.
   Increase the infusion by half of the initial rate; frequently reassess the patient's respiratory status.
   Exclude continued absorption, readministration of opioid, and other etiologies as the cause of the respiratory depression..

are safe to discharge. However, the need for psychosocial intervention in patients with uncontrolled drug use or after a suicide attempt may prevent discharge from the emergency department (ED).

Patients with recurrent or profound poisoning by long-acting opioids, such as methadone, or patients with large GI burdens (eg, "body packers" or those taking sustained-release preparations), may require continuous infusion of naloxone to ensure continued adequate ventilation (Table 38–3). An hourly infusion rate of two-thirds of the initial reversal dose of naloxone is sufficient to prevent recurrence.[57] Titration of the dose may be necessary as indicated by the clinical situation. Although repetitive bolus dosing of naloxone may be effective, it is labor intensive and subject to error.

Despite the availability of long-acting opioid antagonists (eg, naltrexone and nalmefene) that theoretically permit single-dose reversal of methadone poisoning, the attendant risk of precipitating an unrelenting withdrawal syndrome hinders their use as antidotes for initial opioid reversal. However, these opioid antagonists may have a clinical role in the maintenance of consciousness and ventilation in opioid-poisoned patients already awakened by naloxone. Prolonged observation and perhaps antidote readministration may be required to match the pharmacokinetic parameters of the two antagonists. Otherwise, well children who ingest short-acting opioids may be given a long-acting opioid antagonist initially because they are not expected to develop a prolonged, potentially hazardous withdrawal. However, the same caveats remain regarding the need for extended hospital observation periods if ingestion of methadone or other long-acting opioids is suspected.

RAPID AND ULTRARAPID OPIOID DETOXIFICATION

The concept of antagonist-precipitated opioid withdrawal is promoted extensively as a "cure" for opioid dependency, particularly heroin and oxycodone, but has fallen out of favor in recent years. Rather than slow, deliberate withdrawal or detoxification from opioids over several weeks, antagonist-precipitated withdrawal occurs over several hours or days.[59] The purported advantage of this technique is a reduced risk of relapse to opioid use because the duration of discomfort is reduced and a more rapid transition to naltrexone maintenance can be achieved. Although most studies find excellent short-term results, relapse to drug use is very common.[112] Rapid opioid detoxification techniques are usually offered by outpatient clinics and typically consist of naloxone- or naltrexone-precipitated opioid withdrawal tempered with varying amounts of clonidine, benzodiazepines, antiemetics, or other drugs. UROD uses a similar concept but involves the use of deep sedation or general anesthesia for greater patient control and comfort. The risks of these techniques are not fully defined but are of substantial concern. Massive catecholamine release, ALI, renal insufficiency, and thyroid hormone suppression have been reported after UROD, and many patients still manifest opioid withdrawal 48 hours after the procedure. As with other forms of opioid detoxification, the loss of tolerance after successful completion of the program paradoxically increases the likelihood of death from heroin overdose if these individuals relapse. That is, recrudescence of opioid use in pre-detoxification quantities is likely to result in overdose.[160] Both techniques are costly; UROD under anesthesia commonly costs thousands of dollars.

SPECIFIC OPIOIDS

The vast majority of opioid-poisoned patients follow predictable clinical courses that can be anticipated based on our understanding of opioid receptor pharmacology. However, certain opioids taken in overdose may produce atypical manifestations. Therefore, careful clinical assessment and institution of empiric therapy usually are necessary to ensure proper management (Table 38–4).

MORPHINE AND CODEINE

Morphine is poorly bioavailable by the oral route because of extensive first-pass elimination. Morphine is hepatically metabolized primarily to morphine-3-glucuronide (M3G) and, to a lesser extent, to morphine-6-glucuronide (M6G), both of which are cleared renally. Unlike M3G, which is essentially devoid of activity, M6G has μ-agonist effects in the CNS.[2] However, M6G administered peripherally is significantly less potent as an analgesic than is morphine.[146] The polar glucuronide has a limited ability to cross the blood–brain barrier, and P-glycoprotein is capable of expelling M6G from the cerebrospinal fluid. The relative potency of morphine and M6G in the brain is incompletely defined, but the metabolite is generally considered to be several-fold more potent.[2]

Codeine itself is an inactive opioid agonist, and it requires metabolic activation by *O*-demethylation to morphine by CYP2D6 (Fig. 38–3). This typically represents a minor metabolic pathway for codeine metabolism. *N*-demethylation into norcodeine by CYP3A4 and glucuronidation are more prevalent but produce inactive metabolites. The need for conversion to morphine explains why approximately 5% to 7% of white patients, who are devoid of CYP2D6 function, cannot derive an analgesic response from codeine.[76,104] Rarely, ultrarapid CYP2D6 metabolizers produce unexpectedly large amounts of morphine, with resulting life-threatening opioid toxicity.[49]

HEROIN

Heroin is 3,6-diacetylmorphine, and its exogenous synthesis is performed relatively easily from morphine and acetic anhydride. Heroin has a lower affinity for the receptor than does morphine, but it is

TABLE 38–4. Classification, Potency, and Characteristics of Opioids

Opioid (Representative Trade Name)	Type[a]	Derivation	Analgesic Dose (mg) (via route, equivalent to 10 mg morphine SC[b])	Comments[a,c]
Alvimopan (Entereg)	Ant	Synthetic	Nonanalgesic (12mg PO)	Peripherally acting antagonist; reverses opioid constipation
Buprenorphine (Buprenex)	P/AA	Semisynthetic	0.4 IM	Opioid substitution therapy requires 6–16 mg/d
Butorphanol (Stadol)	AA	Semisynthetic	2 IM	
Codeine	Ag	Natural	120 PO	Often combined with acetaminophen; requires demethylation to morphine by CYP2D6
Dextromethorphan (Robitussin DM)	NEC	Semisynthetic	Nonanalgesic (10–30 PO)	Antitussive; psychotomimetic via or NMDA receptor
Diphenoxylate (Lomotil)	Ag	Synthetic	Nonanalgesic (2.5 PO)	Antidiarrheal, combined with atropine; difenoxin is potent metabolite
Fentanyl (Sublimaze)	Ag	Synthetic	0.125 IM	Very short acting (<1 h)
Heroin (Diamorph)	Ag	Semisynthetic	5 SC	Diacetylmorphine, used therapeutically in some countries, Schedule I medication in the United States
Hydrocodone (Vicodin, Hycodan)	Ag	Semisynthetic	10 PO	
Hydromorphone (Dilaudid)	Ag	Semisynthetic	1.3 SC	
LAAM (Orlaam)	Ag	Synthetic	(Flexible oral dosing[d])	Long acting, potent metabolites; no longer distributed in US because of QTc interval prolongation
Levorphanol (Levodromoran)	Ag	Semisynthetic	2 SC/IM	
Loperamide (Imodium)	Ag	Synthetic	Nonanalgesic (2 PO)	Antidiarrheal
Meperidine, pethidine (Demerol)	Ag	Synthetic	75 SC/IM	Seizures caused by metabolite accumulation
Methadone (Dolophine)	Ag	Synthetic	10 IM	Very long acting (24 h)
Methylnaltrexone (Relistor)	Ant	Synthetic	Nonanalgesic (8-12mg SC)	Peripherally acting antagonist; reverses opioid constipation
Morphine	Ag	Natural	10 SC/IM	
Nalbuphine (Nubain)	AA	Semisynthetic	10 IM	
Nalmefene (Revex)	Ant	Semisynthetic	Nonanalgesic (0.1 IM)	Long-acting antagonist (4–6 h)
Nalorphine	AA	Semisynthetic	15 IM	Historically used as an opioid antagonist[a]
Naloxone (Narcan)	Ant	Semisynthetic	Nonanalgesic (0.1–0.4 IV/IM)	Short-acting antagonist (0.5 h)
Naltrexone (Trexan, Revia)	Ant	Semisynthetic	Nonanalgesic (50 PO)	Very long-acting antagonist (24 h)
Oxycodone (Percocet, OxyContin)	Ag	Semisynthetic	10 PO	Often combined with acetaminophen; OxyContin is sustained release
Oxymorphone (Numorphan)	Ag	Semisynthetic	1 SC	
Paregoric (Parapectolin)	Ag	Natural	25 mL PO	Tincture of opium (0.4 mg/mL)
Pentazocine (Talwin)	AA	Semisynthetic	50 SC	Psychotomimetic via receptor
Propoxyphene (Darvon)	Ag	Synthetic	65 PO	Seizures, dysrhythmias; combined with acetaminophen
Tapentadol (Nucynta)	Ag	Synthetic	50-100mg PO	Seizures
Tramadol (Ultram)	Ag	Synthetic	50–100 PO	Seizures possible with therapeutic dosing

[a] Agonist–antagonists, partial agonists, and antagonists may cause withdrawal in tolerant individuals.

[b] Typical dose (mg) for agents without analgesic effects is given in parentheses.

[c] Duration of therapeutic clinical effect 3–6 hours unless noted; likely to be exaggerated in overdose.

[d] Although approximately equipotent with methadone, LAAM is not used as an analgesic.

AA, agonist antagonist (κ agonist, μ antagonist); Ag, full agonist (μ_1, μ_2, κ); Ant, full antagonist (μ_1, μ_2, κ antagonist); NEC, not easily classified; NMDA, *N*-methyl-D-aspartate; P, partial agonist (μ_1, μ_2 agonist, κ antagonist).

rapidly metabolized by plasma cholinesterase and liver human carboxylesterase (hCE)-2 to 6-monoacetylmorphine, a more potent μ agonist than morphine (see Fig. 38–3).[142] Users claim that heroin has an enhanced euphorigenic effect, often described as a "rush." This effect likely is related to the enhanced blood–brain barrier penetration occasioned by the additional organic functional groups of heroin and its subsequent metabolic activation within the CNS. Interestingly, cocaine and heroin compete for metabolism by plasma cholinesterase and the

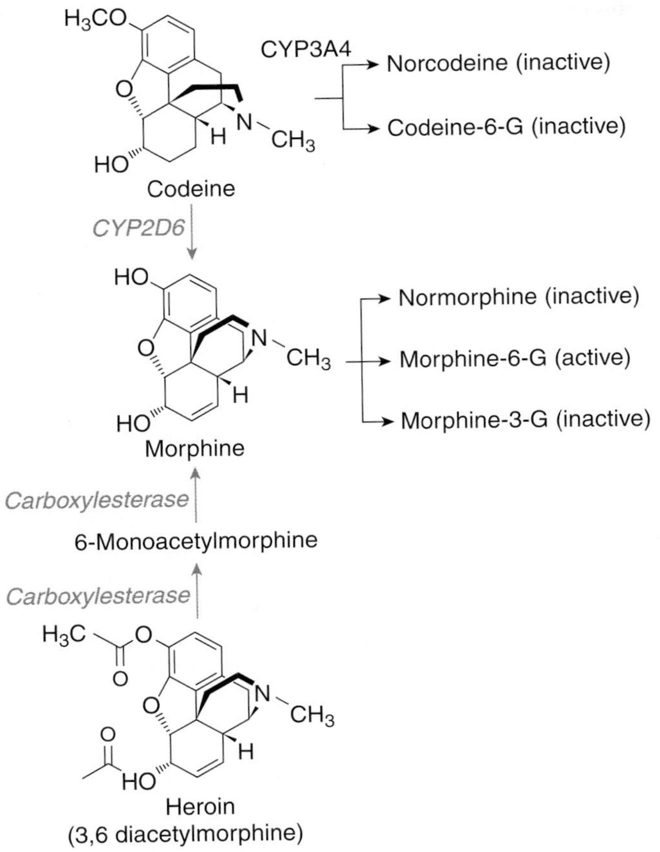

H3CO
Codeine
CYP3A4
Norcodeine (inactive)
Codeine-6-G (inactive)
CYP2D6
Morphine
Normorphine (inactive)
Morphine-6-G (active)
Morphine-3-G (inactive)
Carboxylesterase
6-Monoacetylmorphine
Carboxylesterase
Heroin
(3,6 diacetylmorphine)

FIGURE 38–3. Opiate/opioid metabolism. Codeine can be *O*-methylated to morphine, *N*-demethylated to norcodeine, or glucuronidated to codeine-6-glucuronide (codeine-6-G). Morphine can be *N*-demethylated to normorphine or glucuronidated to either morphine-3-glucuronide (morphine-3-G) or morphine-6-glucuronide (morphine-6-G). Heroin is converted to morphine by a two-step process involving plasma cholinesterase and two human liver carboxylesterases known as human carboxylesterase-1 and human carboxylesterase-2.

two human liver carboxylesterases hCE-1 and hCE-2. This interaction may have pharmacokinetic and clinical consequences in patients who "speedball."[8,83]

Heroin can be obtained in two distinct chemical forms: base or salt. The hydrochloride salt form typically is a white or beige powder and was the common form of heroin available before the 1980s.[81] Its high water solubility allows simple IV administration. Heroin base, on the other hand, now is the more prevalent form of heroin in most regions of the world. It often is brown or black. "Black tar heroin" is one appellation referring to an impure South American import available in the United States. Because heroin base is virtually insoluble in water, IV administration requires either heating the heroin until it liquefies or mixing it with acid. Alternatively, because the alkaloidal form is heat stable, smoking or "chasing the dragon" is sometimes used as an alternative route. Street-level heroin base frequently contains caffeine or barbiturates,[81] which improves the sublimation of heroin and enhances the yield.[74]

Widespread IV use has led to many significant direct and indirect medical complications, particularly endocarditis and AIDS, in addition to fatal and nonfatal overdose. Nearly two-thirds of all long-term (>10 years) heroin users in Australia had overdosed on heroin.[34] Among recent-onset heroin users, 23% had overdosed on heroin, and 48% had been present when someone else overdosed.[58] Risk factors for fatality after heroin use include the concomitant use of other drugs of abuse, particularly ethanol; recent abstinence, as occurs during incarceration[141]; and perhaps unanticipated fluctuations in the purity of available heroin.[33,132] Because most overdoses occur in seasoned heroin users and about half occur in the company of other users,[34] a trial distribution of naloxone to heroin users was initiated. Although earlier administration of antidote could be beneficial, certain issues make this approach controversial. For example, despite the acknowledged injection skills of the other users in the "shooting gallery," their judgment likely is impaired. In one survey, summoning an ambulance was the initial response to overdose of a companion in only 14% of cases.[35] A survey of heroin users suggested they lacked an understanding of the pharmacology of naloxone, which might lead to inappropriate behaviors regarding both heroin and naloxone administration.[140]

Recognition of the efficacy of intranasal heroin administration, or snorting, has fostered a resurgence of heroin use, particularly in suburban communities. The reasons for this trend are unclear, although it is widely suggested that the increasing purity of the available heroin has rendered it more suitable for intranasal use. However, because intranasal administration of a mixture of 3% heroin in lactose produces clinical and pharmacokinetic effects similar to an equivalent dose administered IM, the relationship between heroin purity and price and intranasal use is uncertain.[24,135] Needle avoidance certainly is important, reducing the risk of transmission of various infectious diseases, including HIV. Heroin smoking has also increased in popularity in the United States, albeit not to the extent in other countries (see "Chasing the Dragon" below).

Celebrities and musicians have popularized intranasal heroin use as a "safe" alternative to IV use. This usage is occurring despite a concomitantly reported rise in heroin deaths in regions of the country where its use is prevalent. Although intranasal use may be less dangerous than IV use from an infectious disease perspective, it is clear that both fatal overdose and drug dependency remain common.[166]

Adulterants, Contaminants, and "Heroin" Substitutes The history of heroin adulteration and contamination has been extensively described. Retail (street-level) heroin almost always contains adulterants or contaminants. What differentiates the two is the intent of their admixture. Adulterants typically are benign because inflicting harm on the consumer with their addition would be economically and socially unwise, although adulterants occasionally are responsible for epidemic death. Interestingly, most heroin overdose fatalities do not have serum morphine concentrations that substantially differ from those of living users, raising the possibility that the individual death is related to an adulterant or contaminant.[36]

Historically, alkaloids, such as quinine and strychnine, were used to adulterate heroin to mimic the bitter taste of heroin and to mislead clients. Quinine may have first been added in a poorly reasoned attempt to quell an epidemic of malaria among IV heroin users in New York City in the 1930s.[66] That quinine adulteration was common is demonstrated by the common practice of urine screening for quinine as a surrogate marker for heroin use. However, quinine was implicated as a causative factor in an epidemic of heroin-related deaths in the District of Columbia between 1979 and 1982. Toxicity attributed to quinine in heroin users includes cardiac dysrhythmias (see Chap. 23), amblyopia, and thrombocytopenia. Quinine adulteration currently is much less common than it was in the past. Trend analysis of illicit wholesale and street-level heroin adulteration over a 12-year period in Denmark revealed that although caffeine, acetaminophen, methaqualone, and phenobarbital all were prevalent adulterants, quinine was not found.[81] Recent data on adulteration in the United States are unavailable. Many other adulterants or contaminants, including thallium, lead, cocaine, and amphetamines, have been reported.

Poisoning by scopolamine-tainted heroin reached epidemic levels in the northeastern United States in 1995.[61] Exposed patients presented with acute psychosis and anticholinergic signs. Several patients were treated with physostigmine, with excellent therapeutic results.

Clenbuterol, a β-2 adrenergic agonist with a rapid onset and long duration of action, was found to be a contaminant in street heroin in the Eastern United States in early 2005. Users had, in most cases, insufflated what they believed to be unadulterated street heroin, but they rapidly developed nausea, chest pain, palpitations, dyspnea, and tremor. Physical findings included significant tachycardia and hypotension, as well as hyperglycemia, hypokalemia, and increased lactate concentrations on laboratory evaluation, and a few fatalities occurred.[72,184] Although the patients were initially thought to be cyanide poisoned, laboratory investigation uncovered clenbuterol. Several patients were treated with β-adrenergic antagonists or calcium channel blockers and potassium supplementation with good results (see Chaps. 39 and 44).

"Chasing the Dragon" IV injection and insufflation are the preferred means of heroin self-administration in the United States. In other countries, including the Netherlands, the United Kingdom, and Spain, a prevalent method is "chasing the dragon" whereby users inhale the white pyrolysate that is generated by heating heroin base on aluminum foil using a hand-held flame. This means of administration produces heroin pharmacokinetics similar to those observed after IV administration.[68] Chasing the dragon is not a new phenomenon, but it has gained acceptance recently among both IV heroin users and drug-naïve individuals.[235] The reasons for this shift are diverse but probably are related to the avoidance of injection drug use with its concomitant infectious risks. The increasing availability of the smokable base form of heroin is associated, but whether it is a cause or an effect of this trend is unknown.

In the early 1980s, a group of individuals who smoked heroin in the Netherlands developed spongiform leukoencephalopathy. Other causes of this rare clinicopathologic entity include prion-related infections such as bovine spongiform leukoencephalopathy, hexachlorophene, pentachlorophenol, and metal poisoning, although none appeared responsible for this phenomenon. Since the initial report, similar cases have been reported in other parts of Europe and in the United States.[93,103] Initial findings may occur within 2 weeks of use and include bradykinesia, ataxia, abulia, and speech abnormalities. Of those whose symptoms do not progress, half may recover. However, in others, progression to spastic paraparesis, pseudobulbar palsy, or hypotonia may occur over several weeks. Approximately half of individuals in this group do not develop further deficits or improve, but death occurs in approximately 25% of reported cases. The prominent symmetric cerebellar and cerebral white matter destruction noted on brain computed tomography and magnetic resonance imaging corresponds to that noted at necropsy.[86,122]

The syndrome has the characteristics of a point-source toxic exposure, but no culpable contaminants have been identified, although aluminum concentrations may be elevated.[45] A component or pyrolysis product unique to certain batches of "heroin" is possible.[15] Treatment is largely supportive. Based on the finding of regional mitochondrial dysfunction on functional brain imaging and an elevated brain lactate concentration, supplementation with 300 mg QID of coenzyme Q has purported benefit but has not undergone controlled study.[93]

OTHER OPIOIDS

Fentanyl and Its Analogs Fentanyl is a short-acting, highly potent opioid agonist that is widely used in clinical medicine. Fentanyl has approximately 50 to 100 times the potency of morphine. It is well absorbed by the transmucosal route, accounting for its use in the form of a "lollipop." Fentanyl is widely abused as a heroin substitute and is the controlled substance most often abused by anesthesiologists.[11]

Transdermal fentanyl in the form of a patch (Duragesic) was approved in 1991 and is widely used by patients with chronic pain syndromes. Fentanyl has adequate solubility in both lipid and water for transdermal delivery. The transdermal pharmacokinetics differ markedly from those of the more conventional routes.[90] A single patch contains an amount of drug to provide a transdermal gradient sufficient to maintain a steady-state plasma concentration for approximately 3 days (eg, a 50 μg/h patch contains 5 mg). However, even after the patch is considered exhausted, approximately 50% of the total initial fentanyl dose remains. Interindividual variation in dermal drug penetration and errors in proper use, such as use of excessive patches or warming of the skin, may lead to an iatrogenic fentanyl overdose. Fentanyl patch misuse and abuse occur either by application of one or more patches to the skin or by withdrawal or extraction of the fentanyl from the reservoir for subsequent administration.[165]

Regional epidemics of heroin substitutes with "superpotent" activity occasionally produce a dramatic increase in "heroin-related" fatalities. Epidemic deaths among heroin users first appeared in Orange County, California, in 1979 and were traced to α-methylfentanyl sold under the brand name China White.[91] Similar epidemics of China White poisoning occurred in Pittsburgh in 1988 and in Philadelphia in 1992, although the adulterant in these cases was 3-methylfentanyl, another potent analog. A later epidemic in New York City marked the reappearance of 3-methylfentanyl under the brand name Tango and Cash. Typically, patients present comatose and apneic, with no opioids detected on routine blood and urine analysis. In such cases, unsuspecting users had administered their usual "dose of heroin," measured in 25-mg "bags" that contained variable amounts of the fentanyl analog. Because of the exceptional potency of this fentanyl analog (as much as 6000 times greater than that of morphine), users rapidly developed apnea.

The largest epidemic of more than 1000 fentanyl-related deaths occurred between 2005 and 2007 primarily in the Philadelphia, Chicago, and Detroit regions because of surreptitiously adulterated or substituted heroin. Fentanyl use was identified by postmortem urine and blood testing or through analysis of unused drug found on either the decedent or persons with whom the decedent shared drugs. In response to this large epidemic, drug users and others were counseled in overdose prevention and cardiopulmonary resuscitation and even provided with "take-home" parenteral or intranasal naloxone.[19]

Sufentanil and alfentanil are anesthetic opioids with increased potency compared to fentanyl. In some regions of the country, fentanyl and both licit and illicit fentanyl analogs (eg, 3-methylfentanyl and para-fluorofentanyl) are common drugs of abuse. Experienced heroin users could not easily differentiate fentanyl from heroin, although in one study, heroin was noted to provide a more intense "rush."[94] Although unconfirmed, the xenobiotic used by Russian authorities to overcome terrorists and subdue a hostage situation in Moscow in October 2002 may have been carfentanil,[179] a potent μ-receptor agonist that is commonly used as a positron emission tomography scan radioligand.

Although fentanyl is a more potent opioid agonist than heroin, the dose of naloxone required to reverse respiratory depression appears to be similar to that of other common opioids.[164] This is because the binding affinity (K_d) of fentanyl at the μ opioid receptor is similar to that of both morphine and naloxone.[171] In a typical overdose, the quantity of fentanyl is likely to be equipotent to typical heroin. However, if large quantities of fentanyl are involved in the poisoning, higher than normal doses of naloxone may be required for reversal. Use of other opioids, such as sufentanil and buprenorphine, which have higher affinity for opioid receptors (lower K_d') may lead to the need for larger doses of naloxone to reverse the patient's respiratory depression[101] (see Antidotes in Depth A6: Opioid Antagonists).

Oxycodone and Hydrocodone Although media reports highlight the abuse of these and other prescription opioids by sports figures and other personalities, this trend has reached epidemic levels in regions of the country where heroin is difficult to obtain (thus the term "hillbilly heroin"). The abuse liabilities of these semisynthetic opioids based on their subjective profile are similar.[175] Although many users initially receive oxycodone or hydrocodone as analgesics, the majority of abusers obtain the drugs illicitly or from friends.[13,105] Regulatory agencies, law enforcement, and the drug manufacturer have made tremendous efforts to control drug diversion to illicit use.[52,170] Physicians have been charged criminally with complicity for inappropriate prescriptions for patients with the intent to sell or abuse these drugs.[52] Many of these opioids are sold in fixed combination with acetaminophen (eg, Percocet [oxycodone 5 mg], Vicodin [hydrocodone]), raising concerns about the complications of acetaminophen hepatotoxicity. Unlike most immediate-release prescription opioids, oxycodone can be obtained in a controlled-release form (OxyContin) that contains as much as 80 mg. Abusers typically crush the tablet, which destroys the sustained-release matrix and liberates large amounts of insufflatable or injectable oxycodone. The psychoactive effects of these opioids are similar to other μ-receptor agonists[189] and often are used as a substitute for heroin. Opioid dependence, overdose, and death are common sequelae of oxycodone abuse.

Body Packers In an attempt to transport illicit drugs from one country to another, "mules," or body packers, ingest large numbers of multiple-wrapped packages of concentrated cocaine or heroin. When the authorities discover such individuals or when individuals in custody become ill, they may be brought to a hospital for evaluation and management. Although these patients generally are asymptomatic on arrival, they are at risk for delayed, prolonged, or lethal poisoning as a consequence of packet rupture.[168] In the past, determining the country of origin of the current journey was nearly diagnostic of packet content. However, because most of the heroin imported into the United States now originates from South America, which is also the major source of imported cocaine, the discernment from cocaine on this basis is impossible. Given the current greater revenue potential of heroin, the majority of body packers carry heroin.[56] Details of diagnosis and management are discussed in Special Considerations SC4: Internal Concealment of Xenobiotics.

Agonist–Antagonists The opioid agonists in common clinical use tend to have specific binding affinity toward the μ-opioid–receptor subtype. The agonist–antagonists differ in that they interact with multiple receptor types and may have different effects at each receptor. Thus, although most opioids typically produce either agonist or antagonist effects, the agonist–antagonists generally have agonist effects at the κ-receptor subtype and antagonistic effects at the μ-receptor subtype. Therefore, opioids such as pentazocine (Talwin) may elicit a withdrawal syndrome in a μ-opioid–tolerant individual because of antagonist effects at the μ receptor. This effect forms the basis of the claim offered by many methadone-dependent patients that they are "allergic to Talwin." However, this same drug may act as an analgesic in nonopioid-using patients through its agonist effects at the κ_1-receptor subtype. Although the clinical effects of agonist–antagonists after overdose resemble those of the other opioids, including lethal respiratory depression,[124] they are less likely than the full agonists to produce severe morbidity or mortality because of their ceiling effect on respiratory depression (see Respiratory Depression above).

Pentazocine. Historically, patients abusing pentazocine (Talwin) administered it with tripelennamine, a blue capsule, accounting for the appellation "T's and Blues." Although this mixture has largely fallen out of favor, pentazocine abuse occurs occasionally. The psychotomimetic effects noted with high doses of pentazocine likely are mediated by κ_2 or perhaps σ receptors. Because pentazocine can be readily dissolved, IV injection was a preferred route for its abuse until the commercial formulation was altered to include 0.5 mg naloxone (Talwin NX). When ingested, the naloxone is eliminated by first-pass hepatic metabolism; if injected, naloxone prevents the euphoria sought by users.

AGENTS USED IN OPIOID SUBSTITUTION THERAPY: METHADONE, LAAM, AND BUPRENORPHINE

Two contrasting approaches to the management of patients with chronic opioid use exist: detoxification and maintenance therapy. Detoxification probably is most appropriate for patients motivated or compelled to discontinue opioid use. It can be performed either by tapered withdrawal of an opioid agonist or with the assistance of opioid antagonists. Maintenance therapy may include use of a long-acting opioid antagonist, such as naltrexone, to pharmacologically block the effects of additional opioid use. Alternatively, and more commonly, maintenance therapy involves opioid substitution therapy.[17]

Methadone Methadone is a synthetic μ-opioid–receptor agonist used both for treatment of chronic pain and as a maintenance substitute for opioid dependence. Methadone has been available for the latter use for more than 40 years through methadone maintenance treatment programs (MMTPs).[38] In MMTPs, the opioid in use is replaced by methadone, which is legal, oral, and long acting. This opioid allows patients to abstain from activities associated with procurement and administration of the abused opioid and eliminates much of the morbidity and mortality associated with illicit drug use. Although often successful in achieving opioid abstinence, some methadone users continue to use heroin, other opioids, and other xenobiotics.[84]

Methadone is administered as a chiral mixture of (R,S)-methadone. In humans, methadone metabolism is mediated by several cytochrome P450 (CYP) isozymes, mainly CYP3A4 and CYP2B6, and to a lesser extent CYP2D6. CYP2B6 demonstrates stereoselectivity toward (S)-methadone,[53] and in vivo data show that CYP2B6 slow metabolizer status is associated with high (S)- but not serum (R)-methadone concentrations.[29] In clinical trials, QT prolongation was exacerbated in individuals who were CYP2B6 slow metabolizers, and this population had higher (S)-methadone concentrations.[41] (R)-methadone is used in Germany and is both more effective and safer than the chiral mixture or the (S) enantiomer, but it is not available in the United States at the present time.

Methadone predictably produces QT interval prolongation because of blockade of the hERG (human *ether-a-gogo* related gene) channel. In the human heart, the hERG voltage-gated potassium channel mediates the rapidly activating delayed rectifier current (see Chap 22). Blocking potassium efflux from the cardiac myocyte prolongs cellular repolarization, prolonging the QT interval. Syncope and sudden death caused by ventricular dysrhythmias (such as torsades de pointes) are the result. Initially described in case reports of patients on high doses of methadone, clinical trials now reveal that methadone can prolong the QT interval in a concentration-dependent fashion.[107] Genetic factors in the metabolism of methadone[41] and probably baseline QT status at the initiation of methadone therapy may underlie and potentially predict adverse effects. (S)-methadone binding to hERG is greater than twofold than that of (R)-methadone and is primarily responsible for the drug's cardiotoxicity.[77]

A major difficulty is identification of individuals who are at risk for life threatening dysrhythmias from methadone-induced QT interval prolongation. Expert-derived guidelines recommend questioning patients about intrinsic heart disease or dysrhythmias, counseling patients initiating methadone therapy, and obtaining a pretreatment ECG and a follow-up ECG at 30 days and yearly.[92] Patients who receive methadone doses of greater than 100 mg/day might warrant more frequent ECGs, particularly after dose escalation or change in comorbid disease staus.[92] Although these guidelines are disputed by some and limited data exist on the utility of the ECG as a screening test for persons at risk for torsades de pointes from methadone, given its low cost, easy availability, and minimal invasiveness, the guideline recommendations seem practical and appropriate.

Although therapeutic methadone is generally safe, rapid dose escalation during induction in the treatment program may unintentionally produce toxicity and, rarely, fatal respiratory depression.[17] This adverse effect is generally the result of the long duration of effect of methadone and the time lag for the development of tolerance.

Acute methadone overdose results in clinical findings typical of opioid poisoning, although the duration is substantially longer than expected after overdose of prototypical therapeutic opioids. After a successful therapeutic response to the administration of naloxone, recurrence should be expected because the duration of effect of naloxone is approximately 1 hour. In many cases, continuous infusion of naloxone or possibly administration of a long-acting opioid antagonist is indicated to maintain adequate ventilation.

Unintentional methadone overdosage ironically may be related to the manner in which MMTPs dispense the drug. Most patients attending MMTPs are given doses of methadone greater than needed to simply prevent withdrawal and to prevent surreptitious heroin or other opioid use.[159] Additionally, many MMTPs provide their established patients with sufficient methadone to last through a weekend or holiday without the need to revisit the program. This combination of dose and quantity may allow diversion of portions of the dose without the attendant risk of opioid withdrawal. Furthermore, home storage of this surplus drug in inappropriate containers, such as juice containers or baby bottles,[63] is a cause of unintentional methadone ingestion by children. Such events can be anticipated because methadone is frequently formulated as a palatable liquid and may not be distributed in child-resistant containers. The primary reason for distribution as a liquid, as opposed to the pill form given to patients with chronic pain syndromes, is to ensure dosing compliance at the MMTP. Unfortunately, death is frequent in children who overdose.[102]

Buprenorphine Because prescription of methadone for maintenance therapy is restricted to federally licensed programs, it is inaccessible and inconvenient for many patients. Buprenorphine was approved in 2000 as a schedule III medication for office-based prescription, administered thrice weekly, providing an attractive alternative for patients with substantially broader potential for obtaining outpatient therapy. However, because of the initial limitations on patient volume (subsequently expanded), the requirement for physician certification, and possibly the hesitation on the part of community physicians to welcome patients with substance use problems into their practices, many of the purported benefits of buprenorphine therapy over methadone have not been realized.

Buprenorphine (Subutex), a partial μ-opioid agonist, in doses of 8 to 16 mg sublingually, is effective at suppressing both opioid withdrawal symptoms and the covert use of illicit drugs. Buprenorphine for opioid substitution therapy may be preferred as an alternative to methadone because it has a better safety profile. That is, buprenorphine overdose is associated with markedly less respiratory depression than full agonists such as methadone, and there is no reported effect on the QT interval.

Buprenorphine competes with the extant opioid for the μ receptor; thus, administration of initial doses of buprenorphine in patients taking methadone for opioid substitution therapy can be complicated by opioid withdrawal, particularly in patients on higher doses of methadone. For this reason, the initial dose of buprenorphine typically is administered in the presence of a physician. The use of buprenorphine to assist opioid maintenance is limited in that many patients have difficulty stopping or decreasing their methadone dose. In patients in whom transfer from methadone to buprenorphine is indicated, dose reduction of methadone to 30 mg/day or less can reduce withdrawal symptoms precipitated by buprenorphine.[14] Buprenorphine use has been reported to result in only a mild withdrawal syndrome when abruptly discontinued and for this reason may prove efficacious in opioid detoxification programs.[3] After the initial doses of buprenorphine, sublingual tablets containing both buprenorphine and naloxone (Suboxone) are prescribed to prevent their IV use.

Buprenorphine at therapeutic doses produces nearly complete occupancy of the μ opioid receptors, where it prevents other opioids from binding.[60] Interestingly, naloxone may prevent the clinical effects of buprenorphine, but the reversal of respiratory effects by naloxone appear to be related in a nonlinear fashion. Relatively low bolus doses of IV naloxone had no effect on the respiratory depression induced by buprenorphine, but high doses (5–10 mg) caused only partial reversal of the respiratory effects of buprenorphine. More recently, data in healthy volunteers suggest a bell-shaped dose response to naloxone,[137,169] with a midrange dose of naloxone that is most effective at reversing respiratory depression. Although doses that would reverse other opioids were ineffective (0.2–0.4 mg), increasing the dose of naloxone to 2 to 4 mg caused full reversal of buprenorphine respiratory depression. However, the onset of reversal is usually slower than occurs when antagonizing other opioids.[169] Further increasing the naloxone dose to 5 to 7 mg caused a decline in reversal activity and actually increased the degree of respiratory depression. Although life-threatening respiratory depression from buprenorphine overdose appears to be rare, reversal of respiratory depression should be treated with a starting dose that is slightly higher than used to reverse other opioids and increased slowly and titrate to reversal of respiratory depression. For example, a starting dose of naloxone of 0.02 mg/kg, or between 1 and 2 mg, is reasonable, and upward titration should not provide doses in excess of about 5 mg without careful consideration and monitoring. Furthermore, because respiratory depression from buprenorphine may outlast the reversal effects of naloxone boluses or short infusions, a continuous infusion of naloxone may be required to maintain respiratory function.

As a partial agonist, buprenorphine has a ceiling effect on respiratory depression in healthy volunteers, with minimal plateau in analgesic effect.[31] However, in some patients, despite the ceiling effect, clinically consequential respiratory depression may occur.[167] Data from multiple case series indicate that most buprenorphine-related deaths are associated with concomitant use of other drugs, most often benzodiazepines, or to the IV injection of crushed tablets.[167]

The higher affinity (lower K_d) and partial agonism of buprenorphine should allow it to function as an antagonist to the respiratory depressant effects of heroin and improve spontaneous respiration. Although administration of sublingual buprenorphine for opioid overdose is reportedly successful in some case reports,[182] this practice is largely unstudied. Interestingly, some reported deaths involved patients given buprenorphine tablets intravenously by fellow drug users for the treatment of heroin-induced respiratory depression.[12]

Clonidine Clonidine, a presynaptic α_2-adrenergic agonist of the imidazoline class, is widely used by both clinicians and patients to reduce the disturbing autonomic effects of opioid withdrawal. Although clonidine is not structurally related to any opioid, in overdose, clonidine produces a clinical syndrome identical to that produced by the μ-active opioids. Mechanistically, there is functional overlap between α_2 and μ receptors within the brain (see Fig. 38–1). For these reasons, clonidine is commonly used to ameliorate the autonomic effects of opioid withdrawal. Although the autonomic abnormalities can be normalized with this approach, the psychological aspects of withdrawal, including drug craving and poor judgment, may not be alleviated.

UNIQUE OPIOIDS

Meperidine Meperidine, also called pethidine outside of the United States, is widely used for treatment of chronic and acute pain syndromes. Meperidine produces clinical manifestations typical of the other opioids and may lead to greater euphoria.[188] Pupillary constriction is less pronounced and, if it occurs, is less persistent than that associated with morphine.[54] However, normeperidine, a toxic, renally eliminated hepatic metabolite, accumulates in patients receiving chronic high-dose meperidine therapy, such as those with sickle cell disease or cancer. A similar accumulation occurs in patients with renal insufficiency, in whom the elimination half-life increases from a normal of 14 to 21 hours to 35 hours.[162] Normeperidine causes excitatory neurotoxicity, which manifests as delirium, tremor, myoclonus, or seizures. Based on animal studies, the seizures should not be expected to respond to naloxone.[55] In fact, experimental evidence suggests that naloxone may potentiate normeperidine-induced seizures, presumably by inhibiting an anticonvulsant effect of meperidine.[26] Hemodialysis using a high-efficiency membrane may be of limited clinical benefit but rarely, if ever, is indicated because the toxicity generally is self-limited.

Although primarily an opioid, meperidine is capable of exerting effects at other types of receptors. The most consequential nonopioid-receptor effects occur through the serotonin receptor. Blockade of the presynaptic reuptake of released serotonin may produce the serotonin syndrome, characterized by muscle rigidity, hyperthermia, and altered mental status, particularly in patients using monoamine oxidase inhibitors (MAOIs) (see Chap. 71). However, dextromethorphan (see Dextromethorphan below) also may produce this syndrome. Conversely, the simultaneous use of MAOIs and morphine, fentanyl, or methadone is not expected to produce the serotonin syndrome based on the currently appreciated pharmacology of these drugs. Despite its purported (and likely overstated) beneficial effects on biliary tract physiology, meperidine offers little to support its clinical use and has significant disadvantages. Meperidine use has been dramatically reduced or is closely monitored in many institutions and has been eliminated in other centers because of its adverse risk–benefit profile.

MPTP In 1982, several cases of acute, severe parkinsonian symptoms were identified in IV drug users.[96] The patients were labeled "frozen addicts" because of the severe bradykinesia, and extensive investigations into the etiology of the problem ensued. This ultimately led to the discovery of 1-methyl-4-phenyl-1,2,3,6-tetrahydropyridine (MPTP), an inadvertent product of presumed errors in the attempted synthesis of the illicit meperidine analog MPPP (1-methyl-4-phenyl-4-propionoxy-piperidine). MPTP is metabolized to the ultimate toxicant MPP^+ by monoamine oxidase-B in glial cells. Toxicity is inhibited by pretreatment with deprenyl, a monoamine oxidase-B inhibitor. MPP^+ is a paraquatlike xenobiotic capable of selectively destroying the dopamine-containing cells of the substantia nigra by inhibiting mitochondrial oxidative phosphorylation.[139] The index cases initially responded to standard antiparkinsonian therapy, but none improved substantially, and the effects of the medications waned.[5] Although calamitous for exposed patients, MPTP has proved to be invaluable in the development of experimental models for the study of Parkinson's disease. Several of the original "frozen" patients subsequently underwent stereotactic implantation of fetal adrenal tissue grafts into their basal ganglia, with significant clinical improvement.[97]

Dextromethorphan Dextromethorphan is devoid of analgesic properties altogether, even though it is the optical isomer of levorphanol, a potent opioid analgesic. Based on this structural relationship, dextromethorphan is commonly considered an opioid, although its receptor pharmacology is much more complex and diversified. At high doses, dextromethorphan does bind to opioid receptors to produce miosis, respiratory depression, and CNS depression. Reversal of these opioid effects by naloxone is reported. Binding to the PCP site on the NMDA receptor, and subsequent inhibition of calcium influx through this receptor-linked ion channel, causes sedation. This same activity may account for its antiepileptic properties and for its neuroprotective effects in ischemic brain injury. Because NMDA receptor blockade also enhances the analgesic effects of μ-opioid agonists, combination therapy with morphine and dextromethorphan (MorphiDex) has been introduced.

Blockade of presynaptic serotonin reuptake by dextromethorphan may elicit the serotonin syndrome in patients receiving MAOIs.[154] Movement disorders, described as choreoathetoid or dystonialike, occasionally occur and presumably result from alteration of dopaminergic neurotransmission. Dextrorphan, the active *O*-demethylation metabolite of dextromethorphan, is produced by CYP2D6, an enzyme with a well-described genetic polymorphism.[4] Whereas patients with the "extensive metabolizer" polymorphism appear to experience more drug-related psychoactive effects, poor metabolizers experience more adverse effects related to the parent compound.[190]

Dextromethorphan is available without prescription in cold preparations, primarily because of its presumed lack of significant addictive potential. However, abuse of dextromethorphan is increasing, particularly among high school students.[8] This increase in use likely is related to the easy availability of dextromethorphan and its perceived limited toxicity. Common street names include "DXM," "dex," and "robo-shots." Users often have expectations of euphoria and hallucinations, but a dysphoria comparable to that of PCP commonly ensues. Reports of substantial cold medicine consumption raise several concerns, including acetaminophen poisoning, opioid dependency, and bromide toxicity.[75] This last concern relates to the common formulation of dextromethorphan as the hydrobromide salt. At times, the first clue may be an elevated serum chloride concentration when measured on certain autoanalyzers (see Chaps. 6 and 16).

Tramadol Tramadol (Ultram) is a novel synthetic analgesic with both opioid and nonopioid mechanisms responsible for its clinical effects. Although it binds only weakly to μ opioid receptors, tramadol exhibits cross-tolerance with morphine in rats, suggesting an opioid-mediated mechanism of analgesia.[88] The demethylated tramadol metabolite M1 exhibits higher-affinity binding to receptors in vitro and may be important in patients chronically using the drug. However, the role of M1 as an acute analgesic is not well defined. Naloxone only partially reverses tramadol-induced analgesia in mice and in humans, suggesting that an independent, nonopioid mechanism is also involved in mediating the clinical effects of tramadol. This effect appears to be inhibition of reuptake of biogenic amines, specifically serotonin and norepinephrine. This mechanism is supported by the nearly complete reversal of analgesic efficacy by yohimbine, an α_2-adrenergic antagonist that inhibits release of these neurotransmitters. Patients using MAOIs may be at risk for development of the serotonin syndrome.

A large number of spontaneous reports to the Food and Drug Administration suggest that therapeutic use of tramadol may cause seizures, particularly on the first day of therapy. However, epidemiologic studies have not confirmed this association.[50] Tramadol-related seizures are not responsive to naloxone but are suppressed with benzodiazepines. In fact, the package insert cautions against using naloxone in patients with tramadol overdoses because in animals treated with naloxone, the risk of seizure is increased. Correspondingly, one patient in a prospective series had a seizure that was temporally related to naloxone administration.[155] Acute overdose of tramadol is generally considered non–life threatening, and most fatalities were associated with polysubstance overdose.

Tramadol abuse is reported, but its extent is undefined. In a review of physician drug abuse in several states, tramadol was the second most frequent opioid reported.[148] Opioid users recognized tramadol as an opioid only when given in an amount that was six times the therapeutic dose, but at this dose, the users did not develop opioid-like clinical effects such as miosis. Patients may develop typical opioid manifestations after a large overdose. Significant respiratory depression is uncommon and should respond to naloxone.[155] Generally, urine drug screening for drugs of abuse is negative for opioids in tramadol-exposed patients.

Propoxyphene Propoxyphene is a weak analgesic with limited efficacy data and serious safety concerns. Similar to its structural analog methadone, propoxyphene binds μ-opioid receptors and produces the expected opioid clinical findings. However, unanticipated properties of propoxyphene manifest after overdose. Propoxyphene and its hepatic metabolite, norpropoxyphene, produce myocardial sodium channel blockade identical to the type IA antidysrhythmics. This process results in QRS complex widening and negative inotropy. QRS prolongation was identified in 42 (19%) of 222 propoxyphene-poisoned patients.[149] These symptoms can be corrected with parenteral administration of hypertonic sodium bicarbonate or with lidocaine (see A5 Sodium Bicarbonate). As in patients with tricyclic antidepressant overdose, the sodium ion component of the sodium bicarbonate enhances sodium influx through a partially occluded sodium channel by augmenting the extracellular to intracellular sodium concentration gradient. The paradoxical effect of lidocaine, another sodium channel blocker, can be explained by the very different dissociation constants of these two xenobiotics with the sodium channel. Lidocaine may competitively displace propoxyphene and norpropoxyphene, both more highly toxic sodium channel blockers. Naloxone has never been shown to be effective therapy for the cardiotoxic effects of propoxyphene, although hemodynamic improvement in one reported case probably was related to naloxone-induced propoxyphene withdrawal.[62]

Propoxyphene overdose may produce acute CNS toxicity that usually manifests as seizures. In one study of propoxyphene-overdosed patients, 10% of the subjects developed seizures.[149] Although the exact mechanism is unclear, experimental models demonstrate that propoxyphene, and not norpropoxyphene, is capable of inducing seizures. Therapy for seizures should follow standard management strategies, including benzodiazepines or barbiturates. High-dose naloxone (60 mg/kg intraperitoneally) prevents experimental propoxyphene-induced seizures,[55] but its role in seizure termination is undefined.

Propoxyphene use and overdose in the United States is relatively uncommon compared with the other opioids. However, in the United Kingdom, propoxyphene overdose may account for up to 5% of all suicides.[64] Propoxyphene often is formulated with acetaminophen (Darvocet-N, Coproxamol) or salicylates (Darvon compound) to enhance the analgesic effects. Patients who overdose on the combinations may experience toxicity from either of these two nonopioid analgesics. Because patients consequently may be acetaminophen poisoned yet be asymptomatic or manifest only opioid toxicity, empiric quantitative serum analysis for acetaminophen is indicated. Delayed peak serum acetaminophen concentrations after ingestion of combination opioid products may occur. The precise clinical implication of this delay is unclear (see Chap 34). Furthermore, the respiratory depressant effects of propoxyphene may hinder the ability to detect salicylate poisoning by clinical examination, suggesting a situation in which empiric laboratory testing for salicylates may be indicated.

Diphenoxylate and Loperamide Although diphenoxylate is structurally similar to meperidine, its extreme insolubility limits absorption from the GI tract. This factor may enhance its use as an antidiarrheal agent, which presumably occurs via a local opioid effect at the GI μ receptor. However, the standard adult formulation may result in significant systemic absorption and toxicity in children, and all such ingestions should be deemed consequential. Diphenoxylate is formulated with a small dose (0.025 mg) of atropine (as Lomotil), both to enhance its antidiarrheal effect and to discourage illicit use.

Because both components of Lomotil may be absorbed and their pharmacokinetic profiles differ somewhat, a biphasic clinical syndrome is occasionally noted.[111] Patients may manifest atropine poisoning (anticholinergic syndrome), either independently or concomitantly with the opioid effects of diphenoxylate. Delayed, prolonged, or recurrent toxicity is common and is classically related to the delayed gastric emptying effects inherent to both opioids and anticholinergics. However, these effects are more likely explained by the accumulation of the hepatic metabolite difenoxin, which is a significantly more potent opioid than diphenoxylate and possesses a longer serum half-life. Still, the relevance of gastroparesis is highlighted by the retrieval of Lomotil pills by gastric lavage as late as 27 hours postingestion.

A review of 36 pediatric reports of Lomotil overdoses found that although naloxone was effective in reversing the opioid toxicity, recurrence of CNS and respiratory depression was common.[111] This series included a patient with an asymptomatic presentation 8 hours postingestion who was observed for several hours and then discharged. This patient returned to the ED 18 hours postingestion with marked signs of atropinism. In this same series, children with delayed onset of respiratory depression and other opioid effects were reported, and others describe cardiopulmonary arrest 12 hours postingestion. Naloxone infusion may be appropriate for patients with recurrent signs of opioid toxicity. Because of the delayed and possibly severe consequences, all children, and adult patients with potentially significant ingestions, should be admitted for monitored observation in the hospital.

Loperamide (Imodium) is another insoluble meperidine analog that is used to treat diarrhea. This medication is available without a prescription, and the paucity of adverse patient outcomes reported in the medical literature suggests the safety profile of this agent is good.

CLOSTRIDIAL INFECTIONS

Heroin-related clostridial infections, although uncommon, present in a manner similar to those of conventional botulism or tetanus but may be atypical (see Chap. 46).[16] Interestingly, during the 1950s and early 1960s, users of quinine-adulterated heroin in New York City[21] and Chicago[99] were substantially more likely to develop tetanus than were users of nonquinine-adulterated heroin. This likely is a result of the extensive tissue destruction caused by SC quinine administration, which also occurs in patients receiving therapeutic IM quinine. "Black tar heroin," an impure form of heroin, is implicated in multiple epidemics of wound botulism.[18] Whether the minimally processed heroin was contaminated with *Clostridium botulinum* or whether it led to improved anaerobic growing conditions for the spores is not known. Early antitoxin therapy is associated with improved outcome. Other *Clostridia* species (eg, *C. novyi* and *C. sordellii*) are responsible for epidemics of necrotizing fasciitis that are common among users of black tar heroin. Nearly half of the victims of necrotizing fasciitis die of the disease.

SUMMARY

Opioid use is widespread. Overdose and toxicity, both intentional and unintentional, remain major causes of drug-related morbidity and mortality. Lethality related to opioids is primarily caused by respiratory depression. Thus mechanical ventilation, or administration of a short-acting opioid antagonist such as naloxone, should be adequate initial therapy. An appreciation of the pharmacologic differences between the various opioids allows for the identification and appropriate management of patients poisoned or otherwise adversely affected by these xenobiotics.

REFERENCES

1. Aicher SA, Goldberg A, Sharma S. Co-localization of mu opioid receptor and N-methyl-D-aspartate receptor in the trigeminal dorsal horn. *J Pain.* 2002;3:203-210.
2. Andersen G, Christrup L, Sjogren P. Relationships among morphine metabolism, pain and side effects during long-term treatment: an update. *J Pain Symptom Manage.* 2003;25:74-91.
3. Assadi SM, Hafezi M, Mokri A, et al. Opioid detoxification using high doses of buprenorphine in 24 hours: a randomized, double blind, controlled clinical trial. *J Subst Abuse Treat.* 2004;27:75-82.
4. Bailey B, Daneman R, Daneman N, et al. Discrepancy between CYP2D6 phenotype and genotype derived from post-mortem dextromethorphan blood level. *Forensic Sci Int.* 2000;110:61-70.
5. Ballard PA, Tetrud JW, Langston JW. Permanent human parkinsonism due to 1-methyl-4-phenyl-1,2,3,6-tetrahydropyridine (MPTP): seven cases. *Neurology.* 1985;35:949-956.
6. Barke KE, Hough LB. Opiates, mast cells and histamine release. *Life Sci.* 1993;53:1391-1399.
7. Beckett A, Casy A. Synthetic analgesics: stereochemical considerations. *J Pharm Pharmacol.* 1954;6:986-1001.
8. Bencharit S, Morton CL, Xue Y, et al. Structural basis of heroin and cocaine metabolism by a promiscuous human drug-processing enzyme. *Nat Struct Biol.* 2003;10:349-356.
9. Bodnar RJ, Williams CL, Lee SJ, et al. Role of mu 1-opiate receptors in supraspinal opiate analgesia: a microinjection study. *Brain Res.* 1988;447:25-34.
10. Bonnet U, Banger M, Wolstein J, et al. Choreoathetoid movements associated with rapid adjustment to methadone. *Pharmacopsychiatry.* 1998;31:143-145.
11. Booth JV, Grossman D, Moore J, et al. Substance abuse among physicians: a survey of academic anesthesiology programs. *Anesth Analg.* 2002;95:1024-1030.
12. Boyd J, Randell T, Luurila H, et al. Serious overdoses involving buprenorphine in Helsinki. *Acta Anaesthesiol Scand.* 2003;47:1031-1033.
13. Brands B, Blake J, Sproule B, et al. Prescription opioid abuse in patients presenting for methadone maintenance treatment. *Drug Alcohol Depend.* 2004;73:199-207.
14. Breen CL, Harris SJ, Lintzeris N, et al. Cessation of methadone maintenance treatment using buprenorphine: transfer from methadone to buprenorphine and subsequent buprenorphine reductions. *Drug Alcohol Depend.* 2003;71:49-55.
15. Brenneisen R, Hasler F. GC/MS determination of pyrolysis products from diacetylmorphine and adulterants of street heroin samples. *J Forensic Sci.* 2002;47:885-888.
16. Brett MM, Hood J, Brazier JS, et al. Soft tissue infections caused by spore-forming bacteria in injecting drug users in the United Kingdom. *Epidemiol Infect.* 2005;133:575-582.
17. Center for Substance Abuse Prevention. Methadone-associated mortality: report of a national assessment Rockville, MD: U.S. Dept. of Health and Human Services, Substance Abuse and Mental Health Services Administration, Center for Substance Abuse Treatment; 2004 DHHS publication no (SMA) 04-3904.
18. Centers for Disease Control and Prevention. Wound botulism among black tar heroin users—Washington, 2003. *MMWR Morb Mortal Wkly Rep.* 2003;52:885-886.
19. Centers for Disease Control and Prevention. Nonpharmaceutical fentanyl-related deaths—multiple states, April 2005–March 2007. *MMWR Morb Mortal Wkly Rep.* 2008;57:793-796.
20. Cepeda MS, Gonzalez F, Granados V, et al. Incidence of nausea and vomiting in outpatients undergoing general anesthesia in relation to selection of intraoperative opioid. *J Clin Anesth.* 1996;8:324-328.
21. Cherubin CE. Epidemiology of tetanus in narcotic addicts. *N Y State J Med.* 1970;70:267-271.
22. Christensen O, Christensen P, Sonnenschein C, et al. Analgesic effect of intraarticular morphine. A controlled, randomised and double-blind study. *Acta Anaesthesiol Scand.* 1996;40:842-846.
23. Cohen MR, Cohen RM, Pickar D, et al. Behavioural effects after high dose naloxone administration to normal volunteers. *Lancet.* 1981;2:1110.
24. Cone EJ, Holicky BA, Grant TM, et al. Pharmacokinetics and pharmacodynamics of intranasal "snorted" heroin. *J Anal Toxicol.* 1993;17:327-337.
25. Courteix C, Coudore-Civiale MA, Privat AM, et al. Evidence for an exclusive antinociceptive effect of nociceptin/orphanin FQ, an endogenous ligand for the ORL1 receptor, in two animal models of neuropathic pain. *Pain.* 2004;110:236-245.
26. Cowan A, Geller EB, Adler MW. Classification of opioids on the basis of change in seizure threshold in rats. *Science.* 1979;206:465-467.
27. Crain SM, Shen KF. Modulation of opioid analgesia, tolerance and dependence by Gs-coupled, GM1 ganglioside-regulated opioid receptor functions. *Trends Pharmacol Sci.* 1998;19:358-365.
28. Crain SM, Shen KF. Antagonists of excitatory opioid receptor functions enhance morphine's analgesic potency and attenuate opioid tolerance/dependence liability. *Pain.* 2000;84:121-131.
29. Crettol S, Deglon JJ, Besson J, et al. Methadone enantiomer plasma levels, CYP2B6, CYP2C19, and CYP2C9 genotypes, and response to treatment. *Clin Pharmacol Ther.* 2005;78:593-604.
30. da Silva O, Alexandrou D, Knoppert D, et al. Seizure and electroencephalographic changes in the newborn period induced by opiates and corrected by naloxone infusion. *J Perinatol.* 1999;19:120-123.
31. Dahan A, Yassen A, Romberg R, et al. Buprenorphine induces ceiling in respiratory depression but not in analgesia. *Br J Anaesth.* 2006;96:627-632.
32. Daldrup T. A forensic toxicological dilemma: the interpretation of post-mortem concentrations of central acting analgesics. *Forensic Sci Int.* 2004;142:157-160.
33. Darke S, Hall W, Weatherburn D, et al. Fluctuations in heroin purity and the incidence of fatal heroin overdose. *Drug Alcohol Depend.* 1999;54:155-161.
34. Darke S, Ross J, Hall W. Overdose among heroin users in Sydney, Australia: I. Prevalence and correlates of non-fatal overdose. *Addiction.* 1996;91:405-411.
35. Darke S, Ross J, Hall W. Overdose among heroin users in Sydney, Australia: II. responses to overdose. *Addiction.* 1996;91:413-417.
36. Darke S, Sunjic S, Zador D, et al. A comparison of blood toxicology of heroin-related deaths and current heroin users in Sydney, Australia. *Drug Alcohol Depend.* 1997;47:45-53.
37. Dhawan BN, Cesselin F, Raghubir R, et al. International Union of Pharmacology. XII. Classification of opioid receptors. *Pharmacol Rev.* 1996;48:567-592.
38. Dole VP, Nyswander M. A medical treatment for diacetylmorphine (heroin) addiction. A clinical trial with methadone hydrochloride. *JAMA.* 1965;193:646-650.
39. Drummer OH. Postmortem toxicology of drugs of abuse. *Forensic Sci Int.* 2004;142:101-113.
40. Duberstein JL, Kaufman DM. A clinical study of an epidemic of heroin intoxication and heroin-induced pulmonary edema. *Am J Med.* 1971;51:704-714.
41. Eap CB, Crettol S, Rougier JS, et al. Stereoselective block of hERG channel by (S)-methadone and QT interval prolongation in CYP2B6 slow metabolizers. *Clin Pharmacol Ther.* 2007;81:719-728.
42. Eckenhoff J, Oech S. The effects of narcotics and antagonists upon respiration and circulation in man. *Clin Pharmacol Ther.* 1960;1:483-524.
43. Elman I, D'Ambra MN, Krause S, et al. Ultrarapid opioid detoxification: effects on cardiopulmonary physiology, stress hormones and clinical outcomes. *Drug Alcohol Depend.* 2001;61:163-172.
44. Elvenes J, Andjelkov N, Figenschau Y, et al. Expression of functional mu-opioid receptors in human osteoarthritic cartilage and chondrocytes. *Biochem Biophys Res Commun.* 2003;311:202-207.
45. Exley C, Ahmed U, Polwart A, et al. Elevated urinary aluminium in current and past users of illicit heroin. *Addict Biol.* 2007;12:197-199.
46. Fahnenstich H, Steffan J, Kau N, et al. Fentanyl-induced chest wall rigidity and laryngospasm in preterm and term infants. *Crit Care Med.* 2000;28:836-839.
47. Flacke JW, Flacke WE, Bloor BC, et al. Histamine release by four narcotics: a double-blind study in humans. *Anesth Analg.* 1987;66:723-730.

48. Gan TJ, Ginsberg B, Glass PS, et al. Opioid-sparing effects of a low-dose infusion of naloxone in patient-administered morphine sulfate. *Anesthesiology.* 1997;87:1075-1081.
49. Gasche Y, Daali Y, Fathi M, et al. Codeine intoxication associated with ultrarapid CYP2D6 metabolism. *N Engl J Med.* 2004;351:2827-2831.
50. Gasse C, Derby L, Vasilakis-Scaramozza C, et al. Incidence of first-time idiopathic seizures in users of tramadol. *Pharmacotherapy.* 2000;20:629-634.
51. Gaveriaux-Ruff C, Kieffer BL. Opioid receptor genes inactivated in mice: the highlights. *Neuropeptides.* 2002;36:62-71.
52. General Accounting Office. *Prescription Drugs: OxyContin Abuse and Diversion and Efforts to Address the Problem: Report to Congressional Committees.* Washington, DC: United States General Accounting Office; 2003.
53. Gerber JG, Rhodes RJ, Gal J. Stereoselective metabolism of methadone N-demethylation by cytochrome P4502B6 and 2C19. *Chirality.* 2004;16:36-44.
54. Ghoneim MM, Dhanaraj J, Choi WW. Comparison of four opioid analgesics as supplements to nitrous oxide anesthesia. *Anesth Analg.* 1984;63:405-412.
55. Gilbert PE, Martin WR. Antagonism of the convulsant effects of heroin, d-propoxyphene, meperidine, normeperidine and thebaine by naloxone in mice. *J Pharmacol Exp Ther.* 1975;192:538-541.
56. Gill JR, Graham SM. Ten years of "body packers" in New York City: 50 deaths. *J Forensic Sci.* 2002;47:843-846.
57. Goldfrank L, Weisman RS, Errick JK, et al. A dosing nomogram for continuous infusion intravenous naloxone. *Ann Emerg Med.* 1986;15:566-570.
58. Gossop M, Griffiths P, Powis B, et al. Frequency of non-fatal heroin overdose: survey of heroin users recruited in non-clinical settings. *Br Med J.* 1996;313:402.
59. Gowing L, Ali R, White J. Opioid antagonists under heavy sedation or anaesthesia for opioid withdrawal. *Cochrane Database Syst Rev.* 2006;CD002022.
60. Greenwald MK, Johanson CE, Moody DE, et al. Effects of buprenorphine maintenance dose on mu-opioid receptor availability, plasma concentrations, and antagonist blockade in heroin-dependent volunteers. *Neuropsychopharmacology.* 2003;28:2000-2009.
61. Hamilton RJ, Perrone J, Hoffman R, et al. A descriptive study of an epidemic of poisoning caused by heroin adulterated with scopolamine. *J Toxicol Clin Toxicol.* 2000;38:597-608.
62. Hantson P, Evenepoel M, Ziade D, et al. Adverse cardiac manifestations following dextropropoxyphene overdose: can naloxone be helpful? *Ann Emerg Med.* 1995;25:263-266.
63. Harkin K, Quinn C, Bradley F. Storing methadone in babies' bottles puts young children at risk. *Br Med J.* 1999;318:329-330.
64. Hawton K, Simkin S, Deeks J. Co-proxamol and suicide: a study of national mortality statistics and local non-fatal self poisonings. *Br Med J.* 2003;326:1006-1008.
65. Hayashi T, Su TP. Sigma-1 receptor ligands: potential in the treatment of neuropsychiatric disorders. *CNS Drugs.* 2004;18:269-284.
66. Helpern M, Rho YM. Deaths from narcotism in New York City. Incidence, circumstances, and postmortem findings. *N Y State J Med.* 1966;66:2391-2408.
67. Hemby SE, Martin TJ, Co C, et al. The effects of intravenous heroin administration on extracellular nucleus accumbens dopamine concentrations as determined by in vivo microdialysis. *J Pharmacol Exp Ther.* 1995;273:591-598.
68. Hendriks VM, van den Brink W, Blanken P, et al. Heroin self-administration by means of "chasing the dragon": pharmacodynamics and bioavailability of inhaled heroin. *Eur Neuropsychopharmacol.* 2001;11:241-252.
69. Henriksen G, Willoch F. Imaging of opioid receptors in the central nervous system. *Brain.* 2008;131:1171-1196.
70. Hine CH, Wright JA, Allison DJ, et al. Analysis of fatalities from acute narcotism in a major urban area. *J Forensic Sci.* 1982;27:372-384.
71. Hoffman JR, Schriger DL, Luo JS. The empiric use of naloxone in patients with altered mental status: a reappraisal. *Ann Emerg Med.* 1991;20:246-252.
72. Hoffman RS, Kirrane BM, Marcus SM. A descriptive study of an outbreak of clenbuterol-containing heroin. *Ann Emerg Med.* 2008;52:548-553.
73. Holzer P. Opioids and opioid receptors in the enteric nervous system: from a problem in opioid analgesia to a possible new prokinetic therapy in humans. *Neurosci Lett.* 2004;361:192-195.
74. Huizer H. Analytical studies on illicit heroin. V. Efficacy of volatilization during heroin smoking. *Pharm Weekbl Sci.* 1987;9:203-211.
75. Hung YM. Bromide intoxication by the combination of bromide-containing over-the-counter drug and dextromethorphan hydrobromide. *Hum Exp Toxicol.* 2003;22:459-461.
76. Ingelman-Sundberg M. Genetic polymorphisms of cytochrome P450 2D6 (CYP2D6): clinical consequences, evolutionary aspects and functional diversity. *Pharmacogenomics J.* 2005;5:6-13.
77. Inturrisi CE. Pharmacology of methadone and its isomers. *Minerva Anesthesiol.* 2005;71:435-437.
78. Jackson HC, Nutt DJ. Investigation of the involvement of opioid receptors in the action of anticonvulsants. *Psychopharmacology (Berl).* 1993;111:486-490.
79. Jannetto PJ, Wong SH, Gock SB, et al. Pharmacogenomics as molecular autopsy for postmortem forensic toxicology: genotyping cytochrome P450 2D6 for oxycodone cases. *J Anal Toxicol.* 2002;26:438-447.
80. Joranson DE, Ryan KM, Gilson AM, et al. Trends in medical use and abuse of opioid analgesics. *JAMA.* 2000;283:1710-1714.
81. Kaa E. Impurities, adulterants and diluents of illicit heroin. Changes during a 12-year period. *Forensic Sci Int.* 1994;64:171-179.
82. Kalant H. Opium revisited: a brief review of its nature, composition, non-medical use and relative risks. *Addiction.* 1997;92:267-277.
83. Kamendulis LM, Brzezinski MR, Pindel EV, et al. Metabolism of cocaine and heroin is catalyzed by the same human liver carboxylesterases. *J Pharmacol Exp Ther.* 1996;279:713-717.
84. Karch SB, Stephens BG. Toxicology and pathology of deaths related to methadone: retrospective review. *West J Med.* 2000;172:11-14.
85. Katchman AN, McGroary KA, Kilborn MJ, et al. Influence of opioid agonists on cardiac human ether-a-go-go-related gene K(+) currents. *J Pharmacol Exp Ther.* 2002;303:688-694.
86. Keogh CF, Andrews GT, Spacey SD, et al. Neuroimaging features of heroin inhalation toxicity: "chasing the dragon." *AJR Am J Roentgenol.* 2003;180:847-850.
87. King MA, McDonough MA, Drummer OH, et al. Poppy tea and the baker's first seizure. *Lancet.* 1997;350:716.
88. Klotz U. Tramadol—the impact of its pharmacokinetic and pharmacodynamic properties on the clinical management of pain. *Arzneimittelforschung.* 2003;53:681-687.
89. Koob GF, Ahmed SH, Boutrel B, et al. Neurobiological mechanisms in the transition from drug use to drug dependence. *Neurosci Biobehav Rev.* 2004;27:739-749.
90. Kornick CA, Santiago-Palma J, Moryl N, et al. Benefit-risk assessment of transdermal fentanyl for the treatment of chronic pain. *Drug Saf.* 2003;26:951-973.
91. Kram TC, Cooper DA, Allen AC. Behind the identification of China White. *Anal Chem.* 1981;53:1379A-1386A.
92. Krantz MJ, Martin J, Stimmel B, et al. QTc interval screening in methadone treatment. *Ann Intern Med.* 2009;150:387-395.
93. Kriegstein AR, Shungu DC, Millar WS, et al. Leukoencephalopathy and raised brain lactate from heroin vapor inhalation ("chasing the dragon"). *Neurology.* 1999;53:1765-1773.
94. LaBarbera M, Wolfe T. Characteristics, attitudes and implications of fentanyl use based on reports from self-identified fentanyl users. *J Psychoactive Drugs.* 1983;15:293-301.
95. Lalley PM. Opioidergic and dopaminergic modulation of respiration. *Respir Physiol Neurobiol.* 2008;164:160-167.
96. Langston JW, Ballard P, Tetrud JW, et al. Chronic Parkinsonism in humans due to a product of meperidine-analog synthesis. *Science.* 1983;219:979-980.
97. Langston JW, Palfreman J. *The Case of the Frozen Addicts.* New York: Pantheon Books; 1995.
98. Lee HK, Wang SC. Mechanism of morphine-induced miosis in the dog. *J Pharmacol Exp Ther.* 1975;192:415-431.
99. Levinson A, Marske RL, Shein MK. Tetanus in heroin addicts. *JAMA.* 1955;157:658-660.
100. Levy S, Sherritt L, Vaughan BL, et al. Results of random drug testing in an adolescent substance abuse program. *Pediatrics.* 2007;119:e843-848.
101. Leysen JE, Gommeren W, Niemegeers CJ. [3H]Sufentanil, a superior ligand for mu-opiate receptors: binding properties and regional distribution in rat brain and spinal cord. *Eur J Pharmacol.* 1983;87:209-225.
102. Li L, Levine B, Smialek JE. Fatal methadone poisoning in children: Maryland 1992–1996. *Subst Use Misuse.* 2000;35:1141-1148.
103. Long H, Deore K, Hoffman RS, et al. A fatal case of spongiform leukoencephalopathy linked to "chasing the dragon." *J Toxicol Clin Toxicol.* 2003;41:887-891.

104. Lotsch J, Skarke C, Liefhold J, et al. Genetic predictors of the clinical response to opioid analgesics: clinical utility and future perspectives. *Clin Pharmacokinet.* 2004;43:983-1013.
105. Manchikanti L, Singh A. Therapeutic opioids: a ten-year perspective on the complexities and complications of the escalating use, abuse, and nonmedical use of opioids. *Pain Physician.* 2008;11:S63-88.
106. Marks CE, Jr., Goldring RM. Chronic hypercapnia during methadone maintenance. *Am Rev Respir Dis.* 1973;108:1088-1093.
107. Martell BA, Arnsten JH, Krantz MJ, et al. Impact of methadone treatment on cardiac repolarization and conduction in opioid users. *Am J Cardiol.* 2005;95:915-918.
108. Martin M, Hecker J, Clark R, et al. China White epidemic: an eastern United States emergency department experience. *Ann Emerg Med.* 1991;20:158-164.
109. Martin WR, Eades CG, Thompson JA, et al. The effects of morphine- and nalorphine- like drugs in the nondependent and morphine-dependent chronic spinal dog. *J Pharmacol Exp Ther.* 1976;197:517-532.
110. Matthes HW, Maldonado R, Simonin F, et al. Loss of morphine-induced analgesia, reward effect and withdrawal symptoms in mice lacking the mu-opioid-receptor gene. *Nature.* 1996;383:819-823.
111. McCarron MM, Challoner KR, Thompson GA. Diphenoxylate-atropine (Lomotil) overdose in children: an update (report of eight cases and review of the literature). *Pediatrics.* 1991;87:694-700.
112. McGregor C, Ali R, White JM, et al. A comparison of antagonist-precipitated withdrawal under anesthesia to standard inpatient withdrawal as a precursor to maintenance naltrexone treatment in heroin users: outcomes at 6 and 12 months. *Drug Alcohol Depend.* 2002;68:5-14.
113. McGuire G, El-Beheiry H, Manninen P, et al. Activation of electrocorticographic activity with remifentanil and alfentanil during neurosurgical excision of epileptogenic focus. *Br J Anaesth.* 2003;91:651-655.
114. McNicol E, Boyce DB, Schumann R, et al. Efficacy and safety of mu-opioid antagonists in the treatment of opioid-induced bowel dysfunction: systematic review and meta-analysis of randomized controlled trials. *Pain Med.* 2008;9:634-659.
115. Meissner W, Schmidt U, Hartmann M, et al. Oral naloxone reverses opioid-associated constipation. *Pain.* 2000;84:105-109.
116. Millan MJ, Czlonkowski A, Lipkowski A, et al. Kappa-opioid receptor-mediated antinociception in the rat. II. Supraspinal in addition to spinal sites of action. *J Pharmacol Exp Ther.* 1989;251:342-350.
117. Mills CA, Flacke JW, Flacke WE, et al. Narcotic reversal in hypercapnic dogs: comparison of naloxone and nalbuphine. *Can J Anaesth.* 1990;37:238-244.
118. Mills CA, Flacke JW, Miller JD, et al. Cardiovascular effects of fentanyl reversal by naloxone at varying arterial carbon dioxide tensions in dogs. *Anesth Analg.* 1988;67:730-736.
119. Moeller MR, Hammer K, Engel O. Poppy seed consumption and toxicological analysis of blood and urine samples. *Forensic Sci Int.* 2004;143:183-186.
120. Mule SJ, Casella GA. Rendering the "poppy-seed defense" defenseless: identification of 6-monoacetylmorphine in urine by gas chromatography/mass spectroscopy. *Clin Chem.* 1988;34:1427-1430.
121. Nelson LS. Toxicologic myocardial sensitization. *J Toxicol Clin Toxicol.* 2002;40:867-879.
122. Offiah C, Hall E. Heroin-induced leukoencephalopathy: characterization using MRI, diffusion-weighted imaging, and MR spectroscopy. *Clin Radiol.* 2008;63:146-152.
123. Oldendorf WH, Hyman S, Braun L, et al. Blood-brain barrier: penetration of morphine, codeine, heroin, and methadone after carotid injection. *Science.* 1972;178:984-986.
124. Osifo OD, Aghahowa SE. Hazards of pentazocine for neonatal analgesia: a single-centre experience over 10 years. *Ann Trop Paediatr.* 2008;28:205-210.
125. Osler W. Oedema of left lung-Morphia poisoning. *Montreal Gen Hosp Rep.* 1880;1:291-293.
126. Pert CB, Snyder SH. Opiate receptor: demonstration in nervous tissue. *Science.* 1973;179:1011-1014.
127. Philbin DM, Moss J, Akins CW, et al. The use of H1 and H2 histamine antagonists with morphine anesthesia: a double-blind study. *Anesthesiology.* 1981;55:292-296.
128. Pick CG, Paul D, Pasternak GW. Nalbuphine, a mixed kappa 1 and kappa 3 analgesic in mice. *J Pharmacol Exp Ther.* 1992;262:1044-1050.
129. Prough DS, Roy R, Bumgarner J, et al. Acute pulmonary edema in healthy teenagers following conservative doses of intravenous naloxone. *Anesthesiology.* 1984;60:485-486.
130. Richardson DE, Akil H. Pain reduction by electrical brain stimulation in man. Part 1: acute administration in periaqueductal and periventricular sites. *J Neurosurg.* 1977;47:178-183.
131. Rigg JR, Rondi P. Changes in rib cage and diaphragm contribution to ventilation after morphine. *Anesthesiology.* 1981;55:507-514.
132. Risser D, Uhl A, Stichenwirth M, et al. Quality of heroin and heroin-related deaths from 1987 to 1995 in Vienna, Austria. *Addiction.* 2000;95:375-382.
133. Rohrig TP, Moore C. The determination of morphine in urine and oral fluid following ingestion of poppy seeds. *J Anal Toxicol.* 2003;27:449-452.
134. Romberg R, Sarton E, Teppema L, et al. Comparison of morphine-6-glucuronide and morphine on respiratory depressant and antinociceptive responses in wild type and mu-opioid receptor deficient mice. *Br J Anaesth.* 2003;91:862-870.
135. Rook EJ, Huitema AD, van den Brink W, et al. Pharmacokinetics and pharmacokinetic variability of heroin and its metabolites: review of the literature. *Curr Clin Pharmacol.* 2006;1:109-118.
136. Santiago TV, Pugliese AC, Edelman NH. Control of breathing during methadone addiction. *Am J Med.* 1977;62:347-354.
137. Sarton E, Teppema L, Dahan A. Naloxone reversal of opioid-induced respiratory depression with special emphasis on the partial agonist/antagonist buprenorphine. *Adv Exp Med Biol.* 2008;605:486-491.
138. Schier J. Avoid unfavorable consequences: dextromethorpan can bring about a false-positive phencyclidine urine drug screen. *J Emerg Med.* 2000;18:379-381.
139. Schober A. Classic toxin-induced animal models of Parkinson's disease: 6-OHDA and MPTP. *Cell Tissue Res.* 2004;318:215-224.
140. Seal KH, Downing M, Kral AH, et al. Attitudes about prescribing take-home naloxone to injection drug users for the management of heroin overdose: a survey of street-recruited injectors in the San Francisco Bay Area. *J Urban Health.* 2003;80:291-301.
141. Seaman SR, Brettle RP, Gore SM. Mortality from overdose among injecting drug users recently released from prison: database linkage study. *Br Med J.* 1998;316:426-428.
142. Selley DE, Cao CC, Sexton T, et al. mu Opioid receptor-mediated G-protein activation by heroin metabolites: evidence for greater efficacy of 6-monoacetylmorphine compared with morphine. *Biochem Pharmacol.* 2001;62:447-455.
143. Sgherza AL, Axen K, Fain R, et al. Effect of naloxone on perceived exertion and exercise capacity during maximal cycle ergometry. *J Appl Physiol.* 2002;93:2023-2028.
144. Sheffler DJ, Roth BL, Salvinorin A. The "magic mint" hallucinogen finds a molecular target in the kappa opioid receptor. *Trends Pharmacol Sci.* 2003;24:107-109.
145. Shook JE, Watkins WD, Camporesi EM. Differential roles of opioid receptors in respiration, respiratory disease, and opiate-induced respiratory depression. *Am Rev Respir Dis.* 1990;142:895-909.
146. Skarke C, Darimont J, Schmidt H, et al. Analgesic effects of morphine and morphine-6-glucuronide in a transcutaneous electrical pain model in healthy volunteers. *Clin Pharmacol Ther.* 2003;73:107-121.
147. Skarke C, Jarrar M, Erb K, et al. Respiratory and miotic effects of morphine in healthy volunteers when P-glycoprotein is blocked by quinidine. *Clin Pharmacol Ther.* 2003;74:303-311.
148. Skipper GE, Fletcher C, Rocha-Judd R, et al. Tramadol abuse and dependence among physicians. *JAMA.* 2004;292:1818-1819.
149. Sloth Madsen P, Strom J, Reiz S, et al. Acute propoxyphene self-poisoning in 222 consecutive patients. *Acta Anaesthesiol Scand.* 1984;28:661-665.
150. Smith G, Beecher H. Subjective effects of heroin and morphine in normal subjects. *J Pharmacol Exp Ther.* 1962;136:47-52.
151. Smith ML, Hughes RO, Levine B, et al. Forensic drug testing for opiates. VI. Urine testing for hydromorphone, hydrocodone, oxymorphone, and oxycodone with commercial opiate immunoassays and gas chromatography-mass spectrometry. *J Anal Toxicol.* 1995;19:18-26.
152. Smith NT, Benthuysen JL, Bickford RG, et al. Seizures during opioid anesthetic induction—are they opioid-induced rigidity? *Anesthesiology.* 1989;71:852-862.
153. Sneader W. The discovery of heroin. *Lancet.* 1998;352:1697-1699.
154. Sovner R, Wolfe J. Interaction between dextromethorphan and monoamine oxidase inhibitor therapy with isocarboxazid. *N Engl J Med.* 1988;319:1671.
155. Spiller HA, Gorman SE, Villalobos D, et al. Prospective multicenter evaluation of tramadol exposure. *J Toxicol Clin Toxicol.* 1997;35:361-364.

156. Stein C, Comisel K, Haimerl E, et al. Analgesic effect of intraarticular morphine after arthroscopic knee surgery. *N Engl J Med.* 1991;325:1123-1126.
157. Stein C, Schafer M, Machelska H. Attacking pain at its source: new perspectives on opioids. *Nat Med.* 2003;9:1003-1008.
158. Storrow AB, Magoon MR, Norton J. The dextromethorphan defense: dextromethorphan and the opioid screen. *Acad Emerg Med.* 1995;2:791-794.
159. Strain EC, Bigelow GE, Liebson IA, et al. Moderate- vs high-dose methadone in the treatment of opioid dependence: a randomized trial. *JAMA.* 1999;281:1000-1005.
160. Strang J, McCambridge J, Best D, et al. Loss of tolerance and overdose mortality after inpatient opiate detoxification: follow up study. *Br Med J.* 2003;326:959-960.
161. Streisand JB, Bailey PL, LeMaire L, et al. Fentanyl-induced rigidity and unconsciousness in human volunteers. Incidence, duration, and plasma concentrations. *Anesthesiology.* 1993;78:629-634.
162. Szeto HH, Inturrisi CE, Houde R, et al. Accumulation of normeperidine, an active metabolite of meperidine, in patients with renal failure of cancer. *Ann Intern Med.* 1977;86:738-741.
163. Takahama K, Shirasaki T. Central and peripheral mechanisms of narcotic antitussives: codeine-sensitive and -resistant coughs. *Cough.* 2007;3:8.
164. Takahashi M, Sugiyama K, Hori M, et al. Naloxone reversal of opioid anesthesia revisited: clinical evaluation and plasma concentration analysis of continuous naloxone infusion after anesthesia with high-dose fentanyl. *J Anesth.* 2004;18:1-8.
165. Tharp AM, Winecker RE, Winston DC. Fatal intravenous fentanyl abuse: four cases involving extraction of fentanyl from transdermal patches. *Am J Forensic Med Pathol.* 2004;25:178-181.
166. Thiblin I, Eksborg S, Petersson A, et al. Fatal intoxication as a consequence of intranasal administration (snorting) or pulmonary inhalation (smoking) of heroin. *Forensic Sci Int.* 2004;139:241-247.
167. Tracqui A, Kintz P, Ludes B. Buprenorphine-related deaths among drug addicts in France: a report on 20 fatalities. *J Anal Toxicol.* 1998;22:430-434.
168. Traub SJ, Hoffman RS, Nelson LS. Body packing—the internal concealment of illicit drugs. *N Engl J Med.* 2003;349:2519-2526.
169. van Dorp E, Yassen A, Sarton E, et al. Naloxone reversal of buprenorphine-induced respiratory depression. *Anesthesiology.* 2006;105:51-57.
170. Van Zee A. The promotion and marketing of OxyContin: commercial triumph, public health tragedy. *Am J Public Health.* 2009;99:221-227.
171. Villiger JW, Ray LJ, Taylor KM. Characteristics of [3H]fentanyl binding to the opiate receptor. *Neuropharmacology.* 1983;22:447-452.
172. von Euler M, Villen T, Svensson JO, et al. Interpretation of the presence of 6-monoacetylmorphine in the absence of morphine-3-glucuronide in urine samples: evidence of heroin abuse. *Ther Drug Monit.* 2003;25:645-648.
173. Waldhoer M, Bartlett SE, Whistler JL. Opioid receptors. *Annu Rev Biochem.* 2004;73:953-990.
174. Walker JS. Anti-inflammatory effects of opioids. *Adv Exp Med Biol.* 2003;521:148-160.
175. Walsh SL, Nuzzo PA, Lofwall MR, et al. The relative abuse liability of oral oxycodone, hydrocodone and hydromorphone assessed in prescription opioid abusers. *Drug Alcohol Depend.* 2008;98:191-202.
176. Wanger K, Brough L, Macmillan I, et al. Intravenous vs subcutaneous naloxone for out-of-hospital management of presumed opioid overdose. *Acad Emerg Med.* 1998;5:293-299.
177. Ward CF, Ward GC, Saidman LJ. Drug abuse in anesthesia training programs. A survey: 1970 through 1980. *JAMA.* 1983;250:922-925.
178. Ward JM, McGrath RL, Weil JV. Effects of morphine on the peripheral vascular response to sympathetic stimulation. *Am J Cardiol.* 1972;29:659-666.
179. Wax PM, Becker CE, Curry SC. Unexpected "gas" casualties in Moscow: a medical toxicology perspective. *Ann Emerg Med.* 2003;41:700-705.
180. Weil JV, McCullough RE, Kline JS, et al. Diminished ventilatory response to hypoxia and hypercapnia after morphine in normal man. *N Engl J Med.* 1975;292:1103-1106.
181. Weinhold LL, Bigelow GE. Opioid miosis: effects of lighting intensity and monocular and binocular exposure. *Drug Alcohol Depend.* 1993;31:177-181.
182. Welsh C, Sherman SG, Tobin KE. A case of heroin overdose reversed by sublingually administered buprenorphine/naloxone (Suboxone). *Addiction.* 2008;103:1226-1228.
183. Whipple JK, Quebbeman EJ, Lewis KS, et al. Difficulties in diagnosing narcotic overdoses in hospitalized patients. *Ann Pharmacother.* 1994;28:446-450.
184. Wingert WE, Mundy LA, Nelson L, et al. Detection of clenbuterol in heroin users in twelve postmortem cases at the Philadelphia medical examiner's office. *J Anal Toxicol.* 2008;32:522-528.
185. Yajima Y, Narita M, Takahashi-Nakano Y, et al. Effects of differential modulation of mu-, delta- and kappa-opioid systems on bicuculline-induced convulsions in the mouse. *Brain Res.* 2000;862:120-126.
186. Yealy DM, Paris PM, Kaplan RM, et al. The safety of prehospital naloxone administration by paramedics. *Ann Emerg Med.* 1990;19:902-905.
187. Yuan CS, Foss JF. Oral methylnaltrexone for opioid-induced constipation. *JAMA.* 2000;284:1383-1384.
188. Zacny JP, Lichtor JL, Binstock W, et al. Subjective, behavioral and physiological responses to intravenous meperidine in healthy volunteers. *Psychopharmacology (Berl).* 1993;111:306-314.
189. Zacny JP, Gutierrez S. Characterizing the subjective, psychomotor, and physiological effects of oral oxycodone in non-drug-abusing volunteers. *Psychopharmacology (Berl).* 2003;170:242-254.
190. Zawertailo LA, Kaplan HL, Busto UE, et al. Psychotropic effects of dextromethorphan are altered by the CYP2D6 polymorphism: a pilot study. *J Clin Psychopharmacol.* 1998;18:332-337.

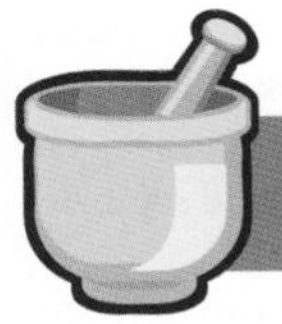

ANTIDOTES IN DEPTH (A6)

OPIOID ANTAGONISTS

Mary Ann Howland and Lewis S. Nelson

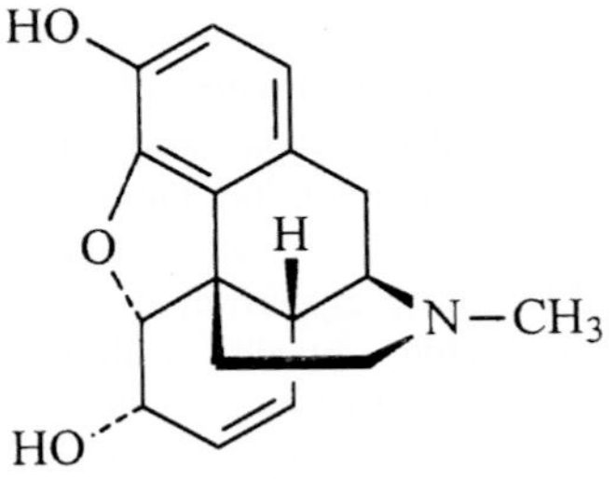

Morphine

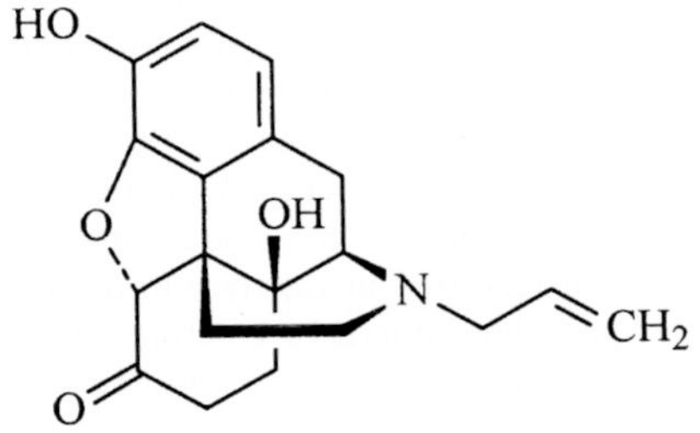

Naloxone

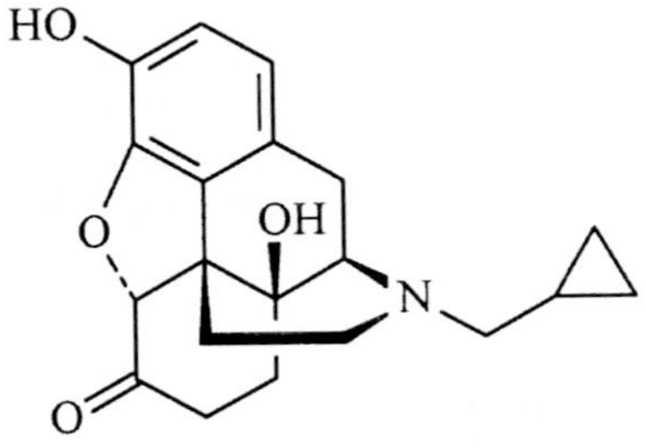

Naltrexone

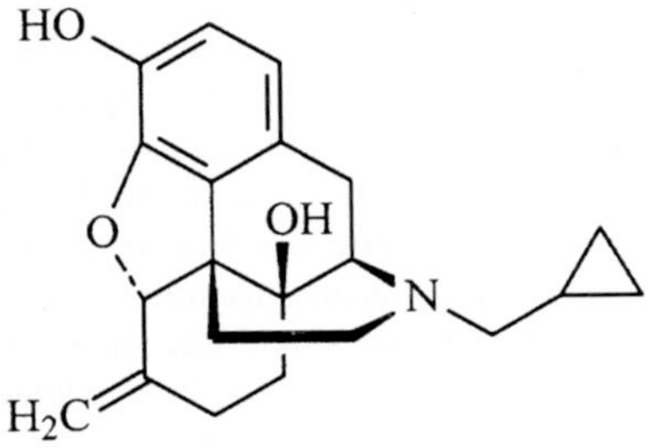

Nalmefene

Naloxone, nalmefene, naltrexone, and methylnaltrexone are pure competitive opioid antagonists at the mu (μ), kappa (κ), and delta (δ) receptors. Opioid antagonists prevent the actions of opioid agonists, reverse the effects of both endogenous and exogenous opioids, and cause opioid withdrawal in opioid-dependent patients. Naloxone is primarily used to reverse respiratory depression in patients manifesting opioid toxicity. The parenteral dose should be titrated to maintain adequate airway reflexes and ventilation. By titrating the dose, beginning with 0.04 mg and increasing as indicated to 0.4 mg, 2 mg, and finally 10 mg, abrupt opioid withdrawal can be prevented. This method of administration limits withdrawal-induced adverse effects, such as vomiting and the potential for aspiration pneumonitis, and a surge in catecholamines with the potential for cardiac dysrhythmias and acute lung injury (ALI). Because of its poor oral bioavailability, oral naloxone may be used to treat patients with opioid-induced constipation. Methylnaltrexone is a parenteral medication and alvimopan an oral capsule that fail to enter the central nervous system (CNS) and are uniquely effective in reversing opioid-induced constipation. Naltrexone is used orally for patients after opioid detoxification to maintain opioid abstinence and as an adjunct to achieve ethanol abstinence. Nalmefene is available for parenteral use with a duration of action between those of naloxone and naltrexone.

HISTORY

The understanding of structure–activity relationships led to the synthesis of many new molecules in the hope of producing potent opioid agonists free of abuse potential. Although this goal has not yet been achieved, opioid antagonists and partial agonists resulted from these investigations. *N*-Allylnorcodeine was the first opioid antagonist synthesized (in 1915), and *N*-allylnormorphine (nalorphine) was synthesized in the 1940s.[39,83] Nalorphine was recognized as having both agonist and antagonist effects in 1954. Naloxone was synthesized in 1960, and naltrexone was synthesized in 1963.

CHEMISTRY

Minor alterations can convert an agonist into an antagonist.[38] The substitution of the *N*-methyl group on morphine by a larger functional group led to nalorphine and converted the agonist levorphanol to the antagonist levallorphan.[35] Naloxone, naltrexone, and nalmefene are derivatives of oxymorphone with antagonist properties resulting from addition of organic or other functional groups.[35,42] Relatedly, nalmefene is a 6-methylene derivative of naltrexone.

PHARMACOLOGY

The μ receptors are responsible for analgesia, sedation, miosis, euphoria, respiratory depression, and decreased gastrointestinal (GI) motility. κ receptors are responsible for spinal analgesia, miosis, dysphoria, anxiety, nightmares, and hallucinations. δ receptors are responsible for analgesia and hunger. The currently available opioid receptor antagonists are most potent at the μ receptor, with higher doses required to affect the κ and δ receptors. They all bind to the opioid receptor in a competitive fashion, preventing the binding of agonists, partial agonists, or mixed agonist–antagonists without producing any independent action. Naloxone, naltrexone, and nalmefene are similar in their antagonistic mechanism but differ primarily in their pharmacokinetics. Both nalmefene and naltrexone have longer durations of action than naloxone, and both have adequate oral bioavailability to produce systemic effects. Methylnaltrexone can be given orally or parenterally but is excluded from the CNS and only produces peripheral effects. Selective antagonists for μ, κ, and δ are available experimentally and are undergoing investigation.[62]

In the proper doses, pure opioid antagonists reverse all of the effects at the μ, κ, and δ receptors of endogenous and exogenous opioid agonists, except for those of buprenorphine, which has a very high affinity for and slow rate of dissociation from the μ receptor.[62,63] Actions of opioid agonists that are not mediated by interaction with opioid receptors, such as direct mast cell liberation of histamine or the sodium channel-blocking effects of propoxyphene, are not reversed by these antagonists.[3] Chest wall rigidity from rapid fentanyl infusion is usually reversed with naloxone.[23] Opioid-induced seizures in animals, such as from propoxyphene, tend to be antagonized by opioid antagonists, though seizures caused by meperidine (normeperidine) and tramadol are exceptions.[6,30] The benefit in humans is less clear. A report of two newborns who developed seizures associated with fentanyl and morphine infusion demonstrated abrupt clinical and electroencephalographic resolution after administration of naloxone.[13]

Opioids operate bimodally on opioid receptors.[10] At low concentrations, μ opioid receptor agonism is excitatory and actually antianalgesic. This antianalgesic effect is modulated through a G_s protein and usually is less important clinically than the well-known inhibitory actions that result from coupling to a G_o protein at usual analgesic doses. For this reason, extremely low doses of opioid antagonists (ie, 0.25 mcg/kg/h of naloxone) enhance the analgesic potency of opioids, including morphine, methadone, and buprenorphine.[11,29,48] Naloxone also attenuates or prevents the development of tolerance and dependence.[10,29] Coadministration of these very low doses of antagonists or derivatives with the opioid also limits opioid-induced adverse effects such as nausea, vomiting, constipation, and pruritus.[97]

Opioid antagonists may reverse the effects of endogenous opioid peptides, including endorphins, dynorphins, and enkephalins. Endogenous opioids are found in tissues throughout the body and may work in concert with other neurotransmitter systems to modulate many physiologic effects.[22,84,86] For instance, during shock, the release of circulating endorphins produces an inhibition of central sympathetic tone by stimulating κ receptors within the locus coeruleus, resulting in vasodilation. Vagal tone is also enhanced through stimulation of opioid receptors in the nucleus ambiguus.

Research investigating the cardioprotective effects of opioid agonists through their action at the sarcolemmal and mitochondrial K^+ ATP (adenosine triphosphate) channels is ongoing.[64,69,73] Nonselective opioid antagonists may negate these protective effects.

PHARMACOKINETICS AND PHARMACODYNAMICS

The bioavailability of sublingual naloxone is only 10%.[5,38] In contrast, naloxone is well absorbed by all parenteral routes of administration, including the intramuscular (IM), subcutaneous (SC), endotracheal, intranasal, intralingual, and inhalational (nebulized) routes. The onset of action with the various routes of administration are as follows: IV, 1-2 minutes; SC, approximately 5.5 minutes; intralingual, 30 seconds; intranasal, 3.4 minutes; inhalational, 5 minutes; endotracheal, 60 seconds; and IM, 6 minutes.[19,43,52,5878,94] The distribution half-life is rapid (~5 minutes) because of its high lipid solubility. The volume of distribution (Vd) is 0.8 to 2.64 L/kg.[31,33]

A naloxone dose of 13 μg/kg in an adult occupies approximately 50% of the available opioid receptors.[54] The duration of action of naloxone is approximately 20 to 90 minutes and depends on the dose of the agonist, the dose and route of administration of naloxone, and the rates of elimination of the agonist and naloxone.[5,21,85] Naloxone is metabolized by the liver to several compounds, including a glucuronide. The elimination half-life is 60 to 90 minutes in adults and approximately two to three times longer in neonates.[60]

Naltrexone is rapidly absorbed with an oral bioavailability of 5% to 60%, and peak serum concentrations occur at 1 hour.[34,89,93] Distribution is rapid, with a Vd of approximately 15 L/kg and low protein binding.[48] Naltrexone is metabolized in the liver to β-naltrexol (with 2%–8% activity) and 2-hydroxy,3-methoxy-β-naltrexol,[88] and undergoes an enterohepatic cycle.[93] The plasma elimination half-life is 10 hours for β-naltrexone and 13 hours for β-naltrexol,[88,92,93] with a terminal phase of elimination of 96 hours and 18 hours, respectively.[89]

Nalmefene has an oral bioavailability of 40%, with peak serum concentrations usually reached within 1 to 2 hours.[17] However, in the United States, it is currently available only in a parenteral formulation. After SC administration, peak concentrations do not occur for more than 2 hours, though therapeutic concentrations are reached within 5 to 15 minutes.[59] A 1-mg parenteral dose blocked more than 80% of opioid receptors within 5 minutes.[59] The apparent Vd is 3.9 L/kg for the central compartment and 8.6 L/kg at steady state.[59] Protein binding is approximately 45%.[16] Nalmefene has a redistribution half-life of 41 ± 34 minutes and a terminal half-life of 10.8 ± 5 hours after a 1-mg intravenous (IV) dose.[59] It is metabolized in the liver to an inactive glucuronide conjugate that probably undergoes enterohepatic recycling, accounting for approximately 17% of drug elimination in the feces. Less than 5% is excreted unchanged in the urine.

Methylnaltrexone is a quaternary amine methylated derivative of naltrexone that is peripherally restricted because of its poor lipid solubility and inability to cross the blood–brain barrier.[97] After SC administration, peak serum concentrations occur in about 30 minutes. The drug has a Vd of 1.1 L/kg and is minimally protein bound (11%–15%).[59] Although there are several metabolites, 85% of the drug is eliminated unchanged in the urine.[97]

ADVERSE DRUG EFFECTS

Pure opioid antagonists produce no clinical effects in opioid naïve or nondependent patients, even when administered in massive doses.[7]

When exposed to opioid antagonists or agonist–antagonists such as pentazocine, patients dependent upon opioid agonists exhibit opioid withdrawal reactions, including yawning, lacrimation, diaphoresis, rhinorrhea, piloerection, mydriasis, vomiting, diarrhea, myalgias, mild elevations in heart rate and blood pressure, and insomnia. Antagonist-precipitated withdrawal may result in an "overshoot" phenomenon, from a transient increase in circulating catecholamines, resulting in hyperventilation, tachycardia, and hypertension. Under these circumstances, there is a potential for related complications such as myocardial ischemia, heart failure, CNS injury.[45,57] Delirium, although rarely reported with gradual withdrawal, may occur when an opioid antagonist is used to reverse effects in patients dependent upon high doses of opioids or during rapid opioid detoxification.[32] Delirium is unique to these circumstances and is not described in patients withdrawing by opioid abstinence. These severe manifestations of precipitated opioid withdrawal may occur with ultrarapid opioid detoxification, and are associated with fatalities occurring in the postadministration period.[37] This rapid form of enforced detoxification differs significantly from the opioid withdrawal associated with volitional opioid abstinence (see Chap. 14).

Case reports describe ALI, hypertension, and cardiac dysrhythmias in association with naloxone administration, generally in opioid-dependent patients.[26,56,66,72,77] The clinical complexities of the setting and case reports make it difficult to analyze and attribute these adverse effects solely to naloxone.[8] ALI occurs after heroin overdose in the absence of naloxone,[20] making the exact contribution of naloxone to the problem unclear. Rather, in certain patients, naloxone may unmask ALI previously induced by the opioid but unrecognized because of the patient's concomitant opioid-induced respiratory depression.[20]

If the patient's airway is unprotected during withdrawal and vomiting occurs, aspiration pneumonitis may complicate the recovery. Given the frequency of polysubstance abuse and overdose associated with altered consciousness, the risk of precipitating withdrawal associated vomiting should always be a concern.

Resedation is a function of the relatively short duration of action of the opioid antagonist compared with the opioid agonist. Most opioid agonists have durations of action longer than that of naloxone and shorter than that of naltrexone; the relationship is variable with nalmefene. A long duration of action is advantageous when the antagonist is used to promote abstinence (naltrexone) but is undesired when inappropriately administered to an opioid-dependent patient.

Unmasking underlying cocaine or other stimulant toxicity may explain some of the cardiac dysrhythmias that develop after naloxone-induced opioid reversal in a patient simultaneously using both opioids and stimulants[55] (see Chap. 76).

Antagonists stimulate the release of hormones from the pituitary, resulting in increased concentrations of luteinizing hormone, follicle-stimulating hormone, and adrenocorticotropic hormone and stimulate the release of prolactin in women.[70]

USE OF OPIOID ANTAGONISTS FOR MAINTENANCE OF OPIOID ABSTINENCE

Opioid dependence is managed by substitution of the abused opioid, typically heroin or a prescription opioid, with methadone or buprenorphine or by detoxification and subsequent abstinence. Maintenance of abstinence is often assisted by naltrexone, although any pure opioid antagonist could be used. Typically, naltrexone is chosen because of its oral absorption and long duration of action compared with that of naloxone or nalmefene.[47,53]

When 1 mg of naloxone is administered IV, it prevents the action of 25 mg of IV heroin for 1 hour, whereas 50 mg of oral naltrexone antagonizes this dose of heroin for 24 hours; 100 mg has a blocking effect for 48 hours, and 150 mg is effective for 72 hours. Nalmefene antagonizes the action of 2 μg/kg of IV fentanyl with a duration of action that is similarly dose dependent: 0.5 mg IV last about 4 hours, 2 mg IV lasts about 8 hours, and 50 mg orally lasts about 50 hours.[27,28]

Before naltrexone can be administered for abstinence maintenance, the patient must be weaned from opioid dependence and be a willing participant. Naloxone should be administered IV to confirm that the patient is no longer opioid dependent and safe for naltrexone. With naloxone, opioid withdrawal, if it occurs, will be short lived instead of prolonged after use of naltrexone or nalmefene. Naltrexone does not produce tolerance, although prolonged treatment with naltrexone produces upregulation of opioid receptors.[96]

USE OF OPIOID ANTAGONISTS FOR ETHANOL ABSTINENCE

Naltrexone, particularly the IM depot form, is used as adjunctive therapy in ethanol dependence, based on the theory that the endogenous opioid system modulates ethanol intake.[65,92] Naltrexone reduces ethanol craving, the number of drinking days, and relapse rates.[68] Naltrexone induces moderate to severe nausea in 15% of these patients, possibly as a result of alterations in endogenous opioid tone induced by prolonged ethanol ingestion.[61,92]

OTHER USES

Poorly orally bioavailable opioid antagonists (eg, naloxone) and peripherally restricted opioid antagonists (eg, methylnaltrexone) are used to prevent or treat the constipation occurring as a side effect of opioid pain management.[1,50,97] Methylnaltrexone administered SC results in laxation within 4 hours in nearly half of those who receive the drug for this indication.[81,98]

Take-home naloxone programs are developing around the world. In these programs, opioid abusers are supplied naloxone to be administered to other users after opioid overdose, generally by the SC or intranasal route.[2,76] These bystander programs are credited with saving numerous lives, although concerns exist regarding proper dosing, relative safety, use in mixed overdose, attempts to overcome precipitated withdrawal, and refusal of Emergency Medical Services involvement.

Opioid antagonists are used infrequently in the management of overdoses with nonopioids such as ethanol,[18,75] clonidine,[74] captopril,[87] and valproic acid.[80] In none of these instances is the reported improvement as dramatic or consistent as in the reversal of an opioid. The mechanisms for each of these, though undefined, may relate to reversal of endogenous opioid peptides at opioid receptors.

Naloxone has been used to reverse the effects of endogenous opioid peptides in patients with septic shock, although the results are variable. Treatment is often ineffective and may result in adverse effects, particularly in patients who are opioid tolerant.[15,82] Naloxone may have a temporizing effect via elevation of mean arterial pressure.[36]

Although promising in animal models of spinal cord injury, an investigation of naloxone at doses approximately 100 times greater than those used in the management of overdoses failed to demonstrate improvement in neurologic recovery in humans.[7]

Opioid antagonists are used for treatment of morphine-induced pruritus resulting from systemic or epidural opioids[41,46] and for treatment of pruritus associated with cholestasis.[14,79]

DOSING

The initial dose of antagonist is dependent on the dose of agonist and the relative binding affinity of the agonist and antagonist at the opioid receptors. The presently available antagonists have a greater affinity for the μ receptor than for the κ or δ receptors. Some opioids, such as buprenorphine (see below), require greater than expected doses of antagonist to reverse the effects at the μ receptor.[85,95] The duration of action of the antagonist depends on many drug and patient variables, such as the dose and the clearance of both antagonist and agonist.

A dose of naloxone 0.4 mg IV will reverse the respiratory depressant effects of most opioids and is an appropriate starting dose in nonopioid- dependent patients. However, this dose in an opioid-dependent patient usually produces withdrawal, which should be avoided if possible. The goal is to produce a spontaneously and adequately ventilating patient without precipitating significant or abrupt opioid withdrawal. Therefore, 0.04 mg is a practical starting dose in most patients, increasing to 0.4 mg, 2 mg, and finally 10 mg. If the patient has no response to 8 to 10 mg, then an opioid is not likely to be responsible for the respiratory depression. The dose in children without opioid dependence is essentially the same as for adults. However, for those with the possibility of withdrawal or recrudescence of severe underlying pain, more gentle reversal with 0.001 mg/kg, with concomitant supportive care, is warranted. Although both the adult and pediatric doses recommended here are lower than those conventionally suggested in other references, the availability of safe and effective interim ventilatory therapy lower the acceptable risk of precipitating withdrawal.

The use of low doses of IV naloxone to reverse opioid overdose may prolong the time to improvement of ventilation, and during this period, assisted ventilation may be required. The same limitation exists with SC naloxone administration, and the absorbed dose is more difficult to titrate than when administered IV.[94] Naloxone can also be administered intranasally, although this route results in the delivery of unpredictable doses. In the prehospital setting, the time to onset of clinical effect of intranasal naloxone is comparable to that of IV or IM naloxone, largely because of the delay in obtaining IV access and slow absorption, respectively.[4,43,] Intranasal naloxone is not currently recommended as first-line treatment by healthcare providers.[44] Nebulized naloxone (2 mg is mixed with 3 mL of 0.9% sodium chloride solution) has similar limitations in dose accuracy and is further limited in patients with severe ventilatory depression, the group most in need of naloxone. These patients are not optimal candidates for inhalation therapy because delivery of a sufficient reversal dose may not occur. Although needleless delivery is a clear prehospital advantage, there is little role for inhospital use of intranasal or nebulized naloxone.

Evaluation for the redevelopment of respiratory depression requires nearly continuous monitoring. Resedation should be treated with either repeated dosing of the antagonist or, in some cases, such as after a long-acting opioid agonist, with another bolus followed by a continuous infusion of naloxone. Two-thirds of the bolus dose of naloxone that resulted in reversal, when given hourly, usually maintains the desired effect.[33] This dose can be prepared for an adult by multiplying the effective bolus dose by 6.6, adding that quantity to 1000 mL, and administering the solution IV at an infusion rate of 100 mL/h. Titration upward or downward is easily accomplished as necessary to both maintain adequate ventilation and avoid withdrawal. A continuous infusion of naloxone is not a substitute for continued vigilance. A period of 12 to 24 hours often is chosen for observation based on the presumed opioid, the route of administration, and the dosage form (eg, sustained release). Body packers are a unique subset of patients who, because the reservoir of drug in the GI tract, require individualized antagonist management strategies (see Special Considerations: SC-4 Internal Concealment of Xenobiotics.

Naloxone is a pregnancy Category C drug.[60] A risk-to-benefit analysis must be considered in pregnant women, particularly those who are opioid tolerant, and their newborns. Inducing opioid withdrawal in the mother probably will induce withdrawal in the fetus and should be avoided. Likewise, administering naloxone to newborns of opioid-tolerant mothers may induce neonatal withdrawal[40] (see Chaps. 30, 31, and 38).

Use of longer-acting opioid antagonists, such as naltrexone and nalmefene, places the patient at substantial risk for protracted withdrawal syndromes. The use of a long-acting opioid antagonist in acute care situations should be reserved for carefully considered special indications, together with extended periods of observation or careful follow-up. An oral dose of 150 mg of naltrexone generally lasts 48 to 72 hours and should be adequate as an antidote for the majority of opioid-intoxicated patients. Discharge of opioid-intoxicated patients after successful administration of a long-acting opioid antagonist, while theoretically attractive, is not well studied. There are concerns about attempts by patients to overcome opioid antagonism by administering high doses of opioid agonist, with subsequent respiratory depression as the effect of the antagonist wanes.

Naltrexone is administered orally in a variety of dosage schedules for treatment of opioid dependence. A common dosing regimen is 50 mg/day Monday through Friday and 100 mg on Saturdays. Alternatively, 100 mg every other day or 150 mg every third day can be administered. The IM extended-release suspension is injected monthly at a recommended dose of 380 mg.[47]

The initial IV dose of nalmefene is 0.1 mg in a 70-kg person in whom opioid dependency is suspected. If withdrawal does not ensue, 0.5 mg can be given, followed by 1 mg in 2 to 5 minutes as necessary. If IV access is unavailable, the IM or SC route can be used, but the onset of action is delayed by 5 to 15 minutes after a 1-mg dose. For reversal of postoperative opioid respiratory depression, a starting dose of 0.25 μg/kg is used followed by incremental doses of 0.25 μg/kg every 2 to 5 minutes to the desired effect or to a total of 1 μg/kg.

Methylnaltrexone SC dosing for opioid-induced constipation is weight based.[98] The dose is 0.15 mg/kg for patients who weigh less than 38 kg and more than 114 kg. For patients who weigh between 38 and less than 62 kg, 8 mg is administered, and for those between 62 and 114 kg, 12 mg is provided. Dosing for patients with renal failure is required at half the recommended dose.

MANAGEMENT OF OVERDOSE

Although the opioid antagonists are all safe in overdose, excessive administration to an opioid-dependent patient will predictably result in opioid withdrawal. When induced by naloxone, all that is generally required is protecting the patient from harm and reassuring the patient that the effects will be short lived. Symptomatic care may be necessary on occasion. After inadvertent administration of nalmefene or naltrexone, the expected duration of the withdrawal syndrome generally mandates the use of pharmacologic intervention.[25,51] Overcoming the opioid receptor antagonism is difficult, but if used in titrated doses, morphine or fentanyl may be successful. Adverse effects from histamine release from morphine and chest wall rigidity from fentanyl should be expected. If more moderate withdrawal is present, the administration of metoclopramide, clonidine, or a benzodiazepine is usually adequate.[45]

What constitutes an appropriate observation period depends on many factors. After IV bolus naloxone, observation for 2 hours should be adequate to determine whether sedation and respiratory depression will return. Although no fatalities were identified in medical examiner records after the rapid prehospital release of patients who had presumably overdosed with heroin and were administered naloxone, the true safety of this practice remains questionable.[9] Although the matched pharmacokinetics of heroin and naloxone suggests potential utility for such a practice, the high frequency of methadone or sustained-release oxycodone use in many communities raises concerns. That is, the pharmacokinetic mismatch of both methadone and sustained-release oxycodone with naloxone results in recurrent opioid toxicity and prevents widespread implementation of this program.[90] Similarly, patients on continuous naloxone infusion must be observed for ≥2 hours after its discontinuation to ensure that respiratory depression does not recur.

The experience with nalmefene is too limited to estimate an adequate observation period, although 24 hours seems prudent to allow sufficient time for underlying opioid toxicity to resurface.

BUPRENORPHINE

Naloxone reverses the respiratory depressant effects of buprenorphine in a bell-shaped dose–response curve.[12,71,85,95] Bolus doses of naloxone between 2 to 3 mg followed by a continuous infusion of 4 mg/h in adults were able to fully reverse the respiratory depression associated with IV buprenorphine administered in a total dose of 0.2 and 0.4 mg over 1 hour.[85] Reversal was not apparent until about 45 to 60 minutes after the infusion. A reappearance of respiratory depression occurred when the naloxone infusion was stopped because the distribution of naloxone out of the brain and its subsequent elimination from the body are much faster than those of buprenorphine. Consistent with a bell-shaped response curve, doses of naloxone greater than 4 mg/h actually led to the recurrence of respiratory depression. It is postulated that buprenorphine has differential effects on the μ opioid receptor subtypes (see Chap. 38), with agonist activity at low doses and antagonist action at high doses. Therefore, excess naloxone antagonizes the antagonistic effects of buprenorphine, worsening respiratory depression.

AVAILABILITY

Naloxone (Narcan) for IV, IM, or SC administration is available in concentrations of 0.02, 0.4, and 1.0 mg/mL, with and without parabens in 1- and 2-mL ampules and in 10-mL multidose vials with parabens. Naloxone can be diluted in 0.9% sodium chloride solution or 5% dextrose to facilitate continuous IV infusion. Naloxone is stable in 0.9% sodium chloride solution at a variety of concentrations for up to 24 hours.[24]

Nalmefene (Revex) is available in a 1-mL ampule containing 100 μg/mL and in a 2-mL ampule containing 1 mg/mL.

Naltrexone (Revia, Trexan) is available as a 50-mg capsule-shaped tablet. It is also available as a 380-mg vial for reconstitution with a carboxymethylcellulose and polysorbate diluent to form an injectable suspension intended for monthly IM administration (Vivitrol).

Methylnaltrexone (Relistor) is available as a 12 mg/0.6 mL solution for SC injection.[67]

ACKNOWLEDGMENT

Richard S. Weisman, PharmD, contributed to this Antidotes in Depth in a previous edition.

REFERENCES

1. Arpino PA, Thompson BT. Safety of enteral naloxone for the reversal of opiate-induced constipation in the intensive care unit. *J Clin Pharm Ther.* 2009;34:171-175.
2. Baca CT, Grant KJ. Take-home naloxone to reduce heroin death. *Addiction.* 2005;100:1823-1831.
3. Barke KE, Hough LB. Opiates, mast cells and histamine release. *Life Sci.* 1993;53:1391-1399.
4. Barton ED, Ramos J, Colwell C, et al. Intranasal administration of naloxone by paramedics. *Prehosp Emerg Care.* 2002;6:54-58.
5. Berkowitz BA. The relationship of pharmacokinetics to pharmacologic activity: morphine, methadone and naloxone. *Clin Pharmacokinet.* 1976;1:219-230.
6. Bonfiglio MF. Naloxone in the treatment of meperidine induced seizures. *Drug Intell Clin Pharm.* 1987;21:174-175.
7. Bracken MB, Shepard MJ, Collins WF, et al. A randomized controlled trial of methylprednisolone or naloxone in the treatment of acute spinal cord injury. *N Engl J Med.* 1990;322:1405-1411.
8. Buajordet I, Naess AC, Jacobsen D, Brors O. Adverse events after naloxone treatment of episodes of suspected acute opioid overdose. *Eur J Emerg Med.* 2004;11:19-23.
9. Christenson J, Etherington J, Grafstein E, et al. Early discharge of patients with presumed opioid overdose: development of a clinical prediction rule. *Acad Emerg Med.* 2000;7:1110-1118
10. Crain S, Shen K. Antagonists of excitatory opioid receptor functions enhance morphine's analgesic potency and attenuate opioid tolerance/dependence liability. *Pain.* 2000;84:121-131.
11. Cruciani RA, Lussier D, Miller-Saultz D, Arbuck DM. Ultra-low dose oral naltrexone decreases side effects and potentiates the effect of methadone. *J Pain Symptom Manage.* 2003;25:491-494.
12. Dahan A. Opioid-induced respiratory effects: new data on buprenorphine. *Palliat Med.* 2006;20(suppl 1):S3-S8.
13. Da Silva O, Alexandrou D, Knoppert D, Yound GB. Seizure and electroencephalographic changes in the newborn period induced by opiates and corrected by naloxone infusion. *J Perinatol.* 1999;19:120-123.
14. Davis M. Cholestasis and endogenous opioids: liver disease and exogenous opioid pharmacokinetics. *Clin Pharmacokinet.* 2007;46:825-850.
15. DeMaria A, Craven DE, Heffernan JJ, et al. Naloxone versus placebo in treatment of septic shock. *Lancet.* 1985;1:1363-1365.
16. Dixon R, Gentile J, Hsu HB, et al. Nalmefene. Safety and kinetics after single and multiple oral doses of a new opioid antagonist. *J Clin Pharmacol.* 1987;27:233-239.
17. Dixon R, Howes J, Gentile J, et al. Nalmefene. Intravenous safety and kinetics of a new opioid antagonist. *Clin Pharmacol Ther.* 1986;39:49-52.
18. Dole VP, Fishman J, Goldfrank L, et al. Arousal of ethanol-intoxicated comatose patients with naloxone. *Alcohol Clin Exp Res.* 1982;6:275-279.
19. Dowling J, Isbister GK, Kirkpatrick CM, et al. Population pharmacokinetics of intravenous, intramuscular, and intranasal naloxone in human volunteers. *Ther Drug Monit.* 2008;30:490-496.
20. Duberstein JL, Kaufman DM. A clinical study of an epidemic of heroin intoxication and heroin induced pulmonary edema. *Am J Med.* 1971;51:704-714.
21. Evans JM, Hogg MJ, Lunn JN, Rosen M. Degree and duration of reversal by naloxone of effects of morphine in conscious subjects. *Br Med J.* 1974;2:589-591.
22. Faden AI, Jacobs TP, Monsey E, et al. Endorphins in experimental spinal injury: therapeutic effect of naloxone. *Ann Neurol.* 1981;10:326-332.
23. Fahnenstich H, Steffan J, Kau N, Bartmenn P. Fentanyl-induced chest wall rigidity and laryngospasm in preterm and term infants. *Crit Care Med.* 2000;28:836-839.
24. Fishman J, Cotter ML, Norton BI. Narcotic antagonists. 2. Preparation and biological stability of naloxone-7,8-3H. *J Med Chem.* 1973;16:556-557.
25. Fishman M. Precipitated withdrawal during maintenance opioid blockade with extended release naltrexone. *Addiction.* 2008;103:1399-1401.
26. Flacke JW, Flacke WE, Williams GD. Acute pulmonary edema following naloxone reversal of high-dose morphine anesthesia. *Anesthesiology.* 1977;47:376-378.
27. Gal TJ, DiFazio CA. Prolonged antagonism of opioid action with intravenous nalmefene in man. *Anesthesiology.* 1986;64:175-180.
28. Gal TJ, DiFazio CA, Dixon R. Prolonged blockade of opioid effect with oral nalmefene. *Clin Pharmacol Ther.* 1986;40:537-542.
29. Gan T, Ginsberg B, Glass P, et al. Opioid-sparing effects of a low-dose infusion of naloxone in patient administered morphine sulfate. *Anesthesiology.* 1997;87:1075-1081.
30. Gilbert PE, Martin WR. Antagonism of the convulsant effects of heroin, d-propoxyphene, meperidine, normeperidine and thebaine by naloxone in mice. *J Pharmacol Exp Ther.* 1975;192:538-541.
31. Glass PS, Jhaveri RM, Smith LR. Comparison of potency and duration of action of nalmefene and naloxone. *Anesth Analg.* 1994;78:536-541.
32. Golden SA, Sakhrani DL. Unexpected delirium during rapid opioid detoxification (ROD). *J Addict Dis.* 2004;23:65-75.
33. Goldfrank LR, Weisman RS, Errick JK, Lo MW. A dosing nomogram for continuous infusion intravenous naloxone. *Ann Emerg Med.* 1986;15:566-570.
34. Gonzalez JP, Brogden RN. Naltrexone: a review of its pharmacodynamic and pharmacokinetic properties and therapeutic efficacy in the management of opioid dependence. *Drugs.* 1988;35:192-213.
35. Goodman AJ, Le Bourdonnec B, Dolle RE. Mu opioid receptor antagonists: recent developments. *Chem Med Chem.* 2007;2:1552-1570.

36. Hackshaw KV, Parker GA, Roberts JW. Naloxone in septic shock. *Crit Care Med.* 1990;18:47-51.
37. Hamilton RJ, Olmedo RE, Shah S, et al. Complications of ultrarapid opioid detoxification with subcutaneous naltrexone pellets. *Acad Emerg Med.* 2002;9:63-68.
38. Harris LS. Narcotic antagonists—Structure-activity relationships. In: Costa E, Greengard P, Braude MC, et al, eds. *Narcotic Antagonists: Advances in Biochemical Psychopharmacology*, vol. 8. New York: Raven Press; 1973:13-20.
39. Hart ER, McCawley EL. The pharmacology of n-allylnormorphine as compared with morphine. *J Pharmacol Exp Ther.* 1944;82:339-348.
40. Herschel M, Khoshnood B, Lass NA. Role of naloxone in newborn resuscitation. *Pediatrics.* 2000;106:831-834.
41. Jeon Y, Hwang J, Kang J, et al. Effects of epidural naloxone on pruritus induced by epidural morphine: a randomized controlled trial. *Int J Obstet Anesth.* 2005;14:22-25.
42. Kane BE, Svensson B, Ferguson DM. Molecular recognition of opioid receptor ligands. *AAPS J.* 2006;8:E126-137.
43. Kelly AM, Kerr D, Dietze P, et al. Randomised trial of intranasal versus intramuscular naloxone in prehospital treatment for suspected opioid overdose. *Med J Aust.* 2005;182:24-27.
44. Kerr D, Dietze P, Kelly AM. Intranasal naloxone for the treatment of suspected heroin overdose. *Addiction.* 2008;103:379-386.
45. Kienbaum P, Heuter T, Michel MC, et al. Sympathetic neural activation evoked by mu-receptor blockade in patients addicted to opioids is abolished by intravenous clonidine. *Anesthesiology.* 2002;96:346-351.
46. Kjellberg F, Tramer MR. Pharmacological control of opioid-induced pruritus: a quantitative systematic review of randomized trials. *Eur J Anaesthesiol.* 2001;18:346-357.
47. Kleber HD, Kosten TR, Gaspari J, Topazian M. Nontolerance to the opioid antagonism of naltrexone. *Biol Psychiatry.* 1985;20:66-72.
48. Kogan MJ,Verebey K,Mule SJ. Estimation of the systemic availability and other pharmacokinetic parameters of naltrexone in man after acute and chronic oral administration. *Res Commun Chem Pathol Pharmacol.* 1977; 18:29-34.
49. La Vincente SF, White JM, Somogyi AA, et al. Enhanced buprenorphine analgesia with the addition of ultra-low-dose naloxone in healthy subjects. *Clin Pharmacol Ther.* 2008;83:144-152.
50. Liu M, Wittbrodt E. Low-dose oral naloxone reverses opioid-induced constipation and analgesia. *J Pain Symptom Manage.* 2002;23:48-53.
51. Lubman D, Koutsogiannis Z, Kronborg I. Emergency management of inadvertent accelerated opiate withdrawal in dependent opiate users. *Drug Alcohol Rev.* 2003;22:433-436.
52. Maio RF, Gaukel B, Freeman B. Intralingual naloxone injection for narcotic-induced respiratory depression. *Ann Emerg Med.* 1987;16:572-573.
53. Martin WR, Jasinski DR, Mansky PA. Naltrexone, an antagonist for the treatment of heroin dependence: effects in man. *Arch Gen Psychiatry.* 1973;28:784-790.
54. Melichar JK, Nutt DJ, Malizia AL. Naloxone displacement at opioid receptor sites measured in vivo in the human brain. *Eur J Pharmacol.* 2003;459:217-219.
55. Merigian KS. Cocaine-induced ventricular arrhythmias and rapid atrial fibrillation temporally related to naloxone administration. *Am J Emerg Med.* 1993;1:96-97.
56. Michaelis LL, Hickey PR, Clark TA, et al. Ventricular irritability associated with the use of naloxone hydrochloride. *Ann Thorac Surg.* 1984;18: 608-624.
57. Mills CA, Flacke JW, Miller JD, et al. Cardiovascular effects of fentanyl reversal by naloxone at varying arterial carbon dioxide tensions in dogs. *Anesth Analg.* 1988;67:730-736.
58. Mycyk MB, Szyszko AL, Aks SE. Nebulized naloxone gently and effectively reverses methadone intoxication. *J Emerg Med.* 2003;24:185-187.
59. Nalmefene (Revex). Prescribing information. Baxter. Available at http://www.fda.gov/cder/foi/label/2000/20459S2lbl.pdf; accessed September 14, 2009.
60. Naloxone package insert. Chadds Ford, PA: Endo Pharmaceuticals Inc; 2003.
61. O'Malley S, Krishinan-Sarin S, Farren C, O'Connor P. Naltrexone-induced nausea in patients treated for alcohol dependence: clinical predictors and evidence for opioid mediated effects. *J Clin Psychopharmacol.* 2000;20:69-76.
62. Pasternak G. Multiple opiate receptors: déjá vu all over again. *Neuropharmacology.* 2004;47:312-323.
63. Pasternak GW. Pharmacological mechanisms of opioid analgesics. *Clin Neuropharmacol.* 1993;16:1-18.
64. Patel HH, Hsu AK, Peart JN, et al. Sarcolemmal K (ATP) channel triggers opioid-induced delayed cardioprotection in the rat. *Circ Res.* 2002;91: 186-188.
65. Pettinati HM, O'Brien CP, Rabinowitz AR, et al. The status of naltrexone in the treatment of alcohol dependence: specific effects on heavy drinking. *J Clin Psychopharmacol.* 2006;26:610-625.
66. Prough DS, Roy R, Bumgarner J. Acute pulmonary edema in healthy teenagers following conservative doses of intravenous naloxone. *Anesthesiology.* 1984;60:485-486.
67. Relistor (Methylnaltrexone). Prescribing Information, Wyeth. Available at http://www.wyeth.com/content/showlabeling.asp?id=499; accessed September 14, 2009.
68. Richardson K, Baillie A, Reid S, et al. Do acamprosate or naltrexone have an effect on daily drinking by reducing craving for alcohol? *Addiction.* 2008;103:953-959.
69. Romano MA, McNish R, Seymour EM, et al. Differential effects of opioid peptides on myocardial ischemic tolerance. *J Surg Res.* 2004;119:46-50.
70. Russell JA, Douglas AJ, Brunton PJ. Reduced hypothalamo-pituitary-adrenal axis stress responses in late pregnancy: central opioid inhibition and noradrenergic mechanisms. *Ann N Y Acad Sci.* 2008;1148: 428-438.
71. Sarton E, Teppema L, Dahan A. Naloxone reversal of opioid-induced respiratory depression with special emphasis on the partial agonist/antagonist buprenorphine. *Adv Exp Med Biol.* 2008;605:486-491.
72. Schwartz JA, Koenigsberg MD. Naloxone-induced pulmonary edema. *Ann Emerg Med.* 1987;16:1294-1296.
73. Schultz JE, Gross GJ. Opioids and cardioprotection. *Pharmacol Ther.* 2001;89:123-137.
74. Seger DL. Clonidine toxicity revisited. *J Toxicol Clin Toxicol.* 2002;40: 145-155.
75. Sorenson SC, Mattison K. Naloxone as an antagonist in severe alcohol intoxication [letter]. *Lancet.* 1978;2:688-689.
76. Strang J, Manning V, Mayet S, et al. Overdose training and take-home naloxone for opiate users: prospective cohort study of impact on knowledge and attitudes and subsequent management of overdoses. *Addiction.* 2008;103:1648-1657.
77. Tanaka GY. Hypertensive reaction to naloxone. *JAMA.* 1974;228:25-26.
78. Tandberg D, Abercrombie D. Treatment of heroin overdose with endotracheal naloxone. *Ann Emerg Med.* 1982;11:443-445.
79. Terg R, Coronel E, Sordà J, et al. Efficacy and safety of oral naltrexone treatment for pruritus of cholestasis, a crossover, double blind, placebo-controlled study. *J Hepatol.* 2002;37:717-722.
80. Thanacoody HK. Chronic valproic acid intoxication: reversal by naloxone. *Emerg Med J.* 2007;24:677-678.
81. Thomas J, Karver S, Cooney GA, et al. Methylnaltrexone for opioid-induced constipation in advanced illness. *N Engl J Med.* 2008;358:2332-2343.
82. Tuggle DW, Horton JW. Effects of naloxone on splanchnic perfusion in hemorrhagic shock. *J Trauma.* 1989;29:1341-1345.
83. Unna K. Antagonistic effect of n-allyl-normorphine upon morphine. *J Pharmacol Exp Ther.* 1943;79:27-31.
84. Van den Berg MH, Van-Giersbergen PL, Cox-Van-Put J, et al. Endogenous opioid peptides and blood pressure regulation during controlled stepwise hemorrhagic hypotension. *Circ Shock.* 1991;35:102-108.
85. van Dorp E, Yassen A, Sarton E, et al. Naloxone reversal of buprenorphine-induced respiratory depression. *Anesthesiology.* 2006;105:51-57.
86. Van Giersbergen PL, Cox-Van-Put J, de-Jong W. Central and peripheral opiate receptors appear to be activated during controlled hemorrhagic hypotension. *J Hypertens.* 1989;7(suppl):2-27.
87. Varon J, Duncan SR. Naloxone reversal of hypotension due to captopril overdose. *Ann Emerg Med.* 1991;20:1125-1127.
88. Verebey K, DePace A, Jukofsky D, et al. Quantitative determination of 2-hydroxy-3-methoxy-6 beta-naltrexol (HMN), naltrexone, and 6 beta-naltrexol in human plasma, red blood cells, saliva, and urine by gas liquid chromatography. *J Anal Toxicol.* 1980;4:33-37.
89. Verebey K, Volavka J, Mule SJ, Resnick RB. Naltrexone: disposition, metabolism, and effects after acute and chronic dosing. *Clin Pharmacol Ther.* 1976;20:315-328.
90. Vilke GM, Sloane C, Smith AM, Chan TC. Assessment for death in out of hospital heroin overdose patients treated with naloxone who refuse transport. *Acad Emerg Med.* 2003;10:893-896.

91. Vivitrol (methylnaltrexone). Prescribing Information. Frazer PA: Cephalon. Available at http://www.vivitrol.com/pdf_docs/prescribing_info.pdf; accessed September 14, 2009.
92. Volpicelli JR, Clay KL, Watson NT, O'Brien CP. Naltrexone in the treatment of alcoholism: predicting response to naltrexone. *J Clin Psychol.* 1995;56(suppl 7):39-44.
93. Wall ME, Brine DR, Perez-Reyes M. Metabolism and disposition of naltrexone in man after oral and intravenous administration. *Drug Metab Dispos.* 1981;9:369-375.
94. Wanger K, Brough L, Macmillan I, et al. Intravenous vs subcutaneous naloxone for out-of-hospital management of presumed opioid overdose. *Acad Emerg Med.* 1998;5:293-299.
95. Yassen A, Olofsen E, van Dorp E, et al. Mechanism-based pharmacokinetic-pharmacodynamic modelling of the reversal of buprenorphine-induced respiratory depression by naloxone: a study in healthy volunteers. *Clin Pharmacokinet.* 2007;46:965-980.
96. Yoburn BC, Markham CL, Pasternak GW, Inturrisi CE. Upregulation of opioid receptor subtypes correlates with potency changes of morphine and DADLE. *Life Sci.* 1988;43:1319-1324.
97. Yuan CS, Doshan H, Charney MR, et al. Tolerability, gut effects, and pharmacokinetics of methylnaltrexone following repeated intravenous administration in humans. *J Clin Pharmacol.* 2005;45:538-546.
98. Yuan CS, Foss JF, O'Connor M, et al. Methylnaltrexone for reversal of constipation due to chronic methadone use. *JAMA.* 2000;283:367-372.

B.

FOODS, DIETARY AND NUTRITIONAL XENOBIOTICS

CHAPTER 39
DIETING AGENTS AND REGIMENS

Jeanna M. Marraffa

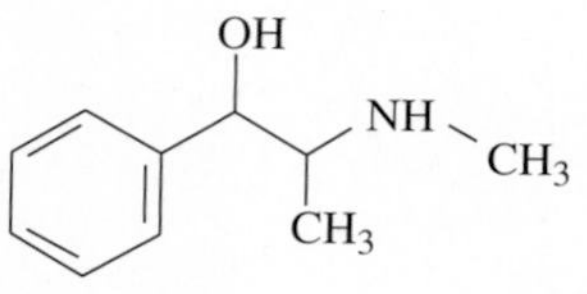

Ephedrine

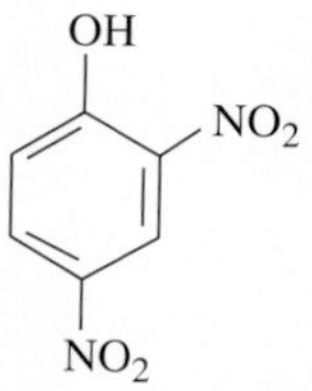

Dinitrophenol

Obesity is a worldwide epidemic. Nearly 60% of Americans are overweight and 30% are obese (body mass index [BMI] >30 kg/m^2).[26,55] Even more alarming, the incidence of obesity in children between the ages of 6 and 19 years has tripled in the past 30 years.[9] Nearly 9 million children and adolescents are now considered overweight.[9] Obesity contributes to 325,000 deaths annually in the United States.[5] Obesity is linked to numerous health risks, including type II diabetes, hypertension, coronary heart disease,[9,19] metabolic syndrome[138] and even low back pain.[119] Because of this, it can be considered a leading preventable health risk, second only to cigarette smoking. In the past several decades, research has been dedicated to the pathophysiology of obesity and to novel therapeutic approaches. Genetic links, including particular gene polymorphisms, have been identified and are being pursued.[3,23,73]

Americans spend $33 billion per year on weight loss therapies and modalities. Dieting and weight loss are attempted by many more people than just those who are overweight and obese by medically defined criteria. Weight loss management is difficult and frequently even the best lifestyle modifications only result in a modest weight loss in a majority of people. Pharmacologic interventions may result in a 5% to 10% weight loss, although a return to baseline upon drug cessation is common.[40] Surgical interventions consistently achieve substantial weight loss, causing up to a 30% reduction in weight, but are not free from complications.[2,16]

Obesity and attempts at weight loss have probably existed since antiquity. One of the earliest accounts of weight loss therapy dates back to 10th-century Spain. King Sancho I, who was obese, underwent successful treatment with a "theriaca," thought to contain plants and possibly opioids, administered with wine and oil. In addition, he was closely supervised and treated by a physician.[60]

Currently, medicinal weight loss therapies (Table 39–1) are available as prescription medications (sibutramine, phentermine); nonprescription dietary supplements (*Citrus aurantium*, chitosan, *Garcinia cambogia,* caffeine); and in late 2007, orlistat, a fat blocker, was approved as a nonprescription diet aid. Acquisition and utilization of natural weight loss remedies have undergone a resurgence since passage of the Dietary Supplement Health and Education Act (DSHEA) of 1994, which created a new category separate from food and drugs. As a result of the DSHEA, numerous botanicals and other substances are offered to consumers as weight loss aids, some with no proven efficacy and some with potentially serious toxicity.

Although dieting aids can be divided into disparate classes, they generally act through one or more of the following mechanisms: (1) appetite suppression, known as *anorectics*; (2) alteration of food absorption or elimination; or (3) increased energy expenditure. The endocannabinoid receptor antagonists such as rimonabant, work in a unique way and have multiple effects, including appetite suppression. Dieting aids that are anorectics are designed to decrease appetite and calorie intake.

The history of dieting agents has a checkered past. A number of weight loss therapies have been withdrawn or banned by the Food and Drug Administration (FDA) because of serious adverse health effects (Table 39–2). For example, phenylpropanolamine (PPA) was withdrawn from the market because of its association with hemorrhagic stroke. Fenfluramine–phentermine (Fen-Phen) was linked to cardiac valvulopathy and primary pulmonary hypertension. γ-Hydroxybutyrate (GHB) and its congeners were initially sold as a dietary supplement (see Chap. 80) and promoted to body builders as a means to "convert fat into muscle" as a result of GHB's effect on growth hormone. Because of overdose toxicity and its association with drug-facilitated sexual assault, GHB is strictly controlled as a Schedule I agent, with limited availability as a Schedule III drug for narcolepsy sodium oxybate (Xyrem). Clenbuterol is a long-acting β_2-adrenergic agonist with β_3-adrenergic agonist effects. Because of its stimulant properties and lipolytic effects, clenbuterol is abused by body builders as an energy source and anoretic agent.[58] Clenbuterol recently has been suggested by celebrities to be an effective diet aid (see Chap. 44).

SYMPATHOMIMETICS

Although controversial, certain sympathomimetic amines still carry official indications for short-term weight reduction (see Table 39-1). Sympathomimetic amines share a β-phenylethylamine parent structure and include phentermine, diethylpropion, and mazindol, which are restricted as Schedule IV agents and carry warnings that advise prescribers to limit use to only a few weeks. Regardless of their source and legal status, sympathomimetics generally share a spectrum of toxicity and produce adverse effects similar to amphetamines (see Chap. 75).

TABLE 39–1. Available Weight Loss Drugs and Dietary Supplements

Drug or Supplement[a]	Mechanism of Action	Regulatory Status	Adverse Effects/Contraindications[b]
Sympathomimetics			
Diethylpropion (Tenuate)	Increased release of norepinephrine and dopamine	Schedule IV prescription drug	Dry mouth, tremor, insomnia, headache, agitation, palpitations, hypertension, stroke, dysrhythmias Contraindications: MAOI use within 14 days, glaucoma, hyperthyroidism
Mazindol (Mazanor, Sanorex)	Increased release of norepinephrine and dopamine	Schedule IV prescription drug	
Phentermine (Fastin, Adipex)	Increased release of norepinephrine and dopamine	Schedule IV prescription drug	
Bitter orange extract (*Citrus aurantium*)	Contains synephrine and octopamine; increases thermogenesis and lipolysis	Dietary supplement	Hypertension, cerebral ischemia, myocardial ischemia, prolonged QT interval
Guarana (*Paullinia cupana*)	Contains caffeine, which may increase thermogenesis	Dietary supplement	Nausea, vomiting, insomnia, diuresis, anxiety, palpitations
Serotonergics			
Sibutramine (Meridia)	Inhibits reuptake of serotonin and norepinephrine	Schedule IV prescription drug	Anxiety, dry mouth, insomnia, headache, hypertension, palpitations, dysmenorrhea Contraindications: Same as sympathomimetics Serotonin syndrome
GI Agents			
Orlistat (Xenical/Alli)	Inhibits gastric and pancreatic lipases	Prescription and nonprescription drug	Abdominal pain, oily stool, fecal urgency or incontinence; fat-soluble vitamin loss Contraindications: Cholestasis, chronic malabsorptive states
Chitosan	Insoluble marine fiber that binds dietary fat	Dietary supplement	Decreased absorption of fat-soluble vitamins Contraindications: Shellfish allergy
Fibers/Other Supplements			
Glucomannan	Expands in stomach to increase satiety	Dietary supplement	GI obstruction with tablet form Contraindications: Abnormal GI anatomy
Garcinia cambogia	Increases fat oxidation (unproven)	Dietary supplement	None reported
Chromium picolinate	Improves blood glucose and lipids; produces fat loss (unproven)	Dietary supplement	Dermatitis, hepatitis, possibly mutagenic in high doses

[a]Trade names or Latin binomials are given in parentheses.

[b]All xenobiotics are contraindicated during pregnancy and lactation.

PHARMACOLOGY

Sympathomimetic amines that act at α- and β-adrenergic receptors are clinically effective in promoting weight loss but have numerous side effects that limit their clinical use. Soon after its introduction as a pharmaceutical for nasal congestion in the 1930s, the prototype sympathomimetic drug amphetamine (Fig. 39-1) was noted to cause weight loss (see Chap. 75). The weight loss effects of amphetamine were also readily apparent in early animal studies, although tolerance to the anorectic effects was also noted.[127] The primary mechanism of action of the weight loss effects of sympathomimetic drugs is central nervous system (CNS) stimulation, resulting from increased release of norepinephrine and dopamine.[125] The effects include direct suppression of the appetite center in the hypothalamus and reduced taste and olfactory acuity, leading to decreased interest in food. Increased energy and the euphoriant effects of the stimulant drugs also contribute to weight loss. However, tachyphylaxis occurs, and the rate of weight loss diminishes within a few weeks of initiating therapy.[44] Significant side effects and abuse potential severely limit the therapeutic use of this class of drugs.

ADVERSE EFFECTS

The absence of polar hydroxyl groups from a sympathomimetic amine increases its lipophilicity; therefore, unsubstituted or predominantly alkyl group–substituted compounds (eg, amphetamine, ephedrine, PPA) have greater CNS activity. Mild cardiovascular and CNS stimulant effects include headache, tremor, sweating, palpitations, and insomnia. More severe effects that may occur after overdose of sympathomimetic amines include anxiety, agitation, psychosis, seizures, palpitations, and chest pain.[43,72,79,90,101,111,132]

Hypertension is common after overdose and occasionally after therapeutic use as well. Patients may present with confusion and altered mental status as a result of hypertensive encephalopathy. Reflex bradycardia after exposure to agents with predominantly α-adrenergic agonist effects may accompany the hypertension and provides a clue to the diagnosis. Children with unintentional ingestions may be at especially high risk for hypertensive episodes because of the relatively significant dose per kilogram of body weight. Other manifestations include chest pain, palpitations, tachycardia, syncope, hypertension, mania, psychosis, convulsions, and coronary vasospasm.[14,20,38,98,144]

TABLE 39–2. Unavailable and Withdrawn Weight Loss Drugs and Dietary Supplements

Drug or Supplement[a]	Mechanism of Action	Adverse Effects	Regulation Status, DEA Schedule, or Withdrawal Date
Amphetamine	Increased release of NE and dopamine	Sympathomimetic effects, psychosis, dependence	Schedule II
Benzphetamine (Didrex)	Increased release of NE and dopamine	Sympathomimetic effects, psychosis, dependence	Schedule III
Clenbuterol	β_3-Adrenergic agonist activity	Tachycardia, headache, nausea, vomiting; may be prolonged	Not approved
Dexfenfluramine (Redux)	Promotes central serotonin release and inhibits its reuptake	Valvular heart disease, primary pulmonary hypertension	Withdrawn September 1997
Dieter's teas (senna, cascara, aloe, buckthorn)	Stimulant laxative herbs that promote colonic evacuation	Diarrhea, vomiting, nausea, abdominal cramps, electrolyte disorders, dependence	FDA required label warning, June 1995
Dinitrophenol	Alters metabolism by uncoupling oxidative phosphorylation	Hyperthermia, cataracts, hepatotoxicity	Not approved
Ma-huang (*Ephedra sinica*)	Increased release of NE and dopamine	Sympathomimetic effects, psychosis	Banned by FDA, April 2004
Fenfluramine (Pondimin)	Increased release and decreased reuptake of serotonin	Valvular heart disease, primary pulmonary hypertension	Withdrawn September 1997
Guar gum (Cal-Ban 3000)	Hygroscopic polysaccharide swells in stomach, producing early satiety	Esophageal and small bowel obstruction, fatalities	Banned by FDA, July 1990
Lipokinetix (sodium usniate, norephedrine, 3,5-diiodothyronine, yohimbine, caffeine)	Unknown	Acute hepatitis	FDA warning, November 2001
Phendimetrazine (Adipost, Bontril)	Increased release of NE and dopamine	Sympathomimetic effects, psychosis	Schedule III
Phenylpropanolamine (Dexatrim, Acutrim)	α_1-Adrenergic agonist	Sympathomimetic effects, headache, hypertension, myocardial infarction, intracranial hemorrhage	Withdrawn November 2000
Rimonabant (Acomplia)	Endocannabinoid receptor antagonist	Anxiety, nausea, diarrhea, dizziness	Phase III clinical trials (yet to be approved by FDA)

[a] Trade names or botanical names as appropriate are given in parentheses.

DEA, Drug Enforcement Administration; FDA, Food and Drug Administration; NE, norepinephrine.

Patients with clinically significant hypertension should be treated aggressively with either phentolamine, a rapidly acting α-adrenergic antagonist, or nitroprusside. Analogous to the management of cocaine toxicity, β-adrenergic antagonists should be avoided in the management because the resultant unopposed α-adrenergic agonist effects may lead to greater vasoconstriction and increased hypertension.[4] Patients with agitation, tachycardia, and seizures should be treated with benzodiazepines.

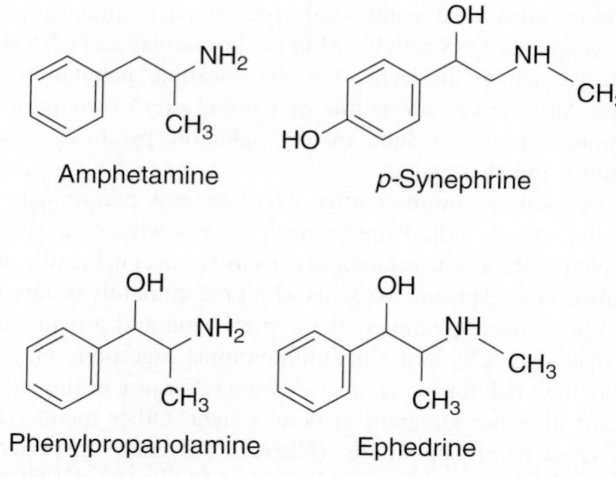

Amphetamine p-Synephrine Phenylpropanolamine Ephedrine

FIGURE 39–1. Sympathomimetic amines formerly and currently used for weight loss.

SPECIFIC SYMPATHOMIMETIC DIETARY SUPPLEMENTS

Phenylpropanolamine PPA, a sympathomimetic amine (see Fig. 39–1), was available until 2000 as a nonprescription diet aid (eg, Dexatrim, Acutrim). It is both a direct-acting agent, via stimulation of α-adrenergic receptors, and an indirect-acting agent, through release of norepinephrine. Both of these actions cause a net increase in blood pressure when given in high doses. PPA-induced anorexia is mediated via α-adrenergic receptors in the hypothalamus.[140] PPA was voluntarily withdrawn after its use was linked to increased risk of hemorrhagic stroke in women.[66]

Reported toxicity associated with PPA generally results from severe hypertension.[41,43,47,53,61,65,90] A comprehensive review of more than 100 case reports of adverse drug effects involving PPA revealed 24 intracranial hemorrhages, eight seizures, and eight fatalities between 1965 and 1990.[52,75] Some adverse events occurred after ingestion of diet preparations that contained both PPA and caffeine, which have pharmacokinetic and pharmacodynamic interactions.[68,76] Cardiac toxicity, although less common, was reported in two young patients who suffered myocardial injury after therapeutic daily dosing in one and acute overdose in the other.[79] Hypertensive emergencies resulting from adverse drug interactions between PPA and drugs such as monoamine oxidase inhibitors (MAOIs) have also been reported.[123]

Ephedrine Ephedra (*Ephedra sinica*), or Ma-huang, is a plant that contains six sympathomimetic amines, known collectively as *ephedra alkaloids*. The two primary alkaloids are ephedrine and pseudoephedrine (see Fig. 39–1). Ephedra was popular as a weight loss dietary supplement until the FDA banned ephedra-containing products in April 2004 because of cases of serious cardiovascular toxicity[14,20,27,38,54,98,132,144] and acute hepatitis.[95] In a review of 140 adverse events reported to MedWatch after use of ephedra, 31% of the cases were considered to be definitely or probably related to the use of ephedra supplements, including four strokes, five cardiac arrests, two myocardial infarctions, and three fatalities.[54] In 2005, there was concern that the FDA ban would be overturned and ephedra would once again be available. But in 2006, the U.S. Court of Appeals upheld the FDA's final rule to ban ephedra. Despite this ban, ephedra still can be obtained from practitioners of complementary medicine as a traditional Chinese herbal medicine for short-term treatment of wheezing and nasal congestion associated with asthma, allergies, and colds. Synthetic ephedrine is still available as the nonprescription medication, such as Primatene for the treatment for asthma.

Since ephedra was banned, herbal weight loss supplements have been reformulated. Many now contain an extract of bitter orange (*C. aurantium*), a natural source of the sympathomimetic amine synephrine, often in combination with caffeine, theophylline, willow bark (containing salicylates), diuretics, and other constituents. The dried fruit peel of bitter orange is a traditional remedy for gastrointestinal (GI) ailments. The predominant constituents, *p*-synephrine (see Fig. 39-1) and octopamine, are structurally similar to epinephrine and norepinephrine. Its isomer *m*-synephrine (phenylephrine or Neo-Synephrine) is used extensively as a vasopressor and nasal decongestant. Although synephrine's physiologic actions are not fully characterized, synephrine appears to interact with amine receptors in the brain and acts at peripheral α_1-adrenergic receptors, resulting in vasoconstriction and increased blood pressure.[48] Some evidence indicates that synephrine may also have β_3-adrenergic agonist activity,[21,48] which could increase lipolysis. β_3-adrenergic agonists were found to have remarkable antiobesity effects in rodents; however, effects in human are not as profound. Octopamine stimulates lipolysis in rats, hamsters, and dogs, but this effect was not seen in human fat cells.[21 48] A recent review described that nearly 2% of 4140 Californians surveyed had used a *C. aurantium*–containing product several times a week.[70] Adverse effects associated with use of *C. aurantium*–containing weight loss products have been reported, including one case of tachydysrhythmia,[46] one case of cerebral ischemia in a 38-year-old man,[12] one case of exercise-induced syncope and QT interval prolongation in a 22-year-old woman,[96] and one possible case of myocardial infarction in a 55-year-old woman.[97]

SEROTONERGIC AGENTS

Xenobiotics that affect central release and reuptake of serotonin are approved for a number of indications, including depression, anxiety, nicotine addiction, migraine, and premenstrual dysphoric syndrome. Although these drugs all reduce food intake to varying degrees, sibutramine (Meridia) is the only FDA-approved serotonergic agent specifically indicated for treatment of obesity.

Sibutramine acts by blocking the reuptake of both serotonin and norepinephrine, but it does not promote neuronal release of serotonin. Its clinical effects include reduced appetite and increased satiety. This xenobiotic is recommended in doses of 10 to 15 mg/day for obese patients with BMIs above 30 kg/m^2 without comorbid conditions and for patients with BMIs above 27 kg/m^2 with comorbid diseases of diabetes mellitus, dyslipidemia, or hypertension. Its effectiveness in producing weight loss was demonstrated in several randomized, double-blind studies.[30,35,78,84] It also decreases binge eating when compared with placebo.[141] Patients receiving intermittent sibutramine therapy have significantly fewer adverse effects than patients who take sibutramine continuously.[142] Clinical use of sibutramine for more than one year is unstudied.

The pharmacologic activity of sibutramine results from hepatic first-pass metabolism by cytochrome P450 (CYP3A4), transforming sibutramine into two active metabolites, mono-desmethylsibutramine and di-desmethylsibutramine, which have half-lives of 14 and 16 hours, respectively. These metabolites are further metabolized and renally excreted. Medications that inhibit CYP3A4, such as cimetidine, erythromycin, and ketoconazole, may slow sibutramine metabolism.[89]

Sibutramine use is associated with psychosis,[10,82,126] hypertension, cardiac ischemia, and death. Since sibutramine was approved in 1998, 397 serious adverse reactions have been reported to the FDA, including 29 deaths. Nineteen of the deaths were attributable to cardiovascular causes, including three deaths in women younger than 30 years.[37] The use of sibutramine as a weight loss agent in the United States and Europe is under scrutiny especially after sibutramine was banned in Italy in March 2002 after two cardiovascular deaths. In a large cohort of patients receiving sibutramine, mania, psychosis, and panic attacks were described, with notable improvement upon drug discontinuation.[103] Cases of dysrhythmias temporally related to sibutramine have also been described.[103]

Because of the concerns with increases in blood pressure and heart rate, a double-blind, placebo-controlled trial in adolescents was performed to evaluate the cardiovascular effects of sibutramine.[30] Although not statically significant, the sibutramine group had a trend toward a slight increase in blood pressure and heart rate compared with those taking placebo. Overall, sibutramine was well tolerated in these patients.[30] However, because sibutramine increases the heart rate and blood pressure, it should not be used in patients with poorly controlled hypertension, coronary artery disease, glaucoma, or previous stroke. Sibutramine taken in combination with MAOIs, selective serotonin reuptake inhibitors, or any xenobiotic that promotes serotonin release or prevents reuptake could induce serotonin syndrome, which is often characterized by agitation, hyperthermia, autonomic instability, and myoclonus. Management should be aimed at treating the specific clinical effects. Benzodiazepines may be useful for tachycardia and hypertension. Rapid identification and management of serotonin syndrome (described in Chap. 72) is essential to prevent associated morbidity and mortality.

Serotonergic drugs used in the past to treat obesity include dexfenfluramine (Redux) and fenfluramine (Pondimin), but these agents were withdrawn because of postmarketing reports of serious cardiac effects associated with their therapeutic use.[13,17,27,37,139] The diet drug combination known as "fen-phen" (fenfluramine with phentermine, an amphetamine derivative) was popular in the 1990s because of the presumed improved side effect profile and efficacy achieved with lower doses of each drug. This drug combination was never approved by the FDA for the treatment of obesity. Because of an unusual and serious cardiac valvulopathy in women taking fen-phen, fenfluramine was withdrawn from the market in 1997.[27] All of the women presented with new heart murmurs and either right- or left-sided valvular abnormalities. Eight of the 24 women also developed newly documented pulmonary hypertension. Several required cardiac surgery and were found to have plaquelike encasement of the leaflets and chordae, with preservation of valvular structure. These pathologic findings are identical to those described in patients with ergotamine-induced valvular disease and in those with carcinoid syndrome. Although subsequent studies confirmed this association, the reported magnitude of risk associated with these drugs has varied.[64,67,139] Cases of regression of these valvular lesions with cessation of the drugs are reported,[18] and limited evidence indicates that the valvular effects are milder than initially described.[50]

Primary pulmonary hypertension has been described in association with fenfluramine and dexfenfluramine since 1981.[7,17,37,88,109] Primary pulmonary hypertension in association with another anorectic drug, aminorex fumarate, was reported earlier in Europe.[53] In one multicenter case control study of patients with primary pulmonary hypertension, use of anorectic drugs such as dexfenfluramine and fenfluramine for more than 3 months was associated with a 30-fold increased risk of primary pulmonary hypertension in these patients compared with nonusers.[1] Several theories are proposed to explain the mechanism of pulmonary toxicity of these agents,[17] namely, serotonin-mediated constriction of pulmonary arteries[87]; serotonin-mediated platelet aggregation; and vasoconstriction in the lungs leading to microembolization, elevated pulmonary vascular resistance, and pulmonary hypertension.[87]

XENOBIOTICS THAT ALTER FOOD ABSORPTION, METABOLISM, AND ELIMINATION

FAT ABSORPTION BLOCKERS

Orlistat (Xenical) was approved by the FDA in 1999 for treatment of obesity. In mid-2007, orlistat (Alli) became available as a nonprescription formulation. The ready availability may pose an abuse potential in patients with eating disorders, and abuse should be considered in patients presenting with adverse events consistent with use of orlistat. Orlistat is the only FDA-approved drug that alters the absorption, distribution, and metabolism of food. Orlistat is a potent inhibitor of gastric and pancreatic lipase, thus reducing lipolysis and increasing fecal fat excretion.[22] The drug is not systemically absorbed but exerts its effects locally in the GI tract. It inhibits hydrolysis of dietary triglycerides and reduces absorption of the products of lipolysis, monoglycerides, and free fatty acids.

Several clinical trials demonstrate that orlistat reduces GI fat absorption by as much as 30%.[145] When taken in association with a slightly calorie-restricted diet, weight loss of approximately 10% body weight can be achieved in 1 year.[121] Moreover, the combination of a very low-energy diet and orlistat is responsible for less weight gain over a 3-year period compared with just a very low-energy diet. The subjects in the orlistat group gained 4.6 kg compared with 7.0 kg in the control group.[108]

Orlistat should be taken only in conjunction with meals that have a high fat content; it should not be consumed in the absence of food intake. Adverse effects correlate with the amount of dietary fat consumption and include abdominal pain, oily stool, fecal incontinence, fecal urgency, flatus, and increased defecation. Systemic effects are rarely reported because of the lack of systemic absorption of orlistat[45,94,130] but include cases of hepatotoxicity secondary to orlistat.[94,130] In a recent cohort of nearly 16,000 patients in England, although there were no cases of serious hepatotoxicity, there were reports of elevations of liver function tests. Two of the cases were deemed as causally related to orlistat, and one had a positive rechallenge result.[103] Because of the increasing use of orlistat, the number of reports of rare adverse events may increase. Concomitant use of natural fibers (6 g of psyllium mucilloid dissolved in water) may reduce the GI side effects of orlistat.[24] Because orlistat reduces absorption of fat-soluble food constituents, daily ingestion of a multivitamin supplement containing vitamins A, D, and K and β-carotene is advised to prevent resultant deficiency. At the time of this writing, there are no reported intentional overdoses of orlistat. In the scenario of overdose and misuse, treatment should be mainly supportive.

Chitosan is a weight loss dietary supplement derived from exoskeletons of marine crustaceans. It is thought to act similarly to orlistat by binding to dietary lipids in the GI tract and reducing breakdown and absorption of fat. Animal models describe an increase fecal fat excretion in rats when they are fed high-fat diets.[34] However, the efficacy of chitosan in humans is disputed.[49,91,92] Some evidence indicates that chitosan may decrease total serum cholesterol concentration in overweight people, but the majority of clinical studies indicate that chitosan is ineffective for weight loss in the absence of dietary and lifestyle modifications.[118] Recently, authors estimated that in the presence of chitosan, it would take more than 7 months to lose 1 lb of body fat.[49] Chitosan is contraindicated in people with shellfish allergy.

DIETARY FIBERS

Guar gum is derived from the bean of the *Cyamopsis psorabides* plant and is a hygroscopic polysaccharide that expands 10- to 20-fold in the stomach, forming a gelatinous mass. The purpose of ingesting guar was to cause gastric distension and create the sensation of satiety, thereby decreasing appetite and food intake. Guar gum resulted in numerous cases of esophageal and small bowel obstruction in patients with both preexisting anatomic lesions such as strictures and in individuals with normal GI anatomy, and it was banned in 1992.[51,80,109,117]

Glucomannan is a dietary fiber consisting of glucose and mannose, which is derived from konjac root, a traditional Japanese food. Edible forms of glucomannan include konjac jelly and konjac flour, which is mixed with liquid before ingestion. Purified glucomannan is available in capsule form and is found in various proprietary products marketed for weight loss. On contact with water, glucomannan swells to approximately 200 times its original dry volume, turning into a viscous liquid. It lowers blood cholesterol and glucose concentrations and decreases systolic blood pressure,[6,136] but significant weight loss benefits have not been demonstrated. After several reports of esophageal obstruction, oral glucomannan tablets were banned in Australia in 1985.[56] Serious adverse effects have not been described with encapsulated glucomannan, presumably because slower dissolution allows for GI transit before expansion. Glucomannan capsules are available as a nutritional supplement in the United States, although adequate safety and efficacy studies have not been published.

DINITROPHENOL

One of the earliest attempts at a pharmaceutical treatment for obesity was 2,4-dinitrophenol (DNP), which was popularized as a weight loss adjuvant in the 1930s.[129] This chemical, which is used in dyes, wood preservatives, herbicides, and explosives, was never approved as a drug product but was legally available as a diet remedy before enactment of the US Federal Food, Drug, and Cosmetic Act of 1938. By increasing metabolic energy expenditure, it reportedly produced weight loss of 1 to 2 lb per week in doses of 100 mg three times per day.[29] DNP increases metabolic work by uncoupling oxidative phosphorylation in the mitochondria. Through this mechanism, the hydrogen ion gradient that allows ATP synthesis is dissipated, preventing the proton motive force from creating high-energy phosphate bonds and thereby inhibiting ATP production (see Chap. 12). Because the energy loss resulting from inefficient substrate utilization is dissipated as heat, elevated temperature and (occasionally) life-threatening hyperthermia may occur.[128] DNP reportedly was administered to Russian soldiers during World War II to keep them warm during winter battles.[74] Symptoms related to DNP toxicity include malaise, skin rash, headache, diaphoresis, thirst, and dyspnea. Severe toxic effects include hyperpyrexia, hepatotoxicity, agranulocytosis, respiratory failure, coma, and death.[11,74,128] Delayed-onset cataract was a frequent and serious complication of DNP use.[11]

Epidemic use of DNP occurred in Texas in the 1980s when industrial DNP was synthesized into tablets by a physician and used at his weight loss center. He distributed DNP under the trade name Mitcal. The death of a wrestler following an intentional overdose of Mitcal in 1984 led a Texas court to stop the use of this chemical for weight loss.[74] DNP continues to reappear sporadically as a weight loss treatment, and cases of serious toxicity are still reported.[86,99] Management should be aimed at aggressive cooling. Benzodiazepines should also be used as an adjunct therapy for management of delirium and seizures and to prevent shivering, which occurs during active cooling.

HYPOCALORIC DIETS AND CATHARTIC AND EMETIC ABUSE

Medication abuse is common among individuals with eating disorders.[15] Starvation, as well as abuse of laxatives, syrup of ipecac, diuretics, and anorectics has led to many fatalities, often in young patients.[47,62] Fad diets and laxative abuse should be strongly considered in young people with unexplained dehydration, syncope, hypokalemia, and metabolic alkalosis. A variety of extreme calorie-restricted diets resulting in profound weight loss were very popular in the late 1970s, but reports of a possible association between these diets and sudden death followed.[120] Myocardial atrophy was a consistent finding on autopsy. Torsades de pointes and other ventricular dysrhythmias are proposed as causes of death as a result of hypokalemia[120,124] and protein-calorie malnutrition of the heart.[39,120,124]

Because of the negative reports and FDA warnings, the enthusiasm for liquid-protein diets waned. Several current diets (Atkin's plan, South Beach diet) advocate intake of high protein, high fat, and low carbohydrates while allowing unlimited amounts of meat, fish, eggs, and cheese. Lack of carbohydrates induces ketosis, which results in diuresis and dehydration, giving the user the appearance of rapid weight loss. With rehydration and resumption of a normal diet, weight gain generally occurs. In addition, dehydration may cause orthostatic hypotension and ureterolithiasis. Atherosclerosis and hypercholesterolemia may occur as a result of substitution of high-calorie, high-fat foods for carbohydrates. Despite the rapid weight loss early on with these diets, as soon as carbohydrates are reintroduced, weight gain occurs rapidly and significantly.[40]

Dieter's teas that contain combinations of herbal laxatives, including senna and *Cascara sagrada*, may produce profound diarrhea, volume depletion, and hypokalemia. They are associated with cases of sudden death, presumably as a result of cardiac dysrhythmias. Despite FDA warnings of the dangers of these weight loss regimens, dieter's teas remain available in retail stores that sell nutritional supplements and are easily accessible to adolescents.

Chronic laxative use can result in an atonic colon ("cathartic bowel") and the development of tolerance, with the subsequent need to increase dosing to achieve catharsis. Because cathartics do not decrease food absorption, they have limited effects on weight control.[8] Various test methods can be used to detect laxative abuse.[32] Phenolphthalein can be detected as a pink or red coloration to stool or urine after alkalinization. Colonoscopy reveals the benign, pathognomonic "melanosis coli," the dark staining of the colonic mucosa secondary to anthraquinone laxative abuse. The combination of misuse and abuse of laxatives in conjunction with use of orlistat has the potential to cause severe diarrhea and subsequent fluid and electrolyte imbalances. Now that orlistat is readily available, the combination of these two agents being abused needs to be considered.[28]

Chronic use of syrup of ipecac to induce emesis by patients with eating disorders, such as bulimia nervosa, leads to the development of cardiomyopathy, subsequent dysrhythmias, and death.[47,100] Emetine, a component of syrup of ipecac, is the alkaloid responsible for the severe myopathy. Chronic administration of syrup of ipecac results in tolerance to the emetic effects and increased systemic absorption of emetine.[100] Emetine can be detected in serum by high-pressure liquid chromatography or thin-layer chromatography. It persists for weeks to months after ingestion. In 2003, an FDA advisory committee recommended that the nonprescription drug status of syrup of ipecac be rescinded because of its use by patients with bulimic disorders.

SURGICAL APPROACHES

Although not a specific toxicologic concern, it is imperative to mention surgical interventions for management of obesity. Surgical interventions to manage obesity have increased in frequency over the past years and may provide a long-term solution for obesity. Roux-en-Y gastric bypass (RYGBP), laparoscopic adjustable gastric banding (LAGB), and biliary-pancreatic diversion with duodenal switch (BPD/DS) are the most commonly described techniques.[2,16,36] Patients undergoing these procedures are of particular concern because absorption of vitamins, minerals, and drugs are altered.[69,93,105,116,135] The pharmacokinetics of orally administered medications may be altered as well.[105,116] Consideration of drug properties should be examined closely before initiation in this patient population.[69]

ENDOCANNABINOID RECEPTOR ANTAGONISTS

In recent years, focus on the endocannabinoid system (ECS) and its involvement in weight loss and gain has increased tremendously. The ECS contributes to the regulation of food intake, body weight, and energy balance. The ECS is also being studied for a role in inflammation and neuropathic pain.[63,113,137,143] The research and potential for novel pharmacologic agents to treat conditions, including obesity, neuropathic pain, diarrhea, and abdominal cramps, is promising and exciting.

It has long been known that *Cannabis sativa* stimulates appetite and is an effective antiemetic.[25,102] Despite this, it was not until nearly 1990 when the first tetrahydrocannabinol (THC) receptor was identified[102] (see Chap. 83). Endocannabinoids have a vast effect on metabolic functions, including decreasing satiety, increasing food intake, decreasing glucose uptake, increasing lipogenesis and fibrosis in the liver, and decreasing adiponectin, which negatively correlate with BMI.[59] The ECS peripherally has been shown to be upregulated in the presence of diabetes.[42]

Rimonabant, a CB1 antagonist at therapeutic doses and a CB2 antagonist at supratherapeutic doses, was first described in the early 1990s. Rimonabant (Acomplia) is available as a pharmaceutical in Europe but yet to be FDA approved in the United States. Rimonabant has been investigated in animal models and has shown to induce a reduction of food intake as well as a sustained reduction in body weight in a diet induced obesity model in a rat.[107] Moreover, there was an improvement in insulin resistance with a decline in plasma leptin, insulin, and free fatty acid levels. To confirm that indeed CB1 was involved, the investigators used a group of CB1 receptor knockout mice; in these animals, rimonabant had no effect on dietary intake.[107]

Numerous human studies have evaluated the effects of rimonabant,[33,104,112,115,133] and many are currently ongoing. The RIO (Rimonabant in Obesity and Related Metabolic Disorders) series is the largest series of human research. It is a four part phase III multinational, randomized, double-blind, placebo-controlled studies in overweight and obese patients with BMIs above 27 kg/m^2. RIO-North America,[104] RIO-Europe,[133] RIO-Lipids,[33] and RIO-Diabetes[115] included nearly 6700 patients. The data from these trials are promising and exciting. In each of the four studies, the rimonabant group had a statistically significant reduction in weight and a more sustainable weight loss compared with the placebo group. Moreover, the individuals in the rimonabant group had a reduction in the incidence of metabolic syndrome; blood pressure, glycosylated hemoglobin, and high-density lipoprotein cholesterol increased.

The most common adverse events include nausea, dizziness, and diarrhea. There is concern that rimonabant increases anxiety and depression. Because of these concerns, the FDA has yet to approve the drug for the U.S. market. In the RIO studies, there was a 30% to 50% dropout rate because of adverse events, including GI distress, anxiety, and depression. The dropout rates were higher in the first year compared with the second and were higher with doses of 20 mg compared with 5 mg.

Little is known regarding the clinical presentation after an overdose of rimonabant. Based on the clinical trials and the pharmacology, however, one might expect anxiety and GI toxicity, including nausea and vomiting. At this point, treatment should be generally considered as supportive. Data from ongoing studies as well as case reports and case series will be insightful as to the expected toxicity.

NOVEL THERAPEUTIC APPROACHES

The desire to identify new biochemical pathways and pharmacologic approaches to weight loss has been around since antiquity. Research continues to evolve in an ongoing effort to determine the underlying etiology of obesity as well as develop new, more advanced pharmacologic interventions.[3,25]

Leptin and the leptin gene have been explored as a basis for obesity and as a therapeutic strategy. Obese patients have depressed plasma leptin concentrations.[57,81,106] Genetically leptin-deficient mice are obese, and leptin replacement produces weight loss. Subcutaneous leptin supplementation appears to induce weight loss in lean and obese adults.[57] In three humans with genetically based obesity caused by a presumed leptin deficiency, leptin replacement therapy resulted in profound weight loss and normalization of endocrine function.[81] Much of the enthusiasm about the potential role for leptin as an anti-obesity therapy has subsided because leptin does not induce the expected response on weight control, suggesting leptin resistance.[106,114]

Ghrelin antagonists have also been suggested as a possible adjunct therapy for weight loss. Ghrelin is a growth hormone–releasing agent produced by the stomach and has been shown to stimulate appetite.[71,73,131] Data suggest that ghrelin and leptin work together.[31,85] Ghrelin antagonists may decrease the increased appetite that often occurs with dietary modifications for weight loss, and such agents are under investigation. Because β_3-adrenergic receptors mediate lipolysis in adipose tissue, β_3-selective agonists are also under investigation as weight loss agents.[110] Neuropeptide Y, a peptide found in the arcuate and paraventricular nucleus of the hypothalamus, is a potent central appetite stimulant. Future drug therapy may target these genes, receptors, and proteins to modify metabolism. As obesity research proceeds and the biologic basis for obesity is defined, new approaches and mechanisms for drug therapy may be identified.

OTHER HERBAL REMEDIES

Several herbal remedies for weight loss have resulted in serious toxicity. In France, germander (*Teucrium chamaedrys*) supplements taken for weight loss resulted in seven cases of hepatotoxicity.[77] A "slimming regimen" first prescribed in a weight loss clinic in Belgium produced an epidemic of progressive renal disease, known as Chinese herb nephropathy, when botanical misidentification led to the substitution of *Stephania tetrandra* with the nephrotoxic plant *Aristolochia fangji*.[134] The toxic constituent, identified as aristolochic acid, has been implicated in numerous cases of renal failure and urothelial carcinoma.[83] A case of profound digitalis toxicity occurred with a laxative regimen contaminated with *Digitalis lanata*.[122] Contamination of herbal products remain a concern today because of the lack of standardization of manufacturing processes. Most recently, a dietary supplement was contaminated with selenium, resulting in nearly 45 serious adverse events (see Chap. 98). Until regulation of herbal products is improved and manufacturing practices worldwide are standardized, sporadic reports of herb-related toxicity likely will continue (see Chaps. 27 and 43).

SUMMARY

Although obesity is a major health concern and a significant cause of preventable diseases and sequelae, unproven weight loss modalities are associated with treatment failure and the potential for significant adverse events. Despite the desire for the "easy" solution, there probably is no appropriate substitute for a balanced weight loss plan that encompasses decreased caloric intake with increased energy expenditure through exercise. Clinicians should be aware of the lack of regulation of most available diet remedies and should report adverse events involving these products to poison centers and to the FDA MedWatch system so that appropriate regulatory actions can be taken to prevent further instances of toxicity. A historical review of compounds used as weight loss agents readily uncovers numerous examples of poorly conceived drug regimens, popular misunderstanding of the benefits and risk of the drugs involved, and relatively poor postmarketing surveillance, leading to unnecessary morbidity and mortality.

ACKNOWLEDGMENT

Christine Haller and Jeanmarie Perrone contributed to this chapter in a previous edition.

REFERENCES

1. Abenhaim L, Moride Y, Brenot F, et al. Appetite-suppressant drugs and the risk of primary pulmonary hypertension. International Primary Pulmonary Hypertension Study Group. *N Engl J Med.* 1996;335:609-616.
2. Adams TD, Gress RE, Smith SC, et al. Long-term mortality after gastric bypass surgery. *N Engl J Med.* 2007;357:753-761.
3. Ahima RS, Osei SY. Adipokines in obesity. *Front Horm Res.* 2008;36:182-197.
4. Albertson TE, Dawson A, de Latorre F, et al. TOX-ACLS: toxicologic-oriented advanced cardiac life support. *Ann Emerg Med.* 2001;37:S78-S90.
5. Allison DB, Fontaine KR, Manson JE, Stevens J, VanItallie TB. Annual deaths attributable to obesity in the United States. *JAMA.* 1999;282:1530-1538.
6. Arvill A, Bodin L. Effect of short-term ingestion of konjac glucomannan on serum cholesterol in healthy men. *Am J Clin Nutr.* 1995;61:585-589.
7. Atanassoff PG, Weiss BM, Schmid ER, Tornic M. Pulmonary hypertension and dexfenfluramine. *Lancet.* 1992;339:436.
8. Baker EH, Sandle GI. Complications of laxative abuse. *Annu Rev Med.* 1996;47:127-134.
9. Bibbins-Domingo K, Coxson P, Pletcher MJ, Lightwood J, et al. Adolescent overweight and future adult coronary heart disease. *N Engl J Med.* 2007;357:2371-2379.

10. Binkley K, Knowles SR. Sibutramine and panic attacks. *Am J Psychiatry.* 2002;159:1793-1794.
11. Boardman WW. Rapidly developing cataract after dinitrophenol. *JAMA.* 1935;105:108-110.
12. Bouchard NC, Howland MA, Greller HA, et al. Ischemic stroke associated with use of an ephedra-free dietary supplement containing synephrine. *Mayo Clin Proc.* 2005;80:541-545.
13. Brenot F, Herve P, Petitpretz P, et al. Primary pulmonary hypertension and fenfluramine use. *Br Heart J.* 1993;70:537-541.
14. Bruno A, Nolte KB, Chapin J. Stroke associated with ephedrine use. *Neurology.* 1993;43:1313-1316.
15. Bulik CM. Abuse of drugs associated with eating disorders. *J Subst Abuse.* 1992;4:69-90.
16. Bult MJ, van Dalen T, Muller AF. Surgical treatment of obesity. *Eur J Endocrinol.* 2008;158:135-145.
17. Cacoub P, Dorent R, Nataf P, et al. Pulmonary hypertension and dexfenfluramine. *Eur J Clin Pharmacol.* 1995;48:81-83.
18. Cannistra LB, Cannistra AJ. Regression of multivalvular regurgitation after the cessation of fenfluramine and phentermine treatment. *N Engl J Med.* 1998;339:771.
19. Capewell S, Critchley JA. Adolescent overweight and coronary heart disease. *N Engl J Med.* 2008;358:1521.
20. Capwell RR. Ephedrine-induced mania from an herbal diet supplement. *Am J Psychiatry.* 1995;152:647.
21. Carpene C, Galitzky J, Fontana E, et al. Selective activation of beta3-adrenoceptors by octopamine: comparative studies in mammalian fat cells. *Naunyn Schmiedebergs Arch Pharmacol.* 1999;359:310-321.
22. Carriere F, Renou C, Ransac S, et al. Inhibition of gastrointestinal lipolysis by orlistat during digestion of test meals in healthy volunteers. *Am J Physiol Gastrointest Liver Physiol.* 2001;281:G16-G28.
23. Cauchi S, Choquet H, Gutierrez-Aguilar R, et al. Effects of TCF7L2 polymorphisms on obesity in European populations. *Obesity (Silver Spring).* 2008;16:476-482.
24. Cavaliere H, Floriano I, Medeiros-Neto G. Gastrointestinal side effects of orlistat may be prevented by concomitant prescription of natural fibers (psyllium mucilloid). *Int J Obes Relat Metab Disord.* 2001;25:1095-1099.
25. Chaput JP, Tremblay A. Current and novel approaches to the drug therapy of obesity. *Eur J Clin Pharmacol.* 2006;62:793-803.
26. Christakis NA, Fowler JH. The spread of obesity in a large social network over 32 years. *N Engl J Med.* 2007;357:370-379.
27. Connolly HM, Crary JL, McGoon MD, et al. Valvular heart disease associated with fenfluramine-phentermine. *N Engl J Med.* 1997;337:581-588.
28. Cumella EJ, Hahn J, Woods BK. Weighing Alli's impact. Eating disorder patients might be tempted to abuse the first FDA-approved nonprescription diet pill. *Behav Healthc.* 2007;27:32-34.
29. Cutting WC, Mehrtens HG, Tainter ML. Actions and uses of dinitrophenol. *JAMA.* 1933;101:195.
30. Daniels SR, Long B, Crow S, et al. Cardiovascular effects of sibutramine in the treatment of obese adolescents: results of a randomized, double-blind, placebo-controlled study. *Pediatrics.* 2007;120:e147-e157.
31. de Luis DA, Sagrado MG, Conde R, et al. Changes of ghrelin and leptin in response to hypocaloric diet in obese patients. *Nutrition.* 2008;24:162-166.
32. de Wolff FA, Edelbroek PM, de Haas EJ, Vermeij P. Experience with a screening method for laxative abuse. *Hum Toxicol.* 1983;2:385-389.
33. Despres JP, Golay A, Sjostrom L, Rimonabant in Obesity-Lipids Study Group. Effects of rimonabant on metabolic risk factors in overweight patients with dyslipidemia. *N Engl J Med.* 2005;353:2121-2134.
34. Deuchi K, Kanauchi O, Shizukuishi M, Kobayashi E. Continuous and massive intake of chitosan affects mineral and fat-soluble vitamin status in rats fed on a high-fat diet. *Biosci Biotechnol Biochem.* 1995;59:1211-1216.
35. Di Francesco V, Sacco T, Zamboni M, et al. Weight loss and quality of life improvement in obese subjects treated with sibutramine: a double-blind randomized multicenter study. *Ann Nutr Metab.* 2007;51:75-81.
36. Dixon JB, O'Brien PE, Playfair J, et al. Adjustable gastric banding and conventional therapy for type 2 diabetes: a randomized controlled trial. *JAMA.* 2008;299:316-323.
37. Douglas JG, Munro JF, Kitchin AH, Muir AL, Proudfoot AT. Pulmonary hypertension and fenfluramine. *Br Med J (Clin Res Ed).* 1981;283:881-883.
38. Doyle H, Kargin M. Herbal stimulant containing ephedrine has also caused psychosis. *Br Med J.* 1996;313:756.
39. Drott C, Lundholm K. Cardiac effects of caloric restriction-mechanisms and potential hazards. *Int J Obes Relat Metab Disord.* 1992;16:481-486.
40. Eckel RH. Clinical practice. Nonsurgical management of obesity in adults. *N Engl J Med.* 2008;358:1941-1950.
41. Edwards M, Russo L, Harwood-Nuss A. Cerebral infarction with a single oral dose of phenylpropanolamine. *Am J Emerg Med.* 1987;5:163-164.
42. Engeli S, Bohnke J, Feldpausch M, et al. Activation of the peripheral endocannabinoid system in human obesity. *Diabetes.* 2005;54:2838-2843.
43. Fallis RJ, Fisher M. Cerebral vasculitis and hemorrhage associated with phenylpropanolamine. *Neurology.* 1985;35:405-407.
44. Fernstrom JD, Choi S. The development of tolerance to drugs that suppress food intake. *Pharmacol Ther.* 2008;117:105-122.
45. Filippatos TD, Derdemezis CS, Gazi IF, et al. Orlistat-associated adverse effects and drug interactions: a critical review. *Drug Saf.* 2008;31:53-65.
46. Firenzuoli F, Gori L, Galapai C. Adverse reaction to an adrenergic herbal extract (*Citrus aurantium*). *Phytomedicine.* 2005;12:247-248.
47. Friedman EJ. Death from ipecac intoxication in a patient with anorexia nervosa. *Am J Psychiatry.* 1984;141:702-703.
48. Fugh-Berman A, Myers A. *Citrus aurantium*, an ingredient of dietary supplements marketed for weight loss: current status of clinical and basic research [see comment]. *Exp Biol Med (Maywood).* 2004;229:698-704.
49. Gades MD, Stern JS. Chitosan supplementation and fat absorption in men and women. *J Am Diet Assoc.* 2005;105:72-77.
50. Gardin JM, Schumacher D, Constantine G, et al. Valvular abnormalities and cardiovascular status following exposure to dexfenfluramine or phentermine/fenfluramine. *JAMA.* 2000;283:1703-1709.
51. Gebhard RL, Albrecht J. The diet pill that worked. *N Engl J Med.* 1990;322:702.
52. Glick R, Hoying J, Cerullo L, Perlman S. Phenylpropanolamine: an over-the-counter drug causing central nervous system vasculitis and intracerebral hemorrhage. Case report and review. *Neurosurgery.* 1987;20:969-974.
53. Gurtner HP. Aminorex and pulmonary hypertension. A review. *Cor Vasa.* 1985;27:160-171.
54. Haller CA, Benowitz NL. Adverse cardiovascular and central nervous system events associated with dietary supplements containing ephedra alkaloids. *N Engl J Med.* 2000;343:1833-1838.
55. Hedley AA, Ogden CL, Johnson CL, et al. Prevalence of overweight and obesity among US children, adolescents, and adults, 1999-2002. *JAMA.* 2004;291:2847-2850.
56. Henry DA, Mitchell AS, Aylward J, et al. Glucomannan and risk of oesophageal obstruction. *Br Med J (Clin Res Ed).* 1986;292:591-592.
57. Heymsfield SB, Greenberg AS, Fujioka K, et al. Recombinant leptin for weight loss in obese and lean adults: a randomized, controlled, dose-escalation trial. *JAMA.* 1999;282:1568-1575.
58. Hoffman RJ, Hoffman RS, Freyberg CL, et al. Clenbuterol ingestion causing prolonged tachycardia, hypokalemia, and hypophosphatemia with confirmation by quantitative levels. *J Toxicol Clin Toxicol.* 2001;39:339-344.
59. Hoffstedt J, Arvidsson E, Sjolin E, et al. Adipose tissue adiponectin production and adiponectin serum concentration in human obesity and insulin resistance. *J Clin Endocrinol Metab.* 2004;89:1391-1396.
60. Hopkins KD, Lehmann ED. Successful medical treatment of obesity in 10th century Spain. *Lancet.* 1995;346:452.
61. Horowitz JD, Lang WJ, Howes LG, et al. Hypertensive responses induced by phenylpropanolamine in anorectic and decongestant preparations. *Lancet.* 1980;1:60-61.
62. Isner JM, Roberts WC, Heymsfield SB, Yager J. Anorexia nervosa and sudden death. *Ann Intern Med.* 1985;102:49-52.
63. Jhaveri MD, Richardson D, Chapman V. Endocannabinoid metabolism and uptake: novel targets for neuropathic and inflammatory pain [see comment]. *Br J Pharmacol.* 2007;152:624-632.
64. Jick H, Vasilakis C, Weinrauch LA, et al. A population-based study of appetite-suppressant drugs and the risk of cardiac-valve regurgitation. *N Engl J Med.* 1998;339:719-724.
65. Kase CS, Foster TE, Reed JE, et al. Intracerebral hemorrhage and phenylpropanolamine use. *Neurology.* 1987;37:399-404.
66. Kernan WN, Viscoli CM, Brass LM, et al. Phenylpropanolamine and the risk of hemorrhagic stroke. *N Engl J Med.* 2000;343:1826-1832.
67. Khan MA, Herzog CA, St Peter JV, et al. The prevalence of cardiac valvular insufficiency assessed by transthoracic echocardiography in obese patients treated with appetite-suppressant drugs. *N Engl J Med.* 1998;339:713-718.
68. Kikta DG, Devereaux MW, Chandar K. Intracranial hemorrhages due to phenylpropanolamine. *Stroke.* 1985;16:510-512.

69. Klockhoff H, Naslund I, Jones AW. Faster absorption of ethanol and higher peak concentration in women after gastric bypass surgery. *Br J Clin Pharmacol.* 2002;54:587-591.
70. Klontz KC, Timbo BB, Street D. Consumption of dietary supplements containing *Citrus aurantium* (bitter orange)—2004 California Behavioral Risk Factor Surveillance Survey (BRFSS). *Ann Pharmacother.* 2006;40:1747-1751.
71. Kojima M, Kangawa K. Ghrelin: structure and function. *Physiol Rev.* 2005;85:495-522.
72. Kokkinos J, Levine SR. Possible association of ischemic stroke with phentermine. *Stroke.* 1993;24:310-313.
73. Kola B, Grossman AB, Korbonits M. The role of AMP-activated protein kinase in obesity. *Front Horm Res.* 2008;36:198-211.
74. Kurt TL, Anderson R, Petty C, et al. Dinitrophenol in weight loss: the poison center and public health safety. *Vet Hum Toxicol.* 1986;28:574-575.
75. Lake CR, Gallant S, Masson E, Miller P. Adverse drug effects attributed to phenylpropanolamine: a review of 142 case reports. *Am J Med.* 1990;89:195-208.
76. Lake CR, Rosenberg DB, Gallant S, et al. Phenylpropanolamine increases plasma caffeine levels. *Clin Pharmacol Ther.* 1990;47:675-685.
77. Larrey D, Vial T, Pauwels A, et al. Hepatitis after germander (*Teucrium chamaedrys*) administration: another instance of herbal medicine hepatotoxicity. *Ann Intern Med.* 1992;117:129-132.
78. Lean ME. Sibutramine—a review of clinical efficacy. *Int J Obes Relat Metab Disord.* 1997;21:S30-S36.
79. Leo PJ, Hollander JE, Shih RD, Marcus SM. Phenylpropanolamine and associated myocardial injury. *Ann Emerg Med.* 1996;28:359-362.
80. Lewis JH. Esophageal and small bowel obstruction from guar gum-containing "diet pills": analysis of 26 cases reported to the Food and Drug Administration. *Am J Gastroenterol* .1992;87:1424-1428.
81. Licinio J, Caglayan S, Ozata M, et al. Phenotypic effects of leptin replacement on morbid obesity, diabetes mellitus, hypogonadism, and behavior in leptin-deficient adults. *Proc Natl Acad Sci U S A.* 2004;101:4531-4536.
82. Litvan L, Alcoverro-Fortuny O. Sibutramine and psychosis. *J Clin Psychopharmacol.* 2007;27:726-727.
83. Lord GM, Cook T, Arlt VM, et al. Urothelial malignant disease and Chinese herbal nephropathy. *Lancet.* 2001;358:1515-1516.
84. Luque CA, Rey JA. Sibutramine: a serotonin-norepinephrine reuptake-inhibitor for the treatment of obesity. *Ann Pharmacother.* 1999;33:968-978.
85. Maestu J, Jurimae J, Valter I, Jurimae T. Increases in ghrelin and decreases in leptin without altering adiponectin during extreme weight loss in male competitive bodybuilders. *Metabolism.* 2008;57:221-225.
86. McFee RB, Caraccio TR, McGuigan MA, et al. Dying to be thin: a dinitrophenol related fatality. *Vet Hum Toxicol.* 2004;46:251-254.
87. McGoon MD, Vanhoutte PM. Aggregating platelets contract isolated canine pulmonary arteries by releasing 5-hydroxytryptamine. *J Clin Invest.* 1984;74:828-833.
88. McMurray J, Bloomfield P, Miller HC. Irreversible pulmonary hypertension after treatment with fenfluramine. *Br Med J (Clin Res Ed).* 1986; 293:51-52.
89. McNeely W, Goa KL. Sibutramine. A review of its contribution to the management of obesity. *Drugs.* 1998;56:1093-1124.
90. Mesnard B, Ginn DR. Excessive phenylpropanolamine ingestion followed by subarachnoid hemorrhage. *South Med J.* 1984;77:939.
91. Mhurchu CN, Dunshea-Mooij C, Bennett D, Rodgers A. Effect of chitosan on weight loss in overweight and obese individuals: a systematic review of randomized controlled trials [see comment]. *Obes Rev.* 2005;6:35-42.
92. Mhurchu CN, Poppitt SD, McGill AT, et al. The effect of the dietary supplement, Chitosan, on body weight: a randomised controlled trial in 250 overweight and obese adults. *Int J Obes Relat Metab Disord.* 2004;28: 1149-1156.
93. Miller AD, Smith KM. Medication use in bariatric surgery patients: what orthopedists need to know. *Orthopedics.* 2006;29:121-123.
94. Montero JL, Muntane J, Fraga E, et al. Orlistat associated subacute hepatic failure. *J Hepatol.* 2001;34:173.
95. Nadir A, Agrawal S, King PD, Marshall JB. Acute hepatitis associated with the use of a Chinese herbal product, ma-huang [see comment]. *Am J Gastroenterol.* 1996;91:1436-1438.
96. Nasir JM, Durning SJ, Ferguson M, et al. Exercise-induced syncope associated with QT prolongation and ephedra-free Xenadrine. *Mayo Clin Proc.* 2004;79:1059-1062.
97. Nykamp DL, Fackih MN, Compton AL. Possible association of acute lateral-wall myocardial infarction and bitter orange supplement. *Ann Pharmacother.* 2004;38:812-816.
98. Pace S. Ma Huang food supplement toxicity in two adolescents [abstract]. *J Toxicol Clin Toxicol.* 1996;34:598.
99. Pace SA, Pace S. Dinitrophenol oral ingestion resulting in death [abstract]. *J Toxicol Clin Toxicol.* 2002;40:683.
100. Palmer EP, Guay AT. Reversible myopathy secondary to abuse of ipecac in patients with major eating disorders. *N Engl J Med.* 1985;313:1457-1459.
101. Pentel P. Toxicity of over-the-counter stimulants. *JAMA.* 1984;252: 1898-1903.
102. Perkins JM, Davis SN. Endocannabinoid system overactivity and the metabolic syndrome: prospects for treatment. *Curr Diab Rep.* 2008;8:12-19.
103. Perrio MJ, Wilton LV, Shakir SA. The safety profiles of orlistat and sibutramine: results of prescription-event monitoring studies in England. *Obesity (Silver Spring).* 2007;15:2712-2722.
104. Pi-Sunyer FX, Aronne LJ, Heshmati HM, Devin J, Rosenstock J, RIO-North America Study G. Effect of rimonabant, a cannabinoid-1 receptor blocker, on weight and cardiometabolic risk factors in overweight or obese patients: RIO-North America: a randomized controlled trial. *JAMA.* 2006;295:761-775.
105. Ponsky TA, Brody F, Pucci E. Alterations in gastrointestinal physiology after Roux-en-Y gastric bypass [see comment]. *J Am Coll Surg.* 2005;201:125-131.
106. Quilliot D, Bohme P, Zannad F, Ziegler O. Sympathetic-leptin relationship in obesity: effect of weight loss. *Metabolism.* 2008;57:555-562.
107. Ravinet Trillou C, Arnone M, Delgorge C, et al. Anti-obesity effect of SR141716, a CB1 receptor antagonist, in diet-induced obese mice. *Am J Physiol Regul Integr Comp Physiol.* 2003;284:R345-R353.
108. Richelsen B, Tonstad S, Rossner S, et al. Effect of orlistat on weight regain and cardiovascular risk factors following a very-low-energy diet in abdominally obese patients: a 3-year randomized, placebo-controlled study. *Diabetes Care.* 2007;30:27-32.
109. Roche N, Labrune S, Braun JM, Huchon GJ. Pulmonary hypertension and dexfenfluramine. *Lancet.* 1992;339:436-437.
110. Rosenbaum M, Leibel RL, Hirsch J. Obesity [see comment] [erratum appears in *N Engl J Med.* 1998;338(3):555]. *N Engl J Med.* 1997;337:396-407.
111. Rostagno C, Caciolli S, Felici M, et al. Dilated cardiomyopathy associated with chronic consumption of phendimetrazine. *Am Heart J.* 1996;131:407-409.
112. Ruilope LM, Despres JP, Scheen A, et al. Effect of rimonabant on blood pressure in overweight/obese patients with/without co-morbidities: analysis of pooled RIO study results. *J Hypertens.* 2008;26:357-367.
113. Sanger GJ. Endocannabinoids and the gastrointestinal tract: what are the key questions? *Br J Pharmacol.* 2007;152:663-670.
114. Scarpace PJ, Matheny M, Tumer N, et al. Leptin resistance exacerbates diet-induced obesity and is associated with diminished maximal leptin signalling capacity in rats. *Diabetologia.* 2005;48:1075-1083.
115. Scheen AJ. Cannabinoid-1 receptor antagonists in type-2 diabetes. *Baillieres Best Pract Res Clin Endocrinol Metab.* 2007;21:535-553.
116. Seaman JS, Bowers SP, Dixon P, Schindler L. Dissolution of common psychiatric medications in a Roux-en-Y gastric bypass model. *Psychosomatics.* 2005;46:250-253.
117. Seidner DL, Roberts IM, Smith MS. Esophageal obstruction after ingestion of a fiber-containing diet pill. *Gastroenterology.* 1990;99:1820-1822.
118. Shields KM, Smock N, McQueen CE, Bryant PJ. Chitosan for weight loss and cholesterol management. *Am J Health-Syst Pharm.* 2003;60:1310-1312.
119. Shiri R, Solovieva S, Husgafvel-Pursiainen K, et al. The association between obesity and the prevalence of low back pain in young adults: the Cardiovascular Risk in Young Finns Study. *Am J Epidemiol.* 2008;167:1110-1119.
120. Singh BN, Gaarder TD, Kanegae T, et al. Liquid protein diets and torsade de pointes. *JAMA.* 1978;240:115-119.
121. Sjostrom L, Rissanen A, Andersen T, et al. Randomised placebo-controlled trial of orlistat for weight loss and prevention of weight regain in obese patients. European Multicentre Orlistat Study Group. *Lancet.* 1998;352:167-172.
122. Slifman NR, Obermeyer WR, et al. Contamination of botanical dietary supplements by Digitalis lanata. *N Engl J Med.* 1998;339:806-811.
123. Smookler S, Bermudez AJ. Hypertensive crisis resulting from an MAO inhibitor and an over-the-counter appetite suppressant. *Ann Emerg Med.* 1982;11:482-484.
124. Sours HE, Frattali VP, Brand CD, et al. Sudden death associated with very low calorie weight reduction regimens. *Am J Clin Nutr.* 1981;34:453-461.
125. Spedding M, Ouvry C, Millan M, et al. Neural control of dieting. *Nature.* 1996;380:488.
126. Taflinski T, Chojnacka J. Sibutramine-associated psychotic episode. *Am J Psychiatry.* 2000;157:2057-2058.
127. Tainter ML. Actions of benzedrine and propadrine in control of obesity. *J Nutr.* 1944;27:89-105.

128. Tainter ML, Cutting WC. Febrile, respiratory and some other actions of dinitrophenol. *J Pharmac Exp Ther*. 1933;48:410-429.
129. Tainter ML, Stockton AB, Cutting WC. Dinitrophenol in the treatment of obesity. *JAMA*. 1935;105:332-337.
130. Thurairajah PH, Syn WK, Neil DA, et al. Orlistat (Xenical)-induced subacute liver failure. *Eur J Gastroenterol Hepatol*. 2005;17:1437-1438.
131. Toussirot E, Streit G, Nguyen NU, et al. Adipose tissue, serum adipokines, and ghrelin in patients with ankylosing spondylitis. *Metabolism*. 2007;56:1383-1389.
132. Traub SJ, Hoyek W, Hoffman RS. Dietary supplements containing ephedra alkaloids. *N Engl J Med*. 2001;344:1096-1097.
133. Van Gaal LF, Rissanen AM, Scheen AJ, et al, RIO-Europe Study G. Effects of the cannabinoid-1 receptor blocker rimonabant on weight reduction and cardiovascular risk factors in overweight patients: 1-year experience from the RIO-Europe study. *Lancet*. 2005;365:1389-1397.
134. Vanherweghem JL, Depierreux M, Tielemans C, et al. Rapidly progressive interstitial renal fibrosis in young women: association with slimming regimen including Chinese herbs. *Lancet*. 1993;341:387-391.
135. Voelker M, Foster TG. Nursing challenges in the administration of oral antidepressant medications in gastric bypass patients. *J Perianesth Nurs*. 2007;22:108-121.
136. Vuksan V, Jenkins DJ, Spadafora P, et al. Konjac-mannan (glucomannan) improves glycemia and other associated risk factors for coronary heart disease in type 2 diabetes. A randomized controlled metabolic trial. *Diabetes Care*. 1999;22:913-919.
137. Wang J, Ueda N. Role of the endocannabinoid system in metabolic control. *Curr Opin Nephrol Hypertens*. 2008;17:1-10.
138. Weiss R, Dziura J, Burgert TS, et al. Obesity and the metabolic syndrome in children and adolescents. *N Engl J Med*. 2004;350:2362-2374.
139. Weissman NJ, Tighe JF Jr, Gottdiener JS, et al. An assessment of heart-valve abnormalities in obese patients taking dexfenfluramine, sustained-release dexfenfluramine, or placebo. Sustained-Release Dexfenfluramine Study Group. *N Engl J Med*. 1998;339:725-732.
140. Wellman PJ. Overview of adrenergic anorectic agents. *Am J Clin Nutr*. 1992;55:193S-198S.
141. Wilfley DE, Crow SJ, Hudson JI, et al. Efficacy of sibutramine for the treatment of binge eating disorder: a randomized multicenter placebo-controlled double-blind study. *Am J Psychiatry*. 2008;165:51-58.
142. Wirth A, Krause J. Long-term weight loss with sibutramine: a randomized controlled trial. *JAMA*. 2001;286:1331-1339.
143. Wright KL, Duncan M, Sharkey KA. Cannabinoid CB2 receptors in the gastrointestinal tract: a regulatory system in states of inflammation. *Br J Pharmacol*. 2008;153:263-270.
144. Zahn KA, Li RL, Purssell RA. Cardiovascular toxicity after ingestion of "herbal ecstasy." *J Emerg Med*. 1999;17:289-291.
145. Zhi J, Melia AT, Eggers H, et al. Review of limited systemic absorption of orlistat, a lipase inhibitor, in healthy human volunteers. *J Clin Pharmacol*. 1995;35:1103-1108.

CHAPTER 40
IRON

Jeanmarie Perrone

Iron		
MW	=	55.85 daltons
Serum normal concentration	=	80–180 μg/dL
	=	14–32 μmol/L

Iron poisoning, once an all-too-frequent tragedy in children, has become uncommon. This may underscore the success of a poisoning that has been prevented by interventions gleaned from poison center data and poison prevention advocacy. Blister packaging, smaller dosages, and education of parents and healthcare providers have led to a great decline in iron poisoning in the past decade. However, significant poisonings still occur, and when they do, they may not be managed as effectively as in the past because they less commonly occur and clinicians are less familiar with the problem. Clinicians must be vigilant for signs of serious iron poisoning and be ready to intervene if gastrointestinal (GI) symptoms are followed by acid–base disturbances, altered mental status, or hemodynamic compromise.

HISTORY AND EPIDEMIOLOGY

Iron salts such as ferrous sulfate have been used therapeutically for thousands of years and continues to be available, both with and without prescription, for the prevention and treatment of iron-deficiency anemia in patients of all ages. Despite this long history of use, the first reports of iron toxicity only occurred in the mid-20th century. Since then, numerous cases of iron poisoning and fatalities have been reported, mostly in children.[56,57] In 1950, the manufacturer of "fersolate" included a package warning: "Excessive doses of iron can be dangerous. Do not leave these tablets within reach of young children, who may eat them as sweets with harmful results."[85]

The incidence of iron exposures continued to increase in the 1980s, ultimately becoming, in the 1990s, the leading cause of poisoning deaths reported to poison centers among children younger than 6 years. This problem was publicized as a result of a case series of tragic fatalities involving five toddlers in Los Angeles during a 6-month period in 1992, all of whom were exposed to prenatal vitamins containing iron.[92] The association between death and prenatal vitamins highlights the availability of these potentially lethal medications in the homes of families with young children, ironically as a result of more attentive prescribing of prenatal iron. A case control study in Canada identified a fourfold increase in the risk of iron poisoning to the older sibling of a newborn during the first postpartum month.[41] The authors concluded that almost half of all hospital admissions of young children for iron poisoning could be prevented by safer storage of iron supplements in the year before and the year after the birth of a sibling.

In 1997, the Food and Drug Administration (FDA) mandated that all iron salt-containing preparations have warning labels on them regarding the dangers of pediatric iron poisoning.[23] In addition to the warning labels, the FDA launched an educational campaign to alert caregivers and prescribers of the potential toxicity of iron supplements.[24] Other preventive initiatives instituted by the FDA in 1997 included unit dosing (blister packs) of prescriptions containing more than 30 mg of elemental iron and limitations on the number of pills dispensed (ie, maximum 30-day supply).[24] These efforts to prevent unintentional exposure dramatically decreased the incidence of poisoning and were pivotal in decreasing morbidity and mortality associated with iron poisoning[79] (see Chap. 135 and associated references). Unfortunately, in 2003, the FDA rescinded the blister packaging requirement in response to a lawsuit charging that the FDA did not have jurisdiction over the packaging of dietary supplements.[22] Although isolated fatalities continue to occur,[55] the trend in the National Poison Data System suggests they are becoming less commonly reported (see Chap. 135 and associated references). Iron poisoning may also occur after ingestion of other iron salts, such as ferric chloride, used in industry.[100]

Iron supplements are available in two nonionic forms, carbonyl iron and iron polysaccharide, both of which appear to be less toxic after overdose than are iron salts.[74] Parenteral iron, such as iron dextran, administered intravenously (IV) to patients with renal failure and chronic anemia, may also result in toxicity, as well as anaphylactoid reactions. Newer parenteral formulations, including iron sucrose and sodium ferrous gluconate, appear to be safer.[21]

PHARMACOLOGY, PHARMACOKINETICS, AND TOXICOKINETICS

Iron is an element critical to organ function. As a transition metal, iron can easily accept and donate electrons, thereby shifting from a ferric (Fe^{3+}) to a ferrous (Fe^{2+}) oxidation state (see Chap. 11). This redox interchange allows iron to fulfill its role in multiple protein and enzyme complexes, including cytochromes and myoglobin, although it is principally incorporated into hemoglobin in erythrocytes. Whereas insufficient iron availability results in anemia, excess total body iron results in hemochromatosis.

The body cannot directly excrete iron, so body iron stores are regulated by controlling iron absorption from the GI tract. Iron absorption, which occurs predominantly in the duodenum, is determined by the body's iron requirements. In iron deficiency, iron uptake into intestinal mucosal cells may increase from a normal 10% to 35% to as much as 80% to 95%. After uptake into the intestinal mucosal cells, iron is either stored as ferritin and lost when the cell is sloughed or released to transferrin, a serum iron binding protein. In therapeutic doses, some of these processes become saturated, and absorption into the intestinal cell may be limited. However, in overdose, the oxidative effects of iron on GI mucosal cells lead to dysfunction of this regulatory balance, and passive absorption of iron increases down its concentration gradient[78] (see Pathophysiology below).

Iron supplements are available as the iron salts ferrous gluconate, ferrous sulfate, and ferrous fumarate and as the nonionic preparations carbonyl iron and polysaccharide iron. Additional sources of significant quantities of iron are vitamin preparations, especially prenatal vitamins (Table 40-2). Toxic effects of iron poisoning occur at doses of 10 to 20 mg/kg elemental iron (elemental iron is a measure of the amount of iron present in an iron salt; see Table 40–1). Significant GI symptoms occurred in human adult volunteers who ingested 10 to 20 mg of elemental iron/kg.[9,49] In one volunteer study, six subjects who ingested 20 mg/kg elemental iron developed nausea and voluminous diarrhea within 2 hours, and five of the six subjects had serum iron concentrations above 300 μg/dL.[9]

Chewable vitamins continue to entice children with their sweet taste and recognizable character shapes, increasing the risk of significant

TABLE 40–1. Common Iron Formulations and Their Elemental Iron Contents

Iron Formulation	Elemental Iron (%)
Ionic	
Ferrous chloride	28
Ferrous fumarate	33
Ferrous gluconate	12
Ferrous lactate	19
Ferrous sulfate	20
Nonionic	
Carbonyl iron	98[a]
Iron polysaccharide	46[a]

[a] Although these nonionic iron formulations contain higher elemental iron content than ionic formulations, carbonyl iron and iron polysaccharide have better therapeutic-to-toxic ratios, due to limited GI absorption.

exposure. Children's chewable multivitamins contain less iron per tablet (10–18 mg of elemental iron) than typical prenatal vitamins (65 mg of elemental iron). Toxicity still results when large quantities are ingested, but fatalities have not been reported.[2] One animal study paradoxically demonstrates higher iron concentrations after ingestion of equivalent elemental iron doses of chewable versus solid iron tablets.[59] This finding was attributed, in part, to the limited gastric irritation associated with the chewable iron preparations, resulting in less vomiting and higher iron concentrations.

Iron polysaccharide and carbonyl iron appear to be safer formulations than iron salts despite their high elemental iron content.[45] Carbonyl iron is a form of elemental iron that is highly bioavailable in therapeutic doses compared to other forms of iron because of its high elemental iron content and its very fine, spherical particle size (5 μm). This delayed oxidation is the rate-limiting step that prevents excess absorption.[33] In a rat model of iron toxicity, carbonyl iron had a median lethal dose (LD_{50}) of 50 g/kg compared with an LD_{50} of 1.1 g/kg for ferrous sulfate.[95] No significant toxicity in humans exposed to carbonyl iron has been reported.[74]

Iron polysaccharide contains approximately 46% elemental iron by weight. It is synthesized by neutralization of a ferric chloride carbohydrate solution. This form of iron also appears to have much lower toxicity than iron salts. The estimated LD_{50} in rats is more than 5 g/kg body weight. Retrospective poison center data have shown little toxicity from either of these products.[45]

PATHOPHYSIOLOGY

As a transition metal, iron can assume one of several different oxidation, or valence, states. It is an active participant in reduction oxidation (redox) reactions. In particular, the participation of iron in the Fenton reaction and Haber-Weiss cycle explains its toxicologic effects as a generator of oxidative stress and inhibitor of several key metabolic enzymes (see Chap. 11). Reactive oxygen species oxidize membrane-bound lipids and cause loss of cellular integrity and tissue injury (see Chap. 11).[68,70]

The initial oxidative damage to the GI epithelium produced by iron-induced reactive oxygen species permits iron ions to enter the systemic circulation. Iron ions are rapidly bound to circulating binding proteins, particularly transferrin. After transferrin is saturated with iron, "free" iron (ie, iron not bound to a transport protein) is widely distributed to the various organ systems, where it promotes damaging oxidative processes. A postmortem series of 11 patients who died from iron ingestion substantiated these findings with measurements of elevated iron concentrations in most major organs examined, including the stomach, liver, brain, heart, lung, small bowel, and kidney.[63] Consistent with gastric and intestinal mucosal oxidative damage, congestion, edema, necrosis, and iron deposition in the gastric and intestinal mucosa as well as hemorrhage and congestion in the lungs, are noted on postmortem examination.[30,31,51]

Iron ions disrupt critical cellular processes such as mitochondrial oxidative phosphorylation. Subsequent buildup of unused hydrogen ions normally incorporated into the synthesis of adenosine triphosphate leads to liberation of H^+ and development of metabolic acidosis (see Chap. 12). In addition, absorption of iron from the GI tract leads to conversion of ferrous iron (Fe^{2+}) to ferric iron (Fe^{3+}). Ferric iron ions exceed the binding capacity of plasma, leading to formation of ferric hydroxide and production of three protons ($Fe^{3+} + 3H_2O \rightarrow Fe(OH)_3 + 3H^+$).[68,78]

Decreased cardiac output contributes to hemodynamic shock in animals.[89,98] Although this finding has been attributed to decreased preload and relative bradycardia,[89] a direct negative inotropic effect of iron on the myocardium has also been demonstrated in animal models.[3] Reports of early coagulopathy unrelated to hepatotoxicity[81] led to the identification of free iron as an inhibitor of thrombin formation and the reduction of the effect of thrombin on fibrinogen.[71]

CLINICAL MANIFESTATIONS

Classic teaching posits five clinical stages of iron toxicity based on the pathophysiology of iron poisoning.[6,40,66] Although these stages are conceptually important, they are of limited benefit to clinicians managing poisoned patients. Although the stages are typically described in approximate postingestion time frames, a clinical stage should never be assigned based solely on the number of hours postingestion because patients do not necessarily follow the same temporal course through these stages.

The first stage of iron toxicity is characterized by nausea, vomiting, abdominal pain, and diarrhea. These "local" toxic effects of iron predominate, and subsequent salt and water depletion contribute to the ill appearance of the iron-poisoned patient. Intestinal ulceration, edema, transmural inflammation, and, in some extreme cases, small-bowel infarction and necrosis may occur.[25,69,83] Hematemesis, melena, or hematochezia may cause hemodynamic instability. GI symptoms always occur after significant overdose. Conversely, the absence of symptoms, specifically vomiting, in the first 6 hours after ingestion, essentially excludes serious iron toxicity.

The second, or "latent," stage of iron poisoning commonly refers to the period 6 to 24 hours after resolution of GI symptoms and before development of overt systemic toxicity. Delineation of this stage may have evolved from early case reports of patients whose GI symptoms had resolved before subsequent deterioration.[85] This second stage is not a true quiescent phase because ongoing cellular organ toxicity occurs during this phase.[6] Although clinicians should be wary of patients who no longer have active GI complaints after iron overdose, most such patients have, in fact, recovered and are not in the latent phase. Patients in the latent phase generally have lethargy, tachycardia, or metabolic acidosis. They should be readily identifiable as clinically ill despite resolution of their GI symptoms. In summary, patients who have remained well since ingestion and who have stable vital signs, a normal mental status, and a normal acid–base balance will have a benign clinical course.

Patients who progress to the third, or "shock," stage of iron poisoning have profound toxicity. This stage may occur in the first few hours after a massive ingestion or 12 to 24 hours after a more moderate ingestion. The etiology of shock may be multifactorial, resulting from hypovolemia, vasodilation, and poor cardiac output,[89,98] with decreased tissue perfusion and an ongoing metabolic acidosis. An iron-induced coagulopathy may worsen bleeding and hypovolemia.[81] Systemic toxicity produces central nervous system effects with lethargy, hyperventilation, seizures, or coma.

The fourth stage of iron poisoning is characterized by hepatic failure, which may occur 2 to 3 days after ingestion.[30] The hepatotoxicity is directly attributed to iron uptake by the reticuloendothelial system in the liver, where it causes oxidative damage.[26,99]

The fifth stage of iron toxicity rarely manifests. Gastric outlet obstruction, secondary to strictures and scarring from the initial GI injury, may develop 2 to 8 weeks after ingestion.[29,35,83]

Patients with chronic iron overload are at increased risk for *Yersinia enterocolitica* infection. Iron is a required growth factor for *Y. enterocolitica*; however, the bacterium lacks the siderophore to solubilize and transport iron intracellularly. Because deferoxamine is a siderophore, it fosters the growth of *Y. enterocolitica*. Patients with chronic iron overload or acute poisoning develop *Yersinia* infection or sepsis as a complication of iron poisoning or deferoxamine therapy.[11,53,55,76] *Yersinia* infection should be suspected in patients who experience abdominal pain, fever, and bloody diarrhea after resolution of iron toxicity. In this setting, cultures should be obtained, fluid and electrolyte repletion accomplished, and fluoroquinolones or third-generation cephalosporin therapy initiated.

DIAGNOSTIC TESTING

RADIOGRAPHY

Iron is available in many forms, and the different preparations vary with respect to radiopacity on abdominal radiography.[75] Factors such as the time since ingestion and elemental iron content of the pills also play roles.[58,75] Liquid iron formulations and chewable iron tablets typically are not radiopaque.[19] A retrospective review of iron ingestions in children revealed that abdominal radiographs were positive in only one of 30 patients who ingested chewable vitamins.[19] Because adult preparations have a higher elemental iron content and do not readily disperse, they tend to be more consistently radiopaque.[58] Finding radiopaque pills on an abdominal radiograph is helpful in guiding and evaluating the success of GI decontamination.[36] However, the absence of radiographic evidence of pills is not a reliable indicator to exclude potential toxicity.[58,62]

LABORATORY STUDIES

Various laboratory studies are used as surrogate markers to assess the severity of iron poisoning. An anion-gap metabolic acidosis and an elevated lactate concentration may develop in patients with serious iron ingestions. Serial electrolyte measurements may be used to assess progression and response to volume replacement. Anemia may result from GI blood loss but may not be evident initially because of hemoconcentration secondary to plasma volume loss.

Although one small retrospective study of iron-poisoned children found that white blood cells (WBC) above 15,000/mm^3 or a blood glucose concentration above 150 mg/dL was 100% predictive of iron concentration above 300 μg/dL,[48] three subsequent similar studies were unable to validate this association.[12,47,62] In practice, an elevated WBC or glucose concentration in the setting of a known or suspected iron ingestion should raise concern about an elevated serum iron concentration; however, assessment of the signs and symptoms of the patient is more reliable.

Although iron poisoning remains a clinical diagnosis, serum iron concentrations can be used effectively to gauge toxicity and the success of treatment.[6] In the previously mentioned human volunteer study of six adults who ingested 20 mg/kg of elemental iron, all six adults demonstrated significant GI toxicity, and the four who required IV fluid resuscitation had peak serum iron concentrations in the range of 300 μg/dL between 2 and 4 hours after ingestion.[9]

In another study of human volunteers who ingested 5 to 10 mg/kg elemental iron in the form of chewable vitamins, peak serum iron concentrations occurred between 4.2 and 4.5 hours in all subjects.[49] In overdose, peak concentrations of iron are thought to occur 2 to 6 hours after ingestion, depending on the iron preparation.[9,49] Serum iron concentrations between 300 and 500 μg/dL usually correlate with significant GI toxicity and modest systemic toxicity. Concentrations between 500 and 1000 μg/dL are associated with pronounced systemic toxicity and shock.[93] Concentrations above 1000 μg/dL are associated with significant morbidity and mortality.[93] Although elevated serum iron concentrations may be an additional indicator of potentially serious toxicity, lower concentrations cannot be used to exclude the possibility of serious toxicity. A single serum iron concentration may not represent a peak concentration or may be falsely lowered by the presence of deferoxamine unless an atomic absorption technique is used for measurement.[28,34]

Total iron-binding capacity (TIBC) is a measurement of the total amount of iron that can be bound by transferrin in a given volume of serum.[20] Previously, clinical iron toxicity was thought not to occur if the serum iron concentration was less than the TIBC because insufficient circulating "free" iron was present to cause tissue damage. Although this may be true conceptually, further research has clarified the limitations of TIBC values. Most importantly, the in vitro value of TIBC factitiously increases as a result of iron poisoning and thus has a tendency to apparently increase above a concurrently measured serum iron concentration.[9,84] Because of many confounding issues, the TIBC as currently determined has no value in the assessment of iron-poisoned patients.

MANAGEMENT

INITIAL APPROACH

As with any serious ingestion, initial stabilization must include supplemental oxygen, airway assessment, and establishment of IV access. Evidence of hematemesis or lethargy after an iron exposure may be a manifestation of significant toxicity. IV volume repletion should begin while orogastric lavage and whole-bowel irrigation (WBI) are considered. In any lethargic patient who likely will deteriorate further, early orotracheal intubation may facilitate safe GI decontamination measures. Abdominal radiography may be used to estimate the iron burden in the GI tract given the caveats discussed earlier. Laboratory values, including chemistries, hemoglobin, iron concentration, coagulation, and hepatic profiles, are necessary in the sickest patients. An arterial or venous blood gas or a lactate concentration rapidly detects a metabolic acidosis. Patients who appear well and had only one or two brief episodes of vomiting can be observed pending discharge. Alternatively, the serum iron concentration can be measured.

LIMITING ABSORPTION

GI decontamination procedures should be initiated after stabilization. Adequate gastric emptying is critical after ingestion of xenobiotics, such as iron, that are not well adsorbed to activated charcoal. Because vomiting is a prominent early symptom in patients with significant toxicity, induced emesis is not recommended. Orogastric lavage is more effective but may be of only limited value because of the large size and poor solubility of most iron tablets, their ability to form adherent masses,[25,88] and their movement into the bowel several hours after ingestion.[42] The presence and location of radiopaque pills on abdominal radiography can help guide orogastric lavage. Orogastric lavage likely will not be successful after iron tablets move past the pylorus, so WBI may be more effective (Figs. 40–1 and 40–2).

Many strategies were used in the past in attempts to improve the efficacy of orogastric lavage. At the present time, no data support the use of oral deferoxamine,[32,39,96,97,102] bicarbonate,[15,16] phosphosoda,[4,27] or magnesium.[13,73,91] Although some of these techniques demonstrate efficacy, avoidance of the associated risks mandates using only 0.9% sodium chloride solution or tap water for orogastric lavage.

The value of WBI in patients with iron poisoning is supported primarily by case reports and one uncontrolled case series.[18,42,80,81] However, the rationale for WBI use is logical, especially considering the limitations of other gastric decontamination modalities. The usual dose of WBI with polyethylene glycol electrolyte lavage solution (PEG-ELS) is 500 mL/h in children and 2 L/h in adults. This rate is best achieved by starting slowly and increasing as tolerated, often using a nasogastric tube and an infusion pump to administer large volumes. Antiemetics such as metoclopramide or serotonin antagonists may be used to treat nausea and vomiting. A large volume (44 L) of WBI was administered safely over a 5-day period to a child who had persistent iron tablets on serial abdominal radiographs[42] (see Antidotes in Depth A3: Whole-Bowel Irrigation) (see Chap. 7).

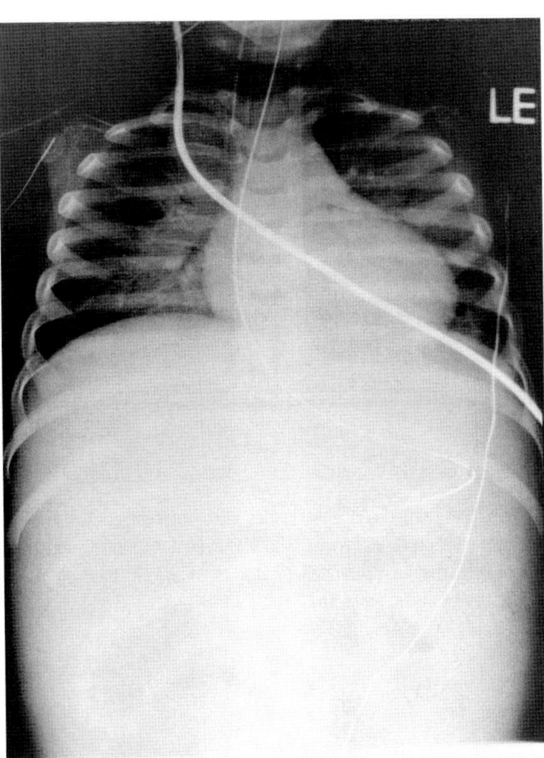

FIGURE 40–2. The same 17 month old child ten hours after ingestion. Persistent iron pills were removed from the stomach by gastrotomy. No further radiopaque fragments can be visualized; however, acute lung injury is now visible.

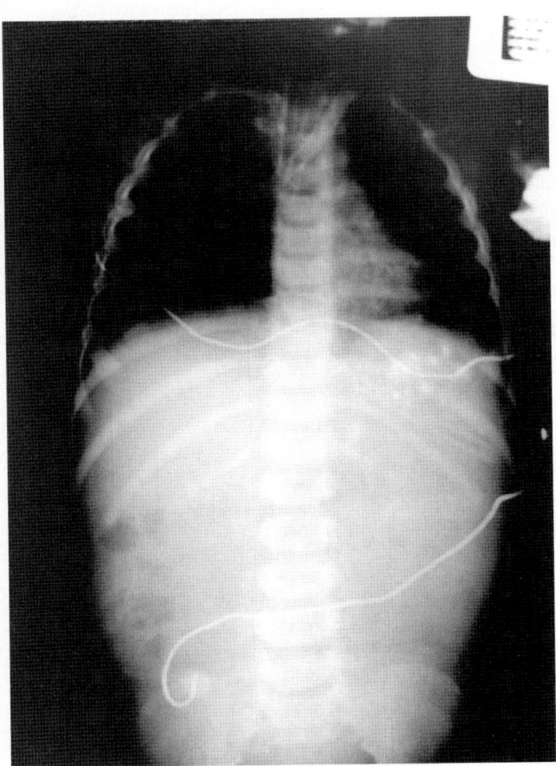

FIGURE 40–1. A 17-month-old boy presented to the hospital with lethargy and hematemesis after a large ingestion of iron supplement pills. Despite orogastric lavage and whole-bowel irrigation, iron pills and fragments can be visualized in the stomach 4 hours after ingestion.

For patients with consequential toxicity who demonstrate persistent iron in the GI tract despite orogastric lavage and WBI, upper endoscopy or gastrotomy and surgical removal of iron tablets adherent to the gastric mucosa may be necessary and lifesaving.[25,64,88]

DEFEROXAMINE

Deferoxamine has been available since the 1960s as a specific chelator for patients with acute iron overdose or chronic iron overload (eg, multiple transfusions). Deferoxamine, which is derived from culture of *Streptomyces pilosus,* has high affinity and specificity for iron. In the presence of ferric iron (Fe^{3+}), deferoxamine forms the complex ferrioxamine, which is excreted by the kidneys,[43] imparting a reddish-brown color to the urine. (See Fig. 40–3) Deferoxamine chelates free iron and the iron transported between transferrin and ferritin[50,65] but not the iron present in transferrin, hemoglobin, hemosiderin, or ferritin.[5,43] Deferoxamine may work by other mechanisms in addition to binding excess systemic iron. Because 100 mg of deferoxamine mesylate chelates approximately 8.5 mg of ferric iron, recommended or typical therapeutic dosing of deferoxamine does not produce significant excretion of chelated iron in the urine, yet it does often result in dramatic clinical benefits (see Antidotes in Depth A7: Deferoxamine). Sufficient evidence suggests that deferoxamine can reach intracytoplasmic and mitochondrial free iron, thereby limiting intracellular iron toxicity.[50]

IV administration of deferoxamine should be considered in iron-poisoned patients with any of the following findings: metabolic acidosis, repetitive vomiting, toxic appearance, lethargy, hypotension, or signs of shock. Deferoxamine administration also should be considered for any patient with an iron concentration above 500 μg/dL. In patients manifesting serious signs and symptoms of iron poisoning,

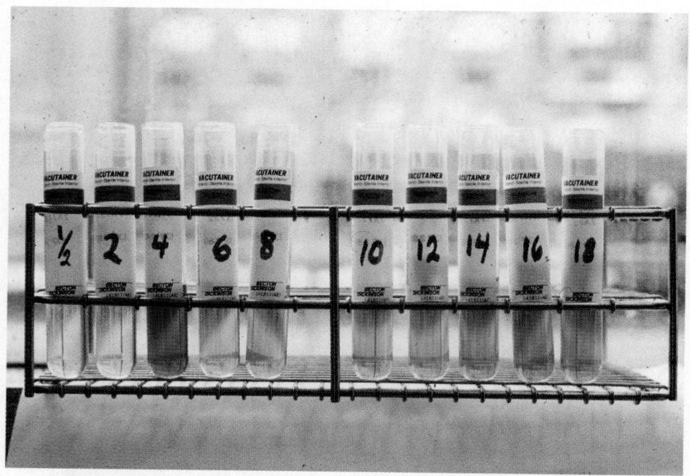

FIGURE 40–3. These timed sequential urines were obtained from a small child with a serum iron concentration of 990 μg/dL who was treated with intravenous deferoxamine. A characteristic color change is illustrated. *(Image contributed by the New York City Poison Center Toxicology Fellowship Program).*

deferoxamine should be initiated as an IV infusion, starting slowly and gradually increasing to a dose of 15 mg/kg/h. Hypotension is the rate-limiting factor as more rapid infusions are used.[37,94,96] Patients who appear toxic or have serum iron concentrations above 500 μg/dL should be treated with IV deferoxamine. Patients who have concentrations below 500 μg/dL or who do not appear toxic should be treated supportively without administration of parenteral deferoxamine (Fig. 40–4).

Clinicians have attempted to define the earliest clear end points for deferoxamine therapy because of possible deferoxamine toxicity. In one report, a urine iron-to-creatinine ratio (U_I/Cr) was used to determine if free iron excretion into the urine continued during deferoxamine therapy.[101] This ratio is a more objective measure of the presence of ferrioxamine in the urine than the less reliable and more subjective use of urinary color change.[17,46,90] This method must be further studied clinically before its use can be advocated. Most authors agree that deferoxamine therapy should be discontinued when the patient appears clinically well, the anion-gap acidosis has resolved, and urine color undergoes no further change.[54] In patients with persistent signs and symptoms of serious toxicity after 24 hours of IV deferoxamine, continuing therapy should be undertaken cautiously, if at all, and perhaps at a lower dose (see Antidotes in Depth A7: Deferoxamine).

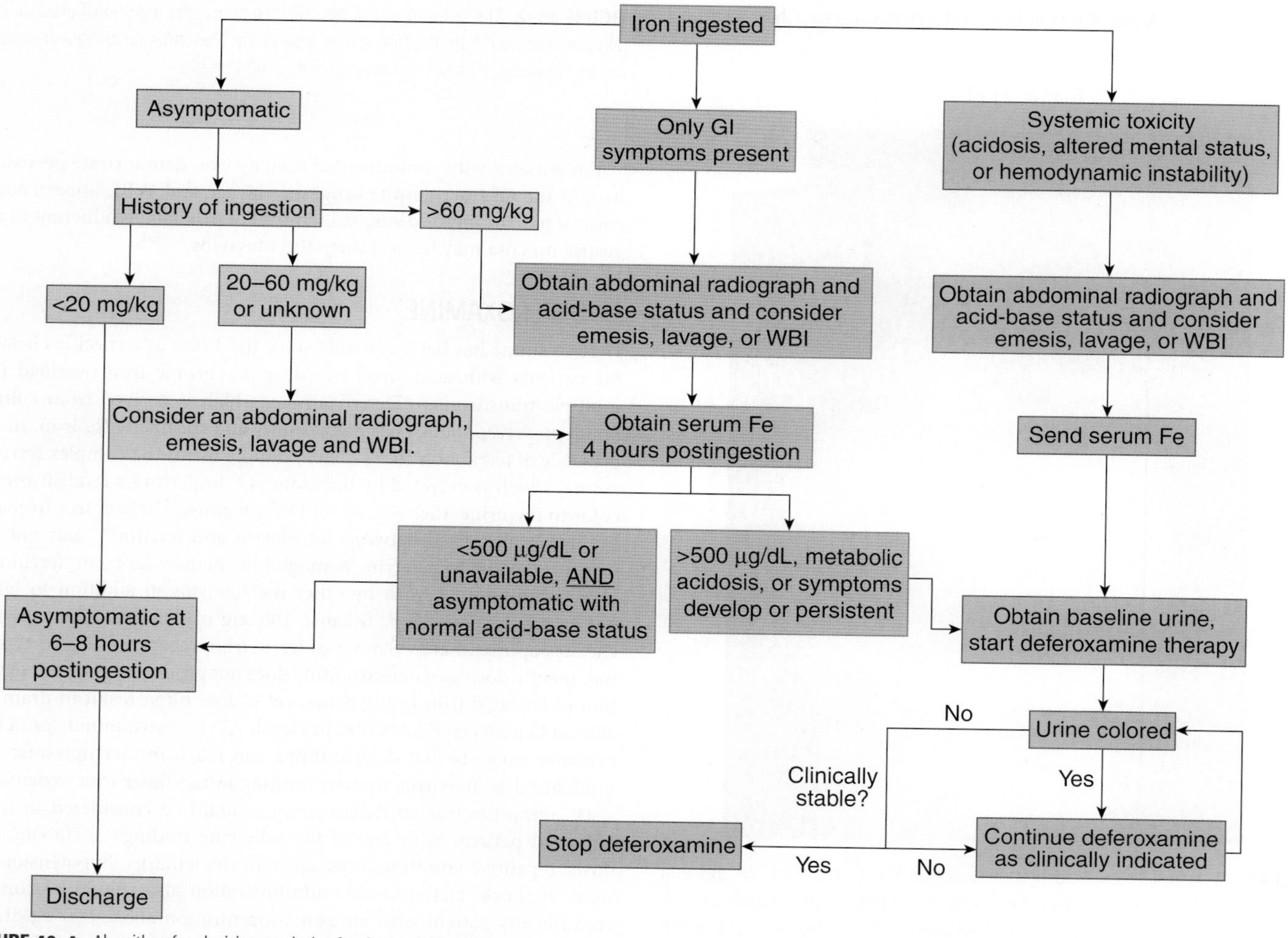

Iron ingested
Asymptomatic
Only GI symptoms present
Systemic toxicity (acidosis, altered mental status, or hemodynamic instability)
History of ingestion
>60 mg/kg
<20 mg/kg
20–60 mg/kg or unknown
Obtain abdominal radiograph and acid-base status and consider emesis, lavage, or WBI
Obtain abdominal radiograph and acid-base status and consider emesis, lavage, or WBI
Consider an abdominal radiograph, emesis, lavage and WBI.
Obtain serum Fe 4 hours postingestion
Send serum Fe
<500 μg/dL or unavailable, AND asymptomatic with normal acid-base status
>500 μg/dL, metabolic acidosis, or symptoms develop or persistent
Asymptomatic at 6–8 hours postingestion
Obtain baseline urine, start deferoxamine therapy
No
Urine colored
Clinically stable?
Yes
Stop deferoxamine
Continue deferoxamine as clinically indicated
Yes
No
Discharge

FIGURE 40–4. Algorithm for decision analysis after iron salt ingestion.

Adverse Effects of Deferoxamine Most adverse effects of deferoxamine are reported in the setting of chronic administration for treatment of hemochromatosis.[38,61,72] The same effects, such as acute lung injury and acute respiratory distress syndrome (ARDS), are also described after treatment for acute iron overdose.[82] Four patients with serum iron concentrations ranging from 430 to 620 μg/dL developed ARDS after IV administration of deferoxamine for 32 to 72 hours.[82] An animal study revealed significantly increased pulmonary toxicity when high-dose deferoxamine therapy was administered in the presence of high concentrations of oxygen (75%–80% FiO_2).[1] The authors suggested that this effect was mediated via an oxygen free radical mechanism (see Antidotes in Depth A7: Deferoxamine).

PATIENT DISPOSITION

Many patients who ingest iron do not develop significant toxic effects. Recommendations for hospital referral of toddlers who ingest iron range from those with potential exposures of 20 mg/kg[6] up to 60 mg/kg.[46] These wide ranges probably result from the interpretation of retrospective studies in possibly "exposed" toddlers for whom the actual doses were estimated. Many authors suggest that doses were overestimated in patients who subsequently did not develop toxicity (see Chap. 135). If a toddler remains asymptomatic or develops minimal or no GI manifestations after a 6-hour observation period in the emergency department (ED), discharge to an appropriate home situation can be considered. Patients who develop GI symptoms and signs of mild poisoning including vomiting and diarrhea can be observed as inpatients outside the ICU. Patients who manifest signs and symptoms of significant iron poisoning, such as metabolic acidosis, hemodynamic instability, or lethargy, should be monitored and treated in an intensive care unit. Except in the case of carbonyl iron, hospital evaluation is recommended for any child with an estimated unintentional ingestion of more than 20 mg/kg of elemental iron. Children who appear well with unintentional ingestions between 10 and 20 mg/kg elemental iron and fewer than two episodes of vomiting should be closely followed at home in consultation with the poison control center.

PREGNANT PATIENTS

The frequent diagnosis of iron-deficiency anemia during pregnancy has led to serious and even fatal iron ingestions in pregnant women.[8,44,60,67,86] In all cases of toxic exposures during pregnancy, maternal resuscitation should always be the primary objective, even if an antidote poses a real or theoretical risk to the fetus. Unproven concerns regarding possible deferoxamine toxicity to fetuses have inappropriately, and at times, disastrously delayed therapy.[60,77] These fears about fetal deferoxamine toxicity are not supported in either human or animal studies,[14,52,87] which have demonstrated that neither iron nor deferoxamine is transferred to fetuses in appreciable quantities. An animal study demonstrated that fetal serum iron concentrations were not elevated and fetal deferoxamine concentrations could not be detected in pregnant near-term ewes poisoned with iron and treated with deferoxamine. Fetal demise under these circumstances presumably results from maternal iron toxicity and not from direct iron toxicity to the fetus. Thus, deferoxamine should be used to treat serious maternal iron poisoning and should never be withheld because of unfounded concern for fetal exposure to deferoxamine.

ADJUNCTIVE THERAPIES

Another modality used experimentally for treatment of iron intoxication is continuous arteriovenous hemofiltration (CAVH). In a study of five iron-poisoned dogs, increased elimination of ferrioxamine in the ultrafiltrate was demonstrated when increasing doses of deferoxamine were infused into the arterial side of the system.[7] This technique is not described in iron-poisoned humans, in whom continuous venovenous hemofiltration (CVVH) is more commonly used. Theoretically, ferrioxamine in the blood could be dialyzable with new high-molecular-weight (large-pore) dialysis filters, but this technique has not been studied.

In toddlers with severe poisoning, exchange transfusion may help to physically remove free iron from the blood while replacing it with normal blood. Exchange transfusion in children is effective for poisonings with theophylline when the volume of drug distribution is small and removal from the blood compartment can be expected. Treatment with exchange transfusion has been suggested in iron poisoning based on early reports and recently reported in the successful treatment of an 18-month-old child with iron poisoning.[10] However, removal of blood volume must be performed cautiously because it may not be well tolerated by iron-poisoned patients with hemodynamic instability.

SUMMARY

Despite FDA-mandated warnings on iron preparations, morbidity and mortality secondary to iron exposures continue. A toddler presenting to the ED after presumed iron exposure who has evidence of GI toxicity and lethargy is at high risk for significant iron toxicity and possibly death. Although iron is available in multiple formulations (eg, prenatal vitamins, ferrous gluconate supplements), toxicity is determined by the amount of elemental iron present; signs and symptoms occur after ingestions of 20 mg/kg of elemental iron. After the patient's condition is stabilized, GI decontamination, including orogastric lavage and WBI using PEG-ELS, should be initiated when indicated because activated charcoal is ineffective in binding iron. Abdominal radiography may be helpful in determining the iron burden in the GI tract with preparations that are radiopaque. After iron is absorbed, GI symptoms of nausea, vomiting, diarrhea, hematemesis, and abdominal pain are prominent. Systemic iron toxicity leads to metabolic acidosis, hypotension, coagulopathy, and multiorgan system failure. Diagnosis and treatment of shock and acidosis, as well as chelation with deferoxamine, may be lifesaving. Education of parents, caregivers, and prescribers may decrease the incidence of serious iron ingestions in the future.

REFERENCES

1. Adamson IY, Sienko A, Tenenbein M. Pulmonary toxicity of deferoxamine in iron poisoned mice. *Toxicol Appl Pharmacol.* 1993;120:13-19.
2. Anderson BD, Turchen SG, Manoguerra AS, Clark RF. Retrospective analysis of ingestions of iron containing products in the United States: are there differences between chewable vitamins and adult preparations? *J Emerg Med.* 2000;19:255-258.
3. Artman M, Olson RD, Boerth RC. Depression of myocardial contractility in acute iron toxicity in rabbits. *Toxicol Appl Pharmacol.* 1982;66:329-337.
4. Bachrach L, Correa A, Levin R, Grossman M. Iron poisoning: complications of hypertonic phosphate lavage therapy. *J Pediatr.* 1979;94:147-149.
5. Balcerzak SP, Jensen WN, Pollack S. Mechanism of action of desferrioxamine on iron absorption. *Scand J Haematol.* 1966;3:205-212.
6. Banner W, Tong TG. Iron poisoning. *Pediatr Clin North Am.* 1986;33:393-409.
7. Banner W, Vernon DD, Ward RM, et al. Continuous arteriovenous hemofiltration in experimental iron intoxication. *Crit Care Med.* 1989;17:1187-1190.
8. Blanc P, Hryhorczuk D, Danel I. Deferoxamine treatment of acute iron intoxication in pregnancy. *Obstet Gynecol.* 1984;64:125-145.
9. Burkhart KK, Kulig KW, Hammond KB, et al. The rise in the total iron-binding capacity after iron overdose. *Ann Emerg Med.* 1991;20:532-535.

10. Carlsson M, Cortes D, Jepsen S, Kanstrup T. Severe iron intoxication treated with exchange transfusion. *Arch Dis Child.* 2008;93:321-322.
11. Chiesa C, Pacifico L, Renzulli F, et al. *Yersinia* hepatic abscesses and iron overload. *JAMA.* 1987;257:3230-3231.
12. Chyka PA, Butler AY. Assessment of acute iron poisoning by laboratory and clinical observations. *Am J Emerg Med.* 1993;11:99-102.
13. Corby DG, McCullen AH. Effect of orally administered magnesium hydroxide in experimental iron intoxication. *J Toxicol Clin Toxicol.* 1985;23:489-499.
14. Curry SC, Bond GR, Raschke R, et al. An ovine model of maternal iron poisoning in pregnancy. *Ann Emerg Med.* 1990;19:632-638.
15. Czajka PA, Konrad JD, Duffy JP. Iron poisoning: an in vitro comparison of bicarbonate and phosphate lavage solutions. *J Pediatr.* 1981;98:491-494.
16. Dean BS, Krenzelok EP. In vivo effectiveness of oral complexation agents in the management of iron poisoning. *J Toxicol Clin Toxicol.* 1987:25:221-230.
17. Eisen TF, Lacouture PG, Woolf A. Visual detection of ferrioxamine color changes in urine. *Vet Hum Toxicol.* 1988;30:369-370.
18. Everson GW, Bertaccini EJ, O'Leary JO. Use of whole-bowel irrigation in an infant following iron overdose. *Am J Emerg Med.* 1991;9:366-369.
19. Everson GW, Oudjhane K, Young LW, Krenzelok EP. Effectiveness of abdominal radiographs in visualizing chewable iron supplements following overdose. *Am J Emerg Med.* 1989;7:459-463.
20. Finch CA, Huebers H. Perspectives in iron metabolism. *N Engl J Med.* 1982;306:1520-1528.
21. Fishbane S. Safety in iron management. *Am J Kid Dis.* 2003;41(suppl 5): S18-S26.
22. Food and Drug Administration. Iron-containing supplements and drugs; label warning statements and 752 unit-dose packaging requirements; removal of regulations for unit-dose packaging 753 requirements for dietary supplements and drugs. Final rule; removal of regulatory 754 provisions in response to court order. *Fed Regist.* 2003;68:59714-59715.
23. Food and Drug Administration. Iron-containing supplements and drugs: label warning statements and unit-dose packaging requirements. *Fed Regist.* 1997;62:2217.
24. Food and Drug Administration. Preventing iron poisoning in children. FDA backgrounder—Current and useful information from the Food and Drug Administration, BG 97-1, amended 1/12/99. Available at http://www.fda.gov/opacom/backgrounders/ironbg.html; accessed December 2, 2005.
25. Foxford R, Goldfrank L. Gastrotomy: a surgical approach to iron overdose. *Ann Emerg Med.* 1985;14:1223-1226.
26. Ganote CE, Nahara G. Acute ferrous sulfate hepatotoxicity in rats. *Lab Invest.* 1973;28:426-436.
27. Geffner ME, Opas LM. Phosphate poisoning complicating treatment for iron ingestion. *Am J Dis Child.* 1980;134:509-510.
28. Gervitz NR, Wasserman LR. The measurement of iron and iron-binding capacity in plasma containing deferoxamine. *J Pediatr.* 1966;68:802-804.
29. Ghandi R, Robarts F. Hourglass stricture of the stomach and pyloric stenosis due to ferrous sulfate poisoning. *Br J Surg.* 1962;49:613-617.
30. Gleason WA, de Mello DE, de Castro FJ, et al. Acute hepatic failure in severe iron poisoning. *J Pediatr.* 1979;95:138-140.
31. Gold H, Cattell M, Hoppe JO, et al. Progress of medical science: a review of the toxicity of iron compounds. *Am J Med.* Sci 1955;230:558-571.
32. Gomez HF, McCLafferty HH, Flory D, et al. Prevention of gastrointestinal iron absorption by chelation from an orally administered premixed deferoxamine charcoal slurry. *Ann Emerg Med.* 1997;30:587-592.
33. Gordeuk VR, Brittenham GM, McLaren CE, et al. Carbonyl iron therapy for iron deficiency anemia. *Blood.* 1986;67:745-752.
34. Helfer RE, Rodgerson DO. The effect of deferoxamine on the determination of serum iron and iron-binding capacity. *J Pediatr.* 1966;68:804-806.
35. Henretig FM, Karl SR, Weintraub WH. Severe iron poisoning treated with enteral and intravenous deferoxamine. *Ann Emerg Med.* 1983;12:306-309.
36. Hosking CS. Radiology in the management of acute iron poisoning. *Med J Aust.* 1969;1:576-579.
37. Howland MA. Risks of parenteral deferoxamine for acute iron poisoning. *J Toxicol Clin Toxicol.* 1996;34:491-497.
38. Ioannides AS, Panisello JM. Acute respiratory distress syndrome in children with acute iron poisoning: the role of intravenous desferrioxamine. *Eur J Pediatr.* 2000;159:158-159.
39. Jackson TW, Ling LJ, Washington V. The effect of oral deferoxamine on iron absorption in humans. *J Toxicol Clin Toxicol.* 1995;33:325-329.
40. Jacobs J, Greene H, Gendel BR. Acute iron intoxication. *N Engl J Med.* 1965;273:1124-1127.
41. Juurlink DN, Tenenbein M, Koren G, Redelmeier DA. Iron poisoning in young children: association with the birth of a sibling. *CMAJ.* 2003;168:1539-1542.
42. Kaczorowski JM, Wax PM. Five days of whole-bowel irrigation in a case of pediatric iron ingestion. *Ann Emerg Med.* 1996:27:258-263.
43. Keberle M. The biochemistry of desferrioxamine and its relation to iron metabolism. *Ann N Y Acad Sci.* 1964;119:758-768.
44. Khoury S, Odeh M, Oettinger M. Deferoxamine treatment for acute iron intoxication in pregnancy. *Acta Obstet Gynecol Scand.* 1995:74:756-757.
45. Klein-Schwartz W. Toxicity of polysaccharide-iron complex exposures reported to poison control centers. *Ann Pharmacother.* 2000;34:165-169.
46. Klein-Schwartz W, Oderda GM, Gorman RL, et al. Assessment of management guidelines: acute iron ingestion. *Clin Pediatr.* 1990;29:316-321.
47. Knasel AL, Collins-Barrow MD. Applicability of early indicators of iron toxicity. *J Natl Med Assoc.* 1986;78:1037-1040.
48. Lacouture PG, Wason S, Temple AR, et al. Emergency assessment of severity in iron overdose by clinical and laboratory methods. *J Pediatr.* 1981;99:89-91.
49. Ling LJ, Hornfeldt CS, Winter JP. Absorption of iron after experimental overdose of chewable vitamins. *Am J Emerg Med.* 1991;9:24-26.
50. Lipschitz D, Dugard J, Simon M, et al. The site of action of desferrioxamine. *Br J Haematol.* 1971;20:395-404.
51. Luongo MA, Bjornson SS. The liver in ferrous sulfate poisoning: a report of three fatal cases in children and an experimental study. *N Engl J Med.* 1954;251:996-999.
52. McElhatton PR, Roberts JC, Sullivan FM. The consequences of iron overdose and its treatment with desferrioxamine in pregnancy. *Hum Exp Toxicol.* 1991;10:251-259.
53. Melby K, Slordahl S, Gutterberg T, et al. Septicemia due to *Yersinia enterocolitica* after oral overdoses of iron. *Br Med J* (Clin Res Ed). 1982;285:467-468.
54. Mills KC, Curry SC. Acute iron poisoning. *Emerg Med Clin North Am.* 1994;12:397-413.
55. Mofenson HC, Caraccio TR, Sharieff N. Iron sepsis: *Yersinia enterocolitica* septicemia possibly caused by an overdose of iron. *N Engl J Med.* 1987;316:1092-1093.
56. Morris CC. Pediatric iron poisonings in the United States. *South Med J.* 2000;93;352-358.
57. Morse SB, Hardwick WE, King WD. Fatal iron intoxication in an infant. *South Med J.* 1997;90:1043-1047.
58. Ng RCW, Perry K, Martin DJ. Iron poisoning: assessment of radiography in diagnosis and management. *Clin Pediatr.* 1979;18:614-616.
59. Nordt SP, Williams SR, Behling C, et al. Comparison of the toxicities of two iron formulations in a swine model. *Acad Emerg Med.* 1999;6:1104-1108.
60. Olenmark M, Biber B, Dottori O, Rybo G. Fatal iron intoxication in late pregnancy. *J Toxicol Clin Toxicol.* 1987;25:347-359.
61. Olivieri NF, Buncic JR, Chew E, et al. Visual and auditory neurotoxicity in patients receiving subcutaneous deferoxamine infusions. *N Engl J Med.* 1986;314:869-873.
62. Palatnick W, Tenenbein M. Leukocytosis, hyperglycemia, vomiting, and positive x-rays are not indicators of severity of iron overdose in adults. *Am J Emerg Med.* 1996;14:454-455.
63. Pestaner JP, Ishak KG, Mullick FG, Centeno JA. Ferrous sulfate toxicity: a review of autopsy findings. *Biol Trace Elem Res.* 1999;69:191-198.
64. Peterson CD, Fifield GC. Emergency gastrotomy for acute iron poisoning. *Ann Emerg Med.* 1980:9:262-264.
65. Propper R, Nathan D. Clinical removal of iron. *Ann Rev Med.* 1982;33:509-519.
66. Proudfoot AT, Simpson D, Dyson EH. Management of acute iron poisoning. *Med Toxicol.* 1986;1:83-100.
67. Rayburn WF, Donn SM, Wolf ME. Iron overdose during pregnancy: successful therapy with deferoxamine. *Am J Obstet Gynecol.* 1983;147:717-718.
68. Reissman KR, Coleman TJ. Acute intestinal iron intoxication. II: metabolic, respiratory and circulatory effects of absorbed iron salts. *Blood.* 1955;10:46-51.
69. Roberts RJ, Nayfield S, Soper R, et al. Acute iron intoxication with intestinal infarction managed in part by small bowel resection. *Clin Toxicol.* 1975;8:3-12.
70. Robotham JL, Troxler RF, Lietman PS. Iron poisoning: another energy crisis. *Lancet.* 1974;2:664-665.

71. Rosenmund A, Haeberli A, Struab PW. Blood coagulation and acute iron toxicity. *J Lab Clin Med.* 1984:103:524-533.
72. Scanderbeg AC, Izzi GC, Butturini A, Benaglia G. Pulmonary syndrome and intravenous high-dose desferrioxamine. *Lancet.* 1990;336:1511.
73. Snyder BK, Clark RF. Effect of magnesium hydroxide administration on iron absorption after a supratherapeutic dose of ferrous sulfate in human volunteers: a randomized controlled trial. *Ann Emerg Med.* 1999;33:400-405.
74. Spiller HA, Wahlen HS, Stephens TL, et al. Multi-center retrospective evaluation of carbonyl iron ingestions. *Vet Hum Toxicol.* 2002;44:28-29.
75. Staple TW, McAlister WH. Roentgenographic visualization of iron preparations in the gastrointestinal tract. *Radiology.* 1964;83:1051-1056.
76. Stein ZL, Barkin RL. Yersiniae and iron intoxication. *Drug Intell Clin Pharm.* 1987:21:661.
77. Strom RL, Schiller P, Seeds AE, ten Bensel R. Fatal iron poisoning in a pregnant female. *Minn Med.* 1976;59:483-489.
78. Tenenbein M. Toxicokinetics and toxicodynamics of iron poisoning. *Toxicol Lett.* 1998;102-103:653-656.
79. Tenenbein M. Unit dose packaging of iron supplements and reduction of iron poisoning in young children. *Arch Pediatr Adolesc Med.* 2005:159:593-595.
80. Tenenbein M. Whole-bowel irrigation in iron poisoning. *J Pediatr.* 1987;111:142-145.
81. Tenenbein M, Israels SJ. Early coagulopathy in severe iron poisoning. *J Pediatr.* 1988;113:695-697.
82. Tenenbein M, Kowalski S, Bowden DH, Adamson IYR. Pulmonary toxic effects of continuous desferrioxamine administration in acute iron poisoning. *Lancet.* 1992;339:699-701.
83. Tenenbein M, Littman C, Stimpson RE. Gastrointestinal pathology in adult iron overdose. *J Toxicol Clin Toxicol.* 1990;28:311-320.
84. Tenenbein M, Yatscoff RW. The total iron-binding capacity in iron poisoning. Is it useful? *Am J Dis Child.* 1991;45:437-439.
85. Thomson J. Ferrous sulphate poisoning: its incidence, symptomatology, treatment and prevention. *Br Med J.* 1950;1:645-646.
86. Tran T, Wax JR, Steinfeld JD, Ingardia CJ. Acute intentional iron overdose in pregnancy. *Obstet Gynecol.* 1998;92:678-680.
87. Turk J, Aks S, Ampuero F, Hryhorczuk DO. Successful therapy of iron intoxication in pregnancy with intravenous deferoxamine and whole-bowel irrigation. *Vet Hum Toxicol.* 1993;35:441-444.
88. Venturelli J, Kwee Y, Morris N, et al. Gastrotomy in the management of acute iron poisoning. *J Pediatr.* 1982;100:768-769.
89. Vernon DD, Banner W Jr, Dean JM. Hemodynamic effects of experimental iron poisoning. *Ann Emerg Med.* 1989;18:863-866.
90. Villalobos D. Reliability of urine-color changes after deferoxamine challenge [abstract]. *Vet Hum Toxicol.* 1992;34:330.
91. Wallace K, Curry SC, LoVecchio F, Raschke RA. Effect of magnesium hydroxide on iron absorption following simulated mild iron overdose in human subjects. *Acad Emerg Med.* 1998;5:961-965.
92. Weiss B, Alkon E, Weindlar F, et al. Toddler deaths resulting from ingestion of iron supplements—Los Angeles, 1992-1993. *MMWR Morb Mortal Wkly Rep.* 1993;42:111-113.
93. Westlin WF. Deferoxamine as a chelating agent. *Clin Toxicol.* 1971;4:597-602.
94. Westlin W. Deferoxamine in the treatment of acute iron poisoning: clinical experiences with 172 children. *Clin Pediatr.* 1966;5:531-535.
95. Whittaker P, Ali SF, Imam SZ, Dunkel VC. Acute toxicity of carbonyl iron and sodium iron EDTA compared with ferrous sulfate in young rats. *Regul Toxicol Pharmacol.* 2002;36:280-286.
96. Whitten CF, Gibson GW, Good MH, et al. Studies in acute iron poisoning. I. Desferrioxamine in the treatment of acute iron poisoning: clinical observations, experimental studies, and theoretical considerations. *Pediatrics.* 1965;36:322-335.
97. Whitten CF, Chen YC, Gibson GW. Studies in acute iron poisoning: II. Further observations on desferrioxamine in the treatment of acute experimental iron poisoning. *Pediatrics.* 1966;38:102-110.
98. Whitten CF, Chen YC, Gibson GW. Studies in acute iron poisoning III. The hemodynamic alterations in acute experimental iron poisoning. *Pediatr Res.* 1968:2:479-485.
99. Witzleben CL, Chaffey NJ. Acute ferrous sulphate poisoning: a histochemical study of its effect on the liver. *Arch Pathol Lab Med.* 1966;82:454-460.
100. Wu ML, Yang CC, Ger J, Deng JF. A fatal case of acute ferric chloride poisoning. *Vet Hum Toxicol.* 1998;40:31-34.
101. Yatscoff RW, Wayne EA, Tenenbein M. An objective criterion for the cessation of deferoxamine therapy in the acutely iron poisoned patient. *J Toxicol Clin Toxicol.* 1991;29:1-10.
102. Yonker J, Banner W, Picchioni A. Absorption characteristics of iron and deferoxamine onto charcoal. *Vet Hum Toxicol.* 1980;22(suppl):75.

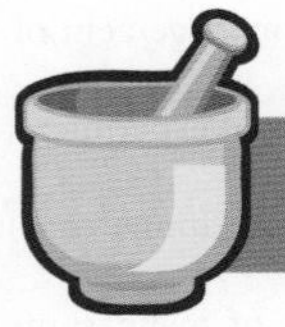

ANTIDOTES IN DEPTH (A7)

DEFEROXAMINE

Mary Ann Howland

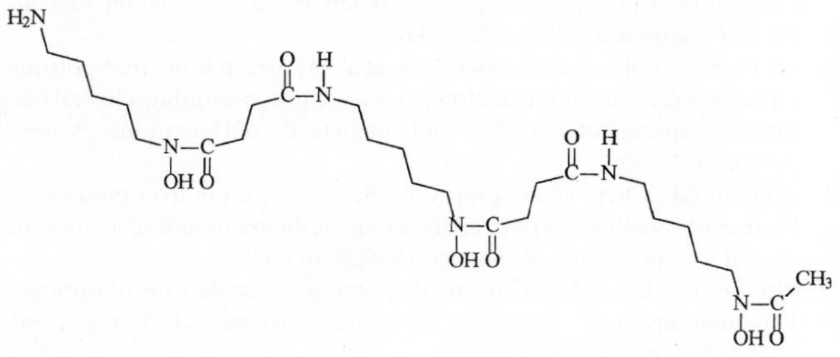

Deferoxamine (DFO) is the parenteral chelator of choice for treatment of acute iron poisoning. Considering that DFO has been used to treat patients with acute iron overdose for a little over 40 years,[30] there is still much that is unknown. No controlled studies have evaluated the efficacy or dosing of DFO. Animal studies and case series from the 1960s and 1970s form the basis for how we use DFO. This information has been supplemented since then by limited case reports and clinical experience. DFO is also used for chelation of aluminum in patients with chronic renal failure. The merits of DFO as a treatment strategy for acute iron overdose is discussed in Chapter 40 and for aluminum toxicity in Chapter 86.

HISTORY AND CHEMISTRY

The development of DFO (or desferrioxamine B) resulted from an analysis of the iron containing metabolites of a species of actinomycetes. DFO is the colorless compound that results when the trivalent iron is chemically removed from ferrioxamine B (Fig. A7–1).[35] Ferrioxamine is a brownish-red compound containing trivalent iron (ferric, Fe^{3+}) and three molecules of trihydroxamic acid isolated from the organism *Streptomyces pilosus*.[35]

DFO is a water-soluble hexadentate chelator with a molecular weight of 561 daltons. The commercial formulation is the mesylate salt with a molecular weight of 657 daltons. One mole of DFO binds 1 mole of Fe^{3+}; therefore, 100 mg DFO as the mesylate salt theoretically can bind 8.5 mg Fe^{3+}.

DFO has a much greater affinity constant for iron (10^{31}) and aluminum (10^{22}) than for zinc, copper, nickel, magnesium, or calcium (10^{2}–10^{14}).[35] Thus, at physiologic pH, DFO complexes almost exclusively with ferric iron.[26,75]

MECHANISM OF ACTION

DFO binds Fe^{3+} at the 3 N–OH sites, forming an octahedral iron complex (see Fig. A7–1). Once bound, the resultant ferrioxamine is very stable. DFO appears to benefit iron-poisoned patients by chelating free iron (nontransferrin plasma iron) and iron in transit between transferrin and ferritin (labile chelatable iron pool)[29,41,58] while not directly affecting the iron of hemoglobin, hemosiderin, or ferritin.[35] Although in vitro studies suggest that DFO removes iron from ferritin and transferrin with only very little from hemosiderin,[46] in vivo experiments demonstrate that DFO cannot remove iron after the iron is bound to transferrin.[4] DFO does bind "free iron" found in the plasma as nontransferrin plasma iron after transferrin saturation, which only occurs acutely after overdose or chronically in iron overload syndromes.[29] In vitro studies demonstrate that DFO chelates and inactivates cytoplasmic, lysosomal, and probably mitochondrial iron, preventing disruption of mitochondrial function and injury.[25,41] An in vitro study suggests that DFO gains access to cytosol and endosomes through endocytosis rather than passive diffusion.[25] In chronic iron overload, DFO chelates iron deposited in the reticuloendothelial cells found in the spleen, liver, and bone marrow and excretes iron in the urine as ferrioxamine.[29] Whether DFO actually chelates the iron within the reticuloendothelial cells or after liberation into the plasma is unclear. In vitro studies demonstrate that the liver can donate iron to DFO, and thus chelation subsequently may also lead to biliary iron excretion and fecal elimination.[29,45]

PHARMACOKINETICS

The volume of distribution of DFO ranges from 0.6 to 1.33 L/kg.[35,38,53] The initial distribution half-life of DFO is 5 to 10 minutes.[37,63] The terminal elimination half-life of DFO is approximately 6 hours in healthy patients[2] but approximately 3 hours in patients with thalassemia. DFO is metabolized in the plasma to several metabolites (A–F), of which metabolite B is believed to be toxic.[35,38,53,55] Unchanged DFO undergoes glomerular filtration and tubular secretion.[45]

In comparison, ferrioxamine has a smaller volume of distribution than DFO. In nephrectomized dogs, the volume of distribution of ferrioxamine was calculated to be 19% of body weight compared with 50% of body weight for DFO.[35] This finding implies that DFO has a more extensive tissue distribution. The different pharmacokinetic patterns may be related to the potential for facilitated penetrance of the straight-chain molecule DFO compared with that of the octahedral ferrioxamine.[55] Experiments in dogs with normal renal function demonstrate that intravenous (IV) ferrioxamine is entirely eliminated by the kidney within 5 hours[33] via glomerular filtration and partial reabsorption.[45]

The pharmacokinetics of DFO and ferrioxamine differ in healthy versus iron-overloaded patients. Whereas plasma DFO concentrations in healthy patients are approximately twice the concentrations noted in patients with thalassemia major, ferrioxamine concentrations are five times greater in patients with thalassemia major compared with healthy patients.[35,65]

Some investigators suggest that DFO can be administered during hemodialysis to remove ferrioxamine.[76] Hemodialysis,[14,63] particularly high-flux hemodialysis [70] and hemoperfusion,[14] are effective in ferrioxamine removal and are indicated in patients with renal failure.

ANIMAL STUDIES

Guinea pigs given oral lethal doses of ferrous sulfate and oral DFO in a dose calculated to bind most of the iron showed dramatically improved survival rates.[46] Mortality rates in this study and in a swine study[18] directly correlated with the delay to DFO administration.[46]

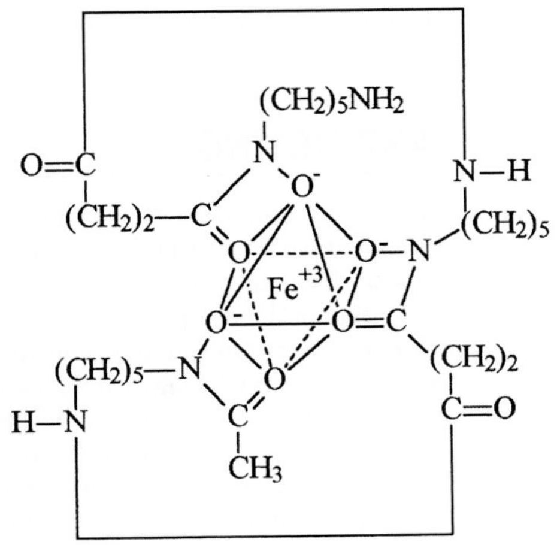

FIGURE A7–1. Ferrioxamine.

In two canine studies, dogs that received the iron–DFO complex orally had a 40% to 100% mortality.[75,76] When both oral and IV DFO were administered, the mortality rate was 67%.[74] A similar follow-up study demonstrated a 50% mortality rate in dogs given a lethal dose (225 mg/kg) of iron, followed by oral DFO (2.6 g) and IV DFO (0.75–1.5 mg/kg/min for 8–12 hours).[76] These studies discouraged further investigation in the use of oral DFO despite the more favorable results in other animal models.[5,31,46,69]

EARLY HUMAN USE AND HISTORY OF DOSING RECOMMENDATIONS

In one of the earliest case series, 172 hemodynamically stable children who were not severely poisoned were treated with 5 to 10 g oral DFO and either 1 or 2 g intramuscular (IM) DFO every 3 to 12 hours.[74] Patients who were in shock or severely ill received 1 g of DFO IV at a maximum of 15 mg/kg/h every 4 to 12 hours for 2 to 3 days as necessary. Of the 28 patients who developed coma, shock, or both, only three died. One of the three patients who died had received late treatment with DFO.

This case series was expanded to 472 patients, and guidelines for DFO dosing were formulated as a result of this clinical experience.[73] The recommended initial dose of DFO was suggested as 1 g IM followed by 0.5 g at 4 and 8 hours later and then every 4 to 12 hours as necessary, not to exceed 6 g in 24 hours. For patients in shock, DFO was recommended at an initial dose not to exceed 1 g IV and a rate not to exceed 15 mg/kg/h followed 4 and 8 hours later by two 0.5-g doses for a total dosage not to exceed 6 g in 24 hours. These recommendations for total dosages were not scientifically developed and appear to be based on arbitrary assumptions. However, the manufacturer continues to recommend these doses.[19]

URINARY COLOR CHANGE

To further define the role of DFO and the quantitative excretion of urinary iron, investigators studied urinary samples.[46] Several reviews of patients with acute iron poisoning who had received DFO[43,78] investigated the correlation between urinary iron concentrations and systemic toxicity. Most data suggest that the absence of a urine color change, often referred to as a *vin rose* color, after DFO administration indicates very little renal excretion of ferrioxamine.[24] However, unless a baseline urine color is obtained before DFO administration, post-DFO administration comparisons of urine color are unreliable. No relationship between urinary iron excretion, clinical iron toxicity, and the effectiveness of DFO has been established.

INTRAMUSCULAR VERSUS INTRAVENOUS ADMINISTRATION

Before 1976, IM DFO was the preferred route of administration, and IV DFO was reserved for patients in shock. However, when transfusion-induced iron overload was studied and IM and IV DFO administration were compared, IV DFO significantly enhanced urinary iron elimination.[59] This study provided compelling arguments against IM dosing, as did data showing higher peak and more stable DFO concentrations with IV infusions. A single patient was given 425 mg/kg IV over 24 hours without incident, although the increase in urinary iron excretion seen when the DFO dose increased from 4 to 16 g/d appeared to be of limited consequence.

DURATION OF DOSING

The optimum duration of DFO administration is unknown. In canine models, serum iron concentrations peak within 3 to 5 hours and then decrease quickly as iron is transported out of the blood into the tissues.[71,77] In one human study, initial iron concentrations of approximately 500 μg/dL decreased to approximately 100 μg/dL within 12 hours.[39] Other case reports also suggest that most of the easily accessible iron is distributed out of the blood compartment by 24 hours.[20] Although severely poisoned patients have received DFO for more than 24 hours, pulmonary toxicity is associated with prolonged DFO infusions.[28,51,67] Intuitively, in patients with acute iron overdose, DFO should be administered early and for a shorter duration while the iron is easily accessible in the blood. In patients with chronic iron overload, prolonged infusions of smaller DFO doses are necessary to act as a sink and to slowly remove iron from the limited labile pool and tissue stores.[32]

ADVERSE EFFECTS

DFO administration to patients with acute iron overdose is associated with rate-related hypotension, hypersensitivity reactions and systemic allergic reactions, pulmonary toxicity, and infection. DFO administration to patients with chronic iron overload is associated with auditory, ocular, and pulmonary toxicity and infection.[9,32]

Significant hypotension was first noted in 1965 in two children who were administered approximately 80 to 150 mg/kg DFO IV over 15 minutes.[75] The mechanism for rate-related hypotension is not fully understood, although histamine release is at least partially implicated. Although elevated histamine concentrations were documented in a canine experiment, pretreatment with diphenhydramine was not protective.[76] Intravascular volume depletion caused by iron toxicity also contributes to hypotension. No experiment has determined the maximum safe rate of DFO administration. Adverse effects of DFO, including tachycardia, hypotension, shock, were reported with rapid infusion.[74] These complications resulted in the current recommendations for less rapid IV infusions of DFO not to exceed 15 mg/kg/h.[74-76] Currently suggested IV infusion rates are somewhat empirical because of the lack of robust evidence. Higher rates were administered successfully in critically ill patients when time was of the essence.[11,15,20]

Acute lung injury (ALI) occurs in patients with acute iron overdoses who have received IV administration of DFO (15 mg/kg/h) therapy for more than 24 hours.[3,34,67] Usually, iron concentrations are normal in these patients within 24 hours, and the rationale for continued administration of DFO was not reported. Examination of the nontoxicologic literature reveals other instances of ALI occurring in patients receiving continuous IV DFO for hemosiderosis and malignancies.[13,23,72] Administration of continuous IV doses of DFO for prolonged (>24 hours) periods was common to all of these patients. The mechanism for development of pulmonary toxicity after DFO is unknown. Pulmonary toxicity may result from excessive DFO chelation of intracellular iron and depletion of catalase, resulting in oxidant damage[27] or generation of free radicals.[1]

DFO therapy may lead to infection with a number of unusual organisms, including *Yersinia enterocolitica*, *Zygomycetes spp*, and *Aeromonas hydrophilia*. The virulence of these organisms is facilitated when the DFO–iron complex acts as a siderophore for their growth.[40,44,47] Most cases of septicemia occurred when DFO was used for treatment of aluminum toxicity in patients receiving chronic hemodialysis.[45] Several cases of *Yersinia* sepsis were reported after acute iron overdose and treatment with DFO.[44,47]

Ocular toxicity characterized by decreased visual acuity, night blindness, color blindness, and retinal pigmentary abnormalities has occurred in patients who received continuous IV DFO for thalassemia and other nonacute iron and aluminum excess conditions.[8,12,17,50,52] Ototoxicity documented by abnormal audiograms indicating partial or total deafness has been reported.[55,56] However, neither ocular toxicity nor ototoxicity has been reported in the setting of acute overdose treatment.

USE IN PREGNANCY

A review of the literature identified 61 cases of intentional iron overdose in pregnant women.[68] Serious iron toxicity with organ involvement was associated with spontaneous abortion, preterm delivery, and maternal death. There is no evidence to indicate that DFO is teratogenic.[68] Neither iron nor DFO appears to cross the ovine placenta.[16] A case report of a pregnant woman with thalassemia and a review of 40 other pregnant patients with thalassemia treated extensively with DFO found no evidence of teratogenicity.[62] Thus, DFO should be administered to pregnant women with acute iron overdose for the same indications as for nonpregnant women and is listed by the Food and Drug Administration (FDA) in pregnancy Category C.

USE IN ALUMINUM TOXICITY

Patients with renal insufficiency are at high risk for aluminum toxicity.[79] Acute aluminum toxicity resulting from bladder irrigations with alum for hemorrhagic cystitis is also reported.[54] Chronic aluminum toxicity is reported from administration of aluminum salts as phosphate binders or from hemodialysis with a water source containing aluminum. DFO binds aluminum to form aluminoxamine, analogous to iron and ferrioxamine. The chelate is a 1:1 octahedral complex with aluminum.[79] Aluminoxamine is excreted renally. In patients with renal insufficiency, hemodialysis (especially with a high-flux membrane) is effective in removing the aluminoxamine and should be used to prevent aluminum redistribution to the CNS and other tissues.[48] The dosing of DFO is unclear but should be tailored to the patient's serum aluminum concentrations, symptomatology, and response.[48] Electroencephalography (EEG) monitoring is recommended. DFO doses of 5 to 15 mg/kg/day, infused over several hours and 6 to 8 hours before a 3- to 4-hour run of high-flux hemodialysis, have been successful and maximize aluminoxamine removal without exacerbating side efects.[48,61] The appropriate duration of this DFO dosing with hemodialysis is unknown and should be based on CNS symptoms, serum aluminum concentrations, and renal function. The correlation of serum aluminum concentrations with toxicity is poorly defined and may depend on the chronicity of aluminum exposure. Patients are treated for days to weeks, with one holiday per week (see Chap. 86).

INDICATIONS AND DOSING

The indications and dosage schedules for DFO administration are largely empirical.[6,60] Systemic toxicity associated with acute iron poisoning manifested by coma, shock, or metabolic acidosis warrants IV infusion of DFO. The duration of therapy probably should be limited to 24 hours to maximize effectiveness while minimizing the risk of pulmonary toxicity. Some investigators have suggested that more than the recommended dose of 15 mg/kg/h be infused during the first 24 hours for life-threatening iron toxicity, but this recommendation remains to be validated experimentally.[32] We recommend starting with 5 mg/kg/h and increasing over 15 minutes if tolerated to 15 mg/kg/h to minimize the risk of hypotension. In adults, after the first 1000 mg is infused, the subsequent doses can be adjusted to infuse the remainder of the 6 to 8 g over the next 23 hours. In a 70-kg patient, this would be about 3 to 4 mg/kg/h for the next 23 hours. Although patients with mild toxicity can be treated with IM injections of 90 mg/kg of DFO (maximum of 1 g in children or 2 g in adults), this volume of antidote cannot be given IM with ease or painlessly in children. Therefore, few clinicians administer IM DFO, and most prefer the IV route (see Chap. 40). The total daily parenteral dose is limited by the infusion rate in children (if the manufacturer's recommendations are followed). Conservative recommendations in adults limit the dose to 6 to 8 g/day, although doses as high as 16 g/day with diverse dosing regimens have been administered without incident.[15,20,42,5159,66]

AVAILABILITY

DFO mesylate (Desferal) is available in vials containing 500 mg or 2 g of sterile, lyophilized powder. Adding 5 or 20 mL of sterile water for injection to either the 500-mg or the 2-g vial, respectively, results in an approximately 100 mg/mL solution. The drug must be completely dissolved before using. The resulting solution is isotonic, clear, and colorless to slightly yellowish[19] and can be diluted further with 0.9% NaCl solution, glucose in water, or Ringer lactate solution for IV administration. For IM administration, a smaller volume of solution is preferred. Adding 2 or 8 mL of sterile water for injection to the 500-mg or 2-g vial, respectively, results in a stronger yellow-colored solution containing approximately 200 mg/mL.

ADDITIONAL IRON CHELATORS

New iron chelators are being investigated. Pyridoxal isonicotinylhydrase and pyridoxal benzoylhydrazone are potent lipophilic chelators. Lipophilicity increases iron mobilization but may also increase toxicity. Deferiprone is a bidentate oral iron chelator. Three moles of deferiprone are required to bind 1 mole of ferric ion to form a stable complex.[29] Inappropriate ratios of drug to iron may be ineffective or even harmful because of the formation of potentially toxic intermediates.[29] Preliminary animal studies of acute toxicity are contradictory.[10,22,33,36] The effectiveness and long-term safety of deferiprone for chronic iron overload associated with thalassemia major have been questioned.[7,37,49] More recently, deferasirox, an oral iron chelator, has been FDA approved to treat chronic iron overload caused by blood transfusions. Deferasirox, a tridentate ligand, is an iron chelator that binds ferric iron in a 2:1 ratio. The soluble iron complexes are predominantly eliminated in the feces. Preliminary short-term studies demonstrate a comparable efficacy and side effect profile to DFO in patients with chronic iron overload. There have been no studies evaluating the use of deferasirox in acute iron overdose. Similar to other oral chelators, concerns exist about increasing oral absorption of the deferasirox iron complex and the toxicity of this complex in the setting of an acute iron overdose.[21,57,64]

SUMMARY

DFO is the parenteral chelator of choice for treatment of iron poisoning. Although DFO has been used to treat acute iron overdose for many years,[30] no controlled studies have evaluated its efficacy or dosing. Much of our knowledge derives from animal studies and case series in the 1960s and early 1970s and from limited case reports throughout the ensuing years. DFO is also used for chelation of aluminum in patients with chronic renal failure.

REFERENCES

1. Adamson I, Sienko A, Tenenbein M. Pulmonary toxicity of deferoxamine in iron-poisoned mice. *Toxicol Appl Pharmacol.* 1993;120:13-19.
2. Allain P, Mauras Y, Chaleil D, et al. Pharmacokinetics and renal elimination of desferrioxamine and ferrioxamine in healthy subjects and patients with hemochromatosis. *Br J Clin Pharmacol.* 1987;24:207-212.
3. Anderson KJ, Rivers PRA. Desferrioxamine in acute iron poisoning. *Lancet.* 1992;339:1602.
4. Balcerzak SP, Jensen WN, Pollack S. Mechanism of action of desferrioxamine on iron absorption. *Scand J Haematol.* 1966;3:205-212.
5. Banner W. Of iron and ancient mariners. *Ann Emerg Med.* 1997;30:687-688.
6. Banner W, Tong T. Iron poisoning. *Pediatr Clin North Am.* 1986;33:393-409.
7. Barman Balfour JA, Foster RH. Deferiprone. A review of its clinical potential in iron overload in beta-thalassaemia major and other trans-fusion-dependent diseases. *Drugs.* 1999;58:553-578.
8. Bene C, Manzler A, Bene D, et al. Irreversible ocular toxicity from a single "challenge" dose of deferoxamine. *Clin Nephron.* 1989;31:45-48.
9. Bentur Y, McGuigan M, Koren G. Deferoxamine (desferrioxamine), new toxicities for an old drug. *Drug Saf.* 1991;6:37-46.
10. Berkovitch M, Livne A, Lushkov G, et al. The efficacy of oral deferiprone in acute iron poisoning. *Am J Emerg Med.* 2000;18:36-40.
11. Berland Y, Charhon SA, Olmer M, et al. Predictive value of desferrioxamine infusion test for bone aluminum deposit in hemodialyzed patients. *Nephron.* 1985;40:433-435.
12. Blake D, Winyard P, Lunec J, et al. Cerebral and ocular toxicity induced by desferrioxamine. *Q J Med.* 1985;219:345-355.
13. Castriota Scanderberg A, Izzi G, Butturini A, Benaglia G. Pulmonary syndrome and intravenous high-dose desferrioxamine. *Lancet.* 1990;336:1511.
14. Chang TMS, Barne P. Effect of desferrioxamine on removal of aluminum and iron by coated charcoal hemoperfusion and hemodialysis. *Lancet.* 1983;2:1051-1053.
15. Cheney K, Gumbiner C, Benson B, et al. Survival after a severe iron poisoning treated with intermittent infusions of deferoxamine. *J Toxicol Clin Toxicol.* 1995;33:61-66.
16. Curry SC, Bond GR, Raschke R, et al. An ovine model of maternal iron poisoning in pregnancy. *Ann Emerg Med.* 1990;19:632-638.
17. Davies S, Hungerford J, Arden G, et al. Ocular toxicity of high-dose intravenous desferrioxamine. *Lancet.* 1983;2:181-184.
18. Dean B, Oehme FW, Krenzelok E, Hines R. A study of iron complexation in a swine model. *Vet Hum Toxicol.* 1988;30:313-315.
19. Desferal [prescribing information]. East Hanover, NJ: Novartis; 2007.
20. Douglas D, Smilkstein M. Deferoxamine-iron induced pulmonary injury and N-acetylcysteine. *J Toxicol Clin Toxicol.* 1995;33:495.
21. Exjade [prescribing information]. East Hanover, NJ: Novartis Pharmaceuticals Corporation; 2008.
22. Fassos FF, Berkovitch M, Daneman N, et al. Efficacy of deferiprone in the treatment of acute iron intoxication in rats. *J Toxicol Clin Toxicol.* 1996;34:279-287.
23. Freedman M, Grisaru D, Oliveri NF, et al. Pulmonary syndrome in patients with thalassemia major receiving intravenous deferoxamine infusions. *Am J Dis Child.* 1990;144:565-569.
24. Freeman DA, Manoguerra AS. Absence of urinary color change in severely iron poisoned child treated with deferoxamine [abstract]. *Vet Hum Toxicol.* 1981;23(suppl 1):49.
25. Glickstein H, El R, Shvartsman M, Cabantchik Z. Intracellular labile iron pools as direct targets of iron chelators. a fluorescence study of chelator action in living cells. *Blood.* 2005;106:3242-3250.
26. Goodwin JF, Whitten CF. Chelation of ferrous sulfate solution by deferoxamine B. *Nature.* 1965;205:281-283.
27. Helson L, Helson C, Braverman S, et al. Desferrioxamine in acute iron poisoning. *Lancet.* 1992;339:1602-1603.
28. Henretig F, Karl S, Weintraub W. Severe iron poisoning treated with enteral and intravenous deferoxamine. *Ann Emerg Med.* 1983;12:306-309.
29. Hershko C, Link G, Cabantchik I. Pathophysiology of iron overload. *Ann N Y Acad Sci.* 1998;850:191-201.
30. Hoppe JO, Marcell GMA, Tainter ML. A review of the toxicity of iron compounds. *Am J Med Sci.* 1955;230:558-571.
31. Hoskin CS. A pharmacologic investigation of acute iron poisoning and its treatment. *Aust Paediatr J.* 1970;6:92-96.
32. Howland MA. Risks of parenteral deferoxamine. *J Toxicol Clin Toxicol.* 1996;34:491-497.
33. Hung O, Manoach S, Howland MA, et al. Deferiprone for acute iron poisoning [abstract]. *J Toxicol Clin Toxicol.* 1997;35:565.
34. Ioannides AS, Panisello JM. Acute respiratory distress syndrome in children with acute iron poisoning. The role of intravenous desferrioxamine. *Eur J Pediatr.* 2000;159:158-159.
35. Keberle M. The biochemistry of desferrioxamine and its relation to iron metabolism. *Ann N Y Acad Sci.* 1964;119:758-768.
36. Kontoghiorgher GJ. New concepts of iron and aluminum chelation therapy with oral L1 (deferiprone) and other chelators. *Analyst.* 1995;120:845-851.
37. Kowdley K, Kaplan M. Iron chelation therapy with oral deferiprone—toxicity or lack of efficacy. *N Engl J Med.* 1998;339:468-469.
38. Lee P, Mohammed N, Marshal L, et al. Intravenous infusion pharmacokinetics of desferrioxamine in thalassemic patients. *Drug Metab Dispos.* 1993;21:640-644.
39. Leikin S, Vossough P, Mochiv-Fatemi F. Chelation therapy in acute iron poisoning. *J Pediatr.* 1969;71:425-430.
40. Lin S, Shieh S, Lin Y, et al. Fatal Aeromonas hydrophilia bacteremia in a hemodialysis patient treated with deferoxamine. *Am J Kidney Dis.* 1996;27:733-735.
41. Lipschitz D, Dugard J, Simon M, et al. The site of action of desferrioxamine. *Br J Haematol.* 1971;20:395-404.
42. Lovejoy F. Chelation therapy in iron poisoning. *J Toxicol Clin Toxicol.* 1982;19:871-874.
43. McEnery J. Hospital management of acute iron ingestion. *Clin Toxicol.* 1971;4:603-613.
44. Melby K, Slordahal S, Gutteberg TJ, Nordbo SA. Septicemia due to *Yersinia enterocolitica* after oral doses of iron. *Br Med J.* 1982;285:487-488.
45. Mersko C, Hersko C, Weatherall D. Iron chelating therapy. *Crit Rev Clin Lab Sci.* 1988;26:303-340.
46. Moeschlin S, Schnider U. Treatment of primary and secondary hemochromatosis and acute iron poisoning with a new potent iron eliminating agent (desferrioxamine-B). *N Engl J Med.* 1963;269:57-66.
47. Mofenson HC, Caraccio TR, Sharieff N. Iron sepsis. *Yersinia enterocolitica* septicemia possibly caused by an overdose of iron. *N Engl J Med.* 1987;316:1092-1093.
48. Nakamura H, Rose PG, Blumer JL, et al. Acute encephalopathy due to aluminum toxicity successfully treated by combined intravenous deferoxamine and hemodialysis. *J Clin Pharmacol.* 2000;40:296-300.
49. Olivieri NF, Brittenham GM, McLaren CE, et al. Long-term safety and effectiveness of iron-chelation therapy with deferiprone for thalassemia major. *N Engl J Med.* 1998;339:417-423.
50. Olivieri N, Buncic J, Chew E, et al. Visual and auditory neuro-toxicity in patients receiving subcutaneous deferoxamine infusions. *N Engl J Med.* 1986;314:869-873.
51. Peck M, Rogers J, Riverbach J. Use of high doses of deferoxamine (Desferal) in an adult patient with acute iron overdosage. *J Toxicol Clin Toxicol.* 1982;19:865-869.
52. Pengloan J, Dantal J, Rossazza M, et al. Ocular toxicity after a single dose of desferrioxamine in two hemodialysis patients. *Nephron.* 1987;46:211-212.
53. Peter G, Keberle M, Schmid K. Distribution and renal excretion of desferrioxamine and ferrioxamine in the dog and in the rat. *Biochem Pharmacol.* 1966;15:93-109.

54. Phelps K, Naylor K, Brien T, et al. Encephalopathy after bladder irrigation with alum. case report and literature review. *Am J Med Soc.* 1999;318:185.
55. Porter JB, Faherty A, Stallibrass L, et al. A trial to investigate the relationship between DFO pharmacokinetics and metabolism and DFO-related toxicity. *Ann N Y Acad Sci.* 1998;30:483-487.
56. Porter J, Jaswon M, Huehns E, et al. Desferrioxamine ototoxicity. Evaluation of risk factors in thalassemic patients and guidelines for safe dosage. *Br J Haematol.* 1989;73:403-409.
57. Porter J, Taher T, Cappellini M, et al. Ethical issues and risk/benefit assessment of iron chelation therapy. Advances with deferiprone/deferoxamine combinations and concerns about the safety, efficacy and costs of deferasirox [letter to editor]. *Hemoglobin.* 2008;32:601-607.
58. Propper R, Nathan D. Clinical removal of iron. *Annu Rev Med.* 1982;33: 509-519.
59. Propper R, Shurn S, Nathan D. Reassessment of the use of desferrioxamine B in iron overload. *N Engl J Med.* 1976;294:1421-1423.
60. Robotham J, Lietman P. Acute iron poisoning. *Am J Dis Child.* 1980;134: 875-879.
61. Sherrard D, Walker J, Boykin J. Precipitation of dialysis dementia by deferoxamine treatment of aluminum related bone disease. *Am J Kid Dis.* 1988;12:126-130.
62. Singer ST, Vichinsky EP. Deferoxamine treatment during pregnancy. Is it harmful? *Am J Hematol.* 1999;60:24-26.
63. Stivelman J, Schulman G, Fosburg M, et al. Kinetics and efficacy of deferoxamine in iron overloaded hemodialysis patients. *Kidney Int.* 1989;36: 1125-1132.
64. Stumpf J. Deferasirox. *Am J Health Sys Pharm.* 2007;64:606-616.
65. Summers MR, Jacobs A, Tudway D, et al. Studies in desferrioxamine and ferrioxamine metabolism in normal and iron loaded subjects. *Br J Haematol.* 1979;42:547-555.
66. Tenenbein M. Benefits of parenteral deferoxamine for acute iron poisoning. *J Toxicol Clin Toxicol.* 1996;34:485-489.
67. Tenenbein M, Kowalski S, Sienko A, et al. Pulmonary toxic effects of continuous administration in acute iron poisoning. *Lancet.* 1992;339:699-701.
68. Tran T, Wax JR, Philput C, et al. Intentional iron overdose in pregnancy—Management and outcome. *J Emerg Med.* 2000;18:225-228.
69. Tripod JA. Pharmacologic comparison of the binding of iron and other metals. In. Gross F, ed. *Iron Metabolism. International Symposium on Iron Metabolism.* Berlin: Springer-Verlag; 1964:503-524.
70. Vasilakakis D, D'Haese P, Lamberts L, et al. Removal of aluminoxamine and ferrioxamine by charcoal hemoperfusion and hemodialysis. *Kidney Int.* 1992;41:1400-1407.
71. Vernon DD, Banner W Jr, Dean JM. Hemodynamic effects of experimental iron poisoning. *Ann Emerg Med.* 1989;18:863-866.
72. Weitman S, Buchanan G, Kamen B. Pulmonary toxicity of deferoxamine in children with advanced cancer. *J Natl Cancer Inst.* 1991;83:1834-1835.
73. Westlin W. Deferoxamine as a chelating agent. *Clin Toxicol.* 1971;4:597-602.
74. Westlin W. Deferoxamine in the treatment of acute iron poisoning. Clinical experiences with 172 children. *Clin Pediatr.* 1966;5:531-535.
75. Whitten C, Gibson G, Good M, et al. Studies in acute iron poisoning. Desferrioxamine in the treatment of acute iron poisoning—clinical observations, experimental studies and theoretical considerations. *Pediatrics.* 1965;36:322-335.
76. Whitten C, Chen YC, Gibson G. Studies in acute iron poisoning. II. Further observations on deferoxamine in the treatment of acute experimental iron poisoning. *Pediatrics.* 1966;38:102-110.
77. Whitten CF, Chen YC, Gibson GW. Studies in acute iron poisoning III. The hemodynamic alterations in acute experimental iron poisoning. *Pediatr Res.* 1968;2:479-485.
78. Yatscoff RW, Wayne EA, Tenenbein M. An objective criterion for the cessation of deferoxamine therapy in the acutely poisoned patient. *J Toxicol Clin Toxicol.* 1991;29:1-10.
79. Yokel R. Aluminum chelation principles and recent advances. *Coord Chem Rev.* 2002;228:97-113.

CHAPTER 41
VITAMINS

Beth Y. Ginsburg

Vitamins are essential for normal human growth and development.[43] By definition, a vitamin is a substance that is present in small amounts in natural foods, is necessary for normal metabolism, and whose lack in the diet causes a deficiency disease.[37] According to the American Medical Association, healthy men and nonpregnant women who eat a varied diet do not need supplemental vitamins.[8] In a recent national survey, 73% of adults in the United States reported use of a dietary supplement within the past year.[202] Eighty-five percent of these supplement users reported use of a multivitamin-multimineral. Many of these individuals share the mistaken beliefs that vitamin preparations provide extra energy or promote muscle growth and regularly ingest quantities of vitamins in great excess of the recommended dietary allowances (RDAs) (Table 41–1). Some vitamins are associated with consequential adverse effects when ingested in very large doses.

Vitamins can be divided into two general classes. Most of the vitamins in the *water-soluble* class have minimal toxicity because they are stored to only a limited extent in the body. Thiamine, riboflavin, cyanocobalamin, pantothenic acid, folic acid, and biotin are not reported to cause any toxicity following oral ingestion.[43] Ascorbic acid (vitamin C), nicotinic acid (vitamin B_3), and pyridoxine (vitamin B_6) are associated with toxicity syndromes. The *fat-soluble* vitamins, however, can bioaccumulate to massive degrees. As a result, the potential for toxicity greatly exceeds that of the water-soluble group. Vitamins A, D, and E but not K are associated with toxicity following very large overdose. The adverse effect secondary to vitamin K is limited to severe, and sometimes fatal, anaphylactoid reactions with rapid administration of the intravenous (IV) preparation.[69]

VITAMIN A

MW = 272.43 daltons
Therapeutic serum concentration = 65–275 IU/dL
16.6–83.3 μg/dL

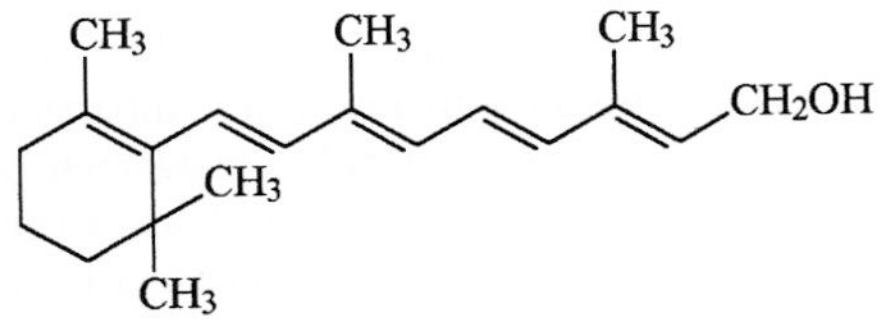

HISTORY AND EPIDEMIOLOGY

Vitamin A is present in two forms. Preformed vitamin A as retinol is derived from retinyl esters, its storage form, in animal sources of food. Provitamin A carotenoids are vitamin A precursors and are found in plants. Among the carotenoids, β-carotene is most efficiently made into retinol. The term *vitamin A* was classically only used to refer to the compound retinol. Currently, it is used to describe all retinoids, compounds chemically related to retinol, that exhibit the biological activity of retinol. Retinol can be converted in the body to the retinoids retinal and retinoic acid. Synthetic retinoids have been developed via chemical modification of naturally occurring retinoids, often for a specific therapeutic purpose. Vitamin A activity is expressed in retinol equivalents (RE). One RE corresponds to 1 μg of retinol or 3.33 international units (IU) of vitamin A activity as retinol. Twelve micrograms of β-carotene is equivalent to 1 RE (3.33 IU).

As a group, retinoids have specific sites of action and varying degrees of biologic potency. Retinoic acid is primarily responsible for maintaining normal growth and differentiation of epithelial cells in mucus-secreting or keratinizing tissue.[137] Vitamin A deficiency results in the disappearance of goblet mucous cells and replacement of the normal epithelium with a stratified, keratinized epithelium. Dermal manifestations are the earliest to develop and include dry skin and hair and broken fingernails. In the cornea, hyperkeratization is called *xerophthalmia* and can lead to permanent blindness. Alterations in the epithelial lining of other organ systems may lead to increased susceptibility to respiratory infections, diarrhea, and urinary calculi. Vitamin A, in the form of 11-*cis*-retinal, plays a critical role in retinal function.[211] Deficiency results in nyctalopia, which is decreased vision in dim lighting, more commonly known as *night blindness*.

Two independent groups discovered vitamin A in 1913.[140,160] They reported that animals fed an artificial diet with lard as the sole source of fat developed a nutritional deficiency characterized by xerophthalmia. They found that this deficiency could be corrected by adding to the diet a factor contained in butter, egg yolks, and cod liver oil. They named this substance "fat soluble vitamin A." The chemical structure of vitamin A was determined in 1930.[111] Vitamin A is also found naturally in liver, fish, cheese, and whole milk. In the United States and other parts of the world, including some developing countries, many cereal, grain, dairy, and other products, as well as infant formulas, are fortified with vitamin A.[6,217] Vitamin A content varies widely among different food types. A 3-oz serving of cooked beef liver contains 30,325 IU (9100 RE) of vitamin A, whereas 1 cup of whole milk contains 305 IU (92 RE) of vitamin A. Fish-liver oils, such as swordfish and black sea bass, have extremely large amounts of vitamin A and may contain more than 180,000 IU (54,050 RE) of vitamin A per gram of oil. Carotenoids are present in yellow and green fruits and vegetables. A raw carrot has a high β-carotene content of approximately 20,250 IU (6080 RE). One half-cup serving of spinach contains approximately 7400 IU (2220 RE) of β-carotene, whereas an apricot or peach contains 500–600 IU (150–180 RE). The average American diet provides about half of its daily vitamin A intake as carotenoids and about half as preformed vitamin A.[41] The RDA of vitamin A is 900 μg RE/d (3000 IU/d) for adult men and 700 μg RE/d (2300 IU/d) for women (Table 41–1).[73] The tolerable upper intake level for adults is 3000 μg RE/d (9900 IU/d).

Vitamin A toxicity can occur in people who ingest large doses of preformed vitamin A in their daily diets. Inuits in the 16th century recognized that ingestion of large amounts of polar bear liver caused a severe illness characterized by headaches and prostration.[70] Arctic explorers in the 1800s knew of the poisonous qualities of polar bear liver and described an acute illness following its ingestion.[77] Explorers also described a condition among the Inuit population known as *pibloktoq*, or "Arctic hysteria," characterized by hysteria, depression, echolalia, insensitivity to extreme cold, and seizures, and believed to be related to ingestion of polar bear liver and other organ meats.[165] Vitamin A toxicity is implicated in the etiology of pibloktoq as some somatic and behavioral effects of vitamin A toxicity closely parallel many of the symptoms reported in Inuit patients diagnosed with pibloktoq.[120] However, the toxic substance in polar bear liver was not identified as vitamin A until 1942.[180] The vitamin A content of polar bear liver is as high as 34,600 IU/g (10,400 RE/g), supporting the view that vitamin A is the toxic factor in liver.[181]

Vitamin A toxicity was reported in an adult who chronically ingested large amounts of beef liver,[103] as well as following ingestion of the liver of the grouper fish *Cephalopholis boenak*, which has a high content of vitamin A.[38] Ingestion of sea whale and seal liver, as well as the livers

TABLE 41–1. Recommended Dietary Daily Allowances/Adequate Daily Intakes*

Age (yr)	Vitamin A (μg RE/IU)	Vitamin D (μg/IU)	Vitamin E (mg α-TE/IU)	Vitamin C (mg)	Vitamin B_6 (mg)	Niacin (mg NE)
Infants						
0.0–0.5	400/1300*	5/200*	4/4*	40*	0.1*	2*
0.5–1.0	500/1700*	5/200*	5/5*	50*	0.3*	4*
Children						
1–3	300/990	5/200*	6/6	15	0.5	6
4–8	400/1300	5/200*	7/7	25	0.6	8
Males						
9–13	600/2000	5/200*	11/11	45	1.0	12
14–18	900/3000	5/200*	15/15	75	1.3	16
19–50	900/3000	5/200*	15/15	90	1.3	16
51–70	900/3000	10/400*	15/15	90	1.7	16
>70	900/3000	15/600*	15/15	90	1.7	16
Females						
9–13	600/2000	5/200*	11/11	45	1.0	12
14–18	700/2300	5/200*	15/15	65	1.2	14
19–50	700/2300	5/200*	15/15	75	1.3	14
51–70	700/2300	10/400*	15/15	75	1.5	14
>70	700/2300	15/600*	15/15	75	1.5	14
Pregnant						
≤18	750/2500	5/200*	15/15	80	1.9	18
19–50	770/2500	5/200*	15/15	85	1.9	18
Lactating						
≤18	1200/4000	5/200*	19/19	115	2.0	17
19–50	1300/4300	5/200*	19/19	120	2.0	17

RE = retinol equivalents; NE = niacin equivalents; TE = tocopherol equivalents.

*Values with an asterisk represent the Adequate Daily Intakes. Values without an * represent the Recommended Dietary Daily Allowances.

Adapted from Food and Nutrition Information Center homepage. http://fnic.nal.usda.gov/nal. Accessed January 12, 2009.

of large fish, such as shark, tuna, and sea bass, also is associated with development of vitamin A toxicity.

Vitamin A toxicity usually is not expected to occur following ingestion of large doses of provitamin A carotenoids. However, vitamin A–induced hepatotoxicity and neurotoxicity was believed to have developed in an 18-year-old woman who maintained a diet nearly limited to foods rich in β-carotene, including pumpkin, carrots, and liver, for several years.[152]

The majority of cases reported of vitamin A toxicity result from inappropriate use of vitamin supplements.[15,18] In the United States, approximately 1.3% of adults take vitamin A alone as a dietary supplement.[175]

Vitamin A is prescribed for some people for dermatologic and ophthalmic conditions. Vitamin A toxicity often occurs in adults who continue to use the vitamin without medical supervision.[78]

Isotretinoin (Accutane), 13-*cis*-retinoic acid, is prescribed for treatment of severe cystic acne. Of great concern is the teratogenicity associated with its use. According to the National Disease and Therapeutic Index, 38% of isotretinoin users are females aged 13–19 years. The likelihood of pregnancy in this group underscores the need to inform all users of the contraindication of the use of this drug during pregnancy and the need to demonstrate the absence of pregnancy prior to initiating treatment. This is mandated through the Food and Drug Administration via a risk management program called the System to Manage Accutane-Related Teratogenicity (SMART).[205] The program attempts to ensure that isotretinoin therapy is not initiated in pregnant women and that pregnancy does not occur in women taking isotretinoin. Prescriber education is required as well as patient informed consent, and all prescribers, patients, and dispensing pharmacies are entered in a registry. Women must have two negative urine or serum pregnancy tests before starting treatment and must have a negative pregnancy test before receiving each monthly prescription. Women who are sexually active must use two forms of contraception for at least 1 month before starting isotretinoin, during therapy, and for 1 month after discontinuation of therapy. Pharmacists may fill prescriptions for isotretinoin only if the prescribing physician and patient have complied with the SMART program. In addition, patients must consider the consequences of unintentional pregnancy while they are taking isotretinoin.

All-*trans*-retinoic acid (ATRA), or tretinoin, is used as a differentiating agent in the treatment of acute promyelocytic leukemia (APL), a disease characterized by the accumulation of promyelocytic blasts in bone marrow due to obstruction of differentiation of granulocytic cells.[122] ATRA, in combination with anthracycline chemotherapy, improves the complete remission rate, often reported to be greater than 90%, and reduces the incidence of relapse to only 10%–15% when used in a maintenance therapy regimen.[65] Arsenic trioxide is also recognized as an effective differentiating agent for the treatment of APL and works synergistically with ATRA.[223,224] APL differentiation syndrome, previously known as ATRA syndrome or retinoic acid syndrome (RAS), is the main adverse effect and occurs in up 14%–16% of patients who receive ATRA with an associated mortality of about 2%.[167] ATRA has also been used for the treatment of myelodysplastic syndrome and acute myelogenous leukemia.

PHARMACOLOGY AND TOXICOKINETICS

Absorption of vitamin A in the small intestine is nearly complete. However, some vitamin A may be eliminated in the feces when large doses are taken. The majority of vitamin A is ingested as retinyl esters, the storage form of retinol.[137] Retinyl esters undergo enzymatic hydrolysis to retinol by digestive enzymes in the intestinal lumen and brush border of the intestinal epithelial wall. A small portion of retinol is absorbed directly into the circulation, where it is bound to retinol-binding protein (RBP) and transported to the liver. Most of the retinol is taken into intestinal epithelial cells by the carrier protein cellular RBP.[157] Subsequently, retinol is re-esterified and incorporated into chylomicrons, which are released into the blood and taken up by the Ito cells of the liver. After large oral doses, significant amounts of retinyl esters coupled to chylomicrons circulate in association with low-density lipoproteins (LDLs) and are delivered to the liver. Approximately 50%–80% of the total vitamin A content of the body is stored in the liver as retinyl esters.[26] The liver releases vitamin A into the bloodstream to maintain a constant plasma retinol concentration and is thus delivered to tissues as needed.

Carotenoid absorption requires bile and absorbable fat in the stomach or intestine. These components combine with carotenoids to form mixed lipid micelles which move into the duodenal mucosal cells via passive diffusion. The majority of β-carotene that is metabolized undergoes central cleavage via oxidation to form retinal which is then reduced to retinol. Retinol is then esterified with fatty acids and incorporated into chylomicrons which are transported to the bloodstream via the lymphatics for delivery to the liver. Massive doses of β-carotene are rarely associated with vitamin A toxicity due to decreased efficiency in absorption secondary to saturation of dissolution in bulk lipid, micellar incorporation, and diffusion due to a reduction in the concentration gradient.[164] Unabsorbed β-carotene is excreted in the feces. In addition, there is a decrease in the rate of conversion of carotenoids to vitamin A.[57] Hypercarotenemia develops when massive doses are ingested. Excess absorbed β-carotene is incorporated with lipoproteins and released into the bloodstream via the lymphatics for delivery to the adipose tissue and adrenals for storage. Hypercarotenemia usually is not associated with morbidity.

The normal plasma retinol concentration is approximately 30–70 μg/dL.[192] Blood concentrations are maintained at the expense of hepatic reserves when insufficient amounts of vitamin A are ingested. A normal adult liver contains enough vitamin A to fulfill the body's requirements for approximately 2 years.[146] Excessive intake of vitamin A is not initially reflected by elevated blood concentrations because vitamin A is soluble in fat but not in water. Instead, hepatic accumulation is increased. This storage system allows for cumulative toxic effects. Although no relationship exists between the magnitude of liver stores and blood concentrations of vitamin A, in chronic vitamin A toxicity serum concentrations are generally >3.49 μmol/L (95 μg/dL).[18] Vitamin A has a half-life of 286 days in the blood.[194,215] Retinoids undergo a variety of metabolic and conjugation pathways and are subsequently eliminated in the feces, urine, or bile.

Clinical toxicity correlates well with total body vitamin A content, which is a function of both dosage and duration of administration. Vitamin A toxicity is rare, with a reported average incidence of <10 cases per year from 1976 to 1987.[18] A randomized double-blind trial, in which 390 women who received 400,000 IU (120,000 RE) of vitamin A as a single dose were compared with 380 women who received placebo, suggested that dosing at this level is well tolerated by postpartum women.[102] Doses of 100,000 IU (30,000 RE) of vitamin A in children aged 6–11 months and 200,000 IU (60,000 RE) of vitamin A every 3 to 6 months for children aged 12–60 months results in few side effects.[17] The minimal dose required to produce toxicity in humans is not established. However, an animal study has shown that the median lethal acute dose in monkeys weighing between 1.0 and 1.8 kg is 560,000 IU (168,000 RE) per kg body weight.[132] In this study, all monkeys receiving >300,000 RE/kg (>999,000 IU/kg) died, whereas none died at a dose of 100,000 RE/kg (333,000 IU/kg). Hepatotoxicity can occur in humans following an acute ingestion of a massive dose of vitamin A (>600,000 IU, 180,000 RE).[117]

Vitamin A toxicity may occur more frequently secondary to chronic ingestions of vitamin A. Hepatotoxicity typically requires vitamin A ingestions of at least 50,000–100,000 IU/d (15,000–30,000 RE/d) for months or years.[6,117] One study found that in patients with vitamin A–induced hepatotoxicity, the average daily vitamin A intake was higher in patients who developed cirrhosis (135,000 IU/d, 40,500 RE/d) compared to patients who developed noncirrhotic liver disease (66,000 IU/d, 20,000 RE/d).[78] However, case reports have documented hepatotoxicity resulting from vitamin A doses as low as 25,000 IU/d (7500 RE/d),[78,117] a dose widely available in nonprescription vitamin A preparations.

PATHOPHYSIOLOGY

The mechanism of action for many of the toxic effects of vitamin A may be at the nuclear level. Retinoic acid influences gene expression by combining with nuclear receptors.[137] Retinoids also influence expression of receptors for certain hormones and growth factors. Thus they are able to influence growth, differentiation, and function of target cells.[130]

In epithelial cells and fibroblasts, retinoids affect changes in nuclear transcription, resulting in enhanced production of proteins such as fibronectin and decreased production of other proteins such as collagenase.[134] Excessive concentrations of retinoids lead where goblet cells are present to the production of a thick mucin layer and inhibition of keratinization. In addition, lipoprotein membranes have increased permeability and decreased stability, resulting in extreme thinning of the epithelial tissue.

In vitro studies in bone demonstrate that high doses of vitamin A are capable of directly stimulating bone resorption and inhibiting bone formation. This effect is secondary to increased osteoclast formation and activity and inhibition of osteoblast growth.[154,159,187]

Hepatotoxicity may develop secondary to an acute overdose or ingestion of "low" or "therapeutic" doses if taken over a prolonged time.[78,117] Ninety percent of hepatic vitamin A stores are located in the Ito, or fat-storing, cells of the liver, which are located in the perisinusoidal space of Disse, and are responsible for maintaining normal hepatic architecture.[88,89] Ito cells undergo hypertrophy and hyperplasia as vitamin A storage increases.[117] This results in transdifferentiation of the Ito cell into a myofibroblast-like cell that secretes a variety of extracellular matrix components, leading to narrowing of the perisinusoidal space of Disse, obstruction to sinusoidal blood flow, and

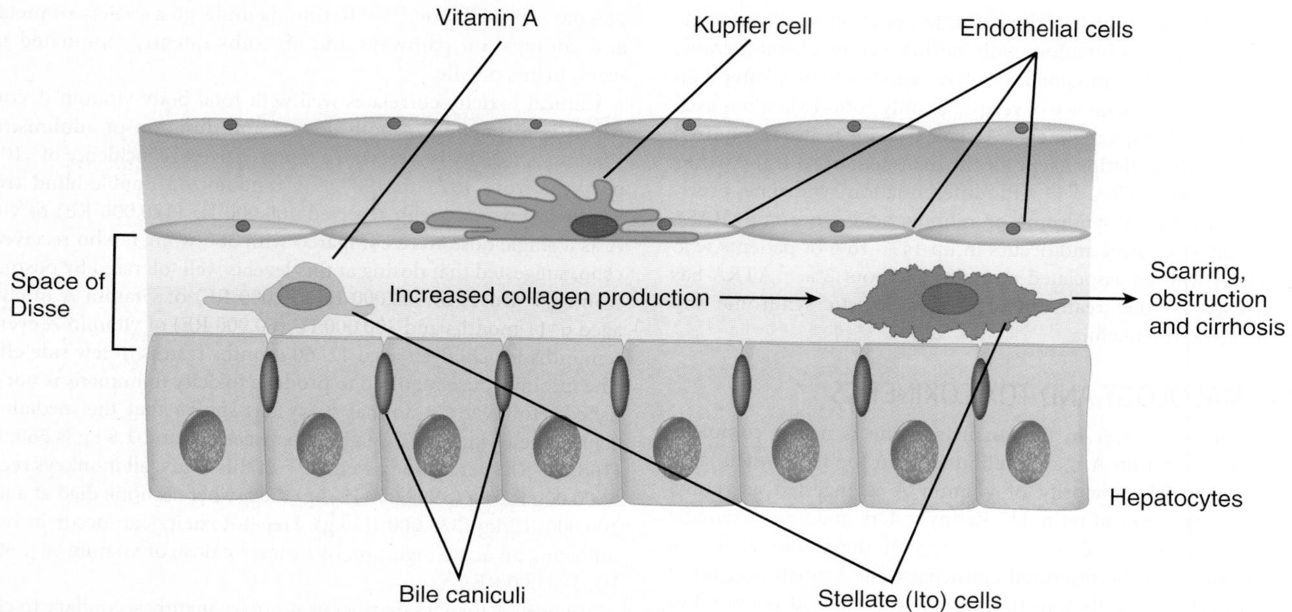

FIGURE 41–1. Schematic demonstration of hepatotoxicity resulting from excessive deposition of vitamin A in the Ito cells of the liver.

noncirrhotic portal hypertension (Fig. 41–1).[48,82,99,112,117,184] Continued ingestion of vitamin A and hepatic storage may lead to obliteration of the space of Disse, sinusoidal barrier damage, perisinusoidal hepatocyte death, fibrosis, and cirrhosis[99,106,117,182] (see Chap. 26). Vitamin A toxicity is associated with idiopathic intracranial hypertension (IIH). Although the role of vitamin A in the development of IIH is not definitively understood, serum concentrations of vitamin A are significantly higher in patients with IIH compared to healthy controls.[104] In addition, cerebrospinal fluid (CSF) concentrations of vitamin A are significantly elevated in patients with IIH compared to patients with normal intracranial pressure (ICP) or patients with other causes of elevated ICP.[214] Unbound, circulating retinol and retinyl esters are proposed to be capable of interacting with cell membranes and producing damage by membranolytic surface-active properties.[104] In the CNS, disruption of cell membrane integrity might lead to disruption of CSF outflow, thereby producing signs and symptoms consistent with IIH.[80,104,115,133]

CLINICAL MANIFESTATIONS

Vitamin A toxicity affects the skin, hair, bones, liver, and brain. The most common skin manifestations include xerosis, which is associated with pruritus and erythema, skin hyperfragility, and desquamation.[54,55,220] Retinoid toxicity may cause hair thinning and even diffuse hair loss in 10%–75% of patients.[72,81,114] In addition, the characteristics of the hair may change after regrowth. Hair sometimes becomes permanently curly or kinky.[10] Nail changes include a shiny appearance, brittleness, softening, and loosening.[66] Dryness of mucous membranes develops with chapped lips and xerosis of nasal mucosa, which sometimes is associated with nasal bleeding.[45]

Findings from epidemiologic studies are consistent with bone loss and a resulting increase in fracture risk. In northern Europe, the region with the highest incidence of osteoporotic fractures, dietary intake of vitamin A is high. A study of this population demonstrated that the risk of first hip fracture was increased by 68% for every 1 mg increase in RE intake.[142] This study also showed that compared to intake <0.5 mg/d, intake >1.5 mg/d reduced bone mineral density by 10% at the femoral neck, 14% at the lumbar spine, and 6% for the total body, and doubled the risk of hip fracture. These findings are supported by other studies demonstrating an increased risk of hip fracture among women with elevated serum vitamin A concentrations and in women ingesting large daily amounts of vitamin A.[67,158] One study found that among women not taking supplemental vitamin A, a diet rich in vitamin A was also associated with an increased fracture risk.[67]

Other musculoskeletal findings include skeletal hyperostoses, most commonly affecting the vertebral bodies of thoracic vertebrae, extraspinal tendon and ligament calcifications, soft tissue ossification, cortical thickening of bone shafts, periosteal thickening, and bone demineralization.[45,146,148] Many of these findings are apparent on radiographs. Patients often complain of bone and joint pain and muscle stiffness or tenderness. Hypercalcemia, with low or normal parathyroid hormone (PTH) concentrations, is thought to be secondary to increased osteoclast activity and bone resorption.[27] Patients with chronic renal failure are at increased risk for developing hypercalcemia at vitamin A doses lower than usual toxic doses secondary to decreased renal metabolism of retinol. This complication occurred in an 8-year-old boy with chronic renal failure following a dose of 12,000 IU/d (3600 RE/d) for at least 2 years.[52] Premature epiphyseal closure in children is reported.[172] Teratogenic effects include interference with skeletal differentiation and growth.[27]

The degree of hepatotoxicity appears to correlate with the dose of vitamin A and chronicity of use. With large doses, cirrhosis develops and may lead to portal hypertension, esophageal varices, jaundice, and ascites.[49,78,117] Hepatotoxicity may be manifested by elevations in bilirubin, aminotransferases, and alkaline phosphatase concentrations.

Idiopathic intracranial hypertension is characterized by elevated ICP in the absence of a structural anomaly. It occurs in patients with altered endocrine function, systemic diseases, impaired cerebral venous drainage, or ingestion of various xenobiotics, including excessive vitamin A (Table 41–2).[5] The syndrome is most common in young obese women, but the etiology remains unknown in the majority of cases. The first case of IIH associated with vitamin A toxicity was described in 1954.[77] However, the symptoms were first described in 1856 by an Arctic explorer who noted vertigo and headache after eating polar bear

TABLE 41–2. Xenobiotics Associated with Intracranial Hypertension

Antibiotics: ampicillin, minocycline, metronidazole, nalidixic acid, nitrofurantoin, sulfamethoxazole, tetracycline
Corticosteroid therapy (oral and intranasal) and cessation
Enflurane
Griseofulvin
Halothane
Ketamine
Lead
Lithium
Oral contraceptives and progestins
Phenothiazines
Phenytoin
Tubocurarine
Vitamin A

liver.[191] Patients typically present with headache and visual disturbances, including sixth nerve palsies, visual field deficits, and blurred vision, and have a normal mental status. Despite severe papilledema, visual loss often is minimal. However, permanent blindness may result from optic atrophy.[131] Other symptoms of neurotoxicity include ataxia, fatigue, depression, irritability, and psychosis.[24]

Isotretinoin is effective in the management of acne. However, its use is associated with teratogenicity. It is thought to interfere with cranial-neural-crest cells, which contribute to the development of both the ear and the conotruncal area of the heart, and may cause malformed or absent external ears or auditory canals and conotruncal heart defects.[119] Although studies have not shown a teratogenic risk with topical preparations, case reports describe fetal malformations associated with topical preparation use during pregnancy.[12,33,107,129,190] In addition, mucocutaneous abnormalities, IIH, corneal opacities, hypercalcemia, hyperuricemia, musculoskeletal symptoms, liver function abnormalities, elevated triglyceride concentrations, and spontaneous abortion are reported.[3,71,76,85,86]

APL differentiation syndrome is the main adverse effect of treatment with ATRA. The syndrome is characterized by dyspnea, pulmonary effusions and infiltrates, fever, weight gain, renal failure, pericardial effusions, and hypotension.[63] Onset of symptoms is typically 2 to 21 days after initiation of ATRA.[167] Elevated leukocyte counts at diagnosis or rapidly increasing counts during ATRA treatment predict the development of APL differentiation syndrome. Its etiology is thought to be related to cytokine release by maturing blast cells. Addition of dexamethasone to the treatment regimen was shown to decrease the incidence of this syndrome to approximately 15% and its mortality to 1%.[64] However, other data demonstrated a 17% occurrence of APL differentiation syndrome despite concurrent use of steroids and not all authors support its use.[167,219]

Symptoms of an acute overdose of vitamin A often develop within hours to 2 days after ingestion.[146] Initial signs and symptoms include headache, papilledema, scotoma, photophobia, seizures, anorexia, drowsiness, irritability, nausea, vomiting, abdominal pain, liver damage, and desquamation.[146] Additional signs and symptoms are associated with chronic toxicity.[146] Nonspecific symptoms include fatigue, fever, weight loss, edema, polydipsia, dysuria, hyperlipidemia, anemia, and menstrual abnormalities.

Hypercarotenemia produces a yellow-orange skin discoloration that can be differentiated from jaundice by the absence of scleral icterus.

DIAGNOSTIC TESTING

The diagnosis of vitamin A-associated hepatotoxicity is supported by histologic evidence of Ito cell hyperplasia with fluorescent vacuoles on liver biopsy.[78] Laboratory testing should also include serum electrolytes including calcium, hepatic enzymes, and a complete blood cell count. Because the liver has a large storage capacity for excess vitamin A, hepatotoxicity may occur prior to an elevation in the serum concentration of vitamin A, which may be normal or even low, in the setting of an acute overdose. As the hepatic storage capacity is overwhelmed, the serum concentration may rapidly rise in a nonlinear fashion. Further evaluation should be guided by the clinical presentation and may include bone radiographs, computed tomography of the brain, and lumbar puncture.

TREATMENT

Management of a recent acute, large overdose should begin with gastrointestinal decontamination. This can be accomplished with a dose of activated charcoal. In extremely large overdoses that are expected to produce significant toxicity, gastric lavage may be considered. Although most signs and symptoms of vitamin A toxicity resolve within 1 week following vitamin A discontinuation and supportive care, papilledema, desquamation, and skeletal abnormalities may persist for several months. Hypercalcemia should be treated with intravenous fluids, loop diuretics, and prednisone 20 mg/d.[23] Bisphosphonates may be beneficial in refractory cases.

Idiopathic intracranial hypertension may require more aggressive therapy, similar to that of other causes of increased ICP. Depending on the severity of the syndrome, patients may require dexamethasone (0.25–0.5 mg/kg/d in children <40 kg and 12–16 mg/d in adults); an initial adult dose of 250 mg acetazolamide, which can be increased to 500 mg 3 times per day; 40 mg IV furosemide; and 1 g/kg mannitol.[191] Tapering doses of hydrocortisone or prednisone are alternatives to dexamethasone. Acetazolamide decreases CSF formation but may be associated with a transient increase in ICP. Patients with extremely high ICP may benefit from daily lumbar punctures with CSF drainage.

Treatment of APL differentiation syndrome involves prompt administration of corticosteroids, commonly dexamethasone 10 mg IV twice daily for at least 3 days.[167] In severe cases, ATRA should be discontinued or another antineoplastic agent, typically cytarabine, should be added to ATRA in patients with high white blood cell counts.[167] ATRA can be reintroduced upon resolution of the differentiation syndrome.

VITAMIN D

MW	= 384.62 daltons
Therapeutic serum concentration	= 10–50 ng/mL

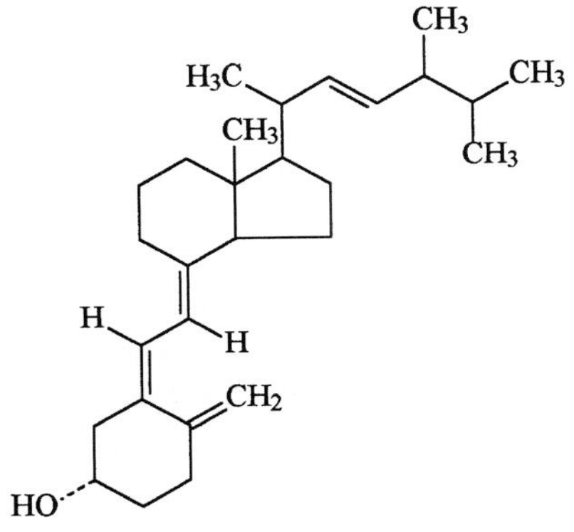

HISTORY AND EPIDEMIOLOGY

Vitamin D is the name given to both ergocalciferol (vitamin D_2) and cholecalciferol (vitamin D_3). In humans, both forms of vitamin D have the same biologic potency. Vitamin D is used for the prophylaxis and treatment of rickets, osteomalacia, and osteoporosis, and for the treatment of hypoparathyroidism and skin conditions including psoriasis. Rickets, a disease of urban children living in temperate zones, was thought to result from the lack of a dietary factor or adequate sunshine. In 1919, two independent groups demonstrated that rickets could be prevented or cured by either the addition of cod liver oil to the diet or exposure to sunlight.[101,143] Vitamin D is found in other foods, including butter, cheese, and cream, which contain 12–40 IU/100 g (0.3–1 μg/100 g); eggs, which contain 25 IU/100 g (0.6 μg/100 g); and fatty fish, such as salmon and mackerel, which contain 150–550 IU/100 g (4–14 μg/100 g) and 1100 IU/100 g (28 μg /100 g), respectively. Some foods typically are fortified with vitamin D, including cereals, bread, and milk.[94] Many dietary supplements, such as multivitamins, contain vitamin D. One microgram of vitamin D is equivalent to 40 IU of vitamin D.

Vitamin D deficiency should not occur in individuals who are exposed to adequate sunlight and eat a well-balanced diet. Casual exposure of cutaneous tissues to ultraviolet light during the summer months should produce adequate vitamin D storage for winter months.[83] Total body sun exposure provides the vitamin D equivalent of 10,000 IU/d (250 μg/d);[207] the body requires only a total vitamin D supply of 4000 IU/d (100 μg/d).[207] Breast-fed infants may require supplemental vitamin D if they have limited exposure to sunlight because the vitamin D content of human milk is extremely low.[43] Other groups susceptible to vitamin D deficiency include the elderly, vegans, and persons without adequate sunlight exposure. The daily adequate intake of vitamin D for nonelderly adults is 200 IU/d (5 μg/d).[73] This dose approximates the vitamin D content of a half-teaspoon of cod liver oil.[163] These doses appear to prevent rickets and osteomalacia. However, larger doses of vitamin D may be required for treatment of osteoporosis or hypoparathyroidism.

Rickets has been eliminated as a major public health concern in children in Europe and North America since the fortification of milk with vitamin D. Outbreaks of vitamin D poisoning subsequently occurred in Europe in the 1950s because of excessive fortification of milk and cereals to compensate for wartime nutritional deprivation of children.[50] This vitamin D poisoning led to a period of prohibition of vitamin D fortification of foods.[94] More recently, a study showed that milk and infant formulas rarely contain the amount of vitamin D stated on the label and may be either significantly underfortified or overfortified, leading to vitamin D deficiency or toxicity.[94] One case series demonstrated vitamin D toxicity in eight patients who drank local dairy milk that was excessively fortified with vitamin D_3.[105] Many cases of vitamin D toxicity result from continued supplementation of vitamin D and calcium initially prescribed for treatment of hypoparathyroidism, osteoporosis, or osteomalacia, due to inadequate patient followup.[47,124,168] Two reports describe vitamin D toxicity in families secondary to use of a highly concentrated vitamin D preparation in nut oil that was not intended for human consumption.[53,169] Another case report describes vitamin D poisoning secondary to contamination of table sugar with crystalline vitamin D_3.[209] Vitamin D toxicity can occur secondary to vitamin D_3 exposure in the form of rodenticides (Chap. 108).

PHARMACOLOGY AND TOXICOKINETICS

Vitamin D itself is not biologically active but must go through extensive metabolism to an active form, whether it is ingested from a food source or synthesized in the body. Vitamin D_3 is synthesized in the skin from 7-dehydrocholesterol (provitamin D_3) in a reaction catalyzed by ultraviolet B irradiation (Fig. 41–2).[124] Vitamin D_3 then is bound to vitamin D-binding protein, a protein that also binds vitamin D from the diet, and afterward enters the circulation. In the endoplasmic reticulum of the liver, vitamin D_3 is metabolized to 25-hydroxyvitamin D [25(OH)D] by vitamin D-25-hydroxylase.[74] Once formed, 25(OH)D is again bound to vitamin D-binding protein and transported to the proximal convoluted tubule in the kidney for hydroxylation to 1,25-dihydroxyvitamin D [1,25$(OH)_2$D], or calcitriol, by 25(OH)D-1α-hydroxylase.[74] Once formed, 1,25$(OH)_2$D is secreted back into circulation, bound to vitamin D-binding protein, and delivered to target cells where it binds to receptors.

Vitamin D might be more appropriately called a hormone rather than a vitamin because it is synthesized in the body, circulates in the blood, and then binds to receptors in order to evoke its biologic action. The primary role of vitamin D is regulation of calcium homeostasis via interactions with the intestines and bones. Protein-bound calcitriol is taken up by cells and then binds to a specific nuclear vitamin D receptor protein that, in turn, binds to regulatory sequences on chromosomal DNA.[124] The result is induction of gene transcription and translation of proteins that carry out the cellular functions of vitamin D. In the intestines, calcitriol increases the production of calcium-binding proteins and plasma membrane calcium pump proteins, thereby increasing

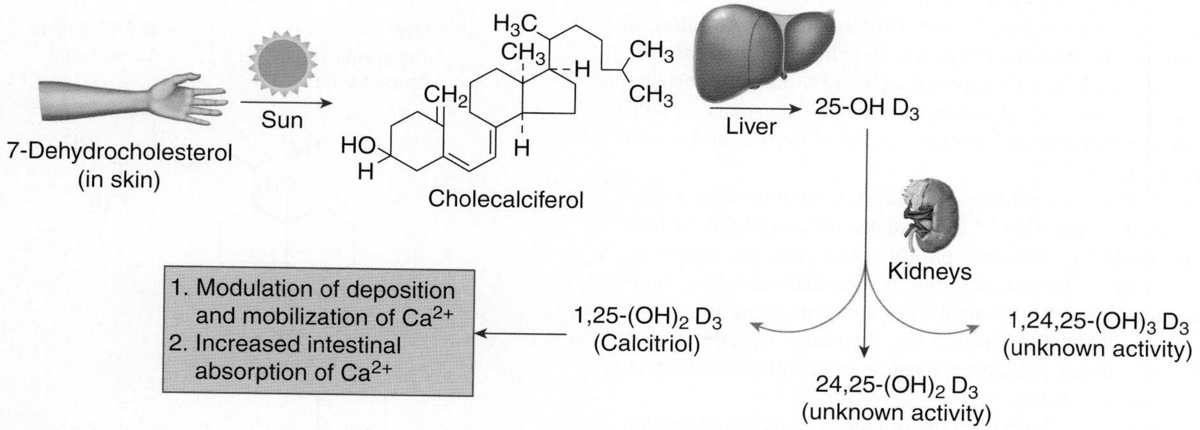

FIGURE 41–2. Schematic representation of the synthesis and physiologic response to Vitamin D.

calcium absorption through the duodenum.[108] In the bone, calcitriol stimulates osteoclastic precursors to differentiate into mature osteoclasts.[95] Mature osteoclasts, together with PTH, lead to mobilization of calcium stores from bone, thereby raising serum concentrations of calcium. Given sufficient serum concentrations of calcium, calcitriol promotes bone mineralization by osteoblasts, resulting in increased deposition of calcium hydroxyapatite into the bone matrix.[95] Calcitriol also binds to a vitamin D receptor in the parathyroid glands, which leads to decreased synthesis and secretion of PTH.[153] The vitamin D receptor is present in most cells of the body including lymphocytes, epidermal skin cells, and tumor cells.[183] The binding of calcitriol can inhibit proliferation and induce terminal differentiation.[171] Although the role of vitamin D has not been elucidated in all cells, abnormalities present during vitamin D deficiency may help identify the function of vitamin D in various tissues.

Vitamin D deficiency results in hypocalcemia, leading to increased secretion of PTH, which acts to restore plasma calcium concentrations at the expense of bone. In children, this situation leads to rickets in which newly formed bone is not adequately mineralized and results in bone deformities and growth defects. Adults develop osteomalacia, a disease characterized by undermineralized bone matrix. Patients typically present with bone pain and tenderness and proximal muscle weakness. Bone deformities are limited to the advanced stages of disease.

The literature varies regarding the toxic dose of vitamin D, with little scientific data available for corroboration. The current "no observed adverse effect level" or tolerable upper intake dose was conservatively set at 2000 IU/d (50 μg/d)[73,207] but this determination occurred without the consideration of studies showing that doses as high as 4400 IU/d (110 μg/d) and 100,000 IU (2500 μg) for 4 days did not result in adverse effects.[196,203,207] Case reports describe toxicity in the setting of vitamin D intake of 50,000–150,000 IU or, simply, doses in the milligram range, daily for prolonged periods.[47,168]

PATHOPHYSIOLOGY

The hallmark of vitamin D toxicity is hypercalcemia. Vitamin D in the form of 1,25$(OH)_2$D promotes calcium absorption from the gut and mobilization of calcium from bone. Vitamin D toxicity may be associated with a plasma concentration of 25(OH)D 20 times higher than normal, whereas the concentration of 1,25$(OH)_2$D remains exceedingly variable.[74,169] 25-Hydroxyvitamin D can mimic the action of 1,25$(OH)_2$D when it is present in excess and can bind to receptors usually specific for 1,25$(OH)_2$D.[74,124] Alternatively, 25(OH)D, which has a higher affinity for vitamin D-binding protein compared to 1,25$(OH)_2$D, may preferentially bind to vitamin D-binding protein when it is present in elevated concentrations, displacing 1,25$(OH)_2$D and allowing it to circulate in an unbound form, or loosely bound to albumin.[208] A study of patients with vitamin D toxicity who had normal or near-normal total 1,25$(OH)_2$D levels had elevated free 1,25$(OH)_2$D levels.[169] The availability of 1,25$(OH)_2$D to its receptors likely is increased, resulting in vitamin D toxicity.

CLINICAL MANIFESTATIONS

Patients with vitamin D toxicity present with signs and symptoms characteristic of hypercalcemia.[124] Early manifestations include weakness, fatigue, somnolence, irritability, headache, dizziness, muscle and bone pain, nausea, vomiting, abdominal cramps, and diarrhea or constipation. As the calcium concentration increases, hypercalcemia may induce polyuria and polydipsia. Diuresis results in salt and water depletion, further impairing calcium excretion. Severe hypercalcemia may present with ataxia, confusion, psychosis, seizures, coma, and renal failure. In addition, cardiac dysrhythmias result from a shortened refractory period and slowed conduction. ECG findings include increased PR intervals, widening of QRS complexes, QT shortening, and flattened T waves.[155] Patients can develop metastatic calcification of the kidneys, blood vessels, myocardium, lung, and skin. Several patients with vitamin D toxicity have presented with anemia.[173,185] Proposed mechanisms for anemia include a direct effect of vitamin D on hematopoietic cells and inhibition of erythropoietin production.[173]

DIAGNOSTIC TESTING

Vitamin D toxicity should be considered in patients presenting with signs and symptoms of hypercalcemia. In addition to an elevated serum calcium, laboratory results may reveal hyperphosphatemia given that vitamin D facilitates phosphate absorption in the small intestine, enhances its mobilization from bone, and decreases its excretion by the kidney.[135] The diagnosis should be suspected in children with nephrocalcinosis and hypercalcuria even if serum calcium and phosphorus concentrations are normal.[149]

MANAGEMENT

Treatment of hypercalcemia in patients with vitamin D toxicity should include discontinuation of both vitamin D and calcium supplementation, maintenance of a low-calcium diet, and administration of adequate volumes of oral or IV fluid to increase renal calcium clearance.[124] Many cases of hypercalcemia will respond to such supportive care. Following rehydration, a loop diuretic, such as furosemide at a standard dose, can be added to promote calcium excretion.[124] Corticosteroids, in doses of hydrocortisone, 100 mg/d, or prednisone, 20 mg/d, improve hypercalcemia and hypercalcuria in vitamin D poisoning. Studies have attempted to explain this effect as being a result of either decreased intestinal calcium absorption or inhibition of bone resorption.[113,198] Bisphosphonates, such as pamidronate, 90 mg IV, and coldronate, 600 mg IV, were used successfully in cases of severe hypercalcemia.[123,178] These drugs inhibit bone resorption via actions on osteoclasts. Their use may preclude the need for hemodialysis in refractory cases of hypercalcemia. Calcitonin, a hypocalcemic hormone secreted by the thyroid gland that directly inhibits osteoclast activity, can be used to decrease bone resorption. Salmon calcitonin was successfully used to treat refractory hypercalcemia in a child with vitamin D poisoning at a dose of 4 U/kg IM twice daily until hypercalcemia resolved at 15 days.[144]

ANTIOXIDANTS (VITAMINS E AND C)

The antioxidants include vitamins E and C, and β-carotene. During the 1990s, the concept that antioxidants had a protective effect against atherosclerosis and carcinogenesis was widely promoted. This notion was based on the "oxidative-modification hypothesis" of atherosclerosis, which proposes that atherogenesis is initiated by lipid peroxidation of LDLs.[51] Unregulated or prolonged production of cellular oxidants leading to oxidant-induced DNA damage is thought to be responsible for carcinogenesis.[116] Epidemiologic evidence seems to support the use of antioxidants for these indications.[118,176,195] However, several prospective, randomized, placebo-controlled clinical trials, designed to test for the effect of antioxidant vitamins on cardiovascular disease and cancer, have consistently shown that commonly used antioxidant regimens do not significantly reduce or prevent overall cardiovascular events or cancer.[31,87,91,156,200,221]

VITAMIN E

MW	= 430.69 daltons
Therapeutic serum concentration	= 0.5–2.0 mg/dL

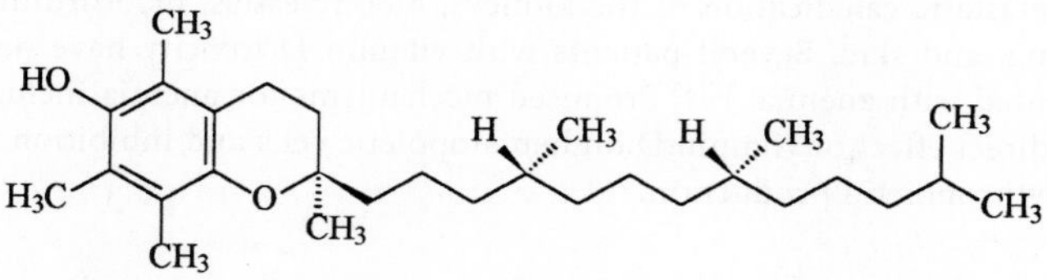

HISTORY AND EPIDEMIOLOGY

Vitamin E includes eight naturally occurring compounds in two classes—tocopherols and tocotrienols—which have differing biologic activities. The most biologically active form is RRR-α-tocopherol, previously known as d-α-tocopherol, which is the most widely available form of vitamin E in food. A synthetic form of α-tocopherol, often used in vitamin supplements, contains a mixture of *d* and *l* isomers and is designated *all-rac*-α-tocopherol (previously *d,l*-α-tocopherol).

The existence of vitamin E was first demonstrated in 1922 by researchers noting that female rats deficient in a dietary principal were unable to sustain a pregnancy.[60] Testicular lesions in male rats were described in deficiency states, and vitamin E was referred to as the "antisterility vitamin."[137] Vitamin E was first isolated from wheatgerm oil in 1936.[59] The richest sources of vitamin E include nuts, wheat germ, whole grains, vegetable and seed oils, including soybean, corn, cottonseed, and safflower, and the products made from these oils. In general, animal products are poor sources of vitamin E. Human milk, in contrast to cow's milk, has sufficient α-tocopherol to meet the needs of breast-fed infants.[137] In the United States, approximately 12.7% of adults take vitamin E alone as a dietary supplement.[175] Supplementation should not be necessary in persons who consume a well-balanced diet. One IU is equivalent to 1 mg α-tocopherol acetate.

Vitamin E deficiency occurs in patients with malabsorption syndromes, which may occur in the presence of pancreatic insufficiency or hepatobiliary disease, such as biliary atresia.[25] Patients with abetalipoproteinemia are at risk for vitamin E deficiency.[13] In this rare disease, absorption and transport of vitamin E are impaired secondary to a lack of chylomicron and β-lipoprotein formation. Manifestations of deficiency are variable but seem to have the most effect in organ systems that rely on vitamin E for normal functioning.[137] The clinical syndrome is primarily manifested by a peripheral neuropathy and spinocerebellar syndrome that improves with supplemental vitamin E.[145] Symptoms include ophthalmoplegia, hyporeflexia, gait disturbances, and decreased sensitivity to vibration and proprioception.[25]

Vitamin E is an essential nutrient. It is believed to be necessary for normal functioning of the nervous, reproductive, muscular, cardiovascular, and hematopoietic systems. Use of vitamin E has been proposed for a wide range of conditions. In most cases, scientific rationale for its use is lacking or is based on in vitro or animal data that have not been validated in humans or have demonstrated equivocal results.[25] As examples, vitamin E has been used for treatment of recurrent abortion, hemolytic anemias, claudication, wound healing, tardive dyskinesia, epilepsy, and adult respiratory distress syndrome. In addition, much research over the past decade has focused on the use of vitamin E for the prevention and treatment of cardiovascular disease and cancer, with disappointing results.[201]

PHARMACOLOGY AND TOXICOKINETICS

Vitamin E absorption is dependent on the ingestion and absorption of fat. The presence of bile also is essential. Vitamin E is passively absorbed in the intestinal tract into the lymphatic circulation by a nonsaturable process. Approximately 45% of a dose is absorbed in this manner and subsequently enters the bloodstream in chylomicrons, which are taken up by the liver. Vitamin E then is secreted back into the circulation, where it is primarily associated with LDLs. Vitamin E is distributed to all tissues, with the greatest accumulation in adipose tissue, liver, and muscle.

The primary biologic function of vitamin E is as an antioxidant. It prevents damage to biologic membranes by protecting polyunsaturated fats within membrane phospholipids from oxidation.[32] It accomplishes this task by preferentially binding to peroxyl radicals and forming the corresponding organic hydroperoxide and tocopheroxyl radical, which, in turn, interacts with other antioxidant compounds, such as ascorbic acid, thereby regenerating tocopherol. Vitamin E may be responsible for cell growth and proliferation by combating the inhibitory effects of lipid peroxidation.[145] Vitamin E may have a negative role in the regulation of cellular proliferation through its nonoxidant properties, such as inhibition of protein kinase C activity.[145]

Large amounts of vitamin E, ranging from 400–800 IU/d (400–800 mg/d) for months to years, were previously thought to be without apparent harm.[43] Vitamin E supplementation results in few obvious adverse effects, even at doses as high as 3200 mg/d (3200 IU/d).[19] In several species, the oral median lethal dose was 2000 mg/kg (2000 IU/kg) or more, and significant adverse effects were observed only when daily doses were >1000 mg/kg (>1000 IU/kg), equivalent to 200–500 mg/kg (200–500 IU/kg) in humans.[146] However, a meta-analysis reveals that all cause mortality may increase at doses ≥400 IU/d (≥400 mg/d).[147]

PATHOPHYSIOLOGY

In vitro studies demonstrate that vitamin E in high doses may have a paradoxical pro-oxidant effect.[2,30,147] The pro-oxidant effect of vitamin E on LDLs is related to the production of α-tocopheroxyl radicals, which normally are inhibited by other antioxidants such as vitamin C. High doses of vitamin E may displace other antioxidants, thereby disrupting the natural balance of the antioxidant system and increasing vulnerability to oxidative damage.[100] High doses of vitamin E may inhibit human cytosolic glutathione *S*-transferases, enzymes that are active in the detoxification of drugs and endogenous toxins.[206]

CLINICAL MANIFESTATIONS

Gastrointestinal symptoms, including nausea and gastric distress, were reported in patients who had received vitamin E 2,000–2,500 IU/d (2000–2500 mg/d).[92,216] Diarrhea and abdominal cramps were reported in patients who received a dose of 3200 IU/d (3200 mg/d).[9] Reports of other adverse effects, including fatigue, weakness, emotional changes, thrombophlebitis, increased serum creatinine concentration, and decreased thyroid hormone concentrations, have not been reproduced in other case series or clinical trials.[146]

The most significant toxic effect of vitamin E, at doses exceeding 1000 IU/d (1000 mg/d), is its ability to antagonize the effects of vitamin K.[43] Vitamin E appears to increase the epoxidation of vitamin K to its inactive form, thereby increasing the vitamin K requirement severalfold.[19,210] Although high oral doses of vitamin E typically do not produce a coagulopathy in normal humans with adequate vitamin K stores, coagulopathy may develop in vitamin K–deficient patients or those taking warfarin.[19,42,62,210] Animal studies demonstrate that absorption of both vitamins A and K is impaired by large doses of vitamin E.[25,179]

Use of an IV vitamin E preparation (E-Ferol) was associated with a severe epidemic of unexplained thrombocytopenia, renal dysfunction, hepatomegaly, cholestasis, ascites, hypotension, and metabolic acidosis in low-birth-weight infants in several neonatal intensive care units in the early 1980s.[29] Use of polysorbate 20 and polysorbate 80 for emulsification of lipids and fat-soluble vitamins in this IV vitamin E product was implicated as the cause of this syndrome, rather than vitamin E.

VITAMIN C

MW = 176.12 daltons
Therapeutic serum concentration = 0.4–2.0 mg/dL

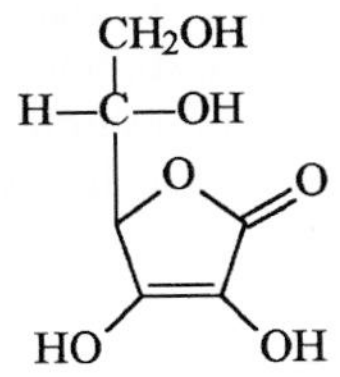

HISTORY AND EPIDEMIOLOGY

Vitamin C alone, also known as *ascorbic acid*, is ingested by approximately 12.4% of the United States adult population.[175] In the United States approximately 80.3% of men and 86.4% of women who take multiple dietary supplements also take vitamin C, making it one of the most widely consumed xenobiotics, in addition to a B-complex preparation, within this group.[28] Vitamin C has long been used as a preventative for the common cold. Interestingly, an extensive review of 14 studies of the role of vitamin C in the treatment of the common cold suggested that only eight were valid investigations, and none of the studies demonstrated any therapeutic benefit.[36] Its function as an antioxidant has led to its use for the prevention and treatment of cardiovascular disease and cancer. Human data from clinical trials have failed to demonstrate that vitamin C significantly reduces or prevents overall cardiovascular events or cancer. Vitamin C may have a role as a reducing agent in the treatment of idiopathic methemoglobinemia. However, it is less effective than standard treatment with methylene blue and therefore not employed.[136] Vitamin C is popularly used to promote wound healing, treat cataracts, combat chronic degenerative diseases, counteract the effects of aging, and increase mental attentiveness and decrease stress.[43,146] However, little, if any, objective data demonstrate a benefit of treatment for any of these indications.[43]

Vitamin C has long been associated with prevention of scurvy.[136] In 1747, James Lind, a physician in the British Royal Navy, analyzed the relationship between diet and scurvy and confirmed the protective and curative effects of citrus fruits. Vitamin C was isolated from cabbage in 1928 and subsequently shown in 1932 to be the active antiscorbutic factor in lemon juice. It was given the name *ascorbic acid* to indicate its role in preventing scurvy. Other dietary sources of vitamin C include tomatoes, strawberries, and potatoes. Today, those at risk for developing scurvy include the elderly, alcoholics, chronic drug users, and others with inadequate diets, including infants fed formula diets with insufficient concentrations of vitamin C.[136] Symptoms include gingivitis, poor wound healing, bleeding, and petechiae and ecchymoses. Musculoskeletal symptoms consisting of arthralgias, myalgias, hemarthrosis, and muscular hematomas develop in 80% of cases.[61] Children experience severe pain in their lower limbs secondary to subperiosteal bleeding.[61]

PHARMACOLOGY AND TOXICOKINETICS

Following ingestion, intestinal absorption of vitamin C occurs via an active transport system that is saturable.[177] The absorptive capacity is reached with ingestions of approximately 3 g/d, and vitamin C dietary supplements are commonly taken in doses of 500 mg/d. When given as a single oral dose, absorption decreases from 75% at 1 g to 20% at 5 g. Vitamin C is distributed from the plasma to all cells in the body. Tissue uptake is also a saturable process.[146] Metabolic degradation of vitamin C to oxalate accounts for 30%–40% of oxalate excreted daily.[84] Because absorption and metabolic conversion are saturable, large ingestions of vitamin C should not significantly increase oxalate production.[189] Only a small amount of vitamin C is filtered through the glomeruli, and tubular resorption, a saturable process that may compete with uric acid, usually is almost complete.[22] Plasma concentrations of vitamin C typically are maintained at approximately 1 mg/dL. The kidney efficiently eliminates excess vitamin C as unchanged ascorbic acid.

Vitamin C is a cofactor in several hydroxylation and amidation reactions by functioning as a reducing agent.[126,127] As a result, vitamin C plays an important role in the synthesis of collagen, carnitine, folinic acid, and norepinephrine. It also influences the processing of hormones such as oxytocin, antidiuretic hormone, and cholecystokinin. Vitamin C reduces iron from the ferric to the ferrous state in the stomach, thereby increasing intestinal absorption of iron. Vitamin C may be involved in steroidogenesis in the adrenals. Vitamin C also has a pro-oxidant effect in vivo.[170] This effect is not believed to occur at doses <500 mg/d but may occur in the setting of overdose.

CLINICAL MANIFESTATIONS

The possibility of oxalate nephrolithiasis is not a significant clinical concern.[76] Nevertheless, conflicting studies and reports regarding the association between vitamin C overdose and the development of oxalosis exist. Some reports of high urine oxalate concentrations likely were erroneous because of conversion of ascorbate to oxalate in alkaline urine samples left standing after collection.[11,213] Individual case reports documenting the presence of oxalate stones in the setting of vitamin C overdose often have involved either IV administration or patients with chronic renal failure.[14,75,121,139,146,199] A prospective study on the risk of kidney stones in men did not support an association between high daily vitamin C intake and stone formation.[44] This was also demonstrated in a study involving daily ingestion of 4 g of ascorbic acid for 5 days in healthy men in which there was no increase in urinary oxalate excretion.[11] Another study did show increased rates of oxalate absorption and endogenous synthesis contributing to hyperoxaluria, but this effect was found in individuals with a prior history of renal calcium oxalate stones and not in individuals without a prior history of calcium oxalate stones.[35] In contrast, other reports show an increase in urinary oxalate and calcium oxalate crystallization following ingestion of high doses of calcium in both stone-formers and non-stone-formers.[16,138] Gastrointestinal tract effects of high doses of vitamin C may include localized esophagitis, given prolonged mucosal contact with ascorbic acid, and an osmotic diarrhea.[98,212]

VITAMIN B_6

MW = 169 daltons
Therapeutic serum concentration = 3.6–18 ng/mL

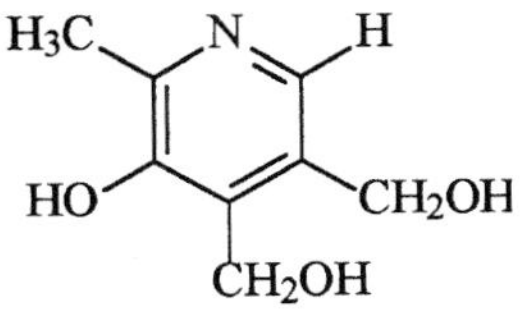

HISTORY

Pyridoxine, pyridoxal, and pyridoxamine are related compounds that have the same physiologic properties. Although all three compounds are included in the term *vitamin B_6*, the vitamin has been assigned the name *pyridoxine*. This vitamin was discovered in 1936 as the water-soluble factor whose deficiency was responsible for the development of dermatitis in rats.[136] In humans, deficiency is characterized by a seborrheic dermatitis around the eyes, nose, and mouth, cheilosis, stomatitis, glossitis, and blepharitis.[193] More importantly, pyridoxine deficiency is associated with seizures.

Pyridoxine is found in several foods, including meat, liver, whole-grain breads and cereals, soybeans, and vegetables.[136] Deficiency should not occur in humans who eat a well-balanced diet.[193]

Pyridoxine is popularly used as a component of bodybuilding regimens and for treatment of premenstrual syndrome and carpal tunnel syndrome.[1,56] High doses have been used for treatment of schizophrenia and autism with variable results.[68,125]

PHARMACOLOGY

All forms of vitamin B_6 are well absorbed from the intestinal tract. Pyridoxine is rapidly metabolized to pyridoxal, pyridoxal phosphate (PLP), and 4-pyridoxic acid.[222] PLP accounts for approximately 60% of circulating vitamin B_6 and is the primary form that crosses cell membranes.[136] Most vitamin B_6 is renally excreted as 4-pyridoxic acid, with only 7% excreted unchanged in the urine.[136,222] Experiments in anephric rats demonstrate an up to 10-fold increase in susceptibility to pyridoxine-induced neurotoxicity, suggesting a need for caution when prescribing pyridoxine to patients with renal failure.[128]

PLP is the active form of vitamin B_6. It is a coenzyme required for the synthesis of γ-aminobutyric acid (GABA), an inhibitory neurotransmitter. Decreased GABA formation in the setting of pyridoxine deficiency may contribute to seizures.[136] Isoniazid and other hydrazines inhibit the enzyme responsible for conversion of pyridoxine to PLP[96] (see Chap. 57). Therefore, pyridoxine should be administered concomitantly with isoniazid. Seizures resulting from isoniazid overdose often are successfully treated with pyridoxine (see A15: Pyridoxine).

PATHOPHYSIOLOGY

Interestingly, like pyridoxine deficiency, pyridoxine toxicity is characterized by neurologic effects. The pathophysiology of pyridoxine neurotoxicity is not well defined. However, studies indicate that the mammalian peripheral sensory nervous system is vulnerable to large doses of pyridoxine.[186] Histopathology in dogs reveals sensory distal axonopathy with relative sparing of the cell body.[97] Peripheral sensory nerves may be particularly vulnerable to circulating xenobiotics because of the permeability of their associated blood vessels.[186] Compared to the CNS, these nerves lack the blood–brain barrier. In addition, the nerves of the CNS may be relatively shielded from pyridoxine toxicity because pyridoxine is transported into the CNS by a saturable mechanism.[186]

CLINICAL MANIFESTATIONS

Chronic overdoses are associated with progressive sensory ataxia and severe distal impairment of proprioception and vibratory sensation. Touch, pain, and temperature sensation may be minimally impaired, and reflexes may be diminished or absent. These findings were first described in 1983 in a case series of seven patients who were taking pyridoxine 2–6 g/d for 2–40 months for premenstrual syndrome.[186] Nerve conduction and somatosensory studies in these patients showed dysfunction in the distal sensory peripheral nerves. Nerve biopsy showed widespread, nonspecific axonal degeneration. This syndrome has since been reported with pyridoxine doses as low as 200 mg/d.[166] Among 26 patients with elevated serum pyridoxine concentrations, the most common symptoms reported were numbness (96%), burning pain (49.9%), tingling (57.7%), balance difficulties (30.7%), and weakness (7.8%).[188] In most cases, symptoms gradually improved over several months with abstinence from pyridoxine. However, symptoms may still progress for 2–3 weeks after pyridoxine discontinuation.[21]

Acute neurotoxicity may occur when a massive amount of pyridoxine is administered as a single dose or given over a few days.[4] Large overdoses of pyridoxine are associated with incoordination, ataxia, seizures, and death.[204] Administration of IV pyridoxine 2 g/kg in two patients for the treatment of mushroom poisoning resulted in permanent dorsal root and sensory ganglia deficits.[4]

NICOTINIC ACID

MW	= 123 daltons
Therapeutic concentration	= not determined

N
COOH

HISTORY

Nicotinic acid, or niacin, was discovered to be an essential dietary component in the early 1900s.[79] A deficiency of this vitamin, also known as vitamin B_3, causes pellagra, which is characterized by dermatitis, diarrhea, and dementia. This disease had been prevalent for centuries in countries that heavily relied on maize as a dietary staple until it was determined that pellagra could be prevented by increasing dietary intake of fresh eggs, milk, and fresh meat, including liver.[136] Other food sources of nicotinic acid include fish, poultry, nuts, legumes, and whole-grain and enriched breads and cereals. Supplementation of flour with nicotinic acid in 1939 probably is responsible for the near eradication of this disease in the United States. Chronic alcohol users still develop pellagra, likely secondary to malnutrition.

Niacin was introduced as a treatment for hyperlipidemia in 1955.[7] Nicotinic acid reduces triglyceride synthesis, with a resultant drop in very-low-density lipoprotein cholesterol and LDL cholesterol and a rise in high-density-lipoprotein cholesterol.[79] Therapy usually is started with single doses of 100–250 mg. Frequency of dose and total daily dose are gradually increased until a dose of 1.5–2.0 g/d is reached. If the LDL cholesterol concentration is not sufficiently decreased with this dosing regimen, the dose is further increased to 3.0 g/d. These doses of niacin are 100-fold higher than the amount necessary to meet adult nutritional needs.[174]

More recently, the nonmedicinal use of niacin for the purpose of altering or masking the results of urine testing for illicit drugs was noted.[34,150] However, there is no evidence that ingestion of niacin is capable of this effect.

PHARMACOLOGY AND TOXICOKINETICS

Nicotinic acid is well absorbed from the intestinal tract and is distributed to all tissues. With therapeutic dosing, little unchanged vitamin is excreted in the urine. When extremely high doses are ingested, the unchanged vitamin is the major urinary component. Nicotinic acid ultimately is converted to nicotinamide adenine dinucleotide (NAD^+) and nicotinamide adenine dinucleotide phosphate ($NADP^+$), which are the physiologically active forms of this vitamin. NADH and NADPH act as coenzymes for proteins that catalyze oxidation–reduction reactions that are essential for tissue respiration.[136]

CLINICAL MANIFESTATIONS

The most common adverse effects associated with niacin use are vasodilatory such as cutaneous flushing and pruritus. These effects may occur at doses of 0.5–1.0 g/d.[141] Symptoms are caused by the production of prostaglandin D2 and E2 via the G protein–coupled receptor, GPR109A.[20] Flushing occurs because of the predilection for the skin as a source of prostaglandin production after niacin ingestion.[197] Prostaglandins D2 and E2 act on receptors DP1 and EP2/4 in dermal capillaries causing vasodilation.[110] Vasodilatory side effects occur in up to 100% of patients, particularly when given an immediate-release form of niacin.[141] Although tolerance to flushing usually develops over several weeks, 25%–40% of patients discontinue niacin use because of vasodilatory symptoms.[46,141,174] A dose of 325 mg of aspirin taken 30 minutes before ingestion of niacin diminishes flushing.[218] This is because aspirin inhibits cyclooxygenase thereby decreasing production of prostaglandins.

Recent in vitro studies demonstrate that methylnicotinate induces serotonin release from human platelets in addition to prostaglandin D2 release from human mast cells.[161] Also, animal studies demonstrate the ability of various serotonin antagonists including cyproheptadine to inhibit the niacin-induced temperature increase, associated with flush, by 90%.[161] Flavanoids are being studied as a potential treatment for niacin flush due to their ability to inhibit both niacin-induced plasma prostaglandin D2 and serotonin increase in a rat model.[162] In a small human study, a dietary supplement containing 150 mg of the flavanoid quercetin decreased the severity and longevity of erythema and burning sensation scores on a visual scale.[109]

Other strategies for reduced flushing include dosing with meals, and avoidance of alcohol, hot beverages, spicy foods, and hot baths or showers close to or after dosing.[46] Flushing may also be decreased by starting at a low dose and gradually increasing to the full dose. Tolerance to flushing may develop after several weeks, but flushing will recur if doses are missed.

Because rapid absorption of niacin seems to be related to development of flushing, modified time-release preparations of niacin were developed. Unfortunately, these preparations are more likely to produce gastrointestinal side effects, such as epigastric distress, nausea, and diarrhea.[141] In addition, niacin-induced hepatotoxicity occurs more frequently and is more severe in patients treated with modified-release niacin rather than immediate-release niacin.[39,174] Elevated liver enzyme concentrations may occur with doses as low as 1 g/d, whereas symptoms of hepatic dysfunction occur at doses of 2–3 g/d.[141] These patients may have elevated serum bilirubin and ammonia concentrations and a prolonged prothrombin time. They may present with fatigue, anorexia, nausea, vomiting, and jaundice. In most cases, liver function improves following niacin withdrawal.[58,141] Severe cases have progressed to fulminant hepatic failure and hepatic encephalopathy.[40,93,151] Niacin also causes amblyopia, hyperglycemia, hyperuricemia, coagulopathy, myopathy, and hyperpigmentation.[90]

SUMMARY

Healthy adults consuming a well-balanced diet do not require vitamin supplementation. However, vitamins are popularly believed to be a panacea and are commonly taken in supraphysiologic doses. Because the therapeutic index is large, toxicity generally does not develop unless very large doses are taken for sustained periods. Physicians should consider hypervitaminosis in the differential diagnosis when patients present with symptomatology consistent with a vitamin toxicity syndrome. A thorough history, with emphasis on diet and prescribed and supplemental vitamin use, is important.

ACKNOWLEDGMENT

Richard J. Hamilton contributed to this chapter in a previous edition.

REFERENCES

1. Abraham GE, Hargrove JT: Effect of vitamin B_6 on premenstrual symptomatology in women with premenstrual tension syndrome: a double-blind crossover study. *Infertility*. 1980;3:155-165.
2. Abudu N, Miller JJ, Attaelmannan M, Levinson SS: Vitamins in human arteriosclerosis with emphasis on vitamin C and vitamin E. *Clin Chim Acta*. 2004;339:11-25.
3. Adverse effects with isotretinoin. *FDA Drug Bull*. 1983;13:1-3.
4. Albin RL, Alpers JW, Greenberg HS, et al: Acute sensory neuropathy from pyridoxine overdose. *Neurology*. 1987;37:1729-1732.
5. Allain HJ, Weintraub M: Drug-induced headache. *Ration Drug Ther*. 1980; 14:1-6.
6. Allen LH, Haskell M: Estimating the potential for vitamin A toxicity in women and young children. *J Nutr*. 2002;132:2907S-2919S
7. Altschul R, Hoffer A, Stephen JD: Influence of nicotinic acid on serum cholesterol in man. *Arch Biochem Biophys*. 1955;54:558-559.
8. AMA Council on Scientific Affairs: Vitamin preparations as dietary supplements and as therapeutic agents. *JAMA*. 1987;257:1929-1936.
9. Anderson TW, Reid DBW: A double-blind trial of vitamin E in angina pectoris. *Am J Clin Nutr*. 1974;27:1174-1178.
10. Archer CB, Cerio R, Griffiths WAD: Etretinate and acquired kinking of the hair. *Br J Dermatol*. 1987;12:239.
11. Auer BL, Auer D, Rodgers AL: The effect of ascorbic acid ingestion on the biochemical and physicochemical risk factors associated with calcium oxalate kidney stone formation. *Clin Chem Lab Med*. 1998;36:143-147.
12. Autret E, Berjot M, Jonville-Bera A, et al: Anophthalmia and agenesis of optic chiasma associated with adapalene gel in early pregnancy. *Lancet*. 1997;350:339.
13. Azizi E, Zaidman JL, Eshchar J, Szeinberg A: Abetalipoproteinemia treated with parenteral and oral vitamins A and E, and with medium chain triglycerides. *Acta Paediatr Scand*. 1978;67:797-801.
14. Balcke P, Schmidt P, Zazzgornik J, et al: Ascorbic acid aggravates secondary hyperoxalemia in patients on chronic hemodialysis. *Ann Intern Med*. 1984;101:344-345.
15. Bauernfeind JC: The safe use of vitamin A. A report of the International Vitamin A Consultative Group. Washington Nutrition Foundation. 1980;1-44.
16. Baxmann AC, De O G Mendonca C, Heilberg IP: Effect of vitamin C supplements on urinary oxalate and pH in calcium stone-forming patients. *Kidney Int*. 2003;63:1066-1071.
17. Beaton GH, Martorell R, L'Abbe KA, et al: Effectiveness of vitamin A supplementation in the control of young child morbidity and mortality in developing countries. ACC/SCN Nutrition Policy Discussion Paper. 1993;13:1-120.
18. Bendich A, Langseth L: Safety of vitamin A. *Am J Clin Nutr*. 1989;49: 358-371.
19. Bendich A, Machlin LJ: Safety of oral intake of vitamin E. *Am J Clin Nutr*. 1998;48:612-619.
20. Benyo Z, Gille A, Kero J, et al: GPR109A (PUMA-G/HM74A) mediates nicotinic acid-induced flushing. *J Clin Invest*. 2005;115:3634-3640.
21. Berger AR, Schaumberg HH, Schroeder C, et al: Dose response, coasting, and differential fiber vulnerability in human toxic neuropathy: a prospective study of pyridoxine neurotoxicity. *Neurology*. 1992;42:1367-1370.
22. Berger L, Gerson CD, Yu T: The effect of ascorbic acid on uric acid excretion with a commentary on the renal handling of ascorbic acid. *Am J Med*. 1977;62:71-76.
23. Bergman SM, O'Mailia J, Krane NK, Wallin JD: Vitamin A-induced hypercalcemia: response to corticosteroids. *Nephron*. 1988;50:362-364.

24. Bernstein AL, Leventhal-Rochon JL: Neurotoxicity related to the use of topical tretinoin (Retin-A). *Ann Intern Med.* 1996;124:227-228.
25. Bieri JG, Corash L, Hubbard VS: Medical uses of vitamin E. *N Engl J Med.* 1983;306:1063-1070.
26. Biesalski HK, Nohr D: New aspects in vitamin A metabolism: the role of retinyl esters as systemic and local sources for retinol in mucous epithelia. *J. Nutr.* 2004;134:3453S-3457S.
27. Binkley N, Krueger D: Hypervitaminosis A and bone. *Nutr Rev.* 2000; 58:138-144.
28. Block G, Jensen CD, Norkus EP, et al: Usage patterns, health, and nutritional status of long-term multiple dietary supplement users: a cross-sectional study. *Nutr J.* 2007; 6:30.
29. Bove KE, Kosmetatos N, Wedig KE, et al: Vasculopathic hepatotoxicity associated with E-Ferol syndrome in low-birth-weight infants. *JAMA.* 1985;254:2422-2430.
30. Bowry VW, Stocker R: Tocopherol-mediated peroxidation. The prooxidant effect of vitamin E on the radical initiated oxidation of human low-density lipoprotein. *J Am Chem Soc.* 1993;115:6029-6044.
31. Brown BG, Crowley J: Is there any hope for vitamin E? *JAMA.* 2005;293: 1387-1390.
32. Burton GW, Joyce A, Ingold KU: Is vitamin E the only lipid-soluble, chain-breaking antioxidant in human blood plasma and erythrocyte membranes? *Arch Biochem Biophys.* 1983;221:281-290.
33. Camera G, Pregliasco P: Ear malformation in baby born to mother using tretinoin cream. *Lancet.* 1992;339:687.
34. Centers for Disease Control and Prevention: Use of niacin in attempts to defeat urine drug testing—five states, January-September 2006. MMWR *Morb Mortal Wkly Rep.* 2007;56:365-366.
35. Chai W, Liebman M, Kynast-Gales S, Massey L: Oxalate absorption and endogenous oxalate synthesis from ascorbate in calcium oxalate stone formers and non-stone formers. *Am J Kidney Dis.* 2004;44:1060-1069.
36. Chalmers TC: Effect of ascorbic in the common cold: an evaluation of the evidence. *Am J Med.* 1975;58:532-536.
37. Chesney RW: Modified vitamin D compounds in the treatment of certain bone diseases. In: Spiller GA, ed: *Nutritional Pharmacology.* New York, AR USS, 1981, pp. 147-201.
38. Chiu YK, Lai MS, Ho JC, Chen JB: Acute fish liver intoxication: report of three cases. *Changgeng Yi Xue Za Zhi.* 1999;22:468-473.
39. Christensen NA, Achor RWP, Berge KG, Mason HL: Nicotinic acid treatment of hypercholesteremia: comparison of plain and sustained-action preparations and report of two cases of jaundice. *JAMA.* 1961;177:546-550.
40. Clementz GL, Holmes AW: Nicotinic acid-induced fulminant hepatic failure. *J Clin Gastroenterol.* 1989;9:582-584.
41. Committee on Recommended Dietary Allowances: Report of Food and Nutritional Board, 10th ed. Washington, DC: National Academy of Sciences, National Research Council; 1989: 62-63.
42. Corrigan JJ: The effect of vitamin E on warfarin-induced vitamin K deficiency. *Ann N Y Acad Sci.* 1982;393:361-368.
43. Council on Scientific Affairs: Vitamin preparations as dietary supplements and as therapeutic agents. *JAMA.* 1987;257:1929-1936.
44. Curhan GC, Willett WC, Rimm EB, Stampfer MJ: A prospective study of the intake of vitamins C and B_6 and the risk of kidney stones in men. *J Urol.* 1996;155:1847-1851.
45. David M, Hodak E, Lowe NJ: Adverse effects of retinoids. *Med Toxicol.* 1988;3:273-288.
46. Davidson MH: Niacin use and cutaneous flushing: mechanisms and strategies for prevention. *Am J Cardiol.* 2008;101:14B-19B.
47. Davies M, Adams PH: The continuing risk of vitamin D intoxication. *Lancet.* 1978;2:621-623.
48. Davis BH, Pratt BM, Madei JA: Retinol and extracellular collagen matrices modulate hepatic Ito cell collagen phenotype and cellular retinal binding protein levels. *J Biol Chem.* 1987;262:280-286.
49. Davis BH, Vucic A: The effect of retinol on Ito cell proliferation in vitro. *Hepatology.* 1988;8:788-793.
50. DeLuca HF: The vitamin D system in the regulation of calcium and phosphorus metabolism. *Nutr Rev.* 1979;37:161-193.
51. Diaz MN, Frei B, Vita JA, Keaney JF Jr: Antioxidants and atherosclerotic heart disease. *N Engl J Med.* 1997;337:408-416.
52. Doireau V, Macher MA, Brun P, et al: Vitamin A poisoning revealed by hypercalcemia in a child with kidney failure. *Arch Pediatr.* 1996;3:888-890.
53. Down PF, Polak A, Regan RJ: A family with massive acute vitamin D intoxication. *Postgrad Med J.* 1979;55:897-902.
54. Elias PM, Williams ML: Retinoids, cancer and the skin. *Arch Dermatol.* 1981;117:160-280.
55. Ellis CN, Voorhees JJ: Etretinate therapy. *J Am Acad Derm.* 1987;16: 267-291.
56. Ellis J, Folkers K, Levy M, et al: Therapy with vitamin B_6 with and without surgery for treatment of patients having the idiopathic carpal tunnel syndrome. *Res Commun Chem Pathol Pharmacol.* 1981;33:331-344.
57. E-Siong T: The medical importance of vitamin A and carotenoids (with particular reference to developing countries) and their determination. *Mal J Nutr.* 1995;1:179-230,
58. Etchason JA, Miller TD, Squires RW, et al: Niacin-induced hepatitis: a potential side effect with low-dose time-release niacin. *Mayo Clin Proc.* 1991;66:23-28.
59. Evans HM, Emerson OH, Emerson GA: The isolation from wheat germ oil of an alcohol, α-tocopherol, having properties of vitamin E. *J Biol Chem.* 1936;113:329-332.
60. Evans HM, Vishop KS: On the relationship between fertility and nutrition. II. The ovulation rhythm in the rat on inadequate nutritional regimes. *J Metab Res.* 1922;1:319-356.
61. Fain O: Musculoskeletal manifestations of scurvy. *Joint Bone Spine.* 2005;72:124-128.
62. Farrell PM, Bieri JC: Megavitamin E supplementation in man. *Am J Clin Nutr.* 1975;18:1381-1386.
63. Fenaux P, Chastang C, Sanx M, et al: ATRA followed by chemotherapy versus ATRA plus chemotherapy and the role of maintenance therapy in newly diagnosed APL: first interim results of APL93 trial. *Blood.* 1997;90(Suppl 1):122a.
64. Fenaux P, De Botton S: Retinoic acid syndrome: recognition, prevention, and management. *Drug Saf.* 1998;18:273-279.
65. Fenaux P, Wang ZZ, Degos L: Treatment of acute promyelocytic leucemia by retinoids. *Curr Top Microbiol Immunol.* 2007;313:101-128.
66. Ferguson MM, Simpson NB, Hammersley N: Severe nail dystrophy associated with retinoid therapy. *Lancet.* 1983;2:974.
67. Feskanich D, Singh V, Willett WC, Colditz GA: Vitamin A intake and hip fractures among postmenopausal women. *JAMA.* 2002;287:47-54.
68. Findling RL, Maxwell K, Scotese-Wojtila L, et al: High-dose pyridoxine and magnesium administration in children with autistic disorder: an absence of salutary effects in a double-blind, placebo-controlled study. *J Autism Dev Disord.* 1997;27:467-478.
69. Fiore LD, Scola MA, Cantillon CE, Brophy MT: Anaphylactoid reactions to vitamin K. *J Thrombosis Thrombolysis.* 2001;11:175-183.
70. Fishman RA: Polar bear liver, vitamin A, aquaporins, and pseudotumor cerebri. *Ann Neurol.* 2002;52:531-533.
71. Flynn WJ, Freeman PG, Wickboldt LG: Pancreatitis associated with isotretinoin-induced hypertriglyceridemia. *Ann Intern Med.* 1987;106:63.
72. Foged EK, Jocobson FK: Side effects due to Ro-9359 (Tigason): a retrospective study. *Dermatologica.* 1982;164:395-403.
73. Food and Nutrition Board, Institute of Medicine—National Academy of Sciences: Dietary reference intakes: vitamins. Available at http://fnic.nal.usda.gov/nal. Last accessed January 12, 2009.
74. Fraser DR: Vitamin D. *Lancet.* 1995;345:104-107.
75. Friedman AL, Chesney RW, Gilchrist KW, et al: Secondary oxalosis as a complication of parenteral alimentation in acute renal failure. *Am J Nephrol.* 1983;3:248-252.
76. Garewal HS, Diplock AT: How "safe" are antioxidant vitamins? *Drug Saf.* 1995;13:8-14.
77. Gerber A, Raab AP, Sobel AE: Vitamin A poisoning in adults with description of a case. *Am J Med.* 1954;16:729-745.
78. Geubel A, De Galocsy C, Alves N, et al: Liver damage caused by therapeutic vitamin A administration. Estimate of dose-related toxicity in 41 cases. *Gastroenterology.* 1991;100:1701-1709.
79. Gibbons LW, Gonzalez V, Gordon N, Grundy S: The prevalence of side effects with regular and sustained-release nicotinic acid. *Am J Med.* 1995;99:378-385.
80. Gjerris F, Sorensen PS, Vorstrup S, Paulson OB: Intracranial pressure, conductance to cerebrospinal fluid outflow, and cerebral blood flow in patients with benign intracranial hypertension (pseudotumor cerebri). *Ann Neurol.* 1985;17:158-162.
81. Goldstein JA, Socha-Szott A, Thomsen RS, et al: Comparative effect of isotretinoin and etretinate on acne and sebaceous gland secretion. *J Am Acad Dermatol.* 1982;6:760-765.
82. Grassnor AM, Bachem MG: Cellular sources of noncollagenous matrix proteins: role of fat-storing cells in fibrogenesis. *Semin Liver Dis.* 1990;10:30-45.

83. Haddad JG: Vitamin D: solar rays, the Milky Way or both? *N Engl J Med.* 1992;326:1213-1215.
84. Hagler L, Herman RH: Oxalate metabolism, II: Urinary oxalate and the diet. *Am J Clin Nutr.* 1973;26:758-765, 882-889.
85. Hall JG: Vitamin A: A newly recognized human teratogen—harbinger of things to come? *J Pediatr.* 1984:105:583-584.
86. Hall JG: Vitamin A teratogenicity. *N Engl J Med.* 1984;311:797-798.
87. Heart Protection Collaborative Study Group: MRC/BHF Heart Protection Study of antioxidant vitamin supplementation in 20,536 "high-risk" individuals: a randomized placebo-controlled trial. *Lancet.* 2002; 360:23-33.
88. Hendriks HF, Bosma A, Brouwer A: Fat-storing cells: hyper- and hypovitaminosis A and the relationships with liver fibrosis. *Semin Liver Dis.* 1993;13:72-79.
89. Hendriks HF, Verhoofstad WA, Brouwer A, et al: Perisinusoidal fat-storing cells are the main vitamin A storage sites in rat liver. *Exp Cell Res.* 1985;160:138-149.
90. Henkin Y, Oberman A, Hurst DC, Segrest JP: Niacin revisited: clinical observations on an important but underutilized drug. *Am J Med.* 1991;91:239-246.
91. Hennekens CH, Buring JE, Manson JE, et al: Lack of effect of long-term supplementation with beta carotene on the incidence of malignant neoplasms and cardiovascular disease. *N Engl J Med.* 1996;334:1145-1149.
92. Hillman RW: Tocopherol excess in man: creatinuria associated with prolonged ingestion. *Am J Clin Nutr.* 1957;5:597-600.
93. Hodis HN: Acute hepatic failure associated with the use of low-dose sustained-release niacin. *JAMA.* 1990;264:181.
94. Holick MF, Shao Q, Liu WW, Chen TC: The vitamin D content of fortified milk and infant formula. *N Engl J Med.* 1992;327:1637-1642.
95. Holick MF: Vitamin D: photobiology, metabolism, and clinical applications. In: DeGroot L, Besser H, Burger HG, et al, eds: *Endocrinology*, 3rd ed. Philadelphia: WB Saunders; 1995: 990-1013.
96. Holtz P, Palm D: Pharmacological aspects of vitamin B_6. *Pharmacol Rev.* 1964;16:113-178.
97. Hoover DM, Carlton WW, Henrikson CK: Ultrastructural lesions of pyridoxine toxicity in beagle dogs. *Vet Pathol.* 1981;18:769-777.
98. Hoyt CJ: Diarrhea from vitamin C. *JAMA.* 1980;244:1674.
99. Hruban Z, Russell RM, Boyer JL: Ultrastructural changes in livers of two patients with hypervitaminosis A. *Am J Pathol.* 1974;76:451-468.
100. Huang HY, Appel LJ: Supplementation of diets with alpha-tocopherol reduces serum concentrations of gamma- and delta-tocopherol in humans. *J Nutr.* 2003;133:3137-3140.
101. Huldschinsky K: Heilung von Rachitis durch Kunstliche Hohensonne. *Dtsch Med Wochenschr.* 1919;14:712-713.
102. Iliff P, Humphrey J, Mahomva A: Tolerance of large doses of vitamin A given to mothers and their babies shortly after delivery. *Nutr Res.* 1999;129:1437-1446.
103. Inkeles SB, Connor WE, Illingworth DR: Hepatic and dermatologic manifestations of chronic hypervitaminosis A in adults. Report of two cases. *Am J Med.* 1986;80:491-496.
104. Jacobson DM, Berg R, Wall M, et al: Serum vitamin A concentration is elevated in idiopathic intracranial hypertension. *Neurology.* 1999;53:1114-1118.
105. Jacobus CH, Holick MF, Shao Q, et al: Hypervitaminosis D associated with drinking milk. *N Engl J Med.* 1992;326:1173-1177.
106. Jacques EA, Buschmann RJ, Layden TJ: The histopathologic progression of vitamin A-induced hepatic injury. *Gastroenterology.* 1979;76:599-602.
107. Jick SS, Terris BZ, Jick H: First trimester topical tretinoid and congenital disorders. *Lancet.* 1993;341:1181-1182.
108. Johnson JA, Kumar R: Renal and intestinal calcium transport. Role of vitamin D and vitamin D-dependent calcium binding proteins. *Semin Nephrol.* 1994;14:119-1128.
109. Kalogeromitros D, Makris M, Chliva D, et al: A quercetin containing supplement reduces niacin-induced flush in humans. *Int J Immunopathol Pharmacol.* 2008; 21:509-514.
110. Kamanna VS, Vo A, Kashyap ML: Nicotinic acid: recent developments. *Curr Opin Cardiol.* 2008; 23:393-398.
111. Karner P, Helfenstein A, Wehrli H, WettsteinA: Pflanzenfabstoffe, XXV: uber die Konstitution des Lycopins und Carotins. *Helv Chim Acta.* 1930;13:1084-1099.
112. Kent G, Gay S, Inouye T: Vitamin A containing lipocytes and formation of type III collagen in liver injury. *Proc Natl Acad Sci USA.* 1976;73: 3719-3722.
113. Kimberg DV, Baerg RD, Gershon E, et al: Effect of cortisone treatment on the active transport of calcium by the small intestine. *J Clin Invest.* 1971;50:1309-1321.
114. Kingston TP, Matt L, Lowe NJ: Etretin therapy for severe psoriasis. *Arch Dermatol.* 1987;123:55-58.
115. Klar FH, Beyer CW, Ramanathan M, et al: Cerebrospinal fluid dynamics in patients with pseudotumor cerebri. *Neurosurgery.* 1979;5:208-216.
116. Klaunig JE, Kamendulis LM: The role of oxidative stress in carcinogenesis. *Annu Rev Pharmacol Toxicol.* 2004;44:239-267.
117. Kowalski TE, Falestiny M, Furth E, Malet PF: Vitamin A hepatotoxicity. A cautionary note regarding 25,000 IU supplements. *Am J Med.* 1994;97:523-528.
118. Kushi LH, Fee RM, Sellers TA, et al: Intakes of vitamins A, C, E and postmenopausal breast cancer. The Iowa Women's Health Study. *Am J Epidemiol.* 1996;144:165-174.
119. Lammer EJ, Chen DT, Hoar RM, et al: Retinoic acid embryopathy. *N Engl J Med.* 1985;313:837-841.
120. Landy D: Pibloktoq (hysteria) and Inuit nutrition: possible implication of hypervitaminosis A. *Soc Sci Med.* 1985;21:173-185.
121. Lawton JM, Conway LT, Crosson JT, et al: Acute oxalate nephropathy after massive ascorbic acid administration. *Arch Intern Med.* 1985;145:950-951.
122. Le-Coco F, Ammatuna E, Montesinos P, Sanz MA: Acute promyelocytic leucemia: recent advances in diagnosis and management. *Semin Oncol.* 2008;35:401-409.
123. Lee DC, Lee GY: The use of pamidronate for hypercalcemia secondary to acute vitamin D intoxication. *Clin Toxicol.* 1998; 36:719-721.
124. Lee KW, Cohen KL, Walters JB, Federman DG: Iatrogenic vitamin D intoxication. Report of a case and review of vitamin D physiology. *Connecticut Med.* 1999;63:399-403.
125. Lerner V, Miodownik C, Kaptsan A, et al: Vitamin B_6 as add-on treatment in chronic schizophrenic and schizoaffective patients: a double-blind, placebo-controlled study. *J Clin Psychiatry.* 2002;63:54-58.
126. Levine M, Cantilena CC, Dhariwal KR: In situ kinetics and ascorbic acid requirements. *World Rev Nutr Diet.* 1993;72:114-127.
127. Levine M: New concepts in the biology and biochemistry of ascorbic acid. *N Engl J Med.* 1986;314:892:902.
128. Levine S, Saltzman A: Pyridoxine (vitamin B_6) toxicity: enhancement by uremia in rats. *Food Chem Toxicol.* 2002;40:1449-1451.
129. Lipson AH, Collins F, Webster WS: Multiple congenital defects associated with maternal use of topical tretinoin. *Lancet.* 1993;341:1352-1353.
130. Love JM, Gudas LJ: Vitamin A, differentiation and cancer. *Curr Opin Cell Biol.* 1994;6:825-831.
131. Lysak WR, Svien HJ: Long term follow-up on patients with diagnosis of pseudotumor cerebri. *J Neurol Surg.* 1966;25:284-287.
132. Macapinlac M, Olson J: A lethal hypervitaminosis A syndrome in young monkeys following a single intramuscular dose of a water-miscible preparation containing vitamins A, D_2 and E. *Int J Vitam Nutr Res.* 1981;51:331-341.
133. Malm J, Kristensen B, Markgren P, Ekstedt J: CSF hydrodynamics in idiopathic intracranial hypertension: a long-term study. *Neurology.* 1992;42:851-858.
134. Mangelsdorf DJ, Umesomo K, Evans RM: The retinoid receptors. In: Sporn MB, Roberts AB, Goodman DS, eds: *The Retinoids: Biology, Chemistry, Medicine*, 2nd ed. New York: Raven Press; 1994: 573-595.
135. Marcus R: Agents affecting calcification and bone turnover: calcium, phosphate, parathyroid hormone, vitamin D, calcitonin, and other compounds. In: Hardman JG, Limbird LE, Gilman AG, eds: *The Pharmacological Basis of Therapeutics*, 10th ed. New York: McGraw-Hill; 2001: 1715-1752.
136. Marcus R, Coulston AM: Water-soluble vitamins: the vitamin B complex and ascorbic acid. In: Hardman JG, Limbird LE, Gilman AG, eds: The *Pharmacological Basis of Therapeutics*, 10th ed. New York: McGraw-Hill; 2001:1753-1771.
137. Marcus R, Coulston AM: Fat-soluble vitamins: vitamins A, K, and E. In: Hardman JG, Limbird LE, Gilman AG, eds: *The Pharmacological Basis of Therapeutics*, 10th ed. New York: McGraw-Hill; 2001:1773-1791.
138. Massey LK, Liebman M, Kynast-Gales SA: Ascorbate increases human oxaluria and kidney stone risk. *J Nutr.* 2005;135:1673-1677.
139. McAllister CJ: Renal failure secondary to massive infusion of vitamin C. *JAMA.* 1984;252:1684.
140. McCollum EV, Davis M: The necessity of certain lipids in the diet during growth. *J Biol Chem.* 1913;15:167-175.
141. McKenney JM, Proctor JD, Harris S, Chinchili VM: A comparison of the efficacy and toxic effects of sustained- vs immediate-release niacin in hypercholesterolemic patients. *JAMA.* 1994;271:672-677.
142. Melhus H, Michaelsson K, Kindmark A, et al: Excessive dietary in-take of vitamin A is associated with reduced bone mineral density and increased risk for hip fracture. *Ann Intern Med.* 1998;129:770-778.

143. Mellanby E: An experimental investigation of rickets. *Lancet.* 1919;1:407-412.
144. Mete E, Dilmen U, Energin M, et al: Calcitonin therapy in vitamin D intoxication. *J Trop Pediatr.* 1997;43:241-242.
145. Meydani M: Vitamin E. *Lancet.* 1995;345:170-175.
146. Meyers DG, Maloley PA, Weeks D: Safety of antioxidant vitamins. *Arch Intern Med.* 1996;156:925-935.
147. Miller, III ER, Pastor-Barriuso R, Dalal D, et al: Meta-analysis: High-dosage vitamin E supplementation may increase all-cause mortality. *Ann Intern Med.* 2005;142:37-46.
148. Mills CM, Marks R: Adverse reactions to oral retinoids: An update. *Drug Saf.* 1993;9:280-290.
149. Misselwitz J, Hesse V, Markestad T: Nephrocalcinosis, hypercalciuria and elevated serum levels of 1,25-dihydrovitamin D in children. *Acta Paediatr Scand.* 1990;79:637-643.
150. Mittal MK, Florin T, Perrone J, et al: Toxicity from the use of niacin to beat urine drug screening. *Ann Emerg Med.* 2007;50:587-590.
151. Mullin GE, Greenson JK, Mitchell MC: Fulminant hepatic failure after ingestion of sustained-release nicotinic acid. *Ann Intern Med.* 1989;111:253-255.
152. Nagai K, Hosaka H, Kubo S, et al: Vitamin A toxicity secondary to excessive intake of yellow-green vegetables, liver and laver. *J Hepatol.* 1999;31:142-148.
153. Naveh-Many T, Silver J: Regulation of parathyroid hormone gene expression by hypocalcemia, hypercalcemia, and vitamin D in the rat. *J Clin Invest.* 1990;86:1313-1319.
154. Ng, KW, Livesey SA, Collier F, et al: Effect of retinoids on the growth, ultrastructure, and cytoskeletal structures of malignant rat osteoblasts. *Cancer Res.* 1985;45:5106-5113.
155. Nordt SP, Williams SR, Clark RF: Pharmacologic misadventure resulting in hypercalcemia from vitamin D intoxication. *J Emerg Med.* 2002;22:302-303.
156. Omenn GS, Goodman GE, Thronquist MD, et al: Effects of a combination of beta-carotene and vitamin A on lung cancer and cardiovascular disease. *N Engl J Med.* 1996;334:1150-1155.
157. Ong D, Newcomer ME, Chytil F: Cellular retinoid binding proteins. In: Sporn MB, Roberts AB, Goodman DS, eds: *The Retinoids: Biology, Chemistry, Medicine*, 2nd ed. New York: Raven Press; 1994: 283-317.
158. Opotowsky AR, Bilezikian JP: Serum vitamin A concentration and the risk of hip fracture among women 50 to 74 years old in the United States: a prospective analysis of the NHANESI follow-up study. *Am J Med.* 2004;117:169-174.
159. Oreffo ROC, Teti A, Triffitt JT, et al: Effect of vitamin A on bone resorption: evidence for direct stimulation of isolated chicken osteoclasts by retinol and retinoic acid. *J Bone Miner Res.* 1988;3:203-209.
160. Osborne TB, Mendel LB: The relation of growth to the chemical constituents of the diet. *J Biol Chem.* 1913;15:311-326.
161. Papaliodis D, Boucher W, Kempuraj D, et al: Niacin-induced "flush" involves release of prostaglandin D2 from mast cells and serotonin from platelets: evidence from human cells in vitro and an animal model. *J Pharmacol Exp Ther.* 2008;327:665-672.
162. Papaliodis D, Boucher W, Kempuraj D, Theoharides TC: The flavanoid luteolin inhibits niacin-induced flush. *Br J Pharmacol.* 2008;153: 1382-1387.
163. Park EA: The therapy of rickets. *JAMA.* 1940;115:370-379.
164. Parker RS: Absorption, metabolism, and transport of carotenoids. *FASEB J.* 1996; 10:542-551.
165. Parker, S: Eskimo psychopathology in the context of Eskimo personality and culture. *Am Anthropol.* 1962;64:76-96.
166. Parry GJ, Bredesen DE: Sensory neuropathy with low dose pyridoxine. *Neurology.* 1985;35:1466-1468.
167. Patatanian E, Thompson DF: Retinoic acid syndrome: a review. *J Clin Pharm Ther.* 2008;33:331-338.
168. Paterson CR: Vitamin-D poisoning. Survey of causes in 21 patients with hypercalcaemia. *Lancet.* 1980;1:1164-1165.
169. Pettifor JM, Bikle DD, Cavaleros M, et al: Serum levels of free 1,25-dihydroxyvitamin D in vitamin D toxicity. *Ann Intern Med.* 1995;122:511-513.
170. Podmore ID, Griffiths HR, Herbert KE, et al: Vitamin C exhibits pro-oxidant properties. *Nature.* 1998;392:559.
171. Pols HA, Birkenhager JC, Foekens JA, van Leeuwen JP: Vitamin D: a modulator of cell proliferation and differentiation. *J Steroid Biochem Mol Biol.* 1990;37:873-876.
172. Prendiville J, Bingham EA, Burrows D: Premature epiphyseal closure—a complication of etretinate therapy in children. *J Am Acad Dermatol.* 1986;15:1259-1262.
173. Puig J, Corcoy R, Rodriguez-Espinosa J: Anemia secondary to vitamin D intoxication. *Ann Intern Med.* 1998;128:602-603.
174. Rader JI, Calvert RJ, Hathcock JN: Hepatic toxicity of unmodified and time-release preparations of niacin. *Am J Med.* 1992;92:77-81.
175. Radimer K, Bindewald B, Hughes J, et al: Dietary supplement use by US adults: data from the National Health and Nutrition Exam Survey, 1999-2000. *Am J Epidemiol.* 2004;160:339-349.
176. Rimm EB, Stampfer MJ, Ascherio A, et al: Vitamin E consumption and the risk of coronary heart disease in men. *N Engl J Med.* 1993;328:1450-1456.
177. Rivers JM: Safety of high-level vitamin C ingestion. *Ann N Y Acad Sci.* 1987;498:445-454.
178. Rizzoli R, Stoermann C, Ammann P, Bonjour J-P: Hypercalcemia and hyperosteolysis in vitamin D intoxication. Effects of clodronate therapy. *Bone.* 1994;15:193-198.
179. Roberts HJ: Perspective of vitamin E as therapy. *JAMA.* 1981;246:129-131.
180. Rodahl K, Moore T: The vitamin A content and toxicity of polar bear and seal liver. *Biochem J.* 1943;37:166-169.
181. Russel FE: Vitamin A content of polar bear liver. *Toxicon.* 1966;5:61-62.
182. Russel RM, Boyer JL, Bagheri SA, Hruban Z: Hepatic injury from chronic hypervitaminosis A resulting in portal hypertension and as-cites. *N Engl J Med.* 1974;291:435-440.
183. Sandgren ME, Bronnegard M, DeLuca HF: Tissue distribution of the 1,25-dihydroxyvitamin D_3 receptor in the male rat. *Biochem Biophys Res Commun.* 1991;181:611-616
184. Schafer S, Zerbe O, Gressner AM: The synthesis of proteoglycans in fat storing cells of rat liver. *Hepatology.* 1987;7:680-687.
185. Scharfman WB, Propp S: Anemia associated with vitamin D intoxication. *N Engl J Med.* 1956;255:1208-1212.
186. Schaumburg H, Kaplan J, Windebank A, et al: Sensory neuropathy from pyridoxine abuse: a new megavitamin syndrome. *N Engl J Med.* 1983;309:445-448.
187. Scheven BAA, Hamilton NJ: Retinoic acid and 1,25-dihydroxyvitamin D_3 stimulate osteoclast formation by different mechanisms. *Bone.* 1990;11:53-59.
188. Scott K, Zeris S, Kethari MJ: Elevated B6 levels and peripheral neuropathies. *Electromyogr Clin Neurophysiol.* 2008;48:219-223.
189. Sestili MA: Possible adverse health effects of vitamin C and ascorbic acid. *Semin Oncol.* 1983;10:299-304.
190. Shapiro L, Pastuszak A, Curto G, Koren G: Safety of first-trimester exposure to topical tretinoin: Prospective cohort study. *Lancet.* 1997;350: 1143-1144.
191. Sharieff GQ, Hanten K: Pseudotumor cerebri and hypercalcemia resulting from vitamin A toxicity. *Ann Emerg Med.* 1996;27:518-521.
192. Silverman AK, Ellis CN, Vorrhees JJ: Hypervitaminosis A syndrome. A paradigm of retinoid side effects. *J Am Acad Dermatol.* 1987;16: 1027-1039.
193. Skelton III, WP, Skelton NK: Deficiency of vitamins A, B, C: something to watch for. *Postgrad Med.* 1990;87:293-310.
194. Smith FR, Goodman DS Vitamin A transport in human vitamin A toxicity. *N Engl J Med.* 1976;294:805-808.
195. Stampfer MJ, Hennekens CH, Manson JE, et al: Vitamin E consumption and the risk of coronary disease in women. *N Engl J Med.* 1993;328: 1444-1449.
196. Stern PH, Taylor AB, Bell NH, Epstein S: Demonstration that circulation 1,25-dihydroxyvitamin D is loosely regulated in normal children. *J Clin Invest.* 1981;68:1374-1377.
197. Stern RH, Spence JD, Freeman DJ, Parbtani A: Tolerance to nicotinic acid flushing. *Clin Pharmacol Ther.* 1991;50:66-70.
198. Streck WF, Waterhouse C, Haddad JG: Glucocorticoid effects in vitamin D intoxication. *Arch Intern Med.* 1979;139:974-977.
199. Swartz RD, Wesley JR, Somermeyer MG, Lau K: Hyperoxaluria and renal insufficiency due to ascorbic acid administration during total parenteral nutrition. *Ann Intern Med.* 1984;100:530-531.
200. The Alpha-Tocopherol, Beta Carotine Cancer Prevention Study Group: The effect of vitamin E and beta carotene on the incidence of lung cancer and other cancers in male smokers. *N Engl J Med.* 1994;330:1029-1035.
201. The HOPE and HOPE-TOO Trial Investigators: Effects of long-term vitamin E supplementation on cardiovascular events and cancer: a randomized controlled trial. *JAMA.* 2005:293:1338-1347.
202. Timbo BB, Ross MP, McCarthy PV, Lin CT: Dietary supplements in a national survery: prevalence of use and reports of adverse events. *J Am Diet Assoc.* 2006; 106:1966-1974.

203. Tjellesen L, Hummer L, Christiansen C, Rodbro P: Serum concentration of vitamin D metabolites during treatment with vitamin D_2 and D_3 in normal premenopausal women. *Bone Miner*. 1986;1:407-413.
204. Unna IC: Studies of the toxicity and pharmacology of vitamin B_6 (2-methyl, 3-hydroxy-4,5-bis-pyridine). *Pharmacol Exp Ther*. 1940;70:400-407.
205. U.S. Food and Drug Administration. Available at http://www.fda.gov/bbs/topics/ANSWERS/2004/ANS01328.html. Last accessed March 31, 2009.
206. van Haaften RI, Haenen GR, van Bladeren PJ, et al: Inhibition of various glutathione S-transferase isoenzymes by RRR-alpha-tocopherol. *Toxicol In Vitro*. 2003;17:245-251.
207. Vieth R: Vitamin D supplementation, 25-hydroxyvitamin D concentrations, and safety. *Am J Clin Nutr*. 1999;69:842-856.
208. Vieth R: The mechanisms of vitamin D toxicity. *Bone Miner*. 1990;11: 267-272.
209. Vieth R, Pinto TR, Reen BS, Wong MM: Vitamin D poisoning by table sugar. *Lancet*. 2002;359:672.
210. Vitamin K, vitamin E and the coumarin drugs. *Nutr Rev*. 1982;40:180-181.
211. Wald G: The molecular basis of visual excitation. *Nature*. 1968;219:800-807.
212. Walta DC, Giddens JD, Johnson LF: Localized proximal esophagitis secondary to ascorbic acid ingestion and esophageal motility disorder. *Gastroenterology*. 1976;70:766-769.
213. Wandzilak TR, D'Andre SD, Davis PA, et al: Effect of high dose vitamin C on urinary oxalate levels. *J Urol*. 1994;151:834-837.
214. Warner JEA, Bernstein PS, Yemelyanov A, et al: Vitamin A in the cerebrospinal fluid of patients with and without idiopathic intracranial hypertension. *Ann Neurol*. 2002;52:647-650.
215. Weber FL, Mitchell GE, Powel DE, et al: Reversible hepatotoxicity associated with hepatic vitamin A accumulation in a protein deficient patient. *Gastroenterology*. 1982;82:118-122.
216. Welch AL: Lupus erythematosus: treatment by combined use of massive amounts of pantothenic acid and vitamin E. *Arch Dermatol Syphilol*. 1954;70:181-198.
217. West CE, Eilander A, van Lieshout M: Consequences of revised estimates of carotenoid bioefficacy for dietary control of vitamin A deficiency in developing countries. *J Nutr*. 2002;132:2920S-2926S.
218. Whelan AM, Price SO, Fowler SF, Hainer BL: The effect of aspirin on niacin-induced cutaneous reactions. *J Fam Pract*. 1992;34:165-168.
219. Wiley JS, Firkin FC: Reduction of pulmonary toxicity by prednisolone prophylaxis during all-transretinoic acid treatment of acute promyelocytic leukemia. *Leukemia*. 1995;, 9:774-778.
220. Windhorst DB, Nigra T: General clinical toxicology of oral retinoids. *J Am Acad Dermatol*. 1982;6:675-682.
221. Yusuf S, Dagenais G, Pogue J, et al: Vitamin E supplementation and cardiovascular events in high-risk patients: The Heart Outcomes Prevention Evaluation Study Investigators. *N Engl J Med*. 2000;342:154-160.
222. Zempleni J, Kubler W: The utilization of intravenously infused pyridoxine in humans. *Clin Chim Acta*. 1994;229:27-36.
223. Zhang TD, Chen GQ, Wang ZG, et al: Arsenic trioxide, a therapeutic agent for APL. *Oncogene*. 2001;20:7146-7153.
224. Zhou GB, Zhang J, Wang ZY, et al: Treatment of acute promyelocitic leukaemia with all-trans retinoic acid and arsenic trioxide: a paradigm of synergistic molecular targeting therapy. *Philos Trans R Soc Lond B Biol Sci*. 2007;362:959-971.

CHAPTER 42
ESSENTIAL OILS

Sarah Eliza Halcomb

Essential oils are a class of polyaromatic hydrocarbons extracted through steam distillation or cold pressed from the leaves, flowers, bark, wood, fruit, or peel of a single parent plant. The term "essential" refers to the essence of a plant, rather than an indispensible component of the oil or a vital biologic function. These organic compounds are a complex mixture of chemicals with structures that give the oil its aroma, therapeutic properties, and occasionally cause toxicity. More than 500 essential oils exist and can be categorized into five chemical groups: terpenes, quinines, substituted benzenes, aromatic/aliphatic esters, and phenols and aromatic/aliphatic alcohols.

HISTORY AND EPIDEMIOLOGY

Use of plant-derived essential oils in the practice of herbal medicine has a long and colorful history, dating back thousands of years. The virtues of these extracts have been mentioned in ancient Egyptian and Greek medical literature and throughout the Bible.

Essential oils were used to treat everything from asthma to snakebites until the early 20th century. In America "Indian doctors" frequently sold these products, claiming they learned medicinal secrets from local Native American tribes. These remedies were advertised at medicine shows and demonstrated by troupes such as the famous Kickapoo Indian Medicine Company. The purpose of these traveling caravans was to sell patent medicines, which typically contained substantial quantities of ethanol, in addition to other xenobiotics of uncertain therapeutic value. A bottle of Kickapoo Oil sold at the beginning of the 20th century purportedly contained "camphor, ether, capsicum, oil of cloves, oil of sassafras and myrrh." Needless to say, the risk-to-benefit ratio for this did not favor the patient, and the "doctors" who sold them quite rightly earned a reputation for quackery.[86]

With the ascent of scientific research, many essential oil remedies fell from use. More recently, however, trends in globalization and natural healing have led to a popular resurgence in the use of essential oils in developed countries. Essential oils currently are marketed for use in aromatherapy and certain complementary medicines. The reintroduction of these xenobiotics into mainstream society has highlighted the need for research and toxicity studies to ensure that appropriate decision making and care can be provided to exposed patients.

ABSINTHE; OIL OF WORMWOOD

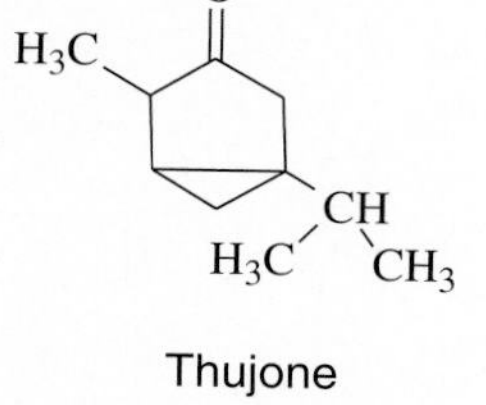

Thujone

History Absinthe is an emerald green liqueur made from the extract of the wormwood plant *Artemisia absinthium*. The earliest references to wormwood date to 1500 B.C., when its antihelminthic properties were described. It is thought that Napoleon's soldiers popularized the drink upon their return from Algeria, where they had added wormwood extract to their wine to avoid helminthic infections during the war.[43]

Absinthe achieved exceptional popularity in the late 19th century in Europe. Famous artists and authors including Lautrec, Van Gogh, Baudelaire, and Wilde sat for hours in the cafes of Paris, drinking the green liqueur and romanticizing its aphrodisiac effects. However, recognition of the devastating side effects led the French, Swiss, and American governments to ban its sale by the early 1900s.[43] It remained off the market in the United States until December of 2007 when a small company, St. George Spirits of Alameda, became the first company to sell absinthe in the United States since 1912. Absinthe is also sold without its toxic ingredient, thujone, as Pernod.

Many people have speculated on the cause of Vincent Van Gogh's bizarre behavior. Some have concluded that his fondness for absinthe may have contributed to his seizures and psychotic episodes. However, it is more likely that his consumption of large amounts of ethanol contributed to his erratic behavior.

Pharmacology The toxic component in oil of wormwood is thujone, a monoterpene ketone, which exists in α- and β-diastereoisomeric forms.[42] After oral absorption, both isomers undergo species-specific hydroxylation reactions by the cytochrome P450 system, followed by glucuronidation in the hepatocyte, leading to production of several renally eliminated nontoxic metabolites.[42]

Pathophysiology The α-stereoisomer is generally accepted to be the more toxic of the two isomers and the parent compound antagonizes the γ-aminobutyric acid $(GABA)_A$ receptor by binding at the picrotoxin site on the chloride channel, leading to neuroexcitation that may manifest as hallucinations or seizures, presumably in a dose-dependent fashion.[42] Interestingly, ethanol enhances GABA activity and may have a protective effect by reducing seizures in mice.[43]

Thujones are implicated in the development of porphyria-like syndromes by inducing the synthesis of 5-aminolevulinic acid synthetase, leading to increased porphyrin production. This finding suggests that individuals with defects in heme synthesis may unmask a porphyria-like syndrome upon ingestion of thujones.[11]

Clinical Features Case reports of toxicity reflect a recent resurgence in the popularity of the absinthe liquor, which has reappeared on the market in Europe and America.[90] Clinical features of acute toxicity are similar to those of ethanol intoxication, including euphoria and confusion, which may progress to restlessness, visual hallucinations, and delirium. Chronic abusers may suffer from seizures, hallucinations, and erratic behavior.[4] Although thujone is the purported agent in the development of these symptoms, the concentrations of thujone make it more likely that ethanol is responsible for the reported toxicity.

Rhabdomyolysis and acute renal failure have occurred following ingestion of oil of wormwood intended for preparation as absinthe.[90] The etiology of the rhabdomyolysis has not been elucidated.[90]

CAMPHOR

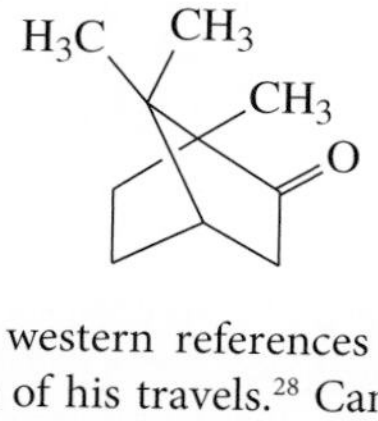

History One of the first western references to camphor is found in Marco Polo's description of his travels.[28] Camphor was traded widely throughout Asia. Historically it was used as a rubefacient, antiseptic, decongestant, and moth repellent. It gained immense popularity as a liniment during the American Civil War, and the US government signed a contract with China to buy the entire camphor output of Formosa (Taiwan).

The French introduced camphor to Europe in 1879.[28] Camphor oil is extracted from an evergreen tree from the Laurel family *Cinnamomum camphora*,[19] which is native to eastern China, Japan, and Taiwan. It is primarily used today in nasal decongestant ointments such as Vicks Vapo-Rub, although in the recent past it was widely used in moth repellents (Chap. 103).

Pharmacology Camphor belongs to the terpene family and is capable of causing CNS toxicity.[19] Camphor is a monoterpene ketone that is rapidly absorbed from the gastrointestinal (GI) tract and then undergoes extensive first-pass metabolism. After hydroxylation and glucuronidation in the liver, its inactive metabolites undergo urinary excretion.[69,82]

Pathophysiology Camphor toxicity is reported after its ingestion, inhalation, and nasal administration. It is rapidly absorbed from the GI tract or through mucous membranes. Camphor is highly lipid soluble and readily crosses the blood–brain barrier and placenta. Seizures are common postingestion, although the specific mechanism of action is not elucidated. Cellular respiration is inhibited by camphor and similar compounds, resulting in increased excitability of neuronal tissue. Children seem particularly prone to hepatotoxicity because of the relative immaturity of their hepatic enzyme systems. They may develop hepatotoxicity resembling Reye syndrome.[47] The fetus is thought to be susceptible to toxicity through the same mechanism. Several cases of camphor use as an abortifacient and a single case of fetal demise after ingestion are reported.[68,91]

Clinical Features Camphor ingestion results in rapid onset of nausea and vomiting, followed by headache, agitation, and seizures.[21] Symptom onset usually occurs within minutes of ingestion. Seizures can occur in isolation without antecedent gastrointestinal effects.[5] Inhalational and dermal exposures typically result in local irritation.

OIL OF CLOVES

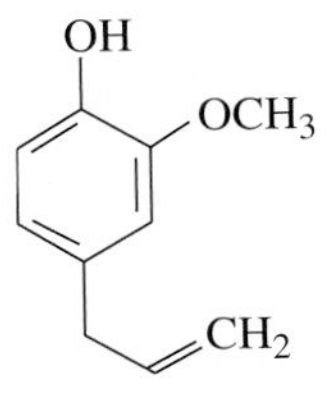

OH
OCH_3
CH_2

Eugenol

History In Medieval and Renaissance Europe, cloves were considered one of the most important commodities in the world second only to nutmeg. Clove oil is extracted from the plant *Syzygium aromaticum*, also known as *Eugenia aromatica*. This evergreen plant is native to the islands of the Malaccan Straits. Its unopened buds, when dried, are known as cloves. Eugenol has been used for centuries as a remedy for toothache and in multiple dental products.[8]

Pharmacology Eugenol, a phenol, is the principal component of clove oil. Very little available data on the metabolism of eugenol is available. An in vitro study found that incubation of isolated rat hepatocytes with eugenol resulted in a glucuronic acid conjugate, although other conjugates with sulfate and glutathione were found.[80]

Pathophysiology Little is known about the pathophysiology of eugenol toxicity. Intravenous infusion and intratracheal instillation of eugenol in rats led to the development of hemorrhagic pulmonary edema, which is thought to result from oxidative damage.[53,93]

In vitro studies of hepatic cell cultures incubated with eugenol demonstrated marked glutathione depletion, covalent bonding of conjugates to cell proteins, and cell death. These findings indicate that a reactive intermediate might be formed, leading to toxicity.[80] Nerve conduction studies performed with frog sciatic nerves demonstrate that eugenol irreversibly blocks impulse conduction. Eugenol has been demonstrated to inhibit peripheral sensory nerve conduction at low doses, but is associated with CNS depression at higher doses.[51]

Clinical Features A case report on the neurotoxicity of eugenol described a 24-year-old woman who spilled a small amount of clove oil on her face in an attempt to relieve a toothache. Permanent infraorbital anesthesia and anhidrosis resulted.[45] Likewise, inhibition of the pharyngeal reflex by inhalation of clove cigarettes is reported to cause aspiration pneumonitis.[30,35]

Inadvertent oral administration of 1–2 teaspoons of clove oil resulted in marked CNS depression, metabolic acidosis, and elevation of aminotransferases in two children.[39,52]

OIL OF EUCALYPTUS

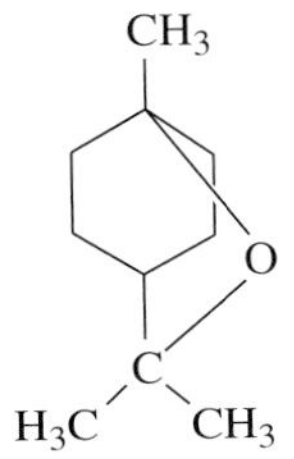

CH_3
O
C
H_3C CH_3

Eucalyptol

History The eucalyptus tree is native to Australia. Its extracts were historically used as an aboriginal fever remedy. In 1778, the Surgeon General of the First Fleet arrived in Australia and noted that these unusual trees produced a gumlike resin, which he distilled into a quart of oil and sent back to England for further examination. The introduction of eucalyptus oil to the West led to an increased demand for the product to relieve the symptoms of the common cold and influenza. Eucalyptol is found in many nonprescription cough preparations and is widely used for treatment of upper respiratory infections because of its purported antiinflammatory effects.[48] Although oral administration of eucalyptol-containing products rarely causes toxicity, ingestion of eucalyptus oil has resulted in morbidity and mortality.

Pharmacology Eucalyptus oil contains up to 70% eucalyptol, a monocyclic terpene compound. Eucalyptol, also known as 1,8-cineole, is rapidly absorbed from the gastrointestinal tract. It undergoes oxidation in the liver to form hydroxycineole, and subsequently undergoes further glucuronidation and excretion.[89] In rats, the main urinary metabolites have been characterized as 2-hydroxycineole, 3-hydroxycineole, and 1,8-dihydroxycineol-9-oic acids.[56,74] Rabbits given oral eucalyptus excrete 2-exo-hydroxycineole and 2-endo-hydroxycineole, as well as 3-exo-hydroxycineole and 3-endo-hydroxycineole in the urine.[62]

Ingestion of less than 1 teaspoon (5 mL) of eucalyptus oil has resulted in severe toxicity.[1,6,27] The lowest lethal doses reported are 4–5 mL[57] in adults and 1.9 g in a 10-year-old boy.[63] However, ingestion of higher doses in another case series caused less severe effects.[88]

Pathophysiology The mechanism of toxicity is unclear because little toxicity seems to be associated with eucalyptol.[24]

Clinical Features Symptoms develop rapidly and include headache and light-headedness progressing to CNS depression. Serious poisoning is marked by respiratory depression and vomiting, which heighten the risk of aspiration.[73,81]

OIL OF LAVENDER

History Lavender has been used as a fragrance and tonic for centuries. The Gospel of Luke mentions its use, referring to it by its ancient name, spikenard, when Mary anointed Jesus' feet with lavender oil and dried them with her hair. Lavender enjoys the distinction of being the most commonly used ingredient in perfume production worldwide.

Pharmacology There are four major species of lavender: *Lavandula latifolia* and *L. augustifolia*, otherwise known as English lavender; *L. stoechus* or French lavender; and *L. intermedis*, a hybrid cross between English and French lavenders. Oil of lavender is derived from the steam distillation of the flowers and leaves of the plant.[17] It is predominately used as a topical agent, and undergoes rapid absorption from the skin, achieving peak serum concentration approximately 20 minutes after application.[46] Linalool, linalyl acetate, and β-caryophyllene are the primary active constituents of the oil. The former two are rapidly oxidized when exposed to air forming hydroperoxides. These highly reactive molecules rapidly cross the epidermis and form protein adducts, initiating a cascade of immunomodulatory events.[36] In an elegant experiment, both lavender and tea tree oil were shown to elicit a dose-dependent increase in estrogen responsivity and antiandrogenic activity in in vitro breast cancer cell cultures similar to the effects of estradiol.[41]

Pathophysiology The constituents of lavender oil undergo auto-oxidation when exposed to air leading to skin sensitization and the development of contact dermatitis.

A case series reported the development of gynecomastia in three prepubertal boys using lavender oil. All three children had extensive endocrine evaluations, with no abnormalities detected, and in each case the gynecomastia resolved when lavender oil was discontinued. One of the children was also using a tea tree oil preparation topically.[41]

Clinical Features The predominant clinical feature of exposure is contact dermatitis. Unexplained or "idiopathic" gynecomastia in prepubertal boys with negative endocrine evaluations should prompt questions regarding the use of essential oils.

OIL OF NUTMEG

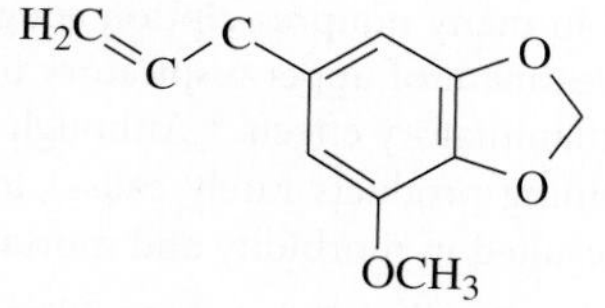

Myristicin

History During the Middle Ages, spices were prized for their medicinal and preservative qualities. Chief among these spices was nutmeg, which, after silver and gold, was the most valued commodity in the western world. In addition to its soporific and emetic properties, nutmeg was purported to be a prophylactic against the plague. Nutmeg has been used unsuccessfully as an abortifacient and used as a hallucinogen.

In 1510, a European explorer named Ludovico de Varthema described seeing the nutmeg tree flourishing in the Indonesian archipelago on the Bandas Islands, which was the only place on Earth that the spice could be found. This discovery led to an intense competition among the great navies of Europe to dominate the spice trade.[71]

Pharmacology Nutmeg oil is extracted from the fruit of the evergreen tree *Myristica fragrans*. Its main active ingredient is thought to be myristicin, although other putative toxins derived from the extraction process include mace, eugenol, and other terpenes.[67] Case reports of toxicity suggest that patients become symptomatic 3–6 hours after ingestion of one to three whole nuts or 1–2 tablespoons of ground nutmeg. Myristicin is oxidized in the hepatic P450 system to 5-allyl-1-methoxy-2,3-dihydroxybenzene,[94] which then undergoes glucuronidation and urinary excretion.

Pathophysiology Animal studies have suggested that myristicin-induced CNS toxicity may result from increased serotonin concentrations in the brain.[83] Myristicin has been known to inhibit monoamine oxidase,[83,84] which theoretically could lead to an adverse reaction if combined with another monoamine oxidase inhibitor. Another in vitro experiment showed that myristicin was converted to the amphetamine derivative 3-methoxy-4,5-methylene dioxyamphetamine,[13] which may explain its euphoric effects. Other animal studies have demonstrated fatty degeneration of the liver.[87]

Clinical Features CNS effects tend to be the predominant clinical features of nutmeg poisoning. Nutmeg toxicity may mimic anticholinergic toxicity, with flushing, dryness, tachycardia, hypertension, agitation, and altered mental status.[66] One feature that may help differentiate anticholinergic toxicity from nutmeg ingestion is that the pupils often are small.

Escalating doses result in increasing drowsiness that may progress to coma. Abdominal pain is frequently reported, but nausea and vomiting are uncommon. The toxic syndrome typically resolves within 24 hours, although resolution may be delayed.[32] A single fatality is reported in the literature.[23]

OIL OF PENNYROYAL

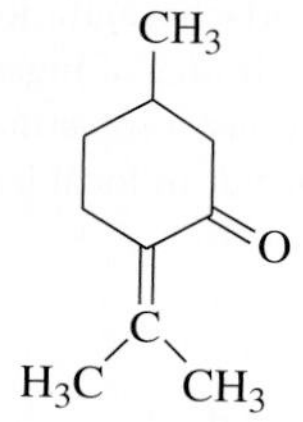

Pulegone

History References to pennyroyal oil date back to antiquity when Pliny the Elder wrote about its insect repellent effects in Book 20 of his masterpiece, *The Natural History*. Its scientific name *Mentha pulegium* is derived from the Latin pulex, which means flea. Both the fresh plant and smoke from the burning leaves were used as early insect repellents. Over the centuries this essential oil also developed a reputation for being an abortifacient and an emmenagogue.[12] The 16th-century English herbalist Gerard noted, "Pennie Royall boiled in wine and drunken, provoketh the monthly terms, bringeth forth the secondine, the deade childe and unnatural birth."[22] An early American 19th-century pamphlet recommended a recipe that included drinking a pint of pennyroyal water to induce abortion.[78] The toxic effects of pennyroyal were first described in a case report to The Lancet in 1897.[2] Today, Internet searches for pennyroyal oil lead to multiple web sites where women relate their experiences with the substance for inducing abortion.

Pharmacology The active ingredient in pennyroyal oil is R(+)-pulegone, a monoterpene commonly found in mint oils. Toxicity predominately results from ingestion of pennyroyal for the purposes of inducing abortion, although cases of oil administration to children with gastrointestinal complaints are reported.[7] Toxicity is noted in mice when 300–500 mg/kg is administered, and a human fatality was reported at an approximate dose of 500 mg/kg.

After ingestion, pulegone is metabolized by the P450 system in the liver to methofuran and other reactive metabolites, which in turn are excreted in the urine.

Pathophysiology The reactive metabolites of pulegone bind to cell proteins, disrupting normal cellular function and resulting in cellular damage.[3] Methofuran also appears to be associated with pennyroyal-induced pulmonary toxicity, which is manifested as bronchiolar necrosis.[31] Electrophilic reactive metabolites of pulegone deplete hepatic glutathione concentrations by reacting with the nucleophilic cysteinyl sulfhydryl group on glutathione, further worsening hepatotoxicity.[79] This hepatotoxicity is manifested as centrilobular necrosis, which occurs in both mouse and human specimens.[31]

Clinical Features Case reports describe a variety of symptoms after ingestion of pennyroyal oil. The most common symptoms of significant toxicity seem to include abdominal discomfort, nausea, vomiting, dizziness, syncope, and coma. Ingestion of 5–10 mL has been associated with coma and seizures, and ingestion of 15 mL may cause death.[3,7,76] Early symptoms are manifested by gastrointestinal and CNS toxicity,[7] followed by the development of hepatic and renal dysfunction.[76,85] In fatal ingestions, patients have developed disseminated intravascular coagulation and hepatic failure manifested as purpuric rash, epistaxis, vaginal bleeding, and oozing at venipuncture sites.[3,76,65]

OIL OF PEPPERMINT

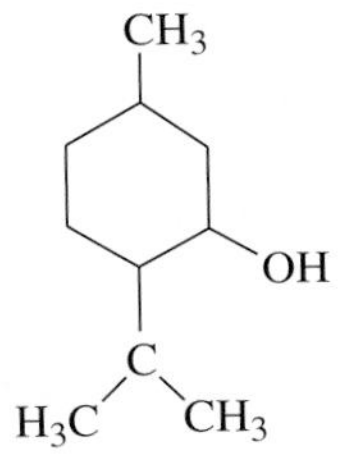

Menthol

History Plants in the mint family have been used as medicinal herbs for centuries. One of the first known references to the medicinal qualities of mint comes from the Ebers Papyrus, an ancient Egyptian pharmacopoeia dating back to 1552 B.C. In this document, mint is mentioned as one of the recommended remedies for indigestion and nausea. According to ancient Greek mythology, Hades, the god of the underworld, fell in love with the beautiful nymph Minthe. The affair was short-lived, however, as Hades' jealous wife Persephone turned Minthe into a plant. Hades tempered the curse on the nymph by making the plant fragrant. Peppermint oil is extracted from the plant *Mentha piperita* and is widely used in flavorings and aromatherapy.

Pharmacology Menthol, the active ingredient in peppermint oil, is a cyclic terpene alcohol that is rapidly absorbed from the GI tract when ingested. In the liver, menthol undergoes hydroxylation to form p-menthane-3,8-diol and 3,8-dihydroxy-p-menthane-7-carboxylic acid by the P450 microsomal enzyme system. These metabolites subsequently are glucuronidated by uridine diphosphate (UDP)-glucuronyl transferase and excreted in the urine.[25]

Pathophysiology The unique cooling property of menthol adds to its commercial value and is one of the most studied features of the oil. Electrophysiologic investigations have shown that menthol has a dose-dependent effect on calcium concentrations across cell membranes. Inhibition of calcium efflux results in depolarization and, in turn, increases electrical discharges from cold receptors.[25] The increased electrical activity in the trigeminal nerve is thought to be responsible for the subjective impression that menthol has a decongestant effect on the nasal passages.[25] Research has shown that menthol actually increases nasal congestion and causes an inhibition of upper airway muscle reflexes.[61]

Clinical Features Rare case reports of menthol toxicity appear in the literature. The reported symptoms include CNS effects such as ataxia, confusion, and coma,[64] nausea, and vomiting.[60,70]

OIL OF PINE AND TURPENTINE

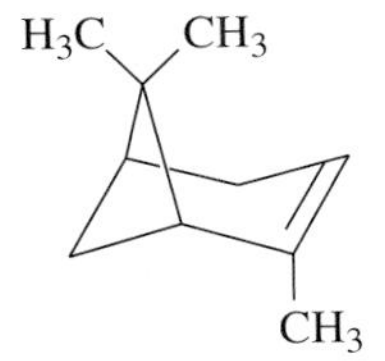

α-Pinene

History Pine oil and turpentine are distilled from the wood of conifer trees particularly of the genus *Pinus*. Turpentine has been historically used as a solvent and paint thinner, whereas pine oil is derived from turpentine and is used as a disinfectant. Turpentine has also been used medicinally in the past as a diuretic and expectorant.

Toxicokinetics The main active ingredient in pine oil is α-pinene, a monoterpene hydrocarbon that is absorbed via the GI tract or through inhalation. The lipophilicity of this compound results in its accumulation in adipose tissue and slow metabolism. The primary modes of metabolism include hydration, hydroxylation, and acetylation reactions, after which inactive metabolites undergo renal excretion.[50] Turpentine also contains α-pinene as its main constituent; however, β-pinene, camphene, and limonene are also found in this product.[34] Like pine oil, these constituents are rapidly absorbed through the GI tract or inhalation and are renally excreted.[72]

Pathophysiology Pine oil and turpentine are volatile hydrocarbon compounds with low viscosity. Aspiration and inhalational injury is common when low-viscosity hydrocarbons are ingested or inhaled, because of inhibited surfactant production in the alveoli[14] (see Chap. 106). Household cleaning products which contain pine oil as an additive to increase the solution's viscosity appear to result in limited inhalational injury when aspiration occurs. However, significant risk of pulmonary injury is associated with turpentine ingestion and aspiration or inhalation.[29] Animal studies suggest that the LD50 for inhalational injury is 5204.8 ppm.[9]

Clinical Features Pine oil ingestion results in a characteristic pine odor on the breath,[92] whereas turpentine ingestion reportedly causes the urine to smell of violets.[65] Significant ingestions may result in CNS depression that progresses from headache, dizziness, and blurry vision to lethargy and coma.[15] Aspiration resulting in pneumonitis, acute lung injury, and acute respiratory distress syndrome reportedly causes subsequent development of pneumatocoeles.[14,92] Inhalational exposure to turpentine fumes causes increased airway resistance and irritation of the oral mucosa in study subjects.[26] Delayed hemorrhagic cystitis has been reported up to 72 hours after a turpentine ingestion.[49] Further details on the management of hydrocarbon aspiration are given in Chap. 106.

OIL OF TEA TREE

History Tea tree oil has been used by Australian aborigines as a topical antimicrobial agent for centuries.[16] Recently, researchers have conducted in vitro studies on the antimicrobial properties of this essential oil and have confirmed that tea tree oil has some microbicidal efficacy.[37,44] Tea tree oil is widely available in over-the-counter topical preparations that claim to have antimicrobial properties.

Pharmacology Tea tree oil is obtained by the steam distillation of the *Melaluca alternifolia* tree which is indigenous to New South Wales, Australia. Very little data exist on the pharmacokinetics of tea tree oil, although the antibacterial properties are thought to be due in part to a disturbance in cellular potassium fluxes.[20] The main active ingredient, terpinen-4-ol, is thought to be the principal antimicrobial component in tea tree oil.[16]

Clinical Features Like lavender oil, tea tree oil has been reported to cause prepubertal gynecomastia in boys, likely secondary to estrogenic effects.[41]

OIL OF WINTERGREEN

Methyl salicylate

History European botanists became fascinated by medicinal plants upon the discovery of the New World. John Bartram established the first botanical garden in the United States in 1728 and was named the "Botanizer Royal for America" in 1765. His collection included the *Gaultheria procumbens*, or the Eastern Teaberry, which is a fragrant ground cover plant whose leaves were steamed. The distilled product, oil of wintergreen, was used topically to relieve the symptoms of rheumatism.[10] Oil of wintergreen is also obtained from the twigs of Sweet Birch, or Betula lenta. It is found in topical preparations worldwide, such as Tiger Balm and Ben-Gay, which are used to treat myalgias. The active ingredient in oil of wintergreen is methyl salicylate, which has a pleasant smell and taste, posing a significant hazard to children. Interestingly enough, there are many other names for this essential oil, including checkerberry oil, sweet birch oil, mountain tea, teaberry, groundberry oil, gaultheria oil, and spicewood oil.

Five milliliters of oil of wintergreen is equivalent in salicylate content to 7 g aspirin, and numerous case reports of fatalities after even small ingestions are reported.[33,58,75]

Pharmacology Methyl salicylate is absorbed both from the GI tract and transdermally,[59] and can cause significant toxicity.[18,40] Once absorbed, methyl salicylate enters the circulation and is transported to the liver, where it undergoes hydrolysis to form salicylic acid. The salicylic acid undergoes conjugation with glycine and glucuronic acid, forming salicyluric acid, salicyl acyl, and phenolic glucuronide.[54] Salicylates are predominantly excreted by the kidney as salicyluric acid (75%), free salicylic acid (10%), salicylic phenol (10%) acyl (5%) glucuronides, and gentisic acid (<1%).[55]

Pathophysiology An extensive discussion of salicylate pathophysiology is given in Chap. 35.

Clinical Features Oil of wintergreen overdose can result in a toxic syndrome of salicylate poisoning, characterized by nausea, vomiting, tinnitus, hyperpnea, and tachypnea. Patients often present with diaphoresis and mental status changes. Severe toxicity is associated with seizures, cerebral edema, acute lung injury, coma, and death. Further details on the laboratory tests and treatment of salicylate toxicity are given in Chap. 35.

DIAGNOSTIC TESTING

Laboratory studies are of limited value in essential oil toxicity. Generally, blood or urine concentrations of the active ingredients are not available in a meaningful time frame. However, the patient's clinical status should determine which laboratory studies are to be ordered. Patients who present with altered mental status or seizures warrant a complete evaluation that may include basic metabolic studies, a head CT and lumbar puncture for serious potential structural or metabolic etiologies, such as hypoglycemia or hyponatremia. In patients who present with respiratory distress, chest radiographs and continuous pulse oximetry are warranted.

A few of the essential oils require specific studies:

Absinthe: Laboratory studies should include a complete blood count (CBC), chemistry panel, creatine phosphokinase concentration, and glucose monitoring in patients who present with seizures. Urinalysis should be performed to evaluate for myoglobinuria.

Camphor, Nutmeg: Useful laboratory studies include a chemistry panel to evaluate hydration status and liver enzyme concentrations.

Pennyroyal: CBC and liver function studies, including the aminotransferases, bilirubin, prothrombin time, and partial thromboplastin time, and a β-HCG in women are indicated.

Wintergreen: Salicylate concentrations and acid–base status should be determined.

TREATMENT

Treatment of symptomatic essential oil toxicity is generally supportive, including administration of intravenous fluids and supplemental oxygen. A dose of activated charcoal may be helpful in alert patients with an intact airway. Benzodiazepines are the mainstay of treatment in patients who present with agitation and seizures.

A few of the essential oils require specific treatment:

Absinthe: If rhabdomyolysis is present, hydration and urinary alkalinization may be appropriate, depending on the clinical severity.

Clove: In patients who exhibit signs of hepatotoxicity, *N*-acetylcysteine (NAC) should be administered. Although no definitive studies on NAC use in this patient population are available, the suggestion that NAC is protective in the rat model,[80] combined with the safety profile of NAC, warrant its use in the setting of eugenol-induced hepatotoxicity.

Pennyroyal: Patients who present with a recent history of pennyroyal ingestion should undergo gastric decontamination with gastric lavage and administration of activated charcoal. NAC therapy is warranted following significant pennyroyal oil ingestions, given the depletion of hepatic glutathione stores.[3,38] Administration of NAC should continue until the patient's clinical status improves or hepatotoxicity resolves. NAC should be administered in the same doses used for acetaminophen toxicity because no trials have demonstrated the optimal dose in the setting of pennyroyal poisoning. If no signs of hepatic or renal toxicity develop, the traditional 21-hour course of intravenous NAC should suffice. If oral NAC is administered, a 24- to 36-hour period of administration should prevent hepatotoxicity, given the 1- to 2-hour half-life of pennyroyal oil and its metabolites.[3] In asymptomatic patients with minimal ingestions, a brief observation period of 3–6 hours is sufficient. An animal study demonstrated that treatment of mice with a combination of disulfiram and cimetidine prior to pennyroyal administration diminished the hepatotoxic effects, but whether these treatments would be beneficial in human toxicity is uncertain.[77]

SUMMARY

Essential oils are increasingly being used as an alternative form of medical therapy. In general, the topical use of these products is associated with minimal toxicity. However, ingestion, prolonged inhalation or massive cutaneous application or application to abraded skin of essential oils may result in significant morbidity and mortality. Suspected cases of essential oil toxicity should be reported to the regional poison center to enhance our epidemiologic data with regard to essential oil toxicity.

REFERENCES

1. Allan J: Poisoning by oil of eucalyptus. *Br Med J*. 1910;1:569.
2. Allen WT: Note of a case of supposed poisoning by pennyroyal. *Lancet*. 1897;1:1022-1023.
3. Anderson IB, Mullen WH, Meeker JE, et al: Pennyroyal toxicity: measurement of toxic metabolite levels in two cases and review of the literature. *Ann Intern Med*. 1996;124:726-734.
4. Arnold WN: Absinthe. *Sci Am*. 1989;260:112-117.
5. Aronow R: Camphor poisoning—Editorial. *JAMA*. 1976;235:1260.
6. Atkinson R: Eucalyptus oil. *Br Med J*. 1909;2:1656.
7. Bakerink JA, Gospe SM Jr, Dimand RJ, Eldridge MW: Multiple organ failure after ingestion of pennyroyal oil from herbal tea in two infants. *Pediatrics*. 1996;98:944-947.
8. Barkin ME, Boyd JP, Cohen S: Acute allergic reaction to eugenol. *Oral Surg*. 1984;57:441-442.
9. Baxter, CS. Alicyclic hydrocarbons. In: Bingham E, Cohrssen B, Powell CH, eds: *Patty's Toxicology*, Vol. 8, 5th ed. New York: John Wiley & Sons; 2001:710-1080.
10. Berkley E, Berkley DS: *The Life and Travels of John Bartram: From Lake Ontario to the River St. John*, reprint edition. Tallahassee: University Presses of Florida; 1990.
11. Bonkovsky H, Cable E, Cable J, et al: Porphyrogenic properties of the terpenes camphor, pinene, and thujone. *Biochem Pharmacol*. 1992;43:2359-2368.
12. Braithewaite PF: A case of poisoning by pennyroyal: recovery. *Br Med J*. 1906;2:865.
13. Braun U, Kalbhen DA: Evidence for the biogenic formation of amphetamine derivatives from components from nutmeg. *Pharmacology*. 1973;9:312-316.
14. Bray A, Pirronti T, Marano P: Pneumatoceles following hydrocarbon aspiration. *Eur Radiol*. 1998;8:262-263.
15. Brook MP, McCarron MM, Mueller JA, et al: Pine oil cleaner ingestion. *Ann Emerg Med*. 1989;18:391-395.
16. Carson CF, Hammer KA, Riley TV: *Melaleuca alternafolia* (tea tree) oil: a review of antimicrobial and other medicinal properties. *Clin Microbiol Rev*. 2006:19(1);50-62.
17. Cavenaugh HM, Wilkinson, JM: Biological activities of lavender essential oil. *Phytother Res*. 2002;16:301-308.
18. Chan TYK: Potential dangers from topical preparations containing methyl salicylate. *Hum Exp Toxicol*. 1996;15:747-750.
19. Clark TL: Fatal case of camphor poisoning. *Br Med J*. 1924;1:467.
20. Cox SD, Gustafson JE, Mann CM, et al: Tea tree oil causes K+_leakage and inhibits respiration in *Escherichia coli*. *Lett Appl Microbiol*. 1998:26;355-358.
21. Craig JO: Poisoning by the volatile oils in childhood. *Arch Dis Child*. 1953;28:475-483.
22. Crellin, JK, Philpott J: *Herbal Medicine Past and Present*, Vol. 2. Durham, NC: Duke University Press; 1990:327-330.
23. Cushny AR: Nutmeg poisoning. *Proc R Soc Med*. 1908;1:39-44.
24. DeVincenzi M, Silano M, De Vincenzi A, et al: Constituents of aromatic plants: eucalyptol. *Fitoterapia*. 2002;73:269-275.
25. Eccles R: Menthol and related cooling compounds. *J Pharm Pharmacol*. 1994;46:618-630.
26. Filipsson AF: Short term inhalation exposure to turpentine: toxicokinetics and acute effects in men. *Occup Environ Med*. 1996;53:100-105.
27. Foggie WE: Eucalyptus oil poisoning. *Br Med J*. 1911;1:359-360.
28. Fox N: Effect of camphor, eucalyptol and menthol on the vascular state of the mucous membrane. *Arch Otolaryngol Head Neck Surg*. 1927;6:112-122.
29. Gerarde HW: Toxicological studies on hydrocarbons. IX. Aspiration hazard and toxicity of hydrocarbons and hydrocarbon mixtures. *AMA Arch Environ Health*. 1963;6:329-34.
30. Gibson DE, Moore GP, Pfaff JA: Camphor ingestion. *Am J Emerg Med*. 1989;7:41-43.
31. Gordon WP, Forte AJ, McMutry RJ, et al: Hepatotoxicity and pulmonary toxicity of pennyroyal oil and its constituent terpenes in the mouse. *Toxicol Appl Pharmacol*. 1982;65:413-424.
32. Green RC: Nutmeg poisoning. *JAMA*. 1959;171:1342.
33. Gross M, Greenberg L: *Salicylates: A Critical Bibliographic View*. New Haven, CT: Hillhouse Press; 1948:380.
34. Gscheidmeier M, Fleig, H: Turpentines. In: Elvers B, Hawkins S, eds: *Ullman's Encyclopedia of Industrial Chemistry*. New York: CH Publishers; 1996:267-280.
35. Guidotti TL, Binder S, Stratton JW, et al: Clove cigarettes: development of the fad and evidence of health effects. In: Hollinger MA, ed: *Current Topics in Pulmonary Pharmacology and Toxicology*, Vol. 2. New York: Elsevier;1987:1-23.
36. Hagvall L, Skold M, Brared-Christensson J, et al: Lavender oil lacks natural protection against autoxidation, forming strong contact allergens on air exposure. *Contact Dermatitis*. 2008;59:143-150.
37. Hammer KA, Carson CF, Riley TV. Antifungal effects of *Melaleuca alternifolia* (tea tree) oil and its components on *Candida albicans*, *Candida glabrata* and *Saccharomyces cerevisiae*. *J Antimicrob Chemother*. 2004:53:1081-1085.
38. Harrison PM, Wendon JA, Gimson AES, et al: Improvement by acetylcysteine of hemodynamics and oxygen transport in fulminant hepatic failure. *N Engl J Med*. 1991;324:1852-1857.
39. Hartnoll G, Moore D, Dovek D: Near fatal ingestion of oil of cloves. *Arch Dis Child*. 1993;69:392-393
40. Heng MC: Local necrosis and interstitial nephritis due to topical methylsalicylate and menthol. *Cutis*. 1987;39:442-444.
41. Henley DV, Lipson N, Korach KS, et al: Prepubertal gynecomastia linked to lavender and tea tree oils. *N Engl J Med*. 2007;356 (5):479-485.
42. Hold K, Sirisoma N, Ikeda T, et al: Alpha-thujone (the active component of absinthe): gamma-aminobutyric acid type A receptor modulation and metabolic detoxification. *Proc Natl Acad Sci USA*. 2000;97:3826-3831.
43. Holstege CP, Baylor MR, Rusyniak DE: Absinthe: return of the green fairy. *Semin Neurol*. 2002;22:89-93.
44. Inouye S, Takizawa T, Yamaguchi A. Antibacterial activity of essential oils and their major constituents against respiratory tract pathogens by gaseous contact. *J Antimicrob Chemother*. 2001:47;565-573.
45. Isaacs G: Permanent local anesthesia and anhidrosis after clove oil spillage. *Lancet*. 1983;1:882.
46. Jager W, BuchbauerG, Jirovetz L et al: Percutaneous absorption of lavender oil from a massage oil. *J Soc Cosmetic Chem*. 1992;43:49-54.
47. Jimenez JF, Brown AL, Arnold WC, et al: Chronic camphor ingestion mimicking Reye's syndrome. *Gastroenterology*. 1983;84:394-398.
48. Juergens UR, Dethlefsen U, Steinkamp G, et al: Anti-inflammatory activity of 1,8-cineol (eucalyptol) in bronchial asthma: a double-blind placebo-controlled trial. *Respir Med*. 2003;97:250-256.
49. Klein FA, Hackler RH. Hemorrhagic cystitis associated with turpentine ingestion. *Urology*. 1984:16:187.
50. Koppel C, Tenczer J, Tonnesmann U, et al: Acute poisoning with pine oil-metabolism of monoterpenes. *Arch Toxicol*. 1981;49:73-78.
51. Kozam G: The effect of eugenol on nerve transmission. *Oral Surg Oral Med Oral Pathol*. 1977;44:799-805.
52. Lane BW, Ellenhorn MJ, Hulbert TV, et al: Clove oil ingestion in an infant. *Hum Exp Toxicol*. 1991;10:291-294
53. LaVoie EJ, Adams JD, Reinhardt J: Toxicity studies on clove cigarette smoke and constituents of clove: determination of the LD 50 of eugenol by intratracheal instillation in rats and hamsters. *Arch Toxicol*. 1986;59:2:78-81.
54. Levy G, Tsuchiya T: Salicylate accumulation kinetics in man. *N Engl J Med*. 1972;287:430-432.
55. Levy G: Clinical pharmacokinetics of aspirin. *Pediatrics*. 1978;62 (Suppl): 867-872.
56. Madyastha KM, Chadha A: Metabolism of 1,8-cineole in rat: its effects on liver and lung microsomal cytochrome P-450 systems. *Bull Environ Contam Toxicol*. 1986;37:759-766.
57. MacPherson, J: The toxicology of eucalyptus oil. *Med J Aust*. 1925;2:108-110
58. MacCready R: Methyl salicylate poisoning. A report of five cases. *N Engl J Med*. 1943;228:155.
59. Martin D, Valdez J, Boren J, et al: Dermal absorption of camphor, menthol, and methyl salicylate in humans. *J Clin Pharmacol*. 2004;44:1151-1157.
60. Martindale W: *The Extra Pharmacopoeia*, 27th ed. London: Pharmaceutical Press; 1977.
61. McBride B, Whitelaw W: A physiological stimulus to upper airway receptors in humans. *J Appl Physiol*. 1981;51:1189-1197.
62. Miyazawa M, Kameoka H, Morinaga K: Hydroxycineole: four new metabolites of 1,8-cineole in rabbits. *J Agric Food Chem*. 1989;37:222-226.
63. Neale A: Case of death following blue gum (eucalyptus Globulus) oil. *Aust Med Gaz*. 1893;12:115-116.
64. O'Mullane NM, Joyce P, Kamath SV, et al: Adverse CNS effects of menthol-containing olbas oil. *Lancet*. 1982;1:1121.

65. Pande TK, Pani S, Hiran S, et al: Turpentine poisoning: a case report. *Forensic Sci Int*. 1994;65:47-49.
66. Payne RB: Nutmeg intoxication. *N Engl J Med*. 1963;269:36-38.
67. Power FB, Salway AH: The constituents of the essential oil of nutmeg. *J Chem Soc*. 1907;91:2037-2058.
68. Riggs J, Hamilton R, Homel S, et al: Camphorated oil intoxication in pregnancy. *Obstet Gynecol*. 1965;25:255-258.
69. Robertson JS, Hussain M: Metabolism of camphors and related compounds. *Biochem J*. 1969;113:57-65.
70. Rogers J, Tay HH, Misiewicz JJ: Peppermint oil. *Lancet*. 1988;2:98-99.
71. Seabrook J: Soldiers and spice: Indonesia. Why the Dutch traded Manhattan for a speck of rock in 1667. *The New Yorker*, August 13, 2001.
72. Sperling, F. In vivo and in vitro toxicology of turpentine. *Clin Toxicol*. 1969. 2:21-35.
73. Spoerke DG, Vandenberg SA, Smolinske SC, et al: Eucalyptus oil: 14 cases of exposure. *Vet Hum Toxicol*. 1989;31:166-168.
74. Steinmetz M, Vial M, Millet Y: Actions de l'huile essentielle de romarin et de certains de ses constituents (eucalyptol et camphre) sur le cortex cérébral de rat in vitro. *J Toxicol Clin Exp*. 1987;7:259-271.
75. Stevenson CS: Oil of wintergreen (methyl salicylate) poisoning. Report of three cases, one with autopsy, and a review of the literature. *Am J Med Sci*. 1937;193:772-788.
76. Sullivan, JB Rumack BH, et al: Pennyroyal oil poisoning and hepatotoxicity. *JAMA*. 1979;242:2873-2874.
77. Sztajnkrycer MD, Otten EJ, Bond GR, et al: Mitigation of pennyroyal oil hepatotoxicity in the mouse. *Acad Emerg Med*. 2003;10:1024-1028.
78. Tennent J: Every Man His Own Doctor, or The Poor Planter's Physician. Philadelphia, 1736, p 40. In: Riddle JM. *Eve's Herbs: A History of Contraception and Abortion in the West*. Cambridge: Harvard University Press; 1997:201.
79. Thomassen D, Pearsin PG, Slattery JT, et al: Partial characterization of biliary metabolites of pulegone by tandem mass spectrometry. Detection of glucuronide, glutathione, and glutathinyl glucuronide conjugates. *Drug Metab Dispos*. 1991;19:997-1003.
80. Thompson DC, Constatin-Teodosio D, Moldeus P: Metabolism and cytotoxicity of eugenol in isolated rat hepatocytes. *Chem Biol Interact*. 1991;77:137-147.
81. Tibballis J: Clinical effects and management of eucalyptus oil ingestion in infants and young children. *Med J Aust*. 1995;163:177-180.
82. Trestrail JH, Spartz ME: Camphorated and castor oil confusion and its toxic results. *Clin Toxicol*. 1977;11:151-158
83. Truitt EB: *The Pharmacology of Myristicin and Nutmeg*. Washington, DC: Public Health Service Publications; 1967;1645:215-222.
84. Truitt EB Jr, Duritz G, Ebersberger EM: Evidence of monoamine oxidase inhibition by myristicin and nutmeg. *Proc Soc Exp Biol Med*. 1963;112: 647-650.
85. Vallence WB: Pennyroyal poisoning. A fatal case. *Lancet*. 1955;2:850-851.
86. Vogel VJ: *American Indian Medicine*. Norman: University of Oklahoma Press; 1970: 130-144.
87. Wallace GB: On nutmeg poisoning. In: *Contributions to Medical Research, Dedicated to Victor Clarence Vaughan*. Ann Arbor, MI: 1903:351-364.
88 Webb NJA, Pitt WR: Eucalyptus oil poisoning in childhood: 41 cases in south-east Queensland. *J Paediatr Child Health*. 1993;29:368-371.
89. Williams RT: *Detoxication Mechanisms*, 2nd ed. London: Chapman & Hall; 1959:528.
90. Weisbord S, Soule J, Kimmel P: Poison on line: acute renal failure caused by oil of wormwood purchased through the internet. *N Engl J Med*. 1997;337:825-827.
91. Weiss J, Catalano P: Camphorated oil intoxication during pregnancy. *Pediatrics*. 1973;52:713-714.
92. Welker JA, Zaloga GP: Pine oil ingestion: a common cause of poisoning. *Chest*. 1999;116:1822-1826.
93. Wright SE, Baron DA, Heffner JE: Intravenous eugenol causes lung edema in rats: proposed oxidant mechanisms. *J Lab Clin Med*. 1995;125: 257-264.
94. Yun CH, Lee HS, Lee HY, et al: Roles of human liver cytochrome P450 3A4 and 1A2 in the oxidation of myristicin. *Toxicol Lett*. 2003;137:143-150.

CHAPTER 43
HERBAL PREPARATIONS

Oliver L. Hung

Although, there is increased awareness of the widespread use of herbal preparations in the United States, frequently physicians seek information about the use of these products only after the patient demonstrates toxicity perhaps not completely attributable to a pharmaceutical product or a disease process. Some historical examples of toxicity from herbal usage include the death a professional baseball pitcher from ephedra in 2003, and its subsequent banning by the FDA in 2004;[183] six cases of anticholinergic poisoning from contaminated Paraguay tea in New York City in 1994;[33,95] three cases of life-threatening bradycardia following consumption of *Jin Bu Huan* tablets in Colorado in 1993;[38] and four cases of agranulocytosis with one death following consumption of *Chui Fong Tou Ku Wan* in San Francisco in 1975.[168] Although few studies have examined this issue, most herbal preparations used in developed countries appear to be safe. From 1983 to 1989, the National Poisons Unit, London, received 1070 inquiries regarding exposures to herbal extracts, of which 270 (25.2%) patients were symptomatic. The investigators were able to demonstrate a probable association between exposure and effect in only 32 of the 270 cases (12%).[159] In Hong Kong, Chinese herbal medicines and proprietary medicines accounted for only 0.2% of all acute medical admissions despite their use by 40%–60% of the population whereas Western medications were responsible for 4.4% of acute medical admissions.[48,49] In the United States, a multicenter poison center study reported in 2003 collected 2253 calls involving dietary supplements including herbals; 493 patient exposures were determined to be caused by dietary supplement and were associated with 5 deaths, 13 seizures, 8 cases of coma, and 9 cases of hepatotoxicity.[154] The overall severity outcome among dietary supplement cases was greater compared to outcomes of other poison center–reported exposures.[154] In developing countries where herbal usage is much greater, reported poisoning from herbal preparation usage appears to be higher. In Southern Africa and in Oman, traditional medicines account for 6%–15% of hospital admissions for acute poisonings.[92,107,127,187]

DEFINITION

The botanical definition of the term *herb* is specific for certain leafy plants without woody stems. However, the term *herbal preparations* often includes nonherb plant materials, even animal and mineral products. Thus, in a broad sense, the term herbals includes any "natural" or "traditional" remedy, but these terms also are poorly defined. Although these products often are also called *medications*, this terminology may be inaccurate and misleading. Many herbal preparations purportedly are used for their nonspecific "adaptogenic" properties by permitting the body return to a normal state by resisting stress, but they lack any specific medicinal effects. Because many herbal users and herbalists do not consider herbal preparations medications, use of the term *herbal medicine* by the clinician may convey a different, and perhaps unintended, meaning. For these reasons, it may be inappropriate and without benefit to refer to these products as medication, but they are xenobiotics.

Herbal preparations are considered to be a subset of "alternative medical therapies." These therapies are defined as interventions that are neither widely taught in medical schools nor generally available in US hospitals.[71] When these alternative medical therapies are used in conjunction with conventional medical therapies, they are also known as *complementary and alternative medicine* (CAM).[143] The National Center for Complementary and Alternative Medicine (NCCAM) groups CAM into five domains: whole medical systems (eg, Ayurveda, homeopathy), mind–body medicine (eg, prayer, hypnosis), biologically based practices (eg, herbal preparations, dietary supplements), manipulative and body-based practices (eg, acupressure, chiropractic, massage), and energy medicine (eg, therapeutic touch).[143]

For regulatory purposes the US government classifies herbal preparations as a type of dietary supplement, which means that the Food and Drug Administration (FDA) classifies them as nutrients with nondrug status.[59] However, many nonherbals, such as vitamins, minerals, nutritional supplements, and food additives, are also dietary supplements (Chaps. 39, 41, and 42).

The study of herbal preparations is complicated by the lack of standardized nomenclature, while the diversity of common, proprietary, and botanical names may increase the confusion. A single plant preparation may have many common names, in addition to its botanical name. For example, *Datura stramonium* is also known as jimson weed, Angel's trumpet, apple of Peru, Jamestown weed, thornapple, and tolguacha. Likewise, a common name for a plant, such as gordolobo, may refer to several botanical plants, such as *Verbascum thapsus* and *Gnaphalium macounii*.[100] The mandrake refers not only to the belladonna-alkaloid–containing *Mandragora officinarum* but also the podophyllum-containing *Podophyllum peltatum*. Thus, accurate classification of herbal preparations is very difficult, which limits effective study and increases the risk of adverse effects.

HISTORICAL BACKGROUND

Since ancient times and perhaps since prehistoric times, people of all cultures have used herbal preparations to treat disease and promote health.[53] A 60,000-year-old Iraqi burial site contained eight different medicinal plants, suggesting very early historical usage.[179] The earliest surviving written account of medicinal plants is the Egyptian Ebers papyrus, circa 1500 B.C., which lists dozens of medicinal plants and their intended uses. In India, the *Vedas*, epic poems written in approximately 1500 B.C., contain references to herbal preparations of the time. In China, the *Divine Husbandman's Classic*, written in the 1st century A.D., lists 252 herbal preparations. In ancient Europe, herbal medicines were the mainstay of healing. In the 1st century, the Greek physician Dioscorides wrote one of the first European herbal books, *De Materia Medica*, which listed 600 herbals and was translated into many languages. Shamans and folk healers from the Americas, Africa, Australia, and Asia continue to include herbals for spiritual and medicinal purposes, based on oral traditions passed from generation to generation.

During the Scientific Revolution, European scientists began to isolate purified extracts of plant products for use as medicinal agents. In 1804 and 1832, morphine and codeine were isolated from the sap of the poppy plant *Papaver somniferum*.[89] In the mid-18th century, Edward Stone described in a letter to the president of the Royal Society of Medicine the successful use of the bark of the willow tree in curing "agues" (fever).[28] In 1829, salicin, the active ingredient of the willow bark, was identified. Its derivative sodium salicylate was marketed in 1875 as a treatment for rheumatic fever and as an antipyretic. The enormous success of this drug led to the synthesis of acetylsalicylic acid in 1899. The original name, aspirin (*acetyl-spiric* acid), is said to have been derived from *Spiraea*, the plant genus from which salicylic acid once was prepared. Even today, plant preparations still are being investigated for the development of modern drugs. Sweet wormwood (*Artemisia annua*, qing hao) was first described as a treatment for malaria in China in 168 B.C.[113] In 1971, the active parent compound artemisinin was first isolated by Chinese investigators. Artemisinin, when used in combination with other antimalarials, is considered the best treatment for drug-resistant malaria.[106,133,170] Prescriptions from plant-derived medicines currently represent approximately 25% of prescriptions dispensed in the United States[4,202] and at least 60% of nonprescription medications still contain one or more natural products as ingredients.[62]

Today, herbal preparations continue to be the dominant form of healing in the developing world because of the high cost of "western" medical treatment and the scarcity of "western"-trained medical personnel.[61,118,121,134] The World Health Organization estimates that 4 billion people, up to 80% of the world population, use herbal preparations for some aspect of primary healthcare.[4,207] In the developed world in recent years there has been a resurgence in herbal preparation usage.[70] In 1991, a US survey determined that 2.5% of respondents had used herbal preparations in the prior year.[70] When the same survey was repeated in 1997 reported herbal usage in the previous year increased to 12.1%.[71] Two studies published in 2002 and 2004 revealed that 14% and 19% of the population used at least one herbal supplement during the preceding week and past 12 months, respectively.[12,110] Factors attributed to this resurgence in use include lower cost and ease of purchase compared to prescription medications; consumer empowerment; dissatisfaction with conventional therapies; and a perception by many users that herbals are better and safer.[44,178]

Herbal preparations and other dietary supplements are no longer sold exclusively in health food stores but are readily available for sale in mainstream retail outlets such as grocery stores, drug stores, complementary medicine practitioners, offices, mail order companies, the Internet, and gasoline stations. In 1999, sales of herbal preparations in the United States were estimated to be approximately $4 billion, with an annual growth rate of 18% per year.[25] In 1998, several US pharmaceutical companies launched a line of herbal products.[6] However, the explosive increase in demand in the 1990s was followed by marked decreases in the early 2000s. Market growth (food, drug, and mass market retailers [FDM]) dropped by 1% in 2000, 21% in 2001, and 14% in 2002.[19-21] The drop in sales was attributed to negative publicity concerning the dangers associated with ephedra and kava kava and the lack of efficacy of some popular herbal preparations, such as ginkgo and St. John's wort.[20,21] By 2005, the US herbal market appeared to have stabilized, and more recently in 2007 total estimated US herbal sales and recorded FDM US herbal sales increased 4.4% and 7.6%, respectively from the previous year.[32] Total US herbal dietary supplement sales were estimated at $4.79 billion in 2007, representing direct sales of $2.501 billion, natural and health food sales of $1.537 billion, and sales of $752 million from mass market retailers.[32]

Although they often are used by consumers in the hope of preventing or treating medical illness, herbals are not classified as medications and therefore, despite reports of toxicity associated with their usage, no systematic evaluation of herbal efficacy or safety is required. Additionally problematic is that patients often do not consider herbal preparations as medications and may not provide a history of usage unless questioned specifically about herbal usage. In an urban emergency department (ED) survey, 21.7% of respondents reported using herbal preparations. For 15.6% of these users, the herbal preparation was being used specifically to treat aspects of the patient's presenting chief complaint. Thirty-seven percent of herbal users reported that their physicians were unaware of their herbal preparation usage.[97] A survey of outpatients in a veteran's administration hospital revealed that 43% of respondents were taking at least one dietary supplement with prescription medications. Of those taking dietary supplements, 45% had a potential for xenobiotic dietary supplement interactions when considered with the respondent's prescription medications.[157] A recent telephone survey by the AARP determined that 63% of respondents 50 years or older admitted to current or prior usage of CAM but that only 22% said they had discussed their CAM use with their physician. Herbal product and dietary supplement usage was reported by 42% of respondents.[2] The most common reasons given for not discussing their use of CAM with their physician were: physician never asked (42%); respondent did not know they should (30%); there was not enough time in the office visit (19%); respondent assumed physician would not know about the topic (17%); and respondent thought doctor would be dismissive (12%).[2]

Herbal preparation use also appears to vary greatly by the community surveyed. Rural areas of Mississippi and southwestern West Virginia reported that 71% and 73% of respondents, respectively, used herbal preparations in the past year.[44,45,58] Among Chinese Americans in New York City and Hispanic Americans in west Texas, herbal preparation use was reported to be 43% and 50%, respectively.[130,158] Use of herbal preparations appears to be higher among people with chronic illness such as AIDS, rheumatoid arthritis, and cancer.[109,111,200] In the United States, increased likelihood of herbal preparation usage is associated with multiple factors, including concurrent illness and diverse socioeconomic and cultural influences.

Unfortunately, the medical profession's response to the widespread usage of herbal preparations appears to be inconsistent with one study suggesting that the medical practitioner's knowledge of current herbal preparation regulations is grossly inadequate.[9] Several studies have attempted to determine how US hospitals regulate herbal preparation use in their facilities.[7,13,55,79] Depending on the study, only 31% to 79% of respondents reported having formal policies governing the usage of herbal preparations in their facilities. Herbal preparation use was completely banned in 11%–22% of facilities. However, the majority of facilities did allow the use of herbal preparations if they were ordered by an authorized prescriber. Identified concerns addressed in these studies included difficulties in identifying products (particularly "home supply" products), and concerns for appropriate dosing, efficacy, safety, and consistency. The conflicting approaches have been attributed to healthcare facilities attempting to balance patient-centered care with their legal and ethical concerns about these products.[24,79]

In 1998, Congress established the National Center for Complementary and Alternative Medicine at the National Institutes of Health to stimulate, develop, and support research in complementary and alternative medicines.[131] The following is a summary of NCCAM-funded studies and their evaluation of the effectiveness of specific herbal preparations. In 2002, St. John's wort was found to be no more effective in treating depression than was placebo.[101] In 2004, hawthorne extract was described as ineffective in treating congestive heart failure.[1] In 2005, echinacea was determined to be ineffective in preventing symptoms of the common cold.[192] In 2006, glucosamine and chondroitin sulfate were considered unable to reduce pain in patients with osteoarthritis of the knee.[54] In 2006, saw palmetto was found not to improve symptoms or objective measures of benign prostatic hypertrophy over a 1-year followup.[15] In 2008, a pilot study failed to demonstrate any benefit of using ginkgo biloba in delaying the onset of dementia in the elderly.[67]

REGULATION OF HERBAL PREPARATIONS

In the US, herbal preparations are not subjected to the same standards and regulations as drugs. The FDA has gradually assumed an increased role in its vigilance over the manufacturing, marketing, and sales of herbal preparations. In 1994, Congress passed the Dietary Supplement Health and Education Act (DSHEA), which reduced the FDA's oversight of products categorized as dietary supplements.[74] Dietary supplements include vitamins, minerals, herbals, amino acids, and any product that had been sold as a "supplement" before October 15, 1994.[59] After October 15, 1994, any new ingredient intended for use in dietary supplements requires notification and approval by the FDA at least 75 days in advance of marketing. The FDA must review and determine whether the proposed ingredient is expected to be safe under the intended conditions for use. However, because most ingredients contained in dietary supplements were in use prior to 1994, the vast majority of dietary supplements are not subject to even this weakened premarket safety evaluation. After marketing, if the FDA determines that a manufactured dietary supplement is unsafe, the agency can warn the public, suggest changes to make the supplement safer, urge the manufacturer to recall the product, recall the product, or ban the product.

On several occasions the FDA has urged manufacturers to stop producing dietary supplements containing unsafe products. In July 2001, the FDA warned dietary supplement manufacturers to stop marketing products containing aristolochic acid because of nephrotoxicity and to remove comfrey products from the market because of hepatotoxicity. In November 2001, the FDA warned the manufacturer of LipoKinetix (containing phenylpropanolamine, caffeine, yohimbine, diiodothyronine, usnic acid) to remove the supplement from the marketplace because of reports of associated hepatotoxicity. In 2002, the FDA warned consumers and healthcare providers of the risk of hepatotoxicity associated with the use of kava-containing products.[197] However, the FDA did not ban the development of kava-containing products or ban their sale in the United States. In March 2004, the FDA warned dietary supplement manufacturers to stop manufacturing androstenedione or face enforcement actions.[196] To ban a dietary supplement from the marketplace, the FDA must prove that the product is unsafe. In April 2004, the FDA banned all sales of dietary supplements containing ephedra. This was the first FDA prohibition of a supplement since 1994.[195]

Because the law requires the FDA to consider dietary supplements as food products, quality control issues and production methods are governed by the Current Good Manufacturing Practices regulations for foods.[194] However, these regulations only ensure that foods, and thus dietary supplements, are produced under sanitary conditions; they do not guarantee the safety or efficacy of the product, as is required for pharmaceuticals. Before the FDA's release of the final rule Current Good Manufacturing Practices in 2007, there had been no attempt to ensure the purity and composition of herbal products.[75] In fact, two studies suggest that many herbal preparations do not even contain appreciable quantities of the listed herb. In one study of 54 ginseng products, 60% of those analyzed contained pharmacologically insignificant amounts of ginseng and 25% contained no ginsenosides at all.[123] A study of echinacea preparations determined that 10% of preparations contained no measurable echinacea, the assayed species was consistent with labeled content in 52% of the sample, and only 43% met the quality standard described by the label.[81] From 2004 to 2008, the FDA investigated online sales of dietary supplements purported to treat erectile dysfunction or enhance sexual performance by purchasing and analyzing the ingredients of these products.[193] One-third of the purchased dietary supplements (6 out of 17) contained undisclosed prescription drug ingredients: sildanafil or substances similar to sildanafil or vardenafil.[193]

Herbal products can be initially marketed without any proof of testing for efficacy or safety. Although packaging that claims to cure or prevent a specific disease is not permitted unless approved by the FDA, claims detailing how a product affects the "body's structure or function" are permissible. Substantiation of these claims is required if challenged by regulators,[194] but their methodology and requirements are not well defined. These findings were corroborated by a study evaluating herbal advertising on the Internet. The study determined that 81% of Web sites marketing dietary supplements made one or more health claims without approval from the FDA, and of these sites, 55% made specific claims to treat, prevent, or cure specific diseases.[139]

In March 1999, the FDA implemented new dietary supplement labeling rules. All dietary supplement labels must provide a statement of identity (eg, ginseng); net quantity of contents (eg, 60 capsules); structure–function claims with disclaimers that the product has not been evaluated by the FDA; directions for use; supplements fact panel (list of serving size, amount, and active ingredients); other ingredients list; and name and place of business of manufacturer, packer, or distributor. In February 2000, the FDA advised dietary supplement manufacturers not to make pregnancy-related claims on their products. In October 2004, the FDA sent warning letters to eight companies for making unsubstantiated claims over the Internet regarding the use of dietary supplement products for weight loss. In addition, it sent letters to major retailers of dietary supplements suggesting that it may take enforcement action against misbranded products and is "intent on starting a program of inspection of retail establishments to identify products bearing unsubstantiated claims in their labeling." The Dietary Supplement and Nonprescription Drug Consumer Protection Act was signed into law in December 2006.[66] Under this law, manufacturers, packers, or distributors of nutritional supplements are required to notify the FDA about serious adverse events related to their products. In 2007, the FDA issued its current good manufacturing practices final rule, effective in June 2008. The final rule is more stringent than previous regulations and it contains sections similar to current good manufacturing practices for drugs. Manufacturers are now required to evaluate the identity, purity, strength, and composition of their dietary supplements. Yet, unlike the FDA regulations for drugs; the final rule still does not require any proof of efficacy or safety. In essence, the FDA, through its regulations, has gradually shifted dietary supplements from a poorly regulated food product into a unique category between a conventional food product and a drug. This has served to increase the philosophical debate on both sides: from proponents who view dietary supplements as more similar to food groups (eg, chamomile tea) and want less government regulation, to proponents who argue that herbs are pharmacologically active drugs (eg, ephedra) that that require greater regulation.[132,140]

PHARMACOLOGIC PRINCIPLES

The pharmacologic activity of herbal preparations (plant containing or derived) can be classified by five active constituent classes: volatile oils, resins, alkaloids, glycosides, and fixed oils.[181]

- **Volatile oils** are aromatic plant ingredients. They are also called ethereal or essential oils, because they evaporate at room temperatures. Many are mucous membrane irritants and have CNS activity. Examples of herbs containing volatile oils include pennyroyal oil (*Mentha pulegium*), catnip (*Nepeta cataria*), chamomile (*Chamomilla recutita*), and garlic (*Allium sativum*) (Chap. 42).
- **Resins** are complex chemical mixtures of acrid resins, resin alcohols, resinol, tannols, esters, and resenes. These substances are often strong gastrointestinal irritants. Examples of resin-containing herbs include dandelion (*Taraxacum officinale*), elder (*Sambucus* spp), and black cohosh root (*Cimicifuga racemosa*).

- **Alkaloids** are a heterogeneous group of alkaline, organic, and nitrogenous compounds. The alkaloid compound usually is found throughout the plant. This class consists of many pharmacologically active and toxic compounds. Examples of alkaloid-containing herbs include aconitum (*Aconitum napellus*), goldenseal (*Hydrastis canadensis*), and jimson weed (*Datura stramonium*).
- **Glycosides** are esters that contain a sugar component (glycol) and a nonsugar (aglycone), which yields one or more sugars during hydrolysis. They include the anthroquinones, saponins, cyanogenic glycosides, and lactone glycosides. The anthroquinones (senna [*Cassia acutifolia*] and aloe [*Aloe vera*]) are irritating cathartics. Saponins (licorice [*Glycyrrhiza lepidota*] and ginseng [*Panax ginseng* and *P. quinquefolius*]) are mucous membrane irritants, cause hemolysis, and have steroid activity. Cyanogenic glycosides found in apricot, cherry, and peach pits release cyanide. Lactone glycosides (tonka beans [*Dipteryx odorata*]) have anticoagulant activities. Cardiac glycosides defined as cardioactive steroids (Chap. 64) are found in foxglove (*Digitalis* spp) and oleander (*Nerium oleander*).
- **Fixed oils** are esters of long-chain fatty acids and alcohols. Herbs containing fixed oils are generally used as emollients, demulcents, and bases for other agents. Generally, they are the least active and least dangerous of all herbal preparations. Examples include olive (*Olea europaea*) and peanut (*Arachis hypogaea*) oils.

FACTORS CONTRIBUTING TO HERBAL TOXICITY

The toxicity of a plant may vary widely and depends on conditions such as the time of year and developmental stage at which the plant is collected.[100] The pyrrolizidine alkaloid content of *Senecio* leaves varies widely from month to month and year to year.[100] In some cases, only selective parts of a plant used to prepare an herbal preparation are responsible for its toxicity. For example, the pyrrolizidine content of comfrey–pepsin capsules varies from 270 to 2900 mg/kg, depending on whether the leaves or roots were used in the preparation.[99] The geographical area in which the plant is collected may affect its toxicity. *Senecio longilobus* from Gardner Canyon, Arizona, may contain up to 18% pyrrolizidine alkaloids by dry weight, the highest level recorded for any *Senecio* plant species (normal concentration is 0.5%). Finally, conditions and duration of storage may affect its toxicity. The toxicity of *Crotalaria* decreases with storage because of the breakdown of pyrrolizidines.

Few poisonings result from the inherent toxicity of the herbal, because of the low concentration of active ingredient and the known safety of the chosen herb (Table 43-1). Instead, poisonings tend to result from the misuse, overuse (including increased concentration in some commercial derivative products), misidentification, misrepresentation, or contamination of the product. Heavy-metal poisonings from lead, cadmium, mercury, copper, zinc, and arsenic are associated with herbal preparation usage.[40,49,60,64,68,155,159,165] High concentrations of these elements sometimes result from contamination during the manufacturing process of some herbal or patent medications (ready-made preparations used by traditional Chinese herbalists). In some cases, as with cinnabar (mercuric sulfide) and calomel (mercurous chloride), these ingredients are intentionally included for purported medicinal benefit.[108] Patent medications may also contain pharmaceutical medications, such as acetaminophen, aspirin, antihistamines, or corticosteroids.[50,64] Many of these medicines are not listed on the packaging and may not even be approved for use in the United States. For example, four cases of agranulocytosis followed consumption of *Chui Fong Tou Ku Wan*, a preparation that contains both aminopyrine (which is not approved for nonprescription sales in the United States) and phenylbutazone (which was withdrawn from the US market), neither of which are listed on the packaging.[168] Both aminopyrine and phenylbutazone are associated with agranulocytosis.

CLASSIFICATION OF TOXICITY

Herbal preparations are associated with a wide variety of toxicologic manifestations (Table 43-2). In addition, many individual herbal preparations are associated with multiple toxicologic effects. To better understand these effects, it is useful to organize herbal toxicity into several general categories.[63]

DIRECT HEALTH RISKS

Direct health risks include pharmacologically predictable and dose-dependent toxic reactions, idiosyncratic toxic reactions, long-term toxic effects, and delayed toxic effects. For example, ingestion of aconite tea, in the suggested dose, causes tachydysrhythmias and hypotension. Idiosyncratic toxic reactions cannot be predicted on the basis of principal pharmacologic properties. For example, ingestion of chamomile tea results in anaphylaxis in a small subset of patients with probable allergies to the Compositae family. Long-term toxic effects occur only after chronic usage. For example, chronic use of herbal anthranoid laxatives results in muscular weakness from hypokalemia. Delayed toxic effects include carcinogenicity and teratogenicity. Another example is urothelial cancers in humans as a result of prolonged consumption of *Aristolochia*.[147]

INDIRECT HEALTH RISKS

Herbal use may adversely impact health by altering previous conventional prescription medication therapy. A patient may discontinue or become less compliant with previous therapy, with untoward consequences. Alternatively, the addition of an herbal preparation may affect the pharmacologic effect, principally by altering the bioavailability or clearance of concurrently used medications. Coadministration of St. John's wort, an inducer of CYP3A4, with the protease inhibitor indinavir, which is metabolized by this enzyme, may result in decreased plasma indinavir concentrations and potentially decreased antiretroviral activity.[162]

MOST WIDELY USED HERBAL SUPPLEMENTS

The most popular herbal supplements (food, drug, and mass-market retail outlets [excluding warehouse buying clubs and convenience store sales]) in the United States in 2007 are listed below in order of sales.[32] The top five represent more than 100 million dollars of sales.[32]

1. **Soy** (*Glycine max*)—Soy contains two popularly advertised ingredients: protein and isoflavones. Diets high in soy protein are associated with decreased cholesterol and low-density lipoprotein concentrations. Soy isoflavone supplements (genisten, daidzen) are phytoestrogens (plant estrogens) that currently are suggested as alternative remedies for treatment of menopausal symptoms. There is current concern regarding how high concentrations of isoflavones will affect the risk of developing breast cancer in postmenopausal women.
2. **Cranberry** (*Vaccinium macrocarpon*)—Cranberry is a popular remedy for treatment of urinary tract infections and they may be effective in preventing recurrent urinary tract infections.[104] Cranberry appears to be safe in appropriate doses.[10]

TABLE 43–1. Laboratory Analysis and Treatment Guidelines for Specific Herbal Preparations

Herbal Preparation	Suggested Laboratory Analysis	Antidote
Cardiac xenobiotics		
Ch'an Su (Bufo Bufo)	Serum digoxin, potassium	Digoxin-specific Fab
Foxglove	Serum digoxin, potassium	Digoxin-specific Fab
Oleander	Serum digoxin, potassium	Digoxin-specific Fab
Squill	Serum digoxin, potassium	Digoxin-specific Fab
Central Nervous System Xenobiotics		
Henbane	None	Physostigmine
Jimson weed (Datura)	None	Physostigmine
Mandrake	None	Physostigmine
Gastrointestinal Xenobiotics		
Aloe	Serum electrolytes	Potassium repletion
Buckthorn	Serum electrolytes	Potassium repletion
Cascara	Serum electrolytes	Potassium repletion
Fo-Ti	Serum electrolytes	Potassium repletion
Senna	Serum electrolytes	Potassium repletion
Metals	Ag, As, Au, Cd, Cr, Cu, Hg, Pb, Th, or Zn Abdominal radiograph (as appropriate)	Metal chelators
Hematologic Xenobiotics		
Dong Quai	PT	Vitamin K_1
Tonka bean	PT	Vitamin K_1
Woodruff	PT	Vitamin K_1
Hepatic xenobiotics		
Pennyroyal oil	AST/ALT	*N*-Acetylcysteine
Pyrrolizidine Alkaloids	AST/ALT	None available
Salicylates		
Medicated oils	Serum salicylate	Sodium bicarbonate, multiple-dose activated charcoal, hemodialysis
Cellular Xenobiotics		
Apricot pits (cyanogenic amygdalin)	Lactate	Cyanide antidote
Autumn crocus (colchicine)	WBC, BUN	? Glutamic acid
Elder (cyanide)	Lactate	Cyanide antidote
Periwinkle (vincristine)	WBC, BUN	? Glutamic acid
Podophyllum (podophyllin)	WBC, BUN	? Glutamic acid
Miscellaneous		
Licorice	Serum potassium	Potassium repletion
Quinine	ECG, serum potassium	Sodium bicarbonate, magnesium

3. **Garlic** (*Allium sativum*)—Garlic has been used as a food and a medicine since ancient times. As a herb, it is used for treatment of infections, hypertension, colic, and cancer.[80] The intact cells of garlic contain the odorless, sulfur-containing amino acid derivative (+)-*S*-allyl-L-cysteine sulfoxide, also known as *alliin*. When crushed, alliin is converted to allicin (diallyl thiosulfinate), which has antibacterial and antioxidant activity and gives the herb its characteristic odor and flavor. Side effects of garlic extracts include contact dermatitis, gastroenteritis, nausea, and vomiting. Several constituents of garlic, such as ajoene, possess antiplatelet effects. Consequently, garlic may increase the risk of bleeding in individuals who are also taking antiplatelet agents or anticoagulants.[80]
4. **Ginkgo** (*Ginkgo biloba*)—This herb contains ginkgo flavone glycosides, known as *ginkgolides*, that are reputed to have antioxidant properties, inhibit platelet aggregation, and increase circulation. It is a popularly used to treat or prevent both Alzheimer disease and peripheral vascular disease. However, two studies in 2002 and 2008 failed to demonstrate any improvement in cognitive function in healthy elderly subjects without cognitive impairment.[67,180] In appropriate doses ginkgo appears to be safe, although it may

TABLE 43–2. Selected Herbal Preparations, Popular Use, and Potential Toxicities

Herbal Preparation	Scientific Name	Other Common Names	Traditional and Popular Usage	Active/Toxic Ingredient(s)	Adverse Effects
Aconite	*Acontium napellus* *Acontium kusnezoffi* *Acontium carmichaelii*	Monkshood, wolfsbane caowu, chuanwu, bushi	Topical analgesic Neuralgia, asthma, heart disease	Aconite alkaloids (C19 diterpenoid esters) aconitine	GI upset, dysrhythmias
Agrimony	*Agrimonia eupatoria*	Cocklebur, stickwort, liverwort	Catarrh, gallbladder disease, astringent		Photodermatitis
Alfalfa	*Medicago sativa*		Arthritis, diabetes	l-canavanine	High doses: lupus, pancytopenia
Aloe	*Aloe vera* and other spp	Cape, Zanzibar, Socotrine, Curacao, Carrisyn	Heals wounds, emollient, laxative, abortifacient	Anthraquinones, barbaloin, isobarbaloin	GI upset, dermatitis, hepatitis
Apricot pits	*Prunus armeniaca*	–	(Laetrile) cancer remedy	Amygdalin	Cyanide poisoning
Aristolochia	*Aristolochia clematis* *Aristolochia reticulata* *Aristolochia fangchi*	Birthwort, heartwort, fangchi	Uterine stimulant, cancer treatment, antibacterial	Aristolochic acid	Nephrotoxin Renal cancer Retroperitoneal fibrosis
Artemisia	*Artemisia vulgaris* *Artemisia dracunculus* *Artemisia lactiflora*	Mugwort, felon herb, moxa, guizhou	Depression, dyspepsia, menstrual disorder, abortifacient	Lactones (sesquiterpenes)	GI upset, allergic reaction (skin, pulmonary)
Astragalus	*Astragalus membranaceus*	Huang qi, milk vetch root	Immune booster, AIDS, cancer, antioxidant, increase endurance	Astrogalasides, trigonoside, and flavonoid constituent	May alter effectiveness immunosuppressives (eg steroids, cyclosporine)
Atractylis	*Atractylis gummifera*	Piney thistle	Chewing gum, antipyretic, diuretic, gastrointestinal remedy	Potassium atractylate and gummiferin: mitochondrial toxin	Hepatitis, altered mental status, seizures, vomiting, hypoglycemia
Atractylodes	*Atractylodes macrocephala*	Baizhu, cangzhu	Appetitie stimulant, diuretic, GI upset	Atractylon, atractylol, atractylenolides	None
Autumn crocus	*Colchicum autumnale*	Crocus, fall crocus, meadow saffron, mysteria, vellorita	Gout, rheumatism, prostate/hepatic disease, cancer, gonorrhea	Colchicine	GI upset, renal disease, agranulocytosis
Bee pollen, royal jelly	Derived from *Apis mellifera*	–	Increase stamina, athletic ability, longevity	Pollen mixture containing hyperallergenic plant pollen or fungi contamination	Allergic reactions, anaphylaxis
Bee venom	Derived from *Apis mellifera*	–	Immunomodulator	Phospholipase A2 and mellitin, hyaluronidases	Allergic reactions, anaphylaxis
Betel nut	*Areca catechu*	Areca nut, pinlang, pinang	Stimulant	Arecholine	Possible bronchospasm, chronic use associated with leukoplakia and oropharyngeal squamous cell carcinoma
Bilberry	*Vaccinium myrtillus*	Whortleberry, black whortles	Diarrhea, night vision, varicose veins	Anthocyanosides	None reported
Bitter orange	*Citrus aurantia*	Changcao, Fructus auranti, green orange, kijitsu, Seville orange, sour orange, Zhi shi	Dyspepsia, increase appetite Weight loss	Synephrines	Cardiovascular toxicity, ephedrine-like effects
Bitter melon	*Momordica charantia*	Balsam pear	Abortifacient, diabetes, GI disorder, cancer, HIV therapy	Polysaccharide MAP-30 (protein)	None reported
Black cohosh	*Cimicifuga racemosa*	Black snakeroot, squawroot, bugbane, baneberry	Abortifacient, menstrual irregularity, astringent, dyspepsia	Triterpene glycosides	Dizziness, nausea, vomiting, headache

TABLE 43–2. Selected Herbal Preparations, Popular Use, and Potential Toxicities (*Continued*)

Herbal Preparation	Scientific Name	Other Common Names	Traditional and Popular Usage	Active/Toxic Ingredient(s)	Adverse Effects
Black currant oil	*Ribes nigrum*	Quinsy berry, squinancy berry	Immunostimulant, premenstrual syndrome	GLA (γ-linolenic acid) ALA (α-linolenic acid)	None reported
Blue cohosh	*Caulophyllum thalictroides*	Squaw root, papoose root, blue ginseng	Abortifacient, dysmenorrhea, antispasmodic	*N*-methylcytisine (2.5% the potency of nicotine)	Nicotinic toxicity
Boneset	*Eupatorium perfoliatum*	Thoroughwort, vegetable antimony, feverwort	Antipyretic	Pyrrolizidine alkaloids	Possible hepatotoxicity, dermatitis, milk sickness
Borage	*Borago officinalis*	Bee plant, bee bread	Diuretic, antidepressant, antiinflammatory	Pyrrolizidine alkaloids, amabiline	Hepatotoxicity
Boron		Boron	Topical astringent, wound remedy	Boron	Dermatitis, GI upset, renal and hepatic toxicity, seizures, coma, death
Broom	*Cytisus scoparius*	Scotch broom, Bannal, broom top	Cathartic, diuretic, induce labor, drug of abuse	l-sparteine	Nicotinic toxicity
Buchu	*Agathosma betulina*	Bookoo, buku, diosma, bucku, bucco	Diuretic, stimulant, carminative, urine infections, insect repellent	Diosmin, hesperidin; pulegone	None reported
Buckthorn	*Rhamnus frangula*		Laxative	Anthraquinones	Diarrhea, weakness
Burdock root	*Arctium lappa* *Arctium minus*	Great burdock, gobo, lappa, beggar's button, hareburr, niu bang zi	Diuretic, cholerectic, induce sweating, skin disorders, burn remedy, diabetes treatment	Atropine (contamination with belladonna alkaloids during harvesting)	Anticholinergic toxicity
Calendula	*Calendula officinalis*	Marigold, garden marigold, pot marigold, gold bloom, holligold	Wounds, dysmenorrhea, "radiation" dermatitis		None reported
Cantharidin	*Cantharis vesicatoria* beetle	Spanish fly, blister beetles	Aphrodisiac, abortifacient, blood purifier	Terpenoid: cantharidin	GI upset, urinary tract and skin irritant, renal toxicity
Caraway	*Umbelliferae carvi*		Antispasmodic, carminative	d-carvone	
Carp bile (raw)	*Ctenopharyngodon idellus*	Grass carp	Improve visual acuity and health	? Cyprinol, C27 bile alcohol	Hepatitis, renal failure
	Cyprinus carpio	Common carp			
Cascara	*Rhamnus purshiana*	Cascara sagrada	Laxative	Anthraquinones	Diarrhea, weakness
Cat's claw	*Uncaria tomentosa* *Uncaria guianensis*	Uña de gato	AIDS, cancer, arthritis, ulcers, dysmenorrhea, wounds, contraceptives	Pentacyclic oxindole alkaloids, tetracyclic oxindole alkaloids	None reported
Catnip	*Nepeta cataria*	Cataria, catnep, catmint	Indigestion, colic, sedative, euphoriant, headaches, emmenagogue	Nepetalactone	Sedative
Ch'an Su	*Bufo bufo gargarizans* *Bufo bufo melanosticus*	Stone, lovestone, black stone, rock hard, chuan wu, kyushin	Topical anesthetic, aphrodisiac, cardiac disease	Bufodienolides, bufotenin	Dysrhythmias, hallucinations
Chamomile	*Matricaria recutita, Chamaemelum nobile*	Manzanilla	Digestive disorders, skin disorders, cramps	Allergens	Contact dermatitis, allergic reaction, anaphylaxis very rare
Chaparral	*Larrea tridentata*	Creosote bush, greasewood, hediondilla	Bronchitis, analgesic, anti-aging, cancer	Nondihydroguaiaretic acid (NDGA)	Hepatotoxicity (chronic)
Chestnut	*Chestnut*	Horse chestnut, California buckeye, Ohio buckeye, buckeye	Arthritis, rheumatism, varicose veins, hemorrhoids	Esculin, nicotine, quercetin, quercitrin, rutin, saponin, shikimic acid	Fasciculations, weakness, incoordination, GI upset, paralysis, stupor
Chuen-Lin	*Coptis chinensis, Coptis japonicum*	Golden thread, Huang-Lien, Ma-Huang	Infant tonic	Berberine: displaces bilirubin from protein	Neonatal hyperbilirubinemia

(*Continued*)

TABLE 43–2. Selected Herbal Preparations, Popular Use, and Potential Toxicities (*Continued*)

Herbal Preparation	Scientific Name	Other Common Names	Traditional and Popular Usage	Active/Toxic Ingredient(s)	Adverse Effects
Clove	*Syzygium aromaticum*	Caryophyllum	Expectorant, antiemetic, counterirritant, antiseptic, carminative euphoriant	Eugenol (4-allyl-2-methoxyphenol)	Pulmonary toxicity (cigarettes)
Coltsfoot	*Tussilago farfara*	Coughwort, horsehoof, kuandong hua	Throat irritation, asthma, bronchitis, cough	Pyrrolizidine alkaloids: tussilagin, senkirkine	Allergy, hepatotoxicity
Comfrey	*Symphytum officinale, Symphytum spp, S. x uplandicum*	Knitbone, bruisewort, blackwort, slippery root, Russian comfrey	Ulcers, hemorrhoids, bronchitis, burns, sprains, swelling, bruises	Pyrrolizidine alkaloids: symphytine, echimidine, lasiocarpine	Hepatic veno-occlusive disease
Compound Q	*Trichosanthes kirilowii*	Gualougen, GLQ-223, Chinese cucumber root	Fevers, swelling, expectorant, abortifacient, diabetes, AIDS	Trichosanthin	Pulmonary injury (ALI), cerebral edema, cerebral hemorrhage, seizures, fevers
Cordyceps {mushroom]	*Cordyceps sinensis*	Dong chong xia cao	General tonic, aphrodisiac, bronchitis, kidney disorders	Cordyceptic acid, Cordycepin	None reported
Damiana	*Turnera diffusa var aphrodisiaca*	–	Stimulant, purgative, aphrodisiac, antidepressant	Caryophyllene oxide, caryophyllene, δ-cadinene, elemene, 1,8-cineol	Genitourinary irritation
Dandelion	*Taraxacum officinale*		Diuretic, detoxifying remedy, bitter	Luteolin	None reported
Deer antler velvet			Erectile dysfunction, infertility immunostimulant, antiinflammatory, athletic performance	Small amounts of androstenedione, dihydroepiandrosterone, and testosterone	None reported
Dong Quai	*Angelica polymorpha*	Tang kuei, dang gui	Blood purifier, dysmenorrhea, improve circulation	Coumarin, psoralens, safrole in essential oil	Anticoagulant effects, photodermatitis, possible carcinogen in oil
Echinacea	*Echinacea angustifolia, Echinacea purpurea*	American cone flower, purple cone flower, snakeroot	Infections, immunostimulant	Echinacoside	CYP 1A2 inhibitor
Elder	*Sambucus* spp	Elderberry, sweet elder, sambucus	Diuretic, laxative, astringent, cancer	Isoquercitrin Cyanogenic glycoside: sambunigrin in leaves	GI upset, weakness if uncooked leaves ingested
Ephedra	*Ephedra* spp	Ma-huang, Mormon tea, yellow horse, desert tea, squaw tea, sea grape	Stimulant, bronchospasm	Ephedrine, pseudoephedrine	Headache, insomnia, dizziness, palpitations, seizures, stroke, myocardial infarction, death
Evening primrose	*Oenothera biennis*	Oil of evening primrose	Coronary disease, multiple sclerosis, cancer, diabetes rheumatoid arthritis, premenstrual syndrome	Cis-γ-linoleic acid	Lower seizure threshold
Fennel	*Foeniculum vulgare*	Common, sweet, or bitter fennel	Gastroenteritis, expectorant, emmenagogue, stimulate lactation	Volatile oils: transanethole, fenchone; estrogens: dianethole, photoanethole	Ingestion of volatile oils: vomiting, seizures, pulmonary injury (ALI), dermatitis, estrogen effects
Fenugreek	*Trigonella foenumgraecum*	Bird's foot, Greek hay seed	Expectorant, demulcent, antiinflammatory, emmenanogue, galactogogue, diabetes	4-hydroxyisoleucine	Hypoglycemia, Hypokalemia

TABLE 43–2. Selected Herbal Preparations, Popular Use, and Potential Toxicities (*Continued*)

Herbal Preparation	Scientific Name	Other Common Names	Traditional and Popular Usage	Active/Toxic Ingredient(s)	Adverse Effects
Feverfew	*Tanacetum parthenium*	Featherfew, altamisa, bachelor's button, featherfoil, febrifuge plant, midsummer daisy, nosebleed, wild quinine	Migraine headache, menstrual pain, asthma, dermatitis, arthritis, antipyretic, abortifacient		Oral ulcerations, "postfeverfew syndrome," rebound of migraine symptoms, anxiety, insomnia following cessation of chronic use
Fo-Ti	*Polygonum multiflorum*	Climbing knotwood, he shou-wu	Scrofula, cancer, constipation therapy, promote longevity	Anthraquinones: chrysophanol, emodin, rhein	Cathartic effects
Foxglove	*Digitalis purpurea, Digitalis lanata, Digitalis lutea, Digitalis* spp	Purple foxglove, throatwort, fairy finger, fairy cap, lady's thimble, scotch mercury, witch's bells, dead man's bells	Asthma, sedative, diuretic/cardiotonic, wounds and burns (India)	Cardioactive steroids (eg, digitoxin, gitoxin, digoxin, digitalin, gitaloxin)	Blurred vision, GI upset, dizziness, muscle weakness, tremors, dysrhythmias
Garcinia	*Garcinia cambogia*	Brindleberry, hydroxycitric acid	Weight loss	Hydroxycitric acid	May lower serum glucose concentration in diabetics
Garlic	*Allium sativum*	Allium, stinking rose, rustic treacle, nectar of the gods, da suan	Infections, coronary artery disease, hypertension	Alliin, Ajoene	Contact dermatitis, gastroenteritis, antiplatelet effects
Gentian	*Gentiana lutea, Gentiana* spp	Bitter root, gall weed Longdancao	Bitter, digestive stimulant, emmenagogue	–	None reported
Germander	*Teucrium chamaedrys*	Wall germander	Antipyretic, abdominal disorders, wounds, diuretic, choleretic	Furano neoclerodane diterpenes	Hepatotoxicity, hepatitis, cirrhosis
Ginger	*Zingiber officinale*		Carminative, diuretic, antiemetic, stimulant, motion sickness	Volatile oil, phenol	Possible increased risk of bleeding when taken with anticoagulants
Ginkgo	*Ginkgo biloba*	Maidenhair tree, kew tree, tebonin, tanakan, rokan, kaveri	Asthma, chilblain, digestive aid, cerebral dysfunction	Ginkgo flavone glycosides and terpene lactones (ginkgolides and bilobalide)	Extracts: GI upset, headache, skin reaction; whole plants: allergic reactions
Ginseng	*Panax ginseng Panax quinquefolius Panax pseudoginseng*	Ren shen	Respiratory illnesses, gastrointestinal disorders, impotence, fatigue, stress, adaptogenic, external demulcent	Ginsenosides: panaxin, ginsenin	Ginseng abuse syndrome
Glucomannan	*Amorphophallus konjac*	Konjac, konjac mannan	Weight-reducing agent: "grapefruit diet," increase viscosity, decrease gastric emptying	Polysaccharides	Esophageal and lower GI obstruction
Glucosamine	2-amino-2-deoxyglucose	Chitosamine	Wound-healing polymer, antiarthritic	Glucosamine	None reported
Goat's rue	*Galega officinalis*	French lilac, French honeysuckle	Antidiabetic	Galegine, paragalegine	Hypoglycemia
Goji	*Lycium barbarum, chinense*	Wolfberry, gou qi zi	Protect liver, improve eyesight, enhance immune system	Carotenoids, lutein, atropine	May inhibit warfarin metabolism
Goldenseal	*Hydrastis canadensis*	Orange root, yellow root, turmeric root	Astringent, GI disorders, dysmenorrhea	Berberine, hydrastine	GI upset, Very high doses: paralysis and respiratory failure

(*Continued*)

TABLE 43–2. Selected Herbal Preparations, Popular Use, and Potential Toxicities (*Continued*)

Herbal Preparation	Scientific Name	Other Common Names	Traditional and Popular Usage	Active/Toxic Ingredient(s)	Adverse Effects
Gordolobo yerba	*Senecio longiloba* *Senecio aureu,* *Senecio vulgaris* *Senecio spartoides*	Groundsel, liferoot	Gargle, cough, emmenagogue	Pyrrolizidine alkaloids	Hepatic veno-occlusive disease
Gotu Kola	*Centella asiatica*	Hydrocotyle, Indian pennywort, talepetrako	Wound healing, tonic, antibacterial	Asiaticoside, asiatic acid, madecassic acid	Contact dermatitis
Grape seed	*Vitis vinifera*		Antioxidant: antiaging, peripheral vascular disease	Proanthocyanidins	None reported
Green tea	*Camillia sinensis*	Green tea	Antioxidant, weight loss, reduce cholesterol	Polyphenols (catechins and epigallocatechin gallate)	Hepatoxicity from green tea extracts
Hawthorn	*Crataegus oxyacantha* *Crataegus laevigata* *Crataegus monogyna*	English hawthorn, haw, maybush, whitethorn	Hypertension, CHF, dysrhythmias, antispasmodic, sedative	Hyperoside, vitexin, procyanidin	Hypotension, sedation
Heliotrope	*Crotalaria specatabilis,* *Heliotropium europaeum*	Rattlebox, groundsel, viper's bugloss, bush tea	Cancer	Pyrrolizidine alkaloids	Hepatic veno-occlusive disease
Henbane	*Hyoscyamus niger*	Fetid nightshade, poison tobacco, insane root, stinky nightshade	Sedative, analgesic, antispasmodic, asthma	Hyoscyamine, hyoscine	Anticholinergic toxicity
Holly	*Ilex aquifolium* *Ilex opaca* *Ilex vomitoria*	English holly, American holly, and yaupon	Tea, emetic, CNS stimulant, coronary artery disease	Saponins	GI upset
Hoodia	*Hoodia gordonii*	Xhooba, khoba, Ghaap, hoodia cactus, South African desert cactus	Weight loss, appetite suppressant	P57	None reported
Horny goat weed	*Epimedium grandiflorum*	Ying yang huo	Aphrodisiac	Icariin	None reported
Hydrangea	*Hydrangea arborescens* *Hydrangea paniculata*	Seven bark, wild hydrangea	Diuretic, stimulant, carminative, cystitis, renal calculi, asthma	Hydrangin, saponin	Dizziness, chest pain, GI upset
Iboga	*Tabernanthe iboga*	Ibogaine	Aphrodisiac, stimulant, hallucinogen, addiction treatment	Indole alkaloid: ibogaine	Hallucinations, cholinergic hyperactivity
Impila	*Callipesis laureola*		Zulu traditional remedy	Potassium atractylate–like compound	Vomiting, hypoglycemia, centrilobular hepatic necrosis
Jalap	*Ipomoea purga*	–	Cathartic	Convolvulin	Profuse watery diarrhea
Jimsonweed	*Datura stramonium*	Datura, stramonium, apple of Peru, Jamestown weed, thornapple, tolguacha	Asthma	Atropine, scopolamine, hyoscyamine, stramonium	Anticholinergic toxicity
Juniper	*Juniperus communis* *Juniperus macropoda*	Oil of sabinol	Tonic, diuretic, urinary antiseptic, emmenogogue, abortifacient	Monoterpenes (terpinen-4-ol)	Renal irritation

TABLE 43–2. Selected Herbal Preparations, Popular Use, and Potential Toxicities (*Continued*)

Herbal Preparation	Scientific Name	Other Common Names	Traditional and Popular Usage	Active/Toxic Ingredient(s)	Adverse Effects
Kava kava	*Piper methysticum*	Awa, kava-kava, kew, tonga	Relaxation beverage, uterine relaxation headaches, colds, wounds, aphrodisiac	Kava lactones Flavokwain A and B	Mild euphoria, muscle weakness Skin discoloration, hepatic failure
KH-3	Procaine HCl	Gerovital-H3, GH-3, Gero-vita	Cerebral atherosclerosis, dementia, arthritis, hair loss, hypertension	Procaine	Procaine toxicity
Khat	*Catha edulis*	Qut, kat, chaat, Kus es Salahin, Tchaad, Gat	CNS stimulant, depression, fatigue, obesity, ulcers	Cathine, cathinone	Euphoria, dysphoria, stimulation, sedation, psychological dependence leukoplakia
Kola nut	*Cola acuminata*	Botu cola, cola nut	Digestive aid, tonic, aphrodisiac, headache, diuretic	Caffeine, theobromine, kolanin	CNS stimulant
Kombucha	Mixture of bacteria and yeast	Kombucha tea, kombucha mushroom, Manchurian tea	Memory loss, premenstrual syndrome, cancer	—	Hepatotoxicity/metabolic acidosis
Levant berry	*Anamirta cocculus*	Fish killer, fishberry, hockle elderberry, Indian berry, louseberry, poisonberry	Vermifuge, malaria	Picrotoxin	CNS stimulant, GI upset
Licorice	*Glycyrrhiza glabra*	Spanish licorice, Russian licorice, gancao	Gastric irritation	Glycoside glycyrrhizin	Flaccid weakness, dysrhythmias, hypokalemia, lethargy
Lipoic acid		α-lipoic acid, thioctic acid	Antioxidant, diabetes, neuropathy, AIDS	Lipoic acid	Hypoglycemia
Lobelia	*Lobelia inflata*	Indian tobacco	Antispasmodic, respiratory stimulant, relaxant	Pyridine-derived alkaloids (lobeline)	Nicotine toxicity
Mace	*Myristica fragrans*	Mace, muscade, seed cover of nutmeg	Diarrhea, mouth sores, insomnia, rheumatism	Myristicin (methoxysafrole)	Hallucinations
Mandrake	*Mandragora officinarum*		Hallucinogen	Atropine, scopolamine, hyoscyamine	Anticholinergic toxicity
Mate	*Ilex paraguayensis*	Paraguay tea	Stimulant	Caffeine	Caffeine toxicity
Milk thistle	*Carduus marianus* *Silybum marinaum*	Mary thistle	Liver disease, antidepressant, HIV	Silymarin	None
Mistletoe	*Viscum album* *Phoradendron leucarpum*	Iscador	Antispasmodic, calmative, cancer, HIV	Viscotoxins, lectins	GI upset, bradycardia, delirium
Morinda	*Morinda citrifolia*	Noni, Indian mulberry, nonu/nono, mengkudu, bajitian	Antioxidant, stress, depression	Polysaccharides, anthraquinone: damnacanthal	None
Morning glory	*Ipomoea purpurea* *I. violacea*	Heavenly blue, blue star, flying saucers	Hallucinogen	Lysergic acid lamide Ergine	LSD-like toxicity
Myrrh	*Commiphora molmol*	Mulmul, ogo, heerabol	Astringent, antiseptic, emmenagogue, antispasmodic, cancer	Sesquiterpenes	None
Nutmeg	*Myristica fragrans*	Mace, rou dou kou	Hallucinogen, abortifacient, aphrodisiac, GI disorders, emmenogogue	Myristicin	Hallucinogen, GI upset

(*Continued*)

TABLE 43–2. Selected Herbal Preparations, Popular Use, and Potential Toxicities (*Continued*)

Herbal Preparation	Scientific Name	Other Common Names	Traditional and Popular Usage	Active/Toxic Ingredient(s)	Adverse Effects
Oleander	*Nerium oleander*	Adelfa, laurier rose, rosa laurel, rose bay, rose francesca	Cardiac disorders, asthma, corns, cancer, epilepsy	Oleandrin, neriin, Gentiobiosyloeandrin, odoroside A	GI upset, diarrhea, dysrhythmias
Olive leaf extract	*Olea europaea*		Immunostimulant	Oleuropein	
Ostrich fern	*Matteuccia struthipteris*	–	Laxative	–	GI upset if eaten undercooked
Parsley	*Petroselinum crispum*	Rock parsley, garden parsley	Diuretic, uterine stimulant, abortifacient	Myristicin, apiol, furocoumarin, psoralen	Uterine stimulant, photosensitization
Passion flower	*Passiflora incarnata*	Passiflora, maypop	Insomnia, analgesic stimulant	Harmala alkaloids	Sedation
Pau d'Arco	*Tabebuia* spp	Ipe roxo, lapacho, taheebo tea	Tonic, "blood builder," cancer, AIDS	Napthoquinone derivative: lapachol	GI upset anemia, bleeding
Pennyroyal oil	*Hedeoma pulegioides* *Mentha pulegium*	American pennyroyal, Squawmint, mosquito plant	Abortifacient, regulate menstruation, digestive tonic	Cyclohexanone: pulegone	Hepatotoxicity
Periwinkle	*Catharanthus roseus*	Red periwinkle, Madagascar or Cape periwinkle, old maid, church-flower, ram-goat rose, "myrtle," magdalena	Hallucinogen, ocular inflammation, diabetes, hemorrhage, insect stings, cancers	Vincristine, vinblastine Indole alkaloid	Vincristine/vinblastine toxicity
Podophyllum	*Podophyllum peltatum* *Podophyllum hexandrum* *Podophyllum emodi*	Mandrake, mayapple, American podophyllum Indian podophyllum guijiu	Cathartic, purgative	Podophyllin	Podophyllin toxicity
Pokeweed	*Phytolacca americana* *Phytolacca decandra*	American nightshade, Cancer jalap, inkberry, poke, scoke	Arthritis, emetic, purgative	Saponins: phytolaccigenin, jaligonic acid, phytolaccagenic acid, pokeweed mitogen	Gastroenteritis, blurry vision, weakness, respiratory distress, seizures, leukocytosis
Pycnogenol (French maritime pine bark extract)	*Pinus pinaster*	Pine bark extract	Antioxidant, hypertension vascular disease, ADHD	Proanthocyanidins	None reported
Pygeum	*Prunus africana*	Pygeum africanum, African prune	Impotence, male infertility, prostate cancer, benign prostatic hypertrophy	β-sitosterol, pentacyclic terpenes, ferulic esters	None reported
Quinine	*Cinchona succirubra* *Cinchona calisya* *Cinchona ledgeriana*	Red bark, Peruvian bark Jesuit's bark, China bark Cinchona bark, quinaquina, fever tree	Malaria, fever, indigestion Cancer Hemorrhoids, varicose veins, abortifacient	Quinine	Cinchonism
Red bush tea	*Aspalathus linearis*	Rooibos tea	Anxiety, allergic dermatitis, indigestion	Aspalathin, isoorientin, orientin, rutin	None reported
Red clover	*Trifolium pratense*	Trefoil, purple clover, wild clover	Bronchitis, cough, eczema, acne, premenstrual syndrome	Isoflavones: biochanin A and formononetin	None reported
Rehmannia	*Rehmannia glutinosa*	Sheng di huang, Chinese foxglove root	Arthritis, asthma, kidney and liver tonic, aplastic anemia, hypopituitarism	Irodoids and iridoid glycosides	None reported
Reishi mushroom	*Ganoderma lucidum*	Ling zhi, lucky fungus	Hepatitis, promote longevity	Polysaccharide peptides, triterpenes (ganoderic acid)	None reported

TABLE 43–2. Selected Herbal Preparations, Popular Use, and Potential Toxicities (*Continued*)

Herbal Preparation	Scientific Name	Other Common Names	Traditional and Popular Usage	Active/Toxic Ingredient(s)	Adverse Effects
Rosavin	*Rhodiola rosea*	Golden root, crenulin	Weight loss, aphrodisiac, adaptogen, improve cognitive function	Loaustralin, rosavin, rosin, rosarin, salidroside	None reported
Rose hips	*Rosa canina*	Hip berry, rose haws, rose heps, wild boar fruit	Vitamin C supplement, Upper respiratory infection, diarrhea	Vitamin C, vitamin K	May interfere with warfarin
Rue	*Ruta graveolens*	Herb of grace, herb grass	Emmenagogue, antispasmodic, abortifacient	Fucocoumarins, bergapten, xanthoxanthin	Photosensitization
Sage	*Salvia officinalis*	Garden sage, true sage, scarlet sage, meadow sage	Antiseptic, astringent, hormonal stimulant, carminative, abortifacient	Camphor, thujone	Seizures
St. John's wort	*Hypericum perforatum*	Klamath weed, John's wort, goatweed, sho-rengyo	Anxiety, depression, gastritis, insomnia, promote healing, AIDS	Hyperforin, Hypericin	Occasional photosensitization, drug interaction: CYP3A4
Salvia	*Salvia divinorum* *Salvia miltiorrhizae*	Sierra mazateca, diviners sage, magic mint, Maria pastora	Hallucinogen, renal disease	Salvinorum A Lithospermate B	Hallucinations
SAM-e	*S*-adenosyl-L-methionine		Antidepressant, osteoarthritis, liver disease	*S*-adenoysl-L-methionine,	None reported
Sassafras	*Sassafras albidum*	Lauraceae	Stimulant, antispasmodic, purifier	sassafras oil (80% Safrole)	Hepatotoxicity, carcinogen (?)
Saw palmetto	*Serenoa repens*	Sabal, American dwarf palm tree, cabbage palm	Genitourinary disorders, increase sperm production, sexual vigor	5-α reductase inhibitor	Diarrhea
Schisandra	*Schisandra chinensis*	Wu zei zi, five flavored seed	Tonic, aphrodisiac, liver treatment, sedative	Schisandrins, nigranoic acid	None reported
Scullcap	*Scutellaria lateriflora*	Skullcap, helmetflower, hood wort	Tranquilizer, tonic, antispasmodic	Flavone glucuronides and flavanone glucuronides	None reported
Senna	*Cassia acutifoli* *Cassia angustifolia*	Alexandrian senna	Stimulant, laxative, diet tea	Anthraquinone, glycosides (sennosides)	Diarrhea, CNS effects
Shark cartilage	*Squalus acanthias* *Sphyrna lewini*	–	Cancer: inhibit tumor angiogenesis	Chondroitin sulfate	None reported
Siberian ginseng	*Eleutherococcus senticos*	Devil's shrub, eleuthra, eleutherococ	Adaptogens, hypertension, immunomodulator	Ginsenosides	None reported
Slippery elm	*Ulmus rubra* *Ulmus fulva*	Elm, elm bark, red elm	Acne, boils, indigestion, abortifacient	Polysaccharide mucilage Oleoresin	Contact dermatitis
Soapwort	*Saponaria officinalis*	Bruisewort, bouncing bet, dog cloves, fuller's herb, latherwort	Acne, psoriasis, eczema, boils, natural soaps	Saponins	IV: highly toxic PO: None
SOD	Superoxide dismutase	Orgotein, ormetein, palosein	Improve health, lengthen lifespan, chronic bladder disease, paraquat poisoning	Superoxide dismutase	None reported
Soy isoflavone	*Glycine max*		Menopausal symptoms, heart disease	Phytoestrogens: genistein, daidzein, glycitein	Cancer
Squill	*Urginea maritima* *Urginea indica*	Sea onion Red Squill	Diuretic, emetic, cardiotonic, expectorant	Cardioactive steroid, scillaren A	Emesis, dysrhythmias

(*Continued*)

TABLE 43–2. Selected Herbal Preparations, Popular Use, and Potential Toxicities (*Continued*)

Herbal Preparation	Scientific Name	Other Common Names	Traditional and Popular Usage	Active/Toxic Ingredient(s)	Adverse Effects
Stephania	*Stephania tetranda*	Han fang ji	Fever, pain, inflammation, decrease water retention	–	None (misidentification of this herb with aristolochia [Guang fang ji] resulted in cases of Chinese herb nephropathy)
Stevia	*Stevia rebaudiana*	Sweet leaf of Paraguay	Sugar-free sweetener, diabetes, hypertension, weight-loss aid	Stevioside	None reported
T'u-san-chi	*Gynura segetum*	–	Tea	Pyrrolizidine alkaloids	Hepatic veno-occlusive disease
Tonka bean	*Dipteryx odorata, Dipteryx oppositifolia*	Tonquin bean, cumaru	Food, cosmetics	Coumarin	Anticoagulant effect
Tung seed	*Aleurites moluccana A. fordii*	Tung, candlenut, candleberry, barnish tree, balucanat, otaheite	Wood preservative (oil), purgative (oil), asthma treatment (seed)	Saponins, phytotoxins	GI upset, hyporeflexia, death; latex: dermatitis
Valerian	*Valeriana officinalis*	Radix valerianae, Indian Valerian, red valerian	Anxiety, insomnia, antispasmodic	– Valepotriates, valerenic acid	Sedation
Vitex	*Vitex agnus-castus*	Chasteberry, chaste tree, agnus castus	Premenstrual syndrome, female infertility	–	None reported
White cohosh	*Actaea alba, Actaea rubra*	Baneberry, snakeberry, doll's eyes, coralberry	Emmenagogue	Protoanemonin	Headache, GI upset, delirium, circulatory failure
White willow bark	*Salix alba*	Common willow, European willow	Fever, pain astringent	Salicin	Salicylate toxicity
Wild lettuce	*Lactuca virosa Lactuca sativa*	Lettuce opium, prickley lettuce	Sedative, cough suppressant, analgesic	–	None reported
Woodruff	*Galium odoratum*	Sweet woodruff	Wound healing, tonic, varicose veins, antispasmodic	Coumarin	None reported
Wormwood	*Artemisia absinthium*	Absinthes	Sedative, analgesic, antihelminthic	Thujone	Psychosis, hallucinations, seizures
Yarrow	*Achillea millefolium*	Bloodwort, carpenter's grass, dog daisy, nosebleed	Heal wounds, viral symptoms, digestive disorder, diuretic	–	Contact dermatitis
Yew	*Texus baccata*	Yew	Antispasmodic, cancer remedy	Taxine (Sodium channel blocker)	Dizziness, dry mouth, bradycardia, cardiac arrest
Yohimbe	*Pausinystalia yohimbe*	Yohimbi, yohimbehe	Body building, aphrodisiac, stimulant	Alkaloid yohimbine from bark	Hypertension, abdominal pain, weakness

increase the risk of bleeding in individuals who are also taking antiplatelet agents or anticoagulants.[77,136,151]

5. **Saw palmetto** (*Serenoa repens*)—Saw palmetto is a popular remedy for benign prostatic hypertrophy. Saw palmetto inhibits 5-α-reductase. However, a recent study observed that saw palmetto did not improve symptoms or objective measures of benign prostatic hypertrophy.[15] Saw palmetto appears to be safe in appropriate doses.[136,151]
6. **Echinacea** (*Echinacea purpurea, angustifolia*)—Echinacea is a reputed immunostimulant and is a popular herbal remedy for cold symptoms. However, a NCCAM-funded study was unable to detect any improvement in preventing these symptoms.[192] Echinacea appears to be safe in appropriate doses.[87] Rare individuals develop allergic reactions when taking echinacea.[141]
7. **Black cohosh** (*Cimicifuga racemosa*)—Black cohosh is a popular remedy for treatment of premenstrual syndrome and as alternative estrogen replacement therapy for relief of perimenopausal symptoms. It also is used as a treatment for arthritis and as a mild sedative. Black cohosh appears to be safe in appropriate doses.[18,98]
8. **Milk thistle** (*Silybum marianum*)—Milk thistle contains silymarin and is a popular remedy for treatment of liver dysfunction. It appears to be safe.

TABLE 43–3. Constituent Psychoactive Xenobiotics in Herbal Preparations

Labeled Ingredient	Scientific Name	Usage	Active Ingredients	Effects
Broom	*Cytisus scoparius*	Smoke for relaxation	L-Sparteine	Sedative-hypnotic
California poppy	*Eschscholtzia californica*	Smoke as marijuana substitute	Alkaloids and glucosides	Euphoriant
Catnip	*Nepeta cataria*	Smoke or tea as marijuana substitute	Nepetalactone	Euphoriant
Ch'an Su	*Bufo bufo gargarizans* *Bufo bufo melanosticus*	Smoke or lick for hallucinations	Bufotenin	Hallucinogen
Cinnamon	*Cinnamomum camphora*	Smoke with marijuana	?	Stimulant
Clove	*Syzgium aromaticum*	Smoke in cigarette/"kreteks"	Eugenol	Euphoriant
Damiana	*Turnera diffusa*	Smoke as marijuana substitute	?	Stimulant/hallucinogen
Goldenseal	*Hydrastis canadensis*	Ingest to mask detection of opioid, marijuana, or cocaine in urinary drug screen	–	No evidence
Hops	*Humulus lupulus*	Smoke or tea as sedative and marijuana substitute	Humulone, lupulone → methylbutenol	Sedative (mild)
Hydrangea	*Hydrangea paniculata*	Smoke as marijuana substitute	Hydrangin, saponin	Stimulant
Ibogaine	*Tabernanthe iboga*	Stimulant, hallucinogen	Ibogaine	Hallucinogen
Juniper	*Juniperus macropoda*	Smoke as hallucinogen	?	Hallucinogen
Kava kava	*Piper methysticum*	Smoke or tea as marijuana substitute	Kava lactones	Hallucinogen
Kola nut	*Cola acuminata*	Smoke, tea, or capsules as stimulant	Caffeine, theobromine, kolanin	Stimulant
Lobelia	*Lobelia inflata*	Smoke or tea as marijuana substitute	Lobeline	Euphoriant
Mandrake	*Mandragora officinarum*	Tea as hallucinogen	Atropine, scopolamine	Hallucinogen
Mate	*Ilex paraguayensis*	Tea as stimulant	Caffeine	Stimulant
Mormon tea	*Ephedra nevadensis*	Tea as stimulant	Ephedrine	Stimulant
Morning glory	*Ipomoea violacea*	Seeds have hallucinogens	D-lysergic acid amide (ergine)	Hallucinogen
Nutmeg	*Myristica fragrans*	Tea as hallucinogen	Myristicin	Hallucinogen
Passion flower	*Passiflora incarnata*	Smoke, tea, or capsules as marijuana substitute	Harmala alkaloids	Stimulant (mild)
Periwinkle	*Catharanthus roseus*	Smoke or tea as euphoriant	Indole alkaloids	Hallucinogen
Prickly poppy	*Argemone mexicana*	Smoke as euphoriant	Protopine, bergerine, isoquinolones	Analgesic
Salvia	*Salvia divinorum*	Smoked, chewed	Salvinorum A	Hallucinogen
Snakeroot	*Rauwolfia serpentina*	Smoke or tea as tobacco substitute	Reserpine	Tranquilizer
Thorn apple	*Datura stramonium*	Smoke or tea as tobacco substitute or hallucinogen	Atropine, scopolamine	Hallucinogen
Tobacco	*Nicotiana* spp	Smoke as tobacco	Nicotine	Stimulant
Valerian	*Valeriana officinalis*	Tea or capsules	Chatinine, velerine alkaloids	Tranquilizer
Wild lettuce	*Lactuca sativa*	Smoke as opium substitute	Unknown	Analgesic (mild)
Wormwood	*Artemisia absinthium*	Smoke or tea as relaxant	Thujone	Analgesic
Yohimbe	*Pausinystalia yohimbe*	Smoke or tea as stimulant	Yohimbine	Hallucinogen (mild)

9. **Ginseng** (*Panax ginseng*)—Ginseng is the common name for deciduous, perennial plants of the genus *Panax*. *Panax ginseng* is native to Korea, China, Japan, and Russia. *Panax quinquefolius* is the common ginseng species in North America and grows abundantly throughout the central and eastern regions of Canada and the United States. Ginseng preparations have been used in China for treatment of respiratory illnesses, gastrointestinal disorders, impotence, fatigue, and stress ("adaptogenic effect"). It is regarded as a tonic and panacea (hence the name *Panax*, meaning "all healing"). Its only recognized use in the United States is as an external demulcent.[82,122,137] Ginseng provides a good example of the complexity of the biochemistry and pharmacologic effects of herbs. The active components of ginseng are called *ginsenosides* and include panaxin, panax acid, panaquilin, panacen, sapogenin,

and ginsenin. Its general metabolic effects include decreasing serum glucose and serum cholesterol concentrations; increasing erythropoiesis, hemoglobin production, and iron absorption from the gut; increasing blood pressure and heart rate; GI motility; and CNS stimulation. Ginseng abuse syndrome (GAS), which consists of hypertension, nervousness, sleeplessness, and morning diarrhea, has been described following long-term use of ginseng.[82,175,176] Ginseng use may reduce the anticoagulant effect of warfarin.[102,210]

10. **St. John's wort** (*Hypericum perforatum*)—St. John's wort is a popular herbal remedy for treatment of depression and is also used as a topical remedy for cuts, bruises, and wounds.[171] It has lost its popularity as an AIDS treatment because of the lack of clinical efficacy.[88] The active ingredients are hyperforin and hypericin. Its antidepressant properties likely derive from the ability of hyperforin to inhibit the reuptake of serotonin, dopamine, norepineprine, γ-aminobutyric acid, and glutamate.[30] A major study in 2002 demonstrated that St. John's wort is ineffective in treating depression.[101] Acute toxicity appears limited to photosensitization reactions. St. John's wort induces CYP3A4 and may interact with medications metabolized by this enzyme (eg, indinavir, oral contraceptives, cycloserine).[128,162] Hyperforin is a weak monoamine oxidase inhibitor, raising concerns about interactions with the selective serotonin reuptake inhibitors.[162]
11. **Green tea**—Green tea is a popular antioxidant used to prevent chronic disease as well as for weight reduction. It is also touted to protect against cancer and decrease cholesterol. A 2006 study in Japan observed that green tea consumption was associated with a decreased mortality from all causes of cardiovascular disease.[117] Polyphenols contained in green tea including catechins and epigallocatechin gallate (EGCG) are responsible for its antioxidant properties. Although green tea consumption is considered to be safe, recent case reports describing the development of acute hepatitis following ingestion of green tea extracts or infusions suggests that idiosyncratic hepatotoxicity may occur in rare individuals.[3,17,22,78,83,103,105,156,164,182,191,201]
12. **Evening primrose** (*Oenothera biennis*)—Evening primrose contain *cis*-γ-linoleic acid (GLA), a prostaglandin E_1 precursor. This herb is a popular remedy for treatment of premenstrual syndrome, diabetes, eczema, and rheumatoid arthritis. Evening primrose appears to be safe in appropriate doses. This herb may lower the seizure threshold in epilepsy.
13. **Valerian** (*Valeriana officinalis*)—Valerian is a popular remedy for treatment of anxiety and is also used as a sleeping aid. Valerian appears to be safe in appropriate doses. Valerian may potentiate sedation in patients taking sedative-hypnotics.[151]

TOXICITY OF SIGNIFICANT HERBAL PREPARATIONS

CARDIOVASCULAR TOXINS

Aconite Aconites (caowu, chuanwu, and fuzi) are the dried rootstocks of the *Aconitum* plant.[185] In China, aconite usually is derived from *Aconitum carmichaelii* (chuan wu) or *A. kuznezoffii* (caowu). In Europe and the United States, aconite is derived from *A. napellus*, commonly known as *monkshood* or *wolfsbane*. The tubers are the most toxic part of the plant, When ingested, both cardiac and neurologic toxicity occur. Aconite poisoning is far more common in Asia, especially China.[52] In Hong Kong, it is responsible for the majority of serious poisonings from Chinese herbal preparations.[47,50,52]

Aconite toxicity is caused by C19 diterpenoid-ester alkaloids, including aconitine, mesaconitine, and hypaconitine.[29] Aconitine increases sodium influx through the sodium channel, increasing inotropy while delaying the final repolarization phase of the action potential and promoting premature excitation.[94] Sinus bradycardia and ventricular dysrhythmias can occur.[51] Symptoms can occur from 5 minutes to 4 hours after ingestion. Paresthesias of the oral mucosa and entire body may be followed by nausea, vomiting, diarrhea, and hypersalivation, and then by progressive skeletal muscle weakness. Fatalities may occur with doses as low as 5 mL aconite tincture, 2 mg pure aconite, or 1 g dried plant. Atropine may be of value in treating bradycardia or hypersalivation.[186] Although no antidote is available, anecdotal reports suggest the use of amiodarone, flecainide, bretylium, lidocaine, and procainamide for ventricular tachydysrhythmias.[186,209] Pharmacologic principles support the use of these sodium channel blockers. One case of aconite-induced refractory tachydysrhythmias was successfully managed with a ventricular assist device.[73] In a case series of two aconite-poisoned patients, reversal of aconite-induced ventricular dysrhythmias was attributed to the use of charcoal hemoperfusion for aconitine removal.[124,125]

Ch'an Su Ch'an su is a traditional herbal remedy derived from the secretions of the parotid and sebaceous glands of the toad Bufo bufo gargarizans or Bufo melanosticus. This remedy is traditionally used as a treatment for congestive heart failure.[115] Ch'an su contains two groups of toxic compounds: digoxin-like cardioactive steroids consisting of bufadienolides and the hallucinogenic compound bufotenin. Clinical findings following ingestion are similar to cardioactive steroid poisoning, including gastrointestinal symptoms and dysrhythmias. It was also marketed as an aphrodisiac for its purported topical anesthetic effects and sold under names such as "Stone," "Love Stone," "Black Stone," and "Rock Hard." Between 1993 and 1996 in New York City, several fatalities were associated with the ingestion of Ch'an su marketed as a topical aphrodisiac.[35] Severe toxic reactions and death are reported after mouthing toads, "toad licking," or eating an entire toad, or ingesting toad soup, or toad eggs.[26] Assays for serum digoxin unpredictably cross-react with bufadienolides, but may qualitatively assist in making a presumptive diagnosis (Table 43-1). Digoxin-specific Fab was successfully used to treat Ch'an su poisoning and should be empirically administered for any suspected case of cardiotoxicity from Ch'an su or other cardioactive steroid[26,177] (Chap. 64).

CENTRAL NERVOUS SYSTEM TOXINS

Absinthe Wormwood (Artemisia absinthium) extract is the main ingredient in absinthe, a toxic liquor that was outlawed in the United States in 1912. This volatile oil is a mixture of α- and β-thujone (Table 43-3).[208] Both tetrahydrocannabinol and thujone have an affinity for a common CNS receptor binding site and for similar oxidative metabolic pathways.[208]

Chronic absinthe use caused "absinthism," characterized by psychosis, hallucinations, intellectual deterioration, and seizures. The most famous victim of absinthism may have been Vincent Van Gogh, who is thought to have suffered from this disorder in the later part of his life.[8] A thujone-free wormwood extract now is used for flavoring vermouth and pastis. A case of wormwood-induced seizures, rhabdomyolysis, and acute renal failure was described involving a patient who purchased from the Internet and consumed approximately 10 mL essential oil of wormwood, assuming it was absinthe liquor.[204] Treatment remains supportive.

Anticholinergic Agents: Henbane, Jimson Weed, Mandrake Many plants contain the belladonna alkaloids atropine (dl-hyoscyamine), hyoscyamine, and scopolamine (l-hyoscine). They may still be used therapeutically for treatment of asthma and occasionally are mistakenly included in herbal teas.[46] Signs and symptoms of anticholinergic poisoning include mydriasis, diminished bowel sounds, urinary retention, dry mouth, flushed skin, tachycardia, and agitation. Mildly poisoned patients usually require only supportive care and sedation with intravenous benzodiazepines. Intravenous physostigmine reverses anticholinergic poisoning; however, its use should be limited to treatment of moderately to severely symptomatic patients because inappropriate use may cause seizures and dysrhythmias.

Ephedra Members of the genus *Ephedra* generally consist of erect evergreen plants resembling small shrubs.[190] Common names include sea grape, ma-huang, yellow horse, desert tea, squaw tea, and Mormon tea. *Ephedra* species have a long history of use as stimulants and for management of bronchospasm. They contain the alkaloids ephedrine and, in some species, pseudoephedrine.[167,190] In large doses, ephedrine causes nervousness, headache, insomnia, dizziness, palpitations, skin flushing, tingling, vomiting, anxiety, restlessness, mania, and psychosis. The treatment is similar to that for other CNS stimulants (Chap. 75). In a published review of 140 reports of adverse events associated with ephedra use submitted to the FDA, 62% of cases (82) were considered "probable" or "possibly" related to ephedra use. Hypertension was the most commonly reported adverse effect (17 cases), followed by palpitations or tachycardia (13 cases), strokes (10 cases), and seizures (7 cases). Ten reported cases resulted in death. Thirteen cases resulted in permanent disability.[91] In 2002, the FDA banned the sale of ephedra-containing dietary supplements.[195] However, other herbal preparations, such as bitter orange (*Citrus aurantia*), contain ephedralike alkaloids (synephrine) and are still widely available.[141,149] Exposures may result in cardiovascular toxicity.[142,150]

Khat A common form of drug abuse in East Africa involves chewing the leaves and stems of the khat (*Catha edulis*) plant and swallowing the juice.[69,126] Khat is used by herbalists to treat depression, fatigue, obesity, and gastric ulcers. The two active compounds in khat are cathine (norpseudoephedrine) and cathinone (α-aminopropiophenone), the more active stimulant (an extensive discussion is given in Chap. 75).

Nicotinic Agents: Betel Nut, Blue Cohosh, Broom, Chestnut, Lobelia, Tobacco Betel (*Areca catechu*) is chewed by an estimated 200 million people worldwide for its euphoric effect. As an herb, it used as a digestive aid and as a treatment for cough and sore throat. Its active ingredient is arecoline, a direct-acting nicotinic agonist. The betel leaf also contains a phenolic volatile oil and an alkaloid capable of producing sympathomimetic reactions. Arecoline is a bronchoconstrictor, although weaker than methacholine, and may exacerbate bronchospasm in asthmatic patients chewing betel nut.[189] Treatment for betel nut toxicity is supportive. Long-term use of betel nut is associated with leukoplakia and squamous cell carcinoma of the oral mucosa.[148]

Many other herbal preparations have nicotinic effects. Examples of plants and their nicotinic ingredient include blue cohosh,[18] methylcytisine; broom, l-sparteine; chestnut, esculin; lobelia, lobeline; and tobacco/nicotine.

Other herbs that have CNS activity include valerian (sedation), kava kava (sedation), Japanese star anise (seizures), nutmeg (hallucinations),[205] mace (hallucinations), and iboga (hallucinations).

GASTROINTESTINAL TOXINS

Goldenseal Goldenseal (*Hydrastis canadensis*) originally was used by the Cherokees and other Native Americans as a dye and an internal remedy.[84] Today, it is used as an astringent, as a remedy for mucous membranes or gastrointestinal tract disorders, and as treatment for menorrhagia. Goldenseal is reputed to mask the presence of illicit drugs on urinary drug screens, although multiple studies indicate goldenseal does not affect the results of urinary drug screens.[56,144,153] This myth originated in the murder-mystery *Stringtown on the Pike* (1900), which was written by the internationally known plant pharmacist Uri Lloyd. In this novel, one of the major characters is accused of murder by poisoning with strychnine but is posthumously exonerated with evidence that hydrastine (the active alkaloid in goldenseal) and morphine cross-react to produce a positive color assay for strychnine.[76] Appropriate usage of this herb is thought to be safe, but ingestion of large amounts can cause vomiting, diarrhea, convulsions, paralysis, and respiratory failure. In cases of large ingestions, the patient should receive supportive and symptomatic care.

HEPATOTOXINS

Pennyroyal Pennyroyal oil is a volatile oil extract from the leaves of Mentha pulegium and Hedeoma pulegioides plants. Herbalists use pennyroyal oil as an abortifacient and to regulate menstruation. It is also used as a flea/mosquito repellant and as a fragrance. The abortive effect is thought to be caused by irritation and contraction of the uterus.[185] Pennyroyal usually is ingested as a strong tea prepared from the leaves or as the oil itself. It is cited as the causative agent in several well-documented cases of hepatic failure following ingestion of as little as 15 mL of the oil.[5,11] The postulated mechanism is direct hepatotoxicity following glutathione depletion from the cyclohexanone pulegone and its cytochrome P450 (CYP1A2, CYP2E1, CYP2C19)-dependent toxic metabolites that include menthofuran.[112] On autopsy, vacuolization of the white matter of the midbrain was reported in both a fatal human exposure and in animal models.[10,152] Because pulegone depletes hepatic glutathione stores, N-acetylcysteine treatment may be beneficial[5,27] (A4: *N*-Acetylcysteine). In an animal model, pretreatment with cytochrome P450 inhibitors cimetidine (CYP1A2, CYP2C19) and disulfiram (CYP2E1) reduced pulegone-induced hepatotoxicity.[184] It may be reasonable to consider use of cytochrome P450 inhibitors in the treatment of pennyroyal-poisoned patients; however, evidence of clinical benefit in humans currently is lacking.

Pyrrolizidine Alkaloids Pyrrolizidine alkaloids are hepatotoxins found in many plants, including *Heliotropium*, *Senecio*, *Crotalaria*, and *Symphytum*.[161,166] Examples of other plants and products containing pyrrolizidine alkaloids include borage (*Borago officinalis*), coltsfoot (*Tussilago farfara*), and T'u-san-chi'i (*Gynura segetum*).[99,116,167]

The alkaloids undergo metabolism to pyrroles, which serve as biologic alkylating agents.[99] The pyrroles cause hepatic sinusoidal hypertrophy and venous occlusion, resulting in hepatic veno-occlusive disease, hepatomegaly, cirrhosis, and possibly hepatic carcinoma. Chronic low doses may cause pulmonary toxicity resulting in pulmonary artery hypertension and right ventricular hypertrophy. Consumption of "bush" tea, prepared from the leaves of the *Crotalaria* plant, is considered an endemic problem in Jamaica. Epidemics have also occurred in Afghanistan and India, where ingestion of contaminated cereals containing *Heliotropium* and *Crotalaria* seeds resulted in reports of 1632 and 60 cases of veno-occlusive disease, respectively.[138,188] In western countries, ingestion of herbal products containing *Senecio* and comfrey have led to several cases of hepatic veno-occlusive disease.[161] Treatment of hepatic veno-occlusive disease is supportive but may require liver transplantation in severe cases.

Several other herbal preparations are associated with hepatotoxicity.[119] These preparations include chaparral (*Larrea tridentata*),[34,85] germander (*Teucrium chamaedrys*),[120] impilia (*Callilepsis laureola*),[116] atractylis (*Atractylis gummifera*), sassafras (*Sassafras albidum*),[175] and kava kava (*Piper methysticum*).[197]

METALS

Poisonings by metals, including arsenic, cadmium, lead, and mercury, may occur following consumption of various types of herbal preparations[39,41,60,167] (Chaps. 88, 90, 94, and 96). Treatment consists of ceasing consumption of the herbal product and use of an appropriate chelating agent when indicated.

Hai-ge-ten (clamshell powder) contamination with copper, chromium, arsenic, or lead is described in several case reports.[93,129] Pay-loo-ah, a red and orange powder used by the Hmong people as a fever and rash remedy, was contaminated with lead.[36] Ayurvedic remedies are either herbal only or *rasa shastra* which, based upon ancient traditional healing of India, deliberately combines metals such as gold, silver, copper, zinc, iron, lead, tin, and mercury and are used by the majority of the Indian population.[40,163,165,173] Ghasard, Bola Goli, Kandu, and Moha Yogran Guggulu, traditional Indian remedies for abdominal pain, are associated with lead poisoning.[39,174] One fatality from lead poisoning from Ghasard, Bola Goli, and Kandu is reported from the United States.[39] In one study, 20% of surveyed Ayurvedic products produced in South Asia and sold on a nonprescription basis in stores in the Boston area contained potentially harmful concentrations of lead, mercury, or arsenic.[172] A followup study determined that a similar percentage 21% of Ayurvedic products sold over the unit also contained potentially harmful levels of lead, mercury, or arsenic irrespective of whether manufacture occurred in the United States or India.

These same investigators recently studied the lead, mercury and arsenic concentrations in US and Indian manufactured Ayurvedic medicines sold via the Internet demonstrating that 20% of these were contaminated with one of these metals, all exceeding one or more standards for acceptable daily intake of a toxic metal.[173] Azarcon (lead tetroxide) and greta (lead oxide) are used by an estimated 7.2%–12.1% of Mexican-Hispanic families for treatment of *empacho*. In Spanish, *empacho* means "blocked intestine," but it refers to any type of chronic digestive problem, including such diverse symptoms as constipation, diarrhea, nausea, vomiting, anorexia, apathy, and lethargy.[42,45] Azarcon and greta are fine powders with total lead contents varying from 70% to >90%.[23,43]

Herbal balls, hand-rolled mixtures of herbs and honey produced in China, are often associated with arsenic and mercury contamination.[72] Examples include An Gong Niu Huang Wan, Da Huo Luo Wan, and Niu Huang Chiang Ya Wan.

RENAL TOXINS

Aristolochia An epidemic of renal failure in Belgium was linked to the substitution of Aristolochia fangchi, also known as birthwort, heartwort, and fangchi, for another Chinese herbal, Stephania tetranda, in the formulation of a weight-loss regimen.[198,199] Of 70 identified cases of renal fibrosis, 30 patients developed chronic renal failure. Aristolochic acid in Aristolochia causes renal fibrosis which typically becomes clinically apparent 12 to 24 months after the initial injury. Patients with Aristolochia-induced nephropathy also have an increased risk for developing urothelial cancer.[147]

MISCELLANEOUS

Chamomile Tea Chamomile tea is a popular herbal drink made from chamomile flower heads. Anaphylactic reactions can occur in patients allergic to ragweed, asters, chrysanthemums, or other members of the Compositae family.[14,31] Such reactions are rare but can be life threatening. The patient need not have severe allergies or be highly atopic to experience a cross-reaction.

Rattlesnake Capsules Rattlesnake capsules are a common Mexican folk remedy used to treat cancer, arthritis, and skin disorders. These capsules contain dried, pulverized rattlesnake powder and are sold under various names, such as vibora de cascabel, polvo de vibora, and carne de vibora, without prescriptions. Infection with Salmonella arizonae is described following ingestion.[16,57,149,169,203]

CHINESE PATENT MEDICATIONS

Chinese patent medicines, a component of traditional Chinese medicine, contain traditional herbals, formulated into tablets, capsules, syrups, powders, ointments, and plasters, for easy use. They are produced by poorly regulated Chinese pharmaceutical agencies and are highly susceptible to adulteration or contamination. They are often sold by nonherbalists at convenience stores in packages with incomplete documentation of ingredients, and, typically, they are not labeled in English. In 1998, the California Department of Health Services investigated 260 Asian patent medications for adulterants and determined that 32% contained undeclared pharmaceutics or heavy metals.[114] A similar study in Taiwan determined that 24% of 2609 samples collected were contaminated by at least one adulterant.[96] In 2007, 90 Chinese patent medicines randomly purchased in New York City's Chinatown identified five samples containing nine western medications including chlormethiazole, chlorpheniramine, diclofenac, chlordiazepoxide, hydrochlorothiazide, triamterene, diphenhydramine, and sildenafil citrate.[135]

Jin Bu Huan is a traditional Chinese preparation used as a sedative and analgesic.[206] The active ingredient, an isoquinoline alkaloid l-tetrahydropalmatine (l-THP), is responsible for the morphine-like properties of Jin Bu Huan. In two case reports, three pediatric patients developed life-threatening bradycardia and seven adult patients developed hepatitis while using Jin Bu Huan.[37,38] Hepatotoxicity may be related to L-THP, which is structurally similar to the hepatotoxic pyrrolizidine alkaloids.[206] Although the package insert for Jin Bu Huan in these cases indicated that *Polygala chinensis* was the plant source for L-THP, *P. chinensis* does not contain L-THP. Plants from the genera *Stephania* and *Corydalis* are also known as Jin Bu Huan and contain appreciable amounts of L-THP. The product implicated in the case reports may have been simply mislabeled by the manufacturer.

Nan Lien Chiu Fong Toukuwan (now withdrawn from the market) was found to variably contain aminopyrine, phenacetin, phenylbutazone, indomethacin, mefenamic acid, diazepam, hydrochlorothiazide, dexamethasone, mercuric sulfide, lead, and cadmium, depending on the manufacturer.[50] Several cases of agranulocytosis were reported following ingestion of this preparation.[168] Dr. Tong Shap Yee's asthma pills were found to contain theophylline.[50] Leng Pui Kee cough pills were found to contain bromhexine.[50]

Tung Shueh (black ball) contains diazepam and mefenamic acid and is associated with acute interstitial nephritis.[65] Gan Mao Tong Pian, an herbal cold remedy, contains phenylbutazone and caused aplastic anemia in one child.[145] Chui Feng Su Ho Wan, which contains *Glycyrrhiza glabra*, was associated with hypokalemia-induced torsade de pointes in an elderly woman.[50]

Several Chinese patent medicines contain the mercurials cinnabar (mercuric sulfide) and calomel (mercurous chloride). Tse Koo Choy and Qing Fen, which contain calomel, are associated with several cases of mercury poisoning.[108]

Many Chinese medicated oils contain oil of wintergreen, which is methylsalicylate. Although these oils are intended for external use, it is a common practice to ingest a few drops undiluted or in a hot drink as a general tonic or specific remedy. Examples of medicated oils include White Flower Medicine Oil (40% oil of wintergreen, 30% menthol, 6% camphor), Red Flower Oil (67% oil of wintergreen, 22% turpentine oil), and Kwan Loong Medicated Oil (menthol 25%, methylsalicylate 15%, camphor 10%).[50]

HERBAL PREPARATIONS AND AIDS THERAPIES

Many patients infected with human immunodeficiency virus (HIV) have turned to alternative treatments in the hope of finding less toxic therapy than the conventional modalities currently available. In a study of 114 HIV-positive patients in a university-based AIDS clinic, 22% used one or more herbal products in a 3-month period.[109] Twenty-four percent of these patients were unable to state which herbs they were taking. Adverse effects included dermatitis, nausea, vomiting, diarrhea, thrombocytopenia, coagulopathies, altered mental status, hepatotoxicity, and electrolyte imbalances. Twenty percent of patients stated their physicians were unaware of their use of herbs. A more recent study reported that more than two thirds of AIDS patients were taking alternative medicines, and 24% of AIDS patients were taking Chinese herbs or other botanicals.[86]

Current popular herbal preparations and dietary supplements for treatment of AIDS or AIDS-related illnesses include *Lactobacillus acidophilus*, adrenal cortex, aloe vera, *Artemisia*, *Astragalus*, bitter melon, bioperine, blue-green algae, cat's claw, *Chlorella*, coenzyme Q10, colloidal silver, curcumin, dehydroepiandrosterone (DHEA), echinacea, elderberry, evening primrose oil, flaxseed oil, garlic, germanium, ginger, *Ginkgo biloba*, glucosamine, glutamine, glutathione, glycyrrhizin, grapeseed, green tea, lipoic acid, *N*-acetylcysteine, saw palmetto, Siberian ginseng, and silymarin, and are used for treatment of HIV infection.[146]

TREATMENT

A specific treatment strategy should emphasize identification of the specific herbal preparation(s) used by the patient, concurrent medication(s), and medical illness(es). Because herbal preparation toxicity varies greatly depending on the preparation used, careful examination may be aided by knowledge of the herbal preparation. In most cases, supportive care and discontinuation of the herbal preparation(s) are sufficient. Some herbal toxicities require specific laboratory analysis and therapy (Table 43-1).

All adverse events associated with herbal preparations should be reported to the local poison control center or to FDA MedWatch by phone at 1-800-FDA-1088 or online at https://www.fda.gov/ medwatch.

SUMMARY

Herbal preparation usage is a popular type of "complementary" or alternative medicine. Although most herb users will suffer no ill effects, both herb users and clinicians should be aware that these preparations are pharmacologically active, have the potential for toxicity, and are not as closely regulated by the FDA (or any governmental agency) as pharmaceuticals. They may interact with prescription medications to increase the toxicity of the medication or decrease its therapeutic effect. Patients with specific medical conditions may have increased risk for toxicity when using herbal preparations.

Herb users should be aware that these preparations are poorly studied with scientific proof of efficacy lacking for most preparations. No standards exist for their manufacture, quality, or control and many herbal products do not contain the purported amount of the active ingredient. Some herbal products do not even contain the correct active ingredient. Some herbal products are reported to be adulterated with prescription medications or contain contaminants such as heavy metals.

Many herbal stores are staffed by untrained personnel who may dispense incorrect medical advice and unfounded claims concerning their products.[160] Herbalists (eg, Chinese herbalists) may dispense traditional remedies with the potential for serious toxicity as the result of improper identification of the correct herb or improper preparation of the herbal product by the herbalist or herb user.[50] Most herb users and many herbalists may be unaware of the potential for toxicity of their product.

Clinicians should be familiar with herbal preparations and their potential for drug interactions and adverse effects. This is especially important because standard herbal reference texts may lack sufficient information on the management of poisoning or other adverse effects.[90] Every patient history should include questions assessing the concurrent or recent past use of herbal preparations.

ACKNOWLEDGMENT

Mary Ann Howland and Neal Lewin contributed to this chapter in previous editions.

REFERENCES

1. Aaronson K. HERB-CHF (Hawthorn Extract Randomized Blinded Chronic HF Study): Late-Breaking and Recent Clinical Trials. Presented at the 8th Annual Scientific Meeting of the Heart Failure Society of America; September 12-15, 2004; Toronto, Ontario, Canada.
2. AARP, NCCAM: What people 50 and older are using and discussing with their physicians. Washington DC: AARP;2007. Available at http://assets.aarp.org/rgcenter/health/cam_2007.pdf. Last accessed on September 1, 2008.
3. Abu el Wafa Y, Benavente Fernandez A, Talavera Fabuel A, et al: Acute hepatitis induced by *Camellia sinensis* (green tea) [Spanish] [letter]. *Anal Med Int.* 2005;22:298.
4. Akerele O: Summary of WHO guidelines for the assessment of herbal medicines. *HerbalGram.* 1993;28:13-20.
5. Anderson IB, Mullen WH, Meeker JE, et al: Pennyroyal toxicity: measurement of toxic metabolite levels in two cases and review of the literature. *Ann Intern Med.* 1996;124:726-734.
6. Annual Industry Overview 1998. *Nutr Business J.* 1998;3:5-6.
7. Ansani NT, Cliberto NC, Freedy T:. Hospital policies regarding herbal medicines. *Am J Health-Syst Pharm.* 2003;60:367-370.
8. Arnold WN: Vincent van Gogh and the thujone connection. *JAMA.* 1988;260:3042-3044.
9. Ashar BH, Rice TN, Sisson SD: Physicians' understanding of the regulation of dietary supplements. *Arch Intern Med.* 2007;167:966-969.
10. Avorn J, Monane M, Gurwitz JH, et al: Reduction of bacteriuria and pyuria after ingestion of cranberry juice. *JAMA.* 1994;271:751-754.
11. Bakerink JA, Gospe SM, Dimand RJ, et al: Multiple organ failure after ingestion of pennyroyal oil from herbal tea in two patients. *Pediatrics.* 1996;98:944-947.
12. Barnes PM, Powell-Griner E, McFann K, et al: Complementary and alternative medicine use among adults: United States, 2002. Rockville, MD: Advance Data from Vital and Health Statistics, US Department of Health and Human Services; 2004.
13. Bazzie KL Witmer DR, Pinto B, et al: National survey of dietary supplement policies in acute care facilities. *Am J Health-Syst Pharm.* 2006;63:65-70.
14. Benner M, Lee H: Anaphylactic reaction of chamomile tea. *J Allergy Clin Immunol.* 1973;52:307-308.
15. Bent S, Kane C, Shinohara K, et al: Saw palmetto for benign prostatic hyperplasia. *N Engl J Med.* 2006;354:557-566.
16. Bhatt BD, Zuckerman MJ, Foland JA, et al: Rattlesnake meat ingestion—a common Hispanic folk remedy. *West J Med.* 1988;149:605.
17. Bjornsson E, Olsson R: Serious adverse liver reactions associated with herbal weight-loss supplements [letter]. *J Hepatol.* 2007;47:295-297.
18. Blue Cohosh. *Review of Natural Products.* Levittown, PA: Pharmaceutical Information Associates; May 1985.
19. Blumenthal M: Herb sales up 1% for all channels of trade in 2000. *HerbalGram.* 2001;53:63.
20. Blumenthal M: Herb sales down in mainstream market, up in natural food stores. *HerbalGram.* 2002;55:60.
21. Blumenthal M: Herbs continue to slide in mainstream market: sales down 14 percent. *HerbalGram.* 2002;58:71.

22. Bonkovsky HL: Hepatotoxicity associated with supplements containing Chinese green tea (Camellia sinensis) [letter]. *Ann Intern Med.* 2006;144:68-71.
23. Bose A, Vashishta K, O'Loughlin BJ: Azarcon por emphacho—another cause of lead toxicity. *Pediatrics.* 1983;72:106-110.
24. Boyer EW. Issues in the management of dietary supplement use among hospitalized patients. *Int Med J Toxicol.* 2002;5(1):1.
25. Breevoort P: The booming US botanical market: a new overview. *HerbalGram.* 1998;44:33-56.
26. Brubacher JR, Ravikumar PR, Bania T, et al: Treatment of toad venom poisoning with digoxin-specific Fab fragments. *Chest.* 1996;110:1282-1288.
27 Buechel DW, Haverlah, VC, Gardner ME: Pennyroyal oil ingestion: report of a case. *J Am Osteopath Assoc.* 1983;82:793-794.
28. Burke AB, Smyth EM, and FitzGerald GA: Analgesic-antiypretic and anti-inflammatory agents; pharmacotherapy of gout. In: Brunston LL, Lazo JS, Parker KL, eds: *Goodman and Gilman's The Pharmacological Basis of Therapeutics*, 11th ed. New York: McGraw-Hill; 2006:671-715.
29. But PP, Tai YT, Young K: Three fatal cases of herbal aconite poisoning. *Vet Hum Toxicol.* 1994;34:212-215.
30. Butterveck V: Mechanism of action of St. John's wort in depression: what is known? *CNS Drugs.* 2003;17:539-562.
31. Casterline C: Allergy to chamomile teas. *JAMA.* 1980;244:330-331.
32. Cavaliere C, Rea P, Blumenthal M: Herbal supplement sales in United States shows growth in all channels. *HerbalGram.* 2008;78:60-63.
33. Centers for Disease Control and Prevention: Anticholinergic poisoning associated with an herbal tea—New York City. *MMWR.* 1995;44:193-195.
34. Centers for Disease Control and Prevention: Chaparral-induced toxic hepatitis—California and Texas. *MMWR.* 1992;41:812-814.
35. Centers for Disease Control and Prevention: Deaths associated with a purported aphrodisiac—New York City. *MMWR.* 1995;44:853-861.
36. Centers for Disease Control and Prevention: Folk remedy-associated lead poisoning in Hmong children. *MMWR.* 1983;32:555-556.
37. Centers for Disease Control and Prevention: Jin Bu Huan toxicity in adults—Los Angeles. *MMWR.* 1993;42:920-922.
38. Centers for Disease Control and Prevention: Jin Bu Huan toxicity in children—Colorado. *MMWR.* 1993;42:633-636.
39. Centers for Disease Control and Prevention: Lead poisoning associated death from Asian Indian folk remedies—Florida. *MMWR.* 1984;33:638-645.
40. CDC: Lead poisoning associated with Ayurvedic medications. *MMWR.* 2004;53:582-584.
41. Centers for Disease Control and Prevention: Lead poisoning associated with traditional ethnic remedies—California, 1991-1992. *MMWR.* 1993;42:521-524.
42. Centers for Disease Control and Prevention: Lead poisoning from lead tetroxide used as a folk remedy—Colorado. *MMWR.* 1982;30:647-648.
43. Centers for Disease Control and Prevention: Lead poisoning from Mexican folk remedies—California. *MMWR* 1983;32:554.
44. Centers for Disease Control and Prevention: Self-treatment with herbal and other plant-derived remedies—rural Mississippi, 1993. *MMWR.* 1995;44:204-207.
45. Centers for Disease Control and Prevention: Use of lead tetroxide as a folk remedy for gastrointestinal illness. *MMWR.* 1981;30:546-547.
46. Chan JCN, Chan TYK, Chan KL, et al: Anticholinergic poisoning from Chinese herbal medicines [letter]. *Aust N Z J Med.* 1994;24:317.
47. Chan TYK: Aconitine poisoning: a global perspective. *Vet Hum Toxicol.* 1994;36:326-328.
48. Chan TYK, Chan AYW, Critchley JAJH: Hospital admissions due to adverse reactions to Chinese herbal medicines. *J Trop Med Hyg.* 1992;95:296-298.
49. Chan TYK, Chan JCN, Tomlinson B, et al: Chinese herbal medicines revisited: a Hong Kong perspective. *Lancet.* 1993;342-1532-1534.
50. Chan TYK, Critchley JAJH: Usage and adverse effects of Chinese herbal medicines. *Hum Exp Toxicol.* 1996;15:5-12.
51. Chan TYK, Tomlinson B, Chan WWM, et al: A case of acute aconitine poisoning caused by chuanwu and caowu. *J Trop Med Hyg.* 1993;96:62-63.
52. Chan TYK, Tse LKK, Chan JCN, et al: Aconitine poisoning due to Chinese herbal medicines: a review. *Vet Hum Toxicol.* 1994;36:452-455.
53. Chevalier A: *The Encyclopedia of Medicinal Plants.* New York: Publishing DK; 1996.
54. Clegg DO, Reda DJ, Harris CL, et al: Glucosamine, chondroitin sulfate, and the two in combination for painful knee osteoarthritis. *N Engl J Med.* 2006;354:795-808.
55. Cohen MH, Hrbek A, Davis RB, Schachter SC, et al: Emerging credentialing practices, malpractice liability policies, and guidelines governing complementary and alternative medical practices and dietary supplement recommendations. *Arch Intern Med.* 2005;165:289-295.
56. Combie J, Nugent TE, Tobin T: Inability of goldenseal to interfere with the detection of morphine in urine. *Equine Vet Sci.* 1982;Jan/Feb:16-21.
57. Cone LA, Boughton WH, Cone LA, et al: Rattlesnake capsule-induced Salmonella arizonae bacteremia. *West J Med.* 1990;153;315-316.
58. Cook C, Baisden D: Ancillary use of folk medicine by patients in primary care clinics in southwestern West Virginia. *South Med J.* 1986;79:1098-1101.
59. Cowley G: Herbal warning. *Newsweek*, May 6, 1996;60-65.
60. D'Arcy PF: Adverse reactions and interactions with herbal medicines. *Adverse Drug React Toxicol Rev.* 1991;10:189-208.
61. Danesi MA, Adetunji JB: Use of alternative medicine by patients with epilepsy: a survey of 265 epileptic patients in a developing country. *Epilepsia.* 1994;35:344-351.
62. Der Marderosian A: Promising practices in the use of medicinal plants in the United States. In: Tomlinson TR, Akerele O, eds: *Medicinal Plants, Their Role in Health and Biodiversity.* Philadelphia, PA: University of Pennsylvania Press; 1998:177-190.
63. DeSmet PA: Health risks of herbal remedies. *Drug Saf.* 1995;13:81-93.
64. DeSmet PA: Toxicological outlook on the quality assurance of herbal remedies. *Adverse Effects Herb Drugs.* 1992;1:1-72.
65. Diamond JR, Pallone PL: Acute interstitial nephritis following use of Tung Shueh pills. *Am J Kidney Dis.* 1994;24:219-221.
66. Dietary Supplement and Nonprescription Drug Consumer Protection Act. *Public Law.* 2006;109-462.
67. Dodge HH, Zitzelberger T, Osken BS, et al: A randomized placebo-controlled trial of Ginkgo biloba for the prevention of cognitive decline. *Neurology.* 2008;70:1809-1817.
68. Dolan G Blumsohn A: Lead poisoning due to Asian ethnic treatment for impotence. *J R Soc Med.* 1991;84:630-631.
69. Duke JA: *CRC Handbook of Medicinal Herbs.* Boca Raton, FL: CRC Press; 1985.
70. Eisenberg DM, Kessler RC, Foster C, et al: Unconventional medicine in the United States. *N Engl J Med.* 1993;328:246-252.
71. Eisenberg DM, Davis RB, Ettner SL: Trends in alternative medicine use in the United States, 1990-1997: results of a follow-up national survey. *JAMA.* 1998;280:1569-1575.
72. Espinoza EO, Mann MJ, Bleasdell B: Arsenic and mercury in traditional Chinese herbal balls [letter]. *N Engl J Med.* 1995;333:803-804.
73. Fitzpatrick AJ, Crawford M, Allan RM, et al: Aconite poisoning managed with a ventricular assist device. *Anaesth Intensive Care.* 1994;22:714-717.
74. Food and Drug Administration: Part II 21 CFR Part 101. Food labeling; final rule and proposed rules. *Fed Reg.* December 28, 1995.
75. Food and Drug Administration: 21 CFR Part 111. Current good manufacturing practice in manufacturing, packaging, labeling, or holding operations for dietary supplements; final rule. *Fed Reg.* June 25, 2007.
76. Foster S: Goldenseal: Masking of drug tests. *HerbalGram.* 1989;21:7-8.
77. Fugh-Berman A: Herb-drug interactions. *Lancet.* 2000;355:134-138.
78. Garcia-Moran S, Saez-Royuela F, Gento E, Lopez Morante A, Arias L. Acute hepatitis associated with Camellia thea and Orthosiphon stamineus ingestion [letter]. *Gastroenterol Hepatol.* 2004;27:559-60.
79. Gardiner P, Phillips RS, Kemper KJ, et al: Dietary supplements: inpatient policies in US children's hospitals. *Pediatrics.* April 1, 2008;121(4):e775-e781.
80. Garlic. *Review of Natural Products.* Levittown, PA: Pharmaceutical Information Associates; April 1994.
81. Gilroy CM, Steiner JF, Byers T, et al: Echinacea and truth in labeling. *Arch Intern Med.* 2003;163:699-704.
82. Ginseng. *Review of Natural Products.* Levittown, PA: Pharmaceutical Information Associates; September 1990.
83. Gloro R, Hourmand-Ollivier I, Mosquet B, et al: Fulminant hepatitis during self-medication with hydroalcoholic extract of green tea. *Eur J Gastroent Hepatol.* 2005;17:1135-1137.
84. Goldenseal. *Review of Natural Products.* Levittown, PA: Pharmaceutical Information Associates; May 1994.
85. Gordon DW, Rosenthal G, Hart J, et al: Chaparral ingestion. *JAMA.* 1995;273:489-490.

86. Gore-Felton C, Vosnick M, Power R, et al: Alternative therapies: a common practice among men and women living with HIV. *J Assoc Nurses AIDS Care*. 2003;14:17-23.
87. Grimm W Muller HH: A randomized controlled trial of the effect of fluid extract of *Echinacea purpurea* on the incidence and severity of colds and respiratory infections. *Am J Med*. 1999;106:138-143.
88. Gullick RM, McAuliffe V, Holden-Wiltse J, et al: Phase I studies of hypericin, the active compound in St. John's wort, as an antiretroviral agent in HIV-infected adults. AIDS Clinical Trials Group Protocols 150 and 258. *Ann Intern Med*. 1999;130:510-514.
89. Gutstein HB, Akil H. Opioid analgesics. In: Brunston LL, Lazo JS, and Parker KL, eds: *Goodman and Gilman's The Pharmacological Basis of Therapeutics*, 11th ed. New York: McGraw-Hill; 2006:547-590.
90. Haller CA, Anderson IB, Kim SY, et al: An evaluation of selected herbal reference texts and comparison to published reports of adverse herbal events. *Adverse Drug React Toxicol*. 2002;21:143-150.
91. Haller CA, Benowitz NL: Adverse cardiovascular and central nervous system events associated with dietary supplements containing ephedra alkaloids. *N Engl J Med*. 2000;343:1833-1838.
92. Hanssens Y, Deleu D, Taqi A. Etiologic and demographic characteristics of poisoning: a prospective hospital-based study in Oman. *J Toxicol Clin Toxicol*. 2001;39(4):371-380.
93. Hill GJ: Lead poisoning due to Hai Ge Fen. *JAMA*. 1995;273:24-25.
94. Honerjager P, Meissner A: The positive inotropic effect of aconitine. *Arch Pharmacol*. 1983;322:49-58.
95. Hsu CK, Leo P, Shastry D, et al: Anticholinergic poisoning associated with herbal tea. *Arch Intern Med*. 1995;155:2245-2248.
96. Huang WF, Wen KC, Hsiao ML: Adulteration by synthetic therapeutic substances of traditional Chinese medicines in Taiwan. *J Clin Pharmacol*. 1997;37:334-350.
97. Hung OL, Shih RD, Chiang WK, et al: Herbal preparation usage among urban emergency department patients. *Acad Emerg Med*. 1997;4:209-213.
98. Huntley A, Ernst E: A systematic review of the safety of black cohosh. *Menopause*. 2003;10:58-64.
99. Huxtable RJ: Herbal teas and toxins: novel aspects of pyrrolizidine poisoning in the United States. *Perspect Biol Med*. 1980;24:1-14.
100. Huxtable RJ: The harmful potential of herbal and other plant products. *Drug Saf*. 1990;5(Suppl 1):126-136.
101. Hypericum Depression Trial Study Group: Effect of *Hypericum perforatum* (St. John's wort) in major depressive disorder: a randomized, controlled trial. *JAMA*. 2002;287:1807-1814.
102. Janetzky K, Morreale AP: Probable interaction between warfarin and ginseng. *Am J Health Syst Pharm*. 1997;54:692-693.
103. Javaid A, Bonkovsky HL: Hepatotoxicity due to extracts of Chinese green tea (*Camellia sinensis*): a growing concern [letter]. *J Hepatol*. 2006;45:334-335.
104. Jepson RG, Craig JC. Cranberries for preventing urinary tract infections. *Cochrane Database Syst Rev*. 2007;(3):CD001321.
105. Jimenez-Saenz M, Martinez-Sanchez M. Acute hepatitis associated with ingestion of green tea infusions [letter]. *J Hepatol*. 2006;44:616-617.
106. Jones KL. Donegan S. Lalloo DG. Artesunate versus quinine for treating severe malaria. *Cochrane Database Syst Rev*. 2007;(4):CD005967.
107. Joubert PH: Poisoning admissions in black South Africans. *J Toxicol Clin Toxicol*. 1990;28:85-94.
108. Kang-Yum E, Oransky SH: Chinese patent medicine as a potential source of mercury poisoning. *Vet Hum Toxicol*. 1992;34:235-238.
109. Kassler WJ, Blanc P, Greenblatt R: The use of medicinal herbs by human immunodeficiency virus-infected patients. *Arch Intern Med*. 1991;151:2281-2288.
110. Kaufman DW, Kelly JP, Rosenberg L, et al: Recent patterns of medication use in the ambulatory adult population of the United States: the Sloan survey. *JAMA*. 2002;287;337-344.
111. Kestin M, Miller L, Littlejohn G, et al: The use of medicinal herbs by human immunodeficiency virus-infected patients. *Arch Intern Med*. 1991;151:2281-2288.
112. Khojasteh-Bakht SC, Chen W, Koenigs LL, Peter RM, Nelson SD: Metabolism of (R)-(+)-pulegone and (R)-(+)-menthofuran by human liver cytochrome P-450s: evidence for formation of a furan epoxide. *Drug Metab Dispos*. 1999;27:574-80.
113. Klayman D: Qinghaosu (Artemisinin): antimalarial drug from China. *Science*. 1985;238:1049-1055.
114. Ko RJ: Adulterants in Asian patent medicines. *N Engl J Med*. 1998;339:847.
115. Ko RJ, Greenwald MS, Loscutoff SM, et al: Lethal ingestion of Chinese herbal tea containing Ch'an Su. *West J Med*. 1996:164:71-75.
116. Kumana CR, Ng M, Lin HJ, et al: Herbal tea induced hepatic venoocclusive disease: quantification of toxic alkaloid in adults. *Gut*. 1985;26: 101-104.
117. Kuriyama S, Shimazu T, Ohmori K, et al: Green tea consumption and mortality due to cardiovascular disease, cancer, and all causes in Japan: the Ohsaki study. *JAMA*. 2006;296(10):1255-1265.
118. Lam CL, Catarivas MG, Munro C, et al: Self-medication among Hong Kong Chinese. *Soc Sci Med*. 1994;39:1641-1647.
119. Larrey D, Pageaux GP: Hepatotoxicity of herbal remedies and mushrooms. *Semin Liver Dis*. 1995;15:183-188.
120. Larrey D, Vial T, Pauwels A, et al: Hepatitis after germander (*Teucrium chamaedrys*) administration: another instance of herbal medicine hepatotoxicity. *Ann Intern Med*. 1992;117:129-132.
121. LeGrand A, Sri-Ngernyuang L, Streefland PH: Enhancing appropriate drug use: the contribution of herbal medicine promotion. *Soc Sci Med*. 1993;36:1023-1035.
122. Lewis W: Ginseng revisited. *N Engl J Med*. 1980;243:31.
123. Liberti LE, DerMarderosian A: Evaluation of commercial ginseng products. *J Pharm Sci*. 1978;67:1487-1489.
124. Lin CC, Chou HL, Lin JL: Acute aconitine poisoned patients with ventricular arrhythmias successfully reversed by charcoal hemoper-fusion. *Am J Emerg Med*. 2002;20:66-67.
125. Lin CC, Chan TY, Deng JF: Clinical features and management of herb-induced aconitine poisoning. *Ann Emerg Med*. 2004;43:574-579.
126. Louman W, Danouske MD: The use of khat (*Catha edulis*) in Yemen social and medical observations. *Ann Intern Med*. 1976;85:246-249.
127. Malangu N. Characteristics of acute poisoning at two referral hospitals in Francistown and Gaborone. *SA Fam Pract*. 2008;50(3):67
128. Markowitz JS, Donovan JL, DeVane CL, et al: Effect of St John's wort on drug metabolism by induction of cytochrome P450 3A4 enzyme. *JAMA*. 2003;290:1500-1504.
129. Markowitz SB, Nunez CM, Klitzman S, et al: Lead poisoning due to Hai Ge Fen. The porphyric content of individual erythrocytes. *JAMA*. 1994;271:932-934.
130. Marsh WW, Hentges K: Mexican folk remedies and conventional medical care. *Am Fam Physician*. 1988;37:257-262.
131. Marwick C: New center director state complementary agenda. *JAMA*. 2000;293:990-991.
132. McGuffin M. Should herbal medicines by regulated as drugs? *Clin Pharmacol Ther*. 2008;83:393-395.
133. McNeil DG: Herbal drug is embraced in treating malaria. *The New York Times*, May 10, 2004. Available at www.nytimes.com. Last accessed September 1, 2008.
134. Michie CA: The use of herbal remedies in Jamaica. *Ann Trop Paediatr*. 1992;12:31-36.
135. Miller GM, Stripp R. A study of western pharmaceuticals contained within samples of Chines herbal/patent medicines collected from New York City's Chinatown. *Legal Med*. 2007;9:258-264.
136. Miller LG: Herbal medicinals: selected clinical considerations focusing on known or potential drug-herb interactions. *Arch Intern Med*. 2000;158:2200-2211.
137. Minor JR: Ginseng: fact or fiction. *Hosp Form*. 1979;186-192.
138. Mohabbat O, Younos MS, Merzad AA, et al: An outbreak of hepatic veno-occlusive disease in northwestern Afghanistan. *Lancet*. 1976;2: 269-271.
139. Morris CA, Avorn J: Internet marketing of herbal products. *JAMA*. 2003;290:1505-1509.
140. Morrow JD. Why the United States still needs improved dietary supplement regulationand oversight. *Clin Pharmacol Ther*. 2008;83:391-393.
141. Mullins RJ, Heddle R: Adverse reactions associated with echinacea: the Australian experience. *Ann Allergy Asthma Immunol*. 2002;88:42-51.
142. Nasir JM, Durning SJ, Ferguson M, et al: Exercise-induced syncope associated with QT prolongation and ephedra-free xenadrine. *Mayo Clin Proc*. 2004;79:1059-1062.
143. National Center for Complementary and Alternative Medicine: Major domains of complementary and alternative medicine. Available at http://nccam.nih.gov/health/whatiscam/. Last accessed September 1, 2008.
144. Nebelkopf E: Herbal therapy in the treatment of drug use. *Int J Addict*. 1987;22:695-717.
145. Nelson L, Shih R, Hoffman R: Aplastic anemia-induced by an adulterated herbal preparation. *J Toxicol Clin Toxicol*. 1995;33:467-470.

146. New York Buyer's Club Members Store Catalog. Available at http://www.nybcsecure.org. Last accessed September 1, 2008.
147. Nortier JL, Martinez MCM, Schmeiser HH, et al: Urothelial carcinoma associated with the use of a Chinese herb (*Aristolochia fangchi*). *N Engl J Med.* 2000;342:1686-1692.
148. Norton SA: Betel: Consumption and consequences. *J Am Acad Dermatol.* 1998;38:81-88.
149. Noskin GA, Clarke JT: Salmonella arizonae bacteremia as the presenting manifestation of human immunodeficiency virus infection following rattlesnake meat ingestion. *Rev Infect Dis.* 1990;12:514-517.
150. Nykamp DL, Fackih MN, Compton AL: Possible association of acute lateral-wall myocardial infarction and bitter orange supplement. *Ann Pharmacother.* 2004;38:812-6.
151. O'Hara MA, Kiefer D, Farrell K, et al: A review of 12 commonly used medicinal herbs. *Arch Fam Med.* 1998;7:523-536.
152. P, Thorup I: Neurotoxicity in rats dosed with peppermint oil and pulegone. *Arch Toxicol.* (Suppl) 1984;7:408-409.
153. Ostrenga UJ, Perry D: Goldenseal. *PharmChem Newsl.* 4, January 1975.
154. Palmer ME, Haller C, McKinney PE, et al: Adverse events associated with dietary supplements: an observational study. *Lancet.* 2003;361:1566.
155. Parsons JS: Contaminated herbal tea as a potential source of chronic arsenic poisoning. *NC Med J.* 1981;42:38-39.
156. Pedros C, Cereza G, Garcia N, et al: Liver toxicity of *Camellia sinensis* dried ethanolic extract [letter]. *Med Clin (Barc).* 2003;121:598-599.
157. Peng CC, Glassman PA, Trilli LE, et al: Incidence and severity of potential drug-dietary supplement interactions in primary care patients: an exploratory study of 2 outpatient practices. *Arch Intern Med.* 2004;164:630-636.
158. Pearl WS, Leo P, Tseng WO: Use of Chinese therapies among Chinese patients seeking emergency department care. *Ann Emerg Med.* 1995;26:735-738.
159. Perharic L, Shaw D, Colbridge M, et al: Toxicological problems resulting from exposure to traditional remedies and food supplements. *Drug Saf.* 1994;11:285-294.
160. Phillips LG, Nichols MH, King WD: Herbs and HIV: the health food industry's answer. *South Med J.* 1995;88:911-913.
161. Pillans PI: Toxicity of herbal products. *N Z Med J.* 1995;108:469-471.
162. Piscitelli SC, Burstein AH, Chaitt D, et al: Indinavir concentrations and St. John's wort. *Lancet.* 2000;355:547-548.
163. Pontifex AH, Gary AK: Lead poisoning from an Asian Indian folk remedy. *CMAJ.* 1985;133:1227-1228.
164. Porcel JM, Bielsa S, Madronero AB. Hepatotoxicity associated with green tea extracts [electronic letter]. May 16, 2005. Available at http://www.annals.org/cgi/eletters/142/6/477#1669. Last accessed on September 1, 2008.
165. Prpic-Majic D, Pizent A, Jurasovic J, et al: Lead poisoning associated with the use of Ayurvedic meta-mineral tonics. *J Toxicol Clin Toxicol.* 1996;34:417-423.
166. Ridker PM, Ohk'uma S, McDermott WV, et al: Hepatic veno-occlusive disease associated with the consumption of pyrrolizidine-containing dietary supplements. *Gastroenterology.* 1985;88:1050-1054.
167. Ridker PM: Toxic effects of herbal teas. *Arch Environ Health.* 1987;42:133-136.
168. Ries CA, Sahud MA: Agranulocytosis caused by Chinese herbal medicines. *JAMA.* 1975;231:352-355.
169. Riley KB, Antoniskis D, Maris R, et al: Rattlesnake capsule-associated *Salmonella arizonae* infections. *Arch Intern Med.* 1988;148:1207-1210.
170. Rosenthal PJ. Artesunate for the treatment of severe falciparum malaria. *N Engl J Med.* 2008; 358:1829-36.
171. Saint John's Wort. *Review of Natural Products.* Levittown, PA: Pharmaceutical Information Associates; January 1995.
172. Saper RB, Kales SN, Paquin J, et al: Heavy metal content of Ayurvedic herbal medicine products. *JAMA.* 2004;292:2868-2873.
173. Saper RB, Phillips RS, Sehgal A, et al: Lead, mercury, and arsenic in US- and Indian-manufactured ayurvedic medicines sold via the internet. *JAMA.* 2008;3300:915-923.
174. Saryan LA: Surreptitious lead exposure from an Asian Indian medication. *J Anal Toxicol.* 1991;15:336-338.
175. Segelman AB, Segelman FP, Karliner J, et al: Sassafras and herb tea: potential health hazards. *JAMA.* 1976;236:477.
176. Siegel RK: Ginseng abuse syndrome. *JAMA.* 1979;241:1614-1615.
177. Slifman NR, Obermeyer WR, Aloi BK: Brief report: contamination of botanical dietary supplements by *Digitalis lanata*. *N Engl J Med.* 1998; 339:806-811.
178. Snow LG: Folk medical beliefs and their implications for care of patients: a review based on studies among black patients. *Ann Intern Med.* 1974;81:82-96.
179. Solecki RS: Shanidar IV, a Neanderthal flower burial of northern Iraq. *Science.* 1975;190:880.
180. Solomon PR, Adams F, Silver A, et al: Ginkgo biloba for memory enhancement: a randomized controlled trial. *JAMA.* 2002;288:835-840.
181. Spoerke DG: Herbal medication: use and misuse. *Hosp Form.* 1980; 941-951.
182. Stevens T, Qadri A, Zein NN. Two patients with acute liver injury associated with use of the herbal weight-loss supplement Hydroxycut [letter]. *Ann Intern Med.* 2005;142:477.
183. Stolberg SG. US to prohibit supplement tied to health risk. *The New York Times.* Dec 31, 2003. Available at www.nytimes.com. Last accessed December 27, 2008.
184. Sztajnkrycer MD, Otten EJ, Bond GR, et al: Mitigation of penny-royal oil hepatotoxicity in the mouse. *Acad Emerg Med.* 2003;10:1024-1028.
185. Sullivan JB, Rumack BH, Thomas H, et al: Pennyroyal oil poisoning and hepatotoxicity. *JAMA.* 1979;242:2873-2874.
186. Tai YT, But PP-H, Young K, et al: Cardiotoxicity after accidental herb-induced aconite poisoning. *Lancet.* 1992;340:1254-1256.
187. Tagwireyi D, Ball DE, Nhachi CF. Poisoning in Zimbabwe: a survey of eight major referral hospitals. *J Appl Toxicol.* 2002;22(2)99-105.
188. Tandon BN, Handon HD, Tandon RK, et al: An epidemic of veno-occlusive disease of liver in central India. *Lancet.* 1976;2:271-272.
189. Taylor RFH, Al-Jarad N, John LME, et al: Betel nut chewing and asthma. *Lancet.* 1992;330:1134-1136.
190. The Ephedras. *Review of Natural Products.* Levittown, PA: Pharmaceutical Information Associates; November 1995.
191. Thiolet C, Mennecier D, Bredin C, et al: Acute cytolysis induced by Chinese tea [letter]. *Gastroenterol Clin Biol.* 2002;26:939-40.
192. Turner RB, Bauer R, Woelkart K, et al: An evaluation of *Echinacea angustifolia* in experimental rhinovirus infections. *N Engl J Med.* 2005;353: 341-348.
193. US Food and Drug Administration. Buying fake ED products online. January 4, 2008. Available at http://www.fda.gov/consumer/updates/erectiledysfunction010408.pdf. Last accessed December 27, 2008.
194. US Food and Drug Administration: Overview of Dietary Supplements. January 3, 2001. http://www.cfsan.fda.gov/~dms/ds-oview.html#what Last accessed September 1, 2008.
195. US Food and Drug Administration: 21 CFR Part 119. Final rule declaring dietary supplements containing ephedrine alkaloids adulterated because they present an unreasonable risk; final rule. April 12, 2004. *Fed Reg.* Available at http://www.cfsan.fda.gov/~lrd/ fr040211.html. Last accessed September 1, 2008.
196. US Food and Drug Administration: FDA warns manufacturers to stop distributing products containing androstenedione. March 11, 2004. Available at http://www.cfsan.fda.gov/~dms/dsandro.html Last accessed. September 1, 2008.
197. US Food and Drug Administration: FDA consumer advisory. Kava-containing dietary supplements may be with severe liver injury. March 25, 2002. Available at http://www.cfsan.fda.gov/~dms/addskava.html. Last accessed September 1, 2008.
198. Vanhaelen M, Vanhaelen-Fastre R, But P, et al: Identification of aristolochic acid in Chinese herbs [letter]. *Lancet.* 1994;343:174.
199. Vanherweghem JL, Depierreux M, Tielemans C, et al: Rapidly progressive interstitial renal fibrosis in young woman: association with slimming regimen including Chinese herbs. *Lancet.* 1993;341:387-391.
200. Verhoef MJ, Sutherland LR, Brkich L: Use of alternative medicine by patients attending a gastroenterology clinic. *CMAJ.* 1990;142:121-125.
201. Vial T, Bernard G, Lewden B, Dumortier J, Descotes J. Acute hepatitis due to Exolise, a *Camellia sinensis*-derived drug [letter]. *Gastroenterol Clin Biol.* 2003;27:1166-1167.
202. Voelker R: Seeds of knowledge grow in urban garden. *JAMA.* 2002;288: 1706-1707.
203[AU: please cite Ref. 203 in text)]. Waterman SH, Juarez G, Carr SJ, et al: *Salmonella arizonae* infections in Latinos associated with rattlesnake folk medicine. *Am J Public Health.* 1990;80:286-289.
204. Weisbord SD, Soule JB, Kimmel PL: Brief report: Poison online—acute renal failure caused by oil of wormwood purchased through the Internet. *N Engl J Med.* 1997;337:825-827.

205. Weiss G: Hallucinogenic and narcotic-like effects of powdered myristica (nutmeg). *Psychiatr Q.* 1960;34:346-356.
206. Woolf GM, Petrovic JM, Rojter SE: Acute hepatitis associated with the Chinese herbal product Jin Bu Huan. *Ann Intern Med.* 1994;121:729-735.
207. World Health Organization. WHO Traditional Medicine Strategy 2002-2005. Geneva: World Health Organization; 2002.
208. Wormwood. Review of Natural Products. Levittown, PA: Pharmaceutical Information Associates; April 1991.
209. Yeih DF, Chiang FT, Huang SKS: Successful treatment of aconitine induced life threatening ventricular tachyarrhythmia with amiodarone. *Heart.* 2000;84:e8.
210. Yuan CS, Wei G, Dey L, et al: Brief communication: American ginseng reduces warfarin's effect in healthy patients: a randomized, controlled trial. *Ann Intern Med.* 2004:141;23-27.

BIBLIOGRAPHY

Chevalier A: *The Encyclopedia of Medicinal Plants.* New York: DK Publishing; 1996.

Foster S, Tyler VE: *Tyler's Honest Herbal: A Sensible Guide to the Use of Herbs and Related Remedies*, 4th ed. New York: Haworth Press; 1999.

The Review of Natural Products Monograph System. Wolters Kluwer Health (http://www.skolar.com/description/rnp.html). Accessed September 1, 2008.

Lewis WH, Elvin-Lewis MP: *Medical Botany: Plant Affecting Man's Health*, 2nd ed. New York: Wiley; 2003.

Robbers, JE, Speedie MK, Tyler VE: *Pharmacognosy and Pharmacobiotechnology.* Philadelphia: Williams & Wilkins; 1996.

Robbers JE, Tyler VE: *Tyler's Herbs of Choice: The Therapeutic Use of Phytomedicinals*, 2nd ed. New York: Haworth Press; 1999.

CHAPTER 44
ATHLETIC PERFORMANCE ENHANCERS

Susi U. Vassallo

Public interest in extraordinary athletic achievement fuels the modern-day science of performance enhancement in sports. The desire to improve athletic performance in a scientific manner is a relatively recent development; at one time, the focus on maximizing human physical and mental potential centered on the importance of manual work and military service. The role of sport was inconsequential, except for its potential in improving military preparedness.[105] Today, "sports doping" refers to the use of a prohibited xenobiotic to enhance athletic performance. The word *doping* comes from the Dutch word *doop,* a viscous opium juice used by the ancient Greeks.[30]

HISTORY AND EPIDEMIOLOGY

Controversy surrounding the systematic use of performance-enhancing xenobiotics by the participating athletes has marred many sporting events. Since the International Olympic Committee (IOC) began testing for xenobiotics during the 1968 Olympic games, prominent athletes have been sanctioned and stripped of their Olympic medals because they tested positive for banned xenobiotics. However, from a public health perspective, the use of performance-enhancing xenobiotics among athletes of all ages and abilities is a far more serious concern than the highly publicized cases involving world-class athletes. The majority of studies on the epidemiology of performance-enhancing xenobiotics have investigated androgenic anabolic steroid use. *Androgenic* means masculinizing and *anabolic* means tissue building. An *anabolic process* stimulates protein synthesis, promotes nitrogen deposition in lean body mass, and decreases protein breakdown.[250] Studies of high school students document that 6.6% of male seniors have used anabolic steroids, and 35% of these individuals were not involved in organized athletics.[32] Other studies find rates of androgenic steroid use in adolescent athletes ranging from 3% to 19%.[114,127,182,246,251,250]

PERFORMANCE ENHANCEMENT AND SUDDEN DEATH IN ATHLETES

Many unexpected deaths in certain groups of young competitors have occurred in the absence of obvious medical or traumatic cause. In some cases, the use of performance-enhancing drugs is linked to the deaths. The use of erythropoietin (EPO), introduced in Europe in 1987, may have contributed to the large number of deaths in young European endurance athletes over the subsequent few years.[67,89,149,173,239] In young healthy athletes experiencing cerebrovascular events or myocardial infarction, the temporal link between the use of cocaine, ephedrine, or performance enhancers such as anabolic androgenic steroids suggests a role for these xenobiotics as precipitants of these adverse events[147] (Chap. 76). Nevertheless, the leading cause of nontraumatic sudden death in young athletes is most often associated with congenital cardiac anomalies.[146] In autopsy studies of athletes in the United States with sudden death, hypertrophic cardiomyopathy is the most common structural abnormality, accounting for more than one-third of the cardiac arrests, followed by coronary artery anomalies.[147] Medical causes of sudden death other than cardiac causes include heat stroke (Chap. 15), sickle cell trait, and asthma.[75,119,132]

PRINCIPLES

Performance enhancers can be classified in several ways for the purposes of study. Some categorize performance enhancers according to the expected effects. For example, some xenobiotics increase muscle mass, whereas others decrease recovery time, increase energy, or mask the presence of other drugs. However, one xenobiotic may have several expected effects. For example, diuretics may be used to mask the presence of other xenobiotics by producing dilute urine, or they may be used to reduce weight. Clenbuterol is an anabolic xenobiotic, but it also is a stimulant because of its β_2-adrenergic agonist effects. Bromontan is another stimulant, but it is used as a masking agent. Depending on the xenobiotic, it is used either during training to improve future performance or during competition to improve immediate results.[30]

According to the World Anti-Doping Agency (WADA) World Anti-Doping Code 2008, a xenobiotic or method constitutes doping and can be added to the prohibited list if it is a masking xenobiotic, or if it meets two of the following three criteria: it enhances performance; its use presents a risk to the athlete's health; and it is contrary to the spirit of sport[248] (Table 44–1).

THERAPEUTIC USE EXEMPTION

Some of the Prohibited Substances and Methods on the WADA 2008 Prohibited List are used to treat legitimate medical conditions encountered in athletes.[247] Athletes with documented medical conditions requiring the use of a prohibited substance or method may request a Therapeutic Use Exemption (TUE). In the Olympics, use of inhaled β_2-adrenergic agonists requires a TUE. Nevertheless, a high salbutamol concentration (free salbutamol concentration plus glucuronide level >1000 ng/mL) is considered a positive test and an adverse finding unless the athlete proves that the abnormal value results from therapeutic use of the drug.[45,247] Many athletes have sought to explain a positive doping test by claiming the substance was prescribed for a medical condition, such as the use of modafinil, a stimulant, for the sleep disorder narcolepsy.

ANABOLIC XENOBIOTICS

ANDROGENIC STEROIDS

Androgenic anabolic steroids (AAS) increase muscle mass, lean body weight, and cause nitrogen retention.[157] Testosterone is the prototypical androgen, and most androgenic anabolic steroids are synthetic testosterone derivatives. The androgenic effects of steroids are responsible for male appearance and secondary sexual characteristics such as increased growth of body hair and deepening of the voice.

In the 1970s and 1980s, federal regulation of anabolic steroids was under the direction of the Food and Drug Administration (FDA). Because of increasing media reports on the use of anabolic steroids in sports, particularly by high school students and amateur athletes, Congress enacted the Anabolic Steroid Control Act of 1990, which

TABLE 44–1. Abbreviated Summary of World Anti-Doping Agency 2008 Prohibited List[247]

Substances (S) and Methods (M) Prohibited at All Times (In- and Out-of-Competition)
- S1. Anabolic Androgenic Agents
  - Clenbuterol
  - Selective androgen receptor modulators (SARMS)
- S2. Hormones and Related Substances
- S3. β_2-Adrenergic Agonists
  - Exceptions require Therapeutic Use Exemption
- S4. Hormone Antagonists and Modulators
  - Myostatin inhibitors
- S5. Diuretics and Other Masking Agents
- M1. Enhancement of Oxygen Transfer
- M2. Chemical and Physical Manipulation
- M3. Gene Doping

Substances and Methods Prohibited In Competition

In addition to S1 to S5 and M1 to M3 above, the following categories are prohibited in competition:
- S6. Stimulants
- S7. Narcotics
- S8. Cannabinoids
- S9. Glucocorticosteroids except topically unless TUE

Substances Prohibited in Particular (P) Sports
- P1. Alcohol
- P2. β-Adrenergic Antagonists

Specified substances[a]
- Ephedrine
- Cannabinoids
- All inhaled β_2-adrenergic agonists, except Clenbuterol
- Probenecid
- All glucocorticosteroids
- All β-adrenergic antagonists
- Alcohol in competition only

[a] In certain circumstances, a doping violation involving specified substances may result in a reduced sanction, provided the athlete establishes that the use was not intended to enhance performance.

TUE = therapeutic use exemption

TABLE 44–2. Synthetic Testosterone Derivatives/Anabolic Androgenic Steroids

Generic Nomenclature		
17α-Alkyl Derivatives (Oral)	**17β-Ester Derivatives (Parenteral)**	**Transdermal Testosterone Preparations**
Ethylestrenol	Boldenone	Buccal gel, sublingual
Fluoxymesterone	Nandrolone decanoate	Dermal gel, ointment
Methandrostenolone	Nandrolone phenpropionate	Transdermal reservoir patch
Methyltestosterone	Testosterone esters	
Oxandrolone	Testosterone cypionate	
Oxymetholone	Testosterone enanthate	
Stanozolol	Testosterone ester combination	
	Testosterone propionate	
	Trenbolone	

amended the Controlled Substances Act and placed anabolic steroids on schedule III. Schedule III states that a xenobiotic has a currently accepted medical use in the United States and has less potential for abuse than the xenobiotics categorized as schedule I or II. The Anabolic Steroid Control Act of 2004 adds certain steroid precursors, such as androstenedione and dihydrotestosterone, to the list of controlled substances that are considered illegal without a prescription. Possession of androstenedione or other metabolic precursors called *prohormone drugs* is considered a federal crime. Nevertheless, anabolic steroids are still available illicitly over the Internet from international marketers, veterinary pharmaceutical companies, and some legitimate US manufacturers.

PHYSIOLOGY AND PHARMACOLOGY

The Leydig cells of the testis produce 95% of endogenous male testosterone; the remainder comes from the adrenal glands. Normally 4–10 mg testosterone and 1–3 mg androstenedione are produced daily in men. Women secrete approximately 0.04–0.12 mg testosterone and 2–4 mg androstenedione daily from their ovaries and adrenal glands.[219]

Testosterone is rapidly degraded in the liver, with a plasma half-life of less than 30 minutes. Therefore, in order to create a medication that is useful clinically, testosterone is esterified at the 17-hydroxy position, forming a hydrophobic compound that can be administered in an oil vehicle for gradual release.[14] Most of these esters of testosterone must be injected intramuscularly to avoid extensive first-pass hepatic metabolism associated with oral administration.[14] Alternatively, alkylation at the 17-hydroxy position produces androgens that can be administered orally because they are more resistant to hepatic metabolism. These agents, more commonly used by athletes, are responsible for the majority of complications associated with AAS use[14] (Table 44–2).

ANTIESTROGENS AND ANTIANDROGENS

In male athletes using androgens, avoiding the unwanted side effects of feminization such as gynecomastia, or in the case of female athletes avoiding masculinization and features such as facial hair and deepening voice, requires manipulation of the metabolic pathways of androgen metabolism. Creating a xenobiotic that completely dissociates the desired from the unwanted effects has not been possible. However, xenobiotics with properties capable of manipulating metabolic pathways associated with undesirable side effects are divided into four main groups, all on the prohibited list: (1) Aromatase inhibitors such as anastrozole and aminoglutethimide prevent the conversion of androstenedione and testosterone into estrogen. (2) The antiestrogen clomiphene blocks estrogen receptors in the hypothalamus, opposing the negative feedback of estrogen, causing an increase in gonadotropin releasing hormone, thereby increasing testosterone release. (3) Selective estrogen receptor modulators (SERMs) such as tamoxifen and raloxifene bind to estrogen receptors and exhibit agonist or antagonist effects at the estrogen receptors. By indirectly increasing gonadotropin release, SERMs restore endogenous testosterone production upon discontinuation of androgenic anabolic steroids.[190] (4) Selective androgen receptor modulators (SARMs) are nonsteroidal tissue-selective anabolic agents that are not yet commercially available. They are not aromatized and are not substrates for 5α-reductase, nor do they undergo the same metabolic pathways to testosterone. Therefore, they have fewer unwanted androgenic side effects.[82,223]

ADMINISTRATION

Approximately 50% of AASs are taken orally. The remainder is administered by intramuscular injection, with one-fourth of intramuscular AAS users sharing needles.[62,163] One-third of the needles and syringes exchanged in a needle-exchange program in Wales were used for anabolic steroids.[171] Unlike therapeutically indicated regimens, which consist of fixed doses at regular intervals, athletes typically use AASs in cycles of 6 to 8 weeks.[14] For example, the athlete may use steroids for 2 months and then abstain for 2 months. Cycling is based on the athlete's individual preferences and not on any validated protocol. *Stacking* implies combining the use of several AASs at one time, often with both oral and intramuscular administration. To prevent *plateauing,* or developing tolerance, to any one drug, some athletes use an average of five different AASs simultaneously. The doses used are frequently hundreds of times in excess of scientifically based therapeutic recommendations.[3,245] *Pyramiding* implies starting the AAS at a low dose, increasing the dose many times, and then tapering once again. Fat-soluble AASs may require several months to be totally eliminated, whereas water-soluble steroids may require only days to weeks to be cleared by the kidney. Water-soluble testosterone esters are used for bridging therapy. *Bridging* refers to the practice of halting the administration of long-lasting alkylated testosterone formulations so that urine analyses at a specific time offer no evidence of use, while injections of shorter-acting testosterone esters are used to replace the orally administered alkylated formulations. This strategy, which was used extensively in the German Democratic Republic, is documented in a review of the subject based on extensive research of previously classified records.[74] Clearance profiles for testosterone congeners were determined for each athlete. In general, the daily injection of testosterone esters was used when termination of the more readily detectable synthetic alkylated testosterone derivatives was necessary to avoid a positive doping test. These daily injections of testosterone propionate were halted 4–5 days before competition. Corrupt officials involved in doping were sure that the values would decrease to acceptable concentrations in time for the event, based on the science of athletes' clearance of testosterone esters.[74]

CLINICAL MANIFESTATIONS OF ANDROGENIC ANABOLIC STEROID USE

Musculoskeletal Supraphysiologic doses of testosterone, when combined with strength training, increase muscle strength and size.[24] The most common musculoskeletal complications of steroid use are tendon and ligament rupture.[76,102,133,138]

Hepatic Hepatic subcapsular hematoma with hemorrhage is reported.[203] Peliosis hepatis, a condition of blood-filled sinuses in the liver that may result in fatal hepatic rupture, occurs most commonly with alkylated androgens and may not improve when androgen use is stopped.[15,104,211,241] This condition is not associated with the dose or duration of treatment.[14,112,214] Cyproterone acetate is a chlorinated progesterone derivative that inhibits 5α-reductase and reportedly causes hepatotoxicity.[14,79,84]

Infectious Local complications from injection include infected joints,[70] cutaneous abscess,[148,187] and *Candida albicans* endophthalmitis.[244] Injection of steroids using contaminated needles has led to transmission of infectious diseases such as HIV and hepatitis B and C.[163,167,185,186,205,210] Severe varicella is reported in long-term AAS users.[114]

Dermatologic/Gingiva Cutaneous side effects are common and include keloid formation, sebaceous cysts, comedones, seborrheic furunculosis, folliculitis, and striae.[206] Acne is associated with steroid use and sometimes is referred to as "gymnasium acne."[44,174] A common triad of acne, striae, and gynecomastia occurs. The production of sebum is an androgen-dependent process, and dihydrotestosterone is active in sebaceous glands.[14] Gingival hyperplasia is reported.[165]

Endocrine Conversion of AAS to estradiol in peripheral tissues results in feminization of male athletes. Gynecomastia may be irreversible. AAS use causes negative feedback inhibition of gonadotropin-releasing hormone, luteinizing hormone, and follicle-stimulating hormone from the hypothalamus. This process results in testicular atrophy and decreased spermatogenesis, which may be reversible. In females, menstrual irregularities and breast atrophy may occur. AAS use causes virilization in females.[219]

Cardiovascular Cardiac complications include acute myocardial infarction and sudden cardiac arrest.[9,73,100,110,140,142,153] Autopsy examination of the heart may reveal biventricular hypertrophy, extensive myocardial fibrosis, and contraction-band necrosis. Myofibrillar disorganization and hypertrophy of the interventricular septum and left ventricle are present.[140] Intense training and use of AAS impair diastolic function by increasing left ventricular wall thickness. Animal models and in vitro myocardial cell studies show similar pathologic changes.[54,126,154,221,230,231] Doppler echocardiography shows that several years after strength athletes discontinue using AAS, concentric left ventricular hypertrophy remains, compared to similar strength athletes not using AAS.[231] Growth hormone may potentiate the effects of AAS and further increase concentric remodeling of the left ventricle.[118] In addition to direct myocardial injury, vasospasm or thrombosis may occur.[154] Alkylated androgens lower the concentration of high-density lipoprotein (HDL) cholesterol and may increase platelet aggregation.[3,73] Thromboembolic complications include pulmonary embolus,[59,81] stroke,[122,123,209] carotid arterial occlusion,[132] cerebral sinus thrombosis, poststeroid balance disorder,[28,130] and popliteal artery entrapment.[137]

Neuropsychiatric Distractibility, depression or mania, delirium, irritability, insomnia, hostility, anxiety, mood lability, and aggressiveness ("roid rage") may occur.[18,178,179,220] These neuropsychiatric effects do not appear to correlate with plasma AAS concentrations.[209,220] Withdrawal symptoms from AAS include decreased libido, fatigue, and myalgias.[121,250]

Cancer An association between AAS use and development of cancer has been observed in experimental animals.[192] Testicular and prostatic carcinomas are reported in more frequent users of AAS.[80,191] Hepatocellular carcinoma,[71,113,164] cholangiocarcinoma,[14,91] Wilms tumor, and renal cell carcinoma are also reported in young AAS users.[33,181] The relationship between the dose of AAS and cancer is unknown.

SPECIFIC ANABOLIC XENOBIOTICS

Dehydroepiandrosterone Dehydroepiandrosterone (DHEA) is a precursor to testosterone (Fig. 44–1). Although banned by the FDA in 1996, this drug subsequently was marketed as a nutritional supplement and is available for purchase without a prescription.[219] DHEA is converted to androstenedione and then to testosterone by the enzyme 17β-hydroxysteroid dehydrogenase.[108,139,143] Administration of androstenedione in dosages of 300 mg/d increases testosterone and estradiol concentrations in some men and women.[136] Women with

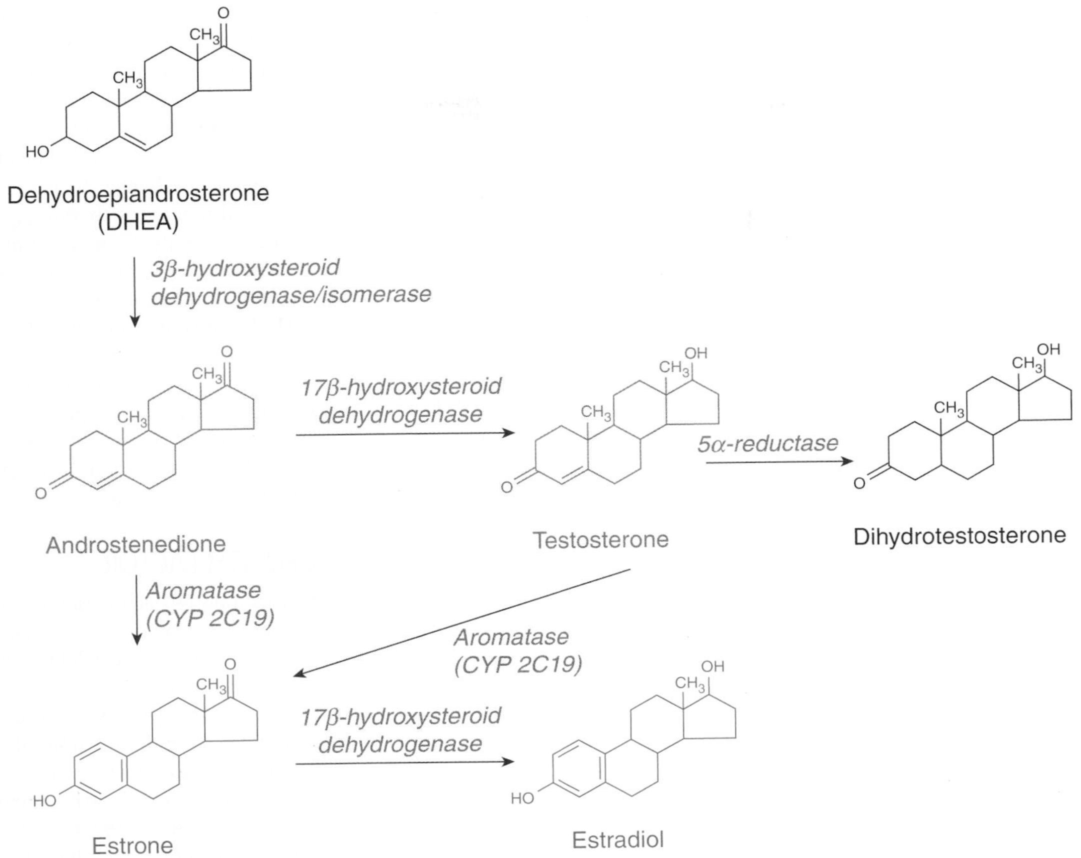

FIGURE 44–1. Metabolic pathways of dehydroepiandrosterone (DHEA).

adrenal insufficiency given DHEA replacement at a dose of 50 mg/d orally for 4 months demonstrated increased serum concentrations of DHEA, androstenedione, testosterone, and dihydrotestosterone. Serum total and HDL cholesterol concentrations simultaneously decreased. Some women experienced androgenic side effects, including greasy skin, acne, and hirsutism.[12] Sense of well-being and sexuality increased in men and women after 4 months of treatment.[12,158,159] The neuropsychiatric effects of DHEA have been demonstrated in animals. Increased hypothalamic serotonin, anxiolytic effects, antagonism at the γ-aminobutyric acid type A ($GABA_A$) receptor, and agonism of the *N*-methyl-D-aspartate receptor are demonstrated.[12,144,155]

Clenbuterol Clenbuterol is a β_2-adrenergic agonist that decreases fat deposition and prevents protein breakdown in animal models.[7,42] Clenbuterol is also a potent *nutrient partitioning agent,* a term implying it can increase the amount of muscle and decrease the amount of fat produced per pound of feed given to cattle and other animals.[77,189] Use of clenbuterol in cattle farming is illegal in many countries. Nevertheless, the consumption of veal liver contaminated with clenbuterol has resulted in sympathomimetic symptoms and positive urine tests in affected individuals.[195] Clenbuterol increases the glycolytic capacity of muscle and causes hypertrophy, enhancing the growth of fast-twitch fibers.[145,253] β_2-Adrenergic receptors are present in skeletal muscle and may mediate the anabolic effect of this class of drugs. Athletes typically use doses of 60–100 μg/d clenbuterol and in some cases as much as 600 μ/d. Clenbuterol overdose is characterized by the typical symptoms of sympathomimetic overdose [41,51,106] (Chap. 65).

PEPTIDES AND GLYCOPROTEIN HORMONES

CREATINE

Creatine is an amino acid formed by combining the amino acids methionine, arginine, and glycine. It is synthesized naturally by the liver, kidneys, and pancreas. Creatine is found in protein-containing foods such as meat and fish. In its phosphorylated form it is involved in the rapid resynthesis of adenosine triphosphate (ATP) from adenosine diphosphate (ADP) by acting as a substrate to donate phosphorous.[218] Because ATP is the immediate source of energy for muscle contraction, creatine is used by athletes to increase energy during short, high-intensity exercise.[234] More than 2.5 million kg of creatine is consumed annually in the United States.[5] Exceptional athletes have admitted to using creatine as part of their training nutritional regimen, leading to interest by athletes at all levels. Numerous studies demonstrate improved performance with creatine supplementation, particularly in sports requiring short, high-intensity effort.[27,34,97,129,152,234] Creatine is found in skeletal muscle and in the heart, brain and kidney. Two-thirds of creatine is stored primarily as phosphorylated creatine (PCr) and the remainder as free creatine (Cr).[16] Consuming carbohydrates with creatine supplements increases total creatine and PCr stores in skeletal muscle.[94] This process explains why creatine is marketed in combination with carbohydrate. Human endogenous creatine production is 1 g/d, and normal diets containing meat and fish offer another 1–2 g/d as dietary intake. One to two grams of creatine is eliminated daily by irreversible conversion to creatinine.[240]

Creatine supplementation is most commonly accomplished with creatine monohydrate. A dose of 20–25 g/d can increase the skeletal muscle total creatine concentration by 20%.[97,111] Creatine stores do not increase in some individuals despite creatine supplementation. Creatine uptake in skeletal muscle occurs via the creatine transporter proteins at the sarcolemma. Creatine transporter expression and activity, as well as exercise and training, influence the uptake of creatine and the effect of creatine loading on athletic performance.[212,213,215]

One adverse effect of creatine supplementation is weight gain, which is thought to result primarily from water retention.[97,152] However, evidence indicates that net protein increase is partially responsible for the weight gain associated with long-term creatine use.[116] Diarrhea was the most commonly reported side effect of creatine use in one study of 52 male college athletes. Other complaints were muscle cramping and dehydration, although many subjects had no complaints.[117]

Creatine supplementation increases urinary creatine and creatinine excretion and may increase serum creatinine concentrations by 20%.[97,116] Long-term and short-term creatine supplementation does not appear to have an adverse effect on renal function.[176,177] One patient who had been taking creatine 5 g/d for 4 weeks developed interstitial nephritis that improved with cessation of creatine use. Whether ingestion of creatine caused the nephritis is unknown.[128] A young man with focal segmental glomerular sclerosis developed an elevated creatinine concentration and a decreased glomerular filtration rate (GFR) when creatine supplementation was started. The values returned to baseline upon cessation of creatine supplementation.[11] The possibility of developing decreased renal function is a theoretical concern. Ingestion of large amounts of creatine may result in formation of the carcinogenic substance *N*-nitrososarcosine, which induces esophageal cancer in rats.[10,11]

HUMAN GROWTH HORMONE

Human growth hormone (hGH) is an anabolic peptide hormone secreted by the anterior pituitary gland. It causes its anabolic effect by stimulating protein synthesis and increasing growth and muscle mass in children. Recombinant human growth hormone has been available since 1984. It is commonly used therapeutically for children with growth hormone deficiency in daily doses of 5–26 μg/kg body weight.[235]

Growth hormone secretion is stimulated by growth hormone–releasing hormone and is inhibited by somatostatin. Growth hormone receptors occur in many tissues, including the liver. Binding of hGH to hepatic receptors causes secretion of insulin-like growth factor-1 (IGF-1), which has potent anabolic effects and is the mediator responsible for many of the actions of hGH.

Human growth hormone is released in a pulsatile manner, mainly during sleep. Exercise stimulates hGH release, and more intense exercise causes proportionately more hGH release.[29,50,219] Amino acids such as ornithine, l-arginine, tryptophan, and L-lysine increase hGH release through an unknown mechanism and often are ingested for this purpose.[50,99]

Human growth hormone stimulates protein synthesis and tissue growth by nitrogen retention and increased movement of amino acids into tissue. The effects on increasing muscle mass and size are well proven in growth hormone–deficient individuals, but some studies do not support a resultant increase in strength related to the increase in muscle size in athletes.[48,141] In a more recent study, lean body mass, strength, and power increased.[93] Human growth hormone improves muscle and cardiac function, increases red cell mass and oxygen-carrying capacity, stimulates lipolysis, normalizes serum lipid concentrations, and decreases subcutaneous fat. It also improves mood and sense of well-being.[48,49,101,197,219,235]

Growth hormone is used by athletes for its anabolic potential. As a xenobiotic of abuse, it is particularly attractive because laboratory detection is difficult. In one survey, 12% of people in gyms used hGH for body building.[69] In another survey of adolescents, 5% of 10th-grade boys had used hGH.[188] Human growth hormone may be illicitly sold as recombinant growth hormone on the black market.

Human growth hormone administration may cause myalgias, arthralgias, carpal tunnel syndrome, and edema.[235] The effects of hGH on skeletal growth depend on the user's age. In preadolescence, excessive hGH may cause increased bony growth and gigantism. In adults, excessive hGH may cause acromegaly.[235] Growth hormone may cause glucose intolerance and hyperglycemia. Skin changes such as increased melanocytic nevi and altered skin texture occur.[175] Lipid profiles may be adversely affected. HDL concentrations are decreased, a change associated with increased risk of coronary artery disease.[254] Because hGH must be given parenterally, there is risk of transmission of infection.[141] The illicit sale of cadaveric human pituitary–derived growth hormone is associated with a risk of Creutzfeldt-Jakob disease.[58] Long-term users of hGH may be at increased risk for prostate cancer because of the complications associated with IGF-1[90] (see next section).

INSULIN-LIKE GROWTH FACTOR

IGF-1 is a peptide chain structurally related to insulin. A recombinant form is available.[188] Parenteral administration of IGF-1 is approved for clinical treatment of dwarfism and insulin resistance. Children who develop antibodies to recombinant growth hormone may respond to IGF-1.

Human growth hormone is the primary stimulus for release of IGF-1, although insulin, DHEA, and nutrition play a role.[194] The actions of IGF-1 can be classified as either anabolic or insulin-like.[194] The effects of growth hormone are primarily mediated by IGF-1. IGF-1 is produced in the liver and many other cell types. IGF-1 binds principally to the type I IGF receptor, which has 40% homology with the insulin receptor and a similar tyrosine kinase subunit.[225] IGF-1 also binds to insulin receptors, but it has only 1% of insulin's affinity for the insulin receptor. IGF-1 increases glucose utilization by causing the movement of glucose into cells, increasing amino acid uptake and stimulating protein synthesis.

Side effects are similar to those associated with use of growth hormone and include acromegaly. Other effects include headache, jaw pain, edema, and alterations in lipid profiles. A potentially serious side effect of IGF-1 is hypoglycemia. High endogenous plasma IGF-1 levels are associated with an increased risk for prostate cancer.[39]

Few studies on the efficacy of IGF-1 in improving the conditioning of athletes are available. IGF-1 is attractive to female athletes because it does not cause virilization.[219]

INSULIN

Insulin is used by body builders for its anabolic properties. Of 20 self-identified anabolic androgenic steroid users in one gym, five (25%) who had no medical reason to take insulin reported using it to increase muscle mass.[184] These individuals stated that they had injected insulin from 20 to 60 times over the 6 months prior to the study.[184] Their practice was to inject 10 U regular insulin and then eat sugar-containing foods after injection. Hypoglycemia has been reported in body builders using insulin.[66,183]

Insulin inhibits proteolysis and promotes growth by stimulating movement of glucose and amino acids into muscle and fat cells. It increases the synthesis of glycogen, fatty acids, and proteins[53] (Chap. 48).

HUMAN CHORIONIC GONADOTROPIN

Human chorionic gonadotropin (hCG) is a glycoprotein that stimulates testicular steroidogenesis in men. In women, hCG is secreted by the placenta during pregnancy. Human chorionic gonadotropin may be used by male athletes to prevent testicular atrophy during and after androgen administration.[124] Analysis of hCG in 740 urinary specimens of male athletes revealed abnormal concentrations in 21 individuals. This finding prompted the IOC ban on hCG use in 1987. Presently, distinguishing exogenous hCG administration from hCG production in early pregnancy is not possible, so the urine samples of women are not tested.[124]

Very small amounts of hCG are normally present in men and non-pregnant women. Currently measurement is made by immunoassay. The decision limit, the concentration at which the test is considered positive, is set at 5 IU/mL urine. Trophoblastic tumors and nontrophoblastic tumors can increase hCG concentrations, and this possibility must be considered in the evaluation of elevated urinary hCG concentration.[57]

Administration of hCG causes an increase in the total testosterone and epitestosterone produced.

OXYGEN TRANSPORT

ERYTHROPOIETIN (EPO)

Human erythropoietin (hEPO) is a hormone that, through a receptor-mediated mechanism, induces erythropoiesis by stimulating stem cells. Erythropoietin has been available since 1988 as recombinant human erythropoietin (rhEPO), and its use in international competition has been prohibited since 1990. While hEPO is produced primarily by the kidneys, rhEPO is produced in hamsters; this results in differing glycosylation patterns, an important piece in the laboratory detection of EPO in sports doping (see Laboratory Detection).[61]

Because EPO increases exercise capacity and hemoglobin production, it is used by athletes, often with additional iron supplementation. The clinical effects of increased hematocrit occur several days after administration.[78,168] EPO increases maximal oxygen uptake by 6%–7%, an effect that lasts approximately 2 weeks after rhEPO administration is completed.[65]

Two EPO analogs exist. Darbopoietin, also known as *new erythropoiesis-stimulating protein* (NESP), differs from EPO by five amino acids. It has a much longer half-life and can be injected weekly.[169] Another protein known as synthetic erythropoiesis protein (SEP) has a similar protein structure to EPO. The protein polymers created in this molecule have less immunogenicity, fewer biologic contaminants, and more predictable pharmacokinetics.[169]

Human erythropoietin is secreted primarily by the kidney, although some is produced by other tissues, including the liver. The mean half-life of rhEPO is 4.5 hours following IV administration and 25 hours after subcutaneous administration.[196]

In patients with renal failure who are on dialysis, a typical dose is approximately 50 U/kg body weight given three times per week.[103,196] EPO enhances endothelial activation and platelet reactivity and increases systolic blood pressure during submaximal exercise.[23,217] These effects, in addition to the increase in hemoglobin, increase the risk for thromboembolic events, hypertension, and hyperviscosity syndromes.[23,151,168] Nineteen Belgian and Dutch cyclists died of uncertain causes between 1987 and 1990.[63] Increases in hematocrit subsequent to EPO use are believed to have contributed to these deaths. The 1998 Tour de France was marred by the discovery of widespread EPO use by members of several different cycling teams.

An EPO overdose occurred in a patient who self-administered 10,000 U/d for an unknown period of time as a result of a dosing error. The patient presented to the hospital with confusion, a plethoric appearance, blackened toes, decreased pulses, and a hematocrit of 72%. Emergent erythropheresis was performed and resulted in rapid reduction of hematocrit and improvement in the patient's condition.[252] Another report of deliberate daily self-administration of an unknown dose of rhEPO resulted in a hematocrit of 70%. The patient was treated emergently with phlebotomy and intravenous hydration and improved.[32]

ARTIFICIAL OXYGEN CARRIERS

Artificial oxygen carriers are blood substitutes that supplement the oxygen-carrying capacity of RBCs.[204] Artificial oxygen carriers fall into two categories: hemoglobin-based oxygen carrier (HBOC) and perfluorocarbon (PFC) emulsions. Athletes may experiment with these substances to increase endurance.

Hemoglobin can be genetically engineered or obtained from cattle or outdated blood. Bovine hemoglobin may serve as a source for human HBOC products. Hemoglobin is composed of four subunits, two α-chains and two β-chains. When removed from erythrocytes, hemoglobin is unstable and dissociates into dimers. The life of HBOCs is much shorter than that of RBCs. In a meta-analysis of 16 trials of HBOCs, there is a 30% statistically significant increased risk of death and 2.7 times greater risk of myocardial infarction, regardless of the product.[162]

The differences in molecular weights of native hemoglobin and stabilized hemoglobin can be determined by size-exclusion high-performance liquid chromatography, which is one of the primary methods of doping analysis for HBOCs.[236]

PERFLUOROCARBONS

Perfluorocarbons are synthetic oxygen-carrying compounds that can be used as RBC substitutes. These liquids, which are composed of eight to ten carbon atoms with fluorine substitution for hydrogen, serve as excellent solvents for gases.[92] In 1966, it was shown that mice could survive when fully submerged in PFCs infused with oxygen.[43] Compared to RBC transfusions, PFCs are without risk of infection, require no cross-matching, and do not increase the viscosity of blood. PFCs are stable at room temperature and have a shelf life of greater than 1 year, attributes that make them convenient to use.

Perfluorocarbons increase vascular tone, which may cause hypertension. Both systemic and pulmonary vascular resistance is increased.[92] For unclear reasons, intravenous infusion of these emulsions can cause cardiac arrest.[227]

Because PFCs are perceived by the immune system as foreign substances, they are rapidly cleared by the reticuloendothelial system. The plasma half-life is approximately 12 hours. PFCs accumulate in the liver and spleen and are slowly transported to the lung. Over a period of months to years, the PFCs are eliminated unchanged in the expired air and can be measured in expired air by thermal conductance or in blood by using gas chromatography-mass spectrometry.[204,227]

AUTOTRANSFUSION

Infusion of autologous blood (the athletes' own) or homologous blood (from a donor, also called *allogeneic* transfusion) for the purpose of increasing the hematocrit is known as *blood doping*. Blood doping was used in the Olympic Games as early as 1972 by a Finnish steeplechaser. During subsequent summer and winter Olympics, distance runners, cyclists, and skiers acknowledged their use of this practice. The US cycling team admitted to using blood transfusions in the 1984 Olympics. Subsequently, the IOC banned the practice.

Blood doping is beneficial in endurance athletes. Infusion of 400 mL packed RBCs into distance runners increased the total RBC concentration and substantially improved performance in 10-km races.[31] Blood doping also increases the speed performance of cross-country skiers.[22] The preparatory technique involves the removal of 1000 mL blood, the immediate replacement of plasma volume, and the freezing and storage of RBCs. After 5–6 weeks (the time needed to return to normocythemia), reinfusion of frozen RBCs resulted in increased hematocrit values from 45% to 49%, 5% increase in oxygen utilization, and increased endurance capacity.[64] Reinfusion of packed RBCs resulted overnight in an increase in maximal exercise work time of 23% and increased maximal oxygen uptake by 9%. These improvements correlated with the increase in hemoglobin concentration.[64]

Detection of homologous blood transfusion is possible based on red blood cell surface antigen typing. The surface of the erythrocyte contains genetically determined complex oligosaccharides and rhesus (Rh) polypeptides. Using flow cytometry complemented by enhanced separation of RBCs using signal amplification, histograms are created which visually represent distinct cell populations. In this way, the blood of one individual athlete may be discriminated from that of a donor.[223,238] Transplantation, transfusion, or a rare event in which an individual known as a chimera has a mixed red blood cell population are reported reasons for the presence of mixed populations of RBCs not due to doping; additionally, RBC agglutination may make interpretation of histograms uncertain. [87]

STIMULANTS

CAFFEINE

Caffeine is a CNS stimulant that causes a feeling of decreased fatigue and increases endurance performance[68,170] (Chap. 65). These changes may occur through several different mechanisms, including increased calcium permeability in the sarcoplasmic reticulum and enhanced contractility of muscle, phosphodiesterase inhibition and subsequent increased cyclic nucleotides, adenosine blockade leading to blood vessel dilation, and inhibited lipolysis. Caffeine is no longer on the 2008 WADA Prohibited List.[247]

AMPHETAMINES

The beneficial effects of amphetamines in sports result from their ability to mask fatigue and pain.[55] Initial studies of soldiers showed they could march longer and ignore pain when they took amphetamines.[228] In one study of college students, resting and maximal heart rates, strength, acceleration, and anaerobic capacity increased. However, although the perception of fatigue decreased, lactic acid continued to accumulate and maximal oxygen consumption was unchanged.[40] Other studies have shown no significant effects on exercise performance[120] (Chap. 75).

SODIUM BICARBONATE

Sodium bicarbonate loading, known as *soda loading,* has a long history of use in horse racing.[17] Sodium bicarbonate may buffer the lactic acidosis caused by exercise, thereby delaying fatigue and enhancing performance.[88]

During high-intensity exercise, metabolism becomes anaerobic and lactic acid is produced. Intracellular acidosis is said to contribute to muscle fatigue by reducing the sensitivity of the muscle contractile apparatus to calcium.[172] Several studies demonstrated improved running performance when sodium bicarbonate was ingested 2–3 hours before competition.[46,193] The study dose was 0.2–0.3 g/kg body weight of sodium bicarbonate, approximately 160 mEq $NaHCO_3$ per day. The effects of sodium bicarbonate are greatest when periods of exercise last longer than 4 minutes because anaerobic metabolism contributes more to total energy production and energy from aerobic metabolism diminishes.[86,88] Adverse effects of bicarbonate loading include diarrhea, abdominal pain, and possible hypernatremia.[86]

An animal model demonstrated that intracellular acidosis, occurring as a consequence of lactate production, reversed muscle fatigue.[4,172] Previously, intracellular acidosis was thought to contribute to muscle fatigue by reducing the sensitivity of the muscle contractile apparatus to calcium, decreasing the force of muscle contraction. However, the mechanism of excitation–contraction is complex. Because it permeates membranes easily, chloride is an ion important for maintaining and stabilizing the muscle fiber resting membrane potential at normal pH. Because of this characteristic, a large sodium current is needed to overcome membrane stabilization and produce an action potential. In intracellular acidosis, membrane permeability to the chloride ion is reduced, the resting membrane potential is no longer stabilized, and less inward sodium influx is needed to produce an action potential. The excitability of the muscle T-tubule system is therefore increased by acidosis, protecting against muscle fatigue.[172]

DIURETICS

The World Anti-Doping Agency bans nonmedical diuretic use.[247] Diuretics are used in sports in which the athlete must achieve a certain weight to compete in discrete weight classes. In addition to weight loss, body builders find that diuretic use gives greater definition to the physique as the skin draws tightly around the muscles.[2] In one report a professional body builder attempted to lose weight using diuretics including bumetanide and spironolactone, and potassium supplements. He presented with hyperkalemia and hypotension[2] (Chap. 62). Diuretics also result in increased urine production, thereby diluting the urine and making more difficult the detection of other banned xenobiotics.[35,56]

MISCELLANEOUS XENOBIOTICS

CHROMIUM PICOLINATE

Chromium acts as a cofactor to enhance the action of insulin.[96] It is found naturally in meats, grains, raisins, apples, and mushrooms.[218] It is sold as chromium picolinate because picolinic acid is thought to enhance chromium absorption.[218] In people who are chromium deficient, chromium supplementation results in increased glycogen synthesis and glucose tolerance. Studies have not shown an increase in strength or a change in body composition or glucose metabolism when chromium is administered in a controlled fashion.[6,52] Anemia may result from chromium picolinate doses greater than 200 μg/d.[47] A 24-year-old body builder developed rhabdomyolysis after ingesting 1200 μg chromium picolinate, 6–24 times the daily recommended dose of 50–200 μg, over 48 hours.[150] Renal failure developed in one patient who took chromium picolinate 600 mcg/d for 6 weeks for weight reduction, which is 12–45 times the usual intake of dietary chromium and 3 times the recommended supplementation dose.[242] Another individual who took 1200–2400 μg/d chromium picolinate for the previous 4–5 months for weight loss presented with renal failure, liver dysfunction, anemia, thrombocytopenia, and hemolysis. Serum chromium concentrations were 2–3 times normal (Chap. 91). Other causes of the abnormalities were excluded, and laboratory parameters improved with cessation of chromium ingestion.[38]

LABORATORY DETECTION

Enormous amounts of energy and money are expended to determine the presence or absence of performance-enhancing substances. Analysis of samples on the international level is performed by a limited number of accredited laboratories. The majority of tests are performed on urine, with careful procedural requirements regarding handling of samples. Attention must be paid to proper storage of specimens, because bacterial metabolism may increase urinary steroid concentrations.[26,60] Upon the sample's arrival at the testing laboratory, the integrity of the sample is checked, including the code, seal, visual appearance, density, and pH. Registration of the sample is completed, and the sample is divided into two aliquots. All testing is done on the first aliquot, and any positive results are confirmed on the second aliquot. The aliquots are commonly referred to as sample A and sample B. Sample preparation is difficult and time consuming.

The complexity of the laboratory testing and continuous attempts to evade detection is illustrated in the discovery of an AAS previously undetectable by standard sport doping tests of urine. In the following situation, there was no preexisting reference data for the unknown xenobiotic. In the summer of 2003, a used syringe was provided anonymously to the United States antidoping authority. Through a painstaking process of analyses, an impurity in the substance in the syringe was identified as a derivative of the AAS norbolethone, a known reference compound, leading to the discovery, synthesis, and detection of tetrahydrogestrinone (THG), a new chemical previously unknown as a pharmaceutical or veterinary compound.[37] Since the discovery of THG, the identity of another designer steroid, madol, or desoxymethyltestosterone (DMT) was similarly discovered and the structure synthesized. [207]

CAPILLARY GAS CHROMATOGRAPHY/ MASS SPECTROMETRY

Capillary gas chromatography allows the determination of approximately 95% of all doping positive results. Gas chromatography typically is combined with mass spectrometry for detection of the majority of substances.[161] Analysis of the urine by gas chromatography-mass spectrophotometry (GC-MS) is the current standard for detection of anabolic androgenic steroids.[35] Such analysis relies on a large amount of previously derived reference data.[37]

TESTOSTERONE-TO-EPITESTOSTERONE (T/E) RATIO

Gas chromatography-mass spectrophotometry cannot distinguish endogenous testosterone from pharmaceutically derived exogenous testosterone. Therefore, other methods of detection are needed. One way of detecting the use of exogenous testosterone is to measure the ratio of testosterone to epitestosterone (T/E). Epitestosterone is not a metabolite of testosterone, but its 17-α epimer, differing from testosterone only in the configuration of the hydroxyl group on C-17. Men produce 30 times more testosterone than epitestosterone; however, 1% of testosterone and 30% of epitestosterone is excreted unchanged in the urine. Therefore, the normal T/E ratio in the urine is about 1:1.[216] A T/E ratio less than 4:1 is considered acceptable; a T/E ratio >greater than 4:1 is considered evidence of doping using testosterone. In order to maintain a normal T/E ratio, an athlete may self-administer both testosterone and epitestosterone.[36]

The overall pattern of the T/E ratio over time is important. Athletes subjected to testing will have previous measurements of their T/E ratios on record with antidoping authorities, or additional tests may be obtained to establish a pattern of T/E ratios. These results are plotted against time. The mean, standard deviation, and confidence values are calculated.[36] The confidence values of three or more samples taken over months will be less than 60% unless the athlete is using testosterone.[36] Sudden variations in an athlete's pattern of T/E ratios over time is a cause for further testing.

In one high-profile doping case where the T/E ratio was elevated, the athlete suggested that ethanol consumption the previous night had caused the elevated T/E ratio. In this regard, there is evidence that at very high doses, for example, 2 g/kg, ethanol increases the T/E ratio, although the T/E ratio did not exceed 6:1.[72] This effect of ethanol is more pronounced in females and is limited to 8 hours postingestion of ethanol. The mechanism of this effect of ethanol may be that it increases the NADH to NAD^+ ratio and many steroid oxidation–reduction reactions are dependent on the relative abundance of NADH to NAD^+.[72] Ketoconazole inhibits testosterone synthesis and may cause a decrease in the T/E ratio within 6 hours of administration.[125]

ISOTOPE RATIO MASS SPECTROMETRY (IRMS)

Carbon is made up of six protons and six neutrons, giving it an atomic weight of 12 (^{12}C). Sometimes carbon has an extra neutron, giving it an atomic weight of 13 (^{13}C). Carbon is derived from carbon dioxide in the atmosphere. Warm-climate plants, such as soy, process carbon dioxide differently than other plants, using different photosynthetic pathways for carbon dioxide fixation, causing the depletion of ^{13}C.[198] Pharmaceutical testosterone is made from plant sterols, primarily soy plants, and therefore has less ^{13}C isotope than endogenous testosterone, made in the body from a typical human diet based in corn and not soy. This difference in isotope ratios is measured by IRMS. An athletes' natural carbon makeup is determined by analysis of an endogenous reference compound such as the testosterone precursor cholesterol. Cholesterol may be called an "autostandard" because it represents the athlete's $^{13}C/^{12}C$ ratio.[21] Finally, it is the difference between the ratio of the athlete's $^{13}C/^{12}C$ ratio and an international standard ratio that is measured and reported.[1] Values are negative because both endogenous and pharmaceutical testosterone contain less ^{13}C than the international standard. [98]

GROWTH HORMONE

Growth hormone testing is plagued by the difficulties inherent in testing for exogenous peptide doping in general; the identical amino acid sequences of both rhGH and hGH; and the fluctuating, pulsatile secretion, short half-life, and variation in normal level depending on sleep, stress, and exercise status, to name a few. Unlike the ability to use the differing pattern of *N*-linked glycosylation in hEPO produced in the human kidney to distinguish it from rhEPO produced in the hamster, hGH has no *N*-linked glycosylation sites.

There are currently two approaches to detection of hGH; the marker approach and the isoform approach.[107] The marker approach uses an immunoassay to measure growth hormone–dependent factors through which growth hormone exerts its effect, such as insulin-like growth factor 1 (IGF-1) and insulin-like growth factor binding proteins (IGFBP), and other markers of bone growth and turnover, such as the N-terminal extension peptide of procollagen type III (PIIIP).[25,180] The isoform approach refers to the measurement of the various forms of growth hormone. Recombinant hGH is primarily a 22-kDa monomeric form; pituitary hGH contains multiple isoforms. In athletes using rhGH, endogenous hGH with its multiple isoforms is suppressed through negative feedback on the pituitary. Therefore, the 22-kDa form characteristic of rhGH becomes predominant. The ratio of isoforms changes, as measured by immunoassay.

ERYTHROPOIETIN

Erythropoietin is directly measured by a monoclonal anti-EPO antibody test, which does not distinguish between endogenously produced and exogenously administered recombinant EPO. Therefore, indirect methods of EPO detection are used, such as measurement of hemoglobin or hematocrit.

Previously, some sports-governing bodies, such as the International Cycling Federation and the International Skiing Federation, selected a hematocrit of 50% in men and 47% in women as the action level above which an athlete may be disqualified for presumed EPO use. However, normal hematocrit values vary greatly among athletes. Several studies have shown that hematocrits above the action values of 50% in men and 47% in women are common in athletes. From 3% to 6% of athletes who did not use EPO had hematocrits greater than 50%.[237] Of those athletes living and training at altitudes between 2000 m and 3000 m above sea level, 20.5% had hematocrit values greater than 50%.[237] Other studies confirm the increased hematocrits of athletes training at altitudes from 1000 m to 6000 m.[20,199,200,237]

Although many endurance athletes may have increased blood volume, the hematocrit may be lowered because of the increased plasma volume, which exceeds the RBC volume. This dilutional pseudoanemia is sometimes called *sports anemia.*[208] Additionally, hematocrit measurements are affected by hydration status, upright versus supine posture, and nutrition, and they demonstrate an approximately 3% diurnal variation.[201] Because of natural variations among individuals, postural effects, and the ease of manipulation through saline infusion, indirect detection of EPO use by hematocrit measurement is fraught with potential for error.[168]

Several methods have been studied to detect the use of recombinant EPO by athletes. The ratio between serum soluble transferrin receptors (sTfr) and ferritin was used as an indirect method for detection of EPO use. Soluble transferrin receptor is released from RBC progenitors. EPO stimulates erythropoiesis and causes an increase in sTfr and a decrease in ferritin.[83] Individuals with other causes of polycythemia or accelerated erythropoiesis also can exhibit increased ratios and be falsely accused of EPO use. An increased hematocrit with sTfr greater than 10 μg/mL and sTfr-to-serum protein ratio greater than 153 has been proposed as an indirect measurement of EPO use.[13]

At the 2000 Olympics in Sydney, Australia, a combination of multiple indirect markers was developed for detection of altered erythropoiesis of rhEPO use.[168] Current EPO use, known as the "ON-model," and recent, but not current, use of EPO, known as the "OFF-model," were identified by measured laboratory values. For example, five variables predict current rhEPO use: reticulocyte count, serum EPO concentration, sTfr, hematocrit, and percentage of macrocytes. The three-variable combination of hematocrit, reticulocyte count, and serum EPO concentration was the best mechanism for detecting recent rhEPO use.[168] A major drawback to this method is the instability of these variables in whole blood so that confirmatory testing of the split blood sample is impossible.[169]

State-of-the-art detection of EPO doping is accomplished with isoelectric focusing and immunoblotting performed on urine samples. The two isoforms of EPO, recombinant and endogenous, have different glycosylation patterns and glycan sizes resulting in differing molecular charges.[169] An immunoblotting procedure takes advantage of these different net charges, and the proteins can be separated by their charges when they are placed in an electric field.[135] Subsequently, isoelectric focusing obtains an image of EPO patterns in the urine.[134] WADA considers a positive urine test result definitive using this method, even without the blood testing of indirect markers.[169] Because of darbopoietin's structural similarity to EPO, these detection techniques also are effective for darbopoietin.[169]

INSULIN

Insulin laboratory detection methods are not yet standardized and accredited by WADA; therefore, athletes are not currently tested for insulin use. The technology for testing for insulin uses immunoaffinity purification followed by liquid chromatography-tandem mass spectrometry to identify analytes including urinary metabolites of insulin.[224] When insulin is modified to improve its receptor selectivity or give it other favorable properties, the change in molecular weight or amino acid profile from human insulin makes it detectable by GCMS.[224]

MASKING XENOBIOTICS

Any chemical or physical manipulation done with the purpose of altering the integrity of a urine or blood sample is prohibited by WADA.[247] For example, use of intravenous fluids for dilution of the sample, or urine substitution, is prohibited. Some agents are added to the urine available for the sole purpose of interfering with urine testing and are easily detected. Examples include Klear, which is 90% methanol, and Golden Seal tea, which produces colored urine.[30] Other commercially available products include Xxtra Clean, which contains pyridinium chlorochromate, and Urine Luck, which contains glutaraldehyde.

Niacin has been used to alter urine test results, although there is no evidence it is effective for this purpose. There are reports of niacin toxicity, including skin reactions such as itching, flushing, and burning, when niacin is used for this purpose.[8,156] More serious symptoms including nausea, elevated liver enzymes, hypoglycemia, and anion gap acidosis are reported as a result of ingesting niacin in large amounts, such as 2.5–5.5 grams over 1–2 days.[8,156]

A significant issue in the analysis of urine for the presence of prohibited peptides such as rhEPO is the masking potential of proteases surreptitiously added to urine specimens slated for doping analysis. The proteases are packaged in grains known as protease granules or "rice grains" and placed in the urethra.[223] Upon urination for the purpose of providing a specimen for doping analysis, the grain flows with urine into the specimen cup. The proteases, including trypsin, chymotrypsin, and papain, will quickly degrade renally excreted peptides, most notably erythropoietin, making them undetectable. By the process of autolysis, proteases may themselves become undetectable over time. In one report, urine with elevated protease concentrations greater than 15 μg/mL underwent further analysis to identify normal urinary proteins such as albumin.[223] Normally, the presence of urinary proteins creates the image of a visible band by gel electrophoresis. However, the urine with elevated protease activity may demonstrate something called *trace of burning*, a term used to describe the appearance of a blank lane with no bands, indicating an absence of proteins.[222] In this report, suspicious specimens were subjected to further testing using liquid chromatography–mass spectrometry (LC-MS). After further molecular sequencing of derived proteins, human proteases can be distinguished from nonhuman proteases, such as bovine chymotrypsin or papain. The addition of a protease inhibitor to urine samples immediately after collection may be a future strategy to control the effectiveness of protease addition as a masking method.[222]

Although a small amount of hEPO is most commonly found in urine, in approximately 15% of urine specimens, hEPO is undetectable. This is due in part to circumstances unrelated to doping, such as physiological variation in EPO production and very low or very high urine-specific gravity. However, doping with exogenous rEPO and inhibition of endogenous hEPO production is another possible cause. In any case, a urine deemed as suspicious based on low urinary proteins or the absence of hEPO may ultimately not result in a positive doping test result.[131,223]

The list of prohibited masking agents includes diuretics, epitestosterone, probenecid, plasma expanders such as albumin, dextran, and hydroxymethyl starch, and α-reductase inhibitors such as finasteride and dutasteride.[247] Probenecid blocks urinary excretion of the glucuronide conjugates of AAS.

GENE DOPING

The discovery of the genetic codes for some diseases has made gene therapy of medical conditions, such as muscular dystrophy, a reality. It is now conceivable that this technology can be used to enhance athletic performance. Gene doping is included on the WADA 2008 Prohibited List. Gene doping is defined as "the non-therapeutic use of cells, genes, genetic elements, or of the modulation of gene expression, having the capacity to enhance athlete performance."[247] For example, insertion of a gene sequence could produce a desired effect, such as large muscles or increased body production of potentially advantageous substances such as testosterone or growth hormone. In animal models, genes for EPO lead to erythropoiesis, and genes for IGF-1 produce increased muscle size and strength.[19] Myostatin, which belongs to a family of proteins that control growth and differentiation of tissues in the body, inhibits skeletal muscle growth.[115,202] Mutations of the myostatin gene may result in muscle hypertrophy. In dogs, the athletic performance of racing whippets is enhanced in those animals with a myostatin gene mutation.[160] In humans, a report of an extremely muscular baby born with a mutation in the myostatin gene illustrates the potential effect of gene alterations on athletic performance. The mother of this infant was a professional athlete, and other members of the family were known for their strength.[202] Monoclonal antibodies capable of inhibiting myostatin gene activity may be useful in the treatment of muscular dystrophy. Several studies associate an increased frequency of polymorphism in the angiotensin-converting enzyme (ACE) gene, particularly the insertion (I-allele) of a 287 base-pair sequence, with increased endurance and power in athletes and high-altitude mountaineers.[85,226] The increased frequency of a single nucleotide change in the α actinin 3 (ACTN3) gene encoding for fast-twitch myofibrils in skeletal muscle is found in Greek Olympic-level power-oriented track and field athletes.[166,249]

Gene doping requires the transfer of genetic material into the athlete by the use of a vector. These vectors include viruses or nonviral synthetic vectors, known as *plasmids*.[229] Plasmid DNA vectors are grown alongside other proteins in bacterial cultures and later purified of contaminants. Gene transfer may take place outside of the body by taking cells from the individual, subsequently genetically altering the cells in culture, and then returning the altered cells to the individual.[243] This is known as *ex vivo* gene transfer and it is the basis of therapy for certain diseases, such as severe combined immunodeficiency.[95] In vivo gene transfer directly delivers the genetic information into the body using a vector. One of the difficulties in applying gene doping has been the dose of vector particles required to treat a human currently exceeds the production capacity of most laboratories. Other limitations to the practical application of gene doping in athletes include the risks of the vectors themselves, the uncontrolled expression of genes, the activation of the immune response to vectors, oncogenesis, and the adverse effects associated with the end product.[243] An example of the latter is the description of autoimmune anemia in macaques genetically altered to increased erythropoietin production.

SUMMARY

Although the press spotlights a few world-class athletes, the vast majority of individuals using performance-enhancing substances are not in the public view. Some individuals suffer adverse consequences. The knowledgeable clinician will identify these health effects when they occur and educate susceptible individuals on the risks of using performance-enhancing substances.

REFERENCES

1. Aguilera R, Becchi M, Casabianca H, et al. Improved method of detection of testosterone abuse by gas chromatography/combustion/isotope ratio mass spectrometry analysis of urinary steroids. *J Mass Spectrom.* 1996;31:169-176.
2. al-Zaki T, Taibot-Stern J. A bodybuilder with diuretic abuse presenting with symptomatic hypotension and hyperkalemia. *Am J Emerg Med.* 1996;14:96-98.
3. Alen M, Reinila M, Vihko R. Response of serum hormones to androgen administration in power athletes. *Med Sci Sports Exerc.* 1985;17:354-359.
4. Allen D, Westerblad H. Physiology. Lactic acid—the latest performance-enhancing drug. *Science.* 2004;305:1112-1113.
5. American College of Sports Medicine. The use of anabolic-androgenic steroids in sports. *Med Sci Sports Exerc.* 1987;19:534-539.
6. Anderson RA, Bryden NA, Polansky MM, et al. Exercise effects on chromium excretion of trained and untrained men consuming a constant diet. *J Appl Physiol.* 1988;64:249-252.
7. Anonymous. Muscling in on clenbuterol. *Lancet.* 1992;340:403.
8. Anonymous. Use of niacin in attempts to defeat urine drug testing—five states, January-September 2006. *MMWR Morb Mortal Wkly Rep.* 2007;56:365-366.
9. Appleby M, Fisher M, Martin M. Myocardial infarction, hyperkalaemia and ventricular tachycardia in a young male body-builder. *Int J Cardiol.* 1994;44:171-174.
10. Archer MC, Clark SD, Thilly JE, et al. Environmental nitroso compounds: reaction of nitrite with creatine and creatinine. *Science.* 1971;174:1341-1343.
11. Archer MC. Use of oral creatine to enhance athletic performance and its potential side effects. *Clin J Sport Med.* 1999;9:119.
12. Arlt W, Callies F, van Vlijmen JC, et al. Dehydroepiandrosterone replacement in women with adrenal insufficiency. *N Engl J Med.* 1999;341:1013-1020.
13. Audran M, Gareau R, Matecki S, et al. Effects of erythropoietin administration in training athletes and possible indirect detection in doping control. *Med Sci Sports Exerc.* 1999;31:639-645.
14. Bagatell CJ, Bremner WJ. Androgens in men—uses and abuses. *N Engl J Med.* 1996;334:707-714.
15. Bagheri SA, Boyer JL. Peliosis hepatis associated with androgenic-anabolic steroid therapy. A severe form of hepatic injury. *Ann Intern Med.* 1974;81:610-618.
16. Balsom PD, Soderlund K, Ekblom B. Creatine in humans with special reference to creatine supplementation. *Sports Med.* 1994;18:268-280.
17. Ban BD. Sodium bicarbonate: speed catalyst or just plain baking soda. *J Am Vet Med Assoc.* 1994;204:1300-1302.
18. Barker S. Oxymethalone and aggression. *Br J Psychiatry.* 1987;151:564.
19. Barton-Davis ER, Shoturma DI, Musaro A, et al. Viral mediated expression of insulin-like growth factor I blocks the aging-related loss of skeletal muscle function. *Proc Natl Acad Sci U S A.* 1998;95:15603-15607.
20. Beard JL, Haas JD, Tufts D, et al. Iron deficiency anemia and steady-state work performance at high altitude. *J Appl Physiol.* 1988;64:1878-1884.
21. Becchi M, Aguilera R, Farizon Y, et al. Gas chromatography/combustion/isotope-ratio mass spectrometry analysis of urinary steroids to detect misuse of testosterone in sport. *Rapid Commun Mass Spectrom.* 1994;8:304-308.
22. Berglund B, Hemmingson P. Effect of reinfusion of autologous blood on exercise performance in cross-country skiers. *Int J Sports Med.* 1987;8:231-233.
23. Berglund B, Ekblom B. Effect of recombinant human erythropoietin treatment on blood pressure and some haematological parameters in healthy men. *J Intern Med.* 1991;229:125-130.
24. Bhasin S, Storer TW, Berman N, et al. The effects of supraphysiologic doses of testosterone on muscle size and strength in normal men. *N Engl J Med.* 1996;335:1-7.
25. Bidlingmaier M, Strasburger CJ. Technology insight: detecting growth hormone abuse in athletes. *Nat Clin Pract Endocrinol Metab.* 2007;3:769-777.
26. Bilton RF. Microbial production of testosterone. *Lancet.* 1995;345:1186-1187.
27. Birch R, Noble D, Greenhaff PL. The influence of dietary creatine supplementation on performance during repeated bouts of maximal isokinetic cycling in man. *Eur J Appl Physiol Occup Physiol.* 1994;69:268-276.
28. Bochnia M, Medras M, Pospiech L, et al. Poststeroid balance disorder—a case report in a body builder. *Int J Sports Med.* 1999;20:407-409.
29. Borer KT. The effects of exercise on growth. *Sports Med.* 1995;20:375-397.
30. Bowers LD. Athletic drug testing. *Clin Sports Med.* 1998;17:299-318.

31. Brien AJ, Simon TL. The effects of red blood cell infusion on 10-km race time. *JAMA*. 1987;257:2761-2765.
32. Brown KR, Carter W, Jr., Lombardi GE. Recombinant erythropoietin overdose. *Am J Emerg Med*. 1993;11:619-621.
33. Bryden AA, Rothwell PJ, O'Reilly PH. Anabolic steroid abuse and renal-cell carcinoma. *Lancet*. 1995;346:1306-1307.
34. Casey A, Constantin-Teodosiu D, Howell S, et al. Creatine ingestion favorably affects performance and muscle metabolism during maximal exercise in humans. *Am J Physiol*. 1996;271:E31-37.
35. Catlin DH, Cowan D, Donike M, et al. Testing urine for drugs. *Ann Biol Clin (Paris)*. 1992;50:359-366.
36. Catlin DH, Hatton CK, Starcevic SH. Issues in detecting abuse of xenobiotic anabolic steroids and testosterone by analysis of athletes' urine. *Clin Chem*. 1997;43:1280-1288.
37. Catlin DH, Sekera MH, Ahrens BD, et al. Tetrahydrogestrinone: discovery, synthesis, and detection in urine. *Rapid Commun Mass Spectrom*. 2004;18:1245-1049.
38. Cerulli J, Grabe DW, Gauthier I, et al. Chromium picolinate toxicity. *Ann Pharmacother*. 1998;32:428-431.
39. Chan JM, Stampfer MJ, Giovannucci E, et al. Plasma insulin-like growth factor-I and prostate cancer risk: a prospective study. *Science*. 1998;279: 563-566.
40. Chandler JV, Blair SN. The effect of amphetamines on selected physiological components related to athletic success. *Med Sci Sports Exerc*. 1980;12:65-69.
41. Chodorowski Z, Sein Anand J. Acute poisoning with clenbuterol—a case report. *Przegl Lek*. 1997;54:763-764.
42. Choo JJ, Horan MA, Little RA, et al. Anabolic effects of clenbuterol on skeletal muscle are mediated by beta 2-adrenoceptor activation. *Am J Physiol*. 1992;263:E50-56.
43. Clark LC, Jr., Gollan F. Survival of mammals breathing organic liquids equilibrated with oxygen at atmospheric pressure. *Science*. 1966;152: 1755-1756.
44. Collins P, Cotterill JA. Gymnasium acne. *Clin Exp Dermatol*. 1995;20:509.
45. Corrigan B, Kazlauskas R. Medication use in athletes selected for doping control at the Sydney Olympics (2000). *Clin J Sport Med*. 2003;13:33-40.
46. Costill DL, Verstappen F, Kuipers H, et al. Acid-base balance during repeated bouts of exercise: influence of HCO_3. *Int J Sports Med*. 1984;5:228-231.
47. Cowart VS. Dietary supplements: alternatives to anabolic steroids? *Physician Sports Med*. 1992;20:189-198.
48. Crist DM, Peake GT, Egan PA, et al. Body composition response to exogenous GH during training in highly conditioned adults. *J Appl Physiol*. 1988;65:579-584.
49. Cuneo RC, Salomon F, Wiles CM, et al. Growth hormone treatment in growth hormone-deficient adults. I. Effects on muscle mass and strength. *J Appl Physiol*. 1991;70:688-694.
50. Cuttler L. The regulation of growth hormone secretion. *Endocrinol Metab Clin North Am*. 1996;25:541-571.
51. Daubert GP, Mabasa VH, Leung VW, et al. Acute clenbuterol overdose resulting in supraventricular tachycardia and atrial fibrillation. *J Med Toxicol*. 2007;3:56-60.
52. Davis JM, Welsh RS, Alerson NA. Effects of carbohydrate and chromium ingestion during intermittent high-intensity exercise to fatigue. *Int J Sport Nutr Exerc Metab*. 2000;10:476-485.
53. Dawson RT, Harrison MW. Use of insulin as an anabolic agent. Br J Sports *Med*. 1997;31:259.
54. De Piccoli B, Giada F, Benettin A, et al. Anabolic steroid use in body builders: an echocardiographic study of left ventricle morphology and function. *Int J Sports Med*. 1991;12:408-412.
55. Dekhuijzen PN, Machiels HA, Heunks LM, et al. Athletes and doping: effects of drugs on the respiratory system. *Thorax*. 1999;54:1041-1046.
56. Delbeke FT, Debackere M. The influence of diuretics on the excretion and metabolism of doping agents—V. Dimefline. *J Pharm Biomed Anal*. 1991;9:23-28.
57. Delbeke FT, Van Eenoo P, De Backer P. Detection of human chorionic gonadotrophin misuse in sports. *Int J Sports Med*. 1998;19:287-290.
58. Deyssig R, Frisch H. Self-administration of cadaveric growth hormone in power athletes. *Lancet*. 1993;341:768-769.
59. Dickerman RD, McConathy WJ, Schaller F, et al. Cardiovascular complications and anabolic steroids. *Eur Heart J*. 1996;17:1912.
60. Donike M, Geyer H, Gotzman A. Recent advances in doping analysis Köln: Sport Buch Strauβ; 1996.
61. Dou P, Liu Z, He J, et al. Rapid and high-resolution glycoform profiling of recombinant human erythropoietin by capillary isoelectric focusing with whole column imaging detection. *J Chromatogr A*. 2008;1190:372-376.
62. DuRant RH, Rickert VI, Ashworth CS, et al. Use of multiple drugs among adolescents who use anabolic steroids. *N Engl J Med*. 1993;328:922-926.
63. Eicher ER. Better dead than second. *J Lab Clin Med*. 1992;120:359-360.
64. Ekblom B, Goldbarg AN, Gullbring B. Response to exercise after blood loss and reinfusion. *J Appl Physiol*.1972;33:175-180.
65. Ekblom B, Berglund B. Effect of erythropoietin administration on maximal aerobic power. *Scand J Med Sci Sports*. 1991;1:88-93.
66. Elkin SL, Brady S, Williams IP. Bodybuilders find it easy to obtain insulin to help them in training. *Br Med J*. 1997;314:1280.
67. Escher S, Maierhofer WJ. Erythropoietin and endurance. *Your Patient Fitness*. 1992:15.
68. Essig D, Costill DL, Van Handel PJ. Effects of caffeine ingestion on utilization of muscle glycogen and lipid during leg ergometer cycling. *Int J Sports Med*. 1980;1:86-90.
69. Evans NA. Gym and tonic: a profile of 100 male steroid users. *Br J Sports Med*. 1997;31:54-58.
70. Evans NA. Local complications of self administered anabolic steroid injections. *Br J Sports Med*. 1997;31:349-350.
71. Falk H, Thomas LB, Popper H, et al. Hepatic angiosarcoma associated with androgenic-anabolic steroids. *Lancet*. 1979;2:1120-1123.
72. Falk O, Palonek E, Bjorkhem I. Effect of ethanol on the ratio between testosterone and epitestosterone in urine. *Clin Chem*. 1988;34:1462-1464.
73. Ferenchick G, Schwartz D, Ball M, et al. Androgenic-anabolic steroid abuse and platelet aggregation: a pilot study in weight lifters. *Am J Med Sci*. 1992;303:78-82.
74. Franke WW, Berendonk B. Hormonal doping and androgenization of athletes: a secret program of the German Democratic Republic government. *Clin Chem*. 1997;43:1262-1279.
75. Franklin B. The tragic death of Korey Stringer: preventing preseason football fatalities. *Am J Med Sports*. 2001;29:267-268.
76. Freeman BJ, Rooker GD. Spontaneous rupture of the anterior cruciate ligament after anabolic steroids. *Br J Sports Med*. 1995;29:274-275.
77. Freidl KE, Moore RJ. Clenbuterol, ma huang, caffeine, L-carnitine, and growth hormone releasers. *Natl Strength Condition Assoc*. 1992:35.
78. Fried W, Johnson C, Heller P. Observations on regulation of erythropoiesis during prolonged periods of hypoxia. *Blood*. 1970;36:607-616.
79. Friedman G, Lamoureux E, Sherker AH. Fatal fulminant hepatic failure due to cyproterone acetate. *Dig Dis Sci*. 1999;44:1362-1363.
80. Froehner M, Fischer R, Leike S, et al. Intratesticular leiomyosarcoma in a young man after high dose doping with Oral-Turinabol: a case report. *Cancer*. 1999;86:1571-1575.
81. Gaede JT, Montine TJ. Massive pulmonary embolus and anabolic steroid abuse. *JAMA*. 1992;267:2328-2329.
82. Gao W, Dalton JT. Ockham's razor and selective androgen receptor modulators (SARMs): are we overlooking the role of 5α-reductase? *Mol Interv*. 2007;7:10-13.
83. Gareau R, Gagnon MG, Thellend C, et al. Transferrin soluble receptor: a possible probe for detection of erythropoietin abuse by athletes. *Horm Metab Res*. 1994;26:311-312.
84. Garty BZ, Dinari G, Gellvan A, et al. Cirrhosis in a child with hypothalamic syndrome and central precocious puberty treated with cyproterone acetate. *Eur J Pediatr*. 1999;158:367-370.
85. Gayagay G, Yu B, Hambly B, et al. Elite endurance athletes and the ACE I allele—the role of genes in athletic performance. *Hum Genet*. 1998;103:48-50.
86. Ghaphery NA. Performance-enhancing drugs. *Orthop Clin North Am*. 1995;26:433-442.
87. Giraud S, Robinson N, Mangin P, et al. Scientific and forensic standards for homologous blood transfusion anti-doping analyses. *Forensic Sci Int*. 2008;179:23-33.
88. Gledhill N. Bicarbonate ingestion and anaerobic performance. *Sports Med*. 1984;1:177-180.
89. Gnarpe H, Gnarpe J. Increasing prevalence of specific antibodies to *Chlamydia pneumoniae* in Sweden. *Lancet*. 1993;341:381.
90. Goldberg M. Dehydroepiandrosterone, insulin-like growth factor-I, and prostate cancer. *Ann Intern Med*. 1998;129:587-588.
91. Goldman B. Liver carcinoma in an athlete taking anabolic steroids. *J Am Osteopath Assoc*. 1985;85:56.
92. Goodnough LT, Scott MG, Monk TG. Oxygen carriers as blood substitutes. Past, present, and future. *Clin Orthop*. 1998:89-100.

93. Graham MR, Baker JS, Evans P, et al. Physical effects of short-term recombinant human growth hormone administration in abstinent steroid dependency. *Horm Res.* 2008;69:343-354.
94. Green AL, Hultman E, Macdonald IA, et al. Carbohydrate ingestion augments skeletal muscle creatine accumulation during creatine supplementation in humans. *Am J Physiol.* 1996;271:E821-826.
95. Hacein-Bey-Abina S, Le Deist F, Carlier F, et al. Sustained correction of X-linked severe combined immunodeficiency by ex vivo gene therapy. *N Engl J Med.* 2002;346:1185-1193.
96. Hallmark MA, Reynolds TH, DeSouza CA, et al. Effects of chromium and resistive training on muscle strength and body composition. *Med Sci Sports Exerc.* 1996;28:139-144.
97. Harris RC, Soderlund K, Hultman E. Elevation of creatine in resting and exercised muscle of normal subjects by creatine supplementation. *Clin Sci (Lond).* 1992;83:367-374.
98. Hatton CK. Beyond sports-doping headlines: the science of laboratory tests for performance-enhancing drugs. *Pediatr Clin North Am.* 2007;54:713-733, xi.
99. Haupt HA. Anabolic steroids and growth hormone. *Am J Sports Med.* 1993;21:468-474.
100. Hausmann R, Hammer S, Betz P. Performance enhancing drugs (doping agents) and sudden death—a case report and review of the literature. *Int J Legal Med.* 1998;111:261-264.
101. Healy ML, Russell-Jones D. Growth hormone and sport: abuse, potential benefits, and difficulties in detection. *Br J Sports Med.* 1997;31:267-268.
102. Hill JA, Suker JR, Sachs K, et al. The athletic polydrug abuse phenomenon. A case report. *Am J Sports Med.* 1983;11:269-271.
103. Hillman RS. Hematopoietic agents: growth factors, minerals and vitamins. In: Goodman LS, Hardman JG, Limbird LE, Gilman AG, eds. *Goodman & Gilman's The Pharmacological Basis of Therapeutics.* 10th ed. New York: McGraw-Hill; 2001:1487-1517.
104. Hirose H, Ohishi A, Nakamura H, et al. Fatal splenic rupture in anabolic steroid-induced peliosis in a patient with myelodysplastic syndrome. *Br J Haematol.* 1991;78:128-129.
105. Hoberman JM. *Mortal Engines: The Science of Performance and the Dehumanization of Sport.* The Free Press; 1992.
106. Hoffman RJ, Hoffman RS, Freyberg CL, et al. Clenbuterol ingestion causing prolonged tachycardia, hypokalemia, and hypophosphatemia with confirmation by quantitative levels. *J Toxicol Clin Toxicol.* 2001;39:339-344.
107. Holt RI, Sonksen PH. Growth hormone, IGF-I and insulin and their abuse in sport. *Br J Pharmacol.* 2008;154:542-556.
108. Horton R, Tait JF. Androstenedione production and interconversion rates measured in peripheral blood and studies on the possible site of its conversion to testosterone. *J Clin Invest.* 1966;45:301-313.
109. Hughes Jr GS, Yancey EP, Albrecht R, et al. Hemoglobin-based oxygen carrier preserves submaximal exercise capacity in humans. *Clin Pharmacol Ther.* 1995;58:434-443.
110. Huie MJ. An acute myocardial infarction occurring in an anabolic steroid user. *Med Sci Sports Exerc.* 1994;26:408-413.
111. Hultman E, Soderlund K, Timmons JA, et al. Muscle creatine loading in men. *J Appl Physiol.* 1996;81:232-237.
112. Ishak KG, Zimmerman HJ: Hepatotoxic effects of the anabolic/androgenic steroids. *Semin Liver Dis.* 1987;7:230-236.
113. Johnson FL, Lerner KG, Siegel M, et al. Association of androgenic-anabolic steroid therapy with development of hepatocellular carcinoma. *Lancet.* 1972;2:1273-1276.
114. Johnson MD. Anabolic steroid use in adolescent athletes. *Pediatr Clin North Am.* 1990;37:1111-1123.
115. Joulia-Ekaza D, Cabello G. The myostatin gene: physiology and pharmacological relevance. *Curr Opin Pharmacol.* 2007;7:310-315.
116. Juhn MS, Tarnopolsky M. Oral creatine supplementation and athletic performance: a critical review. *Clin J Sport Med.* 1998;8:286-297.
117. Juhn MS, O'Kane JW, Vinci DM. Oral creatine supplementation in male collegiate athletes: a survey of dosing habits and side effects. *J Am Diet Assoc.* 1999;99:593-595.
118. Karila TA, Karjalainen JE, Mantysaari MJ, et al. Anabolic androgenic steroids produce dose-dependant increase in left ventricular mass in power atheletes, and this effect is potentiated by concomitant use of growth hormone. *Int J Sports Med.* 2003;24:337-343.
119. Kark JA, Posey DM, Schumacher HR, et al. Sickle-cell trait as a risk factor for sudden death in physical training. *N Engl J Med.* 1987;317:781-787.
120. Karpovich PV. Effect of amphetamine sulfate on athletic performance. *J Am Med Assoc.* 1959;170:558-561.
121. Kashkin KB, Kleber HD. Hooked on hormones? An anabolic steroid addiction hypothesis. *JAMA.* 1989;262:3166-3170.
122. Kennedy MC. Anabolic steroid abuse and toxicology. *Aust N Z J Med.* 1992;22:374-381.
123. Kennedy MC, Corrigan AB, Pilbeam ST. Myocardial infarction and cerebral haemorrhage in a young body builder taking anabolic steroids. *Aust N Z J Med.* 1993;23:713.
124. Kicman AT, Brooks RV, Cowan DA. Human chorionic gonadotrophin and sport. *Br J Sports Med.* 1991;25:73-80.
125. Kicman AT, Oftebro H, Walker C, et al. Potential use of ketoconazole in a dynamic endocrine test to differentiate between biological outliers and testosterone use by athletes. *Clin Chem.* 1993;39:1798-1803.
126. Kinson GA, Layberry RA, Hebert B. Influences of anabolic androgens on cardiac growth and metabolism in the rat. *Can J Physiol Pharmacol.* 1991;69:1698-1704.
127. Korkia P. Use of anabolic steroids has been reported by 9% of men attending gymnasiums. *Br Med J.* 1996;313:1009.
128. Koshy KM, Griswold E, Schneeberger EE. Interstitial nephritis in a patient taking creatine. *N Engl J Med.* 1999;340:814-815.
129. Kreider RB. Effects of creatine supplementation on performance and training adaptations. *Mol Cell Biochem.* 2003;244:89-94.
130. Lage JM, Panizo C, Masdeu J, et al. Cyclist's doping associated with cerebral sinus thrombosis. *Neurology.* 2002;58:665.
131. Lamon S, Robinson N, Sottas PE, et al. Possible origins of undetectable EPO in urine samples. *Clin Chim Acta.* 2007;385:61-66.
132. Laroche GP. Steroid anabolic drugs and arterial complications in an athlete—a case history. *Angiology.* 1990;41:964-969.
133. Laseter JT, Russell JA. Anabolic steroid-induced tendon pathology: a review of the literature. *Med Sci Sports Exerc.* 1991;23:1-3.
134. Lasne F, de Ceaurriz J. Recombinant erythropoietin in urine. *Nature.* 2000;405:635.
135. Lasne F, Martin L, Crepin N, et al. Detection of isoelectric profiles of erythropoietin in urine: differentiation of natural and administered recombinant hormones. *Anal Biochem.* 2002;311:119-126.
136. Leder BZ, Longcope C, Catlin DH, et al. Oral androstenedione administration and serum testosterone concentrations in young men. *JAMA.* 2000;283:779-782.
137. Lepori M, Perren A, Gallino A. The popliteal-artery entrapment syndrome in a patient using anabolic steroids. *N Engl J Med.* 2002;346:1254-1255.
138. Liow RY, Tavares S. Bilateral rupture of the quadriceps tendon associated with anabolic steroids. *Br J Sports Med.* 1995;29:77-79.
139. Longcope C, Kato T, Horton R. Conversion of blood androgens to estrogens in normal adult men and women. *J Clin Invest.* 1969;48:2191-2201.
140. Luke JL, Farb A, Virmani R, et al. Sudden cardiac death during exercise in a weight lifter using anabolic androgenic steroids: pathological and toxicological findings. *J Forensic Sci.* 1990;35:1441-1447.
141. Macintyre JG. Growth hormone and athletes. *Sports Med.* 1987;4:129-142.
142. Madea B, Grellner W. Long-term cardiovascular effects of anabolic steroids. *Lancet.* 1998;352:33.
143. Mahesh VB, Greenblatt RB. In vivo conversion of dehydroepiandrosterone and androstenedione to testosterone in human. *Acta Endocrinol.* 1962;41:400-406.
144. Majewska MD, Demirgoren S, Spivak CE, et al. The neurosteroid dehydroepiandrosterone sulfate is an allosteric antagonist of the $GABA_A$ receptor. *Brain Res.* 1990;526:143-146.
145. Maltin CA, Delday MI, Reeds PJ. The effect of a growth promoting drug, clenbuterol, on fibre frequency and area in hind limb muscles from young male rats. *Biosci Rep.* 1986;6:293-299.
146. Maron BJ, Shirani J, Poliac LC, et al. Sudden death in young competitive athletes. Clinical, demographic, and pathological profiles. *JAMA.* 1996;276:199-204.
147. Maron BJ. Sudden death in young athletes. *N Engl J Med.* 2003;349:1064-1075.
148. Maropis C, Yesalis CE. Intramuscular abscess. Another anabolic steroid danger. *Physician Sports Med.* 1994;22:105-107.
149. Marshall A. Mystery death of orienteers. *The Independent.* November 15, 1992.
150. Martin WR, Fuller RE. Suspected chromium picolinate-induced rhabdomyolysis. *Pharmacotherapy.* 1998;18:860-862.
151. Maschio G. Erythropoietin and systemic hypertension. *Nephrol Dial Transplant.* 1995;10 Suppl 2:74-79.
152. McNaughton LR, Dalton B, Tarr J. The effects of creatine supplementation on high-intensity exercise performance in elite performers. *Eur J Appl Physiol Occup Physiol.* 1998;78:236-240.

153. McNutt RA, Ferenchick GS, Kirlin PC, et al. Acute myocardial infarction in a 22-year-old world class weight lifter using anabolic steroids. *Am J Cardiol.* 1988;62:164.
154. Melchert RB, Herron TJ, Welder AA. The effect of anabolic-androgenic steroids on primary myocardial cell cultures. *Med Sci Sports Exerc.* 1992;24:206-212.
155. Melchior CL, Ritzmann RF. Dehydroepiandrosterone is an anxiolytic in mice on the plus maze. *Pharmacol Biochem Behav.* 1994;47:437-441.
156. Mittal MK, Florin T, Perrone J, et al. Toxicity from the use of niacin to beat urine drug screening. *Ann Emerg Med.* 2007;50:587-590.
157. Mooradian AD, Morley JE, Korenman SG. Biological actions of androgens. *Endocr Rev.* 1987;8:1-28.
158. Morales AJ, Nolan JJ, Nelson JC, et al. Effects of replacement dose of dehydroepiandrosterone in men and women of advancing age. *J Clin Endocrinol Metab.* 1994;78:1360-1367.
159. Morales AJ, Haubrich RH, Hwang JY, et al. The effect of six months treatment with a 100 mg daily dose of dehydroepiandrosterone (DHEA) on circulating sex steroids, body composition and muscle strength in age-advanced men and women. *Clin Endocrinol (Oxf).* 1998;49:421-432.
160. Mosher DS, Quignon P, Bustamante CD, et al. A mutation in the myostatin gene increases muscle mass and enhances racing performance in heterozygote dogs. *PLoS Genet.* 2007;3:e79.
161. Muller RK, Grosse J, Thieme D, et al. Introduction to the application of capillary gas chromatography of performance-enhancing drugs in doping control. *J Chromatogr A.* 1999;843:275-285.
162. Natanson C, Kern SJ, Lurie P, et al. Cell-free hemoglobin-based blood substitutes and risk of myocardial infarction and death: a meta-analysis. *JAMA.* 2008;299:2304-2312.
163. Nemechek PM. Anabolic steroid users—another potential risk group for HIV infection. *N Engl J Med.* 1991;325:357.
164. Overly WL, Dankoff JA, Wang BK, et al. Androgens and hepatocellular carcinoma in an athlete. *Ann Intern Med.* 1984;100:158-159.
165. Ozcelik O, Haytac MC, Seydaoglu G. The effects of anabolic androgenic steroid abuse on gingival tissues. *J Periodontol.* 2006;77:1104-1109.
166. Papadimitriou ID, Papadopoulos C, Kouvatsi A, et al. The ACTN3 gene in elite Greek track and field athletes. *Int J Sports Med.* 2008;29:352-355.
167. Parana R, Lyra L, Trepo C. Intravenous vitamin complexes used in sporting activities and transmission of HCV in Brazil. *Am J Gastroenterol.* 1999;94:857-858.
168. Parisotto R, Gore CJ, Emslie KR, et al. A novel method utilising markers of altered erythropoiesis for the detection of recombinant human erythropoietin abuse in athletes. *Haematologica.* 2000;85:564-572.
169. Pascual JA, Belalcazar V, de Bolos C, et al. Recombinant erythropoietin and analogues: a challenge for doping control. *Ther Drug Monit.* 2004;26:175-179.
170. Pasman WJ, van Baak MA, Jeukendrup AE, et al. The effect of different dosages of caffeine on endurance performance time. *Int J Sports Med.* 1995;16:225-230.
171. Pates R, Temple D. *The Use of Anabolic Steroids in Wales.* Cardiff, Wales: Welsh Committee on Drug Misuse; 1992.
172. Pedersen TH, Nielsen OB, Lamb GD, et al. Intracellular acidosis enhances the excitability of working muscle. *Science.* 2004;305:1144-1147.
173. Pena N. Lethal injection. *Bicycling.* 1991;32:80-81.
174. Pierard GE. [Image of the month. Gymnasium acne: a fulminant doping acne.] *Rev Med Liege.* 1998;53:441-443.
175. Pierard-Franchimont C, Henry F, Crielaard JM, et al. Mechanical properties of skin in recombinant human growth factor abusers among adult bodybuilders. *Dermatology.* 1996;192:389-392.
176. Poortmans JR, Auquier H, Renaut V, et al. Effect of short-term creatine supplementation on renal responses in men. *Eur J Appl Physiol Occup Physiol.* 1997;76:566-567.
177. Poortmans JR, Francaux M. Long-term oral creatine supplementation does not impair renal function in healthy athletes. *Med Sci Sports Exerc.* 1999;31:1108-1110.
178. Pope HG, Katz DL. Affective and psychotic symptoms associated with anabolic steroid use. *Am J Psychiatry.* 1988;145:487-490.
179. Pope HG, Katz DL. Psychiatric and medical effects of anabolic-androgenic steroid use: a controlled study of 160 athletes. *Arch Gen Psychiatry.* 1994;51:375-382.
180. Powrie JK, Bassett EE, Rosen T, et al. Detection of growth hormone abuse in sport. *Growth Horm IGF Res.* 2007;17:220-226.
181. Prat J, Gray GF, Stolley PD, et al. Wilms tumor in an adult associated with androgen abuse. *JAMA.* 1977;237:2322-2323.
182. Radakovich J, Broderick P, Pickell G. Rate of anabolic-androgenic steroid use among students in junior high school. *J Am Board Fam Pract.* 1993;6:341-345.
183. Reverter JL, Tural C, Rosell A, et al. Self-induced insulin hypoglycemia in a bodybuilder. *Arch Intern Med.* 1994;154:225-226.
184. Rich JD, Dickinson BP, Merriman NA. Insulin use by bodybuilders. *JAMA.* 1998;279:1613-1614.
185. Rich JD, Dickinson BP, Merriman NA, et al. Hepatitis C virus infection related to anabolic-androgenic steroid injection in a recreational weight lifter. *Am J Gastroenterol.* 1998;93:1598.
186. Rich JD, Dickinson BP, Feller A, et al. The infectious complications of anabolic-androgenic steroid injection. *Int J Sports Med.* 1999;20:563-566.
187. Rich JD, Dickinson BP, Flanigan TP, et al. Abscess related to anabolic-androgenic steroid injection. *Med Sci Sports Exerc.* 1999;31:207-209.
188. Rickert VI, Pawlak-Morello C, Sheppard V, et al. Human growth hormone: a new substance of abuse among adolescents? *Clin Pediatr (Phila).* 1992;31:723-726.
189. Ricks CA, Dalrymple RH, Baker PK, et al. Use of a beta-agonist to alter fat and muscle deposition in steers. *J Anim Sci.* 1984;59:1247-1255.
190. Riggs BL, Hartmann LC. Selective estrogen-receptor modulators—mechanisms of action and application to clinical practice. *N Engl J Med.* 2003;348:618-629.
191. Roberts JT, Essenhigh DM. Adenocarcinoma of prostate in 40-year-old body-builder. *Lancet.* 1986;2:742.
192. Rosner F, Khan MT. Renal cell carcinoma following prolonged testosterone therapy. *Arch Intern Med.* 1992;152:426, 429.
193. Rupp JC, Bartels RL, Zuelzer W, et al. Effect of sodium-bicarbonate ingestion on blood and muscle pH and exercise performance. *Med Sci Sports Exerc.* 1983;15:115.
194. Russell-Jones DL, Umpleby M. Protein anabolic action of insulin, growth hormone and insulin-like growth factor I. *Eur J Endocrinol.* 1996;135:631-642.
195. Salleras L, Dominguez A, Mata E, et al. Epidemiologic study of an outbreak of clenbuterol poisoning in Catalonia, Spain. *Public Health Rep.* 1995;110:338-342.
196. Salmonson T, Danielson BG, Wikstrom B. The pharmacokinetics of recombinant human erythropoietin after intravenous and subcutaneous administration to healthy subjects. *Br J Clin Pharmacol.* 1990;29:709-713.
197. Salomon F, Cuneo RC, Hesp R, et al. The effects of treatment with recombinant human growth hormone on body composition and metabolism in adults with growth hormone deficiency. *N Engl J Med.* 1989;321:1797-1803.
198. Saudan C, Baume N, Robinson N, et al. Testosterone and doping control. *Br J Sports Med.* 2006;40 (Suppl 1):i21-24.
199. Schmidt W, Dahners HW, Correa R, et al. Blood gas transport properties in endurance-trained athletes living at different altitudes. *Int J Sports Med.* 1990;11:15-21.
200. Schmidt W, Spielvogel H, Eckardt KU, et al. Effects of chronic hypoxia and exercise on plasma erythropoietin in high-altitude residents. *J Appl Physiol.* 1993;74:1874-1878.
201. Schmidt W, Biermann B, Winchenbach P, et al. How valid is the determination of hematocrit values to detect blood manipulations? *Int J Sports Med.* 2000;21:133-138.
202. Schuelke M, Wagner KR, Stolz LE, et al. Myostatin mutation associated with gross muscle hypertrophy in a child. *N Engl J Med.* 2004;350:2682-2688.
203. Schumacher J, Muller G, Klotz KF. Large hepatic hematoma and intraabdominal hemorrhage associated with abuse of anabolic steroids. *N Engl J Med.* 1999;340:1123-1124.
204. Schumacher YO, Ashenden M. Doping with artificial oxygen carriers: an update. *Sports Med.* 2004;34:141-150.
205. Scott MJ, Scott MJ, Jr. HIV infection associated with injections of anabolic steroids. *JAMA.* 1989;262:207-208.
206. Scott MJ, Jr., Scott MJ, 3rd, Scott AM. Linear keloids resulting from abuse of anabolic androgenic steroid drugs. *Cutis.* 1994;53:41-43.
207. Sekera MH, Ahrens BD, Chang YC, et al. Another designer steroid: discovery, synthesis, and detection of 'madol' in urine. *Rapid Commun Mass Spectrom.* 2005;19:781-784.
208. Shaskey DJ, Green GA. Sports haematology. *Sports Med.* 2000;29:27-38.
209. Shiozawa Z, Tsunoda S, Noda A, et al. Cerebral hemorrhagic infarction associated with anabolic steroid therapy for hypoplastic anemia. *Angiology.* 1986;37:725-730.
210. Sklarek HM, Mantovani RP, Erens E, et al. AIDS in a bodybuilder using anabolic steroids. *N Engl J Med.* 1984;311:1701.

211. Smathers RL, Heiken JP, Lee JK, et al. Computed tomography of fatal hepatic rupture due to peliosis hepatis. *J Comput Assist Tomogr.* 1984;8:768-769.
212. Snow RJ, Murphy RM. Creatine and the creatine transporter: a review. *Mol Cell Biochem.* 2001;224:169-181.
213. Snow RJ, Murphy RM. Factors influencing creatine loading into human skeletal muscle. *Exerc Sport Sci Rev.* 2003;31:154-158.
214. Soe KL, Soe M, Gluud C. Liver pathology associated with the use of anabolic-androgenic steroids. *Liver.* 1992;12:73-79.
215. Speer O, Neukomm LJ, Murphy RM, et al. Creatine transporters: a reappraisal. *Mol Cell Biochem.* 2004;256-257:407-424.
216. Starka L. Epitestosterone. *J Steroid Biochem Mol Biol.* 2003;87:27-34.
217. Stohlawetz PJ, Dzirlo L, Hergovich N, et al. Effects of erythropoietin on platelet reactivity and thrombopoiesis in humans. *Blood.* 2000;95:2983-2989.
218. Stricker PR. Other ergogenic agents. *Clin Sports Med.* 1998;17:283-297.
219. Sturmi JE, Diorio DJ. Anabolic agents. *Clin Sports Med.* 1998;17:261-282.
220. Su TP, Pagliaro M, Schmidt PJ, et al. Neuropsychiatric effects of anabolic steroids in male normal volunteers. *JAMA.* 1993;269:2760-2764.
221. Takala TE, Ramo P, Kiviluoma K, et al. Effects of training and anabolic steroids on collagen synthesis in dog heart. *Eur J Appl Physiol Occup Physiol.* 1991;62:1-6.
222. Thevis M, Maurer J, Kohler M, et al. Proteases in doping control analysis. *Int J Sports Med.* 2007;28:545-549.
223. Thevis M, Kohler M, Schanzer W. New drugs and methods of doping and manipulation. *Drug Discov Today.* 2008;13:59-66.
224. Thevis M, Thomas A, Schanzer W. Mass spectrometric determination of insulins and their degradation products in sports drug testing. *Mass Spectrom Rev.* 2008;27:35-50.
225. Thissen JP, Ketelslegers JM, Underwood LE. Nutritional regulation of the insulin-like growth factors. *Endocr Rev.* 1994;15:80-101.
226. Thompson J, Raitt J, Hutchings L, et al. Angiotensin-converting enzyme genotype and successful ascent to extreme high altitude. *High Alt Med Biol.* 2007;8:278-285.
227. Tremper KK. Perfluorochemical "blood substitutes". *Anesthesiology.* 1999;91:1185-1187.
228. Tyler DB. The effect of amphetamine sulfate and some barbiturates on the fatigue produced by prolonged wakefulness. *Am J Physiol.* 1947;150: 253-262.
229. Unal M, Ozer Unal D. Gene doping in sports. *Sports Med.* 2004;34:357-362.
230. Urhausen A, Holpes R, Kindermann W. One- and two-dimensional echocardiography in bodybuilders using anabolic steroids. *Eur J Appl Physiol Occup Physiol.* 1989;58:633-640.
231. Urhausen A, Albers T, Kindermann W. Are the cardiac effects of anabolic steroid abuse in strength athletes reversible? *Heart.* 2004;90:496-501.
232. Van Camp SP, Bloor CM, Mueller FO, et al. Nontraumatic sports death in high school and college athletes. *Med Sci Sports Exerc.* 1995;27:641-647.
233. Van Eenoo P, Delbeke FT. The prevalence of doping in Flanders in comparison to the prevalence of doping in international sports. *Int J Sports Med.* 2003;24:565-570.
234. van Loon LJ, Oosterlaar AM, Hartgens F, et al. Effects of creatine loading and prolonged creatine supplementation on body composition, fuel selection, sprint and endurance performance in humans. *Clin Sci (Lond).* 2003;104:153-162.
235. Vance ML, Mauras N. Growth hormone therapy in adults and children. *N Engl J Med.* 1999;341:1206-1216.
236. Varlet-Marie E, Ashenden M, Lasne F, et al. Detection of hemoglobin-based oxygen carriers in human serum for doping analysis: confirmation by size-exclusion HPLC. *Clin Chem.* 2004;50:723-731.
237. Vergouwen PC, Collee T, Marx JJ. Haematocrit in elite athletes. *Int J Sports Med.* 1999;20:538-541.
238. Voss SC, Thevis M, Schinkothe T, et al. Detection of homologous blood transfusion. *Int J Sports Med.* 2007;28:633-637.
239. Wagner JC, Ulrich LR, McKean DC, et al. Pharmaceutical services at the Tenth Pan American Games. *Am J Hosp Pharm.* 1989;46:2023-2027.
240. Walker JB. Creatine: biosynthesis, regulation, and function. *Adv Enzymol Rel Areas Mol Biol.* 1979;50:177-242.
241. Walter E, Mockel J. Images in clinical medicine. Peliosis hepatis. *N Engl J Med.* 1997;337:1603.
242. Wasser WG, Feldman NS, D'Agati VD. Chronic renal failure after ingestion of over-the-counter chromium picolinate. *Ann Intern Med.* 1997;126:410.
243. Wells DJ. Gene doping: the hype and the reality. *Br J Pharmacol.* 2008;154:623-631.
244. Widder RA, Bartz-Schmidt KU, Geyer H, et al. *Candida albicans* endophthalmitis after anabolic steroid abuse. *Lancet.* 1995;345:330-331.
245. Wilson JD. Androgen abuse by athletes. *Endocr Rev.* 1988;9:181-199.
246. Windsor R, Dumitru D. Prevalence of anabolic steroid use by male and female adolescents. *Med Sci Sports Exerc.* 1989;21:494-497.
247. World Anti-Doping Agency. The 2008 Prohibited List. 2008:1-20, http://www.wada-ama.org/rtecontent/document/2008_List_Format_en.pdf.
248. World Anti-Doping Agency. What is the Code. World Anti-Doping Agency; 2008 http://www.wada-ama.org/en/dynamic.ch2?pageCategory.id=267.
249. Yang N, MacArthur DG, Gulbin JP, et al. ACTN3 genotype is associated with human elite athletic performance. *Am J Hum Genet.* 2003;73:627-631.
250. Yesalis CE, Streit AL, Vicary JR, et al. Anabolic steroid use: indications of habituation among adolescents. *J Drug Educ.* 1989;19:103-116.
251. Yesalis CE, Barsukiewicz CK, Kopstein AN, et al. Trends in anabolic-androgenic steroid use among adolescents. *Arch Pediatr Adolesc Med.* 1997;151:1197-1206.
252. Zelman G, Howland MA, Nelson LS, et al. Erythropoietin overdose treated with emergency erythropheresis. *J Tox Clin Tox.* 1999;37:602-603.
253. Zeman RJ, Ludemann R, Easton TG, et al. Slow to fast alterations in skeletal muscle fibers caused by clenbuterol, a beta 2-receptor agonist. *Am J Physiol.* 1988;254:E726-E732.
254. Zuliani U, Bernardini B, Catapano A, et al. Effects of anabolic steroids, testosterone, and HGH on blood lipids and echocardiographic parameters in body builders. *Int J Sports Med.* 1989;10:62-66.

CHAPTER 45
FOOD POISONING

Michael G. Tunik

There are approximately 76 million cases of food poisoning in the United States every year, resulting in 325,000 hospitalizations and 5000 deaths.[39] Worldwide food distribution, large-scale national food preparation and distribution networks, limited food regulatory practices, and corporate greed place everyone at risk. Food poisoning causes morbidity and mortality by one or more of the following mechanisms: Infectious agents (eg, bacteria, viruses) can be transmitted in food; toxins, produced by organisms can be consumed in food; toxins or chemicals can inadvertently or purposefully contaminate food and be ingested.

This chapter is organized into four major types of food poisoning: foodborne poisoning with neurologic symptoms, foodborne poisoning with gastrointestinal symptoms, foodborne poisoning anaphylaxis-like symptoms, and foodborne poisoning used for bioterrorism.

HISTORY AND EPIDEMIOLOGY

In recent years in the United States *Salmonella* spp and *Escherichia coli* have become the major causes of food poisoning responsible for epidemics that worry millions, poison and hospitalize hundreds, and kill many unsuspecting innocent people.

The most common causes of foodborne disease include bacteria—*Salmonella* spp, *Campylobacter* spp, *Shigella* spp, and *E. coli.*[123] (Table 45–1). In the last decade, large numbers of people have also suffered from food poisoning due to purposeful placement of chemicals in food,[41] and staphyloccal toxin.[154]

FOODBORNE POISONING WITH NEUROLOGIC SYMPTOMS

The differential diagnosis of patients with foodborne poisoning presenting with neurologic symptoms is vast (Tables 45–2 and 45–3). The sources of many of these cases are ichthyosarcotoxic involving toxins from the muscles, viscera, skin, gonads, and mucous surfaces of the fish; rarely, toxicity follows consumption of the fish blood or skeleton. Shellfish poisoning also must be considered. Most episodes of poisoning are not species specific, although particular forms of toxicity from Tetraodontiformes (puffer fish), Gymnothoraces (moray eel), and newts (*Taricha* and other species) are recognized.

In cases of ciguatera poisoning, the major symptoms usually are neurotoxic, and the gastrointestinal (GI) symptoms are minor. Scombroid poisoning, which is exceptionally common, is not associated with focal neurologic manifestations, but facial flushing, headache, and dysphagia are its major signs and symptoms.

Knowing where the fish was caught often helps establish a diagnosis, but refrigerated transport of foods and rapid worldwide travel can complicate that assessment. Travelers to Caribbean and Pacific islands, as well as those traveling within the United States, have suffered from ciguatera poisoning.[94] In geographically disparate regions of Canada,[130] individuals have suffered from domoic acid poisoning due to ingestion of cultivated mussels from Prince Edward Island.

In the differential diagnosis of foodborne poisons presenting with neurologic symptoms, activities other than eating must always be considered. In particular, sport divers often perform their activities in high-risk areas such as Florida, California, and Hawaii, and often during the high-risk periods from May through August. In the process, they may sustain sting from a stingray tail, or laceration (from a deltoid or pectoral fin spine of a lionfish or stonefish) that can cause consequential marine toxicity (Chap. 120).

CIGUATERA POISONING

Ciguatera poisoning is one of the most commonly reported forms of vertebrate fishborne poisonings in the United States accounting for almost half of the reported cases.[123] Ciguatera poisoning is endemic to warm-water, bottom-dwelling shore reef fish living around the globe between 35° north and 35° south latitude, which includes tropical areas such as the Indian Ocean, the South Pacific, and the Caribbean. Hawaii and Florida report 90% of all cases occurring in the United States, most commonly from May through August.[98]

More than 500 fish species have caused human cases of ciguatera poisoning, with the barracuda, sea bass, parrot fish, red snapper, grouper, amber jack, kingfish, and sturgeon the most common sources. The common factor is the comparably large size of the fish involved.

Large fish (4–6 lb or more) become vectors of ciguatera poisoning in accordance with complex feeding patterns inherent in aquatic life. Ciguatoxin can be found in blue-green algae, protozoa, and the free algae dinoflagellates. These plankton members of the phylum Protozoa are single-celled, motile, flagellated, pigmented organisms thriving through photosynthesis. Photosynthetic dinoflagellates such as *Gambierdiscus toxicus* and bacteria within the dinoflagellates are the origins of ciguatoxin.[50,76,102] Dinoflagellates are the main nutritional source for small herbivorous fish which in turn are the major food source for larger carnivorous fish thereby increasing the ciguatoxin concentrations in the flesh, adipose tissue, and viscera of larger and larger fish.[11]

Ciguatoxin is heat stable, lipid soluble, acid stable, odorless, and tasteless. When purified, the toxin is a large (molecular weight 1100 Da) complex ester that does not harm the fish but is stored in its tissues.[98,103] The molecule binds to voltage-sensitive sodium channels in diverse tissues and increases the sodium permeability of the channel.[10,158] The ciguatoxins cause hyperpolarization and a shift in the voltage dependence of channel activation, which opens the sodium channels. Ciguatoxins bind selectively to a particular binding site on the neuron's voltage-sensitive sodium channel protein.[101]

Multiple ciguatoxins are identified in the same fish, perhaps explaining the variability of symptoms and differing severity.[102] People can be afflicted after eating fresh or frozen fish that was prepared by all common methods: boiling, baking, frying, stewing, or broiling. The appearance, taste, and smell of the ciguatoxic fish are usually unremarkable. The majority of symptomatic episodes begin 2–6 hours after ingestion, 75% within 12 hours, and 96% within 24 hours.[11] Symptoms include acute onset of diaphoresis; headaches, abdominal pain with cramps, nausea, vomiting; profuse watery diarrhea; and a constellation of dramatic neurologic symptoms.[175] A sensation of loose, painful teeth may occur. Typically, peripheral dysesthesias and paresthesias predominate. Watery eyes, tingling, and numbness of the tongue, lips, throat, and perioral area occur. A strange metallic taste is frequently reported as is a reversal of temperature discrimination, the pathophysiology of which remains to be elucidated.[28] Myalgias, most often in the lower extremities, arthralgias, ataxia, and weakness are commonly experienced.[11]

Dysuria[63] and symptoms of dyspareunia and vaginal and pelvic discomfort may occur in women after sexual intercourse with men who are ciguatoxic.[93] Vertigo, seizures, and visual disturbances of blurred vision, scotomata, and transient blindness) are reported.

TABLE 45–1. Epidemiology[36] of Foodborne Poisoning Reported to the CDC (1993–1997)

Etiology	Cases	Outbreaks	Deaths
Salmonella *spp*	32,610	357	13
Escherichia coli[a]	3,260	84	8
Clostridium perfringens	2,772	57	0
Other parasitic	2,261	13	0
Other viral	2,104	24	0
Shigella *spp*	1,555	43	0
Staphylococcus aureus	1,413	42	1
Norwalk virus	1,233	9	0
Hepatitis A virus	729	23	0
Bacillus cereus	691	14	0
Other bacterial	609	6	1
Campylobacter *spp*	539	25	1
Scombrotoxin	297	69	0
Ciguatoxin	205	60	0
Streptococcus, group A	122	1	0
Listeria monocytogenes	100	3	2
Clostridium botulinum	56	13	1
Glardia lamblia	45	4	0
Vibrio parahaemolyticus	40	5	0
Other chemical	31	6	0
Yersinia enterocolitica	27	2	1
Mushroom poisoning	21	7	0
Brucella	19	1	0
Trichinella spiralis	19	2	0
Heavy metals	17	4	0
Streptococcus, other	6	1	0
Shellfish	3	1	0
Vibrio cholerae	2	1	0
Monosodium glutamate	2	1	0

[a]The fatality rate of *E. coli* 0157:H7 increased dramatically in the late 1990s.

TABLE 45–2. Differential Diagnosis of Possible Foodborne Poisoning Presenting with Neurologic Symptoms

Anticholinergic poisoning
Bacterial food poisoning
Botulism
Eaton-Lambert syndrome
Metals
MSG (monosodium glutamate)
Organic phosphorous compounds
Plant ingestions (poison hemlock, buckthorn)
Tick paralysis

Bradycardia and orthostatic hypotension are described.[59] The GI symptoms usually subside within 24–48 hours; however, cardiovascular and neurologic symptoms may persist for several days to weeks, depending on the amount of toxin ingested. Delayed symptoms may include protracted itching and hiccoughs. Although internationally deaths are reported, none have been documented in the United States.[123] When it occurs, mortality is a result of respiratory paralysis and seizures not managed with adequate life support. Ciguatoxin may be transmitted in breast milk[20] and can cross the placenta.[128]

Laboratory analysis using an enzyme-linked immunosorbent assay (ELISA) test for ciguatera toxin can be performed; alternatively, high-pressure liquid chromatography (HPLC) is accurate. A dipstick immunobead assay test being developed for field use will allow testing of fish without laboratory processing of the toxin-containing tissues.[10,74,127] A useful approach to diagnosis and management using laboratory testing to exclude other diagnostic possibilities and determine the need for, or extent of, specific therapeutic interventions.

Initial treatment for victims of ciguatoxin poisoning includes standard supportive care for a toxic ingestion.[175] In most patients, elimination of the toxin is accelerated if vomiting (40%) and diarrhea (70%) have occurred. Administration of activated charcoal may be of some benefit. In patients with significant GI fluid loss through vomiting and/or diarrhea, intravenous fluid and electrolyte repletion are essential. The orthostatic hypotension may respond to intravenous fluids and α-adrenergic agonists. Bradycardia may be treated with atropine.[56]

Intravenous mannitol may alleviate neurologic and muscular dysfunctional symptoms associated with ciguatera; however, GI symptoms are not ameliorated.[126,129] In one randomized controlled trial, mannitol failed to produce any greater improvement in symptoms than did IV 0.9% sodium chloride solution.[147] Mannitol should be used with caution because it may cause hypotension. Vascular reexpansion and cardiovascular stability should be initial treatment priorities.

Admission to the hospital for cautious supportive care is essential when the diagnosis is uncertain or when volume depletion or any consequential manifestations are present (Tables 45–2 and 45–3). The etiology of the symptoms must be rapidly identified to provide specific therapy, if available. Diaphoresis is a common clinical finding and an important factor in the differential diagnosis. Late in the course of ciguatera poisoning, amitriptyline 25 mg orally twice daily may alleviate symptoms,[23] which may persist up to 1 year. Victims recovering from ciguatera should avoid alcohol for 3–6 months if exposure exacerbates symptoms.

CIGUATERA-LIKE POISONING

Moray, conger, and anguillid eels carry a ciguatoxin-like neurotoxin in their viscera, muscles, and gonads that does not affect the eel itself. The toxin is a complex ester that may be structurally very similar to ciguatoxin and is heat stable.[122] These same eels also possess an ichthyohemotoxin that is resistant to drying but can be destroyed by heating to >149°F (65°C). Individuals who eat these eels may manifest neurotoxic symptomatology similar to ciguatoxin or may show signs of cholinergic toxicity, such as hypersalivation, nausea, vomiting, and diarrhea. Shortness of breath, mucosal erythema, and cutaneous eruptions may occur. These findings may be present in addition to the neurotoxic symptoms.[69] Management is supportive. Mortality is related to the complications of neurotoxicity, such as seizures and respiratory paralysis.

SHELLFISH POISONING

Healthy mollusks living between 30° north and 30° south latitude ingest and filter large quantities of dinoflagellates. These dinoflagellates are the

TABLE 45–3. Common Toxicologic Foodborne Neurologic Diseases (Primary Presenting Symptoms)

	Onset/Duration*	Symptoms	Toxin Source/Toxin*/Mechanism**	Diagnosis/Therapy*
Ciguatera	2–30 h *Months to years	t, p, n, v, d	Large reef fish: amber jack, barracuda, snapper, parrot, sea bass, moray (dinoflagellate, source) *Ciguatoxin **Increased sodium channel permeability	Clinical, mouse bioassay, immunoassay *Supportive, mannitol, isotonic saline, amitriptyline
Tetrodotoxin	Minutes to hours *Days	p, r, ↓bp	Puffer fish, *fugu*, blue-ringed octopus, newts, horseshoe crab *Tetrodotoxin **Blocks sodium channel	*Clinical *Respiratory support
Neurotoxic shellfish poisoning	15 min to 18 h *Days	b, t, n, v, d, p	Mussels, clams, scallops, oysters, *P. brevis:* "red tide" *Brevetoxin **Increased sodium channel permeability	Clinical, mouse bioassay of food, HPLC
Paralytic shellfish poisoning	30 min *Days	r, p, n, v, d	Mussels, clams, scallops, oysters, *P. catanella, P. tamarensis* *Saxitoxin **Decreases sodium channel permeability	Clinical, mouse bioassay of food, HPLC *Respiratory support
Amnestic shellfish poisoning	15 min to 38 h *Years	a n, v, d, p, r	Mussels, possibly other shellfish; *N. pungens;* *Domoic acid **Glutamate analog	Clinical, mouse bioassay of food, HPLC *Respiratory support
Botulism	12–73 h	v, d, r, w	Home-canned foods, honey, corn syrups, *C. botulinum* *Botulinum toxin **Binds presynaptically, blocks acetylcholine release	Clinical immunoassay *Antitoxin, respiratory support

a = amnesia; b = bronchospasm; d = diarrhea; n = nausea; p = paresthesias; r = respiratory depression; t = temperature reversal sensation; v = vomiting; w = weakness; ↓bp = hypotension.

major source of available ocean food during the "non-R" months (May through August) in the northern hemisphere. During this time, these dinoflagellates are responsible for the "red tides" that may be seen from California to Alaska, from New England to the St. Lawrence, and across the west coast of Europe.[109] The number of toxic dinoflagellates may be so overwhelming that birds and fish die, and humans who walk along the beach may suffer respiratory symptoms caused by aerosolized toxin.[111]

Ingestion of shellfish, including oysters, clams, mussels, and scallops, contaminated by dinoflagellates or algae may cause neurotoxic, paralytic, and amnestic syndromes. The dinoflagellates most frequently implicated are *Karenia brevis* (originally named *Gymnodinium breve* in 1948, renamed *Ptychodiscus brevis* in 1979, and reclassified again to the current nomenclature in 2000). The diatoms causing neurotoxic shellfish poisoning include *Protogonyaulax catanella* and *Protogonyaulax tamarensis*, which cause paralytic shellfish poisoning; and *Nitzschia pungens*, the diatom implicated in amnestic shellfish poisoning. Proliferation of these diatoms may cause a red tide, but shellfish poisoning may occur even in the absence of this extreme proliferation.

Paralytic shellfish poisoning is caused by saxitoxin. Saxitoxin blocks the voltage-sensitive sodium channel in a manner identical to tetrodotoxin (see later). The shellfish implicated usually are clams, oysters, mussels, and scallops, but poisoning has occurred through consumption of crustaceans, gastropods, and fish.

The higher the number of shellfish consumed the more severe the symptoms. Symptoms usually occur within 30 minutes of ingestion. Neurologic symptoms predominate and include paresthesias and numbness of the mouth and extremities, a sensation of floating, headache, ataxia, vertigo, muscle weakness, paralysis, and cranial nerve dysfunction manifested by dysphagia, dysarthria, dysphonia, and transient blindness. GI symptoms are less common and include nausea, vomiting, abdominal pain, and diarrhea. Fatalities may occur as a result of respiratory failure, usually within the first 12 hours after symptom onset. Muscle weakness may persist for weeks.

Treatment is supportive. Early intervention for respiratory failure is indicated. Orogastric lavage and cathartics were used to remove unabsorbed toxin from the GI tract but probably are not necessary or efficacious.[26,99,115,152] Activated charcoal may be given. Antibodies against saxitoxin have reversed cardiorespiratory failure in animals,[14] but this therapy is not yet available for humans. Assays for saxitoxin include a mouse bioassay, ELISA, and HPLC. High-pressure liquid chromatography has good interlaboratory accuracy,[170] but the differences in saxitoxin derivatives make standardization of an analytic test difficult.[9,95]

Neurotoxic shellfish poisoning (NSP) is caused by brevetoxin. Brevetoxin, which is produced by *Karenia brevis* (previously *Gymnodium brevis*, and subsequently *Ptychodiscus brevis*), is a lipid-soluble, heat-stable polyether toxin similar to ciguatoxin. It acts by stimulating sodium flux through the sodium channels of both nerve and muscle.[6,29] NSP is characterized by gastroenteritis with associated neurologic symptoms. GI symptoms include abdominal pain, nausea, vomiting, diarrhea, and rectal burning. Neurologic features include paresthesias, reversal of hot and cold temperature sensation, myalgias, vertigo, and ataxia. Other symptoms may include headache, malaise, tremor, dysphagia, bradycardia, decreased reflexes, and dilated pupils. Paralysis does not occur. The combination of bradycardia and mydriasis is unusual. The incubation period is 3 hours (range 15 minutes to 18 hours). GI and neurologic symptoms appear simultaneously. Other manifestations of brevetoxin poisoning include mucosal irritation, cough, and bronchospasm, which occur when *P. brevis* is aerosolized by wave action during red tides. Duration of symptoms averages 17 hours (range 1–72 hours).[115]

Brevetoxins can be assayed using mouse bioassay, ELISA, and, more recently, antibody radioimmunoassay (RIA) and reconstituted sodium channels.[132,167] Treatment is supportive, and severe respiratory depression is very uncommon. Therapy includes removal of the patient from the environment and the administration of bronchodilators. Neurotoxic shellfish poisoning is not fatal.

Amnestic shellfish poisoning is caused by domoic acid, a structural analogue of glutamic and kainic acids produced by the diatom *N. pungens*. The most extensively documented human outbreak occurred in Canada in 1987, when 107 individuals who had consumed mussels harvested from cultivated river estuaries on Prince Edward Island were affected.[130] Other human outbreaks may have occurred due to a similar diatom—*Pseudonitzschia australis*—which has been isolated in shellfish from other areas.[57] Pelican deaths caused by domoic acid–laden anchovies were reported in 1991 and Canada instituted monitoring for domoic acid after this outbreak.[163] The death of 400 sea lions in California in 1998 was linked to domoic acid from the diatom *N. pungens f multiseries*.[148]

Amnestic shellfish poisoning is characterized by GI symptoms of nausea, vomiting, abdominal cramps, diarrhea, and by neurologic symptoms of memory loss and, less frequently, coma, seizures, hemiparesis, ophthalmoplegia, purposeless chewing, and grimacing. Other signs and symptoms include hemodynamic instability and cardiac dysrhythmias. Symptoms typically begin 5 hours (range 15 minutes to 38 hours) after ingestion of mussels. The mortality rate is 2%, with death most frequently occurring in older patients, who suffer more severe neurologic symptoms. Ten percent of victims may suffer long-term antegrade memory deficits, as well as motor and sensory neuropathy. Postmortem examinations have revealed neuronal damage in the hippocampus and amygdala.[162]

TETRODON POISONING

This type of fish poisoning involves only the order Tetraodontiformes. Although this order of fish is not restricted geographically, it is eaten most frequently in Japan, California, Africa, South America, and Australia.[69] Cases have also occurred in Florida and New Jersey. Approximately 100 freshwater and saltwater species exist in this order, including a number of puffer-like fish such as the globe fish, balloon fish, blowfish, and toad fish.[117] Tetrodotoxin (TTX) found in these fish is also isolated from the blue-ringed octopus[54] and the gastropod mollusk,[177] and has also been responsible for fatalities from ingestion of horseshoe crab eggs.[79] Certain tetrodotoxin-containing newts (*Taricha*, notophthalmus, triturus, and cynops), particularly *Taricha granulosa*, found in Oregon, California, and southern Alaska, can be fatal when ingested. Most newts and salamanders with bright colors and rough skins contain toxins.[24] In Japan, *fugu* (a local variety of puffer fish) is considered a delicacy, but special licensing is required to prepare this exceedingly toxic fish. In 1989, the FDA legalized the importation of puffer fish. However, prior to exportation from Japan, the fish must be laboratory tested and certified by two Japanese organizations to be tetrodotoxin free.

Tetrodotoxin is a heat-stable (except in alkaline milieu), water-soluble nonprotein, found mainly in the fish skin, liver, ovary, intestine, and possibly muscle.[69,143] The ovary has a high concentration of the toxin and is most poisonous if eaten during the spawning season. Tetrodotoxin is detected by mouse bioassay. It is unstable when heated to 212°F (100°C) in acid, distinguishing it from saxitoxin. Tetrodotoxin from fish can be detected using fluorescent spectrometry[9] or from the urine of poisoned patients using a combination of immunoaffinity chromatography and fluorometric HPLC.[82]

Tetrodotoxin and saxitoxin are produced by marine bacteria and likely accumulate in animals higher on the food chain that consume these bacteria.[121] Accumulation of toxins, primarily in the skin, of two species of asian puffer fish has been documented. Whether this accumulation of toxin is simply an evolutionary adaptation, to remove a toxic substance, or one that has evolutionary advantages of protection is unclear.[120]

Neurotoxicity is produced by inhibition of sodium channels and blockade of neuromuscular transmission.[118] The sodium channel is blocked from the external surface of the neuron, by the TTX molecule which contains a guanidinium group that fits into the external orifice of sodium channel. This causes external "plugging" of the sodium channel, though the gating mechanism is functional.[119]

Symptoms of tetrodon poisoning typically occur within minutes of ingestion. Headache, diaphoresis, dysesthesias, and paresthesias of the lips, tongue, mouth, face, fingers, and toes evolve rapidly. Buccal bullae and salivation may develop. Dysphagia, dysarthria, nausea, vomiting, and abdominal pain may ensue. Generalized malaise, loss of coordination, weakness, fasciculations, and an ascending paralysis (with risk of respiratory paralysis) occur in 4–24 hours. Other cranial nerves may be involved. In more severe toxicity, hypotension is present. In some studies, mortality has approached 50%.[155]

Therapy is supportive. Removal of the toxin and prevention of absorption are the essential measures. Supportive respiratory care emphasizing airway protection, including intubation, if necessary, is extremely important.

LESS COMMON POISONINGS: ECHINODERMS

The sea urchin usually causes toxicity by contact with its spinous processes, but this Caribbean delicacy also is toxic upon ingestion. When the sea urchin is prepared as food, the venom-containing gonads should be removed because they contain an acetylcholine-like substance that causes the cholinergic syndrome of profuse salivation, abdominal pain, nausea, vomiting, and diarrhea. The sea star is considered edible by some individuals, although an asteriotoxin with saponin-like activity that produces nausea and vomiting is reported.

PREVENTION OF MARINE FOODBORNE DISEASE

Careful evaluation of the symptoms and meticulous reporting to local and state health departments, as well as to the Centers for Disease Control and Prevention (CDC), will allow for more precise analysis of epidemics of poisoning from contaminated or poisonous food or fish. Many states and countries have developed rigorous health codes with regard to harvesting certain species of fish in certain areas at certain times.

Some examples of actions taken by state and foreign health agencies in controlling epidemics of seafood-borne food poisoning are the following: A 3230-km stretch of Massachusetts coastline was noted to be unsafe for shellfish harvesting due to a red tide bloom. The state declared a health emergency and confiscated shellfish harvested in this area, and prohibited the marketing, export, and serving of shellfish.[109] The health code of Miami, Florida prohibits the sale of barracuda and warns against eating fillets from large and potentially toxic fish containing ciguatoxin. The Japanese closely regulate preparation and selling of the puffer fish (fugu), requiring that preparers receive special training and licensing. The sale of fugu is now also permitted under strict control in the United States as well. The Canadian government marks the location and time of harvesting of mussels, and mussels are tested for the presence of domoic acid.[57,130]

FOODBORNE POISONING ASSOCIATED WITH DIARRHEA

The initial differential diagnosis for acute diarrhea involves several etiologies: infectious (bacterial, viral, parasitic, and fungal), structural (including surgical), metabolic, functional, inflammatory, toxin induced, and food induced. The differential diagnosis is described in greater detail in Chap. 25.

An elevated temperature may be caused by invasive organisms, including *Salmonella* spp, *Shigella* spp, *Campylobacter* spp, invasive *E. coli, Vibrio parahaemolyticus*, and *Yersinia* spp, as well as some viruses. Episodes of acute gastroenteritis not associated with fever can be caused by organisms producing toxins, including *Staphylococcus aureus, Bacillus cereus, Clostridium perfringens*, enterotoxigenic *E. coli*, and viruses.[3]

Fecal leukocytes typically are found in patients with invasive shigellosis, salmonellosis, Campylobacter enteritis, typhoid fever, invasive *E. coli* colitis, *V. parahaemolyticus, Yersinia enterocolitica*, and ulcerative colitis. In all of these conditions, except typhoid fever, the leukocytes are primarily polymorphonuclear; in typhoid fever, they are mononuclear. No stool leukocytes are noted in cholera, viral diarrhea, noninvasive *E. coli* diarrhea, or nonspecific diarrhea.[73]

The timing of diarrhea onset after exposure or the incubation period can be useful in differentiating the cause. Extremely short incubation periods of less than 6 hours are typical for *Staphylococcus, B. cereus* (type I), enterotoxigenic *E. coli*,[3,106,161] and pre-formed enterotoxins, as well as roundworm larvae ingestions. Intermediate incubation periods of 8–24 hours are found with *C. perfringens, B. cereus* (type II enterotoxin), enteroinvasive *E. coli*,[48,113] and salmonella. Longer incubation periods are seen in other bacterial causes of acute gastroenteritis (Table 45–4).

The three most likely etiologies of diarrhea are infectious, xenobiotics, and foodborne. These three etiologies are not mutually exclusive. The differential diagnosis must be made among these groups. When

TABLE 45–4. Common Foodborne Disease: Gastrointestinal (Primary Presenting Symptom)

Etiology	Onset	Symptoms A	V	Di	Dy	F	Source	Pathogenesis	Therapy
Staphylococcus spp	2–6 h	+	+	+	–	–	Prepared foods: meats, pastries, salads	Heat-stable enterotoxin	Supportive, Volume expansion
Bacillus cereus									
Type I	1–6 h	+	+	+	–	–	Fried rice	Heat-labile toxins	Supportive, Volume expansion
Type II	12 h	+	–	+	–	–	Meats, vegetables	Heat-labile toxins	
Anisakiasis	1–12 h	+	+	–	–	–	Raw fish, sushi, Eustrongyloides, minnows, salmon, cod, herring, squid, tuna	Intestinal larvae	Endoscopy Laparotomy Removal
Clostridium perfringens	8–24 h	+	±	+	±	–	Poultry, heat-processed meats	Heat-labile enterotoxin	Volume expansion
Salmonella spp	8–24 h	±	±	+	±	+	Poultry, egg Pets (turtles, lizards, chicks)	Bacteria, endotoxin (bactermia)	Antibiotics
E. coli	24–72 h						Water, food	Enterotoxin, heat stable	
Enterotoxigenic	<6h	+	±	+	–	+	Enteric contact		Volume expansion Electrolytes
Invasive		+	–	+	+	+	Raw produce	Bacteria (invasive)	Antibiotics
Hemorrhagic		+	+	+	+	±	Under cooked beef Unpasteurized milk	Shigalike toxin	Renal, hematologic support
Vibrio cholera	24–72 h	±	±	+	–	±	Water, food Enteric contact	Enterotoxin Heat labile	Electrolyte replacement, antibiotics
Shigella spp	24–72 h	+	±	+	+	±	Institutional food handler Household, preschool, enteric contact	Bacteria Endotoxin	Antibiotics
Campylobacter jejuni	1–7 d	+	+	+	±	+	Milk, poultry Unchlorinated water	Bacteria, Heat-labile enterotoxin	Antibiotics
Yersinia spp	1–7 d	+	+	+	±	+	Pork, milk, pets	Bacteria, Enterotoxin	Antibiotics

A = abdominal pain; Di = diarrhea; Dy = dysentery; F = fever; V = vomiting.

the time from exposure to onset of symptoms is brief, all of the nonbacterial infectious etiologies (viral, parasitic, fungal, and algal) except for upper GI invasion by roundworm larvae can be eliminated. The possibility of a bacterial etiology with enterotoxin production should be considered (Table 45–4).[3,21]

EPIDEMIOLOGY

Epidemiologic analysis is of immediate importance, particularly when GI diseases strike more than one person in a group. The questions raised in Table 45–5 must be answered.[142] If available, an infectious disease consultant or infection control officer should be called for assistance. Alternatively, assistance from state and local health departments should be sought. Often, only the CDC or state health department has the resources to investigate and confirm a presumptive diagnosis in an outbreak. Sophisticated techniques such as toxin detection, matching the organism in the food by phage type with a food handler, matching an organism by phage type with other persons, isolating 10 or more organisms per gram of implicated food,[48,52] or PCR identification of bacterial or plasmid DNA are potentially useful, although generally not possible using the laboratory and personnel available in most hospitals.[27,32,64] Structural, metabolic, and functional causes often can be eliminated. As in these diseases, neither a significant grouping of cases nor a limited clinical history is characteristic. Foodborne parasites such as *Trichinella spiralis* (trichinosis), *Toxoplasma gondii* (toxoplasmosis), and *G. lamblia* (giardiasis) must be considered, although acute GI symptoms are not usually prominent.

SALMONELLA SPECIES

Salmonella enteritidis infections are of great concern in the United States. Two particular outbreaks define very special problems. In the 1980s, recurrent outbreaks associated with grade A eggs or food containing such eggs occurred. In the past, such outbreaks of salmonella enteritis were attributed to infection of the egg with salmonella (from the chicken's GI tract) through cracks in the shell. More recently, outbreaks have involved noncracked, nonsoiled eggs.[114] In these cases, presumably the salmonella has infected the eggs before the shell was formed. In either case, people who consume raw or undercooked eggs are at most risk for salmonella enteritis. Raw eggs can be found as ingredients of chocolate mousse, hollandaise sauce, eggnog, caesar salads, and homemade ice cream. Whole, partially cooked eggs are eaten sunny side up or poached.[37] The second group of outbreaks was associated with raw milk,[133] which has become very popular in certain communities. Inadequate microwave cooking may cause small outbreaks.[52] These outbreaks are of great concern because they frequently involve multiple drug-resistant salmonella infections.[45] Drinking pasteurized milk may not be protective. An outbreak of salmonellosis resulting in more than 16,000 culture-proven cases was traced to one Illinois dairy. The probable cause of the outbreak was a transfer line connecting raw and pasteurized milk containment tanks.[139]

The contamination of food that is widely distributed places thousands at risk. A recent outbreak of salmonella food poisoning from peanut butter caused 529 confirmed illnesses in 48 states and Canada, 116 hospitalizations, and possibly 8 deaths.[40] The CDC estimates that the proportion of salmonella infections that are confirmed by laboratory testing is 3% of the total, so the estimated number of infected people affected by this contamination incident may be more than 15,000. News reports state that the peanut butter contamination with salmonella was known, and that the peanut butter was retested for contamination, until no salmonella was reported. The peanut butter was then distributed nationally.[72]

Additional concern has developed over the widespread use of antibiotics in animal feed, responsible for meats, poultry, and manure-fertilized vegetables now frequently containing resistant bacterial strains to which virtually the entire population may be exposed.[45,139] "Household" pets such as chicks, turtles, and iguanas carry salmonella and frequently transmit the organism to household contacts, including infants, who are at particular risk for invasive diseases, as well as other family members.[1]

TABLE 45–5. Epidemiologic Analysis of Gastrointestinal Disease

1. Is the occurrence of the disease in a large group significant enough to be consistent with foodborne disease (two or more cases)?
2. Is the symptomatology in affected individuals well defined and similar?
3. Is the onset, time, and duration of illness similar among affected group members (incubation)?
4. What are the possible modes of transmission (ie, contact, food, water)?
5. Is there a relationship between the time of exposure of the group and the mode of transmission?
6. Do attack rates differ for age, gender, or occupation?
7. Can it be determined which foods were served and to whom? Can the items which were not eaten by those who did not become ill be identified?
8. What is the food-specific attack rate?
9. How was the food procured? How was it stored?
10. Was cooking technique adequate?
11. Was personal hygiene acceptable?
12. Was there animal contamination?

FOODBORNE POISONING ASSOCIATED WITH GASTROENTERITIS, ANEMIA, THROMBOCYTOPENIA, AND AZOTEMIA

The hemolytic uremic syndrome (HUS) is frequently caused by a bacterial gastroenteritis. The most commonly responsible organism is *E. coli* O157:H7.[66] Other bacteria producing a Shigalike toxin can cause the same findings, and other xenobiotics also implicated in causing HUS include estrogen-containing oral contraceptives, mitomycin C, cyclosporin A, and radiation therapy.[131] Nontoxicologic causes of this same clinical picture include autoimmune disease, Kawasaki syndrome, and bacterial enteritis/sepsis leading to disseminated intravascular coagulopathy and shock.

Laboratory findings typically include microangiopathic hemolytic anemia, thrombocytopenia, and acute renal failure. Hyperkalemia, metabolic acidosis, hyponatremia, and hypocalcemia also are found. Hepatic aminotransferase concentrations may be elevated, and pancreatic involvement may produce hyperamylasemia, elevated lipase concentration, and hyperglycemia.

Most children with HUS are younger than 6 years, and many are younger than 2 years. HUS begins with a prodrome of diarrhea 90% of the time. The diarrhea lasts for 3–4 days and frequently becomes bloody. Abdominal pain due to colitis is common, and vomiting, altered mental status (irritability or lethargy), pallor, and low-grade fever frequently occur. At the time of presentation, many children have oliguria or anuria. Approximately 10% of children present with a generalized seizure at the onset of HUS.[151]

Postdiarrheal HUS is endemic in Argentina.[105] Frequent epidemics occur in North America, and many of these reports describe the association of enterohemorrhagic *E. coli* (EHEC) or *E. coli* O157:H7 with postdiarrheal HUS.[25,108,124,125,137,172] Postdiarrheal HUS occurs most frequently during the summer months, matching the peak incidence of positive stool cultures in cattle (the most common source of the organism).[70] Food products from cattle (ground beef, milk, yogurt, cheese) and water contaminated with fecal material are common sources.[47,70,110] Contaminated water used in gardens and unpasteurized apple cider have caused bloody diarrhea and HUS as a result of EHEC.[16,44]

Enterohemorrhagic *E. coli*, including *E. coli* O157:H7, produces a toxin similar to the toxin produced by *Shigella dysenteriae* type I, referred to as Shigalike toxin (SLT) or verotoxin.[21] The proposed mechanism for SLT damage is intestinal absorption, bloodstream access to renal glomerular endothelium, intracellular adsorption via glycolipid receptors, ribosomal inactivation, and cell death.[160] In animal models, organ damage is more severe if endothelial cells have high concentrations of globotriaosylceramide receptors, which have a high binding affinity for shiga toxin. Other organs with these receptors include the renal, GI, and central nervous systems, which may explain the pattern of organ damage in children with HUS. Endothelial cell damage and other pathologic processes, including platelet and leukocyte activation, triggering of the coagulation cascade, and the production of cytokines, occur.[81,169] More than one type of SLT exists; SLT-1, SLT-2, and variants of SLT-2 structure have been identified.[17]

Detection of *E. coli* O157:H7 through stool culture early in the course of disease is useful. The recovery decreases after the first week of illness.[131,160] *E. coli* O157:H7 almost always produces SLT; therefore, if stool cultures are negative, enzyme immunoassay (EIA) and polymerase chain reaction (PCR) tests can be used to detect SLT in the stool when *E. coli* can no longer be identified by culture.[27]

Treatment of HUS should focus on meticulous supportive care, with fluid and electrolyte balance the priority. Peritoneal dialysis or hemodialysis should be instituted early for azotemia, hyperkalemia, acidosis, and fluid overload. Red blood cells transfusions maintain hemoglobin concentrations greater than 6 g/dL and platelet transfusion may be necessary to maintain hemostasis, especially important measures before invasive procedures are undertaken. Hypertension should be treated with short-acting calcium channel blockers (nifedipine 0.25–0.5 mg/kg/dose orally) and seizures with benzodiazepines. The many therapies used for HUS include heparin, fibrinolytics, IV immunoglobulin, fresh-frozen plasma, vitamin E, and antiplatelet agents. However, none has been obviously beneficial, and some have been deleterious.[165] Plasmapheresis has been used in nondiarrheal HUS and in recurrent HUS after renal transplants. In a controlled trial, antibiotics did not change the course or outcome for children with postdiarrheal HUS.[134] A meta-analysis also found no increased risk from antibiotic therapy.[140] Anti–SLT-2 antibodies have protected mice from SLT-2 toxicity, but IV immunoglobulin with SLT-2 activity has not improved outcome in children with HUS. A double-blind, placebo-controlled study on the use of synthetic SLT receptors attached to an oral carrier found that mortality or serious morbidity of HUS syndrome did not change as a result.[166]

The mortality from HUS with good supportive care is approximately 5%; another 5% of victims suffer end-stage renal disease or cerebral ischemic events and chronic neurologic impairment. Prolonged anuria (>1 week), oliguria (>2 weeks), or severe extrarenal disease may serve as markers for higher mortality and morbidity.[131]

Strategies to prevent the spread of *E. coli* O157:H7 and subsequent HUS include public education on the importance of thorough cooking of beef to a "well-done" temperature of 170°F (77°C), pasteurization of milk and apple cider, and thorough cleaning of vegetables. Public health measures include education of clinicians to consider *E. coli* O157:H7 in patients with bloody diarrhea and insuring the routine capability of microbiology laboratories to culture *E. coli* O157:H7 and provide for EIA or PCR determination of SLT. Public health departments should provide active surveillance systems to identify early outbreaks of *E. coli* O157:H7 infection.

STAPHYLOCOCCUS SPECIES

In cases of suspected food poisoning with a short incubation period, the physician should first assess the risk for staphylococcal causes. The usual foods associated with staphylococcal toxin production include milk products and other proteinaceous foods, cream-filled baked goods, potato and chicken salads, sausages, ham, tongue, and gravy. Pie crust can act as an insulator, maintaining the temperature of the cream filling and occasionally permitting toxin production even during refrigeration.[4] A routine assessment must be made for the presence of lesions on the hands or nose of any food handlers involved. Unfortunately, carriers of enterotoxigenic staphylococci are difficult to recognize because they usually lack lesions and appear healthy.[75] A fixed association between a particular food and an illness would be most helpful epidemiologically but rarely occurs clinically. Factors such as environment, host resistance, nature of the agent, and dose make the results surprisingly variable.

Although patients with staphylococcal food poisoning rarely have significant temperature elevations, 16% of 2992 documented cases in a published review had a subjective sense of fever.[75] Abdominal pain, nausea followed by vomiting, and diarrhea dominate the clinical findings. Diarrhea does not occur in the absence of nausea and vomiting. The mean incubation period is 4.4 hours with a mean duration of illness of 20 hours. Two staphylococcal enterotoxin food poisoning incidents involving large numbers of people have been reported. At a public event in Brazil in 1998, half of the 8000 people who attended suffered nausea, emesis, diarrhea, abdominal pain, and dizziness within hours of consuming food. Of the ill patients, 2000 overwhelmed the capacity of local emergency departments, 396 (20%) were admitted including 81 to intensive care units, and 16 young children and elderly participants died.[154] In another report, 328 individuals became ill with symptoms of diarrhea, vomiting, dizziness, chills, and headache after eating cheese or milk.[153] In both reports, staphylococcus enterotoxin was found in the food consumed.

Most enterotoxins are produced by *S. aureus* coagulase–positive species. The enterotoxins initiate an inflammatory response in GI mucosal cells and lead to cell destruction. The enterotoxins also may exert a sudden explosive effect on the emesis center in the brain and diverse other organ systems. Discrimination of unique *S. aureus* isolates from those found in foodborne outbreaks can be made using restriction fragment length polymorphism analysis by pulsed-field gel electrophoresis and PCR techniques.[173]

CAMPYLOBACTER JEJUNI

Campylobacter jejuni, a curved Gram-negative rod, is a major cause of bacterial enteritis. The organism is most commonly isolated in children younger than 5 years and in adults 20–40 years. Campylobacter enteritis outbreaks are more common in the summer months in temperate climates. Although most cases of *Campylobacter enteritis* are sporadic, outbreaks are associated with contaminated food and water. The most frequent sources of *Campylobacter* in food are raw or undercooked poultry products[53] and unpasteurized milk.[31,167] Birds are a common reservoir, and small outbreaks are associated with contamination of milk by birds pecking on milk-container tops.[156] Contaminated water supplies are also frequent sources of Campylobacter enteritis involving large numbers of individuals.[19] *C. jejuni* is heat labile; cooking of food, pasteurization of milk, and chlorination of water will prevent human transmission.

The incubation period for *Campylobacter enteritis* varies from 1–7 days (mean 3 days). Typical symptoms include diarrhea, abdominal cramps, and fever. Other symptoms may include headache, vomiting, excessive gas, and malaise. The diarrhea may contain gross blood, and leukocytes are frequently present on microscopic examination.[73] Illness usually lasts 5–6 days (range 1–8 days). Rarely, symptoms last for several weeks. Severely affected individuals present with lower GI hemorrhage, abdominal pain mimicking appendicitis, a typhoid-like syndrome, reactive arthritis, or meningitis. The organism may be detected using PCR identification techniques.[61] Treatment is supportive, and consists of volume resuscitation, and possibly quinolone antibiotics for the more severe cases.[3]

GROUP A *STREPTOCOCCUS*

Bacterial infections not usually associated with food or food handling are nevertheless occasionally transmitted by food or food handling. Transmission of streptococcal pharyngitis in food prepared by an individual with streptococcal pharyngitis has been demonstrated.[46] A Swedish food handler caused 153 people to become ill with streptococcal pharyngitis when his infected finger wound contaminated a layer cake served at a birthday party.[7]

CLOSTRIDIUM BOTULINUM

In the last 3 decades, a median of 4 cases of foodborne botulism, 3 cases of wound botulism, and 71 cases of infant botulism have been reported annually to the CDC.[150] Home-canned fruits and vegetables, as well as commercial fish products, are among the common foods causing botulism. The incubation period usually is 12–36 hours; typical symptoms include some initial GI symptoms, followed by malaise, fatigue, diplopia, dysphagia, and rapid development of small muscle incoordination.[96] In botulism, the toxin is irreversibly bound to the neuromuscular junction, where it impairs the presynaptic release of acetylcholine.[90] A patient's survival depends on a rapidly diagnosing botulism and immediate initiation of aggressive respiratory therapy. Establishing the diagnosis early may make it possible to treat the "sentinel" patient and also others who consumed the contaminated food with antitoxin prior to their developing signs and symptoms (Chap. 46 and Antidotes in Depth A8: Botulinum Antitoxin). The differential diagnosis of botulism includes myasthenia gravis, atypical Guillain-Barré syndrome, tick-induced paralysis, and certain chemical ingestions (see Tables 46-1 and 46-2).

YERSINIA ENTEROCOLITICA

Yersinia enterocolitica is a Gram-negative coccobacillus that causes enteritis most frequently in children and young adults. Typical clinical features include fever, abdominal pain, and diarrhea, which usually contains mucus and blood.[8,159,171] Other associated symptoms include nausea, vomiting, anorexia, and weight loss. The incubation period may be 1 day to 1 week or more. Less common features include prolonged enteritis, arthritis, pharyngeal and hepatic involvement, and rash. Yersinia is a common pathogen in many animals, including dogs and pigs. Sources of human infection include milk products, raw pork products, infected household pets, and person-to-person transmission.[22,68,97] Diagnosis may be based on cultures of food, stool, blood, and, less frequently, skin abscesses, pharyngeal cultures, or cultures from other organ tissues (mesenteric lymph nodes, liver). Yersinia may be identified by PCR.[80] Patients receiving the chelator deferoxamine may aquire yersinia infections due to the patients increased susceptibility. The deferoxamine-iron complex acts as a siderophore for the organism growth. Therapy is usually supportive, but patients with invasive disease (eg, bacteremia, bacterial arthritis) should be treated with IV antibiotics. Fluoroquinolones and third-generation cephalosporins are highly bacteriocidal against *Yersinia* spp.

LISTERIA MONOCYTOGENES

Listeriosis transmitted by food usually occurs in pregnant women and their fetuses, the elderly, and immunocompromised individuals using corticosteroids or with malignancies, diabetes mellitus, renal disease, or HIV infection.[15,34,36,146] Typical food sources include unpasteurized milk, soft cheeses such as feta, and undercooked chicken. Individuals at risk should avoid the usual sources and should be evaluated for listeriosis if typical symptoms of fever, severe headache, muscle ache, and pharyngitis develop. Treatment with IV ampicillin or trimethoprim–sulfamethoxazole is indicated for systemic listerial infections.

XENOBIOTIC-INDUCED DISEASES

In addition to the aforementioned saxitoxin tetrodotoxin, domoic acid, and ciguatoxin, many other xenobiotics contaminate our food sources. Careful assessment for possible foodborne pesticide poisoning is essential. For example, aldicarb contamination has occurred in hydroponically grown vegetables and watermelons contaminated with pesticides.[65] Eating malathion-contaminated chapatti and wheat flour resulted in 60 poisonings including a death in one outbreak[42] (Chap. 113). Insecticides, rodenticides, arsenic, lead, or fluoride preparations can be mistaken for a food ingredient. These poisonings usually have a rapid onset of signs and symptoms after exposure.

The possibility of unintentional acute heavy-metal ingestion must also be considered. This type of poisoning most typically occurs when very acidic fruit punch is served in metal-lined containers. Antimony, zinc, copper, tin, or cadmium in a container may be dissolved by an acid food or juice medium.

MUSHROOM-INDUCED DISEASE

Some species produce major GI effects. *Amanita phalloides,* the most poisonous mushroom, usually causes GI symptoms as well as hepatotoxic effects with a delay to clinical manifestations. The rapid onset of symptoms suggests some of the gastroenterotoxic mushrooms (Chap. 117).

INTESTINAL PARASITIC INFECTIONS

The popularity of eating raw fish, a popular form of Japanese cuisine, has led to an increase in reported intestinal parasitic infections. The etiologic agents typically are roundworms (*Eustrongyloides anisakis*) and fish tapeworms (*Diphyllobothrium* spp). Symptoms of anisakiasis, or eustrongylidiasis, that are localized to the stomach typically occur 1–12 hours after eating raw fish, whereas symptoms of lower intestinal involvement may be delayed for days or weeks. Typical gastric or intestinal symptoms include nausea, vomiting, and severe crampy abdominal pain that may mimic a gastric ulcer. Typical lower intestinal symptoms include abdominal cramping and, with perforation of the intestinal wall by the larvae, severe localized abdominal pain, rebound, and guarding, which may mimic an acute abdomen (appendicitis). In some cases, the symptoms include anaphylaxis with or without abdominal pain. Without an adequate dietary history of eating raw fish, the diagnosis may be almost impossible to establish and therapy might instead be directed toward the most likely diagnostic entity such as gastric ulcer or appendicitis. Diagnosis of parasitic infection usually is established by visual inspection of the larvae (on endoscopy, laparotomy, or pathologic examination), which typically are pink or red. Raw fish that may contain *Eustrongyloides* include minnows (*Fundulus* spp) and other bait fish. *Anisakis simplex* and *Pseudoterranova decipiens* are Anisakidae that may be found in several types of frequently consumed raw fish, including mackerel, cod, herring, rockfish, salmon, yellowfin tuna, and squid. Reliable methods of preventing ingestion of live anisakid larvae are freezing −4°F (−20°C) for 60 hours or cooking at 140°F (60°C) for 5 minutes.[31,87,104,138,144,176]

Diphyllobothriasis (fish tapeworm disease) is caused by eating uncooked fish that harbor the parasite. Hosts include, but are not limited to, herring, salmon, pike, and whitefish. The symptoms are less acute than with intestinal roundworm ingestions and usually begin 1–2 weeks after ingestion.[30] Signs and symptoms include nausea, vomiting, abdominal cramping, flatulence, abdominal distension, diarrhea, and megaloblastic anemia. Diagnosis is based on a history of ingesting raw fish and on identification of the tapeworm proglottids in stool. Treatment with niclosamide, praziquantel, or paromomycin usually is effective.[35]

Yet another foodborne toxin with GI symptoms is associated with eating reheated fried rice. *Bacillus cereus* type I is the causative organism, and bacterial overgrowth and toxin production causes consequential early onset nausea and vomiting.[2] Infrequently this toxin causes liver failure.[107] *Bacillus cereus* type II has a delayed onset of similar GI symptoms, including diarrhea.[58]

MONOSODIUM GLUTAMATE

The so-called Chinese restaurant syndrome results from the ingestion of monosodium glutamate (MSG). Affected individuals present with a burning sensation of the upper torso, facial pressure, headache, flushing, chest pain, nausea and vomiting, and, infrequently, life-threatening bronchospasm[3] and angioedema.[157] Intensity and duration of symptoms are generally dose related but with significant variation in individual responses to the amount ingested.[145,178] MSG causes "shudder attacks" or a seizure-like syndrome in young children. Absorption is more rapid following fasting, and the typical burning symptoms rapidly spread over the back, neck, shoulders, abdomen, and occasionally the thighs. GI symptoms are rarely prominent and symptoms can usually be prevented by prior ingestion of food. When symptoms do occur, they tend to last approximately 1 hour. The syndrome is a reaction to MSG, which had traditionally been commonly used in Chinese restaurants in the past but frequently used in many other restaurants. MSG is also marketed as an effective flavor enhancer.[13] Many sausages and canned soups contain heavy doses of MSG.

MSG (regarded as "safe" by the FDA) can cause other acute and bizarre neurologic symptoms. There is evidence that humans have a unique taste receptor for glutamate.[89] This explains its ability to act as a flavor enhancer for foods. Glutamate is also an excitatory neurotransmitter which can stimulate central nervous system neurons through activation of glutamate receptors, and may be the explanation for some of the neurologic symptoms described with ingestion.[179]

ANAPHYLAXIS AND ANAPHYLACTOID PRESENTATIONS

Some foods and foodborne toxins may cause allergic or anaphylacticlike manifestations,[83] also sometimes referred to as "restaurant syndromes"[149] (Table 45-6). The similarity of these syndromes complicates a patient's future approach to safe eating. Isolating the precipitant is essential so that the risk can be effectively assessed. Manufacturers of processed foods should provide an unambiguous listing of ingredients on package labels. Sensitive individuals (or in the cases of children their parents) must be rigorously attentive.[141,180] Those who experience severe reactions should make sure that epinephrine and antihistamines are always available immediately. Attempts to prevent allergic reactions to dairy products by avoiding dairy-containing foods may fail. Nondairy foods may still be processed in equipment used for dairy products or contain flavor enhancers of a dairy origin (eg, partially hydrolyzed sodium caseinate), both of which can cause morbidity and death in allergic individuals.[60] Individuals with known food allergies do not always carry prescribed autoinjectable spring-injected epinephrine

TABLE 45–6. Common Foodborne Disease Symptoms: Flushing, Bronchospasm, Headache (Primary Presenting Symptoms)

	Onset	Symptoms/Signs	Cause	Therapy
Anaphylaxis (anaphylactoid)	Minutes to hours	Urticaria, angioedema, bronchospasm, hypotension	Allergens—nuts, eggs, milk, fish, shellfish, peanuts, soy	Oxygen, epinephrine, β_2-adrenergic agonist, Corticosteroids, volume expansion, H_1, H_2 histamine blockers
MSG (monosodium glutamate)	Minutes	Flushing, hypotension, palpitations, facial pressure, headaches, bronchospasm, shivering (Children)	Flavor enhancer of foods	Oxygen, β_2-adrenergic agonists, volume expansion, avoidance
Metabisulfites	Minutes	Flushing, hypotension, bronchospasm	Preservative in wines, salad (bars), fruit juice, shrimp	See Anaphylaxis, Avoidance
Scombroid	Minutes to hours	Flushing, hypotension urticaria, headache, pruritis, GI symptoms	Large fish—poorly refrigerated; tuna, bonito, albacore, mackerel, mahi mahi (histidine)	See Anaphylaxis, Avoidance
Tyramine	Minutes to hours	Headache, hypertension (INH or MAOI) increases risk	Wines, aged cheeses	Avoidance for those with hypertension, migraines
Tartrazine	Hours	Urticaria, angioedema, brochospasm	Yellow coloring food additive	See Anaphylaxis, Avoidance

INH = isoniazid; MAOI = monoamine oxide inhibitor.

syringes, in some cases from a belief that the allergen is easily identifiable and avoidable.[83] Food additives that can cause anaphylaxis include antibiotics, aspartame, butylated hydroxyanisole (BHA), butylated hydroxytoluene (BHT), nitrates or nitrites, sulfites, and paraben esters.[100] Regulation of these preservatives is limited, and agents such as sulfites are so ubiquitous that predicting which guacamole, cider, vinegar, fresh or dried fruits, wines, or beers contain these sensitizing agents may be impossible.

SCOMBROID POISONING

Scombroid poisoning originally was described with the Scombroidae fish (including the large dark-meat marine tuna, albacore, bonito, mackerel, and skipjack). However, the most commonly ingested vectors identified by the CDC are nonscombroid fish, such as mahi mahi and amber jack.[33] All of the implicated fish species live in temperate or tropical waters. Ingestion of bluefish in New Hampshire was the probable cause of scombroid poisoning in five people,[51] and mackerel was the likely offender in 28 cases reported from a prison.[50] The incidence of this disease is probably far greater than was originally perceived. This type of poisoning differs from other fishborne causes of illness in that it is entirely preventable if the fish is properly stored following removal from the water.

Scombroid poisoning results from eating cooked, smoked, canned, or raw fish. The implicated fish all have a high concentration of histidine in their dark meat. *Morganella morganii, E. coli,* and *Klebsiella pneumoniae,* commonly found on the surface of the fish, contain a histidine decarboxylase enzyme that acts on a warm (not refrigerated), freshly killed fish, converting histidine to histamine, saurine, and other heat-stable substances. Although saurine has been suggested as the causative toxin, chromatographic analysis demonstrates that histamine is found as histamine phosphate and saurine is merely histamine hydrochloride.[55,116] The term *saurine* originated from saury, a Japanese dried fish delicacy often associated with scombroid poisoning. The extent of spoilage usually correlates with histamine concentrations. Histamine concentrations in healthy fish are less than 0.1 mg/100 g fish meat. In fish left at room temperature, the concentration rapidly increases, reaching toxic concentrations of 100 mg/100 g fish within 12 hours.

The appearance, taste, and smell of the fish are usually unremarkable.[5] Rarely, the skin has an abnormal "honeycombing" character or a pungent, peppery taste that may be a clue to its toxicity (Chap. 20). Within minutes to hours after eating the fish, the individual experiences numbness, tingling, or a burning sensation of the mouth, dysphagia, headache, and, of particular significance for scombroid poisoning, a unique flush characterized by an intense diffuse erythema of the face, neck, and upper torso.[84] Rarely, pruritus, urticaria, angioedema, or bronchospasm ensues. Nausea, vomiting, dizziness, palpitations, abdominal pain, diarrhea, and prostration may develop.[43,62,84,112]

The prognosis is good with appropriate supportive care and parenteral antihistamines such as diphenhydramine. H_2-receptor antagonists such as cimetidine or ranitidine may also be useful in alleviating gastrointestinal symptoms.[18] The toxic substance should be removed or absorbed from the gut. Inhaled β_2-adrenergic agonists and epinephrine may be necessary if bronchospasm is prominent. Patients usually show significant improvement within a few hours.

Elevated serum or urine histamine concentrations can confirm the diagnosis, but are usually unnecessary. If any uncooked fish remains, isolation of causative bacteria from the flesh is suggestive, but not diagnostic. A capillary electrophoretic assay makes rapid histamine detection possible.[108] Histamine concentrations greater than 50 mg/100 g fish meat are considered hazardous by the US Food and Drug Administration (FDA). Isoniazid may increase the severity of the reaction to scombroid fish by inhibiting enzymes that break down histamine.[77,168]

Patients may be reassured that they are not allergic to fish if other individuals experience a similar reaction to eating the same fish at the same time, or if any remaining fish can be preserved and tested for elevated histamine concentrations. If this information is not available, an anaphylactic reaction to the fish must be considered. Table 45-4 lists the differential diagnosis of flushing, bronchospasm, and headache. Because many people often consume alcohol with fish, alcohol must be considered an independent variable.

The differential diagnosis of the scombrotoxic flush apart from a disulfiram-like reaction includes ingestion of niacin or nicotinic acid, and pheochromocytoma. The history and clinical evolution usually establish the diagnosis quickly.

GLOBAL FOOD DISTRIBUTION, ILLEGAL FOOD ADDITIVES

Xenobiotics are given to animals to increase their health and growth. Clenbuterol, a β_3 agonist, has been administered to cattle raised for human consumption. The substance can cause toxicity in humans who eat contaminated animal meat. Tachycardia, tremors, nausea, epigastric pain, headache, muscle pain, and diarrhea were present in 50 poisoned patients. Other findings included hypertension and leukocytosis.[136] No deaths have been reported. The use of antibiotics, β_3 agonists, and other growth enhancers continues, despite safety concerns and laws against their use, because these practices increase yield and profit.

The globalization of food supplies and international agricultural trade has created a new global threat, the apparent purposeful contamination of food for profit. In 2008, almost 300,000 children in China were affected by melamine contamination of milk. Of these 50,000 were hospitalized and 6 reported deaths occurred.

The melamine-contaminated milk was sold in China as powdered infant formula, with over 22 brands containing melamine. The contamination was not limited to China, as melamine has been found in candy, chocolate, cookies, and biscuits sold in the United States, likely due to the adulteration of milk used in preparation of these products.

Melamine is a non-nutritious nitrogen-containing compound, usually used in glues, plastics, and fertilizers. To increase profits, milk sold in China had previously been diluted, causing protein malnutrition in children. Because the nitrogen content of milk (a surrogate measure for protein content) is now carefully monitored to detect dilution and to prevent another episode of malnutrition, melamine was added to increase the measured nitrogen content and hide the dilution. This purposeful addition of melamine is suspected to be the cause of the melamine contamination of powdered milk in China.

Melamine and its metabolite cyanuric acid are excreted in the kidneys. Renal stones containing melamine and uric acid were found in 13 children with acute renal failure, who had consumed melamine containing milk formula.[67] Both melamine and cyanuric acid appear necessary to cause renal stones in animals. The combination alone caused renal crystals in cats.[135] Melamine found in wheat gluten that was added to pet food in 2007, and resulted in thousands of complaints, and dozens of suspected animal deaths in the United States.

The full extent of the melamine milk contamination, and the number of people affected is not yet known.[41,78]

Food products from all over the world find their way into our foods. Increased vigilance by the agencies responsible for food safety, both in countries where the food originates and in countries that import the food are needed to prevent other events such as the melamine contaminations.

VEGETABLES AND PLANTS

Plants, vegetables, and their diverse presentations often are involved in food poisonings.[71,85,86,91,92] Edible plants and plant products may be poorly cooked or prepared, or they may be contaminated. Extensive discussion of this may be found in Chap. 118.

FOOD POISONING AND BIOTERRORISM

The threat of terrorist assaults has received increased attention and is discussed in Chaps. 131 and 132. The use of food as a vehicle for intentional contamination with the intent of causing mass suffering or death has already occurred in the United States.[38,88,164] In the first report, 12 laboratory workers suffered GI symptoms, primarily severe diarrhea, after consuming food purposefully contaminated with *Shigellla. dysenteriae* type II[88] served in a staff break room. Four workers were hospitalized; none had reported long-term sequelae. This *Shigella* strain rarely causes endemic disease. Nevertheless an identical strain, identified by pulsed-field gel electrophoresis, was found in 8 of the 12 symptomatic workers, as well as in the pastries served in the break room, and in the laboratory stock culture of *S. dysenteriae.* This finding suggests purposeful poisoning of food eaten by laboratory personnel. The person responsible and the motive remain unknown.

The second case series describes a large community outbreak of food poisoning caused by *Salmonella typhimurium.*[164] The outbreak occurred in the Dalles, Oregon area during the fall of 1984; a total of 751 people suffered salmonella gastroenteritis. The outbreak was traced to the intentional contamination of restaurant salad bars and coffee creamer by members of a religious commune using a culture of *S. typhimurium* purchased before the outbreak of food poisoning. A criminal investigation found a salmonella culture on the religious commune grounds that contained *S. typhimurium* identical to the salmonella strain found in the food poisoning victims. It was identified by using antibiotic sensitivity, biochemical testing, and DNA restriction endonuclease digestion of plasmid DNA. Only after more than 1 year of investigation was this salmonella outbreak linked to terrorist activity. Reasons for the delay in identifying the outbreak as a purposeful food poisoning included (1) no apparent motive; (2) no claim of responsibility; (3) no pattern of unusual behavior in the restaurants; (4) no disgruntled restaurant employees identified; (5) multiple time points for contamination indicated by epidemic exposure curves, suggesting a sustained source of contamination and not a single act; (6) no previous event of similar nature as a reference; (7) the likeliness of other possibilities (eg, repeated unintentional contamination by restaurant workers); and (8) fear that the publicity necessary to aid the investigation might generate copycat criminal activity.

Publication of the event was delayed by almost 10 years out of fear of unintentionally encouraging copycat activity. On the other hand, use of biological weapons by the Japanese cult Aum Shinrikyo appears to have motivated authorities to release this publication in the hopes of quickly identifying similar deliberate food poisoning patters in the future.

A third report describes a disgruntled employee who contaminated 200 lb of meat at a supermarket with a nicotine-containing insecticide.[38] Ninety-two people became ill, and four sought medical care. Symptoms included vomiting, abdominal pain, rectal bleeding, and one case of atrial tachycardia.

In another case of human greed, a Chinese restaurant owner poisoned the food in his neighbor's restaurant with tetramine. Tetramine or tetramethylenedisulfotetramine is a highly lethal neurotoxic rodenticide, once used worldwide, now illegal in the United States. The snack shop owner caused hundreds to become ill and 38 deaths by spiking his competitors breakfast offerings (fried dough sticks, sesame cakes, and sticky rice balls). Tetramethylenedisulfotetramine is odorless and tasteless white crystal that is water soluble. The mechanism of action is noncompetitive irreversible binding to the chloride channel on the γ-aminobutyric acid receptor complex, which blocks the influx of chloride, and alters the neurons potential. It is referred to as a "cage convulsant" because of its globular structure. Severe intoxication presents with tachycardia, arrhythmias, agitation as well as status epilepticus and coma. Immediate or early treatment with sodium-(RS)-2,3-dimercaptopropane-1-sulfonate and pyridoxine (vitamin B6) appears to be effective in a mouse model.[12,49,174]

The capacity of foodborne xenobiotics that are easy to obtain and disburse to infect large numbers of people is clearly exemplified by two specific outbreaks: (1) the purposeful salmonella outbreak in Oregon, (2) the apparently unintentional salmonella outbreak that resulted in more than 16,000 culture-proven cases traced to contamination in an Illinois dairy. The probable cause of the outbreak was a contaminated transfer pipe connecting the raw and pasteurized milk containment tanks.[139] These events emphasize the vulnerability of our food supply and the importance of ensuring its safety and security.

SUMMARY

The diverse etiologies of food poisoning involve almost all aspects of toxicology. Our concerns center around the natural toxicity of plant or animal, the contamination of which can occur in the field, during factory processing, subsequent transport and distribution, or during home preparation or storage. Whether these events are intentional or unintentional, they alter our approaches to general nutrition and society. Issues in food safety include government's role in food preparation and protection, bacteria such as salmonella and *E. coli* 0157:H7, prions in Creutzfeldt-Jacob disease (bovine encephalopathy), and genetically altered materials such as corn. Future discussions of food poisonings and interpretations of the importance of these problems may dramatically alter our food sources and their preparation and monitoring.

REFERENCES

1. Ackman DM, Drabkin P, Birkhead G, et al. Reptile-associated salmonellosis in New York State. *Pediatr Infect Dis J.* 1995;14:955.
2. Agata N, Ohta M, Yokoyama K. Production of *Bacillus cereus* emetic toxin (cereulide) in various foods. *Int J Food Microbiol.* 2002;73:23.
3. American Medical Association, American Nurses Association-American Nurses Foundation, Centers for Disease Control and Prevention, et al. Diagnosis and management of foodborne illnesses: a primer for physicians and other health care professionals. *MMWR Morbid Wkly Rep.* 2004;53:1.
4. Anunciacao LL, Linardi WR, do Carmo LS, et al. Production of staphylococcal enterotoxin A in cream-filled cake. *Int J Food Microbiol.* 1995;26:259.
5. Arnold SH, Brown WD. Histamine (?) toxicity from fish products. *Adv Food Res.* 1978;24:113.
6. Asai S, Krzanowski JJ, Lockey RF, et al. The site of action of *Ptychodiscus brevis* toxin within the parasympathetic axonal sodium channel h gate in airway smooth muscle. *J Allergy Clin Immunol.* 1984;73:824.
7. Asteberg I, Andersson Y, Dotevall L, et al. A food-borne streptococcal sore throat outbreak in a small community. *Scand J Infect Dis.* 2006;38:988-994.
8. Attwood SE, Mealy K, Cafferkey MT, et al. Yersinia infection and acute abdominal pain. *Lancet.* 1987;1:529.
9. Baden DG, Fleming LE, Bean JA. Marine toxins. In: deWolff FA, Vinken PJ, eds. *Handbook of Clinical Neurology: Intoxication of the Nervous System.* Amsterdam: Elsevier; 1994:141-175.
10. Baden DG, Melinek R, Sechet V, et al. Modified immunoassays for polyether toxins: implications of biological matrixes, metabolic states, and epitope recognition. *J AOAC Int.* 1995;78:499.
11. Bagnis R, Kuberski T, Laugier S. Clinical observations on 3,009 cases of ciguatera (fish poisoning) in the South Pacific. *Am J Trop Med Hyg.* 1979;28:1067.
12. Barrueto F, Jr., Furdyna PM, Hoffman RS, et al. Status epilepticus from an illegally imported Chinese rodenticide: "tetramine". *J Toxicol Clin Toxicol.* 2003;41:991-994.
13. Bellisle F. Effects of monosodium glutamate on human food palatability. *Ann N Y Acad Sci.* 1998;855:438.

14. Benton BJ, Rivera VR, Hewetson JF, et al. Reversal of saxitoxin-induced cardiorespiratory failure by a burro-raised alpha-STX antibody and oxygen therapy. *Toxicol Appl Pharmacol.* 1994;124:39.
15. Berenguer J, Solera J, Diaz MD, et al. Listeriosis in patients infected with human immunodeficiency virus. *Rev Infect Dis.* 1991;13:115.
16. Besser RE, Lett SM, Weber JT, et al. An outbreak of diarrhea and hemolytic uremic syndrome from *Escherichia coli* O157:H7 in fresh-pressed apple cider. *JAMA.* 1993;269:2217.
17. Bitzan M, Ludwig K, Klemt M, et al. The role of *Escherichia coli* O 157 infections in the classical (enteropathic) haemolytic uraemic syndrome: results of a Central European, multicentre study. *Epidemiol Infect.* 1993;110:183.
18. Blakesley ML. Scombroid poisoning: prompt resolution of symptoms with cimetidine. *Ann Emerg Med.* 1983;12:104.
19. Blaser MJ, Reller LB. *Campylobacter* enteritis. *N Engl J Med.* 1981;305:1444-1452.
20. Blythe DG, de Sylva DP. Mother's milk turns toxic following fish feast. *JAMA.* 1990;264:2074.
21. Bokete TN, O'Callahan CM, Clausen CR, et al. Shiga-like toxin-producing *Escherichia coli* in Seattle children: a prospective study. *Gastroenterology.* 1993;105:1724.
22. Bottone EJ. Yersinia enterocolitica: the charisma continues. *Clin Microbiol Rev.* 1997;10:257.
23. Bowman PB. Amitriptyline and ciguatera. *Med J Aust.* 1984;140:802.
24. Bradley SG, Klika LJ. A fatal poisoning from the Oregon rough-skinned newt (*Taricha granulosa*). *JAMA.* 1981;246:247.
25. Brandt JR, Fouser LS, Watkins SL, et al. *Escherichia coli* O 157:H7-associated hemolytic-uremic syndrome after ingestion of contaminated hamburgers. *J Pediatr.* 1994;125:519.
26. Brett MM. Food poisoning associated with biotoxins in fish and shellfish. *Curr Opin Infect Dis.* 2003;16:461.
27. Brian MJ, Frosolono M, Murray BE, et al. Polymerase chain reaction for diagnosis of enterohemorrhagic *Escherichia coli* infection and hemolytic-uremic syndrome. *J Clin Microbiol.* 1992;30:1801.
28. Cameron J, Capra MF. The basis of the paradoxical disturbance of temperature perception in ciguatera poisoning. *J Toxicol Clin Toxicol.* 1993;31:571.
29. Catterall WA, Trainer V, Baden DG. Molecular properties of the sodium channel: a receptor for multiple neurotoxins. *Bull Soc Pathol Exot.* 1992;85:481.
30. Centers for Disease Control and Prevention. Diphyllobothriasis associated with salmon. *MMWR Morb Mortal Wkly Rep.* 1981;30:331-338.
31. Centers for Disease Control and Prevention. Intestinal perforation caused by larval Eustrongylides—Maryland. *MMWR Morb Mortal Wkly Rep.* 1982;31:383.
32. Centers for Disease Control and Prevention. Surveillance for epidemics—United States. *MMWR Morb Mortal Wkly Rep.* 1989;38:694.
33. Centers for Disease Control and Prevention. Scombroid fish poisoning—Illinois, South Carolina. *MMWR Morb Mortal Wkly Rep.* 1989;38:140.
34. Centers for Disease Control and Prevention. Update: foodborne listeriosis—United States, 1988-1990. *MMWR Morb Mortal Wkly Rep.* 1992;41:251, 257.
35. Centers for Disease Control and Prevention. Drugs for parasitic infections. *Med Lett Drugs Ther.* 1998;40:1.
36. Centers for Disease Control and Prevention. Multistate outbreak of listeriosis—United States, 1998. *MMWR Morb Mortal Wkly Rep.* 1998;47:1085.
37. Centers for Disease Control and Prevention. Outbreaks of Salmonella serotype enteritidis infection associated with eating raw or undercooked shell eggs—United States, 1996-1998. *MMWR Morb Mortal Wkly Rep.* 2000;49:73.
38. Centers for Disease Control and Prevention. Nicotine poisoning after ingestion of contaminated ground beef—Michigan, 2003. *MMWR Morb Mortal Wkly Rep.* 2003;52:413.
39. Centers for Disease Control and Prevention. Foodborne Illness, Frequently asked questions. http://www.cdc.gov/ncidod/dbmd/diseaseinfo/foodborneinfections_g.htm, 2005.
40. Centers for Disease Control and Prevention. Multistate outbreak of Salmonella infections associated with peanut butter and peanut butter-containing products—United States, 2008-2009. *MMWR Morb Mortal Wkly Rep.* 2009;58:85-90.
41. Chan EY, Griffiths SM, Chan CW. Public-health risks of melamine in milk products. *Lancet.* 2008;372:1444-1445.
42. Chaudhry R, Lall SB, Mishra B, et al. A foodborne outbreak of organophosphate poisoning. *Br. Med J. (Clin Res Ed).* 1998;317:268.
43. Chen KT, Malison MD. Outbreak of scombroid fish poisoning, Taiwan. *Am J Public Health.* 1987;77:1335.
44. Cieslak PR, Barrett TJ, Griffin PM, et al. *Escherichia coli* O157:H7 infection from a manured garden. *Lancet.* 1993;342:367.
45. Cody SH, Abbott SL, Marfin AA, et al. Two outbreaks of multidrug-resistant *Salmonella* serotype typhimurium DT104 infections linked to raw-milk cheese in Northern California. *JAMA.* 1999;281:1805.
46. Decker MD, Lavely GB, Hutcheson RH, Jr., et al. Food-borne streptococcal pharyngitis in a hospital pediatrics clinic. *JAMA.* 1985;253:679.
47. Deschenes G, Casenave C, Grimont F, et al. Cluster of cases of haemolytic uraemic syndrome due to unpasteurised cheese. *Pediatr Nephrol.* 1996;10:203.
48. DuPont HL, Formal SB, Hornick RB, et al. Pathogenesis of *Escherichia coli* diarrhea. *N Engl J Med.* 1971;285:1.
49. Eckholm E. Man Admits Poisoning Food in Rival's Shop, Killing 38 in China. *The New York Times.* 2002; A.5. http://query.nytimes.com/gst/abstract.html?res=F40E11FE3E540C7B8DDDA00894DA404482.
50. Endean R, Monks SA, Griffith JK, et al. Apparent relationships between toxins elaborated by the cyanobacterium *Trichodesmium erythraeum* and those present in the flesh of the narrow-barred Spanish mackerel *Scomberomorus commersoni. Toxicon.* 1993;31:1155.
51. Etkind P, Wilson ME, Gallagher K, et al. Bluefish-associated scombroid poisoning. An example of the expanding spectrum of food poisoning from seafood. *JAMA.* 1987;258:3409.
52. Evans MR, Parry SM, Ribeiro CD. Salmonella outbreak from microwave cooked food. *Epidemiol Infect.* 1995;115:227.
53. Finch MJ, Blake PA. Foodborne outbreaks of campylobacteriosis: the United States experience, 1980-1982. *Am J Epidemiol.* 1985;122:262.
54. Flachsenberger WA. Respiratory failure and lethal hypotension due to blue-ringed octopus and tetrodotoxin envenomation observed and counteracted in animal models. *J Toxicol Clin Toxicol.* 1986;24:485.
55. Foo LY. Scombroid poisoning. Isolation and identification of "saurine". *J Sci Food Agric.* 1976;27:807.
56. Friedman MA, Fleming LE, Fernandez M, et al. Ciguatera fish poisoning: treatment, prevention and management. *Mar Drugs.* 2008;6:456-479.
57. Fritz L, Quilliam M, Wright J, et al. An outbreak of domoic acid poisoning attributed to the pinnate diatom pseudonitzchia australis. *J Phycol.* 1992;28:439-442.
58. Gaulin C, Viger YB, Fillion L. An outbreak of *Bacillus cereus* implicating a part-time banquet caterer. *Can J Public Health.* 2002;93:353.
59. Geller RJ, Benowitz NL. Orthostatic hypotension in ciguatera fish poisoning. *Arch Intern Med.* 1992;152:2131.
60. Gern JE, Yang E, Evrard HM, et al. Allergic reactions to milk-contaminated "nondairy" products. *N Engl J Med.* 1991;324:976.
61. Giesendorf BA, Quint WG. Detection and identification of *Campylobacter* spp. using the polymerase chain reaction. *Cell Mol Biol* (Noisy-le-grand). 1995;41:625.
62. Gilbert RJ, Hobbs G, Murray CK, et al. Scombrotoxic fish poisoning: features of the first 50 incidents to be reported in Britain (1976-9). *Br Med J.* 1980;281:71.
63. Gillespie NC, Lewis RJ, Pearn JH, et al. Ciguatera in Australia. Occurrence, clinical features, pathophysiology and management. *Med J Aust.* 1986;145:584.
64. Goossens H, Giesendorf BA, Vandamme P, et al. Investigation of an outbreak of *Campylobacter upsaliensis* in day care centers in Brussels: analysis of relationships among isolates by phenotypic and genotypic typing methods. *J Infect Dis.* 1995;172:1298.
65. Green MA, Heumann MA, Wehr HM, et al. An outbreak of watermelon-borne pesticide toxicity. *Am J Public Health.* 1987;77:1431.
66. Griffin PM, Tauxe RV. The epidemiology of infections caused by *Escherichia coli* O157:H7, other enterohemorrhagic *E. coli*, and the associated hemolytic uremic syndrome. *Epidemiol Rev.* 1991;13:60.
67. Guan N, Fan Q, Ding J, et al. Melamine-contaminated powdered formula and urolithiasis in young children. *N Engl J Med.* 2009; 360:1067-1074.
68. Gutman LT, Ottesen EA, Quan TJ, et al. An inter-familial outbreak of *Yersinia enterocolitica* enteritis. *N Engl J Med.* 1973;288:1372.
69. Halstead BW, Halstead LG. *Poisonous and Venomous Marine Animals of the World.* Rev. ed. Princeton, NJ: Darwin Press; 1978 International Oceanographic Foundation selection; Variation: International Oceanographic Foundation selection.
70. Hancock DD, Besser TE, Kinsel ML, et al. The prevalence of *Escherichia coli* O157.H7 in dairy and beef cattle in Washington State. *Epidemiol Infect.* 1994;113:199.

71. Hardin JW, Arena JM. *Human Poisoning from Native and Cultivated Plants*. Chapel Hill, NC: Duke University Press; 1969:69-73.
72. Harris G. Salmonella Was Found at Peanut Plant Before. *The New York Times*. 2009. http://www.nytimes.com/2009/01/28/us/29Peanut.html?_r=1&scp=1&sq=salmonella%20peanut%20butter&st=cse.
73. Harris JC, Dupont HL, Hornick RB. Fecal leukocytes in diarrheal illness. *Ann Intern Med*. 1972;76:697.
74. Hokama Y, Asahina AY, Shang ES, et al. Evaluation of the Hawaiian reef fishes with the solid phase immunobead assay. *J Clin Lab Anal*. 1993;7:26.
75. Holmberg SD, Blake PA. Staphylococcal food poisoning in the United States. New facts and old misconceptions. *JAMA*. 1984;251:487.
76. Holmes MJ, Lewis RJ, Poli MA, et al. Strain dependent production of ciguatoxin precursors (gambiertoxins) by *Gambierdiscus toxicus* (Dinophyceae) in culture. *Toxicon*. 1991;29:761.
77. Hui JY, Taylor SL. Inhibition of in vivo histamine metabolism in rats by foodborne and pharmacologic inhibitors of diamine oxidase, histamine N-methyltransferase, and monoamine oxidase. *Toxicol Appl Pharmacol*. 1985;81:241.
78. Ingelfinger JR. Melamine and the global implications of food contamination. *N Engl J Med*. 2008;359:2745-2748.
79. Kanchanapongkul J, Krittayapoositpot P. An epidemic of tetrodotoxin poisoning following ingestion of the horseshoe crab *Carcinoscorpius rotundicauda*. *Southeast Asian J Trop Med Public Health*. 1995;26:364.
80. Kapperud G, Vardund T, Skjerve E, et al. Detection of pathogenic Yersinia enterocolitica in foods and water by immunomagnetic separation, nested polymerase chain reactions, and colorimetric detection of amplified DNA. *Appl Environ Microbiol*. 1993;59:2938.
81. Karpman D, Andreasson A, Thysell H, et al. Cytokines in childhood hemolytic uremic syndrome and thrombotic thrombocytopenic purpura. *Pediatr Nephrol*. 1995;9:694.
82. Kawatsu K, Shibata T, Hamano Y. Application of immunoaffinity chromatography for detection of tetrodotoxin from urine samples of poisoned patients. *Toxicon*. 1999;37:325.
83. Kemp SF, Lockey RF, Wolf BL, et al. Anaphylaxis. A review of 266 cases. *Arch Intern Med*. 1995;155:1749.
84. Kim R. Flushing syndrome due to mahimahi (scombroid fish) poisoning. *Arch Dermatol*. 1979;115:963.
85. Kingsbury JM. *Poisonous Plants of the United States and Canada*. Englewood Cliffs, NJ: Prentice Hall; 1964.
86. Kingsbury JM. Phytotoxicology. I. Major problems associated with poisonous plants. *Clin Pharmacol Ther*. 1969;10:163.
87. Kliks MM. Human anisakiasis: an update. *JAMA*. 1986;255:2605.
88. Kolavic SA, Kimura A, Simons SL, et al. An outbreak of Shigella dysenteriae type 2 among laboratory workers due to intentional food contamination. *JAMA*. 1997;278:396.
89. Kurihara K, Kashiwayanagi M. Physiological studies on umami taste. *J Nutr*. 2000;130:931S-934S.
90. Lamanna C, Carr CJ. The botulinal, tetanal, and enterostaphylococcal toxins: a review. *Clin Pharmacol Ther*. 1967;8:286.
91. Lampe KF, McCann MA. *AMA Handbook of Poisonous and Injurious Plants*. Chicago, IL: American Medical Association; 1985.
92. Lampe KF. Rhododendrons, mountain laurel, and mad honey. *JAMA*. 1988;259:2009.
93. Lange WR, Lipkin KM, Yang GC. Can ciguatera be a sexually transmitted disease? *J Toxicol Clin Toxicol*. 1989;27:193.
94. Lange WR, Snyder FR, Fudala PJ. Travel and ciguatera fish poisoning. *Arch Intern Med*. 1992;152:2049.
95. Laycock MV, Thibault P, Ayer SW, et al. Isolation and purification procedures for the preparation of paralytic shellfish poisoning toxin standards. *Nat Toxins*. 1994;2:175.
96. Lecour H, Ramos H, Almeida B, et al. Food-borne botulism. A review of 13 outbreaks. *Arch Intern Med*. 1988;148:578-580.
97. Lee LA, Gerber AR, Lonsway DR, et al. Yersinia enterocolitica O:3 infections in infants and children, associated with the household preparation of chitterlings. *N Engl J Med*. 1990;322:984.
98. Lehane L, Lewis RJ. Ciguatera: recent advances but the risk remains. *Int J Food Microbiol*. 2000;61:91.
99. Levin RE. Paralytic shellfish toxins: their origin, characteristics and methods of detection: a review. *J Food Biochem*. 1991;15:405-417.
100. Levine AS, Labuza TP, Morley JE. Food technology. A primer for physicians. *N Engl J Med*. 1985;312:628.
101. Lewis RJ, Sellin M, Poli MA, et al. Purification and characterization of ciguatoxins from moray eel (*Lycodontis javanicus*, Muraenidae). *Toxicon*. 1991;29:1115-1127.
102. Lewis RJ, Sellin M. Multiple ciguatoxins in the flesh of fish. *Toxicon*. 1992;30:915.
103. Lewis RJ, Holmes MJ. Origin and transfer of toxins involved in ciguatera. *Comp Biochem Physiol C*. 1993;106:615.
104. Lopez-Serrano MC, Gomez AA, Daschner A, et al. Gastroallergic anisakiasis: findings in 22 patients. *J Gastroenterol Hepatol*. 2000;15:503.
105. Lopez EL, Contrini MM, Devoto S, et al. Incomplete hemolytic-uremic syndrome in Argentinean children with bloody diarrhea. *J Pediatr*. 1995;127:364.
106. Lumish RM, Ryder RW, Anderson DC, et al. Heat-labile enterotoxigenic *Escherichia coli* induced diarrhea aboard a Miami-based cruise ship. *Am J Epidemiol*. 1980;111:432-436.
107. Mahler H, Pasi A, Kramer JM, et al. Fulminant liver failure in association with the emetic toxin of *Bacillus cereus*. *N Engl J Med*. 1997;336:1142-1148.
108. Martin DL, MacDonald KL, White KE, et al. The epidemiology and clinical aspects of the hemolytic uremic syndrome in Minnesota. *N Engl J Med*. 1990;323:1161-1167.
109. Massachusetts Department of Health. The red tide—a public health emergency. *N Engl J Med*. 1973;288:1126-1127.
110. McCarthy TA, Barrett NL, Hadler JL, et al. Hemolytic-uremic syndrome and *Escherichia coli* O121 at a lake in Connecticut, 1999. *Pediatrics*. 2001;108:E59.
111. McCollum JP, Pearson RC, Ingham HR, et al. An epidemic of mussel poisoning in North-East England. *Lancet*. 1968;2:767-770.
112. Merson MH, Baine WB, Gangarosa EJ, et al. Scombroid fish poisoning. Outbreak traced to commercially canned tuna fish. *JAMA*. 1974;228:1268-1269.
113. Merson MH, Morris GK, Sack DA, et al. Travelers' diarrhea in Mexico. A prospective study of physicians and family members attending a congress. *N Engl J Med*. 1976;294:1299-1305.
114. Mishu B, Griffin PM, Tauxe RV, et al. Salmonella enteritidis gastroenteritis transmitted by intact chicken eggs. *Ann Intern Med*. 1991;115:190-194.
115. Morris PD, Campbell DS, Taylor TJ, et al. Clinical and epidemiological features of neurotoxic shellfish poisoning in North Carolina. *Am J Public Health*. 1991;81:471-474.
116. Morrow JD, Margolies GR, Rowland J, et al. Evidence that histamine is the causative toxin of scombroid-fish poisoning. *N Engl J Med*. 1991;324:716-720.
117. Mosher HS, Fuhrman FA, Buchwald HD, et al. Tarichatoxin–tetrodotoxin: a potent neurotoxin. *Science*. 1964;144:1100-1110.
118. Narahashi T. Mechanism of action of tetrodotoxin and saxitoxin on excitable membranes. *Fed Proc*. 1972;31:1124-1132.
119. Narahashi T. Tetrodotoxin—a brief history. *Proc Jpn Acad Ser B*. 2008;84:147-154.
120. Ngy L, Tada K, Yu CF, et al. Occurrence of paralytic shellfish toxins in Cambodian Mekong pufferfish *Tetraodon turgidus*: selective toxin accumulation in the skin. *Toxicon*. 2008;51:280-288.
121. Noguchi T, Arakawa O, Takatani T. TTX accumulation in pufferfish. *Comp Biochem Physiol D*. 2006;1:145-152.
122. Nukina M, Koyanagi LM, Scheuer PJ. Two interchangeable forms of ciguatoxin. *Toxicon*. 1984;22:169-176.
123. Olsen SJ, MacKinnon LC, Goulding JS, et al. Surveillance for foodborne-disease outbreaks—United States, 1993-1997. *Morbid Mortal Wkly Rep*. CDC Surveillance Summaries, 2000;49:1-62.
124. Orr P, Lorencz B, Brown R, et al. An outbreak of diarrhea due to verotoxin-producing *Escherichia coli* in the Canadian Northwest Territories. *Scand J Infect Dis*. 1994;26:675-684.
125. Ostroff SM, Kobayashi JM, Lewis JH. Infections with *Escherichia coli* O157:H7 in Washington State. The first year of statewide disease surveillance. *JAMA*. 1989;262:355-359.
126. Palafox NA, Jain LG, Pinano AZ, et al. Successful treatment of ciguatera fish poisoning with intravenous mannitol. *JAMA*. 1988;259:2740-2742.
127. Park DL. Evolution of methods for assessing ciguatera toxins in fish. *Rev Environ Contam Toxicol*. 1994;136:1-20.
128. Pearn J, Harvey P, De Ambrosis W, et al. Ciguatera and pregnancy. *Med J Aust*. 1982;1:57-58.
129. Pearn JH, Lewis RJ, Ruff T, et al. Ciguatera and mannitol: experience with a new treatment regimen. *Med J Aust*. 1989;151:77-80.
130. Perl TM, Bedard L, Kosatsky T, et al. An outbreak of toxic encephalopathy caused by eating mussels contaminated with domoic acid. *N Engl J Med*. 1990;322:1775-1780.

131. Pickering LK, Obrig TG, Stapleton FB. Hemolytic-uremic syndrome and enterohemorrhagic *Escherichia coli*. *Pediatr Infect Dis J*. 1994;13:459-475; quiz 476.
132. Poli MA, Rein KS, Baden DG. Radioimmunoassay for PbTx-2-type brevetoxins: epitope specificity of two anti-PbTx sera. *J AOAC Int*. 1995;78:538-542.
133. Potter ME, Kaufmann AF, Blake PA, et al. Unpasteurized milk. The hazards of a health fetish. *JAMA*. 1984;252:2048-2052.
134. Proulx F, Turgeon JP, Delage G, et al. Randomized, controlled trial of antibiotic therapy for *Escherichia coli* O157:H7 enteritis. *J Pediatr*. 1992;121:299-303.
135. Puschner B, Poppenga RH, Lowenstine LJ, et al. Assessment of melamine and cyanuric acid toxicity in cats. *J Vet Diagn Invest*. 2007;19:616-624.
136. Ramos F, Silveira I, Silva JM, et al. Proposed guidelines for clenbuterol food poisoning. *Am J Med*. 2004;117:362.
137. Rowe PC, Orrbine E, Wells GA, et al. Epidemiology of hemolytic-uremic syndrome in Canadian children from 1986 to 1988. The Canadian Pediatric Kidney Disease Reference Centre. *J Pediatr*. 1991;119:218-224.
138. Ruttenberg M. Safe sushi. *N Engl J Med*. 1989;321:900-901.
139. Ryan CA, Nickels MK, Hargrett-Bean NT, et al. Massive outbreak of antimicrobial-resistant salmonellosis traced to pasteurized milk. *JAMA*. 1987;258:3269-3274.
140. Safdar N, Said A, Gangnon RE, et al. Risk of hemolytic uremic syndrome after antibiotic treatment of Escherichia coli O157:H7 enteritis: a meta-analysis. *JAMA*. 2002;288:996-1001.
141. Sampson HA, Mendelson L, Rosen JP. Fatal and near-fatal anaphylactic reactions to food in children and adolescents. *N Engl J Med*. 1992;327:380-384.
142. Sartwell PE. *Maxcy-Rosenau Preventive Medicine and Public Health*. 10th ed. Norwalk, CT: Appleton & Lange; 1992.
143. Schantz EJ, Johnson EA. Properties and use of botulinum toxin and other microbial neurotoxins in medicine. *Microbiol Rev*. 1992;56:80-99.
144. Schantz PM. The dangers of eating raw fish. *N Engl J Med*. 1989;320: 1143-1145.
145. Schaumburg HH, Byck R, Gerstl R, et al. Monosodium L-glutamate: its pharmacology and role in the Chinese restaurant syndrome. *Science*. 1969;163:826-828.
146. Schlech WF, III. Foodborne listeriosis. *Clin Infect Dis*. 2000;31:770-775.
147. Schnorf H, Taurarii M, Cundy T. Ciguatera fish poisoning: a double-blind randomized trial of mannitol therapy. *Neurology*. 2002;58:873-880.
148. Scholin CA, Gulland F, Doucette GJ, et al. Mortality of sea lions along the central California coast linked to a toxic diatom bloom. *Nature*. 2000;403:80-84.
149. Settipane GA. The restaurant syndromes. *Arch Intern Med*. 1986;146:2129-2130.
150. Shapiro RL, Hatheway C, Swerdlow DL. Botulism in the United States: a clinical and epidemiologic review. *Ann Intern Med*. 1998;129:221-228.
151. Siegler RL, Pavia AT, Christofferson RD, et al. A 20-year population-based study of postdiarrheal hemolytic uremic syndrome in Utah. *Pediatrics*. 1994;94:35-40.
152. Sierra-Beltran AP, Cruz A, Nunez E, et al. An overview of the marine food poisoning in Mexico. *Toxicon*. 1998;36:1493-1502.
153. Simeao Do Carmo L, Dias R, Linardi V, et al. Food poisoning due to enterotoxigenic strains of Staphylococcus present in Minas cheese and raw milk in Brazil. *Food Microbial*. 2002;19:9-14.
154. Simeao Do Carmo LS, Cummings C, Linardi VR, et al. A case study of a massive staphylococcal food poisoning incident. *Foodborne Pathog Dis*. 2004;1:241-246.
155. Sims JK, Ostman DC. Pufferfish poisoning: emergency diagnosis and management of mild human tetrodotoxication. *Ann Emerg Med*. 1986;15:1094-1098.
156. Southern JP, Smith RM, Palmer SR. Bird attack on milk bottles: possible mode of transmission of *Campylobacter jejuni* to man. *Lancet*. 1990;336: 1425-1427.
157. Squire EN, Jr. Angio-oedema and monosodium glutamate. *Lancet*. 1987;1:988.
158. Swift AE, Swift TR. Ciguatera. *J Toxicol Clin Toxicol*. 1993;31:1-29.
159. Tacket CO, Ballard J, Harris N, et al. An outbreak of *Yersinia enterocolitica* infections caused by contaminated tofu (soybean curd). *Am J Epidemiol*. 1985;121:705-711.
160. Tarr PI, Neill MA, Clausen CR, et al. *Escherichia coli* O157:H7 and the hemolytic uremic syndrome: importance of early cultures in establishing the etiology. *J Infect Dis*. 1990;162:553-556.
161. Taylor WR, Schell WL, Wells JG, et al. A foodborne outbreak of enterotoxigenic *Escherichia coli* diarrhea. *N Engl J Med*. 1982;306:1093-1095.
162. Teitelbaum JS, Zatorre RJ, Carpenter S, et al. Neurologic sequelae of domoic acid intoxication due to the ingestion of contaminated mussels. *N Engl J Med*. 1990;322:1781-1787.
163. Todd E. Domoic acid and amnesic shellfish poisoning: a review. *J Food Prot*. 1993;56:68-83.
164. Torok TJ, Tauxe RV, Wise RP, et al. A large community outbreak of salmonellosis caused by intentional contamination of restaurant salad bars. *JAMA*. 1997;278:389-395.
165. Trachtman H, Christen E. Pathogenesis, treatment, and therapeutic trials in hemolytic uremic syndrome. *Curr Opin Pediatr*. 1999;11:162-168.
166. Trachtman H, Cnaan A, Christen E, et al. Effect of an oral Shiga toxin-binding agent on diarrhea-associated hemolytic uremic syndrome in children: a randomized controlled trial. *JAMA*. 2003;290:1337-1344.
167. Trainer VL, Baden DG, Catterall WA. Detection of marine toxins using reconstituted sodium channels. *J AOAC Int*. 1995;78:570-573.
168. Uragoda CG, Kottegoda SR. Adverse reactions to isoniazid on ingestion of fish with a high histamine content. *Tubercle*. 1977;58:83-89.
169. van de Kar NC, van Hinsbergh VW, Brommer EJ, et al. The fibrinolytic system in the hemolytic uremic syndrome: in vivo and in vitro studies. *Pediatr Res*. 1994;36:257-264.
170. van Egmond HP, van den Top HJ, Paulsch WE, et al. Paralytic shellfish poison reference materials: an intercomparison of methods for the determination of saxitoxin. *Food Addit Contam*. 1994;11:39-56.
171. Vantrappen G, Geboes K, Ponette E. Yersinia enteritis. *Med Clin North Am*. 1982;66:639-653.
172. Waters JR, Sharp JC, Dev VJ. Infection caused by *Escherichia coli* O157:H7 in Alberta, Canada, and in Scotland: a five-year review, 1987-1991. *Clin Infect Dis*. 1994;19:834-843.
173. Wei HL, Chiou CS. Molecular subtyping of *Staphylococcus aureus* from an outbreak associated with a food handler. *Epidemiol Infect*. 2002;128:15-20.
174. Whitlow KS, Belson M, Barrueto F, et al. Tetramethylenedisulfotetramine: old agent and new terror. *Ann Emerg Med*. 2005;45:609-613.
175. Withers NW. Ciguatera fish poisoning. *Annu Rev Med*. 1982;33:97-111.
176. Wittner M, Turner JW, Jacquette G, et al. Eustrongylidiasis—a parasitic infection acquired by eating sushi. *N Engl J Med*. 1989;320:1124-1126.
177. Yang CC, Han KC, Lin TJ, et al. An outbreak of tetrodotoxin poisoning following gastropod mollusc consumption. *Hum Exp Toxicol*. 1995;14:446-450.
178. Yang WH, Drouin MA, Herbert M, et al. The monosodium glutamate symptom complex: assessment in a double-blind, placebo-controlled, randomized study. *J Allergy Clin Immunol*. 1997;99:757-762.
179. Yu L, Zhang Y, Ma R, et al: Potent protection of ferulic acid against excitotoxic effects of maternal intragastric administration of monosodium glutamate at a late stage of pregnancy on developing mouse fetal brain. *Eur Neuropsychopharmacol*. 2006;16:170-177.
180. Yunginger JW, Sweeney KG, Sturner WQ, et al. Fatal food-induced anaphylaxis. *JAMA*. 1988;260:1450-1452.

CHAPTER 46
BOTULISM

Howard L. Geyer

Botulism, a potentially fatal neuroparalytic illness, has been recognized since the 18th century. It results from botulinum neurotoxin (BoNT), the most potent toxin known, which is produced by *Clostridium botulinum* and other *Clostridium* species. The toxin interferes with release of acetylcholine from presynaptic motor and autonomic nerve terminals, thereby disrupting neuromuscular transmission and autonomic synapses, resulting in flaccid paralysis and autonomic dysfunction. In adults, most cases are foodborne, resulting from ingestion of toxin, while most cases in infants result from ingestion of bacterial spores which proliferate and produce toxin in the gastrointestinal tract. Less common forms of botulism include wound botulism, in which spores are inoculated into a wound and locally produce toxin, and inhalational botulism due to aerosolized BoNT, potentially used as a weapon of bioterrorism. Therapeutic injections of BoNT may result in transient adverse effects, but serious sequelae are rare when BoNT is properly prepared and administered.

HISTORY AND EPIDEMIOLOGY

The earliest cases of botulism were described in Europe in 1735 and were attributed to improperly preserved German sausage; the name of the disease alludes to this association, *botulus* being Latin for *sausage.* Emile van Ermengem identified the causative organism in 1897 and named it *Bacillus botulinum*; it was later renamed *Clostridium botulinum*.[25] These Gram-positive, spore-forming bacteria produce seven serotypes of BoNT, denoted A through G. All clostridial species are ubiquitous, and the bacteria and spores are present in soil, seawater, and air.[130] Botulism outbreaks can occur anywhere in the world[118] and have been reported from such diverse areas as Iran,[106] Japan,[100] Thailand,[73] France,[1] Portugal,[77] and Canada.[94]

In 2007, a total of 144 cases of botulism were reported to the Centers for Disease Control and Prevention (CDC). Foodborne botulism constituted 18% of cases, infant botulism 63% of cases, and wound botulism 15%.[42] In this analysis, toxin type A accounted for the majority of cases of both foodborne (58%) and wound (82%) botulism, while infant botulism was due to toxin type A in 43% and to toxin type B in 56% of cases.[42] Six deaths were confirmed: three in patients with foodborne botulism and three in patients with wound botulism. The case fatality rate has improved for all botulism toxin types, probably due to increasing awareness of the problem and consequent earlier diagnosis, appropriate and early use of antitoxin, and better and more accessible life support techniques.

In the last 50 years, home-processed food has accounted for 65.1% of outbreaks, with commercial food processing constituting only 7% of reported cases; in the other 27.9% of outbreaks the origin remains unknown.[38] Common home-canning errors responsible for botulism include failure to use a pressure cooker and allowing food to putrefy at room temperature. Minimally processed foods such as soft cheeses may lack sufficient quantities of intrinsic barriers to BoNT production, such as salt and acidifying agents.[112] These foods become high-risk sources of botulism when refrigeration standards are violated. The US Food and Drug Administration (FDA) continuously reviews recommendations for appropriate measures to process such foods.[142,143]

Outbreaks of botulism have been associated with specialty foods consumed by different ethnic groups: chopped garlic in soy oil by Chinese in Vancouver, British Columbia;[94,136] uneviscerated salted fish—called *kapchunka*—eaten by Russian immigrants in New York City;[34,140] and the same fish—called *faseikh*—eaten by Egyptians in Egypt.[151] The incidence of botulism is high in Alaska where traditional foods include fermented fish and fish eggs, seal, beaver, and whale; between 1990 and 2000, 39% of cases of foodborne botulism occurred in Alaska.[133] Approximately 90% of toxin type E outbreaks have occurred in Alaska because of home-processed fish or meat from marine animals,[41,48,79,150] while one incident occurred in New Jersey.[35] In the 1990s, three cases of botulism involved members of a Native American church after they ingested a ceremonial tea made from the buttons of dried, alkaline-ground peyote cactus that were prepared in a water-covered refrigerated jar. The resultant alkaline and anaerobic milieu presumably fostered the growth of toxin from naturally occurring spores.[66] In 1996, eight cases of foodborne botulism in Italy were linked to mascarpone cream cheese eaten either alone or in tiramisu contaminated with BoNT type A.[14] In 2006, carrot juice was implicated in four cases in Georgia and Florida.[37] Ten cases in California, Indiana, Ohio, and Texas were linked to commercially processed chili sauce in 2007.[44] Awareness of evolving trends and unusual presentations or locations of botulism permits the establishment of preventive education programs.

Among cases attributed to commercial food processing, vegetables (peppers, beans, mushrooms, tomatoes, and beets, with or without meat) were thought to be the causative agents in approximately 70%, meat in 17%, and fish in 13% of cases.[38] Although only 4% of foodborne botulism is associated with food purchased in restaurants, restaurant-related outbreaks usually affect large numbers of individuals.[79]

Of 26 reported cases of botulism in 2007, 16 occurred in multicase outbreaks.[42] Among hundreds of outbreaks from 1975 to 1988 totaling more than 400 persons, approximately 70% involved only one person, 20% involved two persons, and only 10% involved more than two persons (mean 2.7 cases per outbreak).[155] Single affected patients were more severely ill, with 85% requiring intubation, compared to only 42% requiring intubation in multiperson outbreaks.[155] It may be that diagnosis in the index case leads to more rapid therapeutic intervention for associated cases.

Infant botulism is most common in certain geographic areas, presumably due to higher concentrations of botulinum spores in soil. Raw honey is a potential source of spores.[95] Most affected infants are younger than 6 months of age. Of 91 cases reported in 2007, most were from California (40%), Pennsylvania (14%), and New Jersey (11%). The median age was 15 weeks, and no deaths were reported.[42] With appropriate support and treatment, a favorable outcome is achieved in the majority of cases.

In 2007, 22 cases of wound botulism were reported; 20 of those cases occurred in California. Ages ranged from 23 to 58 years, with a median of 42 years. All but two were known to be injection drug users. Three patients died, and outcome information was unavailable for three others.[42]

Since 2001, concern about the use of inhalational BoNT as a biologic weapon has increased. In ways unimaginable when the first edition of this chapter was published, medical and public health realities associated with terrorism in the 21st century unfortunately have resulted in increased relevance of botulism to medical practitioners (Chap. 132). Concern regarding potential adverse consequences of therapeutic BoNT injections also has developed.[11]

BACTERIOLOGY

The genus *Clostridium* comprises a group of four spore-forming anaerobic Gram-positive bacillary species that produce seven different neurotoxic proteins: *C. botulinum,* which produces all BoNT serotypes A through G; *Clostridium baratii,* which produces toxin type F; *Clostridium butyricum,* which produces toxin type E; and *Clostridium argentinense,* which produces toxin type G.[67,124,129] Rare instances of both adult and infant botulism are attributed to *C. baratii* and *C. butyricum.*[65,88,101,108] The reported incidence of cases due to BoNT type F may be underestimated because of the only recent capacity of most laboratories to determine the presence of *C. baratii* and other clostridial species producing toxin type F.[65]

Toxin types A through G, with Cα and Cβ subtypes, have been identified to date. In the United States, toxin type A is found in soil west of the Mississippi,[81] type B is found east of the Mississippi, particularly in the Allegheny range, and type E is found in the Pacific northwest and the Great Lakes states.[36,130] Toxin types A and B typically are found in poorly processed meats and vegetables. Toxin type E is commonly found in raw or fermented marine fish and mammals. Toxin types C and D cause disease in birds and mammals. Toxin type G has not been associated with naturally occurring disease. Although botulinum toxins differ in the cellular molecules they target, the ultimate pathophysiology and clinical syndromes are identical.

All botulinum spores are dormant and highly resistant to damage. They can withstand boiling at 212°F (100°C) for hours, although they usually are destroyed by 30 minutes of moist heat at 248°F (120°C). Factors that promote germination of spores in food are pH greater than 4.5, sodium chloride content less than 3.5%, or a low nitrite concentration. Most viable organisms produce toxin in an anaerobic milieu with temperatures greater than 80.6°F (27°C), although some strains produce toxins even when conditions are not optimal. *C. botulinum* organisms can produce toxin type E at temperatures as low as 41°F (5°C). To prevent spore germination, acidifying agents such as phosphoric or citric acid are added to canned or bottled foods that have a low acid content, such as green beans, corn, beets, asparagus, chili peppers, mushrooms, spinach, figs, olives, and certain nonacidic tomatoes. Unlike the spores, the toxin itself is heat labile and can be destroyed by heating to 176°F (80°C) for 30 minutes or to 212°F (100°C) for 10 minutes. At high altitudes, where the boiling point of water may be as low as 202.5°F (94.7°C), a minimum of 30 minutes of boiling may be required to destroy the toxin. Under high-altitude conditions, pressure cooking at 13–14 lb of pressure often is necessary to achieve appropriate temperatures to destroy the toxin.

Food contaminated with *C. botulinum* toxin types A and B may look or smell putrefied because of the action of proteolytic enzymes.[64] In contrast, because toxin type E organisms are saccharolytic and not proteolytic, food contaminated with toxin type E may look and taste normal.[18]

PHARMACOKINETICS AND TOXICOKINETICS

BoNT is the most poisonous substance known. The LD_{50} for mice is 3 million molecules injected intraperitoneally. The human oral lethal dose is 1 μg/kg.[117]

Foodborne botulism results from ingestion of preformed BoNT from food contaminated with *Clostridium* spores. The toxin is complexed to associated proteins (hemagglutinins and a nontoxic nonhemagglutin)[129] which protect it from the acidic and proteolytic environment in the stomach. In the intestine, the alkaline pH dissociates the toxin from the associated proteins, allowing for subsequent absorption into the bloodstream.[92] Because the toxin is often demonstrated only in the stool, determining what percentage of the toxin actually is absorbed is difficult.[52,54] The median incubation period for all patients is 1 day, but ranges from 0–7 days for toxin type A, 0–5 days for toxin type B, and 0–2 days for toxin type E.[155]

Infant botulism results not from ingestion of preformed BoNT but from ingestion of *C. botulinum* spores, which germinate in the gastrointestinal tract and produce toxin. The immaturity of the bacterial flora in the infant GI tract facilitates colonization by the *Clostridia.* Adults with altered GI flora can also develop botulism in the same way; onset of symptoms typically follows ingestion by a month or two. A single case of foodborne botulism associated with home-canned baby food has been reported in a 6-month-old infant.[6]

In wound botulism, spores proliferate in a wound or abscess and locally elaborate toxin. The incubation period is typically less than 2 weeks but may be as long as 51 days.[70]

The duration of action of the BoNT types may vary, depending on the components of the neurotransmitter release apparatus that are disrupted (see Pathophysiology). The persistence of clinical effect may result from the individual cleavage target, the intraneuronal biological half-life of the toxin, or both. Current evidence indicating intraneuronal toxin metabolism or elimination is inadequate.[128]

PATHOPHYSIOLOGY

BoNT is produced as a protein consisting of a single polypeptide chain with a molecular weight of 900 kDa, which includes a 750-kDa nontoxic protein and a 150-kDa neurotoxic component. To become fully active, the single-chain polypeptide 150-kDa neurotoxin must undergo proteolytic cleavage to generate a dichain structure consisting of a heavy chain (100 kDa) linked by a disulfide bond to a light chain (50 kDa). The dichain form of the molecule is responsible for all clinical manifestations.[67,28] It appears that both the single polypeptide chain toxin and the dichain form both are resistant to gastrointestinal degradation.[82]

The ingested toxin binds to serotype-specific receptors on the mucosal surfaces of gastric and small intestinal epithelial cells, where endocytosis followed by transcytosis permits release of the toxin on the serosal (basolateral) cell surface.[75,83] The dichain form travels intravascularly to peripheral cholinergic nerve terminals, where it binds rapidly and irreversibly to the cell membrane and is taken up by endocytosis. The heavy chain is responsible for cell-specific membrane binding to acetylcholine-containing neurons.[104]

Once inside the cell, the light chain acts as a zinc-dependent endopeptidase to cleave presynaptic membrane polypeptides that are essential components of the soluble *N*-ethylmaleimide-sensitive factor attachment receptor (SNARE) apparatus which subserves acetylcholine exocytosis, thereby inhibiting release.[117] BoNT types specifically cleave different proteins belonging to the SNARE family, and these differences may be responsible for their variable toxicity.[126] SNARE proteins targeted by proteolysis include vesicle-associated membrane protein (VAMP, also known as synaptobrevin) localized on synaptic vesicles, syntaxin found on the presynaptic membrane, and synaptosomal-associated protein (SNAP)-25 which is attached to syntaxin and to the presynaptic membrane. Toxin types A and E cleave SNAP-25; types B, D, F, and G act on VAMP/synaptobrevin; and type C cleaves both syntaxin and SNAP-25 (Fig. 46–1).[75] All BoNT types impair transmission at acetylcholine-dependent synapses in the peripheral nervous system, but cholinergic synapses in the central nervous system are not thought to be affected. Very high concentrations of BoNT can also impair release of other neurotransmitters including norepinephrine and serotonin.[63]

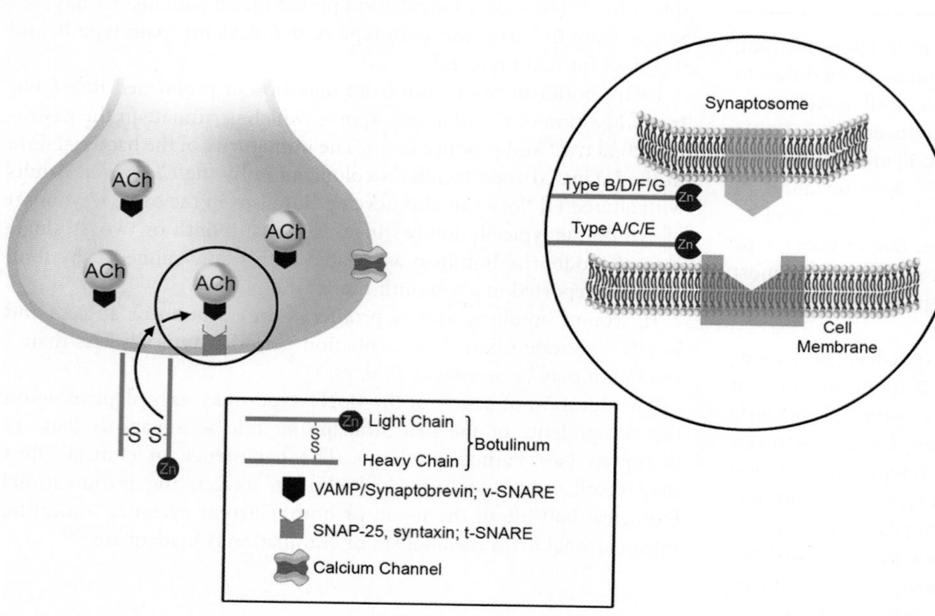

FIGURE 46–1. Botulinum toxin consists of two peptides linked by disulfide bonds. The heavy chain is responsible for specific binding to acetylcholine (ACh)-containing neurons. Following binding to the cell surface, the entire complex undergoes endocytosis and subsequent translocation of the light chain into the nerve cell cytoplasm. The light chain contains a zinc-requiring endopeptidase that cleaves proteins required by the docking/fusion complex critical to neuroexocytosis. Botulinum toxin types B , D, F, and G target the vesicle-associated soluble NSF (N-ethylmaleimide sensitive factor) attachment protein receptor (v-SNARE) protein synaptobrevin, a docking protein located on the acetylcholine-containing synaptic vesicles (synaptosome). Botulinum toxins types A , C and and E proteolyse the target associated soluble NSF attachment protein receptors (t-SNAREs) synaptosomal associated protein (SNAP)-25 and syntaxin, a component of the presynaptic cell-membrane docking complex (associated with syntaxin). After these components of the docking complex are cleaved by the endopeptidase, acetylcholine will not be released, resulting in impaired neuromuscular transmission.

CLINICAL MANIFESTATIONS

FOODBORNE BOTULISM

Although botulism is the most dreaded of all food poisonings, the initial phase of the disease (which typically occurs the day following ingestion) often is so subtle that it goes unnoticed. Botulism often is misdiagnosed on the first visit to a physician.[30,156] When gastrointestinal symptoms are striking and food poisoning is suspected, the differential diagnosis should include other acute poisonings, such as metals, plants, mushrooms, and the common bacterial, viral, and parasitic agents discussed in Chap. 45.

Early gastrointestinal signs and symptoms of botulism include nausea, vomiting, abdominal distension, and pain. A time lag (from 12 hours to several days, but typically not more than 24 hours) may be observed before neurologic signs and symptoms appear. Common findings include diplopia (often with lateral rectus palsy), blurred vision with impaired accommodation, and bilaterally symmetric flaccid paralysis which typically begins in cranial muscles and descends to the limbs. Constipation due to smooth muscle involvement is frequent, and urinary retention and ileus may also occur. Dry mouth, dysphagia, and dysarthria/dysphonia (manifested by a nasal quality to the voice) may be severe, and many patients exhibit fixed mydriatic pupils and ptosis. Deep tendon reflexes are usually reduced or absent. Hypotension and bradycardia sometimes develop, but temperature regulation is normal.

Weakness of respiratory muscles may necessitate intubation and mechanical ventilation. Approximately 67% of patients with toxin type A require intubation, compared to 52% of patients with toxin type B, and 39% with toxin type E botulism.[155]

Importantly, mental status and sensation remain normal. These negatives, along with the absence of tachycardia, distinguish botulism from the anticholinergic syndrome, which shares many features with botulism.

The differential diagnosis of botulism includes a variety of toxicologic and nontoxicologic conditions (Tables 46–1A and 46–1B). The most difficult and frequently encountered diagnostic challenge is differentiating between botulism and the Miller Fisher variant of the Guillain-Barré syndrome (Table 46–2). Because physicians so rarely encounter botulism (especially compared to other much more common diseases in the differential diagnosis), initiation of appropriate management often is seriously delayed. The index case of an epidemic or an isolated case often is misdiagnosed at a stage when the risk of morbidity and mortality still could be substantially diminished. This is particularly true of toxin type E botulism, which typically initially causes much more prominent gastrointestinal signs than neurologic signs.[18] The differences in the initial clinical symptoms associated with the various serotypes may be related to the presence of proteolytic enzymes in toxin types A and B and saccharolytic enzymes in toxin types E and C botulism.

INFANT BOTULISM

First described in California[10,68,71] in 1976, several thousand cases of infant botulism have now been confirmed across the world. Interestingly, 95% of these cases are reported in the United States.[49,101] Although infant botulism is reported from approximately half of the states in the United States and all inhabited continents except Africa,[49] 50% of reported cases originate from California, Utah, Pennsylvania, and New Mexico.[154] In California, aggressive surveillance and educational efforts have been practiced since 1976, which may help to explain the disproportionate distribution of reported cases.[7]

Infant botulism is the most common form of botulism in the United States, and 99% of cases are due to BoNT type A or B.[42] Affected children are younger than 1 year (median of 15 weeks) and characteristically have normal gestation and birth. The first signs of infant botulism are constipation; difficulty with feeding, sucking, and swallowing; feeble cry; and diffusely decreased muscle tone ("floppy baby").[40] The hypotonia is particularly apparent in the limbs and neck. Ophthalmoplegia, loss of facial grimacing, dysphagia, diminished gag reflex, poor anal sphincter tone, and respiratory failure are often

TABLE 46–1A. Differential Diagnosis of Botulism: Toxicologic Conditions

Condition	Associated Findings
Aminoglycoside poisoning	Postanesthetic paralysis, exposure to aminoglycoside antibiotics
Anticholinergic poisoning	Mydriasis, vasodilation, fever, tachycardia, ileus, dry mucosa, altered mental status
Buckthorn (*Karwinskia humboldtiana*) poisoning	Rapidly progressive ascending paralytic neuropathy with quadriplegia
Carbon monoxide poisoning	Headache, nausea, altered sensorium, tachypnea, elevated carboxyhemoglobin concentration
Diphtheria (demyelinating neuropathy)	Exudative pharyngitis, cranial polyneuropathy (late), cardiac manifestations, hypotension
Elapid (coral snake) envenomation	Euphoria, light-headedness, fasciculations, tremor, weakness, salivation, nausea, vomiting followed by bulbar palsy and paralysis including slurred speech, diplopia, ptosis, dysphagia, dyspnea, respiratory compromise
Organic phosphorus compound poisoning	Salivation, lacrimation, urination, defecation, fasciculations, bronchorrhea, delayed neuropathy
Paralytic shellfish poisoning	Incubation <1 h, dysesthesias, paresthesias, impaired mentation, respiratory paralysis
Thallium poisoning	Constipation, cranial neuropathy, ascending sensory neuropathy, Mees' lines, alopecia

present, but fever does not occur. Mydriasis is typical, and hypotension may occur. The differential diagnosis of infant botulism initially includes dehydration, failure to thrive, sepsis, and a viral syndrome. Because the toxin in infant botulism is absorbed gradually as it is produced, the onset of clinical manifestations may be less abrupt than in severe cases of foodborne botulism which are caused by large amounts of preformed toxin absorbed over a brief period of time.

Infant botulism may result from ingestion of *C. botulinum* organisms in food or following the inhalation or ingestion of organism-laden aerosolized dust. A number of factors determine a child's susceptibility to development of botulism. While bile acids and gastric acid in the gastrointestinal tract may inhibit clostridial growth in older children and adults, gastric acidity is reduced in the infant during the first few months of life.[84] Also, some infants may be deficient in immunologic mechanisms for spore control, resulting in a permissive environment for spore germination and toxin development within their gastrointestinal tracts and subsequent gut absorption. Approximately 70% of infant botulism cases occur in breastfed infants, even though only 45%–50% of all infants are breastfed. Formula-fed infants are rapidly colonized by *Coliforme* spp, *Enterococcus* spp, and *Bacteroides* spp,

TABLE 46–1B. Differential Diagnosis of Botulism: Nontoxicologic Conditions

Condition	Associated Findings
Lambert-Eaton myasthenic syndrome	Neoplasm (especially small cell lung cancer), limb weakness exceeding ocular/bulbar weakness , increased strength following sustained contractions, postexercise facilitation on repetitive nerve stimulation, antibodies to voltage-gated calcium channels
Encephalitis	Fever, mental status abnormalities, seizures CSF: elevated protein and pleocytosis
Food "poisoning" (other bacterial)	Rapid onset of disease, absence of cranial nerve findings
Guillain-Barré syndrome/ acute inflammatory demyelinating polyneuropathy (and Miller Fisher variant)	Areflexia, paresthesias, ataxia CSF: elevated protein without pleocytosis, slowed nerve conduction velocity
Hypermagnesemia	Respiratory compromise, diffuse flushing, weakness, thirst
Inflammatory myelopathies	Complete (transverse) or incomplete spinal syndrome with paraparesis and/or sensory level, back pain, may be preceded by viral illness, CSF pleocytosis
Myasthenia gravis	Aggravation of fatigue with exercise, fluctuating weakness, positive edrophonium (Tensilon) test, acetylcholine receptor antibodies, decremental response on rapid repetitive nerve stimulation
Poliomyelitis	Fever, GI symptoms, asymmetric neurologic findings CSF: elevated protein and pleocytosis
Polymyositis	Insidious onset, proximal limb weakness, dysphagia, muscle tenderness sometimes present, elevated CK, aldolase, c-reactive protein and ESR, fibrillations and sharp waves on electromyography
Stroke	Asymmetric paralysis, abnormal brain imaging
Tetanus	Rigidity, cranial nerve defects (rare)
Tick paralysis (*Dermacentor* species)	Rapidly evolving paralysis, ptosis, absence of paresthesias, normal CSF analysis, presence of an embedded tick with resolution upon removal

CK = creatine kinase; CSF = cerebrospinal fluid; ESR = erythrocyte sedimentation rate; GI = gastrointestinal.

TABLE 46–2. Differentiating Botulism from Guillain-Barré Syndrome

	Botulism	Guillain-Barré Syndrome	Miller Fisher Variant of Guillain-Barré Syndrome
Fever	Absent (except in wound botulism)	Occasionally present	Occasionally present
Pupils	Dilated or unreactive (50%)	Normal	Normal
Ophthalmoplegia	Present (early)	May be present (late)	Present (early)
Paralysis	Descending	Ascending (classically, but not necessarily)	Descending
Deep tendon reflexes	Diminished	Absent	Absent
Ataxia	Absent	Often present	Present
Paresthesias	Absent	Present	Present
CSF protein	Normal	Elevated (late)	Elevated (late)

CSF = cerebrospinal fluid.

which may inhibit *C. botulinum* proliferation; conversely, the absence of these typical organisms in breastfed infants may facilitate *C. botulinum* multiplication.[68]

Epidemiologic studies in Europe have found that ingestion of honey was associated with 59% of cases of infant botulism.[15] When *C. botulinum* spores were isolated from honey implicated in cases of infant botulism, the same toxin type was isolated from the infant and, as expected, no preformed toxin was isolated from the honey.[10] Honey is the only food generally considered likely to be a risk factor for infant botulism,[10] although a recent report from the United Kingdom implicated a milk formula in the development of infant botulism.[97] It is possible that spoiled pollen and nectar carried by worker bees results in contamination of honey with spores of *Clostridia* found in soil.[95] In addition, the oxidative metabolism of *Bacillus alvei*, another common contaminant of honey, may promote spore germination by creating a anaerobic microenvironment.[92]

Previous studies suggested a correlation between the presence of both *C. botulinum* organisms and toxin and sudden infant death syndrome (SIDS).[9,134] However, in a prospective study of 248 infants with SIDS, *C. botulinum* was not found on stool culture of any of the children.[31]

Cases of infant botulism must be managed in the hospital, preferably in a pediatric intensive care unit for at least the first week, when the risk of respiratory arrest is greatest. In one study, approximately 80% of children with botulism required intubation for reduced vital capacity, and 25% of these children had frank respiratory compromise.[119] In a group of 57 affected infants 18 days to 7 months of age managed during the decade ending in the mid-1980s, 77% were intubated and 68% required mechanical ventilation. In the subsequent decade, investigators from the same institution found that 61.7% of 60 infants required endotracheal intubation (for a mean duration of 21 days).[4] The apparent decrease in intubations and complications was ascribed to better understanding of disease progression and closer observation of patients. However, a similar study at another institution revealed that 54% of 24 infants admitted between 1985 and 1994 required ventilatory support, compared to 75% of 20 infants admitted in the subsequent decade.[144] All but one patient in this study required nasogastric feeding. Airway complications of intubation such as stridor, granuloma formation, and subglottic stenosis are common, yet tracheotomy is infrequently performed.[3] The survival rate in infant botulism is approximately 98%.[120]

WOUND BOTULISM

Wound contamination previously was considered an uncommon cause of botulism. The first case of wound botulism was not reported until 1943. The classic presentation of wound botulism is that of a patient injured in a motor vehicle who sustains a deep muscle laceration, crush injury, or compound fracture treated with open reduction. The wound typically is dirty and associated with inadequate débridement, subsequent purulent drainage, and local tenderness, although in some cases the wound appears unremarkable. Four to 18 days later, cranial nerve palsies and other neurologic findings typical of botulism may appear.[90] Other manifestations characteristic of food-related botulism, such as gastrointestinal symptoms, usually are absent.

In wound botulism, fever may be prominent and associated with abscess, sinusitis, or other tissue infection presumed to harbor the clostridial organisms. Although some patients may require management for wound-related problems, in other cases the wounds appear clean and uninfected. Recognition of botulism as a potential complication of wound infections is essential for appropriate early and aggressive therapy.

The prevalence of wound botulism has risen in recent years, predominantly in association with injection of illicit drugs, although the number of cases identified by the CDC decreased from 45 in 2006 to 22 in 2007.[42] In 2007, BoNT type A accounted for 91% of cases, while 9% were type B.[42] Use of heroin, particularly subcutaneous injection ("skin-popping") of black tar heroin, is associated with an increasing number of wound botulism cases.[43,103,115,152] This increased frequency associated appears to be related, at least in part, to the physical characteristics of black tar heroin such as its viscosity, its potential to facilitate anaerobic growth and spore germination, and its ability to devitalize tissue or inhibit wound resolution.[21] Wound botulism also has been reported in association with subcutaneous,[107] intraveneous,[137] and intranasal [74,110] cocaine use. The first case of wound botulism with BoNT type E was reported recently, affecting a drug user in Sweden.[13]

In a small series of parenteral drug-using patients with botulism in New York City, the most prominent symptoms were dysphagia, dysarthria, and dry mouth. BoNT type A toxin was detected in the serum of one patient, and in another patint *C. botulinum* was isolated from an abscess. In four other drug abusers with clinically comparable presentations, CDC investigators were not able to find any organism or toxin in serum, stool, or skin lesions.[80]

ADULT INTESTINAL COLONIZATION BOTULISM

While gastrointestinal colonization is the typical pathogenetic mechanism responsible for infant botulism, it is rare in adults. Prior to 1997 only 15 cases had been reported.[62,88] Patients invariably have anatomic or functional gastrointestinal abnormalities. Risk factors favoring organism persistence and *C. botulinum* colonization include achlorhydria (surgically or pharmacologically induced), previous intestinal surgery, and probably recent antibiotic therapy. Cases of adult infectious botulism have occurred in patients after ileal bypass surgery and Crohn disease,[22] jejunoileal bypass for obesity,[58,87] gastroduodenostomy,[87] vagotomy and pyloroplasty,[87] and necrotic volvulus.[79]

There is a well-documented case of botulism resulting from the ingestion of a food source contaminated with *C. botulinum* type A organisms and no preformed toxin.[47] In this case, the long incubation period with toxin present in the serum and stool for 3 weeks after exposure in combination with the absence of disease in the patient's spouse who shared the food suggested *in vivo* intraluminal elaboration of toxin. This patient was a very unusual host in that she had a history of peptic ulcer disease treated with truncal vagotomy, antrectomy, and a Billroth I anastomosis. She had received perioperative antibiotics 5 weeks prior to the development of botulism. All of these factors may have compromised the gastric and bile acid barrier, gut flora, and motility, thus allowing spore germination, altered bacterial growth, and toxin development.

In another case report,[62] a 67-year-old man with long-standing Crohn disease who had undergone terminal ileum and right colonic resection presented with abdominal pain. Prior to admission, the patient had experienced several episodes of diplopia. After admission, systemic paralysis developed. The patient had a prolonged recovery after receiving two courses of equine trivalent (ABE) botulinum antitoxin and 81 days of antibiotic treatment. Of note, a high concentration of endogenously produced antibody to toxin type A was identified. This finding highlights a distinct characteristic of adult intestinal colonization botulism, as endogenous antitoxin immunity does not develop in patients with foodborne botulism.[117]

IATROGENIC BOTULISM

Two preparations of BoNT are available in the United States: botulinum toxin type A (Botox [also available in Europe as Dysport]) and botulinum toxin type B (Myobloc). The therapeutic use of BoNT injections in humans was first investigated in the 1970s, and the FDA approved BoNT type A for the treatment of strabismus and blepharospasm in 1989. Subsequently, both types A and B were approved for treatment of cervical dystonia. A 1990 consensus statement by the National Institutes of Health recommended treatment with BoNT for patients with blepharospasm, adductor spasmodic dysphonia, jaw-closing oromandibular dystonia, and cervical dystonia.[96] BoNT type A is approved by the FDA for treatment of cervical dystonia, facial nerve disorders, strabismus, axillary hyperhidrosis, and for cosmetic use to minimize wrinkles; BoNT type B is FDA-approved for cervical dystonia. BoNTs are also used off-label for treatment of a variety of conditions such as spasticity, migraine, achalasia, and anal fissure.

These xenobiotics are thought to exert their therapeutic effect in most cases by causing temporary weakness in muscles whose overactivity results in the clinical condition. Doses range widely depending on the size of the muscle to be treated, the degree of weakness required, and the commercial preparation of the toxin. The injected toxin blocks the local neuromuscular junction by inhibiting release of acetylcholine. The "chemodenervated" muscles recover within 2–4 months as nerve transmission is restored through sprouting of new nerve endings and formation of functional connections at motor endplates,[2,117] necessitating repeated injections of BoNT for prolonged clinical efficacy.

Doses of BoNT are measured in functional units corresponding to the median intraperitoneal lethal dose (LD_{50}) in female Swiss-Webster mice weighing 18–20 grams.[102] The units of each marketed xenobiotic are distinctly different and may confuse the clinician, leading to inadvertent overdosing.[33] The potential for confusion may be substantial when switching between type A and type B BoNT, because their relative potencies are quite different.[98,113,122] As an approximation,

TABLE 46–3. Botulinum Toxin Type A (OnabotulinumtoxinA®)[11,56,115,120] Approximate Human LD_{50}

Route of Exposure	Approximate LD_{50} in Humans
Intravenous	0.09–0.15 μg ≅ 36–60 Units
Inhaled	0.70–0.90 μg ≅ 280–360 Units
Intramuscular	7.0 μg ≅ 2800 Units
Intraperitoneal	7.5 μg ≅ 3000 Units
Oral	70 μg ≅ 28,000 Units

1 Unit Botox® ≅ 2.5 ng botulinum toxin type A.

1 Unit of Botox (onabotulinumtoxinA) is roughly equivalent to 50 Units of Myobloc (rimabotulinumtoxinB) or 3–5 Units of Dysport (abobotulinumtoxinA).[29,141] Estimated quantities of type A BoNT lethal to humans by different routes of administration are given in Table 46–3.

Although one early marketing assumption was that the neurotoxin does not diffuse from the injection site, BoNT does diffuse into adjacent tissues and produce local adverse effects.[111] Systemic manifestations are of concern when an inadvertent, excessive, or misdirected dose of toxin is administered, or in the setting of a neuromuscular disorder which may be previously undiagnosed, as in one case in which injection of BoNT type A unmasked Lambert-Eaton myasthenic syndrome[53]. In addition, a number of studies demonstrate that even appropriately injected doses result in neuromuscular junction abnormalities throughout the body, occasionally producing autonomic dysfunction without muscle weakness.[59,76,99] Several cases of iatrogenic botulism-like symptoms, including diplopia and severe generalized muscle weakness with widespread electromyographic abnormalities, have resulted from therapeutic doses of intramuscular BoNT injections.[19,24,145] A very recent report raised the possibility that BoNT type A may undergo retrograde axonal transport and transcytosis to afferent neurons,[5] suggesting a potential mechanism for such generalized effects. However, the reproducibility and clinical significance of these findings have yet to be established.

In a large series of 139 patients with cervical dystonia randomized to treatment with BoNT type A or BoNT type B, no difference in efficacy was found between serotypes; the groups were also equivalent in frequency of adverse effects such as neck pain and neck weakness, but dry mouth and dysphagia were more common in the group treated with BoNT type B.[50]

Following repeated injections of therapeutic doses of BoNT, patients may develop neutralizing antibodies that subsequently may limit the toxin's efficacy; this situation should prompt a clinician to switch to use of a different toxin type.[28] In Japan and the United Kingdom, a preparation of BoNT type F is available for use when antibodies to type A develop.[125] Some studies suggest that animals receiving BoNT type F have more transient and reversible weakness than that associated with types A and B.[26] In 1998, the formulation of Botox was changed to reduce the amount of potentially antigenic protein, and studies in rabbits demonstrate a much lower rate of development of anti-BoNT antibodies with the new batch compared with the previous preparation.[23]

In a well-publicized case in late 2004, four patients in Florida developed paralysis after being injected with BoNT type A. An FDA investigation revealed that these patients were injected by an unlicensed physician who obtained raw toxin (not approved for medical purposes) and administered it at a dose 2000 to 100,000 times greater than that used in clinical practice.[3] These events were not felt to be relevant to the approved uses of medicinal BoNT. In February 2008, the FDA issued an Early Communication stating that it is reviewing safety data on Botox (onabotulinumtoxinA) and Myobloc (rimabotulinumtoxinB) after receiving reports of hospitalization or death in patients injected with these agents, mostly in children treated for cerebral palsy–associated spasticity;[147] this review is ongoing as of the time of this writing.

INHALATIONAL BOTULISM

Inhaled BoNT is estimated to be 100 times more potent than orally ingested BoNT; a single gram of toxin, if disseminated evenly, could kill more than 1 million people.[11] A 1962 report from West Germany described three veterinary workers who inhaled BoNT type A from the fur of animals they were handling; on the third day after exposure they developed mucus in the throat, dysphagia, and dizziness, while on the next day they developed ophthalmoparesis, mydriasis, dysarthria, gait dysfunction, and weakness.[11] Use of aerosolized BoNT as a bioweapon has been attempted by terrorists in Japan, and Iraq has developed BoNT (along with anthrax and aflatoxin) as part of a biological warfare program.[11,157] (see Chap. 132)

DIAGNOSTIC TESTING

The CDC case definition for foodborne botulism is established in a patient with a neurologic disorder manifested by diplopia, blurred vision, bulbar weakness, and symmetric paralysis in whom[36]

- BoNT is detected in serum, stool, or implicated food samples; or
- *C. botulinum* is isolated from stool; or
- A clinically compatible case is epidemiologically linked to a laboratory-confirmed case of botulism.

Routine laboratory studies, including CSF analysis, are normal in patients with botulism. Specific tests that can be helpful in diagnosing botulism are discussed below.

TENSILON TESTING

Edrophonium (Tensilon) is a rapidly acting and short-acting cholinesterase inhibitor that can be useful in the diagnosis of myasthenia gravis. It is occasionally used to differentiate myasthenia gravis from botulism. This drug inhibits the metabolism of acetylcholine located in synapses, permitting continued binding with the reduced number of postsynaptic acetylcholine receptors in myasthenia gravis.

A syringe containing 10 mg of edrophonium is prepared, and then a test dose of 1–2 mg is administered intravenously. A positive result (ie, consistent with myasthenia gravis) consists of dramatic improvement in the strength of weak muscles within 30–60 seconds, lasting 3–5 minutes. If there is no effect, the remainder of the edrophonium is given and the same effect sought. Ideally, a second syringe is filled with saline and the test performed under double-blind conditions.

Because release of acetylcholine is impaired in botulism, preventing its metabolism has little clinical effect. In rare cases, early in the course of botulism injection of edrophonium results in limited improvement in strength that is far less dramatic than occurs in patients with myasthenia gravis.[105] Anticholinesterase drugs such as edrophonium have no effect on the action of BoNT but may affect patients clinically if some cells can still release acetylcholine.

ELECTROPHYSIOLOGIC TESTING

In all forms of botulism, sensory nerve action potentials are normal. Motor potentials are typically reduced in amplitude (although this reduction may not be appreciated unless severely affected muscles are studied), but conduction velocity is not affected. Repetitive nerve stimulation at high frequencies would be expected to result in an increment of the amplitude of the motor potential, given the presynaptic localization of the defect, but this finding is neither sensitive nor specific; it may be more common in disease due to BoNT type B than with type A.[46,85] A marked incremental response is more likely to suggest Lambert-Eaton myasthenic syndrome (LEMS) than botulism. Likewise, a decremental response to low-frequency repetitive nerve stimulation is characteristic of LEMS but is not consistently present in botulism.[85]

The needle electromyography (EMG) examination in botulism is characterized by low-amplitude, short-duration motor unit action potentials (MUAPs), due to blockade of neuromuscular transmission in many muscle fibers (Fig. 46–2). Polyphasic MUAPs are also common. Recruitment is usually normal but may be reduced in severely affected muscles if all muscle fibers of a motor unit are blocked. Spontaneous activity, including positive sharp waves and fibrillation potentials, is often seen.

Although these electrodiagnostic abnormalities can support the diagnosis of botulism, they can be subtle. Nerve conduction studies and EMG are most useful in their ability to exclude differential diagnostic considerations, including Guillain-Barré syndrome and other neuropathies (both demyelinating and axonal), poliomyelitis, and myasthenia gravis. Moreover, there are no pathognomonic electrophysiologic findings in botulism; in particular, the findings can closely resemble those of a myopathic process, and muscle biopsy may be necessary to exclude such a condition.[85]

LABORATORY TESTING

Samples of serum, stool, vomitus, gastric contents, and suspected foods should be subjected to anaerobic culture (for *C. botulinum*) and mouse bioassay (for BoNT) (Table 46–4). A list of the patient's medications should accompany each sample to exclude other xenobiotics that might interfere with the assay (eg, pyridostigmine) or be toxic to the mice. The serum samples must be collected prior to initiation of antitoxin therapy. If wound botulism is suspected, serum, stool, exudate, débrided tissue, and swab samples should be collected. For infant botulism, feces and serum samples also should be obtained. Infants who are constipated may require an enema with nonbacteriostatic sterile

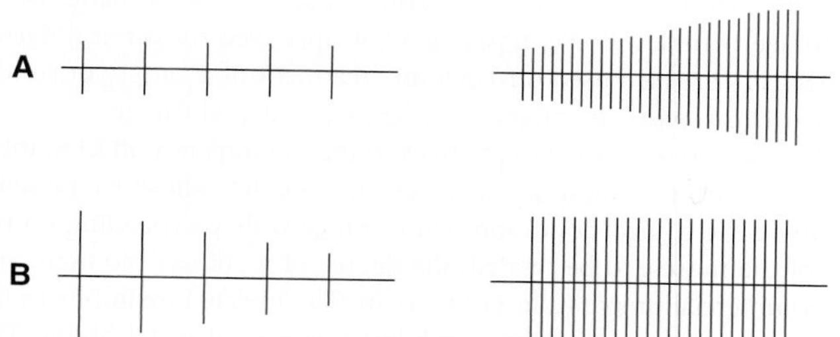

FIGURE 46–2. Electromyographic findings. Schematic representations of repetitive nerve stimulation at low (5/sec) and high (50/sec) frequencies. In botulism (**A**), repetitive stimulation produces a small-muscle action potential that facilitates (increases in amplitude) at higher frequencies. This effect (which, although classic, is not found in all cases of botulism) results from increased acetylcholine release with high-frequency stimulation because of intracellular calcium accumulation. In contrast, myasthenia gravis (**B**) is associated with a normal muscle action potential amplitude and a decremental response at low-frequency stimulation with a normal response at high-frequency stimulation. Myasthenia gravis, a disorder of the muscle end plate, produces this decremental response at low frequencies because the natural reduction in acetylcholine response with subsequent stimulation falls below threshold.[105,148]

TABLE 46–4. Epidemiologic and Laboratory Assessment of Botulism

Classification	Foodborne	Infant	Wound	Adult Intestinal Colonization
Toxin type	A, B, E, F, G in humans; C, D in animals	A, B, C, F	A, B	A
Route	Ingestion of toxin	Ingestion of bacteria and spores	Wound, abscess (sinusitis)	Ingestion of bacteria and spores
Specimens	Stool: positive for bacteria/spores and toxin	Stool: positive for bacteria/spores and toxin for up to 8 weeks after recovery	Wound site: Gram stain, aerobic and anaerobic cultures; positive for bacteria/spores	Stool: positive for bacteria/spores and toxin
Botulinum toxin in serum	Yes	Yes	Yes	Yes
Bacteria/spores in food	Yes	Yes	No	Yes
Botulinum toxin in food	Yes	No	No	No

"Toxin" refers to botulinum toxin. "Bacteria/spores" refers to *C. botulinum*.

water to facilitate collection. All enema fluid and stool should be sent for analysis. The specimens should be refrigerated (not frozen) and examined as soon as possible after collection. Detailed information on specimen collection and examination is available online from the CDC (http://www.cdc.gov/ncidod/dbmd/diseaseinfo/files/botulism.pdf).[38]

In the mouse lethality assay, the standard test for detecting BoNT, the sample (serum, stool, or food) is injected intraperitoneally into mice which are then observed for development of signs of botulism. Control mice are injected with the sample as well as antitoxin. This test is very sensitive, with a detection limit of 0.01 ng/mL of sample eluate. However, it is laborious, expensive, and a positive result may not appear for several days, reducing its usefulness in early diagnosis of botulism.[78] Alternative methods for detecting BoNT, including immunological methods (eg, enzyme-linked immunosorbent assay [ELISA]) and endopeptidase assays, are being explored.[78]

C. botulinum can be cultured under strict anaerobic conditions. Stool specimens are incubated anaerobically and then subcultured on egg yolk agar to assess for lipase production, although this test is not specific as other clostridia also produce lipase. Numerous protocols using polymerase chain reaction and probe hybridization to detect and identify *C. botulinum* are described but these have not yet been applied widely in clinical practice.[78]

MANAGEMENT

SUPPORTIVE CARE

Respiratory compromise is the usual cause of death from botulism. To prevent or treat this complication, hospital admission of the patient and of all individuals with suspected exposure is mandatory. Careful continuous monitoring of respiratory status using parameters such as vital capacity, peak expiratory flow rate, negative inspiratory force (NIF), pulse oximetry, and the presence or absence of a gag reflex is essential to determine the need for intubation or tracheostomy, as the patient begins to manifest signs of bulbar paralysis.[119] The most reliable, readily obtainable test is the NIF, which can be used in most institutions to determine the need for intubation. When suspicion of disease is high, and the vital capacity is less than 30% of predicted or the NIF is less than –30 cm H_2O, intubation should be strongly considered.[89,139]

Reverse Trendelenburg positioning at 20°–25° with cervical support has been suggested to be beneficial by enhancing diaphragmatic function, but the clinical application to seriously ill patients has not been validated.[11] This approach may reduce the risk of aspiration while decreasing the pressure of abdominal viscera on the diaphragm, with resultant improvement in ventilatory effort.

In addition to attention to respiratory issues, patients require nutrition (enteral or parenteral) and prompt recognition and treatment of secondary infections.

GASTRIC DECONTAMINATION

An attempt should be made to remove the spores and toxin from the gut. Although most patients present after a substantial time delay, the etiologic agent may still be present hours or even days later. Activated charcoal should be a routine part of supportive care, because in vitro it adsorbs BoNT type A and probably also the other BoNT types.[60] Gastric lavage or emesis should be initiated only for an asymptomatic person who has very recently ingested a known contaminated food. If a cathartic is chosen, sorbitol is the preferable agent because others such as magnesium salts may exacerbate neuromuscular blockade. Theoretically, whole-bowel irrigation may have a role in decontamination, particularly if there is concern about initiating emesis, but interventions other than activated charcoal have not been evaluated under these circumstances.

WOUND CARE

Thorough wound débridement is the most critical aspect in the management of wound botulism and should be performed promptly.[70,79] Antibiotic therapy alone is inadequate, as evidenced by several case reports of disease despite antibiotic therapy. Aminoglycoside antibiotics[116] and clindamycin[121] should not be used because they may interfere with neuromuscular transmission.

Penicillin G is one of many drugs with excellent in vitro antimicrobial efficacy against *C. botulinum* and is useful for wound management.[138] However, penicillin has no role in the management of botulism caused by preformed toxin, nor does it prevent gut spores from germinating. For these reasons, penicillin is not considered useful in infant and adult infectious botulism, and it is not by itself considered adequate for wound botulism.

GUANIDINE, 4-AMINOPYRIDINE, AND 3,4-DIAMINOPYRIDINE

Guanidine is no longer recommended for treatment of botulism, because its merits were not substantiated.[55,72] (See previous editions of this text for a more extensive discussion.) Several studies[114] and case reports[51] have proposed that 4-aminopyridine and 3,4-diaminopyridine are effective in improving neuromuscular transmission by enhancing acetylcholine release from the motor nerve terminal.[114] In a rat BoNT type A model, 3,4-diaminopyridine restored neuromuscular function and enhanced animal survival.[127] The therapeutic efforts for those with LEMS and the successful animal results all suggest that further investigative efforts are necessary. The potential of 4-aminopyridine to induce seizures at therapeutic doses limits its clinical usefulness. The fact that 3,4-diaminopyridine does not substantially cross the blood–brain barrier, resulting in limited CNS manifestations, makes this xenobiotic appropriate for further investigation.

BOTULINUM ANTITOXIN

Since the 1960s, passive immunization with antitoxin has been used to neutralize unbound BoNT. In the United States, the CDC supplies equine-derived antitoxin through state and (except in California and Alaska) local health departments. It is indicated for patients with foodborne or wound botulism. Currently, the CDC formulary includes a bivalent antitoxin effective against BoNT types A and B, and an antitoxin against type E is available as an investigational product.[39] A trivalent (ABE) antitoxin that was used in the past is not currently available. A heptavalent (ABCDEFG) antitoxin has been developed by the US Army on an investigational basis; its efficacy has yet to be elucidated.[11,69] Although the antitoxins are highly serotype specific, type E antitoxin may have partial neutralizing potential against BoNT type F; in disease due to type F, use of type E antitoxin may be warranted.[65,88,108]

In a review of 132 cases of type A foodborne botulism, a lower fatality rate and a shorter course of illness were demonstrated for patients who received trivalent antitoxin, even after controlling for age and incubation period.[139] The earlier a patient received antitoxin, the shorter was the clinical course. In addition, no respiratory arrests occurred more than 5 hours after antitoxin was administered. Two studies on the use of antitoxin in the presence of wound botulism demonstrated that the longer the delay to antitoxin administration, the more prolonged the requirement for ventilatory support and the poorer the outcome.[45] Consequently, antitoxin should be requested from the CDC at the time the diagnosis of botulism is first suspected.

Unless the BoNT serotype is known, permitting type-specific therapy, combined therapy with both bivalent AB antitoxin (7500 U type A, 5500 U type B) and E antitoxin (5000 U type E) should be used for foodborne botulism. Bivalent antitoxin AB should be used for presumptive wound botulism. The entire 10-mL vial of antitoxin should be given intravenously as a 1:10 vol/vol dilution in 0.9% sodium chloride over several minutes. Because antitoxin is an equine globulin preparation, hypersensitivity skin testing for horse serum should be performed prior to treatment, with desensitization of patients who exhibit a wheal-and-flare response (as described in the antitoxin package insert[16,17]). Epinephrine and diphenhydramine should always be readily available to treat anaphylaxis or hypersensitivity reactions. The overall rate of adverse reactions, including hypersensitivity and serum sickness,[27] is reported as 9%–17%, with an incidence of anaphylaxis as high as 1.9%.[18,91] In recent years, the frequency of serious reactions in patient treated with a single vial of antitoxin is less than 1%.[132] Because the amount of antibody in each vial far exceeds the quantity needed to neutralize all BoNT in the serum, and because the antitoxin has a circulating half-life of 5 to 8 days, repeat treatment is usually not needed.[38]

BoNT antitoxin neutralizes only unbound toxin, and consequently can prevent paralysis but does not affect already paralyzed muscles.[57] Due to the high mortality rate associated with foodborne botulism, the antitoxin should be given to patients in whom the diagnosis is suspected; treatment should not be delayed while awaiting laboratory confirmation of the diagnosis. In the event of a potential outbreak of foodborne botulism, asymptomatic individuals should be closely monitored for early signs of illness so that antitoxin can be administered promptly.[124] (see A8 Botulinum Antitoxin)

TREATMENT OF INFANT BOTULISM

Like adults, infants with botulism require intensive care, with meticulous monitoring for respiratory compromise. Autonomic dysfunction may also occur. Constipation may be severe.

Equine-derived antitoxin is not recommended in infant botulism because of doubtful efficacy as well as safety concerns.[38,71,77,118] In October 2003 the FDA licensed human-derived botulism immune globulin (BIG) as BabyBIG for treatment of infant botulism.[8] A randomized trial of 122 cases of infant botulism showed that treatment with intravenous BIG significantly reduced the length of hospital stay and intensive care, duration of mechanical ventilation and tube or intravenous feeding, and cost of hospitalization relative to placebo, without causing serious adverse effects.[12,56] Similar results were seen in a recent retrospective chart review.[146] BabyBIG is available from the California Department of Health Services Infant Botulism Treatment and Prevention Program.[32]

PREVENTION

Measures used to prevent infant botulism include limiting exposure to spores by thoroughly washing foods and objects that might be placed in a child's mouth. In addition, honey should not be given to infants younger than 6 months.

A pentavalent (ABCDE) botulinum toxoid is available as an investigational new drug; the CDC recommends immunization for laboratory personnel working with *C. botulinum* or BoNTs, as well as military personnel at risk of exposure.[39] Numerous vaccination strategies are under investigation, including several recombinant vaccines that have shown promise in protecting against botulism in animal and human trials.[20,131]

PROGNOSIS

The prolonged and variable period of recovery that occurs after exposure to BoNT is directly related to the extent of neuromuscular blockade and neurogenic atrophy as well as the regeneration rates of nerve endings and presynaptic membranes.[86] If the patient has excellent respiratory support during the acute phase and receives adequate parenteral nutrition, residual neurologic disability may not occur. Although the initial course may be protracted, near-total functional recovery can follow within several months to 1 year. Common long-term sequelae include dysgeusia, dry mouth, constipation, dyspepsia, arthralgia, exertional dyspnea, tachycardia, and easy fatigability.

The status of 13 patients who survived a toxin type B botulinum outbreak was characterized 2 years later by persistent dyspnea and fatigue, although surprisingly, pulmonary function tests had returned to normal in all patients.[152] Inspiratory muscle weakness persisted in 4 of 13 patients. Maximal oxygen consumption and maximal workload during exercise were diminished in all patients, and all had more rapid shallow breathing and a higher dyspnea score than controls. The reasons for premature exercise termination may be multifactorial. Although persistent respiratory muscle weakness may be an explanation, most dyspnea and fatigue appeared to be related to reduced cardiovascular fitness, leg fatigue, and diminished nutrition.[153]

A recent case-control series reported long-term outcomes in 217 adults with foodborne botulism in the Republic of Georgia. Six patients died; the remaining 211 were interviewed a median of 4.3 years after onset of disease. They were significantly more likely than control subjects to report ongoing fatigue, dizziness, weakness, dry mouth, difficulty lifting things, and difficulty breathing with moderate exertion.[61]

PREGNANCY

At least three cases of botulism occurring during pregnancy have been reported. One case occurred during the second trimester,[109] and two cases occurred during the third trimester.[135] Although in two cases BoNT or *C. botulinum* was isolated from the mother prior to administration of antitoxin therapy, no detectable toxin was isolated from the neonates in either of the third-trimester cases. The large molecular weight of the neurotoxin (150 kDa) makes passive diffusion through the placenta unlikely,[67] and, although theoretically possible, no active transport system has been identified.[135] None of the three neonates had neurologic evidence of botulism. Appropriate care of the mother and preparation for maternal complications of delivery appear to assure the best potential outcome for the infant.

A recent survey of physicians identified 16 women who were treated with BoNT type A during 19 pregnancies. (One patient was injected while carrying twins, and another was treated during three separate singleton pregnancies.) One patient who received a single session of 300 U of BoNT for cervical dystonia miscarried; she had a history of previous miscarriages. Another patient underwent a therapeutic abortion. No other complications occurred. Nevertheless, the authors "do not recommend injection of pregnant women … until more data are available."[93] Botox (onabotulinumtoxinA) and Myobloc (rimabotulinumtoxinB) are both FDA pregnancy category C. Additionally, it is unknown whether BoNT is excreted in breast milk.

EPIDEMIOLOGIC AND THERAPEUTIC ASSISTANCE

Whenever botulism is suspected or proven, the local health department should be contacted. The health department should report to the CDC Emergency Operations Center at 770-488-7100. The CDC can provide or facilitate diagnostic, consultative, and laboratory testing services, access to botulinum antitoxin, and assistance in epidemiologic investigations. All foods that are potentially responsible for the illness should be refrigerated and preserved for epidemiologic investigation. The merits of this surveillance and antitoxin release system were demonstrated in Argentina,[149] where the CDC assisted in establishing nation-specific principles, including local stocking of antitoxin and establishing mechanisms for distribution, emergency identification, response, and laboratory confirmation of suspected cases. Expansion of this system to other nations will enhance worldwide botulism surveillance for foodborne botulism and for potential terrorist dissemination of BoNT.[123]

SUMMARY

Botulism remains one of the rarest poisonings, yet its etiologies have become increasingly diverse. The incidence of wound botulism has increased dramatically. Previously unrecognized complications of therapeutic BoNT use now permit a better understanding of the effects of the toxin and an appreciation of its risks. The international experience with botulism epidemics has allowed the CDC to enhance epidemiologic surveillance and to prepare for the possible use of BoNT as a biologic weapon. Promising treatment strategies currently being developed include recombinant vaccines and other creative advances.

ACKNOWLEDGMENT

Neal E. Flomenbaum contributed to this chapter in previous editions.

REFERENCES

1. Abgueguen P, Delbos V, Chennebault JM, et al. Nine cases of foodborne botulism type B in France and literature review. *Eur J Clin Microbiol Infect Dis.* 2003;22:749-752.
2. Alderson K, Holds JB, Anderson RL. Botulinum-induced alteration of nerve-muscle interactions in human orbicularis oculi following treatment for blepharospasm. *Neurology.* 1991;41:1800-1805.
3. Allergan. Allergan's BOTOX — botulinum toxin type A — not the cause of botulism in Florida patients. http://agn360.client.shareholder.com/releasedetail.cfm?ReleaseID=150344. Accessed June 1, 2008.
4. Anderson TD, Shah UK, Schreiner MS, et al. Airway complications of infant botulism: ten-year experience with 60 cases. *Otolaryngol Head Neck Surg.* 2002;126:234-239.
5. Antonucci F, Rossi C, Gianfranceschi L, et al. Long-distance retrograde effects of botulinum neurotoxin A. *J Neurosci.* 2008;28:3689-3696.
6. Armada M, Love S, Barrett E, et al. Foodborne botulism in a six-month-old infant caused by home-canned baby food. *Ann Emerg Med.* 2003;42:226-229.
7. Arnon SS. Infant botulism. In: Feigen RD, Cherry JD, eds. *Textbook of Infectious Diseases,* 4th ed. Philadelphia: WB Saunders;, 1998;1570-1577.
8. Arnon SS. Creation and development of the public service orphan drug Human Botulism Immune Globulin. *Pediatrics.* 2007;119;785-789.
9. Arnon SS, Damus K, Chin J. Infant botulism: epidemiology and relation to sudden infant death syndrome. *Epidemiol Rev.* 1981;3:45-66.
10. Arnon SS, Midura TF, Damus K, et al. Honey and other environmental risk factors for infant botulism. *J Pediatr.* 1979;94:331-336.
11. Arnon SS, Schechter R, Inglesby TV, et al. Botulinum toxin as a biological weapon: medical and public health management. *JAMA.* 2001;285:1059-1070.
12. Arnon SS, Schechter R, Maslanka SE, et al. Human Botulism Immune Globulin for the treatment of infant botulism. *N Engl J Med.* 2006;354:462-71.
13. Artin I, Björkman P, Cronqvist J, et al. First case of type E wound botulism diagnosed using real-time PCR. *J Clin Microbiol.* 2007;4:3589-3594.
14. Aureli P, Di Cunto M, Maffei A, et al. An outbreak in Italy of botulism associated with a dessert made with mascarpone cream cheese. *Eur J Epidemiol.* 2000;16:913-918.
15. Aureli P, Franciosa G, Fenicia L. Infant botulism and honey in Europe: a commentary. *Ped Inf Dis J.* 2002;21:866-868.
16. Aventis Pasteur. Botulinum antitoxin bivalent (equine) types A and B (package insert). 1997.
17. Aventis Pasteur. Botulinum antitoxin (equine) type E (package insert). 1999.
18. Badhey H, Cleri DJ, D'Amato RF, et al. Two fatal cases of type E adult foodborne botulism with early symptoms and terminal neurologic signs. *J Clin Microbiol.* 1986;23:616-618.
19. Bakheit AMO, Ward CD, McLellan DL. Generalised botulism-like syndrome after intramuscular injections of botulinum toxin type A: a report of two cases. *J Neurol Neurosurg Psychiatry.* 1997;62:198.
20. Baldwin MR, Tepp WH, Przedpelski A. Subunit vaccine against the seven serotypes of botulism. *Infect Immun.* 2008;76:1314-1318.
21. Bamberger J, Terplan M. Wound botulism associated with black tar heroin. *JAMA.* 1998;280:1479-1480.
22. Bartlett JC. Infant botulism in adults. *N Engl J Med.* 1986;315:254-255.
23. Benedetto, AV. The cosmetic uses of Botulinum toxin type A. *Int J Dermatol.* 1999;38:641-655.
24. Bhatia KP, Münchau A, Thompson PD, et al. Generalised muscular weakness after botulinum toxin injections for dystonia: a report of three cases. *J Neurol Neurosurg Psychiatry.* 1999;67:90-93.

25. Bieri PL. Botulinum neurotoxin. In: Spencer PS, Schaumburg HH, eds.: *Experimental and Clinical Neurotoxicology*, 2nd ed. New York: Oxford University Press; 2000:243-253.
26. Billante CR, Zealear DL, Billante M, et al. Comparison of neuromuscular blockade and recovery with botulinum toxins A and F. *Muscle Nerve.* 2002;26:395-403.
27. Black RE, Gunn RA. Hypersensitivity reactions associated with botulinal antitoxin. *Am J Med.* 1980;69:567-570.
28. Borodic GE, Pearce LB. New concepts in botulinum toxin therapy. *Drug Saf.* 1994;11:145-152.
29. Brashear A, Lew MF, Dykstra DD, et al. Safety and efficacy of NeuroBloc (botulinum toxin type B) in type A-responsive cervical dystonia. *Neurology.* 1999;53:1439-1446.
30. Burningham MD, Walter FG, Mechem C, et al. Wound botulism. *Ann Emerg Med.* 1994;24:1184-1187.
31. Byard RW, Moore L, Bourne AJ, et al. *Clostridium botulinum* and sudden infant death syndrome: a 10-year prospective study. *J Paediatr Child Health.* 1992;28:157-157.
32. California Department of Health Services Infant Botulism Treatment and Prevention Program. http://www.infantbotulism.org. Accessed June 1, 2008.
33. Callaway JE, Arezzo JC, Grethlein AJ. Botulinum toxin type B: an overview of its biochemistry and preclinical pharmacology. *Semin Cutan Med Surg.* 2001;20:127-136.
34. Centers for Disease Control and Prevention. International outbreak of type E botulism associated with ungutted, salted white fish. *MMWR Morb Mortal Wkly Rep.* 1987;36:812-813.
35. Centers for Disease Control and Prevention. Outbreak of type E botulism associated with an uneviscerated, salt-cured fish product: New Jersey, 1992. *MMWR Morb Mortal Wkly Rep.* 1992;41:521-522.
36. Centers for Disease Control and Prevention. Case definitions for infectious conditions under public health surveillance—recommendations and report. *MMWR Morb Mortal Wkly Rep.* 1997;46(RR10):1-55.
37. Centers for Disease Control and Prevention. Botulism associated with commercial carrot juice—Georgia and Florida, September 2006. *MMWR Morb Mortal Wkly Rep.* 2006;55:1098-1099.
38. Centers for Disease Control and Prevention. Botulism in the United States, 1899-1996. *Handbook for Epidemiologists, Clinicians and Laboratory Workers.* Atlanta: Centers for Disease Control and Prevention; 1998.
39. Centers for Disease Control and Prevention. Drug Service: Formulary: Products distributed by the Centers for Disease Control and Prevention. http://www.cdc.gov/ncidod/srp/drugs/formulary.html. Accessed January 14, 2009.
40. Centers for Disease Control and Prevention. Infant Botulism—New York City, 2001-2002. *MMWR Morb Mortal Wkly Rep.* 2003;52: 21-24.
41. Centers for Disease Control and Prevention. Outbreak of botulism type E associated with eating a beached whale—Western Alaska, July 2002. *MMWR Morb Mortal Wkly Rep.* 2003;52:24-26.
42. Centers for Disease Control and Prevention. Summary of botulism cases reported in 2007. http://www.cdc.gov/nationalsurveillance/PDFs/Botulism_CSTE_2007.pdf. Accessed January 14, 2009.
43. Centers for Disease Control and Prevention. Wound botulism among black tar heroin users—Washington, 2003. *MMWR Morb Mortal Wkly Rep.* 2003;52:885-886.
44. Centers for Disease Control and Prevention. Botulism associated with commercially canned chili sauce—Texas and Indiana, July 2007. *MMWR Morb Mortal Wkly Rep.* 2007;56:767-769.
45. Chang GY, Ganguly G. Early antitoxin treatment in wound botulism results in better outcome. *Eur Neurol.* 2003;49:151-153.
46. Cherington M. Electrophysiologic methods as an aid in the diagnosis of botulism: a review. *Muscle Nerve.* 1982;5(suppl):S28-S29.
47. Chia JK, Clark JB, Ryan CA, et al. Botulism in an adult associated with foodborne intestinal infection with *Clostridium botulinum. N Engl J Med.* 1986;315:239-241.
48. Chiou LA, Hennessy TW, Horn A, et al. Botulism among Alaska natives in the Bristol Bay area of Southwest Alaska. *Int J Circumpolar Health.* 2002;61:50-60.
49. Cochran DP, Appleton RE. Infant botulism—is it that rare? *Dev Med Child Neurol.* 1995;37:274-278.
50. Comella CL, Jankovic J, Shannon KM, et al. Comparison of botulinum toxin serotypes A and B for the treatment of cervical dystonia. *Neurology.* 2005;65:1423-1429.
51. Dock M, Ben-Ali A, Karras A, et al. Traitement d'un botulisme grave par la 3,4-diaminopyridine. *Presse Med.* 2002;31:601-602.
52. Dowell Jr. UR, McCroskey LM, Hatheway CL, et al. Coproexamination for botulinal toxin and *Clostridium botulism. JAMA.* 1977;238: 1829-1832.
53. Erbguth F, Claus D, Engelhardt A, et al. Systemic effect of local botulinum toxin injections unmasks subclinical Lambert-Eaton myasthenic syndrome. *J Neurol Neurosurg Psychiatry.* 1993;56:1235-1236.
54. Fach P, Gilbert M, Griffais R, et al. PCR and gene probe identification of botulinum neurotoxin A-, B-, E-, F-, and G-producing *Clostridium* spp. and evaluation in food samples. *Appl Environ Microbiol.* 1995;61: 1389-1392.
55. Faich GA, Graebner RW, Sato S. Failure of guanidine therapy in botulism A. *N Engl J Med.* 1971;285:773-776.
56. Frankovich TL, Arnon SS. Clinical trial of botulism immune globulin for infant botulism. *West J Med.* 1991;154:103.
57. Franz DR, Pitt LM, Clayton MA, et al. Efficacy of prophylactic and therapeutic administration of antitoxin for inhalation botulism. In: Das-Gupta BR, ed. *Botulinum and Tetanus Neurotoxins: Neurotransmission and Biomedical Aspects.* New York: Plenum Press; 1993; 473–476.
58. Freedman M, Armstrong RM, Killian JM, Boland D. Botulism in a patient with jejunoileal bypass. *Ann Neurol.* 1986;20:641-643.
59. Girlanda P, Vita G, Nicolosi C, et al. Botulinum toxin therapy: distant effects on neuromuscular transmission and autonomic nervous system. *J Neurol Neurosurg Psychiatry.* 1992;55:844-845.
60. Gomez HF, Johnson R, Guven H, et al. Adsorption of botulinum toxin to activated charcoal with a mouse bioassay. *Ann Emerg Med.* 1995;25: 818-822.
61. Gottlieb SL, Kretsinger K, Tarkhashvili N, et al. Long-term outcomes of 217 botulism cases in the Republic of Georgia. *Clin Infect Dis.* 2007;45:174-80.
62. Griffin PM, Hatheway CL, Rosenbaum RB, et al. Endogenous antibody production to botulinum toxin in an adult with intestinal colonization botulism and underlying Crohn's disease. *J Infect Dis.* 1997;175:633-637.
63. Habermann E, Dreyer F. Clostridial neurotoxins: handling and action at the cellular and molecular level. *Curr Top Microbiol Immunol.* 1986;129: 94-179.
64. Hallett M. One man's poison—clinical applications of botulinum toxin. *N Engl J Med.* 1999;341:118-120.
65. Harvey SM, Sturgeon J, Dassey DE. Botulism due to *Clostridium baratii* type F toxin. *J Clin Microbiol.* 2002;40:2260-2262.
66. Hashimoto H, Clyde VJ, Parko KL. Botulism from peyote. *N Engl J Med.* 1998;339:203-204.
67. Hatheway CL. Toxigenic clostridia. *Clin Microbiol Rev.* 1990;3:66-98.
68. Hentges D. The intestinal flora and infant botulism. *Rev Infect Dis.* 1979;1:668-673.
69. Hibbs RG, Weber JT, Corwin A, et al. Experience with the use of an investigational F(ab')2 heptavalent botulism immune globulin of equine origin during an outbreak of type E botulism in Egypt. *Clin Infect Dis.* 1996;23:337-340.
70. Hikes DC, Manoli A II. Wound botulism. *J Trauma.* 1981;21:68-71.
71. Johnson RO, Clay SA, Arnon SS. Diagnosis and management of infant botulism. *Am J Dis Child.* 1979;133:586-593.
72. Kaplan JE, Davis LE, Narayan V, et al. Botulism, type A, and treatment with guanidine. *Ann Neurol.* 1979;6:69-71.
73. Kongsaengdao S, Samintarapanya K, Rusmeechan S, et al. An outbreak of botulism in Thailand: clinical manifestations and management of severe respiratory failure. *Clin Infect Dis.* 2006;43:1247-1256.
74. Kudrow DB, Henry DA, Haake DA, et al. Botulism associated with *Clostridium botulinum* sinusitis after intranasal cocaine abuse. *Ann Intern Med.* 1988;109:984-985.
75. Lalli G, Bohnert S, Deinhardt K, et al. The journey of tetanus and botulinum neurotoxins in neurons. *Trends Microbiol.* 2003;11:431-437.
76. Lange DJ, Brin MF, Warner CL, et al. Distant effects of local injection of botulinum toxin. *Muscle Nerve.* 1987;10:552-555.
77. LeCour H, Ramos H, Almeida B, et al. Food borne botulism: a review of 13 outbreaks. *Arch Intern Med.* 1988;148:578-580.
78. Lindström M, Korkeala H. Laboratory diagnostics of botulism. *Clin Microbiol Rev.* 2006;19:298-314.
79. MacDonald KL, Cohen ML, Blake PA. The changing epidemiology of adult botulism in the United States. *Am J Epidemiol.* 1986;124: 794-799.
80. MacDonald KL, Rutherford GW, Friedman SM, et al. Botulism and botulism-like illness in chronic drug users. *Ann Intern Med.* 1985;102: 616-618.

81. MacDonald KL, Spengler RF, Hatheway CL, et al. Type A botulism from sauteed onions: clinical and epidemiologic observations. *JAMA*. 1985;253:1275-1278.
82. Maksymowych AB, Simpson LL. Binding and transcytosis of botulinum neurotoxin by polarized human colon carcinoma cells. *J Biol Chem*. 1998;273:21950-21957.
83. Maksymowych AB, Reinhard M, Malizio CJ, et al. Pure botulinum neurotoxin is absorbed from the stomach and small intestine and produces peripheral neuromuscular blockade. *Infect Immun*. 1999;67: 4708-4712.
84. Maples HD, James LP, Stowe CD. Special pharmacokinetic and pharmacodynamic considerations in children. In: Burton ME, Shaw LM, Schentag JJ, Evans WE, eds. *Applied Pharamacokinetics and Pharmacodynamics: Principles of Therapeutic Drug Monitoring*, 4th ed. Philadelphia: Lippincott Williams and Wilkins; 2005:213-230.
85. Maselli RA, Bakshi N. AAEE Case Report #16: Botulism. *Muscle Nerve*. 2000;23:1137-1144.
86. Maselli RA, Ellis W, Mandler RN, et al. Cluster of wound botulism in California: clinical, electrophysiologic, and pathologic study. *Muscle Nerve*. 1997;20:1284-1295.
87. McCroskey LM, Hatheway CL. Laboratory findings in four cases of adult botulism suggest colonization of the intestinal tract. *J Clin Microbiol*. 1988;26:1052-1054.
88. McCroskey LM, Hatheway CL, Woodruff, et al. Type F botulism due to neurotoxigenic *Clostridium baratii* from an unknown source in an adult. *J Clin Microbiol*. 1991;29:2618-2620.
89. Mehta S. Neuromuscular disease causing acute respiratory failure. *Respir Care*. 2006 Sep;51(9):1016-1021.
90. Merson MH, Dowel VR. Epidemiologic, clinical and laboratory aspects of wound botulism. *N Engl J Med*. 1973;289:1005-1010.
91. Metzger JF, Lewis GE Jr. Human derived immune globulin for the treatment of botulism. *Rev Infect Dis*. 1979;1:689-692.
92. Montecucco C, Schiavo G, Tugnoli V, et al. Botulinum neurotoxins: mechanism of action and therapeutic applications. *Molec Med Today*. 1996;2:418-424.
93. Morgan JC, Iyer SS, Moser ET. Botulinum toxin A during pregnancy: a survey of treating physicians. *J Neurol Neurosurg Psychiatry*. 2006;77: 117-119.
94. Morse DL, Pichard LK, Guzewich JT, et al. Garlic in oil associated botulism: episode leads to product modification. *Am J Public Health*. 1990;80:1372-1373.
95. Nakano H, Kizaki H, Sakaguchi G. Multiplication of Clostridium botulinum in dead honey-bees and bee pupae, a likely source of heavy contamination of honey. *Int J Food Microbiol*. 1994; 21: 247-252.
96. National Institutes of Health. Botulinum toxin. Consensus Statement 1990;8:1-20.
97. O'Brien S. Case of infant botulism in the United Kingdom. *Eurosurveillance Weekly*. 2001;33:16.
98. Odergren T, Hjaltason H, Kaakkola S, et al. A double-blind, randomised, parallel group study to investigate the dose equivalence of Dysport¯ and Botox¯ in the treatment of cervical dystonia. *J Neurol Neurosurg Psychiatry*. 1998;64:6-12.
99. Olney RK, Aminoff MJ, Gelb DJ, et al. Neuromuscular effects distant from the site of botulinum neurotoxin injection. *Neurology*. 1988;38:1780-1783.
100. Otofugi T, Tokiwa H, Takahashi K. A food-poisoning incident caused by *Clostridium botulinum* toxin A in Japan. *Epidemiol Infect*. 1987; 99: 167-172.
101. Paisley JW, Lauer BA, Arnon RS. A second case of infant botulism type F caused by *Clostridium baratii*. *Pediatr Infect Dis J*. 1995;14: 912-914.
102. Parish JL. Commercial preparations and handling of botulinum toxin type A and type B. *Clin Dermatol*. 2003;21:481-484.
103. Passaro DJ, Werner B, McGee J, et al. Wound botulism associated with black tar heroin among injecting drug users. *JAMA*. 1998;279: 859-863.
104. Pellizzari R, Rossetto O, Schiavo G, et al. Tetanus and botulinum neurotoxins: mechanism of action and therapeutic uses. *Phil Trans R Soc Lond B*. 1999;354:259-268.
105. Pickett JB, III. AAEE case report #16: Botulism. *Muscle Nerve*. 1988;11: 1201-1205.
106. Pourshafie MR, Saifie M, Shafiee A, et al. An outbreak of food-borne botulism associated with contaminated locally made cheese in Iran. *Scand J Infect Dis*. 1998;30:92-94.
107. Rapoport S, Watkins PB. Descending paralysis resulting from occult wound botulism. *Ann Neurol*. 1984;16:359-361.
108. Richardson WH, Frei SS, Williams SR. A case of type F botulism in Southern California. *J Toxicol Clin Toxicol*. 2004;42:383-387.
109. Robin L, Herman D, Redett R. Botulism in a pregnant woman. *N Engl J Med*. 1996;335:823-824.
110. Roblot F, Popoff M, Carlier JP. Botulism in patients who inhale cocaine: the first cases in France. *Clin Infect Dis*. 2006;43:e51-52.
111. Ross MH, Charness ME, Sudarsky L, et al. Treatment of occupational cramp with botulinum toxin: diffusion of toxin to adjacent noninjected muscles. *Muscle Nerve*. 1997;20:593-598.
112. Sacks HS. The botulism hazard. *Ann Intern Med*. 1997;126: 918-919.
113. Sampaio C, Ferreira JJ, Simões F, et al. DYSBOT: a single-blind, randomized parallel study to determine whether any differences can be detected in the efficacy and tolerability of two formulations of botulinum toxin type A—Dysport and Botox—assuming a ratio of 4:1. *Mov Disord*. 1997;12:1013-1018.
114. Sanders DB, Massey JM, Sanders LL, et al. A randomized trial of 2,3-diaminopyridine in Lambert-Eaton myasthenic syndrome. *Neurology*. 2000;54:603-607.
115. Sandrock CE, Murin S. Clinical predictors of respiratory failure and long-term outcome in black tar heroin-associated wound botulism. *Chest*. 2001;120:562-566.
116. Santos JI, Swensen P, Glasgow LA. Potentiation of clostridium botulinum toxin by aminoglycoside antibiotics: clinical and laboratory observations. *Pediatrics*. 1981;68:50-54.
117. Schantz EJ, Johnson EA. Properties and use of botulinum toxin and other microbial neurotoxins in medicine. *Microbiol Rev*. 1992;56: 80-99.
118. Schmidt RD, Schmidt TW. Infant botulism: a case series and a review of the literature. *J Emerg Med*. 1992;10:713-718.
119. Schmidt-Nowara WW, Samet JM, et al. Early and late pulmonary complications of botulism. *Arch Intern Med*. 1983;143:451-456.
120. Schreiner MS, Field E, Ruddy R. Infant botulism: a review of 12 years' experience at the Children's Hospital of Philadelphia. *Pediatrics*. 1991;87: 159-165.
121. Schulze J, Toepfer M, Schroff KC, et al. Clindamycin and nicotinic neuromuscular transmission. *Lancet*. 1999;354:1792-1793.
122. Scott AB, Suzuki D. Systemic toxicity of botulinum toxin by intramuscular injection in the monkey. *Mov Disord*. 1988;3:333-335.
123. Shapiro RL, Hatheway C, Becher J, Swerdlow DL. Botulism surveillance and emergency response. *JAMA*. 1997;278:433-435.
124. Shapiro RL, Hatheway C, Swerdlow DL. Botulism in the United States: a clinical and epidemiologic review. *Ann Intern Med*. 1998; 129:221-228.
125. Sheean GL, Lees AJ. Botulinum toxin F in the treatment of torticollis clinically resistant to botulinum toxin A. *J Neurol Neurosurg Psychiatry*. 1995;59:601-607.
126. Sheridan RE. Gating and permeability of ion channels produced by *Botulinum* toxin types A and E in PC12 cell membranes. *Toxicon*. 1998;36:703-717.
127. Siegel LS, Johnson-Winegar AD, Sellin LC. Effect of 3,4-diaminopyridine on the survival of mice injected with botulinum neurotoxin type A, B, E or F. *Toxicol Appl Pharmacol*. 1986;84:255-263.
128. Simpson LL. Botulinum toxin: a deadly poison sheds its negative image. *Ann Intern Med*. 1996;125:616-617.
129. Simpson LL. Identification of the major steps in botulinum toxin action. *Ann Rev Pharmacol Toxicol*. 2004;44:167-193.
130. Smith LDS. The occurrence of *Clostridium botulinum* and *Clostridium tetani* in the soil of the United States. Health Lab Sci. 1978;15: 74-80.
131. Smith LA, Rusnak JM. Botulinum neurotoxin vaccines: past, present, and future. *Crit Rev Immunol*. 2007;27(4):303-318.
132. Sobel J. Botulism. *Clin Infect Dis*. 2005:41:1167-1173.
133. Sobel J, Tucker N, Sulka A, et al. Foodborne botulism in the United States, 1990-2000. *Emerg Infec Dis*. 2004;10:1606-1611.
134. Sonnabend OAR, Sonnabend WFF, Krech V, et al. Continuous microbiological and pathological study of 70 sudden and unexpected infant deaths: Toxigenic intestinal *Clostridium botulinum* infection in 9 cases of sudden infant death. *Lancet*. 1985;1:237-241.
135. St. Clair EH, DiLiberti JH, O'Brien ML. Observations of an infant born to a mother with botulism. *J Pediatr*. 1975;87:658.
136. St. Louis ME, Peck SHS, Bowering D, et al. Botulism from chopped garlic, delayed recognition of a major outbreak. *Ann Intern Med*. 1988;108: 363-368.
137. Swedberg J, Wendel TH, Deiss F. Wound botulism. *West J Med*. 1987; 147:335-338.

138. Swenson JM, Thornsberry C, McCroskey LM, et al. Susceptibility of *Clostridium botulinum* to thirteen antimicrobial agents. *Antimicrob Agents Chemother.* 1980;18:13-19.
139. Tacket CO, Shandera WX, Mann JM, et al. Equine antitoxin use and other factors that predict outcome in type A foodborne botulism. *Am J Med.* 1984;76:794-798.
140. Telzak EE, Bell EP, Kauter DA, et al. An international outbreak of type E botulism due to uneviscerated fish. *J Infect Dis.* 1990;161: 340-342.
141. Terranova W, Palumbo JN, Breman JG. Ocular findings in botulism type B. *JAMA.* 1979;241:475-477.
142. Townes JM, Cieslak PR, Hatheway CL, et al. An outbreak of Type A botulism associated with a commercial cheese sauce. *Ann Intern Med.* 1996;125:558-563.
143. Townes JM, Solomon HM, Griffin PM. The botulism hazard. *Ann Intern Med.* 1997;126:919.
144. Tseng-Ong L, Mitchell WG. Infant botulism: 20 years' experience at a single institution. *J Child Neurol.* 2007;22:1333-1337.
145. Tugnoli V, Eleopra R, Quatrale R, et al. Botulism-like syndrome after botulinum toxin type A injections for focal hyperhidrosis. *Br J Dermatol.* 2002;147:808.
146. Underwood K, Rubin S, Deakers T, et al. Infant botulism: a 30-year experience spanning the introduction of botulism immune globulin intravenous in the intensive care unit at Childrens Hospital Los Angeles. *Pediatrics.* 2007;120:e1380-e1385.
147. U.S. Food and Drug Administration. Early communication about an ongoing safety review of Botox and Botox Cosmetic (botulinum toxin type A) and Myobloc (botulinum toxin type B). http://www.fda.gov/CDER/Drug/early_comm/botulinium_toxins.htm. Accessed June 1, 2008.
148. Valli G, Barbieri S, Scarlato G. Neurophysiological tests in human botulism. *Electromyogr Clin* . 1983;23:3-11.
149. Villar RG, Shapiro RL, Busto S, et al. Outbreak of type A botulism and development of a botulism surveillance and antitoxin release system in Argentina. *JAMA.* 1999;281:1334-1340.
150. Wainwright RB, Heyward WL, Middaugh JP, et al. Foodborne botulism in Alaska, 1947-1985: epidemiology and clinical findings. *J Infect Dis.* 1988;157:1158-1162.
151. Weber JT, Hibbs RG, Darwish A, et al. A massive outbreak of type E botulism associated with traditional salted fish in Cairo. *J Infect Dis.* 1993;167:451-454.
152. Werner SB, Passaro D, McGee J, et al. Wound botulism in California 1951-1998: recent epidemic in heroin injectors. *Clin Infect Dis.* 2000;31: 1018-1024.
153. Wilcox P, Andofatto G, Fairbain MS, Pardy RL. Long-term follow-up of symptoms, pulmonary function, respiratory muscle strength and exercise performance after botulism. *Am Rev Respir Dis.* 1989;139:157-163.
154. Wilson R, Morris JG, Snyder JD, Feldman RA. Clinical characteristics of infant botulism in the United States: a study of the non-Californian cases. *Pediatr Infect Dis.* 1982;1:148-150.
155. Woodruff BA, Griffin PM, McCroskey LM, et al. Clinical and laboratory comparison of botulism form toxin types A, B, E in the United States, 1975-1988. *J Infect Dis.* 1992;166:1281-1286.
156. Wolfe L. Death by botulism: a medical mystery story. *New York Magazine.* 1980;13:56-60.
157. Zilinskas RA. Iraq's biological weapons. The past as future? *JAMA.* 1997;278:418-24.

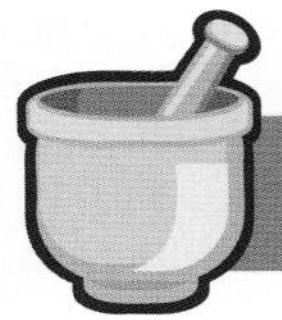

ANTIDOTES IN DEPTH (A8)

BOTULINUM ANTITOXIN

Lewis R. Goldfrank and Howard L. Geyer

Type-specific botulinum antitoxins are available as immunoglobins derived from equine and human sources. Various forms of monovalent to pentavalent botulinum antitoxins are available for the various serotypes of clostridium botulinum. Antitoxins may be beneficial for most clinical forms of botulism, but evidence has demonstrated preventive benefits rather than the reversal of clinical manifestations.

EQUINE IMMUNOGLOBULINS

The production of antitoxin is complex, requiring almost 2 years to immunize healthy horses against botulinum toxin. The resultant immunoglobulin product, which is then defibrinated, digested, dialyzed, and purified as a 20% protein antitoxin,[10] can be lyophilized and preserved.[27] Bivalent (serotypes A and B) and serotype E botulinum antitoxin are the equine immunoglobulin preparations available in the United States, the latter as an investigational new drug.[9] Whereas the bivalent (AB) preparation is used for patients with presumed wound botulism, both AB and E antitoxins should be administered to patients with foodborne botulism. The trivalent (serotypes A, B, and E) product is no longer available.

Botulinum antitoxin is distributed from the nine regional centers of the Centers for Disease Control and Prevention (CDC) on a named-patient basis after a probable diagnosis of botulism has been established. Each vial of the bivalent botulinum antitoxin contains 7500 IUnits (2381 US units) of type A botulinum antitoxin and 5500 IUnits (1839 US units) of type B antitoxin.[2] The type E product contains 5000 IUnits of antitoxin.[3] If both are given, each should be administered separately.[3]

Evidence substantiating the efficacy of types A and E antitoxin is available,[17,31] but the efficacy of type B antitoxin has not been established in clinical trials.

Currently, only limited data are available on the relationship of dose and route of administration, the amount of circulating antitoxin found in treated patients, the toxin-neutralizing capacity of this material, and the half-life of the antitoxin. Peak serum concentrations of antitoxin are 10 to 1000 times higher than the concentrations of antitoxin calculated to be necessary to achieve toxin neutralization.[14] Ninety percent of the activity of the equine antitoxin administered was detected when all the circulating toxin was neutralized.[10,19] The half-lives for antitoxin persistence in a single patient treated with trivalent antitoxin were calculated at 6.5, 7.6, and 5.3 days for antitoxin types A, B, and E, respectively.[14] The prolonged half-life of the antitoxin and the exceedingly small quantities of toxin measured explain the limited decrease in antitoxin titers after toxin–antitoxin binding.

In the presence of disease, 1 vial of the antitoxin is administered slowly intravenously (IV) over several minutes as a 1:10 vol/vol dilution in 0.9% sodium chloride solution. Subsequent doses can be given IV every 2 to 4 hours if there is progression of clinical findings.[2,3,10,13]

For prevention, 20% of a vial of the type A/type B bivalent botulinum antitoxin and 20% of a vial of the type E botulinum antitoxin can be given intramuscularly (IM) followed by a full dose (IV) if signs and symptoms occur.[2,3]

As is the case with many other heterologous proteins, administration of this horse serum-derived preparation results in significant adverse effects.[18] Each patient who was treated with antitoxin during the first decade during which it was available (1967–1977) was studied to determine both hypersensitivity reaction rates and the efficacy of the treatment of botulism. The overall rate of adverse reactions, including hypersensitivity and serum sickness, was 9% to 17%, with an incidence of anaphylaxis as high as 1.9%.[4,5,21] However, the doses of antitoxin used in that era were substantially larger than those currently used. Because of the lethality of botulinum toxin, the risk of adverse drug reaction for the antitoxin is considered acceptable for anyone with presumed illness and for anyone potentially exposed to the toxin. Pregnancy is not a contraindication to antitoxin administration, and antitoxin has been used successfully in these circumstances.[26,30]

Anaphylaxis should be anticipated, and the clinician should be prepared to treat this complication immediately with epinephrine. However, the smaller quantities of botulinum antitoxin used for botulism present a far smaller risk for serum sickness[4] than do the larger amounts of antivenom used to treat snake envenomation. The risk of serum sickness from the refined serum proteins in botulinum antitoxin is approximately 4% to 10%.[5,13]

Patients who received antitoxin within the first 24 hours after exposure had a shorter clinical course of botulism without regression of symptoms but a comparable mortality rate to those who received antitoxin later.[31] Reduced mortality can only be demonstrated in animal models.[23] Morbidity and mortality studies are difficult to perform for a disorder that is so rare and often recognized at a delayed stage, when the toxin already is tightly bound to the neuromuscular junction. Also, most of the reported case series involve patients who received varying degrees of supportive care, further making evaluation or comparison unreliable.

INVESTIGATIONAL ANTITOXINS

$F(ab')_2$ "despeciated" heptavalent (against toxin types A, B, C_1, D, E, F, and G) botulism immune globulin (dBIG) was previously available from the CDC.[25] This equine immune globulin[11] is extensively purified to eliminate fibrinogen, plasminogen, and other proteins. Pepsin is used to remove the Fc fragment of the immunoglobulin to reduce the potential for allergic manifestations if reexposure to equine protein occurs.[16] It contains 4000 IU of types A, B, C, E, and F and 500 IU of types D and G.[16,25] Although 10 of 45 patients given dBIG in the Egyptian type E botulism outbreak manifested adverse reactions, nine were considered mild and one episode was classified as serum sickness.[16] In this botulism epidemic, the incidence of adverse effects of dBIG was comparable to those of numerous other internationally available botulinal antitoxins. Although follow-up of individuals was limited, the antitoxin appeared to be as safe as other commercially available antitoxins.

HUMAN IMMUNOGLOBULINS

Human-derived preparations of type E antitoxin were developed as 5000 IUnits per 2-mL vials for IM use. This human-derived type E botulinum antitoxin was dosed between 1000 and 5000 IU based on the estimated quantity of botulinum toxin ingested by the 100 Egyptians who presumably had eaten (or consumed) toxin-contaminated, uneviscerated, salted mullet fish.[12,34] The safety of the human-derived preparation allowed for repetitive dosing in any individual who developed clinical findings.[11] This regimen was based on the premise that effective treatment could be achieved by delivering small antitoxin doses before tissue binding of circulating toxin.

Human-derived botulism immune globulin (BIG) was developed for use in the treatment of botulism in infants. This pentavalent (types A, B, C, D, and E) immune globulin is harvested by plasmapheresis from human donors who received multiple immunizations with pentavalent botulinum toxoid.[24,32] Use of a human immune globulin obviously avoids the risk of hypersensitivity that is associated with equine proteins. It is indicated in treatment of patients younger than 1 year of age with infant botulism caused by toxin type A or B. The half-life is approximately 28 days. Treatment with IV BIG significantly reduces the length of both overall hospital stay and intensive care, the duration of mechanical ventilation and tube or IV feeding, and the cost of hospitalization.[1]

A single-dose vial contains 100 mg ± 20 mg of lyophilized powder, which should be reconstituted with 2 mL of sterile water, which results in a 50- to 60-mg/mL solution. The reconstituted product contains antibody titers against botulinum toxin type A of at least 15 IUnits/mL and titers of antibodies against botulinum toxin type B of at least 2.7 IUnits/mL. BIG should be infused at 0.5 mL/kg/hr IV. If there are no untoward reactions within 15 minutes, the rate can be decreased to 1 mL/kg/hr. The principal adverse effect is erythematous rash on the face or trunk that is mild and transient.[8]

OTHER INVESTIGATIONAL TREATMENTS

A pentavalent toxoid vaccine (types A, B, C, D, and E) was developed at the US Army Medical Research Institute of Infectious Diseases (USAMRID) at Fort Detrick, Maryland, and has been under study for more than 40 years.[6,19] Its use remains investigational and is suggested only for laboratory personnel who work with *Clostridium botulinum* or who might be first responders in cases of terrorism.[9,28] It is available for these laboratory personnel in 5-mL multidose vials. Each dose is 0.5 mL and contains 5 μg of inactivated toxin (toxoid).[9] An additional monovalent toxoid type F vaccine was manufactured for the US Army and remains under study by USAMRID.[15,20]

Recombinant vaccines,[6,29] recombinant monoclonal antibodies, recombinant oligoclonal antibodies,[22] and drugs that act as metalloproteinase inhibitors (thereby preventing toxin uptake) are all currently under investigation by the Department of Defense.[11] Humanized monoclonal antibodies, small peptides and peptide mimetics, receptor mimics, and small molecules targeting the endopeptidase activity are all promising avenues being explored for treatment of botulism.[7]

SUMMARY

Consultation with a regional poison center and local health department and ultimately between the health department and the CDC at 770-488-7100, 24 hours per day, 7 days per week (or other comparable agencies in other parts of the world) provides improved access to rapid diagnostic tests for botulism and effective therapeutic modalities. Earlier disease recognition and the currently organized public health approach appear to be responsible for decreasing morbidity and increasing survival after typical foodborne botulism.[27,33] Since 2003, IV BIG has been licensed by the FDA for treatment of infant botulism and is an effective therapy for this form of the disease.

REFERENCES

1. Arnon SS, Schechter R, Maslanka SE, et al. Human botulism immune globulin for the treatment of infant botulism. *N Engl J Med.* 2006;354:462-471.
2. Aventis Pasteur. Botulinum antitoxin bivalent (equine) types A and B (package insert); 1997.
3. Aventis Pasteur. Botulinum antitoxin (equine) type E (package insert); 1999.
4. Badhey H, Cleri DJ, D'Amato RF, et al. Two fatal cases of type E adult foodborne botulism with early symptoms and terminal neurologic signs. *J Clin Microbiol.* 1986;23:616-618.
5. Black RE, Gunn RA. Hypersensitivity reactions associated with botulinal antitoxin. *Am J Med.* 1980;69:567-570.
6. Byrne MP, Smith LA. Development of vaccines for prevention of botulism. *Biochimie.* 2000;82:955-966.
7. Cai S, Singh BR. Strategies to design inhibitors of *Clostridium botulinum* neurotoxins. *Infect Disord Drug Targets.* 2007;7:47-57.
8. California Department of Health Services. BabyBIG, Botulism immune globulin intravenous (human) (package insert); 2008.
9. Centers for Disease Control and Prevention. Drug Service: Formulary: Products distributed by the Centers for Disease Control and Prevention. Available at http://www.cdc.gov/ncidod/srp/drugs/formulary.html; accessed January 14, 2009.
10. Food and Drug Administration. Biological products, bacterial vaccines and toxoids: implementation of efficacy review: proposed rule. *Fed Reg.* 1985;50:51002-51117.
11. Franz DR, Jahrling PB, Friedlander AM, et al. Clinical recognition and management of patients exposed to biological warfare agents. *JAMA.* 1997;278:399-411.
12. Goldsmith MF. Defensive biological warfare researchers prepare to counteract "natural enemies" in battle, at home. *JAMA.* 1991;266:2522-2523.
13. Grabenstein JD. Immunoantidotes: II. One hundred years of antitoxins. *Hosp Pharm.* 1992;27:637-646.
14. Hatheway CH, Snyder JD, Seals JE, et al. Antitoxin levels in botulism patients treated with trivalent equine botulism antitoxin to toxin types A, B, and E. *J Infect Dis.* 1984;150:407-412.
15. Hatheway CL. Toxoid of Clostridium botulinum type F: purification and immunogenicity studies. *Appl Environ Microbiol.* 1976;31:234-242.
16. Hibbs RG, Weber JT, Corwin A, et al. Experience with the use of an investigational $F(ab')_2$ heptavalent botulism immune globulin of equine origin during an outbreak of type E botulism in Egypt. *Clin Infect Dis.* 1996;23:337-340.
17. Koenig MG, Spickard A, Cardella MA, Rogers DE. Clinical and laboratory observations on type E botulism in man. *Medicine.* 1964;43:517-545.
18. Merson MH, Hughes JM, Dowell VR. Current trends in botulism in the United States. *JAMA.* 1974;229:1305-1308.
19. Metzger JR, Lewis LE. Human-derived immune globulins for the treatment of botulism. *Rev Infect Dis.* 1979;1:689-692.
20. Montgomery VA, Makuch RS, Brown JE, Hack DC. The immunogenicity in humans of a botulinum type F vaccine. *Vaccine.* 2000;18:728-735.
21. Morris JG Jr, Hatheway CL. Botulism in the United States, 1979. *J Infect Dis.* 1980;142:302-305.
22. Nowakowski A, Wang C, Powers DB, et al. Potent neutralization of botulinum neurotoxin by recombinant oligoclonal antibody. *Proc Natl Acad Sci U S A.* 2002;99:11346-11350.
23. Oberst FW, Crook JW, Cresthull P, House MJ. Evaluation of botulinum antitoxin, supportive therapy, and artificial respiration in monkeys with experimental botulism. *Clin Pharmacol Ther.* 1968;9:209-214.
24. Pickett J, Berg B, Chaplin E, Brunstetter-Shafer MA. Syndrome of botulism in infancy: clinical and electrophysiologic study. *N Engl J Med.* 1976;295:770-772.
25. Richardson WH, Frei SS, Williams SR. A case of type F botulism in Southern California. *J Toxicol Clin Toxicol.* 2004;42:383-387.

26. Robin L, Herman D, Redett R. Botulism in a pregnant woman. *N Engl J Med.* 1996;335:823-824.
27. Shapiro RL, Hatheway C, Becher J, Swerdlow DL. Botulism surveillance and emergency response. *JAMA.* 1997;278:433-435.
28. Siegel LS. Human immune response to botulinum pentavalent (ABCDE) toxoid determined by a neutralization test and by an enzyme linked immunosorbent assay. *J Clin Microbiol.* 1988;26:2351-2356.
29. Smith LA. Development of recombinant vaccines for botulinum neurotoxin. *Toxicon.* 1998;36:1539-1548.
30. St. Clair EH, DiLiberti JH, O'Brien ML. Observations of an infant born to a mother with botulism. *J Pediatr.* 1975;87:658.
31. Tacket CO, Shandera WX, Mann JM, et al. Equine antitoxin use and other factors that predict outcome in type A foodborne botulism. *Am J Med.* 1984;76:794-798.
32. Thilo EH, Townsend SF, Deacon J. Infant botulism at 1 week of age: report of two cases. *Pediatrics.* 1993;92:151-153.
33. Villar RG, Shapiro RL, Busto S, et al. Outbreak of type A botulism and development of a botulism surveillance and antitoxin release system in Argentina. *JAMA.* 1999;281:1334-1338,1340.
34. Weber JT, Hibbs RG, Darwish A, et al. A massive outbreak of type E botulism associated with traditional salted fish in Cairo. *J Infect Dis.* 1993;167:451-454.

C.
PHARMACEUTICALS

CHAPTER 47
ANTICONVULSANTS

Suzanne Doyon

Therapeutic serum concentrations		
Xenobiotic	**mg/L**	**μmol/L**
Carbamazepine	4–12	17–51
Ethosuximide	40–100	283–708
Gabapentin	12–20	12–88
Lamotrigine	3–14	≤19.5
Phenobarbital	15–40	65–172
Phenytoin	10–20	40–79
Valproic acid	50–120	347–833

A seizure is defined as the clinical manifestation of excessive neuronal activity within the central nervous system (CNS). It is accompanied by varying degrees of motor, sensory, and cognitive dysfunction. Seizures result from one of four possible cellular mechanisms: sustained repeated firing of the sodium channels, excessive calcium conductance, increased excitatory neurotransmission (eg, glutamate), or loss inhibitory neurotransmitter control (eg, γ-aminobutyric acid [GABA]).

HISTORY AND EPIDEMIOLOGY

Historically, seizures were treated by a variety of methods, including ketogenic diets, fluid restriction, and surgical excision of scars or irritable cortical foci. The first effective anticonvulsant therapy was introduced in 1857, when administration of bromides was noted to sedate patients and significantly reduce their seizures. Phenobarbital, another sedative-hypnotic, was first used to treat seizures in 1912. Most of the subsequently introduced anticonvulsants, such as primidone, had chemical structures similar to that of phenobarbital, and sedation was erroneously believed to be an essential component of anticonvulsant therapy.

The search for nonsedating anticonvulsants led to the introduction of phenytoin in 1938.[114] After 1965, benzodiazepines, carbamazepine, and valproic acid (VPA) were introduced and gained wide use as anticonvulsants. These were the only anticonvulsants available until the 1990s, when new anticonvulsants became available for clinical use: gabapentin, lamotrigine, levetiracetam, oxcarbazepine, tiagabine, topiramate, felbamate, vigabatrin, lacosamide and zonisamide.

Anticonvulsants are also currently used for treating mood disorders, refractory pain syndromes such as trigeminal neuralgia, bruxism, migraine headaches, drug withdrawal syndromes, and social phobias.

In a review of more than 5000 patient suicides, anticonvulsants were implicated in 8.2% of cases, suggesting a fairly high rate of suicidal ideation among people with access to these medications.[71,73] In the last decade, as reported in the American Association of Poison Control Centers (AAPCC) National Poison Data System (NPDS), a shift occurred from predominantly carbamazepine and phenytoin exposures to VPA and newer anticonvulsants (Chap. 135).

This chapter reviews the toxicity and management of overdoses with anticonvulsants other than the benzodiazepines and barbiturates, which are discussed in Chap. 74.

PHARMACOLOGY

The mechanisms of action of anticonvulsants correspond to one of four categories: sodium channel inhibition, calcium channel inhibition, inhibition of excitatory amines, and GABA agonism. Frequently, more than one mechanism accounts for the anticonvulsive action of a drug.

Electrophysiologic analyses demonstrate that a high-frequency pattern of neuronal firing occurs during seizure activity. This pattern is not observed during normal neuronal activity. Voltage-activated sodium and calcium channels are primarily responsible for this high-frequency firing. Sodium-channel blocking anticonvulsants preferentially bind to inactivated conformations of the voltage-activated sodium channels hindering recovery and preventing them from firing at high frequencies. Phenytoin, carbamazepine, VPA, lamotrigine, topiramate, oxcarbazepine, zonisamide, and felbamate all bind to the batrachotoxin site (or adjacent area) on the sodium channel and reduce its ability to recover from inactivation.[187,189] At therapeutic concentrations, effects on sodium channels are selective and no effect on spontaneous activity is noted. At toxic concentrations, selectivity is lost and both high-frequency firing and spontaneous sodium channel activity are inhibited.[113] Voltage-activated calcium channels are multisubunit complexes that are broadly classified into low-voltage and high-voltage groups. The low-voltage group encompasses the T-type calcium channels. Zonisamide, VPA, and ethosuximide inhibit flow of calcium through these channels, thus reducing the T current, also known as the *pacemaker current.*[59,131,142] The high-voltage group consists of the L, R, P/Q, and N subtypes. These channels regulate calcium entry. Levetiracetam inhibits the N-type calcium channels.[106,142]

The *N*-methyl-D-aspartate (NMDA) receptor is the glutamate receptor of greatest clinical importance with respect to development of seizures. When stimulated by glutamate, the NMDA receptor activates a ligand-gated ion channel that permits entry of Na^+ and Ca^{2+} into the neuronal cells. Suppression of the glutamate–NMDA interaction protects against seizures.[113] Felbamate and possibly VPA are competitive glutamate antagonists at the NMDA receptors.[65] More specifically, felbamate acts at the strychnine-insensitive glycine recognition site on the NMDA receptor (Chap. 13). Lamotrigine and possibly high-dose phenytoin inhibit glutamate release by binding to presynaptic Na^+ channels.[60] Topiramate binds to kainate, another excitatory amino acid receptor subtype, and blocks Na^+ entry into the neuronal cell.[135]

GABA acts through fast chloride-permeable ionotropic $GABA_A$ receptors and slower G protein–coupled $GABA_B$ receptors. Vigabatrin irreversibly inhibits GABA transaminase, the enzyme primarily responsible for GABA metabolism.[73,113] VPA may have similar effects.[113] Tiagabine inhibits the GABA transporter GAT-1 and thereby prevents reuptake of GABA into presynaptic neurons following its release.[73,113] Despite its structural similarities to GABA, the mechanism of action of gabapentin is poorly understood.[73,113] Figure 47–1 summarizes these mechanisms.

Broad spectrum antiepileptics treat all seizure types. This group includes lamotrigine, leveritacetam, topiramate, and valproic acid. Narrow spectrum antiepileptics treat specific seizure types or syndromes such as localization-related (focal) epilepsy with partial and secondarily generalized seizures. Narrow spectrum antiepileptics are less effective than broad spectrum antiepileptics in treating the idiopathic generalized epilepsy syndromes and may exacerbate certain seizure types.[53] The terms *anticonvulsant* and *antiepileptic* are used interchangeably in this chapter. The anticonvulsants will be discussed in alphabetical order.

CARBAMAZEPINE

Carbamazepine is structurally related to the cyclic antidepressants. It is a narrow spectrum anticonvulsant. Carbamazepine is a first-line anticonvulsant for seizures and may be especially useful for the management of epilepsy in pregnancy.[53]

PHARMACOKINETICS AND TOXICOKINETICS

Carbamazepine is lipophilic, with slow and unpredictable absorption following oral administration, and rapid distribution to all tissues. Peak concentrations are reached as late as 12–24 hours postingestion, especially after large ingestion of sustained-release preparations.[44,190] Carbamazepine also possesses weak anticholinergic properties and can decrease gastrointestinal motility, delaying its own absorption. Hence, no simple relationship exists between the dose and the serum concentration of carbamazepine.

Carbamazepine is metabolized primarily by CYP3A4 to carbamazepine 10,11-epoxide, which is pharmacologically active. This quantifiable metabolite is further degraded by epoxide hydrolase to carbamazepine-diol, a largely inactive compound.[85] Elimination of carbamazepine increases over the first few weeks of therapy because of autoinduction,

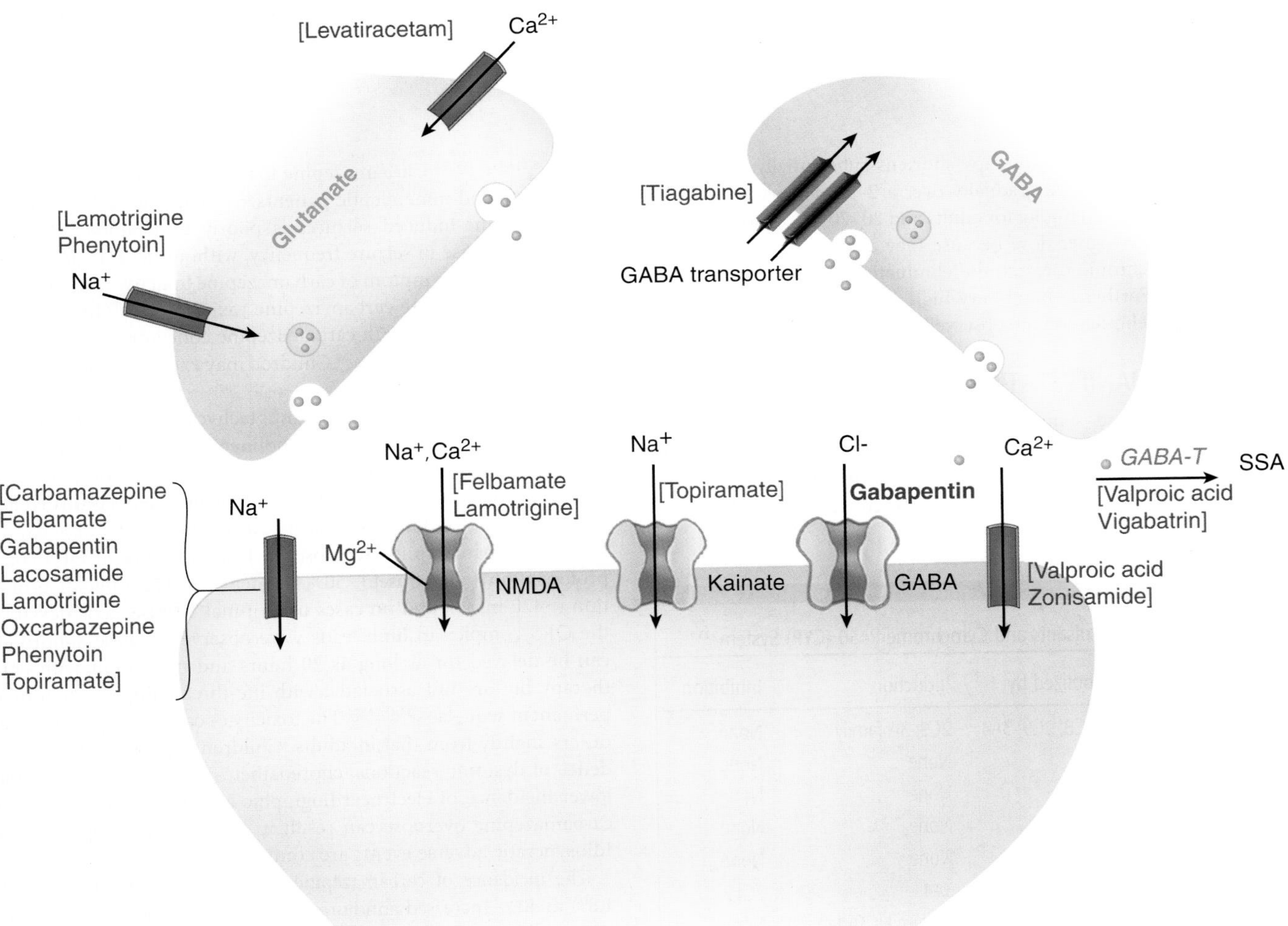

FIGURE 47–1. The mechanisms of action of anticonvulsants can generally be placed into one of four categories: sodium channel inhibition, calcium channel inhibition, inhibition of excitatory amines, and GABA agonism. SSA = succinic acid semialdehyde; GABA-T = GABA transaminase; NMDA = N-Methyl-D-Aspartate; GABA = γ-Aminobutyric acid.

TABLE 47–1. Pharmacokinetics of Anticonvulsants.[12,73,53,113,123]

	Time to Max Serum Concentration (h)	Therapeutic Serum Concentration (mg/L)	Vd (L/kg)	Protein Binding (%)	Urinary Elimination Unchanged (%)	Active Metabolite	Elimination Half-life (h)
Carbamazepine	3–24 in overdose	4–12	0.8–1.8	75	1–2	CBZ 10, 11-epoxide	6–20 acute 5–12 chronic
Gabapentin	3	12–20	0.8–1.3	0	100	None	5–7
Lacosamide	1-4		0.6	15	40	None	13
Lamotrigine	1–3	3–14	0.9–1.2	55	10	None	15–35
Levetiracetam	1–2	10–40	0.6	10	95	None	5–8
Oxcarbazepine	1–5	1–3	0.7	67	1	MHD	1–2
(MHD)		3–40		47	27		9
Phenytoin	5–24 in overdose	10–20	0.6	>90	<5	None	6–60
Tiagabine	1–2	0.01–0.1	0.8–2.1	95	<5	None	5–9
Topiramate	1–4	5–25	0.5–0.8	15	60	None	20–30
Valproic acid	1–24 in overdose	50–120	0.1–0.4	>90**	<5	None	6–18
Vigabatrin	1	20–80	0.8	0	70	None	6–8
Zonisamide	2–6	10–40	1.7–1.8	40–60	85	None	60

[a] After therapeutic oral administration.

** Saturable

CBZ = carbamazepine, MHD = monohydroxycarbazepine, VPA = valproic acid.

and the half-life on chronic therapy shortens substantially. Therefore, the dose must be increased gradually over a 2- to 4-week period to a final daily dose of 10–20 mg/kg for adults and 20–70 mg/kg for children. Children require a higher dose because they eliminate the drug more rapidly. During chronic therapy, the elimination half-life ranges from 10–20 hours.[100] Furthermore, at very high serum concentrations, zero order kinetics of elimination are observed[190] (Tables 47–1 and 47–2).

CLINICAL MANIFESTATIONS

Neurologic signs and symptoms and possibly some cardiovascular effects characterize acute carbamazepine toxicity. The initial neurologic disturbances include nystagmus, ataxia, and dysarthria. In patients with large overdoses, fluctuations in level of consciousness and coma occur.[38,44,69,151,155,188] Carbamazepine toxicity may cause seizures in both in epileptic and nonepileptic patients.[22,107] The mechanism underlying carbamazepine-induced seizures is poorly understood.[69,131] In some cases, an increase in seizure frequency, without neurologic symptoms, is the presenting symptom of carbamazepine toxicity. Status epilepticus may complicate acute carbamazepine toxicity.[157,164,182] In a case series, 55% of adult patients with carbamazepine concentrations greater than 40 mg/L developed seizures.[69] Children may experience seizures at even lower concentrations.[163]

TABLE 47–2. Anticonvulsants and Cytochrome P450 (CYP) System[5,73,113]

	Metabolized by	Induction	Inhibition
Carbamazepine	1A2; 2C8; 2C9; 3A4	2C9; 3A family	None
Gabapentin	None	None	None
Lacosamide	2C19	None	None
Lamotrigine	None	None	None
Levetiracetam	None	None	None
Oxcarbazepine	?	3A4	2C19
Phenytoin	2C9; 2C19; 3A4	2C family; 3A family	None
Tiagabine	3A4	None	None
Topiramate	None	None	2C19
Valproic acid	2C9; 2C19	None	2C19
Zonisamide	3A4	None	None

Cardiovascular effects include sinus tachycardia, which occurs in 35% of overdoses as a result of an anticholinergic mechanism, hypotension with myocardial depression, and cardiac conduction abnormalities.[58,69,98] High concentrations of carbamazepine may cause depression of phases 0, 2, and 4 of the action potential in cardiac tissue.[32,167] In a large case series of carbamazepine overdoses, a 15% incidence of QRS complex prolongation (>100 msec), 50% incidence of QT interval prolongation (>420 msec), and no cases of terminal 40-msec axis deviation of the QRS complex in limb leads were observed.[7] These abnormalities can be delayed for as long as 20 hours and may occur with chronic therapy but are not associated with life-threatening dysrhythmias or permanent sequelae.[7,32,43,79,171] The toxicity of carbamazepine in children differs slightly from that in adults. Children experience a higher incidence of dystonic reactions, choreoathetosis, and seizures and have a lower incidence of electrocardiographic abnormalities.[16,163,170] Chronic carbamazepine overdose can result in headaches, diplopia, or ataxia. Idiosyncratic adverse events are common.[146]

The incidence of carbamazepine-induced hyponatremia ranges from 1.8% to 40%. Increased antidiuretic hormone secretion or increased sensitivity of peripheral osmoreceptors to antiduretic hormone are suggested mechanisms.[56,93,113] (Chap. 16).

DIAGNOSTIC TESTING

Serum carbamazepine concentrations should be obtained in all cases of moderate-to-severe carbamazepine overdose. Because of erratic absorption, the concentrations should be repeated every 4–6 hours and closely monitored until a downward trend is observed. In one case report, peak concentrations were reached 106 hours postingestion in a patient who ingested a sustained release preparation.[22] Serum concentrations greater than 40 mg/L are associated with coma, seizures, respiratory depression, and prolongation of the QRS and QT intervals.[69] Carbamazepine may cross-react with toxicology screening for cyclic antidepressants (Chap. 73).[51]

Patients receiving multiple anticonvulsants, especially combination therapy with VPA and lamotrigine, may develop carbamazepine toxicity at serum concentrations within the therapeutic reference range due to elevated concentrations of the circulating carbamazepine-10,11-epoxide metabolite (Table 47–3). This finding is attributed to the additive inhibitory effects of VPA and lamotrigine on the enzyme epoxide hydrolase. Carbamazepine-10,11-epoxide concentrations in the 1–4 mg/L range are detected at therapeutic doses of carbamazepine and in the 1–10 mg/L range in overdoses.[134,190]

MANAGEMENT

Cardiac monitoring for occurrence of QRS or QT abnormalities is recommended. Although not formally studied, sodium bicarbonate should be administered if the QRS duration exceeds 100 msec. Carbamazepine-induced seizures are treated with benzodiazepines. Multiple-dose activated charcoal (MDAC) reduces enterohepatic and enteroenteric circulation of carbamazepine.[14,76,107,125,182] In a randomized trial, MDAC was associated with a reduction in the elimination half life of carbamazepine from 28 to 13 hours, a decrease in need for mechanical ventilation, a shorter coma, and a shorter length of stay in the intensive care unit.[14] Hemodialysis and charcoal hemoperfusion both effectively lower serum carbamazepine concentrations.[22,58,133] Clearance rates with high flux hemodialysis rival those obtained by charcoal hemoperfusion.[154] Continuous venovenous hemofiltration and hemodialfiltration were used successfully in 2 children.[8,192]

TABLE 47–3. Anticonvulsant Drug Interactions[53,73]

	Toxicity Increased by	Anticonvulsant Effect Decreased by	Increases Concentrations of	Decreases Concentrations of
Carbamazepine	Allopurinol, cimetidine, danazol, diltiazem, fluoxetine, fluvoxamine, gemfibrozil, INH, ketoconazole, lamotrigine, macrolides, nefazodone, nicotine, propoxyphene, protease inhibitors, verapamil	Benzodiazepines, felbamate, isotretinoin, phenobarbital, phenytoin, primidone, succinimides, valproic acid	None	Doxycycline, felbamate, haloperidol, lamotrigine, ?methadone, OCP, phenytoin, primidone, tiagabine, VPA, warfarin
Gabapentin	Cimetidine	Antacids	Felbamate	None
Lamotrigine	Sertraline, valproic acid	Antituberculous agents, CBZ, phenobarbital, phenytoin	CBZ epoxide	None
Levetiracetam	None	None	Phenytoin	None
Oxcarbazepine	None	CBZ, phenobarbital, phenytoin	Phenytoin	Lamotrigine, OCP
Phenytoin	Allopurinol, amiodarone, chloramphenicol, chlorpheniramine, clarithromycin, cloxacillin, cimetidine, disulfiram, ethosuxamide, felbamate, fluconazole, fluoxetine, fluvoxamine, imipramine, INH, methylphenidate, metronidazole, miconazole, omeprazole, phenylbutazone, sulfonamides, trimethaprim, tolbutamide, tolazamide, topiramate, VPA warfarin	Antacids, antineoplastics CBZ, calcium, diazepam, diazoxide, ethanol (chronic), folic acid, influenza vaccine, loxapine, nitrofurantoin, phenobarbital, phenylbutazone, pyridoxine, rifampin, salicylates, sulfisoxazole, sulcrafate, theophylline, tolbutamide, VPA vigabatrin	Phenobarbital, primidone, warfarin	Amiodarone, CBZ, cardioactive steroids, corticosteroids, cyclosporine, disopyramide, dopamine, doxycycline, furosemide, haloperidol, influenza vaccine, levodopa, methadone, mexilitene, OCP phenothiazines, quinidine, tacrolimus, theophylline, tiagabine, tolbutamide, VPA
Tiagabine	None	CBZ, phenobarbital, phenytoin	None	VPA
Topiramate	None	CBZ, phenobarbital, phenytoin	Phenytoin	OCP, digoxin
Valproic acid	Cimetidine, felbamate, ranitidine	Antacids, CBZ, chitosan, chlorpromazine, felbamate, INH, methotrexate, phenobarbital, phenytoin, primidone, salicylates	Felbamate, lamotrigine, phenobarbital, primidone	CBZ, tiagabine
Vigabatrin	None	None	None	Phenytoin
Zonisamide	None	CBZ, phenobarbital, phenytoin	?CBZ	?CBZ

CBZ = carbamazepine, VPA = valproic acid, INH = isoniazid, OCP = oral contraceptives.

Extracorporeal drug removal techniques should be reserved for severe life-threatening overdoses. MDAC is safer, easier, and produces similar outcomes to hemodialysis and hemoperfusion.

FELBAMATE

Felbamate is structurally similar to meprobamate, a sedative hypnotic rarely used today (see Chap. 74). Because of potential adverse effects, including hepatic failure and aplastic anemia, it is reserved as a therapy of last resort for management of seizures. It is absorbed quickly, and 50% of an ingested dose is excreted unchanged in the urine.[65] Mild lethargy and gastrointestinal symptoms are reported following acute overdose.[122] Crystalluria and reversible renal failure following an acute overdose are reported.[140] Treatment of felbamate overdose is largely supportive.

GABAPENTIN

Gabapentin, a derivative of GABA, is approved as adjunctive therapy for the management of seizures in adults and children and postherpetic neuralgia. It is also currently used as a treatment for posttraumatic stress disorder, behavioral disorders, mood disorders, bruxism, migraine prophylaxis, idiopathic trigeminal neuralgia, neuropathic pain, and a number of other neurologic disturbances. Pregabalin is a gabapentin prodrug. Both gabapentin and pregabalin are narrow spectrum antiepileptics.[53]

PHARMACOKINETICS AND TOXICOKINETICS

The bioavailability of gabapentin is approximately 60% with therapeutic dosing. Absorption kinetics may be dose dependent with decreasing bioavailability at increased dose, possibly due to a saturable transport system. It is highly lipophilic and easily crosses the blood–brain barrier. Dosage adjustments are necessary in patients with decreased renal function (creatinine clearance <60 mL/min). It is not metabolized by, and does not affect, the CYP450 system[113] (Table 47–1).

CLINICAL MANIFESTATIONS

Sedation, ataxia, movement disorders,[136] and gastrointestinal symptoms are observed following acute overdose.[67,91,137,183] Similar symptoms occur in patients with renal failure after initial dosing.[41,70,183] In a case series of 20 patients with overdose, lethargy, ataxia, and gastrointestinal symptoms resolved within 4–24 hours.[91]

Catatonia following abrupt withdrawal of gabapentin is described.[145] Pregabalin-induced psychosis is reported.[128]

DIAGNOSTIC TESTING

Consensus regarding a precise therapeutic range is not available. Because gabapentin is not appreciably protein bound, serum concentrations essentially represent free gabapentin.

MANAGEMENT

Treatment is largely supportive. Although activated charcoal (AC) may limit absorption, the lack of severe toxicity and rapidity of CNS depression generally makes the administration of AC both unnecessary and unwise. No specific antidote exists. Patients with persistent neurologic symptoms should be admitted to the hospital. Hemodialysis and hemoperfusion are not generally required, except in patients with significant renal impairment, because supportive care is sufficient in most instances.[21,41,70,137]

LAMOTRIGINE

Lamotrigine, a broad spectrum anticonvulsant, is approved as an adjunctive medication for treatment of seizures in adults and children. It also is approved for maintenance treatment of bipolar mood disorder.[108]

PHARMACOKINETICS AND TOXICOKINETICS

The bioavailability of lamotrigine is 98%. It is predominantly glucuronidated to lamotrigine 2-*N*-glucuronide. The elimination half-life is approximately 25 hours but can be halved in the presence of phenytoin and carbamazepine and doubled in the presence of VPA. Phenytoin and carbamazepine induce glucuronidation. VPA competes with lamotrigine for the same step in the glucuronidation process. Significantly reduced clearance of lamotrigine occurs in patients with Gilbert syndrome (a syndrome of defective glucuronidation). Lamotrigine does not affect the CYP450 system or the metabolism of other drugs except when it is administered concomitantly with carbamazepine, where it is associated with accumulation of the carbamazepine epoxide metabolite.[60]

CLINICAL MANIFESTATIONS

Neurologic manifestations such as lethargy, ataxia, nystagmus, and gastrointestinal symptoms are described following overdose. Coma, seizures, and QRS prolongation may occur.[15,20,102,126,130,139,153]

A chronic overdose presented with a rash, rhabdomyolysis, and elevation of hepatic aminotransferases and serum creatinine phosphokinase concentrations, suggesting a hypersensitivity reaction.[150] All abnormalities resolved upon withdrawal of the drug.[121]

DIAGNOSTIC TESTING

Lamotrigine concentrations greater than 14 mg/L are potentially toxic.

MANAGEMENT

Activated charcoal should be administered. Supportive care and ECG monitoring are recommended. Lamotrigine-induced seizures should be treated with benzodiazepines.[20,178] Data on hemodialysis and hemoperfusion are not available, but based on its size, relatively low protein binding, and volume of distribution (1.4 L/kg), lamotrigine should be removed by hemodialysis. However, hemodialysis should be reserved for severe life-threatening overdoses.

LEVETIRACETAM

Levetiracetam was approved in 1999 as an "add-on" medication for the management of intractable epilepsy. Its mechanism of action remains incompletely understood, although it is known to inhibit N-type calcium channels. Research has illustrated both a neuroprotective and an antiinflammatory effect.[66,109] Levetiracetam is a broad spectrum antiepileptic medication with a wide margin of safety in administration and very favorable pharmacokinetics.[66]

PHARMACOKINETICS AND TOXICOKINETICS

The bioavailability of levetiracetam approaches 100%. The major metabolic pathway involves enzymatic hydrolysis of the acetamide group. This reaction is not dependent on hepatic CYP450 activity. There are no active metabolites. Dosage adjustments are necessary in patients with decreased renal function (creatinine clearance <60 mL/min).[73]

CLINICAL MANIFESTATIONS

In one report of overdose, lethargy, coma, and respiratory depression were noted. Symptoms persisted for 24 hours.[11] Two children receiving supratherapeutic doses developed only mild effects such as decrease in muscle tone, which reversed immediately after the doses were adjusted.[9]

DIAGNOSTIC TESTING

Therapeutic concentrations are 10–40 mg/L. Because of its large therapeutic window, routine monitoring of serum levetiracetam concentrations may not be necessary.[73]

MANAGEMENT

Activated charcoal should be considered. Supportive care is recommended.

OXCARBAZEPINE

Oxcarbazepine is an analog of carbamazepine that functions as a prodrug. Presystemic 10-ketoreduction metabolizes oxcarbazepine to monohydroxycarbazepine (MHD), which is pharmacologically active.[113] MHD is subsequently conjugated and renally eliminated. It is a less potent inducer of CYP3A4 than carbamazepine, and has minimal effects on its own metabolism.[113] Somnolence, tinnitus, bradycardia and hypotension occur following acute single overdose.[75,181] In these cases, serum oxcarbazepine concentrations reached 12–31.6 mg/L (approximately 10-fold therapeutic concentrations), yet concentrations of MHD were only 59–65 mg/L, less than 2-fold the therapeutic concentrations (10–35 mg/L). These findings suggest that the formation of MHD is rate limited.[55,181]

Activated charcoal should be administered and supportive care should be provided. The rate-limited enzymatic conversion from inactive prodrug to active metabolite may limit its toxicity. Hemodialysis does not increase the clearance of oxcarbazepine or its metabolite and is not useful. [55]

PHENYTOIN/FOSPHENYTOIN

Phenytoin is still widely considered a first-line anticonvulsant for treatment of most seizure disorders, except absence seizures. It is a narrow spectrum antiepileptic agent that is nonsedating in therapeutic doses and therefore often used successfully for long-term management of epilepsy. [53]

Introduced in 1997, fosphenytoin is a water soluble phosphate ester prodrug of phenytoin. Advantages include availability for intramuscular administration and low potential for tissue injury at injection sites.[17,113]

PHARMACOKINETICS AND TOXICOKINETICS

Phenytoin is rapidly distributed to all tissues. Oral loading doses of 20 mg/kg phenytoin are well tolerated and yield therapeutic (>10 mg/L) serum concentrations at 5.6 ± 0.2 hours.[173] In very large oral overdoses, gastrointestinal absorption can be delayed even more for up to several days.[25,34] Some authors suggest that phenytoin absorption may continue in the colon because of its lipophilic properties.[168] Additionally, phenytoin occasionally forms concretions in the gastrointestinal tract.[25,34]

Phenytoin is extensively bound to serum proteins, mainly albumin. Only the unbound free fraction can traverse biologic membranes and become pharmacologically active. A significant fraction of phenytoin remains unbound in neonates, uremic patients, and other patients with hypoalbuminemia, such as patients in the intensive care unit.[37,62]

Less than 5% of a given dose of phenytoin is excreted unchanged in the urine. The remainder is metabolized in the liver. The major phenytoin metabolite, a parahydroxylphenyl derivative, is inactive but is the putative metabolite responsible for the hypersensitivity reaction associated with phenytoin administration.[92] The Michaelis-Menten model of saturable enzyme kinetics explains the relationship between phenytoin doses and serum concentrations at steady state. At phenytoin concentrations below 10 mg/L, elimination usually is first order, and elimination half-life ranges between 6 and 24 hours. At higher concentrations, zero-order elimination occurs as a result of saturation of the hydroxylation reaction, and the apparent elimination half-life increases to 20–60 hours.[28,113] Therefore, the apparent half-life of elimination of phenytoin is progressively prolonged as plasma concentration increases (Chap. 8).

Fosphenytoin is metabolized by tissue and blood phosphatases to phenytoin, phosphate, and formaldehyde. The bioavailability of the derived phentyoin is 100% when compared to intravenously administered phenytoin regardless of the route of administration (intravenous or intramuscular). The half-life of conversion of fosphenytoin to phenytoin is 7–15 minutes. After administration of an intravenous loading dose, time to therapeutic serum concentration of phenytoin (>10 mg/L) is approximately 0.2 hours whether fosphenytoin 150 mg/min or phenytoin 50 mg/min is administered.[173] Faster rates of intravenous infusion and displacement of phenytoin from protein binding sites by fosphenytoin compensate for the conversion-related delay in appearance of phenytoin in serum.[50] The dose of fosphenytoin is expressed in phenytoin equivalents (PE).

CLINICAL MANIFESTATIONS

Acute toxicity produces predominantly neurologic dysfunction that typically affects the cerebellar and vestibular systems. Phenytoin concentrations greater than 15 mg/L are associated with nystagmus, concentrations greater than 30 mg/L are associated with ataxia and poor coordination, and concentrations exceeding 50 mg/L are associated with lethargy, slurred speech, and pyramidal and extrapyramidal manifestations.[34,95,115,117] Toxic concentrations rarely cause de novo seizures.[169] Young children and the elderly may present with atypical manifestations of toxicity. Decreased appetite, poor feeding, diminished activity, abdominal distension, chorea, and opisthotonic posturing are reported following oral overdoses in children.[104,115]

Cardiotoxicity resulting from oral overdoses of phenytoin is not reported.[45,191] However, IV phenytoin impairs myocardial contractility, decreases peripheral vascular resistance, and depresses myocardial conduction. In a large case series, IV phenytoin was associated with a 3.5% incidence of hemodynamic complications.[45] Deaths following IV administration of phenytoin are reported.[61,147,186,193] Hypotension, dysrhythmias and cardiac arrest correlate with rate of administration and total dose infused. All can be at least partially attributed to propylene glycol (40%) and ethanol (10%), the diluents used in the IV preparation of phenytoin.[118] Propylene glycol in particular depresses myocardial tissue and decreases peripheral vascular resistance (Chap. 55). Fosphenytoin, available only as a parenteral preparation, does not contain propylene glycol, but the metabolism of this prodrug releases phosphate and formaldehyde. Two reports describe bradycardia, hypotension, and asystole following 5- to 10-fold dosing errors in young infants suffering from status epilepticus.[97,144] One infant had a serum phenytoin concentration of 77.2 mg/L and marked hyperphosphatemia (serum phosphate of 25.9 mg/L), although the serum calcium, magnesium, and blood urea nitrogen were normal.[144] Another report describes hyperphosphatemia without hemodynamic instability or electrocardiographic abnormality 9 hours after the administration of fosphenytoin 667 mg PE intravenously to a patient with end stage renal failure; the serum phosphate was 12.1 mg/dL and serum calcium was

8.2 mg/dL. A third report describes hypocalcemia and prolongation of the QT interval following the administration of fosphenytoin 1500 mg PE intravenously to an adult patient with normal renal function, however, no phosphate measurements were obtained.[84]

Intravenous phenytoin is commonly associated with local irritation. Extravasation may lead to local skin necrosis, possibly necessitating surgical intervention.[30,45,89] The risk of fosphenytoin-induced skin necrosis is lower because of its high water solubility.

Chronically elevated phenytoin concentrations occasionally results in gingival hyperplasia, frontal bossing, cerebellar effects, behavioral changes, and encephalopathy. Hyperactivity, confusion, lethargy, and hallucinations characterize the behavioral changes. Chronic use of phenytoin is also associated with agranulocytosis. Phenytoin may produce hepatotoxicity. The drug rash with eosinophilia and systemic symptoms (DRESS) syndrome is discussed later in this chapter.

DIAGNOSTIC TESTING

Serum phenytoin concentrations should be obtained in all cases of moderate-to-severe phenytoin overdose. Because of unpredictable absorption, phenytoin concentrations should be repeatedly monitored. Therapeutic concentrations are 10–20 mg/L. Because of zero-order elimination, high serum phenytoin concentrations may take days or weeks to return to the therapeutic range.[34,104,117]

Patients with impaired or decreased protein-binding capacity can develop symptoms at total phenytoin concentrations within the therapeutic range. Patients at greatest risk include neonates, the elderly, hypoalbuminemic, hyperbilirubinemic, and uremic patients, and patients undergoing combination therapy with VPA, salicylates, and sulfonamides because these xenobiotics displace phenytoin from its albumin binding sites. In such patients, determination of the free phenytoin concentration is helpful because it compares more reliably with the CSF concentrations than does the total phenytoin concentration.[37] Therapeutic free phenytoin concentrations are 1.0–2.1 mg/L.[13]

Equation 47–1 approximates the total phenytoin concentration that would be experience based on a given measured serum phenytoin concentration and measured albumin concentration.[35]

$$[\text{Phenytoin}] = \frac{[\text{Measured phenytoin}]}{(0.25 \times [\text{Measured albumin}]) + 0.1} \qquad (47\text{–}1)$$

MANAGEMENT

The treatment of patients with acute or chronic phenytoin overdoses remains largely supportive. Phenytoin-related deaths are rare, even after massive overdoses. MDAC reduces the elimination half-life of intravenously administered phenytoin from 44.5 to 22.3 hours. It is recommended in patients in whom serial serum concentrations are increasing or persistently elevated irrespective of route of exposure.[110] Hemodialysis, charcoal hemoperfusion, and other techniques including molecular adsorbents recirculating systems (MARS) are of little benefit in the management of phenytoin overdose and do not improve outcomes.[37,81,95,117,152] Otherwise healthy patients admitted to the hospital after isolated oral phenytoin overdoses require neurologic assessments but do not require routine cardiac monitoring because they do not experience dysrhythmias or cardiovascular complications.[46,191] Phenytoin-induced agranulocytosis can be treated successfully with administration of granulocyte colony-stimulating factor.[172]

Hypotension, cardiac dysrhythmias, and dyskinesias during IV administration of phenytoin are generally transient and usually resolve in 30–60 minutes unless complications occur. Stopping the phenytoin infusion for a few minutes and administering a bolus of 250–500 mL 0.9% sodium chloride solution generally is sufficient to treat the hypotension. Restarting the infusion at half the initial rate is recommended.

Electocardiographic abnormalities, especially a prolonged QT interval temporally related to fosphenytoin infusions, may be due to hyperphosphatemia and hypocalcemia and those electrolyte abnormalities should be rapidly corrected. In one case hemodialysis was required to correct the hyperphosphatemia.[112] Life-threatening dysrhythmias may require prolonged periods of cardiopulmonary resuscitation.[97,144]

The management of extravasation is discussed in Special Considerations: Extravasation.

TIAGABINE

Tiagabine inhibits GABA reuptake and is approved as an adjunctive treatment of seizures. It is also prescribed for a variety of psychiatric disorders. Tiagabine is a narrow spectrum antiepileptic medication.[53]

PHARMACOKINETICS AND TOXICOKINETICS

Tiagabine is quickly and completely absorbed within 2–3 hours of ingestion. It is widely distributed and easily crosses the blood–brain barrier.[90] It is metabolized by the CYP3A4 system to inactive metabolites. The elimination half-life is reduced by 50% in patients taking enzyme-inducing anticonvulsive agents.[105] It has no effect on the CYP450 system.[96,105]

CLINICAL MANIFESTATIONS

Lethargy, facial myoclonus (grimacing), nystagmus, and posturing are described following overdose.[24,165] Seizures and status epilepticus are reported at therapeutic doses as well as in overdose.[54,72,83,129] A previously healthy toddler developed three seizures after an unintentional overdose of tiagabine; serum concentrations were 0.53 mg/L.[83] A patient presented in status epilepticus and was believed to be noncompliant with therapy until a tiagabine concentration of 1.87 mg/L was obtained and an acute overdose determined.[72,129] Stimulation of the presynaptic $GABA_B$ receptors in the thalamus is suggested as the underlying mechanism for tiagabine-induced seizures.[141] Symptoms generally persist for 12–24 hours, and permanent neurologic sequelae usually are not found.[24,83,129,165]

DIAGNOSTIC TESTING

Therapeutic tiagabine concentrations are 5–70 ng/mL.

MANAGEMENT

Activated charcoal and supportive care are recommended. Seizures respond to administration of benzodiazepines even though the beneficial effects of the GABA agonists like benzodiazepines seem paradoxical when treating seizures from tiagabine.[54,72,83,129] Status epilepticus should be treated with barbiturates or propofol. Posturing and grimacing are treated with benzodiazepines as well.[24] Data on the use of hemodialysis and hemoperfusion are not available, but because of high protein binding, hemodialysis will likely not be effective.

TOPIRAMATE

Topiramate is approved as adjunctive therapy for seizures in adults, as well as for migraine prophylaxis, infantile spasms, and other refractory seizure disorders in infants and children. Topiramate is a broad spectrum antiepileptic. Its sulfamate moiety weakly inhibits carbonic anhydrase, specifically the carbonic anhydrase II and IV isoforms present in the kidney and CNS.[40,156]

PHARMACOKINETICS AND TOXICOKINETICS

Topiramate is readily bioavailable. Only 20% of the dose is hepatically metabolized via hydroxylation, hydrolysis, and glucuronidation;

the remaining 80% of the drug is eliminated unchanged in the urine (Table 47–1).

CLINICAL MANIFESTATIONS

Lethargy, ataxia, nystagmus, myoclonus, coma, seizures, and status epilepticus are all reported following topiramate overdose.[29,49,103,162] Lethargy may be accompanied by abnormal speech patterns, such as echolalia, and word-finding difficulties following acute overdose.[29,179] Nonanion gap metabolic acidosis resulting from inhibition of renal cortical carbonic anhydrase may be present (lowest reported bicarbonate concentration 12 mEq/L) along with hyperchloremia (range 110–120 mEq/L). The nonanion gap metabolic acidosis typically appears within hours of ingestion and can persist for days.[29,49,132,179]

DIAGNOSTIC TESTING

A death with a postmortem concentration of 170 mg/L is reported.[94] Serum chemistry and/or arterial blood gas analysis should be adequate to evaluate for hyperchloremia, hypokalemia, and metabolic acidosis.

MANAGEMENT

Activated charcoal and supportive care are recommended. Severe hyperchloremic metabolic acidosis should be treated with sodium bicarbonate 1–2 mEq/kg intravenously. However, systemic administration of sodium bicarbonate may impair the anticonvulsive effect of topiramate.[29,49] Hemodialysis can increase topiramate clearance 4- to 6-fold.[57] Hemodialysis is generally recommended in patients with life-threatening topiramate overdoses presenting with significant neurologic impairment, intractable electrolyte abnormalities, or renal insufficiency.

VALPROIC ACID

Valproic acid (di-*n*-propylacetic acid [VPA]) is a simple branched chain carboxylic acid that is used for treatment of seizure disorders, mania associated with bipolar disorder, and in migraine prophylaxis. It is a broad spectrum antiepileptic agent.

PHARMACOKINETICS, TOXICOKINETICS, AND PATHOPHYSIOLOGY

Valproic acid is almost 100% absorbed from the gastrointestinal tract. Peak concentrations usually are reached in 6 hours, except for enteric-coated and extended-release preparations, where peak concentrations are delayed for up to 24 hours.[18,47,64,87,116] VPA is 90% protein bound at therapeutic concentrations, but the percentage decreases to 35% as the VPA concentration exceeds 300 mg/L[174] (Table 47–1).

VPA metabolism is complex and involves conjugation by glucuronic acid or oxidation. Glucuronidation accounts for 80% of VPA metabolism.[174] Oxidation can occur in mitochondria or in cytosolic microsomes. Mitochondrial β-oxidation accounts for 14% of VPA metabolism and cytosolic ω-oxidation the remaining 6%.

β-oxidation occurs in the mitochondrial matrix and begins with the transport of VPA across the double-layered mitochondrial membrane using acetyl CoA and L-carnitine[101,174] (Fig. 47-2 and Table 47–4). β-oxidation of VPA depletes both carnitine and acetyl CoA stores through a number of different mechanisms. VPA increases carnitine excretion via formation of valproylcarnitine, which can be renally excreted. Second, valproylcarnitine inhibits the ATP-dependent carnitine transporter located on the plasma membrane. Third, VPA metabolites trap mitochondrial CoA. Mitochondrial CoA trapping (or depletion) decreases ATP production, which in turn negatively affects the carnitine transporter.[101,138] Depletion of carnitine will halt

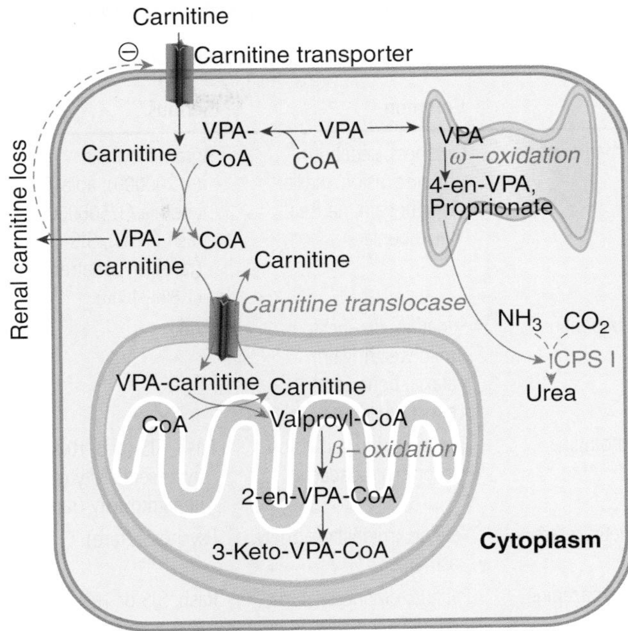

FIGURE 47–2. Valproic acid metabolism by the hepatocyte. Valproic acid is linked to coenzyme A (CoA) by acyltransferase I and subsequently transferred to carnitine. Valproylcarnitine (VPA-carnitine) is shuttled into the mitochondrion where, after transfer back to CoA by acyltransferase II, it undergoes β-oxidation yielding several metabolites. These metabolites sequester CoA, preventing its use in the β-oxidation of other fatty acids. This process may lead to a Reyelike syndrome of hepatic steatosis. Alternatively, valproylcarnitine may diffuse from the cell and be renally eliminated, or it may inhibit cellular uptake of carnitine. In either case, the cellular depletion of carnitine shifts valproate metabolism toward microsomal ω-oxidation, which occurs in the endooplasmic reticulum. This pathway forms 4-en-valproate, a putative hepatotoxin. ω-Oxidation products also interfere with carbamoylphosphate synthase I (CPS I), the initial step in the urea cycle, resulting in hyperammonemia.

β-oxidation. Subsequent fatty acid accumulation in the cytoplasm may cause steatosis.[86]

Depletion of acetyl CoA also halts the formation of *N*-acetylglutamate, a required cofactor for carbamoylphosphate synthetase I (CPS I). CPS I is the primary enzyme responsible for incorporation of ammonia into the urea cycle. The result of CoA depletion is impaired ureogenesis and hyperammonemia.[2,101] Ammonia can damage muscle and brain.[10]

CLINICAL MANIFESTATIONS

Overdoses of VPA result in symptoms varying from lethargy to coma and can be associated with cerebral edema. In one large case series, 100% of patients with serum VPA concentrations greater than 850 mg/L manifested coma, 63% manifested respiratory depression requiring intubation and mechanical ventilation, and 25% developed hypotension.[160,166]

Metabolic complications following acute VPA overdoses include hypernatremia, hypocalcemia, anion gap metabolic acidosis and hyperammonemia.[6,47,161,166] Anion gap metabolic acidosis following overdose is a poor prognostic sign.[48,120] It results from accumulation of ketoacids, lactic, carboxylic, and proprionic acids.[6,31,63,119,143]

Bone marrow suppression occurs 3–5 days following acute massive overdoses of VPA and is characterized by pancytopenia.[6,166] These hematopoietic disturbances usually resolve spontaneously within a few days.

Pancreatitis, hepatotoxicity, and renal insufficiency are rare manifestations of acute toxicity.[5,31,88] Chronic VPA therapy may lead to

TABLE 47–4. Adverse Events Associated with Anticonvulsants

	Common	Serious
Carbamazepine	Dizziness, sedation, blurred vision, ataxia, weight gain, nausea, leukopenia	Agranulocytosis (1/200000), aplastic anemia (1/500000), rash (10%), SJS (rare), hyponatremia (1.8%–40%)
Gabapentin	Sedation, dizziness, mild weight gain, ataxia, behavioral effect (children)	None
Lamotrigine	Dizziness, blurred vision, insomnia, headache	Rash, SJS (1–3/1000), hypersensisivity (rare), hepatotoxicity (rare)
Levetiracetam	Fatigue, irritability, anxiety, asthenia	Psychosis (rare)
Oxcarbazepine	Fatigue, dizziness, ataxia, diplоplia, nausea, headache	Rash, SJS or TEN (0.5–6/million), hyponatremia (2.5%), anaphylaxis (rare)
Phenytoin	Fatigue, dizziness, ataxia, nausea, headache, gingival hypertrophy, hirsutism, osteopenia	Blood dyscrasia (rare), rash, SJS or TEN (2–4/10000), hepatotoxicity (rare), lupus-like syndrome
Tiagabine	Fatigue, dizziness, ataxia, somnolence, anxiety	Seizures
Topiramate	Sedation, ataxia, word-finding difficulty, slowed speech, difficulty concentrating, anorexia, weight loss, paresthesias, oligohydrosis (children)	Metabolic acidosis (3%), nephrolithiasis (1.5%), acute glaucoma (rare), heat stroke
Valproic acid	Sedation, ataxia, weight gain, nausea, tremor, hair loss	Hepatotoxicity (1/20000), thrombocytopenia, hyperammonemia, aplastic anemia (rare), pancreatitis (1/3000)
Vigabatrin	Fatigue, headache, dizziness, weight gain	Vision loss, psychosis
Zonisamide	Sedation, ataxia, difficulty concentrating, irritability, nausea, headache	Aplastic anemia, nephrolithiasis (0.2%–4%), rash (1%–2%), SJS or TEN (rare), heat stroke (rare)

SJS = Stevens-Johnson syndrome TEN = toxic epidermolysis.

Data from Ref: 53.

hepatotoxicity and microvesicular steatosis secondary to the aforementioned metabolic aberration in fatty acid metabolism rather than, as with other anticonvulsants, a hypersensitivity reaction.[19,42,86] Clinical findings may vary from asymptomatic elevation of aminotransferase concentrations to fatal hepatitis.

Valproate-induced hyperammonemic encephalopathy is characterized by impaired consciousness with confusion or lethargy, focal or bilateral neurologic signs, and increased seizure frequency. It is not always accompanied by elevated VPA concentrations. The etiology is uncertain, but elevated ammonia concentrations coupled with elevated concentrations of some of the more neurotoxic VPA metabolites may be responsible.[23,47]

DIAGNOSTIC TESTING

Serum VPA concentrations should be obtained in all cases of moderate-to-severe VPA overdose, and repeated every 4–6 hours until a downward trend is observed. Therapeutic concentrations are 50–100 mg/L, although some clinicians use higher concentrations.

All nine VPA metabolites can be measured in the urine. In large overdoses the 4-en-VPA concentration may be elevated, indicating a shift toward ω-oxidation. The β-oxidation metabolite 2-en-VPA may be low or absent, indicating inhibition of β-oxidation and/or carnitine depletion. Concentrations of the 2-en-VPA metabolite increased 1–3 days following acute ingestion, signaling the return to normal β-oxidation.[120]

Electrolytes, blood gases, liver function tests, platelets and serum lactate, and serum ammonia concentrations should be monitored in all patients with severe VPA overdose with evidence of neurologic impairment. Hyperammonemia (>80 μg/dL or >35 μmol/L) occurs in 16%–52% of patients receiving chronic VPA therapy.[33,127,184]

MANAGEMENT

Supportive management is sufficient to ensure complete recovery in most patients with VPA overdoses. Discontinuation of all medications that likely affect VPA metabolism is also recommended (Table 47-2).

MDAC is useful in preventing absorption of VPA, especially in overdoses of enteric-coated or extended-release preparations.[3,49] As expected, naloxone is not effective in VPA-induced CNS or respiratory depression.[26,77,180]

L-Carnitine should be administered if evidence indicates the presence of hyperammonemia or hepatotoxicity.[36,80] Intravenous carnitine is preferred in symptomatic patients whereas oral L-carnitine is sufficient in asymptomatic patients. The intravenous loading dose is 100 mg/kg over 30 minutes (maximum 6 g) followed by 15 mg/kg IV over 10–30 minutes every 4 hours until clinical improvement occurs (Antidotes in Depth A9: L-Carnitine).

Published data on extracorporeal removal of VPA are limited. Hemodialysis alone reduced the elimination half-life of VPA to 2.2–2.9 hours.[18,39,68,74,78,159] Charcoal hemoperfusion alone and in combination with hemodialysis were not superior to hemodialysis alone.[52,63,161,176] Continuous venovenous hemodialfiltration did not significantly improve elimination in one patient with a serum valproic acid concentration of 1402 mg/L.[82] Since hemodialysis will additionally remove ammonia it is also recommended for hemodynamically or neurologically unstable patients or patients who have severe metabolic disturbances such as life-threatening hyperammonemia following VPA overdose.[4]

VIGABATRIN

Vigabatrin, or vinyl GABA, is a stereospecific irreversible inhibitor of GABA-transaminase. Although vigabatrin has a short elimination half-life, its duration of action is 24 hours. Dosage adjustments are necessary in patients with impaired renal function.[113] Agitation, coma, and long-term psychosis are reported after acute ingestion.[35,99]

Chronic toxicity may result in psychosis, dizziness, vision loss and tremor, which usually is mild and transient, as well as depression and psychosis.[99] Treatment of vigabatrin toxicity is largely supportive. Severe agitation is best treated with IV benzodiazepines. Some cases of mild vigabatrin-induced psychosis resolve simply by withdrawal of the medication.[99]

ZONISAMIDE

Zonisamide is a sulfonamide derivative that inhibits sodium channels, low-voltage T-type calcium channels, and possibly also inhibits carbonic anhydrase similarly to topiramate.[113] Somnolence is a commonly reported adverse effect. Overdose experience with zonisamide is limited. In one case report, status epilepticus, coma, and death were attributed to zonisamide overdose despite a minimally elevated concentration of 44 mg/L (therapeutic 10–40 mg/L).[175] Activated charcoal should be considered. Supportive care is recommended.

DRESS SYNDROME OR ANTICONVULSANT HYPERSENSITIVITY SYNDROME

Drug rash with eosinophilia and systemic symptoms (DRESS) syndrome, previously named "drug hypersensitivity syndrome," is a severe adverse drug event that was first described in 1950.[177] DRESS syndrome is a distinct severe adverse drug reaction triad characterized by fever, rash, and internal organ involvement. DRESS occurs in approximately 1 of every 1000–10,000 uses of anticonvulsants, usually aromatic anticonvulsants such as phenytoin, carbamazepine, phenobarbital, primidone, and lamotrigine. Literature also supports the inclusion of oxcarbazepine as a causative agent. The incidence remains the same regardless of the patient's gender and ethnic origin. Data suggest a genetic defect in drug metabolism as the causative lesion. First-degree relatives of patients with DRESS have a 25% risk of developing this syndrome.[92,185]

DRESS occurs most frequently within the first 2 months of therapy and is not related to dose or serum concentration. The pathophysiology is related to the accumulation of reactive arene oxide metabolites resulting from decreased epoxide hydrolase enzyme activity. These metabolites bind to macromolecules and cause cellular apoptosis and necrosis. They also form neoantigens that may trigger immunologic responses. Interestingly, the same metabolite is believed to cause other serious dermatologic reactions, such as Stevens-Johnson syndrome and toxic epidermal necrolysis (see Chap. 29 and Figure 29–4).

Initial symptoms also include malaise and pharyngitis (including tonsillitis). A skin eruption characterized by macular erythema evolves into a pruritic and confluent papular rash primarily involving the face, trunk, and later the extremities. A tender lymphadenopathy usually follows. The rash usually spares the mucous membranes but severely affected cases develop toxic epidermal necrolysis. Multiorgan involvement usually occurs 1–2 weeks into the syndrome. The liver is the most frequently affected organ, although involvement of the CNS (encephalitis), cardiac muscle (myocarditis), lungs (pneumonitis), renal system (nephritis), and thyroid (hyperthyroid thyroiditis followed by hypothyroidism) are possible. Eosinophilia and mononucleosis-type atypical lymphocytosis are common. Liver disturbances range from mildly elevated aminotransferase concentrations to fulminant hepatic failure.[92,185] Fatality rates are reportedly as high as 10%.[177]

Skin biopsies reveal nonspecific perivascular lymphocytic infiltration, spongiotic or lichenoid dermatitis, and variable degrees of edema.[185] Lymph node histology reveals benign hyperplasia, atypical lymphoid cells, or lymphoma. Other laboratory abnormalities include a positive rheumatoid factor, antinuclear antibodies, anti–double-stranded DNA smooth muscle antibodies, cold agglutinins, and hypogammaglobinemia or hypergammaglobulinemia. A novel, easy, fast, objective lymphocyte toxicity assay is being studied.[124]

Prompt discontinuation of the offending agent is essential to prevent symptom progression. Patients should be admitted to the hospital and receive methylprednisolone 0.5–1 mg/kg/d divided in four doses.[27,185] Other promising therapies include use of IV immunoglobulin.[111,149,185]

In one case series, 90% of patients with DRESS showed in vitro cross-reactivity to other aromatic antiepileptics.[1] Based on this evidence, avoidance of phenytoin, carbamazepine, phenobarbital, primidone, lamotrigine, and oxcarbazepine is recommended whereas benzodiazepines, levetiracetam, VPA, gabapentin, topiramate, and tiagabine are safe alternatives.[158]

SUMMARY

All anticonvulsant drugs produce CNS symptoms when taken in overdose and therefore differentiation based on clinical findings is difficult. Lethargy, sedation, ataxia, and nystagmus occur following overdoses of almost all the anticonvulsants. Coma occurs following substantial overdose of all anticonvulsants with the exception of gabapentin. Seizures, including status epilepticus, may occur with carbamazepine, lamotrigine, tiagabine, topiramate and zonisamide overdoses.

Hemodynamic instability and abnormal electrocardiograms are rare findings. Carbamazepine, lamotrigine, and possibly topiramate can cause QRS prolongation. Electrolyte abnormalities occur following overdoses with carbamazepine, oxcarbezipine, VPA and topiramate. Topiramate is uniquely associated with hyperchloremic metabolic acidosis.

Except for VPA overdoses there are no specific antidotes or overdoses of anticonvulsants. Supportive care alone usually yields beneficial outcomes. Administration of activated charcoal is generally recommended because of its safety and efficacy. Anticonvulsant-induced seizures are treated with benzodiazepines, barbiturates, or propofol. Patients with severe VPA overdoses or VPA-induced hyperammonemia should be treated with carnitine. Extracorporeal drug removal is rarely necessary and should be reserved for severe carbamazepine, VPA, or topiramate overdose patients with concurrent electrolyte abnormalities, hemodynamic instability, and/or clinical deterioration. Data on overdoses with the newer anticonvulsants are limited.

REFERENCES

1. Allam JP, Paus T, Reichel C, et al. DRESS syndrome associated with carbamazepine and phenytoin. *Eur J Dermatol.* 2004;14(5):339-342.
2. Alonso E, Girbes J, Garcia-Espana A, et al. Changes in urea cycle-related metabolites in the mouse after combined administration of valproic acid and an amino acid load. *Arch Biochem Biophys.* 1989;272:267-273.
3. Al-Shareef A, Buss DC, Shetty HG, et al. The effect of repeated-dose activated charcoal on the pharmacokinetics of sodium valproate in healthy volunteers. *Br J Clin Pharmacol.* 1997;43:109-111.
4. Aly ZA, Yalamanchili P, Gonzalez E. Extracorporeal management of valproic acid toxicity: a case report and review of the literature. *Semin Dial.* 2005:18:62-66.
5. Andersen GD. A mechanistic approach to antiepileptic drug interactions. *Ann Pharmacother.* 1998;32:554-563.
6. Andersen GO, Ritland S. Life-threatening intoxication with sodium valproate. *J Toxicol Clin Toxicol.* 1995;33:279-284.
7. Apfelbaum JD, Caravati EM, Kerns WP, et al. Cardiovascular effects of carbamazepine toxicity. *Ann Emerg Med.* 1995;25:631-635.
8. Askenazi DJ, Goldstein SL, Chang IF, et al. Management of a severe carbamazepine overdose using albumin enhanced continuous venovenous hemodialysis. *Pediatrics.* 2004;113:406-409.
9. Awaad Y. Accidental overdosage of levetiracetam in two children caused no side effects. *Epilepsy Behav.* 2007;11:247.
10. Bachman C, Braissant O, Villard AM, et al. Ammonia toxicity to the brain and creatine. *Mol Genet Metab.* 2004;81:Suppl 1:S52-S57.
11. Barrueto F, Williams K, Howland MA, et al. A case of levetiracetam (Keppra) poisoning with clinical and toxicokinetic data. *J Toxicol Clin Toxicol.* 2002;40:881-884.
12. Baselt RC, ed. *Disposition of Toxic Drugs and Chemicals in Man*, 7th ed. Foster City, CA: Biomedical Publications; 2004.
13. Booker HE, Darcey B. Serum concentrations of free diphenylhydantoin and their relationship to clinical intoxication. *Epilepsia.* 1973;14:177-184.

14. Brahmi K, Kouraic N, Thabet N, Amamou N. Influence of activated charcoal on pharmacokinetics and clinical features of carbamazepine poisoning. *Am J Emerg Med.* 2006;24:440-443.
15. Briassoulis G, Kalabalikis P, Tamiolaki M. Lamotrigine childhood overdose. *Pediatr Neurol.* 1998;19:239-242.
16. Bridge TA, Norton RL, Robertson WO. Pediatric carbamazepine overdoses. *Pediatr Emerg Care.* 1994;10:260-263.
17. Browne TR, Kugler AR, Eldon MA. Pharmacology and pharmacokinetics of fosphenytoin. *Neurology.* 1996;46:S3-S7.
18. Brubacher JR, Dahghani P, McKnight D. Delayed toxicity following ingestion of enteric-coated divalproex sodium (Epival). *J Emerg Med.* 1999;17:463-467.
19. Bryant AE, Dreifuss FE. Valproic acid hepatic fatalities: US experience since 1986. *Neurology.* 1996;46:465-469.
20. Buckley NA, Whyte IM, Dawson AH. Self-poisoning with lamotrigine. *Lancet.* 1993;342:1552-1553.
21. Butler TC, Rosen RM, Wallace AL, Amsden G. Flumazenil and dialysis for gabapentin-induced coma. *Ann Pharmacother.* 2003;37:74-76.
22. Cameron RJ, Hungerford P, Dawson AH. Efficacy of charcoal hemoperfusion in massive carbamazepine poisoning, *J Toxicol Clin Toxicol.* 2002;40:507-512.
23. Camilleri C, Albertson T, Offerman S. Fatal cerebral edema after moderate valproic acid overdose. *Ann Emerg Med.* 2005;45:337-338.
24. Cantrell FL, Ritter M, Himes E. Intentional overdose with tiagabine: an unusual clinical presentation. *J Emerg Med.* 2004;27:271-272.
25. Chaikin P, Adir J. Unusual absorption profile of phenytoin in a massive overdose case. *J Clin Pharmacol.* 1987;27:70-73.
26. Chan YC, Tse ML, Lau FL. Two cases of valproic acid poisoning treated with L-carnitine. *Hum Exp Toxicol.* 2007;26:967-969.
27. Chopra S, Levell NJ, Cowley G, et al. Systemic corticosteroids in the phenytoin hypersensitivity syndrome. *Br J Dermatol.* 1996;134:1109-1112.
28. Chua HC, Venketasubramanian N, Tjia H, et al. Elimination of phenytoin in toxic overdose. *Clin Neurol Neurosurg.* 2000;102:6-8.
29. Chung AM, Reed MD. Intentional topiramate ingestion in an adolescent female. *Ann Pharmacother.* 2004;38:1439-1442.
30. Comer JB. Extravasation from intravenous phenytoin. *Intrav Ther Clin Nutr.* 1984;11:23-29.
31. Connacher AA, Macnab JP, Jung RT. Fatality due to massive overdose of sodium valproate. *Scott Med J.* 1987;32:85-86.
32. Corday E, Enescu V, Vyden JK, et al. Antiarrhythmic properties of carbamazepine. *Geriatrics.* 1971;26:78-81.
33. Coulter DL, Allen RJ. Secondary hyperammonemia: a possible mechanism for valproate encephalopathy. *Lancet.* 1980;1:1310-1311.
34. Craig S. Phenytoin poisoning. *Neurocrit Care.* 2005;3:161-170.
35. Davie MB, Cook MJ, Ng C. Vigabatrin overdose. *Med J Aust.* 1996;165:403.
36. DeVivo DC, Bohan TP, Coulter DL, et al. L-Carnitine supplementation in childhood epilepsy: current perspectives. *Epilepsia.* 1998;39:1216-1225.
37. De Schoenmakere G, De Waele J, Terryn W, et al. Phenytoin intoxication in critically ill patients. *Am J Kidney Dis.* 2005;45:189-192.
38. De Zeuw R, Westemberg H, Van der Kleijn E. An unusual case of carbamazepine poisoning with a near fatal relapse after two days. *J Toxicol Clin Toxicol.* 1979;14:263-269.
39. Dharnidherka VR, Fennell RS 3rd, Richard GA. Extracorporeal removal of toxic valproic acid levels in children. *Pediatr Nephrol.* 2002;17:312-315.
40. Dodgson SJ, Shank RP, Maryanoff BE. Topiramate as an inhibitor of carbonic anhydrase isoenzymes. *Epilepsia.* 2000;41:S35-S39.
41. Dogukan A, Aygen B, Berilgen MS. Gabapentin-induced coma in a patient with renal failure. *Hemodial Int.* 2006;10:168-169.
42. Dreifuss FE, Langer DH, Moline KA, et al. Valproic acid hepatic fatalities. *Neurology.* 1989:39:201-207.
43. Drenck NE, Risbo A. Carbamazepine poisoning, a surprisingly severe case. *Anesth Intens Care.* 1980;8:203-204.
44. Durelli L, Massazza V, Cavallo R. Carbamazepine toxicity and poisoning. Incidence, clinical features and management. *Med Toxicol Adv Drug Exp.* 1989;4:95-107.
45. Earnest MP, Marx JA, Drury LR. Complications of intravenous phenytoin for acute treatment of seizures. *JAMA.* 1983;249:762-765.
46. Evers ML, Ishar A, Agil A. Cardiac monitoring after phenytoin overdose. *Heart Lung.* 1997;26:325-328.
47. Eyer F, Flegenhauer N, Gempel K, et al. Acute valproate poisoning: pharmacokinetics, alterations of fatty acid metabolism and changes during therapy. *J Clin Psychopharmacol.* 2005;25:376-380.
48. Farrar HC, Harold DA, Reed MD. Acute valproic acid intoxication: enhanced drug clearance with oral-activated charcoal. *Crit Care Med.* 1993;21:299-301.
49. Fakhoury T, Murray L, Seger D, et al. Topiramate overdose: clinical and laboratory features. *Epilepsy Behav.* 2002:3:185-189.
50. Fischer JH, Patel TV, Fischer PA. Fosphenytoin clinical pharmacokinetics and comparative advantages in acute treatment of seizures. *Clin Pharmacol.* 2003;42(1):33-58.
51. Fleishman A, Chiang VW. Carbamazepine overdose recognized by a tricyclic antidepressant assay. *Pediatrics.* 2001;107:176-177.
52. Franssen EJ, van Essen GG, Portman AT, et al. Valproic acid toxicokinetics serial hemodialysis and hemoperfusion. *Ther Drug Monit.* 1999;21: 289-292.
53. French JA, Pedley TA. Initial management of epilepsy. *N Engl J Med.* 2008;359:166-176.
54. Fulton JA, Hoffman RS, Nelson LS. Tiagabine overdose: a case of status epilepticus in a non-epileptic individual. *Clin Toxcol.* 2005;43:869-871.
55. Furlanat M, Franceshi L, Poz D, et al. Acute oxcarbazepine, benazepril and hydrochlorothiazide overdose with alcohol. *Ther Drug Monit.* 2006;28:267-268.
56. Gandelman MS. Review of carbamazepine-induced hyponatremia. *Prog Neuropsychopharmacol Biol Psychiatry.* 1994;18:211-233.
57. Garnett WR. Clinical pharmacology of topiramate: a review. *Epilepsia.* 2000;41:61-65.
58. Gary NE, Byra WM, Eisinger RP. Carbamazepine poisoning: treatment by hemoperfusion. *Nephron.* 1981;27:202-203.
59. Gee NS, Brown JP, Dissanayake VU, et al. The novel anticonvulsant drug gabapentin (Neurontin) binds to the alpha-2-delta subunit of a calcium channel. *J Biol Chem.* 1996;271:5768-5776.
60. Gilman JT. Lamotrigine: an antiepileptic agent for the treatment of partial seizures. *Ann Pharmacother.* 1993;29:144-151.
61. Goldschlager AW, Karliner JS. Ventricular standstill after intravenous diphenylhydantoin. *Am Heart J.* 1967;74:410-412.
62. Gordon MF, Gerstenblitt D. The use of free phenytoin levels in averting phenytoin toxicity. *N Y State J Med.* 1990;90:469-470.
63. Graudins A, Aaron CK. Delayed peak serum valproic acid in massive divalproex overdose: treatment with charcoal hemoperfusion. *J Toxicol Clin Toxicol.* 1996;34:335-341.
64. Graudins A, Peden GD, Owsett RP. Massive overdose with controlled-release carbamazepine resulting in delayed peak serum concentrations and life-threatening toxicity. *Emerg Med.* 2002;14:89-94.
65. Graves NM. Felbamate. *Ann Pharmacother.* 1993;27:1073-1081.
66. Grunewald R. Levetiracetam in treatment of idiopathic epilepsies. *Epilepsia.* 2005;46(Suppl9):154-160.
67. Heckman JG, Ultrich K, Dutsch M, et al. Pregabalin associated asterixis. *Am J Phys Med Rehabil.* 2006;84:724.
68. Hicks LK, McFarlane PA. Valproic acid overdose and haemodialysis. *Nephrol Dial Transplant.* 2001;16:1483-1486.
69. Hojer J, Malmlund HO, Berg A. Clinical features in 28 consecutive cases of laboratory confirmed massive poisoning with carbamazepine alone. *J Toxicol Clin Toxicol.* 1993;31:449-458.
70. Hung TY, Seow VK, Chong CF, et al. Gabapentin toxicity: an important cause of altered consciousness in patients with uraemia. *Emerg Med J.* 2008;25:178-179.
71. Isacsson G, Holmgren P, Druid H, Bergman U. Psychotropics and suicide prevention. Implication from toxicological screening of 5281 suicides in Sweden 1992–1994. *Br J Psychiatry.* 1999;174:259-265.
72. Jette N, Cappell J, VanPassel L, et al. Tiagabine-induced nonconvulsive status epilepticus in an adolescent without epilepsy. *Neurology.* 2006;67:1514-1515.
73. Johannessen SI, Battino D, Berry DJ, et al. Therapeutic drug monitoring of the newer antiepileptic drugs. *Ther Drug Monit.* 2003;25:347-363.
74. Johnson LZ, Martinez I, Fernandez MC, et al. Successful treatment of valproic acid overdose with hemodialysis. *Am J Kidney Dis.* 1999;33:786-789.
75. Jolliff Ha, Fehrenbacher N, Dart RC. Bradycardia, hypotension and tinnitus after accidental oxcarbazepine overdose. *Clin Toxicol.* 2001;39:316-317 [abstract].
76. Jones AL, Proudfoot AT. Features and management of poisoning with modern drugs used to treat epilepsy. *Q J Med.* 1998;91:325-332.
77. Jung J, Eo E, Ahn K. A case of hemoperfusion and L-carnitine management in valproic acid overdose. *Am J Emerg Med.* 2008;26:388e3-388e4.
78. Kane SL, Constantine M, Staubus AE, et al. High flux hemodialysis without hemoperfusion is effective in acute valproic acid overdose. *Ann Pharmacother.* 2000;34:1146-1151.

79. Karsarkis EJ, Kuo CS, Berger R, et al. Carbamazepine-induced cardiac dysfunction. Characterization of two distinct clinical syndromes. *Arch Intern Med.* 1992;152:186-191.
80. Katiyar A, Aaron C. Case files of the Children's Hospital of Michigan Regional Poison Control Center: the use of carnitine for the management of acute valproic acid toxicity. *J Med Toxicol.* 2007;3:129-138.
81. Kawasaki C, Nishi R, Vekihara S, et al. Charcoal hemoperfusion in the treatment of phenytoin overdose. *Am J Kidney Dis.* 2000;35:323-326.
82. Kay TD, Playford HR, Johnson DW. Hemodialysis versus continuous venovenous hemodialfiltration in the management of severe valproate overdose. *Clin Nephrol.* 2003;59(1):56-58.
83. Kazzi Z, Jones C, Morgan B. Seizures in a pediatric patient with tiagabine overdose. *J Med Toxicol.* 2006;2:160-162.
84. Keegan MT, Bondy LR, Blackshear JL, et al. Hypocalcemia-like electrocardiographic changes after administration of intravenous fosphenytoin. *Mayo Clinic Proc.* 2002;77:584-586.
85. Kerr BM, Thummel KE, Wurden CJ, et al. Human liver carbamazepine metabolism. Role of CYP3A4 and CYP2C8 in 10,11epoxide formation. *Biochem Pharmacol.* 1994;47:1969-1979.
86. Kesterson JW, Granneman GR, Machinist JM. The hepatotoxicity of valproic acid and its metabolites in rats: I. Toxicologic, biochemical and histopathologic studies. *Hepatology.* 1984,4:1143-1152.
87. Khan E, Huggan P, Celi L, et al. Sustained low-efficiency dialysis with filtration (SLEDD-f) in the management of acute sodium valproate intoxication. *Hemodial Inter.* 2008;12:211-214.
88. Khoo SH, Layland MJ. Cerebral edema following acute sodium valproate overdose. *J Toxicol Clin Toxicol.* 1992;30:209-214.
89. Kilarski DJ, Buchanan C, Von Behren L. Soft-tissue damage associated with intravenous phenytoin. *N Engl J Med.* 1984;311:1186-1187.
90. Kilvienen R. Long-term safety of tiagabine. *Epilpesia.* 2001;42:46-48.
91. Klein-Scwartz W, Shepherd JG, Gorman S, Dahl B. Characterization of gabapentin overdose using a poison center case series. *J Toxicol Clin Toxicol.* 2003;41:11-15.
92. Knowles SR, Shapiro LE, Shear NH. Anticonvulsant hypersensitivity syndrome: incidence, prevention and management. *Drug Saf.* 1999;21:489-501.
93. Kuz GM, Manssourian A. Carbamazepine-induced hyponatremia: assessment of risk factors. *Ann Pharmacother.* 2005;39:1943-1945.
94. Langman LJ, Kaliciak HA, Boone SA. Fatal acute topiramate toxicity. *J Anal Toxicol.* 2003;27:323-324.
95. Larsen JR, Larsen LS. Clinical features and management of poisoning due to phenytoin. *Med Toxicol Adv Drug Exp.* 1989;4:229-245.
96. Leach JP, Brodie MJ. Tiagabine. *Lancet.* 1998;351:203-207.
97. Leiber BL, Snodgrass WR. Cardiac arrest following large intravenous fosphenytoin overdose in an infant [abstract]. *J Toxicol Clin Toxicol.* 1998:36:473.
98. Leslie PJ, Heyworth R, Prescott LF. Cardiac complications of carbamazepine intoxication: treatment by haemoperfusion. *Br Med J.* 1983;286:1018.
99. Levinson DF, Devinsky O. Psychiatric adverse events during vigabatrin therapy. *Neurology.* 1999;53:1503-1511.
100. Levy RH, Pitlick WHJ, Troupin AS, et al. Pharmacokinetics of carbamazepine in normal man. *Clin Pharmacol Ther.* 1975;17:657–668.
101. Li J, Norwood DL, Li-Feng M, Schulz H. Mitochondrial metabolism of valproic acid. *Biochemistry.* 1991;30:388–394.
102. Lofton AL, Klein-Schwartz W. Evaluation of lamotrigine toxicity reported to poison centers. *Ann Pharmacother.* 2004;38:1-5.
103. Lofton Al, Klein-Schwartz W. Evaluation of toxicity of topiramate exposures reported to poison centers. *Hum Exp Toxicol.* 2005;24:591-595.
104. Lowry JA, Vandover JC, DeGreeff J, et al. Unusual presentation of iatrogenic phenytoin toxicity in a newborn. *J Med Toxicol.* 2005;1:26-29.
105. Luer MS, Rhoney DH. Tiagabine: a novel antiepileptic drug. *Ann Pharmacother.* 1998;32:1173-1180.
106. Lukyanetz EA, Shryl VM, Kostyuk PG. Selective blockade of N type calcium channels by levetiracetam. *Epilepsia.* 2002;43:9-18.
107. Lurie Y, Bentur Y, Levy Y, et al. Limited efficacy of gastrointestinal decontamination in severe slow-release carbamazepine overdose. *Ann Pharmacother.* 2007;41:1539-1543.
108. Mackey FJ, Wilton GL, Pearce SN, et al. Safety of long-term lamotrigine in epilepsy. *Epilepsia.* 1997;38:881-886.
109. Marini H, Costa C, Passaniti M. Levetiracetam protects against kainic acid-induced toxicity. *Life Sci.* 2004;74:1253-1264.
110. Mauro LS, Mauro V, Brown D, et al. Enhancement of phenytoin elimination by multiple-dose activated charcoal. *Ann Emerg Med.* 1987;16:1132-1135.
111. Mayorga C, Torres MJ, Corzo JL, et al. Improvement of toxic epidermal necrolysis after the early administration of a single high dose of intravenous immunoglobulin. *Ann Allergy Asthma Immunol.* 2003; 91:86-91.
112. McBride KD, Wilcox J, Kher KK. Hyperphosphatemia due to fosphenytoin in a pediatric ESRD patient. *Pediatr Nephrol.* 2005;20:1182-1185.
113. McNamara JO. Pharmacotherapy of the Epilepsies. Brunton LL, Lazo JS, Parker KL, eds. *Goodman and Gilman's The Pharmacological Basis of Therapeutics,* 11th ed. New York: McGraw-Hill; 2005;501-525.
114. Merritt HH, Putnam TJ. Sodium diphenylhydantoinate in treatment of convulsive disorders. *JAMA.* 1938;111:1068-1073.
115. Mellick LB, Morgan JA, Mellick GA. Presentations of acute phenytoin overdose. *Ann Emerg Med.* 1989;7:61-67.
116. Meyer S, Kuhlmann MK, Peters FT, et al. Severe valproic acid intoxication is associated with atrial tachycardia: secondary detoxification by hemoperfusion. *Klin Pediatr.* 2005;217:82-85.
117. Miller MA, Crystal CS, Patel MM. Hemodialysis and hemoperfusion in a patient with an isolated phenytoin overdose. *Am J Emerg Med.* 2006;24:748-749.
118. Mixter CG, Moran JM, Austen WG. Cardiac and peripheral vascular effects of diphenylhydantoin sodium. *Am J Cardiol.* 1966;17:332-338.
119. Mortensen PB, Hansen HE, Pedersen B, et al. Acute valproate intoxication: biochemical investigations and hemodialysis treatment. *Int J Clin Pharmacol Ther Toxicol.* 1983;21:64-68.
120. Murakami K, Sugimoto T, Woo M, et al. Effect of L-carnitine supplementation on acute valproate intoxication. *Epilepsia.* 1996;37:687-689.
121. Mylonakis E, Vittorio CC, Hollick DA, et al. Lamotrigine overdose presenting as anticonvulsant hypersensitivity syndrome. *Ann Pharmacother.* 1999;33:557-559.
122. Nagel TR, Schunk JE. Felbamate overdose: a case report and discussion of a new antiepileptic drug. *Pediatr Emerg Care.* 1995;11:369-371.
123. Neels HM, Sierens AC, Naelerts K, et al. Therapeutic drug monitoring of old and newer anti-epileptic drugs. *Clin Chem Lab Med.* 2004;42:1228-1255.
124. Neuman MG, Mlakiewicz IM, Shear NH. A novel lymphocyte assay to assess drug hypersensitivity syndromes. *Clin Biochem.* 2000;33:517-524.
125. Neuvonen PJ, Elonen E. Effect of activated charcoal on absorption and elimination of phenobarbitone, carbamazepine and phenylbutazone in man. *Eur J Clin Pharmacol.* 1980;17:51-57.
126. O'Donnell John, Bateman ND. Lamotrigine overdose in an adult. *J Toxicol Clin Toxicol.* 2000;38:659-660.
127. Ohtani Y, Endo F, Matsuda I. Carnitine deficiency and hyperammonemia associated with valproic acid therapy. *J Pediatr.* 1982;101:782-785.
128. Olaizola I, Ellger T, Young P, et al. Pregabalin-associated acute psychosis and epileptiform EEG-changes. *Seizure.* 2006;15:208-210.
129. Ostovskiy D, Spanaki MV, Morris GL. Tiagabine overdose can induce convulsive status epilepticus. *Epilepsia.* 2002;43:773-774.
130. Paopairochanakorn C, White S, Malafa MJ. Cardiac and neurologic toxicity from lamortigine ingestion. *J Toxicol Clin Toxciol.* 2002;40:620-621.
131. Perucca E, Gram L, Avanzini G, Dulac O. Antiepileptic drugs as a cause of worsening seizures. *Epilepsia.* 1998;39:5-17.
132. Philippi H, Boor R, Reitter B. Topiramate and metabolic acidosis in infants and toddlers. *Epilepsia.* 2002;43:744-747.
133. Pilapil M, Petersen J. Efficacy of hemodialysis and charcoal hemoperfusion in carbamazepine overdose. *Clin Toxicol.* 2008;46:342-343.
134. Potter JM, Donnelly A. Carbamazepine-10,11-epoxide in therapeutic drug monitoring. *Ther Drug Monit.* 1998;20:652-657.
135. Privitera MD. Topiramate: a new antiepileptic drug. *Ann Pharmacother.* 1997;31:1164-1173.
136. Raju PM, Waller RW, Lee MA. Dyskinesia induced by gabapentin in idiopathic Parkinson's disease. *Mov Disord.* 2007;22:288-289.
137. Randinitis EJ, Posvar EL, Alvey CW, et al. Pharmacokinetics of pregabalin in subjects with various degrees of renal function. *J Clin Pharmacol.* 2003;43:277-283.
138. Raskind JY, El-Chaar GM. The role of carnitine supplementation during valproic acid therapy. *Ann Pharmacother.* 2000;34:630-638.
139. Reimers A, Reinholt G. Acute lamotrigine overdose in an adolescent. *Ther Drug Monit.* 2007;29:669-670.
140. Rengstroff DS, Milstone AP, Seger DL, et al. Felbamate overdose complicated by massive crystalluria and acute renal failure. *J Toxicol Clin Toxicol.* 2000;38:666-667.
141. Richards DA, Lemos T, Whitton PS, et al. Extracellular GABA in the ventrolateral thalamus of rats exhibiting spontaneous absence epilepsy: a microdialysis study. *J Neurochem.* 1995;65:1674-1680.

142. Rogawski MA, Loscher W. The neurobiology of antiepileptic drugs. *Nat Rev Neurosci.* 2004;5:553-564.
143. Roodhooft AM, Van Dam K, Haentjens D, et al. Acute sodium valproate intoxication: occurrence of renal failure and treatment with haemoperfusion-haemodialysis. *Eur J Pediatr.* 1990;149:363-364.
144. Rose R, Cisek J, Michell J. Fosphenytoin-induced bradyasystole arrest in an infant treated with charcoal hemofiltration [abstract]. *J Toxicol Clin Toxicol.* 1998;36:473.
145. Rosebush PI, MacQueen GM, Mazurek MF. Catatonia following gabapentin withdrawal. *J Clin Psychopharmacol.* 1999;19:188-189.
146. Rush JA, Beran RG. Leucopenia as an adverse reaction to carbamazepine therapy. *Med J Aust.* 1984;140:426-428.
147. Russell MA, Bousvaros G. Fatal results from diphenylhydantoin administered intravenously. *JAMA.* 1968;20:2118-2119.
148. Schaub JEM, Williamson PJ, Barnes EW, Trewby PN. Multisystem adverse reaction to lamotrigine. *Lancet.* 1994;344:481.
149. Scheuerman O, Nofech-Moses Y, Rachmel A, et al. Successful treatment of antiepileptic drug hypersensitivity with intravenous immune globulin. *Pediatrics.* 2000;107:E14.
150. Schlienger RG, Knowles SR, Shear NH. Lamotrigine-associated anticonvulsant hypersensitivity syndrome. *Neurology.* 1998;51:1172-1175.
151. Schmidt S, Schmitz-Buhl M. Signs and symptoms of carbamazepine overdose. *J Neurol.* 1995;242:169-173.
152. Sen S, Ratnaraj N, Davies NA, et al. Treatment if phenytoin toxicity by the molecular adsorbents recirculating system (MARS). *Epilepsia.* 2003;44:265-267.
153. Schwartz MD, Geller RJ. Seizures and altered mental status after lamotrigine overdose. *Ther Drug Monit.* 2007;29:843-844.
154. Schuerer DJE, Brophy PD, Maxvold NJ, et al. High-efficiency dialysis for carbamazepine overdose. *J Toxicol Clin Toxicol.* 2000;38:321-323.
155. Seymour JF. Carbamazepine overdose. Features of 33 cases. *Drug Saf.* 1993;8:81-88.
156. Shank RP, Gardocki JF,Vaught JL, et al. Topiramate: preclinical evaluation of structurally novel anticonvulsant. *Epilepsia.* 1994;35:450-460.
157. Sharma P, Gupta RC, Bhardwaja B, et al. Status epilepticus and death following acute carbamazepine poisoning. *J Assoc Physicians India.* 1992;40:561-562.
158. Shear N, Spielberg S. Anticonvulsant hypersensitivity syndrome, in vitro assessment of risk. *J Clin Invest.* 1988;82:1826-1832.
159. Shih VE. Alternative-pathway therapy for hyperammonemia. *N Engl J Med.* 2007;356:2321-2322.
160. Sikma M, Mier JC, Meulenbelt J. Massive valproic acid overdose a misleading case. *Am J Emerg Med.* 2008;26:110e3-6.
161. Singh SM, McCormick BB, Mustata S, et al. Extracorporeal management of valproic acid overdose: a large regional experience. *J Nephrol.* 2004;17:43-49.
162. Smith AG, Brauer HR, Catalano G, Catalano MC. Topiramate overdose: a case report and literature review. *Epilepsy Behav.* 2001;2: 603-607.
163. Soman P, Jain S, Rajsekhar V, et al. Dystonia—a rare manifestation of carbamazepine toxicity. *Postgrad Med J.* 1994;70:54-56.
164. Spiller HA, Carlisle RD. Status epilepticus after massive carbamazepine overdose. *J Toxicol Clin Toxicol.* 2002;40:81-90.
165. Spiller HA, Winter ML, Ryan M, et al. Retrospective evaluation of tiagabine overdoses. *Clin Toxicol.* 2005;43:855-859.
166. Spiller HA, Krenzelok P, Klein-Schwartz W, et al. Multicenter case series of valproic acid ingestion: serum concentrations and toxicity. *J Toxicol Clin Toxicol.* 2000;38:755-760.
167. Steiner C, Wit AL, Weiss MB, et al. The antiarrhythmic actions of carbamazepine. *J Pharmacol Exp Ther.* 1970;173:323-335.
168. Stevenson CM, Kim J, Felischer D. Colonic absorption of antiepileptic agents. *Epilepsia.* 1997;38:63-67.
169. Stilman N, Masdeu JC. Incidence of seizures with phenytoin toxicity. *Neurology.* 1985;35:1769-1772.
170. Stremski ES, Brady W, Prasad K, et al. Pediatric carbamazepine intoxication. *Ann Emerg Med.* 1995;25:624-630.
171. Sullivan JB, Rumack BH, Peterson RG. Acute carbamazepine toxicity resulting from overdose. *Neurology.* 1981;31:621-624.
172. Sung SF, Chiang PC, Tung HH, Ong CT. Charcoal hemoperfusion in an elderly man with life-threatening adverse reactions due to poor metabolism of phenytoin. *J Formos Med Assoc.* 2004;103:648-652.
173. Swadron SP, Rudis MI, Azimian K et al. A comparison of phenytoin-loading techniques in the emergency department. *Acad Emerg Med.* 2004;11:244-252.
174. Sztajnkrycer MD. Valproic acid toxicity: overview and management. *J Toxicol Clin Toxicol.* 2002;40:789-801.
175. Sztajinkrycer MD, Huang EE, Bond GR. Acute zonisamide overdose: a death revisited. *Vet Hum Toxicol.* 2003;45:154-156.
176. Tank JE, Palmer BF. Simultaneous "in series" hemodialysis and hemoperfusion in the management of valproic acid overdose. *Am J Kidney Dis.* 1993;22:341-344.
177. Tas S, Simonart T. Management of drug rash with eosinophilia and systemic symptoms (DRESS syndrome): an update. *Dermatology.* 2003;206:353-356.
178. Thundiyil JG, Anderson I, Stewart PJ, et al. Lamotrigine-induced seizures in a child: case report and literature review. *Clin Toxicol.* 2007:45:169-172.
179. Traub SJ, Howland MA, Hoffman RS, Nelson LS. Acute topiramate toxicity. *J Toxicol Clin Toxicol.* 2003;41:987-990.
180. Unal E, Kaya U, Aydin K. Fatal valproate overdose in a newborn baby. *Human Exp Toxicol.* 2007;26:453-456.
181. VanOpstal M, Jankneg TR, Cilissen J. Severe overdosage with the antiepileptic drug oxcarbazepine. *Br J Pharmacol.* 2004;58:329-31.
182. Vale JA. Carbamazepine overdose. *J Toxicol Clin Toxicol.* 1992;30:481-482.
183. Verma A, St Clair EW, Radtke RA. A case of sustained massive gabapentin overdose without serious side effects. *Ther Drug Monit.* 1999;21:615-617.
184. Verrotti A, Trotta D, Morgese G, et al. Valproate-induced hyperammonemic encephalopathy. *Metab Brain Dis.* 2002;17:367-373.
185. Verrotti A, Trotta D, Salladini C, Chiarelli F. Anticonvulsant hypersensitivity syndrome in children. *CNS Drugs.* 2002;16:197-205.
186. Voigt GC. Death following intravenous sodium diphenylhydantoin (Dilantin). *Johns Hopkins Med J.* 1968;123:153-157.
187. Wang SY, Wang GK. Voltage-gated sodium channels as primary targets of diverse lipid soluble neutotoxins. *Cell Signal.* 2003;15:151-159.
188. Weaver DF, Camfield P, Fraser A. Massive carbamazepine overdose: clinical and pharmacologic observation in five episodes. *Neurology.* 1988;38:755-759.
189. Willow M, Gonoi R, Catterall WA. Voltage clamp analysis of the inhibitory actions of diphenylhydantoin and carbamazepine on voltage sensitive sodium channels in neuroblastoma cells. *Mol Pharmacol.* 1985;27: 549-558.
190. Winnicka RI, Lopacinski B, Szymczak WM, Szymanska B. Carbamazepine poisoning: elimination kinetics and quantitative relationship with carbamazepine 10,11 epoxide. *J Toxicol Clin Toxicol.* 2002;40:759-765.
191. Wyte CD, Berk WA. Severe oral phenytoin overdose does not cause cardiovascular morbidity. *Ann Emerg Med.* 1991;20:508-512.
192. Yildiz TS, Toprak GD, Arisoy ES, Solak M, Toker K. Continuous venovenous hemodialfiltration to treat controlled-release carbamazepine overdose in a pediatric patient. *Ped Anes.* 2006;16:1176-1178.
193. Zoneraich S, Zoneraich O, Seigel J. Sudden death following intravenous sodium diphenylhydantoin. *Am Heart J.* 1976;91:375-377.

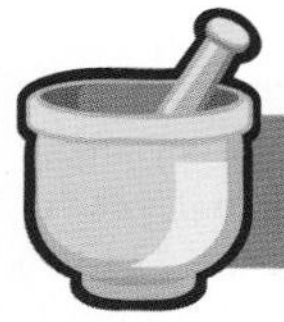

ANTIDOTES IN DEPTH (A9)

L-CARNITINE

Mary Ann Howland

$$H_3C-N^{+}(CH_3)_2-CH_2-CH(OH)-CH_2-C(=O)O^{-}$$

L-Carnitine

L-Carnitine (levocarnitine) is an amino acid that is vital to mitochondrial utilization of fatty acids. It is an orphan drug approved by the Food and Drug Administration for treatment of L-carnitine deficiency that results from inborn errors of metabolism, is associated with hemodialysis, occurs secondary to valproic acid toxicity, and for zidovudine (AZT)-induced mitochondrial myopathy[10,11,20] and pediatric cardiomyopathy.[17]

L-Carnitine decreases valproic acid–induced hyperammonemia and limits valproic acid–induced hepatic toxicity. L-Carnitine should be administered intravenously (IV) to symptomatic patients because of the limited bioavailability after oral (PO) administration.

HISTORY

L-Carnitine is found in mammals, in many bacteria, and in very small amounts in most plants.[37] Carnitine was first discovered in 1905 in extracts of muscle, and its name is derived from *carnis*, the Latin word for flesh.[21] Over the next 25 years, its chemical formula and structure were identified, and in 1997, its enantiomeric properties were confirmed.[37] Carnitine was formerly known as vitamin BT.

CHEMISTRY

Carnitine is a water-soluble amino acid that can exist as either the D or L form; however, the L isomer, which is found endogenously, is active and should be used therapeutically. L-Carnitine ($C_7H_{15}NO_3$) has a molecular weight of 161 daltons. At physiologic pH, L-carnitine contains both a positively charged quaternary nitrogen ion and a negatively charged carboxylic acid group.[15]

Fatty acids provide 9 kcal/g and are an important source of energy for the body, especially for the liver, heart, and skeletal muscle. The utilization of fatty acids as an energy source requires L-carnitine–mediated passage through both the outer and inner mitochondrial membranes to reach the mitochondrial matrix where β-oxidation occurs (see Figs. 47-2 and 12-8). Enzymes in the outer and inner mitochondrial membranes (carnitine palmitoyltransferase and carnitine acylcarnitine translocase) catalyze the synthesis, translocation, and regeneration of L-carnitine.[33] Binding of L-carnitine to fatty acids occurs through esterification at the hydroxyl group on the chiral carbon.[15] The L-carnitine regenerated in the mitochondrial matrix can also translocate in the opposite direction, from the matrix and through the inner membrane back to the space between the outer and inner membrane. Acyl-coenzyme A (CoA) is transported by carnitine from the cytosol to the mitochondria and undergoes β-oxidation in the mitochondrial matrix, generating acetyl-CoA, which then enters the citric acid cycle for the generation of adenosine triphosphate (ATP).

L-CARNITINE HOMEOSTASIS

Approximately 54% to 87% of the body stores of L-carnitine is derived primarily from meat and dairy products in the diet; the remainder is synthesized.[37] Although most plants supply very little L-carnitine, avocado and fermented soy products are exceptionally rich in this amino acid. The remainder of the carnitine needed by the body is synthesized from trimethyllysine. This amino acid, found largely in skeletal muscle, is converted to trimethylammoniobutanoate (γ-butyrobetaine) and then carried to the liver and kidney for hydroxylation to L-carnitine.[21] Synthesis of L-carnitine in the liver and kidney occurs at a rate of approximately 2 μmol/kg/d and is regulated by the amount of diet-derived trimethyllysine.[21,37] L-Carnitine is filtered by the kidneys, and tubular reabsorption maintains serum L-carnitine concentrations in the normal range.

PHARMACOKINETICS OF EXOGENOUS L-CARNITINE

Our current understanding of L-carnitine pharmacokinetics is largely derived from three major studies.[9,19,43] L-Carnitine is not bound to plasma proteins. Its volume of distribution of the central compartment (Vc) is 0.15 L/kg, approximating extracellular fluid volume. Its volume of distribution (Vd) is 0.7 L/kg. Both vary depending on the compartment model analyzed. The α half life is 0.6 to 0.7 hours with a terminal elimination half-life of 10 to 23 hours but may be 25% to 50% shorter. Baseline serum concentrations for L-carnitine are 40 μmol/L but increase to 1600 μmol/L after administration of 40 mg/kg IV over 10 minutes. Whereas 2 g of L-carnitine administered IV produces a peak plasma concentration of 1000 μmol/L, PO administration of 2 g produces peaks of only 15 to 70 μmol/L. The time to peak concentrations after PO administration occurs at 2.5 to 7.0 hours, indicating slow uptake by intestinal mucosal cells. After a 2-g carnitine dose, PO absorption is rapidly saturated, and no further absorption occurs after administration of 6 g PO. After a radiolabeled dose, most L-carnitine is metabolized to trimethylamine *N*-oxide and butyrobetaine, with only approximately 4% to 8% remaining unchanged. The metabolites trimethylamine and trimethylamine *N*-oxide may accumulate after chronic high-dose PO therapy in patients with severely compromised renal function.[9] Fecal excretion of L-carnitine is less than 1% of the total dose.

Carnitor (levocarnitine) tablets are bioequivalent to the Carnitor PO solution, with an absolute bioavailability of approximately 15%. After 4 days of dosing at 1980 mg (6 × 330-mg tablets) twice daily or 2 g twice daily of the PO solution, the maximum serum concentration was 80 μmol/L.

VALPROIC ACID AND HYPERAMMONEMIA

Valproic acid may cause hyperammonemia (defined as serum ammonia concentration >80 μg/dL or >35 μmol/L) regardless of symptoms or liver function. Hyperammonemia and hepatic toxicity may be associated either with therapeutic dosing or an acute overdose. Approximately 35% of patients receiving valproic acid demonstrate hyperammonemia, often with corresponding reduced serum L-carnitine concentrations.[7] In the absence of hepatic dysfunction, the postulated mechanisms for hyperammonemia are unclear but may result from interference with hepatic synthesis of urea or a small increase in ammonia production by the kidney.[27,45] Valproic acid induces both carnitine and acetyl-CoA deficiencies by combining with L-carnitine as valproylcarnitine and with acetyl CoA as valproyl-CoA. Ultimately, β-oxidation of all fatty acids is reduced, resulting in decreased energy production. Valproylcarnitine formation may inhibit the renal reabsorption of L-carnitine.[32]

Valproic acid stimulates glutaminase, favoring glutamate uptake and ammonia release from the kidney. Reduced glutamate concentrations lead to impaired production of *N*-acetylglutamate (NAGA), a cofactor for carbamoyl phosphate synthetase I (CPS I), which is used in the liver to synthesize urea from ammonia.

In humans taking valproic acid, L-carnitine supplementation reduces ammonia concentrations.[1,3,5,7,18,25,31,34,35,39,46] The exact time frame for normalization of ammonia concentrations is unknown, but a preliminary report suggests hastening of ammonia elimination with L-carnitine (3–15 h) compared with published controls (11–90 h), although the difference was not statistically significant.[41,42]

VALPROIC ACID AND HEPATOTOXICITY

Valproic acid therapy is commonly associated with a transient dose-related asymptomatic increase in liver enzyme concentrations and a rare symptomatic, life-threatening, idiosyncratic hepatotoxicity similar to Reye syndrome.[4] Liver histology of the latter demonstrates microvesicular steatosis, similar to that described in both hypoglycin-induced Jamaican vomiting sickness (see Chap. 118) and Reye syndrome. This occurrence presumably results from L-carnitine and acetyl-CoA deficiency, which inhibits mitochondrial β-oxidation of valproic acid and other fatty acids, causing them to accumulate in the hepatocyte. One study compared valproic acid administration in mice bred to have decreased carnitine stores with normal mice and found that the mice with decreased carnitine stores developed microvesicular steatosis of the liver. In addition, evaluation of their isolated liver mitochondria demonstrated decreased oxidative capacity.[23]

Evidence for the benefit of L-carnitine treatment in improving survival from valproic acid–induced hepatotoxicity comes from the retrospective analysis of patients identified by the International Registry for Adverse Reactions to valproic acid.[6] When 50 patients with acute, symptomatic hepatic dysfunction who were not treated with L-carnitine were compared with 42 similar patients treated with L-carnitine, only 10% of the untreated patients survived but 48% of the L-carnitine–treated patients survived.[6] Early diagnosis of patients, prompt discontinuance of valproic acid, and administration of IV rather than PO L-carnitine resulted in the greatest survival.[6] Most patients received 50 to 100 mg/kg/d of L-carnitine regardless of the route of administration.[6] Additionally, case reports and animal studies[40] offer both support[38,44] and lack of support for the beneficial effects of L-carnitine in the presence of valproic acid–induced hepatotoxicity.[24,25,30,41]

L-CARNITINE CONCENTRATIONS

In the serum, 80% of L-carnitine is free, and the rest is acylated.[14] In adults who eat all food groups and children older than 1 year of age, the normal serum concentrations of free L-carnitine are 22 to 66 μmol/L and of total L-carnitine concentrations are 28 to 84 μmol/L. Vegetarians have L-carnitine concentrations 12% to 30% lower than omnivores.[36]

Studies in patients taking valproic acid demonstrate decreases in both free and total serum L-carnitine concentrations[35] and decreases in both total and free muscle carnitine concentrations.[2]

Case studies demonstrate reduced serum free L-carnitine concentrations and abnormal valproic acid metabolite profiles that normalize with L-carnitine supplementation.[22,28,29] All of these data support the use of L-carnitine and provide a potential mechanism for its beneficial effects in valproic acid–induced hepatotoxicity.

ADVERSE EFFECTS AND CONTRAINDICATIONS TO L-CARNITINE

L-Carnitine administration is well tolerated.[26] Transient nausea and vomiting are the most common side effects reported, with diarrhea and a fishy body odor noted at higher doses.[9] After chronic high doses of L-carnitine in patients with severely compromised renal function, the potentially toxic L-carnitine metabolites trimethylamine and methylamine *N*-oxide accumulate. The importance of this accumulation is unknown. Trimethylamine and its metabolite dimethylamine may contribute to cognitive abnormalities and the fishy odor.[13] In a pharmacokinetic study after IV administration of 6 g of L-carnitine over 10 minutes, two of six subjects complained of transient visual blurring; one subject also complained of headache and lightheadedness. The manufacturer of L-carnitine has received case reports of convulsive episodes after L-carnitine use by patients with or without a preexisting seizure disorder. These reports are currently noted in the package insert. No reports of seizures related to L-carnitine use can be found in the human literature. The only data suggesting carnitine-related seizures are found in a rat model.[16]

There are no known contraindications to the use of L-carnitine. However, only the L isomer and not the racemic mixture should be used because the DL mixture may interfere with mitochondrial utilization of L-carnitine. L-carnitine is considered FDA pregnancy Category B.

OVERDOSE OF L-CARNITINE

No cases of toxicity from overdose have been reported, although large PO doses may cause diarrhea.[9] The LD_{50} in rats is 5.4 g/kg IV and 19.2 g/kg PO.[9]

DOSAGE AND ADMINISTRATION

The optimal dosing of L-carnitine for valproic acid–induced hyperammonemia or hepatotoxicity has not been established. Recommendations for IV L-carnitine administration to patients with acute metabolic disorders resulting from L-carnitine deficiency range from 50 to 500 mg/kg/d.[9,12] A loading dose equal to the daily dose may be given initially, followed by the daily dose divided into every 4 hourly doses. The 500-mg/kg/d dose was intended for children[8] and did not list a maximum dose After the loading dose, we suggest a maximal daily dose of 6 g . The PO dosing of L-carnitine usually is 50 to 100 mg/kg/d up to 3 g/d and should be reserved for patients who are not acutely ill.

For patients with end-stage renal disease undergoing hemodialysis, the package insert recommends an IV starting dose of 10 to 20 mg/kg dry body weight as a slow IV bolus over 2 to 3 minutes after completion of dialysis followed by a dose adjustment according to L-carnitine trough (predialysis) serum concentrations (normal, 40–50 μmol/L).

For patients with an acute overdose of valproic acid and without hepatic enzyme abnormalities or symptomatic hyperammonemia, L-carnitine administration can be considered prophylactic, and enteral doses of 100 mg/kg/d divided every 6 hours up to 3 g/d are appropriate. For patients with valproic acid–induced symptomatic hepatotoxicity or symptomatic hyperammonemia, IV L-carnitine should be administered. We suggest a dose of 100 mg/kg IV up to 6 g administered over 30 minutes as a loading dose followed by 15 mg/kg every 4 hours administered over 10 to 30 minutes.

AVAILABILITY

L-Carnitine (Carnitor) is available as a sterile injection for IV use in 1 g/5 mL single-dose vials.[9] L-Carnitine is supplied without a preservative. After the vial is opened, the unused portion should be discarded. Carnitor injection is compatible with and stable when mixed with normal saline or lactated Ringer solution in concentrations as high as 8 mg/mL for as long as 24 hours.[9] L-Carnitine (Carnitor) is also available as a 330-mg tablet; as an PO solution with artificial cherry flavoring, malic acid, sucrose syrup, and methylparaben and propylparaben as preservatives; and as a sugar-free PO solution (Carnitor SF) at a concentration of 100 mg/mL.[8] The PO solution may be consumed without diluting, or it may be dissolved in other drinks to mask the taste. Slow consumption reduces gastrointestinal side effects.[9]

REFERENCES

1. Altunbasak S, Baytok V, Tasouji M, et al. Asymptomatic hyperammonemia in children treated with valproic acid. *J Child Neurol.* 1997;12:461-463.
2. Anil M, Helvaci M, Ozbal E et al. Serum and muscle carnitine levels in epileptic children receiving sodium valproate. *J Child Neurol.* 2009;24:80-86.
3. Barrueto F Jr, Hack JB. Hyperammonemia and coma without hepatic dysfunction induced by valproate therapy. *Acad Emerg Med.* 2001;8:999-1001.
4. Berthelot-Moritz F, Chadda K, Chanavaz I, et al. Fatal sodium valproate poisoning. *Intensive Care Med.* 1997;23:599.
5. Beversdorf D, Allen C, Nordgren R. Valproate induced encephalopathy treated with carnitine in an adult. *J Neurol Neurosurg Psychiatry.* 1996;61:211.
6. Bohan TP, Helton E, McDonald I, et al. Effect of L-carnitine treatment for valproate-induced hepatotoxicity. *Neurology.* 2001;56:1405-1409.
7. Böhles H, Sewell AC, Wenzel D. The effect of carnitine supplementation in valproate-induced hyperammonaemia. *Acta Paediatr.* 1996;85:446-449.
8. Carnitor (levocarnitine) tablets, Carnitor Oral Solution, and Carnitor SF Sugar Free Oral solution (package insert). Gaithersburg, MD: Sigma-Tau; June 2006.
9. Carnitor® (levocarnitine) Injection (product information). Gaithersburg, MD: Sigma-Tau; March 2004.
10. Carter R, Singh J, Archambault C, et al. Severe lactic acidosis in association with reverse transcriptase inhibitors with potential response to L-carnitine in a pediatric HIV positive patient. *AIDS Patient Care.* 2004;18:131-134.
11. Claessens Y, Chiche J, Mira J, et al. Bench to bedside review: severe lactic acidosis in HIV patients treated with nucleoside analogue reverse transciptase inhibitors. *Crit Care.* 2003;7:226-232.
12. De Vivo DC, Bohan TP, Coulter DL, et al. L-carnitine supplementation in childhood epilepsy: current perspectives. *Epilepsia.* 1998;39:1216-1225.
13. Eknoyan G, Latos DL, Lindberg J. Practice recommendations for the use of L-carnitine in dialysis-related carnitine disorder. National Kidney Foundation Carnitine Consensus Conference. *Am J Kidney Dis.* 2003;41:868-876.
14. Evangeliou A, Vlassopoulos D. Carnitine metabolism and deficit—when supplementation is necessary? *Curr Pharm Biotechnol.* 2003;4:211-219.
15. Evans A. Dialysis-related carnitine disorder and levocarnitine pharmacology. *Am J Kidney Dis.* 2003;41(suppl):S13-S26.
16. Fariello RG, Zeeman E, Golden GT, et al. Transient seizure activity induced by acetylcarnitine. *Neuropharmacology.* 1984;23:585-587.
17. Ferrari R, Cicchitelli D, Fucili M, et al. Therapeutic effects of L-carnitine and propionyl-L-carnitine on cardiovascular disease: a review. *Ann NY Acad Sci.* 2004;1033:79-91.
18. Gidal BE, Inglese CM, Meyer JF, et al. Diet- and valproate-induced transient hyperammonemia: effect of L-carnitine. *Pediatr Neurol.* 1997;16:301-305.
19. Harper P, Elwin CE, Cederblad G. Pharmacokinetics of intravenous and oral bolus doses of L-carnitine in healthy subjects. *Eur J Clin Pharmacol.* 1988;35:555-562.
20. Hoffman R, Currier J. Management of antiretroviral treatment related complications *Infect Dis Clinics North Am.* 2007;21:103-132.
21. Hoppel C. The role of carnitine in normal and altered fatty acid metabolism. *Am J Kidney Dis.* 2003;41:S4-S12.
22. Ishikura H, Matsue N, Matsubara M, et al. Valproic acid overdose and L-carnitine therapy. *J Anal Toxicol.* 1996;20:55-58.
23. Knapp A, Todesco L, Beier K, et al. Toxicity of valproic acid in mice with decreased plasma and tissue carnitine stores. *J Pharm Exp Ther.* 2008;324:568-575.
24. Laub MC, Paetzke-Brunner I, Jaeger G. Serum carnitine during valproic acid therapy. *Epilepsia.* 1986;27:559-562.
25. Lheureux P, Hantson P. Carnitine in the treatment of valproic acid induced toxicity. *Clin Toxicol.* 2009;47:101-111.
26. LoVecchio F, Shriki J, Samaddar R. L-carnitine was safely administered in the setting of valproic acid toxicity. *Am J Emerg Med.* 2005;23:321-322.
27. Marini AM, Zaret BS, Beckner RR. Hepatic and renal contributions to valproic acid-induced hyperammonemia. *Neurology.* 1988;38:365-371.
28. Murakami K, Sugimoto T, Nishida, et al. Alterations of urinary acetylcarnitine in valproate-treated rats: the effect of L-carnitine supplementation. *J Child Neurol.* 1992;7:404-407.
29. Murakami K, Sugimoto T, Woo M, et al. Effect of L-carnitine supplementation on acute valproate intoxication. *Epilepsia.* 1996;37:687-689.
30. Murphy JV, Groover RV, Hodge C. Hepatotoxic effects in a child receiving valproate and carnitine. *J Pediatr.* 1993;123:318-320.
31. Ohtani Y, Endo F, Matsuda I. Carnitine deficiency and hyperammonemia associated with valproic acid. *J Pediatr.* 1982;101:782-785.
32. Okamura N, Ohnishi S, Shimaoka H et al. Involvement of recognition and interaction of carnitine transporter in the decrease of L-carnitine concentration induced by pivalic acid and valproic acid. *Pharm Res.* 2006;23:1729-1735.
33. Pande SV. Carnitine-acylcarnitine translocase deficiency. *Am J Med Sci.* 1999;318:22-27.
34. Raby WN. Carnitine for valproic acid-induced hyperammonemia. *Am J Psychiatry.* 1997;154:158.
35. Raskind JY, El-Chaar M. The role of carnitine supplementation during valproic acid therapy. *Ann Pharmacother.* 2000;34:630-638.
36. Rebouche CJ. Carnitine function and requirements during the life cycle. *FASEB J.* 1992;6:3379-3386.
37. Rebouche CJ, Seim H. Carnitine metabolism and its regulation in microorganisms and mammals. *Annu Rev Nutr.* 1998;18:39-61.
38. Romero-Falcón A, de la Santa Belda E, García-Contreras R, Varela JM. A case of valproate-associated hepatotoxicity treated with L-carnitine. *Eur J Intern Med.* 2003;14:338-340.
39. Segura-Bruna N, Rodriguez-Campello A, Puente V et al. Valproate induced hyperammonemic encephalopathy. *Acta Neurol Scand.* 2006;114:1-7.
40. Sugimoto T, Araki A, Nishida N, et al. Hepatotoxicity in rat following administration of valproic acid: effect of L-carnitine supplementation. *Epilepsia.* 1987;28:373-377.
41. Sztajnkrycer M. Valproic acid toxicity: overview and management. *J Toxicol Clin Toxicol.* 2002;40:789-801.
42. Sztajnkrycer MD, Scaglione JM, Bond GR. Valproate-induced hyperammonemia: preliminary evaluation of ammonia elimination with carnitine administration. *J Toxicol Clin Toxicol.* 2001;39:497.
43. Uematsu T, Itaya T, Nishimoto M, et al. Pharmacokinetics and safety of L-carnitine infused I.V. in healthy subjects. *Eur J Clin Pharmacol.* 1988;34:213-216.
44. Vance CK, Vance WH, Winter SC, et al. Control of valproate-induced hepatotoxicity with carnitine. *Ann Neurol.* 1989;26:456.
45. Verrotti A, Trotta D, Morgese G, Chiarelli F. Valproate-induced hyperammonemic encephalopathy. *Metab Brain Dis.* 2002;17:367-373.
46. Wadzinski J, Franks R, Roane D, et al. Valproate associated hyperammonemic encephalopathy. *J Am Board Fam Med.* 2007;20:499-502.

CHAPTER 48
ANTIDIABETICS AND HYPOGLYCEMICS

George M. Bosse

Glucose

MW	=	180 daltons
Normal fasting range (blood)	=	60–100 mg/dL
	=	3.3–5.6 mmol/L

Although various xenobiotics and medical conditions may cause hypoglycemia, this chapter focuses on the medications used for treatment of diabetes mellitus. These medications include insulin, incretin mimetics, and oral agents: the sulfonylureas, biguanides, α-glucosidase inhibitors, thiazolidinediones, meglitinides, and gliptins. Some of the medications in these chemically heterogeneous groups of xenobiotics can cause unique toxic effects in addition to hypoglycemia.

In general, neurohormonal control of glucose production in healthy individuals maintains a fasting serum glucose concentration in the range of 60–100 mg/dL. In diabetes mellitus, the body fails to maintain normal blood glucose concentrations. The two glycemic complications of diabetes mellitus and its therapy are hyperglycemia and hypoglycemia.

Most patients with diabetes mellitus are classified as having either insulin-dependent diabetes mellitus (IDDM), also known as type I diabetes, or non–insulin-dependent diabetes mellitus (NIDDM), also known as type II diabetes. This classification scheme for diabetes mellitus is not perfect. For example, some patients with type II diabetes may require insulin in addition to oral hypoglycemics. Early in the course of type I diabetes, patients may enter a remission period during which exogenous insulin is not required.

HISTORY AND EPIDEMIOLOGY

Insulin first became available for use in 1922 after Banting and colleagues successfully treated diabetic patients with pancreatic extracts.[10] In an attempt to more closely simulate physiologic conditions, additional "designer" insulins with unique kinetic properties have been developed, including an ultrashort-acting preparation known as *lispro*.[62,130] Several oral delivery systems for insulin have been studied.[87] Development of an oral delivery system for use in humans has not been successful because of poor intestinal absorption and degradation of the oral form of insulin by digestive enzymes. Using zonula occludens toxin, modulation of intestinal tight junctions in animal models has resulted in significant increases in enteral absorption of insulin.[38] An inhaled form of insulin had recently become available, but has been withdrawn from the market due to poor sales.[83]

The hypoglycemic activity of a sulfonamide derivative used for typhoid fever was noted during World War II.[70] This discovery was verified later in animals. The sulfonylureas in use today are chemical modifications of that original sulfonamide compound. In the mid-1960s, the first-generation sulfonylureas were widely used. Newer second-generation drugs differ primarily in their potency.

Although insulin is widely used for treating diabetes mellitus, sulfonylurea exposures are much more commonly reported to poison centers than are insulin exposures, based on 15 years of data from 1993 to 2007 (Chap. 135). These data likely reflect a significant percentage of intentional overdose cases. In a review of 1418 medication-related cases of hypoglycemia, sulfonylureas (especially the long-acting chlorpropamide and glyburide) alone or with a second hypoglycemic accounted for the largest percentage of cases (63%).[120] Only 18 of the sulfonylurea cases in this series involved overdose with suicidal intent. However, hypoglycemia is reported in as many as 20% of patients using sulfonylureas.[55] Despite the lack of evidence reported in the literature, we speculate that insulin-induced hypoglycemia occurs frequently in settings other than volitional overdose. Besides sulfonylurea use, advanced age and fasting are identified as major risk factors for hypoglycemia. Other causes of hypoglycemia are listed in Table 48–1.

The biguanides metformin and phenformin were developed as derivatives of *Galega officinalis,* the French lilac, recognized in medieval Europe as a treatment for diabetes mellitus.[8] Phenformin was used in the United States until 1977, when it was removed from the market because of its association with life-threatening metabolic acidosis with hyperlactatemia (64 cases/100,000 patient-years). However, phenformin still is available outside the United States.[101]

Development of the α-glucosidase inhibitors began in the 1960s when an α-amylase inhibitor was isolated from wheat flour.[116] Acarbose was discovered more than 10 years later and approved for use in the United States in 1995. Troglitazone and repaglinide were approved for use in the United States in 1997. The FDA subsequently directed the manufacturer of troglitazone to withdraw the product from the US market in 2000 because of associated liver toxicity. Exenatide, a synthetic form of a compound found in the saliva of the Gila monster, is an incretin mimetic. Incretins are endogenous compounds in humans which stimulate insulin secretion in response to an oral glucose load. Most recently, the gliptins, which inhibit the enzyme responsible for the inactivation of incretins, have been introduced.

PHARMACOLOGY

Insulin is synthesized as a precursor polypeptide in the β-islet cells of the pancreas. Proteolytic processing results in the formation of proinsulin, which is cleaved, giving rise to C-peptide and insulin itself, a double-chain molecule containing 51 amino acid residues. Glucose concentration plays a major role in the regulation of insulin release.[107] Glucose is phosphorylated after transport into the β-islet cell of the pancreas. Further metabolism of glucose-6-phosphate results in the formation of ATP. ATP inhibition of the K^+ channel results in cell depolarization, inward calcium flux, and insulin release. After release, insulin binds to specific receptors on cell surfaces in insulin-sensitive tissues, particularly the hepatocyte, myocyte, and fat cells. The action of insulin on these cells involves various phosphorylation and dephosphorylation reactions.

Figure 48–1 depicts the chemical structures of oral agents representing the major classes of antidiabetic and hypoglycemic agents. The sulfonylureas stimulate the β cells of the pancreas to release insulin; therefore, they are ineffective in type I diabetes mellitus resulting from islet cell destruction (Fig. 48–2). This stimulatory effect diminishes with chronic therapy. All the sulfonylureas bind to high-affinity receptors on the pancreatic β-cell membrane, resulting in closure of K^+ channels.[36,43,44] Inhibition of potassium ion efflux mimics the effect of naturally elevated intracellular ATP and results in insulin release. High-affinity sulfonylurea receptors also present within pancreatic β cells are postulated to be either located on granular membranes or part of a regulatory exocytosis kinase. Binding to these receptors promotes exocytosis by direct interaction with secretory machinery not involving closure of the plasma membrane K^+ channels.[36,43,44]

TABLE 48–1. Causes of Hypoglycemia

Artifactual	**Miscellaneous**	**Neoplasms**	Disopyramide
Chronic myelogenous leukemia	Acquired immunodeficiency syndrome (AIDS)	Carcinomas (diverse extrapancreatic)	Ethanol
Polycythemia vera	Anorexia nervosa	Hematologic	Hypoglycin (Ackee)
Endocrine disorders	Autoimmune disorders	Insulinoma	Pentamidine
Addison disease	Burns	Mesenchymal	Propoxyphene
Glucagon deficiency	Diarrhea (childhood)	Multiple endocrine adenopathy type 1 (Werner syndrome)	Quinidine
Panhypopituitarism (Sheehan syndrome)	Graves disease	**Reactive hypoglycemia**	Quinine
Hepatic disease	Leucine sensitivity	**Renal disease**	Ritodrine
Acute hepatic atrophy	Muscular activity (excessive)	Chronic hemodialysis	Salicylates
Alcoholism	Postgastric surgery (including gastric bypass)	Chronic renal insufficiency	Streptozocin
Cirrhosis	Pregnancy	**Xenobiotics**	Sulfonamides
Galactose or fructose intolerance	Protein calorie malnutrition	β-Adrenergic antagonists	Vacor
Glycogen storage disease	Rheumatoid arthritis	Alloxan	Valproic acid
Neoplasia	Septicemia	Antidiabetics (insulin, sulfonylureas, miglitinides)	
	Shock		
	SLE		

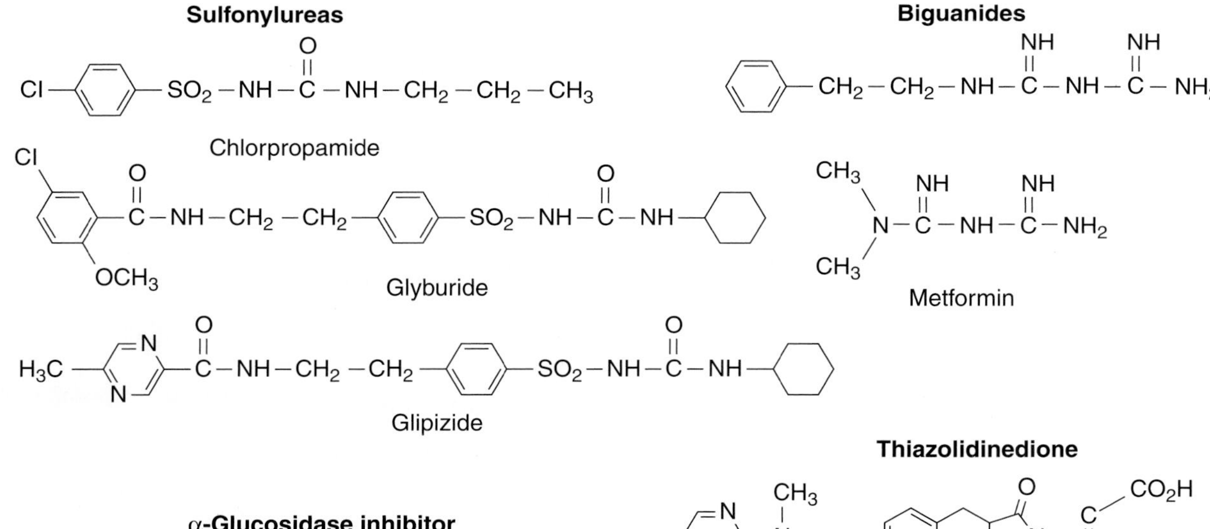

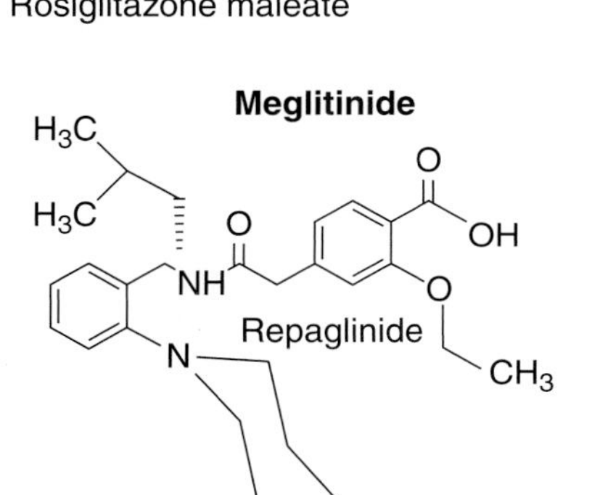

FIGURE 48–1. Chemical structures of representative oral antidiabetics.

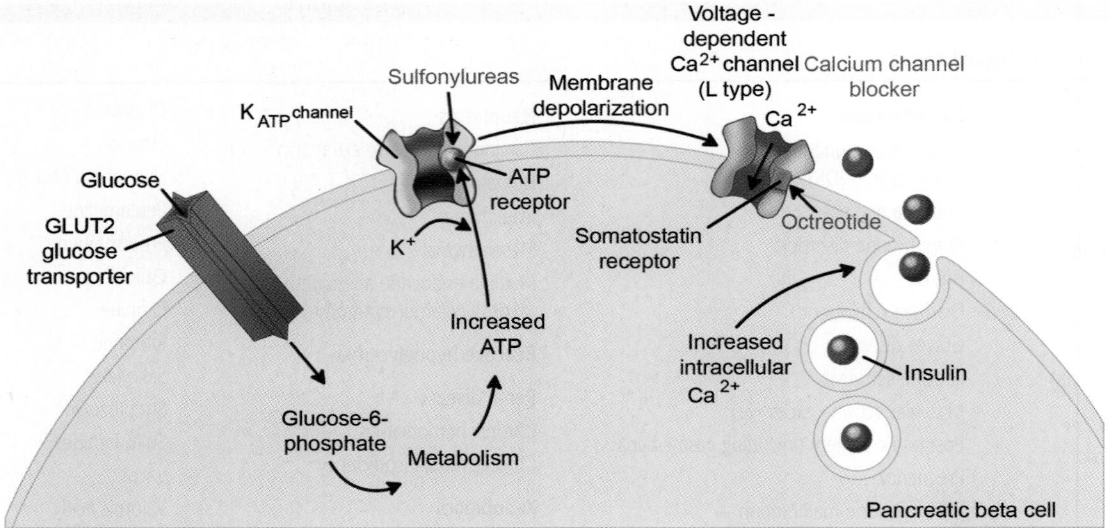

FIGURE 48–2. Under normal conditions, cells release insulin in response to elevation of intracellular ATP concentrations. Sulfonylureas potentiate the effects of ATP at its "sensor" on the ligand-gated K^+ channels and prevent efflux of K^+. The subsequent rise in intracellular potential opens voltage-gated Ca^{2+} channels, which increases intracellular calcium concentration through a series of phosphorylation reactions. The increase in intracellular calcium results in the release of insulin. Release of insulin is also caused by binding of sulfonylureas to postulated receptor sites on regulatory exocytosis kinase and insulin granular membranes.

Repaglinide and nateglinide are oral agents of the meglitinide class and differ structurally from the sulfonylureas.[111] However, they also bind to K^+ channels on pancreatic cells, resulting in increased insulin secretion. Compared to the sulfonylureas, the hypoglycemic effects of the meglitinides are shorter in duration.

The linkage of two guanidine molecules forms the biguanides. Metformin is an oral compound approved for treatment of type II diabetes mellitus. Its glucose-stabilizing effect is caused by several mechanisms, the most important of which appears to involve inhibition of gluconeogenesis and subsequent decreased hepatic glucose output. Enhanced peripheral glucose uptake also plays a significant role in maintaining euglycemia. Metformin's ability to lower blood glucose concentrations also occurs as a result of decreased fatty acid oxidation and increased intestinal use of glucose.[9,132] In skeletal muscle and adipose cells, metformin causes enhanced activity and translocation of glucose transporters. Although the details are unclear, the mechanism by which this process occurs involves an interaction between metformin and tyrosine kinase on the intracellular portion of the insulin receptor. Figure 48–3 depicts the mechanism of action of metformin.

Insulin resistance in patients with type II diabetes mellitus may occur because of secretion of biologically defective insulin molecules, circulating insulin antagonists, or target tissue defects in insulin action.[96] The thiazolidinedione derivatives decrease insulin resistance by potentiating insulin sensitivity in the liver, adipose tissue, and skeletal muscle. Uptake of glucose into adipose tissue and skeletal muscle is enhanced, while hepatic glucose production is reduced.[17,54]

Acarbose and miglitol are oligosaccharides that inhibit α-glucosidase enzymes such as glucoamylase, sucrase, and maltase in the brush border of the small intestine. As a result, postprandial elevations in blood glucose concentrations after carbohydrate ingestion are blunted.[139] Delayed gastric emptying may be another mechanism for the antihyperglycemic effect of these oligosaccharides.[110]

Exenatide is structurally similar to glucagon-like peptide-1 (GLP-1), a human gut hormone that is released in response to an oral glucose

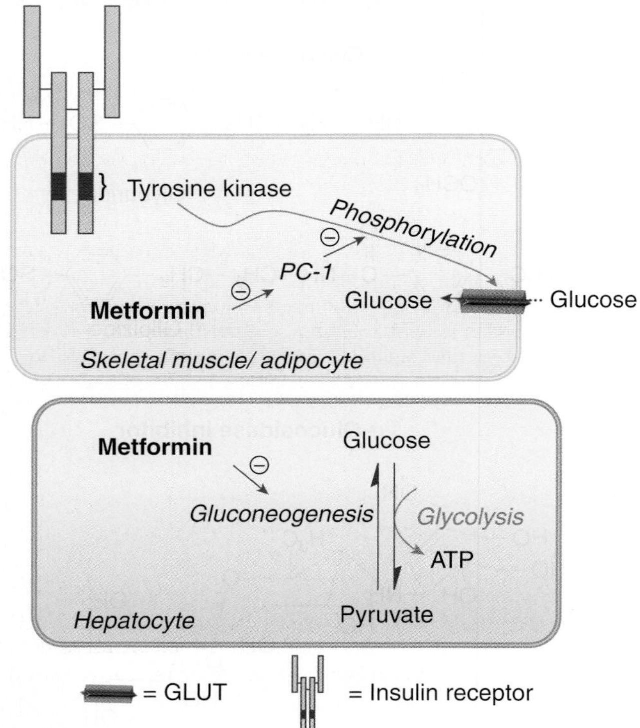

FIGURE 48–3. Under normal conditions, insulin binding to its receptor on myocytes and adipocytes activates tyrosine kinase, resulting in phosphorylation and activation of the membrane-bound glucose transporter GLUT. Non–insulin-dependent diabetes mellitus is causally associated with an increased activity of PC-1, a glycoprotein that inhibits tyrosine kinase activity and thus reduces myocyte and adipocyte glucose uptake. Metformin reduces PC-1 activity in these cells, enhancing peripheral glucose utilization. In addition, gluconeogenesis in hepatic cells is reduced through interference with pyruvate carboxylase, the enzyme responsible for conversion of pyruvate to oxaloacetate.

TABLE 48–3. Characteristics of Routinely Used Forms of Insulin

Insulin	Onset of Action (h)	Duration of Action (h)	Peak Glycemic Response (h)
Rapid and Ultrashort-acting			
Aspart	0.25	3–5	0.75–1.5
Glulusine	0.5	<5	1.5–2
Lispro	0.25–0.5	<5	0.5–2.5
Short-acting			
Regular	0.5–1	5–8	2.5–5
Intermediate-acting			
Lente	1–3	18–24	6–14
NPH	1–2	18–24	6–14
Long-acting			
Detemir	1.5	24	No true peak
Glargine	1.1	24	No true peak
Ultralente	4–6	20–36	8–20

glucagon and epinephrine secretion. These counterregulatory defenses against hypoglycemia are defective in most people with type I diabetes mellitus and in many with type II diabetes mellitus.

Although various xenobiotics can cause hypoglycemia (Table 48–1), salicylates and ethanol are particularly notable for their unintended hypoglycemic effects. The mechanism of ethanol-induced hypoglycemia is discussed in Chap. 77. Salicylate inhibition of prostaglandin synthesis in the β cell of the pancreas is postulated to result in enhanced insulin secretion.[11] Salicylates may also cause hypoglycemia by poorly defined mechanisms that do not involve enhanced insulin secretion.

Besides decreasing glucose concentrations, the hypoglycemics can produce a number of adverse effects, both in overdose and in therapeutic doses. The sulfonylureas, predominantly chlorpropamide, can cause a syndrome of inappropriate antidiuretic hormone secretion.[57] Concomitant use of sulfonylureas, predominantly chlorpropamide and ethanol can cause a disulfiram–ethanol reaction, as sulfonylureas inhibit aldehyde dehydrogenase.[104]

TABLE 48–4. Xenobiotics Known to React with Hypoglycemics Resulting in Hypoglycemia

Angiotensin-converting enzyme (ACE) inhibitors	Methotrexate
Allopurinol	Monamine oxidase inhibitors
Anabolic steroids	Pentamidine
β-Adrenergic antagonists	Phenylbutazone
Chloramphenicol	Probenecid
Clofibrate	Quinine
Disopyramide	Salicylates
Ethanol	Sulfonamide
Fluoroquinolones	Trimethoprim sulfamethoxazole
Haloperidol	Warfarin

See Table 48–1 for list of xenobiotics that cause hypoglycemia independently.

CLINICAL MANIFESTATIONS

Hypoglycemia and its secondary effects on the CNS (neuroglycopenia) are the most common adverse effects related to insulin and the sulfonylureas. It is essential to remember that hypoglycemia is primarily a clinical and not a numerical disorder. Clinical hypoglycemia is the failure to maintain a serum glucose concentration that prevents signs or symptoms of glucose deficiency. The clinical presentations of patients with hypoglycemia are extremely variable. Hypoglycemia must be considered to be the etiology of any neuropsychiatric abnormality, whether persistent or transient, focal or generalized. The cerebral cortex usually is most severely affected. Categorization of these findings is as follows:[106]

- Delirium with subdued, confused, or manic behavior.
- Coma with multifocal brainstem abnormalities, including decerebrate spasms and respiratory abnormalities, with preservation of the oculocephalic (doll's eyes), oculovestibular (cold-caloric), and pupillary responses.
- Focal neurologic deficits simulating a cerebrovascular accident (CVA) with or without the presence of coma. During a 12-month study period, 3 (2.4%) of 125 hypoglycemic patients presented with hemiplegia.[76] There are numerous reports[4,125] and series[119,138] of patients with focal neurologic deficits.
- Solitary or multiple seizures.

These neuropsychiatric symptoms are usually reversible if the hypoglycemia is corrected promptly. The morbidity resulting from undiagnosed hypoglycemia is related partly to the etiology and partly to the duration and severity of the hypoglycemia. Because the etiologies of hypoglycemia encompass both severe diseases such as fulminant hepatic failure and benign problems such as a missed meal by an insulin-requiring diabetic, the literature with regard to outcome is confusing. Although a study of 125 emergency department (ED) cases of symptomatic hypoglycemia reported an 11% mortality rate,[76] only 1 death (0.8%) was attributed directly to hypoglycemia. In that same study, nine patients (7.2%) presented with seizures (focal in one case), three patients (2.4%) presented with hemiparesis, and four survivors (3.2%) suffered residual neurologic deficits. In one tertiary care medical center, 1.2% of all admitted patients had hypoglycemia (defined as a glucose concentration less than 50 mg/dL). The overall mortality was 27% for this group of 94 patients.[40] The longer and more profound the hypoglycemic episode, the more likely permanent CNS damage will occur.[7]

No absolute criteria available from the physical examination or history distinguish one form of metabolic coma from another. Moreover, the findings classically associated with hypoglycemia, such as tremor, sweating, tachycardia, confusion, coma, and seizures, frequently may not occur.[52] The glycemic threshold is the glucose concentration below which clinical manifestations develop, a threshold that is host variable. In one study, the mean glycemic threshold for hypoglycemic symptoms was 78 mg/dL in patients with poorly controlled Type 1 diabetes compared to 53 mg/dL in nondiabetics.[15]

Patients with well-controlled Type 1 diabetes may be unaware of hypoglycemia. It appears that even in the presence of numerical hypoglycemia, diabetic individuals with near-normal glycosylated hemoglobin values maintain near-normal glucose uptake by the brain, thereby preserving cerebral metabolism and limiting the response of counterregulatory hormones. The result of this limited response is unawareness of hypoglycemia.[14,15] A threshold level likely is achieved below which the glucose concentration is inadequate, but this may be a concentration so close to that causing serious neuroglycopenia that patients have limited opportunity for corrective action.[14] Hypoglycemia unawareness is most likely in diabetics with chronic exposure to hypoglycemics because of hypoglycemia-associated autonomic failure.[28] Acute ingestion of hypoglycemic agents in nondiabetic patients likely would cause classic signs and symptoms.

Sinus tachycardia, atrial fibrillation, and ventricular premature contractions are the most common dysrhythmias associated with hypoglycemia.[69,95] An outpouring of catecholamines, hypoglycemia itself, transient electrolyte abnormalities, and underlying heart disease appear to be the most likely etiologies. Based on their mechanisms of action, both insulin and the sulfonylureas are expected to promote the shift of potassium into cells, and hypokalemia after insulin overdose is well documented.[6,129] Other cardiovascular manifestations include angina and ischemia, which rarely may be the sole manifestations of hypoglycemia.[35] Both are directly related to hypoglycemia.[12,103] Increased release of catecholamines during hypoglycemia increases myocardial oxygen demand and may decrease supply by causing coronary vasoconstriction.

Hypothermia may occur in hypoglycemic patients.[41,59,131] If present, hypothermia usually is mild (90°–95°F [32°–35°C]), unless coexisting conditions such as environmental exposure, infection, head injury, or hypothyroidism are present. In a study comparing two groups of patients with depressed mental status, hypothermia was almost exclusively limited to the hypoglycemic patients; of these patients, 53% with demonstrated hypoglycemia showed hypothermia.[131] The central hypothalamic response to hypoglycemia stimulated by the sympathetic nervous system may actually "overshoot" normal temperatures, resulting in hyperthermia following recovery.[25]

Hypoglycemia is reported in two cases of metformin overdose.[134] In both cases, metabolic acidosis with hyperlactatemia was evident on initial presentation. Hypoglycemia was present initially in one of the cases but did not develop until 7 hours later in the second case. Hypoglycemia and metabolic acidosis with hyperlactatemia are reported in a case of overdose with metformin, atenolol, and diclofenac.[48] Hypoglycemia is reported in a case of metformin-associated metabolic acidosis with hyperlactatemia related to therapeutic use.[64] Insufficient evidence supports the concept that metformin-associated hypoglycemia can develop in a patient who is not critically ill without metabolic acidosis. Because many patients receiving metformin also take sulfonylureas, hypoglycemia should be anticipated after overdose. Phenformin is similar to metformin in that ingestion alone rarely causes hypoglycemia, in overdose or following therapeutic use.[120]

The α-glucosidase inhibitors, thiazolidinediones, meglitinides, exenatide, and gliptins, are newer agents for which overdose data are limited. Acarbose and miglitol are not likely to cause hypoglycemia based on their mechanism of action of inhibiting α-glucosidase. The most common adverse effects associated with therapeutic use of these xenobiotics are gastrointestinal, including nausea, bloating, abdominal pain, flatulence, and diarrhea. Elevated aminotransferase concentrations were noted after use of acarbose in clinical trials.[53] Most patients were asymptomatic, and the aminotransferase concentrations returned to normal after the drug was discontinued. The therapeutic use of acarbose in some cases reportedly led to hepatotoxicity that resolved after the drug was discontinued.[5,23]

Although hypoglycemia would not be expected after thiazolidinedione overdose, experience is limited. The most serious adverse effect of troglitazone is the development of liver toxicity with therapeutic doses, which in some cases was severe enough to require liver transplantation.[45,92] Liver toxicity related to therapeutic use of rosiglitazone[3,42] and pioglitazone is also reported.[75,78] Therapeutic use of pioglitazone and rosiglitazone may precipitate fluid retention in patients with underlying congestive heart failure.[91] A meta-analysis concluded that rosiglitazone therapy is associated with an increased risk of myocardial infarction and death from cardiovascular causes.[94]

Hypoglycemia should be anticipated after repaglinide and nateglinide ingestion. Hypoglycemia has been reported after nateglinide overdose,[89] and a case of intentionally self-induced hypoglycemia secondary to repaglinide is reported.[51] Hypoglycemia did not occur in a recently published case of intentional overdose with a total of 90 μg exenatide.[27] "Severe hypoglycemia" was reported in a phase III clinical trial after inadvertent administration of ten times the normal dose of exenatide. The specific glucose concentration is not noted in the report.[21] Sitagliptin was recently released in the United States and overdose data are lacking.

HYPOGLYCEMIC POTENTIAL OF ANTIDIABETICS

Hypoglycemia may not occur until 18 hours after lente insulin overdose,[88] may persist for up to 53 hours after insulin glargine overdose,[18] and may persist up to 6 days after ultralente insulin overdose.[77] Death after insulin overdose cannot be correlated directly with either the dose or preparation type. Some patients have died with doses estimated in the hundreds of units, whereas others have survived doses in the thousands of units.[117] Mortality and morbidity may correlate better with delay in recognition of the problem, duration of symptoms, onset of therapy, and type of complications, as opposed to the absolute degree of hypoglycemia or persistence of elevated insulin concentrations. A significant correlation exists between the amount of insulin injected and either the total amount of dextrose used for treatment or the duration of dextrose infusion.[129] In a retrospective study of insulin overdose, 7 (41%) of 17 cases developed recurrent hypoglycemia between 5 and 39 hours after overdose despite oral feeding and intravenous dextrose infusion ranging from 5 to 17 g of dextrose per hour.

In a retrospective review of 40 sulfonylurea overdose cases, the time from ingestion to the onset of hypoglycemia, when known, was variable.[98] The longest delay was 21 hours after ingestion of glyburide and 48 hours after ingestion of chlorpropamide. In a retrospective poison center review of 93 cases of sulfonylurea exposures in children, 25 patients (27%) developed hypoglycemia, with a time of onset ranging from 0.5 to 16 hours and a mean of 4.3 hours.[108] In a prospective poison center study of sulfonylurea exposures in children, 56 (30%) of 185 patients developed hypoglycemia, with a time of onset ranging from 1 to 21 hours and a mean of 5.3 hours.[126] Single-tablet ingestions of chlorpropamide 250 mg, glipizide 5 mg, and glyburide 2.5 mg can result in hypoglycemia in young children,[108] and the hypoglycemia may be delayed.[133]

DIAGNOSTIC TESTING

Suspicion of possible hypoglycemia, particularly neuroglycopenia, is important in the patient with an abnormal neurologic examination. The most frequent reasons for failure to diagnose hypoglycemia and mismanaging patients are the erroneous conclusions that the patient is not hypoglycemic but rather is psychotic, epileptic, experiencing a CVA, or intoxicated because of an "odor of alcohol" on the breath (Chap. 77). Compounding the problem of misdiagnosis is the erroneous assumption that a single bolus of 0.5–1 g/kg of dextrose 50% in water ($D_{50}W$) for an adult will always be sufficient.

Serum glucose concentrations are accurate, but treatment cannot be delayed pending the results of laboratory testing. Glucose reagent strip testing can be performed at the bedside. The sensitivity of these tests for detecting hypoglycemia is excellent, but these tests are not perfect. Bedside glucose testing is discussed in more detail in Antidotes in Depth A10: Dextrose.

Diagnostic studies other than determinations of glucose concentrations may be indicated, depending on the clinical situation. In some instances, determination of serum ethanol concentration may be helpful in confirming alcohol as a contributing or sole etiologic factor. Renal function tests may indicate the presence of renal impairment as a causative factor of hypoglycemia. This commonly occurs in diabetics taking insulin, who often develop renal failure after they have had the disease for several years. Insulin half-life increases as renal function declines. Measures of hepatic function may be a clue to liver disease as a cause of hypoglycemia, although liver disease may also be evident on physical examination. Seizures are commonly associated with hypoglycemia, but other studies, such as electrolytes, calcium, magnesium, and computed tomographic scanning of the brain, may be indicated if doubt about the etiology exists.

In the majority of overdose cases, laboratory testing for specific antidiabetics is not helpful. Exceptions might include malicious, surreptitious, or unintentional overdoses (discussed in the next section). Metformin concentrations in the setting of overdose and metformin-associated metabolic acidosis with hyperlactatemia are variable and do not necessarily correlate with the clinical condition.[2,65,66]

For known diabetics in whom overdose is not suspected, the clinician must search diligently for the cause of hypoglycemia. Sometimes it is as simple as a missed meal in an insulin user or an unusually strenuous exercise routine, but in many cases the cause cannot be clearly defined. Numerous medical conditions, as well as a variety of medications, may be involved (Table 48–1), and diagnostic testing must be individualized for each episode depending on the clinical suspicion. Diagnosing the etiology as "idiopathic" is never acceptable.

EVALUATION OF MALICIOUS, SURREPTITIOUS, OR UNINTENTIONAL INSULIN OVERDOSE

The physical examination may provide helpful clues to the evaluation of a suspected malicious, surreptitious, or unintentional insulin overdose. A meticulous search may reveal a site that is erythematous, hemorrhagic, atypically boggy in nature, or even painful if the subcutaneous (or intramuscular) injection of insulin was particularly large. A simple unexplained needle puncture mark in the appropriate clinical setting may suggest insulin injection.

An understanding of how the β cells of the pancreas secrete insulin in response to glucose concentrations in the blood is essential to understanding the investigation of fasting hypoglycemia.[29] When the plasma glucose concentration is less than 45 mg/dL, insulin secretion should be almost completely suppressed, so plasma insulin concentrations should be minimal or absent.[105] Moreover, insulin is secreted as proinsulin, which is cleaved in vivo to form insulin (a double-stranded peptide) and C-peptide, which are released into the blood in equimolar quantities. Insulin is biologically active, whereas proinsulin has limited activity, and C-peptide has no activity. Although insulin is normally cleared during hepatic transit, C-peptide is not. For this reason, C-peptide can be utilized as a quantitative marker of *endogenous* insulin secretion. Commercially available exogenous human insulin does not contain C-peptide fragments (Table 48–5). When plasma glucose concentration falls to hypoglycemic concentrations (usually less than 60 mg/dL), insulin concentration should fall to less then 6 μUnits /mL. If hypoglycemia is caused by exogenous insulin administration, plasma C-peptide concentrations should be less than 0.2 nmol/L in the presence of insulin concentrations that are substantially higher than insulin concentrations resulting from an insulinoma. With insulinoma, insulin concentrations generally are greater than 6 μUnits /mL in the presence of hypoglycemia. Insulinoma results in elevations of both C-peptide and insulin concentrations. Sulfonylurea overdose is expected to have similar effects, but concentrations in reported cases of sulfonylurea-induced hypoglycemia vary considerably.[33] In the face of uncertainty, sulfonylurea concentrations are readily available from reference laboratories. Animal insulin can be distinguished from human insulin by high-performance liquid chromatography.[46] However, this technique has limited use because of the virtually exclusive use of human insulin at present.

In summary, patients with chronic insulin-induced hypoglycemia will have high insulin concentrations, the presence of insulin-binding antibodies,[39] and low C-peptide concentrations. Those who have taken sulfonylureas will have high insulin concentrations, absent insulin-binding antibodies, high C-peptide concentrations, and presence of urinary sulfonylurea metabolites (Table 48–5). The issues of evidence collection that are appropriate to document malicious or surreptitious use of insulin successfully have been described[73] (Chap. 140).

TABLE 48–5. Laboratory Assessment of Fasting Hypoglycemia

Clinical State	Insulin[a] (Plasma) (μUnit/mL)	C-Peptide (Plasma) (nmol/L)	Proinsulin (pmol/L)	Antiinsulin Antibodies[b]
Normal	<6	<0.2	<5	–
Exogenous insulin	Very high	Low (suppressed)	Absent	Present[c]
Insulinoma	High	High	Present	Absent
Sulfonylurea ingestion[d]	High	High	Present	Absent
Autoimmune	Very high (artifact)	Low (or) high (artifact)	Present	Present
Decreased glucose production	Low	Low	Present	Absent
Neoplasia (non–β-cell)	Low	Low	Present	Absent

[a]Insulin concentrations are determined during fasting hypoglycemia at low concentrations, preferably <60 mg/dL of blood glucose.

[b]The antiinsulin antibodies produced spontaneously differ from those of treated (exposed to exogenous insulin) and those of untreated insulin-dependent diabetics.

[c]The presence of antiinsulin antibodies occurs less frequently in those exposed only to human insulin.

[d]Sulfonylurea ingestion is diagnosed by detection of the drugs or their metabolites in plasma or urine.

MANAGEMENT

Treatment centers on the correction of hypoglycemia and the anticipation that hypoglycemia may recur. Symptomatic patients with hypoglycemia require immediate treatment with 0.5–1 g/kg concentrated intravenous dextrose in the form of $D_{50}W$ in adults, $D_{25}W$ in children, and $D_{10}W$ in neonates. Occasionally, patients require a larger dose to achieve an initial response. If hypoglycemia is suspected but not confirmed, as in the absence of rapid reagent strip availability or when such readings are "borderline," dextrose should be administered. Theoretical risks are associated with use of concentrated dextrose in the setting of cerebral ischemia, but failure to rapidly correct hypoglycemia may lead to deleterious neurologic effects. Appropriate emergency and toxicologic uses of hypertonic dextrose are covered in detail in Antidotes in Depth A10: Dextrose.

Glucagon should not be considered as an antihypoglycemic agent except in the uncommon situation where intravenous access cannot be obtained. Glucagon has a delay to onset of action and may be ineffective in patients with depleted glycogen stores, as in the elderly, cancer patients, or alcoholics. Glucagon also stimulates insulin release from the pancreas, which may lead to prolonged hypoglycemia in settings such as sulfonylurea ingestion and insulinoma.[135]

Numerous studies have evaluated approaches for treating insulin reactions with carbohydrates in tablet, solution, or gel forms in a well-defined diabetic population.[123] None of these forms is appropriate for the undefined, possibly hypoglycemic patient if IV access is available. Patients who have significant clinical symptoms of hypoglycemia are at risk for grave CNS complications unless they are treated quickly and adequately with glucose.

A common occurrence involves symptomatic hypoglycemic patients who receive intravenous dextrose in the prehospital setting and subsequently refuse transport to the hospital. The authors of a retrospective review of 571 paramedic runs involving hypoglycemic patients concluded that out-of-hospital treatment of hypoglycemic diabetic patients is safe and effective even when transport is refused.[124] However, of the 159 patients who agreed to hospital transport, 40% were admitted. The admitted group was older than those released from the Emergency Department (ED). The admission rate for transported patients on oral hypoglycemics was higher than those on insulin. The reasons for admission are not otherwise detailed. The authors of a prospective study involving 132 hypoglycemic diabetic patients who refused transport after therapy concluded that most such patients have good short-term outcome, but they still encouraged transport because of the risk of recurrent hypoglycemia.[84] One patient died in each of these two studies. A prospective study in 35 patients with 38 hypoglycemic events related to insulin use concluded that most patients were successfully treated in the prehospital setting without transport.[71] However, two patients developed recurrent hypoglycemia that they treated themselves, and one of these patients required placement in a long-term care facility for posthypoglycemic encephalopathy. We *emphatically* encourage the further education of paramedics and restructuring of their protocols, emphasizing the importance of transporting all hypoglycemic patients to EDs if their approach differs from these recommendations.

Emesis, lavage, and catharsis are of limited benefit in the management of patients who overdose on antidiabetics and hypoglycemics. The extensive affinity between chlorpropamide, tolazamide, tolbutamide, glyburide, glipizide, and activated charcoal is demonstrated in vitro.[58] The affinities ranged from 0.45 to 0.52 g/g activated charcoal at pH 7.5 and were higher at pH 4.9. Single-dose activated charcoal should be beneficial in the management of these overdoses. Although affinity studies are lacking for the other antidiabetics and hypoglycemics, their chemical characteristics are such that single-dose activated charcoal is expected to be beneficial for these overdoses as well. Multiple-dose activated charcoal and whole-bowel irrigation may be of benefit and should be considered after overdose of modified-release antidiabetics and hypoglycemics, but outcome studies are not available.

In patients who overdose on insulin, case reports describe the use of surgical excision of the injection site.[22,72,80] However, this technique has not been studied in a systematic fashion, so further data are necessary before this approach can be recommended. Needle aspiration of a depot site is less invasive and should be considered.

Urinary alkalinization to a pH of 7–8 can reduce the half-life of chlorpropamide from 49 hours to approximately 13 hours. Urinary alkalinization is not useful for other oral antidiabetics, because of their limited renal excretion.[93]

MAINTAINING EUGLYCEMIA AFTER INITIAL CONTROL

After the patient is awake and alert, further therapy depends on the xenobiotic involved and pancreatic islet cell function. Some patients, particularly those with prolonged hypoglycemia, may have persistent altered mental status despite euglycemia. Whether the event was unintentional or intentional with suicidal or homicidal intent must be determined. One problem associated with dextrose administration occurs in individuals who can produce insulin via glucose-stimulated insulin release (nondiabetics and those with type II diabetes mellitus), placing them at substantial risk for recurrent hypoglycemia. This complication can occur with insulin overdose but is particularly problematic with overdoses of sulfonylurea or meglitinide because these hypoglycemics stimulate insulin release. Treatment with hypertonic dextrose solutions can be expected to result in dramatic yet only transient increases in glucose concentrations, with a subsequent fall in serum glucose concentration possibly back to hypoglycemic concentrations.

For diabetic patients who unintentionally inject an excessive amount of insulin and are not neuroglycopenic, feeding should be initiated and intravenous access maintained while avoiding routine dextrose infusion. In the event of recurrent hypoglycemia, a concentrated dextrose bolus should be used. Overdose in the setting of suicidal or homicidal intent likely involves significant quantities of insulin. Nondiabetics may be particularly prone to significant hypoglycemia because they lack insulin resistance. Feeding should be initiated and glucose concentrations maintained in the 100–150 mg/dL range using a concentrated dextrose infusion ($D_{10}W$).

Some patients may require even more concentrated dextrose infusions, such as 20% dextrose in water ($D_{20}W$) augmented by repeated doses of $D_{50}W$. Central venous lines should be used when $D_{20}W$ infusion is instituted, because concentrated dextrose solutions are substantial venous irritants. The presence of glycosuria is not an adequate indicator of euglycemia; frequent serial blood or reagent strip glucose concentrations should be obtained. The appropriate timing of glucose monitoring varies depending on the clinical situation. Mental status must be observed. As a rough guide, glucose monitoring every 1–2 hours after initial control is reasonable, with subsequent spacing of the intervals to once every 4–6 hours. Phosphate concentrations should be monitored because glucose loading may lead to hypophosphatemia.[85] Potassium concentrations should be monitored because glucose administration may lead to hypokalemia in nondiabetics and hyperkalemia in patients with impaired insulin secretion.[26] The duration of sampling necessary depends on the stability of the patient, the underlying metabolic disorders, the extent of overdose, and the rate of improvement. When the patient begins to eat an adequate diet and the initial hypoglycemia is controlled, the serum glucose concentration will rise, and the concentration and rate of dextrose infusion can be tapered. Many patients may actually develop significant hyperglycemia.

The therapeutic approach differs for patients who overdose on sulfonylureas or meglitinides. After initial control of hypoglycemia with concentrated dextrose, the patient should be fed. Intravenous access is necessary, but routine dextrose infusion should be avoided. As with insulin overdose, frequent monitoring of glucose concentrations and mental status is critical. We recommend early use of octreotide in this setting because of the significant risk of glucose-stimulated insulin release.

Octreotide, a semisynthetic long-acting analog of somatostatin with an intravenous half-life of 72 minutes, inhibits glucose-stimulated β-cell insulin release via receptors coupled to G proteins on β-islet cells.[13] Somatostatin is present in diverse tissues such as the hypothalamus, pancreas, and GI tract. It alters the secretion of growth hormone and thyroid-stimulating hormone, gastrointestinal secretions, and the endocrine pancreas (glucagon and insulin).[112,113] Octreotide was compared to intravenous hypertonic dextrose and to diazoxide and concomitant dextrose in normal subjects brought to hypoglycemia using glipizide.[13] Fewer episodes of recurrent hypoglycemia occurred after octreotide therapy, and overall dextrose requirements were lower than in the dextrose-alone and dextrose-plus-diazoxide groups. Several successful clinical experiences with octreotide are reported with quinine-induced hypoglycemia resulting from malaria therapy,[102] insulinoma,[50] nesidioblastosis of infancy,[32] hypoglycemia related to therapeutic use of gliclazide,[16] and tolbutamide overdose.[13] In a retrospective study of nine patients with hypoglycemia resulting from either glyburide or glipizide, octreotide effectively reduced the risk of recurrent hypoglycemia.[81]

Octreotide appears to be relatively free of serious side effects. The most likely adverse effects are injection-site discomfort if the agent is administered subcutaneously and gastrointestinal symptoms such as nausea, bloating, diarrhea, and constipation.[74] The suggested adult octreotide dose is 50 μg subcutaneously every 6 hours (Antidotes in Depth A11: Octreotide). The patient should be monitored for 24 hours after the last dose of octreotide to assure that recurrence of hypoglycemia does not occur. Like octreotide, diazoxide may be effective in patients with refractory sulfonylurea-induced hypoglycemia.[56,98] However, because of its potential to cause hypotension, diazoxide should be considered only if octreotide is ineffective or unavailable.

ADMITTING PATIENTS TO THE HOSPITAL

The decision to admit a patient may be complex, but several guidelines can be followed. Admission is required for hypoglycemia related to sulfonylureas, ethanol, starvation, hepatic failure, and renal failure and for hypoglycemia of unknown etiology. The decision to admit a patient often depends on finding an etiology for hypoglycemia, particularly in the setting of insulin use. In most cases, if a diabetic patient on therapeutic doses of insulin develops hypoglycemia after a missed meal, the patient can be discharged after a 4-6-hour observation period during which the individual eats a meal and remains asymptomatic with no evidence of hypoglycemia. Patients receiving therapeutic doses of insulin require inpatient evaluation of recurrent and unexplained hypoglycemic episodes. All patients with hypoglycemia after unintentional overdose with long-acting insulin should be admitted. Hospitalization is recommended after unintentional overdose with ultrashort-acting, short-acting, or intermediate-acting insulin if hypoglycemia is persistent or recurrent during a 4-6-hour observation period in the ED. Many factors may be responsible for unintentional insulin overdose, such as patient error because of impaired vision, syringe structure, and prescription error, and hospital admission may be warranted. Admission is indicated for any patient, regardless of serum glucose concentration or presence or absence of symptoms, who intentionally overdoses on a sulfonylurea or any form of injected insulin, because delayed, profound, and protracted hypoglycemia may result. Although insulin overdose by the intravenous route is expected to result in more immediate symptoms, experience with this scenario is limited. Admission in this setting is advised unless short-acting insulin is involved. Hypoglycemia related to sulfonylurea use in any setting requires hospitalization.[19]

Patients with possible intentionally self-induced hypoglycemia should be admitted. Intentionally self-induced hypoglycemia is most commonly recognized by members of the medical profession. Administration of insulin to a nondiabetic child is a form of child abuse or an attempt at homicide[34] (see Chap. 31. Children who have been given an inappropriate dose of insulin, as well as any patient who may be a victim of attempted homicide, should be admitted.

A 4 to 6-hour observation period is recommended after metformin overdose. Further observation or hospital admission is not required for patients who remain asymptomatic during this period with no evidence of metabolic acidosis or hypoglycemia. Patients who overdose on α-glucosidase inhibitors are not expected to have delayed or serious systemic toxicity, and routine medical admission is unnecessary. There is limited study of the risk of hypoglycemia and other adverse events after thiazolidinedione ingestion. Based on the mechanism of action and existing clinical experience, hypoglycemia after thiazolidinedione overdose is possible but uncommon. Delayed onset of hypoglycemia or other serious clinical manifestations is unlikely. A 4 to 6-hour observation period after thiazolidinedione overdose is recommended. Significant hypoglycemia is reported with nateglinide overdose,[89] and with repaglinide used in a setting of intentionally self-induced hypoglycemia.[51] Meglitinides are expected to behave pharmacologically like sulfonylureas. For this reason alone, hospital admission after meglitinide overdose is advisable, even when the patient is asymptomatic. Admission after exenatide, sitagliptin, and saxagliptin overdose is advised until more overdose data are obtained. Delays in onset of clinical manifestations, particularly hypoglycemia, are not expected, but there is currently limited clinical experience with regard to overdose.

Children who unintentionally ingest one or more sulfonylurea tablets should be observed for 24 hours. Although this recommendation may be controversial and some authors suggest shorter observation periods[20] or even home monitoring in some cases,[114] we believe that delayed hypoglycemic effects of sulfonylurea ingestion in children are well documented in the literature[108,126,133] and convincing enough to support admission in all cases. Asymptomatic children with single-tablet exposures to sulfonylureas are best managed without prophylactic intravenous dextrose, which could contribute to delayed onset of hypoglycemia.[20] Elevations in glucose concentrations stimulate insulin release by the pancreas. Such patients instead are best managed by early feeding, frequent checks of glucose concentrations, and observation of mental status.

METFORMIN-ASSOCIATED METABOLIC ACIDOSIS WITH HYPERLACTATEMIA

Throughout this chapter, the term *metabolic acidosis with hyperlactatemia* is employed rather than *metformin-associated lactic acidosis*. The biochemical and pathophysiologic processes involving lactate are complex, but a few points are worth summarizing. Hyperlactatemia occurs in various disease states, and can be present in the absence of acidosis. The production of lactic acid does not result in a net increase in hydrogen ion concentration unless there is associated impairment of oxidative metabolism. Impaired oxidative metabolism leads to an increase in hydrogen ion production through the hydrolysis of ATP.[86]

The biguanides are uniquely associated with the occurrence of metabolic acidosis with hyperlactatemia. Phenformin causes lactic acid production by several mechanisms including interference with cellular aerobic metabolism and subsequent enhanced anaerobic metabolism.

Phenformin suppresses hepatic gluconeogenesis from pyruvate and causes a decrease in hepatocellular pH, resulting in decreased lactate consumption and hepatic lactate uptake. Metformin-associated metabolic acidosis with hyperlactatemia occurs 20 times less commonly than that occurring with phenformin. In isolated perfused rat liver, metformin inhibits both hepatic lactate uptake and conversion of lactate to glucose.[109] Metabolic acidosis with hyperlactatemia related to metformin usually occurs in the presence of an underlying condition, particularly renal impairment.[24,64] In this setting, increased tissue burden of metformin, which is renally eliminated, probably occurs. Other risk factors include cardiorespiratory insufficiency, septicemia, liver disease, history of metabolic acidosis with hyperlactatemia, advanced age, alcohol abuse, and use of radiologic contrast media.[9,24] Iodinated contrast material may induce acute renal failure, leading to accumulation of metformin and subsequent risk for development of metabolic acidosis with hyperlactatemia. However, the risk of developing metabolic acidosis with hyperlactatemia after contrast administration is low in patients taking metformin who have normal renal function and no other risk factors.[79,90]

Severe metabolic acidosis with hyperlactatemia occurs after metformin overdose[66,82,97,134] but appears to be uncommon. In one case,[82] metabolic acidosis was not diagnosed until 14 hours after metformin overdose. The patient had early symptoms of repeated vomiting at 1 hour postingestion. In a series of 13 metformin overdose cases reported to a French pharmaceutical company, 7 patients presented with metabolic acidosis with hyperlactatemia.[66] The 13 cases were selected based on the overdose history and for whom arterial pH, arterial lactate, and serum metformin concentrations were obtained. The authors do not document the number of overdose cases not included in the study. In a larger poison center series of 65 adult cases of metformin overdose, 2 patients developed significant metabolic acidosis with hyperlactatemia, 1 of whom died.[127] One patient developed disseminated intravascular coagulation, and hypoglycemia occurred in seven patients with concomitant insulin or sulfonylurea overdose. The remaining cases were described as having minimal toxicity. In a poison center series of 55 children exposed to metformin, metabolic acidosis with hyperlactatemia was not reported, and no significant adverse effects were noted.[128] The doses reportedly ingested ranged from 250 mg to 16.5 g, with a median of 500 mg.

A systematic review from the Cochrane Library concluded that therapeutic use of metformin is not associated with an increased risk of metabolic acidosis with hyperlactatemia compared with other antidiabetic treatments if no contraindications are present.[115] This conclusion was based on a review of prospective comparative trials and observational cohort studies. However, the risk of metformin-associated metabolic acidosis with hyperlactatemia in the setting of overdose setting or renal insufficiency was not assessed. Although metabolic acidosis with hyperlactatemia after overdose is not common, it does occur with sufficient frequency to require vigilance on the part of the treating physician. Case reports were not used in the Cochrane review, and a few cases of metformin-associated metabolic acidosis with hyperlactatemia in the setting of therapeutic use with no underlying risk factors are reported.[24,100,137]

Metformin-associated metabolic acidosis with hyperlactatemia is a potentially lethal condition. Recognition and awareness of this disorder are important. Symptoms may be nonspecific and include abdominal pain, nausea, vomiting, malaise, myalgia, and dizziness. However, gastrointestinal symptoms are common adverse effects associated with therapeutic use of metformin and do not necessarily require discontinuation of the drug. More severe clinical manifestations of metformin-associated metabolic acidosis with hyperlactatemia include confusion, mental status depression, hypothermia, respiratory insufficiency, and hypotension. Serum metformin concentrations can be obtained as a diagnostic aid, but may not correlate with the clinical state in both the acute overdose setting and in the setting of therapeutic metformin use. In a series of 13 cases with metformin overdose, 6 of 7 patients with metabolic acidosis with hyperlactatemia had elevated metformin concentrations.[66] Of the six patients without acidosis, three had markedly elevated metformin concentrations. In a series of cases of metabolic acidosis with hyperlactatemia related to therapeutic use, 10 of 14 patients had elevated serum metformin concentrations.[65]

Aggressive airway management and vasopressor therapy may be required. Indications for use of intravenous sodium bicarbonate in critically ill patients with metabolic acidosis with hyperlactatemia of various etiologies are poorly defined and controversial. Rather than using an arterial pH cutoff, we recommend using sodium bicarbonate given evidence of impaired buffering capacity based on a serum bicarbonate concentration of less than 5 mEq/L. Based on case reports, hemodialysis using a sodium bicarbonate buffer may be effective in improving acid–base status and clinical outcome in patients with significant metabolic acidosis with hyperlactatemia.[49,64,67] In some of these cases, metformin concentrations were measured and remained abnormally high after dialysis. Clinical improvement despite inadequate removal of metformin may be related to correction of acid–base status.

SUMMARY

Numerous xenobiotics and medical conditions may cause hypoglycemia. Hypoglycemia is the predominant adverse effect related to therapeutic use and overdose of the drugs used for treatment of diabetes mellitus. Various clinical manifestations, particularly neurologic, may occur and can be confused with conditions such as ethanol intoxication, psychosis, epilepsy, and cerebrovascular accidents. The potential for delayed and prolonged hypoglycemia must be recognized in overdose situations. Although several treatment options exist, rapid intravenous administration of dextrose is the most important measure. Octreotide is useful for patients with recurrent hypoglycemia following sulfonylurea or meglitinide overdose.

REFERENCES

1. Ahren B. Dipeptidyl peptidase-4 inhibitors: clinical data and clinical implications. *Diabetes Care.* 2007;30:1344-1350.
2. Al-Jebawi AF, Lassman MN, Abourizk NN. Lactic acidosis with therapeutic metformin blood levels in a low-risk diabetic patient. *Diabetes Care.* 1998;21:1364-1365.
3. Al-Salman J, Arjomand H, Kemp D, et al. Hepatocellular injury in a patient receiving rosiglitazone: a case report. *Ann Intern Med.* 2000;132:121-124.
4. Andrade R, Mathew V, Morgenstern MJ, et al. Hypoglycemic hemiplegic syndrome. *Ann Emerg Med.* 1984;13:529-531.
5. Andrade RJ, Lucena M, Vega JL, et al. Acarbose-associated hepatotoxicity. *Diabetes Care.* 1998;21:2029-2030.
6. Arem R, Zoghbi W. Insulin overdose in eight patients: insulin pharmacokinetics and review of the literature. *Medicine (Baltimore).* 1985;64:323-332.
7. Arky RA, Veverbrants E, Abramson EA. Irreversible hypoglycemia. A complication of alcohol and insulin. *JAMA.* 1968;206:575-578.
8. Bailey CJ, Day C. Traditional plant medicines as treatments for diabetes. *Diabetes Care.* 1989;12:553-564.
9. Bailey CJ, Turner RC. Metformin. *N Engl J Med.* 1996;334:574-579.
10. Banting FG, Best CH, Collip JB, et al. Pancreatic extracts in the treatment of diabetes mellitus: preliminary report. *CMAJ.* 1922;12:141-146.
11. Baron SH. Salicylates as hypoglycemic agents. *Diabetes Care.* 1982;5:64-71.
12. Bowman CE, MacMahon DG, Mourant AJ. Hypoglycaemia and angina. *Lancet.* 1985;1:639-640.

13. Boyle PJ, Justice K, Krentz AJ, et al. Octreotide reverses hyperinsulinemia and prevents hypoglycemia induced by sulfonylurea overdoses. *J Clin Endocrinol Metab*. 1993;76:752-756.
14. Boyle PJ, Kempers SF, O'Connor AM, et al. Brain glucose uptake and unawareness of hypoglycemia in patients with insulin-dependent diabetes mellitus. *N Engl J Med*. 1995;333:1726-1731.
15. Boyle PJ, Schwartz NS, Shah SD, et al. Plasma glucose concentrations at the onset of hypoglycemic symptoms in patients with poorly controlled diabetes and in nondiabetics. *N Engl J Med*. 1988;318:1487-1492.
16. Braatvedt GD. Octreotide for the treatment of sulphonylurea induced hypoglycaemia in type 2 diabetes. *N Z Med J*. 1997;110:189-190.
17. Bressler R, Johnson D. New pharmacological approaches to therapy of NIDDM. *Diabetes Care*. 1992;15:792-805.
18. Brvar M, Mozina M, Bunc M. Poisoning with insulin glargine [letter]. *Clin Toxicol*. 2005:43;219-220.
19. Burge MR, Schmitz-Fiorentino K, Fischette C, et al. A prospective trial of risk factors for sulfonylurea-induced hypoglycemia in type 2 diabetes mellitus. *JAMA*. 1998;279:137-143.
20. Burkhart KK. When does hypoglycemia develop after sulfonylurea ingestion? *Ann Emerg Med*. 1998;31:771-772.
21. Calara F, Taylor K, Han J, et al. A randomized, open-label, crossover study examining the effect of injection site on bioavailability of exenatide (synthetic exendin-4). *Clin Ther*. 2005;27:210-215.
22. Campbell IW, Ratcliffe JG. Suicidal insulin overdose managed by excision of insulin injection site. *Br Med J (Clin Res Ed)*. 1982;285:408-409.
23. Carrascosa M, Pascual F, Aresti S. Acarbose-induced severe hepatotoxicity. *Lancet*. 1997;349:698-699.
24. Chan NN, Brain HP, Feher MD. Metformin-associated lactic acidosis: a rare or very rare clinical entity. *Diabet Med*. 1999;16:273-281.
25. Chochinov R, Daughaday WH. Marked hyperthermia as a manifestation of hypoglycemia in long-standing diabetes mellitus. *Diabetes*. 1975;24: 859-860.
26. Clark BA, Brown RS. Potassium homeostasis and hyperkalemic syndromes. *Endocrinol Metab Clin North Am*. 1997;26:553-573.
27. Cohen V, Teperikidis E. Acute exenatide (Byetta®) poisoning was not associated with significant hypoglycemia [letter]. *Clin Toxicol*. 2008;46:346-347.
28. Cryer PE. Diverse causes of hypoglycemia-associated autonomic failure in diabetes. *N Engl J Med*. 2004;350:2272-2279.
29. Cryer PE. Glucose homeostasis and hypoglycemia. In: Kronenberg HM, Melmed S, Polonsky KS, Larsen PR, eds. *Williams Textbook of Endocrinology*, 11th ed. Philadelphia: WB Saunders; 2008:1503-1533.
30. DCCT Research Group. Epidemiology of severe hypoglycemia in the diabetes control and complications trial. *Am J Med*. 1991;90:450-459.
31. DCCT Research Group. The effect of intensive treatment of diabetes on the development and progression of long-term complications in insulin-dependent diabetes mellitus. *N Engl J Med*. 1993;329:977-986.
32. Delemarre-van de Waal HA, Veldkamp EJ, Schrander-Stumpel CT. Long-term treatment of an infant with nesidioblastosis using a somatostatin analogue. *N Engl J Med*. 1987;316:222-223.
33. DeWitt CR, Heard K, Waksman JC. Insulin and c-peptide levels in sulfonylurea-induced hypoglycemia: a systematic review. *J Med Toxicol*. 2007;3:107-118.
34. Dine MS, McGovern ME. Intentional poisoning of children—an overlooked category of child abuse: report of seven cases and review of the literature. *Pediatrics*. 1982;70:32-35.
35. Duh E, Feinglos M. Hypoglycemia-induced angina pectoris in a patient with diabetes mellitus. *Ann Intern Med*. 1994;121:945-946.
36. Eliasson L, Renstrom E, Ammala C, et al. PKC-dependent stimulation of exocytosis by sulfonylureas in pancreatic beta cells. *Science*. 1996;271:813-815.
37. Fahy BG, Coursin DB. Critical glucose control: the devil is in the details. *Mayo Clin Proc*. 2008;83:394-397.
38. Fasano A, Uzzau S. Modulation of intestinal tight junctions by zonula occludens toxin permits enteral administration of insulin and other macromolecules in an animal model. *J Clin Invest*. 1997;99:1158-1164.
39. Fineberg SE, Galloway JA, Fineberg NS, et al. Immunogenicity of recombinant DNA human insulin. *Diabetologia*. 1983;25:465-469.
40. Fischer KF, Lees JA, Newman JH. Hypoglycemia in hospitalized patients. Causes and outcomes. *N Engl J Med*. 1986;315:1245-1250.
41. Fitzgerald FT. Hypoglycemia and accidental hypothermia in an alcoholic population. *West J Med*. 1980;133:105-107.
42. Forman LM, Simmons DA, Diamond RH. Hepatic failure in a patient taking rosiglitazone. *Ann Intern Med*. 2000;132:118-121.
43. Gaines KL, Hamilton S, Boyd AE. Characterization of the sulfonylurea receptor on beta cell membranes. *J Biol Chem*. 1988;263:2589-2592.
44. Gerich JE. Oral hypoglycemic agents. *N Engl J Med*. 1989;321:1231-1245.
45. Gitlin N, Julie NL, Spurr CL, et al. Two cases of severe clinical and histologic hepatotoxicity associated with troglitazone. *Ann Intern Med*. 1998;129:36-38.
46. Given BD, Ostrega DM, Polonsky KS, et al. Hypoglycemia due to surreptitious injection of insulin. Identification of insulin species by high-performance liquid chromatography. *Diabetes Care*. 1991;14:544-547.
47. Grajower MM, Walter L, Albin J. Hypoglycemia in chronic hemodialysis patients: association with propranolol use. *Nephron*. 1980;26:126-129.
48. Harvey B, Hickman C, Hinson G, et al. Severe lactic acidosis complicating metformin overdose successfully treated with high-volume venovenous hemofiltration and aggressive alkalinization. *Pediatr Crit Care Med*. 2005;6:598-601.
49. Heaney D, Majid A, Junor B. Bicarbonate haemodialysis as a treatment of metformin overdose. *Nephrol Dial Transplant*. 1997;12:1046-1047.
50. Hearn PR, Ahmed M, Woodhouse NJ. The use of SMS 201-995 (somatostatin analogue) in insulinomas. Additional case report and literature review. *Horm Res*. 1988;29:211-213.
51. Hirshberg B, Skarulis MC, Pucino F, et al. Repaglinide-induced factitious hypoglycemia. *J Clin Endocrinol Metab*. 2001;86:475-477.
52. Hoffman JR, Schriger DL, Votey SR, et al. The empiric use of hyper-tonic dextrose in patients with altered mental status: a reappraisal. *Ann Emerg Med*. 1992;21:20-24.
53. Hollander P. Safety profile of acarbose an alpha-glucosidase inhibitor. *Drugs*. 1992;44(Suppl 2):47-53.
54. Iwamoto Y, Kosaka K, Kuzuya T, et al. Effects of troglitazone: a new hypoglycemic agent in patients with NIDDM poorly controlled by diet therapy. *Diabetes Care*. 1996;19:151-156.
55. Jennings AM, Wilson RM, Ward JD. Symptomatic hypoglycemia in NIDDM patients treated with oral hypoglycemic agents. *Diabetes Care*. 1989;12:203-208.
56. Johnson SF, Shade DS, Peake GT. Chlorpropamide-induced hypoglycemia: successful treatment with diazoxide. *Am J Med*. 1977;63:799-804.
57. Kadowaki T, Hagura R, Kajinuma H, et al. Chlorpropamide-induced hyponatremia: incidence and risk factors. *Diabetes Care*. 1983;6:468-471.
58. Kannisto H, Neuvonen PJ. Adsorption of sulfonylureas onto activated charcoal in vitro. *J Pharm Sci*. 1984;73:253-256.
59. Kedes LH, Field JB. Hypothermia: a clue to hypoglycemia. *N Engl J Med*. 1964;271:785-787.
60. Kerr D, MacDonald IA, Heller SR, et al. Beta-adrenoceptor blockade and hypoglycaemia. A randomised double-blind placebo controlled comparison of metoprolol CR atenolol and propranolol LA in normal subjects. *Br J Clin Pharmacol*. 1990;29:685-693.
61. Kitabchi AE. Low-dose insulin therapy in diabetic ketoacidosis: fact or fiction? *Diabetes Metab Rev*. 1989;5:337-363.
62. Koivisto VA. The human insulin analogue insulin lispro. *Ann Intern Med*. 1998;30:260-266.
63. Krinsley JS. Association between hyperglycemia and increased hospital mortality in a heterogeneous population of critically ill patients. *Mayo Clin Proc*. 2003;78:1471-1478.
64. Kruse JA. Metformin-associated lactic acidosis. *J Emerg Med*. 2001; 20: 267-272.
65. Lalau JD, Lacroix C, Compagnon P, et al. Role of metformin accumulation in metformin-associated lactic acidosis. *Diabetes Care*. 1995; 18:779-784.
66. Lalau JD, Mourlhon C, Bergeret A, et al. Consequences of metformin intoxication. *Diabetes Care*. 1998;21:2036-2037.
67. Lalau JD, Westeel PF, Debussche X, et al. Bicarbonate haemodialysis: an adequate treatment for lactic acidosis in diabetics treated by metformin. *Intensive Care Med*. 1987;13:383-387.
68. Langley AK, Suffoletta TJ, Jennings HR. Dipeptidyl peptidase IV inhibitors and the incretin system in type 2 diabetes mellitus. *Pharmacotherapy*. 2007;27:1163-1180.
69. Leak D, Starr P. The mechanism of arrhythmias during insulin-induced hypoglycemia. *Am J Heart*. 1962;63:688-691.
70. Lebovitz HE. The oral hypoglycemic agents. In: Porte D Jr, Sherwin RS, eds. *Ellenberg & Rifkin's Diabetes Mellitus*, 5th ed. Stamford, CT: Appleton & Lange; 1997: 761-788.
71. Lerner EB, Billittier AJ, Daniel DR, et al. Can paramedics safely treat and discharge hypoglycemic patients in the field? *Am J Emerg Med*. 2003;21:115-120.

72. Levine DF, Bulstrode C. Managing suicidal insulin overdose. *Br Med J.* 1982;285:974-975.
73. Levy WJ, Gardner D, Moseley J, et al. Unusual problems for the physician in managing a hospital patient who received a malicious insulin overdose. *Neurosurgery.* 1985;17:992-996.
74. Longnecker SM. Somatostatin and octreotide: literature review and description of therapeutic activity in pancreatic neoplasia. *Drug Intell Clin Pharm.* 1988;22:99-106.
75. Maeda K. Hepatocellular injury in a patient receiving pioglitazone. *Ann Intern Med.* 2001;135:306.
76. Malouf R, Brust JC. Hypoglycemia: causes, neurological manifestations, and outcome. *Ann Neurol.* 1985;17:421-430.
77. Martin FI, Hansen N, Warne GL. Attempted suicide by insulin overdose in insulin-requiring diabetics. *Med J Aust.* 1977;1:58-60.
78. May LD, Lefkowitch JH, Kram MT, et al. Mixed hepatocellularcholestatic liver injury after pioglitazone therapy. *Ann Intern Med.* 2002;136:449-452.
79. McCartney MM, Gilbert FJ, Murchison LE, et al. Metformin and contrast media—a dangerous combination? *Clin Radiol.* 1999;54:29-33.
80. McIntyre AS, Woolf VJ, Burnham WR. Local excision of subcutaneous fat in the management of insulin overdose. *Br J Surg.* 1986;73:538.
81. McLaughlin SA, Crandall CS, McKinney PE. Octreotide: an antidote for sulfonylurea-induced hypoglycemia. *Ann Emerg Med.* 2000;36:133-138.
82. McLelland J. Recovery from metformin overdose. *Diabet Med.* 1985;2: 410-411.
83. McMahon GT, Arky RA. Inhaled insulin for diabetes mellitus. *N Engl J Med.* 2007;356:497-502.
84. Mechem CC, Kreshak AA, Barger J, et al. The short-term outcome of hypoglycemic diabetic patients who refuse ambulance transport after out-of-hospital therapy. *Acad Emerg Med.* 1998;5:768-772.
85. Miller DW, Slovis CM. Hypophosphatemia in the emergency department therapeutics. *Am J Emerg Med.* 2000;18:457-461.
86. Mizock BA. Controversies in lactic acidosis—implications in critically ill patients. *JAMA.* 1987;258:497-501.
87. Morcol T, Nagappan P, Nerenbaum L, et al. Calcium phosphate-PEG-insulin-casein (CAPIC) particles as oral delivery systems for insulin. *Int J Pharm.* 2004;277:91-97.
88. Munck O, Quaade F. Suicide attempted with insulin. *Dan Med Bull.* 1963;10:139-141.
89. Nakayama S, Hirose T, Watada H, et al. Hypoglycemia following a nateglinide overdose in a suicide attempt [letter]. *Diabetes Care.* 2005;28:227.
90. Nawaz S, Cleveland T, Gaines PA, et al. Clinical risk associated with contrast angiography in metformin treated patients: a clinical review. *Clin Radiol.* 1998;53:342-344.
91. Nesto RW, Bell D, Bonow RO, et al. Thiazolidinedione use, fluid retention, and congestive heart failure: a consensus statement from the American Heart Association and American Diabetes Association: October 7, 2003. *Circulation.* 2003;108:2941-2948.
92. Neuschwander-Tetri BA, Isley WL, Oki JC, et al. Troglitazone-induced hepatic failure leading to liver transplantation. A case report. *Ann Intern Med.* 1998;129:38-41.
93. Neuvonen PJ, Karkkainen S. Effects of charcoal sodium bicarbonate and ammonium chloride on chlorpropamide kinetics. *Clin Pharm Ther.* 1983;33:386-393.
94. Nissen SE, Wolski K. Effect of rosiglitazone on the risk of myocardial infarction and death from cardiovascular causes. *N Engl J Med.* 2007;356:2457-2471.
95. Odeh M, Oliven A, Bassan H. Transient atrial fibrillation precipitated by hypoglycemia. *Ann Emerg Med.* 1990;19:565-567.
96. Olefsky JM, Kruszynska YT. Insulin resistance. In: Porte JD, Sherwin RS, Baron A, eds. *Ellenberg & Rifkin's Diabetes Mellitus*, 6th ed. New York: McGraw-Hill; 2003:367-400.
97. Palatnick W, Meatherall R, Tenenbein M. Severe lactic acidosis from acute metformin overdose [abstract]. *J Toxicol Clin Toxicol.* 1999;37: 638-639.
98. Palatnick W, Meatherall RC, Tenenbein M. Clinical spectrum of sulfonylurea overdose and experience with diazoxide therapy. *Arch Intern Med.* 1991;151:1859-1862.
99. Peitzman SJ, Agarwal BN. Spontaneous hypoglycemia in end-stage renal failure. *Nephron.* 1977;19:131-139.
100. Pepper GM, Schwartz M. Lactic acidosis associated with glucophage use in man with normal renal and hepatic function. *Diabetes Care.* 1997;20: 232-233.
101. Phenformin hydrochloride. In: Sweetman S, ed. *Martindale: The Complete Drug Reference.* [Internet database]. London: Pharmaceutical Press; Electronic version, Greenwood, CO: Thomson Healthcare: updated periodically.
102. Phillips RE, Warrell DA, Looareesuwan S, et al. Effectiveness of SMS 201–995, a synthetic long-acting somatostatin analogue in treatment of quinine-induced hyperinsulinaemia. *Lancet.* 1986;1:713-716.
103. Pladziewicz DS, Nesto RW. Hypoglycemia-induced silent myocardial ischemia. *Am J Cardiol.* 1989;63:1531-1532.
104. Podgainy H, Bressler R. Biochemical basis of the sulfonylurea-induced Antabuse syndrome. *Diabetes.* 1968;17:679-683.
105. Polonsky KS. A practical approach to fasting hypoglycemia. *N Engl J Med.* 1992;326:1020-1021.
106. Posner JB, Saper CB, Schiff ND, Plum F. *Plum and Posner's Diagnosis of Stupor and Coma,* 4th ed. New York: Oxford University Press; 2007.
107. Powers AC. *Diabetes Mellitus.* In Fauci AS, Kasper DL, Longo DL, Braunwald E, Hauser SL, Jameson JL, Loscalzo J, eds. *Harrison's Principles of Internal Medicine*, 17th ed. New York: McGraw-Hill; 2008:2275-2304.
108. Quadrani DA, Spiller HA, Widder P. Five-year retrospective evaluation of sulfonylurea ingestion in children. *J Toxicol Clin Toxicol.* 1996;34:267-270.
109. Radziuk J, Zhang Z, Wiernsperger N, et al. Effects of metformin on lactate uptake and gluconeogenesis in the perfused rat liver. *Diabetes.* 1997;46:1406-1413.
110. Ranganath L, Norris F, Morgan L, et al. Delayed gastric emptying occurs following acarbose administration and is a further mechanism for its anti-hyperglycaemic effect. *Diabet Med.* 1998;15:120-124.
111. Rendell MS, Kirchain WR. Pharmacotherapy of type 2 diabetes mellitus. *Ann Pharmacother.* 2000;34:878-895.
112. Reichlin S. Somatostatin (Part I). *N Engl J Med.* 1983;309:1495-1501.
113. Reichlin S. Somatostatin (second of two parts). *N Engl J Med.* 1983;309: 1556-1563.
114. Robertson WO. Sulfonylurea ingestions: hospitalization not mandatory. *J Toxicol Clin Toxicol.* 1997;35:115-118.
115. Saltpeter S, Greyber E, Pasternak G, et al. Risk of fatal and nonfatal lactic acidosis with metformin use in type 2 diabetes mellitus [systematic review]. Cochrane Metabolic and Endocrine Disorders Group. Cochrane Database Syst Rev. 2, 2004.
116. Salvatore T, Giugliano D. Pharmacokinetic-pharmacodynamic relationships of acarbose. *Clin Pharmacokinet.* 1996;30:94-106.
117. Samuels MH, Eckel RH. Massive insulin overdose: detailed studies of free insulin levels and glucose requirements. *J Toxicol Clin Toxicol.* 1989;27:157-168.
118. Scheen AJ, Lefebvre PJ. Oral antidiabetic agents. A guide to selection. *Drugs.* 1998;55:225-236.
119. Seibert DG. Reversible decerebrate posturing secondary to hypoglycemia. *Am J Med.* 1985;78:1036-1037.
120. Seltzer HS. Drug-induced hypoglycemia. A review of 1418 cases. *Endocrinol Metab Clin North Am.* 1989;18:163-183.
121. Service FJ. Hypoglycemic disorders. *N Engl J Med.* 1995;332:1144-1152.
122. Shulman GI, Barrett EJ, Sherwin RS. Integrated fuel metabolism. In: Porte JD, Sherwin RS, Baron A, eds. *Ellenberg & Rifkin's Diabetes Mellitus*, 6th ed. New York: McGraw-Hill; 2003:1-13.
123. Slama G, Traynard PY, Desplanque N, et al. The search for an optimized treatment of hypoglycemia. Carbohydrates in tablets, solution or gel for the correction of insulin reactions. *Arch Intern Med.* 1990;150:589-593.
124. Socransky SJ, Pirrallo RG, Rubin JM. Out-of-hospital treatment of hypoglycemia: refusal of transport and patient outcome. *Acad Emerg Med.* 1998;5:1080-1085.
125. Spiller HA, Schroeder SL, Ching DS. Hemiparesis and altered mental status in a child after glyburide ingestion. *J Emerg Med.* 1998;16:433-435.
126. Spiller HA, Villalobos D, Krenzelok EP, et al. Prospective multicenter study of sulfonylurea ingestion in children. *J Pediatr.* 1997;131:141-146.
127. Spiller HA, Weber J, Hofman M, et al. Multicenter case series of adult metformin ingestion [abstract]. *J Toxicol Clin Toxicol.* 1999;37:639.
128. Spiller HA, Weber JA, Winter ML, et al. Multicenter case series of pediatric metformin ingestion. *Ann Pharmacother.* 2000;34:1385-1388.
129. Stapczynski JS, Haskell RJ. Duration of hypoglycemia and need for intravenous glucose following intentional overdoses of insulin. *Ann Emerg Med.* 1984;13:505-511.
130. Stocks AE. Insulin lispro: experience in a private practice setting. *Med J Aust.* 1999;170:364-367.
131. Strauch BS, Felig P, Baxter JD, et al. Hypothermia in hypoglycemia. *JAMA.* 1969;210:345-346.

132. Stumvoll M, Nurjhan N, Perriello G, et al. Metabolic effects of metformin in non-insulin-dependent diabetes mellitus. *N Engl J Med.* 1995;333: 550-554.
133. Szlatenyi CS, Capes KF, Wang RY. Delayed hypoglycemia in a child after ingestion of a single glipizide tablet. *Ann Emerg Med.* 1998;31:773-776.
134. Teale KF, Devine A, Stewart H, et al. The management of metformin overdose. *Anaesthesia.* 1998;53:698-701.
135. Thoma ME, Glauser J, Genuth S. Persistent hypoglycemia and hyperinsulinemia: caution in using glucagon. *Am J Emerg Med.* 1996;14:99-101.
136. Todd JF, Bloom SR. Incretins and other peptides in the treatment of diabetes. *Diabet Med.* 2007;24:223-232.
137. Tymms DJ, Leatherdale BA. Lactic acidosis due to metformin therapy in a low risk patient. *Postgrad Med J.* 1988;64:230-231.
138. Wallis WE, Donaldson I, Scott RS, et al. Hypoglycemia masquerading as cerebrovascular disease (hypoglycemic hemiplegia). *Ann Neurol.* 1985;18: 510-512.
139. Welborn TA. Acarbose, an alpha-glucosidase inhibitor for non-insulin-dependent diabetes. *Med J Aust.* 1998;168:76-78.
140. Van den Berghe G, Wilmer A, Hermans G, et al. Intensive insulin therapy in the medical ICU. *N Engl J Med.* 2006;354:449-461.
141. Van den Berghe G, Wouters P, Weekers F, et al. Intensive insulin therapy in critically ill patients. *N Engl J Med.* 2001;345:1359-1367.

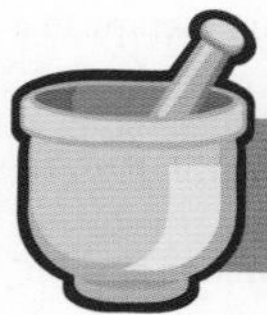

ANTIDOTES IN DEPTH (A10)

DEXTROSE

Larissa I. Velez and Kathleen A. Delaney

$$\text{CH}_2\text{OH}$$

Dextrose (D-glucose)

Hypoglycemia is a common cause of altered mental status. Although classically associated with tachycardia, tremor, and diaphoresis, the predictive value of these manifestations is too low to be relied upon. As a result, all patients with altered consciousness require either rapid point-of-care testing of their glucose concentrations or empiric treatment for presumed hypoglycemia. When rapidly diagnosed and treated, hypoglycemic patients typically recover without sequelae. Delayed or incomplete therapy may lead to permanent neurologic dysfunction.

PHYSIOLOGY

Adenosine triphosphate (ATP) provides the metabolic energy that fuels all critical cellular processes in all organs. In the adult brain, the anaerobic and aerobic metabolism of glucose through glycolysis and the citric acid cycle, respectively, are the primary sources of ATP (see Chap. 12). Although the adult brain can use fatty acids, amino acids, and ketones as alternate substrates for ATP synthesis, these are not adequate to sustain normal cerebral function in the setting of glucose deprivation. In the brain of fetuses and neonates, glucose is the only substrate for ATP production.[81,99] Hypoglycemia is defined by organ dysfunction in the setting of inadequate concentrations of glucose; it cannot be safely defined by strict numerical values. The onset of hypoglycemia in both adults and children is followed rapidly by global cerebral dysfunction. In individuals with diabetes, the density of neuronal insulin receptors varies as a function of glycemic control so that diabetics with poor glycemic control have fewer neuronal glucose receptors and may experience hypoglycemic symptoms at much higher concentrations of glucose than those who are normally euglycemic. An important study of diabetics demonstrated that the mean blood glucose concentration for symptomatic hypoglycemia in poorly controlled diabetics was 78 ± 5 mg/dL compared with 53 ± mg/dL in normal control subjects.[11] Hypoglycemia may cause neuropsychiatric sequelae effects that are clinically indistinguishable from those of other toxic-metabolic and structural brain injuries, which may include focal stroke syndromes, movement disorders, seizures, irritability, confusion, delirium, coma, and irreversible encephalopathy.[3,33,59,67,69,70,85,103,108] The heart is partially dependent on glucose for energy production. Hypoglycemia causes myocardial stress that may manifest as angina and or dysrhythmias. This is aggravated by the systemic catecholamine response to hypoglycemia.[34,62,68,71,72]

THE PHYSICAL EXAMINATION IN HYPOGLYCEMIA

The history and physical examination do not reliably detect patients who are hypoglycemic.[47] Tachycardia, diaphoresis, pallor, hypertension, tremors, hunger, and restlessness tend to predominate when the decline in blood glucose concentration is rapid. These signs and symptoms may be blunted or absent from the use of β-adrenergic antagonists. Central nervous system signs of neuroglycopenia are nonspecific. They include visual disturbances, psychiatric disturbances, confusion, stupor, coma, seizures, and focal neurologic findings.[67,86] In children, the only sign of neuroglycopenia may be lethargy or irritability.[110]

TREATMENT

In most cases, the rapid correction of hypoglycemia by the administration of 0.5 to 1.0 g/kg of concentrated intravenous (IV) dextrose (Table A10–1) immediately reverses these neurologic and cardiac effects. However, prolonged or severe hypoglycemia may result in permanent brain injury, myocardial infarction, and death.[15,35,70] Because of the myriad presentations of hypoglycemia, the difficulties inherent in making the clinical diagnosis, and the serious consequences of failure to treat the condition, the empirical administration of hypertonic dextrose to all patients with altered mental status was once a standard prehospital and emergency department practice.[13,47,48]

COMPLICATIONS OF DEXTROSE ADMINISTRATION

The most serious complication associated with hypoglycemia is the failure to recognize and treat it. Most complications that are attributed to the administration of concentrated IV dextrose are either clinically insignificant or exceedingly rare. Phlebitis and sclerosis of veins may occur, and tissue necrosis may occur after soft tissue infiltration of $D_{50}W$ and after inadvertent intra-arterial injection.[4,31] Inappropriately large boluses of $D_{50}W$ in children have been associated with seizures, brain hemorrhage, and hyperosmolar coma.[87]

Concerns Regarding Elevated Blood Glucose Concentrations In Patients With Cerebral Ischemia Controlled laboratory investigations of ischemic brain injury in a variety of animal models consistently demonstrate that higher blood glucose concentrations are associated with more extensive cerebral injury. Most of these studies use animal models of global cerebral ischemia that include cardiac arrest, four-vessel ligation, or models of focal ischemia that used one- or two-vessel ligation.[27,77] These studies showed deleterious effects of hyperglycemia on a variety of outcomes, such as death, evidence of cerebral edema, and neurologic recovery.[23,25,26,28,42,49,60,79,89,90] The most severe injuries are evident when ischemia is incomplete or focal so that a small amount of blood flow is present, as when collateral circulation

TABLE A 10-1. Dosing of Dextrose

Age	Concentration	Bolus
Adult	$D_{50}W$ (50% = 0.5 g/mL)	0.5–1.0 g/kg
Child	$D_{25}W$ (25% = 0.25 g/mL)	0.5–1.0 g/kg
Infant	$D_{10}W$ (10% = 0.1 g/mL)	0.5–1.0 g/kg

is present near an area of focal infarction.[24,52,78] Hyperglycemia has not been shown to be detrimental in fetal and neonatal animal models of anoxia.[17,97,98]

The cellular biochemical changes that occur in the setting of ischemia have been extensively investigated. Global ischemia is associated with rapid depletion of brain glucose, ATP, and phosphocreatine, followed by a rapid increase in intracellular lactate, disruption of energy-dependent electrolyte gradients, increased intracellular calcium, activation of phospholipase, activation of inflammatory pathways, and generation of destructive free radicals such as superoxide and peroxynitrite.[10,51,91,102,105,106] Hyperglycemia is associated with increased capillary permeability in ischemic tissue and delays in resolution of intracellular calcium elevation during recovery from ischemia.[5,32] Significant increases in neutrophil deposition are demonstrated in areas of focal brain injury associated with hyperglycemia, suggesting a role in injury production.[64] Hyperglycemia may interfere with membrane repair systems by suppressing the synthesis of "heat shock" proteins in injured cells.[21,106] Administration of insulin to control hyperglycemia decreases the extent of ischemic injury in rat models of cerebral ischemia.[28,29,46,63,104,105] Because insulin promotes the synthesis of "heat shock" protein in ischemic cells, it may have a protective effect that is independent of its effect on blood glucose. Insulin also increases hippocampal γ-aminobutyric acid (GABA) concentrations in animal models, which may be neuroprotective.[88,96,100,101]

The clinical literature demonstrates that the presence of hyperglycemia upon admission is associated with poorer outcomes in patients with acute cerebrovascular accidents.[13,30,37,50,74,80,105] Complications include increased rates of hemorrhagic conversion,[14] larger infarction volumes,[7,20,37] a higher incidence of cerebral edema,[92] and increased mortality.[16,20,111] In several studies, the magnitudes of blood glucose concentration elevation that persisted after an acute stroke were positively correlated with larger infarction volumes, poorer functional outcome, and increased mortality.[7,20,111] The association is stronger in those having acute ischemic strokes but has also been observed in patients with subarachnoid and intracerebral hemorrhages.[43,55,75] A poor prognosis is also demonstrated in animal models of head trauma and hyperglycemia and in head trauma patients with hyperglycemia upon admission.[39,59,112]

The largest study to date is from the second European Cooperative Acute Stroke Study (ECASS-II). In this study, persistent and delayed hyperglycemia were associated with worse outcomes, even in nondiabetic patients.[111] Another study confirms the particularly negative association of hyperglycemia with poor outcome in nondiabetics.[94] An older study of thrombolysis in acute stroke from the National Institute of Neurological Disorders and Stroke (NINDS) showed a strong association of admission hyperglycemia with a worse outcome in thrombotic stroke. Hyperglycemic patients also had an increased risk for subsequent intracranial hemorrhage, whether or not they received thrombolytic therapy.[14] Examination of these data could not prove a cause-and-effect relationship between hyperglycemia and a poorer outcome in stroke.

In clinical studies of global ischemia in patients with cardiac arrest, admission hyperglycemia is a poor prognostic indicator. In 430 prehospital patients resuscitated from cardiac arrest, 276 patients who awakened had significantly lower blood glucose concentrations than 154 patients who did not (mean, 262 mg/dL vs. 341 mg/dL, $P = 0.0005$). In 90 awake patients with persistent neurologic deficits, the mean blood glucose concentration was 286 mg/dL compared with 250 mg/dL in patients who recovered fully ($P = 0.02$).[65] In a prospective study of 295 patients with intracerebral hemorrhage, an 18-mg/dL increase in serum glucose was associated with a 33% mortality increase (P: <0.0001).[43]

Methods in these studies have not delineated the primary effect of hyperglycemia on the ischemic brain from hyperglycemia that occurs after an intense sympathetic "stress" response to more severe brain injury. Hyperglycemia may also simply be a marker for poor microcirculation in patients with diabetes.[14,20,43,73,109]

The GIST-UK (Glucose Insulin in Stroke Trial—United Kingdom) was designed to answer the question regarding the importance of glycemic control in stroke patients. Unfortunately, it was stopped prematurely because of slow enrollment. Although underpowered, it failed to show any mortality benefit from treatment of hyperglycemia in acute stroke patients.[44,83]

Clinical Implications of Studies of Hyperglycemia and Cerebral Ischemia The clinical and laboratory studies cited above led to a reassessment of the standard practice of routine inclusion of $D_{50}W$ in the cocktail antidote for patients with altered mental status.[13,47,48] A thoughtful assessment of the literature recognizes the possible detriment of increasing blood glucose concentrations in a patient whose altered mental status or focal neurologic symptoms are caused by a cerebrovascular accident. This must be weighed against the risk of failure to treat hypoglycemia and the potential resultant permanent neurologic injury. This dilemma remains particularly consequential in the prehospital setting, where reliable testing of blood glucose concentration is limited. Without question, the reversal of hypoglycemia is a sound clinical intervention in the patient who is hypoglycemic, and the failure to administer dextrose in a timely fashion to a patient with significant hypoglycemia may result in permanent neurologic injury.

The new guidelines for management of patients with stroke recommend the avoidance of glucose-containing fluids and advocate for aggressive control of hyperglycemia while still avoiding hypoglycemia.[1,12]

BEDSIDE BLOOD GLUCOSE DETERMINATIONS

The bedside diagnosis of hypoglycemia is limited by the sensitivity and specificity of reagent strips, which do not have the reliability and accuracy of the chemistry laboratory.[76] Sensitivities of commonly available reagent strips for detection of hypoglycemia range between 92% and 97% in various studies.[18,19,53,61,66,84] The accuracy of these point-of-care testing methods is affected by the source of blood, whether venous or capillary, and by the poor perfusion associated with shock and cardiac arrest.[6,22,41,54,57,58,95] With reagent strip testing, variations in hematocrit and the presence of isopropyl alcohol in the sample may also alter the accuracy of the test.[9,45] In some specific tests, such as the one using glucose dehydrogenase pyrroloquinolinequinone (GDH-PQQ), accuracy may be affected by a number of interfering substances and xenobiotics, such as serum acetaminophen concentrations above 8 mg/dL, a serum bilirubin concentration above 20 mg/dL, a serum galactose concentration above 10 mg/dL, a maltose concentration above 16 mg/dL, a serum uric acid above 10 to 16 mg/dL, serum triglycerides above 5000 mg/dL, and the presence of D-xylose in the sample. All of these result in falsely elevated glucose measurements.[36] Notably, icodextrin, an ingredient in peritoneal dialysis, may result in overestimation of glucose measurements because it is metabolized to maltose. In several case reports and at least 18 cases reported in a review, this resulted in excess insulin administration and subsequent hypoglycemia.[36,40,56,82] Maltose is also contained in some immunoglobulin solutions, and the same interference can be expected.[38,93] Glucose measurements by the GDH-PQQ method are also affected by the hematocrit. Whereas hematocrits lower than 20% may result in a falsely elevated glucose measurements, hematocrits above 55% may result in falsely low measured glucose concentrations.[36] In a retrospective review of patients admitted to a hospital over a 12-month period, 1.2% were identified as having interfering substances. Of these, 36% had active orders for insulin products. The most common interferences identified were a low hematocrit (44% of patients) and a high serum uric acid (29% of patients).[36]

A study of 66 critically ill newborns that defined critical hypoglycemia as below 30 mg/dL found a sensitivity of 100% for the detection of critical hypoglycemia for each of two different reagent strips.[66] False-positive capillary determinations of hypoglycemia have been demonstrated in patients in shock and cardiac arrest. Hypoglycemia was identified by capillary samples in eight of 50 patients with cardiac arrest. Three of these were confirmed to be hypoglycemic by the laboratory. Reagent strip testing of venous blood correctly classified these patients. There were no false-negative results.[95] A critical care unit study that evaluated patients in shock showed that 32% were incorrectly diagnosed as euglycemic when capillary blood was used. Results of reagent strip tests of venous blood correlated well with laboratory results, correctly classifying all patients. No cases of hypoglycemia were missed.[6] Therefore, capillary determinations of glucose should be used with caution in the critically ill population, recognizing that false-positive detections of hypoglycemia are common. When feasible, reagent stick testing of venous blood rather than capillary samples is preferable.

Several studies have compared the accuracy of standard reagent strips for the detection of hypoglycemia from capillary and venous blood compared with the gold standard of the laboratory. Two studies, one with 97 subjects[41] and one with 270 subjects,[57] evaluated the agreement between reagent strip determinations of capillary and venous blood glucose in healthy normoglycemic volunteers. In the larger study, 18% of subjects had a more than 15-mg/dL difference between capillary and venous reagent strip tests. In this study, capillary measurements were better correlated with the laboratory values. Whether these results have any clinical significance is not clear because none of the subjects fell out of the euglycemic range. However, the results suggest that the capillary blood glucose test has greater accuracy in the euglycemic range and in healthy individuals.

The "safe" number at which no cases of symptomatic hypoglycemia are missed by reagent strip testing is a subject of debate because of the inherent risk of error from lack of sensitivity. In one study in which hypoglycemia was defined as a blood glucose concentration below 60 mg/dL, two of 33 hypoglycemic patients were not detected at the bedside. A cutoff of 90 mg/dL would have detected 100% of numerically hypoglycemic patients.[61] Based on these studies, it can be argued that a bedside reagent measurement of 90 mg/dL is a conservative cutoff for assurance of clinical euglycemia in all patients.

PHARMACOKINETICS OF DEXTROSE

Accurate prediction of the amount of dextrose required to effectively treat patients with hypoglycemia is difficult. At equilibrium, 25 g of dextrose distributed in total body water in a 70-kg adult is calculated to increase the serum glucose concentration by about 60 mg/dL.[48] In the few clinical studies performed, the magnitude of glucose elevation after oral (PO) or IV dextrose loading was unpredictable. In one study, 25 g (50 mL) of $D_{50}W$ administered to adults (both diabetics and nondiabetics) resulted in a mean blood glucose elevation of 166 mg/dL when measured in the opposite extremity 3 to 5 minutes after the bolus; however, the range of this elevation was 37 to 370 mg/dL above baseline.[2] In a human model of insulin-induced hypoglycemia, PO administration of 20 g of PO dextrose increased the serum blood glucose concentration from 60 to 120 mg/dL over 1 hour, but 10 g also raised the concentration from 60 to 100 mg/dL.[107] Another study used 25 volunteers and administered 25 g of IV dextrose as $D_{50}W$. Glucose concentrations were then measured at 5, 15, 30, and 60 minutes. Volume of distribution formulas could not accurately predict postinfusion glucose concentrations. The serum glucose elevation was statistically significant from baseline at 5 and 15 minutes, with glucose concentrations returning to baseline at 30 minutes postinfusion.[8]

It is important to remember that rapid increases in serum glucose are sufficient to cause insulin release from the pancreas. This may result in reactive hypoglycemia. Therefore, glucose concentrations must be closely followed after a bolus of concentrated glucose solutions.

CONCLUSION: A RATIONAL CLINICAL SOLUTION

An ideal clinical solution to the management of patients with altered mental status or focal neurologic symptoms misses no cases of significant symptomatic hypoglycemia but avoids the administration of dextrose to patients with brain ischemia who are not hypoglycemic. A realistic approach can be fashioned from our understanding of the reliability of reagent test strips and a risk-to-benefit assessment of the presenting problem.

Infants and neonates should receive dextrose when clinically indicated without concern for associated ischemia or anoxia because the detrimental effect of hyperglycemia seems to be absent in this age group. Patients with coma or status epilepticus from hypoglycemia benefit greatly from empiric treatment with dextrose and experience the greatest morbidity if not promptly treated. Furthermore, a patient who is comatose from a major stroke has a very limited chance for recovery, and the acute administration of dextrose likely will not impact heavily on the prognosis compared with the impact of a missed diagnosis of significant hypoglycemia. Administering $D_{50}W$ to patients in coma who have a measured blood glucose less than 90 mg/dL determined by bedside reagent strip testing is rational. Similarly, although confusion and delirium without focal neurologic findings may occur as manifestations of structural brain injury, toxic-metabolic causes are much more common. These patients should receive dextrose if the glucose concentration determined by bedside test is 90 mg/dL or less. When a reliable bedside glucose determination is not readily available, all of these patients should receive $D_{50}W$ empirically.

As previously discussed, rapid reagent glucose samples of capillary blood are especially unreliable in patients with hypotension or cardiac arrest. Bedside reagent strip testing of venous blood appears to be more reliable.[6,84,95] Patients in shock or cardiac arrest should undergo reagent testing using a venous blood sample and should receive dextrose if results indicate they are numerically hypoglycemic (<90 mg/dL). Empiric administration of dextrose to a patient with a cardiac arrest who is euglycemic as determined by reagent strip testing of venous blood should be considered only if the patient is diabetic.

Patients with focal neurological deficits due to ischemia constitute a population that is reasonably expected to derive great benefit from maintenance of euglycemia. Although focal presentations of hypoglycemia are not rare, they are infrequent relative to the numbers of patients with focal presentations who have had strokes. In one study,

3% of patients with hypoglycemia presented with focal symptoms.[67] In patients with a history of diabetes who present with focal symptoms, symptomatic hypoglycemia must be strongly considered when the reagent strip shows a blood glucose concentration below 90 mg/dL.

Patients with a clear history and evidence of significant head injury preceded by normal activity should not be treated unless the bedside test indicates numerical hypoglycemia (<90 mg/dL). Diabetic patients may suffer unintentional injuries predisposed by hypoglycemic episodes. The treating physician must use his or her best judgment of the mechanism and evidence of injury, witness reports, available medical history, and result of bedside glucose determination to decide whether to administer $D_{50}W$ to a traumatized patient with an altered level of consciousness.

SUMMARY

Studies have indicated that the currently available reagent strips reliably demonstrate the absence of significant hypoglycemia at readings above 90 mg/dL. Profound neurologic impairment likely is not the result of hypoglycemia when such concentrations are demonstrated, even in diabetic patients. Dextrose should be administered to all patients with altered levels of consciousness and numerical hypoglycemia (glucose concentration <90 mg/dL measured by reagent strips). Concerns regarding the negative effects of elevated blood glucose concentration on cerebral ischemia should not cause a physician to withhold dextrose in patients with neurologic impairment when symptomatic hypoglycemia cannot be promptly and reliably excluded. Dextrose should be empirically administered to patients with altered mental status when bedside reagent strips are not readily available.

REFERENCES

1. Adams HP Jr., del Zoppo G, Alberts MJ, et al. Guidelines for the early management of adults with ischemic stroke: a guideline from the American Heart Association/American Stroke Association Stroke Council, Clinical Cardiology Council, Cardiovascular Radiology and Intervention Council, and the Atherosclerotic Peripheral Vascular Disease and Quality of Care Outcomes in Research Interdisciplinary Working Groups: the American Academy of Neurology affirms the value of this guideline as an educational tool for neurologists. *Stroke.* 2007;38:1655-1711.
2. Adler PM. Serum glucose changes after administration of 50% dextrose solution: pre- and in-hospital calculations. *Am J Emerg Med.* 1986;4:504-506.
3. Andrade R, Mathew V, Morgenstern MJ, et al. Hypoglycemic hemiplegic syndrome. *Ann Emerg Med.* 1984;13:529-531.
4. Arad I, Benady S. Gangrene following intraumbilical injection of hypertonic glucose [letter]. *J Pediatr.* 1976;89:327-328.
5. Araki N, Greenberg JH, Sladky JT, et al. The effect of hyperglycemia on intracellular calcium in stroke. *J Cereb Blood Flow Metab.* 1992;12:469-476.
6. Atkin SH, Dasmahapatra A, Jaker MA, et al. Fingerstick glucose determination in shock. *Ann Intern Med.* 1991;114:1020-1024.
7. Baird TA, Parsons MW, Phanh T, et al. Persistent poststroke hyperglycemia is independently associated with infarct expansion and worse clinical outcome. *Stroke.* 2003;34:2208-2214.
8. Balentine JR, Gaeta TJ, Kessler D, et al. Effect of 50 milliliters of 50% dextrose in water administration on the blood sugar of euglycemic volunteers. *Acad Emerg Med.* 1998;5:691-694.
9. Barreau PB, Buttery JE. The effect of the haematocrit value on the determination of glucose levels by reagent-strip methods. *Med J Aust.* 1987;147:286-288.
10. Bemeur C, Ste-Marie L, Montgomery J. Increased oxidative stress during hyperglycemic cerebral ischemia. *Neurochem Int.* 2007;50:890-904.
11. Boyle PJ, Schwartz NS, Shah SD, et al. Plasma glucose concentrations at the onset of hypoglycemic symptoms in patients with poorly controlled diabetes and in nondiabetics. *N Engl J Med.* 1988;318:1487-1492.
12. Broderick J, Connolly S, Feldmann E, et al. Guidelines for the management of spontaneous intracerebral hemorrhage in adults: 2007 update: a guideline from the American Heart Association/American Stroke Association Stroke Council, High Blood Pressure Research Council, and the Quality of Care and Outcomes in Research Interdisciplinary Working Group. *Stroke.* 2007;38:2001-2023.
13. Browning RG, Olson DW, Stueven HA, et al. 50% dextrose: antidote or toxin? *Ann Emerg Med.* 1990;19:683-687.
14. Bruno A, Levine SR, Frankel MR, et al. Admission glucose level and clinical outcomes in the NINDS rt-PA Stroke Trial. *Neurology.* 2002;59:669-674.
15. Burns CM, Rutherford MA, Boardman JP, et al. Patterns of cerebral injury and neurodevelopmental outcomes after symptomatic neonatal hypoglycemia. *Pediatrics.* 2008;122:65-74.
16. Capes SE, Hunt D, Malmberg K, et al. Stress hyperglycemia and prognosis of stroke in nondiabetic and diabetic patients: a systematic overview. *Stroke.* 2001;32:2426-2432.
17. Chang YS, Park WS, Lee M, et al. Effect of hyperglycemia on brain cell membrane function and energy metabolism during hypoxia-ischemia in newborn piglets. *Brain Res.* 1998;798:271-280.
18. Cheeley RD, Joyce SM. A clinical comparison of the performance of four blood glucose reagent strips. *Am J Emerg Med.* 1990;8:11-15.
19. Choubtum L, Mahachoklertwattana P, Udomsubpayakul U, et al. Accuracy of glucose meters in measuring low blood glucose levels. *J Med Assoc Thai.* 2002;85(suppl 4):S1104-1110.
20. Christensen H, Boysen G. Blood glucose increases early after stroke onset: a study on serial measurements of blood glucose in acute stroke. *Eur J Neurol.* 2002;9:297-301.
21. Combs DJ, Dempsey RJ, Donaldson D, et al. Hyperglycemia suppresses c-fos mRNA expression following transient cerebral ischemia in gerbils. *J Cereb Blood Flow Metab.* 1992;12:169-172.
22. Critchell CD, Savarese V, Callahan A, et al. Accuracy of bedside capillary blood glucose measurements in critically ill patients. *Intensive Care Med.* 2007;33:2079-2084.
23. D'Alecy LG, Lundy EF, Barton KJ, et al. Dextrose containing intravenous fluid impairs outcome and increases death after eight minutes of cardiac arrest and resuscitation in dogs. *Surgery.* 1986;100:505-511.
24. de Courten-Myers G, Myers RE, Schoolfield L. Hyperglycemia enlarges infarct size in cerebrovascular occlusion in cats. *Stroke.* 1988;19:623-630.
25. de Courten-Myers GM, Kleinholz M, Wagner KR, et al. Fatal strokes in hyperglycemic cats. *Stroke.* 1989;20:1707-1715.
26. de Courten-Myers GM, Myers RE, Wagner KR. Effect of hyperglycemia on infarct size after cerebrovascular occlusion in cats. *Stroke.* 1990;21:357-358.
27. de Courten-Myers GM, Wagner KR. Stroke models: strengths and pitfalls. *Resuscitation.* 1992;23:91-100.
28. de Courten-Myers GM, Kleinholz M, Wagner KR, et al. Normoglycemia (not hypoglycemia) optimizes outcome from middle cerebral artery occlusion. *J Cereb Blood Flow Metab.* 1994;14:227-236.
29. de Courten-Myers GM, Wagner KR, Myers RE. Insulin reduction of cerebral infarction. *J Neurosurg.* 1996;84:146-148.
30. de Falco FA, Sepe Visconti O, Fucci G, et al. Correlation between hyperglycemia and cerebral infarct size in patients with stroke. A clinical and X-ray computed tomography study in 104 patients. *Schweiz Arch Neurol Psychiatr.* 1993;144:233-239.
31. DeLorenzo RA, Vista JP. Another hazard of hypertonic dextrose. *Am J Emerg Med.* 1994;12:262-263.
32. Dietrich WD, Alonso O, Busto R. Moderate hyperglycemia worsens acute blood-brain barrier injury after forebrain ischemia in rats. *Stroke.* 1993;24:111-116.
33. Duarte J, Perez A, Coria F, et al. Hypoglycemia presenting as acute tetraplegia. *Stroke.* 1993;24:143.
34. Duh E, Feinglos M. Hypoglycemia-induced angina pectoris in a patient with diabetes mellitus. *Ann Intern Med.* 1994;121:945-946.
35. Duvanel CB, Fawer CL, Cotting J, et al. Long-term effects of neonatal hypoglycemia on brain growth and psychomotor development in small-for-gestational-age preterm infants. *J Pediatr.* 1999;134:492-498.
36. Eastham JH, Mason D, Barnes DL, et al. Prevalence of interfering substances with point-of-care glucose testing in a community hospital. *Am J Health Syst Pharm.* 2009;66:167-170.
37. Els T, Klisch J, Orszagh M, et al. Hyperglycemia in patients with focal cerebral ischemia after intravenous thrombolysis: influence on clinical outcome and infarct size. *Cerebrovasc Dis.* 2002;13:89-94.

38. Epstein JS, Gaines A, Kapit R, et al. Important drug information: immune globulin intravenous (human). *Int J Trauma Nurs.* 1999;5:139-140.
39. Feldman Z, Zachari S, Reichenthal E, et al. Brain edema and neurological status with rapid infusion of lactated Ringer's or 5% dextrose solution following head trauma. *J Neurosurg.* 1995;83:1060-1066.
40. Flore K, Delanghe J. Icodextrin: a major problem for glucose dehydrogenase-based glucose point of care testing systems. *Acta Clin Belg.* 2006;61:351-354.
41. Funk DL, Chan L, Lutz N, et al. Comparison of capillary and venous glucose measurements in healthy volunteers. *Prehosp Emerg Care.* 2001;5:275-277.
42. Ginsberg MD, Welsh FA, Budd WW. Deleterious effect of glucose pretreatment on recovery from diffuse cerebral ischemia in the cat. I. Local cerebral blood flow and glucose utilization. *Stroke.* 1980;11:347-354.
43. Godoy DA, Pinero GR, Svampa S, et al. Hyperglycemia and short-term outcome in patients with spontaneous intracerebral hemorrhage. *Neurocrit Care.* 2008;9:217-229.
44. Gray CS, Hildreth AJ, Sandercock PA, et al. Glucose-potassium-insulin infusions in the management of post-stroke hyperglycaemia: the UK Glucose Insulin in Stroke Trial (GIST-UK). *Lancet Neurol.* 2007;6:397-406.
45. Grazaitis DM, Sexson WR. Erroneously high Dextrostix values caused by isopropyl alcohol. *Pediatrics.* 1980;66:221-223.
46. Hamilton MG, Tranmer BI, Auer RN. Insulin reduction of cerebral infarction due to transient focal ischemia. *J Neurosurg.* 1995;82:262-268.
47. Hoffman JR, Schriger DL, Votey SR, et al. The empiric use of hypertonic dextrose in patients with altered mental status: a reappraisal. *Ann Emerg Med.* 1992;21:20-24.
48. Hoffman RS, Goldfrank LR. The poisoned patient with altered consciousness. Controversies in the use of a "coma cocktail." *JAMA.* 1995;274:562-569.
49. Hoffman WE, Braucher E, Pelligrino DA, et al. Brain lactate and neurologic outcome following incomplete ischemia in fasted, nonfasted, and glucose-loaded rats. *Anesthesiology.* 1990;72:1045-1050.
50. Horowitz SH, Zito JL, Donnarumma R, et al. Clinical-radiographic correlations within the first five hours of cerebral infarction. *Acta Neurol Scand.* 1992;86:207-214.
51. Hoxworth JM, Xu K, Zhou Y, et al. Cerebral metabolic profile, selective neuron loss, and survival of acute and chronic hyperglycemic rats following cardiac arrest and resuscitation. *Brain Res.* 1999;821:467-479.
52. Ibayashi S, Fujishima M, Sadoshima S, et al. Cerebral blood flow and tissue metabolism in experimental cerebral ischemia of spontaneously hypertensive rats with hyper-, normo-, and hypoglycemia. *Stroke.* 1986;17:261-266.
53. Jones JL, Ray VG, Gough JE, et al. Determination of prehospital blood glucose: a prospective, controlled study. *J Emerg Med.* 1992;10:679-682.
54. Kanji S, Buffie J, Hutton B, et al. Reliability of point-of-care testing for glucose measurement in critically ill adults. *Crit Care Med.* 2005;33:2778-2785.
55. Kimura K, Iguchi Y, Inoue T, et al. Hyperglycemia independently increases the risk of early death in acute spontaneous intracerebral hemorrhage. *J Neurol Sci.* 2007;255:90-94.
56. Kroll HR, Maher TR. Significant hypoglycemia secondary to icodextrin peritoneal dialysate in a diabetic patient. *Anesth Analg.* 2007;104:1473-1474, table of contents.
57. Kumar G, Sng BL, Kumar S. Correlation of capillary and venous blood glucometry with laboratory determination. *Prehosp Emerg Care.* 2004;8:378-383.
58. Lacara T, Domagtoy C, Lickliter D, et al. Comparison of point-of-care and laboratory glucose analysis in critically ill patients. *Am J Crit Care.* 2007;16:336-346; quiz 347.
59. Lam AM, Winn HR, Cullen BF, et al. Hyperglycemia and neurological outcome in patients with head injury. *J Neurosurg.* 1991;75:545-551.
60. Lanier WL, Stangland KJ, Scheithauer BW, et al. The effects of dextrose infusion and head position on neurologic outcome after complete cerebral ischemia in primates: examination of a model. *Anesthesiology.* 1987;66:39-48.
61. Lavery RF, Allegra JR, Cody RP, et al. A prospective evaluation of glucose reagent teststrips in the prehospital setting. *Am J Emerg Med.* 1991;9:304-308.
62. Leak D, Starr P. The mechanism of arrhythmias during insulin-induced hypoglycemia. *Am Heart J.* 1962;63:688-691.
63. LeMay DR, Gehua L, Zelenock GB, et al. Insulin administration protects neurologic function in cerebral ischemia in rats. *Stroke.* 1988;19:1411-1419.
64. Lin B, Ginsberg MD, Busto R, et al. Hyperglycemia triggers massive neutrophil deposition in brain following transient ischemia in rats. *Neurosci Lett.* 2000;278:1-4.
65. Longstreth WT Jr, Inui TS. High blood glucose level on hospital admission and poor neurological recovery after cardiac arrest. *Ann Neurol.* 1984;15:59-63.
66. Maisels MJ, Lee CA. Chemstrip glucose test strips: correlation with true glucose values less than 80 mg/dl. *Crit Care Med.* 1983;11:293-295.
67. Malouf R, Brust JC. Hypoglycemia: causes, neurological manifestations, and outcome. *Ann Neurol.* 1985;17:421-430.
68. Meinhold J, Heise T, Rave K, et al. Electrocardiographic changes during insulin-induced hypoglycemia in healthy subjects. *Horm Metab Res.* 1998;30:694-697.
69. Montgomery BM, Pinner CA. Transient hypoglycemic hemiplegia. *Arch Intern Med.* 1964;114:680-684.
70. Mori F, Nishie M, Houzen H, et al. Hypoglycemic encephalopathy with extensive lesions in the cerebral white matter. *Neuropathology.* 2006;26:147-152.
71. Navarro-Gutierrez S, Gonzalez-Martinez F, Fernandez-Perez MT, et al. Bradycardia related to hypoglycaemia. *Eur J Emerg Med.* 2003;10:331-333.
72. Odeh M, Oliven A, Bassan H. Transient atrial fibrillation precipitated by hypoglycemia. *Ann Emerg Med.* 1990;19:565-567.
73. O'Neill PA, Davies I, Fullerton KJ, et al. Stress hormone and blood glucose response following acute stroke in the elderly. *Stroke.* 1991;22:842-847.
74. Parsons MW, Barber PA, Desmond PM, et al. Acute hyperglycemia adversely affects stroke outcome: a magnetic resonance imaging and spectroscopy study. *Ann Neurol.* 2002;52:20-28.
75. Pasternak JJ, McGregor DG, Schroeder DR, et al. Hyperglycemia in patients undergoing cerebral aneurysm surgery: its association with long-term gross neurologic and neuropsychological function. *Mayo Clin Proc.* 2008;83:406-417.
76. Petersen JR, Graves DF, Tacker DH, et al. Comparison of POCT and central laboratory blood glucose results using arterial, capillary, and venous samples from MICU patients on a tight glycemic protocol. *Clin Chim Acta.* 2008;396:10-13.
77. Plum F. What causes infarction in ischemic brain? The Robert Wartenberg Lecture. *Neurology.* 1983;33:222-233.
78. Prado R, Ginsberg MD, Dietrich WD, et al. Hyperglycemia increases infarct size in collaterally perfused but not end-arterial vascular territories. *J Cereb Blood Flow Metab.* 1988;8:186-192.
79. Pulsinelli WA, Levy DE, Duffy TE. Regional cerebral blood flow and glucose metabolism following transient forebrain ischemia. *Ann Neurol.* 1982;11:499-502.
80. Pulsinelli WA, Levy DE, Sigsbee B, et al. Increased damage after ischemic stroke in patients with hyperglycemia with or without established diabetes mellitus. *Am J Med.* 1983;74:540-544.
81. Rehncrona S, Rosen I, Siesjo BK. Brain lactic acidosis and ischemic cell damage: 1. Biochemistry and neurophysiology. *J Cereb Blood Flow Metab.* 1981;1:297-311.
82. Riley SG, Chess J, Donovan KL, et al. Spurious hyperglycaemia and icodextrin in peritoneal dialysis fluid. *Br Med J.* 2003;327:608-609.
83. Scott JF, Robinson GM, French JM, et al. Glucose potassium insulin infusions in the treatment of acute stroke patients with mild to moderate hyperglycemia: the Glucose Insulin in Stroke Trial (GIST). *Stroke.* 1999;30:793-799.
84. Scott PA, Wolf LR, Spadafora MP. Accuracy of reagent strips in detecting hypoglycemia in the emergency department. *Ann Emerg Med.* 1998;32:305-309.
85. Seibert DG. Reversible decerebrate posturing secondary to hypoglycemia. *Am J Med.* 1985;78:1036-1037.
86. Seltzer HS. Drug-induced hypoglycemia. A review of 1418 cases. *Endocrinol Metab Clin North Am.* 1989;18:163-183.
87. Shah A, Stanhope R, Matthew D. Hazards of pharmacological tests of growth hormone secretion in childhood. *Br Med J.* 1992;304:173-174.
88. Shuaib A, Ijaz MS, Waqar T, et al. Insulin elevates hippocampal GABA levels during ischemia. This is independent of its hypoglycemic effect. *Neuroscience.* 1995;67:809-814.
89. Siemkowicz E, Hansen AJ. Clinical restitution following cerebral ischemia in hypo-, normo- and hyperglycemic rats. *Acta Neurol Scand.* 1978;58:1-8.

90. Siemkowicz E. Hyperglycemia in the reperfusion period hampers recovery from cerebral ischemia. *Acta Neurol Scand*. 1981;64:207-216.
91. Siesjo BK. Basic mechanisms of traumatic brain damage. *Ann Emerg Med.* 1993;22:959-969.
92. Song EC, Chu K, Jeong SW, et al. Hyperglycemia exacerbates brain edema and perihematomal cell death after intracerebral hemorrhage. *Stroke.* 2003;34:2215-2220.
93. Souza SP, Castro MC, Rodrigues RA, et al. False hyperglycemia induced by polivalent immunoglobulins. *Transplantation*. 2005;80:542-543.
94. Stead LG, Gilmore RM, Bellolio MF, et al. Hyperglycemia as an independent predictor of worse outcome in non-diabetic patients presenting with acute ischemic stroke. *Neurocrit* Care. 2009;10(2):181-186.
95. Thomas SH, Gough JE, Benson N, et al. Accuracy of fingerstick glucose determination in patients receiving CPR. *South Med J.* 1994;87:1072-1075.
96. Ting LP, Tu CL, Chou CK. Insulin-induced expression of human heat-shock protein gene hsp70. *J Biol Chem*. 1989;264:3404-3408.
97. Vannucci RC. Cerebral carbohydrate and energy metabolism in perinatal hypoxic-ischemic brain damage. *Brain Pathol*. 1992;2:229-234.
98. Vannucci RC, Mujsce DJ. Effect of glucose on perinatal hypoxic-ischemic brain damage. *Biol Neonate*. 1992;62:215-224.
99. Vannucci RC, Yager JY. Glucose, lactic acid, and perinatal hypoxic-ischemic brain damage. *Pediatr Neurol*. 1992;8:3-12.
100. Voll CL, Auer RN. The effect of postischemic blood glucose levels on ischemic brain damage in the rat. *Ann Neurol*. 1988;24:638-646.
101. Voll CL, Auer RN. Insulin attenuates ischemic brain damage independent of its hypoglycemic effect. *J Cereb Blood Flow Metab*. 1991;11:1006-1014.
102. Wagner KR, Kleinholz M, de Courten-Myers GM, et al. Hyperglycemic versus normoglycemic stroke: topography of brain metabolites, intracellular pH, and infarct size. *J Cereb Blood Flow Metab*. 1992;12:213-222.
103. Wallis WE, Donaldson I, Scott RS, et al. Hypoglycemia masquerading as cerebrovascular disease (hypoglycemic hemiplegia). *Ann Neurol.* 1985;18:510-512.
104. Warner DS, Gionet TX, Todd MM, et al. Insulin-induced normoglycemia improves ischemic outcome in hyperglycemic rats. *Stroke*. 1992;23:1775-1780; discussion 1781.
105. Wass CT, Lanier WL. Glucose modulation of ischemic brain injury: review and clinical recommendations. *Mayo Clin Proc*. 1996;71:801-812.
106. White BC, Krause GS. Brain injury and repair mechanisms: the potential for pharmacologic therapy in closed-head trauma. *Ann Emerg Med.* 1993;22:970-979.
107. Wiethop BV, Cryer PE. Alanine and terbutaline in treatment of hypoglycemia in *IDDM*. *Diabetes Care*. 1993;16:1131-1136.
108. Winer JB, Fish DR, Sawyers D, et al. A movement disorder as a presenting feature of recurrent hypoglycaemia. *Mov Disord*. 1990;5:176-177.
109. Woo E, Ma JT, Robinson JD, et al. Hyperglycemia is a stress response in acute stroke. *Stroke*. 1988;19:1359-1364.
110. Yealy DM, Wolfson AB. Hypoglycemia. *Emerg Med Clin North Am.* 1989;7:837-848.
111. Yong M, Kaste M. Dynamic of hyperglycemia as a predictor of stroke outcome in the ECASS-II trial. *Stroke*. 2008;39:2749-2755.
112. Young B, Ott L, Dempsey R, et al. Relationship between admission hyperglycemia and neurologic outcome of severely brain-injured patients. *Ann Surg*. 1989;210:466-472; discussion 463-472.

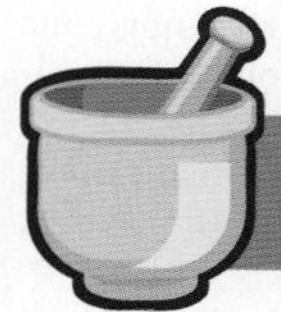

ANTIDOTES IN DEPTH (A11)

OCTREOTIDE

Mary Ann Howland

OH

H_3C OH

DPhe–Cys–Phe–DTrp–Lys–Thr–Cys–NH

Octreotide is a long-acting, synthetic octapeptide analog of somatostatin that inhibits pancreatic insulin secretion. It currently is the essential complement to dextrose for the treatment of refractory hypoglycemia induced by overdoses of oral hypoglycemics (eg, sulfonylureas) and quinine. Octreotide currently is used in toxicology for the treatment of xenobiotic-induced endogenous secretion of insulin.

HISTORY

Somatostatin is a collective term for shorter fragments (SRIF-28, SRIF-25, and SRIF-14) cleaved by tissue-specific enzymes from pre-prosomatostatin (116 amino acids) and prosomatostatin (92 amino acids).[11] Somatostatin was identified in 1973, during the search for growth hormone releasing factor.[6] In addition to its effects on growth hormone and insulin secretion, somatostatin has far-reaching effects as a central nervous system (CNS) neurotransmitter and as a modulator of hormonal release.[32,40] The importance of somatostatin on insulin secretion led to the need to create an analog as a therapeutic tool as somatostatin is limited because of its short duration of action.

Octreotide was synthesized in 1982 in an effort to develop a longer-acting analog of somatostatin.[5] Octreotide is currently FDA approved for the treatment of acromegaly, carcinoid tumors and vasoactive intestinal peptide tumors. It is also used therapeutically for the treatment of pituitary adenomas, pancreatic islet cell tumors, portal hypertension, esophageal varices, and secretory diarrhea.[32] Octreotide is being investigated for its inhibitory effects on tumor cell proliferation through stimulation of apoptosis, antiangiogenesis, immunomodulatory effects, and the suppression of tumor-stimulating growth factors.[31,32,41] Lanreotide and vapreotide are other long-acting somatostatin analogs that are FDA approved.

RECEPTOR AFFINITY

The effects of somatostatin are mediated by high-affinity binding to membrane receptors on target tissues. Five different somatostatin receptor subtypes that belong to a superfamily of G-protein–coupled receptors have been identified and assigned numbers (SSTR1–SSTR5) according to their order of discovery.[11] Octreotide, lanreotide, and vapreotide have high binding affinity for subtype SSTR2, a lower affinity for SSTR5 and SSTR3, and almost no affinity for SSTR1 and SSTR4.[32] The pancreas contains all 5 subtypes but SSTR5 and SSTR1 are more prevalent in the beta cells and SSTR2 is more prevalent in the alpha cells.[49] SSTR5 is found in many tissues including the brain, pituitary, stomach, intestine, thyroid, and adrenal gland; SSTR2 is found in the brain, pituitary, stomach, liver, kidney, lung, intestine, spleen, thymus, uterus, prostate, and adrenal gland.[32,36,43,49] A variety of pituitary and gastroenteropancreatic tumors contain varying percentages of the SSTR subtypes.

EFFECTS ON INSULIN SECRETION AND OTHER HORMONES

Experiments in both healthy human volunteers and an isolated perfused canine pancreas model demonstrate the ability of somatostatin to inhibit glucose-stimulated insulin release.[1,19] Experiments using a whole-cell patch clamp technique on a hamster β-cell line suggest that somatostatin inhibits insulin secretion by a G-protein–mediated decrease in calcium entry through voltage-dependent Ca^{2+} channels.[25] No evidence indicates that somatostatin inhibits insulin release by promoting K^+ efflux through K^+ channels at physiologic concentrations as do the oral hypoglycemics. (Fig. 48-2).[15,33,42] Instead somatostatin, like epinephrine, stimulates a pertussis-toxin sensitive Gi-coupled receptor that inhibits adenylate cyclase and production of cyclic adenosine monophosphate (cAMP), decreasing intracellular calcium and thereby reducing insulin secretion.[23] Simultaneous distal reduction in phosphorylation of specific proteins may also be involved in reducing insulin secretion.[15,23] This latter mechanism appears to be independent of Ca^{2+}.[15,23] Activation of SSTR5 on the β-cell of the pancreas also reduces insulin biosynthesis.[15] One study in human volunteers confirms the ability of somatostatin to inhibit the increased insulin response to both glucose and glucagon.[19] Intravenous (IV) infusion of 1 g tolbutamide over 2 minutes caused insulin concentrations to rise and serum glucose concentration to drop sharply. Similarly, in the presence of somatostatin and tolbutamide, administration of IV glucagon caused a rise in glucose concentration without the expected subsequent glucose-stimulated rise in insulin. The effects of somatostatin were short lived. Within 5 minutes of stopping the somatostatin, the insulin-releasing effects of tolbutamide continued, and within 15 minutes the serum glucose concentration fell. Peak insulin concentrations were achieved within 25 minutes.

Studies comparing octreotide to somatostatin in rats and monkeys demonstrate that octreotide is 1.3 times as potent as somatostatin in inhibiting insulin secretion by 50%. Likewise, compared with somatostatin, octreotide was 45 times more potent in inhibiting growth hormone secretion and 11 times more potent in inhibiting glucagon release.[5] Comparable results were found using a hyperglycemic glucose clamp technique.[28] Octreotide blocks the counterregulatory response to the effects of 0.1 unit/kg IV insulin by preventing an increase in glucagon and growth hormone. The effects of octreotide on the responses of adrenocorticotropin, cortisol, prolactin, luteinizing hormone, and follicle- stimulating hormone to insulin-induced hypoglycemia, all remained intact.[33] In contrast, growth hormone[14] and thyroid-stimulating hormone are significantly inhibited.[33]

PHARMACOKINETICS

The pharmacokinetics of IV and subcutaneous (SC) octreotide were studied in 8 healthy adult volunteers.[30] Subjects received 25, 50, 100, and 200 μg IV octreotide over 3 minutes and 50, 100, 200, and 400 μg SC octreotide in random order. Following IV administration, the distribution half-life averaged 12 minutes, and the elimination half-life ranged from 72 ± 22 minutes to 98 ± 37 minutes and was linear. Vi (volume of distribution of the central compartment) was dose dependent and increased from approximately 5.7 L at 25, 50, and 100 μg IV to 10 L at 200-μg IV doses.[30] The Vd (volume of distribution determined by area under the curve) ranged from 18 ± 6 L to 30 ± 30 L and showed no dose dependency.[30] Renal elimination accounted for approximately 30% of the elimination and was reduced in the elderly and in those with severe renal failure.[40]

After SC administration, bioavailability was 100%, and peak concentrations were achieved within 30 minutes with an absorption half-life of 5–12 minutes. The elimination half-life was 88–102 minutes. Peak plasma concentrations after SC administration ranged from 2.4 ng/mL at doses of 50 μg to 23.5 ng/mL at doses of 400 μg. After IV administration peak plasma concentrations ranged from 9.6 ng/mL at doses of 50 μg to 27.8 ng/mL at doses of 200 μg.[30]

The pharmacokinetics in patients with pathologic conditions may differ from the pharmacokinetics in healthy volunteers as exemplified by a lower peak concentration and a higher steady-state Vd in patients with acromegaly.[40]

The duration of action is variable. When used for tumor suppression, the duration may last up to 12 hours.[40] The duration of action for inhibition of insulin secretion is unknown.

CLINICAL USE FOR INSULIN SUPPRESSION

Octreotide was studied in several clinical conditions, including insulinomas and hypoglycemia of infancy.[2,20,27,46,47] In most instances, octreotide suppressed insulin concentrations, and glucose concentrations rose. However, worsening hypoglycemia is reported when glucagon suppression outlasts insulin suppression.[6,10,18,24,39,46] Another reason for variable effects in these conditions include absence of octreotide susceptible SSTR receptor subtypes.[48] Octreotide currently is used in toxicology for treatment of xenobiotic-induced endogenous secretion of insulin.

In controlled studies of healthy volunteers, octreotide suppressed the release of insulin associated with quinine.[44] Life-threatening hypoglycemia is a well-recognized complication of quinine treatment of *Plasmodium falciparum* malaria. In this setting, hypertonic dextrose and diazoxide therapy are frequently inadequate, with ensuing refractory hypoglycemia. In an investigation of the potential hypoglycemia-sparing effect of octreotide given for treatment of quinine-induced hypoglycemia, healthy adults were given 50 μg/h octreotide or placebo as a continuous IV infusion for 4 hours, followed at the first hour by infusion of 490 mg quinine base.[44] In the control subjects, plasma insulin concentrations rose and serum glucose concentrations fell significantly, whereas in the octreotide group, insulin concentrations fell and glucose concentrations remained constant. This effect of octreotide began within 30 minutes and persisted for 2 hours after octreotide was stopped. Octreotide was used successfully to treat refractory hypoglycemia in a woman receiving 600 mg quinine dihydrochloride IV for malaria.[44]

The efficacy of octreotide against sulfonylurea induced hypoglycemia was demonstrated in an early experimental study. Eight healthy volunteers were given 1.43 mg/kg glipizide orally and randomized to receive either a variable dextrose infusion to remain euglycemic, diazoxide 300 mg IV over 30 minutes and repeated every 4 hours with dextrose, or octreotide 30 ng/kg/min IV continuously.[7] Following administration of glipizide, hypoglycemia of 50 mg/dL was achieved within 30–165 minutes.[7] Insulin concentrations in the diazoxide group were comparable with those in the glipizide group and were 4-5 times higher than in the octreotide group. Four of the 8 patients in the octreotide group did not require supplemental dextrose. At the 5th hour of the protocol, an IV bolus of 50 mL 50% dextrose was given to the octreotide group to study the response to hyperglycemia. Approximately 6.5 hours was necessary for the serum glucose concentration to drop to 85 mg/dL, whereas only 3 hours was necessary in the dextrose and diazoxide groups.[7] Diazoxide infusion was associated with higher norepinephrine concentrations, and epinephrine concentrations were similar in all groups.[7] All xenobiotics were stopped at 13 hours, and serum glucose concentrations fell to < 65 mg/dL within 1.5 hours in subjects who received the dextrose and diazoxide, whereas the serum glucose concentrations remained > 65 mg/dL in 6 of the 8 octreotide subjects for the 4-hour observation period. Without additional octreotide, hypoglycemia continued to recur for as long as 30 hours after the initial glipizide administration.

Several case studies and two case series of 15 patients support the efficacy of octreotide following overdoses of glipizide, glyburide, gliclazide, glimepiride, tolbutamide, and nateglinide. These cases encompass both intentional and unintentional overdoses in children and adults with and without diabetes.[7,9,12,13,16,17,21,22,26,28,34,37,38,45] In these case reports, therapeutic doses ranged considerably, and the most frequent doses were 50–100 μg subcutaneously repeated every 8–12 hours in the adult patients.

ADVERSE DRUG EFFECTS

Octreotide is generally well tolerated, but experience in the toxicologic setting is limited. Adverse reactions occurring with short-term administration usually are local or gastrointestinal. Stinging at the injection site occurs in approximately 7% of patients but rarely lasts more than 15 minutes.[50] Healthy volunteers receiving octreotide noted no side effects when given IV doses of 25 or 50 μg or SC doses of 50 or 100 μg. At higher doses, early transient nausea and later appearing but longer-lasting diarrhea and abdominal pain frequently occur.[29,30] Healthy volunteers were given IV bolus doses of octreotide as high as 1000 μg and infusion doses of 30,000 μg over 20 minutes and 120,000 μg over 8 hours without serious adverse effects. Single doses in healthy volunteers resulted in decreased biliary contractility and bile secretion.[40] Long-term therapy lasting weeks to months results in biliary tract abnormalities.[40,51] Product information warns of the potential for acute cholecystitis, ascending cholangitis, biliary obstruction, cholestatic hepatitis, and pancreatitis.[40]

Octreotide alters the balance among insulin, glucagon, and growth hormone. Serum glucose concentrations must be serially monitored. Hyperglycemia often occurs, but cases of hypoglycemia are reported. A revision in the precautions section of the package labeling states that symptomatic hypoglycemia has occurred in patients with type I diabetes and their insulin requirements will likely be reduced. The most likely explanation is suppression of counter regulatory hormones, in particular when glucagon suppression, is more persistent than insulin suppression.[40]

Other adverse effects reported with long-term administration of octreotide or for octreotide in circumstances other than sulfonylurea induced hypoglycemia include hypothyroidism, cardiac conduction abnormalities, worsening congestive heart failure (in at-risk patients with acromegaly), bradycardia, pancreatitis, substantial hyperglycemia and bradycardia in an infant with congenital hyperinsulinemia, hypoxemia and pulmonary hypertension in premature neonates, altered fat absorption, and decreased vitamin B_{12} concentrations.[3,4,40] Anaphylactoid reactions are also rarely reported.[40]

Drug interactions are expected with xenobiotics that affect glucose regulation. Octreotide may significantly decrease oral absorption of cyclosporine and increase the bioavailability of bromocriptine. Because octreotide may suppress the activity of the CYP450 enzymes, and in particular 3A4, drugs with a narrow therapeutic indices metabolized by these enzymes should be monitored more closely.[40]

ADMINISTRATION

Both SC and IV administration are acceptable, although the usual route is SC.[40] The SC administration sites should be rotated. For IV infusion, octreotide can be diluted in sterile 0.9% sodium chloride solution or D_5W and infused over 15–30 minutes or by IV bolus over 3 minutes.[40] Rapid IV bolus may be indicated for carcinoid crisis.[40] Refrigeration of octreotide is recommended for prolonged storage, although octreotide is stable at room temperature for 14 days when protected from light. Active warming of refrigerated octreotide is not recommended, although passive warming to room temperature prior to administration is suggested and may reduce the pain of SC administration.[35] Using the smallest volume possible also reduces the pain with SC administration. A depot formula designed to last for 4 weeks is available (Sandostatin LAR Depot). Vapreotide (Sanvar IR) and lanreotide (Somatuline Depot) are analogs of somatostatin which are available in the United States, but are inappropriate for use in the setting of xenobiotic-induced insulin secretion. Although the depot formula is useful for patients with insulinomas, its duration of action far exceeds that of any oral hypoglycemic, making it an inappropriate and unnecessary choice for management of xenobiotic-induced hypoglycemia.

DOSING

No controlled trials have evaluated the optimal dose of octreotide for the management of sulfonylurea overdose. In adults, a 50-μg SC dose of octreotide given every 6 hours is suggested. In children, a dose of 4–5 μg/kg/d SC divided every 6 hours, up to the adult dose, can be used for initial therapy. This pediatric dose is derived from the literature on treatment of persistent hyperinsulinemic hypoglycemia of infancy.[20] In situations where compromised peripheral blood flow is expected, octreotide should be administered intravenously in the same dose but every 4 hours instead of every 6 hours. Further experience in the toxicologic setting should permit a better delineation of dosing recommendations. Several days of therapy may be required, depending on the duration of the offending xenobiotic. All patients must be carefully monitored for recurrent hypoglycemia during octreotide therapy and perhaps for 24 hours following termination of octreotide therapy before discharge. Octreotide is considered a category B drug (Table 30-2), but pregnant women must be carefully monitored for recurrent hypoglycemia. Use of octreotide should not diminish this vigilance.

AVAILABILITY

Octreotide acetate (Sandostatin) injection is available in ampules and multidose vials ranging in concentration from 50–1000 μg/mL. The multidose vials contain phenol.

SUMMARY

Octreotide is useful for treating hypoglycemia induced by xenobiotics such as sulfonylureas and quinine that cause endogenous release of insulin. Octreotide is more effective than diazoxide in suppressing insulin and is much better tolerated.

REFERENCES

1. Alberti KGMM, Christensen NJ, Christensen S, et al. Inhibition of insulin secretion by somatostatin. *Lancet.* 1973;2:1299-1301.
2. Alberts AS, Falkson G. Rapid reversal of life-threatening hypoglycemia with a somatostatin analogue (octreotide). *S Afr Med J.* 1988;74:75-76.
3. Arevalo R, Bullabh P, Krauss A, et al. Octreotide induced hypoxemia and pulmonary hypertension in premature neonates. *J Ped Surg.* 2003;38: 251-253.
4. Batra Y, Rajeev S, Samra T, et al. Octreotide induced severe paradoxical hyperglycemia and bradycardia during subtotal pancreatectomy for congenital hyperinsulinemia in an infant. *Ped Anesthesia.* 2007;17:1117-1121.
5. Bauer W, Briner U, Doepfner W, et al. SMS 201–995: A very potent and selective octapeptide analogue of somatostatin with prolonged action. *Life Sci.* 1982;3:1133-1140.
6. Boden G, Ryan IG, Shuman CR. Ineffectiveness of SMS 201–995 in severe hyperinsulinemia. *Diabetes Care.* 1988;11:664-668.
7. Boyle PJ, Justice K, Krentz AJ, et al. Octreotide reverses hyperinsulinemia and prevents hypoglycemia induced by sulfonylurea overdoses. *J Clin Endocrinol Metab.* 1993;76:752-756.
8. Bradeau P, Vale W, Burgus R, et al. Hypothalamic polypeptide that inhibits the secretion of immunoreactive pituitary growth hormone. *Science.* 1973;179:77-79.
9. Braatvedt GD. Octreotide for the treatment of sulphonylurea-induced hypoglycemia in type 2 diabetes. *N Z Med J.* 1997;110:189-190.
10. Brunner JE, Kruger DF, Basha MA, et al. Hypoglycemia after administration of somatostatin analog in metastatic carcinoid. *Henry Ford Hosp Med J.* 1989;37:60-62.
11. Bruns C, Weckbecker G, Raulf F, et al. Molecular pharmacology of somatostatin-receptor subtypes. *Ann N Y Acad Sci.* 1994;733:138-146.
12. Carr R, Zed PJ. Octreotide for sulfonylurea-induced hypoglycemia following overdose. *Ann Pharmacother.* 2002;36:1727-1732.
13. Crawford BA, Perera C. Octreotide treatment for sulfonylurea-induced hypoglycaemia. *Med J Aust.* 2004;180:540-541.
14. del Pozo E. Endocrine profile of a long-acting somatostatin derivative. *Acta Endocrinol.* 1986;111:433-439.
15. Doyle ME, Egan JM. Pharmacological agents that directly modulate insulin secretion. *Pharmacol Rev.* 2003;55:105-131.
16. Fasano C, O'Malley G, Dominici P, et al. Comparison of octreotide and standard therapy versus standard therapy alone for the treatment of sulfonylurea-induced hypoglycemia. *Ann Emerg Med.* 2008;51:400-406.
17. Fleseria M, Skugor M, Chinnappa P, et al. Successful treatment of sulfonylurea-induced prolonged hypoglycemia with use of cotreotide. *Endocrine Pract.* 2006;12:635-640.
18. Gama R, Marks V, Wright J, Teale JD. Octreotide exacerbated fasting hypoglycemia in a patient with a proinsulinoma: The glucostatic importance of pancreatic glucagons. *Clin Endocrinol.* 1995;43:117-120.
19. Gerich J, Lorenzi M, Schneider V, Forsham P. Effect of somatostatin on plasma glucose and insulin to responses to glucagon and tolbutamide in man. *J Clin Endocrinol Metab.* 1974;39:1057-1060.
20. Glaser B, Hirsch H, Landau H. Persistent hyperinsulinemic hypoglycemia of infancy: Long-term octreotide treatment without pancreatectomy. *J Pediatr.* 1993;123:644-650.
21. Graudins A, Linden C, Ferm R. Diagnosis and treatment of sulfonylurea-induced hyperinsulinemic hypoglycemia. *Am J Emerg Med.* 1997;15:95-96.
22. Green RS, Palatnick W. Effectiveness of octreotide in a case of refractory sulfonylurea-induced hypoglycemia. *J Emerg Med.* 2003;25:283-287.
23. Hansen JB, Arkhammar PO, Bodvarsdottir TB, et al. Inhibition of insulin secretion as a new drug target in the treatment of metabolic disorders. *Curr Med Chem.* 2004;11:1595-1615.
24. Healy M, Dawson S, Murray R, et al. Severe hypoglycemia after long acting octreotide in a patient with an unrecognized malignant insulinoma. *Internal Med J.* 2007;37:406-409.

25. Hsu W, Xiang H, Rajan A, et al. Somatostatin inhibits insulin secretion by a G-protein-mediated decrease in Ca^2 entry through voltage dependent Ca^2 channels in the beta cell. *J Biol Chem.* 1991;206:837-843.
26. Hung O, Eng J, Ho J, et al. Octreotide as an antidote for refractory sulfonylurea hypoglycemia [abstract]. *J Toxicol Clin Toxicol.* 1997;35:540.
27. Kane C, Lindley K, Johnson P, et al. Therapy for persistent hyperinsulinemic hypoglycemia of infancy. *J Clin Invest.* 1997;100:1888-1893.
28. Krentz AJ, Boyle PJ, Justice KM, et al. Successful treatment of severe refractory sulfonylurea-induced hypoglycemia with octreotide. *Diabetes Care.* 1993;16:184-186,189-190.
29. Krentz AJ, Boyle PJ, Mavdonald LM, Schade DS. Octreotide: A long-acting inhibitor of endogenous hormone secretion for human metabolic investigations. *Metabolism.* 1994;43:24-31.
30. Kutz K, Nuesch E, Rosenthaler J. Pharmacokinetics of SMS 201–995 in healthy subjects. *Scand J Gastroenterol.* 1986;21(Suppl 119):65-72.
31. Kvols L, Woltering E. Role of somatostatin analogs in the clinical management of non-neuroendocrine solid tumors. *Anticancer Drugs.* 2006;17: 601-608.
32. Lamberts SWJ, Vaanderlely AJ, DeHerder WW, Hofland LJ. Octreotide. *N Engl J Med.* 1996;334:246-254.
33. Lightman SL, Fox P, Dunne MJ. The effects of SMS 201–995, a long-acting somatostatin analogue, on anterior pituitary function in healthy male volunteers. *Scand J Gastroenterol.* 1986;21(Suppl 119):84-95.
34. McLaughlin SA, Crandall CS, McKinney PE: Octreotide: An antidote for sulfonylurea-induced hypoglycemia. Ann Emerg Med 2000;36:133-138.
35. Mercadante S. The role of octreotide in palliative care. *J Pain Symptom Manage.* 1994;9:406-411.
36. Moldovan S, Atiya A, Adrian T, et al. Somatostatin inhibits b-cell secretion via a subtype-2 somatostatin receptor in the isolated perfused human pancreas. *J Surg Res.* 1995;59:85-90.
37. Mordel A, Sivilotti MLA, Old AC, Ferm RP. Octreotide for pediatric sulfonylurea poisoning [abstract]. *J Toxicol Clin Toxicol.* 1998;36:437.
38. Nakayama S, Hirose T, Watada H, et al. Hypoglycemia following a nateglinide overdose in a suicide attempt. *Diabetes Care.* 2005;28:227-228.
39. Navascues I, Gil J, Pascau C, et al. Severe hypoglycemia as a sort term side effect of the somatostatin analog SMS 201-995 in insulin dependent diabetes mellitus. *Horm Metab Res.* 1988;20:749-750.
40. Octreotide [package insert]. East Hanover, NJ: Novartis Pharmaceuticals Corp, 2005.
41. Olias G, Viollet C, Kusserow H, et al. Regulation and function of somatostatin receptors. *J Neurochem.* 2004;89:1057-1091.
42. Pace CS, Tarvin JT. Somatostatin: mechanism of action in pancreatic islet cells beta cells. *Diabetes.* 1981;30:836-842.
43. Patel YC. Somatostatin and its receptor family. *Front Neuroendocrinol.* 1999;20:157-198.
44. Philips RE, Looareesuwan S, Bloom SR, et al. Effectiveness of SMS 201–995, a synthetic, long-acting somatostatin analogue, in treatment of quinine-induced hyperinsulinemia. *Lancet.* 1986;1:713-715.
45. Rath S, Bar-Zeev N, Anderson K, et al. Octreotide in children with hypoglycemia due to sulfonylurea ingestion. *J Peds Child Health.* 2008;44: 383-384.
46. Stehouwer CDA, Lems WF, Fischer HRA, et al. Aggravation of hypoglycemia in insulinoma patients by the long-acting somatostatin analogue octreotide (Sandostatin). *Acta Endocrinol.* 1989;121:34-40.
47. Thorton P, Alter C, Levitt-Katz L, et al. Short- and long-term use of octreotide in the treatment of congenital hyperinsulinism. *J Pediatr.* 1993;123:637-643.
48. de Sá SV, Corrêa-Giannella ML, Machado MC, et al. Somatostatin receptor subtype 5 (SSTR5) mRNA expression is related to histopathological features of cell proliferation in insulinomas. *Endocr Relat Cancer.* 2006;13:69-78.
49. van der Hoek J, Hofland L, Lamberts W. Novel subtype specific and universal somatostin analogs: Clinical potential and pitfalls. *Curr Pharmaceutical Des.* 2005;11:1573-1592.
50. Verschoor L, Uitterlinden P, Lamberts J, del Pozo E. On the use of a new somatostatin analogue in the treatment of hypoglycemia in patients with insulinoma. *Clin Endocrinol (Oxf).* 1986;25:555-560.
51. Waas JAH, Popovic V, Chayvialle JA. Proceedings of the discussion, tolerability and safety of Sandostatin. *Metabolism.* 1992;41(Suppl 2):80-82.

CHAPTER 49
THYROID AND ANTITHYROID MEDICATIONS

Nicole C. Bouchard

Hypothyroidism and hyperthyroidism are relatively common endocrine disorders. The global incidence of neonatal hypothyroidism is 1 per 3000–4500 births. It is estimated that hypothyroidism affects 1%–5% of US adults. It is more prevalent in whites than people of Hispanic or African American descent. In the elderly, the prevalence of hypothyroidism increases to 15% by age 75. Worldwide, iodine deficiency is the leading cause of hypothyroidism. According to US retail pharmaceutical statistics for prescription drugs, levothyroxine (both generic and Synthroid combined) (T_4) has consistently ranked in the top five for overall total prescription count, with an average 67 million per year. Many cases of intentional and unintentional overdoses with thyroid hormone are reported in both adults and children.[60] Despite the profound effects of thyroid hormones on physiologic homeostasis and the widespread use and access to exogenous thyroid hormone, morbidity, and mortality from overdose is very low.

HISTORY AND EPIDEMIOLOGY

Long before the thyroid was recognized as a functional endocrine gland, it was believed to serve a cosmetic function, especially in women. Egyptian paintings often emphasize the full and beautiful necks of women with enlarged thyroid glands. Early theories on the physiologic function of the thyroid gland included lubrication of the trachea, diversion of blood flow from the brain and protection of women from "irritation" and "vexation" from men.[34] Although poorly defined in historical accounts, symptoms resembling hypothyroidism and myxedema that were successfully treated with ground sheep thyroid were described 500 years ago. In the 16th century, Paracelus described the association between goiter (thyroid gland enlargement) and cretinism.[64] A syndrome of cardiac hyperactivity, goiter, and exophthalmos was first described in 1786.[76] Graves and von Basedow further detailed this syndrome and its relationship to the thyroid gland 50 years later.[31,34,60,64,76,104]

In 1891, injection of ground sheep thyroid extract was formally described as a treatment for myxedema.[34] Shortly afterward, oral therapy was determined to be equally effective. Seaweed, which contains large amounts of iodine, was used to treat goiter (hypothyroidism) in Chinese medicine as early as the 3rd century A.D. In 1863, Trousseau[100] fortuitously discovered a treatment for Graves disease when he inadvertently prescribed daily tincture of iodine instead of tincture of digitalis to a tachycardic, thyrotoxic young woman.

Sir Charles R. Harington described the chemical structure and performed the first synthesis of thyroxine (tetraiodothyronine [T_4]) in 1926.[78] Triiodothyronine (T_3) was not isolated and synthesized until the 1950s.[34] Prior to this, desiccated thyroid gland from animal sources was commonly used to treat hypothyroidism. Despite becoming essentially obsolete in the modern medical community, unprocessed, desiccated thyroid can be easily purchased via the Internet and in health food stores as a thyroid supplement.[89] Armour, a pharmaceutical grade porcine-derived thyroid supplement, is still available by prescription. Unfortunately, the misguided use of both organic and synthetic thyroid supplements as vitality agents, stimulants, and weight-loss aids has become increasingly common. Two epidemics of *hamburger thyrotoxicosis* that occurred in the United States in the mid 1980s secondary to consumption of ground beef contaminated with bovine thyroid gland demonstrated the potential widespread toxicologic sequelae after a community unknowingly ingests thyroid hormone.[39,49] Clinically significant overdose with thyroid hormone preparations are uncommon.

PHARMACOLOGY

PHYSIOLOGY

To properly understand the impact of thyroid supplements and antithyroid xenobiotics on the function of the human body, an understanding of thyroid physiology is required. Thyroid function is influenced by the following: (1) the hypothalamus, (2) the pituitary gland, (3) the thyroid gland, and (4) the target organs for the thyroid hormones (Fig. 49–1).

The hypothalamus, viewed by some as the "master gland," is an intermediate between cerebral centers and the pituitary gland. When the hypothalamus receives specific neurotransmitter stimulation, thyroid-releasing hormone (TRH) is produced. TRH is transported through the venous sinusoids to the pituitary gland, which then release thyroid-stimulating hormone (TSH). TSH enters the circulation and stimulates the production and release of the thyroid hormones T_3 and T_4 from the thyroid gland. Thyroid physiology exhibits classic autoregulation or "negative biofeedback" of hormonal function. When adequate thyroid hormones are present, they exert an inhibitory effect on the pituitary gland, leading to diminished production of TSH (Fig. 49–1). Suppression or upregulation of TSH production is a frequently used laboratory marker in the evaluation of hyperthyroidism and hypothyroidism, respectively.

Thyroid hormones are tyrosine molecules with iodine substitutions. Two forms of the hormone are physiologically active: T_3 and T_4 (Table 49–1). Synthesis of thyroid hormones is a multistep process. The amino acid tyrosine is concentrated in the follicles of the thyroid gland, which consist of an epithelial layer surrounding a proteinaceous colloidal substance called thyroglobulin. Thyroglobulin thus contains a large amount of tyrosine. After absorption, iodide (I^-) is concentrated in thyroid cells by an active transport process called *iodide trapping*. Absorbed I^- is then oxidized to iodine (I_2) by thyroid (iodide) peroxidase. Iodine rapidly iodinates tyrosine residues to form monoiodotyrosine (MIT) and diiodotyrosine (DIT). These substituted tyrosine molecules then combine to form T_3 and T_4. The ratio of T_3 to T_4 in thyroglobulin is 1:5. T_3 and T_4 (thyroxine) ultimately are released into circulation from the thyroglobulin matrix.

Iodide trapping can be inhibited pharmacologically by monovalent anions such as thiocyanate (SCN^-), pertechnetate (TcO_4^-), and perchlorate (ClO_4^-). Thyroid peroxidase is inhibited by high concentrations of intrathyroidal iodide and by thioamide drugs. High intrathyroidal iodide concentrations also can inhibit the release of thyroid hormone into circulation (Table 49–2).

Approximately 95% of circulating or peripheral thyroid hormone is T_4; the remainder is T_3. Only 15% of the peripheral T_3 is secreted directly by the thyroid; the balance results from the peripheral conversion of T_4 to T_3. When circulating T_4 enters the cell, it is deiodinated to T_3. Deiodination of the T_4 molecule occurs by monodeiodination of either the outer ring or the inner ring by 5′-deiodinase or 5-deiodinase, yielding 3,5,3′-T_3 and 3,3′,5′-triiodothyronine (reverse

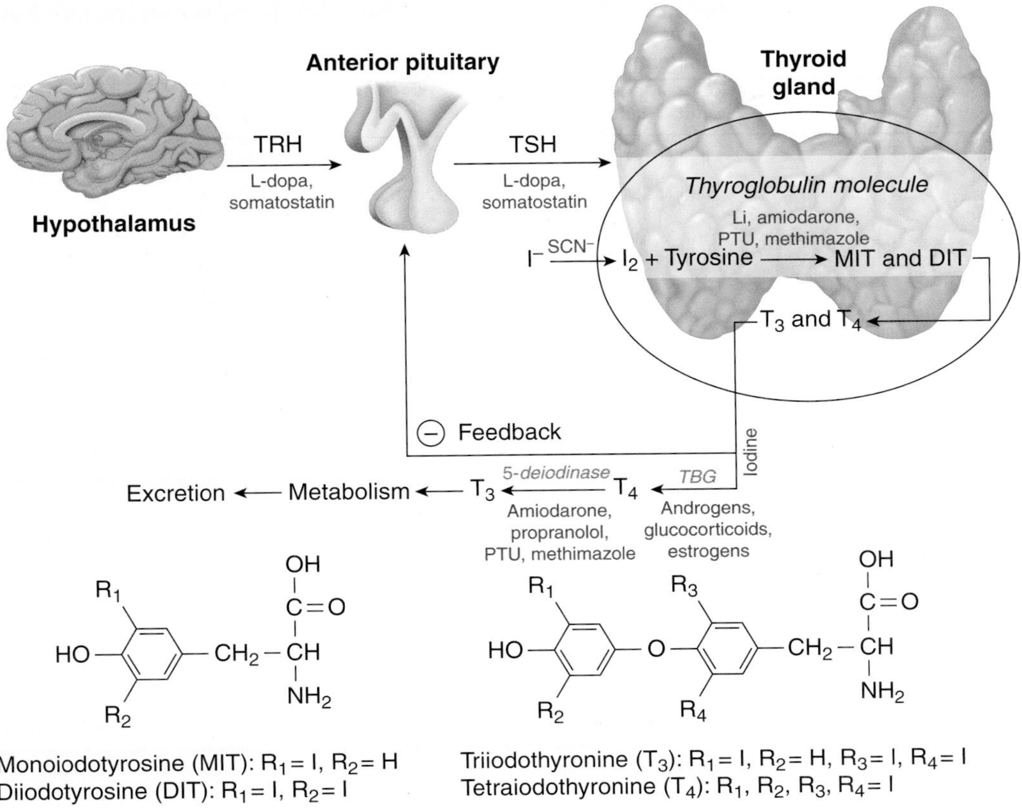

FIGURE 49–1. Thyroid hormone synthesis: its control, metabolism, and molecular structures. PTU = propylthiouracil; SCN^- = thiocyanate; TBG = thyroxine binding globulin; TRH = thyrotropin releasing hormone; TSH = thyroid stimulating hormone.

T_3[rT_3]), respectively.[56] T_3 has approximately four times greater hormonal activity than T_4, whereas rT_3 is metabolically inactive. T_3 exerts its effects by binding to thyroid hormone receptors inside the nucleus. This interaction with nuclear receptors regulates gene transcription and protein synthesis, which ultimately increases oxygen consumption and underlies the thermogenic effects of thyroid hormones.

Propranolol, corticosteroids, ipodate (contrast agent), starvation, and severe illness inhibit 5′-deiodinase, which results in decreased production of metabolically active T_3 and preferential monodeiodination to metabolically inactive rT_3 leading to a syndrome known as "sick euthyroid" (Table 49–2). This energy-conserving effect allows attenuation of the thermogenic effects of thyroid hormones in times of physiologic stress.[94]

TABLE 49–1. Pharmacokinetic Properties of Thyroid Hormones

Pharmacokinetic Property	T_3	T_4
Oral bioavailability (exogenous drug)	95%	80%
Volume of distribution (L/kg)	40	10
Half-life (days)	1	7
Protein binding (normal adult)	99.96%	99.6%
Relative potency	4	1

T_4 AND T_3

Thyroid supplementation for treatment of hypothyroidism is in widespread use both in human and veterinary medicine. Thyroid hormones historically were derived from animal origin, but now are largely produced synthetically. Desiccated and processed porcine thyroid (Armour) contains both T_3 and T_4. Because it is less pharmacologically stable and carries a risk of allergic reaction and thyrotoxicity from T_3, its use has largely been supplanted by the safer synthetic alternatives. Levothyroxine is the preparation of choice because of its low immunogenicity, 7-day half-life, easy dosing regimen and is available IV. Synthroid is the commercial name of the most commonly prescribed form of T_4. Liothyronine (T_3 preparation, Cytomel or Triostat, available PO and IV) and liotrix (combination T_3/T_4 preparations, preparations of Thyrolar, available PO) are synthetic preparations that are seldom used clinically because of their short half-lives, high cost, unique therapeutic indication, and increased risk of thyrotoxicosis.

Steady state with regard to suppression of TSH and elevation of T_4 is reached approximately 6–8 weeks after initiation of therapy. Doses usually are titrated in increments of 12.5 or 25 μg/d after 2–6 weeks based on TSH measurements (see Table 49–3 for typical levothyroxine doses). Different sources suggest that bioequivalence of Synthroid versus generic levothyroxine may or may not be equivalent.[17] As a result, thyroid hormone concentrations and the patient's clinical status should be followed when transitioning between levothyroxine formulations because the switch may present an opportunity for an adverse drug event.

TABLE 49–2. Xenobiotic Interactions: Effects on Thyroid Hormones and Function[6]

Xenobiotic	Interaction	Effect
Dopamine, levodopa, somatostatin	Inhibit TRH and TSH synthesis	No clinical hypothyroidism
Iodides (including amiodarone), lithium, aminoglutethimide	Inhibit thyroid hormone synthesis or release	Hypothyroidism
Monovalent anions (SCN^-, TcO_4^-, ClO_4^-)	Inhibit iodide uptake to thyroid gland	Hypothyroidism
Estrogens, tamoxifen, heroin, methadone, mitotane	Increase TBG	Altered thyroid hormone transport in serum ↑Total measured thyroid hormone (vs. *free* hormone)
Androgens, glucocorticoids	Decreased TBG	Altered thyroid hormone transport in serum ↓Total measured thyroid hormone (vs. *free* hormone)
Salicylates, mefenamic acid, furosemide	Displace T_3 or T_4 from TBG	Transient hyperthyroxinemia
Thioamides (methimazole, propylthiouracil)	Inhibit thyroid peroxidase	Decrease thyroid hormone synthesis
Phenytoin, carbamazepine, phenobarbital, rifampin, rifabutin	Induction of hepatic enzymes	↓Total thyroid hormone measurements
Iopanoic acid, ipodate, amiodarone, propranolol, corticosteroids, propylthiouracil	Inhibition of 5′-deiodinase	Decrease peripheral conversion of T_4 (↓T_3, ↑rT_3)
Cholestyramine, colestipol, aluminum hydroxide, sucralfate, ferrous sulfate, some calcium preparations, infant soy formula	Interfere with GI absorption of T_4	Decreased oral bioavailability of T_4
Interleukin-α, interleukin-2	Induction of autoimmune thyroid disease	Hyperthyroidism or hypothyroidism

TRH = thyroid-releasing hormone; TSH = thyroid-stimulating hormone; TBG = thyroid-binding globulin; GI = gastrointestinal.

TABLE 49–3. Typical Levothyroxine Doses

Age Group	Dose (μg/kg/d)	Total Daily Dose (μg/d)
Infants <6 mos	8–10	25–50
Infants 6–12 mos	6–8	50–75
Children 1–5 years	5–6	75–100
Children 6–12 years	4–5	100–150
Children >12 years	2–3	Until 150 (adult dose reached)
Adults	1.7	120–150
Elderly	Enhanced sensitivity to thyroxine excess	12.5

PHARMACOKINETICS AND TOXICOKINETICS

Gastrointestinal absorption is thought to occur primarily in the duodenum and ileum. Gastrointestinal absorption can be decreased by variations in intestinal flora and binding by xenobiotics (Table 49–2). In circulation, T_3 and T_4 both are highly but reversibly bound to plasma proteins—approximately 99.6% and 99.97%, respectively, in nonpregnant adults. Thyroxine-binding globulin (TBG) binds approximately two-thirds of the circulating thyroid hormones; albumin and other proteins bind the remainder. It is estimated that only 0.4% of T_3 and 0.04% of T_4 exist in the free form. Exogenously derived thyroid hormones exhibit similar binding characteristics when dosed in a physiologic range. The amount of thyroid hormone bound to proteins varies greatly with different physiologic and pharmacologic conditions, for example, increasing in pregnancy and levothyroxine overdose and decreasing in chronic disease. These changes in protein binding must be considered when measuring total thyroid hormone concentrations in the blood (see Diagnostic Testing). Table 49–1 lists some important pharmacokinetic properties of thyroid hormones.

Thyroid hormones undergo their ultimate metabolism peripherally. Intracellular sequential deiodination accounts for approximately two-thirds of inactivation. Most of the remaining third undergoes hepatic metabolism by glucuronidation or sulfation. Xenobiotics that induce hepatic microsomal metabolism, such as rifampin, phenobarbital, phenytoin, and carbamazepine, increase the metabolic clearance of T_3 and T_4 (Table 49–2).

PATHOPHYSIOLOGY

Thyroid hormones are critical for optimal physiologic growth and function. Thyroid function is the most important determinant of basal metabolic rate (BMR). In addition, the thyroid exercises a permissive effect on many hormones, notably catecholamines and insulin.

Hyperthyroidism is a condition characterized by excess active thyroid hormone. Most aspects of carbohydrate, protein, and lipid metabolism are increased in the presence of thyroid hormone excess. The disorder is characterized by manifestations of increased metabolism such as fever, weight loss, diarrhea, heat intolerance, and diaphoresis, along with tachycardia, widened pulse pressure, tremor, anxiety, other behavioral changes, and sometimes tachydysrhythmias such as rapid atrial fibrillation and high output congestive heart failure.[23,51,86] This constellation of symptoms, called *thyrotoxicosis,* may result from overproduction of the hormone, increased conversion from T_4 to T_3, or excess exogenous hormone. Graves disease (diffuse toxic goiter), an autoimmune disorder, is the most common cause of excess thyroid hormone secretion. It accounts for approximately two-thirds of cases and often is accompanied by exophthalmos and diffusely enlarged, nontender thyroid gland. Toxic multinodular goiter, toxic thyroid adenoma, iodine or amiodarone exposure (can also cause hypothyroidism, see Table 49–4), thyrotoxicosis factitia, and thyroiditis (eg, postpartum, Hashimoto, DeQuervain) are some other etiologies of hyperthyroidism.[32] Severe thyrotoxicosis accompanied by decompensation is referred to as *thyroid storm* or *thyrotoxic crisis*. Thyroid storm typically occurs when untreated or undertreated hyperthyroidism occurs simultaneously with a physiologic stressor such as trauma, infection, diabetic ketoacidosis or surgery. In early stages patients appear febrile and markedly tachycardic, tremulous, agitated, or psychotic with nausea, vomiting, and diarrhea. As the disease progresses, stupor, coma, and hypotension may ensue. General treatment strategies include early airway control, crystalloid fluid resuscitation, β-adrenergic antagonist administration (mainstay of treatment, propranolol preferred for the added effect of decreased peripheral conversion of T_4 to T_3), parenteral glucocorticoids if adrenal insufficiency is suspected, and antithyroid medications such as propylthiouracil and methimazole. Mortality in thyroid storm, even with treatment, can approach 20%.[23,84]

As plasma catecholamine concentrations are well established to be normal or decreased in hyperthyroid states, an increase in sensitivity to catecholamines is thought to be responsible for the increased inotropy and chronotropy produced by thyroid hormones.[14,82] Several general mechanisms are proposed for the direct cardiac effects of thyroid hormones, although their relative contributions are uncertain.[3,16,50,99] (1) T_3 increases the number of β-adrenergic receptors in various tissues, including cardiac cells.[16] This process occurs via upregulation of β-adrenergic receptor synthesis at the level of the β-adrenergic gene.[4] (2) T_3 modulates myocyte intracellular signaling mechanisms that lead to increased catecholamine effects. Enhancement of intracellular signaling activity involving protein kinase A, cyclic adenosine monophosphate, G proteins, and increased phosphorylation of thyroid hormone receptor proteins all are implicated to varying degrees.[22,51,80,81,85,92,101] (3) Enhancement of myocardial transmembrane and sarcoplasmic reticulum ion channel function, L-type voltage-gated Ca^{2+} channels,

TABLE 49–4. Common Xenobiotics That Alter Thyroid Function and Cause Clinically Important Effects

Xenobiotic	Effect	Mechanism
Lithium	Goiter (in 37% of patients) Hypothyroidism (in 5%–15% of patients)	Mechanism unclear
Amiodarone (37% iodine by weight)	1. Hypothyroidism (in 25% of patients) 2. Hyperthyroidism, type 1: in patients with preexisting goiters from low iodine intake 3. Hyperthyroidism, type 2: in patients with previously normal thyroid function	1. Inhibition of 5′-deiodinase 2. Type 1: iodine excess stimulates thyroid hormone production 3. Type 2: causes thyroid inflammation
Propranolol	↓Peripheral conversion of T_4 to T_3	Inhibition of 5′-deiodinase
PTU (propylthiourea) or methimazole	Decreased thyroid hormone synthesis ↓Peripheral conversion of T_4 to T_3	Inhibition of thyroid peroxidase Inhibition of 5′-deiodinase
Corticosteroids	↓Peripheral conversion of T_4 to T_3	Inhibition of 5′-deiodinase
Iodine	1. Low dose: transient or no effect 2. High doses (>10 μg/d): ↓thyroid hormone secretion 3. Transient thyrotoxicosis (ie, Jod-Basedow effect) With rapid correction of hypothyroidism from iodine deficiency From topical iodine 4. Delirium 5. Caustic injury	1. Transiently stimulates thyroid hormone secretion 2. Inhibition of thyroid hormone synthesis 3. Increases thyroid hormone synthesis 4. Mechanism unclear 5. Direct cytotoxic injury to cells
Iodinated contrast material	1. Rapid ↓ peripheral conversion of T_4 to T_3 (adjunctive treatment in thyroid storm) 2. Prolonged suppression of T_4 to T_3 3. Causes thyrotoxicosis and thyroid storm 4. Iodide mumps	1. Inhibition of 5′-deiodinase 2. Mechanism unclear 3. Mechanism unclear 4. Idiopathic, toxic accumulation of iodide
Radioactive iodine	Treatment of hyperthyroidism, causes hypothyroidism	Uptake into thyroid follicles causes local destruction
Anion inhibitors[a]	↓Iodine uptake into thyroid follicle, used in iodide-induced hyperthyroidism	Blocks uptake of iodide into the thyroid gland by competitive inhibition

[a] Also referred to as monovalent anions, ie, thiocyanate (SCN^-), pertechnetate (TcO_4^-), and perchlorate (ClO_4^-).

and accelerated Ca^{2+} entry into the sarcoplasmic reticulum also are suggested.[47,48,69,91] Whether the effects on intracellular signaling represent a direct effect of T_3 on intracellular signaling mediators or T_3 induced-augmentation of the individual β-adrenergic receptor response to catecholamines with a secondary change in postreceptor signaling is unclear.[3]

In addition to these mechanisms, T_3 upregulates synthesis of cardiac thyroid hormone receptors (at TRα and TRβ genes), and the thermogenic effects of thyroid hormones can cause decreased systemic vascular resistance leading to a reflex (and indirect) increase in cardiac output. Comprehensive reviews on this topic explore the more complex cellular aspects of thyroid hormones and their effects on the cardiovascular system.[15,51,74]

Hypothyroidism, a condition characterized by decreased BMR and decreased catecholamine effects, is a common disorder, especially in women and the elderly. Worldwide, dietary iodine deficiency remains the leading cause of hypothyroidism. In certain parts of the world, particularly mountainous regions such as the Andes, Alps, and Himalayas, goitrous hypothyroidism still is endemic. Untreated congenital thyroid deficiency and severe dietary iodine deficiency (goitrous hypothyroidism) in young children result in profound, irreversible mental retardation and dwarfism (also referred to as cretinism). In developed nations, the iodization of salt has essentially eliminated dietary iodine deficiency as a cause of hypothyroidism. In developed nations, hypothyroidism often is autoimmune related, although thyroid function diminishes significantly with age in many patients. Treatment of Graves disease with radioactive iodine typically results in hypothyroidism within 1 year. Thyroiditis (eg, postpartum, Hashimoto, DeQuervain) may cause hypothyroidism (as well as hyperthyroidism) as may exposure to certain xenobiotics such as amiodarone and lithium (see Table 49–4). Myxedema and myxedema coma are potentially life-threatening emergencies that represent extremes of hypothyroidism. Hypothyroidism is not discussed in more detail in this chapter, except to note that treatment of hypothyroid emergencies, especially with T_3, can result in thyrotoxic symptoms. Comprehensive reviews of hypothyroidism are available.[88]

CLINICAL MANIFESTATION

The widespread availability and use of thyroid supplements make thyroid hormone a common xenobiotic in acute intentional and unintentional overdoses. In addition, chronic excess thyroid hormone ingestion is a relatively frequent occurrence. Symptoms of toxicity from exogenous thyroid hormone resemble those of catecholamine excess. Pronounced catecholamine-like effects occur in the cardiovascular system, especially tachycardia, tachydysrhythmias (usually atrial fibrillation or flutter), thromboembolism (from both atrial fibrillation and endothelial activation), and cardiac failure.[23,51,86] Interestingly, although hyperthyroid patients typically are anxious, restless, or agitated, patients with thyroid storm may present with a decreased level of consciousness or even coma.[8,43,54,83,90] Hyperthermia can occur secondary to the thermogenic effects of thyroid hormones and psychomotor agitation. Hyperthermia can be extreme (ie, >106°F [>41°C]). The tachycardia associated with thyrotoxicosis often is disproportionate to the temperature elevation.

ACUTE TOXICITY

Acute overdoses with thyroid hormone preparations most commonly occur with oral levothyroxine. Significant ingestions of levothyroxine usually do not manifest clinically until 7–10 days after exposure, but rarely are reported to manifest as early as 2–3 days postingestion.[33,57,84] The delay of peripheral conversion of T_4 to the metabolically active T_3 and the time required to activate nuclear receptors and protein synthesis account for this clinical latency. Acute overdoses involving preparations containing T_3 can manifest in the first 12–24 hours after exposure.[59]

In children, acute thyroxine overdoses almost universally are benign because of their typically unintentional nature and lower doses ingested. Most children remain asymptomatic or develop only mild symptoms. No deaths have been reported.[20,27,45,55,57,60,95] In a series of 15 patients with unintentional overdose, only 3 children developed mild symptoms 12–48 hours postingestion.[58] Similarly, a case series that involved 41 children (ages 1–5 years) with unintentional ingestions of thyroxine (estimated doses ranged from 40 to 800 μg) found mild symptoms (hyperactive behavior, tachycardia, fever, vomiting, diarrhea, diaphoresis, and flushing) in only 27%. All children had good clinical outcomes. The degree of symptoms did not correlate with the amount ingested or measured serum thyroxine concentrations (measured 1–5 hours postingestion) for most cases in that series (see Diagnostic Testing).[27] Two other series involving 78 and 92 cases of unintentional ingestions in children found that mild symptoms developed in only 4 and 8 patients, respectively.[57,102] A report involving an intentional ingestion of 9900 μg in a 13-year-old boy treated empirically with activated charcoal, dexamethasome, and oral propranolol described only mild tremors and anxiety.[93] Only two cases of severe toxicity in children are reported: one child without a history of a seizure disorder had two seizures 7 days after a levothyroxine ingestion (18,000 μg),[53] and another child became gravely ill for a 12-hour period (blood pressure, 120/68 mm Hg; pulse, 200 beats/min; temperature 104°F [40°C]) 6 hours after ingesting a large amount (3.2 g, or 50 grains) of a desiccated thyroid preparation containing both T_3 and T_4.[58]

Ingestions in adults have a wide range of toxicity. Many patients are asymptomatic or mildly symptomatic.[29,61,72] Severe sequelae occur more frequently in adults than in children. Symptoms resemble thyrotoxicosis and, in extreme cases, thyroid storm. Hyperthermia,[33,55,90] dysrhythmias,[5,55,90] and severe agitation[33] are well described. Hemiparesis,[8] muscle weakness,[8,90] coma,[8,55,90] respiratory failure,[25] sudden death,[7] myocardial infarction,[7] cardiac failure,[8] focal myocarditis,[7] rhabdomyolysis with muscle necrosis,[8] delayed palmar desquamation (>2 weeks postingestion),[8,90] and hematuria[33] are also described. Because patients are expected to be asymptomatic shortly after ingestion and laboratory tests correlate poorly with the degree of symptoms, clinical and laboratory findings early in the course of the ingestion are not reliable indicators of which patients will become ill (see Diagnostic Testing).

CHRONIC TOXICITY

Following chronic excessive thyroid hormone ingestion, patients may present with thyrotoxicosis or a have a more subtle and insidious presentation. Classically, chronic ingestion of excess thyroid hormone occurs in patients with hypothyroidism, psychiatric disorders, and eating disorders. Persons who ingest thyroid hormones chronically may develop significant weight loss, anxiety, and accelerated osteoporosis.[71] More severe manifestations, such as cardiac dysrhythmias, tachycardia, cardiac failure, and psychosis, also occur. As in patients with hyperthyroidism, intercurrent illness and physiologic stressors can trigger thyroid storm in these patients.

Numerous miniepidemics of hyperthyroidism and thyrotoxicosis have resulted from the consumption of ground meat containing neck muscle contaminated with thyroid gland.[18,39,49] Investigators in one of these epidemics had three volunteers consume a single large portion of "well-cooked" epidemic-implicated ground beef that previously had been frozen. Although all volunteers remained asymptomatic, the mean serum peak T_4 (8–12 hours postingestion) was elevated ~15 μg/dL, and TSH remained undetectable for 4–17 days.[39] The practice of gullet trimming (using larynx muscles for beef) that led to these outbreaks has since been prohibited in US slaughter houses. However, the risk for sporadic cases remains, especially when laryngeal muscles are used or when farmers and hunters butcher their own meat.[75] Until an exogenous source of thyroid hormone is suspected or identified, such patients often are misdiagnosed with painless thyroiditis or thyrotoxicosis factitia.

Thyrotoxicosis factitia is a symptomatic disorder that mimics physiologic disease. It occurs with intentional chronic ingestion of exogenous thyroid hormone. The pattern of ingestion typically is surreptitious and maladaptive. Patients frequently have comorbid psychiatric disorders, such as Munchausen syndrome or eating disorders, or are taking thyroid hormone for secondary gain.[35] Patients with thyrotoxicosis factitia tend to be either healthcare professionals with access to medications or prescriptions or persons with access to thyroid medications being taken by relatives or friends.[28,35,65]

In recent years, thyroid hormones have gained popularity among dieters and athletes who use the hormones as weight-loss aids and as stimulants. Severe consequences can occur. Sudden death was reported in three patients suspected of chronic ingestion of thyroid hormone for weight loss and energy enhancement.[7] In 2002, the heavily promoted Singaporean diet pill (Slim 10) was linked to hepatotoxicity and hyperthyroidism in numerous patients.[38] Investigators found the proprietary herbal preparation was adulterated with significant amounts of the undeclared ingredients T_4, T_3 (from thyroid gland extract), and fenfluramine (an FDA-banned drug). The medication was promptly withdrawn and the manufacturers convicted under the Singapore Poisons Act.[38] Similar cases were reported from Hong Kong, Japan, and France following ingestion of "slimming pills" containing animal thyroid extract.[73,79] Unfortunately, thyroid hormone–containing supplements are promoted and are readily available to the general public without a prescription through the Internet and in stores selling nutritional supplements (Chap. 44).[89]

TABLE 49–5. Diagnostic Tests for Thyroid Hormone and Thyroid Function

Diagnostic Test	Normal Values[a]	Comments
TSH	0.5–5.0 μIUnits/mL	Available assays with respective detection limits: First generation 1.0 IUnits/L; Second generation 0.1 IUnits/L; Third generation 0.01 IUnits/L
Total T_4 by RIA	5–12 μg/dL (64–153 nmol/L)	↑In pregnancy, estrogens, oral contraceptives
Total T_3 by RIA	40–132 ng/dL (1.1–2.0 nmol/L)	↑In pregnancy, estrogens, oral contraceptives
Free T_4	0.7–1.86 ng/dL (9–24 pmol/L)	↑In hyperthyroidism, exogenous thyroxine ingestion
Free T_3	0.2–0.52 ng/dL (3–8 pmol/L)	↑In hyperthyroidism, exogenous thyroid hormone (T_3 or T_4)

[a] Interlaboratory and interassay variations may occur.

RIA = radioimmunoassay; TSH = thyroid-stimulating hormone.

DIAGNOSTIC TESTING

Traditionally, thyroid testing involved combinations of measurement of total T_4 and some measurement of hormone binding (T_3 uptake). Free T_4 and T_3 also can be measured by equilibrium dialysis (*free* T_4), analogue assays (ie, competitive analogs of either free T_3 or free T_4 that competitively bind for spaces on the serum-binding proteins), and antibody capture assays (ie, sequential assays that capture a representative portion of the free fraction of thyroid hormone). Assessment of pituitary production of TSH has improved greatly in recent years. Supersensitive TSH assays can readily detect suppression of TSH production. TSH is now the primary test for screening thyroid function. Suppressed or elevated concentrations of TSH can be reflexively followed up with a free T_4 assay and, if necessary, a free T_3 assay (Table 49–5).

The clinical manifestations of thyrotoxicosis and thyroid storm are well known to occur at normal, low, moderate, and high concentrations of T_3 and T_4.[10] This lack of correlation between symptoms and serum concentrations is also true for exogenous thyroid hormone ingestion.[8,27,33,39,53,57,66,72,105] In a large case series of children with unintentional ingestions of thyroxine estimated to be between 40 and 800 μg, serum T_4 concentrations were drawn in 11 (1–5 hours postingestion). Serum T_4 concentrations were normal in five of these children and were slightly elevated in six (mean 16 μg/dL). In this series, one infant who was estimated to have ingested 4500 μg had a significantly higher concentration (55 μg/dL at 4.5 hours) but developed only a transient episode of diaphoresis and a "staring spell" 7 days postingestion. Another child who ingested an estimated 4200 μg had a concentration of 12 μg/dL and developed significant tachycardia and hyperthermia.[28] A young child (estimated ingestion 18,000 μg levothyroxine) had a serum T_4 concentration of 117 μg/dL 8 hours postingestion and 38 μg/dL on day 7, when he was symptomatic.[53] In an adult with a massive ingestion of levothyroxine (720,000 μg), serum T_4 concentrations were greater than 30 μg/dL and free T_4 greater than 13 ng/dL (normal 0.7–1.86 ng/dL). In this case, TSH remained undetectable until day 32 postingestion.[33] Overall, the observed symptoms following thyroid hormone ingestion correlate poorly with the amount ingested or with measured serum T_4 concentrations. Prolonged suppression of TSH is common following ingestion of excess thyroid hormone.

Routine analysis of laboratory thyroid function tests in the setting of acute thyroid hormone overdose likely will not affect management. Analysis of thyroid hormone concentrations is indicated only if confirmation of a suspected ingestion is desired and in massive ingestions when early and severe symptoms may occur. Suppression of TSH and elevated thyroid hormone concentrations with a low serum thyroglobulin concentration may help to differentiate between thyrotoxicosis factitia and true endogenous disease.[65]

MANAGEMENT

GENERAL

Based on the existing literature, conservative management is adequate in most cases of acute unintentional thyroxine ingestions in both adults and children. Most children with acute overdose are managed with home observation and follow-up appointments. In cases where the acute thyroxine dose is estimated to be greater than 4000 μg, patient follow-up by regular telephone contact for 10 days is suggested.[27] Historically, most children with unintentional ingestions have been treated with GI decontamination with activated charcoal and/or syrup of ipecac, or by gastric lavage,[27,45,53,55,57,60] but these procedures probably are unnecessary. Based on two large series of unintentional ingestions in children in which no toxicity was observed in the vast majority of cases, clinically significant toxicity is not expected with estimated ingestions less than 4000 μg.[27,102] Because children almost uniformly develop no more than minor symptoms, activated charcoal administration should be considered only if the ingestion is greater than 5000 μg thyroxine. Aspiration risks are minimal in awake, alert children who are able to protect their airways and take activated charcoal orally, without nasogastric tube placement.[55,102] By extension, adults with acute ingestions greater than 5000 μg thyroxine also should be treated with activated charcoal. Except in early presentations with massive thyroxine ingestions (>10,000–50,000 μg) in suicidal adults or ingestions of preparations containing large amounts of T_3, gastric emptying procedures such as induced emesis and orogastric lavage are unwarranted.[8,33] Similarly, patients with massive ingestions (>10,000–50,000 μg) or ingestion of T_3-containing products should be admitted for observation in anticipation of developing significant symptoms.[8,33,53,58]

Treatment should be based on the development of symptoms and should include rehydration, airway protection, and control of sympathomimetic symptoms, mental status alterations, and hyperpyrexia. β-Adrenergic antagonism with propranolol has been used for sympathomimetic symptoms in numerous cases.[24,45,53,57,72,95] Empirical treatment with β-adrenergic antagonists is not recommended. Treatment is only indicated for clinically significant tachycardia, dysrhythmias, and other symptoms of catecholamine-like excess.[24]

AGITATION

If sedation is required, parenteral benzodiazepines and barbiturates are recommended. Rapid-acting benzodiazepines such as midazolam, or diazepam should be used to control severely agitated or symptomatic patients. Phenobarbital should be considered as a sole agent in intubated patients or as an adjunct in patients requiring sedation because it offers the added theoretical benefit of inducing enhanced hepatic elimination of thyroxine (Table 49–2). Because of the general risks of sedation and the lack of evidence regarding the clinical use of enhanced hepatic elimination from phenobarbital, sedation with phenobarbital for the sole purpose of enhanced elimination is not indicated. Sedation with antipsychotics such as haloperidol and droperidol should be avoided because their significant anticholinergic properties can exacerbate thyrotoxic symptoms. In addition, the tendency for this class of drugs to prolong the QT interval and predispose to malignant dysrhythmias is of concern in the already catecholaminergic patient. Antipsychotics should be reserved for medically stable patients with psychiatric behavior.

CATECHOLAMINE-LIKE EXCESS AND CARDIOVASCULAR SYMPTOMS

The principal therapeutic role of β-adrenergic antagonists in hyperthyroidism is antagonism of β-receptor–mediated effects.[71] In addition to these sympatholytic effects, β-adrenergic antagonists inhibit 5′-deiodinase, thereby decreasing peripheral conversion of T_4 to T_3 (Table 49–2). The clinical significance of decreased peripheral conversion in the setting of overdose is unknown. Propranolol is the most frequently used β-adrenergic antagonist in thyrotoxic patients.[27,45,53,57,72,95] Parenteral β-adrenergic antagonists should be used when symptoms are severe or when rapid control of heart rate is required. Starting doses of 1–2 mg IV propranolol every 10–15 minutes are recommended. High doses have been reported in massive thyroxine overdose, where a patient received 23 mg propranolol IV over 1 hour on initial presentation, then required an average of 30 mg/d IV for 5 more days.[33] Oral propranolol can be used for persistent symptoms in patients who are both hemodynamically and medically stable and are not acutely agitated. High oral doses in the range of 20–120 mg every 6 hours may be required. Other β-adrenergic antagonists likely will be effective, provided they *do* have intrinsic sympathomimetic activity (ie, partial agonism at β-adrenergic receptors), such as acebutolol, oxprenolol, penbutolol, and pindolol (Chap. 61). Continuous electrocardiographic and hemodynamic monitoring are indicated when parenteral β-adrenergic antagonists are used or when patients require hospitalization.

When β-adrenergic antagonists are contraindicated, as in patients with asthma or severe congestive heart failure, calcium channel blockers can be used as an alternative. Among calcium channel blockers, diltiazem is the most studied for the management of thyrotoxicosis.[68,87] A double-blind, crossover trial that compared propranolol to diltiazem for thyrotoxic symptoms found that diltiazem was well tolerated and appeared as effective as propranolol.[68] Another study successfully used diltiazem as the sole agent for treatment of cardiovascular symptoms in 11 thyrotoxic patients.[87] Oral doses of 60–120 mg diltiazem 3–4 times daily or 5–10 mg/h parenterally have been used.[68,87] A possible explanation for the efficacy of calcium channel blockers in thyrotoxicosis is that thyroid hormone enhances Ca^{2+} uptake by L-type voltage-gated Ca^{2+} channels, accelerates Ca^{2+} entry into the sarcoplasmic reticulum, and increases cellular Ca^{2+} storage capacity.[47,48,69,91] The net effect of these changes is increased inotropy and chronotropy. Calcium channel blockers, particularly diltiazem and verapamil, attenuate these effects. Use of parenteral β-adrenergic antagonists in combination with parenteral calcium channel blockers is contraindicated because of the risk for profound hypotension and cardiovascular collapse (Chap. 61).

HYPERTHERMIA

Antipyretics are recommended for hyperpyrexia, with acetaminophen being the drug of choice. Aspirin, particularly high doses (1.5–3 g/d), should be avoided because it carries a theoretical risk of increased thyrotoxicity from displacement of T_3 and T_4 from TBG (Table 49–2). Note, however, that hyperthermia, especially extreme hyperthermia (>106°F [>41°C]), most likely is secondary to psychomotor agitation and excess heat production from the hypermetabolic, catecholaminergic, thyrotoxic state. Extreme hyperthermia should be considered a medical emergency and should be rapidly and aggressively treated with active external cooling with ice baths and with β-adrenergic antagonism, sedation with benzodiazepines and/or barbiturates, and endotracheal intubation with paralysis if necessary (Chap. 15).

OTHER THERAPIES

Bile acid sequestrants, such as cholestyramine and colestipol, and aluminum hydroxide (antacids) and sucralfate bind to exogenous T_4 and decrease GI absorption (Table 49–2). Because the evidence supporting their effectiveness is poor, they are not routinely recommended for thyroid hormone overdose.[55]

Oral iodine-containing contrast media is known to decrease peripheral conversion of T_4 to T_3. Doses of 1–2.5 mg/kg iodine PO daily are routinely used for thyroid storm (oral drops commonly referred to as saturated solution KI [SSKI]). Thioamides, such as propylthiouracil (PTU) and methimazole, and the corticosteroids are thyroid gland inhibitors that are used for treatment of non–drug-related hyperthyroidism. In addition, thioamides inhibit peripheral conversion of T_4 to T_3. Evidence from limited case reports suggests poor efficacy of both thioamides and corticosteroids in acute overdose[8,25,55] (see Thioamides and Iodides).

Although use of antithyroid drugs such as PTU, corticosteroids, and iodine contrast media in thyroxine overdose has theoretical benefits, these drugs are unvalidated, potentially harmful, and unlikely to offer additional benefit, or be superior to conventional therapy with activated charcoal, β-adrenergic antagonism, and sedation. These treatments are not recommended as adjunctive therapies for treatment of exogenous thyroxine overdose.

EXTRACORPOREAL DRUG REMOVAL

Extracorporeal drug removal procedures, such as plasma exchange or plasmapheresis, exchange transfusion (in children), and charcoal hemoperfusion, have been used in extreme cases of thyroid hormone overdose and thyroid storm.[1,8,9,25,40,55,59,66,70,97,103] Overall, results regarding improvement of clinical condition and plasma clearances of thyroid hormones with these methods are conflicting. The largest series of acute ingestions involved six patients who became critically ill after massive thyroxine ingestions of prescribed capsules containing a 1000-fold concentration excess of thyroxine (dose range 50,000–125,000 μg/d for 2–12 days). Charcoal hemoperfusion and plasmapheresis were used in all patients. Plasmapheresis was found to be more effective than hemoperfusion in the extraction of thyroxine. The authors suggest this intervention may shorten the duration of thyrotoxicosis. Rebound elevations in plasma concentrations occurred 24 hours later, suggesting redistribution between extravascular and intravascular compartments.[8] This redistribution is expected given the large volume of distribution for thyroid hormones (Table 49–1). There may be a role for early plasmapheresis in the exceptional situation of a known massive ingestion of thyroid hormone. Because the outcomes from most ingestions of thyroid hormone will be favorable with good supportive care, sedation, and β-adrenergic antagonism, the risks of plasmapheresis should be evaluated on a case-by-case basis after consultation with a medical toxicologist.

XENOBIOTICS WITH ANTITHYROID EFFECTS

THIOAMIDES

Antithyroid drugs are used to decrease the amount of thyroid hormone in hyperthyroid states, most commonly in Graves disease. Thioamides are a group of chemicals with the basic structure of R-SCN. Methimazole and propylthiouracil (PTU) are the two principal thioamides used for treatment of hyperthyroidism. Carbimazole, which is bioactivated methimazole, is available in Europe and China. Methimazole and PTU both inhibit the activity of thyroid peroxidase in the thyroid gland.[98] PTU has the added effect of inactivating 5′-deiodinase, which decreases the peripheral conversion of T_4 to the metabolically more active T_3.[19,56] Because thioamides act primarily by decreasing thyroid hormone synthesis (vs. release), a lag time of 3–4 weeks may occur before T_4 is depleted. The oral bioavailability of PTU is 50%–80%. It is rapidly absorbed from the GI tract and may undergo first-pass effect by the liver. Although its plasma half-life is only 1.5 hours, its effects are long-lasting because of accumulation in the thyroid gland. PTU is inactivated by glucuronidation and is renally eliminated. Methimazole is completely absorbed, is concentrated in the thyroid, and is more slowly eliminated than PTU (48 vs. 24 hours). Doses of PTU are in the range of 100 mg orally every 6–8 hours. Methimazole can be given 30 mg PO daily. Although PTU is 10 times less potent than methimazole, it is more commonly used. The indications for its use are mild-to-moderate hyperthyroidism.

The two thioamides traverse the placenta (methimazole more than PTU) and should not be administered during pregnancy. However, they are minimally secreted in breast milk. Adverse effects occur in 3%–12% of patients taking thioamides. The most common adverse effect is a maculopapular pruritic rash. Methimazole, PTU, and, to a lesser extent, carbimazole can cause immune-mediated, dose-related, and age-related agranulocytosis and neutrophil dyscrasias.[58,62,67,77] This potentially life-threatening adverse effect can be treated by administration of granulocyte colony-stimulating factor.[5] Premature withdrawal of thioamides can lead to rebound symptoms and thyrotoxic states.[52]

There are little data regarding overdose with thioamides. A 12-year-old girl with a previous thyroidectomy, who was estimated to have ingested 5000–13,000 mg PTU, developed only a transient decreased T_3 concentration and elevated alkaline phosphatase concentration (7350 mU/mL).[44] The absence of a functioning thyroid gland may have contributed to the benign course in this patient. No other serious sequelae have been associated with acute overdose of thioamides.

IODIDES

Prior to the development of thioamides, iodide salts were the principal treatment for hyperthyroidism. Iodides decrease thyroid hormone concentrations by inhibiting formation and release. In thyroid storm, high-dose iodides (>2 g/d) decrease thyroid hormone release and produce substantial improvements by 2–7 days. Common sources of iodides include calcium iodide, sodium iodide, potassium iodide (KI; pharmaceutical preparations, iopanoic acid, Lugol's solution [iodine + KI solution], oral drops [SSKI]), and methyl iodide (industrial preparations).

The adverse reaction to chronic ingestion of small or excessive amounts of iodide salts, termed *iodism,* is characterized by cutaneous rash, laryngitis, bronchitis, esophagitis, conjunctivitis, drug fever, metallic taste, salivation, headache, and bleeding diathesis. Immune-mediated hypersensitivity symptoms consisting of urticaria, angioedema, eosinophilia, vasculitis, arthralgia, lymphadenitis, and rarely anaphylactoid reactions may occur. Chronic iodide therapy has produced goiters, hypothyroidism, and rarely hyperthyroidism. As much as 10 g sodium iodide has been administered IV without development of signs or symptoms of toxicity.

Iodide (I^-), unlike iodine (I_2) (Chap. 102), is not a caustic. Potassium iodide is added to table salt to form iodized salt for prevention of goiter. It also is used as a prophylactic agent after exposure to large amounts of nuclear fallout to prevent uptake of radioactive iodine into the thyroid gland (see Antidotes in Depth A42: Potassium Iodide) and is the most commonly used iodide for thyroid suppression in hyperthyroidism. Iodide mumps is a well-described but rare disorder characterized by severe sialadenitis (or parotitis),[46] allergic vasculitis, and/or conjunctivitis following administration of ionic and nonionic iodine-containing contrast media and oral iodide salts (Table 49–4).[12,13,45] Although the mechanism remains unclear, it is thought to be idiosyncratic or secondary to iodide accumulation and subsequent inflammation in the ductal systems of the salivary gland. Symptoms tend to occur within 12 hours and resolve spontaneously within 48–72 hours.[12]

Iodides should be avoided in pregnancy because they readily cross the placenta. Severe fetal complications, such as cretinism and death from respiratory failure secondary to obstructive goiter, are reported.[21,41,63] Iodide salts adsorb to activated charcoal.

Methyl iodide is a methylating agent used in the chemical and pharmaceutical industry, as a reagent in microscopy, as a catalyst in production of organic lead compounds, as an etching agent, as a component in fire extinguishers, and formerly as a soil fumigant. Methyl iodide toxicity from inhalation is associated with early pulmonary congestion, lethargy, and renal failure. It also is associated with delayed cerebellar degeneration, multifocal neuropathies (cranial nerve and spinal), parkinsonian symptoms, and late and persistent psychiatric symptoms (months to years).[2,42] Chronic repeated overexposures have led to misdiagnoses such as multiple sclerosis. The toxicity is similar to that of the monohalomethanes (Chap. 116).

SUMMARY

Despite the prevalence of thyroid disorders in the general population and the widespread use of levothyroxine, remarkably little morbidity and mortality associated with overdose from thyroid hormones is reported. Most unintentional ingestions in children are benign, and they can be observed as outpatients for 5–10 days. Intentional ingestions in adults may result in severe symptoms that require ICU management. Supportive care with sedation, cooling measures, and β-adrenergic antagonism are adequate in most cases. Chronic ingestions may produce more severe symptoms as they may present more insidiously or are complicated by thyroid storm. Unregulated dietary supplements containing thyroid hormone used for weight loss and athletic enhancement are becoming increasingly available to consumers via the Internet and in health food or supplement stores. Clinicians should suspect exogenous thyroid hormone exposure in patients with thyrotoxicosis and suppressed TSH concentrations.

ACKNOWLEDGMENT

Christopher Keyes contributed to this chapter in previous editions.

REFERENCES

1. Aghini-Lombardi F, Mariotti S, Fosella PV, et al. Treatment of amiodarone iodine-induced thyrotoxicosis with plasmapheresis and methimazole. *J Endocrinol Invest.* 1993;16:823-826.
2. Appel GB, Galen R, O'Brien J. Methyl iodide intoxication: a case report. *Ann Intern Med.* 1975;82:534-536.
3. Bachman ES, Hampton TG, Dhillon H, et al. The metabolic and cardiovascular effects of hyperthyroidism are largely independent of beta-adrenergic stimulation. *Endocrinology.* 2004;145:2767-2774.
4. Bahouth SW, Cui X, Beauchamp MJ, Park EA. Thyroid hormone induces beta1-adrenergic receptor gene transcription through a direct repeat separated by five nucleotides. *J Mol Cell Cardiol.* 1997;29:3223-3237.
5. Bartalena L, Bogazzi F, Martino E. Adverse effects of thyroid hormone preparations and antithyroid drugs. *Drug Saf.* 1996;15:53-63.
6. Bartalena L, Brogioni S, Grasso L, et al. Treatment of amiodarone-induced thyrotoxicosis, a difficult challenge: results of a prospective study. *J Clin Endocrinol Metab.* 1996;81:2930-2933.
7. Bhasin S, Wallace W, Lawrence JB, et al. Sudden death associated with thyroid hormone abuse. *Am J Med.* 1981;71:887-890.
8. Binimelis J, Bassas L, Marruecos L, et al. Massive thyroxine intoxication: evaluation of plasma extraction. *Intensive Care Med.* 1987;13:33-38.
9. Braithwaite SS, Brooks MH, Collins S, Bermes EW. Plasmapheresis: an adjunct to medical management of severe hyperthyroidism. *J Clin Apheresis.* 1986;3:119-123.
10. Brooks MH, Waldstein SS, Bronsky D, et al. Serum triiodothyronine concentrations in thyroid storm. *J Clin Endocrinol Metab.* 1975;40:339-341.
11. Cappiello E, Boldorini R, Tosoni A, et al. Ultrastructural evidence of thyroid damage in amiodarone-induced thyrotoxicosis. *J Endocrinol Invest.* 1995;18:862-868.
12. Carter JE. Iodide "mumps." *N Eng J Med.* 1961:61;987-988.
13. Christensen J. Iodide mumps after intravascular administration of a nonionic contrast medium. Case report and review of the literature. *Acta Radiol.* 1995;36:82-84.
14. Coulombe P, Dussault JH, Walker P. Plasma catecholamine concentrations in hyperthyroidism and hypothyroidism. *Metabolism.* 1976;25:973-979.
15. Danzi S, Klein I. Thyroid hormone and the cardiovascular system. *Minerva Endocrinol.* 2004;29:130-150.
16. Das DK, Bandyopadhyay D, Bandyopadhyay S, Neogi A. Thyroid hormone regulation of beta-adrenergic receptors and catecholamine sensitive adenylate cyclase in foetal heart. *Acta Endocrinol (Copenh).* 1984;106: 569-576.
17. Dong BJ, Hauck WW, Gambertoglio JG, et al. Bioequivalence of generic and brand-name levothyroxine products in the treatment of hypothyroidism. *JAMA.* 1997;277:1205-1213.
18. Dymling JF, Becker DV. Occurrence of hyperthyroidism in patients receiving thyroid hormone. *J Clin Endocinol Metab.* 1967;27:1487-1491.
19. Farwell AP, Braverman LE. Thyroid and antithyroid drugs. In: Hardman JG, Limbird LE, Molinoff PB, Ruddon RW, eds. *Goodman & Gilman's The Pharmacological Basis of Therapeutics,* 9th ed. New York: McGraw-Hill; 1996:1383-1409.
20. Funderburk SK, Spaulding JS. Sodium levothyroxine intoxications in a child. *Pediatrics.* 1970;45:298-301.
21. Galina MP, Avnet NL, Einhorn A. Iodides during pregnancy: an apparent cause of neonatal death. *N Engl J Med.* 1962;267:1124-1127.
22. Gardner LA, Delos Santos NM, Matta SG, et al. Role of the cyclic AMP-dependent protein kinase in homologous resensitization of the beta1-adrenergic receptor. *J Biol Chem.* 2004;279:21135-21143.
23. Gavin LA. Thyroid crisis. *Med Clin North Am.* 1991;75:179-193.
24. Geffner DL, Hershman JM. Beta-adrenergic blockade for the treatment of hyperthyroidism. *Am J Med.* 1992;93:61-68.
25. Gerard P, Malvaux PG, de Vischer M. Accidental poisoning with thyroid extract treated by exchange transfusion. *Arch Child.* 1972;47:981-982.
26. Gittoes NJ, Franklyn JA. Drug-induced thyroid disorders. *Drug Saf.* 1995;13: 46-55.
27. Golightly LK, Smolinske SC, Kulig KW, et al. Clinical effects of accidental levothyroxine ingestion in children. *Am J Dis Child.* 1985;141:1025-1027.
28. Gorman CA, Wahner HW, Tauxe WN. Metabolic malingerers. Patients who deliberately induce or perpetuate a hypermetabolic or hypometabolic state. *Am J Med.* 1970;48:708-714.
29. Gorman RL, Chamberlain JM, Rose SR, Oderda GM. Massive levothyroxine overdose: high anxiety-low toxicity. *Pediatrics.* 1988;82:666-669.
30. Greenspan FS, Dong BJ. Thyroid and antithyroid drugs. In: Katzung BG, ed. *Basic and Clinical Pharmacology.* New York: McGraw-Hill/Appleton Lange; 2003:644-659.
31. Graves RJ. Newly observed affection of the thyroid gland in females. *Lond Med Surg J,* p. 516. Reprinted in Major RH. *Classic Descriptions of Disease.* Springfield, IL: Charles C Thomas; 1978.
32. Guyetant S, Wion-Barbot N, Rousselet MC. C-cell hyperplasia associated with chronic lymphocytic thyroiditis: a retrospective quantitative study of 112 cases. *Hum Pathol.* 1994;25:514-521.
33. Hack, JB, John AL, Nelson LS, Hoffman RS. Severe symptoms following massive intentional L-thyroxine ingestion. *Vet Human Toxicol.* 1999;41: 323-326.
34. Hamdy RC. The thyroid gland: a brief historical perspective. *South Med J.* 2002;95:471-473.
35. Hamolsky MW. Truth is stranger than factitious. *N Engl J Med.* 1982;307: 436-437.
36. Harjai KJ, Licata AA. Effects of amiodarone on thyroid function. *Ann Intern Med.* 1997;126:63-73.
37. Haynes RC. Thyroid and antithyroid drugs. In: Gilman AG, Rall TW, Nies AS, Taylor P, eds. *Goodman & Gilman's The Pharmacological Basis of Therapeutics,* 8th ed. New York: McGraw-Hill; 1990:1361-1383.
38. Health Science Authority, Singapore. Annual Report 2002-2003, pp 34-35.
39. Hedberg CW. An outbreak of thyrotoxicosis caused by the consumption of bovine thyroid gland in ground beef. *N Engl J Med.* 1987;316:993-998.
40. Henderson A, Hickman P, Ward G, Pond SM. Lack of efficacy of plasmapheresis in a patient overdosed with thyroxine. *Anaesth Intensive Care.* 1994;22:463-464.
41. Herbst AL, Selenkow HA. Hyperthyroidism during pregnancy. *N Engl J Med.* 1965;273:627.
42. Hermouet C, Garnier R, Efthymiou M, Fournier P. Methyl iodide poisoning: report of two cases. *Am J Ind Med.* 1996;30:759-764.
43. Howton JC. Thyroid storm presenting as coma. *Ann Emerg Med.* 1988;17:343-345.
44. Jackson GL, Flickinger FW, Wells LW. Massive overdosage of propylthiouracil. *Ann Intern Med.* 1979;91:418-419.
45. Jahr HM. Thyroid "poisoning" in children. *Nebr S Med J.* 1936;21:388.
46. Kalaria VG, Porsche R, Ong LS. Iodide mumps: acute sialadenitis after contrast administration for angioplasty. *Circulation.* 2001;104:2384.
47. Kim D, Smith TW. Effects of thyroid hormone on calcium handling in cultured chick ventricular cells. *J Physiol.* 1985;364:131-149.
48. Kim D, Smith TW, Marsh JD. Effect of thyroid hormone on slow calcium channel function in cultured chick ventricular cells. *J Clin Invest.* 1987;80:88-94.
49. Kinney JS, Hurwitz ES, Fishbein DB, et al. Community outbreak of thyrotoxicosis: epidemiology, immunogenetic characteristics, and long-term outcome. *Am J Med.* 1988;84:10-18.

50. Klein I, Becker DV, Levey GS. Treatment of hyperthyroid disease. *Ann Intern Med.* 1994;121:281-288.
51. Klein I, Ojamaa K. Thyroid hormone and the cardiovascular system. *N Engl J Med.* 2001;344:501-509.
52. Kubota S, Tamai H, Ohye H, et al. Transient hyperthyroidism after withdrawal of antithyroid drugs in patients with Graves' disease. *Endocr J.* 2004;51:213-217.
53. Kulig KW, Golightly LK, Rumak BH. Levothyroxine overdose associated with seizures in a young child. *JAMA.* 1985;254:2109-2110.
54. Laman DM, Bergough A, Enditz LJ. Thyroid crisis presenting as coma. *Clin Neurol Neurosurg.* 1984;86:295-298.
55. Lehrner LM, Weir MR. Acute ingestions of thyroid hormone. *Pediatrics.* 1984;71:313-317.
56. Leonard JL, Visser TJ. Biochemistry of iodination. In: Hennemann G, ed. *Thyroid Hormone Metabolism.* New York: Marcel Dekker; 1986:189-230.
57. Lewander WJ, Lacoutre PG, Silva JE, et al. Acute thyroxine ingestions in pediatric patients. *Pediatrics.* 1989;84:262-265.
58. Levy RP, Gilger WG. Acute thyroid poisoning. *N Engl J Med.* 1957;256: 459-460.
59. Liel Y, Weksler N. Plasmapheresis rapidly eliminates thyroid hormones from the circulation, but does not affect the speed of TSH recovery following prolonged suppression. *Horm Res.* 2003;60:252-254.
60. Litovitz TL, White J. Levothyroxine ingestions in children: an analysis of 78 cases. *Am J Emerg Med.* 1985;3:297-300.
61. Lo DK, Szeto CC, Chan TY. Mild symptoms of toxicity following deliberate ingestion of thyroxine. *Vet Hum Toxicol.* 2004;46:193.
62. Luther AL, Wade JS, Slaughter JM. Agranulocytosis secondary to methimazole therapy: report of two cases. *South Med J.* 1976;69:1356-1357.
63. Malcom, MM, Rento RD. Iodide goiter with hypothyroidism in two newborn infants. *J Pediatr.* 1962;61:94-99.
64. Major RH. *Classic Descriptions of Disease.* Springfield, IL: Charles C Thomas; 1978.
65. Mariotti S, Marino E, Cupin C, et al. Low serum thyroglobulin as a clue to the diagnosis of thyrotoxicosis factitia. *N Engl J Med.* 1982;307:410-412.
66. May ME, Mintz PD, Lowry P, et al. Plasmapheresis in thyroid overdose: a case report. *J Toxicol Clin Toxicol.* 1983;20:517-520.
67. Meyer-Gessner M, Bender G, Lederbogen S, et al. Antithyroid drug-induced agranulocytosis: clinical experience with ten patients treated at one institution and review of the literature. *J Endocrinol Invest.* 1994;17: 29-36.
68. Milner MR, Gelman KM, Phillips RA, et al. Double-blind crossover trial of diltiazem versus propranolol in the management of thyrotoxic symptoms. *Pharmacotherapy.* 1990;10:100-106.
69. Muller A, Zuidwijk MJ, Simonides WS, van Hardeveld C. Modulation of SERCA2 expression by thyroid hormone and norepinephrine in cardiocytes: role of contractility. *Am J Physiol.* 1997;272:H1876-H1885.
70. Nenov VD, Marinov P, Sabeva J, Nenov DS. Current applications of plasmapheresis in clinical toxicology. *Nephrol Dial Transplant.* 2003;18(Suppl 5): 56-58.
71. Nuovo J, Ellsworth A, Christensen DB, et al. Excessive thyroid hormone replacement therapy. *J Am Board Fam Pract.* 1995;8:435-439.
72. Nystrom E, Lindstedt G, Lundberg P. Minor signs and symptoms of toxicity on a young woman in spite of massive thyroid ingestion. *Acta Med Scand.* 1980;207:135-136.
73. Ohye H, Kukata S, Kanoh, et al. Thyrotoxicosis caused by weight-reducing herbal medicines. *Arch Intern Med.* 2005;165;831-834.
74. Pantos C, Malliopoulou V, Varonos DD, Cokkinos DV. Thyroid hormone and phenotypes of cardioprotection. *Basic Res Cardiol.* 2004;99:101-120.
75. Parmar MS, Sturge C. Recurrent hamburger thyrotoxicosis. *CMAJ.* 2003;169: 415-417.
76. Parry CH. *Collections from the Unpublished Medical Writings.* Underwoods: London; 1825:2:1-120. Reprinted in Major RH: *Classic Descriptions of Disease.* Springfield, IL: Charles C Thomas; 1978.
77. Pearce SH. Spontaneous reporting of adverse reactions to carbimazole and propylthiouracil in the UK. *Clin Endocrinol (Oxf).* 2004;61:5895-5894.
78. Pitt-Rivers R. Sir Charles Harington and the structure of thyroxine. *Mayo Clin Proc.* 1964;39:553-559.
79. Poon WT, Ng SW, Lai CK et al. Factitious thyrotoxicosis and herbal dietary supplement for weight reduction. *Clin Tox.* 2008;46:290-292.
80. Pracyk JB, Slotkin TA. Thyroid hormone differentially regulates development of beta-adrenergic receptors, adenylate cyclase and ornithine decarboxylase in rat heart and kidney. *J Dev Physiol.* 1991;16:251-261.
81. Pracyk JB, Slotkin TA. Thyroid hormone regulates ontogeny of beta adrenergic receptors and adenylate cyclase in rat heart and kidney: effects of propylthiouracil-induced perinatal hypothyroidism. *J Pharmacol Exp Ther.* 1992;261:951-958.
82. Premel-Cabic A, Getin F, Turcant A, et al. Plasma noradrenaline in hyperthyroidism and hypothyroidism [in French]. *Presse Med.* 1986;15:1625-1627.
83. Pugh S, Lalwani K, Awal A. Thyroid storm as a cause of loss of consciousness following anaesthesia for emergency Caesarean section. *Anaesthesia.* 1994;49:35-37.
84. Rennie D. Thyroid storm. *JAMA.* 1997;277:1238-1243.
85. Ririe DG, Butterworth JF 4th, Royster RL. Triiodothyronine increases contractility independent of beta-adrenergic receptors or stimulation of cyclic-3′,5′-adenosine monophosphate. *Anesthesiology.* 1995;82:1004-1012.
86. Roffi M, Cattaneo F, Topol EJ. Thyrotoxicosis and the cardiovascular system: subtle but serious effects. *Cleve Clin J Med.* 2003;70:57-63.
87. Roti E, Montermini M, Roti S, Gardini E, et al. The effect of diltiazem, a calcium channel-blocking drug, on cardiac rate and rhythm in hyperthyroid patients. *Arch Intern Med.* 1988;148:1919-1921.
88. Sawin CT. Hypothyroidism. *Med Clin North Am.* 1985;69:989-1004.
89. Sawin CT, London MH. "Natural" desiccated thyroid. A "health-food" thyroid preparation. *Arch Intern Med.* 1989;149:2117-2118.
90. Schottsaedt ES, Smoller M. "Thyroid storm" produced by a thyroid hormone poisoning. *Ann Intern Med.* 1966;64:847-849.
91. Seppet EK, Kolar F, Dixon IM, et al. Regulation of cardiac sarcolemmal Ca2 channels and Ca2 transporters by thyroid hormone. *Mol Cell Biochem.* 1993;129:145-159.
92. Seppet EK, Kaasik A, Minajeva A, et al. Mechanisms of thyroid hormone control over sensitivity and maximal contractile responsiveness to beta-adrenergic agonists in atria. *Mol Cell Biochem.* 1998; 184:419-442.
93. Shilo L, Kovatz S, Hadari R, et al. Massive thyroid hormone overdose kinetics, clinical manifestations and management. *Isr Med Assoc J.* 2002;4: 298-299.
94. Silva JE. The thermogenic effect of thyroid hormone and its clinical implications. *Ann Intern Med.* 2003;139:205-213.
95. Singh GK, Winterborn MH. Massive overdose with thyroxine, toxicity and treatment. *Pediatrics.* 1991;150:217.
96. Surks MI, Sievert R. Drugs and thyroid function. *N Engl J Med.* 1995;333:1688-1694.
97. Tajiri J, Katsuya H, Kiyokawa T, et al. Successful treatment of thyrotoxic crisis with plasma exchange. *Crit Care Med.* 1984;12:536-537.
98. Taurog A, Dorris ML. Peroxidase-catalyzed bromination of tyrosine, thyroglobulin, and bovine serum albumin: comparison of thyroid peroxidase and lactoperoxidase. *Arch Biochem Biophys.* 1991;287:288-296.
99. Tielens ET, Forder JR, Chatham JC, et al. Acute L-triiodothyronine administration potentiates inotropic responses to beta-adrenergic stimulation in the isolated perfused rat heart. *Cardiovasc Res.* 1996;32:306-310.
100. Trousseau A. Exophthalmic goitre of Graves' disease. In: *Lectures on Clinical Medicine.* vol. 1, lecture XIX. New Sydenham Society: London; 1868:586.
101. Tse J, Gandhi A, Yan L, He YQ, Weiss HR. Effects of triiodothyronine pretreatment on beta-adrenergic responses in stunned cardiac myocytes. *J Cardiothorac Vasc Anesth.* 2003;17:486-490.
102. Tunget CL, Clark RF, Turchen SG, et al. Raising the decontamination level for thyroid hormone ingestions. *Am J Emerg Med.* 1995;13:9-13.
103. Van Huekelom S, Kinderen LH, der Vingerhoeds PJ. Plasmapheresis in L-thyroxine intoxication. *Vet Hum Toxicol.* 1979;S21:7.
104. Von Basedow CA. Exophthlmos durch hypertrophie des zellgewebes in der augenhohle. *Wochenschrif fur die Gesammte Heilkunde*, Berlin: 1840. Reprinted in Major RH: *Classic Descriptions of Disease.* Springfield, IL: Charles C Thomas; 1978.
105. Von Hofe SE, Young RL. Thyrotoxicosis after a single ingestion of levothyroxine. *JAMA.* 1977;237:1361.
106. Wiersinga WM. Amiodarone and the thyroid: In: Weetmen AP, Grossman A, eds. *Handbook of Pharmacology*, Vol. 128: *Pharmacotherapeutics of the Thyroid Gland.* Berlin: Springer-Verlag; 1997:225-287.
107. Yamasaki K, Morimoto N, Gion T, Yanaga K. Delirium and a subclavian abscess. *Lancet.* 1997:390;1294.

CHAPTER 50
ANTIHISTAMINES AND DECONGESTANTS

Anthony J. Tomassoni and Richard S. Weisman

Antihistamines and decongestants rank highly among the top 40 prescription and nonprescription xenobiotics used in the United States. Inappropriate use and unrecognized dangers associated with their use have posed significant public health problems. Their ready availability, singly and in combination with each other and with analgesics and antipyretics, coupled with widespread public impression that nonprescription and herbal xenobiotics are "safe," contributes to their frequent use, misuse, and potential abuse.

HISTORY AND EPIDEMIOLOGY

Recreational use of antihistamines and decongestants as "legal highs" has gained in notoriety over the past several years, and nonprescription sympathomimetics have been used as precursors in the synthesis of illegal stimulants. While the rates of potential adverse events are perceived as low, the issue takes on added significance when the magnitude of the exposure rates for these xenobiotics is considered: in a survey of 2590 participants distributed across the Unied States, 8.1% of adult participants reported taking pseudoephedrine within the past week, and 4.4% reported the use of diphenhydramine within the same time period[47] (Table 50–1).

Despite well-designed and carefully monitored studies prior to US Food and Drug Administration (FDA) approval of medications, only half of newly discovered serious adverse drug events (ADEs) are detected and reported in the Physicians' Desk Reference within 7 years of drug approval.[52] This suggests that increased efforts to detect and report ADEs via improved postmarketing surveillance are required. The quality and timeliness of current toxicovigilance efforts may be hampered by many variables including low reporting rates, variable data quality in reports, and the effects of media attention on spontaneous reporting systems—factors well-known to clinical toxicologists and poison centers. The potential impact of surveillance system inadequacies on public health is dramatically illustrated by the delayed recognition of the risk of intracranial hemorrhage associated with the use of phenylpropanolamine.[48]

Recent information regarding potential hazards of antihistamine or decongestant use has catalyzed new review, regulations and withdrawal of some xenobiotics from the market. The Combat Methamphetamine Act signed into law in 2006 limiting methamphetamine precursor availability and additional precautions in pharmacies (such as dispensing limits for nonprescription quantities and storage of the medications behind pharmacy counters) has attempted to reduce potential harm associated with these xenobiotics.

ANTIHISTAMINES

HISTORY AND EPIDEMIOLOGY

What subsequently became known as H_1 receptor antagonists were introduced into clinical use in the early 1940s with pyrilamine as the first medication. Antihistamines are available worldwide, and many do not require a prescription. The class of medications continues to find widespread application in the treatment of anaphylaxis, allergic rhinitis, urticaria, and other histamine-mediated disorders. They are often used for symptomatic relief of allergy symptoms and are included in many combination cold and cough preparations. First-generation (sedating) antihistamines are also marketed as sleep aids, sometimes in combination with analgesics such as acetaminophen. First-generation H_1 receptor antagonists are commonly ingested in suicide attempts, most likely because of their ready availability and because of the many formulations marketed as "sleeping pills."[65] Second- and third-generation H_1 receptor antagonists, marketed beginning in the mid-1980s, are not sedating and less frequently implicated in suicide attempts.

Both poison center and clinical experiences suggest that recreational use of antihistamines may be increasing. It is unclear whether the increased use results simply from inclusion of antihistamines in cold preparations containing the widely abused cough suppressant dextromethorphan (Chap. 38). The second-generation (nonsedating) antihistamines terfenadine and astemizole are associated with cardiac dysrhythmias and are no longer approved for use in the United States (Chap. 138). Absolute risk of developing ventricular dysrhythmias as a result of nonsedating antihistamine use has been estimated to be 1 in 57,000 prescriptions.[17]

Unintentional exposures to antihistamine-containing preparations are common. Review of the annual reports of the American Association of Poison Control Centers underscores the frequency of antihistamine exposures. Of a total of 2,482,041 human exposure calls voluntarily reported in 2007, antihistamines alone accounted for 79,157 making antihistamines 15th among classes of poison exposures overall and 10th among children (39,686 exposure calls).[8] Additional exposures related to cough and cold medications will be considered in the decongestants section. While reporting is not comprehensive, poison center data suggest that the prevalence of unintentional antihistamine exposure is increasing: antihistamines ranked 13th among children in 2001 accounting for only 67,053 of 2,267,979 human exposure calls.[55] National Association of Medical Examiners data reported 14,000 fatalities involving children younger than 6 years annually.[44] Liquid formulations attractive to children are available, and diphenhydramine or another antihistamine is occasionally administered as a sedative by parents and daycare workers.[3] Although ingestion is the usual route of exposure, exposure to topical preparations containing antihistamines can also cause toxicity.[39]

ANATOMY AND PHYSIOLOGY OF THE HISTAMINE RECEPTOR SYSTEM

The numerous functions of histamine and its receptors in the nervous system, immune system, and other organ systems are continually being appreciated. Four types of histamine receptors are recognized and designated H_1, H_2, H_3, and H_4. All are helical transmembrane molecules that transduce extracellular signals via G proteins to intracellular second-messenger systems.[70]

H_1 receptors are most commonly associated with mediation of inflammation. These receptors are located in the CNS, heart, vasculature, airways, sensory nerves, gastrointestinal smooth muscle cells, immune cells, and adrenal medulla. The functions of histamine and the H_1 receptor include control of the sleep–wake cycle, cognition, memory, and endocrine homeostasis. H_1 receptor stimulation also causes vasodilation, increases vascular permeability and bronchoconstriction, and decreases atrioventricular nodal conduction when histamine is present.

Through H_1 receptors, histamine interacts with G proteins in the plasma membranes. Stimulation of H_1 receptors results in increased synthesis by phospholipases A_2 and C, inositol-1,4,5-triphosphate and several diacylglycerols (DAGs) from phospholipids located in cell membranes.

TABLE 50–1. Antihistamines and Decongestants among the 40 Most Commonly Used Prescription and Nonprescription Drugs (Adult Use in the United States) in 1998 and 1999

Rank	Drug	1-Week Prevalence (%)
4	Pseudoephedrine HCl	8.1
6	Diphenhydramine HCl	4.4
13	Chlorpheniramine maleate/tannate	2.9
17	Loratidine	2.5
35	Fexofenadine	1.3
36	Doxylamine succinate	1.2

From Kaufman DW, Kelly JP, Rosenberg L, et al. Recent patterns of medication use in the ambulatory adult population of the United States. The Slone Survey. *JAMA*. 2002;287:337-344. With permission.

Inositol-1,4,5-triphosphate causes release of calcium, which then activates calcium–calmodulin-dependent myosin light-chain kinase, resulting in enhanced cross-bridging and smooth muscle contraction. The active and inactive forms of this receptor subtype are in equilibrium at baseline, and histamine shifts the equilibrium to the active conformation.[70]

H_2 receptors are located in cells of the gastric mucosa, heart, lung, CNS, uterus, and immune cells. H_2 receptor stimulation is mediated by adenyl cyclase activation of cyclic adenosine monophosphate (cAMP)-dependent protein kinase in smooth muscle and in parietal cells of the stomach and results in increased gastric acidity through stimulation of the H^+-K^+-ATPase pump causing release of H^+ into the gastric lumen.[37,70] The action of histamine on H_2 receptor results in increased gastric acid secretion, increased vascular permeability, and other effects.

H_3 receptors are found in neurons of the central and peripheral nervous systems, airways, and the GI tract. The action of histamine on H_3 receptors of the CNS decreases further release of histamine, acetylcholine, dopamine, and serotonin.[82] H_3 receptors partly act to prevent excessive bronchoconstriction and also are implicated in control of neurogenic inflammation and proinflammatory activity.[53] No H_3 receptor antagonists are commercially available. Some prototypical drugs include clobenpropit, ciproxifan, and thioperamide. Due to nootropic (cognitive enhancement) and stimulant effects it has been suggested that H_3 antihistamines might play a future role in the treatment of ADHD, depression, or dementia.

H_4 receptors are located in leukocytes, bone marrow, spleen, lung, liver, colon, and hippocampus. The H_4 receptor has apparent roles in the differentiation of myeloblasts and promyelocytes, and in eosinophil chemotaxis.[37,70] Due to their association with mast cells and eosinophils, future H_4 antagonists may play a part in the treatment of allergic rhinitis, asthma and rheumatoid arthritis.

This chapter focuses on H_1 and H_2 antihistamines, since no H_3 or H_4 receptor active pharmaceuticals are presently in clinical use.

PHARMACOLOGY

Histamine Antagonists All known H_1 histamine antagonists function as inverse agonists and not simply reversible competitive antagonists.[70] Rather than preventing the binding of histamine to its receptor as in a classical competitive antagonist model, H_1 histamine antagonists stabilize the inactive form of the H_1 receptor and shift the equilibrium to this inactive conformation.[70] However, for consistency with the medical literature and the current clinical use of these drugs, we use the terms H_1 antihistamine and histamine antagonist rather than inverse agonist to describe agents of this class.

Agonists and antagonists that act at each of the four histamine-modulated receptor sites have been identified. Antiallergic and antiinflammatory activities of the H_1 antihistamines involve multiple mechanisms. For example, inhibition of the release of mediators from mast cells or basophils may involve a direct inhibitory effect on calcium-ion channels, thereby reducing the inward calcium current activated when intracellular stores of calcium are depleted. Inhibition of the expression of cell adhesion molecules and eosinophil chemotaxis may involve downregulation of the H_1 receptor-activated nuclear factor (κB) which binds to promoter or enhancer regions of genes that regulate the synthesis of proinflammatory cytokines and adhesion proteins.[70]

Six major classes of H_1 antihistamines are traditionally recognized based on molecular structure. The classes were initially populated by first-generation derivatives of ethylenediamine, ethanolamine, alkylamines, phenothiazines, piperazines, and piperidines (Fig. 50–1).[70]

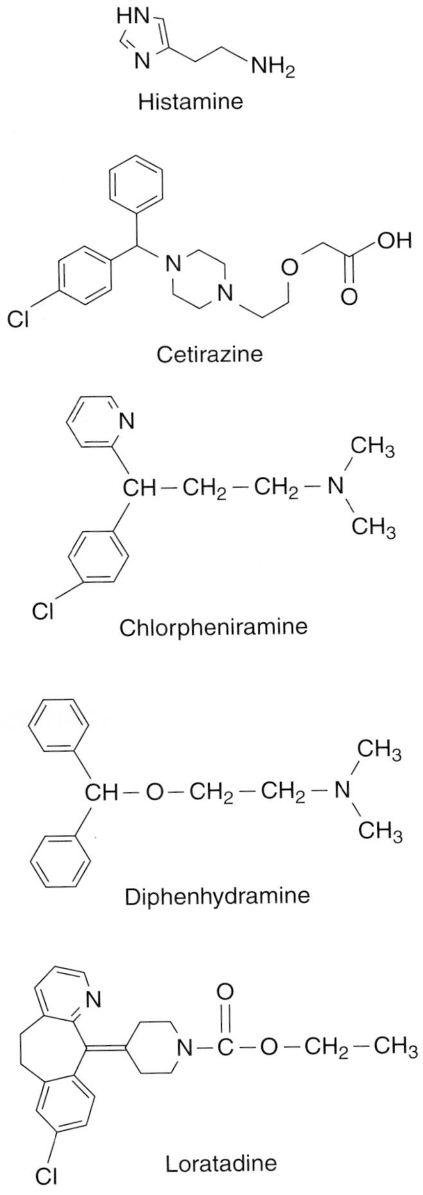

HN, N, NH_2

Histamine

N, O, OH, N, O, Cl

Cetirazine

N, CH_3, $CH-CH_2-CH_2-N$, CH_3, Cl

Chlorpheniramine

CH_3, $CH-O-CH_2-CH_2-N$, CH_3

Diphenhydramine

N, O, $N-C-O-CH_2-CH_3$, Cl

Loratadine

FIGURE 50–1. Structures of histamine and diverse H_1 receptor antagonists.

Many of the classic antihistamines are substituted ethylamine structures with a tertiary amino group linked by a two- or three-carbon chain with two aromatic groups. This structure differs from histamine by the absence of a primary amino group and the presence of a single aromatic moiety.

In some respects, a more functional classification stratifies H_1 antihistamines by sedating properties and ability to cross the blood–brain barrier. So-called first-generation antihistamines readily penetrate the blood–brain barrier and produce CNS effects including sedation and performance impairment. In contrast, second-generation or nonsedating H_1 antihistamines are peripherally selective and have a higher therapeutic index. Central effects of the first-generation H_1 antihistamines likely result from their high lipophilicity or lack of recognition by the P-glycoprotein efflux pump on the luminal surfaces of vascular endothelial cells in the CNS.[13,70] Some first-generation H_1 antihistamines also bind to muscarinic and perhaps to α-adrenergic receptors (Table 50–2).

Second-generation H_1 antihistamines do not penetrate the CNS well because of their hydrophilicity, their relatively high molecular weight, and recognition by the P-glycoprotein efflux pump on the luminal surfaces of vascular endothelial cells in the CNS. Furthermore, the second-generation H_1 antihistamines cetirizine, fexofenadine, loratadine, azelastine (nasal spray), and ebastine have lower binding affinities for the cholinergic, α-adrenergic, and β-adrenergic receptor sites than do the first-generation antihistamines.

Careful prescribing practice may lead to a preference for second-generation H_1 antihistamines in patients whose activities are safety-critical and may be affected by any psychomotor impairment, for example, those who operate motor vehicles.[33,58] Despite this seemingly straightforward precaution, care must be exercised in the selection and use of second-generation H_1 antihistamines since some subjective or objective sedation may still result from their use. Furthermore, it has been posited after meta-analysis that the line between sedating and nonsedating H_1 antihistamines may be blurry, with some studies suboptimally constructed and lacking in distinction between medication side effects and the effects of the condition being treated.[5,78] Overall, it appears that the relative incidence of anticholinergic and CNS adverse effects caused by second-generation H_1 antihistamines may be similar to that produced by placebo.[16] However, some patients report sedation, especially if higher-than-recommended dosages are taken, particularly with cetirizine.[16,78] Table 50–3 lists the peripheral selectivity of the antihistamine that is principally defined by the relative absence of anticholinergic and sedative properties of the H_1 antihistamines.

Using recommended doses of antihistamines, PET scanning shows that first-generation antihistamines occupy more than 70% of the H_1 receptors in the frontal cortex, temporal cortex, hippocampus, and pons. In contrast, the second-generation antihistamines occupy less than 20%–30% of the available CNS H_1 receptors.[77,78] Given the relatively limited anticholinergic effects of the second-generation antihistamines, antihistamine therapy for patients with seasonal asthma has been reintroduced and has proved efficacious.

Some H_1 antihistamines have relatively unique properties that may lead to special uses or marketing. Diphenhydramine and promethazine have local anesthetic properties although higher concentrations are necessary to achieve this effect. Diphenhydramine and doxylamine find frequent application in nonprescription sleeping medications due to their sedative effects. Diphenhydramine and dimenhydrinate have relatively strong antimuscarinic activity and have been used for the management of motion sickness. Oxatomide, a sedating H_1 antihistamine, may possess mast-cell stabilizing properties possibly mediated via calcium-channel blockade and has been associated with dyskinesia. In a test of wheal suppression, fexofenadine had the earliest onset of action while levocetirizine showed maximal inhibition of wheal response at 3 and 6 hours.[18]

H_2 Receptor Antagonists These structural analogs of histamine are highly selective and competitively inhibit the H_2 receptor site. Cimetidine is the original antihistamine in this class; it retains the imidazole ring of histamine (Fig. 50–2). Although newer antihistamines such as ranitidine and famotidine have replaced this ring with a furan or thiazole group, respectively, they retain significant structural similarity to histamine.

The effectiveness of H_2 receptor antagonists in the treatment of gastroesophageal reflux disease is improved further by their concomitant alteration in the response of parietal cells to acetylcholine and gastrin, two other stimulants for gastric acid secretion (Fig. 50–3). Of note, H_2 receptor antagonists have little effect elsewhere in the body, and they have weak CNS penetration secondary to their hydrophilic properties. Though effective in the treatment of *H. pylori*-mediated disease when used in conjunction with appropriate antibiotics, a proton pump inhibitor was used in lieu of an H_2 blocker.

TABLE 50–2. Common Effects of H_1 Antihistamines

Effector	Effect	Comment
H_1 receptors	Decreased CNS neurotransmission resulting in increased appetite, potential weight gain, sedation, impaired psychomotor and cognitive function, dyskinesia, agitation	Observed with first-generation drugs; cetirizine 10 mg or greater dose is associated with sedation in some patients
Ion channels	Electrocardiographic QT interval prolongation; sodium channel blockade; resultant ventricular dysrhythmias; I_{Kr}, I_{Na} and other channels may be affected	Terfenadine and astemizole withdrawn from the US market for this reason Diphenhydramine has CA like effects
Muscarinic receptors	Antimuscarinic (anticholinergic) effects including flushing, hyperthermia via impaired cooling/sweating, dry mouth, dry eyes, sinus tachycardia, mydriasis, agitation/hallucination, reduced GI motility, urinary retention, sinus tachycardia	Insignificant with second-generation agents
α-Adrenergic receptors	Hypotension, orthostasis and reflex tachycardia	No serious effect likely
Serotonin receptors	Increased appetite	

TABLE 50–3. Pharmacologic Characteristics of H_1 Antihistamines

Antihistamine	Anticholinergic Class	Sedation	Duration of Action (h)	Typical Adult Dose
Acrivastine	Alkylamine	+	6–8	8 mg tid
Brompheniramine	Alkylamine	++	4–6	4 mg qid
Chlorpheniramine	Alkylamine	++	4–6	4 mg qid
Dexbrompheniramine	Alkylamine	++	12	3–12 mg bid
Dexchlorpheniramine	Alkylamine	++	3–6	4–6 mg tid
Dimethindene	Alkylamine	++	8	1–2 mg tid
Pheniramine	Alkylamine	++	4–6	5–15 mg q4h
Triprolidine	Alkylamine	++	4–6	2.5 mg qid
Carbinoxamine	Ethanolamine	++++	3–6	4–8 mg qid
Clemastine	Ethanolamine	++++	12–24	2 mg bid
Dimenhydrinate	Ethanolamine	++++	4–6	50–100 mg qid
Diphenhydramine	Ethanolamine	++++	4–6	25–50 mg qid
Doxylamine	Ethanolamine	++++	6	7.5–12.5 mg qid
Phenyltoloxamine	Ethanolamine	++++	4–8	7.5–25 mg tid
Tripelennamine	Ethylenediamine	+++	4–6	25–50 mg qid
Promethazine	Phenothiazine	++++	4–6	12.5–25 mg qid
Trimeprazine	Phenothiazine	++++	4–6	2.5 mg qid
Buclizine	Piperazine	++	4–6	50 mg bid
Cetirizine	Piperazine	+	12	5–10 mg qid
Hydroxyzine	Piperazine	++	6–8	25 mg qid
Levocetirizine	Piperazine	0	24	5 mg daily
Meclizine	Piperazine	++	6–8	25 mg tid
Azatadine	Piperidine	+	12	1–2 mg bid
Desloratadine	Piperidine	0	24	5 mg daily
Fexofenadine	Piperidine	+	12	60 mg bid
Loratadine	Piperidine	+	8–12	10 mg daily

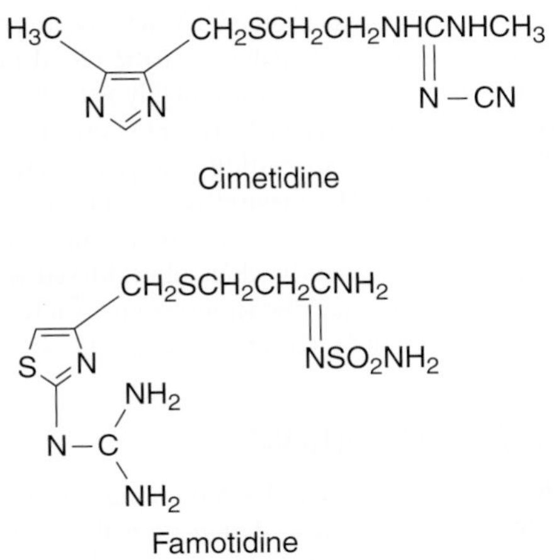

H_3C — $CH_2SCH_2CH_2NHCNHCH_3$ (=N–CN)

Cimetidine

$CH_2SCH_2CH_2CNH_2$ (=NSO_2NH_2); N–C(NH_2)(NH_2)

Famotidine

FIGURE 50–2. Structures of H_2 receptor antagonists.

Reports on the effect of H_2 antihistamines on ethanol metabolism yield conflicting results. Definitive studies have not been performed, but at this time any effect at clinically relevant doses of alcohol appears insignificant.[31] Questions remain regarding the effect of H_2 antagonist induced accelerated gastric emptying time on ethanol kinetics as well as their effects on gastric alcohol dehydrogenase and hepatic cytochromes. Interindividual variability of the effects of H_2 antagonists on ethanol metabolism and the magnitude of the effect caused by different H_2 antagonists remain to be elucidated.[31,76]

PHARMACOKINETICS AND TOXICOKINETICS

H_1 Receptor Antagonists The antihistamines are generally well absorbed following oral administration, and most achieve peak plasma concentrations within 2–3 hours. Although less well studied, dermal absorption appears to be consequential, especially with extensive or prolonged application to abnormal skin.[60] The maximum antihistaminic effect

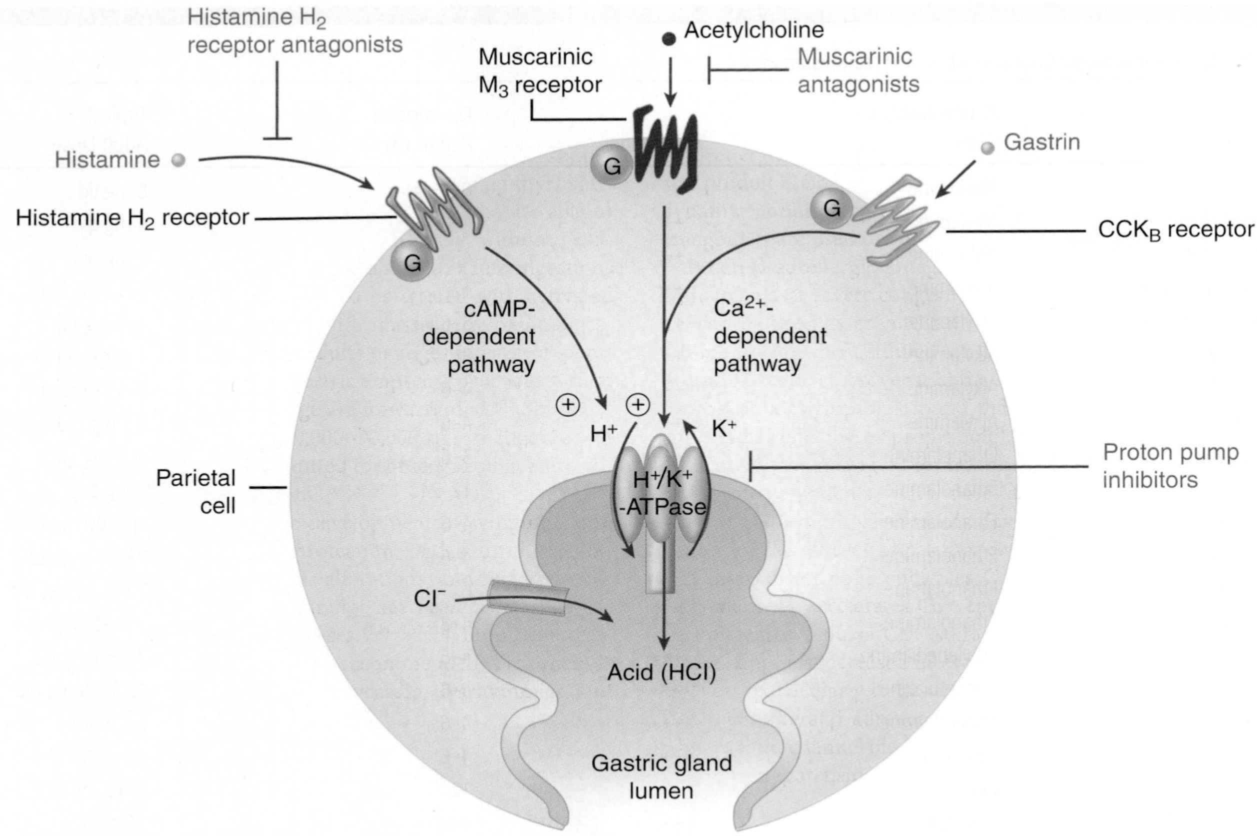

FIGURE 50–3. Schematic representation of a gastric parietal cell demonstrating the mechanism of hydrogen ion secretion into the lumen. Gastric acid is modulated by both calcium-dependent and cyclic adenosine monophosphate (cAMP)-dependent pathways. Histamine binding to the H_2 receptor increases gastric acidity by increasing cAMP. Both acetylcholine and gastrin increase gastric acidity by increasing the influx of calcium. Acetylcholine binds at the muscarinic$_3$ (M_3) receptor, whereas gastrin binds at the cholecystokinin B (CCK_B) receptor.

occurs several hours after peak serum concentrations. The duration of action ranges from 3 hours to 24 hours, which is much longer than predicted from the serum elimination half-lives of the antihistamines. Hepatic metabolism is the primary route of metabolism for antihistamines.[63] Many Asian patients can acetylate therapeutic concentrations of diphenhydramine to a nontoxic metabolite twice as rapidly as Caucasian patients, making Asians much less sensitive to both the psychomotor and sedative effects.[74] Alterations in usual dosages may be required for patients taking other medications, those with hepatic or renal dysfunction, the young, and the elderly. Such modifications often must be made empirically because formal studies and recommendations for many agents are lacking. In a recent study, desloratidine doses of 1 and 1.25 mg in children between the ages of 6 months and 2 years were found to provide a single dose target exposure (AUC) comparable with that experienced by adults receiving the recommended 5 mg dose.[31] Recognized pharmacokinetic drug interactions involving the H_1 antihistamines are generally caused by modulation of CYP450 metabolism (most often CYP2D6 or CYP3A4), or via interference with active transport mechanisms such as P-glycoprotein or organic anion transporter polypeptide (OATP).[4,70] The currently available second-generation H_1 antihistamines undergo fewer clinically relevant pharmacokinetic interactions than the first-generation H_1 antihistamines.

H_2 Receptor Antagonists Cimetidine is the prototypical H_2 receptor antagonist. Cimetidine is rapidly and completely absorbed following oral administration. Cimetidine has a volume of distribution of approximately 2 L/kg, with 13%–25% protein binding.[1] Up to 75% of cimetidine is eliminated unchanged in the urine, 15% is metabolized by the liver, and 10% is eliminated unchanged in the stool. The elimination half-life in patients with normal renal function is approximately 2 hours, but the half-life is substantially prolonged with impaired renal function.[1] Cimetidine is responsible for numerous drug–drug interactions because it can inhibit cytochrome P450 activity, thereby impairing hepatic drug metabolism. It can reduce hepatic blood flow, resulting in decreased clearance of drugs that are highly extracted by the liver. None of the other currently available H_2 receptor antagonists inhibit the cytochrome P450 oxidase system.[59] Additionally, by altering gastric pH, cimetidine and all the other H_2 antagonists may alter the absorption of acid-labile xenobiotics. Finally, cimetidine and ranitidine are associated with myelosuppression particularly when administered with xenobiotics capable of causing bone marrow suppression.[2] Table 50–4 lists the pharmacologic properties of H_2 receptor antagonists.

CLINICAL MANIFESTATIONS

H_1 Receptor Antagonists Although dry mouth and mydriasis are common adverse therapeutic effects, sedation is of the greatest concern. Therapeutic antihistamine use has been described by investigators to be as incapacitating as ethanol intoxication when operating motor

TABLE 50–4. Pharmacology of Histamine H_2 Receptor Antagonists

Drug	Typical Adult Dose (mg)	Half-Life (hours)	Urinary Elimination (%)
Cimetidine	800	2.0	62
Ranitidine	300	2.1	69
Nizatidine	300	1.3	61
Famotidine	40	2.6	67

vehicles.[33] Compared with adults, children may more commonly present with excitation and irritability and may be more prone to hallucinations and seizures. Chlorpheniramine is both a serotonin reuptake inhibitor and a postsynaptic 5-HT_{1A} receptor agonist.[45] Agonism of 5-HT_{1A} receptors has been associated with seizures. Though uncommon, metabolic acidosis followed by seizure has resulted from abuse of a chlorpheniramine-containing cold medication.[61]

The clinical manifestations of H_1 antihistamine overdose are largely extensions of their therapeutic and adverse effects. Following overdose with a first-generation H_1 antihistamine, patients typically present with CNS depression and an anticholinergic syndrome (Chap. 3). Findings typically include mydriasis, tachycardia, hyperthermia, dry mucous membranes, urinary retention, diminished bowel sounds, and altered mental status including disorientation and hallucinations (Table 50–3). The skin may appear flushed, warm, and dry. Hyperthermia correlates with the extent of agitation, ambient temperature and humidity, and length of time during which the patient cannot dissipate heat because of anticholinergic-mediated reduction in sweating.

Some patients with high therapeutic dosing or following overdose develop the central anticholinergic syndrome, in which CNS anticholinergic effects, such as hallucinations, outlast peripheral anticholinergic effects. At a later stage of ingestion the lack of tachycardia, skin changes, or other peripheral anticholinergic manifestations complicates obtaining the correct diagnosis for antihistamine-poisoned patients unless there is a clear exposure history.[29,83] Ingestion of second-generation H_1 antihistamines usually does not result in significant CNS depression or anticholinergic effects.

Cardiotoxicity associated with terfenadine and astemizole may result from accumulation of drug in cardiac tissue after inhibition of drug elimination (eg, terfenadine–ketoconazole interaction) and may be exacerbated by electrolyte (eg, Ca^{2+}) imbalances or concomitant use of another ion channel blocker.[6,35] Newer second-generation H_1 antihistamines are less dysrhythmogenic.

In a review of 136 patients with diphenhydramine overdose, somnolence, lethargy, or coma occurred in approximately 55% of patients, whereas 15% experienced a catatonic stupor.[49] Several reports suggest that young children experience more respiratory complications, CNS stimulation, anticholinergic effects, and seizures than do adult patients.[62] In a placebo-controlled study comparing the CNS effects of first- and second-generation H_1 antihistamines, the second-generation antihistamines caused less cognitive dysfunction and somnolence.[16,36] Results of a study of 100 patients in a sample of 2074 antihistamine users reporting excessive daytime sleepiness after use of H_1 antihistamines (predominantly chlorpheniramine) suggest that the presence of the CYP2D6*10 allele is a risk factor for development of H_1 antihistamine–induced ADEs.[67] A retrospective review of 146 adults and children found that cetirizine overdose is relatively free of CNS or cardiotoxicity when compared with older generation H_1 antagonists.[75] This finding was corroborated in the simulated driving model, in which loratadine produced significantly less impairment than diphenhydramine.[33] Use of diphenhydramine compared with loratadine in a work setting results in significantly higher injury rates.[25]

Sinus tachycardia is a consistent finding following overdose with an H_1 antihistamine with anticholinergic effects. Both hypotension and hypertension may occur.[56] These findings probably relate more to the patient's age, volume status, and vascular tone than to a specific class of antihistamines. As a result of sodium channel blockade following a large diphenhydramine overdose, prolongation of both the QRS complexes and QT intervals may occur.[43,68,79] Of note, postmortem findings are generally limited to pulmonary and visceral edema, suggesting cardiogenic causes of death.[46]

Mydriasis develops at both therapeutic and toxic doses, with most patients describing blurred vision and/or diplopia. Both vertical and horizontal nystagmus may occur in patients with diphenhydramine overdose. Other CNS effects include seizures, hallucinations, acute extrapyramidal movement disorders,[24] and psychoses.

Rhabdomyolysis can occur in patients with extreme agitation or seizures following an H_1 antihistamine overdose.[27] Rhabdomyolysis is commonly noted in patients who overdose with doxylamine, even in the absence of trauma or any of the other common etiologies such as seizures, shock, or crush injuries.[41,50,54] The mechanism remains undefined. A prospective study found that 87% of patients who ingested more than 20 mg/kg of doxylamine developed rhabdomyolysis, and this dose was the best predictor of this complication.[41] Rhabdomyolysis is reported as a rare adverse event following diphenhydramine overdose.[22]

Topical application of some antihistamines, particularly to children with skin lesions such as varicella, may produce classic systemic anticholinergic toxicity.[60] Promethazine and other H_1 antihistamines are associated with sudden infant death syndrome, although causality is not yet proven.[64] Cetirizine, a second-generation H_1 antihistamine, is suggested as safer for infant use, but further study is warranted.[71] Other adverse effects include pancytopenia and jaundice.

Elderly patients are more susceptible to adverse events because renal and hepatic dysfunction, which are more common in the elderly, delay antihistamine metabolism.[36] Several infants who died of diphenhydramine overdose had serum concentrations lower than expected for fatality in adults suggesting a reduced threshold for toxicity.[3] All H_1 antihistamines cross the placenta, and some are teratogenic in animals. First- and second-generation agents fall into FDA categories B and C and should be individually addressed, avoiding or minimizing exposure when possible (see Chap. 30). Because of their antimuscarinic effects, first-generation antihistamines are generally contraindicated in patients with glaucoma or benign prostatic hypertrophy.

Rare effects include fixed-drug rash, urticaria, photosensitivity, hyperthermia, transaminitis, or agranulocytosis.

H_2 Receptor Antagonists Acute toxic effects appear to be extremely rare, even after large (20 g) oral ingestions of H_2 receptor antagonists.[40] Patients may develop tachycardia, dilated and sluggishly reactive pupils, slurred speech, and confusion.[73,80] Bradycardia, hypotension, and cardiac arrest follow rapid intravenous administration of cimetidine in seriously ill patients.[69] Famotidine and ranitidine produce even fewer dose-related toxicities in overdose. In addition, they are less likely than cimetidine to induce or inhibit the cytochrome P450 enzyme system, thereby producing fewer drug–drug interactions.[38]

MANAGEMENT

Patients who will develop severe complications may be initially indistinguishable from those who will have a benign course. The patient's vital signs and mental status must be monitored. The individual should be attached to a cardiac monitor and observed for signs of sodium channel blockade (increased QRS complex duration), potassium channel blockade (prolonged QT interval), and related dysrhythmias, as well as for seizures. Assessment of the serum acetaminophen concentration is important because many analgesics and cough and cold products contain acetaminophen. Other laboratory studies should be obtained as indicated by history or physical signs and symptoms, such as creatine kinase in patients with seizures or doxylamine overdose. Measurement of antihistamine concentrations in body fluid is not readily available and is generally unnecessary for clinical assessment and management. Serum pregnancy tests should be obtained after ingestions by women of childbearing age.

Gastrointestinal decontamination should be undertaken with care to avoid aspiration. The use of oral activated charcoal, while effective if administered immediately, may be considered even after a short delay.[30] Orogastric lavage is rarely indicated except in patients presenting rapidly after a massive overdose of a first-generation H_1 antihistamine. Serial assessments of the patient's vital signs, particularly temperature, and mental status should be made. The potential for clinical deterioration necessitates management of symptomatic patients in a monitored environment.

SPECIFIC THERAPY

H_1 Receptor Antagonists Hypotension generally responds to isotonic fluids (0.9% sodium chloride solution or lactated Ringer solution). If the desired increase in blood pressure is not attained, dopamine or norepinephrine can be titrated to achieve an acceptable blood pressure. In one instance, cardiogenic shock and myocardial depression resulting from a 10-g ingestion of pyrilamine maleate could only be reversed with an intraaortic balloon counterpulsation device.[28] This approach is a rarely needed but potentially useful intervention. Agitation, psychosis, or seizure generally responds readily to titration of a benzodiazepine such as diazepam or lorazepam. Cooling via evaporative methods (tepid mist via spray bottle or similar device; fan) is generally sufficient, but patients with severe hyperthermia should receive more rapid cooling using an ice bath. Hyperthermic patients should be monitored for development of disseminated intravascular coagulation and other complications. Seizures should be treated with an intravenous benzodiazepine such as lorazepam 1–2 mg (0.05–0.1 mg/kg in children) or diazepam 10 mg (0.2–0.5 mg/kg in children) with repeated dosing as necessary. Recurrent seizures refractory to the benzodiazepine should be treated with propofol or general anesthesia. In addition, proper fluid management and urinary alkalinization may be necessary to prevent myoglobin-induced nephrotoxicity.

The sodium channel–blocking (type IA antidysrhythmic) properties of diphenhydramine and other antihistamines may lead to wide-complex dysrhythmias that resemble those that occur after cyclic antidepressant overdose (Chap. 73). Hypertonic sodium bicarbonate may reverse diphenhydramine or other antihistamine-associated conduction abnormalities[68] (see Antidote in Depth A5: Sodium Bicarbonate). Type IA (quinidine, procainamide, disopyramide), IC (flecainide), and III (amiodarone, sotalol) antidysrhythmics are contraindicated because of their capacity to prolong the QT interval.

Physostigmine may effectively reverse the peripheral or central anticholinergic syndrome if clinically indicated. In a retrospective comparison of physostigmine and benzodiazepines, physostigmine was found to be safer and more effective for treating anticholinergic agitation and delirium.[9] Physostigmine can reverse both peripheral and central anticholinergic effects. Contraindications to physostigmine use include wide QRS complexes or bradycardia noted by electrocardiography, asthma, and pulmonary disease.

The primary benefits of physostigmine use in patients with antihistamine overdose include restoration of gastrointestinal motility, elimination of agitation, and possible obviation of the need for CT scan or lumbar puncture if the patient regains a normal mental status and can provide a clear history. The anticipated benefits of physostigmine must outweigh the potential risks prior to its use.

Prior to administering physostigmine, the patient should be attached to a cardiac monitor, and secure intravenous access should be established. Physostigmine (1–2 mg in adults; 0.5 mg in children) should be administered by *slow* intravenous push with continuous monitoring of vital signs, electrocardiogram, breath sounds, and oxygen saturation by pulse oximetry. The initial dose of physostigmine can be repeated at 5- to 10-minute intervals if anticholinergic symptoms are not reversed and cholinergic symptoms such as salivation, diaphoresis, bradycardia, lacrimation, urination, or defecation do not develop. When improvement occurs as a result of physostigmine, readministration of physostigmine at 30- to 60-minute intervals may be necessary. Alternatively, sedation with benzodiazepines may be preferable once the diagnosis is confirmed. A dose of intravenous atropine that is half the dose of physostigmine should be available at the patient's bedside to treat cholinergic toxicity if it occurs (Antidotes in Depth A12: Physostigmine Salicylate).

H_2 Receptor Antagonists Patients who overdose on an H_2 antihistamine in general require no formal gastrointestinal decontamination given their uniformly good outcome. Administration of oral activated charcoal 1 g/kg is acceptable, particularly if co-ingestants are suspected. Monitoring for uncommon complications and assessment for co-ingestants, particularly acetaminophen, should be performed as clinically indicated.

DECONGESTANTS

HISTORY AND EPIDEMIOLOGY

Decongestants are sympathomimetics that act on α-adrenergic receptors, producing vasoconstriction, shrinking swollen mucous membranes, and improving bronchiolar air movement. Ephedrine, the first xenobiotic of this class to be used pharmaceutically, is derived from *Ephedra* spp plants. Ephedrine was used in China for at least 2000 years before it was introduced into Western medicine in 1924. Phenylephrine was introduced into clinical medicine in the 1930s (see Fig. 50–4). Several topical imidazoline decongestants have since been developed for clinical use.

Despite many years of widespread decongestant use in the United States and sporadic case reports of adverse effects, the magnitude and public health significance of adverse effects of this class of medications has only recently been appreciated. Premarketing studies of medications lack the power to detect rare adverse effects. Since 1969, 22 spontaneous reports of hemorrhagic stroke associated with phenylpropanolamine use were received by the FDA. Additionally, over

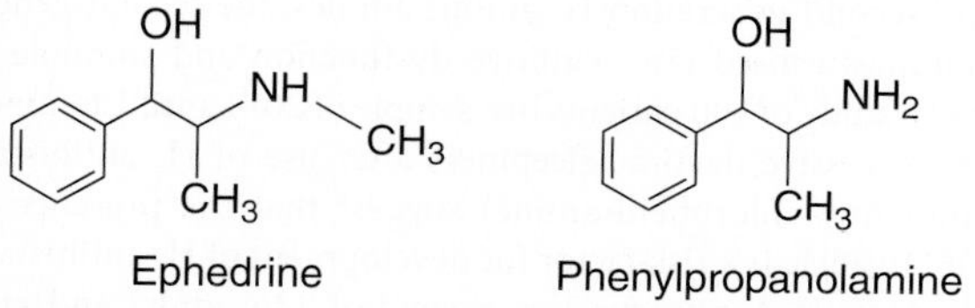

OH NH CH_3 CH_3 Ephedrine

OH NH_2 CH_3 Phenylpropanolamine

FIGURE 50–4. Structures of ephedrine and phenylpropanolamine.

30 cases were reported in the literature since 1979. Statistical analysis published in 2000 confirmed that PPA is an independent risk factor for hemorrhagic stroke in women.[48] The FDA recommended removal of phenylpropanolamine (PPA) from the market in 2000 due to its association with intracranial hemorrhages. Many manufacturers took steps to remove or reformulate PPA-containing products well before the FDA's rulemaking process could be completed.

Recreational use of ephedrine-containing stimulants is common, and combinations of these xenobiotics with caffeine or other herbs may be marketed as "herbal ecstasy" (Chap. 39). The sale of dietary supplements containing Ephedra (ephedrine alkaloids) was banned by the FDA in 2004 because of concerns over their cardiovascular effects, including hypertension, seizures, stroke, and dysrhythmias.[32] Xenobiotics that contain chemically synthesized ephedrine, traditional Chinese herbal remedies, and herbal teas are not covered by the rule.[26]

In children, intentional and unintentional exposures to cough and cold medicines are common with approximately 10% of US children taking a decongestant, antitussive, expectorant or a combination medication in any week,[81] probably driven by caregivers' desire to improve comfort and sleep for those under their care and for themselves as well. Popular mythology suggests that expectorants or decongestants will depress cough and relieve congestion while antihistamines will promote sleep. In reality, these medications have not been shown to be effective and increase the frequency of adverse events related to exposure. In an effort to retain selected drugs on the nonprescription market, the FDA developed a nonprescription monograph rule allowing some medications in use before 1972 to remain on the market without new clinical trials. As such, many nonprescription decongestants, antihistamines, and expectorants have remained available for children, without adequate safety or efficacy data in those under the age of 6 years. More recently, decongestants and cough and cold medicines have come under scrutiny.[15] Despite their widespread use, reviews of nonprescription medications for cough in adults and children by the Cochrane Collaboration in 2008 found no evidence for the effectiveness of non prescription medications in acute cough.[72] Conclusions are similar regarding the use of antihistamines or decongestants in otitis media.[14] It has also been suggested that the majority of any perceived benefit of cough suppressants may be due to sensory impact of sweetness and the placebo effect.[20]

In one study, three deaths in children under 2 years of age were associated with the use of cough and cold medications resulting in high pseudoephedrine concentrations. Additional nonfatal adverse events also occurred in the children during that study period.[12] In another study postmortem analysis of unexpected infant fatalities yielded ten deaths (ages 17 days to 10 months) associated with the use of cough and cold medicines.[66] In response to new information and concerns, the FDA has taken enforcement action to stop the production of unapproved medications and has required labeling changes on other medications aimed toward young children.

PHARMACOLOGY AND PHARMACOKINETICS

Decongestants are pharmacologically active following topical or oral administration. Absorption from the gastrointestinal tract is rapid, with peak blood concentrations occurring within 2–4 hours of ingestion. Oral decongestants can affect the cardiovascular, urinary, central nervous, and endocrine systems. The decongestants phenylephrine, pseudoephedrine, ephedrine, and phenylpropanolamine reduce nasal congestion by stimulating the α-adrenergic receptor sites on vascular smooth muscle.[42] This process constricts dilated arterioles and reduces blood flow to engorged nasal vascular beds. The α_1-adrenergic-mediated decrease in volume ultimately lowers resistance to airflow. Prolonged topical administration may produce rebound congestion upon discontinuation; possible mechanisms include desensitization of receptors and mucosal damage. This damage is thought to be caused by α_2-adrenergic-mediated arteriolar constriction resulting in decreased nutritional supply to the mucosa. Therefore, selective α_1-adrenergic agonists may cause less mucosal damage.

Phenylephrine is a powerful $\alpha_{1,2}$-adrenergic receptor agonist with very little β-adrenergic agonist activity. Pseudoephedrine and ephedrine are mixed-acting (Idirect and indirect) nonspecific $\alpha_{1,2}$- and $\beta_{1,2}$-adrenergic receptor agonists. Pseudoephedrine is the D-isomer of ephedrine and has only 25% of the adrenergic receptor activity of ephedrine.[19] Phenylpropanolamine is an $\alpha_{1,2}$-adrenergic receptor stimulant devoid of β-adrenergic receptor activity. Phenylpropanolamine can directly stimulate $\alpha_{1,2}$ receptors and can indirectly stimulate these receptors by causing norepinephrine release (Table 50–5).

The imidazoline (I) category of sympathomimetics is generally reserved for topical application and the imidazolines are used for their local effects in the nasal passages and the eye. The more common medications include oxymetazoline hydrochloride, tetrahydrozoline hydrochloride, and naphazoline hydrochloride (Fig. 50–5). The imidazolines are rapidly absorbed from the gastrointestinal tract and mucous membranes. The elimination half-lives range from 2 to 4 hours. Their vasoconstrictor effects are mediated by their actions as α-adrenergic agonists, with binding to α_2 receptors on blood vessels. The α_1-mediated vasoconstriction is complemented by an additive effect of preferential binding to α_2 receptors located on resistance vessels regulating blood flow. In addition, these medications show high affinity for imidazoline receptors, which are located in the ventrolateral medulla and some peripheral tissues. Stimulation of imidazoline receptors produces a sympatholytic effect that results in bradycardia and hypotension. All imidazoline preparations have a relatively rapid onset of action, with 60% of maximum effectiveness after only 20 minutes. Oxymetazoline is the only medication with a duration of action more than 8 hours. The other preparations have an average duration of action of approximately 4 hours.

The imidazoline decongestants such as oxymetazoline and naphazoline are pure central and peripheral α_2-adrenergic receptor agonists; tetrahydrozoline stimulates α_2 receptors and H_2 receptors. These medications are primarily used as nasal decongestants. Tetrahydrozoline is available without a prescription as an ophthalmic preparation to decrease conjunctival injection.

TABLE 50–5. Pharmacologic Characteristics of Decongestants

Decongestant	Class	Duration of Action	Receptor Activity
Naphazoline	Imidazoline (I)	8 h	α_2, and I
Oxymetazoline	Imidazoline	6–7 h	α_2, and I
Tetrahydrozoline	Imidazoline	4–8 h	α_2, and I
Xylometazoline	Imidazoline	5–6 h	α_2, and I
Ephedrine	Sympathomimetic	3–5 h	$\alpha_{1,2}$ and $\beta_{1,2}$
Phenylephrine	Sympathomimetic	1 h	$\alpha_{1,2}$
Phenylpropanolamine	Sympathomimetic	12 h (sustained release)	$\alpha_{1,2}$
Pseudoephedrine	Sympathomimetic	3–4 h	$\alpha_{1,2}$ and $\beta_{1,2}$

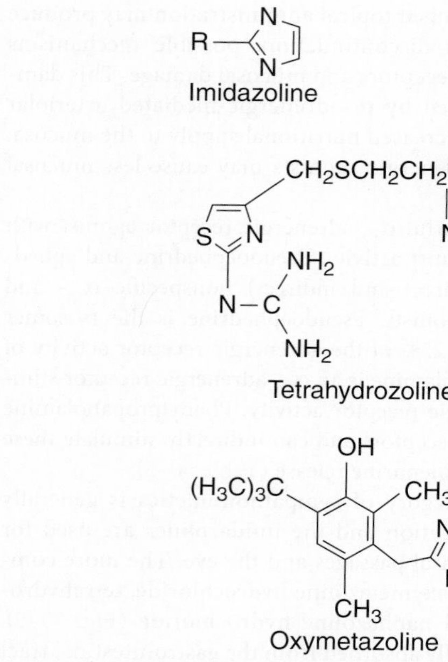

FIGURE 50–5. Structures of imidazoline and the imidazoline decongestants, tetrahydrozoline, and oxymetazoline.

DRUG OVERDOSE

CLINICAL MANIFESTATIONS

Following a decongestant overdose, most patients present with CNS stimulation, hypertension, tachycardia, or reflex bradycardia (in response to pure α_1-adrenergic agonist-induced hypertension only). Approximately 4–5 times the recommended dose of pseudoephedrine,[19] but less phenylpropanolamine, may be required to cause hypertension.[21] An increase in sinus dysrhythmias is reported in adults with ingestion of 120 mg pseudoephedrine and moderate exercise.[7] Headache was the most common initial symptom (39%) reported by patients who later developed severe toxicity.[51] In 45 patients who developed hypertensive encephalopathy from phenylpropanolamine ingestion, 24 patients developed intracranial hemorrhages, 15 developed seizures, and 6 died.[51] Seizures, myocardial infarction, bradycardia, atrial and ventricular dysrhythmias, ischemic bowel infarction, and cerebral hemorrhages are reported, even with therapeutic dosing.[10,23,57] In a review of 500 reports of adverse reactions from patients who had ingested ephedrine and associated stimulants as dietary supplements, 8 fatalities from myocardial infarction and cerebral hemorrhage were reported.[11] Symptoms of toxicity from decongestants usually resolve within 8–16 hours. However, symptoms may persist for more than 24 hours if a sustained-release product is ingested. Little organized information is available regarding the use of decongestants by those with hypertension; these agents are best avoided in patients with hypertension.

When ingested, the imidazoline decongestants naphazoline, oxymetazoline, tetrahydrozoline, and xylometazoline are potent central and peripheral α_2-adrenergic and imidazoline receptor agonists. In overdose, they can cause CNS depression, and initial brief hypertension followed by hypotension, bradycardia, and respiratory depression.[34] Children are particularly sensitive to the effects of the imidazoline decongestants.

MANAGEMENT

Extreme agitation, seizures, tachycardia, hypertension, and psychosis should initially be treated with administration of oxygen and intravenous benzodiazepines, expeditiously titrated upward to effect. A patient who remains hypertensive or is believed to have chest pain of ischemic origin (ECG indicated) should be treated with phentolamine, an α-adrenergic antagonist, or nicardipine, but β-adrenergic antagonists should be avoided due to concern for unopposed α-adrenergic effects.

A patient with a focal neurologic deficit or an abnormal neuropsychiatric examination following decongestant ingestion should be evaluated for cerebral hemorrhage by noncontrast head CT scan and, if indicated, subsequent lumbar puncture to exclude subarachnoid hemorrhage.[51]

Patients who have overdosed on a decongestant generally should receive 1 g of activated charcoal per kilogram body weight as a single dose. Activated charcoal administration may be beneficial several hours after ingestion of sustained-release decongestant preparations, and serial doses of activated charcoal may be considered in this context.

Ventricular dysrhythmias from decongestants should be treated with standard doses of lidocaine or amiodarone. Refractory dysrhythmias may require antiadrenergic therapy with propranolol, but only after pretreatment with phentolamine or another vasodilator, if possible, or with strict expectant management of the patient's blood pressure. Patients who develop hypertension following propranolol should immediately receive phentolamine. Phenylpropanolamine may cause hypertension with a reflex bradycardia and atrioventricular block that is responsive to standard doses of atropine. Atropine must be used with caution because it can cause a dangerous increase in blood pressure as the reflex bradycardia reverses. Therefore, a direct-acting vasodilator such as phentolamine is preferred because the stimulus for the bradycardia is corrected with reversal of the hypertension. Imidazoline-induced hypertension rarely requires therapy, but in the setting of symptomatic hypertension a short-acting α-adrenergic antagonist such as phentolamine may be administered.[84] However, the hypertension is generally transient and followed by hypotension that raises the risk of antihypertensive therapy.

SUMMARY

The popularity and availability of antihistamines and decongestants make them readily accessible for deliberate or unintentional ingestions in both adults and children. Recreational use of these agents may lead to exposure to substantial doses of these medications. Fortunately, nearly all patients exposed to excessive doses of members of these classes of xenobiotics that are currently available in the United States do well if they receive treatment early in the course of ingestion. While serious complications and deaths do result from exposure to these medications, nearly all exposed patients treated with activated charcoal, continuous assessment, supportive care, management of abnormal vital signs, electrocardiography, cardiac monitoring, and continuous observation of mental status generally have an excellent outcome with little risk of adverse sequelae. Familiarity with the more severe complications of antihistamine and decongestant overdoses results in early and appropriate interventions to reduce both morbidity and mortality from these exposures.

REFERENCES

1. Abate MA, Hyneck ML, Cohen IA, Berardi RR. Cimetidine pharmacokinetics. *Clin Pharm.* 1982;1:225-233.
2. Aymard JP, Aymard B, Netter P, et al. Haematological adverse effects of histamine H2-receptor antagonists. *Med Toxicol Adverse Drug Exp.* 1988;3:430-448.
3. Baker AM, Johnson DG, Levisky JA, et al. Fatal diphenhydramine intoxication in infants. *J Forensic Sci.* 2003;48:425-428.
4. Bartra J, Valero AL, del Cuvillo A, et al. Interactions of the H1 antihistamines. *J Investig Allergol Clin Immunol.* 2006;16 Suppl 1:29-36.

5. Bender BG, Berning S, Dudden R, et al. Sedation and performance impairment of diphenhydramine and second-generation antihistamines: a meta analysis. *J Allergy Clin Immunol.* 2003;111:770-776.
6. Berul CI, Morad M. Regulation of potassium channels by nonsedating antihistamines. *Circulation.* 1995(Apr 15);91(8):2220-2225.
7. Bright TP, Sandage BW Jr, Fletcher HP. Selected cardiac and metabolic responses to pseudoephedrine with exercise. *J Clin Pharmacol.* 1981;21:488-492.
8. Bronstein AC, Spyker DA, Cantilena LR Jr, et al. American Association of Poison Control Centers. 2007 Annual Report of the American Association of Poison Control Centers' National Poison Data System (NPDS). *Clin Toxicol.* 2008;46:927-1057.
9. Burns MJ, Linden CH, Graudins A, et al. A comparison of physostigmine and benzodiazepines for the treatment of anticholinergic poisoning. *Ann Emerg Med.* 2000;35:374-381.
10. Cantu C, Arauz A, Murillo-Bonilla LM, et al. Stroke associated with sympathomimetics contained in over-the-counter cough and cold drugs. *Stroke.* 2003;34:1667-1672.
11. Centers for Disease Control and Prevention. Adverse events associated with ephedrine-containing products—Texas, December 1993–September 1995. *MMWR Morb Mortal Wkly Rep.* 1996;45:689-693.
12. Centers for Disease Control and Prevention (CDC). Infant deaths associated with cough and cold medications–two states. *MMWR Morb Mortal Wkly Rep.* 2007;56:1-4.
13. Chen C, Hanson E, Watson JW, Lee JS. P-glycoprotein limits the brain penetration of nonsedating but not sedating H1-antagonists. *Drug Metab Dispos.* 2003;31:312-318.
14. Coleman C, Moore M. Decongestants and antihistamines for acute otitis media in children. *Cochrane Database Syst Rev.* 2008;3:CD001727.
15. Dart RC, Paul IM, Bond GR, et al. Pediatric fatalities associated with over the counter (nonprescription) cough and cold medications. *Ann Emerg Med.* 2009;53:411-417.
16. Day J. Pros and cons of the use of antihistamines in managing allergic rhinitis. *J Allergy Clin Immunol.* 1999;103:S395-399.
17. deAbajo FJ, Rodriguez LA. Risk of ventricular arrhythmias associated with non-sedating antihistamine drugs. *Br J Clin Pharmacol.* 1999;47:307-313.
18. Dhanya NB, Thasleem Z, Rai R, et al. Comparative efficacy of levocetirizine, desloratidine and fexofenadine by histamine wheal suppression test. *Indian J Dermatol Venereol Leprol.* 2008;74:361-363.
19. Drew CD, Knight GT, Hughes DT, Bush M. Comparison of the effects of D-(–)-ephedrine and L-(+)-pseudoephedrine on the cardiovascular and respiratory systems in man. *Br J Clin Pharmacol.* 1978;6:221-225.
20. Eccles R. Mechanisms of the placebo effect of sweet cough syrups. *Respir Physiol Neurobiol.* 2006;152:340-348.
21. Ekins BR, Spoerke DG Jr: An estimation of the toxicity of non-prescription diet aids from seventy exposure cases. *Vet Hum Toxicol.* 1983;25:81-85.
22. Emadian SM, Caravati EM, Herr RD. Rhabdomyolysis: a rare adverse effect of diphenhydramine overdose. *Am J Emerg Med.* 1996;14: 574-576.
23. Ernst ME, Hartz A. Phenylpropanolamine and hemorrhagic stroke. *N Engl J Med.* 2001;344:1094.
24. Etzel JV. Diphenhydramine-induced acute dystonia. *Pharmacotherapy.* 1994;14:492-496.
25. Finkle WD, Adams JL, Greenland S, Melmon KL. Increased risk of serious injury following an initial prescription for diphenhydramine. *Ann Allergy Asthma Immunol.* 2002;89:244-250.
26. Food and Drug Administration. Final rule declaring dietary supplements containing ephedrine alkaloids adulterated because they present an unreasonable risk. Final rule. *Fed Reg.* 2004;69:6787-6854.
27. Frankel D, Dolgin J, Murray BM. Non-traumatic rhabdomyolysis complicating antihistamine overdose. *J Toxicol Clin Toxicol.* 1993;31:493-496.
28. Freedberg RS, Friedman GR, Palu RN, Feit F. Cardiogenic shock due to antihistamine overdose. Reversal with intra-aortic balloon counter-pulsation. *JAMA.* 1987;257:660-661.
29. Garza MB, Osterhoudt KC, Rutstein R. Central anticholinergic syndrome from orphenadrine in a 3 year old. *Pediatr Emerg Care.* 2000;16:97-98.
30. Guay DR, Meatherall RC, Macaulay PA, Yeung C. Activated charcoal adsorption of diphenhydramine. *Int J Clin Pharmacol Ther Toxicol.* 1984;22:395-400.
31. Gupta AM, Baraona E, Lieber CS. Significant increase of blood alcohol by cimetidine after repetitive drinking of small alcohol doses. *Alcohol Clin Exp Res.* 1995;19:1083-1087.
32. Haller C, Benowitz NL. Adverse cardiovascular and central nervous system events associated with dietary supplements containing ephedra alkaloids. *N Engl J Med.* 2000;343:1833-1838.
33. Hennessy S, Strom BL. Nonsedating antihistamines should be preferred over sedating antihistamines in patients who drive. *Ann Intern Med.* 2000;132:405-407.
34. Higgins GL, 3rd, Campbell B, Wallace K, Talbot S. Pediatric poisoning from over-the-counter imidazoline-containing products. *Ann Emerg Med.* 1991;20:655-658.
35. Honig PK, Wortham DC, Zamani K, et al. Terfenadine-ketoconazole interaction. Pharmacokinetic and electrocardiographic consequences. *JAMA.* 1993;269:1513-1518.
36. Horak F, Stubner UP. Comparative tolerability of second-generation antihistamines. *Drug Saf.* 1999;20:385-401.
37. Huang JF, Thurmond RL. The new biology of histamine receptors. *Curr Allergy Asthma Rep.* 2008;8:21-27.
38. Humphries TJ, Merritt GJ. Drug interactions with agents used to treat acid-related diseases. *Aliment Pharmacol Ther.* 1999;13(Suppl 3):18-26.
39. Huston RL, Cypcar D, Cheng GS, Foulds DM. Toxicity from topical administration of diphenhydramine in children. *Clin Pediatr (Phila).* 1990;29:542-545.
40. Illingworth RN, Jarvie DR. Absence of toxicity in cimetidine overdosage. *Br Med J.* 1979;1:453-454.
41. Jo YI, Song JO, Park JH, Koh SY, et al. Risk factors for rhabdomyolysis following doxylamine overdose. *Hum Exp Toxicol.* 2007;26:617-621.
42. Johnson DA, Hricik JG. The pharmacology of alpha-adrenergic decongestants. *Pharmacotherapy.* 1993;13:110S-115S.
43. Joshi AK, Sljapic T, Borghei H, Kowey PR. Case of polymorphic ventricular tachycardia in diphenhydramine poisoning. *J Cardiovasc Electrophysiol.* 2004;15:591-593.
44. Jumbelic MI, Hanzlick R, Cohle S. Alkylamine antihistamine toxicity and review of Pediatric Toxicology Registry of the National Association of Medical Examiners. Report 4: Alkylamines. *Am J Forensic Med Pathol.* 1997;18:65-69.
45. Karamanakos PN. Comment: intoxication with over-the-counter antitussive medication containing dihydrocodeine and chlorpheniramine causes generalized convulsion and mixed acidosis. *Intern Med.* 2008;47:1821.
46. Karch SB: Diphenhydramine toxicity: comparisons of postmortem findings in diphenhydramine-, cocaine-, and heroin-related deaths. *Am J Forensic Med Pathol.* 1998;19:143-147.
47. Kaufman DW, Kelly JP, Rosenberg L, et al. Recent patterns of medication use in the ambulatory adult population of the United States. The Slone Survey. *JAMA.* 2002;287:337-344.
48. Kernan WN, Viscoli CM, Brass LM, et al. Phenylpropanolamine and the risk of hemorrhagic stroke. *N Engl J Med.* 2000;343:1826-1832.
49. Koppel C, Ibe K, Tenczer J. Clinical symptomatology of diphenhydramine overdose: an evaluation of 136 cases in 1982 to 1985. *J Toxicol Clin Toxicol.* 1987;25:53-70.
50. Koppel C, Tenczer J, Ibe K. Poisoning with over-the-counter doxylamine preparations: an evaluation of 109 cases. *Hum Toxicol.* 1987;6:355-359.
51. Lake CR, Gallant S, Masson E, Miller P. Adverse drug effects attributed to phenylpropanolamine: a review of 142 case reports. *Am J Med.* 1990;89:195-208.
52. Lasser KE, Allen PD, Woolhandler SJ, et al. Timing of new black box warnings and withdrawals for prescription medications. *JAMA.* 2002:287:2215-2220.
53. Leurs R, Bakker RA, Timmerman H, de Esch IJ. The histamine H3 receptor: from gene cloning to H3 receptor drugs. *Nat Rev Drug Discov.* 2005;4:107-120.
54. Leybishkis B, Fasseas P, Ryan KF. Doxylamine overdose as a potential cause of rhabdomyolysis. *Am J Med Sci.* 2001;322:48-49.
55. Litovitz TL, Klein-Schwartz W, Rodgers GC Jr, et al. Annual Report of the American Association of Poison Control Centers Toxic Exposure Surveillance System. *Am J Emerg Med.* 2002;20:391-452.
56. Llenas J, Cardelus I, Heredia A, et al. Cardiotoxicity of histamine and the possible role of histamine in the arrhythmogenesis produced by certain antihistamines. *Drug Saf.* 1999;21(Suppl 1):33-38.
57. Manini AF, Kabrhel C, Thomsen TW. Acute myocardial infarction after over-the-counter use of pseudoephedrine. *Ann Emerg Med.* 2005;45:213-216.
58. Mann RD, Pearce GL. Dunn N, et al. Sedation with "non-sedating" antihistamines: four prescription-event monitoring studies in general practice. *Br Med J.* 2000;320:1184-1187.
59. Martinez C, Albet C, Agundez JA, et al. Comparative in vitro and in vivo inhibition of cytochrome P450 CYP1A2, CYP2D6, and CYP3A by H3-receptor antagonists. *Clin Pharmacol Ther.* 1999;65:369-376.

60. McGann KP, Pribanich S, Graham JA, Browning DG. Diphenhydramine toxicity in a child with varicella. A case report. *J Fam Pract.* 1992;35:210, 213-214.
61. Murao S, Manabe H, Yamashita T, et al. Intoxication with over-the-counter antitussive medication containing dihydrocodeine and chlorpheniramine causes generalized convulsion and mixed acidosis. *Intern Med.* 2008;47:1013-1015.
62. Nine JS, Rund CR. Fatality from diphenhydramine monointoxication: a case report and review of the infant, pediatric, and adult literature. *Am J Forensic Med Pathol.* 2006;27:36-41.
63. Paton DM, Webster DR. Clinical pharmacokinetics of H1-receptor antagonists (the antihistamines). *Clin Pharmacokinet.* 1985;10:477-497.
64. Ponsonby AL, Dwyer T, Couper D. Factors related to infant apnoea and cyanosis: a population-based study. *J Paediatr Child Health.* 1997;33:317-323.
65. Pragst F, Herre S, Bakdash A. Poisonings with diphenhydramine—a survey of 68 clinical and 55 death cases. *Forensic Sci Int.* 2006 Sep 12;161(2-3): 189-197.
66. Rimsza ME, Newberry S. Unexpected infant deaths associated with use of cough and cold medications. *Pediatrics.* 2008;122:e318–22.
67. Saruwatari J, Matsunaga M, Ikeda K, et al. Impact of CYP2D6*10 on H1-antihistamine-induced hypersomnia. *Eur J Clin Pharmacol.* 2006;62: 995-1001.
68. Sharma AN, Hexdall AH, Chang EK, et al. Diphenhydramine-induced wide complex dysrhythmia responds to treatment with sodium bicarbonate. *Am J Emerg Med.* 2003;21:212-215.
69. Shaw RG, Mashford ML, Desmond PV: Cardiac arrest after intravenous injection of cimetidine. *Med J Aust.* 1980;2:629-630.
70. Simons FE: Advances in H1-antihistamines. *N Engl J Med.* 2004;351:2203-2217.
71. Simons FE, Silas P, Portnoy JM, et al. Safety of cetirizine in infants 6 to 11 months of age: a randomized, double-blind, placebo-controlled study. *J Allergy Clin Immunol.* 2003;111:1244-1248.
72. Smith SM, Schroeder K, Fahey T. Over-the-counter medications for acute cough in children and adults in ambulatory settings. *Cochrane Database Syst Rev.* 2008;(1):CD001831.
73. Sonnenblick M, Rosin AJ, Weissberg N. Neurological and psychiatric side effects of cimetidine—Report of 3 cases with review of the literature. *Postgrad Med J.* 1982;58:415-418.
74. Spector R, Choudhury AK, Chiang CK, et al. Diphenhydramine in Orientals and Caucasians. *Clin Pharmacol Ther.* 1980;28:229-234.
75. Spiller HA, Villalobos D, Benson BE, et al. Retrospective evaluation of cetirizine (Zyrtec®) ingestion. *Clin Tox.* 2002;40:525-526.
76. Stone CL, Hurley TD, Peggs CF, et al. Cimetidine inhibition of human gastric and liver alcohol dehydrogenase isoenzymes: identification of inhibitor complexes by kinetics and molecular modeling. *Biochemistry.* 1995;34:4008-4014.
77. Tagawa M, Kano M, Okamura N, et al. Neuroimaging of histamine H1-receptor occupancy in human brain by positron emission tomography (PET): a comparative study of ebastine, a second-generation anti-histamine, and (+)-chlorpheniramine, a classical antihistamine. *Br J Clin Pharmacol.* 2001;52:501-509.
78. Tashiro M, Mochizuki H, Iwabuchi K, et al. Roles of histamine in regulation of arousal and cognition: functional neuroimaging of histamine H1 receptors in human brain. *Life Sci.* 2002;72:409-414.
79. Thakur AC, Aslam AK, Aslam AF, et al. QT interval prolongation in diphenhydramine toxicity. *Int J Cardiol.* 2005;98:341-343.
80. Van Sweden B, Kamphuisen HA. Cimetidine neurotoxicity. EEG and behaviour aspects. *Eur Neurol.* 1984;23:300-305.
81. Vernacchio L, Kelly JP, Kaufman DW, et al. Pseudoephedrine use among US children, 1999-2006: results from the Slone survey. *Pediatrics.* 2008;122:1299-1304.
82. Vohora D. Histamine-selective H3 receptor ligands and cognitive functions: an overview. *IDrugs.* 2004;7:667-673.
83. Watemberg NM, Roth KS, Alehan FK, Epstein CE. Central anticholinergic syndrome on therapeutic doses of cyproheptadine. *Pediatrics.* 1999;103: 158-160.
84. Wenzel S, Sagowski C, Laux G, et al. Course and therapy of intoxication with imidazoline derivate naphazoline. *Int J Pediatr Otorhinolaryngol.* 2004;68:979-983.

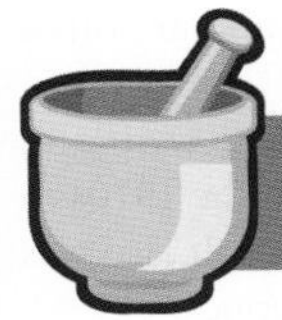

ANTIDOTES IN DEPTH (A12)

PHYSOSTIGMINE SALICYLATE

Mary Ann Howland

Physostigmine is a carbamate that reversibly inhibits cholinesterases in both the peripheral nervous system and the central nervous system (CNS).[45] The tertiary amine structure of physostigmine permits CNS penetration and differentiates it from neostigmine and pyridostigmine, from the quaternary amines that have limited ability to enter the CNS. The inhibition of cholinesterases prevents the metabolism of acetylcholine, allowing acetylcholine to accumulate and antagonize the anticholinergic effects of xenobiotics such as atropine, scopolamine,[53] and diphenhydramine. Although physostigmine previously was used as an antagonist to the anticholinergic effects of the cyclic antidepressants and the phenothiazines, this use is no longer recommended because of a poor risk-to-benefit ratio given the potential for exacerbation of life-threatening cardiotoxicity. A review of 30 years of the literature reassessed and questioned the contraindication to physostigmine use for cyclic antidepressant ingestions. The review concluded that the safety of physostigmine use for seizures or cardiotoxicity was difficult to predict, but the author still did not recommend physostigmine use in the setting of cyclic antidepressant toxicity.[44] Similarly, physostigmine has a poor risk-to-benefit ratio in the management of presumed γ-hydroxybutyrate (GHB) toxicity.[47,54] A study in rats given GHB revealed that physostigmine did not effect arousal but increased the risk of physostigmine-induced toxicities of fasciculations and seizures.[4]

Atypical antipsychotics have complex pharmacologic effects. Although some atypical antipsychotics such as olanzapine have significant antimuscarinic side effects, the benefit of treating these anticholinergic effects with physostigmine in the often confusing overdose setting must be weighed against the potential risks of exacerbating cardiotoxicity.[46,52]

HISTORY

The history of physostigmine dates to antiquity and the Efik people of Old Calabar in Nigeria.[17,20,23,45] The chiefs in this area used a poisonous concoction made from the beans of an aquatic leguminous perennial plant found in the area to deliver the *esere ordeal.* Esere was the word used to represent both the bean and the ritual used to test the innocence or guilt of an accused person. They also believed that the esere had the power to detect and kill those persons practicing witchcraft. Supposedly, innocent persons quickly swallowed the poison, which caused immediate emesis.[23] Vomiting allowed them to survive without therapy or to be given an antidote of excrement in water. The guilty, however, hesitated swallowing, leading to speculation that sublingual absorption led to severe systemic symptoms without the benefit of vomiting. These persons were noted to develop mouth fasciculations and died foaming at the mouth. Daniell, a British medical officer stationed in Calabar, brought samples of the bean and the plant back to England in 1840.[23] John Balfour, a professor of medicine and botany at the Edinburgh Medical School, is credited with characterizing the plant, which became known as *Physostigma venenosum Balfour* (family Leguminoseae) in 1857. The active alkaloid was isolated by Jobst and Hesse in 1864 and was named physostigmine. Independently, one year later Vee and Leven also isolated the active alkaloid and named it eserine.

Christison performed the first toxicologic studies, including self-experimentation with increasing doses of the seed. Fraser, Christison's student and successor, originated the concept of antagonism from his experiments with physostigmine and atropine. Fraser plotted the dose relationships between the effects of atropine versus physostigmine on various organs such as the eye and the heart, demonstrating the antidotal effects of atropine for the lethal effects of physostigmine.[17] Subsequent experiments with physostigmine led to the development of the theory of neurohumoral transmission.[20] By the 1930s physostigmine was already used as a miotic for patients with glaucoma, a treatment for myasthenia gravis, for reversal of the paralytic effects of curare, an antidote to atropine, and an insecticide.

CHEMISTRY AND AFFINITY FOR CHOLINESTERASE

Figure 113–4 shows the general formula for carbamate inhibitors. Figure A12-1A through C shows the chemical structures of physostigmine ($C_{15}H_{21}O_2N_3$), a tertiary amine, and neostigmine, a quaternary amine. Like acetylcholine, physostigmine is a substrate for the cholinesterases (choline ester hydrolases), erythrocyte acetylcholinesterase and plasma cholinesterase. Both acetylcholine and physostigmine bind to cholinesterases to form a complex. Then a part of the substrate known as the *leaving group* (ie, choline for acetylcholine) is removed, and the remaining acetylated (for acetylcholine) or carbamoylated (for physostigmine) enzyme is hydrolyzed, regenerating the enzyme and freeing the acetate or carbamate groups, respectively (Figs. 113-2 and 113-3). For acetylcholine, the process is extremely quick, with a turnover time of 150 msec. In contrast, the half-life for hydrolysis of the carbamoylated enzyme is 15 to 30 minutes.[45] The I_{50} (molar concentration that inhibits 50% of the enzyme) of physostigmine is 2.3×10^{-7} M for acetylcholinesterase, which is much weaker than for other carbamates at 1×10^{-10} M or many organic phosphorus compounds at 1×10^{-11} M.[21] Only the S-isomer inhibits cholinesterases, with plasma cholinesterase just a little more sensitive than acetylcholinesterase.[3] Newer pharmaceuticals used in patients with Alzheimer disease[11] show selectivity for the CNS and for acetylcholinesterase. They include tacrine, donepezil, and galantamine, which are reversible cholinesterase inhibitors, and rivastigmine, a pseudo-irreversible or slowly reversible inhibitor. These pharmaceuticals and neostigmine[22] have undergone limited study for reversal of anticholinergic poisoning.[11,22,26,39]

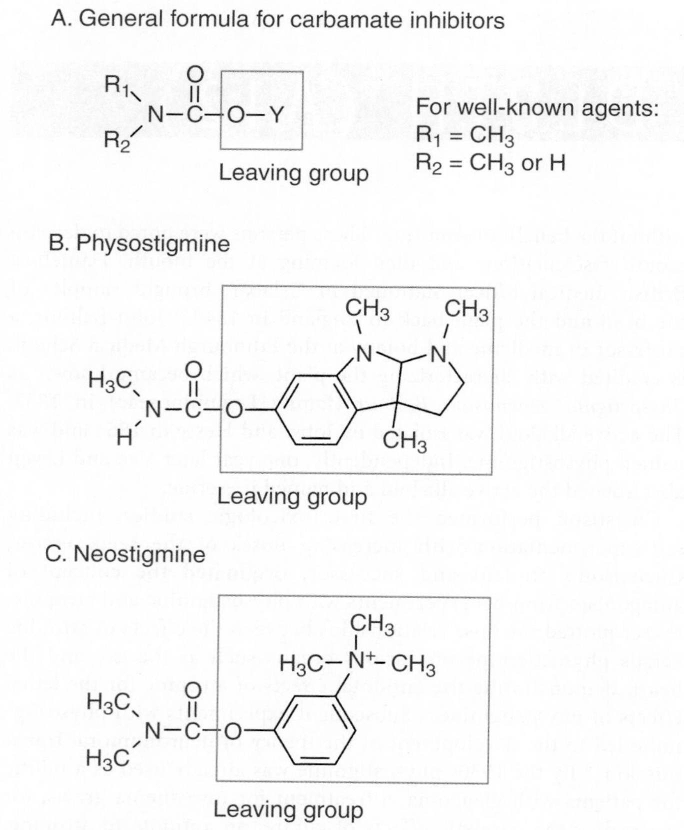

A. General formula for carbamate inhibitors

Leaving group

For well-known agents:
$R_1 = CH_3$
$R_2 = CH_3$ or H

B. Physostigmine

Leaving group

C. Neostigmine

Leaving group

FIGURE A12-1 (A) General formula for carbamate inhibitors. (B) Structure of physostigmine. (C) Structure of neostigmine.

PHARMACOKINETICS

Physostigmine is poorly absorbed orally, with a bioavailability of less than 5% to 12%.[1,31] Cholinesterases cleave the ester linkage, and very little physostigmine is eliminated unchanged in the urine. Pharmacokinetic parameters following IV administration of 1.5 mg over 60 minutes in nine patients with Alzheimer disease demonstrated the following: Vd 2.4 ± 0.6 L/kg; $t_{1/2}$ 16.4 ± 3.2 minutes; peak serum concentration 3 ± 0.5 ng/mL; clearance 0.1 L/min/kg (7.7 L/min). There was a threefold interindividual variability in plasma physostigmine concentrations. Plasma cholinesterase concentrations demonstrated inhibition within 2 minutes of initiating the physostigmine infusion. The half-life of plasma cholinesterase inhibition was 83.7 ± 5.2 minutes, with full recovery within 3 hours of termination of physostigmine infusion. The effects on plasma cholinesterase inhibition lasted approximately five times longer than the half-life of physostigmine.[25] All patients experienced varying degrees of diaphoresis, nausea, vomiting, headache, and generalized fatigue despite pretreatment with 2.5 mg methscopolamine.[2,25]

CLINICAL USE

Physostigmine was first used as an antidote in 1864 to counteract severe atropine poisoning.[33] Today its role is primarily in the treatment of antimuscarinic poisoning. More than 600 xenobiotics respond to physostigmine.[12] Anticholinergics fall into the categories of antimuscarinic (atropine, scopolamine, propantheline, benztropine, trihexyphenidyl), neuromuscular blockers (exemplified by curare), and ganglionic blockers (eg, trimethaphan). Other xenobiotics (eg, antihistamines, antipsychotics, and antidepressants) have anticholinergic properties that are not their primary therapeutic actions and are often considered adverse drug effects.

The clinical use of physostigmine has varied over time.[41] Owing to its ability to cause CNS arousal physostigmine was used in the 1970s to reverse the CNS effects of a large number of anticholinergics. It also was used inappropriately to treat toxicity from nonanticholinergics.[18,30,32,34,37] The success with regard to anticholinergics is directly antidotal by virtue of its inhibition of cholinesterase. Effects of physostigmine on xenobiotics such as the benzodiazepines, opioids,[27,38,50] and GHB[4,47] result from either acetylcholine's direct action on the reticular activating system or interdependence of central neurotransmitters.[34] Few serious adverse effects are reported.[49] However, asystole followed administration of physostigmine in two patients with tricyclic antidepressant overdose.[35] This occurrence led to the realization that toxicity from tricyclic antidepressants is complex and consists of more than just anticholinergic effects.[35] Cyclic-antidepressant-induced sodium channel blockade causes myocardial depression, QRS interval prolongation, and ventricular dysrhythmias. Physostigmine probably augments vagal effects, thus contributing to decreased cardiac output and cardiac conduction defects. A reevaluation must conclude that the risks of physostigmine use for xenobiotics that are not primarily antimuscarinic often outweigh any benefit.

This analysis appears to hold true for reversing the effects of GHB (Chap. 80) as well.[47] GHB is rarely used alone, and its effects are highly variable.[54] Recovery from GHB typically occurs spontaneously in approximately 2 hours (16 min-6 h).[7,8,14,28,47,48] Three patients in whom a presumptive diagnosis of GHB toxicity was made were treated with physostigmine.[7] The three patients had an improved mental status within 5 to 15 minutes. One of these patients relapsed and then fully awakened 40 minutes later. This patient was incontinent of feces, an adverse effect likely caused by the physostigmine.[7] A closer look at the patient descriptions reveals that all three improved with stimulation prior to physostigmine. Furthermore, justification for use based upon a study performed in the 1970s in the operating room at a time when GHB was first being evaluated as an anesthetic appears illogical when caring for those who illicitly use GHB.[19]

However, in cases of anticholinergic overdose, physostigmine use clearly is beneficial. A study of 52 patients showed that physostigmine controlled agitation and reversed delirium in 96% and 87% of patients, respectively,[6] whereas benzodiazepines controlled agitation in 24% of patients but were ineffective in reversing delirium. A shorter time to recovery following agitation was observed in those treated with physostigmine. No significant differences between these groups with regard to side effects and length of stay were noted.[6]

INDICATIONS

Indications for physostigmine use include the presence of peripheral or central anticholinergic manifestations without evidence of significant QRS or QT prolongation. Peripheral manifestations include dry mucosa, dry skin, flushed face, mydriasis, hyperthermia, decreased bowel sounds, urinary retention, and tachycardia. Central manifestations include agitation, delirium, hallucinations, seizures, and coma.[16,29] The peripheral and central findings usually occur simultaneously. In the early phases of overdose, finding only central manifestations is uncommon, although they often are more remarkable.[1,5,9,13,15,21,40,43] The central findings may persist longer than the peripheral findings, particularly when a patient is recovering from an overdose of an antimuscarinic xenobiotic.

ADVERSE EFFECTS

An excess of physostigmine results in accumulation of acetylcholine at peripheral muscarinic receptors, nicotinic receptors (skeletal muscle, autonomic ganglia, adrenal glands), and CNS sites.[24] Muscarinic effects produce stimulation of smooth muscle and glandular secretions in the respiratory, gastrointestinal, and genitourinary tracts and inhibition of contraction of most vascular smooth musculature. Nicotinic effects are stimulatory at low doses and depressant at high doses. For example, acetylcholine excess at the neuromuscular junction produces fasciculations followed by weakness and paralysis. Its effect on the CNS results in anxiety, dizziness, tremors, confusion, ataxia, coma, and seizures.[24] Electroencephalograms (EEGs) demonstrate desynchronous discharges followed by higher-voltage discharges and a pattern similar to tonic clonic seizures.[24] The cardiovascular effects are dose dependent and directly related to the presence of the diverse muscarinic and nicotinic effects.[24] In addition to its inhibition of cholinesterase, physostigmine has a direct action on the nicotinic acetylcholine receptor ionic channel.[42]

Physostigmine toxicity results when physostigmine is used in the absence of antimuscarinic toxicity or when excess is administered with regard to the antimuscarinic xenobiotic. Patients overdosed with physostigmine should be managed with intensive supportive care, including mechanical ventilation if needed, intravenous atropine[51] titrated to reverse bronchial secretions, and, rarely, pralidoxime to reverse skeletal muscle effects.[10]

Relative contraindications to physostigmine use include reversible airway disease, peripheral vascular disease, intestinal or bladder obstruction, intraventricular conduction defects, and atrioventricular block. Little information is available regarding the effects of physostigmine in pregnancy. Transient muscular weakness occurred in 10% to 20% of neonates whose mothers received anticholinesterase treatment for myasthenia gravis.[31]

Drug interactions with cholinergic agonists (eg, ophthalmic pilocarpine), depolarizing neuromuscular blockers, or other anticholinesterases such as carbamates, organic phosphorous compounds, and pyridostigmine are expected to be at least additive when taken concomitantly with physostigmine. The actions of xenobiotics metabolized by plasma cholinesterases such as cocaine, succinylcholine, or mivacurium are expected to be prolonged.

DOSING

The dose of physostigmine is 1 to 2 mg in adults and 0.02 mg/kg (maximum 0.5 mg) in children intravenously infused over at least 5 minutes. The onset of action usually is within minutes.[21] The dose can be repeated after 10 to 15 minutes if an adequate response is not achieved and muscarinic effects are not noted. Rapid administration may cause bradycardia, hypersalivation leading to respiratory difficulty, and seizures. Although the half-life of physostigmine is approximately 16 minutes, its duration of action usually is much longer (often >1 hour) and is directly related to the duration of cholinesterase inhibition.[2] After reversal of anticholinergic symptoms is achieved, additional doses may be required if clinical relapse occurs. The effective dose depends upon the ingested dose and duration of action of the antimuscarinic xenobiotic. Although a total of 4 mg in divided doses usually is sufficient in most clinical situations,[16] significant interindividual variability exists. Atropine should be available at the bedside and titrated to effect should excessive cholinergic toxicity develop. A dose of atropine administered at half the physostigmine dose is often recommended.

Physostigmine is available as an ophthalmic ointment that can be applied topically to the conjunctival sac to produce miosis as treatment of acute angle-closure glaucoma. Miosis occurs within 10 to 30 minutes and persists for 12 to 48 hours.[31]

AVAILABILITY

Physostigmine is available in 2-mL ampules, with 1 mL containing 1 mg physostigmine salicylate. The vehicle contains sodium metabisulfite and benzyl alcohol.[36]

SUMMARY

Physostigmine has been used extensively in the fields of anesthesiology, emergency medicine, and medical toxicology. The only evidence-based use of physostigmine is for the management of patients with an anticholinergic syndrome, particularly those without cardiovascular compromise who have an agitated delirium and a normal QRS duration. In this population, physostigmine has an excellent risk-to-benefit profile.

REFERENCES

1. Aquilonius S, Hartvig P: Clinical pharmacokinetics of cholinesterase inhibitors. *Clin Pharmacokinet.* 1986;11:236-249.
2. Asthana S, Greig NH, Hegedus L, et al: Clinical pharmacokinetics of physostigmine in patients with Alzheimer's disease. *Clin Pharmacol Ther.* 1995;58:299-309.
3. Atack JR, Yu Q-S, Soncrant TT, Brossi I, Rapoport SI: Comparative inhibitory effects of various physostigmine analogs against acetyl and butyrocholinesterases. *J Pharmacol Exp Ther.* 1989;249:194-202.
4. Bania TC, Chu J: Physostigmine does not effect arousal but produces toxicity in an animal model of severe -hydroxybutyrate intoxication. *Acad Emerg Med.* 2005;12:185-189.
5. Beaver KM, Gavin TJ: Treatment of acute anticholinergic poisoning with physostigmine. *Am J Emerg Med.* 1998;16:505-507.
6. Burns MJ, Linden CH, Graudins A, Brown RM, Fletcher KE: A comparison of physostigmine and benzodiazepines for the treatment of anticholinergic poisoning. *Ann Emerg Med.* 2000;35:374-381.
7. Caldicott DGE, Kuhn M: Gamma-hydroxybutyrate overdose and physostigmine: teaching new tricks to an old drug? *Ann Emerg Med.* 2001;37:99-102.
8. Chin RL, Sporer KA, Cullison B, Dyer JE, Wu TD: Clinical course of γ-hydroxy-butyrate overdose. *Ann Emerg Med.* 1998;31:716-722.
9. Crowell EB, Ketchum JS: The treatment of scopolamine-induced delirium with physostigmine. *Clin Pharmacol Ther.* 1967;8:409-414.
10. Cumming G, Harding LK, Prowse K: Treatment and recovery after massive overdose of physostigmine. *Lancet.* 1968;20:147-149.
11. Darreh-Shori T, Hellström-Lindahl E, Flores-Flores C, et al: Long-lasting acetylcholinesterase splice variations in anticholinesterase-treated Alzheimer's disease patients. *J Neurochem.* 2004;88:1102-1113.
12. Daunderer M: Physostigmine salicylate as an antidote. *Int J Clin Pharmacol Ther Toxicol.* 1980;18:523-535.
13. Duvoisin R, Katz R: Reversal of central anticholinergic syndrome in man by physostigmine. *JAMA.* 1968;206:1963-1965.
14. Eckstein M, Henderson SO, DelaCruz P, Newton E: Gamma-hydroxybutyrate (GHB): report of a mass intoxication and review of the literature. *Prehosp Emerg Care.* 1999;3:357-361.
15. El-Yousef MK, Janowsky D, Davis JM, Sekerke HJ: Reversal of antiparkinsonian drug toxicity by physostigmine: a controlled study. *Am J Psychiatry.* 1973;130:141-145.
16. Forrer GR, Miller JJ: Atropine coma—a somatic therapy in psychiatry. *Am J Psychiatry.* 1958;115:455-458.
17. Fraser TR: On the characters, action and therapeutic uses of the bean of Calabar. *Edinburgh Med J.* 1863;9:36-56; 235-245.
18. Giannini AJ, Castellani S: A case of phenylcyclohexylpyrolidine (PHP) intoxication treated with physostigmine. *J Toxicol Clin Toxicol.* 1982;19: 505-508.
19. Henderson RS, Holmes CM: Reversal of the anaesthetic action of sodium gamma-hydroxybutyrate. *Anaesth Intensive Care.* 1976;4:351-354.
20. Holmstedt BO: The ordeal bean of old Calabar: the pageant of *Physostigmine venenosum* in medicine. In: Swain T, ed. *Plants in the Development of Modern Medicine.* Cambridge, MA: Harvard University Press; 1975:303-360.
21. Holzgrate RE, Vondrell JJ, Mintz SM: Reversal of postoperative reactions to scopolamine with physostigmine. *Anesth Analg.* 1973;52:921-925.
22. Isbister GK, Oakley P, Whyte I, Dawson A: Treatment of anticholinergic-induced ileus with neostigmine. *Ann Emerg Med.* 2001;38:689-693.
23. Karczmar AG: History of the research with anticholinesterase agents. In: Karczmar AG, ed. *International Encyclopedia of Pharmacology and Therapeutics, Vol. I.* Oxford: Pergamon Press; 1970:1-44.
24. Karczmar AG: Pharmacology of anticholinesterase agents. In: Karczmar AG, ed. *International Encyclopedia of Pharmacology and Therapeutics, Vol. I.* Oxford: Pergamon Press; 1970:45, 363.

25. Knapp S, Wardlow ML, Albert K, Waters D, Thal LJ: Correlation between plasma physostigmine concentrations and percentage of acetylcholinesterase inhibition over time after controlled release of physostigmine in volunteer subjects. *Drug Metab Dispos.* 1991;19:400-404.
26. Krall WJ, Sramck JJ, Cutler NR: Cholinesterase inhibitors: a therapeutic strategy for Alzheimer disease. *Ann Pharmacother.* 1999;33:441-450.
27. Larson GF, Hurbert BJ, Wingard DW: Physostigmine reversal of diazepam-induced depression. *Anesth Analg.* 1977;56:348-351.
28. Li J, Stokes SA, Woeckener A: A tale of novel intoxication: seven cases of γ-hydroxybutyric acid overdose. *Ann Emerg Med.* 1998;31:723-728.
29. Longo VG: Behavioral and electroencephalographic effects of atropine and related compounds. *Pharmacol Rev.* 1966;18:965-996.
30. Manoguerra AS: Poisoning with tricyclic antidepressant drugs. *Clin Toxicol.* 1977;10:149-158.
31. Physostigmine sulfate. In: McEvoy CK, ed. American Hospital Formulary Service (AHFS). Bethesda, MD: American Society of Health-System Pharmacists; 2004:2705.
32. Nattel S, Bayne L, Ruedy J: Physostigmine in coma due to drug overdose. *Clin Pharmacol Ther.* 1979;25:96-102.
33. Nickalls RWD, Nickalls EA: The first use of physostigmine in the treatment of atropine poisoning. *Anesthesiology.* 1988;43:776-779.
34. Nilsson E: Physostigmine treatment in various drug-induced intoxications. *Ann Clin Res.* 1982;14:165-172.
35. Pentel P, Peterson CD: Asystole complicating physostigmine treatment of tricyclic antidepressant overdose. *Ann Emerg Med.* 1980;9:588-590.
36. Physostigmine Salicylate Injection [package insert]. Decatur, IL: Taylor Pharmaceuticals; 2006.
37. Rumack BH: 707 cases of anticholinergic poisoning treated with physostigmine [abstract]. Presented at: Annual Meeting of American Academy of Clinical Toxicology; 1975; Montreal, Quebec, Canada.
38. Rupreht J, Dworacek B, Oosthoek H, et al: Physostigmine versus naloxone in heroin overdose. *J Toxicol Clin Toxicol.* 1983-1984;21:387-397.
39. Shepherd G, Klein-Schwartz W, Edwards R: Donepezil overdose: a tenfold dosing error. *Ann Pharmacother.* 1999;33:812-815.
40. Smiler BG, Bartholomew EG, Sivak BJ, Alexander GD, Brown EM: Physostigmine reversal of scopolamine delirium in obstetric patients. *Am J Obstet.* 1973;116:326-329.
41. Smilkstein MJ: Physostigmine [editorial]. *J Emerg Med.* 1991;9:275-277.
42. Somani SM, Dube SN: Physostigmine—an overview as pretreatment drug for organophosphate intoxication. *Int J Clin Pharmacol Ther Toxicol.* 1989;27:367-387.
43. Sopchak CA, Stork CM, Cantor RM, O'Hara PE: Central anticholinergic syndrome due to Jimson Weed physostigmine: therapy revisited? *J Toxicol Clin Toxicol.* 1998;36:42-45.
44. Suchard JR: Assessing physostigmine's contraindication in cyclic antidepressant ingestions. *J Emerg Med.* 2003;25:185-191.
45. Taylor P: Anticholinesterase agents. In: Hardman JG, Limbird CE eds. *Goodman and Gilman's The Pharmacologic Basis of Therapeutics.* 10th ed. New York: McGraw-Hill; 2001:175-191.
46. Titier K, Girodet PO, Verdoux H, et al: Atypical antipsychotics: from potassium channels to torsade de pointes and sudden death. *Drug Saf.* 2005;28:35-51.
47. Traub SJ, Nelson LS, Hoffman RS: Physostigmine as a treatment for gamma-hydroxybutyrate toxicity: a review. *J Toxicol Clin Toxicol.* 2002;40:781-787.
48. Viera AJ, Yates SW: Toxic ingestion of gamma-hydroxybutyric acid. *South Med J.* 1999;92:404-405.
49. Walker WE, Levy RC, Hanenson IB: Physostigmine—its use and abuse. *JACEP.* 1976;5:436-439.
50. Weinstock M, Davidson JT, Rosin AJ, Schnieden H: Effect of physostigmine on morphine-induced postoperative pain and somnolence. *Br J Anesth.* 1982;54:429-443.
51. Weiss S: Persistence of action of physostigmine and the atropinephysostigmine antagonism in animals and in man. *J Pharmacol Exp Ther.* 1925;27:181-188.
52. Weizberg M, Su M, Mazzola J, et al: Altered mental status from olanzapine overdose treated with physostigmine. *Clin Tox.* 2006;44:319-325.
53. Young SE, Ruiz RS, Falletta J: Reversal of systemic toxic effects of scopolamine with physostigmine salicylate. *Am J Ophthalmol.* 1971;72:1136-1138.
54. Zvosec D, Smith S, Litonjua R, et al: Physostigmine for gamma-hydroxybutyrate coma: inefficacy, adverse events, and review. *Clin Tox.* 2007;l45:261-265.

CHAPTER 51
ANTIMIGRAINE MEDICATIONS

Jason Chu

A migraine headache is a neurovascular disorder often initiated by a trigger and characterized by a headache, which 20% of the time is preceded by a visual aura. The headache may be accompanied by a variety of multiple organ system symptoms, such as allodynia, nausea, vomiting and urinary frequency. There are various types of migraine, the diagnostic criteria for which have been established by the International Headache Society.[77] The types of migraine are divided into two groups: migraine without aura ("common migraine") and migraine with aura ("classic migraine"). Further subdivisions include migraine with typical aura with or without headache, familial hemiplegic migraine, sporadic hemiplegic migraine, basilar type migraine, and retinal migraine.[77] Treatment of migraines encompasses a wide variety of xenobiotics and can be broadly classified as prophylactic or abortive therapies (Table 51–1).

PATHOPHYSIOLOGY OF MIGRAINE HEADACHES

The initiation of migraines is not fully understood, but likely involves genetic abnormalities in central nervous system (CNS) ion channels that predispose sufferers to specific triggers. Patients with familial hemiplegic migraine, an autosomal dominant disorder, have missense mutations in the $\alpha 1$ subunit of brain specific P/Q voltage gated calcium channels resulting in altered function of these channels. During migraines, the upper brainstem has increased blood flow and is implicated as a "migraine generator." After activation, a wave of cortical depression spreads across the cortex from a caudal to rostral fashion followed by a spreading wave of oligemia, which can produce the auras that occur in 20% of migraineurs.[23,34,83] Current theories suggest that this spreading wave occurs in patients who do not experience visual auras and spares the visual cortex.

Cephalagia begins during vasoconstriction prior to vasodilation unlike previous vascular theory suggested prior to cerebral blood flow studies. Antidromic activation of the afferent neurons of the ophthalmic division of the trigeminal nerve and branches of the C1 and C2 nerves (first order neurons) located on dural arteries at the base of the brain releases inflammatory neuropeptides such as calcitonin gene related polypeptide, VIP and neurokinase A. Vasoactive neuropeptides, including serotonin, vasoactive intestinal peptide, nitric oxide, substance P, neurokinin A, and calcitonin gene-related peptide (CGRP), are released during this process, which exacerbates the vasodilation and irritates the meninges at the base of the brain, causing further pain. CGRP from trigeminal Aδ-fibers produces dural vasodilation, while substance P and neurokinin A from trigeminal C-fibers increase dural vessel permeability.[23,33] Pain impulses are relayed orthodromically to the trigeminal nucleus caudalis (second order neurons) in the lower medulla and upper cervical spinal cord, then to the thalamus (third order neurons) via the quintothalamic tract, and finally to higher cortical areas (fourth order neurons probably located in the limbi cortex).[23,31] The trigeminocervical complex also produces retrograde parasympathetic impulses from sphenopalatine ganglion and the superior salivatory nucleus in the pons through the pterygopalatine, otic, and carotid ganglia to the cerebral vessels.[31] abort migraines when administered intravenously, but it is too dangerous to utilize clinically. Migraineurs have increased serotonin release during migraine attacks.[23,83] Abortive and prophylactic therapy ideally target these processes (see Table 51–1). Current abortive therapies include analgesics (nonsteroidal anti-inflammatory drugs [NSAIDs], acetaminophen, opioids), antiemetics, ergots alkaloids, triptans, oxygen, magnesium sulfate and intranasal lidocaine. Triptans are considered the drugs of choice for migraine therapy. Newer therapies such as CGRP antagonists are currently in phase 2 and 3 trials.

Toxicity of many of these xenobiotics is discussed in depth elsewhere in the text (see Table 51–1).

ERGOT ALKALOIDS

HISTORY AND EPIDEMIOLOGY

Ergot is the product of *Claviceps purpurea*, a fungus that contaminates rye and other grains. The spores of the fungus are both wind borne and transported by insects to young rye, where they germinate into hyphal filaments. When a spore germinates, it destroys the grain and hardens into a curved body called the sclerotium, which remains the major commercial source of ergot alkaloids.[68] The *C. purpurea* fungus can elaborate diverse substances, including ergotamine, histamine, lysergic acid, tyramine, isomylamine, acetylcholine, and acetaldehyde.

In 600 BC, an Assyrian tablet mentioned grain contamination believed to be by *C. purpurea*. In the Middle Ages, epidemics causing gangrene of the extremities, with mummification of limbs, were depicted in the literature as blackened limbs resembling the charring from fire and caused a burning sensation expressed by its victims. The disease was called holy fire or St. Anthony's fire, but the improvement that reportedly occurred when victims went to visit the shrine of St. Anthony were probably the result of a diet free of contaminated grain on the journey.[35] Abortion and seizures were also reported to result from this poisoning. On the other hand, as early as 1582, midwives used ergot to assist in the childbirth process. In 1818, Desgranges was the first physician to use ergot for obstetric care, and in 1822 Hosack reported that ergot could be used for the control of postpartum hemorrhage.[81] Since 1950, the clinical use of ergot derivatives is almost entirely limited to the treatment of vascular headaches. Ergonovine, another ergot derivative, is used in obstetric care for its stimulant effect on uterine smooth muscle and was used in cardiac stress tests. Methylergonovine is used for postpartum uterine atony and hemorrhage. Ergot derivatives have also been used as "cognition enhancers,"[84] to help manage orthostatic hypotension,[74] and to prevent the secretion of prolactin.[68]

Currently in the United States, ergot grain infections are prevented by government inspections of grain fields. If a grain field contains more than 0.3% infected grain, it is rejected for commercial sale; in some years as much as 36% of the grain was rejected.[68] However, elsewhere in the world ergot toxicity remains a problem predominantly in animals.[7,45]

PHARMACOLOGY AND PHARMACOKINETICS

All ergot alkaloids are derivatives of the tetracyclic compound 6-methylergoline.They can be divided into three groups: amino acid alkaloids (ergotamine, ergotoxine), dihydrogenated amino acid alkaloids, and amine alkaloids (Fig. 51–1).

The pharmacokinetics of the ergot alkaloids are well defined by controlled human volunteer studies, whereas the toxicokinetics are essentially unknown (Table 51–2). Almost all of the ergots are poorly absorbed orally and there is considerable first-pass hepatic

TABLE 51–1. Xenobiotics Used in Migraine Treatment*

Prophylactic	Abortive
β adrenergic antagonists	Acetaminophen
Butterbur root	Antiemetics: metoclopramide, ondansetron, prochlorperazine
Calcium channel blockers	Aspirin
Candesartan	Butalbital
Coenzyme Q10	Caffeine
Cyclic antidepressants	Corticosteroids
Enalapril	Ergots
Feverfew	Lidocaine (intranasal)
Flunarizine	Magnesium (IV)
Gabapentin	Metoclopramide
Isometheptene/dichloraphenazone/acetaminophen (midrin)	NSAIDs
Lamotrigine	Opioids
Levetiracetam	Oxygen
Lisinopril	Sedative-hypnotics
Magnesium (oral)	Triptans
MAO inhibitors	Valproic acid
Memantine	
Nefazadone	
Onabotulinumtoxin/A (Botox A)	
Pizotifen	
Riboflavin	
Selective serotonin reuptake inhibitors	
Topiramate	
Valproic acid	

MAO, monoamine oxidase; NSAIDs, nonsteroidal anti-inflammatory drugs.

* Prophylatic xenobiotics are usually taken to prevent triggering of migraines, and abortive xenobiotics are usually taken to stop the clinical manifestations of migraines once they are triggered. However, the separation between the two groups of xenobiotics is not strict, and some xenobiotics may be used in both roles. Triptans are currently considered the drug class of choice for migraine treatment.

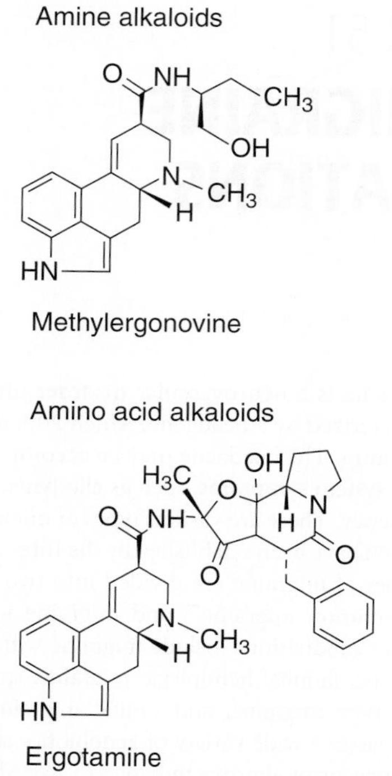

metabolism, resulting in highly variable bioavailability. Intramuscular absorption is unpredictable and actions are often delayed.[60] Peak plasma concentrations with oral ergotamine occur within 45 to 60 minutes.[60] The volume of distribution of ergotamine is approximately 2 L/kg and the half-life varies from 1.4 to 6.2 hours. Ergot alkaloids are metabolized in the liver, probably by CYP3A4, and the metabolites are excreted in the bile.[6,68]

The pharmacologic effects of the ergot alkaloids are complex and can be mutually antagonistic.[68] These actions can be subdivided into central and peripheral effects (Table 51–3). In the CNS, ergotamine stimulates serotonergic (tryptaminergic) receptors, potentiates serotonergic effects, blocks neuronal serotonin reuptake, and has central sympatholytic actions.[35,68] The ergot alkaloids interact with all known 5-HT_1 and 5-HT_2 receptor subtypes.[68] The result is increased intrasynaptic serotonin activity in the median raphe neurons of the brainstem.[65] Ergotamine and dihydroergotamine are thought to decrease the neuronal firing rate and stabilize the cerebrovascular smooth musculature, which make them useful drugs for both acute and prophylactic treatment of migraine headaches.

Amine alkaloids

Methylergonovine

Amino acid alkaloids

Ergotamine

FIGURE 51–1. Chemical structures of 2 ergot derivatives representative of the amine and amino acid alkaloids.

Peripherally, ergotamine acts as a partial α-adrenergic agonist or as an antagonist at adrenergic, dopaminergic, and serotonergic (tryptaminergic) receptors.[68] The amino acid ergot alkaloids (ergotamine, ergotoxine) exhibit α-adrenergic agonism, and dehydrogenation (dihydroergotamine) of the lysergic acid nucleus increases the potency of this effect.[68] However, the peripheral vasoconstrictive effects predominate over the α-adrenergic antagonist effects, and there may be an additional vasoconstrictive effect caused by the direct action of ergotamine on the media of the arterioles.[68] Table 51–3 summarizes the pharmacologic actions of selected ergot alkaloids currently used in clinical medicine. The spectrum of effects depends on dosage, host response, and physiologic conditions.

The clinical effects following overdose are an extension of the therapeutic effects. At toxic doses, extreme vasoconstriction produces the characteristic ischemic changes that occur in ergotism.

The cerebrovascular effects of ergot alkaloids are not as clearly understood. In migraine treatment, for example, therapeutic doses of ergotamine produce mild vasoconstriction via α-adrenergic agonism. This may be more pronounced in intracranial vessels that are already dilated during a migraine. In toxic doses cephalic vasodilation may occur, but the mechanism for this effect is unknown. One hypothesis is that toxic doses of the drug initially produce cerebral vasoconstriction and ischemia, just as it does in the periphery, but since the cerebral vasculature cannot tolerate hypoxia and hypercapnia, rapid vasodilation then ensues to improve local perfusion. Also α-adrenergic receptors in the CNS function differently from those in the periphery, and it may be that CNS vascular tone cannot be maintained in the setting of local tissue hypoxia.

CLINICAL MANIFESTATIONS

Ergotism, a toxicologic syndrome resulting from excessive use of ergot alkaloids, is characterized by intense burning of the extremities, hemorrhagic vesiculations, pruritus, formications, nausea, vomiting,

TABLE 51–2. Pharmacokinetics of Ergots

Ergot Derivative	Clinical Use	t ½ (hours)	Duration of Action (hours)	Bioavailability (%)	Metabolism/ Elimination
Bromocriptine	Parkisonism, amenorrhea/ prolactinemia syndrome	60 (PO)	1 week (suppression of prolactin)	28 (PO)	Liver
Dihydroergotamine	Migraine	2.4	3–4 (IM)	100 (IM) 40 (Nasal) <5 (PO)	Liver metabolism Bile excretion
Ergonovine	Testing for coronary vasospastic angina	1.9	3	?	Liver
Ergotamine	Migraine	2 (1.4–6.2)	22 (IV)	100 (IV) 47 (IM) <5 (PO)	Liver metabolism Bile excretion
Methylergonovine	Postpartum hemorrhage	1.4–2.0	3	78 (IM) 60 (PO)	Liver
Methysergide	Migraine	1 (PO)	–	13 (PO)	Liver–metabolized to methylergonovine

and gangrene (Table 51–4). Headache, fixed miosis, hallucinations, delirium, cerebrovascular ischemia, and convulsions are also associated with this condition, which has been called "convulsive" ergotism.[35] Chronic ergotism usually presents with peripheral ischemia of the lower extremities, although ischemia of cerebral, mesenteric, coronary, and renal vascular beds are well documented.[3,24,25,66,67] Ergotism can also result from interactions of ergot derivatives with P450 CYP3A4 inhibitors such as macrolide antibiotics and protease inhibitors, which increase the area under the curve (AUC) of ergots.[5,6]

The vascular effects ascribed to ergot alkaloids are complex and sometimes conflicting (see Table 51–3). Subintimal and medial fibrosis, vasospasm, and arteriolar and venous thrombi (stasis related) are all reported.[52] Angiography can demonstrate distal, segmental vessel spasm with increased collateralization in patients with chronic

TABLE 51–3. Pharmacology of Ergot Derivatives

Ergot Derivative	Interactions With Tryptaminergic (Serotonergic) Receptors	Interactions with Dopaminergic Receptors	Interactions With α-Adrenergic Receptors
Bromocriptine (amino acid alkaloid)	Weak antagonist	CNS: Partial agonist/antagonist; inhibits prolactin secretion; emetic (high)	Vasculature: Antagonist
Dihydroergotamine (dihydrogenated group)	Smooth muscles: Partial agonist/ antagonist CNS: Agonist lateral geniculate nucleus	CNS: Emetic (mild) Sympathetic ganglia: Antagonism	Vasculature: Partial agonist (veins); antagonist (arteries) Smooth muscles: Antagonism CNS/PNS: Antagonism
Ergonovine and methyl ergonovine (amine alkaloid)	Smooth muscles: Potent antagonist Vasculature: Agonist in umbilical and placental vessels CNS: Partial antagonist/agonist	CNS: Emetic (mild); inhibits prolactin (weak); partial agonist/antagonist Vasculature: Weak antagonist	Vasculature: Partial agonist
Ergotamine (amino acid aklaloid)	Vasculature: Partial agonist Smooth muscles: Nonselective antagonist CNS: Poor agonist/antagonist	CNS: Emetic (potent)	Vasculature: Partial agonist/antagonist Smooth muscles: Partial agonist/antagonist CNS: Antagonist PNS: Antagonist
Methysergide (amine alkaloid)[59]	Vasculature: Partial agonist CNS: Potent antagonist	None	None

CNS, central nervous system; PNS, peripheral nervous system.

TABLE 51–4. Clinical Manifestations of Ergotism

Central Effects	Peripheral Effects
Agitation	Angina
Cerebrovascular ischemia	Bradycardia
Hallucinations	Gangrene
Headaches	Hemorrhagic vesiculations and skin bullae
Miosis (fixed)	Mesenteric infarction
Nausea	Myocardial infarction
Seizures	Renal infarction
Twitching (facial)	
Vomiting	

ergotism. The coronary, renal, cerebral, ophthalmic, and mesenteric vasculature,[67] as well as the vessels of the extremities, may also be affected.[71] Neuropathic changes may be secondary to ischemia of the vasa nervorum.

Bradycardia is a characteristic effect of the ergot alkaloids, and is believed to be a reflex baroreceptor-mediated phenomenon associated with vasoconstriction, but a reduction in sympathetic tone, direct myocardial depression, and increased vagal activity may also be factors.[68]

Myocardial valvular abnormalities are reported with ergot alkaloids. Ergotamine and methysergide both cause mitral and aortic valve leaflet thickening and immobility resulting in valvular regurgitation.[26,66] This finding is particularly striking considering that a similar phenomenon from a class of weight loss agents recently resulted in their withdrawal.

TREATMENT

The treatment for a patient with ergot alkaloid toxicity depends on the nature of the clinical findings. Gastric emptying should rarely be used, if at all, because vomiting is a common early occurrence, and the ingestion may be complicated by seizures. If the patient is not vomiting shortly after an acute oral overdose, activated charcoal should be administered. If emesis is present, metoclopramide a promotility dopamine antagonist or a 5-HT_3 antagonist can be used as an antiemetic to facilitate the administration of activated charcoal. In mild cases, characterized by minimal pain of the extremities, nausea, or headache, supportive measures such as hydration and analgesia are all that are needed. With more serious cases, severe peripheral vasoconstriction may produce ischemic changes that include angina, myocardial infarction, cerebral ischemia, intermittent claudication, and internal organ/mesenteric ischemia. Intravenous vasodilators, such as sodium nitroprusside,[3,10,58] nitroglycerin,[40] and phentolamine, are indicated to reverse the ischemia. Methylprednisolone was reported to reverse ergotamine-induced lower extremity arterial vasospasm.[63] Prazosin,[12] captopril,[86] and nifedipine[14] have also been used to achieve peripheral vasodilation in cases with mild signs and symptoms of vasospasm, such as dysesthesias and minimal ischemic pain of the digits.

Although sympathetic block, epidural block, or sympathectomy—all of which have been used in the past—may relieve vasoconstriction mediated via the CNS, these modalities are not expected to antagonize the direct action of the ergot alkaloids on arteriolar smooth muscle.[3] Heparin, corticosteroids, or low-molecular-weight dextran[70] may be used to prevent sludging and subsequent clot formation. The use of thrombolytic agents in this setting has not been evaluated, but has theoretical utility. Arteriotomy may be necessary to remove large clots. Hyperbaric oxygen may correct local tissue hypoxia, but is not generally indicated.[22] Benzodiazepines should be used to treat seizures or hallucinations.

TRIPTANS

In 1974 investigations began on a new class of compounds that produced vasoconstrictive effects via 5-HT receptors. The first compound successfully use in this way was 5-carboxamidotryptamine (5-CT). When applied to an isolated dog saphenous vein, 5-CT caused potent venoconstriction and induced significant hypotension in vivo. The next compound developed, AH25086 [(3–2-aminoethyl)-N-methyl-1-H-indole-5-acetamide], also constricted saphenous veins in dogs but had more 5-HT receptor selectivity. AH25086 was effective against acute migraine in human volunteers, but further research was stopped because it was deemed less suitable for development in humans, possibly owing to the fact that it was highly lipophobic and unsuitable for oral use.[38,69] In 1984, sumatriptan was synthesized and its clinical success led to the rapid development of six other triptans currently including naratriptan, zolmitriptan, rizatriptan, eletriptan, almotriptan, and frovatriptan (Fig. 51–2 and Table 51–5).

PHARMACOLOGY

The triptans are all primarily 5-HT_{1B} and 5-HT_{1D} receptor agonists and have less activity at 5-HT_{1A} and 5-HT_{1F} receptors[27] (Chap. 13). In the CNS, 5-HT_{1B} receptors are located on cerebral vessels.[32] Stimulation of these receptors results in cerebral vasoconstriction,[15] reversing abnormal cerebral vasodilation. In contrast, the 5-HT_{1D} receptors are located presynaptically on trigeminal neurons, and act as "autoreceptors" to decrease neurotransmitter release from central trigeminal nerve terminals.[43] The triptans also inhibit dural neurogenic inflammation by preventing the release of vasodilating neuropeptides from peripheral trigeminal nerves.[54,72] Peripherally, triptans cause vasoconstriction systemically through the 5-HT_{1B} receptor.[17,49]

Sumatriptan has poor oral bioavailability but good subcutaneous bioavailability (96%), and is therefore preferentially given by this route. The newer triptans differ substantially from sumatriptan with regard to oral bioavailability, plasma half-life, time to maximum effect, and recurrence rate of headaches. All triptans are pharmacodynamically the same but pharmacokinetically different (see Table 51–5).

CLINICAL MANIFESTATIONS

With appropriate therapeutic use, the common adverse effects associated with the triptans are minor and include nausea, vomiting, dyspepsia, flushing, and paresthesias.[16,68] However, the most consequential adverse effects are chest pressure and vasoconstriction. Chest pressure symptoms are reported in up to 15% of sumatriptan users.[9,62] Although triptans reduce coronary artery diameter by 10% to 15%, chest pressure symptoms are not believed to be secondary to cardiac ischemia. Alternate hypotheses for the chest pressure sensations include a

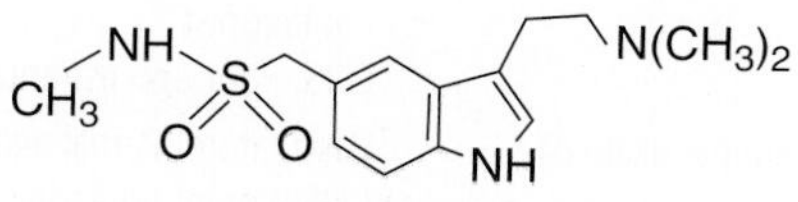

NH CH3 S O O N(CH3)2 NH

Sumatriptan

FIGURE 51–2. Representative chemical structure of the triptans.

TABLE 51–5. Pharmacokinetics of Triptans

Triptan	t ½ (hours)	Duration of Action (hours)	Lipophilicity	Bioavailability (%)	Metabolism/ Elimination
Almotriptan	3.0–3.7	24	Unknown	70–80	CYP3A4, CYP2D6 MAO-A (minor)
Eletriptan	3.6–6.9	14–16	High	50	CYP3A4
Frovatriptan	25	24	Low	24–30	CYP1A2 Renal elimination
Naratriptan	4.5–6.6	Unknown	High	63–74	Renal (major) P450
Rizatriptan	1.8–3.0	25	Moderate	40–45	MAO-A
Sumatriptan	2.0–2.5	4	Low	14 (PO); 96 (SQ)	MAO-A
Zolmitriptan	1.5–3.6	18	Moderate	40–49	CYP1A2 MAO-A (minor)

MAO, monoamine oxidase.

generalized vasospastic disorder in migraineurs, esophageal spasm, bronchospasm, alterations of skeletal muscle energy metabolism, and central sensitization of pain pathways.[18] Although the triptans show some degree of coronary artery constriction in vitro, recent studies demonstrate, and hence recommendations state, that there is no need for routine stress tests in low-risk patients prior to therapy with triptans.[19,48,80]

However, triptans can cause ischemia due to vasoconstriction. Therapeutic sumatriptan use is also associated with myocardial ischemia and or infarction, dysrhythmias, renal infarction, splenic infarction, and ischemic colitis.[1,4,13,44,50,55,57,61] Cephalic vasoconstriction is the desired effect of sumatriptan, but there are reports of adverse neurologic events ranging from transient ischemic attacks to cerebral vascular events, hemorrhages, or infarctions.[11,42,47,53] Extrapyramidal symptoms such as akathisia and dystonia may also occur.[46] Spinal cord infarction is reported after therapeutic zolmitriptan use,[82] and renal infarction is reported after therapeutic rizatriptan use.[29] These complications have not been reported to date with the other triptans but are possible given their similar mechanisms of action.

Animal studies showed a wide margin of safety with oral sumatriptan. Subcutaneous administration of 2 g/kg of sumatriptan to rats was lethal. Death was preceded by erythema, inactivity, and tremor.[39] Dogs survived 20 mg/kg and 100 mg/kg subcutaneous doses, but developed hind limb paralysis, erythema, tremor, salivation, and loss of vocalization.[38] Reactions in other animals include seizures, inactivity, reduced respiratory rate, cyanosis, ptosis, ataxia, mydriasis, salivation, and lacrimation.[39,75]

Excessive triptan usage is associated with vascoconstrictive symptoms. A 43-year-old man who used 23 (25 mg) tablets of sumatriptan and 32 tablets of Midrin (a combination xenobiotic with isometheptene 65 mg, dichloraphenazone 100 mg, and acetaminophen 325 mg) over 7 days for headaches developed a left occipital infarction with a right hemianopsia. Digital subtraction angiography revealed segmental narrowing in multiple cerebral vessels. The hemianopsia and vessel findings resolved after cessation of the sumatriptan and Midrin and treatment with nicardipine.[53] Two patients who received four times and 10 times the recommended dose of naratriptan developed severe hypertension.[56] However, not all triptan overdosages result in toxicity. One 36-year-old man reportedly used 66 (6 mg) doses of sumatriptan subcutaneously over 4 weeks for his cluster headaches and had no adverse effects.[78] The maximum recommended dosage of sumatriptan is 12 mg subcutaneously in a 24-hour period. Patients who took single doses of 100 to 150 mg of almotriptan did not have any adverse effects.[2]

In 2006, the FDA issued an alert, warning of an increased risk of serotonin syndrome with triptans used in combination with selective serotonin reuptake inhibitors (SSRIs) or selective serotonin-norepinephrine reuptake inhibitors. The alert was based on 27 cases reported to the FDA Adverse Events Reporting System between 1998 and 2002. The cases involved triptan use in conjunction with SSRIs that were coded as serotonin syndrome or symptoms indicative of serotonin syndrome.[73] A case series of serotonin syndrome from migraine medications described three cases of serotonin syndrome with sumatriptan use alone, sumatriptan with sertraline, and sumatriptan with methysergide, lithium, and sertraline.[51] Other medications that might precipitate serotonin syndrome when used in conjunction with triptans include monoamine oxidase (MAO) inhibitors (see Chaps. 71 and 72).

TREATMENT

Treatment of triptan-induced vasoconstriction is dependent on the route of exposure and the organ system affected. Decontamination is not feasible after subcutaneous exposures, but can be effective following overdose of oral preparations. Gastrointestinal (GI) decontamination should be performed with activated charcoal. Since vomiting is not as prominent with triptan exposure as with exposure to the ergot alkaloids, gastric emptying procedures such as orogastric lavage may be considered early, but only following massive ingestion. The oral forms of rizatriptan and zolmitriptan are formulated to dissolve on the tongue, limiting the effectiveness of gastrointestinal decontamination.

Triptan-induced vasoconstriction and ischemia should be reversed with a calcium channel blocker or intravenous vasodilators, such as sodium nitroprusside, nitroglycerin, or phentolamine.[53] Cases of sumatriptan-associated myocardial ischemia were effectively treated with aspirin, heparin, and intravenous nitroglycerin.[61] Thrombolytic therapy has not been investigated in this setting but should be instituted if clinically warranted.

ISOMETHEPTENE

Isometheptene is a mild vasoconstrictor marketed as a combination preparation (Midrin) that includes dichloraphenazone, a muscle relaxant, and acetaminophen. It has indirect α- and β-adrenergic agonist effects as well as minor direct α-adrenergic agonist effects on the peripheral vasculature.[79] When administered early during a migraine exacerbation, it is as effective as sumatriptan in relieving migraine headache.[28] Cerebral vasoconstriction is reported after therapeutic and excessive isometheptene use.[55,64] Autonomic dysreflexia, which presented with hypertension, headache, diaphoresis, and flushing, was also reported in a man with spinal cord injury who used isometheptene for treatment of a migraine headache.[85] Treatment of isometheptene-induced vasoconstriction should include discontinuation of the medication and reversal of the vasoconstriction with calcium channel blockers or vasodilators, such as sodium nitroprusside, nitroglycerin, or phentolamine.

CGRP ANTAGONISTS

During migraines, calcitonin gene-related peptide is among the many vasoactive peptides released from activated trigeminal nerves.[30] Treatment of active migraine with sumatriptan decreased CGRP levels to normal.[30] CGRP is a potent vasodilator[8] and is involved in the transmission of nociceptive signals from cerebral vessels to the central nervous system.[20] CGRP receptors are found in nerve fibers in cerebral and dural vessels and in multiple areas of the central nervous system postulated in migraine genesis—the cerebral cortex, periaqueductal gray, locus coeruleus, dorsal raphe nuclei, solitary tractus nucleus, spinal dorsal horn, dorsal root ganglia, and trigeminal ganglia.[76]

Two CGRP antagonists for migraine therapy were recently developed—olcegepant and telcagepant. Olcegepant is available in parenteral form while telcagepant is available as an oral preparation. Based on two high dosing administrations, olcegepant has a volume of distribution of 20 L with a terminal half-life of 2.5 hours and minor renal excretion.[41] Adverse events reported with olcegepant included paresthesia, flushing, fatigue, headache, abdominal pain, diarrhea, flatulence, rhinitis, dry mouth, and abnormal vision.[21,41] Adverse effects reported with telcagepant included nausea, dizziness, somnolence, dry mouth, fatigue, paresthesia, and asthenia.[36,37] Systemic vasoconstrictive adverse effects did not occur in the phase 2 and 3 trials with either olcegepant or telcagepant.

SUMMARY

Although epidemic ergotism is no longer a common concern because of widespread systemic inspection of grain in the United States, ergot poisoning by both unintentional and intentional ingestions continues to be reported. Knowledge of the complex pharmacologic and physiologic actions of these agents and the use of appropriate pharmacologic antidotes enable the clinician to minimize the morbidity and mortality previously associated with ergot alkaloids. The introduction of the triptans for the treatment of migraine has decreased the use and subsequently the toxicity of ergot alkaloids. Ergots, triptans, and isometheptene all share toxicities related to vasoconstriction. CGRP antagonists do not cause vasoconstriction but are currently too new for its toxicities to be characterized.

ACKNOWLEDGMENT

Neal A. Lewin contributed to this chapter in a previous edition of this text.

REFERENCES

1. Abbrescia VD, Pearlstein L, Kotler M. Sumatriptan-associated myocardial infarction: report of case with attention to potential risk factors: *J Am Osteopath Assoc.* 1997;97:162-164.
2. Almotriptan malate tablets product information. Toronto: Janssen-Ortho Inc.; 2003.
3. Andersen PK, Christensen KN, Hole P, et al. Sodium nitroprusside and epidural blockade in the treatment of ergotism. *N Engl J Med.* 1977;296:1271-1273.
4. Arora A, Arora S. Spontaneous splenic infarction associated with sumatriptan use. *J Headache Pain.* 2006;7:214-216.
5. Ausband SC, Goodman PE. An unusual case of clarithromycin associated ergotism. *J Emerg Med.* 2001;21:411-413.
6. Baldwin ZK, Ceraldi CC. Ergotism associated with HIV antiviral protease inhibitor therapy. *J Vasc Surg.* 2003;37:676-678.
7. Botha CJ, Naude TW, Moroe ML, Rottinghaus GE. Gangrenous ergotism in cattle grazing fescue (Festuca elatior L.) in South Africa. *J S Afr Vet Assoc.* 2004;75:45-48.
8. Brain SD, Williams TJ, Tippins JR, Morris HR, MacIntyre I. Calcitonin gene-related peptide is a potent vasodilator. *Nature.* 1985;313:54-56.
9. Brown EG, Endersby CA, Smith RN, Talbot JC. The safety and tolerability of sumatriptan: an overview. *Eur Neurol.* 1991;31:339-344.
10. Carliner N, Denune DP, Finch CS, Goldberg LI. Sodium nitroprusside treatment of ergotamine-induced peripheral ischemia. *JAMA.* 1974;227:308-309.
11. Cavazos JE, Caress JB, Chilukuri VR, et al. Sumatriptan-induced stroke in sagittal sinus thrombosis. *Lancet.* 1994;343:1105-1106.
12. Cobaugh DS. Prazosin treatment of ergotamine-induced peripheral ischemia. *JAMA.* 1980;244:1360.
13. Curtin T, Brooks AP, Roberts JA. Cardiorespiratory distress after sumatriptan given by injection. *BMJ.* 1992;305:713-714; author reply 714.
14. Dagher FJ, Pais SO, Richards W, Queral LA. Severe unilateral ischemia of the lower extremity caused by ergotamine: treatment with nifedipine. *Surgery.* 1985;97:369-373.
15. Dechant KL, Clissold SP. Sumatriptan. A review of its pharmacodynamic and pharmacokinetic properties, and therapeutic efficacy in the acute treatment of migraine and cluster headache. *Drugs.* 1992;43:776-798.
16. Deleu D, Hanssens Y. Current and emerging second-generation triptans in acute migraine therapy: a comparative review. *J Clin Pharmacol.* 2000;40:687-700.
17. Dixon RM, Meire HB, Evans DH, et al. Peripheral vascular effects and pharmacokinetics of the antimigraine compound, zolmitriptan, in combination with oral ergotamine in healthy volunteers. *Cephalalgia.* 1997;17:639-646.
18. Dodick D, Lipton RB, Martin V, et al. Consensus statement: cardiovascular safety profile of triptans (5-HT agonists) in the acute treatment of migraine. *Headache.* 2004; 44:414-425.
19. Dodick DW, Martin VT, Smith T, Silberstein S. Cardiovascular tolerability and safety of triptans: a review of clinical data. *Headache.* 2004;44(Suppl 1):S20-30.
20. Durham PL. Calcitonin gene-related peptide (CGRP) and migraine. *Headache.* 2006;46(Suppl 1):S3-8.
21. Edvinsson L. Clinical data on the CGRP antagonist BIBN4096BS for treatment of migraine attacks. *CNS Drug Rev.* 2005;11:69-76.
22. Eloff SJ, Brummelkamp WH, Boerema I. A case of "Ergot Foot" treated with hyperbaric oxygen drenching. *J Cardiovasc Surg (Torino).* 1963;4:747-751.
23. Ferrari MD. Migraine. *Lancet.* 1998;351:1043-1051.
24. Fincham RW, Perdue Z, Dunn VD. Bilateral focal cortical atrophy and chronic ergotamine abuse. *Neurology.* 1985;35:720-722.
25. Fisher PE, Silk DB, Menzies-Gow N, Dingle M. Ergotamine abuse and extra-hepatic portal hypertension. *Postgrad Med J.* 1985;61:461-463.
26. Flaherty KR, Bates JR. Mitral regurgitation caused by chronic ergotamine use. *Am Heart J.* 1996;131:603-606.
27. Fowler PA, Lacey LF, Thomas M, et al. The clinical pharmacology, pharmacokinetics and metabolism of sumatriptan. *Eur Neurol.* 1991;31:291-294.
28. Freitag FG, Cady R, DiSerio F, et al. Comparative study of a combination of isometheptene mucate, dichloralphenazone with acetaminophen and sumatriptan succinate in the treatment of migraine. *Headache.* 2001;41:391-398.
29. Fulton JA, Kahn J, Nelson LS, Hoffman RS. Renal infarction during the use of rizatriptan and zolmitriptan: two case reports. *Clin Toxicol (Phila).* 2006;44:177-180.
30. Goadsby PJ, Edvinsson L. The trigeminovascular system and migraine: studies characterizing cerebrovascular and neuropeptide changes seen in humans and cats. *Ann Neurol.* 1993;33:48-56.

31. Goadsby PJ, Lipton RB, Ferrari MD. Migraine—current understanding and treatment. *N Engl J Med.* 2002;346:257-270.
32. Hamel E. The biology of serotonin receptors: focus on migraine pathophysiology and treatment. *Can J Neurol Sci.* 1999;26(Suppl 3):S2-6.
33. Hargreaves R. New migraine and pain research. *Headache.* 2007;47 Suppl 1:S26-S43. Review.
34. Hargreaves RJ, Shepheard SL. Pathophysiology of migraine—new insights. *Can J Neurol Sci.* 1999;26(Suppl 3):S12-19.
35. Harrison TE. Ergotaminism. *JACEP.* 1978;7:162-169.
36. Ho TW, Ferrari MD, Dodick DW, et al. Efficacy and tolerability of MK-0974 (telcagepant), a new oral antagonist of calcitonin gene-related peptide receptor, compared with zolmitriptan for acute migraine: a randomised, placebo-controlled, parallel-treatment trial. *Lancet.* 2009;372:2115-2123.
37. Ho TW, Mannix LK, Fan X, et al. Randomized controlled trial of an oral CGRP receptor antagonist, MK-0974, in acute treatment of migraine. *Neurology.* 2008;70:1304-1312.
38. Humphrey PP, Apperley E, Feniuk W, Perren MJ. A rational approach to identifying a fundamentally new drug for the treatment of migraine. In: Saxena PR, Wallis DI, Wouters W, et al., eds. Cardiovascular Pharmacology of 5-Hydroxytryptamine. Dordrecht: Kluwer Academic Publishers; 1990: 417-431.
39. Humphrey PP, Feniuk W, Marriott AS, et al. Preclinical studies on the antimigraine drug, sumatriptan. *Eur Neurol.* 1991;31:282-290.
40. Husum B, Metz P, Rasmussen JP. Nitroglycerin infusion for ergotism. *Lancet.* 1979;2:794-795.
41. Iovino M, Feifel U, Yong CL, Wolters JM, Wallenstein G. Safety, tolerability and pharmacokinetics of BIBN 4096 BS, the first selective small molecule calcitonin gene-related peptide receptor antagonist, following single intravenous administration in healthy volunteers. *Cephalalgia.* 2004;24:645-656.
42. Jayamaha JE, Street MK. Fatal cerebellar infarction in a migraine sufferer whilst receiving sumatriptan. *Intensive Care Med.* 1995;21:82-83.
43. Kaube H, Hoskin KL, Goadsby PJ. Inhibition by sumatriptan of central trigeminal neurones only after blood-brain barrier disruption. *Br J Pharmacol.* 1993;109:788-792.
44. Knudsen JF, Friedman B, Chen M, Goldwasser JE. Ischemic colitis and sumatriptan use. *Arch Intern Med.* 1998;158:1946-1948.
45. Lopez TA, Campero CM, Chayer R, de Hoyos M. Ergotism and photosensitization in swine produced by the combined ingestion of Claviceps purpurea sclerotia and Ammi majus seeds. *J Vet Diagn Invest.* 1997;9:68-71.
46. Lopez-Alemany M, Ferrer-Tuset C, Bernacer-Alpera B. Akathisia and acute dystonia induced by sumatriptan. *J Neurol.* 1997;244:131-132.
47. Luman W, Gray RS. Adverse reactions associated with sumatriptan. *Lancet.* 1993;341:1091-1092.
48. MaassenVanDenBrink A, Reekers M, Bax WA, Ferrari MD, Saxena PR. Coronary side-effect potential of current and prospective antimigraine drugs. *Circulation.* 1998;98:25-30.
49. MacIntyre PD, Bhargava B, Hogg KJ, Gemmill JD, Hillis WS. Effect of subcutaneous sumatriptan, a selective 5HT1 agonist, on the systemic, pulmonary, and coronary circulation. *Circulation.* 1993;87:401-405.
50. Main ML, Ramaswamy K, Andrews TC. Cardiac arrest and myocardial infarction immediately after sumatriptan injection. *Ann Intern Med.* 1998;128:874.
51. Mathew NT, Tietjen GE, Lucker C. Serotonin syndrome complicating migraine pharmacotherapy. *Cephalalgia.* 1996;16:323-327.
52. Merhoff GC, Porter JM. Ergot intoxication: historical review and description of unusual clinical manifestations. *Ann Surg.* 1974;180:773-779.
53. Meschia JF, Malkoff MD, Biller J. Reversible segmental cerebral arterial vasospasm and cerebral infarction: possible association with excessive use of sumatriptan and Midrin. *Arch Neurol.* 1998;55:712-714.
54. Moskowitz MA. Neurogenic versus vascular mechanisms of sumatriptan and ergot alkaloids in migraine. *Trends Pharmacol Sci.* 1992;13:307-311.
55. Mueller L, Gallagher RM, Ciervo CA. Vasospasm-induced myocardial infarction with sumatriptan. *Headache.* 1996;36:329-331.
56. Naratriptan product information. GlaxoSmithKline, Inc.; 2006.
57. O'Connor P, Gladstone P. Oral sumatriptan-associated transmural myocardial infarction. *Neurology.* 1995;45:2274-2276.
58. O'Dell CW, Davis GB, Johnson AD, et al. Sodium nitroprusside in the treatment of ergotism. *Radiology.* 1977;124:73-74.
59. Orlando RC, Moyer P, Barnett TB. Methysergide therapy and constrictive pericarditis. *Ann Intern Med.* 1978;88:213-214.
60. Orton DA, Richardson RJ. Ergotamine absorption and toxicity. *Postgrad Med J.* 1982;58:6-11.
61. Ottervanger JP, Paalman HJ, Boxma GL, Stricker BH. Transmural myocardial infarction with sumatriptan. *Lancet.* 1993;341:861-862.
62. Ottervanger JP, van Witsen TB, Valkenburg HA, Stricker BH. Postmarketing study of cardiovascular adverse reactions associated with sumatriptan. *BMJ.* 1993;307:1185.
63. Rahman A, Yildiz M, Dadas E, et al. Reversal of ergotamine-induced vasospasm following methylprednisolone. *Clin Toxicol (Phila).* 2008;46: 1074-1076.
64. Raroque HG Jr, Tesfa G, Purdy P. Postpartum cerebral angiopathy. *Is there a role for sympathomimetic drugs? Stroke.* 1993;24:2108-2110.
65. Raskin N, Appenzeller O. Migraine pathogenesis. In: Raskin N, Appenzeller O, eds. Major Problems in Internal Medicine. Philadelphia: WB Saunders; 1980:84-104.
66. Redfield MM, Nicholson WJ, Edwards WD, Tajik AJ. Valve disease associated with ergot alkaloid use: echocardiographic and pathologic correlations. *Ann Intern Med.* 1992;117:50-52.
67. Rogers DA, Mansberger JA. Gastrointestinal vascular ischemia caused by ergotamine. *South Med J.* 1989;82:1058-1059.
68. Sanders-Bush E, Mayer SE. 5-Hydroxytryptamine (serotonin) receptor agonists and antagonists. In: Brunton LL, Lazo JS, Parker KL, eds. Goodman and Gilman's The Pharmacological Basis of Therapeutics. New York: McGraw-Hill; 2006:297-315.
69. Saxena PR, Ferrari MD. 5-HT(1)-like receptor agonists and the pathophysiology of migraine. *Trends Pharmacol Sci.* 1989; 10:200-204.
70. Semb BK, Molster A, Halvorsen JF, Tvete S. Ergot-induced vasospasm of the lower extremities treated with epidural anaesthesia. *Scand J Thorac Cardiovasc Surg.* 1975;9:254-258.
71. Senter HJ, Lieverman AN, Pinto R. Cerebral manifestations of ergotism. Report of a case and review of the literature. *Stroke.* 1976;7:88-92.
72. Shepherd SL, Williamson DJ, Beer MS, Hill RG, Hargreaves RJ. Differential effects of 5-HT1B/1D receptor agonists on neurogenic dural plasma extravasation and vasodilation in anaesthetized rats. *Neuropharmacology.* 1997;36:525-533.
73. Soldin OP, Tonning JM. Serotonin syndrome associated with triptan monotherapy. *N Engl J Med.* 2008;358:2185-2186.
74. Stumpf JL, Mitrzyk B. Management of orthostatic hypotension. *Am J Hosp Pharm.* 1994;51:648-660.
75. Sumatriptan. Product information and personal communication. Glaxo Wellcome, Inc.
76. Tepper SJ, Stillman MJ. Clinical and preclinical rationale for CGRP-receptor antagonists in the treatment of migraine. *Headache.* 2008;48:1259-1268.
77. The International Classification of Headache Disorders. 2nd ed. *Cephalalgia.* 2004;24(Suppl 1):9-160.
78. Turhal NS. Sumatriptan overdose in episodic cluster headache: a case report of overuse without event. *Cephalalgia.* 2001;21:700.
79. Valdivia LF, Centurion D, Perusquia M, et al. Pharmacological analysis of the mechanisms involved in the tachycardic and vasopressor responses to the antimigraine agent, isometheptene, in pithed rats. *Life Sci.* 2004;74: 3223-3234.
80. van den Broek RW, MaassenVanDenBrink A, de Vries R, et al. Pharmacological analysis of contractile effects of eletriptan and sumatriptan on human isolated blood vessels. *Eur J Pharmacol.* 2000;407:165-173.
81. van Dongen PW, de Groot AN. History of ergot alkaloids from ergotism to ergometrine. *Eur J Obstet Gynecol Reprod Biol.* 1995;60:109-116.
82. Vijayan N, Peacock JH. Spinal cord infarction during use of zolmitriptan: a case report. *Headache.* 2000;40:57-60.
83. Villalon CM, Centurion D, Valdivia LF, de Vries P, Saxena PR. Migraine: pathophysiology, pharmacology, treatment and future trends. *Curr Vasc Pharmacol.* 2003;1:71-84.
84. Wadworth AN, Chrisp P. Co-dergocrine mesylate. A review of its pharmacodynamic and pharmacokinetic properties and therapeutic use in age-related cognitive decline. *Drugs Aging.* 1992;2:153-173.
85. Wineinger MA, Basford JR. Autonomic dysreflexia due to medication: misadventure in the use of an isometheptene combination to treat migraine. *Arch Phys Med Rehabil.* 1985;66:645-646.
86. Zimran A, Ofek B, Hershko C. Treatment with captopril for peripheral ischaemia induced by ergotamine. *Br Med J (Clin Res Ed).* 1984;288:364.

CHAPTER 52
ANTINEOPLASTICS OVERVIEW

Richard Y. Wang

Although overdoses of antineoplastics are infrequent, these events are of greater consequence than overdoses of many other xenobiotics because of their narrow therapeutic index. This is evident from survey data from poison centers in the United States. From 1988 to 2007, the median annual number of people exposed to antineoplastics reported to US poison centers was about 1000. In the last 5 years, the number of annual exposures to these agents has steadily increased to slightly over 1500 (see Chap. 135). These exposures represent about one per 1000 cases of exposures to pharmaceutical agents, or one per 2000 cases of all exposures annually reported to US poison centers. Approximately two-thirds of the people exposed to antineoplastic agents in these reports were adults, one-fourth of the group was young children, and the remainder was adolescents. The annual trend for the proportion of exposures among adults and children appears to have remained at 70% and 20%, respectively, from 2001 to 2007. Children and adolescents between the ages of 6 and 19 years accounted for approximately 7% of the population annually exposed, and this frequency did not change between these years. Although these differences among age groups can represent the incidence of cancer in these populations, further analysis is warranted to better define the reasons for these observations because they are not apparent.

From 2001 to 2007, the annual prevalence of exposures to antineoplastics reported to US poison centers that resulted in toxicity that was defined as moderate or major in severity has declined from approximately 10% to 5% in the last 2 years. The mortality was about two per 1000 exposures in this same period. This frequency of significant morbidities was higher than expected because unintentional exposures to antineoplastics occurred eight times more frequently than intentional exposures. This observation is consistent with a hospital-based survey and is attributed to the increased toxicity of these agents.[21] The prevalence of the exposure to antineoplastic agents is expected to increase over the next few years because of the increased availability of oral formulations, such as capecitabine, etoposide, vinorelbine, erlotinib and sorafenib, and their expanding therapeutic indications.

MEDICATION ERRORS WITH ANTINEOPLASTICS

The importance of understanding the occurrence of medication errors is to prevent future events of a similar nature. Fortunately, medical errors related to the use of antineoplastics occur infrequently. The reported medical error rate for the antineoplastics ranges from 0.06% to 5.5% based on data from US centers,[12,21,59] although the true prevalence of this event remains unknown. The rates reported by international centers are similar.[35,36,54] These reported estimates vary by the clinical setting, hospital versus outpatient, and the patient population, adults versus children. The outpatient setting and the treatment of children present several unique challenges to the healthcare system: increased volumes, decreased control measures, increased workload, and unique dosing schemes such as dose based on body surface area.[21,59] In a satellite pharmacy setting, two of the potentially lethal overdoses of cisplatin were a result of errors in duration of administration (100 mg/m^2 for 3–4 consecutive days instead of for 1 day).[18] Lack of healthcare provider familiarity with the antineoplastics and its dosing was a major cause of these events.

The factors contributing to the occurrence of medication errors with antineoplastics and the measures identified to prevent these events, such as centralization of services (medical oncology, pharmaceutical) and the use of standardized protocols, are similar to those for other pharmaceutical agents and they are discussed elsewhere (see Chap. 139).[5,7,54] The centralization of services and the institution of information technology, such as electronic prescribing protocols, production, and bedside scanning, can reduce medication error rates with antineoplastics by approximately 25% and 10%, respectively,[7] although drug labeling errors can continue to occur.[35,36] Additional strategies to reduce these errors include tracking and following up on errors, and increased patient education and participation. Many of these features to prevent errors can also improve worker safety by reducing occupational exposures. As more antineoplastics become available and their indications broaden, unintentional exposures and unintended dosing regimens (see Chap. 139) will increase in number and frequency.

Aside from unintentional exposures, additional factors leading to increased toxicity associated with antineoplastics include age, gender, comorbidities, compromised host state, and diminished renal and hepatic function. Diminished hepatic clearance caused by altered enzyme expression can be accounted for by age, gender, smoking status, and the concurrent use of other xenobiotics. Differences in gender can contribute to varying pharmacokinetic parameters, including bioavailability, distribution, metabolism, and elimination. In a study, women treated with 5-fluorouracil (5-FU) for colon cancer were found to have a twofold higher frequency of drug-related toxicity than men.[61] The manifestations included leukopenia, diarrhea, and stomatitis, which also were observed in other reports.[42,56] Although the basis for this difference in toxicity between genders is not known, it may be because of decreased 5-FU clearance from diminished dihydropyrimidine dehydrogenase activity in women.[37,42] Dihydropyrimidine dehydrogenase inactivates more than 80% of fluorouracil by metabolizing it to 5-fluorodihydrouracil, and low activity of this enzyme can result in hematologic and gastrointestinal (GI) toxicity.

At an individual level, genetic polymorphisms can contribute to differences in xenobiotic response with resultant toxicity by altering targets, transporters, and enzyme complexes. Such variations have been characterized for several enzymes that are involved in the metabolism of antineoplastics. Irinotecan and amonafide are two examples that are associated with toxicity. Irinotecan is a topoisomerase I inhibitor that works through its active metabolite, SN-38, which can cause diarrhea and neutropenia at elevated concentrations.[63] A genetic variant of uridine diphosphate glucuronosyltransferase (UGT1A1) containing the T7 allele glucuronidates SN-38 at a slower rate than other variants, which results in increased SN-38 concentrations and increased toxicity.[3,25] Another example is amonafide, which is a topoisomerase II inhibitor, and its active metabolite, *N*-acetyl amonafide is formed by *N*-acetyltransferase 2 (NAT2). Patients capable of "rapid acetylation" have a genetic variation of NAT2 and are more likely to develop myelotoxicity than are slow acetylators.[43] There are additional polymorphisms in metabolism associated with antineoplastics; however, further work is necessary to define their clinical significance. Because of the narrow therapeutic index of the antineoplastics, the significance of such findings demonstrates the benefit of individual drug monitoring and genetic screening for use to maximize the therapeutic efficacy of these agents while limiting host toxicity.

CLASSES OF ANTINEOPLASTICS

Most antineoplastics can be grouped into one of four categories: alkylating agents, antimetabolites, antimitotics, and antibiotics (Table 52–1). There are new antineoplastics that target specific proteins located on the cell membrane, such as growth factor receptors, to inhibit the proliferation of tumor cells.[30,44] These antineoplastics can be categorized as monoclonal antibodies and protein kinase inhibitors based on their therapeutic approach. The antimetabolites are grouped by the substrates with which they interfere. Methotrexate is a folate antagonist; other pharmaceuticals with similar but lesser toxicity include trimethoprim and pyrimethamine. The antimitotics are plant alkaloids and they exert toxic effects by interrupting microtubule assembly. Others are naturally derived and include the antibiotics and the enzyme L-asparaginase, which can be isolated from bacteria. The alkylating agents are more commonly used than other antineoplastics and cause covalent binding to nucleic acids, which inhibits DNA activity (replication and transcription). The more notable antineoplastics in this class, including

TABLE 52–1. Classification of Antineoplastics, Their Adverse Effects and Antidotal Therapy

Class	Antineoplastic	Adverse Effects	Overdose	Antidotes
Alkylating, alkylating like	Busulphan	Hyperpigmentation, pulmonary fibrosis, hyperuricemia	Myelosuppression	
	Dacarbazine	Hypotension, hepatocellular toxicity, influenza-like syndrome		
	Nitrogen mustards			
	Chlorambucil, cyclophosphamide, ifosfamide, mechlorethamine, melphalan	Hemorrhagic cystitis, encephalopathy, pulmonary fibrosis	Seizures, encephalopathy, myocardial necrosis, renal failure, hyponatremia	MESNA; methylene blue
	Nitrosoureas			
	Carmustine, lomustine, semustine	Pulmonary fibrosis, hepatocellular toxicity, renal insufficiency	Myelosuppression (delayed onset and prolonged duration)	
	Platinoids			
	Cisplatin, carboplatin, iproplatin	Renal failure, peripheral neuropathy, hypomagnesemia, hypocalcemia, hyponatremia, ototoxicity, myelosuppression	Seizures, encephalopathy, ototoxicity, retinal toxicity, myelosuppression	Amifostine; thiosulfate
	Procarbazine	MAOI activity		
	Temozolomide		Myelosuppression	
Antimetabolites	Methotrexate	Mucositis, nausea, diarrhea, hepatocellular toxicity	Mucositis, myelosuppression, renal failure	Leucovorin (folinic acid); Glucarpidase (carboxypeptidase G2)
	Purine analogs			
	Fludarabine	Encephalopathy, muscle weakness		
	Mercaptopurine	Hyperuricemia, pancreatitis, cholestasis		
	Pentostatin	Hepatocellular toxicity		
	Thioguanine	Hyperuricemia		
	Pyrimidine analogs			
	Cytarabine	Acute lung injury, neuropathy, cerebellar ataxia		
	Fluorouracil	Cardiogenic shock, cardiomyopathy, neuropathy, cerebellar ataxia		
Antimitotics	Taxenes			
	Docetaxel, paclitaxel	GI perforation, peripheral neuropathy, dysrhythmias		
	Vinca alkaloids			
	Vinblastine, vincristine, vindesine	Peripheral neuropathy, hyponatremia SIADH	Encephalopathy, seizures, autonomic instability, paralytic ileus, myelosuppression	

(*Continued*)

TABLE 52–1. Classification of Antineoplastics and Their Effects (*Continued*)

Class	Antineoplastic	Adverse Effects	Overdose	Antidotes
Antibiotics	Anthracycline			
	Daunorubicin, doxorubicin, epirubicin, idarubicin	Dilated congestive cardiomyopathy	Dysrhythmias, cardiomyopathy, CHF	Dexrazoxane
	Bleomycin	Pulmonary fibrosis		
	Dactinomycin	Hepatocellular toxicity		
	Mitomycin C	Hemolytic uremic syndrome		
	Mitoxantrone	Congestive dilated cardiomyopathy	Cardiomyopathy, CHF	None
Enzyme	L-asparaginase	Hypersensitivity, pancreatitis	No reports	None
Monoclonal antibodies	Alemtuzumab (CD52)	Hypersensitivity, and specific to the site of action	No reports	None
	Bevacizumab (VGFR)			
	Cetuximab (EGFR)			
	Gemtuzumab ozogamicin (CD33, conjugated to calicheamicin)			
	Ibritumomab tiuxetan (CD20, conjugated to yttrium-90)			
	Panitumumab (EGFR)			
	Rituximab (CD20)			
	Tositumomab (CD20, conjugated to iodine-131)			
	Trastuzumab (HER2)			
Protein kinase inhibitors	Dasatinib (bcr-Abl, c-KIT, PDGFR) Erlotinib (EGFR) Gefitinib (EGFR) Imatinib (bcr-Abl, PDGFR, c-KIT) Lapatinib (EGFR, HER2) Sorafenib (VEGFR, PDGFR, Raf-1, c-KIT, FLT3, BRAF) Sunitinib (VEGFR, PDGFR, RET, CSF1R, FLT3)	Gastrointestinal (nausea, diarrhea), acneiform rash (folliculitis), nail fragility, and xerosis (EGFR inhibitor), interstitial lung disease (erlotinib, gefitinib), hypertension (inhibitors of VEGF and PDGF), and hypothyroidism (sunitinib)	Nausea, vomiting, facial rash	None
Topoisomerase inhibitor	Camptothecins	Neutropenia, mucositis, diarrhea, early onset cholinergic syndrome (irinotecan)	Myelosuppression	None
	Irinotecan			
	Topotecan			
	Epipodophyllotoxins			
	Etoposide, teniposide	CHF, hypotension		

bcr-Abl, breakpoint cluster region-Abelson, fusion oncogene; B-RAF; B-RAF murine sarcoma viral oncogene homolog B1; c-KIT, murine leukemia viral oncogene homolog 1; CSF1R, colony-stimulating factor 1 receptor; EGFR, epidermal growth factor receptor; FLT3, FMS-related tyrosine kinase 3; HER2, human epidermal growth factor receptor 2; MESNA, mercaptoethane sulfonate; MOAI, monoamine oxidase inhibitor; PDGFR, platelet-derived growth factor receptor; Raf-1, murine leukemia viral oncogene homolog 1; RET, rearranged during transfection; VEGFR, vascular endothelial growth factor.

those with similar activity, are the nitrogen mustards, platinoids, and nitrosoureas. The antimetabolites and the alkylating agents are cell-cycle active, meaning that they only affect cells undergoing cell division. Some xenobiotics are phase specific; that is, they affect the cell only at a period during cell division. The cell cycle consists of the S phase (DNA replication) and the M phase (mitosis). DNA regulation and chromosomal separation occur during mitosis. Vincristine is M-phase specific and cytarabine is S-phase specific, in their sites of action. Other antineoplastics inhibit topoisomerase, which is necessary for DNA replication because it allows for reversible DNA strand breaks.

Because the majority of the cases of antineoplastic overdoses involve methotrexate, vincristine, mitoxantrone (related to the anthracyclines),[53] nitrogen mustards, and cisplatin, the discussion in this section focuses on these xenobiotics (see Chap. 37 for Vinca alkaloids).

MECHANISMS OF ACTION

The mechanisms responsible for the cytotoxic effects of the antineoplastics are the disruption of cellular replication and proliferation. The former category impairs DNA function by causing strand breaks, inhibiting strand relaxation, and serving as inhibitory analogs of essential cofactors and nitrogenous bases of nucleic acids. For example, alkylating agents form reactive intermediates that covalently bind to nitrogenous bases on the DNA structure, which leads to the formation of strand breaks and mispairings. Cross-linkages between strands can occur with the nitrogen mustards because they contain two reactive chloroethyl side chains. The planar anthracycline antibiotics can intercalate with DNA to alter replication and cause strand breaks through oxidative damage induced by a reactive semiquinone intermediate. DNA strand relaxation can be impaired by topoisomerase inhibitors, such as topotecan. Topotecan is derived from camptothecin, which is isolated from the tree *Camptotheca acuminata*. Single methyl transfer reactions and base pairings are essential activities during DNA synthesis that are affected by the antimetabolites, which include structural analogs to folate, pyrimidines, and purines.

Recent cancer therapy includes antineoplastics that limit cellular proliferation by inhibiting growth factor receptor activation and enhancing cell lysis by antibody-dependent cell-mediated cytotoxicity and complement-dependent cytotoxicity. Monoclonal antibodies to tumor cell surface antigens, such as CD20, CD52, and CD33, and the C1q complement are used to direct host defense mechanisms or deliver antineoplastics to these sites. For example, gemtuzumab ozogamicin is an antibody conjugated to the antibiotic, calicheamicin, and it is directed at CD33-positive leukemic blast cells. Other conjugates under investigation include radiolabeled isotopes (131-iodine, 225-actinium, 177-lutetium) and toxins, such as diphtheria, pseudomonal, ricin-A, saporin, staphylococcal, and enterotoxin A. In addition to the above, monoclonal antibodies against tumor growth factor receptors are available.

Tumor growth factors promote cell progression, proliferation, and differentiation (by angiogenesis). Their receptors located at the cell membrane are characterized for certain tumors, such as epidermal growth factor receptor (EGFR) (lung, renal, and gastrointestinal tumors) and human epidermal growth factor receptor 2 (HER2) (breast). Vascular endothelial growth factor receptor (VEGFR) and platelet derived growth factor receptor (PDGFR) are active in angiogenesis. Inactivation of these receptors can be accomplished with therapeutic monoclonal antibodies (MAB) and protein kinase inhibitors. Monoclonal antibodies prevent the activation of these receptors by inhibiting substrate binding to the receptor located at the extracellular surface. Kinase inhibitors are considered to be small molecule therapeutics that impair the ATP activation of growth factor receptors, tyrosine kinase inhibitors and certain signal transduction proteins responsible for tumor cell division serine/threonine kinase inhibitors. The disruption of the proliferation of keratinocytes, and GI mucosa and epithelial cells at these tissue sites can account for the anticipated toxic effects from the use of MABs and kinase inhibitors directed at EFGR. The therapeutic use of the protein kinase inhibitors of VEGFR and PDGFR, such as sunitib and sorafenib, is associated with hypertension, which can be due to endotheilial dysfunction and diminished microvascular regrowth.

The monoclonal antibodies are derivitized from human and chimeric (human and murine) sources, which contributes to the toxicity. Immunogenic effects from the presence of foreign proteins include rigors, nausea, vomiting, and rashes. Some organ-specific effects include bone marrow, skin (via EGFR), kidney (hypomagnesemia via EGFR), gastrointestinal (via EFGR), and cardiac (via HER2, trastuzumab).

MANIFESTATIONS OF TOXICITY

The antineoplastics are known for their toxicity to cells with a high level of mitotic activity, such as malignant cells. This characteristic feature accounts for their common clinical manifestations of toxicity, including mucositis, alopecia, and bone marrow suppression. They can also cause protracted vomiting because of their ability to stimulate the chemoreceptor trigger zone in the medulla by vagal and sympathetic pathways either directly or indirectly through the GI tract. The likelihood for vomiting depends on the dose, the route of administration, and the type of antineoplastic. Although the onset of emesis typically occurs within 6 hours and lasts for 24 hours, emesis developing beyond this period can occur (ie, cisplatin cyclophosphamide, carboplatin, and doxorubicin). The time of onset for the other manifestations is typically in the first week following treatment, with mucositis preceding leukopenia, which varies depending on the agent and dose. For example, the nadir and recovery for neutropenia is about 7 to 13 days and 21 to 24 days, respectively, but it can be more delayed for busulfan and carmustine, and when high doses are used. Antineoplastics likely to cause severe neutropenia include anthracyclines and platinum-based antineoplastics, and those likely to cause mucositis include methotrexate, 5-fluorouracil, bleomycin, and doxorubicin. Because of the amount of GI fluid loss associated with diarrhea and vomiting, patients can develop dehydration. Death is usually from overwhelming sepsis due to enteric organisms that enter the blood stream through compromised GI epithelium and attack a host with neutropenia from bone marrow suppression. For example, an overdose with topotecan has resulted in bone marrow suppression with overwhelming sepsis and death.[47] Some of the unique manifestations for certain antineoplastics involve the skin, heart, central and peripheral nervous systems, and kidneys.

Dermatologic manifestations caused by antineoplastics can be due to hypersensitivity reactions, extravasations (see Special Considerations SC3: Extravasation of Xenobiotics), or cytotoxicity from the use of tyrosine kinase inhibitors for the EGFR (eg, gefitinib, erlotinib).[67] Patients commonly develop pruritus, xerosis, erythema, and folliculitis or an acneiform rash that can desquamate during therapy. The time of onset is within the first week of treatment and it intensifies at about 2 to 3 weeks. The folliculitis is a dose-dependent response and typically resolves within weeks after treatment. The dermal response appears to be more intense with monoclonal antibodies than the kinase inhibitors for the EFGR. The other kinase inihibitors (ie, sunitinib, sorafenib) involved with growth factor receptors for angiogenesis (ie, VEGFR, PDGFR) are associated with a "hand-foot" skin reaction, which is a painful erythema and edema of the palm and sole that leads to desquamation.

The cardiovascular manifestations of toxicity depend on the antineoplastic, and the common ones include congestive heart failure (CHF), dysrhythmias, and hypertension. The anthracyclines, cyclophosphamide, and 5-fluorouracil can cause cardiac toxicity (Table 52–2). Although

TABLE 52–2. Cardiovascular Manifestations of Toxicity of Selected Antineoplastics

Antineoplastic	Time of Onset Since Treatment	Manifestation
Anthracycline	<24 hours	Dysrhythmias, ST segment and T wave changes on ECG; diminished left ventricular ejection fraction leading to congestive heart failure (CHF), pericarditis, myocarditis, and sudden death
	Months to years, typically at 1–4 months	Dilated congestive cardiomyopathy
Cyclophosphamide	Days	CHF, hemorrhagic pericarditis, tamponade, and death
5-Fluorouracil	Hours to days	Myocardial ischemia and cardiogenic shock

the anthracyclines are known for their late-onset cardiomyopathy, they can also cause acute cardiac manifestations. Those occurring within 24 hours of therapy include dysrhythmias, ST segment and T wave changes on electrocardiogram (ECG), diminished left ventricular ejection fraction leading to congestive heart failure, pericarditis, myocarditis, and sudden death.[8,50,51,58,66] Myocardial ischemia leading to cardiogenic shock can occur from the high dose infusion of 5-fluorouracil.[62] The metabolite fluoroacetate[4] is purported to cause endothelial damage and result in vasospasm.[23] Normalization of ECG findings, including diminished QRS voltage and abnormal ventricular wall motion, are expected by 48 hours after the discontinuation of infusion therapy.[14] Within a few days of exposure, cyclophosphamide can cause CHF, hemorrhagic pericarditis, tamponade, and death at high doses from therapy during bone marrow transplant or the overdose setting. The cardiomyopathy from anthracyclines involves biventricular failure and its onset is variable, from months to years, depending on the agent. Although this period is usually 1 to 4 months, it tends be longer for the less toxic anthracycline analogs.[22,26,54] Trastuzumab is associated with a slight increase in cardiac dysfunction among patients previously treated with anthracyclines or with underlying heart disease. A potential mechanism for the enhanced cardiac toxicity from the drug interaction is that trastuzumab disrupts the HER2-neuregulin compensatory response by the heart to the exposure to anthracyclines.[15]

The neurologic toxicities of antineoplastics include central and peripheral manifestations. The acute manifestations of toxicity include altered mental status and seizures, which occur from the systemic administration of high doses of nitrogen mustards (cyclophosphamide, ifosfamide, and chlorambucil), nitrosureas (lomustine), methotrexate, and vincristine (see Special Considerations SC–2: Intrathecal Administration of Xenobiotics). Also, the inappropriate intrathecal administration of vincristine and methotrexate can cause central nervous system toxicity (see Special Considerations SC–2: Intrathecal Administration of Xenobiotics). Patients with prior seizure disorders, delayed drug clearance, and altered drug pharmacokinetics (eg, nephrotic syndrome)[48] are at increased risk for seizures. L-asparaginase, 5-fluorouracil, and procarbazine are associated with altered mental status.[64] Cerebellar ataxia has been described in 5% of patients treated with 5FU,[41] and high frequency ototoxicity can occur with cisplatin toxicity. The late-onset manifestations of neurotoxicity from antineoplastics include leukoencephalopathy and peripheral neuropathies. Leukoencephalopathy from methotrexate typically presents as the late-onset of behavioral and progressive dementia and it is irreversible at this stage. Peripheral neuropathy involving both sensory and motor findings is seen with the Vinca alkaloids (vincristine), and only with sensory involvement with cisplatin and paclitaxel.[33]

Renal insufficiency due to tubulointerstitial pathology can occur from methotrexate, cisplatin, or nitrosureas in a dose-dependent manner. Also, the nitrosureas (semustine) can cause glomerular injury leading to sclerosis. Renal damage from these agents is attributed to the formation of insoluble intratubular precipitates of drug metabolites (ie, 7-OH MTX metabolite for MTX) or reactive intermediates (eg, cisplatin, nitrosureas) that lead to cell death. The nitrosureas can also form isocyanate, which can impair DNA repair enzymes and lead to irreversible renal damage.[32] The onset, severity, and reversibility of renal toxicity depend on the administered dose and the particular agent in the drug class. For example, streptozocin is more nephrotoxic than the other nitrosureas: semustine, lomustine, and carmustine. Patients at increased risk for worsening renal function from the therapeutic use of these agents include those with prior renal disease, increased age, salt and water depletion, hypotension, and concomitant use of nephrotoxic xenobiotics, such as aminoglycosides. Also, patients with third space fluid, such as ascites and pleural effusions, and aciduria are at increased risk for MTX-induced renal toxicity because of the drug's prolonged half-life and the increased likelihood for the formation of insoluble precipitates in the renal tubules at a low urinary pH. The renal failure due to methotrexate, cisplatin, and streptozocin typically presents in an acute fashion within 1 to 2 weeks unlike that for semustine. Patients treated with semustine can present with elevated serum creatinine in a delayed fashion, months to years, following exposure.[65]

DIAGNOSTIC TESTING

The determination of the antineoplastic concentration in clinical specimens is not routinely available, except for methotrexate. At certain research centers,[9] the testing for specific xenobiotics can be available: busulfan,[57] cisplatin (platinum),[17] vincristine,[16] and topotecan. These concentrations can be used to assist in confirming exposure and monitoring drug clearance, but should not be relied upon to determine initial management because of the difficulty in obtaining these tests and ability to correlate the concentrations with clinical toxicity.

For certain antineoplastics, the presence of typical clinical manifestations can strongly suggest their toxicity. For example, cisplatin (renal insufficiency and ototoxicity), Vinca alkaloids (peripheral neuropathy, central autonomic instability, and syndrome of inappropriate antidiuretic hormone secretion), anthracyclines (CHF and dilated cardiomyopathy), ifosfamide (encephalopathy and seizures), and methotrexate (renal insufficiency, mucositis, and pancytopenia). The diagnosis of a patient with toxicity from these xenobiotics is based on a historical evidence for exposure, clinical manifestations, and laboratory findings that support toxicity or exposure. For patients presenting with delayed or late-onset symptoms, the association between toxicity and exposure requires an increased level of awareness to establish the causation.[22] Additional studies can be obtained to evaluate for specific disorders noted on the clinical examination, such as electromyography and nerve conduction studies for peripheral neuropathies, electroretinogram for retinopathies, and echocardiography for cardiac dysfunction.

GENERAL MANAGEMENT

The initial management of these patients includes stabilization of the hemodynamic status, decontamination, institution of antidotal therapy, and enhanced elimination. Maximal benefits from antidotes and enhanced elimination can be obtained through their timely institution. Hypotension can result from dehydration, cardiac dysfunction, or sepsis. Patients with myocardial ischemia from 5-FU can be treated with coronary vasodilators, such as nitrates and calcium channel blockers. Seizures are treated with benzodiazepines, barbiturates, and propofol. Encephalopathy from high-dose ifosfamide has been treated with methylene blue (adult: 50 mg intravenously [IV] as a 1% solution).[40] Patients with blood dyscrasias, including neutropenia and thrombocytopenia, should be evaluated for gastrointestinal bleeding and infections. Those at risk for overwhelming sepsis should be started on broad-spectrum antibiotics and granulocyte colony stimulating factor as indicated. Oral activated charcoal can be administered to patients soon after an oral exposure to limit the gut bioavailability of the agent. Repeat oral doses of activated charcoal can enhance the clearance of methotrexate in patients with renal insufficiency.[20]

Patients with vomiting are typically difficult to manage. Combination therapy involving multiple antiemetics are needed to treat patients exposed to antineoplastics with high emetogenic potential (eg, cisplatin, doxorubicin, cyclophosphamide, lomustine) or excessive doses of antineoplastics with low emetogenic potential (eg, Vinca alkaloids, fluorouracil). Therapy can include a serotonin receptor antagonist, glucocorticoid, dopamine receptor antagonist, a neurokinin-1 receptor antagonist (eg, aprepitant), or a benzodiazepine.[34] Serotonin receptor antagonists are effective for acute onset vomiting (circa within 6 hours of exposure) and are used with dexamethasone and aprepitant in patients with protracted vomiting. Once the serotonin receptors are saturated, additional doses of these agents are no longer effective. Aprepitant, when used in combination with a glucocorticoid (eg, dexamethasone), is effective for managing delayed-onset vomiting, which can last for 5 days. Dopamine receptor antagonists, serotonin receptor antagonists, or dexamethasone at a higher dose can be used to treat breakthrough vomiting. Also, benzodiazepines can be used in this setting, but they are most effective for the treatment of anticipatory vomiting. A comprehensive serum chemistry panel, complete blood count (CBC), urinalysis, and electrocardiogram should be obtained for patients with a significant overdose to evaluate for extent of toxicity and for establishing baseline values and performance parameters. The patient's peripheral blood count should be followed for up to 2 weeks after antineoplastics administration because the onset of myelosuppression can be delayed.

Gastrointestinal fluid losses from vomiting, diarrhea, and mucosal ulcerations can lead to dehydration, which needs to be treated with intravenous fluids. Also, intravenous fluids are important for patients with cisplatin and methotrexate toxicity to promote the renal elimination of toxic metabolites. Patients with cisplatin toxicity should be treated with normal saline with an osmotic diuretic to maintain an adequate chloride gradient to promote the renal elimination of cisplatin. Urinary alkalinization is indicated for patients with MTX toxicity to limit the precipitation of drug metabolites in the renal tubules.

Antidotal therapy is available for only a few xenobiotics, including anthracyclines (dexrazoxane), methotrexate (leucovorin, glucarpidase), cisplatin (amifostine, thiosulfate), 5-FU (vistinuridine) and ifosfamide (methylene blue, mercaptoethane sulfonate). They are used in medical therapy to allow higher dose therapies of antineoplastics in cancer patients. However, patients with overdoses from antineoplastics can also benefit from these therapies, which should be initiated soon after the decision to treat has been made. Additional information regarding them can be found in chapters 53 and 54 and Antidotes A 13, A 14).

Information on the use of enhanced elimination to remove these agents is limited to case reports in the literature. The effectiveness of these procedures is based on principles similar to other xenobiotics, including molecular size, extent of protein binding, and volume of distribution. Patients with diminished endogenous clearance due to inherent disorders, such as renal failure, or third spacing of fluid, can benefit from these procedures as well. For example, cisplatin is highly protein bound and favored for removal by plasmaperesis, but patients with renal failure can also benefit from hemodialysis. Hemoperfusion has been used for doxorubicin and it appears to be more effective than hemodialysis. For the nitrogen mustards and the alkyl sulfonates, hemodialysis has been used. The early institution of these procedures can maximize the potential benefits to the patient.

The decision to use myeloid growth factors in patients with agranulocytosis depends on the severity and nature of the neutropenia, the anticipated speed of recovery, and the tumor type. Granulocyte-macrophage colony-stimulating factor (GM-CSF) has been used in several patients with antineoplastic overdoses that included cisplatin, melphalan, bleomycin, and methotrexate.[13,24,27-29,31,39,55] Typically, if promyelocytes and myelocytes are present in the bone marrow, neutrophil recovery will occur spontaneously in 4 to 7 days, following the withdrawal of the offending antineoplastic.[19] However, when granulopoiesis is completely absent, neutrophil recovery cannot be expected for at least 14 days. Using granulocyte colony-stimulating factor (G-CSF) or GM-CSF can accelerate neutrophil recovery during cytotoxic antineoplastic therapy. When myeloid precursors are present in the bone marrow, G-CSF can accelerate neutrophil recovery in 1 to 4 days. If myeloid precursors are absent, neutrophil recovery with G-CSF may take longer, but can be expected to occur sooner than without G-CSF therapy. GM-CSF is indicated for use in neutropenic patients following induction antineoplastic therapy for acute myelogenous leukemia because this agent enhances the response of macrophages, neutrophils, and eosinophils. Serum concentrations of the antineoplastic should be below detection before institution of G-CSF to gain maximal response; typically, G-CSF is initiated 24 hours after the completion of the treatment cycle. The initial dose is 5 μg/kg/d IV or subcutaneously, and it is continued beyond the expected white blood cell (WBC) nadir. This is usually a 2-week course; however, it can be prolonged with lomustine overdoses.[1,60] The dose may be adjusted, depending on the patient's WBC response. Therapy can be discontinued when the post-nadir absolute neutrophil count is greater than 10×10^3 cells/mm^3. Bone pain can be anticipated from the use of colony-stimulating factors, presumably because of the increase in cellularity in the marrow space. Additional side effects can be expected from GM-CSF therapy, including myalgia, fevers, and pericarditis.

GM-CSF might produce a transient beneficial response in the WBCs in patients with aplastic anemia.[11] However, when the anemia was severe, the GM-CSF therapy was not effective. Another hematopoietic growth factor is erythropoietin (epoetin alfa and darbepoetin alfa), which is approved for use in patients with anemia associated with cancer chemotherapy treatment.[6,46] Although the purpose of this therapy is to decrease the need for red blood cell transfusions, it does not replace the need for red blood cell transfusion when indicated.

ANTINEOPLASTICS IN THE WORKPLACE

A variety of workers are at risk for increased exposure to antineoplastics, including pharmacists, nurses, physicians, and others involved in the preparation and dispensing of these antineoplastics, and who may be exposed to the body fluids of patients treated with these agents. Several studies demonstrate that these agents can be detected in the work environment and measured in workers,[49] and there is concern about the possible genotoxic effects from these exposures.[52] The worker may absorb these xenobiotics by either the dermal, inhalational, or gastrointestinal route. The factors determining the amount of worker exposure include the nature of the work, the amount of drug used, the frequency and duration of exposure, the physical and chemical nature of the drug, and the use of ventilated cabinets and personal protection equipment during the handling of these agents. The workplace guidelines for antineoplastics fall under the broader category of hazardous xenobiotics. A sample list of drugs considered to be hazardous agents by the National Institute for Occupational Safety and Health (NIOSH) is available for further information.[10] The NIOSH defines a "drug" as a "hazardous agent" if it is carcinogenic, teratogenic, genotoxic, associated with developmental or reproductive toxicity, or toxic to organs at low dose.

Regulatory and workplace recommendations for exposure levels and the waste management of these xenobiotics are available from various agencies and organizations. These recommendations are limited in scope because only a small number of xenobiotics or adverse health effects have been adequately studied, and many xenobiotics do not meet the current definition for inclusion. US Environmental Protection Agency (Resource Conservation and Recovery Act, 40 CFR §§260–279)[45] regulates nine antineoplastics (arsenic trioxide, chlorambucil, cyclophosphamide, daunomycin, melphalan, mitomycin C, naphthylamine mustard, streptozocin, and uracil mustard) and the equipment and devices associated with their preparation or delivery, as well as their disposal, as hazardous waste.[45] The current recommendations for worker safety with these xenobiotics in the workplace include the proper management of the work environment (eg, storage, handling, preparation, administration, use of personal protection equipment, decontamination, waste disposal) and the institution of a medical surveillance program with approved laboratory testing.[2,38,52]

SUMMARY

The antineoplastics are a unique therapeutic class because their cytotoxicity is a direct effect. Medicine is challenged to carefully balance this measure so that there is limited damage to native cells, and thus the patient. Over the years, the number of antineoplastic exposures reported to the American Association of Poison Control Centers National Poison Data System has remained small; however, the consequences of toxicity to the patients in these reports were great. The majority of these occurrences were iatrogenic, involving misreading of the product label, and errors in dosing and transcription of orders (see Chap. 139). A key element was the lack of familiarity of the healthcare provider with the use of these select xenobiotics. The number of antineoplastics and their indicated use has increased over the years and will continue in this fashion into the future, increasing the chance for medical error and patient toxicity. The clinical manifestations of toxicity can develop in various organ systems and are primarily determined by the mechanism of action, route of administration, and duration of exposure. The gut epithelium and bone marrow are extremely susceptible to toxicity because of their high mitotic activity. They are important because their failure will lead to overwhelming sepsis and death. Treatment remains primarily supportive in nature. The early institution of cytoprotectants, such as glucarpidase for methotrexate, amifostine for cisplatin, vistonuridine for 5-FU, and dexrazone for anthracyclines, as antidotal therapy in overdosed patients can limit further toxicity. However, further work is needed to better define their use in these situations. Although cytoprotectants will continue to be developed, they cannot be relied on to rescue patients from exposures, because their number will be few in comparison to the quantity of available antineoplastics and their effectiveness limited to pretreatment. Thus, prevention is the best treatment, which can be accomplished by maintaining a heightened awareness when working with these xenobiotics, educating the patient and healthcare provider regarding their use, and providing increased skilled care.

ACKNOWLEDGMENT

This chapter was written by Richard Y. Wang in his private capacity. No official support or endorsement by the Centers for Disease Control and Prevention is intended or should be inferred. Paul Calabresi, MD contributed to this chapter in a previous edition.

REFERENCES

1. Abele M, Leonhardt M, Dichgans J, Weller M. CCNU overdose during PCV chemotherapy for anaplastic astrocytoma. *J Neurol.* 1998;245:236-238.
2. American Society of Hospital Pharmacists. ASHP technical assistance bulletin on handling cytotoxic and hazardous drugs. *Am J Hosp Pharm.* 1990; 47:1033-1049.
3. Ando Y, Saka H, Ando M, et al. Polymorphisms of UDP-glucuronosyltransferase gene and irinotecan toxicity: a pharmacogenetic analysis. *Cancer Res.* 2000;60:6921-6926.
4. Arellano M, Malet-Martino M, Martino R, Gires P. The anti-cancer drug 5-fluorouracil is metabolized by the isolated perfused rat liver and in rats into highly toxic fluoroacetate. *Br J Cancer.* 1998;77:79-86.
5. Baldo P, Bertola A, Basaglia G, et al. A centralized Pharmacy Unit for cytotoxic drugs in accordance with Italian legislation. *J Eval Clin Pract.* 2007;13:265-271.
6. Bokemeyer C, Aapro MS, Courdi A, et al. EORTC guidelines for the use of erythropoietic proteins in anaemic patients with cancer: 2006 update. *Eur J Cancer.* 2007;43:258-270.
7. Bonnabry P, Cingria L, Ackermann M, et al. Use of a prospective risk analysis method to improve the safety of the cancer chemotherapy process. *Int J Qual Health Care.* 2006;18:9-16.
8. Bristow MR. Toxic cardiomyopathy due to doxorubicin. *Hosp Pract (Off Ed).* 1982;17:101-108, 110-101.
9. Centers for Disease Control and Prevention. National Institute for Occupational Safety and Health. Occupational exposure to antineoplastic to antineoplastic agents. Atlanta, GA: Centers for Disease Control and Prevention; 2008. http://www.cdc.gov/niosh/topics/antineoplastic/monitoring.html. Accesed January 16, 2009.
10. Centers for Disease Control and Prevention. *The NIOSH Alert: Preventing Occupational Exposures to Antineoplastic and Other Hazardous Drugs in Healthcare Settings (Pub. No. 2004–165).* Cincinnati, OH: NIOSH—Publications Dissemination, September; 2004. http://www.cdc.gov/niosh/docs/2004–165/. Accessed January16, 2009.
11. Champlin RE, Nimer SD, Ireland P, Oette DH, Golde DW. Treatment of refractory aplastic anemia with recombinant human granulocyte-macrophage-colony-stimulating factor. *Blood.* 1989;73:694-699.
12. Chen CS, Seidel K, Armitage JO, et al. Safeguarding the administration of high-dose chemotherapy: a national practice survey by the American Society for Blood and Marrow Transplantation. *Biol Blood Marrow Transplant.* 1997;3:331-340.
13. Chu G, Mantin R, Shen YM, Baskett G, Sussman H. Massive cisplatin overdose by accidental substitution for carboplatin. Toxicity and management. *Cancer.* 1993;72:3707-3714.
14. de Forni M, Malet-Martino MC, Jaillais P, et al. Cardiotoxicity of high-dose continuous infusion fluorouracil: a prospective clinical study. *J Clin Oncol.* 1992;10:1795-1801.
15. de Korte MA, de Vries EG, Lub-de Hooge MN, et al. 111Indium-trastuzumab visualises myocardial human epidermal growth factor receptor 2 expression shortly after anthracycline treatment but not during heart failure: a clue to uncover the mechanisms of trastuzumab-related cardiotoxicity. *Eur J Cancer.* 2007;43:2046-2051.
16. Desai ZR, Van den Berg HW, Bridges JM, Shanks RG. Can severe vincristine neurotoxicity be prevented? *Cancer Chemother Pharmacol.* 1982;8: 211-214.
17. Erdlenbruch B, Pekrun A, Schiffmann H, Witt O, Lakomek M. Topical topic: accidental cisplatin overdose in a child: reversal of acute renal failure with sodium thiosulfate. *Med Pediatr Oncol.* 2002;38:349-352.
18. Favier M, de Cazanove F, Saint-Martin F, Bressolle F. Preventing medication errors in antineoplastic therapy. *Am J Hosp Pharm.* 1994;51:832-833.
19. Fleischman RA. Southwestern Internal Medicine Conference: clinical use of hematopoietic growth factors. *Am J Med Sci.* 1993;305:248-273.
20. Gadgil SD, Damle SR, Advani SH, Vaidya AB. Effect of activated charcoal on the pharmacokinetics of high-dose methotrexate. *Cancer Treat Rep.* 1982;66:1169-1171.
21. Gandhi TK, Bartel SB, Shulman LN, et al. Medication safety in the ambulatory chemotherapy setting. *Cancer.* 2005;104:2477-2483.
22. Gbadamosi J, Munchau A, Weiller C, Schafer H. Severe heart failure in a young multiple sclerosis patient. *J Neurol.* 2003;250:241-242.
23. Gorgulu S, Celik S, Tezel T. A case of coronary spasm induced by 5-fluorouracil. *Acta Cardiol.* 2002;57:381-383.
24. Gratwohl A, Dazzi H, Tichelli A, et al. [Emergency therapy with granulocyte-macrophage colony-stimulating factor (GM-CSF)]. *Schweiz Med Wochenschr.* 1991;121:413-417.
25. Innocenti F, Iyer L, Ramirez J, Green MD, Ratain MJ. Epirubicin glucuronidation is catalyzed by human UDP-glucuronosyltransferase 2B7. *Drug Metab Dispos.* 2001;29:686-692.
26. Jensen BV, Skovsgaard T, Nielsen SL. Functional monitoring of anthracycline cardiotoxicity: a prospective, blinded, long-term observational study of outcome in 120 patients. *Ann Oncol.* 2002;13:699-709.
27. Jirillo A, Gioga G, Bonciarelli G, Dalla Valle G. Accidental overdose of melphalan per os in a 69-year-old woman treated for advanced endometrial carcinoma. *Tumori.* 1998;84:611.
28. Jost LM. [Overdose with melphalan (Alkeran): symptoms and treatment. A review]. *Onkologie.* 1990;13:96-101.

29. Jung HK, Lee J, Lee SN. A case of massive cisplatin overdose managed by plasmapheresis. *Korean J Intern Med.* 1995;10:150-154.
30. Karamouzis MV, Grandis JR, Argiris A. Therapies directed against epidermal growth factor receptor in aerodigestive carcinomas. *JAMA.* 2007;298:70-82.
31. Kim IS, Gratwohl A, Stebler C, et al. Accidental overdose of multiple chemotherapeutic agents. *Korean J Intern Med.* 1989;4:171-173.
32. Kramer RA, Schuller HM, Smith AC, Boyd MR. Effects of buthionine sulfoximine on the nephrotoxicity of 1-(2-chloroethyl)-3-(trans-4-methylcyclohexyl)-1-nitrosourea (MeCCNU). *J Pharmacol Exp Ther.* 1985;234:498-506.
33. Krarup-Hansen A, Helweg-Larsen S, Schmalbruch H, Rorth M, Krarup C. Neuronal involvement in cisplatin neuropathy: prospective clinical and neurophysiological studies. *Brain.* 2007;130:1076-1088.
34. Kris MG, Hesketh PJ, Somerfield MR, et al. American Society of Clinical Oncology guideline for antiemetics in oncology: update 2006. *J Clin Oncol.* 2006;24:2932-2947.
35. Limat S, Drouhin JP, Demesmay K, et al. Incidence and risk factors of preparation errors in a centralized cytotoxic preparation unit. *Pharm World Sci.* 2001;23:102-106.
36. Martin F, Legat C, Coutet J, et al. [Prevention of preparation errors of cytotoxic drugs in centralized units: from epidemiology to quality assurance]. *Bull Cancer.* 2004;91:972-976.
37. Milano G, Etienne MC, Cassuto-Viguier E, et al. Influence of sex and age on fluorouracil clearance. *J Clin Oncol.* 1992;10:1171-1175.
38. Occupational Safety and Health Administration. Sec VI, Chapt II: Categorization of drugs as hazardous. TED 1–0.15A. OSHA Technical manual, 1999. http://www.osha.gov/dts/osta/otm/ otm_vi/otm_vi_2.html#2. Accessed January 10, 2009.
39. Pecherstorfer M, Zimmer-Roth I, Weidinger S, et al. High-dose intravenous melphalan in a patient with multiple myeloma and oliguric renal failure. *Clin Investig.* 1994;72:522-525.
40. Pelgrims J, De Vos F, Van den Brande J, et al. Methylene blue in the treatment and prevention of ifosfamide-induced encephalopathy: report of 12 cases and a review of the literature. *Br J Cancer.* 2000;82:291-294.
41. Pirzada NA, Ali, II, Dafer RM. Fluorouracil-induced neurotoxicity. *Ann Pharmacother.* 2000;34:35-38.
42. Port RE, Daniel B, Ding RW, Herrmann R. Relative importance of dose, body surface area, sex, and age for 5-fluorouracil clearance. *Oncology.* 1991;48:277-281.
43. Ratain MJ, Mick R, Berezin F, et al. Paradoxical relationship between acetylator phenotype and amonafide toxicity. *Clin Pharmacol Ther.* 1991;50:573-579.
44. Reichert JM, Rosensweig CJ, Faden LB, Dewitz MC. Monoclonal antibody successes in the clinic. *Nat Biotechnol.* 2005;23:1073-1078.
45. Resource Conservation and Recovery Act, 40 CFR §§ 260–279 (1996).
46. Rizzo JD, Somerfield MR, Hagerty KL, et al. Use of epoetin and darbepoetin in patients with cancer: 2007 American Society of Hematology/American Society of Clinical Oncology clinical practice guideline update. *Blood.* 2008;111:25-41.
47. Royal W 3rd, Dupont B, McGuire D, et al. Topotecan in the treatment of acquired immunodeficiency syndrome-related progressive multifocal leukoencephalopathy. *J Neurovirol.* 2003;9:411-419.
48. Salloum E, Khan KK, Cooper DL. Chlorambucil-induced seizures. *Cancer.* 1997;79:1009-1013.
49. Schreiber C, Radon K, Pethran A, et al. Uptake of antineoplastic agents in pharmacy personnel. Part II: study of work-related risk factors. *Int Arch Occup Environ Health.* 2003;76:11-16.
50. Schwartz CL, Hobbie WL, Truesdell S, Constine LC, Clark EB. Corrected QT interval prolongation in anthracycline-treated survivors of childhood cancer. *J Clin Oncol.* 1993;11:1906-1910.
51. Schwartz RG, McKenzie WB, Alexander J, et al. Congestive heart failure and left ventricular dysfunction complicating doxorubicin therapy. Seven-year experience using serial radionuclide angiocardiography. *Am J Med.* 1987;82:1109-1118.
52. Sessink PJ, Bos RP. Drugs hazardous to healthcare workers. Evaluation of methods for monitoring occupational exposure to cytostatic drugs. *Drug Saf.* 1999;20:347-359.
53. Siegert W, Hiddemann W, Koppensteiner R, et al. Accidental overdose of mitoxantrone in three patients. *Med Oncol Tumor Pharmacother.* 1989;6:275-278.
54. Stahl M, Schweers K, Muller C, Köster W, Wilke H. Application of adjuvant chemotherapy in colorectal cancer—a survey in the region of Essen, Germany. *Onkologie.* 2005;28:7-10.
55. Steger GG, Mader RM, Gnant MF, et al. GM-CSF in the treatment of a patient with severe methotrexate intoxication. *J Intern Med.* 1993;233:499-502.
56. Stein BN, Petrelli NJ, Douglass HO, et al. Age and sex are independent predictors of 5-fluorouracil toxicity. Analysis of a large scale phase III trial. *Cancer.* 1995;75:11-17.
57. Stein J, Davidovitz M, Yaniv I, et al. Accidental busulfan overdose: enhanced drug clearance with hemodialysis in a child with Wiskott-Aldrich syndrome. *Bone Marrow Transplant.* 2001;27:551-553.
58. Steinberg JS, Cohen AJ, Wasserman AG, Cohen P, Ross AM. Acute arrhythmogenicity of doxorubicin administration. *Cancer.* 1987;60:1213-1218.
59. Taylor JA, Winter L, Geyer LJ, Hawkins DS. Oral outpatient chemotherapy medication errors in children with acute lymphoblastic leukemia. *Cancer.* 2006;107:1400-1406.
60. Trent KC, Myers L, Moreb J. Multiorgan failure associated with lomustine overdose. *Ann Pharmacother.* 1995;29:384-386.
61. Tsalic M, Bar-Sela G, Beny A, Visel B, Haim N. Severe toxicity related to the 5-fluorouracil/leucovorin combination (the Mayo Clinic regimen): a prospective study in colorectal cancer patients. *Am J Clin Oncol.* 2003;26:103-106.
62. Tsavaris N, Kosmas C, Vadiaka M, et al. Cardiotoxicity following different doses and schedules of 5-fluorouracil administration for malignancy—a survey of 427 patients. *Med Sci Monit.* 2002;8:PI51-57.
63. Wasserman E, Myara A, Lokiec F, et al. Severe CPT-11 toxicity in patients with Gilbert's syndrome: two case reports. *Ann Oncol.* 1997;8:1049-1051.
64. Weiss HD, Walker MD, Wiernik PH. Neurotoxicity of commonly used antineoplastic agents (second of two parts). *N Engl J Med.* 1974;291:127-133.
65. Weiss RB, Posada JG Jr, Kramer RA, Boyd MR. Nephrotoxicity of semustine. *Cancer Treat Rep.* 1983;67:1105-1112.
66. Wortman JE, Lucas VS Jr, Schuster E, Thiele D, Logue GL. Sudden death during doxorubicin administration. *Cancer.* 1979;44:1588-1591.
67. Wyatt AJ, Leonard GD, Sachs DL. Cutaneous reactions to chemotherapy and their management. *Am J Clin Dermatol.* 2006;7:45-63.

CHAPTER 53
ANTINEOPLASTICS: METHOTREXATE

Richard Y. Wang

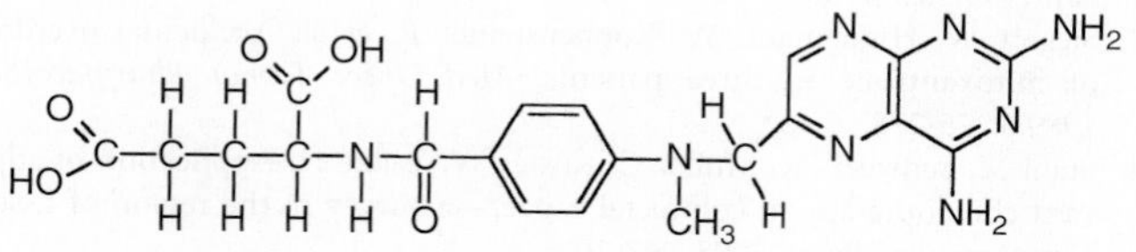

Methotrexate (MTX) is commonly used for a substantial number of therapeutic cancerous and noncancerous indications. Its immunosuppressive activity allows it to also be used for rheumatoid arthritis, organ transplantation, psoriasis, trophoblastic diseases, and therapeutic abortion.[10,29]

Risk factors for MTX toxicity include impaired renal function (primary route of drug elimination); third compartment spacing: ascites and pleural effusions; use of nephrotoxins, such as nonsteroidal anti-inflammatory drugs (NSAIDs) and aminoglycosides[37] and certain intravenous radiologic contrast agents[16,24]; age; folate deficiency; and concurrent infection.[60] MTX toxicity depends more on the duration of exposure than the dose itself.

PHARMACOLOGY

The therapeutic and toxic effects of methotrexate are based on its ability to limit DNA and RNA synthesis by inhibiting dihydrofolate reductase (DHFR) and thymidylate synthetase (Fig. 53–1). Thymidylate synthesis is inhibited by polyglutamic derivatives of methotrexate. DHFR reduces folic acid to tetrahydrofolate (FH4), which serves as an essential cofactor in the synthesis of purine nucleotides. These reduced folates are also required by thymidylate synthetase to serve as methyl donors in the formation of thymidylate. Thymidylate is then used for DNA synthesis. MTX is a structural analog of folate and competitively inhibits DHFR by binding to this enzyme's site of action. This stops reduced folate production, which is necessary for nucleotide formation and DNA/RNA synthesis.

The bioavailability of methotrexate appears to be limited by a saturable intestinal absorption mechanism. At oral doses less than 30 mg/m^2, the absorption is 90%; at doses greater than 80 mg/m^2, the absorption is less than 10% to 20%.[8] The weekly adult dose used for the treatment of psoriasis and rheumatoid arthritis is low and can be administered orally. However, the dose used to induce abortion is higher (50 mg/m^2) and must be administered parenterally to achieve effective drug concentrations. MTX dosing regimens for chemotherapy are variable, but can be generally classified as low (40 mg/m^2), moderate, and high doses (1000 mg/m^2). Conventional intravenous doses of up to 100 mg/m^2 can be administered without leucovorin rescue. Doses of 1000 mg/m^2 are considered potentially lethal. Much higher doses (2 to 3 g/m^2) can be given when MTX is followed by leucovorin in order to prevent life-threatening toxicity. Mortality from high-dose MTX is approximately 6%, and occurs primarily when patients' MTX concentrations are not monitored.[60,63]

MTX has a triphasic plasma clearance. The initial plasma distribution half-life is short—0.75 hours. The second half-life is 2 to 3.4 hours and represents renal clearance of the drug. The third phase has a half-life of about 8 to 10.4 hours and represents tissue redistribution into the plasma. This third phase can be prolonged in the setting of renal failure and is associated with bone marrow and gastrointestinal (GI) toxicity. The volume of distribution is 0.6 to 0.9 L/kg and protein beveling is 50%. Healthy kidneys eliminate 50% to 80% of MTX unchanged within 48 hours of administration. When the creatinine clearance is less than 60 mL/min, MTX clearance is delayed.[53,65]

PATHOPHYSIOLOGY

At high doses, drug and insoluble drug metabolites 7-hydroxy methotrexate and 2,4-diamino-10-methyl pteroic acid accumulate and may precipitate in the renal tubules, causing reversible acute tubular necrosis. MTX is one-tenth as soluble at a pH of 5.5 as it is at a pH of 7.5.[8,54] Expressed another way, the serum concentration threshold for nephrotoxicity is 2.2 mmol/L when the urine pH is 5.5, and 22 mmol/L when the urine pH is 6.9. Thus, patients who are either inadequately hydrated or not alkalinized are at risk for acute renal failure from high-dose MTX treatment.[2,30] MTX is excreted unchanged in the urine by both glomerular filtration and active tubular secretion. Folic acid blocks MTX renal reabsorption and can enhance elimination during leucovorin rescue.[25] A small amount of MTX is metabolized intracellularly to polyglutamate derivatives, which inhibit DHFR and thymidylate synthetase and are believed to be responsible for the persistent cytotoxic effect of MTX because they do not easily diffuse outside of the cell.

CLINICAL MANIFESTATIONS

In the course of MTX therapy, a variety of disorders can occur, resulting from either increased patient susceptibility to toxicity or excessive administration. The clinical manifestations of MTX toxicity include stomatitis, esophagitis, renal failure, myelosuppression, hepatitis, and central neurologic system dysfunction. In a group of 23 patients who received 45 courses of high-dose MTX therapy with leucovorin rescue, the commonly observed signs included increased aspartate aminotransferase (AST)/alanine aminotransferase (ALT) (81%), nausea and vomiting (66%), mucositis (33%), dermatitis (18%), leukopenia (11%), thrombocytopenia (9%), and creatinine elevation (7%).[50]

Nausea and vomiting, considered rare after low-dose cancer therapy (40 mg/m^2), typically begin 2 to 4 hours after high-dose therapy (1000 mg/m^2) and last for about 6 to 12 hours. Mucositis, characterized by mouth soreness, stomatitis, or diarrhea, usually occurs 1 to 2 weeks after therapy and can last for 4 to 7 days. Other gastrointestinal symptoms resulting from MTX therapy include pharyngitis, anorexia, gastrointestinal hemorrhage, and toxic megacolon.[5] Hepatocellular toxicity, as described by increased AST (>1000 IU/L ALT >1000 IU/L), and hyperbilirubinemia, can be observed with both acute and chronic therapy.[42,44] It is usually associated with high-dosage regimens. Laboratory abnormalities improve within 1 to 2 weeks of discontinuation of MTX. The mechanism is incompletely understood, but toxicity is attributed to reduced liver folate stores.[6] Factors associated with hepatotoxicity are sustained high serum concentrations, increased cumulative dosages, chronic therapy, and host factors such as increase in age, obesity, diabetes, and alcoholism.[66]

Pancytopenia usually occurs within the first 2 weeks after an acute exposure. There are several reports demonstrating the occurrence of pancytopenia in individuals receiving chronic MTX therapy for rheumatoid arthritis and psoriasis.[14,36,42,52]

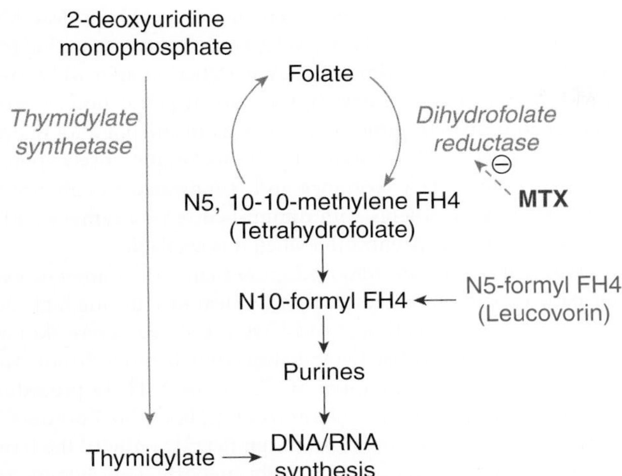

FIGURE 53–1. Mechanism of MTX toxicity. Methotrexate inhibits DHFR activity, which is necessary for DNA and RNA synthesis. Leucovorin bypasses blockade to allow for continued synthesis.

When used in low-dose intravenous (IV) doses of 40 to 60 mg/m^2, MTX is not associated with appreciable nephrotoxicity. However, at doses greater than 5000 mg/m^2 (approximately 130 mg/kg for an adult), several investigators report severe kidney damage, with oliguria, azotemia, and renal failure.[7] The renal function can normalize over time. Patients at risk for nephrotoxicity include the elderly, those with underlying renal disease defined as a glomerular filtration rate of less than 50 mL/min, and those who receive concurrent drug therapy that can delay MTX excretion, which includes agents that reduce renal blood flow such as NSAIDs, the nephrotoxins such as cisplatin, and the aminoglycosides, or weak organic acids such as salicylates and piperacillin which inhibit renal secretion.[28,60]

The neurologic complications associated with either high-dose systemic MTX therapy or intrathecal administration are the most consequential manifestations. The incidence of neurologic toxicity from high-dose MTX therapy is approximately 5% to 15%.[31] The manifestations usually occur from hours to days after the initiation of therapy and include hemiparesis, paraparesis, quadraparesis, seizures, and dysreflexia.[15,41,64,61] These events are reversible to varying degrees.[1] Clinical findings occurring within several hours (usually within 12 hours) of therapy are attributed to chemical arachnoiditis, and they include acute onset of fever, meningismus, pleocytosis, and increased cerebrospinal fluid (CSF) protein concentration.[26] Leukoencephalopathy is associated with the onset of behavioral disorders and progressive dementia from months to years after treatment and is irreversible, although manifestations presenting soon after treatment can be reversible depending on the extent of involvement.[4,69] Patients with increased age and prior cranial radiation are at risk for this disorder.[21] They have findings consistent with edema, and demyelination or necrosis of the white matter on computed tomography (CT) and magnetic resonance imaging (MRI) of the brain.[4]

DIAGNOSTIC TESTING

Serum methotrexate concentrations are monitored during therapy to help limit clinical toxicity. For example, patients with a serum concentration greater than 1.0 μmol/L at 48 hours posttreatment are considered at risk for bone marrow and gastrointestinal mucosal toxicity.[60] The measurement of methotrexate concentrations in the clinical setting is routinely conducted using an immunoassay technique, such as enzyme immunoassay or fluorescence polarization immunoassay (FPIA). These measurements can be performed on serum, plasma, and cerebrospinal fluid. The presence of MTX metabolites, such as 7-OH-MTX and DAMPA (2,4-diamino-N*10*-methylpteroic acid), folic acid, and certain drugs, such as trimethoprim and aminopterin, can diminish the specificity of the method for MTX.[3,9,17,48,55] The amount by which these xenobiotics affect the MTX concentration depends on the assay. The advantages of the high performance liquid chromatography (HPLC) method over these other methods include improved sensitivity, specificity, and ability to detect metabolites; however, it takes longer to run than the routine clinical methods because it is not an automated procedure. When patients are treated with carboxypeptidase G2, (see Antidote in Depth A-14) it is preferable to use the HPLC method to measure MTX because of the presence of metabolites during therapy. The FPIA method with monoclonal antibodies is not recommended for use in patients who have developed antibodies to mouse monoclonal antibodies or elevated concentrations of DAMPA.

An elevated serum methotrexate concentration (greater than 100 μmol/L) is indicative of an excessive intrathecal dose or delayed cerebrospinal fluid outflow obstruction.[46] Radiological imaging of the brain, such as computed tomography and magnetic resonance imaging, can be obtained to evaluate for meningeal inflammation, demyelination and necrosis of the white matter, or other pathologies such as a cerebrovascular accident.

MANAGEMENT

In the event of an oral overdose of methotrexate, the initial concern should be gastrointestinal decontamination. Activated charcoal adsorbs methotrexate and should be administered as soon as possible to limit absorption.[22] The administration of multiple-dose activated charcoal and cholestyramine[15,57] can significantly decrease the elimination half-life of methotrexate by interrupting the enterohepatic circulation.[19,22] This approach can increase MTX clearance but is of most benefit to patients with diminished creatinine clearance.

Adequate hydration with 0.9% sodium chloride solution as well as urinary alkalinization with IV sodium bicarbonate (to urine pH 7 to 8) (see Antidotes in Depth A 5: Sodium Bicarbonate) is also important to prevent renal failure from the precipitation of drug and metabolites in patients who receive inadvertent high doses.[11] The complete blood count (CBC) should be monitored on days 7, 10, and 14 to assess the impact on the bone marrow.[38] Granulocyte-macrophage colony-stimulating factor (GM-CSF) was used in a patient with a chronic MTX overdose and pancytopenia.[59] The patient had a serum MTX concentration of 1.25 μmol/L on admission and was in renal failure. Bone marrow biopsy showed promyelocytes, but no mature white cells, and a marked reduction of megakaryocytes. Because of deteriorating conditions, GM-CSF (125 μg/m^2/d) was administered when the MTX concentration fell below the reference limit for toxicity. Seven days after the initiation of GM-CSF, the white blood cell (WBC) count rose and reached normal values within 10 days.

Patients presenting with meningismus or altered mental status following MTX therapy require an initial MRI of the brain and then CSF analysis for infection.[34] Although not considered standard, the CSF may be assayed for MTX if excessive exposure to this compartment is suspected. The CSF methotrexate concentration is about 0.1 mol/L (1×10^5 μmol/L) and lasts for 48 hours after an IV MTX dose of 1500 mg/m^2, and 100 mol/L (1×10^8 μmol/L) for the peak therapeutic concentration after a 12-mg intrathecal MTX dose.[45] MRI of the brain may demonstrate a high signal throughout the pachymeningeal (dura mater) region, which is consistent with a chemical meningitis,[18] or a high signal of the white matter with a decreased diffusion coefficient in a diffusion weighted image to indicate the presence of edema, which is an early finding of leukoencephalopathy.

ANTIDOTES

The available rescue agents for methotrexate toxicity include folinic acid (leucovorin) (see Antidotes in Depth A–13: Leucovorin [Folinic Acid] and Folic Acid) and glucarpidase (carboxypeptidase G_2) (see Antidotes in Depth A–14: Glucarpidase [Carboxypeptidase G_2]). The effectiveness of these therapies depends on both the timing of administration and the dose, which warrants the monitoring of serum MTX concentrations during the use of these antidotes. Folinic acid rescue therapy limits methotrexate bone marrow and gastrointestinal toxicity by allowing for the continuation of essential biochemical processes that are dependent on reduced folates. The purpose of the initial dose of leucovorin is to achieve a serum concentration equal to the MTX and subsequent doses should be adjusted according to serum MTX concentrations at 12, 24, and 48 hours postexposure (see Fig. A13–1).[35,55] Leucovorin treatment is continued until the MTX concentration is less than 0.01 μmol/L.[10] In patients with marrow toxicity and no cancer, leucovorin therapy should be considered until marrow recovery occurs, even if serum MTX is no longer detectable,[40] because intracellular MTX activity may still be ongoing because of the presence of cytosolic MTX polyglutamates. Among 71 patients undergoing MTX therapy for rheumatoid arthritis (average 6.1 mg MTX per week), 75% of these patients had indirectly detectable MTX polyglutamates in red blood cells and nondetectable MTX in the serum (FPIA, monoclonal antibody).

Glucarpidase (carboxypeptidase G_2, Voraxaze™) is a recombinant bacterial enzyme that is used as a rescue therapy to inactivate MTX. Glucarpidase is available for use as an adjunctive therapy in patients receiving high dose MTX and experiencing MTX toxicity, or are at risk for MTX toxicity: diminished renal function or delayed MTX clearance based on serum MTX concentrations (Clinicaltrials.gov Identifier: NCT00481559; http://clinicaltrials.gov/ct2/show/NCT00481559). Following glucarpidase therapy, serum MTX concentrations need to be monitored because residual levels of MTX in the blood after initial enzymatic therapy can result from an inadequate dose of glucarpidase in patients with large MTX exposures or the redistribution of MTX from tissue stores to the blood compartment.[9,55,67] Glucarpidase has been successfully administered intrathecally to reduce elevated MTX concentrations in the cerebrospinal space (see SC Intrathecal Administration of Xenobiotics).[68]

EXTRACORPOREAL ELIMINATION

There are several reports of the use of hemodialysis and/or hemoperfusion for patients with MTX toxicity.[33,43,51,62,65] Although the volume of distribution (0.6 to 0.9 L/kg) and protein binding (50%) suggest that methotrexate is dialyzable, older clinical evidence suggests otherwise.[59] In one report, less than 10% of an initial 0.7 g dose of methotrexate was cleared in 12 sessions of hemodialysis.[62] The measured clearance was only 38 mL/min, which can be compared to 5 mL/min for peritoneal dialysis,[23] 0.28 to 24 mL/min for continuous venovenous hemodiafiltration,[32,35] and 180 mL/min for normal renal clearance.[39] Using plasma exchange transfusion to remove MTX is not recommended because of the drug's low degree of protein binding, which limits the efficacy of this procedure.[7,35,47,62]

Acute intermittent hemodialysis with a high-flux dialyzer membrane yielded an effective mean serum MTX clearance of 92 mL/min in six patients with renal failure that was a result of either chronic disease or high-dose MTX therapy.[65] These patients received high-dose MTX therapy and had predialysis plasma MTX concentrations ranging from 1.45 to 1813 μmol/L. The time of dialysis initiation after MTX treatment was from 1 hour to 6 days in this patient population. A serum MTX concentration of 0.3 μmol/L was used as an end point for dialysis. The reported serum MTX clearance by this technique closely approximates normal renal MTX clearance and is indicated to enhance the clearance of MTX in patients with diminished renal clearance and an elevated serum MTX concentration when it is available.[53]

Charcoal hemoperfusion removed more than 50% of methotrexate in four patients with impaired renal MTX clearance during high-dose MTX therapy.[13] This was thought to have prevented severe skin and mucosal toxicity. Sequential hemodialysis and hemoperfusion were used for a patient with substantial MTX toxicity.[22] These procedures decreased the half-life of elimination from 45 hours to 7.6 hours. In experimental animals, hemoperfusion significantly reduced the terminal half-life of methotrexate. In surgically anephric dogs, hemoperfusion decreased the half-life from more than 20 hours to 1.3 hours.[27] Consequently, hemoperfusion is recommended over hemodialysis when it is available; otherwise, high-flux hemodialysis is preferred.[51]

In vitro studies indicate that the toxic effects of 100 μmol/L of MTX cannot be reversed by 1000 μmol/L of folinic acid.[49] This suggests the need for extracorporeal elimination, such as high-flux hemodialysis, and enzymatic cleavage to lower persistent serum MTX concentrations of greater than 100 mol/L.[51] It is important to perform high-flux hemodialysis early, prior to distribution into tissues. Rebound of MTX concentrations from tissues may be expected after hemodialysis, which can begin at 2 hours postdialysis and plateau at 16 hours.[20,23,65] Patients who are at the greatest risk for developing MTX toxicity despite folinic acid treatment should be considered for glucarpidase therapy and extracorporeal elimination because they are most likely to benefit from this procedure. This includes patients with progressively diminishing renal clearance.[60] High-flux hemodialysis can offer the additional benefit of correcting fluid and electrolyte disorders resulting from renal failure. Other treatment options to limit additional organ toxicity, including leucovorin and urinary alkalinization, should be continued during extracorporeal MTX removal. Folic acid is water-soluble and can be removed by hemodialysis.[12,51,56,58] This is probably also applicable for folinic acid, and replacement doses of leucovorin postdialysis should be considered.

SUMMARY

The number of patients with methotrexate exposures and resultant toxicity is anticipated to increase due to the expanding therapeutic indications and available multiple formulations of this antineoplastic. Thus, clinicians need to understand the clinical presentations, acute and chronic, and management of methotrexate toxicity to improve the patient's outcome. Patients with associated chronic illnesses, diminished renal clearance, and chronic toxicity are at greatest risk for increased morbidity from overwhelming sepsis. Management includes supportive care, monitoring serum methotrexate concentrations, enhanced elimination (urinary alkalinization), and antidotal therapy with leucovorin and enzymatic cleavage. The early recognition of these patients and institution of these therapies can offer the patient the best outcome.

ACKNOWLEDGMENT

This chapter was written by Richard Y. Wang in his private capacity. No official support or endorsement by the Centers for Disease Control and Prevention is intended or should be inferred. Paul Calabresi contributed to this chapter in a previous edition.

REFERENCES

1. Abelson HT. Methotrexate and central nervous system toxicity. *Cancer Treat Rep.* 1978;62:1999-2001.
2. Abelson HT, Fosburg MT, Beardsley GP, et al. Methotrexate-induced renal impairment: clinical studies and rescue from systemic toxicity with high-dose leucovorin and thymidine. *J Clin Oncol.* 1983;1:208-216.
3. Albertioni F, Rask C, Eksborg S, et al. Evaluation of clinical assays for measuring high-dose methotrexate in plasma. *Clin Chem.* 1996;42:39-44.
4. Allen JC, Rosen G, Mehta BM, Horten B. Leukoencephalopathy following high-dose IV methotrexate chemotherapy with leucovorin rescue. *Cancer Treat Rep.* 1980;64:1261-1273.
5. Atherton LD, Leib ES, Kaye MD. Toxic megacolon associated with methotrexate therapy. *Gastroenterology.* 1984;86:1583-1588.
6. Barak AJ, Tuma DJ, Beckenhauer HC. Methotrexate hepatotoxicity. *J Am Coll Nutr.* 1984;3:93-96.
7. Benezet S, Chatelut E, Bagheri H, et al. Inefficacy of exchange-transfusion in case of a methotrexate poisoning. *Bull Cancer.* 1997;84:788-790.
8. Bleyer WA. The clinical pharmacology of methotrexate: new applications of an old drug. *Cancer.* 1978;41:36-51.
9. Buchen S, Ngampolo D, Melton RG, et al. Carboxypeptidase G2 rescue in patients with methotrexate intoxication and renal failure. *Br J Cancer.* 2005;92:480-487.
10. Chabner BA, Young RC. Threshold methotrexate concentration for in vivo inhibition of DNA synthesis in normal and tumorous target tissues. *J Clin Invest.* 1973;52:1804-1811.
11. Christensen ML, Rivera GK, Crom WR, Hancock ML, Evans WE. Effect of hydration on methotrexate plasma concentrations in children with acute lymphocytic leukemia. *J Clin Oncol.* 1988;6:797-801.
12. Cunningham J, Sharman VL, Goodwin FJ, Marsh FP. Do patients receiving haemodialysis need folic acid supplements? *Br Med J (Clin Res Ed).* 1981;282:1582.
13. Djerassi I, Ciesielka W, Kim JS. Removal of methotrexate by filtration-adsorption using charcoal filters or by hemodialysis. *Cancer Treat Rep.* 1977;61:751-752.
14. Doolittle GC, Simpson KM, Lindsley HB. Methotrexate-associated, early-onset pancytopenia in rheumatoid arthritis. *Arch Intern Med.* 1989;149:1430-1431.
15. Erttmann R, Landbeck G. Effect of oral cholestyramine on the elimination of high-dose methotrexate. *J Cancer Res Clin Oncol.* 1985;110:48-50.
16. Fong CM, Lee AC. High-dose methotrexate-associated acute renal failure may be an avoidable complication. *Pediatr Hematol Oncol.* 2006;23:51-57.
17. Fotoohi K, Skarby T, Soderhall S, Peterson C, Albertioni F. Interference of 7-hydroxymethotrexate with the determination of methotrexate in plasma samples from children with acute lymphoblastic leukemia employing routine clinical assays. *J Chromatogr B Analyt Technol Biomed Life Sci.* 2005;817:139-144.
18. Fukushima T, Sumazaki R, Koike K, et al. A magnetic resonance abnormality correlating with permeability of the blood-brain barrier in a child with chemical meningitis during central nervous system prophylaxis for acute leukemia. *Ann Hematol.* 1999; 78:564-567.
19. Gadgil SD, Damle SR, Advani SH, Vaidya AB. Effect of activated charcoal on the pharmacokinetics of high-dose methotrexate. *Cancer Treat Rep.* 1982;66:1169-1171.
20. Gibson TP, Reich SD, Krumlovsky FA, Ivanovich P, Gonczy C. Hemoperfusion for methotrexate removal. *Clin Pharmacol Ther.* 1978;23:351-355.
21. Gowan GM, Herrington JD, Simonetta AB. Methotrexate-induced toxic leukoencephalopathy. *Pharmacotherapy.* 2002;22:1183-1187.
22. Grimes DJ, Bowles MR, Buttsworth JA, et al. Survival after unexpected high serum methotrexate concentrations in a patient with osteogenic sarcoma. *Drug Saf.* 1990;5:447-454.
23. Hande KR, Balow JE, Drake JC, Rosenberg SA, Chabner BA. Methotrexate and hemodialysis. *Ann Intern Med.* 1977;87:495-496.
24. Harned TM, Mascarenhas L. Severe methotrexate toxicity precipitated by intravenous radiographic contrast. *J Pediatr Hematol Oncol.* 2007;29:496-499.
25. Huang KC, Wenczak BA, Liu YK. Renal tubular transport of methotrexate in the rhesus monkey and dog. *Cancer Res.* 1979;39:4843-4848.
26. Hughes PJ, Lane RJ. Acute cerebral oedema induced by methotrexate. *BMJ.* 1989;298:1315.
27. Isacoff W. Effects of extracorporeal charcoal hemoperfusion on plasma methotrexate [abstract]. *Proc Am Assoc Cancer Res.* 1977;18:1.
28. Iven H, Brasch H. The effects of antibiotics and uricosuric drugs on the renal elimination of methotrexate and 7-hydroxymethotrexate in rabbits. *Cancer Chemother Pharmacol.* 1988;21:337-342.
29. Jackson RC GG. The biochemical basis for methotrexate cytotoxicity. In: Sirotnak FM, ed. *Folate Antagonists as Therapeutic Agents.* New York: Academic Press; 1984:289-315.
30. Jacobs SA, Stoller RG, Chabner BA, Johns DG. 7-Hydroxymethotrexate as a urinary metabolite in human subjects and rhesus monkeys receiving high dose methotrexate. *J Clin Invest.* 1976;57:534-538.
31. Jaffe N, Takaue Y, Anzai T, Robertson R. Transient neurologic disturbances induced by high-dose methotrexate treatment. *Cancer.* 1985;56:1356-1360.
32. Jambou P, Levraut J, Favier C, et al. Removal of methotrexate by continuous venovenous hemodiafiltration. *Contrib Nephrol.* 1995;116:48-52.
33. Kawabata K, Makino H, Nagake Y, et al. A case of methotrexate-induced acute renal failure successfully treated with plasma perfusion and sequential hemodialysis. *Nephron.* 1995;71:233-234.
34. Kelkar R, Gordon SM, Giri N, et al. Epidemic iatrogenic *Acinetobacter* spp. meningitis following administration of intrathecal methotrexate. *J Hosp Infect.* 1989;14:233-243.
35. Kepka L, De Lassence A, Ribrag V, et al. Successful rescue in a patient with high dose methotrexate-induced nephrotoxicity and acute renal failure. *Leuk Lymphoma.* 1998;29:205-209.
36. Kevat SG, Hill WR, McCarthy PJ, Ahern MJ. Pancytopenia induced by low-dose methotrexate for rheumatoid arthritis. *Aust N Z J Med.* 1988;18:697-700.
37. Kremer JM, Hamilton RA. The effects of nonsteroidal antiinflammatory drugs on methotrexate (MTX) pharmacokinetics: impairment of renal clearance of MTX at weekly maintenance doses but not at 7.5 mg. *J Rheumatol.* 1995;22:2072-2077.
38. Langslow A. Nursing and the law. Deadly doses of methotrexate. *Aust Nurs J.* 1995;2:32-34.
39. Liegler DG, Henderson ES, Hahn MA, Oliverio VT. The effect of organic acids on renal clearance of methotrexate in man. *Clin Pharmacol Ther.* 1969;10:849-857.
40. MacKinnon SK, Starkebaum G, Willkens RF. Pancytopenia associated with low dose pulse methotrexate in the treatment of rheumatoid arthritis. *Semin Arthritis Rheum.* 1985;15:119-126.
41. Massenkeil G, Spath-Schwalbe E, Flath B, et al. Transient tetraparesis after intrathecal and high-dose systemic methotrexate. *Ann Hematol.* 1998;77:239-242.
42. McIntosh S, Davidson DL, O'Brien RT, Pearson HA. Methotrexate hepatotoxicity in children with leukemia. *J Pediatr.* 1977;90:1019-1021.
43. Molinari A, Oliva A, Aguilera N, et al. New antineoplastic prenylhydroquinones. Synthesis and evaluation. *Bioorg Med Chem.* 2000;8:1027-1032.
44. Nesbit M, Krivit W, Heyn R, Sharp H. Acute and chronic effects of methotrexate on hepatic, pulmonary, and skeletal systems. *Cancer.* 1976;37:1048-1057.
45. Olver IN, Aisner J, Hament A, et al. A prospective study of topical dimethyl sulfoxide for treating anthracycline extravasation. *J Clin Oncol.* 1988;6:1732-1735.
46. O'Marcaigh AS, Johnson CM, Smithson WA, et al. Successful treatment of intrathecal methotrexate overdose by using ventriculolumbar perfusion and intrathecal instillation of carboxypeptidase G_2. *Mayo Clin Proc.* 1996;71:161-165.
47. Park ES, Han KH, Choi HS, Shin HY, Ahn HS. Carboxypeptidase-G_2 resuce in a patient with a high dose methotrexate-induced nephrotoxicty. *Cancer Res Treat.* 2005;37:2.
48. Pesce MA, Bodourian SH. Enzyme immunoassay and enzyme inhibition assay of methotrexate, with use of the centrifugal analyzer. *Clin Chem.* 1981;27:380-384.
49. Pinedo HM, Zaharko DS, Bull JM, Chabner BA. The reversal of methotrexate cytotoxicity to mouse bone marrow cells by leucovorin and nucleosides. *Cancer Res.* 1976;36:4418-4424.
50. Reggev A, Djerassi I. The safety of administration of massive doses of methotrexate (50 g) with equimolar citrovorum factor rescue in adult patients. *Cancer.* 1988;61:2423-2428.
51. Relling MV, Stapleton FB, Ochs J, et al. Removal of methotrexate, leucovorin, and their metabolites by combined hemodialysis and hemoperfusion. *Cancer.* 1988;62:884-888.
52. Roenigk HH Jr, Maibach HI, Weinstein GP. Methotrexate therapy for psoriasis. Guideline revisions. *Arch Dermatol.* 1973;108:35.
53. Saland JM, Leavey PJ, Bash RO, et al. Effective removal of methotrexate by high-flux hemodialysis. *Pediatr Nephrol.* 2002;17:825-829.

54. Sasaki K, Tanaka J, Fujimoto T. Theoretically required urinary flow during high-dose methotrexate infusion. *Cancer Chemother Pharmacol.* 1984;13:9-13.
55. Schwartz S, Borner K, Muller K, et al. Glucarpidase (carboxypeptidase G_2) intervention in adult and elderly cancer patients with renal dysfunction and delayed methotrexate elimination after high-dose methotrexate therapy. *Oncologist.* 2007;12:1299-1308.
56. Sheikh-Hamad D, Timmins K, Jalali Z. Cisplatin-induced renal toxicity: possible reversal by N-acetylcysteine treatment. *J Am Soc Nephrol.* 1997;8:1640-1644.
57. Shinozaki T, Watanabe H, Tomidokoro R, et al. Successful rescue by oral cholestyramine of a patient with methotrexate nephrotoxicity: nonrenal excretion of serum methotrexate. *Med Pediatr Oncol.* 2000;34:226-228.
58. Skoutakis VA, Acchiardo SR, Meyer MC, Hatch FE. Folic acid dosage for chronic hemodialysis patients. *Clin Pharmacol Ther.* 1975;18:200-204.
59. Steger GG, Mader RM, Gnant MF, et al. GM-CSF in the treatment of a patient with severe methotrexate intoxication. *J Intern Med.* 1993;233:499-502.
60. Stoller RG, Hande KR, Jacobs SA, Rosenberg SA, Chabner BA. Use of plasma pharmacokinetics to predict and prevent methotrexate toxicity. *N Engl J Med.* 1977;297:630-634.
61. Teh HS, Fadilah SA, Leong CF. Transverse myelopathy following intrathecal administration of chemotherapy. *Singapore Med J.* 2007;48:e46-49.
62. Thierry FX, Vernier I, Dueymes JM, et al. Acute renal failure after high-dose methotrexate therapy. Role of hemodialysis and plasma exchange in methotrexate removal. *Nephron.* 1989;51:416-417.
63. Von Hoff DD, Penta JS, Helman LJ, Slavik M. Incidence of drug-related deaths secondary to high-dose methotrexate and citrovorum factor administration. *Cancer Treat Rep.* 1977;61:745-748.
64. Walker RW, Allen JC, Rosen G, Caparros B. Transient cerebral dysfunction secondary to high-dose methotrexate. *J Clin Oncol.* 1986;4:1845-1850.
65. Wall SM, Johansen MJ, Molony DA, et al. Effective clearance of methotrexate using high-flux hemodialysis membranes. *Am J Kidney Dis.* 1996;28:846-854.
66. Weinstein GD. Methotrexate. *Ann Intern Med.* 1977;86:199-204.
67. Widemann BC, Balis FM, Murphy RF, et al. Carboxypeptidase-G_2, thymidine, and leucovorin rescue in cancer patients with methotrexate-induced renal dysfunction. *J Clin Oncol.* 1997;15:2125-2134.
68. Widemann BC, Balis FM, Shalabi A, et al. Treatment of accidental intrathecal methotrexate overdose with intrathecal carboxypeptidase G_2. *J Natl Cancer Inst.* 2004;96:1557-1559.
69. Ziereisen F, Dan B, Azzi N, et al. Reversible acute methotrexate leukoencephalopathy: atypical brain MR imaging features. *Pediatr Radiol.* 2006;36:205-212.

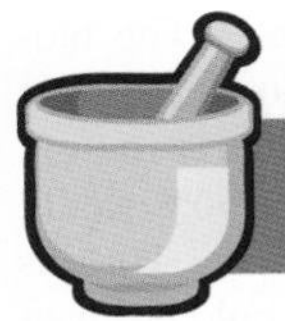

ANTIDOTES IN DEPTH (A13)

LEUCOVORIN (FOLINIC ACID) AND FOLIC ACID

Mary Ann Howland

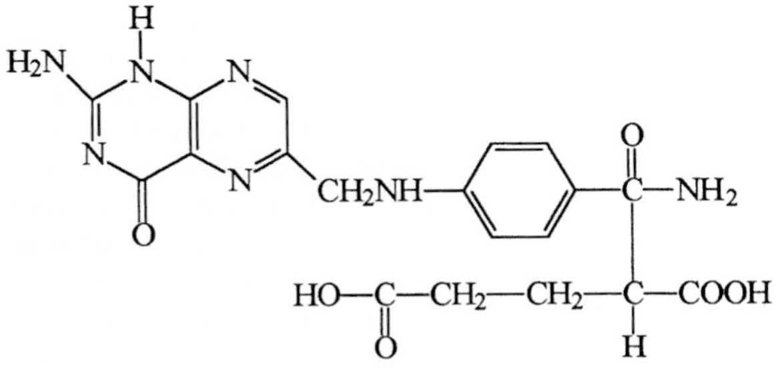

Folic Acid

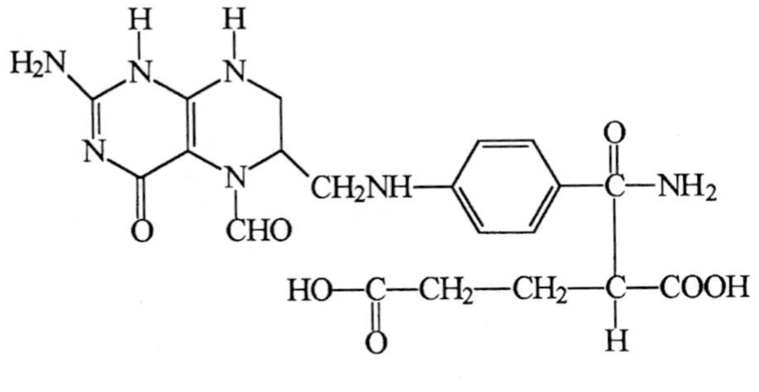

Folinic Acid

Leucovorin (folinic acid) is the primary antidote for a patient who receives an overdose of methotrexate. Methotrexate prevents the conversion of inactive folic acid to the biologically active reduced form of folic acid, known as leucovorin or folinic acid. Only leucovorin is an acceptable antidote for a patient with methotrexate toxicity. Following a methanol overdose, folic acid enhances the metabolism of formate. Since methanol does not interfere with the synthesis of folinic acid, either folic acid or leucovorin is acceptable for a patient poisoned by methanol.

PHARMACOLOGY

Folic acid, an essential water-soluble vitamin, consists of a pteridine ring joined to PABA (*para*-aminobenzoic acid) and glutamic acid.[7] Folic acid is the most common pharmaceutical preparation of the many folate congeners that exist in nature and perform essential cellular metabolic functions. After absorption, folic acid is reduced by dihydrofolic acid reductase (DHFR) to tetrahydrofolic acid, which accepts one-carbon groups. Tetrahydrofolic acid serves as the precursor for several biologically active forms of folic acid, including 5-formyltetrahydrofolic acid, which is best known as folinic acid, leucovorin, and citrovorum factor. These biologically active forms of folate are enzymatically interconvertible and function as cofactors, providing the one-carbon groups necessary for many intracellular metabolic reactions, including the synthesis of thymidylate and purine nucleotides, which are essential precursors of DNA.[23,25,29,31,36] The minimum daily requirement of folate is normally 50 μg, but in pregnant women and nutritionally deprived, acutely ill patients, 100 to 200 μg may be required.[7,8]

ROLE IN METHOTREXATE TOXICITY

Methotrexate, an antimetabolite, is a structural analog of folic acid, differing only in the substitution of an amino group for a hydroxyl group at the number 4 position of the pteridine ring (see Chap. 53). Methotrexate binds to the active site of DHFR, rendering it incapable of reducing folic acid to its biologically active forms, and incapable of regenerating the necessary active forms required for the synthesis of purine nucleotides and thymidylate.[30] At physiologic pH the binding between methotrexate and DHFR is competitive, with an inhibition constant of about 1 μmol/L.[27] Leucovorin is a reduced, active form of folate. As such, it does not require DHFR for enzymatic interconversion to the form required for purine nucleotide and thymidylate formation. Folic acid is unable to counteract methotrexate toxicity because following methotrexate therapy, DHFR is unavailable to convert folic acid to the active reduced forms. *Leucovorin rescue* is the term used to describe the practice of limiting the toxic effects of high-dose methotrexate therapy.

ROLE IN METHANOL TOXICITY

Monkeys experimentally made folate deficient develop methanol toxicity at lower methanol concentrations.[19] Administering folic acid to normal monkeys accelerates formate metabolism.[19] Pretreatment with folic acid or leucovorin decreased both formate concentrations and the accompanying metabolic acidosis, without affecting the rate of methanol elimination.[19] Leucovorin remained effective in hastening the metabolism of formate when given 10 hours after methanol administration.[21]

The hepatic concentrations of total folate, leucovorin, and folate dehydrogenase (which increases leucovorin concentrations) are all diminished in methanol-poisoned humans.[12] In an analysis of a single methanol-poisoned patient who was given folate and ethanol and hemodialyzed, the half-life of formate was 1.1 hours.[22] In another methanol-poisoned patient treated without folate, the formate half-life was 2.8 hours.[9] These comparative data are inadequate to draw definitive conclusions, but may support the therapeutic role of folate, in addition to that of fomepizole and hemodialysis.

LEUCOVORIN PHARMACOKINETICS

Leucovorin is naturally formed in the body as the active (*l* or −) isomer, whereas the commercial preparation is the racemic mixture, which means it consists of equal amounts of the inactive (*d* or +) and active (*l* or −) isomers. The pharmacokinetics of the racemic mixture of leucovorin and its active metabolite were studied after intravenous (IV) infusion, and as a constant infusion in normal human volunteers.[32,33] During constant infusion of 500 mg/m^2/d, the steady-state concentration for the active isomer was 2.33 μM, the half-life was 35 minutes, and the volume of distribution was 13.6 L. The active isomer is metabolized to an active metabolite (L-5-CH3-THF) that achieved a steady-state concentration of 4.85 μM and a half-life of 227 minutes. Similar values were achieved for half-life and volume of distribution after single IV doses ranging from 25 to 100 mg. The inactive d isomer achieved higher concentrations and had a much longer half-life with oral administration which is saturable and stereoselective, resulting in absorption of the active isomer that is four to five times greater than that of the inactive isomer. Studies of stereospecific oral absorption demonstrate that 100% of the l-leucovorin is absorbed whereas only 20% of the d-leucovorin is absorbed at this dose.[15] One study detected no adverse effects of the inactive isomer on the intracellular uptake of the active isomer and concluded that giving the active isomer provided no pharmacokinetic advantage over the racemic mixture.[28]

The pharmacokinetics of IV leucovorin was compared to intramuscular (IM) and oral administration in male volunteers given 25 mg. The mean peak of the active L-5-CH3-THF concentration was 258 ng/mL at 1.3 hours after IV administration compared with 226 ng/mL at 2.8 hours for IM and 367 ng/mL at 2.4 hours for oral administration.

The pharmacokinetics of orally administered leucovorin was studied in healthy, fasted, male volunteers in single doses ranging from 20 to 100 mg, and 200 mg IV over 5 minutes as compared with 200 mg orally.[18,24] Bioavailability decreased from 100% for the 20-mg dose to 78% for the 40-mg dose, and ultimately to 31% for the 200-mg dose. A microbiologic assay was used to measure total tetrahydrofolates (reduced and active folates). Normal serum folate concentrations are approximately 0.05 μmol/L.[10] The 200-mg oral dose produced a peak serum concentration of 1.82 μmol/L, compared to 0.66 μmol/L for the 20-mg oral dose and 27.1 μmol/L for the 200-mg IV dose.[18,24]

LEUCOVORIN DOSING FOR METHOTREXATE OVERDOSES

When a patient overdoses on methotrexate, a dose of leucovorin estimated to produce the same plasma concentration as the methotrexate dose should be given as soon as possible and, preferably, within 1 hour. One mole of methotrexate weighs 455 D and 1 mol of leucovorin calcium weighs 511 D, with the molecular weight of the leucovorin portion equal to 471 D. Because of the safety of leucovorin and because of the toxicity of methotrexate, underdosing leucovorin should be avoided. Although serum methotrexate concentrations are often closely followed in patients on diverse oncologic regimens,[2,3] in the overdose setting, or in the treatment of methotrexate toxicity related to treatment for tubal pregnancies, it is inappropriate to wait for a serum methotrexate concentration before initiating treatment with leucovorin.[1] The toxic threshold for methotrexate is reported to be 1×10^{-8} mol/L (0.01 μmol/L or 10 nmol/L).[4] Normal serum folate concentrations are in the range of 13 to 43 nmol/L. In a patient who is not receiving methotrexate therapeutically, there is no need to permit any methotrexate to remain unantagonized by leucovorin.

For example, if a child unintentionally ingests one hundred 2.5-mg methotrexate tablets for a total dose of 250 mg, only part of this dose is absorbed because methotrexate absorption is saturable.[6] The bioavailability of methotrexate decreases from 100% with doses less than 30 mg/m^2 to approximately 10% to 20% with doses greater than 80 mg/m^2. In this case, it is safe to assume that a bioavailability of 50% would result in an absorbed dose of methotrexate of less than 125 mg. For this substantial exposure an IV dose of 125 mg of leucovorin could be given over 15 to 30 minutes. This dose of IV leucovorin would be expected to produce serum concentrations in excess of that of the methotrexate, given that the volume of distribution of leucovorin is about 25% less than methotrexate and the molecular weights are similar. This dose of IV leucovorin should be repeated every 3 to 6 hours until the serum methotrexate concentration is less than 1×10^{-8} mol/L, and preferably zero. The methotrexate half-life may vary from 5 to 45 hours, depending on the dose and the patient's renal function. For this reason, leucovorin therapy should be continued for 12 to 24 doses (3 days) or longer if methotrexate concentrations are unavailable. Patients who may develop third-space storage in ascites or pleural effusions may also require leucovorin dosing for an extended period of time. Patients with bone marrow toxicity require more prolonged dosing because plasma half-lives of methotrexate do not reflect persistent intracellular concentrations.

Unintentional overdose with intrathecal methotrexate is potentially quite serious and is dose dependent.[11,16] In these cases, IV leucovorin should be administered. Intrathecal leucovorin was considered a major factor in the death of a child given a slightly higher dose of intrathecal methotrexate than was prescribed.[14] Not all intrathecal methotrexate overdoses require aggressive intervention, but consultation with experienced hematologists/oncologists and medical toxicologists is warranted (see Special Considerations SC2: Intrathecal Administration of xenobiotics).[13]

An IV leucovorin dose of 100 mg/m^2 every 3 to 6 hours should be effective, in all but the most severe overdoses. A constant intravenous infusion of 21 mg/m^2/h has been safely administered for 5 days. See Figure A13-1, which offers a nomogram for pharmacokinetically guided rescue after high-dose methotrexate.[2] A transition to the oral administration of leucovorin depends on the serum concentration of the methotrexate and whether adequate serum concentrations of leucovorin can be achieved by that route. In adults, a 200-mg oral dose of leucovorin produces a peak serum concentration of 1.82 μmol/L as compared with 27.1 μmol/L with a 200-mg IV dose.

Levoleucovorin, the active *l* isomer of folinic acid, is available and should be dosed at half the dose of the racemate leucovorin.[5]

Administration of activated charcoal precludes the subsequent administration of oral leucovorin. In addition to leucovorin, other

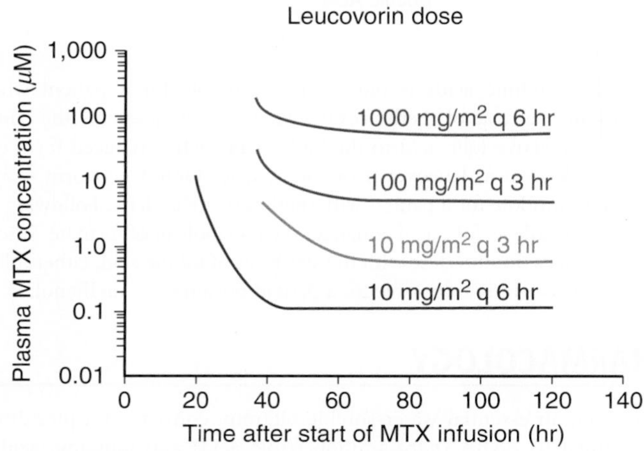

FIGURE A13–1. Example of a nomogram developed by Bleyer[2] for pharmacokinetically guided leucovorin rescue after high-dose methotrexate (MTX) administration.

modalities to treat patients with methotrexate overdoses include activated charcoal and urinary alkalinization, and glucarpidase (carboxypeptidase G) and extracorporeal removal should be considered (see Chap. 53).

ADVERSE EFFECTS AND SAFETY ISSUES

Reports of adverse reactions to parenteral injections of folic acid or leucovorin are uncommon; however, adverse reactions may include allergic or anaphylactoid reactions.[7] Seizures are rarely associated with leucovorin administration.[20] The calcium content of leucovorin warrants a slow intravenous infusion at a rate not faster than 160 mg/min in adults. Leucovorin should never be administered intrathecally.[11,14,26,35]

Leucovorin is not an antidote to 5-fluorouracil (5-FU) and can enhance the therapeutic and toxic effects of fluoropyrimidines such as 5-FU.[15,17]

Many protocols recommended separating leucovorin from glucarpidase by 2 hours (see Antidotes in Depth A14: Glucarpidase [Carboxypeptidase G_2]).

DOSING

The routine dose of leucovorin for "leucovorin rescue" ranges from 10 to 25 mg/m^2 IM or IV every 6 hours for 72 hours to 100 mg/m^2 every 3 hours in patients with renal compromise. If administration to neonates is necessary, a benzyl-alcohol-free preparation must be used because of the toxicity of benzyl alcohol in neonates (see Chap. 55).[34] For methotrexate overdoses, equimolar serum leucovorin concentrations should provide adequate protection, but precise determinations are invariably delayed, and the administration of leucovorin should not be delayed until a serum methotrexate concentration is determined.

As a rough guide, a single dose of IV 25 mg leucovorin in an adult produces a peak concentration of the active L-5-CH3-THF metabolite of approximately 258 ng/mL which is 5.5×10^{-7} M.[15] A dose of about 150 mg every 4 hours in an adult achieves a steady-state concentration of about 4.85×10^{-6} M.[32] And although the dose of leucovorin can be as high as 1000 mg/m^2 every 6 hours, this is rarely warranted and cannot adequately compete with serum concentrations of methotrexate above 10^{-4} M; under these circumstances glucarpidase should be strongly considered. An IV leucovorin dose of 100 mg/m^2 every 3 to 6 hours should be effective in all but the most severe overdoses and should be administered IV as soon as possible over 15 to 30 minutes, but not faster than 160 mg/min in adults due to the calcium content. This dose should be continued for at least several days, or until the serum methotrexate concentration falls below 1×10^{-8} mol/L in the absence of bone marrow toxicity.

Either folic acid or leucovorin (folinic acid) should be administered parenterally at the first suspicion of methanol poisoning. No complications are reported with the use of 50 to 70 mg of IV folic acid every 4 hours for the first 24 hours in the treatment of methanol-poisoned patients.[22] The precise dose necessary is unknown, but 1 to 2 mg/kg every 4 to 6 hours is probably sufficient. The folic acid should be continued until the methanol and formate are eliminated. As the first dose is usually administered prior to hemodialysis, a second dose should be administered at the completion of hemodialysis, because hemodialysis will remove this highly water-soluble vitamin.

AVAILABILITY

Leucovorin (folinic acid) powder for injection is available in 50-, 100-, 200-, and 350-mg vials. Each mg of leucovorin contains 0.004 mEq of calcium. Reconstitution with sterile water for injection—5 mL to the 50-mg vial, 10 mL to the 100-mg vial, or 20 mL to the 200-mg vial—results in a final concentration of 10 mg/mL. Adding 17.5 mL of sterile water for injection to the 350-mg vial results in a final concentration of 20 mg/mL. Leucovorin is also available in a single-use vial as a solution for injection at a concentration of 10 mg/mL in a 50-mL vial. Because of the calcium content, the rate of intravenous administration should not be faster than 160 mg/min in adults.[15] Leucovorin is also available orally in a variety of strengths, including 5-, 10-, 15-, and 25-mg tablets.

Levoleucovorin (Fusilev) lyophilized powder for injection is available in a single-use 50-mg vial containing the equivalent of 50 mg of levoleucovorin as the calcium pentahydrate salt and 50 mg mannitol. Reconstitution with 5.3 mL of 0.9% sodium chloride injection, USP, yields a concentration of 10 mg/mL. Because of the calcium content, the rate of IV administration should not be faster than 160 mg/min (16 mL of reconstituted solution/min).[5]

Folic acid is available parenterally in 10-mL multidose vials with 1.5% benzyl alcohol in concentrations of 5 or 10 mg/mL from a variety of manufacturers. Once opened, this vial must be kept refrigerated.

TABLE A13–1. Rapid Calculations

1 mole = 1 gram molecular weight
1 Molar = 1 mole/L = 1 gram molecular weight/L
1×10^{-3} moles = 1 millimole = 1 mmole
1×10^{-6} moles = 1 micromole = 1 μmole
1×10^{-9} moles = 1 nanomole = 1 nmole
1 mole of methotrexate weighs 455 daltons; 1 mole methotrexate = 455 grams
1 Molar methotrexate = 455 grams/L = 455 mg/mL
1×10^{-8} Molar methotrexate = 455×10^{-8} g/L = 455×10^{-8} mg/mL = 455×10^{-5} μg/mL = 455×10^{-2} ng/mL = 4.55 ng/mL

SUMMARY

Leucovorin (folinic acid) is the primary antidote for a patient who receives an overdose of methotrexate. Leucovorin is the biologically active, reduced form of folic acid, the synthesis of which is prevented by methotrexate. Only leucovorin (folinic acid) is an acceptable antidote for a patient with methotrexate toxicity, but either folic acid or leucovorin is acceptable for a patient poisoned by methanol. Following a methanol overdose, folic acid enhances the elimination of formate (Table A13-1).

REFERENCES

1. American College of Obstetricians and Gynecologists practice bulletin. Medical management of tubal pregnancy. Number 3, December 1998. Clinical management guidelines for obstetrician-gynecologists. *Int J Gynaecol Obstet.* 1999;65:97-103.
2. Bleyer WA. New vistas for leucovorin in cancer chemotherapy. *Cancer.* 1989;63:995-1007.
3. Booser DJ, Walters RS, Holmes FA, Hortobagyi GN. Continuous-infusion high-dose leucovorin with 5-fluorouracil and cisplatin for relapsed metastatic breast cancer: a phase II study. *Am J Clin Oncol.* 2000;23:40-41.
4. Chabner BA, Young RC. Threshold methotrexate concentration for in vivo inhibition of DNA synthesis in normal and tumorous target tissues. *J Clin Invest.* 1973;52:1804-1811.
5. Fusilev [package insert]. Irvine, CA: Manufactured by Chesapeake Biological Labs Inc for Spectrum Pharmaceuticals Inc; 2008.

6. Gibbon BN, Manthey DE. Pediatric case of accidental oral overdose of methotrexate. *Ann Emerg Med.* 1999;34:98-100.
7. Hillman RS. Hematopoetic agents: growth factors, minerals and vitamins. In: Hardman JG, Limbird CE, eds. *Goodman and Gilman's The Pharmacologic Basis of Therapeutics.* 10th ed. New York: McGraw-Hill; 2001:1487-1517.
8. Houben PF, Hommes OR, Knaven PJ. Anticonvulsant drugs and folic acid in young mentally retarded epileptic patients. A study of serum folate, fit frequency and IQ. *Epilepsia.* 1971;12:235-247.
9. Jacobsen D, McMartin KE. Methanol and ethylene glycol poisonings: mechanism of toxicity, clinical course, diagnosis and treatment. *Med Toxicol.* 1986;1:309-334.
10. Janinis J, Papakostas P, Samelis G, et al. Second-line chemotherapy with weekly oxaliplatin and high-dose 5-fluorouracil with folinic acid in metastatic colorectal carcinoma: a Hellenic Cooperative Oncology Group (HeCOG) phase II feasibility study. *Ann Oncol.* 2000;11:163-167.
11. Jardine LF, Ingram LC, Bleyer WA. Intrathecal leucovorin after intrathecal methotrexate overdose. *J Pediatr Hematol Oncol.* 1996;18:302-304.
12. Johlin F, Fortman C, Nghiem D, Tephly TR. Studies on the role of folic acid and folate dependent enzymes in human methanol poisoning. *Mol Pharmacol.* 1987;31:557-561.
13. Lampkin BC, Wells R. Intrathecal leucovorin after intrathecal methotrexate. *J Pediatr Hematol Oncol.* 1996;18:249.
14. Lee ACW, Wong KW, Fong KW, So KT. Intrathecal methotrexate overdose. *Acta Pediatr.* 1997;86:434-437.
15. Leucovorin Calcium Injection, USP [package insert]. Bedford, OH: Manufactured by Ben Venue Labs Inc for Bedford Labs; 2008.
16. Levitt M, Nixon PF, Pincus JH, Bertino JR. Transport characteristics of folates in cerebrospinal fluid; a study utilizing doubly labeled 5-methyltetrahydrofolate and 5-formyltetrahydrofolate. *J Clin Invest.* 1971; 50:1301-1308.
17. Lonardi F, Jirillo A, Bonciarelli G, Pavanato G, Balli M. Toxicity of laevo-leucovorin and dose lowering. *Eur J Cancer.* 1992;28A:1007-1008.
18. McGuire BW, Sia LL, Haynes JD, et al. Absorption kinetics of orally administered leucovorin calcium. *NCI Monogr.* 1987;5:47-56.
19. McMartin KE, Martin-Amat G, Makar AB, Tephly TR. Methanol poisoning. V: role of formate metabolism in the monkey. *J Pharmacol Exp Ther.* 1977;201:564-572.
20. Metropol NJ, Creaven PJ, Petrelli N, White RM, Arbuck SG. Seizures associated with leucovorin administration in cancer patients. *J Natl Cancer Inst.* 1995;87:56-58.
21. Noker PE, Eells MS, Tephly TR. Methanol toxicity: treatment with folic acid and 5-formyltetrahydrofolic acid. *Alcohol Clin Exp Res.* 1980;4:378-383.
22. Osterloh J, Pond S, Grady S, Becker CE. Serum formate concentrations in methanol intoxication as a criterion for hemodialysis. *Ann Intern Med.* 1986;104:200-203.
23. Patel R, Newman EM, Villacorte DG, et al. Pharmacology and phase I trial of high-dose oral leucovorin plus 5-fluorouracil in children with refractory cancer: A report from the Children's Cancer Study Group. *Cancer Res.* 1991;51:4871-4875.
24. Priest DG, Schmitz JC, Bunni MA, Stuart RK. Pharmacokinetics of leucovorin metabolites in human plasma as a function of dose administered orally and intravenously. *J Natl Cancer Inst.* 1991;83:1806-1812.
25. Reynolds EH. Effects of folic acid on the mental state and fit-frequency of drug-treated epileptic patients. *Lancet.* 1967;1:1086-1088.
26. Riva L, Conter V, Rizzari C, et al. Successful treatment of intrathecal methotrexate overdose with folinic acid rescue: a case report. *Acta Paediatr.* 1999;88:780-782.
27. Salmon SE, Sartorelli AC. Cancer chemotherapy. In: Katzung BG, ed. *Basic and Clinical Pharmacology.* 7th ed. Norwalk, CT: Appleton & Lange; 1998:889-891.
28. Schleyer E, Rudolph KL, Braess J, et al. Impact of the simultaneous administration of the (+)- and (−)-forms of formyl-tetrahydrofolic acid on plasma and intracellular pharmacokinetics of (−)-tetrahydrofolic acid. *Cancer Chemother Pharmacol.* 2000;45:165-171.
29. Smith DB, Racusen LC. Folate metabolism and the anticonvulsant efficacy of phenobarbital. *Arch Neurol.* 1973;28:18-22.
30. Smith S, Nelson L. Case files of the New York City Poison Control Center: Antidotal strategies for the management of methotrexate toxicity. *J Med Tox.* 2008;4:132-140.
31. Stover P, Schirch V. The metabolic role of leucovorin. *Trends Biochem Sci.* 1993;18:102-106.
32. Straw JA, Newman EM, Doroshow JH. Pharmacokinetics of leucovorin (*dl*-5 formyltetrahydrofolate) after intravenous injection and constant intravenous infusion. *NCI Monogr.* 1987;5:41-45.
33. Straw JA, Szapary D, Wynn W. Pharmacokinetics of the diastereoisomers of leucovorin after intravenous and oral administration to normal subjects. *Cancer Res.* 1984;44:3114-3119.
34. Tenenbein M. Recent advancements in pediatric toxicology. *Pediatr Clin North Am.* 1999;46:1179-1788.
35. Trinkle R, Wu JK. Intrathecal leucovorin after intrathecal methotrexate overdose. *J Pediatr Hematol Oncol.* 1997;19:267-268.
36. Weh HJ, Bittner S, Hoffknecht M, Hossfeld DK. Neurotoxicity following weekly therapy with folinic acid and high-dose 5-fluorouracil 24h infusion in patients with gastrointestinal malignancies. *Eur J Cancer.* 1993;29A:1218-1219.

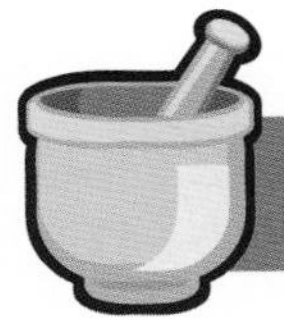

ANTIDOTES IN DEPTH (A14)

GLUCARPIDASE (CARBOXYPEPTIDASE G_2)

Silas W. Smith

Glucarpidase (carboxypeptidase G_2, $CPDG_2$) is indicated for the management of methotrexate (MTX) toxicity. When given intravenously or intrathecally it rapidly enzymatically inactivates intravascular or intrathecal MTX, respectively as well as folates and folate analogues. It is not a substitute for and must be used in conjunction with leucovorin (see Antidotes in Depth A13: Leucovorin [Folinic Acid] and Folic Acid). In most cases glucarpidase administration should precede or follow the use of leucovorin by at least 2 to 4 hours, unless a carefully considered benefit-risk analysis suggests the need to more rapidly eliminate MTX and risk leucovorin inactivation.

HISTORY AND DEVELOPMENT

Soon after the discovery of the structure and synthesis of folate,[7] a *Flavobacterium* species capable of removing the glutamate moiety of folate was described.[34] This was followed by additional reports of *Bacillus* species with glutamyl peptidase activity.[33,68] From 1955 to 1996 a series of experiments demonstrated the inactivation of folate analogues (including chemotherapeutic aminopterin) by bacteria and yeasts.[49,74] Other bacteria with similar folate glutamate-cleaving ability were later identified.[41,56,72] In 1967 purification of "carboxypeptidase G," a pseudomonad derived zinc-dependent enzyme responsible for MTX cleavage, was reported.[25,35] Carboxypeptidases from other bacterial species which differed in their substrate specificity and kinetics were later isolated and purified in 1971 (*Pseudomonas stutzeri* carboxypeptidase G_1),[40] 1978 (*Flavobacterium* carboxypeptidase),[6] and 1992 (*Pseudomonas* sp. M-27 carboxypeptidase G_3).[82] By 1976 carboxypeptidase G_1 was scaled to pilot manufacturing production.[17] The carboxypeptidase currently used in clinical practice (carboxypeptidase G_2) was cloned from *Pseudomonas* strain R-16 and sequenced, characterized, and expressed in *Escherichia coli* in the early 1980s.[44-46,63] A preliminary crystal structure was provided in 1991, with a complete characterization (at 2.5 Å), description of the active site, and biochemical mechanism of action was presented in 1997.[36,58,70]

Carboxypeptidase G_1 was initially explored as an anticancer agent because of its ability to deprive growing tumors of folate.[9,10,15,30] Human usage of $CPDG_1$ for this purpose was reported in 1974.[10] The antidotal potential of carboxypeptidase was suggested in 1972—carboxypeptidase G_1 rapidly decreased MTX levels and improved survival in mice injected with lethal MTX doses.[16] $CPDG_1$ was subsequently used to selectively eliminate systemic MTX in patients treated with high dosages targeting central nervous system (CNS) malignancy.[1,2] $CPDG_1$ was first used for rescue in a patient receiving MTX with renal failure in 1978.[28] Unfortunately, the enzyme source of $CPDG_1$ was then lost.[5,84] Following the revival of the recombinant $CPDG_2$ product, it underwent nonhuman primate testing for both intravenous (IV) and intrathecal (IT) rescue for MTX overdose.[4,5] Reports of successful use in human IV and IT MTX overdose rapidly emerged.[8,14,18,20,26,28,31,32,37,47,50,51,53,59-62,64,66,67,73,76,77,79,80,84] The US FDA designated glucarpidase as an approved Orphan Product in 2003 for treatment of patients at risk of MTX toxicity.[71]

MECHANISM OF ACTION

Glucarpidase is a dimerized protein structure with two domains—a beta-sheet interaction site and a zinc-dependent catalytic domain.[58] The catalytic domain hydrolyzes C-terminal glutamate residues of folate and folate analogues such as MTX. MTX and its metabolite 7-hydroxy-MTX are thus split into inactive DAMPA and hydroxy-DAMPA plus glutamate.[80,81] Glucarpidase similarly inactivates leucovorin (folinic acid) and folate by cleavage of terminal glutamate residues (Fig. A14–1), although to a lesser degree.[6] Several clinical studies supported the mechanism of action of glucarpidase as rapid cleavage of MTX.[14,26,32,61,77]

PHARMACOKINETICS AND PHARMACODYNAMICS

In a manufacturer-sponsored study, 50 Units/kg of glucarpidase IV was given to eight volunteer subjects with normal renal function and four volunteers with severely impaired renal function.[54] In those with normal renal function the mean maximum serum concentration of glucarpidase was 3.1 μg/mL, with a mean half-life of 9.0 hours. These values were essentially unaffected by compromised renal function.

Following glucarpidase administration, a rapid decline of serum MTX concentrations by 71% to 99% occurs within minutes, with the concurrent appearance of DAMPA.[14,32,62,64,75-77] However, $CPDG_2$ does not cross the blood-brain barrier, cannot cross the cell membrane to act intracellularly, and does not act on MTX in the gut lumen.[1,16,18] Intracellular MTX is polyglutamated, which hinders transmembrane transport and increases its intracellular half-life. This MTX pool, inaccessible to $CPDG_2$ (and hemodialysis), can persist for greater than 24 hours to cause cytotoxicity and a rebound in serum MTX concentrations.[24,79]

INDICATIONS AND ROLE IN METHOTREXATE TOXICITY

Patients receiving high-dose MTX therapy are routinely "rescued" with leucovorin (eg, 10 mg orally every 6 hours).[83] Treatment nomograms and institutional algorithms recommend higher leucovorin doses when MTX concentrations are excessive or prolonged.[11,75,83] However, at MTX concentrations above 100 μmol/L (and perhaps even lower), data suggest that adequate leucovorin concentrations cannot be achieved for competitive and complete reversal of toxicity.[14,32,38,55] Also, high-dose leucovorin therapy leads to the administration of 0.004 mEq calcium per mg of leucovorin and may be associated with hypercalcemia.[84]

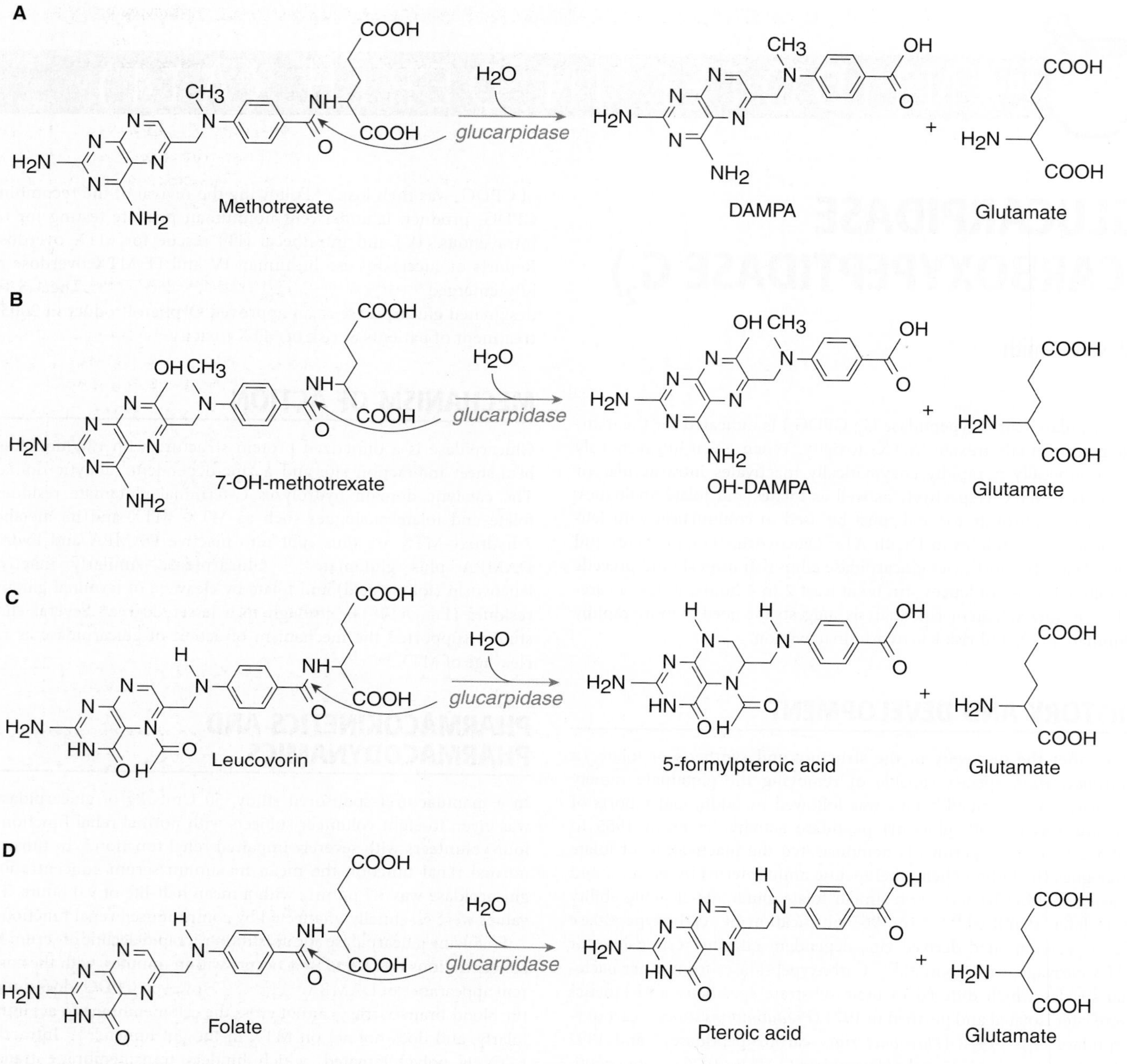

FIGURE A14–1. MECHANISM OF ACTION: Glucarpidase is a dimerized protein structure with two domains–a beta-sheet interaction site and a zinc-dependent catalytic domain. The catalytic domain hydrolyzes C-terminal glutamate residues of folate and folate analogues such as MTX. (A+B) MTX and its metabolite 7-hydroxy-MTX are thus split into inactive DAMPA and hydroxy-DAMPA plus glutamate. (C) Glucarpidase similarly inactivates leucovorin (folinic acid) and folate (D) by cleavage of terminal glutamate residues, although to a lesser degree.

Studies support the use of glucarpidase to treat patients who are at risk of toxicity from MTX due to either persistently elevated MTX concentrations or renal dysfunction.[14,26,61,76] As glucarpidase has not yet received marketing approval at the time of writing in either the United States or Europe, it lacks definitive administration indications. Table A14-1 summarizes the indications used in selected clinical trials and reviews, which vary by malignancy, degree of renal impairment, initial MTX dose, and serum MTX concentration. Mucositis, gastrointestinal distress, myelosuppression, hepatitis, or neurotoxicity should prompt consideration of glucarpidase in addition to aggressive leucovorin therapy. Patients with significant, persistent serum MTX concentration (essentially less than or equal to 50% the normal clearance rate), or MTX concentrations requiring high-dose leucovorin rescue or renal impairment (oliguria or creatinine greater than 1.5 times baseline) following high-dose MTX, should be candidates for glucarpidase.

Since leucovorin is contraindicated for IT administration,[22,29,69] IT glucarpidase provides an effective means to rapidly lower cerebrospinal fluid (CSF) MTX concentrations in cases of overdose or persistence.[50,79] Inadvertent or intentional MTX exposure[48,65] would also be amenable to glucarpidase, particularly prior to drug distribution. Additionally,

TABLE A14–1. Indications for Glucarpidase Use in Clinical Trials and Reviews

Trial/Review	Malignancy	Creatinine/Creatinine Clearance	Methotrexate Concentration
NCT00001298[3,76]	Various	Unspecified	≥10 μmol/L beyond 42 h
	Various	Cr ≥1.5 times the ULN or Cr_{CL} <60 mL/m²/min	≥ 2 standard deviations above the mean MTX elimination curve beyond 12 h
NCT00219791[61]	ALL, NHL, or a solid tumor (eg, osteosarcoma)	Unspecified	>5 μmol/L beyond 42 h
	ALL, NHL or a solid tumor (eg, osteosarcoma)	Cr >1.5 times the ULN and/or urine output <500 mL/24 h	>1 μmol/L beyond 42 h or >0.4 μmol/L beyond 48 h
NCT00424645	Solid tumors and hematologic malignancies	Unspecified	≥ 0.1 μmol/L at 72 ± 2 h (for MTX doses 1–3.5 g/m²) or ≥0.3 μmol/L at 72 ± 2 h (for MTX doses >3.5 g/m²)
NCT00481559	Osteosarcoma	Cr increase >2 times baseline	>50 μmol/L at 24 h, >5 μmol/L at 48 h, or >2 standard deviations above the mean MTX elimination curve beyond 12 h
	Various	Cr >1.5 times the ULN or Cr_{CL} <60 mL/min beyond 12 h	>10 μmol/L beyond 42 h or >2 standard deviations above the mean MTX elimination curve beyond 2 h
Reference 14	Various	Cr >1.5 times the ULN or diuresis of <50% of input hydration	>10 μmol/L at 36 h, >5 μmol/L at 42 h, or >3 μmol/L at 48 h
Reference 75	Various	Unspecified	>10 μmol/L beyond 42 h
		Renal dysfunction	>10 μmol/L beyond 42 h; consider if 1–10 μmol/L beyond 42 h

Where time-specific methotrexate concentrations are given, these indicate time following the initiation of the MTX infusion. Cr, creatinine; Cr_{CL}, creatinine clearance; ALL, acute lymphoblastic leukemia; NHL, non-Hodgkin lymphoma; ULN, upper limit of normal.

glucarpidase has been proposed as an antidote for pemetrexed (a folate antimetabolite) toxicity.[12] In international patent applications, the manufacturer disclosed experiments that demonstrated glucarpidase cleavage of additional antifolates in clinical and experimental use including AAGI 13-161, edatrexate, lometrexol, pemetrexed, and raltitrexed.[42,43]

MONITORING

False elevations of MTX have been reported clinically with all of the various immunoassay techniques following glucarpidase administration.[20,27,32,53,80,84] The DAMPA product of MTX cleavage significantly cross-reacts with both the MTX radioimmunoassay (RIA) and the competitive dihydrofolate reductase binding assays.[19] Both MTX metabolites (7-hydroxy-MTX and DAMPA), appreciably interfere with the newer fluorescence polarization immunoassay (FPIA) and enzyme multiplied immunoassay technique (EMIT) assays. For DAMPA, the cross-reactivity rates are 100% (EMIT) and 36% to 44% (FPIA).[52] 7-OH-MTX cross-reactivity using EMIT is 4% to 31%, and 0.6% to 3% with FPIA.[23,52] Clinically, the concentrations of DAMPA detected are comparable to that of MTX following administration of $CPDG_2$.[18] Thus, the use of high performance liquid chromatography (HPLC) to determine actual MTX concentrations is mandated when glucarpidase is given.[13]

ADVERSE EFFECTS AND OTHER SAFETY ISSUES

Initial studies reported adverse effects in four of nine patients treated with $CPDG_1$, including development of inactivating antibodies, "sensitization" to $CPDG_1$, and anaphylactoid reactions.[1,2,10,28] Studies with the current recombinant enzyme glucarpidase ($CPDG_2$) report a much lower incidence of adverse effects than with the initial $CPDG_1$ enzyme. These typically include warmth, tingling, head pressure, flushing, shaking, and burning of the face and extremities.[77] The current manufacturer reports that 8% of patients (25 of 329) reported a total of 50 possibly related adverse events.[57] One-third of these were "allergic" reactions (burning sensation, flushing, hot flush, allergic dermatitis, feeling hot, pruritus, and hypersensitivity). Two of the adverse events were considered serious (hypertension and dysrhythmia), but both were considered more likely to be associated with MTX itself. In one recent study with glucarpidase, three of seven patients tested produced antiglucarpidase antibodies.[61] In patients administered $CPDG_2$ fused to a murine single-chain Fv antibody, 36% (11 of 30) developed anti-$CPDG_2$ antibodies, while no antimurine antibodies were detected.[39] Although antiglucarpidase antibodies might decrease clinical efficacy or predispose to allergic reaction upon re-exposure,[2,5,21,61] many patients have been successfully treated with more than one dose of glucarpidase for persistently elevated MTX concentrations.[14,18,32,51,53,61,66,80,84] Clinical trials will explore planned repeated use (eg, NCT00727831). Late glucarpidase administration, more then 96 hours after MTX initiation may not prevent significant MTX toxicity.[3]

Since "inactive" DAMPA has a urinary solubility eight to ten times less than MTX (depending on pH),[27,76] alkalinization and saline diuresis must be continued to prevent DAMPA precipitation and further renal compromise. Because of the inability of glucarpidase to access intracellular MTX, rebound may occur.[79] Significant delayed rebound of MTX may occur up to 85 hours after glucarpidase is administered.[61] This slow egress of persistent intracellular MTX requires continued leucovorin therapy at 250 mg/m^2 IV every 6 hours for 48 hours after the last dose of carboxypeptidase. Then, leucovorin is continued until the MTX concentration is less than 50 nmol/L (0.05 μmol/L).[75]

Carboxypeptidase has a 10- to 15-fold higher affinity for MTX than for leucovorin, although its affinity for its active metabolite 5-methyltetrahydrofolate and folate are similar.[6,21,63] Leucovorin is commonly provided as a racemate, although the active enantiomer is now an approved pharmaceutical. Since glucarpidase cleaves the active *levo-(6S)*-leucovorin about 50% faster than the inactive *dextro-(6R)*-isomer,[27] glucarpidase may compromise leucovorin rescue if both antidotes are administered at similar times. Fifteen minutes post $CPDG_2$, median leucovorin and active 5-methyltetrahydrofolate concentrations dropped by 8% and greater than 97%; the remaining leucovorin was likely the inactive d-isomer.[75,78] When provided at 2 or 26 hours after a glucarpidase dose to healthy volunteers, "exposures to" active leucovorin and activated levo-5-methyl-tetrahydrofolate were 50% and 0% (administration after 2 hours) and 80% and 25% (administration after 26 hours) of anticipated, respectively.[21] Thus, because leucovorin and 5-methyltetrahydrofolate can act as competitive substrates for glucarpidase, most protocols recommend that leucovorin should not be administered for 2 to 4 hours before, and for up to 2 to 4 hours after glucarpidase is provided. Administration of glucarpidase more proximate to leucovorin would require a thoughtful benefit-risk assessment. The exigency to rapidly eliminate MTX—ascertained by the patient's clinical status, renal function, and MTX concentration—would be weighed against the risks of inactivating leucovorin and 5-methyltetrahydrofolate, particularly in cases of prolonged exposure to MTX, in which intracellular MTX inaccessible to glucarpidase would be expected.

In the setting of oral MTX overdose, gastrointestinal decontamination should be considered, as glucarpidase has no intraluminal activity. The supplied product contains lactose and Tris-HCl with zinc buffer. Lactose intolerant patients can receive glucarpidase. In those who have previously experienced allergic reactions to lactose-containing xenobiotics or the other excipients, or patients with rare hereditary problems of fructose intolerance, galactose intolerance, galactosemia, or glucose-galactose malabsorption, the anticipated clinical benefit of glucarpidase would need to be weighed against the risk of adverse effects.

DOSING

Glucarpidase is dosed in units per kilogram in both children and adults. One unit of enzyme activity catalyzes the hydrolysis of 1 μmol of MTX per minute at 37°C.[4] After reconstituting each 1000-Units vial with 1 mL of sterile sodium chloride (0.9%), a single dose of 50 U/kg is administered immediately by bolus IV injection over 5 minutes. A second dose can be administered 24 to 48 hours later if there is evidence of persistent MTX. In cases of IT MTX overdose, a fixed dose of glucarpidase (2000 Units) reconstituted in sterile 0.9% sodium chloride is administered intrathecally over 5 minutes.[50,79] With excessive MTX dosing, the glucarpidase could be given IV and IT simultaneously. As compatibility studies have not been performed, glucarpidase should not be mixed with other agents. Glucarpidase should be refrigerated (2°C to 8°C), but not frozen.

AVAILABILITY

Glucarpidase is available in single-use glass vials containing glucarpidase (1000 Units) with lactose (10 mg), buffered to pH 6.5 to 8.0 with Tris-HCl and zinc buffer. At the time of writing, glucarpidase has not yet received US FDA or European marketing approval. Glucarpidase for IV administration may be obtained in the United States under an open-label treatment protocol (ClinicalTrials.gov identifier: NCT00481559). US emergency inquiries, supply details, and procedural details can be directed to AAIPharma: 866-918-1731 (for intravenous emergencies) or BTG: 888-327-1027 (for intrathecal emergencies). Points of contact for other countries, IRB approval, IRB emergency exemption, and intrathecal emergency-use IND procedures are detailed at the manufacturer's and FDA's websites (www.btgplc.com/BTGPipeline/273/Voraxaze.html; http://www.btgplc.com/Voraxaze/284/VoraxazeUSSupplies.html; www.fda.gov/cder/cancer/singleIND.htm.).[57] Ongoing or anticipated clinical trials (eg, ClinicalTrials.gov identifiers: NCT00481559, NCT00634322, NCT00634504, NCT00727831) or specialty cancer centers that may have access to this antidote might also serve as a resource, particularly after hours or on weekends.

SUMMARY

Glucarpidase is a bacterially derived metalloenzyme used in the treatment of MTX toxicity. It cleaves MTX in the serum compartment to rapidly reduce serum MTX concentrations. Ongoing studies are addressing the extent and consequences of concurrent enzymatic destruction of folate and leucovorin and product immunogenicity. Glucarpidase does not substitute for leucovorin, which counteracts persistent intracellular and CNS MTX. In most cases glucarpidase administration should be separated from the leucovorin administration by 2 to 4 hours.

REFERENCES

1. Abelson HT, Ensminger W, Rosowsky A, Uren J. Comparative effects of citrovorum factor and carboxypeptidase G_1 on cerebrospinal fluid-methotrexate pharmacokinetics. *Cancer Treat Rep.* 1978;62:1549-1552.
2. Abelson HT, Kufe DW, Skarin AT, et al. Treatment of central nervous system tumors with methotrexate. *Cancer Treat Rep.* 1981;65(Suppl 1):137-140.
3. Adamson PC, Balis FM, Boron M, et al. Carboxypeptidase-G_2 ($CPDG_2$) and leucovorin (LV) rescue with and without addition of thymidine (Thd) for high-dose methotrexate (HDMTX) induced renal dysfunction [abstract]. *J Clin Oncol (Meeting Abstracts).* 2005;23(16S):2076.
4. Adamson PC, Balis FM, McCully CL, et al. Rescue of experimental intrathecal methotrexate overdose with carboxypeptidase-G_2. *J Clin Oncol.* 1991;9:670-674.
5. Adamson PC, Balis FM, McCully CL, Godwin KS, Poplack DG. Methotrexate pharmacokinetics following administration of recombinant carboxypeptidase-G_2 in rhesus monkeys. *J Clin Oncol.* 1992;10:1359-1364.
6. Albrecht AM, Boldizsar E, Hutchison DJ. Carboxypeptidase displaying differential velocity in hydrolysis of methotrexate, 5-methyltetrahydrofolic acid, and leucovorin. *J Bacteriol.* 1978;134:506-513.
7. Angier RB, Boothe JH, Hutchings BL, et al. The structure and synthesis of the liver *L. casei* factor. *Science.* 1946;103:667-669.
8. Anoop P, Vaidya SJ, Mycroft J. Methotrexate rechallenge following delayed clearance and life-threatening toxicity. *Pediatr Hematol Oncol.* 2008;25:119-121.

9. Bertino JR, O'Brien P, McCullough JL. Inhibition of growth of leukemia cells by enzymic folate depletion. *Science.* 1971;172:161-162.
10. Bertino JR, Skeel R, Makulu D, Gralla EJ, Bertino JR. Initial clinical studies with carboxypeptidase G_1 (CPG_1), a folate depleting enzyme. *Clin Res.* 1974;22:483A.
11. Bleyer WA. Methotrexate: clinical pharmacology, current status and therapeutic guidelines. *Cancer Treat Rev.* 1977;4:87-101.
12. Brandes JC, Grossman SA, Ahmad H. Alteration of pemetrexed excretion in the presence of acute renal failure and effusions: presentation of a case and review of the literature. *Cancer Invest.* 2006;24:283-287.
13. Brandsteterova E, Seresova O, Miertus S, Reichelová V. HPLC determination of methotrexate and its metabolite in serum. *Neoplasma.* 1990;37:395-403.
14. Buchen S, Ngampolo D, Melton RG, et al. Carboxypeptidase G_2 rescue in patients with methotrexate intoxication and renal failure. *Br J Cancer.* 2005;92:480-487.
15. Chabner BA, Chello PL, Bertino JR. Antitumor activity of a folate-cleaving enzyme, carboxypeptidase G_1. *Cancer Res.* 1972;32:2114-2119.
16. Chabner BA, Johns DG, Bertino JR. Enzymatic cleavage of methotrexate provides a method for prevention of drug toxicity. *Nature.* 1972;239:395-397.
17. Cornell R, Charm SE. Purification of carboxypeptidase G-1 by immunoadsorption. *Biotechnol Bioeng.* 1976;18:1171-1173.
18. DeAngelis LM, Tong WP, Lin S, Fleisher M, Bertino JR. Carboxypeptidase G_2 rescue after high-dose methotrexate. *J Clin Oncol.* 1996;14:2145-2149.
19. Donehower RC, Hande KR, Drake JC, Chabner BA. Presence of 2,4-diamino-N10-methylpteroic acid after high-dose methotrexate. *Clin Pharmacol Ther.* 1979;26:63-72.
20. Estève M-, Devictor-Pierre B, Galy G, et al. Severe acute toxicity associated with high-dose methotrexate (MTX) therapy: use of therapeutic drug monitoring and test-dose to guide carboxypeptidase G_2 rescue and MTX continuation. *Eur J Clin Pharmacol.* 2007;63:39-42.
21. European Medicines Agency (EMEA). Pre-authorisation Evaluation of Medicines for Human Use. Withdrawal Assessment Report for Voraxaze. EMEA/CHMP/171907/2008. London, UK: European Medicines Agency (EMEA); 2008. http://www.emea.europa.eu/humandocs/PDFs/EPAR/voraxaze/H-681-WAR-en.pdf. Accessed September 17, 2008.
22. Finkelstein Y, Zevin S, Raikhlin-Eisenkraft B, et al. Intrathecal methotrexate neurotoxicity: clinical correlates and antidotal treatment. *Environ Toxicol Pharmacol.* 2005;19:721-725.
23. Fotoohi K, Skarby T, Soderhall S, Peterson C, Albertioni F. Interference of 7-hydroxymethotrexate with the determination of methotrexate in plasma samples from children with acute lymphoblastic leukemia employing routine clinical assays. *J Chromatogr B Analyt Technol Biomed Life Sci.* 2005;817:139-144.
24. Genestier L, Paillot R, Quemeneur L, Izeradjene K, Revillard JP. Mechanisms of action of methotrexate. *Immunopharmacology.* 2000;47:247-257.
25. Goldman P, Levy CC. Carboxypeptidase G: purification and properties. *PNAS.* 1967;58:1299-1306.
26. Green MR, Chamberlain MC. Renal dysfunction during and after high-dose methotrexate. *Cancer Chemother Pharmacol.* 2009;63(4):599-604.
27. Hempel G, Lingg R, Boos J. Interactions of carboxypeptidase G_2 with 6S-leucovorin and 6R-leucovorin in vitro: implications for the application in case of methotrexate intoxications. *Cancer Chemother Pharmacol.* 2005;55:347-353.
28. Howell SB, Blair HE, Uren J, Frei E 3rd. Hemodialysis and enzymatic cleavage of methotrexate in man. *Eur J Cancer.* 1978;14:787-792.
29. Jardine LF, Ingram LC, Bleyer WA. Intrathecal leucovorin after intrathecal methotrexate overdose. *J Pediatr Hematol Oncol.* 1996;18:302-304.
30. Kalghatgi KK, Moroson BA, Horvath C, Bertino JR. Enhancement of antitumor activity of 2,4-diamino-5-(3',4'-dichlorophenyl)-6-methylpyrimidine and Baker's antifol (Triazinate) with carboxypeptidase G_1. *Cancer Res.* 1979;39:3441-3445.
31. Krackhardt A, Schwartz S, Korfel A, Thiel E. Carboxypeptidase G_2 rescue in a 79 year-old patient with cranial lymphoma after high-dose methotrexate induced acute renal failure. *Leuk Lymphoma.* 1999;35:631-635.
32. Krause AS, Weihrauch MR, Bode U, et al. Carboxypeptidase-G_2 rescue in cancer patients with delayed methotrexate elimination after high-dose methotrexate therapy. *Leuk Lymphoma.* 2002;43:2139-2143.
33. Kream J, Borek BA, DiGrado CJ, Bovarnick M. Enzymatic hydrolysis of γ-glutamyl polypeptide and its derivatives. *Arch Biochem Biophys.* 1954;53:333-340.
34. Lemon J, Sickels JP, Hutchings BL, et al. Conversion of pteroylglutamic acid to pteroic acid by bacterial degradation. *Arch Biochem.* 1948;19:311-316.
35. Levy CC, Goldman P. The enzymatic hydrolysis of methotrexate and folic acid. *J Biol Chem.* 1967;242:2933-2938.
36. Lloyd LF, Collyer CA, Sherwood RF. Crystallization and preliminary crystallographic analysis of carboxypeptidase G_2 from *Pseudomonas* sp. strain RS-16. *J Mol Biol.* 1991;220:17-18.
37. Mantadakis E, Rogers ZR, Smith AK, et al. Delayed methotrexate clearance in a patient with sickle cell anemia and osteosarcoma. *J Pediatr Hematol Oncol.* 1999;21:165-169.
38. Matherly LH, Barlowe CK, Goldman ID. Antifolate polyglutamylation and competitive drug displacement at dihydrofolate reductase as important elements in leucovorin rescue in L1210 cells. *Cancer Res.* 1986;46:588-593.
39. Mayer A, Francis RJ, Sharma SK, et al. A phase I study of single administration of antibody-directed enzyme prodrug therapy with the recombinant anti-carcinoembryonic antigen antibody-enzyme fusion protein MFECP1 and a bis-iodo phenol mustard prodrug. *Clin Cancer Res.* 2006;12:6509-6516.
40. McCullough JL, Chabner BA, Bertino JR. Purification and properties of carboxypeptidase G 1. *J Biol Chem.* 1971;246:7207-7213.
41. McNutt S. The enzymic deamination and amide cleavage of folic acid. *Arch Biochem Biophys.* 1963;101:1-6.
42. Melton R, Atkinson A. Cleavage of antifolate compounds [patent application]. Application number PCT/GB2005/003297. Publication number WO/2007/023243. World Intellectual Property Organization; 2007. http://www.wipo.int/pctdb/en/wo.jsp?IA=GB2005003297&DISPLAY=STATUS. Accessed September 17, 2008.
43. Melton R, Atkinson A. Use of carboxypeptidase G for combating antifolate toxicity [patent application]. Application number PCT/GB2005/000751. Publication number WO/2005/084695. World Intellectual Property Organization; 2005. http://www.wipo.int/pctdb/en/wo.jsp?IA=GB2005000751&DISPLAY=STATUS. Accessed September 17, 2008.
44. Minton NP, Atkinson T, Bruton CJ, Sherwood RF. The complete nucleotide sequence of the *Pseudomonas* gene coding for carboxypeptidase G_2. *Gene.* 1984;31:31-38.
45. Minton NP, Atkinson T, Sherwood RF. Molecular cloning of the *Pseudomonas* carboxypeptidase G_2 gene and its expression in *Escherichia coli* and *Pseudomonas putida. J Bacteriol.* 1983;156:1222-1227.
46. Minton NP, Clarke LE. Identification of the promoter of the *Pseudomonas* gene coding for carboxypeptidase G_2. *J Mol Appl Genet.* 1985;3:26-35.
47. Mohty M, Peyriere H, Guinet C, et al. Carboxypeptidase G_2 rescue in delayed methotrexate elimination in renal failure. *Leuk Lymphoma.* 2000;37:441-443.
48. Moisa A, Fritz P, Benz D, Wehner HD. Iatrogenically related, fatal methotrexate intoxication: a series of four cases. *Forensic Sci Int.* 2006;156:154-157.
49. Nickerson WJ, Webb M. Effects of folic acid analogues on growth and cell division of nonexacting microorganisms. *J Bacteriol.* 1956;71:129-139.
50. O'Marcaigh AS, Johnson CM, Smithson WA, et al. Successful treatment of intrathecal methotrexate overdose by using ventriculolumbar perfusion and intrathecal instillation of carboxypeptidase G_2. *Mayo Clin Proc.* 1996;71:161-165.
51. Park ES, Han KH, Choi HS, et al. Carboxypeptidase-G_2 rescue in a patient with high dose methotrexate-induced nephrotoxicity. *Cancer Res Treat.* 2005;37:133-135.
52. Pesce MA, Bodourian SH. Evaluation of a fluorescence polarization immunoassay procedure for quantitation of methotrexate. *Ther Drug Monit.* 1986;8:115-121.
53. Peyriere H, Cociglio M, Margueritte G, et al. Optimal management of methotrexate intoxication in a child with osteosarcoma. *Ann Pharmacother.* 2004;38:422-427.
54. Phillips M, Smith W, Balan G, Ward S. Pharmacokinetics of glucarpidase in subjects with normal and impaired renal function. *J Clin Pharmacol.* 2008;48:279-284.
55. Pinedo HM, Zaharko DS, Bull JM, Chabner BA. The reversal of methotrexate cytotoxicity to mouse bone marrow cells by leucovorin and nucleosides. *Cancer Res.* 1976;36:4418-4424.
56. Pratt AG, Crawford EJ, Friedkin M. The hydrolysis of mono-, di-, and triglutamate derivatives of folic acid with bacterial enzymes. *J Biol Chem.* 1968;243:6367-6372.
57. Protherics Inc (a BTG Company). Voraxaze" glucarpidase. Voraxaze" Emergency Enquires. BTG; 2009. http://www.btgplc.com/BTGPipeline/273/Voraxaze.html. Accessed May 25, 2009.
58. Rowsell S, Pauptit RA, Tucker AD, et al. Crystal structure of carboxypeptidase G_2, a bacterial enzyme with applications in cancer therapy. *Structure.* 1997;5:337-347.

59. Saland JM, Leavey PJ, Bash RO, et al. Effective removal of methotrexate by high-flux hemodialysis. *Pediatr Nephrol.* 2002;17:825-829.
60. Schwartz S, Borner K, Korfel A, et al. Effects of carboxypeptidase G_2 (CPG_2) rescue in 30 lymphoma patients with high-dose methotrexate (HD-MTX) induced renal failure [abstract]. *Ann Oncol.* 2005;16(Suppl 5):136-137.
61. Schwartz S, Borner K, Müller K, et al. Glucarpidase (carboxypeptidase g2) intervention in adult and elderly cancer patients with renal dysfunction and delayed methotrexate elimination after high-dose methotrexate therapy. *Oncologist.* 2007;12:1299-1308.
62. Schwartz S, Müller K, Fischer L, et al. Favorable outcome in excessive methotrexate (MTX) intoxication after high-dose (HD) MTX therapy by early use of carboxypeptidase G_2 (CPG2) [abstract]. *J Clin Oncol (Meeting Abstracts).* 2005;23(16S):8255.
63. Sherwood RF, Melton RG, Alwan SM, Hughes P. Purification and properties of carboxypeptidase G_2 from *Pseudomonas* sp. strain RS-16. Use of a novel triazine dye affinity method. *Eur J Biochem.* 1985;148:447-453.
64. Sieniawski M, Rimpler M, Herrmann R, et al. Successful carboxypeptidase G_2 rescue of a high-risk elderly Hodgkin lymphoma patient with methotrexate intoxication and renal failure. *Leuk Lymphoma.* 2007;48:1641-1643.
65. Sinicina I, Mayr B, Mall G, Keil W. Deaths following methotrexate overdoses by medical staff. *J Rheumatol.* 2005;32:2009-2011.
66. Smith SW, Nelson LS. Case files of the New York City Poison Control Center: antidotal strategies for the management of methotrexate toxicity. *J Med Toxicol.* 2008;4:132-140.
67. Snyder RL. Resumption of high-dose methotrexate after methotrexate-induced nephrotoxicity and carboxypeptidase G_2 use. *Am J Health Syst Pharm.* 2007;64:1163-1169.
68. Thorne CB, Gomez CG, Noyes HE, Housewright RD. Production of glutamyl polypeptide by bacillus subtilis. *J Bacteriol.* 1954;68:307-315.
69. Trinkle R, Wu JK. Intrathecal leukovorin after intrathecal methotrexate overdose. *J Pediatr Hematol Oncol.* 1997;19:267-269.
70. Tucker AD, Roswell S, Melton RG, Paupitt RA. A new crystal form of carboxypeptidase G_2 from *Pseudomonas* sp. strain RS-16 which is more amenable to structure determination. *Acta Crystallogr D Biol Crystallogr.* 1996;52:890-892.
71. US FDA. Cumulative List of All Orphan Designated and or Approved Products. FDA; 2008. http://www.fda.gov/orphan/designat/alldes.rtf. Accessed September 17, 2008.
72. Volcani BE, Margalith P. A new species (*Flavobacterium polyglutamicum*) which hydrolyzes the γ-L-glutamyl bond in polypeptides. *J Bacteriol.* 1957; 74:646-655.
73. von Poblozki A, Dempke W, Schmoll HJ. Carboxypeptidase-G_2-rescue in a woman with methotrexate-induced renal failure. *Med Klin (Munich).* 2000;95:457-460.
74. Webb M. Inactivation of analogues of folic acid by certain non-exacting bacteria. *Biochim Biophys Acta.* 1955;17:212-225.
75. Widemann BC, Adamson PC. Understanding and managing methotrexate nephrotoxicity. *Oncologist.* 2006;11:694-703.
76. Widemann BC, Balis FM, Kempf-Bielack B, et al. High-dose methotrexate-induced nephrotoxicity in patients with osteosarcoma. *Cancer.* 2004; 100:2222-2232.
77. Widemann BC, Balis FM, Murphy RF, et al. Carboxypeptidase-G_2, thymidine, and leucovorin rescue in cancer patients with methotrexate-induced renal dysfunction. *J Clin Oncol.* 1997;15:2125-2134.
78. Widemann BC, Balis FM, O'Brien M, et al. Rescue with carboxypeptidase-G_2 ($CPDG_2$) and leucovorin (LV) for patients with high-dose methotrexate (HDMTX) induced renal failure. *Proc Am Soc Clin Oncol.* 1998;17:222a.
79. Widemann BC, Balis FM, Shalabi A, et al. Treatment of accidental intrathecal methotrexate overdose with intrathecal carboxypeptidase G_2. *J Natl Cancer Inst.* 2004;96:1557-1559.
80. Widemann BC, Hetherington ML, Murphy RF, Balis FM, Adamson PC. Carboxypeptidase-G_2 rescue in a patient with high dose methotrexate-induced nephrotoxicity. *Cancer.* 1995;76:521-526.
81. Widemann BC, Sung E, Anderson L, et al. Pharmacokinetics and metabolism of the methotrexate metabolite 2, 4-diamino-N(10)-methylpteroic acid. *J Pharmacol Exp Ther.* 2000;294:894-901.
82. Yasuda N, Kaneko M, Kimura Y. Isolation, purification, and characterization of a new enzyme from *Pseudomonas* sp. M-27, carboxypeptidase G_3. *Biosci Biotechnol Biochem.* 1992;56:1536-1540.
83. Zelcer S, Kellick M, Wexler LH, Gorlick R, Meyers PA. The Memorial Sloan-Kettering Cancer Center experience with outpatient administration of high dose methotrexate with leucovorin rescue. *Pediatr Blood Cancer.* 2008;50:1176-1180.
84. Zoubek A, Zaunschirm HA, Lion T, et al. Successful carboxypeptidase G_2 rescue in delayed methotrexate elimination due to renal failure. *Pediatr Hematol Oncol.* 1995;12:471-477.

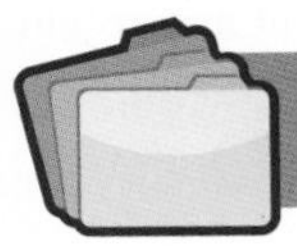

SPECIAL CONSIDERATIONS (SC3)

EXTRAVASATION OF XENOBIOTICS

Richard Y. Wang

Extravasational injuries are among the most consequential local toxic events. When an antineoplastic leaks into the perivascular space, significant necrosis of skin, muscles, and tendons can occur with resultant loss of function. The initial manifestations may include swelling, pain, and a burning sensation that can last for hours. Days later, the area may become erythematous and indurated and can either resolve or proceed to ulceration and necrosis.[30] These early findings may sometimes be difficult to distinguish from other forms of local drug toxicity, such as irritation and hypersensitivity where either the antineoplastic or its vehicle (ethanol, propylene glycol) can cause local irritation as defined by an inflammatory response. Some of the therapeutics associated with local irritation include fluorouracil, carmustine, cisplatin, and dacarbazine. The local irritation and hypersensitivity manifestations are self-limiting and typified by an immediate onset of a burning sensation, pruritus, erythema, and a flare reaction of the vein being infused. Pretreatment with an antihistamine can prevent some of the hypersensitivity manifestations.[38] Drugs reported to cause hypersensitivity reactions include daunorubicin, doxorubicin, idarubicin, and mitoxantrone. When local reactions cannot be differentiated, it is always best to presume extravasation and manage the situation accordingly.

The occurrence of these extravasational events appears to be about 50 times more frequent in the hands of the inexperienced clinician.[14] Several factors are associated with extravasational injuries from peripheral intravenous lines, including (a) patients with poor vessel integrity and blood flow, such as the elderly, those who undergo numerous venipunctures, and those who have received radiation therapy to the site; (b) limited venous and lymphatic drainage caused by either obstruction or surgical resection; and (c) the use of venous access overlying a joint, which increases the risk of dislodgments because of movement.[13,30] Extravasational injuries from implanted ports in central venous vessels can occur from inadequate placement of the needle, needle dislodgment, fibrin sheath formation around the catheter, perforation of the superior vena cava, and fracture of the catheter.[32] When extravasation from a port is suspected and radiographic studies are not diagnostic, a CT scan of the chest with contrast is necessary for evaluation.[1]

The factors associated with a poor outcome from extravasational injuries include (a) areas of the body with little subcutaneous tissue, such as the dorsum of the hand, volar surface of the wrist, and the antecubital fossa, where healing is poor and vital structures are more likely to be involved; (b) increasing concentrations of extravasate; (c) increased volume and duration of contact with tissue; and (d) the type of chemotherapeutic.[30,31] Vesicants, such as doxorubicin, daunorubicin, dactinomycin, epirubicin, idarubicin, mechlorethamine, mitomycin, and the vinca alkaloids, result in more significant local tissue destruction. Mitomycin infusions can cause dermal ulcerations at venipuncture sites remote from the location of administration.[28] The anthracycline antibiotics are associated with a higher incidence of significant injuries and delayed healing, which may be a result of their slow release from bound tissue into surrounding viable tissue. Doxorubicin extravasation is associated with local tissue necrosis in approximately 25% of cases. The extravasational injuries from taxanes appear similar to the vesicants, but are milder in response and more delayed in presentation.[3,29] Prevention is the best form of therapy for these injuries. Specialized nursing care and the use of indwelling central venous catheters limit the extent of these injuries.

MANAGEMENT

The treatment for extravasational injuries is somewhat controversial, varying from conservative care to early surgical debridement and the use of selective antidotes.[33] This uncertainty is a result of the limited number of clinical cases available for study and the discordance between animal studies and human experience. However, general management guidelines for an extravasation and their theoretical foundations exist (Table SC3-1).[6,9]

Once extravasation is suspected, the infusion should be immediately halted. A physician should be notified and the xenobiotic, its concentration, and the approximate amount infused should be noted. The venous access should be maintained so that aspiration of as much of the infusate as possible can be performed and an antidote can be administered, if indicated. Injection of normal saline into the catheter to dilute the extravasate may be beneficial.[17,33] The intermittent local application of ice and elevation of the extremity should be done for 48 to 72 hours so as to limit further progression of the xenobiotic and the development of dependent edema. Cooling the area is believed to prevent cell injury by reducing the amount of xenobiotic absorbed by the tissue and lowering the cellular metabolic rate.[18,37] With just cold application and strict elevation, only 13 (11%) of 119 patients with mild extravasations required surgical intervention for their injuries.[22] In the past, heat was recommended to disperse the agent, but investigations with mice treated with intradermal doxorubicin demonstrated that this practice increased the area of skin ulceration.[11,22] However, dry, warm compresses are still recommended for the vinca alkaloids and etoposide to promote systemic uptake.[6] This is combined with the immediate and local infiltration with hyaluronidase to enhance absorption (Table SC3–1). The amount of hyaluronidase administered at the site ranges from 150 to 900 Units, and the chosen concentration of the solution depends on the area to be treated. For extravasational injuries involving a small area, the initial solution of 150 Units/mL may be adequate. Otherwise, the solution may be diluted by 10-fold with 0.9% NaCl to increase the amount of volume that would be needed to treat a larger surface area. If the intravenous cannula is still accessible, 1 mL of hyaluronidase can be administered through the catheter. Wounds that are either cancerous or infected should not be treated with hyaluronidase stored in a refrigerator. Patients treated with hyaluronidase need to be monitored for allergic reactions, such as anaphylaxis, although the newer human recombinant form (Hylener) is less allergenic than previous animal derivatives.

The wound should be observed closely for the first 7 days, and a surgeon consulted if either pain persists or evidence of ulceration

TABLE SC3–1. Management of Extravasational Injuries[6,16]

Therapy		Purpose/Mechanism
General	Stop infusion and maintain intravenous cannula at the site.	
	Aspirate extravasate from the site by accessing the original intravenous cannula.	Minimizes amount of antineoplastic localized at the site.
	Irrigation of subcutaneous tissue at the site with 0.9% sodium chloride by accessing the original intravenous cannula.	
	Apply dry cool compresses for 1 hour, every 8 hours for 3 days.	Localizes area of involvement and diminishes cellular uptake of the antineoplastic.
	Elevate extremity and administer analgesia.	Promotes drainage, prevents dependent edema, and provides comfort.
Specific		
Anthracyclines	Dexrazoxane 1000 mg/m², daily (max. 2000 mg per day), on days 1 and 2, and 500 mg/m² on day 3 (max. 1000 mg).	Limits free radical formation.
Mechlorethamine	IV sodium thiosulfate: Take 4mL of 25% sodium thiosulfate and add to 21mL of sterile water for injection to make an isotonic (4%) concentration.	Prevents tissue alkylation
	Infiltrate the site of extravasation.	
Mitomycin	Dimethyl sulfoxide (DMSO): 55%–99%. Applied topically and allowed to dry.	Free radical scavenger.
Vinca alkaloids and epipodophyllotoxins	Hyaluronidase: Inject, intradermally or subcutaneously, 150–900 Units into the site.	Degrades hyaluronic acid to enhance systemic absorption
	Dry warm compresses.	Promotes systemic absorption.

appears.[30] However, in severe extravasations—where there is a high incidence of necrosis because of the type of drug (doxorubicin), the volume or concentration, and any area in which there may be significant long-term morbidity (over joints)—early surgical consultation is warranted. If tissue ulceration occurs, initial management may be restricted to sterile dressings to prevent secondary infections. After the area of necrotic skin has evolved to the point where it can be clearly delineated from surviving tissue, surgical debridement may be beneficial to limit secondary infection. The use of intravenous fluorescein or other dye indicators can aid in identifying viable tissue.[2] The patient may require surgical reconstruction or skin grafts depending on the extent of the injury.

ANTIDOTES

Antidotal therapy should be considered when the extravasate is known to respond poorly to conservative care. The vesicants are associated with a significantly worse outcome, and when the exposure is large, a more aggressive approach should be initiated. Otherwise, conservative supportive management may be adequate. The specific antidotal treatments can be divided into several categories based upon their mechanism of action, one of which is the reduction of the inflammatory response through the application of steroids. Hydrocortisone has been used in varying concentrations (50–200 mg) as either subcutaneous or intradermal injections for doxorubicin and the vinca alkaloids,[4,14,23,36] and as a topical cream.[17] Corticosteroids may have only a limited role in doxorubicin-induced lesions because inflammatory cells do not predominate at the wound site.[8] Corticosteroids should not be added to doxorubicin infusions, because the drugs are chemically incompatible.[35] A prophylactic approach is to inactivate the drug by affecting the pH of the environment. The administration of 5 mL of 8.4% sodium bicarbonate through the same IV line to decrease the DNA binding of doxorubicin was advocated in 1980.[5] The use of sodium bicarbonate should not be considered as a routine treatment because its intrinsic hyperosmolarity can cause tissue necrosis.[12] Sodium thiosulfate is recommended for mechlorethamine extravasations, and is believed to work by inactivating the xenobiotic by reacting with the active ethylenimmonium ring.[13,27] The site should be infiltrated with 2 mL of a sterile sodium thiosulfate 0.17 M solution for each mg of mechlorethamine and then ice compresses are applied intermittently for 48 to 72 hours.[6]

Finally, there are antidotes, such as dimethyl sulfoxide (DMSO), that scavenge the free radicals that are believed to cause tissue damage from doxorubicin. Dimethyl sulfoxide has been shown to be beneficial for anthracycline extravasations in both animal and human clinical trials.[7,10,23,27,34] The concentration of DMSO used ranged from 55–99% and was applied topically with intermittent cool compresses.[7,23,26] Some of the other beneficial properties of DMSO are its antiinflammatory, analgesic, and vasodilatory effects, and its ability to promote systemic absorption of the chemotherapeutic at local sites.[24] However, the role for DMSO in the treatment of anthracycline extravasations has become secondary because of the efficacy of dexrazoxane for these exposures and the preparations necessary to make DMSO available in the clinical setting.[21] Also, DMSO is not recommended with the use of dexrazoxane for the treatment of anthracycline extravasations. The systemic administration of dexrazoxane limits anthracycline-induced skin lesions in a murine model[19] and used successfully in patients following doxorubicin[20] and epirubicin[15,19] extravasations. Dexrazoxane was given to these patients over 3 days intravenously at a starting dose of 1000 mg/m². In two prospective, open-label, single-arm, multicenter clinical trials, the systemic administration of dexrazoxane within 6 hours of anthracycline extravasation resulted in the need for surgical resection of the wound site in only 1 of 54 (1.8%) patients.[25] Dexrazoxane (Totect) is approved by the FDA for use in the treatment of anthracycline extravasation.[16] This antidote is administered as an infusion over 15-30 min. at a site distant to that of the extravasation because of its irritating property. Cool compress at the site of the extravastion is discontinued for 15 minutes prior to therapy to promote the antidote's perfusion at the site. The dose of dexrazoxane (see Table SC3–1) is decreased for patients with diminished renal function (creatinine clearance < 40 mL/min). Patients need to be monitored with CBC and serum AST/ALT because dexrazoxane can cause reversible bone marrow suppression and elevated concentrations of these liver enzymes. Additional clinical evidence needs to be gathered to better define the medical management of other antineoplastic extravasations. Although the overall incidence of extravasations with antineoplastics is small, the associated morbidity may be significant. Prevention is the best form of therapy.

ACKNOWLEDGMENT

This chapter was written by Richard Y. Wang in his private capacity. No official support or endorsement by the Centers for Disease Control and Prevention is intended or should be inferred.

REFERENCES

1. Anderson CM, Walters RS, Hortobagyi GN. Mediastinitis related to probable central vinblastine extravasation in a woman undergoing adjuvant chemotherapy for early breast cancer. *Am J Clin Oncol.* 1996;19:566-568.
2. Argenta LC, Manders EK. Mitomycin C extravasation injuries. *Cancer.* 1983;51:1080-1082.
3. Bailey WL, Crump RM. Taxol extravasation: a case report. *Can Oncol Nurs J.* 1997;7:96-99.
4. Barlock AL, Howsen DM, Hubbard SM. Nursing management of Adriamycin extravasation. *Am J Nurs.* 1979;79:94-96.
5. Bartowski-Dodds L, Daniels JR. Use of sodium bicarbonate as a means of ameliorating doxorubicin-induced dermal necrosis in rats. *Cancer Chemother Pharmacol.* 1980;4:179-181.
6. Bertelli G. Prevention and management of extravasation of cytotoxic drugs. *Drug Saf.* 1995a;12:245-255.
7. Bertelli G, Gozza A, Forno GB, et al. Topical dimethylsulfoxide for the prevention of soft tissue injury after extravasation of vesicant cytotoxic drugs: a prospective clinical study. *J Clin Oncol.* 1995b;13:2851-2855.
8. Bhawan J, Petry J, Rybak ME. Histologic changes induced in skin by extravasation of doxorubicin (adriamycin). *J Cutan Pathol.* 1989;16:158-163.
9. Boyle DM, Engelking C. Vesicant extravasation: myths and realities. *Oncol Nurs Forum.* 1995;22:57-67.
10. Desai MH, Teres D. Prevention of doxorubicin-induced skin ulcers in the rat and pig with dimethyl sulfoxide (DMSO). *Cancer Treat Rep.* 1982;66:1371-1374.
11. Dorr RT, Alberts DS, Stone A. Cold protection and heat enhancement of doxorubicin skin toxicity in the mouse. *Cancer Treat Rep.* 1985;69:431-437.
12. Gaze NR. Tissue necrosis caused by commonly used intravenous infusions. *Lancet.* 1978;2:417-419.
13. Ignoffo RJ, Friedman MA. Therapy of local toxicities caused by extravasation of cancer chemotherapeutic drugs. *Cancer Treat Rev.* 1980;7:17-27.
14. Ignoffo RJ. Neoplastic disorders. In: Lloyd Y. Young and Mary Anne Koda-Kimble, eds. *Applied Therapeutics: The Clinical Use of Drugs.* 4th ed. Vancouver, WA: Applied Therapeutics. 1988;1197-1201.
15. Jensen JN, Lock-Andersen J, Langer SW, Mejer J. Dexrazoxane-a promising antidote in the treatment of accidental extravasation of anthracyclines. *Scand J Plast Reconstr Surg Hand Surg.* 2003;37:174-175.
16. Kane RC, McGuinn WD Jr, Dagher R, et al. Dexrazoxane (Totect): FDA review and approval for the treatment of accidental extravasation following intravenous anthracycline chemotherapy. *Oncologist.* 2008;13:445-450.
17. Khan MS, Holmes JD. Reducing the morbidity from extravasation injuries. *Ann Plast Surg.* 2002;48:628-632.
18. Kleiter MM, Yu D, Mohammadian LA, et al. A tracer dose of technetium-99m-labeled liposomes can estimate the effect of hyperthermia on intratumoral doxil extravasation. *Clin Cancer Res.* 2006;12:6800-6807.
19. Langer SW, Sehested M, Jensen PB. Dexrazoxane is a potent and specific inhibitor of anthracycline induced subcutaneous lesions in mice. *Ann Oncol.* 2001;12:405-410.
20. Langer SW, Sehested M, Jensen PB, et al. Dexrazoxane in anthracycline extravasation. *J Clin Oncol.* 2000;18:3064.
21. Langer SW, Thougaard AV, Sehested M, Jensen PB. Treatment of anthracycline extravasation in mice with dexrazoxane with or without DMSO and hydrocortisone. *Cancer Chemother Pharmacol.* 2006;57:125-128.
22. Larson DL. Treatment of tissue extravasation by antitumor agents. *Cancer.* 1982;49:1796-1799.
23. Lawrence HJ, Goodnight SH Jr. Dimethyl sulfoxide and extravasation of anthracycline agents. *Ann Intern Med.* 1983; 98:1025.
24. Lopez AM, Wallace L, Dorr RT, et al. Topical DMSO treatment for pegylated liposomal doxorubicin-induced palmar-plantar erythrodysesthesia. *Cancer Chemother Pharmacol.* 1999;44:303-306.
25. Mouridsen HT, Langer SW, Buter J, et al. Treatment of anthracycline extravasation with Savene (dexrazoxane): results from two prospective clinical multicentre studies. *Ann Oncol.* 2007;18:546-550.
26. Olver IN, Aisner J, Hament A, et al. A prospective study of topical dimethyl sulfoxide for treating anthracycline extravasation. *J Clin Oncol.* 1988;6:1732-1735.
27. Olver IN, Schwarz MA. Use of dimethyl sulfoxide in limiting tissue damage caused by extravasation of doxorubicin. *Cancer Treat Rep.* 1983;67:407-408.
28. Patel JS, Krusa M. Distant and delayed mitomycin C extravasation. *Pharmacotherapy.* 1999;19:1002-1005.
29. Raley J, Geisler JP, Buekers TE, Sorosky JI. Docetaxel extravasation causing significant delayed tissue injury. *Gynecol Oncol.* 2000;78:259-260.
30. Rudolph R, Larson DL. Etiology and treatment of chemotherapeutic agent extravasation injuries: a review. *J Clin Oncol.* 1987;5:1116-1126.
31. Rudolph R, Suzuki M, Luce JK. Experimental skin necrosis produced by adriamycin. *Cancer Treat Rep.* 1979;63:529-537.
32. Schulmeister L, Camp-Sorrell D. Chemotherapy extravasation from implanted ports. *Oncol Nurs Forum.* 2000;27:531-538.
33. Scuderi N, Onesti MG. Antitumor agents: extravasation, management, and surgical treatment. *Ann Plast Surg.* 1994;32:39-44.
34. Svingen BA, Powis G, Appel PL, Scott M. Protection against adriamycin-induced skin necrosis in the rat by dimethyl sulfoxide and alpha-tocopherol. *Cancer Res.* 1981;41:3395-3399.
35. Trissel LA. *Handbook of Injectable Drugs.* Bethesda, MD: American Society of Hospital Pharmacists; 1988.
36. Tsavaris NB, Karagiaouris P, Tzannou I, et al. Conservative approach to the treatment of chemotherapy-induced extravasation. *J Dermatol Surg Oncol.* 1990;16:519-522.
37. van der Heijden AG, Verhaegh G, Jansen CF, et al. Effect of hyperthermia on the cytotoxicity of 4 chemotherapeutic agents currently used for the treatment of transitional cell carcinoma of the bladder: an in vitro study. *J Urol.* 2005;173:1375-1380.
38. Vogelzang NJ. "Adriamycin flare": a skin reaction resembling extravasation. *Cancer Treat Rep.* 1979;63:2067-2069.

CHAPTER 54
MISCELLANEOUS ANTINEOPLASTICS

Richard Y. Wang

The anthracyclines,[31,70,118] nitrogen mustards,[1,27,45,64,65,70,95,112,118,129] and platinum-based antineoplastics[23,24,41,44,57,68,73,76,80,88,97,108] are discussed in this chapter because of their increased likelihood for overdose based on past reports and current clinical use.

ANTHRACYCLINES

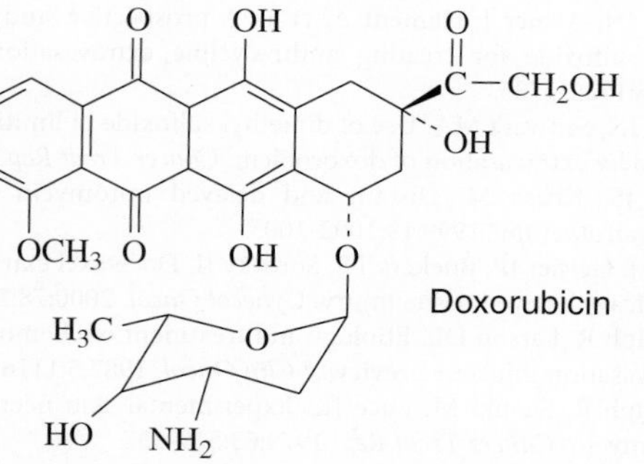

Doxorubicin

Daunorubicin and doxorubicin share many common indications for cancer therapy, but they differ in that doxorubicin is used in solid tumors such as breast carcinoma. The clinical toxicity of the anthracyclines is limited by the use of structural analogs (eg, epirubicin, idarubin) and liposomal encapsulated formulations (pegylated liposomal doxorubicin).

PHARMACOLOGY

The antineoplastics derived from the bacterium *Streptomyces* are dactinomycin, daunorubicin, doxorubicin, bleomycin, mitomycin, and plicamycin. Only plicamycin crosses the blood–brain barrier. The terminal elimination half-life for doxorubicin is about 30 hours.[50] Doxorubicin and daunorubicin are both eliminated by the liver and patients with hepatic dysfunction should have their dosage decreased. Delayed drug elimination contributes to increased drug area under the drug concentration versus time curve (AUC) and peak concentration, which are associated with myelosuppression and cardiac toxicity, respectively.[75] The mechanism of therapeutic action of the anthracyclines is attributed to DNA intercalation[101] and inactivation of topoisomerase II.[117] These xenobiotics are metabolized to active metabolites, which have lesser degrees of activity than their parent compounds. A typical dose schedule for daunorubicin is 30 to 60 mg/m^2 daily for 3 days; for doxorubicin, 45 to 60 mg/m^2 every 18 to 21 days.

PATHOPHYSIOLOGY

The red anthracycline antibiotics—dactinomycin and doxorubicin—can be associated with cardiotoxicity, which limits their therapeutic use. The mechanism responsible for their therapeutic effects is different from that which causes cardiotoxicity.[117] The purported mechanism of cardiac toxicity is from the formation of free radicals and impaired intracellular calcium.[89,96] Doxorubicin and dactinomycin are quinone derivatives and can be reduced to free radicals. These metabolites are extremely cytotoxic through the promotion of lipid peroxidation. Paraquat and bleomycin have similar mechanisms of toxicity. The limited efficacy of free radical scavengers (α-tocopherol, *N*-acetylcysteine) for anthracycline cardiotoxicity led to an understanding of the importance of iron as a cofactor for these radical-producing reactions.[90] The anthracyclines have a high affinity for metal ions. Doxorubicin has an iron (Fe^{3+}) binding constant of 10^{41}, which is comparable to deferoxamine.[48] The heart's increased susceptibility to free radicals is attributed to its lack of sufficient enzyme activity responsible for free radical scavenging.[38]

CLINICAL MANIFESTATIONS

The cardiotoxic manifestations can be divided into acute and late-onset categories. The various findings described with acute toxicity include dysrhythmias, ST and T-wave changes on the electrocardiogram (ECG), diminished ejection fraction that usually resolves over 24 hours, and sudden death.[16,114] Abnormal findings on ECG are present in 41% of patients receiving doxorubicin.[7,54,74,103,114,125,130,132] They are neither dose related nor associated with the development of cardiomyopathy. Acute pericarditis and myocarditis resulting in conduction defects and congestive heart failure are also reported.[15] Animal studies with doxorubicin demonstrate beneficial effects of adrenergic antagonists for toxicity because of elevated concentrations of catecholamines,[15] although the use of β-adrenergic antagonists in the potential setting of diminished cardiac output needs to be considered.

Significant cardiotoxicity results from elevated peak serum concentrations and accounts for continuous and periodic infusions practiced in therapy. In cumulative doses, the anthracycline antibiotics cause a congestive cardiomyopathy that typically presents at 1 to 4 months after exposure depending on the toxicity of the xenobiotic.[62] The condition is irreversible and is associated with a 48% mortality.[98] This drug-induced congestive heart failure is associated with pathognomonic changes on electron microscopy that can distinguish it from infectious and ischemic etiologies. These histologic changes include reduced number of myocardial fibrils, and mitochondrial and cellular degeneration.[13] The incidence of late-onset cardiotoxicity for doxorubicin is between 1% and 10% when the cumulative dose is less than 450 mg/m^2, and becomes greater than 20% when more than 550 mg/m^2 (comparable to dactinomycin, 950 mg/m^2, and epirubicin, 720 mg/m^2) is administered.[84,124] Daunorubicin and mitoxantrone are associated with a 2% incidence at the cumulative doses of 600 mg/m^2 and 140 mg/m^2, respectively.

The best way of monitoring cardiac function during therapy is to use radionuclide cineradiography to measure the left ventricular ejection fraction.[3] Therapy should be discontinued when the ejection fraction falls below 50%. Two-dimensional echocardiography can demonstrate left ventricular wall thickening and fractional shortening from anthracycline overexposure. Newer approaches used to assess for early or subclinical signs of cardiac dysfunction from these agents include cardiac-specific contractile protein, troponin, cardiac natriuretic peptide, and radionuclide-tagged monoclonal antibody imaging.[21,25,37,69]

Factors associated with an increased risk for cardiotoxicity include mediastinal irradiation, preexisting cardiac disease in children, age more than 70 years, and the concomitant use of cyclophosphamide, paclitaxel, and other anthracyclines.[15] Also, the proximate therapeutic use of the monoclonal antibody to human epidermal growth factor receptor 2 (HER2), trastuzumab, with anthracyclines appears to enhance cardiac toxicity.[33] Children are at risk for developing increased left ventricular afterload from doxorubicin toxicity because of the drug's ability to inhibit myocardial growth, which can lead to a disproportionate ratio of left ventricular wall thickness to left ventricular chamber size.[77] Fatalities are reported with minimum doses of 150 to 333 mg/m^2, and occur within 1 to 16 days after exposure.[31]

Myelosuppression and mucositis are other effects associated with the use of the anthracycline agents. They typically occur in 1 to 2 weeks, and patients recover.[10] The white cells are affected more than either the red cells or platelets. Patients with diminished drug clearance due to hepatic failure are at risk for the development of these findings.

Mitoxantrone is recognized to be less toxic than doxorubicin and daunorubicin. Major organs of toxicity remain the heart, bone marrow, and gut. Gastrointestinal effects are less severe and less frequent with mitoxantrone than with doxorubicin.[110] Four cases of mitoxantrone overdose are reported in the literature.[53,110] Common to these events is a 10-fold error in dosing (100 mg/m^2 instead of 10 mg/m^2), early onset of nausea with vomiting, and myelosuppression with fever. Acute decreased cardiac contractility was observed by echocardiography in one patient who was asymptomatic.[53] Otherwise, no patients developed dysrhythmias, congestive failure, ECG changes, or elevated creatine phosphokinase levels early after exposure. Three patients developed fatal congestive heart failure (CHF) from 1 to 4 months later.[110]

MANAGEMENT

Dexrazoxane is a specific antidote for doxorubicin; otherwise, management is largely supportive. Monitoring for cardiotoxicity and pancytopenia is necessary. A baseline chest radiograph, electrocardiogram, and echocardiogram to determine left ventricular ejection fraction (at rest and/or with stress) are required. Endomyocardial biopsy and cardiac catheterization can assist in distinguishing other causes of cardiac dysfunction. Left ventricular function is the best predictor for cardiomyopathy.[43,104] A 10% absolute decrease in the left ventricular ejection fraction (LVEF) or a drop in LVEF of 50% from baseline is a significant finding for the discontinuation of further anthracycline therapy.[104] Although digoxin and furosemide should be used to manage acute CHF, a variable response can be expected.[110] Digoxin and low-dose verapamil benefit patients treated with doxorubicin; however, this benefit may be limited by the severity of the disorder.[47,126] At higher doses of verapamil, hypotension and heart block were observed, which limited further use.[92,116] The role for angiotensin-converting enzyme inhibitor (enalapril) as an effective treatment for congestive cardiomyopathy remains investigatory.[61,111]

Dexrazoxane is a cardioprotectant that limits the adverse cardiac effects of doxorubicin by chelating intracellular iron, which mediates the formation of free radical cellular damage. In clinical trials, patients receiving dexrazoxane had smaller decreases in LVEF per dose of doxorubicin, had fewer histologic changes on cardiac biopsy, were better able to tolerate doxorubicin doses greater than 600 mg/m^2, and had a lower occurrence of serum cardiac troponin T elevations than did patients who were not pretreated with dexrazoxane.[77,78,113] The current role of this chelator is to limit cardiotoxicity in patients receiving more than 300 mg/m^2 of doxorubicin.[106] It is administered 30 minutes before doxorubicin in a 10:1 ratio. Dexrazoxane increased the systemic clearance of epirubicin in a clinical trial, which may be an added benefit to patients with increased exposure.[8] Further investigations are required to determine the optimal use of dexrazoxane in children receiving anthracycline therapy and in patients with overdose exposures. Another cardioprotectant under investigation is monohydroxyethylrutoside. Monohydroxyethylrutoside is a semisynthetic flavonoid that can chelate iron and scavenge free radicals, although the contribution of this action to its cardioprotective effects against doxorubicin-induced toxicity remains unclear.[9] In experimental models, monohydroxyethylrutoside decreased doxorubicin-induced cardiotoxicity as measured by ST segment elevation on ECG[119] and left ventricular function.[60] Clinical trials are lacking for this agent.

ENHANCED ELIMINATION

The anthracyclines are highly protein bound and have a large volume of distribution, which makes them unlikely candidates for hemodialysis. However, the early institution of hemoperfusion may enhance elimination. In an animal model, serum doxorubicin clearance could be enhanced up to 20-fold with hemoperfusion.[128] Factors determining this were duration of therapy, rate of flow, and the use of a 2% acrylic hydrogel-coated cartridge. Three patients with a doxorubicin overdose were treated with hemoperfusion, one with an Amberlite cartridge, and all had a rapid reduction in their serum levels.[31] One survived a 10-fold error in dosing. In a patient with a mitoxantrone overdose of 98 mg intravenously (IV), hemoperfusion was begun within hours, but in two trials, only 0.287 and 0.236 mg of drug were removed.[53]

NITROGEN MUSTARDS

$$H_3C{-}N(CH_2{-}CH_2{-}Cl)_2$$

Mechlorethamine

PHARMACOLOGY

The nitrogen mustards are cyclophosphamide, ifosfamide, chlorambucil, mechlorethamine, and melphalan. Their indicated uses include immunosuppression (eg, controlling graft-versus-host rejection, collagen vascular diseases) and chemotherapy. The tumoricidal activity of these xenobiotics is the result of the formation of reactive intermediates that bind to nucleophilic moieties on DNA, which inactivates DNA synthesis. Unlike the other xenobiotics, cyclophosphamide and ifosfamide require P450 isoenzymes to achieve their alkylating properties. Mechlorethamine is the original compound from which all of the others were derived. It is highly reactive when it comes in contact with water and undergoes rapid chemical transformation. Local reactions caused by mechlorethamine spillage (eg, extravasation) include tissue injury and thrombophlebitis (see Special Considerations SC 3–Extravasation of Xenobiotics). Nonenzymatic hydrolysis is the major route by which the nitrogen mustards are metabolized, thus accounting for their relatively short elimination half-lives (ie, less than 3 hours).[12] Cyclophosphamide, ifosfamide, and chlorambucil have active metabolites, which prolongs their alkylating activity after administration.[66]

CLINICAL MANIFESTATIONS

Chlorambucil and ifosfamide can produce altered mental status and seizures from therapeutic use or from an overdose.[19,45] Both antineoplastics undergo hepatic N-dechloroethylation to produce chloroacetaldehyde, which is purported to be a nervous system toxin.[72] Encephalopathy occurs in 9% of patients receiving 5 g/m^2 of ifosfamide, and is more frequent with oral than with IV administration because of the first-pass effect and increased chloroacetaldehyde production.[81] Seizures are more commonly associated with chlorambucil. Acute overdoses reported in the literature are all from the oral route, and range in dosing from 1.5 to 6.8 mg/kg (therapeutic is 0.1 to 0.2 mg/kg).[5,20] The seizures occur within 6 hours, may appear as generalized tonic–clonic activity or staring spells, and can last for 24 hours. However, in one instance in which therapeutic dosing was increased, seizures occurred 17 hours later. This delay may be attributed to a lower serum concentration or a slower time to peak than in the overdose setting. A similar reasoning would explain why a patient with a chronic overdose of 4.1 mg/kg over 5 days did not sustain central nervous system (CNS) toxicity.[40] Patients with increased likelihood for seizures include those with underlying seizure disorders or with nephrotic syndrome, which can alter pharmacokinetics.[102] Electroencephalograms (EEGs) demonstrated multiple paroxysms of bilaterally symmetric 2 to 3-Hz spikes and slow high-voltage rhythmic slowing that progressed to slower bursts of rhythmic spike and wave discharge in a child with an acute overdose.[20] Myelosuppression occurs in patients with both acute and chronic overdoses, and can present as late as 41 days postexposure. Recovery is expected within 1 week of the nadir, and granulocyte colony-stimulating factor (G-CSF) treatment may be necessary.[64] Renal failure from an acute overdose with ifosfamide is reversible following the immediate institution of hemodialysis.[45]

Cyclophosphamide and its analog ifosfamide induce hemorrhagic cystitis from their irritating metabolite acrolein. This occurs in approximately 5% to 10% of patients who receive therapy.[18,30] The incidence of cystitis does not appear to be related to the total dose and administration route, age, or gender. The course is usually self-limiting, although blood transfusions may be required. Water retention is observed in patients receiving more than 50 mg/kg of cyclophosphamide.[34] This effect is attributed to the activity of the alkylating metabolite on the renal tubule and is observed at 6 to 8 hours after administration. The patient typically develops decreased urinary output, increased urine osmolality, and decreased serum osmolality, which is self-limiting, lasting for about 12 to 16 hours.

In the overdose setting, cyclophosphamide can cause dysrhythmias, myocardial necrosis, hemorrhagic pericarditis, and death. ECG changes are noted at doses of 120 mg/kg and heart failure and myocarditis at doses greater than 150 mg/kg.[6,86] Diminished QRS voltage has been noted on the ECG, which is attributed to myocardial swelling from edema or hemorrhage. An ordering error led to the death of one patient and to irreversible cardiac damage in another patient from cyclophosphamide overdose. These two patients received 6520 mg daily for 4 consecutive days, when the amount was to be divided over 4 days.[100] The onset of heart failure can be sudden and patients older than 50 years of age, and those with a history of cardiac dysfunction or prior treatment with anthracyclines, are at greatest risk for cardiac toxicity.[115]

MANAGEMENT

Recommendations for patients with an acute chlorambucil exposure include routine gastrointestinal decontamination, a 6-hour observation, a determination of a complete blood count (CBC) and hepatic enzymes, and a follow-up CBC weekly for 4 weeks.[121] Ifosfamide-induced encephalopathy can be managed with methylene blue (50 mg IV as a 1% solution), although the mechanism by which methylene blue acts is unknown.[72,131] Seizures are reported to be more effectively managed with benzodiazepines and barbiturates than with phenytoin.[5,129]

When gross hematuria from cyclophosphamide or ifosfamide therapy persists, treatments reported to be effective in the literature can be considered. These treatments include electrocauterization, systemic vasopressin,[99] intravesical administration of silver nitrate,[72] formalin,[46,107] prostaglandin F2,[109] and hydrostatic pressure.[58] Some of the preventive therapies that seem to reduce this occurrence include adequate hydration for dilution effect, frequent bladder emptying, IV administration of 2-mercaptoethane sulfonate sodium (MESNA), and intravesical administration of *N*-acetylcysteine.[18] The thiol group of *N*-acetylcysteine is believed to directly interact with acrolein to limit its irritating effect on the bladder epithelium. MESNA is believed to work by inactivating acrolein to an inert thioether.[59] The IV dose of MESNA is 20% of the cyclophosphamide or ifosfamide amount (wt/wt) and administered during therapy and again at 4 and 8 hours. MESNA is used during standard-dose therapy for ifosfamide and high-dose therapy for cyclophosphamide. In the overdose setting, MESNA does not protect patients from the renal toxic effects of these agents and hemodialysis is indicated. Hemodialysis effectively enhances the elimination of ifosfamide and its metabolites when instituted soon after exposure, and it is more effective than hemoperfusion (Adsorba 300 C, Gambro 300 g active carbon) in removing ifosfamide.[45]

Patients with large exposures to cyclophosphamide require baseline ECGs and echocardiograms. Intravenous fluid restriction, digoxin, and furosemide were successfully used to treat a patient with cyclophosphamide-induced congestive cardiomyopathy.[123]

PLATINOIDS

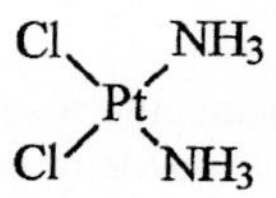

Cisplatin

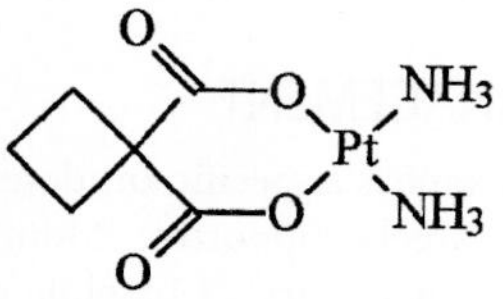

Carboplatin

PHARMACOLOGY

The cytotoxic effects of the platinum-containing compounds were first recognized in 1965. Since then, many types have been derived. The ones of clinical significance are cisplatin, carboplatin, and oxaliplatin.[87] The latter two agents were designed to reduce the incidence of nephrotoxicity and to counter drug resistance to cisplatin. Differences in chemical structure exist among these antineoplastics. Most notably, cisplatin is an inorganic and carboplatin an organic compound. Similarities exist in their mechanism of toxicity, which is the binding of platinum to DNA to form inter- and intrastrand bonds, which lead to DNA dysfunction and strand breakage. These xenobiotics are eliminated from the body primarily in the urine and at varying rates. The amount eliminated at 24 hours is 25% for cisplatin and 90% for carboplatin. Patients with decreased creatinine clearance (< 30 mL/min) will have prolonged elimination half-lives of platinoids.[39]

PATHOPHYSIOLOGY

Renal failure from renal tubular necrosis occurs with cisplatin in a dose-dependent manner. Upon entering the cell, cisplatin forms a cationic complex when the chloride ions are nonenzymatically displaced by water molecules. The reactive complex covalently binds to DNA to disrupt replication and transcription, resulting in cell death. The formation of the hydrated platinum complex is favored by a low chloride concentration in the environment; thus, a sodium chloride infusion promotes the native state of cisplatin by preventing hypochloremia. The presence of alanine aminopeptidase and *N*-acetyl-D-glucosaminidase in the urine can be early indicators of renal tubular damage.[32,36,49]

The sensory neuropathy associated with these platinum-containing antineoplastics can be attributed to their accumulation and toxicity at the dorsal root ganglion, which depends on the water solubility and chemical reactivity of these xenobiotics.[105] Clinical pathologic evaluation demonstrates increased platinum content at the dorsal root ganglion following cisplatin therapy, which suggests that the increased vascularity and fenestration of the endothelium at this tissue site contributes to the uptake of cisplatin.[51,63]

CLINICAL MANIFESTATIONS

The more common manifestations of toxicity with cisplatin during therapy are renal dysfunction, auditory impairment, and peripheral sensory neuropathy. The other antineoplastics recognized to cause a peripheral neuropathy are the Vinca alkaloids and the taxoids. Oxaliplatin-induced neuropathy is triggered or enhanced by exposure to cold and can subside over several months.[42] Myelosuppression is a dose-limiting factor for carboplatin and iproplatin, which does not occur with cisplatin. At a carboplatin dose of 800 mg/m^2, 25% of patients develop marrow toxicity.[93] The marrow effects are delayed, with nadir occurring 3 to 5 weeks after the start of therapy. Patients developing an anemia within the first week of cisplatin therapy should be evaluated for hemolytic anemia.[26]

The sources of error associated with cisplatin are frequency of administration (total dose versus over a period of time), mistaking it for carboplatin, and writing the wrong dose.[28,97] Manifestations in the overdose setting involve neurologic, visual, hearing, bone marrow, pancreatic, and renal disorders.[108] The most common renal disorder is renal failure, which is dose-related and begins at 50 mg/m^2. At this dose, approximately 30% of patients treated with cisplatin develop renal failure and a rise in serum BUN and creatinine typically occurs at 1 to 2 weeks posttreatment. Attributed to the renal toxicity is electrolyte disorders, include hypomagnesemia, hypocalcemia, and hyponatremia.[41] Hyponatremia is an uncommon finding with cisplatin exposure and is attributed to either sodium-wasting nephropathy from renal tubular dysfunction or syndrome of inappropriate secretion of antidiuretic hormone (SIADH). At doses greater than 200 mg/m^2, the development of seizures, encephalopathy, and irreversible peripheral sensory neuropathy is of concern.[11,29,56,92,93,94] At this dose, visual impairment may occur within the first week of exposure.[24,80,127] This can include temporary visual loss, with permanent loss of color discrimination. Physical examination of the anterior chamber and fundus of the eye will be normal; however, an electroretinogram will demonstrate a disorder with the postphotoreceptor neural function.[68] Some other ocular disorders are papilledema and retrobulbar neuritis. High-frequency (2000 Hz) hearing loss is evident 2 to 3 days after exposure to doses greater than 500 mg/m^2.[22]

MANAGEMENT

Renal protection and enhanced elimination of platinum are the two primary goals in the management of a cisplatin overdose. Expectant management for myelosuppression and neurotoxicity can follow. Hydration with 0.9% NaCl solution and an osmotic diuretic (eg, mannitol) should be administered to achieve a high urine output (eg, 1 to 3 mL/kg/h) for 6 to 24 hours postexposure. Sodium chloride diuresis both promotes the inactive state of cisplatin and decreases the urine platinum concentration to limit nephrotoxicity during therapy.[4,122] In the setting of nonoliguric renal failure, careful hydration is recommended to maintain urinary output, because platinum renal excretion is directly related to urinary flow and independent of creatinine clearance.[24] Aside from evaluating BUN and creatinine, assessment of renal function can include glomerular filtration, filtration fraction, and renal plasma flow.[52,82,83,91]

Amifostine (Ethyol™) and sodium thiosulfate are effective nephroprotectants. Amifostine's role is more preventative and its use is approved by the US Food and Drug Administration (FDA) to protect against cisplatin-induced nephrotoxicity. However, additional benefits can include the limitation of myelosuppression, mucositis, and neurotoxicity.[2] Unlike thiosulfate, amifostine is activated intracellularly by alkaline phosphatase to scavenge free radicals, regenerate glutathione, prevent cisplatin-DNA adduct formation, and facilitate DNA repair.[71] The patient requires adequate hydration during amifostine infusion because hypotension can occur. Sodium thiosulfate is effective postexposure. Thiosulfate remains in the extracellular space to bind free platinum and limit cellular damage at the renal tubules. Little or no renal toxicity occurred in patients receiving as much as 270 mg/m^2 of cisplatin when thiosulfate was given as an IV bolus of 4 g/m^2 followed by infusion of 12 g/m^2 over 6 hours.[55,95] In a 14-year-old patient with renal failure, thiosulfate was continued at 2.7 g/m^2 a day until urinary platinum concentration was below 1 µg/mL.[41] Thiosulfate may offer the additional benefit of limiting neurotoxicity and should be administered to all patients after an overdose.[79,120] The effectiveness of thiosulfate is limited by the time in which it needs to be administered after exposure (ie, 1 to 2 hours). *N*-acetylcysteine and BNP7787 (2,2′-dithio-bis-ethanesulfonate) are being investigated as alternative rescue agents for cisplatin toxicity.[14,35,85] Also, BNP7787 is under clinical investigation to limit peripheral neuropathy from paclitaxel therapy.

Hemodialysis is ineffective in patients with cisplatin overdoses, likely as a result of high protein binding.[17] However, in patients with renal failure, hemodialysis may be beneficial when plasmapheresis is not available. Plasmapheresis was performed in four adults and there was a fall in blood serum platinum concentrations with clinical improvement.[23,24,57,67] In one incident, a patient received an overdose of 280 mg/m^2 and was plasmapheresed on day 12 of exposure.[24] After three daily treatments, the serum platinum concentration decreased from 2900 to 200 ng/mL and the patient had noticeable improvement in gastrointestinal and visual symptoms. On day 20, the serum platinum concentration rebounded to 700 ng/mL and the symptoms worsened. Further plasmapheresis lowered the concentration to 290 ng/mL by day 27 and symptoms improved. In another event, a patient received 300 mg/m^2 of cisplatin and received four daily treatments of plasmapheresis starting on day 6 postexposure.[67] The serum platinum concentration declined from 2979 to 430 ng/mL and the patient became more awake and less nauseous. On day 11, platinum concentrations rebounded to 834 ng/mL and fell to 279 ng/mL on reinstitution of plasmapheresis. The amount of platinum removed by three trials in this patient was approximately 4.6 mg. The author of the paper contends that plasmapheresis prevented the need for hemodialysis in renal failure. Other reports have noted an improvement in patients' mental status and hearing loss following the decline in the serum cisplatin (platinum) concentration from plasmapheresis.[23,57] Thus, plasmapheresis appears to be effective in cisplatin overdose and should be instituted immediately after exposure. Patients who remain symptomatic days later also may benefit.

SUMMARY

Anthracyclines, nitrogen mustards, and the platinum-based antineoplastics are some of the antineoplastic agents reported as overdoses in patients undergoing therapy. The primary clinical manifestations of toxicity for these agents include congestive dilated cardiomyopathy (anthracyclines), encephalopathy and seizures (nitrogen mustards), and renal failure (platinum-based agents). The management for these overdoses includes supportive care, enhanced elimination using plasmapheresis for cisplatin, and antidotal therapy, such as dexrazoxane for anthracyclines and amifostine for platinum-based agents. Although rescue agents are available, their effectiveness is markedly diminished in the postexposure period. Specialists in poison information and medical toxicologists need to maintain a current level of understanding of these exposures so they can better assist their patients and interact with other healthcare professionals.

ACKNOWLEDGMENT

This chapter was written by Richard Y. Wang in his private capacity. No official support or endorsement by the Centers for Disease Control and Prevention is intended or should be inferred. Paul Calabresi contributed to this chapter in a previous edition.

REFERENCES

1. Aguiar Bujanda D, Cabrera Suarez MA, Bohn Sarmiento U, Aguiar Morales J. Successful recovery after accidental overdose of cyclophosphamide. *Ann Oncol.* 2006;17:1334.
2. Alberts DS, Bleyer WA. Future development of amifostine in cancer treatment. *Semin Oncol.* 1996;23:90-99.
3. Alexander J, Dainiak N, Berger HJ, et al. Serial assessment of doxorubicin cardiotoxicity with quantitative radionuclide angiocardiography. *N Engl J Med.* 1979;300:278-283.
4. Al-Sarraf M, Fletcher W, Oishi N, et al. Cisplatin hydration with and without mannitol diuresis in refractory disseminated malignant melanoma: a Southwest Oncology Group study. *Cancer Treat Rep.* 1982;66:31-35.
5. Ammenti A, Reitter B, Muller-Wiefel DE. Chlorambucil neurotoxicity: report of two cases. *Helv Paediatr Acta.* 1980;35:281-287.
6. Appelbaum F, Strauchen JA, Graw RG Jr, et al. Acute lethal carditis caused by high-dose combination chemotherapy. A unique clinical and pathological entity. *Lancet.* 1976;1:58-62.
7. Arena E, D'Allesandro N, Dusonchet L, et al. Influence of pharmacokinetic variations on the pharmacologic properties of Adriamycin. In: Carter SK, ed. *International Symposium on Adriamycin.* Berlin ed. New York: Springer-Verlag; 1972:96-116.
8. Basser RL, Sobol MM, Duggan G, et al. Comparative study of the pharmacokinetics and toxicity of high-dose epirubicin with or without dexrazoxane in patients with advanced malignancy. *J Clin Oncol.* 1994;12:7.
9. Bast A, Kaiserova H, den Hartog GJ, Haenen GR, van der Vijgh WJ. Protectors against doxorubicin-induced cardiotoxicity: flavonoids. *Cell Biol Toxicol.* 2007;23:39-47.
10. Benjamin RS, Wiernik PH, Bachur NR. Adriamycin chemotherapy—efficacy, safety, and pharmacologic basis of an intermittent single high-dosage schedule. *Cancer.* 1974;33:19-27.
11. Berman IJ, Mann MP. Seizures and transient cortical blindness associated with cis-platinum (II) diamminedichloride (PDD) therapy in a thirty-year-old man. *Cancer.* 1980;45:764-766.
12. Betcher DL, Burnham N. Melphalan. *J Pediatr Oncol Nurs.* 1990;7:35-36.
13. Billingham ME, Mason JW, Bristow MR, Daniels JR. Anthracycline cardiomyopathy monitored by morphologic changes. *Cancer Treat Rep.* 1978;62:865-872.
14. Boven E, Westerman M, van Groeningen CJ, et al. Phase I and pharmacokinetic study of the novel chemoprotector BNP7787 in combination with cisplatin and attempt to eliminate the hydration schedule. *Br J Cancer.* 2005;92:1636-1643.
15. Bristow MR, Minobe WA, Billingham ME, et al. Anthracycline-associated cardiac and renal damage in rabbits. Evidence for mediation by vasoactive substances. *Lab Invest.* 1981;45:157-168.
16. Bristow MR. Toxic cardiomyopathy due to doxorubicin. *Hosp Pract (Off Ed).* 1982;17:101-108, 110-101.
17. Brivet F, Pavlovitch JM, Gouyette A, et al. Inefficiency of early prophylactic hemodialysis in cis-platinum overdose. *Cancer Chemother Pharmacol.* 1986;18:183-184.
18. Brock N, Pohl J. Prevention of urotoxic side effects by regional detoxification with increased selectivity of oxazaphosphorine cytostatics. *IARC Sci Publ.* 1986;269-279.
19. Brock N, Stekar J, Pohl J, Niemeyer U, Scheffler G. Acrolein, the causative factor of urotoxic side-effects of cyclophosphamide, ifosfamide, trofosfamide and sufosfamide. *Arzneimittelforschung.* 1979;29:659-661.
20. Byrne TN, Jr., Moseley TA 3rd, Finer MA. Myoclonic seizures following chlorambucil overdose. *Ann Neurol.* 1981;9:191-194.
21. Carrio I, Lopez-Pousa A, Estorch M, et al. Detection of doxorubicin cardiotoxicity in patients with sarcomas by indium-111-antimyosin monoclonal antibody studies. *J Nucl Med.* 1993;34:1503-1507.
22. Chiuten D, Vogl S, Kaplan B, Camacho F. Is there cumulative or delayed toxicity from cis-platinum? *Cancer.* 1983;52:211-214.
23. Choi JH, Oh JC, Kim KH, et al. Successful treatment of cisplatin overdose with plasma exchange. *Yonsei Med J.* 2002;43:128-132.
24. Chu G, Mantin R, Shen YM, Baskett G, Sussman H. Massive cisplatin overdose by accidental substitution for carboplatin. Toxicity and management. *Cancer.* 1993;72:3707-3714.
25. Cil T, Kaplan AM, Altintas A, et al. Use of *N*-terminal pro-brain natriuretic peptide to assess left ventricular function after adjuvant doxorubicin therapy in early breast cancer patients: a prospective series. *Clin Drug Investig.* 2009;29:131-137.
26. Cinollo G, Dini G, Franchini E, et al. Positive direct antiglobulin test in a pediatric patient following high-dose cisplatin. *Cancer Chemother Pharmacol.* 1988;21:85-86.
27. Coates TD. Survival from melphalan overdose. *Lancet.* 1984;2:1048.
28. Cohen MR. Medication errors. Cisplatin death. *Nursing.* 1998;28:18.
29. Cohen RJ, Cuneo RA, Cruciger MP, Jackman AE. Transient left homonymous hemianopsia and encephalopathy following treatment of testicular carcinoma with cisplatinum, vinblastine, and bleomycin. *J Clin Oncol.* 1983;1:392-393.
30. Cox PJ. Cyclophosphamide cystitis—identification of acrolein as the causative agent. *Biochem Pharmacol.* 1979;28:2045-2049.
31. Curran CF. Acute doxorubicin overdoses. *Ann Intern Med.* 1991;115:913-914.
32. Daugaard G, Abildgaard U, Holstein-Rathlou NH, et al. Renal tubular function in patients treated with high-dose cisplatin. *Clin Pharmacol Ther.* 1988;44:164-172.
33. de Korte MA, de Vries EG, Lub-de Hooge MN, et al. ^{111}Indium-trastuzumab visualises myocardial human epidermal growth factor receptor 2 expression shortly after anthracycline treatment but not during heart failure: a clue to uncover the mechanisms of trastuzumab-related cardiotoxicity. *Eur J Cancer.* 2007;43:2046-2051.
34. DeFronzo RA, Braine H, Colvin M, Davis PJ. Water intoxication in man after cyclophosphamide therapy. Time course and relation to drug activation. *Ann Intern Med.* 1973;78:861-869.
35. Dickey DT, Muldoon LL, Doolittle ND, et al. Effect of *N*-acetylcysteine route of administration on chemoprotection against cisplatin-induced toxicity in rat models. *Cancer Chemother Pharmacol.* 2008;62:235-241.
36. Diener U, Knoll E, Langer B, et al. Urinary excretion of *N*-acetyl-beta-D-glucosaminidase and alanine aminopeptidase in patients receiving amikacin or cis-platinum. *Clin Chim Acta.* 1981;112:149-157.
37. Dodos F, Halbsguth T, Erdmann E, Hoppe UC. Usefulness of myocardial performance index and biochemical markers for early detection of anthracycline-induced cardiotoxicity in adults. *Clin Res Cardiol.* 2008;97:318-326.
38. Doroshow JH, Locker GY, Myers CE. Enzymatic defenses of the mouse heart against reactive oxygen metabolites: alterations produced by doxorubicin. *J Clin Invest.* 1980;65:128-135.
39. Egorin MJ, Van Echo DA, Tipping SJ, et al. Pharmacokinetics and dosage reduction of cis-diammine(1,1-cyclobutanedicarboxylato)platinum in patients with impaired renal function. *Cancer Res.* 1984;44:5432-5438.
40. Enck RE, Bennett JM. Inadvertent chlorambucil overdose in adult. *N Y State J Med.* 1977;77:1480-1485.
41. Erdlenbruch B, Pekrun A, Schiffmann H, Witt O, Lakomek M. Topical topic: accidental cisplatin overdose in a child: reversal of acute renal failure with sodium thiosulfate. *Med Pediatr Oncol.* 2002;38:349-352.
42. Extra JM, Marty M, Brienza S, Misset JL. Pharmacokinetics and safety profile of oxaliplatin. *Semin Oncol.* 1998;25:13-22.
43. Fantine EO, Garnier-Suillerot A. Interaction of 5-iminodaunorubicin with Fe(III) and with cardiolipin-containing vesicles. *Biochim Biophys Acta.* 1986;856:130-136.
44. Fassoulaki A, Pavlou H. Overdosage intoxication with cisplatin—a cause of acute respiratory failure. *J R Soc Med.* 1989;82:689.
45. Fiedler R, Baumann F, Deschler B, Osten B. Haemoperfusion combined with haemodialysis in ifosfamide intoxication. *Nephrol Dial Transplant.* 2001;16:1088-1089.
46. Firlit CF. Intractable hemorrhagic cystitis secondary to extensive carcinomatosis: management with formalin solution. *J Urol.* 1973;110:57-58.
47. Garbrecht M, Mullerleile U. Verapamil in the prevention of adriamycin-induced cardiomyopathy. *Klin Wochenschr.* 1986;64(Suppl 7):132-134.
48. Garnier-Suillerot A. Metal anthracycline and anthracenedione complexes as a new class of anticancer agents. In: Lown JW, ed. *Anthracycline and Anthracenedione-Based Anticancer Agents.* Amserdam ed. Amsterdam: Elsevier; 1988:129-157.

49. Goren MP, Wright RK, Horowitz ME. Cumulative renal tubular damage associated with cisplatin nephrotoxicity. *Cancer Chemother Pharmacol.* 1986;18:69-73.
50. Greene RF, Collins JM, Jenkins JF, Speyer JL, Myers CE. Plasma pharmacokinetics of adriamycin and adriamycinol: implications for the design of in vitro experiments and treatment protocols. *Cancer Res.* 1983;43:3417-3421.
51. Gregg RW, Molepo JM, Monpetit VJ, et al. Cisplatin neurotoxicity: the relationship between dosage, time, and platinum concentration in neurologic tissues, and morphologic evidence of toxicity. *J Clin Oncol.* 1992;10:795-803.
52. Groth S, Nielsen H, Sorensen JB, et al. Acute and long-term nephrotoxicity of cis-platinum in man. *Cancer Chemother Pharmacol.* 1986;17:191-196.
53. Hachimi-Idrissi S, Schots R, DeWolf D, Van Belle SJ, Otten J. Reversible cardiopathy after accidental overdose of mitoxantrone. *Pediatr Hematol Oncol.* 1993;10:35-40.
54. Herman E, Mhatre R, Lee IP, Vick J, Waravdekar VS. A comparison of the cardiovascular actions of daunomycin, adriamycin and *N*-acetyldaunomycin in hamsters and monkeys. *Pharmacology.* 1971;6:230-241.
55. Hirosawa A, Niitani H, Hayashibara K, Tsuboi E. Effects of sodium thiosulfate in combination therapy of cis-dichlorodiammineplatinum and vindesine. *Cancer Chemother Pharmacol.* 1989;23:255-258.
56. Hitchins RN, Thomson DB. Encephalopathy following cisplatin, bleomycin and vinblastine therapy for non-seminomatous germ cell tumour of testis. *Aust N Z J Med.* 1988;18:67-68.
57. Hofmann G, Bauernhofer T, Krippl P, et al. Plasmapheresis reverses all side-effects of a cisplatin overdose—a case report and treatment recommendation. *BMC Cancer.* 2006;6:1.
58. Holstein P, Jacobsen K, Pedersen JF, Sorensen JS. Intravesical hydrostatic pressure treatment: new method for control of bleeding from the bladder mucosa. *J Urol.* 1973;109:234-236.
59. Hows JM, Mehta A, Ward L, et al. Comparison of mesna with forced diuresis to prevent cyclophosphamide induced haemorrhagic cystitis in marrow transplantation: a prospective randomised study. *Br J Cancer.* 1984;50:753-756.
60. Husken BC, de Jong J, Beekman B, et al. Modulation of the in vitro cardiotoxicity of doxorubicin by flavonoids. *Cancer Chemother Pharmacol.* 1995; 37:55-62.
61. Jensen BV, Nielsen SL, Skovsgaard T. Treatment with angiotensin-converting-enzyme inhibitor for epirubicin-induced dilated cardiomyopathy. *Lancet.* 1996;347:297-299.
62. Jensen BV, Skovsgaard T, Nielsen SL. Functional monitoring of anthracycline cardiotoxicity: a prospective, blinded, long-term observational study of outcome in 120 patients. *Ann Oncol.* 2002;13:699-709.
63. Jimenez-Andrade JM, Herrera MB, Ghilardi JR, et al. Vascularization of the dorsal root ganglia and peripheral nerve of the mouse: implications for chemical-induced peripheral sensory neuropathies. *Mol Pain.* 2008;4:10.
64. Jirillo A, Gioga G, Bonciarelli G, Dalla Valle G. Accidental overdose of melphalan per os in a 69-year-old woman treated for advanced endometrial carcinoma. *Tumori.* 1998;84:611.
65. Jost LM. [Overdose with melphalan (Alkeran): symptoms and treatment. A review]. *Onkologie.* 1990;13:96-101.
66. Juma FD, Rogers HJ, Trounce JR. The pharmacokinetics of cyclophosphamide, phosphoramide mustard and nor-nitrogen mustard studied by gas chromatography in patients receiving cyclophosphamide therapy. *Br J Clin Pharmacol.* 1980;10:327-335.
67. Jung HK, Lee J, Lee SN. A case of massive cisplatin overdose managed by plasmapheresis. *Korean J Intern Med.* 1995;10:150-154.
68. Katz BJ, Ward JH, Digre KB, Creel DJ, Mamalis N. Persistent severe visual and electroretinographic abnormalities after intravenous Cisplatin therapy. *J Neuroophthalmol.* 2003;23:132-135.
69. Kilickap S, Barista I, Akgul E, et al. cTnT can be a useful marker for early detection of anthracycline cardiotoxicity. *Ann Oncol.* 2005;16:798-804.
70. Kim IS, Gratwohl A, Stebler C, et al. Accidental overdose of multiple chemotherapeutic agents. *Korean J Intern Med.* 1989;4:171-173.
71. Korst AE, van der Sterre ML, Eeltink CM, et al. Pharmacokinetics of carboplatin with and without amifostine in patients with solid tumors. *Clin Cancer Res.* 1997;3:697-703.
72. Kupfer A, Aeschlimann C, Wermuth B, Cerny T. Prophylaxis and reversal of ifosfamide encephalopathy with methylene-blue. *Lancet.* 1994;343:763-764.
73. Lagrange JL, Cassuto-Viguier E, Barbe V, et al. Cytotoxic effects of long-term circulating ultrafiltrable platinum species and limited efficacy of haemodialysis in clearing them. *Eur J Cancer.* 1994;30A:2057-2060.
74. Lefrak EA, Pitha J, Rosenheim S, Gottlieb JA. A clinicopathologic analysis of adriamycin cardiotoxicity. *Cancer.* 1973;32:302-314.
75. Legha SS, Benjamin RS, Mackay B, et al. Reduction of doxorubicin cardiotoxicity by prolonged continuous intravenous infusion. *Ann Intern Med.* 1982;96:133-139.
76. Liem RI, Higman MA, Chen AR, Arceci RJ. Misinterpretation of a Calvert-derived formula leading to carboplatin overdose in two children. *J Pediatr Hematol Oncol.* 2003;25:818-821.
77. Lipshultz SE, Colan SD, Gelber RD, et al. Late cardiac effects of doxorubicin therapy for acute lymphoblastic leukemia in childhood. *N Engl J Med.* 1991;324:808-815.
78. Lipshultz SE, Rifai N, Dalton VM, et al. The effect of dexrazoxane on myocardial injury in doxorubicin-treated children with acute lymphoblastic leukemia. *N Engl J Med.* 2004;351:145-153.
79. Markman M, Cleary S, Pfeifle CE, Howell SB. High-dose intracavitary cisplatin with intravenous thiosulfate. Low incidence of serious neurotoxicity. *Cancer.* 1985;56:2364-2368.
80. Marmor MF. Negative-type electroretinogram from cisplatin toxicity. *Doc Ophthalmol.* 1993;84:237-246.
81. Meanwell CA, Blake AE, Kelly KA, Honigsberger L, Blackledge G. Prediction of ifosfamide/mesna associated encephalopathy. *Eur J Cancer Clin Oncol.* 1986;22:815-819.
82. Meijer S, Mulder NH, Sleijfer DT, et al. Influence of combination chemotherapy with cis-diamminedichloroplatinum on renal function: long-term effects. *Oncology.* 1983;40:170-173.
83. Meijer S, Sleijfer DT, Mulder NH, et al. Some effects of combination chemotherapy with cis-platinum on renal function in patients with nonseminomatous testicular carcinoma. *Cancer.* 1983;51:2035-2040.
84. Michelotti A, Venturini M, Tibaldi C, et al. Single agent epirubicin as first line chemotherapy for metastatic breast cancer patients. *Breast Cancer Res Treat.* 2000;59:133-139.
85. Miller AA, Wang XF, Gu L, et al. Phase II randomized study of dose-dense docetaxel and cisplatin every 2 weeks with pegfilgrastim and darbepoetin alfa with and without the chemoprotector BNP7787 in patients with advanced non-small cell lung cancer (CALGB 30303). *J Thorac Oncol.* 2008;3:1159-1165.
86. Mills BA, Roberts RW. Cyclophosphamide-induced cardiomyopathy: a report of two cases and review of the English literature. *Cancer.* 1979;43:2223-2226.
87. Misset JL. Oxaliplatin in practice. *Br J Cancer.* 1998;77(Suppl 4):4-7.
88. Munoz A, Barcelo R, Viteri A, et al. Oxaliplatin overdosage successfully recovered with mild toxicities. *Acta Oncol.* 2006;45:621-622.
89. Myers C. Organ directed toxicities of anticancer drugs: proceedings of the First International Symposium on the Organ Directed Toxicities of Anticancer Drugs, Burlington, Vermont, USA, June 4-6, 1987. In: *Developments in Oncology 53.* Edition Boston, MA: Kluwer Academic Publishers; 1988;17-30.
90. Myers C, Bonow R, Palmeri S, et al. A randomized controlled trial assessing the prevention of doxorubicin cardiomyopathy by *N*-acetylcysteine. *Semin Oncol.* 1983;10:53-55.
91. Offerman JJ, Meijer S, Sleijfer DT, et al. Acute effects of cis-diamminedichloroplatinum (CDDP) on renal function. *Cancer Chemother Pharmacol.* 1984;12:36-38.
92. Ozols RF, Cunnion RE, Klecker RW Jr, et al. Verapamil and adriamycin in the treatment of drug-resistant ovarian cancer patients. *J Clin Oncol.* 1987;5:641-647.
93. Ozols RF, Ostchega Y, Curt G, Young RC. High-dose carboplatin in refractory ovarian cancer patients. *J Clin Oncol.* 1987;5:197-201.
94. Panici PB, Greggi S, Scambia G, et al. High-dose (200 mg/m^2) cisplatin-induced neurotoxicity in primary advanced ovarian cancer patients. *Cancer Treat Rep.* 1987;71:669-670.
95. Pecherstorfer M, Zimmer-Roth I, Weidinger S, et al. High-dose intravenous melphalan in a patient with multiple myeloma and oliguric renal failure. *Clin Investig.* 1994;72:522-525.
96. Pessah IN, Durie EL, Schiedt MJ, Zimanyi I. Anthraquinone-sensitized Ca2+ release channel from rat cardiac sarcoplasmic reticulum: possible receptor-mediated mechanism of doxorubicin cardiomyopathy. *Mol Pharmacol.* 1990;37:503-514.
97. Pike IM, Arbus MH. Cisplatin overdosage. *J Clin Oncol.* 1992;10:1503-1504.
98. Pratt CB, Ransom JL, Evans WE. Age-related adriamycin cardiotoxicity in children. *Cancer Treat Rep.* 1978;62:1381-1385.
99. Pyeritz RE, Droller MJ, Bender WL, Saral R. An approach to the control of massive hemorrhage in cyclophosphamide-induced cystitis by intravenous vasopressin: a case report. *J Urol.* 1978;120:253-254.

100. Roush W. Dana-Farber death sends a warning to research hospitals. *Science*. 1995;269:295-296.
101. Rusconi A, Calendi E. Action of daunomycin on nucleic acid metabolism in HeLa cells. *Biochim Biophys Acta*. 1966;119:413-415.
102. Salloum E, Khan KK, Cooper DL. Chlorambucil-induced seizures. *Cancer*. 1997;79:1009-1013.
103. Schwartz CL, Hobbie WL, Truesdell S, Constine LC, Clark EB. Corrected QT interval prolongation in anthracycline-treated survivors of childhood cancer. *J Clin Oncol*. 1993;11:1906-1910.
104. Schwartz RG, McKenzie WB, Alexander J, et al. Congestive heart failure and left ventricular dysfunction complicating doxorubicin therapy. Seven-year experience using serial radionuclide angiocardiography. *Am J Med*. 1987;82:1109-1118.
105. Screnci D, McKeage MJ, Galettis P, et al. Relationships between hydrophobicity, reactivity, accumulation and peripheral nerve toxicity of a series of platinum drugs. *Br J Cancer*. 2000;82:966-972.
106. Seymour L, Bramwell V, Moran LA. Use of dexrazoxane as a cardioprotectant in patients receiving doxorubicin or epirubicin chemotherapy for the treatment of cancer. The Provincial Systemic Treatment Disease Site Group. *Cancer Prev Control*. 1999;3:145-159.
107. Shah BC, Albert DJ. Intravesical instillation of formalin for the management of intractable hematuria. *J Urol*. 1973;110:519-520.
108. Sheikh-Hamad D, Timmins K, Jalali Z. Cisplatin-induced renal toxicity: possible reversal by *N*-acetylcysteine treatment. *J Am Soc Nephrol*. 1997;8:1640-1644.
109. Shurafa M, Shumaker E, Cronin S. Prostaglandin F2-alpha bladder irrigation for control of intractable cyclophosphamide-induced hemorrhagic cystitis. *J Urol*. 1987;137:1230-1231.
110. Siegert W, Hiddemann W, Koppensteiner R, et al. Accidental overdose of mitoxantrone in three patients. *Med Oncol Tumor Pharmacother*. 1989;6:275-278.
111. Silber JH, Cnaan A, Clark BJ, et al. Enalapril to prevent cardiac function decline in long-term survivors of pediatric cancer exposed to anthracyclines. *J Clin Oncol*. 2004;22:820-828.
112. Slimowitz R. Thoughts on a medical disaster. *Am J Health Syst Pharm*. 1995;52:1464-1465.
113. Speyer JL, Green MD, Kramer E, et al. Protective effect of the bispiperazinedione ICRF-187 against doxorubicin-induced cardiac toxicity in women with advanced breast cancer. *N Engl J Med*. 1988;319:745-752.
114. Steinberg JS, Cohen AJ, Wasserman AG, Cohen P, Ross AM. Acute arrhythmogenicity of doxorubicin administration. *Cancer*. 1987;60:1213-1218.
115. Steinherz LJ, Steinherz PG, Mangiacasale D, et al. Cardiac changes with cyclophosphamide. *Med Pediatr Oncol*. 1981;9:417-422.
116. Stephens LC, Wang YM, Schultheiss TE, Jardine JH. Enhanced cardiotoxicity in rabbits treated with verapamil and adriamycin. *Oncology*. 1987;44:302-306.
117. Tewey KM, Chen GL, Nelson EM, Liu LF. Intercalative antitumor drugs interfere with the breakage-reunion reaction of mammalian DNA topoisomerase II. *J Biol Chem*. 1984;259:9182-9187.
118. Uner A, Ozet A, Arpaci F, Unsal D. Long-term clinical outcome after accidental overdose of multiple chemotherapeutic agents. *Pharmacotherapy*. 2005;25:1011-1016.
119. van Acker FA, van Acker SA, Kramer K, et al. 7-monohydroxyethylrutoside protects against chronic doxorubicin-induced cardiotoxicity when administered only once per week. *Clin Cancer Res*. 2000;6:1337-1341.
120. van Rijswijk RE, Hoekman K, Burger CW, Verheijen RH, Vermorken JB. Experience with intraperitoneal cisplatin and etoposide and i.v. sodium thiosulphate protection in ovarian cancer patients with either pathologically complete response or minimal residual disease. *Ann Oncol*. 1997;8:1235-1241.
121. Vandenberg SA, Kulig K, Spoerke DG, et al. Chlorambucil overdose: accidental ingestion of an antineoplastic drug. *J Emerg Med*. 1988;6:495-498.
122. Vogl SE, Zaravinos T, Kaplan BH. Toxicity of cis-diamminedichloroplatinum II given in a two-hour outpatient regimen of diuresis and hydration. *Cancer*. 1980;45:11-15.
123. von Bernuth G, Adam D, Hofstetter R, et al. Cyclophosphamide cardiotoxicity. *Eur J Pediatr*. 1980;134:87-90.
124. Von Hoff DD, Layard MW, Basa P, et al. Risk factors for doxorubicin-induced congestive heart failure. *Ann Intern Med*. 1979;91:710-717.
125. Von Hoff DD, Rozencweig M, Piccart M. The cardiotoxicity of anticancer agents. *Semin Oncol*. 1982;9:23-33.
126. Whittaker JA, Al-Ismail SA. Effect of digoxin and vitamin E in preventing cardiac damage caused by doxorubicin in acute myeloid leukaemia. *Br Med J (Clin Res Ed)*. 1984;288:283-284.
127. Wilding G, Caruso R, Lawrence TS, et al. Retinal toxicity after high-dose cisplatin therapy. *J Clin Oncol*. 1985;3:1683-1689.
128. Winchester JF, Rahman A, Tilstone WJ, et al. Will hemoperfusion be useful for cancer chemotherapeutic drug removal? *Clin Toxicol*. 1980;17:557-569.
129. Wolfson S, Olney MB. Accidental ingestion of a toxic dose of chlorambucil;report of a case in a child. *J Am Med Assoc*. 1957;165:239-240.
130. Zbinden G, Brandle E. Toxicologic screening of daunorubicin (NSC-82151), adriamycin (NSC-123127), and their derivatives in rats. *Cancer Chemother Rep*. 1975;59:707-715.
131. Zulian GB, Tullen E, Maton B. Methylene blue for ifosfamide-associated encephalopathy. *N Engl J Med*. 1995;332:1239-1240.
132. Zweier JL. Iron-mediated formation of an oxidized adriamycin free radical. *Biochim Biophys Acta*. 1985;839:209-213.

CHAPTER 55
PHARMACEUTICAL ADDITIVES

Sean P. Nordt and Lisa E. Vivero

This chapter summarizes the available literature on commonly used additives associated with direct toxicities. Data on pharmacokinetics and mechanism of toxicity are presented where data are available. Although many additives are associated with hypersensitivity reactions, including anaphylaxis, these are not discussed because of their nonpharmacologic basis. However, excipients should always be considered as possible causative agents in patients developing hypersensitivity reactions (Table 55–1).

HISTORY AND EPIDEMIOLOGY

During the last century there were several US outbreaks of toxicity associated with pharmaceutical additives (Chap. 1). The 1937 Massengill sulfanilamide disaster is the most notorious of these epidemics. Diethylene glycol, an excellent solvent that is a nephrotoxin, was substituted for the additives propylene glycol and glycerin in the liquid formulation of a new sulfanilamide antibiotic because of lower cost.[24,58,65] As a result, more than 100 people died from acute renal failure.[24] More recently, outbreaks of acute renal failure occurred when diethylene glycol was used to solubilize acetaminophen in South Africa, Bangladesh, Nigeria, and Haiti; cough syrup in Panama; and teething powder in Nigera.[19,27,29,67,76,115,126]

In December 1983, E-Ferol, a new parenteral vitamin E formulation, was introduced. It contained 25 Units/mL of α-tocopherol acetate, 9% polysorbate 80, 1% polysorbate 20, and water for injection. At the time, no premarketing testing was required for new formulations of an already approved xenobiotic. Several months after its release, a fatal syndrome in low-birth-weight infants, characterized by thrombocytopenia, renal dysfunction, cholestasis, hepatomegaly, and ascites, was described.[1,102] Thirty-eight deaths and 43 cases of severe symptoms were attributed to E-Ferol. Vitamin E was thought to be the cause and E-Ferol was recalled from the market 4 months after its release. It is now believed that the polysorbate emulsifiers were responsible.[1]

There has been concern over potential mercury toxicity from the preservative thimerosal, a mercury derivative that has been used in parenteral vaccines for 70 years. Although there are a few reports of toxicity from both large oral and injectable thimerosal dosages, no evidence has yet shown toxicity to result from routine vaccination. Potential concerns of toxicity, particularly autism, have spurred ongoing efforts to eliminate thimerosal from vaccines wherever possible.

Although these additive-related occurrences are rare, relative to the frequency of pharmaceutical additive use, they illustrate the potential of pharmaceutical additive toxicity.

Pharmaceuticals are labeled specifically to focus attention on the active ingredient(s) of a product, thus giving the misimpression that additive ingredients are inert and unimportant. Additives, or excipients as they are more properly termed, are necessary to act as vehicles, add color, improve taste, provide consistency, enhance stability and solubility, and impart antimicrobial properties to medicinal formulations. Although it is true that most cases of excipient toxicity involve exposure to large quantities, or to prolonged or improper use, these adverse events are nonetheless related to the toxicologic properties of the excipient.

Prior to selecting the specific additives and quantity necessary for a drug formulation, the drug manufacturer must consider several factors, including the active ingredient's physical form, its solubility and stability, the desired final dosage form and route of administration, and compatibility with the dispensing container materials. The same active ingredient may require different excipients to impart appropriate pharmacokinetic characteristics to different dosage forms, such as in long-acting and immediate-release formulations. Similarly, multiple-dose injection vials containing the same active ingredients as single-dose vials specifically require the addition of a bacteriostatic agent not necessary for single-dose vials.

Unlike requirements for active ingredients, there is no specific US Food and Drug Administration (FDA) approval system for pharmaceutical excipients. As such, the FDA determines the amount and type of data necessary to support the use of a specific excipient on a case-by-case basis. Under current practice, only excipients that were previously permitted for use in foods or pharmaceuticals are defined as *generally recognized as safe* (GRAS), or "GRAS listed." All components of a pharmaceutical product, including excipients, must be produced in accordance with current good manufacturing practice standards to ensure purity. The Safety Committee of the International Pharmaceutical Excipients Council developed guidelines for the toxicologic testing of new excipients.[150] Because of patent protection laws, it was not until very recently that manufacturers were required to provide a list of inactive ingredients contained in all pharmaceutical products. Although it is becoming easier to identify pharmaceutical additives in products, information on their effects and the mechanisms by which they cause adverse responses are often unknown or difficult to obtain.

BENZALKONIUM CHLORIDE

$$\left(C_6H_5-CH_2-\overset{CH_3}{\underset{CH_3}{N^+}}-R \right) Cl^-$$

Benzalkonium chloride (BAC), or alkyldimethyl (phenylmethyl) ammonium chloride, is a quaternary ammonium cationic surfactant composed of a mixture of alkyl benzyl dimethyl ammonium chlorides. Although it is the most widely used ophthalmic preservative in the United States, it is also considered the most cytotoxic (Table 55–2).[82,88] Benzalkonium chloride is also used in otic and nasal formulations, and in some small-volume parenterals. The antimicrobial activity of BAC includes gram-positive and gram-negative bacteria, and some viruses, fungi, and protozoa. Because of its rapid onset of action, good tissue penetration, and long duration of action, BAC is preferred over other preservatives. The concentration of BAC in ophthalmic medications usually ranges from 0.004% to 0.01%.[88] Strong BAC solutions (greater than 0.1%) can be caustic (Chap. 104).

OPHTHALMIC TOXICITY

Corneal epithelial cells harvested from human cadavers within 12 hours of death were exposed to a medium containing 0.01% BAC.[148] The surfactant properties of BAC resulted in intracellular matrix

TABLE 55–1. Potential Systemic Toxicity of Various Pharmaceutical Excipients

Cardiovascular	Ophthalmic
Chlorobutanol	Benzalkonium chloride
Propylene glycol	Chlorobutanol
Fluid and electrolyte	Renal
Polyethylene glycol	Polyethylene glycol
Propylene glycol	Propylene glycol
Sorbitol	
Gastrointestinal	
Sorbitol	
Neurologic	
Benzyl alcohol	
Chlorobutanol	
Polyethylene glycol	
Propylene glycol	
Thimerosal	

dissolution and loss of epithelial superficial layers. Following exposure to the medium, mitotic activity ceased and degenerative changes to corneal epithelium were noted. During a 24-hour observation period, epithelial cell cytokinetic or mitotic activity did not occur. Patients with a compromised corneal epithelium may be at increased risk for the adverse corneal effects of BAC.[148]

TABLE 55–2. Benzalkonium Chloride Concentrations of Common Ophthalmic Medications

Medication	Percent (%)
Artificial tears (various)	0.005-0.01
Acular (ketorolac)	0.01
Betagan (levobunolol)	0.004
Betoptic (betaxolol)	0.01
Ciloxan (ciprofloxacin)	0.006
Cyclogyl (cyclopentolate)	0.01
Decadron (dexamethasone)	0.02
Garamycin (gentamicin)	0.01
Glaucon (epinephrine)	0.01
Isopto Carpine (pilocarpine)	0.01
Murocoll-2 (scopolamine/phenylephrine)	0.01
Mydriacyl (tropicamide)	0.01
Phenylephrine (various)	0.005-0.01
Ocuflox (ofloxacin)	0.005
Ocupress (carteolol)	0.005
Polytrim (polymyxin B sulfate/trimethoprim)	0.004
Timoptic (timolol)	0.01
Tobrex (tobramycin)	0.01
Visine (tetrahydrozoline)	0.01

Two case reports demonstrate the potential toxicity of BAC and the difficulty in recognizing it. A 36-year-old woman complained of decreased vision when she inadvertently switched from Lensrins, a contact lens cleaning solution, to Dacriose, an isotonic boric acid solution preserved with BAC. After 3 days, she had inflammation, pain, and decreased visual acuity. Examination of the cornea revealed many superficial punctate erosions of the epithelium. An in vitro experiment identified significant binding of BAC to soft contact lenses.[53] In the second case, a 56-year-old man diagnosed with keratoconjunctivitis sicca was treated with topical antibiotics and artificial tears containing BAC. Following 1 year of continual use, the patient developed intractable pain, photophobia, and extensive breakdown of the corneal epithelium. Not suspecting the BAC-containing products, the patient continued to use the artificial tears solution for another 9 years despite continued pain and decreasing visual acuity. Replacement with a preservative-free saline solution resulted in resolution of pain, photophobia, and corneal changes.[88]

There was a case series of the inadvertent intraocular use of balanced salt solution (BSS) preserved with BAC instead of preservative-free BSS in 12 patients undergoing phacoemulsification, a surgical technique to remove cataract lenses. The BSS was instilled in the anterior chamber. The operating room had run out of preservative-free BSS and, unbeknownst to the surgeon, it was replaced with the BAC-containing BSS, which contained 0.013% BAC. This is in excess of recommended concentration for intraocular use and is associated with corneal endothelial injury and edema. At 6-months follow-up, only one patient had slight improvement in visual acuity with the other 11 limited to only being able to count fingers from a distance of 2 feet.[89]

NASOPHARYNGEAL AND OROPHARYNGEAL TOXICITY

Human adenoidal tissue was exposed to oxymetazoline nasal spray preserved with BAC at concentrations ranging from 0.005 to 0.15 mg/mL for 1 to 30 minutes.[14] Irregular and broken epithelial cells occurred with all concentrations; however, it developed earlier and more frequently with the higher concentrations. The number of beating ciliary bodies also decreased as the duration and the concentrations increased. Benzalkonium chloride may decrease the viscosity of the normal protective mucous lining of the naso- and oropharynx, resulting in cytotoxicity.

Administration of one of three nasal steroid sprays preserved with either 0.031% or 0.022% BAC in the right nostril of rats twice daily for 21 days caused squamous cell metaplasia and a decrease in the number of goblet cells, cilia, and mucus.[15] No histologic changes occurred in rats receiving the preservative-free steroid or in tissue exposed to 0.9% sodium chloride solution administered into the left nostril as the control. Similarly, in another study, epithelial desquamation, inflammation, and edema occurred when 0.05% and 0.10% BAC was applied hourly to the nasal cavities of rats for 8 hours.[85] No lesions developed in the nasal cavities of rats receiving 0.01% BAC.

In an in vitro study, cultured human nasal epithelial cells were exposed to varying concentrations of BAC compared with another preservative, potassium sorbate (PS), with phosphate-buffered saline (PBS) as a control. Cell viability was greatly reduced at the higher concentrations of BAC compared with no decrease in cell viability in the PS or PBS groups. Additionally, at concentrations used clinically loss of microvilli, destruction of cell membranes, and poor cytoskeletal alignment demonstrated by electron microscope occurred.[74]

An in vitro study of human nasal mucosa exposed mucosa to either fluticasone or mometasone preserved with either BAC or PS at various concentrations measuring ciliary beat frequency. While PS did not affect ciliary beat frequency at any concentration, BAC adversely affected ciliary beat frequency. At lower concentrations, BAC slowed ciliary beat frequency and brought it to standstill at higher concentrations.[75]

BENZYL ALCOHOL

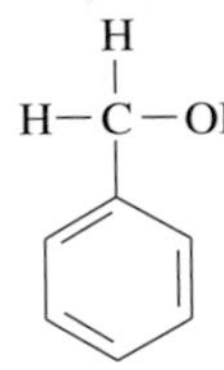

Benzyl alcohol (benzene methanol) is a colorless, oily liquid with a faint aromatic odor that is most commonly added to pharmaceuticals as a bacteriostatic agent (Table 55-3). In 1982, a "gasping" syndrome, which included hypotension, bradycardia, gasping respirations, hypotonia, progressive metabolic acidosis, seizures, cardiovascular collapse, and death, was first described in low-birth-weight neonates in intensive care units.[20,60,94] All the infants had received either bacteriostatic water or sodium chloride solution containing 0.9% benzyl alcohol to flush intravenous catheters or in parenteral medications reconstituted with bacteriostatic water or saline.[20,60] The syndrome occurred in infants who had received greater than 99 mg/kg of benzyl alcohol (range, 99 to 234 mg/kg).[60] The World Health Organization (WHO) currently estimates the acceptable daily intake of benzyl alcohol to be not more than 5 mg/kg body weight.[22]

PHARMACOKINETICS

In adults, benzyl alcohol is oxidized to benzoic acid, conjugated in the liver with glycine, and excreted in the urine as hippuric acid. The immature metabolic capacities of infants diminish their ability to metabolize and excrete benzyl alcohol.[60] Preterm babies have a greater ability to metabolize benzyl alcohol to benzoic acid than do term babies, but are unable to convert benzoic acid to hippuric acid, possibly because of glycine deficiency. This results in the accumulation of benzoic acid (Fig. 55-1).[60] A fatal case of metabolic acidosis was reported in a 5-year-old girl who had received 2.4 mg/kg/h diazepam preserved with benzyl alcohol for 36 hours to control status epilepticus. Elevated benzoic acid concentrations were identified in serum and urine samples. The estimated daily dosage of benzyl alcohol was 180 mg/kg.[60,90]

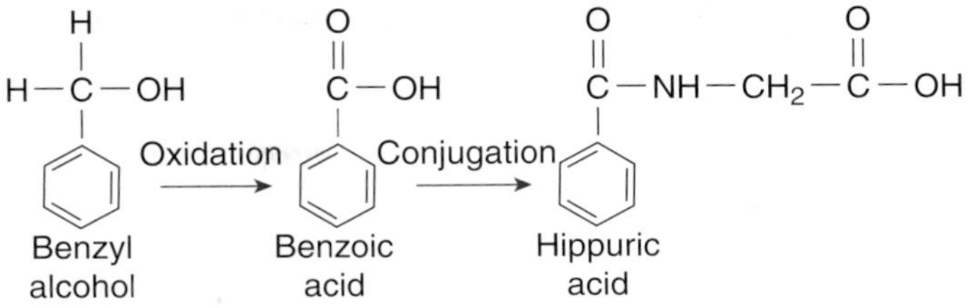

FIGURE 55–1. The oxidative metabolism of benzyl alcohol.

TABLE 55–3. Benzyl Alcohol Concentration of Common Medications

Medication	Percent (%)	mL/Average Dose[a]
Ativan (lorazepam)	2.0	0.02
Bacteriostatic water for injection	1.5	–
Bacteriostatic saline for injection	1.5	–
Bactrim, Septra (trimethoprim-sulfamethoxazole)	1.0	0.61[b]
Bumex (bumetanide)	1.0	0.03
Compazine (prochlorperazine)	0.75	0.01
Cordarone (amiodarone)	2.0	0.42[b]
Lasix (furosemide)	0.9	0.04
Librium (chlordiazepoxide)	1.5	0.03
Methotrexate	0.9	0.01
Norcuron (vecuronium)	0.9	0.01
Tracrium (atracurium)	0.9	0.03
Valium (diazepam)	1.5	0.03
Vasotec (enalapril)	0.9	0.01
VePesid (etoposide)	3.0	0.14
Versed (midazolam)	1.0	0.01
Vistaril (hydroxyzine)	0.9	0.01

[a]Based on dosage for a 70-kg person.

[b]Based on 24-hour dosage.

NEUROLOGIC TOXICITY

Benzyl alcohol is believed to have a role in the increased frequency of cerebral intraventricular hemorrhages and mortality reported in very-low-birth-weight (VLBW) infants (weight less than 1000 g) who received flush solutions preserved with benzyl alcohol.[73] An increased incidence of developmental delay and cerebral palsy was also noted in the same VLBW patients, suggesting a secondary damaging effect of benzyl alcohol.[12]

There are several case reports of transient paraplegia following the intrathecal or epidural administration of antineoplastics or analgesics containing benzyl alcohol as a preservative.[8,37,66,132] The local anesthetic effects are most likely responsible for the immediate paraparesis and limited duration of effects, rather than actual demyelination of nerve roots. In a study in rats, lumbosacral dorsal root action potential amplitudes were measured after exposure to 0.9% or 1.5% benzyl alcohol solutions in either 0.9% sodium chloride solution or distilled water.[66] Rats exposed to all benzyl alcohol solutions for less than 1 minute had inhibited dorsal root action potentials. This was attributed to the local anesthetic effects of benzyl alcohol. Nerve function was 50% to 90% restored after rinsing the nerves with 0.9% sodium chloride solution. Chronic intrathecal exposure to benzyl alcohol 0.9% over 7 days resulted in scattered areas of demyelinization and early remyelinization. The 1.5% benzyl alcohol solution–exposed dorsal nerve roots showed greater changes with widespread areas of demyelinization and fatty degeneration of nerve fibers.

CHLOROBUTANOL

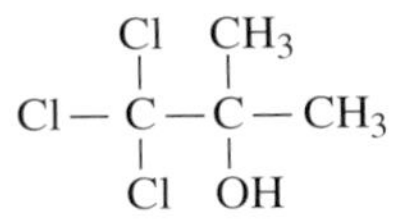

Chlorobutanol, or chlorbutol (1,1,1-trichloro-2-methyl-2-propanol) is available as volatile, white crystals with an odor of camphor. Chlorobutanol has antibacterial and antifungal properties and is widely used as a preservative in injectable, ophthalmic, otic, and cosmetic preparations at concentrations up to 0.5% (Table 55-4). Chlorobutanol also has mild sedative and local anesthetic properties and was formerly used therapeutically as a sedative-hypnotic.[18] Because chlorobutanol is a halogenated hydrocarbon, theoretically it can sensitize the myocardium

TABLE 55–4. Chlorobutanol Concentrations of Common Medications

Medication	Percent (%)	mg/Dose
Adrenaline chloride (epinephrine) injection	0.5	5
Aquasol A (vitamin A)	0.5	5
Chloroptic (chloramphenicol) ophthalmic solution	0.5	–
Dolophine (methadone) injection	0.5	10
Epinephrine ophthalmic solution	0.5	–
Novocaine (procaine) injection	0.25	87
Phospholine iodide (echothiophate iodide) ophthalmic solution	0.55	–
Pyridoxine HCl	0.5	5
Rhinall (phenylephrine) nasal spray	0.14	–
Tobrex (tobramycin) ophthalmic ointment	0.5	–
Vasopressin 20 Units/mL injectable	0.5	5

to catecholamines, although no cases of ventricular dysrhythmias are described in the literature to date. The lethal human chlorobutanol dose is estimated to be 50 to 500 mg/kg.[110]

CENTRAL NERVOUS SYSTEM TOXICITY

Chlorobutanol has a chemical structure similar to trichloroethanol (Fig. 74–1), the active metabolite of chloral hydrate, and is believed to exhibit similar pharmacologic properties. Central nervous system depression was reported in a 40-year-old alcoholic man who chronically abused Seducaps, formerly available in Australia and several other countries, a nonprescription hypnotic containing chlorobutanol as the active ingredient.[18] On admission to the emergency department (ED) he had drowsiness, dysarthria, slurred speech, and occasional episodes of myoclonic movements. His peak serum chlorobutanol concentration was 100 μg/mL, decreasing to 48 μg/mL over 2 weeks, with a half-life of 13 days. His speech abnormality resolved over 4 weeks. Only chlorobutanol was detected in the patient's urine or serum. In a second case, a possible central nervous system depressant effect from chlorobutanol was suggested in a 19-year-old woman treated with high doses of intravenous morphine preserved with chlorobutanol.[42] She received approximately 90 mg/h of chlorobutanol for several days. Her peak serum chlorobutanol concentration was 83 μg/mL, a concentration similar to that in the previous case report[18]; however, the coadministration of morphine precludes the effects being attributed to chlorobutanol alone.

Ketamine is neurotoxic when administered intrathecally to animals.[99,100] The potential neurotoxic effects of chlorobutanol as a preservative in ketamine compared with preservative-free ketamine was studied in rabbits.[100] Forty rabbits were given 0.3 mL intrathecally of 1% preservative-free ketamine, 1% ketamine, 0.05% chlorobutanol, or 1% lidocaine as control. The rabbits were observed and hemodynamically monitored for 8 days then euthanized. Histological evaluation of the spinal cord as well as for blood–brain barrier (BBB) lesions was performed. Seven of 10 rabbits given intrathecal chlorobutanol showed both white and grey matter histologic changes as well as diffuse BBB injury. No histologic changes were seen in either ketamine groups or the lidocaine group, and only one rabbit in each ketamine group had BBB injury. These results suggest chlorobutanol should not be administered intrathecally.[100]

A case series of five patients were given intraarterial papaverine preserved with 0.5% chlorobutanol, which is used to prevent cerebral vasospasm in patients with subarachnoid hemorrhage. Immediately after administration of papaverine in either left, right, or bilateral anterior cerebral arteries, patients had an acute decrease in neurologic status. Subsequent brain magnetic resonance images (MRIs) identified selective grey matter toxicity in the territories treated with papaverine. Postmortem brain histology analysis in one patient identified grey matter changes as well. These authors state the absence of white matter changes is not consistent with ischemic infarction but suggest direct toxic effect of either the papaverine or chlorobutanol. The manufacturer of the papaverine stated that no other reports had been made and the papaverine used came from two different lots; therefore, it is unclear if an unidentified independent variable caused these effects, but authors caution using intraarterial papaverine in patients with subarachnoid hemorrhage.[137]

OPHTHALMIC TOXICITY

Chlorobutanol is a commonly used preservative in ophthalmic preparations and is less toxic to the eye than benzalkonium chloride.[114] Chlorobutanol increases the permeability of cells by impairing cell membrane structure.[148] An in vitro experiment using corneal epithelial cells harvested from human cadavers demonstrated arrested mitotic activity following chlorobutanol exposure.[148]

LIPIDS

In general, there are three types of commercial intravenous lipid drug-delivery systems available: lipid emulsion, liposomal, and lipid complex (Table 55-5). Lipid emulsions are immiscible lipid droplets dispersed in an aqueous phase stabilized by an emulsifier (eg, egg or soy lecithin). Liposomes differ from emulsion lipid droplets in that they are vesicles comprised of one or more concentric phospholipid bilayers surrounding an aqueous core. Lipophilic drugs can be formulated for intravenous administration by partitioning them into the lipid phase of either an emulsion or liposome. Liposomes are capable of encapsulating hydrophilic therapeutic agents within their aqueous core to exploit lipid pharmacokinetic properties.[144] Attaching a therapeutic drug to a lipid to form a lipid complex is another way to take advantage of lipid pharmacokinetics.

TABLE 55–5. Lipid Carrier Formulations of Common Medications

Medication	Lipid Carrier
Propofol (Diprivan)	Emulsion
Cytarabine (DepoCyt)	Liposome
Daunorubicin (DaunoXome)	Liposome
Doxorubicin (Doxil)	Liposome (stealth)
Amphotericin B (AmBisome)	Liposome
Amphotericin B (Abelcet)	Lipid complex
Amphotericin B (Amphotec)	Cholesteryl complex

Lipid carriers are biocompatible because of their similarity to endogenous cell membranes. They can be used to stabilize labile drugs against hydrolysis or oxidation, to decrease toxicity, and to enhance therapeutic efficacy by altering drug pharmacokinetic and pharmacodynamic parameters. The biodistribution, and the rate of release and metabolism of a drug incorporated in a lipid formulation can be regulated by the type and concentration of oil and emulsifier used, pH, drug concentration dispersed in the medium, the size of the lipid particle, and the manufacturing process.[116,144] Intravenous formulations are usually isotonic and have a pH of 7 to 8.[144]

The rate of clearance of a lipid carrier from the blood depends on its physiochemical properties and the molecular weight of the emulsifier. Electrically charged lipid carriers are removed faster than neutral particles.[23,116] Smaller lipid particle size and high-molecular-weight emulsifiers decrease clearance. Stealth liposome formulations incorporate a polyethylene glycol coating that prevents rapid detection and clearance of liposomes by the reticuloendothelial system prolonging circulation time.[116] Active drug targeting can be achieved by conjugating antibodies or vectors to side chains on the emulsifier.[23,116] For a therapeutic drug available in more than one lipid-carrier formulation (eg, amphotericin B) it is important to note that any change in the lipid formulation can alter the drug's pharmacokinetic, pharmacodynamic, and safety parameters; consequently, they are not equivalent dosage formulations (see Chap. 56).

The physiochemical properties of lipid emulsions not only affect the therapeutic drugs carried by them, but the lipids themselves may also have direct pharmacologic effects on the central nervous[159] and immune systems.[87] Lipid fatty acid mediators can affect the membrane receptor channels of *N*-methyl-D-aspartate (NMDA) receptors, potentiating synaptic transmission. This is supported by one animal[103] and several in vitro[104,119,147] studies. Dogs given a medium-chain triglyceride emulsion intravenous infusion developed dose-related central nervous system metabolic and neurologic effects, accompanied by electroencephalographic changes consistent with encephalopathy observed when serum octanoate concentration reached 0.5 to 0.9 mM.[103] In an in vitro model, three of nine lipid emulsions tested (Abbolipid, 20% soya and safflower oil; Intralipid, 20% soya oil; and Structolipid, 20% structured triglycerides) demonstrated a dose-related activation of cortical neuronal NMDA receptor channels.[159] The lipid source for all but one (Omegaven, 10% fish oil) of the emulsions tested was made up solely or partially by soya oil. The authors could not explain why the other six lipid emulsions did not induce membrane currents. Adequate control for the nonlipid constituent contribution of these emulsions is lacking. In another in vitro study, the same authors found that NMDA-induced neuronal currents are reduced by an unknown factor in the aqueous portion of Abbolipid.[160] This suggests that lipid emulsions may pharmacologically enhance the anesthetic effect of hypnotics such as propofol. The clinical relevance of these studies remains to be assessed.

Triglycerides in parenteral nutrition emulsions are implicated in altering the immune system, leading to an increased susceptibility to infection,[52,157] and altering lung function and hemodynamics in patients with acute respiratory distress syndrome (ARDS).[87] Phospholipid activation of phospholipase A_2 may be an initiating cause.[52,87,157] However, it is not clear if these immunologic effects are a consequence of factors other than the lipid in the emulsion.

More recently, lipid emulsions have been employed in the treatment of poisonings in both animal models and human case reports (see Antidotes in Depth A 21:Intravenous Fat Emulsion).[10,118,136] Although no toxicity has been reported in these cases, all of the patients were seriously ill and any adverse effects may have been attributed to their primary exposures.

PARABENS

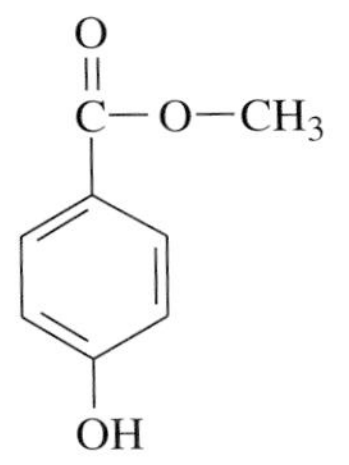

$$\text{HO}-\text{C}_6\text{H}_4-\text{C}(=\text{O})-\text{O}-\text{CH}_3$$

Methylparaben

The parabens, or parahydroxybenzoic acids, are a group of compounds widely employed as preservatives in cosmetics, food, and pharmaceuticals because of their bacteriostatic, fungistatic, and antioxidant properties (Table 55-6).[133] A survey conducted by the FDA identified the parabens as the second most common ingredients in cosmetic formulations, with water being the most common.[91] Parabens are often used in combination, because the presence of two or more parabens are synergistic.[91] Methylparabens and propylparabens are most commonly used.[133] Pharmaceutical parabens concentrations usually range from 0.1% to 0.3%.[127]

Widespread usage of parabens since the 1920s has shown that they have a relatively low order of toxicity.[91] However, because of their allergenic potential they are currently considered less suitable for injectable and ophthalmic preparations.[127] Based on long-term animal studies, the WHO has set the total acceptable daily intake of ethyl-, methyl-, and propylparabens to be 10 mg/kg body weight.[127]

In addition to allergic reactions, parabens have the potential to cause other adverse effects. Bilirubin displacement from albumin binding sites occurred with administration of methyl- and propylparabens preserved gentamicin when serum parabens concentrations were 3 to 15 μg/mL.[39]

TABLE 55–6. Paraben Concentrations of Common Medications

Medication	Percent (%)	mg/Dose
Aldomet (methyldopa) injection	0.17	8
Brofed (pseudoephedrine/brompheniramine) elixir	0.2	20
Bupivicaine HCl 0.25% injection[a]	0.1	–
Haldol (haloperidol) injection	0.2	2
Inapsine (droperidol) injection	0.2	2
Isopto Cetamide (sulfacetamide) ophthalmic solution	0.06	–
Narcan (naloxone) injection	0.2	2
Oncovin (vincristine) injection	0.15	4
Prolixin HCl (fluphenazine) injection	0.11	1
Prostigmin (neostigmine) injection	0.2	2
Romazicon (flumazenil) injection	0.2	4
Talwin (pentazocine) injection	0.1	1
Trandate (labetalol) injection	0.09	4
Xylocaine (lidocaine) injection	0.1	–
Zofran (ondansetron) injection	0.14	3

[a]Amount varies depending on volume used (contains 1mg/mL paraben)

Gentamicin alone has no effect on bilirubin displacement.[92] Spermicidal activity was demonstrated in an in vitro study of human semen specimens exposed to local parabens concentrations of 1 to 8 mg/mL.[141] Possible interference with conception and potential adverse effects on fertility were not investigated.

More recently concern has arisen regarding the potential estrogenic and antiandrogenic effects of the parabens and their common metabolite, *p*-hydroxybenzoic acid. Substances with these effects are commonly referred to as *endocrine disrupting substances.* However, the clinical significance of these effects has not been elucidated.[31,40,124,125,153]

PHENOL

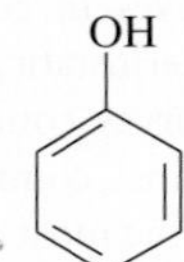

Phenol (carbolic acid, hydroxybenzene, phenylic acid, phenylic alcohol) is a commonly used preservative in injectable medications (Table 55-7). Phenol is a colorless to light pink, caustic liquid with a characteristic odor. When exposed to air and light, phenol turns a red or brown color.[36] Phenol exerts antimicrobial activity against a wide variety of microorganisms, such as gram-negative and gram-positive bacteria, mycobacteria, and some fungi and viruses.[36] Phenol is well absorbed from the gastrointestinal tract, skin, and mucous membranes, and is excreted in the urine as phenyl glucuronide and phenyl sulfate metabolites.[36] Although there are numerous reports of phenol toxicity following intentional ingestions or unintentional dermal exposures (Chap. 104), adverse reactions to its use as a pharmaceutical excipient are uncommon, most likely because of the small quantities used.[36]

CUTANEOUS ABSORPTION

Systemic toxicity from cutaneous absorption of phenol is reported. Ventricular tachycardia was observed in an 11-year-old boy following application of a chemical peel solution containing 88% phenol in water and liquid soap. The solution was applied to 15% of his body surface area for the treatment of xeroderma pigmentosum. Immediately following the onset of the ventricular tachycardia, the phenol-treated areas were irrigated, an infusion of 0.9% sodium chloride solution was begun, and two intravenous lidocaine boluses were given followed by a lidocaine infusion. The dysrhythmia persisted for 3 hours. The urinary phenol concentration the following day was 58.9 mg/dL.[151] In a similar case, multifocal premature ventricular contractions (PVCs) were observed in a 10-year-old boy after application of a chemical peeling solution of 40% phenol, 0.8% croton oil in hexachlorophene soap, and water for the treatment of a giant hairy nevus.[158] The PVCs were refractory to intravenous lidocaine but resolved with intravenous bretylium. No phenol concentrations were obtained to confirm systemic absorption.

Drowsiness, respiratory depression, and blue-colored urine were noted in a 6-month-old infant 12 hours after topical application of magenta paint over most of the body for seborrheic eczema.[129] Magenta paint (also known as Castellani paint) was widely used for seborrheic eczema and contained 4% phenol, magenta, boric acid, resorcinol, acetone, and methylated spirit. Further investigation found that phenol was detected in urine samples of four of 16 other infants with seborrheic eczema who had approximately 11% to 15% of their body surface area painted with magenta paint for 2 days.

TABLE 55–7. Phenol Concentration of Common Medications

Medication	Percent (%)	mg/Dose
Antivenom (Crotaline)	0.25	25 (per vial)
Antivenom (*Micrurus fulvius*)	0.25	25 (per vial)
Dryvax (smallpox) vaccine	0.25	2.5
Pneumovax 23 (pneumococcal) vaccine	0.25	1.25
Prostigmin (neostigmine) injection	0.45	4.5
Quinidine gluconate injection	0.25	18.75

POLYETHYLENE GLYCOL

Polyethylene glycols (PEGs, Carbowax, Macrogol) include several compounds with varying molecular weights (MWs) (200 to 40,000 D).[123] They are typically available as mixtures designated by a number denoting their average molecular weight. Polyethylene glycols are stable, hydrophilic substances, making them useful excipients for cosmetics, and pharmaceuticals of all routes of administration (Table 55-8). Pegylation, a process that modifies the pharmacokinetics of therapeutic liposomes and proteins (eg, peginterferon-α), is the most recent application of PEG. At room temperature, PEGs with molecular weights less than 600 are clear, viscous liquids with a slight characteristic odor and bitter taste. PEGs with molecular weights greater than 1000 are soluble solids and range in consistency from pastes and waxy flakes to powders.[123] Commercially available products used for bowel cleansing preparations and whole bowel irrigation are solutions of PEG 3350 that are sometimes combined with electrolytes and known as polyethylene glycol electrolyte lavage solutions (PEG-ELS) (see Antidotes in Depth A3: Whole Bowel Irrigation and Other Intestinal Evacuants).

The solid, high-molecular-weight PEGs are essentially nontoxic. Conversely, low-molecular-weight PEG exposures have caused adverse effects similar to the chemically related toxic alcohols ethylene and diethylene glycol[27] (see Special Considerations SC5: Diethylene Glycol).

TABLE 55–8. Common Medications Containing Polyethylene Glycol (PEG)

Medication	PEG Molecular Weight (Daltons)
Chloroptic (chloramphenicol) ointment	300
Furacin (nitrofurazone) ointment	300
VePesid (etoposide) injection	300
Ativan (lorazepam) injection	400
Decadron (dexamethasone) ophthalmic ointment	400
Depo-Provera (medroxyprogesterone)	3350
Polyethylene glycol electrolyte solution	3350
Peginterferon alfa-2a (PEGASYS)	40,000

PHARMACOKINETICS

High-molecular-weight PEGs (greater than 1000) are not significantly absorbed from the gastrointestinal tract, but low-molecular-weight PEGs may be absorbed when taken orally.[44,138,139] Topical absorption can occur when PEGs are applied to damaged skin.[21,145] The pharmacokinetics of intravenously administered PEG 3350 has not been studied; however, it did not appear to have any systemic effects when unintentionally given by this route.[128] Once in the systemic circulation, PEGs are mainly excreted unchanged in the urine[44]; however, low-molecular-weight PEGs are metabolized by alcohol dehydrogenase to hydroxyacid and diacid metabolites. PEG may also be partially broken down to ethylene glycol, although the clinical consequence of this is unknown.[21,146]

NEPHROTOXICITY

In rats fed various PEGs (200, 300, and 400) in their drinking water for 90 days, a solution of 8% PEG 200 produced renal tubular necrosis in all of the animals, followed by death within 15 days; however, a 4% PEG 200 solution resulted in only two of nine rats dying within 80 days. A 16% PEG 400 solution killed all animals within 13 days; however, both 8% and 4% PEG 400 solutions had no observable effect except for a decrease in kidney weight when compared to control animals.[140]

Acute tubular necrosis with oliguria, azotemia, and high anion gap metabolic acidosis has been reported after oral and topical exposures to low-molecular-weight PEGs (200 and 300). Acute renal failure occurred in a 65-year-old man with a history of alcohol abuse and seizure disorder after ingestion of the contents of a lava lamp containing 13% PEG 200.[45] Forty-eight hours after admission (approximately 50 to 72 hours postingestion), the patient became oliguric with an anion gap metabolic acidosis and acute renal failure. Blood sample analysis confirmed traces of the lava lamp fluid; no traces were detected in the urine. After clinical complications from ethanol withdrawal and aspiration pneumonitis, the patient was discharged 3 months later with residual kidney dysfunction attributed to the PEG component of the lamp contents. Acute tubular necrosis was noted on autopsy of six burn patients treated with a topical antibiotic cream in a PEG 300 base.[21,145] Mass spectrometry detected hydroxyacid and diacid metabolites in serum and urine samples. Oxalate crystals were seen in two cases. These effects were reproduced with the topical application of PEG for 7 days to rabbits with full-thickness skin defects.[145]

NEUROTOXICITY

There are reports of neurologic complications, such as paraplegia and transient bladder paralysis, following intrathecal steroidal injections containing 3% PEG as a vehicle.[13,17] In an in vitro experiment, rabbit vagus nerves were exposed to concentrations of PEG 3350 ranging from 3% to 40% for 1 hour.[13] Three percent and 10% PEG had no effect on nerve action potential amplitude or conduction velocity. Twenty percent and 30% PEG significantly slowed nerve conduction and had varying effects on the amplitudes of action potentials. Forty percent PEG completely abolished action potentials. These changes were reversible and thought to be related to PEG-induced osmotic effects.

FLUID, ELECTROLYTE, AND ACID–BASE DISTURBANCES

Hyperosmolality was reported in three patients with burn surface areas ranging from 20% to 56% following repeated applications of Furacin, a topical antibiotic dressing containing 63% PEG 300, 32% PEG 4000, and 5% PEG 1000.[21] Polyethylene glycol produces an osmotic effect that is greater than expected for its molecular weight.[134] It is theorized that PEG increases osmolality by sequestering water through hydrogen binding, reducing the availability of water to interact with solutes, thus increasing the chemical and osmotic activity of the solute. Hyperosmolality following the administration of a PEG-containing substance may suggest systemic PEG absorption.

Two cases of metabolic acidosis were reported following administration of therapeutic dosages of an intravenous nitrofurantoin solution containing PEG 300.[146] Similarly, an otherwise unexplained increased anion gap was reported in three patients being treated with a topical PEG-based burn cream.[21] Metabolism of PEG by alcohol dehydrogenase to hydroxyacid and diacid metabolites can explain the metabolic acidosis.[70]

PROPYLENE GLYCOL

$$\begin{array}{ccc} \text{OH} & \text{OH} & \\ | & | & \\ \text{CH}_2- & \text{CH}- & \text{CH}_3 \end{array}$$

Propylene glycol (PG), or 1,2-propanediol, is a clear, colorless, odorless, sweet, viscous liquid employed in numerous pharmaceuticals (Table 55-9), foods, and cosmetics. Propylene glycol is used as a solvent and preservative with antiseptic properties similar to ethanol. The WHO has set the daily allowable intake of PG at a maximum of 25 mg/kg,[161] or 17.5 g/d for a 70-kg person.

PHARMACOKINETICS

Propylene glycol is rapidly absorbed from the gastrointestinal (GI) tract following oral administration and has a volume of distribution of approximately 0.6 L/kg.[101,142] When applied to intact epidermis, the absorption of PG is minimal. Percutaneous absorption may occur following application to damaged skin (eg, extensive burn surface areas). Approximately 12% to 45% of PG is excreted unchanged in

TABLE 55–9. Propylene Glycol Concentration of Common Medications

Medication	Percent (%)	Grams (g)/ Average Dose[a]
Agenerase (amprenavir) oral solution	55	57.75
Amidate (etomidate)	35	3.6
Ativan (lorazepam) injection	80	0.64
Bactrim, Septra (trimethoprim-sulfamethoxazole) injection	40	10.0[b]
Brevibloc (esmolol) injection	25	2.5
Dilantin (phenytoin) injection	40	4.8
Lanoxin (digoxin) injection	40	0.4
Librium (chlordiazepoxide) injection	20	0.08
Luminal (phenobarbital sodium) injection	67.8	0.7
MVI-12 (multivitamins) injection	30	0.45
Nembutal (pentobarbital)	40	1.2
Tridil (nitroglycerin) injection	30	0.3
Valium (diazepam) injection	40	0.4

[a]Based on dosage for 70-kg person.

[b]Based on 24-hour dosage.

the urine[43]; the remainder is hepatically metabolized sequentially by alcohol dehydrogenase to lactaldehyde, which is metabolized further by aldehyde dehydrogenase to lactic acid. Lactic acid is also formed by another metabolite, methylglyoxal.[113] Lactic acid may be additionally oxidized to pyruvic acid and then to carbon dioxide and water.[113] The terminal half-life of propylene glycol is reported to be between 1.4 and 5.6 hours in adults, and as long as 16.9 hours in neonates.[43,144]

CARDIOVASCULAR TOXICITY

Intravenous preparations of phenytoin contain 40% PG to facilitate the solubility of phenytoin. Nine years after intravenous phenytoin became available, several deaths were attributed to the rapid administration of phenytoin used for the treatment of cardiac dysrhythmias.[59,149,171]

Cardiovascular effects reported in these cases included hypotension, bradycardia, widening of the QRS interval, increased amplitude of T waves with occasional inversions, and transient ST elevations. Studies in cats[93] and calves[63] confirmed PG as the cardiotoxin. Bradycardia and depression of atrial conduction were not observed in cats pretreated with atropine, or in those with vagotomy following rapid intravenous infusion of PG, suggesting that these effects are vagally mediated.[93] Amplification of the QRS complex was noted in these same pretreated cats, also suggesting a direct cardiotoxic effect of PG. Similar results were reported in calves pretreated with atropine that received oxytetracycline in a PG vehicle.[63]

NEUROTOXICITY

Smaller infants appear to have a decreased ability to clear PG when compared with older children and adults.[94] An increased frequency of seizures was reported in low-birth-weight infants who received PG 3 g daily in a parenteral multivitamin preparation.[94] Seizures developed in an 11-year-old boy receiving long-term oral therapy with vitamin D dissolved in PG.[6] Serum calcium, magnesium, electrolytes, and blood glucose were normal. Seizures abated after the product was discontinued. Propylene glycol possesses inebriating properties similar to ethanol. Central nervous system depression was reported following an intentional oral ingestion of a PG-containing product.[101]

A black-box warning was added to the product information for amprenavir (Agenerase), an oral protease inhibitor solution, because of concerns over its high PG (550 mg/mL) vehicle content.[131] The recommended daily dosage of amprenavir supplies 1650 mg/kg/d of PG. A 61-year-old man experienced visual hallucinations, disorientation, tinnitus, and vertigo after receiving a 750-mg dose (474 mg/kg PG) of amprenavir solution.[80]

OTOTOXICITY

Otic preparations can contain up to 94% PG in solutions and 10% in suspensions as part of their vehicles.[48] In animal studies, application of high concentrations of PG (greater than 10%) to the middle ear can produce hearing impairment[106,107,155] and morphologic changes, including tympanic membrane perforation, middle ear adhesions, and cholesteatoma.[106,154,166] Although the effects of PG in the human middle ear have not been studied, all medications applied to the external ear canal are contraindicated in patients with perforated tympanic membranes.

FLUID, ELECTROLYTE, AND ACID–BASE DISTURBANCES

Patients receiving continuous or large intermittent quantities of medications containing PG can develop high PG concentrations, particularly those with renal or hepatic insufficiency.[26,43] Propylene glycol electrolyte and metabolic disturbances are evidenced by hyperosmolarity, and an elevated osmolar gap attributed to the osmotically active properties of PG. In most cases, an elevated anion gap, with an otherwise unexplained elevated lactate concentration, is also present. Metabolic acidosis and hyperlactatemia produced from PG metabolism.[25] These adverse effects have been reported with intravenous preparations such as lorazepam,[5,168] diazepam,[162] etomidate,[152] nitroglycerin,[43] pediatric multivitamins,[61] and topical silver sulfadiazine.[11,49,84]

Systemic absorption of PG from topical application of silver sulfadiazine cream[49] resulted in hyperosmolality in patients with burn surface areas greater than 35% of their body.[11,49,84] In one study, nine of 15 burn patients had osmolar gaps (greater than 12) after application of the cream.[84]

Hyperosmolarity occurred in five infants receiving a parenteral multivitamin that provided a daily PG dose of 3 g.[61] After 12 days, one premature infant had a PG concentration of 930 mg/dL and an osmolar gap of 136. Anion gap and lactic acid concentrations were normal. In a study of 11 intubated pediatric patients, aged 1 to 15 months, who were receiving continuous lorazepam infusions over 3 to 14 days, accumulated serum PG concentrations of 17 to 226 mg/dL did not result in significant increases in osmolar gap or serum lactate concentrations from baseline.[32] This was attributed to normal renal function and the low cumulative PG doses received (mean 60 g).

Several small studies have found a strong correlation between elevated PG concentrations and increased osmolar gap measurements in critically ill patients receiving intravenous lorazepam and/or diazepam.[5,163,167,168] An osmolar gap greater than 10 has been suggested as a marker for potential PG toxicity and also indicates when to consider obtaining a serum PG concentration.[167] An osmolar gap of 20 corresponds to a serum PG concentration of approximately 48 mg/dL.[5] This equation should be used cautiously, as larger, more comprehensive studies are needed to validate it. There are rare cases where PG accumulation did not result in an osmolar gap.[62,168] In addition, elevated anion gap measurements and lactate concentrations are seen. As PG toxicity can mimic sepsis in these critically ill patients, sepsis should always be considered as the potential etiology of increased lactate, hypotension, and worsening renal function when considering PG toxicity. Both hemodialysis and fomepizole have been used to treat PG toxicity.[117,170]

NEPHROTOXICITY

Human proximal tubular cells exposed in vitro to PG concentrations of 500 to 2000 mg/dL exhibited significant cellular injury and membrane damage within 15 minutes of exposure.[109] Repeated exposure for up to 6 days produced dose-dependent toxic effects at lower concentrations (76, 190, and 380 mg/dL).[108]

The chronic administration of PG may contribute to proximal tubular cell damage and subsequent decreased renal function. In a retrospective study of eight patients who developed elevations in serum creatinine concentration while receiving continuous lorazepam infusions, serum creatinine rose within 3 to 60 days (median, 9 days).[168] The magnitude of serum creatinine rise was found to correlate with the serum PG concentration and duration of infusion. Serum creatinine decreased within 3 days of discontinuing the infusion. Patients with renal dysfunction are at greater risk for accumulating PG because 45% of PG is eliminated unchanged by the kidneys[43]; the remainder is metabolized by the liver. Caution should be used when prolonged administration of a PG-containing medication is necessary in the presence of renal or hepatic dysfunction.[109]

Propylene glycol-induced renal tubular necrosis has been reported in several cases. Daily PG-vehicle dosages of 11 to 90 g/d over 14 days was associated with rising serum creatinine concentrations (from 0.7 mg/dL to 2.1 mg/dL), elevated serum lactate concentrations, osmolar and anion gaps, and a serum PG concentration of 21 mg/dL.[169] Urine sediment analysis revealed numerous granular, muddy-brown-colored casts and no eosinophils, suggesting an acute renal tubular necrosis. A renal biopsy and electron microscopy showed extensive dilation of the proximal renal tubules, with swollen epithelial cells and mitochondria. Numerous vacuoles containing debris were also noted. A renal biopsy of another case with a serum PG concentration of 30 mg/dL showed disrupted brush borders of the proximal renal tubules after a sudden rise in serum creatinine concentration (3.1 mg/dL), nonoliguric renal failure, and metabolic acidosis. This was attributed to an average daily PG dose of 70 g for 17 days.[68]

SORBITOL

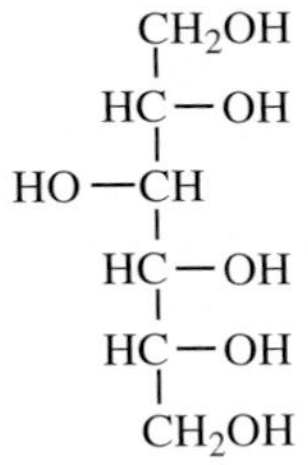

$$\begin{array}{c} CH_2OH \\ | \\ HC-OH \\ | \\ HO-CH \\ | \\ HC-OH \\ | \\ HC-OH \\ | \\ CH_2OH \end{array}$$

Sorbitol (D-glucitol) is widely used in the pharmaceutical industry as a sweetening agent, moistening agent, and a diluent (Table 55-10). Sorbitol occurs naturally in the ripe berries of many fruits, trees, and plants, and was first isolated in 1872 from the berries of the European mountain ash (*Sorbus aucuparia*).[111] It is particularly useful in chewable tablets because of its pleasant taste. In addition, it is widely used by the food industry in chewing gums, dietetic candies, foods, and enteral nutrition formulations. Sorbitol is approximately 50% to 60% as sweet as sucrose.[111]

TABLE 55–10. Common Medications Containing Sorbitol

Medication	Percent (%)	Grams (g)/Dose
Aluminum hydroxide/ magnesium hydroxide	10	3
Brofed elixir (brompheniramine and pseudoephedrine)	20	2
Calcium carbonate suspension	28	1.4
Chloral hydrate syrup	40	2
Fer-In-Sol drops (ferrous sulfate)	31	0.2
Guaifenisin/dextromethorphan syrup	64	6.4
Lanoxin (digoxin) elixir	21	0.1
Lasix (furosemide) solution	35	1.75
Methadone HCl solution	14	5.6
Potassium chloride solution	17.5	1.35
Sudafed (pseudoephedrine) syrup	35	1.75
Symmetrel syrup (amantadine HCl)	64	6.4
Tagamet (cimetidine) syrup	46	2.3
Tegretol (carbamazepine) syrup	17	0.85
Triaminic syrup (chlorpheniramine and pseudoephedrine)	7	0.7

PHARMACOKINETICS

Unlike sucrose, sorbitol is not readily fermented by oral microorganisms and is poorly absorbed from the gastrointestinal tract. Any absorbed sorbitol is metabolized in the liver to fructose and glucose.[111] Sorbitol has a caloric value of 4 kcal/g and is better tolerated by diabetics than sucrose; however, because some of it is metabolized to glucose, it is not unconditionally safe for diabetics.[111]

There is a concern of potentially fatal toxicity for individuals with hereditary fructose intolerance (HFI) receiving sorbitol-containing xenobiotics.[50] HFI is an autosomal recessive disorder caused by a deficiency of fructose-1,6-bisphosphonate aldolase in the liver, kidney, cortex, and small intestine.[81] This results in the accumulation of fructose-1-phosphate, which prevents glycogen breakdown and glucose synthesis causing hypoglycemia. The prevalence of HFI is most commonly reported to be one in 20,000 persons, but can range between one in 11,000 and one in 100,000.[2,79,81]

In individuals with HFI, the prolonged administration of sorbitol, fructose, or sucrose can result in death from liver or renal failure.[35,135] Dietary exclusion of fructose, sucrose, and sorbitol prevents the adverse effects. This condition should not be confused with the more common disorder of dietary fructose intolerance (DFI), which is caused by a defect in the glucose-transport protein 5 (GLUT5) system. This leads to the breakdown of fructose to carbon dioxide, hydrogen, and short-chain fatty acids by colonic bacteria, resulting in abdominal pain and bloating.[86] Dietary fructose intolerance symptoms are minimized by limiting sorbitol, fructose, and sucrose in the diet.

GASTROINTESTINAL TOXICITY

In large dosages, sorbitol can cause abdominal cramping, bloating, flatulence, vomiting, and diarrhea. Sorbitol exerts its cathartic effects by its osmotic properties, resulting in fluid shifts within the gastrointestinal tract. Iatrogenic osmotic diarrhea is reported following administration of many different liquid medication formulations containing sorbitol.[72,95] In a human volunteer study, 42 healthy adults ingested 10 g of a sorbitol solution. Sorbitol intolerance was detected in up to 55% of subjects.[78] One theoretical explanation for why all subjects did not experience the gastrointestinal adverse effects is unrecognized DFI. Diarrhea resulting from sorbitol-containing medications is common and often overlooked as a possible etiology.[30,69] Ingestion of large quantities of sorbitol (more than 20 g/d in adults) is not recommended (see Antidotes in Depth A3: Whole-Bowel Irrigation and Other Intestinal Evacuants).[111]

THIMEROSAL

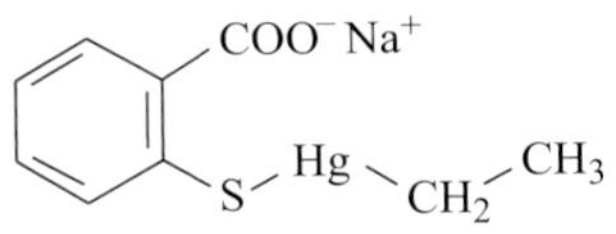

$$C_6H_4(COO^-Na^+)-S-Hg-CH_2-CH_3$$

Thimerosal (Merthiolate, Mercurothiolate), or sodium ethylmercurithiosalicylate, is an organic mercury compound that is approximately 49% elemental mercury (Hg) by weight.[130,156] It is metabolized to ethylmercury and thiosalicylate. Thimerosal has a wide spectrum of antibacterial activity at concentrations ranging from 0.01% to 0.1%; however, higher concentrations are sometimes also used.[83,105] Thimerosal has been widely used as a preservative since the 1930s in contact lens solutions, biologics, and vaccines, particularly those in multidose containers (Table 55-11). The use of thimerosal, which is necessary for the production process of some vaccines (eg, pertussis, influenza), may leave

TABLE 55–11. Thimerosal Concentration of Common Medications

Medication	Percent (%)	Milligrams (mg)/Dose
Injectable		
Antivenom (Crotaline polyvalent immune) Fab	0.001	0.11 (per vial)
Antivenom (*Lactrodectus mactans*)	0.01	0.25 (per vial)
Antivenom (*Micrurus fulvius*)	0.005	0.5 (per vial)
Diphtheria and tetanus toxoids[a]	0.01	0.05
DTaP (all products)	0.01	0.05
Fluzone[a] (influenza virus vaccine)	0.01	0.025
HibTITER (Haemophilus B conjugate vaccine)[a]	0.01	0.05
Menomune-A/C/Y/W-135[a] (meningococcal vaccine)	0.01	0.05
Tetanus toxoid (adsorbed)	0.01	0.05
Topical		
Mersol (thimerosal tincture)	0.1	–
Neosporin (triple antibiotic) ophthalmic solution	0.001	–
Ocufen (flurbiprofen) ophthalmic solution	0.005	–
Sulf-10 (sulfacetamide) ophthalmic solution	0.01	–

[a]Multidose.

trace amounts in the final product.[9] High-dose thimerosal exposure has resulted in neurotoxicity and nephrotoxicity. Although concerns exist regarding infant exposure to low-dose thimerosal through vaccinations and its effects on neurodevelopment, including possible links to causes of autism,[16] these concerns have never been substantiated (see Chap. 96).[41]

Because specific guidelines for ethylmercury exposure have not been developed, regulatory guidelines for dietary methylmercury exposure were applied to monitor ethylmercury exposure from injected thimerosal-containing vaccines. Methylmercury is a similar, but more toxic, organic mercury compound (Chap. 96). Maximum daily recommended methylmercury exposures range from 0.1 μg Hg/kg (US Environmental Protection Agency [EPA]) to 0.47 μg Hg/kg (WHO).[3,29,34]

An FDA review of thimerosal-containing vaccines revealed that some infants, depending on the immunization schedule, vaccine formulations, and infant's weight, might be exceeding the EPA exposure limit of 0.1 μg Hg/kg/d for methylmercury. Over the first 6 months of life, a total cumulative dose of up to 187.5 μg Hg total from thimerosal-containing vaccines was possible. The US Public Health Service (USPHS) and the American Academy of Pediatrics (AAP) responded jointly by recommending the preemptive reduction or removal of thimerosal from vaccines wherever possible.[3,28] The WHO and European regulatory bodies have made similar recommendations.[51] To date, thimerosal has been removed from most US-licensed immunoglobulin products. All vaccines routinely recommended for children younger than 7 years of age are either thimerosal-free or contain only trace amounts (less than 0.5 μg Hg per dose), with the exception of some inactivated influenza vaccines. Multidose vials requiring thimerosal preservative remain important for immunization programs in developing countries. Although efforts continue to eliminate all sources of mercury exposure, complete elimination of thimerosal from all vaccines is unlikely in the near future.[9] When a thimerosal-containing vaccine is the only alternative, the benefits of vaccination far exceed any theoretical risk of mercury toxicity.[112]

Prior to thimerosal use in pharmaceuticals, evidence for its safety and effectiveness was provided in several animal species and in 22 humans.[122] Only limited data exist on infant mercury exposure from thimerosal-containing vaccines. Clinical studies that assess the effects of thimerosal exposure on neurodevelopment and renal and immunologic function are lacking. Based on a comprehensive review of epidemiologic data from the United States,[33,54-57,156] Denmark,[77,96] Sweden,[143] and the United Kingdom,[4,71] the Institute of Medicine's (IOM's) Immunization Safety Review Committee,[112] the Global Advisory Committee on Vaccine Safety (GACVS),[165] and the European Agency for the Evaluation of Medicinal Products (EMEA)[46] have all concluded that there is no causal relationship between thimerosal-containing vaccines and autism. Continued surveillance of autistic spectrum disorders as thimerosal use declines will be conducted to evaluate any associated trends.

PHARMACOKINETICS

Limited pharmacokinetic data exist for thimerosal and ethylmercury. Once absorbed, thimerosal breaks down to form ethylmercury and thiosalicylate. Some ethylmercury further decomposes into inorganic mercury in the blood, and the remainder distributes into kidney and, to a lesser extent, brain tissue.[97,98] Because of its longer organic chain, ethylmercury is less stable and decomposes more rapidly than methylmercury, leaving less ethylmercury available to enter kidney and brain tissue.[97] Ethylmercury crosses the blood–brain barrier by passive diffusion.[98] Intracellular ethylmercury decomposes to inorganic mercury, which accumulates in kidney and brain tissues.[98] The half-life of thimerosal is estimated to be about 18 days.[99] Thimerosal is eliminated in the feces as inorganic mercury (see Chap. 96).[121]

MERCURIAL TOXICITY

Oral Administration A case report described a 44-year-old man who ingested 5 g (83 mg/kg) of thimerosal in a suicide attempt; within 15 minutes he began vomiting spontaneously. Gastric lavage was performed and chelation therapy begun with dimercaptopropane sulfonate (DMPS). Gastroscopy revealed a hemorrhagic gastritis. Polyuric acute renal failure was noted on the day of admission and persisted for 40 days. Four days after admission the patient developed a fever and a maculopapular exanthem attributed to thimerosal. The patient also developed an autonomic and ascending peripheral polyneuropathy that persisted for 13 days. Chelation therapy was continued for a total of 50 days with DMPS followed by succimer. Elevated blood and urine mercury concentration persisted for more than 140 days. The patient was discharged 148 days following the ingestion with only sensory defects in his toes. No other neurologic sequelae were noted.[120]

Oral absorption of thimerosal resulted in the fatal poisoning of an 18-month-old girl from the intra-otic instillation of a solution containing 0.1% thimerosal and 0.14% sodium borate. Tympanostomy tubes placed 1 year earlier allowed the irrigation solution to flow through the auditory tube into the nasopharynx, and subsequently to be swallowed and absorbed through the oral mucosa and gastrointestinal tract. A total of 1.2 L of solution (500 mg Hg) was instilled over a 4-week period, resulting in severe mercury poisoning. Four days after admission, the serum mercury concentration was 163 μg/dL. The patient also received 1.7 g of boric acid. It is unclear what contribution, if any, the boric acid made to the serum mercury concentration. Chelation therapy with *N*-acetyl-D-penicillamine was initiated on day 51. Despite increased urinary mercury concentrations following administration of the *N*-acetyl-D-penicillamine, her neurologic function and blood mercury concentrations remained unchanged. The child died 3 months after admission. An autopsy was not performed.[130]

Intramuscular Administration Urine mercury concentrations of 26 patients with hypogammaglobulinemia, who received weekly intramuscular IgG replacement therapy preserved with 0.01% thimerosal were studied. The dosages of IgG ranged from 25 to 50 mg/kg, containing 0.6 to 1.2 mg of mercury per dose.[64] The total estimated dose of mercury administered ranged from 4 to 734 mg over a period of 6 months to 17 years. Urine mercury concentrations were elevated in 19 patients, ranging from 31 to 75 μg/L; however, no patients had clinical evidence of chronic mercury toxicity.[64]

Six cases of severe mercury poisoning resulting in four deaths were reported following the intramuscular administration of chloramphenicol preserved with thimerosal. A manufacturing error produced vials containing 510 mg of thimerosal (250 mg Hg) instead of 0.51 mg per vial. Two adults received 4 g and 5.5 g of mercury each and four children received 0.2 to 1.8 g each. All six patients had extensive tissue necrosis at the site of injection. Fever, altered mental status, slurred speech, and ataxia were noted. Autopsy identified widespread degeneration and necrosis of the renal tubules; however, creatine kinase concentrations were not reported, so pigment-induced nephrotoxicity cannot be excluded. Elevated mercury concentrations were found in the injection site tissues, and in the kidneys, livers, and brains.[7]

Topical Administration Thirteen infants were exposed to 9 to 48 topical applications of a 0.1% thimerosal tincture for the treatment of exomphalos. Analysis for elevated mercury concentrations was performed in 10 of 13 infants who unexpectedly died. Mercury concentrations were determined in various tissues from six of the infants. Mean tissue concentrations in fresh samples of liver, kidney, spleen, and heart ranged from 5152 to 11,330 ppb, suggesting percutaneous absorption from these repeated topical applications.[47]

Ophthalmic Administration Nine patients undergoing keratoplasty were exposed to a contact lens stored in a solution containing 0.002% thimerosal.[164] After 4 hours, the lens was removed and mercury concentrations of the aqueous humor and excised corneal tissues were determined. Mercury concentrations were elevated in both aqueous humor (range, 20 to 46 ng/mL higher) and corneal tissues (range, 0.6 to 14 ng higher) as compared with eyes that had not been fitted with contact lenses. Only residual amounts of mercury remained on the contact lenses after 4 hours of wear. The authors noted that although the aqueous humor concentrations were in the same range as those measured in 10 patients with vision loss from systemic mercury poisoning (11 to 104 ng/mL), adverse effects did not occur.

A possible drug interaction between orally administered tetracyclines and thimerosal was reported to result in acute, varying degrees of eye irritation in contact lens wearers using thimerosal-containing contact lens solutions who started treatment with tetracycline.[38]

SUMMARY

The benefits of pharmaceutical excipients include improved drug solubility, stability and palatability, antimicrobial activity, the availability of various dosage forms, the provision of products with long-term storage, and the availability of multiple-dose packaging. Excipients are often termed "inert," implying that they possess no pharmacologic or toxicologic properties of their own. While excipients are essential and efficacious, they may also be responsible for severe, and sometimes fatal, adverse effects.

The toxicity of pharmaceutical excipients should be considered for patients requiring high doses or prolonged administration of any medication containing excipients, particularly those additives known to have toxicities. Individuals with decreased renal or hepatic function or patients at the extremes of age may be at an increased risk of accumulating excipients. Under circumstances in which there is no option but to continue treating a patient with a particular xenobiotic, switching to a preservative-free product, or to another brand without the offending excipient, may obviate the need for discontinuation of an effective agent. In addition to inherent toxicities, many excipients may also be responsible for allergic reactions. Their prevalence in numerous pharmaceuticals, cosmetics, and foods may allow for sensitization. However, in the majority of cases, pharmaceutical excipients are safe and effective, and their benefits far exceed their potential for adverse effects when administered properly.

REFERENCES

1. Alade SL, Brown RE, Paquet A. Polysorbate 80 and E-Ferol toxicity. *Pediatrics.* 1986;77:593-597.
2. Ali M, Rellos P, Cox TM. Hereditary fructose intolerance. *J Med Genet.* 1998;35:353-365.
3. American Academy of Pediatrics. Committee on Infectious Diseases and Committee on Environmental Health. Thimerosal in vaccines—an interim report to clinicians (RE9935). *Pediatrics.* 1999;104:570-574.
4. Andrews N, Miller E, Grant A, et al. Thimerosal exposure in infants and developmental disorders. A retrospective cohort study in the United Kingdom does not support a causal association. *Pediatrics.* 2004;114:584-591.
5. Arroliga AC, Shehab N, McCarthy K, Gonzales JP. Relationship of continuous infusion lorazepam to serum propylene glycol concentration in critically ill adults. *Crit Care Med.* 2004;32:1709-1714.
6. Arulanantham K, Genel M. Central nervous system toxicity associated with ingestion of propylene glycol. *J Pediatr.* 1978;93:515-516.
7. Axton JH. Six cases of poisoning after parenteral organic mercurial compound (Merthiolate). *Postgrad Med J.* 1972;48:417-421.
8. Bagshawe KD, Magrath IT, Golding PR. Intrathecal methotrexate. *Lancet.* 1969;2:1258.
9. Ball LK, Ball R, Pratt RD. An assessment of thimerosal use in childhood vaccines. *Pediatrics.* 2001;107:1147-1154.
10. Bania TC, Chu J, Perez E, Su M, Hahn IH. Hemodynamic effects of intravenous fat emulsion in an animal model of severe verapamil toxicity resuscitated with atropine, calcium, and saline. *Acad Emerg Med.* 2007;4:105-111.
11. Bekeris L, Baker C, Fenton J, Kimball D, Bermes E. Propylene glycol as a cause of an elevated serum osmolality. *Am J Clin Pathol.* 1979;72:633-636.
12. Benda GI, Hiller JL, Reynolds JW. Benzyl alcohol toxicity. Impact on neurologic handicaps among surviving very-low-birth-weight infants. *Pediatrics.* 1986;77:507-512.
13. Benzon HT, Gissen AJ, Strichartz GR, Avram MJ, Covino BG. The effect of polyethylene glycol on mammalian nerve impulses. *Anesth Analg.* 1987;66:553-559.
14. Berg ØH, Henriksen RN, Steisvåg SK. The effect of a benzalkonium chloride-containing nasal spray on human respiratory mucosa in vitro as a function of concentration and time of action. *Pharmacol Toxicol.* 1995;76:245-249.
15. Berg ØH, Lie K, Steisvåg SK. The effects of topical nasal steroids on rat respiratory mucosa in vivo, with special reference to benzalkonium chloride. *Allergy.* 1997;52:627-632.
16. Bernard S, Enayati A, Redwood L, et al. Autism. A novel form of mercury poisoning. *Med Hypotheses.* 2001;56:462-471.
17. Bernat JL. Intraspinal steroid therapy. *Neurology.* 1981;31:168-171.
18. Borody T, Chinwah PM, Graham GG, Wade DN, Williams KM. Chlorobutanol toxicity and dependence. *Med J Aust.* 1979;1:288.

19. Bowie MD, McKenzie D. Diethylene glycol poisoning in children. *S Afr Med J.* 1972;46:931-934.
20. Brown WJ, Buist WJ, Cory Gipson HT, et al. Fatal benzyl alcohol poisoning in an neonatal intensive care unit. *Lancet.* 1982;1:1250.
21. Bruns DE, Herold DA, Rodheaver GT, Edlich RF. Polyethylene glycol intoxication in burn patients. *Burns.* 1982;9:49-52.
22. Brunson EL. Benzyl alcohol. In: Rowe RC, Sheskey PJ, Weller PJ, eds. *Handbook of Pharmaceutical Excipients*, 4th ed. Washington, DC: American Pharmaceutical Association; 2003:53-55.
23. Buszello K, Muller BW. Emulsions as drug delivery systems. In: Nielloud F, Marti-Mestres G, eds. *Drugs and the Pharmaceutical Sciences. Pharmaceutical Emulsions and Suspensions.* New York: Marcel Dekker; 2000:191-224.
24. Calvery HO, Klumpp TG. The toxicity for human beings of diethylene glycol with sulfanilamide. *South Med J.* 1939;32:1105-1109.
25. Cate JC, Hedrick R. Propylene glycol intoxication and lactic acidosis. *N Engl J Med.* 1980;303:1237.
26. Cawley MJ. Short-term lorazepam infusion and concern for propylene glycol toxicity. Case report and review. *Pharmacotherapy.* 2001;21:1140-1144.
27. Centers for Disease Control and Prevention. Fatalities associated with ingestion of diethylene glycol-contaminated glycerin used to manufacture acetaminophen syrup—Haiti, November 1995-June 1996. *MMWR Morb Mortal Wkly Rep.* 1996;45:649-650.
28. Centers for Disease Control and Prevention. Recommendations regarding the use of vaccines that contain thimerosal as preservative. *MMWR Morb Mortal Wkly Rep.* 1999;48:996-998.
29. Centers for Disease Control and Prevention. Thimerosal in vaccines. A joint statement of the American Academy of Pediatrics. and the Public Health Service. *MMWR Morb Mortal Wkly Rep.* 1999;48:563-565.
30. Chassany O, Michaux A, Bergmann JF. Drug-induced diarrhoea. *Drug Saf.* 2000;22:53-72.
31. Chen J, Ahn KC, Gee NA, et al. Antiandrogenic properties of parabens and other phenolic containing small molecules in personal care products. *Toxicol Appl Pharmacol.* 2007;221:278-284.
32. Chicella M, Jansen P, Parthiban A, et al. Propylene glycol accumulation associated with continuous infusion of lorazepam in pediatric intensive care patients. *Crit Care Med.* 2002;30:2752-2756.
33 The evidence for the safety of thiomersal in newborn and infant vaccines. *Vaccine.* 2004;22:1854-1861.
34. Clements CJ, Ball LK, Ball R, Pratt D. Thiomersal in vaccines. *Lancet.* 2000;355:1279-1280.
35. Collins J. Time for fructose solutions to go. *Lancet.* 1993;341:600.
36. Conway V, Mulski M. Phenol. In: Rowe RC, Sheskey PJ, Weller PJ, eds. *Handbook of Pharmaceutical Excipients.* 4th ed. Washington, DC: American Pharmaceutical Association; 2003:426-428.
37. Craig DB, Habib GG. Flaccid paraparesis following obstetrical epidural anesthesia. Possible role of benzyl alcohol. *Anesth Analg.* 1977;56: 219-221.
38. Crook TG, Freeman JJ. Reactions induced by the concurrent use of thimerosal and tetracycline. *Am J Optom Physiol Optics.* 1983;60:759-761.
39. Cukier JO, Seungdamrong S, Odell JL, et al. The displacement of albumin bound bilirubin by gentamicin. *Pediatr Res.* 1974;8:399.
40. Darbre PD, Harvey PW. Paraben esters: review of recent studies of endocrine toxicity, absorption, esterase and human exposure, and discussion of potential human health risks. *J Appl Toxicol.* 2008;28:561-578.
41 Davidson PW, Myers GJ, Weiss B. Mercury exposure and child development outcomes. *Pediatrics.* 2004;113:1023-1029.
42. DeChristoforro R, Corden BJ, Hood JC, Narang PK, Magrath IT. High-dose morphine complicated by chlorobutanol-somnolence. *Ann Intern Med.* 1983;98:335-336.
43. Demey HE, Daelemans RA, Verpooten GA, et al. Propylene glycol induced side effects during intravenous nitroglycerin therapy. *Intensive Care Med.* 1988;14:221-226.
44. DiPiro JT, Michael KA, Clark BA, et al. Absorption of polyethylene glycol after administration of a PEG-electrolyte lavage solution. *Clin Parm.* 1986;5: 153-155.
45. Erickson TB, Aks SE, Zabaneh R, Reid R. Acute renal toxicity after ingestion of lava light liquid. *Ann Emerg Med.* 1996;27:781-784.
46. European Agency for the Evaluation of Medicinal Products. EMEA public statement on thiomersal in vaccines for human use-recent evidence supports safety of thimerosal-containing vaccines. Doc Ref. EMEA/CMP/VEG/1194/04/Adopted. London, England, 2004. http://www.eu.int/pdfs/human/press/pus/119404en.pdf. Accessed December 4, 2004.
47. Fagan DG, Pritchard JS, Clarkson TW, Greenwood MR. Organ mercury levels in infant with omphaloceles treated with organic mercurial antiseptic. *Arch Dis Child.* 1977;52:962-964.
48. FDA Center for Drug Evaluation and Research. Inactive Ingredient Guide (Redacted) January 1996. Rockville, MD; 2001. http://www.fda.gov/cder/drug/iig/default.htm. Accessed February 24, 2005.
49. Fligner CL, Jack R, Twiggs GA, Raisys VA. Hyperosmolality induced by propylene glycol, a complication of silver sulfadiazine therapy. *JAMA.* 1985;253:1606-1609.
50. Florence AT, Salole EG, eds. *Formulation Factors in Adverse Reactions.* London: Wright; 1990:11.
51. Freed GL, Andreae MC, Cowan AE, Katz SL. Vaccine safety policy analysis in three European countries. The case of thimerosal. *Health Policy.* 2002; 62:291-307.
52. Garnacho-Montero J, Ortiz-Leyba C, Garnacho-Montero MC, et al. Effects of three intravenous lipid emulsions on the survival and mononuclear phagocytes function of septic rats. *Nutrition.* 2002;18:751-754.
53. Gassett AR. Benzalkonium chloride toxicity to the human cornea. *Am J Ophthamol.* 1977;84:169-171.
54. Geier DA, Geier MR. A comparative evaluation of the effects of MMR immunization and mercury doses from thimerosal-containing childhood vaccines on the population prevalence of autism. *Med Sci Monit.* 2004;10:PI33-PI39.
55. Geier DA, Geier MR. An assessment of the impact of thimerosal on childhood neurodevelopmental disorders. *Pediatr Rehabil.* 2003;6:97-102.
56. Geier DA, Geier MR. Thimerosal in childhood vaccines, neurodevelopmental disorders, and heart disease in the United States. *J Am Phys Surg.* 2003;8:6-11.
57. Geier MR, Geier DA. Neurodevelopmental disorders after thimerosal containing vaccines. A brief communication. *Exp Biol Med.* 2003;228:660-664.
58. Geiling EM, Cannon PR. Pathologic effects of elixir of sulfanilamide (diethylene glycol) poisoning. *JAMA.* 1938;111:919-926.
59. Gellerman GL, Martinez C. Fatal ventricular fibrillation following intravenous sodium diphenylhydantoin therapy. *JAMA.* 1967;200:337-338.
60. Gershanik J, Boecler B, Ensley H, McCloskey S, George W. The gasping syndrome and benzyl alcohol poisoning. *N Engl J Med.* 1982:1384-1388.
61. Glasgow AM, Boeckx RL, Miller MK, et al. Hyperosmolality in small infants due to propylene glycol. *Pediatrics.* 1983;72:353-355.
62. Glover ML, Reed MD. Propylene glycol. The safe diluent that continues to cause harm. *Pharmacotherapy.* 1996;16:690-693.
63. Gross DR, Kitzman JV, Adams HR. Cardiovascular effects of intravenous administration of propylene glycol and oxytetracycline in propylene glycol in calves. *Am J Vet Res.* 1979;40:783-791.
64. Haeney MR, Carter GF, Yeoman WB, Thompson RA. Long-term parenteral exposure to mercury in patients with hypogammaglobulinaemia. *Br Med J.* 1979;2:12-14.
65. Hagebusch OE. Necropsies of four patients following administration of elixir sulfanilamide—Massengill. *JAMA.* 1937;109:1537-1539.
66. Hahn AF, Feasby TE, Gilbert JJ. Paraparesis following intrathecal chemotherapy. *Neurology.* 1983;33:1032-1038.
67. Hanif M, Mobarak MR, Ronan A. Fatal renal failure by diethylene glycol in paracetamol elixir. The Bangladesh epidemic. *BMJ.* 1995;311:88-91.
68. Hayman M, Seidl EC, Ali M, Malik K. Acute tubular necrosis associated with propylene glycol from concomitant administration of intravenous lorazepam and trimethoprim-sulfamethoxazole. *Pharmacotherapy.* 2003;23:1190-1194.
69. Henley E. Sorbitol-based elixirs, diarrhea and enteral tube feeding. *Am Fam Physician.* 1997;55:2084-2086.
70. Herold DA, Keil K, Bruns DE. Oxidation of polyethylene glycols by alcohol dehydrogenase. *Biochem Pharmacol.* 1989;38:73-76.
71. Heron J, Golding J, ALSPAC Study Team. Thimerosal exposure in infants and developmental disorders. A prospective cohort study in the United kingdom does not support a causal association. *Pediatrics.* 2004;114: 577-583.
72. Hill DB, Henderson LM, McClain CJ. Osmotic diarrhea by sugar-free theophylline solution in critically ill patients. *J Parenter Enteral Nutr.* 1991;15:332-336.
73. Hiller JL, Benda GI, Rahatzad M, et al. Benzyl alcohol toxicity. Impact on mortality and intraventricular hemorrhage among very-low birth-weight infants. *Pediatrics.* 1986;77:500-506.
74. Ho CY, Wu MC, Lan MY, Tan CT, Yang AH. In vitro effects of preservatives in nasal sprays on human nasal epithelial cells. *Am J Rhinol.* 2008;22:125-129.

75. Hofmann T, Gugatschga M, Koidl B, Wolf G. Influence of preservatives and topical steroids on ciliary beat frequency in vitro. *Arch Otolaryngol Head Neck Surg.* 2004;130:440-445.
76. http://www.ajc.com/services/content.shared-gen/ap/Africa/AF_Nigeria_Fatal_Formula.html?cxntlid=inform_sr. Nigeria:84 children dead from teething formula. Associated Press Article.
77. Hviid A, Stellfeld M, Wohlfahrt J, Melbye M. Association between thimerosal containing vaccine and autism. *JAMA.* 2003;290:1763-1766.
78. Jain NK, Patel VP, Pitchumoni CS. Sorbitol intolerance in adults. *Am J Gastroenterol.* 1985;80:678-681.
79. James CL, Rellos P, Alli M, et al. Neonatal screening for HFI. Frequency of the most common mutant aldolase B allele (A149P) in the British population. *J Med Genet.* 1996;33:837-841.
80. James CW, McNelis KC, Matalia MD, Cohen DM, Szabo S. Central nervous system toxicity and amprenavir oral solution. *Ann Pharmacother.* 2001;35:174.
81. Jorde LB, Carey JC, Bamshad MJ, White RL. Biochemical genetics. Disorders of metabolism. In: Jorde LB, Carey JC, Bamshad MJ, White RL, eds. *Medical Genetics.* 2nd ed. St. Louis: Mosby; 2000:136-155.
82. Kibbe AH. Benzalkonium chloride. In: Rowe RC, Sheskey PJ, Weller PJ, eds. *Handbook of Pharmaceutical Excipients.* 4th ed. Washington, DC: American Pharmaceutical Association; 2003:45-47.
83. Kibbe AH, Weller PJ. Thimerosal. In: Rowe RC, Sheskey PJ, Weller PJ, eds. *Handbook of Pharmaceutical Excipients.* 4th ed. Washington, DC: American Pharmaceutical Association; 2003:648-650.
84. Kulick MI, Lewis NS, Bansal V, Warpeha R. Hyperosmolality in the burn patient. Analysis of an osmolal discrepancy. *J Trauma.* 1980;20:223-228.
85. Kuoyama Y, Suzuki K, Hara T. Nasal lesion induced by intranasal administration of benzalkonium chloride in rats. *J Toxicol Sci.* 1997;22:153-160.
86. Ledochowski M, Widner B, Bair H, Probst T, Fuchs D. Fructose and sorbitol-reduced diet improves mood and gastrointestinal disturbances in fructose malabsorbers. *Scand J Gastroenterol.* 2000;35:1048-1052.
87. Lekka ME, Liokatis S, Nathanail C, Galani V, Nakos G. The impact of intravenous fat emulsion administration in acute lung injury. *Am J Respir Crit Care Med.* 2004;169:638-644.
88. Lemp MA, Zimmerman LE. Toxic endothelial degeneration in ocular surface disease treated with topical medications containing benzalkonium chloride. *Am J Ophthamol.* 1988;105:670-673.
89. Liu H, Routley I, Teichmann KD. Toxic endothelial cell destruction from intraocular benzalkonium chloride. *J Cataract Refract Surg.* 2001;27:1746-1750.
90. Lopez-Herce J, Bonet C, Meana A, Albajara L. Benzyl alcohol poisoning following diazepam intravenous infusion. *Ann Pharmacother.* 1995;29:632.
91. Lorenzetti OJ, Wernet TC. Topical parabens. Benefits and risks. *Dermatologica.* 1977;154:244-250.
92. Loria CJ, Echeverria P, Smith AL. Effect of antibiotic formulations in serum protein. Bilirubin interaction of newborn infants. *J Pediatr.* 1976;89:479-482.
93. Louis S, Kutt H, McDowell F. The cardiovascular changes caused by intravenous Dilantin and its solvent. *Am Heart J.* 1967;74:523-529.
94. MacDonald MG, Getson PR, Glasgow AM, et al. Propylene glycol. Increased incidence of seizures in low-birth-weight infants. *Pediatrics.* 1987;79:622-625.
95. Madigan SM, Courtney DE, Macauley D. The solution was the problem. *Clin Nutr.* 2002;21:531-532.
96. Madsen KM, Lauritsen MB, Pedersen CB, et al. Thimerosal and the occurrence of autism. Negative ecological evidence from Danish population-based data. *Pediatrics.* 2003;112:604-606.
97. Magos L. Neurotoxic character of thimerosal and the allometric extrapolation of adult clearance half-time to infants. *J Appl Toxicol.* 2003;23:263-269.
98. Magos L, Brown AW, Sparrow S, et al. The comparative toxicology of ethyl and methylmercury. *Arch Toxicol.* 1985;57:260-297.
99. Malinovsky JM, Cozian A, Lepage JY, Pinaud M. Ketamine and midazolam neurotoxicity in the rabbit. *Anesthesiology.* 1991;75:91-97.
100. Malinovsky JM, Lepage JY, Cozian A, et al. Is ketamine or its preservative responsible for neurotoxicity in the rabbit? *Anesthesiology.* 1993;78:109-115.
101. Martin G, Finberg L. Propylene glycol. A potentially toxic vehicle in liquid dosage form. *J Pediatr.* 1970;77:877-878.
102. Martone WJ, Williams WW, Mortensen ML, et al. Illness with fatalities in premature infants. Association with intravenous vitamin E preparation, E-Ferol. *Pediatrics.* 1986;78:591-600.
103. Miles JM, Cattalini M, Sharbrough FW, et al. Metabolic and neurologic effects of an intravenous medium-chain triglyceride emulsion. *JPEN J Parenter Enteral Nutr.* 1991;15:37-41.
104. Miller B, Traynelis SF, Attwell D. Potentiation of NMDA receptor currents by arachidonic acid. *Nature.* 1992;355:722-725.
105. Möller H. Merthiolate allergy. A nationwide iatrogenic sensitization. *Acta Derm Venereol.* 1977;57:509-517.
106. Morizono T. Toxicity of ototopical drugs. Animal modeling. *Ann Otol Rhinol Laryngol Suppl.* 1990;148:42-45.
107. Morizono T, Paparella MM, Juhn SK. Ototoxicity of propylene glycol in experimental animals. *Am J Otolaryngol.* 1980;1:393-399.
108. Morshed KM, Jain SK, McMartin KE. Propylene glycol-mediated injury in a primary cell culture of human proximal tubule cells. *Toxicol Sci.* 1998;46:410-417.
109. Morshed KM, Jain SK, McMartin KE. Acute toxicity of propylene glycol. An assessment using cultured proximal tubule cells of human origin. *Fundam Appl Toxicol.* 1994;23:38-43.
110. Nash RA. Chlorbutanol. In: Rowe RC, Sheskey PJ, Weller PJ, eds. *Handbook of Pharmaceutical Excipients.* 4th ed. Washington, DC: American Pharmaceutical Association; 2003:141-143.
111. Nash RA. Sorbitol. In: Rowe RC, Sheskey PJ, Weller PJ, eds. *Handbook of Pharmaceutical Excipients.* 4th ed. Washington, DC: American Pharmaceutical Association; 2003:596-599.
112. National Academy of Sciences. Immunization Safety Review Committee. Immunization Safety Review. Vaccines and Autism (Free Executive Summary). ISBN: 0-309-53275-2. Washington, DC: Author; 2004. See http://www.nap.edu/catalog/10997.html for ordering information; accessed December 5, 2004.)
113. Neale BW, Mesler EL, Young M, Rebuck JA, Weise WJ. Propylene glycol-induced lactic acidosis in a patient with normal renal function: a proposed mechanism and monitoring recommendations. *Ann Pharmacother.* 2005;39:1732-1736.
114. Neville R, Dennis, P, Sens D, Crouch R. Preservative cytotoxicity to cultured corneal epithelial cells. *Curr Eye Res.* 1986;5:367-372.
115. Okuonghae HO, Ighogboja IS, Lawson JO, Nwana EJ. Diethylene glycol poisoning in Nigerian children. *Ann Trop Paediatr.* 1992;12:235-238.
116. Papahadjopoulos D. Steric stabilization an overview. In: Janoff SA, ed. *Liposomes Rational Design.* New York: Marcel Dekker; 1999:1-12.
117. Parker MG, Fraser GL, Watson DM, Riker RR. Removal of propylene glycol and correction of increased osmolar gap by hemodialysis in a patient on high dose lorazepam infusion therapy. *Intens Care Med.* 2002;28:81-81.
118. Perez E, Bania TC, Medlej K, Chu J. Determining the optimal dose of intravenous fat emulsion for the treatment of severe verapamil toxicity in a rodent model. *Acad Emerg Med.* 2008;15:1284-1289.
119. Petrou S, Ordway RW, Hamilton JA, Walsh JV Jr, Singer JJ. Structural requirements for charged lipid molecules to directly increase or suppresses K^+ channel activity in smooth muscle cells. *J Gen Physiol.* 1994;103:471-486.
120. Pfab R, Mückter H, Roider G, Zilker T. Clinical course of severe poisoning with thimerosal. *J Toxicol Clin Toxicol.* 1996;34:453-460.
121. Pichichero ME, Cernichiari E, Lopreiato J, Treanor J. Mercury concentrations and metabolism in infants receiving vaccines containing thimerosal. A descriptive study. *Lancet.* 2002;360:1737-1741.
122. Powell HM, Jamieson WA. Merthiolate as a germicide. *Am J Hygiene.* 1931;13:296-310.
123. Price JC. Polyethylene glycol. In: Rowe RC, Sheskey PJ, Weller PJ, eds. *Handbook of Pharmaceutical Excipients.* 4th ed. Washington, DC: American Pharmaceutical Association; 2003:454-459.
124. Prusakiewicz JJ, Harville HM, Zhang Y, Ackermann C, Voorman RL. Parabens inhibit human skin estrogen sulfotransferase activity: possible link to paraben estrogenic effects. *Toxicology.* 2007;232:248-256.
125. Pugazhendhi D, Pope GS, Darbre PD. Oestrogenic activity of p-hydroxybenzoic acid (common metabolite of paraben esters) and methylparaben in human breast cancer cell lines. *J Appl Toxicol.* 2005;25:301-309.
126. Rentz ED, Lewis L, Mujica OJ, et al. Outbreak of acute renal failure in Panama in 2006: a case-control study. *Bull World Health Organ.* 2008;86:749-756.
127. Rieger MM. Methylparaben. In: Rowe RC, Sheskey PJ, Weller PJ, eds. *Handbook of Pharmaceutical Excipients.* 4th ed. Washington, DC: American Pharmaceutical Association; 2003:390-394.
128. Rivera W, Velez LI, Guzman DD, Shepherd G. Unintentional intravenous infusion of GoLYTELY in a 4-year-old girl. *Ann Pharmacother.* 2004;38:1183-1185.
129. Rogers SC, Burrows D, Neill D. Percutaneous absorption of phenol and methyl alcohol in magenta paint BPC. *Br J Dermatol.* 1978;98:559-560.

130. Rohyans J, Walson PD, Wood GA, MacDonald WA. Mercury toxicity following Merthiolate ear irrigations. *J Pediatr.* 1984;104:311-313.
131. Rubin M. Dear Health Care Professional Letter. Agenerase. Research Triangle Park, NC: Glaxo Wellcome; May 2000.
132. Saiki JH, Thompson S, Smith F, Atkinson R. Paraplegia following intrathecal chemotherapy. *Cancer.* 1972;29:370-374.
133. Schamberg IL. Allergic contact dermatitis to methyl and propyl paraben. *Arch Dermatol.* 1967;95:626-328.
134. Schiller LR, Emmett M, Santa CA, et al. Osmotic effects of polyethylene glycol. *Gastroenterology.* 1988;94:933-941.
135. Schulte MJ, Lenz W. Fatal sorbitol infusion in patient with fructose sorbitol intolerance. *Lancet.* 1977;2:188.
136. Sirianni AJ, Osterhoudt KC, Calello DP, et al. Use of lipid emulsion in the resuscitation of a patient with prolonged cardiovascular collapse after overdose of bupropion and lamotrigine. *Ann Emerg Med.* 2008;51:412-415.
137. Smith WS, Dowd CF, Johnston SC, et al. Neurotoxicity of intra-arterial papaverine preserved with chlorobutanol used for the treatment of cerebral vasospasm after aneurysmal subarachnoid hemorrhage. *Stroke.* 2004;35:2518-2522.
138. Smyth HF, Carpenter CP, Shaffer CB. The toxicity of high-molecular-weight polyethylene glycols: chronic oral and parenteral administration. *J Am Pharm Assoc (Wash).* 1947;36:157-160.
139. Smyth HF, Carpenter CP, Weil CS. The chronic oral toxicity of the polyethylene glycols. *J Am Pharm Assoc (Wash).* 1955;44;27-30.
140. Smyth HF, Carpenter CP, Weil CS. The toxicology of the polyethylene glycols. *J Am Pharm Assoc (Wash).* 1950;39:349-354.
141. Song BL, Li HY, Peng DR. In vitro spermicidal activity of parabens against human spermatozoa. *Contraception.* 1989;39:331-335.
142. Speth PA, Vree TB, Neilen NF, et al. Propylene glycol pharmacokinetics and effect after intravenous infusion in humans. *Ther Drug Monit.* 1987;9:255-258.
143. Stehr-Green P, Tull P, Stellfeld M, Mortenson PB, Simpson D. Autism and the thimerosal containing vaccines. Lack of consistent evidence for an association. *Am J Prev Med.* 2003;25:101-106.
144. Strickley RG. Solubilizing excipients in oral and injectable formulations. *Pharm Res.* 2004;21:201-230.
145. Sturgill BC, Herold DA, Bruns DE. Renal tubular necrosis in burn patients treated with topical polyethylene glycol. *Lab Invest.* 1982;46:81A.
146. Sweet AY. Fatality from intravenous nitrofurantoin. *Pediatrics.* 1958;22:1204.
147. Tabuchi S, Kume K, Aihara M, et al. Lipid mediators modulate NMDA receptor currents in a *Xenopus* oocyte expression system. *Neurosci Lett.* 1997;237:13-16.
148. Tripathi BJ, Tripathi RC. Cytotoxic effects of benzalkonium chloride and chlorobutanol on human corneal epithelial cells in vitro. *Lens Eye Toxic Res.* 1989;6:395-403.
149. Unger AH, Sklaroff HJ. Fatalities following intravenous use of sodium diphenylhydantoin for cardiac arrhythmias. *JAMA.* 1967;200:35-36.
150. United States Pharmacopeia 24/National Formulary 19. Rockville, MD: United States Pharmacopeial Convention; 2000.
151. Unlu RE, Alagoz MS, Uysai AC, et al. Phenol intoxication in a child. *J Craniofac Surg.* 2004;15:1010-1013.
152. Van de Wiele B, Rubinstein E, Peacock W, Martin N. Propylene glycol toxicity caused by prolonged infusion of etomidate. *J Neurosurg Anesthesiol.* 1995;7:259-262.
153. van Meeuwen JA, van Son O, Piersma AH, de Jong PC, van den Berg M. Aromatase inhibiting and combined estrogenic effects of parabens and estrogenic effects of other additives in cosmetics. *Toxicol Appl Pharmacol.* 2008;230:372-382.
154. Vassalli L, Harris DM, Gradini R, Applebaum EL. Propylene glycol-induced cholesteatoma in chinchilla middle ears. *Am J Otolaryngol.* 1988;9:180-188.
155. Vernon J, Brummett R, Walsh T. The ototoxic potential of propylene glycol in guinea pigs. *Arch Otolaryngol.* 1978;104:726-729.
156. Verstraeten T, Davis RL, DeStefano F, et al. Safety of thimerosal-containing vaccines. A two-phased study of computerized health maintenance organization databases. *Pediatrics.* 2003;112:1039-1048.
157. Wanten GJ, Netea MG, Naber TH, et al. Parenteral administration of medium-but not long-chain lipid emulsions may increase the risk for infections by candida albicans. *Infect Immun.* 2002;70:6471-6474.
158. Warner MA, Harper JV. Cardiac dysrhythmias associated with chemical peeling with phenol. *Anesthesiology.* 1985;62:366-367.
159. Weigt HU, Georgieff M, Beyer C, Föhr KJ. Activation of neuronal *N*-methyl-D-aspartate receptor channels by lipid emulsions. *Anesth Analg.* 2002;94:331-337.
160. Weigt HU, Georgieff M, Beyer C, et al. Lipid emulsions reduce NMDA-evoked currents. *Neuropharmacology.* 2004;47:373-380.
161. Weller PJ. Propylene glycol. In: Rowe RC, Sheskey PJ, Weller PJ, eds. *Handbook of Pharmaceutical Excipients.* 4th ed. Washington, DC: American Pharmaceutical Association; 2003:521-523.
162. Wilson KC, Reardon C, Farber HW. Propylene glycol toxicity in a patient receiving intravenous diazepam. *N Engl J Med.* 2000;343:815.
163. Wilson KC, Reardon C, Theodore AC, Farber HW. Propylene glycol toxicity: a severe iatrogenic illness in ICU patients receiving IV benzodiazepines. a case series and prospective, observational pilot study. *Chest.* 2005; 128:1674-1681.
164. Winder AF, Astbury NJ, Sheraidah GA, Ruben M. Penetration of mercury from ophthalmologic preservatives into the human eye. *Lancet.* 1980;2:237-239.
165. World Health Organization Global Advisory Committee on Vaccine Safety. Statement on Thiomersal. Geneva, Switzerland; August 2003. http://www.who.int/vaccine_safety/topics/thiomersal/statement200308/en/print.html. Accessed December 4, 2004.
166. Wright CG, Bird LL, Meyerhoff WL. Tympanic membrane microstructure in experimental cholesteatoma. *Acta Otolaryngol.* 1991;111: 101-111.
167. Yahwak JA, Riker RR, Fraser GL, Subak-Sharpe S. Determination of a lorazepam dose threshold for using the osmol gap to monitor for propylene glycol toxicity. *Pharmacotherapy.* 2008;28:984-991.
168. Yaucher NE, Fish JF, Smith HW, et al. Propylene glycol-associated renal toxicity from lorazepam infusion. *Pharmacotherapy.* 2003;23: 1094-1099.
169. Yorgin PD, Theodorou AA, Al-Uzri A, et al. Propylene glycolinduced proximal tubule cell injury. *Am J Kidney Dis.* 1997;30:134-139.
170. Zar T, Yusufzai I, Sullivan A, Graeber C. Acute kidney injury, hyperosmolality and metabolic acidosis associated with lorazepam. *Nat Clin Pract Nephrol.* 2007;3:515-520.
171. Zoneraich S, Zoneraich O, Siegel, J. Sudden death following intravenous sodium diphenylhydantoin. *Am Heart J.* 1976;91:375-377.

D.

ANTIMICROBIALS

CHAPTER 56

ANTIBACTERIALS, ANTIFUNGALS, AND ANTIVIRALS

Christine M. Stork

Antimicrobials in the forms of antibacterials, antifungals, and antivirals have added significantly to the clinical care of infected patients since the introduction of penicillin in the 1940s. The development of drug-resistant strains of these pathogens has greatly expanded the number of antimicrobials necessary, and this has increased the overall potential for toxicity after use. Fortunately, toxicity due to acute overdose and even chronic therapeutic doses does not preclude their appropriate use in the majority of patients.

HISTORY AND EPIDEMIOLOGY

The majority of the adverse effects related to antimicrobials occur as a result of iatrogenic complications rather than intentional overdose. The diverse origins of these complications include dosing, route and decision errors, allergic reactions, adverse drug effects, and drug-drug interactions. Prevention in the form of process improvements and information regarding populations at risk for adverse drug effects is required to minimize these untoward events. Dosing errors are common in neonates and infants, necessitating careful and constant diligence on the part of all healthcare providers.

Antimicrobials are more commonly associated with anaphylactic reactions than are other xenobiotics. The reason for this is unclear, but it may be a result of their high frequency of use, repeated interrupted exposures caused by intermittent prescriptive use, or environmental contamination. A complete and clear allergy history is essential to minimize these adverse events in patients being considered for antimicrobial therapy.

Many adverse effects attributed to antimicrobials are difficult to predict even when given patient- and population-specific parameters. In some cases, a diluent or an excipient is responsible for the adverse effect, as recognized with the use of procaine penicillin G in patients with procaine allergy. Antimicrobials are involved in many of the common and severe drug interactions, primarily through the inhibition of metabolic enzymes. Patients being considered for antimicrobial therapy should be carefully assessed for the use of concomitant drug therapy that may be pharmacokinetically or pharmacodynamically affected by the chosen antimicrobial.

PHARMACOLOGY AND TOXICOLOGY

Antimicrobial pharmacology is aimed at the destruction of microorganisms through the inhibition of cell-cycle reproduction or the altering of a critical function within a microorganism. Table 56–1 lists antimicrobials and their associated mechanisms of activity. Often the mechanisms for toxicologic effects following acute overdose differ from the therapeutic mechanisms. Table 56–1 also lists the toxicologic effects and related mechanisms. Table 56–2 lists the pharmacokinetics of each class of drugs.

ANTIBACTERIALS

AMINOGLYCOSIDES

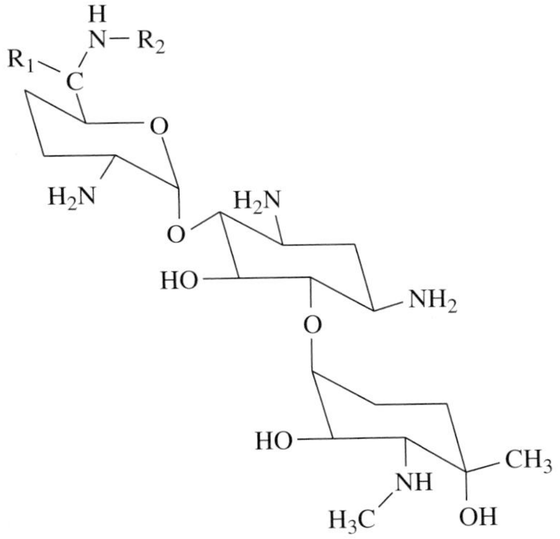

H
N— R_2
R_1 C
O
H_2N H_2N
O
HO NH_2
O
HO CH_3
NH
H_3C OH

Gentamicin C_1: $R_1 = R_2 = CH_3$
Gentamicin C_2: $R_1 = CH_3$, $R_2 = H$
Gentamicin C_{1a}: $R_1 = R_2 = H$

Aminoglycoside antimicrobials that are in current use in the United States include amikacin, gentamicin, kanamycin, neomycin, netilmicin, streptomycin, and tobramycin.

Since aminoglycosides are only available in parenteral, topical, and ophthalmic forms, overdoses are almost exclusively the result of dosing errors. Fortunately, overdoses are rarely life threatening, and most patients can be safely managed with minimal intervention.[28,136] The adverse effects of aminoglycosides are generally class based, although subtle differences may exist in the potency with which the adverse effects occur (Table 56–3).

Large intravenous doses of aminoglycosides are both sufficiently effective and safe for use in single daily doses.[4] Rarely, acute aminoglycoside overdose results in nephrotoxicity, ototoxicity, or vestibular toxicity.[131,157] In one reported case, postmortem analysis confirmed complete loss of hair cells in the inner and outer cochlear (Chap. 20).

TABLE 56–1. Antimicrobial Pharmacology and Adverse Effects

Antimicrobial	Antimicrobial Mechanism of Action	Acute Overdose	Chronic Administration
Antibacterials			
Aminoglycosides	Inhibits 30s ribosomal subunit	Neuromuscular blockade—inhibits the release of acetylcholine from presynaptic nerve terminals and acts as an antagonist at acetylcholine receptors	*Nephrotoxicity/ototoxicity*—forms an iron complex that inhibits mitochondrial respiration and causes lipid peroxidation
Penicillins, cephalosporins, and other β-lactams	Inhibits cell wall mucopeptide synthesis	Seizures—agonist at picrotoxin binding site causing GABA antagonism	*Hypersensitivity*—immune *Other*—see text
Chloramphenicol	Inhibits 50s ribosomal subunit and inhibits protein synthesis in rapidly dividing cells	Cardiovascular collapse	"Gray baby syndrome" Same as mechanism of action
Fluoroquinolones	Inhibits DNA topoisomerase and DNA gyrase	Same as mechanism of action; binds to cations (Mg^{2+}), seizures	Not entirely known; binds to cations (Mg^{2+}), tendon rupture, hyper- and hypoglycemia
Linezolid	Inhibits bacterial protein synthesis through inhibition of *N*-formylmethionyl-t RNA	None clinically relevant	MAOI activity: vasopressor response to tyramine; serotonin syndrome with SSRI and possibly meperidine
Macrolides, lincosamides, and ketolides	Inhibit 50s ribosomal subunit in multiplying cells	Prolong QT; block delayed rectifier potassium channel	Not entirely known; cytotoxic effect; exacerbation of myasthenia gravis
Nitrofurantoin	Bacterial enzymatic inhibitor	Gastritis	Dermatologic, hematologic, pancreatitis, partotitis, hepatitis, crystaluria, pulmonary fibrosis
Sulfonamides	Inhibit *para*-aminobenzoic acid and/or *para*-amino glutamic acid in the synthesis of folic acid	None clinically relevant	*Hypersensitivity*—metabolite acts as hapten leading to hemolysis/methemoglobinemia—exposure to UVB causes free radical formation
Tetracycline	Inhibits 30s and 50s ribosomal subunits; binds to aminoacyl transfer RNA	None clinically relevant	Unknown
Vancomycin	Inhibits glycopeptidase polymerase in cell wall synthesis	"Red-man syndrome"—anaphylactoid	Unknown
Antifungal			
Amphotericin B	Binds with ergosterol on cytoplasmic membrane to cause pores to facilitate organelle leak	Same as mechanism of action	*Nephrotoxicity*—vehicle deoxycholate may be involved; nephrocalcinosis
Triazoles and imidazoles	Increases permeability of cell membranes	None clinically relevant	None clinically relevant ?CYP inhibition

γ-aminobutyric acid; MAOI, monoamine oxidase inhibitor; SSRI, selective serotonin reuptake inhibitor; UVB, ultraviolet B.

Aminoglycosides may exacerbate neuromuscular blockade, particularly at times corresponding to high-peak serum aminoglycoside concentrations (Chap. 68).[187] Aminoglycosides inhibit the release of acetylcholine from presynaptic nerve terminals by antagonism of the aminoglycoside of the presynaptic calcium channel. Risk factors for enhanced neuromuscular blockade include patients with abnormal neuromuscular junction function, such as those with myasthenia gravis and botulism.

Adverse Effects Associated With Therapeutic Use Adverse effects, including nephrotoxicity and ototoxicity, correlate more closely with elevated trough serum concentrations than with elevated peak concentrations.[120,166] Less common adverse effects associated with chronic use include electrolyte abnormalities, allergic reactions, hepatotoxicity, anemia, granulocytopenia, thrombocytopenia, eosinophilia, retinal toxicity, reproductive dysfunction, tetany, and psychosis.[62,125,142,229,244] When aminoglycosides are administered at high doses or during once-daily dosing, sepsis-like reactions, including chills and malaise, can occur.[51] This is likely a result of excipients that are delivered to the patient during the infusion.

Nephrotoxicity The mechanism of nephrotoxicity and ototoxicity is incompletely understood, but appears to include the formation of reactive oxygen species in the presence of iron. Mitochondrial respiration is inhibited, lipid peroxidation occurs, and stimulation of

TABLE 56–2. Antimicrobial Pharmacokinetics

Xenobiotic	Absorption	Volume of Distribution (L/kg)	Elimination Route	$t_{1/2}$ (h)
Antibacterial				
Aminoglycosides	Parenteral	0.25	Renal	2–3
Penicillins, cephalosporins, and other β-lactams	Oral, parenteral	Variable	Renal (predominant)	Variable
Chloramphenicol	Oral, parenteral, otic	0.5–1.0	90% hepatic, 10% renal	1.6–3.3
Fluoroquinolones	Oral, parenteral	Variable	Renal	3–5
Ketolides	Oral	2.9 L/kg	63% renal, 37% hepatic (50% of which is CYP3A4)	10–13
Macrolides	Oral, parenteral	Variable	Hepatic	Variable
Sulfonamides	Oral, parenteral	Variable	Hepatic	Variable
Tetracyclines	Oral	Variable	Hepatic	6–26
Vancomycin	Parenteral	0.2–1.25	Renal	4–6
Antifungal				
Triazoles and imidazoles	Oral	Variable	Hepatic	Variable
Amphotericin B	Parenteral	4.0	Hepatic	360
Antiviral				
Acyclovir	Parenteral, oral, topical	0.8	Renal	2.2–20

glutamate activated *N*-methyl-D-aspartate (NMDA) receptors may play a role.[108,253] The incidence of nephrotoxicity with aminoglycoside therapy is estimated at 5% to 10%.[9] Although the aminoglycosides are almost completely excreted prior to biotransformation in the kidney, a small fraction of filtered aminoglycoside is transported by absorptive endocytosis across the apical membrane of proximal tubular cells where it becomes sequestered within lysosomes. The aminoglycoside then binds to and destroys phospholipids contained on brush border membranes in the proximal renal tubule.[9]

When this happens, acute tubular necrosis occurs after 7 to 10 days of standard-dose therapy. Laboratory abnormalities include granular casts, proteinuria, elevated urinary sodium, and increased fractional excretion of sodium. Usually renal dysfunction is reversible; however, irreversible toxicity is reported. Functional renal injury occurs days prior to elevations in serum creatinine concentration, and for this reason a delay in diagnosis is common.[217] Risk factors for the development of nephrotoxicity include increasing age, renal dysfunction, female sex, previous aminoglycoside therapy, liver dysfunction, large total dose, long duration of therapy, frequent doses, high trough concentrations, presence of other nephrotoxic drugs, and shock.[9,170] Because the uptake of aminoglycosides into organs is saturable, appropriate once-daily high-dose regimens are less problematic than several lesser doses given in a single day.

TABLE 56–3. Predominant Aminoglycoside Toxicity

Cochlear	Cochlear and Vestibular	Vestibular	Renal
Kanamycin	Amikacin	Streptomycin	Amikacin
Neomycin	Gentamicin		Gentamicin
	Tobramycin		Kanamycin
			Neomycin
			Streptomycin
			Tobramycin

Ototoxicity Ototoxicity can occur after acute or prolonged exposure to aminoglycosides.[105] Both cochlear and vestibular dysfunction are correlated with high trough aminoglycoside concentrations. Because aminoglycosides bioaccumulate in the endolymph and perilymph spaces, they have prolonged contact time with sensory hair cells. Vestibular toxicity, caused by destruction of sensory receptor portions of the inner ear or destruction of hair cells in the utricle and saccule, occurs in 0.4% to 10% of patients. Symptoms include vertigo or tinnitus. Table 56–3 details the relative characteristic toxicity of various aminoglycosides.

Full-tone audiometric testing may first show high-frequency hearing loss, which may subsequently progress. Given the inability of cochlear hair cells to regenerate, all hearing loss that develops is permanent. Electronystagmography is the diagnostic tool of choice for vestibular dysfunction, and up to 63% of patients with early findings of vestibular dysfunction may improve after discontinuation of the drug.[124] Simultaneous administration of other ototoxic xenobiotics enhances the ototoxicity of aminoglycosides (Chap. 20).

Withdrawal of the offending xenobiotic is indicated in patients with either nephrotoxicity or ototoxicity caused by an aminoglycoside antibiotic. Supportive care is the mainstay of therapy. Experimental treatments in animal models include the use of deferoxamine, glutathione, and NMDA receptor antagonists in an attempt to chelate and/or detoxify a reactive intermediate.[181,231] The antibiotic ticarcillin forms a renally eliminated complex with aminoglycosides in the blood to provide protection against tobramycin-induced renal toxicity. In humans, ticarcillin removes 50% more tobramycin in 48 hours than two hemodialysis sessions.[79] However, ticarcillin therapy is generally of limited value because in most instances the serum concentration of the aminoglycoside has decreased before any therapeutic measures can be used. The use of ticarcillin should be considered only early after large overdose in patients with either demonstrated toxicity or renal failure where the risks of toxicity are significant.

PENICILLINS

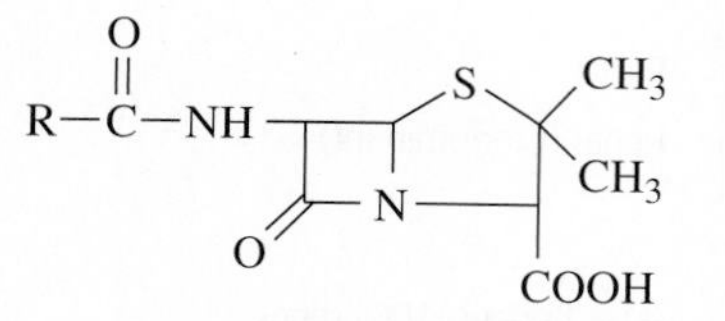

$$\mathrm{R{-}C(=O){-}NH}\text{–[β-lactam ring fused to thiazolidine ring with S, N, } CH_3, CH_3, COOH]$$

Penicillin nucleus

Penicillin is derived from the fungus *Penicillium* and many semisynthetic derivatives have clinical utility. Penicillins, as a class, contain a 6-aminopenicillanic acid nucleus, composed of a β-lactam ring fused to a five-member thiazolidine ring. Classic available penicillins include penicillin G, penicillin V, and the antistaphylococcal penicillins (nafcillin, oxacillin, cloxacillin, and dicloxacillin). Penicillins developed to enhance the spectrum of antibiotic efficacy, particularly against gram-negative bacilli, include the second-generation penicillins (ampicillin, amoxicillin, bacampicillin, and mezlocillin), third-generation penicillins (carbenicillin and ticarcillin), and fourth-generation penicillins (piperacillin). Table 56–1 lists the pharmacologic mechanism of penicillins and Table 56–2 lists their pharmacokinetic properties.

Acute oral overdoses of penicillin-containing drugs are usually not life threatening.[237] The most frequent complaints following acute overdose are nausea, vomiting, and diarrhea.

Seizures occur in persons given large intravenous or intraventricular doses of penicillins.[40,127,139,164] More than 50 million units intravenously in less than 8 hours are generally required to produce seizures in adults.[222] Penicillin-induced seizures appear to be mediated through an interaction of the drug with the picrotoxin-binding site on the neuronal chloride channel near the γ-aminobutyric acid (GABA) binding site (Chap. 13). Binding of the penicillin produces an allosteric change in the receptor that prevents GABA from binding, resulting in a relative lack of inhibitory tone.[66] Penicillin analogs (such as imipenem) also cause seizures, presumably through a similar mechanism.

Treatment of patients who develop penicillin-induced seizures include GABA agonists such as the benzodiazepines and barbiturates, if needed. Patients who receive an intraventricular overdose may require cerebrospinal fluid exchange or perfusion to attenuate seizure activity (see Special Considerations SC 2: Intrathecal Administration of Xenobiotics).[139] There are rare reports of hyperkalemia resulting in electrocardiographic abnormalities after the rapid intravenous infusion of potassium penicillin G to patients with renal failure and amoxicillin overdose resulting in frank hematuria and renal failure.[37,94] There is also a single case report of penicillin-associated hearing loss.[33]

Adverse Effects Associated With Therapeutic Use Penicillins are associated with a myriad of adverse effects after therapeutic use, the most common of which are allergic reactions. Penicillins are commonly implicated in immune-related reactions such as bone marrow suppression, cholestasis, hemolysis, interstitial nephritis, and vasculitis.[6,92,114,230] Rare effects include pemphigus after penicillin use and corneal damage after the use of methicillin.[23,263]

Acute Allergy Penicillins are the pharmaceuticals most commonly implicated in the development of acute anaphylactic reactions. Anaphylactic reactions are severe life-threatening immune-mediated (IgE) reactions involving multiple organ systems that occur most often immediately after exposure to a trigger. Table 56–4 lists the classifications of anaphylactic reactions. Anaphylaxis to penicillin typically occurs after IgE antibody formation, which requires prior exposure. Life-threatening clinical manifestations include angioedema, tongue and airway swelling, bronchospasm, bronchorrhea, dysrhythmias, cardiovascular collapse, and cardiac arrest.[80] The pathophysiology of systemic anaphylaxis is complex and involves multiple pathways. IgE antibodies are cross-linked on the surface of mast cells and basophils, resulting in local and systemic release of preformed mediators of anaphylactic response, including leukotrienes C_4 and D_4, histamine, eosinophilic chemotactic factor, and other vasoactive substances, such as bradykinin, kallikrein, prostaglandin D_2, and platelet-activating factor.

TABLE 56–4. Classification of Anaphylactic Reactions

Grade	Description
I	Large local contiguous reaction (>15 cm)
II	Pruritus (urticaria) generalized
III	Asthma, angioedema, nausea, vomiting
IV	Airway (asthma, lingual swelling, dysphagia, respiratory distress, laryngeal edema)
	Cardiovascular (hypotension, cardiovascular collapse)

The incidence of penicillin hypersensitivity is 5% overall, with 1% of penicillin reactions resulting in anaphylaxis. The risk for a fatal hypersensitivity reaction after penicillin administration is two per 100,000 (0.002%) patient exposures.[251] All routes of penicillin administration can result in anaphylaxis; however, it occurs most commonly after intravenous administration.

Treatment is supportive with careful attention to airway, breathing, and circulation. If the penicillin was ingested, the patient may theoretically benefit from oral activated charcoal 1 g/kg. This is unlikely to prevent anaphylaxis, as only a few molecules need be absorbed to trigger the immunologic response. Initial drug therapy for anaphylaxis includes epinephrine 0.01 mg/Kg (up to 0.5 mL) of 1:1000 dilution subcutaneously (SC) every 10 to 20 minutes. Through β-receptor stimulation, epinephrine bronchodilates and increases cardiac output. In addition, β-receptor stimulation results in decreased peripheral vascular tone. Oxygen and inhaled β_2-adrenergic agonists are warranted in severe cases, as are corticosteroids. H_1-receptor antagonists may be sufficient in patients with mild allergic reactions who do not have pulmonary manifestations or airway concerns.

H_2-receptor antagonism as a treatment for anaphylaxis is controversial. H_2-receptors, when stimulated in the peripheral vasculature, cause vasodilation; in the heart, they cause positive inotropy, positive chronotropy, and coronary vasodilation; and in the lung, they cause increased mucus production.[212] Theoretically, H_2-receptor antagonists can lead to a decrease in myocardial activity at a time when H_1-receptor stimulation is causing hypotension, coronary vasoconstriction, and bronchospasm. However, in vitro and animal models demonstrate decreases in coronary circulation and decreases in the overall anaphylactic response following administration of H_1 blockers.[16,27] Cimetidine and ranitidine are useful for the treatment of pruritus and flushing after acute allergic reactions involving the skin.[154,168] Cimetidine use following anaphylaxis may result in clinical improvement, particularly hypotension and tachycardia.[72,264] There is one case, however, of chronic ranitidine administration, which was postulated to result in heart block after an anaphylactic response to latex.[189] Available data indicate that treatment using H_2-receptor antagonists should only be considered when other therapies have failed and the patient is adequately H_1-receptor blocked. Aminophylline, although mentioned in some references for the treatment of anaphylaxis, is inadequately studied and should not be routinely used. Finally, glucagon may be of some benefit, particularly in patients who are maintained on β-adrenergic antagonists (Chap. 61 and A-19).

Amoxicillin-Clavulanic Acid and Hepatitis Cholestatic hepatitis occurs 1 to 6 weeks after initiation of therapy with amoxicillin-clavulanate.[7] The incidence of hepatotoxicity typically is estimated at 1.1 to 2.7 per 100,000 prescriptions.[91] The mechanism of hepatotoxicity is not clear, but may be related to clavulanate, a β-lactamase inhibitor used to prevent the bacterial destruction of β-lactam antimicrobials, or one of its metabolites. Treatment is supportive and clinical findings typically resolve after the discontinuation of therapy. However, prolonged hepatitis, ductopenia (vanishing bile duct syndrome), and pancreatitis rarely occur.[53,199] Behavorial disturbance with disorientation, agitation, and visual hallucinations is also reported temporally related to use.[19]

Hoigne Syndrome and Jarisch-Herxheimer Reaction The most common adverse effects occurring after administration of large intramuscular or intravenous doses of procaine penicillin G are the Hoigne syndrome and the Jarisch-Herxheimer reaction.[12,90,102,122,163] Hoigne syndrome is characterized by extreme apprehension and fear, illusions, or hallucinations; changes in auditory and visual perception; tachycardia; systolic hypertension; and, occasionally, seizures that begin within minutes of injection.[250] These effects occur in the absence of signs or symptoms of anaphylaxis. The cause of this syndrome is unknown. Procaine is implicated as the causative agent because of this syndrome's similarity to events that occur after the administration of other pharmacologically similar local anesthetics.[214,223,246] Hoigne syndrome is six times more common in men than women.[226] The reason for this increased prevalence is unclear, but autosomal dominance and influences of prostaglandin and thromboxane A_2 activity in this population may be responsible.[12]

The Jarisch-Herxheimer reaction is a self-limited reaction that develops within a few hours of antibiotic therapy for the treatment of early syphilis or Lyme disease. Clinical findings include myalgias, chills, headache, rash, and fever, which spontaneously resolve within 18 to 24 hours, even with continued antibiotic therapy.[169] The pathogenesis of this reaction is likely an acute antigen release by lysed bacteria.[178]

CEPHALOSPORINS

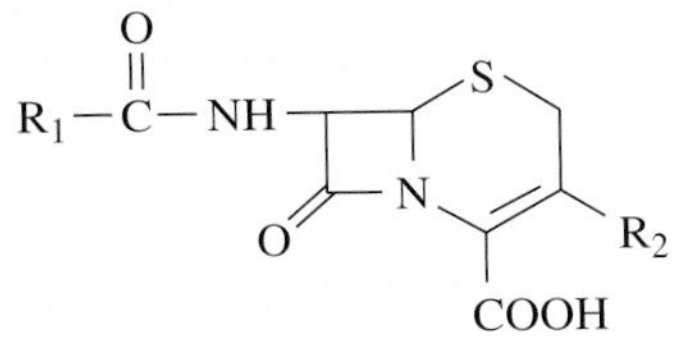

Cephem nucleus

Cephalosporins are semisynthetic derivatives of cephalosporin C produced by the fungus *Acremonium*, previously called *Cephalosporium*. Cephalosporins have a ring structure similar to that of penicillins. Cephalosporins are generally divided into first, second, third, and fourth generations based on their antimicrobial spectrum. First-generation cephalosporins include cefadroxil, cefazolin, cephalexin, cephapirin, and cephradine. Second-generation cephalosporins include cefaclor, cefamandole, cefonicid, cefotetan, cefoxitin, cefprozil, and cefuroxime. Third-generation cephalosporins include cefdinir, ceftazidime, cefixime, ceftibuten, cefoperazone, ceftizoxime, cefotaxime, ceftriaxone, and cefpodoxime. Finally, of the fourth-generation cephalosporins, cefepime was the first to be marketed.

Effects occurring after acute overdose of cephalosporins resemble those occurring after penicillin exposure. Some cephalosporins also have epileptogenic potential similar to penicillin.[255] Case reports demonstrate seizures after inadvertent intraventricular administration.[39,146,265] Management of cephalosporin overdose is similar to that of penicillin overdose. Table 56–1 lists the pharmacologic mechanism of cephalosporins and Table 56–2 lists their pharmacokinetic properties.

Adverse Effects Associated With Therapeutic Use Cephalosporins rarely cause an immune-mediated acute hemolytic crisis.[78] Cefaclor is the cephalosporin most commonly reported to cause serum sickness, although this can occur with other cephalosporins.[132,156] Also like penicillins, first-generation cephalosporins are associated with chronic toxicity, including interstitial nephritis and hepatitis.[262] Cefepime is reported in a single case to cause reversible coma and electroencephalogram (EEG) confirmed nonconvulsive seizures.[2]

Cross-Hypersensitivity The cephalosporins contain a six-member dihydrithiazine ring instead of the five-member thiazolidine penicillin ring. The extent of cross-reactivity between penicillins and cephalosporins in an individual patient is largely determined by the type of penicillin allergic response experienced by the patient. The incidence of anaphylaxis to cephalosporins is between 0.0001% and 0.1%, with a threefold increase in patients with previous penicillin allergy.[133] Ten percent of patients with prior penicillin-related anaphylactic reactions will have positive skin test for cephalosporin hypersensitivity.[205] A negative skin test predicts a negative allergic response on oral cephalosporin challenge in penicillin-allergic patients. Finally, the incidence of delayed hypersensitivity reactions after cephalosporin use is 1% to 2.8% in the general population and 8.1% in those with prior penicillin delayed hypersensitivity. Cross-reactivity may be greater with the first- and second-generation cephalosporins that are more structurally similar to penicillin or that are contaminated by penicillin.[8] Antibody binding after cephalosporin exposure occurs at the determinants located on the side-chain groups of the cephalosporin.[14] In fact, IgE directed against a methylene substituent linking the side chain to the penicillin molecule is identified.[107] These determinants are quite distinct among cephalosporins, which cause the pattern of cross-hypersensitivity among cephalosporins to be much less well defined than among the penicillins. Caution should be used when considering cephalosporins in penicillin- or cephalosporin-allergic patients; however, if a risk-to-benefit analysis demonstrates a clear benefit to the patient without equivalent alternatives, the cephalosporin should be given.

***N*-methylthiotetrazole Side-Chain Effects** Cephalosporins containing an *N*-methylthiotetrazole (nMTT) side chain (moxalactam, cefazolin, cefoperazone, cefmetazole, cefamandole, cefotetan) have toxic effects unique to their group structure. As these cephalosporins undergo metabolism, they release free nMTT, which is responsible for their effects (Fig. 56–1).[165] Free nMTT inhibits the enzyme aldehyde dehydrogenase and, in conjunction with ethanol, can cause a disulfiram-like reaction (Chap. 79).[43]

The nMTT side chain is also associated with hypoprothrombinemia, although a causal relationship is controversial.[101] It is thought that nMTT depletes vitamin K-dependent clotting factors by inhibition of vitamin K epoxide reductase.[183] In a study of children 1 month to 1 year of age who were maintained on a prolonged antibiotic regimen, a significant degree of vitamin K depletion was found.[25] Treatment of patients suspected of hypoprothrombinemia caused by these cephalosporins consists of fresh-frozen plasma, if bleeding is evident, and vitamin K_1 in doses required to resynthesize vitamin K cofactors (Chap. 59).

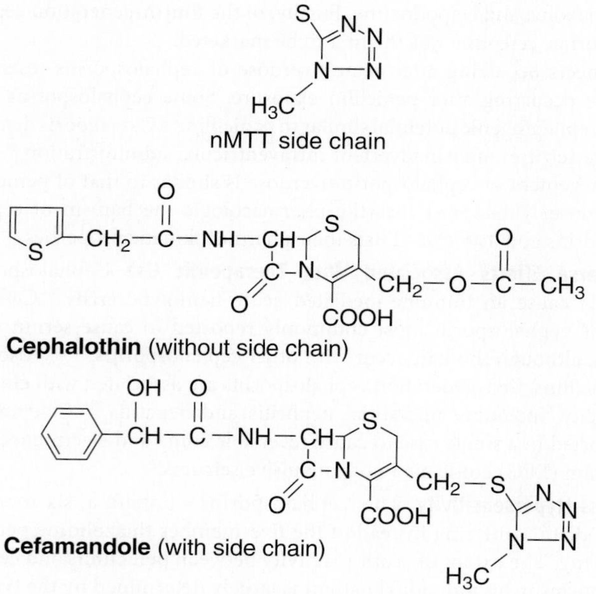

nMTT side chain

Cephalothin (without side chain)

Cefamandole (with side chain)

FIGURE 56-1. Characteristic structures of cephalosporins emphasizing the nMTT side chain.

OTHER β-LACTAM ANTIMICROBIALS

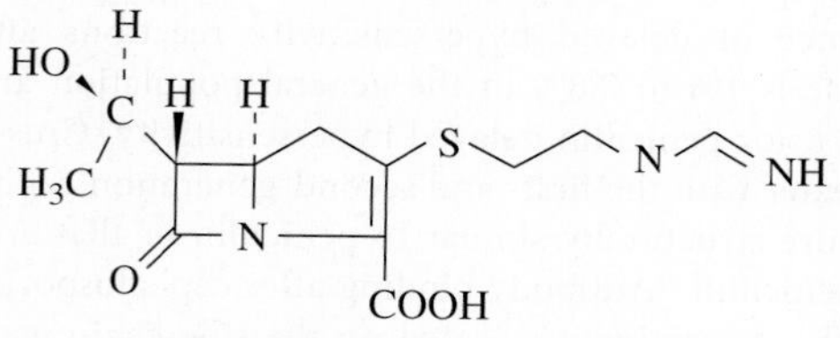

Imipenem

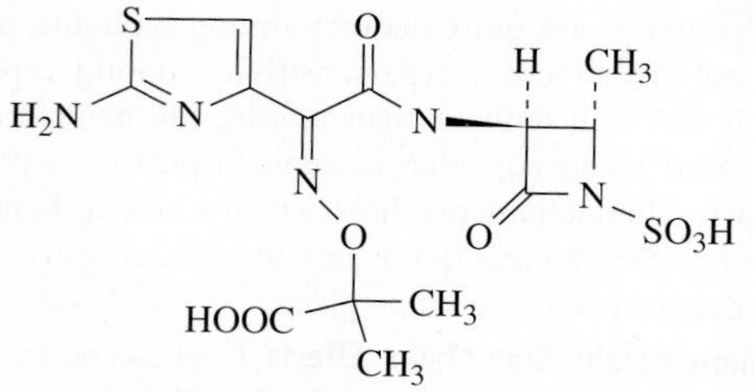

Aztreonam

Included in this group are monobactams such as aztreonam and carbapenems such as imipenem and meropenem. Table 56–1 lists the pharmacologic mechanism of these drugs, and Table 56–2 lists their pharmacokinetic properties.

Effects occurring after acute overdose of other β-lactam antimicrobials resemble those occurring after penicillin exposure. Imipenem has epileptogenic potential in both overdose and therapeutic dosing (see section Adverse Effects Associated With Therapeutic Use).[48,148] Management guidelines for other β-lactam overdoses are similar to those for penicillin overdoses.

Adverse Effects Associated With Therapeutic Use The risk factors for imipenem-related seizures include central nervous system disease, prior seizure disorders, and abnormal renal function.[190] The mechanism for seizures appears to be GABA antagonism (similar to the penicillins) in conjunction with enhanced activity of excitatory amino acids.[67,235]

Cross-Hypersensitivity Aztreonam is a monobactam that does not contain the antigenic components required for cross-allergy with penicillins, and generalized cross-allergenicity is not expected.[215] However, aztreonam cross-reacts in vitro with ceftriaxone, thought to be the result of the similarity in their side-chain structure.[192] Cross-allergenicity has also been noted between imipenem and penicillin, although the incidence has yet to be determined.

TRIMETHOPRIM-SULFAMETHOXAZOLE

Trimethoprim and sulfamethoxazole work as antibacterials in tandem effectively preventing tetrahydrofolic acid synthesis in bacterial cells. Significant toxicity after acute overdose is not expected; however, a myrid of effects occur after chronic therapeutic use. Trimethoprim/sulfamethoxazole combinations are commonly reported to result in cutaneous allergic reactions, hematologic disorders, methemoglobinemia, hypoglycemia, rhabdomyolysis, and psychosis.[134,135,234,254,260]

CHLORAMPHENICOL

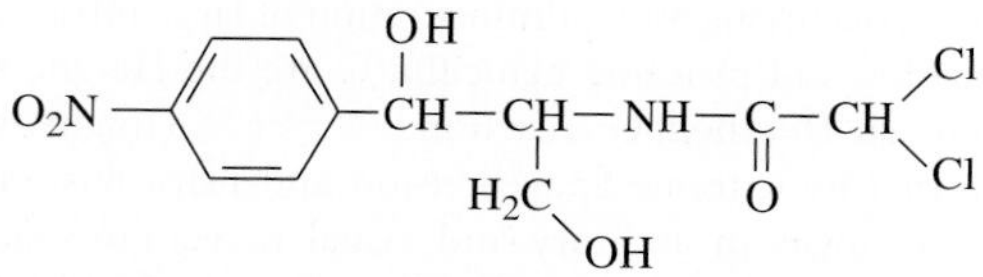

Chloramphenicol was originally derived from *Streptomyces venezuelae* and is now produced synthetically. Antimicrobial activity exists against many gram-positive and gram-negative aerobes and anaerobes. Table 56–1 lists the pharmacologic mechanism of chloramphenicol, and Table 56–2 lists its pharmacokinetic properties.

Acute overdose of chloramphenicol commonly causes nausea and vomiting. Effects are caused by its ability to inhibit protein synthesis in rapidly proliferating cells. Metabolic acidosis occurs as a result of the inhibition of mitochondrial enzymes, oxidative phosphorylation, and mitochondrial biogenesis.[88] Infrequently, sudden cardiovascular collapse can occur 5 to 12 hours after acute overdoses. In case series, cardiovascular compromise was more frequent in patients with serum concentrations greater than 50 μg/mL.[88,172,242] Because concentrations are not readily available, all poisoned patients should be closely observed for at least 12 hours after exposure. Orogastric lavage may be useful for recent ingestions when the patient has not vomited, and activated charcoal 1 g/kg should be given orally.

Extracorporeal means of eliminating chloramphenicol are not usually required because of its rapid metabolism (see Table 56–2). However, both hemodialysis and charcoal hemoperfusion decrease elevated serum chloramphenicol concentrations and may be of benefit in patients with large overdoses, or in patients with severe hepatic or renal dysfunction.[87,167,227] Exchange transfusion also lowers chloramphenicol serum concentrations in neonates.[233] Surviving patients should be closely monitored for signs of bone marrow suppression.

Adverse Effects Associated With Therapeutic Use Chronic toxicity of chloramphenicol is similar to that which occurs following acute poisoning. The classic description of chronic chloramphenicol toxicity is the "gray baby syndrome."[87,88,167,233] Children with this syndrome exhibit vomiting, anorexia, respiratory distress, abdominal distension, green stools, lethargy, cyanosis, ashen color, metabolic acidosis, hypotension, and cardiovascular collapse.

The majority (90%) of a dose of chloramphenicol is metabolized via glucuronyl transferase, forming a glucuronide conjugate. The remainder is excreted renally unchanged. Infants, in particular, are predisposed to the gray baby syndrome because they have a limited capacity to form a glucuronide conjugate of chloramphenicol and, concomitantly, a limited ability to excrete unconjugated chloramphenicol in the urine.[97,261]

There are two types of bone marrow suppression that occur after use of chloramphenicol. The most common type is dose dependent and occurs with high serum concentrations of chloramphenicol.[118,119,221] Clinical manifestations usually occur within several weeks of therapy and include anemia, thrombocytopenia, leukopenia, and very rarely, aplastic anemia. Bone marrow suppression is generally reversible on discontinuation of therapy. A second type of bone marrow suppression caused by chloramphenicaol occurs through this inhibition of protein synthesis in the mitochondria of marrow cell lines.[175] This type causes the development of aplastic anemia, which is not dose related and generally occurs in susceptible patients within 5 months of treatment and has an approximately 50% mortality rate (Chap. 24).[77,268] The dehydro and nitroso bacterial metabolites of chloramphenicol injure human bone marrow cells through inhibition of myeloid colony growth, inhibition of DNA synthesis, and inhibition of mitochondrial protein synthesis.[129]

Other adverse effects associated with chloramphenicol include peripheral neuropathy[195]; neurologic abnormalities, such as confusion and delirium[150]; optic neuritis[59]; nonlymphocytic leukemia[225]; and contact dermatitis.[140]

FLUOROQUINOLONES

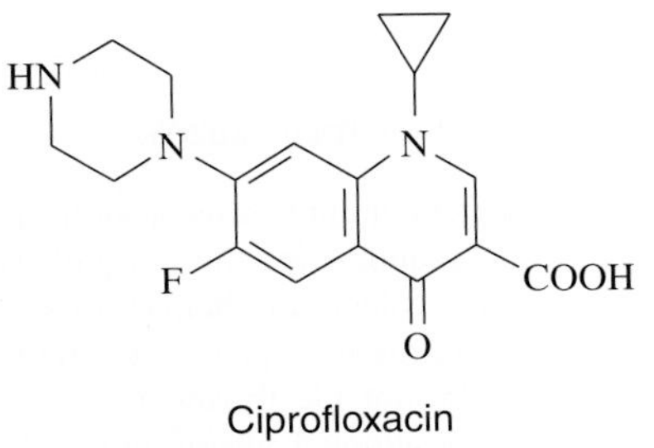

Ciprofloxacin

The fluoroquinolones are a structurally similar, synthetically derived group of antimicrobials that have diverse antimicrobial activities. They include balofloxacin, ciprofloxacin, clinafloxacin, enoxacin, fleroxacin, gatifloxacin, gemifloxacin, grepafloxacin, levofloxacin, lomefloxacin, moxifloxacin, nadifloxacin, nalidixic acid, norfloxacin, ofloxacin, pefloxacin, rufloxacin, sparfloxacin, temafloxacin, tosufloxacin, and trovafloxacin. Like other antimicrobials, the fluoroquinolones rarely produce life-threatening effects following acute overdose, and most patients can be safely managed with minimal intervention.[11] Table 56–1 lists the pharmacologic mechanism of fluoroquinolones, and Table 56–2 lists their pharmacokinetic properties.

Rarely, acute overdose of a fluoroquinolone results in renal failure or seizures.[143] The mechanism of renal failure after fluoroquinolone exposure is controversial. In animals, ciprofloxacin and norfloxacin cause nephrotoxicity, especially in the setting of neutral or alkaline urine.[61,218] In humans, renal failure is reported after both acute and chronic exposure to fluoroquinolones. A hypersensitivity reaction is postulated to explain pathologic changes consistent with interstitial nephritis.[116,202] Treatment includes discontinuation of the fluoroquinolone and supportive care. Improvement in renal function is usually noticed within several days.

Seizures are reported with ciprofloxacin and may be a result of the inhibition of GABA.[228,245] Others postulate that seizures result from the ability of fluoroquinolones to bind efficiently to cations, particularly magnesium. This hypothesis is related to the inhibitory role of magnesium at the excitatory NMDA-gated ion channel (Chap. 13).[68,219] Treatment is supportive, using benzodiazepines and, if necessary, barbiturates to increase inhibitory tone.

Adverse Effects Associated With Therapeutic Use Several fluoroquinolones are substrates and/or inhibitors of cytochrome CYP isozymes. This can result in drug interactions, which are especially important with drugs that have a narrow therapeutic index.

Serious adverse effects related to fluoroquinolone use consist of central nervous system toxicity, as discussed, cardiovascular toxicity,[126] hepatotoxicity, and notable musculoskeletal toxicity.

Fluoroquinolones cause prolongation of the QT interval and may cause torsades de pointes.[40,126,213] Although the mechanism is unclear, sequestering of magnesium, resulting in clinical hypomagnesemia, is postulated.[219] Treatment of patients presenting with QT prolongation is supportive, with careful attention to magnesium supplementation if necessary.

The fluoroquinolones rarely result in potentially fatal hepatotoxicity.[54,89,99,144,158,206] This adverse effect is most notable with trovafloxacin. In vitro models show trovafloxacin to be uniquely capable of altering gene expression that regulates oxidative stress and RNA processing leading to mitochondrial damage.[152] Consequently, trovafloxacin (Trovan) is now reserved only for the treatment of patients with life-threatening infections in whom the benefits are thought to outweigh the risks. In addition, the manufacturer has initiated a limited distribution system that allows drug shipment only to pharmacies within inpatient healthcare facilities.

Fluoroquinolones should be used with caution in children and pregnant women because of their potential adverse effects on developing cartilage and bone. Damage to articular cartilage is demonstrated in young dogs and rats, although the extent varies among different fluoroquinolones.[45,238] There are very limited data regarding damage to articular cartilage as a result of using fluoroquinolones in humans; however, children given ciprofloxacin on a compassionate basis developed complaints of swollen, painful, and stiff joints after 3 weeks of therapy.[128] All signs and symptoms abated within 2 weeks of discontinuation of therapy. However, 29 additional children treated with ofloxacin or ciprofloxacin showed no differences with respect to cartilage thickness, cartilage structure, edema, cartilage-bone borderline, or synovial fluid.[65] Women who received quinolones during pregnancy had larger babies and more caesarean deliveries because of fetal distress than did controls.[22] However, there were no congenital malformations, delay to developmental milestones, or musculoskeletal abnormalities found.

Fluoroquinolones are also implicated as a cause of tendon rupture, which is reported to occur up to 120 days after the start of treatment and even after the discontinuation of therapy.[191] The fluoroquinolone should be discontinued in patients, particularly athletes who complain of symptoms consistent with painful and swollen tendons.

Other adverse effects include acute psychosis, dysglycemia (hyper- and hypoglycemia), rash, tinnitus, eosinophilia, serum sickness, and photosensitivity.[44,103,173,188,232]

MACROLIDES AND KETOLIDES

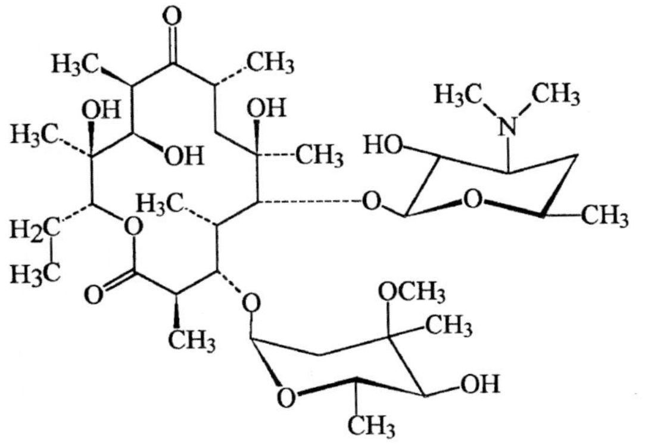

Erythromycin

The macrolide antimicrobials include various forms of erythromycin (base, estolate, ethylsuccinate, gluceptate, lactobionate, stearate), azithromycin, clarithromycin, troleandomycin, and dirithromycin. Ketolides are similar in pharmacology to macrolides; telithromycin is the only available agent at this time. Table 56–1 lists the pharmacologic mechanism of macrolides and ketolides, and Table 56–2 lists their pharmacokinetic properties.

Acute oral overdoses of macrolide antimicrobials are usually not life threatening and symptoms, which are generally confined to the gastrointestinal tract, include nausea, vomiting, and diarrhea. A single case of pancreatitis is reported.[241] Erythromycin lactobionate causes QT prolongation and torsades de pointes after intravenous use.[184] Oral erythromycin is also implicated in causing prolongation of the QT and torsades de pointes, especially in patients concurrently taking cytochrome P450 (CYP) 3A4 inhibitors.[196] In vitro models demonstrate erythromycin's ability to slow repolarization in a concentration-dependent manner.[177] The cause of prolonged QT interval was once thought to be from hypokalemia-induced promotion of intracellular efflux of potassium.[197] Data, however, demonstrate that the QT interval prolongation results from blockade of delayed rectifier potassium currents (Chaps. 22 and 23).[208] QT prolongation and torsades de pointes are common after intravenous erythromycin lactobionate.[184] More pronounced prolongation occurs in patients with underlying heart disease and correlates with the infusion rate.[106] Epidemiologic studies note an increased incidence of ventricular dysrhythmias in women treated with erythromycin.[75]

Although there are no acute overdose data regarding ketolide antimicrobials, effects are expected to be similar to macrolide antimicrobials. Therapeutic use of telithromycin is reported to result in QT prolongation, hepatotoxicity, toxic epidermal necrolysis and anaphylaxis.[1,17,27,29,74,185]

Adverse Events Associated With Therapeutic Use *Drug Interactions.* Erythromycin is the prototypical macrolide and, as such, has received the most attention with respect to potential and documented drug interactions. [115] Clarithromycin, erythromycin, and troleandomycin are all potent inhibitors of the CYP3A4 enzyme system; azithromycin does not inhibit this enzyme.[64] Erythromycin inhibits cytochrome P450 after metabolism to a nitroso intermediate, which then forms an inactive complex with the iron (II) of cytochrome P450. Chapter 12 (Appendix) lists substrates for the CYP3A4 system. Clinically significant interactions occur with erythromycin and warfarin, carbamazepine, terfenadine or cyclosporine.[46,111,115,194] Inhibition of cisapride metabolism results in increased concentrations of the parent drug, which is capable of causing prolongation of the QT interval and causing torsades de pointes.[35] Cases of carbamazepine toxicity are documented when combined with the use of erythromycin.[111] Erythromycin also inhibits CYP1A2, producing clinically significant interactions with clozapine, theophylline, and warfarin.[204]

Macrolides may also interact with the absorption and renal excretion of drugs that are amenable to intestinal P-glycoprotein excretion, or interfere with normal gut flora responsible for metabolism. This may be part of the underlying mechanism of cases of macrolide-induced digoxin toxicity (Chap. 64).[182]

End-Organ Effects The most common toxic effect of macrolides after chronic use is hepatitis, which may be immune mediated.[49] Erythromycin estolate is the agent most frequently implicated in causing cholestatic hepatitis.[96,123]

Large doses (more than 4 g/d) of macrolide antimicrobials are also associated with reversible high-frequency sensorineural hearing loss.[41] Renal impairment may be a risk factor.[211,236] There are rare case reports in which ototoxicity did not resolve following discontinuation of therapy.[149] There are insufficient data concerning the ototoxic potential of the other macrolide antimicrobials. Other, rare toxic effects associated with macrolides include cataracts after clarithromycin use in animals and acute pancreatitis in humans.[82,249] Allergy is rare and reported at a rate of 0.4% to 3%.[70] Telithromycin contains a carbamate side chain that may interfere with the normal function of neuronal cholinesterase. It should be used cautiously in patients with myasthenia gravis, particularly patients receiving pyridostigmine because of the risk of cholinergic crisis.[240]

Clindamycin is a lincosamide with similar structure and clinical effects to macrolides. Clindamycin phosphate is commonly used topically while clindamycin hydrochloride is available for intravenous use. Data regarding acute overdose is limited and the majority of the chronic toxicity is seen after use of systemic doses of clindamycin phosphate. The most consequental toxicity is gastrointestinal resulting in esophageal ulcers, diarrhea, and colitis.[203]

SULFONAMIDES

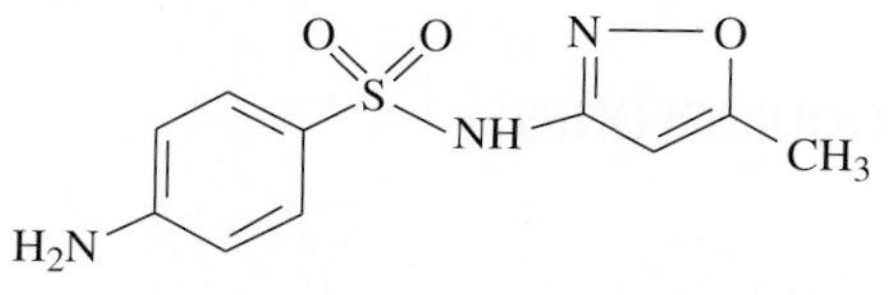

O O N—O
S NH CH$_3$
H$_2$N

Sulfamethoxazole

Sulfonamides antagonize *para*-aminobenzoic acid or *para*-aminobenzyl glutamic acid, which are required for the biosynthesis of folic acid. Table 56–1 lists the pharmacologic mechanism of sulfonamides, and Table 56–2 lists their pharmacokinetic properties. Acute oral overdoses of sulfonamides are usually not life threatening, and symptoms are generally confined to nausea, although allergy and methemoglobinemia occur rarely.[86] Treatment is similar to acute oral penicillin overdoses.

Adverse Effects Associated With Therapeutic Use The most common adverse effects associated with sulfonamide therapy are nausea and cutaneous hypersensitivity reactions. Hypersensitivity reactions are thought to be caused by the formation of hapten sulfamethoxazole metabolites, *N*-hydroxy-sulfamethoxazole and nitroso-sulfamethoxazole. The degree of hapten binding is mitigated in vitro by cysteine and glutathione.[176] The incidence of adverse reactions to sulfonamides, including allergy, is increased in HIV-positive patients and is positively correlated to the number of previous opportunistic infections experienced by the patient.[147] This may be caused by a decrease in the mechanisms available for detoxification of free radical formation, as cysteine and glutathione levels are low in these patients.[257] Whether supplementation with a glutathione precursor such as *N*-acetylcysteine will reduce the incidence of these reactions is unknown.[3]

Methemoglobinemia and hemolysis also rarely occur.[76,155] The mechanism for adverse reactions is not entirely clear. However, when sulfamethoxazole is exposed to ultraviolet B (UVB) radiation in vitro, free radicals are formed that can participate in the development of tissue peroxidation and hemolysis.[268] This finding may be of particular importance in treating patients with glucose-6-phosphate dehydrogenase (G6PD) deficiency associated with decreased in reducing capabilities.[5]

The sulfonamides are associated with many chronic adverse effects. Bone marrow suppression is rare, but the incidence is increased in patients with folic acid or vitamin B12 deficiency, and in children, pregnant women, alcoholics, dialysis patients, and immunocompromised patients, as well as in patients who are receiving other folate antagonists. Other adverse effects include hypersensitivity pneumonitis, stomatitis, aseptic meningitis, hepatotoxicity, renal toxicity, and central nervous system toxicity.[30]

TETRACYCLINES

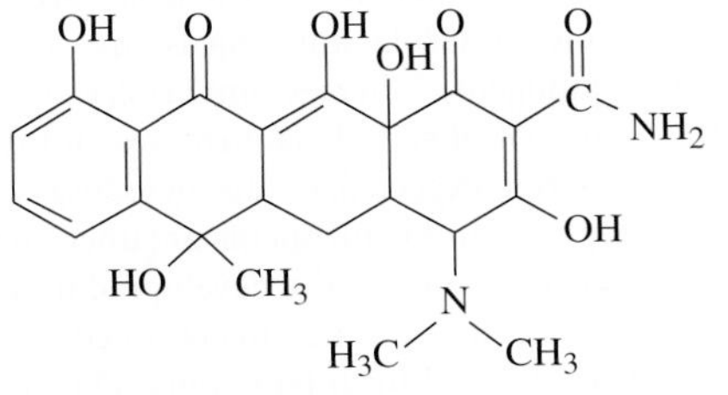

Tetracycline

Tetracyclines are derivatives of *Streptomyces* cultures. Currently available tetracyclines include demeclocycline, doxycycline, methacycline, minocycline, oxytetracycline, and tetracycline. Table 56–1 lists the pharmacologic mechanism of tetracyclines, and Table 56–2 lists their pharmacokinetic properties. Significant toxicity after acute overdose of tetracyclines is unlikely. Gastrointestinal effects consisting of nausea, vomiting, and epigastric pain have been reported.[42]

Adverse Effects Associated With Therapeutic Use Tetracycline should not be used in children during the first 6 to 8 years of life or by pregnant women after the 12th week of pregnancy because of the risk of development of secondary tooth discoloration in children or developing children in utero.

Other effects associated with tetracyclines include nephrotoxicity, hepatotoxicity, skin hyperpigmentation in sun-exposed areas, and hypersensitivity reactions.[49,100,121,239] More severe hypersensitivity reactions, drug-induced lupus, and pneumonitis are reported after minocycline use, as are cases of necrotizing vasculitis of the skin and uterine cervix, and lymphadenopathy with eosinophilia.[160,220,224] Demeclocycline rarely causes nephrogenic diabetes insipidus (Chap. 16).[50] Of historical interest, outdated older formulations of tetracycline were reported to cause hypouricemia, hypokalemia, and a proximal and distal renal tubular acidosis.[57]

VANCOMYCIN

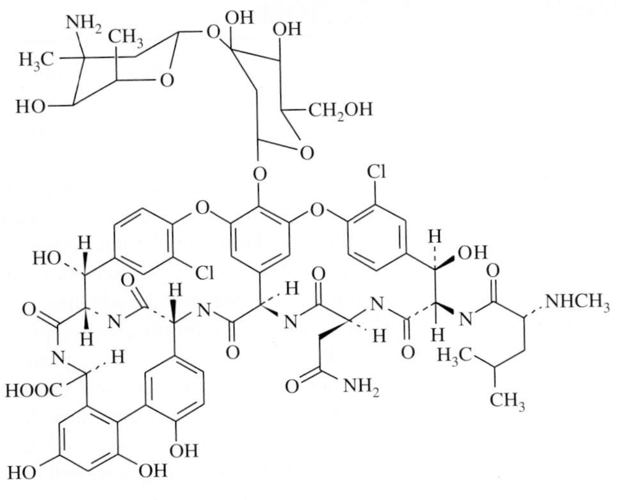

Vancomycin

Vancomycin is obtained from cultures of *Nocardia orientalis* and is a tricyclic glycopeptide. Vancomycin is biologically active against numerous gram-positive organisms. Table 56–1 lists the pharmacologic mechanism of vancomycin, and Table 56–2 lists its pharmacokinetic properties.

Acute oral overdoses of vancomycin rarely cause significant toxicity and most cases can be treated with supportive care alone. Multiple-dose activated charcoal and potentially high-flux hemodialysis can be considered for patients with large overdoses when the patient is expected to have prolonged clearance.[141,248]

Adverse Effects Associated With Therapeutic Use Patients who receive intravenous vancomycin may develop the "red man syndrome" through an anaphylactoid reaction.[93] Symptoms include chest pain, dyspnea, pruritus, urticaria, flushing, and angioedema.[207] Signs and symptoms spontaneously resolve, typically within 15 minutes. Other symptoms attributable to red man syndrome include hypotension, cardiovascular collapse, and seizures.[13,179]

The incidence of red man syndrome appears to be related to the rate of infusion and is approximately 14% when 1 g is given over 10 minutes, whereas it is 3.4% when given over 1 hour.[179,186] A trial in 11 healthy persons studied the relationship between intradermal skin hypersensitivity and the development of red man syndrome. Each of the 11 subjects underwent skin testing that was followed 1 week later by an intravenous dose of vancomycin 15 mg/kg over 60 minutes. Following intravenous vancomycin, all subjects developed dermal flare responses and erythema, and 10 of 11 subjects developed pruritus within 20 to 45 minutes. After the infusion was terminated, symptoms resolved within 60 minutes.[193]

The signs and symptoms of red man syndrome are related to the rise and fall of histamine concentrations.[110,151] Tachyphylaxis occurs in patients given multiple doses of vancomycin.[109,256] Animal models demonstrated a direct myocardial depressant and vasodilatory effect of vancomycin.[60] More serious reactions result when vancomycin is given via intravenous bolus, further supporting a rate-related anaphylactoid mechanism.[24]

Patients most often experience red man syndrome after vancomycin is administered intravenously. In rare cases, oral administration of vancomycin can also result in the syndrome.[21] Treatment includes increasing the dilution of vancomycin and slowing intravenous administration. Antihistamines may be useful as pretreatment, especially prior to the first dose.[198] A placebo-controlled trial in adult patients studied the incidence of these symptoms in patients given 1 g of vancomycin over 1 hour, as well as the effect of diphenhydramine in the prevention of the syndrome.[256] There was a 47% incidence of reaction without diphenhydramine and a 0% incidence with diphenhydramine.

Chronic use of vancomycin may cause reversible nephrotoxicity, particularly in patients with prolonged excessive steady-state se rum levels.[10,201] Concomitant administration of aminoglycoside antimicrobials may increase the risk of nephrotoxicity.[209] Vancomycin also causes, though rarely, thrombocytopenia and neutropenia.[56,58,73]

ANTIFUNGALS

Numerous antifungals are available. Toxicity related to the use of antifungals is variable and is based generally on their mechanism of action.

AMPHOTERICIN B

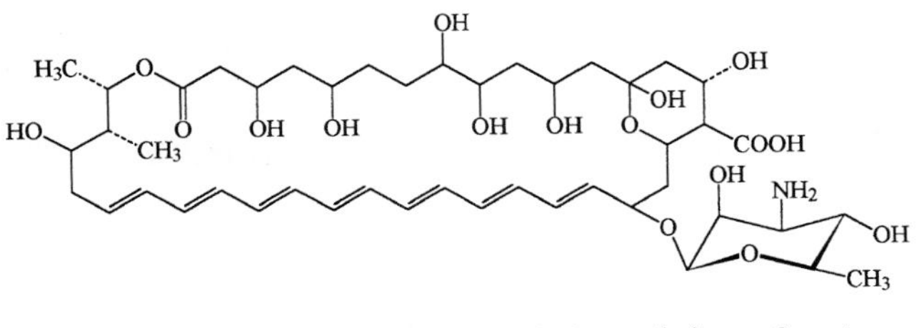

Amphotericin B is a potent antifungal derived from *Streptomyces nodosus*. Amphotericin B is generally fungistatic against fungi that contain sterols in their cell membrane. Table 56–1 lists the pharmacologic mechanism of amphotericin B, and Table 56–2 lists its pharmacokinetic properties. Development of lipid and colloidal formulations of amphotericin B attenuate the adverse effects associated with amphotericin B.[104] In these preparations, the amphotericin B is complexed with either a lipid or cholesteryl sulfate. On contact with a fungus, lipases are released to free the complexed amphotericin B, resulting in focused cell death.[113]

There are several case reports of amphotericin B overdose in infants and children. Significant clinical findings include hypokalemia, increased aspartate aminotransferase concentrations, and cardiac complications. Dysrhythmias and cardiac arrest have occurred following doses of 5 to 15 mg/kg of amphotericin B.[36,58,137] Care should be used in the doses of amphotericin B administered according to dosage form, as these are not interchangeable. For example, intravenous therapy for fungal infections includes a usual dose of 0.25 to 1 mg/kg/d of amphotericin B or 3 to 4 mg/kg/d of amphotericin B cholesteryl. The potential for significant dosage errors and their sequelae is readily apparent in this comparison.

Adverse Effects Associated With Therapeutic Use Infusion of amphotericin B results in fever, rigors, headache, nausea, vomiting, hypotension, tachycardia, and dyspnea.[161] Pretreatment with acetaminophen, diphenhydramine, ibuprofen, and hydrocortisone is helpful in alleviating the febrile symptoms, as are slower rates of infusion and lower total daily doses.[95,247] Doses greater than 1 mg/kg/d and rapid administration of drug in less than 1 hour are not recommended. Infusion concentrations of amphotericin B greater than 0.1 mg/mL can result in localized phlebitis. Slower infusion rates, hot packs, and frequent line flushing with dextrose in water may help to alleviate symptoms.

Eighty percent of patients exposed to amphotericin B will sustain some degree of renal insufficiency (Chap. 27).[47] Initial distal renal tubule damage causes renal artery vasoconstriction ultimately resulting in azotemia.[83] Studies in animals show depressed renal blood flow and glomerular filtration rate, and increased renal vascular resistance. It is unclear why this occurs, but at this time, renal nerves, angiotensin II, nitric oxide, and tubuloglomerular feedback are excluded.[210,216] The toxic effects associated with amphotericin B may also be caused by the deoxycholate vehicle.[267] After large total doses of amphotericin B, residual decreases in glomerular filtration rate may occur even after discontinuation of therapy. This is hypothesized to be the result of nephrocalcinosis. Potassium and magnesium wasting, proteinuria, decreased renal concentrating ability, renal tubular acidosis, and hematuria also occur (Chap. 16).[15,161] Strategies to reduce renal toxicity after amphotericin B include intravenous saline or magnesium and potassium supplementation.[34,84,112] Liposomal formulations of amphotericin B resulted in fewer patients with breakthrough fungal infections, infusion-related fever, rigors, or nephrotoxicity.[258] However, chest pain is uniquely reported after use of the liposomal agent.[130]

Other adverse effects reported after treatment with amphotericin B include normochromic, normocytic anemia secondary to decreased erythropoietin release;[159] respiratory insufficiency with infiltrates; and, rarely, dysrhythmias, tinnitus, thrombocytopenia, peripheral neuropathy, and leukopenia.[153,159,161]

Exchange transfusion may be useful in neonates and infants and should be considered after large intravenous exposures. In adults, extracorporeal elimination is not expected to be useful because of the low water solubility and high blood-protein binding of the drug.

AZOLE ANTIFUNGALS: TRIAZOLE AND IMIDAZOLES

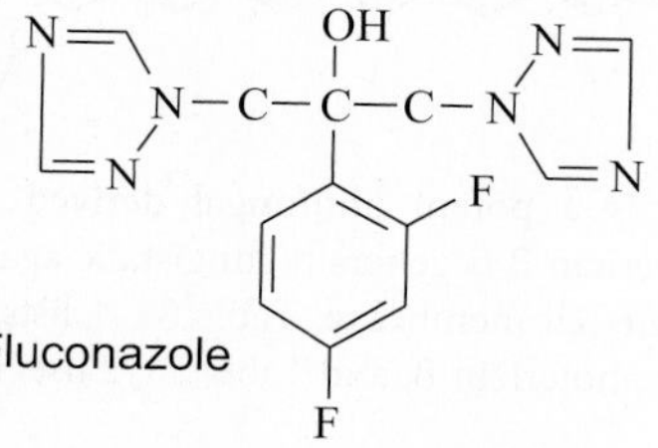

Fluconazole

Common triazole antifungals include fluconazole, itraconazole, and voriconazole. Common imidazoles include clotrimazole, econazole, ketoconazole, and miconazole. Triazole antifungals are active to treat an array of fungal pathogens, whereas imidazoles are used almost exclusively in the treatment of superficial mycoses and vaginal candidiasis. Severe toxicity is not expected in the overdose setting. Hepatotoxicity, thrombocytopenia, and neutropenia are uncommon.[31] Rare case reports implicate voriconazole in the development of toxic epidermal necrolysis.[117] The majority of toxic effects noted after the use of these drugs result from their drug interactions. Fluconazole, itraconazole, ketoconazole, and miconazole competitively inhibit CYP3A4, the enzyme system responsible for the metabolism of many drugs. Table 56–5 lists other organ system manifestations associated with antifungal agents and other antimicrobials.

ANTIPARASITICS

Antiparasitics such as thiabendazole, mebendazole, albendazole, diethylcarbazine, ivermectin, metrifonate, niclosamide, oxamniquine, piperazine, priziquantel, and pyrantel pamoate generally have a low level of toxicity in the overdose setting. Common symptoms after therapeutic use are gastrointestinal in nature and include abdominal pain, nausea, vomiting, and diarrhea. A single case of ivermectin-associated hepatic failure is reported 1 month after a single dose.[252]

ANTIVIRAL

Acyclovir is well tolerated in therapeutic doses and overdoses, although data are limited. In 105 dogs ingesting 40 to 2195 mg/kg, gastrointestinal symptoms were most common with one dog developing mild creatinine increases.[200] Depressed mental status and nephrotoxicity are also reported after therapeutic use in humans.[32]

ANTIMICROBIALS SPECIFIC TO THE TREATMENT OF HUMAN IMMUNODEFICIENCY VIRUS AND RELATED INFECTIONS

The evaluation and management of patients infected with the human immunodeficiency virus (HIV) and associated acquired immune deficiency syndrome (AIDS) is ever evolving at a rapid and progressive pace. Medications used to manage this disorder have dramatically increased life expectancy as new, more powerful antiviral agents and drug combinations become available. Drug therapy for HIV commonly consists of a combination of drugs from different classes (nucleoside reverse transcriptase inhibitor [NRTI], nonnucleoside reverse transcriptase inhibitor [NNRTI], and protease inhibitor) in order to take advantage of the unique mechanism that each drug offers in inhibiting viral replication and minimizing drug resistance. Resistance patterns to the typical drugs used in attenuating viral replication and proliferation are a substantial issue and will continue to be addressed with yet more evolution in management in the foreseeable future. This section focuses on overdoses and major toxic effects from HIV-directed antiviral therapy, as well as from drugs that are specifically used in the management of opportunistic infections.[20] Table 56–6 lists the common antibiotic agents used to treat HIV-related opportunistic infections, and Table 56–7 lists common adverse drug effects and overdose effects, if known, for antimicrobials that are specific in their use for HIV-related infections.

SPECIFIC ANTIRETROVIRAL CLASSES

Nucleoside Analog Reverse Transcriptase Inhibitors The nucleoside analog reverse transcriptase inhibitors inhibit the reverse transcription

TABLE 56–5. Consequential Organ System Manifestations Associated With Antimicrobials

Antimicrobial	System	Signs, Symptoms, Laboratory
Antibacterials		
Bacitracin	Immune	Hypersensitivity reactions
Clindamycin	Immune	Hypersensitivity reactions
	Gastrointestinal	Nausea, vomiting, diarrhea
	Nervous	Dizziness, headache, vertigo
Colistimethate (colistin sulfate)	Renal	Decreased function, acute tubular necrosis
	Nervous	Peripheral paresthesias, confusion, coma, seizures, neuromuscular blockade
Lincomycin	Gastrointestinal	Nausea, vomiting, diarrhea
	Immune	Hypersensitivity reactions
Metronidazole	Neurologic	Peripheral neuropathy, seizures
	Gastrointestinal	Nausea, vomiting
	Other	Disulfiram reactions
Nitrofurazone	Immune	Hypersensitivity reactions
	Other	Ointment contains polyethylene glycols (renal dysfunction)
Nitrofurantoin	Gastrointestinal	Nausea, vomiting, diarrhea
	Hepatic	Jaundice
	Immune	Rash, acute and chronic pulmonary hypersensitivity
	Neurologic	Peripheral neuropathy
Novobiocin	Immune	Rash
	Gastrointestinal	Nausea, vomiting, diarrhea
	Hematologic	Pancytopenia, hemolytic anemia
Polymyxin B sulfate	Neurologic	Muscle weakness, seizures
	Renal	Azotemia, proteinuria
Selenium sulfide	Cutaneous	Contact dermatitis, alopecia (rare)
Silver sulfadiazine	Cutaneous	Contact dermatitis
	Hematologic	Anemia, aplastic anemia
Spectinomycin	Immune	Rash (rare)
Antifungals		
Benzoic acid	Gastrointestinal	Nausea, vomiting, diarrhea
Carbol-fuchsin solution (phenol/ resorcinol/ fuchsin)	Gastrointestinal	Nausea, vomiting, diarrhea
Gentian violet	Gastrointestinal	Nausea, vomiting, diarrhea
	Immune	Rash (rare)
Griseofulvin	Renal	Proteinuria, nephrosis
	Hepatic	Increased enzymes
	Gastrointestinal	Nausea, vomiting, diarrhea
	Immune	Granulocytopenia
	Other	Disulfiram reactions, increased porphyrins
Nystatin	Gastrointestinal	Nausea, vomiting, diarrhea
Salicylic acid	Gastrointestinal and dermal	Higher concentrations are caustic
Undecylenic acid and undecylenate salt	Gastrointestinal	Nausea, vomiting, diarrhea

TABLE 56–6. Antimicrobials Used to Treat Common Opportunistic Infections[20]

Antimicrobial	Opportunistic Infection
Albendazole	Microsporidiosis
Amphotericin B	Aspergillosis
	Coccidioidomycosis
	Cryptococcosis
	Histoplasmosis
	Leishmaniasis
	Paracoccidioidomycosis
	Penicilliosis
Antimony (pentavalent)	Leishmaniasis
Atovaquone	*Pneumocystis jiroveci*
Azithromycin	*Mycobacterium avium* complex
Clarithromycin	Mycobacterium avium complex
Caspofungin	Aspergillosis
Clindamycin	*Pneumocystis jiroveci*
	Toxoplasma gondii
Dapsone	*Pneumocystis jiroveci*
Ethambutol	*Mycobacterium avium* complex
Fluconazole	Coccidioidomycosis
	Histoplasmosis
Flucytosine	Cryptococcosis
Foscarnet	Cytomegalovirus
Fumagillin	Microsporidiosis
Ganciclovir	Cytomegalovirus
Itraconazole	Histoplasmosis
Leucovorin	*Pneumocystis jiroveci*
	Toxoplasma gondii
Nitazoxanide	Cryptosporidiosis
	Microsporidiosis
Paromomycin	Cryptosporidiosis
Pentamidine	*Pneumocystis jiroveci*
Primaquine	*Pneumocystis jiroveci*
Pyrimethamine	*Toxoplasma gondii*
Rifabutin	*Mycobacterium avium* complex
Sulfadiazine	*Toxoplasma gondii*
Trimethoprin-sulfamethoxazole	*Pneumocystis jiroveci* *Toxoplasma gondii*
	Isosporiasis
Trimetrexate	*Pneumocystis jiroveci*
Valganciclovir	Cytomegalovirus
Voriconazole	Aspergillosis

of viral RNA into proviral DNA. Currently available drugs include abacavir (ABC), emtricitabine (FTC), didanosine (ddI), lamivudine (3TC), stavudine (d4T), tenofovir (TDF), zidovudine (AZT, ZDV), and zalcitabine (ddC).

Acute Overdose Effects. Many intentional overdoses of reverse transcriptase inhibitors occur without major toxicologic effect. The most serious adverse effect anticipated after acute overdose of an NRTI is

TABLE 56–7. Antimicrobials Used in the Treatment of HIV-Related Infections[20]

Antimicrobial	Overdose Effects	Common Adverse Drug Effects
Albendazole	No reported cases	Increased AST/ALT, nausea, vomiting, and diarrhea. Hematologic, rare—encephalopathy, renal failure, rash
Antimony (pentavalent)	Acute tubular necrosis	Acute tubular necrosis. Multiorgan system failure
Atovaquone	No clinical relevant effects in reported cases[55]	Rashes, anemia, leukopenia, increased AST/ALT
Caspofungin	No reported cases	Phlebitis, headache, hypokalemia, increased AST/ALT, fever
Flucytosine	No reported cases	Bone marrow suppression, hepatotoxicity, nausea, vomiting, diarrhea, and rash
Foscarnet	No reported cases	Azotemia, hypocalcemia and renal failure (common); anemia, leukopenia, thrombocytopenia, fever, headache, seizures, genital and oral ulcers, fixed-drug eruptions, nausea, vomiting, diarrhea, headaches, seizures, coma, diabetes insipidus, hypophosphatemia, hypokalemia, and hypomagnesemia
Fumagillin	No reported cases	Neutropenia and thrombocytopenia
Ganciclovir	No clinical relevant effects in reported cases[138]	Leukopenia, worsening of renal function; can also cause nausea, vomiting, diarrhea, increased AST/ALT, anemia, thrombocytopenia, headache, dizziness, confusion, seizures
Nitazoxzanide	No reported cases	Hypotension, headache, abdominal pain, nausea, vomiting; may cause green-yellow urine discoloration
Pentamidine	40 times dosing error in a 17-month-old child resulted in cardiac arrest[259]	Hypoglycemia (early) followed by hyperglycemia, azotemia; can cause hypotension, torsades de pointes, phlebitis, rash, Stevens-Johnson syndrome, hypocalcemia, hypokalemia, anorexia, nausea, vomiting, metallic taste, leukopenia, and thrombocytopenia
Primaquine	No reported cases	Granulocytopenia, hemolytic anemia, methemoglobinemia, leukocytosis; hypertension
Pyrimethamine	No reported cases	Agranulocytosis, aplastic anemia, thrombocytopenia, and leukopenia
Rifabutin	High doses (>1 g daily): arthralgia/arthritis	Nausea, vomiting, diarrhea; can cause hepatotoxicity, neutropenia, thrombocytopenia, and hypersensitivity reactions
Sulfadiazine	Acute renal failure and hypoglycemia[63]	Rash, Stevens-Johnson syndrome, toxic epidermal necrolysis, erythema multiforme; headaches, depression, hallucinations, ataxia, tremor, crystalluria, hematuria, proteinuria, and nephrolithiasis
Trimetrexate	No reported cases; treat similar to methotrexate (Chap. 53)	Myelosuppression, nausea, vomiting, histaminergic reactions
Valganciclovir	No reported cases; expect to be similar to ganciclovir	Anemia, neutropenia, thrombocytopenia; nausea, vomiting, headache, peripheral neuropathy

AST/ALT, serum alanine aminotransferase or serum aspartate aminotransferase.

the development of a lactic acidemia, which appears to be more common in women.[52,81,162] Following incorporation of the nucleoside analog into mitochondrial DNA by RNA polymerase, DNA polymerase γ is inhibited. This results in decreased production of mitochondrial DNA electron transport proteins, which ultimately inhibits oxidative phosphorylation (Chap. 12). Organ system toxicity follows in addition to the development of acidemia. The reported mortality in patients with NRTI-associated metabolic acidosis associated with elevated lactate is 33% to 57%.[81] Resolution of symptoms in survivors is 1 to 24 weeks. Patients with NRTI-associated acidemia may recover more quickly after the use of cofactors such as thiamine, riboflavin, L-carnitine, vitamin C, and antioxidants.[38,71] The indications for the use of these drugs are unclear at this time; however, because of the relative lack of toxicity, they may be considered.

Chronic Effects. Development of acidemia is more commonly associated with therapeutic use of reverse transcriptase inhibitors than with acute overdose. The mechanism is likely identical to that described above. Other common adverse effects are somewhat agent specific and include hematologic toxicity after zidovidine,[71,98] pancreatitis with didanosine,[145] hypersensitivity after abacavir,[70] and sensory peripheral neuropathy after zalcitabine, stavudine, and didanosine.[171]

Nonnucleoside Reverse Transcriptase Inhibitors NNRTI bind directly to reverse transcriptase enzymes enabling allosteric inhibition of enzymatic function.[243] Delavirdine (Rescriptor), etravirine (Intelence), efavirenz (Sustiva), and nevirapine (Viramune) comprise the currently available agents.

There are no substantial acute overdose data on these drugs, although they generally appear to be safe in overdose. Treatment should include supportive care until more information is available. The NNRTIs are also limited in toxicity after chronic use. Nevirapine and delavirdine use commonly results in hypersensitivity reactions such as rash.[69] Efavirenz is reported to result in dizziness and dysphoria. Otherwise, toxicity can result from the ability of these drugs to either inhibit or enhance CYP isozymes in the metabolism of other drugs.

Protease Inhibitors Protease inhibitors inhibit the vital enzyme (proteinase), which is required for viral replication.[85] Currently available drugs include ataznavir (Reyatax), darunavir (Prezista), fosamprenavor (Lexiva), indinavir (Crixivan), lopinavir (Kaletra), nelfinavir (Viracept), ritonavir (Norvir), saquinavir mesylate (Invirase), and tipranavir (Aptivus).

Data after protease inhibitor overdose are limited. A review of data submitted to the manufacturer of indinavir found that of 79 reports, the complaints were nausea, vomiting, abdominal pain, and nephrolithiasis. Protease inhibitors as a class commonly result in gastrointestinal symptoms and rash.[85] A unique finding is an altered fat distribution pattern that, over time, results in lymphodystrophy central obesity, "buffalo hump," breast enlargement, cushingoid appearance, and peripheral wasting.[85]

Entry/Fusion Inhibitors This class of drugs interferes with the binding or entry of the HIV viron into the cell.[26] No acute overdose data are available for this class, but after chronic use, hypersensitivity, hepatotoxicity, and infusion reactions seem to be of greatest concern.[18,174,180] The currently available agents include enfuvirtide (Fuzeon) and maraviroc (Selzentry).

Integrace Inhibitor This class of drugs prevents the activity of the enzyme in HIV to function normally. This enzyme is responsible for the incorporation of the virus into DNA. The currently available agent is raltegravir (Isentress). No information is currently available regarding its toxicity.

SUMMARY

Adverse effects attributable to antimicrobials are largely related to chronic administration, although rarely acute toxicity does occur. Acute toxic effects of antimicrobials are more common following intravenous administration, drug interactions, or iatrogenic overdose. Vigilance on the part of the healthcare provider will prevent the majority of acute toxic manifestations following antimicrobial use.

REFERENCES

1. [No authors listed.] Telithromycin. QT prolongation. *Prescrire Int.* 2007; 16:71.
2. Abanades S, Nolla J, Rodriguez-Campello A, et al. Reversible coma secondary to cefepime neurotoxicity. *Ann Pharmacother.* 2004;38:606-608.
3. Akerlund B, Tynell E, Bratt G, Bielenstein M, Lidman C. *N*-Acetylcysteine treatment and the rise of toxic reactions to trimethoprim-sulfamethoxazole in primary *Pneumocystis carinii* prophylaxis in HIV-infected patients. *J Infect.* 1997;35:143-147.
4. Ali MZ, Goetz MB. A meta-analysis of the relative efficacy and toxicity of single daily dosing versus multiple daily dosing of aminoglycosides. *Clin Infect Dis.* 1997;24:796-809.
5. Ali NA, Al-Naama LM, Khalid LO. Haemolytic potential of three chemotherapeutic agents and aspirin in glucose-6-phosphate dehydrogenase deficiency. *East Mediterr Health J.* 1999;5:457-464.
6. Andrade RJ, Guilarte J, Salmeron FJ, Lucean MI, Bellot V. Benzylpenicillin-induced prolonged cholestasis. *Ann Pharmacother.* 2001;35:783-784.
7. Andrade RJ, Lucena MI, Fernandez MC, Vega JL, Camargo R. Hepatotoxicity in patients with cirrhosis, an often unrecognized problem. Lessons from a fatal case related to amoxicillin/clavulanic acid. *Dig Dis Sci.* 2001;46: 1416-1419.
8. Anne S, Reisman RE. Risk of administering cephalosporin antibiotics to patients with history of penicillin allergy. *Ann Allergy Asthma Immunol.* 1995;74:167-170.
9. Appel GB. Aminoglycoside nephrotoxicity. *Am J Med.* 1990;88(Suppl 3C): 16S-20S.
10. Appel GB, Given DB, Levine LR, Cooper GL. Vancomycin and the kidney. *Am J Kidney Dis.* 1986;8:75-80.
11. Arcieri GM, Becker N, Esposito B, et al. Safety of intravenous ciprofloxacin. *Am J Med.* 1989;87(Suppl 5A):92S-97S.
12. Backon J. Hoigne's syndrome. Relevance of anomalous dominance and prostaglandins. *Am J Dis Child.* 1986;140:1091-1092.
13. Bailie GR, Yu R, Morton R, Waldek S. Vancomycin, red neck syndrome and fits. *Lancet.* 1985;2:279-280.
14. Balso BA, Pham NH. Invited review. Structure-activity studies on drug-induced anaphylactic reactions. *Chem Res Toxicol.* 1994;7:703-721.
15. Barton CH, Pahl M, Vaziri ND. Renal magnesium wasting associated with amphotericin B therapy. *Am J Med.* 1984;77:471-474.
16. Baumann G, Loher U, Felix SB, et al. Deleterious effects of cimeti-dine in the presence of histamine on coronary circulation. *Res Exp Med.* 1982;180: 209-213.
17. Bedard MS, Gilbert M. Telithromycin-induced TEN. report of a case. *Arch Dermatol.* 2007;143:427-428.
18. Beilke MA. Acute hypersensitivity reaction to enfuvurtide upon re-challenge. *Scand J Infect Dis.* 2004;36:778.
19. Bell CL, Watson B, Waring WS. Acute psychosis caused by co-amoxiclav. *BMJ.* 2008;337:a2117.
20. Benson CA, Kaplan JE, Masur H, et al. Treatment opportunistic infections among HIV infected adults and adolescents. Centers for Disease Control and Prevention. *MMWR Morb Mortal Wkly Rep.* 2004;53:1-112.
21. Bergeron L, Boucher FD. Possible red-man syndrome associated with systemic absorption of oral vancomycin in a child with normal renal function. *Ann Pharmacother.* 1994;28:581-584.
22. Berkovitch M, Pastuszak A, Gazarian M, Lewis M, Koren G. Safety of the new quinolones in pregnancy. *Obstet Gynecol.* 1994;84:535-538.
23. Berry M, Gurung A, Easty DL. Toxicity of antibiotics and antifungals on cultured human corneal cells. Effect of mixing, exposure and concentration. *Eye.* 1995;9:110-115.
24. Best CJ, Ewart M, Sumner E. Perioperative complications following the use of vancomycin during anaesthesia. Two clinical reports. *Br J Anaesth.* 1989;62:567-577.
25. Bhat RV, Deshmukh CT. A study if vitamin K status in children on prolonged antibiotic therapy. *Indian Pediatr.* 2003;40:36-40.
26. Biswas P, Tambussi G, Lazzarin A. Access denied? The status of co-receptor inhibition to counter HIV entry. *Expert Opin Pharmacother.* 2007;8:923-933.
27. Blandana P, Brunelleschi S, Fantozzi R, et al. The antianaphylactic action of histamine H2-receptor agonists in the guinea pig isolated heart. *Br J Pharmacol.* 1987;90:459-466.
28. Bolam DL, Jenkins SA, Nelson RM Jr. Aminoglycoside overdose in neonates. *J Pediatr.* 1982;100:835.
29 Bottenberg MM, Wall GC, Hicklin GA. Apparent anaphylactoid reaction after treatment with a single dose of telithromycin. *Ann Allergy Asthma Immunol.* 2007;98:89-91.
30. Bovino JA, Marcus DF. The mechanism of transient myopia induced by sulfonamide therapy. *Am J Ophthamol.* 1982;94:99-102.
31. Bradbury BD, Jick SS. Itraconazole and fluconazole and certain rare, serious adverse events. *Pharmacotherapy.* 2002;22:697-700.
32. Bradley J, Forero N, Pho H, Escobar B, Kasinath BS, Anzueto A. Progressive somnolence leading to coma in a 68-year-old man. *Chest.* 1997;112:538-540.
33. Brahams D. Penicillin overdose and deafness. *Lancet.* 1987;1:1445.
34. Branch RA. Prevention of amphotericin B-induced renal impairment. *Arch Intern Med.* 1988;148:2389-2394.
35. Brandriss MW, Richardson WS, Barold SS. Erythromycin-induced QT prolongation and polymorphic ventricular tachycardia (torsades de pointes). Case report and review. *Clin Infect Dis.* 1994;18:995-998.
36. Brent J, Hunt M, Kulig K, Rumack B. Amphotericin B overdoses in infants. Is there a role for exchange transfusion? *Vet Hum Toxicol.* 1990;32:124-125.
37. Bright DA, Gaupp FB, Becker LJ, Schiffert MG, Ryken TC. Amoxicillin overdose with gross hematuria. *West J Med.* 1989;150:698-699.
38. Brinkman K, ter Hofstede HJM. Mitochondrial toxicity of nucleo-side analogue reverse transcriptase inhibitors. Lactic acidosis, risk factors and therapeutic options. *AIDS Rev.* 1999;1:140-146.

39. Brossner G, Engelhardt K, Beer R, et al. Accidental intrathecal infusion of cefotiam. Clinical presentation and management. *Eur J Clin Pharmacol.* 2004; 60:373-375.
40. Brozanski BS, Scher MS, Albright AL. Intraventricular nafcillin-induced seizures in a neonate. *Pediatr Neurol.* 1988;4:188-190.
41. Brummett RE. Ototoxic liability of erythromycin and analogues. *Otolaryngol Clin North Am.* 1993;26:811-819.
42. Bryant SG, Fisher S, Kluge RM. Increased frequency of doxycycline side effects. *Pharmacotherapy.* 1987;7:125-129.
43. Buening MK, Wold JS, Israel KS, Kammer RB. Disulfiram-like reaction to beta-lactams. *JAMA.* 1980;245:2027-2028.
44. Burdge DR, Nakielna EM, Rabin HR. Photosensitivity associated with ciprofloxacin use in adult patients with cystic fibrosis. *Antimicrob Agents Chemother.* 1995;39:793.
45. Burkhardt JE, Hill MA, Lamar CH, Smith GN Jr, Carlton WW. Effects of difloxacin on the metabolism of glycosaminoglycans and collagen in organ cultures of articular cartilage. *Fundam Appl Toxicol.* 1993;20:257-263.
46. Bussey HI, Knodel LC, Boyle DA. Warfarin-erythromycin interaction. *Arch Intern Med.* 1985;145:1736-1737.
47. Butler WT, Bennett JE, Hill GJ 2nd. Electrocardiographic and electrolyte abnormalities caused by amphotericin B in dog and man. *Proc Soc Exp Biol Med.* 1964;116:857-863.
48. Calandra GB, Wang C, Aziz M, Brown KR. The safety profile of imipenem/cilastatin. Worldwide experience base on 3,470 patients. *J Antimicrob Chemother.* 1986;18(Suppl E):193-202.
49. Carson JL, Strom BL, Duff A, et al. Acute liver disease associated with erythromycins, sulfonamides, and tetracyclines. *Ann Intern Med.* 1993;119:576-583.
50. Castell DO, Sparks HA. Nephrogenic diabetes insipidus due to demethylchlortetracycline hydrochloride. *JAMA.* 1965;193:237.
51. Centers for Disease Control. Endotoxin-like reactions associated with intravenous gentamicin—California, 1998. *MMWR Morb Mortal Wkly Rep.* 1998;47:877-880.
52. Chattha G, Arieff AI, Cummings C, Tierney LM. Lactic acidosis complicating the acquired-immunodeficiency syndrome. *Ann Intern Med.* 1993;118:37-39.
53. Chawla A, Kahn E, Yunis EJ, Daum F. Rapidly progressive cholestasis. An unusual reaction to amoxicillin/clavulanic acid therapy in a child. *J Pediatr.* 2000;136:121-123.
54. Chen HJ, Bloch KL, Maclean JA. Acute eosinophilic hepatitis from trovafloxacin. *N Engl J Med.* 2000;342:359-360.
55. Cheung TW. Overdose of atovaquone in a patient with AIDS. *AIDS.* 1999;13:1984.
56 Christie DJ, Van Buren N, Lennon SS, Putnam JL. Vancomycin-dependent antibodies associated with thrombocytopenia and refractoriness to platelet transfusion in patients with leukemia. *Blood.* 1990;75:518-525.
57. Chusil S, Tungsanga K, Wathanavaha A, Pansin P. Hypouricemia, hypokalemia, proximal and distal tubular acidification defect following administration of outdated tetracycline. A case report. *J Med Assoc Thai.* 1994;77:98-102.
58. Cleary JD, Hayman J, Sherwood J, Lasala GP, Piazza-Hepp T. Amphotericin B overdose in pediatric patients with associated cardiac arrest. *Ann Pharmacother.* 1993;27:715-719.
59. Cocke JG, Brown RE, Geppert LJ. Optic neuritis with prolonged use of chloramphenicol. *J Pediatr.* 1966;68:27-31.
60. Cohen LS, Wechsler AS, Mitchell JH, Glick G. Depression of cardiac function by streptomycin and other antimicrobial agents. *Am J Cardiol.* 1970;26:505-511.
61. Connor JP, Curry JM, Selby TL, Perlmutter AD. Acute renal failure secondary to ciprofloxacin use. *J Urol.* 1994;154:975-976.
62. Covinsky JO. Aminoglycoside-induced electrolyte imbalance. *Hosp Ther.* 1986;5:17-29.
63. Craft AW, Brocklebank JT, Jackson RH. Acute renal failure and hypoglycaemia due to sulphadiazine poisoning. *Postgrad Med J.* 1977;53:103-104.
64. Danan G, Descatoire V, Pessayre D. Self-induction of erythromycin by its own transformation into a metabolite forming an inactive complex with reduced cytochrome P-450. *J Pharmacol Exp Ther.* 1989;250:746-751.
65 Danisovicova A, Brezina M, Belan S, et al. Magnetic resonance imaging in children receiving quinolones. No evidence of quinolone-induced arthropathy. A multicenter survey. *Chemotherapy.* 1994;40:209-214.
66. De Boer T, Stoof JC, Van Duyn H. Effect of penicillin on neurotransmitter release from rat cortical tissue. *Brain Res.* 1980;192:296-300.
67. De Sarro A, Ammendola D, De Sarro G. Effects of some quinolones on imipenem-induced seizures in DBA/2 mice. *Gen Pharmacol.* 1994;25:369-379.
68. De Sarro G, Nava F, Calapai G, De Sarro A. Effects of some excitatory amino acid antagonists and drugs enhancing gamma-amino butyric acid neurotransmission on pefloxacin-induced seizures in DBA/2 mice. *Antimicrob Agents Chemother.* 1997;41:427-434.
69. Deeks SG, Volberding PA. Antiretroviral therapy. In: Sande MA, Volberding PA, eds. *The Medical Management of AIDS*, 6th ed. Philadelphia: WB Saunders; 1999:97-115.
70. Demoly P, Benahmed S, Valembois M, et al. Allergy to macrolide antibiotics. Review of the literature [French]. *Presse Med.* 2000;29:321-326.
71 DeRay G, Diquet B, Martinez F, et al. Pharmacokinetics of zidovudine in a patient on maintenance hemodialysis. *N Engl J Med.* 1988;319:1606-1607.
72. DeSoto H. Cimetidine in anaphylactic shock refractory to standard therapy. *Anesth Analg.* 1989;69:260-269.
73. Domen RE, Horowitz S. Vancomycin-induced neutropenia associated with anti-granulocyte antibodies. *Immunohematology.* 1990;6:41-43.
74. Dore DD, DiBello JR, Lapane KL. Telithromycin use and spontaneous reports of hepatotoxicity. *Drug Saf.* 2007;30:697-703.
75. Drici MD, Knollmann BC, Wang WX, Woosley RL. Cardiac actions of erythromycin. Influence of female sex. *JAMA.* 1998;280:1774-1776.
76. Dunn RJ. Massive sulfasalazine and paracetamol ingestion causing acidosis, hyperglycemia, coagulopathy and methemoglobinemia. *J Toxicol Clin Toxicol.* 1998;36:239-242.
77. Durosinmi MA, Ajayi AA. A prospective study of chloramphenicol-induced aplastic anaemia in Nigerians. *Trop Geogr Med.* 1993;45:159-161.
78. Ehmann WC. Cephalosporin-induced hemolysis. A case report and review of the literature. *Am J Hematol.* 1992;40:121-125.
79. English J, Gilbert DN, Kohlhepp S, et al. Attenuation of experimental tobramycin nephrotoxicity by ticarcillin. *Antimicrob Agents Chemother.* 1985;27:897-902.
80. Engrav MB, Zimmerman M. Electrocardiographic changes associated with anaphylaxis in a patient with anaphylaxis in a patient with normal coronary arteries. *West J Med.* 1994;161:602.
81. Falco V, Rodriguez D, Ribera E, et al. Severe nucleoside-associated lactic acidosiss in human immunodeficiency virus-infected patients. Report of 12 cases and review of the literature *Clin Infect Dis.* 2002;34:838-846.
82. Fang CC, Wang HP, Lin JT. Erythromycin-induced acute pancreatitis. *J Toxicol Clin Toxicol.* 1996;34:93-95.
83. Fanos V, Cataldi L. Amphotericin-B induced nephrotoxicity. A review. *J Chemother.* 2000;12:463-470.
84. Fisher MA, Talbot GH, Maislin G, et al. Risk factors for amphotericin B associated nephrotoxicity. *Am J Med.* 1989;87:547-552.
85. Flexner C. HIV-protease inhibitors. *N Engl J Med.* 1998;338:1281-1292.
86. Fraser DG. Suicide attempt with Azo Gantanol resulting in methemoglobinemia. *Mil Med.* 1969;134:679-681.
87. Freundlich M, Cynamon H, Tames A, et al. Management of chloramphenicol intoxication in infancy by charcoal hemoperfusion. *J Pediatr.* 1983;103:485-487.
88. Fripp RR, Carter MC, Werner JC. Cardiac function and acute chloramphenicol toxicity. *J Pediatr.* 1983;103:487-490.
89. Fuchs S, Simon Z, Brezis M. Fatal hepatic failure associated with ciprofloxacin. *Lancet.* 1994;343:738-739.
90. Galpin JE, Chow AW, Yoshikawa TT, Guze LB. Pseudoanaphylactic reactions for inadvertent infusion of procaine penicillin G. *Ann Intern Med.* 1974;81:358-359.
91. Garica RLA, Stricker BH, Zimmerman HJ. Risk of acute liver injury associated with the combination of amoxicillin and clavulanic acid. *Arch Intern Med.* 1996;156:1327-1332.
92. Garratty G. Immune cytopenia associated with antibiotics. *Transfus Med Rev.* 1993;7:255-267.
93. Garrelts JC, Peterie JD. Vancomycin and the "red man's syndrome." *N Engl J Med.* 1985;312:245.
94 Geller RJ, Chevalier RL, Spyker DA. Acute amoxicillin nephrotoxicity following an overdose. *J Toxicol Clin Toxicol.* 1986;24:175-182.
95. Gigliotti F, Shenep JL, Lott L, Thornton D. Induction of prostaglandin synthesis as the mechanism responsible for the chills and fever produced by infusing amphotericin B. *J Infect Dis.* 1987;156:784-789.
96. Gilbert FI Jr. Cholestatic hepatitis caused by esters of erythromycin and oleandomycin 1962 (classical article). *Hawaii Med J.* 1995;54:603-605.
97. Glazko AJ. Identification of chloramphenicol metabolites and some factors affecting metabolic disposition. *Antimicrob Agents Chemother.* 1966;6:655-665.

98 Gold JWM. The diagnosis and management of HIV infection. In: Gold JWM, Telzak EE, White DA, eds. *The Diagnosis and Management of the HIV-Infected Patient, Part 1. Med Clin North Am.* 1996;80:1283-1307.
99. Gonzolez CP, Huidobro ML, Zabala AP, Vicente EM. Fatal subfulminant hepatic failure with ofloxacin. *Am J Gastroenterol.* 2000;95:1606.
100. Gordon G, Sparano BM, Iatripoulos MJ. Hyperpigmentation of the skin associated with minocycline therapy. *Arch Dermatol.* 1985;121:618-623.
101. Goss TF, Walawander CA, Grasela TH, et al. Prospective evaluation of risk factors for antibiotic-associated bleeding in critically ill patients. *Pharmacotherapy.* 1992;12:283-291.
102. Green RL, Lewis JE, Kraus ST, et al. Elevated plasma procaine concentration after administration of procaine penicillin G. *N Engl J Med.* 1979;291:223-226.
103. Guharoy SR. Serum sickness secondary to ciprofloxacin use. *Vet Hum Toxicol.* 1994;36:540-541.
104. Gurwith M, Mamelok R, Pietrelli L, DuMond C. Renal sparing by amphotericin B colloidal dispersion. Clinical experience in 572 patients. *Chemotherapy.* 1999;45(Suppl 1):39-47.
105. Guthrie OW. Aminoglycoside induced ototoxicity. *Toxicology.* 2008;249: 91-96.
106. Haefeli WE, Schoenberger RA, Weiss PH, Ritz R. Possible risk for cardiac arrhythmias related to intravenous erythromycin. *Intensive Care Med.* 1992;18:469-473.
107. Harle DG, Baldo BA. Drugs as allergens. An immunoassay for detecting IgE antibodies to cephalosporins. *Int Arch Allergy Appl Immunol.* 1990;92:439-444.
108. Harvey SC, Li X, Skolnick P, Kirst HA. The antibacterial and NMDA receptor activating properties of aminoglycosides are dissociable. *Eur J Pharmacol.* 2000;387:1-7.
109. Healy DP, Polk RE, Garson ML, Rock DT, Comstock TJ. Comparison of steady-state pharmacokinetics of two dosage regimens of vancomycin in normal volunteers. *Antimicrob Agents Chemother.* 1987;31:393-397.
110. Healy DP, Sahai JV, Fuller SH, Polk RE. Vancomycin-induced histamine release and "red man's syndrome". Comparison of 1- and 2-hour infusions. *Antimicrob Agents Chemother.* 1990;34:550-554.
111. Hedrick R, Williams F, Morin R, Lamb WA, Cate JC 4th. Carbamazepine-erythromycin interaction leading to carbamazepine toxicity in four epileptic children. *Ther Drug Monit.* 1983;5:405-407.
112. Heidemann HT, Gerkens JF, Spickard WA, Jackson EK, Branch RA. Amphotericin B nephrotoxicity in humans decreased by salt repletion. *Am J Med.* 1983;75:476-481.
113. Hiemenz JW, Walsh TJ. Lipid formulation of amphotericin B. Recent progress and future directions. *Clin Infect Dis.* 1996;22:S133-S144.
114. Ho WK, Martinelli A, Duggan JC. Severe immune haemolysis after standard doses of penicillin. *Clin Lab Haematol.* 2004;26:153-156.
115 Honig PK, Woolsley RL, Zamani K, Connor DP, Cantilena LR Jr. Changes in the pharmacokinetics and electrocardiographic pharmacodynamics of terfenadine with concomitant administration of erythromycin. *Clin Pharmacol Ther.* 1992;52:231-238.
116. Hootkins R, Fenves AZ, Stephens MK. Acute renal failure secondary to oral ciprofloxacin therapy. A presentation of three cases and a review of the literature. *Clin Nephrol.* 1989;32:75-78.
117. Huang DB, Wu JJ, LaHart CJ. Toxic epidermal necrolysis as a complication of treatment with voriconazole. *S Med J.* 2004;97:1116-1117.
118. Hughes DW. Studies on chloramphenicol I. Assessment of hemopoietic toxicity. *Med J Aust.* 1968;2:436-438.
119. Hughes DW. Studies on chloramphenicol II. Possible determinants and progress of hemopoietic toxicity during chloramphenicol therapy. *Med J Aust.* 1973;2:1142-1146.
120. Humes HD. Aminoglycoside nephrotoxicity. *Kidney Int.* 1988;33:900-901.
121. Hunt CM, Washington K. Tetracycline-induced bile duct paucity and prolonged cholestasis. *Gastroenterology.* 1994;107:1844-1847.
122. Ilechukwu STC. Acute psychotic reactions and stress response syndromes following intramuscular aqueous procaine penicillin. *Br J Psychiatry.* 1990;156:554-559.
123. Inman WH, Rawson NS. Erythromycin estolate and jaundice. *Br Med J.* 1983;286:1954-1955.
124. Jackson GG, Arcieri G. Ototoxicity of gentamicin in man. A survey and controlled analysis of clinical experience in the United States. *J Infect Dis.* 1971;124:S130-S137.
125. Jackson TL, Williamson TH. Amikacin retinal toxicity. *Br J Ophthalmol.* 1999;83:1199-1200.
126 Jaillon P, Morganroth J, Brumpt I, Talbot G. Overview of the electrocardiographic and cardiovascular safety data for sparfloxacin. Sparfloxacin safety group. *J Antimicrob Chemother.* 1996;37(Suppl A):161-167.
127. Jalbert EO. Seizures after penicillin administration. *Am J Dis Child.* 1985; 139:1075.
128. Jawad ASM. Cystic fibrosis and drug induced arthropathy. *Br J Rheumatol.* 1989;28:179-180.
129. Jimenez JJ, Arimura GK, Abou-Khalil WH, Isildar M, Yunis AA. Chloramphenicol-induced bone marrow injury. Possible role of bacterial metabolites of chloramphenicol. *Blood.* 1987;70(4):1180-1185.
130. Johnson MD, Drew RH, Perfect JR. Chest discomfort associated with liposomal amphotericin B. Report of three cases and review of the literature. *Pharmacotherapy.* 1998;18:1053-1061.
131. Johnsson LG, Hawkins JE, Weiss JM, Federspil P. Total deafness from aminoglycoside overdose. Histopathologic study. *Am J Otolaryngol.* 1984;5:118-126.
132. Kearns OL, Wheeler JO, Childress SH, Letzig LU. Serum sickness-like reactions to cefaclor. Role of hepatic metabolism and individual susceptibility. *J Pediatr.* 1994;125:805-811.
133. Kelkar PS, Li JTC. Cephalosporin allergy. *N Engl J Med.* 2001;345:804-809.
134. Kocak Z, Hatipoglu CA, Ertem G, et al. Trimethoprim-sulfamethoxazole induced rash and fatal hematologic disorders. *J Infect.* 2006;52:e49-e52.
135. Koirala J. Trimethoprim-sulfamethoxazole--induced methemoglobinemia in an HIV-infected patient. *Mayo Clin Proc.* 2004;79:829-830.
136. Koren G, Barzilay Z, Greenwald M. Tenfold errors in administration of drug doses. A neglected iatrogenic disease in pediatrics. *Pediatrics.* 1986;77:848-849.
137. Koren G, Lau A, Kenyon CF, Kroppert D, Klein J. Clinical course and pharmacokinetics following a massive overdose of amphotericin B in a neonate. *J Toxicol Clin Toxicol.* 1990;28:371-378.
138. Kostis EB, Nanas JN, Moulopoulos SD. Absence of toxicity after overdose of ganciclovir in a cardiac transplant recipient. *Eur J Cardiothaorac Surg.* 1999;15:876.
139. Kristof RA, Clusmann H, Koehler W, Fink KB, Schramm J. Treatment of accidental high-dose intraventricular mezlocillin application by cerebrospinal fluid exchange. *J Neurol Neurosurg Psychiatry.* 1998;64:379-381.
140. Kubo Y, Nonaka S, Yoshida H. Contact sensitivity to chloramphenicol. *Contact Dermatitis.* 1987;17:245-247.
141. Kucukguclu S, Tuncok Y, Ozkan H, et al. Multiple-dose activated charcoal in an accidental vancomycin overdose. *J Toxicol Clin Toxicol.* 1996;34:83-87.
142. Kumar A, Dada T. Preretinal hemorrhages. An unusual manifestation of intravitreal amikacin toxicity. *Aust N Z J Ophthalmol.* 1999;27:435-436.
143. Kushner JM, Peckman HJ, Snyder CR. Seizures associated with fluoroquinolones. *Ann Pharmacother.* 2001;35:1194-1198.
144. Labowitz JK, Silverman WB. Cholestatic jaundice induced by ciprofloxacin. *Dig Dis Sci.* 1997;42:192-194.
145. Lambert JS, Seidlin M, Reichman RV, et al. 2',3' -dideoxyinosine (ddI) in patient with acquired immunodeficiency syndrome or AIDS-related complex. A phase I trial. *N Engl J Med.* 1990;322:1333-1340.
146. Lang EW, Weinhart D, Behneke A, et al. A massive intrathecal cefazoline overdose. *Eur J Anaesthesiol.* 1999;16:204-205.
147. Lehmann DF, Liu A, Newman N, Blair DC. The association of opportunistic infections with the occurrence of trimethoprim/sulfamethoxazole hypersensitivity in patients infected with human immunodeficiency virus. *J Clin Pharmacol.* 1999;39:533-537.
148. Leo RJ, Ballow CH. Seizure activity associated with imipenem use. Clinical case reports and review of the literature. *Ann Pharmacother.* 1991;25:351-354.
149. Levin G, Behrenth E. Irreversible ototoxic effect of erythromycin. *Scand Audiol.* 1986;15:41-42.
150. Levine PH, Regelson W, Holland JF. Chloramphenicol-associated encephalopathy. *Clin Pharmacol Ther.* 1970;11:194-199.
151. Levy JH, Kettlekamp N, Goertz P, Hermens J, Hirshman CA. Histamine release by vancomycin. A mechanism for hypotension in man. *Anaesthesia.* 1987;67:122-125.
152. Liguori MJ, Anderson MG, Bukofzer S, et al. Microarray analysis in human hepatocytes suggests a mechanism for hepatotoxicity induced by trovafloxacin. *Hepatology.* 2005;41:177-86.
153. Lin AC, Goldwasser E, Bernard EM, Chapman SW. Amphotericin B blunts erythropoietin response to anemia. *J Infect Dis.* 1990;161:348-351.
154. Lin RY, Curry A, Pesola GR, et al. Improved outcomes in patients with acute allergic syndromes who are treated with combined H_1 and H_2 antagonists. *Ann Emerg Med.* 2000;36:462-468.

155. Lopez A, Bernado B, Lopez-Herce J, Cristina AI, Carrillo A. Methaemoglobinaemia secondary to treatment with trimethoprim and sulfamethoxazole associated with inhaled nitric oxide. *Acta Paediatr.* 1999;88:915-916.
156. Lowery N, Kearns GL, Young RA, Wheeler JG. Serum sickness-like reactions associated with cefprozil therapy. *J Pediatr.* 1994;125:325-328.
157. Lu CMC, James SH, Lien YHH. Acute massive gentamicin intoxication in a patient with end-stage renal disease. *Am J Kidney Dis.* 1996;28:767-771.
158. Lucena MI, Andrake RJ, Rodrigo L, et al. Trovafloxacin-induced acute hepatitis. *Clin Infect Dis.* 2000;30:400-401.
159 MacGregor RR, Bennett JE, Erslev AJ. Erythropoietin concentration in amphotericin B induced anemia. *Antimicrob Agents Chemother.* 1978;14:270-273.
160. MacNeil M, Haase DA, Tremaine R, Marrie TJ. Fever, lymph-adenopathy, eosinophilia, lymphocytosis, hepatitis and dermatitis. A severe adverse reaction to minocycline. *J Am Acad Dermatol.* 1997;36:347-350.
161. Maddux MS, Barriere SL. A review of complications of amphotericin therapy. Recommendations for prevention and management. *DICP.* 1980;14:177-180.
162. Maignen F, Meglio S, Bidault I, Castot A. Acute toxicity of zidovu-dine. Analysis of the literature and number of cases at the Paris poison control center [French]. *Therapie.* 1993;48:129-131.
163. Malone JD, Lebar RD, Hilder R. Procaine-induced seizures after intramuscular procaine penicillin G. *Mil Med.* 1988;153:191-192.
164. Marks C, Cummins BH. Rescue after 2 megaunits of intrathecal penicillin. *Lancet.* 1981;1:658-659.
165. Matsubara T, Otsubo S, Ogawa A, et al. Effects of beta-lactam antibiotics and *N*-methyltetrazolethiol on the alcohol-metabolizing system in rats. *Jpn J Pharmacol.* 1987;45:303-315.
166. Mattle H, Craig WA, Pechere PC. Determinants of efficacy and toxicity of aminoglycosides. *J Antimicrob Chemother.* 1989;24:281-293.
167. Mauer SM, Chavers BM, Kjellstrand CM. Treatment of an infant with severe chloramphenicol intoxication using charcoal-column hemoperfusion. *J Pediatr.* 1980;96:136-139.
168. Mayumi H, Kimura S, Asano M, et al. Intravenous cimetidine as an effective treatment for systemic anaphylaxis and acute allergic skin reactions. *Ann Allergy.* 1987;58:447-450.
169. Meislin HW, Bremer JC. Jarisch-Herxheimer reaction case report. *JACEP.* 1976;5:779-781.
170. Moore RD, Smith CR, Lipsky JJ, Mellits ED, Lietman PS. Risk factors for nephrotoxicity in patients treated with aminoglycosides. *Ann Intern Med.* 1984;100:352-357.
171. Moyle GJ, Sadler M. Peripheral neuropathy with nucleoside antiretrovirals. Risk factors, incidence and management. *Drug Saf.* 1998;19:34-40.
172. Mulhall A, deLouvois J, Hurley R. Chloramphenicol toxicity in neonates. Its incidence and prevention. *Br Med J.* 1983;287:1424-1427.
173. Mulhall JP, Bergmann LS. Ciprofloxacin-induced acute psychosis. *Urology.* 1995;46:102-103.
174. Myers SA, Selim AA, McDaniel MA, et al. A prospective clinical and pathological examination of injection site reactions with the HIV-1 fusion inhibitor enfuvirtide. *Antivir Ther (Lond).* 2006;11:935-939.
175. Nahtha MC. Serum concentrations and adverse effects of chloramphenicol in pediatric patients. *Chemotherapy.* 1987;33:322-327.
176. Naisbitt DJ, Hough SJ, Gill HJ, et al. Cellular deposition of sulphamethoxazole and its metabolites. Implications for hypersensitivity. *Br J Pharmacol.* 1999;126:1393-1407.
177. Nattel S, Ranger S, Talajic M, Lemery R, Rogy D. Erythromycin-induced prolonged QT syndrome. Concordance with quinidine and underlying cellular electrophysiologic mechanism. *Am J Med.* 1990;89:235-238.
178. Negussie Y, Remick DG, De Forge LE, et al. Detection of plasma tumour necrosis factor, interleukins 6 and 8 during Jarisch-Herxheimer reaction of relapsing fever. *J Exp Med.* 1992;175:1207-1212.
179. Newfield P, Roizen MF. Hazards of rapid administration of vancomycin. *Ann Intern Med.* 1979;91:58.
180. Nichols WG, Steel HM, Bonny T, et al. Hepatotoxicity observed in clinical trials of aplaviroc (GW873140). *Antimicrob Agents Chemother.* 2008;52:858-865.
181. Nishidi I, Takumida M. Attenuation of aminoglycoside ototoxicity by glutathione. *ORL J Otorhinolaryngol Relat Spec.* 1996;58:68-73.
182. Nordt SP, Williams SR, Manoguerra AS, Clark RF. Clarithromycin induced digoxin toxicity. *J Accid Emerg Med.* 1998;15:194-195.
183. Obata H, Iizuka B, Uchida K. Pathogenesis of hypoprothrombinemia induced by antibiotics. *J Nutr Sci Vitaminol (Tokyo).* 1992;S13-S15:421-424.
184. Oberg KC, Bauman JL. QT prolongation and torsades de pointes due to erythromycin lactobionate. *Pharmacotherapy.* 1995;15:687-692.
185. Onur O, Guneysel O, Denizbasi A, Celikel C. Acute hepatitis attack after exposure to telithromycin. *Clin Ther.* 2007;29:1725-1729.
186. O'Sullivan TL, Ruffing MJ, Lamp KC, Warbasse LH, Rybak MJ. Prospective evaluation of red man syndrome in patients receiving vancomycin. *J Infect Dis.* 1993;168:773-776.
187. Paradelis AG. Aminoglycoside antibiotics and neuromuscular blockade. *J Antimicrob Chemother.* 1979;5:737-738.
188. Park-Wyllie LY, Juurlink DN, Kopp A, et al. Outpatient gatifloxacin therapy and dysglycemia in older adults. *N Engl J Med.* 2006;354:1352-1361.
189. Patterson LJ, Milne B. Latex anaphylaxis causing heart block. Role of ranitidine. *Can J Anesth.* 1999;46:776-778.
190. Pestotnik SL, Classen DC, Evans RS, Stevens LE, Burke JP. Prospective surveillance of imipenem/cilastatin use and associated seizures using a hospital information system. *Ann Pharmacother.* 1993;27:497-501.
191. Pierfitte C, Gillet P, Royer RJ. More on fluoroquinolone antibiotics and tendon rupture. *N Engl J Med.* 1995;332:193.
192. Pimiento PA, Martinez GM, Mena MA, et al. Aztreonam and ceftazidime. Evidence of in vivo cross allergenicity. *Allergy.* 1998;53:624-625.
193. Polk RE, Israel D, Wang J, et al. Vancomycin skin tests and prediction of "red man syndrome" in healthy volunteers. *Antimicrob Agents Chemother.* 1993;37:2139-2143.
194. Ptachainski RJ, Carpenter BJ, Burckart GJ, Venkataramanan R, Rosenthal JT. Effect of erythromycin on cyclosporine levels. *N Engl J Med.* 1985;313:1416-1417.
195. Ramilo O, Kinane BT, McCracken GH. Chloramphenicol neurotoxicity. *Pediatr Infect Dis J.* 1988;7:358-359.
196. Ray WA, Murray KT, Meredity S, et al. Oral erythromycin and the risk of sudden death from cardiac causes. *N Engl J Med.* 2004;351:1089-1096.
197. Regan TJ, Khan MI, Olde IHA, Passannant AJ. Antibiotic effect on myocardial K transport and the production of ventricular tachycardia [abstract]. *J Clin Invest.* 1969;48:66A.
198. Renz CL, Thurn JD, Finn HA, Lynch JP, Moss, J. Antihistamine prophylaxis permits rapid vancomycin infusion. *Crit Care Med.* 1999;27:1732-1737.
199. Richardet JP, Mallat A, Zafrani ES, et al. Prolonged cholestasis with ductopenia after administration of amoxicillin/clavulanic acid. *Dig Dis Sci.* 1999;44: 1997-2000.
200. Richardson JA. Accidental ingestion of acyclovir in dogs. 105 reports. *Vet Hum Toxicol.* 2000;42:370-371.
201. Riley HD Jr. Vancomycin and novobiocin. *Med Clin North Am.* 1970;54: 1277-1289.
202. Rippelmeyer DJ, Synhavsky A. Ciprofloxacin and allergic interstitial nephritis. *Ann Intern Med.* 1988;109:170.
203. Rivera Vaquerizo PA, Santisteban Lopez Y, Blasco Colmenarejo M, et al. Clindamycin-induced esophageal ulcer. *Revista Espanola de Enfermedades Digestivas.* 2004;96:143-145.
204. Rockwood RP, Embardo LS. Theophylline, ciprofloxacin, erythromycin. A potentially harmful regimen. *Ann Pharmacother.* 1993;27:651-652.
205. Romano A, Gueant-Rodriguez RM, Viola M, Pettinato R, Gueant JL. Cross-reactivity and tolerability of cephalosporins in patients with immediate hypersensitivity to penicillins. *Ann Intern Med.* 2004;141:16-22.
206. Romero-Gomez M, Suarez GE, Fernandez MC. Norfloxacin-induced acute cholestatic hepatitis in a patient with alcoholic liver cirrhosis. *Am J Gastroenterol.* 1999;94:2324-2325.
207. Rothenberg HJ. Anaphylactoid reaction to vancomycin. *JAMA.* 1959;171: 1101-1102.
208. Rubart M, Pressler ML, Pride HP, Zipes DP. Electrophysiological mechanisms in a canine model of erythromycin-associated long QT syndrome. *Circulation.* 1993;88(Pt 1):1832-1844.
209. Rybak MJ, Boike SC. Additive toxicity in patients receiving vancomycin and aminoglycosides. *Clin Pharm.* 1983;2:508.
210. Sabra R, Takahashi K, Branch RA, Badr KF. Mechanisms of amphotericin B-induced reduction of glomerular filtration rate. A micro-puncture study. *J Pharmacol Exp Ther.* 1990;253:34-37.
211. Sacristan JA, Soto JA, deCos MA. Erythromycin-induced hypoacusis. 11 new cases and literature review. *Ann Pharmacother.* 1993;27:950-955.
212. Sage DJ. Management of acute anaphylactoid reactions. *Int Anesthesiol Clin.* 1985;23:175-186.
213. Samaha FF. QTC interval prolongation and polymorphic ventricular tachycardia in association with levofloxacin. *Am J Med.* 1999;107:528-529.
214. Saraway SM, Marke J, Steinberg M, et al. Doom anxiety and delirium in lidocaine toxicity. *Am J Psychiatry.* 1987;144:159-163.

215. Saxon A, Swabb EA, Adkinson NF Jr. Investigation into the immunologic cross-reactivity of aztreonam with other beta lactam antibiotics. *Am J Med.* 1985;78(Suppl A):19-26.
216. Sayawa BP, Weihprecht H, Cambell WR, et al. Direct vasoconstriction as a possible cause for amphotericin B-induced nephrotoxicity in rats. *J Clin Invest.* 1991;87:2079-2107.
217. Schentag JJ, Plaut ME. Patterns of beta-2-microglobulin excretion in patients treated with aminoglycosides. *Kidney Int.* 1980;16:654-661.
218. Schluter G. Ciprofloxacin. Review of potential toxicologic effects. *Am J Med.* 1987;82(Suppl 4A):91-93.
219. Schmuck G, Schurmann A, Schluter G. Determination of the excitatory potencies of fluoroquinolones in the central nervous system by an in vitro model. *Antimicrob Agents Chemother.* 1998;42:1831-1836.
220. Schrodt BJ, Kulp-Shorten CL, Callen JP. Necrotizing vasculitis of the skin and uterine cervix associated with minocycline therapy for acne vulgaris. *South Med J.* 1999;92:502-504.
221. Scott JL, Finegold SM, Belkins GA, Lawrence JS. A controlled double-blind study of the hematologic toxicity of chloramphenicol. *N Engl J Med.* 1965;272:1137.
222. Seamans KB, Gloor P, Dobell RAR, Wyant JD. Penicillin-induced seizures during cardiopulmonary bypass. A clinical and electroencephalographic study. *N Engl J Med.* 1968;278:861-868.
223. Seldon R, Sasahara AA. Central nervous system toxicity induced by lidocaine. *JAMA.* 1967;202:908-909.
224. Shapiro LE, Knowles SR, Shear N. Comparative safety of tetracycline, minocycline and doxycycline. *Arch Dermatol.* 1997;133:1224-1230.
225. Shu XO, Gao YT, Linet MS, et al. Chloramphenicol use and childhood leukaemia in Shanghai. *Lancet.* 1987;2:934-937.
226. Silber T, D'Angelio L. Doom, anxiety, and Hoigne's syndrome. *Am J Psychiatry.* 1987;144:1365.
227. Slaughter RL, Cerra FB, Koup JR. Effect of hemodialysis on total body clearance of chloramphenicol. *Am J Hosp Pharm.* 1980;37:1083-1086.
228. Slavich IL, Gleffe RF, Haas EJ. Grand mal epileptic seizures during ciprofloxacin therapy. *JAMA.* 1989;261:558-559.
229. Slayton W, Anstine D, Lakhdir F, Sleasman J, Neiberger R. Tetany in a child with AIDS receiving intravenous tobramycin. *South Med J.* 1996; 89:1108-1110.
230. Somer T, Finegold SM. Vasculitis associated with infections, immunization, and antimicrobial drugs. *Clin Infect Dis.* 1995;20:1010-1036.
231. Song BB, Sha SH, Schacht J. Iron chelators protect from aminoglycoside-induced cochleo- and vestibulo-toxicity. *Free Radic Biol Med.* 1998;25:189-195.
232. Stahlmann R, Lode H. Toxicity of quinolones. *Drugs.* 1999;58(Suppl 2):37-42.
233. Stevens DC, Kleiman MB, Lietman PS, Schreiner RL. Exchange transfusion in acute chloramphenicol toxicity. *J Pediatr.* 1981;99:651-653.
234. Strevel EL, Kuper A, Gold WL. Severe and protracted hypoglycaemia associated with co-trimoxazole use. *Lancet Infect Dis.* 2006;6:178-182.
235. Sunagawa M, Matsumura H, Sumita Y, Nouda H. Structural features resulting in convulsive activity of carbapenem compounds. Effect of C-2 side chain. *J Antibiot (Tokyo).* 1995;48:408-416.
236. Swanson DJ, Sung RJ, Fine MJ, et al. Erythromycin ototoxicity. Prospective assessment with serum concentrations and audiograms in a study of patients with pneumonia. *Am J Med.* 1992;92:61-68.
237. Swanson-Biearman B, Dean BS, Lopez G, Krenzelok EP. The effects of penicillin and cephalosporin ingestions in children less than six years of age. *Vet Hum Toxicol.* 1988;30:66-67.
238. Takada S, Kato M, Takayama S. Comparison of lesions induced by intra-articular injections of quinolones and compounds damaging cartilage components in rat femoral condyles. *J Toxicol Environ Health.* 1994;42:73-88.
239. Teitelbaum JE, Perez-Atayde AR, Cohen M, Bousvaros A, Jonas MM. Minocycline-related autoimmune hepatitis. Case series and literature review. *Arch Pediatr Adolesc Med.* 1998;152:1132-1136.
240. Telithromycin Product Information. Kansas City, MO: Aventis Pharmaceuticals; 2004.
241. Tenenbein MS, Tenenbein M. Acute pancreatitis due to erythromycin overdose. *Pediatr Emerg Care.* 2005;21:675-676.
242. Thompson WL, Anderson SE Jr, Lipsky JJ, et al. Overdose of chloramphenicol. *JAMA.* 1975;234:149-150.
243. Threlkeld SC, Hirsch MS. Antiviral therapy. The epidemiology of HIV and AIDS. Current trends. In: Gold JWM, Telzak EE, White DA, eds. *The Diagnosis and Management of the HIV-Infected Patient, Part 1. Med Clin North Am.* 1996;80:1263-1283.
244. Timmermans L. Influence of antibiotics on spermatogenesis. *J Urol.* 1974; 112:348-349.
245. Tsuji A, Sato H, Kume Y, et al. Inhibitory effects of quinolone antibacterial agents on gamma-aminobutyric acid binding to receptor sites in rat brain membranes. *Antimicrob Agents Chemother.* 1988;32:190-194.
246. Turner WM. Lidocaine and psychotic reactions. *Ann Intern Med.* 1982;97:149-150.
247. Tynes BS, Utz JP, Bennett JE, Alling DW. Reducing amphotericin B reactions. *Am Rev Respir Dis.* 1963;87:264-268.
248. Ulinski T, Deschenes G, Bensman A. Large-pore haemodialysis membranes. an efficient tool for rapid removal of vancomycin after accidental overdose. *Nephrol Dial Transplant.* 2005;20:1517-1518.
249. Unal M, Peyman GA, Liang C, et al. Ocular toxicity of intravitreal clarithromycin. *Retina.* 1999;19:442-446.
250. Utley PM, Lucas JB, Billings TE. Acute psychotic reactions to aqueous procaine penicillin. *South Med J.* 1966;59:1271-1274.
251. Van Arsdel PP Jr. The risk of penicillin reactions. *Ann Intern Med.* 1968;69:1071-1073.
252. Veit O, Beck B, Steuerwald M, Hatz C. First case of ivermectin-induced severe hepatitis. *Trans R Soc Trop Med Hyg.* 2006;100:795-797.
253. Walker PD, Barri Y, Shah SV. Oxidant mechanisms in gentamicin nephrotoxicity. *Ren Fail.* 1999;21:433-442.
254. Walker S, Norwood J, Thornton C, Schaberg D. Trimethoprim-sulfamethoxazole associated rhabdomyolysis in a patient with AIDS: case report and review of the literature. *Am J Med Sci.* 2006;331:339-341.
255. Wallace KL. Antibiotic-induced convulsions. *Med Toxicol.* 1997;13:741-762.
256. Wallace MR, Mascola JR, Oldfield EC 3rd. Red man syndrome. Incidence, etiology and prophylaxis. *J Infect Dis.* 1991;164:1180-1185.
257. Walmsley SL, Winn LM, Harrison ML, Uetrecht JP, Wells PG. Oxidative stress and thiol depletion in plasma and peripheral blood lymphocytes from HIV-infected patients. Toxicological and pathological implications. *AIDS.* 1997;11:1689-1697.
258. Walsh TJ, Finberg RW, Arndt C, et al. Liposomal amphotericin B for empirical therapy in patients with persistent fever and neutropenia. *N Engl J Med.* 1999;340:764-771.
259. Watts RG, Conte JE, Zurlinden E, Waldo FB. Effect of charcoal hemoperfusion on clearance of pentamidine isethionate after accidental overdose. *J Toxicol Clin Toxicol.* 1997;35:89-92.
260. Weis S, Karagulle D, Kornhuber J, Bayerlein K. Cotrimoxazole-induced psychosis. a case report and review of literature. *Pharmacopsychiatry.* 2006;39:236-237.
261. Weisberger AS, Wessler S, Avioli LV. Mechanisms of action of chloramphenicol. *JAMA.* 1969;209:97-103.
262. Westphal JF, Vetter D, Brogard JM. Hepatic side-effects of antibiotics. *J Antimicrob Chemother.* 1994;33:387-401.
263. Wolf R, Brenner DS. An active amide group in the molecule of drugs that induce pemphigus. A casual or causal relationship? *Dermatology.* 1994;189:1-4.
264. Yarbrough JA, Moffitt JE, Brown DA, Stafford C. Cimetidine in the treatment of refractory anaphylaxis. *Ann Allergy.* 1989;63:235-238.
265. Yoshioka H, Nambu H, Fujia M, Uehara H. Convulsion following intrathecal cephaloridine. *Infection.* 1975;2:123-124.
266. Yunis AA. Chloramphenicol-induced bone marrow suppression. *Semin Hematol.* 1973;10:255-234.
267. Zager RA, Bredl CR, Schimpf BA. Direct amphotericin B-mediated tubular toxicity. Assessments of selected cytoprotective agents. *Kidney Int.* 1992; 42:1588-1594.
268. Zhou W, Moore DE. Photosensitizing activity of the anti-bacterial drugs sulfamethoxazole and trimethoprim. *J Photochem Photobiol.* 1997; 39:63-72.

CHAPTER 57
ANTITUBERCULOUS MEDICATIONS

Christina H. Hernon and Edward W. Boyer

Tuberculosis and antituberculous therapy have ever increasing global implications. More and more people are exposed to more combinations of antituberculous and antiretroviral drugs throughout the world. Vigilance for depression and suicide risk are particularly important to evaluate as complications of the diseases under treatment and as complications of the therapy. Isoniazid remains the most commonly used and the most consequential in overdose.

HISTORY AND EPIDEMIOLOGY

The global burden of tuberculosis is enormous. Approximately two billion people, one-third of the total population of the world, are infected with *Mycobacterium tuberculosis.* An estimated 8.8 million new cases of disease are diagnosed and 1.6 million persons die from tuberculosis annually.[3] In 2007, the incidence of tuberculosis (TB) in the United States was the lowest recorded (13,000 cases) since the inception of national reporting in 1953.[22] The introduction of isoniazid (INH) into clinical practice in 1952 produced a steady decline in the number of TB cases in the United States over the subsequent 30 years. However, between 1985 and 1991, there was a resurgence in TB cases in the United States resulting primarily from the effects of human immunodeficiency virus (HIV), homelessness, deterioration in the healthcare infrastructure, and an increased presence of foreign-born persons. With the initiation and implementation of containment strategies, the spread of the infection has been slowed by aggressive case identification and patient-centered management, including directly observed therapy, social support, housing, and substance abuse treatment. These methods have decreased the incidence rate in the United States as well as worldwide. In 2005, the tuberculosis incidence was stable or declining worldwide, although the total number of new TB cases continues to increase slowly. Also in that year, extensively-drug-resistant tuberculosis (XDR-TB) was recognized, with between 4% and 19% of multidrug resistant tuberculosis (MDR-TB) strains being resistant to both INH and rifampin, all fluoroquinolones, and at least one of three injectable drugs (capreomycin, kanamycin, and amikacin).[7,21,94] At present, populations that remain at risk for tuberculosis include HIV-positive patients, the homeless, injection drug users, healthcare workers, prisoners, prison workers, and Native Americans. In addition, the tuberculosis rate in foreign-born persons is nearly 10 times higher than in US-born persons. In the US population, countries of birth generating the highest number of tuberculosis cases are Mexico, the Philippines, India, and Vietnam.[7,21] The use of second-line (reserve) drugs and multidrug antituberculous regimens for MDR-TB and XDR-TB resulted in an increased incidence of adverse drug effects, increasing to 40-70% and sometimes requiring discontinuation of the treatment. Hepatotoxicity, peripheral neuropathy, and ocular neuropathy are often irreversible and potentially fatal. Psychosocial conditions, chronic illness, and adverse drug effects involving anxiety, depression, and psychosis all contribute to an escalated risk of suicidality, intentional overdose, and noncompliance with therapy.[128]

ISONIAZID

PHARMACOLOGY

Isoniazid (INH, or isonicotinic hydrazide) is structurally related to nicotinic acid (niacin, or vitamin B_3), nicotinamide-adenosine dinucleotide (NAD), and pyridoxine (vitamin B_6) (Fig. 57–1). The pyridine ring is essential for antituberculous activity. Isoniazid itself does not have direct antibacterial activity. It is a prodrug that undergoes metabolic activation by KatG, a catalase-peroxidase in *M. tuberculosis* that produces a highly reactive intermediate,[95,130] which in turn interacts with InhA, a mycobacterial enzyme that functions as an enoyl-acyl carrier protein (enoyl-ACP) reductase.[92,93] This activated form of INH is either an anion or radical that is stabilized by the pyridine ring. Enoyl-ACP reductase catalyzes the NADH-dependent reduction of the double bonds in the growing fatty acid chain linked to acyl carrier proteins. InhA is required for the synthesis of very-long-chain lipids, mycolic acids (containing between 40 and 60 carbons) that are important components of mycobacterial cell walls.

This INH metabolite enters the binding site of InhA where it reacts with the reduced form of nicotinamide adenine dinucleotide (NADH).[95] The covalently linked INH-NADH complex remains bound to the active site of InhA, irreversibly inhibiting the enzyme.[76,92]

PHARMACOKINETICS AND TOXICOKINETICS

When therapeutic doses of 300 mg are administered orally, INH is rapidly absorbed, reaching peak serum concentrations typically within 2 hours.[60,87,88] Isoniazid diffuses into all body fluids with a volume of distribution of approximately 0.6 L/kg and has negligible binding to serum proteins. After the drug penetrates infected tissue, it persists in concentrations well above those generally required for bacteriocidal activity.[88]

Isoniazid is metabolized via a cytochrome P450—mediated process, with approximately 75% to 95% of INH renally eliminated in the form of its hepatic metabolites within 24 hours of administration.[89] The primary metabolic pathway for INH is via *N*-acetylation performed by hepatocytes and mucosal cells in the small intestine. Polymorphic *N*-acetyltransferase-2 (NAT2), the enzyme responsible for this conversion, exhibits Michaelis-Menten kinetics, although the activity of an individual's enzymes is determined by an autosomal dominant inheritance pattern, with homozygous fast acetylators (FF), heterozygous fast acetylators (FS), and homozygous slow acetylators (SS). Patients are distinguishable phenotypically as slow and fast acetylators. The fast acetylation isoform is found in 40% to 50% of American whites and African Americans, whereas the fast acetylator isoenzymes are found in 80% to 90% of Asians and Inuits.[35,39] These isoforms are distinguishable by the following characteristics: (1) slow acetylators have less presystemic clearance, or first-pass effect, than do fast acetylators; (2) fast acetylators metabolize INH five to six times faster than slow acetylators; and (3) serum INH concentrations are 30% to 50% lower in fast acetylators than in slow acetylators. The elimination half-life of INH is approximately 70 minutes in fast acetylators, and 180 minutes in slow acetylators. Twenty-seven percent of INH is excreted unchanged in urine by slow acetylators, as compared with 11% excretion in fast acetylators. The clearance of INH averages 46 mL/min.[10,122] Isoniazid is acetylated into acetylisoniazid and then hydrolyzed into isonicotinic acid and acetylhydrazine. Subsequent acetylation of acetylhydrazine into diacetylhydrazine or hydrolysis into hydrazine occurs.

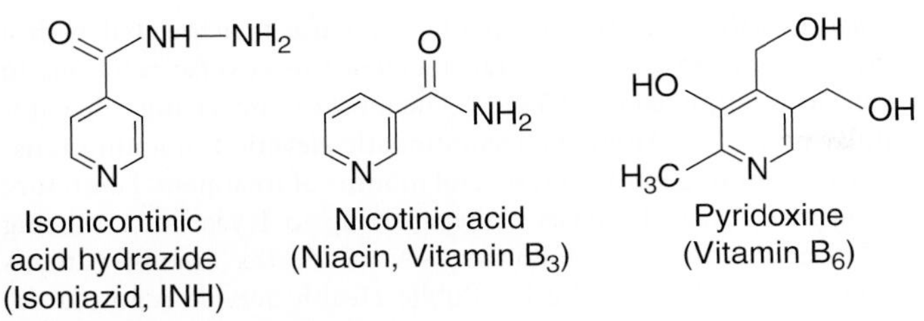

Isonicontinic acid hydrazide (Isoniazid, INH)

Nicotinic acid (Niacin, Vitamin B_3)

Pyridoxine (Vitamin B_6)

FIGURE 57–1. INH and related compounds.

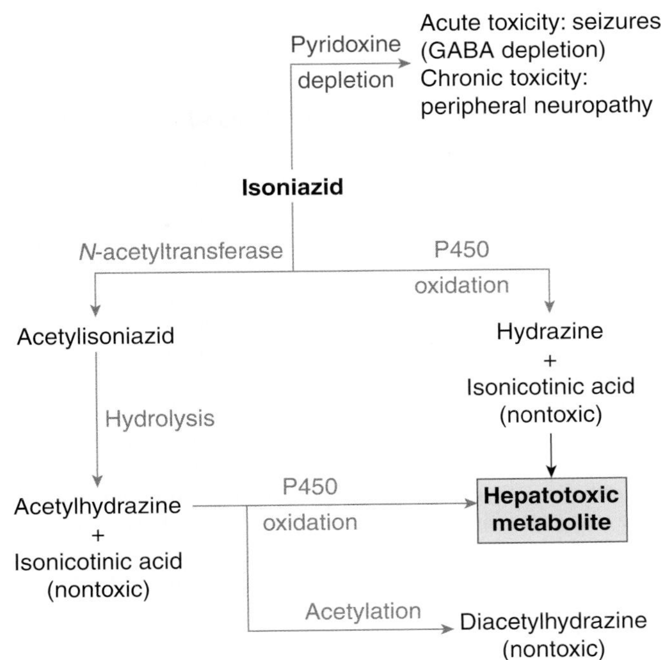

FIGURE 57–2. Metabolism of INH. Acetylator status is determined by polymorphism in *N*-acetyltransferase.

Additionally, a small portion of isoniazid is directly hydrolyzed into isonicotinic acid and hydrazine, and this pathway is of greater quantitative significance in slow acetylators than in rapid acetylators. Hepatic microsomal oxidation of the acetylhydrazine intermediate into reactive intermediates has been proposed as the cause of hepatotoxicity, but continuing research suggests that hydrazine plays perhaps an even greater role in hepatic injury.[46,80,119] Figure 57–2 illustrates the metabolism of INH.

PATHOPHYSIOLOGY

Mechanism of Toxicity Toxic effects of INH are caused by two additive mechanisms. First, INH alters the metabolism of pyridoxine (vitamin B_6), the coenzyme needed for transamination, transketolization, and decarboxylation biotransformation reactions. Isoniazid creates a functional deficiency of pyridoxine by at least two mechanisms (Fig. 57–3). Hydrazone INH metabolites inhibit pyridoxine phosphokinase, the enzyme that converts pyridoxine to its active form, pyridoxal-5'-phosphate.[25,59,78] In addition, INH reacts with pyridoxal phosphate to produce an inactive hydrazone complex that is renally excreted.[78,122] Urinary excretion of pyridoxine and its metabolites increases with increasing INH dosage, reflecting the effect of INH on pyridoxine metabolism. The consequences of pyridoxine depletion include impaired activity of pyridoxine-dependent enzyme systems, as well as a decrease in catecholamine synthesis. In addition, INH either replaces nicotinic acid in the synthesis of NAD or reacts with NAD to form inactive hydrazones. Isoniazid disrupts cellular reduction/oxidation capabilities through both of these mechanisms.

Second, isoniazid interferes with the synthesis and metabolism of γ-aminobutyric acid (GABA), the primary inhibitory neurotransmitter in the central nervous system (CNS). Two pyridoxine-dependent enzymes control GABA metabolism: glutamic acid decarboxylase (GAD) and GABA aminotransferase. The former catalyzes GABA synthesis from glutamate, while the latter degrades the neurotransmitter. The inhibitory effects are greater on GAD, which leads to both decreased GABA and elevated glutamate concentrations.[124] Depletion of GABA is thought to be the etiology of INH-induced seizures.[5] Structurally similar chemicals exert similar acute toxic effects. Monomethylhydrazine, a metabolite produced from gyromitrin isolated from the *Gyromitra* species ("false morel") mushroom, and the hydrazines used in liquid rocket fuel have a similar mechanism of action (see Chap. 117).

The use of isoniazid in pregnancy is of concern since it is a class C drug, crosses the placenta, and produces umbilical cord serum concentrations comparable to maternal serum concentrations.[13,14,61] Mammalian teratogen studies suggest that isoniazid is not a human teratology, although fetal deformities following acute overdose of INH have been reported.[70,122] Administration of INH to pregnant women was not associated with cancer in their offspring. Although isoniazid

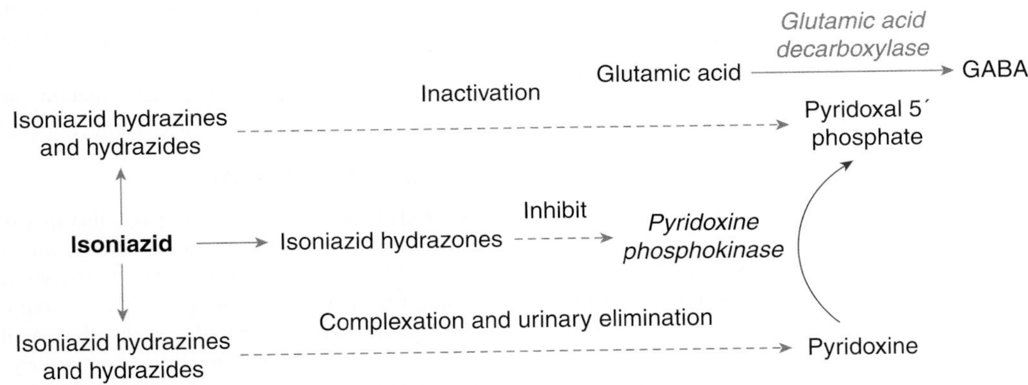

FIGURE 57–3. The effect of isoniazid on γ-aminobutyric acid (GABA) synthesis.

readily enters breast milk, breast-feeding during therapy is considered acceptable.[100,122]

INTERACTIONS WITH OTHER DRUGS AND FOODS

Drug—drug interactions associated with isoniazid are mediated through alteration of hepatic metabolism of several cytochrome P450 (CYP) isoenzymes. The majority of these interactions are inhibitory, with decreased (CYP)-mediated transformations—particularly demethylation, oxidation, and hydroxylation (see Chap. 12 Appendix). Clinically relevant adverse effects with elevated concentrations of theophylline (CYP1A2), phenytoin (CYP2C9/CYP2C19), warfarin (CYP2C9/CYP2C19), valproic acid, and carbamazepine (CYP3A4) are due to decreased hepatic metabolism of these drugs.[33,106,126] The CYP2E1 cytochrome subtype, however, exhibits a complex response to isoniazid; a therapeutic dose of INH induces expression of CYP2E1, but simultaneously binds, stabilizes, and inhibits its metabolic activity. Eventual dissociation of isoniazid from the isoenzyme active site creates an increased intracellular concentration of CYP2E1 available to metabolize potential substrates. The formation of the acetaminophen metabolite responsible for toxicity, NAPQI (*N*-acetyl-*p*-benzoquinoneimine), is catalyzed by CYP2E1. Isoniazid-mediated effects in acetaminophen-induced hepatotoxicity are uncertain because of differences in acetylator status (fast, slow) and variations in CYP2E1 activity.[24,106]

Isoniazid interacts with numerous foods. Isoniazid is a weak monoamine oxidase inhibitor, and tyramine reactions to foods (aged cheeses, wines) and serotonin syndrome from meperidine are reported in patients taking INH. Clinical effects include flushing, tachycardia, and hypertension.[32,45,69,112] Furthermore, INH inhibits the enzyme histaminase, leading to exacerbated reactions following the ingestion of histamine in scombrotoxic fish.[56,77,106] Table 57–1 summarizes additional INH drug and food interactions.

CLINICAL MANIFESTATIONS OF INH TOXICITY

Acute Toxicity Isoniazid produces the triad of seizures refractory to conventional therapy, severe metabolic acidosis, and coma. These clinical manifestations may appear as soon as 30 minutes following ingestion.[54,58,117] The case fatality rate of a single acute ingestion may be as high as 20%.[15,18] Although vomiting, slurred speech, dizziness, and tachycardia may represent early manifestations of toxicity, seizures may be the initial sign of acute overdose.[72] Seizures may occur following the ingestion of greater than 20 mg/kg of INH, and invariably occur with ingestions greater than 35 to 40 mg/kg. Patients with underlying seizure disorders may develop seizures at lower doses.[15] Hyperreflexia or areflexia may herald INH-induced seizures. Consciousness may return between seizures or status epilepticus can occur.[30,83] Because GABA, the primary inhibitory neurotransmitter, is depleted in acute INH toxicity, seizure activity may persist until GABA concentrations are restored, even with anticonvulsant therapy.

Acute INH toxicity is often associated with seizures and an anion gap metabolic acidosis associated with a high serum lactate concentration. Typically, arterial pH ranges between 6.80 and 7.30, although survival in the setting of an arterial pH of 6.49 was reported.[54] Paralyzed animals poisoned with INH do not develop elevated lactate concentrations, a finding that suggests the lactate arises from intense muscular activity.[25,84]

Protracted coma typically occurs with acute severe INH toxicity. Coma may last as long as 24 to 36 hours and persist beyond the termination of seizure activity as well as the resolution of acidemia. The etiology of coma is unknown.[11,54] Additional sequelae from acute INH toxicity include rhabdomyolysis, renal failure, hyperglycemia, glycosuria, and ketonuria, along with hypotension and hyperpyrexia.[4,8,19,85,122,123]

Chronic Toxicity. Chronic therapeutic INH use is associated with a variety of adverse effects. Overall incidence of adverse reactions to isoniazid is estimated to be 5.4%.[89] The most disconcerting is hepatocellular necrosis.[41] Although asymptomatic elevation of aminotransferases is common in the first several months of treatment, laboratory testing may reveal the onset of hepatitis up to 1 year after starting INH therapy. In 1978, following several deaths among patients receiving INH therapy, the US Public Health Service reported the incidence of clinically evident hepatitis as 1% of those taking INH; of that subgroup, 10% died, for an overall mortality of 0.1%.[17,66] Research performed since the resurgence of TB, however, identified a considerably lower rate of hepatotoxicity. Clinically relevant hepatitis occurred in only 11 patients in a population of 11,141 persons receiving INH and close monitoring, an incidence of 0.1%.[82] Additional studies suggest that the death rate from INH hepatotoxicity is only 0.001% (two of 202,497 treated patients).[98] Hepatotoxicity is associated with chronic overdosage, increasing age, comorbid conditions such as malnutrition, and combinations of antituberculous drugs that may serve as cytochrome inducers. Overt hepatic failure often occurs if INH therapy is continued after onset of hepatocellular injury in both adults and children.[37,38,51,74,109,125] The incidence of hepatitis is two to four times higher in pregnant women than in nonpregnant women.[43]

Isoniazid-induced hepatitis can arise via two pathways.[37,127] The first involves an immunologic mechanism resulting in hepatic injury that is thought to be idiopathic.[103,122] The association of hepatitis with lupus erythematosus, hemolytic anemia, thrombocytopenia, arthritis, vasculitis, and polyserositis supports an immunologic process.[102,122] However, symptoms commonly found in autoimmune disorders such as fever, rash, and eosinophilia are usually absent with drug-induced lupus erythematosus, and rechallenge with isoniazid often fails to provoke recurrence of hepatocellular injury.[37,102,127] The second, more common mechanism involves direct hepatic injury by INH or its metabolites. The metabolites believed responsible for hepatic injury are acetylhydrazine and hydrazine (see Figure 57–2).[46,80,118]

Peripheral neuropathy and optic neuritis are known adverse drug effects of chronic INH use. Neurotoxicity is probably caused by pyridoxine deficiency aggravated by the formation of pyridoxine-INH hydrazones.[39] Peripheral neuropathy, the most common complication of INH therapy, presents in a stocking-glove distribution that progresses proximally. Although primarily sensory in nature, myalgias and weakness may occur.[110] Peripheral neuropathy is generally observed in severely malnourished, alcoholic, uremic, or diabetic patients; it is also associated with slow acetylator status, an effect that leads to increased INH concentrations and, consequently, increased pyridoxine depletion.[48] Optic neuritis may occur with isoniazid therapy, usually concurrent with other medications such as ethambutol or etarencept, and presents as decreased visual acuity, eye pain, and dyschromatopsia; visual field testing may reveal central scotomata and bitemporal hemianopsia.[49,58,64] Isoniazid is also associated with such findings of CNS toxicity as ataxia, psychosis, hallucinations, and coma.[1,9,47,97]

DIAGNOSTIC TESTING

Acute INH toxicity is a clinical diagnosis that may be inferred by history and confirmed by measuring serum INH concentrations.[105] Acute toxicity from INH has been defined as a serum INH concentration greater than 10 mg/L 1 hour after ingestion, greater than 3.2 mg/L 2 hours after ingestion, or greater than 0.2 mg/L 6 hours after the ingestion.[83] Because serum INH concentration measurements are not widely available, clinicians cannot rely on serum concentrations to confirm the diagnosis or initiate therapy. Because of the risk of hepatitis associated with chronic INH use,

TABLE 57–1. Adverse Reactions and Drug Interactions of Antituberculous Drugs

Drug	Major Adverse Reactions	Drug Interactions Clinical Effect	Monitoring	Comments
Isoniazid (INH)	*Acute:* seizures, acidosis, coma, hyperthermia, oliguria, anuria *Chronic:* elevation of liver enzyme concentrations autoimmune hepatitis, arthritis, anemia, hemolysis, eosinophilia, peripheral neuropathy, optic neuritis, vitamin B_6 deficiency (pellagra)	Rifampin, PZA, ethanol: hepatic necrosis Acetaminophen: hepatic necrosis Warfarin: increased INR Theophylline: tachycardia, vomiting, seizures, acidosis Phenytoin: increased phenytoin concentrations Carbamazepine: altered mental status Meperidine: hypertension Lactose: decreased INH absorption Antacids: decreased INH absorption Red wine/soft cheese: tyramine reaction Fish (scombroid): flushing, pruritus	Liver enzymes, ANA, CBC	HIV enteropathy may decrease absorption; INH should not be given with lactose-containing drug formulations because lactose can form hydrazones and lower INH concentrations
Rifampin	*Acute:* diarrhea, periorbital edema *Chronic:* hepatitis, reddish discoloration of body fluids	Protease inhibitors: decreased serum concentration of protease inhibitor Delavirdine: increased HIV resistance Cyclosporine: graft rejection Warfarin: decreased INR Oral contraceptives: ineffective contraception Methadone: opioid withdrawal Phenytoin: higher frequency of seizures Theophylline: decreased theophylline concentrations Verapamil: decreased cardiovascular effect	If administered with HIV antiretrovirals, viral titers should be followed. Liver enzymes; monitor serum concentrations of drugs (i.e., phenytoin, cyclosporine) or clinical markers of efficacy (i.e., coagulation times)	Interactions of rifampin with several HIV medications are very poorly described; changes in dosing or dosing interval for both rifampin and antiretroviral drugs may be required; teratogenic
Ethambutol	*Chronic:* optic neuritis, loss of red-green discrimination, loss of peripheral vision		Visual acuity, color discrimination	Contraindicated in children too young for formal ophthalmologic examination
Pyrazinamide (PZA)	*Chronic:* hepatitis, decreased urate excretion	INH: increased rates of hepatotoxicity (when extended courses or high dose pyrazinamide used)	Liver enzymes	Courses of therapy of 2 months or less recommended
Cycloserine	*Chronic:* depression, paranoia, seizures, megaloblastic anemia	INH: increased frequency of seizures	CBC, psychiatric monitoring	
Ethionamide	*Chronic:* orthostatic hypotension, depression	Cycloserine: may increase CNS effects	Blood pressure, pulse, orthostasis	
para-Aminosalicylic acid	*Chronic:* malaise, GI upset, elevated liver enzymes, hypersensitivity reactions, thrombocytopenia		Liver enzymes, CBC	
Capreomycin	*Chronic:* hearing loss, tinnitus, proteinuria, sterile abscess at IM injection sites		Audiometry, renal function tests	

ANA, antinuclear antibodies; HIV, human immunodeficiency virus.

hepatic aminotransferases should be regularly monitored once therapy is started. In critically ill patients, serum should be assessed for acidosis, renal function, creatine phosphokinase (CPK), and urine myoglobin indicating rhabdomyolysis and possible renal failure.

MANAGEMENT

Acute Toxicity The initial management requires termination of seizure activity with pyridoxine, benzodiazepines, fluid resuscitation, stabilization and correction of vital signs and maintenance of a patent airway. Gastrointestinal (GI) decontamination should be performed by administering activated charcoal to patients who are awake and able to comply with therapy.[108] Orogastric lavage is relatively contraindicated because of the risk of seizures, unless the patient is intubated. Delayed absorption of INH has not been observed, suggesting that late GI decontamination with activated charcoal will probably be ineffective in preventing toxicity.[104]

The antidote for INH-induced neurologic dysfunction is pyridoxine. Pyridoxine rapidly terminates seizures, corrects metabolic acidosis, and reverses coma. The efficacy of pyridoxine is correlated with the administered dose; one study identified recurrent seizures in 60% of patients who received no pyridoxine and in 47% of those who received 10% of the ideal pyridoxine dose, and no seizures in patients who received the full dose of pyridoxine.[121] To treat acute toxicity, the pyridoxine dose in grams should equal the amount of INH ingested in grams, with a first dose of up to 5 g intravenously in adults. Unknown quantities of ingested INH warrant initial empiric treatment with a pyridoxine dose of no more than 5 g (pediatric dose: 70 mg/kg to a maximum of 5 g). Pyridoxine should be administered at a rate of 1 g every 2 to 3 minutes. Seizures that persist beyond administration of the initial dose should receive an additional similar dose of pyridoxine (see Antidotes in Depth A15—Pyridoxine).[6]

Hospital pharmacies may stock insufficient quantities of intravenous pyridoxine to treat even a single patient with a large INH ingestion.[101] In the event that intravenous formulations are unavailable in sufficient quantities, pyridoxine tablets may be crushed and administered with fluids via nasogastric tube.[101]

Conventional anticonvulsants, although generally used as first-line agents, demonstrate variable effectiveness in terminating INH-induced seizures. Benzodiazepines may be used to potentiate the antidotal efficacy of pyridoxine, particularly if optimal doses of the antidote are unavailable. The benzodiazepines act synergistically with pyridoxine, as well as possess inherent GABA-agonist activity, but as single agents they may be ineffective in the treatment of acute INH poisoning because of their reliance on GABA to exert their activity.[26,27,58,121] Phenytoin has no intrinsic GABAergic effect and is not recommended as therapy for patients with INH-induced seizures.[58,83,96] Barbiturates, which have potent GABA-agonist activity, are expected to be as effective as the benzodiazepines, although the risk of respiratory depression is greater with this class of anticonvulsant. The efficacy of propofol in terminating INH-induced seizures has not been evaluated in humans.

Although hemodialysis has been used to enhance elimination of INH in acute overdose, with clearance rates reported as high as 120 mL/min, hemodialysis is rarely indicated for initial management. It is usually reserved for patients who develop INH-overdose-induced renal failure.[19,122]

Asymptomatic patients who present to the emergency department (ED) within 2 hours of ingestion of toxic amounts of INH should receive prophylactic administration of 5 g of oral or intravenous pyridoxine. This recommendation is based on the observation that INH reaches its peak serum concentration within 2 hours of ingestion of therapeutic doses. Asymptomatic patients may be observed for a 6-hour period for signs of toxicity. Acute toxicity is unlikely to manifest more than 6 hours beyond ingestion.

Chronic Toxicity Hepatitis (defined as aminotransferase concentrations two to three times baseline concentrations) resulting from therapeutic INH administration mandates termination of therapy; malnourished patients may require nutritional support. After resolution of liver injury, INH may be restarted, provided aminotransferase concentrations are closely monitored.[37,109] Pyridoxine does not reverse hepatic injury; consequently, surveillance for and recognition of hepatocellular injury remains essential. Cases of hepatitis refractory to medical therapy may require liver transplantation.[40,55,125]

Neurologic toxicity, including peripheral neuropathies, cerebellar findings, and psychosis, is commonly treated with as much as 50 mg/d of oral pyridoxine, although doses as low as 6 mg/d appear to be effective.[1,9,97,113] Because of its effectiveness in preventing neurologic toxicity, pyridoxine is often used concurrently with INH therapy.

RIFAMYCINS

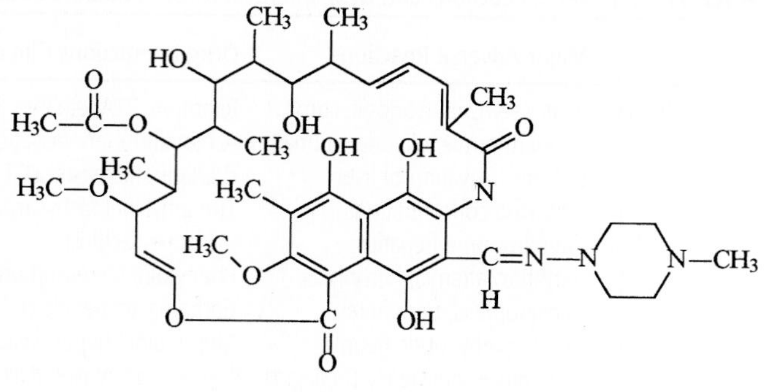

Rifampin

PHARMACOLOGY

Rifamycins are a class of macrocyclic antibiotics derived from *Amycolatopsis mediterranei*. Xenobiotics in this class include rifampin (a semisynthetic derivative), rifabutin, and rifapentine, of which the first two are most commonly used.[89] Rifampin inhibits the initial steps in RNA chain polymerization through the formation of a stable drug-enzyme complex with RNA polymerase. Disruption of RNA synthesis interrupts protein synthesis, leading to cell death. Whereas mycobacterial RNA polymerase is susceptible to rifampin, eukaryotic RNA polymerase is not. High concentrations of rifamycin antibiotics, however, can affect mammalian mitochondrial RNA synthesis, as well as reverse transcriptases and viral DNA-dependent RNA polymerases.[89]

PHARMACOKINETICS AND TOXICOKINETICS

When administered orally, rifampin reaches peak serum concentrations in 0.25 to 4 hours; foods, but not antacids, interfere with absorption.[88] Rifampin is secreted into the bile and undergoes enterohepatic recirculation. Although the recirculating antibiotic is deacetylated, the metabolite retains antimicrobial activity. The half-life of rifampin, which is normally between 1.5 and 5 hours, increases in the setting of hepatic dysfunction. After therapy is started, however, rifampin induces its own metabolism to shorten its half-life by approximately 40%. Rifampin is distributed widely into body compartments, and imparts a reddish color to all body fluids, including the cerebrospinal fluid (CSF),[89] and in this setting has been erroneously identified as xanthochromia suggesting subarachnoid hemorrhage to the clinician.[58] Because mycobacteria rapidly develop resistance to rifampin, it should not be used as single-agent therapy against tuberculosis.[89]

Rifampin therapy carries greater teratogenic risk than other antituberculous therapies, with 4.4% incidence of malformation. Anencephaly, hydrocephalus, and congenital limb abnormality and dislocations have been reported.[14,115] Rifampin is associated with hemorrhagic disease of the newborn[14] but is nevertheless compatible with breast-feeding, as only minute amounts of rifampin are secreted into breast milk.[14,114]

DRUG–DRUG INTERACTIONS

Rifamycins are potent inducers of CYP isoenzymes, which result in numerous drug interactions (Chap. 12 (Appendix)). Of the rifamycins, rifampin has greater activity in inducing CYP3A4 than rifapentine; rifabutin has the least inductive activity of the class.[71] Rifampin also induces CYP1A2, CYP2C9, and CYP2C19.[126] Additionally, the ability of rifampin to induce CYP3A4 is strongly correlated with p-glycoprotein concentrations. P-glycoprotein is a transmembrane protein that functions as a cellular efflux pump of endogenous and exogenous xenobiotics; variations in expression of p-glycoprotein significantly affects the bioavailability of many drugs and subsequent drug—drug interactions (see Chap. 12 Appendix).[42] Concurrent administration of rifampin thus affects the metabolism of an array of drugs such as warfarin, cyclosporine, phenytoin, opioids, and oral contraceptives.[42,107,126] Enzyme and p-glycoprotein induction by rifampin therefore may be responsible for a variety of pathophysiologic processes, including insufficient anticoagulation in patients receiving oral anticoagulants, acute graft rejection in transplant patients, graft-versus-host disease, difficulty controlling phenytoin concentrations, methadone withdrawal, and unplanned pregnancy. Effects arising from CYP3A4 induction begin within 5 to 6 days after rifampin is started, and persist for up to 7 days after therapy is stopped.[89]

RIFAMYCINS AND HIV

There is an increased risk of tuberculosis in patients with HIV, and concurrent highly active antiretroviral therapy (HAART) and antituberculous therapy decreases mortality. However, there are many factors that influence the efficacy and feasibility of treating these illnesses. There is decreased absorption of nearly all antituberculous drugs in patients with advanced HIV due to chronic diarrhea, intestinal pathogens, and general malabsorption. Also, there are many drug—drug interactions between antituberculous and HIV medications due to alterations in absorption, cytochrome isoenzymes, p-glycoprotein transporters, and noncytochrome metabolism.[42,52,119]

Rifampin accelerates the clearance of protease inhibitors (such as saquinavir, lopinavir) thereby decreasing the serum concentration, resulting in lower trough concentrations, which correlate with antiviral effect, increased frequency of drug-resistant mutations in the protease gene, and promotion of outgrowth of drug-resistant HIV strains.[16,116,119] The reduction of serum concentrations of protease inhibitors is of such magnitude that coadministration of rifampin with protease inhibitors could lead to loss of HIV suppression and to the emergence of resistant HIV strains.[16] Increasing the dose of protease inhibitor is associated with significant adverse drug effects and therapeutic intolerance, and cannot overcome the significant clearance of protease inhibitors, even when combined with the standard "boosting strategy" of adding ritonavir, a potent CYP3A4 inhibitor that can increase the concentration of other protease inhibitors 20-fold to attain a therapeutic effect.[20,90,119] It may be possible that "super boosted protease inhibitors" with high-dose ritonavir may be tolerable and effective. Research is ongoing.

Rifampin also induces the metabolism and clearance of nucleoside reverse transcriptase inhibitors (NRTIs, such as stavudine, lamivudine, zidovudine) without influencing cytochrome P450 mechanisms. Resulting decreased serum concentrations of NRTIs, however, do not significantly interfere with drug efficacy. The efficacy of NRTIs is not related to the serum concentration of drug, but is instead related to the intracellular concentration of the active metabolite, a triphosphate derivative. Even though rifampin decreases serum zidovudine concentrations by 47%, active metabolite is present within cells in sufficient levels for activity. Rifampin, therefore, has minimal effect on the efficacy of nucleoside reverse transcriptase inhibitors.[16] Table 57-1 lists the drug interactions of rifampin.

Combining rifampin with nonnucleoside reverse transcriptase inhibitors (NNRTIs, such as efavirenz, nevirapine) should be considered on a case-by-case basis, as NNRTIs vary widely in their role as substrates, inducers, or inhibitors of cytochome P450 systems, particularly CYP3A4. As a result, it is often difficult to anticipate the degree and effect of drug—drug interactions with rifamycins. It is clear, however, that rifamycins have a role in the treatment of HIV-associated tuberculosis, and that drug interactions are often modest and surmountable with dose adjustment or drug substitution.[90]

Rifampin suppresses the transformation of antigen-stimulated lymphocytes, as well as normal T-cell function, leading to decreased sensitivity to tuberculin, in turn resulting in false-negative purified protein derivative (PPD) test results.

CLINICAL MANIFESTATIONS

Acute Toxicity The most common side effects of acute rifampin overdose are GI symptoms consisting of epigastric pain, nausea, vomiting, and diarrhea.[37,89] The presence of diarrhea distinguishes rifampin ingestion from overdose of other antimycobacterial agents. Three reported deaths have been described from rifampin or rifampicin ingestion; an autopsy performed on one of these patients demonstrated the presence of pulmonary edema, although no causation was implied.[12,62,91] Other effects include flushing, angioedema, and obtundation. Children who receive an overdose of rifampin can develop facial or periorbital edema. Anterior uveitis is occasionally observed, as are neurologic effects consisting of generalized numbness, extremity pain, ataxia, and muscular weakness.[50] Isolated rifamycin overdose infrequently produces serious acute effects.

CHRONIC TOXICITY

When rifampin was originally introduced as an antituberculous drug, hepatitis was more frequently observed in patients taking combination therapy of rifampin and INH than in those taking INH alone. These findings potentially arise from the ability of rifampin to induce cytochromes responsible for INH hepatotoxicity and not from direct hepatic injury by rifampin itself. Liver injury, when attributable to rifampin alone, is predominantly cholestatic, suggesting that clinical surveillance for hepatic injury is important as is regular biochemical monitoring.[37,86] Rifampin alters the metabolism of other xenobiotics, such as INH, pyrazinamide, and acetaminophen, to increase their potential for hepatotoxicity.[37,81] Although some reports highlight increased compliance and typically mild and transient hepatotoxicity with combined rifampin and pyrazinamide treatment for latent tuberculosis infection, other recent studies suggest a significant risk of fatal hepatotoxicity, and the Centers for Disease Control and Prevention (CDC) recommends generally avoiding this combination of drugs.[75]

A condition similar to a viral syndrome may result from a hypersensitivity reaction that is associated with rifampin therapy. The syndrome, which occurs in 20% of patients receiving high doses or intermittent (less than twice weekly) dosing, includes fever, chills, and myalgias. Eosinophilia, hemolytic anemia, thrombocytopenia, and interstitial nephritis can develop in severe cases, and acute renal injury is likely related to hypersensitivity. Renal failure is rarely oliguric and is usually self-limited; patients usually recover with supportive care, although rechallenge with rifampin should be undertaken only with caution.[86]

The concomitant administration of rifampin and protease inhibitors results in increased rates of arthralgias, uveitis, leukopenia, and skin discoloration. Identical side effects occurred during the simultaneous administration of rifampin and CYP3A4 inhibitors such as clarithromycin, suggesting that toxic effects arise from elevated serum rifampin concentrations.[16] Current recommendations are that rifampin not be given with protease inhibitors, except for ritonavir in rare circumstances. In patients already on protease inhibitors, rifabutin may be used in place of rifampin.[90]

THERAPEUTIC TESTING AND MANAGEMENT

Management of patients with acute rifampin overdose is primarily supportive. Stabilization of vital signs and administration of activated charcoal are usually adequate, although clinicians should remain vigilant for coingestants. For chronic toxicity, recognition of interactions between rifampin and other drugs is critical. Hepatic function should be monitored because of the ability of rifampin to augment the hepatotoxicity of other xenobiotics. Treatment for hepatic injury involves withholding rifampin therapy and reassessing the appropriateness of other xenobiotics administered to the patient. Supportive care for hepatotoxicity may be required. Influenza-like symptoms and renal failure secondary to rifampin may respond to decreasing the interval between administration of the drug.[86] Although rifampin interacts with protease inhibitors, the utility of therapeutic drug monitoring is uncertain because the correlation of clinical events with serum concentrations of rifampin and antiretroviral drugs is unknown.[16]

ETHAMBUTOL

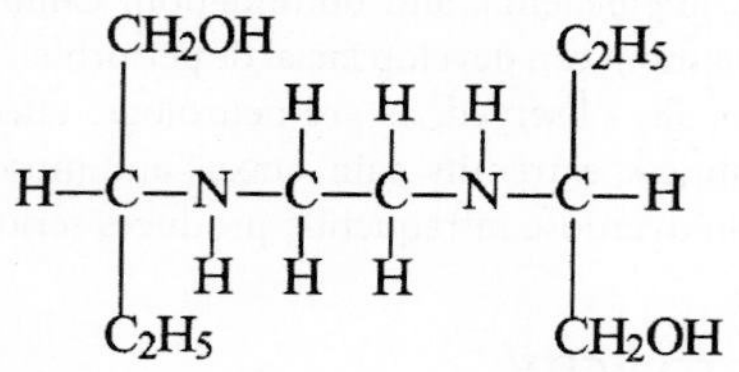

```
    CH2OH                 C2H5
    |       H    H    H    |
    |       |    |    |    |
H — C — N — C  — C  — N — C — H
    |       |    |         |
    |       H    H    H    |
    C2H5                  CH2OH
```

PHARMACOLOGY

Ethambutol is effective against *Mycobacterium tuberculosis* and *Mycobacterium kansasii* as well as some strains of Mycobacterium avium complex; however, it has no effect on other bacteria. Ethambutol inhibits arabinosyl transferases, interfering with biosynthesis of arabinogalactan and liparabinomannan, which are required for polymerization of arabinan within mycobacterial cell walls.[63,89]

PHARMACOKINETICS AND TOXICOKINETICS

Only the D(+) isomer is used therapeutically, but both enantiomers are bacteriocidal.[58] The drug is taken up rapidly by growing cells, where bacteriostatic effects appear approximately 24 hours after ethambutol is incorporated by mycobacteria.[89] About 80% of an oral dose is absorbed gastrointestinally, but both foods and antacids decrease absorption.[16,89] Maximum serum concentrations are reached within 4 hours of oral administration and are proportional to the dose. Ethambutol is approximately 20% to 30% protein bound and has a half-life of between 4 and 6 hours.[68,89] Three-fourths of a standard dose is excreted unchanged into the urine by a combination of glomerular filtration and tubular secretion. Consequently, ethambutol accumulates in patients with renal compromise, making adjustments in dosing necessary.[89] Increasingly, mutations in the Mycobacterium embB gene confer resistance to ethambutol, as high as 14.2%, with acquired resistance reaching nearly 40%.[63]

Ethambutol is considered safe for use during pregnancy as a first-line drug. Although a 2.2% incidence of congenital abnormalities was identified in women undergoing ethambutol therapy, no consistent pattern of abnormalities occurred in their offspring.[14] Ethambutol is excreted into breast milk in approximately a 1:1 ratio with serum, but is considered to be compatible with breast-feeding.[14]

CLINICAL MANIFESTATIONS AND MANAGEMENT

Acute overdose of ethambutol is generally well tolerated, although a death has been reported.[62] More commonly, nausea, abdominal pain, confusion, visual hallucinations, and optic neuropathy occur following acute ingestions of greater than 10 g.[36] Although stabilization of vital signs and GI decontamination with activated charcoal remain the hallmarks of therapy, clinicians must remain vigilant for coingestants, particularly INH. Hemodialysis is rarely used as treatment for multidrug ingestions including ethambutol.[36]

Although peripheral neuropathy and cutaneous reactions occur with chronic therapy, the most significant effect of the therapeutic use of ethambutol is unilateral or bilateral ocular toxicity presenting as painless blurring of vision, decreased perception of color, and loss of peripheral vision. These effects are largely dose and duration related, and are typically reversible with drug discontinuation.[23,29] Optic neuritis develops in approximately 15% of patients receiving 50 mg/kg/d, 5% of patients receiving 25 mg/kg/d, and fewer than 1% of those receiving 15 mg/kg/d.[86] Patients may develop subclinical ocular disease within 30 days of starting ethambutol.[129] The loss of peripheral vision and color discrimination that accompanies the optic neuropathy caused by ethambutol distinguishes this condition from the optic neuropathy secondary to INH.[58,86]

Management of chronic toxicity from ethambutol involves cessation of therapy, although improvement may be hastened by treatment with hydroxocobalamin.[58,89] Recovery is less likely in older patients and is related to the degree of visual impairment.[120]

Ethambutol is a strong metal-chelator and inactivation of zinc and copper may be related to its induction of retinal cell vacuoles and enlarged lysosomes, which interfere with membrane permeabilization, possibly causing abnormal cell function and cell death.[29,65] The visual abnormalities induced by ethambutol are similar to those caused by a hereditary condition known as Leber optic neuropathy. Both ethambutol and Leber hereditary optic neuropathy can affect oxidative phosphorylation through impairment of mitochondrial function.[28,65] Ethambutol is suspected of mimicking this condition by binding intracellular copper, altering mitochondrial function, and producing neuronal injury.[57,65] Alternatively, optic neuritis may be related to zinc metabolism. Ethambutol chelates intracellular zinc to induce reversible vacuolar degeneration in retinal cultures. Progressive degeneration leads to irreversible neuronal destruction.[29] The effect of this injury is a shift in the threshold for wavelength discrimination without changing the absolute sensitivity of the cone system, which leads to a loss of red-green discrimination.[111]

DIAGNOSTIC TESTING

All patients should receive neuro-ophthalmic testing prior to ethambutol therapy. The use of visual-evoked potentials is especially useful in identifying subclinical optic nerve disease. Furthermore, patients should receive regular visual acuity examinations, and clinicians should encourage patients to report any visual subjective symptoms. The use of ethambutol may be relatively contraindicated in children who are unable to comply with an ophthalmic examination.[58,86]

PYRAZINAMIDE

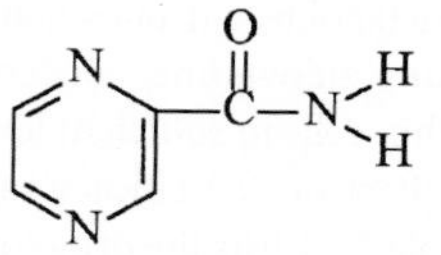

```
                 O
                 ‖      H
   N             |     /
 /   \  ——————   C — N
|     |               \
 \   /                 H
   N
```

PHARMACOLOGY AND PHARMACOKINETICS

Pyrazinamide (PZA) is a structural analog of nicotinamide with a mechanism of action similar to that of isoniazid (INH). Like INH, PZA is a prodrug. Pyrazinamide requires deamidation to anionic pyrazinoic acid by pyrazinamidase, an endogenous cytoplasmic bacterial enzyme. In this form, PZA has no antibacterial activity, but once exposed to acidic conditions, it becomes protonated to the uncharged, active form of the drug, 5-hydroxypyrazinoic acid, which enters the cell, accumulates, and kills the bacteria by disruption of mycolic acid biosynthesis.

28. Chowdhury B, Nagpaul AK, Chowdhury D. Leber's hereditary optic neuropathy masquerading as ethambutol-induced optic neuropathy in a young male. *Indian J Ophthalmol.* 2006;54:218-219.
29. Chung H, Yoon Y, Hwang J, et al. Ethambutol-induced toxicity is mediated by zinc and lysosomal membrane permeabilization in cultured retinal cells. *Toxicol Applied Pharmacol.* 2009;235:163-170.
30. Coyer J, Nicholson D. Isoniazid-induced seizures. Part I—clinical. Part II—cxperimental. *South Med J.* 1972;69:294-297.
31. Cycloserine [package insert]. Indianapolis, IN: Eli Lilly and Company; 2005.
32. DiMartini A. Isoniazid, tricyclics and the "cheese reaction." *Int Clin Psychopharmacol.* 1995;10:197-198.
33. Dockweiler U. Isoniazid-induced valproate toxicity, or vice versa. *Lancet.* 1987;18(2):152.
34. Dolgikh-Litt N. Attempted of suicide with ethionamide. *Klin Med (Mosk).* 1967;45:148-150.
35. Donald P, Parkin D, Seifart H, et al. The influence of dose and *N*-acetyltransferase-2 (NAT2) genotype and phenotype on the pharmacokinetics and pharmacodynamics of isoniazid. *Eur J Clin Pharmacol.* 2007;63:633-639.
36. Ducobu J, Dupont P, Laurent M. Acute isoniazid/ethambutol/rifampin overdosage. *Lancet.* 1982;1:632.
37. Durand F, Jebrak G, Pessayre D, Fournier M, Bernau J. Hepatotoxicity of antitubercular treatments: Rationale for monitoring liver status. *Drug Saf.* 1996;15:394-405.
38. Durand F, Pessayre D, Fournier M, et al. Antituberculous therapy and acute liver failure. *Lancet.* 1995;345:1170.
39. Ellard G. The potential clinical significance of the isoniazid acetylator phenotype in the treatment of pulmonary tuberculosis. *Tubercle.* 1984;65:211-227.
40. Farrell FJ, Keeffe EB, Man KM, Imperial JC, Esquivel CO. Treatment of hepatic failure secondary to isoniazid hepatitis with liver transplantation. *Dig Dis Sci.* 1994;39:2255-2259.
41. Farrell G. Drug-Induced *Acute Hepatitis. Drug-Induced Liver Disease.* Edinburgh: Churchill Livingstone; 1994:247-299.
42. Finch C, Chrisman C, Baciewicz A, Self TH. Rifampin and rifabutin drug interactions: an update. *Arch Intern Med.* 2002;162:985-989.
43. Franks A, Binkin N, Snider D. Isoniazid hepatitis in pregnant an postpartum Hispanic patients. *Public Health Rep.* 1989;104:151-155.
44. Fu LM, Shinnick TM. Genome-wide exploration of the drug action of capreomycin in Mycobacterium tuberculosis using Affymetrix oligonucleotide gene chips. *J Infection.* 2007;54:277-284.
45. Gannon R, Pearsall W, Rowley R. Isoniazid, meperidine, and hypotension. *Ann Intern Med.* 1983;99:415.
46. Gent W, Seifart H, Parkin D, Donald PR, Lamprecht JH. Factors in hydrazine formation from isoniazid by paediatric and adult tuberculosis patients. *Eur J Clin Pharmacol.* 1992;43:131-136.
47. Gnam W, Flint A, Goldbloom D. Isoniazid-induced hallucinosis: response to pyridoxine. *Psychosomatics.* 1993;34:537-539.
48. Goel U, Baja S, Gupta O, Dwiedi N. Isoniazid-induced neuropathy in slow versus rapid acetylators. *J Assoc Physicians India.* 1992;40:671-672.
49. Gonzalez-Gay MA, Sanchez-Andrade A, Aguero JJ, et al. Optic neuritis following treatment with isoniazid in a hemodialyzed patient. *Nephron.* 1993;63:360.
50. Griffith D, Brown B, Girard W, Wallace R. Adverse events associated with high-dose rifabutin in macrolide-containing regimens for treatment of *Mycobacterium avium* complex lung disease. *Clin Infect Dis.* 1995;21:594-598.
51. Gurumurthy P, Krishnamurthy M, Nazareth O. Lack of relationship between hepatic toxicity and acetylator phenotype and in South Indian patients during treatment with isoniazid for tuberculosis. *Am Rev Respir Dis.* 1984;129:58-61.
52. Gurumurthy P, Ramachandran G, Kumar AK, et al. Decreased bioavailability of rifampin and other antituberculosis drugs in patients with advanced human immunodeficiency virus disease. *Antimicrob Agents Chemother.* 2004;48:4473-4475.
53. Halouska S, Chacon O, Fenton R, et al. Use of NMR metabolomics to analyze the targets of D-cycloserine in Mycobacteria: role of D-alanine racemase. *J Proteome Res.* 2007;6:4608-4614.
54. Hankinns DG, Saxena K, Faville RJ, Warren BJ. Profound acidosis caused by isoniazid ingestion. *Am J Emerg Med.* 1987;5:165-166.
55. Hasagawa T, Reyes J, Nour B, et al. Successful liver transplantation for isoniazid-induced hepatic failure—a case report. *Transplantation.* 1994;57:1274-1277.
56. Hauser M, Baier H. Interactions of isoniazid with foods. *Clin Pharmacokinet.* 1982;16:617-618.
57. Heng J, Vorwerk C, Lessell E, et al. Ethambutol is toxic to retinal ganglion cells via an excitotoxic pathway. *Invest Ophthalmol Vis Sci.* 1999;40: 190-196.
58. Holdiness MR. Neurological manifestations and toxicities of the antituberculosis drugs—a review. *Med Toxicol.* 1987;2:33-51.
59. Holtz P, Palm D. Pharmacological aspects of vitamin B_6. *Pharmacol Rev.* 1964;16:113-178.
60. Hurwitz A, Schlozman DL. Effects of antacids on gastrointestinal absorption of isoniazid in rat and man. *Am Rev Respir Dis.* 1974;109:41-47.
61. Isoniazid [package insert]. Princeton, NJ: Sandoz Inc; 2006.
62. Jack D, Knepil J, McLay W, Fergie R. Fatal rifampicin-ethambutol overdose. *Lancet.* 1978;2:1107-1108.
63. Jain A, Mondal R, Srivastava S, et al. Novel mutations in embB gene of ethambutol-resistant isolates of Mycoplasma tuberculosis: A preliminary report. *Indian J Med Res.* 2008;128:134-139.
64. Kocabay G, Erelel M, Tutkun I, Ecder T. Optic neuritis and bitemporal hemianopsia associated with isoniazid-treatment in end-stage renal failure. *Int J Tuberc Lung Dis.* 2006;10:1418-1419.
65. Kozak S, Inderlied C, Hsu H, Heller KB, Sadun AA. The role of copper on ethambutol's antimicrobial action and implications for ethambutol-induced optic neuropathy. *Diagn Microbiol Infect Dis.* 1998;30:83-87.
66. Kozanoff D, Snider D, Caras G. Isoniazid hepatitis: a US Public Health Service cooperative surveillance study. *Am Rev Respir Dis.* 1978;117:991-1001.
67. Kwon HM, Kim HK, Cho J, Hong YH, Nam H. Cycloserine-induced encephalopathy: evidence on brain MRI. *Eur J Neurology.* 2008;15:e60-e61.
68. Lee C, Gambertoglio J, Brater D, Benet L. Kinetics of oral ethambutol in the normal subject. *Clin Pharmacol Ther.* 1977;22:615-621.
69. Lejonc J, Schaeffer A, Brochard P, Portos JL. Paroxystic hypertension after ingestion of gruyere cheese during isoniazid treatment: a report of two cases. *Ann Med Interne (Paris).* 1980;131:346-348.
70. Lenke R, Turkel S, Monsen R. Severe fetal deformities associated with ingestion of excessive isoniazid in early pregnancy. *Acta Obstet Gynecol Scand.* 1985;64:281-282.
71. Li A, Reith M, Rasmussen A, et al. Primary human hepatocytes as a tool for the evaluation of structure-activity relationship in cytochrome P450 induction potential of xenobiotics: evaluation of rifampin, rifapentine, and rifabutin. *Chem Biol Interact.* 1997;107:17-30.
72. Lopez-Samblas A, Tsiligiannis T. Isoniazid intoxication in three adolescent patients. *Hosp Pharm.* 1991;26:119-121.
73. Malone R, Fish D, Spiegel D, Childs JM, Peloquin CA. The effect of hemodialysis on cycloserine, ethionamide, *para*-aminosalicylic acid, and clofazimine. *Chest.* 1999;116:984-990.
74. Martinez-Roig A, Cami J, Llorens-Terol J. Acetylation phenotype and hepatotoxicity in the treatment of tuberculosis in children. *Pediatrics.* 1986;77:912-915.
75. McElroy PD, Ijaz K, Lambert LA, et al. National survey to measure rates of liver injury, hospitalization, and death associated with rifampin and pyrazinamide for latent tuberculosis infection. *Clin Infect Dis.* 2005;41:1125-1133.
76. Mdluli K, Slayden R, Zhu Y, et al. Inhibition of *a Mycobacterium tuberculosis* beta-ketoacyl ACP synthetase by isoniazid. *Science.* 1998;280:1607-1610.
77. Miki M, Ishikawa T, Okayama H. An outbreak of histamine poisoning after ingestion of the ground saury paste in eight patients taking isoniazid in tuberculosis ward. *Int Med.* 2005;44:1133-1136.
78. Miller J, Robinson A, Percy AL. Acute isoniazid poisoning in childhood. *Am J Dis Child.* 1980;134:290-292.
79. Mitnick CD, Shin SS, Seung KW, et al. Comprehensive treatment of extensively drug-resistant tuberculosis. *N Engl J Med.* 2008;359:563-574.
80. Nelson S, Mitchell J, Timbrell J, Snodgrass W. Isoniazid activation of metabolites to toxic intermediates in man and rat. *Science.* 1975;193:901-903.
81. Nicod L, Villon C, Regnier A, et al. Rifampicin and isoniazid increase acetaminophen and isoniazid cytotoxicity in human HapG2 hepatoma cells. *Hum Exp Toxicol.* 1997;16:28-34.
82. Nolan C, Goldberg S, Buskin S. Hepatotoxicity associated with isoniazid preventive therapy: a 7-year survey from a public health tuberculosis clinic. *JAMA.* 1999;281:1014-1081.
83. Orlowski JP, Paganini EP, Pippenger CE. Treatment of a potentially lethal dose isoniazid ingestion. *Ann Emerg Med.* 1988;17:73-76.
84. Pahl MV, Vaziri ND, Ness R, Nathan R, Maksy M. Association of beta-hydroxybutyric acidosis with isoniazid intoxication. *J Toxicol Clin Toxicol.* 1984;22:167-176.

85. Panganiban L, Makalinao I, Cortes-Maramba N. Rhabdomyolysis in isoniazid poisoning. *Clin Tox.* 2001;39:143-151.
86. Patel A, McKeon J. Avoidance and management of adverse reactions to antituberculosis drugs. *Drug Saf.* 1995;12:1-25.
87. Paulsen O, Hoglund P, Nilsson LG, Gredeby H. No interaction between H_2 blockers and isoniazid. *Eur J Respir Dis.* 1986;68:286-290.
88. Peloquin C, Namdar R, Dodge A, Nix DE. Pharmacokinetics of isoniazid under fasting conditions, with food, and with antacids. *Int J Tuberc Lung Dis.* 1999;3(8):703-710.
89. Petri WA. Antimicrobial agents: chemotherapy of tuberculosis, *Mycobacterium avium* complex disease and leprosy. In: Brunton LL, Lazo JS, Parker KL, eds. *Goodman and Gilman's the Pharmcological Basis of Therapeutics*, 11th ed. New York: McGraw-Hill; 2006: 1203-1223.
90. Piscitelli SC, Gallicano KD. Interactions among drugs for HIV and opportunistic infections. *N Engl J Med.* 2001;344:984-996.
91. Plomp T, Battista H, Unterdorfer H. A case of fatal poisoning by rifampicin. *Arch Toxicol.* 1981;48:245-248.
92. Quemard A, Dessen A, Sugantino M, et al. Binding of catalaseperoxidase activated isoniazid to wild-type and mutant *Mycobacterium tuberculosis* enoyl-ACP reductases. *J Am Chem Soc.* 1996;118:1561-1562.
93. Quemard A, Sacchettini J, Dessen A, et al. Enzymatic characterization of the target for isoniazid in *Mycobacterium tuberculosis. Biochemistry.* 1995;34:8235-8241.
94. Raviglione M, Smith I. XDR-Tuberculosis—implications for global public health. *New Engl J Med.* 2007;356:656-659.
95. Rawat R, Whitty A, Tonge P. The isoniazid-NAD adduct is a slow, tight-binding inhibitor of InhA, the *Mycobacterium tuberculosis* enoyl reductase: adduct affinity and drug resistance. *Proc Natl Acad Sci U S A.* 2003;100:13881-13886.
96. Saad S, el Masry A, Scott P. Influence of certain anticonvulsants on the concentration of GABA in the cerebral hemispheres of mice. *J Am Chem Soc.* 1954;76:300-304.
97. Salkind A, Hewitt C. Coma from long-term overingestion of isoniazid. *Arch Intern Med.* 1997;157:2518-2520.
98. Salpeter SR. Fatal isoniazid-induced hepatitis—its risk during chemoprophylaxis. *West J Med.* 1993;159:560-564.
99. Sanchez-Albisua I, Vidal L, Joya-Verde F, et al. Tolerance of pyrazinamide in short course chemotherapy for pulmonary tuberculosis in children. *Pediatr Infect Dis J.* 1997;16:760-763.
100. Sanders B, Draper G. Childhood cancer and drugs in pregnancy. *Br Med J.* 1979;1:717-718.
101. Santucci K, Shah B, Linakis J. Acute isoniazid exposures and antidote availability. *Pediatr Emerg Care.* 1999;15:99-101.
102. Sarzi-Puttini P, Atzeni F, Capsoni F, Lubrano E, Doria A. Drug-induced lupus erythematosus. *Autoimmunity.* 2005;38:507-518.
103. Schreiber J, Zissel G, Greinert U, Schlaak M, Müller-Quernhim J. Lymphocyte transformation test for the evaluation of adverse effects of antituberculous drugs. *Eur J Med Res.* 1999;4:67-71.
104. Scolding N, Ward M, Hutchings A, Routledge P. Charcoal and isoniazid pharmacokinetics. *Hum Toxicol.* 1986;5:285-286.
105. Scott E, Wright R. Fluorometric determination of INH in serum. *J Lab Clin Med.* 1967;70:355-360.
106. Self T, Chrisman C, Baciewicz A, Bronze M. Isoniazid drug and food interactions. *Am J Med Sci.* 1999;317:304-311.
107. Shenfield G. Oral contraceptives. Are drug interactions of clinical significance? *Drug Saf.* 1993;9:211-237.
108. Siefkin A, Albertson T, Corbett M. Isoniazid overdose: pharmacokinetics and effects of oral charcoal in treatment. *Hum Toxicol.* 1987;6:497-501.
109. Singh J, Garg P, Tandon R. Hepatotoxicity due to antituberculosis therapy: clinical profile and reintroduction of therapy. *J Clin Gastroenterol.* 1996;22:211-214.
110. Siskind MS, Thienemann D, Kirlin L. Isoniazid-induced neurotoxicity in chronic dialysis patients: report of three cases and a review of the literature. *Nephron.* 1993;64:303-306.
111. Sjoerdsma T, Kamermans M, Spekreijse H. Modulating wavelength discrimination in goldfish with ethambutol and stimulus intensity. *Vision Res.* 1996;36:3519-3525.
112. Smith C, Durack D. Isoniazid and reaction to cheese. *Ann Intern Med.* 1979;88:520-521.
113. Snider D. Pyridoxine supplementation during isoniazid therapy. *Tubercle.* 1980;61:191-196.
114. Snider D, Pwell K. Should women taking antituberculosis drugs breastfeed? *Arch Intern Med.* 1984;144:589-590.
115. Steen J, Stainton-Ellis D. Rifampicin in pregnancy. *Lancet.* 1977; 2:604-605.
116. Stein D, Fish D, Bilello J, et al. A 24-week open-label phase I/II evaluation of the HIV protease inhibitor MK-639 (indinavir). *AIDS.* 1996;10:485-492.
117. Terman DS, Teitelbaum DT. Isoniazid self-poisoning. *Neurology.* 1970;20:299-304.
118. Timbrell J, Mitchell J, Snodgrass W. Isoniazid hepatotoxicity: the relationship between covalent binding and metabolism in vivo. *J Pharmacol Exp Ther.* 1980;213:364-369.
119. Tobairo J, Losso M. Pharmacokinetics interaction studies between rifampin and protease inhibitors: methodological problems. *AIDS.* 2008;22: 2046-2047.
120. Tsai RK, Lee Y. Reversibility of ethambutol optic neuropathy. *J Ocul Pharmacol Ther.* 1997;13:473-477.
121. Wason S, Lacouture PG, Lovejoy F. Single high-dose pyridoxine treatment for isoniazid overdose. *JAMA.* 1981;246:1102-1104.
122. Weber WW, Hein DW. Clinical pharmacokinetics of isoniazid. *Clin Pharmacol.* 1979;4:401-422.
123. Whitefield C, Klein R. Isoniazid overdose: report of 40 patients with a critical analysis of treatment and suggestions for prevention. *Am Rev Respir Dis.* 1971;103:887-893.
124. Wood JD, Paesker SJ. The effect on GABA metabolism in brain of isonicotinic acid hydrazide and pyridoxine as a function of time after administration. *J Neurochem.* 1972;19:1527-1537.
125. Wu S, Chao C, Vargas J, et al. Isoniazid-related hepatic failure in children: a survey of liver transplantation centers. *Transplantation.* 2007;84:173-179.
126. Yew W. Clinically significant interactions with drugs used in the treatment of tuberculosis. *Drug Saf.* 2002;25:111-133.
127. Yew W, Leung C. Antituberculous drugs and hepatotoxicity. *Respirology.* 2006;11:699-707.
128. Yew W, Leung C. Management of multidrug-resistant tuberculosis: update 2007. *Respirology.* 2008;13:21-46.
129. Yiannidas C, Walsh J, McLeod J. Visual evoked potentials in the detection of subclinical optic toxic effects secondary to ethambutol. *Arch Neurol.* 1983;40:645-648.
130. Zabinski R, Blanchard J. Activation of INH by KatG. *J Am Chem Soc.* 1997;1999:2331-2332.
131. Zhang Y, Mitchison D. The curious characteristics of pyrazinamide: a review. *Int J Tuberc Lung Dis.* 2003;7:6-21.

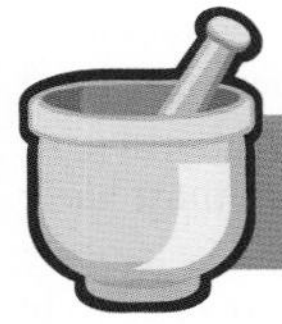

ANTIDOTES IN DEPTH (A15)

PYRIDOXINE

Mary Ann Howland

$$\text{pyridoxine: pyridine ring with } H_3C\text{ and N, H; HO, } CH_2OH\text{; } CH_2OH$$

Pyridoxine (vitamin B_6), a water-soluble vitamin, is administered as an antidote for overdoses of isonicotinic acid hydrazide (isoniazid, INH), *Gyromitra esculenta* mushrooms, hydrazine, methylated hydrazines, and ethylene glycol. With the exception of ethylene glycol, all of these xenobiotics produce seizures by the competitive inhibition of pyridoxal-5′-phosphate (PLP). Pyridoxine overcomes this inhibition and may also enhance the less-toxic pathway of ethylene glycol metabolism to form benzoic and hippuric acid, instead of oxalic acid.[6] Hydrazine and methylated hydrazines (1,1-dimethylhydrazine [UDMH], monomethylhydrazine [MMH]) are used as rocket fuels, and MMH is also found in *Gyromitra esculenta* mushrooms.[3]

HISTORY

Pyridoxine deficiency characterized by seborrheic dermatitis, cheilosis, stomatitis, and glossitis was first identified in 1926 but was mistakenly attributed to the absence of vitamin B_2 (see Chap. 41).[31] Ten years later, the deficiency was fully characterized and correctly recognized as a deficiency to vitamin B_6.[31] A rare genetic abnormality that produced pyridoxine-responsive seizures in newborns was first described in 1954.[5]

CHEMISTRY

The active form of pyridoxine is PLP.[31] The alcohol pyridoxine, the aldehyde pyridoxal, and the aminomethyl pyridoxamine are all naturally occurring, related compounds that are metabolized by the body to PLP.[31] Pyridoxine was chosen by the Council on Pharmacy and Chemistry to represent vitamin B_6.[31] Pyridoxine hydrochloride was chosen as the commercial preparation because of its stability.[53]

PHARMACOLOGY

Pyridoxal-5′-phosphate is an important cofactor in more than 100 enzymatic reactions, including decarboxylation and transamination of amino acids, and the metabolism of tryptophan to 5-hydroxytryptamine [serotonin] and methionine to cysteine.[23,31] Iatrogenic pyridoxine deficiency in animals produces seizures associated with reduced brain concentrations of PLP, glutamic acid decarboxylase, and γ-aminobutyric acid (GABA).[16]

PHARMACOKINETICS

Pyridoxine is not protein bound, has a volume of distribution of 0.6 L/kg, and easily crosses cell membranes; in contrast, PLP is nearly entirely plasma protein bound and essential for the synthesis and metabolism of GABA.[53] At extrahepatic sites pyridoxine is rapidly metabolized to pyridoxal, PLP, and 4-pyridoxic acid, with only 7% excreted unchanged in the urine.[53] After intravenous infusion of 100 mg of pyridoxine over 6 hours, PLP concentration increases rapidly in serum and in erythrocytes.[53] Pyridoxal-5'-phosphate rises from 37 nmol/L to 2183 nmol/L in serum and from undetectable to 5593 nmol/L in erythrocytes, with peak concentrations achieved at the end of the infusion.[53] Oral pyridoxine, in doses of 600 mg, is 50% absorbed within 20 minutes of ingestion by a first-order process with rapid achievement of peak serum concentrations of pyridoxine, PLP, and pyridoxal.[52] The concentration of PLP appears to be tightly controlled in the serum and related to alkaline phosphatase activity.[24,52] Oral doses of pyridoxine from 10 to 800 mg result in PLP concentrations of 518 to 732 nmol/L 4 hours after ingestion.[52] Chronic alcoholic patients have lower baseline serum PLP concentrations, as acetaldehyde enhances the degradation of PLP in erythrocytes, through stimulation of an erythrocyte membrane-bound phosphatase that hydrolyzes phosphate-containing B_6 compounds.[30]

MECHANISM OF HYDRAZIDE- AND HYDRAZINE-INDUCED SEIZURES

The role of pyridoxine as an antidote to poisoning from INH and methylated hydrazines like MMH is based on overcoming the interference of these xenobiotics with the normal function of pyridoxine as a coenzyme. INH produces a syndrome resembling cerebral vitamin B_6 deficiency, which results in seizures.[43] Specifically, INH and other hydrazides and hydrazines inhibit the enzyme pyridoxine phosphokinase that converts pyridoxine to PLP (see Fig. 57–3).[23] In addition, hydrazides directly combine with PLP, causing inactivation through the production of hydrazones that are rapidly excreted by the kidney.[23,49] PLP is a coenzyme for L-glutamic acid decarboxylase, which facilitates the synthesis of GABA from L-glutamic acid. Animal studies suggest that interference with PLP disrupts the formation of GABA.[23,49,50] The decreased GABA formation and increased glutamic acid reduces cerebral inhibition, which may contribute in part to the seizures resulting from exposure to INH and methylated hydrazines.[41,51]

ANIMAL STUDIES

In a dog model of INH-induced toxicity, pyridoxine reduced the severity of seizures, increased the duration of seizure-free periods, and prevented the mortality of a previously lethal dose of INH in a dose-dependent fashion.[13,14] Lower molar ratios prevented deaths and higher molar ratios prevented both deaths and seizures.[14] When used as single treatments for INH-induced seizures phenobarbital, pentobarbital, phenytoin, ethanol, and diazepam were ineffective in controlling seizures and mortality, but when combined with pyridoxine, each protected the animals from seizures and death.[13] Other small-animal experiments have documented the effectiveness of pyridoxine against MMH-induced seizures when used alone[23,34,46] and when used in combination with diazepam.[20] Anticonvulsant efficacy is also demonstrated in cat[42] and monkey[44] models.

Rat studies with intraperitoneal UDMH also demonstrate the protective effects of pyridoxine given intraperitoneally 90 minutes after exposure.[15] Pyridoxine prevented seizures and death in a model that produced 94% mortality and 100% seizures without pyridoxine.[15] When intraperitoneal UDMH was followed in 20 minutes by pyridoxine intravenously (IV) in rats, 17% died at 24 hours, compared with a 100% mortality without pyridoxine.[15] Other studies in dogs and monkeys also demonstrate the effectiveness of pyridoxine in preventing seizures and mortality, and in treating seizures.[4] Pyridoxine intramuscularly (IM) protected the monkeys from death and stopped the seizures caused by IV UDMH.

HUMAN DATA

Clinical experience with the use of pyridoxine for INH overdose in humans demonstrates favorable results.[2,11] Rapid seizure control with no morbidity or mortality was achieved when the ratio in grams of pyridoxine administered to INH ingested ranged from 0.14 to 1.3, although in practice, most patients receive approximately gram-for-gram amounts. In five patients, the use of gram-for-gram amounts of pyridoxine resulted in the complete control of seizures and a resolution of the metabolic acidosis.[48] In eight patients with intentional INH overdoses, basic poison management, intensive supportive care, and a mean dose of 5 g of pyridoxine IV resulted in no fatalities.[8] Seizures were controlled in a 22-month-old boy given 100 mg of IV pyridoxine, after an estimated INH ingestion of 5 g.[43] Variable results are reported when relatively small doses of pyridoxine are used.[32] Seizures were reported in two patients following the ingestion of INH-pyridoxine combination tablets, although the actual amount of pyridoxine ingested was not noted.[45]

In addition to controlling seizures, the administration of pyridoxine also appears to restore consciousness. Two patients, who remained obtunded for as long as 72 hours after the apparent resolution of the seizures, were reported to awaken immediately after 3 to 10 g of IV pyridoxine was administered.[10] A third patient who was lethargic awakened with IV pyridoxine. This suggests that mental status abnormalities associated with INH overdose, and possibly hydrazine overdoses, may be responsive to pyridoxine and also may require repetitive dosing.[11,48] Patients treated with large doses of pyridoxine awaken more rapidly even after experiencing sustained seizure activity or status epilepticus.

Monomethylhydrazine poisoning can be encountered in a variety of clinical situations. In the aerospace industry, where MMH is used as a rocket propellant, percutaneous or inhalational poisoning may occur. Ingestion of the false morel mushroom, *G. esculenta*, can also produce toxicity when its major toxic compound, gyromitrin, is metabolized to MMH[3,18] (Chap. 117).

The neurologic effects of MMH poisoning are similar to those of INH toxicity and include seizures and respiratory failure.[16] Severe liver damage similar to INH-induced hepatotoxicity is also described.[9] As in the case of INH hepatotoxicity, there is no evidence that MMH-induced hepatotoxicity can be treated by administration of pyridoxine.[9]

A patient who was exposed to hydrazine became comatose 14 hours later and remained comatose for 60 hours until 25 mg/kg of pyridoxine aroused him.[25] Another case report describes improvement in the mental status of a confused, lethargic, and restless man who had ingested a mouthful of hydrazine and was treated with a 10-g dose of pyridoxine.[22] This improvement developed over 24 hours and may have been unrelated to pyridoxine therapy. A severe sensory peripheral neuropathy lasting for 6 months developed 1 week following the overdose and was most likely a result of the hydrazine ingestion and not the pyridoxine. Six patients exposed to an Aerozine-50 (hydrazine and UDMH) spill were effectively treated with pyridoxine after developing twitching, clonic movements, hyperactivity, or gastrointestinal (GI) symptoms.[19] A patient exposed to UDMH during an explosion developed extensive burns, diverse neurologic manifestations and electroencephalogram (EEG) findings that resolved rapidly with the delayed administration of IV pyridoxine.[17]

ETHYLENE GLYCOL

PLP is a cofactor in the conversion of glycolic acid to nonoxalate compounds (Chap. 107). Patients poisoned with ethylene glycol should receive 100 mg/d of pyridoxine IV in an attempt to shunt metabolism preferentially away from the production of oxalic acid. This approach is supported by an animal model[6] and by the study of primary hyperoxaluria,[21] but has not been studied adequately in humans with ethylene glycol poisoning.[36]

SAFETY ISSUES

Pyridoxal-5′-phosphate is clearly neurotoxic to animals and humans when administered chronically in supraphysiologic doses.[25,27,37] Delayed peripheral neurotoxicity occurred in patients taking daily doses of 200 mg to 6 g of pyridoxine for 1 month.[35,40,41] Healthy volunteers given 1 or 3 g/d developed a small- and large-fiber distal axonopathy, with sensory findings and quantitative sensory threshold abnormalities occurring after 1.5 months in the high-dose and 4.5 months in the low-dose regimens. Once symptoms occurred, the pyridoxine was immediately stopped, but symptoms progressed for 2 to 3 weeks, leading to speculation that it took time for the reversal of neuronal metabolic manifestations (see chapter 18).[7]

Pyridoxine may also induce a sensory neuropathy when massive doses are administered, either as a single dose or over several days.[1,26,47] Ataxia occurred in dogs receiving 1 g/kg of pyridoxine.[47] Larger doses of pyridoxine produce incoordination, ataxia, seizures, and death.[47] Death after pyridoxine administration was sometimes delayed for 2 to 3 days.[47] Two patients treated with 2 g/kg of IV pyridoxine (132 and 183 g, respectively) over 3 days developed severe and crippling sensory neuropathies.[1] One year later, both patients were unable to walk. Inadequate information is available to determine the maximal single acute nontoxic dose in humans; however, there appears to be a wide margin of safety. Doses of pyridoxine ranging from 70 to 375 mg/kg or doses equivalent to the milligram-per-kilogram historical dose of ingested INH have been administered without adverse effects.[28,48]

The 0.5% chlorobutanol preservative in IV pyridoxine, which equates to doses of 250 to 500 mg of chlorobutanol when 5 and 10 g doses of pyridoxine are administered, might produce CNS depression.[12] However, a dose of 5 g IV pyridoxine administered over 5 min to five healthy volunteers produced only a transient minor increase in base deficit, without any CNS depression noted.[29]

DOSING

Considering all of the available data, a safe and effective pyridoxine regimen for INH overdoses in adults is 1 g of pyridoxine for each gram of INH ingested, to a maximum of 5 g or 70 mg/kg in a child.[48]

These doses are sufficient in the majority of patients, but the dose can be repeated if necessary. The best way to administer pyridoxine in a patient after an INH overdose has not been established. For a patient who is actively seizing, pyridoxine may be given by slow IV infusion at approximately 0.5 g/min until the seizures stop or the maximum dose has been reached. When the seizures stop, the remainder of the dose should be infused over 4 to 6 hours to maintain pyridoxine availability while the INH is being eliminated. The dose should be repeated if seizures persist or recur, or if the patient exhibits mental status depression. If IV pyridoxine is unavailable, oral pyridoxine should be administered.[39]

For hydrazine and methylated hydrazines (ie, MMH, UDMH) poisoning, there is no established dose.[51] Using the same dosage regimen as for INH is theoretically reasonable, but has never been tested in humans.

AVAILABILITY

Pyridoxine HCl is available parenterally at a concentration of 100 mg/mL with 1 mL in a 2 mL vial with 0.5% chlorobutanol as the preservative and 1.4 µg/1 mL aluminum from APP Pharmaceuticals.[38] Thus, a 5 g IV dose of pyridoxine requires fifty 100 mg/mL vials. This is an exception to the rule that appropriate doses of medications rarely require multiple dosages of this magnitude and also emphasizes the necessity of keeping an adequate supply available in the emergency department, as well as in the pharmacy.[33] Oral pyridoxine is available in many tablet strengths from 10 to 500 mg depending on the manufacturer.

SUMMARY

Pyridoxine should not be the sole therapy used for INH or MMH poisoning. A benzodiazepine should be used with pyridoxine in an attempt to achieve synergistic control of seizures. If the seizures do not respond to both of these measures, they can be repeated, followed by IV agents such as propofol, pentobarbital, or phenobarbital, and, if necessary, neuromuscular blockade and general anesthesia. When neuromuscular blockade is achieved without extinguishing the seizure activity, irreversible neuronal damage may result. Although metabolic acidosis is probably a result of the seizures and should therefore resolve once the underlying condition is controlled, severe or refractory metabolic acidosis may require titration of blood pH using IV sodium bicarbonate.

REFERENCES

1. Albin R, Albers J, Greenberg H, et al. Acute sensory neuropathy-neuronopathy from pyridoxine overdose. *Neurology.* 1987;37:1729-1732.
2. Alvarez EG, Guntupalli KK. Isoniazid overdose: four case reports and review of the literature. *Intensive Care Med.* 1995;21:641-644.
3. Andary C, Bourrier MJ. Variations in the monomethylhydrazine content in *Gyromitra esculenta. Mycologia.* 1985;77:259-264.
4. Back KC, Pinkerton MK, Thomas AA. Therapy of acute UDMH intoxication. *Aerosp Med.* 1963;34:1001-1004.
5. Baxter P. Pyridoxine-dependent seizures: a clinical and biochemical conundrum. *Biochim Biophys Acta.* 2003;1647:36-41.
6. Beasley UR, Buck WB. Acute ethylene glycol toxicosis: a review. *Vet Hum Toxicol.* 1980;22:255-263.
7. Berger AR, Schaumberg HH, Schroeder C, et al. Dose response, coasting, and differential fiber vulnerability in human toxic neuropathy: a prospective study of pyridoxine neurotoxicity. *Neurology.* 1992;42:1367-1370.
8. Blanchard P, Yao J, McAlpine D, et al. Isoniazid overdose in the Cambodian population of Olmsted County, Minnesota. *JAMA.* 1986;256:3131-3133.
9. Braun R, Greeff U, Netter KJ. Liver injury by the false morel poison gyromitrin. *Toxicology.* 1979;12:155-163.
10. Brent J, Vo N, Kulig K, Rumack BH. Reversal of prolonged isoniazid-induced coma by pyridoxine. *Arch Intern Med.* 1990;150:1751-1753.
11. Brown CV. Acute isoniazid poisoning. *Am Rev Respir Dis.* 1972;105:206-216.
12. Burda A, Sigg T, Wahl M. Possible adverse reactions in preservatives in high-dose pyridoxine hydrochloride IV injection. *Am J Health Syst Pharm.* 2002;59:1886-1887.
13. Chin L, Sievers ML, Herrier RN, Picchioni AL. Potentiation of pyridoxine by depressants and anticonvulsants in the treatment of acute isoniazid intoxication in dogs. *Toxicol Appl Pharmacol.* 1981;58:504-509.
14. Chin L, Sievers ML, Laird HE, Herrier RN, Picchioni AL. Evaluation of diazepam and pyridoxine as antidotes to isoniazid intoxication in rats and dogs. *Toxicol Appl Pharmacol.* 1978;45:713-722.
15. Cornish HH. The role of B_6 in toxicity of hydrazines. *Ann N Y Acad Sci.* 1969;166:136-145.
16. Dakshinamurti K, Paulose CS, Viswanathan M, et al. Neurobiology of pyridoxine. *Ann N Y Acad Sci.* 1990;585:128-144.
17. Dhennin C, Vesin L, Feauveaux J. Burns and the toxic effects of a derivative of hydrazine. *Burns Incl Therm Inj.* 1988;14:130-134.
18. Franke S, Freimuth U, List PH. Uber die Giftigkeit der fruhjahrslorchel *Gyromitra (Helvella) esculenta. Fr Arch Toxicol.* 1967;22:293-332.
19. Frierson WB. Use of pyridoxine HCl in acute hydrazine and UDMH intoxication. *Ind Med Surg.* 1965;34:650-651.
20. George ME, Pinkerton MK, Bach KC. Therapeutics of monomethylhydrazine intoxication. *Toxicol Appl Pharmacol.* 1982;63:201-208.
21. Gibbs DA, Watts RWE. The action of pyridoxine in primary hyperoxaluria. *Clin Sci.* 1970;38:277-286.
22. Harati Y, Niakan E. Hydrazine toxicity, pyridoxine therapy and peripheral neuropathy. *Ann Intern Med.* 1986;104:728-729.
23. Holtz P, Palm D. Pharmacological aspects of vitamin B_6. *Pharmacol Rev.* 1964;16:113-178.
24. Jang YM, Kim DW, Kang TC, et al. Human pyridoxal phosphatase. Molecular cloning, functional expression, and tissue distribution. *J Biol Chem.* 2003;278:50040-50046.
25. Kirlin JK. Treatment of hydrazine induced coma with pyridoxine. *N Engl J Med.* 1976;294:938-939.
26. Krinke G, Naylor DC, Skorpil V. Pyridoxine megavitaminosis: an analysis of the early changes induced with massive doses of vitamin B_6 in rat primary sensory neurons. *J Neuropathol Exp Neurol.* 1985;44:117-129.
27. Krinke G, Schaumburg HH, Spencer PS, et al. Pyridoxine megavitaminosis produces degeneration of peripheral sensory neurons (sensory neuropathy) in the dog. *Neurotoxicology.* 1980;2:13-24.
28. Lheureux P, Penaloza A, Gris M. Pyridoxine in clinical toxicology: a review. *Eur J Emerg Med.* 2005;12:78-85.
29. Lo Vecchio F, Curry S, Graeme K, et al. Intravenous pyridoxine-induced metabolic acidosis. *Ann Emerg Med.* 2001;38:62-64.
30. Lumeng L, Li T. Vitamin B_6 metabolism in chronic alcohol abuse. *J Clin Invest.* 1974;53:693-704.
31. Marcus R, Coulston AM. Water-soluble vitamins. In: Hardman JG, Limbird LE, Molinoff PB, Ruddon RW, eds. *Goodman and Gilman's the Pharmacological Basis of Therapeutics*, 10th ed. New York: McGraw-Hill; 2001:1760-1761.
32. Miller J, Robinson A, Percy AK. Acute isoniazid poisoning in childhood. *Am J Dis Child.* 1980;134:290-292.
33. Morrow LE, Wear RE, Schuller D, Malesker M. Acute isoniazid toxicity and the need for adequate pyridoxine supplies. *Pharmacotherapy.* 2006;26:1529-1532.
34. O'Brien RD, Kirkpatrick M, Miller PS. Poisoning of the rat by hydrazine and alkylhydrazines. *Toxicol Appl Pharmacol.* 1964;84:371-377.
35. Parry G, Bredesen D. Sensory neuropathy with low dose pyridoxine. *Neurology.* 1985;35:1466-1468.
36. Parry MF, Wallach R. Ethylene glycol poisoning. *Am J Med.* 1974;57:143-150.
37. Perry TA, Weerasuriya A, Mouton PR, Holloway HW, Greig NH. Pyridoxine-induced toxicity in rats: A stereological quantification of the sensory neuropathy. *Exp Neurol.* 2004;190:133-144.
38. Pyridoxine Hydrochloride Injection, USP [package insert]. Schaumburg, IL: APP Pharmaceuticals, LLC; 2008.
39. Scharman EJ, Rosencrance JG. Isoniazid toxicity: a survey of pyridoxine availability. *Am J Emerg Med.* 1994;12:386-388.
40. Schaumburg H. Sensory neuropathy from pyridoxine abuse. *N Engl J Med.* 1984;310:198.
41. Schaumburg H, Kaplan J, Windebank A, et al. Sensory neuropathy from pyridoxine abuse: a new megavitamin syndrome. *N Engl J Med.* 1983;309:445-448.

42. Shouse MN. Acute effects of pyridoxine hydrochloride on monomethylhydrazine seizure latency and amygdaloid kindled seizure thresholds in cats. *Exp Neurol.* 1982;75:79-88.
43. Starke H, Williams S. Acute poisoning from overdose of isoniazid: a case report. *Lancet.* 1963;83:406-408.
44. Sterman MB, Kovalesky RA. Anticonvulsant effects of restraint and pyridoxine on hydrazine seizures in the monkey. *Exp Neurol.* 1979;65:78-86.
45. Terman DS, Teitelbaum DT. Isoniazid self-poisoning. *Neurology.* 1970;20:299-304.
46. Toth B, Erickson J. Reversal of the toxicity of hydrazine an analogues by pyridoxine hydrochloride. *Toxicology.* 1977;7:31-36.
47. Unna IC. Studies of the toxicity and pharmacology of vitamin B_6 (2-methyl, 3-hydroxy-4,5-*bis*-pyridine). *Pharmacol Exp Ther.* 1940;70:400-407.
48. Wason S, Lacouture PG, Lovejoy FH. Single high-dose pyridoxine treatment for isoniazid overdose. *JAMA.* 1981;246:1102-1104.
49. Wood JD, Peesker SJ. A correlation between changes in GABA metabolism and isonicotinic acid. Hydrazide-induced seizures. *Brain Res.* 1972;45:489-498.
50. Wood JD, Peesker SJ. The effect on GABA metabolism of isonicotinic acid hydrazide and pyridoxine as a function of time after administration. *J Neurochem.* 1972;19:1527-1537.
51. Zelnick SD, Mattie DR, Stepaniak PC. Occupational exposure to hydrazines: Treatment of acute central nervous system toxicity. *Aviat Space Environ Med.* 2003;74:1285-1291.
52. Zempleni J. Pharmacokinetics of vitamin B_6 supplements in humans. *J Am Coll Nutr.* 1995;14:579-586.
53. Zempleni J, Kubler W. The utilization of intravenously infused pyridoxine in humans. *Clin Chim Acta.* 1994;229:27-36.

CHAPTER 58
ANTIMALARIALS

J. Dave Barry

The malaria parasite has caused untold grief throughout human history. The name originated from Italian *mal aria* (bad air), since the ancient Romans believed the disease was caused by the decay in marshes and swamps, and was carried by the malodorous "foul" air emanating from these areas.[5] In the 1880s both the Plasmodium protozoa as well as its mosquito vector were identified.[5] Today, 40% of world's population lives in areas where malaria is endemic. More than 500 million people suffer acute malaria infection, and one to three million die from the infection each year.[5,41,129] Included among those at risk of becoming infected are 50 million travelers from industrialized countries who visit the developing countries each year. Despite using prophylactic medications (Table 58–1), 30,000 of these travelers will acquire malaria.[97]

HISTORY AND EPIDEMIOLOGY

The bark of the cinchona tree, the first effective remedy for malaria, was introduced to Europeans more than 350 years ago.[114] The toxicity of its active ingredient, quinine, was noted from the inception of its use. Pharmaceutical advances occurred, funded largely by the military during World War II (chloroquine, proguanil, amodiaquine, pyrimethamine) and later during the Vietnam conflict (mefloquine, halofantrine).[109,114] Chloroquine, hydroxychloroquine, primaquine, amodiaquine, mefloquine, and halofantrine are all related to quinine, but have different patterns of toxicity. Other drugs used to treat malaria include the folate inhibitors proguanil and pyrimethamine (frequently used in combination with atovaquone), the sulfonamide sulfadoxine, or the sulfone dapsone, as well as tetracyclines and the macrolides (Chap. 56).

With the introduction of each new drug, resistance developed, particularly in Oceania, Southeast Asia, and Africa.[109,114] In some places, quinine is once again the first-line therapy for some types of malaria.[58] In the last two decades, the search for active xenobiotics has returned to a natural product, the Chinese herb qinghaosu.[86,110] The active ingredient, artemisinin, in the form of an artemisinin-based combination therapy (ACT), is recommended by the World Health Organization (WHO) as the preferred treatment of malaria in drug-resistant areas.[5,129] With increased leisure travel, a greater number of North Americans are taking prophylactic medications with potential toxicity.

QUINOLINE DERIVATIVES

QUININE

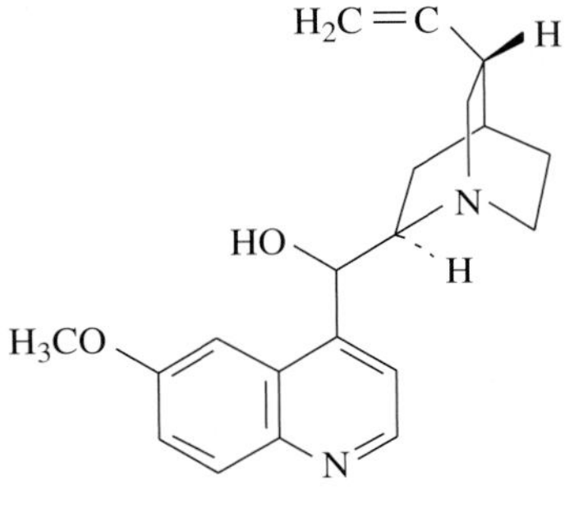

The therapeutic benefits of the bark of the cinchona tree have been known for centuries. As early as 1633, cinchona bark was used for its antipyretic and analgesic effects,[73] and in the 1800s it was used for the treatment of "rebellious palpitations."[114] Quinine, the primary alkaloid in cinchona bark, was the first effective treatment for malaria. Due to a reported curare-like action, quinine has been used as a treatment for muscle cramps. Due to its extremely bitter taste similar to that of heroin, quinine is used as an adulterant in drugs of abuse. Small quantities of quinine can be also found in some tonic waters.

High doses of quinine and other cinchona alkaloids are oxytocic, potentially leading to abortion or premature labor in pregnant women. Because of this, quinine has been used as an abortifacient (Chap. 28).[74] Chloroquine continues to be used for this purpose in some parts of the developing world.[7,90] Neither is safe for this purpose because of their narrow toxic-to-therapeutic ratio.

Pharmacokinetics and Toxicokinetics See Table 58–2 for the pharmacokinetic properties of quinine. Quinine and quinidine are optical isomers and share similar pharmacologic effects as class IA antidysrhythmics and antimalarials. Both are extensively metabolized in the liver, kidneys, and muscles to a variety of hydroxylated metabolites. Quinine undergoes transplacental distribution and is secreted in breast milk.

Pathophysiology Quinine overdose affects multiple organ systems through a number of different pathophysiologic mechanisms. Studies evaluating mechanisms of toxicity have focused on those organ systems primarily affected. Outcomes appear to be most closely related to the degree of cardiovascular dysfunction.[38]

Quinine and quinidine share anti- and prodysrhythmic effects primarily from an inhibiting effect on the cardiac sodium channels and potassium channels (Chaps. 23 and 63).[39] Blockade of the sodium channel in the inactivated state decreases inotropy, slows the rate of depolarization, slows conduction, and increases action potential duration. Inhibition of this rapid inward sodium current is increased at higher heart rates (called *use-dependent blockade*), leading to a rate-dependent widening of the QRS complex.[114,123]

Inhibition of the potassium channels suppresses the repolarizing delayed rectifier potassium current, particularly the rapidly activating component,[123] leading to prolongation of the QT interval. The resultant increase in the effective refractory period is also rate dependent, causing greater repolarization delay at slower heart rates and predisposing to torsades de pointes. As a result, syncope and sudden dysrhythmogenic death may occur. An additional α-adrenergic blocking effect contributes to the syncope and hypotension occuring in quinine toxicity.

Inhibition of the adenosine triphosphate (ATP)-sensitive potassium channels of the pancreatic β cells results in the release of insulin, similar to the action of sulfonylureas (Chap. 48).[30] Patients at increased risk of quinine-induced hyperinsulinemia include those patients receiving high-dose intravenous (IV) quinine, intentional overdose, and patients with other metabolic stresses, such as concurrent malaria, pregnancy, malnutrition, and alcohol consumption.[18,59,81,84,85,94]

The mechanism of quinine-induced inhibition of hearing appears to be multifactorial.[109] Microstructural lengthening of the outer hair cells of the cochlea and organ of Corti occurs.[43] Additionally, vasoconstriction and local prostaglandin inhibition within the organ of Corti may contribute to decreased hearing.[109] Inhibition of the potassium channel may impair hearing and produce vertigo, as it is known that the homozygous absence of gene products that form part of some potassium channels (Jervell and Lange-Nielson syndrome) causes deafness and prolonged QT intervals (Chap. 20 and 22).[108]

Although older theories suggested that quinine caused retinal ischemia, the preponderance of evidence points to a direct toxic effect on the retina.[40,44] Electroretinographic studies demonstrate a rapid and direct effect on the retina (decreased potentials) within minutes after doses of

TABLE 58–1. Common Adult Doses of Antimalarials Used Worldwide

Drug	Prophylactic Dose	Upper Dose Range, Treatment[a]
Amodiaquine	Not used	10 mg of base/kg/d × 3 days
Artemether/lumefantrine	Not used	80 mg artomether + 480 mg lumefantrine bid × 3 days
Artesunate/amodiaquine	Not used	200 mg arteunate + 612 mg amodiaquine × 3 days
Artesunate/mefloquine	Not used	200 mg artesunate × 3 days, 1000 mg mefloquine on day 2, 500 mg mefloquine on day 3
Artesunate/pyrimethamine/sulfadozine	Not used	200 mg artesunate × 3 days, 75 mg pyrimethamine + 1500 mg sulfadoxine as single dose
Chloroquine phosphate (Aralen)	500 mg/wk as single dose	1000 mg STAT then 500 mg at 6 h, 24 h, and 48 h
Doxycycline (Vibramycin)	100 mg/day	100 mg bid[d]
Halofantrine	Not used	500 mg q6h × 3 doses, repeat in 7 days
Hydroxychloroquine sulfate (Plaquenil)	400 mg/wk as single dose	Rarely used
Mefloquine (Lariam)	250 mg/wk as single dose	750 mg STAT, then 500 mg 8 h later
Primaquine phosphate	30 mg of base/d × 14 days[c]	30 mg of base/d × 14 days
Proguanil/atovaquone (Malarone)	100 mg proguanil + 250 mg atovaquone once per day	400 mg proguanil 1000 mg atovaquone per day × 3 days
Proguanil/chloroquine	200 mg proguanil + 100 mg chloroquine once per day	Not used
Pyrimethamine/sulfadoxine (Fansidar)	Not used	75 mg pyrimethamine + 1500 mg sulfadoxine as single dose
Quinine sulfate (Qualaquin)	Not used	650 mg tid × 7 days[b]

[a] Choice, duration, and dosage may vary with malarial species and frequency of drug resistance in the geographic area.

[b] Usually with doxycycline, tetracycline, or clindamycin for chloroquine-resistant cases.

[c] After leaving *Plasmodium vivax* or *Plasmodium ovale* area.

[d] With quinine sulfate for chloroquine-resistant cases.

quinine.[40] These early retinographic changes, as well as histologic lesions in photoreceptor and ganglion cell layers, provide evidence of direct damage.[40] Changes in the electrooculogram suggest changes in the retinal pigment epithelium, and parallel changes in visual acuity. In contrast, no electrophysiologic, angiographic, or morphologic experimental evidence for retinal ischemia has been found.[40,44] Quinine may also antagonize cholinergic neurotransmission in the inner synaptic layer.

Quinine has direct irritant effects on the gastrointestinal (GI) tract and stimulates the center in the brainstem responsible for nausea and emesis.[114]

Clinical Manifestations Quinine overdose typically leads to GI complaints, tinnitus, and visual symptoms within hours, but the time course varies with the formulation ingested, coingestants, patient characteristics, and other case-specific details. Significant overdose is heralded by cardiovascular and central nervous system toxicity. Death can occur within hours to days, usually from a combination of shock, ventricular dysrhythmias, respiratory arrest, or renal failure.

Patients receiving even therapeutic doses often experience a syndrome known as "cinchonism," which typically includes GI complaints, headache, vasodilation, tinnitus, and decreased hearing acuity.[73,114] Vertigo, syncope, dystonia, tachycardia, diarrhea, and abdominal pain are also described.[47,63,81,114]

Quinine toxicity is closely correlated with total serum concentrations, but only the non-protein-bound portion is likely responsible for toxic effects. However, since free and total quinine concentrations vary widely from person to person,[35] a single quinine concentration may not always correlate with clinical toxicity. In general, serum concentrations of greater than 5 μg/mL may cause cinchonism, greater than 10 μg/mL visual impairment, greater than 15 μg/mL cardiac dysrhythmias, and greater than 22 μg/mL death.[2] Similar concentrations in individuals who are severely ill with malaria do not necessarily result in as severe toxicity because of the increase α_1-acid glycoprotein and consequent reduction in free fraction of quinine present.[98,103]

The margin between therapeutic and toxic dosing of quinine is very small. It is not surprising that patients taking therapeutic doses frequently develop toxicity since the recommended range of serum quinine concentrations for treatment of falciparum malaria is 5 to 15 μg/mL, well above the concentration reported to cause cinchonism.

The average oral lethal dose of quinine is 8 g, although a dose as small as 1.5 g has been reported to cause death.[36,47] Delirium, coma, and seizures are less common, usually occurring only after severe overdoses.[14]

Cardiovascular manifestations of quinine use are related to myocardial drug concentrations.[11] They manifest on the electrocardiogram (ECG) as prolongation of the PR interval; prolongation of the QRS complex, QT interval, and ST depression with or without T-wave inversion also occurs.[11] Patients may develop complete heart block or dysrhythmias.[11] Patients on high doses of quinine must be monitored for torsades de pointes, ventricular tachycardia, and ventricular fibrillation. Quinine toxicity can also result in significant hypotension.

Although mild hyperinsulinemia may occur, hypoglycemia is not commonly described in cases of oral quinine overdose.[14,18,38,59,102,122,126] Hypoglycemia with elevated serum insulin concentrations following therapeutic dosing was seen in case reports complicated by severe congestive heart failure and significant ethanol consumption. Hypoglycemia was also noted in a healthy patient following overdose.[59,121]

TABLE 58–2. Pharmacokinetic Properties of Antimalarials

Antimalarial	Bioavailability (%)	Time to Peak Hours (oral)	Protein Bound (%)	Volume of Distribution (L/kg)	Half-Life	Urinary Excretion (%)	Comments
Artemisinin	Limited	–	Large	–	2–5 h	–	Metabolism largely through cytochrome p450 system.
Chloroquine	80	2–5	50-65	>100	40–55 d	55	–
Dapsone	90	3–6	70–80	0.5–1	21–30 h	20	–
Halofantrine	Low, varies	4–7	–	>100	1–6 d	–	Active metabolite.
Mefloquine	>85	8–24	98	15–40	15–27 d	<1	Hepatic metabolism. Inactive metabolite.
Primaquine	74	1–3	–	2.9	5–7 h	4	Metabolites primarily responsible for therapeutic and toxic effects.
Pyrimethamine	>95	2–6	87	3	3–4 d	16-32	–
Quinine	76	1–3	93	1.8–4.6	9–15 h	20	Protein binding increased in alkaline environments. Urinary excretion increased with acidic urine.

–, poorly studied or unknown.

Eighth-nerve dysfunction results in tinnitus and deafness. The decreased acuity is not usually clinically apparent, although the patient recognizes tinnitus.[95] These findings usually resolve within 48 to 72 hours, and permanent hearing impairment is unlikely.

Ophthalmic presentations include blurred vision, visual field constriction, tunnel vision, diplopia, altered color perception, mydriasis, photophobia, scotomata, and sometimes complete blindness.[14,32,40] Onset of blindness is invariably delayed and usually follows the onset of other manifestations by at least 6 hours. The pupillary dilation that occurs is usually nonreactive and correlates with the severity of visual loss. Funduscopic examination may be normal, but usually demonstrates extreme arteriolar constriction associated with optic disc and retinal edema. Normal arteriolar caliber may be initially present, but funduscopic manifestations such as vessel attenuation and disc pallor may develop as clinical improvement occurs. Improvement in vision can occur rapidly, but is usually slow, occurring over a period of months after a severe exposure. Initially, improvement occurs centrally and is followed later by improvement in peripheral vision. The pupils may remain dilated even after return to normal vision.[36] Patients with the greatest exposure may develop optic atrophy.

Hypokalemia is often described in the setting of quinine poisoning,[102] although the mechanism is unclear. An intracellular shift of potassium rather than a true potassium deficit is the predominant theory behind the hypokalemia associated with chloroquine,[68,70] and the mechanism may be similar with quinine.

A number of hypersensitivity reactions are described. These are the result of antiquinine or antiquinine-hapten antibodies cross-reacting with a variety of membrane glycoproteins.[15,51] Asthma, and dermatologic manifestations including urticaria, photosensitivity dermatitis, cutaneous vasculitis, lichen planus, and angioedema also occur.[94]

Hematologic manifestations of hypersensitivity are rare, but include thrombocytopenia (Chap. 24), agranulocytosis, microangiopathic hemolytic anemia, and disseminated intravascular coagulation (DIC), which can lead to jaundice, hemoglobinuria, and renal failure.[47,51] Hemolysis may also occur in patients with glucose-6-phosphate dehydrogenase (G6PD) deficiency. Immunogenic drug-platelet complex interactions can occur even after low doses of quinine, such as those in tonic drinks. This self-limited interaction has previously been termed "cocktail purpura."[73,114]

A hepatitis hypersensitivity reaction,[34] acute respiratory distress syndrome (ARDS), and a sepsis-like syndrome are also reported.[55]

Diagnostic Testing Urine thin-layer chromatography is sensitive enough to confirm the presence of quinine, even following the ingestion of tonic water.[126] Quinine immunoassay techniques are also available. Quantitative serum testing is not rapidly or widely available.

Management Patients may frequently vomit spontaneously. Emetics should not be used in the absence of vomiting since seizures, dysrhythmias, and hypotension can occur rapidly. Orogastric lavage should only be considered for patients with recent, substantial (potentially life-threatening) ingestions with no spontaneous emesis. Activated charcoal effectively adsorbs quinine and may additionally decrease serum concentrations by altering enteroenteric circulation.[3,62]

Supportive care should be initiated including oxygen, cardiac and hemodynamic monitoring, IV fluid resuscitation, and frequent ECG and blood glucose measurements.

Cardiac. Prolonged QRS should be treated with sodium bicarbonate alkalinization to achieve a serum pH of 7.45 to 7.50, as would be done in patients with cardiotoxicity associated with cyclic antidepressant overdoses (see Antidotes in Depth A5: Sodium Bicarbonate). The cardiotoxic manifestations of quinine and increased protein binding in the setting of alkalosis make the choice of serum alkalinization a logical therapeutic intervention. Sodium bicarbonate therapy has been successful in case reports,[11,38,73] but has not been specifically studied. Hypertonic sodium bicarbonate may result in or worsen existing hypokalemia, potentially exacerbating the effect of potassium channel blockade.

Potassium supplementation for quinine-induced hypokalemia is controversial since experimental data from the 1960s suggest that hypokalemia is protective against cardiotoxicity and prolongs survival.[17,68,102] Since hypokalemia can also lead to lethal dysrhythmias, supplementation for hypokalemia is presently recommended.

The QT interval should be carefully monitored for prolongation. If necessary, interventions for torsades de pointes, including magnesium administration, potassium supplementation, and overdrive pacing, should be initiated (Chap. 22).

Class IA, IC, or III antidysrhythmics and other xenobiotics with sodium-channel- and/or potassium-channel-blocking activity should not be used to treat a quinine overdosed patient because they may exacerbate quinine-induced conduction disturbances or dysrhythmias. Type IB antidysrhythmics, such as lidocaine, have been used with reported success, but no clinical trials have been performed (Chap. 63).

Hypotension refractory to IV crystalloid boluses should be treated with vasopressors. Although not directly studied, direct-acting vasopressors such as epinephrine, norepinephrine, or phenylephrine are recommended. An intraaortic balloon pump was successfully used for the treatment of refractory hypotension in one case report.[102]

Ophthalmic. Funduscopic examination, visual field examination, and color testing may be appropriate bedside diagnostic studies. Electroretinography, electrooculogram, visual-evoked potentials, and dark adaptation may be helpful in assessing the injury, but are not practical because they require equipment that is not portable or readily available in most clinical settings. There is no specific, effective treatment for quinine retinal toxicity,[40,42] although hyperbaric oxygen (HBO) was used in three patients who recovered vision, but the role of HBO in that recovery was not established.[40,127]

Hypoglycemia. A low serum glucose concentration should be supported with an adequate infusion of dextrose. Serum potassium concentration and the QT interval should be monitored during correction and maintenance. Octreotide has been successfully used to correct quinine-induced hyperinsulinemia in adult malaria victims.[84,85] In volunteers, quinine-induced hyperinsulinemia was suppressed within 15 minutes following a 100 μg intramuscular dose of octreotide (see Antidotes in Depth A11: Octreotide).[85] Octreotide should be used for cases of refractory hypoglycemia in a fashion similar to that recommended in sulfonylurea toxicity which is 50 μg subcutaneously (SC) every 6 hours (Chap. 48).

Enhanced Elimination The effect of multiple-dose activated charcoal (MDAC) on quinine elimination was studied in an experimental human model as well as in symptomatic patients.[88] In these patients, MDAC decreased the half-life of quinine from approximately 8 hours to about 4.5 hours, and increased clearance by 56%.[88] Although numerous studies show that activated charcoal decreases quinine half-life,[9,62,88] evidence of clinical benefit is lacking. Nevertheless, because ophthalmic, central nervous system (CNS), and cardiovascular toxicity are related to serum concentration, it is prudent to reduce concentrations as quickly as practicable; thus, activated charcoal (0.5 g/kg) should be administered every 2 to 4 hours, unless otherwise contraindicated, for about four doses.

There is conflicting evidence about a benefit of urinary acidification in enhancing clearance.[9,98] But because of the increased potential for cardiotoxicity associated with acidification, this technique is never recommended.

Because quinine has a relatively large volume of distribution and is highly protein bound, hemoperfusion, hemodialysis, and exchange transfusion have only a limited effect on drug removal.[9,14,67,98,114,119] Although the blood compartment can be cleared with these techniques, total body clearance is only marginally altered. After rapid tissue distribution occurs, there is little impact on the total body burden because of the large volume of distribution and extensive protein binding.

Extracorporeal membrane oxygenation (ECMO) was used in one case of severe quinidine poisoning with bradydysrhythmias and refractory hypotension to stabilize the cardiovascular system while a quinidine-activated charcoal bezoar was removed, and the patient metabolized the remaining quinidine.[112] A similar approach should be considered for intractable quinine toxicity.

CHLOROQUINE, HYDROXYCHLOROQUINE, AND AMODIAQUINE

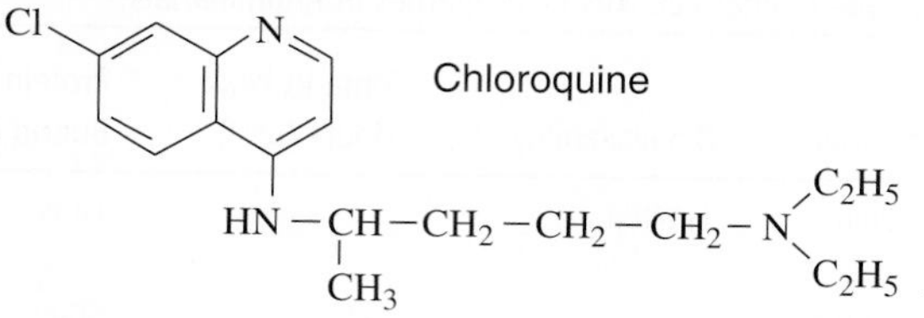

Chloroquine

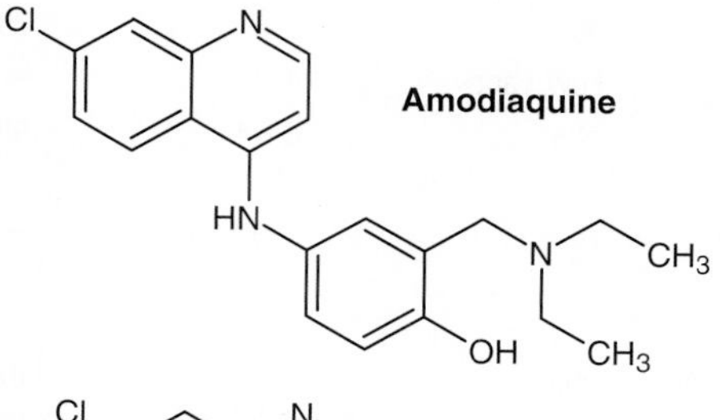

Cl; N; HN−CH−CH$_2$−CH$_2$−CH$_2$−N; CH$_3$; C$_2$H$_5$; C$_2$H$_5$

Amodiaquine

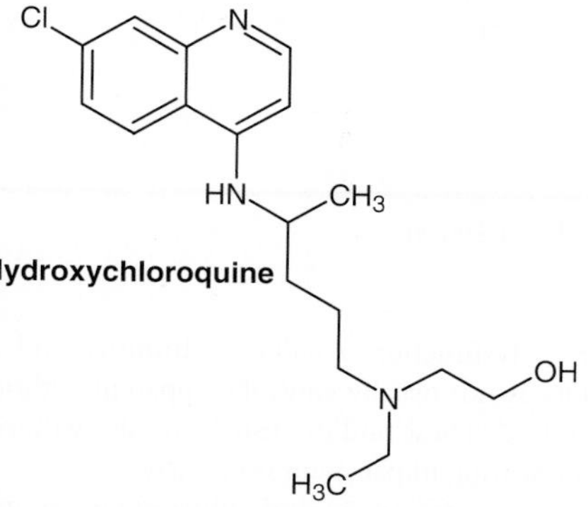

Cl; N; HN; N; CH$_3$; OH; CH$_3$

Hydroxychloroquine

Cl; N; HN; CH$_3$; N; OH; H$_3$C

The structurally related compounds chloroquine and amodiaquine were once used extensively for malaria prophylaxis. However, with the development of resistance, they are used in fewer geographic regions. Amodiaquine is associated with a higher incidence of hepatic toxicity and agranulocytosis. In general, these xenobiotics have low toxicity when used in therapeutic doses. Because of its low toxicity, chloroquine remains the first-line drug for malaria prophylaxis and treatment in areas where *Plasmodium* remains sensitive.

Hydroxychloroquine is similar to chloroquine in therapeutic, pharmacokinetic, and toxicologic properties.[67] The side-effect profiles of the two are slightly different, favoring chloroquine use for malarial prophylaxis and hydroxychloroquine use as an antiinflammatory agent.[63,114] Hydroxychloroquine is used in the treatment of rheumatic diseases such as rheumatoid arthritis and lupus erythematosus. In animal studies, chloroquine is two to three times more toxic than hydroxychloroquine.[49]

Piperaquine is structurally similar to chloroquine but is primarily used in conjunction with artemisinin compounds as a component of an artemisinin-based combination therapy (ACT). Piperaquine is discussed in more detail in the Artemisinin and Derivatives section.

Pharmacokinetics and Toxicodynamics See Table 58–2 for the pharmacokinetic properties of chloroquine. Oral chloroquine is rapidly and completely absorbed and is ultimately sequestered in many different organs, particularly the kidney, liver, and lung, as well as erythrocytes.[13,43]

Chloroquine is slowly distributed from the blood compartment to the larger central compartment, leading to transiently high whole blood concentrations shortly after ingestion.[90,104] It is the initial high blood concentrations that are thought to be responsible for the rapid development of profound cardiorespiratory collapse, which is typical of chloroquine toxicity. These whole-blood chloroquine concentrations correlate with mortality.[26]

Pathophysiology With structural similiarity to quinine, the pathophysiologic mechanisms of chloroquine and hydroxychloroquine are also similar. Most notably, sodium and potassium channel blockade are the proposed primary mechanisms of cardiovascular toxicity.[123]

Although less common in quinine toxicity, hypokalemia is extremely common in chloroquine overdose. The mechanism appears to be a shift of potassium from the extracellular to the intracellular space and not a true potassium deficit.[68,90,102]

Clinical Manifestations Like quinine, chloroquine has a small toxic-to-therapeutic margin. Severe chloroquine poisoning is usually associated with ingestions of 5 g or more in adults, systolic blood pressure less than 80 mm Hg, QRS duration of more than 120 milliseconds, ventricular fibrillation, hypokalemia, and serum chloroquinine concentrations exceeding 25 μmol/L (8 μg/mL).[24,92]

Symptoms usually occur within 1 to 3 hours of ingestion.[92] The range of symptoms associated with chloroquine toxicity are similar to quinine, but the frequencies of various manifestations differ and other features such as cinchonism, are uncommon. Nausea, vomiting, diarrhea, and abdominal pain occur less commonly than with quinine.[47,63] In contrast, respiratory depression is common and apnea, hypotension, and cardiovascular compromise can be precipitous.[47]

The cardiovascular effects of chloroquine and hydroxychloroquine are similar to those of quinine, including QRS prolongation, atrioventricular (AV) block, ST- and T-wave depression, increased U waves, and QT interval prolongation. Hypotension is more prominent in chloroquine toxicity than with quinine.[47]

Significant hypokalemia in chloroquine toxicity is invariably associated with cardiac manifestations.[25,47] In fact, the extent of hypokalemia is a good indicator of the severity of chloroquine overdose.[24]

Neurologic manifestations include CNS depression, dizziness, headache, and convulsions.[47] Rarely, dystonic reactions occur.[82] Transient parkinsonism has been reported following excessive dosing.[82]

Ophthalmic manifestations are infrequent in acute chloroquine toxicity and transient in nature.[47,63] More severe and irreversible vision and hearing changes are described in association with the chronic use of chloroquine and hydroxychloroquine as antiinflammatory agents.[63,75] Myopathy, neuropathy, and cardiomyopathy also occur in this context.[5,120] Dermatologic findings and hypersensitivity reactions are similar to those associated with quinine.[31] Likewise, red blood cell (RBC) oxidant stress from chloroquine may result in hemolysis in patients with G6PD deficiency (Chap. 24).

Acute hydroxychloroquine toxicity is similar to chloroquine toxicity.[49] Side effects from therapeutic doses include nausea and abdominal pain, hemolysis in G6PD-deficient patients and, rarely, retinal damage, sensorineural deafness, and hypoglycemia.[10,48,101] Hypersensitivity reactions, including myocarditis and hepatitis, are described.[37,66]

One report of amodiaquine toxicity suggests that involuntary movements, muscle stiffness, dysarthria, syncope, and seizures may occur.[47] Amodiaquine is associated with hypersensitivity hepatitis and neutropenia in prophylactic use, but not therapeutic use.[18] There is no overdose experience reported.

Management Aggressive supportive care should be initiated including oxygen, cardiac and hemodynamic monitoring, and large-bore IV access, and serial blood glucose concentrations should be obtained. Orogastric lavage could be considered for life-threatening ingestions presenting early, but there is little evidence of efficacy. Activated charcoal adsorbs chloroquine well, binding 95% to 99% when administered within 5 minutes of ingestion.[54] The frequent development of precipitous cardiovascular and CNS toxicity should be considered before initiating any type of GI decontamination.

Early aggressive management of severe chloroquine toxicity decreases mortality.[92] This includes early endotracheal intubation and mechanical ventilation. There is evidence to suggest barbiturates may *not* be the best agent for induction in chloroquine overdose. When thiopental was used to facilitate intubation, its use immediately preceded sudden cardiac arrest in seven of 25 patients after chloroquine overdose.[26] An adequate FiO_2, tidal volume and ventilatory rate should be ensured.

Although theoretically any direct-acting pressor would be beneficial in the setting of hypotension not responsive to fluid resuscitation, epinephrine is the pressor that has been studied the most and is considered the vasopressor of choice. High doses of epinephrine were used in the original studies describing the benefits of early mechanical ventilation and the administration of diazepam and epinephrine in chloroquine poisoning.[92,93] The epinephrine doses used in these studies are still recommended today.[92,93] The recommended dose is 0.25 μg/kg/min, increasing by 0.25 μg/kg/min until an adequate systolic blood pressure (greater than 90 mm Hg) is achieved.[28,70,92,93] Clinicians should be mindful that high doses of epinephrine could exacerbate preexisting hypokalemia.

The use of diazepam to augment the treatment of dysrhythmias and hypotension is a unique use of this drug. Initial observations with regard to patients with mixed overdoses of chloroquine and diazepam suggested less cardiovascular toxicity and a potential benefit of high-dose diazepam.[24,68] Animal and human studies that followed also showed a potential benefit.[28,92,93] When early mechanical ventilation was combined with the administration of high-dose diazepam and epinephrine in patients severely poisoned by chloroquine, a dramatic improvement in survival compared with historical controls (91% versus 9% survival) occurred.[92] Studies in moderately poisoned patients failed to show similar benefit,[24] and a rat model failed to show an inotropic effect. Although the definitive study has yet to be done, high-dose diazepam therapy (2 mg/kg IV over 30 minutes, followed by 1 to 2 mg/kg/d for 2 to 4 days) seems warranted for serious toxicity. Diazepam or an equivalent benzodiazepine should also be used to treat seizures and for sedation.

The mechanism for a potential benefit of diazepam is unclear, but multiple theories have been postulated: (1) a central antagonistic effect, (2) anticonvulsant effect, (3) antidysrhythmic effect by an electrophysiologic action inverse to chloroquine, (4) pharmacokinetic interaction between diazepam and chloroquine, and (5) decrease in chloroquine-induced vasodilation.[68,90,92,93] (see Antidotes in Depth A24: Benzodiazepines).

The use of sodium bicarbonate for correction of QRS prolongation is also controversial. Although alkalinization would be expected to counteract the effects of sodium channel blockade, it could also exacerbate preexisting hypokalemia. Although case reports describe the successful use of sodium bicarbonate in conjunction with other agents for massive hydroxychloroquine overdose, no clinical trials have been performed.[60,130] Before using sodium bicarbonate in the setting of chloroquine toxicity clinicians should consider the overall clinical status of the patient, including the suspected degree of cardiac toxicity and severity of hypokalemia.

Hypokalemia in the setting of chloroquine toxicity correlates with the severity of the intoxication.[24,68] This hypokalemia is thought to be due to intracellular shift, not total-body potassium depletion.[25,47,49] Potassium replacement in this setting is, again, controversial since it has not been shown that potassium supplementation will improve cardiac toxicity. In fact, several reports suggest a possible protective effect of hypokalemia in acute chloroquine toxicity.[24,68,90] This should be balanced against the fact that severe hypokalemia can itself result in lethal dysrhythmias and data suggesting severe hypokalemia (less than 1.9 mEq/L) is associated with severe, life-threatening ingestion.[22,47,68,104] Hypokalemia could not be directly attributed as the cause of death in most cases, however.[24] Based on the available evidence, potassium replacement for significant hypokalemia seems warranted, but it is essential to anticipate rebound hyperkalemia as chloroquine toxicity resolves and redistribution of intracellular potassium occurs. Cases of hyperkalemia-related complications after aggressive potassium supplementation have been reported.[49,60,68]

Because chloroquine and hydroxychloroquine have high volumes of distribution and significant protein binding, enhanced elimination procedures are not beneficial.[13,47]

PRIMAQUINE

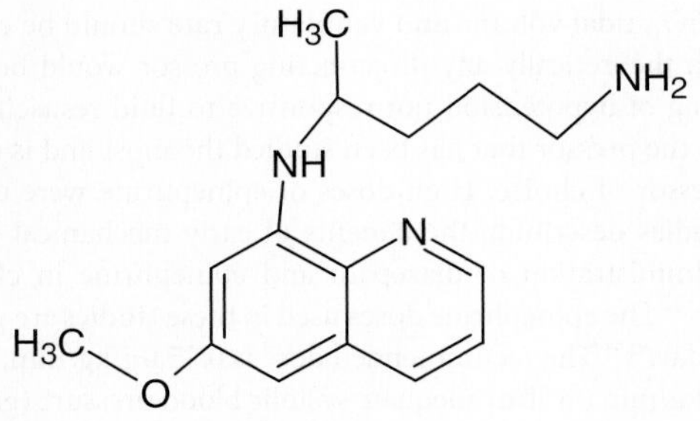

Pharmacokinetics and Toxicodynamics See Table 58–2 for the pharmacokinetic properties of primaquine.

Pathophysiology Primaquine blocks sodium channels both in vitro and animal models.[47,123] Significant cardiovascular toxicity has not been reported, although experience with primaquine overdose is limited primarily to case reports.

The predominant clinical toxicity of primaquine relates to its ability to cause RBC oxidant stress and resultant hemolysis or methemoglobinemia (metHb). Methemoglobinemia and hemolysis can even occur in normal individuals given high doses as well as those with the autosomal recessive disorder nicotinamide adenine dinucleotide (NADH) methemoglobin reductase deficiency.[63,111]

The major complication of primaquine in therapeutic use has been hemolysis in G6PD-deficient individuals.[29] Primaquine is contraindicated in pregnant women because of the risk of metHb or hemolysis in the fetus. Reversible bone marrow suppression can occur.

Clinical Manifestations Gastrointestinal irritation is also common and dose related.

The extent of hemolysis in G6PD-deficient individuals is dependent on the extent of enzyme activity, those with higher levels of enzyme activity having less severe hemolysis than those with less enzyme activity (see Chap. 24). Other variables include the dose of primaquine and comorbid conditions, such as infection, liver disease, and administration of other drugs with hemolytic activity.

Overdose with primaquine is rarely reported and unintentional overdoses have led to metHb requiring IV methylene blue.[111] Acute liver failure has occurred following unintentional overdose and fatal hepatotoxicity is described in animal models.[61]

Management Therapy should be directed at minimizing absorption with appropriate decontamination, and diagnosing then treating significant metHb or hemolysis. Because of structural similarities with other quinolone antimalarials and animal model evidence of sodium channel blockade, cardiovascular toxicity should be anticipated with continuous monitoring and resuscitative interventions initiated as needed.

Activated charcoal would be expected to bind primaquine well if given early (see Antidotes in Depth A2: Activated Charcoal). Methylene blue (Chap. 127 and Antidotes in Depth A41: Methylene Blue) should be administered for patients who are symptomatic with methemoglobinemia. Treatment of hemolysis necessitates avoiding further exposure to primaquine and possibly exchange transfusion in severe cases. Adequate hydration should be ensured to protect against hemoglobin-induced renal injury. Urinary alkalinization with sodium bicarbonate is controversial in this setting but may have some benefit (see Antidotes in Depth A5—Sodium Bicarbonate).

Although no clinical studies have been performed, primaquine's large volume of distribution makes it an unlikely candidate for benefit from extracorporeal removal.

MEFLOQUINE

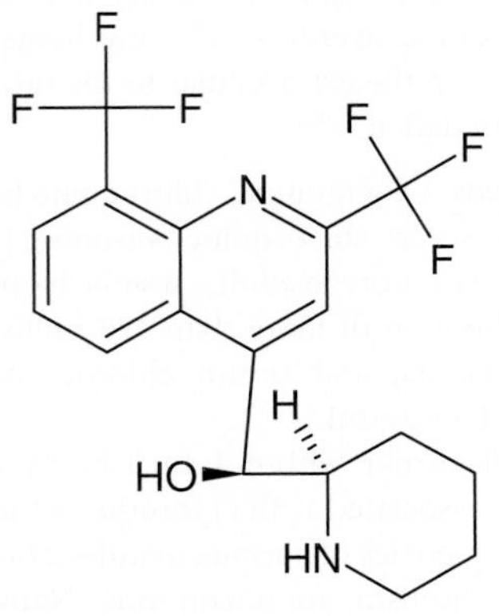

Pharmacokinetics and Toxicodynamics See Table 58–2 for the pharmacokinetic properties of mefloquine.

Clinical Manifestations Common effects with prophylactic and therapeutic dosing include nausea, vomiting, and diarrhea.[78] These effects are noted particularly in the extremes of age and with high therapeutic dosing. Similar symptoms should be expected in acute overdose.[94,124]

Mefloquine has a mild cardiodepressant effect—less than that of quinine or quinidine—which is not clinically significant in prophylactic dosing or with therapeutic administration. Bradycardia is commonly reported.[22,63,78] With prophylactic use, neither the PR interval nor the QRS complex is prolonged, but QT prolongation has been reported.[31,63] Reports of torsades de pointes are rare, but the increase in QT and risk of torsades de pointes are increased when mefloquine is used concurrently with quinine, chloroquine or, most particularly, with halofantrine.[63,78,79,123] The long half-life of mefloquine means that particular care must be taken with therapeutic use of other antimalarials when breakthrough malaria occurs during mefloquine prophylaxis or within 28 days of mefloquine therapy to avoid potential drug—drug interactions. This risk may increase with acute overdose, although there is little clinical experience.

Mefloquine commonly has neuropsychiatric side effects. During prophylactic use, 10% to 40% of patients experience insomnia and bizarre or vivid dreams, and complain of dizziness, headache, fatigue, mood alteration, and vertigo.[99,117] Only 2% to 10% of these complications necessitate the traveler to seek medical advice or change normal activities.[22,46,100] Predisposing factors include a past history of neuropsychiatric disorders, recent prior exposure to mefloquine (within 2 months), previous mefloquine-related neuropsychiatric adverse effects, and previous treatment with psychotropic drugs.[111] Women appear to be more likely than men to experience neuropsychiatric adverse effects.[111,117]

The risk of serious neuropsychiatric adverse effects during prophylaxis is estimated to be 1:10,600, but is reported to be as high as 1:200 with therapeutic dosing.[29,94,111] Seizures occur rarely with prophylaxis and therapeutic use.[87,96] In many of these cases, there is a history of previous seizures, seizures in a first-degree relative, or other seizure risk factors. Other neuropsychiatric symptoms include dysphoria, "clouded" consciousness, encephalopathy, anxiety, depression, giddiness, and an agitated delirium with psychosis. Although there is a suggestion that the severity of neuropsychiatric events is dose dependant, there does not seem to be a correlation with serum or tissue concentrations.[51] In one case report, the severe neuropsychiatric manifestations of mefloquine were reversed with physostigmine, leading the authors to suggest a possible central anticholinergic etiology.[107] A self-resolving postmalaria neurologic syndrome including confusion, seizures, and/or tremor is associated with therapeutic use of mefloquine for severe malaria.[65,96]

The effect of mefloquine on the pancreatic potassium channel is much less than that of quinine, resulting in only a mild increase in insulin secretion.[30,31] Symptomatic hypoglycemia has not been reported as an effect of mefloquine alone in healthy individuals, but has occurred with concomitant use of ethanol and in a severely malnourished patient with acquired immune deficiency syndrome (AIDS).[6,31,63] In overdose, particularly when accompanied by alcohol use or starvation, hypoglycemia could be severe.

Rare events such as hypersensitivity reactions reported with prophylaxis include urticaria, alopecia, erythema multiforme, toxic epidermal necrolysis, myalgias, mouth ulcers, neutropenia, and thrombocytopenia.[69,78,99,105] It is unclear which, if any, would be significant following overdose. ARDS was linked to therapeutic dosing in one case.[115]

In therapeutic use, mefloquine is associated with an increased incidence of stillbirth compared with quinine and a group of other antimalarial medications.[80] Mefloquine was not, however, linked to an increased incidence of abortion, low birth weight, mental retardation, or congenital malformations. The implications of overdose in the absence of malaria are unknown, but fetal monitoring should be instituted.

The consequences of excessive dosing and overdose are not only severe, but also prolonged and potentially permanent. Mefloquine overdose led to acute hearing loss and gradual resolution of acute symptoms over one year in one case and persistent symptoms even after one year in another.[61] After ingesting 5.25 g of mefloquine over 6 days, a man suffered prolonged prothrombin time and weakness persisting for two months after resolution of the acute symptoms.[16] A fourth case involved coingestion of 2.5 times the usual therapeutic dose of mefloquine, chloroquine, and sulfadoxine-pyrimethamine over 3 days. The man suffered encephalopathy that had not resolved 8 months later.[20]

Management In overdose, treatment is primarily supportive with monitoring for potential adverse effects. Decontamination with activated charcoal is indicated if the patient presents soon after the ingestion. Specific monitoring for ECG abnormalities, hypoglycemia, and liver injury should be provided. Patients should also be followed for CNS and cranial nerve complications.

In two patients with renal failure who received mefloquine, prophylactic hemodialysis did not remove mefloquine.[27] Given the large volume of distribution and high degree of protein binding of mefloquine, extracorporeal elimination techniques are unlikely to be effective.

PHENANTHRENE METHANOLS

HALOFANTRINE

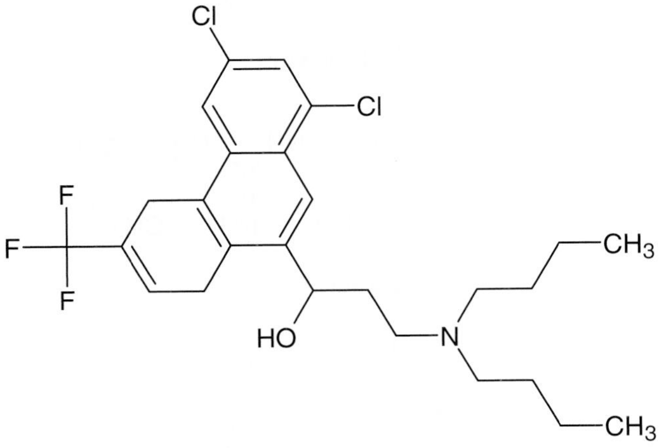

Cl Cl F F F HO N CH_3 CH_3

Because of erratic absorption, potential for lethal cardiotoxicity, and concern for cross-resistance with mefloquine, halofantrine is not presently recommended for malaria prophylaxis by the WHO.[111] Lumefantrine is structurally similar to halofantrine. Since lumefantrine is primarily used as a partner drug in an ACT, it is discussed in more detail in the Artemisinin and Derivatives section.

Pharmacokinetics and Toxicodynamics See Table 58–2 for the pharmacokinetic properties of halofantrine.[19]

Clinical Manifestations The primary toxicity from therapeutic and supratherapeutic doses is prolongation of the QT interval and the risk of torsades de pointes and ventricular fibrillation.[79,113] Palpitations, hypotension, and syncope may occur. First-degree heart block is common, but bradycardia is rare.[79] Dysrhythmias are also likely in the context of combined overdose, or combined or serial therapeutic use with other xenobiotics that cause QT interval prolongation, particularly mefloquine.[52] Because the QT interval duration is directly related to serum halofantrine concentration, dysrhythmias should be expected in overdose.[22,79,111] Fifty percent of children receiving a therapeutic course of halofantrine will have a QT interval greater than 440 milliseconds.[106]

Other side effects, including nausea, vomiting, diarrhea, abdominal cramps, headache, and light-headedness, which frequently occur in therapeutic use, are also expected in overdose.[63] Less frequently described side effects include pruritus, myalgias, and rigors. Seizures, minimal liver enzyme abnormalities, and hemolysis are described.[63,72,116] Whether these manifestations are related to halofantrine or to the underlying malaria is not clear.

Management Management of halofantrine overdose should focus on decontamination, supportive care, monitoring for QT interval prolongation, and treatment of any associated dysrhythmias.

ARTEMISININ AND DERIVATIVES

CH_3 H_3C O O O O CH_3 O

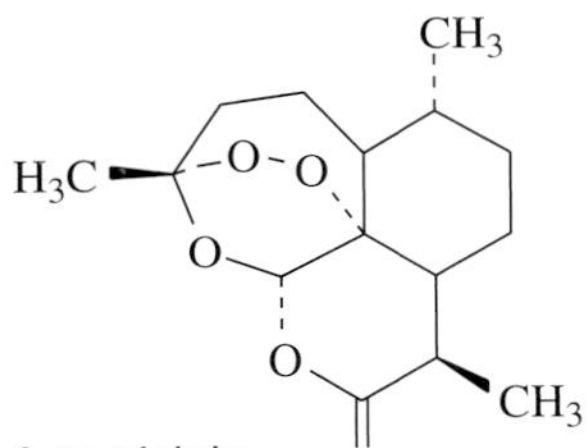

Artemisinin

The medicinal value of natural artemisinin, the active ingredient of *Artemisia annua* (sweet wormwood or quinghao), has been known for thousands of years. Its antimalarial properties were first recognized by Chinese herbalists in 340 AD, but the primary active component of qinghaosu, now known as artemisinin, was not isolated until 1974.[5,114] Artemisinin and its semisynthetic derivatives, artesunate, artemether, arteether, and dihydroartemisinin, are the most potent and rapidly acting of all antimalarial drugs. They were introduced in the 1980s in China for the treatment of malaria, and since then millions of doses have been used in Asia and Africa. Because of their extremely short half-lives, artemisinins are now used in combination with longer half-life drugs to delay or prevent the emergence of resistance. Artemisinin-based combination therapies (ACTs) are currently recommended by the WHO for the treatment of uncomplicated malaria,[5,128] but have not been licensed for use in the United States. Only four ACTs are currently recommended by the WHO. These include artesunate plus mefloquine, artesunate plus pyrimethamine/sulfadoxine, artesunate plus amodiaquine, and artemether plus lumefantrine.

Pharmacokinetics and Toxicodynamics See Table 58–2 for the pharmacokinetic properties of artemisinin. The efficacy and toxicity of artemisinin is thought to be a result of the ability of the trioxane molecular core to form intracellular free radicals, particularly in the presence of heme. In animals, damage to brainstem nuclei is consistently produced following prolonged, high-dose, and parenteral administration.[111] Sustained CNS exposure from slowly absorbed or eliminated artemisinins is considered markedly more neurotoxic than intermittent brief exposure seen after oral dosing.[94] Embryonic loss has also been observed in animals.[94]

Clinical Manifestations In contrast to the experience with animals, the experience of more than 8000 human study participants shows that these drugs have a very low incidence of side effects.[94] Uncommon side effects include nausea, vomiting, abdominal pain, diarrhea, and dizziness.

Prospective studies have failed to identify adverse neurologic outcomes.[53,94] Rare reports of adverse CNS effects during therapeutic use suggest the possibility of CNS depression, seizures, or cerebellar symptoms following intentional self-poisoning. In children with cerebral malaria, a higher incidence of seizures and a delay to recovery from coma were noted in a comparison with quinine.[12] No neurologic difference was noted in long-term follow-up. In an artemether—quinine comparative trial of adults with severe malaria, recovery from coma was also prolonged in the artemether group.[45] Rare patients receiving an artemisinin derivative in two other studies experienced transient dizziness or cerebellar signs.[71,89] Most recovered within days. One patient in each study suffered prolonged symptoms, 1 month and 4 months, respectively, but both ultimately recovered.[71,89]

When serial ECGs were obtained, a small but statistically significant fall in heart rate was noted, coincident with peak drug concentrations.[71] In one therapeutic trial, 7% of adult patients receiving artemether had an asymptomatic QT interval prolongation of at least 25%.[45] Changes in the QRS are not reported.

Although uncommon, neutropenia, reticulocytopenia, anemia, eosinophilia, and elevated concentrations of aminotransferases are reported.[94]

Two of the ACT partner drugs frequently being used today have not been previously discussed: lumefantrine, in the ACT artemether-lumefantrine (AL), and piperaquine, in the ACT dihydroartemisinin-piperaquine (DP).

Lumefantirine Lumefantrine is pharmacologically related to mefloquine and halofantrine. Little toxicity of lumefantrine alone or in combination is reported.[125] Studies do not show an increase in QT or evidence of cardiac toxicity related to lumefantrine.[33,118] Cough and angioedema were described in one case.[56] As with all antimalarials there is difficulty in differentiating drug-related adverse events from those of malaria, comorbid diseases, or other ingested drugs, which confounds the study of potential complications.

lumefantrine

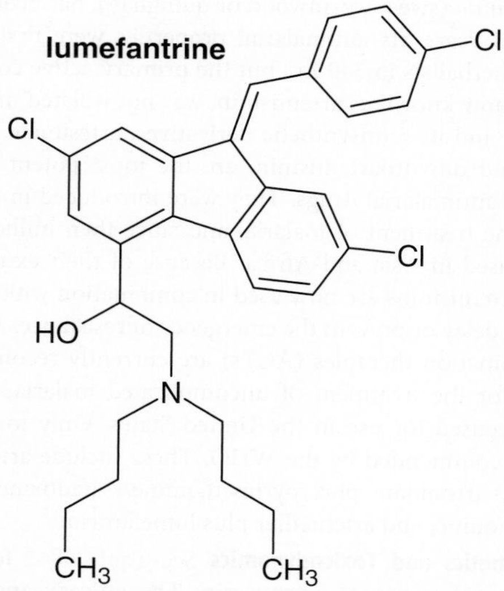

Piperaquine Piperaquine, a bisquinolone with a structure similar to chloroquine, was used extensively in China and Indonesia as an antimalarial until the development of piperaquine-resistant strains led to the use of better alternatives. Piperaquine has since undergone a rediscovery as a viable combination with atremisinin derivatives in ACT DP therapy. Animal studies show piperaquine to be substantially less toxic than chloroquine, with cumulative doses of piperaquine associated with cardiovascular toxicity about fivefold higher than that for chloroquine. Hepatotoxicity occurs following chronic exposure in animals. In a human study, no significant ECG, changes in serum glucose concentration, or postural hypotension was seen following therapeutic doses of DP.

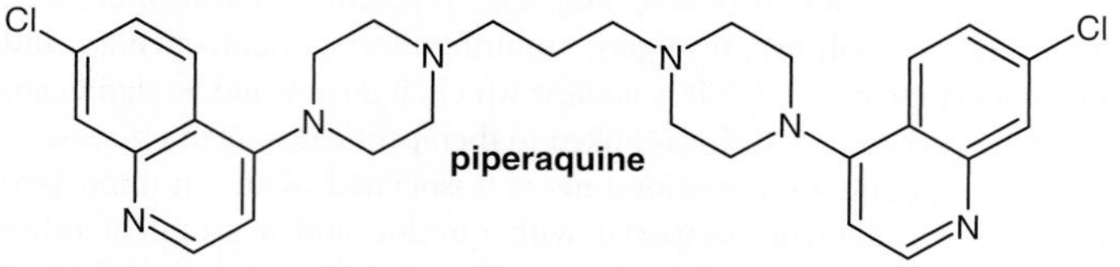

piperaquine

Management Patients with overdose should be managed with supportive measures and expectant observation including cardiovascular and CNS monitoring.

OTHER ANTIMALARIALS

ATOVAQUONE/PROGUANIL, PYRIMETHAMINE/SULFADOXINE, AND DAPSONE

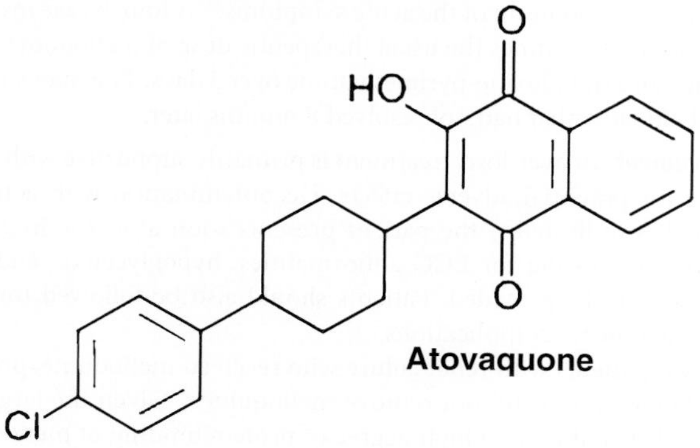

Atovaquone

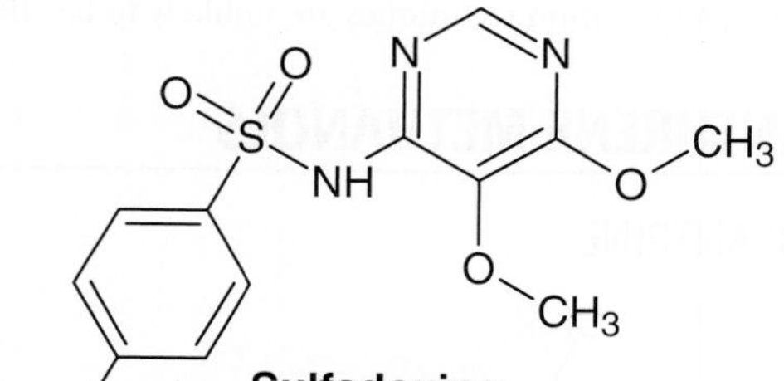

Sulfadoxine

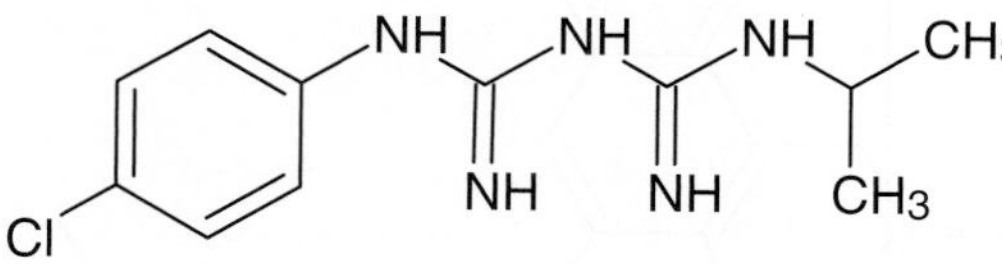

Proguanil

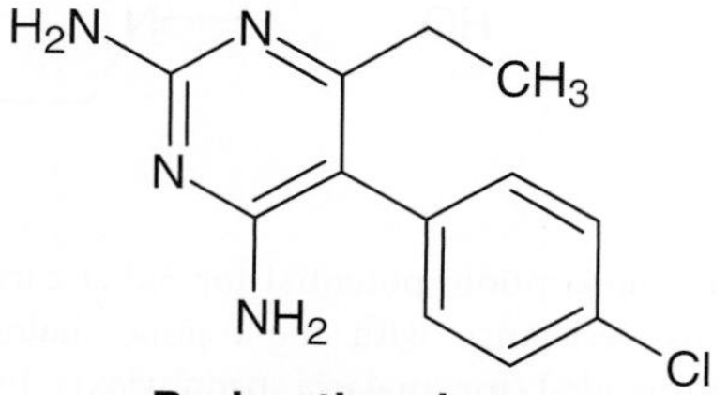

Pyrimethamine

Pharmacokinetics and Toxicodynamics Proguanil, pyrimethamine, sulfadoxine, and dapsone all interfere with malarial folate metabolism at concentrations far lower than that required to produce comparable inhibition of mammalian enzymes.[114] Slow onset of action and concerns for the development of resistance have led to the use of these agents in synergistic combinations. Proguanil (chloroguanide) may be used alone, but is most often used with dapsone (Lapdap), chloroquine, or the antiparasitic atovaquone (Malarone) for prophylaxis. Atovaquone inhibits the de novo pyrimidine synthesis that is necessary for protozoal survival and replication, but is unnecessary in mammalian cells. Based on its beneficial side-effect profile, many North American physicians are switching from mefloquine to atovaquone/proguanil for routine antimalarial prophylaxis for travelers. Atovaquone and proguanil may now be the most common antimalarials used in North America. The price of this combination limits its use mainly to treatment and prevention in travelers from affluent countries.[22]

Pyrimethamine is used synergistically in combination with sulfonamides such as sulfadoxine (Fansidar) or dapsone (Maloprim), but growing malarial resistance and unfavorable toxicity profiles have limited the usefulness of these drug combinations (see Table 58–2 for pharmacokinetic profile). Neither combination is recommended for antimalarial use by the US Centers for Disease Control and Prevention (CDC).

Genetic polymorphism is described in the metabolism of proguanil and dapsone.[50,91] This may be the cause of the significant hypersensitivity reactions noted with dapsone.[91]

Clinical Manifestations The side effects of proguanil during prophylaxis include nausea, diarrhea, and mouth ulcers.[63] Because of the interference with folate metabolism, megaloblastic anemia is a rare complication. Megaloblastic bone marrow toxicity has been reported in renal failure patients.[111] Folate supplementation may be required in pregnancy and renal failure to avoid this complication.[29] Rarely, neutropenia, thrombocytopenia, rash, and alopecia are also noted.[29] In a single case report, hypersensitivity hepatitis was described.[29] When used to treat malaria, atovaquone/proguanil causes vomiting, sometimes severe, in a significant portion of patients (15% to 45%).[94] This combination is also associated with aminotransferase elevations.[94] Unintentional or deliberate overdose has caused little serious toxicity.[111]

Atovaquone alone, primarily used to treat *Pneumocystis jiroveci* in AIDS patients, is relatively well tolerated.[83] Side effects include maculopapular rash, erythema multiforme (rarely), GI complaints, and mild aminotransferase elevations. Three cases of three- to 42-fold overdose or excess dosing have been reported.[23] No symptoms occurred in one case (at three times therapeutic serum concentration). Rash occurred in another, and in the third case metHb was attributed to a simultaneous overdose of dapsone.

Overdose of pyrimethamine alone is rare. In children, it results in nausea, vomiting, the rapid onset of seizures, fever, and tachycardia.[1,47] Blindness, deafness, and mental retardation have followed.[1,47] Seizures were attributed to sulfadoxine-pyrimethamine in an overdose of 12 tablets over 2 days (usual dose is three tablets taken once).[77] It is unclear whether the chronic neurologic deficits described in case reports are due to direct toxicity of pyrimethamine on the central nervous system or to complications of toxicity such as status epilepticus.[1,47] Chronic high-dose use may be associated with a megaloblastic anemia, requiring folate replacement.[1]

The sulfonamides, including the sulfone dapsone, have a long history of causing idiosyncratic reactions, including neutropenia, thrombocytopenia, eosinophilic pneumonia, aplastic anemia, neuropathy, and hepatitis.[63,94] The rare occurrence of life-threatening erythema multiforme major and toxic epidermal necrolysis, associated with pyrimethamine-sulfadoxine prophylaxis, has limited the use of this combination for prophylaxis.

Acute ingestion of dapsone may result in nausea, vomiting, and abdominal pain.[47] Following overdose, dapsone produces RBC oxidant stress leading to metHb and, to a much lesser extent, sulfhemoglobinemia through formation of an active metabolite (Chap. 127).[21,64] The onset of hemolysis may be either immediate or delayed. Dapsone, in particular, is known for its tendency to cause prolonged metHb. Other symptoms, particularly tachycardia, dyspnea, dizziness, visual hallucinations, seizure, syncope, and coma resulting from end-organ hypoxia, can occur.[21,47] Additional effects described in overdose include hepatitis and peripheral neuropathy.[47]

Management Folate supplementation should be considered after overdose of proguanil or pyrimethamine (Antidotes in Depth A13: Leucovorin [Folinic Acid] and Folic Acid). Other efforts should include supportive care.

Following dapsone ingestion, clinically significant metHb should be treated with methylene blue and possibly cimetidine (Chap. 127 and Antidotes in Depth A41: Methylene Blue). There is no antidote for sulfhemoglobinemia, but it constitutes an insignificant portion of total hemoglobin. Both hemodialysis and multidose activated charcoal enhance elimination of dapsone during therapy.[76] Multidose activated charcoal is routinely recommended in the treatment of dapsone overdose.[64] Required support may include RBC transfusion and urinary alkalinization if hemolysis is extensive (Antidotes in Depth A5: Sodium Bicarbonate).

SUMMARY

A variety of xenobiotics are used in the prevention and treatment of malaria. The optimal choices and, consequently, the most widely available xenobiotics, change rapidly with shifting patterns of parasite resistance. Most antimalarials have significant toxicity in acute overdose. Although many toxic effects are related to quinine, even within the quinine group, the pattern of predominant symptoms is xenobiotic dependent. Effects at the low doses associated with prophylaxis and therapy include nausea, vomiting, headache, and confusion. Autoimmune-mediated idiosyncratic reactions are described with most of the antimalarials. In overdose, cardiovascular, neurologic, and hematologic symptoms predominate. Dysrhythmias are the effects that are the most life threatening, particularly with quinine derivatives and especially with chloroquine. These result from sodium channel blockade effect, potassium channel blockade, and myocardial depression. Other significant effects are coma, seizures, and neurologic injury, particularly to the special senses. Primaquine and dapsone produce significant oxidant stress resulting in metHb and often hemolysis. Little is known of the acute toxicity of the newest agent, artemisinin.

Decontamination, including the administration of activated charcoal, should be considered. Multidose activated charcoal is particularly important for quinine and dapsone ingestions. When xenobiotic-specific symptoms are anticipated and specific management strategies followed, improved outcome has resulted, particularly for chloroquine poisoning.

ACKNOWLEDGMENT

G. Randall Bond, MD contributed to this chapter in previous editions.

REFERENCES

1. Akinyanju O, Goddell JC, Ahmed I. Pyrimethamine poisoning. *Lancet.* 1973;4:147-148.
2. AlKadi HO. Antimalarial drug toxicity: a review. *Chemotherapy.* 2007;53(6):385-391.

3. American Academy of Clinical Toxicology, European Association of Poisons Centres and Clinical Toxicologists. Position statement and practice guidelines on the use of multi-dose activated charcoal in the treatment of acute poisoning. *J Toxicol Clin Toxicol.* 1999;37:731-751.
4. Assan R, Perronne C, Chotard L, Larger E, Vilder JL. Mefloquine-associated hypoglycemia in a cachectic AIDS patient. *Diabete Metab.* 1995;21:54-57.
5. Aweeka FT, German PI. Clinical pharmacology of artemisinin-based combination therapies. *Clin Pharmacokinet.* 2008;47(2):91-102.
6. Baguet JP, Tremel F, Fabre M. Chloroquine cardiomyopathy with conduction disorders. *Heart.* 1999;81:221-223.
7. Ball De, Tagwireyi D, Nhachi CFB. Chloroquine poisoning in Zimbabwe: a toxicoepidemiological study. *J Appl Toxicol.* 2002;22:311-315.
8. Baselt RC. Quinine. In *Disposition of Toxic Drugs and Chemicals in Man*, 7th ed. Foster City, CA: Biomedical Publications; 2004:981-983.
9. Bateman DN, Blain PG, Woodhouse KW, et al. Pharmacokinetics and clinical toxicity of quinine overdose: lack of efficacy of techniques intended to enhance elimination. *Q J Med.* 1985;54:125-131.
10. Block JA. Hydroxychloroquine and retinal safety. *Lancet.* 1998;351:1388.
11. Bodenhamer JE, Smilkstein MJ. Delayed cardiotoxicity following quinine overdose: a case report. *J Emerg Med.* 1993;11:279-285.
12. Boele van Hensbroek M, Onyiorah E, Jaffar E, et al. A trial of artemether or quinine in children with cerebral malaria. *N Engl J Med.* 1996;335:65-75.
13. Boereboom F, Ververs FF, Meulenbelt J, van Dijk A. Hemoperfusion is ineffectual in severe chloroquine poisoning. *Crit Care Med.* 2000;28:3346-3350.
14. Boland ME, Roper SMB, Henry JA. Complications of quinine poisoning. *Lancet.* 1985;1(8425):384-385.
15. Bougie DW, Wilker PR, Aster RH. Patients with quinine-induced immune thrombocytopenia have both "drug-dependent" and "drug-specific" antibodies. *Blood.* 2006;108(3):922-927.
16. Bourgeade A, Tonin V, Keudjian F, Levy PY, Faugere B. Intoxication accidentale a la mefloquine. *Presse Med.* 1990;19:1903.
17. Brandfonbrener M, Kronholm J, Jones HR. The effect of serum potassium concentration on quinidine toxicity. *J Pharmacol Exp Ther.* 1966;154(2):250-254.
18. Breckenridge AM, Winstanley PA. Clinical pharmacology and malaria. *Ann Trop Med Parasitol.* 1997;91:727-733.
19. Bryson HM, Goa KL. Halofantrine: a review of its antimalarial activity, pharmacokinetic properties and therapeutic potential. *Drugs.* 1992;43:236-258.
20. Burgmann H, Winkler S, Uhl F, et al. Mefloquine and sulfadoxine/pyrimethamine overdose in malaria tropica. *Wien Klin Wochenschr.* 1993;105:61-63.
21. Carrazza MA, Carrazza FR, Oga S. Clinical and laboratory parameters in dapsone acute intoxication. *Rev Saude Publica.* 2000;4:396-401.
22. Chattopadhyay R, Mahajan B, Kumar S. Assessment of safety of the major antimalarial drugs. *Expert Opin Drug Saf.* 2007;6(5):505-521.
23. Cheung TW. Overdose of atovaquone in a patient with AIDS. *AIDS.* 1999;13:1984-1985.
24. Clemessy JL, Angel G, Borron SW, et al. Therapeutic trial of diazepam versus placebo in acute chloroquine intoxications of moderate gravity. *Intensive Care Med.* 1996;22(12):1400-1405.
25. Clemessy JL, Favier C, Borron SW, et al. Hypokalemia related to acute chloroquine ingestion. *Lancet.* 1995;346:877-880.
26. Clemessy JL, Taboulet P, Hoffman JR, et al. Treatment of acute chloroquine poisoning: a 5-year experience. *Crit Care Med.* 1996;24:1189-1195.
27. Crevoisier C, Joseph I, Fischer M, Graf H. Influence of hemodialysis on plasma concentration-time profiles of mefloquine in two patients with end stage renal disease: a prophylactic drug monitoring study. *Antimicrob Agents Chemother.* 1995;39:1892-1895.
28. Crouzette J, Vicaut E, Palombo J, et al. Experimental assessment of the protective activity of diazepam on the acute toxicity of chloroquine. *J Toxicol Clin Toxicol.* 1983;20(3):271-279.
29. Davis TME. Adverse effects of antimalarial prophylactic drugs: an important consideration in the risk-benefit equation. *Ann Pharmacother.* 1998;22:1104-1106.
30. Davis TME. Antimalarial drugs and glucose metabolism. *Br J Clin Pharmacol.* 1997;44:1-7.
31. Davis TME, Dembo LG, Kaye-Eddie SA, et al. Neurological, cardiovascular, and metabolic effects of mefloquine in healthy volunteers: a double-blind placebo-controlled trial. *Br J Clin Pharmacol.* 1996;42:415-421.
32. Dyson EH, Proudfoot AT, Bateman DN. Quinine amblyopia: is current management appropriate? *J Toxicol Clin Toxicol.* 1985;23:571-578.
33. Ezzet F, van Vugt M, Nosten F, Looareesuwan S, White NJ. Pharmacokinetics and pharmacodynamics of lumefantrine (benflumetol) in acute falciparum malaria. *Antimicrob Agents Chemother.* 2000;44:697-704.
34. Farver DK, Lavin MN. Quinine-induced hepatotoxicity. *Ann Pharmacother.* 1999;33:32-34.
35. Flanagan KL, Budkley-Sharp M, Doherty T, Whitty CJ. Quinine levels revisited: the value of routine drug level monitoring for those on parenteral therapy. *Acta Trop.* 2006;97(2):233-237.
36. Gangitano JL, Keltner JL. Abnormalities of the pupil and visual-evoked potential in quinine amblyopia. *Am J Ophthalmol.* 1980;89:425-430.
37. Getz MA, Subramian R, Logeman R, Bellantyne F. Acute necrotizing eosinophilic myocarditis as a manifestation of severe hypersensitivity myocarditis. *Ann Intern Med.* 1991;115:201-202.
38. Goldenberg AM, Wexler LF. Quinine overdose: review of toxicity and treatment. *Clin Cardiol.* 1988;11(10):716-718.
39. Grace AA, Camm AJ. Quinidine. *N Engl J Med.* 1998;338:35-45.
40. Grant WM, Schuman JS. Quinine sulfate. In *Toxicology of the Eye, Vol. II: Effects on the Eyes and Visual System from Chemicals, Drugs, Metals and Minerals, Plants, Toxins and Venoms*, 4th ed. Springfield, IL: Charles C. Thomas; 1993:1225-1233.
41. Guinovart C, Navia MM, Tanner M, Alonso PL. Malaria: burden of disease. *Curr Mol Med.* 2006;6(2):137-140.
42. Guly U, Driscoll P. The management of quinine induced blindness. *Arch Emerg Med.* 1992;9:317-322.
43. Gustafsson LI, Walker O, Alvan G, et al. Disposition of chloroquine in man after single intravenous and oral doses. *Br J Clin Pharmacol.* 1983;15:471-479.
44. Hall A, Williams S, Rajkumar K, Galloway R. Quinine-induced blindness. *Br J Ophthalmol.* 1997;81:1-4.
45. Hein TT, Day NPJ, Phu NH, et al. A controlled trial of artemether or quinine in Vietnamese adults with severe falciparum malaria. *N Engl J Med.* 1996;335:76-83.
46. Ingram RJH, Ellis-Pegler RB. Malaria, mefloquine and the mind. *N Z Med J.* 1997;110:137-138.
47. Jaeger A, Sauder P, Kopferschmitt J, Flesch F. Clinical features and management of poisoning due to antimalarial drugs. *Med Toxicol.* 1987;2:242-273.
48. Johansen PB, Gran JT. Ototoxicity due to hydroxychloroquine: report of two cases. *Exp Rheumatol.* 1998;16:472-474.
49. Jordan P, Brookes JG, Nickolic G, LeCouteur DG. Hydroxychloroquine overdose, toxicokinetics and management. *J Toxicol Clin Toxicol.* 1999;37:861-864.
50. Kaneko A, Bergqvist Y, Taleo G, et al. Proguanil disposition and toxicity in malaria patients from Vanuatu with high frequencies of CYP2C19 mutations. *Pharmacogenetics.* 1999;9:317-326.
51. Karbwang J, White NJ. Clinical pharmacokinetics of mefloquine. *Clin Pharmacokinet.* 1990;19:264-279.
52. Karbwang J, Na Bangchang K, Bunnag D, Harinasuta T, Laothavorn P. Cardiac effect of halofantrine. *Lancet.* 1993;342:501.
53. Kissinger E, Hien TT, Hung NT, et al. Clinical and neurophysiological study of the effects of multiple doses of artemisinin on brain-stem function in Vietnamese patients. *Am J Trop Med Hyg.* 2000;63:48-55.
54. Kivisto KT, Neuvonen PJ. Activated charcoal for chloroquine poisoning. *BMJ.* 1993;307(6911):1068.
55. Krantz MJ, Dart RC, Mehler PS. Transient pulmonary infiltrates possibly induced by quinine sulfate. *Pharmacotherapy.* 2002;22:775-778.
56. Krippner R, Staples J. Suspected allergy to artemether-lumefantrine treatment of malaria. *J Travel Med.* 2003;10:303-305.
57. Krishna S, White NJ. Pharmacokinetics of quinine, chloroquine and amodiaquine: clinical implications. *Clin Pharmacokinet.* 1996;30:263-299.
58. Lalloo, DG, Shineadia D, Pasvol G, et al. UK malaria treatment guidelines. *J Infect.* 2007;54(2):111-121.
59. Limburg PJ. Katz H, Grant CS, Service FJ. Quinine-induced hypoglycemia. *Ann Intern Med.* 1993;119:218-219.
60. Ling Ngan Wong A, Tsz Fung Cheung I, Graham CA. Hydroxychloroquine overdose: case report and recommendations for management. *Eur J Emerg Med.* 2008;15(1):16-18.
61. Lobel Ho, Coyne PE, Rosenthal PJ. Drug overdoses with antimalarial agents: prescribing and dispensing errors. *JAMA.* 1998;280:1483.
62. Lockey D, Bateman DN. Effect of oral activated charcoal on quinine elimination. *Br J Clin Pharmacol.* 1989;27:92-94.

63. Luzzi GA, Peto TWA. Adverse effects of antimalarials. *Drug Saf.* 1993;8: 295-311.
64. MacDonald RD, McGuigan MA. Acute dapsone intoxication: a pediatric case report. *Pediatr Emerg Care.* 1997;13:127-129.
65. Mai N, Day N, Van Chuong L, et al. Post-malaria neurological syndrome. *Lancet.* 1996;348:917-921.
66. Makin AJ, Wendon J, Fitt S, Portmann BC, Williams R. Fulminant hepatic failure secondary to hydroxychloroquine. *Gut.* 1994;35:569-571.
67. Markham TN, Dodson VN, Eckberg DL. Peritoneal dialysis in quinine sulfate intoxication. *JAMA.* 1967;202:1102-1103.
68. Marquardt K, Albertson TE. Treatment of hydroxychloroquine overdose. *Am J Emerg Med.* 2001;19(5):420-424.
69. McBride SR, Lawrence CM, Pape SA, Reid CA. Fatal toxic epidermal necrolysis associated with mefloquine antimalarial prophylaxis. *Lancet.* 1997;349:101.
70. Meeran K, Jacobs MG, Scott J, et al. Chloroquine poisoning. Rapidly fatal without treatment. *BMJ.* 1993;307:49-50.
71. Miller LG, Panosian CB. Ataxia and slurred speech after artesunate treatment for falciparum malaria. *N Engl J Med.* 1997;336:1328.
72. Monlun E, Le Metayer P, Szwandt S, et al. Cardiac complications of halofantrine: a prospective study of 20 patients. *Trans R Soc Trop Med Hyg.* 1995;89:430-433.
73. Morrison LD, Velez LI, Shepherd G, et al. Death by quinine. *Vet Hum Toxicol.* 2003;45(6):303-306.
74. Netland K, Martinez J. Abortifacients: toxidromes, ancient to modern—a case series and review of the literature. *Acad Emerg Med.* 2000;7: 824-829.
75. Neubauer AS, Stiefelmeyer S, Berninger T, Arden GB, Rudolph G. The multifocal pattern electroretinogram in chloroquine retinopathy. *Ophthalmic Res.* 2004;36:106-113.
76. Neuvonen PJ, Elonen E, Haapenen EJ. Acute dapsone poisoning: clinical findings and effect of oral activated charcoal and haemodialysis on dapsone elimination. *Acta Med Scand.* 1983;214:215-220.
77. Nicolas X, Granier H, Laborde JP, Martin J, Talarmin F. Danger of malaria self-treatment. Acute neurologic toxicity of mefloquine and its combination with pyrimethamine-sulfadoxine. *Presse Med.* 2001;30:1349-1350.
78. Nosten F, Price RN. New antimalarials: a risk-benefit analysis. *Drug Saf.* 1995:12:264-272.
79. Nosten F, Ter Kuile FO, Luxemburger C, et al. Cardiac effects of antimalarial treatment with halofantrine. *Lancet.* 1993;341:1054-1056.
80. Nosten F, Vincenti M, Simpson J, et al. The effects of mefloquine treatment in pregnancy. *Clin Infect Dis.* 1999;28:808-815.
81. Okitolonda W, Delacollette C, Malengreau M, Henquin JC. High incidence of hypoglycemia in African patients treated with intravenous quinine for severe malaria. *Br Med J.* 1987;295:716-718.
82. Parmar RC, Valvi CV, Kamat JR, Vaswani RK. Chloroquine induced parkinsonism. *J Postgrad Med.* 2000;46:29-30.
83. Peters BS, Carlin E, Weston RJ, et al. Adverse effects of drugs used in the management of opportunistic infections associated with HIV infection. *Drug Saf.* 1994;10:439-454.
84. Phillips RE, Looareesuwan S, Bloom SR, et al. Effectiveness of SMS 201-995, a synthetic long-acting somatostatin analogue, in treatment of quinine-induced hyperinsulinemia. *Lancet.* 1986;i:713-716.
85. Phillips RE, Looareesuwan S, Molyneux ME, Hatz C, Warrell DA. Hypoglycemia and counterregulatory hormone responses in severe falciparum malaria: treatment with Sandostatin. *Q J Med.* 1993;86:233-240.
86. Ploypradith P. Development of artemisinin and its structurally simplified trioxane derivatives as antimalarial drugs. *Acta Trop.* 2003;89:329-342.
87. Pous E, Gascon J, Obach J, Corachan M. Mefloquine-induced grand mal seizure during malaria chemoprophylaxis in a non-epileptic subject. *Trans R Soc Trop Med Hyg.* 1995;89:434.
88. Prescott LF, Hamilton AR, Heyworth R. Treatment of quinine overdose with repeated oral charcoal. *Br J Clin Pharmacol.* 1989;27:95-97.
89. Price R, van Vugt M, Phaipun L, et al. Adverse effects in patients with acute falciparum malaria treated with artemisinin derivatives. *Am J Trop Med Hyg.* 1999;60:547-555.
90. Reddy VG, Sinna S. Chloroquine poisoning: report of two cases. *Acta Anaesthesiol Scand.* 2000;44:1017-1020.
91. Reilly TP, Woster PM, Swensson CK. Methemoglobin formation by hydroxylamine metabolites of sulfamethoxazole and dapsone: implications for differences in adverse drug reactions. *J Pharmacol Exp Ther.* 1999;288:951-959.
92. Riou B, Barriot P, Rimailho A, Baud FJ. Treatment of severe chloroquine poisoning. *N Engl J Med.* 1988;318:1-7.
93. Riou B, Rimailho A, Galliot M, Bourdon R, Huet Y. Protective cardiovascular effects of diazepam in experimental acute chloroquine poisoning. *Intensive Care Med.* 1988;14:610-616.
94. Robert W, Taylor J, White NJ. Antimalarial drug toxicity: a review. *Drug Saf.* 2004;27:25-61.
95. Roche RJ, Silamut K, Pukrittayakamee S, et al. Quinine induces reversible high tone hearing loss. *Br J Clin Pharmacol.* 1990;29:780-782.
96. Rouviex B, Bricaire F, Michon C, et al. Mefloquine and an acute brain syndrome. *Ann Intern Med.* 1989;110:577-578.
97. Ryan ET, Kain KC. Health advice and immunizations for travelers. *N Engl J Med.* 2000;342:1716-1725.
98. Sabto J, Pierce RM, West RH, Gurr FW. Haemodialysis, peritoneal dialysis, plasmapheresis and forced diuresis for the treatment of quinine overdose. *Clin Nephrol.* 1981;16:264-268.
99. Schlagenhauf P. Mefloquine for malaria prophylaxis: a review. *J Travel Med.* 1999;6:122-133.
100. Schlagenhauf P, Tschopp A, Johnson R, et al. Tolerability of malaria chemoprophylaxis in non-immune travelers to sub-Saharan Africa: multicentre, randomized, double blind, four arm study. *BMJ.* 2003;327: 1078-1082.
101. Shojania K, Koehler BE, Elliot T. Hypoglycemia induced by hydroxychloroquine in a type II diabetic treated for polyarthritis. *J Rheumatol.* 1999;26:195-196.
102. Shub C, Gau GT, Sidell PM, Brennan LA Jr. The management of acute quinidine intoxication. *Chest.* 1978;73(2):173-178.
103. Sialmut K, Molunto P, Ho M, Davis JM, White NJ. Alpha 1-acid glycoprotein (orosomucoid) and plasma protein binding of quinine in falciparum malaria. *Br J Clin Pharmacol.* 1991;32:311-315.
104. Smith ER, Klein-Schwartz W. Are 1-2 dangerous? Chloroquine and hydroxychloroquine exposure in toddlers. *J Emerg Med.* 2005;28(4):437-443.
105. Smith HR, Croft AM, Black MM. Dermatological adverse effects with the antimalarial drug mefloquine: a review of 74 published case reports. *Clin Exp Dermatol.* 1999;24:249-254.
106. Sowunmi A, Fehintola FA, Ogundahansi AT, et al. Comparative cardiac effects of halofantrine and chloroquine plus chlorpheniramine in children with acute uncomplicated falciparum malaria. *Trans R Soc Trop Med Hyg.* 1999;93:78-83.
107. Speich R, Haller A. Central anticholinergic syndrome with the anti-malarial drug mefloquine. *N Engl J Med.* 1994;331:57-58.
108. Splawski I, Timothy KW, Vincent GM, Atkinson DL, Keating MT. Molecular basis of the long-QT syndrome associated with deafness. *N Engl J Med.* 1997;336:1562-1567.
109. Tange RA. Ototoxicity. *Adverse Drug React Toxicol Rev.* 1998;17:75-89.
110. Taylor S, Berridge V. Medicinal plants and malaria: an historical case study of research at the London School of Hygiene and Tropical Medicine in the twentieth century. *Trans R Soc Trop Med Hyg.* 2006;100(8):707-714.
111. Taylor WR, White NJ. Antimalarial drug toxicity: a review. *Drug Saf.* 2004;27(1):25-61.
112. Tecklenburg FW, Thomas NJ, Webb SA, Case C, Habib DM. Pediatric ECMO for severe quinidine cardiotoxicity. *Pediatr Emerg Care.* 1997;13:111-113.
113. Touze JE, Keundjian BA, Viguier PIA, et al. Electrocardiographic changes and halofantrine plasma level during acute falciparum malaria. *Am J Trop Med Hyg.* 1996;54:225-228.
114. Tracy JW, Webster LT. Drugs used in the chemotherapy of protozoal infection: malaria. In Hardman JG, Limbird LE, Molinoff PB, et al., eds. *Goodman and Gilman's the Pharmacological Basis of Therapeutics*, 10th ed. New York: McGraw-Hill; 2001:1059-1095.
115. Udry E, Bailly F, Dusmet M, et al. Pulmonary toxicity with mefloquine. *Eur Respir J.* 2000;18:890-892.
116. Vachon F, Fajac I, Gachot B, Coulaud JP, Charmot G. Halofantrine and acute intravascular haemolysis. *Lancet.* 1992;340:909-910.
117. Van Riemsdijk MM, Sturkenboom MC, Ditters JM, et al. Atovaquone plus chloroguanide versus mefloquine for malaria prophylaxis: a focus on neuropsychiatric adverse events. *Clin Pharmacol Ther.* 2002;72:294-301.
118. Van Vugt M, Ezzet F, Nosten F, et al. No evidence of cardiotoxicity during antimalarial treatment with artemether-lumefantrine. *Am J Trop Med Hygiene.* 1999;61:964-967.
119. Wanwimolruk S, Denton JR. Plasma protein binding of quinine: binding to human serum albumin, α_1-acid glycoprotein and plasma from patients with malaria. *J Pharm Pharmacol.* 1992;44:806-811.

120. Wasay M, Wolfe GI, Herrold JM, Burns DK, Barohn RJ. Chloroquine myopathy and neuropathy with elevated CSF protein. *Neurology.* 1998;51:1226-1227.
121. Wenstone R, Bell M, Mostafa SM. Fatal adult respiratory distress syndrome after quinine overdose. *Lancet.* 1989;1:1143-1144.
122. Winek CL, Davis ER, Collom WD, Shanor SP. Quinine fatality—case report. *Clin Toxicol.* 1974;7(2):129-132.
123. White NJ. Cardiotoxicity of antimalarial drugs. *Lancet Infect Dis.* 2007;7(8):549-558.
124. White NJ. The treatment of malaria. *N Engl J Med.* 1996;335:800-806.
125. White NJ, van Vugt M, Ezzet F. Clinical pharmacokinetics and pharmacodynamics of artemether-lumefantrine. *Clin Pharmacokinet.* 1999;37:105-125.
126. Wolf LR, Otten EJ, Spadafora MP. Cinchonism: two case reports and review of acute quinine toxicity and treatment. *J Emerg Med.* 1992;10:295-301.
127. Wolff RS, Wirtschafter D, Adkinson C. Ocular quinine toxicity treated with hyperbaric oxygen. *Undersea Hyperb Med.* 1997;24:131-134.
128. World Health Organization. Facts on ACTs (Atreminisinin-based combination therapies). http://www.searo.who.int/LinkFiles/Drug_Policy_RBMInfosheet_9.pdf. Published January 2006 [cited].
129. World Health Organization. Malaria fact sheet. http://www.who.int/mediacentre/factsheets/fs094/en/. Published May 2007 [cited].
130. Yanturali S. Diazepam for treatment of massive chloroquine intoxication. *Resuscitation.* 2004;63(3):347-348.

E.

CARDIOPULMONARY MEDICATIONS

CHAPTER 59
ANTICOAGULANTS

Mark Su

Anticoagulants have numerous clinical applications, including in the treatment of coronary artery disease, cerebrovascular events, deep venous thrombosis, and pulmonary embolism. The anticoagulants are a diverse group of xenobiotics that are widely studied and constantly in the process of therapeutic evolution. Bleeding is a major complication of these xenobiotics. Knowledge of anticoagulants will be of ever-increasing utility for clinicians as their use increases.

HISTORY AND EPIDEMIOLOGY

The origins and discovery of anticoagulants are extraordinary.[2,16,73,131] The discovery of modern-day oral anticoagulants originated following investigations of a hemorrhagic disorder in Wisconsin cattle in the early 20th century that resulted from the ingestion of spoiled sweet clover silage. The hemorrhagic agent, eventually identified as bishydroxycoumarin, would be the precursor to its synthetic congener warfarin (named after the *W*isconsin *A*lumni *R*esearch *F*oundation). This knowledge also led to the use of warfarin as a rodenticide. "Superwarfarins" were subsequently developed as selective pressure caused rats to develop genetic resistance to warfarin. These potent anticoagulants permitted either small, repetitive ingestions or single, larger ingestions to successfully function as rodenticides.

As in the case of warfarin, the origins of the anticoagulant heparin are equally fascinating. A medical student initially attempting to study ether-soluble procoagulants derived from porcine intestines serendipitously found that, over time, these apparent "procoagulants" actually prevented normal blood coagulation. The phospholipid anticoagulant responsible for this effect would later be identified as an early form of heparin. Shortly thereafter, the water-soluble mucopolysaccharide termed *heparin* (because of its abundance in the liver) was then discovered. *Unfractionated* heparin is a mixture of polysaccharide chains with varying molecular weights. Following the identification of the active pentasaccharide segment of heparin in the 1970s, multiple *low-molecular-weight* heparins were isolated and synthetic forms created.

In the late 19th century, human urine was noted to have proteolytic activity with a specificity for fibrin. A substance found to be an activator of endogenous plasminogen leading to the consumption of fibrin, fibrinogen, and other coagulation proteins was isolated and purified and given the name *urokinase*. Streptokinase, a protein produced by β-hemolytic streptococci, tissue plasminogen activator (t-PA), and other synthetic thrombolytics were later discovered. Although known to exist for many years, ancrod (a purified derivative of snake venom) and hirudin (a product of leeches) only recently gained attention as naturally occurring antithrombotic therapeutic agents.

The diversity of these anticoagulants and fibrinolytics has led to ever-increasing use in many fields of medicine. Warfarin is the most common oral anticoagulant in use today because of its utility in patients with cerebrovascular disease, cardiac dysrhythmias, and thromboembolic disease. During the period of 2005 to 2007, the total number of cases of reported warfarin exposures to the American Association of Poison Control Centers was 10,508 with eight deaths (Chap. 135). Throughout this time, there was a general trend toward an increasing number of reports. Additionally, because the common problem of excessive warfarin effects leading to hemorrhage is poorly quantitated as an adverse drug reaction, it frequently goes unrecorded. Thus, as long as warfarin continues to be routinely prescribed, it is likely that the incidence of adverse drug events will continue. Physicians must be cognizant of the complications of warfarin and other anticoagulants, as well as their various therapeutic modalities, while balancing the potential for their risk and benefits.

PHYSIOLOGY

BALANCE BETWEEN COAGULATION AND ANTICOAGULATION

An understanding of the normal function of the coagulation pathways is essential to appreciate the etiology of a coagulopathy. This section summarizes the critical steps of the coagulation cascade. For additional details, the reader is referred to Chap. 24 and several reviews.[63,129,155]

Coagulation consists of a series of events that prevent blood loss and assist in the restoration of blood vessel integrity. Although the traditional understanding of the events that occur in the coagulation cascade,[48,114] as discussed below, adequately describe in vitro events, the current understanding emphasizes some distinct differences that occur in vivo.[63,129,155] Despite these differences, an understanding of the traditional model is most useful for interpreting the results of diagnostic tests of coagulation.

Within the cascade, coagulation factors exist as inert precursors and are transformed into enzymes when activated. Activation of the cascade occurs through one of two distinct pathways, the *intrinsic* and *extrinsic* systems (Fig. 59–1).[48,114] Once activated, these enzymes catalyze a series of reactions that ultimately converge and lead to the generation of thrombin and the formation of a fibrin clot.

The intrinsic pathway is activated by the complexation of factor XII (Hageman factor) with high-molecular-weight kininogen (HMWK) and prekallikrein, or vascular subendothelial collagen. This results in sequential activation of factor XII, active kallikrein, active factors IX to XI, and prothrombin (factor II) (Fig. 59–2). Prothrombin is converted to thrombin in the presence of factor V, calcium, and phospholipid. The integrity of this system is usually evaluated by determining the partial thromboplastin time (PTT).

In the extrinsic or tissue-factor-dependent pathway, a complex is formed between factor VII, calcium, and tissue factor, which is released following injury. A calcium and lipid-dependent complex is then created between factors VII and X. The factor VII–X complex subsequently converts prothrombin to thrombin, which promotes the formation of fibrin from fibrinogen (see Fig. 59–1). The integrity of this pathway is usually assessed by determining the prothrombin time (PT or international normalized ratio [INR]).

Activation of factor X provides the important link between the intrinsic and extrinsic coagulation pathways. Additional evidence that tissue factors can activate both factors IX and X suggests that there are more interrelations between the two pathways.[143] Furthermore, cell surfaces facilitate the process of clotting. Platelets are also known to interact with proteins of the coagulation cascade through surface receptors for factors V, VIII, IX, and X.[66,118,169] As a final step, factor XIII assists in the cross-linking of fibrin to form a stable thrombus.

Antithrombin III (now known simply as AT), protein C, protein S, and protein Z serve as inhibitors, maintaining the homeostasis that is required to prevent spontaneous clotting and keep blood fluid. Protein C, when aided by protein S, inactivates two plasma factors, V and VIII.[27,40,63] Protein Z is a glycoprotein molecule that forms a complex with the protein Z-dependent protease inhibitor (ZPI) which, in turn, inhibits the activated factor X (Xa)[184] AT complexes with all the serine protease coagulation factors (factor Xa, factor IXa, and contact factors, including XIIa, kallikrein, and HMWK), except factor VII.[27,63,155]

Thrombolytics such as streptokinase, urokinase, anistreplase, and recombinant tissue plasminogen activator (rt-PA) enhance the normal processes that lead to clot degradation.[129]

Thrombosis is initiated when exposed endothelium or released tissue factors leads to platelet adherence and aggregation, the formation of thrombin, and cross-linking of fibrinogen to form fibrin strands.[63,129,155] This results in a hemostatic plug or thrombus formation. Thrombus formation, in turn, leads to generation of plasmin from plasminogen, which causes fibrinolysis and eventual dissolution of the hemostatic plug.[42,43] Thus the fibrinolytic system may be thought of as a natural balance against unregulated coagulation. Thrombolytic therapy increases fibrinolytic activity by accelerating the conversion of plasminogen to plasmin, which actively degrades fibrin.[42,43] Following the administration of thrombolytics, a drug-induced coagulopathy ensues, and fibrin degradation products are elevated secondary to the rapid turnover of clot.

DEVELOPMENT OF COAGULOPATHY

Impaired coagulation results from decreased production or enhanced consumption of coagulation factors, the presence of inhibitors of coagulation, activation of the fibrinolytic system, or abnormalities in platelet number or function. Platelets are involved in the initial phases of clotting following blood vessel injury by assisting in the formation of the fibrin plug. For the purposes of this chapter, a discussion of platelet-related abnormalities is excluded. Some of this information can be found in Chap. 24.

Decreased production of coagulation factors results from congenital and acquired etiologies. Although congenital disorders of factor VIII (hemophilia), factor IX (Christmas factor), factor XI, and factor XII (Hageman factor) are all reported, their overall incidence is still quite low. Clinical conditions that result in acquired factor deficiencies are much more common and result from either a decrease in synthesis or activation. Factors II, V, VII, and X are entirely synthesized in the liver,[63,129,155] making hepatic dysfunction a common cause of acquired coagulopathy. In addition, factors II, VII, IX, and X require postsynthetic activation by an enzyme that uses vitamin K as a cofactor,[174,179,180] such that vitamin K deficiency (from malnutrition, changes in gut flora secondary to xenobiotics, or malabsorption), or inhibition of vitamin K cycling (from warfarin, as will be described) is capable of impairing coagulation.

Excessive consumption of coagulation factors usually results from massive activation of the coagulation cascade. Massive activation occurs during severe hemorrhage or disseminated intravascular coagulation. The latter results from infection, such as sepsis, and from conditions that introduce tissue factor into the blood, such as neoplasms, snake envenomations, stagnant blood flow, diffuse endothelial injury secondary to hyperthermia, ruptured aortic aneurysm, or aortic dissection. The hallmark of a consumptive coagulopathy is a depressed concentration of fibrinogen with an elevation of fibrin-degradation products. This combination suggests the rapid turnover of fibrin in the coagulation process. In the other coagulopathic conditions, the failure to activate the coagulation cascade is associated with normal or high fibrin concentrations and low fibrin-degradation products because of limited clot formation.

Inhibitors of the coagulation cascade (circulating anticoagulants) are of two types: immunoglobulin and nonimmunoglobulin. Immunoglobulins, which are often antibodies to existing coagulation factors, may occur without obvious cause. They may be part of a systemic autoimmune disorder or as a result of repeated transfusions with exogenous factors (as occurs in hemophilia).[77,106,165] The clinical syndromes associated with antibody inhibitors are similar to those associated with deficiencies of the particular coagulation factors involved. Antibodies to factors V, VII to XI, and XIII are described.[20,165] Alternatively, nonimmunoglobulin neutralizers of coagulation occur in conditions associated with rapid white blood cell turnover.[20] These lysosomal cationic proteins are neutralizers that compete with coagulation factors for negatively charged phospholipid membrane surfaces. Although they prolong in vitro coagulation times, they are rarely responsible for clinical coagulopathy because of the excess of phospholipid surface area available in vivo.[77,106]

ORAL ANTICOAGULANTS

WARFARIN AND "WARFARINLIKE" ANTICOAGULANTS

Oral anticoagulants can be divided into two groups: (1) hydroxycoumarins, including warfarin (commonly called by its trade name Coumadin), difenacoum, panwarfarin, warficide, coumachlor, coumafuryl, fumasol, prolin, ethyl biscoumacetate (Tromexan), phenprocoumon, dicumarol bishydroxycoumarin, and acenocoumarin (Sintrom); and (2) indanediones, including chlorophacinone, pindone, pivalyn, diphacinone, diphenadione, phenindione, and anisindione. Regardless of the classification, their mechanism of action involves inhibition of the vitamin K cycle. Vitamin K is a cofactor in the postribosomal synthesis of clotting factors II, VII, IX, and X (Fig. 59–2). The vitamin K–sensitive enzymatic step that occurs in the liver involves the γ-carboxylation of 10 or more glutamic acid residues at the amino terminal end of the precursor proteins, to form a unique amino acid γ-carboxyglutamate.[53,174,179,180] These amino acids chelate calcium in vivo, which allows the binding of the four vitamin K–dependent clotting factors to phospholipid membranes during activation of the coagulation cascade.[195]

Vitamin K is inactive until it is reduced from its quinone form to a quinol (or hydroquinone) form in hepatic microsomes. This reduction of vitamin K must precede the carboxylation of the precursor factors. The carboxylation activity is coupled to an epoxidase activity for

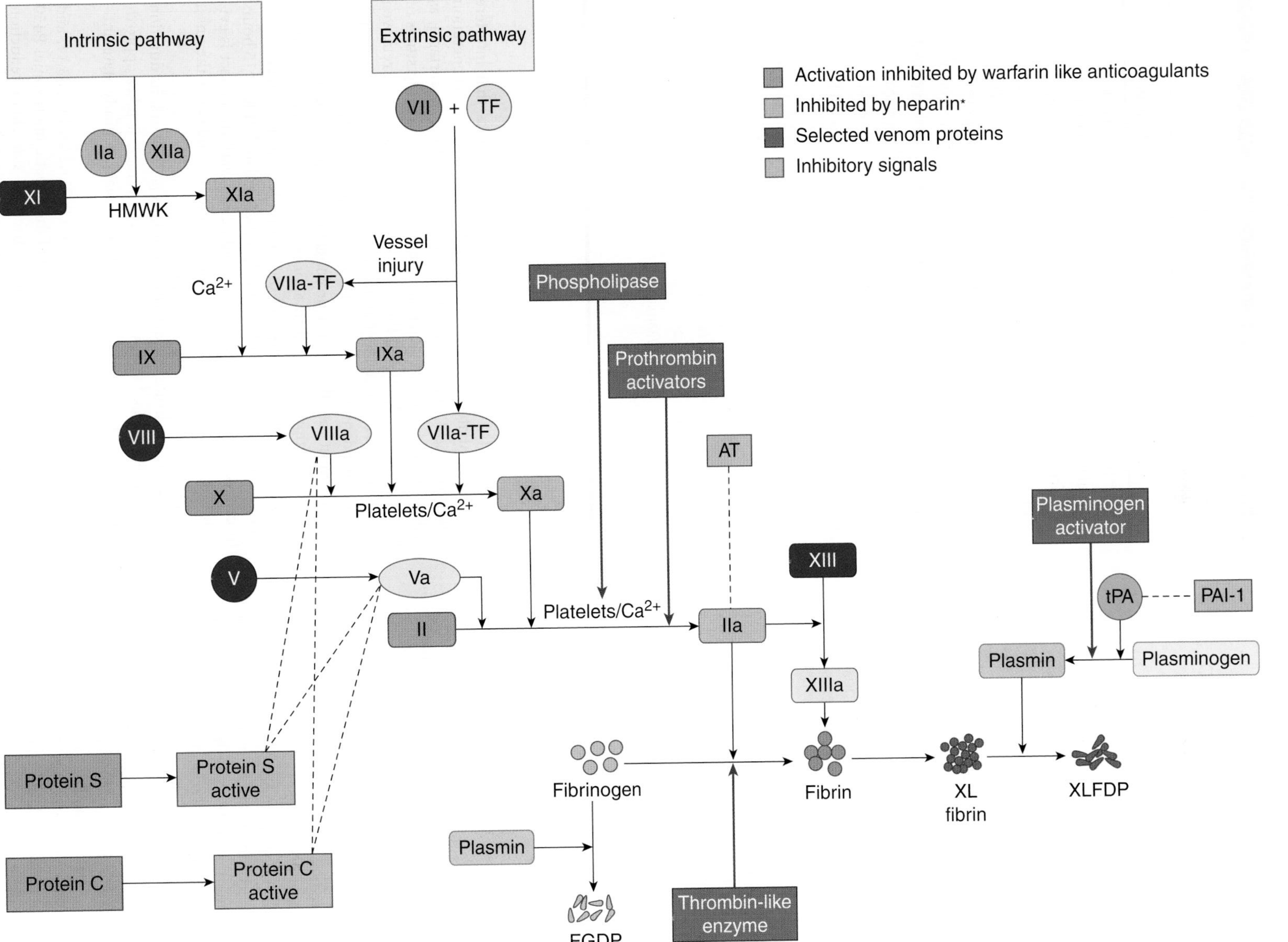

FIGURE 59–1. A schematic overview of the coagulation and fibrinolytic pathways indicating where phospholipids on the platelet surface interact with the coagulation pathway intermediates. Arrows are not shown from platelets to phospholipids involved in the tissue factor VIIa and the factor IXa to VIIIa interactions to avoid confusion. Interactions of selected venom proteins are indicated in the purple boxes. The diagram is not complete with reference to the multiple sites of interaction of the SERPINS (serine protease inhibitors) to avoid overcrowding.[115]; XL cross-linked. FDP, fibrin degredation products FGDP, fibrinogen degredation products. HMWK = high molecular-weight kininogen. Dashed lines indicate inhibitory effects.

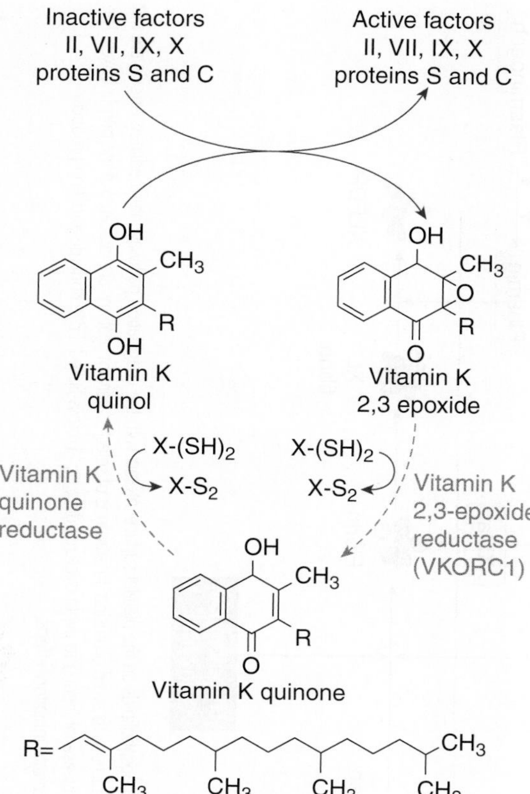

FIGURE 59–2. The vitamin K cycle. Dotted lines represent pathways that can be blocked with warfarin and warfarinlike anticoagulants. The aliphatic side chain (R) of vitamin K is shown below the metabolic pathway. VKORC1=Vitamin K reductase complex 1.

TABLE 59–1. Common Xenobiotic Interactions With Warfarin Anticoagulation

Potentiation		Antagonism
Acetaminophen	Isoniazid	Antacids
Allopurinol	Ketoconazole	Barbiturates
Amiodarone	Metronidazole	Carbamazepine
Anabolic steroids	Nonsteroidal antiinflammatory drugs	Cholestyramine
Aspirin		Colestipol
Carbenicillin	Omeprazole	Corticosteroids
Clarithromycin	Phenytoin	Griseofulvin
Cephalosporins	Propafenone	Oral contraceptives
Chloral hydrate	Propoxyphene	Phenytoin
Cimetidine	Quinidine	Rifampin
Clofibrate	Quinolones	Vitamin K
Cyclic antidepressants	Sulfonylureas	
Disulfiram	Tamoxifen	
Erythromycin	Tetracycline	
Ethanol	Thyroxine	
Fluconazole	Trimethoprim-Sulfamethoxazole	
fluoroquinolone antibiotics	Vitamin E	
HMG-CoA reductase Inhibitors		

vitamin K, whereby vitamin K is oxidized simultaneously to vitamin K 2,3-epoxide (see Fig. 59–2).[179,195] This inactive form of the vitamin is converted back to the active form by two successive reductions.[53,116,146] In the first step, an epoxide reductase (known as vitamin K 2,3-epoxide reductase) uses reduced nicotinamide adenine dinucleotide (NADH) as a cofactor to convert vitamin K 2,3-epoxide to a quinone form.[139,179] Subsequently, the quinone is reduced to the active vitamin K quinol form (see Antidotes in Depth A16–Vitamin K_1).

Warfarin is a racemic mixture of R warfarin and S warfarin enantiomers. In rodents, S warfarin is three to six times more potent than R warfarin at producing hypoprothrombinemia.[29] In humans, S warfarin may only be about 1.5 times as potent as R warfarin.[30] Warfarin and all warfarinlike compounds inhibit the activity of vitamin K 2,3-epoxide reductase, as can be demonstrated by the observation of elevated concentrations of vitamin K 2,3-epoxide in orally anticoagulated subjects.[39,198] Additional evidence suggests that another enzyme, vitamin K quinone reductase, is also inhibited by warfarin and its related compounds (Fig. 59–2).[53,57] This reduction in the cyclic activation of vitamin K subsequently inhibits the formation of activated clotting factors.

Pharmacology of Warfarin Orally ingested warfarin is virtually completely absorbed, and peak serum concentrations occur approximately 3 hours after administration.[178] Because only the free warfarin is therapeutically active, concurrent administration of xenobiotics that alter the concentration of free warfarin, either by competing for binding to albumin or by inhibiting warfarin metabolism, may markedly influence the anticoagulant effect.[12,61,178] The pharmacologic response to warfarin is a polygenic trait with approximately 30 genes contributing to its therapeutic effects.[101] Table 59–1 lists the xenobiotics that interfere with or potentiate warfarin's effects. Although vitamin K regeneration is altered almost immediately, the anticoagulant effect of warfarin, as well as other oral anticoagulants, is delayed until the existing stores of vitamin K are depleted and the active coagulation factors are removed from circulation. Because vitamin K turnover is rapid, this effect is largely dependent on factor half-life ($t_{1/2}$), with factor VII ($t_{1/2}$ ~5 hours) depleted most rapidly.[61] For a prolongation of the INR to occur, factor concentrations must fall to approximately 25% of normal values. Assuming complete inhibition of the vitamin K cycle, this suggests that in most patients who are not originally anticoagulated, at least 15 hours (three factor VII half-lives) are required before warfarin's effect is evident.[59] In fact, complete inhibition does not occur, and hence the onset of coagulation is even further delayed.

Because the half-life of warfarin in humans is 35 hours, its duration of action may be as long as 5 days.[29,178] On average, it takes approximately 6 days of warfarin administration to reach a steady-state anticoagulant effect.

R warfarin is metabolized by isozymes CYP1A2 and CYP3A4, and S warfarin is metabolized by CYP2C9 of the hepatic microsomal P450 enzyme system. R warfarin is metabolized by side-chain reduction to secondary alcohols that are subsequently excreted by the kidney, whereas S warfarin is metabolized by hydroxylation to 7-hydroxy warfarin, which is excreted into the bile.[178] The elimination of S warfarin is more rapid than that of R warfarin.[30]

The therapeutic dose of warfarin is established for both adults and children. Typical adult recommendations are to give a starting dose of 5 mg/d with subsequent doses based on nomograms, computer programs, and/or clinical experience.[64] Previous recommendations of initiating with a "loading" dose appear to be unnecessary.[5] Wide variability of maintenance dosing also exists, depending on, for example, individual responsiveness, comorbid health conditions, and age. For children, the suggested starting dose of warfarin is 0.2 mg/kg, followed by continued loading over 3 days, followed by a daily maintenance dose to maintain the INR between 2 and 3.[127,152] For patients with mechanical heart valves, depending on the type of valve, an increased intensity of anticoagulation (INR 3.0 to 4.0) may be recommended.[54]

Dosing of warfarin and other vitamin K antagonists is potentially problematic in certain individuals. In one study, genetic polymorphisms of the vitamin K epoxide reductase complex 1 (VKORC1) and CYP2C9 genes appear to be the strongest predictors of interindividual variability in the anticoagulant effect of warfarin.[101] Furthermore, pharmacogenomic research with complex xenobiotics, such as warfarin, may improve the treatment of patients and predict or prevent interactions with other xenobiotics. In fact, the US Food and Drug Administration (FDA) has recently approved a commercially available test to identify variants within these genes.[97]

PHARMACOLOGY OF LONG-ACTING ANTICOAGULANTS

Within the coumarin group are two 4-hydroxycoumarin derivatives—difenacoum and brodifacoum differ from warfarin by their longer, higher-molecular-weight polycyclic hydrocarbon side chains (Fig. 59–3). Together with chlorophacinone, an indandione derivative, they are known as "superwarfarins," or long-acting anticoagulants.

Long-acting anticoagulants were designed to be effective rodenticides in warfarin-resistant rodents.[113] Their mechanism of action is identical to that of the traditional warfarinlike anticoagulants, as demonstrated by the measurement of increased concentrations of vitamin K 2,3-epoxide after long-acting anticoagulant administration.[28,31,32,107,145] The ability of these xenobiotics to perform as superior rodenticides is attributed to their high lipid solubility and concentration in the liver.[107,113,145] They also may saturate hepatic enzymes at very low concentrations, as demonstrated by zero-order elimination following overdose.[32] These factors make them about 100 times more potent than warfarin on a molar basis.[107,113,145] In addition, they have a longer duration of action than the traditional warfarins.[107,113,145] For example, to obtain 100% lethality in a mouse, more than 21 days of feeding with a warfarin-containing rodenticide (0.025% anticoagulant by weight of bait) is required.[113] Similar efficacy can be achieved with a single ingestion of brodifacoum (0.005% anticoagulant by weight of bait).[113]

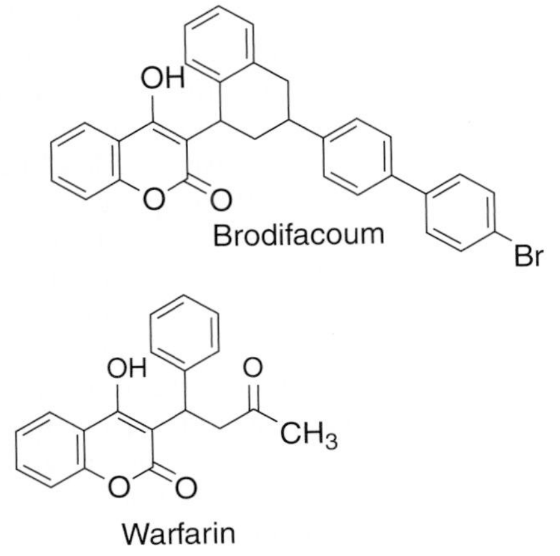

FIGURE 59–3. Structural comparison of prototypical short-acting (warfarin) and long-acting (brodifacoum) anticoagulants.

Many animals have been poisoned with long-acting anticoagulants, either secondary to the unintentional ingestion of rodenticides or intentionally for scientific investigation. In rats, the half-life of brodifacoum is reported to be 156 hours.[9] The half-life in dogs is reported to be between 6 and 120 days.[200] Horses intentionally poisoned with brodifacoum had a half-life of 1.22 days.[23] The veterinary literature is replete with reports of fatalities and of animals that remained anticoagulated in excess of 1 month.[130,176]

Likewise, many cases of intentional overdose of long-acting anticoagulants in humans are also described in the literature. These patients' clinical courses are characterized by a severe coagulopathy that may last weeks to months, often accompanied by consequential blood loss. The most common sites of bleeding are the gastrointestinal and genitourinary tracts. Although initial parenteral vitamin K_1 doses as high as 400 mg have been required for reversal,[33] daily oral vitamin K_1 requirements may be in the range of 50 to 100 mg. Recent experience in both animals and humans suggests that parenteral vitamin K_1 therapy might not be required (see Antidotes in Depth A16: Vitamin K_1).[32,200] It should also be noted that although ingestions of these xenobiotics are the most common route of exposure and subsequent cause of toxicity, dermal absorption can occur also resulting in coagulopathy.[172]

Patients with unintentional ingestions must be distinguished from those with intentional ingestions, because the former individuals demonstrate a low likelihood of producing coagulation abnormalities and have only rare morbidity or mortality. Prolongation of the INR is unlikely with a single small ingestion of a superwarfarin rodenticide. Clinically significant anticoagulation is even rarer. In a combined pediatric case series, prolongation of the INR occurred in only eight of 142 children (5.6%) reported with single small ingestions of long-acting anticoagulants.[15,94,95,171] Only one child in this group was reported to have "abnormal prolonged bleeding," but this required no medical attention.[171] In a single case report, a 36-month-old child developed a coagulopathy manifested by epistaxis and hematuria, with anticoagulation persisting for more than 100 days after a presumed, but unwitnessed, single unintentional ingestion of brodifacoum.[182] Clinically significant coagulopathy can result, however, following small repeated ingestions. Two children reportedly became poisoned by repeated ingestions of a long-acting anticoagulant. One child presented with a neck hematoma that compromised his airway, and the other with a hemarthrosis.[69] Similarly, a 7-year-old girl required multiple hospitalizations over a 20-month period following repeated nonsuicidal ingestions of brodifacoum.[192] Finally, a 24-month-old child who presented with unexplained bruising and a PT greater than 125 seconds was the victim of brodifacoum poisoning because of a Munchausen syndrome by proxy.[8]

Most patients (usually children) are entirely asymptomatic and have a normal coagulation profile following an acute unintentional exposure. Knowing that the risk of coagulopathy is low and that it takes days to develop, most authors recommend supportive care only.[93,171] Despite the fact that significant toxicity from superwarfarins is rare, it should be recognized that the reported benign courses of pediatric exposures may be misleading. Multiple retrospective studies suggest that children with unintentional acute exposures do not require any follow-up coagulation studies.[128,132,147,166] However, this conclusion and approach to management may be an unjustified attempt to decrease the cost of "unnecessary" coagulation studies. There are clearly insufficient data to justify this conclusion, as many of these "exposed" children were never documented to have ingested long-acting anticoagulants (see Chap. 135). We recommend that clinicians continue to manage these children as possible significant exposures, and that all children be followed up with at least a single INR at least 48 hours after the exposure.

A baseline INR is usually unnecessary but may be performed if there is a suspicion of chronic ingestion.

CLINICAL MANIFESTATIONS

Typical warfarin rodenticides contain only small concentrations of anticoagulant, 0.025% (or 25 mg of warfarin per 100 g of product). Using the data previously listed, a 10-kg child would require an initial dose of 2.5 mg of warfarin (or 10 g of rodenticide). These quantities are far greater than those that occur in typical "tastes." Thus, single small unintentional ingestions of warfarin-containing rodenticides pose a minimal threat to normal patients.[93] In contrast, intentional and large unintentional ingestions of pharmaceutical-grade anticoagulants have the potential to produce a coagulopathy and bleeding. In one study describing 12 patients with surreptitious ingestion of oral anticoagulants, nine were healthcare professionals.[140] These patients presented with bruising, hematuria, hematochezia, and menorrhagia, the typical manifestations of impaired coagulation. Hemorrhage into the neck with resultant airway compromise is a rare but life-threatening complication that has occurred.[24]

Although intentional ingestions of warfarin-containing products are uncommon, adverse drug events resulting in excessive anticoagulation and bleeding frequently occur. The risk of hemorrhage during oral anticoagulant therapy depends on a myriad of factors, including the intensity of anticoagulation, patient characteristics, and comorbid conditions such as hypertension, renal insufficiency, hepatic dysfunction, malignancy, length of anticoagulant therapy, and indications for anticoagulation—cerebrovascular disease, prosthetic heart valves, atrial fibrillation, ischemic heart disease, and venous and arterial thromboembolism. Although the significance of each of these clinical conditions varies among different reports, most studies demonstrate that there is a greater incidence of bleeding complications with increasing INR,[41] increasing intensity (or variation) of coagulation, advanced age, a history of previous bleeding episodes while on therapeutic warfarin, drug interactions, impaired liver function, and dietary changes.[59,61,71,76,150,197] Clearly, the most serious complication of excessive anticoagulation is intracranial hemorrhage, which is reported to occur in as many as 2% of patients on long-term therapy.[61] This complication is associated with a fatality rate as high as 77%.[121] A recent study of patients with intracranial hemorrhage found that decreased level of consciousness and increased size of hemorrhage were predictors of poor prognosis.[203] Somewhat surprisingly, the degree of INR elevation was not associated with worse outcome.[203]

An Outpatient Bleeding Risk Index was created and shown to be more accurate than physician judgment in classifying patients according to the risk of major bleeding.[18] The index was based on independent risk factors: age 65 years or older; history of cerebrovascular accident; history of gastrointestinal bleeding; and history of recent myocardial infarction, hematocrit less than 30%, serum creatinine greater than 1.5 mg/dL, or diabetes mellitus. The sum of the number of risk factors successfully predicted major bleeding at 48 months to be 3% in low-risk (zero risk factors), 12% in intermediate risk (one to two risk factors), and 53% in high-risk (three to four risk factors) patients. Because physicians are often unable to accurately estimate the probability of bleeding, use of the Outpatient Bleeding Risk Index seems appropriate to improve awareness and treatment of these high-risk patients and was validated in at least one subsequent study.[193]

In a study of 32 patients who developed life-threatening hemorrhage while on warfarin therapy, most patients had multiple risk factors including excessive anticoagulation.[197] The gastrointestinal tract was identified as the source of bleeding in 67% of the patients.[197] Sixty-six percent of patients were given vitamin K_1, 50% were given fresh-frozen plasma (FFP), and 7% were given both therapies.[197]

LABORATORY ASSESSMENT

Established screening tests are helpful for diagnosis. Four studies—PT (INR), PTT, thrombin time, and fibrinogen concentration—are usually adequate. Prothrombin time is calculated by adding standardized thromboplastin reagent (phospholipid and tissue factor) to a sample of the patient's citrated plasma (the citrate removes calcium to prevent clotting). Calcium is then introduced and the time to clotting measured. With the exception of factor X, the PT is unaffected by the presence or absence of factors VIII to XIII, platelets, prekallikrein, and HMWK. An individual's PT was formerly expressed as a ratio (PT observed to PT control). Because this ratio is directly affected by both laboratory methodology and the source of the thromboplastin reagent used, the generated results suffered from significant variability. Thus, a standard, the INR, was developed in an attempt to limit interlaboratory variability.[78,136] The INR is derived by raising the PT ratio to a power value known as the International Sensitivity Index (ISI): $(\text{PT ratio})^{\text{ISI}}$. The ISI is a measure of responsiveness of the particular thromboplastin to warfarin. Although the use of the INR does not completely eliminate variability,[80,135] it does improve the potential for standardized interpretation and limits interinstitutional variations. It should be noted that in patients taking oral anticoagulants, specifically warfarin, the INR is extremely effective at monitoring the extent of anticoagulation. However, use of the INR measurement in the setting of fulminant hepatic failure, as in the recently developed Model for End-Stage Liver Disease (MELD) score, a tool to predict the need for liver transplantation, is unwarranted.[35] In these patients the INR is extremely variable and inaccurate as a consequence of the variability in thromboplastins.[154] This problem may be mitigated in the United States because of the use of recombinant human preparations of thromboplastin, which results in greater consistency.[36]

The partial thromboplastin time is measured by adding kaolin or celite to citrated plasma in order to activate the "contact" components of the intrinsic system. This mixture is then recalcified and the time to clotting observed. Some tests use phospholipids in the reagent to activate the remaining coagulation factors, thereby giving rise to the term *activated partial thromboplastin time* (aPTT). Because the PTT and aPTT are essentially interchangeable, the term PTT is used hereafter to represent the concept. The PTT is not affected by alterations in factors VII, XIII, or platelets.

The thrombin time, determined by adding exogenous thrombin to citrated plasma, evaluates the ability to convert fibrinogen to fibrin, and is thus unaffected by abnormalities of factors II, V, VII to XIII, platelets, prekallikrein, or HMWK. Finally, either a fibrinogen concentration or a determination of fibrin degradation products will help distinguish between problems with clot formation and consumptive coagulopathy (disseminated intravascular coagulation). An evaluation of the combination of normal and abnormal results of these tests usually determines a patient's clotting abnormality (Table 59–2).

Inhibitors can be diagnosed by "mixing studies," because only a small percentage of the coagulation factors present in normal plasma are necessary to have normal clotting studies. If the patient with an abnormal PT or PTT suffers from even a severe factor deficiency, restoration of that factor activity to 50% of normal will completely normalize the PT or PTT. Thus the presence of an abnormal PT or PTT that will not correct by incubation of the patient's plasma with an equal volume of normal plasma is diagnostic of an inhibitor of coagulation. Heparin-induced anticoagulation results in an elevated PTT that corrects when mixing studies are performed. More sophisticated studies can be used to identify specific coagulation-factor deficiencies. The reader is referred to one of several standard references for a more detailed discussion of the approach to patients with abnormal coagulation studies.[156]

TABLE 59–2. Evaluation of Abnormal Coagulation Times

PT normal, PTT prolonged, bleeding
Deficiencies of factors VIII, IX, XI
von Willebrand disease
PT normal, PTT prolonged, no bleeding
Deficiencies of factor XII, prekallikrein, high-molecular-weight kininogen inhibitor syndrome
PT prolonged, PTT normal
Deficiency of factor VII
Warfarin therapy (early)
Vitamin K deficiency (mild)
Liver disease (mild)
PT and PTT prolonged, thrombin time normal, fibrinogen normal
Deficiencies of factors II, V, IX; vitamin K deficiency (severe)
Warfarin therapy (late)
PT and PTT prolonged, thrombin time abnormal, fibrinogen normal
Heparin effect
Dysfibrinogenemia
PT and PTT prolonged, thrombin time abnormal, fibrinogen abnormal
Liver disease
Disseminated intravascular coagulation
Fibrinolytic therapy
Crotaline envenomation

PT, prothrombin time; PTT, partial thromboplastin time.

Although warfarin concentrations may be useful to confirm the diagnosis in unknown cases and to study drug kinetics,[72,138] the routine use of simple and inexpensive measures such as INR determination seems more appropriate.

LABORATORY EVALUATION OF LONG-ACTING ANTICOAGULANTS

For patients who have ingested long-acting anticoagulants and who are considered likely to develop a coagulopathy, baseline coagulation studies are not usually helpful, but they may provide information about chronic exposures. If the history is reliable and the patient is healthy, baseline studies can be avoided. A single INR at 48 hours should identify all patients at risk of coagulopathy.[171] Depending on the social situation, these studies can be obtained while the patient remains in the home setting.

In contrast, all patients with intentional ingestion of long-acting anticoagulants should be presumed to be at risk for a severe coagulopathy. In fact, most patients do not seek medical care until bruising or bleeding is evident.[11,32,33,38,56,82,95,100,133,181] These events often occur many days after ingestion, which obviates the need for gastric decontamination unless there is a suggestion of repetitive ingestion. These patients should be managed as described below.

For patients who have suspected long-acting anticoagulant overdose, daily or twice-daily INR evaluations for 2 days should be adequate to identify most patients at risk for coagulopathy. Early detection through coagulation factor analysis may be preferred,[72,82] however, and concentrations of long-acting anticoagulants can now be measured.[102,138]

GENERAL MANAGEMENT AND ANTIDOTAL TREATMENT

Gastrointestinal decontamination should be performed on patients who are believed to have potentially significant life-threatening ingestions unless they already present with significant bleeding. For patients who present after a few hours of ingestion, gastric emptying is not indicated (see Chap. 7). Although convincing data on the efficacy of either single- or multiple-dose activated charcoal (AC; possible enterohepatic circulation) are lacking, at least a single dose of AC should be administered unless it is contraindicated. Oral cholestyramine can also be used to enhance warfarin elimination,[151] but no studies are available that compare these two therapies or evaluate the role of combined activated charcoal and cholestyramine therapy. Although in animal models phenobarbital also enhances elimination, it is relatively contraindicated in humans because of the decreased ability to reliably monitor the mental status of a patient who has the possibility of spontaneous intracranial hemorrhage and subsequent increased risk of falling. In addition to general supportive measures, the patient should be placed in a supervised medical and psychiatric environment that offers protection against external or self-induced trauma, and permits observation for the onset of coagulopathy.

Blood transfusion is required for any patient with a history of blood loss or active bleeding who is hemodynamically unstable, has impaired oxygen transport, or is expected to become unstable. Although a transfusion of packed red blood cells is ideal for replacing lost blood, it cannot correct a coagulopathy, and thus patients will continue to bleed. Whole blood contains both the cellular elements the patient is losing and the necessary coagulation factors to reverse the coagulopathy. Transfusion of whole blood may be considered in severe cases because whole blood contains many components, including platelets, white blood cells, and non–vitamin-K-dependent factors. However, because whole blood contains only relatively small amounts of vitamin K–dependent factors, selective use of specific blood products is generally preferred. These products include packed red blood cells, FFP, cryoprecipitate, or other factor concentrates, such as factor IX complex (Konyne 80), recombinant factor VIIa (rFVIIa), and prothrombin complex concentrate.

Life-threatening hemorrhage secondary to oral anticoagulant toxicity should be immediately reversed with FFP, followed by vitamin K_1. FFP is rich in active vitamin K–dependent coagulation factors and will reverse oral anticoagulant-induced coagulopathy in most patients. In general, approximately 15 mL/kg of FFP should be adequate to reverse any coagulopathy.[47] However, the specific factor quantities and volume of each unit may be varied, leading to an unpredictable response.[117] A study comparing the efficacy of FFP and various clotting factor concentrates (prothrombin complex concentrate, factor VII concentrate, and Prothromplex T [factors II, VII, IX, and X]) in rapid reversal of anticoagulation, showed that despite significant reduction in the INR, FFP had an extremely varied effect on factor IX repletion. These clotting factor concentrates not only significantly decreased the INR, but completely corrected it, and factor IX replacement was much more consistent.[117] Additionally, multiple FFP transfusions may also be required because of the rapid degradation of coagulation factors in the absence of vitamin K. Administration of FFP to patients with intracerebral hemorrhage may also result in volume overload.[1] Prothrombin complex concentrates (PCCs) are likely to produce complete INR reversal faster than FFP and appear to be associated with fewer adverse effects.[50] One group in the United Kingdom reports success with its use for the reversal of oral anticoagulation.[92] Consequently, prothrombin complex concentrates may be preferable to FFP if readily available.

Preliminary data using rVIIa demonstrates it to be a useful pharmacologic therapy for bleeding secondary to warfarin-induced excessive anticoagulation.[51,126] There is also a single case report demonstrating efficacy at reversing severe bleeding caused by enoxaparin,[86] and a recent case series showing beneficial effects in four patients with superwarfarin toxicity.[204] Since a possible complication of its use may be thrombosis, further experience with rVIIa is necessary to determine its safety and efficacy in anticoagulant-induced hemorrhage. It should also be noted that if rVIIa is used, assays based on PT may be inaccurate and should be avoided when administering rVIIa.[96]

Several issues influence the decision to administer vitamin K_1 to a patient with a suspected overdose of a warfarinlike anticoagulant. Answers to the following questions should always be considered. Does the ingestion involve a warfarin-containing rodenticide or a pharmaceutical preparation? Is the ingestion unintentional or intentional? Does the patient require maintenance of therapeutic anticoagulation? Moreover, although vitamin K_1 administration is required to reverse the blockade of coagulation factor activation, it cannot be relied on for the patient with acute and consequential hemorrhage (see Antidotes in Depth A16: Vitamin K_1). Treatment with vitamin K_1 takes several hours to activate enough factors to reverse the patient's coagulopathy,[117,146] and this delay may be potentially fatal.

Repetitive, large doses of vitamin K_1 (on the order of 60 mg/d) may be required in some patients.[72,140] If complete reversal of INR prolongation occurs or is desirable (as in most cases of life-threatening bleeding), and the patient's underlying medical condition still requires some degree of anticoagulation, they can then receive anticoagulation with heparin once the bleeding is controlled and they are otherwise stable. Heparin anticoagulation was used without apparent bleeding complications in 25% of patients in one cross-sectional study.[197]

Vitamin K_1 is preferable over the other forms of vitamin K; the other forms are ineffective[90,133,139,183] and are potentially toxic.[10] (Vitamins K_3 [menadione] and K_4 [menadiol sodium diphosphate] can cause oxidative stress on neonatal erythrocytes and produce hemolysis, hyperbilirubinemia, and kernicterus.) Parenteral administration of vitamin K_1 (phytonadione) is traditionally preferred as initial therapy by many authors, but success can also be achieved with early oral therapy, especially when the coagulopathy is not severe.[32] In most cases, the patient can be switched to oral vitamin K_1 for long-term care. Vitamin K_1 can be administered intramuscularly, subcutaneously, intradermally, or intravenously. Although intravenous therapy has the most rapid onset of action of all routes of delivery, its use as the sole therapeutic agent is still associated with a delay of several hours[116,146] and carries the added risk of anaphylactoid reactions.[153] The use of low doses and slow rate of administration reduces this risk[168] (see Antidotes in Depth A16–Vitamin K_1). In cases where oral administration is undesirable, for example, with significant gastrointestinal hemorrhage, the subcutaneous route may be used, realizing that absorption may be erratic. Furthermore, if a patient is anticoagulated or overanticoagulated, administration of vitamin K_1 by the intramuscular route may result in a large hematoma. Caution should be exercised if this route of administration is chosen.

For patients with non–life-threatening hemorrhage, the clinician must consider whether anticoagulation is required for long-term care. In patients not requiring chronic anticoagulation, even small elevations of the INR may be treated with vitamin K_1 alone to prevent deterioration in coagulation status and reduce the risk of bleeding. Because in most cases of warfarin ingestion coagulopathy persists only for several days, there may be a rationale for prophylactic vitamin K_1 administration in known warfarinlike anticoagulant ingestions in patients not requiring anticoagulation. In contrast to ingestions of warfarin, prophylactic vitamin K_1 should never be given to asymptomatic patients with unintentional ingestions of long-acting anticoagulants because (1) if the patient develops a coagulopathy, it will last for weeks, and the one or two doses of vitamin K_1 given will not prevent complications; (2) a gradual decline in coagulation factors occurs over the first day of anticoagulation, so no one would be expected to develop a life-threatening coagulopathy in 1 or 2 days; and (3) after vitamin K_1 is administered, the onset of an INR abnormality will be delayed, which could impair the clinician's ability to diagnose any coagulation abnormality, possibly requiring the patient to undergo an unnecessarily prolonged observation period.

For patients requiring chronic anticoagulation, the American College of Chest Physicians has issued guidelines for the management of patients with elevated INRs (Table 59–3). Moreover, the use of a regression formula may assist in calculating the amount of oral vitamin K_1 necessary to partially correct the INR, without completely discontinuing the oral anticoagulant. Although it remains unvalidated, it would be extremely useful prior to minor surgery or dental procedures in patients requiring chronic anticoagulation, while theoretically decreasing the likelihood of thromboembolism.[194] It should also be noted that low-dose vitamin K may be safely administered to patients with mildly elevated INRs (4 to 10) to decrease the INR more

TABLE 59–3. Recommendations for Management of Elevated INRs or Bleeding in Patients Receiving Vitamin K Antagonists[5]

INR	Recommendations[a]
<5.0; no significant bleeding	Lower dose or omit next dose of warfarin
>5.0 but <9.0; no significant bleeding	Omit warfarin for next one or two doses. Alternatively, omit next dose and give oral vitamin K_1 (1-2.5 mg) especially if at increased risk of bleeding. If more rapid reversal is necessary, give oral vitamin K_1 (≤5 mg) and wait 24 hours. Give additional vitamin K_1 orally (1-2 mg) as needed.
>9.0; no significant bleeding	Hold warfarin therapy and give a higher dose of oral vitamin K_1 (2.5-5 mg) and wait 24 hours. Give additional vitamin K_1 if necessary.
Serious bleeding at any INR concentration or life-threatening bleeding	Hold warfarin therapy and give FFP, PCC, or rVIIa[b] supplemented with vitamin K_1 (10 mg by slow parenteral[c] infusion). Vitamin K_1 administration may need to be repeated q12h.
Administration of vitamin K	Patients with mildly to moderately elevated INRs without bleeding should be given vitamin K orally rather than subcutaneously.

FFP, fresh-frozen plasma; INR, international normalized ratio; PCC, prothrombin complex concentrate; rVIIa, recombinant factor VIIa.

[a] If continued warfarin therapy is indicated after high doses of vitamin K_1, then anticoagulation with heparin or low-molecular-weight heparin can be concomitantly given. INR values greater than 4.5 are also less reliable than values at or near the therapeutic range.

[b] rVIIa may cause thrombosis and we do not advocate its routine use at this time.

[c] Although parenteral infusion of vitamin K_1 is recommended, we urge caution with this route of administration because there may not be an appreciable difference in onset of therapeutic effect and, although rare, it may cause severe anaphylactoid reactions.

rapidly; however, one study did not demonstrate decreased bleeding in the treatment group.[46] Furthermore, simply omitting warfarin doses may be adequate for the patient without active hemorrhage who has an INR between 4 and 9.[46]

It is often unclear why patients with consistent therapeutic dosing have seemingly random elevations in their INR. A recent case-control study identified the following risk factors associated with overcoagulation from vitamin K antagonists: previous medical history of increased INR levels, antibiotic therapy, fever and concomitant use of amiodarone and proton pump inhibitors.[34] Clinicians should pay particular attention to patients with these conditions and close monitoring of coagulation profiles should be performed.[34]

TREATMENT OF LONG-ACTING ANTICOAGULANT OVERDOSES

Treatment of a patient with a long-acting anticoagulant overdose is essentially the same as the treatment of oral anticoagulant toxicity with certain exceptions.

Long-acting anticoagulants are metabolized by the hepatic mixed-function oxidase system (cytochrome P450 [CYP]).[9,139] In a rat model, the duration of coagulopathy was shortened by administering phenobarbital, a CYP3A4 inducer.[9] Although a phenobarbital effect has never been systematically studied in humans, this approach was used by several authors in isolated human cases of long-acting anticoagulant toxicity.[33,90,110,182,192] Although these anecdotal reports suggest some improvement with phenobarbital therapy, the risks of producing sedation in a patient who might be prone to bleeding complications appear consequential.

Patients with long-acting anticoagulant overdose should be followed until their coagulation studies remain normal while off therapy for several days. This usually requires daily or even twice-daily INR measurements until the INR is at the lower limit of the therapeutic range. Monitoring of serial INR measurements should allow for a gradual decrease in vitamin K_1 requirement over time. Periodic coagulation factor analysis, however, may provide an early clue to the resolution of toxicity.[82] The patient may require weeks to months of close observation for both psychiatric and medical management. Emphasis has been placed on determining a critical superwarfarin concentration below which anticoagulation does not occur.[33] In one case report, brodifacoum was observed to follow zero-order elimination kinetics.[32] If this type of toxicokinetics is consistent in the analysis of other long-acting anticoagulants, these laboratory measurements may prove more reliable than the current empiric end points of therapy.

OTHER ORAL ANTICOAGULANTS

Because of the potential therapeutic limitations of warfarin (eg, dosing, risk of hemorrhage, narrow therapeutic window, etc) novel oral anticoagulants have been developed with directed activity against specific clotting factors. Ximelagatran was one of the first direct thrombin inhibitors that appeared to be as effective as warfarin in the treatment of stroke prevention, nonvalvular atrial fibrillation, and deep venous thrombosis, and was shown to be more effective than aspirin alone for patients who have had a recent myocardial infarction.[81] Ximelagatran had many advantages over warfarin, including rapidity of onset, fixed dosing, stable absorption, decreased risk of drug interactions, and lack of necessity for therapeutic monitoring.[81] However, because of its major side effect of heptatotoxicity, it has been removed from the world market by its manufacturer. Since then, new anticoagulants including factor Xa inhibitors (eg, rivaroxaban, apixaban) and direct thrombin inhibitors (eg, argatroban, dabigatran) are gaining in popularity for their therapeutic effects.[173] Argatroban binds noncovalently to the active site of thrombin to function as a competitive inhibitor.[79] It is metabolized by CYP3A4/5 in the liver and is particularly useful in patients with renal impairment.[79] These medications show tremendous promise and may revolutionize the treatment of thromboembolic disease. Limited data are currently available regarding toxicity of these agents; however, overdose of argatroban was successfully treated with FFP in one recent case report.[201]

PARENTERAL ANTICOAGULANTS

HEPARIN

Conventional or unfractionated heparin is a heterogeneous group of molecules within the class of glycosaminoglycans.[89] The heparin precursor molecule is composed of long chains of mucopolysaccharides, a polypeptide, and carbohydrates. The main carbohydrate components of heparin molecules include uronic acids and amino sugars in polysaccharide chains. Heparin for pharmaceutical use is extracted from bovine lung tissue and porcine intestines.[163]

Heparin inhibits thrombosis by accelerating the binding of AT to thrombin (factor II) and other serine proteases involved in coagulation.[115,157] Thus, factors IX to XII, kallikrein, and thrombin are inhibited. Heparin also affects plasminogen activator inhibitor, protein C inhibitor, and other components of coagulation. Heparin's therapeutic effect is usually measured through the activated PTT. The activated blood coagulation time (ACT) may be more useful for monitoring large therapeutic doses or in the overdose situation.[103]

Low-molecular-weight heparins (LMWHs) are 4000- to 6000-dalton fractions obtained from conventional (unfractionated) heparin.[62] As such, they share many of the pharmacologic and toxicologic properties of conventional heparin.[26] The various LMWHs (eg, fraxiparine, enoxaparin, dalteparin) are prepared by different methods of depolymerization of heparin; consequently, they each differ to a certain extent regarding their pharmacokinetic properties and anticoagulant profiles. The major differences between LMWHs and conventional heparin are greater bioavailability, longer half-life, more predictable anticoagulation with fixed dosing, targeted activity against activated factor X, and less targeted activity against activated factor II.[26,62] As a result of this targeted factor X activity, LMWHs have minimal effect on the activated PTT, thereby eliminating either the need for, or the usefulness of, monitoring. They are therefore administered on a fixed-dose schedule. However, in certain instances (eg, patients with impaired renal function, pregnancy, etc), monitoring of anti–factor Xa activity may be performed to assess adequacy of anticoagulation and prevent risk of bleeding.[75] Controversy exists as to whether such testing is clinically necessary.[25]

LMWHs have been investigated for prevention of thromboembolic disease after hip surgery and trauma, in patients with stroke or deep venous thrombosis, in pregnancy, and in other conditions where anticoagulation with heparin would otherwise be indicated (eg, at the onset of oral anticoagulation therapy). Although these xenobiotics are presumed to have a minimal risk in pregnancy[124] because they do not cross the placenta,[60,177] they are not yet approved for treatment or prophylaxis of thromboembolic disease in pregnancy. Most studies demonstrate a lower incidence of embolization; however, there is still a trend toward increased bleeding.[17,70,109]

PHARMACOLOGY

Because of the large size of heparin and negative charge it is unable to cross cellular membranes. These factors prevent oral administration, and heparin must be administered by either subcutaneous injection or continuous intravenous infusion. Following parenteral administration, heparin remains in the intravascular compartment, in part bound to globulins, fibrinogen, and low-density lipoproteins, resulting in a volume of distribution of 0.06 L/kg in humans.[55,141] Because of its rapid metabolism in the liver by a heparinase, heparin has a short duration of effect.[115] Although the half-life of elimination is dose dependent and ranges from 1 to 2.5 hours,[115,122,141] the duration of anticoagulant effect is usually reported as 1 to 3 hours.[115] Dosing errors or drug interactions with thrombolytic agents, antiplatelet drugs, or nonsteroidal antiinflammatory drugs may increase the risk of hemorrhage.[76] LMWHs are nearly 90% bioavailable following subcutaneous administration and have an elimination half-life of 3 to 6 hours.[79] Anti–factor Xa activity peaks between 3 and 5 hours after dosing.[79] LMWHs are renally eliminated and patients with severe renal insufficiency (creatinine clearance less than 30 mL/min) or end-stage renal disease are at increased risk of toxicity.[187]

CLINICAL MANIFESTATIONS

Intentional overdoses with heparin are rare.[120] Most reported cases involve unintentional poisoning in hospitalized patients.[65,67,120,144,162] These cases have involved the administration of large amounts of heparin as a consequence of misidentification of heparin vials, during the process of flushing intravenous lines, and secondary to intravenous pump malfunction. Significant bleeding complications occurred in several cases, including one fatality.[65]

Similar adverse effects to unfractionated heparins are also reported with LMWHs and include epidural/spinal hematoma, intrahepatic hemorrhage,[84] abdominal wall hematomas,[6] psoas hematoma after lumbar plexus block,[98] and intracranial hemorrhage in patients with malignancy in the brain.[52] These complications were all reported in patients who received the LMWH enoxaparin.

EVALUATION AND TREATMENT

After stabilization of the airway and breathing, and circulation are assured, the physician should be prepared to replace blood loss and reverse the coagulopathy, if indicated. Because of the relatively short duration of action of heparin, observation alone might be indicated if significant bleeding has not occurred. For the patient requiring anticoagulation, serial PTT determinations will indicate when it is safe to resume therapy. If significant bleeding occurs, either removal of the heparin or reversal of its anticoagulant effect is indicated. Because heparin has a very small volume of distribution, it can be effectively removed by exchange transfusion.[162] Although this technique has been used successfully in neonates, it is not generally applicable to older children and adults.

When severe bleeding occurs, heparin may be effectively neutralized by protamine sulfate.[3] Protamine is a low-molecular-weight protein found in the sperm and testes of salmon, which forms ionic bonds with heparin and renders it devoid of anticoagulant activity.[115] One milligram of protamine sulfate injected intravenously neutralizes 100 Units of heparin.[115] The dose of protamine should be calculated from the dose of heparin administered if known and assuming heparin's approximate half-life to be 60 to 90 minutes; the amount of protamine should not exceed the amount of heparin expected to be found intravascularly at the time of infusion. As with other foreign proteins, protamine administration is associated with numerous adverse effects such as hypotension, bradycardia, and allergic reactions. Because approximately 0.2% of patients receiving protamine experience anaphylaxis, a complication that carries a 30% mortality rate, most authors commonly recommend that protamine be reserved for patients with life-threatening hemorrhage (see Antidotes in Depth A17–Protamine).[83] It should also be noted that excess protamine administration may result in paradoxical anticoagulation.

Because of the severe adverse effects associated with protamine, research has focused on safer methods to reverse heparin anticoagulation. These agents include heparinase,[125] synthetic protamine variants,[188,189] and platelet factor 4, but these therapies are not widely available.

If life-threatening bleeding occurs following LMWH administration, patients should be treated with protamine. In a case report of a 10-fold dosing error of enoxaparin, protamine effectively reversed the anticoagulant effects.[199] Current recommendations are to administer 1 mg protamine per 100 anti–factor Xa units where 1 mg enoxaparin equals 100 anti–factor Xa units if within 8 hours of the LMWH.[79] A second dose of 0.5 mg protamine should be administered per 100 anti–factor Xa units if bleeding continues.[79] If more than 8 hours has elapsed, then a smaller dose of protamine can be administered. The appropriate dosages for protamine are described in detail in the Antidotes in Depth A17: Protamine. The newer experimental protamine variants appear to be effective against LMWHs but are not yet available.[188,189] Interestingly, there is one case report of recombinant activated factor VII reversing the effects of LMWH in the setting of postoperative renal failure.[134]

NONBLEEDING COMPLICATIONS OF ANTICOAGULANTS

Warfarin therapy is associated with three nonhemorrhagic lesions of the skin: urticaria,[161] purple toe syndrome,[58] and warfarin skin necrosis.[44,99,104,123,186] Although warfarin skin necrosis was once thought to be a rare and idiosyncratic reaction,[99,104] more recent evidence suggests a link between this disorder and protein C deficiency.[104,186] Protein C activation is also dependent on vitamin K.[40] Patients who are homozygotes for protein C deficiency have an increased incidence of thrombosis and embolic events, such that they often require long-term anticoagulant therapy.[40] Because the half-life of protein C is shorter than that of many of the vitamin K–dependent coagulation factors, protein C concentrations fall rapidly during the first hours of warfarin therapy. In the protein C–deficient patient, protein C concentrations fall dramatically prior to a reduction in coagulation factors. This results in an imbalance that actually favors coagulation, and skin necrosis results due to microvascular thrombosis in dermal vessels.[123,186] Although warfarin skin necrosis is more common in patients with protein C deficiency, this disorder is also described in patients with protein S and AT deficiencies.[44] Unfortunately, these deficiencies are neither necessary nor sufficient to account for the incidence of warfarin necrosis.[44] If necrosis occurs, warfarin should be discontinued and heparin should be initiated to decrease thrombosis of postcapillary venules. Some patients may also require surgical débridement.[158] The purple toe syndrome, in contrast to warfarin-induced skin necrosis, is presumed to result from small atheroemboli that are no longer adherent to their plaques by clot (see Fig. 29–7).

An additional major nonhemorrhagic complication of warfarin therapy relates to its use in pregnant women. Most warfarin-induced fetal abnormalities occur during weeks 6 to 12 of gestation, but central nervous system (CNS) and ocular abnormalities can develop at any time during gestation (see Chap. 30 for further details).[74,175]

Heparin therapy is associated with a transient and mild thrombocytopenia called heparin-induced thrombocytopenia (HIT) that occurs in approximately 25% of patients during the first few days of therapy.[191] Although this syndrome results from heparin-induced platelet aggregation, a more severe form of thrombocytopenia, heparin-induced thrombocytopenia and thrombosis syndrome (HITT; formerly known as HIT-2 or the white clot syndrome), occurs in 1% to 5% of patients between days 7 and 14 of therapy.[116] In patients who were previously treated with heparin, these events can occur earlier than 7 days. Heparin stimulates platelets to release platelet factor 4, which subsequently complexes with heparin to provoke an IgG response. These antibodies against the heparin–platelet factor 4 complex activate platelets, which may lead to platelet–fibrin thrombotic events.[7,202] Patients may present with either hemorrhagic or thromboembolic complications. LMWH may also be associated with thrombocytopenia (isolated HIT), and less frequently with HITT.[190] Consequently, once HITT occurs, LMWH is contraindicated.[190] Treatment of HIT includes discontinuation of heparin or LMWH and immediate use of alternative anticoagulant such as danaparoid, lepirudine, or argatroban.[37] (Danaparoid is currently unavailable in the United States.[79]) In addition to HIT and HITT, necrotizing skin lesions[149] and hyperkalemia from aldosterone suppression[142] also rarely occur in patients receiving heparin therapy. These patients should not receive heparin or LMWH again, not even in low doses to keep veins open.

Some additional complications of heparin use include osteoporosis, which mostly occurs in patients on long-term therapy with unfractionated heparin.[85] A small percentage of these patients may develop bone fractures if treated continuously for more than 3 months. Data for LMWHs are limited and the incidence of osteoporosis may be less compared with unfractionated heparin.[85] In 2008, an outbreak of adverse events was linked to heparin contaminated with oversulfated chondroitin sulfate.[111] The contaminated heparin, which was found in at least 10 countries, originated in China.[22] Many patients developed anaphylactoid-type reactions with at least 100 reported deaths.[111]

HIRUDIN

Hirudin, a 65-amino-acid polypeptide produced by the salivary glands of the medicinal leech (*Hirudo medicinalis*), irreversibly blocks thrombin without the need for AT.[164] Unlike heparin, the small size of hirudin allows it to enter clots and inhibit clot-bound thrombin, offering the distinct advantage of restricting further thrombus formation. Hirudin demonstrates enhanced bioavailability and a longer half-life than unfractionated heparin. In addition, there are no known natural inhibitors of hirudin, such as platelet factor 4. Desirudin is a recombinant hirudin that is used in acute coronary syndrome, in the prevention of thromboembolic disease, and in patients with heparin-induced thrombocytopenia.[21,160,164] Both of these xenobiotics appear to be at least as effective as unfractionated heparin, and without increased bleeding or thrombocytopenia. However, in the Global Use of Strategies to Open Occluded Coronary Arteries (GUSTO) IIb study of patients with unstable angina/non–Q wave myocardial infarction, there was an increase in the number of blood transfusions in patients who received desirudin as compared with those who received heparin.[4]

FIBRINOLYTICS

THROMBOLYTICS

The fibrinolytic system is designed to remove unwanted clots, while leaving those clots protecting sites of vascular injury intact. Plasminogen exists as a proenzyme and is converted to the active form, plasmin, by various plasminogen activators.[42,43] t-PA is released from the endothelium and is under the inhibitory control of two inactivators known as tissue plasminogen activator inhibitors 1 and 2 (t-PAI-1 and t-PAI-2).[42,43,116,129] Plasmin's actions are nonspecific in that it degrades not only fibrin clots but also some plasma proteins and coagulation factors.[116] Inhibition of plasmin occurs through α_2-antiplasmin.

With their diverse indications in acute myocardial infarction, unstable angina, arterial and venous thrombosis and embolism, and cerebrovascular disease, the thrombolytic agents (streptokinase, urokinase, alteplase, and anistreplase) are commonly used.[14] The reader is referred to a number of reviews for specific indications and dosing regimens.[45,105,116,148,170,196] Although all xenobiotics enhance fibrinolysis, they differ in their specific sites of action and durations of effect. t-PA is specific for clot (it does not increase fibrinolysis in the absence of a thrombus), whereas streptokinase, urokinase, and anistreplase are not clot specific. t-PA has the shortest half-life and duration of effect (5 minutes and 2 hours, respectively), and anistreplase the longest (90 minutes and 18 hours, respectively).[148,170] Streptokinase has the additional risk of severe allergic reaction on rechallenge, limiting its use to once in a lifetime.

Newer thrombolytic drugs such a reteplase, and some non–commercially available agents, including monteplase, lanoteplase, pamiteplase, and desmoteplase, are being evaluated for therapeutic use.[112] These fibrinolytics have a longer half-life and may be administered via single or repeated bolus injections. They also have increased fibrin selectivity, but no improvement in mortality is demonstrated when compared to t-PA.[91] Although the incidence of bleeding requiring transfusion may be as high as 7.7% following high-dose (150 mg) t-PA and 4.4% following low-dose t-PA,[45] the incidence of intracranial hemorrhage with t-PA appears to be similar to the newer agents (monteplase, tenecteplase, reteplase, and lanoteplase).[185] The addition of heparin to the thrombolytic regimen increases the risk of bleeding. Reviews of multiple trials suggest that life-threatening events such as intracranial hemorrhage occur in 0.30% to 0.58% of patients receiving anistreplase, 0.42% to 0.73% of patients receiving alteplase, and 0.08% to 0.30% of patients receiving streptokinase.[196] Regardless of the thrombolytic agent used the frequency of bleeding events is similar even with the newer agents, with the exception that lanoteplase may have a decreased incidence of significant bleeding.[49] Supportive care is indicated for patients with minor bleeding complications; however, for patients with significant bleeding, fibrinogen and coagulation factor replacement with cryoprecipitate and FFP should be administered.[159]

SNAKE VENOMS

A detailed discussion of snake envenomations is found in Chap. 121; only a few specific issues are discussed here. Snake venoms may be composed of a vast number of complex proteins and peptides that interact with components of the human hemostatic system. In general, their functions may be thought of as being procoagulant, anticoagulant, fibrinolytic, vessel wall interactive, platelet active, or as protein inactivators. Additionally, they may more specifically also be classified based on their specific biologic activity; some of the various mechanisms include individual factor activation, inhibition of protein C and thrombin, fibrinogen degradation, platelet aggregation, and inhibition of serine protease inhibitors (SERPINS). Currently, there are more than 100 different snake venoms that affect the hemostatic system[87,88]; Fig. 59–2 is an overview of their multiple interactions with the coagulation and fibrinolytic systems.[119]

Some of these venom proteins are being used as therapeutic agents for human diseases. Ancrod, a purified derivative of the Malayan pit viper, *Calloselasma rhodostoma* (formerly known as *Agkistrodon rhodostoma*), is therapeutically used because of its defibrinogenating property.[13] The mechanism of action of ancrod and other similar agents is to link fibrinogen end to end and subsequently prevent cross-linking. It has been investigated in the treatment of deep vein thrombosis, myocardial infarction, pulmonary embolus, acute cerebrovascular thrombosis, HIT, and warfarin-related vascular complications. In a multicenter study of 500 patients with acute or progressing ischemic neurologic events, ancrod showed a favorable benefit-to-risk ratio compared with placebo.[167] As expected, an increased risk of hemorrhage is observed; however, the risk appears to be less than that with thrombolytic agents.[167] Monitoring of fibrinogen levels is essential to avoid potential complications, as no specific antidote exists. For envenomation of other snake venoms (such as from the Crotalinae family) that induce hemorrhage, antivenin treatment may be required.

PENTASACCHARIDES

Pentasaccharides are recently developed synthetic anticoagulants that possess activity exclusively against factor Xa and are used for the prevention and treatment of venous thromboembolic disorders. Although other agents are currently being studied, fondaparinux is the only pentasaccharide currently available for clinical use.[108] The pentasaccharides have long half-lives and have no reliable antidote if bleeding occurs; they do not bind to protamine.[79] They are also contraindicated in patients with renal failure (CrCl less than 30 mL/min).[79] No controlled trials are available yet, but rVIIa may be effective, as demonstrated in one study of healthy volunteers.[19]

ANTICOAGULANT APTAMERS

Aptamer anticoagulants are small nucleic acid molecules that are currently under development to target specific blood coagulation proteins.[137] They are direct protein inhibitors and function similarly to monoclonal antibodies.[137] Specific aptamers that are currently being studied include the anti–factor IX aptamer, the anti–activated protein C aptamer, and the anti–factor VIIa aptamer.[68] These xenobiotics may have clinical utility in the future as their anticoagulant effects appear to be easier to control, and consequently safer, compared with the anticoagulants currently most used.

SUMMARY

The ever-increasing frequency of anticoagulant therapeutic use is associated with complications and adverse outcomes. A complete understanding of the normal mechanisms of coagulation, anticoagulation, and thrombolysis, combined with an understanding of the pharmacology of the agent and the patient's clinical needs, will allow the clinician to better choose among the complex therapies currently available. Supportive care is often adequate for certain complications associated with these therapies; however, occasionally, more aggressive interventions and specific antidotes are necessary depending on the particular agent and medical condition of the patient.

ACKNOWLEDGMENTS

Teresa Kierenia, MD (deceased), and Robert S. Hoffman contributed to this chapter in a previous edition.

REFERENCES

1. Aiyagari V, Testai FD. Correction of coagulopathy in warfarin associated cerebral hemorrhage. *Curr Opin Crit Care.* 2009;15:87-92.
2. Ancalmo N, Ochsner J. Heparin, the miracle drug: a brief history of its discovery. *J La State Med Soc.* 1990;142:22-24.
3. Andersen MN NM, Alfano GA. Experimental studies of heparin-protamine activity with special reference to protamine inhibition clotting. *Surgery.* 1959; 46:1060-1068.
4. Anonymous. A comparison of recombinant hirudin with heparin for the treatment of acute coronary syndromes. The Global Use of Strategies to Open Occluded Coronary Arteries (GUSTO) IIb investigators. *N Engl J Med.* 1996;335:775-782.
5. Ansell J, Hirsh J, Hylek E, et al. Pharmacology and management of the vitamin K antagonists. American College of Chest Physicians Evidence-Based Clinical Practice Guidelines (8th Edition). *Chest.* 2008;133:160S-198S.
6. Antonelli D, Fares L 2nd, Anene C. Enoxaparin associated with hugh abdominal wall hematomas. a report of two cases. *Am Surg.* 2000;66:797-800.
7. Aster RH. Heparin-induced thrombocytopenia and thrombosis. *N Engl J Med.* 1995;332:1374-1376.
8. Babcock J, Hartman K, Pedersen A, et al. Rodenticide-induced coagulopathy in a young child. A case of Munchausen syndrome by proxy. *Am J Pediatr Hematol Oncol.* 1993;15:126-130.
9. Bachmann KA, Sullivan TJ. Dispositional and pharmacodynamic characteristics of brodifacoum in warfarin-sensitive rats. *Pharmacology.* 1983; 27:281-288.
10. Badr M, Yoshihara H, Kauffman F, et al. Menadione causes selective toxicity to periportal regions of the liver lobule. *Toxicol Lett.* 1987;35:241-246.
11. Barlow AM, Gay AL, Park BK. Difenacoum (Neosorexa) poisoning. *Br Med J (Clin Res Ed).* 1982;285:541.
12. Becker RC. Seminars in thrombosis, thrombolysis, and vascular biology. Part 2. Coagulation and thrombosis. *Cardiology.* 1991;78:257-266.
13. Bell WR Jr. Defibrinogenating enzymes. *Drugs.* 1997;54(Suppl 3):18-30; discussion 30-11.
14. Benedict CR, Mueller S, Anderson HV, et al. Thrombolytic therapy: a state of the art review. *Hosp Pract (Off Ed).* 1992;27:61-72.
15. Bennett DL CD, Veltri JC. Long-acting anticoagulant ingestion. A prospective study [abstract]. *Vet Hum Toxicol.* 1987;29:472.
16. Beretz A, Cazenave JP. Old and new natural products as the source of modern antithrombotic drugs. *Planta Med.* 1991;57:S68-72.
17. Bergqvist D, Benoni G, Bjorgell O, et al. Low-molecular-weight heparin (enoxaparin) as prophylaxis against venous thromboembolism after total hip replacement. *N Engl J Med.* 1996;335:696-700.
18. Beyth RJ, Quinn LM, Landefeld CS. Prospective evaluation of an index for predicting the risk of major bleeding in outpatients treated with warfarin. *Am J Med.* 1998;105:91-99.
19. Bijsterveld NR, Moons AH, Boekholdt SM, et al. Ability of recombinant factor VIIa to reverse the anticoagulant effect of the pentasaccharide fondaparinux in healthy volunteers. *Circulation.* 2002;106:2550-2554.
20. Bithell T. Acquired coagulation disorders. In: Lee GR BT, Foerster J, et al., eds. *Wintrobe's Clinical Hematology*, 9th ed. Philadelphia: Lea & Febiger; 1993.
21. Bittl JA, Strony J, Brinker JA, et al. Treatment with bivalirudin (Hirulog) as compared with heparin during coronary angioplasty for unstable or postinfarction angina. Hirulog Angioplasty Study Investigators. *N Engl J Med.* 1995;333:764-769.
22. Blossom DB, Kallen AJ, Patel PR, et al. Outbreak of adverse reactions associated with contaminated heparin. *N Engl J Med.* 2008;359:2674-2684.
23. Boermans HJ, Johnstone I, Black WD, et al. Clinical signs, laboratory changes and toxicokinetics of brodifacoum in the horse. *Can J Vet Res.* 1991;55:21-27.
24. Boster SR, Bergin JJ. Upper airway obstruction complicating warfarin therapy—with a note on reversal of warfarin toxicity. *Ann Emerg Med.* 1983;12:711-715.
25. Bounameaux H, de Moerloose P. Is laboratory monitoring of low-molecular-weight heparin therapy necessary? No. *J Thromb Haemost.* 2004;2: 551-554.
26. Bounameaux H, Goldhaber SZ. Uses of low-molecular-weight heparin. *Blood Rev.* 1995;9:213-219.
27. Bowen KJ, Vukelja SJ. Hypercoagulable states. Their causes and management. *Postgrad Med.* 1992;91:117-118, 123-115, 128 passim.
28. Braithwaite GB. Vitamin K and brodifacoum. *J Am Vet Med Assoc.* 1982;181:531, 534.
29. Breckenridge A, Orme ML. The plasma half lives and the pharmacological effect of the enantiomers of warfarin in rats. *Life Sci II.* 1972;11:337-345.
30. Breckenridge A, Orme M, Wesseling H, et al. Pharmacokinetics and pharmacodynamics of the enantiomers of warfarin in man. *Clin Pharmacol Ther.* 1974;15:424-430.
31. Breckenridge AM, Leck JB, Park BK, et al. Mechanisms of action of the anticoagulants warfarin, 2-chloro-3-phytylnaphthoquinone (Cl-K), acenocoumarol, brodifacoum and difenacoum in the rabbit [proceedings]. *Br J Pharmacol.* 1978;64:399P.

32. Bruno GR, Howland MA, McMeeking A, et al. Long-acting anticoagulant overdose: brodifacoum kinetics and optimal vitamin K dosing. *Ann Emerg Med.* 2000;36:262-267.
33. Burucoa C, Mura P, Robert R, et al. Chlorophacinone intoxication. A biological and toxicological study. *J Toxicol Clin Toxicol.* 1989;27:79-89.
34. Cadiou G, Varin R, Levesque H, et al. Risk factors of vitamin K antagonist overcoagulation. A case-control study in unselected patients referred to an emergency department. *Thromb Haemost.* 2008;100:685-692.
35. Caldwell S, Shah N. The prothrombin time-derived international normalized ratio. great for warfarin, fair for prognosis and bad for liver-bleeding risk. *Liver Int.* 2008;28:1325-1327.
36. Chazouilleres O, Robert A. Normalizing the prothrombin time. *Hepatology.* 2000;32:881.
37. Chong BH, Isaacs A. Heparin-induced thrombocytopenia: what clinicians need to know. *Thromb Haemost.* 2009;101:279-283.
38. Chong LL, Chau WK, Ho CH. A case of 'superwarfarin' poisoning. *Scand J Haematol.* 1986;36:314-315.
39. Choonara IA, Scott AK, Haynes BP, et al. Vitamin K_1 metabolism in relation to pharmacodynamic response in anticoagulated patients. *Br J Clin Pharmacol.* 1985;20:643-648.
40. Clouse LH, Comp PC. The regulation of hemostasis: the protein C system. *N Engl J Med.* 1986;314:1298-1304.
41. Coccheri S, Palareti G, Cosmi B. Oral anticoagulant therapy: efficacy, safety and the low-dose controversy. *Haemostasis.* 1999;29:150-165.
42. Collen D. On the regulation and control of fibrinolysis. Edward Kowalski Memorial Lecture. *Thromb Haemost.* 1980;43:77-89.
43. Collen D, Lijnen HR. Basic and clinical aspects of fibrinolysis and thrombolysis. *Blood.* 1991;78:3114-3124.
44. Comp PC. Coumarin-induced skin necrosis. Incidence, mechanisms, management and avoidance. *Drug Saf.* 1993;8:128-135.
45. Conti CR. Brief overview of the end points of thrombolytic therapy. *Am J Cardiol.* 1991;68:8E-10E.
46. Crowther MA, Ageno W, Garcia D, et al. Oral vitamin K versus placebo to correct excessive anticoagulation in patients receiving warfarin: a randomized trial. *Ann Intern Med.* 2009;150:293-300.
47. Cruickshank J, Ragg M, Eddey D. Warfarin toxicity in the emergency department. recommendations for management. *Emerg Med (Fremantle).* 2001;13:91-97.
48. Davie EW, Ratnoff OD. Waterfall sequence for intrinsic blood clotting. *Science.* 1964;145:1310-1312.
49. den Heijer P, Vermeer F, Ambrosioni E, et al. Evaluation of a weight-adjusted single-bolus plasminogen activator in patients with myocardial infarction: a double-blind, randomized angiographic trial of lanoteplase versus alteplase. *Circulation.* 1998;98:2117-2125.
50. Dentali F, Crowther MA. Management of excessive anticoagulant effect due to vitamin K antagonists. *Hematology Am Soc Hematol Educ Program.* 2008; 2008:266-270.
51. Deveras RA, Kessler CM. Reversal of warfarin-induced excessive anticoagulation with recombinant human factor VIIa concentrate. *Ann Intern Med.* 2002;137:884-888.
52. Dickinson LD, Miller LD, Patel CP, et al. Enoxaparin increases the incidence of postoperative intracranial hemorrhage when initiated preoperatively for deep venous thrombosis prophylaxis in patients with brain tumors. *Neurosurgery.* 1998;43:1074-1081.
53. Dowd P, Ham SW, Naganathan S, et al. The mechanism of action of vitamin K. *Annu Rev Nutr.* 1995;15:419-440.
54. Emery RW, Emery AM, Raikar GV, et al. Anticoagulation for mechanical heart valves: a role for patient based therapy. *J Thromb Thrombolysis.* 2008;25:18-25.
55. Estes JW, Poulin PF. Pharmocokinetics of heparin. Distribution and elimination. *Thromb Diath Haemorrh.* 1975;33:26-37.
56. Exner DV, Brien WF, Murphy MJ. Superwarfarin ingestion. *CMAJ.* 1992; 146:34-35.
57. Fasco MJ, Hildebrandt EF, Suttie JW. Evidence that warfarin anticoagulant action involves two distinct reductase activities. *J Biol Chem.* 1982;257: 11210-11212.
58. Feder W, Auerbach R. "Purple toes": an uncommon sequela of oral coumarin drug therapy. *Ann Intern Med.* 1961;55:911-917.
59. Fihn SD, Callahan CM, Martin DC, et al. The risk for and severity of bleeding complications in elderly patients treated with warfarin. The National Consortium of Anticoagulation Clinics. *Ann Intern Med.* 1996;124: 970-979.
60. Forestier F, Daffos F, Capella-Pavlovsky M. Low molecular weight heparin (PK 10169) does not cross the placenta during the second trimester of pregnancy study by direct fetal blood sampling under ultrasound. *Thromb Res.* 1984;34:557-560.
61. Freedman MD, Olatidoye AG. Clinically significant drug interactions with the oral anticoagulants. *Drug Saf.* 1994;10:381-394.
62. Frydman A. Low-molecular-weight heparins: an overview of their pharmacodynamics, pharmacokinetics and metabolism in humans. *Haemostasis.* 1996;26(Suppl 2):24-38.
63. Furie B, Furie BC. Molecular and cellular biology of blood coagulation. *N Engl J Med.* 1992;326:800-806.
64. Gage BF, Fihn SD, White RH. Management and dosing of warfarin therapy. *Am J Med.* 2000;109:481-488.
65. Galant SP. Accidental heparinization of a newborn infant. *Am J Dis Child.* 1967;114:313-319.
66. Gilbert GE, Sims PJ, Wiedmer T, et al. Platelet-derived microparticles express high affinity receptors for factor VIII. *J Biol Chem.* 1991;266:17261-17268.
67. Glueck HI, Light IJ, Flessa H, et al. Inadvertent sodium heparin administration to a newborn infant. *JAMA.* 1965;191:1031-1032.
68. Gopinath SC. Anti-coagulant aptamers. *Thromb Res.* 2008;122:838-847.
69. Greeff MC, Mashile O, MacDougall LG. "Superwarfarin" (bromodialone) poisoning in two children resulting in prolonged anticoagulation. *Lancet.* 1987;2:1269.
70. Green D, Hirsh J, Heit J, et al. Low molecular weight heparin: a critical analysis of clinical trials. *Pharmacol Rev.* 1994;46:89-109.
71. Gurwitz JH, Avorn J, Ross-Degnan D, et al. Aging and the anticoagulant response to warfarin therapy. *Ann Intern Med.* 1992;116:901-904.
72. Hackett LP, Ilett KF, Chester A. Plasma warfarin concentrations after a massive overdose. *Med J Aust.* 1985;142:642-643.
73. Haines ST, Bussey HI. Thrombosis and the pharmacology of antithrombotic agents. *Ann Pharmacother.* 1995;29:892-905.
74. Hall JG, Pauli RM, Wilson KM. Maternal and fetal sequelae of anticoagulation during pregnancy. *Am J Med.* 1980;68:122-140.
75. Harenberg J. Is laboratory monitoring of low-molecular-weight heparin therapy necessary? Yes. *J Thromb Haemost.* 2004;2:547-550.
76. Harrington R, Ansell J. Risk-benefit assessment of anticoagulant therapy. *Drug Saf.* 1991;6:54-69.
77. Harris EN, Gharavi AE, Asherson RA, et al. Antiphospholipid antibodies: a review. *Eur J Rheumatol Inflamm.* 1984;7:5-8.
78. Hirsh J. Substandard monitoring of warfarin in North America. Time for change. *Arch Intern Med.* 1992;152:257-258.
79. Hirsh J, Bauer KA, Donati MB, et al. Parenteral anticoagulants. American College of Chest Physicians Evidence-Based Clinical Practice Guidelines (8th edition). *Chest.* 2008;133:141S-159S.
80. Hirsh J, Poller L. The international normalized ratio. A guide to understanding and correcting its problems. *Arch Intern Med.* 1994;154:282-288.
81. Ho SJ, Brighton TA. Ximelagatran: direct thrombin inhibitor. *Vasc Health Risk Manag.* 2006;2:49-58.
82. Hoffman RS, Smilkstein MJ, Goldfrank LR. Evaluation of coagulation factor abnormalities in long-acting anticoagulant overdose. *J Toxicol Clin Toxicol.* 1988;26:233-248.
83. Holland CL, Singh AK, McMaster PR, et al. Adverse reactions to protamine sulfate following cardiac surgery. *Clin Cardiol.* 1984;7:157-162.
84. Houde JP, Steinberg G. Intrahepatic hemorrhage after use of low-molecular-weight heparin for total hip arthroplasty. *J Arthroplasty.* 1999;14: 372-374.
85. Hovanessian HC. New-generation anticoagulants: the low molecular weight heparins. *Ann Emerg Med.* 1999;34:768-779.
86. Hu Q, Brady JO. Recombinant activated factor VII for treatment of enoxaparin-induced bleeding. *Mayo Clin Proc.* 2004;79:827.
87. Iyaniwura TT. Snake venom constituents: biochemistry and toxicology (part 1). *Vet Hum Toxicol.* 1991;33:468-474.
88. Iyaniwura TT. Snake venom constituents: biochemistry and toxicology (part 2). *Vet Hum Toxicol.* 1991;33:475-480.
89. Jacques LB. Heparin: an old drug with a new paradigm. *Science.* 1979;206: 528-533.
90. Jones EC, Growe GH, Naiman SC. Prolonged anticoagulation in rat poisoning. *JAMA.* 1984;252:3005-3007.
91. Jones JB, Docherty A. Non-invasive treatment of ST elevation myocardial infarction. *Postgrad Med J.* 2007;83:725-730.
92. Junagade P, Grace R, Gover P. Fixed dose prothrombin complex concentrate for the reversal of oral anticoagulation therapy. *Hematology.* 2007;12:439-440.

93. Katona B, Wason S. Superwarfarin poisoning. *J Emerg Med.* 1989;7:627-631.
94. Katona B SL, Wason S. Anticoagulant rodenticide poisoning [abstract]. *Vet Hum Toxicol.* 1986;28:478.
95. Katona B WS. Anticoagulant rodenticide poisoning. *Clin Toxicol Rev.* 1986;8:1-2.
96. Keeney M, Allan DS, Lohmann RC, et al. Effect of activated recombinant human factor 7 (Niastase) on laboratory testing of inhibitors of factors VIII and IX. *Lab Hematol.* 2005;11:118-123.
97. Kim JH, Schwinn DA, Landau R. Pharmacogenomics and perioperative medicine—implications for modern clinical practice. *Can J Anaesth.* 2008; 55:799-806.
98. Klein SM, D'Ercole F, Greengrass RA, et al. Enoxaparin associated with psoas hematoma and lumbar plexopathy after lumbar plexus block. *Anesthesiology.* 1997;87:1576-1579.
99. Koch-Weser J. Coumarin necrosis. *Ann Intern Med.* 1968;68:1365-1367.
100. Kruse JA, Carlson RW. Fatal rodenticide poisoning with brodifacoum. *Ann Emerg Med.* 1992;21:331-336.
101. Krynetskiy E, McDonnell P. Building individualized medicine: prevention of adverse reactions to warfarin therapy. *J Pharmacol Exp Ther.* 2007;322:427-434.
102. Kuijpers EA, den Hartigh J, Savelkoul TJ, et al. A method for the simultaneous identification and quantitation of five superwarfarin rodenticides in human serum. *J Anal Toxicol.* 1995;19:557-562.
103. Kunert M, Sorgenicht R, Scheuble L, et al. Value of activated blood coagulation time in monitoring anticoagulation during coronary angioplasty. *Z Kardiol.* 1996;85:118-124.
104. Lacy JP, Goodin RR. Letter. Warfarin-induced necrosis of skin. *Ann Intern Med.* 1975;82:381-382.
105. Lawrence PF, Goodman GR. Thrombolytic therapy. *Surg Clin North Am.* 1992;72:899-918.
106. Lechner K, Pabinger-Fasching I. Lupus anticoagulants and thrombosis. A study of 25 cases and review of the literature. *Haemostasis.* 1985;15:254-262.
107. Leck JB, Park BK. A comparative study of the effects of warfarin and brodifacoum on the relationship between vitamin K_1 metabolism and clotting factor activity in warfarin-susceptible and warfarin-resistant rats. *Biochem Pharmacol.* 1981;30:123-128.
108. Levi M. Emergency reversal of antithrombotic treatment. *Intern Emerg Med.* 2009;4:137-145.
109. Levine M, Gent M, Hirsh J, et al. A comparison of low-molecular-weight heparin administered primarily at home with unfractionated heparin administered in the hospital for proximal deep-vein thrombosis. *N Engl J Med.* 1996;334:677-681.
110. Lipton RA, Klass EM. Human ingestion of a 'superwarfarin' rodenticide resulting in a prolonged anticoagulant effect. *JAMA.* 1984;252:3004-3005.
111. Liu H, Zhang Z, Linhardt RJ. Lessons learned from the contamination of heparin. *Nat Prod Rep.* 2009;26:313-321.
112. Longstaff C, Williams S, Thelwell C. Fibrin binding and the regulation of plasminogen activators during thrombolytic therapy. *Cardiovasc Hematol Agents Med Chem.* 2008;6:212-223.
113. Lund M. Comparative effect of the three rodenticides warfarin, difenacoum and brodifacoum on eight rodent species in short feeding periods. *J Hyg (Lond).* 1981;87:101-107.
114. Macfarlane RG. An enzyme cascade in the blood clotting mechanism, and its function as a biochemical amplifier. *Nature.* 1964;202:498-499.
115. MacLean JA, Moscicki R, Bloch KJ. Adverse reactions to heparin. *Ann Allergy.* 1990;65:254-259.
116. Majerus PW BG, Miletich JP, et al. Anticoagulant, thrombolytic, and antiplatelet drugs. In: Hardiman JG LL, Molinoff PB, Ruddon RW, eds. *Goodman and Gilman's the Pharmacological Basis of Therapeutics*, 9th ed. New York: McGraw-Hill; 1996.
117. Makris M, Greaves M, Phillips WS, et al. Emergency oral anticoagulant reversal. the relative efficacy of infusions of fresh frozen plasma and clotting factor concentrate on correction of the coagulopathy. *Thromb Haemost.* 1997;77:477-480.
118. Marcus A. Hemorrhagic disorders. Abnormalities of platelet and vascular function. In: Wyngaarden JB SL, ed. *Cecil Textbook of Medicine*, 18th ed. Philadelphia: WB Saunders; 1988.
119. Markland FS. Snake venoms and the hemostatic system. *Toxicon.* 1998;36: 1749-1800.
120. Martin CM, Engstrom PF, Barrett O Jr. Surreptitious self-administration of heparin. *JAMA.* 1970;212:475-476.
121. Mathiesen T, Benediktsdottir K, Johnsson H, et al. Intracranial traumatic and non-traumatic haemorrhagic complications of warfarin treatment. *Acta Neurol Scand.* 1995;91:208-214.
122. McAvoy TJ. Pharmacokinetic modeling of heparin and its clinical implications. *J Pharmacokinet Biopharm.* 1979;7:331-354.
123. McGehee WG, Klotz TA, Epstein DJ, et al. Coumarin necrosis associated with hereditary protein C deficiency. *Ann Intern Med.* 1984;101:59-60.
124. Melissari E, Parker CJ, Wilson NV, et al. Use of low molecular weight heparin in pregnancy. *Thromb Haemost.* 1992;68:652-656.
125. Michelsen LG, Kikura M, Levy JH, et al. Heparinase I (neutralase) reversal of systemic anticoagulation. *Anesthesiology.* 1996;85:339-346.
126. Midathada MV, Mehta P, Waner M, et al. Recombinant factor VIIa in the treatment of bleeding. *Am J Clin Pathol.* 2004;121:124-137.
127. Monagle P, Chalmers E, Chan A, et al. Antithrombotic therapy in neonates and children. American College of Chest Physicians Evidence-Based Clinical Practice Guidelines (8th edition). *Chest.* 2008;133:887S-968S.
128. Morrissey B, Burgess JL, Robertson WO. Washington's experience and recommendations re: anticoagulant rodenticides. *Vet Hum Toxicol.* 1995;37: 362-363.
129. Mosher DF. Blood coagulation and fibrinolysis: an overview. *Clin Cardiol.* 1990;13:VI5-11.
130. Mount ME. Diagnosis and therapy of anticoagulant rodenticide intoxications. *Vet Clin North Am Small Anim Pract.* 1988;18:115-130.
131. Mueller RL, Scheidt S. History of drugs for thrombotic disease. Discovery, development, and directions for the future. *Circulation.* 1994;89:432-449.
132. Mullins ME, Brands CL, Daya MR. Unintentional pediatric superwarfarin exposures: do we really need a prothrombin time? *Pediatrics.* 2000;105: 402-404.
133. Murdoch DA. Prolonged anticoagulation in chlorphacinone poisoning. *Lancet.* 1983;1:355-356.
134. Ng HJ, Koh LP, Lee LH. Successful control of postsurgical bleeding by recombinant factor VIIa in a renal failure patient given low molecular weight heparin and aspirin. *Ann Hematol.* 2003;82:257-258.
135. Ng VL, Levin J, Corash L, et al. Failure of the international normalized ratio to generate consistent results within a local medical community. *Am J Clin Pathol.* 1993;99:689-694.
136. Nichols WL, Bowie EJ. Standardization of the prothrombin time for monitoring orally administered anticoagulant therapy with use of the international normalized ratio system. *Mayo Clin Proc.* 1993;68:897-898.
137. Nimjee SM, Rusconi CP, Harrington RA, et al. The potential of aptamers as anticoagulants. *Trends Cardiovasc Med.* 2005;15:41-45.
138. O'Bryan SM, Constable DJ. Quantification of brodifacoum in plasma and liver tissue by HPLC. *J Anal Toxicol.* 1991;15:144-147.
139. O'Reilly R. Vitamin K antagonists. In: Colman RW HJ, Marder VJ, Salzman EW, eds. *Hemostasis and Thrombosis.* Philadelphia: Lippincott; 1987.
140. O'Reilly RA, Aggeler PM. Surreptitious ingestion of coumarin anticoagulant drugs. *Ann Intern Med.* 1966;64:1034-1041.
141. Olsson P, Lagergren H, Ek S. The elimination from plasma of intravenous heparin. An experimental study on dogs and humans. *Acta Med Scand.* 1963;173:619-630.
142. Oster JR, Singer I, Fishman LM. Heparin-induced aldosterone suppression and hyperkalemia. *Am J Med.* 1995;98:575-586.
143. Osterud B, Rapaport SI. Activation of factor IX by the reaction product of tissue factor and factor VII: additional pathway for initiating blood coagulation. *Proc Natl Acad Sci U S A.* 1977;74:5260-5264.
144. Pachman DJ. Accidental heparin poisoning in an infant. *Am J Dis Child.* 1965;110:210-212.
145. Park BK, Leck JB. A comparison of vitamin K antagonism by warfarin, difenacoum and brodifacoum in the rabbit. *Biochem Pharmacol.* 1982;31:3635-3639.
146. Park BK, Scott AK, Wilson AC, et al. Plasma disposition of vitamin K_1 in relation to anticoagulant poisoning. *Br J Clin Pharmacol.* 1984;18:655-662.
147. Parsons BJ, Day LM, Ozanne-Smith J, et al. Rodenticide poisoning among children. *Aust N Z J Public Health.* 1996;20:488-492.
148. Paspa PA, Movahed A. Thrombolytic therapy in acute myocardial infarction. *Am Fam Physician.* 1992;45:640-648.
149. Platell CF, Tan EG. Hypersensitivity reactions to heparin: delayed onset thrombocytopenia and necrotizing skin lesions. *Aust N Z J Surg.* 1986;56:621-623.
150. Raskob GE. Oral anticoagulant therapy. *Curr Opin Hematol.* 1996;3:361-364.
151. Renowden S, Westmoreland D, White JP, et al. Oral cholestyramine increases elimination of warfarin after overdose. *Br Med J (Clin Res Ed).* 1985;291:513-514.

152. Revel-Vilk S, Chan AK. Anticoagulation therapy in children. *Semin Thromb Hemost.* 2003;29:425-432.
153. Rich EC, Drage CW. Severe complications of intravenous phytonadione therapy. Two cases, with one fatality. *Postgrad Med.* 1982;72:303-306.
154. Robert A, Chazouilleres O. Prothrombin time in liver failure: time, ratio, activity percentage, or international normalized ratio? *Hepatology.* 1996;24:1392-1394.
155. Roberts HR, Lozier JN. New perspectives on the coagulation cascade. *Hosp Pract (Off Ed).* 1992;27:97-105, 109-112.
156. Rodgers GM BT. The diagnostic approach to bleeding disorders. In: Lee GR FJ, et al., eds. *Wintrobe's Clinical Hematology,* 10th ed. Baltimore: Williams & Wilkins; 1999.
157. Rosenberg RD. Actions and interactions of antithrombin and heparin. *N Engl J Med.* 1975;292:146-151.
158. Sallah S, Thomas DP, Roberts HR. Warfarin and heparin-induced skin necrosis and the purple toe syndrome: infrequent complications of anticoagulant treatment. *Thromb Haemost.* 1997;78:785-790.
159. Sane DC, Califf RM, Topol EJ, et al. Bleeding during thrombolytic therapy for acute myocardial infarction: mechanisms and management. *Ann Intern Med.* 1989;111:1010-1022.
160. Schiele F, Vuillemenot A, Mouhat T, et al. [Anticoagulant therapy with recombinant hirudin in patients with thrombopenia induced by heparin]. *Presse Med.* 1996;25:757-760.
161. Schiff BL, Kern AB. Cutaneous reactions to anticoagulants. *Arch Dermatol.* 1968;98:136-137.
162. Schreiner RL, Wynn RJ, McNulty C. Accidental heparin toxicity in the newborn intensive care unit. *J Pediatr.* 1978;92:115-116.
163. Schwartz BS. Heparin: what is it? How does it work? *Clin Cardiol.* 1990;13:VI12-15.
164. Serruys PW, Herrman JP, Simon R, et al. A comparison of hirudin with heparin in the prevention of restenosis after coronary angioplasty. Helvetica Investigators. *N Engl J Med.* 1995;333:757-763.
165. Shapiro S. Acquired anticoagulants. In: Williams WJ BE, Erslev AJ, Rundles RW, eds. *Hematology,* 2nd ed. New York: McGraw-Hill; 1973.
166. Shepard G K-SW, Anderson B. Acute pediatric brodifacoum ingestion [abstract]. *J Toxicol Clin Toxicol.* 1998;36:464.
167. Sherman DG, Atkinson RP, Chippendale T, et al. Intravenous ancrod for treatment of acute ischemic stroke: the STAT study: a randomized controlled trial. Stroke Treatment with Ancrod Trial. *JAMA.* 2000;283:2395-2403.
168. Shields RC, McBane RD, Kuiper JD, et al. Efficacy and safety of intravenous phytonadione (vitamin K_1) in patients on long-term oral anticoagulant therapy. *Mayo Clin Proc.* 2001;76:260-266.
169. Sims PJ, Faioni EM, Wiedmer T, et al. Complement proteins C5b-9 cause release of membrane vesicles from the platelet surface that are enriched in the membrane receptor for coagulation factor Va and express prothrombinase activity. *J Biol Chem.* 1988;263:18205-18212.
170. Smitherman TC. Considerations affecting selection of thrombolytic agents. *Mol Biol Med.* 1991;8:207-218.
171. Smolinske SC, Scherger DL, Kearns PS, et al. Superwarfarin poisoning in children: a prospective study. *Pediatrics.* 1989;84:490-494.
172. Spiller HA, Gallenstein GL, Murphy MJ. Dermal absorption of a liquid diphacinone rodenticide causing coagulaopathy. *Vet Hum Toxicol.* 2003;45:313-314.
173. Spyropoulos AC. Brave new world: the current and future use of novel anticoagulants. *Thromb Res.* 2008;123(Suppl 1):S29-35.
174. Stenflo J, Suttie JW. Vitamin K-dependent formation of gamma-carboxyglutamic acid. *Annu Rev Biochem.* 1977;46:157-172.
175. Stevenson RE, Burton OM, Ferlauto GJ, et al. Hazards of oral anticoagulants during pregnancy. *JAMA.* 1980;243:1549-1551.
176. Stowe CM, Metz AL, Arendt TD, et al. Apparent brodifacoum poisoning in a dog. *J Am Vet Med Assoc.* 1983;182:817-818.
177. Sturridge F, de Swiet M, Letsky E. The use of low molecular weight heparin for thromboprophylaxis in pregnancy. *Br J Obstet Gynaecol.* 1994;101:69-71.
178. Sutcliffe FA, MacNicoll AD, Gibson GG. Aspects of anticoagulant action: a review of the pharmacology, metabolism and toxicology of warfarin and congeners. *Rev Drug Metab Drug Interact.* 1987;5:225-272.
179. Suttie JW. Warfarin and vitamin K. *Clin Cardiol.* 1990;13:VI16-18.
180. Suttie JW, Jackson CM. Prothrombin structure, activation, and biosynthesis. *Physiol Rev.* 1977;57:1-70.
181. Swigar ME, Clemow LP, Saidi P, et al. "Superwarfarin" ingestion. A new problem in covert anticoagulant overdose. *Gen Hosp Psychiatry.* 1990;12:309-312.
182. Travis SF, Warfield W, Greenbaum BH, et al. Spontaneous hemorrhage associated with accidental brodifacoum poisoning in a child. *J Pediatr.* 1993;122:982-984.
183. Udall JA. Don't use the wrong vitamin K. *Calif Med.* 1970;112:65-67.
184. Vasse M. Protein Z, a protein seeking a pathology. *Thromb Haemost.* 2008;100:548-556.
185. Verstraete M. Third-generation thrombolytic drugs. *Am J Med.* 2000;109:52-58.
186. Vigano S, Mannucci PM, Solinas S, et al. Decrease in protein C antigen and formation of an abnormal protein soon after starting oral anticoagulant therapy. *Br J Haematol.* 1984;57:213-220.
187. Von Visger J, Magee C. Low molecular weight heparins in renal failure. *J Nephrol.* 2003;16:914-916.
188. Wakefield TW, Andrews PC, Wrobleski SK, et al. Effective and less toxic reversal of low-molecular weight heparin anticoagulation by a designer variant of protamine. *J Vasc Surg.* 1995;21:839-849; discussion 849-850.
189. Wakefield TW, Andrews PC, Wrobleski SK, et al. A [+18RGD] protamine variant for nontoxic and effective reversal of conventional heparin and low-molecular-weight heparin anticoagulation. *J Surg Res.* 1996;63:280-286.
190. Warkentin TE, Greinacher A, Koster A, et al. Treatment and prevention of heparin-induced thrombocytopenia. American College of Chest Physicians Evidence-Based Clinical Practice Guidelines (8th Edition). *Chest.* 2008;133:340S-380S.
191. Warkentin TE, Levine MN, Hirsh J, et al. Heparin-induced thrombocytopenia in patients treated with low-molecular-weight heparin or unfractionated heparin. *N Engl J Med.* 1995;332:1330-1335.
192. Watts RG, Castleberry RP, Sadowski JA. Accidental poisoning with a superwarfarin compound (brodifacoum) in a child. *Pediatrics.* 1990;86:883-887.
193. Wells PS, Forgie MA, Simms M, et al. The outpatient bleeding risk index: validation of a tool for predicting bleeding rates in patients treated for deep venous thrombosis and pulmonary embolism. *Arch Intern Med.* 2003;163:917-920.
194. Wentzien TH, O'Reilly RA, Kearns PJ. Prospective evaluation of anticoagulant reversal with oral vitamin K_1 while continuing warfarin therapy unchanged. *Chest.* 1998;114:1546-1550.
195. Wessler S, Gitel SN. Warfarin. From bedside to bench. *N Engl J Med.* 1984;311:645-652.
196. White HD. Comparative safety of thrombolytic agents. *Am J Cardiol.* 1991;68:30E-37E.
197. White RH, McKittrick T, Takakuwa J, et al. Management and prognosis of life-threatening bleeding during warfarin therapy. National Consortium of Anticoagulation Clinics. *Arch Intern Med.* 1996;156:1197-1201.
198. Whitlon DS, Sadowski JA, Suttie JW. Mechanism of coumarin action: significance of vitamin K epoxide reductase inhibition. *Biochemistry.* 1978;17:1371-1377.
199. Wiernikowski JT, Chan A, Lo G. Reversal of anti-thrombin activity using protamine sulfate. Experience in a neonate with a 10-fold overdose of enoxaparin. *Thromb Res.* 2007;120:303-305.
200. Woody BJ, Murphy MJ, Ray AC, et al. Coagulopathic effects and therapy of brodifacoum toxicosis in dogs. *J Vet Intern Med.* 1992;6:23-28.
201. Yee AJ, Kuter DJ. Successful recovery after an overdose of argatroban. *Ann Pharmacother.* 2006;40:336-339.
202. Young MA, Ehrenpreis ED, Ehrenpreis M, et al. Heparin-associated thrombocytopenia and thrombosis syndrome in a rehabilitation patient. *Arch Phys Med Rehabil.* 1989;70:468-470.
203. Zubkov AY, Mandrekar JN, Claassen DO, et al. Predictors of outcome in warfarin-related intracerebral hemorrhage. *Arch Neurol.* 2008;65:1320-1325.
204. Zupancic-Salek S, Kovacevic-Metelko J, Radman I. Successful reversal of anticoagulant effect of superwarfarin poisoning with recombinant activated factor VII. *Blood Coagul Fibrinolysis.* 2005;16:239-244.

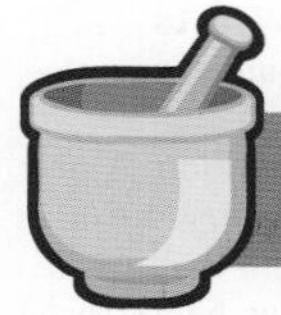

ANTIDOTES IN DEPTH (A16)

VITAMIN K_1

Mary Ann Howland

Vitamin K_1 (phytonadione) is the commercial preparation of the natural form of vitamin K (phylloquinone) that is indicated for the reversal of elevated prothrombin times (PTs) and international normalized ratios (INRs) in patients with xenobiotic-induced vitamin K deficiency. Acquired vitamin K deficiency is typically induced following the therapeutic administration of warfarin, or following the overdose of warfarin or the long-acting anticoagulant rodenticides (LAARs), such as brodifacoum. The optimal dosage regimen of vitamin K_1 to treat patients who develop an elevated INR while receiving warfarin has been reviewed and a revised guideline regarding the dose and route of administration published.[1,7] Oral administration of vitamin K_1 is used safely and successfully. Because intravenous administration of vitamin K_1 may be associated with anaphylactoid reactions, it should be avoided unless serious or life-threatening bleeding is present. Subcutaneous administration should only be considered when a patient is unable to tolerate oral vitamin K therapy yet is not clinically compromised enough to necessitate intravenous vitamin K_1.[7]

HISTORY

It was noted in 1929 that chickens fed a poor diet developed spontaneous bleeding. In 1935, Dam and coworkers discovered that incorporating a fat-soluble substance defined as a "koagulation factor," into the diet could correct the bleeding. Hence the name vitamin K was developed.[20,30,35]

CHEMISTRY

Vitamin K is an essential fat-soluble vitamin encompassing at least two distinct natural forms. Vitamin K_1 (phytonadione, phylloquinone) is the only form synthesized by plants and algae. Vitamin K_2 (menaquinones) is actually a series of compounds with the same 2-methyl-1, 4-naphthoquinone ring structure as phylloquinone, but with a variable number (1-13) of repeating 5-carbon units on the side chain. Bacteria synthesize vitamin K_2 (menaquinones). Most of the vitamin K ingested in the diet is phylloquinone (vitamin K_1).

DAILY REQUIREMENT

The human daily requirement for vitamin K is small; the Food and Nutrition Board set the recommended daily allowance at 1 μg/kg/d of phylloquinone for adults, although 10 times that amount is required for infants to maintain normal hemostasis.[29] Extrahepatic enzymatic reactions that are vitamin K dependent relate to carboxylation of proteins in the bone, kidney, placenta, lung, pancreas, and spleen, and include the synthesis of osteocalcin, matrix Gla protein, plaque Gla protein, and one or more renal Gla proteins.[29,30,34] Variations in an individual's dietary vitamin K intake while receiving therapeutic oral anticoagulation can significantly result in either over- or under-anticoagulation.[1,13]

PHARMACOKINETICS OF DIETARY VITAMIN K

Dietary vitamin K in the forms of phylloquinone and menaquinones is solubilized in the presence of the bile salts, free fatty acids, and monoglycerides, which enhance absorption. Vitamin K is incorporated into chylomicrons, entering the circulation through the lymphatic system in transit to the liver.[30] In the plasma, vitamin K is primarily in the phylloquinone form, whereas liver stores are 90% menaquinones and 10% phylloquinone.[30] Within 3 days of a low vitamin K diet, a group of surgical patients showed a fourfold decrease of liver vitamin K concentrations.[33] Rats given a vitamin K—deficient diet develop severe bleeding within 2 to 3 weeks.

PHARMACOLOGY

Activation of coagulation factors II, VII, IX, and X, and proteins S and C and Z require γ-carboxylation of the glutamate residues in a vitamin K—dependent process. Only the reduced (K_1H_2, hydroquinone) form of vitamin K manifests biologic activity. During the carboxylation step, the active reduced vitamin K_1 is converted to an epoxide. This 2,3-epoxide is reduced and recycled to the active K_1H_2 in a process that is inhibited by warfarin (Fig. 59-3). For further details, the reader is referred to an in-depth model of the chemical basis of this reaction.[9,39] The phytonadione form of vitamin K can be activated to the reduced, vitamin K_1H_2 form directly by nicotinamide adenine dinucleotide (phosphate) (NAD(P)H)-dehydrogenase (DT-diaphorase)—dependent pathway that is relatively insensitive to warfarin, while the vitamin K 2,3-epoxide form cannot be activated through this pathway.[30,34,35,36]

VITAMIN K DEFICIENCY AND MONITORING

Vitamin K deficiency can result from inadequate intake, malabsorption, or interference with the vitamin K cycle. Malnourishment and any condition in which bile salts or fatty acids are inadequate, such as extrahepatic cholestasis or severe pancreatic insufficiency, can lead to vitamin K deficiency. Additionally, multifactorial etiologies place newborns at risk for hemorrhage. Phylloquinone does not readily cross the placenta, and breast milk contains less phylloquinone than vitamin K—fortified formula. Fetal hepatic stores of phylloquinone are low and therapy such as maternal anticonvulsant therapy may lead to increased vitamin K metabolism.[30,34] Although menaquinones are produced in the colon by bacteria, it is unlikely that enteric production contributes significantly to vitamin K stores or that eradication of the bacteria with antibiotics, without a coexistent dietary deficiency of vitamin K, results in deficiency.[30] Determination of vitamin K deficiency is usually established on the basis of a prolonged PT or INR, which are surrogate markers of specific coagulation factors. Measurement of the vitamin K—dependent factors, II, VII, IX, and X, appears to be an effective way to determine the adequacy of vitamin K_1 dosing.[16] Serial measurements of factor VII, the factor with the shortest half-life, allows for the early detection of inadequate vitamin K in the diet or a therapeutic regimen.[6] Direct measurement of serum vitamin K concentrations is done by high-performance liquid chromatography (HPLC) analysis. The human serum vitamin K concentration required for adequate production of activated clotting factors in the presence of LAARs is still unclear. A single study in a patient who overdosed on brodifacoum suggested that a serum vitamin K concentration of 0.2 to 0.4 μg/mL was sufficient, to achieve a normal coagulation profile. Prior studies suggested 1.0 μg/mL was necessary in rabbits.[6,25]

MECHANISM OF ACTION FOR XENOBIOTIC-INDUCED VITAMIN K DEFICIENCY

Oral anticoagulants are vitamin K antagonists that interfere with the vitamin K cycle, causing the accumulation of vitamin K 2,3-epoxide, an inactive metabolite. Warfarin is a strong irreversible inhibitor of the vitamin K 2,3 epoxide reductase, which regenerates vitamin K into its active (K_1H_2, hydroquinone) form.[3] The superwarfarins are even more potent vitamin K reductase inhibitors. Without exogenous interference, vitamin K is recycled and only 1 μg/kg/d is required in adults to maintain adequate coagulation. NAD(P)H-dehydrogenases (DT-diaphorases) are warfarin-insensitive enzymes capable of reducing vitamin K_1 to its active hydroquinone form, but it is incapable of regenerating vitamin K from vitamin K 2,3-epoxide following carboxylation of the coagulation factor (Fig. 59-3).[3] Thus, in the presence of warfarin or superwarfarin, additional vitamin K_1 must be administered to supply this active cofactor for each and every carboxylation step, as it can no longer be recycled.[6] The minimum vitamin K_1 requirement in the presence of a LAAR is unknown. Other compounds have varying degrees of vitamin K antagonistic activity and include the *N*-methylthiotetrazole side-chain-containing antibiotics such as moxalactam and cefamandole (Chap. 56), as well as salicylates (Chap. 35).[30]

AVAILABILITY OF DIFFERENT FORMS OF VITAMIN K

Vitamin K_1 (phytonadione) is the only vitamin K preparation that should be used to reverse anticoagulant-induced vitamin K deficiency or to treat infants or pregnant women. In addition, patients with glucose-6-phosphate dehydrogenase (G6PD) deficiency have an increased risk of hemolysis with other vitamin K preparations. Vitamin K_1 is superior to the other previously commercially available vitamin K preparations because it is more active, thus requiring comparatively smaller doses, because it works more rapidly (6 vs. 12 hours), and because it has fewer associated risks.[14,32]

Vitamins K_3 (menadione) and K_4 (menadiol sodium diphosphate) (no longer FDA approved in the US) can produce hemolysis, hyperbilirubinemia, and kernicterus in neonates, and hemolysis in G6PD-deficient patients. The only advantage that menadione and menadiol sodium diphosphate have is that these preparations are absorbed directly from the intestine by a passive process that does not require the presence of bile salts. Theoretically, they are advantageous for patients with cholestasis or severe pancreatic insufficiency. However, they are neither interchangeable with vitamin K_1, nor a substitute for vitamin K_1, when anticoagulants such as warfarin or LAAR are responsible for coagulation deficits. Therefore, for a patient deficient in bile salts who requires vitamin K_1, exogenous bile salts, such as ox bile extract 300 mg or dehydrocholic acid 500 mg, should be given with each dose of oral vitamin K_1.[26]

PHARMACOKINETICS AND PHARMACODYNAMICS OF ADMINISTERED VITAMIN K_1

There are only a limited number of pharmacokinetic studies of vitamin K_1.[6,15,25,40] One study evaluated the pharmacokinetics of vitamin K_1 in healthy volunteers, brodifacoum-anticoagulated rabbits, and a patient poisoned with brodifacoum.[25] In the volunteers and the poisoned patient, a 10-mg intravenous (IV) dose of vitamin K_1 had a half-life of 1.7 hours. After oral administration of doses of 10 and 50 mg of vitamin K_1, peak concentrations of 100 to 400 ng/mL and 200 to 2000 ng/mL, respectively, occurred at 3 to 5 hours. Bioavailability varied significantly between patients (10% to 65%) for both doses, and in individual patients with the 50-mg dose. Oral vitamin K_1 is absorbed in an energy-dependent saturable process in the proximal small intestine, and this likely contributes to the variability.[25] In maximally brodifacoum-anticoagulated rabbits, IV vitamin K_1 (10 mg/kg) increased prothrombin complex activity (PCA) from 14% to 50% by 4 hours, and to 100% by 9 hours, after which it declined with a half-life of 6 hours.[25] High doses of oral vitamin K_1 were effectively used to treat a patient anticoagulated with brodifacoum.[6]

The pharmacokinetics of oral and intramuscular (IM) vitamin K_1 were compared in eight healthy female volunteers. Baseline serum vitamin K concentrations were 0.23 ng/mL. Following the oral administration of 5 mg of vitamin K, peak serum concentrations of 90 ng/mL were achieved between 4 and 6 hours. These concentrations dropped to a steady state of 3.8 ng/mL, and exhibited a half-life of about 4 hours.

The pharmacokinetics were distinctly different and quite variable after IM administration. IM administration of 5 mg of vitamin K resulted in peak serum concentrations of only 50 ng/mL with delays from 2 to 30 hours following administration and with the maintenance of a plateau for about 30 hours.[15] Consequently, IM administration is not recommended; either oral or IV is more appropriate and the route will be defined by the severity of bleeding. Only in the case of acute gastrointestinal disease in a patient without life-threatening over-anticoagulation is the subcutaneous route an appropriate alternative to the oral route (see Table 59-3).

ROUTES OF ADMINISTRATION AND ADVERSE EFFECTS

Although vitamin K_1 can be administered orally, subcutaneously, intramuscularly, or intravenously, the oral route is preferred for maintenance therapy. When administered orally, vitamin K_1 is virtually free of adverse effects, except for overcorrection of the INR for a patient who requires maintenance anticoagulation. The preparations available for IV administration are rarely associated with anaphylactoid reactions. Because of the lipid solubility of vitamin K these preparations are not available in solution, but rather as an aqueous colloidal suspension of a polyoxyethylated fatty acid derivative, dextrose, and benzyl alcohol. IV administration has resulted in death secondary to anaphylactoid reactions, probably as a result of the colloidal formulation of the preparation.[4,8,21] Numerous anaphylactoid reactions are reported, even when the preparation is properly diluted and administered slowly.[12,24,38] Rarely non-IV routes of administration may also result in an anaphylactoid reaction.[12] New liposomal preparations are under development, which may become safer alternatives.

ONSET OF EFFECT

The time necessary for the INR to return to a safe or normal range is variable and dependent on the rate of absorption of vitamin K_1, the serum concentration achieved, and the time necessary for the synthesis of activated clotting factors. A decrease in the INR can often occur within several hours, although it may take 8 to 24 hours to reach target values.[5,11,22,27] Maintenance of a normal INR depends on the half-life of the vitamin K_1, maintenance of an effective serum concentration, and the half-life of the anticoagulant involved. The IV route is unpredictably faster than the oral route in restoring the INR to a safe range.[15,19] A comparison of oral versus IV vitamin K_1 therapy for excessive anticoagulation, without major bleeding, demonstrated that individuals with INRs of 6 to 10 had similarly improved INRs at 24 hours and that the IV group was more often overcorrected to an INR of less than two.[19]

DOSING AND ADMINISTRATION

The optimal dosage regimen for vitamin K_1 remains unclear. Variables include the vitamin K_1 pharmacokinetics and the amount and type of anticoagulant ingested.[28] Reported cases of LAAR poisoning have required as much as 50 to 250 mg of vitamin K_1 daily for weeks to months.[2,6,10,17,18,31,37] A reasonable starting approach for a patient who has overdosed on LAAR is 25 to 50 mg of vitamin K_1 orally three to four times a day for 1 to 2 days. The INR should be monitored and the vitamin K_1 dose adjusted accordingly. Once the INR is less than 2, a downward titration in the dose of vitamin K_1 can be made on the basis of factor VII analysis. For an ingestion of brodifacoum, serial serum concentrations of brodifacoum may be helpful in determining the ultimate duration of treatment.[6,23]

The management of patients with elevated INRs secondary to excessive warfarin is described in Table 59-3. IV administration of vitamin K_1 should be reserved for life-threatening bleeding and serious bleeding at any elevation of INR.[1] Under these circumstances, patients may be supplemented with prothrombin complex concentrate, fresh-frozen plasma (FFP), or recombinant factor VIIa based on a risk to benefit analysis. A starting dose of 10 mg of vitamin K_1 is recommended. To minimize the risk of an anaphylactoid reaction, the preparation should be diluted with preservative-free 5% dextrose, 0.9% sodium chloride, or 5% dextrose in 0.9% sodium chloride, and administered slowly, at a rate not to exceed 1 mg/min in adults. Precautions should be anticipated in the event of an anaphylactoid reaction.

Because the duration of action of vitamin K_1 is short-lived, the dose must be repeated two to four times daily. The onset of the effect of vitamin K_1 is not immediate, regardless of the route of administration.

AVAILABILITY

Vitmain K_1 is available for IV and subcutaneous administration as AquaMEPHYTON and phytonadione injection emulsion in 2 mg/mL and 10 mg/mL concentrations. The preparation should be diluted with preservative-free 5% dextrose, 0.9% sodium chloride, or 5% dextrose in 0.9% sodium chloride, and administered slowly, at a rate not to exceed 1 mg/min in adults to minimize the risk of an anaphylactoid reaction. These preparations contain benzyl alcohol (0.9%) as a preservative. Oral vitamin K_1 is available as Mephyton in 5 mg tablets.

SUMMARY

Vitamin K_1 (phytonadione) is indicated for the reversal of elevated prothrombin times (PTs) and international normalized ratios (INRs) in patients with xenobiotic-induced vitamin K deficiency. IV administration is reserved for patients with serious or life-threatening bleeding. Vitamin K_1 is administered with other therapies such as prothrombin complex, recombinant factor VIIa, and FFP that have rapid onsets of action. The onset of action of vitamin K_1 is delayed for several hours regardless of the route of administration. The parenteral route of administration is rarely associated with consequential adverse events.

REFERENCES

1. Ansell J, Hirsh J, Hylek E, et al. The pharmacology and management of the vitamin K antagonists. The eighth ACCP conference on antithrombotic and thrombolytic therapy. *Chest.* 2008;133:160S-198S.
2. Babcock J, Hartman K, Pedersen A, Murphy M, Alving B. Rodenticide induced coagulopathy in a young child. *Am J Pediatr Hematol Oncol.* 1993;15:126-130.
3. Baglin T. Management of warfarin (Coumadin) overdose. *Blood Rev.* 1998;12:91-98.
4. Barash P, Kitahata LM, Mandel S. Acute cardiovascular collapse after intravenous phytonadione. *Anesth Analg.* 1976;55:304-306.
5. Brophy M, Fiore L, Deykin D. Low-dose vitamin K therapy in excessively anticoagulated patients: a dose finding study. *J Thromb Thrombolysis.* 1997;4:289-292.
6. Bruno GR, Howland MA, McMeeking A, Hoffman RS. Long-acting anticoagulant overdose: brodifacoum kinetics and optimal vitamin K_1 dosing. *Ann Emerg Med.* 2000;36:262-267.
7. Crowther MA, Douketis JD, Schnurr T, et al. Oral vitamin K reversed warfarin-associated coagulopathy faster than subcutaneous vitamin K. *Ann Intern Med.* 2002;137:251-254.
8. De la Rubia J, Grau E, Montserrat I, Zuazu I, Payá A. Anaphylactic shock and vitamin K_1. *Ann Intern Med.* 1989;110:943.
9. Dowd P, Ham SW, Naganathan S, Hershline R. The mechanism of action of Vitamin K. *Annu Rev Nutr.* 1995;15:419-440.
10. Exner DV, Brien WF, Murphy MJ. Superwarfarin ingestion. *CMAJ.* 1992;146:34-35.
11. Fetrow CW, Overlock T, Leff L. Antagonism of warfarin induced hypoprothrombinemia with use of low-dose subcutaneous vitamin K_1. *J Clin Pharmacol.* 1997;37:751-757.
12. Fiore L, Scola M, Cantillon C. Anaphylactoid reactions to Vitamin K. *J Thromb Thrombolysis.* 2001;11:175-183.
13. Franco V, Polanczyk CA, Clausell N, Rohde LE. Role of dietary vitamin K intake in chronic oral anticoagulation: prospective evidence from observational and randomized protocols. *Am J Med.* 2004;116:651-656.
14. Gamble JR, Dennis EW, Coon WW, et al. Clinical comparison of vitamin K_1 and water-soluble vitamin K. *Arch Intern Med.* 1955;5:52-58.
15. Hagstrom JN, Bovill EG, Soll R, Davidson KW, Sadowksi JA. The pharmacokinetics and lipoprotein fraction distribution of intramuscular versus oral vitamin K_1 supplementation in women of childbearing age: effects on hemostasis. *Thromb Haemost.* 1995;74:1486-1490.
16. Hoffman R, Smilkstein M, Goldfrank L. Evaluation of coagulation factor abnormalities in long-acting anticoagulant overdose. *J Toxicol Clin Toxicol.* 1998;26:233-248.
17. Hollinger B, Pastoor T. Case management and plasma half-life in a case of brodifacoum poisoning. *Arch Intern Med.* 1993;153:1925-1928.
18. La Rosa F, Clarke S, Lefkowitz J. Brodifacoum intoxication with marijuana smoking. *Arch Pathol Lab Med.* 1997;121:67-69.
19. Lubetsky A, Yonath H, Olchovsky D, et al. Comparison of oral vs intravenous phytonadione (vitamin K_1) in patients with excessive anticoagulation: a prospective randomized controlled study. *Arch Intern Med.* 2003;163:2469-2473.

20. Majerus P, Tollefsen D. Blood coagulation and anticoagulant, thrombolytic, and antiplatelet drugs. In: Brunton L, Lazo J, Parker K eds. *Goodman and Gilman's the Pharmacological Basis of Therapeutics*, 11th ed. New York: McGraw-Hill; 2006:1467-1488.
21. Mattea E, Quinn K. Adverse reactions after intravenous phytonadione administration. *Hosp Pharm.* 1981;16:230-235.
22. Nee R, Doppenschmidt, Donovan D, Andrews T. Intravenous versus subcutaneous vitamin K_1 in reversing excessive oral anticoagulation. *Am J Cardiol.* 1999;83:286-288.
23. Olmos V, Lopez C. Brodifacoum poisoning with toxicokinetic data. *Clin Tox.* 2007;45:487-489.
24. O'Reilly R, Kearns P. Intravenous vitamin K_1 injections: dangerous prophylaxis. *Arch Intern Med.* 1995;155:2127-2128.
25. Park BK, Scott AK, Wilson AC, et al. Plasma disposition of vitamin K_1 in relation to anticoagulant poisoning. *Br J Clin Pharmacol.* 1984;18: 655-662.
26. Phytonadione. In: GK McEvoy, ed. *AHFS Drug Information*. Bethesda, MD: American Society of Health System Pharmacists; 2004:3525-3527.
27. Raj G, Kumar R, Mckinney P. Time course of reversal of anticoagulant effect of warfarin by intravenous and subcutaneous phytonadione. *Arch Intern Med.* 1999;159:2721-2724.
28. Routh CR, Triplett DA, Murphy MJ, et al. Superwarfarin ingestion and detection. *Am J Hematol.* 1991;36:50-54.
29. Shearer MJ. Vitamin K. *Lancet.* 1995;345:229-233.
30. Shearer MJ. Vitamin K metabolism and nutrition. *Blood Rev.* 1992;6:92-104.
31. Sheen S, Spiller H. Symptomatic brodifacoum ingestion requiring high-dose phytonadione therapy. *Vet Hum Toxicol.* 1994;36:216-217.
32. Udall JA. Don't use the wrong vitamin K. *West J Med.* 1970;112:65-67.
33. Usuri Y, Taminura M, Nishimura N, et al. Vitamin K concentrations in the plasma and liver of surgical patients. *Am J Clin Nutr.* 1990;51:846-852.
34. Vermeer C, Hamulyak K. Pathophysiology of vitamin K deficiency and oral anticoagulants. *Thromb Haemost.* 1991;66:153-159.
35. Vermeer C, Schurgers L. A comprehensive review of vitamin K and vitamin K antagonists. *Hem Onc Clin N Am.* 2000;15:339-353.
36. Wallin R, Hutson S. Warfarin and the vitamin K dependent γ-carboxylation system. *Trends Molec Med.* 2004;10:299-302.
37. Weitzel J, Sadowski J, Furie BC, et al. Surreptitious ingestion of a long-acting vitamin K antagonist/rodenticide, brodifacoum: clinical and metabolic studies of three cases. *Blood.* 1990;76:2555-2559.
38. Wjasow C, McNamara R. Anaphylaxis after low dose intravenous vitamin K. *J Emerg Med.* 2003;24:169-172.
39. Wilson CR, Sauer J, Carlson GP, et al. Species comparison of vitamin K_1 2,3-epoxide reductase activity in vitro: kinetics and warfarin inhibition. *Toxicology.* 2003;189:191-198.
40. Winn MJ, Cholerton S, Park BK. An investigation of the pharmacological response to vitamin K_1 in the rabbit. *Br J Pharmacol.* 1988;94:1077-1084.

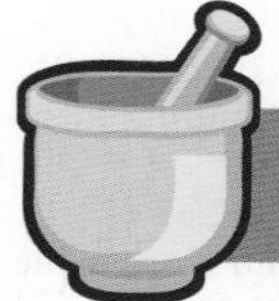

ANTIDOTES IN DEPTH (A17)

PROTAMINE

Mary Ann Howland

Protamine is a rapidly acting antidote that is used primarily to reverse the anticoagulant effects of unfractionated heparin (UFH). It also can partially reverse the effects of low-molecular-weight heparin (LMWH).

HISTORY

The antidotal property of protamine was recognized in the late 1930s, leading to its approval as an antidote for heparin overdose in 1968.[57] However, the largest body of literature pertaining to protamine originates from its use in neutralizing heparin following cardiopulmonary bypass and dialysis procedures.

PHARMACOLOGY

The protamines are a group of simple basic cationic proteins found in fish sperm that bind to heparin to form a stable neutral salt, rapidly inactivating heparin and reversing its anticoagulant effect.[62] Commercially available protamine sulfate is derived from the sperm of mature testes of salmon and related species. On hydrolysis, it yields basic amino acids, particularly arginine, proline, serine, and valine, but not tyrosine and tryptophan. The effects of protamine sulfate and protamine chloride appear to be comparable.[43] The molecular weight of heparins ranges from 3000 to 30,000 daltons and is composed of approximately 45 monosaccharide chains. One milligram of protamine will neutralize approximately 100 U (1 mg) of standard UFH (mean molecular weight [MW]~12,000 daltons).

In contrast to the case of heparin there is no proven method for neutralizing LMWH. Protamine neutralizes the anti-IIa activity of LMWH and a variable portion of the anti-Xa activity of LMWH.[28] Because the interaction of protamine and heparin is dependent on the MW of heparin, LMWH (mean MW 4500 daltons) has reduced protamine binding. The protamine-resistant fraction in LMWH is an ultralow-molecular-weight fraction with low sulfide charge.[15] It is suggested that 1 mg of enoxaparin equals approximately 100 antifactor-Xa units. To reverse the antithrombotic effects of LMWH within the first 8 hours following administration, the recommendation is to administer 1 mg protamine per 100 antifactor-Xa units of LMWH followed by administration of a second dose of 0.5 mg protamine per 100 anti factor-Xa units if bleeding continues.[28]

No human studies offer convincing evidence either demonstrating or disputing a beneficial effect of protamine as treatment for hemorrhage following LMWH use.[28] Case studies demonstrating both failure and success exist.[10,50,52,80] In animal studies, synthetic protamine variants were effective in reversing the anticoagulant effects of LMWH and are reported to be less toxic than protamine. These xenobiotics are not available for clinical use.[5,28,33,71,72]

MECHANISM OF ACTION

Heparins are large electronegative xenobiotics that are rapidly complexed by the electropositive protamine, forming an inactive salt. Heparin is an indirect anticoagulant, requiring a cofactor. This cofactor, AT, was formerly called antithrombin III.[28] Heparin alters the stereochemistry of AT, thereby catalyzing the subsequent inactivation of thrombin and other clotting factors.[24] Only about one-third of an administered dose of unfractionated heparin binds to AT, and this fraction is responsible for most of its anticoagulant effect.[3,45] LMWH has a reduced ability to inactivate thrombin as a result of lesser AT binding, but the smaller fragments of LMWH inactivate factor Xa almost as well as the larger molecules of UFH, allowing for equal efficacy.[28] Immunoelectrophoretic studies demonstrate that because of the net positive charge of protamine it has a greater affinity for heparin than AT, producing a dissociation of the heparin–AT complex in favor of a protamine–heparin complex.[59]

ADVERSE EFFECTS, RISK FACTORS, AND SAFETY ISSUES

Protamine is routinely used in the neutralization of heparin at the completion of cardiopulmonary bypass surgery. Millions of patients are exposed to protamine each year and approximately 100 deaths are reported in total with the use of protamine under these circumstances. It is largely in this setting that the adverse effects of protamine are also documented and studied.[30,31,49,58] It is often difficult to separate the adverse effects caused by protamine from those of the protamine–heparin complex or those actually related to heparin. Adverse effects associated with protamine include both rate- and non–rate-related hypotension,[12,18-21,23,35,38,65,68] anaphylaxsis[34,48] and anaphylactoid reactions,[37,53,55] bradycardia,[1] thrombocytopenia,[76] thrombogenicity,[14] leukopenia, decreased oxygen consumption,[73,75] acute lung injury,[4,70] pulmonary hypertension and pulmonary vasoconstriction,[7,27] cardiovascular collapse,[46,63] and anticoagulant effects.[2]

The mechanisms for these adverse effects are multifactorial. The significant electropositivity of protamine may be responsible for some of the adverse effects and probably directly injures a variety of organelles, including platelets.[9,77] The protamine–heparin complex activates the arachidonic acid pathway and the production of thromboxane is at least partly responsible for some of the hemodynamic changes, including pulmonary hypertension.[7,13,29,54,77] Pretreatment with indomethacin limits these effects.[13,29,54,77] Free protamine or protamine complexed with heparin can convert L-arginine to nitric oxide (formerly called endothelium-derived relaxing factor), which in turn causes vasodilation and inhibits platelet aggregation and adhesion.[60] Protamine administered in the absence of heparin, or in an amount exceeding that necessary for heparin neutralization, can act as an anticoagulant and may inhibit platelet function, resulting in weaker clot formation.[36,73] This anticoagulant effect may result from effects on factor VII and/or AT. Protamine in excess of heparin can enter the myocardium and decrease cyclic adenosine monophosphate (cAMP), causing myocardial depression.[7,67] Protamine and protamine–heparin complexes can activate the complement pathway and contribute to vasoactive events.[7,61] Protamine stimulates mast cells in the human heart and skin to release histamine.[7] Risk factors for protamine-induced adverse reactions include prior exposure to protamine in insulin or during previous surgery with protamine reversal or a previous vasectomy, as well as an allergy to fish or a rapid rate of protamine infusion.[46,61] A prospective study reported a 0.06% incidence of anaphylactic reactions to protamine in all patients undergoing coronary artery bypass, but a 2% incidence in diabetics using neutral protamine Hagedorn (NPH) insulin.[6] A recent systematic review of the literature revealed an incidence of 1% but expressed caution in interpreting the results because of the heterogeneity of the studies.[58] The resultant elevation of histamine concentrations, the activation of complement, and elevated IgE, IgA, and IgG concentrations are also suggested as possible mechanisms for the adverse effects.[44,69,78,79] Diabetic patients receiving daily subcutaneous injections of a protamine-containing insulin (NPH) have a 40% to 50% increased risk of immune-mediated adverse reactions.[22,25,34,42,68]

Occasionally, patients manifesting a protamine allergy are incorrectly presumed to have insulin allergy.[41] In diabetic patients receiving protamine insulin injections, the presence of serum antiprotamine IgE antibody is a significant risk factor for acute protamine reactions. Only patients with previous exposure to protamine insulin injections had serum antiprotamine IgE antibodies. However, in the group without previous protamine insulin exposure, antiprotamine IgG antibody was noted as a risk factor for protamine reactions.[79] Either naturally occurring cross-reacting antibodies, or perhaps previously unrecognized protamine exposure, was responsible for the generation of these IgG antibodies.

ALTERNATIVES TO PROTAMINE FOR PATIENTS AT HIGH RISK FOR AN ADVERSE DRUG REACTION

There are limited options to replace protamine for the reversal of heparin in patients who have previously experienced anaphylaxis following protamine therapy, or in patients who are suspected of being at high risk. Clotting factors may be replaced, or exchange transfusion instituted in neonates, and protamine avoided, or protamine may be used while being prepared to treat anaphylaxis expectantly. Several alternatives under investigation include the placement of heparin removal devices in the coronary artery bypass extracorporeal circuit, as well as the use of hexadimethrine, methylene blue, platelet factor 4, and heparinase as antidotes.[6,40] Pretreatment with antihistamines and corticosteroids may be sufficient for immune-mediated mechanisms, but will probably not be beneficial for pulmonary vasoconstriction and non–immune-mediated anaphylactoid reactions.[32]

DOSING IN CARDIOPULMONARY BYPASS

Protamine is most frequently used at the conclusion of cardiopulmonary bypass operations to reverse the effects of heparin. There are many regimens used for protamine dosing, including (1) administration of an arbitrary amount of protamine (eg, greater than 2 mg/kg); (2) administration of protamine in a ratio of 0.6 to 1.5:1 times the initial heparin dose that results in an activated coagulation time (ACT) of about 480 seconds; and (3) giving protamine in a ratio of 0.75 to 2:1 times the total operative heparin dose.[81] Two additional methods of calculating the protamine dose to improve accuracy and avoid excess protamine have been proposed.[36,81] One advocates an initial protamine dose based on ACT, with subsequent doses based on the ratio of the change in thrombin time to the heparin-neutralized thrombin time. If this ratio is greater than 12 seconds, then 10-mg incremental protamine doses should be administered.[36] The other uses a nomogram based on heparin activity in milligrams per kilograms versus ACT.[81] Both methods demonstrate efficacy with 2 mg/kg doses of protamine, about one-half of the dose previously used. With these approaches, the ACT responded to protamine within 5 minutes, decreasing in value from between 550 and 700 seconds to a control of 150 seconds. Other investigators suggest a variety of monitoring methods and dosing schemas in this setting.[16,26,47,66]

HEPARIN REBOUND AND REDOSING OF PROTAMINE

A heparin anticoagulant rebound effect is noted after cardiopulmonary bypass and is attributed to the presence of detectable circulating heparin several hours after apparently adequate heparin neutralization with protamine. The incidence of heparin rebound and the need for additional protamine range from 4% to 42% depending on the neutralization protocol.[24,51,64] It is likely that larger heparin doses may prolong the clearance of heparin, contributing to higher than expected heparin concentrations.[64] When 300 Units/kg of body weight doses of heparin were reversed with 3 mg/kg of protamine at the conclusion of cardiopulmonary bypass a 14% incidence of small but detectable concentrations of circulating heparin was noted at 2 hours, which lasted less than 1 hour in all but one case.[51] A prolonged prothrombin time and thrombocytopenia occurred without increase in hemorrhage.

DOSING CONSIDERATIONS

Approximately 1 mg of protamine will neutralize about 100 Units (1 mg) of heparin (UFH). A limited number of studies suggest incomplete neutralization by protamine of the LMWHs enoxaparin, dalteparin, and tinzaparin. Current recommendations are to administer 1 mg protamine per 100 anti-factor Xa units, where 1 mg enoxaparin equals 100 anti–factor Xa units if administered within 8 hours of the LMWH.[28] A second dose of 0.5 mg protamine should be administered per 100 anti–factor Xa units if bleeding continues.[17,28] If more than 8 hours have elapsed, then a smaller dose of protamine can be administered.

A number of tests directly measure heparin concentrations or indirectly measure the effect of heparin on the clotting cascade.[8,11,16] These tests may be helpful in determining the appropriate dose of protamine. Because excessive protamine can act as an anticoagulant, the dose chosen should always be an underestimation of that which is needed. In the case of unintentional overdose, the half-life of heparin should be considered, because half of the administered dose of heparin is eliminated within 60 to 90 minutes. In the case of an unintentional overdose without hemorrhage, the short half-life of heparin and the potential risks of protamine administration limit the need for and benefit from protamine reversal of anticoagulation. If protamine use is necessary to treat active hemorrhage, the dose must be administered very slowly intravenously either undiluted or diluted in D_5W or 0.9% NaCl over 10 to 15 minutes to limit rate-related hypotension.[39,62,74]

DOSING IN THE OVERDOSE SETTING

When a patient is believed to have received an overdose of an unknown quantity of heparin, the decision to use protamine should be determined by the presence of a prolonged activated partial thromboplastin time (aPTT) and the presence of persistent hemorrhage. The risks of protamine use, especially in those who have had a prior life-threatening reaction to protamine as well as in a diabetic receiving protamine-containing insulin, and the risks of continued heparin anticoagulation must be evaluated. A baseline ACT, thrombin time, heparin-neutralized thrombin time, heparin activity, platelets, prothrombin time, partial thromboplastin time, hemoglobin, and hematocrit should be obtained. Because of the routine nature of heparin reversal following cardiopulmonary bypass, consultation with members of the bypass team may be helpful. An empiric dose of protamine may be suggested by the baseline ACT: (1) an ACT of 150 seconds necessitates no protamine; (2) an ACT of 200 to 300 seconds necessitates 0.6 mg/kg; and (3) an ACT of 300 to 400 seconds necessitates 1.2 mg/kg. These doses have not been tested outside the operating room. The ACT should be repeated 5 to 15 minutes following the protamine dose and in 2 to 8 hours to evaluate the potential for heparin rebound. Further dosing should be based on these values.

When the ACT is not available, 25 to 50 mg of protamine can be administered to an adult and adjusted accordingly. The initial dose should not be more than 50 mg in an adult.[62] Repeat dosing in several hours may be necessary if heparin rebound occurs. The dose should be administered slowly intravenously over 15 minutes with resuscitative equipment immediately available. Neonates should not receive protamine that has been diluted with bacteriostatic water containing benzyl alcohol.

Future interventions for bleeding following heparin may include activated factor VII. Activated factor VII therapy was recently shown to be successful in treating postoperative bleeding in a patient with renal failure who was given LMWH and aspirin.[56] Adenosine triphosphate, an experimental nucleotide, completely reversed clinical bleeding related to LMWH in a rat model.[17] Other substances or devices include hexadimethrine, heparinase, PF4, synthetic protamine variants, and extracorporeal heparin-removal devices.[24] These xenobiotics have not been approved by the Food and Drug Administration (FDA) for clinical use in this setting.[17,28]

AVAILABILITY

Protamine is available as a parenteral solution ready for injection in a concentration of 10 mg/mL in either a 5-mL or 25-mL vial containing totals of 50 mg and 250 mg, respectively.[62]

SUMMARY

Protamine is an effective, rapidly acting antidote used to reverse the anticoagulant effect of unfractionated heparin, while its ability to reverse the effects of LMWH is less clear. This antidote should only be used for a prolonged aPTT in the presence of persistent hemorrhage, since potential risks of its use include hypotension, anaphylaxis, dysrhythmias, leukopenia, thrombocytopenia, and acute lung injury.

REFERENCES

1. Alvarez J, Alvarez L, Escudero C, Olivares JLC. Sinus node function and protamine sulfate. *J Cardiothorac Anesth.* 1989;3:44-51.
2. Andersen MN, Mendelow M, Alfano GA. Experimental studies of heparin-protamine activity with special reference to protamine inhibition of clotting. *Surgery.* 1959;46:1060-1068.
3. Andersson LO, Barrowcliffe TW, Holmer E, et al. Anticoagulant properties of heparin fractionated by affinity chromatography on matrix-bound antithrombin III and by gel filtration. *Thromb Res.* 1976;6:575-583.
4. Brooks JC. Noncardiogenic pulmonary edema immediately following rapid protamine administration. *Ann Pharmacother.* 1999;33:927-930.
5 Byun Y, Singh VK, Yang VC. Low molecular weight protamine: a potential nontoxic heparin antagonist. *Thromb Res.* 1999;94:53-61.
6. Carr JA, Silverman N. The heparin-protamine interaction. A review. *J Cardiovasc Surg (Torino).* 1999;40:659-666.
7. Carr ME, Carr, SL. At high heparin concentrations, protamine concentrations which reverse heparin anticoagulant effects are insufficient to reverse heparin antiplatelet effects. *Thromb Res.* 1994;75:617-630.
8. Castellani WJ, Hodges ED, Bode AP. Effect of protamine sulfate on the ACA heparin assay. *Clin Chem.* 1991;37:1119-1120.
9. Chang SW, Westcott JY, Henson JE, Voelkel NF. Pulmonary vascular injury by polycations in perfused rat lungs. *J Appl Physiol.* 1987;62:1932-1943.
10. Chawla L, Moore G, Seneff M. Incomplete reversal of enoxaparin toxicity by protamine: implications of renal insufficiency, obesity and low molecular weight heparin sulfate content. *Obesity Surgery.* 2004;14:695-698.
11. Chen W, Yang V. Versatile non-clotting based heparin assay requiring no instrumentation. *Clin Chem.* 1991;37:832-837.
12 Chilukuri K, Henrikson C, Dalal D, et al. Incidence and outcomes of protamine reactions in patients undergoing catheter ablation of atrial fibrillation. *J Interv Card Electrophysiol.* 2009;25:175-181.
13. Conzen PF, Habazettl H, Gutmann R, et al. Thromboxane mediation of pulmonary hemodynamic responses after neutralization of heparin by protamine in pigs. *Anesth Analg.* 1989;68:25-31.
14. Cosgrove J, Qasim A, Latib A, et al. Protamine usage following implantation of drug-eluting stents: a word of caution. *Cath Cardiovas Interv.* 2008; 71:913-914.
15. Crowther MA, Berry LR, Monagle PT, Chan AKC. Mechanisms reponsible for the failure of protamine to inactivate low-molecular-weight heparin. *Br J Haematol.* 2002;116:178-186.
16. Despotis GJ, Gravlee G, Filos K, Levy J. Anticoagulation monitoring during cardiac surgery: a review of current and emerging techniques. *Anesthesiology.* 1999;91:1122-1151.
17. Dietrich CP, Shinjo SK, Moraes FA, et al. Structural features and bleeding activity of commercial low-molecular-weight heparins: neutralization by ATP and protamine. *Semin Thromb Hemost.* 1999;3:43-50.
18. Fadali MA, Ledbetter M, Papacostas CA, et al. Mechanism responsible for the cardiovascular depressant effect of protamine sulfate. *Ann Surg.* 1974;180:232-235.
19. Fadali MA, Papacostas CA, Duke JJ, et al. Cardiovascular depressant effect of protamine sulfate. *Thorax.* 1976;31:320-323.
20. Frater RMW, Oka Y, Hong Y, et al. Protamine-induced circulatory changes. *J Thorac Cardiovasc Surg.* 1984;87:687-692.
21. Goldman BS, Joison J, Austen WG. Cardiovascular effects of protamine sulfate. *Ann Thorac Cardiovasc Surg.* 1969;7:459-471.
22. Gottschlich GM, Gravlee GP, Georgitis JW. Adverse reactions to protamine sulfate during cardiac surgery in diabetic and nondiabetic patients. *Ann Allergy.* 1988;61:277-281.
23. Gourin A, Streisand RL, Greineder JK, Stuckey JH. Protamine sulfate administration and the cardiovascular system. *J Thorac Cardiovasc Surg.* 1971;62:193-204.
24. Gundry SR, Drongowski RA, Klein MD, et al. Postoperative bleeding in cardiovascular surgery: does heparin rebound really exist? *Am Surg.* 1989;55:162-165.
25. Gupta SK, Veith FJ, Wengerter KR, et al. Anaphylactoid reactions to protamine: an often lethal complication in insulin-dependent diabetic patients undergoing vascular surgery. *J Vasc Surg.* 1989;9:342-350.
26. Hall RI. Protamine dosing—the quandary continues. *Can J Anaesth.* 1998; 45:1-5.
27. Hiong Y, Tang Y, Chui W, et al. A case of catastrophic pulmonary vasoconstriction after protamine administration in cardiac surgery: role of intraoperative transesophageal echocardiography. *J Cardiothoracic and Vascular Anesth.* 2008;22:727-731.
28. Hirsh J, Bauer K, Donati M, et al. Parenteral anticoagulants. The Eighth ACCP Conference on Antithrombotic and Thrombolytic Therapy. *Chest.* 2008;133:141S-198S.
29. Hobbhahn J, Conzen PF, Zenker B, et al. Beneficial effect of cyclooxygenase inhibition on adverse hemodynamic responses after protamine. *Anesth Analg.* 1988;67:253-260.
30. Holland CL, Singh AK, McMaster PRB, Fang W. Adverse reactions to protamine sulfate following cardiac surgery. *Clin Cardiol.* 1984;7:157-162.
31. Horrow JC. Protamine: a review of its toxicity. *Anesth Analg.* 1985;64:348-361.
32. Hughes C, Haddock M. Protamine reaction in a patient undergoing coronary artery bypass grafting. *CRNA.* 1995;6:172-176.
33. Hulin MS, Wakefield TW, Andrews PC, et al. Comparison of the hemodynamic and hematologic toxicity of a protamine variant after reversal of low-molecular-weight heparin anticoagulation in a canine model. *Lab Anim Sci.* 1997;47:153-160.

34. Jackson DR. Sustained hypotension secondary to protamine sulfate. *Angiology.* 1970;21:295-298.
35. Jastrebski MK, Sykes MK, Woods DG. Cardiorespiratory effects of protamine after cardiopulmonary bypass in man. *Thorax.* 1974;20:534-538.
36. Jobes DR, Aitken GL, Shaffer GW. Increased accuracy and precision of heparin and protamine dosing reduces blood loss and transfusion in patients undergoing primary cardiac operations. *J Thorac Cardiovasc Surg.* 1995;110:36-45.
37. Kambam JR, Merrill WH, Smith BE. Histamine$_2$ receptor blocker in the treatment of protamine-related anaphylactoid reactions: two case reports. *Can J Anaesth.* 1989;36:463-465.
38. Katz NM, Kim YD, Siegelman R, et al. Hemodynamics of protamine administration. *J Thorac Cardiovasc Surg.* 1987;94:881-886.
39. Kien ND, Quam DD, Reitan JA, White DA. Mechanism of hypotension following rapid infusion of protamine sulfate in anesthetized dogs. *J Cardiothorac Vasc Anesth.* 1992;6:143-147.
40. Kikura M, Lee MK, Levy JH. Heparin neutralization with methylene blue, hexadimethrine, or vancomycin after cardiopulmonary bypass. *Anesth Analg.* 1996;83:223-227.
41. Kim R. Anaphylaxis to protamine masquerading as an insulin allergy. *Del Med J.* 1993;65:17-23.
42. Kimmel SE, Sekers MA, Berlin JA, et al. Risk factors for clinically important adverse events after protamine administration following cardiopulmonary bypass. *J Am Coll Cardiol.* 1998;32:1916-1922.
43. Kuitunen AH, Salmenpera MT, Heinonen J, et al. Heparin rebound: a comparative study of protamine chloride and protamine sulfate in patients undergoing coronary artery bypass surgery. *J Cardiothorac Vasc Anesth.* 1991;5:221-226.
44. Lakin JD, Blocker TJ, Strong DM, Yocum MW. Anaphylaxis to protamine sulfate mediated by a complement dependent IgG antibody. *J Allergy Clin Immunol.* 1978;61:102-107.
45. Lam LH, Silbert JE, Rosenberg RD. The separation of active and inactive forms of heparin. *Biochem Biophys Res Commun.* 1976;69:570-577.
46. Levy J, Adkinson N. Anaphylaxis during cardiac surgery: implications for clinicians. *Anesth Anal.* 2008;106:392-403.
47. Levy J, Tanaka K. Anticoagulation and reversal paradigms: is too much of a good thing bad? *Anesth Anal.* 2009;108:692-694.
48. Lieberman P, Kemp S, Oppenheimer J, et al. The diagnosis and amanagement of anaphylaxis: an updated practice parameter. *J Allergy Clin Immunol.* 2005;115:S483-S523.
49. Lindblad B. Protamine sulphate: a review of its effects—hypersensitivity and toxicity. *Eur J Vasc Surg.* 1989;3:195-201.
50. Makris M, Hough RE, Kitchen S. Poor reversal of low molecular weight heparin by protamine. *Br J Hematol.* 2000;108:884-885.
51. Martin P, Horkay F, Gupta NK, et al. Heparin rebound phenomenon: much ado about nothing. *Blood Coagul Fibrinolysis.* 1992;3:187-191.
52. Massonnet-Castel S, Pelissier E, Bara L, et al. Partial reversal of low molecular weight heparin (PK 10169) anti-Xa activity by protamine sulfate: in vitro and in vivo study during cardiac surgery with extracorporeal circulation. *Hemostais.* 1986;16:139-146.
53. Moorthy SS, Pond W, Rowland RG. Severe circulatory shock following protamine (an anaphylactoid reaction). *Anesth Analg.* 1980;59:77-78.
54. Morel DR, Zapol WM, Thomas SJ, et al. C5a and thromboxane generation associated with pulmonary vaso- and broncho-constriction during protamine reversal of heparin. *Anesthesiology.* 1987;66:597-604.
55. Neidhart PP, Meier B, Polla BS, et al. Fatal anaphylactoid response to protamine after percutaneous transluminal coronary angioplasty. *Eur Heart J.* 1992;13:856-858.
56. Ng HJ, Koh LR, Lee LH. Successful control of postsurgical bleeding by recombinant factor VIIa in a renal failure patient given low molecular weight heparin and aspirin. *Ann Hematol.* 2003;82:257-258.
57. New Drug Application. Washington, DC: Food and Drug Administration; 1968, 6460, log 775.
58. Nybo M, Madsen S. Serious anaphylaxis reactions to protamine sulfate: a systematic literature review. *Basic Clin Pharmacol Toxicol.* 2008;103:192-196.
59. Okajirna Y, Kanayama S, Maeda Y, et al. Studies on the neutralizing mechanism of antithrombin activity of heparin by protamine. *Thromb Res.* 1981;24:21-29.
60. Pearson PJ, Evora PRB, Ayrancioglu K, Schaff HV. Protamine releases endothelium-derived relaxing factor from systemic arteries. *Anesth Prog.* 1991; 38:99-100.
61. Porsche R, Brenner ZR. Allergy to protamine sulfate. *Heart Lung.* 1999;28: 418-428.
62. Protamine sulfate injection, USP [package insert]. Schaumberg, IL: APP Pharmaceuticals, LLP; 2008.
63. Pugsley M, Kalra V, Froebel-Wilson S. Protamine is a low molecular weight polycationic amine that produces actions on cardiac muscle. *Life Sci.* 2002; 72:293-305.
64. Raul TK, Crow MJ, Rajah SM, et al. Heparin administration during extracorporeal circulation: heparin rebound and postoperative bleeding. *J Thorac Cardiovasc Surg.* 1979;78:95-102.
65. Shapira N, Schaff HV, Piehler JM, et al. Cardiovascular effects of protamine sulfate in man. *J Thorac Cardiovasc Surg.* 1982;84:505-514.
66. Shore-Lesserson L, Reich DL, DePerio M. Heparin and protamine titration do not improve haemostasis in cardiac surgical patients. *Can J Anaesth.* 1998;45:10-18.
67 Stefaniszyn HJ, Novick RJ, Salerno TA. Toward a better understanding of the hemodynamic effects of protamine and heparin interaction. *J Thorac Cardiovasc Surg.* 1984;87:678-686.
68. Stewart WJ, McSweeney SM, Kellett MA, et al. Increased risk of severe protamine reactions in NPH insulin-dependent diabetics undergoing cardiac catheterization. *Circulation.* 1984;70:788-792.
69. Stoelting RK, Henry DD, Verburg KM. Hemodynamic changes and circulating histamine concentrations following protamine administration to patients and dogs. *Can Anaesth Soc J.* 1984;31:534-540.
70. Urdaneta F, Lobato EB, Kirby RR, Horrow JC. Noncardiogenic pulmonary edema associated with protamine administration during coronary artery bypass graft surgery. *J Clin Anesth.* 1999;11:675-681.
71. Wakefield TW, Andrews PC, Wrobleski SK. A [18RGD] protamine variant for nontoxic and effective reversal of conventional heparin and low-molecular-weight heparin anticoagulation. *J Surg Res.* 1996;63:280-296.
72. Wakefield TW, Andrews PC, Wrobleski SK, et al. Effective and less toxic reversal of low-molecular weight heparin anticoagulation by a designer variant of protamine. *J Vasc Surg.* 1995;21:839-849.
73. Wakefield TW, Bies LE, Wrobleski SK, et al. Impaired myocardial function and oxygen utilization due to protamine sulfate in an isolated rabbit heart preparation. *Ann Surg.* 1990;212:387-393.
74. Wakefield TW, Mantler CB, Wrobleski SK, et al. Effects of differing rates of protamine reversal of heparin anticoagulation. *Surgery.* 1996;119:123-128.
75. Wakefield TW, Ucros I, Kresowik TF, et al. Decreased oxygen consumption as a toxic manifestation of protamine sulfate reversal of heparin anticoagulation. *J Vasc Surg.* 1989;9:772-777.
76. Wakefield TW, Wrobleski SK, Nichol BJ, et al. Heparin-mediated reduction of the toxic effects of protamine sulfate on rabbit myocardium. *J Vasc Surg.* 1992;16:47-53.
77. Wakefield TW, Wrobleski BS, Wirthlin DJ, et al. Increased prostacyclin and adverse hemodynamic responses to protamine sulfate in an experimental canine model. *J Surg Res.* 1991;50:449-456.
78. Weiss ME, Chatham F, Kagey Sobotka A, Adkinson NF. Serial immunological investigations in a patient who had a life-threatening reaction to intravenous protamine. *Clin Exp Allergy.* 1990;20:713-720.
79. Weiss ME, Nyhan D, Zhikang P, et al. Association of protamine IgE and IgG antibodies with life-threatening reactions to intravenous protamine. *N Engl J Med.* 1989;320:886-892.
80. Wiernikowski J, Chan A, Lo G. Reversal of anti-thrombin activity using protamine sulfate. Experience in a neonate with a 10-fold overdose of enoxaparin. *Thromb Res.* 2007;120:303-305.
81. Wright SJ, Murray WB, Hampton WA, et al. Calculating the protamine-heparin reversal ratio: a pilot study investigating a new method. *J Cardiothorac Vasc Anesth.* 1993;7:416-421.

CHAPTER 60
CALCIUM CHANNEL BLOCKERS

Francis Jerome DeRoos

Since calcium channel blockers (CCBs) were first introduced experimentally in the 1960s, their use has steadily risen to make them among the most frequently prescribed cardiovascular medications. Mirroring this widespread use, poisonings involving CCBs have also risen. The combination of sustained-release formulations to improve compliance and the potent hemodynamic effects complicates the management of patients poisoned with CCBs. The hallmarks of CCB toxicity include hypotension and bradydysrhythmias. Unfortunately, in severely poisoned patients, no therapeutic intervention is demonstrated to be consistently effective. Management decisions must be made on an individual patient basis with careful assessment of the physiologic response to each treatment.

HISTORY AND EPIDEMIOLOGY

CCBs were first introduced commercially in the United States in the late 1970s. Currently, there are 10 individual CCBs available in either immediate or sustained-release formulations (Table 60–1), plus several combination products. They are used for a variety of medical conditions, including hypertension, stable angina, dysrhythmias, migraine headache, Raynaud phenomenon, and subarachnoid hemorrhage.

In 1986, more than 1200 exposures and seven deaths related to CCBs were reported to the American Association of Poison Control Centers. In 2007, those figures increased to 10,084 exposures with 435 of moderate to major toxicity, including 17 deaths (Chap. 135). This reported rise in fatalities is most likely the result of the increased use and access to these drugs, along with the introduction of sustained-release preparations in 1988.

PHARMACOLOGY

There are many types of calcium channels, including L, N, P, T, Q, and R types, that can be found either intracellularly on the sarcoplasmic reticulum or on cell plasma membranes, particularly in neuronal and secretory tissue.[91]

All CCBs commercially available in the United States exert their physiologic effects by antagonizing L-type voltage-sensitive calcium channels and are classified into three structural groups (see Table 60–1).[50,107] Each group binds a slightly different region of the alpha$_{1c}$ subunit of the calcium channel and thus has different affinities for the various L-type calcium channels, both in the myocardium and the vascular smooth muscle.[1,28] Verapamil and diltiazem have profound inhibitory effects on the sinoatrial (SA) and atrioventricular (AV) nodal tissue, whereas the dihydropyridines as a class have little, if any, direct myocardial effects at therapeutic doses.[51,107] A fourth class of CCBs, sometimes referred to as "nonselective," includes mibefradil and bepridil, which are no longer available in the United States because of adverse drug events.

These receptor-binding differences among the CCB classes determine their potential therapeutic role. Verapamil and diltiazem are used in the management of hypertension, to reduce myocardial oxygen demand, to achieve rate control in atrial flutter and atrial fibrillation, and to abolish supraventricular reentrant tachycardias.[1] Dihydropyridines are typically used to treat diseases with increased peripheral vascular tone such as hypertension, Raynaud phenomenon, Prinzmetal angina, esophageal spasm, vascular headaches, and post-subarachnoid hemorrhage vasospasm, but not for rhythm disturbances.

PHARMACOKINETICS AND TOXICOKINETICS

All CCBs are well-absorbed orally and undergo hepatic oxidative metabolism predominantly via the CYP3A4 subgroup of the cytochrome P450 (CYP) isoenzyme system.[68] Norverapamil, formed by *N*-demethylation of verapamil, is the only active metabolite and retains 20% of the activity of the parent compound.[46] Diltiazem is predominantly deacetylated into minimally active deacetyldiltiazem, which is then eliminated via the biliary tract.[39] After repeated doses, as well as overdose, these hepatic enzymes become saturated, reducing the potential of the first-pass effect and increasing the quantity of active drug absorbed systemically.[116] Saturation metabolism contributes to the prolongation of the apparent half-lives reported following overdose of various CCBs.[84] All CCBs are highly protein bound.[68] Volumes of distribution are large for verapamil (5.5 L/kg) and diltiazem (5.3 L/kg), and somewhat smaller for nifedipine (0.8 L/kg). Although not well studied, the substantial protein binding and the large volumes of distribution make it unlikely that extracorporeal drug removal with hemodialysis or hemoperfusion would be of any value in overdose. Several case reports offer clinical support for this conclusion.[89,104]

One interesting aspect of the pharmacology of CCBs is their potential for drug–drug interactions. CYP3A4, which metabolizes most CCBs, is also responsible for the initial oxidation of numerous other xenobiotics. Verapamil and diltiazem specifically compete for this isoenzyme and can decrease the clearance of many drugs including carbamazepine, cisapride, quinidine, various β-hydroxy-β-methylglutaryl-coenzyme A (HMG-CoA) reductase inhibitors, cyclosporine, tacrolimus, most HIV-protease inhibitors, and theophylline (see Chap. 12 Appendix).[33,78] In June 1998, mibefradil, a structurally unique CCB, was voluntarily withdrawn following several reports of serious adverse drug interactions caused in part by its potent inhibition of CYP3A4.[58] Other inhibitors of CYP3A4, such as cimetidine, fluoxetine, some antifungals, macrolide antibiotics, and even the flavinoids in grapefruit juice, raise serum concentrations of several CCBs and may result in toxicity.[32,93]

In addition to affecting CYP3A4, verapamil and diltiazem also inhibit P-glycoprotein–mediated drug transport into peripheral tissue—an inhibition that results in elevated serum concentrations of xenobiotics such as cyclosporine and digoxin that use this transport system (Chap. 12 Appendix). Unlike diltiazem and verapamil, nifedipine and the other dihydropyridines do not appear to affect the clearance of other xenobiotics via CYP3A4 or P-glycoprotein–mediated transport.[1]

PHYSIOLOGY AND PATHOPHYSIOLOGY

Calcium initiates excitation-contraction coupling and myocardial conduction (Fig. 60–1; see Chap. 22 and 23). Ca^{2+} enters the cardiac myocyte through L-type calcium channels and follows electrochemical gradients.[66] The alpha$_{1c}$ subunit is the pore-forming portion of this channel and is where all CCBs bind to prevent Ca^{2+} transport.[12,83] In myocardial cells, this Ca^{2+} influx is slower relative to the initial sodium influx that initiates cellular depolarization, and prolongs this

TABLE 60–1. Classification of Calcium Channel Blockers Available in the United States

Phenylalkylamine
Verapamil (Calan, Isoptin, Verelan)
Benzothiazepine
Diltiazem (Cardizem, Dilacor, Tiazac)
Dihydropyridines
Nifedipine (Adalat, Procardia)
Amlodipine (Norvasc)
Clevidipine (Cleviprex)
Felodipine (Plendil)
Isradipine (DynaCirc)
Nicardipine (Cardene)
Nimodipine (Nimotop)
Nisoldipine (Sular)

depolarization, creating the plateau phase (phase 2) of the action potential. The Ca^{2+} subsequently stimulates a receptor-operated calcium channel on the sarcoplasmic reticulum, known as the ryanodine receptor (RyR2), releasing Ca^{2+} from the vast stores of the sarcoplasmic reticulum into the cytosol.[74] This is often termed calcium-dependent calcium release. Calcium then binds troponin C, which causes a conformational change that displaces troponin and tropomyosin from actin, allowing actin and myosin to bind, resulting in a contraction (see Fig. 23–2).[16,24]

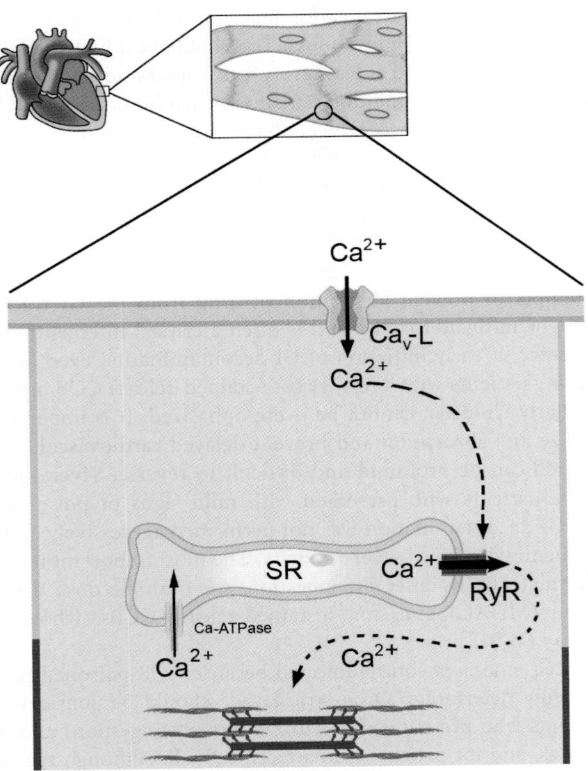

FIGURE 60–1. Normal contraction of myocardial cells. The L-type voltage sensitive calcium channels (Ca_V-L) open to allow calcium ion influx during myocyte depolarization. This causes the concentration-dependent release of more calcium ions from the ryanodyne receptor (RyR) of the sarcoplasmic reticulum (SR) that ultimately produce cardiac contraction.

In addition to its role in myocardial contractility, Ca^{2+} influx is also important in myocardial conduction. Calcium influx plays an important role in the spontaneous depolarization (phase 4) of the action potential in the SA node. This Ca^{2+} influx also allows normal propagation of electrical impulses via the specialized myocardial conduction tissues, particularly the AV node.[85] After opening, the rate of recovery of these slow calcium channels, in both the SA and AV nodal tissue, determines rate of conduction.[107]

In smooth muscle, calcium influx stimulates myosin light-chain kinase activity through calmodulin.[66] The myosin light-chain kinase phosphorylates, and thus activates, myosin, which subsequently binds actin, causing a contraction to occur.[66]

The life-threatening toxicities of CCBs are manifested largely within the cardiovascular system and are an extension of their therapeutic effects. Inhibition of L-type-voltage–sensitive calcium channels is particularly significant in the myocardium and smooth muscle, which are dependant on this influx for normal function. In the myocardium, this impaired Ca^{2+} flow results in a decreased force of contraction. In addition, the delay in recovery of the slow calcium channels in the SA and AV nodal tissue results in decreased heart rate and conduction. In the vascular smooth muscle, the cytosolic Ca^{2+} concentration maintains basal tone and any decrease of Ca^{2+} influx results in relaxation and arterial vasodilation.[45]

The pharmacological differences among CCBs on the myocardium and the vascular smooth muscle is the result of their different affinities for the various L-type calcium channels.[1,28] In the myocardium, verapamil has the most marked effects, while diltiazem has less and dihydropyridines have little, if any, effect at therapeutic doses.[51] In fact, in several experimental models, nifedipine does not alter the recovery of myocardial calcium channels.[57] In addition, not only do verapamil and, to a lesser extent, diltiazem impede Ca^{2+} influx and channel recovery in the myocardium, but their blockade is potentiated as the frequency of channel opening increases.[34,75] Therefore, in a frequently contracting tissue, such as the myocardium, the blockade of verapamil and diltiazem would be augmented. In the peripheral vascular tissue, dihydropyridines have the most potent vasodilatory effects; verapamil is the next most potent, followed by diltiazem. Dihydropyridines bind the calcium channel best at less-negative membrane potentials. Because the resting potential for myocardial muscle (–90 mV) is lower than that of vascular smooth muscle (–70 mV), dihydropyridines bind preferentially in the peripheral vascular tissue.[75]

Consequently, verapamil is the most effective at decreasing heart rate, cardiac output, and blood pressure, whereas the dihydropyridines produce the greatest decrease in systemic vascular resistance. Because dihydropyridines have limited myocardial effect at therapeutic concentrations, the baroreceptor reflex remains intact and a slight increase in heart rate and cardiac output may occur. Isradipine is the only dihydropyridine whose inhibitory effect on the SA node is significant enough to blunt any reflex tachycardia.

CLINICAL MANIFESTATIONS

Myocardial depression and peripheral vasodilation occur, producing bradycardia and hypotension.[90] Myocardial conduction may be impaired, producing AV conduction abnormalities, idioventricular rhythms, and complete heart block.[8,29,41,44,63,77] Junctional escape rhythms frequently occur in patients with significant poisonings.[20,27] The negative inotropic effects may be so profound, particularly with verapamil, that ventricular contraction may be completely inhibited.[11,27,36] Patients may initially be asymptomatic but deteriorate rapidly and develop cardiogenic shock.[95,109]

Hypotension is the most common abnormal vital sign finding following a CCB overdose.[81] The associated clinical findings represent the degree of cardiovascular compromise and hypoperfusion of the central nervous system (CNS). Early or mild symptoms include dizziness, fatigue, and lightheadedness, whereas more severely poisoned patients may manifest lethargy, syncope, altered mental status, coma, and death.[41,76] Seizures,[38,41] cerebral ischemic events,[87,92] ischemic bowel,[98,110] and renal failure,[77] occurring in the presence of CCB-induced cardiogenic shock, also are reported. Severe CNS depression is distinctly uncommon, and if respiratory depression or coma is present without severe hypotension, coingestants or other causes of altered mental status must be considered. Gastrointestinal (GI) symptoms, such as nausea and vomiting, are also uncommon.[42]

Although receptor selectivity is lost in overdose, and all CCBs can produce severe bradycardia, hypotension, and death, there are some subtle variations in presentation, depending on the xenobiotic. The CCBs with the most significant myocardial effects, verapamil and, to a lesser extent, diltiazem, are associated with more negative inotropic and chronotropic effects.[72] In a prospective, poison center–based study, AV nodal block occurred much more frequently in the setting of verapamil poisoning.[80] In contrast, nifedipine, and likely the other dihydropyridines because of their limited myocardial binding, may produce tachycardia or a "normal" heart rate initially, with bradycardia developing only in patients with more substantial ingestions.[19,112] While deaths are much more commonly associated with verapamil and diltiazem, they nevertheless occur with the dihydropyridines.

Numerous reports document hyperglycemia in patients with severe CCB poisoning.[38,41,61] Insulin release from the β-islet cells in the pancreas is dependent on calcium influx via an L-type calcium channel. In CCB overdose, this channel is blocked, reducing insulin release.[23] This may be due to dysregulation of the insulin-dependent phosphatidylinositol 3-kinase pathway.[9] The hyperglycemic effect may be exacerbated in a diabetic patient, or if glucagon is used as inotropic therapy (Chap. 48).[105]

Acute pulmonary injury is also associated with CCB poisoning.[43,49,60] Although the mechanism is unknown, precapillary vasodilation may cause an increase in transcapillary hydrostatic pressure.[43] The elevated pressure gradient results in increased pulmonary capillary transudates and, ultimately, interstitial edema.

Several factors, including the CCB involved, the dose ingested, the product formulation, and the patient's underlying cardiovascular health, may play a role in the ultimate degree of toxicity. Coingestion with other cardioactive xenobiotics, such as β-adrenergic antagonists and digoxin, may potentiate conduction abnormalities.[15,47,118]

The product formulation (immediate or regular versus sustained release) affects the onset of symptoms and duration of toxicity. With regular-release formulations, toxicity is often present within 2 to 3 hours of ingestion.[10,81] With sustained-release products, however, initial signs or symptoms may be delayed for 6 to 8 hours, and delays of up to 15 hours are reported.[10,81,97] In addition, with ingestion of sustained-release products, the apparent half-life is prolonged and toxicity may last longer than 48 hours.[3,8,27]

Comorbidity and age are two factors that negatively impact both morbidity and mortality in patients with CCB poisoning. Elderly patients, and those with underlying cardiovascular disease such as congestive heart failure, are much more sensitive to the myocardial depressant effects of CCBs.[67] Even at therapeutic doses, these individuals more frequently develop symptoms of mild hypoperfusion, such as dizziness and fatigue.[37,70] One or two tablets of any of the CCBs may produce significant poisoning in toddlers.[10,82]

DIAGNOSTIC TESTING

All patients with suspected CCB ingestions should have continuous cardiac monitoring and a 12-lead electrocardiogram (ECG) performed to assess heart rate and rhythm, as well as any conduction abnormalities. Careful assessment of the degree of hypoperfusion, if any, may include pulse oximetry and serum chemistry analysis for metabolic acidosis. Assays for various CCB serum concentrations are not routinely available and are not used to manage patients after overdose. If a patient presents with bradydysrhythmias of unclear origin, assessment of electrolytes, particularly potassium and magnesium, renal function, and a digoxin concentration, may be helpful, although careful history taking often provides the most valuable clues. If hyperkalemia is present, cardioactive steroid poisoning should be considered, particularly in the absence of renal failure. Acute lung injury can be initially assessed by auscultation, pulse oximetry, and chest radiography.

Because calcium channel blocker poisoning can impair insulin secretion from the pancreas, hyperglycemia may be detected. A recent retrospective study suggests that serum glucose concentrations correlate with the severity of the poisoning. The initial mean serum glucose concentration in patients who required vasopressors or a pacemaker, or who died, was 188 mg/dL versus 122 mg/dL in those not requiring intervention. Peak serum glucose concentrations were also significantly different.[61] This finding may become a useful early sign of severity and an indicator for when to initiate hyperinsulinemia-euglycemia therapy.

MANAGEMENT

Any patient with a suspected CCB ingestion should be immediately evaluated, even if there are no abnormal clinical findings and the initial vital signs are normal. Intravenous access should be initiated. A 12-lead ECG should be repeated at least every 1 to 2 hours for the first several hours. If the patient's condition remains normal (or normalizes), ECGs can be repeated subsequently at longer intervals. Initial treatment should begin with adequate oxygenation and airway protection (as clinically indicated), and aggressive GI decontamination. For a patient who is hypotensive with no evidence of congestive heart failure or acute lung injury, an initial fluid bolus of 10 to 20 mL/kg of crystalloid should be given, and repeated as needed.

Attempts to prevent absorption of drug from the GI tract may prevent or mitigate toxicity and is often a critical intervention. The importance of early initiation of GI decontamination even for well-appearing patients with a history of sustained-release CCB ingestion, particularly children, cannot be overemphasized. It is imperative to minimize any absorption and prevent delayed cardiovascular toxicity, which can be profound and difficult to reverse. Several reports describe patients who presented with mild signs of poisoning, in whom GI decontamination was not performed aggressively and who subsequently displayed severe toxicity. The most important measures to eliminate CCBs after an ingestion are multiple-dose activated charcoal (MDAC) and, for sustained-release CCBs, whole-bowel irrigation (WBI).

Induced emesis is contraindicated because CCB-poisoned patients can rapidly deteriorate. Orogastric lavage should be considered for all patients who present early (1 to 2 hours postingestion) after large ingestions, and for patients who are critically ill. Although the effects of orogastric lavage following overdose of a sustained-release CCB have not been specifically studied, and although most of these formulations tend to be large and poorly soluble, because of their significant danger in overdose, orogastric lavage should still be strongly considered. When performing orogastric lavage in a CCB-poisoned patient, it is important to remember that lavage may increase vagal tone and potentially exacerbate any bradydysrhythmias.[106] Pretreatment with a therapeutic dose of atropine may prevent this.

All patients with CCB ingestions should receive 1 g/kg of activated charcoal orally. Multiple doses (0.5 g/kg) of activated charcoal (MDAC) without a cathartic should be administered to nearly all patients with either sustained-release pill ingestions or signs of continuing absorption. Although data are limited, there is no evidence that MDAC increases CCB clearance from the serum.[84] Rather, its efficacy may be a result of the continuous presence of activated charcoal throughout the GI tract, which adsorbs any active xenobiotic from its slow-release formulation. MDAC should not be administered to a patient with inadequate GI function (eg, hypotensive, no bowel sounds; see Antidotes in Depth A2–Activated Charcoal).

WBI with polyethylene glycol solution (1 to 2 L/h orally or via nasogastric tube in adults, up to 500 mL/h in children) should be initiated for patients who ingest sustained-release products.[14] Administration should be continued until the rectal effluent is clear (see Antidotes in Depth A3–Whole-Bowel Irrigation and Other Intestinal Evacuants).

There are no data to clearly support extracorporeal removal, and its use is generally limited by the hemodynamic effects of the CCBs.[86]

Pharmacotherapy should focus on maintenance or improvement of both cardiac output and peripheral vascular tone. Although atropine, calcium, insulin, glucagon, isoproterenol, dopamine, epinephrine, norepinephrine, and phosphodiesterase inhibitors, have been used with reported success in CCB-poisoned patients, no single intervention has consistently demonstrated total efficacy. Little prospective or basic research specifically evaluates effective treatment modalities.

Therapy should begin with crystalloids and atropine, but more critically poisoned patients will not respond to these initial efforts, and inotropes and vasopressors will be needed. Although it would be ideal to initiate each therapy individually and monitor the patient's hemodynamic response, in the most critically ill patients, multiple therapies should be administered simultaneously. A reasonable treatment sequence includes calcium followed by a catecholamine such as epinephrine or norepinephrine, hyperinsulinemia-euglycemia therapy, glucagon, and perhaps a phosphodiesterase inhibitor. In addition, in the event of a cardiac arrest, a 20% intravenous fat emulsion may be administered.

ATROPINE

Atropine is considered by many to be the drug of choice for patients with symptomatic bradycardia. In an early dog model of verapamil poisoning, atropine improved heart rate and cardiac output.[31] In one prospective study, two of eight bradycardic CCB-poisoned patients also had an improvement in heart rate with atropine therapy.[80] Clinical experience, however, demonstrates atropine to be largely ineffective in improving heart rate in severe CCB-poisoned patients.[76,95] Initial treatment with calcium might improve the efficacy of atropine.[42] Given its availability, familiarity, efficacy in mild poisonings, and safety profile, atropine should still be considered as initial therapy in patients with symptomatic bradycardia. Dosing should begin with 0.5 to 1.0 mg (0.02 mg/kg in children) minimum 0.1mg) intravenously (IV) every 2 or 3 minutes up to a maximum dose of 3 mg in all patients with symptomatic bradycardia. However, because of its limited efficacy in severely poisoned patients, treatment failures should be anticipated. In patients in whom WBI or MDAC will be used, the use of atropine must be carefully considered, weighing the potential benefits of improved heart rate, and thus cardiac output, against the anticholinergic effects, potentially decreasing GI motility.

CALCIUM

Pharmacologically, Ca^{2+} appears to be a logical choice to treat patients with CCB toxicity. Pretreatment with intravenous Ca^{2+}, prior to verapamil use for supraventricular tachydysrhythmias, prevents hypotension without diminishing the antidysrhythmic efficacy.[25,94] This is also observed in the overdose setting where Ca^{2+} tends to improve blood pressure more than it does the heart rate. Although the exact mechanism is unclear, boluses of Ca^{2+} increase the extracellular Ca^{2+} concentration and increase the transmembrane concentration gradient. Calcium salts are beneficial in experimental models of CCB poisoning.[31,36] In verapamil-poisoned dogs, improvement in inotropy and blood pressure was demonstrated after increasing the serum Ca^{2+} concentration by 2 mEq/L with an intravenous infusion of 10% calcium chloride ($CaCl_2$) at 3 mg/kg/min.[36]

Calcium ion reverses the negative inotropy, impaired conduction, and hypotension in humans poisoned by CCBs.[14,59,62,70] Unfortunately, this effect is often short lived and more severely poisoned patients may not improve significantly with Ca^{2+} administration.[18,21,84,89] Although some authors believe that these failures might represent inadequate dosing,[14,42,59] optimal effective dosing of Ca^{2+} is unclear. Moreover, if there is any suspicion that a cardioactive steroid such as digoxin is involved in an overdose, Ca^{2+} should be avoided until after digoxin-specific Fab is administered because of concerns that it may worsen digoxin toxicity (Chap. 64 and A 20).[13] Reasonable recommendations for poisoned adults include an initial intravenous infusion of approximately 13 to 25 mEq of Ca^{2+} (10 to 20 mL of 10% calcium chloride or 30 to 60 mL of 10% calcium gluconate) followed by either repeat boluses every 15 to 20 minutes up to three to four doses or a continuous infusion of 0.5 mEq/kg/h of Ca^{2+} (0.2 to 0.4 mL/kg/h of 10% calcium chloride or 0.6 to 1.2 mL of 10% calcium gluconate; see Antidotes in Depth A19–Glucagon).[72] Careful selection and attention to the type of calcium salt used is critical for dosing. Although there is no difference in efficacy of calcium chloride or calcium gluconate, 1 g of calcium chloride contains 13.4 mEq of Ca^{2+}, which is more than three times the 4.3 mEq found in 1 g of calcium gluconate. Consequently, to administer equal doses of Ca^{2+}, three times the volume of calcium gluconate compared with that of calcium chloride is required. The main limitation of using calcium chloride, however, is that it has significant potential for causing tissue injury if extravasated, so administration should ideally be via central venous access. If repeat dosing or continuous infusions are necessary serum Ca^{2+} and PO_4^{-3} concentrations should be closely monitored to detect developing hypercalcemia or hypophosphatemia. These concerns are not unfounded, and may in fact significantly limit Ca^{2+} therapy. Other adverse effects of intravenous Ca^{2+} include nausea, vomiting, flushing, constipation, confusion, and angina.

INOTROPES AND VASOPRESSORS

Catecholamines are the next line of therapy in the treatment of CCB poisoning. Numerous case reports describe the success or failure of a wide variety of vasopressors, including epinephrine (success,[18] failure[38,63]), norepinephrine (success,[41] failure[63]), dopamine (success,[3] failure[18,38,63]), isoproterenol (success,[77] failure[38]), dobutamine (success,[77] failure[21,63]), and vasopressin.[31,48,101] Experimentally, no single therapy is consistently effective. This is not surprising, given the significant variability in both the CCBs and the patients involved. Mechanistically, however, stimulation of either β_1-adrenergic receptors on the myocardium or α_1-adrenergic receptors on the peripheral vascular smooth muscle is the most logical target, but which one depends upon the etiology of the hypotension.

β-Adrenergic agonists activate adenylate cyclase via G_s protein, resulting in formation of cyclic adenosine monophosphate (cAMP), which stimulates protein kinase A to phosphorylate the α_1 subunit of various calcium channels (Fig. 60–2).[96] It is unclear whether this phosphorylation allows calcium channels to remain open longer,[19] or if

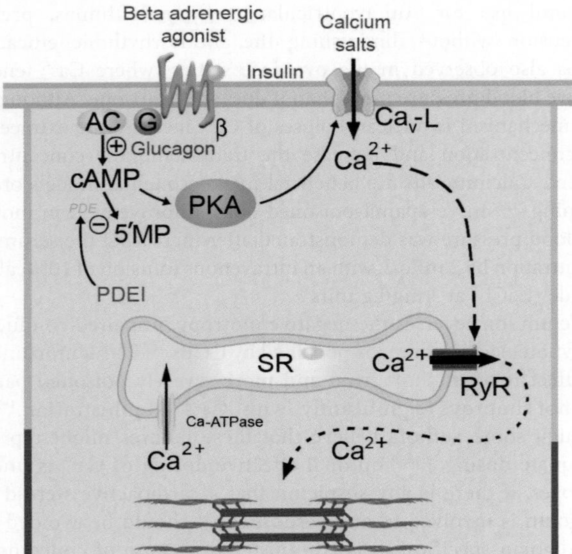

FIGURE 60–2. Myocardial toxicity of calcium channel blockers and use of antidotal therapies. Calcium channel blockers reduce calcium ion influx through the L-type calcium channel (Ca$_V$-L) and thus reduce contractility. Mechanisms to increase intracellular calcium include recruitment of new or dormant calcium channels by increasing cyclic adenosine monophosphate (cAMP) either by stimulating its formation by adenyl cyclase (AC) with catecholamines or glucagon (see text), or by inhibiting its degradation to 5′-monophosphate with phosphodiesterase inhibitors (PDEI) such as amrinone. Increasing the calcium concentration gradient across the cellular membrane to further its influx may improve contractility. The mechanism by which insulin therapy enhances inotropy is not fully known. PKA, protein kinase A; RyR = ryanodyne receptor.

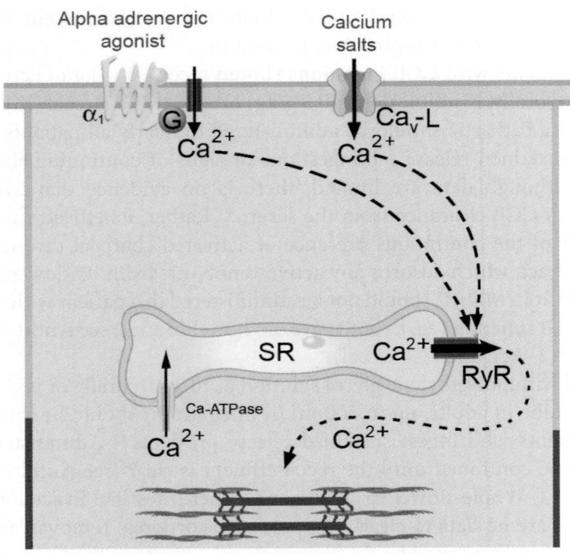

FIGURE 60–3. Vascular toxicity of calcium channel blockers and antidotal therapies. Calcium's entry via voltage-sensitive channels (Ca$_V$-L) initiates a cascade of events that result in actin-myosin coupling and contraction; this is inhibited by calcium channel blockers. Mechanisms to increase intracellular calcium include activation of receptor-operated calcium channels with α_1-adrenergic agonists or increasing the calcium ion gradient across the cellular membrane to further its influx; RyR = ryanodyne receptor.

it opens dormant channels within the plasma membrane. In addition, protein kinase A also phosphorylates phospholamban, which improves calcium release from troponin after contraction.[100] In the myocardium, this multifactorial increase in intracellular calcium results in improved chronotropy, dromotropy, and inotropy.

In the peripheral vascular smooth muscle, α_1-adrenergic receptor agonists activate receptor-operated calcium channels. This opening of nonpoisoned calcium channels allows calcium influx (Fig. 60–3), which makes α_1-adrenergic agonists such as norepinephrine and phenylephrine logical choices if the hypotension is primarily the result of peripheral vasodilation, as would occur most typically with the dihydropyridine CCBs. Based on these pharmacologic mechanisms, and on experimental data epinephrine, or perhaps norepinephrine, appears to be the most an appropriate initial catecholamine to use in hypotensive CCB-poisoned patients. The significant β_1-adrenergic activity of both catecholamines combat the myocardial depressant effects, while the α_1-adrenergic agonist effects of norepinephrine (more so than epinephrine) increase peripheral vascular resistance if desired. There is some theoretical concern about using pure β-adrenergic receptor agonists, such as isoproterenol and, to a lesser extent, dobutamine, because β_2-adrenergic receptor agonist–induced peripheral vasodilation may worsen hypotension, particularly at high doses.

Dopamine is predominantly an indirect acting pressor that acts by stimulating the release of norepinephrine from the distal nerve terminal, and not by direct α- and β-adrenergic receptor stimulation. This may limit its effectiveness in severely stressed patients who may have catecholamine depletion.[109] Published clinical experience of patients with severe CCB poisonings support these concerns.[20,38,63,109] Improvement in blood pressure may be noted with dopamine at high dosing, when it has additional direct α- and β-adrenergic effects.

The choice of a catecholamine is based on numerous factors, including the individual pharmacologic profile, the patient's underlying physiologic condition, and the physician's familiarity and comfort with the medication. If one catecholamine is unsuccessful, determining the cardiac output and systemic vascular resistance may be helpful in assessing whether the myocardial depressant or peripheral vasodilatory effects are responsible for the hypotension.[76] This knowledge will help guide the subsequent choice of pharmacologic agents.

GLUCAGON

Glucagon is an endogenous polypeptide hormone secreted by the pancreatic α cells in response to hypoglycemia and catecholamines. In addition, it has significant inotropic and chronotropic effects (see Antidotes in Depth A19–Glucagon).[17,99] Glucagon is a therapy of choice for β-adrenergic antagonist poisoning (Chap. 61) because of its ability to bypass the β-adrenergic receptor and activate adenylate cyclase via a G_s protein in the myocardium.[115] Thus, glucagon is unique in that it is functionally a "pure" β_1 agonist, with no peripheral vasodilatory effects. However, in CCB poisoning, because the cellular lesion is "downstream" from adenylate cyclase, glucagon offers no pharmacologic advantage over more traditional β-adrenergic agents (see Fig. 60–2).[4] There are reports of both successes[26] and failures[20,38] of glucagon in CCB-poisoned patients who failed to respond to fluids, Ca^{2+}, or dopamine and dobutamine.

Dosing for glucagon is not well established.[4] An initial dose of 3 to 5 mg IV, slowly over 1 to 2 minutes, is reasonable in adults, and if there is no hemodynamic improvement within 5 minutes, retreatment with a dose of 4 to 10 mg may be effective. The initial pediatric dose is 50 μg/kg.

Because of the short half-life of glucagon repeat doses may be useful. A maintenance infusion should be initiated once a desired effect is achieved (see Antidotes in Depth A19–Glucagon). Adverse effects include vomiting and hyperglycemia, particularly in diabetics or during continuous infusion.[105]

INSULIN AND GLUCOSE

Hyperinsulinemia euglycemia (HIE) therapy has become the treatment of choice for patients who are severely poisoned by CCBs.[61,69] Healthy myocardial tissue relies predominantly on free fatty acids for their metabolic needs and CCB poisoning forces them to become more carbohydrate dependent.[52,55,56] At the same time, CCBs inhibit calcium-mediated insulin secretion from the β-islet cells in the pancreas,[23,71] resulting in glucose uptake in myocardial cells becoming dependent upon concentration gradients rather than insulin-mediated active transport.[53] In addition, there is evidence that the CCB-poisoned myocardium also becomes insulin resistant possibly by dysregulation of the phosphatidylinositol 3 kinase pathway.[9,54] This may not allow normal recruitment of insulin-responsive glucose transporter proteins.[9] The combination of inhibition of insulin secretion and impaired glucose utilization may explain why severe CCB toxicity often produces significant hyperglycemia and may be a marker for the severity of poisoning (see Antidotes in Depth A18–Insulin-Euglycemia Therapy).[61]

There are now several reported cases of CCB-poisoned patients in whom adjuvant HIEG therapy successfully improved hemodynamic function mainly by improving contractility, with little effect on heart rate.[65,108,117] There are reports of the failure of this treatment,[22] but this may represent initiation of therapy in terminally ill patients with multiple organ failure.

Although the dose of insulin is not definitively established, therapy typically begins with a bolus of 1 Unit/kg of regular human insulin along with 0.5 g/kg of dextrose. If blood glucose is greater than 400 mg/dL (22.2 mmol/L), the dextrose bolus is not necessary. An infusion of regular insulin should follow the bolus starting at 0.5 Units/kg/h titrated up to 2 Units/kg/h if no improvement after 30 minutes. A continuous dextrose infusion, beginning at 0.5 g/kg/h should also be started. Glucose should be monitored every half hour for the first 4 hours and titrated to maintain euglycemia. The response to insulin is typically delayed for 15 to 60 minutes so it will usually be necessary to start a catecholamine infusion before the full effects of insulin are apparent.[35,69]

PHOSPHODIESTERASE INHIBITORS

Another class of therapeutics that has some demonstrated usefulness in treating CCB poisoning is the cardiac and vascular phosphodiesterase 3 inhibitors: inamrinone, milrinone, and enoximone. These agents inhibit the breakdown of cAMP by phosphodiesterase, thereby increasing intracellular cAMP concentrations. These noncatecholamine inotropic agents do not disproportionately increase myocardial oxygen demand and have been traditionally used for congestive heart failure (see Fig. 60–2).[5] This inhibition results in increased cAMP, increased intracellular calcium, and improved inotropy. Inamrinone improved myocardial contractility in two canine models of verapamil poisoning.[2,64] In addition, phosphodiesterase inhibitors have been reported to be clinically successful in patients with CCB poisoning when used in combination with another inotrope, such as isoproterenol or glucagon.[88,113,114] This "two-pronged" approach of increasing myocardial cAMP concentrations, by stimulating its formation and inhibiting its breakdown, is pharmacologically rational. However, because of the nonselective inhibition of phosphodiesterase 3 by these inhibitors, cAMP is also increased in the vascular smooth muscle. This causes smooth muscle relaxation, peripheral vasodilation and, unfortunately often, hypotension, which may severely limit its usefulness in many CCB-poisoned patients. Phosphodiesterase inhibitors should be used only as second-line agents, in combination with another inotrope and preferably in patients with hemodynamic monitoring. Dosing in the treatment of CCB-poisoned patients is not well defined, but should be based on traditional dosing for congestive heart failure. For inamrinone, the experimental data and the case reports suggest that an initial bolus of 1 mg/kg over 2 minutes followed by a continuous infusion of 5 to 20 μg/kg/min is appropriate.[2,113]

EXPERIMENTAL ANTIDOTES

In animal models intravenous fat emulsions (IFE) decreases the toxicity of a few lipid-soluble drugs, most notably bupivacaine. Other models suggest that IFE is an effective therapy for CCB-poisoned patients.[7,73,102,111] This mechanism is most likely pharmacokinetic in nature, in that IFE incorporates these highly cardiotoxic drugs and thus lower the free or effective serum drug concentrations.[7,111] Until more data are available, IFE should be considered adjuvant therapy for critically ill, preterminal CCB-poisoned patients (see Antidotes in Depth A21–Intravenous Fat Emulsion).

Digoxin has been experimentally evaluated in CCB poisoning since inhibiting the sodium/potassium adenosine triphosphatase (ATPase), the cardioactive steroids raise the intracellular Ca^{2+} concentration.[6] In a canine model of verapamil poisoning, digoxin, in conjunction with atropine or calcium, improved both systolic blood pressure and myocardial inotropy.[6,79] However, because digoxin requires a significant amount of time to distribute into tissue, and because limited efficacy data and no safety data have yet been collected, more work is needed before digoxin is administered to patients with CCB poisoning.

ADJUNCTIVE HEMODYNAMIC SUPPORT

The most severely CCB-poisoned patients may not respond to any pharmacologic intervention.[27,38] Transthoracic or intravenous cardiac pacing may be required to improve heart rate, as several case reports demonstrate.[95,109] However, in a prospective cohort of CCB poisonings, two of four patients with significant bradycardia requiring electrical pacing had no electrical capture.[80] In addition, even if electrical pacing is effective in increasing the heart rate, blood pressure often remains unchanged.[40,41]

Intraaortic balloon counterpulsation is another invasive supportive option to be considered in CCB poisoning refractory to pharmacologic therapy. Intraaortic balloon counterpulsation was used successfully to improve cardiac output and blood pressure in a patient with a mixed verapamil and atenolol overdose.[30] The synchronized inflation and deflation is dependent on regular cardiac electrical activity, so cardiac pacing is often required in addition to the intraaortic balloon. It is important to remember that CCB-poisoned patients typically have a much better prognosis than patients with severe left ventricular failure from ischemic heart disease, in whom this technology is traditionally used. Between 24 and 48 hours of assisted cardiac output allows metabolism and elimination of the CCBs and a return of baseline myocardial function.

Severely CCB-poisoned patients have also been supported for days and subsequently recovered fully with much more invasive and technologically demanding extracorporeal membrane oxygenation (ECMO) and emergent open and percutaneous cardiopulmonary bypass.[27,38,40] The major limitation of all these technologies, however, is that they are available only at tertiary care facilities.

DISPOSITION

Every patient who manifests any signs or symptoms of toxicity should be admitted to an intensive care setting. Because of the potential for delayed toxicity, despite some recommendations to the contrary,[10] any patient ingesting sustained-release products should be admitted for 24 hours to a monitored setting, even if asymptomatic. This is particularly important for toddlers and small children in whom just one or a few tablets may produce significant toxicity.[10,38,82] All admitted patients should be treated with activated charcoal, and those with a history of sustained-release product ingestion should be treated with WBI. Only patients with a reliable history of an "immediate-release" preparation ingestion who have received adequate gastrointestinal decontamination, have serial ECGs over 6 to 8 hours that have remained unchanged, and are asymptomatic can be "medically cleared" for disposition. Patients with unintentional overdose may be discharged at this point, and those whose poisoning is intentional typically receive psychiatric evaluation.

SUMMARY

Calcium channel blockers are commonly used to treat hypertension, stable and vasospastic angina, dysrhythmias, migraine headaches, Raynaud phenomenon, and subarachnoid hemorrhage. Hallmarks of toxicity include bradydysrhythmias and hypotension, which are an extension of the pharmacologic effects of these agents. Although most patients develop symptoms of hypoperfusion, such as lightheadedness, nausea, or fatigue, within hours of a significant ingestion, sustained-release formulations may significantly delay any and all hemodynamic consequences and certainly may prolong toxicity.

Because of the significant lethality of large ingestions of sustained-release CCBs, it is imperative to make GI decontamination with WBI a high priority. Aggressive decontamination of patients with exposures to sustained-release products should begin as soon as possible and should not be delayed by waiting for signs of toxicity.[103] Once hemodynamic toxicity develops, in addition to supportive care, pharmacologic treatment with HIE and calcium salt boluses should be initiated. Traditional catecholamines are also typically needed, but their use alone may not be sufficient for the most critically poisoned patients. Other therapeutic options include the use of glucagon, phosphodiesterase inhibitors, and possibly IFE. Patients who fail to respond to all pharmaceutical interventions should be considered for extracorporeal mechanical support whenever available.

REFERENCES

1. Abernethy DR, Schwartz JB. Calcium-antagonist drugs. *N Engl J Med.* 1999; 341:1447-1457.
2. Alousi AA, Canter JM, Fort DJ. The beneficial effect of amrinone on acute drug-induced heart failure in the anaesthetised dog. *Cardiovasc Res.* 1985;19:483-494.
3. Ashraf M, Chaudhary K, Nelson J, Thompson W. Massive overdose of sustained-release verapamil: a case report and review of literature. *Am J Med Sci.* 1995;310:258-263.
4. Bailey B. Glucagon in β-blocker and calcium channel blocker overdoses: a systematic review. *J Toxicol Clin Toxicol* 2003;41:595-602.
5. Baim DS. Effect of phosphodiesterase inhibition on myocardial oxygen consumption and coronary blood flow. *Am J Cardiol.* 1989;63:23A-26A.
6. Bania TC, Chu J, Almond G, Perez E. Dose-dependent hemodynamic effect of digoxin therapy in severe verapamil toxicity. *Acad Emerg Med.* 2004;11:221-227.
7. Bania TC, Chu J, Perez, E, Su M, Hahn IH. Hemodynamic effects of intravenous fat emulsion in an animal model of severe verapamil toxicity resuscitated with atropine, calcium, and saline. *Acad Emerg Med.* 2007;14: 105-111.
8. Barrow PM, Houston PL, Wong DT. Overdose of sustained-release verapamil. *Br J Anaesth.* 1994;72:361-365.
9. Bechtel LK, Haverstick DM, Holstege CP. Verapamil toxicity dysregulates the phophotidylinosotil 3-kinase pathway. *Acad Emerg Med.* 2008;15:368-374.
10. Belson MG, Gorman SE, Sullivan K, Geller RJ. Calcium channel blocker ingestions in children. *Am J Emerg Med* 2000;18:581-586.
11. Beniam ME. Asystole after verapamil. *Br Med J.* 1972;2:169-170.
12. Bodi I, Mikala G, Koch SE, Akhter SA, Schwartz A. The L-type calcium channel in the heart. the beat goes on. *J Clin Invest.* 2005;115:3306-3317.
13. Bower JO, Mengle HAK. The additive effects of calcium and digitalis: a warning with a report of two deaths. *JAMA.* 1936;106:1151-1153.
14. Buckley N, Dawson AH, Howarth D, Whyte IM. Slow-release verapamil poisoning. Use of polyethylene glycol whole-bowel lavage and high-dose calcium. *Med J Aust.* 1993;158:202-204.
15. Carruthers SG, Freeman DJ, Gailey DG. Synergistic adverse hemo-dynamic interaction between oral verapamil and propranolol. *Clin Pharmacol Ther.* 1989;46:469-477.
16. Chakraborti S, Das S, Kar P, et al. Calcium signaling phenomena in heart diseases: a perspective. *Mol Cell Biochem.* 2007;298:1-40.
17. Chernow B, Zagola GP, Malcolm D, et al. Glucagon's chronotropic action is calcium dependent. *J Pharmacol Exp Ther.* 1987;241:833-837.
18. Chimienti M, Previtali M, Medici A, Piccinini M. Acute verapamil poisoning: successful treatment with epinephrine. *Clin Cardiol.* 1982;5: 219-222.
19. Clifton DG, Booth DC, Hobbs S, et al. Negative inotropic effect of intravenous nifedipine in coronary artery disease. Relation to plasma levels. *Am Heart J.* 1990;119:283-290.
20. Connolly DL, Nettleton MA, Bastow MD. Massive diltiazem overdose. *Am J Cardiol.* 1993;72:742-743.
21. Crump BJ, Holt DW, Vale JA. Lack of response to intravenous calcium in severe verapamil poisoning. *Lancet.* 1982;2:939-940.
22. Cumpston K, Mycyk M, Pallasch E, et al. Failure of hyperinsulinemia/euglycemia therapy in severe overdose [abstract]. *J Toxicol Clin Toxicol.* 2002;40:618.
23. Devis G, Somers G, Van Obberghen E, Malaisse WJ. Calcium antagonists and islet function. I: inhibition of insulin release by verapamil. *Diabetes.* 1975;24:547-551.
24. Dibb KM, Graham HK, Venetucci LA, Eisner DA, Trafford AW. Analysis of cellular calcium fluxes in cardiac muscle to understand calcium homeostasis in the heart. *Cell Calcium.* 2007;42(4-5):503-512.
25. Dolan DL. Intravenous calcium before verapamil to prevent hypotension. *Ann Emerg Med.* 1991;20:588-589.
26. Doyon S, Roberts JR. The use of glucagon in a case of calcium channel blocker overdose. *Ann Emerg Med.* 1993;22:1229-1233.
27. Durward A, Guerguerian AM, Lefebvre M, Shemien SD. Massive diltiazem overdose treated with extracorporeal membrane oxygenation. *Pediatr Crit Care Med.* 2003;4:372-376.
28. Eisenberg MJ, Brox A, Bestawros AN. Calcium channel blockers: an update. *Am J Med.* 2004;116:35-43.
29. Fauville JP, Hantson P, Honore P, et al. Severe diltiazem poisoning with intestinal pseudo-obstruction: case report and toxicological data. *J Toxicol Clin Toxicol.* 1995;33:273-277.
30. Frierson J, Bailly D, Shultz T, et al. Refractory cardiogenic shock and complete heart block after unsuspected verapamil-SR and atenolol overdose. *Clin Cardiol.* 1991;14:933-935.
31. Gay R, Angeo S, Lee R, et al. Treatment of verapamil toxicity in intact dogs. *J Clin Invest.* 1986;77:1805-1811.
32. Geronimo-Pardo M, Cuartero-del-Pozo AB, Jimenez-Vizuete JM, et al. Clarithromycin-nifedipine interaction as possible cause of vasodilatory shock. *Ann Pharmacother.* 2005;39:538-542.
33. Gladding P, Pilmore H, Edwards C. Potentially fatal interaction between diltiazem and statins. *Ann Intern Med.* 2004;140:W31.
34. Grace AA, Camm AJ. Voltage-gated calcium-channels and antiar-rhythmic drug action. *Cardiovasc Res.* 2000;45:43-51.
35. Greene SL, Gawarammana I, Wood DM, et al. Relative safety of hyperinsulinaemia/euglycaemia therapy in the management of calcium channel blocker overdose: a prospective observational study. *Intensive Care Med.* 2007;33:2019-2024.
36. Hariman RJ, Mangiardi LM, McAllister RG, et al. Reversal of the cardiovascular effects of verapamil by calcium and sodium: differences between electrophysiologic and hemodynamic responses. *Circulation.* 1979;59:797-804.
37. Hattori VT, Mandel WJ, Peter T. Calcium for myocardial depression from verapamil. *N Engl J Med.* 1982;306:238.
38. Hendren WC, Schreiber RS, Garretson LK. Extracorporeal bypass for the treatment of verapamil poisoning. *Ann Emerg Med.* 1989;18:984-987.

39. Hermann PH, Rodger SD, Remones G, et al. Pharmacokinetics of diltiazem after intravenous and oral administration. *Eur J Clin Pharmacol.* 1983;24:349-352.
40. Holzer M, Sterz F, Schoerkhuber W, et al. Successful resuscitation of a verapamil-intoxicated patient with percutaneous cardiopulmonary bypass. *Crit Care Med.* 1999;27:2818-2823.
41. Horowitz BZ, Rhee KJ. Massive verapamil ingestion: a report of two cases and a review of the literature. *Am J Emerg Med.* 1989;7:624-631.
42. Howarth DM, Dawson AH, Smith AJ, Buckley N, Whyte IM. Calcium channel blocking drug overdose: an Australian series. *Hum Exp Toxicol.* 1994;13:161-166.
43. Humbert VH, Munn NJ, Hawkins RF. Noncardiogenic pulmonary edema complicating massive diltiazem overdose. *Chest.* 1991;99:258-260.
44. Ishikawa T, Imamura T, Koiwaya Y, Tanaka K. Atrioventricular dissociation and sinus arrest induced by oral diltiazem. *N Engl J Med.* 1983;309:1124-1125.
45. Johns A, Leijten P, Yamamoto H, et al. Calcium regulation in vascular smooth muscle contractility. *Am J Cardiol.* 1987;59:18A-23A.
46. Johnson KE, Balderston SM, Pieper JA, Mann E, Reiter MJ. Electrophysiologic effects of verapamil metabolites in the isolated heart. *J Cardiovasc Pharmacol.* 1991;17:830-837.
47. Jolly SR, Kipnis JN, Lucchesi BR. Cardiovascular depression by verapamil: reversal by glucagon and interactions with propranolol. *Pharmacology.* 1987;35:249-255.
48. Kanagarajan K, Marraffa JM, Bouchard NC, et al. The use of vasopressin in the setting of recalcitrant hypotension due to calcium channel blocker overdose. *Clin Toxicol.* 2007;45:56-59.
49. Karti S, Ulusoy H, Yandi M, et al. Non-cardiogenic pulmonary oedema in the course of verapamil intoxication. *Emerg Med J.* 2002;19:458-459.
50. Katz AM. Calcium channel diversity in the cardiovascular system. *J Am Coll Cardiol.* 1996;28:522-529.
51. Kawai C, Konishi T, Matsuyama E, Okazaki H. Comparative effects of three calcium antagonist, diltiazem, verapamil, and nifedipine, on the sinoatrial and atrioventricular nodes. *Circulation.* 1981;63:1035-1042.
52. Kline JA, Leonova E, Raymond RM. Beneficial myocardial metabolic effects of insulin during verapamil toxicity in the anesthetized canine. *Crit Care Med.* 1995;23:1251-1263.
53. Kline JA, Leonova E, Williams TC, et al. Myocardial metabolism during graded intraportal verapamil infusion in awake dogs. *J Cardiovasc Pharmacol.* 1996;27:719-726.
54. Kline JA, Raymond RM, Leonova E, et al. Insulin improves heart function and metabolism during non-ischemic cardiogenic shock in awake canines. *Cardiovasc Res.* 1997;34:289-298.
55. Kline JA, Raymond RM, Schroeder JD, Watts JA. The diabetogenic effects of acute verapamil poisoning. *Toxicol Appl Pharmacol.* 1997;145:357-362.
56. Kline JA, Tomaszewski CA, Schroeder JD, Raymond RM. Insulin is a superior antidote for cardiovascular toxicity induced by verapamil in the anesthetized canine. *J Pharm Exp Ther.* 1993;267:744-750.
57. Kochegarov AA. Pharmacological modulators of voltage-gated calcium channels and their therapeutical application. *Cell Calcium.* 2003;33:145-162.
58. Krayenbuhl JC, Vozeh S, Kondo-Oestreicher M, Dayer P. Drug-drug interactions of new active substances: Mibefradil example. *Eur J Clin Pharmacol.* 1999;55:559-565.
59. Lam YM, Tse HF, Lau CP. Continuous calcium chloride infusion for massive nifedipine overdose. *Chest.* 2001;119:1280-1282.
60. Leesar MA, Martyn R, Talley JD, Frumin H. Noncardiogenic pulmonary edema complicating massive verapamil overdose. *Chest.* 1994;105:606-607.
61. Levine M, Boyer EW, Pozner CN, et al. Assessment of hyperglycemia after calcium channel blocker overdoses involving diltiazem or verapamil. *Crit Care Med.* 2007;35:2071-2075.
62. Luscher TF, Noll G, Sturmer T, et al. Calcium gluconate in severe verapamil intoxication. *N Engl J Med.* 1994;330:718-720.
63. MacDonald D, Alguire PC. Case report: fatal overdose with sustained-release verapamil. *Am J Med Sci.* 1992;303:115-117.
64. Makela HMV, Kapur PA. Amrinone and verapamil-propranolol induced cardiac depression during isoflurane anesthesia in dogs. *Anesthesiology.* 1987;66:792-797.
65. Marques I, Gomes E, de Oliveira J. Treatment of calcium channel blocker intoxication with insulin infusion: case report and literature review. *Resuscitation.* 2003;57:211-213.
66. Marston S, El-Mezgueldi M. Role of tropomyosin in the regulation of contraction in smooth muscle. *Adv Exp Med Biol.* 2008;644:110-123.
67. Materne P, Legrand V, Vandormael M, et al. Hemodynamic effects of intravenous diltiazem with impaired left ventricular function. *Am J Cardiol.* 1984;54:733-737.
68. McAllister RG, Hamann SR, Blouin RA. Pharmacokinetics of calcium-entry blockers. *Am J Cardiol.* 1985;55:30B-40B.
69. Megarbane, B, Karyo S, Baud FJ. The role of insulin and glucose (hyperinsulinemia/euglycaemia) therapy in acute calcium channel antagonist and β-blocker poisoning. *Toxicol Rev.* 2004;23:215-222.
70. Morris DL, Goldschlager N. Calcium infusion for reversal of adverse effects of intravenous verapamil. *JAMA.* 1981;249:3212-3213.
71. Ohta M, Nelson D, Nelson J, et al. Effect of Ca channel blockers on energy level and stimulated insulin secretions in isolated rat islets of Langerhans. *J Pharmacol Exp Ther.* 1993;264:35-40.
72. Pearigen PD, Benowitz NL. Poisoning due to calcium antagonists. *Drug Saf.* 1991;6:408-430.
73. Perez E, Bania TC, Medlej K, Chu J. Determining the optimal dose of intravenous fat emulsion for the treatment of severe verapamil toxicity in a rodent model. *Acad Emerg Med.* 2008;15:1-6.
74. Petrovic MM, Vales K, Putnikovic B, Djulejic V, Mitrovic DM. Ryanodine receptors, voltage-gated calcium channels and their relationship with protein kinase A in the myocardium. *Physiol Res.* 2008;57:141-149.
75. Pitt B. Diversity of calcium antagonists. *Clin Ther.* 1997;19(Suppl A):3-17.
76. Proano L, Chiang WK, Wang RY. Calcium channel blocker overdose. *Am J Emerg Med.* 1995;13:444-450.
77. Quezado Z, Lippmann M, Wertheimer J. Severe cardiac, respiratory, and metabolic complications of massive verapamil overdose. *Crit Care Med.* 1991;19:436-438.
78. Quinn DI, Day RO. Drug interactions of clinical importance. *Drug Saf.* 1995;12:393-452.
79. Ramo MP, Grupp I, Pesola MK, et al. Cardiac glycosides in the treatment of experimental overdose with calcium-blocking agents. *Res Exp Med.* 1992;192:335-343.
80. Ramoska EA, Spiller HA, Myers A. Calcium channel blocker toxicity. *Ann Emerg Med.* 1990;19:649-653.
81. Ramoska EA, Spiller HA, Winter M, Borys D. A one-year evaluation of calcium channel blocker overdoses: toxicity and treatment. *Ann Emerg Med.* 1993;22:196-200.
82. Ranniger C, Roche C. Are one of two dangerous? Calcium channel blocker exposure in toddlers. *J Emerg Med.* 2007;33:145-154.
83. Ravens U, Wettwer E, Hála O. Pharmacological modulation of ion channels and transporters. *Cell Calcium.* 2004;35:575-582.
84. Roberts D, Honcharik N, Sitar DS, Tenenbein M. Diltiazem overdose: pharmacokinetics of diltiazem and its metabolites and effect of multiple dose charcoal therapy. *J Toxicol Clin Toxicol.* 1991;29:45-52.
85. Roden DM, George AL. The cardiac ion channels: relevance to management of arrhythmias. *Annu Rev Med.* 1996;47:135-148.
86. Rosansky SJ. Verapamil toxicity—treatment with hemoperfusion. *Ann Intern Med.* 1991;114:340-341.
87. Samniah N, Schlaeffer F. Cerebral infarction associated with oral verapamil overdose. *J Toxicol Clin Toxicol.* 1988;26:365-369.
88. Sandroni C, Cavallaro F, Addario C, et al. Successful treatment with enoximone for severe poisoning with atenolol and verapamil: a case report. *Acta Anaesthesiol Scand.* 2004;48:790-792.
89. Schiffl H, Ziupa J, Schollmeyer P. Clinical features and management of nifedipine overdosage in a patient with renal insufficiency. *J Toxicol Clin Toxicol.* 1984;22:387-395.
90. Schoffstall JM, Spivey WH, Gambone LM, et al. Effects of calcium channel blocker overdose-induced toxicity in the conscious dog. *Ann Emerg Med.* 1991;20:1104-1108.
91. Schwartz A. Molecular and cellular aspects of calcium channel antagonism. *Am J Cardiol.* 1992;70:6F-8F.
92. Shah AR, Passalacqua BR. Case report: sustained-released verapamil overdose causing stroke: an unusual complication. *Am J Med Sci.* 1992;304:257-359.
93. Sica DA. Interaction of grapefruit juice and calcium channel blockers. *AJH.* 2006;19:768-773.
94. Singh NA. Intravenous calcium and verapamil—when the combination may be indicated. *Int J Cardiol.* 1983;4:281-284.
95. Snover SW, Bocchino V. Massive diltiazem overdose. *Ann Emerg Med.* 1986;15:1221-1224.
96. Sperelakis N. Cyclic AMP and phosphorylation in regulation of calcium influx into myocardial cells and blockade by calcium antagonist drugs. *Am Heart J.* 1984;107:347-357.

97. Spiller HA, Meyers A, Ziemba T, Riley M. Delayed onset of cardiac arrhythmias from sustained-release verapamil. *Ann Emerg Med.* 1991;20:201-203.
98. Sporer KA, Manning JJ. Massive ingestion of sustained-release verapamil with a concretion and bowel infarction. *Ann Emerg Med.* 1993;22:603-605.
99. Stone CK, May WA, Carroll R. Treatment of verapamil overdose with glucagon in dogs. *Ann Emerg Med.* 1995;25:369-374.
100. Sulakhe MV, Vox T. Regulation of phospholamban and troponin 1 phosphorylation in the intact rat cardiomyocytes by adrenergic and cholinergic stimuli: roles of cyclic nucleotides, calcium, protein kinases, and phosphatases and depolarization. *Mol Cell Biochem.* 1995;149-150:103-126.
101. Sztajnkrycer MD, Bond GR, Johnson SB, Weaver AM. Use of vasopressin in a canine model of severe verapamil poisoning: a preliminary descriptive study. *Acad Emerg Med.* 2004;11:1253-1261.
102. Tebbutt S, Harvey M, Nicholson T, Cave G. Intralipid prolongs survival in a rat model of verapamil toxicity. *Acad Emerg Med.* 2006;13:134-139.
103. Tenenbein M, Cohen S, Sitar DS. Whole bowel irrigation as a decontamination procedure after acute drug overdose. *Arch Intern Med.* 1987;147: 905-907.
104. Ter Wee PM, Kremer Hovinga TK, Uges DRA, van der Geest S. 4-aminopyridine and haemodialysis in the treatment of verapamil intoxication. *Hum Toxicol.* 1985;4:327-329.
105. Thomas SH, Stone K, May WA. Exacerbation of verapamil-induced hyperglycemia with glucagon. *Am J Emerg Med.* 1995;13:27-29.
106. Thompson AM, Robbins, JP, Prescott JL. Changes in cardiorespiratory function during gastric lavage for drug overdose. *Hum Toxicol.* 1987;6:215-218.
107. Triggle DJ. L-type calcium channels. *Curr Pharm Des.* 2006;12:443-457.
108. Verbrugge LB, va Wezel HB. Pathopysiology of verapamil overdose: new insights in the role of insulin. *J Cardiothoracic Vasc Anesth.* 2007;21:406-409.
109. Watling SM, Crain JL, Edwards TD, Stiller RA. Verapamil overdose: case report and review of the literature. *Ann Pharmacother.* 1992;26: 1373-1377.
110. Wax P. Intestinal infarction due to nifedipine overdose. *J Toxicol Clin Toxicol.* 1995;33:725-728.
111. Weinberg GL, Ripper R, Feinstein DL, Hoffman W. Lipid emulsion infusion rescues dogs from bupivacaine-induced cardiac toxicity. *Reg Anesth Pain Med.* 2003;28:198-202.
112. Whitebloom D, Fitzharris J. Nifedipine overdose. *Clin Cardiol.* 1988;11: 505-506.
113. Wolf LR, Spadafora MP, Otten EJ. Use of amrinone and glucagon in a case of calcium channel blocker overdose. *Ann Emerg Med.* 1993;22: 1225-1228.
114. Wood DM, Wright KD, Jones AL, Dargan PI. Metaraminol (Aramine) in the management of a significant amlodipine overdose. *Human Exp Toxicol.* 2005;24:377-381.
115. Yagami T. Differential coupling of glucagon and beta-adrenergic receptors with the small and large forms of the stimulatory G protein. *Mol Pharmacol.* 1995;48:849-854.
116. Yeung PKF, Alcos A, Tang J, Tsui B. Pharmacokinetics and metabolism of diltiazem in rats: comparing single vs repeated subcutaneous injections. *Biopharm Drug Dispos.* 2007;28:403-407.
117. Yuan TH, Kerns WP, Tomaszewski CA, et al. Insulin-glucose as adjunctive therapy for severe calcium channel antagonist poisoning. *J Toxicol Clin Toxicol.* 1999;37:463-474.
118. Yust I, Hoffman M, Aronson RJ. Life-threatening bradycardic reactions due to beta blocker-diltiazem interactions. *Isr J Med Sci.* 1992;28: 292-294.

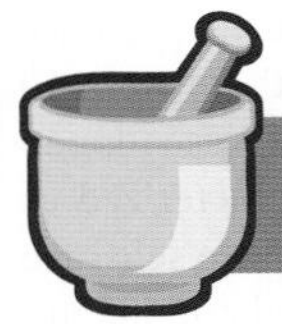

ANTIDOTES IN DEPTH (A18)

INSULIN-EUGLYCEMIA THERAPY

William Kerns

In the last decade, insulin has gained increased attention and importance in the management of a spectrum of critical illnesses including sepsis, heart failure, and cardiac drug toxicity. The benefits of insulin go well beyond simple control of hyperglycemia. In xenobiotic-induced myocardial depression the use of high-dose insulin along with sufficient glucose to maintain euglycemia can restore normal hemodynamics.

BACKGROUND

To understand the role of insulin specifically for resuscitating cardiac drug toxicity, it is useful to briefly review the altered myocardial physiology that occurs during drug-induced shock.

The hallmark of severe beta-adrenergic antagonist (BAA) and calcium channel blocker (CCB) toxicity is cardiogenic shock with bradycardia, vasodilation, and decreased contractility.[7] This is due to direct β-adrenergic receptor antagonism and calcium channel blockade. In addition to direct receptor or ion channel effects, metabolic derangements may occur that closely resemble diabetes with acidemia, hyperglycemia, and insulin deficiency.

In the nonstressed state, the heart primarily catabolizes free fatty acids for its energy needs. On the other hand, the stressed myocardium switches preference for energy substrates to carbohydrates, as demonstrated in models of both BAA and CCB toxicity.[19,35] The greater the degree of shock, the greater the demand for carbohydrates.[20] The liver responds to stress by making more glucose available via glycogenolysis. As a result, blood glucose concentrations are elevated. Hyperglycemia is noted both in animal models and in human cases of cardiac drug overdose.[4,9,22,36] Hyperglycemia is especially evident with CCB toxicity. This is because CCBs interfere with carbohydrate use by inhibiting pancreatic insulin release that is necessary to transport glucose across cell membranes. Insulin release from the islet cell requires functioning L-type or voltage-gated calcium channels similar to those found in myocardial and vascular tissue. Calcium channel blocking drugs directly inhibit pancreatic calcium channels.[6] In models of verapamil toxicity, circulating glucose increases without an associated increase in insulin.[20] There is additional evidence that CCBs interfere with phosphotidyl inositol 3-kinase–mediated glucose transport into cells.[1] As a result of diminished circulating insulin and inhibited enzymatic glucose uptake, glucose movement into cells becomes concentration dependent and may not sufficiently support the myocardial demand. Calcium channel blockers further contribute to metabolic abnormalities by inhibiting lactate oxidation.[19,23] This likely occurs through inhibition of pyruvate dehydrogenase, the enzyme responsible for conversion of pyruvate to acetylcoenzyme A (acetyl-CoA). As a result, pyruvate is preferentially converted to lactate, rather than the acetyl-CoA that would ordinarily enter the Krebs cycle; lactate then accumulates. Lactate accumulation and acidemia are consistent manifestations of CCB toxicity.[7,23]

PROPOSED MECHANISM

Initially, insulin's ability to improve cardiac function was attributed to increased catecholamine release. However, there is evidence that this is not the mechanism. For example, β-receptor antagonism does not inhibit improved myocardial performance that followed insulin administration.[24,35] In a CCB toxic model that measured circulating hormone concentrations, insulin therapy improved function and survival without increasing catecholamines.[22] In contrast, evidence demonstrates that insulin works via altered calcium, potassium, and sodium ion homeostasis.[8,24] However, the preponderant evidence demonstrates that insulin's positive inotropic effects occur because of metabolic support of the heart during hypodynamic shock.

Insulin facilitates myocardial utilization of carbohydrate that is favored during stress. A number of studies demonstrate a direct correlation between carbohydrate metabolism and the improved indices of cardiac function that occur with insulin therapy. Despite β-adrenergic antagonism by propranolol, insulin increased myocardial glucose uptake with subsequent increased contractility.[35] In a model of verapamil toxicity, insulin increased glucose uptake with resultant improved contractility.[19] Insulin therapy also increased lactate uptake, most likely by restoring pyruvate dehydrogenase activity.[21] In this way, lactate serves as an energy source following conversion to pyruvate and then acetyl-CoA that can then enter the Krebs cycle. Insulin-mediated improved contractility appears to be a critical factor to survival from hypodynamic shock. In models of BAA and CCB toxicity, survival is directly due to improved contractility, as insulin neither affected drug-induced hypotension nor bradycardia.[19,23]

In studies comparing insulin to more traditional therapies for drug-induced cardiogenic shock such as epinephrine and glucagon, insulin improved cardiac function and work efficiency.[21] Epinephrine and glucagon did not perform as well because they promoted free fatty acid utilization. As such, epinephrine and glucagon afforded limited increases in contractility at the expense of less efficient work due to increased oxygen demand.

CLINICAL EXPERIENCE

Insulin-euglycemia therapy for drug-induced shock was first reported in 1999.[39] This case series included four patients who overdosed on verapamil and one with combined amlodipine-atenolol overdose. All failed traditional antidote therapy, but responded to rescue insulin therapy. Since the initial case series, the author's institution has treated six additional patients with rescue insulin therapy following inadequate response to standard antidotes, five of the six with good outcome. Sixty-seven cases appear in the literature that were treated at other institutions.[2,3,5,10-13,16,25-29,31,33,34,36-38] Thus, there is an aggregate of 78 cases in which insulin was used. Of these cases, 72 primarily involved CCBs, five combined CCBs-BAAs, and one BAA. Various regimens of standard antidotes were used prior to insulin therapy and no case received insulin alone. Although no direct outcome comparisons can be made between insulin and standard therapies in these 78 cases, overall survival was 88% when insulin was included in resuscitation. Further review of these cases yields important clinical information that can be used to guide insulin therapy.

Experimental models suggest that large doses of insulin (2.5 to 10 units of regular insulin/kg/h) may be necessary to provide inotropic support.[1,18,21,23] However, humans appear to respond to less insulin. The most common doses given were 0.5 (n = 31) and 1.0 Units/kg/h (n = 19) of regular insulin in 62 patients where dose was reported. A few patients were treated with higher rates of infusion, up to 2.6 Units/kg/h in one case.[36] Sixteen patients received an insulin bolus (10 to 100 Units) prior to continuous infusion. The theoretical advantage to giving an initial insulin bolus is to rapidly saturate insulin receptors to enhance the physiological response. Interestingly, one report noted that patients receiving an insulin bolus prior to the infusion showed a better blood pressure response than patients who received only a continuous infusion.[10] Three patients received bolus insulin without continuous infusion, including a patient who inadvertently received 1000 units.[34] In this case, hemodynamics improved and there was no adverse event related to the extreme insulin dose. The mean duration of insulin infusion in 24 patients was 33 hours with a range of 0.75 to 96 hours. The need for prolonged infusion likely reflects the prolonged effects and kinetics of cardiovascular drugs typically observed following overdose.

The predominant clinical effect of insulin was increased contractility with subsequent blood pressure improvement. Contractility typically increased within 15 to 60 minutes after initiating insulin and often allowed a decrease in concurrent vasopressor requirements. The timing of increased contractility is consistent with the observed response times in animal models.[18,23] Other salutary effects were observed during insulin therapy. In two cases, blood pressure increased directly because of increased vascular resistance rather than increased cardiac function.[28,37] Two patients converted from third-degree heart block to normal sinus rhythm with increased pulse in temporal relationship to insulin.[40] Except for these two patients, insulin therapy did not significantly affect heart rate in other reports.

In four cases, authors reported a lack of response to insulin. Reasons for no response in three of these reports may include inadequate dose and excessive delay to insulin therapy.[5]

ADVERSE EVENTS

The major anticipated adverse event associated with the use of large amounts of insulin, especially in insulin-naïve patients, is hypoglycemia, defined here as blood glucose less than 60 mg/dL (3.3 mmol/L) regardless of the presence or absence of symptoms. Because of potential hypoglycemia, all experimental animals received sufficient dextrose during insulin infusion to maintain euglycemia. In the aggregate human cases, patients typically received empiric supplemental dextrose as well as frequent glucose monitoring. The mean dextrose dose was 23 g/h, but requirements varied widely from 0.5 to 75 g/h (actual data only available in 14 cases). The duration of exogenous dextrose averaged 43 hours, but like the dextrose dose, also varied significantly from patient to patient (9-100 hours). Dextrose supplementation was sometimes necessary beyond cessation of insulin. In seven of 10 cases with evaluable data, dextrose was continued an average of 10 hours after stopping insulin. Despite empiric dextrose and blood glucose monitoring (albeit not standardized), hypoglycemia occurred in some patients. In 58 cases where authors specifically document the presence or absence of complications related to insulin therapy, there were 10 patients with hypoglycemia. In five cases, insulin therapy was stopped because of hypoglycemia.[27] These five patients were characterized as mildly hypotensive. If mildly toxic, they may have been more sensitive to insulin. In the remaining cases, euglycemia was restored and insulin treatment continued.

Another anticipated consequence of insulin treatment is lowered serum potassium concentration. Although serum concentrations may at times fall below normal laboratory ranges, this change simply reflects shifting of potassium from the extracellular to intracellular space that occurs as a result of the action of insulin. In other words, patients maintain normal total body potassium stores and do not experience true deficiency unless they have other reasons for potassium loss. In the initial case series, three patients had a nadir of potassium ranging from 2.2 to 2.8 mEq/L without sequelae.[39] There is a theoretical risk of excessive potassium replacement in the instance of lowered serum potassium, but normal total body stores, as hyperkalemia may worsen verapamil-induced myocardial depression.[15,30]

Other observed ion changes during insulin therapy include hypomagnesemia and hypophosphatemia. Similar to action on potassium, insulin causes an intracellular shift of both phosphorus and magnesium.[17,32] Insulin (0.6 Units/kg/hr) for diabetic ketoacidosis is likewise associated with a marked decline of serum magnesium and phosphorus.[14] In the initial series of drug-induced shock treated with insulin, four patients had lowered magnesium (0.4 to 0.6 mmol/L; normal 0.8 to 1.2 mmol/L) and phosphorus (0.2 to 0.5 mmol/L; normal 1 to 1.4 mmol/L) concentrations. No symptoms were attributed to lowered serum concentrations, but three patients received supplementation of both electrolytes. No other insulin-treated CCB cases address these two electrolytes.

INSULIN-EUGLYCEMIA TREATMENT GUIDELINES

Based on the experimental studies and aggregate human cases, insulin-euglycemia is most likely going to benefit patients with cardiac drug-induced myocardial depression. Insulin-euglycemia may also be considered for those patients with hypotension due to poor vascular resistance without myocardial depression that does not respond to standard vasopressor treatment. Lastly, it is reasonable to initiate empiric insulin-euglycemia if a delay to cardiac diagnostic studies is expected. The experimental evidence and human case experience is strongest for CCB toxicity. Animal studies and limited human experience also support its use for BAA intoxication.

Myocardial function can be estimated at the bedside via emergency department ultrasonography or more formally via echocardiography or placement of a pulmonary artery catheter. When decreased myocardial function is present, insulin therapy can be used by first administering a 1 Unit/kg bolus of regular human insulin along with 0.5 g/kg of dextrose. If blood glucose is greater than 400 mg/dL (22.2 mmol/L), the dextrose bolus is not necessary. An infusion of regular insulin should follow the bolus starting at 0.5 to 1 Unit/kg/h. A continuous dextrose infusion, beginning at 0.5 g/kg/h should also be started. Dextrose is best delivered as $D_{25}W$ or $D_{50}W$ via central venous access to lessen large fluid volumes that would otherwise be necessary with administration of more dilute dextrose solutions. Patients with markedly elevated blood glucose may not require dextrose support at the start of insulin therapy.

If possible, cardiac function should be reassessed every 20 to 30 minutes after starting insulin-euglycemia therapy. If cardiac function remains depressed or there is persistent hypotension, the insulin dose can be increased. Doses up to 2.5 Units/kg/h have been used, although the maximum dose is not established in humans. The blood glucose should be monitored every 30 minutes until stable and then every 1 to 2 hours. The dextrose infusion should be titrated to keep blood glucose between 100 and 250 mg/dL (5.5 to 14 mmol/L).

The serum potassium concentration should be measured during insulin-euglycemia therapy. If it is low, especially when potassium loss is suspected, then supplementation to maintain the concentration in the "mildly hypokalemic" range (2.8 to 3.2 mEq/L) can be given. Magnesium and phosphorus can also be measured and supplemented as medically indicated. However, unless there is reason for loss of these three electrolytes, lowered serum concentrations likely reflect compartmental shifts, not depletion.

The ultimate goal of insulin-euglycemia is improvement in organ perfusion as demonstrated by increased blood pressure, improved mental status, and adequate urine output. Other markers of effective insulin-euglycemia therapy are reversal of acidemia and decreasing lactate concentrations. An increase in dextrose infusion to maintain euglycemia often accompanies hemodynamic and metabolic improvements. This is due to drug metabolism and loss of the drug-induced diabetogenic influences, and can be regarded as a favorable prognostic indicator.

REFERENCES

1. Bechtel LK, Haverstick DM, Holstege CP. Verapamil toxicity dysregulates the phosphatidylinositol 3-kinase pathway. *Acad Emerg Med.* 2008;15:368-374.
2. Boyer EW, Duic PA, Evans A. Hyperinsulinemia/euglycemia therapy for calcium channel blocker poisoning. *Pediatr Emerg Care.* 2002;18:36-37.
3. Boyer EW, Shannon M. Treatment of calcium-channel-blocker intoxication with insulin infusion. *N Engl J Med.* 2001;344:1721-1722.
4. Buiumsohn A, Eisenberg ES, Jacob H, Rosen N, Bock J, Frishman WH. Seizures and intraventricular conduction defect in propranolol poisoning. A report of two cases. *Ann Intern Med.* 1979;91:860-862.
5. Cumpston K, Mycyk M, Pallasch E, et al. Failure of hyperinsulinemia/euglycemia therapy in severe diltiazem overdose. *J Toxicol Clin Toxicol.* 2002;40:618 (abstract).
6. Devis G, Somers G, Obberghen E, Malaisse WJ. Calcium antagonists and islet function. I. Inhibition of insulin release by verapamil. *Diabetes.* 1975;24:247-251.
7. DeWitt CR, Waksman JC. Pharmacology, pathophysiology, and management of calcium channel blocker and beta-blocker toxicity. *Toxicol Rev.* 2004;23:223-238.
8. Draznin B. Intracellular calcium, insulin secretion, and action. *Am J Med.* 1988;85:44-58.
9. Enyeart JJ, Price WA, Hoffman DA, Woods L. Profound hyperglycemia and metabolic acidosis after verapamil overdose. *J Am Coll Cardiol.* 1983;2:1228-1231.
10. Greene SL, Gawarammana IB, Wood DM, Jones AE, Dargan PI. Relative safety of hyperinsulinaemia/euglycaemia in the management of calcium channel blocker overdose: a prospective observational study. *Intensive Care Med.* 2007;33:2019-2024.
11. Harris NS. Case records of the Massachusetts General Hospital. Case 24-2006. A 40-year-old woman with hypotension after an overdose of amlodipine. *N Engl J Med.* 2006;355:602-611.
12. Hasin T, Lebowitz D, Antopolsky M. The use of low-dose insulin in cardiogenic shock due to combined overdose of verapamil, enalapril and metoprolol. *Cardiology.* 2006;106:233-236.
13. Herbert JX, O'Malley C, Tracey JA, Dwyer R, Power M. Verapamil overdosage unresponsive to dextrose/insulin therapy. *J Toxicol Clin Toxicol.* 2001;39:293-294 (abstract).
14. Ionescu-Tirgoviste C, Bruckner I, Mihalache N, Ionescu C. Plasma phosphorus and magnesium values during treatment of severe diabetic ketoacidosis. *Med Intern.* 1981;19:66-68.
15. Jolly SR, Keaton N, Movahed A, Rose GC, Reeves WC. Effect of hyperkalemia on experimental myocardial depression by verapamil. *Am Heart J.* 1991;121:517-523.
16. Kanagarajan K, Marraffa JM, Bouchard NC, Krishnan P, Hoffman RS, Stork CM. The use of vasopressin in the setting of recalcitrant hypotension due to calcium channel blocker overdose. *Clin Toxicol.* 2007;45:56-59.
17. Kebler R, McDonald FD, Cadnapaphornchai P. Dynamic changes in serum phosphorus levels in diabetic ketoacidosis. *Am J Med.* 1985;79:571-576.
18. Kerns W, Schroeder JD, Williams C, Tomaszewski CA, Raymond RM. Insulin improves survival in a canine model of acute beta-blocker toxicity. *Ann Emerg Med.* 1997;29:748-757.
19. Kline J, Leonova E, Raymond RM. Beneficial myocardial metabolic effects of insulin during verapamil toxicity in the anesthetized canine. *Crit Care Med.* 1995;23:1251-1263.
20. Kline JA, Leonova E, Williams TC, Schroeder JD, Watts JA. Myocardial metabolism during graded intraportal verapamil infusion in awake dogs. *J Cardiovasc Pharmacol.* 1996;27:719-726.
21. Kline JA, Raymond RM, Leonova E, Winter M, Watts JA. Insulin improves heart function and metabolism during non-ischemic cardiogenic shock in awake canines. *Cardiovasc Res.* 1997;34:289-298.
22. Kline JA, Raymond RM, Schroeder JD, Watts JA. The diabetogenic effects of acute verapamil poisoning. *Toxicol Appl Pharmacol.* 1997;145:357-362.
23. Kline JA, Tomaszewski CA, Schroeder JD, Raymond RM. Insulin is a superior antidote for cardiovascular toxicity induced by verapamil in the anesthetized canine. *J Pharmacol Exp Ther.* 1993;267:744-750.
24. Lucchesi BR, Medina M, Kniffen FJ. The positive inotropic actions of insulin in the canine heart. *Eur J Pharmacol.* 1972;18:107-115.
25. Marques M, Gomes E, de Oliviera J. Treatment of calcium channel blocker intoxication with insulin infusion: case report and literature review. *Resuscitation.* 2003;57:211-213.
26. Masters TN, Glaviano VV. Effects of d,l-propranolol on myocardial free fatty acid and carbohydrate metabolism. *J Pharmacol Exp Ther.* 1969;167:187-193.
27. Meyer M, Stremski E, Scanlon M. Verapamil-induced hypotension reversed with dextrose-insulin. *J Toxicol Clin Toxicol.* 2001;39:500 (abstract).
28. Miller AD, Maloney GE, Kanter MZ, DesLauriers CM, Clifton JC. Hypoglycemia in patients treated with high-dose insulin for calcium channel blocker poisoning. *J Toxicol Clin Toxicol.* 2006;44:782-783 (abstract).
29. Min L, DeshPande K. Diltiazem overdose haemodynamic response to hyperinsulinaemia-euglycemia therapy: a case report. *Crit Care Resusc.* 2004;6:28-30.
30. Morris-Kukoski CL, Biswas AK, Parra M, Smith C. Insulin "euglycemia" therapy for accidental nifedipine overdose. *J Toxicol Clin Toxicol.* 2000;38:577 (abstract).
31. Nugent M, Tinker JH, Moyer TP. Verapamil worsens rate of development and hemodynamic effects of acute hyperkalemia in halothane-anesthetized dogs: effects of calcium therapy. *Anesthesiology.* 1984;60:435-439.
32. Ortiz-Munoz L, Rodriguez-Ospina LF, Figeroa-Gonzalez M. Hyperinsulinemia-euglycemia therpay for intoxication with calcium channel blockers. *Boletin Associacion Medica de Puerto Rico.* 2005;97:182-189.
33. Paolisso G, Sgambato S, Passariello N, et al. Insulin induces opposite changes in plasma and erythrocyte magnesium concentrations in man. *Diabetologia.* 1986;29:644-647.
34. Place R, Carlson A, Leiken J, Hanashiro P. Hyperinsulin therapy in the treatment of verapamil overdose. *J Toxicol Clin Toxicol.* 2000;38:576-577 (abstract).
35. Rasmussen L, Husted SE, Johnsen SP. Severe intoxication after an intentional overdose of amlodipine. *Acta Anaesthesiol Scand.* 2003;47:1038-1040.
36. Reikeras O, Gunnes P, Sorlie D, Ekroth R, Jorde R, Mjos OD. Metabolic effects of high doses of insulin during acute left ventricular failure in dogs. *Eur Heart J.* 1985;6:451-457.
37. Smith SW, Ferguson KL, Hoffman RS, Nelson LS, Greller HA. Prolonged severe hypotension following combined amlodipine and valsartan ingestion. *Clin Toxicol.* 2008;46:470-474.
38. Verbrugge LB, van Wezel HB. Pathophysiology of verapamil overdose: new insights in the role of insulin. *J Cardiothorac Vasc Anesth.* 2007;21:406-409.
39. Vogt S, Mehlig A, Hunziker P, et al. Survival of severe amlodipine intoxication due to medical intensive care. *Forensic Sci Int.* 2006;161:216-220.
40. Yuan TH, Kerns WP, Tomaszewski CA, Ford MD, Kline JA. Insulin-glucose as adjunctive therapy for severe calcium channel antagonist poisoning. *J Toxicol Clin Toxicol.* 1999;37:463-467.

CHAPTER 61

β-ADRENERGIC ANTAGONISTS

Jeffrey R. Brubacher

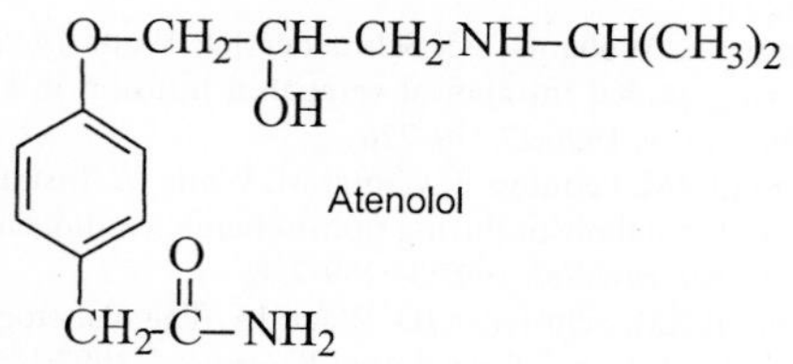

$O-CH_2-CH(OH)-CH_2-NH-CH(CH_3)_2$ / $CH_2-C(=O)-NH_2$

Atenolol

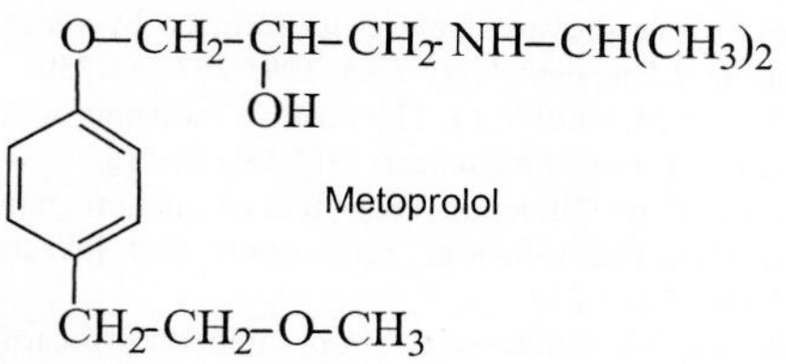

$O-CH_2-CH(OH)-CH_2-NH-CH(CH_3)_2$ / $CH_2-CH_2-O-CH_3$

Metoprolol

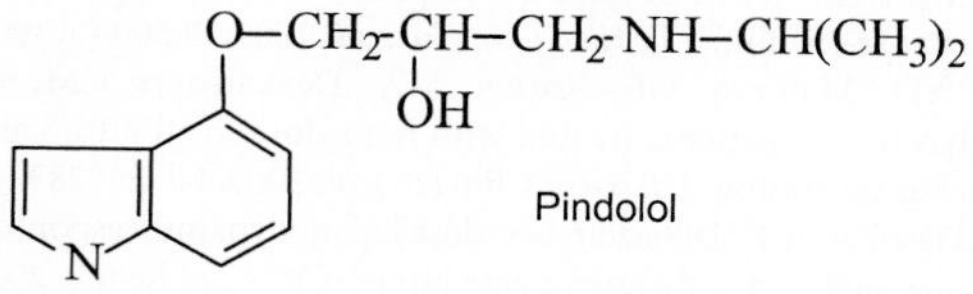

$O-CH_2-CH(OH)-CH_2-NH-CH(CH_3)_2$ / N

Pindolol

$O-CH_2-CH(OH)-CH_2-NH-CH(CH_3)_2$

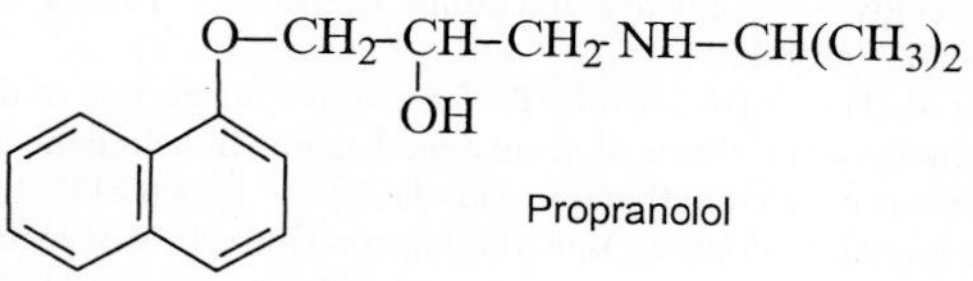

Propranolol

The pharmacology, toxicology, and poison management issues discussed in this chapter are applicable to all of the β-adrenergic antagonists. They are commonly used in the treatment of patients with cardiovascular disease, including hypertension, coronary artery disease, and tachydysrhythmias. Additional indications for β-adrenergic antagonists include congestive heart failure, migraine headaches, benign essential tremor, panic attack, stage fright, and hyperthyroidism. Ophthalmic preparations containing β-adrenergic antagonists are used in the treatment of glaucoma.[56] The diverse indications have led to complex toxicologic emergencies from intentional and unintentional overdoses as well as adverse drug reactions and drug–drug interactions. The management of patients with β-adrenergic antagonist overdoses is complicated by the lack of a routine strategy or a simple antidote. It is for these reasons that this class of xenobiotics remains intensely under study.

HISTORY

In 1948, Raymond Alquist postulated that epinephrine's cardiovascular actions of hypertension and tachycardia were best explained by the existence of two distinct sets of receptors that he generically named α and β receptors. At that time, the contemporary "antiepinephrines," such as phenoxybenzamine, reversed the hypertension but not the tachycardia associated with epinephrine. According to Alquist's theory, these drugs acted at the α-adrenergic receptors. The β-adrenergic receptors, in his schema, mediated catecholamine-induced tachycardia. The British pharmacist Sir James Black was influenced by Alquist's work and recognized the potential clinical benefit of a β-adrenergic antagonist. In 1958, Black synthesized the first β-adrenergic antagonist, pronethalol. This drug was briefly marketed as Alderlin, named after Alderly Park, the research headquarters of ICI Pharmaceuticals. Pronethalol was discontinued because it produced thymic tumors in mice. Propranolol was soon developed and marketed as Inderal (an incomplete anagram of Alderlin) in the United Kingdom in 1964[17,146] and in the United States in 1973.

Before the introduction of β-adrenergic antagonists, the management of angina was limited to medications such as nitrates that reduced preload through dilatation of the venous capacitance vessels and increased myocardial oxygen delivery by vasodilation of the coronary arteries. Propranolol gave clinicians the ability to decrease myocardial oxygen utilization. This new approach proved to decrease morbidity and mortality in patients with ischemic heart disease.[74] New drugs soon followed, and by 1979 there were ten β-adrenergic antagonists available in the United States.[37] Unfortunately it soon became apparent that these medications were dangerous when taken in overdose, and by 1979 cases of severe toxicity and death from β-adrenergic overdose were reported.[37] Today 19 β-adrenergic antagonists are approved by the Food and Drug Administration (FDA), and other β-adrenergic antagonists are available worldwide (Table 61–1).

EPIDEMIOLOGY

Intentional β-adrenergic antagonist overdose, although relatively uncommon, continues to account for a number of deaths annually. From 1985 to 1995, there were 52,156 β-adrenergic antagonist exposures reported to the American Association of Poison Control Centers (see Chap. 135). These exposures accounted for 164 deaths of which β-adrenergic antagonists were implicated as the primary cause of death in 38. The other fatalities could not be clearly ascribed to β-adrenergic antagonists because of cardioactive co-ingestants such as calcium channel blockers or other factors. Children younger than age 6 years accounted for 19,388 exposures, but no fatalities were reported in this age group. The youngest fatality reported in this series was 7 years old. It is interesting to note that more than 50% of the patients who died developed cardiac arrest after reaching healthcare personnel.[91] The number of exposures to β-adrenergic antagonists reported to the National Poison Data System (NPDS) has increased annually from 9500 in 1999 to nearly 20,000 in 2007. Each year in this period, β-adrenergic antagonist exposures resulted in 200 to 400 cases with a "major toxic effect" and 20 to more than 40 deaths. This changed in 2006, when deaths and major morbidity were only tabulated for single-substance exposures. In 2007, β-adrenergic antagonists were the sole ingestant in 61 exposures, with major morbidity and three deaths (see Chap. 135).

Compared with the other β-adrenergic antagonists, propranolol accounts for a disproportionate number of cases of self-poisoning[25,117] and deaths.[72,91] This may be explained by the fact that propranolol is frequently prescribed to patients with diagnoses such as anxiety, stress, and migraine who may be more prone to suicide attempts.[117] Propranolol is also more lethal because of its lipophilic and membrane stabilizing properties.[51,117]

TABLE 61–1. Pharmacologic Properties of the β-adrenergic Antagonists[38,51,109,154,101,165]

	Adrenergic Antagonist Activity	Partial Agonist Activity (ISA)	Membrane Stabilizing Activity	Vasodilating Property	Lipid Solubility	Protein Binding (%)	Oral Bio-availability (%)	Half-Life (h)	Metabolism	Volume of Distribution (L/kg)
Acebutolol*	β_1	Yes	Yes	No	Low	25	40	2–4	Hepatic or renal	1.2
Atenolol	β_1	No	No	No	Low	<5	40–50	5–9	Renal	1
Betaxolol (tablets and ophthalmic)	β_1	No	Yes	Yes (Calcium channel blockade)	Low	50	80–90	14–22	Hepatic or renal	NA
Bisoprolol	β_1	No	No	No	Low	30	8	9–12	Hepatic or renal	NA
Bucindolol[a]	β_1, β_2	No		Yes (β_2-agonism and α_1 blockade)	Moderate		30	8 ± 4.5	Hepatic	NA
Carteolol (ophthalmic)	β_1, β_2	Yes	No	Yes (β_2-agonism and nitric oxide mediated)	Low	30	85	5–6	Renal	NA
Carvedilol	β_1, β_2, α_1	No	Yes	Yes (α_1 blockade; calcium channel blockade)	Moderate	~98	25–35	6–10	Hepatic	115
Celiprolol[a]	α_2, β_1	No		Yes (β_2 agonism, nitric oxide mediated)	Low	22–24	30–70	5	Hepatic	NA
Esmolol	β_1	No	No	No	Low	50	NA	~8 min	RBC esterases	2
Labetalol	α_1, β_1, β_2	β_2	Low	Yes (α_1 blockade, β_2 agonism)	Moderate	50	20–33	4–8	Hepatic	9
Levobunolol (ophthalmic)	β_1, β_2	No	No	No	NA	NA	NA	6	NA	NA
Metipranolol (ophthalmic)	β_1, β_2	No	No	No	NA	NA	NA	3–4	NA	NA
Metoprolol (long-acting form available)	β_1	No	Low	No	Moderate	10	40–50	3–4	Hepatic	4
Nadolol	β_1, β_2	No	No	No	Low	20–30	30–35	10–24	Renal	2
Nebivolol[a]	β_1	No		Yes (nitric oxide mediated)	Moderate	98	12–96	8–32	Hepatic	10–40
Oxprenolol	β_1, β_2	Yes	Yes	No	Moderate	80	20–70	1–3	Hepatic	1.3
Penbutolol	β_1, β_2	Yes	No	No	High	90	~100	5	Hepatic or renal	NA
Pindolol	β_1, β_2	Yes	Low	No	Moderate	50	75–90	3–4	Hepatic or renal	2
Propranolol (long-acting form available)	β_1, β_2	No	Yes	No	High	90	30–70	3–5	Hepatic	4
Sotalol*	β_1, β_2	No	No	No	Low	0	90	9–12	Renal	2
Timolol (tablets and ophthalmic)	β_1, β_2	No	No	No	Moderate	60	75	3–5	Hepatic or renal	2

[a] Not approved by the Food and Drug Administration.

NA, information not available; ISA, intrinsic sympathomimetic activity.

* Also inhibits K channels.

PHYSIOLOGY AND PHARMACOLOGY

THE CARDIAC CYCLE

Normal cardiac electrical activity involves a complex series of ion fluxes that result in myocyte depolarization and repolarization. Cardiac electrical activity is coupled to myocyte contraction and relaxation respectively by increases and decreases in intracellular calcium concentrations that is closely regulated by the autonomic nervous system. In normal conditions, heart rate is determined by the rate of spontaneous discharge of specialized pacemaker cells that comprise the sinoatrial (SA) node (Fig. 61–1). Pacemaker cell depolarization is caused by either inward cation current through "pacemaker channels"[2,29] or through rhythmic release of calcium from the sarcoplasmic reticulum (SR).[99,100] β-adrenergic stimulation significantly increases the rate of pacemaker cell depolarization by phosphorylating SR proteins and by a direct phosphorylation-independent action of cyclic AMP (cAMP) at the pacemaker channels.[2,20,21,99] Depolarization of cells in the SA node initiates an electric current that spreads from cell to cell along specialized pathways to depolarize the entire heart. This depolarization, referred to as *cardiac excitation*, is linked to mechanical activity of the heart by the process of electrical–mechanical coupling described below (see Chap. 22 and 23).

Myocyte Calcium Flow and Contractility During systole, voltage sensitive slow L-type calcium channels on the myocyte membrane open in response to cell depolarization allowing calcium to flow down its concentration gradient into the myocyte (Fig. 61–2). Invaginations of the myocyte membrane (T-tubules) place L-type calcium channels in close proximation to calcium release channels (ryanodine receptors: RyR) on the SR. The local increase in calcium concentration that occurs after the opening of these L-type calcium channels (couplons) triggers the opening of the associated RyR channels, resulting in a large release of calcium from the SR, a phenomenon known as calcium-dependent calcium release.[45,167] Myocyte contraction requires synchronized release of calcium from numerous couplons throughout the myocyte. After its release from the SR, cytostolic calcium binds to troponin C and allows actin-myosin interaction and subsequent myocyte contraction. The strength of contraction is proportional to the amount of calcium release from the SR during depolarization, which depends, in part, on the magnitude of SR calcium stores. Actin–myosin interaction is also modulated by β-adrenergic–mediated troponin phosphorylation, ischemia, intracellular pH, and myofilament stretch.[11,13,15,127,153]

During diastole, several ion pumps actively remove calcium from the cytoplasm (Fig. 61–2). The most important of these are the SR calcium ATPase that pumps cytosolic calcium into the SR and the calcium–sodium transporter that exchanges one calcium ion for three sodium ions. The SR calcium ATPase is important for maintaining SR calcium stores and is modulated by β-adrenergic stimulation (see below). When calcium concentrations decrease during diastole, calcium dissociates from troponin, and relaxation occurs.[11,13,14,15,136]

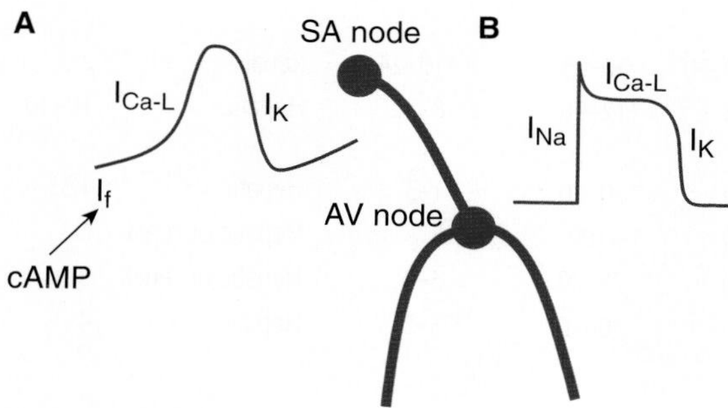

FIGURE 61–1. Cardiac conduction system. (**A**) The cardiac cycle begins when pacemaker cells in the sinoatrial node depolarize spontaneously. Traditionally, this depolarization has been attributed to inward "pacemaker" currents (I_f). Recent evidence suggests that that pacemaker cell depolarization may be driven by cyclical calcium release from a "calcium clock" in the sarcoplasmic reticulum (SR) and modulated by the "pacemaker" currents (I_f). β-adrenergic stimulation increases both the frequency of the "calcium clock" by a protein kinase Cav-L = L type voltage dependent calcium channel A (PKA)–mediated effect and the magnitude of the pacemaker current secondary to a direct effect of cAMP. These effects both increase the heart rate. Cholinergic stimulation has the opposite effects and results in bradycardia. Pacemaker cells lack fast sodium channels. Pacemaker cell depolarization triggers the opening of voltage sensitive L-type calcium channels (I_{Ca}-L), and the impulse is transmitted to surrounding cells. (**B**) Coordinated sinoatrial nodal depolarization generates an impulse sufficient to open fast sodium channels in surrounding atrial tissue, and the impulse spreads along specialized pathways to depolarize the atria and ventricles.

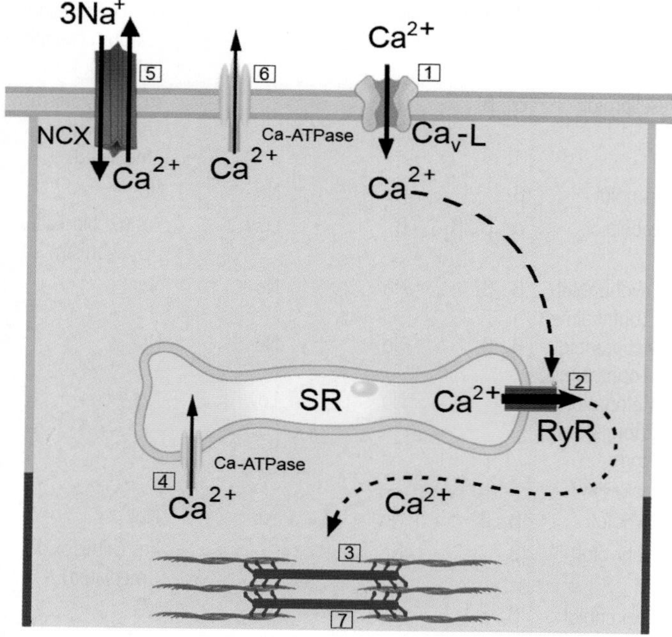

FIGURE 61–2. Fluctuations in calcium concentrations couple myocyte depolarization with contraction and myocyte repolarization with relaxation. 1. Depolarization opens voltage-sensitive calcium channels (Ca_V-L) and calcium flows down its concentration gradient into the myocyte. 2. This calcium current triggers the opening of ryanodyne calcium release channels (RyR) in the sarcoplasmic reticulum (SR), and calcium pours out. The amount of calcium released is proportional to the initial inward calcium current and to the amount of calcium stored in the SR. 3. At rest, the actin-myosin interaction is prevented by troponin. When calcium binds to troponin, this inhibition is removed, actin and myosin slide relative to each other, and the cell contracts. 4. After contraction, calcium is actively pumped back into the SR primarily by a calcium ATPase (Ca-ATPase) to allow relaxation. Calcium stored in the SR is thus available for release during subsequent depolarizations. 5. Additionally, the sodium-calcium antiporter (NCX) couples the flow of three molecules of sodium in one direction to that of a single molecule of calcium in the opposite direction. This transporter is passively driven by electrochemical gradients, which usually favors the extrusion of calcium. However, the extrusion of calcium is inhibited by high intracellular sodium or extracellular calcium concentrations and by cell depolarization. Under these conditions, the pump may "run in reverse." 6. Some calcium is actively pumped from the cell by a calcium ATPase. 7. As myocyte calcium concentrations decrease, calcium is released from troponin, and the myocyte relaxes.

β-adrenergic Receptors and the Heart β-adrenergic receptors are divided into β_1, β_2, and β_3 subtypes. In the healthy heart, approximately 80% of human cardiac β-adrenergic receptors are β_1, and 20% are β_2. Human hearts may also contain a small number of β_3-adrenergic receptors.[23,40,126] The relative density of cardiac β_2-adrenergic receptors increases with heart failure.[23,147] β_1-adrenergic receptors mediate increased inotropy by a well-described pathway involving cAMP and protein kinases (Fig. 61–3). β_1-adrenergic receptors are coupled to G_s proteins that activate adenylate cyclase when the receptor is stimulated. This increases intracellular production of cAMP, which binds to and activates protein kinase A and other cAMP-dependent protein kinases.[81] Protein kinase A, in turn, phosphorylates important myocyte proteins, including phospholamban, the voltage-sensitive calcium channels, the SR Ca^{2+} release (RyR) channels, and troponin.[13,23,48,136,150,153] Phosphorylation of the L-type calcium channel increases contractility by increasing the influx of Ca^{2+} during each cell depolarization, triggering greater release of Ca^{2+} from the SR.[118,138,144] Phospholamban inhibits the SR calcium ATPase. Phosphorylation of phospholamban removes this inhibition and increases the activity of the sarcoplasmic calcium ATPase, resulting in increased SR Ca^{2+} stores and hence enhanced contractility.[27,150] Improved activity of the SR calcium ATPase also results in more rapid removal of cytoplasmic Ca^{2+} during diastole and aids in myocyte relaxation. Phosphorylation of the RyR channels results in more rapid release of Ca^{2+} from SR stores.[13,136,153] Troponin phosphorylation facilitates Ca^{2+} unbinding and thus improves cardiac performance by enhancing myocyte relaxation.[3,11,82,150] β_1-adrenergic receptors increase chronotropy by an incompletely understood mechanism that may involve phosphorylation of SR proteins, resulting in an increased rate of Ca^{2+} discharge from the SR[99,100] in addition to direct cAMP interaction with membrane-bound pacemaker channels.[2,21] Although β-adrenergic stimulation acutely improves cardiac function, chronic β-adrenergic stimulation results in a number of detrimental effects, including Ca^{2+} related increased risk of dysrhythmias, impaired excitation–contraction coupling, and possibly myocyte apoptosis.[13,23]

Cardiac β_2-adrenergic receptors also mediate increased inotropy and chronotropy; however, the mechanisms are less well understood than for β_1-adrenergic receptors. Under normal conditions, human cardiac β_2-adrenergic receptors, similar to β_1-adrenergic receptors, appear to be linked to excitatory G_s proteins so that β_2-adrenergic stimulation improves cardiac contractility, relaxation, and chronotropy through the protein kinase A pathway described above. In the failing heart, β_2-adrenergic receptors are also linked to inhibitory G_i proteins that, when stimulated by receptor binding, inhibit adenyl cyclase and reduce cAMP formation. β_2-adrenergic receptor stimulation may also improve contractility by increasing cytoplasmic pH independent of G-protein activation.[23,136,170]

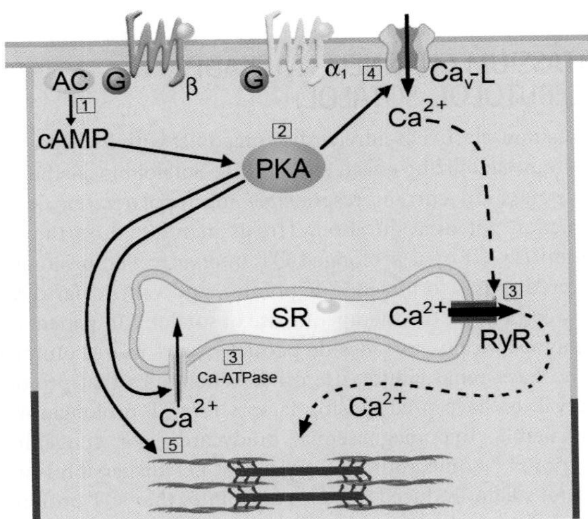

FIGURE 61–3. β_1-adrenergic agonists are positive inotropes. 1. β_1 -adrenergic receptors are coupled to G_S proteins, which activate adenyl cyclase when catecholamines bind to the receptor. This increases formation of cyclic adenosine monophosphate (cAMP) from adenosine triphosphate. 2. Increased cAMP levels activate protein kinase A (PKA), which mediates the ultimate effects of β-adrenergic receptor stimulation by phosphorylating key intracellular proteins. 3. Phosphorylation of phospholamban disinhibits the sarcoplasmic reticulum (SR) calcium ATPase, resulting in increased SR calcium stores available for release during subsequent depolarizations, and phosphorylation of SR calcium release channels (RyR) enhances calcium release from the SR during contraction. 4. Phosphorylation of voltage-sensitive calcium channels increases calcium influx through these channels during systole. 5. Troponin phosphorylation improves cardiac performance by facilitating calcium unbinding during diastole. β_2 receptors are also coupled to G_S proteins and mediate positive inotropy through a cAMP mechanism (see text). Increased cAMP directly increases the heart rate (see Fig. 61–1A).

Noncardiac Effects of β-Adrenergic Receptor Activation β-adrenergic agonists have important noncardiac effects. β–adrenergic receptors mediate smooth muscle relaxation in several organs. Relaxation of arteriolar smooth muscle predominately by β_2-adrenergic stimulation reduces peripheral vascular resistance and decreases blood pressure. This counteracts α-adrenergic–mediated arteriolar constriction. In the lungs, β_2-adrenergic receptors mediate bronchodilation. Third trimester uterine tone and contractions are inhibited by β_2-adrenergic agonists, and gut motility is decreased by both β_1- and β_2-adrenergic stimulation.

β-adrenergic receptors play a role in the immune system. Mast cell degranulation is inhibited by β_2-adrenergic stimulation, explaining the role of epinephrine in aborting and treating severe allergic reactions. Polymorphonuclear leukocytes demarginate in response to β-adrenergic stimulation, resulting in the increased white blood cell counts with catecholamine infusions or with increased endogenous release of epinephrine seen with pain or physiological stress.

β-adrenergic agonists also have important metabolic effects. Insulin secretion is increased by β_2-adrenergic receptor stimulation. Despite increased insulin concentrations, the net effect of β_2-adrenergic receptor stimulation is to increase glucose concentrations because of increased skeletal muscle glycogenolysis and hepatic gluconeogenesis and glycogenolysis. β_2-adrenergic receptors also cause glucagon secretion from pancreatic α cells.[73] β-adrenergic agonists act at fat cells, causing lipolysis and thermogenesis. Stimulation of adipocyte β-adrenergic receptors results in breakdown of triglycerides and release of free fatty acids. Skeletal muscle potassium uptake is increased by β_2-adrenergic stimulation, resulting in hypokalemia, explaining the role of β_2-adrenergic agonists in the treatment of hyperkalemia. Finally, renin secretion is increased by β_1-adrenergic stimulation, resulting in increased blood pressure.

ACTION OF β-ADRENERGIC ANTAGONISTS

β-adrenergic antagonists competitively antagonize the effects of catecholamines at β-adrenergic receptors and blunt the chronotropic and inotropic response to catecholamines. Bradycardia and hypotension may be severe in patients who take other xenobiotics that impair cardiac conduction or contractility and in those with underlying cardiac or medical conditions that make them reliant on sympathetic stimulation. In addition to slowing the rate of SA node discharge, β-adrenergic antagonists inhibit ectopic pacemakers and slow conduction through atrial and AV nodal tissue. β-adrenergic antagonists block the detrimental effects of chronic overstimulation and have become the standard of care for patients with all stages of compensated chronic heart failure, including patients with stable New York Heart Association class III or IV disease.[1,44,169] Unfortunately, β-adrenergic antagonism may acutely exacerbate symptoms in patients with decompensated congestive heart failure.[108,159]

The antihypertensive effect of β-adrenergic antagonists is counteracted by a reflex increase in peripheral vascular resistance. This effect is augmented by the β_2-adrenergic antagonism of nonselective β-adrenergic antagonists. By causing increased peripheral vascular resistance, β_2-adrenergic antagonists may rarely worsen peripheral vascular disease.

Patients with reactive airways disease may experience severe bronchospasm after using β-adrenergic antagonists because of a loss of β_2-adrenergic–mediated bronchodilation. Catecholamines inhibit mast cell degranulation through a β_2-adrenergic mechanism. Interference with this may predispose to life-threatening effects after anaphylactic reactions in atopic individuals.[61] β_2-adrenergic antagonists impair the ability to recover from hypoglycemia and may mask the sympathetic discharge that serves to warn of hypoglycemia. This combination of effects is dangerous for diabetic patients at risk for hypoglycemic episodes.[165]

β_2-adrenergic antagonism inhibits catecholamine-mediated K^+ uptake at skeletal muscle. This may cause slight elevations in serum K^+, concentrations, especially after exercise. Although β_2-adrenergic stimulation augments insulin release, β-adrenergic antagonists seldom lower insulin concentrations and may actually cause hypoglycemia by interference with glycogenolysis and gluconeogenesis. As mentioned above, these effects are important in diabetics at risk for hypoglycemia. β-adrenergic antagonists also alter lipid metabolism. Although the release of free fatty acids from adipose tissue is inhibited, patients taking nonselective β-adrenergic antagonists typically have increased serum concentrations of triglycerides and decreases in high-density lipoproteins.[165]

PHARMACOKINETICS

The pharmacokinetic properties of the β-adrenergic antagonists depend in large part on their lipophilicity. Propranolol is the most lipid soluble, and atenolol is the most water soluble. The oral bioavailability ranges from approximately 25% for propranolol to almost 100% for pindolol and penbutolol.

The highly lipid soluble drugs cross lipid membranes rapidly and concentrate in adipose tissue. These properties allow rapid entry into the central nervous system (CNS) and typically result in large volumes of distribution. In contrast, highly water-soluble drugs cross lipid membranes slowly, distribute in total body water, and tend to have less CNS toxicity. Volumes of distribution range from about 1 L/kg for atenolol to more than 100 L/kg for carvedilol.

The highly lipid-soluble β-adrenergic antagonists are highly protein bound and are therefore poorly excreted by the kidneys. They require hepatic biotransformation before they can be eliminated and tend to accumulate in patients with liver failure. In contrast, the water-soluble β-adrenergic antagonists tend to be slowly absorbed, poorly protein bound, and renally eliminated. They tend to accumulate in patients with renal failure. Esmolol, although water soluble, is rapidly metabolized by red blood cell esterases and does not accumulate in renal failure. The half life of esmolol is about 8 minutes. Half lives of the other β-adrenergic antagonists range from about 2 hours for oxprenolol to as much as 32 hours for nebivolol. The β-adrenergic antagonists also differ in their β_1-adrenergic selectivity, intrinsic sympathomimetic activity (ISA), and vasodilatory properties[109,116,119,151,165] (see Table 61–1 and below).

β_1 SELECTIVITY (ACEBUTOLOL, ATENOLOL, BETAXOLOL, BISOPROLOL, CELIPROLOL, ESMOLOL, METOPROLOL, NEBIVOLOL)

β_1-selective antagonists may avoid some of the adverse effects of the nonselective antagonists. Short-term use of β_1-adrenergic selective antagonists appears to be safe in patients with mild to moderately severe reactive airways.[131] These drugs may be safer for patients with diabetes mellitus or peripheral vascular disease and may be more effective antihypertensive agents. Their β_1-adrenergic selectivity, however, is incomplete, and adverse reactions secondary to β_2-adrenergic antagonism may occur with therapeutic dosage as well as in overdose.[83,165]

MEMBRANE-STABILIZING EFFECTS (ACEBUTOLOL, BETAXOLOL, CARVEDILOL, OXPRENOLOL, PROPRANOLOL)

β-adrenergic antagonists that inhibit fast sodium channels (also known as type I antidysrhythmic activity) are said to possess membrane-stabilizing activity. No significant membrane stabilization occurs with therapeutic use of β-adrenergic antagonists, but this property contributes to toxicity in overdose.

INTRINSIC SYMPATHOMIMETIC ACTIVITY (ACEBUTOLOL, CARTEOLOL, OXPRENOLOL, PENBUTOLOL, PINDOLOL)

These antagonists act as partial agonists at β-adrenergic receptors and are said to have ISA. This property avoids the severe decrease in resting heart rate that occurs with β-adrenergic antagonism in susceptible patients, but the clinical benefit is not demonstrated in controlled trials.[35]

POTASSIUM CHANNEL BLOCKADE (ACEBUTOLOL, SOTALOL)

Sotalol is a nonselective β-adrenergic antagonist with low lipophilicity, no membrane stabilizing effect, and no ISA. Sotalol blocks the delayed rectifier potassium current responsible for repolarization, prolonging the action potential duration. This is manifested on the electrocardiogram (ECG) by a prolonged QT interval.[57] The prolonged QT interval predisposes to torsades de pointes, and ventricular dysrhythmias may complicate the therapeutic use of sotalol.[71] In patients taking sotalol therapeutically, torsades de pointes occurs more commonly in those who have renal failure, use other xenobiotics that prolong the QT interval, or have predisposing factors for QT prolongation such as hypokalemia, hypomagnesemia, bradycardia, or congenital QT prolongation.[26,57] Some authors suggest that QT dispersion is a better predictor of sotalol-induced torsades de pointes than QT prolongation alone. A difference between the longest and shortest QT interval on the 12-lead ECG of more than 100 msec indicates an increased risk of torsade de pointes.[26] Acebutolol also prolongs the QT interval presumably secondary to blockade of outward potassium channels.[88]

VASODILATION (BETAXOLOL, BUCINDOLOL, CARTEOLOL, CARVEDILOL, CELIPROLOL, LABETALOL, NEBIVOLOL)

Labetalol and the newer "third-generation" β-adrenergic antagonists (betaxolol, bucindolol, carteolol, carvedilol, celiprolol, nebivolol) are also vasodilators. Labetalol and carvedilol are nonselective β-adrenergic antagonists that also possess α-adrenergic antagonist activity. Nebivolol is a selective β_1-adrenergic antagonist that causes vasodilation by release of nitric oxide.[101] Bucindolol, carteolol, and celiprolol vasodilate because they are agonists at the β_2-adrenergic receptors. Celiprolol and carteolol also vasodilate because of nitric oxide–mediated effects. Bucindolol and celiprolol are not FDA approved. Carteolol is currently available as an ocular preparation. Betaxolol and carvedilol also have calcium channel blocking properties that result in vasodilation (see Table 61–1). β-adrenergic antagonists with vasodilating properties may be particularly beneficial for patients with congestive heart failure.[114] These medications may also have a role in managing patients with coronary artery disease or peripheral vascular disease. Those drugs with β_2-adrenergic agonist activity may prove useful for patients with reactive airways.

β-adrenergic antagonists should not be given without appropriate α-adrenergic blockade in situations of catecholamine excess such as pheochromocytoma or cocaine use. In these conditions, β_2-adrenergic mediated vasodilation is essential to counteract α-adrenergic mediated vasoconstriction. Administration of β-adrenergic antagonists would result in an "unopposed α" adrenergic effect, causing dangerous increases in vascular resistance. Even the β-adrenergic antagonists with combined α-adrenergic antagonism may cause this problem. Labetalol, for example, is five- to 10-fold more potent as a β-adrenergic antagonist than as an α-adrenergic antagonist. Theoretically, medications with β_2-adrenergic agonist properties may avoid the "unopposed α" effect, but their availability is limited, and use in this situation has not yet been investigated.[33,42,101,154,165]

OTHER PREPARATIONS (OPHTHALMIC PREPARATIONS, SUSTAINED-RELEASE PRODUCTS, COMBINED PRODUCTS)

Therapeutic use of ophthalmic solutions containing β-adrenergic antagonists may cause systemic adverse effects such as bradycardia, high-grade atrioventricular (AV) block, heart failure, and bronchospasm.[38,104,139,165] An extended-release tablet containing a combination of the calcium channel blocker felodipine and metoprolol has been studied as an antihypertensive medication.[47] This medication (Logimax, Astra-Zeneca) is marketed in more than 35 countries worldwide but is not available in the United States or Canada. Another combined β-adrenergic antagonist and calcium channel blocker containing atenolol and nifedipine (Nif-Ten, Astra-Zeneca) is also used as an antihypertensive agent.[31]

PATHOPHYSIOLOGY

Most of the toxicity of β-adrenergic antagonists is because of their ability to competitively antagonize the action of catecholamines at cardiac β-adrenergic receptors. The peripheral effects of β-adrenergic antagonism are less prominent in overdose. β-adrenergic antagonists also appear to have toxic effects independent of their action at catecholamine receptors. In catecholamine-depleted, spontaneously beating isolated rat hearts, propranolol, timolol, and sotalol all decreased heart rate and contractility.[28] Surprisingly, these effects were similar in catecholamine-depleted and nondepleted hearts.[77] A membrane depressant effect likely contributes to the cardiac depressant effects of propranolol but not to that of timolol or sotalol. It may be concluded that β-adrenergic antagonists cause myocardial depression at least in part by an action independent of catecholamine antagonism or membrane depressant activity.[77]

Other investigators studied the role of extracellular ions and cardiac membrane potential in modulating β-adrenergic antagonist toxicity. β-adrenergic antagonists interfere with Ca^{2+} uptake into intracellular organelles. This interference with cytosolic Ca^{2+} handling may stimulate Ca^{2+} sensitive outward potassium channels and result in myocyte hyperpolarization and subsequent refractory bradycardia. Decreasing extracellular potassium or increasing extracellular Na^+ concentrations was conjectured to counteract this effect and, in fact, partially reversed propranolol and atenolol toxicity in isolated rat hearts.[64] In another series of experiments with isolated rat hearts, calcium improved the function of rat hearts poisoned with β-adrenergic antagonists. This may have been caused by a nonspecific positive inotropic action of Ca^{2+}.[75] Although cardiovascular effects are most prominent in overdose, β-adrenergic antagonists also cause respiratory depression.[76] This effect is centrally mediated and appears to be an important cause of death in spontaneously breathing animal models of β-adrenergic antagonism toxicity.[75] Propranolol may interfere with synaptic transmission, which may explain some of the CNS effects noted in propranolol overdose.

CLINICAL MANIFESTATIONS

Symptoms of toxicity generally occur within 2 hours after immediate-release β-adrenergic antagonist overdose. Propranolol overdose, in particular, may be complicated by the rapid development of hypoglycemia, seizures, coma, and dysrhythmias. In a retrospective review of published reports of adult β-adrenergic antagonist overdose, there were 39 symptomatic patients with well-documented times from ingestion to symptom onset. Only one patient had ingested a sustained-release product. Thirty-one patients were symptomatic at 2 hours, all but one developed symptoms by 4 hours, and all of the patients developed symptoms within the first 6 hours. The authors concluded that there have been no well-documented reports of immediate-release β-adrenergic antagonist overdose resulting in toxicity delayed more than 6 hours after ingestion.[85] In 58 patients with β-adrenergic antagonist overdose, all major symptoms began within 6 hours of ingestion.[117] These observations do not apply to sotalol, which is well known to cause delayed toxicity in overdose, nor to sustained-release preparations.

Isolated β-adrenergic antagonist overdose in healthy people is often benign. In several series, one-third or more of patients reporting a β-adrenergic overdose remained asymptomatic.[32,87,151] This is partially explained by the fact that β-adrenergic antagonism is often well tolerated in healthy persons who do not rely on sympathetic stimulation to maintain cardiac output. In particular, unintentional ingestions in children rarely result in significant toxicity.[12] In fact, a recent review of published cases found a few reports of hypoglycemia but no deaths or serious cardiovascular morbidity after β-adrenergic antagonist ingestion in children younger than age 6 years.[93] This finding should be interpreted with caution because actual ingestion of a β-adrenergic antagonist was not confirmed in most cases.

β-adrenergic antagonists severely impair the heart's ability to respond to peripheral vasodilation, bradycardia, or decreased contractility caused by other toxins. Therefore, even relatively benign vasoactive xenobiotics may cause catastrophic toxicity when co-ingested with β-adrenergic antagonists. Thus, an important predictor of toxicity in β-adrenergic antagonist overdose is likely to be the presence of a cardioactive co-ingestant.[84] Isolated β-adrenergic antagonist overdose is most likely to cause symptoms in persons with congestive heart failure, sick sinus syndrome, or impaired AV conduction who rely on sympathetic stimulation to maintain heart rate or cardiac output. Nevertheless, severe toxicity and death may still occur in healthy persons who have ingested β-adrenergic antagonists alone.[37,117,145] This may be explained by an increased susceptibility of certain persons to β-adrenergic antagonism or by special properties that increase the toxicity of certain β-adrenergic antagonists (see below). In patients without a co-ingestant, toxicity is most likely to occur in those who ingest a β-adrenergic antagonist with membrane-stabilizing activity.[84]

Patients with symptomatic β-adrenergic antagonist overdose will most often be hypotensive and bradycardic. Decreased SA node function results in sinus bradycardia, sinus pauses, or sinus arrest. Impaired

AV conduction manifested as prolonged PR interval or high-grade AV block occurs rarely. Prolonged QRS and QT intervals may occur, and severe poisonings may result in asystole. Congestive heart failure often complicates β-adrenergic antagonist overdose. Delirium, coma, and seizures occur most commonly in the setting of severe hypotension but may also occur with normal blood pressure, especially with exposure to the more lipophilic agents such as propranolol.[37,117] Respiratory depression and apnea may have an additional role in toxicity.[6] In a review of reported cases, 18% of patients with propranolol toxicity and 6% of those with atenolol toxicity had a respiratory rate less than 12 breaths/min.[117] Respiratory depression after β-adrenergic antagonist overdose typically occurs in patients who are hypotensive and comatose but is also reported in awake patients.[105] Hypoglycemia may complicate β-adrenergic antagonist poisoning in children[55,93] but is uncommon in acutely poisoned adults. In a series of 15 cases of β-adrenergic antagonist overdose, none of the 13 adults were hypoglycemic, but both of the two children had symptomatic hypoglycemia.[37] Bronchospasm is relatively uncommon after β-adrenergic antagonist overdose and appears to occur only in susceptible patients. In the series mentioned above, only two of the 15 patients developed bronchospasm,[37] and in a recent review of 39 cases of symptomatic adults with β-adrenergic antagonist overdose, only one patient developed bronchospasm.[85] Clinical use of β-adrenergic antagonists slightly increases serum K^+, concentration[94] but significant hyperkalemia is rare.

β_1 SELECTIVITY

In overdose, cardioselectivity is largely lost, and deaths attributable to the β_1-adrenergic selective agents, including acebutolol,[51] atenolol,[91] betaxolol, and metoprolol,[121,145] have been reported. There have been single reports of minor toxicity after overdose with bisoprolol[154] and nebivolol.[50]

MEMBRANE-STABILIZING EFFECTS

Propranolol possesses the most membrane-stabilizing activity of this class, and propranolol poisoning is characterized by coma, seizures, hypotension, bradycardia, impaired AV conduction, and prolonged QRS interval. Ventricular tachydysrhythmias may also occur.[4,91] Hypotension may be out of proportion to bradycardia, and deaths from propranolol overdose are well reported.[37,51,91] Acebutolol, betaxolol, and oxprenolol also possess significant membrane-stabilizing activity and have caused fatalities when taken in overdose.[51,109,115]

LIPID SOLUBILITY

In overdose, the more lipophilic β-adrenergic antagonists may cause delirium, coma, and seizures even in the absence of hypotension.[37,117] Atenolol, the least lipid soluble of the β-adrenergic antagonists, appears to be one of the safer β-adrenergic antagonists when taken in overdose.[51] In fact, in one series of β-adrenergic antagonist overdoses, none of the 18 patients with atenolol overdose had seizures compared with eight of 28 patients with propranolol overdose.[117] Nevertheless, atenolol overdose may result in severe toxicity and cardiovascular death.[91,112,148]

INTRINSIC SYMPATHOMIMETIC ACTIVITY

There is little experience with overdose of these medications, but ISA would theoretically make them safer than the other β-adrenergic antagonists. Sympathetic stimulation with mild tachycardia or hypertension often predominates in patients with pindolol overdose.[37,72,116] In addition to ISA, acebutolol and oxprenolol have significant membrane-stabilizing activity, making them dangerous in overdose; deaths have been reported.[37,51,88,115] Overdose with carteolol or penbutolol has not been reported.

POTASSIUM CHANNEL BLOCKADE

In six patients with sotalol overdose, the average QT interval was 172% of normal, and five patients had ventricular dysrhythmias, including multifocal ventricular extrasystoles, ventricular tachycardia, and ventricular fibrillation.[107] Sotalol overdose may also be complicated by hypotension, bradycardia, and asystole,[5,107] and fatalities are well documented.[111]

Sotalol overdose may cause delayed and prolonged toxicity, although ECG changes appear to occur early. In a series of six patients with sotalol overdose, all had prolonged QT interval noted on the initial ECG taken 30 minutes to 4.5 hours after ingestion. The authors do not specify whether these patients were taking sotalol therapeutically before the overdose, so it is possible that the prolonged QT on the initial ECG was present before the overdose.[107] The greatest QT prolongation occurred 4 to 15 hours after ingestion, and the risk of ventricular dysrhythmias was highest between 4 and 20 hours. All four patients who developed ventricular tachycardia did so after 4 hours, and in two patients, ventricular dysrhythmias first occurred 9 hours after ingestion. One patient continued to have ventricular dysrhythmias at 48 hours, and abnormally prolonged QT intervals were noted as long as 100 hours after ingestion. In this series, the average sotalol half-life was 13 hours, and the average time until normalization of the QT interval was 82 hours.[107] Acebutolol-induced QT interval prolongation may partially explain the ventricular tachydysrhythmias that occur with severe acebutolol toxicity.[30,88,91]

VASODILATION

The vasodilatory properties of these antagonists would theoretically act in synergy with β-adrenergic antagonism to increase toxicity. Conversely, the low membrane-stabilizing effect of these drugs may make them relatively safe in overdose. Betaxolol is the sole drug in this class with membrane-stabilizing properties. Overdose with labetalol appears to be similar to that of other β-adrenergic antagonists, with hypotension and bradycardia as prominent features.[67,68] Experience with overdose of the newer vasodilating β-adrenergic antagonists is extremely limited. There have been two reports of carvedilol overdose, and clinical manifestations were similar to those caused by poisoning with conventional β-adrenergic antagonists. One patient developed hypotension and bradycardia responsive to dopamine.[46] The second patient chewed carvedilol tablets and developed a rapid onset of hypotension and bradycardia responsive to glucagon and dopamine.[18] Both patients had full recoveries. In a single case report from Germany, nebivolol overdose was complicated by bradycardia, lethargy, and hypoglycemia. The patient received standard treatment and had a benign outcome.[50] Severe toxicity and death have occurred after betaxolol[16] and celiprolol[125] poisoning. Overdoses with bucindolol or carteolol have not been reported.

OTHER PREPARATIONS

There is very little published experience with overdoses of the sustained release β-adrenergic antagonists, but it is reasonable to expect that overdose with these agents will result in both a delayed onset and prolonged duration of toxicity. Acute overdose of ophthalmic β-adrenergic antagonists has not been reported. Patients who take mixed overdoses with calcium channel blockers and β-adrenergic antagonists are difficult to manage because of synergistic toxicity.[130,137,142] Overdoses with combined β-adrenergic antagonist and calcium channel blocker preparations such as Logimax (felodipine and metoprolol) or Nif-Ten (atenolol and nifedipine) have not been reported, but these combinations would be expected to be quite dangerous in overdose.

DIAGNOSTIC TESTING

All patients with an intentional overdose of a β-adrenergic antagonist should have a 12 lead ECG and continuous cardiac monitoring performed. Serum glucose concentration should be measured regardless of the patient's mental status because β-adrenergic antagonists may cause hypoglycemia. A chest radiograph and measurement of oxygen saturation should be obtained if the patient is at risk for or experiencing symptoms of congestive heart failure. For patients with bradycardia of uncertain etiology, measurement of thyroid function, serum K^+ concentration, renal function, cardiac enzymes, and digoxin concentration may prove helpful. Serum concentrations of β-adrenergic antagonists are not readily available for routine clinical use but may prove helpful in making a retrospective diagnosis in selected cases.

MANAGEMENT

The airway and ventilation should be maintained with endotracheal intubation if necessary. Because laryngoscopy may induce a vagal response, it is reasonable to give atropine before intubation of patients with bradycardia. This is particularly true for children, who are more susceptible to this complication. The initial treatment of bradycardia and hypotension consists of atropine and fluids. These measures will likely be insufficient in patients with severe toxicity but may suffice in patients with mild poisoning or other causes of bradycardia.

Gastrointestinal (GI) decontamination is warranted for all persons who have ingested significant amounts of a β-adrenergic antagonist. Induction of emesis is contraindicated because of the potential for catastrophic deterioration of mental status and vital signs in these patients and because vomiting increases vagal stimulation and may worsen bradycardia.[143] Orogastric lavage is recommended for patients with significant symptoms such as seizures, hypotension, or bradycardia if the drug is still expected to be in the stomach. Orogastric lavage is also recommended for all patients who present shortly after ingestion of large (gram amount) ingestions of propranolol or one of the other more toxic β-adrenergic antagonists (ie, acebutolol, betaxolol, metoprolol, oxprenolol, sotalol). Orogastric lavage causes vagal stimulation and carries the risk of worsening bradycardia, so it is reasonable to pretreat patients with standard doses of atropine. We recommend activated charcoal alone for persons with minor symptoms after an overdose with one of the more water-soluble β-adrenergic antagonists who present later than 1 hour after ingestion. Whole-bowel irrigation with polyethylene glycol should be considered in patients who have ingested sustained-release preparations (see Antidotes in Depth: Whole Bowel Irrigation).

Seizures or coma associated with cardiovascular collapse are treated by attempting to restore circulation. Seizures in a patient with relatively normal vital signs should be treated with benzodiazepines followed by propofol if benzodiazepines fail. Refractory seizures are rare in β-adrenergic antagonist overdose.

Patients who fail to respond to atropine and fluids require management with the inotropes discussed below (Fig. 61–4). When time permits, it is preferable to introduce new medications sequentially so that the effects of each may be assessed. We recommend glucagon followed by calcium, high-dose insulin euglycemia therapy, a catecholamine pressor, and if this fails, phosphodiesterase inhibitors. In critically ill patients, there may not be enough time for this approach, and multiple treatments may be started simultaneously. Advanced hemodynamic monitoring, when available, is advisable to guide therapy for all patients receiving catecholamine pressors or phosphodiesterase inhibitors. Intravenous fat emulsion should be considered for patients

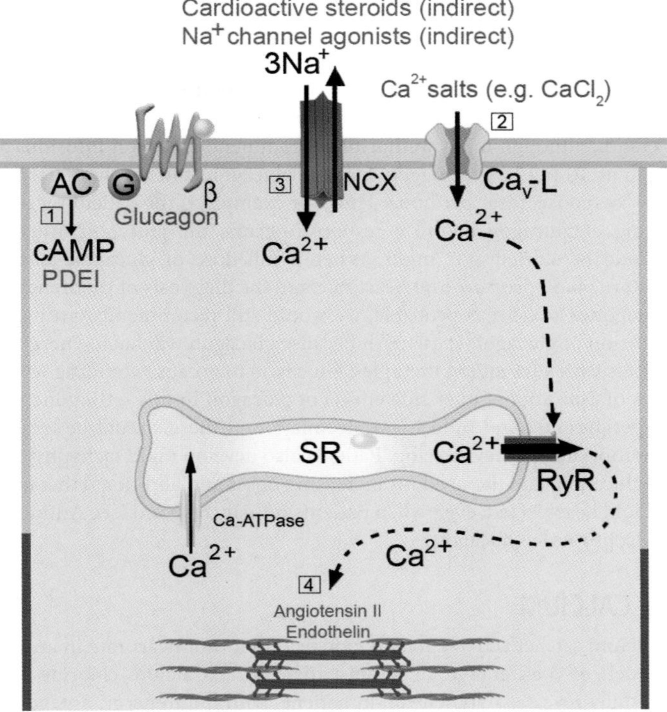

FIGURE 61–4. Positive inotropes improve cardiac function by a number of mechanisms, which usually result in increased intracellular calcium. 1. Xenobiotics that increase cyclic adenosine monophosphate (cAMP): Glucagon receptors and β-adrenergic receptors are coupled to Gs proteins; receptor binding increases cAMP by activation of adenyl cyclase. Phosphodiesterase inhibitors (PDEI) increase cAMP by inhibiting its breakdown. 2. Calcium salts increase calcium influx through the L-type voltage dependent calcium channel (Ca_V-L) during cell depolarization and result in higher intracellular calcium stores. 3. Xenobiotics that inhibit extrusion of calcium via the sodium-calcium exchange pump (NCX), including xenobiotics that increase intracellular sodium, such as cardioactive steroids and sodium channel agonists (eg, aconitine). 4. Xenobiotics that increase the sensitivity of the contractile elements to calcium: Angiotensin II and endothelin do this by inducing an intracellular alkalosis. The calcium sensitizers levosimendan and pimobendan (not shown) can be used to treat heart failure.

who fail this therapy. Mechanical life support with intra-aortic ballon pump or extracorporeal circulation may be lifesaving when medical management fails.

GLUCAGON

Cardiac glucagon receptors, similar to β-adrenergic receptors, are coupled to G_s proteins. Glucagon binding increases adenyl cyclase activity independent of β-adrenergic receptor binding.[171] The inotropic effect of glucagon is enhanced by its ability to inhibit phosphodiesterase and thereby prevent cAMP breakdown.[103]

No controlled trials of glucagon in human cases of β-adrenergic antagonist poisoning have been conducted.[9,19] Nevertheless, with more than 30 years of clinical use,[70,161] glucagon is still recognized as a useful treatment of choice for severe β-adrenergic antagonist toxicity.[63,113,151,164] This is supported by animal models[41,69,90] and a case series suggesting that glucagon is also effective in correcting symptomatic bradycardia and hypotension secondary to therapeutic β-adrenergic antagonist use.[92] Glucagon is a vasodilator, and in animal models of propranolol poisoning, it is more effective in restoring contractility, cardiac output, and heart rate than in restoring blood pressure.[9,90]

The initial adult dose of glucagon for β-adrenergic antagonist toxicity is 3 to 5 mg given slowly over 1 to 2 minutes. The initial pediatric dose is 50 μg/kg. If there is no response to the initial dose, higher doses up to a total of 10 mg may be used. When a response occurs, a glucagon infusion is started. Most authors recommend using an infusion of 2 to 5 mg/h, although many authorities recommend glucagon infusions as high as 10 mg/h. We suggest that the glucagon infusion be started at the "response dose" per hour. Thus, for example, if the patient receives 7 mg of glucagon before a response occurs, the glucagon infusion should be started at 7 mg/h. When a full dose of glucagon fails to restore blood pressure and heart rate and the diagnosis of β-adrenergic antagonist toxicity is probable, we would still recommend starting an infusion of glucagon at 10 mg/h because glucagon will have synergistic effects with subsequent therapies. Glucagon may cause vomiting with a risk of aspiration. Other side effects of glucagon in this setting include hyperglycemia and mild hypocalcemia,[60] and these should be treated appropriately if they develop. Patients also develop rapid tachyphylaxis to glucagon, and the need for increasing doses and additional therapies should be expected, even when patients initially respond (see Antidotes in Depth A19: Glucagon).

CALCIUM

Calcium salts effectively treat hypotension but not heart rate in animal models of β-adrenergic antagonist toxicity.[75,86] Calcium chloride successfully reverses hypotension in patients with β-adrenergic antagonist overdose[22,112] and in combined calcium channel blocker and β-adrenergic antagonist toxicity.[52] The adult starting dose of calcium gluconate is 3 g of the 10% solution given intravenously (IV). We recommend using up to 9 g of calcium gluconate if needed. The initial dose of calcium gluconate in children is 60 mg/kg up to 3 g. This may be repeated up to a total of 180 mg/kg (see Antidotes in Depth A30: Calcium).

INSULIN AND GLUCOSE

High-dose insulin, euglycemia therapy improves cardiac function after cardiac surgery[43] and survival after myocardial infarction.[34,96-98] There is evidence that high-dose insulin combined with sufficient glucose to maintain euglycemia is beneficial in patients with β-adrenergic antagonist poisoning. In a canine model of propranolol toxicity, all six animals treated with insulin and glucose survived compared with 4 of six in the glucagon group, one of six in the epinephrine group, and no survivors in the sham treatment group.[65] Insulin plus glucose was markedly more effective than vasopressin plus epinephrine in a porcine model of propranolol toxicity. In that experiment, all five animals in the insulin group survived the 4-hour protocol, and all five in the vasopressin plus epinephrine group died within 90 minutes.[58] A patient who ingested atenolol and amlodipine had a beneficial response to high-dose insulin.[173] High-dose insulin is simple to use, safe (with appropriate monitoring of glucose and potassium), and does not require invasive monitoring. For these reasons and despite limited clinical experience, we recommend using high-dose insulin and glucose infusions for patients with β-adrenergic antagonist toxicity who have not responded to fluids, atropine, and glucagon. Although the dose of insulin is not definitively established, therapy typically begins with a bolus of 1 Unit/kg of regular human insulin along with 0.5 g/kg of dextrose. If blood glucose is greater than 400 mg/dL (22.2 mmol/L), the dextrose bolus is not necessary. An infusion of regular insulin should follow the bolus starting at 0.5 Unit/kg/h titrated up to 2 Unit/kg/h if there is no improvement after 30 minutes. A continuous dextrose infusion beginning at 0.5 g/kg/h should also be started. Glucose should be monitored every half hour for the first 4 hours and titrated to maintain euglycemia. The response to insulin is typically delayed for 15 to 60 minutes, so it is usually necessary to start a catecholamine infusion before the full effects of insulin are apparent. It is important to continue monitoring glucose and electrolytes for several hours after insulin is discontinued (see Antidotes in Depth A18: Insulin-Euglycemia Therapy).

CATECHOLAMINES

Patients who do not respond to the preceding therapies usually require a catecholamine infusion. The choice of catecholamine is somewhat controversial. Theoretically, the pure β-adrenergic agonist isoproterenol would seem to be ideal because it can overcome β-adrenergic blockade without causing any α-adrenergic effects. Unfortunately, this therapy has several potential drawbacks that limit its efficacy. In the presence of β-adrenergic antagonism, extraordinarily high doses of isoproterenol and other catecholamines are frequently required.[25,115,120,151,158] Individual case reports document isoproterenol infusions as high as 800 μg/min.[116] At these high doses, the β_2-adrenergic effects of isoproterenol cause peripheral vasodilation and may actually lower blood pressure.[120] Nevertheless, in some animal models, isoproterenol is the most effective catecholamine and is even more effective than glucagon in reversing β-adrenergic antagonist toxicity.[149,162] Clinical experience, however, has not shown this to be the case.

In a review of reported cases, glucagon increased heart rate 67% of the time and blood pressure 50% of the time. In contrast, isoproterenol was effective in increasing heart rate only 11% of the time and blood pressure only 22% of the time. Epinephrine was more effective than isoproterenol.[164] The selective β_1-adrenergic agonist prenalterol may avoid some of the problems associated with isoproterenol and was used successfully to treat patients with β-adrenergic antagonist overdose.[36,72] However, prenalterol is not FDA approved, and its relatively long half life (~2 hours) makes titration difficult.[123] Dobutamine is a β_1-adrenergic agonist with relatively little effect on vascular resistance that may be useful in this setting. However, experience is limited, and dobutamine is not always effective in patients with β-adrenergic antagonist overdose.[115,141] In the setting of β-adrenergic antagonism, catecholamines with substantial α-adrenergic agonist properties may increase peripheral vascular resistance without improving contractility, resulting in acute cardiac failure.

Severe hypertension caused by a lack of β_2-adrenergic–mediated vasodilation is another potential adverse reaction from this so called "unopposed α" adrenergic effect.[39] Because of these potential problems, we recommend that catecholamine use be guided by hemodynamic monitoring using clinical criteria, noninvasive techniques such as bioimpedance or echocardiographic monitoring, or direct invasive measures of determining cardiac performance. Catecholamine infusions should be started at the usual rates and then increased rapidly until a clinical effect is obtained. If advanced monitoring is impossible and the diagnosis of β-adrenergic antagonist overdose is fairly certain, it is reasonable to begin an isoproterenol or epinephrine infusion with careful monitoring of the patient's blood pressure and clinical status. The infusion should be stopped immediately if the patient becomes more hypotensive or develops congestive heart failure.

PHOSPHODIESTERASE INHIBITORS

The phosphodiesterase inhibitors inamrinone, milrinone, and enoximone are theoretically beneficial in β-adrenergic antagonist overdose because they inhibit the breakdown of cAMP by phosphodiesterase and hence increase cAMP independently of β-adrenergic receptor stimulation. Phosphodiesterase inhibitors increase inotropy in the presence of β-adrenergic antagonism in both animal models[78] and in humans.[156] Although these therapies appear to be as effective as glucagon in animal models of β-adrenergic antagonist toxicity,[90,134] controlled dog models were unable to demonstrate an additional benefit of over glucagon.[89,135] Phosphodiesterase inhibitors might be useful in selected patients who fail glucagon therapy and have been used clinically to treat β-adrenergic antagonist–poisoned patients.[67,132,133] Therapy with phosphodiesterase inhibitors is often limited by hypotension secondary to peripheral vasodilation. Furthermore, these medications are difficult to titrate because of relatively long half-lives (ie, 30 to 60 minutes for milrinone, 2 to 4 hours for inamrinone, and approximately 2 hours for enoximone).[106] For these reasons, the phosphodiesterase inhibitors should generally only be considered for patients who have arterial or pulmonary artery pressure monitoring.

VENTRICULAR PACING

Ventricular pacing is not a particularly useful intervention in patients with β-adrenergic antagonist toxicity, but it increases the heart rate in some patients.[62] Unfortunately, there will frequently be failure to capture or pacing may increase the heart rate with no increase in cardiac output or blood pressure.[4,72,151] In fact, some authors have noticed that ventricular pacing occasionally decreases blood pressure perhaps secondary to loss of organized atrial contraction or because of impaired ventricular relaxation.[151]

EXTRACORPOREAL REMOVAL

Extracorporeal removal is ineffective for the lipid-soluble β-adrenergic antagonists because of their large volumes of distribution. Hemodialysis may remove water-soluble, renally eliminated β-adrenergic antagonists such as atenolol[129] and acebutolol.[124] Because hemodialysis is often technically difficult in poisoned patients because of hypotension and bradycardia, it is rarely used in patients with β-adrenergic antagonist overdose but may be considered in selected cases.

MECHANICAL LIFE SUPPORT

It is important to remember that patients with severe hypotension from an acute overdose typically recover without sequelae if ventilation and circulation can be maintained until the xenobiotic is eliminated. When the preceding medical treatment fails, it is appropriate to consider the use of an intra-aortic balloon pump or extracorporeal circulation. Several case reports describe remarkable recoveries after the use of these therapies for refractory β-adrenergic antagonist toxicity[16,102] or combined β-adrenergic antagonist and calcium channel blocker overdose.[66,128,168] A case series documents experience with extracorporeal membrane oxygenation (ECMO) for patients with cardiac arrest caused by cardiovascular drug poisoning. In this series of six patients, two deaths were attributed to the delay to institution of ECMO. The other four patients survived without sequelae.[8]

EXPERIMENTAL TREATMENT

Intravenous fat emulsion (IFE) is a promising new antidote that may have a role in selected cases of severe β-adrenergic antagonist overdose. IV administration of lipid emulsion is hypothesized to reduce the toxicity of lipid-soluble agents by lowering free serum concentrations of these xenobiotics as they partition into the lipemic component of blood and improve the bioenergetics of the heart. Although clinical experience is lacking, it is reasonable based on animal models to consider the use of IV fat emulsion in patients with toxicity from a lipid-soluble β-adrenergic antagonist that does not respond to usual therapy.[24,49] The optimal dose and formulation of intravenous fat emulsion for this purpose is unknown. One protocol for the use of lipid emulsion for severe local anesthetic toxicity calls for a 1.5 mL/kg of 20% IFE followed by an infusion of 0.25 mL/kg/min. The bolus can be repeated in 3 to 5 minutes if necessary. The total dose should be less than 8 mL/kg[163] (see Antidotes in Depth A21: Intravenous Fat Emulsion).

Aminophylline increases the heart rate and contractility by several mechanisms, including catecholamine release, adenosine antagonism, and at supratherapeutic doses, phosphodiesterase inhibition. Aminophylline has been used in cases of refractory bradycardia[160] and was effective in a dog model of propranolol poisoning.[168] Aminophylline was used with good effect in a mixed overdose involving atenolol, quinapril, and fluvoxamine.[120] Because aminophylline has a narrow therapeutic index and other therapies are generally effective, we cannot currently recommend its use unless all other treatment options have failed.

Vasopressin is a hypothalamic hormone that acts at G-protein–coupled receptors to mediate vasoconstriction (at V_1 receptors), water retention (at V_2 receptors), and corticotropin secretion (at V_3 receptors) and may also increase the response to catecholamines. Vasopressin analogues have been used as vasopressors clinically in shock states and for patients in cardiopulmonary arrest.[10,157] Even though vasopressin is a weak or even negative inotrope,[59] it was as effective as glucagon in a porcine model of propranolol toxicity.[58] There have been no reports of vasopressin use for human β-adrenergic antagonist toxicity.

The calcium sensitizers levosimendan and pimobendan interact with the contractile proteins to improve cardiac function and are used clinically to treat patients with heart failure. Levosimendan is both a positive inotrope and a vasodilator and has a better safety profile than pimobendan. It is approved in Europe for use in heart failure patients and is as effective as dobutamine in increasing contractility. Levosimendan infusions allow up-titration of β-adrenergic antagonists in patients with severe heart failure. Calcium sensitizers may prove to have a role in managing patients poisoned with β-adrenergic antagonists.[7,79,80,110]

Pyruvate has been shown to be an effective and apparently safe inotrope when given via the coronary arteries to patients with heart failure.[53,54] Pyruvate acts alone or in synergy with catecholamines to improve both systolic and diastolic function of the heart.[95] The action of pyruvate is poorly understood but likely involves improved cardiac energy delivery. Unfortunately, pyruvate is taken up rapidly in tissues, and some researchers have concluded that intracoronary infusions are required to attain sufficient delivery of pyruvate to the heart.[53,54] However, other researchers have shown that IV pyruvate infusions improve ventricular contractility in intact dogs[172] and in a canine model of cardiac arrest.[140] IV or intracoronary pyruvate infusions may have a place in the management of patients with severe β-adrenergic antagonist poisoning.

SPECIAL CIRCUMSTANCES

The preceding discussion applies to the generic management of β-adrenergic antagonists. Certain β-adrenergic antagonists have unique properties that modify their toxicity. The management considerations for these unique agents are discussed below.

SOTALOL

Sotalol toxicity may result in a prolonged QT interval and ventricular dysrhythmias, including torsades de pointes in addition to bradycardia and hypotension. Sotalol-induced bradycardia and hypotension should be managed as with other β-adrenergic antagonists. Specific management of patients with sotalol overdose includes correction of hypokalemia and hypomagnesemia. Overdrive pacing, magnesium infusion, or lidocaine may be effective for sotalol-induced torsade de pointes. In the future, potassium channel openers such as the cardioprotective drug nicorandil may prove effective for sotalol-induced torsade de pointes.[152]

PERIPHERAL VASODILATION

Treatment of patients who have overdosed with one of the vasodilating β-adrenergic antagonists is similar to that for patients who ingest other β-adrenergic antagonists. Decisions about the need for vasopressors should be guided by clinical findings. If vasodilation is a prominent feature, then high doses of pressors with α-adrenergic agonist properties (eg, norepinephrine or phenylephrine) may be required. Conversely, if β-adrenergic antagonism is prominent, then xenobiotics that act to increase intracellular cAMP, such as glucagon, may be needed.[50,67]

MEMBRANE-STABILIZING EFFECTS

It might be expected that hypertonic sodium bicarbonate would be beneficial in treating the ventricular dysrhythmias that occur with these xenobiotics. Unfortunately, there is limited experience with the use of hypertonic sodium bicarbonate in this situation, and the experimental data are mixed. Bicarbonate was not beneficial in a canine model of propranolol toxicity, although there was a trend toward QRS interval narrowing in the hypertonic sodium bicarbonate group.[88] In models with propranolol-poisoned isolated rat hearts, however, hypertonic sodium proved beneficial.[64,65] Perhaps most compelling is the fact that hypertonic sodium bicarbonate appeared to reverse ventricular tachycardia in a human case of acebutolol poisoning.[30] Because hypertonic sodium bicarbonate is a relatively safe and simple intervention, we recommend that it be used in addition to standard therapy for β-adrenergic antagonist–poisoned patients with QRS widening, ventricular dysrhythmias, or severe hypotension. Hypertonic sodium bicarbonate would not be expected to be beneficial in sotalol-induced ventricular dysrhythmias and, by causing hypokalemia, may actually increase the risk of torsade de pointes. The usual dose of hypertonic sodium bicarbonate is 1 to 2 mEq/kg given as an IV bolus. This may be followed by an infusion or repeated boluses may be given as needed. Care should be taken to avoid severe alkalosis or hypokalemia (see Antidotes in Depth: Bicarbonate).

OBSERVATION

All patients who have bradycardia, hypotension, abnormal ECGs, or CNS toxicity after a β-adrenergic antagonist overdose should be observed in a intensive care unit (ICU) until these findings resolve. Toxicity from regular-release β-adrenergic antagonist poisoning other than with sotalol almost always occurs within the first 6 hours.[85,88,117] Therefore, patients without any findings of toxicity after an overdose of a regular-release β-adrenergic antagonist other than sotalol may be discharged from medical care after an observation time of 6 to 8 hours if they remain asymptomatic with normal vital signs and a normal ECG and have had GI decontamination with activated charcoal. Ingestion of extended-release preparations may cause delayed toxicity, and these patients should be observed for 24 hours in an ICU. Patients who may have delayed absorption because of a mixed overdose or underlying GI disease may also require longer observation. Sotalol toxicity may also be delayed with ventricular dysrhythmias first occurring as late as 9 hours after ingestion.[107] We recommend that all patients with sotalol overdose be monitored for at least 12 hours. Patients who remain stable without QT prolongation may then be discharged from a monitored setting.

SUMMARY

β-adrenergic antagonists are commonly used to treat hypertension, angina, tachydysrhythmias, tremor, migraine, and panic attacks. Overdoses of β-adrenergic antagonists are relatively uncommon but continue to cause deaths worldwide. Patients who develop symptoms after ingesting regular release β-adrenergic antagonists do so within the first 6 hours. Patients with sotalol ingestions are an exception to this and may cause delayed and prolonged toxicity. Extended-release formulations may also result in delayed toxicity and patients who overdose require 24 hours of observation. Patients with β-adrenergic antagonist overdose, when symptomatic, typically develop bradycardia and hypotension. Propranolol and other β-adrenergic antagonists with membrane-stabilizing properties and high lipid solubility are the most toxic in overdose. These drugs cause prolongation of the QRS interval, severe hypotension, coma, seizures, and apnea. Hypoglycemia is rare in adults after β-adrenergic antagonist ingestions but may complicate overdose in children. Bronchospasm may occur in acute β-adrenergic antagonist toxicity in susceptible persons. Sotalol is unique in its ability to prolong the QT interval, and sotalol toxicity often results in refractory ventricular dysrhythmias, which may respond to overdrive pacing or to magnesium infusions. In addition to supportive care, the most important therapy for β-adrenergic antagonist toxicity is glucagon. High doses of insulin together with glucose provide another important early treatment modality. Catecholamine infusions may also be helpful but should be closely monitored, and large doses are typically required. Patients who fail treatment with glucagon, insulin, and catecholamines are critically ill and may respond to phosphodiesterase inhibitors, intravenous fat emulsion, or mechanical support of circulation. Fortunately, most patients respond to simpler measures, and this aggressive therapy is rarely required.

REFERENCES

1. Abraham WT. Beta-blockers. the new standard of therapy for mild heart failure. *Arch Intern Med.* 2000;160:1237-1247.
2. Accili EA, Proenza C, Baruscotti M, DiFrancesco D. From funny current to HCN channels. 20 years of excitation. *News Physiol Sci.* 2002;17:32-37.
3. Adelstein RS, Eisenberg E. Regulation and kinetics of the actin-myosin-ATP interaction. *Annu Rev Biochem.* 1980;49:921-956.
4. Agura ED, Wexler LF, Witzburg RA. Massive propranolol overdose. Successful treatment with high-dose isoproterenol and glucagon. *Am J Med.* 1986;80:755-757.
5. Alderfliegel F, Leeman M, Demaeyer P, Kahn RJ. Sotalol poisoning associated with asystole. *Intensive Care Med.* 1993;19:57-58.
6. Annane D. Beta-adrenergic mediation of the central control of respiration. myth or reality. *J Toxicol Clin Exp.* 1991;11:325-336.
7. Archan S, Toller W. Levosimendan. current status and future prospects. *Curr Opin Anaesthesiol.* 2008;21:78-84.
8. Babatasi G, Massetti M, Verrier V, Lehoux P, Le Page O, Bruno PG, et al. Severe intoxication with cardiotoxic drugs. value of emergency percutaneous cardiocirculatory assistance. *Arch Mal Coeur Vaiss.* 2001;94:1386-1392.
9. Bailey B. Glucagon in beta-blocker and calcium channel blocker overdoses. a systematic review. *J Toxicol Clin Toxicol.* 2003;41:595-602.
10. Barrett LK, Singer M, Clapp LH. Vasopressin. mechanisms of action on the vasculature in health and in septic shock. *Crit Care Med.* 2007;35:33-40.
11. Barry WH, Bridge JH. Intracellular calcium homeostasis in cardiac myocytes. *Circulation.* 1993;87:1806-1815.
12. Belson MG, Sullivan K, Geller RJ. Beta-adrenergic antagonist exposures in children. *Vet Hum Toxicol.* 2001;43:361-365.
13. Bers DM. Calcium cycling and signaling in cardiac myocytes. *Annu Rev Physiol.* 2008;70:23-49.
14. Bers DM. Calcium fluxes involved in control of cardiac myocyte contraction. *Circ Res.* 2000;87:275-81.
15. Bers DM. Cardiac excitation-contraction coupling. *Nature.* 2002;415:198-205.
16. Bilbault P, Pynn S, Mathien C, Mazzucotelli JP, Schneider F, Jaeger A. Near-fatal betaxolol self-poisoning treated with percutaneous extracorporeal life support. *Eur J Emerg Med.* 2007;14:120-122.
17. Black JW, Duncan WA, Shanks RG. Comparison of some properties of pronethalol and propranolol. 1965. *Br J Pharmacol.* 1997;120:285-299.

18. Bouchard NC, Forde J, Hoffman RS. Carvedilol overdose with quantitative confirmation. *Basic Clin Pharmacol Toxicol.* 2008;103:102-103.
19. Boyd R, Ghosh A. Towards evidence based emergency medicine: best bets from the Manchester royal infirmary. Glucagon for the treatment of symptomatic beta blocker overdose [review]. *Emerg Med J.* 2003;20:266-267.
20. Boyett MR, Dobrzynski H, Lancaster MK, Jones SA, Honjo H, Kodama I. Sophisticated architecture is required for the sinoatrial node to perform its normal pacemaker function. *J Cardiovasc Electrophysiol.* 2003;14:104-106.
21. Boyett MR, Honjo H, Kodama I. The sinoatrial node, a heterogeneous pacemaker structure. *Cardiovasc Res.* 2000;47:658-687.
22. Brimacombe JR, Scully M, Swainston R. Propranolol overdose—a dramatic response to calcium chloride. *Med J Aust.* 1991;155:267-268.
23. Brodde O-E, Bruck H, Leineweber K. Cardiac adrenoceptors: physiological and pathophysiological relevance. *J Pharm Sci.* 2006;100:323-337.
24. Cave G, Harvey MG, Castle CD. The role of fat emulsion therapy in a rodent model of propranolol toxicity. a preliminary study. *J Med Toxicol.* 2006;2:4-7.
25. Critchley JA, Ungar A. The management of acute poisoning due to beta-adrenoceptor antagonists. *Med Toxicol Adverse Drug Exp.* 1989;4:32-45.
26. Dancey D, Wulffhart Z, McEwan P. Sotalol-induced torsades de pointes in patients with renal failure. *Can J Cardiol.* 1997;13:55-58.
27. Davis BA, Edes I, Gupta RC, Young EF, Kim HW, Steenaart NA, et al. The role of phospholamban in the regulation of calcium transport by cardiac sarcoplasmic reticulum. *Mol Cell Biochem.* 1990;99:83-88.
28. de Wildt D, Sangster B, Langemeijer J, de Groot G. Different toxicological profiles for various beta-blocking agents on cardiac function in isolated rat hearts. *J Toxicol Clin Toxicol.* 1984;22:115-132.
29. DiFrancesco D, Borer JS. The funny current. cellular basis for the control of heart rate. *Drugs.* 2007;67(suppl 2):15-24.
30. Donovan KD, Gerace RV, Dreyer JF. Acebutolol-induced ventricular tachycardia reversed with sodium bicarbonate. *J Toxicol Clin Toxicol.* 1999;37:481-484.
31. Duckett GK, Cheadle B. Hypertension in the elderly. a study of a combination of atenolol and nifedipine. *Br J Clin Pract.* 1990;44:52-54.
32. Elkharrat D, Bismuth C, Davy JM. [Beta adrenergic receptor blockade. a self-limited phenomenon explaining the benignancy of acute poisoning with beta adrenergic inhibitors. Report of a series of 40 patients seen at the Fernand-Widal toxicology center, with a 0% mortality rate]. *Sem Hop.* 1982;58:1073-1076.
33. Fareed FN, Chan G, Hoffman RS. Death temporally related to the use of a beta adrenergic receptor antagonist in cocaine associated myocardial infarction. *J Med Toxicol.* 2007;3:169-172.
34. Fath-Ordoubadi F, Beatt KJ. Glucose-insulin-potassium therapy for treatment of acute myocardial infarction. an overview of randomized placebo-controlled trials. *Circulation.* 1997;96:1152-1156.
35. Fitzgerald JD. Do partial agonist beta-blockers have improved clinical utility? *Cardiovasc Drugs Ther.* 1993;7:303-310.
36. Freestone S, Thomas HM, Bhamra RK, Dyson EH. Severe atenolol poisoning. treatment with prenalterol. *Hum Toxicol.* 1986;5:343-345.
37. Frishman W, Jacob H, Eisenberg E, Ribner H. Clinical pharmacology of the new beta-adrenergic blocking drugs. Part 8. Self-poisoning with beta-adrenoceptor blocking agents. recognition and management. *Am Heart J.* 1979;98:798-811.
38. Frishman WH, Kowalski M, Nagnur S, Warshafsky S, Sica D. Cardiovascular considerations in using topical, oral, and intravenous drugs for the treatment of glaucoma and ocular hypertension. focus on beta-adrenergic blockade. *Heart Dis.* 2001;3:386-397.
39. Gandy W. Severe epinephrine-propranolol interaction. *Ann Emerg Med.* 1989;18:98-99.
40. Gauthier C, Seze-Goismier C, Rozec B. Beta 3-adrenoceptors in the cardiovascular system. *Clin Hemorheol Microcirc.* 2007;37:193-204.
41. Glick G, Parmley WW, Wechsler AS, Sonnenblick EH. Glucagon. Its enhancement of cardiac performance in the cat and dog and persistence of its inotropic action despite beta-receptor blockade with propranolol. *Circ Res.* 1968;22:789-799.
42. Gold EH, Chang W, Cohen M, Baum T, Ehrreich S, Johnson G, et al. Synthesis and comparison of some cardiovascular properties of the stereoisomers of labetalol. *J Med Chem.* 1982;25:1363-1370.
43. Gradinac S, Coleman GM, Taegtmeyer H, Sweeney MS, Frazier OH. Improved cardiac function with glucose-insulin-potassium after aortocoronary bypass grafting. *Ann Thorac Surg.* 1989;48:484-489.
44. Guyatt GH, Devereaux PJ. A review of heart failure treatment. *Mt Sinai J Med.* 2004;71:47-54.
45. Gyorke I, Gyorke S. Regulation of the cardiac ryanodine receptor channel by luminal Ca^{2+} involves luminal Ca^{2+} sensing sites. *Biophys J.* 1998;75: 2801-2810.
46. Hantson P, Lambermont JY, Simoens G, Mahieu P. Carvedilol overdose. *Acta Cardiol.* 1997;52:369-371.
47. Haria M, Plosker GL, Markham A. Felodipine/metoprolol. a review of the fixed dose controlled release formulation in the management of essential hypertension. *Drugs.* 2000;59:141-157.
48. Hartzell HC, Hirayama Y, Petit-Jacques J. Effects of protein phosphatase and kinase inhibitors on the cardiac l-type Ca current suggest two sites are phosphorylated by protein kinase a and another protein kinase. *J Gen Physiol.* 1995;106:393-414.
49. Harvey MG, Cave G. Intralipid infusion ameliorates propranolol-induced hypotension in rabbits. *J Med Toxicol.* 2008;4:71-76.
50. Heinroth KM, Kuhn C, Walper R, Busch I, Winkler M, Prondzinsky R. [Acute beta 1-selective beta-receptor blocker nebivolol poisoning in attempted suicide]. *Dtsch Med Wochenschr.* 1999;124:1230-4.
51. Henry JA, Cassidy SL. Membrane stabilising activity. a major cause of fatal poisoning. *Lancet.* 1986;1:1414-1417.
52. Henry M, Kay MM, Viccellio P. Cardiogenic shock associated with calcium-channel and beta blockers. reversal with intravenous calcium chloride. *Am J Emerg Med.* 1985;3:334-336.
53. Hermann HP. Energetic stimulation of the heart. *Cardiovasc Drugs Ther.* 2001;15:405-411.
54. Hermann HP, Arp J, Pieske B, et al. Improved systolic and diastolic myocardial function with intracoronary pyruvate in patients with congestive heart failure. *Eur J Heart Fail.* 2004;6:213-218.
55. Hesse B, Pedersen JT. Hypoglycaemia after propranolol in children. *Acta Med Scand.* 1973;193:551-552.
56. Hoffman BB. Catecholamines, sympathomimetic drugs, and adrenergic receptor antagonists. In: Hardman JG, Limbird LE, Gilman AG, Eds. *Goodman and Gilman's The Pharmacological Basis of Therapeutics.* 10th ed. New York: McGraw-Hill; 2001:215-268.
57. Hohnloser SH, Woosley RL. Sotalol. *N Engl J Med.* 1994;331:31-38.
58. Holger JS, Engebretsen KM, Fritzlar SJ, Patten LC, Harris CR, Flottemesch TJ. Insulin versus vasopressin and epinephrine to treat beta-blocker toxicity. *Clin Toxicol.* 2007;45:396-401.
59. Holmes CL, Landry DW, Granton JT. Science review. Vasopressin and the cardiovascular system part 2—clinical physiology. *Crit Care.* 2004;8: 15-23.
60. Illingworth RN. Glucagon for beta-blocker poisoning. *Lancet.* 1980;2:86.
61. Javeed N, Javeed H, Javeed S, Moussa G, Wong P, Rezai F. Refractory anaphylactoid shock potentiated by beta-blockers. *Cathet Cardiovasc Diagn.* 1996;39:383-384.
62. Kenyon CJ, Aldinger GE, Joshipura P, Zaid GJ. Successful resuscitation using external cardiac pacing in beta adrenergic antagonist-induced bradyasystolic arrest. *Ann Emerg Med.* 1988;17:711-713.
63. Kerns W 2nd. Management of beta-adrenergic blocker and calcium channel antagonist toxicity. *Emerg Med Clin North Am.* 2007;25:309-331; abstract viii.
64. Kerns W 2nd, Ransom M, Tomaszewski C, Kline J, Raymond R. The effects of extracellular ions on beta-blocker cardiotoxicity. *Toxicol Appl Pharmacol.* 1996;137:1-7.
65. Kerns W 2nd, Schroeder D, Williams C, Tomaszewski C, Raymond R. Insulin improves survival in a canine model of acute beta-blocker toxicity. *Ann Emerg Med.* 1997;29:748-757.
66. Kolcz J, Pietrzyk J, Januszewska K, Procelewska M, Mroczek T, Malec E. Extracorporeal life support in severe propranolol and verapamil intoxication. *J Intensive Care Med.* 2007;22:381-385.
67. Kollef MH. Labetalol overdose successfully treated with amrinone and alpha-adrenergic receptor agonists. *Chest.* 1994;105:626-627.
68. Korzets A, Danby P, Edmunds ME, Feehally J, Walls J. Acute renal failure associated with a labetalol overdose. *Postgrad Med J.* 1990;66:66-67.
69. Kosinski EJ, Malindzak GS, Jr. Glucagon and isoproterenol in reversing propranolol toxicity. *Arch Intern Med.* 1973;132:840-843.
70. Kosinski EJ, Stein N, Malindzak GS, Jr., Boone E. Glucagon and propranolol (Inderal) toxicity. *N Engl J Med.* 1971;285:1325.
71. Krapf R, Gertsch M. Torsade de pointes induced by sotalol despite therapeutic plasma sotalol concentrations. *Br Med J Clin Res Ed.* 1985;290:1784-1785.
72. Kulling P, Eleborg L, Persson H. Beta-adrenoceptor blocker intoxication: epidemiological data. Prenalterol as an alternative in the treatment of cardiac dysfunction. *Hum Toxicol.* 1983;2:175-181.

73. Lacey RJ, Berrow NS, Scarpello JH, Morgan NG. Selective stimulation of glucagon secretion by beta 2-adrenoceptors in isolated islets of Langerhans of the rat. *Br J Pharmacol.* 1991;103:1824-1828.
74. Lambert DM. Effect of propranolol on mortality in patients with angina. *Postgrad Med J.* 1976;52(suppl 4):57-60.
75. Langemeijer J, de Wildt D, de Groot G, Sangster B. Calcium interferes with the cardiodepressive effects of beta-blocker overdose in isolated rat hearts. *J Toxicol Clin Toxicol.* 1986;24:111-133.
76. Langemeijer J, de Wildt D, de Groot G, Sangster B. Respiratory arrest as main determinant of toxicity due to overdose with different beta-blockers in rats. *Acta Pharmacol Toxicol (Copenh).* 1985;57:352-6.
77. Langemeijer JJ, de Wildt DJ, de Groot G, Sangster B. Centrally induced respiratory arrest. main cause of death in beta-adrenoceptor antagonist intoxication. *Hum Toxicol.* 1986;5:65.
78. Lee KC, Canniff PC, Hamel DW, Pagani ED, Ezrin AM. Cardiovascular and renal effects of milrinone in beta-adrenoreceptor blocked and non-blocked anaesthetized dogs. *Drugs Exp Clin Res.* 1991;17:145-158.
79. Lehmann A, Boldt J, Kirchner J. The role of Ca^{++}-sensitizers for the treatment of heart failure. *Curr Opin Crit Car.* 2003;9:337-344.
80. Lehtonen L, Poder P. The utility of levosimendan in the treatment of heart failure. *Ann Med.* 2007;39:2-17.
81. Levitzki A, Marbach I, Bar-Sinai A. The signal transduction between beta-receptors and adenylyl cyclase. *Life Sci.* 1993;52:2093-2100.
82. Li L, Desantiago J, Chu G, Kranias EG, Bers DM. Phosphorylation of phospholamban and troponin I in beta-adrenergic-induced acceleration of cardiac relaxation. *Am J Physiol Heart Circ Physiol.* 2000;278:H769-H779.
83. Lofdahl CG, Svedmyr N. Cardioselectivity of atenolol and metoprolol. A study in asthmatic patients. *Eur J Respir Dis.* 1981;62:396-404.
84. Love JN. Acebutolol overdose resulting in fatalities. *J Emerg Med.* 2000; 18:341-344.
85. Love JN. Beta blocker toxicity after overdose. when do symptoms develop in adults? *J Emerg Med.* 1994;12:799-802.
86. Love JN, Hanfling D, Howell JM. Hemodynamic effects of calcium chloride in a canine model of acute propranolol intoxication. *Ann Emerg Med.* 1996;28:1-6.
87. Love JN, Enlow B, Howell JM, Klein-Schwartz W, Litovitz TL. Electrocardiographic changes associated with beta-blocker toxicity. *Ann Emerg Med.* 2002;40:603-610.
88. Love JN, Howell JM, Litovitz TL, Klein-Schwartz W. Acute beta blocker overdose: factors associated with the development of cardiovascular morbidity. *J Toxicol Clin Toxicol.* 2000;38:275-281.
89. Love JN, Leasure JA, Mundt DJ. A comparison of combined amrinone and glucagon therapy to glucagon alone for cardiovascular depression associated with propranolol toxicity in a canine model. *Am J Emerg Med.* 1993;11:360-363.
90. Love JN, Leasure JA, Mundt DJ, Janz TG. A comparison of amrinone and glucagon therapy for cardiovascular depression associated with propranolol toxicity in a canine model. *J Toxicol Clin Toxicol.* 1992;30:399-412.
91. Love JN, Litovitz TL, Howell JM, Clancy C. Characterization of fatal beta blocker ingestion: a review of the American Association of Poison Control Centers data from 1985 to 1995. *J Toxicol Clin Toxicol.* 1997;35:353-359.
92. Love JN, Sachdeva DK, Bessman ES, Curtis LA, Howell JM. A potential role for glucagon in the treatment of drug-induced symptomatic bradycardia. *Chest.* 1998;114:323-326.
93. Love JN, Sikka N. Are 1-2 tablets dangerous? Beta-blocker exposure in toddlers. *J Emerg Med.* 2004;26:309-314.
94. Lundborg P. The effect of adrenergic blockade on potassium concentrations in different conditions. *Acta Med Scand Suppl.* 1983;672:121-126.
95. Mallet RT, Sun J, Knott EM, et al. Metabolic cardioprotection by pyruvate: recent progress. *Exp Biol Med.* 2005;230:435-443.
96. Malmberg K. Prospective randomised study of intensive insulin treatment on long term survival after acute myocardial infarction in patients with diabetes mellitus. DIGAMI (Diabetes Mellitus, Insulin Glucose Infusion in Acute Myocardial Infarction) study group. *Br Med J.* 1997;314:1512-1515.
97. Malmberg K. Role of insulin-glucose infusion in outcomes after acute myocardial infarction: the Diabetes and Insulin-Glucose Infusion in Acute Myocardial Infarction (DIGAMI) study. *Endocr Pract.* 2004;10(suppl 2):13-16.
98. Malmberg K, Ryden L, Efendic S, Herlitz J, Nicol P, Waldenstrom A, et al. Randomized trial of insulin-glucose infusion followed by subcutaneous insulin treatment in diabetic patients with acute myocardial infarction (DIGAMI study). effects on mortality at 1 year. *J Am Coll Cardiol.* 1995;26:57-65.
99. Maltsev VA, Lakatta EG. Normal heart rhythm is initiated and regulated by an intracellular calcium clock within pacemaker cells. *Heart Lung Circ.* 2007;16:335-348.
100. Maltsev VA, Vinogradova TM, Lakatta EG. The emergence of a general theory of the initiation and strength of the heartbeat. *J Pharm Sci.* 2006; 100:338-369.
101. Mangrella M, Rossi F, Fici F. Pharmacology of nebivolol. *Pharmacol Res.* 1998;38:419-431.
102. McVey FK, Corke CF. Extracorporeal circulation in the management of massive propranolol overdose. *Anaesthesia.* 1991;46:744-746.
103. Mery PF, Brechler V, Pavoine C, Pecker F, Fischmeister R. Glucagon stimulates the cardiac Ca^{2+} current by activation of adenylyl cyclase and inhibition of phosphodiesterase. *Nature.* 1990;345:158-161.
104. Miki A, Tanaka Y, Ohtani H, Sawada Y. Betaxolol-induced deterioration of asthma and a pharmacodynamic analysis based on beta-receptor occupancy. *Int J Clin Pharmacol Ther.* 2003;41:358-364.
105. Montgomery AB, Stager MA, Schoene RB. Marked suppression of ventilation while awake following massive ingestion of atenolol. *Chest.* 1985;88:920-921.
106. Morita S, Sawai Y, Heeg JF, Koike Y. Pharmacokinetics of enoximone after various intravenous administrations to healthy volunteers. *J Pharm Sci.* 1995;84:152-157.
107. Neuvonen PJ, Elonen E, Vuorenmaa T, Laakso M. Prolonged QT interval and severe tachyarrhythmias, common features of sotalol intoxication. *Eur J Clin Pharmacol.* 1981;20:85-89.
108. Nohria A, Lewis E, Stevenson LW. Medical management of advanced heart failure. *JAMA.* 2002;287:628-40.
109. Olin BR, Blasing S, Bastean JN. Beta-adrenergic blocking agents. In: Short RM, Snitker JA, eds. *Drug Facts and Comparisons.* CliniSphere v. 2, The Electronic Drug Information Library. St. Louis, Mo: Facts and Comparisons; 2000.
110. Perrone SV, Kaplinsky EJ. Calcium sensitizer agents. a new class of inotropic agents in the treatment of decompensated heart failure [see comment]. *Int J Cardiol.* 2005;103:248-255.
111. Perrot D, Bui-Xuan B, Lang J, Bouffard Y, Delafosse B, Faucon G, et al. A case of sotalol poisoning with fatal outcome. *J Toxicol Clin Toxicol.* 1988;26:389-396.
112. Pertoldi F, D'Orlando L, Mercante WP. Electromechanical dissociation 48 hours after atenolol overdose. usefulness of calcium chloride. *Ann Emerg Med.* 1998;31:777-781.
113. Pollack CV Jr. Utility of glucagon in the emergency department. *J Emerg Med.* 1993;11:195-205.
114. Poole-Wilson PA, Swedberg K, Cleland JG, Di Lenarda A, Hanrath P, Komajda M, et al. Comparison of carvedilol and metoprolol on clinical outcomes in patients with chronic heart failure in the carvedilol or metoprolol European trial (COMET). *Lancet.* 2003;362:7-13.
115. Prichard BN, Battersby LA, Cruickshank JM. Overdosage with beta-adrenergic blocking agents. *Adverse Drug React Acute Poisoning Rev.* 1984;3:91-111.
116. Pritchard BN, Thorpe P. Pindolol in hypertension. *Med J Aust.* 1971;58:1242.
117. Reith DM, Dawson AH, Epid D, Whyte IM, Buckley NA, Sayer GP. Relative toxicity of beta blockers in overdose. *J Toxicol Clin Toxicol.* 1996;34: 273-278.
118. Reuter H, Porzig H. Beta-adrenergic actions on cardiac cell membranes. *Adv Myocardiol.* 1982;3:87-93.
119. Reynolds RD, Gorczynski RJ, Quon CY. Pharmacology and pharmacokinetics of esmolol. *J Clin Pharmacol.* 1986;(26 suppl A):A3-A14.
120. Richards DA, Prichard BN. Self-poisoning with beta-blockers. *Br Med J.* 1978;1:1623-1624.
121. Riker CD, Wright RK, Matusiak W, de Tuscan BE. Massive metoprolol ingestion associated with a fatality—a case report. *J Forensic Sci.* 1987;32: 1447-1452.
122. Roberge RJ, Rossetti ML, Rosetti JM. Aminophylline reversal of antihypertensive agent toxicity. *Vet Hum Toxicol.* 2001;43:285-287.
123. Ronn O, Graffner C, Johnsson G, Jordo L, Lundborg P, Wikstrand J. Haemodynamic effects and pharmacokinetics of a new selective beta 1-adrenoceptor agonist, prenalterol, and its interaction with metoprolol in man. *Eur J Clin Pharmacol.* 1979;15:9-13.
124. Rooney M, Massey KL, Jamali F, Rosin M, Thomson D, Johnson DH. Acebutolol overdose treated with hemodialysis and extracorporeal membrane oxygenation. *J Clin Pharmacol.* 1996;36:760-763.
125. Roussel O, Burnod A, Perrin M, Belhadj-Tahar H, Delaitre D, Sadeg N. [Celiprolol poisoning: two case reports]. *Therapie.* 2005;60:81-84.
126. Rozec B, Gauthier C. Beta3-adrenoceptors in the cardiovascular system. putative roles in human pathologies. *Pharmacol Ther.* 2006;111:652-673.

127. Ruegg JC. Cardiac contractility: how calcium activates the myofilaments. *Naturwissenschaften.* 1998;85:575-582.
128. Rygnestad T, Moen S, Wahba A, Lien S, Ingul CB, Schrader H, et al. Severe poisoning with sotalol and verapamil: recovery after 4 h of normothermic CPR followed by extra corporeal heart lung assist. *Acta Anaesthesiol Scand.* 2005;49:1378-1380.
129. Saitz R, Williams BW, Farber HW. Atenolol-induced cardiovascular collapse treated with hemodialysis. *Crit Care Med.* 1991;19:116-118.
130. Sakurai H, Kei M, Matsubara K, Yokouchi K, Hattori K, Ichihashi R, et al. Cardiogenic shock triggered by verapamil and atenolol: a case report of therapeutic experience with intravenous calcium. *Jpn Circ J.* 2000;64:893-896.
131. Salpeter SR. Cardiovascular safety of beta(2)-adrenoceptor agonist use in patients with obstructive airway disease. a systematic review. *Drugs Aging.* 2004;21:405-414.
132. Sandroni C, Cavallaro F, Addario C, Ferro G, Gallizzi F, Antonelli M. Successful treatment with enoximone for severe poisoning with atenolol and verapamil: a case report. *Acta Anaesthesiol Scand.* 2004;48:790-792.
133. Sandroni C, Cavallaro F, Caricato A, Scapigliati A, Fenici P, Antonelli M. Enoximone in cardiac arrest caused by propranolol: two case reports. *Acta Anaesthesiol Scand.* 2006;50:759-761.
134. Sato S, Tsuji MH, Okubo N, Naito H. Milrinone versus glucagon. Comparative hemodynamic effects in canine propranolol poisoning. *J Toxicol Clin Toxicol.* 1994;32:277-289.
135. Sato S, Tsuji MH, Okubo N, Nishimoto C, Naito H. Combined use of glucagon and milrinone may not be preferable for severe propranolol poisoning in the canine model. *J Toxicol Clin Toxicol.* 1995;33:337-342.
136. Schaub MC, Hefti MA, Zaugg M. Integration of calcium with the signaling network in cardiac myocytes. *J Mol Cell Cardiol.* 2006;41:183-214.
137. Schier JG, Howland MA, Hoffman RS, Nelson LS. Fatality from administration of labetalol and crushed extended-release nifedipine. *Ann Pharmacother.* 2003;37:1420-1423.
138. Scoote M, Poole-Wilson PA, Williams AJ. The therapeutic potential of new insights into myocardial excitation-contraction coupling. *Heart.* 2003; 89:371-376.
139. Sharifi M, Koch JM, Steele RJ, Adler D, Pompili VJ, Sopko J. Third degree AV block due to ophthalmic timolol solution. *Int J Cardiol.* 2001;80:257-259.
140. Sharma AB, Knott EM, Bi J, et al. Pyruvate improves cardiac electromechanical and metabolic recovery from cardiopulmonary arrest and resuscitation. *Resuscitation.* 2005;66:71-81.
141. Shore ET, Cepin D, Davidson MJ. Metoprolol overdose. *Ann Emerg Med.* 1981;10:524-527.
142. Snook CP, Sigvaldason K, Kristinsson J. Severe atenolol and diltiazem overdose. *J Toxicol Clin Toxicol.* 2000;38:661-665.
143. Soni N, Baines D, Pearson IY. Cardiovascular collapse and propranolol overdose. *Med J Aust.* 1983;2:629-30.
144. Sperelakis N. Regulation of calcium slow channels of cardiac muscle by cyclic nucleotides and phosphorylation. *J Mol Cell Cardiol.* 1988;20(suppl 2): 75-105.
145. Stajic M, Granger RH, Beyer JC. Fatal metoprolol overdose. *J Anal Toxicol.* 1984;8:228-230.
146. Stapleton MP. Sir James Black and propranolol. The role of the basic sciences in the history of cardiovascular pharmacology. *Tex Heart Inst J.* 1997;24:336-342.
147. Steinberg SF. The molecular basis for distinct beta-adrenergic receptor subtype actions in cardiomyocytes. *Circ Res.* 1999;85:1101-1111.
148. Stinson J, Walsh M, Feely J. Ventricular asystole and overdose with atenolol. *Br Med J.* 1992;305:693.
149. Strubelt O. Evaluation of antidotes against the acute cardiovascular toxicity of propranolol. *Toxicology.* 1984;31:261-270.
150. Sulakhe PV, Vo XT. Regulation of phospholamban and troponin-i phosphorylation in the intact rat cardiomyocytes by adrenergic and cholinergic stimuli. roles of cyclic nucleotides, calcium, protein kinases and phosphatases and depolarization. *Mol Cell Biochem.* 1995;149-150:103-126.
151. Taboulet P, Cariou A, Berdeaux A, Bismuth C. Pathophysiology and management of self-poisoning with beta-blockers. *J Toxicol Clin Toxicol.* 1993; 31:531-551.
152. Takahashi N, Ito M, Saikawa T, et al. Clinical suppression of bradycardia dependent premature ventricular contractions by the potassium channel opener nicorandil. *Heart.* 1998;79:64-68.
153. Taur Y, Frishman WH. The cardiac ryanodine receptor (RyR2) and its role in heart disease. *Cardiol Rev.* 2005;13:142-146.
154. Toda N. Vasodilating beta-adrenoceptor blockers as cardiovascular therapeutics. *Pharmacol Ther.* 2003;100:215-334.
155. Tracqui A, Kintz P, Mangin P, Lenoir B. Self-poisoning with the beta-blocker bisoprolol. *Hum Exp Toxicol.* 1990;9:255-256.
156. Travill CM, Pugh S, Noble MI. The inotropic and hemodynamic effects of intravenous milrinone when reflex adrenergic stimulation is suppressed by beta-adrenergic blockade. *Clin Ther.* 1994;16:783-92.
157. Treschan TA, Peters J. The vasopressin system. physiology and clinical strategies. *Anesthesiology.* 2006;105:599-612.
158. Tynan RF, Fisher MM, Ibels LS. Self-poisoning with propranolol. *Med J Aust.* 1981;1:82-83.
159. Van Bakel AB, Chidsey G. Management of advanced heart failure. *Clinical Cornerstone.* 2002;4:42-52.
160. Viskin S, Belhassen B, Roth A, Reicher M, Averbuch M, Sheps D, et al. Aminophylline for bradyasystolic cardiac arrest refractory to atropine and epinephrine. *Ann Intern Med.* 1993;118:279-281.
161. Ward DE, Jones B. Glucagon and beta-blocker toxicity. *Br Med J.* 1976;2:151.
162. Wei J, Spotnitz HM, Spotnitz WD, Benvenisty AI, Haasler GB, Malm JR, et al. Pharmacologic antagonism of propranolol in dogs: effects of dopamine-isoproterenol and glucagon on hemodynamics and myocardial oxygen consumption in ischemic hearts during chronic propranolol administration. *J Thorac Cardiovasc Surg.* 1984;87:732-742.
163. Weinberg G. LipidRescue™ resuscitation for cardiac toxicity. *Treatment Regimens.* 2007. Available from http://lipidrescue.squarespace.com/links-to-literature/accessed September 15, 2009.
164. Weinstein RS. Recognition and management of poisoning with beta-adrenergic blocking agents. *Ann Emerg Med.* 1984;13:1123-1131.
165. Westfall TC, Westfall DP. Adrenergic agonists and antagonists. In: Brunton LL, Lazo JS, Parker KL, Eds. *Goodman and Gilman's The Pharmacological Basis of Therapeutics* (electronic edition). 11th ed. New York: McGraw-Hill; 2006:237-295.
166. Whitehurst VE, Vick JA, Alleva FR, Zhang J, Joseph X, Balazs T. Reversal of propranolol blockade of adrenergic receptors and related toxicity with drugs that increase cyclic AMP. *Proc Soc Exp Biol Med.* 1999;221:382-385.
167. Wier WG, Balke CW. Ca$^{(2+)}$ release mechanisms, Ca$^{(2+)}$ sparks, and local control of excitation-contraction coupling in normal heart muscle. *Circ Res.* 1999;85:770-776:237-295.
168. Wnek W. The use of intra-aortic balloon counterpulsation in the treatment of severe hemodynamic instability from myocardial depressant drug overdose. *Przegl Lek.* 2003;60:274-276.
169. Wu AH, Cody RJ. Medical and surgical treatment of chronic heart failure. *Curr Probl Cardiol.* 2003;28:229-260.
170. Xiao RP, Cheng H, Zhou YY, Kuschel M, Lakatta EG. Recent advances in cardiac beta(2)-adrenergic signal transduction. *Circ Res.* 1999;85: 1092-1100.
171. Yagami T. Differential coupling of glucagon and beta-adrenergic receptors with the small and large forms of the stimulatory G protein. *Mol Pharmacol.* 1995;48:849-854.
172. Yanos J, Patti MJ, Stanko RT. Hemodynamic effects of intravenous pyruvate in the intact, anesthetized dog. *Crit Care Med.* 1994;22:844-850.
173. Yuan TH, Kerns WP, 2nd, Tomaszewski CA, Ford MD, Kline JA. Insulin-glucose as adjunctive therapy for severe calcium channel antagonist poisoning. *J Toxicol Clin Toxicol.* 1999;37:463-474.

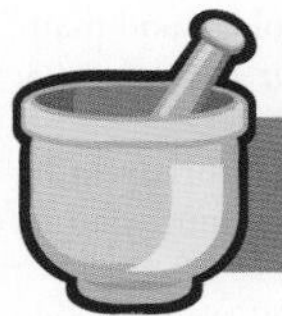

ANTIDOTES IN DEPTH (A19)

GLUCAGON

Mary Ann Howland

Glucagon is a polypeptide counterregulatory hormone with a molecular weight of 3500 daltons, secreted by the α-cells of the pancreas. Glucagon was discovered in 1923, just 2 years after the discovery of insulin.[9] Previously animal derived, and possibly contaminated with insulin, the current Food and Drug Administration (FDA)-approved form has been synthesized by recombinant DNA technology since 1998.[29] Its traditional role was to reverse life-threatening hypoglycemia in diabetic patients who were unable to ingest dextrose in the outpatient setting. In medical toxicology, however, glucagon is used in the management of β-adrenergic antagonist and calcium channel blocker toxicity.

PHARMACOKINETICS AND PHARMACODYNAMICS

The volume of distribution of glucagon is 0.25 L/kg.[19] The plasma, liver, and kidney extensively metabolize glucagon with an elimination half-life of 8 to 18 minutes.[19] In human volunteers following a single intravenous (IV) bolus, the cardiac effects of glucagon begin within 1 to 3 minutes, are maximal within 5 to 7 minutes, and persist for 10 to 15 minutes.[50] The time to maximal glucose concentration is 5 to 20 minutes, with a duration of action of 60 to 90 minutes.[20] Smooth muscle relaxation begins within 1 minute and lasts 10 to 20 minutes.[20] The onset of action following intramuscular and subcutaneous administration occurs in about 10 minutes, with a peak at about 30 minutes.[19]

Tachyphylaxis or desensitization of receptors may occur with repetitive dosing. Experimental heart preparations exposed to glucagon for varying lengths of time demonstrated a decrease in the amount of cyclic adenosine monophosphate (cAMP) generated.[28,74] Possible explanations for tachyphylaxis include uncoupling from the glucagon receptor and/or increased phosphodiesterase (PDE) hydrolysis of cAMP.[28,70,74,77] Other experiments demonstrated a transient effect of glucagon on contractility and hyperglycemia, also suggesting tachyphylaxis.[24,30]

MECHANISM OF ACTION

Glucagon receptors are demonstrated in animal and human hearts and brains as well as the pancreas, and binding is closely correlated with activation of cardiac adenylate cyclase.[26,37,68] A large number of glucagon binding sites are demonstrated, and as little as 10% occupancy produces near maximal stimulation of adenylate cyclase. The binding of glucagon to its receptor results in coupling with two isoforms of the G_s protein, catalyzing the exchange of guanosine triphosphate (GTP) for guanosine diphosphate (GDP) on the α subunit of the G_s protein.[25,56,73] One isoform is coupled to β agonists, while both isoforms are coupled to glucagon.[73] The GTP-G_s units stimulate adenylate cyclase to convert adenosine triphosphate (ATP) to cAMP.[36,44] In frog, mouse, and guinea pig hearts, glucagon also inhibits the cyclic guanosine monophosphate (cGMP)-inhibited, milrinone-sensitive phosphodiesterase, PDE-3.[4,47] Selective inhibition of PDE-4 potentiated the cAMP response to glucagon in adult rat ventricular myocytes.[55] Glucagon, along with β_2 agonists, histamine, and serotonin (but not β_1 agonists), also activates G_i, which inhibits cAMP formation in human atrial heart tissue.[31]

Stimulation of glucagon receptors in the liver and adipose tissue increases cAMP synthesis, resulting in glycogenolysis, gluconeogenesis, and ketogenesis.[36] Other properties of glucagon include relaxation of smooth muscle in the lower esophageal sphincter, stomach, small and large intestines, common bile duct, and ureters.[22,25,34]

CARDIOVASCULAR EFFECTS

Investigations of the mechanism of action of glucagon on the heart have been performed on cardiac tissue obtained from patients during surgical procedures and in a variety of in vivo and ex vivo animal studies. The results are often species specific and are affected by the presence or absence of congestive heart failure. The inotropic action of glucagon appears to be related to an increase in cardiac cAMP concentrations.[14,36,44] Both the positive inotropic[2,18,42,50] and chronotropic[2,14,18,32,34,42,44,50,71] actions of glucagon are very similar to those of the β-adrenergic agonists, except that they are not blocked by β-adrenergic antagonists.[73] Although in some canine experiments glucagon was associated with ventricular tachycardia, glucagon was not found to be dysrhythmogenic in studies in patients with severe chronic congestive heart failure or myocardial infarction–related acute congestive heart failure, or in postoperative patients with myocardial depression.[30,38,43,46] The effects of glucagon are also markedly diminished as the severity and chronicity of congestive heart failure increases.[50]

Evidence now suggests an additional mechanism of action for glucagon, independent of cAMP, and dependent on arachidonic acid.[61] Cardiac tissue metabolizes glucagon, liberating mini-glucagon, an apparently active smaller terminal fragment.[61,70] Mini-glucagon stimulates phospholipase A_2, releasing arachidonic acid. Arachidonic acid acts to increase cardiac contractility through an effect on calcium. The effect of arachidonic acid, and therefore of mini-glucagon, is synergistic with the effect of glucagon and cAMP.[62]

VOLUNTEER STUDIES

Cardiovascular effects were extensively studied in 21 patients with heart failure who were given varied doses and durations of glucagon therapy.[51] Eleven patients who received 3 to 5 mg via IV bolus had increases in the force of contraction, as measured by maximum dP/dT (upstroke pattern on apex cardiogram), heart rate, cardiac index, blood pressure, and stroke work. There was no change in systemic vascular resistance, left ventricular end-diastolic pressure (LVEDP), or stroke index. Additionally, glucose concentrations increased by 50% and the potassium concentrations fell. A study of nine patients demonstrated a 30% increase in coronary blood flow following a 50 μg/kg IV dose.[46] Patients who received 1 mg via IV bolus also had an increase in cardiac index, but systemic vascular resistance fell, probably secondary to splanchnic and hepatic vascular smooth muscle relaxation.[51] Patients who received an infusion of 2 to 3 mg/min for 10 to 15 minutes responded similarly to those who received the 3-5 mg IV boluses, but patients receiving boluses experienced significant dose-limiting nausea and vomiting.[51]

ROLE IN THE MANAGEMENT OF OVERDOSES WITH β-ADRENERGIC ANTAGONISTS

Overdoses with β-adrenergic antagonists are particularly dangerous and are manifested by hypotension, bradycardia, prolonged atrioventricular conduction times, depressed cardiac output, and cardiac failure. Other noncardiovascular effects include alterations in consciousness, seizures and, rarely, hypoglycemia.[1,12,15,17,23,69] Management is often complicated and many therapies, including atropine, isoproterenol, epinephrine, norepinephrine, dopamine, dobutamine, and various combinations, are used with variable success.[16,17] Recently high-dose insulin with glucose, and in the event of a cardiac arrest, intravenous fat emulsion, have been added to the armamentarium. Animal studies document the ability of glucagon to increase contractility, restore the sinus node function after sinus node arrest, increase atrioventricular (AV) conduction, and improve survival.[40,50,59] Glucagon has successfully reversed bradydysrhythmias and hypotension in patients unresponsive to the aforementioned traditional xenobiotics, and should be administered early in the management of patients with severe overdoses.[10,12,15,32,58,67] By increasing myocardial cAMP concentrations independent of the β receptor,[36,44] glucagon is able to increase inotropy[2,18,42,50] and chronotropy.[2,18,32,42,50,71]

Glucagon successfully reversed the bradycardia, low-output heart failure, and hypotension that developed in a premature newborn, presumably as a result of an inappropriately large prenatal dose of labetalol given to the mother. This neonate, delivered at 32 weeks gestation and weighing 1.8 kg, received 0.3 mg/kg glucagon intravenously initially and five additional doses of 0.3 to 0.6 mg/kg over the next 5 hours, with improvement in heart rate, blood pressure, and perfusion. Epinephrine and diuretics were also used.[63]

COMBINED EFFECTS WITH PHOSPHODIESTERASE INHIBITORS AND CALCIUM

Strategies for enhancing the effects of glucagon have involved combining it with the PDE-3 inhibitor amrinone (inamrinone) and its derivative milrinone and most recently rolipram PDE-4 inhibitor. In a canine model of propranolol toxicity, both amrinone (inamrinone) and milrinone alone were comparable to glucagon,[40,60] but the combination of amrinone and glucagon resulted in a decrease in mean arterial pressure.[39] A tachycardia occurred when milrinone was used with glucagon.[59] In an ex vivo model using strips of rat ventricular heart, rolipram enhanced the inotropic effect of glucagon and limited glucagon tachyphylaxis.[28]

The relationship between calcium and the chronotropic effects of glucagon was demonstrated in rats.[7] Maximal chronotropic effects of glucagon are dependent on a normal circulating ionized calcium. Both hypocalcemia and hypercalcemia blunt the maximal chronotropic response.[6,7]

ROLE IN CALCIUM CHANNEL BLOCKER OVERDOSE

Calcium channel blocker overdoses produce a constellation of clinical findings similar to those recognized with β-adrenergic antagonist overdoses, including hypotension, bradycardia, heart block, and myocardial depression. Animal studies[27,57,64,65,75,76] demonstrate the ability of glucagon to reverse the myocardial depression produced by nifedipine, diltiazem, and verapamil. Human case reports demonstrate similar benefit.[11,13,45,48,49,66] Some authors suggest that the addition of amrinone to glucagon therapy is beneficial.[72]

REVERSAL OF HYPOGLYCEMIA

Glucagon was once proposed as part of the initial treatment for all comatose patients.[54] Glucagon stimulates glycogenolysis in the liver. The theoretical rationale for this approach is only partially sound in that hypoglycemic patients may present in coma or with an altered mental status and hypoglycemia can be present concomitantly with a drug overdose. Immediately restoring the patient's blood glucose concentration may be life-saving; however, glucagon requires time to act and may be ineffective in a patient with depleted glycogen stores. Patients with type 2 diabetes are more likely to respond than are patients with type 1 diabetes. The IV administration of 0.5 to 1.0 g/kg of 50% dextrose in adults rapidly reverses hypoglycemia and does not rely on glycogen stores for its effect. IV dextrose, therefore, is preferred over glucagon as the initial substrate to be given to all patients with an altered mental status presumed to be related to hypoglycemia (see Antidotes in Depth A10: Dextrose). Glucagon retains a role as a temporizing measure, until medical help can be obtained, in settings such as in the home where IV dextrose is not an option.

In patients with insulinoma, after an initial hyperglycemic response glucagon may actually worsen hypoglycemia, as the result of a feedback rise in insulin.

ADVERSE EFFECTS AND SAFETY ISSUES

Side effects associated with glucagon include dose-dependent nausea, vomiting,[43] hyperglycemia, hypoglycemia, and hypokalemia; relaxation of the smooth muscle of the stomach, duodenum, small bowel, and colon; and, rarely, urticaria, respiratory distress, and hypotension.[19] The hyperglycemia is followed by an immediate rise in insulin, which causes an intracellular shift in potassium, resulting in hypokalemia.[24,43,50] It is unclear whether stimulation of the Na^+-K^+-adenosine triphosphatase (ATPase) in skeletal muscle also contributes to the hypokalemia as occurs with β-adrenergic agonists.[33,53]

Glucagon can also increase the release of catecholamines in a patient with a pheochromocytoma, resulting in a hypertensive crisis,[24] which can be treated with phentolamine.[19] Continuous prolonged treatment with glucagon might lead to a dilated cardiomyopathy, as was reported in a patient with a glucagonoma.[5] Glucagon is a pregnancy category B drug.

DOSING

An initial IV bolus of 50 μg/kg, infused over 1 to 2 minutes, is recommended (3-5 mg in a 70-kg person).[17] If clinically acceptable, a longer duration of infusion may be used to limit vomiting. Higher doses may be necessary if the initial bolus is ineffective, and up to 10 mg can be used in an adult.[26] Using too small a dose can potentially decrease systemic vascular resistance.[51] In many cases, the bolus dose has been followed by a continuous infusion of 2-5 mg/h (up to 10 mg/h) in 5% dextrose in water, which can be tapered as the patient improves.[1,25,26,52,58,69] This dosing regimen has never been studied and is based on case reports. Experimental heart preparations clearly demonstrate tachyphylaxis with continuous administration. Whether this occurs in humans is unclear, but might plead for repeated bolus infusions over 1 to 5 minutes rather than continuous infusion.[28,74] In addition, the smooth muscle relaxation associated with a continuous infusion would be assumed to impede attempts at gastrointestinal decontamination with multiple-dose activated charcoal (MDAC) or whole-bowel irrigation (WBI).

AVAILABILITY

Glucagon (rDNA origin) by Eli Lilly and Company is available as a 1 mg (1-Unit) lyophilized powder for injection, with an accompanying 1 mL of diluent in a disposable syringe.[19] The diluent contains 12 mg/mL of glycerin, water for injection, and hydrochloric acid, if needed, for pH adjustment. Phenol is not longer used in the diluent.[3,21] Glucagon (rDNA origin) as GlucaGen by Novo Nordisk A/S is available as a 1-mg (1-Unit) lyophilized powder for injection. It should be reconstituted with 1 mL of sterile water for injection.[20] Concentrations greater than 1 mg/mL should not be used. An adequate supply of glucagon in the emergency department is at least 20 1 mg vials, with assurance of another 30 mg in the pharmacy.[8,41]

SUMMARY

Glucagon can produce positive inotropic and chronotropic effects despite β-adrenergic antagonism and calcium channel blockade. Glucagon is often beneficial in the treatment of patients with severe overdoses of β-adrenergic antagonists and calcium channel blockers. The effects of glucagon may not persist and other therapies, such as insulin and dextrose, should also be considered (Chaps. 60 and 61). The relatively benign character of an IV bolus of glucagon in the patient with a serious overdose of a β-adrenergic antagonist or calcium channel blocker should lead the clinician to use glucagon early in patient management.

REFERENCES

1. Agura E, Wexler L, Witzburg R. Massive propranolol overdose. *Am J Méd.* 1986;80:755-757.
2. Benvenisty A, Spotnitz H, Rose EA, et al. Antagonism of chronic canine beta-adrenergic blockage with dopamine, isoproterenol, dobutamine, and glucagon. *Surg Forum.* 1979;30:187-188.
3 Brancato DJ. Recognizing potential toxicity of phenol. *Vet Hum Toxicol.* 1982;24:29-30.
4. Brechlert V, Pavoine C, Hanf R, et al. Inhibition by glucagon of the cGMP-inhibited low Km cAMP phosphodiesterase in the heart is medicated by a pertussis toxin-sensitive G-protein. *J Biolog Chem.* 1992;267:15496-15501.
5. Chang-Chretien K, Chew JT, Judge DP. Reversible dilated cardiomyopathy associated with glucagonoma. *Heart.* 2004;90:e44.
6. Chernow B, Reed L, Geelhoed G, et al. Glucagon endocrine effects and calcium involvement in cardiovascular actions in dogs. *Circ Shock.* 1986;19: 393-407.
7. Chernow B, Zaloga G, Malcolm D, et al. Glucagon's chronotropic action is calcium dependent. *J Pharm Exp Ther.* 1987;241:833-837.
8. Dart RC, Goldfrank LR, Chyka PA. Combined evidence-based literature analysis and consensus guidelines for stocking of emergency antidotes in the United States. *Ann Emerg Med.* 2000;36:126-132.
9. Davis S, Granner D. Insulin, oral hypoglycemic agents and the pharmacology of the pancreas. In: Hardman JG, Limbird LE, eds. *Goodman and Gilman's the Pharmacologic Basis of Therapeutics*, 10th ed. New York: McGraw-Hill; 2001:1707-1708.
10. DeLima L, Khararasch E, Butler S. Successful pharmacologic treatment of massive atenolol overdose: sequential hemodynamics and plasma atenolol levels. *Anesthesiology.* 1995;83:204-207.
11. Doyon S, Roberts JR. The use of glucagon in a case of calcium channel blocker overdose. *Ann Emerg Med.* 1993;22:1229-1233.
12. Ehgartner GR, Zelinka MA. Hemodynamic instability following intentional nadolol overdose. *Arch Intern Med.* 1988;148:801-802.
13. Fant JS, James LP, Fiser RT, Kearns GL. The use of glucagon in nifedipine poisoning complicated by clonidine ingestion. *Pediatr Emerg Care.* 1997; 13:417-419.
14. Farah A. Glucagon and the circulation. *Pharm Rev.* 1983;35:181-217.
15. Fernandes CMB, Daya MR. Sotalol-induced bradycardia reversed by glucagon. *Can Fam Physician.* 1995;41:659-665.
16. Frishman W. Beta-adrenoceptor antagonists: new drugs and new indications. *N Engl J Med.* 1980;305:500-506.
17. Frishman W, Jacob H, Eisenberg E, Ribner H. Clinical pharmacology of the new beta-adrenergic blocking drugs. Part 8. Self-poisoning with beta-adrenoceptor blocking agents: recognition and management. *Am Heart J.* 1979;98:798-811.
18. Glick G, Parmley W, Wechsler AS, Sonnenblick EH. Glucagon. *Circ Res.* 1968;22:798-799.
19. Glucagon [package insert]. Indianapolis, IN: Eli Lilly; 2003.
20. Glucagon [package insert]. Princeton, NJ: Novo Nordisk A/S; 2003.
21 Golightly L, Smolinske S, Bennett M, et al. Pharmaceutical excipients. *Med Toxicol.* 1988;3:128-165.
22. Hall-Boyer K, Zaloga G, Chernow B. Glucagon: hormone or therapeutic agent. *Crit Care Med.* 1984;12:584-589.
23. Heath A. β-Adrenoreceptor blocker toxicity: clinical features and therapy. *Am J Emerg Med.* 1984;2:518-526.
24. Hendy GN, Tomlinson S, O'Riordan J. Impaired responsiveness to the effects of glucagon on plasma adenosine 3 5 -cyclic monophosphate in normal man. *Eur J Clin Invest.* 1977;7:155-160.
25. Homcy CJ. The beta adrenergic signaling pathway in the heart. *Hosp Pract.* 1991;26:43-50.
26. Illingworth RN. Glucagon for beta-blocker poisoning. *Practitioner.* 1979;223: 683-685.
27. Jolly S, Kipnis J, Lucchesi B. Cardiovascular depression by verapamil: reversal by glucagon and interactions with propanolol. *Pharmacology.* 1987;35:249-255.
28. Juan-Fita M, Vargas M, Kaumann A. Rolipram reduces the inotropic tachyphylaxis of glucagon in rat ventricular myocardium. *Naunyn Schmiedebergs Arch Pharmacol.* 2004;370:324-329.
29. Kerns W II. Management of beta-adrenergic blocker and calcium channel antagonist toxicity. *Emerg Med Clin North Am.* 2007;25:309-331.
30. Kerns W II, Schroeder D, Williams C, et al. Insulin improves survival in a canine model of acute β-blocker toxicity. *Ann Emerg Med.* 1997;29: 748-757.
31. Kilts JD, Gerhardt MA, Richardson MD, et al. β_2-Adrenergic and several other G protein-coupled receptors in human atrial membranes activate both G_s and G_i. *Circ Res.* 2000;87:635-637.
32. Kosinski EJ, Malidzak GS. Glucagon and isoproterenol in reversing propanolol toxicity. *Arch Intern Med.* 1973;132:840-843.
33. Kraus-Friedmann N, Hummel L, Radominska-Pyrek A, et al. Glucagon stimulation of hepatic Na^+, K^+-ATPase. *Mol Cell Biochem.* 1982;44:173-180.
34. Larner J. Insulin and oral hypoglycemic drugs: glucagon. In: Gilman AG, Goodman LS, Gilman A, eds. *The Pharmacologic Basis of Therapeutics*, 6th ed. New York: Macmillan; 1980:1497-1523.
35 Lawrence AM. Glucagon provocative test for pheochromocytoma. *Ann Intern Med.* 1967;66:1091-1096.
36. Levey G, Epstein S. Activation of adenyl cyclase by glucagon in cat and human heart. *Circ Res.* 1969;24:151-156.
37. Levey GS, Fletcher MA, Klein I, et al. Characterisation of I-glucagon binding in a solubilized preparation of cat myocardial adenylate cyclase. *J Biol Chem.* 1974;249:2665-2673.
38. Lipski JI, Kaminsky D, Donoso E, Friedberg CK. Electrophysiological effects of glucagon on the normal canine heart. *Am J Physiol.* 1972;222:1107-1112.
39. Love JN, Leasure JA, Mundt DJ. A comparison of combined amrinone and glucagon therapy to glucagon alone for cardiovascular depression associated with propranolol toxicity in a canine model. *Am J Emerg Med.* 1993;11:360-363.
40. Love JN, Leasure JA, Mundt DJ, Janz TG. A comparison of amrinone and glucagon therapy for cardiovascular depression associated with propanolol toxicity in a canine model. *J Toxicol Clin Toxicol.* 1992;30:399-412.
41. Love JN, Tandy TK. β-Adrenoreceptor antagonist toxicity: a survey of glucagon availability. *Ann Emerg Med.* 1993;22:151-152.
42. Lucchesi B. Cardiac actions of glucagon. *Circ Res.* 1968;22:777-787.
43. Lvoff R, Wilcken D. Glucagon in heart failure and in cardiogenic shock—experience in 50 patients. *Circulation.* 1972;45:534-542.

44. MacLeod K, Rodgers R, McNeil J. Characterization of glucagon-induced changes in rate, contractility, and cyclic AMP levels in isolated cardiac preparations of the rat and guinea pig. *J Pharmacol Exp Ther.* 1981;217:798-804.
45. Mahr NC, Valdes A, Lamas G. Use of glucagon for acute intravenous diltiazem toxicity. *Am J Cardiol.* 1997;79:1570-1571.
46. Manchester JH, Parmley WW, Matloff JM, et al. Effects of glucagon on myocardial oxygen consumption and coronary blood flow in man and in dog. *Circulation.* 1970;41:579-588.
47. Méry PF, Brechler V, Pavoine C, et al. Glucagon stimulates the cardiac Ca^{2+} current by activation of adenyl cyclase and inhibition of phosphodiesterase. *Nature.* 1990;345:158-161.
48. Mullen JT, Walter FG, Ekins BR, Khasigian PA. Amelioration of nifedipine poisoning associated with glucagon therapy. *Vet Hum Toxicol.* 1991;33:358.
49. Papadopoulos J, O'Neil M. Utilization of a glucagon infusion in the management of a massive nifedipine overdose. *J Emerg Med.* 2000;18:453-455.
50. Parmley WW. The role of glucagon in cardiac therapy. *N Engl J Med.* 1971; 285:801-802.
51. Parmley W, Glick G, Sonnenblick E. Cardiovascular effects of glucagon in man. *N Engl J Med.* 1968;279:12-17.
52. Peterson C, Leeder S, Sterner S. Glucagon therapy for beta-blocker overdose. *Drug Intell Clin Pharm.* 1984;18:394-398.
53. Pettit GW, Vick RL, Kastello MD. The contribution of renal and extrarenal mechanisms to hypokalemia induced by glucagon. *Eur J Pharmacol.* 1977;41:437-441.
54. Rappolt R, Inaba D, Gay G. NAGD regime (Naloxone [Narcan], activated charcoal, glucagon, doxapram [Dopram]) for the coma of drug related overdoses. *Clin Toxicol.* 1980;16:395-396.
55. Rochais F, Abi-Gerges A, Horner K, et al. A specific pattern of phosphodiesterases controls the cAMP signals generated by different G_s-coupled receptors in adult rat ventricular myocytes. *Circ Res.* 2006;98:1081-1088.
56. Rodell M. The role of hormone receptors and GTP-regulatory proteins in membrane transduction. *Nature.* 1980;284:17-22.
57. Sabatier J, Pouyet T, Shelvey G, Cavero I. Antagonistic effects of epinephrine, glucagon and methylatropine but not calcium chloride against atrioventricular conduction of disturbances produced by high doses of diltiazem, in conscious dogs. *Fundam Clin Pharmacol.* 1991;5:93-106.
58. Salzberg M, Gallagher EJ. Propranolol overdose. *Ann Emerg Med.* 1980;9: 26-27.
59. Sato S, Tsuhi MH, Okubo N, et al. Combined use of glucagon and milrinone may not be preferable for severe propanolol poisoning in the canine model. *J Toxicol Clin Toxicol.* 1995;33:337-342.
60. Sato S, Tsuhi MH, Okubo N, et al. Milrinone versus glucagons: comparative effects in canine propranolol poisoning. *J Toxicol Clin Toxicol.* 1994;32: 277-289.
61. Sauvadet A, Rohn T, Pecker F, Pavione C. Arachidonic acid drives miniglucagon action in cardiac cells. *J Biol Chem.* 1997;272:12437-12445.
62. Sauvadet A, Rohn T, Pecker F, Pavione C. Synergistic actions of glucagons and miniglucagon on Ca^2 mobilization in cardiac cells. *Cir Res.* 1996;78: 102-109.
63. Stevens T, Guillet R. Use of glucagon to treat neonatal low-output congestive heart failure after maternal labetalol therapy. *J Pediatr.* 1995;127:151-153.
64. Stone CK, May WA, Carroll R. Treatment of verapamil overdose with glucagon. *Ann Emerg Med.* 1995;25:369-374.
65. Stone CK, Thomas SH, Koury SI, Low RB. Glucagon and phenylephrine combination vs glucagon alone in experimental verapamil overdose. *Acad Emerg Med.* 1996;3:120-125.
66. Walter FG, Frye G, Mullen JT, et al. Amelioration of nifedipine poisoning associated with glucagon therapy. *Ann Emerg Med.* 1993;22:1234-1237.
67. Ward DE, Jones B. Glucagon and beta-blocker toxicity. *Br Med J.* 1976; 2:151.
68. Wei Y, Mojsov S. Tissue-specific expression of the human receptor for glucagon-like peptide-I: brain, heart and pancreatic forms have the same deduced amino acid sequences. *FEBS Lett.* 1995;358:219-224.
69. Weinstein R. Recognition and management of poisoning with beta-blocking agents. *Ann Emerg Med.* 1984;13:1123-1131.
70. White CM. A review of potential cardiovascular uses of intravenous glucagon administration. *J Clin Pharmacol.* 1999;39:442-447.
71. Whitehouse F, James T. Chronotropic action of glucagon on the sinus node. *Proc Soc Exp Biol Med.* 1966;122:823-826.
72. Wolf LR, Spadafora MP, Otten EJ. Use of amrinone and glucagon in a case of calcium channel blocker overdose. *Ann Emerg Med.* 1993;22: 1225-1228.
73. Yagami T. Differential coupling of glucagon and beta adrenergic receptors with the small and large forms of the stimulatory G protein. *Mol Pharmacol.* 1995;48:849-854.
74. Yao L, Macleod KM, McNeill JH. Glucagon-induced desensitization: correlation between cyclic AMP levels and contractile force. *Eur J Pharmacol.* 1982;9:147-150.
75. Zaloga G, Malcolm D, Holaday J, et al. Glucagon reverses the hypotension and bradycardia of verapamil overdose in rats. *Crit Care Med.* 1985; 13:273.
76. Zaritsky A, Morowitz M, Chernow B. Glucagon antagonism of calcium blocker-induced myocardial dysfunction. *Crit Care Med.* 1988;16:246-251.
77. Zeiders JL, Seidler FJ, Iaccarino G, et al. Ontogeny of cardiac beta-adrenoceptor desensitization mechanisms: agonist treatment enhances receptor/G-protein transduction rather than eliciting uncoupling. *J Mol Cell Cardiol.* 1999;31:413-423.

CHAPTER 62
OTHER ANTIHYPERTENSIVES

Francis Jerome DeRoos

Hypertension is one of the most common chronic medical problems and one of the most readily amenable to pharmacotherapy. Beginning in the 1960s, when asymptomatic hypertension was linked to significant adverse effects such as stroke and sudden death, antihypertensive pharmacotherapeutics began being used. The first generation included centrally acting, sympatholytics, direct vasodilators, sodium nitroprusside, and diuretics. Unfortunately, these often had significant side effects, leading to the development of not only β-adrenergic antagonists and calcium channel blockers (CCBs) and more recently, angiotensin-converting enzyme inhibitors (ACEIs), and angiotensin receptor blockers (ARBs). This chapter reviews the first-generation antihypertensives, as well ACEIs and ARBs. In general, the majority of antihypertensives manifest clinical signs and symptoms in terms of the degree of hypotension produced. Particular attention will be placed on mechanisms of action and unique toxicologic considerations for each of these xenobiotics.

CLONIDINE AND OTHER CENTRALLY ACTING ANTIHYPERTENSIVES

Clonidine is an imidazoline compound that was synthesized in the early 1960s. Because of its potent peripheral α_2-adrenergic agonist effects, it was initially studied as a potential topical nasal decongestant. However, hypotension was a common side effect, which redirected its consideration for other therapeutic applications.[95] Clonidine is the best understood and the most commonly used of all the centrally acting antihypertensives, a group that includes methyldopa, guanfacine, and guanabenz. Although these drugs differ chemically and structurally, they all decrease blood pressure in a similar manner—by reducing the sympathetic outflow from the central nervous system (CNS). The imidazoline compounds oxymetazoline and tetrahydrozoline, which are used as ocular topical vasoconstrictors and nasal decongestants, produce similar systemic effects when ingested[95] (see Chap. 50).

Since 1985, the increased efficacy and improved side effect profiles of the newer antihypertensives have diminished the use of the α_2-adrenergic agonists in routine hypertension management. However, clonidine use is increasing as a result of a wide variety of applications, including attention-deficit hyperactivity disorder (ADHD); peripheral nerve and spinal anesthesia; and as an adjunct in the management of opioid, ethanol, and nicotine withdrawal.[110,116,120,202] In addition, abuse of clonidine may be a growing problem in opioid-dependent patients, and it has been used in criminal acts of chemical submission.[17,134]

Although centrally acting α_2-adrenergic agonist exposure is relatively uncommon, it may cause significant toxicity, particularly in children. One report from two large pediatric hospitals identified 47 children requiring hospitalization for unintentional clonidine ingestions over a 5-year period.[241] Significant clonidine poisoning has also resulted from formulation and dosing errors in children.[189,219] Imidazolines used as ocular vasoconstrictors have resulted in significant systemic toxicity as well.[95,138,126,180]

PHARMACOLOGY

Clonidine and the other centrally acting antihypertensives exert their hypotensive effects primarily via stimulation of presynaptic α_2-adrenergic receptors in the brain.[174,196,233] This central α_2-adrenergic receptor agonism enhances the activity of inhibitory neurons in the vasoregulatory regions of the CNS, notably the nucleus tractus solitarius in the medulla, resulting in decreased norepinephrine release. This results in decreased sympathetic outflow from the intermediolateral cell columns of the thoracolumbar spinal tracts into the periphery[1,232] and reduces the heart rate; vascular tone; and ultimately, arterial blood pressure.[175,245] This centrally mediated sympatholytic effect is modulated by nitric oxide and γ-aminobutyric acid (GABA), which may explain some of the clinical variability that occurs among patients who have overdosed with clonidine.[32,76,212,237]

PHARMACOKINETICS

Clonidine is well absorbed from the gastrointestinal (GI) tract (~75%) with an onset of action within 30 to 60 minutes. The peak serum concentration occurs at 2 to 3 hours and lasts as long as 8 hours.[53] Clonidine has 20% to 40% protein binding and an apparent volume of distribution of 3.2 to 5.6 L/kg.[132] The majority of clonidine is eliminated unchanged via the kidneys.[132]

Guanabenz and guanfacine are structurally and pharmacologically very similar to each other. They are well absorbed orally, achieving peak concentrations within 3 to 5 hours, and both have large volumes of distribution (4-6 L/kg for guanfacine; 7-17 L/kg for guanabenz).[100,214] Whereas guanabenz is metabolized predominantly in the liver and undergoes extensive first-pass effect, guanfacine is eliminated equally by the liver and kidney.[100,214] The metabolism of neither drug results in the production of significant active metabolites.

Whereas clonidine, guanabenz, and guanfacine are all active drugs with direct α_2-adrenergic agonist effects, methyldopa is a prodrug. It enters the CNS, probably by an active transport mechanism, before it is converted into its pharmacologically active degradation products.[19] α-Methylnorepinephrine is the most significant of its metabolites, although α-methyldopamine and α-methylepinephrine may also be important.[66,91,188] These metabolites are direct α_2-adrenergic agonists and impart their hypotensive effect as do the other centrally acting antihypertensives. Approximately 50% of an oral dose of methyldopa is absorbed, and peak serum concentrations are achieved in 2 to 3 hours.[156] However, because methyldopa requires metabolism into its active form, these concentrations have little correlation with its clinical effects. Methyldopa has a small volume of distribution (0.24 L/kg) and little protein binding (15%).[156] It is eliminated in the urine, both as parent compound and after hepatic sulfation.[163]

Clonidine is available in both oral and patch form. The patch, referred to as the clonidine transdermal therapeutic system, allows slow, continuous delivery of drug over a prolonged period of time, typically 1 week. This formulation, however, offers unique clinical challenges. Each patch contains significantly more drug than is typically delivered during the prescribed duration of use. For example, whereas a patch that delivers 0.1 mg/day of clonidine contains 2.5 mg total, the product that delivers 0.3 mg/day contains 7.5 mg.[31] Even after 1 week of use, between 35% and 50% and, in some instances, as much as 70%, of the drug remains in the patch.[31,88] Puncturing the outer membrane layer or backing opens the drug reservoir and allows a significant amount of the drug to be released rapidly. In addition, patients do not perceive this delivery system as a medication, and they may not exercise appropriate precautions. For example, discarding a used patch in an open wastebasket provides toddlers, who often are fascinated with stickers and other adhesive objects, an opportunity to remove the patch and apply, taste, or ingest it. Numerous reports of toxicity in both adults and children have resulted from dermal exposure, mouthing, or ingesting one clonidine patch, emphasizing this concern.[31,88,92,113,182,183]

PATHOPHYSIOLOGY

In therapeutic oral dosing, clonidine and the other centrally acting antihypertensives have little effect on the peripheral α_2 receptors, the peripheral sympathetic nervous system, or the normal circulatory responses that occur with exercise or the Valsalva maneuver.[155,167] However, when serum concentrations increase above 2 ng/mL, as in the setting of intravenous (IV) administration or oral overdose, peripheral postsynaptic α_2-adrenergic stimulation may occur, causing increased norepinephrine release and producing vasoconstriction and hypertension.[39,47,158,221] This hypertension is short-lived, however, because the potent centrally mediated sympathetic inhibition becomes the predominant effect, and hypotension ensues.[3,142,200]

Imidazoline-specific binding sites are identified both in the ventrolateral medulla of the brain and in other tissues and may be important in the clinical effects of these xenobiotics.[200,226] Direct stimulation of these receptors appears to lower blood pressure independent of central α_2-adrenergic effects.[21] Therefore, although their precise physiologic relationship has not been clearly elucidated, more evidence supports the concept that both imidazoline and α_2-adrenergic receptors modulate the ability of clonidine, and presumably other centrally acting antihypertensives, to inhibit central norepinephrine release and the cardiovascular effects.[22,89,151]

CLINICAL MANIFESTATIONS

Although the majority of the published cases involve clonidine, the signs and symptoms of poisoning with any centrally acting antihypertensive are similar. The CNS and cardiovascular toxicity reflect an exaggeration of their pharmacologic action. Common signs include CNS depression, bradycardia, hypotension, and (occasionally) hypothermia.[5,172,205,229] Most patients who ingest clonidine or the other similarly acting drugs manifest symptoms rapidly, typically within 30 to 90 minutes.[241] The exception may be methyldopa, which requires metabolism to be activated, possibly delaying toxicity for hours.[205,245]

CNS depression is the most frequent clinical finding and may vary from mild lethargy to coma.[137,142,166,181] In addition, severely obtunded patients may experience decreased ventilatory effort and hypoxia.[3] Respirations may be slow and shallow, with intermittent deep, sighing breaths. Various other terms are used to describe this phenomenon, including *gasping*, *Cheyne-Stokes respirations*, and *periodic apnea*.[5,9,113,142] This hypoventilation is typically responsive to tactile stimuli alone, although mechanical ventilation may be required in severe cases.[3,5,93,113] The associated CNS depression typically resolves over 12 to 36 hours.[9,166] Other manifestations of this CNS depression include hypotonia, hyporeflexia, and irritability.[39,142,217] The cranial nerve examination often demonstrates miotic pupils that may remain reactive to light.[3,5,223] Two unusual case reports describe seizures in the setting of clonidine poisoning,[39,135] the mechanism of which is unclear.

Hypothermia is associated with overdoses involving centrally acting antihypertensives.[5,142,172] This is thought to be a consequence of α-adrenergic effects within the thermoregulatory center, although other authors suggest that these drugs activate central serotonergic pathways that alter normal thermoregulation.[127,149] Although this phenomenon may last several hours, it rarely requires treatment and responds well to passive rewarming.[39,172]

Sinus bradycardia may occur in up to 50% of patients who ingest clonidine.[217,241] Although usually associated with hypotension, it may be an isolated finding. Plausible explanations for this bradycardia include an exaggerated centrally mediated sympatholytic effect, a centrally mediated increase in vagal tone, or a direct stimulation of α_2-adrenergic receptors on the myocardium.[49,122,232,242]

Other conduction abnormalities, including first-degree heart block, Mobite Type I and II atrioventricular block, and complete heart block, have been described both in overdose and after therapeutic dosing.[112,166,196,199,230,242] It appears that very young patients and patients who have underlying sinus node dysfunction, concurrent sympatholytic drug therapy, or renal insufficiency are at greatest risk of developing bradydysrhythmias after central antihypertensive agent ingestion.[26,217,225]

Hypotension is the major cardiovascular manifestation of central antihypertensive toxicity.[5,31,166,217,241] This typically occurs within the first few hours after exposure.[62] Paradoxically, severe hypertension may be noted early in dosing, particularly during IV administration, or in massive overdoses.[3,47,52,142,221] This is the result of peripheral α_2-adrenergic agonism. Typically, as the central sympatholytic effects become predominant, the hypertensive effect is short lived.[93] However, in patients with massive ingestions, hypertension may be protracted and require pharmacologic intervention.[3,52,142,217]

A recent study suggested a dose–response relationship between the history of the quantity of the centrally acting antihypertensive ingested and the severity of the clinical manifestations in children.[15] Others suggest that the age of the patient exposed may be a critical variable as well.[215] Although these observations seem intuitive, it is always important to remember that clonidine ingestions as small as 0.2 mg have resulted in clinically severe poisoning, so it is necessary to assess each exposure individually; the presence of any symptoms should prompt immediate medical evaluation.[166] Fatalities from any of these xenobiotics are rare, with few published reports from the American Association of Poison Control Centers (AAPCC) database[205] (see Chap. 135). This may be because these xenobiotics effectively block all sympathetic outflow from the CNS, and this physiologic effect is not essential for life. The CNS depression resulting in hypoventilation, hypoxia, and poor airway protection may be more pronounced in fatalities.

As a result of Food and Drug Administration (FDA) postmarketing surveillance and a case report that identified four deaths of children who received clonidine, a question was raised about whether there was an association between patients with ADHD who were being treated with combination clonidine–methylphenidate therapy and sudden death.[30,63] However, close scrutiny of these cases revealed significant confounders, and an investigation by the FDA concluded that there was inadequate evidence to confirm this association.[63,178,220,241]

WITHDRAWAL

Abrupt cessation of central antihypertensive therapy may result in withdrawal that is characterized by excessive sympathetic activity. Symptoms include agitation, insomnia, tremor, palpitations, and hypertension that begins between 16 and 48 hours after cessation of therapy.[85,184] Ventricular tachycardia and myocardial infarction may occur in patients with clonidine withdrawal.[16,157,173] The frequency and severity of symptoms appear to be greater in patients treated with higher doses for several months and in those with the most severe pretreatment hypertension.[184] However, cases occur even when the dosing is gradually reduced.[27,234] Although this phenomenon is associated with all centrally acting α_2-agonists, it appears to be more prominent with shorter-acting drugs such as clonidine and guanbenz.[25,72,179,244] The mechanism for this hyperadrenergic phenomenon appears to involve an increase in CNS noradrenergic activity in the setting of decreased α_2-receptor sensitivity.[58] Reasonable treatment strategies include administering clonidine or benzodiazepines, via either the oral or IV route followed by a closely monitored tapering of the dosing over several weeks. Animal and human data suggest that β-adrenergic antagonists, including labetalol, are harmful in the setting of clonidine withdrawal, and their use is contraindicated.[8,107]

DIAGNOSTIC TESTING

Clonidine and other centrally acting antihypertensives are not routinely included in serum or urine toxicologic assays. Consequently, management decisions should be based on clinical parameters. No electrolyte or hematologic abnormalities are associated with this exposure. Because of the potential for bradydysrhythmias and hypoventilation, a 12-lead electrocardiogram (ECG) and continuous cardiac and pulse oximetry monitoring are strongly recommended during the assessment.

MANAGEMENT

Appropriate therapy begins with particular focus on the patient's respiratory and hemodynamic status. Administration of activated charcoal (AC) is the primary mode of GI decontamination in most ingestions. However, in patients manifesting significant toxicity, the risks of placing a nasogastric tube and instilling AC may not exceed the potential benefits. Induction of emesis is contraindicated because of the possibility of rapid deterioration in mental status. Orogastric lavage has limited utility because these drugs are rapidly absorbed. Patients often present after the onset of symptoms rather than immediately after ingestion, and patients respond well to supportive care. In cases involving clonidine patch ingestions, whole-bowel irrigation appears to be an effective intervention.[92]

All patients with CNS depression should be evaluated for hypoxia and hypoglycemia. Those with respiratory compromise, including apnea, often respond well to simple auditory or tactile stimulation.[3,5,93,113] Significant arousal during preparation for intubation often precludes the need for mechanical ventilation.[3] Endotracheal intubation may be required, however, for the most severely poisoned patients.

Patients with isolated hypotension should initially be treated with standard doses of IV boluses of crystalloid. Bradycardia is typically mild and usually does not require any therapy if adequate peripheral perfusion exists. If the bradycardia is severe, however, atropine is often effective, but redosing may be required.[3,5,137,217] Dopamine may be beneficial in patients with recalcitrant bradycardia or hypotension.[3,5,31,77,137]

Naloxone was probably first used in patients with clonidine poisoning because of the similarity of its clinical findings to those of opioid toxicity, namely CNS and respiratory depression and miosis. Several clonidine-poisoned patients have had significant arousal after naloxone administration, as well as increased respiratory effort, heart rate, and blood pressure.[9,118,223] However, the exact reason for this physiologic response remains unclear. Animal models suggest that endogenous CNS opioids may modulate sympathetic outflow.[62,106,200]

This concept is supported by a clinical study in which clonidine administration to hypertensive patients for 3 days resulted in a significant decrease in blood pressure. Subsequent administration of 0.4 mg of naloxone parenterally reversed the decrease in blood pressure and heart rate in almost 60% of the patients.[61] Because of the short duration of effects of naloxone (20–60 minutes), redosing or continuous infusion may be required. As with some synthetic opioids, such as propoxyphene and fentanyl, clinical improvement may occur only after high doses (4–10 mg) of naloxone,[113,140] and some patients have no response regardless of dosing.[10,137,241] If, in fact, naloxone acts as a nonspecific sympatholytic agent, it may also be beneficial in poisoning involving other α-adrenergic agents; however, there is a paucity of published clinical experience. In one adult with severe guanabenz poisoning, 7 mg of naloxone failed to improve her clinical status.[172] Rarely, naloxone administration in the setting of clonidine overdose may precipitate significant hypertension, so continuous hemodynamic monitoring is indicated.[113,241]

The use of α-adrenergic antagonists such as tolazoline and yohimbine as specific antidotes for patients with α_2-adrenergic agonist overdoses is controversial. Although some patients have had significant clinical improvement,[166,197] tolazoline was ineffective in others.[3,217] The adult dose of tolazoline is 5 to 10 mg IV infusion every 15 minutes, up to a total maximum of 40 mg.[39] Given that tolazoline treatment is variably successful and that most physicians are unfamiliar with it, it cannot be recommended in the primary management strategy for centrally acting antihypertensive poisoning.

Early-onset hypertension is typically self-limited, and therapy should be cautiously undertaken, with the expectation that the hypertension will be self-limited. If hypertension is severe or prolonged, treatment with an infusion of sodium nitroprusside is appropriate.[142] Other short-acting antihypertensives, such as esmolol, may exacerbate this paradoxical hypertension in a manner similar to that which occurs when these xenobiotics are used in cocaine toxicity by inducing unopposed α_1-receptor stimulation (see Chap. 76). Although oral nifedipine has been used,[52] its lack of titratability and its unpredictable efficacy make its use inappropriate as well.

OTHER SYMPATHOLYTIC ANTIHYPERTENSIVES

Several other xenobiotics also exert their antihypertensive effect by decreasing the effects of the sympathetic nervous system. Often termed *sympatholytics*, they can be classified as ganglionic blockers, presynaptic adrenergic blockers, or α_1-adrenergic antagonists, depending on their mechanism of action. These drugs are rarely used clinically, and little is known about their effects in overdose.

GANGLIONIC BLOCKERS

Ganglionic blockers, such as trimethaphan, inhibit impulse transmission down both the postganglionic sympathetic and parasympathetic nerves, decreasing vascular tone, cardiac output, and blood pressure. These xenobiotics were used more frequently in the 1950s and 1960s in Europe, but because of their significant side effects, they were quickly replaced. Side effects stem from the unpredictable degree of sympathetic, as well as additional parasympathetic, blockade and include paralytic ileus, constipation, urinary retention, impotence, dry mouth, and blurred vision.[163] Trimethaphan is the only ganglionic blocker available in the United States, and it is administered IV. Although there have been no reported cases of intentional overdose, there have been cases of cardiopulmonary arrest associated with administration of continuous doses and with a 10-fold dosing error in a child while treating a hypertensive crisis.[46,84] In overdose, the exaggerated hypotensive response should respond well to IV crystalloid boluses and, if needed, a direct-acting vasopressor such as norepinephrine.

PRESYNAPTIC ADRENERGIC ANTAGONISTS

N–CH_2–CH_2–NH–C(=NH)–NH_2

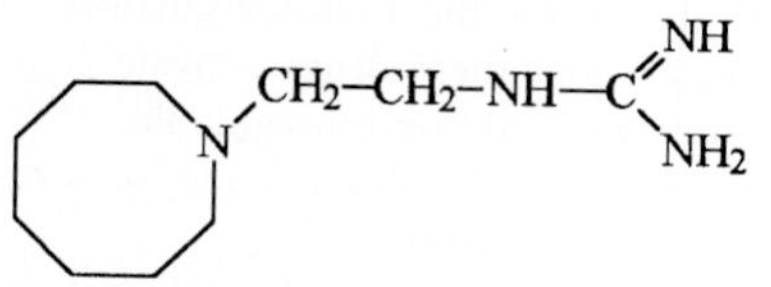

Guanethidine

These xenobiotics exert their sympatholytic action by decreasing norepinephrine release from presynaptic nerve terminals. Whereas guanethidine and guanadrel interfere with the action potential that triggers norepinephrine release,[202] reserpine depletes norepinephrine and other catecholamines from the presynaptic nerve terminals, probably by direct binding and inactivation of catecholamine storage vesicles.[73] Adverse effects limit their clinical usefulness. These effects include a high incidence of orthostatic and exercise-induced hypotension, diarrhea, increased gastric secretions, and impotence.[163] In addition, this hypotensive effect may be prolonged for as long as 1 week.[109,203] Because of its ability to cross the blood–brain barrier, reserpine may also deplete central catecholamines and produce drowsiness, extrapyramidal symptoms, hallucinations, or depression.[131] In overdose, an extension of their pharmacologic effects is expected. Patients with severe orthostatic hypotension should be anticipated and treated with IV crystalloid boluses and a direct-acting vasopressor. If reserpine is involved, significant CNS depression should also be anticipated.[131]

PERIPHERAL α_1-ADRENERGIC ANTAGONISTS

The selective α_1-adrenergic antagonists include prazosin, terazosin, and doxazosin. The α_1 receptor is a postsynaptic receptor primarily located on vascular smooth muscle, although they are also found in the eye and in the GI and genitourinary tracts.[43] In fact, these xenobiotics provide first-line pharmacologic therapy for patients with urinary dysfunction secondary to benign prostatic hyperplasia. They produce arterial smooth muscle relaxation, vasodilation, and a reduction of the blood pressure. Although better tolerated than ganglionic blockers and peripheral adrenergic neuron blockers, they may still produce significant symptoms of postural hypotension, including lightheadedness, syncope, or palpitations, particularly after the first dose or if the dosing is rapidly increased.[14] Hypotension and CNS depression ranging from lethargy to coma have been reported in overdose.[125,129,194] In addition, priapism may occur.[129,186] Treatment with supportive care, including IV fluid boluses and a vasopressor such as dopamine, was effective in the few overdose cases reported.[125,129,144]

DIRECT VASODILATORS

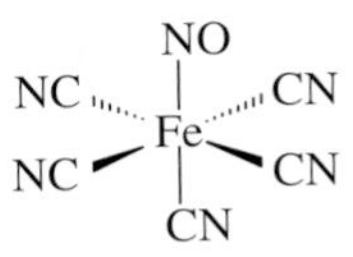

NO, NC, CN, Fe, NC, CN, CN

Nitroprusside

Hydralazine, Minoxidil, and Diazoxide These xenobiotics produce vascular smooth muscle relaxation independent of innervation or known pharmacologic receptors.[54,108,115] This vasodilatory effect has been attributed to stimulation of nitric oxide release from vascular endothelial cells. The nitric oxide then diffuses into the underlying smooth muscle cells, stimulating guanylyl cyclase to produce cyclic guanosine monophosphate (cGMP). This second messenger indirectly inhibits calcium entry into the smooth muscle cells, producing vasodilation.[193] Minoxidil, however, also has direct potassium channel activation effects.[123,161] It has been proposed that the opening of these adenosine triphosphate–linked potassium channels results in potassium influx and cell depolarization, thereby reducing calcium influx and ultimately relaxing vascular smooth muscle.[28]

As this vasodilation occurs, the baroreceptor reflexes, which remain intact, produce an increased sympathetic outflow to the myocardium, resulting in an increase in heart rate and contractile force. Typically, these xenobiotics are used therapeutically in patients with severe, refractory hypertension and in conjunction with a β-adrenergic antagonist to diminish reflex tachycardia. Hydralazine, minoxidil, and diazoxide are effective orally, but sodium nitroprusside is only used IV. Minoxidil is also used topically in a 2% solution to promote hair growth, and significant poisoning has occurred in suicidal adults who have ingested this formulation.[148] Diazoxide, although previously used to rapidly reduce blood pressure in hypertensive emergencies, is rarely used for this indication now as a consequence of its poor titratability and its variable, and occasionally profound, hypotensive effect.[114]

Adverse effects associated with daily hydralazine use include several immunologic phenomenon such as hemolytic anemia; vasculitis; acute glomerulonephritis; and most notably, a lupuslike syndrome.[176] Minoxidil may cause ECG changes, both in therapeutic doses and in overdose. Sinus tachycardia, ST segment depression, and T-wave inversion have all been reported.[83,177,210] There also appears to be an association with supratherapeutic doses of minoxidil and left ventricular multifocal, subacute necrosis, and subsequent fibrosis.[86,87] The significance of either of these changes is unknown; they typically resolve with either continued therapy or as other toxic manifestations resolve.[83,87,210]

The common toxic manifestations of these xenobiotics in overdose are an extension of their pharmacologic action. Symptoms may include lightheadedness, syncope, palpitations, and nausea.[2,136] Signs may be isolated to tachycardia alone,[177,210] flushing, or alterations in mental status, which is related to the degree of hypotension.[148] Based on AAPCC annual poison data, it appears that in recent years, the majority of reported exposures to this class of drugs involve the topical formulation of minoxidil[60] (see Chap. 135).

After appropriate GI decontamination, routine supportive care should be performed, with special consideration to maintaining adequate mean arterial pressure. If IV crystalloid boluses are insufficient, a peripherally acting α-adrenergic agonist, such as norepinephrine or phenylephrine, is an appropriate next therapy. Dopamine and epinephrine should be avoided to prevent an exaggerated myocardial response and tachycardia from β-adrenergic stimulation.

Nitroprusside Sodium nitroprusside is effectively a prodrug, exerting its vasodilatory effects only after its breakdown and the release of nitric oxide. The nitroprusside molecule also contains five cyanide radicals that, although gradually released, occasionally produce cyanide or thiocyanate toxicity.[162,198] Physiologic methemoglobin can bind the liberated cyanide. The binding capacity of physiologic methemoglobin is about 175 μg/kg of cyanide, corresponding to a little less than 500 μg/kg of infused sodium nitroprusside. These cyanide moieties are rapidly cleared, both by interacting with various sulfhydryl groups in the surrounding tissues and blood and enzymatically in the liver by rhodanese, which couples them to thiosulfate-producing thiocyanate.[67] This cyanide detoxification process in healthy adults occurs at a rate of about 1 μg/kg/min, which corresponds to a sodium nitroprusside infusion rate of 2 μg/kg/min.[44,198] It is limited by the sulfur donor availability, so factors that reduce these stores, such as poor nutrition in infants and toddlers, critical illness, surgery, and diuretic use, place patients at risk for developing cyanide toxicity.[35,44] The hemolysis associated with cardiopulmonary bypass may place the patient at particular risk because the elevated free hemoglobin may accelerate the release of cyanide from the sodium nitroprusside moiety.[35] Therefore, depending on the balance of cyanide release (eg, the rate of sodium nitroprusside infusion) and the rate of cyanide detoxification (eg, the sulfur donor stores), cyanide toxicity may develop within hours. Infusion of nitroprusside at a rate of more than 1.5 mg/kg administered over a few hours or more than 4 μg/kg/min for more than 12 hours may overwhelm the capacity of rhodanese for detoxifying cyanide.[185] Signs and symptoms of cyanide toxicity include alteration in mental status; anion gap metabolic acidosis; and in late stages, hemodynamic instability (see Chap. 126). Hydroxycobalamin is rapidly becoming the drug of choice for known cyanide poisonings.

One method of preventing cyanide toxicity from sodium nitroprusside is to expand the thiosulfate pool available for detoxification by the concomitant administration of sodium thiosulfate.[44,81,198] Dosing of 1 g sodium thiosulfate for every 100 mg of nitroprusside is typically sufficient to prevent cyanide accumulation[185] infusing 500 mg sodium thiosulfate (A standard 50-mL bottle of 25% sodium thiosulfate found in the Cyanide Antidote kit contains 12.5 gm).[185] Unfortunately, the thiocyanate that is formed may accumulate, particularly in patients with renal insufficiency, and may produce thiocyanate toxicity.[67,198]

Thiocyanate is almost exclusively renally eliminated, with an elimination half-life of 3 to 7 days. It is postulated that a continuous sodium nitroprusside infusion of 2.5 μg/kg/min in patients with normal renal function could produce thiocyanate toxicity within 7 to 14 days, although it may be as short as 3 to 6 days or as little as 1 μg/kg/min in patients with chronic renal insufficiency who are not receiving hemodialysis.[198] The symptoms of thiocyanate toxicity begin to appear at serum concentrations of 60 μg/mL (1 mmol/L); are very nonspecific; and may include nausea, vomiting, fatigue, dizziness, confusion, delirium, and seizures.[67] Thiocyanate toxicity may produce life-threatening effects, such as hemodynamic and intracranial pressure elevation, when serum concentrations are above 200 μg/mL.[44,67,81,227] Anion gap metabolic acidosis and hemodynamic instability do not occur with thiocyanate toxicity. Although cyanide or thiocyanate concentrations are not typically useful in the management of patients with cyanide toxicity, they may be beneficial for monitoring critically ill patients who are at risk of thiocyanate poisoning. Hemodialysis clears thiocyanate from the serum and should be strongly considered in patients with severe clinical manifestations of thiocyanate toxicity.[57,141,160]

Another therapeutic used to prevent cyanide toxicity from sodium nitroprusside is a simultaneous infusion of hydroxocobalamin. Although only available in the United States since 2007, hydroxocobalamin has been studied and successfully used in Europe to prevent cyanide poisoning from sodium nitroprusside infusions.[42,96,117,246] Similar to thiosulfate, when simultaneously infused, hydroxocobalamine does not interfere with the vasodilatory effects of sodium nitroprusside.[94] Dosing of 25 mg/h has successfully reduced cyanide poisoning in humans.[42,246] Because of the relative cost, and interactions with some laboratory tests of hydroxocobalamin, however, thiosulfate should remain the mainstay of prophylaxis against sodium nitroprusside-induced cyanide toxicity (see Antidotes in Depth A39 and A40: Hydroxocobalamin and Sodium Thiosulfate).

DIURETICS

Diuretics can be divided into three main groups: (1) the thiazides and related compounds, including hydrochlorothiazide and chlorthalidone; (2) the loop diuretics, including furosemide, bumetanide, and ethacrynic acid; and (3) the potassium-sparing diuretics, including amiloride, triamterene, and spironolactone. Two other groups of diuretics—the carbonic anhydrase inhibitors, such as acetazolamide, and osmotic diuretics, such as mannitol—are not used as antihypertensive agents.

The thiazides produce their diuretic effect by inhibition of sodium and chloride reabsorption in the distal convoluted tubule. Loop diuretics, in contrast, inhibit the coupled transport of sodium, potassium, and chloride in the thick ascending limb of the loop of Henle. Although their exact antihypertensive mechanism is unclear, an increased urinary excretion of sodium, potassium, and magnesium results from the use of loop diuretics. Potassium-sparing diuretics act either as aldosterone antagonists, such as spironolactone, or as renal epithelial sodium channel antagonists, such as triamterene, in the late distal tubule and collecting duct.[104]

The majority of toxicity associated with diuretics is metabolic and occurs during chronic therapy or overuse.[240] Hyponatremia develops within the first 2 weeks of initiation of therapy in more than 67% of susceptible patients.[213] Patients who are elderly, female, malnourished, or taking thiazides are at greatest risk.[7] With severe hyponatremia (<120 mEq/L), symptoms may include headache, nausea, vomiting, confusion, seizures, or coma. The osmotic demyelination syndrome has been reported during rapid correction of severe hyponatremia secondary to diuretic abuse[40] (see Chap. 16).

Other electrolyte abnormalities associated with diuretic use include hypokalemia and hypomagnesemia, which may precipitate ventricular dysrhythmias and sudden death. This is an extremely controversial topic, with several excellent studies providing conflicting results.[18,68,169,206,208] Although it is unclear how great a risk, if any, diuretic use may be, it remains prudent to monitor and correct the patient's potassium concentration.[99,206,239] This is particularly important in elderly patients and for those patients who concomitantly use digoxin, in which setting hypokalemia is clearly associated with dysrhythmias (see Chap. 64).[24,218] Potassium-sparing diuretics may cause hyperkalemia, particularly in the setting of renal insufficiency or when combined with other hyperkalemia-producing drugs such as ACEIs.[108]

Thiazide diuretics are associated with inducing hyperglycemia, particularly in patients with diabetes mellitus. This is a result of depletion of total-body potassium stores. Because insulin secretion is dependent on transmembrane potassium fluxes, this decrease in potassium concentration reduces the amount of insulin secreted.[133] This effect is dose dependent and reversible either by potassium supplementation or discontinuation of the thiazide diuretic.[34,90] This association has lead to significant work and discussion about the routine use of thiazide diuretics as first-line antihypertensives in the treatment of uncomplicated patients.[45,79,153]

Thiazide diuretics are also associated with inducing hyperuricemia, uric acid, renal calculi, and gout. Uric acid is the end product of purine metabolism, and its renal elimination is significantly dependent on intravascular and urinary volume. Diuretic-induced volume depletion decreases uric acid filtration and increases its reabsorption in the proximal tubule.[204,216] Several studies support the association with hyperuricemia and the development of gout.[29,82] One study found a link between thiazide diuretic use and the likelihood of the need for subsequent antigout therapy.[80]

Several unusual reactions are associated with thiazide diuretic use, including pancreatitis; cholecystitis; and hematologic abnormalities such as hypercoagulability, thrombocytopenia, and hemolytic anemia.[55,56,190,192,228,238]

Despite the widespread use of these xenobiotics, acute overdoses are distinctly rare.[128] Major signs and symptoms include GI distress, brisk diuresis, possible hypovolemia and electrolyte abnormalities, and altered mental status.[128] Typically, the diuresis is short lived because of the limited duration of effect and the rapid clearance of the majority of diuretics. Assessment should focus on fluid and electrolyte status, which should be corrected as needed. If hyperkalemia is unexpectedly discovered, either the ingestion of a potassium-sparing xenobiotic or, more likely, an overdose of potassium supplements, which are frequently prescribed in conjunction with thiazide and loop diuretics, should be considered.[101,102] Altered mental status, including coma, may result from diuretic overdose without evidence of any fluid or electrolyte abnormalities.[15,128,191] Postulated mechanisms include a direct drug effect and induction of transient cerebral ischemia.[164]

ANGIOTENSIN-CONVERTING ENZYME INHIBITORS

ACEIs are among the most widely prescribed antihypertensive drugs. At the time of this writing, there are 10 ACEIs approved by the US FDA

TABLE 62–1. Classification of Antihypertensives Available in the United States

β-Adrenergic antagonists (see Chap. 61)
Calcium channel blockers (see Chap. 60)
Sympatholytics
- Central α_2-adrenergic agonists
  - Clonidine, guanabenz, guanfacine, methyldopa
- Ganglionic blockers
  - Trimethaphan
- Peripheral adrenergic neuron antagonists
  - Guanethidine, guanadrel, metyrosine, reserpine
- Peripheral α_1-adrenergic antagonists
  - Prazosin, terazosin, doxazosin

Diuretics
- Thiazides
  - Bendroflumethiazide, chlorthalidone, chlorothiazide, hydrochlorothiazide, hydroflumethiazide, indapamide, methyclothiazide, metolazone, polythiazide, trichlormethiazide
- Loop diuretics
  - Bumetanide, ethacrynic acid, furosemide, torsemide
- Potassium-sparing diuretics
  - Amiloride, eplerenone, spironolactone, triamterene

Vasodilators
- Hydralazine, minoxidil, diazoxide, nitroprusside

Angiotensin-converting enzyme inhibitors
- Benazepril, captopril, enalapril, fosinopril, lisinopril, moexipril, perindopril, quinapril, ramipril, spirapril, trandolapril

Angiotensin II receptor blockers
- Candesartan, cilexetil, eprosartan, irbesartan, losartan, telmisartan, valsartan, olmesartan

for the treatment of hypertension (Table 62–1). In general, these drugs are well absorbed from the GI tract, reaching peak serum concentrations within 1 to 4 hours. Enalapril and ramipril are prodrugs and require hepatic metabolism to produce their active forms. These drugs are primarily eliminated via the kidneys.

All ACEIs have a common core structure of a 2-methylpropanolol-L-proline moiety.[71] This structure binds directly to the active site of ACE, which is found in the lung and vascular endothelium, preventing the conversion of angiotension I to angiotensin II. Because angiotensin II is a potent vasoconstrictor and stimulant of aldosterone secretion, vasodilation; decreased peripheral vascular resistance; decreased blood pressure; increased cardiac output; and a relative increase in renal, cerebral, and coronary blood flow occur.[71] This hypotensive response may be severe in select patients after their initial dose, resulting in syncope and cardiac ischemia.[37,97] Patients with renovascular-induced hypertension and patients who are hypovolemic from concomitant diuretic use appear to be at greatest risk.[97] Overall, however, these drugs are well tolerated and have a very low incidence of side effects. Some reported adverse effects include rash, dysgeusia, neutropenia, hyperkalemia, chronic cough, and angioedema.[51,71,224] Because of their interference with the renin–angiotensin system, ACEIs are potential teratogens and should never be used by pregnant women or women who intend to become pregnant.[12]

ACEI-Induced Angioedema Angioedema is an inflammatory reaction in which there is increased capillary blood flow and permeability, resulting in an increase in interstitial fluid. If this process is confined to the superficial dermis, urticaria develops; if the deeper layers of the dermis or subcutaneous tissue are involved, angioedema results. Angioedema most commonly involves the periorbital, perioral, or oropharyngeal tissues.[187] This swelling may progress rapidly over minutes and result in complete airway obstruction and death.[70,74,201] The pathogenesis of acquired angioedema involves multiple vasoactive substances, including histamine, prostaglandin D_2, leukotrienes, and bradykinin. Because ACE also inactivates bradykinin and substance P, ACE inhibition results in elevations in bradykinin concentrations that appear to be the primary cause of both ACEI-induced angioedema and cough (Fig. 62–1).[4,103] There is no evidence that the ACEI-induced angioedema phenomenon is IgE mediated.[4]

Although the literature is replete with reports of ACEI-induced angioedema, the overall incidence is only approximately 0.1%, and it is idiosyncratic.[64,103,105,209] One-third of these reactions occur within hours of the first dose, and another third occur within the first week.[139,209] It is important to remember that the remaining third of cases may occur at any time during therapy, even after years.[36] Women, African Americans, and patients with a history of idiopathic angioedema appear to be at greater risk.[139,168]

Treatment varies depending on the severity and rapidity of the swelling. Because of its propensity to involve the tongue, face, and oropharynx, the airway must remain the primary focus of management. A nasopharygeal airway is often helpful. If there is any potential for or suggestion of airway compromise, endotracheal intubation should be performed. Severe tongue and oropharyngeal swelling may make orotracheal or nasotracheal intubation extremely difficult, if not impossible. If this is a concern, fiberoptic nasal intubation may be an attractive option, provided that the resources are available. Other techniques, including retrograde intubation over a guidewire that was passed through the cricothyroid membrane and emergent cricothyrotomy, should also be considered.[187] The most important aspect of airway management in patients experiencing ACEI-induced angioedema, however, is early risk assessment for airway obstruction and rapid intervention before the development of severe and obstructive swelling.

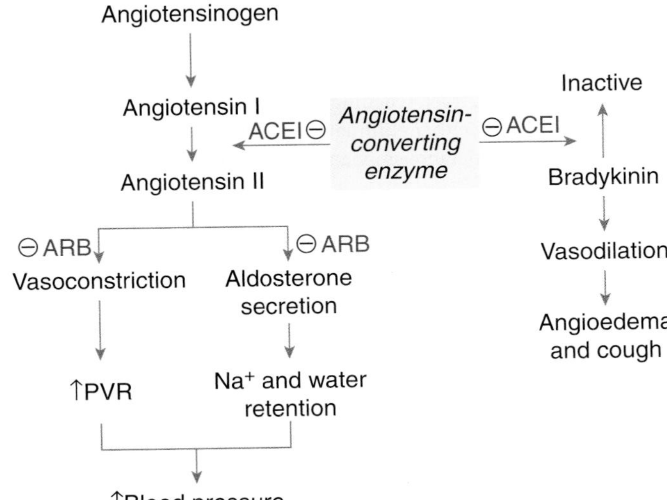

FIGURE 62–1. An overview of the normal function of angiotensin II and the mechanisms of action of angiotensin-converting enzyme inhibitors (ACEI) and the angiotensin II receptor blockers (ARB). PVR, peripheral vascular resistance. ACEIs are often implicated in angioedema and cough.

Because ACEI-induced angioedema is not an IgE-mediated phenomenon pharmacologic therapy targeting an allergic cascade, such as epinephrine, diphenhydramine, and steroids, should not be expected to be effective. However, when the history is unclear, these medications should not be withheld for fear of withholding life-saving therapy from someone having a severe IgE-mediated allergic reaction.

All patients with mild or quickly resolving angioedema should be observed for several hours to ensure that the swelling does not progress or return. Outpatient therapy with a short course of oral antihistamines and corticosteroids is appropriate. Such patients should be instructed to discontinue ACEI therapy permanently and to consult their primary care physicians about other antihypertensive options. Because this is a mechanistic and not allergic adverse effect, the use of any other ACEIs is contraindicated.

Angiotensin-Converting Enzyme Inhibitor Overdose The toxicity of ACEIs in overdose appears to be limited.[38,130] Although several reports of overdoses involving ACEIs have been published, the majority of the cases reported manifested toxicity of a coingestant.[48,78,239] Hypotension may occur in select patients,[12,117] but deaths are rarely reported in isolated ACEI ingestions.[170,236] Other patients may remain asymptomatic despite high serum drug concentrations.[124]

Treatment should focus on supportive care and on identifying any coingestants that may be more toxic, particularly other antihypertensives such as β-adrenergic antagonists and CCBs. In most cases, AC alone is sufficient GI decontamination. IV crystalloid boluses are often effective in correcting hypotension, although in rare cases, catecholamines may be required.[6]

Naloxone may also be effective in reversing the hypotensive effects of ACEIs. ACEIs may inhibit the metabolism of enkephalins and potentiate their opioid effects, which include lowering blood pressure.[50,154] In a controlled human volunteer study, continuous naloxone infusion effectively blunted the hypotensive response of captopril.[1] In one case report, naloxone appeared to be effective in reversing symptomatic hypotension secondary to a captopril overdose.[235] In another published case, naloxone was ineffective.[11] Although its role in the setting of ACEI overdose remains unclear, naloxone may obviate the need for large quantities of crystalloid or vasopressors and should therefore be considered.

ANGIOTENSIN II RECEPTOR BLOCKERS

ARBs were first introduced in 1995, and currently, six members of this class are marketed in the United States. These drugs are rapidly absorbed from the GI tract, reaching peak serum concentrations in 1 to 4 hours, and then are either eliminated unchanged in the feces or after undergoing hepatic metabolism via the mixed function oxidase system eliminated in the bile.[143,145-147,165]

Although these drugs are similar to ACEIs in that they decrease the effects of angiotensin II rather than decrease the formation of angiotensin II, they act by antagonizing angiotensin II at the type 1 angiotensin (AT-1) receptor (see Fig. 62–1).[111] This allows the drugs to inhibit the vasoconstrictive- and aldosterone-promoting effects of angiotensin II and reduce blood pressor by blunting both the sympathetic as well as the rennin–angiotensin systems.[143] In addition, they do not interfere with bradykinin degradation, thus reducing the risk of adverse effects, such as cough or angioedema, when compared to ACEI therapy.[119,139,171,222] However, cases of angioedema associated with ARB therapy have been reported.[33,139,231]

Similar to ACEIs, ARBs should never be used by pregnant patients because of their teratogenic potential.[12,207] In addition, when starting the drug, up to 1% develop of patients first-dose orthostatic hypotension.[75]

There have been few published reports of overdoses involving these drugs. Adverse signs and symptoms reflect orthostatic or absolute hypotension and include palpitations, diaphoresis, dizziness, lethargy, or confusion.[65,150,211] In mildly poisoned patients, this hypotension may be treated with IV crystalloid alone. However, in the most severe cases, hypotension may require pressor therapy.[150,211] Patients who are chronically taking ARBs have exhibited significant hypotension during induction of general anesthesia that is often refractory to traditional vasoconstrictor therapy, such as norepinephrine, ephedrine, and phenylephrine, but appear to respond rapidly to vasopressin.[20,23,59]

SUMMARY

Numerous xenobiotics are currently marketed for the treatment of chronic hypertension, including centrally acting drugs, other sympatholytics, direct vasodilators, diuretics, ACEIs, and ARBs. Although these xenobiotics are not typically associated with severe poisonings, either because of limited use, as with many of the sympatholytics and direct vasodilators, or because of limited toxicity, as with diuretics, ACEIs, and ARBs, severe poisonings may occur. Although centrally acting antihypertensives, such as clonidine, may produce significant CNS depression and bradycardia, as well as hypotension and the signs and symptoms associated with the degree of the hypoperfusion. Management of ingestions involving these antihypertensives should focus on appropriate GI decontamination, typically oral AC, and hemodynamic monitoring and support with IV crystalloids and catecholamines. Naloxone may be used in clonidine- or ACEI-poisoned patients, but its efficacy is variable. Sodium nitroprusside use may result in cyanide toxicity if the infusion rate exceeds the body's thiosulfate stores. Although cyanide toxicity may be prevented with concomitant infusion of sodium thiosulfate, thiocyanate toxicity may develop, particularly in patients with renal dysfunction.

REFERENCES

1. Ajayi AA, Campbell BC, Rubin PC, Reid JL. Effect of naloxone on the actions of captopril. *Clin Pharmacol Ther.* 1985;38:560-565.
2. Allon M, Hall WD, Macon EJ. Prolonged hypotension after initial minoxidil dose. *Arch Intern Med.* 1986;146:2075-2076.
3. Anderson FJ, Hart GR, Crumpler CP, Lerman MJ. Clonidine overdose. Report of six cases and review of the literature. *Ann Emerg Med.* 1981;10:107-112.
4. Anderson MW, deShazo RD. Studies of the mechanism of ACE inhibitor-associated angioedema: the effect of an ACE inhibitor on cutaneous responses to bradykinin, codeine, and histamine. *J Allergy Clin Immunol.* 1990;85:856-858.
5. Artman M, Boerth RC. Clonidine poisoning. *Am J Dis Child.* 1983;137:171-174.
6. Augenstein WL, Kulig KW, Rumack BH. Captopril overdose resulting in hypotension. *JAMA.* 1988;259:3302-3305.
7. Baglin A, Boulard JC, Hanslink T, Prinseau J. Metabolic adverse reactions to diuretics. *Drug Saf.* 1995;12:161-167.
8. Bailey RR, Neale TJ. Rapid clonidine withdrawal with blood pressure overshoot exaggerated by beta-blockade. *Br Med J.* 1976;1:942-943.
9. Bamshad MJ, Wasserman GS. Pediatric clonidine intoxications. *Vet Hum Toxicol.* 1990;32:220-223.
10. Banner WJR, Lund ME, Clawson L. Failure of naloxone to reverse clonidine toxic effect. *Am J Dis Child.* 1983;137:1170-1171.
11. Barr CS, Payne R, Newton RW. Profound prolonged hypotension following captopril overdose. *Postgrad Med J.* 1991;67:953-954.
12. Barr M Jr. Teratogen update: angiotensin-converting enzyme inhibitors. *Teratology.* 1994;50:399-409.
13. Bass JW, Beisel WR. Coma due to acute chlorothiazide intoxication *Am J Dis Child.* 1973;106:620-623.

14. Bendall MJ, Baloch KH, Wilson PB. Side effects due to treatment of hypertension with prazosin. *Br Med J.* 1975;2:727-729.
15. Benson BE, Spyker DA, Troutman WG, Watson WA. TESS-based dose-response using pediatric clonidine exposures. *Toxicol Appl Pharmacol.* 2006;213:145-151.
16. Berge KH, Lanier WL. Myocardial infarction accompanying acute clonidine withdrawal in a patient without a history of ischemic coronary artery disease. *Anesth Analg.* 1991;72:259-261.
17. Beuger M, Tommasello A, Schwartz R, Clinton M. Clonidine use and abuse among methadone program applicants and patients. *J Subst Abuse Treat.* 1998;15:589-593.
18. Bigger TJ. Diuretic therapy, hypertension, and cardiac arrest. *N Engl J Med.* 1994;330:1899-1900.
19. Bobik A, Jennings G, Jackman G, et al. Evidence for a predominantly central hypotensive effect of alpha-methyldopa in humans. *Hypertension.* 1986;8:16-23.
20. Boccara G, Ouattara A, Godet G, et al. Terlipressin vs norepinephrine to correct refractory arterial hypotension after general anesthesia in patients chronically treated with rennin angiotensin system inhibitors. *Anesthesiology.* 2003;98:1338-1344.
21. Bousquet P, Feldman J, Tibirica E, et al. A new concept in central regulation of the arterial blood pressure. *Am J Hypertens.* 1992;4(suppl): 47S-50S.
22. Bousquet P, Brauban V, Schann S, et al. Participation of imidazo-line receptor and alpha$_2$-adrenoceptors in the central hypotensive effects of imidazoline-like drugs. *Ann NY Acad Sci.* 1999;881:272-278.
23. Brabant SM, Eyraud D, Bertrand M, Coriat P. Refractory hypotension after induction of anaesthesia in a patient chronically treated with angiotensin receptor antagonists. *Anesth Analg.*1999;89:887-889.
24. Brater DC, Morrelli HF. Digoxin toxicity in patients with normokalaemic potassium depletion. *Clin Pharmacol Ther.* 1978;22:21-33.
25. Burden AC, Alexander CPT. Rebound hypertension after acute methyldopa withdrawal. *Br Med J.* 1976;2:1056-1057.
26. Byrd BF III, Collins HW, Primm RK. Risk factors for severe bradycardia during oral clonidine therapy for hypertension. *Arch Intern Med.* 1988;148:729-733.
27. Cairns SA, Marshall AJ. Clonidine withdrawal. *Lancet.* 1976;1:268.
28. Campese VM. Minoxidil: a review of its pharmacological properties and therapeutic us. *Drugs.* 1981;22:257-278.
29. Campion EW, Glynn RJ, DeLabry LO. Asymptomatic hyperuricemia. Risks and consequences in the Normative Aging Study. *Am J Med.* 1987;82: 421-426.
30. Cantwell D, Swanson J, Connor D. Case study. Adverse response to clonidine. *J Am Acad Child Adolesc Psychiatry.* 1997;36:539-544.
31. Caravati EM, Bennett DL. Clonidine transdermal patch poisoning. *Ann Emerg Med.* 1988;17:175-176.
32. Castro JL, Ricci D, Taira C, et al. Central benzodiazepine involvement in clonidine cardiovascular actions. *Can J Physiol Pharmacol.* 1995;77: 844-851.
33. Cha YJ, Pearson VE. Angioedema due to losartan. *Ann Pharmacother.* 1999; 33:936-938.
34. Chan JC, Cockram CS, Critchley JA. Drug-induced disorders of glucose metabolism. Mechanisms and management. *Drug Saf.* 1996;15:135-157.
35. Cheung AT, Cruz-Shiavone GE, Meng QC, et al. Cardiopulmonary bypass, hemolysis and nitroprusside-induced cyanide production. *Anesth Analg.* 2007;105:29-33.
36. Chin HL, Buchan DA. Severe angioedema after long term use of an angiotensin-converting enzyme inhibitor. *Ann Intern Med.* 1990;112:312-313.
37. Cleland JGF, Dargie HJ, McAlpine, et al. Severe hypotension after first dose of enalapril in heart failure. *Br Med J.* 1985;291:1309-1312.
38. Cobaugh DJ, Everson GW, Normann SA, et al. Angiotensin converting enzyme inhibitor overdoses: a multi-centre study. *Vet Hum Toxicol.* 1990;32:352.
39. Conner CS, Watanabe AS. Clonidine overdose: a review. *Am J Hosp Pharm.* 1979;36:906-911.
40. Copeland PM. Diuretic abuse and central pontine myelinolysis. *Psychother Psychosom.* 1989;52:101-105.
41. Corneli HM, Banner WW, Vernon DD, Swenson PH. Toddler eats clonidine patch and nearly quits smoking for life. *JAMA.* 1989;261:42.
42. Cottrell JE, Casthely P, Brodie JD, et al. Prevention of nitroprusside-induced cyanide toxicity with hydroxocobalamin. *N Engl J Med.* 1978;298: 809-811.
43. Cubeddu LX. New alpha$_1$-adrenergic receptor antagonists for the treatment of hypertension: role of vascular alpha receptors in the control of peripheral resistance. *Am Heart J.* 1988;116:133-162.
44. Curry SC, Arnold-Capell P. Nitroprusside, nitroglycerin, and angiotensin-converting enzyme inhibitors. *Crit Care Clin.* 1991;7:555-581.
45. Cutler JA, Davis BR. Thiazide-type diuretics and β-adrenergic blockers as first-line drug treatments for hypertension. *Circulation.* 2008;117:2691-2705.
46. Dale RC, Schroeder ET. Respiratory paralysis during treatment of hypertension with trimethaphan camsylate. *Arch Intern Med.* 1976;126:816-818.
47. Davies DS, Wing MH, Reid JL, et al. Pharmacokinetics and concentration-effect relationships of intravenous and oral clonidine. *Clin Pharmacol Ther.* 1976;21:593-601.
48. Dawson AH, Harvey D, Smith AJ, et al. Lisinopril overdose. *Lancet.* 1990;335:487-488.
49. De Jonge A, Timmermans PB, van Zwieten PA. Qualitative aspects of α-adrenergic effects induced by clonidine-like imidazolidines: II. Central and peripheral bradycardia activities. *J Pharmacol Exp Ther.* 1982;222:712-719.
50. Di Nicolantonia R, Hutchinson JS, Takata Y, Veroni M. Captopril potentiates the vasodepressor action of metenkephalin in anaesthetised dogs. *Br J Pharmacol.* 1983;80:405-408.
51. DiBianco R. Adverse reactions with angiotensin converting enzyme (ACE) inhibitors. *Med Toxicol.* 1986;1:122-141.
52. Dire DJ, Kuhns DW. The use of sublingual nifedipine in a patient with a clonidine overdose. *J Emerg Med.* 1988;6:125-128.
53. Dollery CT, Davies DS, Draffan GH, et al. Clinical pharmacology and pharmacokinetics of clonidine. *Clin Pharmacol Ther.* 1976;19:11-17.
54. DuCharme DW, Freyburger WA, Graham BE, Carlson RG. Pharmacologic properties of minoxidil: a new hypertensive agent. *J Pharmacol Exp Ther.* 1973;184:662-670.
55. Eckhauser ML, Dokler MA, Imbembo AL. Diuretic-associated pancreatitis: a collective review and illustrative cases. *Am J Gastroenterol.* 1987;82:865-870.
56. Eisner EV, Crowell EB. Hydrochlorothiazide-dependent thrombocytopenia due to IgM antibodies. *JAMA.* 1971;215:480-482.
57. Elberg AJ, Gorman HM, Baker R, et al. Prolonged nitroprusside and intermittent hemodialysis as therapy for intractable hypertension. *Am J Dis Child.* 1978;132:988-989.
58. Engberg G, Elam M, Svensson TH. Clonidine withdrawal: activation of brain noradrenergic neurons with specifically reduced alpha 2-receptor sensitivity. *Life Sci.* 1982;30:235-243.
59. Eyraud D, Brabant S, Nathalie D, et al. Treatment of intraoperative refractory hypotension with terlipressin in patients chronically treated with an antagonist of the rennin-angiotensin system. *Anesth Analg.*1999;88:980-984.
60. Farrell SE, Epstein SK. Overdose of Rogaine Extra Strength for Men topical minoxidil preparation. *J Toxicol Clin Toxicol.* 1999;37:781-783.
61. Farsang C, Kapocsi J, Vajda L, et al. Reversal of naloxone of the antihypertensive action of clonidine: involvement of the sympathetic nervous system. *Hypertension.* 1984;69:461-467.
62. Farsang C, Ramirez MDR, Mucci L, Kunos G. Possible role of an endogenous opiate in the cardiovascular effects of central alpha adrenoceptor stimulation in spontaneously hypertensive rats. *J Pharmacol Exp Ther.* 1980;214:203-208.
63. Fenichel RR. Post-marketing surveillance identifies three case of sudden death in children during treatment with clonidine and methylphenidate. *J Child Adolesc Psychopharmacol.* 1995;5:157-166.
64. Finley CJ, Silverman MA, Nunez AE. Angiotensin converting enzyme inhibitor-induced angioedema: still unrecognized. *Am J Emerg Med.* 1992;10:550-552.
65. Forrester MB. Valsartan ingestions among adults reported to Texas poison control centers 2000-2005. *J Med Toxicol.* 2007;3:157-163.
66. Freed CR, Quintero E, Murphy RC. Hypotension and hypothalamic amine metabolism after long-term alpha-methyldopa infusions. *Life Sci.* 1978;23: 313-322.
67. Friederich JA, Butterworth JF. Sodium nitroprusside: twenty years and counting. *Anesth Analg.* 1995;81:152-162.
68. Freis ED. Adverse effects of diuretics. *Drug Saf.* 1992;7:364-373.
69. Frohlich ED, Messerli FH, Pegram BL, Kardon MB. Hemodynamic and cardiac effects of centrally acting antihypertensive drugs. *Hypertension.* 1984;6(suppl II):76-81.
70. Gannon TH, Eby Tl. Angioedema for angiotensin-converting enzyme inhibitors: a cause of upper airway obstruction. *Laryngoscope.* 1990;100: 1156-1160.
71. Gavras H, Gavras I. Angiotensin converting enzyme inhibitors: properties and side effects. *Hypertension.* 1988;11(suppl II):37-41.

72. Geyskes GG, Boer P, Dorhout MEJ. Clonidine withdrawal. Mechanism and frequency of rebound hypertension. *Br J Clin Pharmacol.* 1979;7:55-62.
73. Giachetti A, Shore PA. The reserpine receptor. *Life Sci.* 1978;23:89-92.
74. Giannoccaro PJ, Wallace GJ, Higginson LAJ, et al. Fatal angioedema associated with enalapril. *Can J Cardiol.* 1989;5:335-336.
75. Goldberg AJ, Dunlay MC, Sweet CS. Safety and tolerability of losartan potassium, an angiotensin II receptor antagonist, compared with hydrochlorothiazide, atenolol, felodipine ER, and angiotensin converting enzyme inhibitors for the treatment of systemic hypertension. *Am J Cardiol.* 1995;75:793-795.
76. Gozliniska B, Czyzewska-Szafran H. Clonidine action in spontaneously hypertensive rats (SHR) depends on the GABAergic system function. *Amino Acids.* 1999;17:131-138.
77. Grabert B. Clonidine. Recurrent apnea following overdose. *Drug Intell Clin Pharm.* 1979;13:1778-1780.
78. Graham SR, Day RO, Hardy M. Captopril overdose. *Med J Aust.* 1989;151:111.
79. Gress TW, Nieto FJ, Shahar, et al. Hypertension and antihypertensive therapy as risk factors for type 2 diabetes mellitus. *N Engl J Med.* 2000;342:904-912.
80. Gurwitz JH, Kalish SC, Bohn RL, et al. Thiazide diuretics and the initiation of anti-gout therapy. *J Clin Epidemiol.* 1997;50:953-959.
81. Hall AH, Rumack BH. Hydroxocobalamin/sodium thiosulfate as a cyanide antidote. *J Emerg Med.* 1987;5:115-121.
82. Hall AP, Barry PE, Dawber TR, McNamara PM. Epidemiology of gout and hyperuricemia: a long-term population study. *Am J Med.* 1967;42:27-37.
83. Hall D, Charocopos F, Froer KL, Rudolph W. ECG changes during long term minoxidil therapy for severe hypertension. *Arch Intern Med.* 1979;139:790-794.
84. Hammer GB. Ultra-high dose trimethaphan in an infant with severe hypertension. *Clin Toxicol.* 1996;34:227-229.
85. Hansson L. Clinical aspects of blood pressure crisis due to withdrawal of centrally acting antihypertensive drugs. *Br J Clin Pharmacol.* 1983;15:485-490.
86. Hanton G, Gautier M, Bonnet P. Use of M-mode and Doppler echocardiography to investigate the cardiotoxicity of minoxidil in beagle dogs. *Arch Toxicol.* 2004;78:40-48.
87. Hanton G, Sobry C, Dagues N, et al. Cardiovascular toxicity of minoxidil in the marmoset. *Toxicol Lett.* 2008:180;157-165.
88. Harris JM. Clonidine patch toxicity. *Ann Pharmacother.* 1990;24:1191-1194.
89. Head GA, Chan CKS, Burke SL. Relationship between imidazoline and α_2-adrenoceptors involved in the sympatho-inhibitory actions of centrally acting antihypertensive agents. *J Auton Nerv Syst.* 1998;72;163-169.
90. Helderman JH, Elahi D, Anderson DK, et al. Prevention of the glucose intolerance of thiazide diuretics by maintenance of body potassium. *Diabetes.* 1983;32:106-111.
91. Henning M, Rubenson A. Evidence that the hypotensive action of alpha-methyl-DOPA is mediated by central actions of methylnoradrenaline. *J Pharm Pharmacol.* 1971;23:407-411.
92. Henretig F, Wiley J, Brown L. Clonidine patch toxicity: the proof is in the poop [abstract]. *J Toxicol Clin Toxicol.* 1995;33:520.
93. Henretig F. Clonidine and central acting antihypertensives. In: Ford M, Delaney DA, Ling L, Erickson T, eds. *Clinical Toxicology.* Philadelphia: WB Saunders; 2001:391-396.
94. Henwick DS, Butler AR, Glidewell C, McIntosh AS. Sodium nitroprusside. pharmacological aspects of its interaction with hydroxocobalamin and thiosulphate. *J Pharm Pharmacol.* 1987;39:113-117.
95. Higgins GL, Campbell B, Wallace K, et al. Pediatric poisoning from over-the-counter imidazoline-containing products. *Ann Emerg Med.* 1991;20:655-658.
96. Hobel M, Engeser, P. Nemeth, L. Pill, J. The antidote effect of thiosulphate and hydroxocobalamin in formation of nitroprusside intoxication of rabbits. *Arch Toxicol.* 1980;46:207-213.
97. Hodsman GP, Isles CG, Murray GD, et al. Factors related to first dose hypotensive effect of captopril: prediction and treatment. *Br Med J.* 1993;286: 832-834.
98. Hoffman BB, Lefkowitz RJ. Catecholamines, sympathomimetic drugs, and adrenoceptor antagonists. In: Hardman JG, Limbird LE, Molinoff PB, Ruddon RW, eds. *Goodman and Gilman's The Pharmacological Basis of Therapeutics*, 9th ed. New York: McGraw-Hill; 1996:199-248.
99. Holland OB, Nixon JV, Kuhnet L. Diuretic induced ventricular ectopic activity. *Am J Med.* 1981;70:762-765.
100. Holmes B, Brogden RN, Heel RC. Guanabenz: a review of its pharmacodynamic properties and therapeutic efficacy in hypertension. *Drugs.* 1983;26:212-229.
101. Hume L, Forfar JC: Hyperkalaemia and overdose of antihypertensive agents. *Lancet.* 1977;2:1182.
102. Illingworth RN, Proudfoot AT. Rapid poisoning with slow-release potassium. *Br Med J.* 1980;2:485-486.
103. Israili ZH, Hall WD. Cough and angioneurotic edema associated with angiotensin-converting enzyme inhibitor therapy. *Ann Intern Med.* 1992;117:234-242.
104. Jackson EK. Diuretics. In: Hardman JG, Limbird LE, eds. Goodman and Gilman's *The Pharmacological Basis of Therapeutics*, 10th ed. New York: McGraw-Hill; 2001:757-787.
105. Jett KG. Captopril-induced angioedema. *Ann Emerg Med.* 1984;13;489-490.
106. Jin CM, Rockhold RW. Sympathoadrenal control by paraventricular hypothalamic β-endorphin in hypertension. *Hypertension.* 1991;18:503-515.
107. Jonkman FA, Man PW, Breurkes R, van Zwieten PA. Beta 2-adrenoceptor antagonists intensify clonidine withdrawal syndrome in conscious rats. *J Cardiovasc Pharmacol.* 1989;14:886-891.
108. Juurlink DN, Mamdani MM, Lee DS, et al. Rates of hyperkalemia after publication of the Randomized Aldactone Evaluation Study. *N Engl J Med.* 2004;351:543-551.
109. Kalmanovitch DVA. Hypotension after guanethidine block. *Anaesthesia.* 1988;43:256.
110. Kambibayashi T, Maze M. Clinical uses of α_2-adrenergic agonists. *Anesthesiology.* 2000;93:1345-1349.
111. Kang PM, Landau AJ, Eberhardt RT, Frishman WH. Angiotensin II receptor antagonists: a new approach to blockade of the renin-angiotensin system. *Am Heart J.* 1994;127:1388-1401.
112. Kibler LE, Gazes PC. Effect of clonidine on atrioventricular conduction. *JAMA.* 1977;238:1930-1932.
113. Knapp JF, Fowler MA, Wheeler CA, Wasserman GS. Case 01-1995: a two-year-old female with alteration of consciousness. *Pediatr Emerg Care.* 1995;11:62-65.
114. Koch-Weser J. Diazoxide. *N Engl J Med.* 1976;294:1271-1274.
115. Koch-Weser J. Hydralazine *N Engl J Med.* 1976;295:320-323.
116. Kosten TR, O'Connor PG. Management of drug and alcohol withdrawal. *N Engl J Med.* 2003;348:1786-1795.
117. Krapez JR, Vesey CJ, Adams L, Cole PV. Effects of cyanide antidotes used with sodium nitroprusside infusions: sodium thiosulphate and hydroxocobalamin given prophylactically to dogs. *Br J Anaesth.* 1981;53:793-804.
118. Kulig K, Duffy J, Rumack BH, et al. Naloxone for treatment of clonidine overdose. *JAMA.* 1982;247:1697.
119. Lacourciere Y, Lefebvre J, Nakhle G, et al. Association between cough and angiotensin converting enzyme inhibitors versus angiotensin II antagonists: the design of a prospective, controlled study. *J Hypertens.* 1994;12(suppl):S49-S53.
120. Landau R, Schiffer E, Morales M, et al. The dose-sparing effect of clonidine added to ropivacaine for labor epidural analgesia. *Anesth Analg.* 2002;95:728-734.
121. Lau CP. Attempted suicide with enalapril. *N Engl J Med.* 1986;315:197.
122. Laubie M, Schmitt H, Drouillat M. Action of clonidine on the baroreceptor pathway and medullary sites mediating vagal bradycardia. *Eur J Pharmacol.* 1976;38:293-303.
123. LeBlanc N, Wilde, DW, Keff, KD, Hume JR. Electrophysiological mechanisms of minoxidil-induced vasodilation of rabbit portal vein. *Circ Res.* 1989;65:1102-1111.
124. Lechleitner P. Uneventful self-poisoning with a very high dose of captopril. *Toxicology.* 1990;64:325-329.
125. Lenz K, Druml W, Kleinberger G, et al. Acute intoxication with prazosin: a case report. *Hum Toxicol.* 1985;4:53-56.
126. Lev R, Clark RF. Visine overdose: case report of an adult with hemodynamic compromise. *J Emerg Med.* 1995;5:649-652.
127. Lin MT, Chandra A, Ko WC, Chen YM. Serotonergic mechanisms of clonidine-induced hypothermia in rats. *Neuropharmacology.* 1981;20:15-21.
128. Lip GYH, Ferner RE. Poisoning with anti-hypertensive drugs: diuretics and potassium supplements. *J Hum Hypertens.* 1995;9:295-301.
129. Lip GYH, Ferner RE. Poisoning with anti-hypertensive drugs: alphaadrenoreceptor antagonists. *J Hum Hypertens.* 1995;9:523-526.
130. Lip GYH, Ferner RE. Poisoning with anti-hypertensive drugs: angiotensin converting enzme inhibitors. *J Hum Hypertens.* 1995;9:711-715.
131. Loggie JMH, Saito H, Kahn I, et al. Accidental reserpine poisoning: clinical and metabolic effects. *Clin Pharmacol Ther.* 1967;8:692-695.
132. Lowenthal DT. Pharmacokinetics of clonidine. *J Cardiovasc Pharmacol.* 1980;2(suppl):529-537.

133. Luna B, Feinglos MN. Drug-induced hyperglycemia. *JAMA*. 2001;286:945-1948.
134. Lusthof KJ, Lameijer W, Zweipfenning PGM. Use of clonidine for chemical submission. *Clin Toxicol*. 2000;38:329-332.
135. MacFaul R, Miller G. Clonidine poisoning in children. *Lancet*. 1979;1:1266-1267.
136. MacMillan AR, Warshawski FJ, Steinberg RA. Minoxidil overdose. *Chest*. 1993;103:1290-1291.
137. Maggi JC, Iskra MK, Nussbaum E. Severe clonidine overdose in children requiring critical care. *Clin Paediatr*. 1986;25:453-455.
138. Mahieu LM, Rooman RP, Goossens E. Imidazoine intoxication in children. *Eur J Pediatr*. 1993;152:944-946.
139. Malde B, Regalado J, Greenberger PA. Investigation of angioedema associated with the use of angiotensin-converting enzyme inhibitors and angiotensin receptor blockers. *Ann Allergy Asthma Immunol*. 2007;98:57-63.
140. Mannelli M, Maggi M, DeFeo ML, et al. Naloxone administration releases catecholamines. *N Engl J Med*. 1983;308:654-655.
141. Marbury TC, Sheppard JE, Gibbons K, Lee CS. Combined antidotal and hemodialysis treatments for nitroprusside-induced cyanide toxicity *J Toxicol Clin Toxicol*. 1982;19:475-482.
142. Marruecos L, Roglan A, Frati ME, Artigas A. Clonidine overdose. *Crit Care Med*. 1983;11:959-960.
143. Mazzolai L, Burnier M. Comparative safety and tolerability of angiotensin II receptor antagonists. *Drug Saf*. 1999;21:23-33.
144. McClean WJ. Prazosin overdose. *Med J Aust*. 1976;1:592.
145. McClellan KJ, Balfour JA. Eprosartan. *Drugs*. 1997;55:713-720.
146. McClellan KJ, Goa KL. Candesartan cilexetil: a review of its use in essential hypertension. *Drugs*. 1998;56:847-869.
147. McClellan KJ, Markham A. Telmisartan. *Drugs*. 1998;56:1039-1046.
148. McCormick MA, Forman MH, Manoguerra AS. Severe toxicity from ingestion of a topical minoxidil preparation. *Am J Emerg Med*. 1989;7:419-421.
149. McLennan PL. The hypothermic effect of clonidine and other imidazolidines in relation to their ability to enter the central nervous system in mice. *Eur J Pharmacol*. 1981;69:477-482.
150. McNamee JJ, Trainor D, Michalek P. Terlipressin for refractory hypotension following angiotensin II receptor antagonist overdose. *Anaesthesia*. 2006;61:408-409.
151. Meana JJ, Herrera-Marschitz M, Goiny M, Silveira R. Modulation of catecholamine release by α_2-adrenoceptors and I_1-imidazoline receptors in rat brain. *Brain Res*. 1997;744:216-226.
152. Megarbane B, Delahaye A. Goldgran-Toledano D, et al. Antidotal treatment of cyanide poisoning. *J Chin Med Assoc*. 2003;66:193-203.
153. Messerli FH, Bangalore S, Julius S. Risk/benefit assessment of β-blockers and diuretics precludes their use for first-line therapy in hypertension. *Circulation*. 2008:117:2706-2715.
154. Millar JA, Sturani A, Rubin PC, Reid JL. Attenuation of the antihypertensive effect of captopril by the opioid receptor antagonist naloxone. *Clin Exp Pharmacol Physiol*. 1983;10:253-259.
155. Muir AL, Burton JL, Lawrie DM. Circulatory effects at rest and exercise of clonidine, an imidazoline derivative with hypotensive properties. *Lancet*. 1969;2:181-185.
156. Myhre E, Rugstad HE, Hansen T. Clinical pharmacokinetics of methyldopa. *Clin Pharmacokinet*. 1982;7:221-223.
157. Nakagawa S, Yamamoto Y, Koiwaya Y. Ventricular tachycardia induced by clonidine withdrawal. *Br Heart J*. 1985;53:654-658.
158. Nayler WG, Price JM, Swann JB, et al. Effect of the hypotensive drug ST 155 (Catapres) on the heart and peripheral circulation. *J Pharmacol Exp Ther*. 1968;164:45-59.
159. Neimann JT, Getzug T, Murphy W. Reversal of clonidine toxicity by naloxone. *Ann Emerg Med*. 1986;15:1229-1231.
160. Nessim SJ, Richardson RMA. Dialysis for thiocyanate intoxication: a case report and review of the literature. *ASAIO Journal*. 2006;52:479-481.
161. Newgreen DH, Bray KM, McHarg AD, et al. The actions of diazoxide and minoxidil sulphate on rat blood vessels: a comparison with cromakalin. *Br J Pharmacol*. 1990;100:605-613.
162. Norris JC, Hume AS. In vivo release of cyanide from sodium nitroprusside. *Br J Anaesth*. 1987;59:236-239.
163. Oates JA, Brown NJ. Antihypertensive agents and the drug therapy of hypertension. In. Hardman JG, Limbird LE, eds. *Goodman and Gilman's The Pharmacological Basis of Therapeutics*, 10th ed. New York: McGraw-Hill; 2001:871-900.
164. O'Doherty NJ. Thiazides and cerebral ischaemia. *Lancet*. 1965;2:1297.
165. Ohtawa M, Takayama F, Saitoh K, et al. Pharmacokinetics and biochemical efficacy after single and multiple oral administration of losartan, an orally active nonpeptide angiotensin II receptor antagonist, in humans. *Br J Clin Pharmacol*. 1993;35:290-297.
166. Olsson JM, Pruitt AW. Management of clonidine ingestion in children. *J Pediatr*. 1983;103:646-650.
167. Onesti G, Schwartz AB, Kim KE, et al. Pharmacodynamic effects of a new antihypertensive drug: Catapres (ST-155). *Circulation*. 1969;34:219-228.
168. Orfan N, Patterson R, Dykewicz MS. Severe angioedema related to ACE inhibitor in patients with a history of idiopathic angioedema. *JAMA*. 1990;264:1287-1290.
169. Papademetriou V, Burris JF, Notargiacomo A, et al. Thiazide therapy is not a cause of arrhythmia in patients with systemic hypertension. *Arch Intern Med*. 1988;148:1272-1276.
170. Park H, Purnell GV, Mirchandani HG. Suicide by captopril overdose. *J Toxicol Clin Toxicol*. 1990;28:379-382.
171. Paster RZ, Snaely DB, Sweet AR, et al. Use of losartan in the treatment of hypertensive patients with a history of cough induced by angiotensin-converting enzyme inhibitors. *Clin Ther*. 1998;20:978-989.
172. Perrone J, Hoffman RS, Jones B, Hollander JE. Guanabenz induced hypothermia in a poisoned elderly female. *J Toxicol Clin Toxicol*. 1994;32:445-449.
173. Peters RW, Hamilton BP, Hamilton J, et al. Cardiac arrhythmias after abrupt clonidine withdrawal. *Clin Pharmacol Ther*. 1983;34:435-439.
174. Pettinger WA. Clonidine, a new antihypertensive drug. *N Engl J Med*. 1975;293:1179-1180.
175. Pettinger WA. Pharmacology of clonidine. *J Cardiovasc Pharmacol*. 1980;2:521-528.
176. Pettinger WA, Mitchell HC. Side effects of vasodilator therapy. *Hypertension*. 1988;11(suppl II):34-36.
177. Poff SW, Rose SR. Minoxidil overdose with ECG changes: case report and review. *Am J Emerg Med*. 1992;10:53-57.
178. Popper CW. Combined methylphenidate and clonidine: news reports about sudden death. *J Child Adolesc Psychopharmacol*. 1995;5;155-166.
179. Ram VCS, Holland B, Fairchild C, Gomez-Sanchez CE. Withdrawal syndrome following cessation of guanabenz therapy. *J Clin Pharmacol*. 1979;19:148-150.
180. Rangan C, Everson G, Cantrell FL. Central α-2 adrenergic eye drops: case series of 3 pediatric systemic poisonings. *Ped Emerg Care*. 2008;24:197-169.
181. Raper JH, Shinar C, Finkelstein S. Clonidine patch ingestion in an adult. *Ann Pharmacother*. 1993;27:719-722.
182. Rapko DA, Rastegar DA. Intentional clonidine patch ingestion by 3 adults in a detoxification unit. *Arch Intern Med*. 2003;163:367-368.
183. Reed MT, Hamburg EL. Person to person transfer of transdermal drug-delivery systems: a case report. *N Engl J Med*. 1986;314:1120-1121.
184. Reid JL, Campbell BC, Hamilton CA. Withdrawal reactions following cessation of central α-adrenergic receptor agonists. *Hypertension*. 1984;6(suppl II):71-75.
185. Rindone JP, Sloane EP. Cyanide toxicity from sodium nitroprusside: risks and management. *Ann Pharmacother*. 1992;26:515-519.
186. Robbins DN, Crawford ED, Lackner LH. Priapism secondary to prazosin overdose. *J Urol*. 1983;130:975.
187. Roberts JR, Wuerz RC. Clinical characteristics of angiotensin-converting enzyme inhibitor-induced angioedema. *Ann Emerg Med*. 1991;20:555-558.
188. Robertson D, Tung C, Goldberg MR, et al. Antihypertensive metabolites of -methyldopa. *Hypertension*. 1984;6(suppl II);45-50.
189. Romano MJ, Dinh A. A 1000-fold overdose of clonidine caused by a compounding error in a 5-year-old child with attention-deficit/ hyperactivity disorder. *Pediatrics*. 2001;108:471-472.
190. Rosenberg L, Shapiro S, Slone D, et al. Thiazides and acute cholecystitis. *N Engl J Med*. 1980;303:546-548.
191. Rougraff ME. Chlorothiazide overdosage effects in two-year-old child. *Penn Med J*. 1959;62:694.
192. Rubinstein I. Fatal thrombosis of left internal carotid artery following diuretic abuse. *Ann Emerg Med*. 1985;14:275.
193. Rybalkin SD, Yan C, Bornfeldt KE, Beavo JA. Cyclic GMP phosphodiesterases and regulation of smooth muscle function. *Circ Res*. 2003;93:280-291.
194. Rygnestad TK, Dale O. Self-poisoning with prazosin. *Acta Med Scand*. 1983;213:157-158.
195. Saunders C, Limbird, LE. Localization and trafficking of α_2-adrenergic receptor subtypes in cells and tissues. *Pharmacol Ther*. 1999;84:193-205.
196. Scheinman MM, Strauss HC, Evans GT, et al. Adverse effects of sympatholytic agents in patients with hypertension and sinus node dysfunction. *Am J Med*. 1978;64:1013-1020.

197. Schieber RA, Kaufman ND. Use of tolazoline in massive clonidine poisoning. *Am J Dis Child.* 1981;135:77-78.
198. Schulz V. Clinical pharmacokinetics of nitroprusside, cyanide, thiosulphate and thiocyanate. *Clin Pharmacokinet.* 1984;9:239-251.
199. Schwartz E, Friedman E, Mouallem M, Farfel Z. Sinus arrest associated with clonidine therapy. *Clin Cardiol.* 1987;11:53-54.
200. Seger D. Clonidine toxicity revisited. *Clin Toxicol.* 2002;40:145-155.
201. Self F, Bates GHEM, Drake-Lee A. Severe angioneurotic oedema causing acute airway obstruction. *J Royal Soc Med.* 1988;81:544-545.
202. Shand DG, Morgan DH, Oates JA. The release of guanethidine and bethanidine by splenic nerve stimulation: a quantitative evaluation showing dissociation from adrenergic blockade. *J Pharmacol Exp Ther.* 1973;184:73-80.
203. Sharpe E, Milaszkiewicz R, Carli R. A case of prolonged hypotension following intravenous guanethidine blockade. *Anaesthesia.* 1987;42:1081-1084.
204. Shekarriz B, Stoller ML. Uric acid nephrolithiasis. Current concepts and controversies. *J Urol.* 2002;168:1307-1314.
205. Shnaps Y, Almog S, Halkin H, Tirosh M. Methyldopa poisoning. *Clin Toxicol.* 1982;19:501-503.
206. Siegel D, Hulley SB, Black DM, et al. Diuretics, serum and intracellular electrolyte levels, and ventricular arrhythmias in hypertensive men. *JAMA.* 1992;267:1083-1089.
207. Simonetti GD, Baumann T, Pachlopnik JM, et al. Non-lethal fetal toxicity of the angiotensin receptor blocker candesartan. *Pediatr Nephrol.* 2006;21:1329-1330.
208. Siscovick DS, Raghunathan TE, Psaty BM, et al. Diuretic therapy for hypertension and the risk of primary cardiac arrest. *N Engl J Med.* 1994;330:1852-1857.
209. Slater EE, Merril DD, Guess HA, et al. Clinical profile of angioedema associated with angiotensin converting enzyme inhibition. *JAMA.* 1988;260:967-970.
210. Smith BA, Ferguson DB. Acute hydralazine overdose: marked ECG abnormalities in a young adult. *Ann Emerg Med.* 1992;21:326-330.
211. Smith SA, Ferguson KL, Hoffman RS, et al. Prolonged severe hypotension following combined amlodipine and valsartan ingestion. *Clin Toxicol.* 2008;46:470-474.
212. Soares de Moura R, Leao MC, Resende C, et al. Actions of L-NAME and methylene blue on the hypotensive effects of clonidine and rilmenidine in the anesthetized rat. *J Cardiovasc Pharmacol.* 2000;35:791-795.
213. Sonnenblick M, Friedlander Y, Rosin AJ. Diuretic-induced hyponatremia: reproducibility by single dose rechallenge and an analysis of pathogenesis. *Chest.* 1993;103:601-606.
214. Sorkin EM, Heel RC. Guanfacine: a review of its pharmacodynamic and pharmacokinetic properties and therapeutic efficacy in the treatment of hypertension. *Drugs.* 1986;31:301-336.
215. Spiller HA, Klein-Schwartz W, Colvin JM, et al. Toxic clonidine ingestions in children. *J Pediatr.* 2005;146:263-266.
216. Steele TH, Oppenheimer S. Factors affecting urate excretions following diuretic administration in man. *Am J Med.* 1969;47:564-567.
217. Stein B, Volans GN. Dixarit overdose. The problem of attractive tablets. *Br Med J.* 1978;2:667-668.
218. Steiners E. Diuretics, digitalis, and arrhythmias. *Acta Med Scand.* 1981; 647(suppl):75-78.
219. Suchard JR, Graeme KA. Pediatric clonidine poisoning as a result of pharmacy compounding error. *Pediatr Emerg Care.* 2002;18:295-296.
220. Swanson J, Flockhart D, Udrea D, et al. Clonidine in the treatment of ADHD. questions about safety and efficacy. *J Child Adolesc Psychopharmacol.* 1995;5: 301-304.
221. Talke PO, Caldwell JE, Richardson CA, Heier T. The effects of clonidine on human digital vasculature. *Anesth Analg.* 2000;91:793-797.
222. Tanaka H, Teramoto S, Oashi K, et al. Effects of candesartan on cough and bronchial hyperresponsiveness in mildly and moderately hypertensive patients with symptomatic asthma. *Circulation.* 2001;104:281-285.
223. Tenenbein M. Naloxone in clonidine toxicity. *Am J Dis Child.* 1984;138:1084.
224. Textor SC, Bravo EL, Fouad FM, Tarazi RC. Hyperkalemia in azotemic patients during angiotensin-converting enzyme inhibition and aldosterone reduction with captopril. *Am J Med.* 1982;73:719-725.
225. Thormann J, Neuss H, Schlepper M, Mitrovic V. Effects of clonidine on sinus node function in man. *Chest.* 1981;80:201-206.
226. Tibirica E, Feldman J, Mermet C, et al. An imidazoline-specific mechanism for the hypotensive effect of clonidine: a study with yohimbine and idazoxan. *J Pharmacol Exp Ther.* 1991;256:606-613.
227. Tinker JH, Michenfelder JD. Sodium nitroprusside. pharmacology, toxicology, and therapeutics. *Anesthesiology.* 1976;45:340-354.
228. Van der Linden W, Ritter B, Edlund G. Acute cholecystitis and thiazides. *Br Med J.* 1984;289:654-655.
229. Van Dyke MW, Bonace AL, Ellenhorn MJ. Guanfacine overdose in a pediatric patient. *Vet Hum Toxicol.* 1990;32:46-47.
230. van Etta L, Burchell H. Severe bradycardia with clonidine. *JAMA.* 1978; 240:2047.
231. van Rijnsoever EW, Kwee-Zuiderwijk WJ, Feenstra J. Angioneurotic edema attributed to the use of losartan. *Arch Intern Med.* 1998;158:2063-2065.
232. van Zweiten PA. Antihypertensive drugs with a central action. *Prog Pharmacol.* 1975;1:1-66.
233. van Zwieten PA, Thoolen MJ, Timmermans PB. The hypotensive activity and side effects of methyldopa, clonidine, and guanfacine. *Hypertension.* 1984;6(suppl II):28-33.
234. Vanholder R, Carpentier J, Schurgers M, Clement DL. Rebound phenomenon during gradual withdrawal of clonidine. *Br Med J.* 1977;1:1138.
235. Varon J, Duncan SR. Naloxone reversal of hypotension due to captopril overdose. *Ann Emerg Med.* 1991;20:1125-1127.
236. Varughese A, Taylor AA, Neslon EB. Consequences of angiotensin converting enzyme inhibitor overdose. *Am J Hypertens.* 1989;2:355-357.
237. Venturini G, Colasanti M, Persichini T, et al. Selective inhibition of nitric oxide synthase type I by clonidine, an antihypertensive drug. *Biochem Pharmacol.* 2000;60:539-544.
238. Vila JM, Blum L, Dosik H. Thiazide-induced immune hemolytic anemia. *JAMA.* 1976;236:1723-1724.
239. Waeber B, Nussberger J, Brunner HR. Self-poisoning with enalapril. *Br Med J.* 1984;288:287-288.
240. Weinberger MH. Diuretics and their side effects. *Hypertension.* 1988;11 (suppl II):16-20.
241. Wiley JF, Wiley CC, Torrey SB, Henretig FM. Clonidine poisoning in young children. *J Pediatr.* 1990;116:654-658.
242. Williams PL, Krafcik JM, Potter BB, et al. Cardiac toxicity of clonidine. *Chest.* 1977;72:784-785.
243. Yeh BK, Natel A, Goldberg LI. Antihypertensive effect of clonidine. *Arch Intern Med.* 1971;127:233-237.
244. Zamboulis C, Reid JL. Withdrawal of guanfacine after long term treatment in essential hypertension. *Eur J Clin Pharmacol.* 1981;19:19-24.
245. Zarifis J, Lip GYH, Ferner RE. Poisoning with anti-hypertensive drugs: methyldopa and clonidine. *J Hum Hypertens.* 1995;9:787-790.
246. Zerbe NF, Wagner KJ. Use of vitamin B_{12} in the treatment and prevention of nitroprusside-induced cyanide toxicity. *Crit Care Med.* 1993;21:465-467.

CHAPTER 63
ANTIDYSRHYTHMICS

Lewis S. Nelson and Neal A. Lewin

The term *dysrhythmia* encompasses an array of abnormal cardiac rhythms that range in clinical significance from merely annoying to instantly life threatening. Antidysrhythmics include all xenobiotics that are used to treat any of these various dysrhythmias. The importance of dysrhythmia management in the modern practice of medicine cannot be overstated because dysrhythmias are among the most common causes of preventable sudden cardiac death.[30,53] Despite an incomplete understanding of the underlying mechanisms of dysrhythmia formation, an abundance of antidysrhythmics have been developed, each attempting to alter specific electrophysiologic components of the cardiac impulse generating or conducting system. In addition to the predictable, mechanism-based adverse effect of each xenobiotic, unique and often unanticipated effects also occur.[96] Experience with overdose of many of these xenobiotics is limited, and management is generally based on the underlying pharmacologic principles, existing case reports, and the experimental literature.

HISTORY AND EPIDEMIOLOGY

For a long time, antidysrhythmics were considered among the most rational of the available cardiac medications. This well-earned reputation was related to their high efficacy at reducing the incidence of malignant dysrhythmias. Similarly, they are effective at controlling nuisance rhythm disorders. However, this approach changed dramatically after publication of the Cardiac Arrhythmia Suppression Trials (CAST and CAST II)[1,3,29] and, more recently, with the rise of mechanical interventions, such as ablation therapy and implantable defibrillators. CAST assessed the ability of three antidysrhythmics to suppress asymptomatic ventricular dysrhythmias known to be harbingers of sudden death. The original CAST study was discontinued in 1989 before completion, when encainide and flecainide not only failed to prevent sudden death but actually increased overall mortality. The CAST II trial noted similar problems with moricizine.[1] It has since become clear that the enhanced mortality associated with many antidysrhythmics is a result of their dysrhythmogenic effects and that virtually all xenobiotics of this group carry such a risk.[95] More recently, it has been demonstrated that for patients with atrial fibrillation, there is no benefit to rhythm conversion compared with controlling the ventricular response rate.[99]

This chapter focuses on the xenobiotics that serve primarily as antidysrhythmics that, with the exception of lidocaine, have few other medicinal indications. Chapters 22 and 23 provide a more detailed description of the electrophysiology of dysrhythmias and a discussion of their genesis. In addition, the toxicities from calcium channel blockers and β-adrenergic antagonists, which have indications in addition to dysrhythmia control, are discussed separately in Chapters 60 and 61.

CLASSIFICATION OF ANTIDYSRHYTHMICS

Antidysrhythmics modify impulse generation and conduction by interacting with various membrane sodium, potassium, and calcium ion channels. Generally, antidysrhythmics affect electrophysiologic effects either through alteration of the channel pore or, more commonly, by modification of its gating mechanism (Fig. 63–1).[56] Unfortunately, given their exceedingly complex mechanisms of action, the descriptive terms used to explain their molecular actions are not always completely accurate. For example, the description of an antidysrhythmic as a specific "channel blocker," although representative of the conceptual action of that drug, is inaccurate because in most cases, the molecule does not actually block the channel but rather prevents the channel from opening properly. Furthermore, many of these drugs are active nonspecifically at other channels or on other cells, resulting in divergent clinical actions of similarly classified drugs.

The Vaughan-Williams classification of antidysrhythmics by electrophysiologic properties emphasizes the connection between the basic electrophysiologic actions and the antidysrhythmic effects.[115] Although initially proposed as a descriptive model for electrophysiologic actions and not for clinical effects, the Vaughan-Williams classification is commonly invoked as a user-friendly guide to clinical therapy. In 1991, a competing system known as "the Sicilian Gambit" was constructed by a task force of European cardiologists based on the mechanisms by which antidysrhythmics modify dysrhythmogenic mechanisms.[2] Although perhaps more contemporary in theory, this latter classification system is complex and is therefore not widely implemented. An even more rational classification would match the electrophysiologic effects of the antidysrhythmics with their molecular interactions on different regions of the various ion channels, such as channel gating and pore conductance.[56]

This discussion of antidysrhythmics uses the Vaughan-Williams classification, recognizing the shortcomings delineated above.[113] The pharmacokinetic properties of the various drugs are summarized in Table 63–1.

CLASS I ANTIDYSRHYTHMICS

All antidysrhythmics in Vaughan-Williams class I (A, B, and C) alter Na^+ conductance through cardiac voltage-gated, fast inward Na^+ channels (see Table 63–1). These drugs bind to the Na^+ channels and slow their recovery from the open or inactivated state to the resting, or closed, state (see Fig. 63–1). This conversion must occur before the channel can reopen and participate in another depolarization. Consequently, as the proportion of drug-bound Na^+ channels increases, fewer of these channels are capable of reactivation on the arrival of the next depolarizing impulse. As a result, by reducing the excitability of the myocardium, abnormal rhythms are both prevented and terminated.

Blockade of these sodium channels slows the rise of phase 0 of the cellular action potential, which correlates with a reduction in the rate of depolarization of the myocardial cell (or V_{max}). Similarly, conduction through the myocardium is slowed, producing a measurable prolongation of the QRS complex on the surface electrocardiogram (ECG). Correspondingly, slowed intramyocardial conduction is associated with reduced contractility, manifesting as negative inotropy. Myocardial depression also results from effects of reduced intracellular Na^+ on Na^+-Ca^{2+} exchange.[76] This in turn reduces the intracellular Ca^{2+} concentration, normal concentrations of which are required for adequate contractility.

The differences among class I drugs are directly related to their pharmacologic relationships with the Na^+ channel. However, it is noteworthy that the original subdivision of class I drugs was based on clinical observations, not current pharmacologic awareness, accounting for the somewhat illogical ordering of the class I subdivisions.[113] Type IB drugs have their highest affinity for inactivated Na^+ channels. This occurs at the end of depolarization, during early repolarization, and during periods of myocardial ischemia, all situations in which

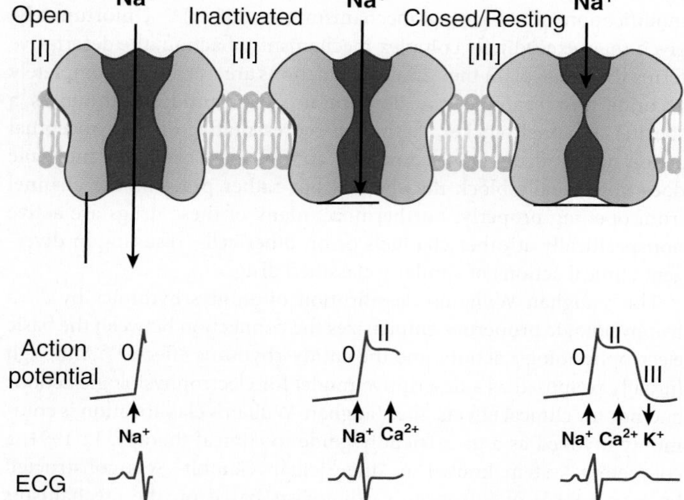

FIGURE 63–1. Sodium channel blockade. On appropriate signal, sodium channel activation occurs, at which time the sodium channel converts from the resting (III) state to the open state (I). This allows sodium ion influx to initiate phase 0 of the action potential, or cellular depolarization. The sodium channels subsequently assume the inactivated state by closure of an inactivation gate; this is a voltage-dependent phenomena and occurs concomitantly with, although more slowly than, channel activation. Cellular depolarization is maintained for a period of time by other ion channels that form the plateau of the action potential. Before reactivating, sodium channels must convert back to the resting state, which also occurs in a voltage-dependent fashion. Many antidysrhythmics stabilize the inactivated state of the channel and, by slowing conversion to the resting state, prevent its reopening, reducing the excitability of the cell. Because this is a population phenomena, there are dose-dependent effects on channel blockade; thus, more drug interferes with more channels. Interestingly, certain xenobiotics, such as ciguatoxin and aconitine, stabilize the open state of the sodium channel and produce persistent depolarization.

the myocardium is partially depolarized. These drugs also have rapid "on–off" binding kinetics (rapid $\tau_{recovery}$) and are thus bound only briefly, during late electrical systole, the period during which the Na^+ channels are predominantly in the inactivated form. They are almost exclusively unbound during electrical diastole, which is the major portion of the cardiac cycle at normal heart rates. However, the degree of binding increases as the heart rate accelerates because the duration of diastole decreases and the relative proportion of time spent in systole increases; this is termed *use dependence*. Because all IB drugs do not bind to activated sodium channels, in therapeutic doses, they do not affect the rate of rise of phase 0 of the action potential, or V_{max}, and have no effect on the ECG.[114] Alternatively, the class IC drugs either act preferentially on activated Na^+ channels or they release from the Na^+ channels very slowly (slow $\tau_{recovery}$) and thus are still bound during the next cardiac cycle. This prolonged channel blockade and reduced channel reactivation results in both greater pharmacologic effects and toxicity, even at slow heart rates. These drugs reduce V_{max} and prolong the QRS complex. Class IA drugs fall between the other two subclasses.

Although in the Vaughan-Williams classification, class I drugs are considered primarily sodium channel blockers, many, particularly those in class IA, have important effects on cardiac potassium channels. These channels are critical to maintenance of the cardiac action potential and repolarization of the myocardial cell. Slowing of potassium efflux prolongs the duration of the action potential and accounts for the persistence of refractoriness, or the time during which the cell is incapable of re-depolarization. This effect produces QT prolongation on the surface ECG, and predisposes to the triggering of polymorphic ventricular tachycardia.[94] Because class IB drugs have no effect on myocardial potassium channels, they do not alter refractoriness or the QT interval. In fact, class IB drugs often reduce the action potential duration, shortening refractoriness. Further discussion of potassium channel blockade is found in Chapter 22 and below in the discussion of class III antidysrhythmics.

CLASS IA ANTIDYSRHYTHMICS: PROCAINAMIDE, QUINIDINE, AND DISOPYRAMIDE

Procainamide Procainamide (Fig. 63–2) can be used to suppress either atrial or ventricular tachydysrhythmias. Importantly, procainamide undergoes hepatic biotransformation by acetylation to *N*-acetylprocainamide (NAPA), the rate of which is genetically determined.[79] Although NAPA lacks the Na^+ channel-blocking activity of procainamide, it prolongs the action potential duration through blockade of the K^+ rectifier currents, and for this reason, it is available as the class III antidysrhythmic acecainide.[47]

Rapid intravenous (IV) dosing of procainamide is potentially dangerous because its initial volume of distribution is smaller than its final volume of distribution. Because this initial compartment includes the heart, adverse myocardial effects may be unexpectedly pronounced. Thus, to prevent toxicity during drug infusion, the IV loading dose is generally administered by slow infusion with ECG monitoring. Both procainamide and NAPA are renally eliminated and may accumulate in patients with renal insufficiency.[28,69]

Although the chronic use of procainamide may be accompanied by the development of antinuclear antibodies or drug-induced systemic lupus erythematosis,[50] this syndrome is not associated with acute poisoning. Furthermore, NAPA has less propensity than procainamide to produce this syndrome.[47] Other reported adverse effects include seizures and antimuscarinic effects with acute overdose and myopathic pain, thrombocytopenia, and agranulocytosis after long-term use.

Serum concentrations of both procainamide and NAPA should be determined as part of therapeutic drug monitoring (therapeutic dose, 5–20 μg/mL) and in patients with procainamide overdose. Because the elimination half-life of procainamide is 3 to 4 hours, which is substantially shorter than that of NAPA (6–10 hours), chronic overdosing typically results in NAPA toxicity.[7] In this situation, the QT interval, a reflection of K^+ channel blockade, correlates directly—and blood pressure correlates inversely—with the degree of poisoning. Severe effects usually do not occur until total (procainamide plus NAPA) serum concentrations are greater than 60 μg/mL.[8] Because of its structural similarity with amphetamine, patients with procainamide overdose may have a false-positive urine enzyme-multiplied immunoassay test (EMIT) result for amphetamines.[116]

Quinidine Quinidine (see Fig. 63–2), the *d*-isomer of quinine, is derived from the bark of the cinchona tree. Because it is a weak base, it is typically formulated as the sulfate or gluconate salt. Quinidine undergoes hydroxylation by the liver, and both active and inactive metabolites are renally eliminated.

Quinidine was once widely used for the management of patients with atrial or ventricular dysrhythmias but has largely fallen out of favor because of its adverse effects. Quinidine has substantial cardiotoxicity that includes intraventricular conduction abnormalities and an increased QT interval. Many of the ECG changes mimic those of hypokalemia. "Quinidine syncope," in which patients on therapeutic doses of quinidine experience paroxysmal, transient loss of consciousness, is most frequently a result of torsade de pointes.[54]

TABLE 63–1. Antidysrhythmics: Pharmacology, Pharmacokinetics, and Adverse Effects

Drug	Route	Primary Route of Elimination	Elimination Half-Life	Channel Blockade	Volume Distribution (L/kg)	Protein Binding (%)	Adverse Effects and Complicating Factors	Other
Class IA								
Disopyramide	PO	Liver, kidney	4-10 h	Na^+, ($\tau = 9$ s), K^+, Ca^{2+}	0.59 ± 0.15	35–95 depending on serum concentration	CHF, negative inotropic effects, anticholinergic, torsades de pointes, heart block, hypoglycemia	
Procainamide (PA)	IV, PO	50%–60% unchanged in kidney; active hepatic metabolite (NAPA)	PA: 3–4 h ↑ renal disease NAPA: 6–10 h ↑ renal disease	Na^+ ($\tau = 1.8$ s), K^+	1.9 ± 0.3	16 ± 9	Hypotension (ganglionic blockade), QRS widening, fever, SLE-like syndrome, torsades de pointes	NAPA: active metabolite, renally eliminated, K^+ channel blocker; half-life: 6–10 h; a sustained-release PA preparation is available
Quinidine	PO	Liver, kidney, 10%–20% unchanged	6–8 hours ↑ liver disease (to >50 hours) and renal failure (to 9–12 h).	Na^+ ($\tau = 3$ s), K^+, Ca^{2+}	2.7 ± 1.2	87 ± 3	Heart block, sinus node dysfunction, prolonged QT, hypotension, hypoglycemia, torsades de pointes, thrombocytopenia, ↑ digoxin concentrations	
Class IB								
Lidocaine	SC, IV, PO	Liver, active metabolite (MEGX CYP3A4) (30% BA)	8 min after bolus 2 h terminal	Na^+ ($\tau = 0.1$ s)	1.1 ± 0.4	70 ± 5	Fatigue, agitation, paresthesias, seizures, hallucinations, rarely bundle branch block	Metabolites: GX and MEGX, are less potent as Na^+ channel blockers than lidocaine
Mexiletine	IV, PO	Liver (CYP 2D6)	6-17 h	Na^+($\tau = 0.3$ s)	4.9 ± 0.5	63 ± 3	See lidocaine	
Phenytoin	IV, PO	Liver	7-42 h	Na^+($\tau = 0.2$ s)	0.64 ± 0.04	89 ± 23	Hypotension and asystole related in part to IV propylene glycol (diluent) infusion, nystagmus, ataxia	
Tocainide	IV, PO	Kidney, liver	11-22.8 h ↑ renal disease	Na^+($\tau = 0.4$ s)	3.0 ± 0.2	10 ± 15	See lidocaine, aplastic anemia, interstitial pneumonia	
Class IC								
Flecainide	IV, PO	Liver (CYP2D6) 75%, kidney 25%	Long half-life	Na^+ ($\tau = 11$ s), Ca^{2+}, K^+	4.9 ± 0.4	61 ± 10	Negative inotropic effects, bradycardia, heart block, ventricular fibrillation, ventricular tachycardia, neutropenia	Two metabolites, one active
Moricizine	PO	Liver		Na^+($\tau = 10$ s)	NA	95	↑ Mortality after MI, bradycardia, CHF, ventricular fibrillation, ventricular tachycardia	
Propafenone	IV, PO	Liver (CYP2D6) (extensive first pass)	5-8 h	Na^+ ($\tau = 1$ s), K^+	3.6 ± 2.1	85 ± 95	Asthma, CHF, hypoglycemia, AV block, QRS prolongation, bradycardia, ventricular fibrillation, ventricular tachycardia	Active metabolite 5-OH-propafenone

(*Continued*)

TABLE 63–1. Antidysrhythmics: Pharmacology, Pharmacokinetics, and Adverse Effects (continued)

Drug	Route	Primary Route of Elimination	Elimination Half-Life	Channel Blockade	Volume Distribution (L/kg)	Protein Binding (%)	Adverse Effects and Complicating Factors	Other
Class II								
β-Adrenergic antagonists	IV, PO	Variable	Variable	β-adrenergic receptor	Variable	Variable	CHF, asthma, hypoglycemia, Raynaud disease Asystole (if used IV with IV calcium channel blocker)	
Class III								
Amiodarone	IV, PO	Liver (100%) (CYP 3A4)	2 months	Na^+, Ca^{2+}	66 ± 44	99.98 ± 0.01	Negative inotropic effects, pulmonary fibrosis, corneal microdeposits, thyroid abnormalities, hepatitis photosensitivity, ↑ diltiazem, quinidine, procainamide, flecainide, digoxin concentrations	Desethylamiodarone, has comparable activity to the parent compound
Dofetilide	IV, PO	Kidney	7.5-10 h	K^+	3.6 ± 0.8	64	Torsades de pointes	
Ibutilide	IV	Kidney	2–12; average, 6 h	K^+, Na^+ opener	11	40	Torsades de pointes, heart block	
Class IV								
Calcium channel blockers	IV, PO	Variable	Variable	Ca^{2+}	Variable	Variable	Asystole (if used IV with IV β-adrenergic antagonists), AV block, hypotension, CHF, constipation, ↑ digoxin levels	
Not classified								
Adenosine	IV	All cells (intracellular adenosine deaminase)	Seconds	Nucleoside-specific G protein-coupled adenosine receptors, ↑Ca^{2+} currents activates ACh-sensitive K^+ current	–	–	Transient asystole <5 s, chest pain, dyspnea, atrial fibrillation, ↓ BP, effects potentiated by dipyridamole and in heart transplant patients, ↑ dose needed with methylxanthine use	

[a] $\tau_{recovery}$ describes the time it takes for the sodium channel to recover from blockade

AV, atrioventricular; BA, bioavailable; BP, blood pressure; CHF, congestive heart failure; GX, glycine xylidide; MEGX, monoethyl glycine xylidide; NAPA, *N*-acetylprocainamide; SLE; systemic lupus erythematosus.

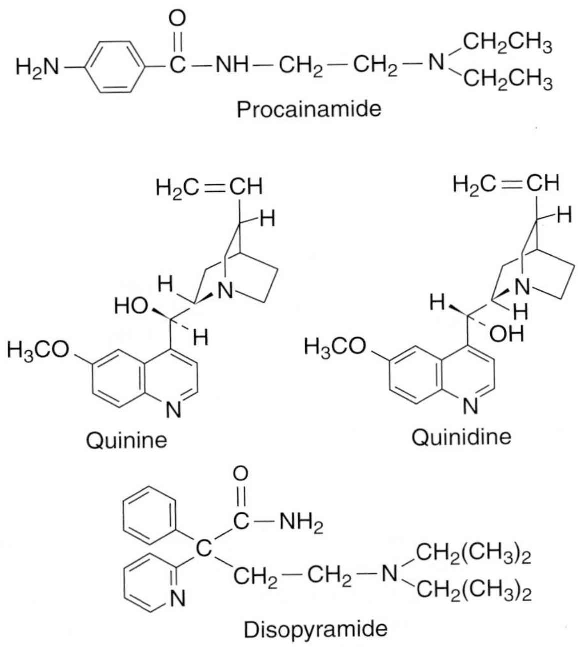

Procainamide

Quinine

Quinidine

Disopyramide

FIGURE 63–2. Structures of class IA antidysrhythmics and quinine.

Because quinidine shares many pharmacologic properties with quinine (see Chap. 58), patients may occasionally experience cinchonism after either chronic or acute quinidine overdose. This syndrome includes abdominal symptoms, tinnitus, and altered mental status. Quinidine also produces both peripheral and cardiac antimuscarinic effects, which enhances conduction via the atrioventricular (AV) node. Furthermore, as with quinine, quinidine-induced blockade of K^+ channels in pancreatic islet cells may cause uncontrolled insulin release, leading to hypoglycemia.[86]

Serum quinidine concentrations greater than 14 μg/mL are associated with cardiotoxicity,[61] as evidenced by a 50% increase in either the QRS or QT interval.

Disopyramide Disopyramide (see Fig. 63–2) is more likely than other class IA antidysrhythmics to produce negative inotropy and congestive heart failure. This effect may be noted both in patients receiving therapeutic dosing[108] and in those who overdose, and may be related to the blockade of myocardial calcium channels caused by disopyramide.[51] The mono-*N*-dealkylated metabolite of disopyramide produces the most pronounced anticholinergic effects of the class,[88,100] accounting for the occasional use of disopyramide to treat patients with neurocardiogenic syncope. Lethargy, confusion, or hallucinations may be prominent in overdose.

Electrophysiologic abnormalities similar to those associated with poisoning from other class IA drugs can occur, including intraventricular conduction abnormalities, torsades de pointes, and other ventricular dysrhythmias. Disopyramide frequently causes hyperinsulinemic hypoglycemia through its antagonism of K^+ channels in the pancreatic islet cells.[48]

Management of Class IA Antidysrhythmic Toxicity Management centers on assessment and correction of cardiovascular dysfunction. Following airway evaluation and IV line placement, 12-lead ECG and continuous ECG monitoring are of paramount importance. Appropriate gastrointestinal decontamination is recommended when the patient is sufficiently stabilized and should include whole-bowel irrigation if a sustained-release preparation is involved.

For patients who have widening of the QRS complex duration, bolus administration of IV hypertonic sodium bicarbonate is indicated. [see Antidotes In Depth A5, Sodium Bicarbonate] Depolarization is accelerated and the QRS complex duration is reduced, by enhancing rapid sodium ion influx through the myocardial sodium channels.[14] However, hypokalemia from the use of sodium bicarbonate may further prolong the QT interval, requiring careful monitoring of the serum K^+ concentration and ECG. Class IA antidysrhythmic-induced hypotension is treated primarily with rapid infusion of 0.9% NaCl, in order to expand the patient's intravascular volume and to simultaneously increase myocardial contractility (i.e., enhanced Starling force). Hypotension in the setting of QRS complex duration prolongation may respond favorably to hypertonic sodium bicarbonate, which enhances inotropy by both accelerating depolarization and raising intravascular volume. Dopamine, dobutamine, isoproterenol, norepinephrine, and intraaortic balloon pump insertion may also be required, but their use has not been systematically evaluated. Because disopyramide also blocks calcium channels, calcium administration is reportedly beneficial,[4] although evidence to support this antidotal effect is lacking. Glucagon effectively reversed myocardial depression in canine models, but it has not been evaluated in humans.[78]

Patients with stable ventricular dysrhythmias occurring in the setting of class IA antidysrhythmic poisoning are usually treated with hypertonic sodium bicarbonate or lidocaine. Although it may seem counterintuitive to administer another class I antidysrhythmic to a patient already poisoned by a class I antidysrhythmic, there is sound theoretical and experimental literature to support the use of lidocaine in this setting.[118] Because lidocaine is a class IB drug with rapid on-off receptor kinetics, it may displace the "slower" class IA drug from the binding site on the sodium channel, effectively reducing channel blockade. Sodium bicarbonate enhances conduction through the myocardium, promoting spontaneous termination of the ventricular dysrhythmia. Magnesium sulfate and overdrive pacing may be helpful in treating torsades de pointes. Xenobiotics that must be avoided in treating patients with dysrhythmias associated with class IA poisoning include other class IA and IC antidysrhythmics, as well as the β-adrenergic antagonists and calcium channel blockers, all of which may exacerbate conduction abnormalities or produce hypotension.

The roles of activated charcoal hemoperfusion, hemofiltration, and continuous arteriovenous hemodiafiltration are inadequately defined, but may be most beneficial for removing NAPA.[8,16,69] There is no clinical evidence to support the use of hemodialysis or hemoperfusion for quinidine or disopyramide poisoning.[55]

CLASS IB ANTIDYSRHYTHMICS: LIDOCAINE, TOCAINIDE, MEXILETINE, AND MORICIZINE

Lidocaine Lidocaine (Fig. 63–3) is an aminoacyl amide that is a synthetic derivative of cocaine. Its predominant clinical uses are as a local anesthetic and, for mechanistically similar reasons, to control ventricular dysrhythmias. The high frequency of lidocaine-related medication errors relates in part to its wide use as well as the availability of multiple diverse "amps" of lidocaine designed for varying indications including resuscitation, preparation of infusions, and local anesthesia.[57] Lidocaine may prevent myocardial reentry by preferentially suppressing conduction in compromised tissue.[109] Following an IV bolus, lidocaine rapidly enters the central nervous system but quickly redistributes into the peripheral tissue with a distribution half-life of approximately 8 minutes.[15,71] Lidocaine is 95% dealkylated by hepatic CYP 3A4 to an active metabolite, monoethylglycylxylidide (MEGX) and, subsequently, to the inactive glycine xylidide (GX). GX is further metabolized to monoethylglycine and xylidide. MEGX, although less

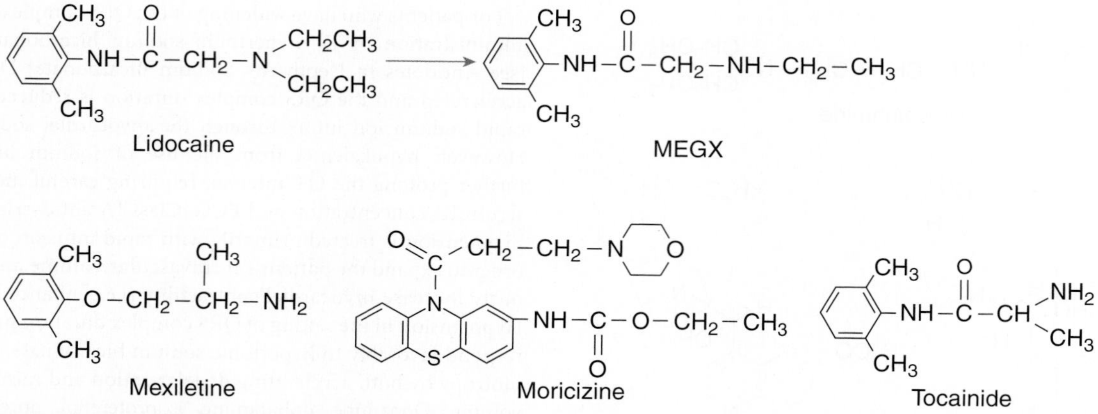

FIGURE 63–3. Structures of the class IB antidysrhythmics lidocaine (and metabolite [MEGX]), tocainide, mexiletine, and moricizine.

potent as a Na^+ channel blocker than the parent drug, may bioaccumulate because of its substantially longer half-life.[12]

Patients with lidocaine toxicity develop both central nervous system and cardiovascular effects, generally in that order. Because of its rapid entry into the brain, acute lidocaine poisoning typically produces central nervous system dysfunction, particularly seizures, as its initial manifestation.[34,93,103] Concomitant respiratory arrest generally occurs. Shortly following the central nervous system effects, depression in the intrinsic cardiac pacemakers leads to sinus arrest, AV block, intraventricular conduction delay, hypotension, and/or cardiac arrest.[23] If the patient is supported through this period, the drug rapidly distributes away from the heart, and spontaneous cardiac function returns.

Acute lidocaine toxicity from nonmassive amounts is generally related to excessive or inappropriate therapeutic dosing. Common settings include inadvertent IV administration instead of the intended route and excessive subcutaneous administration during laceration repair. Acute lidocaine toxicity may occur also with topical tracheal application of lidocaine used for bronchoscopy,[120] during cirumcision,[93] as well as intraureteral application during ureteroscopic stone extraction.[83] The typical CNS manifestations of nonmassive acute lidocaine poisoning include drowsiness, weakness, a sensation of "drifting away," euphoria, diplopia, decreased hearing, paresthesias, muscle fasciculations, and seizures. The more severe of these effects develop when serum lidocaine concentrations exceed 5 μg/mL and are often preceded by paresthesias or somnolence. Any of these symptoms should, therefore, prompt the clinician to examine the patient's medication administration history or drug-infusion rate. Apnea and seizures, as well as hypotonia in neonates, are reported to result from nonmassive acute lidocaine toxicity.[92]

A related form of toxicity and death results from subcutaneous and adipose administration of lidocaine during tumescent liposuction.[90] In this technique, a large volume of dilute lidocaine is used to distend subcutaneous fat prior to liposuction. Although in some reports the cause of death was controversial,[87] postmortem lidocaine concentrations were commonly elevated, and it is likely that lidocaine metabolites were also involved in the adverse events.[58,90] Interestingly, proponents of this procedure suggest that lidocaine doses up to a maximum of 55 mg/kg are safe,[81] whereas the conventional recommended limit for subcutaneous lidocaine with epinephrine is only 5–7 mg/kg. Of significant concern is that the recommended doses used for liposuction procedures do not consider the ability of lidocaine to saturate the CYP3A4 enzymes. When saturation occurs, elimination lags behind absorption and lidocaine toxicity may result.

Numerous publications unequivocally demonstrate the toxicity associated with orally administered lidocaine despite its poor bioavailability.[23, 121] Some of the toxicity may be due to MEGX. Because of the relatively high concentration of viscous lidocaine (typically 4%), this preparation is overrepresented in reports of oral lidocaine poisoning.[49] As little as 15 mL of 2% viscous lidocaine in a 3-year-old child (estimate, 300 mg or 21.4 mg/kg/dose) may cause seizures.

Chronic lidocaine toxicity most commonly occurs as a result of therapeutic misadventure in patients receiving lidocaine infusions, generally in a critical care unit. Toxicity following appropriate dosing is most likely to occur in patients with reduced hepatic blood flow (e.g., congestive heart failure), liver disease, or concomitant therapy with CYP3A4 and CYP1A2 inhibitors (see Chap. 12 Appendix).[80,111] Adverse reactions to lidocaine also increase with advancing age, decreasing body weight, and increasing infusion rate. Chronic lidocaine toxicity occurs in 6–15% of patients receiving infusions at 3 mg/min for several days.[101] Partly for this reason, lidocaine is no longer routinely used to prevent dysrhythmias in the immediate postmyocardial infarction period. The clearance of lidocaine falls after approximately 24 hours of the start of an infusion, and this effect may be due to competition for hepatic metabolism between lidocaine and its metabolites.

Tocainide Tocainide is indicated for the oral treatment of ventricular dysrhythmias; it is no longer available in the US. Although a lidocaine analog, it does not undergo first-pass metabolism and is therefore almost 100% orally bioavailable.[65] Both renal failure and congestive heart failure prolong its half-life considerably. The few overdoses reported with tocainide are associated with CNS and cardiovascular complications similar to those that occur with lidocaine overdose.[10,107] Therapeutic dosing is associated with rash, hepatotoxicity and blood dyscrasias, which, although rare, have limited its widespread use.

Mexiletine Mexiletine, originally developed as an anorectic agent, was found to have antidysrhythmic, local anesthetic, and anticonvulsant activity.[20] It is currently available in oral form for the management of ventricular dysrhythmias. Its chemical structure and electrophysiologic properties are similar to those of lidocaine. Mexiletine, a base, is absorbed in the small intestine; therefore, its absorption is increased when the gastric contents are alkalinized. Congestive heart failure and cirrhosis, as well as therapy with cimetidine or disulfiram, decrease the clearance of mexiletine.[64] Its metabolism, predominantly through CYP2D6, is accelerated by concomitant use of phenobarbital, rifampin, and phenytoin.[64]

Adverse therapeutic effects are primarily neurologic and are similar to those that occur with lidocaine. The few reported cases of mexiletine overdose describe prominent cardiovascular effects such as complete heart block, torsade de pointes, and asystole.[26,38] Neurotoxicity resulting from overdose includes self-limited seizures, generally in the setting of cardiotoxicity. Moreover, a single case report described a patient with mexiletine poisoning who experienced status epilepticus without any hemodynamic or electrocardiographic abnormalities.[77] Mexiletine may produce a false-positive result on the amphetamine immunoassay of the urine.[26,62]

Moricizine Moricizine possesses the general qualities of class I drugs but is difficult to specifically subclassify because it has properties that place the drug in either classes IB or IC.[25] Historically, it has been discussed as a class IB drug, as it is here. The parent drug undergoes extensive and rapid metabolism. Dose-related lengthening of PR and QRS intervals are expected, as are hemiblocks, bundle blocks, and sustained ventricular tachydysrhythmias. Experience with moricizine during the CAST II trial in the setting of myocardial infarction suggests that it is a prodysrhythmic.[1] Clinical experience with overdose is limited, but it is expected to be similar to that of other class I antidysrhythmics.

Management of Class IB Antidysrhythmic Toxicity The focus of the initial management for IV lidocaine-induced cardiac arrest is continuous cardiopulmonary resuscitation to allow lidocaine to redistribute away from the heart. Apart from this setting, management of hemodynamic compromise includes fluid replacement and other conventional strategies. Resistant hypotension may require dopamine or norepinephrine administration, insertion of an intraaortic balloon assist pump, or bypass.[40] Cardiopulmonary bypass, which does not directly enhance elimination, maintains hepatic perfusion, thereby allowing the lidocaine to be metabolized.[40] Bradydysrhythmias typically do not respond to atropine, requiring the administration of a chronotrope such as dopamine, norepinephrine, or isoproterenol. External pacing or insertion of a transvenous pacemaker may be useful, but the myocardium is often refractory to electrical capture. Lidocaine-induced seizures and those related to lidocaine analogs are generally brief in nature and do not require specific therapy. For patients requiring treatment, an IV benzodiazepine generally suffices; rarely, a barbiturate is required. Similarly, although IV lipid emulsion is often described as useful for the resuscitation of patients with life-threatening local anesthetic overdose, its use for lidocaine-poisoned patients is unstudied and likely unnecessary given the rapid time course of recovery (see Antidotes in Depth: A21: Intravenous Fat Emulsion). Enhanced elimination techniques are limited after IV poisoning because of the rapid time course of poisoning.

After oral poisoning by a class IB drug, activated charcoal should be administered as appropriate. Hemoperfusion or hemodialysis may increase the clearance of tocainide, but its indications remain unclear, and its benefit is likely very limited.[117] The extensive distribution and rapid metabolism of mexiletine make it a poor candidate for extracorporeal drug removal.

CLASS IC ANTIDYSRHYTHMICS: FLECAINIDE AND PROPAFENONE

Flecainide Flecainide, a derivative of procainamide, is orally administered to maintain sinus rhythm in patients with structurally normal hearts who have atrial fibrillation or supraventricular tachycardia.[11] Renal insufficiency, drug interactions, and congestive heart failure all decrease the clearance of flecainide and its active metabolite. Additionally, alkaluria reduces its clearance, presumably by enhanced tubular reuptake of nonionized drug. Patients using therapeutic doses may develop left ventricular dysfunction with worsening congestive heart failure. This is presumably a result of the negative inotropic effect of flecainide, which itself may relate to its antagonistic effects on calcium channels. Furthermore, sudden dysrhythmic death may occur, particularly in patients with underlying ischemic heart disease.[89]

A 50% increase in QRS duration, a 30% prolongation of the PR interval, or a 15% prolongation of the QT interval occurs with flecainide toxicity, a combined complex that may mimic Brugada syndrome.[45,52] The expected consequences of these electrophysiologic disturbances include bradycardia, premature ventricular contractions, and ventricular fibrillation. The combination of marked QRS and PR interval changes, associated with minimal QT interval prolongation, is characteristic of flecainide toxicity and contrasts with those described with other antidysrhythmic agents.[24]

Propafenone Propafenone bears a structural resemblance to propranolol,[36] as well as similar qualitative, but not quantitative, electrophysiologic properties.[73] Propafenone blocks fast inward sodium channels, is a weak β-adrenergic antagonist, and is an L-type calcium channel blocker.[33,104] Its long half-life allows the accumulation of parent compound, particularly in patients with the slow metabolizer pharmacogenetic variant of CYP2D6, which may cause excessive β-adrenergic antagonism.[66] Propafenone overdose produces sinus bradycardia, as well as ventricular dysrhythmias and negative inotropy.[36]

Acute overdose of propafenone typically produces wide complex tachycardia, right bundle-branch block, first-degree AV block, and prolongation of the QT interval, as well as generalized seizures.[59] Massive overdose in a young adult may be related to the subsequent development of a mild cardiomyopathy and a left bundle-branch block.[59]

Management of Class IC Antidysrhythmic Toxicity Initial stabilization should include standard management strategies for hypotension and seizures. Additionally, therapy for hypotension and the electrocardiographic manifestations of class IC poisoning includes IV hypertonic sodium bicarbonate to overcome the Na^+ channel blockade.[60] An animal study documented the beneficial effects of hypertonic sodium bicarbonate on flecainide-induced ventricular dysrhythmias, and three reports of human overdose verify QRS complex narrowing in response to hypertonic sodium bicarbonate administration.[17,42,68] Although sodium loading with hypertonic saline may be similarly effective, it remains unproven. The renal elimination of flecainide is reduced by urinary alkalinization, suggesting that sodium chloride, in equimolar doses, may ultimately prove superior to sodium bicarbonate.[74] The administration of other class IC or IA antidysrhythmics is contraindicated because of their additive blockade of the Na^+ channel. Similarly, the administration of phenytoin to a child with propafenone poisoning was associated with a prolongation of the QRS interval, which initially responded to sodium bicarbonate, but the patient subsequently developed a bradyasystolic arrest.[72] However, amiodarone has been successful in the setting of flecainide-induced ventricular fibrillation refractory to other therapy.[105] The efficacy of an external or internal pacemaker may be limited because of the drug-induced increased electrical pacing threshold of the ventricle.[31] Successful therapy with cardiopulmonary bypass or extracorporeal membrane oxygenation (ECMO) has been reported and should be considered if available.[9,27]

Extracorporeal removal is not expected to be beneficial for patients with flecainide poisoning. Although hemodialysis was successful in removing propafenone after overdose, additional studies are needed to determine its clinical benefit.[18]

CLASS III ANTIDYSRHYTHMICS: AMIODARONE, DOFETILIDE, AND IBUTILIDE

The class III antidysrhythmics prevent and terminate reentrant dysrhythmias by prolonging the action potential duration and effective refractory period without slowing conduction velocity during

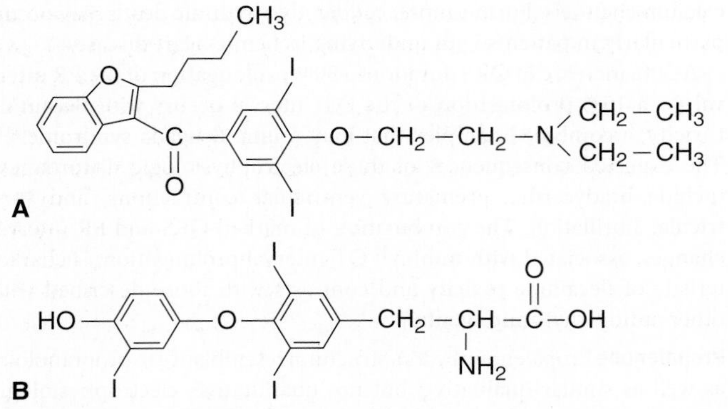

FIGURE 63–4. Structures of amiodarone (A) compared with triiodothyronine (T_3) (B). Amiodarone is nearly 40% iodine (I) by weight.

phase 0 or 1 of the action potential. This drug-induced effect on the action potential is generally caused by blockade of the rapidly activating component of the delayed rectifier potassium current, which is responsible for repolarization.

The class III antidysrhythmics in use today prolong repolarization of both the atria and the ventricles. Thus, common electrocardiographic effects at therapeutic doses include prolongation of the PR and QT intervals and abnormal T and U waves. Chapters 22 and 23 contain a detailed discussion of the pharmacologic mechanisms of class III antidysrhythmics. Also, Chapters 23 and 61 discuss sotalol.

Amiodarone Amiodarone (Fig. 63–4) is an iodinated benzofuran derivative that is structurally similar to both thyroxine and procainamide. Forty percent of its molecular weight is iodine. The 2005 revision of the Advanced Cardiac Life Support (ACLS) guidelines placed tremendous emphasis on the early IV administration of amiodarone. This, along with the ability of amiodarone to terminate or prevent atrial fibrillation, has lead to the increased use of this drug despite its association with potentially severe adverse effects.[112]

Although amiodarone has multiple pharmacologic effects, its efficacy as an antidysrhythmic agent is primarily the result of its class III antidysrhythmic effects. It also has weak α- and β-adrenergic antagonist activity and can block both L-type calcium channels and inactivated sodium channels. Amiodarone is slowly absorbed by the oral route and concentrates in the liver, lung, and adipose tissue. Steady-state pharmacokinetics may not occur until after 1 month of use.

The ECG effects of amiodarone differ based on the route of drug administration. Therapeutic oral doses prolong PR and QT intervals but not the QRS complex. IV dosing may produce a prolongation of the PR interval but has few other ECG manifestations. Ventricular dysrhythmias and sinus bradycardia are the most serious cardiac complications of therapeutic doses of amiodarone.[119] Monomorphic and polymorphic ventricular tachycardias may be resistant to cardioversion and pharmacologic interventions[13,35] but are surprisingly uncommon, given the frequency and extent to which the QT interval prolongation occurs. The ability of amiodarone to compete for P-glycoprotein is responsible for several consequential drug effects, including elevated digoxin and cyclosporin concentrations and an enhanced anticoagulation effectiveness of warfarin[63,122] (see Chap. 8 and 12).

The diverse complications associated with long-term therapy do not occur after short-term IV use. Chronic therapy with oral amiodarone is associated with substantial pulmonary, thyroid, corneal, hepatic, and cutaneous toxicity because of bioaccumulation in these organs. Many of these effects appear to be dose related, but because of the wide range of bioavailabilities and metabolic patterns among different patients, as well as the overlap between therapeutic and toxic serum concentrations, therapeutic drug monitoring is of limited benefit.[43] Pneumonitis, the most consequential extracardiac adverse effect, affects up to 5% of patients taking amiodarone therapeutically. Amiodarone pneumonitis may develop within days of initiating therapy but typically occurs only after years of therapy. Its occurrence may be dose related: a daily dose of more than 400 mg is a risk factor, and pneumonitis is rare in those taking less than 200 mg daily. The recent focus on using the minimal effective dose has reduced the incidence of pneumonitis.[32,82] Oxygen supplementation may speed the development of pneumonitis, which may explain the initial belief that patients with chronic lung disease are at increased risk for amiodarone pneumonitis. Manifestations of pneumonitis include dyspnea, cough, hemoptysis, crackles, hypoxia, and radiographic changes.[21] Computed tomography scanning is the most helpful initial diagnostic test for pneumonitis, but is not useful for monitoring purposes (monitoring is often done with diffusing capacity of CO).[43] Bronchoalveolar lavage typically reveals interstitial pneumonitis with many macrophages and a characteristic finely vacuolated foamy cytoplasm, but confirmation of the diagnosis requires open lung biopsy.

Thyroid dysfunction, either amiodarone-induced thyrotoxicosis (AIT) or amiodarone-induced hypothyroidism (AIH), occurs in approximately 4% of patients.[22] AIH is more common than AIT when iodine intake is sufficient.[43] AIH is likely caused by an exaggerated Wolff-Chaikoff effect, in which iodine, in this case from amiodarone, inhibits the organification and release of thyroid hormone. AIT appears to exist in two distinct forms: type I AIT, which occurs in patients with abnormal thyroid glands and iodine-induced excessive thyroid hormone synthesis and release, and type II AIT, in which destructive thyroiditis leads to release of thyroid hormone from the damaged follicular cells. The relative prevalence of the two forms of AIT is unknown, but it may depend on the ambient iodine intake. Amiodarone may also reduce the effect of thyroid hormone on peripheral tissue.[37] The diagnosis is confirmed with standard thyroid function testing[110] (see Chap. 49).

Corneal microdeposits are extremely common during chronic therapy and may lead to vision loss.[70] Abnormal elevation of hepatic enzymes occurs in more than 30% of those on long-term therapy, and hepatotoxicity may be associated with progression to cirrhosis. Periodic monitoring of aminotransferases is typically recommended.[43] Hepatotoxicity may occur after initial loading of amiodarone.[91] Slate gray or bluish discoloration of the skin is common, particularly in sun-exposed portions of the body.[97]

Dofetilide Dofetilide is approved for conversion of atrial fibrillation or atrial flutter to a normal sinus rhythm. Dofetilide increases the effective refractory period more substantially in atrial tissue than in ventricular fibers, accounting for this clinical indication.[98] Unlike many of the other antidysrhythmics, it may reduce the morbidity of atrial fibrillation in patients with congestive heart failure, and it is still used despite the emphasis on rate control instead of rhythm control in treating atrial fibrillation. Dofetilide has no known effect on calcium or sodium channels, nor does it result in β-adrenergic antagonism. Dofetilide increases the QT interval but does not change either the PR interval or the QRS complex in humans. Heart rate and blood pressure are also not appreciably affected.

Although limited data are available, the expected and reported adverse cardiac events include ventricular tachycardia, particularly torsade de pointes.[119] The approximate incidence of torsade de pointes in patients receiving high therapeutic doses of the drug is 3%.[5] For this reason, the Food and Drug Administration has in place strict requirements for the use of dofetilide, such as an individualized dose initiation algorithm and mandatory hospitalization for initial therapy.[6,85]

Overdose data reported by the manufacturer include two cases. Whereas one patient reportedly ingested 28 capsules and experienced no events, a second patient inadvertently received two supratherapeutic doses 1 hour apart and experienced fatal ventricular fibrillation after the second dose.[85] A 33-year-old man ingested 5 mg (20 capsules) and developed QT prolongation within 1 hour of ingestion but had no dysrhythmia during his 4-day hospital stay.

Ibutilide Ibutilide is an antidysrhythmic with predominant class III activity used for the rapid conversion of atrial fibrillation and flutter to normal sinus rhythm. Because of its extensive first-pass metabolism, ibutilide can only be administered parenterally. Its metabolic pathways are not well understood but do not involve the isoenzymes CYP3A4 or CYP2D6. Pharmacokinetic data thus far do not indicate that age, gender, hepatic, or renal dysfunction necessitates adjustment of recommended dosage of ibutilide. In addition to its effects on the delayed rectifier current, ibutilide activates a slow inward sodium current.[75]

Ibutilide may increase the QT interval and cause torsades de pointes, especially in patients with congenital long-QT syndrome and in women.[44] Although ibutilide may enhance the efficacy of transthoracic cardioversion for atrial fibrillation, its use in patients with ejection fractions below 20% is associated with an increased incidence of sustained polymorphic ventricular tachycardia. Acute renal failure, including biopsy-identified crystals, has been reported in association with ibutilide cardioversion, but a causal relationship is not yet definitive.[39] Acute overdose information, only available in limited form (four patients) through the manufacturer, suggests that ventricular dysrhythmias and high-degree AV conduction abnormalities should be expected.[84]

Management of Class III Antidysrhythmic Toxicity Treatment experience with class III drug overdose is limited. Isoproterenol and overdrive pacing have been used successfully to treat patients with amiodarone-induced torsades de pointes.[102] Administration of class IB antidysrhythmics or propranolol for the control of monomorphic ventricular tachycardia cannot be recommended on theoretical grounds. Paradoxically, amiodarone may reduce the "torsadogenic" effects of the other class III antidysrhythmics.[106] This effect is likely mediated by the beneficial effects of amiodarone on the dispersion of myocardial repolarization and its calcium channel–blocking activity.

Multiple-dose activated charcoal may be helpful if used shortly after overdose. Hemodialysis is not expected to be beneficial in general, either because of extensive protein binding or because of large volumes of distribution (see Table 63–1). A neonate survived cardiovascular collapse with the use of ECMO after an iatrogenic IV amiodarone overdose.[46]

UNCLASSIFIED: ADENOSINE

Adenosine, a nucleoside found in all cells, is released from myocardial cells under physiologic and pathophysiologic conditions. It is administered as a rapid IV bolus to terminate reentrant supraventricular tachycardia. The effects of adenosine are mediated by its interaction with specific G protein–coupled adenosine (A_1) receptors that activate acetylcholine-sensitive outward K^+ current in the atrium, sinus nodes, and AV nodes. The resultant hyperpolarization reduces the rate of cellular firing. Adenosine also reduces the Ca^{2+} currents, and its antidysrhythmic activity results from its effect in increasing AV nodal refractoriness and from inhibiting delayed afterdepolarizations elicited by sympathetic stimulation.[67]

The adverse effects of adenosine administration are very common and include transient asystole, dyspnea, chest tightness, flushing, hypotension, and atrial fibrillation. Although bronchospasm occurs after intrapulmonary administration, it has not been reported after IV use. Dyspnea, and probably chest tightness, is related to adenosine stimulation of the pulmonary vagal C fibers.[19] Fortunately, most of the adverse effects of adenosine are transient because of its rapid metabolism to inosine by both extracellular and intracellular deaminases. The clinical effects are potentiated by dipyridamole, an adenosine uptake inhibitor,[41] and by denervation hypersensitivity in cardiac transplant recipients. Methylxanthines may produce adenosine receptor blockade (see Chap. 65). In this setting, larger-than-usual doses of adenosine are required to produce an antidysrhythmic effect. Overdose of adenosine has not been reported. Treatment is supportive because of the rapid elimination of the drug.

SUMMARY

Many antidysrhythmics are currently available for clinical use. In the overdose setting, the class IA, B, and C drugs are all associated with sodium channel blockade, which may cause profound cardiac dysrhythmias and morbidity if not treated judiciously. The class IC drugs are considerably more toxic than the other class I drugs, although even the class IB drugs may be lethal in overdose. The class III antidysrhythmics in overdose may cause malignant dysrhythmias, particularly torsades de pointes. Amiodarone has many noncardiac effects, particularly pneumonitis and thyroid effects, that limit its therapeutic usefulness. Clinical effects after overdose are poorly described for class III drugs but will likely manifest as exaggerations of therapeutic pharmacologic effects. Proper management of both adverse effects and overdose can be accomplished only by understanding the pharmacokinetics and toxicokinetics of these drugs.

ACKNOWLEDGMENTS

Mary Ann Howland, PharmD, and Harold Osborn, MD, contributed to this chapter in a previous edition.

REFERENCES

1. Effect of the antiarrhythmic agent moricizine on survival after myocardial infarction. The Cardiac Arrhythmia Suppression Trial II Investigators. *N Engl J Med.* 1992;327:227-233.
2. The Sicilian gambit. A new approach to the classification of antiarrhythmic drugs based on their actions on arrhythmogenic mechanisms. Task Force of the Working Group on Arrhythmias of the European Society of Cardiology. *Circulation.* 1991;84:1831-1851.
3. Preliminary report: effect of encainide and flecainide on mortality in a randomized trial of arrhythmia suppression after myocardial infarction. The Cardiac Arrhythmia Suppression Trial (CAST) Investigators. *N Engl J Med.* 1989;321:406-412.
4. Accornero F, Pellanda A, Ruffini C, Bonelli S, Latini R. Prolonged cardiopulmonary resuscitation during acute disopyramide poisoning. *Vet Hum Toxicol.* 1993;35:231-232.
5. Aktas MK, Shah AH, Akiyama T. Dofetilide-induced long QT and torsades de pointes. *Ann Noninvasive Electrocardiol.* 2007;12:197-202.
6. Allen LaPointe NM, Chen A, Hammill B, DeLong E, Kramer JM, Califf RM. Evaluation of the dofetilide risk-management program. *Am Heart J.* 2003; 146:894-901.
7. Atkinson AJ Jr, Ruo TI, Piergies AA. Comparison of the pharmacokinetic and pharmacodynamic properties of procainamide and N-acetylprocainamide. *Angiology.* 1988;39:655-667.
8. Atkinson AJ Jr, Krumlovsky FA, Huang CM, del Greco F. Hemodialysis for severe procainamide toxicity: clinical and pharmacokinetic observations. *Clin Pharmacol Ther.* 1976;20:585-592.
9. Auzinger GM, Scheinkestel CD. Successful extracorporeal life support in a case of severe flecainide intoxication. *Crit Care Med.* 2001;29:887-890.

10. Barnfield C, Kemmenoe AV. A sudden death due to tocainide overdose. *Hum Toxicol.* 1986;5:337-340.
11. Benijts T, Borrey D, Lambert WE, et al. Analysis of flecainide and two metabolites in biological specimens by HPLC: application to a fatal intoxication. *J Anal Toxicol.* 2003;27:47-52.
12. Bennett PB, Woosley RL, Hondeghem LM. Competition between lidocaine and one of its metabolites, glycylxylidide, for cardiac sodium channels. *Circulation.* 1988;78:692-700.
13. Bonati M, D'Aranno V, Galletti F, Fortunati MT, Tognoni G. Acute overdosage of amiodarone in a suicide attempt. *J Toxicol Clin Toxicol.* 1983; 20:181-186.
14. Bou-Abboud E, Nattel S. Relative role of alkalosis and sodium ions in reversal of class I antiarrhythmic drug-induced sodium channel blockade by sodium bicarbonate. *Circulation.* 1996;94:1954-1961.
15. Boyes RN, Scott DB, Jebson PJ, Godman MJ, Julian DG. Pharmacokinetics of lidocaine in man. *Clin Pharmacol Ther.* 1971;12:105-116.
16. Braden GL, Fitzgibbons JP, Germain MJ, Ledewitz HM. Hemoperfusion for treatment of N-acetylprocainamide intoxication. *Ann Intern Med.* 1986; 105:64-65.
17. Brubacher J. Bicarbonate therapy for unstable propafenone-induced wide complex tachycardia. *CJEM.* 2004;6:349-356.
18. Burgess ED, Duff HJ. Hemodialysis removal of propafenone. *Pharmacotherapy.* 1989;9:331-333.
19. Burki NK, Dale WJ, Lee LY. Intravenous adenosine and dyspnea in humans. *J Appl Physiol.* 2005;98:180-185.
20. Campbell RW. Mexiletine. *N Engl J Med.* 1987;316:29-34.
21. Camus P, Martin WJ 2nd, Rosenow EC 3rd. Amiodarone pulmonary toxicity. *Clin Chest Med.* 2004;25:65-75.
22. Cardenas GA, Cabral JM, Leslie CA. Amiodarone induced thyrotoxicosis: diagnostic and therapeutic strategies. *Cleve Clin J Med.* 2003;70:624-6, 628-31.
23. Centini F, Fiore C, Riezzo I, Rossi G, Fineschi V. Suicide due to oral ingestion of lidocaine: a case report and review of the literature. *Forensic Sci Int.* 2007;171:57-62.
24. Chung PK, Tuso P. The electrocardiographic changes in a case of flecainide overdose. *Conn Med.* 1990;54:183-185.
25. Clyne CA, Estes NA 3rd, Wang PJ. Moricizine. *N Engl J Med.* 1992;327: 255-260.
26. Cocco G, Strozzi C, Chu D, Pansini R. Torsades de pointes as a manifestation of mexiletine toxicity. *Am Heart J.* 1980;100:878-880.
27. Corkeron MA, van Heerden PV, Newman SM, Dusci L. Extracorporeal circulatory support in near-fatal flecainide overdose. *Anaesth Intensive Care.* 1999;27:405-408.
28. Domoto DT, Brown WW, Bruggensmith P. Removal of toxic levels of N-acetylprocainamide with continuous arteriovenous hemofiltration or continuous arteriovenous hemodiafiltration. *Ann Intern Med.* 1987;106: 550-552.
29. Echt DS, Liebson PR, Mitchell LB, et al. Mortality and morbidity in patients receiving encainide, flecainide, or placebo: the Cardiac Arrhythmia Suppression Trial. *N Engl J Med.* 1991;324:781-788.
30. Eckart RE, Scoville SL, Campbell CL, et al. Sudden death in young adults: a 25-year review of autopsies in military recruits. *Ann Intern Med.* 2004;141:829-834.
31. Eray O, Fowler J. Severe propafenone poisoning responded to temporary internal pacemaker. *Vet Hum Toxicol.* 2000;42:289.
32. Ernawati DK, Stafford L, Hughes JD. Amiodarone-induced pulmonary toxicity. *Br J Clin Pharmacol.* 2008;66:82-87.
33. Faber TS, Camm AJ. The differentiation of propafenone from other class Ic agents, focusing on the effect on ventricular response rate attributable to its beta-blocking action. *Eur J Clin Pharmacol.* 1996;51:199-208.
34. Finkelstein F, Kreeft J. Massive lidocaine poisoning. *N Engl J Med.* 1979; 301:50.
35. Foley P, Kalra P, Andrews N. Amiodarone—avoid the danger of torsade de pointes. *Resuscitation.* 2008;76:137-141.
36. Fonck K, Haenebalcke C, Hemeryck A, et al. ECG changes and plasma concentrations of propafenone and its metabolites in a case of severe poisoning. *J Toxicol Clin Toxicol.* 1998;36:247-251.
37. Forini F, Nicolini G, Balzan S, et al. Amiodarone inhibits the 3,5,3′-triiodothyronine-dependent increase of sodium/potassium adenosine triphosphatase activity and concentration in human atrial myocardial tissue. *Thyroid.* 2004;14:493-499.
38. Frank SE, Snyder JT. Survival following severe overdose with mexiletine, nifedipine, and nitroglycerine. *Am J Emerg Med.* 1991;9:43-46.
39. Franz M, Geppert A, Kain R, Horl WH, Pohanka E. Acute renal failure after ibutilide. *Lancet.* 1999;353:467.
40. Freed CR, Freedman MD. Lidocaine overdose and cardiac bypass support. *JAMA.* 1985;253:3094-3095.
41. Gamboa A, Abraham R, Diedrich A, et al. Role of adenosine and nitric oxide on the mechanisms of action of dipyridamole. *Stroke.* 2005;36: 2170-2175.
42. Goldman MJ, Mowry JB, Kirk MA. Sodium bicarbonate to correct widened QRS in a case of flecainide overdose. *J Emerg Med.* 1997;15:183-186.
43. Goldschlager N, Epstein AE, Naccarelli GV, et al. A practical guide for clinicians who treat patients with amiodarone: 2007. *Heart Rhythm.* 2007;4: 1250-1259.
44. Gowda RM, Khan IA, Punukollu G, Vasavada BC, Sacchi TJ, Wilbur SL. Female preponderance in ibutilide-induced torsade de pointes. *Int J Cardiol.* 2004; 95:219-222.
45. Greig J, Groden BM. Persistent electrocardiographic changes after flecainide overdose. *Br J Clin Pract.* 1995;49:218-219.
46. Haas NA, Wegendt C, Schaffler R, et al. ECMO for cardiac rescue in a neonate with accidental amiodarone overdose. *Clin Res Cardiol.* 2008; 97(12):878-881.
47. Harron DW, Brogden RN. Acecainide (N-acetylprocainamide): a review of its pharmacodynamic and pharmacokinetic properties, and therapeutic potential in cardiac arrhythmias. *Drugs.* 1990;39:720-740.
48. Hasegawa J, Mori A, Yamamoto R, Kinugawa T, Morisawa T, Kishimoto Y. Disopyramide decreases the fasting serum glucose level in man. *Cardiovasc Drugs Ther.* 1999;13:325-327.
49. Hess GP, Walson PD. Seizures secondary to oral viscous lidocaine. *Ann Emerg Med.* 1988;17:725-727.
50. Heyman MR, Flores RH, Edelman BB, Carliner NH. Procainamide-induced lupus anticoagulant. *South Med J.* 1988;81:934-936.
51. Hiraoka M, Kuga K, Kawano S, Sunami A, Fan Z. New observations on the mechanisms of antiarrhythmic actions of disopyramide on cardiac membranes. *Am J Cardiol.* 1989;64:15J-19J.
52. Hudson CJ, Whitner TE, Rinaldi MJ, Littmann L. Brugada electrocardiographic pattern elicited by inadvertent flecainide overdose. *Pacing Clin Electrophysiol.* 2004;27:1311-1313.
53. Huikuri HV, Castellanos A, Myerburg RJ. Sudden death due to cardiac arrhythmias. *N Engl J Med.* 2001;345:1473-1482.
54. Jenzer HR, Hagemeijer F. Quinidine syncope. torsade de pointes with low quinidine plasma concentrations. *Eur J Cardiol.* 1976;4:447-451.
55. Kaji T, Nojima Y, Arisaka H, Naruse T. Clinical pharmacokinetics and effects of an oral sustained-release preparation of disopyramide prescribed for patients undergoing maintenance hemodialysis. *Blood Purif.* 2000; 18:55-58.
56. Katz AM. Selectivity and toxicity of antiarrhythmic drugs: molecular interactions with ion channels. *Am J Med.* 1998;104:179-195.
57. Kempen PM. Lethal/toxic injection of 20% lidocaine: a well-known complication of an unnecessary preparation? *Anesthesiology.* 1986;65:564-565.
58. Kenkel JM, Lipschitz AH, Shepherd G, et al. Pharmacokinetics and safety of lidocaine and monoethylglycinexylidide in liposuction: a microdialysis study. *Plast Reconstr Surg.* 2004;114:516-524; discussion 525-526.
59. Kerns W 2nd, English B, Ford M. Propafenone overdose. *Ann Emerg Med.* 1994;24:98-103.
60. Keyler DE, Pentel PR. Hypertonic sodium bicarbonate partially reverses QRS prolongation due to flecainide in rats. *Life Sci.* 1989;45:1575-1580.
61. Kim SY, Benowitz NL. Poisoning due to class IA antiarrhythmic drugs: quinidine, procainamide and disopyramide. *Drug Saf.* 1990;5:393-420.
62. Kozer E, Verjee Z, Koren G. Misdiagnosis of a mexiletine overdose because of a nonspecific result of urinary toxicologic screening. *N Engl J Med.* 2000; 343:1971-1972.
63. Kurnik D, Loebstein R, Farfel Z, Ezra D, Halkin H, Olchovsky D. Complex drug-drug-disease interactions between amiodarone, warfarin, and the thyroid gland. *Medicine (Baltimore).* 2004;83:107-113.
64. Labbe L, Turgeon J. Clinical pharmacokinetics of mexiletine. *Clin Pharmacokinet.* 1999;37:361-384.
65. Lalka D, Meyer MB, Duce BR, Elvin AT. Kinetics of the oral antiarrhythmic lidocaine congener, tocainide. *Clin Pharmacol Ther.* 1976;19:757-766.
66. Lee JT, Kroemer HK, Silberstein DJ, et al. The role of genetically determined polymorphic drug metabolism in the beta-blockade produced by propafenone. *N Engl J Med.* 1990;322:1764-1768.
67. Lerman BB, Belardinelli L. Cardiac electrophysiology of adenosine: basic and clinical concepts. *Circulation.* 1991;83:1499-1509.

68. Lovecchio F, Berlin R, Brubacher JR, Sholar JB. Hypertonic sodium bicarbonate in an acute flecainide overdose. *Am J Emerg Med.* 1998;16:534-537.
69. Low CL, Phelps KR, Bailie GR. Relative efficacy of haemoperfusion, haemodialysis and CAPD in the removal of procainamide and NAPA in a patient with severe procainamide toxicity. *Nephrol Dial Transplant.* 1996; 11:881-884.
70. Mantyjarvi M, Tuppurainen K, Ikaheimo K. Ocular side effects of amiodarone. *Surv Ophthalmol.* 1998;42:360-366.
71. Mazoit JX, Dalens BJ. Pharmacokinetics of local anaesthetics in infants and children. *Clin Pharmacokinet.* 2004;43:17-32.
72. McHugh TP, Perina DG. Propafenone ingestion. *Ann Emerg Med.* 1987;16: 437-440.
73. McLeod AA, Stiles GL, Shand DG. Demonstration of beta adrenoceptor blockade by propafenone hydrochloride: clinical pharmacologic, radioligand binding and adenylate cyclase activation studies. *J Pharmacol Exp Ther.* 1984;228:461-466.
74. Muhiddin KA, Johnston A, Turner P. The influence of urinary pH on flecainide excretion and its serum pharmacokinetics. *Br J Clin Pharmacol.* 1984;17:447-451.
75. Murray KT. Ibutilide. *Circulation.* 1998;97:493-497.
76. Nelson LS. Toxicologic myocardial sensitization. *J Toxicol Clin Toxicol.* 2002;40:867-879.
77. Nelson LS, Hoffman RS. Mexiletine overdose producing status epilepticus without cardiovascular abnormalities. *J Toxicol Clin Toxicol.* 1994;32:731-736.
78. O'Keeffe B, Hayler AM, Holt DW, Medd RK. Cardiac consequences and treatment of disopyramide intoxication: experimental evaluation in dogs. *Cardiovasc Res.* 1979;13:630-634.
79. Okumura K, Kita T, Chikazawa S, Komada F, Iwakawa S, Tanigawara Y. Genotyping of N-acetylation polymorphism and correlation with procainamide metabolism. *Clin Pharmacol Ther.* 1997;61:509-517.
80. Olkkola KT, Isohanni MH, Hamunen K, Neuvonen PJ. The effect of erythromycin and fluvoxamine on the pharmacokinetics of intravenous lidocaine. *Anesth Analg.* 2005;100:1352-1366, table of contents.
81. Ostad A, Kageyama N, Moy RL. Tumescent anesthesia with a lidocaine dose of 55 mg/kg is safe for liposuction. *Dermatol Surg.* 1996;22:921-927.
82. Ott MC, Khoor A, Leventhal JP, Paterick TE, Burger CD. Pulmonary toxicity in patients receiving low-dose amiodarone. *Chest.* 2003;123:646-651.
83. Pantuck AJ, Goldsmith JW, Kuriyan JB, Weiss RE. Seizures after ureteral stone manipulation with lidocaine. *J Urol.* 1997;157:2248.
84. Pfizer Inc, New York. Corvert (Ibutilide) Prescribing information. February 2006.
85. Pfizer Inc, New York. Tikosyn Prescribing information. March 2004.
86. Phillips RE, Looareesuwan S, White NJ, et al. Hypoglycaemia and antimalarial drugs. quinidine and release of insulin. *Br Med J (Clin Res Ed).* 1986;292:1319-1321.
87. Platt MS, Kohler LJ, Ruiz R, Cohle SD, Ravichandran P. Deaths associated with liposuction: case reports and review of the literature. *J Forensic Sci.* 2002;47:205-207.
88. Powell F, Smith P, Carey O. Fatal disopyramide overdose. *Ir Med J.* 1978; 71:552.
89. Ranger S, Nattel S. Determinants and mechanisms of flecainide-induced promotion of ventricular tachycardia in anesthetized dogs. *Circulation.* 1995;92:1300-1311.
90. Rao RB, Ely SF, Hoffman RS. Deaths related to liposuction. *N Engl J Med.* 1999;340:1471-1475.
91. Ratz Bravo AE, Drewe J, Schlienger RG, Krahenbuhl S, Pargger H, Ummenhofer W. Hepatotoxicity during rapid intravenous loading with amiodarone: description of three cases and review of the literature. *Crit Care Med.* 2005;33:128-134; discussion 245-246.
92. Resar LM, Helfaer MA. Recurrent seizures in a neonate after lidocaine administration. *J Perinatol.* 1998;18:193-195.
93. Rezvani M, Finkelstein Y, Verjee Z, Railton C, Koren G. Generalized seizures following topical lidocaine administration during circumcision. establishing causation. *Paediatr Drugs.* 2007;9:125-127.
94. Roden DM. Drug-induced prolongation of the QT interval. *N Engl J Med.* 2004;350:1013-1022.
95. Roden DM. Mechanisms and management of proarrhythmia. *Am J Cardiol.* 1998;82:49I-57I.
96. Roden DM. Risks and benefits of antiarrhythmic therapy. *N Engl J Med.* 1994;331:785-791.
97. Rogers KC, Wolfe DA. Amiodarone-induced blue-gray syndrome. *Ann Pharmacother.* 2000;34:1075.
98. Roukoz H, Saliba W. Dofetilide: a new class III antiarrhythmic agent. *Expert Rev Cardiovasc Ther.* 2007;5:9-19.
99. Roy D, Talajic M, Nattel S, et al. Rhythm control versus rate control for atrial fibrillation and heart failure. *N Engl J Med.* 2008;358:2667-2677.
100. Sathyavagiswaran L. Fatal disopyramide intoxication from suicidal/accidental overdose. *J Forensic Sci.* 1987;32:1813-1818.
101. Sawyer DR, Ludden TM, Crawford MH. Continuous infusion of lidocaine in patients with cardiac arrhythmias: unpredictability of plasma concentrations. *Arch Intern Med.* 1981;141:43-45.
102. Sclarovsky S, Lewin RF, Kracoff O, Strasberg B, Arditti A, Agmon J. Amiodarone-induced polymorphous ventricular tachycardia. *Am Heart J.* 1983;105:6-12.
103. Shimizu K, Shiono H, Matsubara K, et al. The tissue distribution of lidocaine in acute death due to overdosing. *Leg Med (Tokyo).* 2000;2:101-105.
104. Siddoway LA, Thompson KA, McAllister CB, et al. Polymorphism of propafenone metabolism and disposition in man: clinical and pharmacokinetic consequences. *Circulation.* 1987;75:785-791.
105. Siegers A, Board PN. Amiodarone used in successful resuscitation after near-fatal flecainide overdose. *Resuscitation.* 2002;53:105-108.
106. Singh BN, Wadhani N. Antiarrhythmic and proarrhythmic properties of QT-prolonging antianginal drugs. *J Cardiovasc Pharmacol Ther.* 2004; 9(suppl 1):S85-S97.
107. Sperry K, Wohlenberg N, Standefer JC. Fatal intoxication by tocainide. *J Forensic Sci.* 1987;32:1440-1446.
108. Takada Y, Isobe S, Okada M, et al. Effects of antiarrhythmic agents on left ventricular function during exercise in patients with chronic left ventricular dysfunction. *Ann Nucl Med.* 2004;18:209-219.
109. Takeo S, Tanonaka K, Hayashi M, et al. A possible involvement of sodium channel blockade of class-I-type antiarrhythmic agents in postischemic contractile recovery of isolated, perfused hearts. *J Pharmacol Exp Ther.* 1995; 273:1403-1409.
110. Tanda ML, Piantanida E, Lai A, et al. Diagnosis and management of amiodarone-induced thyrotoxicosis: similarities and differences between North American and European thyroidologists. *Clin Endocrinol (Oxf).* 2008;69(5):812-818.
111. Thomson PD, Melmon KL, Richardson JA, et al. Lidocaine pharmacokinetics in advanced heart failure, liver disease, and renal failure in humans. *Ann Intern Med.* 1973;78:499-508.
112. Vassallo P, Trohman RG. Prescribing amiodarone: an evidence-based review of clinical indications. *JAMA.* 2007;298:1312-1322.
113. Vaughan Williams EM. Classifying antiarrhythmic actions: by facts or speculation. *J Clin Pharmacol.* 1992;32:964-977.
114. Vaughan Williams EM. Significance of classifying antiarrhythmic actions since the cardiac arrhythmia suppression trial. *J Clin Pharmacol.* 1991; 31:123-135.
115. Vaughan EM, Williams DM. Classification of antidysrhythmic drugs. *Pharmacol Ther [B].* 1975;1:115-138.
116. White SR, Dy G, Wilson JM. The case of the slandered Halloween cupcake: survival after massive pediatric procainamide overdose. *Pediatr Emerg Care.* 2002;18:185-188.
117. Wiegers U, Hanrath P, Kuck KH, et al. Pharmacokinetics of tocainide in patients with renal dysfunction and during haemodialysis. *Eur J Clin Pharmacol.* 1983;24:503-507.
118. Winecoff AP, Hariman RJ, Grawe JJ, Wang Y, Bauman JL. Reversal of the electrocardiographic effects of cocaine by lidocaine: part 1. Comparison with sodium bicarbonate and quinidine. *Pharmacotherapy.* 1994;14: 698-703.
119. Wolbrette DL. Risk of proarrhythmia with class III antiarrhythmic agents: sex-based differences and other issues. *Am J Cardiol.* 2003;91:39D-44D.
120. Wu FL, Razzaghi A, Souney PF. Seizure after lidocaine for bronchoscopy: case report and review of the use of lidocaine in airway anesthesia. *Pharmacotherapy.* 1993;13:72-78.
121. Yamashita S, Sato S, Kakiuchi Y, Miyabe M, Yamaguchi H. Lidocaine toxicity during frequent viscous lidocaine use for painful tongue ulcer. *J Pain Symptom Manage.* 2002;24:543-545.
122. Yamreudeewong W, DeBisschop M, Martin LG, Lower DL. Potentially significant drug interactions of class III antiarrhythmic drugs. *Drug Saf.* 2003;26:421-438.

CHAPTER 64
CARDIOACTIVE STEROIDS

Jason B. Hack

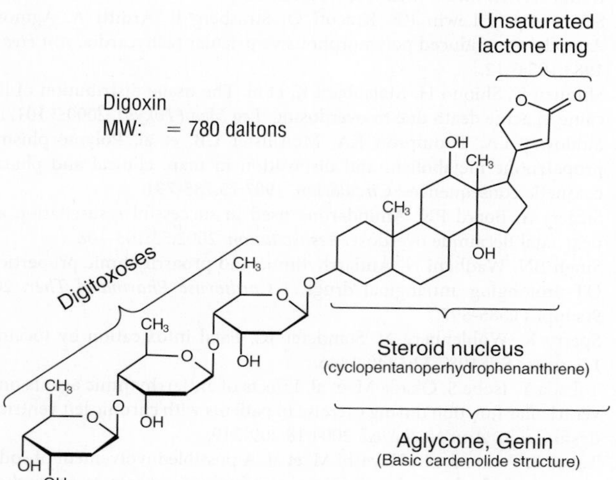

Unsaturated lactone ring
Digoxin
MW: = 780 daltons
Digitoxoses
Steroid nucleus
(cyclopentanoperhydrophenanthrene)
Aglycone, Genin
(Basic cardenolide structure)

Cardioactive steroids (CAS) remain in wide use throughout the world, although their benefits have become more and more restricted. Some of the most remarkable poisonings occur with exposures to plants such as *Digitalis purpurea* and *Nerium oleander* containing CAS, which are used by herbalists for varied disorders. Recent abuse of dried toad secretions from *Bufo* spp has lead to deaths with typical CAS morbidity and very high mortality. Rapid recognition of the CAS toxidrome and appropriate use of digoxin-specific antibody fragments can prove lifesaving.

HISTORY AND EPIDEMIOLOGY

There is evidence in the *Ebers Papyrus* (Papyrus Smith) that the Egyptians used plants containing CAS at least 3000 years ago. However, it was not until 1785, when William Withering wrote the first systemic account about the effects of the foxglove plant, that the use of CAS was more widely accepted into the Western apothecary. Foxglove was initially used as a diuretic and for the treatment of "dropsy" (edema), and Withering eloquently described its "power over the motion of the heart, to a degree yet unobserved in any other medicine."[124]

Subsequently, CAS became the mainstay of treatment for congestive heart failure and to control the ventricular response rate in atrial tachydysrhythmias. Because of their narrow therapeutic index and widespread use, both acute and chronic toxicity remain important problems.[84] According to the American Association of Poison Control Centers data, between the years 2002 and 2006, there were approximately 8000 exposures to CAS-containing plants with no attributable deaths and about 14,000 exposures to CAS-containing xenobiotics resulting in 100 deaths (see Chap. 135).

Toxicity is typically encountered in very young and very old individuals. In children, most acute overdoses are unintentional, resulting from dosing errors (this is particularly pertinent with the use of digoxin because the submilligram doses make dose calculations subject to 10-fold [decimal point] errors), or mistakenly ingesting an adult's medication. Older adults are at particular risk for toxicity, either from interactions of the CAS with other medications in their chronic regimen or indirectly as a consequence of an alteration in the absorption or elimination kinetics. Drug–drug interactions from an adult's polypharmacy or from additional acute care xenobiotics that change CAS clearance in the liver or kidney, may alter protein binding and may result in increased bioavailability.

The most commonly prescribed CAS in the United States is digoxin; other internationally available but much less commonly used preparations are digitoxin, ouabain, lanatoside C, deslanoside, and gitalin. CAS toxicity may also result from exposure to certain plants or animals. Documented plant sources of CAS include oleander (*Nerium oleander*); yellow oleander (*Thevetia peruviana*), which has been implicated in the suicidal deaths of thousands of patients in Southeast Asia[26], foxglove (*Digitalis* spp), lily of the valley (*Convallaria majalis*), dogbane (*Apocynum cannabinum*), and red squill (*Urginea maritima*). CAS poisoning may result from teas containing seeds of these plants and water and herbal products contaminated with plant CAS (see Chap. 43).[16,19,52,79,90,97,116] Toxicity also results from ingestion, instead of the intended topical application, of a purported aphrodisiac derived from the dried secretion of toads from the *Bufo* species, which contains a bufadienolide-class CAS.[10,12,13] Although there have been no reported human exposures, fireflies of the *Photinus* species (*P. ignitus*, *P. marginellus*, and *P. pyralis*) contain the CAS lucibufagin that is structurally a bufadienolides.[30,65]

CHEMISTRY

CAS contain an aglycone or "genin" nucleus structure with a steroid core and an unsaturated lactone ring attached at C-17. Cardiac glycosides contain additional sugar groups attached to C-3. The sugar residues confer increased water solubility and enhance the ability of the molecule to enter cells. Cardenolides are primarily plant-derived aglycones with a five-member unsaturated lactone ring. The bufadienolide and lucibufagin groups of CAS molecules are mainly animal derived (with such notable exceptions as scillaren from red squill) and contain a six-member unsaturated lactone ring. When the aglycone digoxigenin is linked to one or more hydrophilic sugar (digitoxoses) moieties at C-3, it forms digoxin, a cardiac glycoside. The aglycone of digitoxin differs from that of digoxin by the lack of a hydroxyl group on C-12, and ouabain differs from digoxin by both the absence of a hydroxyl group on C-12 and the addition of hydroxyl groups on C-1, -5, -10, and -11. The cardioactive components in toad secretions are genins and lack sugar moieties.

PHARMACOKINETICS

The correlation between clinical effects and serum concentrations is based on steady-state concentrations, which are dependent on many absorption, distribution, and elimination factors (Table 64–1). Although not proven, other CAS likely follow the distribution pattern of digoxin or digitoxin such that obtaining a serum concentration before 6 hours after ingestion (the time at which tissue concentration peak) gives a misleadingly high serum concentration resulting from its bimodal distribution. After therapeutic dosing, the intravascular distribution and elimination of digoxin from the plasma are best described using a two-compartment model that is achieved over approximately 36 to 48 hours in patients with normal renal function. The distribution or α-phase represents the rapid decrease of drug concentration intravascularly and is dependent on whether the method of administration

TABLE 64–1. Pharmacology of Selected Cardioactive Steroids

Pharmacology	Digoxin	Digitoxin
Onset of Action		
PO	1.5–6 h	3–6 h
IV	5–30 min	30 min–2 h
Maximal effect		
PO	4–6 h	6–12 h
IV	1.5–3 h	4–8 h
Intestinal absorption	40%–90% (mean, 75%)	>95%
Plasma protein binding	25%	97%
Volume of distribution	5–7 L/kg (adults) 16 L/kg (infants) 10 L/kg (neonates) 4–5 L/kg (adults with renal failure)	0.6 L/kg (adults)
Elimination half-life	1.6 days	6–7 days
Route of elimination	Renal (60%–80%), with limited hepatic metabolism	Hepatic metabolism (80%)
Enterohepatic circulation	7%	26%.

is intravenous (IV) or oral (PO). An exponential decline occurs as the drug is rapidly distributed from the blood to the peripheral tissues, with a 30-minute distribution half-life. During the distribution phase, most of the intravascular CAS leaves the blood and is found in the tissues, resulting in a large volume of distribution (Vd) (eg, the Vd of digoxin is 5–7 L/kg with therapeutic use). The β or elimination phase with a half-life (for digoxin) of approximately 36 hours represents the drug's total-body clearance, which is achieved primarily by the kidneys (70% in a person with normal renal function).[17,46]

After a massive acute digoxin overdose, the half-life may be shortened to as little as 13 to 15 hours because elevated serum concentrations result in greater renal clearance before distribution to the tissues.[51,111] Even with therapeutic administration of CAS, adjustments to the dosing regimen must be made to avert toxicity caused by the physiologic changes associated with aging, including hypothyroidism, chronic hypoxemia with alkalosis, and decreased creatinine clearance. Physiologic changes in CAS kinetics occur with functional decline of the liver, kidney, and heart and dynamics with electrolyte abnormalities, including hypomagnesemia, hypercalcemia, hypernatremia, and commonly hypokalemia. Therefore, serum concentrations should be monitored to avoid inadvertent toxicity. Hypokalemia resulting from a variety of mechanisms, such as the use of loop diuretics, poor dietary intake, diarrhea, and the administration of potassium-binding resins, enhances the effects of CAS on the myocardium and is associated with dysrhythmias at lower serum CAS concentrations. Chronic hypokalemia reduces the number of Na^+-K^+-adenosine triphosphatase (ATPase) units in skeletal muscle, which may alter drug effects.[63]

Drug interactions between digoxin and quinidine, verapamil, diltiazem, carvedilol, amiodarone, and spironolactone are common.[20,23,45,68,93] These interactions occur because of a reduction in the protein binding of the CAS, increasing availability to the tissues; a reduction in excretion as a consequence of a decrease in renal perfusion; or as a result of interference with secretion by the kidneys and intestines because of inactivation of P-glycoproteins. In approximately 10% to 15% of patients receiving digoxin, a significant amount of digoxin is inactivated in the gastrointestinal (GI) tract by enteric bacterium, primarily *Eubacterium lentum*. Inhibition of this inactivation by the alteration of the GI flora by many antibiotics, particularly the macrolide antibiotics, may result in increased bioavailability[73] and therefore may produce as much as a twofold increase in serum CAS concentration.[92]

MECHANISMS OF ACTION AND PATHOPHYSIOLOGY

ELECTROPHYSIOLOGIC EFFECTS ON INOTROPY

Although incompletely understood, it appears that CAS increase the force of contraction of the heart (positive inotropic effect) by increasing cytosolic Ca^{2+} during systole. Both Na^+ and Ca^{2+} ions enter and exit cardiac muscle cells during each cycle of depolarization and contraction–repolarization and relaxation. Sodium entry heralds the start of the action potential (phase 0) and carries the inward, depolarizing positive charge. Calcium subsequently enters the cardiac myocyte through L-type calcium channels during late phase 0 and the plateau phase of the action potential, and this Ca^{2+} triggers the release of more Ca^{2+} into the cytosol from the sarcoplasmic reticulum. During repolarization and relaxation (diastole), Ca^{2+} is both pumped back into the sarcoplasmic reticulum by a local Ca^{2+}-ATPase and is pumped extracellularly by an Na^+-Ca^{2+} antiporter (Fig. 64–1; see Chap. 23).[78]

CAS inhibit active transport of Na^+ and K^+ across the cell membrane during repolarization by binding to a specific site on the extracellular face of the α-subunit of the membrane Na^+-K^+-ATPase. This inhibits the cellular Na^+ pump activity, which decreases Na^+ extrusion and increases Na^+ in the cytosol, thereby decreasing the transmembrane Na^+ gradient. Because the Na^+-Ca^{2+} antiporter derives its power not from adenosine triphosphate (ATP) but rather from the Na^+ gradient generated by the Na^+-K^+ transport mechanism,[29] the dysfunction of the Na^+-K^+-ATPase pump reduces Ca^{2+} extrusion from the cell. The additional cytoplasmic Ca^{2+} enhances the Ca^{2+}-induced Ca^{2+} release from the sarcoplasmic reticulum during systole and by this mechanism increases the force of contraction of the cardiac muscle. Additional mechanisms of action are being explored and include creation of transmembrane calcium channels by cardioactive glycosides.[1]

EFFECTS ON CARDIAC ELECTROPHYSIOLOGY

At therapeutic serum concentrations, CAS increase automaticity and shorten the repolarization intervals of the atria and ventricles (Table 64–2). There is a concurrent decrease in the rate of depolarization and conduction through the sinoatrial (SA) and atrioventricular (AV) nodes, respectively. This is mediated both indirectly via an enhancement in vagally mediated parasympathetic tone and directly by depression of myocardial tissue. These changes in nodal conduction are reflected on the electrocardiogram (ECG) by a decrease in ventricular response rate to suprajunctional rhythms and by PR interval prolongation (the latter is part of digitalis effect). The effects of CAS on ventricular repolarization are related to the elevated intracellular resting potential caused by the enhanced availability of Ca^{2+} and manifest on the ECG as QT interval shortening and ST segment and T-wave forces opposite in direction to the major QRS forces. The last effect results in the characteristic scooping of the ST segments (referred to as the *digitalis effect*) (Fig. 64–2).

Excessive increases in intracellular Ca^{2+} caused by toxic CAS effects result in delayed afterdepolarizations. These are fluxes in membrane potential caused by spontaneous Ca^{2+}-induced Ca^{2+} release, which is caused by the excess intracellular Ca^{2+} and appear on the ECG like

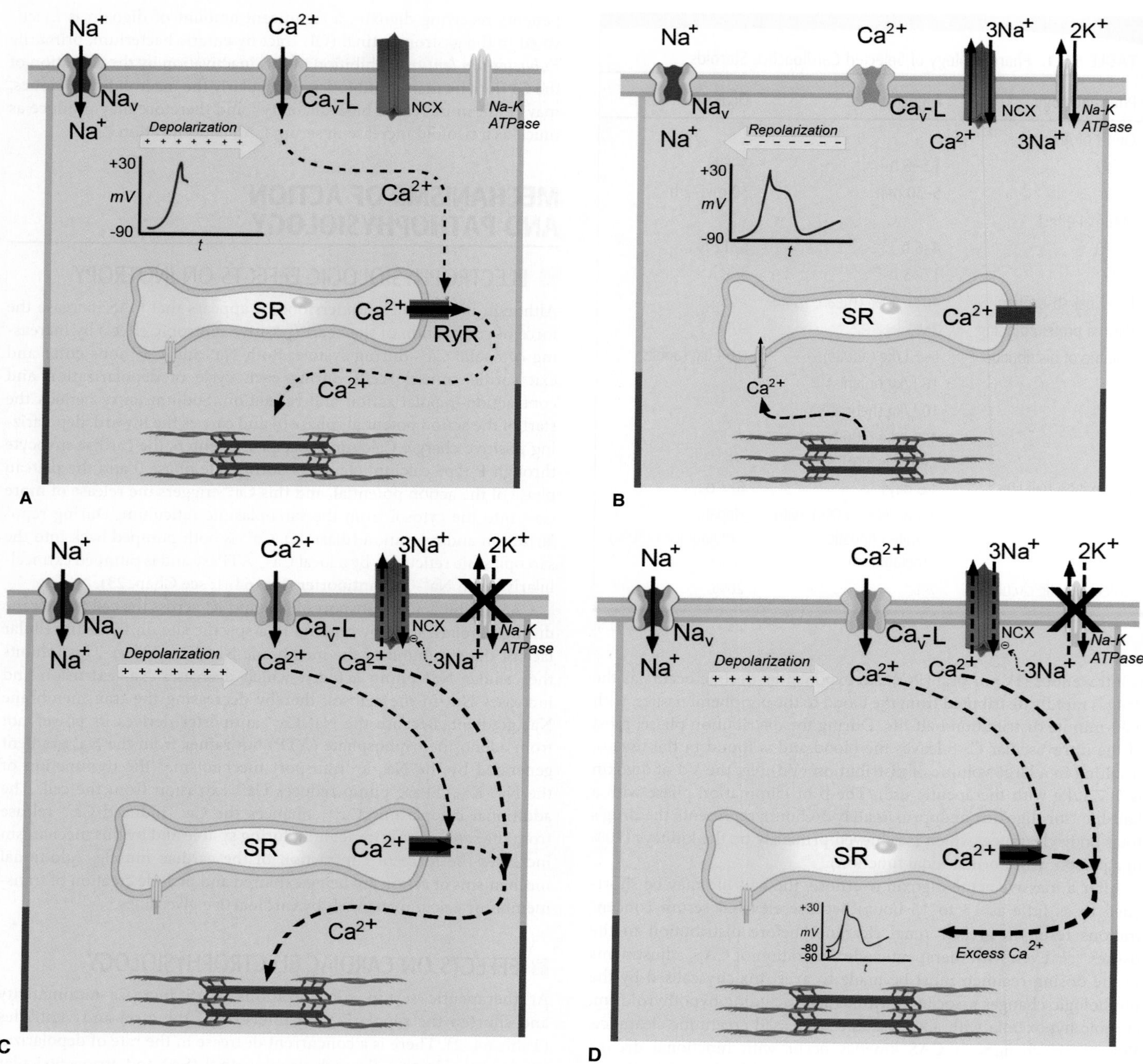

FIGURE 64–1. Pharmacology and toxicology of the cardioactive steroids (CAS). (**A**) Normal depolarization. Depolarization occurs after the opening of fast Na^+ channels; the increase in intracellular potential opens voltage-dependent Ca^{2+} channels, and the influx of Ca^{2+} induces the massive release of Ca^{2+} from the sarcoplasmic reticulum, producing contraction. (**B**) Normal repolarization. Repolarization begins with active expulsion of Na^+ ions in exchange for K^+ using an ATPase. This electrogenic (3 Na^+ for 2 K^+) pump creates an Na^+ gradient that is used to expel Ca^{2+} via an antiporter (NCX). The sarcoplasmic reticulum resequesters its Ca^{2+} load via a separate ATPase. (**C**) Pharmacologic CAS. Digitalis inhibition of the Na^+-K^+-ATPase raises the intracellular Na^+ content, preventing the antiporter from expelling Ca^{2+} in exchange for Na^+. The net result is an elevated intracellular Ca^{2+}, resulting in enhanced inotropy through enhanced SR calcium release. (**D**) Toxic CAS. Excessive elevation of the intracellular Ca^{2+} elevates the resting potential, producing myocardial sensitization, and predisposing to dysrhythmias. The addition of exogenous Ca^{2+} may overwhelm the capacity of the sarcoplasmic reticulum to sequester this ion, resulting in dysrhythmia or myocardial dysfunction.

U waves. Occasionally, these may initiate a cellular depolarization that manifests as a premature ventricular contraction (see Chap. 23).[28,60]

Hypokalemia inhibits Na^+-K^+-ATPase activity and contributes to the pump inhibition induced by CAS, enhances myocardial automaticity, and increases myocardial susceptibility to CAS-related dysrhythmias. This may be partly a result of decreased competitive inhibition between the CAS and potassium at the Na^+-K^+-ATPase exchanger.[95] Severe hypokalemia (<2.5 mEq/L) reduces the rate of sodium-potassium pump function, slowing the pump and exacerbating concomitant sodium-potassium pump inhibition by the CAS.[60]

TABLE 64–2. Electrophysiologic Effects of Cardioactive Steroids on the Myocardium

	Atria and Ventricles	AV Node	Electrocardiogram
Excitability	↑	–	Extrasystoles, tachydysrhythmias
Automaticity	↑	–	Extrasystoles, tachydysrhythmias
Conduction velocity	↓	↓	↑ PR interval, AV block
Refractoriness	↓	↑	↑ PR interval, AV block, decreased QT interval

AV, atrioventricular.

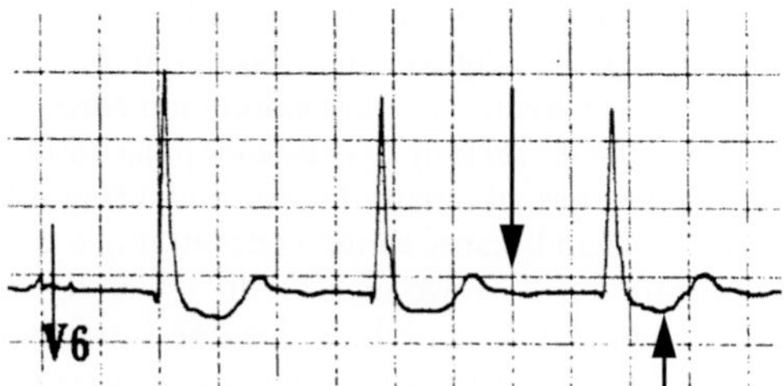

FIGURE 64–2. Digitalis effect noted in the lateral precordial lead, V6. Note the prolonged PR interval (long arrow) and the repolarization abnormality (scooping of the ST segment) (short arrow).

EFFECTS OF CARDIOACTIVE STEROIDS ON THE AUTONOMIC NERVOUS SYSTEM

CAS affect the parasympathetic system by increasing the release of acetylcholine from vagal fibers,[75,114] possibly through augmentation of intracellular calcium. CAS affect the sympathetic system by increasing efferent sympathetic discharge,[85,109] which may exacerbate dysrhythmias.

CLINICAL MANIFESTATIONS

Although there are differences in the signs and symptoms of acute and chronic CAS poisoning, adults and children have similar manifestations when poisoned.

NONCARDIAC MANIFESTATIONS

Acute Toxicity An asymptomatic period of several minutes to several hours may follow a single administered toxic dose of CAS. The first symptom is typically nausea, vomiting, or abdominal pain. Central nervous system effects of acute toxicity may include lethargy, confusion, and weakness that are not caused by hemodynamic changes.[16] The absence of nausea and vomiting several hours after exposure makes acute CAS poisoning unlikely.

Chronic Toxicity Chronic toxicity is often difficult to diagnose as a result of its insidious development and protean manifestations, including weakness, anhedonia, and loss of appetite. Symptoms may also include those that occur with acute poisonings; however, they are often less obvious. GI findings include nausea, vomiting, abdominal pain, and weight loss. Neuropsychiatric disorders include delirium, confusion, drowsiness, headache, hallucinations, and (rarely) seizures.[16,38,40] Visual disturbances include transient amblyopia, photophobia, blurring, scotomata, photopsia, decreased visual activity, and aberrations of color vision (chromatopsia), such as yellow halos (xanthopsia) around lights.[69,70]

Electrolyte Abnormalities Elevated serum potassium concentrations frequently occur in patients with acute CAS poisoning.[60,63] Hyperkalemia has important prognostic implications because the serum potassium concentration is a better predictor of lethality than either the initial ECG changes or the serum CAS concentration.[5,6] In a study of 91 acutely digitoxin poisoned patients conducted before digoxin-specific Fab was available, approximately 50% of the patients with serum potassium concentrations of 5.0 to 5.5 mEq/L died. Although a serum potassium concentration lower than 5.0 mEq/L was associated with no deaths, all of the 10 patients with serum potassium concentration above 5.5 mEq/L died.[5] Elevation of the serum potassium concentration after administration of CAS is a result of CAS inhibition of the Na^+-K^+-ATPase pump, which results in the inhibition of potassium uptake in exchange for Na^+ by skeletal muscle (the largest potassium reservoir). Hyperkalemia probably causes further hyperpolarization of myocardial conduction tissue, increasing AV nodal block, thereby exacerbating CAS-induced bradydysrhythmias and conduction delays.[60] However, correction of the hyperkalemia alone does not increase patient survival;[5] it is a marker for, but not the cause of, the morbidity and mortality associated with CAS poisoning. The interrelationships between intracellular and extracellular potassium and CAS therapy are complex and incompletely understood.

CARDIAC MANIFESTATIONS

General The alterations in cardiac rate and rhythm occurring with CAS poisoning may result in nearly any dysrhythmia. The exception is that a rapidly conducted supraventricular tachydysrhythmia is not likely attributable to the prominent depressive effect of CAS on the AV node. In 10% to 15% of cases, the first sign of toxicity is the appearance of an ectopic ventricular rhythm.[94] Although no single dysrhythmia is pathognomonic of CAS toxicity, toxicity should be suspected when there is evidence of increased automaticity in combination with impaired conduction through the SA and AV nodes.[60] Bidirectional ventricular tachycardia is nearly diagnostic, although it may also occur with poisoning by aconitine and other uncommon xenobiotics[105] (see Fig. 22–19). Dysrhythmias result from the complex electrophysiologic influences on both the myocardium and conduction system of the heart resulting from direct, vagotonic, and other autonomic actions of the CAS.

The effects of digoxin vary with dose and differ depending on the type of cardiac tissue involved. The atrial and ventricular myocardial tissues exhibit increased automaticity and excitability, resulting in extrasystoles and tachydysrhythmias. Conduction velocity is reduced in both the atrial conducting system and nodal tissue, resulting in an increased PR interval and AV nodal block. Indeed, AV junctional blocks of varying degrees associated with increased ventricular automaticity are the most common cardiac manifestations, occurring in 30% to 40%, of patients with CAS toxicity.[76] AV dissociation may result from suppression of the dominant pacemaker with escape of a secondary pacemaker or from inappropriate acceleration of a ventricular pacemaker. Hypotension, shock, and cardiovascular collapse may ensue. Table 64–3 summarizes these phenomena.

Acute Toxicity Many cardiac dysrhythmias are associated with CAS toxicity. These dysrhythmias are unified by a sensitized myocardium and a depressed AV node (see Table 64–3). The initial bradydysrhythmia results from increased vagal tone at the SA and AV nodes and is often responsive to atropine.

TABLE 64–3. Cardiac Dysrhythmias Associated with Cardioactive Steroid Poisoning

Myocardial irritability causing dysrhythmias
Atrial flutter and atrial fibrillation with atrioventricular (AV) block
Bidirectional ventricular tachycardia
Delayed after no space depolarizations
Nonparoxysmal atrial tachydysrhythmias with AV block
Nonsustained ventricular tachycardia
Premature and sustained ventricular contractions
Ventricular bigeminy
Ventricular fibrillation
Primary conduction system dysfunction causing dysrhythmias
AV dissociation
Exit blocks
High-degree AV block
His-Purkinje dysfunction
Junctional tachycardia
Sinoatrial (SA) nodal arrest
Sinus bradycardia.

Chronic Toxicity Bradydysrhythmias that appear later in acute poisonings and with chronic CAS toxicity occur by direct actions on the heart and often are minimally responsive to atropine, if at all. Ventricular tachydysrhythmias are more common in patients with chronic or late acute poisoning.

DIAGNOSTIC TESTING

Properly obtained and interpreted serum digoxin concentrations aid significantly in the management of patients with suspected digoxin toxicity, as well as in the management of patients poisoned by several other CAS. Although most institutions report a therapeutic range for serum digoxin concentration from 0.5 to 2.0 ng/mL (SI units, 1.0-2.6 nmol/mL), current research suggests lowering the upper limit to 1.0 ng/mL maintains benefit while decreasing the risk of toxicity.[98,107] In addition to determining a serum CAS concentration, care must be taken to interpret the concentration as a correlate with the clinical condition of the patient; the interval between the last dose and the time the blood sample was taken; and the presence of other metabolic abnormalities, including hypokalemia, hypomagnesemia, hypercalcemia, hypernatremia, alkalosis, hypothyroidism, and hypoxemia and the use of xenobiotics such as amiodarone, calcium channel blockers, catecholamines, quinidine, and diuretics.

Although CAS poisoning is multifactorial and it is inappropriate to use the upper limit of the therapeutic range of digoxin as the sole indicator of toxicity,[101] there is a significant correlation between a patient's clinical condition and their serum concentration. In general, patients with pharmaceutical CAS toxicity have mean serum concentrations above 2 ng/mL for digoxin and above 40 ng/mL for digitoxin measured 6 hours after the last dose.[59] The significance of a serum concentration depends on when the value is obtained in relation to an acute ingestion and the distribution phase of the drug; a value of 15 ng/mL of digoxin is more ominous 6 hours after an ingestion than 1 hour after an ingestion. Additionally, there is often an overlap in serum digoxin concentrations between toxic and nontoxic patients.

In most hospitals, "digoxin levels" are the only estimation available to physicians in the acute setting when evaluating a patient for presumed non-digoxin CAS poisoning. The polyclonal assays typically used in most institutions frequently, but unpredictably, cross-react with other plant- or animal-derived CAS. Although a monoclonal digoxin immunoassay accurately quantifies serum digoxin, an elevated digoxin concentration in the correct clinical setting may qualitatively assist in making a presumptive diagnosis of non-digoxin CAS exposure (see Chaps. 43 and 118).[14,88] For example, using various techniques, including high-performance liquid chromatography (HPLC) and monoclonal and polyclonal antibody analysis, "digoxin" concentrations are recorded from serum to which has been added oleandrin and oleandrigenin from *Nerium oleander* or from patients exposed to *Thevetia peruviana* (yellow oleander) or toad-secreted bufadienolides.[10,26,54] With the use of more specific analytic technology, patients with CAS poisoning from plant- or animal-derived CAS may have low or nonexistent digoxin concentrations (see Chaps. 43 and 118).

Serum concentrations of digoxin are measured in one of two ways: free digoxin and total digoxin. The most common method of quantifying total digoxin in the serum is by fluorescence polarization immunoassay (FPIA). Under normal circumstances, measuring total digoxin in the serum is sufficient because serum concentrations are predictive of cardiac concentrations.[24] However, after the use of digoxin-specific Fab (which remains almost entirely within the intravascular space [Vd, 0.40 L/kg]), there is a large elevation in total CAS concentrations because the CAS is drawn from the tissues and complexes with the antibody fragment, thus trapping the CAS in the intravascular space. When this bulk movement is achieved by binding with Fab fragments, a tremendous increase, often approaching an order of magnitude, in total serum digoxin concentrations occurs. In this situation, laboratory manipulation methods to detect only the unbound digoxin and allow the quantification of free digoxin in the serum include ultrafiltration and equilibrium dialysis.[36] Paradoxically, excess digoxin antibody may cause a false elevation in digoxin concentration (see Chap. 6).

ENDOGENOUS DIGOXIN-LIKE IMMUNOREACTIVE SUBSTANCE

Some patients who are not receiving a CAS may nevertheless have a positive digoxin assay result as a result of an endogenous substance that is structurally and functionally similar to the prescribed CAS.[45] This finding is described in patients with increased inotropic need or reduced renal clearance, including neonates[117]; patients with renal insufficiency,[11,41,53] liver disease,[81] subarachnoid hemorrhage,[123] congestive heart failure,[39,102] insulin-dependent diabetes,[35] stress,[40,118] acromegaly,[26] or hypothermia[117]; after strenuous exercise[118]; and in pregnancy.[32,42,50] An endogenous Na^+-K^+-ATPase inhibiting dihydropyrone-substituted bufadienolide CAS has been isolated from human placenta.[33] It differs from the toad bufadienolides solely by a single double-bond pyrone ring. Because bufadienolides are not normally found in either healthy humans or edible plants, a synthetic pathway to produce dihydropyrone-substituted steroids in humans may be responsible for this endogenous digoxin-like immunoreactive substance (EDLIS). Further research is necessary to confirm this pathway.[50] The clinician suspecting this problem should consult the clinical laboratory.[34] Clinical observations indicate that the serum digoxin concentration contributed by EDLIS is usually less than 2 ng/mL. Other endogenous substances, such as bilirubin,[81] and exogenous substances, such as spironolactone,[103] may also cross-react with the digoxin assay and cause a false-positive result.

THERAPY

ACUTE MANAGEMENT OVERVIEW

Initial treatment of a patient with acute CAS poisoning includes providing general care, (eg, GI decontamination, monitoring for dysrhythmias, measuring electrolyte and digoxin concentrations) and definitive care (eg, administering digoxin-specific antibody fragments). Secondary care includes treating complications such as dysrhythmias and electrolyte abnormalities.

GASTROINTESTINAL DECONTAMINATION

The initial treatment should be directed toward prevention of further GI absorption. Only rarely should emesis or lavage may be considered because efficacy is limited secondary to rapid absorption from the gut and to the emetic effects of the drug itself. Patients with chronic ingestion also do not usually benefit from these GI decontamination techniques because of the limited availability of drug in the GI tract for removal. Because many CAS, such as digitoxin and digoxin, are recirculated enterohepatically and enteroenterically, both late and repeated activated charcoal administration (1 g/kg of body weight every 2–4 hours for up to four doses) may be beneficial in reducing serum concentrations.[17,21,67,71,86,121] Similar to activated charcoal, steroid-binding resins, such as cholestyramine and colestipol,[49,91] may prevent reabsorption of CAS from the GI tract and reduce the serum half-life by interrupting both enteroenteric and enterohepatic circulation, and they may be used when digoxin-specific Fab is not immediately available or when renal function is inadequate.[21,49]

ADVANCED MANAGEMENT

Digoxin-Specific Antibody Fragments The definitive therapy for patients with life-threatening CAS toxicity is to administer digoxin-specific antibody fragments.[2,34,36,87,90,97,106,112,125] Purified digoxin-specific Fab causes a sharp decrease in free serum digoxin concentrations; a concomitant but clinically unimportant, massive increase in total serum digoxin; an increase in renal clearance of CAS; and a decrease in the serum potassium concentration.[2] In addition, the administration of digoxin-specific Fab is pharmacoeconomically advantageous.[22] Although the xenobiotic itself is relatively expensive, its expense is far outweighed by obviating the need, risk, and expense of long-term intensive care unit stays and of repetitive evaluation of potassium and digoxin concentrations. Table 64–4 lists the indications for administering digoxin-specific Fab. Extensive discussion is found in Antidotes in Depth A20: Digoxin-Specific Antibody Fragments (Fab).

TABLE 64–4. Indications for Administration of Digoxin-Specific Antibody Fragments (DSFab)

Any digoxin-related life-threatening dysrhythmias, regardless of digoxin concentration

Potassium concentration >5 mEq/L in setting of acute digoxin poisoning

Chronic elevation of serum digoxin concentration (SDC) associated with dysrhythmias, significant GI symptoms, or altered mental status

SDC ≥15 ng/mL at any time or ≥10 ng/mL 6 h postingestion, regardless of symptoms

Acute ingestion of 10 mg of digoxin in an adult

Acute ingestion of 4 mg of digoxin in a child

Poisoning with a non-digoxin cardioactive steroid

Digoxin-specific Fab dosing (round up to number of whole vials in calculation)

$$\text{No. of vials} = \frac{\text{SDC(ng/mL)} \times \text{Patient Weight(kg)}}{100}$$

$$\text{No. of vials} = \frac{\text{Amount ingested(mg)}}{0.5\text{(mg/vial)}} \times 80\%\ \text{bioavailability}$$

Empiric therapy for acute poisoning:
- 10–20 vials (adult or pediatric)

Empiric therapy for chronic poisoning:
- Adults: 3–6 vials
- Children: 1–2 vials.

Other Cardiac Therapeutics Secondary xenobiotics used in patients with symptomatic CAS exposures include the use of atropine for supraventricular bradydysrhythmias or high degrees of AV block. Atropine dosing is 0.5 mg administered IV to an adult or 0.02 mg/kg with a minimum of 0.1 mg to a child. Atropine should be titrated to block the vagotonic effects of the CAS. The dose may be repeated at 5-minute intervals if necessary. Therapeutic success is unpredictable because the depressant actions of CAS are mediated only partly through the vagus nerve.

Phenytoin and lidocaine are other drug therapies that are rarely used (secondary to Fab fragments obviating their utility) for the management of CAS-induced ventricular tachydysrhythmias and ventricular irritability. These xenobiotics depress the enhanced ventricular automaticity without significantly slowing, and perhaps enhancing, AV nodal conduction.[96] In fact, phenytoin may reverse digitalis-induced prolongation of AV nodal conduction while suppressing digitalis-induced ectopic tachydysrhythmia without diminishing myocardial contractile forces.[48] In addition, phenytoin may terminate supraventricular dysrhythmias induced by digitalis more effectively than lidocaine.[96] Underlying atrial fibrillation and flutter typically do not convert to a normal sinus rhythm with administration of phenytoin or lidocaine. When used, phenytoin should be infused slowly IV (~50 mg/min) or in boluses of 100 mg repeated every 5 minutes until control of the dysrhythmias is achieved or a maximum of 1000 mg has been given in adults or 15–20 mg/kg in children.[9,80] Fosphenytoin has not been evaluated in this setting. Maintenance PO doses of phenytoin (300 to 400 mg/d in adults and 6–10 mg/kg/d in children) should be continued until digoxin toxicity is resolved. Lidocaine is given as a 1-1.5-mg/kg IV bolus followed by continuous infusion at 1 to 4 mg/min in adults or as a 1-1.5-mg/kg IV bolus followed by 30 to 50 μg/kg/min in children as required to control the rhythm disturbance (see Chap. 63).

Class IA antidysrhythmics are contraindicated in the setting of CAS poisoning because they may induce or worsen AV nodal block and decrease His-Purkinje conduction at slow heart rates and because their α-adrenergic receptor blockade and vagal inhibition may induce significant hypotension and tachycardia. Class IA antidysrhythmics are also prodysrhythmogenic, and their safety in the setting of CAS poisoning is unstudied. Additionally, quinidine reduces renal clearance of digoxin and digitoxin. The use of isoproterenol should be avoided in CAS-induced conduction disturbances because there may be an increased incidence of ventricular ectopic activity in the presence of toxic concentrations of CAS.

PACEMAKERS AND CARDIOVERSION

External or transvenous pacemakers have had limited indications in the management of patients with CAS poisoning. In one retrospective study of 92 digitalis-poisoned patients, 51 patients were treated with cardiac pacing, digoxin-specific Fab, or both; the overall mortality rate was 13%.[113] Prevention of life-threatening dysrhythmias failed in 8% of patients treated with immunotherapy and 23% of patients treated with internal pacemakers. The main reasons for failure of digoxin-specific Fab were pacing-induced dysrhythmias and delayed or insufficient doses of digoxin-specific Fab. Iatrogenic complications of pacing occurred in 36% of patients. Thus, overdrive suppression with a temporary transvenous pacemaker should not be used to abolish ventricular tachydysrhythmias in the presence of CAS poisoning.[6,113] In the setting of digoxin poisoning, administration of transthoracic electrical cardioversion for atrial tachydysrhythmias has been associated with the development of potentially lethal ventricular dysrhythmias. The dysrhythmias were related to the degree of toxicity and the amount of administered current in cardioversion.[99] In CAS-poisoned patients with unstable rhythms, such as hemodynamically unstable ventricular tachycardia and ventricular fibrillation, cardioversion and defibrillation, respectively, are indicated.

ELECTROLYTE THERAPY

Potassium Hypokalemia and hyperkalemia may exacerbate CAS cardiotoxicity even at "therapeutic digoxin concentrations." When hypokalemia is noted in conjunction with tachydysrhythmias or bradydysrhythmias, potassium replacement should be administered with serial monitoring of the serum potassium concentration. Digoxin-specific Fab administration generally should not be used unless the hypokalemia is corrected and the patient continues to have life-threatening manifestations of CAS cardiotoxicity.

Hyperkalemia may also exacerbate CAS-induced cardiotoxicity, at "therapeutic digoxin concentrations." In this setting, therapies directed at reducing potassium concentrations should be judiciously initiated with care to avoid hypokalemia. Any exacerbation of CAS cardiotoxicity despite this correction should be treated immediately with Fab fragments.

In the presence of acute CAS toxicity, when potassium exceeds 5 mEq/L, digoxin-specific antibody fragments are indicated. When marked hyperkalemia develops in conjunction with ECG evidence of hyperkalemia and if digoxin-specific Fab is not available immediately, an attempt should be made to lower the serum potassium with IV insulin, dextrose, sodium bicarbonate, and PO administration of the ion-exchange resin sodium polystyrene sulfonate. Caution should be applied to the subsequent administration of digoxin-specific Fab because of concern for profound hypokalemia.

Calcium is beneficial in most hyperkalemic patients, but in the setting of CAS poisoning, calcium salts administration is considered to be potentially dangerous. A number of experimental studies cite the additive or synergistic actions of calcium and CAS on the heart (because intracellular hypercalcemia is already present), resulting in dysrhythmias,[37,83,104] cardiac dysfunction[61] (eg, hypercontractility, or the so-called "stone heart," hypocontractility), and cardiac arrest.[72,104,119] Although a 2004 study was unable to show an adverse effect,[43] there exist three case reports[8,64] of CAS-poisoned patients who died at various intervals after calcium administration, which supports the withholding of calcium administration in the setting of hyperkalemia.

The purported mechanism is augmented intracellular cytoplasmic Ca^{2+}, which results from an increased transmembrane concentration gradient that further inhibits calcium extrusion through the Na^+-Ca^{2+} exchange or increased intracytoplasmic stores.[59] This additional cytoplasmic calcium may result in altered contraction of myofibril organelles,[61] less negative intracellular resting potential that allows delayed afterdepolarizations to reach firing threshold,[47,59,83] altered function of the sarcoplasmic reticulum,[61,95] or increased calcium interfering with myocardial mitochondrial function (see Chap. 22 and 23).[61] Although some investigators suspect that the rate of administration of the calcium may be a factor in the subsequent cardiac toxicity,[72,83] calcium administration should be avoided because better, safer, alternative treatments, such as digoxin-specific Fab, insulin, and sodium bicarbonate, are available for CAS-induced hyperkalemia.[8,37,64,83,104]

Magnesium Hypomagnesemia may also occur in CAS-poisoned patients secondary to the contributory factors mentioned with hypokalemia, such as long-term diuretic use to treat congestive heart failure. The theoretical benefits of magnesium therapy include blockade of the transient inward calcium current, antagonism of calcium at intracellular binding sites, decreased CAS-related ventricular irritability, and blockade of potassium egress from CAS-poisoned cells.[4,31,55,89,100,110,122] Although hypomagnesemia increases myocardial digoxin uptake and decreases cellular Na^+-K^+-ATPase activity, there is conflicting evidence on whether magnesium "reactivates" the CAS-bound Na^+-K^+-ATPase activity.[81,100,110]

The successful use of IV magnesium sulfate in the treatment of patients with ventricular tachydysrhythmias caused by digoxin toxicity has been reported, even in the presence of elevated serum magnesium concentrations.[62] The mechanism of efficacy of magnesium may be its ability to suppress delayed afterdepolarizations, prolong refractory period by decreasing calcium uptake and potassium efflux,[110] activate Na^+-K^+-ATPase as an essential metallo-coenzyme, or antagonize digoxin at the sarcolemma Na^+-K^+-ATPase pump. However, this treatment is only temporizing until digoxin-specific Fab is available for definitive therapy, and it is not advocated as first-line therapy. The precise dosing of magnesium sulfate in CAS-poisoned patients has not been established.[4,31,55,62,89,100,122] A common regimen uses 2 g of magnesium sulfate IV over 20 minutes in adults (25–50 mg/kg/dose to a maximum of 2 g in children). After stabilization, adult patients with severe hypomagnesemia may require a magnesium infusion of 1–2 g/h (25–50 mg/kg/h to a maximum of 2 g in children), with serial monitoring of serum magnesium concentrations, telemetry, respiratory rate (observing for bradypnea), deep tendon reflexes (observing for hyporeflexia), and monitoring of blood pressure. Magnesium is contraindicated in the setting of bradycardia or AV block, preexisting hypermagnesemia, and renal insufficiency or failure.

EXTRACORPORAL REMOVAL OF CARDIOACTIVE STEROIDS

Forced diuresis,[66] hemoperfusion,[79,120] and hemodialysis[120] are ineffective in enhancing the elimination of digoxin because of its large volume of distribution (4–10 L/kg), which makes it relatively inaccessible to these techniques. Because of its high affinity for tissue proteins, approximately 10% of the amount of digoxin is found in the serum than is found at the tissue level, and of that amount, approximately 20% to 40% is protein bound.[57]

Various investigations into new methods of extracorporeal removal are under investigation. Plasmapheresis may have a role in removing retained Fab–digoxin complexes to prevent rebound toxicity after digoxin overdose treatment in anuric patients, but its usefulness has not been clearly defined.[15,87] Additionally, there is a suggestion that hemoperfusion through a β_2-microglobulin adsorptive column might be useful as a second line measure for treating patients with acute digoxin toxicity.[55,115]

SUMMARY

Digoxin and digitoxin are the most commonly prescribed members of the drugs classified as CAS. These share common structural similarities and functions at the cellular level. CAS has a narrow therapeutic index. Signs and symptoms of CAS toxicity range from subtle to profound. Both cardiac and noncardiac effects occur after CAS poisoning. Patients with acute toxicity often have a higher serum concentration of the drug and may present with profound nausea, vomiting, bradycardia, atrial and ventricular ectopy with block, or hyperkalemia. Patients with chronic toxicity often have a lower serum concentration of CAS and may present similarly, but more often the symptoms are more protean and include loss of appetite, headache, weakness, nausea, alteration in mental status, all of which may be combined with similar ectopic rhythms as with acute toxicity.

In addition to overt overdose, an elevation in the serum CAS concentrations and an exacerbation of the clinical drug effect leading to toxicity may occur from drug interactions or from deteriorating metabolic processes such as with declining renal function or from electrolyte abnormalities such as hypokalemia and hypomagnesemia. A systematic approach toward treating patients using basic supportive and decontamination management techniques supplemented by the early administration of digoxin-specific Fab immunotherapy may significantly reduce morbidity and mortality in these high-risk patients.

ACKNOWLEDGEMENT

Neal A. Lewin contributed to this chapter in previous editions.

REFERENCES

1. Arispe N, Diaz JC, Simakova O, Pollard HB. Heart failure drug digoxin induces calcium uptake into cells by forming transmembrane calcium channels. *Proc Natl Acad Sci.* 2008;105:2610-2615.
2. Banner W, Bach P, Burk B, et al. Influence of assay methods on serum concentrations of digoxin during Fab fragment treatments. *J Toxicol Clin Toxicol.* 1992;30:259-267.
3. Bayer MJ. Recognition and management of digitalis intoxication: implications for emergency medicine. *Am J Emerg Med.* 1991;9(suppl 1):29-32.
4. Beller GA, Hood WB, Smith TW, et al. Correlation of serum magnesium level and cardiac digitalis intoxication. *Am J Cardiol.* 1974;33:225-229.
5. Bismuth C, Gaultier M, Conso F, Efthymiou ML. Hyperkalemia in acute digitalis poisoning: prognostic significance and therapeutic implications. *Clin Toxicol.* 1973;6:153-162.
6. Bismuth C, Motte G, Conso F, Chauvin M. Acute digitoxin intoxication treated by intracardiac pacemaker: experience in sixty-eight patients. *Clin Toxicol.* 1977;10:443-456.
7. Blaustein MP. Physiologic effects of endogenous ouabain: control of intracellular Ca^{2+} stores and cell responsiveness. *Am J Physiol.* 1993; 264: C1367-C1387.
8. Bower JO, Mengle HAK. The additive effect of calcium and digitalis. *JAMA.* 1936;106:1151-1153.
9. Bristow MR, Port JD, Kelly RA. Treatment of heart failure: pharmacologic methods. In: Braunwald E, Zipes D, Libby P, eds. *Heart Disease. A Textbook of Cardiovascular Medicine*, 6th ed. New York: WB Saunders; 2001:573-575.
10. Brubacher JR, Ravikumar PR, Bania T, et al. Treatment of toad venom poisoning with digoxin-specific Fab fragments. *Chest.* 1996;110:1282-1288.
11. Carver JL, Valdes R. Anomalous serum digoxin concentrations in uremia. *Ann Intern Med.* 1983;98:483-484.
12. Centers for Disease Control and Prevention. Deaths associated with a purported aphrodisiac. New York City, February 1993–May 1995. *MMWR Morb Mortal Wkly Rep.* 1995;44:853-855.
13. Chern MS, Ray CY, Wu DL. Biological intoxication due to digitalis-like substance after ingestion of cooked toad soup. *Am J Cardiol.* 1991;67: 443-444.
14. Cheung K Hinds JA, Duffy P. Detection of poisoning by plant-origin cardiac glycoside with the Abbot TDx analyzer. *Clin Chem.* 1989;35:295-297.
15. Chillet P, Korach JM, Vincent N, et al. Digoxin poisoning and anuric acute renal failure: efficiency of the treatment associating digoxin-specific antibodies (Fab) and plasma exchanges. *Int J Artif Organs.* 2002;25:538-541.
16. Cooke D. The use of central nervous system manifestations in the early detection of digitalis toxicity. *Heart Lung.* 1993;22:477-481.
17. Critchley JA, Critchley LA. Digoxin toxicity in chronic renal failure: treatment by multiple-dose activated charcoal intestinal dialysis. *Hum Exp Toxicol.* 1997;16:733-735.
18. Cummins RO, Haulman J, Quan L. Near-fatal yew berry intoxication treated with external cardiac pacing and digoxin-specific Fab antibody fragments. *Ann Emerg Med.* 1990;19:38-43.
19. Dasgupta A, Wu S, Actor J, et al. Effect of Asian and Siberian ginseng on serum digoxin measurement by five digoxin immunoassays. Significant variation in digoxin-like immunoreactivity among commercial ginsengs. *Am J Clin Pathol.* 2003;119:298-303.
20. De-Mey C, Brendel E, Enterling D. Carvedilol increases the systemic bioavailability of oral digoxin. *Br J Clin Pharmacol.* 1990;29:486-490.
21. de Silva HA, Fonseka MMD, Pathmeswaran A, et al. Multiple-dose activated charcoal for treatment of yellow oleander poisoning: a single-blind randomised, placebo-controlled trial. *Lancet.* 2003;361:1935-1938.
22. DiDomenico RJ, Walton SM, Sanoski CA, et al. Analysis of the use of digoxin immune Fab for the treatment of non-life-threatening digoxin toxicity. *J Cardiovasc Pharmacol Ther.* 2000;5:77-85.
23. Doering W. Quinidine-digoxin interaction: pharmacokinetics, underlying mechanism and clinical implications. *N Engl J Med.* 1979;301:400-404.
24. Doherty JE, Perkins WH, Flanigan WJ. The distribution and concentration of tritiated digoxin in human tissues. *Ann Intern Med.* 1967;66:116-124.
25. Doolittle MH, Lincoln K, Graves SW. Unexplained increase in serum digoxin: a case report. *Clin Chem.* 1994;40:487-492.
26. Eddelston M, Ariaratnam CA, Sjostrom L, et al. Acute yellow oleander (*Thevetia peruviana*) poisoning: cardiac arrhythmias, electrolyte disturbances, and serum cardiac glycoside concentrations on presentation to hospital. *Heart.* 2000;83:301-306.
27. Eddleston M, Sheriff MHR, Hawton K. Deliberate self harm in Sri Lanka: an overlooked tragedy in the developing world. *Br Med J.* 1998; 317:133-135.
28. Eisner DA, Lederer WJ, Vaughan-Jones RD. The quantitative relationship between twitch tension and intracellular sodium activity in sheep cardiac Purkinje fibers. *J Physiol.* 1984;355:251-266.
29. Eisner DA, Smith TW. The Na-K pump and its effect in cardiac muscle. In: Fozzard HA, ed. *The Heart and Cardiovascular System*, 2nd ed. New York: Raven Press; 1991:863-902.
30. Eisner T, Wiemer DF, Haynes LW, Meinwald J. Lucibufagins: defensive steroids from the fireflies *Photinus ignitus* and *P. marginellus* (*Coleoptera: Lampyridae*). *Proc Natl Acad Sci U S A.* 1978;75:905.
31. French JH, Thomas RG, Siskind AP, et al. Magnesium therapy in massive digoxin intoxication. *Ann Emerg Med.* 1984;13:562-566.
32. Friedman HS, Abramowitz I, Nguyen T, et al. Urinary digoxin-like immunoreactive substance in pregnancy. *Am J Med.* 1987;83:261-264.
33. Gao S, Chen Z, Xu Y. The source of endogenous digitalis-like substance in normal pregnancy. *Zhonghua Fu Chan Ke Za Zhi.* 1998; 33:539-41.
34. George S, Brathwaite RA, Hughes EA. Digoxin measurements following plasma ultrafiltration in two patients with digoxin toxicity treated with specific Fab fragments. *Ann Clin Biochem.* 1994;31:380-381.
35. Giampietro O, Clerico A, Gregori G, et al. Increased urinary excretion of digoxin-like immunoreactive substance by insulin-dependent diabetic patients: a linkage with hypertension? *Clin Chem.* 1988;34:2418-2422.
36. Gibb T, Adams PC, Parnham AJ, Jennings K. Plasma digoxin: assay anomalies in Fab-treated patients. *Br J Clin Pharmacol.* 1983;16:445-447.
37. Gold H, Edwards DJ. The effects of ouabain on heart in the presence of hypercalcemia. *Am Heart J.* 1927;3:45-50.
38. Gorelick DA, Kussin SZ, Kahn I. Paranoid delusions and auditory hallucinations associated with digoxin intoxication. *J Nerv Ment Dis.* 1978;166: 817-819.
39. Graves SW. Endogenous digitalis-like factors. *Crit Rev Clin Lab Sci.* 1986;23:177-200.
40. Graves SW, Adler G, Stuenkel C, et al. Increases in plasma digitalis-induced hypoglycemia. *Neuroendocrinology.* 1989;49:586-591.
41. Graves SW, Brown BA, Valdes R. Digoxin-like substances measured in patients with renal impairment. *Ann Intern Med.* 1983;99:604-608.
42. Graves SW, Valdes R, Brown BA, et al. Endogenous immunoreactive digoxin-like substance in human pregnancies. *J Clin Endocrinol Metab.* 1984; 58:748-751.
43. Hack JB, Woody JH, Lewis DE, et al. The effect of calcium chloride in treating hyperkalemia due to acute digoxin toxicity in a porcine model. *J Toxicol Clin Toxicol.* 2004;42:337-342.

44. Haddy FJ. Endogenous digitalis-like factor or factors. *N Engl J Med.* 1987; 316:621-622.
45. Hager WD, Fenster P, Mayersohn M, et al. Digoxin-quinidine interaction: pharmacokinetic evaluation. *N Engl J Med.* 1979;300:1238-1241.
46. Hastreiter AR, John EG, van der Horst RL. Digitalis, digitalis antibodies, digitalis-like immunoreactive substances, and sodium homeostasis: a review. *Clin Perinatol.* 1988;15:491-522.
47. Hauptman PJ, Kelly RA. Digitalis. *Circulation.* 1999;99:1265-1270.
48. Helfant RH, Scherlac BJ, Damata AN. Protection from digitalis toxicity with the prophylactic use of diphenylhydantoin sodium an arrhythmic-inotropic dissociation. *Circulation.* 1967:36:119-124.
49. Henderson RP, Solomon CP. Use of cholestyramine in the treatment of digoxin intoxication. *Arch Intern Med.* 1988;148:745-746.
50. Hilton PJ, White G, Lord A, et al. An inhibitor of the sodium pump obtained from human placenta. *Lancet.* 1996;348:303-305.
51. Hobson J, Zettner A. Digoxin serum half-life following suicidal digoxin poisoning. *JAMA.* 1973;223:147-149.
52. Hollman A. Plants and cardiac glycosides. *Br Heart J.* 1985;54:258-261.
53. Isensee L, Solomon RJ, Weinberg MS, et al. Digoxin levels in dialysis patients. *Hosp Physician.* 1988;24:50-52.
54. Jortani SA, Helm RA, Valdes R. Inhibition of Na,K-ATPase by oleandrin and oleandrigenen, and their detection by digoxin immunoassays. *Clin Chem.* 1996;42:1654-1658.
55. Kaneko T, Kudo M, Okumura T, et al. Successful treatment of digoxin intoxication by hemoperfusion with specific columns for β_2-microglobulin adsorption (Lixelle) in a maintenance haemodialysis patient. *Nephrol Dial Transplant.* 2001;16;195-196.
56. Karkal SS, Ordog G, Wasserberg J. Digitalis intoxication: dealing rapidly and effectively with a complex cardiac toxidrome. *Emerg Med Rep.* 1991;12:29-44.
57. Katzung BG, Parmley WM. Cardiac glycosides & other drugs used in congestive heart failure. In: Katzung BG, ed. *Basic and Clinical Pharmacology,* 7th ed. Stamford, CT: Appleton & Lange; 1998:197-215.
58. Kelly RA, Smith TW. Endogenous cardiac glycosides. *Adv Pharmacol.* 1994;25:263-288.
59. Kelly RA, Smith TW. Pharmacological treatment of heart failure. In: Hardman JG, Limbird LE, Molinoff PB, Ruddon RW, eds. *Goodman and Gilman's The Pharmacological Basis of Therapeutics,* 9th ed. New York: McGraw-Hill; 1996:809-838.
60. Kelly RA, Smith TW. Recognition and management of digitalis toxicity. *Am J Cardiol.* 1992;69:108-109.
61. Khatter JC, Agbanyo M, Navaratnam S, et al. Digitalis cardiotoxicity: cellular calcium overload as a possible mechanism. *Basic Res Cardiol.* 1989;84:553-563.
62. Kinlay S, Buckley N. Magnesium sulfate in the treatment of ventricular arrhythmias due to digoxin toxicity. *J Toxicol Clin Toxicol.* 1995;33:55-59.
63. Klausen T, Kjeldsen K, Norgaard A. Effects of denervation on sodium, potassium and [3H] ouabain binding in muscles of normal and potassium depleted rats. *J Physiol.* 1983;345:123-124.
64. Kne T, Brokaw M, Wax P. Fatality from calcium chloride in a chronic digoxin toxic patient (abstract). *J Toxicol Clin Toxicol.* 1997;5:505.
65. Knight M, Glor R, Smedley SR, et al. Firefly toxicosis in lizards. *J Chem Ecol.* 1999;25:1981-1986.
66. Koren G, Klein J. Enhancement of digoxin clearance by mannitol diuresis: in vivo studies and their clinical implications. *Vet Hum Toxicol.* 1988;30:25-27.
67. Lalonde RL, Deshpande R, Hamilton PP, et al. Acceleration of digoxin clearance by activated charcoal. *Clin Pharmacol Ther.* 1985;37:367-371.
68. Leahy EB Jr, Reiffel JA, Drusin RE, et al. Interaction between quinidine and digoxin. *JAMA.* 1978;240:533-534.
69. Lee TC. Van Gogh's vision. *JAMA.* 1981;245:727-729.
70. Lely AH, van Enter CH. Large-scale digitoxin intoxication. *Br Med J.* 1970; 3:737-740.
71. Levy G. Gastrointestinal clearance of drugs with activated charcoal. *N Engl J Med.* 1982;307:676-678.
72. Lieberman AL. Studies on calcium VI: some interrelationships of the cardiac activities of calcium gluconate and scillaren-B. *J Pharmacol Exp Ther.* 1933;47:183-192.
73. Lindenbaum J, Rund DG, Butler VP. Inactivation of digoxin by the gut flora: reversal by antibiotic therapy. *N Engl J Med.* 1981;305:789-794.
74. Lown B, Byatt NF, Levine HD. Paroxysmal atrial tachycardia with block. *Circulation.* 1960;21:129-143.
75. Madan BR, Khanna NK, Soni RK. Effect of some arrhythmogenic agents upon the acetylcholine content of the rabbit atria. *J Pharm Pharmacol.* 1970;22:621-622.
76. Mahdyoon H, Battilana G, Rosman H, et al. The evolving pattern of digoxin intoxication: observations at a large urban hospital from 1980 to 1988. *Am Heart J.* 1990;120:1189-1194.
77. Marbury T, Mahoney J, Juncos L, et al. Advanced digoxin toxicity in renal failure: treatment with charcoal hemoperfusion. *South Med J.* 1979;72: 279-282.
78. McGary SJ, Williams AJ. Digoxin activates sarcoplasmic reticulum Ca^{2+} release channels: a possible role in cardiac inotropy. *Br J Pharmacol.* 1993; 108:1043-1050.
79. McRae S. Elevated serum digoxin levels in a patient taking digoxin and Siberian ginseng. *CMAJ.* 1996;155:292-295.
80. Miller JM, Zipes DP. Management of the patient with cardiac arrhythmias. In: Braunwald E, Zipes D, Libby P, eds. *Heart Disease. A Textbook of Cardiovascular Medicine,* 6th ed. New York: WB Saunders; 2001:726-727.
81. Nanji AA, Greenway DC. Falsely raised plasma digoxin concentrations in liver disease. *Br Med J.* 1985;290:432-433.
82. Neff MS, Mendelssohn S, Kim KS, et al. Magnesium sulfate in digitalis toxicity. *Am J Cardiol.* 1974;62:377-382.
83. Nola GT, Pope S, Harrison DC. Assessment of the synergistic relationship between serum calcium and digitalis. *Am Heart J.* 1970;79:499-507.
84. Ordog GJ, Benaron S, Bhasin V, et al. Serum digoxin levels and mortality in 5,100 patients. *Ann Emerg Med.* 1987;16:32-39.
85. Pace DG, Gillis RA. Neuroexcitatory effects of digoxin in the cat. *J Pharmacol Exp Ther.* 1976;199:583-600.
86. Pond S, Jacos M, Marks J, et al. Treatment of digitoxin overdose with oral activated charcoal. *Lancet.* 1981;2:1177-1178.
87. Rabetoy GM, Price CA, Findlay JWA, et al. Treatment of digoxin intoxication in a renal failure patient with digoxin-specific antibody fragments and plasmapheresis. *Am J Nephrol.* 1990;10:518-521.
88. Radford DJ, Cheung K, Urech R, et al. Immunologic detection of cardiac glycosides in plants. *Aust Vet J.* 1994;71:236-238.
89. Reisdorff EJ, Clark MR, Walter BL. Acute digitalis poisoning: the role of intravenous magnesium sulfate. *J Emerg Med.* 1986;4:463-469.
90. Rich SA, Libera JM, Locke RJ. Treatment of foxglove extract poisoning with digoxin-specific Fab fragments. *Ann Emerg Med.* 1993;22:1904-1907.
91. Roberge RJ. Congestive heart failure and toxic digoxin levels: role of cholestyramine. *Vet Hum Toxicol.* 2000;42:172-173.
92. Rodin SM, Johnson BF. Pharmacokinetic interactions with digoxin. *Clin Pharmacokinetic.* 1988;15:227-244.
93. Rose AM, Valdes R. Understanding the sodium pump and its relevance to disease. *Clin Chem.* 1994;40:1674-1685.
94. Rosen MR, Wit AL, Hoffman BF. Cardiac antiarrhythmic and toxic effects of digitalis. *Am Heart J.* 1975;89:391-399.
95. Rosen MR. Cellular electrophysiology of digitalis toxicity. *J Am Coll Cardiol.* 1985;2:22A-34A.
96. Rumack BH, Wolfe RR, Gilfinch H. Diphenylhydantoin treatment of massive digoxin overdose. *Br Heart J.* 1974;36:405-408.
97. Safadi R, Levy T, Amitai Y, et al. Beneficial effect of digoxin-specific Fab antibody fragments in oleander intoxication. *Arch Intern Med.* 1995;155:2121-2125.
98. Sameri RM, Soberman JE, Finch CK, et al. Lower serum digoxin concentrations in heart failure and reassessment of laboratory report forms. *Am J Med Sci.* 2002;324:10-13.
99. Sarubbi B, Ducceschi V, D'Antonello A, et al. Atrial fibrillation: what are the effects of drug therapy on the effectiveness and complications of electrical cardioversion? *Can J Cardiol.* 1998;14:1267-1273.
100. Seller RH. The role of magnesium in digitalis toxicity. *Am Heart J.* 1971; 82:551-556.
101. Selzer A. Role of serum digoxin assay in patient management. *J Am Coll Cardiol.* 1985;5:106A-110A.
102. Shilo LM, Adawi A, Solomon G, Shenkman L. Endogenous digoxinlike immunoreactivity in congestive heart failure. *Br Med J.* 1987;295:415-416.
103. Silber B, Sheiner LB, Powers JL, et al. Spironolactone-associated digoxin radioimmunoassay interference. *Clin Chem.* 1979;25:48-54.
104. Smith PK, Winkler AW, Hoff HE. Calcium and digitalis synergism: the toxicity of calcium salts injected intravenously into digitalized animals. *Arch Intern Med.* 1939;64:322-328.
105. Smith SW, Shah RR, Herzog CA. Bidirectional ventricular tachycardia resulting from herbal aconite poisoning. *Ann Emerg Med.* 2005;45:100.

106. Smith TW, Haber E, Yeatman L, et al. Reversal of advanced digoxin intoxication with Fab fragments of digoxin-specific antibodies. *N Engl J Med.* 1976;294:797-800.
107. Smith TW. Pharmacokinetics, bioavailability and serum levels of cardiac glycosides. *J Am Coll Cardiol.* 1985;5:43A-50A.
108. Smith TW. Digitalis. *N Engl J Med.* 1988;318:358-365.
109. Somberg JC, Bounous H, Levitt B. The antiarrhythmic effects of quinidine and propranolol in the ouabain-intoxicated spinally transected cat. *Eur J Pharmacol.* 1979;54:161-166.
110. Spechter MJ, Schweizer E, Goldman RH. Studies on magnesium's mechanism of action in digitalis-induced arrhythmias. *Circulation.* 1975;52: 1001-1005.
111. Springer M, Olson KR, Feaster W. Acute massive digoxin overdose: survival without use of digitalis-specific antibodies. *Am J Emerg Med.* 1986;4:364-369.
112. Sullivan JB. Immunotherapy in the poisoned patient. *Med Toxicol.* 1986;1: 47-60.
113. Taboulet P, Baud FJ, Bismuth C, et al. Acute digitalis intoxication: is pacing still appropriate? *J Toxicol Clin Toxicol.* 1993;31:261-273.
114. Torsti P. Acetylcholine content and cholinesterase activities in the rabbit heart in experimental heart failure and the effect of g-strophanthin treatment on them. *Ann Med Exp Biol Fenn.* 1959;37(suppl 4):4-9.
115. Tsuruoka S, Osono E, Nishiki K, et al. Removal of digoxin by column for specific adsorption of β_2-microglobulin: a potential use for digoxin intoxication. *Clin Pharmacol Ther.* 2001;69:422-30.
116. Tuncok Y, Kozan O, Cavdar C, et al. Urginea maritima (squill) toxicity. *J Toxicol Clin Toxicol.* 1995;33:83-86.
117. Valdes R, Graves SW, Brown BA, et al. Endogenous substances in newborn infants causing false-positive digoxin measurements. *J Pediatr.* 1983;102:947-950.
118. Valdes R, Hagberg JM, Vaughan TE, et al. Endogenous digoxin-like immunoreactivity in blood is increased during prolonged strenuous exercise. *Life Sci.* 1988;42:103-110.
119. Wagner J, Salzer WW. Calcium-dependent toxic effects of digoxin in isolated myocardial preparations. *Arch Int Pharmacodyn.* 1976;223:4-14.
120. Warren SE, Fanestil DD. Digoxin overdose: limitations of hemoperfusion-hemodialysis treatment. *JAMA.* 1979;242:2100-2101.
121. Watson WA. Factors influencing the clinical efficacy of activated charcoal. *Drug Intell Clin Pharm.* 1987;21:160-166.
122. Whang R, Aikawa J. Magnesium deficiency and refractoriness to potassium repletion. *J Chron Dis.* 1977;30:65-68.
123. Wildicks EFM, Vermeulen M, van Brummelen P, et al. Digoxin-like immunoreactive substance in patients with aneurysmal subarachnoid hemorrhage. *Br Med J.* 1987;294:729-732.
124. Withering W. An account of the foxglove and some of its medical uses: with practical remarks on dropsy and other diseases. *Med Classics.* 1937; 2:295-443.
125. Woolf AD, Wenger T, Smith TW, et al. The use of digoxin-specific Fab fragments for severe digitalis intoxication in children. *N Engl J Med.* 1992; 326:1739-1744.

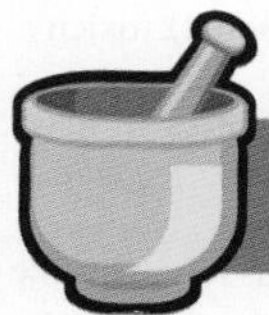

ANTIDOTES IN DEPTH (A20)

DIGOXIN-SPECIFIC ANTIBODY FRAGMENTS

Mary Ann Howland

Digoxin-specific antibody fragments (DSFab) are indicated for the management of patients with toxicity related to digoxin and digitoxin, as well as oleander, squill, and toad venom which contain other cardioactive steroids. DSFab have an excellent record of efficacy and safety, and should be administered early in both established and suspected cardioactive steroid poisoning.

HISTORY

The production of antibody fragments to treat patients poisoned with digoxin followed the development of digoxin antibodies for measuring serum digoxin concentrations by radioimmunoassay (RIA).[11] This RIA technique permitted the correlation between serum digoxin concentration and clinical digoxin toxicity.[4,18,24,57]

In 1967, Butler and Chen suggested that purified antidigoxin antibodies with a high affinity and specificity should be developed to treat digoxin toxicity in humans.[11] The digoxin molecule alone, with a molecular weight of 780 daltons, was too small to be immunogenic. But digoxin could function as a hapten when joined to an immunogenic protein carrier such as albumin. These investigators immunized sheep with this conjugate to generate antibodies.[77,79] The immunized sheep subsequently produced a mixture of antibodies that included antialbumin antibodies and antidigoxin antibodies. The antibodies were separated and highly purified to retain the digoxin antibodies, while removing the antibodies to the albumin and all other extraneous proteins. The antibodies that were developed have a high affinity for digoxin, and sufficient cross-reactivity with digitoxin and other cardioactive steroids to be clinically useful for the treatment of all cardioactive steroid poisonings.[13,69,70]

Intact IgG antidigoxin antibodies reversed digoxin toxicity in dogs.[12] Unfortunately, the urinary excretion of digoxin was delayed, and free digoxin was released after antibody degradation occurred. Furthermore, there was significant concern for developing hypersensitivity reactions. To make such antibodies both safe and effective in humans, whole IgG antidigoxin antibodies were cleaved with papain, yielding two antigen-binding fragments (Fab), with a molecular weight of 50,000 daltons each, and one Fc fragment of 50,000 daltons.[12] Affinity chromatography is used to isolate and purify the DSFab following papain digestion. Since the Fc fragment does not bind antigen and increases the potential for hypersensitivity reactions, it was eliminated. When compared with whole IgG antibodies the advantages of DSFab include a larger volume of distribution, more rapid onset of action, smaller risk of adverse immunologic effects, and more rapid elimination.[12,45,48,50] Ultimately, in 1976 Digibind was first used successfully,[78] and in 1986—it became commercially available,[22] Digibind, a relatively pure, very safe, and extremely effective Fab product, was produced. Another commercial product, DigiFab, approved by the US Food and Drug Administration (FDA) in 2001 is also currently available.[23] It is very similar to Digibind except that it is prepared using a digoxin derivative (digoxin-dicarboxymethoxylamine) as the hapten.

PHARMACOLOGY

Immediately following intravenous (IV) administration, DSFab antibody fragments bind intravascular unbound digoxin. Uncomplexed antibodies then diffuse into the interstitial space, binding free digoxin there. A concentration gradient is then established, which facilitates movement into the interstitial or intravascular spaces of both the free intracellular digoxin and digoxin that is dissociated from its binding sites (the external surface of Na^+-K^+-adenosine triphosphatase [ATPase] enzyme) in the heart and in skeletal muscle.[71] The dissociation rate constant of digoxin for Na^+-K^+-ATPase, therefore, affects the time course for binding to DSFab and, consequently, the onset of action.[52,72]

The binding affinities of DSFab for digoxin and digitoxin are about 10^9 to 10^{11} M^{-1} and 10^8 to 10^9 M^{-1}, and are greater than the affinities of digoxin or digitoxin for the Na^+-K^+-ATPase pump receptor.[22]

PHARMACOKINETICS

The pharmacokinetics of Digibind versus DigiFab (previously named DigiTAb) were compared in human volunteers, in a study financed by Protherics.[88] Each subject received 1 mg of digoxin intravenously as a 5-minute bolus, followed 2 hours later by a 30-minute IV infusion of 76 mg (an equimolar neutralizing dose) of either Digibind or DigiFab. Free and total digoxin (free plus DSFab bound) were assayed using an ultrafiltration method over 48 hours. At 30 minutes after infusion of either DSFab, the serum free digoxin concentration was below the level of detection of the assay and remained so for several hours. A few patients in both groups had free digoxin concentrations rebound to peak concentrations of 0.5 ng/mL at approximately 18 hours and the area under the plasma drug concentration versus time curve (AUC) for 2 to 48 hours, for free digoxin, was similar for both treatment groups. The elimination half-life of total digoxin averaged 18 hours for DigiFab and 21 hours for Digibind, while the distribution half-life was 1 hour for each. The volumes of distribution were 0.3 L/kg for DigiFab versus 0.4 L/kg for Digibind.[22,23] The systemic clearance of DigiFab was higher than Digibind, accounting for the shorter elimination half-life of DigiFab (15 hours versus 23 hours).[88] Urine sampling over the first 24 hours demonstrated mostly free digoxin and very little free DSFab for both groups. The authors postulate that during renal excretion, the DSFab digoxin complex is metabolized in the kidney by the proximal tubular cells, releasing free digoxin and unmeasured DSFab metabolites.[88]

Similar findings were first described by Smith and associates in 1976, following the first clinical use of Digibind in a patient who gave a history of ingesting 90 (0.25 mg) digoxin tablets.[78] Total serum digoxin concentration, which was 17.6 ng/mL before Digibind were given, rose to 226 ng/mL 1 hour after the start of the Digibind infusion and remained there for 11 hours, before falling off the next 44 hours, with a half-life of 20 hours.[78] Fab concentrations peaked at the end of the infusion and then apparently exhibited a biphasic or triphasic decline, probably reflecting distribution into different compartments, as well as excretion and catabolism. Free serum digoxin concentrations were undetectable for the first 9 hours, then rose to a peak of 2 ng/mL at 16 hours, and fell to 1.5 ng/mL at both 36 hours and 56 hours at which time sampling stopped. An analysis of renal elimination based on an incomplete collection suggested that digoxin was excreted only in the bound form during the first 6 hours, but by 30 hours after Fab administration all digoxin in the urine was free digoxin.

In order to better match availability of DSFab to liberated digoxin, one study compared a loading dose of DSFab followed by an infusion to the total DSFab dose infused over a short amount of time.[68] The former strategy increased the ratio of digoxin bound to uncomplexed DSFab in the plasma from 50% to 70%.[68] The authors hypothesized that a too rapid infusion regimen would result in the elimination of DSFab before the fragments could optimally bind the digoxin redistributing from tissue sites.[68]

Digoxin takes several hours to distribute from the blood to the tissue compartment. As expected, a rodent model demonstrated that DSFab were more effective when administered prior to complete distribution of digoxin.[65] Once distribution is complete, increasing the dose of DSFab improved efficacy, as measured by comparing the AUC of digoxin to that of the Fab-digoxin complex.[65]

Pharmacokinetic studies in patients with renal failure demonstrate that the half-life of DSFab is prolonged 10-fold, with no change in the apparent volume of distribution (Vd).[82] In this situation serum DSFab concentrations remain detectable for 2 to 3 weeks. Total serum digoxin concentrations generally follow DSFab. Case reports demonstrate that free digoxin concentrations reappear up to 10 days following administration of DSFab to patients with severe renal dysfunction, as compared with 12 to 24 hours in patients with normal renal function.[16,25,28,43,54,55,74,76,82–84,89] In one series of patients with end-stage renal disease, the maximum average concentration of free digoxin was 1.30 ± 0.7 ng/mL and occurred at 127 ± 40 hours.[84] The mechanism for this rebound is unclear. Following the peak, there is a slow decline that parallels the elimination of DSFab.

EFFICACY

A large study evaluating adults and children with acute and chronic digoxin toxicity established the efficacy of Digibind.[1] Of the 150 patients treated, 148 were evaluated for cardiovascular manifestations of toxicity prior to treatment: 79 patients (55%) had high-grade atrioventricular (AV) block, 68 (46%) had refractory ventricular tachycardia, 49 (33%) had ventricular fibrillation, and 56 (37%) had hyperkalemia. Ninety percent of patients had a response to DSFab within minutes to several hours of Digibind administration. Complete resolution of all signs and symptoms of digoxin toxicity occurred in 80% of cases. Partial response was observed in 10% of patients, and of the 15 patients who did not respond, 14 were moribund or later found to not be digoxin toxic. The spectacular success of DSFab for patients with digoxin toxicity is demonstrated by the fact that of the 56 patients who had cardiac arrest caused by digoxin, 54% survived hospitalization, as compared with 100% mortality before the availability of these antibody fragments for treatment.[1,5] Newborns, infants, and children have all been successfully treated with Digibind.[5,29,41,73]

ADVERSE EFFECTS AND SAFETY

DSFab are generally safe and effective. Reported adverse effects include hypokalemia as a consequence of reactivation of the Na^+-K^+-ATPase; withdrawal of the inotropic or atrioventricular nodal blocking effects of digoxin, leading to congestive heart failure or a rapid ventricular rate in patients with atrial fibrillation; and, rarely, allergic reactions.[22,23] In the multicenter study of 150 patients treated with Digibind, the only acute adverse clinical manifestations were hypokalemia in six patients (4%), worsening of congestive heart failure in four patients (3%), and transient apnea in a several hours old neonate.[1] There were no other reactions reported in any of the patients in this series. In a postmarketing surveillance study of Digibind that included 451 patients, two patients with a prior history of allergy to antibiotics reportedly developed rashes.[59] One of these patients developed a total body rash, facial swelling, and a flush during the infusion. The other experienced a pruritic rash. Two other reported adverse reactions were thrombocytopenia and rigors and were probably unrelated to the use of Digibind.[59] One patient received Digibind on three separate occasions over the course of 1 year for multiple suicide attempts, with no adverse effects.[8]

During the clinical trials with DigiFab, one patient developed pulmonary edema, bilateral pleural effusions, and renal failure, most likely caused by the loss of the inotropic and chronotropic digoxin effects.[23] Phlebitis and postural hypotension were related to the infusion of DigiFab in two healthy volunteers.[23]

Both products warn that patients with allergies to papain, chymopapain, or other papaya extracts may be at risk for an allergic reaction because trace amounts of these residues may remain in the DSFab.[23,50] Manufacturers of DigiFab state that because some literature suggests a resemblance between both dust mite allergens and some latex allergens with the antigenic structures of papain, patients may exhibit cross-allergenicity amongst all three. Patients with an allergy to sheep protein or those who have previously received ovine antibodies or ovine Fab may also be at risk for allergic reactions, although this is not reported.

INDICATIONS FOR DSFab

DSFab are indicated for life-threatening, or potentially life-threatening, toxicity from any cardioactive steroid.[22] Patients with known or suggestive cardioactive steroid exposure with progressive bradydysrhythmias, including symptomatic sinus bradycardia, or second- or third-degree heart block unresponsive to atropine, and patients with severe ventricular dysrhythmias, such as ventricular tachycardia or ventricular fibrillation, should also be treated with DSFab. Ventricular tachycardia with a fascicular block is likely to be a digoxin-toxic rhythm.[26,49] Any patient with a potassium concentration exceeding 5 mEq/L in the setting of an acute or chronic overdose that is attributable to a cardioactive steroid in the presence of other manifestations of digoxin toxicity should also be treated.[6] Acute ingestions greater than 4 mg in a healthy child (or more than 0.1 mg/kg), or 10 mg in a healthy adult, may require DSFab, with the threshold lower in patients with significant medical illness. Serum digoxin concentrations are not representative of myocardial concentrations until tissue distribution takes place. Following ingestion, a time delay of 4 to 6 hours is usually required for digoxin to achieve an equilibrium distribution from the serum to the myocardium. Serum concentrations of ≥10 ng/mL soon after an acute ingestion may predict the need for treatment with DSFab. Because the elderly appear to be at greatest risk of lethality, the threshold for treating patients older than 60 years of age should be lower.[7] Before the advent of DSFab, mortality in patients older than 60 years of age was 58%, as compared to 8% in patients younger than 40 years of age, and 34% in patients between 40 and 50 years of age.[7] A rapid progression of clinical signs and symptoms, such as cardiac and gastrointestinal toxicity and an elevated or rising potassium concentration, in the presence of an acute overdose, suggests a potentially life-threatening exposure and the need for DSFab.

Cardioactive steroid toxicity causes intracellular myocardial hypercalcemia, and the administration of exogenous calcium may further exacerbate conduction abnormalities and potentially result in cardiac arrest, unresponsive to further resuscitation. Thus, in a patient with an unknown exposure who is clinically ill with characteristics suggestive of poisoning by a cardioactive steroid, a calcium channel blocker, or a β-adrenergic antagonist, DSFab should be administered early in the management, and always prior to calcium use. If digoxin or another cardioactive steroid is involved, the toxic effects can be reversed, obviating the need to administer calcium and avoiding the danger of giving calcium to a cardioactive-steroid-toxic patient. Also, as it may be difficult to distinguish clinically between digoxin poisoning and intrinsic cardiac disease, the administration of DSFab can help establish the diagnosis.

A recent computer-based simulation model compared the treatment of non–life-threatening digoxin toxicity with standard therapy. The authors concluded that treatment with DSFab could decrease length of hospitalization by 1.5 days.[21]

ONSET OF RESPONSE

In the multicenter study of 150 patients, the mean time to initial response from the completion of the Digibind infusion (accomplished over 15 minutes to 2 hours) was 19 minutes (range, 0–60 minutes), and the time to complete response was 88 minutes (range, 30–360 minutes).[17] Time to response was not affected by age, concurrent cardiac disease, or presence of chronic or acute ingestion.[1]

DOSING

The dose of DSFab depends on the total body load (TBL) of digoxin. Adults and children receiving digoxin therapeutically who develop chronic digoxin toxicity require small doses of DSFab because their total body burden of digoxin is smaller when toxicity develops. Children with acute overdoses require DSFab doses based on the amount of digoxin ingested, in a manner similar to adults with acute ingestions.

Estimates of digoxin TBL can be made in three ways: (1) estimate the quantity of digoxin acutely ingested and assume 80% bioavailability (milligrams ingested × 0.8 equals TBL); (2) obtain a serum digoxin concentration (SDC) and, using a pharmacokinetic formula, incorporate the apparent Vd of digoxin and the patient's body weight (in kilograms); or (3) use an empiric dose based on the average requirements for an acute or chronic overdose in an adult or child.

Each of these methods of estimating the dose of DSFab has limitations. History of ingestion is often unreliable, and empiric doses based on averages may overestimate or underestimate Fab requirements. Using the pharmacokinetic formula assumes a steady-state Vd of 5 L/kg. This is not accurate in the acute setting. In addition, the 5 L/kg Vd is a population average that varies both with each individual and in certain diseases, such as the decreases that occur in patients with renal disease (thought to be due to displaced tissue binding) and hypothyroidism.[87]

Sample calculations for each of these methods are shown in Tables A20–1, A20–2, and A20–3. Each vial of DSFab contains 38 mg (Digibind) or 40 mg (DigiFab) of purified DSFab that will bind

TABLE A20–1. Sample Calculation Based on History of Acute Digoxin Ingestion

Adult	Child
Weight: 70 kg Ingestion: 50 (0.25-mg) digoxin tablets Calculation: 0.25 mg × 50 = 12.5 mg ingested dose 12.5 mg × 0.80 (assume 80% bioavailability) = 10 mg (absorbed dose) $\frac{10\text{ mg}}{0.5\text{ mg/vial}} = 20$ vials	Weight: 10 kg Ingestion: 50 (0.25-mg) digoxin tablets Calculation: Same as for adult. Child will require 20 vials.

TABLE A20–2. Sample Calculations Based on the Serum Digoxin Concentration (SDC)

Adult	Child	Quick Estimation (for Adults and Children)
Weight: 70 kg SDC = 10 ng/mL Volume of distribution = 5 L/kg Calculation[a]: $\text{No. of vials} = \frac{\text{Total body load (mg)}}{0.5\text{ mg/vial}}$ $= \frac{\text{SDC} \times V_d \times \text{Patient Wt (Kg)}}{1000 \times 0.5\text{ mg/vial}}$ $\text{No. of vials} = \frac{10\text{ ng/mL} \times 5\text{ L/kg} \times 70\text{ kg}}{1000 \times 0.5\text{ mg/vial}}$ (Roundup) No. of vials = 7	Weight: 10 kg Serum digoxin concentration: 10 ng/mL Volume of distribution: 5 L/kg Calculation[a]: $\text{No. of vials} = \frac{10\text{ ng/mL} \times 5\text{ L/kg} \times 10\text{ kg}}{1000 \times 0.5\text{ mg/vial}}$ (Roundup) No. of vials = 1	$\text{No. of vials} = \frac{\text{SDC (ng/mL)} \times \text{Patient Wt (kg)}}{100}$ (Roundup)

[a]1000 is a conversion factor to change ng/mL to mg/L.

TABLE A20–3. Empiric Dosing Recommendations

Acute Ingestion	Chronic Toxicity
Adult: 10–20 vials	Adult: 3–6 vials
Child[a]: 10–20 vials	Child[b]: 1–2 vials

[a]Monitor for volume overload in very small children.

[b]The prescribing information contains a table for infants and children, with corresponding serum concentrations.

approximately 0.5 mg of digoxin or digitoxin. If the quantity of ingestion cannot be reliably estimated, it is safest to use the largest calculated estimate. The clinician should always be prepared to increase the dose, should symptom resolution be incomplete.

ADMINISTRATION

Digibind should be administered intravenously over 30 minutes via a 0.22-μm membrane filter.[22] The 38-mg vial (which binds 0.5 mg digoxin) must be reconstituted with 4 mL of sterile water for IV injection, furnishing an isoosmotic solution containing 9.5 mg/mL of DSFab. This preparation can be further diluted with sterile isotonic saline for injection (for small infants, addition of 34 mL to the 4 mL [for 38 mL total] achieves 1 mg/mL). After Digibind is reconstituted, it should be used immediately, or if refrigerated, it should be used within 4 hours.[22] Although slow IV infusion over 30 minutes is preferable, Digibind may be given by IV bolus to a critically ill patient.

Each 40-mg vial of DigiFab (which binds 0.5 mg digoxin) should be reconstituted with 4 mL of sterile water for IV injection and gently mixed to provide a solution containing 10 mg/mL of DSFab.[23] The reconstituted product should be used promptly or, if refrigerated, it should be used within 4 hours. This preparation can be further diluted with sterile isotonic saline for injection. DigiFab should be administered slowly as an IV infusion over at least 30 minutes unless the patient is critically ill, in which case the DigiFab can be given by IV bolus. If a rate-related infusion reaction occurs, the infusion should be stopped and restarted at a slower rate. For infants and small children, the manufacturer recommends diluting the 40-mg vial with 4 mL of sterile water for IV injection and administering the dose undiluted using a tuberculin syringe. For very small doses, this preparation can be further diluted with an additional 36 mL of sterile isotonic saline for injection (for a total of 40 mL) to achieve a 1 mg/mL concentration.

AVAILABILITY

DSFab are available as Digibind or DigiFab. Vials contain 38 mg or 40 mg of purified lyophilized digoxin-immune ovine immunoglobulin fragments, respectively, with each vial binding 0.5 mg digoxin.

MEASUREMENT OF SERUM DIGOXIN CONCENTRATION AFTER DSFab ADMINISTRATION

Many laboratories are not equipped to determine free serum digoxin concentrations and it is important to remember that after DSFab are administered, total serum digoxin concentrations are no longer clinically useful, because they represent free plus bound digoxin.[2,22,33,38,46,80] The type of test for total digoxin concentrations used can either result in falsely high or falsely low serum concentrations, depending on which phase (solid or supernatant) is sampled.[37,51] If the correct dose of DSFab is administered, the free serum digoxin concentrations should be near zero. Free digoxin concentrations begin to reappear 5 to 24 hours or longer after Fab administration, depending on the antibody dose, infusion technique, and the patient's renal function. Newer commercial methods, using ultrafiltration or immunoassays, make free digoxin concentration measurements easier to perform and, therefore, more clinically useful, but they remain associated with errors in the underestimation or overestimation of the free digoxin level.[32,39,56,63,81,85] Free digoxin concentrations are particularly useful in patients with severe renal dysfunction. Independent of the availability of these data, the patient's cardiac status must be carefully monitored for signs of recurrent toxicity.

Other pitfalls in the measurement and utility of serum digoxin concentrations include endogenous and exogenous factors. Endogenous digoxinlike immunoreactive substances (EDLISs) have been described in infants, in women in the third trimester of pregnancy, and in patients with renal and hepatic failure.[31,34,36,40,42,52,86,87] When EDLISs are free or weakly bound, as in these circumstances, they are measurable by the typical RIA and can account for factitiously high reported serum digoxin concentrations in the absence of digoxin treatment. The role of EDLISs in the body has not been fully elucidated, but they have an effect on both the Na^+-K^+-ATPase pump and the cardioactive steroid receptor site.[35] EDLISs are implicated as a causative factor in hypertension and renal disease.[53] Exogenous factors relate primarily to measurement techniques and interpretation.[44] Digoxin metabolites have varying degrees of cardioactivity.[47] Some metabolites cross-react and are measured by RIA, while others are not. The in vivo production of these metabolites varies in patients, and may depend on intestinal metabolism by gut flora as well as renal and liver clearance.

ROLE OF DSFab WITH OTHER CARDIOACTIVE STEROIDS

DSFab were designed to have high-affinity binding for digoxin and digitoxin. There are structural similarities, however, among all cardioactive steroids. In fact, RIA-determined digoxin concentrations have been reported in patients following poisoning with many nondigoxin cardioactive steroids,[28,49,58,64] suggesting that there is also cross-reactivity between DSFab and other cardioactive steroids. Thus, DSFab may have variable efficacy for all natural cardioactive steroid poisonings, including those unique cardioactive steroids in oleander, yellow oleander, squill, and toad venom.[3,9,10,15,27,30,66] In vitro studies also suggest the binding affinity of Digibind for cardioactive steroids.[19,20,60] One recent GlaxoSmithKline-funded in vitro study demonstrated that although both Digibind and DigiFab bound digoxin equally well, a small difference in the amount of ouabain binding to Fab subpopulations was identified with twice as much bound to Digibind as DigiFab.[61]

The successful reversal, by Digibind, of cardiotoxicity resulting from ingestion of *Nerium oleander* and *Thevetia peruviana* are reported.[14,75] One adult and one child each responded to five vials (200 mg) of Fab, but larger doses may be required in other cardioactive steroid poisonings because of the lower affinity binding of Digibind for these toxins. DigiFab is expected to have similar affinity binding toward cardioactive steroids. Both products are polyclonal, contributing to their broad spectrum of affinity for nondigoxin cardioactive steroids. Treatment decisions should be based on empirical grounds, with initial therapy consisting of 10 to 20 vials. Subsequent doses can be based on clinical response.

SUMMARY

Digoxin-specific antibody fragments have dramatically advanced the care of patients poisoned with cardioactive steroids. In the more than 30 years since the release DSFab, a lethal overdose has become manageable allowing the clinician ease in treatment with almost no risk to the patient.

REFERENCES

1. Antman EM, Wenger TL, Butler VP, et al. Treatment of 150 cases of life-threatening digitalis intoxication with digoxin specific Fab antibody fragments: final report of multicenter study. *Circulation.* 1990;81:1744-1752.
2. Argyle JC. Effect of digoxin antibodies on TDX digoxin assay. *Clin Chem.* 1986;32:1616-1617.
3. Barrueto F Jr, Jortani SA, Valdes R Jr, et al. Cardioactive steroid poisoning from an herbal cleansing preparation. *Ann Emerg Med.* 2003;41:396-399.
4. Beller GA, Smith TW, Abelmann WH, et al. Digitalis intoxication: a prospective clinical study with serum level correlations. *N Engl J Med.* 1971;284:989-997.
5. Berkovitch M, Akilesh MR, Gerace R, et al. Acute digoxin overdose in a newborn with renal failure: use of digoxin immune Fab and peritoneal dialysis. *Ther Drug Monit.* 1994;16:531-533.
6. Bismuth C, Gaultier M, Conso F, et al. Hyperkalemia in acute digitalis poisoning: prognostic significance and therapeutic implications. *Clin Toxicol.* 1973;6:153-162.
7. Borron S, Bismuth C, Muszynski J. Advances in the management of digoxin toxicity in the older patient. *Drugs Aging.* 1997;10:18-33.
8. Bosse GM, Pope TM. Recurrent digoxin overdose and treatment with digoxin- specific Fab antibody fragments. *J Emerg Med.* 1994;12:179-185.
9. Brubacher J, Lachmanen D, Ravikumar PR, Hoffman RS. Efficacy of digoxin specific Fab fragments (Digibind) in the treatment of toad venom poisoning. *Toxicon.* 1999;37:931-942.
10. Brubacher J, Ravikumar P, Bania T, et al. Treatment of toad venom poisoning with digoxin-specific Fab fragments. *Chest.* 1996;110:1282-1288.
11. Butler VP, Chen J. Digoxin specific antibodies. *Proc Natl Acad Sci U S A.* 1967; 57:71-78.
12. Butler VP, Schmidt DH, Smith TW, et al. Effects of sheep digoxin specific antibodies and their Fab fragments on digoxin pharmacokinetics in dogs. *J Clin Invest.* 1977;59:345-359.
13. Butler VP, Smith TW, Schmidt DH, et al. Immunological reversal of the effects of digoxin. *Fed Proc.* 1977;36:2235-2241.
14. Camphausen C, Haas N, Mattke A. Successful treatment of oleander intoxication (cardiac glycosides) with digoxin-specific Fab antibody fragments in a 7-year-old child. *Z Kardiol.* 2005;94:817-823.
15. Cheung K, Urech R, Taylor L, et al. Plant cardiac glycosides and digoxin Fab antibody. *J Pediatr Child Health.* 1991;27:312-313.
16. Colucci R, Choses M, Kluger J, et al. The pharmacokinetics of digoxin immune Fab, total digoxin and free digoxin in patients with renal impairment [abstract]. *Pharmacotherapy.* 1989;9:175.
17. Curd J, Smith TW, Jaton J, et al. The isolation of digoxin specific antibody and its use in reversing the effects of digoxin. *Proc Natl Acad Sci U S A.* 1971;68:2401-2406.
18. D'Angio RG, Stevenson JG, Lively BT, et al. Therapeutic drug monitoring: improved performance through educational intervention. *Ther Drug Monit.* 1990;12:173-181.
19. Dasgupta A, Emerson L. Neutralization of cardiac toxins oleandrin, oleandrigenin, bufalin, and cinobufotalin by Digibind: monitoring the effect by measuring free digitoxin concentrations. *Life Sci.* 1998;63:781-788.
20. Dasgupta A, Lopez AE, Wells A, et al. The Fab fragment of antidigoxin antibody (Digibind) binds digitoxin-like immunoreactive components of Chinese medicine Chan Su: monitoring the effect by measuring free digitoxin. *Clin Chim Acta.* 2001;309:91-95.
21. DiDomenico RJ, Walton SM, Sanoski CA, Bauman JL. Analysis of the use of digoxin immune Fab for the treatment of non-life-threatening digoxin toxicity. *J Cardiovasc Pharmacol Ther.* 2000;5:77-85.
22. Digibind [package insert]. Research Triangle Park, NC: GlaxoSmithKline; 2003.
23. DigiFab [package insert]. Brentwood, TN: Protherics; 2005.
24. Duhme DW, Greenblatt DJ, Kock-Weser J. Reduction of digoxin toxicity associated with measurement of serum levels: a report from the Boston Collaborative Drug Surveillance Program. *Ann Intern Med.* 1974;80:516-519.
25. Durham G, Califf RM. Digoxin toxicity in renal insufficiency treated with digoxin immune Fab. *Prim Cardiol.* 1988;1:31-34.
26. Eagle KA, Haber E, DeSanctis RW, et al., eds. *The Practice of Cardiology*, 2nd ed. Boston: Little, Brown; 1989.
27. Eddleston M, Rajapakse S, Rajakanthan, et al. Anti-digoxin Fab fragments in cardiotoxicity induced by ingestion of yellow oleander: a randomized controlled trial. *Lancet.* 2000;355:967-972.
28. Erdmann E, Mair W, Knedel M, et al. Digitalis intoxication and treatment with digoxin antibody fragments in renal failure. *Klin Wochenschr.* 1989;67:16-19.
29. Eyal D, Molczan K, Carroll L. Digoxin toxicity: pediatric survival after asystolic arrest. *Clin Tox.* 2005;1:51-54.
30. Flanagan RJ, Jones AL. Fab antibody fragments: some applications in clinical toxicology. *Drug Saf.* 2004;27:1115-1133.
31. Frisolone J, Sylvia LM, Gelwan J, et al. False-positive serum digoxin concentrations determined by three digoxin assays on patients with liver disease. *Clin Pharm.* 1988;7:444-449.
32. George S, Braithwaite RA, Hughes EA. Digoxin measurements following plasma ultrafiltration in two patients with digoxin toxicity treated with specific Fab fragments. *Ann Clin Biochem.* 1994;31:380-381.
33. Gibb I, Adams PC, Parnham AJ, et al. Plasma digoxin: assay anomalies in Fab treated patients. *Br J Clin Pharmacol.* 1983;16:445-447.
34. Graves SW, Brown B, Valdes R. An endogenous digoxin like substance in patients with renal impairment. *Ann Intern Med.* 1983;99:604-608.
35. Hastreiter AR, John EG, Nander Hoist RL. Digitalis, digitalis antibodies, digitalis-like immunoreactive substances, and sodium homeostasis: a review. *Clin Perinatol.* 1988;15:491-522.
36. Haynes BE, Bessen HA, Wightman WD, et al. Oleander tea: herbal draught of death. *Ann Emerg Med.* 1985;14:350-353.
37. Honda SAA, Rios CN, Murakami L, et al. Problems in determining levels of free digoxin in patients treated with digoxin immune Fab. *J Clin Lab Anal.* 1995;9:407-412.
38. Hursting MJ, Raisys VA, Opheim KE, et al. Determination of free digoxin concentrations in serum for monitoring Fab treatment of digoxin overdose. *Clin Chem.* 1987;33:1652-1655.
39. Jortani S, Pinar A, Johnson N, Valdes R. Validity of unbound digoxin measurements by immunoassays in presence of antidote (Digibind). *Clin Chim Acta.* 1999;283:159-169.
40. Karboski JA, Godley PJ, Frohna PA, et al. Marked digoxin like immunoreactive factor interference with an enzyme immunoassay. *Drug Intell Clin Pharm.* 1988;2:703-705.
41. Kaufman J, Leikin J, Kendzierski D, Polin K. Use of digoxin Fab immune fragments in a seven-day-old infant. *Pediatr Emerg Care.* 1990;6:118-121.
42. Kelly RA, O'Hara DS, Canessa MG, et al. Characterization of digitalis like factors in human plasma. *J Biol Chem.* 1985;260:11396-11405.
43. Koren G, Deatie D, Soldin S. Agonal elevation in serum digoxin concentrations in infants and children long after cessation of therapy. *Crit Care Med.* 1988;16:793-795.
44. Koren G, Parker R. Interpretation of excessive serum concentrations of digoxin in children. *Am J Cardiol.* 1985;55:1210-1214.
45. Lechat P, Mudgett-Hunter M, Margolies M, et al. Reversal of lethal digoxin toxicity in guinea pigs using monoclonal antibodies and Fab fragments. *J Pharmacol Exp Ther.* 1984;229:210-215.
46. Lemon M, Andrews DJ, Binks AM, et al. Concentrations of free serum digoxin after treatment with antibody fragments. *Br Med J.* 1987;295:1520-1521.
47. Lindenbaum J, Rund D, Butler VP, et al. Inactivation of digoxin by the gut flora: reversal by antibiotic therapy. *N Engl J Med.* 1981;305:789-794.
48. Lloyd BL, Smith TW. Contrasting rates of reversal of digoxin toxicity by digoxin: specific IgG and Fab fragments. *Circulation.* 1978;58:280-283.
49. Marchlinski FE, Hook BG, Callans DJ. Which cardiac disturbances should be treated with digoxin immune Fab (ovine) antibody? *Am J Emerg Med.* 1991; 9:24-34.
50. Marcus L, Margel S, Savin H, et al. Therapy of digoxin intoxication in dogs by specific hemoperfusion through agarose polyacrolein microsphere beads: antidigoxin antibodies. *Am Heart J.* 1985;110:30-39.
51. McMillin GA, Owen WE, Lambert TL, et al. Comparable effects of Digibind and DigiFab in thirteen digoxin immunoassays. *Clin Chem.* 2002;48:1580-1584.
52. Nabauer M, Erdmann E. Reversal of toxic and non-toxic effects of digoxin by digoxin-specific Fab fragments in isolated human ventricular myocardium. *Klin Wochenschr.* 1987;65:558-561.

53. Naomi S, Graves S, Lazarus M, et al. Variation in apparent serum digitalis-like factor levels with different digoxin antibodies: the "immunochemical fingerprint." *Am J Hypertens.* 1991;4:795-800.
54. Nollet H, Verhaaren H, Stroobandt R, et al. Delayed elimination of digoxin antidotum determined by RIA. *J Clin Pharmacol.* 1989;29:41-45.
55. Nuwayhid N, Johnson G. Digoxin elimination in a functionally anephric patient after digoxin specific Fab fragment therapy. *Ther Drug Monit.* 1989;11:680-685.
56. Ocal I, Green T. Serum digoxin in the presence of Digibind: determination of digoxin by the Abbott AxSYM and Baxter Stratus II immunoassays by direct analysis without pretreatment of serum samples. *Clin Chem.* 1998;44:1947-1950.
57. Ordog GJ, Benaron S, Bhasin V. Serum digoxin levels and mortality in 5100 patients. *Ann Emerg Med.* 1987;16:32-39.
58. Osterloh J, Herold S, Pond S. Oleander interference in the digoxin radioimmunoassay in a fatal ingestion. *JAMA.* 1982;247:1596-1597.
59. *Postmarketing Surveillance Study of Digibind: Interim Report to Contributors.* Research Triangle Park, NC: Burroughs Wellcome; July 1986-July 1987.
60. Pullen MA, Brooks DP, Edwards RM. Characterization of the neutralizing activity of digoxin-specific Fab toward ouabain-like steroids. *J Pharmacol Exp Ther.* 2004;310:319-325.
61. Pullen M, Harpel M, Danoff T, Brooks D. Comparison of non-digitalis binding properties of digoxin-specific Fabs using direct binding methods. *J Immunolog Methods.* 2008;336:235-241.
62. Quaife EJ, Banner W, Vernon D, et al. Failure of CAVH to remove digoxin Fab complex in piglets. *J Toxicol Clin Toxicol.* 1990;28:61-68.
63. Rainey P. Digibind and free digoxin. *Clin Chem.* 1999;5:719-721.
64. Renard C, Grene-Lerouge N, Beau N, et al. Pharmacokinetics of digoxin-specific Fab: effects of decreased renal function and age. *Br J Clin Pharmacol.* 1997;44:135-138.
65. Renard C, Weinling E, Pau B, Schermann JM. Time and dose-dependent digoxin redistribution by digoxin-specific antigen binding fragments in a rat model. *Toxicology.* 1999;137:117-127.
66. Safadi R, Levy I, Amitai Y, Caraco Y. Beneficial effect of digoxin-specific Fab antibody fragments in oleander intoxication. *Arch Intern Med.* 1995;155:2121-2125.
67. Savin H, Marcus L, Margel S, et al. Treatment of adverse digitalis effect by hemoperfusion through columns with antidigoxin antibodies bound to agarose polyacrolein microsphere beads. *Am Heart J.* 1987;113:1078-1084.
68. Schaumann W, Kaufmann B, Neubert P, et al. Kinetics of the Fab fragments of digoxin antibodies and of bound digoxin in patients with severe digoxin intoxication. *Eur J Clin Pharmacol.* 1986;30:527-533.
69. Schmidt DH, Butler VP. Immunological protection against digoxin toxicity. *J Clin Invest.* 1971;50:866-871.
70. Schmidt DH, Butler VP. Reversal of digoxin toxicity with specific antibodies. *J Clin Invest.* 1971;50:1738-1744.
71. Schmidt TA, Holm-Nielsen P, Kjeldsen K. Human skeletal muscle digitalis glycoside receptors (Na,K-ATPase)—importance during digitalization. *Cardiovasc Drugs Ther.* 1993;7:175-181.
72. Schmidt TA, Kjeldsen K. Enhanced clearance of specifically bound digoxin from human myocardial and skeletal muscle samples by specific digoxin antibody fragments: subsequent complete digitalis glycoside receptor (Na,K-ATPase) quantification. *J Cardiovasc Pharmacol.* 1991;17:670-677.
73. Schmitt K, Tulzer G, Hackel F, et al. Massive digitoxin intoxication treated with digoxin-specific antibodies in a child. *Pediatr Cardiol.* 1994;15:48-49.
74. Sherron PA, Gelband H. *Reversal of digoxin toxicity with Fab fragments in a pediatric patient with acute renal failure.* Paper presented at Management of Digitalis Toxicity: The Role of Digibind. San Francisco, July 26-28, 1985. Burroughs Wellcome, sponsor.
75. Shumaik GM, Wu AU, Ping AC. Oleander poisoning: treatment with digoxin-specific Fab antibody fragments. *Ann Emerg Med.* 1988;17:732-735.
76. Sinclair AJ, Hewick DS, Johnston PC, et al. Kinetics of digoxin and anti-digoxin antibody fragments during treatment of digoxin toxicity. *Br J Clin Pharmacol.* 1989;28:352-356.
77. Smith TW. New advances in the assessment and treatment of digitalis toxicity. *J Clin Pharmacol.* 1985;25:522-528.
78. Smith TW, Haber E, Yeatman L, et al. Reversal of advanced digoxin intoxication with Fab fragments of digoxin-specific antibodies. *N Engl J Med.* 1976;294:797-800.
79. Smith TW, Lloyd BL, Spicer N, et al. Immunogenicity and kinetics of distribution and elimination of sheep digoxin specific IgG and Fab fragments in the rabbit and baboon. *Clin Exp Immunol.* 1979;36:384-396.
80. Soldin S. Digoxin: issues and controversies. *Clin Chem.* 1986;32:5-12.
81. Ujhelyi MR, Colucci RD, Cummings DM, et al. Monitoring serum digoxin concentrations during digoxin immune Fab therapy. *Ann Pharmacother.* 1991;25:1047-1049.
82. Ujhelyi MR, Robert S. Pharmacokinetic aspects of digoxin-specific Fab therapy in the management of digitalis toxicity. *Clin Pharmacokinet.* 1995;28:483-493.
83. Ujhelyi MR, Robert S, Cummings DM, et al. Disposition of digoxin immune Fab in patients with kidney failure. *Clin Pharmacol Ther.* 1993;54:388-394.
84. Ujhelyi MR, Robert S, Cummings DM, et al. Influence of digoxin immune Fab therapy and renal dysfunction on the disposition of total and free digoxin. *Ann Intern Med.* 1993;119:273-277.
85. Valdes R, Jortani S. Monitoring of unbound digoxin in patients treated with antidigoxin antigen-binding fragments: a model for the future? *Clin Chem.* 1998;44:1883-1885.
86. Vasdev S, Johnson E, Longerich L, et al. Plasma endogenous digitalis-like factors in healthy individuals and in dialysis dependent and kidney transplant patients. *Clin Nephrol.* 1987;27:169-174.
87. Vinge E, Ekman R. Partial characterization of endogenous digoxin-like substance in human urine. *Ther Drug Monit.* 1988;10:8-15.
88. Ward SB, Sjostrom L, Ujhelyi MR. Comparison of the pharmacokinetics and in vivo bioaffinity of DigiTAb versus Digibind. *Ther Drug Monit.* 2000;22:599-607.
89. Wenger TL. Experience with digoxin immune Fab (ovine) in patients with renal impairment. *Am J Emerg Med.* 1991;9:21-23.
90. Winter ME. Digoxin. In: Koda-Kimble MA, Young LY, eds. *Basic Clinical Pharmacokinetics*, 3rd ed. Vancouver, WA: Applied Therapeutics; 1994:198-235.

CHAPTER 65
METHYLXANTHINES AND SELECTIVE β_2 ADRENERGIC AGONISTS

Robert J. Hoffman

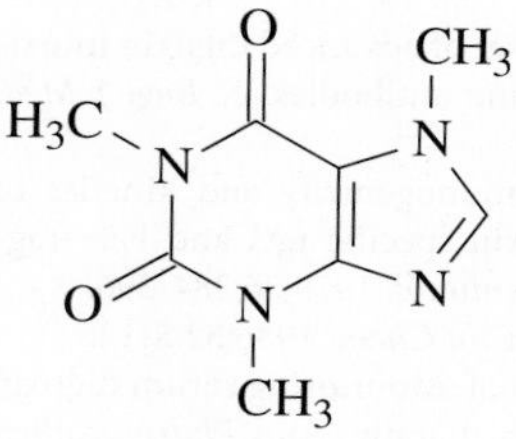

Caffeine
(1,3,7-trimethylxanthine)

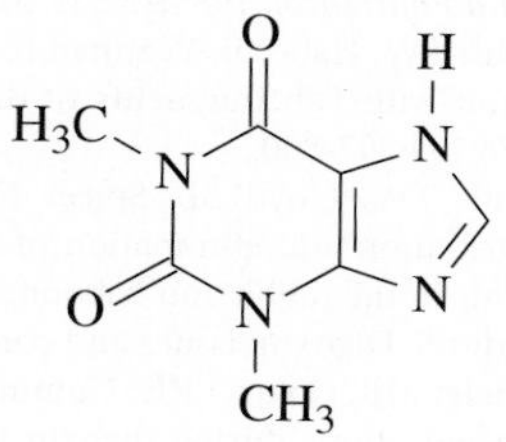

Theophylline
(1,3-dimethylxanthine)

Caffeine

MW	= 194.19 daltons
Therapeutic serum concentration	= 1–10 μg/mL

Theophylline

MW	= 180.17 daltons
Therapeutic serum concentration	= 5–15 μg/mL
	= 10 μg/mL
	= 55.5 μmol/L

Methylxanthines are plant-derived alkaloids that include caffeine (1,3,7 trimethylxanthine), theobromine (3,7-dimethylxanthine), and theophylline (1,3-dimethylxanthine). They are so named because they are methylated derivatives of xanthine. Members of this group have very similar pharmacologic properties and clinical effects. Methylxanthines are used ubiquitously throughout the world, most commonly in beverages imbibed for their stimulant, mood elevating, and fatigue abating effects. *Coffea arabica* and related species are used to make coffee, a beverage rich in caffeine. Cocoa and chocolate are derived from the seeds of *Theobroma cacao*, which contains theobromine and to a lesser extent caffeine. *Thea sinensis*, a bush native to China but now cultivated worldwide, produces leaves from which various teas, rich in caffeine and containing small amounts of theophylline and theobromine, are brewed. *Paullinia* spp, commonly known as guarana, is a South American plant that produces berries with a caffeine content much greater than that of coffee beans. Guarana is widely used as an additive in herbal energy drinks.

Selective β_2 adrenergic agonists (β_2AA) have been developed for the treatment of bronchoconstriction. Their selectivity has improved therapy for bronchoconstriction, allowing avoidance of the adverse effects of the previously used therapies: epinephrine, an α-and β-adrenergic agonist, as well as isoproterenol, a β_1 and β_2AA. All β_2AAs have nearly identical clinical effects; the principal differences are their pharmacokinetics. This chapter does not examine each β_2AA individually but instead discusses them as a class. The β_2AAs include albuterol, bitolterol, formoterol, pirbuterol, salmeterol, terbutaline, and ritodrine. Clenbuterol, a long-acting agonist at β_2 and β_3 adrenergic receptors, used for the purpose of treating bronchoconstriction in countries outside the United States, has emerged as an abused anabolic xenobiotic in recent years.

EPIDEMIOLOGY

The American Association of Poison Control Centers reported the following trends in methylxanthine exposures. Theophylline exposures decreased from 2609 involving 20 deaths in 1998 to 413 exposures and four deaths in 2006. Caffeine exposures decreased from 7390 exposures and no deaths in 1998 to 5696 exposures of pharmaceutical and herbal caffeine but involving seven deaths in 2006. The decrease in theophylline exposures presumably reflects continued decrease in use of theophylline in the treatment of patients with pulmonary disease. The number of caffeine exposures has essentially remained stable, reflecting steady use of caffeine, particularly caffeine in substances other than coffee, tea, and soft drinks.

There were 11,397 selective β_2AA exposures and one death in 1998 and 9564 and one death in 2006. The number of selective β_2AA exposures has remained relatively stable, presumably from consistent use of these agents, but death has remained uncommon. See Chap. 135 for a discussion of poison exposure data.

The overwhelming preponderance of caffeine consumed is in beverages, and a lesser portion is consumed in foods and tablets or capsules. Users typically seek the stimulant and psychoactive effects of caffeine. Caffeine, particularly in herbal forms such as guarana or cola nut, is also increasingly advocated for use as a weight loss agent.[76,15] The use of guarana, a plant with very high caffeine content, for weight loss and athletic performance enhancement has increased dramatically in recent years. With some scientific evidence demonstrating benefit in athletic performance, caffeine is advocated as a concentration[101,163] and "energy" booster and as an athletic performance enhancer.[34,100] Energy drinks typically containing caffeine and other stimulant ingredients are increasingly popular, particularly with adolescents and athletes.[122]

Despite the limited experience with overdose from these combination preparations, formulations containing caffeine and guarana combined with ephedrine and ma huang cause illnesses such as myocardial infarctions and death.[83] Formulations containing phenylpropanolamine and caffeine, also once marketed as an anorexiant diet aid, were removed from U.S. markets because of adverse drug events and a demonstrated lack of benefit from the inclusion of caffeine and a sympathomimetic xenobiotic for the purpose of appetite suppression.[86] (See Chap. 39 for more discussion of dietary supplements). Energy drinks are, not unexpectedly, revealing themselves as having adverse side effects.[42]

Medicinally, caffeine is used to treat neonatal apnea and bradycardia syndrome, as an analgesic adjuvant, particularly when combined with relatively mild analgesics such as acetaminophen, aspirin, and ibuprofen, and as an adjuvant treatment for headaches.

Theophylline or its water-soluble salt, aminophylline, is used to treat varied respiratory conditions, but is most well studied for its use in reversible bronchospastic airway disease, particularly asthma and chronic obstructive pulmonary disease (COPD). Theophylline was once the mainstay of therapy for such diseases, but more selective β_2aAs with fewer adverse effects, such as albuterol and other selective β_2aA, are now generally used. However, antiinflammatory and other beneficial effects of theophylline continue to be described.[107] In neonates, theophylline and aminophylline are used similarly to caffeine to treat apnea and bradycardia syndrome. The result of such treatment is increased respiratory rate, decreased apnea, increased cardiac chronotropy and inotropy, and increased cardiac output.[32]

Caffeine toxicity is generally classified as acute, acute on chronic, or chronic in nature. Neonates receiving caffeine therapy may develop either acute or chronic caffeine toxicity.[7,17]

Chronic toxicity from caffeine is most typically described as a result of the frequent self-administration of excessive caffeine. A particular syndrome associated with chronic caffeine use consisting of headache, palpitations, tachycardia, insomnia, and delirium is termed *caffeinism*.

Theophylline toxicity results from the use of theophylline as a medicinal therapeutic agent and may develop as acute, chronic, or acute-on-chronic toxicity.

Acute-on-chronic toxicity may occur with caffeine or theophylline and is the circumstance of acute overdose in a patient already receiving chronic therapy.

Most reported cases of theobromine poisoning occur in the veterinary literature and typically result from small animals ingesting cocoa or chocolate.[57,84] Theobromine has become an ingredient of numerous "energy" drinks used for stimulation and athletic enhancement. No reports of human toxicity currently exist, but it is probable that toxicity from these sources will be reported.

Use of β_2AAs is widespread. Adverse effects are associated with both therapeutic dosing and overdose. Excessive use of β_2AAs may result in tachyphylaxis, a phenomenon in which downregulation of receptors occurs and the effects from this drug diminish as a result of excessive use.[46,96] Consequently, patients may require higher doses to achieve the same clinical effects previously experienced at lower doses, resulting in more profound systemic side effects. The most common selective β_2AA toxicity results from children ingesting oral (PO) albuterol. Toxicity of terbutaline and ritodrine are infrequent but well reported. Epidemic clenbuterol exposures have occurred in recent years, which are the result of both admixture of this substance with illicit xenobiotics as well as by intentional use for bodybuilding purposes in the United States.[53] Food poisoning by consumption of animal meat from livestock treated with clenbuterol has occurred in Europe.[18]

PHARMACOLOGY

METHYLXANTHINES

Methylxanthines cause the release of endogenous catecholamines, resulting in stimulation of β_1 and β_2 receptors. The resulting adrenergic agonism is important in both the therapeutic effects and of toxicity.[187] Endogenous catecholamine concentrations are extremely elevated in patients with methylxanthine poisoning.[22]

Methylxanthines are structural analogs of adenosine and function pharmacologically as adenosine antagonists. Adenosine is believed to modulate histamine release and cause bronchoconstriction, which may explain the primary therapeutic efficacy of adenosine antagonists in the treatment of bronchospasm. Additionally, adenosine antagonism results in release of norepinephrine, and to a lesser extent epinephrine, through blockade of presynaptic A2 receptors. The additional methyl group possessed by caffeine (1,3,7 trimethylxanthine) affords this agent greater central nervous system (CNS) penetration relative to theophylline and theobromine, which are dimethylxanthines. Caffeine is an effective analgesic adjuvant, possibly because of the stimulant properties of the drug.[129,131,161,162]

Methylxanthines also inhibit phosphodiesterase, the enzyme responsible for degradation of intracellular cyclic AMP (cAMP), which has many effects, including an increase in intracellular calcium concentrations. Phosphodiesterase inhibition was long considered to be the primary therapeutic mechanism of the methylxanthines, but clinically significant elevations in cAMP levels are not achieved until serum methylxanthine concentrations are well above the therapeutic range. This likely occurs as a result of the structural similarity of the adenosine moiety of cAMP and the methylxanthines. cAMP is involved in the postsynaptic second messenger system of β-adrenergic stimulation. Thus, elevated cAMP levels cause clinical effects similar to adrenergic stimulation, including smooth muscle relaxation, peripheral vasodilation, myocardial stimulation, skeletal muscle contractility, and CNS excitation.

SELECTIVE β_2 ADRENERGIC AGONISTS

Selective β_2AAs act quite specifically at β_2 adrenergic receptors, resulting in an increase in intracellular cAMP. The effects of β_2 agonism include relaxation of vascular, bronchial, and uterine smooth muscle; glycogenolysis in skeletal muscle; and hepatic glycogenolysis and gluconeogenesis. These receptors are located on other cells such as type II alveolar cells, mast cells, and lymphocytes, but their significance is unknown. Selective β_2AAs have been characterized as either directly activating the β_2 receptor, such as albuterol, being taken up into a membrane depot, such as formoterol, or interacting with a receptor-specific auxiliary binding site, such as salmeterol. These differences do not appear to be relevant in acute toxicity.[91] However, emerging evidence suggests that prolonged overuse of long-acting β_2AAs may have severe or fatal adverse effects.[159]

PHARMACOKINETICS AND TOXICOKINETICS

CAFFEINE PHARMACOKINETICS

Caffeine is bioavailable by PO, intravenous (IV), subcutaneous, intramuscular, and rectal routes of administration. PO administration, which is by far the most common route of exposure, results in nearly 100% bioavailability of the drug. The presence of food in the gut does little to affect peak concentration. However, food in the gut does delay time until the peak serum concentration is reached, which is typically 30 to 60 minutes in the absence of food. Caffeine rapidly diffuses into the total body water and all tissues and readily crosses the blood–brain barrier and into the placenta. The volume of distribution (Vd) is 0.6 L/kg, and 36% is protein bound. Caffeine is secreted in breast milk with concentrations of 2 to 4 μg/mL in breast milk after 100 mg PO dosing in a breastfeeding mother.[180] Consumption of very large caffeine doses or chronic caffeine use might result in breast milk concentrations capable of causing clinical effects in the breastfeeding child, but this is not typical.

When taken in amounts greater than the typical therapeutic dose in a caffeinated beverage, caffeine exhibits Michaelis-Menten kinetics and is metabolized via the microsomal cytochrome P450 system, primarily by the isoenzyme CYP1A2. The major pathway involves demethylation to 1,7 dimethylxanthine (paraxanthine) followed by hydroxylation or repeated demethylation followed by hydroxylation. To a lesser extent, caffeine is also metabolized to theobromine and theophylline. Neonates demethylate caffeine, producing theophylline, and possess the unique ability to convert theophylline to caffeine by methylation.[1,11,12,31,71] By approximately 4 to 7 months of age, infants metabolize and eliminate caffeine in a manner similar to adults.[10] All patients demethylate some quantity of caffeine to active metabolites, including theophylline and theobromine. The degree to which this occurs is dependent on the patient's age, cytochrome P450 enzyme induction status, and other factors.

Less than 5% of caffeine is excreted in the urine unchanged. The half-life of caffeine is highly variable and dependent on several factors. Generally speaking, younger patients, particularly infants as well as patients with cytochrome P450 inhibition, such as pregnant patients and patients with cirrhosis, have longer caffeine half-lives than the 4.5 hour half-life in healthy, adult, nonsmoking patients.[33,50,54,179]

Caffeine Toxicokinetics Caffeine toxicity is a dose-dependent phenomenon. Unfortunately, the range of toxic concentrations reported in different references varies greatly, and no definite conclusions can be drawn regarding the relationship between serum concentrations and symptomatology in overdose. Therapeutic dosing in neonates is typical loading dose is 20 mg/kg, with daily maintenance dosing of 5 mg/kg. Based on case reports and series, lethal dosing in adults is estimated at 150 to 200 mg/kg, and death may be associated with serum concentrations above 80 μg/mL. Numerous fatalities are reported with serum concentrations under 200 μg/mL; survival of a patient with an acute caffeine overdose and a serum concentration over 400 μg/mL has been reported.[184] Infants survive toxicity with greater serum concentrations of caffeine than are tolerated by children and adults.

THEOPHYLLINE PHARMACOKINETICS

Theophylline is approximately 100% bioavailable by the PO and IV routes. Many of the available PO preparations are sustained release designed to provide stable serum concentrations over a prolonged period of time with less frequent dosing. Peak absorption for immediate-release preparations is 60 to 90 minutes and sustained-release preparations generally occurs 6 to 10 hours after ingestion.

Similar to caffeine, theophylline rapidly diffuses into the total body water and all tissues, readily crosses the blood–brain barrier, and crosses into the placenta and breast milk.[14,109,197,199] Theophylline's Vd is 0.5 L/kg, and 56% of it is protein bound at therapeutic concentrations.

Theophylline is metabolized via the microsomal cytochrome P450 system, primarily by the isozyme CYP1A2. The major pathway is demethylation to 3-methylxanthine in addition to being demethylated or oxidized to other metabolites. Less than 10% of theophylline is excreted in the urine unchanged.

Similar to caffeine, the half-life of theophylline is highly variable and is dependent on several factors. In healthy, adult, nonsmoking patients, the half-life is 4.5 hours. Infants and the elderly as well as patients with cytochrome P450 inhibition, pregnant patients, and patients with cirrhosis have longer theophylline half-lives than healthy children and adult nonsmoking patients.[92,123,178] Factors that induce cytochrome P450, such as cigarette smoking, or others that inhibit cytochrome P450, such as exposure to cimetidine, erythromycin, and PO contraceptives, can significantly alter theophylline clearance.[79,121,137,138,153,189] Cessation of smoking, such as when a COPD patient develops bronchitis, leads to a reversal of P450 induction and predisposes to the development of chronic toxicity.

Theophylline Toxicokinetics As in the case of caffeine, theophylline exhibits Michaelis-Menten kinetics, presumably when greater than a single therapeutic dose is taken.[152] At higher doses and in overdose, it undergoes zero-order elimination, and only a fixed amount of the drug can be eliminated in a given time because of saturation of metabolic enzymes.[150]

Therapeutic serum concentrations of theophylline are 5 to 15 μg/mL. Although morbidity and mortality are not always predictable based on serum levels, life-threatening toxicity are associated with serum concentrations of 80 to 100 μg/mL in acute overdoses and of 40 to 60 μg/mL in chronic toxicity.

THEOBROMINE TOXICOKINETICS AND PHARMACOKINETICS

As is the case with the other methylxanthines, theobromine is well absorbed from the gut and is 80% bioavailable when administered in solution. It is bioavailable PO and rectally. Theobromine has 21% protein binding, a Vd of 0.62 L/kg and a plasma half-life of 6 to 10 hours.[58,147] Theobromine undergoes hepatic metabolism by the CYP1A2 and CYP2E1.[30] Similar to the other methylxanthines, theobromine is excreted in breast milk. Toxic concentrations of theobromine in animals are known, but comparable human data are lacking.

SELECTIVE β_2 ADRENERGIC AGONIST PHARMACOKINETICS

The β_2AAs are bioavailable by both the inhalational and enteral route, and much of "inhaled" β_2AAs may actually be swallowed and absorbed from the gastrointestinal (GI) tract. Absorption, distribution, and elimination vary among these agents. The half-life of albuterol is approximately 4 hours, less than 5% crosses the blood–brain barrier, it is metabolized extensively in the liver, and it is excreted in urine and feces as albuterol and metabolites.[3]

Terbutaline is partially metabolized in the liver, mainly to inactive conjugates. With parenteral administration, 60% of a given dose is excreted in the urine unchanged.[2]

Clenbuterol has a terminal half-life of approximately 22 hours and a prolonged duration of action. Additionally, it is more potent than other β_2AA, with a typical therapeutic dose of 20 to 40 μg, as opposed to milligram doses for other β_2AAs.

Selective β_2AA Toxicokinetics Overdose of albuterol, which typically happens predominantly in young children treated with PO albuterol preparations, may cause significant symptomatology.[106] For PO albuterol poisoning, 1 mg/kg appears to be the dose threshold for developing clinically significant toxicity.[194]

Clenbuterol toxicity occurs from use by a variety of routes, generally as a result of the varied route of illicit drug use. Ingestion, intranasal use, and IV use of clenbuterol or clenbuterol-tainted street drug have been reported.

METHYLXANTHINE AND β_2AA TOXICITY

Caffeine, theobromine, and theophylline affect the same organ systems and cause qualitatively similar effects.

It should be noted, however, that there are distinct differences in the activity and effects of the various methylxanthines, particularly in therapeutic dose. Toxicity affects the GI, cardiovascular, central nervous, and musculoskeletal systems in addition to causing a constellation of metabolic derangements. A putative cause for toxicity involves the increase in metabolism that occurs with methylxanthine toxicity, particularly in the setting of a decreased ability to meet the increased demand by way of impaired perfusion.

Polypharmacy poisoning with other xenobiotics that result in adrenergic stimulation, such as pseudoephedrine, ephedrine, amphetamines, or cocaine, may be particularly severe.[55,192]

Gastrointestinal In overdose, methylxanthines cause nausea, and most significant acute overdoses result in severe and protracted emesis. Whereas emesis occurs in 75% of cases of acute theophylline poisoning, only 30% of cases of chronically poisoned patients have emesis.[171] When it occurs, the emesis is often quite severe and may be difficult to control despite the use of potent antiemetics. This is especially evident with sustained-release theophylline preparations.[4] Emesis is less common with β_2AA, and when it does occur, it is uncommonly as severe as is associated with methylxanthines.

Methylxanthines cause an increase in gastric acid secretion and smooth muscle relaxation. These factors contribute to the gastritis and esophagitis reported in chronic methylxanthine users.[45] Gastritis is noted in drinkers of decaffeinated coffee, so some adverse gastric effects associated with coffee drinking may be caused by ingredients other than caffeine.

Cardiovascular Methylxanthines are cardiac stimulants and result in positive inotropy and chronotropy even with therapeutic dosing. Dysrhythmias, particularly tachydysrhythmias, are common in patients with methylxanthines overdose. Tachydysrhythmias, particularly ventricular extrasystoles, are more common after overdose of methylxanthines.[41,130,164] Cardiac dysrhythmias, although described with β_2AA poisoning, are most frequently supraventricular in origin and clinically inconsequential. Dysrhythmias other than sinus tachycardia associated with β_2AA toxicity are not routinely noted with toxicity from other β_2AAs, but clenbuterol may result in atrial fibrillation.[53] Palpitations, tachycardia, and chest pain are common presenting complaints for patients with clenbuterol toxicity.

In the setting of acute poisoning, generally benign sinus tachycardia is nearly universal in patients without antecedent cardiac disease. In any patient, particularly those with underlying cardiac disease, sinus tachycardia may degenerate to a more severe rhythm disturbance, and these represent the most common causes of fatality associated with methylxanthines poisoning. Both atrial and ventricular dysrhythmias, including supraventricular tachycardia (SVT), multifocal atrial tachycardia, atrial fibrillation, premature ventricular contractions, and ventricular tachycardia, may all result from methylxanthine toxicity.[21,168] Electrolyte disturbances, particularly hypokalemia, may be a contributing factor in the development of dysrhythmias. Dysrhythmias occur more commonly and at lower serum concentrations in cases of chronic poisoning with methyxanthines. Consequential dysrhythmias occur in 35% of patients with chronic theophylline poisoning but in only 10% of acute poisoning.[168] Ventricular dysrhythmias occur at serum concentrations of 40 to 80 μg/mL in patients with chronic theophylline overdoses and most commonly at serum levels greater than 80 μg/mL in patients with acute overdoses. Neonates born to mothers who consumed more than 500 mg/day of caffeine are more likely to have dysrhythmias compared with cohorts born to mothers consuming less than 250 mg/day of caffeine.[80] For reference, a cup of coffee or bottle of cola may contain 50 to 100 mg of caffeine.

Myocardial ischemia and myocardial infarction may result from acute caffeine or theophylline poisoning.[64,85,125] Myocardial infarction has been associated with both albuterol [61] and more recently clenbuterol.[105] Isoproterenol, once a common asthma therapy before widespread use of selective β_2AAs, has both β_1- and β_2-adrenergic agonist activity and is a well-reported cause of myocardial infarction. Given the frequency of use of selective β_2AAs as well as toxicity and adverse effects, it seems as though myocardial infarction is unlikely to occur. The same cannot be presumed about clenbuterol because the toxicity profile for this drug is still emerging.

Elevation of creatine phosphokinase muscle (CPK-MM) and cardiac (CPK-MB) fractions after large doses of β_2AA, particularly terbutaline infusions and continuous albuterol nebulization, have been well described.[47,48,183] In the absence of electrocardiographic (ECG) changes suggestive of ischemia, the clinical significance of increased CPK-MB and cardiac troponins in patients receiving terbutaline infusions, particularly children, is unclear and has not been demonstrated to correlate with clinically adverse effects.[43]

In therapeutic doses, methylxanthines cause cerebral vasoconstriction, which is a desirable effect when caffeine is used to treat a migraine headache. However, in overdose, this effect likely exacerbates CNS toxicity by diminishing cerebral perfusion.[125] Tolerance to the vasopressor effects of methylxanthines develops after several days of use and rapidly disappears after relatively brief periods of abstinence.

It has been noted that dietary caffeine use is associated with a slight but significant increase in blood pressure that may contribute to population levels of morbidity and mortality.[95] At elevated serum concentrations, patients with methylxanthine or β_2AA poisoning often develop a characteristic widened pulse pressure or divergence of the systolic and diastolic blood pressures. This is caused by enhanced inotropy (β_1), resulting in systolic hypertension combined with peripheral vasodilation (β_2), resulting in diastolic hypotension. In cases of acute theophylline overdose, serum concentrations greater than 100 μg/mL are usually associated with severe hypotension.

Methylxanthines cause renal vasodilation that, in addition to the increased cardiac output, results in a mild diuresis.[139]

Pulmonary Methylxanthines stimulate the CNS respiratory center, causing an increase in respiratory rate. For this reason, caffeine and theophylline are used to treat neonatal apnea syndromes. Caffeine and theophylline overdose may cause hyperventilation, respiratory alkalosis, respiratory failure, respiratory arrest, and acute lung injury.

Neuropsychiatric The stimulant and psychoactive properties of methylxanthines, particularly caffeine, elevate mood and improve performance of manual tasks.[25,35,94] These stimulant effects are typically considered desirable and are one reason caffeine is so widely used. CNS stimulation is an effect sought by users of coffee, tea, cocoa, and chocolate, but CNS stimulation resulting from therapeutic use of theophylline is generally considered to be an undesirable side effect. Although at low doses methylxanthines improve cognitive performance and elevate mood, with increasing doses they result in adverse effects. Headache, anxiety, agitation, insomnia, tremor, irritability, hallucinations, and seizures may result from caffeine or theophylline poisoning. In adults, caffeine doses of 50 to 200 mg result in increased alertness, decreased drowsiness, and lessened fatigue, and caffeine doses of 200 to 500 mg produce adverse effects such as tremor, anxiety, diaphoresis, and palpitations. Children tend to develop CNS symptoms at lower serum theophylline concentrations than adults, and such excitation is a significant clinical disadvantage of theophylline use.

Seizures are a major complication of methylxanthine poisoning. Caffeine's ability to both promote and prolong seizures is well recognized, and caffeine has been used to prolong therapeutically induced seizures in electroconvulsive therapy (ECT).[52,103] Seizures resulting from methylxanthine overdose tend to be severe and recurrent and may be refractory to conventional treatment. Antagonism of adenosine, the endogenous neurotransmitter responsible for halting seizures, contributes to the profound seizures associated with methylxanthine overdose.[59,65,169,198] When studied prospectively, whereas chronic theophylline toxicity results in seizures in 14% of patients, 5% of acutely poisoned patients experience seizures. In cases of chronic and acute-on-chronic toxicity, seizures are more likely to occur, and they occur at lower serum concentrations.[141] Patients at extremes of age—those younger than age 3 years and older than age 60 years—are more likely to experience seizures with overdose.

Musculoskeletal Methylxanthines increase striated muscle contractility, secondarily decreasing muscle fatigue. They also increase muscle oxygen consumption and increase the basal metabolic rate. These effects are sought by users of methylxanthines to enhance or improve athletic performance or weight loss.[9,19,44,60,74,75] Theobromine has the most potent activity to increase muscle contractility—more than 100 times that of caffeine—and theophylline has the least muscle-stimulating activity. All methylxanthines cause smooth muscle relaxation.

Tremor is the most common adverse effect of methylxanthines. Skeletal muscle excitation, which may include fasciculation, hypertonicity, myoclonus, or even rhabdomyolysis, may occur with methylxanthine overdose.[110,120,155,197] Mechanisms by which rhabdomyolysis may result include increased muscle activity, particularly from seizures, and direct cytotoxicity from excessive sequestered intracytoplasmic calcium. Interestingly, there have been multiple case reports of compartment syndrome with rhabdomyolysis resulting from theophylline overdose.[119,185]

Metabolic Numerous metabolic derangements result from acute methylxanthine toxicity and are similar to those in other hyperadrenergic situations.[79,82,159,170]

Severe hypokalemia may result from β_2 adrenergic stimulation.[186] This results from influx of extracellular potassium into the intracellular compartment despite normal total body potassium content. Both ECG and neuromuscular complications of hypokalemia may develop. Other metabolic effects of methylxanthine and β_2AA poisoning include hypomagnesemia and hypophosphatemia.[29,106,191]

Transient hypokalemia resulting from β-adrenergic agonism occurs in 85% of patients with acute theophylline overdose, and typically the serum potassium decreases to approximately 3 mEq/L.[5,173] Stimulation of Na^+-k^+ ATPase results in a shift of serum potassium to the intracellular compartment of skeletal muscle. Total body potassium stores are unchanged. The significance of hypokalemia in patients with methylxanthine overdose is unclear. Vomiting and renal losses do not contribute significantly to hypokalemia, but these may result in fluid loss. Hyperkalemia may result from rhabdomyolysis and overly aggressive repletion of potassium.

Metabolic acidosis with increased serum lactate levels is commonly noted as a complication of theophylline overdose.[24,114] Tachypnea and respiratory alkalosis secondary to stimulation of the respiratory center are also common. Clenbuterol is unique among β_2AAs in that its toxicity is associated with anion gap metabolic acidemia in some cases.

Hyperglycemia, with serum glucose of approximately 200 mg/dL in nondiabetics, is common and occurs in 75% of patients with acute theophylline overdose. Hyperthermia caused by increased metabolic activity and increased muscle activity may result from caffeine and theophylline overdose. Leukocytosis, probably secondary to the high levels of circulating catecholamines, results from acute methylxanthine overdose. This phenomenon apparently lacks clinical significance. In the absence of seizures or protracted emesis, chronic methylxanthine poisoning does not typically lead to metabolic derangements because such toxicity is an ongoing, compensated process.

CHRONIC METHYLXANTHINE TOXICITY

The major difference between acute and chronic toxicity is the duration of exposure to the xenobiotic. Patients with chronic toxicity may manifest subtle signs such as anorexia, nausea, palpitations, or emesis, although they may also present with seizures or dysrhythmias.

Patients chronically receiving theophylline or caffeine have higher total body stores and often underlying medical disorders, and they may develop toxicity with a smaller amount of additional theophylline or caffeine. Chronic methylxanthine poisoning typically occurs in the setting of therapeutic use of theophylline and may occur with iatrogenic administration of caffeine or from frequent, chronic consumption of caffeinated products. Patients often manifest subtle signs of illness, such as anorexia, nausea, palpitations, or emesis. However, the initial presentation in these patients, even with serum concentrations in the 40 to 60 μg/mL range, may be a seizure. In children chronically overdosed with theophylline, the peak serum theophylline concentration may fail to identify those who will progress to life-threatening toxicity. In the absence of protracted emesis or seizures, the initial electrolytes and blood gases are expected to be normal in patients with chronic methylxanthine toxicity.

CHRONIC METHYLXANTHINE USE

An inconclusive link to cancer, heart disease, osteoporosis, hyperlipidemia, and hypercholesterolemia is associated with caffeine use.[63,66,78,151,195] Excessive consumption of caffeine-containing beverages may cause hypokalemia.[154]

Debate centers on the psychiatric and cognitive effects of chronic theophylline use, particularly in children.[118] To date, evidence suggests that although theophylline may acutely result in excessive CNS stimulation and hyperactivity, chronic use of methylxanthines does not adversely affect children's cognitive development.[20]

CAFFEINE WITHDRAWAL

Caffeine induces tolerance, and a withdrawal syndrome, including headache, yawning, nausea, drowsiness, rhinorrhea, lethargy, irritability, nervousness, a disinclination to work, and depression may result upon abstinence.[182] Caffeine withdrawal symptoms are described in neonates born to mothers with consequential caffeine use.[127] The onset of caffeine withdrawal symptoms begins 12 to 24 hours after cessation and lasts up to 1 week.[77] In a double-blind trial, 52% of adults with low to moderate caffeine intake, defined as 2.5 cups of coffee daily, developed a withdrawal syndrome upon caffeine abstinence.[176]

REPRODUCTION

Massive doses of methylxanthines are teratogenic, but the doses of typical use are not associated with birth defects. Decreased fecundity and adverse fetal outcome are noted in animals with chronic exposure to methylxanthines.[67,72,126] Human studies of fertility, fetal loss, and fetal outcome produce divergent results, and the effects of methylxanthines use during gestation are unclear.[91,98,132,136]

DIAGNOSTIC TESTING

An ECG, serum electrolytes, and a serum caffeine or theophylline concentration as appropriate are indicated in cases of suspected methylxanthine toxicity. Because toxicity is dose related in acute overdose, serum concentrations of caffeine and theophylline may be loosely applied as a correlate with toxicity.

Hospitals in which caffeine is used therapeutically, usually for treatment of apnea of prematurity, typically have the capability to assay serum caffeine concentration within the institution. Overdose of caffeine may result in a spuriously elevated serum theophylline concentration.[62,99]

Theophylline concentrations, and to a lesser extent, caffeine concentrations, may be used prognostically to guide management of poisoning. Proper interpretation requires insight into the context of poisoning, that is, whether acute or chronic. In the setting of toxicity, serum methylxanthines concentrations should be obtained immediately and then serially every 1 to 2 hours until a downward trend is evident. In neonates there may be a role for assessment of serum theophylline concentration in the management of suspected caffeine overdose, but such a role is not clearly defined.

Likewise, serum electrolytes, particularly potassium, should be monitored serially as long as the poisoned patient remains symptomatic and such values are in a range that may warrant treatment. Cardiac monitoring should continue until the patient is free of dysrhythmias other than sinus tachycardia, the patient has a decreasing serum methylxanthine concentration, and the patient is clinically stable. In patients with systemic illness, hyperthermia, or increased muscle tone, assessing serum CPK and urinalysis to detect rhabdomyolysis is also indicated.

MANAGEMENT

GENERAL PRINCIPLES AND GASTROINTESTINAL DECONTAMINATION

After assuring adequacy of airway, breathing, and circulation, supportive care and maintenance of vital signs within acceptable limits are the mainstays of therapy for patients with methylxanthine and selective

β_2AA toxicity. Decisions regarding GI decontamination, including orogastric lavage, administration of activated charcoal (AC), or whole-bowel irrigation (WBI), depends on the dosage and type of preparation involved, the time since exposure, and the patient's physical condition. AC is the only GI decontamination that should be routinely considered for selective β_2AA ingestion.

Emesis Induced emesis is not indicated for selective β_2AA ingestion or methylxanthine ingestion. A simulated overdose controlled volunteer study with sustained-release theophylline was unable to demonstrate reduction of absorption of theophylline in patients treated with syrup of ipecac.[136] Seizures are possible with any significant methylxanthine poisoning, and emesis in a patient experiencing a seizure is contraindicated. Because the benefits of emetics are undemonstrated and emesis interferes with administration of AC, induced emesis is rarely considered for those with methylxanthine poisoning.[6,165]

Orogastric Lavage Orogastric lavage may be considered for patients with potentially toxic methylxanthine ingestions who reach medical care immediately after ingestion. Selective β_2AA liquid ingestion that occurs within 1 hour before treatment may warrant aspiration through a nasogastric tube.

Ingestion of sustained-release theophylline tablets is associated with the formation of bezoars that may be difficult to remove or dislodge. Treatment in such cases has included endoscopic removal.[39]

Activated Charcoal AC may play an important role in the treatment of methylxanthine poisoning. AC can adsorb methylxanthines and selective β_2AA present in the GI tract and limit their absorption. Multiple-dose AC (MDAC) is helpful to enhance the elimination of methylxanthine toxicity but is not indicated for selective β_2AA ingestion. MDAC may be useful for any sustained-release preparations of methylxanthine. Additionally, MDAC enhances elimination of theophylline by "gut dialysis" (see Antidote in Depth A2: Activated Charcoal). Such enhanced elimination by gut dialysis is not demonstrated experimentally or otherwise, for caffeine or theobromine toxicity. Because caffeine is to some extent metabolized to theophylline, in cases of caffeine poisoning, MDAC would at the very least enhance elimination of theophylline metabolites. The pharmacologic similarity of the methylxanthines and the relative safety of MDAC therapy warrant the use of such treatment for patients with any methylxanthine toxicity. MDAC is used for enhanced elimination.

Whole-Bowel Irrigation Treatment of patients with significant ingestions of sustained-release pills may include WBI with a balanced electrolyte solution to enhance GI elimination (see Antidotes in Depth A3: Whole-Bowel Irrigation and Other Intestinal Evacuants). Polyethylene glycol electrolyte solution used for WBI may displace theophylline already bound to charcoal.[88] This may be a particular problem in patients who have taken several doses of AC before WBI, in which desorption of methylxanthines from AC may result in a bolus of methylxanthines available for GI absorption. Also, WBI is experimentally demonstrated to provide no additional benefit to AC in treatment of sustained-released theophylline ingestion.[37] Despite these data, WBI with MDAC remains the preferred and recommended treatment of a patient with ingestion of sustained-release theophylline.

Selecting a Method of Decontamination The use of decontamination methods that involve more than minimal risk, specifically orogastric lavage, should only occur after careful consideration of the indications. Patients with potentially life-threatening acute ingestions occurring no more than 1 hour previously may be treated with orogastric lavage (see Chap. 7).

TREATMENT

Gastrointestinal Toxicity Phenothiazine antiemetics are contraindicated in those with methylxanthine poisoning because they are typically ineffective and may lower the seizure threshold. Metoclopramide may be used, but a more potent 5HT$_3$ antagonist antiemetic, such as ondansetron or granisetron, may be required.[51,148,158] Histamine (H$_2$) blockers or proton pump inhibitors may be administered to any patient with hematemesis. Cimetidine is contraindicated because it inhibits CYP450, delaying clearance of methylxanthines.

Cardiovascular Toxicity Hypotension should initially be treated by administration of isotonic IV fluid, such as 0.9% sodium chloride or lactated Ringer solution, in bolus volumes of 20 mL/kg. If acceptable blood pressure cannot be maintained despite several fluid boluses or if there are contraindications to fluid bolus, vasopressor therapy should be considered.

Methylxanthines and selective β_2AA toxicity may cause hypotension via β-adrenergic agonism; therefore, administration of vasopressors with β-adrenergic agonist effects, such as epinephrine, dobutamine, or isoproterenol, are not optimal. An α-adrenergic agonist such as phenylephrine is the first-line pressor of choice in such a situation, although norepinephrine is also acceptable (Table 65–1).

In rare cases of refractory hypotension, the administration of a β-adrenergic antagonist may be warranted.[56] Administration of a β-adrenergic antagonist to a hypotensive patient may seem counterintuitive, but it may reverse β_2-adrenergic mediated vasodilation. In addition, β_1-adrenergic blockade treats tachycardia and any decreased cardiac output that may result from inefficient tachycardiac activity. In dogs with aminophylline-induced tachycardia and hypotension, administration of esmolol results in a return to normal heart rate and blood pressure, and it does not exacerbate hypotension.[68] Propranolol, esmolol, and metoprolol have been used successfully to treat methylxanthine-induced hypotension.[26,145] It is most appropriate to use a β-adrenergic blocker with a brief duration of action, such as esmolol, at least initially, in such circumstances. In the event of an adverse reaction or side effect such as hypotension or bronchospasm, the duration of such will be relatively brief. Any β-adrenergic blocker therapy should ideally be preceded and accompanied by assessment of cardiac output and central venous blood pressure, either directly or noninvasively.[104]

When drug toxicity is not in question, adenosine or electrical cardioversion are the preferred treatment for SVT, but this is not so for SVT resulting from methylxanthine toxicity. Because of the antagonist effects at the adenosine receptor, administration of adenosine should not be expected to convert a methylxanthine-induced SVT. However, even if adenosine is successfully used to convert an SVT, the effect is likely to be transient. Because methylxanthine toxicity has a global effect on the myocardium and methylxanthine concentrations do not change rapidly, cardioversion, which is effective in electrically "reorganizing" depolarization, is unlikely to sustain a normal rhythm.

The primary treatment for methylxanthine-induced SVT includes administration of benzodiazepines, which work to abate CNS stimulation and concomitant release of catecholamines. More focused pharmacologic therapy to treat SVT would be through cautious administration of a conduction-attenuating calcium channel blocker such as diltiazem or verapamil.

In animal models, treatment of acute theophylline toxicity with the calcium channel blockers diltiazem, verapamil, and nifedipine each results in decreased cardiac-related deaths and prevention of dysrhythmias, hypotension, myocardial necrosis, and seizures.[193] In addition to the cardiovascular benefit of calcium channel blockers, they may also afford neurologic protection and prevention of seizure. In non-asthmatic patients, methylxanthine-induced SVT and other tachydysrhythmias may be treated by administration of β-adrenergic antagonist.

Central Nervous System Toxicity Administration of a benzodiazepine, such as diazepam or lorazepam, is appropriate treatment for anxiety, agitation, or seizure. The seizures associated with methylxanthine

TABLE 65–1. Therapeutic Interventions for Methylxanthines and Selective β_2 Adrenergic Agonist Poisoning

System	Indication	Therapeutic Agent	Comments
Cardiovascular	Hypotension	Vasopressors	
		Phenylephrine	
		Norepinephrine	
		β-adrenergic antagonists	Relatively contraindicated in asthmatic patients
		Esmolol	Requires hemodynamic monitoring
		Metoprolol	Hypotension unresponsive to IV fluid
		Propranolol	
	Supraventricular dysrhythmias	Calcium channel blockers	
		Diltiazem	
		Verapamil	
		β-adrenergic antagonists	Relatively contraindicated in asthmatic patients
		Esmolol	Requires hemodynamic monitoring
		Metoprolol	
		Propranolol	
	Ventricular dysrhythmias	Antidysrhythmics	
		Lidocaine	
		β-adrenergic antagonists	Relatively contraindicated in asthmatic patients
		Esmolol	Requires hemodynamic monitoring
		Metoprolol	
		Propranolol	
Gastrointestinal	Emesis	Antiemetics	
		Metoclopramide	
		Ondansetron	
		Granisetron	
	Hematemesis	Proton pump inhibitors	
		Esomeprazole or others	
		H_2 antagonists	Cimetidine is not recommended as it may decrease clearance of methylxanthines and prolong toxicity
		Ranitidine	
		Famotidine	
Central nervous system	Agitation	Benzodiazepines	
	Anxiety	Diazepam	
		Lorazepam	
	Seizure prophylaxis	Benzodiazepines	
	Seizures	Diazepam	
		Lorazepam	
		Barbiturates	
		Phenobarbital	
		Pentobarbital	
		Propofol	
Metabolic	Metabolic acidosis	Sodium bicarbonate (controversial)	Not routinely recommended for this purpose
	Hypokalemia	Potassium chloride	
		β-adrenergic antagonists	Relatively contraindicated in asthmatic patients
		Esmolol	Requires hemodynamic monitoring
		Metoprolol	
		Propranolol	

toxicity are severe and often refractory to treatment. Seizures not controlled with one or two therapeutic doses of a benzodiazepine should be treated with a barbiturate such as phenobarbital or pentobarbital or another suitable sedative–hypnotic such as propofol. No delay should occur before administering such medications. Unsuccessful treatment of methylxanthine-induced seizures with any particular agent should quickly be abandoned in favor of treatment with an additional or more efficacious anticonvulsant. The administration of barbiturates may result in or exacerbate hypotension. Treatment of any aforementioned problem with benzodiazepines, barbiturates, or other sedative–hypnotic may require repeated dosing until clinical effect is achieved.

Administration of phenobarbital to prevent seizures in theophylline-poisoned rabbits and mice increases survival by decreasing the incidence of seizures.[49,73] Although historically, phenobarbital was the recommended drug for such prophylaxis, use of a benzodiazepine such as lorazepam seems preferable based on pharmacokinetic and practical considerations. Patients at risk for seizure include those identified earlier in this chapter—patients older than age 60 years or younger than age 3 years , those with chronic overdose and a serum concentration above 40μg/mL, and acutely overdosed patients with serum levels greater than 100 μg/mL.

Phenytoin and fosphenytoin are of no benefit in controlling methylxanthine-induced seizures and they have no role in such treatment.[87,124] Retrospective review of human cases demonstrated phenytoin to be ineffective in treating seizures in 21 of 22 cases.[93] Phenytoin results in the occurrence of seizures at an earlier time after overdose and results in higher mortality when administered to theophylline-poisoned mice.[27]

Metabolic Derangements Patients with symptomatic hypocalcemia should be treated with electrolyte repletion. Most cases of mild hypokalemia are well tolerated, but any patient with symptomatic hypokalemia, particularly those associated with ECG changes of T waves or QTc prolongation, should be treated. The frequency of ventricular dysrhythmias in methylxanthine poisoning is exacerbated by hypokalemia coupled with increased intrinsic catecholamine release. Correction of hypokalemia may be crucial in methylxanthine poisoning associated with ventricular dysrhythmias.

There is no specific level of hypokalemia that absolutely necessitates treatment. In the absence of associated dysrhythmia, the clinical significance of such hypokalemia is unclear. Although correction is generally performed with the administration of IV or PO potassium, hypokalemia has been experimentally demonstrated to respond to treatment with β-adrenergic antagonist.

Cautious administration of potassium to treat symptomatic hypokalemia may be indicated, but this is distinct from higher doses of potassium used in total body potassium repletion. In cases of hypokalemia secondary to β-adrenergic agonism, after the β-adrenergic agonism returns to baseline level, an efflux of potassium from the intracellular compartment occurs. A concomitant increase of the serum potassium concentration occurs at that time. Overly aggressive attempts to correct hypokalemia may result in hyperkalemia after the β-adrenergic agonist effects abate. Acute methylxanthine-induced hypokalemia may be treated with potassium supplementation, but because of the nature of the problem with excess β-adrenergic agonism, potassium supplementation is typically unnecessary.

Experimentally, administration of propranolol to theophylline-poisoned dogs prevented or partially reversed hypokalemia, hypophosphatemia, hyperglycemia, and metabolic acidosis as well as hypotension.[102] Prevention or correction of the metabolic derangements associated with theophylline toxicity by administration of a β-adrenergic antagonists is congruent with the fact that these derangements, particularly hypokalemia, are the consequence of β-adrenergic agonism. The efficacy of β-adrenergic antagonists as therapy for hypokalemia resulting from acute methylxanthine poisoning in humans is unstudied.

The importance of treating hypomagnesemia, hypophosphatemia, and hypocalcemia is not evident, and these phenomena should be treated as they would for other patients. As with hypokalemia, QTc prolongation is an absolute indication to treat these derangements.

Hyperglycemia, likely resulting from increased circulating catecholamines, is common. This hyperglycemia does not necessitate treatment with any type of hypoglycemic agent, both because it is a transient effect and because in other situations of hyperglycemia resulting from adrenergic agonism, rebound hypoglycemia may occur.

Musculoskeletal Toxicity The use of benzodiazepines is appropriate treatment for fasciculations, hypertonicity, myoclonus, and rhabdomyolysis. Rhabdomyolysis necessitates aggressive IV fluid therapy, possibly with sodium bicarbonate (see Antidotes in Depth: Sodium Bicarbonate).

Enhanced Elimination Fortunately, methylxanthine toxicity lends itself well to several methods of enhanced elimination, including gastrointestinal dialysis with MDAC, charcoal hemoperfusion, and hemodialysis, as well as lesser-used methods such as continuous arteriovenous hemoperfusion (CAVHP), continuous venovenous hemoperfusion (CVVH), and plasmapheresis.[16,111,117]

Infants with methylxanthine poisoning may be too ill, unstable, or small to be treated with hemodialysis or hemoperfusion. Both MDAC and exchange blood transfusion are effective methods of enhanced elimination in infants and may be the preferred method of treatment in these patients if hemodialysis is unavailable.[142,144,172,174]

The therapeutic effects of AC in such cases are much greater than simply limiting absorption of ingested methylxanthines. AC, particularly MDAC, allows elimination of theophylline by way of GI dialysis.[13] MDAC is extremely effective at enhancing elimination of theophylline.[23,69,116,140] Experimentally in dogs, rabbits, and human volunteers, AC administered after IV aminophylline administration results in increased systemic clearance and decreased half-life of theophylline.[90,108,128,146] The pharmacologic similarity of the methylxanthines suggests that MDAC may be effective in GI dialyzing of caffeine or theobromine, and MDAC certainly will be effective in eliminating any theophylline generated from metabolism of caffeine or theobromine. The efficacy of MDAC combined with the safety and ease with which this therapy can be administered make MDAC the mainstay of enhanced elimination in methylxanthine toxicity. Severe emesis associated with methylxanthine poisoning may result in intolerance of MDAC[166] (see Antidotes in Depth: Activated Charcoal).

Charcoal hemoperfusion is the single most effective method of enhanced elimination of methylxanthines, decreasing theophylline's half-life to 2 hours and increasing its clearance possibly up to sixfold.[36,135,156,196] Variations of charcoal hemoperfusion, including albumin colloid hemoperfusion, resin hemoperfusion, and charcoal hemoperfusion in series with hemodialysis, have been reported.[40,89,112,149,181]

If hemoperfusion is available, it is preferable, but because charcoal hemoperfusion is typically unavailable,[167] hemodialysis is acceptable therapy.

Hemodialysis is less efficient than hemoperfusion in the extracorporeal removal of methylxanthines.[8,113,115,177] The ability of hemodialysis to correct fluid and electrolyte imbalances, the greater availability of hemodialysis, greater technical ease, and lower complication rates have resulted in a paradigm shift from considering charcoal hemoperfusion to be the definitive treatment for significant methylxanthine toxicity to one in which charcoal hemoperfusion and hemodialysis are considered equivalent treatment options.[175]

In the treatment of patients with methylxanthine poisoning, the specific indications for hemodialysis are not agreed upon. Several

TABLE 65–2. Methylxanthine Poisoning: Indications for Charcoal Hemoperfusion or Hemodialysis

1. Acute serum theophylline or caffeine concentration >90 μg/mL and any symptom
2. Serum theophylline or caffeine concentration >40 μg/mL and
   A. Seizures
   B. Hypotension unresponsive to intravenous fluid or
   C. Ventricular dysrhythmias

studies and clinical experience are the basis for the following suggested indications for extracorporeal elimination by charcoal hemoperfusion, hemodialysis, combined charcoal hemoperfusion and hemodialysis, or combined hemodialysis and MDAC.

Many recommendations regarding hemoperfusion and hemodialysis for theophylline toxicity use serum theophylline concentration as a guideline. Serum levels may not be available in instances of caffeine poisoning and do not exist for theobromine poisoning. Thus, the clinical aspects of theophylline management guidelines can be generalized to all methylxanthine toxicities.

When indicated, hemodialysis preferably should be initiated while the patient is still hemodynamically stable. Hemodialysis therapy should be used for patients with consequential chronic theophylline poisoning associated with a serum theophylline concentration above 40 to 60 μg/mL or with a deteriorating clinical status.

Hemodialysis should be strongly considered any time a methylxanthine exposure results in a serum theophylline or caffeine concentration of greater than 90 μg/mL and symptoms, regardless of clinical stability (Table 65–2). Any patient with a symptomatic methylxanthine poisoning that is associated with ventricular dysrhythmias, seizures, hypotension unresponsive to fluids, or emesis unresponsive to antiemetics should also be treated with charcoal hemoperfusion, hemodialysis, or both.

The fact that a patient experiences seizure or dysrhythmias or becomes extremely ill is not a contraindication for extracorporeal drug removal. To the contrary, these events make administration of such therapy more critical to ensure survival of the patient.

TREATMENT OF CHRONIC METHYLXANTHINE TOXICITY

Treatment of chronic methylxanthine toxicity is determined by the patient's clinical status and by the efficacy of MDAC. The precise serum theophylline or caffeine concentration at which patients with chronic theophylline or caffeine toxicity should receive hemodialysis is controversial. For a hemodynamically stable patient without signs of life-threatening methylxanthine toxicity such as ventricular dysrhythmias or seizure, therapy with MDAC may be sufficient. If the serum theophylline or caffeine concentration does not decline after the administration of AC or if the patient's clinical status deteriorates, hemodialysis is indicated.

TREATMENT OF ACUTE-ON-CHRONIC METHYLXANTHINE TOXICITY

Patients chronically receiving theophylline or caffeine who acutely overdose should be initially managed in the same manner as patients with acute overdose, although action concentrations for dialysis are the same for chronic toxicity. Total body stores of the methylxanthines are higher in patients who are chronically exposed, and the threshold for toxicity may be reached at lower serum concentrations.

SUMMARY

Selective β_2AAs were widely used for the treatment of bronchospasm. Selective β_2AA toxicity typically results from excessive therapeutic use of these agents, but illicit use of clenbuterol or admixture of clenbuterol with drugs of abuse has become prominent. Methylxanthine toxicity results from both the use of medicinal and therapeutic agents as well as from consumption of methylxanthine-containing foods and beverages. There are significant differences in the clinical presentation and management of patients with acute and chronic methylxanthine poisoning. Supportive care and treatment of GI, cardiovascular, CNS, metabolic, and musculoskeletal toxicities are the mainstay of therapy. The unique properties of methylxanthines necessitate specific therapies for the GI, cardiovascular, and CNS toxicities of methylxanthines. With some unique exceptions, selective β_2AA toxicity is usually well tolerated and only requires supportive care. Clenbuterol is such an exception, and toxicity from this substance is typically more severe than that from other β_2AA. For this reason, clenbuterol toxicity should be managed with greater caution and cognizance for the potential for severe morbidity and possible mortality from this substance.

Methods of enhanced elimination, particularly extracorporeal elimination by charcoal hemoperfusion, hemodialysis, or charcoal hemoperfusion and hemodialysis in series, as well as gut dialysis with MDAC, are effective treatments for patients with methylxanthine toxicity. Supportive care is typically the management strategy for β_2AAs.

REFERENCES

1. Aldridge A, Aranda JV, Neims AH. Caffeine metabolism in the newborn. *Clin Pharmacol Ther.* 1979;25:447-453.
2. American Society of Health-System Pharmacists. Albuterol. In: McEvoy GK, ed. *AHFS Drug Information 2004*. Bethesda, MD: American Society of Health-System Pharmacists, Inc; 2004.
3. American Society of Health-System Pharmacists. Terbutaline. In: McEvoy GK, ed. *AHFS Drug Information 2004*. Bethesda, MD: American Society of Health-System Pharmacists, Inc; 2004.
4. Amitai Y, Lovejoy FH Jr. Characteristics of vomiting associated with acute sustained release theophylline poisoning: implications for management with oral activated charcoal. *J Toxicol Clin Toxicol.* 1987;25:539-554.
5. Amitai Y, Lovejoy FH Jr. Hypokalemia in acute theophylline poisoning. *Am J Emerg Med.* 1988;6:214-218.
6. Amitai Y, Yeung AC, Moye J, Lovejoy FH Jr. Repetitive oral activated charcoal and control of emesis in severe theophylline toxicity. *Ann Intern Med.* 1986;105:386-387.
7. Anderson BJ, Gunn TR, Holford NH, Johnson R. Caffeine overdose in a premature infant: clinical course and pharmacokinetics. *Anaesth Intensive Care.* 1999;27:307-311.
8. Anderson JR, Poklis A, McQueen RC, et al. Effects of hemodialysis on theophylline kinetics. *J Clin Pharmacol.* 1983;23:428-432.
9. Anselme F, Collomp K, Mercier B, et al. Caffeine increases maximal anaerobic power and blood lactate concentration. *Eur J Appl Physiol Occup Physiol.* 1992;65:188-191.
10. Aranda JV, Collinge JM, Zinman R, Watters G. Maturation of caffeine elimination in infancy. *Arch Dis Child.* 1979;54:946-949.
11. Aranda JV, Cook CE, Gorman W, et al. Pharmacokinetic profile of caffeine in the premature newborn infant with apnea. *J Pediatr.* 1979;94:663-668.
12. Aranda JV, Sitar DS, Parsons WD, et al. Pharmacokinetic aspects of theophylline in premature newborns. *N Engl J Med.* 1976;295:413-416.
13. Arimori K, Nakano M. Transport of theophylline from blood to the intestinal lumen following i.v. administration to rats. *J Pharmacobiodyn.* 1985;8:324-327.
14. Arwood LL, Dasta JF, Friedman C. Placental transfer of theophylline: two case reports. *Pediatrics.* 1979;63:844-846.

15. Astrup A. Thermogenic drugs as a strategy for treatment of obesity. *Endocrine.* 2000;13:207-212.
16. Bania TC, Hoffman RS, Howland MA, et al. Plasmapheresis for theophylline intoxication. *Vet Hum Toxicol.* 1992;34:330.
17. Banner W Jr, Czajka PA. Acute caffeine overdose in the neonate. *Am J Dis Child.* 1980;134:495-498.
18. Barbosa J, Cruz C, Martins J, et al. Food poisoning by clenbuterol in Portugal. *Food Additives & Contaminants.* 2005;22:563-566.
19. Bell DG, Jacobs I, Zamecnik J. Effects of caffeine, ephedrine and their combination on time to exhaustion during high-intensity exercise. *Eur J Appl Physiol Occup Physiol.* 1998;77:427-433.
20. Bender BG, Ikle DN, DuHamel T, Tinkelman D. Neuropsychological and behavioral changes in asthmatic children treated with beclomethasone dipropionate versus theophylline. *Pediatrics.* 1998;101:355-360.
21. Bender PR, Brent J, Kulig K. Cardiac arrhythmias during theophylline toxicity. *Chest.* 1991;100:884-886.
22. Benowitz NL, Osterloh J, Goldschlager N, et al. Massive catecholamine release from caffeine poisoning. *JAMA.* 1982;248:1097-1098.
23. Berlinger WG, Spector R, Goldberg MJ, et al. Enhancement of theophylline clearance by oral activated charcoal. *Clin Pharmacol Ther.* 1983;33:351-354.
24. Bernard S. Severe lactic acidosis following theophylline overdose. *Ann Emerg Med.* 1991;20:1135-1137.
25. Bernstein GA, Carroll ME, Crosby RD, et al. Caffeine effects on learning, performance, and anxiety in normal school-age children. *J Am Acad Child Adolesc Psychiatry.* 1994;33:407-415.
26. Biberstein MP, Ziegler MG, Ward DM. Use of beta-blockade and hemoperfusion for acute theophylline poisoning. *West J Med.* 1984;141:485-490.
27. Blake KV, Massey KL, Hendeles L, et al. Relative efficacy of phenytoin and phenobarbital for the prevention of theophylline-induced seizures in mice. *Ann Emerg Med.* 1988;17:1024-1028.
28. Bloss JD, Hankins GD, Gilstrap LC 3rd, Hauth JC. Pulmonary edema as a delayed complication of ritodrine therapy. A case report. *J Reprod Med.* 1987;32:469-471.
29. Bodenhamer J, Bergstrom R, Brown D, et al. Frequently nebulized beta-agonists for asthma: effects on serum electrolytes. *Ann Emerg Med.* 1992;21:1337-1342.
30. Bonati M, Latini R, Sadurska B, et al. Kinetics and metabolism of theobromine in male rats. *Toxicology.* 984;30:327-341.
31. Bory C, Baltassat P, Porthault M, et al. Metabolism of theophylline to caffeine in premature newborn infants. *J Pediatr.* 1979;94:988-993.
32. Brouard C, Moriette G, Murat I, et al. Comparative efficacy of theophylline and caffeine in the treatment of idiopathic apnea in premature infants. *Am J Dis Child.* 1985;139:698-700.
33. Brown CR, Jacob P 3rd, Wilson M, Benowitz NL. Changes in rate and pattern of caffeine metabolism after cigarette abstinence. *Clin Pharmacol Ther.* 1988;43:488-491.
34. Bruce CR, Anderson ME, Fraser SF, et al. Enhancement of 2000-m rowing performance after caffeine ingestion. *Med Sci Sports Exerc.* 2000;32:1958-1963.
35. Bryant CA, Farmer A, Tiplady B, et al. Psychomotor performance: investigating the dose-response relationship for caffeine and theophylline in elderly volunteers. *Eur J Clin Pharmacol.* 1998;54:309-313.
36. Burgess E, Sargious P. Charcoal hemoperfusion for theophylline overdose: case report and proposal for predicting treatment time. *Pharmacotherapy.* 1995;15:621-624.
37. Burkhart KK, Wuerz RC, Donovan JW. Whole-bowel irrigation as adjunctive treatment for sustained-release theophylline overdose. *Ann Emerg Med.* 1992;21:1316-1320.
38. Centers for Disease Control and Prevention. Atypical reactions associated with heroin use—five states, January–April 2005. *MMWR Morbid Mortal Wkly Rep.* 2005;54:793-796.
39. Cereda JM, Scott J, Quigley EM. Endoscopic removal of pharmacobezoar of slow release theophylline. *Br Med J (Clin Res Ed).* 1986;293:1143.
40. Chang TM, Espinosa-Melendez E, Francoeur TE, Eade NR. Albumin-collodion activated charcoal hemoperfusion in the treatment of severe theophylline intoxication in a 3-year-old patient. *Pediatrics.* 1980;65:811-814.
41. Chazan R, Karwat K, Tyminska K, et al. Cardiac arrhythmias as a result of intravenous infusions of theophylline in patients with airway obstruction. *Int J Clin Pharmacol Ther* 1995;33:170-175.
42. Chelben J, Piccone-Sapir A, Ianco J, et al. Effects of amino acid energy drinks leading to hospitalization in individuals with mental illness. *Gen Hosp Psychiatry.* 2008;30:187-189.
43. Chiang VW, Burns JP, Rifai N, et al. Cardiac toxicity of intravenous terbutaline for the treatment of severe asthma in children: a prospective assessment. *J Pediatr.* 2000;137:73-77.
44. Cohen BS, Nelson AG, Prevost MC, et al. Effects of caffeine ingestion on endurance racing in heat and humidity. *Eur J Appl Physiol Occup Physiol.* 1996;73:358-363.
45. Cohen S, Booth GH, Jr. Gastric acid secretion and lower-esophageal-sphincter pressure in response to coffee and caffeine. *N Engl J Med.* 1975;293:897-899.
46. Conolly ME, Tashkin DP, Hui KK, et al. Selective subsensitization of beta-adrenergic receptors in central airways of asthmatics and normal subjects during long-term therapy with inhaled salbutamol. *J Allergy Clin Immunol.* 1982;70:423-431.
47. Craig TJ, Smits W, Soontornniyomkiu V. Elevation of creatine kinase from skeletal muscle associated with inhaled albuterol. *Ann Allergy Asthma Immunol.* 1996;77:488-490.
48. Craig VL, Bigos D, Brilli RJ. Efficacy and safety of continuous albuterol nebulization in children with severe status asthmaticus. *Pediatr Emerg Care.* 1996;12:1-5.
49. Czuczwar SJ, Janusz W, Wamil A, Kleinrok Z. Inhibition of aminophylline-induced convulsions in mice by antiepileptic drugs and other agents. *Eur J Pharmacol.* 1987;144:309-315.
50. Dalvi RR. Acute and chronic toxicity of caffeine: a review. *Vet Hum Toxicol.* 1986;28:144-150.
51. Daly D, Taylor JN. Ondansetron in theophylline overdose. *Anaesth Intensive Care.* 1993;21:474-475.
52. Datto C, Rai AK, Ilivicky HJ, Caroff SN. Augmentation of seizure induction in electroconvulsive therapy: a clinical reappraisal. *J ECT.* 2002;18:118-125.
53. Daubert GP, Mabasa VH, Leung VW, Aaron C. Acute clenbuterol overdose resulting in supraventricular tachycardia and atrial fibrillation. *J Med Toxicol.* 2007;3:56-60.
54. Denaro CP, Wilson M, Jacob P,3rd, Benowitz NL. The effect of liver disease on urine caffeine metabolite ratios. *Clin Pharmacol Ther.* 1996;59:624-635.
55. Derlet RW, Tseng JC, Albertson TE. Potentiation of cocaine and d-amphetamine toxicity with caffeine. *Am J Emerg Med.* 1992;10:211-216.
56. Dettloff RW, Touchette MA, Zarowitz BJ. Vasopressor-resistant hypotension following a massive ingestion of theophylline. *Ann Pharmacother.* 1993;27:781-784.
57. Drolet R, Arendt TD, Stowe CM. Cacao bean shell poisoning in a dog. *J Am Vet Med Assoc.* 1984;185:902.
58. Drouillard DD, Vesell ES, Dvorchik BH. Studies on theobromine disposition in normal subjects: alterations induced by dietary abstention from or exposure to methylxanthines. *Clin Pharmacol Ther.* 1978;23:296-302.
59. Eldridge FL, Paydarfar D, Scott SC, Dowell RT. Role of endogenous adenosine in recurrent generalized seizures. *Exp Neurol.* 1989;103:179-185.
60. Falk B, Burstein R, Ashkenazi I, et al. The effect of caffeine ingestion on physical performance after prolonged exercise. *Eur J Appl Physiol Occup Physiol.* 1989;59:168-173.
61. Fisher AA, Davis MW, McGill DA. Acute myocardial infarction associated with albuterol. *Ann Pharmacother.* 2004;38:2045-2049.
62. Fligner CL, Opheim KE. Caffeine and its dimethylxanthine metabolites in two cases of caffeine overdose: a cause of falsely elevated theophylline concentrations in serum. *J Anal Toxicol.* 1988;12:339-343.
63. Folsom AR, McKenzie DR, Bisgard KM, et al. No association between caffeine intake and postmenopausal breast cancer incidence in the Iowa Women's Health Study. *Am J Epidemiol.* 1993;138:380-383.
64. Forman J, Aizer A, Young CR. Myocardial infarction resulting from caffeine overdose in an anorectic woman. *Ann Emerg Med.* 1997;29:178-180.
65. Fredholm BB. Theophylline actions on adenosine receptors. *Eur J Respir Dis Suppl.* 1980;109:29-36.
66. Fried RE, Levine DM, Kwiterovich PO, et al. The effect of filtered-coffee consumption on plasma lipid levels. results of a randomized clinical trial. *JAMA.* 1992;267:811-815.
67. Friedman L, Weinberger MA, Farber TM, et al. Testicular atrophy and impaired spermatogenesis in rats fed high levels of the methylxanthines caffeine, theobromine, or theophylline. *J Environ Pathol Toxicol.* 1979;2:687-706.
68. Gaar GG, Banner W Jr, Laddu AR. The effects of esmolol on the hemodynamics of acute theophylline toxicity. *Ann Emerg Med.* 1987;16:1334-1339.

69. Gal P, Miller A, McCue JD. Oral activated charcoal to enhance theophylline elimination in an acute overdose. *JAMA*. 1984;251:3130-3131.
70. Gartrell BD, Reid C. Death by chocolate: a fatal problem for an inquisitive wild parrot. *N Z Vet J*. 2007;55:149-151.
71. Giacoia G, Jusko WJ, Menke J, Koup JR. Theophylline pharmacokinetics in premature infants with apnea. *J Pediatr*. 1976;89:829-832.
72. Gilbert SG, Rice DC. Somatic development of the infant monkey following in utero exposure to caffeine. *Fundam Appl Toxicol*. 1991;17:454-465.
73. Goldberg MJ, Spector R, Miller G. Phenobarbital improves survival in theophylline-intoxicated rabbits. *J Toxicol Clin Toxicol*. 1986;24:203-211.
74. Graham TE, Rush JW, van Soeren MH. Caffeine and exercise: metabolism and performance. *Can J Appl Physiol*. 1994;19:111-138.
75. Graham TE, Spriet LL. Metabolic, catecholamine, and exercise performance responses to various doses of caffeine. *J Appl Physiol*. 1995;78:867-874.
76. Greenway FL. The safety and efficacy of pharmaceutical and herbal caffeine and ephedrine use as a weight loss agent. *Obes Rev*. 2001;2:199-211.
77. Griffiths RR, Woodson PP. Caffeine physical dependence: a review of human and laboratory animal studies. *Psychopharmacology (Berl)*. 1988;94:437-451.
78. Grobbee DE, Rimm EB, Giovannucci E, et al. Coffee, caffeine, and cardiovascular disease in men. *N Engl J Med*. 1990;323:1026-1032.
79. Grygiel JJ, Birkett DJ. Cigarette smoking and theophylline clearance and metabolism. *Clin Pharmacol Ther*. 1981;30:491-496.
80. Hadeed A, Siegel S. Newborn cardiac arrhythmias associated with maternal caffeine use during pregnancy. *Clin Pediatr (Phila)*. 1993;32:45-47.
81. Hagley MT, Traeger SM, Schuckman H. Pronounced metabolic response to modest theophylline overdose. *Ann Pharmacother*. 1994;28:195-196.
82. Hall KW, Dobson KE, Dalton JG, et al. Metabolic abnormalities associated with intentional theophylline overdose. *Ann Intern Med*. 1984;101:457-462.
83. Haller CA, Benowitz NL. Adverse cardiovascular and central nervous system events associated with dietary supplements containing ephedra alkaloids. *N Engl J Med*. 2000;343:1833-1838.
84. Hanington E, Bell H. Suspected chocolate poisoning of calves. *Vet Rec*. 1972;90:408-409.
85. Hantson P, Gautier P, Vekemans MC, et al. Acute myocardial infarction in a young woman: possible relationship with sustained-release theophylline acute overdose? *Intensive Care Med*. 1992;18:496.
86. Hayes AH. New drug status of OTC combination products containing caffeine, phenylpropanolamine, and ephedrine. *Fed Reg*. 1982;47:35344-35346.
87. Hoffman A, Pinto E, Gilhar D. Effect of pretreatment with anticonvulsants on theophylline-induced seizures in the rat. *J Crit Care*. 1993;8:198-202.
88. Hoffman RS, Chiang WK, Howland MA, et al. Theophylline desorption from activated charcoal caused by whole bowel irrigation solution. *J Toxicol Clin Toxicol*. 1991;29:191-201.
89. Hootkins RS, Lerman MJ, Thompson JR. Sequential and simultaneous "in series" hemodialysis and hemoperfusion in the management of theophylline intoxication. *J Am Soc Nephrol*. 1990;1:923-926.
90. Huang JD. Kinetics of theophylline clearance in gastrointestinal dialysis with charcoal. *J Pharm Sci*. 1987;76:525-527.
91. Infante-Rivard C, Fernandez A, Gauthier R, et al. Fetal loss associated with caffeine intake before and during pregnancy. *JAMA*. 1993;270:2940-2943.
92. Jackson SH, Johnston A, Woollard R, Turner P. The relationship between theophylline clearance and age in adult life. *Eur J Clin Pharmacol*. 1989;36:29-34.
93. Jacobs MH, Senior RM. Theophylline toxicity due to impaired theophylline degradation. *Am Rev Respir Dis*. 1974;110:342-345.
94. Jacobson BH, Thurman-Lacey SR. Effect of caffeine on motor performance by caffeine-naive and familiar subjects. *Percept Mot Skills*. 1992;74:151-157.
95. James JE. Critical review of dietary caffeine and blood pressure: a relationship that should be taken more seriously. *Psychosom Med*. 2004;66:63-71.
96. January B, Seibold A, Whaley B, et al. Beta2-adrenergic receptor desensitization, internalization, and phosphorylation in response to full and partial agonists. *J Biol Chem*. 1997;272:23871-23879.
97. Jenny RW, Jackson KY. Two types of error found with the seralyzer ARIS assay of theophylline. *Clin Chem*. 1986;32:2122-2123.
98. Jensen TK, Henriksen TB, Hjollund NH, et al. Caffeine intake and fecundability: a follow-up study among 430 Danish couples planning their first pregnancy. *Reprod Toxicol*. 1998;12:289-295.
99. Johnson M. The β adrenoreceptor. *Am J Respir Crit Care Med*. 1998;58:S146-S153.
100. Juhn M. Popular sports supplements and ergogenic aids. *Sports Med*. 2003;33:921-939.
101. Kamimori GH, Penetar DM, Headley DB, et al. Effect of three caffeine doses on plasma catecholamines and alertness during prolonged wakefulness. *Eur J Clin Pharmacol*. 2000;56:537-544.
102. Kearney TE, Manoguerra AS, Curtis GP, Ziegler MG. Theophylline toxicity and the beta-adrenergic system. *Ann Intern Med*. 1985;102:766-769.
103. Kelsey MC, Grossberg GT. Safety and efficacy of caffeine-augmented ECT in elderly depressives: a retrospective study. *J Geriatr Psychiatry Neurol*. 1995;8:168-172.
104. Kempf J, Rusterholtz T, Ber C, Gayol S, et al. Haemodynamic study as guideline for the use of beta blockers in acute theophylline poisoning. *Intensive Care Med*. 1996;22:585-587.
105. Kierzkowska B, Stanczyk J, Kasprzak JD. Myocardial infarction in a 17 year-old body builder using clenbuterol. *Circulation*. 2005;69:1144-1146.
106. King WD, Holloway M, Palmisano PA. Albuterol overdose: a case report and differential diagnosis. *Pediatr Emerg Care*. 1992;8:268-271.
107. Kraft M, Torvik JA, Trudeau JB, et al. Theophylline. Potential antiinflammatory effects in nocturnal asthma. *J Allergy Clin Immunol*. 1996;97:1242-1246.
108. Kulig KW, Bar-Or D, Rumack BH. Intravenous theophylline poisoning and multiple-dose charcoal in an animal model. *Ann Emerg Med*. 1987;16:842-846.
109. Labovitz E, Spector S. Placental theophylline transfer in pregnant asthmatics. *JAMA*. 1982;247:786-788.
110. Laurence AS, Wight J, Forrest AR. Fatal theophylline poisoning with rhabdomyolysis. *Anaesthesia*. 1992;47:82.
111. Laussen P, Shann F, Butt W, Tibballs J. Use of plasmapheresis in acute theophylline toxicity. *Crit Care Med*. 1991;19:288-290.
112. Lawyer C, Aitchison J, Sutton J, Bennett W. Treatment of theophylline neurotoxicity with resin hemoperfusion. *Ann Intern Med*. 1978;88:516-517.
113. Lee CS, Marbury TC, Perrin JH, Fuller TJ. Hemodialysis of theophylline in uremic patients. *J Clin Pharmacol*. 1979;19:219-226.
114. Leventhal LJ, Kochar G, Feldman NH, et al. Lactic acidosis in theophylline overdose. *Am J Emerg Med*. 1989;7:417-418.
115. Levy G, Gibson TP, Whitman W, Procknal J. Hemodialysis clearance of theophylline. *JAMA*. 1977;237:1466-1467.
116. Lim DT, Singh P, Nourtsis S, Dela Cruz R. Absorption inhibition and enhancement of elimination of sustained-release theophylline tablets by oral activated charcoal. *Ann Emerg Med*. 1986;15:1303-1307.
117. Lin JL, Jeng LB. Critical, acutely poisoned patients treated with continuous arteriovenous hemoperfusion in the emergency department. *Ann Emerg Med*. 1995;25:75-80.
118. Lindgren S, Lokshin B, Stromquist A, et al. Does asthma or treatment with theophylline limit children's academic performance? *N Engl J Med*. 1992;327:926-930.
119. Lloyd DM, Payne SP, Tomson CR, et al. Acute compartment syndrome secondary to theophylline overdose. *Lancet*. 1990;336:312.
120. Macdonald JB, Jones HM, Cowan RA. Rhabdomyolysis and acute renal failure after theophylline overdose. *Lancet*. 1985;1:932-933.
121. Maddux MS, Leeds NH, Organek HW, et al. The effect of erythromycin on theophylline pharmacokinetics at steady state. *Chest*. 1982;81:563-565.
122. Malinauskas BM, Aeby VG, Overton RF, Carpenter-Aeby T, Barber-Heidal K. A survey of energy drink consumption among college students. *Nutr J*. 2007;6:35.
123. Mangione A, Imhoff TE, Lee RV, et al. Pharmacokinetics of theophylline in hepatic disease. *Chest*. 1978;73:616-622.
124. Marquis JF, Carruthers SG, Spence JD, et al. Phenytoin-theophylline interaction. *N Engl J Med*. 1982;307:1189-1190.
125. Mathew RJ, Wilson WH. Caffeine induced changes in cerebral circulation. *Stroke*. 1985;16:814-817.
126. Matsuoka R, Uno H, Tanaka H, et al. Caffeine induces cardiac and other malformations in the rat. *Am J Med Genet Suppl*. 1987;3:433-443.
127. McGowan JD, Altman RE, Kanto WP, Jr. Neonatal withdrawal symptoms after chronic maternal ingestion of caffeine. *South Med J*. 1988;81:1092-1094.
128. McKinnon RS, Desmond PV, Harman PJ, et al. Studies on the mechanisms of action of activated charcoal on theophylline pharmacokinetics. *J Pharm Pharmacol*. 1987;39:522-525.

129. McQuay HJ, Angell K, Carroll D, et al. Ibuprofen compared with ibuprofen plus caffeine after third molar surgery. *Pain*. 1996;66:247-251.
130. Mehta A, Jain AC, Mehta MC, Billie M. Caffeine and cardiac arrhythmias: an experimental study in dogs with review of literature. *Acta Cardiol.* 1997;52:273-283.
131. Migliardi JR, Armellino JJ, Friedman M, et al. Caffeine as an analgesic adjuvant in tension headache. *Clin Pharmacol Ther*. 1994;56:576-586.
132. Mills JL, Holmes LB, Aarons JH, et al. Moderate caffeine use and the risk of spontaneous abortion and intrauterine growth retardation. *JAMA*. 1993;269:593-597.
133. Minton NA, Glucksman E, Henry JA. Prevention of drug absorption in simulated theophylline overdose. *Hum Exp Toxicol*. 1995;14:170-174.
134. Muro M, Shono H, Oga M, et al. Ritodrine-induced agranulocytosis. *Int J Gynaecol Obstet*. 1991;36:329-331.
135. Nagesh RV, Murphy KA Jr. Caffeine poisoning treated by hemoperfusion. *Am J Kidney Dis*. 1988;12:316-318.
136. Nehlig A, Debry G. Potential teratogenic and neurodevelopmental consequences of coffee and caffeine exposure: a review on human and animal data. *Neurotoxicol Teratol*. 1994;16:531-543.
137. Nicot G, Charmes JP, Lachatre G, et al. Theophylline toxicity risks and chronic renal failure. *Int J Clin Pharmacol Ther Toxicol*. 1989;27:398-401.
138. Nix DE, Di Cicco RA, Miller AK, et al. The effect of low-dose cimetidine (200 mg twice daily) on the pharmacokinetics of theophylline. *J Clin Pharmacol.* 1999;39:855-865.
139. Nobel PA, Light GS. Theophylline-induced diuresis in the neonate. *J Pediatr*. 1977;90:825-826.
140. Ohning BL, Reed MD, Blumer JL. Continuous nasogastric administration of activated charcoal for the treatment of theophylline intoxication. *Pediatr Pharmacol (New York)*. 1986;5:241-245.
141. Olson KR, Benowitz NL, Woo OF, Pond SM. Theophylline overdose: acute single ingestion versus chronic repeated overmedication. *Am J Emerg Med.* 1985;3:386-394.
142. Osborn HH, Henry G, Wax P, et al. Theophylline toxicity in a premature neonate—elimination kinetics of exchange transfusion. *J Toxicol Clin Toxicol*. 1993;31:639-644.
143. Parr MJ, Willatts SM. Fatal theophylline poisoning with rhabdomyolysis. A potential role for dantrolene treatment. *Anaesthesia*. 1991;46:557-559.
144. Perrin C, Debruyne D, Lacotte J, et al. Treatment of caffeine intoxication by exchange transfusion in a newborn. *Acta Paediatr Scand*. 1987;76:679-681.
145. Price KR, Fligner DJ. Treatment of caffeine toxicity with esmolol. *Ann Emerg Med*. 1990;19:44-46.
146. Radomski L, Park GD, Goldberg MJ, et al. Model for theophylline overdose treatment with oral activated charcoal. *Clin Pharmacol Ther*. 1984;35:402-408.
147. Resman BH, Blumenthal P, Jusko WJ. Breast milk distribution of theobromine from chocolate. *J Pediatr*. 1977;91:477-480.
148. Roberts JR, Carney S, Boyle SM, Lee DC. Ondansetron quells drug-resistant emesis in theophylline poisoning. *Am J Emerg Med*. 1993;11:609-610.
149. Rongved G, Westlie L. Hemoperfusion/hemodialysis in the treatment of acute theophylline poisoning—description of a fatal case. *Int J Clin Pharmacol Ther Toxicol*. 1986;24:85-87.
150. Rosenberg J, Benowitz NL, Pond S. Pharmacokinetics of drug overdose. *Clin Pharmacokinet*. 1981;6:161-192.
151. Ross PD. Osteoporosis: frequency, consequences, and risk factors. *Arch Intern Med*.1996;156:1399-1411.
152. Rovei V, Chanoine F, Strolin Benedetti M. Pharmacokinetics of theophylline: a dose-range study. *Br J Clin Pharmacol*. 1982;14:769-778.
153. Roy AK, Cuda MP, Levine RA. Induction of theophylline toxicity and inhibition of clearance rates by ranitidine. *Am J Med*. 1988;85:525-527.
154. Rudy DR, Lee S. Coffee and hypokalemia. *J Fam Pract*. 1988;26:679-680.
155. Rumpf KW, Wagner H, Criee CP, et al. Rhabdomyolysis after theophylline overdose. *Lancet*. 1985;1:1451-1452.
156. Russo ME. Management of theophylline intoxication with charcoal-column hemoperfusion. *N Engl J Med*. 1979;300:24-26.
157. Ryan T, Coughlan G, McGing P, Phelan D. Ketosis, a complication of theophylline toxicity. *J Intern Med*. 1989;226:277-278.
158. Sage TA, Jones WN, Clark RF. Ondansetron in the treatment of intractable nausea associated with theophylline toxicity. *Ann Pharmacother*. 1993;27:584-585.
159. Saltpeter SR, Buckley NS, Ormiston TM, et al. Meta-analysis: effect of long-acting beta agonists on severe asthma exacerbations and asthma-related deaths. *Ann Intern Med*. 2006;144:904-912.
160. Sawyer WT, Caravati EM, Ellison MJ, Krueger KA. Hypokalemia, hyperglycemia, and acidosis after intentional theophylline overdose. *Am J Emerg Med*. 1985;3:408-411.
161. Sawynok J, Yaksh TL. Caffeine as an analgesic adjuvant: a review of pharmacology and mechanisms of action. *Pharmacol Rev*. 1993;45:43-85.
162. Schachtel BP, Fillingim JM, Lane AC, et al. Caffeine as an analgesic adjuvant. A double-blind study comparing aspirin with caffeine to aspirin and placebo in patients with sore throat. *Arch Intern Med*. 1991;151:733-737.
163. Seidl R, Peyrl A, Nicham R, Hauser E. A taurine and caffeine-containing drink stimulates cognitive performance and well-being. *Amino Acids*. 2000;19:635-642.
164. Sessler CN, Cohen MD. Cardiac arrhythmias during theophylline toxicity. A prospective continuous electrocardiographic study. *Chest*. 1990;98:672-678.
165. Sessler CN. Poor tolerance of oral activated charcoal with theophylline overdose. *Am J Emerg Med*. 1987;5:492-495.
166. Sessler CN, Glauser FL, Cooper KR. Treatment of theophylline toxicity with oral activated charcoal. *Chest*. 1985;87:325-329.
167. Shalkham AS, Kirrane BM, Hoffman RS, et al. The availability and use of charcoal hemoperfusion in the treatment of poisoned patients. *Am J Kidney Dis*. 2006;48:239-241.
168. Shannon M. Life-threatening events after theophylline overdose: a 10-year prospective analysis. *Arch Intern Med*. 1999;159:989-994.
169. Shannon M, Maher T. Anticonvulsant effects of intracerebroventricular adenocard in theophylline-induced seizures. *Ann Emerg Med*. 1995;26:65-68.
170. Shannon M. Hypokalemia, hyperglycemia and plasma catecholamine activity after severe theophylline intoxication. *J Toxicol Clin Toxicol.* 1994;32:41-47.
171. Shannon M. Predictors of major toxicity after theophylline overdose. *Ann Intern Med*. 1993;119:1161-1167.
172. Shannon M, Wernovsky G, Morris C. Exchange transfusion in the treatment of severe theophylline poisoning. *Pediatrics*. 1992;89:145-147.
173. Shannon M, Lovejoy FH Jr. Hypokalemia after theophylline intoxication: the effects of acute vs chronic poisoning. *Arch Intern Med*. 1989;149:2725-2729.
174. Shannon M, Amitai Y, Lovejoy FH Jr. Multiple dose activated charcoal for theophylline poisoning in young infants. *Pediatrics*. 1987;80:368-370.
175. Shannon MW. Comparative efficacy of hemodialysis and hemoperfusion in severe theophylline intoxication. *Acad Emerg Med*. 1997;4:674-678.
176. Silverman K, Evans SM, Strain EC, Griffiths RR. Withdrawal syndrome after the double-blind cessation of caffeine consumption. *N Engl J Med*. 1992;327:1109-1114.
177. Slaughter RL, Green L, Kohli R. Hemodialysis clearance of theophylline. *Ther Drug Monit*. 1982;4:191-193.
178. Staib AH, Schuppan D, Lissner R, et al. Pharmacokinetics and metabolism of theophylline in patients with liver diseases. *Int J Clin Pharmacol Ther Toxicol*. 1980;18:500-502.
179. Statland BE, Demas TJ. Serum caffeine half-lives. healthy subjects vs. patients having alcoholic hepatic disease. *Am J Clin Pathol*. 1980;73:390-393.
180. Stavchansky S, Combs A, Sagraves R, Delgado M, Joshi A. Pharmacokinetics of caffeine in breast milk and plasma after single oral administration of caffeine to lactating mothers. *Biopharm Drug Dispos*. 1988;9:285-299.
181. Stegmayr BG. On-line hemodialysis and hemoperfusion in a girl intoxicated by theophylline. *Acta Med Scand*. 1988;223:565-567.
182. Strain EC, Mumford GK, Silverman K, Griffiths RR. Caffeine dependence syndrome. evidence from case histories and experimental evaluations. *JAMA*. 1994;272:1043-1048.
183. Sykes AP, Lawson N, Finnegan JA, Ayres JG. Creatine kinase activity in patients with brittle asthma treated with long term subcutaneous terbutaline. *Thorax*. 1991;46:580-583.
184. Tisdell R, Iacobucci M, Snodgrass WR. Caffeine poisoning in an adult-survival with a serum concentration of 400 mg/L and need for adenosine agonist antidotes. *Vet Hum Toxicol*. 1986;28:492.
185. Titley OG, Williams N. Theophylline toxicity causing rhabdomyolysis and acute compartment syndrome. *Intensive Care Med*. 1992;18:129-130.
186. Udezue E, D'Souza L, Mahajan M. Hypokalemia after normal doses of neubulized albuterol (salbutamol). *Am J Emerg Med*. 1995;13:168-171.
187. Vestal RE, Eiriksson CE, Jr, Musser B, et al. Effect of intravenous aminophylline on plasma levels of catecholamines and related cardiovascular and metabolic responses in man. *Circulation*. 1983;67:162-171.

188. Victor BS, Lubetsky M, Greden JF. Somatic manifestations of caffeinism. *J Clin Psychiatry*. 1981;42:185-188.
189. Vozeh S, Powell JR, Riegelman S, et al. Changes in theophylline clearance during acute illness. *JAMA*. 1978;240:1882-1884.
190. Wang-Cheng R, Davidson BJ. Ritodrine-induced neutropenia. *Am J Obstet Gynecol*. 1986;154:924-925.
191. Wasserman D, Amitai Y. Hypoglycemia following albuterol overdose in a child. *Am J Emerg Med*. 1992;10:556-557.
192. Weinberger M, Bronsky E, Bensch GW, et al. Interaction of ephedrine and theophylline. *Clin Pharmacol Ther*. 1975;17:585-592.
193. Whitehurst VE, Joseph X, Vick JA, et al. Reversal of acute theophylline toxicity by calcium channel blockers in dogs and rats. *Toxicology*. 1996;110:113-121.
194. Wiley JF 2nd, Spiller HA, Krenzelok EP, Borys DJ. Unintentional albuterol ingestion in children. *Pediatr Emerg Care*. 1994;10:193-196.
195. Willett WC, Stampfer MJ, Manson JE, et al. Coffee consumption and coronary heart disease in women. A ten-year follow-up. *JAMA*. 1996;275:458-462.
196. Woo OF, Pond SM, Benowitz NL, Olson KR. Benefit of hemoperfusion in acute theophylline intoxication. *J Toxicol Clin Toxicol*. 1984;22:411-424.
197. Wrenn KD, Oschner I. Rhabdomyolysis induced by a caffeine overdose. *Ann Emerg Med*. 1989;18:94-97.
198. Yeh TF, Pildes RS. Transplacental aminophylline toxicity in a neonate. *Lancet*. 1977;1:910.
199. Young D, Dragunow M. Status epilepticus may be caused by loss of adenosine anticonvulsant mechanisms. *Neuroscience*. 1994;58:245-261.
200. Yurchak AM, Jusko WJ. Theophylline secretion into breast milk. *Pediatrics*. 1976;57:518-520.

F.

ANESTHETICS AND RELATED MEDICATIONS

CHAPTER 66

LOCAL ANESTHETICS

David R. Schwartz and Brian Kaufman

Local anesthetics are xenobiotics that block excitation of, and transmission along, a nerve axon in a predictable and reversible manner. The anesthesia produced is selective to the chosen body part in contrast to the nonselective effects of a general anesthetic. Local anesthetics do not require the circulation as an intermediate carrier, and they usually are not transported to distant organs. Therefore, the actions of local anesthetics are largely confined to the structures with which they come into direct contact. Local anesthetics may provide analgesia in various parts of the body by topical application, injection in the vicinity of peripheral nerve endings and major nerve trunks, or via instillation within the epidural or subarachnoid spaces. The various local anesthetics differ with regard to their potency, duration of action, and degree of effects on sensory and motor fibers. Toxicity may be local or systemic. With systemic toxicity, the central nervous system (CNS) and cardiovascular systems typically are affected.

HISTORY

Until the 1880s, the only xenobiotics available for pain relief were centrally acting depressants such as alcohol and opioids, which blunted the perception of pain rather than attacking the root cause. The coca shrub (*Erythroxylon coca*) was brought back to Europe from Peru by Karl Von Scherzer, an Austrian explorer, in the mid-1800s. Some of the coca leaves were analyzed by the chemist Albert Niemann, who in 1860 successfully extracted and named the active principle, the alkaloid *cocaine* (see Chap. 76). Sigmund Freud studied the use of cocaine to cure morphine addiction. Koller at the Ophthalmological Clinic at the University of Vienna dissolved coca powder in distilled water; instilled the solution in the conjunctival sacs of a frog, a rabbit, a dog, and himself; and noted that their corneas as well as his own could be touched without any evidence of a reflex blink. In 1884, Koller performed an operation for glaucoma with topical cocaine anesthesia, and the news spread rapidly, leading to diversification of use.[42]

Although the clinical benefits of cocaine anesthesia were significant, so were its toxic and addictive potential. At least 13 deaths were reported in the first 7 years after the introduction of cocaine in Europe, and within 10 years after the introduction of cocaine as a regional anesthetic, reviews of "cocaine poisoning" appeared in the literature.[66,84] The toxicity of cocaine, coupled with the tremendous advantages it provided for surgery, led to a search for less toxic substitutes.

After the elucidation of the chemical structure of cocaine (the benzoic acid methyl ester of the alkaloid ecgonine) in 1895, other amino esters were examined. Synthetic compounds with local anesthetic activity were introduced, but they were either highly toxic or irritating or had an impractically brief clinical effectiveness. In 1904, Einhorn synthesized procaine, but its short duration of action limited its clinical utility. Research then focused on synthesis of xenobiotics with more prolonged durations of action.

The potent, long-acting local anesthetics dibucaine and tetracaine were synthesized in 1925 and 1928, respectively, and were introduced into clinical practice. However, these anesthetics were not safe for regional anesthetic techniques because of systemic toxicity secondary to the large volumes of drug that were required to ensure distribution throughout the entire neuronal sheath. On the other hand, these drugs were very useful for spinal anesthesia, which required much smaller volumes.

Lofgren synthesized the prototypical local anesthetic lidocaine from a series of aniline derivatives in 1943. This amino amide combined high tissue penetrance and a moderate duration of action with acceptably low systemic toxicity. Additionally, the metabolites of lidocaine did not include *para*-aminobenzoic acid (PABA), which was the reported cause of allergic reactions to the amino ester anesthetics. Subsequent to the release of lidocaine in 1944, several other amino amide compounds were synthesized and introduced into clinical practice. These include mepivacaine in 1956, prilocaine in 1959, bupivacaine in 1963, etidocaine in 1971, and ropivacaine in 1996.

EPIDEMIOLOGY

Considering how frequently local anesthetics are administered, both within and outside healthcare facilities, clinically significant toxic reactions are few, and most are iatrogenic. In reports of fatalities resulting from toxic exposures reported to U.S. poison centers, local anesthetics are rare, representing less than 0.5% of cases (see Chap. 135). Most poisonings result from inadvertent injection of a therapeutic dose into a blood vessel, repeated use of a therapeutic dose, or unintentional administration of a toxic dose. The amide local anesthetics have largely replaced the esters in clinical use because of their increased stability and relative absence of hypersensitivity reactions (see Pharmacology below). Poisoning from topical benzocaine is relatively common because of the large number of nonprescription products available for treatment of teething and hemorrhoids and because of the widespread use of benzocaine, mostly as a spray, for topical mucosal anesthesia before intubation, upper endoscopy, and transesophageal echocardiography. With nonprescription use, toxic effects after exposure are typically mild, and death rarely occurs. Toxicity usually occurs as a therapeutic misadventure, but child abuse or neglect should be considered if the patient is younger than 2 years, and suicide should be considered in older children and adults.

Benzocaine spray may be the most important cause of severe acquired methemoglobinemia in the hospital setting[3] (see Chap. 127). Between November 1997 and March 2002, the U.S. Food and Drug

Administration (FDA) received 198 reported adverse events secondary to benzocaine products. A total of 132 cases (66.7%) involved definite or probable methemoglobinemia; most were serious adverse events, and two deaths occurred.[75] In these cases, a single spray of unspecified duration of 20% benzocaine was the dose most commonly reported. Because of the difficulty in limiting the dose to the manufacturer's recommendation given the current formulations available, these authors recommend a metered-dosing preparation and prominent package warnings.

PHARMACOLOGY

CHEMICAL STRUCTURE

Local anesthetics fall into one of two chemically distinct groups: amino esters and amino amides (Fig. 66–1). The basic structure of all local anesthetics consists of three major components. A lipophilic, aromatic ring is connected by an ester or amide linkage to a short alkyl, intermediate chain that is bound to a hydrophilic tertiary (or, less commonly, secondary) amine. The amine is a base (proton acceptor) that is partially charged in the physiologic pH range.

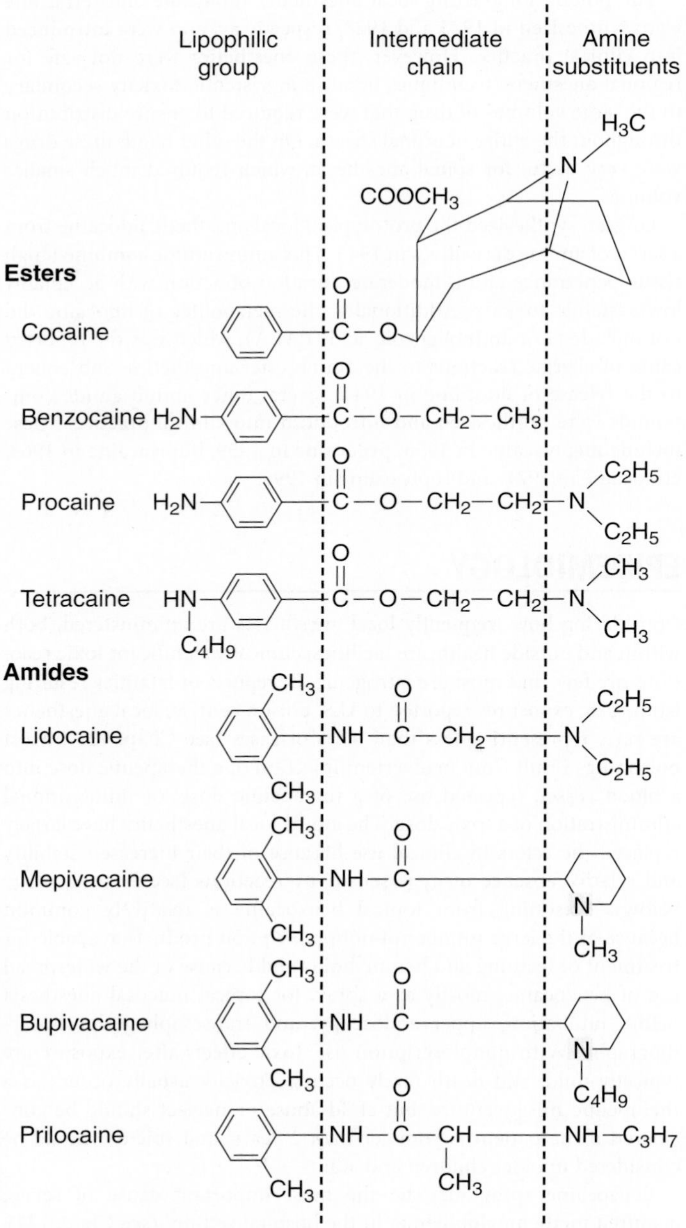

Lipophilic group | Intermediate chain | Amine substituents

Esters

Cocaine: $COOCH_3$, H_3C–N (tropane ring), C(=O)–O

Benzocaine: H_2N–C₆H₄–C(=O)–O–CH_2–CH_3

Procaine: H_2N–C₆H₄–C(=O)–O–CH_2–CH_2–N(C_2H_5)₂

Tetracaine: HN(C_4H_9)–C₆H₄–C(=O)–O–CH_2–CH_2–N(CH_3)₂

Amides

Lidocaine: (CH_3)₂C₆H₃–NH–C(=O)–CH_2–N(C_2H_5)₂

Mepivacaine: (CH_3)₂C₆H₃–NH–C(=O)–(piperidine N–CH_3)

Bupivacaine: (CH_3)₂C₆H₃–NH–C(=O)–(piperidine N–C_4H_9)

Prilocaine: (CH_3)C₆H₄–NH–C(=O)–CH(CH_3)–NH–C_3H_7

FIGURE 66–1. Representative local anesthetics in common clinical use.

MODE OF ACTION

All local anesthetics function by reversibly binding to specific receptor proteins within the membrane-bound sodium channels of conducting tissues. These receptors can be reached only via the cytoplasmic side of the cell membrane, that is, by intracellular drug. Blockade of ion conductance through the sodium channel eventually leads to failure to form and propagate action potentials (Fig. 66–2). The analgesic effect results from inhibiting axonal transmission of the nerve impulse in small-diameter myelinated and unmyelinated nerve fibers carrying pain and temperature sensation. Conduction block of these fibers occurs at lower concentrations than in the larger fibers responsible for touch, motor function, and proprioception.[22] This likely occurs in myelinated nerves because smaller fibers have closer spacing of the nodes of Ranvier. Given that a fixed number of nodes must be blocked for conduction failure to occur, the shorter critical length of nerve is reached sooner by the locally placed anesthetic in small fibers.[36] For unmyelinated fibers, the smaller diameter limits the distance that such fibers can passively propagate the electrical impulse. In addition, differential nerve block may relate to voltage and time dependence of the affinity of local anesthetics to the sodium channels.

The sodium channel may exist in three states (see Chap. 23). At resting membrane potential or in the hyperpolarized membrane, the channel is closed to sodium conductance. With an appropriate activating stimulus, the channel opens, allowing rapid sodium influx and membrane depolarization. Milliseconds later, the channel is inactivated, terminating the fast sodium current. Blockade is much stronger for channels that are activated (open) or inactivated than for channels that are resting. Pain fibers have a higher firing rate and longer action potential (ie, more time with the sodium channel open or inactivated) than other fiber types and therefore are more susceptible to local anesthetic action.[48]

These effects also occur in other conductive tissues in the heart and brain that rely on sodium current. Although sodium channel

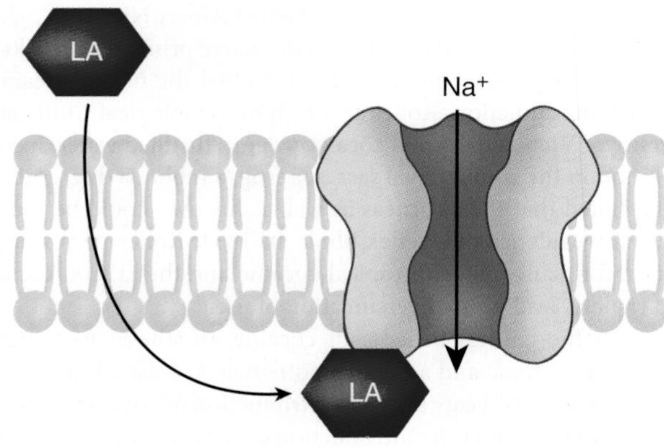

FIGURE 66–2. The multi-unit sodium channel is embedded in the nerve cell membrane. Local anesthetics (LA) enter the nerve cell at the exposed membranes of the Nodes of Ranvier and bind to the cytoplasmic side of the sodium channel (also located at the Node of Ranvier) and alter sodium conductance.

blockade initially was believed to be the sole cause of systemic toxicity, the mechanisms are more complex, especially in the heart, and may occur at systemic concentrations lower than previously thought.[68] Local anesthetics may interact with other cellular systems at clinically relevant concentrations. For example, lidocaine inhibited muscarinic signaling in *Xenopus* oocytes at less than 50% of the concentration required for sodium channel blockade.[47] Growing evidence indicates that local anesthetics can directly affect many other organ systems and functions such as the coagulation, immune, and respiratory systems at concentrations much lower than those required to achieve sodium channel blockade.[16,46,47] Study of these less well-described effects may help elucidate both therapeutic and toxic phenomenon that are incompletely explained.

PHYSICOCHEMICAL PROPERTIES

The primary determinant of the onset of action of a local anesthetic is its pK_a, which affects the lipophilicity of a drug (Table 66–1). All of the local anesthetics are weak bases, with a pK_a between 7.8 and 9.3. At physiologic pH (7.4), xenobiotics with a lower pK_a have more uncharged molecules that are free to cross the nerve cell membrane, producing a faster onset of action than xenobiotics with a higher pK_a. The onset of action also is influenced by the total dose of local anesthetic administered, which affects the concentration available for diffusion.

Local anesthetic potency is highly correlated with the lipid solubility of the xenobiotic. Therefore, the aromatic side of the anesthetic is the primary determinant of potency. The hydrophilic amine is important in occupying the sodium channel, which involves an ionic interaction with the charged form of the tertiary amine. The length of the intermediate chain is another determinant of local anesthetic activity, with three to seven carbon-equivalents providing maximal activity.[22] Shorter or longer intermediate chain lengths are associated with rapid loss of local anesthetic action, suggesting that a critical length of separation of the aromatic group from the tertiary amine is required for sodium channel blockade to occur.

The degree of protein binding influences the duration of action of a local anesthetic. Anesthetics with greater protein binding remain associated with the neural membrane for a longer time interval and therefore have longer durations of action.[22] When high serum concentrations are achieved, a higher degree of protein binding increases the risk for cardiac toxicity.

PHARMACOKINETICS

A distinction must be made between local disposition (distribution and elimination) and systemic disposition. Local distribution is influenced by several factors, including spread of local anesthetic by bulk flow, diffusion, transport via local blood vessels, and binding to local tissues. Local elimination occurs through systemic absorption, transfer into the general circulation, and local hydrolysis of amino ester anesthetics. Systemic absorption decreases the amount of local anesthetic that is available for anesthetic effect, thereby limiting the duration of the block. Systemic absorption is dependent on the avidity of binding of local anesthetics to tissues near the site of injection and on local perfusion. Both of these factors vary with the site of injection. In general, areas with greater blood flow will have more rapid and complete systemic uptake of local anesthetic therfore, intravenous (IV) > tracheal > intercostal > paracervical > epidural > brachial plexus > sciatic > subcutaneous.

Because of their lipophilicity, local anesthetics readily cross cell membranes, the blood–brain barrier, and the placenta. Once absorbed, systemic tissue distribution is highly dependent on tissue perfusion. After local anesthetics enter into the venous circulation, they pass through the lungs, where significant uptake may occur, thereby lowering peak arterial concentrations. Thus, the lungs may serve as a buffer against systemic toxicity.[59] This mechanism, however, has saturable kinetics. Part of the reason why most local anesthetic–induced seizures result from unintentional intravascular injection rather than absorptive uptake is that lung uptake of these drugs appears to exceed 90%.

TABLE 66–1. Pharmacologic Properties of Local Anesthetics[48,100]

	pK_a	Protein Binding (%)	Relative Potency	Duration of Action	Approximate Maximum Allowable Subcutaneous Dose (mg/kg)
Esters					
Chloroprocaine	9.3	Unknown	Intermediate	Short	10
Cocaine	8.7	92	Low	Medium	3
Procaine	9.1	5	Low	Short	10
Tetracaine	8.4	76	High	Long	3
Amides					
Bupivacaine	8.1	95	High	Long	2
Etidocaine	7.9	95	High	Long	4
Lidocaine	7.8	70	Low	Medium	4.5
Mepivacaine	7.9	75	Intermediate	Medium	4.5
Prilocaine	8.0	40	Intermediate	Medium	8
Ropivacaine	8.2	95	Intermediate	Long	3.

The very high peak venous concentrations produced by rapid injection usually are necessary to produce toxic arterial concentrations.

All local anesthetics, except cocaine, cause peripheral vasodilation by direct relaxation of vascular smooth muscle. Vasodilation enhances vascular absorption of the local anesthetic. Addition of epinephrine (5 μg/mL or 1:200,000) to the local anesthetic solution decreases the rate of vascular absorption, thereby improving the depth and prolonging the duration of local action. An epinephrine local anesthetic mixture also decreases bleeding into the surgical field and serves as a marker for inadvertent intravascular injection (by producing tachycardia) when a test dose of the mixture is injected through a needle or catheter.[72]

Significant drawbacks to epinephrine use include uncomfortable side effects such as palpitations and tremors, local tissue ischemia, and life-threatening systemic adverse reactions in susceptible patients, such as myocardial ischemia and hypertensive crisis. Inadvertent intravascular injection of local anesthetics mixed with epinephrine can be fatal, although generally, the epinephrine in these mixtures is very dilute.[63]

The two classes of local anesthetics undergo metabolism by different routes (see Chap. 76). The amino esters are rapidly metabolized by plasma cholinesterase to the major metabolite, PABA. The amino amides are metabolized more slowly in the liver to a variety of metabolites that do not include PABA.[21] Patients with atypical or low concentrations of plasma cholinesterase are at increased risk for systemic toxicity from ester local anesthetics. Factors that decrease hepatic blood flow or impair hepatic function increase the risk for toxic reactions to the amino amides and make management of serious reactions more difficult. The patient's age, as it relates to liver enzyme activity and plasma protein binding, influences the rate of metabolism of local anesthetics. Whereas the lidocaine terminal half-life after IV administration averaged 80 minutes in volunteers ages 22 to 26 years, the half-life was 138 minutes in those ages 61 to 71 years[80] (see Chap. 63). Newborn infants with immature hepatic enzyme systems have prolonged elimination of amino amides, which is associated with seizures when high continuous infusion rates are used.[1,69] Lidocaine elimination is reduced by congestive heart failure or coadministration of xenobiotics that reduce hepatic blood flow, thus explaining the increased risk of toxicity with cimetidine and propranolol.[90] Propranolol and cimetidine also potentially decrease lidocaine clearance by inhibiting hepatic mixed-function oxidase enzymes.

Local anesthetics are often mixed to take advantage of desirable pharmacokinetics. Ideally, rapid-acting, relatively short-duration local anesthetics such as chloroprocaine or lidocaine can be combined with the longer latency, long-acting tetracaine or bupivacaine. In practice, the advantages of the mixtures are small, and toxicities are additive.[5] Administration of one local anesthetic increases the free plasma fraction of another by displacement from protein-binding sites.[51]

Local anesthetics usually cannot penetrate intact skin in sufficient quantities to produce reliable anesthesia.[11] Efficient skin penetration requires the combination of a high water content and a high concentration of the water-insoluble base form of the local anesthetic. This combination of properties has been achieved by mixing lidocaine and prilocaine in their base forms in a 1:1 ratio (eutectic mixture of local anesthetics [EMLA]).[14] Application for at least 45 minutes is required to achieve adequate dermal analgesia. Local anesthetic uptake continues for several hours during application. A liposomal formulation of 4% lidocaine (ELA-Max) facilitates skin absorption. It is as effective as EMLA for topical anesthesia.[31] In addition, a 4% tetracaine gel preparation has been used in children for topical skin anesthesia with an onset of action and efficacy at least as good as EMLA and without any systemic side effects.

CLINICAL MANIFESTATIONS OF TOXICITY

TOXIC REACTIONS

Regional Side Effects and Tissue Toxicity At some concentration, all local anesthetics are directly cytotoxic to nerve cells. However, in clinically relevant doses, they rarely produce localized nerve damage.[55,79] Significant direct neurotoxicity may result from intrathecal injection or infusion of local anesthetics for spinal anesthesia. In this setting, studies suggest lidocaine has an increased risk for both persistent lumbosacral neuropathy and a syndrome of painful but self-limited postanesthesia buttock and leg pain or dysesthesia referred to as *transient neurologic symptoms.*[50] Nerve damage often is attributed to use of excessively concentrated solutions or inappropriate formulations. Several reports of cauda equina syndrome have been associated with use of hyperbaric 5% lidocaine solutions for spinal anesthesia. Hyperbaric solutions are more dense than cerebrospinal fluid. This neurotoxicity appears to be a phenomena that occurs when the anesthetic is injected through narrow-bore needles or through continuous spinal catheters. This process may result in very high local concentrations of the anesthetic that might pool around the sacral roots because of inadequate mixing.[91] The mechanism of this neurotoxic effect is unknown but is believed to be independent of sodium channel blockade.[50] Because an equally effective block can be achieved with injection of larger volumes of lower concentration, 5% lidocaine should be avoided and bupivacaine used instead.

Similar severe neurotoxic reactions have occurred after massive subarachnoid injection of chloroprocaine during attempted epidural anesthesia.[88] The neurotoxicity initially appeared to be associated with use of the antioxidant sodium bisulfite and the low pH of the commercial solution rather than use of the anesthetic itself.[108] Although chloroprocaine has been reformulated without bisulfite, new animal data suggest that it is the anesthetic that may be responsible for the neurotoxicity.[104] Skeletal muscle changes are observed after intramuscular injection of local anesthetics, especially the more potent, longer-acting xenobiotics. The effect is reversible, and muscle regeneration is complete within 2 weeks after injection of local anesthetics.[8]

SYSTEMIC SIDE EFFECTS AND TOXICITY

Allergic Reactions Allergic reactions to local anesthetics are extremely rare. Fewer than 1% of all adverse drug reactions caused by local anesthetics are immunoglobulin (Ig)E-mediated.[39] In one study designed to determine the prevalence of true local anesthetic allergy in patients referred to an allergy clinic for suspected hypersensitivity, skin prick and intradermal testing results were negative for all 236 subjects tested.[9] As noted, the amino esters are responsible for the majority of true allergic reactions. When hydrolyzed, the amino ester local anesthetics produce PABA, a known allergen (see Chap. 55). Cross-sensitivity to other amino ester anesthetics is common. Some multidose commercial preparations of amino amides may contain the preservative methylparabens, which is chemically related to PABA and is the most likely cause of the much rarer allergic reaction to amino amides or seeming allergic responses to both the amides and esters. Preservative-free amino amides, including lidocaine, can be used safely in patients who have reactions to drug preparations containing methylparabens unless the patient is specifically sensitive to lidocaine. Again, if the patient with a history of allergic reaction to a particular drug requires a local anesthetic, a paraben preservative-free drug from the opposite class can be chosen because there is no cross-reactivity between the amides and esters.

Methemoglobinemia Methemoglobinemia is reported frequently as an adverse effect of topical and oropharyngeal benzocaine use and occasionally with lidocaine, tetracaine, or prilocaine use. The diagnosis can be established by direct measurement of methemoglobin percent with a cooximeter. Most reports of methemoglobinemia associated with local anesthetics are the result of an excessive dose, a break in the normal mucosal barrier for topical anesthetics, or a deficiency of a congenital reducing enzyme such as methemoglobin reductase (see Chap. 127).

Benzocaine is metabolized to aniline and then further metabolized to phenylhydroxylamine and nitrobenzene, which are both potent oxidizing agents (see Chap. 127). Although reports describe methemoglobinemia resulting from standard doses of benzocaine topical oropharyngeal spray given for laryngoscopy or gastrointestinal upper endoscopy,[29,75] affected patients commonly have abnormal mucosal integrity, as occurs with thrush or mucositis. Prilocaine is an amino ester local anesthetic primarily used in obstetric anesthesia because of its rapid onset of action and low systemic toxicity in both the mother and fetus. Use of large doses of prilocaine may lead to the development of methemoglobinemia.[45,61] Prilocaine is an aniline derivative that, when metabolized in the liver, produces *ortho*-toluidine, another oxidizing agent.[45] A direct relationship exists between the amount of epidural prilocaine administered and the incidence of methemoglobinemia. A dose greater than approximately 8 mg/kg is generally necessary to produce symptoms, which may not become apparent until several hours after epidural administration of the drug. Standard doses of EMLA cream used for circumcision in term neonates are associated with minimal production of methemoglobin, but risks may be increased in neonates with metabolic disorders.[102] EMLA-associated methemoglobinemia has been reported in children and rarely in adults.[41] When clinically indicated, affected patients with symptomatic methemoglobinemia should be treated with IV methylene blue (see Chap. 127 and Antidotes in Depth A41: Methylene Blue).

Other Reactions The most common adverse reactions to local anesthetics are vasovagal reactions.[106]

Systemic Toxicity Systemic toxicity for all local anesthetics correlates with serum concentrations. Factors that determine the concentration include (1) dose; (2) rate of administration; (3) site of injection (absorption occurs more rapidly and completely from vascular areas, such with neck blocks and intercostal blocks); (4) the presence or absence of a vasoconstrictor; and (5) the degree of tissue–protein binding, fat solubility, and pK_a of the local anesthetic.[73] The brain and heart are the primary target organs for systemic toxicity because of their rich perfusion, moderate tissue–blood partition coefficients, lack of diffusion limitations, and presence of cells that rely on voltage-gated sodium channels to produce an action potential.

Recommendations for maximal local anesthetic doses designed to minimize the risk for systemic toxic reactions have been published.[100] These maximal recommended doses aim to prevent infiltration of excessive drug. However, because most episodes of systemic toxicity from local anesthetics, with the exception of methemoglobinemia from topical drug, occur secondary to unintentional intravascular injection rather than from overdosage, limiting the maximal dose will not prevent most toxic systemic reactions.[97]

Toxicity is also related to the metabolism for a given local anesthetic. The rapidity of elimination from the plasma influences the total dose delivered to the CNS or heart. The amino esters are rapidly hydrolyzed in the plasma and eliminated, explaining their relatively low potential for systemic toxicity. The amino amides have a much greater potential for producing systemic toxicity because termination of the therapeutic effect of these drugs is achieved through redistribution and slower metabolic inactivation.[35] Another factor that creates difficulty in specifying the minimal toxic plasma concentration of lidocaine results from the fact that its *N*-dealkylated metabolites are pharmacologically active. Although these factors make it difficult to establish safe doses of local anesthetics, Table 66–2 summarizes the estimates of minimal toxic intravenous doses of various local anesthetics.

TABLE 66–2. Toxic Doses of Local Anesthetics

Local Anesthetic	Minimum IV Toxic Dose of Local Anesthetic in Humans (mg/kg)
Procaine	19.2
Chloroprocaine	22.8
Tetracaine	2.5
Lidocaine	6.4
Mepivacaine	9.8
Bupivacaine	1.6
Etidocaine	3.4

IV, intravenous.

Central Nervous System Toxicity Systemic toxicity in humans usually presents as CNS abnormalities. IV infusion studies in volunteers have demonstrated an inverse relationship between the anesthetic potency of various local anesthetics and the dosage required to induce signs of CNS toxicity.[98] A similar relationship exists between the convulsive concentration of various local anesthetics and their relative anesthetic potency. In humans, seizures are reported at serum concentrations of approximately 2 to 4 μg/mL for bupivacaine and etidocaine. Concentrations in excess of 10 μg/mL are usually required for production of seizures when less-potent drugs such as lidocaine are administered. Despite the strong relationship between local anesthetic potency and CNS toxicity, several other factors influence the CNS effects, including the rate of injection, drug interactions, and acid–base status.[24]

The rapidity with which a particular serum concentration is achieved influences the toxicity of the anesthetic. Volunteers could tolerate an average dose of 236 mg of etidocaine and a serum concentration of 3 μg/mL before onset of CNS symptoms when the anesthetic was infused at a rate of 10 mg/min. However, when the infusion rate was increased to 20 mg/min, the same individuals could tolerate only an average of 161 mg of the drug, which produced a serum concentration of approximately 2 μg/mL.[96]

Centrally acting local anesthetics can modify the clinical presentation of a systemic toxic reaction. In general, whereas CNS-depressant drugs minimize the signs and symptoms of CNS excitation, they increase the threshold for local anesthetic–induced seizures. Flumazenil increases the sensitivity of the CNS to the amino amide anesthetics.[13]

Both metabolic and respiratory acidoses increase local anesthetic–induced CNS toxicity. Acidemia decreases plasma protein binding, increasing the amount of free drug available for CNS diffusion despite promoting the charged form of the amine. The convulsive threshold of various local anesthetics is inversely related to arterial PCO_2.[26,32,33] Hypercarbia may lower the seizure threshold by several mechanisms: (1) increased cerebral blood flow, which increases drug delivery to the CNS; (2) increased conversion of the drug base to the active cation in the presence of decreased intracellular pH; and (3) decreased plasma protein binding, which increases the amount of free drug available for diffusion into the brain.[15,26,32,33]

A gradually increasing serum lidocaine concentration produces a common pattern of symptoms and signs (Fig. 66–3). In an awake patient, the initial symptoms are subjective and include tinnitus, lightheadedness, circumoral numbness, disorientation, confusion, auditory and visual disturbances, and lethargy. Subjective side effects occur at serum concentrations between 3 and 6 μg/mL. Significant

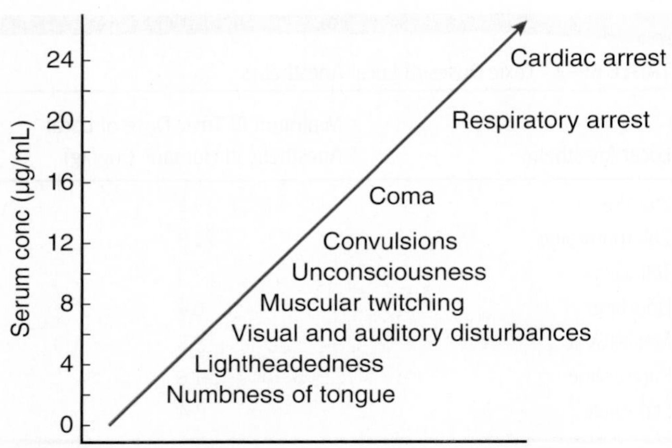

FIGURE 66–3. Relationship of signs and symptoms of toxicity to serum lidocaine concentrations.

psychological effects of local anesthetics have also been reported. Near-death experiences and delusions of actual death are described as specific symptoms of local anesthetic toxicity.[64] Thus, the appearance of psychologic symptoms during administration of local anesthetics should not be disregarded as unrelated nervous reactions or effects of sedatives given as premedication but rather as a possible early sign of CNS toxicity.

Objective signs, usually excitatory, then develop and include shivering, tremors, and ultimately generalized tonic–clonic seizures. Objective CNS toxicity usually is evident at concentrations between 5 and 9 µg/mL. Seizures may occur at concentrations above 10 µg/mL, with higher concentrations producing coma, apnea, and cardiovascular collapse. The excitatory phase has a wide range of intensity and duration, depending on the chemical properties of the local anesthetic. With the highly lipophilic, highly protein-bound drugs, the excitement phase is brief and mild. Toxicity from a large IV bolus of bupivacaine may present without any CNS excitement and with bradycardia, cyanosis, and coma as the first signs.[93] Rapid intravascular injection of lidocaine may produce a brief excitatory phase followed by generalized CNS depression with respiratory arrest. Seizures may follow even a small dose injected into the vertebral or carotid artery (as may occur during stellate ganglion block).[54] A relative overdose produces a slower onset of symptoms (usually within 5–15 minutes of drug injection), with irritability progressing into seizures.

The mechanism of the initial CNS excitation involves a selective block of cerebral cortical inhibitory pathways in the amygdala.[103,107] The resulting increase in unopposed excitatory activity leads to seizures. As the concentration increases further, both inhibitory and excitatory neurons are blocked, and generalized CNS depression ensues.

TREATMENT OF LOCAL ANESTHETIC CENTRAL NERVOUS SYSTEM TOXICITY

At the first sign of possible CNS toxicity, administration of the drug must be discontinued. One hundred percent oxygen should be supplied immediately, and ventilation should be supported if necessary. Patients with minor symptoms usually do not require treatment, provided adequate respiratory and cardiovascular functions are maintained. The patient must be followed closely so that progression to more severe effects can be detected.

Although most seizures caused by local anesthetics are self-limited, they should be treated quickly because the hypoxia and acidosis produced by prolonged seizures may increase both CNS and cardiovascular toxicity.[76,78] Intubation is not mandatory, and the decision to intubate must be individualized. Maintaining adequate ventilation is of proven value, but modest hyperventilation in theory might decrease CNS toxicity. By decreasing CNS extraction of drug, lowering extracellular potassium, and hyperpolarizing the neuronal cell membrane, normalizing (lowering) PCO_2 may decrease the affinity or accelerate separation of the local anesthetic from the sodium channel. Barbiturates and benzodiazepines have been used for treatment of local anesthetic–induced seizures. An induction dose of thiopental, which is readily available to the anesthesiologist or an IV benzodiazepine such as lorazepam, can rapidly terminate a seizure, but either of these medication groups can also exacerbate circulatory and respiratory depression.[24,71] Propofol 1 mg/kg IV was as effective as thiopental 2 mg/kg IV in stopping bupivacaine-induced seizures in rats and has been used successfully in a patient with uncontrolled muscle twitching secondary to local anesthetic toxicity.[10,43] However, propofol may cause significant bradydysrhythmias and even asystole, especially when used with other xenobiotics that cause bradycardia. Whether propofol interacts with local anesthetics to enhance their bradydysrhythmic effects is not known, and it is not possible to generally recommend propofol over barbiturates and benzodiazepines for treatment of local anesthetic CNS toxicity. Neuromuscular blocking agents have been proposed as adjunctive treatment for local anesthetic–induced seizures. They block muscular activity, decreasing oxygen demand and lactic acid production. However, neuromuscular blocking agents should never be used to treat seizures per se because they have no anticonvulsant effect and can make clinical diagnosis of ongoing seizures problematic by abolishing muscle contractions. To avoid this potentially lethal complication, chemical paralysis should be used only to facilitate endotracheal intubation if needed. Use of short-acting neuromuscular blockers is desirable to allow for subsequent repeated neurologic assessments. Succinylcholine may not be ideal because of its significant side effects, including hyperkalemia and dysrhythmias. Newer short-acting nondepolarizing neuromuscular blockers with less potential for cardiac side effects, such as rocuronium, should be considered (see Chap. 68).

When severe systemic toxicity occurs, the cardiovascular system must be monitored closely because cardiovascular depression may go unnoticed while the seizures are being treated. Because local anesthetic–induced myocardial depression may occur even with preserved blood pressure, it is important to be aware of early signs of cardiac toxicity, including electrocardiographic (ECG) changes.

If toxicity results from an oral ingestion, activated charcoal is generally indicated, but its benefits are unproven. If the patient has presented for care immediately after ingestion, orogastric lavage with a nasogastric tube may be considered. Induction of emesis is contraindicated even after oral administration because of the risk of seizures and aspiration. Contaminated mucous membranes should be washed off. Hemodialysis is not of proven utility and may be impractical, as is hemoperfusion.

Cardiovascular Toxicity Cardiovascular side effects are the most feared manifestations of local anesthetic toxicity. Shock and cardiovascular collapse may be related to effects on vascular tone, inotropy, and dysrhythmias related to indirect CNS and direct cardiac and vascular effects of the local anesthetic. Animal studies and clinical observations clearly demonstrate that for most local anesthetics, CNS toxicity develops at lower serum concentrations (exception: bupivacaine) than those needed to produce cardiac toxicity, that is, they have a high CV:CNS toxicity ratio.[54,77,78,93] When cardiac toxicity occurs, management may be exceedingly difficult. Some of the discrepancy between the incidence of CNS and cardiac toxicity may result from a detection bias. Not only can the treating physicians fail to recognize cardiac effects because of preoccupation with CNS manifestations of toxicity, but significant early cardiac toxicity may be quite subtle. An experimental study attempting to identify early warning signs of bupivacaine-induced cardiac toxicity in pigs evaluated bupivacaine-induced changes in cardiac output, heart rate, blood pressure, and ECG.[83] A 40% reduction in cardiac output was not associated without significant change in heart rate or blood pressure, the latter secondary to a direct vasoconstrictive effect of bupivacaine at the concentrations produced. [17]

Changes in systemic vascular tone induced by local anesthetics may be mediated by direct effect on vascular smooth muscle or indirectly via effects on spinal cord sympathetic outflow. Predictably, sympathetic blockade after spinal anesthesia or epidural anesthesia above the T5 dermatome results in peripheral venodilation and arterial dilation. Shock may result when high doses of anesthetic are used in hypovolemic patients. Local anesthetics have a biphasic effect on peripheral vascular smooth muscle. Whereas lower doses produce direct vasoconstriction, higher doses are associated with severe cardiovascular toxicity and cause vasodilation, contributing to cardiovascular collapse.

All local anesthetics directly produce a dose-dependent decrease in cardiac contractility, with the effects roughly proportional to their peripheral anesthetic effect. Although the classic anesthetic action of sodium channel blockade in heart muscle accounts in large part for the negative inotropy by affecting excitation–contraction coupling, it does not explain the entire difference in myocardial depression produced by different anesthetics.[28] Poorly understood effects on calcium handling or effects of the intracellular drug directly on contractile proteins or mitochondrial function may be operable.[28]

Blockade of the fast sodium channels of cardiac myocytes decreases maximum upstroke velocity (V_{max}) of the action potential (see Chap. 22 and 23 and Fig. 63–1). This effect slows impulse conduction in the sinoatrial and atrioventricular (AV) nodes, the His-Purkinje system, and atrial and ventricular muscle.[20] These changes are reflected on ECG by increases in PR interval and QRS duration. At progressively higher anesthetic concentrations, hypotension, sinus arrest with junctional rhythm, and eventually cardiac arrest occur.[4] Asystole has been described in patients who received unintentional IV bolus injections of 800 to 1000 mg of lidocaine.[4,34] Cardiovascular toxicity of local anesthetics usually occurs after a sudden increase in serum concentration, as in unintentional intravascular injection. Cardiovascular toxicity is rare in other circumstances because large doses are necessary to produce this effect and because CNS toxicity precedes cardiovascular events, thus providing a warning. Cardiac toxicity usually is not observed with lidocaine use in humans until the serum lidocaine concentration greatly exceeds 10 μg/mL unless the patient is also receiving xenobiotics that depress sinus and AV nodal conduction such as calcium channel blockers, β-adrenergic antagonists, or cardioactive steroids.

Bupivacaine is significantly more cardiotoxic than most other local anesthetics commonly used. Inadvertent intravascular injection produces near-simultaneous signs of CNS and cardiovascular toxicity.

Animal studies have compared the dosage or serum concentrations of local anesthetics required to produce irreversible circulatory collapse with those necessary to produce seizures.[25,77,78] This cardiovascular collapse/CNS toxicity (CC/CNS) ratio for lidocaine is approximately 7; therefore, CNS toxicity should become evident well before potentially cardiotoxic concentrations are reached. In contrast, the CC/CNS ratio for bupivacaine is 3.7. Bupivacaine produces myocardial depression out of proportion to its anesthetic potency and, more importantly, may cause refractory ventricular dysrhythmias.[95] Enhanced cardiovascular toxicity may relate to enhanced CNS effects at cardiovascular centers,[105] direct effects on myocyte metabolism, and important differences related to sodium channel blockade. Although lidocaine and bupivacaine both block sodium channels in the open or inactivated states lidocaine quickly dissociates from the channel at diastolic potentials, allowing rapid recovery from block during diastole (fast on–fast off). Therefore, sodium channel blockade with lidocaine is much more pronounced at rapid heart rates (accounting for the antidysrhythmic effects for ventricular tachycardia).[63] On the other hand, at high concentrations, bupivacaine rapidly binds to and slowly dissociates from sodium channels (fast on–slow off), with significant block accumulating at all physiologic heart rates.[20] Accordingly, at heart rates of 60 to 150 beats/min, approximately 70 times more lidocaine is needed than bupivacaine to produce an equal effect on V_{max}. Enhanced conduction block in Purkinje fibers and ventricular muscle cells can set up a reentrant circuit responsible for the ventricular tachydysrhythmias induced by bupivacaine.[70]

Bupivacaine, a potent and long-acting amide anesthetic, has the highest potential for cardiovascular toxicity, which can be refractory to conventional therapy. Inadvertent intravascular injection produces near-simultaneous signs of CNS and cardiovascular toxicity. Bupivacaine has an asymmetrically substituted carbon, and the kinetics of sodium channel binding are stereospecific.[56] The S (levo)-enantiomer levobupivacaine is significantly less cardiotoxic than the R (dextro)-enantiomer despite having similar anesthetic properties.[6,68] Consequently, bupivacaine, the racemic mixture of both enantiomers, is more cardiotoxic than levobupivacaine, which contains only the levo-enantiomer.[40] The stereospecific effect on sodium channels seems to differ between the heart and the peripheral nerves because the local anesthetic potency of levobupivacaine is the same as, or perhaps even greater than, that of bupivacaine.[30,81] Ropivacaine is a pure enantiomer and is less cardiotoxic than bupivacaine, but it is also slightly less potent as an analgesic.[85,86]

Effects other than sodium channel blockade may contribute to cardiotoxicity. Lipophilic local anesthetics such as bupivacaine may directly impair mitochondrial energy transduction via two mechanisms: (1) uncoupling of oxygen consumption and adenosine triphosphate (ATP) synthesis and (2) inhibition of complex I in the respiratory chain.[101] This effect is related to the lipophilic properties of the drug rather than to stereospecific effects on ion channels. Lidocaine has no effect on mitochondrial respiration, and ropivacaine has less effect than bupivacaine.[114] There is no difference between the two bupivacaine enantiomers. These effects occur with higher concentrations of the local anesthetic, as occur after unintentional intravascular injection.

Low-dose bupivacaine-induced cardiotoxic effects have been described in humans under certain circumstances and at concentrations that are not associated with seizure activity in pigs.[52,113] Severe cardiac toxicity is described after injection of a small subcutaneous dose of bupivacaine in a patient with secondary carnitine deficiency.[113] Myocytes are highly dependent on oxidation of fatty acids for energy turnover. Interference with this mechanism via bupivacaine-induced inhibition of carnitine-acylcarnitine translocase has been proposed to contribute to the cardiotoxicity of lipophilic local anesthetics[113] (see Chap. 47 and Fig. 47–2 and Antidote in Depth A21: Intravenous Fat Emulsion). Bupivacaine may produce dysrhythmias by blocking GABAergic neurons that tonically inhibit the autonomic nervous system.[44] In addition to its other effects on the heart, bupivacaine may induce a marked decrease in cardiac contractility by altering Ca^{2+} release from sarcoplasmic reticulum.[62]

In a large series of patients receiving bupivacaine, systemic toxicity occurred in only 15 of 11,080 nerve blocks.[74] Of these patients, 80% convulsed; the other 20% had milder symptoms. A series of cases was described in which bupivacaine use, particularly at 0.75% concentration, was associated with severe cardiovascular depression, ventricular dysrhythmias, and even death. Pregnant women were disproportionately affected. Some of these patients required prolonged and difficult resuscitation.[89] In 1983, 49 incidents of cardiac arrest or ventricular tachycardia that occurred over a 10-year period were presented to the U.S. FDA Anesthetic and Life Support Advisory Committee. Among these cases, 0.75% bupivacaine was used in 27 obstetric patients with 10 deaths, and 0.5% bupivacaine was used in eight obstetric patients

TABLE 66–3. Types of Local Anesthetic Reactions

Cause	Major Clinical Features
Local anesthetic toxicity (intravascular injection)	Immediate seizure or cardiac toxicity
Reaction to catecholamine	Tachycardia, hypertension, headache
Vasovagal reaction	Bradycardia, rapid onset and recovery, hypotension, pallor
Allergic reaction	Anaphylaxis
High spinal or epidural block	Bradycardia, hypotension, respiratory distress, respiratory arrest

with six deaths. Among the 14 nonobstetric patients, five died. The overall mortality was 21 of 49 (43%). Partly as a result of these reports, in 1984, the U.S. FDA withdrew approval of bupivacaine 0.75% for use as obstetric anesthesia.[89]

Acid–base and electrolyte status influence the cardiac toxicity of a given drug because all depressant properties are potentiated by acidosis, hypoxia, or hypercarbia.[12] Table 66–3 outlines the spectrum of acute local anesthetic reactions.

LABORATORY STUDIES

In cases of possible local anesthetic toxicity, an ECG should be obtained to detect dysrhythmias and conduction disturbances. Serum electrolytes, blood urea nitrogen (BUN), creatinine, and arterial blood gas analysis should be obtained to help assess the cause of cardiac dysrhythmias. A methemoglobin percent should be obtained in patients in whom methemoglobinemia is suspected clinically. Rapid, sensitive assays are available for measuring concentrations of lidocaine and its monoethylglycylxylidide (MEGX) metabolite. When properly interpreted, the results of these assays may be used to prevent lidocaine toxicity and to identify lidocaine toxicity in the nontherapeutic setting. Assays for determining serum concentrations of other local anesthetics are not routinely available. Treatment should never be delayed while waiting for results of xenobiotic concentration determinations.

TREATMENT

TREATMENT OF LOCAL ANESTHETIC CARDIAC TOXICITY

Treatment of cardiovascular complications of local anesthetics is complicated by the complex effects of local anesthetics on the heart. Initial therapy should focus on correcting the physiologic derangements that may potentiate the cardiac toxicity of local anesthetics, including hypoxemia, acidosis, and hyperkalemia.[12,92] Prompt support of ventilation and circulation limits hypoxia and acidosis. Early recognition of potential cardiac toxicity is critical to achieving a good outcome because patients with cardiac toxicity that goes unrecognized for any interval are more difficult to resuscitate.[7] If a potentially massive intravascular local anesthetic injection is suspected, maximizing oxygenation of the patient before cardiovascular collapse occurs is critical.

INTRAVENOUS FAT EMULSIONS

While investigating the relationship between lipid metabolism and bupivacaine toxicity (described above), a rat study of bupivacaine-induced asystolic arrest showed that pretreatment with IV fat emulsion (IFE) increased the toxic dose of bupivacaine by 50%. In addition, a dose of bupivacaine that was uniformly fatal in control rats showed universal survival in animals that also received fat emulsion.[117] Subsequent studies with experimental models of local anesthetic toxicity have demonstrated accelerated return of cardiac function after IFE both in intact animals and the isolated heart.[115,116]

In clinical reports, epinephrine has limited efficacy in the treatment of cardiac arrest that occurs from bupivacaine toxicity. This could possibly be secondary to inhibition of intracellular cyclic adenosine monophosphate production by bupivacaine. The efficacy of IFE was compared with epinephrine for resuscitation of bupivacaine-induced cardiovascular collapse in a rodent model.[112] IFE led to improved recovery.

A 20% IFE was successfully used to resuscitate a patient from a prolonged cardiac arrest caused by bupivacaine toxicity. The patient rapidly stabilized with IFE after failing to improve with 20 minutes of advanced cardiopulmonary resuscitation (CPR).[94] Subsequently, several case reports have been published describing successful use of IFE (in various formulations) to treat patients in cardiac arrest after regional anesthesia with various local anesthetic agents, including bupivacaine, ropivacaine, and levobupivacaine.[49,58,109]

The mechanism by which IFE reverses local anesthetic toxicity is uncertain. One of the hypotheses is that the exogenous fat emulsion provides a competing source for binding of lipid-soluble local anesthetics, a circulating lipid sink. This view is supported by a study that demonstrated decreased cardiac bupivacaine concentrations after IFE.[116] Another possibility is that the fat emulsion load might overwhelm the inhibition of the carnitine acylcarnitine translocase by mass action and thereby increase the myocardial energy supply, making the heart more likely to respond to resuscitation. In addition, IFE has positive inotropic effects in isolated heart preparations and reversed bupivacaine-induced cardiac depression at lipid levels less than those needed to reduce aqueous bupivacaine concentration.[99]

The limited clinical data suggest that an IV bolus of fat emulsion may be lifesaving in patients with refractory cardiovascular collapse secondary to local anesthetic overdose. Optimal dosing is uncertain.[110] Suggested dosing for a patient in cardiac arrest is 1.5 mL/kg bolus of 20% IFE over 1 minute while continuing chest compressions followed by 15 mL/kg/min for 30 to 60 minutes. If there is evidence of recovery, dosing should be changed to a continuous infusion of 20% IFE at a rate of 0.25 mL/kg/min [15 mL/kg/h] given until hemodynamic recovery, which can be increased as indicated.[111] IFE should be given after signs of local anesthetic toxicity become manifest[110] (see Antidote in Depth A21: Intravenous Fat Emulsion).

In addition to lipid therapy, standard advanced cardiac life support (ACLS) protocols should be generally followed when dealing with most episodes of local anesthetic cardiac toxicity. Hypotension in sinus rhythm results from both peripheral vasodilation and myocardial depression and should be treated with α- and β-adrenergic agonists. Vasopressin may be administered during CPR in addition to epinephrine. Atropine supplemented with electrical pacing should be used to treat bradycardia. The effectiveness of epinephrine in reversing local anesthetic–induced cardiac depression is inconsistent in various animal models. The dysrhythmic effects of epinephrine are of particular concern. Amrinone, a phosphodiesterase III inhibitor, was evaluated for treatment of bupivacaine-induced cardiac toxicity.[38,57] Anesthetized pigs with cardiovascular collapse induced by bupivacaine infusion survived when they were treated with amrinone; all of the control animals died of irreversible cardiac arrest.[57] A phosphodiesterase III inhibitor would be a good choice for reversing bupivacaine-induced cardiac depression.[96]

Bupivacaine-induced dysrhythmias often are refractory to cardioversion, defibrillation, and pharmacologic treatment. Lidocaine, phenytoin, magnesium, bretylium, amiodarone, calcium channel blockers, and combined therapy with clonidine and dobutamine have all been used in animal models with variable results.[27,65,67] Therapy for bupivacaine toxicity should be directed toward dissociating bupivacaine from the myocardial sodium channel, thereby reversing the drug's effects on cardiac conduction. Lidocaine competes with bupivacaine for cardiac sodium channels and at high doses may displace it. Anecdotal reports suggest that lidocaine has occasionally helped in this application.[23] However, concern persists about additive CNS effects when lidocaine is used to treat bupivacaine cardiac toxicity, and we do not recommend its routine use.

With toxicity from the longer-acting, highly lipid-soluble, protein-bound amide local anesthetics (bupivacaine and etidocaine), if the patient does not respond promptly to therapy, CPR can be expected to be difficult and prolonged (1–2 hours) before depression of the cardiac conduction system spontaneously reverses as a result of redistribution and metabolism of the drugs.[2,87] Vital organ perfusion is seriously compromised during CPR despite optimal chest compression. The significance of this problem increases with the duration of resuscitation; therefore, rapid initiation of cardiopulmonary bypass should be considered, if practical. Its use has resulted in a successful outcome in some cases of lidocaine and bupivacaine overdose.[37,60] Cardiopulmonary bypass provides circulatory support that is far superior to that provided by closed-chest cardiac massage. The improved perfusion prevents tissue hypoxia and the development of metabolic acidosis, which in turn decreases the binding of local anesthetics to myocardial sodium channel receptors. Hepatic blood flow is better maintained, enhancing local anesthetic metabolism, and increased myocardial blood flow helps redistribute local anesthetics out of the myocardium.[60]

Cardiac pacing was used successfully for treatment of cardiac arrest after unintentional administration of a 2 g bolus of lidocaine into a cardiopulmonary bypass circuit as the patient was being removed from bypass.[82] Pharmacologic therapy was unsuccessful, and resumption of bypass was necessary. Forty-five minutes after the injection, AV pacing restored perfusion and permitted discontinuation of bypass.

Use of sodium bicarbonate early in resuscitation to prevent acidosis-mediated potentiation of cardiac toxicity may have been beneficial in some cases,[23] but paradoxical effects on intracellular pH during CPR suggest against its use in the absence of strong experimental or clinical data. In another canine model, an infusion of 2 mL/kg 50% dextrose plus 1 Unit/kg insulin was superior to saline or dextrose alone in reversing bupivacaine-induced cardiac depression.[19] (see A18: Insulin Euglycemia) Effects on potassium current, calcium handling, and myocardial energy utilization all may have contributed to the salutatory effects of the insulin infusion.

PREVENTION OF SYSTEMIC TOXICITY OF LOCAL ANESTHETICS

Despite the development of new, relatively less toxic amide local anesthetics such as levobupivacaine and ropivacaine, severe CNS and cardiovascular effects are not eliminated. Several cases of ropivacaine-induced cardiac arrest have been reported.[18,49,53] In these cases, patients with both asystolic arrest and ventricular fibrillation–associated arrest were successfully resuscitated. Nonetheless, it is clear that prevention is more prudent and effective than treatment of toxicity. The keys to prevention are to use the lowest possible anesthetic concentration and volume consistent with effective anesthesia and to avoid a significant intravascular injection. The latter is accomplished by careful, slow aspiration of a needle or catheter before injection; injection of a small test dose of anesthetic mixed with epinephrine to assess a cardiovascular response if injection is intravascular; and use of slow, fractional dosing of large-volume injections with vigilance for early signs of CNS and cardiac toxicity.

SUMMARY

Local anesthetics are frequently used xenobiotics that provide surgical analgesia and acute and chronic pain relief. The analgesic effect of local anesthetics is primarily caused by inhibition of neural conductance secondary to sodium channel blockade. Systemic toxicity, which primarily affects the heart and brain, is also largely related to sodium channel blockade. Severe systemic toxicity usually occurs secondary to inadvertent intravascular injection. In most cases of systemic toxicity, CNS manifestations precede cardiovascular events. If cardiovascular collapse and cardiac arrest occur, resuscitation may be difficult and prolonged. A novel therapy of IV fat emulsion is shown to reverse, by uncertain mechanisms, local anesthetic toxicity. Cardiopulmonary bypass may be useful because it provides cardiovascular support, limits exacerbating factors such as tissue hypoxia and acidosis, and improves hepatic blood flow, thereby increasing local anesthetic metabolism. Avoidance of intravascular injection and vigilance for early signs of CNS and cardiac toxicity are keys to preventing serious adverse events.

ACKNOWLEDGMENT

Staffan Wahlander contributed to this chapter is a previous edition.

REFERENCES

1. Agarwal R, Gutlove D, Lockhart C. Seizures occurring in pediatric patients receiving continuous infusion of bupivacaine. *Anesth Analg.* 1992;75: 284-286.
2. Albright G. Cardiac arrest following regional anesthesia with etidocaine or bupivacaine. *Anesthesiology.* 1979;51:285-287.
3. Ash-Bernal R, Wise R, Wright S. Acquired methemoglobinemia—a retrospective series of 138 cases at 2 teaching hospitals. *Medicine.* 2004;83: 265-273.
4. Babui E, Garcia-Rubi D, Estanol B. Inadvertent massive lidocaine overdose causing temporary complete heart block in myocardial infarction. *Am Heart J.* 1981;102:801-803.
5. Badgwell J. Cardiovascular and central nervous system effects of co-administered lidocaine and bupivacaine in piglets. *Reg Anesth.* 1991;16:89-94.
6. Bardsley H, Gristwood R, Baker H, et al. A comparison of the cardiovascular effects of levobupivacaine and rac-bupivacaine following intravenous administration to healthy volunteers. *Br J Clin Pharmacol.* 1998;46: 245-249.
7. Batra MS, Bridenbaugh LD, Caldwell RD, Hecker BR. Bupivacaine cardiotoxicity in a pregnant patient with mitral valve prolapse: an example of an improperly administered epidural block. *Anesthesiology.* 1984;60:170-171.
8. Benoit P, Belt WD. Some effects of local anesthetic agents on skeletal muscle. *Exp Neurol.* 1972;34:264–278.
9. Berkun Y, Ben-Zvi A, Levy Y, et al. Evaluation of adverse reactions to local anesthetics: experience with 236 patients. *Ann Allergy Asthma Immunol.* 2003;91:342-345.
10. Bishop D, Johnstone R. Lidocaine toxicity treated with low-dose propofol. *Anesthesiology.* 1993;78:788-789.
11. Bonadio W. TAC: a review. *Pediatr Emerg Care.* 1989;5:128-130.
12. Bosnjak Z, Stowe D, Kampine J. Comparison of lidocaine and bupivacaine depression of sinoatrial node activity during hypoxia and acidosis in adult and neonatal guinea pigs. *Anesth Analg.* 1986;65:911-917.
13. Bruguerolle B, Emperaire N. Local anesthetic-induced toxicity may be modified by low-dose flumazenil. *Life Sci.* 1992;50:185-187.
14. Buckley MM, Benfield P. Eutectic lidocaine/prilocaine cream: a review of the topical anaesthetic/analgesic efficacy of a eutectic mixture of local anaesthetics (EMLA). *Drugs.* 1993;46:126-151.
15. Burney R, DiFazio C, Foster J. Effects of pH on protein binding of lidocaine. *Anesth Analg.* 1978;57:478-480.
16. Butterworth JF, Strichartz G. Molecular mechanisms of local anesthesia: a review. *Anesthesiology.* 1990;72:711-734.
17. Chang KS, Morrow DR, Kuzume K, et al. Bupivacaine inhibits baroreflex control of heart rate in conscious rats. *Anesthesiology.* 2000; 92:197-207.

18. Chazalon P, Tourtier J, Villevielle T, et al. Ropivacaine-induced cardiac arrest after peripheral nerve block: successful resuscitation. *Anesthesiology.* 2003; 99:1253-1254.
19. Cho H, Lee J, Chung I, et al. Insulin reverses bupivacaine-induced cardiac depression in dogs. *Anesth Analg.* 2000;91:1096-1102.
20. Clarkson C, Hondeghem LM. Mechanism for bupivacaine depression of cardiac conduction: fast block of sodium channels during the action potential with slow recovery from block during diastole. *Anesthesiology.* 1985;62:396-405.
21. Covino BG. New developments in the field of local anesthetics and the scientific basis for their clinical use. *Acta Anaesth Scand.* 1982;26:242-249.
22. Covino BG. Pharmacology of local anesthetic agents. *Br J Anaesth.* 1986;58: 701-716.
23. Davis N, de Jong R. Successful resuscitation following massive bupivacaine overdose. *Anesth Analg.* 1982;61:62-64.
24. de Jong R, Heavner J. Local anesthetic seizure prevention: diazepam versus pentobarbital. *Anesthesiology.* 1972;36:449-457.
25. de Jong R, Ronfeld R, DeRosa R. Cardiovascular effects of convulsant and supraconvulsant doses of amide local anesthetics. *Anesth Analg.* 1982;61:3-9.
26. de Jong R, Wagman I, Prince D. Effect of carbon dioxide on the cortical seizure threshold to lidocaine. *Exp Neurol.* 1967;17:221-232.
27. de la Coussaye J, Bassoul B, Brugada J, et al. Reversal of electrophysiologic and hemodynamic effects induced by high-dose of bupivacaine by the combination of clonidine and dobutamine in anesthetized dogs. *Anesth Analg.* 1992;74:703-711.
28. de la Coussaye J, Bassoul B, Albat B, et al. Experimental evidence in favor of role of intracellular actions of bupivacaine in myocardial depression. *Anesth Analg.* 1992;74:698-702.
29. Dinneen S, Mohr D, Fairbanks V. Methemoglobinemia from topically applied anesthetic spray. *Mayo Clin Proc.* 1994;69:886-888.
30. Dyhre H, Lang M, Wallin R, et al. The duration of action of bupivacaine, levobupivacaine, ropivacaine, and pethidine in peripheral nerve block in the rat. *Acta Anaesthesiol Scand.* 1997;41:1345-1352.
31. Eichenfeld LA. clinical study to evaluate the efficacy of ELA-Max (4% liposomal lidocaine) as compared with eutectic mixture of local anesthetics cream for pain reduction of venipuncture in children. *Pediatrics.* 2002;109:1093-1099.
32. Englesson S. The influence of acid-base changes on central nervous system toxicity of local anesthetic agents. I. An experimental study in cats. *Acta Anaesthesiol Scand.* 1974;18:79-87.
33. Englesson S. The influence of acid-base changes on central nervous system toxicity of local anesthetic agents: II. *Acta Anaesthesiol Scand.* 1974;18: 88-103.
34. Finkelstein F, Kreeft J. Massive lidocaine poisoning. *N Engl J Med.* 1979;301:50.
35. Foldes FF, Davidson GM, Duncalf D, Kuwabara S. The intravenous toxicity of local anesthetic agents in man. *Clin Pharm Ther.* 1965;6:328-335.
36. Franz D, Perry R. Mechanisms for differential block among single myelinated and nonmyelinated axons by procaine. *J Physiol.* 1974;236:193-210.
37. Freedman M, Gal J, Freed C. Extracorporeal pump assistance—novel treatment for acute lidocaine poisoning. *Eur J Clin Pharmacol.* 1982;22:129-135.
38. Fujita Y. Amrinone reverses bupivacaine-induced regional myocardial dysfunction. *Acta Anaesthesiol Scand.* 1996;40:47-52.
39. Giovannitti JA, Bennett CR. Assessment of allergy to local anesthetics. *J Am Dent Assoc.* 1979;98:701-706.
40. Graf BM, Martin E, Bosnjak ZJ, et al. Stereospecific effect of bupivacaine isomers on atrioventricular conduction in the isolated perfused guinea pig heart. *Anesthesiology.* 1997;86:410-419.
41. Hahn I, Hoffman RS, Nelson LS. EMLA-induced methemoglobinemia (metHb) and systemic topical anesthetic toxicity. *J Emerg Med.* 2004; 26: 85-88.
42. Halsted WS. Practical comments on the use and abuse of cocaine suggested by its invariably successful employment in more than a thousand minor surgical operations. *N Y Med J.* 1885;42:294.
43. Heavner J, Arthur J, Zou J, et al. Comparison of propofol with thiopentone for treatment of bupivacaine-induced seizures in rats. *Br J Anaesth.* 1993;71:715-719.
44. Heavner JE. Cardiac dysrhythmias induced by infusion of local anesthetics into the lateral ventricle of cats. *Anesth Analg.* 1986;65:133-138.
45. Hjelm M, Holmdahl M. Biochemical effects of aromatic amines II. Cyanosis methemoglobinemia and Heinz-body formation induced by a local anaesthetic agent (prilocaine). *Acta Anaesthesiol Scand.* 1965; 2:99-120.
46. Hollmann MW, Durieux ME. Local anesthetics and the inflammatory response: a new therapeutic indication? *Anesthesiology.* 2000;93:858-875.
47. Hollmann MW, Fisher LG, Byforf AM, et al. Local anesthetic inhibition of m1 muscarinic acetylcholine signaling. *Anesthesiology.* 2000; 93:497-509.
48. Hondeghem L, Miller R. *Local Anesthetics, Basic and Clinical Pharmacology*, 4th ed. Stamford, CT: Appleton and Lange; 1989:315-322.
49. Huet O, Eyrolle L, Mazoit J, et al. Cardiac arrest after injection of ropivacaine for posterior lumbar plexus blockade. *Anesthesiology.* 2003;99: 1451-1453.
50. Johnson M. Potential neurotoxicity of spinal anesthesia with lidocaine. *Mayo Clin Proc.* 2000;75:921-932.
51. Jorfeldt L, Lewis DH, Lofstrom JB, Post C. Lung uptake of lidocaine in man as influenced by anaesthesia, mepivacaine infusion or lung insufficiency. *Acta Anaesth Scand.* 1983;27:5-9.
52. Kasten G, Martin S. Successful cardiovascular resuscitation after massive intravenous bupivacaine overdosage in anesthetized dogs. *Anesth Analg.* 1985;64:491-497.
53. Klein S, Pierce T, Rubin Y, et al. Successful resuscitation after ropivacaine-induced ventricular fibrillation. *Anesth Analg.* 2004;97:901-903.
54. Kozody R, Ready L, Barsa J, Murphy T. Dose requirements of local anesthetic to produce grand mal seizure during stellate ganglion block. *Can Anaesth Soc J.* 1982;29:489-491.
55. Lambert L, Lambert D, Strichartz G. Irreversible conduction block in isolated nerve by high concentrations of local anesthetics. *Anesthesiology.* 1994;80:1082-1093.
56. Lee-Son S, Wang GK, Concus A, et al. Stereoselective inhibition of neuronal sodium channels by local anesthetics: evidence for two sites of action? *Anesthesiology.* 1992;77:324-335.
57. Lindgren L, Randell T, Suzuki N, et al. The effect of amrinone on recovery from severe bupivacaine intoxication in pigs. *Anesthesiology.* 1992;77: 309-315.
58. Litz RJ, Roessel T, Heler AR, Stehr SN. Reversal of central nervous system and cardiac toxicity after local anesthetic intoxication by lipid emulsion injection. *Anesth Analg.* 2008;106:1575-1577.
59. Lofstrom JB. Physiologic disposition of local anesthetics. *Reg Anesth.* 1982;7:33-38.
60. Long W, Rosenblum S, Grady I. Successful resuscitation of bupivacaine-induced cardiac arrest using cardiopulmonary bypass. *Anesth Analg.* 1989;69: 403-406.
61. Lund P, Cwik J. Propitocaine (citanest) and methemoglobinemia. *Anesthesiology.* 1965;26:569-571.
62. Lynch C III. Depression of myocardial contractility in vitro by bupivacaine, etidocaine, and lidocaine. *Anesth Analg.* 1986;65:551-559.
63. Mallampati SR, Liu P, Knapp RM. Convulsions and ventricular tachycardia from bupivacaine with epinephrine: successful resuscitation. *Anesth Analg.* 1984;63:856-859.
64. Marsch SCU, Schaefer HG, Castelli I. Unusual psychological manifestation of systemic local anesthetic toxicity. *Anesthesiology.* 1998;88:531-533.
65. Matsuda F, Kinney W, Wright W, Kambam J. Nicardipine reduces the cardio-respiratory toxicity of intravenously administered bupivacaine in rats. *Can J Anaesth.* 1990;37:920-923.
66. Mattison JB. Cocaine poisoning. *Med Surg Rep.* 1891;60:645-650.
67. Maxwell L, Martin L, Yaster M. Bupivacaine-induced cardiac toxicity in neonates: successful treatment with intravenous phenytoin. *Anesthesiology.* 1994;80:682-686.
68. Mazoit JX, Decaux A, Bouaziz H, et al. Comparative ventricular electrophysiologic effect of racemic bupivacaine, levobupivacaine, and ropivacaine on the isolated rabbit heart. *Anesthesiology.* 2000;92:784-792.
69. McCloskey J, Haun S, Deshpande J. Bupivacaine toxicity secondary to continuous caudal epidural infusion in children. *Anesth Analg.* 1992;75:287-290.
70. Moller R, Covino B. Cardiac electrophysiologic effects of lidocaine and bupivacaine. *Anesth Analg.* 1988;67:107-114.
71. Moore D, Balfour R, Fitzgibbons D. Convulsive arterial plasma levels of bupivacaine and the response to diazepam therapy. *Anesthesiology.* 1979;50:454-456.
72. Moore DC, Batra M. The components of an effective test dose prior to epidural block. *Anesthesiology.* 1981;55:693-696.
73. Moore DC, Bridenbaugh LD, Thompson GE, et al. Factors determining dosages of amide-type local anesthetic drugs. *Anesthesiology.* 1977;47: 263-268.
74. Moore DC, Bridenbaugh LD, Thompson GE, et al. Bupivacaine: a review of 11,080 cases. *Anesth Analg.* 1978;57:42-53.

75. Moore T, Walsh C, Cohen M. Reported adverse event cases of methemoglobinemia associated with benzocaine products. *Arch Intern Med.* 2004;164: 1192-1196.
76. Morishima H, Corvino B. Toxicity and distribution of lidocaine in nonasphyxiated and asphyxiated baboon fetuses. *Anesthesiology.* 1981;54:182-186.
77. Morishima H, Pederson H, Finster M, et al. Bupivacaine toxicity in pregnant and nonpregnant ewes. *Anesthesiology.* 1985;63:134-139.
78. Morishima H, Pederson H, Finster M, et al. Toxicity of lidocaine in adult, newborn, and fetal sheep. *Anesthesiology.* 1981;55:57-61.
79. Myers RR, Kalichman MW, Reisner LS, et al. Neurotoxicity of local anesthetics: altered perineural permeability, edema, and nerve fiber injury. *Anesthesiology.* 1986;64:29-35.
80. Nation R, Triggs E, Selig M. Lignocaine kinetics in cardiac and aged subjects. *Br J Clin Pharmacol.* 1977;4:439-445.
81. Nau C, Vogel W, Hempelmann G, et al. Stereoselectivity of bupivacaine in local anesthetic-sensitive ion channels of peripheral nerve. *Anesthesiology.* 1999;91:786-795.
82. Noble J, Kennedy D, Latimer R, et al. Massive lignocaine overdose during cardiopulmonary bypass: successful treatment with cardiac pacing. *Br J Anaesth.* 1984;56:1439-1441.
83. Nystrom EUM, Heavner JE, Buffington CW. Blood pressure is maintained despite profound myocardial depression during acute bupivacaine overdose in pigs. *Anesth Analg.* 1999;88:1143-1148.
84. Peterson RC. History of cocaine. *NIDA Res Monogr.* 1977;13:17-34.
85. Pitkanen M, Feldman HS, Arthur GR, et al. Chronotropic and inotropic effects of ropivacaine, bupivacaine, and lidocaine in the spontaneously beating and electrically paced isolated perfused rabbit heart. *Reg Anesth Pain Med.* 1992;17:183-192.
86. Polley LS, Columb MO, Naughton NN, et al. Relative analgesic potencies of ropivacaine and bupivacaine for epidural analgesia in labor: implications for therapeutic indexes. *Anesthesiology.* 1999;90:944-950.
87. Prentiss J. Cardiac arrest following caudal anesthesia. *Anesthesiology.* 1979;50:51-53.
88. Reisner LS, Hochman BN, Plumer MH. Persistent neurologic deficit and adhesive arachnoiditis following intrathecal 2-chloroprocaine injection. *Anesth Analg.* 1980;59:452-454.
89. Reiz S, Nath S. Cardiotoxicity of local anesthetic agents. *Br J Anaesth.* 1986;58:736-746.
90. Reynolds F. Adverse effects of local anaesthetics. *Br J Anaesth.* 1987;59:78-95.
91. Rigler M, Drasner K, Krejcie T, et al. Cauda equina syndrome after continuous spinal anesthesia. *Anesth Analg.* 1991;72:275-281.
92. Rosen M, Thigpen J, Schnider S, et al. Bupivacaine-induced cardiotoxicity in hypoxic and acidotic sheep. *Anesth Analg.* 1985;64:1089-1096.
93. Rosenberg PH, Kalso EA, Tuominen MK, Linden HB. Acute bupivacaine toxicity as a result of venous leakage under the tourniquet cuff during a bier block. *Anesthesiology.* 1983;58:95-98.
94. Rosenblatt MA, Abel M, Fischer GW, et al. Successful use of a 20% lipid emulsion to resuscitate a patient after a presumed bupivacaine-related cardiac arrest. *Anesthesiology.* 2006;105:217-218.
95. Saitoh K, Hirabayashi Y, Shimizu R, Fukuda H. Amrinone is superior to epinephrine in reversing bupivacaine-induced cardiovascular depression in sevoflurane-anesthetized cats. *Anesthesiology.* 1995;83:127-133.
96. Scott DB. Evaluation of the toxicity of local anaesthetic agents in man. *Br J Anaesth.* 1975;47:56-61.
97. Scott DB. "Maximal recommended doses" of local anaesthetic drugs. *Br J Anaesth.* 1989;63:373-374.
98. Scott DB. Toxicity caused by local anaesthetic drugs. *Br J Anaesth.* 1981;53: 553-554.
99. Stehr SN, Pexa A, Hannack S, et al. The effects of lipid infusion on myocardial function and bioenergetics in l-bupivacaine toxicity in the isolated rat heart. *Anesth Analg.* 2007;104:186-192.
100. Strichartz GR, Berde CB. Local anesthetics. In: Miller RD, ed. *Anesthesia,* 4th ed. New York: Churchill Livingstone; 1994:489-521.
101. Sztark F, Malgat M, Dabadie P, et al. Comparison of the effects of bupivacaine and ropivacaine on heart cell mitochondrial bioenergetics. *Anesthesiology.* 1998;88:1340-1349.
102. Taddio A, Stevens B, Craig K, et al. Efficacy and safety of lidocaine prilocaine cream for pain during circumcision. *N Engl J Med.* 1997; 336:1197-1201.
103. Tanaka K, Yamasaki M. Blocking of cortical inhibitory synapses by intravenous lidocaine. *Nature.* 1966;209:207-208.
104. Taniguchi M, Bollen A, Drasner K. Sodium bisulfite: scapegoat for chloroprocaine neurotoxicity? *Anesthesiology.* 2004;100:85-91.
105. Thomas R, Behbehani M, Coyle D, et al. Cardiovascular toxicity of local anesthetics: an alternative hypothesis. *Anesth Analg.* 1986;65: 444-450.
106. Verrill PJ. Adverse reactions to local anesthetics and vasoconstrictor drugs. *Practitioner.* 1975;214:380-387.
107. Wagman IH, de Jong RH, Prince DA. Effects of lidocaine on the central nervous system. *Anesthesiology.* 1967;28:155-172.
108. Wang BC, Hillman DE, Spielholz NI, et al. Chronic neurologic deficits and Nesacaine: an effect of the anesthetic 2-chloroprocaine or the antioxidant sodium bisulfite? *Anesth Analg.* 1984;63:445-447.
109. Warren JA, Thoma RB, Georgescu A, Shah SJ. Intravenous lipid infusion in the successful resuscitation of local anesthetic-induced cardiovascular collapse after supraclavicular brachial plexus block. *Anesth Analg.* 2008;106:1578-1580.
110. Weinberg GL. Lipid infusion therapy. Translation to clinical practice. *Anesth Analg.* 2008;106:1340-1342.
111. Weinberg GL. Lipid rescue—caveats and recommendations for the "Silver Bullet." [letter]. *Reg Anesth Pain Med.* 2004;29:74-75.
112. Weinberg GL, Gregorio GD, Ripper R, et al. Resuscitation with lipid versus epinephrine in a rat model of bupivacaine overdose. *Anesthesiology.* 2008; 108:907-913.
113. Weinberg GL, Laurito C, Geldner P, et al. Malignant ventricular dysrhythmias in a patient with isovaleric acidemia receiving general and local anesthesia for suction lipectomy. *J Clin Anesth.* 1997;9:668-670.
114. Weinberg GL, Palmer JW, VadeBoncourer TR, et al. Bupivacaine inhibits acylcarnitine exchange in cardiac mitochondria. *Anesthesiology.* 2000;92: 523-528.
115. Weinberg G, Ripper R, Feinstein D, et al. Lipid emulsion infusion rescues dogs from bupivacaine-induced cardiac toxicity. *Reg Anesth Pain Med.* 2003; 28:198-202.
116. Weinberg G, Ripper R, Murphy P, et al. Lipid infusion accelerates removal of bupivacaine and recovery from bupivacaine toxicity in the isolated rat heart. *Reg Anesth Pain Med.* 2006;31:296-303.
117. Weinberg GL, VadeBoncouer T, Ramaraju GA, et al. Pretreatment or resuscitation with a lipid infusion shifts the dose-response to bupivacaine-induced asystole in rats. *Anesthesiology.* 1998:88:1071-1075.

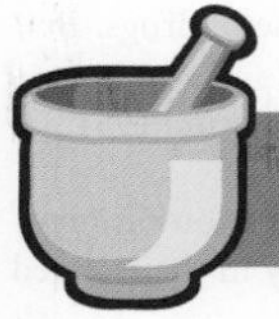

ANTIDOTES IN DEPTH (A21)

INTRAVENOUS FAT EMULSIONS

Theodore C. Bania

Intravenous fat emulsion (IFE) has been used as a source of parenteral nutrition for over 40 years. More recently, IFE has also been used as a diluent for intravenous drug delivery of highly lipophilic xenobiotics such as propofol and liposomal amphotericin. The use of IFE as an antidote is most extensively studied for the treatment of local anesthetic toxicity, specifically from bupivacaine, but new applications that are being investigated and reported on include the treatment of overdose from lipophilic drugs such as calcium channel blockers, cyclic antidepressants, clomipramine, and beta adrenergic antagonists, to name a few.

PHARMACOLOGY

Intravenous fat emulsion is composed of two types of lipids, triglycerides and phospholipids. Triglycerides are hydrophobic molecules that are formed when three fatty acids are linked to one glycerol. The fatty acid chain length varies, producing different triglycerides. The main triglycerides in IFE are linoleic, linolenic, oleic, palmitic, and stearic acids, and concentrations of these vary slightly in the different commercially available fat emulsions. These long-chain triglycerides (12 or more carbons) are extracted from safflower oil and/or soybean oil depending on the brand of the emulsion.[42] Newer fat emulsions contain long-chain triglycerides in addition to medium-chain triglycerides (6–12 carbons) derived from coconut, olive, and fish oils but are currently not available in the United States.[46]

Phospholipids contain two fatty acids bound to glycerol along with a phosphoric acid moiety at the third hydroxyl (Fig A21–1). Phospholipids are amphipathic, that is, the nonpolar fatty acids are hydrophobic while the polar phosphate head is hydrophilic. This imparts important pharmacological properties to this carrier molecule, allowing it to solubilize nonpolar xenobiotics into the aqueous serum. The phospholipids in IFE are extracted from egg yolks.

The lipids in IFE are dispersed in the serum by forming an emulsion of small lipid droplets. To create the emulsion droplets, the phospholipids form a layer around a triglyceride core. The hydrophobic fatty acid component of the phospholipid molecule is directed toward the triglycerides while the hydrophilic glycerol component is directed outward away from the triglyceride core. The presence of small amounts of glycerol, which is hydrophilic, allows the lipid droplets to be suspended as an emulsion in water and serum.

Intravenous fat emulsion is a white, milky liquid. It is sterile and nonpyrogenic with a pH of about 8 (range 6 to 9). IFEs are isotonic solutions (260–310 mOsm/L) and are available in 5%, 10%, 20%, and 30% solutions. The 30% solution should be diluted before administration. IFE can be delivered through a peripheral or central vein.[42]

Intravenous fat emulsions have different globule sizes depending on their uses.[7] Microemulsions (mean droplet size less than 0.1 μm) are used for drug delivery. Mini-emulsions (mean droplet size greater than 0.1 μm but less than 1.0 μm) are used for parenteral nutrition. Droplet sizes in commercially available nutritional IFEs range from 0.4 to 0.5 μm. After intravenous administration, IFEs are found in the serum as chylomicron-like lipid droplets that turn the serum turbid or milky. Macro-emulsions (mean droplet size greater than 1.0 μm) are used for chemoembolization. These macro-emulsions contain antineoplastics that are delivered intraarterially directly into the tumor blood supply. The lipid droplets occlude the artery and slowly release the antineoplastic.

Lipid droplets that are less than 1 μm are primarily removed from circulation as they pass through the capillaries of adipose tissue and the liver. The capillary endothelium in these tissues contains lipoprotein lipase, which hydrolyzes triglycerides releasing fatty acids and glycerol that then diffuses into the cells. Fatty acids also enter the cardiac myocyte either by passive diffusion or protein-mediated transport.[39]

Once inside the cells, fatty acids are used as energy or resynthesized into triglycerides and stored. For use as energy, triglycerides are transported into the mitochondria by carnitine palmitoyl transferase, where they undergo β oxidation sequentially releasing acetylcoenzyme A (acetyl-CoA) as the fatty acid chain is reduced in length. These acetyl-CoA molecules enter the Krebs cycle, where they ultimately generate adenosine triphosphate (ATP) (see Fig. 12-3 and 12-8). Although glucose, lactate, and fatty acid metabolism may ultimately lead to the production of acetyl-CoA, fatty acid metabolism produces the largest amount of energy. For example, 1 mol of glucose produces 38 ATP while 1 mol of stearic acid produces 146 ATPs[55] and the metabolism of longer fatty acid chains may produce more ATP.

The half-life of IFE is 30 to 60 minutes, and can vary substantially depending on the patient's clinical state, dose of IFE, and droplet size.[8] Larger droplet sizes have slower clearances, and are removed by reticuloendothelial phagocytosis. These larger droplets are more likely to induce an inflammatory response, obstruct the microvasculature, and produce capillary fat emboli.

MECHANISM OF ACTION

The mechanisms of action of IFE in toxicology are not clearly understood. There are currently three proposed mechanisms of action of IFE in toxicology: modulation of intracellular metabolism, a lipid sink or sponge mechanism, and activation of ion channels.

In experimental models of poisoning from xenobiotics that alter intracellular energy metabolism, toxicity was successfully treated with IFE, suggesting that repairing or circumventing this dysfunction may be involved. Bupivacaine blocks carnitine-dependent mitochondrial lipid transport and inhibits adenosine triphosphatase (ATPase) synthetase in the electron transport chain.[6,51] Verapamil also inhibits intracellular processing of fatty acids,[20,21] but it inhibits insulin release and produces insulin resistance as well.[21] The cyclic antidepressant amitriptyline depresses human myocardial contraction independent of an effect on conduction[16] and inhibits medium- and short-chain fatty acid metabolism.[48] Propranolol changes intracellular energy from primarily fatty acid to carbohydrate-dependent metabolism.[28]

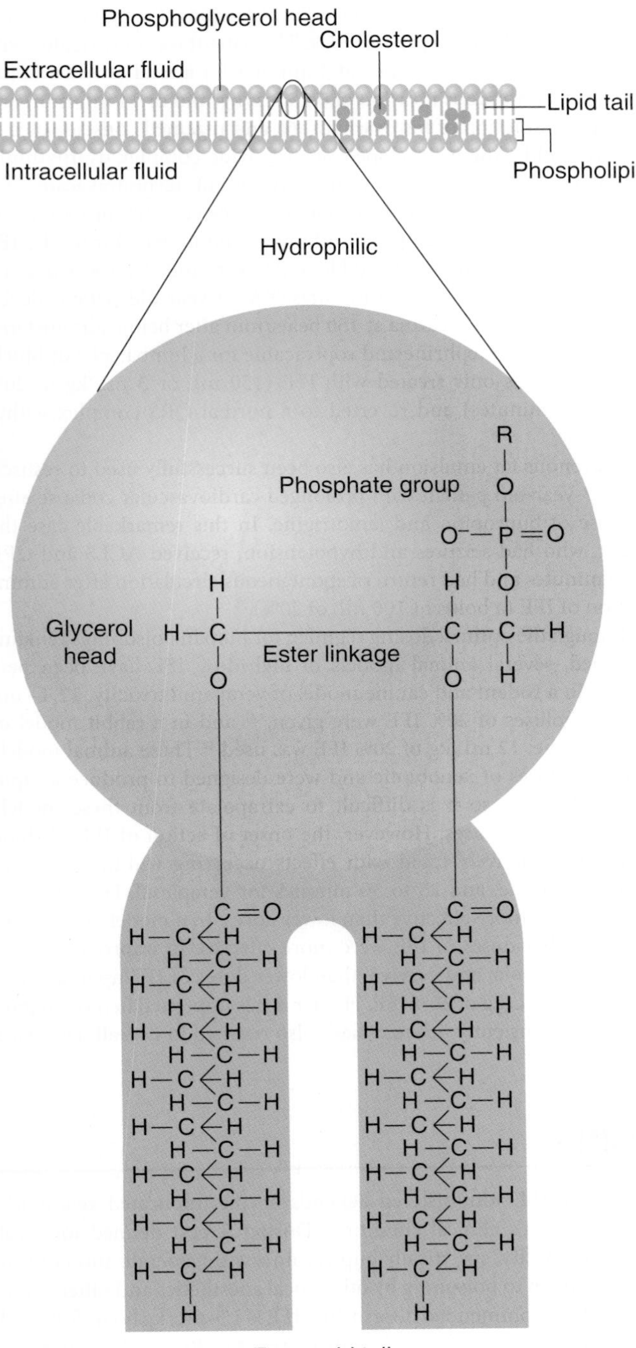

FIGURE A21–1. Biologic membranes are comprised of phospolipids that have a hyrophilic phosphoglycerol "head" and hydrophobic fatty acid "tails." .

Theoretically, adding excess fatty acids may overcome blocked or inhibited enzymes by mass action, providing energy to an energy "starved" heart, reversing toxicity. There is limited experimental evidence to support a modulation of intracellular energy metabolism as the mechanism of action of the IFE for poisoning. The only evidence to support this mechanism comes from IFE effect in reversing myocardial depression resulting from myocardial ischemia.[43] In a canine model of 10 minutes of regional myocardial ischemia, treatment with IFE after ischemia resulted in improved systolic wall thickening. In the same canine model, pretreatment with oxfenicine, which blocks carnitine palmitoyl transferase one blocked the beneficial effect of IFE.[20] This implies that the effects of IFE on myocardial contraction following ischemia are mediated by mitochondrial metabolism. To determine if this is the mechanism of action in verapamil toxicity, rodents were pretreated with oxfenicine or control solution and had verapamil toxicity induced. Both groups were then resuscitated with IFE.[1] There was no significant difference in survival time and mean arterial pressure between the oxfenicine-treated and control groups. This implies that in verapamil toxicity IFE works by a mechanism other than supplying energy to the mitochondria.

In the lipid sink/sponge mechanism, IFE soaks up lipid-soluble xenobiotic and removes it from the site of toxicity. In a slight variation of this mechanism, IFE may pull the xenobiotic out of the aqueous plasma, which bathes the tissue, and into a nonaqueous part of the plasma that is not in contact with the site of toxicity. IFE may also change the distribution of lipid-soluble xenobiotics and deposit them away from the site of toxicity into an area with high lipid content. There is some experimental support for this lipid/sponge mechanism. In an isolated heart model, hearts were perfused with bupivacaine until asystole and then treated with control or IFE. The IFE-treated hearts had a faster recovery from asystole, lower concentration of bupivacaine in the tissue, and higher concentrations of bupivacaine in the venous effluent.[52] In a successful resuscitation from bupropion overdose, bupropion concentrations increased dramatically after administration of IFE.[36] These findings in the experimental model and case report can be explained by the lipid sink/sponge model, where IFE pulls a xenobiotic out of tissue stores. However, the increased concentrations in both could also be explained by an increased perfusion of tissues with the return of circulation and release of the drug. Stronger evidence for the lipid sink/sponge mechanism comes from a pharmacokinetic study of clomipramine concentrations following infusion of IFE. In a rabbit model of clomipramine-induced hypotension, IFE resulted in a more rapid increase in blood pressure compared with saline.[15] These hemodynamic effects were associated with an increased concentration and decreased volume of distribution of clomipramine.

Additionally, IFE may activate ion, particularly Ca^{2+}, channels. Fatty acids directly activate myocardial calcium channels and induce a dose-dependent increase in the Ca^{2+} current. Oleic, linoleic, and linolenic acids act directly on the Ca^{2+} channel to increase Ca^{2+} current.[18] Unfortunately, there is no direct support for this mechanism of action of IFE.

Despite the lack of studies on mechanisms of action, the lipid sink/sponge model is the most likely hypothesis since beneficial effects from IFE are most frequently noted for lipid-soluble xenobiotics. Other mechanisms may be consequential and the mechanism of action may vary for different xenobiotics.

EFFICACY IN POISONING

EXPERIMENTAL MODELS

IFE was first studied as an antidote to bupivacaine toxicity and then evaluated for calcium channel blockers, cyclic antidepressants, and β-adrenergic antagonist toxicity. In a rodent model, pretreatment with IFE (10%–30%) followed by a continuous infusion of bupivacaine (10 mg/kg/min) increased the dose of bupivacaine needed to induce asystole.[53] In the second part of this study, bupivacaine was infused into rodents until the development of cardiac arrest. Rodents were resuscitated with IFE (30% IFE, 7.5 mL/kg bolus then 3 mL/kg/min for 2 minutes) or an equivalent volume of saline. Animals were more successfully resuscitated with IFE from a larger dose of bupivacaine then when saline treated. The LD_{50} for saline resuscitation was 12.5 mg/kg, whereas the LD_{50} for IFE resuscitation was 18.5 mg/kg. In a larger animal model, bupivacaine was administered until cardiac arrest and then the animal was resuscitated with IFE (20% IFE, 4 mL/kg bolus, then 0.5 mL/kg/min for 10 minutes) or saline. Intravenous fat emulsion resulted in a dramatic improvement in survival as six of six survived following IFE versus none in the control (zero of six).[49,50]

In a controlled study of rodents given a continuous infusion of verapamil, treatment with 12.4-mL/kg bolus of 20% IFE resulted in an increase in heart rate and survival compared with control.[41] In a larger animal model of verapamil toxicity where animals were also treated with calcium and atropine, 7 mL/kg of 20% IFE over 30 minutes resulted in improved blood pressure and survival.[2]

In an experimental model of clomipramine toxicity,[14] rabbits were given clomipramine until mean arterial pressure decreased to 50% of baseline. They were then treated with sodium bicarbonate (3 mL/kg of 8.4%), IFE (12 mL/kg of 20%), or sodium chloride (12 mL/kg of 0.9%). Intravenous fat emulsion resulted in an increase in mean arterial pressure over sodium chloride and $NaHCO_3$. In a second part of this study, clomipramine was administered until cardiovascular collapse followed by resuscitation with $NaHCO_3$ (2 mL/kg of 8.4%) or IFE (8 mL/kg of 20%) delivered over 2 minutes. Intravenous fat emulsion resulted in improved survival (four of four) whereas $NaHCO_3$ resulted in no resuscitations (zero of four).

In a rodent model with a constant infusion of propranolol, IFE decreased QRS prolongation, but the study was underpowered to detect an effect on heart rate or survival.[5] In another rodent and rabbit model of propranolol toxicity, IFE resulted in an increase in blood pressure.[4,13]

CLINICAL CASE REPORTS

Based upon the experimental evidence in bupivacaine toxicity, IFE was subsequently successfully used in several reported human cases of cardiovascular collapse from local anesthetic overdose. Previously, cardiopulmonary bypass was the only effective treatment for these patients, as most cases were refractory to standard cardiac resuscitative measures (see Chap. 66). The first reported case occurred in a patient who developed cardiac arrest after the inadvertent intravenous administration of bupivacaine and mepivacaine during an interscalene block.[32] The patient was treated with cardiopulmonary resuscitation (CPR) and advanced cardiac life support (ACLS) for 20 minutes, but only had return of spontaneous circulation after administration of the first dose of IFE (100 mL of 20% IFE followed by 0.5 mL/kg/min for 2 hours). The second successfully treated case occurred when a patient developed asystole after inadvertent intravenous administration of ropivacaine during an axillary plexus block.[25] The patient received CPR and ACLS and had return of spontaneous circulation 10 minutes after administration of IFE (100 mL of 20% or 2 mL/kg followed by an infusion at 10 mL/min for an additional dose of 100 mL of IFE). Additionally, a 60-year-old man with diabetes, coronary artery disease, and end-stage renal failure became unresponsive and developed ventricular fibrillation and torsades de pointes after administration of mepivacaine and bupivacaine for a supraclavicular brachial plexus block. The patient was treated with CPR and ACLS for 10 minutes and then was treated with IFE (250 mL of 20% over 30 minutes). He had return of pulse and blood pressure 11 minutes later.[47]

In addition to its use during resuscitation, IFE has been used to treat milder symptoms of local anesthetic toxicity such as central nervous system symptoms and dysrhythmias without loss of pulse. A patient developed agitation, dizziness, unresponsiveness, and atrial premature contractions and bigeminy after administration of mepivacaine and prilocaine for a brachial plexus block. The patient was only treated with IFE (1 mL/kg of 20%, repeated at 3 minutes for a total of 100 mL, followed by a continuous infusion of 0.25 mL/kg/min or 14 mL/min) and had rapid resolution of his dysrhythmia and regained consciousness.[26] A 75-year-old patient developed seizure, wide complex dysrhythmia, and hypotension following administration of levobupivacaine for a lumbar plexus block. The patient was treated with propofol and metaraminol and IFE (20%, 100 mL over 5 minutes). During the IFE infusion, the QRS narrowed and blood pressure and electrocardiogram (ECG) normalized within 10 minutes.[10] A 13-year-old patient developed ventricular tachycardia at 150 beats/min after being administered lidocaine with epinephrine and ropivacaine for a lumbar plexus block. The patient was only treated with IFE (150 mL or 3 mL/kg of 20% IFE over 3 minutes) and reverted to a normal QRS complex within 2 minutes.[27]

Intravenous fat emulsion has also been successfully used to resuscitate a 17-year-old patient with prolonged cardiovascular collapse after overdose of bupropion and lamotrigine. In this remarkable case the patient, who had seizures and hypotension, received ACLS and CPR for 70 minutes and had return of spontaneous circulation after administration of IFE (a bolus of 100 mL of 20%).[36]

Although the optimal dosing regimen for human poisonings remains undefined, several animal models of high-dose IFE have been performed. In a rodent and canine model of verapamil toxicity, 12.4- and 7-mL/kg boluses of 20% IFE were given,[3,41] and in a rabbit model of clomipramine, 12 mL/kg of 20% IFE was used.[42] These animal models used large doses of xenobiotic and were designed to produce a rapid onset of toxicity, so it is difficult to extrapolate from these models to typical human cases. However, the onset of action of IFE in these models was relatively rapid with effects occurring within 5 minutes for clomipramine, and 25 to 30 minutes for verapamil. Higher doses of IFE also are more effective than lower doses. In a model of verpamil toxicity, higher doses of IFE were more effective in improving blood pressure, acidemia, and survival than lower doses of IFE up to a maximum of 18.6 mL/kg of 20% IFE. Higher doses improved hemodynamic parameters transiently but may have also resulted in overall decreased survival times.[31]

DOSING

The dose of IFE administered depends on the implicated xenobiotic and the patient's clinical condition. Dosing is best defined for local anesthetic toxicity, specifically bupivacaine, with generalization of this dosing regimen to poisoning by other local anesthetics and other xenobiotics. The recommended dose of 20% IFE is 1.5-mL/kg bolus followed by 0.25 mL/kg/min or 15 mL/kg/h to run for 30 to 60 minutes.[11,49] The bolus can be repeated several times for persistent asystole, and the infusion rate can be increased if blood pressure decreases. For local anesthetic poisoning, earlier recommendations limited use of IFE only if standard resuscitative measures failed. As a result of the experimental evidence and many successful case reports, some authors are recommending adding IFE at the first signs of local anesthetic toxicity or, in the setting of cardiovascular collapse, to use IFE concomitantly with CPR and ACLS.[54] Generalization of this practice to other xenobiotics is not currently studied or recommended. Some authors are also recommending that IFE be stored for easy and rapid access in operating rooms or in areas where local anesthetics are frequently used.[33] Most case reports documenting successful treatment of local anesthetic toxicity with lipids have been with Intralipid®; however, other parenteral lipid formulations such as Medialipid® (a mixture of 50%

long-chain triglycerides and 50% medium-chain triglycerides; Braun, Germany)[27] and Liposyn III® (Hospira Inc., Lake Forest, IL)[47] have also been successful, suggesting that all currently available parenteral lipid products will be as effective.

Propofol is formulated as a 10% lipid emulsion, but it is not recommended for use a lipid rescue agent[50] because of the adverse effect of the propofol from the dose needed as a lipid rescue agent. For bupivacaine toxicity, 1.5-mL/kg bolus of 20% IFE is recommended which equates to 3 mL/kg of the 10% lipid emulsion in the propofol solution. As normal dose of propofol (1%) for general anesthesia is 2.5 mg/kg or 0.25 mL/kg.[34] Using propofol as a lipid rescue agent would deliver a bolus of 12 times the recommended dose of propofol. This would exacerbate any drug-induced hypotension and bradycardia.

Experimental evidence indicates that IFE may be potentially beneficial in verapamil,[2,31,41] clomipramine,[14,15] and propranolol[4,13] toxicity and this may be extrapolated to other lipid-soluble calcium channel blockers, cyclic antidepressants, or β-adrenergic antagonists. These xenobiotics will usually demonstrate continued absorption, longer duration of toxicity, severe hypotension, and either dysrhythmias or bradycardia over several hours or days. The precise indications and dose of IFE for these situations has not been studied.

It may occasionally be necessary to administer a continuous infusion of IFE following initial resuscitation. The dose of IFE used for nutrition is generally considered a safe dose, except for the potential complications described above. Currently, the nutritional dose of IFE is 1 to 2 g/kg/d or 5 to 10 mL/kg/d of 20% IFE, which is administered over 6 to 24 hours.[8,33] The dose can be increased daily up to 3 g/kg/d. This dose and rate is less than the dose recommended for bupivacaine toxicity (1.5 mL/kg bolus of 20% IFE followed by 15 mL/kg/h for 30 to 60 minutes)[11] and less than the doses used in experimental models for other xenobiotic toxicity. Based on the current data available from animal models, if IFE is used for severe xenobiotic-induced toxicity other than for that of local anesthetics, the safest dosing would be to start with the low dose suggested for bupivacaine toxicity and titrate up, every hour, if hemodynamic parameters continue to worsen.

ADVERSE EFFECTS AND CONTRAINDICATIONS

There have been no reported adverse effects attributed to IFE in the case reports of IFE use in local anesthetic or bupropion toxicity. With the doses used in these cases and the short durations of administration, most patients recovered fully without any significant adverse effects.[10,25-27,33,36,47] Based on these case reports, a dose of 1.5-mL/kg bolus of 20% IFE followed by 0.25 mL/kg/min or 15 mL/kg/h to run for 30 to 60 minutes appears to be safe in bupivacaine-induced cardiac arrest and severe toxicity.

Because of the limited number of case reports, toxicity from IFE remains a concern. Pulmonary toxicity has been reported when IFE is used as a source of parenteral nutrition. In patients with acute respiratory distress syndrome (ARDS), 500 mL of 20% IFE administered over 8 hours resulted in an increase in pulmonary artery pressures, pulmonary shunting, pulmonary vascular resistance, and a decrease in partial pressure of oxygen in the alveoli/fraction of inspired oxygen (PAO_2/FIO_2).[45] Similar results were found in patients with ARDS administered 500 mL of 10% IFE over 4 hours resulting in an increase in pulmonary shunting and a decrease in the fraction of PAO_2/FIO_2.[19] The pulmonary effect of IFE in ARDS may be related to the rate of infusion. In patients with ARDS, 500 mL of 20% IFE infused over 5 hours resulted in an increase in pulmonary pressures, and slower infusion over 10 hours had no effect on pulmonary pressures.[29] There are conflicting results of the effects of IFE in patients without ARDS. In septic and nonseptic patients without ARDS, 500 mL of 20% IFE administered over 10 hours resulted in an increase in pulmonary artery pressures and pulmonary shunting.[44] In patients with chronic obstructive pulmonary disease (COPD) and pneumonia, 500 mL of 10% IFE administered over 4 hours did not have any pulmonary effects, and in a group of healthy postoperative patients this dose actually decreased pulmonary shunting and increased PAO_2/FIO_2 ratio.[19]

In these studies, when pulmonary effects occurred they were mild and resolved after the IFE infusion was stopped or within 3 to 4 hours. Larger doses may result in clinically significant toxicity and more prolonged effect. However, studies using fat emulsions with medium-chain triglycerides have shown less pulmonary toxicity.[9,37]

There are two mechanisms by which IFE may cause pulmonary toxicity. IFE may occlude the pulmonary vasculature with micro–fat emboli. This is supported by the finding of macrophages containing lipid droplets in the bronchial alveolar lavage fluid of ARDS patients treated with IFE.[24] Experimental evidence also supports the possibility that the high concentrations of linoleic acid in IFE are converted to arachidonic acid and then into vasoactive prostaglandins. Indomethacin, an inhibitor of prostaglandin synthesis, prevented any pulmonary vascular effect caused by IFE in a sheep model.[30]

In addition to pulmonary toxicity, large dose and/or more rapid infusion of IFE have the potential to induce a fat overload syndrome. The fat overload syndrome is characterized by hyperlipemia, fever, fat infiltration, hepatomegaly, jaundice, splenomegaly, anemia, leukopenia, thrombocytopenia, coagulation disturbances, seizures, and coma. Multiple end-organ dysfunction is attributed to inadequate clearance of lipids and sludging in the lungs, brain, kidney, retina, and liver.[7,8,12,17,22,24,34,35,40] Because of the rapid redistribution of most local anesthetics, prolonged IFE infusion should not be required (see Chap. 66). However, many other lipid-soluble xenobiotics have a long duration of toxicity and prolonged IFE infusions may be recommended, resulting in a fat overload syndrome.

Intravenous fat emulsion has the potential to increase gastrointestinal absorption of lipid-soluble xenobiotics. Although this is only currently a theoretical concern, the excessive xenobiotic would likely be partitioned into the IFE and thus be unlikely to result in additional toxicity. Intravenous fat emulsion also has the potential to interact with other antidotes being used. If an antidote is lipid soluble, it may be incorporated by the IFE and result in decreased effectiveness. This is a theoretical concern, and there are no clinical data supporting this concern. IFE has been used with several medications during resuscitation from bupivacaine toxicity including epinephrine, atropine, amiodarone, vasopressin, sodium bicarbonate, magnesium sulfate, calcium chloride, naloxone, and metaraminol.[10,25,32,36,47]

The combined use of IFE and high-dose insulin-euglycemia was evaluated in a model of severe verapamil toxicity and there was no improvement in hemodynamics, metabolic parameters, or survival.[3] Therefore, while other resuscitative drugs should be used as indicated, there is no evidence yet to support or refute the simultaneous use of IFE and high-dose insulin-euglycemia therapy.

IFE is contraindicated in patients with egg allergy, soybean allergy, disorders of fat metabolism, and liver disease. It is contraindicated in patients with myocardial ischemia and infarction because in animal models it increased dysrhythmias and impaired cardiac pump performance when administered during ischemia,[23,38] but was of benefit when administered after ischemia. In an ischemic myocardial cell, fatty acid metabolism is thought to result in lipid peroxidation and free radical production, which increases dysrhythmias and impairs myocardial performance.[43]

SUMMARY

IFE should be used for local-anesthetic-induced cardiac arrest and severe toxicity such as persistent ventricular dysrhythmias. IFE can be used with standard resuscitation and should be stored where local anesthetics are used. A bolus dose of 1.5 mL/kg of 20% IFE should be followed by an infusion for 30 to 60 minutes of 0.25 mL/kg/min or 15 mL/kg/h. Repeat boluses of IFE can be used for persistent asystole.

The use of IFE for other xenobiotics is unclear at this time, though animal data support its use for several lipid-soluble xenobiotics such as verapamil, clomipramine, and β-adrenergic antagonists.

REFERENCES

1. Bania TC, Chu J, Lyon T, Yoon JT. The role of cardiac free fatty acid metabolism in verapamil toxicity treated with intravenous fat emulsion. *Acad Emerg Med.* 2007;14:S196-S197.
2. Bania TC, Chu J, Perez E, et al. Hemodynamic effects of intravenous fat emulsion in an animal model of severe verapamil toxicity resuscitated with atropine, calcium, and saline. *Acad Emerg Med.* 2007;14:105-111.
3. Bania TC, Chu J, Perez E, et al. Hemodynamic effects of intravenous fat emulsion plus standard therapy in a model of severe verapamil toxicity. *Acad Emerg Med.* 2007;14:S49.
4. Bania TC, Chu J, Wesolowski M. The hemodynamic effect of intralipid on propranolol toxicity. *Acad Emerg Med.* 2006;13:S108-S109.
5. Cave G, Harvey MG, Castle CD. The role of fat emulsion therapy in a rodent model of propranolol toxicity: a preliminary study. *J Med Toxicol.* 2006;2:4-7.
6. Chazotte B, Vanderkooi G. Multiple sites of inhibition of mitochondrial electron transport by local anesthetics. *Biochim Biophys Acta.* 1981l;636:153-161.
7. Driscoll DF. Lipid injectable emulsions: pharmacopeial and safety issues. *Pharm Res.* 2006;23:1959-1969.
8. Fat emulsion. Drug information. www.uptodate.com. Accessed March 23, 2009.
9. Faucher M, Bregeon F, Gainnier M, et al. Cardiopulmonary effects of lipid emulsions in patients with ARDS. *Chest.* 2003;124:285-291.
10. Foxall G, McCahon R, Lamb J, et al. Levobupivacaine-induced seizures and cardiovascular collapse treated with Intralipid. *Anaesthesia.* 2007;62:516-518.
11. Getting started, treatment regimen. http://www.lipidrescue.org. Accessed March 24, 2009.
12. Haber LM, Hawkins EP, Seilheimer DK, Saleem A. Fat overload syndrome. An autopsy study with evaluation of the coagulopathy. *Am J Clin Pathol.* 1988;90:223-227.
13. Harvey MG, Cave GR. Intralipid infusion ameliorates propranolol-induced hypotension in rabbits. *J Med Toxicol.* 2008;4:71-76.
14. Harvey M, Cave G. Intralipid outperforms sodium bicarbonate in a rabbit model of clomipramine toxicity. *Ann Emerg Med.* 2007;49:178-185.
15. Harvey M, Cave G, Hoggett K. Correlation of plasma and peritoneal diasylate clomipramine concentration with hemodynamic recovery after intralipid infusion in rabbits. *Acad Emerg Med.* 2009;16:151-156.
16. Heard K, Cain BS, Dart RC, Cairns CB. Tricyclic antidepressants directly depress human myocardial mechanical function independent of effects on the conduction system. *Acad Emerg Med.* 2001;8:1122-1127.
17. Hessov I, Melsen F, Haug A. Postmortem findings in three patients treated with intravenous fat emulsions. *Arch Surg.* 1979;114:66-69.
18. Huang JM, Xian H, Bacaner M. Long-chain fatty acids activate calcium channels in ventricular myocytes. *Proc Natl Acad Sci USA.* 1992;89:6452–6456.
19. Hwang TL, Huang SL, Chen MF. Effects of intravenous fat emulsion on respiratory failure. *Chest.* 1990;97:934-938.
20. Kline JA, Leonova E, Williams TC, et al. Myocardial metabolism during graded intraportal verapamil infusion in awake dogs. *J Cardiovasc Pharmacol.* 1996;27:719-726.
21. Kline JA, Raymond RM, Schroeder JD, Watts JA. The diabetogenic effects of acute verapamil poisoning. *Toxicol Appl Pharmacol.* 1997;145:357-362.
22. Kollef MH, McCormack MT, Caras WE, et al. The fat overload syndrome: successful treatment with plasma exchange. *Ann Intern Med.* 1990;112:545-546.
23. Kurien VA, Yates PA, Oliver MF. The role of free fatty acids in the production of ventricular arrhythmias after acute coronary artery occlusion. *Eur J Clin Invest.* 1971;1:225-241.
24. Lekka ME, Liokatis S, Nathanail C, et al. The impact of intravenous fat emulsion administration in acute lung injury. *Am J Respir Crit Care Med.* 2004;169:638-644.
25. Litz RJ, Popp M, Stehr SN, Koch T. Successful resuscitation of a patient with ropivacaine-induced asystole after axillary plexus block using lipid infusion. *Anaesthesia.* 2006;61:800-801.
26. Litz RJ, Roessel T, Heller AR, Stehr SN. Reversal of central nervous system and cardiac toxicity after local anesthetic intoxication by lipid emulsion injection. *Anesth Analg.* 2008;106:1575-1577.
27. Ludot H, Tharin JY, Belouadah M, et al. Successful resuscitation after ropivacaine and lidocaine-induced ventricular arrhythmia following posterior lumbar plexus block in a child. *Anesth Analg.* 2008;106:1572-1574.
28. Masters TN, Glaviano VV. Effects of dl-propranolol on myocardial free fatty acid and carbohydratemetabolism. *J Pharmacol Exp Ther.* 1969;167:187-193.
29. Mathru M, Dries DJ, Zecca A, et al. Effect of fast vs slow intralipid infusion on gas exchange, pulmonary hemodynamics, and prostaglandin metabolism. *Chest.* 1991;99:426-429.
30. McKeen CR, Brigham KL, Bowers RE, Harris TR. Pulmonary vascular effects of fat emulsion infusion in unanesthetized sheep. Prevention by indomethacin. *J Clin Invest.* 1978;61:1291-1297.
31. Perez E, Bania TC, Medlej K, Chu J. Determining the optimal dose of intravenous fat emulsion for the treatment of severe verapamil toxicity in a rodent model. *Acad Emerg Med.* 2008;15:1284-1289.
32. Rosenblatt MA, Abel M, Fischer GW, et al. Successful use of a 20% lipid emulsion to resuscitate a patient after a presumed bupivacaine-related cardiac arrest. *Anesthesiology.* 2006;105:217-218.
33. Rowlingson JC. Lipid rescue: a step forward in patient safety? Likely so! *Anesth Analg.* 2008;106:1333-1336.
34. Rxlist.com. www.rxlist.com. Accessed March 24, 2009.
35. Schulz PE, Weiner SP, Haber LM, et al. Neurological complications from fat emulsion therapy. *Ann Neurol.* 1994;35:628-630.
36. Sirianni AJ, Osterhoudt KC, Calello DP, et al. Use of lipid emulsion in the resuscitation of a patient with prolonged cardiovascular collapse after overdose of bupropion and lamotrigine. *Ann Emerg Med.* 2008;51:412-415.
37. Smirniotis V, Kostopanagiotou G, Vassiliou J, et al. Long-chain versus medium-chain lipids in patients with ARDS: effects on pulmonary haemodynamics and gas exchange. *Intensive Care Med.* 1998;24:1029-1033.
38. Smiseth OA, Mjøs OD. Haemodynamic and metabolic consequences of elevated plasma free fatty acids during acute ischaemic left ventricular failure in dogs. *Scand J Clin Lab Invest.* 1985;45:515-520.
39. Stanley WC, Recchia FA, Lopaschuk GD. Myocardial substrate metabolism in the normal and failing heart. *Physiol Rev.* 2005;85:1093-1129.
40. Stock JG, Pope J Jr, Enzenauer RW. Retinal findings in the fat overload syndrome. *Arch Ophthalmol.* 1990;108:329.
41. Tebbutt S, Harvey M, Nicholson T, Cave G. Intralipid prolongs survival in a rat model of verapamil toxicity. *Acad Emerg Med.* 2006;13:134-139.
42. Trissel L. Fat emulsion, intravenous. In: *Handbook of Injectable Drugs,* 15th ed. Bethesda, MD: American Society of Health-System Pharmacists; 2009:653-674.
43. Van de Velde M, Wouters PF, Rolf N, et al. Long-chain triglycerides improve recovery from myocardial stunning in conscious dogs. *Cardiovasc Res.* 1996;32:1008-1015.
44. Venus B, Prager R, Patel CB, et al. Cardiopulmonary effects of Intralipid infusion in critically ill patients. *Crit Care Med.* 1988;16:587-590.
45. Venus B, Smith RA, Patel C, Sandoval E. Hemodynamic and gas exchange alterations during Intralipid infusion in patients with adult respiratory distress syndrome. *Chest.* 1989;95:1278-1281.
46. Waitzberg DL, Torrinhas RS, Jacintho TM. New parenteral lipid emulsions for clinical use. *J Parenter Enteral Nutr.* 2006;30:351-367.
47. Warren JA, Thoma RB, Georgescu A, Shah SJ. Intravenous lipid infusion in the successful resuscitation of local anesthetic-induced cardiovascular collapse after supraclavicular brachial plexus block. *Anesth Analg.* 2008;106:1578-1580.
48. Weinbach EC, Costa JL, Nelson BD, et al. Effects of tricyclic antidepressant drugs on energy-linked reactions in mitochondria. *Biochem Pharmacol.* 1986;35:1445-1451.
49. Weinberg G, Hertz P, Newman J. Lipid, not propofol, treats bupivacaine overdose. *Anesth Analg.* 2004;99:1875-1876.

50. Weinberg G, Ripper R, Feinstein DL, Hoffman W. Lipid emulsion infusion rescues dogs from bupivacaine-induced cardiac toxicity. *Reg Anesth Pain Med.* 2003;28:198-202.
51. Weinberg GL, Palmer JW, VadeBoncouer TR, et al. Bupivacaine inhibits acyl-carnitine exchange in cardiac mitochondria. *Anesthesiology.* 2000;92:523-528.
52. Weinberg GL, Ripper R, Murphy P, et al. Lipid infusion accelerates removal of bupivacaine and recovery from bupivacaine toxicity in the isolated rat heart. *Reg Anesth Pain Med.* 2006;31:296-303.
53. Weinberg GL, VadeBoncouer T, Ramaraju GA, et al. Pretreatment or resuscitation with a lipid infusion shifts the dose–response to bupivacaine-induced asystole in rats. *Anesthesiology.* 1998;88:1071-1075.
54. Weinberg GL. Lipid infusion therapy: translation to clinical practice. *Anesth Analg.* 2008;106:1340-1342.
55. Yudkin M, Offord R, Harrison K. Synthesis of ATP-fat breakdown. In: *A Guidebook to Biochemistry*, 4th ed. Cambridge, MA: Cambridge University Press; 1980:140-145.

CHAPTER 67
INHALATIONAL ANESTHETICS

Brian Kaufman and Martin Griffel

General anesthesia occurs as a result of reversible changes in neurologic function caused by xenobiotics that modulate synaptic neurotransmission. The commonly accepted elements of general anesthesia include hypnosis, amnesia, analgesia, inhibition of noxious reflexes, and skeletal muscle relaxation.[8] However, precise definitions for some of these terms are lacking. In addition, different effects occur at varying concentrations of inhaled anesthetics. Side effects may be redefined as toxicity, depending on the clinical situation.

HISTORY

The earliest description of the use of an inhalational anesthetic was made by Paracelsus, a Swiss physician and alchemist who prepared a mixture of diethyl ether, alcohol, and water called sweet oil of vitriol. He described the administration of this preparation to hens that fell into a deep sleep from which they recovered unharmed. In 1735, Wilhelm Froben gave this substance its modern name of "ether." Ether was used topically, particularly via the intranasal route, as a treatment of headache, nervous diseases, and fits.

Modern anesthetic practice often is stated to have begun in 1846 at the Massachusetts General Hospital, when the dentist William Morton gave the first public demonstration of the ability of inhaled ether vapor to alleviate the pain of surgery. Oliver Wendell Holmes chose the Greek-related noun *anesthesia* (without feeling) to characterize the process.

Observations on circulatory and respiratory physiology eventually led to an understanding of the effects of inhalation gases and vapors. In the last decade of the 18th century, centers for the pneumatic treatment of disease were established in Birmingham and Bristol, England. Experiments with ether that was inhaled via a funnel and with nitrous oxide were conducted at these institutions. After Humphry Davy described his own pleasurable and exhilarating experience when he inhaled the "laughing" gas, many of his colleagues and friends inhaled nitrous oxide to experience its inebriating effects. Davy also described how inhalation of nitrous oxide relieved headache and the pain of an erupting molar tooth. Although Davy recognized the analgesic properties of nitrous oxide and its possible application for surgery, he failed to pursue the idea.

The public soon took up the use of nitrous oxide in the form of nitrous oxide frolics. Audiences to itinerant medicine shows volunteered to experience the exhilarating effects of nitrous oxide inhalation. At one such show in 1844 in Hartford, Connecticut, a man under the influence of nitrous oxide injured his leg but did not feel any pain. Dr. Horace Wells, a dentist in the audience that day, inhaled nitrous oxide the following day and had his partner painlessly remove a troublesome tooth. A subsequent public demonstration of the use of nitrous oxide for dental extraction caused concern, impeding its general acceptance as a surgical anesthetic.

In Great Britain in 1847, James Simpson, an obstetrician, first used ether to relieve the pain of labor. He subsequently adopted chloroform for this purpose because of its more pleasant odor and more rapid induction and emergence. The clergy and other physicians opposed the concept of relieving pain during childbirth, but the method ultimately was accepted after Queen Victoria gave birth to Prince Leopold with chloroform given by John Snow.

Over the next century, several volatile anesthetics were introduced, including ethyl chloride in 1848, divinyl ether in 1933, trichloroethylene in 1934, and ethyl vinyl ether in 1947. All had significant safety problems associated with their use, including combustibility and direct organ toxicity.

Advances in fluorine chemistry led to the cost-effective incorporation of fluorine into molecules used in the development of modern anesthetics. Fluroxene was the first of the new fluorinated anesthetics to be widely used clinically. However, this anesthetic was flammable and hepatotoxic. It was largely replaced by the nonflammable halothane, which was synthesized in 1951 and introduced into clinical practice in 1956. Methoxyflurane was evaluated in humans in 1960 but is no longer used because of nephrotoxicity and hepatotoxicity. Other halogenated hydrocarbons with improved clinical properties have been introduced, including enflurane, isoflurane, desflurane, and sevoflurane (Fig. 67–1). The inert gas xenon has been shown to be a useful anesthetic and is being studied. It is both cardio- and neuroprotective in experimental studies.[38] The clinical use of xenon is limited both by its cost and difficulty to manufacture. Although xenon is environmentally friendly compared with presently used anesthetics, its toxicity is relatively unknown but is believed to be minimal.

PHARMACOLOGY

Because a wide range of chemically distinct xenobiotics can produce anesthesia, a unique receptor for the inhaled anesthetics is improbable. More likely, the volatile anesthetics cause general anesthesia by modulating synaptic function from within cell membranes. Anesthetics are known to interact with many proteins. The most likely, but not yet proven, targets for the inhalational anesthetics are the ion channels that control ion flow across the cytoplasmic membrane. An in-depth discussion is beyond the scope of this chapter, but several concepts are important to consider. First, more than 20 different ion channels have been identified, each controlling various anion and cation flows. The results of these ion channel effects include release of inhibitory neurotransmitters and inhibition of excitatory neurotransmitters. In fact, each anesthetic type has variable actions. The receptor for γ-aminobutyric acid type A ($GABA_A$) is the best studied and plays an important role because $GABA_A$ is an inhibitory neurotransmitter. The interaction of all of these receptor effects produces the condition we refer to as *general anesthesia.* Many of the side effects of the inhalational anesthetics result directly from ion channel effects in nonneural tissue, primarily cardiac cell membranes.

Reversible changes in neurologic function cause loss of perception and reaction to pain, unawareness of immediate events, and loss of memory of those events. The common pharmacologic mechanisms for general anesthesia include the physical–chemical behavior of volatile hydrocarbons within the hydrophobic regions of biologic membrane lipids and proteins.

The potency of the various inhaled anesthetics correlates with their physicochemical properties. The dominant theories of the molecular mechanisms by which volatile anesthetics affect membrane function are based on the lipid solubility of the drugs and experimental demonstration of pressure reversal of anesthesia. Anesthetic potency correlates directly with the relative lipid solubility of each drug, suggesting that the primary molecular actions of anesthetics occur in the lipid portion of cell membranes. This mechanism is known as the

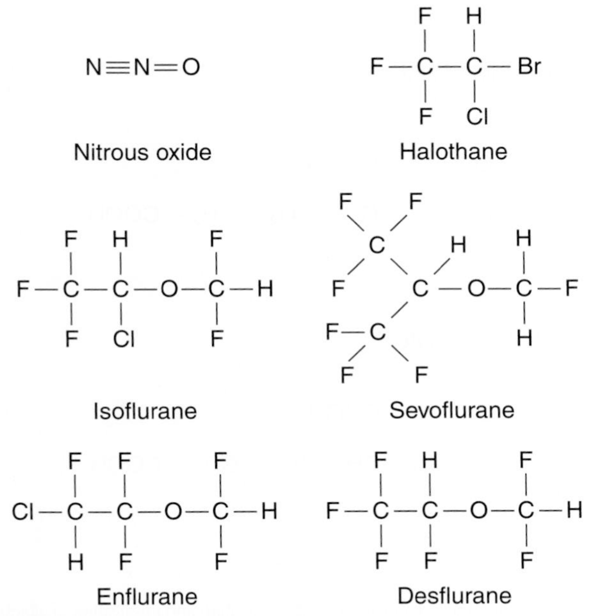

N≡N=O

Nitrous oxide

Halothane

Isoflurane

Sevoflurane

Enflurane

Desflurane

FIGURE 67–1. The inhalational anesthetics.

Meyer-Overton lipid solubility theory. Potential membrane regions for anesthetic action include the hydrophobic areas of proteins and protein–lipid interface regions, as well as the phospholipid matrix. High pressures (100–200 atm) can reverse the anesthetic effects of several drugs, suggesting that the drugs cause anesthesia by increasing membrane volume at normal atmospheric pressure, an effect known as the *volume expansion theory*.

PHARMACOKINETICS

Because the inhaled anesthetics enter the body through the lungs, the factors that influence their absorption by blood and distribution to other tissues, particularly the brain, include the solubility of the drug in blood, blood flow through the lungs, blood flow distribution to the various organs, solubility of the anesthetic in tissue, and the mass of the tissue. The goal of inhalation anesthesia is to develop and maintain a satisfactory partial pressure of anesthetic in the brain, the primary site of action.

The pharmacokinetics of anesthetics can be linked to their pharmacodynamics by considering anesthetic potency. The linkage exists because anesthesia strives to achieve and maintain a desired alveolar concentration. For the inhaled anesthetics, potency is commonly referred to as the *minimum alveolar concentration* (MAC) of the anesthetic. MAC is the alveolar concentration at 1 atm that prevents movement in 50% of subjects in response to a painful stimulus. MAC is used when comparing the effects of equipotent doses of anesthetics on various organ functions.

NITROUS OXIDE

Nitrous oxide is the most commonly used inhalational anesthetic in the world. Recently, clinicians have questioned its continued use. In a recent exhaustive review,[39] the toxicity of nitrous oxide was reviewed both from its chemical perspective and its clinical activity. The authors concluded that a ban on its use is not required. Its advantages include a mild odor, absence of airway irritation, rapid induction and emergence, potent analgesia, and minimal respiratory and circulatory effects. When administered in a modern operating room using current standards of monitoring to prevent unintentional hypoxia, nitrous oxide is a remarkably safe xenobiotic. Unfortunately, nitrous oxide also has a potential for abuse, particularly among hospital and dental personnel.[26] Death and permanent brain damage have been reported but do not generally result from direct toxic effects; instead, they are secondary to hypoxia as a result of simple asphyxiation[13] (see Chap. 124).

Death may occur when patients receive commercially prepared nitrous oxide from tanks contaminated with impurities such as nitric oxide or nitrogen dioxide. Pulmonary toxicity resulting from similar contaminants has been reported after illicit preparation of nitrous oxide from the combustion of ammonium nitrate fertilizer.[32]

Injury may result from the physical properties of this anesthetic. Nitrous oxide is 35 times more soluble in blood than is nitrogen. When nitrous oxide is inhaled, any compliant air-containing space, such as bowel, increases in size; noncompliant spaces, such as the eustachian tubes, exhibit an increase in pressure. These effects occur because nitrous oxide diffuses along the concentration gradient from the blood into a closed space much more rapidly than nitrogen can be transferred in the opposite direction. Clinical consequences include rapid progression of a pneumothorax to a tension pneumothorax, tympanic membrane rupture with hearing loss, bowel distension, and tracheal or laryngeal trauma caused by increased endotracheal cuff pressure resulting from replacement of air by a larger volume of nitrous oxide. Nitrous oxide may be particularly dangerous in patients who have suffered air emboli, and its use should be immediately discontinued upon recognition of these events. When intracranial or neuraxial air is injected during placement of an epidural catheter, it also can theoretically expand upon subsequent exposure to nitrous oxide.

HEMATOLOGIC EFFECTS

Bone marrow depression was first recognized as a complication of long-term nitrous oxide exposure in the 1950s, when the gas was used to sedate intubated patients who had severe tetanus.[25] Leukopenia with hypoplastic bone marrow and megaloblastic erythropoiesis typically developed 3 to 5 days after initial exposure and was followed by thrombocytopenia. Recovery usually occurred within 4 days after the anesthetic was discontinued. Healthy patients undergoing routine surgical procedures demonstrate mild megaloblastic bone marrow changes within 12 hours of exposure to 50% nitrous oxide and marked changes within 24 hours.[36] Critically ill patients may be more sensitive to the effects of nitrous oxide on the bone marrow, with megaloblastic changes described after only 1 hour of exposure.[3]

The hematologic effects of exposure to nitrous oxide strongly resemble the biochemical characteristics of pernicious anemia.[2,34,35] Vitamin B_{12}, or cyanocobalamin, is a bound coenzyme of cytoplasmic methionine synthase. The cobalt moiety in the enzyme functions as a methyl carrier in its transfer from 5-methyltetrahydrofolate to homocysteine to form methionine (Fig. 67–2). Nitrous oxide oxidizes the cobalt, converting vitamin B_{12} from the active monovalent form (Co^{+}) to the inactive divalent form (Co^{2+}), which irreversibly inhibits methionine synthase.[34] The metabolic consequences of this inhibition are significant because methionine and tetrahydrofolate are required for both DNA synthesis and myelin production. This interference is responsible for the development of bone marrow depression and polyneuropathy resembling the characteristic findings that occur in pernicious anemia.[34]

NEUROLOGIC EFFECTS

Disabling polyneuropathy in healthcare workers who habitually abused nitrous oxide was first described in 1978.[26] The neurologic disorder improved slowly when the patients abstained from further nitrous oxide

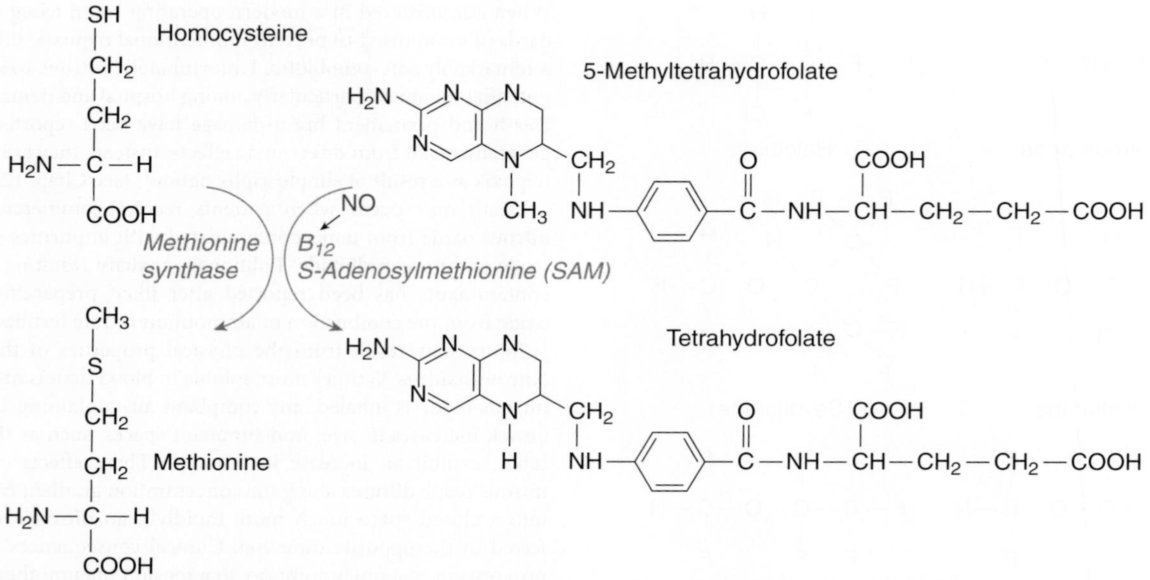

Homocysteine
5-Methyltetrahydrofolate
NO
Methionine synthase
B_{12}
S-Adenosylmethionine (SAM)
Tetrahydrofolate
Methionine

FIGURE 67–2. Hematologic effects of exposure to nitrous oxide (NO) resemble those characteristic of pernicious anemia and are related to oxidation and inactivation of vitamin B_{12}. The irreversible blockade of methionine synthase is consequential with regard to DNA synthesis and myelin production.

abuse. As discussed, this neuropathy is clinically indistinguishable from subacute combined degeneration of the spinal cord associated with pernicious anemia. The syndrome of nitrous oxide neuropathy is characterized by sensorimotor polyneuropathy, often combined with signs of posterior and lateral spinal cord involvement. Signs and symptoms include numbness and paresthesias in the extremities, weakness, and truncal ataxia. Neurologic changes develop only after several months of frequent exposure to nitrous oxide. Those at risk include individuals who chronically abuse the gas and those who are occupationally exposed for prolonged periods to environments contaminated with high concentrations of nitrous oxide.[4] Animal studies demonstrate that methionine synthase may be inactivated by exposure to greater than 1000 parts per million (ppm) of nitrous oxide, a concentration often exceeded in dental procedure rooms. This scenario is highly unlikely in the modern operating room, where inhalational anesthetics are scavenged, but it may occur in poorly ventilated dental offices, where personnel are exposed to concentrations greater than 1000 ppm nitrous oxide. This problem probably is markedly underdiagnosed because the neurologic changes that occur in mild cases mimic other more common neurologic conditions.[7]

CHRONIC EXPOSURE TO TRACE LEVELS OF NITROUS OXIDE

Dentists and dental assistants are often exposed to greater concentrations of waste anesthetic gases than are individuals working in well-vented operating rooms. An epidemiologic survey compared 15,000 dentists who used with 15,000 dentists who did not use nitrous oxide in their practices.[7] A 1.2- to 1.8-fold increase in liver, kidney, and neurologic disease was found in the dentists and their chairside assistants who were chronically exposed to trace concentrations of nitrous oxide. For those with heavy office use of nitrous oxide, a fourfold increase in the incidence of neurologic complaints compared with the nonexposed group was observed. Female dental assistants who were exposed to nitrous oxide had a two- to threefold increase in spontaneous abortion rates, reduced fertility, and a higher rate of congenital abnormalities in their offspring.[7]

TREATMENT

General Removal of the acutely affected person from the toxic environment should be the initial intervention. Individuals who have developed toxicity from abuse of the gas should be educated about the relationship between their recreational activities and their clinical findings.

Specific Vitamin B_{12} may help patients with a vitamin B_{12} deficiency who develop megaloblastic anemia and neurologic dysfunction after brief exposure to nitrous oxide, but it is not beneficial in patients who have toxicity resulting from more chronic exposure.[40] The reason for the ineffectiveness of vitamin B_{12} in this situation is uncertain.

The bone marrow abnormalities associated with nitrous oxide toxicity may be reversed by administration of a single 30-mg intravenous (IV) dose of folinic acid (the active form of folate)[31] (see Antidotes in Depth A13: Leucovorin and Folic Acid). In primates, a methionine-supplemented diet greatly reduced demyelination and neurologic damage from chronic exposure to 15% nitrous oxide.[41]

HALOGENATED HYDROCARBONS

The inhaled anesthetics were initially considered biochemically inert. Initial reports of toxicity after their administration were poorly explained and were attributed to direct effects on susceptible organs. It now is clear that the inhalational anesthetics are metabolized in vivo and that their metabolites are responsible for acute and chronic toxicity. Much of the toxicity relates to predictable responses that are dose related.

HALOTHANE HEPATITIS

Two distinct types of hepatotoxicity are associated with halothane use. The first is a mild dysfunction that develops in approximately 20% of exposed patients. Patients often are asymptomatic but exhibit modestly elevated serum aminotransferase concentrations within a few days of anesthetic exposure. Recovery is complete.[32] In contrast, a life-threatening hepatitis occurs in approximately one in 10,000 exposed patients and produces fatal massive hepatic necrosis in one in 35,000 patients.[44] Because the histologic findings of massive hepatocellular necrosis are indistinguishable from many of the causes of viral hepatitis,[48] differentiating halothane hepatitis from other causes of hepatitis in the postoperative period is difficult without positive serologic studies. Jaundice, which is common after anesthesia and surgery, usually results from factors such as preexisting liver disease, blood transfusion, sepsis, or other causes of hepatitis. Thus halothane hepatitis is a diagnosis of exclusion or inclusion based on the chemical history.

Several studies report an association between multiple exposures to halothane and subsequent development of hepatitis.[33,47,52] In one study, 95% of cases of halothane hepatitis occurred after repeat exposures, 55% of which involved reexposure within 4 weeks.[52] Under these circumstances, liver dysfunction usually is more severe, and the latency before clinical presentation usually is shorter than when the syndrome develops after initial exposure to halothane.[47]

Obesity is a risk factor commonly implicated in halothane hepatotoxicity.[1,49] Increased fat stores may act as a "reservoir" for halothane, with slow and prolonged release into the circulation and subsequent increase in production of potentially hepatotoxic metabolites.

Most cases of halothane hepatitis occur in middle-aged patients, with women having twice the risk.[22] Genetic factors may play a role in some patients, as indicated by a report of this syndrome in three pairs of related Mexican women.[21]

Mechanism of Toxicity Halothane is the most extensively metabolized inhalational anesthetic (Fig. 67–3). Approximately 20% of the absorbed anesthetic undergoes oxidative metabolism, principally by cytochrome P450 2E1 in the liver, to trifluoroacetic acid. Reduction to trifluorochloroethane and difluorochloroethylene is a minor route of halothane metabolism that requires the absence of oxygen and the presence of an electron donor. These volatile metabolites are free radicals, which may directly produce acute hepatic toxicity by irreversibly binding to and destroying hepatocellular structures. Alternatively, by acting as haptens, they may trigger an immune-mediated hypersensitivity response.[37,50] The high percentage of patients with halothane hepatitis who had recent exposure to the xenobiotic is most consistent with the latter mechanism in which the first exposure primes the development of antibodies to a haptenized protein.[22]

Enflurane, which was used extensively in North America since 1966, is rarely used now. It is too weakly associated with hepatotoxicity. Some authorities believe the evidence does not support the existence of enflurane-induced hepatic necrosis.[14,16,43] Isoflurane, desflurane, and sevoflurane all appear to have low hepatotoxic potential. The immune form of hepatitis has been reported with all anesthetics except sevoflurane. Cross-sensitivity may be applicable, such that prior exposure to one anesthetic triggers hepatotoxicity upon subsequent exposure to a different anesthetic.

NEPHROTOXICITY

The kidneys are the only other organ at risk for toxicity from modern inhalational anesthetics. Methoxyflurane is an anesthetic that was introduced in 1962. By 1966, it was linked to the development of vasopressin-resistant polyuric renal insufficiency (nephrogenic diabetes insipidus) in 16 of 94 patients receiving prolonged methoxyflurane anesthesia for abdominal surgery[11] (see Chap. 16). Polyuria was associated with a negative fluid balance, elevations of serum sodium and urea nitrogen concentrations; osmolality, and a fixed urinary osmolality close to that of serum. Renal abnormalities lasted from 10 to 20 days in most patients but persisted for more than 1 year in three patients. Subsequent studies demonstrated that renal toxicity was caused by inorganic fluoride (F^-) released during biotransformation of methoxyflurane.[46] The risk of toxicity was highly correlated with both the total dose of methoxyflurane (concentration times duration) and the peak serum F^- concentration.[10,31] The nephrotoxic serum fluoride concentration is 50 to 60 μmol/L.[10] The factors that enhance biotransformation such as obesity and enzyme induction also increase the risk of toxicity. Although the precise mechanism by which fluoride produces its toxic effect on the kidneys is not clear, one hypothesis is that fluoride inhibits adenylate cyclase, thereby interfering with the normal action of antidiuretic hormone on the distal convoluted tubules.

Although methoxyflurane is no longer used, lessons learned regarding its toxicity are applied when evaluating the nephrotoxic potential of other fluorinated anesthetics. Of the currently used anesthetics: halothane, isoflurane, enflurane, desflurane, sevoflurane; only enflurane and sevoflurane undergo biotransformation by defluorination.

Approximately 5% of sevoflurane is metabolized. This process occasionally results in sufficient serum fluoride concentrations to produce transient decreases in urine-concentrating ability.[24] However, clinically evident renal impairment almost never occurs with use of

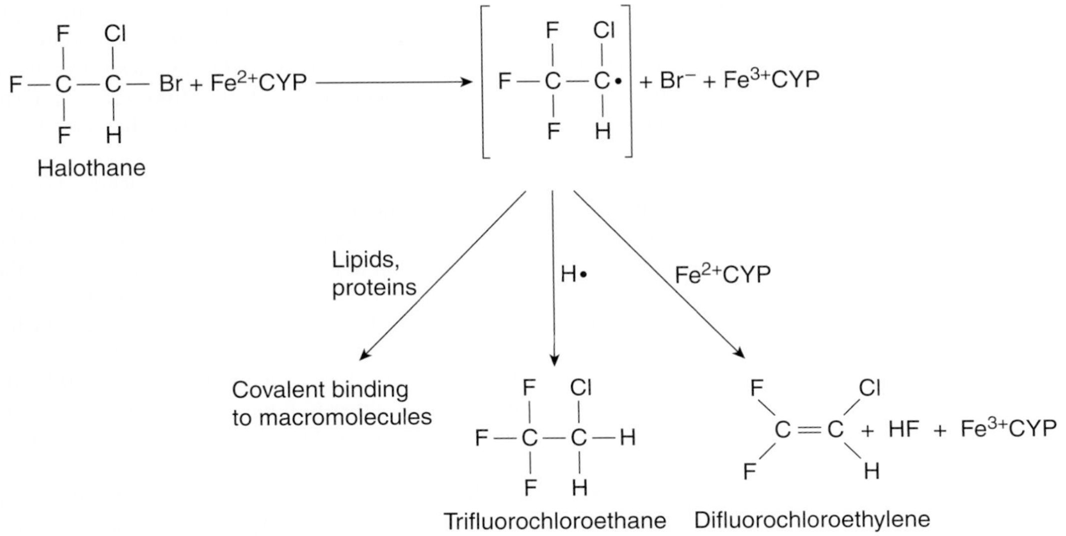

Halothane: $CF_3CHClBr + Fe^{2+}CYP \rightarrow [CF_3CHCl\cdot] + Br^- + Fe^{3+}CYP$

Lipids, proteins → Covalent binding to macromolecules

$H\cdot$ → Trifluorochloroethane (CF_3CH_2Cl)

$Fe^{2+}CYP$ → Difluorochloroethylene ($CF_2{=}CHCl$) + HF + $Fe^{3+}CYP$

FIGURE 67–3. Reductive metabolism of halothane results in formation of a reactive metabolite that may directly bind macromolecules and create neoantigens, or undergo further metabolism to trifluorochloroethane and difluorochloroethylene. CYP = cytochrome P450

either enflurane or sevoflurane.[18] In addition, volunteer studies failed to show any urine-concentrating defect after exposure to sevoflurane that resulted in high serum fluoride concentrations. In patients with preexisting renal insufficiency, the risk of postoperative renal dysfunction is believed to be worse with exposure to inhalational anesthetics. However, studies demonstrate that deterioration of renal function does not occur after exposure to desflurane and isoflurane,[28] possibly because intrarenal fluoride concentrations are more important than serum fluoride concentrations in the development of nephrotoxicity.

PHARMACOKINETICS

Chronic use of isoniazid induces CYP2E1, the enzyme responsible for enflurane metabolism. This induction results in elevated serum fluoride concentrations in approximately 50% of isoniazid-treated patients who receive an enflurane anesthetic.[31] The fluoride concentrations, however, are neither high enough nor sustained enough to produce clinically significant renal dysfunction. Nonetheless, a prudent course is to avoid prolonged use of enflurane in patients taking isoniazid or other xenobiotics, such as ethanol, phenobarbital, or phenytoin, which elevate the activity of cytochrome P450 2E1 (see Chap. 12).

Unusually high serum fluoride concentrations are reported in morbidly obese patients anesthetized with enflurane.[9] This finding may be related to a large storage capacity for fat-soluble anesthetics. Although prolonged postoperative release and metabolism of enflurane may occur, renal dysfunction has not been reported with enflurane use even in obese patients.

Sevoflurane reacts with the alkali within carbon dioxide absorbers to produce several degradation products, including a vinyl ether called compound A ($CF_2C(CF_3)OCH_2F$), which is nephrotoxic and hepatotoxic in rats.[23,51] The site of compound A–induced nephrotoxicity in rats is the renal tubule, especially at the corticomedullary junction.[23] The extent of nephrotoxicity is determined by both the concentration of compound A and the duration of exposure. Compound A is also conjugated, and its breakdown products are nephrotoxic.

Technical Issues Extensive clinical experience with several million patients who were exposed to sevoflurane and 4000 closely studied volunteers failed to demonstrate nephrotoxicity.[30] Higher concentrations of compound A are generated during low-flow anesthesia, use of high concentrations of sevoflurane, fresh calcium hydroxide and barium hydroxide use, and increased temperature conditions. A high fresh-gas flow rate dilutes the concentration of compound A. Concern that higher compound A concentrations are generated when a low fresh-gas flow rate (eg, <2 L/min) is used in a closed circuit led to the current sevoflurane package labeling, which warns the anesthesia provider against fresh-gas flow rates below 2 L/min in a circle absorber system.[29]

Some controversy exists regarding the safety of low-flow sevoflurane anesthesia. Although there have been no clinical reports of sevoflurane-induced nephrotoxicity as measured by changes in blood urea nitrogen (BUN), serum creatinine, or creatinine clearance, clinical data demonstrate transient nephrotoxicity when more subtle measurements of glomerular and tubular function are used.[15,20] For example, when young, healthy patients without underlying renal disease were anesthetized with low-flow sevoflurane for a mean of 6.7 hours, transient but statistically significant increases in urinary glucose and protein excretion were documented without any changes in BUN, creatinine, or creatinine clearance.[20] The clinical significance of such transient abnormalities in renal function is uncertain. Regardless, it seems prudent to not use low-flow sevoflurane in patients with preexisting renal disease until clinical data document the safety of this practice. Newer carbon dioxide absorbents that are free of strong alkali have been identified and studied in an attempt to find products that generate less compound A.

INHALATIONAL ANESTHETIC–RELATED CARBON MONOXIDE POISONING

PHARMACOLOGY

Desflurane, enflurane, and isoflurane contain a difluoromethoxy moiety that can be degraded to carbon monoxide (CO). This process occasionally results in patient exposure to toxic CO concentrations and, in rare instances, severe CO poisoning.[6] The true incidence of CO exposure during clinical anesthesia is unknown. Routine detection of intraoperative CO exposure is not currently used, but newer pulse oximeters will permit continuous carboxyhemoglobin evaluations.

CO production is inversely proportional to the water content of CO_2 absorbents. Calcium hydroxide and barium hydroxide (Baralyme) and soda lime, the two most frequently used CO_2 absorbents, are sold wet (13%–15% water by weight), but wet absorbents may dry with high gas-inflow rates. Higher concentrations of CO are most apt to be present during the first case after a weekend because of drying of CO_2 absorbent from a continuous inflow of dry oxygen over the weekend.[17]

Other factors influence the concentration of CO that may result from anesthetic degradation, including temperature (higher temperature increases CO formation), type of absorbent, choice of anesthetic, and concentration of anesthetic. Strong alkalis, such as potassium and sodium hydroxide, initiate the reaction that forms CO. Baralyme, which contains potassium hydroxide, forms more CO than does soda lime, which contains a combination of both.

In one experiment, Baralyme was exposed to 48 hours of dry gas flowing at 10 L/min. Nine swine were then anesthetized with desflurane. Three of the animals died of cardiac arrest within 20 minutes; the other six were successfully resuscitated with IV epinephrine and discontinuation of desflurane.[19] Extremely high concentrations of CO (mean peak concentration, 37,000 ppm) were detected in the circuit within 15 minutes of initiating desflurane anesthesia. All the animals had carboxyhemoglobin concentrations above 80%, with a concentration above 90% in seven of the swine. Lower CO concentrations were detected when the CO_2 absorbent was exposed to only 24 hours of dry gas and when soda lime was substituted for Baralyme.

Clinical monitors routinely used in the operating room cannot detect CO. Mass spectrometry (available in some operating rooms) cannot directly detect CO because its molecular weight is equivalent to that of nitrogen, a gas usually present in much greater amounts. In addition, detection of CO by fragmentation products is not possible by mass spectrometry because CO_2 is present in greater amounts and has similar fragmentation products. However, the presence of CO should be suspected if the mass spectrometer shows the presence of enflurane when it is not being administered.

Trifluoromethane is produced by degradation of isoflurane and desflurane and is responsible for the false readings for enflurane.[56] Simultaneous production of trifluoromethane and CO during chemical decomposition of isoflurane and desflurane allows the false reading of the former as enflurane by mass spectrometry to serve as a gross CO monitor and allows for interventions to prevent further CO production and enhance CO elimination. The overall incidence of CO exposure from anesthetic degradation was six of 1372 (0.44%) first cases of the day in which either isoflurane or desflurane was administered.[56] Mass spectrometry is a useful monitor for indirect detection of CO poisoning in the clinical setting.[55]

Although no case reports document patient morbidity or mortality from intraoperative CO exposures, carboxyhemoglobin reportedly as high as 36% may cause morbidity and mortality in patients with concurrent disease.[6] Unfortunately, the diagnosis of CO poisoning during anesthesia is difficult because the main clinical features of toxicity are masked by anesthesia, and no routinely available means can identify CO within the breathing circuit or detect when the CO_2 absorbent has been desiccated. Delayed neurologic sequelae from intraoperative CO poisoning are likely missed on the anesthesiologist's postoperative patient evaluation.[54]

The product labels of desflurane and isoflurane have been altered to include a precaution that the CO_2 absorbent should be replaced if a practitioner suspects the absorbent is desiccated. However, the problem associated with this warning is the lack of a reliable method for determining when the absorbent is fully or partially desiccated.

If an anesthetic machine is found with the fresh-gas flow "on" at the beginning of the day, a reasonable practice is to replace the absorbent. Changing from Baralyme to soda lime use also should be considered as a protective measure. Newer CO_2 absorbents that are less likely to degrade anesthetics are being evaluated but are not yet available in the United States.

Extreme heat and fires within the anesthesia circuits have been reported in a warning distributed by the manufacturer of sevoflurane. The cases involved desiccated carbon dioxide absorbents, high sevoflurane concentrations, and primarily but not exclusively Baralyme adsorbent. The exact mechanisms have not been entirely elucidated but again point to the need to change absorbent when it is dry or routinely every Monday morning before the first case.

ABUSE OF HALOGENATED VOLATILE ANESTHETICS

Fatal or life-threatening complications occur when halogenated inhalational anesthetics are used for nonanesthetic purposes such as suicide attempts, mood elevation, and topical treatment of herpes simplex labialis. When ingested, halothane usually produces gastroenteritis with vomiting followed by depressed consciousness, hypotension, shallow breathing, bradycardia with extrasystoles, and acute lung injury (ALI). Coma usually resolves within 72 hours.[12,53] The diagnosis should be suspected when these features occur in a patient with the sweet or fruity odor of halothane on the breath. Supportive care, including endotracheal intubation and nasogastric lavage, should be provided with protection for potentially exposed staff. Full recovery can occur without permanent organ injury.

IV injections of halothane may occur as a suicide attempt or unintentionally during anesthesia induction. A young patient who was found unconscious and hypotensive with ALI after self-administered IV injection of halothane was not successfully resuscitated.[5] A 16-year-old girl received an unintentional IV injection of 2.5 mL of halothane during anesthesia induction.[45] She became unconscious and apneic within 30 seconds but began to awaken within 2 to 3 minutes. Four hours later, she developed respiratory distress from ALI but subsequently made a full recovery.

Transient coma and apnea probably are secondary to a halothane bolus reaching the brain on its first pass through the bloodstream. Redistribution then occurs, explaining the rapid awakening. The ALI that develops after injection of halothane may result from a direct toxic effect of high concentrations of this hydrocarbon drug on the pulmonary vascular bed. After injection, the anesthetic likely travels as a bolus during the first passage through the pulmonary circulation because of its poor solubility in blood.

Hospital personnel are involved in most reported cases of halothane abuse by inhalation.[42] Inhalation of halothane produces a pleasurable sensation similar to that described with glue sniffing. Death may result from upper airway obstruction after loss of consciousness or from dysrhythmias. Death occurred in a student nurse anesthetist suggested to have applied a full 250-mL bottle of enflurane over 3 hours to "cold sores" on her lower lip.[27]

SUMMARY

Inhalational anesthetics remain popular choices for maintenance of general anesthesia. Their advantage over IV drugs is that their drug concentration within the body can be rapidly increased or decreased at will. Toxicity with use of these drugs may result from a variety of mechanisms, including excessive physiologic drug effect, direct drug effects on metabolic pathways, and toxic effects of drug metabolites. Although life-threatening adverse reactions occur infrequently, physicians who use these drugs should be knowledgeable about their pharmacology and potential toxicity.

REFERENCES

1. Abernathy D, Greenblatt D. Pharmacokinetics of drugs in obesity. *Clin Pharmacokinet.* 1982;7:108-124.
2. Amess J, Burman J, Rees G, et al. Megaloblastic haemopoieses in patients receiving nitrous oxide. *Lancet.* 1978;2:339-342.
3. Amos R, Amess J, Hinds C, Mollin D. Incidence and pathogenesis of acute megaloblastic bone marrow change in patients receiving intensive care. *Lancet.* 1982;2:835-839.
4. Baird P. Occupational exposure to nitrous oxide—not a laughing matter. *N Engl J Med.* 1992;327:1026-1027.
5. Berman P, Tattersall M. Self-poisoning with intravenous halothane. *Lancet.* 1982;1:340.
6. Berry PD, Sessler DI, Larson MD. Severe carbon monoxide poisoning during desflurane anesthesia. *Anesthesiology.* 1999;90:613-616.
7. Brodsky J, Cohen E, Brown B, et al. Exposure to nitrous oxide and neurologic disease among dental professionals. *Anesth Analg.* 1981;60:297-301.
8. Campagna JA, Miller KW, Forman SA. Mechanisms of inhaled anesthetics. *N Engl J Med.* 2003;348:2110-2124.
9. Cousins M, Greenstein L, Hitt B, Mazze R. Metabolism and renal effects of enflurane in man. *Anesthesiology.* 1976;44:44-53.
10. Cousins M, Mazze R. Methoxyflurane nephrotoxicity: a study of dose-response in man. *JAMA.* 1973;225:1611-1616.
11. Crandell W, Pappas S, MacDonald A. Nephrotoxicity associated with methoxyflurane anesthesia. *Anesthesiology.* 1966;27:591-607.
12. Curelaru I, Stanciu S, Nicolau V, et al. A case of recovery from coma produced by the ingestion of 250 mL of halothane. *Br J Anaesth.* 1968;40:283-288.
13. Di Maio V, Garriott J. Four deaths resulting from abuse of nitrous oxide. *J Forensic Sci.* 1978;23:169-172.
14. Dykes M. Is enflurane hepatotoxic? *Anesthesiology.* 1984;61:235-237.
15. Eger EI, Gong D, Koblin DD, et al. Dose-related biochemical markers of renal injury after sevoflurane versus desflurane anesthesia in volunteers. *Anesth Analg.* 1997;85:1154-1163.
16. Eger E, Smuckler E, Ferrell L, et al. Is enflurane hepatotoxic? *Anesth Analg.* 1986;65:21-30.
17. Fang ZX, Eger EL, Laster MJ, et al. Carbon monoxide production from degradation of desflurane, enflurane, isoflurane, halothane, and sevoflurane by soda lime and Baralyme. *Anesth Analg.* 1995;80:1187-1193.
18. Frink EJ, Malan TP, Isner RJ et al. Renal concentrating function with prolonged sevoflurane or enflurane anesthesia in volunteers. *Anesthesiology.* 1994;80:1019-1025.
19. Frink EJ, Nogami WM, Morgan SE, Salmon RC. High carboxyhemoglobin concentrations occur in swine during desflurane anesthesia in the presence of partially dried carbon dioxide absorbents. *Anesthesiology.* 1997;87:308-316.
20. Higuchi H, Sumita S, Wada H, et al. Effects of sevoflurane and isoflurane on renal function and on possible markers of nephrotoxicity. *Anesthesiology.* 1998;89:307-322.
21. Hoft R, Bunker J, Goodman H. Halothane hepatitis in three pairs of closely related women. *N Engl J Med.* 1981;304:1023-1024.
22. Inman W, Mushlin W. Jaundice after repeat exposure to halothane: a further analysis of reports to the committee on safety of medicines. *Br Med J.* 1978;2:1455-1456.

23. Kandel L, Laster MJ, Eger EL, et al. Nephrotoxicity in rats undergoing a one-hour exposure to compound A. *Anesth Analg.* 1995;81:559-563.
24. Kobayashi Y, Ochiai R, Takeda J, et al. Serum and urinary inorganic fluoride concentrations after prolonged inhalation of sevoflurane in man. *Anesth Analg.* 1992;74:753-757.
25. Lassen H, Henriksen E, Neukirch F, Kristensen H. Treatment of tetanus: severe bone marrow depression after prolonged nitrous-oxide anaesthesia. *Lancet.* 1956;1:527-530.
26. Layzer R, Fishman R, Schafer J. Neuropathy following abuse of nitrous oxide. *Neurology.* 1978;28:504-506.
27. Lingenfelter R. Fatal misuse of enflurane. *Anesthesiology.* 1981;55:603.
28. Litz RJ, Hubler M, Lorenz W, et al. Renal responses to desflurane and isoflurane in patients with renal insufficiency. *Anesthesiology.* 2002;97:1133-1136.
29. Marie-Paule LAB, Versichelen LFM, Struys MMRF, et al. No Compound A formation with Superia® during minimal flow sevoflurane anesthesia: a comparison with Sofnolime®. *Anesth Analg.* 2002;95:1680-1685.
30. Mazze R, Jamison R. The renal effects of sevoflurane. *Anesthesiology.* 1995;83:443-445.
31. Mazze R, Woodruff R, Heerdt M. Isoniazid-induced enflurane defluorination in humans. *Anesthesiology.* 1982;57:5-8.
32. Messina F, Wynne J. Homemade nitrous oxide: no laughing matter. *Ann Intern Med.* 1982;96:333-334.
33. Neuberger J, Williams R. Halothane hepatitis. *Dig Dis.* 1988;6:52-64.
34. Nunn J. Clinical aspects of the interaction between nitrous oxide and vitamin B_{12}. *Br J Anaesth.* 1987;59:3-13.
35. Nunn J, Chanarin I, Tanner A, Owen E. Megaloblastic bone marrow changes after repeated nitrous oxide anaesthesia. *Br J Anaesth.* 1986;58:1469-1470.
36. O'Sullivan H, Jennings F, Ward K, et al. Human bone marrow biochemical function and megaloblastic hematopoiesis after nitrous oxide anesthesia. *Anesthesiology.* 1981;55:645-649.
37. Pohl L, Gillette JR. A perspective on halothane-induced hepatotoxicity. *Anesth Analg.* 1982;61:809-811.
38. Preckel B, Weber NC, Sanders RD, et al. Molecular mechanisms transducing the anesthetic, analgesic, and organ-protective actions of xenon. *Anesthesiology.* 2006;105:187-197.
39. Sanders RD, Weimann J, Maze M. Biologic effects of nitrous oxide. *Anesthesiology.* 2008;109:707-722.
40. Schilling R. Is nitrous oxide a dangerous anesthetic for vitamin B_{12}-deficient subjects? *JAMA.* 1986;255:1605-1606.
41. Scott J, Dinn J, Wilson P, Weir D. Pathogenesis of subacute combined degeneration: a result of methyl group deficiency. *Lancet.* 1981;2:334-337.
42. Spencer J, Raasch F, Trefny F. Halothane abuse in hospital personnel. *JAMA.* 1976;235:1034-1035.
43. Stock J, Strunin L. Unexplained hepatitis following halothane. *Anesthesiology.* 1985;63:424-439.
44. Subcommittee on the National Halothane Study of the Committee on Anesthesia National Academy of Sciences—National Research Council: summary of the national halothane study: possible association between halothane anesthesia and postoperative hepatic necrosis. *JAMA.* 1966;197:121-134.
45. Suton J, Harrison G, Hickie J. Accidental intravenous injection of halothane: case report. *Br J Anaesth.* 1971;43:513-520.
46. Taves D, Fry B, Freeman R, Gillies A. Toxicity following methoxyflurane anesthesia. II. Fluoride concentrations and nephrotoxicity. *JAMA.* 1970;214:91-95.
47. Touloukian J, Kaplowitz N. Halothane-induced hepatic disease. *Semin Liver Dis.* 1981;1:134-142.
48. Uzunalimoglu B, Yardley J, Boitnott J. The liver in mild halothane hepatitis: light and electron microscopic findings with special reference to the mononuclear cell infiltrate. *Am J Pathol.* 1970;61:457-478.
49. Vaughn R. Biochemical and biotransformation alterations in obesity. *Contemp Anesth Pract.* 1982;5:55-70.
50. Vergani D, Tsantoulas D, Eddleston A, et al. Sensitization to halothane-altered liver components in severe hepatic necrosis after halothane anesthesia. *Lancet.* 1978;2:801-803.
51. Versichelen LFM, Marie-Paule LAB, Rolly G, et al. Only carbon dioxide absorbents free of both NaOH and KOH do not generate Compound A during *in vitro* closed system sevoflurane. *Anesthesiology.* 2001;95:750-755.
52. Walton B, Simpson B, Strunin L, et al. Unexplained hepatitis following halothane. *Br Med J.* 1976;1:1171-1176.
53. Wig J, Chakravarty S, Krishnamurthy K, Mehta D. Coma following ingestion of halothane: its successful management. *Anaesthesia.* 1983;38:552-555.
54. Woehick HJ, Dunning M, Connolly LA. Reduction in the incidence of carbon monoxide exposures in humans undergoing general anesthesia. *Anesthesiology.* 1997;87:228-234.
55. Woehick HJ, Dunning M, Gandhi S, et al. Indirect detection of intra-operative carbon monoxide exposure by mass spectrometry during isoflurane anesthesia. *Anesthesiology.* 1995;83:213-217.
56. Woehick HJ, Dunning M, Nithpatikom K, et al. Mass spectrometry provides warning of carbon monoxide exposure via trifluoromethane. *Anesthesiology.* 1996;84:1489-1493.

CHAPTER 68
NEUROMUSCULAR BLOCKERS

Kenneth M. Sutin

These remarkably powerful xenobiotics have evolved throughout history from essential weapons for hunting to critical adjuncts to modern anesthesia. Understanding the pharmacokinetics of the depolarizing and nondepolarizing neuromuscular blockers (NDNMBs) improves care in the emergency department, intensive care unit (ICU), and operating room. Understanding and early recognition of the complications of each NMB limit associated morbidity and mortality.

HISTORY

Curare is the generic term for the resinous arrowhead poisons used to paralyze hunted animals.[100] The curare alkaloids are derived from the bark of the *Strychnos* vine, and the most potent alkaloids, the toxiferines, are derived from *Strychnos toxifera*. Fortunately for the hunters who used curare, ingestion of their prey did not cause paralysis. Sir Walter Raleigh discovered the use of curare in Guyana in 1595, and he was the first person to bring curare to Europe. The use of curare (d-tubocurarine) in anesthesia spanned almost 60 years and has been replaced by superior agents (with less histamine release and hypotension). Curare played a pivotal role in the discovery of the mechanism of neuromuscular transmission. In 1844, Claude Bernard placed a small piece of dry curare under the skin of a live frog and observed that the frog became limp and died.[7] He performed an immediate autopsy and discovered that the heart was beating. Because direct muscle stimulation produced contraction but nerve stimulation did not, Bernard concluded that curare paralyzed the motor nerves. He later observed, however, that bathing the isolated nerve did not affect neuromuscular transmission, leading him to conclude: "Curare must act on the terminal plates of motor nerves."[12] Curare was also used by Nobel Laureate physiologists Charles Sherrington, John Eccles, and Bernard Katz to further elucidate neuromuscular physiology. Its first clinical use was described in 1878 when Hunter used curare to treat patients with tetanus and seizures.[100] In 1932, Raynard West used curare to reduce the muscular rigidity of hemiplegia.[100]

More recent nonmedical uses of succinylcholine have been less benign.[2] The anesthesiologist Dr. Carl Coppolino was accused of murdering his wife in 1965 by succinylcholine injection.[65] In 1983, shortly after Dr. Michael Swango began his internship at Ohio State University Hospital, patients began dying inexplicably, and he was relieved of his duties.[92] After multiple residencies and jobs over 14 years, extending as far as Mnene Hospital in Zimbabwe, the prosecution secured Swango's guilty plea for the murder of three victims. The toxicologic analysis of the 7-year-old remains of Thomas Sammarco revealed succinylcholine in the liver and gallbladder and its metabolite succinylmonocholine in multiple organs which assisted in the conviction.

With the advent of new modalities of drug delivery, toxicologists must be attuned to possible malicious intent. Emergency personnel responding to a 911 call observed the widow removing an insulin pump reservoir from her dead husband's body with the stated intent to donate the costly equipment.[4] A natural cause of death was presumed, yet surprisingly, forensic analysis revealed etomidate and laudanosine (a metabolite of atracurium) in the victim's liver.

MECHANISM OF NEUROMUSCULAR TRANSMISSION AND BLOCK

The purpose of a NMB is to selectively and reversibly inhibit transmission at the skeletal neuromuscular junction (NMJ). All NMBs possess at least one positively charged quaternary ammonium moiety that binds to the postsynaptic nicotinic acetylcholine (nACh) receptor at the NMJ, inhibiting its normal activation by acetylcholine (ACh). The nACh receptor is a ligand-gated ion channel that consists of four different protein subunits in a pentameric structure surrounding a central channel. The nACh receptor found in human skeletal muscle is present in two primary forms: a mature type found at the NMJ ($\alpha\alpha\beta\varepsilon\delta$) or as a fetal (immature) type found on muscle at extrajunctional regions of the muscle fiber ($\alpha\alpha\beta\gamma\delta$). Before discussing the mechanism of neuromuscular block, it is first helpful to understand normal neuromuscular transmission and excitation–contraction coupling (Fig. 68–1).

Therapeutic and toxicologic skeletal muscle paralysis may occur by several mechanisms. For example, tetrodotoxin blocks voltage-sensitive sodium channels, preventing action potential conduction by the motor neuron. On the other hand, botulinum toxin blocks ACh release from the presynaptic neuron by inhibiting the binding of ACh-containing vesicles to the neuronal membrane in the region of the synaptic cleft. Modulation of postsynaptic ACh receptor activity at the NMJ may produce paralysis by one of two mechanisms: depolarizing (phase I block) and nondepolarizing (phase II block). Succinylcholine is the only depolarizing neuromuscular blocker (DNMB) in current clinical use. Nicotine at high doses may also cause a depolarizing block. All other drugs discussed are NDNMBs.

The process of DNMB requires several steps. First, two molecules of succinylcholine must bind to each α site of the nACh receptor. This action causes a prolonged open state of the nACh receptor ion channel. The initial depolarization generates a muscle action potential and usually causes brief contractions (fasciculations). In contrast to ACh, succinylcholine is not hydrolyzed efficiently by junctional (true) acetylcholinesterase (AChE); thus, the effect of succinylcholine lasts much longer than ACh. Persistence of succinylcholine at the ACh receptor causes a sustained local muscle endplate depolarization that, in turn, causes the voltage-gated sodium channel in the perijunctional region to remain in a prolonged inactive state, inducing a desensitization block. The muscle is temporarily refractory to presynaptic release of ACh (phase I block).

The NDNMBs cause skeletal muscle paralysis by competitively inhibiting the effects of ACh and thus preventing muscle depolarization. One molecule of an NDNMB bound to a single nACh receptor (on the α site) is sufficient to competitively inhibit normal channel activation. Because the NDNMBs do not block voltage-gated sodium channels on the skeletal muscle membrane, direct electrical stimulation with a current sufficient to cause membrane depolarization will still elicit a muscular contraction. The NDNMBs are classified by duration of action as ultrashort, short, intermediate, and long. They are also classified by chemical structure as either a synthetic benzylisoquinolinium or an aminosteroid (Table 68–1).

NDNMBs also block nACh receptors on the prejunctional nerve terminal and inhibit ACh-stimulated ACh production and release[83] by blocking local autoregulation of available ACh. This effect reduces the available pool of ACh and augments the extent of neuromuscular block.[9]

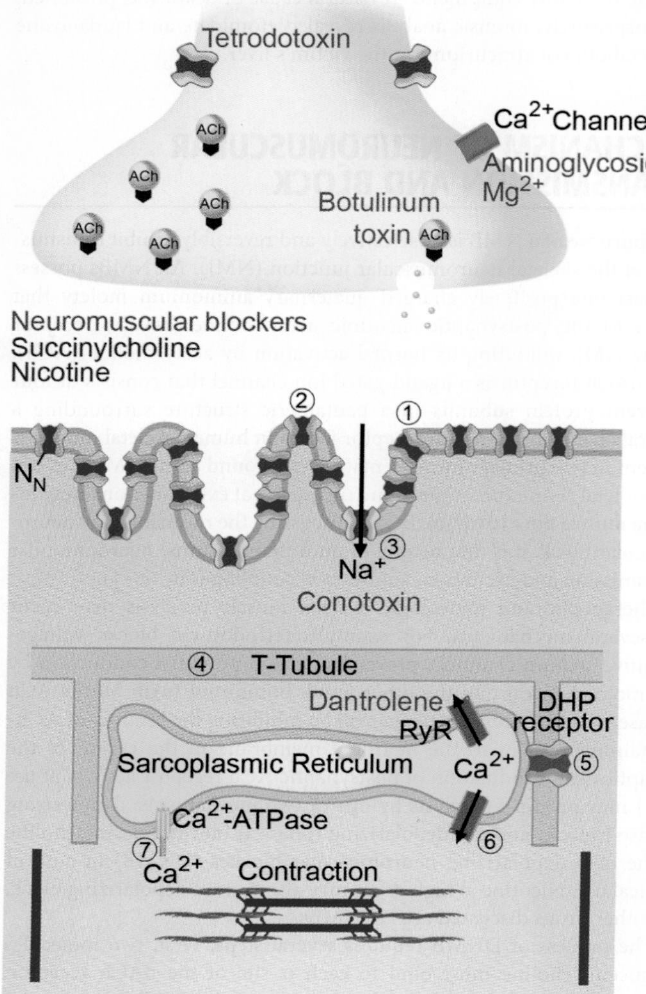

FIGURE 68–1. Excitation–contraction coupling in skeletal muscle. At the neuromuscular junction, acetylcholine (◎) released from the presynaptic nerve terminal crosses the 50-nm synaptic cleft to reach the nicotinic acetylcholine (nACh) receptor. When agonist simultaneously occupies both receptor sites this ion channel opens, becoming nonselectively permeable to monovalent cations, resulting in an influx of Na^+ and an efflux of K^+. This produces local membrane depolarization (end plate potential), which, in turn, opens voltage-activated Na^+ channels. A depolarization of sufficient amplitude generates a propagated muscle action potential (MAP), which is conducted along the muscle membrane and down the transverse (T) tubules. In the T tubule, the MAP triggers a voltage-activated calcium channel (the dihydropyridine receptor) which then activates the skeletal muscle ryanodine receptor/channel. To allow the fastest activation of mammalian skeletal muscle, calcium diffusion is not necessary for activation of RYR-1; instead, there is a direct electrical (protein) linkage between the dihydropyridine receptor and the ryanodine receptor.[26] Active ATPase driven calcium reuptake terminates muscle contraction. Many factors influence the activity of the RYR-1 channel, including Ca^{2+}, Mg^{2+}, and anesthetic drugs such as inhalation agents that accelerate Ca^{2+} release in persons susceptible to malignant hyperthermia. Antagonists such as conotoxin are red and agonists such as nicotine are green.

PHARMACOKINETICS

The NMBs are highly water soluble and relatively insoluble in lipids. Thus, they are rapidly distributed in the extracellular space and very slowly permeate lipid membranes such as the gut, placenta, and the normal blood–brain barrier. For this reason, they are devoid of central nervous system (CNS) effects. Because these drugs distribute in the extracellular space, their dosage is based on ideal body mass. In obese patients, estimation of drug requirement according to total body mass results in the administration of an excessive dose.

The speed of onset of an NMB is inversely related to its molar potency (ie, ED_{95} expressed as moles NMB drug per kilogram body weight).[48,49] Stated differently, the greater the affinity of the NDNMB for the ACh receptor, the fewer molecules per kilogram of tissue are required to produce a given degree of ACh receptor occupancy. Atracurium is the only drug that does not follow this generalization because it is a mixture of 10 isomers each having a different receptor affinity (cisatracurium consists of only one isomer).

In general, small, fast-contracting muscles such as the extraocular muscles are more susceptible to neuromuscular block than are larger, slower muscles such as the diaphragm. This is the so-called *respiratory sparing effect.* After an intravenous (IV) bolus of NDNMB, paralysis of the diaphragm is coincident with paralysis of laryngeal muscles because high tissue perfusion results in rapid drug distribution and diffusion into the NMJ of all tissues.[18] However, recovery from NMB is fastest for the diaphragm and intercostal muscles; intermediate for the large muscles of the trunk and extremities; and slowest for the adductor pollicis, larynx, pharynx, and extraocular muscles.[18]

COMPLICATIONS OF NEUROMUSCULAR BLOCKERS

Complications associated with the use of NMBs include (1) problems associated with the care of a paralyzed patient (eg, undetected hypoventilation resulting from ventilator or airway problems, impaired ability to monitor neurologic function, unintentional patient awareness, peripheral nerve injury, deep vein thrombosis, and skin breakdown), (2) immediate side effects, and (3) effects occurring after prolonged drug exposure.[72,73]

CONSCIOUSNESS

Even though NMB drugs do not affect consciousness, misconceptions about these drugs persist.[62] The pupillary light reflex, an important indicator of midbrain function, is preserved in healthy subjects who receive NDNMBs[35] because pupillary function is mediated by muscarinic cholinergic receptors, for which the NMBs have no affinity.

HISTAMINE RELEASE

Muscle relaxants may elicit dose- and injection rate-related nonimmunologic (non IgE-mediated) histamine release from tissue mast cells by an uncertain mechanism (see Table 68–1). The drugs most commonly associated with histamine release are atracurium and succinylcholine.[68]

ANAPHYLAXIS

Of the anaphylactic reactions occurring during general anesthesia, approximately 60% are the result of NMBs, but only 17% are the result of latex.[68] Rocuronium is responsible for 43% and succinylcholine for 23% of all NMB-associated anaphylaxis. In up to half of these patients,

TABLE 68–1. Pharmacology of Selected Neuromuscular Blockers

Generic Name	Class	Duration	Initial Dose (mg/kg)[A,B]	Onset (min)[C]	Clinical Duration (min)[D]
Succinylcholine	Depolarizer	Ultrashort	0.6–1	1–1.5	3–7
Atracurium	Nondepolarizer, benzylisoquinolinium	Intermediate	0.4	2–4	20–40
Cisatracurium		Intermediate	0.1	2–4	20–40
Mivacurium		Short	0.25	2–3	12–20
Pancuronium	Nondepolarizer, aminosteroid	Long	0.1	3–6	60–90
Rocuronium		Intermediate	0.6	1–3	30–40
Vecuronium		Intermediate	0.1	2–4	20–40

	Renal Excretion (%)[E]	Biliary Excretion (%)[F]	Metabolite	Histamine Release	Effect on Heart Rate
Succinylcholine	<10	Minimal	Succinic acid	Minimal	Bradycardia (rare)
Atracurium	5–10	Minimal	Laudanosine	Minimal	No
Cisatracurium	10–20	Minimal	Laudanosine	No	No
Mivacurium	<10	Minimal	Several	Minimal	No
Pancuronium	40–60	10–20	3-Desacetyl-pancuronium[G]	No	Tachycardia
Rocuronium	10–20	50–70	No	No	Tachycardia at high dose
Vecuronium	15–25	40–70	3-Desacetyl-vecuronium[G]	No	No

[A] Cisatracurium is labeled as milligram of base per milliliter. Other drugs are labeled and packaged as milligram of salt per milliliter.

[B] Typical initial dose is approximately 2 × ED_{95}(mg/kg).

[C] Onset = time from bolus to 100% block.

[D] Clinical duration = time from drug injection until 25% recovery of single twitch height.

[E] Percent renal excretion in the first 24 hours of unchanged drug; if high, associated with prolongation of clinical effect.

[F] Percent Biliary excretion in first 24 hours of unchanged drug; if high, associated with prolongation of clinical effect.

[G] Active metabolite.

Data adapted from Donati F. Neuromuscular blocking drugs for the new millennium: current practice, future trends–Comparative pharmacology of neuromuscular blocking drugs. *Anesth Analg*. 2000;90(suppl):S2-S6; McManus MC. Neuromuscular blockers in surgery and intensive care, part 1. *Am J Health Syst Pharm.* 2001;58:2287-2299; and Murray MJ, Cowen J, DeBlock H, et al. Clinical practice guidelines for sustained neuromuscular blockade in the adult critically ill patient. *Crit Care Med.* 2002:30:142-156.

there is no prior exposure to an NMB, and cross-sensitization by another allergen is the likely explanation.[55] Pancuronium is the drug that is least associated with serious allergic reactions.[99]

CONTROL OF RESPIRATION

At subparalyzing doses, NDNMBs blunt the hypoxic ventilatory response (HVR) but not the ventilatory response to hypercapnia.[23,24] HVR returns to normal when chemical paralysis is completely reversed. Hypoventilation resulting from blunting of the HVR, especially when combined with the residual effects of other drugs used during anesthesia (eg, opioids or inhalational anesthetics), may cause delayed respiratory failure (eg, after general anesthesia).

AUTONOMIC SIDE EFFECTS

Nicotinic ACh receptors found in autonomic ganglia, similar to those at the NMJ, are pentamers composed of α and β subunits. In general, they are less susceptible to block by NMBs.[63] There is one notable exception. At the same dose that produces neuromuscular block, tubocurarine also blocks nACh receptors at the parasympathetic ganglia, causing tachycardia, and at the sympathetic ganglia, blunting the sympathetic response.[87] In combination with tubocurarine-related histamine release, the sympathetic block may cause significant hypotension, especially in patients with heart failure or hypovolemia.[9] This is an important reason why tubocurarine is no longer available in the United States.

The muscarinic receptors (M_1–M_5) are members of the seven-transmembrane G-protein–coupled receptor family. As such, they are structurally unique and mostly unaffected by NMBs. At clinical doses, pancuronium elicits dose- and injection rate–related increases in heart rate, blood pressure, cardiac output, and sympathetic tone.[19,88,93] This is attributed to a selective block of parasympathetic transmission at the cardiac muscarinic receptors (atropine-like effect),[88] block of presynaptic (feedback) muscarinic receptors at sympathetic nerve terminals, and perhaps an indirect norepinephrine-releasing effect at postganglionic fibers.[19]

Dysrhythmias, including bradycardia, junctional rhythms, ventricular dysrhythmias, and cardiac arrest, occur rarely after use of succinylcholine. Dysrhythmias most likely result from stimulation of the cardiac muscarinic receptors and can be prevented by pretreatment with 15 to 20 μg/kg IV of atropine. Bradycardia is uncommon, but it may be especially severe in children during anesthetic induction when large or repeated doses of succinylcholine are given.

INTERACTIONS OF NEUROMUSCULAR BLOCKERS WITH OTHER XENOBIOTICS AND PATHOLOGIC CONDITIONS

NMBs have significant interactions with many xenobiotics and coexisting medical conditions. These interactions may affect the neuromuscular system at any level from the CNS to the muscle itself[79,98] (Table 68–2). In most neuromuscular diseases, such as muscular dystrophy, Guillain-Barré syndrome, myasthenia gravis, and postpolio syndrome, the sensitivity to NDNMB is increased, so a small dose of NMB produces a profound degree of block.[1,10,37] However, persons with myasthenia gravis typically demonstrate resistance to the effects of succinylcholine.[1,10] In individuals with myopathy in whom the specific cause is not yet known, it is prudent to avoid succinylcholine because of the possible sensitivity to malignant hyperthermia (MH), hyperkalemia, or rhabdomyolysis; in place of succinylcholine, a short-acting NDNMB can be used (to lessen the chance of prolonged weakness).

Many pathologic conditions potentiate the duration or intensity of NDNMB, such as respiratory acidosis, hypokalemia, hypocalcemia, hypermagnesemia, hypophosphatemia, hypothermia, shock, and liver or kidney failure.[82] Alternatively, acute sepsis and inflammatory states are associated with mild resistance to the effect of NDNMB.[74]

PHARMACOLOGY OF SUCCINYLCHOLINE

Succinylcholine is a bis-quaternary ammonium ion composed of two molecules of ACh joined end to end at the acetate groups.[21] After a conventional IV induction dose (1 mg/kg), typical serum concentrations are approximately 62 μg/mL.[76]

Succinylcholine is hydrolyzed primarily by plasma cholinesterase (ChE) and to a slight extent by alkaline hydrolysis. Hydrolysis is a two-step reaction; first succinylmonocholine and choline are formed, and then succinic acid and choline are formed (the latter two are normal products of intermediary metabolism). The first reaction is approximately six times faster than the second reaction. Less than 3% of the administered dose is excreted unchanged in the urine.[33] After an IV bolus, the serum succinylcholine concentration increases abruptly, and there is a rapid onset of NMJ block. Later, the serum succinylcholine concentration undergoes a rapid decline as a result of drug redistribution to extravascular tissues and hydrolysis in the serum. Finally, succinylcholine leaves the NMJ to reenter the serum as a result of reversal of the concentration gradient.[32,44]

Succinylcholine 1 mg/kg IV usually increases cerebral blood flow, cortical electrical activity, intracranial pressure,[50] and intraocular pressure, especially in lightly anesthetized patients. These effects, when they occur, are usually modest and of no clinical significance.

TOXICITY OF SUCCINYLCHOLINE

The important adverse drug reactions associated with succinylcholine include anaphylaxis, prolonged drug effect, hyperkalemia, acute rhabdomyolysis in patients with muscular dystrophy, MH in susceptible patients, muscle spasms or trismus in patients with myotonia congenita, and cardiac dysrhythmias.

PROLONGED EFFECT

The effects of succinylcholine may last for several hours if metabolism is slowed because of decreased plasma ChE concentration, abnormal plasma ChE activity (genetic variant or drug inhibition), or a phase II block.[14] Acquired plasma ChE deficiency may be caused by hepatic disease, malnutrition, plasmapheresis, or pregnancy.[14] Inactivation of plasma ChE may be caused by fluoride poisoning, organic phosphorus compounds, and carbamates. However, even with only 20% to 30% of normal plasma ChE activity, the clinical duration of succinylcholine is less than doubled.[28]

Many genetic variants of plasma ChE are known. The most common atypical plasma ChE (atypical type, homozygous; incidence, one in 3000) can be assayed by its resistance to inhibition by the local anesthetic dibucaine.[80] A history of uneventful exposure to succinylcholine *excludes* the possibility of atypical plasma ChE except in the case of hepatic transplantation. Dibucaine inhibits the ability of normal plasma ChE to hydrolyze benzoylcholine by more than 70% (ie, dibucaine number >70), heterozygous atypical enzyme by 40% to 60%, and homozygous atypical enzyme by 30% or less. Fresh-frozen plasma or plasma ChE concentrates may be infused to hasten recovery in the case of a genetic enzyme defect or an acquired ChE deficiency. However, to avoid the risks of transfusion, it is best to simply keep the patient sedated, intubated, and ventilated until the drug is metabolized. In this setting, spontaneous reversal usually occurs within 3 to 4 hours, although in rare cases, full recovery requires up to 12 hours.[14] When the duration of succinylcholine is very prolonged, blood samples should be drawn for measurement of plasma ChE concentration and activity.

Prolonged nondepolarizing block may occur when unusually large IV doses of succinylcholine (3–5 mg/kg) are given over minutes.[57] This is called *phase II block*, and it can be partially reversed by neostigmine.

HYPERKALEMIA

Succinylcholine 1 mg/kg IV typically causes serum K^+ to increase within minutes by approximately 0.5 mEq/L both in normal individuals and in persons with renal failure. The acute hyperkalemic response to succinylcholine is exaggerated with coexisting myopathy or proliferation of extrajunctional muscle ACh receptors. However, the mortality is highest (30%) when rhabdomyolysis is present.[36] Severe, precipitous, potentially life-threatening hyperkalemia also occurs after succinylcholine administration in several conditions associated with proliferation of ACh receptors. These conditions include denervation (head or spinal cord injury, stroke, neuropathy, prolonged use of NDNMBs), muscle pathology (direct trauma, crush or compartment syndrome, muscular dystrophy), critical illness (hemorrhagic shock, neuropathy, myopathy, prolonged immobility), thermal burn or cold injury, and sepsis lasting several days (eg, intraabdominal infections). After a neurologic injury, susceptibility to hyperkalemia begins within 4 to 7 days and may persist indefinitely. In patients who have been in the ICU for more than 1 week, a prudent course is to avoid succinylcholine altogether because of the risk of hyperkalemic cardiac arrest, which is associated with a mortality rate of at least 19%.[6,8,36] Severe hyperkalemia is modified, but not prevented, by a dose of an NDNMB sufficient to prevent succinylcholine-induced muscle fasciculations.

Severe or even fatal hyperkalemia has been reported in a few patients who received succinylcholine immediately after exsanguinating hemorrhage or massive trauma. The mechanism for this condition is not the same as that after neurologic injury because of inadequate time for proliferation of extrajunctional ACh receptors. Succinic acid, a tricarboxylic acid cycle intermediate (which is also a metabolite of succinylcholine), facilitates activation of voltage-gated sodium channels in a dose-dependent fashion, increasing skeletal muscle excitability.[38] In hemorrhagic shock, accumulation of succinic acid as a result of cell breakdown and anaerobic metabolism possibly augments the potassium-releasing effect of succinylcholine.

TABLE 68–2. Effect of Prior Administration of Xenobiotics on Subsequent Response to Succinylcholine or Nondepolarizing Neuromuscular Blockers

Xenobiotic	Response to Succinylcholine	Response to Nondepolarizer	Comments
Aminoglycosides (eg, amikacin, gentamicin)	Potentiates	Potentiates	Dose-related decrease in presynaptic ACh release. May decrease postjunctional response to ACh. Partially reversible with calcium supplementation. Effect of neostigmine unpredictable.
Anticholinesterase, peripheral acting: neostigmine, edrophonium	Prolongs succinylcholine (except edrophonium)	No effect	Neostigmine, pyridostigmine, and physostigmine inhibit plasma AChE and prolong succinylcholine block. Edrophonium does not inhibit plasma cholinesterase.
Anticholinesterase, centrally acting: donepezil	Potentiates	Potentiates mivacurium	Inhibits AChE (junctional >> plasma); long half-life (70 h).
β-Adrenergic antagonist: propranolol	Potentiates in cats, effects in humans uncertain	Potentiates	When given alone, may unmask myasthenic syndrome. Blocks ACh binding at postsynaptic membrane. Reversal of block with neostigmine may cause severe bradycardia.
β-Adrenergic antagonist: esmolol	? Mild prolongation	Slows onset of rocuronium	Competes for plasma AChE.
Botulinum toxin	?	Early potentiation, delayed resistance	Single case report: acutely, subclinical systemic denervation leads to vecuronium hypersensitivity. Subsequent NMJ remodeling and ACh receptor upregulation lead to vecuronium resistance.
CAs			Pancuronium and CA may cause cardiac dysrhythmias because of sympathetic effects.
Calcium channel blockers: nifedipine, verapamil	Potentiates	Potentiates	Causes calcium channel block pre- and postjunctionally. Verapamil has local cholinesterase inhibitor effect on nerve. May inhibit block reversal by cholinesterase inhibitor.
Carbamazepine	?	Inhibits, shortened duration	Chronic therapy causes resistance to NDNMB, except for atracurium.
Cardioactive steroids	More prone to cardiac dysrhythmias	Pancuronium increases catecholamines and may cause dysrhythmias	
Dantrolene	?	Potentiates	Blocks excitation–contraction coupling by blocking ryanodine calcium channel in sarcoplasmic reticulum of skeletal muscle.
Furosemide <10 μg/kg 1–4 mg/kg	Potentiates/Inhibits	Potentiates/Inhibits	Biphasic dose response in cats; protein kinase inhibition at low doses and phosphodiesterase inhibition at high doses. Diuretic-related hypokalemia potentiates pancuronium in cats.
Glucocorticoids	?	Inhibits	Chronic steroid use induces resistance to pancuronium and decrease plasma cholinesterase activity by 50%. Steroids ± NDNMB associated with myopathies.
Inhalational anesthetics: isoflurane	Potentiates	Potentiates	Decrease CNS activity and potentiates NMB in anesthetic doses: dependent fashion (postsynaptic and muscle effects). Halothane causes less muscle relaxation than isoflurane.
Lidocaine	Potentiates	Low-dose potentiates block. High-dose inhibits nerve terminals and blocks ACh binding site at postsynaptic membrane.	The fast Na^+ channel blockers decrease action potential propagation, ACh release, postsynaptic membrane sensitivity, and muscle excitability. Weak inhibitor of plasma cholinesterase.
Lithium carbonate	Prolongs onset and duration	Prolongs effect of pancuronium	Inhibits synthesis and release of ACh. Lithium alone may cause myasthenic reaction.
Magnesium	Potentiates; may block fasciculations	Potentiates; may also prolong block	Decreases prejunctional ACh release, postjunctional membrane sensitivity, and muscle excitability.

(Continued)

TABLE 68–2. Effect of Prior Administration of Xenobiotics on Subsequent Response to Succinylcholine or Nondepolarizing Neuromuscular Blockers (*Continued*)

Xenobiotic	Response to Succinylcholine	Response to Nondepolarizer	Comments
NDNMB : pancuronium vecuronium rocuronium	"Precurarization" with NDNMB shortens the onset and decreases side effects of succinylcholine. Pancuronium increases block duration.	Chronic NDNMB induces resistance to their effect. Mixing different NDNMBs may cause greater than additive effects, especially combining pancuronium with tubocurarine or metocurine	Prior NDNMB inhibits plasma AChE and prolongs mivacurium and succinylcholine block. Rank order: pancuronium > vecuronium > atracurium. Heterozygote for atypical plasma AChE may develop phase II block when given succinylcholine and pancuronium.
Organic phosphorus compounds	Potentiates	?	Irreversible plasma AChE inhibitor. May totally block enzyme activity.
Phenelzine (MAOI)	Prolongs	?	Decreases plasma AChE activity.
Phenytoin	?	Resistant, shortened duration	Acutely, potentiates NDNMB paralysis. With chronic use (except for atracurium), phenytoin induces resistance to NDNMB and increases drug metabolism. This increases the initial dose and decreases the repeat dosing interval.
Polypeptide antibiotics: polymyxin	Potentiates	Potentiates	May cause severe weakness. May induce postsynaptic neuromuscular block. Neostigmine increases block.
Succinylcholine	Self-taming dose of succinylcholine may be used to limit muscular fasciculations	Pancuronium and vecuronium slightly prolonged by prior succinylcholine	
Theophylline		Inhibits	Pancuronium and theophylline may increase cardiac dysrhythmias.

ACh, acetylcholine; AChE, acetylcholinesterase; MAOI, monoamine oxidase inhibitor; NMJ, neuromuscular junction; NDNMB, nondepolarizing neuromuscular blocker; CA, cyclic antidepressant.

Data adapted from Crowe S, Collins L. Suxamethonium and donepezil: a cause of prolonged paralysis. *Anesthesiology.* 2003;98:574-575; Flacchino F, Grandi L, Soliven P, et al. Sensitivity to vecuronium after botulinum toxin administration. *J Neurosurg Anesthesiol.* 1997;9:1491153; Fleming NW, Macres S, Antognini JF, Vengco J. Neuromuscular blocking action of suxamethonium after antagonism of vecuronium by edrophonium, pyridostigmine or neostigmine. *Br J Anaesth*. 1996;77:492-495; Kaeser HE: Drug-induced myasthenic syndromes. *Acta Neurol Scand Suppl.* 1984;100:39-47; Kato M, Hashimoto Y, Horinouchi T, et al. Inhibition of human plasma cholinesterase and erythrocyte acetylcholinesterase by nondepolarizing neuromuscular blocking agents. *J Anesth*. 2000;14:30-34; Ostergaard D, Engback J, Viby-Mogensen J. Adverse reactions and interactions of the neuromuscular blocking drugs. *Med Toxicol Adverse Drug Exp*. 1989; 4:351-368; and Viby-Mogensen J. Interaction of other drugs with muscle relaxants. In: Katz RL, ed. *Muscle Relaxants: Basic and Clinical Aspects*. New York, Grune and Stratton; 1985:233-256.

RHABDOMYOLYSIS

Severe hyperkalemia rarely occurs in the absence of a clinical history that readily discloses an obvious risk factor, with one important exception. Acute or delayed onset of rhabdomyolysis, hyperkalemia, ventricular dysrhythmias, cardiac arrest, and death have been reported in apparently healthy children who subsequently were found to have a myopathy.[53] Since March 1995, a black box warning on the package insert has stated that succinylcholine should be avoided in elective surgery in children, particularly in children younger than 8 years of age, because of the small risk of a previously undiagnosed skeletal myopathy, especially Duchenne muscular dystrophy. Sudden cardiac arrest occurring immediately after succinylcholine administration should always be assumed to be caused by hyperkalemia. If fever, muscle rigidity, hyperlactatemia, or metabolic and respiratory acidosis also is present, the presumptive diagnosis of MH should prompt immediate therapy with dantrolene.

MALIGNANT HYPERTHERMIA

MH is a syndrome characterized by extreme skeletal muscle hypermetabolism; it is initiated after exposure to an anesthetic that triggers abnormal calcium release from the skeletal muscle sarcoplasmic reticulum, and it can have a variable presentation.[85] Although MH is associated with certain myopathies (including Duchenne muscular dystrophy, central core disease, King-Denborough syndrome, hypokalemic periodic paralysis, and certain sodium channel forms of myotonia), the disorder typically affects individuals who are otherwise healthy. It is inherited as an autosomal dominant trait with variable penetrance.[64] Triggering xenobiotics that can precipitate an attack of MH include succinylcholine and volatile inhalational anesthetics (the prototypical agent is halothane). In individuals considered MH susceptible, xenobiotics that can be administered safely include NDNMBs, nitrous oxide, propofol, ketamine, etomidate, benzodiazepines, barbiturates, opioids, and local anesthetics.

In human MH, there is a causal association with several unique defects involving a skeletal muscle receptor/regulatory protein, especially defects involving the calcium-activated calcium release channel found in skeletal muscle; the type 1 ryanodine receptor (or RYR-1, chromosome 19q13.1). Mutations of the RYR-1 receptor are detected in more than 50% of patients with MH, and more than 40 different mutations have been described[94] (see Fig. 68–1). The structurally distinct type 2 ryanodine receptor (RYR-2) is the primary type expressed in cardiac muscle, and this could explain why the myocardium is relatively spared in the early phase of MH (with the exception that the heart is hyperdynamic).[84] Of practical importance, the existence of multiple mutations across multiple alleles means that genetic testing is not likely to prove useful in detecting all individuals who are MH susceptible.

Although the prevalence of a genetic disorder associated with MH is one in 3000 to one in 8500, the observed incidence of MH reactions in patients exposed to general anesthesia (with triggering anesthetic agents) is one in 5000 to one in 60,000.[78,85] Each year in the United States, there are an estimated 700 cases of MH.[52] In patients who are MH susceptible, clinical manifestations develop less than half the time after exposure to triggering agents. For this reason, a previous uneventful anesthetic exposure does not preclude development of MH on a subsequent exposure.[3] In the operating room, MH most often presents abruptly soon after initial exposure to a triggering anesthetic agent, but the onset of MH may be delayed several hours into general anesthesia[71] or it may occur as long as 12 hours after surgery. In addition, MH can recur 24 to 36 hours after an initial episode.

The immediate systemic manifestations of MH result from extreme skeletal muscle hypermetabolism. The uncontrolled release of calcium from the terminal cisternae of the sarcoplasmic reticulum causes skeletal muscle contraction. Although muscular rigidity is a specific sign of MH, it is not consistently observed. Futile calcium cycling by sarcoplasmic Ca^{2+}-ATPase rapidly depletes intracellular ATP and leads to anaerobic metabolism. Clinically, MH presents as skeletal muscle hypermetabolism, increased CO_2 production (respiratory acidosis), increased O_2 consumption (mixed venous O_2 saturation far below normal of 75%, arterial hypoxemia, anaerobic metabolism, metabolic acidosis with elevated lactate concentration, cyanosis and skin mottling), and excess heat production (hyperthermia).[39] Other clinical findings include tachycardia, cardiac dysrhythmias, hyperkalemia, rhabdomyolysis, and disseminated intravascular coagulopathy.

The earliest signs of MH include an early and rapid increase in CO_2 production, causing an increase in arterial, venous, and end-tidal CO_2; tachycardia; tachypnea; hypertension or labile blood pressure; and skeletal and jaw muscle rigidity. Despite the name of the syndrome, hyperthermia is not a universal finding in MH, and moreover, it is often a late sign.[97] Acute potassium release from skeletal muscle cells may produce life-threatening hyperkalemia. Subsequent rhabdomyolysis may exacerbate the elevation of potassium by causing renal failure. In late-stage MH, cardiac decompensation results from hyperkalemia, heart failure, vascular collapse, or myocardial ischemia (especially with coexisting coronary artery disease). A standardized clinical grading scale has been published ranking the qualitative likelihood (ranging from "almost never" to "almost certain") that an adverse event represents a true episode of MH.[51]

The differential diagnosis of MH includes neuroleptic malignant syndrome, propofol infusion syndrome, serotonin syndrome, thyroid storm, pheochromocytoma, baclofen withdrawal, malignant syndrome in Parkinson's disease, tetanus, meningitis, poisoning by salicylates, amphetamines, cocaine, or antimuscarinics, unintentional intraoperative hyperthermia, heat stroke, and transfusion reactions. Of note, early septic shock is also associated with hypermetabolism, increased cardiac output, and fever, however, in contrast to MH, early septic shock is associated with an elevated mixed venous O_2 saturation (typically >75%).

Rarely, MH is triggered by severe exercise in a hot climate, IV potassium (which depolarizes the muscle membrane), antipsychotic drugs, or infection.[17,43] Some patients with hypermetabolism or rhabdomyolysis have responded favorably to dantrolene, but this does not necessarily confirm the diagnosis of MH. Such confirmation requires a muscle biopsy.

One theory of the pathogenesis of MH suggests that MH-triggering xenobiotics interact with an abnormal RYR-1 channel, causing it to stay in a prolonged open state and leading to rapid efflux of calcium from the skeletal muscle sarcoplasmic reticulum into the myoplasm. Succinylcholine prolongs muscle depolarization, leading to elevated myoplasmic calcium concentration. This action initiates accelerated calcium-activated calcium release from the myoplasmic reticulum.[36] However, not all cases of MH can be explained by an RYR-1 mutation.[29] For example, MH is also associated with defects in the CACNA1S protein that encodes a subunit of the skeletal muscle L-type calcium channel (known as the dihydropyridine receptor) and possibly with certain disorders of sodium channels (observed in the myotonic disorders).[29,70]

The antidote for MH is dantrolene, and the key aspects of MH therapy are rapid initial diagnosis, discontinuation of triggering anesthetics, and immediate therapy with dantrolene (within minutes). By partially blocking calcium release from skeletal muscle sarcoplasmic reticulum, dantrolene rapidly reverses the signs and symptoms of hypermetabolism. Before the introduction of dantrolene, the mortality rate of MH was 64%.[52] When patients with acute MH are treated immediately with dantrolene, removal of triggering agents, and supportive measures (volume resuscitation, active cooling, control of hyperkalemia), the mortality rate is less than 5%.[52] Factors associated with an increase in mortality are a muscular body habitus, development of disseminated intravascular coagulation, and a longer duration of anesthesia before the peak in end-tidal carbon dioxide.[52] Even if administration is delayed for hours or days, dantrolene may still improve survival after an acute episode. Patients with significant dysrhythmias can be treated with standard antidysrhythmics; however, calcium channel blockers must *not* be given with dantrolene because they may precipitate hyperkalemia and severe hypotension[86] (Table 68–3).

Persons who have experienced a possible episode of MH or have a positive family history may be considered for muscle biopsy and muscle testing. The fresh tissue specimen is placed in a tissue bath perfused with Krebs solution, and halothane or caffeine is added. According to the North America Malignant Hyperthermia Group, an MH-susceptible individual is one who demonstrates a positive muscle contraction in response to either halothane or caffeine.

MUSCLE SPASMS

Masseter muscle rigidity (MMR) was observed in 0.3% to 1.0% of pediatric patients when general anesthesia was induced with succinylcholine and halothane (a technique now obsolete), and, at present, it is much less frequently encountered. MMR is clinically significant because it may complicate airway management and herald the onset of MH.[77]

When administered to persons genetically predisposed to myotonia, succinylcholine may precipitate tonic muscular contractions, ranging from trismus (which may prevent orotracheal intubation) to severe generalized myoclonus and chest wall rigidity[25] (which may prevent ventilation). Because the myotonic contractions are independent of neural activity, they cannot be aborted by an NDNMB. Usually the contractions are self-limited, but occasionally they can be life-threatening if an airway cannot be established and hypoxemia ensues.

PHARMACOLOGY OF NONDEPOLARIZING NEUROMUSCULAR BLOCKERS

Table 68–1 summarizes the pharmacology and toxicity of the NDNMB drugs.[42,66,67,73] Whereas atracurium is composed of 10 different isomers, each having its unique pharmacokinetic and pharmacodynamic profile, cisatracurium contains only the 1R-*cis* and 1′R-*cis* isomers. Both

TABLE 68–3. Suggested Therapy for Malignant Hyperthermia

Acute Phase Treatment of Malignant Hyperthermia (MH)

1. **Call for help.** Immediately summon experienced help when MH is suspected.
2. **Stop triggers such as xenobiotics,** volatile inhalational anesthetics, and succinylcholine.
3. **Mildly hyperventilate with 100% O_2** with flows ≥10 L/min and monitor end-tidal CO_2.
4. **Administer dantrolene sodium.** Give the initial IV bolus of 2.5 mg/kg rapidly followed by additional boluses (every 15 min), until signs of MH are controlled (tachycardia, rigidity, increased end-tidal CO_2, hyperthermia). Typically, a total dose of 10 mg/kg IV controls symptoms, but occasionally 30 mg/kg may be required.
5. **Monitor core temperature closely.**
6. **Actively cool the patient** with core temperature >39°C simultaneously with the above.
   - Immersion in ice-water slurry is best. Peritoneal or gastric lavage can also be useful.
   - Surface cool with ice and hypothermia blanket.
7. **Aggressively treat hyperkalemia.** Hyperkalemia is common and should be treated with hyperventilation, sodium bicarbonate, IV calcium gluconate or chloride, IV dextrose and insulin. Those with hypokalemia should be treated with great caution because hyperkalemia may occur because of rhabdomyolysis.
8. **Sodium bicarbonate.** Consider correcting metabolic acidosis guided by arterial blood gas analysis (Not currently recommended).
9. **Monitor** arterial and mixed venous blood gases, serum potassium and calcium, clotting studies, and urine output.
10. **Dysrhythmias** usually respond to dantrolene and correction of acidosis and hyperkalemia. If dysrhythmias persist or are life threatening, standard antidysrhythmics may be used.
    - **Calcium channel blockers are not to be used (especially verapamil) to treat dysrhythmias** because they may cause hyperkalemia and cardiac arrest.
11. Ensure adequate urine output by hydration and/or administration of mannitol or furosemide. Insert a urinary bladder catheter and consider central venous or pulmonary artery catheterization.
12. **For emergency consultation, refer to the Malignant Hypertension Association of the United States** at http://www.mhaus.org/. **Call the MH Emergency Hotline:**
    - Inside United States or Canada, call **800-MH-HYPER (800-644-9737)**
    - Outside the United States and Canada, call **001 315-464-7079**

Postacute Phase Treatment of Malignant Hyperthermia

1. **Observe the patient in an ICU setting for at least 24 hours** because recrudescence of MH occurs in 25% of cases, particularly after a fulminant case resistant to treatment.
2. **Administer dantrolene 1 mg/kg IV q4–6h or 0.25 mg/kg/hr by infusion for at least 24 hours after the episode.**
3. Follow arterial blood gases, creatine phosphokinase, potassium, calcium, phosphorus, urine and serum myoglobin, PT, PTT, platelet count, and core body temperature until they return to normal values (eg, q6h). Central temperature (eg, rectal, esophageal) should be monitored continuously.
4. Counsel the patient and family regarding MH and further precautions.
   - For nonemergency patient referrals, contact MHAUS at 800-986-4287, 11 East State Street, PO Box 1069, Sherburne, NY 13460-1069.
   - Report patients who have had an acute MH episode to the **North American MH Registry of MHAUS** at **412-692-5464.**
   - Alert family members to the possible dangers of MH and anesthesia.
5. Recommend an MH medical ID tag or bracelet for the patient, which should be worn at all times.

Notes:

1. Each vial of dantrolene contains 20 mg of dantrolene and 3 g of mannitol (to improve water solubility). Each vial should be reconstituted with at least 60 mL of sterile, preservative-free water. Dissolution of the lyophilized dantrolene in water is slow and requires thorough mixing. Prewarming the water to 38°C speeds dissolution.
2. The guideline above may not apply to every patient and of necessity must be altered according to specific patient needs.
3. Sudden unexpected cardiac arrest in children: Children younger than about 10 years old who experience sudden cardiac arrest after succinylcholine administration in the absence of hypoxemia and anesthetic overdose should be treated for acute hyperkalemia first. In this situation, calcium chloride should be administered along with means to reduce serum potassium. They should be presumed to have subclinical muscular dystrophy, and a pediatric neurologist should be consulted.

ICU, intensive care unit; IV, intravenous; PT, prothrombin time; PTT, partial thromboplastin time.

atracurium and cisatracurium exhibit organ-independent elimination and are rapidly metabolized by spontaneous (nonenzymatic) temperature- and pH-dependent Hoffmann degradation and, to a lesser extent, by ester hydrolysis. The latter is catalyzed by nonspecific plasma esterases distinct from the plasma ChE that hydrolyzes succinylcholine. In addition, significant drug metabolism or elimination occurs in the liver and kidney.[27]

TOXICITY OF NONDEPOLARIZING NEUROMUSCULAR BLOCKERS

The most important toxic effects of the NDNMBs are accumulation of laudanosine and persistent weakness. In general, limiting the drug dose and monitoring the drug effect with a portable nerve stimulator reduce the incidence of prolonged weakness.

LAUDANOSINE

Metabolism of atracurium and cisatracurium generates laudanosine which crosses the blood–brain and placental barriers and may cause neuroexcitation but has no neuromuscular blocking activity.[22] Metabolism of each atracurium molecule generates one molecule of laudanosine.[75] Cisatracurium is an improvement over atracurium because it produces one-third as much laudanosine (and is three times more potent).[31,47]

In the CNS, laudanosine has an inhibitory effect at the γ-aminobutyric acid, nACh, and opioid receptors. At high serum concentrations in experimental animals, laudanosine causes dose-related neuroexcitation, myoclonic activity (>14 μg/mL), and generalized seizures[11,31] (>17 μg/mL). In humans, the toxic serum laudanosine concentration is unknown, and seizures directly attributable to atracurium have not been observed even after prolonged infusion in the ICU.[31,101] In ICU patients who received a 72-hour infusion of atracurium (1 mg/kg/h), the highest serum laudanosine concentrations (10–20 μg/mL) were observed in patients with renal insufficiency.[58] Laudanosine is excreted primarily in the bile, and its elimination is prolonged in patients with liver disease, biliary obstruction, and renal insufficiency.[81]

PERSISTENT WEAKNESS ASSOCIATED WITH NONDEPOLARIZING NEUROMUSCULAR BLOCKERS

Short-term blockade with a NDNMB usually resolves promptly upon discontinuation. When an NDNMB is administered for more than 48 hours, there is a risk that weakness will persist longer than anticipated based on the kinetics of drug elimination. In addition, critical illness is associated with dysfunction of the peripheral nerve, NMJ, and muscle (Table 68–4). For instance, in the ICU, persistent weakness is observed in 68% to 100% of patients with sepsis or multiple organ failure[16,30,96] and in 20% to 30% of patients who receive NDNMB for only 48 to 72 hours.[60] Persistent weakness is multifactorial and associated with illness severity, sepsis, acute respiratory distress syndrome, multiorgan failure, hyperglycemia, NDNMB, use of systemic glucocorticoids, muscle injury, thermal injury, and electrolyte, endocrine, and nutritional disorders.[15,20,40,59] Many xenobiotics given to patients in the ICU can cause weakness by themselves or potentiate the effects of NDNMB.[41,79] Progressive weakness and acute respiratory failure have even been described after discharge from the ICU and may be life threatening if not immediately recognized.[54] Patients who develop persistent weakness have a 2.5- to 3.5-fold increase in ICU mortality[60] and ICU stay.

TABLE 68–4. Acute Neuromuscular Pathology Associated with Critical Illness or NDNMB

	Critical Illness Polyneuropathy	Residual Neuromuscular Block	Disuse (Cachectic) Myopathy	Critical Illness Myopathy
Sensory	Moderate to severe, distal > proximal	Normal	Normal	Normal
Motor	Symmetric weakness, lower > upper extremity, proximal > distal or diffuse, respiratory failure	Diffuse symmetric weakness, respiratory failure	Diffuse weakness, proximal > distal	Symmetric weakness, proximal > distal or diffuse, respiratory failure
Creatine phosphokinase	Normal	Normal	Normal	Elevated in ≤50%
Electrodiagnostic studies (EMG, NCV)	Axonal degeneration of motor > sensory, reduced sensory and motor compound action potentials, normal NCV	Fatigue at NMJ assessed by fade on repetitive nerve stimulation	Normal EMG and NCV	Myopathic changes, muscle membrane inexcitability, normal NCV
Muscle biopsy	Denervation atrophy	Normal	Atrophy of type 2 fibers, no myosin loss, no necrosis	Atrophy of type 2 (fast-twitch) fibers, myosin loss, mild myonecrosis, no inflammatory infiltration

Data adapted from Bolton CF. Critical illness polyneuropathy and myopathy. *Crit Care Med.* 2001;29:2388-2390; Lacomis D. Critical illness myopathy. *Curr Rheumatol Rep.* 2002;4:403-408; Lacomis D, Campellone JV. Critical illness neuromyopathies. *Adv Neurol.* 2002;88:325-335; and Leijten FSS, de Weerd AW: Critical illness polyneuropathy: a review the literature, definition and pathophysiology. *Clin Neurol Neurosurg.* 1994;96:10-19.

EMG, electromyography; NCV, nerve conduction velocity; NMJ, neuromuscular junction.

TABLE 68–5. Pharmacology of Intravenous Neuromuscular Blockade Reversal Drugs and Coadministered Antimuscarinics

Anticholinesterases			
	Neostigmine	Pyridostigmine	Edrophonium
Initial dose (mg/kg)	0.04–0.08	0.2–0.4	0.5–1.0
Onset (min)	7–11	10–16	1–2
Duration (min)	60–120	60–120	60–120
Recommended antimuscarinic	Glycopyrrolate	Glycopyrrolate	Atropine
Antimuscarinics			
	Glycopyrrolate	Atropine	
Structure	Quaternary ammonium	Tertiary amine	
Initial dose (mg/kg)	0.01–0.02	0.02–0.03	
Onset (min)	2–3	1	
Duration (min)	30–60	30–60	
Elimination	Renal	Renal	
Crosses blood-brain barrier	No	Yes	

PHARMACOLOGY OF REVERSAL DRUGS

Termination of NMB effect initially results from drug redistribution and later from drug elimination, metabolism, or chemical antagonism. Pharmacologic antagonism of a partial NDNMB is achieved by giving a reversal agent that inhibits junctional AChE and increases ACh at the NMJ. This increase in ACh can overcome the competitive inhibition caused by residual NDNMB. The commonly used anti-ChEs are polar molecules that possess a quaternary ammonium (Table 68–5). Neostigmine and pyridostigmine are hydrolyzed by ChE and form short-lived carbamyl complexes (half-life, 15–20 minutes) with the esteratic site of the enzyme.[5] In contrast, edrophonium is not hydrolyzed by ChE; rather, it forms an electrostatic interaction and a hydrogen bond with the cationic site of ChE that is both competitive and reversible. Neostigmine and pyridostigmine, but not edrophonium, inhibit plasma ChE and thus prolong the effects of drugs metabolized by this enzyme, such as succinylcholine.[28]

TOXICOLOGY OF REVERSAL AGENTS

The most common and troublesome clinical side effect of ChE inhibition is bradycardia, which usually is prevented by coadministration of an antimuscarinic drug.[13] Bradydysrhythmias may be severe and lead to nodal or idioventricular rhythm, complete heart block, or even asystole.[61] These side effects occur more frequently in patients with preexisting bradycardia and those receiving chronic β-adrenergic antagonist therapy. They are not necessarily prevented by prior administration of atropine.[91] Other problems that may result from excess ChE inhibition are hypersalivation, bronchospasm, increased bronchial secretions, abdominal cramping from intestinal hyperperistalsis, cell division, tearing, and increased bladder tone. After general anesthesia, use of AChE may increase the incidence of nausea, vomiting, and abdominal cramps.[46] Because atropine crosses the blood–brain barrier, it may produce central anticholinergic syndrome.

DIAGNOSTIC TESTING

Quantitative methods for analysis of blood and tissue NDNMB and metabolite concentrations using high-performance liquid chromatography and mass spectrometry are described.[45,89]

Succinylcholine and succinylmonocholine can be assayed by gas chromatography and mass spectrometry in blood, urine, or the site of intramuscular injection.[76,90] Less than 3% of administered succinylcholine and 10% of its metabolite succinylmonocholine are excreted in the urine. However, both the parent drug and the metabolite undergo spontaneous hydrolysis, especially in alkaline conditions.[95] Historically, detection of succinylcholine has proven difficult because of its rapid hydrolysis. However, techniques for detecting this parent compound in tissues even after embalming have been described.[34] Because succinic acid is a product of intermediary metabolism, assay of this metabolite is not useful for positive identification of prior succinylcholine exposure.[69] Surprisingly, the presence of succinylmonocholine in forensic samples also cannot prove prior exposure to succinylcholine. Succinylmonocholine in concentrations of 0.01 to 0.20 μg/g has been detected in tissues of six autopsy cases with no history of succinylcholine exposure.[56]

SUMMARY

Succinylcholine is the only DNMB in current clinical use. Its immediate adverse effects include dose- and rate-related histamine release and modulation of autonomic tone. Acute and potentially fatal hyperkalemia may occur after succinylcholine administration, particularly in patients with certain myopathies (eg, Duchenne muscular dystrophy). The effect of succinylcholine is prolonged when there is an atypical genetic variant of plasma ChE, when it is inhibited (eg, organic phosphorus compounds, or donezepil), or when it is deficient (eg, from liver disease or plasmapheresis). In MH, acute onset of severe hypermetabolism causing acidosis, rhabdomyolysis, hyperkalemia, and death occurs if treatment with dantrolene and aggressive cooling is not rapidly administered.

The most important complications associated with use of NDNMBs are undetected hypoventilation and prolonged drug effect. NDNMBs have clinically important interactions with many xenobiotics and coexisting medical conditions. In most neuromuscular diseases, sensitivity to NDNMB is increased. In renal failure, active metabolites of pancuronium and vecuronium may accumulate and cause prolonged block.

REFERENCES

1. Azar I. The response of patients with neuromuscular disorders to muscle relaxants: a review. *Anesthesiology.* 1984;61:173-187.
2. Bailey FL. *Defense Never Rests.* New York: Signet Books; 1972.
3. Bendixen D, Skovgaard LT, Ording H. Analysis of anaesthesia in patients suspected to be susceptible to malignant hyperthermia before diagnostic in vitro contracture test. *Acta Anaesthesiol Scand.* 1997;41:480-484.
4. Benedict B, Keyes R, Sauls FC. The insulin pump as murder weapon: a case report. *Am J Forensic Med Pathol.* 2004;25:159-160.
5. Bevan DR, Donati F, Kopman AF. Reversal of neuromuscular blockade. *Anesthesiology.* 1992;77:785-805.
6. Biccard BM, Hughes M. Succinylcholine in the intensive care unit. *Anesthesiology.* 2002;96:253-254.
7. Black J. Claude Bernard on the action of curare. *Br Med J.* 1999;319:622.
8. Booij LH. Is succinylcholine appropriate or obsolete in the intensive care unit? *Crit Care.* 2001;5:245-246.
9. Bowman WC. Non-relaxant properties of neuromuscular blocking drugs. *Br J Anaesth.* 1982;54:147-160.
10. Briggs ED, Kirsch JR. Anesthetic implications of neuromuscular disease. *J Anesth.* 2003;17:177-185.
11. Chapple DJ, Miller AA, Ward JB, Wheatley PL. Cardiovascular and neurological effects of laudanosine. Studies in mice and rats, and in conscious and anaesthetized dogs. *Br J Anaesth.* 1987;59:218-225.
12. Conti F. Claude Bernard's des fonctions du cerveau: an ante litteram manifesto of the neurosciences? *Nat Rev Neurosci.* 2002;3:979-985.
13. Cronnelly R, Morris RB. Antagonism of neuromuscular blockade. *Br J Anaesth.* 1982;54:183-194.
14. Davis L, Britten JJ, Morgan M. Cholinesterase. Its significance in anaesthetic practice. *Anaesthesia.* 1997;52:244-260.
15. de Letter MA, Schmitz PI, Visser LH, et al. Risk factors for the development of polyneuropathy and myopathy in critically ill patients. *Crit Care Med.* 2001;29:2281-2286.
16. Deem S, Lee CM, Curtis JR. Acquired neuromuscular disorders in the intensive care unit. *Am J Respir Crit Care Med.* 2003;168:735-739.
17. Denborough M. Malignant hyperthermia. *Lancet.* 1998;352:1131-1136.
18. Dhonneur G, Kirov K, Slavov V, Duvaldestin P. Effects of an intubating dose of succinylcholine and rocuronium on the larynx and diaphragm: an electromyographic study in humans. *Anesthesiology.* 1999;90:951-955.
19. Domenech JS, Garcia RC, Sastain JM, et al. Pancuronium bromide: an indirect sympathomimetic agent. *Br J Anaesth.* 1976;48:1143-1148.
20. Douglass JA, Tuxen DV, Horne M, et al. Myopathy in severe asthma. *Am Rev Respir Dis.* 1992;146:517-519.
21. Durant NN, Katz RL. Suxamethonium. *Br J Anaesth.* 1982;54:195-208.
22. Eddleston JM, Harper NJ, Pollard BJ, et al. Concentrations of atracurium and laudanosine in cerebrospinal fluid and plasma during intracranial surgery. *Br J Anaesth.* 1989;63:525-530.
23. Eriksson LI. Reduced hypoxic chemosensitivity in partially paralysed man. A new property of muscle relaxants? *Acta Anaesthesiol Scand.* 1996;40:520-523.
24. Eriksson LI. The effects of residual neuromuscular blockade and volatile anesthetics on the control of ventilation. *Anesth Analg.* 1999;89:243-251.
25. Farbu E, Softeland E, Bindoff LA. Anaesthetic complications associated with myotonia congenita: case study and comparison with other myotonic disorders. *Acta Anaesthesiol Scand.* 2003;47:630-634.
26. Fill M, Copello JA. Ryanodine receptor calcium release channels. *Physiol Rev.* 2002;82:893-922.
27. Fisher DM, Canfell PC, Fahey MR, et al. Elimination of atracurium in humans: contribution of Hofmann elimination and ester hydrolysis versus organ-based elimination. *Anesthesiology.* 1986;65:6-12.
28. Fleming NW, Macres S, Antognini JF, Vengco J. Neuromuscular blocking action of suxamethonium after antagonism of vecuronium by edrophonium, pyridostigmine or neostigmine. *Br J Anaesth.* 1996;77:492-495.
29. Fletcher JE, Wieland SJ, Karan SM, et al. Sodium channel in human malignant hyperthermia. *Anesthesiology.* 1997;86:1023-1032.
30. Fletcher SN, Kennedy DD, Ghosh IR, et al. Persistent neuromuscular and neurophysiologic abnormalities in long-term survivors of prolonged critical illness. *Crit Care Med.* 2003;31:1012-1016.
31. Fodale V, Santamaria LB. Laudanosine, an atracurium and cisatracurium metabolite. *Eur J Anaesthesiol.* 2002;19:466-473.
32. Foldes FF. Distribution and biotransformation of succinylcholine. *Int Anesthesiol Clin.* 1975;13:101-115.
33. Foldes FF, Norton S. The urinary excretion of succinyldicholine and succinylmonocholine in man. *Br J Pharmacol Chemother.* 1954;9:385-388.
34. Forney RB Jr, Carroll FT, Nordgren IK, et al. Extraction, identification and quantitation of succinylcholine in embalmed tissue. *J Anal Toxicol.* 1982;6:115-119.
35. Gray AT, Krejci ST, Larson MD. Neuromuscular blocking drugs do not alter the pupillary light reflex of anesthetized humans. *Arch Neurol.* 1997;54:579-584.
36. Gronert GA, Mott J, Lee J. Aetiology of malignant hyperthermia. *Br J Anaesth.* 1988;60:253-267.
37. Gyermek L. Increased potency of nondepolarizing relaxants after poliomyelitis. *J Clin Pharmacol.* 1990;30:170-173.
38. Haeseler G, Petzold J, Hecker H, et al. Succinylcholine metabolite succinic acid alters steady state activation in muscle sodium channels. *Anesthesiology.* 2000;92:1385-1391.
39. Heffron JJ. Malignant hyperthermia. biochemical aspects of the acute episode. *Br J Anaesth.* 1988;60:274-278.
40. Herridge MS, Cheung AM, Tansey CM, et al. One-year outcomes in survivors of the acute respiratory distress syndrome. *N Engl J Med.* 2003;348:683-693.
41. Kaeser HE. Drug-induced myasthenic syndromes. *Acta Neurol Scand Suppl.* 1984;100:39-47.
42. Kampe S, Krombach JW, Diefenbach C. Muscle relaxants. *Best Pract Res Clin Anaesthesiol.* 2003;17:137-146.
43. Kasamatsu Y, Osada M, Ashida K, et al. Rhabdomyolysis after infection and taking a cold medicine in a patient who was susceptible to malignant hyperthermia. *Intern Med.* 1998;37:169-173.
44. Kato M, Shiratori T, Yamamuro M, et al. Comparison between in vivo and in vitro pharmacokinetics of succinylcholine in humans. *J Anesth.* 1999;13:189-192.
45. Kerskes CH, Lusthof KJ, Zweipfenning PG, Franke JP. The detection and identification of quaternary nitrogen muscle relaxants in biological fluids and tissues by ion-trap LC-ESI-MS. *J Anal Toxicol.* 2002;26:29-34.
46. King MJ, Milazkiewicz R, Carli F, Deacock AR. Influence of neostigmine on postoperative vomiting. *Br J Anaesth.* 1988;61:403-406.
47. Kisor DF, Schmith VD. Clinical pharmacokinetics of cisatracurium besilate. *Clin Pharmacokinet.* 1999;36:27-40.
48. Kopman AF, Klewicka MM, Kopman DJ, Neuman GG. Molar potency is predictive of the speed of onset of neuromuscular block for agents of intermediate, short, and ultrashort duration. *Anesthesiology.* 1999;90:425-431.
49. Kopman AF, Klewicka MM, Neuman GG. Molar potency is not predictive of the speed of onset of atracurium. *Anesth Analg.* 1999;89:1046-1049.
50. Kovarik WD, Mayberg TS, Lam AM, et al. Succinylcholine does not change intracranial pressure, cerebral blood flow velocity, or the electroencephalogram in patients with neurologic injury. *Anesth Analg.* 1994;78:469-473.
51. Larach M, Localio A, Allen G, et al. A clinical grading scale to predict malignant hyperthermia susceptibility. *Anesthesiology.* 1994;80:771-779.
52. Larach MG, Brandom BW, Allen GC, et al. Cardiac arrests and deaths associated with malignant hyperthermia in North America from 1987 to 2006: a report from the North American Malignant Hyperthermia Registry of the Malignant Hyperthermia Association of the United States. *Anesthesiology.* 2008;108:603-611.
53. Larach MG, Rosenberg H, Gronert GA, Allen GC. Hyperkalemic cardiac arrest during anesthesia in infants and children with occult myopathies. *Clin Pediatr (Phila).* 1997;36:9-16.
54. Latronico N, Guarneri B, Alongi S, et al. Acute neuromuscular respiratory failure after ICU discharge. Report of five patients. *Intensive Care Med.* 1999;25:1302-1306.
55. Laxenaire MC. Neuromuscular blocking drugs and allergic risk. *Can J Anaesth.* 2003;50:429-433.
56. LeBeau M, Quenzer C. Succinylmonocholine identified in negative control tissues. *J Anal Toxicol.* 2003;27:600-601.

57. Lee C. Dose relationships of phase II, tachyphylaxis and train-of-four fade in suxamethonium-induced dual neuromuscular block in man. *Br J Anaesth.* 1975;47:841-845.
58. Lefrant JY, Farenc C, De la Coussaye JE, et al. Pharmacodynamics and atracurium and laudanosine concentrations during a fixed continuous infusion of atracurium in mechanically ventilated patients with acute respiratory distress syndrome. *Anaesth Intensive Care.* 2002;30:422-427.
59. Leijten FS, De Weerd AW, Poortvliet DC, et al. Critical illness polyneuropathy in multiple organ dysfunction syndrome and weaning from the ventilator. *Intensive Care Med.* 1996;22:856-861.
60. Leijten FS, Harinck-de Weerd JE, Poortvliet DC, de Weerd AW. The role of polyneuropathy in motor convalescence after prolonged mechanical ventilation. *JAMA.* 1995;274:1221-1225.
61. Lonsdale M, Stuart J. Complete heart block following glycopyrronium/neostigmine mixture. *Anaesthesia.* 1989;44:448-449.
62. Loper KA, Butler S, Nessly M, Wild L. Paralyzed with pain: the need for education. *Pain.* 1989;37:315-316.
63. Lukas RJ, Changeux JP, Le Novere N, et al. International Union of Pharmacology. XX. Current status of the nomenclature for nicotinic acetylcholine receptors and their subunits. *Pharmacol Rev.* 1999;51:397-401.
64. MacLennan DH, Phillips MS. Malignant hyperthermia. *Science.* 1992;256:789-794.
65. Maltby JR. Criminal poisoning with anaesthetic drugs: murder, manslaughter, or not guilty. *Forensic Sci.* 1975;6:91-108.
66. McManus MC. Neuromuscular blockers in surgery and intensive care, Part 1. *Am J Health Syst Pharm.* 2001;58:2287-2299.
67. McManus MC. Neuromuscular blockers in surgery and intensive care, Part 2. *Am J Health Syst Pharm.* 2001;58:2381-2395.
68. Mertes PM, Laxenaire MC. Adverse reactions to neuromuscular blocking agents. *Curr Allergy Asthma Rep.* 2004;4:7-16.
69. Meyer E, Lambert WE, De Leenheer A. Succinic acid is not a suitable indicator of suxamethonium exposure in forensic blood samples. *J Anal Toxicol.* 1997;21:170-171.
70. Monnier N, Kozak-Ribbens G, Krivosic-Horber R, et al. Correlations between genotype and pharmacological, histological, functional, and clinical phenotypes in malignant hyperthermia susceptibility. *Hum Mutat.* 2005;26:413-425.
71. Morrison AG, Serpell MG. Malignant hyperthermia during prolonged surgery for tumour resection. *Eur J Anaesthesiol.* 1998;15:114-117.
72. Murphy GS, Vender JS. Neuromuscular-blocking drugs. Use and misuse in the intensive care unit. *Crit Care Clin.* 2001;17:925-942.
73. Murray MJ, Cowen J, DeBlock H, et al. Clinical practice guidelines for sustained neuromuscular blockade in the adult critically ill patient. *Crit Care Med.* 2002;30:142-156.
74. Narimatsu E, Nakayama Y, Sumita S, et al. Sepsis attenuates the intensity of the neuromuscular blocking effect of d-tubocurarine and the antagonistic actions of neostigmine and edrophonium accompanying depression of muscle contractility of the diaphragm. *Acta Anaesthesiol Scand.* 1999;43:196-201.
75. Nigrovic V, Fox JL. Atracurium decay and the formation of laudanosine in humans. *Anesthesiology.* 1991;74:446-454.
76. Nordgren IK, Forney RB, Jr., Carroll FT, et al. Analysis of succinylcholine in tissues and body fluids by ion-pair extraction and gas chromatography-mass spectrometry. *Arch Toxicol Suppl.* 1983;6:339-350.
77. O'Flynn RP, Shutack JG, Rosenberg H, Fletcher JE. Masseter muscle rigidity and malignant hyperthermia susceptibility in pediatric patients. An update on management and diagnosis. *Anesthesiology.* 1994;80:1228-1233.
78. Ording H. Incidence of malignant hyperthermia in Denmark. *Anesth Analg.* 1985;64:700-704.
79. Ostergaard D, Engbaek J, Viby-Mogensen J. Adverse reactions and interactions of the neuromuscular blocking drugs. *Med Toxicol Adverse Drug Exp.* 1989;4:351-368.
80. Pantuck EJ. Plasma cholinesterase: gene and variations. *Anesth Analg.* 1993;77:380-386.
81. Parker CJ, Jones JE, Hunter JM. Disposition of infusions of atracurium and its metabolite, laudanosine, in patients in renal and respiratory failure in an ITU. *Br J Anaesth.* 1988;61:531-540.
82. Prielipp RC, Coursin DB. Applied pharmacology of common neuromuscular blocking agents in critical care. *New Horiz.* 1994;2:34-47.
83. Riker W. Pre-junctional effects of neuromuscular blocking and facilitatory drugs. In: Katz R, ed. Muscle Relaxants. Amsterdam, Netherlands: North-Holland Publishing Co.; 1975:59-102.
84. Roewer N, Dziadzka A, Greim CA, et al. Cardiovascular and metabolic responses to anesthetic-induced malignant hyperthermia in swine. *Anesthesiology.* 1995;83:141-159.
85. Rosenberg H, Davis M, James D, et al. Malignant hyperthermia. *Orphanet J Rare Dis.* 2007;2:21.
86. Saltzman LS, Kates RA, Corke BC, et al. Hyperkalemia and cardiovascular collapse after verapamil and dantrolene administration in swine. *Anesth Analg.* 1984;63:473-478.
87. Savarese JJ. The autonomic margins of safety of metocurine and d-tubocurarine in the cat. *Anesthesiology.* 1979;50:40-46.
88. Saxena PR, Bonta IL. Mechanism of selective cardiac vagolytic action of pancuronium bromide. Specific blockade of cardiac muscarinic receptors. *Eur J Pharmacol.* 1970;11:332-341.
89. Sayer H, Quintela O, Marquet P, et al. Identification and quantitation of six non-depolarizing neuromuscular blocking agents by LC-MS in biological fluids. *J Anal Toxicol.* 2004;28:105-110.
90. Somogyi G, Varga M, Prokai L, et al. Drug identification problems in two suicides with neuromuscular blocking agents. *Forensic Sci Int.* 1989;43:257-266.
91. Sprague DH. Severe bradycardia after neostigmine in a patient taking propranolol to control paroxysmal atrial tachycardia. *Anesthesiology.* 1975;42:208-210.
92. Stewart JB. *Blind Eye: How the Medical Establishment Let a Doctor Get Away with Murder.* New York: Simon & Schuster; 1999.
93. Stoelting RK. The hemodynamic effects of pancuronium and d-tubocurarine in anesthetized patients. *Anesthesiology.* 1972;36:612-615.
94. Tammaro A, Bracco A, Cozzolino S, et al. Scanning for mutations of the ryanodine receptor (RYR1) gene by denaturing HPLC: detection of three novel malignant hyperthermia alleles. *Clin Chem.* 2003;49:761-768.
95. Tsutsumi H, Nishikawa M, Katagi M, Tsuchihashi H. Adsorption and stability of suxamethonium and its major hydrolysis product succinylmonocholine using liquid chromatography-electrospray ionization mass spectrometry. *J Health Sci.* 2003;49:285-291.
96. van Mook WN, Hulsewe-Evers RP. Critical illness polyneuropathy. *Curr Opin Crit Care.* 2002;8:302-310.
97. Verburg MP, Oerlemans FT, van Bennekom CA, et al. In vivo induced malignant hyperthermia in pigs. I. Physiological and biochemical changes and the influence of dantrolene sodium. *Acta Anaesthesiol Scand.* 1984;28:1-8.
98. Viby-Mogensen J. Interaction of other drugs with muscle relaxants. In: Katz R, ed. *Muscle Relaxants: Basic and Clinical Aspects.* New York: Grune & Stratton; 1985:233-256.
99. Watkins J. Adverse reaction to neuromuscular blockers: frequency, investigation, and epidemiology. *Acta Anaesthesiol Scand Suppl.* 1994;102:6-10.
100. West R. Curare in man. *Proc Royal Soc Med.* 1932;25:1107-1116.
101. Yate PM, Flynn PJ, Arnold RW, et al. Clinical experience and plasma laudanosine concentrations during the infusion of atracurium in the intensive therapy unit. *Br J Anaesth.* 1987;59:211-217.

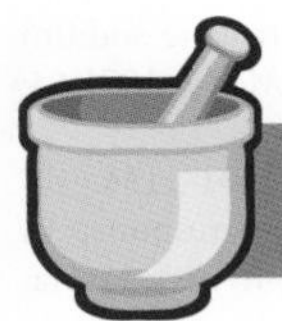

ANTIDOTES IN DEPTH (A22)

DANTROLENE SODIUM

Kenneth M. Sutin

Dantrolene produces relaxation of skeletal muscle without causing complete paralysis, and is the only xenobiotic proven to be effective for both treatment and prophylaxis of malignant hyperthermia (MH). Although dantrolene is a hydantoin derivative that is structurally similar to local anesthetics and anticonvulsants, it possesses none of their properties.[14,29] The drug is available as Dantrium® and in generic forms.

MH should be considered when hyperthermia is associated with severe hypermetabolism, increased CO_2 production, metabolic acidosis with elevated lactate, hyperkalemia, and/or rhabdomyolysis, especially when the course is fulminating and refractory to supportive therapy.

HISTORY AND EPIDEMIOLOGY

Dantrolene was first synthesized in 1967.[25] Four years later, the xenobiotic was first used clinically to treat muscular spasticity caused by neurological disorders.[4] The ability of dantrolene to reverse MH was first reported in swine in 1975[8] and in humans in 1982.[13] The delay from dantrolene discovery to clinical use was in part because of the difficulty encountered in formulating a parenteral (water-soluble) solution of the lipid-soluble drug.

PHARMACOKINETICS

Dantrolene is highly lipophilic and relatively insoluble in water. Dantrolene exhibits variable absorption by the small intestine. Oral bioavailability is up to 70% and peak blood concentrations are achieved 3 to 6 hours after ingestion.[14] In plasma, dantrolene is reversibly bound to plasma proteins, especially albumin. Most of the drug is eliminated by the liver; however, dantrolene is first metabolized in the liver by 5-hydroxylation of the hydantoin ring or by reduction of the nitro group to an amine.[29] Up to 20% of administered dantrolene is excreted in the urine as the 5-hydroxydantrolene metabolite, which is half as potent as the parent drug.[29] In adults, elimination half-life is 6 to 9 hours for dantrolene and 15.5 hours for the 5-hydroxydantrolene metabolite.[29] In one study of children aged 2 to 7 years, the dantrolene elimination half-life was 10 hours and that for 5-hydroxydantrolene was 9 hours.[16]

Quantitative analysis of dantrolene and its metabolites has been performed using high-performance liquid chromatography.[15] After a 2.4 mg/kg intravenous (IV) dose, the mean serum dantrolene concentration is 4.2 μg/mL,[6] which results in a 75% reduction in skeletal muscle with contraction.[6] The therapeutic serum concentration in humans is estimated at 2.8 to 4.2 μg/mL.[6]

MECHANISM

At therapeutic concentrations, dantrolene inhibits binding of [^{3}H] ryanodine to the ryanodine receptor type 1 (RYR-1).[7] [^{3}H]Dantrolene and [^{3}H]ryanodine appear to bind to the same sites on sarcoplasmic reticulum membrane fractions.[20] Dantrolene acts primarily at skeletal muscle RYR-1, causing a dose-dependent inhibition of both the steady and peak components of sarcoplasmic calcium release.[26] This reduces the free myoplasmic calcium, thereby directly inhibiting excitation–contraction coupling.[17] Dantrolene causes skeletal muscle weakness but not complete paralysis, and this plateau effect may be related to its low water solubility. This plateau effect occurs at approximately a 75% reduction of skeletal muscle twitch contraction.[6] Dantrolene does not change the electrical properties or excitation of nerve, neuromuscular junction (NMJ), or muscle, and it does not alter sarcoplasmic calcium reuptake. Because dantrolene does not bind to the cardiac ryanodine receptor (RYR-2), it has minimal cardiac effects[7,28,32] and no effect on smooth muscle.

INDICATIONS

Dantrolene is indicated for treatment of skeletal muscle hypermetabolism characteristic of MH and following an acute episode of MH to prevent recrudescence. Long-term oral dantrolene therapy is used rarely to treat chronic spasticity.[12] Historically, dantrolene was used prophylactically in MH-susceptible individuals; however, current practice is simply to avoid exposure to MH triggers during anesthesia in this patient population.

Dantrolene should be considered for patients who present with severe hyperthermia when the diagnosis of MH cannot be excluded with certainty, especially when there is coexisting respiratory or metabolic acidosis, coagulopathy, or rhabdomyolysis.[5] In typical fulminant MH, the diagnosis is not subtle, and the course of treatment is obvious once the diagnosis is considered. Atypical clinical presentations of MH in the presence or absence of triggering anesthetics are reported, especially in MH susceptible individuals.

Dantrolene has been used to treat acute hyperthermia other than that caused by MH, including neuroleptic malignant syndrome,[21] heat stroke,[1] serotonin syndrome,[9] monoamine oxidase inhibitor overdose,[10] methylenedioxymethamphetamine ("ecstasy") overdose,[18,23] intrathecal baclofen withdrawal,[11] and thyroid storm.[3] Given the lack of evidence-based support, dantrolene therapy is not recommended for indications other than MH. However, given that (1) the differential diagnosis of a hyperthermic syndrome does not necessarily exclude (and often includes) that of MH, (2) the definitive diagnosis of a hyperthermic syndrome may be subtle or delayed, and (3) MH may occur simultaneously with another hyperthermic syndrome,[19] consideration should be given to dantrolene therapy when MH cannot be specifically excluded since its use may be life-saving. It bears emphasizing that dantrolene given for hyperthermia is not a substitute for aggressive cooling.

DOSING

Dantrolene is supplied as a sterile lyophilized powder in a 70-mL vial that contains 20 mg dantrolene sodium, 3 g mannitol (to maintain tonicity), and sodium hydroxide (to maintain alkalinity). The dantrolene powder must be reconstituted in preservative-free sterile water for injection (and not NaCl or dextrose-containing solutions) as this hastens dissolution and prevents precipitation. Prewarming the sterile water to less than or equal to 38°C may decrease the time to dissolve the powder. After addition of 60 mL sterile water, the dantrolene bottles are shaken until the solution becomes clear (indicating the powder is fully dissolved). The final solution is isotonic and has a pH of approximately 9.5. The alkalinity of the reconstituted solution can corrode glass and thus must not be transferred into a glass bottle.

The initial dose of dantrolene for treatment of acute MH is an IV bolus of 2.5 mg/kg in adults and children.[16] For a typical adult, 10 bottles of dantrolene may need to be reconstituted for the initial dose. The pharmacokinetics of dantrolene in obese patients are not determined.[6] Redosing of 2 to 3 mg/kg IV is repeated every 15 minutes until the signs of hypermetabolism are reversed or until a total dose of approximately 10 mg/kg has been administered. Occasionally, however, doses in excess of 10 mg/kg are required. The key point is that the total dose of dantrolene is determined by titration to a metabolic end point—resolution of skeletal muscle hypermetabolism. When an effective dose of dantrolene is given, signs of muscle hypermetabolism generally begin to resolve within 30 minutes.[13]

Following the initial treatment, it is recommended that dantrolene therapy be continued 1 mg/kg IV every 4 to 6 hours for at least for 24 hours to prevent recrudescence.

SIDE EFFECTS AND TOXICITY

The alkaline pH of the reconstituted dantrolene causes venous irritation (pain) and thrombophlebitis. Unintended extravasation can cause tissue necrosis, highlighting that dantrolene should only be given through a central vein or a large peripheral vein. There is no evidence to suggest allergic cross-reactivity with dantrolene in patients with prior phenytoin allergy.

Dantrolene and verapamil should not be used in combination because of the risk of hyperkalemia and hypotension; however, the mechanistic details of this drug interaction remain unclear.[14,22,24] Intravenous calcium salts are safe to administer with dantrolene if needed, such as for the treatment of cardiac dysrhythmias or hyperkalemia (during an episode of MH).

When given to healthy persons or for MH prophylaxis or treatment, dantrolene causes dizziness, skeletal muscle weakness (but not paralysis), and diaphragm weakness (dyspnea).[30,31] In healthy volunteers, dantrolene 2.5 mg/kg does not reduce respiratory rate, vital capacity, or peak expiratory flow rate.[6] However, in patients with diminished respiratory reserve (e.g., end-stage pulmonary disease or neuromuscular disease), dantrolene may precipitate respiratory failure.[14] Oral dantrolene may cause gastrointestinal upset, nausea, and vomiting. Other reported side effects include light-headedness, ptosis, difficulty focusing, and difficulty swallowing.[6,31]

When dantrolene is given orally for more than 2 months to treat skeletal muscle spasticity, there is a 1.8% risk of dose- and duration-related chronic hepatitis, including elevated aminotransferase concentrations, hyperbilirubinemia, or jaundice[27] that may not be fully reversible after dantrolene is discontinued.[2]

REFERENCES

1. Bouchama A, Dehbi M, Chaves-Carballo E. Cooling and hemodynamic management in heatstroke: practical recommendations. *Crit Care.* 2007;11:R54.
2. Chan CH. Dantrolene sodium and hepatic injury. *Neurology.* 1990;40:1427-1432.
3. Christensen PA, Nissen LR. Treatment of thyroid storm in a child with dantrolene. *Br J Anaesth.* 1987;59:523.
4. Chyatte SB, Birdsong JH, Bergman BA. The effects of dantrolene sodium on spasticity and motor performance in hemiplegia. *South Med J.* 1971;64:180-185.
5. Denborough M. Malignant hyperthermia. *Lancet.* 1998;352:1131-1136.
6. Flewellen EH, Nelson TE, Jones WP, et al. Dantrolene dose response in awake man: implications for management of malignant hyperthermia. *Anesthesiology.* 1983;59:275-280.
7. Fruen BR, Mickelson JR, Louis CF. Dantrolene inhibition of sarcoplasmic reticulum Ca^{2+} release by direct and specific action at skeletal muscle ryanodine receptors. *J Biol Chem.* 1997;272:26965-26971.
8. Harrison GG. Control of the malignant hyperpyrexic syndrome in MHS swine by dantrolene sodium. *Br J Anaesth.* 1975;47:62-65.
9. John L, Perreault MM, Tao T, Blew PG. Serotonin syndrome associated with nefazodone and paroxetine. *Ann Emerg Med.* 1997;29:287-289.
10. Kaplan RF, Feinglass NG, Webster W, Mudra S. Phenelzine overdose treated with dantrolene sodium. *JAMA.* 1986;255:642-644.
11. Khorasani A, Peruzzi WT. Dantrolene treatment for abrupt intrathecal baclofen withdrawal. *Anesth Analg.* 1995;80:1054-1056.
12. Kita M, Goodkin DE. Drugs used to treat spasticity. *Drugs.* 2000;59:487-495.
13. Kolb ME, Horne ML, Martz R. Dantrolene in human malignant hyperthermia. *Anesthesiology.* 1982;56:254-262.
14. Krause T, Gerbershagen MU, Fiege M, et al. Dantrolene—a review of its pharmacology, therapeutic use and new developments. *Anaesthesia.* 2004;59:364-373.
15. Lalande M, Mills P, Peterson RG. Determination of dantrolene and its reduced and oxidized metabolites in plasma by high-performance liquid chromatography. *J Chromatogr.* 1988;430:187-191.
16. Lerman J, McLeod ME, Strong HA. Pharmacokinetics of intravenous dantrolene in children. *Anesthesiology.* 1989;70:625-629.
17. Lopez JR, Gerardi A, Lopez MJ, Allen PD. Effects of dantrolene on myoplasmic free [Ca2+] measured in vivo in patients susceptible to malignant hyperthermia. *Anesthesiology.* 1992;76:711-719.
18. Moon J, Cros J. Role of dantrolene in the management of the acute toxic effects of ecstasy (MDMA). *Br J Anaesth.* 2007;99:146.
19. Nishiyama K, Kitahara A, Natsume H, et al. Malignant hyperthermia in a patient with Graves' disease during subtotal thyroidectomy. *Endocr J.* 2001;48:227-232.
20. Paul-Pletzer K, Yamamoto T, Bhat MB, et al. Identification of a dantrolene-binding sequence on the skeletal muscle ryanodine receptor. *J Biol Chem.* 2002;277:34918-34923.
21. Reulbach U, Dutsch C, Biermann T, et al. Managing an effective treatment for neuroleptic malignant syndrome. *Crit Care.* 2007;11:R4.
22. Rubin AS, Zablocki AD. Hyperkalemia, verapamil, and dantrolene. *Anesthesiology.* 1987;66:246-249.
23. Rusyniak DE, Banks ML, Mills EM, Sprague JE. Dantrolene use in 3,4-methylenedioxymethamphetamine (ecstasy)-mediated hyperthermia. *Anesthesiology.* 2004;101:263; author reply, 264.
24. Saltzman LS, Kates RA, Corke BC, et al. Hyperkalemia and cardiovascular collapse after verapamil and dantrolene administration in swine. *Anesth Analg.* 1984;63:473-478.
25. Snyder HR Jr, Davis CS, Bickerton RK, Halliday RP. 1-[(5-arylfurfurylidene)amino]hydantoins. A new class of muscle relaxants. *J Med Chem.* 1967;10:807-810.
26. Szentesi P, Collet C, Sarkozi S, et al. Effects of dantrolene on steps of excitation-contraction coupling in mammalian skeletal muscle fibers. *J Gen Physiol.* 2001;118:355-375.
27. Utili R, Boitnott JK, Zimmerman HJ. Dantrolene-associated hepatic injury. Incidence and character. *Gastroenterology.* 1977;72:610-616.
28. Van Winkle WB. Calcium release from skeletal muscle sarcoplasmic reticulum: site of action of dantrolene sodium. *Science.* 1976;193:1130-1131.
29. Ward A, Chaffman MO, Sorkin EM. Dantrolene. A review of its pharmacodynamic and pharmacokinetic properties and therapeutic use in malignant hyperthermia, the neuroleptic malignant syndrome and an update of its use in muscle spasticity. *Drugs.* 1986;32:130-168.
30. Watson CB, Reierson N, Norfleet EA. Clinically significant muscle weakness induced by oral dantrolene sodium prophylaxis for malignant hyperthermia. *Anesthesiology.* 1986;65:312-314.
31. Wedel DJ, Quinlan JG, Iaizzo PA. Clinical effects of intravenously administered dantrolene. *Mayo Clin Proc.* 1995;70:241-246.
32. Zhao F, Li P, Chen SR, et al. Dantrolene inhibition of ryanodine receptor Ca^{2+} release channels. Molecular mechanism and isoform selectivity. *J Biol Chem.* 2001;276:13810-13816.

G.

PSYCHOTROPIC MEDICATIONS

CHAPTER 69
ANTIPSYCHOTICS

David N. Juurlink

Most antipsychotics produce toxicity by one of two mechanisms—dose related and idiosyncratic. Overdose, whether intentional or unintentional, causes dose-related toxicity, which reflects an extension of the pharmacologic effects of the drug on neurotransmitter systems and other biologic processes. Such features of antipsychotic overdose are therefore generally predictable. Idiosyncratic adverse reactions may also occur in the context of routine therapeutic use resulting from individual susceptibility, which usually is pharmacogenetic in nature and only partially correlated with dose. In both instances, the severity of illness may range from minor to life threatening, depending on a number of other factors, including concomitant drug exposures, comorbidity, and access to medical care.

HISTORY AND EPIDEMIOLOGY

Before the introduction of chlorpromazine in 1950, patients with schizophrenia were treated with nonspecific sedatives such as barbiturates. Highly agitated patients were housed in large mental institutions and often placed in physical restraints. By 1955, approximately 500,000 patients with psychotic disorders were hospitalized in the United States. The advent of antipsychotics in the 1950s revolutionized care. Originally termed *major tranquilizers* and subsequently *neuroleptics*, these drugs dramatically reduced the hallucinations, delusions, and paranoia, which are "positive" symptoms that characterize schizophrenia.

Shortly after their introduction, however, it became apparent that the xenobiotics had potential danger in an overdose and were also associated with serious adverse effects, principally involving the endocrine and nervous systems, even when properly prescribed. Neurological sequelae included the extrapyramidal syndromes (EPS), a constellation of disorders that were relatively common, sometimes irreversible, and occasionally life threatening.

The search for antipsychotics led to the development of new types of xenobiotics from several different chemical classes characterized by varying potencies and markedly different adverse effect profiles. One novel antipsychotic, clozapine, was first synthesized in 1959 but did not enter widespread clinical use until the early 1970s. Clozapine was unique in that it was not only relatively free of EPS, but it was also an extremely effective antipsychotic even in patients who had not responded well to other drugs. Moreover, unlike other antipsychotics available at the time, it often improved the "negative" symptoms of schizophrenia, such as avolition, alogia, and social withdrawal, symptoms that are not as readily apparent as the positive symptoms but that also cause significant disability. Reports of agranulocytosis, sometimes fatal, led to the withdrawal of clozapine from the market in 1974, although it was reintroduced in 1990.[9] The unique therapeutic and pharmacologic properties of clozapine make it an *atypical* antipsychotic, the forerunner and prototype of more than a dozen compounds that have collectively become the most widely used antipsychotics over the past decade.

Unfortunately, the true incidence of antipsychotic drug reactions is not known with certainty with some patients not seeking medical attention, and others may be misdiagnosed. Even among those who seek medical attention and are correctly diagnosed, notification of poison centers or other adverse event reporting systems is discretionary and incomplete (see Chaps. 135 and 139). With these limitations in mind, a few observations can be made.

In 2007, antipsychotic exposures were reported in combination with sedative–hypnotics, but these collectively represented 154,602 exposures annually. This group of xenobiotics was associated with more fatalities than any other ($n = 377$ deaths), and most antipsychotic exposures involved the atypical antipsychotics.[16] The vast majority of poison center calls for antipsychotics involve intentional overdoses in patients ages 19 years and older. Although most of these patients have a good outcome, dozens of fatalities were reported in 2007, and the majority of these occurred in patients with concomitant xenobiotic exposures (see Chap. 135). A substantial body of clinical experience and some observational data suggest that the older low-potency, typical antipsychotics, such as thioridazine, chlorpromazine, and mesoridazine, are associated with greater toxicity than other antipsychotics.[17,19] Inferences regarding relative toxicity derived from aggregated population data should be extrapolated to individual patients with caution,[17,39] but at least one study supports the notion that thioridazine is associated with greater cardiovascular toxicity than other antipsychotics.[19]

PHARMACOLOGY

CLASSIFICATION

Antipsychotics can be classified according to their chemical structure, their receptor binding profiles, or as "typical" or "atypical" antipsychotics. Table 69–1 outlines the taxonomy of some commonly used antipsychotics. Classification by chemical structure was most useful before the 1970s, when phenothiazines and butyrophenones constituted most of the antipsychotics in clinical use. Currently, the surfeit of different compounds and their structural heterogeneity renders this scheme cumbersome and of limited use to clinicians. It is worth noting, however, that the phenothiazine antipsychotics bear a high degree of structural similarity to the tricyclic antidepressants (TCAs) (Fig. 69–1) and share many of their manifestations in overdose. The phenothiazines can be further subclassified according to the substituent on the nitrogen atom at position 10 of the center ring as aliphatic, piperazine, or piperidine compounds.

TABLE 69–1. Classification of Commonly Used Antipsychotics

Classification	Compound	Usual Daily Adult Dose (mg)	Volume of Distribution (L/kg)	Half-Life (Range, h)	Protein Binding (%)	Active Metabolite
Typical Antipsychotics						
Butyrophenones	Droperidol	1.25–30	2–3	2–10	85–90	N
	Haloperidol	1–20	18–30	14–41	90	Y
Diphenylbutylpiperidines	Pimozide	1–20	11–62	28–214	99	Y
Phenothiazines						
Aliphatic	Chlorpromazine	100–800	10–35	18–30	98	Y
	Methotrimeprazine	2–50	23–42	17–78	NR	Y
	Promazine	50–1000	30–40	8–12	98	N
	Promethazine	25–150	9–25	9–16	93	Y
Piperazine	Fluphenazine	0.5–20	220	13–58[b]	99	NR
	Perphenazine	8–64	10–35	8–12	>90	NR
	Prochlorperazine	10–150	13–32	17–27	>90	NR
	Trifluoperazine	4–50	NR	7–18	>90	Y
Piperidine	Mesoridazine	100–400	3–6	2–9	98	Y
	Thioridazine	200–800	18	26–36	96	Y
	Pipotiazine	25–250 (monthly IM depot)	7.5	3–11	NR	N
Thioxanthenes	Chlorprothixene	30–300	11–23	8–12	NR	NR
	Flupenthixol	3–6	7–8	7–36	NR	NR
	Thiothixene	5–30	NR	12–36	>90	NR
	Zuclopenthixol	20–100	10	20	NR	NR
Atypical Antipsychotics						
Benzamides	Amisulpride	50–1200	5.8	12	16	N
	Raclopride	3–6	1.5	12–24	NR	N
	Remoxipride	150–600	0.7	3–7	80	Y
	Sulpride	200–1200	0.6–2.7	4–11	14–40	N
Benzepines						
Dibenzodiazepine	Clozapine	50–900	15-30	6–17	95	Y
Dibenzooxazepine	Loxapine[a]	20–250	NR	2–8	90–99	Y
Thienobenzodiazepine	Olanzapine	5–20	10–20	21–54	93	N
Dibenzothiazepine	Quetiapine	150–750	10	3–9	83	N
Indoles						
Benzisoxazole	Risperidone	2–16	0.7–2.1	3–20	90	Y
Imidazolidinone	Sertindole	12–24	20–40	24–200	99	Y
Benzisothiazole	Ziprasidone	40–160	2	4–10	99	N
Quinolinones	Aripiprazole	10–30	5	47–68	99	Y

[a]Loxapine's atypical profile is lost at doses >50 mg/d; hence it is sometimes categorized as a typical antipsychotic.

[b]For hydrochloride salt; enanthate and decanoate have ranges of 3–4 days and 5–12 days, respectively.

IM, intramuscular; NR, not reported.

Data adapted from Baldessarini RJ, Tarazi FI. Pharmacotherapy of psychosis and mania. Brunton LL, Lazo JS, Parker KL, eds. *Goodman and Gilman's The Pharmacological Basis of Therapeutics*, 11th ed. New York, McGraw-Hill: 2006, pp 461-500. Baselt RC. *Disposition of Toxic Drugs and Chemicals in Man*, 8th ed. Foster City, CA: Biomedical Publications; Borison RL. Recent advances in the pharmacotherapy of schizophrenia. *Harv Rev Psychiatry.* 1997;4:255-271; Ereshefsky L. Pharmacologic and pharmacokinetic considerations in choosing an antipsychotic. *J Clin Psychiatry.* 1999;60(suppl 10):20-30:20-30; Jibson MD, Tandon R. New atypical antipsychotic medications. *J Psychiatr Res.* 1998;32:215-228; and Keck PE Jr, McElroy SL. Clinical pharmacodynamics and pharmacokinetics of antimanic and mood-stabilizing medications. *J Clin Psychiatry.* 2002;63(suppl 4): 3-11:3-11.

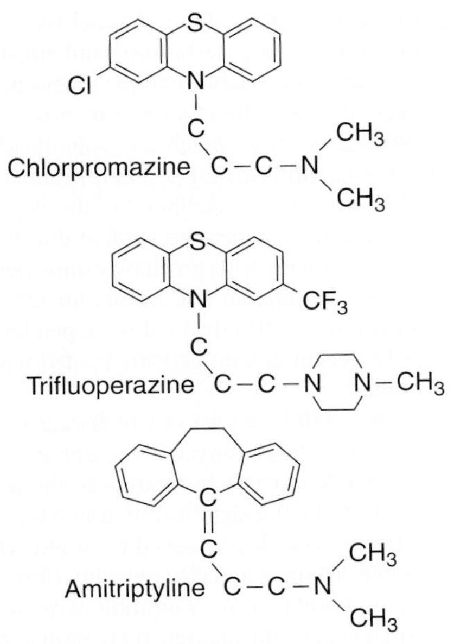

FIGURE 69–1. Structural similarity between phenothiazines and cyclic antidepressants.

Of greater clinical utility is the classification of antipsychotics according to their binding affinities for various receptors (Table 69–2). However, by far, the most widely used classification system categorizes antipsychotics as either *typical* or *atypical*. Typical, *traditional* or *conventional* antipsychotics dominated the first 40 years of antipsychotic therapy. They were subcategorized according to their affinity for the D_2 receptor as either low potency exemplified by thioridazine and chlorpromazine or high potency exemplified by haloperidol. These xenobiotics ameliorated the "positive symptoms" of schizophrenia, such as hallucinations, delusions, paranoia, and disorganization of thought, but they were of little benefit for the also disabling "negative symptoms" of schizophrenia, which are avolition, alogia, flattening of affect, and social withdrawal. Moreover, they were associated with acute, subacute, and long-term motor disturbances collectively referred to as EPS.

The notion of antipsychotic atypicality has evolved over time with the introduction of new xenobiotics[83,102] and connotes different properties to pharmacologists and clinicians. From a clinical perspective, atypical antipsychotics or *second-generation antipsychotics* treat both the positive and negative symptoms of schizophrenia, are less likely than traditional antipsychotics to produce EPS at clinically effective doses, and cause little or no elevation of serum prolactin concentration.[53] From a pharmacologic perspective, most atypical antipsychotics also inhibit the action of serotonin at the 5-HT_{2A} receptor. More than a

TABLE 69–2. Toxic Manifestations of Selected Antipsychotics

	α_1-Adrenergic Antagonism	Muscarinic Antagonism	Fast Sodium Channel (I_{Na}) Blockade	Delayed Rectifier (I_{Kr}) Current Blockade
Clinical Effect	Hypotension	Central and Peripheral Anticholinergic Effects	QRS Widening; Rightward T40 msec; Myocardial Depression	QT Prolongation; Torsades de Pointes
Typical Antipsychotics				
Chlorpromazine	+++	++	++	++
Fluphenazine	–	–	+	+
Haloperidol	–	–	+	++
Loxapine	+++	++	++	+
Mesoridazine	+++	+++	+++	++
Perphenazine	+	–	+	++
Pimozide	+	–	+	++
Thioridazine	+++	+++	+++	+++
Trifluoperazine	+	–	+	++
Atypical Antipsychotics				
Aripiprazole	++	–	–	–
Clozapine	+++	+++	–	+
Olanzapine	++	+++	–	–
Quetiapine	+++	+++	+	– to +
Remoxipride	–	–	–	–
Risperidone	++	–	–	–
Sertindole	+	–	–	++
Ziprasidone	++	–	–	+++

+++ = very significant effort; + = minimal effect; – = no effect.

Data adapted from Buckley NA, Sanders P. Cardiovascular adverse effects of antipsychotic drugs. *Drug Saf.* 2000;23:215-228; Burns MJ. The pharmacology and toxicology of atypical antipsychotic agents. *J Toxicol Clin Toxicol.* 2001;39:1-14; Haddad PM, Anderson IM. Antipsychotic-related QT prolongation, torsades de pointes and sudden death. *Drugs.* 2002;62:1649-1671; Richelson E, Nelson A. Antagonism by antidepressants of neurotransmitter receptors of normal human brain in vitro. *J Pharmacol Exp Ther.* 1984;230:94-102; and Robinson K, Smith RN. Radioimmunoassay of tricyclic antidepressant and some phenothiazine drugs in forensic toxicology. *J Immunoassay.* 1985;6:11-22.

dozen atypical antipsychotics are now in clinical use or under development. Despite their considerably higher cost, these drugs have largely supplanted traditional antipsychotics because of their effectiveness in treating the negative symptoms of schizophrenia and their more favorable adverse effect profile, in addition to the perception that they cause fewer long-term adverse effects than conventional antipsychotics, a belief that may result, in part, from the use of higher doses of older drugs in studies comparing the tolerability of typical and atypical antipsychotics.[45] It is worth noting that the use of antipsychotics for unapproved (off-label) indications is extremely common, particularly as adjunctive therapies for the management of agitation association with cognitive impairment in the elderly.

ANTIPSYCHOTIC MECHANISMS OF ACTION

Of the many contemporary theories of schizophrenia, the most enduring has been the *dopamine hypothesis*.[96] First advanced in 1967 and supported by in vivo data,[1] this theory holds that the "positive symptoms" of schizophrenia (hallucinations, delusions, paranoia, and disorganization of thought) result from excessive dopaminergic signaling in the mesolimbic and mesocortical pathways.[66] This hypothesis resulted in part from the observation that hallucinations and delusions could be produced in otherwise normal individuals by drugs that increase dopaminergic transmission, such as cocaine and amphetamine, and that these effects could be blunted by dopamine antagonists.

There are five subtypes of dopamine receptors (D_1 through D_5), but schizophrenia principally involves excess signaling at the D_2 subtype,[96] and antagonism of D_2 neurotransmission is the *sine qua non* of antipsychotic activity. Antipsychotics have different potencies at this receptor, reflected by the dissociation constant (K_d), which in turn reflects release from the D_2 receptor. For example, the receptor releases clozapine and quetiapine more rapidly than it does any other drugs.[94,96]

Dopamine receptors are present in many other areas of the central nervous system (CNS), including the nigrostriatal pathway (substantia nigra, caudate, and putamen, which collectively govern the coordination of voluntary movement); tuberoinfundibular pathway; hypothalamus and pituitary; and area postrema of the brainstem, which contains the chemoreceptor trigger zone (CTZ). Antipsychotic-related blockade of D_2 neurotransmission in these areas is associated with many of the beneficial and adverse effects of these xenobiotics. For example, whereas D_2 antagonism in the CTZ alleviates nausea and vomiting, blockade of hypothalamic D_2 receptors increases prolactin release by the pituitary, resulting in breast tenderness and galactorrhea. Blockade of nigrostriatal D_2 receptors underlies many of the movement disorders associated with antipsychotic therapy.[107,119]

Antipsychotics also interfere with signaling at other receptors, including acetylcholine M_1 and M_2 muscarinic receptors, H_1 histamine receptors, and α-adrenergic receptors. The extent to which these other receptors are blocked at doses that effectively block D_2 transmission varies among antipsychotics but can be used to predict the adverse effect profile of each drug.[21] For example, drugs that antagonize muscarinic receptors at clinically effective doses (primarily the aliphatic and piperidine phenothiazines along with clozapine, loxapine, olanzapine, and quetiapine) often cause bothersome anticholinergic effects with routine use and may produce pronounced anticholinergic manifestations after overdose (see Table 69–2). Similarly, blockade of peripheral α_1-adrenergic receptors by the aliphatic and piperidine phenothiazines, clozapine, risperidone, and several other drugs renders them more likely to cause postural hypotension during therapy and supine hypotension after overdose.

Several antipsychotics also block voltage-gated fast sodium channels (I_{Na}). Although this effect is of little consequence during therapy, in the setting of overdose, this sodium channel blockade may slow cardiac conduction (phase 0 depolarization) and impair myocardial contractility. This effect, most notable with the phenothiazines, is both rate and voltage dependent and therefore is more pronounced at faster heart rates and less negative transmembrane potentials.[18] Blockade of the delayed rectifier potassium current (I_{Kr}) may produce prolongation of the QT interval, increasing the likelihood of developing torsade de pointes.[70] QT prolongation is sometimes evident during maintenance therapy, particularly in patients with previously unrecognized repolarization abnormalities or additional risk factors for QT prolongation. This effect is thought to contribute to dose-dependent increase in risk of sudden cardiac death among patients treated with typical and atypical antipsychotics.[81,82]

Several antipsychotics exhibit a relatively high degree of antagonism at the $5\text{-}HT_{2A}$ receptor, which conveys two important therapeutic properties: (1) greater effectiveness in treating of the negative symptoms of schizophrenia and (2) a significantly lower incidence of EPS. Several antipsychotics are also distinguished by unique effects at other receptors. For example, loxapine and clozapine interfere with reuptake of catecholamines and antagonize γ-aminobutyric acid $(GABA)_A$ receptors,[101] which may explain the apparent increase in seizures reported with these agents.[78]

Clozapine binds to dopamine receptors (D_1–D_5) and serotonin receptors ($5\text{-}HT_{1A/1C}$, $5\text{-}HT_{2A/2C}$, $5\text{-}HT_3$, and $5\text{-}HT_6$) with moderate to high affinity.[9,79,87] It also antagonizes α_1-adrenergic, α_2-adrenergic, and H_1 histamine receptors and has the highest binding affinity of any atypical antipsychotic at M_1 muscarinic receptors.[86] Despite this feature, clozapine paradoxically activates the M_4 genetic subtype of the muscarinic receptor and frequently produces sialorrhea during therapy.[85]

Olanzapine, binds avidly to serotonin ($5\text{-}HT_{2A/2C}$, $5\text{-}HT_3$, and $5\text{-}HT_6$) and dopamine receptors (D_1, D_2, and D_4), although its potency at D_2 receptors is lower than that of most traditional antipsychotics.[56,87] It is an exceptionally potent H_1 antagonist, binding more avidly than pyrilamine (see Chap. 50), which is a widely used antihistamine. It also has a high affinity for M_1 receptors and is a relatively weak α_1 antagonist.

Risperidone has high affinity for several receptors, including serotonin receptors ($5\text{-}HT_{2A/2C}$), D_2 dopamine receptors, and α_1 and H_1 receptors.[56,85,87] It has no appreciable activity at M_1 receptors. Its primary metabolite (9-hydroxyrisperidone) is nearly equipotent compared with the parent compound at D_2 and $5\text{-}HT_{2A}$ receptors.[56]

Quetiapine is a weak antagonist at D_2, M_1, and $5\text{-}HT_{1A}$ receptors, but it is a relatively potent antagonist of α_1-adrenergic and H_1 receptors.[56] Of its 11 different metabolites, at least two are pharmacologically active. However, they circulate at very low concentrations and likely contribute little to the clinical effect of the drug. A considerable proportion of fatalities involving antipsychotics reported to North American poison control centers involve quetiapine, usually in combination with other drugs (see Chap. 135).

Ziprasidone is a potent antagonist at dopaminergic D_2 and several serotonin ($5\text{-}HT_{2A/2C}$, $5\text{-}HT_{1D}$, and $5\text{-}HT_7$) receptors, but it also displays agonist activity at $5\text{-}HT_{1A}$ receptors.[56,57,87] Its α_1 antagonist activity is particularly strong, with a binding affinity approximately one-tenth that of prazosin. In addition, it exhibits considerable inhibition of the cardiac delayed rectifier channel and may significantly prolong repolarization.[57,64]

Aripiprazole is a novel compound that binds avidly to dopamine D_2 and D_3 receptors and serotonin $5\text{-}HT_{1A}$, $5\text{-}HT_{2A}$, and $5\text{-}HT_{2B}$ receptors.[69,87] Some evidence suggests that its efficacy in the treatment of schizophrenia and its lower propensity for EPS may reflect partial agonist activity at dopamine D_2 receptors. Aripiprazole also acts as a partial agonist at serotonin $5\text{-}HT_{1A}$ receptors but is an antagonist at serotonin $5\text{-}HT_{2A}$ receptors. Its principal active metabolite, dehydroaripiprazole, has affinity for dopamine D_2 receptors and thus has some pharmacologic activity similar to that of the parent compound.[69]

Similar to aripiprazole, bifeprunox is a partial agonist at D_2 and 5-HT_{1A} receptors. It has been characterized as a third-generation antipsychotic and has no appreciable affinity for serotonin 5-HT_{2A} and 5-HT_{2C}, histaminergic, or muscarinic receptors.[28,72,95] Clinical experience with this drug is limited.

Amisulpride an investigational drug preferentially binds to dopamine receptors in limbic rather than striatal structures. At low doses, it blocks presynaptic D_2 and D_3 receptors, thereby accentuating dopamine release, but at high doses, it blocks postsynaptic D_2 and D_3 receptors. It has relatively low affinity for serotonergic, histaminergic, adrenergic, and cholinergic receptors.

Sertindole is a second-generation antipsychotic that was recently reintroduced into the market after being voluntarily withdrawn in 1998 because of concerns about its effects on the QT interval. It binds to striatal D_2 receptors, although less avidly than olanzapine, and also exhibits antagonism at 5-HT_{2A} and α-adrenergic receptors.[55,76,100]

PHARMACOKINETICS AND TOXICOKINETICS

With a few exceptions, the antipsychotics have similar pharmacokinetic characteristics regardless of their chemical classification. Most are lipophilic, have a large volume of distribution, and are generally well absorbed, although anticholinergic effects may delay absorption of some antipsychotics. Serum concentrations generally peak within 2 to 3 hours after a therapeutic dose, but this can be prolonged after overdose.

Most antipsychotics are substrates for various isoenzymes of the hepatic cytochrome P450 (CYP) enzyme system. For example, haloperidol, perphenazine, thioridazine, sertindole, and risperidone are extensively metabolized by the CYP2D6 system, which is functionally absent in approximately 7% of white patients and overexpressed in 1–25% of other patients, depending on their ethnicity.[53] These polymorphisms appear to influence the tolerability and efficacy of treatment with these antipsychotics during therapeutic use[15,29,30,52,112] but are unlikely to significantly alter the severity of acute antipsychotic overdose.

Drugs that inhibit CYP2D6 (eg, paroxetine, fluoxetine, bupropion) may increase the concentrations of these antipsychotics and increase the risk of adverse effects. In contrast, metabolism of clozapine is primarily mediated by CYP1A2, and increased clozapine concentrations may result after exposure to CYP1A2 inhibitors, such as fluvoxamine macrolide and fluoroquinolone antibiotics, as well as after smoking cessation because smoking induces CYP1A2.[34] The kidney plays a relatively small role in the elimination of antipsychotics, and dose adjustment is generally not necessary for patients with renal disease.

PATHOPHYSIOLOGY AND CLINICAL MANIFESTATIONS

Table 69–3 lists the adverse effects of antipsychotics. Some of these effects develop primarily after overdose, but others may occur during the course of therapeutic use.

ADVERSE EFFECTS DURING THERAPEUTIC USE

The Extrapyramidal Syndromes The EPS (Table 69–4) are a heterogeneous group of disorders that share the common feature of abnormal muscular activity. Among the typical antipsychotics, the incidence of EPS appears to be highest with the more potent drugs, such as haloperidol and flupentixol, and lower with less potent drugs, such as chlorpromazine and thioridazine. Atypical antipsychotics are associated with an even

TABLE 69–3. Adverse Effects of Antipsychotics

Cardiovascular	
Clinical	Tachycardia
	Hypotension (orthostatic or resting)
	Myocardial depression
Electrocardiographic	QRS complex widening
	Right deviation of terminal 40 msec of frontal plane axis
	QT interval prolongation
	Torsades de pointes
	Nonspecific repolarization changes
Central nervous system	Somnolence, coma
	Respiratory depression
	Hyperthermia
	Seizures
	Extrapyramidal syndromes
	Central anticholinergic syndrome
Dermatologic	Impaired sweat production
	Cutaneous vasodilation
Endocrine	Amenorrhea, oligomenorrhea, or metrorrhagia
	Breast tenderness, galactorrhea
Gastrointestinal	Impaired peristalsis
	Dry mouth
Genitourinary	Urinary retention
	Ejaculatory dysfunction
	Priapism
Ophthalmic	Mydriasis or miosis, visual blurring

lower incidence of EPS. Although the physiologic mechanisms for this observation are not fully understood, several hypotheses have been put forth. In addition to the aforementioned antagonism of 5-HT_{2A} receptors, some atypical drugs dissociate more rapidly from the D_2 receptor and incite a lower degree of nigrostriatal dopaminergic hypersensitivity during chronic use.[53,54,65] However, it is important to note that EPS may occur during treatment with any of the antipsychotics, typical or atypical, regardless of potency.

Acute Dystonia. Acute dystonia is a movement disorder characterized by sustained involuntary muscle contractions, often involving the muscles of the head and neck, including the extraocular muscles and the tongue but occasionally involving the extremities. These contractions are sometimes referred to as *limited reactions*, reflecting their transient nature rather than their severity. All of the currently available antipsychotics are associated with the development of acute dystonic reactions.[107] Spasmodic torticollis, facial grimacing, protrusion of the tongue, and oculogyric crisis are among the more common manifestations. Laryngeal dystonia is a rare but potentially life-threatening variant that is easily misdiagnosed because it may present with throat pain, dyspnea, stridor, and dysphonia rather than the more characteristic features of dystonia.[37]

Acute dystonia typically develops within a few hours of starting treatment but may be delayed for several days. Left untreated, dystonia resolves slowly over several days after the offending xenobiotic is

TABLE 69–4. The Extrapyramidal Syndromes

Disorder	Time of Maximal Risk	Features	Postulated Mechanism	Possible Treatments
Acute dystonia	Hours to a few days	Sustained, involuntary muscle contraction; torticollis, lingual protrusion, blepharospasm, oculogyric crisis	Imbalance of dopaminergic/cholinergic transmission	Anticholinergics, benzodiazepines
Akathisia	Hours to days	Restlessness and unease, inability to sit still	Mesocortical D_2 antagonism	Dose reduction, trial of alternate drug, propranolol, benzodiazepines, anticholinergics
Parkinsonism	Weeks	Bradykinesia, rigidity, shuffling gait, masklike facies, resting tremor	Postsynaptic striatal D_2 antagonism	Dose reduction, anticholinergics, dopamine agonists
Neuroleptic malignant syndrome	2–10 days	Altered mental status, motor symptoms, hyperthermia, autonomic instability (see Table 69-5)	D_2 antagonism in striatum, hypothalamus, and mesocortex	Cooling, benzodiazepines, supportive care, consider dantrolene, bromocriptine, or other direct-acting dopamine agonists
Tardive dyskinesia	3 months–years	Late-onset involuntary choreiform movements, orobuccal, lingual, masticatory stereotypic movements	Excess dopaminergic activity	Recognize early and stop offending drug; addition of other antipsychotics; cholinergics

Data adapted from Pierre JM. Extrapyramidal symptoms with atypical antipsychotics: incidence, prevention and management. *Drug Saf.* 2005;28:191-208 and van Harten PN, Hoek HW, Kahn RS. Acute dystonia induced by drug treatment. *Br Med J.* 1999;319:623-626.

withdrawn. Risk factors for acute dystonia include male gender, young age (children are particularly susceptible), a previous episode of acute dystonia, and recent cocaine use.[108,119] Although the reaction may appear dramatic and sometimes is mistaken for seizure activity, it is rarely life threatening. Of note, xenobiotics other than antipsychotics, particularly metoclopramide, the antidepressants, some antimalarials, histamine H_2 receptor antagonists, anticonvulsants, and cocaine, may sometimes cause acute dystonia.[108]

Treatment of Acute Dystonia. Acute dystonia is generally more distressing than serious, but in rare cases, it may compromise respiration, necessitating supplemental oxygen and, occasionally, assisted ventilation.[37,108] The response to parenteral anticholinergics often is rapid and dramatic, and every effort should be made to administer benztropine as the first-line agent (2 mg intravenously [IV] or intramuscularly [IM] in adults; 0.05 mg/kg up to 2.0 mg in children). Often, diphenhydramine is more readily available and can be used instead (50 mg IV or IM in adults; 1 mg/kg up to 50 mg in children). Parenteral benzodiazepines such as lorazepam (0.05–0.10 mg/kg IV or IM) or diazepam (0.1 mg/kg IV) should be considered if patients do not respond to anticholinergics, but it may also be used effectively as initial therapy. It is important to recognize that because the elimination half-lives of most anticholinergics are shorter than those of most antipsychotics, dystonia may recur, and administering additional doses of anticholinergics may be necessary over the subsequent 48 to 72 hours.[27] Patients in whom acute dystonia jeopardizes respiration should be observed for at least 12 to 24 hours after initial resolution.

Akathisia. Akathisia (from the Greek phrase "not to sit") is characterized by a feeling of inner restlessness, anxiety, or sense of unease, often in conjunction with the objective finding of an inability to sit still. Patients with akathisia frequently appear uncomfortable or fidgety. They may rock back and forth while standing or may repeatedly cross and uncross their legs while seated. Akathisia can be difficult to diagnose and is easily misinterpreted as a manifestation of the underlying psychiatric disorder rather than an adverse effect of therapy.

Akathisia is common and may be an important determinant of a failure to adhere to therapy. Similar to acute dystonia, akathisia tends to occur relatively early in the course of treatment and coincides with peak serum antipsychotic concentrations.[119] The incidence appears highest with typical, high-potency antipsychotics and lowest with atypical antipsychotics. Although most cases develop within days to weeks after initiation of treatment or an increase in dose, a delayed-onset (tardive) variant is also recognized.

The pathophysiology of akathisia is incompletely understood but appears to involve antagonism of postsynaptic D_2 receptors in the mesocortical pathways.[65,107] Interestingly, a similar phenomenon has been described in patients after the initiation of treatment with antidepressants, particularly the selective serotonin reuptake inhibitors.[8,62]

Treatment of Akathisia. Akathisia may be difficult to treat. A reduction in the antipsychotic dose is sometimes helpful, as is substitution of another (generally atypical) antipsychotic. Treatment with lipophilic β-adrenergic antagonists such as propranolol may reduce the symptoms of akathisia, but there is little evidence supporting their use.[60,77] Benzodiazepines produce short-term relief, and anticholinergics such as benztropine or procyclidine may reduce symptoms of akathisia, but they are more likely to be effective for akathisia induced by antipsychotics with little or no intrinsic anticholinergic activity.[20,61]

Parkinsonism. Parkinsonism is thought to result from antagonism of postsynaptic D_2 receptors in the striatum[107] and is characterized by rigidity, akinesia or bradykinesia, and postural instability. It is similar to idiopathic Parkinson's disease, although the classic "pill-rolling" tremor is often less pronounced.[77] The syndrome typically develops during the first few months of therapy, particularly with high-potency antipsychotics. It is more common among older women, and in some patients, it may represent iatrogenic unmasking of latent Parkinson's disease.

Treatment of Xenobiotic-Induced Parkinsonism. The risk of xenobiotic-induced parkinsonism may be minimized by using the lowest effective dose of an antipsychotic. The addition of an anticholinergic often attenuates symptoms at the expense of additional side effects. This strategy often is effective in younger patients, although the routine use of prophylactic anticholinergics is not recommended. Addition of a dopamine agonist, such as amantadine, is sometimes used, particularly in older patients who may be less tolerant of anticholinergics, but this may aggravate the underlying psychiatric disturbance.[63]

Tardive Dyskinesias. The term *tardive dyskinesia* was coined in 1952 to describe the delayed onset of persistent orobuccal masticatory movements occurring in three women after several months of antipsychotic therapy.[107] The adjective *tardive*, or late, was used to distinguish these movement disorders from the parkinsonian movements described above. The incidence of tardive dyskinesia in younger patients is approximately 3% to 5% per year but increases considerably with age. A prospective study of older patients treated with high-potency typical antipsychotics identified a 60% cumulative incidence of tardive dyskinesia after 3 years of treatment.[50] Potential risk factors for tardive dyskinesia include alcohol use, affective disorder, prior electroconvulsive therapy (ECT), diabetes mellitus, and various genetic factors.[107]

Several distinct tardive syndromes are recognized, including the classic orobuccal lingual masticatory stereotypy, chorea, dystonia, myoclonus, blepharospasm, and tics. The atypical antipsychotics are generally believed to be responsible for a lower incidence of tardive dyskinesia and other drug-related movement disorders. However, whether this is true of all atypical antipsychotics is unclear. Among the atypical antipsychotics, clozapine is associated with the lowest incidence of tardive dyskinesia and risperidone with the highest incidence (when higher doses are used), but the reasons for this observation are uncertain.[104,105,107]

Treatment of Tardive Dyskinesia. Tardive dyskinesia is highly resistant to the usual pharmacologic treatments for movement disorders. Anticholinergics do not alleviate tardive dyskinesia and may worsen it. Calcium channel blockers, β-adrenergic antagonists, benzodiazepines, and vitamin E have all been used with only limited supporting evidence.[35] Clozapine appears to temporarily suppress tardive dyskinesia. Although discontinuation of the causative drug may not produce total relief of symptoms, when possible, the antipsychotic should be discontinued as soon as signs or symptoms begin.

Neuroleptic Malignant Syndrome. Neuroleptic malignant syndrome (NMS) is a potentially life-threatening drug-induced emergency. First described in 1960 in patients treated with haloperidol, this syndrome has been associated with virtually every antipsychotic [31] because the reported incidence of NMS ranges from 0.2% to 1.4% of patients receiving antipsychotics,[2,23,103] but less severe episodes may go undiagnosed or unreported. As a result, much of the epidemiology and treatment of NMS is speculative and based only on case reports and case series.

The pathophysiology of NMS is incompletely understood but appears to involve abrupt reductions in central dopaminergic neurotransmission in the striatum and hypothalamus, altering the core temperature "set point"[41] and leading to impaired thermoregulation and other manifestations of autonomic dysfunction. Blockade of striatal D_2 receptors contributes to muscle rigidity and tremor.[13,25,109] In some cases, a direct effect on skeletal muscle may play a role in the pathogenesis of hyperthermia.[41] Altered mental status is multifactorial and may reflect hypothalamic and spinal dopamine receptor antagonism, a genetic predisposition, or the direct effects of hyperthermia and other drugs.[42] Serotonin also appears to play a role in the pathogenesis of NMS because antipsychotics that antagonize 5-HT_{2A} receptors seem to be associated with a lower incidence of NMS.[4]

Although NMS most often occurs during treatment with a D_2 receptor antagonist, withdrawal of dopamine agonists may produce an indistinguishable syndrome. The latter typically occurs in patients with long-standing Parkinson's disease who abruptly change or discontinue treatment with dopamine agonists such as levodopa/carbidopa, amantadine, or bromocriptine.[13] The resulting disorder is sometimes referred to as the *parkinsonian-hyperpyrexia syndrome*, and mortality rates of up to 4% are reported.[71] Hospitalization for aspiration pneumonia, a common occurrence in older patients with Parkinson's disease, is a particularly high-risk setting for this complication and is particularly dangerous because the cardinal manifestations of NMS are easily misattributed to the combined effects of pneumonia and the underlying movement disorder.

The vast majority of NMS cases occur in the context of therapeutic use of antipsychotics rather than after overdose. Postulated risk factors for the development of NMS include young age, male gender, extracellular fluid volume contraction, use of high-potency antipsychotics, use of depot preparations, cotreatment with lithium, use of multiple drugs in combination, and rapid dose escalation.[2,24,58]

The manifestations of NMS include the tetrad of altered mental status, muscular rigidity or "lead pipe" rigidity, hyperthermia, and autonomic dysfunction. These symptoms may appear in any sequence, although in a review of 340 NMS cases, mental status changes and rigidity usually preceded the development hyperthermia and autonomic instability.[110] Signs typically evolve over a period of several days, with the majority occurring within 2 weeks of starting treatment. However, it is important to recognize that NMS may occur even after prolonged use of an antipsychotic, particularly after a dose increase, the addition of another xenobiotic, or the development of intercurrent illness. It is also worth noting that the clinical course of NMS may fluctuate with remarkable rapidity, sometimes waxing and waning dramatically over a few hours.

There are no universally accepted criteria for the diagnosis of NMS, and at least four different sets of criteria have been proposed.[3,23,33,58] The operating characteristics of these criteria have not been formally evaluated partly because of the absence of a gold standard. The criteria set forth by the *Diagnostic and Statistical Manual of Mental Disorders*, 4th edition (DSM-IV) are perhaps the most widely cited, but their principal limitation is that they make no provision for a causal relationship with xenobiotics other than antipsychotics.[33] Because NMS is an uncommon and potentially life-threatening disorder with highly variable clinical manifestations, an algorithmic approach to diagnosis in inadvisable. Rather, clinicians should be aware of its many possible clinical and laboratory features (Table 69–5) and entertain the possibility of NMS in any unwell patient receiving an antipsychotic, particularly when altered mentation, unexplained fever, or muscle rigidity is present, particularly in the setting of recent modifications to the antipsychotic regimen.

It may be difficult to distinguish NMS from other toxin-induced hyperthermia syndromes, such as the anticholinergic (antimuscarinic) syndrome (see Chap. 50) and the serotonin syndrome (see Chap. 72), all of which share the common features of elevated temperature, altered mental status, and neuromuscular abnormalities. The most important differentiating feature is the medication history, with dopamine antagonists, antimuscarinics, and direct or indirect serotonin agonists (often in combination) as the most likely causes, respectively. Other helpful distinguishing features include the time course (NMS typically develops more gradually than serotonin syndrome and the antimuscarinic syndrome, both of which are characterized by a rapid onset) and the nature of neuromuscular abnormalities. Specifically, serotonin syndrome is characterized by myoclonus (spontaneous or inducible), shivering, and hyperreflexia, which occur rarely in patients with NMS. Because skeletal muscle contraction is governed by nicotinic rather than muscarinic acetylcholine receptors, patients with the

TABLE 69–5. Clinical and Laboratory Features of the Neuroleptic Malignant Syndrome[2,24,58,110]

Feature	Potential Manifestations
Altered mental status	Delirium, lethargy, confusion, stupor, catatonia, coma
Motor symptoms	"Lead pipe" rigidity, cogwheeling, dysarthria or mutism, parkinsonian syndrome, akinesia, tremor, dystonic posture, dysphagia, dysphonia, choreiform movements
Hyperthermia	Temperature >100.4°F (38°C)
Autonomic instability	Tachycardia, diaphoresis, sialorrhea, incontinence, respiratory irregularities, cardiac dysrhythmias, hypertension or hypotension
Laboratory findings	Increased muscle enzymes (creatine phosphokinase, lactate dehydrogenase, aldolase), leukocytosis, renal insufficiency (reflecting volume contraction and pigment nephropathy), acidemia, myoglobinuria, aminotransferase elevation, hypoxia, hyponatremia, increased prothrombin time/partial thromboplastin time

antimuscarinic syndrome have few muscular abnormalities. However, patients with prominent CNS features may be highly resistant to physical restraint, giving the appearance of increased muscle tone.

Treatment of Neuroleptic Malignant Syndrome: General Measures. Treatment recommendations are largely based on general physiologic principles, case reports, and case series. Therapy should be individualized according to the severity and duration of illness and the modifying influences of comorbidity.[13,84,111]

Good supportive care is the cornerstone of treatment of NMS. It is essential to recognize the condition as an emergency and to withdraw the offending xenobiotic immediately. When NMS ensues after abrupt discontinuation of a dopamine agonist such as levodopa, the drug should be reinstituted promptly. All patients with NMS should be admitted to an intensive care unit. Supplemental oxygen should be administered, and assisted ventilation may be necessary in cases of respiratory failure, which may result from central hypoventilation, loss of protective airway reflexes, or rigidity of the chest wall muscles.

The hyperthermia associated with NMS is multifactorial in origin and, when present, should be treated aggressively. For patients with severe hyperthermia, it is difficult to overstate the importance of normalizing body temperature. Submersion in an ice-water bath is the most rapidly efficient technique, although this may be impractical in some settings (see Chap. 15). Other strategies include the use of active cooling blankets; the placement of ice packs in the groin and axillae; or evaporative cooling, which can be accomplished by removing the patient's clothing and exposing the patient to cooled water or towels immersed in ice water while maintaining constant air circulation with the use of fans.[115]

Hypotension should be treated initially with volume resuscitation with 0.9% sodium chloride solution followed by vasopressors if necessary. Alkalinization of the urine with sodium bicarbonate may reduce the incidence of myoglobinuric renal failure in patients with high creatine phosphokinase concentrations, but maintenance of intravascular volume and adequate renal perfusion are of far greater importance. Tachycardia does not require specific treatment, but bradycardia may necessitate the use of transcutaneous or transvenous electrical pacing. Venous thromboembolism is a major cause of morbidity and mortality in patients with NMS, and prophylactic doses of low-molecular-weight heparin should be considered in patients who likely will be immobilized for more than 12 to 24 hours.

Pharmacologic Treatment of Neuroleptic Malignant Syndrome. Benzodiazepines are the most widely used pharmacologic adjuncts for treatment of NMS and are considered first line-therapy. Despite the length of time that they have been available and recommended by many, dantrolene and bromocriptine are not well studied, and their incremental benefit over good supportive care is debated.[84,89] However, these drugs are associated with relatively little toxicity, and the absence of definitive evidence should not preclude their use, particularly in patients with moderate or severe NMS.

Benzodiazepines are frequently used in the management of patients with NMS because of their rapid onset of action, which is particularly important when patients are agitated or restless. Benzodiazepine actions are nonspecific in nature, but they presumably attenuate the sympathetic hyperactivity that characterizes NMS by facilitating GABA-mediated chloride transport and producing neuronal hyperpolarization in a fashion analogous to their beneficial effects in cocaine toxicity.[42] The primary disadvantage of benzodiazepines is that they may cloud the assessment of mental status.

Dantrolene reduces skeletal muscle activity by inhibiting ryanodine receptor calcium release channels, thereby interfering with calcium release from the sarcoplasmic reticulum. In theory, this process should reduce body temperature and total oxygen consumption and lessen the risk of myoglobinuric renal failure. Dantrolene may be particularly useful when muscular rigidity is a prominent feature of NMS.[13] It may be given by mouth (50–100 mg/d) or by IV infusion (2–3 mg/kg/d or ≤10 mg/kg/d in severe cases), although the latter requires laborious reconstitution. A recent review of 271 published cases of NMS that included information regarding drug treatment found that combination therapy including dantrolene was associated with a prolonged clinical recovery but also found that dantrolene monotherapy was associated with higher mortality rate than other treatment modalities including supportive care.[84] However, it is extremely difficult to draw meaningful conclusions regarding the effectiveness of dantrolene from this study in light of its design. Dantrolene is a relatively nontoxic drug suggested by some to be a reasonable therapeutic agent in patients with NMS, particularly those with prominent rigidity, although there is inadequate supportive evidence (see Antidote in Depth A22: Dantrolene).

Bromocriptine is a centrally acting dopamine agonist that is given orally or by nasogastric tube at doses of 2.5 to 10 mg three to four times a day. The rationale for its use rests in the belief that reversal of antipsychotic-related striatal D_2 antagonism will ameliorate the manifestations of NMS. Other dopamine agonists anecdotally associated with success include levodopa[74,99] and amantadine.[40,49,103] An important consideration with dopaminergic agents, however, is that their use may be associated with exacerbation of the underlying psychiatric illness. There is no current evidence to support their use at this time.

Electroconvulsive Therapy. ECT has been reported to dramatically improve the manifestations of NMS, presumably by enhancing central dopaminergic transmission. In one report, five patients received an average of 10 ECT treatments, and resolution generally occurred after the third or fourth session.[73] Whether this result represents a true effect of ECT or simply the natural course of NMS with good supportive care alone is not clear. As with drug therapies for NMS, the efficacy of ECT remains unclear and its indications speculative, but its use seems reasonable in patients with severe, persistent, or treatment-resistant NMS and for those with residual catatonia or psychosis after resolution of other manifestations.[13,74]

Adverse Effects on Other Organ Systems. Sedation, dry mouth, and urinary retention occur commonly with the antipsychotics, particularly during the initial period of therapy. These symptoms occur most commonly with drugs that have potent antihistaminic and antimuscarinic activity. All antipsychotics can lower the seizure threshold, but seizures rarely complicate therapeutic use in patients without additional risk factors. Because hypothalamic dopamine normally inhibits prolactin release by the pituitary gland, hyperprolactinemia and galactorrhea may occur, although these are more common with atypical antipsychotic drugs.

All antipsychotics are associated with weight gain, dyslipidemia, steatohepatitis, and rare but dramatic instances of glucose intolerance, including fatal cases of diabetic ketoacidosis.[6,44,80,106] The mechanisms of the lipid and carbohydrate effects are incompletely understood and not adequately explained solely by the weight gain associated with antipsychotic therapy because glucose disturbances often develop shortly after therapy is instituted. Other idiosyncratic reactions reported with use of antipsychotics include photosensitivity, skin pigmentation and cholestatic hepatitis (which occur with the phenothiazines), myocarditis, and agranulocytosis (which occurs with several drugs but most notably clozapine, ie, between 0.38% and 2% of patients).[68] Most of these conditions result from an immunologically based hypersensitivity reaction and develop during the first month of therapy.

ACUTE OVERDOSE

Antipsychotic overdose may produce a spectrum of manifestations affecting multiple organ systems, but most serious toxicity involves the CNS and cardiovascular system. Some of these manifestations are present to a minor degree during therapeutic use. They tend to be most pronounced during the early period of therapy but dissipate with continued use.

Impaired consciousness is a common and dose-dependent feature of antipsychotic overdose, ranging from somnolence to coma. It may be associated with impaired airway reflexes, but significant respiratory depression is uncommon. Many antipsychotics, including several of the atypical drugs, are potent muscarinic antagonists and may produce dramatic anticholinergic manifestations in overdose.[11,21,26] Peripheral manifestations include tachycardia, decreased production of sweat and saliva, flushed skin, urinary retention, diminished bowel sounds, and mydriasis, although miosis also occurs. These findings may be present in isolation or coexist with central manifestations, which may be highly variable and may be mistakenly attributed to the underlying psychiatric illness. These manifestations include agitation, delirium, psychosis, hallucinations, and coma.

Mild elevations in body temperature are common and reflect impaired heat dissipation because of impaired sweating and increased heat production in agitated patients. Elevations in body temperature should always prompt a search for other manifestations of NMS. Tachycardia is a common finding in patients with antipsychotic overdose and reflects peripheral anticholinergic effects as well as a compensatory response to hypotension. Bradycardia is distinctly uncommon. Although it may be a preterminal event, its presence should prompt a search for alternate causes, including β-adrenergic antagonists, calcium channel blockers, cardioactive steroids, opioids, and myocardial ischemia. Hypotension is a common feature of antipsychotic overdose. Peripheral α_1-adrenergic blockade reduces vasomotor tone. Central maintenance of vasomotor tone may be impaired, albeit by an unknown mechanism.

The electrocardiographic (ECG) manifestations of antipsychotic overdose are similar to those of CA toxicity (see Chaps. 22 and 73) and include prolongation of the QRS complex and a rightward deflection of the terminal 40 msec of the QRS complex (T_{40}msec, a tall, broad terminal component of the QRS complex in lead aVR). These changes reflect blockade of the inward sodium current (I_{Na}). Prolongation of the QT interval results from blockade of the delayed rectifier potassium current (I_{Kr}), creating a substrate for development of torsades de pointes.[70] This situation is sometimes evident during maintenance therapy and may underlie the apparent increase in sudden cardiac death among users of antipsychotics.[81,83] A published meta-analysis of the operating characteristics of the ECG in patients with cyclic antidepressant toxicity found the ECG was a relatively poor predictor of seizures, dysrhythmia, and death.[7] However, the ECG is a dynamic instrument, particularly in the initial hours after overdose, and few studies have evaluated longitudinal changes in the ECG.[59]

DIAGNOSTIC TESTS

The diagnosis of antipsychotic poisoning is supported by the clinical history, the physical examination, and a limited number of adjunctive tests. Both the clinical and ECG findings are nonspecific and can occur after overdose of several different drug classes, including CAs, skeletal muscle relaxants, carbamazepine, and first-generation antihistamines such as diphenhydramine. Moreover, the absence of typical ECG changes does not exclude a significant antipsychotic ingestion, particularly early after overdose, and at least one additional ECG should be performed in the following 2 to 3 hours.

Serum concentrations of antipsychotics are not widely available, do not correlate well with clinical signs and symptoms, and do not help guide therapy. Comprehensive urine drug screens using high-performance liquid chromatography, gas chromatography–mass spectrometry, or tandem mass spectrometry may indicate the presence of antipsychotics, but these tests are available at only a few hospitals and in most instances provide only a qualitative result. Blood and urine immunoassays for CAs may yield a false-positive result in the presence of phenothiazines.[5,88]

MANAGEMENT

The care of a patient with an antipsychotic overdose should proceed with the recognition that other drugs, particularly other psychotropic agents, may have been prescribed and coingested and may confound both the clinical presentation and management. Regularly encountered coingestants include other psychotropic drugs such as antidepressants, sedative–hypnotics, anticholinergics, valproic acid, and lithium, as well as ethanol and nonprescription analgesics such as acetaminophen and aspirin.

Supportive care is the cornerstone of treatment for patients with antipsychotic overdose. Supplemental oxygen should be administered if hypoxia is present. Patients with altered mental status should receive thiamine and parenteral dextrose as clinically indicated. Intubation and ventilation are rarely required for patients with single drug ingestions but may be necessary for patients with very large overdoses of antipsychotic agents or ingestion of other CNS depressants. All symptomatic patients should undergo continuous cardiac monitoring. In addition, an ECG should be recorded upon presentation and reliable venous access obtained. Asymptomatic patients with a normal ECG 6 hours after overdose have an exceedingly low risk of complications and no longer require cardiac monitoring. Symptomatic patients and those with an abnormal ECG should be continuously monitored for a minimum of 24 hours.

GASTROINTESTINAL DECONTAMINATION

Gastrointestinal decontamination with activated charcoal (1 g/kg by mouth or nasogastric tube) should be considered for patients who present after a large or polydrug overdose. Although this intervention is time sensitive, many antipsychotics exhibit significant antimuscarinic activity and slow gastric emptying, thereby increasing the likelihood that activated charcoal will be beneficial. Although improvement in clinically important, outcomes cannot be attributed to activated charcoal at present. A Bayesian analysis of pharmacokinetic data from 54 quetiapine overdoses (19 of whom received activated charcoal) concluded that charcoal reduced absorption by 35%.[47] Orogastric lavage and whole-bowel irrigation likely will not improve clinical outcomes and should not be routinely used in the management of those with antipsychotic overdoses. Induction of emesis using syrup of ipecac is absolutely contraindicated because of the high potential for pulmonary aspiration.

TREATMENT OF CARDIOVASCULAR COMPLICATIONS

Vital signs should be monitored closely. Hypotension may result from peripheral α-adrenergic blockade and is most likely to occur with older, low-potency antipsychotics such as thioridazine. The hypotension should be treated initially with appropriate titration of 0.9% sodium chloride solution (30–40 mL/kg). If vasopressors are required, direct-acting agonists such as norepinephrine or phenylephrine are preferred over dopamine, which is an indirect agonist and likely will be ineffective. Vasopressin or its analogs may also be used, although direct-acting vasopressors should be used with great caution in patients who have coingested a negative inotropic drug such as a β-adrenergic antagonist or calcium channel blocker. Continuous, intraarterial blood pressure monitoring may be warranted in such cases. Central venous pressure monitoring and pulmonary artery catheterization rarely influence treatment decisions and should be used only if the patient's clinical status is obfuscated by significant coingestion or comorbidity.

Sodium bicarbonate (1–2 mEq/kg) is the first-line therapy for ventricular dysrhythmias and should be considered for patients with dysrhythmias or QRS prolongation above 0.12 seconds. The rationale for this strategy is based on the treatment of cyclic antidepressant overdose (see Antidotes in Depth A5: Sodium Bicarbonate and Chap. 73). At least two mechanisms underlie the beneficial effects of sodium bicarbonate: (1) the degree of sodium channel blockade is partially overcome by an increase in extracellular sodium; indeed, hypertonic saline alone may be beneficial and (2) the binding of these drugs to the sodium channel is pH dependent, with less extensive binding at higher pH.

Repeated boluses of bicarbonate may be administered to achieve a target blood pH of 7.5, although many toxicologists recommend continuous infusions.[98] If the patient is intubated, hyperventilation may also be used but is not comparably efficacious and should not be used for alkalinization. When significant conduction abnormalities or ventricular dysrhythmias persist despite the use of sodium bicarbonate, lidocaine (1–2 mg/kg followed by continuous infusion) is a reasonable second-line antidysrhythmic agent. Although lidocaine is also a sodium channel antagonist, it exhibits rapid on/off sodium channel binding with preferential binding in the inactivated state and may lessen the cardiotoxicity associated with antipsychotic drug overdose.[97] Class IA antidysrhythmics (procainamide, disopyramide, and quinidine), class IC antidysrhythmics (propafenone, encainide, and flecainide), and class III antidysrhythmics (amiodarone, sotalol, and bretylium) may all aggravate cardiotoxicity and should not be used. When administering sodium bicarbonate to patients with antipsychotic overdose, caution must be taken to avoid hypokalemia because many of these antipsychotics block cardiac potassium channels, thereby prolonging the QT interval. Hypokalemia may exacerbate this blockade, potentially leading to torsade de pointes.

Sinus tachycardia related to anticholinergic activity should not be treated unless it is associated with ischemia. Prolongation of the QT interval requires no specific treatment other than monitoring and correction of potential contributing causes such as hypokalemia and hypomagnesemia. Torsade de pointes should be treated with IV magnesium sulfate, taking care to prevent hypotension, which is dose and rate dependent. Overdrive pacing with isoproterenol or transcutaneous or transvenous pacing should be considered if the patient does not respond to magnesium sulfate, although in theory this therapy may worsen the rate-dependent sodium channel blockade.

Many antipsychotics, including olanzapine, quetiapine, and sertindole, exhibit a high degree of lipophilicity in addition to significant cardiovascular toxicity. Recently, considerable enthusiasm has emerged for the use of high-dose lipid emulsion therapy for patients with significant overdoses of drugs displaying these characteristics. The rationale for this therapy depends, in part, in the concept that highly lipophilic drugs will selectively partition into the exogenous lipid, thereby minimizing toxicity at the biophase. This treatment has been extensively studied in animal models of bupivacaine toxicity,[32,113,114] but published experience with antipsychotic drugs is extremely limited.[38] Dosing for lipid "rescue" is not well established, but the current recommended protocol involves 20% lipid emulsion given as a bolus (1.5 mL/kg) followed by an infusion of 0.25 mL/kg/min for 30 to 60 minutes with adjustment of therapy according to the individual response (see Antidote in Depth: A22: Intravenous Fat Emulsion).

TREATMENT OF SEIZURES

Seizures associated with an antipsychotic overdose are generally short lived and often require no pharmacologic treatment. Multiple or refractory seizures should prompt a search for other causes, including hypoglycemia and ingestion of other proconvulsants. When treatment is necessary, benzodiazepines such as lorazepam or diazepam generally suffice, although phenobarbital may be necessary. Although phenytoin may be part of the standard algorithm for treating those with status epilepticus, it is of limited effectiveness for xenobiotic-induced seizures; and in this situation, barbiturates are preferred. Patients with refractory seizures typically respond to propofol infusion or general anesthesia. Seizures complicated by hyperthermia are considerably more ominous and warrant aggressive lowering of body temperature with aggressive rapid cooling measures. Finally, seizures may abruptly lower serum pH and may abruptly increase the cardiotoxicity of these drugs; therefore, an ECG should be obtained after resolution of seizure activity.

TREATMENT OF THE CENTRAL ANTIMUSCARINIC SYNDROME

Many of the older- and newer-generation antipsychotics have pronounced anticholinergic properties. Case reports and observational studies suggest that the cholinesterase inhibitor physostigmine (see Antidotes in Depth A12: Physostigmine Salicylate) can safely and effectively ameliorate the agitated delirium associated with the central anticholinergic syndrome by indirectly increasing synaptic acetylcholine levels.[25,91-93] Although benzodiazepines control agitation, they further impair alertness, obfuscating the assessment of mental status and increasing the risk of complications.[22]

Physostigmine has been used successfully in patients with antipsychotic overdose[22,90,93,116,117] but should be used with caution and not in patients with dysrhythmias, any degree of heart block, or widening of the QRS complex. If physostigmine is used, it should be given in 0.5-mg increments every 3 to 5 minutes with close observation of the patient. Subsequent bradycardia, bronchospasm, or bronchorrhea can be treated with 0.2 to 0.4 mg of IV glycopyrrolate. Although atropine is often more widely available and could be used, it crosses the blood–brain barrier and may aggravate any associated delirium. The clinical effects of physostigmine are transient, typically ranging in duration from 30 to 90 minutes, and additional doses are often necessary. Physostigmine does not prevent other complications of antipsychotic overdose, particularly those involving the cardiovascular system.

Other commonly used cholinesterase inhibitors, such as edrophonium, neostigmine, or pyridostigmine, should not be used to treat anticholinergic delirium because they do not cross the blood–brain barrier. Case reports involving other anticholinergics suggest that cholinesterase inhibitors used for treatment of dementia (eg, tacrine, donepezil, and galantamine) may be alternatives to physostigmine for patients who are able to take medications orally.[48,67,75]

ENHANCED ELIMINATION

No pharmacologic rationale supports the use of multiple-dose charcoal or manipulation of urinary pH to increase the clearance of antipsychotics. One volunteer study found that urinary acidification may increase remoxipride elimination,[118] but this practice is impractical and possibly dangerous. Because most antipsychotics exhibit large volumes of distribution and extensive protein binding (see Table 69–1), neither hemodialysis nor hemoperfusion is warranted. These modalities should be considered only if the patient has concomitantly ingested other xenobiotics amenable to extracorporeal removal, such as lithium.

SUMMARY

Over the past decade, the atypical antipsychotics have largely supplanted traditional (typical) antipsychotics, which are associated with greater toxicity in overdose and a higher incidence of EPS.

However, significant toxicity may occur either during the course of therapy or after overdose with both typical and atypical antipsychotics. Of the various toxicities that arise during therapeutic use, NMS is the most dangerous. Its manifestations are protean, and it may be difficult to recognize. Altered mental status, muscle rigidity, fever, and autonomic instability are its hallmarks, but the diagnosis should be considered in any unwell patient treated with antipsychotics, particularly in the 2 weeks after a change in therapy or in a patient with severe intercurrent illness. Treatment of NMS is largely supportive and often involves the use of benzodiazepines. Dantrolene, dopamine agonists such as bromocriptine or entacopone, and ECT are anecdotally associated with dramatic clinical improvement.

The principal manifestations of antipsychotic overdose involve the CNS and cardiovascular system. Depressed mental status, hypotension, and anticholinergic signs are nonspecific features that support the diagnosis of antipsychotic overdose, particularly in conjunction with typical ECG findings of sodium channel blockade and QT prolongation. However, these signs and symptoms vary considerably among the available antipsychotics. Most fatalities after antipsychotic overdose occur in the setting of coingestions of other CNS depressants or cardiotoxic medications. Supportive care is the mainstay of therapy for patients with antipsychotic overdose, although selective use of nonspecific antidotes, such as activated charcoal, sodium bicarbonate, and physostigmine, may improve outcomes in some patients. Particularly severe or refractory cardiovascular toxicity may warrant a trial of lidocaine or IV lipid emulsion, although these interventions are not well studied in the context of antipsychotic drug overdose.

ACKNOWLEDGMENTS

Frank LoVecchio and Neal A. Lewin contributed to this chapter in a previous edition.

REFERENCES

1. Abi-Dargham A, Rodenhiser J, Printz D, et al. Increased baseline occupancy of D_2 receptors by dopamine in schizophrenia. *Proc Natl Acad Sci U S A.* 2000;97:8104-8109.
2. Addonizio G, Susman VL, Roth SD. Neuroleptic malignant syndrome: review and analysis of 115 cases. *Biol Psychiatry.* 1987;22:1004-1020.
3. Adnet P, Lestavel P, Krivosic-Horber R. Neuroleptic malignant syndrome. *Br J Anaesth.* 2000;85:129-135.
4. Ananth J, Parameswaran S, Gunatilake S, et al. Neuroleptic malignant syndrome and atypical antipsychotic drugs. *J Clin Psychiatry.* 2004;65:464-470.
5. Asselin WM, Leslie JM. Use of the EMITtox serum tricyclic antidepressant assay for the analysis of urine samples. *J Anal Toxicol.* 1990;14:168-171.
6. Avella J, Wetli CV, Wilson JC, et al. Fatal olanzapine-induced hyperglycemic ketoacidosis. *Am J Forensic Med Pathol.* 2004;25:172-175.
7. Bailey B, Buckley NA, Amre DK. A meta-analysis of prognostic indicators to predict seizures, arrhythmias or death after tricyclic antidepressant overdose. *J Toxicol Clin Toxicol.* 2004;42:877-888.
8. Baldassano CF, Truman CJ, Nierenberg A, et al. Akathisia: a review and case report following paroxetine treatment. *Compr Psychiatry.* 1996;37:122-124.
9. Baldessarini RJ, Frankenburg FR. Clozapine. A novel antipsychotic agent. *N Engl J Med.* 1991;324:746-754.
10. Baldessarini RJ, Tarazi FI. Drugs and the treatment of psychiatric disorders: psychosis and mania. In *Goodman and Gilman's The Pharmacological Basis of Therapeutics*, 10th ed. Hardman JG, Limbird LE, eds. New York, McGraw-Hill 2001, pp 485-520.
11. Balit CR, Isbister GK, Hackett LP, Whyte IM. Quetiapine poisoning: a case series. *Ann Emerg Med.* 2003;42:751-758.
12. Baselt RC. *Disposition of Toxic Drugs and Chemicals in Man*, 8th ed. Foster City, CA: Biomedical Publications.
13. Bhanushali MJ, Tuite PJ. The evaluation and management of patients with neuroleptic malignant syndrome. *Neurol Clin.* 2004;22:389-411.
14. Borison RL. Recent advances in the pharmacotherapy of schizophrenia. *Harv Rev Psychiatry.* 1997;4:255-271.
15. Brockmoller J, Kirchheiner J, Schmider J, et al. The impact of the CYP2D6 polymorphism on haloperidol pharmacokinetics and on the outcome of haloperidol treatment. *Clin Pharmacol Ther.* 2002;72:438-452.
16. Bronstein AC, Spyker DA, Cantilena LR Jr, et al. 2007 Annual report of the American Association of Poison Control Centers' National Poison Data System (NPDS): 25th annual report. *Clin Toxicol (Phila).* 2008;46:927-1057.
17. Buckley N, McManus P. Fatal toxicity of drugs used in the treatment of psychotic illnesses. *Br J Psychiatry.* 1998;172:461-4:461-464.
18. Buckley NA, Sanders P. Cardiovascular adverse effects of antipsychotic drugs. *Drug Saf.* 2000;23:215-228.
19. Buckley NA, Whyte IM, Dawson AH. Cardiotoxicity more common in thioridazine overdose than with other neuroleptics. *J Toxicol Clin Toxicol.* 1995;33:199-204.
20. Burgyone K, Aduri K, Ananth J, Parameswaran S. The use of antiparkinsonian agents in the management of drug-induced extrapyramidal symptoms. *Curr Pharm Des.* 2004;10:2239-2248.
21. Burns MJ. The pharmacology and toxicology of atypical antipsychotic agents. *J Toxicol Clin Toxicol.* 2001;39:1-14.
22. Burns MJ, Linden CH, Graudins A, et al. A comparison of physostigmine and benzodiazepines for the treatment of anticholinergic poisoning. *Ann Emerg Med.* 2000;35:374-381.
23. Caroff SN, Mann SC. Neuroleptic malignant syndrome. *Med Clin North Am.* 1993;77:185-202.
24. Caroff SN, Mann SC. Neuroleptic malignant syndrome and malignant hyperthermia. *Anaesth Intensive Care.* 1993;21:477-478.
25. Caroff SN, Mann SC, Campbell EC, Sullivan KA. Movement disorders associated with atypical antipsychotic drugs. *J Clin Psychiatry.* 2002;63(suppl 4):12-9:12-19.
26. Chue P, Singer P. A review of olanzapine-associated toxicity and fatality in overdose. *J Psychiatry Neurosci.* 2003;28:253-261.

27. Corre KA, Niemann JT, Bessen HA. Extended therapy for acute dystonic reactions. *Ann Emerg Med.* 1984;13:194-197.
28. Dahan L, Husum H, Mnie-Filali O, et al. Effects of bifeprunox and aripiprazole on rat serotonin and dopamine neuronal activity and anxiolytic behaviour. *J Psychopharmacol.* 2009;23:177-189.
29. Dahl ML. Cytochrome p450 phenotyping/genotyping in patients receiving antipsychotics: useful aid to prescribing? *Clin Pharmacokinet.* 2002;41: 453-470.
30. Dahl-Puustinen ML, Liden A, Alm C, et al. Disposition of perphenazine is related to polymorphic debrisoquin hydroxylation in human beings. *Clin Pharmacol Ther.* 1989;46:78-81.
31. Delay J, Pichot P, LemperiereT, et al. A non-phenothiazine and non-reserpine major neuroleptic, haloperidol, in the treatment of psychoses. *Ann Med Psychol (Paris).* 1960;118:145-152.
32. Di Gregorio G, Schwartz D, Ripper R, et al. Lipid emulsion is superior to vasopressin in a rodent model of resuscitation from toxin-induced cardiac arrest. *Crit Care Med.* 2009;37:993-999.
33. *Diagnostic and Statistical Manual of Mental Disorders (DSM-IV)*, 4th ed. Washington, DC: American Psychiatric Press; 1994:739-742.
34. Dresser GK, Bailey DG. A basic conceptual and practical overview of interactions with highly prescribed drugs. *Can J Clin Pharmacol.* 2002;9:191-198.
35. Egan MF, Apud J, Wyatt RJ. Treatment of tardive dyskinesia. *Schizophr Bull.* 1997;23:583-609.
36. Ereshefsky L. Pharmacologic and pharmacokinetic considerations in choosing an antipsychotic. *J Clin Psychiatry.* 1999;60(suppl 10):20-30:20-30.
37. Fines RE, Brady WJ Jr, Martin ML. Acute laryngeal dystonia related to neuroleptic agents. *Am J Emerg Med.* 1999;17:319-320.
38. Finn SD, Uncles DR, Willers J, Sable N. Early treatment of a quetiapine and sertraline overdose with Intralipid. *Anaesthesia.* 2009;64:191-194.
39. Frey R, Schreinzer D, Stimpfl T, et al. Fatal poisonings with antidepressive drugs and neuroleptics. Analysis of a correlation with prescriptions in Vienna 1991 to 1997. *Nervenarzt.* 2002;73:629-636.
40. Gangadhar BN, Desai NG, Channabasavanna SM. Amantadine in the neuroleptic malignant syndrome. *J Clin Psychiatry.* 1984;45:526.
41. Gurrera RJ, Chang SS. Thermoregulatory dysfunction in neuroleptic malignant syndrome. *Biol Psychiatry.* 1996;39:207-212.
42. Gurrera RJ, Romero JA. Sympathoadrenomedullary activity in the neuroleptic malignant syndrome. *Biol Psychiatry.* 1992;32:334-343.
43. Haddad PM, Anderson IM. Antipsychotic-related QTc prolongation, torsade de pointes and sudden death. *Drugs.* 2002;62:1649-1671.
44. Henderson DC. Atypical antipsychotic-induced diabetes mellitus: how strong is the evidence? *CNS Drugs.* 2002;16:77-89.
45. Hugenholtz GW, Heerdink ER, Stolker JJ, et al. Haloperidol dose when used as active comparator in randomized controlled trials with atypical antipsychotics in schizophrenia: comparison with officially recommended doses. *J Clin Psychiatry.* 2006;67:897-903.
46. Iqbal MM, Rahman A, Husain Z, et al. Clozapine: a clinical review of adverse effects and management. *Ann Clin Psychiatry.* 2003;15:33-48.
47. Isbister GK, Friberg LE, Hackett LP, Duffull SB. Pharmacokinetics of quetiapine in overdose and the effect of activated charcoal. *Clin Pharmacol Ther.* 2007;81:821-827.
48. Isbister GK, Oakley P, Dawson AH, Whyte IM. Presumed Angel's trumpet (Brugmansia) poisoning: clinical effects and epidemiology. *Emerg Med (Fremantle).* 2003;15:376-382.
49. Jee A. Amantadine in neuroleptic malignant syndrome. *Postgrad Med J.* 1987;63:508-509.
50. Jeste DV, Caligiuri MP, Paulsen JS, et al. Risk of tardive dyskinesia in older patients. A prospective longitudinal study of 266 outpatients. *Arch Gen Psychiatry.* 1995;52:756-765.
51. Jibson MD, Tandon R. New atypical antipsychotic medications. *J Psychiatr Res.* 1998;32:215-228.
52. Kakihara S, Yoshimura R, Shinkai K, et al. Prediction of response to risperidone treatment with respect to plasma concentrations of risperidone, catecholamine metabolites, and polymorphism of cytochrome P450 2D6. *Int Clin Psychopharmacol.* 2005;20:71-78.
53. Kapur S, Mamo D. Half a century of antipsychotics and still a central role for dopamine D_2 receptors. *Prog Neuropsychopharmacol Biol Psychiatry.* 2003;27:1081-1090.
54. Kapur S, Seeman P. Does fast dissociation from the dopamine D(2) receptor explain the action of atypical antipsychotics? A new hypothesis. *Am J Psychiatry.* 2001;158:360-369.
55. Kasper S, Tauscher J, Kufferle B, et al. Sertindole and dopamine D_2 receptor occupancy in comparison to risperidone, clozapine and haloperidol—a 123I-IBZM SPECT study. *Psychopharmacology (Berl).* 1998;136:367-373.
56. Keck PE Jr, McElroy SL. Clinical pharmacodynamics and pharmacokinetics of antimanic and mood-stabilizing medications. *J Clin Psychiatry.* 2002;63(suppl 4):3-11:3-11.
57. Keck PE Jr, McElroy SL, Arnold LM. Ziprasidone: a new atypical antipsychotic. *Expert Opin Pharmacother.* 2001;2:1033-1042.
58. Levenson JL. Neuroleptic malignant syndrome. *Am J Psychiatry.* 1985;142: 1137-1145.
59. Liebelt EL, Ulrich A, Francis PD, Woolf A. Serial electrocardiogram changes in acute tricyclic antidepressant overdoses. *Crit Care Med.* 1997;25:1721-1726.
60. Lima AR, Bacalcthuk J, Barnes TR, Soares-Weiser K. Central action beta-blockers versus placebo for neuroleptic-induced acute akathisia. *Cochrane Database Syst Rev.* 2004;CD001946.
61. Lima AR, Weiser KV, Bacaltchuk J, Barnes TR. Anticholinergics for neuroleptic-induced acute akathisia. *Cochrane Database Syst Rev.* 2004;CD003727.
62. Lipinski JF Jr, Mallya G, Zimmerman P, Pope HG Jr. Fluoxetine-induced akathisia: clinical and theoretical implications. *J Clin Psychiatry.* 1989;50:339-342.
63. Mamo DC, Sweet RA, Keshavan MS. Managing antipsychotic-induced parkinsonism. *Drug Saf.* 1999;20:269-275.
64. Manini AF, Raspberry D, Hoffman RS, Nelson LS. QT prolongation and torsades de pointes following overdose of ziprasidone and amantadine. *J Med Toxicol.* 2007;3:178-181.
65. Marsden CD, Jenner P. The pathophysiology of extrapyramidal side-effects of neuroleptic drugs. *Psychol Med.* 1980;10:55-72.
66. Meltzer HY, Stahl SM. The dopamine hypothesis of schizophrenia: a review. *Schizophr Bull.* 1976;2:19-76.
67. Mendelson G. Pheniramine aminosalicylate overdosage. Reversal of delirium and choreiform movements with tacrine treatment. *Arch Neurol.* 1977;34:313.
68. Miller DD. Review and management of clozapine side effects. *J Clin Psychiatry.* 2000;61(suppl 8):14-7; discussion 18-9:14-17.
69. Naber D, Lambert M. Aripiprazole: a new atypical antipsychotic with a different pharmacological mechanism. *Prog Neuropsychopharmacol Biol Psychiatry.* 2004;28:1213-1219.
70. Nelson LS. Toxicologic myocardial sensitization. *J Toxicol Clin Toxicol.* 2002;40:867-879.
71. Newman EJ, Grosset DG, Kennedy PG. The parkinsonism-hyperpyrexia syndrome. *Neurocrit Care.* 2009;10:136-140.
72. Newman-Tancredi A, Cussac D, Depoortere R. Neuropharmacological profile of bifeprunox: merits and limitations in comparison with other third-generation antipsychotics. *Curr Opin Investig Drugs.* 2007;8: 539-554.
73. Nisijima K, Ishiguro T. Electroconvulsive therapy for the treatment of neuroleptic malignant syndrome with psychotic symptoms: a report of five cases. *JECT.* 1999;15:158-163.
74. Nisijima K, Noguti M, Ishiguro T. Intravenous injection of levodopa is more effective than dantrolene as therapy for neuroleptic malignant syndrome. *Biol Psychiatry.* 1997;41:913-914.
75. Noyan MA, Elbi H, Aksu H. Donepezil for anticholinergic drug intoxication: a case report. *Prog Neuropsychopharmacol Biol Psychiatry.* 2003;27:885-887.
76. Perquin L, Steinert T. A review of the efficacy, tolerability and safety of sertindole in clinical trials. *CNS Drugs.* 2004;18(suppl 2):19-30; discussion 41-3:19-30.
77. Pierre JM. Extrapyramidal symptoms with atypical antipsychotics: incidence, prevention and management. *Drug Saf.* 2005;28:191-208.
78. Pisani F, Oteri G, Costa C, et al. Effects of psychotropic drugs on seizure threshold. *Drug Saf.* 2002;25:91-110.
79. Pope HG Jr, Keck PE Jr, McElroy SL. Frequency and presentation of neuroleptic malignant syndrome in a large psychiatric hospital. *Am J Psychiatry.* 1986;143:1227-1233.
80. Ragucci KR, Wells BJ. Olanzapine-induced diabetic ketoacidosis. *Ann Pharmacother.* 2001;35:1556-1558.
81. Ray WA, Chung CP, Murray KT, et al. Atypical antipsychotic drugs and the risk of sudden cardiac death. *N Engl J Med.* 2009;360:225-235.
82. Ray WA, Meredith S, Thapa PB, et al. Antipsychotics and the risk of sudden cardiac death. *Arch Gen Psychiatry.* 2001;58:1161-1167.
83. Remington G. Understanding antipsychotic "atypicality": a clinical and pharmacological moving target. *J Psychiatry Neurosci.* 2003;28:275-284.

84. Reulbach U, Dutsch C, Biermann T, et al. Managing an effective treatment for neuroleptic malignant syndrome. *Crit Care.* 2007;11:R4.
85. Richelson E. Receptor pharmacology of neuroleptics: relation to clinical effects. *J Clin Psychiatry.* 1999;60(suppl 10):5-14:5-14.
86. Richelson E, Nelson A. Antagonism by antidepressants of neurotransmitter receptors of normal human brain in vitro. *J Pharmacol Exp Ther.* 1984;230:94-102.
87. Richelson E, Souder T. Binding of antipsychotic drugs to human brain receptors focus on newer generation compounds. *Life Sci.* 2000;68:29-39.
88. Robinson K, Smith RN. Radioimmunoassay of tricyclic antidepressant and some phenothiazine drugs in forensic toxicology. *J Immunoassay.* 1985;6:11-22.
89. Rosebush PI, Stewart T, Mazurek MF. The treatment of neuroleptic malignant syndrome. Are dantrolene and bromocriptine useful adjuncts to supportive care? *Br J Psychiatry.* 1991;159:709-12:709-712.
90. Ross SR, Rodgers SR. Physostigmine in amoxapine overdose. *Am J Hosp Pharm.* 1981;38:1121-1122.
91. Schneir AB, Offerman SR, Ly BT, et al. Complications of diagnostic physostigmine administration to emergency department patients. *Ann Emerg Med.* 2003;42:14-19.
92. Schuster MA, Stein BD, Jaycox L, et al. A national survey of stress reactions after the September 11, 2001, terrorist attacks. *N Engl J Med.* 2001;345: 1507-1512.
93. Schuster P, Gabriel E, Kufferle B, et al. Reversal by physostigmine of clozapine-induced delirium. *Clin Toxicol.* 1977;10:437-441.
94. Seeman P. Atypical antipsychotics: mechanism of action. *Can J Psychiatry.* 2002;47:27-38.
95. Seeman P. Dopamine D2 High receptors moderately elevated by bifeprunox and aripiprazole. *Synapse.* 2008;62:902-908.
96. Seeman P, Kapur S. Schizophrenia: more dopamine, more D_2 receptors. *Proc Natl Acad Sci U S A.* 2000;97:7673-7675.
97. Seger DL. A critical reconsideration of the clinical effects and treatment recommendations for sodium channel blocking drug cardiotoxicity. *Toxicol Rev.* 2006;25:283-296.
98. Seger DL, Hantsch C, Zavoral T, Wrenn K. Variability of recommendations for serum alkalinization in tricyclic antidepressant overdose: a survey of U.S. Poison Center medical directors. *J Toxicol Clin Toxicol.* 2003;41:331-338.
99. Shoop SA, Cernek PK. Carbidopa/levodopa in the treatment of neuroleptic malignant syndrome. *Ann Pharmacother.* 1997;31:119.
100. Spina E, Zoccali R. Sertindole: pharmacological and clinical profile and role in the treatment of schizophrenia. *Expert Opin Drug Metab Toxicol.* 2008;4:629-638.
101. Squires RF, Saederup E. Mono N-aryl ethylenediamine and piperazine derivatives are GABAA receptor blockers: implications for psychiatry. *Neurochem Res.* 1993;18:787-793.
102. Stahl SM. Introduction: what makes an antipsychotic atypical? *J Clin Psychiatry.* 1999;60(suppl 10):3-4.
103. Strawn JR, Keck PE Jr, Caroff SN: neuroleptic malignant syndrome. *Am J Psychiatry.* 2007;164:870-876.
104. Tarsy D. Movement disorders with neuroleptic drug treatment. *Psychiatr Clin North Am.* 1984;7:453-471.
105. Tarsy D, Baldessarini RJ, Tarazi FI. Effects of newer antipsychotics on extrapyramidal function. *CNS Drugs.* 2002;16:23-45.
106. Torrey EF, Swalwell CI. Fatal olanzapine-induced ketoacidosis. *Am J Psychiatry.* 2003;160:2241.
107. Trosch RM. Neuroleptic-induced movement disorders: deconstructing extrapyramidal symptoms. *J Am Geriatr Soc.* 2004;52:S266-S271.
108. van Harten PN, Hoek HW, Kahn RS. Acute dystonia induced by drug treatment. *Br Med J.* 1999;319:623-626.
109. Velamoor VR. Neuroleptic malignant syndrome. Recognition, prevention and management. *Drug Saf.* 1998;19:73-82.
110. Velamoor VR, Norman RM, Caroff SN, et al. Progression of symptoms in neuroleptic malignant syndrome. *J Nerv Ment Dis.* 1994;182:168-173.
111. Velamoor VR, Swamy GN, Parmar RS, et al. Management of suspected neuroleptic malignant syndrome. *Can J Psychiatry.* 1995;40:545-550.
112. von Bahr C, Movin G, Nordin C, et al. Plasma levels of thioridazine and metabolites are influenced by the debrisoquin hydroxylation phenotype. *Clin Pharmacol Ther.* 1991;49:234-240.
113. Weinberg G, Hertz P, Newman J. Lipid, not propofol, treats bupivacaine overdose. *Anesth Analg.* 2004;99:1875-1876.
114. Weinberg G, Ripper R, Feinstein DL, Hoffman W. Lipid emulsion infusion rescues dogs from bupivacaine-induced cardiac toxicity. *Reg Anesth Pain Med.* 2003;28:198-202.
115. Weiner JS, Khogali M. A physiological body-cooling unit for treatment of heat stroke. *Lancet.* 1980;1:507-509.
116. Weisdorf D, Kramer J, Goldbarg A, Klawans HL. Physostigmine for cardiac and neurologic manifestations of phenothiazine poisoning. *Clin Pharmacol Ther.* 1978;24:663-667.
117. Weizberg M, Su M, Mazzola JL, et al. Altered mental status from olanzapine overdose treated with physostigmine. *Clin Toxicol (Phila).* 2006;44:319-325.
118. Widerlov E, Termander B, Nilsson MI. Effect of urinary pH on the plasma and urinary kinetics of remoxipride in man. *Eur J Clin Pharmacol.* 1989;37: 359-363.
119. Wirshing WC. Movement disorders associated with neuroleptic treatment. *J Clin Psychiatry.* 2001;62(suppl 21):15-8:15-18.

CHAPTER 70
LITHIUM

Howard A. Greller

MW	=	6.94 daltons
Lithium concentration (serum):		
Therapeutic concentration for bipolar depression	=	0.6–1.2 mEq/L (mmol/L)

Lithium is the most efficient long-term therapy for treatment and prevention of bipolar affective disorders,[57,89,211] with a demonstrated antisuicidal effect and an ability to improve both the manic and depressive symptoms of the illness.[15–17,51,59,86,87,145,192,212] Investigations on the use of lithium for compulsive gambling have also demonstrated beneficial results.[99] In most industrialized nations, approximately one in 1000 persons is prescribed one or more of the various lithium formulations.[8,187]

HISTORY

The Swedish chemistry student Arfwedson discovered lithium in 1817.[145] Lithium derives its name from the Greek word for stone, *lithos*, from which it was first isolated. Lithium has a long history of therapeutic use beginning in the mid 19th century, when lithium salts were used to treat individuals with gout. The therapy also improved symptoms of mania and depression.[16,120,212] The soft drink 7-Up was originally formulated with lithium as its "active ingredient."[5] During the 1930s and 1940s, lithium was used as a salt substitute ("Westsal") for patients with heart failure but was discontinued after several cases of acute lithium poisoning were described.[61,68,92,188] The beneficial effects of lithium on bipolar disorder were "rediscovered" by Cade in 1949, when he noticed the calming effect of lithium carbonate on guinea pigs.[48,49] The same year, however, the Food and Drug Administration (FDA) banned the use of lithium in response to reported poisonings.[48,172,188] The FDA lifted the ban in 1970 and approved the use of lithium for the treatment of mania.

PHARMACOLOGY

The simplicity of the lithium molecule belies the complexity of its mechanism of action. Although lithium has been used therapeutically for almost 50 years, the precise pharmacology of its therapeutic effects has not yet been fully elucidated.[80] Part of the difficulty in defining the precise mechanism of lithium is the difficulty in defining the precise pathophysiology of bipolar disorder.[192] Early efforts focused on dysfunctional neurotransmitter systems, particularly the role of biogenic amines. Lithium increases basal and stimulation-induced serotonin release and receptor sensitivity to serotonin.[45,213] Lithium modulates the effect of norepinephrine through its interactions with the G-protein–mediated β-adrenergic receptor, stabilizing fluctuations in the intracellular pool of cyclic adenosine monophosphate (cAMP). It performs this function by inhibiting not only the inhibitory subunit G_i, which increases basal concentrations of cAMP but also the stimulatory subunit, G_s, preventing fluctuations from adrenergic stimulation.[45]

Clinically, the therapeutic effects of lithium and other mood-stabilizing pharmaceuticals become evident only after chronic administration, so their mechanism of action is likely not solely the result of acute biochemical interactions. Postulated mechanisms go beyond simple neurotransmitter function or dysfunction and focus on altered cellular signaling, neuronal plasticity, and neurogenesis. Rather than trying to identify any single neurotransmitter system as responsible for the complexity of depressive illness, efforts now are directed at elucidating the functional balance between interacting systems. Additionally postulated is a neuroprotective effect of lithium, with evidence to support benefit in neurodegenerative illnesses such as Alzheimer's disease.[26] Along with these advances, a clearer understanding of the action of lithium is developing.[22,45,80,95,120,121,192]

Among the first proposed mechanisms of action of lithium is the inositol-depletion hypothesis. Inositol is a six-carbon sugar that forms the backbone of a number of cellular signaling mechanisms. Lithium treatment results in decreased myoinositol (the most biologically active stereoisomer of inositol) concentration in the cerebral cortex.[6,26,95,114] Abnormalities in regional brain myoinositol concentrations are thought to occur in bipolar patients. This theory is partially supported by experimental magnetic resonance spectroscopy data.[195,229] Myoinositol is phosphorylated to form phosphatidyl inositol (PIP), which is further phosphorylated and combined with diacylglycerol (DAG) to form phosphatidyl 4,5 bisphosphate (PIP_2). Upon stimulation of a cell, G-protein–coupled receptors activate phospholipase C (PLC), which hydrolyzes PIP_2 to release the secondary messengers DAG and inositol 1,4,5 trisphosphate (IP_3).[95,191,195,229] Each of these secondary messengers in turn initiates a cascade of events, including activation of protein kinase C (PKC), which is important for calcium homeostasis and neurotransmitter release,[140,142,157,195] as well as independent mobilization and regulation of intracellular calcium.[18,55,152,174,195] Many extracellular signals, including some serotonin receptor subtypes, activate PLC to exert their actions.[88,139,162]

Serial dephosphorylation of IP_3 leads to regeneration of myoinositol and recycling of the inositol pool. Two enzymes involved in this pathway are inhibited by lithium. The first enzyme, inositol 1,4-bisphosphate 1-phosphatase (IPPase), dephosphorylates the bisphosphate to inositol monophosphate (IMP). The second enzyme, inositol-1-monophosphatase (IMPase), dephosphorylates IMP to myoinositol.

The inhibition of IMPase is interesting and important. First, the mechanism of inhibition is uncommon. Lithium noncompetitively inhibits IMPase by binding to the enzyme–substrate complex and preventing the release of a phosphate. It performs this function by displacing a magnesium ion from the active site after hydrolysis. Essentially, noncompetition means the higher the concentration of the substrate, the more the enzyme is inhibited.[9] This supports a theory about the pathophysiology of bipolar disorder involving an excess of myoinositol and is one reason why the mood-stabilizing effects of lithium are thought to occur only in bipolar patients.[95] That is, the noncompetitive nature of the action of lithium serves as a regulator to preferentially block pathologic signaling caused by excessive myoinositol while leaving the normal signaling intact. As described, IMPase is an important step in the cellular recycling of the inositol pool. Lithium inhibits the last step in this cycle.

Myoinositol is also generated de novo from glucose-6-phosphate by inositol synthase, which forms IMP. The inhibition of IMPase by lithium subsequently leads to myoinositol depletion by preventing the conversion of the newly synthesized IMP to inositol. Interestingly, valproic acid (VPA) also inhibits inositol synthase, illustrating a potential mechanism for the synergy of these complementary mood stabilizers.[160] A third mechanism of intracellular diminution of inositol by lithium (as well as VPA and carbamazepine) is the effect of lithium on reducing activity and transcription of the sodium myoinositol transporter (SMIT), preventing the uptake of exogenous myoinositol by the cell. This mechanism of inhibition may be overcome by increased extracellular concentration of myoinositol.[95,224]

The result of these effects is depletion of the inositol pool available to the cell, causing a series of events at different points in the signal transduction cascade that leads to differential gene transcription and expression. This sequence ultimately is responsible for the observed clinical effects of lithium on the central nervous system (CNS).[45,191] Experimental data using dextroamphetamine as a model for clinical mania demonstrate increased regional inositol signaling in the human brain, that is, attenuated by pretreatment with lithium, lending support to the hypothesis.[35]

The inositol depletion hypothesis represents an original attempt to explain in molecular terms the therapeutic effects of lithium. However, experimentally, this model does not fully elucidate nor replicate the clinical disease or response to therapy. In vivo studies with more drastic inositol depletion than from lithium therapy fail to replicate predicted behavioral patterns. Studies in knockout mice lacking various isoforms of inositol monophosphatase fail to replicate the antidepressant or antimanic effects of lithium. The model remains an attractive one, and the flaws may represent species variation with validity more in humans with bipolar disorder than the mouse model illustrates.[25,26,145]

A second compelling mechanism for the action of lithium is inhibition of the family of glycogen synthase kinase-3 (GSK3) kinases. GSK-3β overactivity is associated with neuronal degeneration and sensitivity to apoptotic stimulation. Dysregulation of GSK-3β is implicated in tumor growth and the neurofibrillary tangles of Alzheimer's disease.[225,226] GSK-3β is a key regulator of neuronal cell fate, with a proapoptotic effect in many settings.[3,25,27,62,73,98,107-109,145,178] GSK-3β is involved in regulating the activity of β-catenin, Jun and cAMP response element-binding protein (CREB), transcription factors important in embryonic patterning, cell proliferation, neuronal modeling and plasticity, neuronal signal transduction, and cytoskeletal remodeling. Lithium inhibits GSK-3β enzymatic activity directly through magnesium mimicry. Lithium also leads to indirect inhibition of GSK-3β through its interaction with the serine/threonine kinase Akt, which phosphorylates and inhibits GSK-3β. Lithium seems to accomplish this disparate inhibition by preventing the formation of a protein complex that is involved in G-protein–coupled receptor signaling. Dopaminergic neurotransmission through G-protein–coupled receptors is mediated through a protein complex that involves Akt, β-arrestin, and protein phosphatase 2A (Fig. 70–1). The complex, when active, dephosphorylates (deactivates) Akt in response to dopamine, leading to the activation of GSK-3β. Lithium disrupts assembly of the complex, which has the downstream effect of inactivation of GSK-3β, and the disruption of dopaminergic signaling. Lithium appears to be specific for this particular protein complex and seems to exert its inhibitory influence through displacement of the magnesium cofactor required for complex assembly. Evidence for this pathway is derived from in vivo models of mood-altering xenobiotics, such as phencyclidine models of schizophrenia, as opposed to in vitro biochemical studies.[31,159,165,228]

Inhibition of GSK-3β by lithium is thought to be neuroprotective.[3,26,45,91,96,169,179,180,231] Lithium is implicated in the neuroprotective modulation of the *bcl-2* gene, which is known for its role in preventing apoptosis and in downregulation of the proapoptotic protein *p53*. Lithium increases *bcl-2* levels in cultured nervous tissue of both rats and humans.[53,141,147] Additional support comes from patients undergoing long-term therapy with either lithium or VPA who show prefrontal cortex volumes significantly greater than in patients not treated with

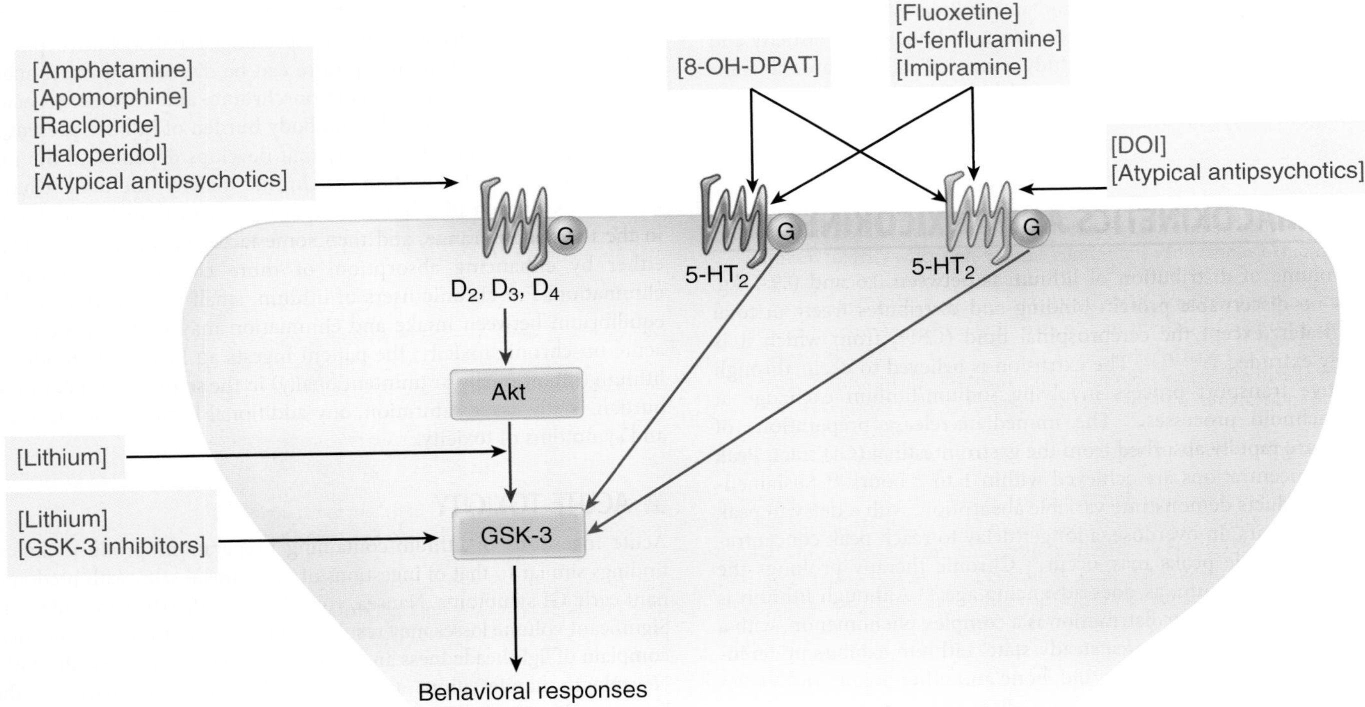

FIGURE 70–1. Lithium influences myriad signals of commonly encountered xenobiotics that affect the dopamine (D) and serotonin (5-HT) neurotransmitter systems through the common pathway of Akt/GSK-3 signaling, cumulating in an observable behavioral response. Lithium exerts these effects through direct inhibition of GSK-3 signaling and indirectly through upstream disruption of the Akt Pathway. 8-OH-DPAT = 8-Hydroxy-N,N-dipropyl-2-aminotetralin; DOI = 2,5-dimethoxy-4-iodoamphetamine; D2, D3, D4 = dopamine receptors; Akt = serine/threonine kinase Akt; GSK-3 = glycogen synthesis kinase -3.

either agent, suggesting a protective effect in humans.[45,56,66] Further evidence points toward a protective effect of lithium and possible therapeutic role in such neurodegenerative conditions as Parkinson's disease (in a mice model of Parkinson's disease using N-methyl-4-pheynyl-1, 2, 3, 6-tetrahydropyridine [MPTP]),[230] Huntington's disease,[52,190] amyotrophic lateral sclerosis (ALS),[77] and Alzheimer's disease.[3,22,23,26,47,122,123,135,145,149,158,170,206]

A link between GSK-3β activity and bipolar disorder and depression is supported by the finding that serotonergic activity inhibits GSK-3β in vivo.[125] Additional evidence of an interaction between serotonergic neurotransmission and inhibition of GSK-3β by specific serotonin reuptake inhibitors (SSRIs), monoamine oxidase inhibitors (MAOIs), and atypical antipsychotic agents lends further behavioral support to this theory.[27,124,125] Evidence from in vivo models of depression and mania implicate that GSK-3β is involved in regulation of behavioral stimulus by dopaminergic and serotoninergic neurotransmission.[25–33] Hypoxia contributes to increased GSK-3β activity, which may be counteracted or inhibited through mood-stabilizing drugs. Vascular depression, or depression after stroke, is an organic model of major depression.[148] The finding that this depressive state responds similarly to intervention with mood stabilizers lends further support to the GSK-3β hypothesis.[110] Thus, the diminished serotonergic activity associated with depression, or the hypoxic-induced activation of GSK-3β, may lead to impaired inhibition of GSK-3β. Mood stabilizers counteract this dysregulation and may explain their effectiveness in depression.[45,88,95,96,169,222]

In summary, although the precise mechanism of action is unknown, some common features of investigation have emerged. The potential targets, widely found and disparate in function, all seem to be inhibited by lithium in a noncompetitive fashion, most commonly through displacement of a divalent cation, usually Mg^{2+}. The systems affected by this inhibition vary widely. Downstream targets seem to modulate secondary cell messengers and intracellular signal transduction, transcription factors and gene expression, and neuronal plasticity and cellular differentiation. Further study is needed to elucidate the complex interaction of these pathways with the action of lithium to form an integrated hypothesis.

PHARMACOKINETICS AND TOXICOKINETICS

The volume of distribution of lithium is between 0.6 and 0.9 L/kg. It has no discernable protein binding and distributes freely in total body water, except the cerebrospinal fluid (CSF), from which it is actively extruded.[69,163,182,197] The extrusion is believed to occur through an active transport process involving sodium/lithium exchange at the arachnoid processes.[70] The immediate-release preparations of lithium are rapidly absorbed from the gastrointestinal (GI) tract. Peak serum concentrations are achieved within 1 to 2 hours.[105] Sustained-release products demonstrate variable absorption, with a delay to peak of 6 to 12 hours. In overdose, a longer delay to reach peak concentrations or multiple peaks may occur.[67] Chronic therapy prolongs the elimination of lithium, as does advancing age.[163] Although lithium is rapidly absorbed, tissue distribution is a complex phenomenon, with a significant delay in reaching a steady-state. Lithium exhibits preferential uptake into the kidney, thyroid, bone and other organs and tissues such as the liver and muscle. Lithium distribution into the brain can take up to 24 hours to reach equilibrium. Lithium is concentrated in red blood cells (RBCs) by both passive diffusion and active transport. The RBC concentration may correlate closely with the brain concentration, although this does not appear to be clinically useful.[50,71,173] The pharmacokinetic profile of lithium is described as an open, two-compartment model.[76,106]

Each 300-mg lithium carbonate tablet contains 8.12 mEq of lithium.[212] Ingestion of a single 300-mg tablet is expected to acutely increase the serum lithium concentration by approximately 0.1 to 0.3 mEq/L (assuming a volume of distribution of approximately 0.6–0.9 L/kg and a patient weight 50–100 kg).

Lithium is eliminated almost entirely (95%) by the kidneys, with a small amount eliminated in the feces.[105] Lithium is also found in sweat, saliva, and breast milk.[64,102,153] In an adult with normal renal function, lithium clearance ranges from 25 to 35 mL/min.[34,208,209] At steady-state equilibrium, total body clearance equals renal clearance.

Lithium is handled by the kidneys much in the same way as sodium. Lithium is freely filtered, and more than 60% is reabsorbed by the proximal tubule. Evidence also indicates a small amount of reabsorption by the loop of Henle and distal tubule.[10,40,41,65,79,119,163,212] Lithium excretion is therefore dependent on factors that affect the glomerular filtration rate (GFR) or decrease sodium concentration. Any condition that makes the kidney sodium avid such as volume depletion or salt restriction increases lithium reabsorption in the proximal tubule.[10] Thus, risk factors for development of lithium toxicity include advanced age with its decrease in GFR; use of thiazide diuretics, nonsteroidal antiinflammatory drugs (NSAIDs, or angiotensin-converting enzyme (ACE) inhibitors; decreased sodium intake; and low-output heart failure.[105,119]

The therapeutic to toxic index of lithium is narrow. The generally accepted steady-state therapeutic range of serum lithium concentrations is 0.6 to 1.2 mmol/L, although much disagreement exists about whether this serum concentration truly reflects therapeutic efficacy.[83,84,181] Both in therapeutic and overdose situations, clinical signs and symptoms seem to be a more valuable indicator of brain lithium concentrations.[181]

CLINICAL MANIFESTATIONS

Similar to other substances having prolonged redistributive phases and tissue burdens, lithium exposure can be divided into three main categories of toxicity: acute, acute-on-chronic, and chronic. In acute lithium toxicity, the patient has no body burden of lithium present at the time of ingestion. The toxicity that develops depends on the rate of absorption and distribution. In chronic toxicity, the patient has a stable body burden of lithium as serum concentration is maintained in the therapeutic range, and then some factor disturbs this balance, either by enhancing absorption, or more commonly, decreasing elimination. For chronic users of lithium, small perturbations in the equilibrium between intake and elimination may lead to toxicity. In acute-on-chronic toxicity, the patient ingests an increased amount of lithium (intentionally or unintentionally) in the setting of a stable body burden. With tissue saturation, any additional lithium leads to signs and symptoms of toxicity.

ACUTE TOXICITY

Acute ingestions of lithium-containing preparations produce clinical findings similar to that of ingestions of other metal salts, with predominant early GI symptoms. Nausea, vomiting, and diarrhea are prevalent. Significant volume losses may result from these symptoms. Patients may complain of lightheadedness and dizziness, and they may be orthostatic. Neurologic manifestations are a late finding in acute toxicity as the lithium redistributes slowly into the CNS.

Lithium is associated with a number of electrocardiographic (ECG) abnormalities, although the evidence for significant effects is lacking. Most reports are uncontrolled case reports without corroborating experimental data or biologic plausibility. The most commonly reported manifestation has been T-wave flattening or inversion, primarily in the precordial leads.[44,167,211] Lithium is also associated with prolongation of the QT interval.[227] One study associated elevated serum lithium concentrations with QT prolongation above 440 msec, although the number of patients studied was small.[101] Associations have been made between lithium and sinoatrial dysfunction, with resultant bradycardia.[85,166,194,205] Theoretically, this condition may result from the effect of lithium on G-protein–mediated cAMP generation and subsequent modification of calcium channel opening and calcium influx in the pacemaker cells.[44,101,167,211] Additional reports attempt to link lithium therapy with cardiomyopathy and unmasking of a Brugada pattern.[4,63,111] For the most part, lithium has few consequential effects on cardiac function, even in overdose, and malignant dysrhythmias or significant dysfunction is uncommon.[133,155,163]

CHRONIC TOXICITY

Lithium is primarily a neurotoxin. The earliest case reports of lithium toxicity described predominantly neurologic symptoms.[61,220] Of note, neurotoxicity does not correlate with serum concentrations. The initial clinical condition of the patient and the duration of exposure to an elevated concentration seem to be more closely predictive of outcome than the initial serum lithium concentration.[2,8,20,93,117,155,186,217]

Tremor, a common finding in patients undergoing chronic therapy, may increase with toxicity. Other findings of chronic toxicity include fasciculations, hyperreflexia, choreoathetoid movements, clonus, dysarthria, nystagmus, and ataxia.[163,212] Mental status is often altered and may progress from confusion to stupor, coma, and seizures.[46] Electroencephalographic changes are most frequently reported as "slowing."[193] The progression of these symptoms follows no order, and any patient undergoing chronic therapy may have one or any combination of these features.

The syndrome of irreversible lithium-effectuated neurotoxicity (SILENT) is a descriptive syndrome of the irreversible neurologic and neuropsychiatric sequelae of lithium toxicity.[2,171] SILENT is defined as neurologic dysfunction caused by lithium in the absence of prior neurologic illness, persists for at least 2 months after cessation of the drug. Case reports in the literature support these findings and this definition. However, as is true in most case reports, confounders make wide applicability of the findings difficult. Because of the polypharmacy prevalent in psychiatric treatment, long-term neurologic sequelae attributed to lithium are frequently described in patients using lithium in combination with other xenobiotics, such as haloperidol, chlorpromazine, carbamazepine, phenytoin, aspirin, VPA, amitriptyline, β-adrenergic antagonists, calcium channel blockers, ACE inhibitors, diuretics, and NSAIDs.[2,12,58,75,76,94,138,151,217] However, there are reports of patients using lithium without coingestants who had no comorbid illness and sustained lasting dysfunction as a result of lithium toxicity.[8,115,154,164,186,217] Cerebellar findings seem to predominate in patients with SILENT.[2,90,112,115,143] One of the predictors of persistent neurologic dysfunction seems to be the concomitant finding of hyperpyrexia, an ominous finding in patients with lithium toxicity.[90,143] The mechanism of the persistent dysfunction is unclear, but demyelination and cellular loss are proposed.[2,143,155,185]

ACUTE-ON-CHRONIC TOXICITY

Patients undergoing chronic therapy who acutely ingest an additional amount of lithium (either intentionally or unintentionally) are at risk for signs and symptoms of both acute and chronic toxicity. These patients may display prominent GI and neurologic symptoms and may be difficult to diagnose and manage. Serum lithium concentrations in cases of acute or chronic toxicity may be difficult to interpret, and therapy should be guided by the patient's clinical status.

OTHER SYSTEMIC MANIFESTATIONS OF CHRONIC LITHIUM THERAPY

The most common adverse effect of chronic lithium therapy is the development of nephrogenic diabetes insipidus. The process thought to be involved is the interference of lithium on magnesium-dependent G proteins that activate vasopressin-sensitive adenylate cyclase, leading to decreased generation of cAMP in the cell membranes of distal tubular cells.[54,143,198,218] Decreased cAMP leads to reduced expression and translocation of the vasopressin-regulated water channel aquaporin-2 (AQP2), making the distal tubules resistant to the action of vasopressin.[7,60,113,144,146,184,221] Lithium also inhibits the transport of sodium through the amiloride-sensitive Na^+ channel.[208]

Another theory proposed for the mechanism of lithium-induced nephrogenic diabetes insipidus suggests that lithium inhibits GSK-3β directly and through a phosphorylation pathway. GSK-3β exhibits tonic inhibition of cyclooxygenase-2 (COX-2). When this inhibition is removed by lithium, COX-2 activity leads to increased prostaglandin expression in the renal medulla. Increased prostaglandin expression is believed to be important in nephrogenic diabetes insipidus through regulation of glomerular blood flow.[136,175]

Chronic lithium therapy is also associated with chronic tubulointerstitial nephropathy, as manifested by the development of renal insufficiency with little or no proteinuria and biopsy findings of tubular cysts. This association was demonstrated in a biopsy-based study of 24 chronically treated patients, although the overall prevalence of this condition is low.[144]

Lithium is associated with a number of endocrine disorders. The most prevalent endocrine manifestation of chronic lithium therapy is hypothyroidism.[38,39,81,154] The causative etiology is multifactorial. Lithium is selectively concentrated in the thyroid gland and impairs iodine uptake, synthesis of triiodothyronine (T_3), responsiveness of the gland to thyroid-stimulating hormone (TSH), release of T_3 and tetraiodothyronine (T_4), and peripheral conversion of T_4 to T_3. Additionally, lithium decreases responsiveness of peripheral tissues to T_3 and leads to the development of antithyroglobulin antibodies (see Fig. 49-1).[13,161,223] Although hypothyroidism is most common, hyperthyroidism and frank thyrotoxicosis are also reported.[19] However, hyperthyroidism, by altering proximal tubule function, leads to decreased lithium excretion.[24] Thus, hyperthyroidism may lead to chronic lithium toxicity through impaired elimination, and the elevated lithium concentrations may mask the manifestations of hyperthyroidism.[161]

The combination of hyperparathyroidism and hypercalcemia is frequently reported with chronic lithium therapy, most commonly in women. The mechanism is thought to be modification of calcium feedback on parathyroid hormone release, although stimulation of parathyroid hyperplasia and adenomas is suggested.[1,11,37,118,196,212]

Developmentally, in utero exposure to lithium increases the incidence of congenital heart defects, specifically Ebstein anomaly.[102,169,196] Additionally, many effects similar to those that occur in patients undergoing chronic therapy are found in infants exposed in utero, including thyroid disease and neurotoxicity.[102]

Lithium causes a leukocytosis and an increase in neutrophils. It has been proposed as an adjunct to chemotherapy-induced neutropenia, other marrow suppressive therapies, and acquired immunodeficiency syndrome (AIDS). Although lithium increases the total neutrophil count, no improved clinical outcomes are documented, and its use has been superseded by recombinant colony-stimulating factors.[42,169,177,196,200]

DIAGNOSTIC TESTING

Because of the prevalence of lithium use, therapeutic drug monitoring is ready available in most settings, and concentrations should be readily obtainable. A lithium concentration should be requested upon patient presentation and serial measurements requested or considered in most instances, especially after ingestion of sustained-release preparations. Emphasis should be placed on the lithium concentration as a marker of exposure and response to therapy but not necessarily as a determinant of toxicity or treatment. The history, clinical signs, and symptoms rather than the absolute lithium concentration should guide therapy. The sample must be sent in an appropriate lithium-free tube, because use of lithiated-heparin tubes may lead to clinically false-positive results. Serum electrolyte concentrations and renal function should be monitored because renal function is important in determining the need for more aggressive therapy, including enhanced elimination techniques such as hemodialysis. If the patient is hypernatremic, nephrogenic diabetes insipidus should be suspected, and determinations of serum and urine osmolarity and electrolytes help confirm the diagnosis (see Chap. 16). If clinical thyroid disease is suspected, thyroid function tests should be obtained. If a deliberate ingestion, a serum acetaminophen concentration should be obtained. An ECG is also indicated. The complete blood count may indicate a leukocytosis, as a stress response or due to the hematologic effects of lithium.

MANAGEMENT

The initial management and stabilization should begin with assessment and, if necessary, support of airway, breathing, and circulation. Lithium rarely, if ever, affects the patient's airway or breathing, although coingestants may. Emesis, which occurs with significant frequency after acute exposure, may lead to aspiration and respiratory compromise. After the patient is stable, the characteristics of the exposure should be determined while the physical examination and laboratory assessment commence. The formulation and nature of the product should be ascertained and most importantly, identified as immediate-release or sustained-release. Also, whether or not lithium is part of the patient's medication regimen may help determine whether the ingestion is acute, acute-on-chronic, or chronic.

GASTROINTESTINAL DECONTAMINATION

For patients who present after an acute overdose or an acute-on-chronic overdose, a risk benefit analysis of GI decontamination must be undertaken. Two factors should be considered. With an acute overdose and predominance of early GI symptoms, including emesis, self-decontamination may already have started. Second, immediate-release preparations are often rapidly absorbed and may not lend themselves to GI evacuation.

Few GI decontamination options are available. Although syrup of ipecac is no longer generally recommended as a standard decontamination choice, because activated charcoal is not an effective adsorbent for lithium, emesis may still be useful in certain instances after ingestion of sustained-release lithium preparations when care may be delayed or is distant, as in remote or rural areas. Whereas immediate-release preparations of lithium are rapidly absorbed and typically produce emesis, sustained-release formulations of lithium (ie, controlled-release tablets) compounded in a slowly dissolving film-coated formulation often make the tablet too large to fit through even the largest lavage tube. Thus, orogastric lavage has essentially no role in the acute management of a patient with an lithium overdose unless indicated for a coingestant.

Lithium is a monovalent cation that does not bind readily to activated charcoal.[130] Because no beneficial effect from activated charcoal is expected, the danger of a depressed level of consciousness, potential loss of protective airway reflexes, and prominent emesis and the possible need for subsequent endoscopy for a coingestant-related problem contraindicate activated charcoal use except for treatment of a potential coingestant.

Sodium polystyrene sulfonate (SPS) is a cationic exchange resin often used for the treatment of severe hyperkalemia. It binds potassium in exchange for sodium, allowing elimination of excess potassium in the feces. Because of the similarity between potassium and lithium, use of SPS has been proposed for decontamination of patients being treated for lithium toxicity. A number of models have examined the effectiveness of this technique.[126–134] Use of SPS has many theoretical benefits, including demonstrated effectiveness of lithium binding compared with activated charcoal and the ability of orally administered SPS to reduce serum concentrations of intravenously administered lithium in mice.[128–130] Unfortunately, the finding that doses used to increase lithium elimination also lead to significant hypokalemia in human subjects limits the application of this technique.[129,183] In a murine model, potassium supplementation with SPS was found to mitigate this process but only at the expense of elevating lithium concentrations.[134] Two reports in the literature demonstrate increased lithium elimination with SPS, one in a healthy volunteer and another in a patient with an acute overdose. However, the serum potassium concentration was not reported in either case.[82,176] At present, use of SPS in the management of the lithium-poisoned patient cannot be routinely recommended.

Whole-bowel irrigation (WBI) is the only GI decontamination modality that has shown any efficacy in eliminating lithium from human subjects. In one of the few clinical trials of WBI, the serum lithium concentrations of 10 normal volunteers who had ingested sustained-release lithium carbonate were plotted against time over a 72-hour period. In the second phase of the trial, the volunteers received 2 L/h of polyethylene glycol solution 1 hour after the ingestion with a significant reduction (67%) in the serum concentration, even as early as 1 hour after the therapeutic intervention.[199] Thus, use of WBI is recommended for sustained-release preparations.

FLUID AND ELECTROLYTES

The critical initial management of the lithium-poisoned patient should focus on restoration of intravascular volume, both in acute poisonings with GI losses and in chronic poisonings with toxic effects that are often the result of disturbances of renal function and lithium elimination. Many patients with lithium toxicity have volume-responsive decreases in renal function,[163] which can be managed by infusion of 0.9% sodium chloride solution at 1.5 to two times the maintenance rate. This therapy increases renal perfusion, increases the GFR, and lithium elimination. Urine output must be closely monitored and any electrolyte abnormalities corrected. Caution must be used in patients with renal insufficiency, renal failure, and congestive heart failure. Monitoring for the development of hypernatremia in patients suspected of having nephrogenic diabetes insipidus is critical.[212]

Lithium-induced nephrogenic diabetes insipidus may be reversed by discontinuation of the drug and repletion of electrolytes and free water. However, nonreversible effects have been reported.[137,144,207] Clinical application of amiloride to mitigate lithium-induced polyuria has been described, although the potential for volume contraction and stimulation of lithium reabsorption limits recommendation of this drug as a routine adjunct to acute care.[21,74,78,116]

Any attempt to enhance elimination of lithium by forced diuresis using loop diuretics (furosemide), osmotic agents (mannitol), carbonic anhydrase inhibitors (acetazolamide), or phosphodiesterase inhibitors (aminophylline) should be avoided. An initial small increase in elimination may be achieved, but typically salt and water depletion subsequently develop followed by increased lithium retention. Sodium bicarbonate for urinary alkalinization should also be avoided because it does not significantly increase elimination over volume expansion with sodium chloride and may lead to hypokalemia, alkalemia, and fluid overload.

EXTRACORPOREAL DRUG REMOVAL

Debate surrounds the efficacy and practicality of using enhanced elimination techniques in cases of lithium poisoning. Lithium does have physiochemical properties that make it amenable to extracorporeal removal,[97,104,105,119] and with these characteristics, it would seem to be an ideal candidate for hemodialysis. In fact, hemodialysis is often recommended for treatment of acute, acute-on-chronic, and chronic lithium toxicity.[14,103–105,143,168,204,212,219] However, some characteristics of lithium make extracorporeal elimination difficult. Lithium is predominantly localized intracellularly and diffuses slowly across cell membranes.[163] When traditional intermittent hemodialysis is used for chronic exposures, clearance of the blood compartment is often followed by a rebound phenomenon of redistribution from tissue stores, leading to increased serum concentrations, in some cases approaching predialysis concentrations.[43] An additional complicating factor is that the brain, the "target organ" of toxicity, is not amenable to a rapid artificial elimination process. Attempts have been made to correlate the serum concentration with the lithium concentration in the CSF and brain. But in the few studies where CSF concentrations were obtained, although serum and CSF lithium concentrations seemed to correlate, brain concentrations and toxicity did not.[105,189] Magnetic resonance spectroscopy studies of bipolar patients with steady-state lithium concentrations demonstrated a significant variability between brain and serum concentrations, especially within the therapeutic range.[105,181,189] No consensus recommendation on the appropriate time to initiate therapy is available.[14,105,183] In addition, because of the toxicokinetic profile of lithium, serum concentrations do not correlate well with toxicity.[68,105,201,212]

Hemodialysis or an alternative extracorporeal technique is clearly indicated for three groups of patients. The first group consists of patients who are manifesting severe signs and symptoms of neurotoxicity, such as alterations in mental status. The second group consists of patients who have renal failure and show signs or symptoms of lithium toxicity. Such patients are unable to eliminate their lithium burden on their own and should undergo hemodialysis. The third group consists of patients who show little or no sign of toxicity but who cannot tolerate sodium repletion therapy; these patients who should be considered for early hemodialysis includes patients with congestive heart failure or such "redistributive diseases" as liver failure, pancreatitis, or sepsis.

For a patient who belongs to this last group, the next step is to determine the probability that the patient will develop toxicity if elimination is not enhanced. Although serum concentrations do not necessarily correlate with toxicity, they can nevertheless be a useful aid to making the decision for hemodialysis. As an adjunct to the clinical presentation, an absolute lithium concentration above 4.0 mEq/L (mmol/L) with any type of overdose or a concentration of greater than 2.5 mEq/L with chronic toxicity should prompt dialysis. These criteria originate from a case series of 23 patients and a review of 100 other patients published in 1978, which was before the introduction of sustained-release products.[93] Although this recommendation has never been prospectively evaluated (or subsequently reevaluated), it still can serve as a useful guide in the management of lithium-poisoned patients.[14,34]

The dialysate bath should contain bicarbonate rather than acetate to help lessen the intracellular sequestration of lithium that occurs from the activation of the sodium/potassium antiporter and preferential intracellular transport of lithium.[168,204]

Whether hemodialysis diminishes or enhances the risk of permanent neurologic sequelae is a subject of debate.[202,203] Although no controlled studies have analyzed this important management question, the preponderance of evidence suggests a reduced risk.[2,8,14,73,100,105,143,150,163,168,186,212]

Continuous venovenous hemodialysis and continuous venovenous hemodiafiltration are two continuous renal replacement therapies (CRRTs) commonly used in the treatment of patients with acute renal failure or volume overload and for elimination of xenobiotics.[34,119,214–216] Both techniques are effective in patients who are hemodynamically unstable because blood flow through the filter is pump driven and is not dependent on the arterial blood pressure.[97] Other continuous techniques that use patient blood pressure as the basis of flow through the system also may have application here.[215] Traditional intermittent hemodialysis offers clearance rates that vary between 50 and 170 mL/min.[34,36,119,163,168,215] Although CRRT techniques offer lower clearance per hour than does intermittent hemodialysis, their overall daily clearances are similar.[34,119] With continued improvements in techniques, use of high volumes, and high dialysate flow rates, clearances are improving, approaching more than half the clearance per hour achieved by intermittent hemodialysis in some studies.[34,97,119,215] Although one case of a rebound concentration was reported in a patient treated with continuous arteriovenous hemodiafiltration,[36] no cases with use of the venovenous techniques have been reported, offering a clear advantage over intermittent hemodialysis. Unfortunately, CRRT requires prolonged anticoagulation with its inherent risks. Nevertheless, these techniques may be beneficial in patients who are hemodynamically unstable, or they may be used in series with traditional dialysis in other patients to prevent redistribution of lithium and rebound of serum concentrations (see Chap. 9).

Peritoneal dialysis (PD) offers no increased efficacy of clearance of lithium over the natural clearance of normal kidneys.[14,97,105,183] Although recommended in the past, given its lack of efficacy coupled with its infrequent use and potential for serious complications such as bowel perforation, PD has no role in the management of lithium-poisoned patients.

SUMMARY

Lithium is a simple ion with extensive current usage and extremely varied and complex clinical and pathophysiologic effects. It is available in multiple formulations, both immediate release and sustained release, and is an essential part of the pharmacologic arsenal of clinical psychiatry. Because of the complexity of the pharmacokinetic profile of lithium, toxicity may develop in a wide range of conditions and may be precipitated by both intentional overdose and therapeutic misadventure. The care of lithium-poisoned patients should be predicated on rapid clinical evaluation of the patient's condition coupled with identification of the poisoning and followed by management that includes the use of volume resuscitation and, when indicated, WBI and hemodialysis or other extracorporeal techniques to prevent or treat severe neurologic morbidity and to prevent mortality.

REFERENCES

1. Abdullah H, Bliss R, Guinea AI, et al. Pathology and outcome of surgical treatment for lithium-associated hyperparathyroidism. *Br J Surg.* 1999;86:91-93.
2. Adityanjee, Munshi KR, Thampy A. The syndrome of irreversible lithium-effectuated neurotoxicity. *Clin Neuropharmacol.* 2005;28:38-49.
3. Aghdam SY, Barger SW. Glycogen synthase kinase-3 in neurodegeneration and neuroprotection: lessons from lithium. *Curr Alzheimer Res.* 2007;4:21-31.
4. Aichhorn W, Huber R, Stuppaeck C, et al. Cardiomyopathy after long-term treatment with lithium—more than a coincidence? *J Psychopharmacol.* 2006;20:589-591.

5. Aita JF, Aita JA, Aita VA. 7-Up anti-acid lithiated lemon soda or early medicinal use of lithium. *Nebr Med J.* 1990;75:277-279.
6. Allison JH, Stewart MA. Reduced brain inositol in lithium-treated rats. *Nat New Biol.* 1971;233:267-268.
7. Anai H, Ueta Y, Serino R, et al. Upregulation of the expression of vasopressin gene in the paraventricular and supraoptic nuclei of the lithium-induced diabetes insipidus rat. *Brain Res.* 1997;772:161-166.
8. Apte SN, Langston JW. Permanent neurological deficits due to lithium toxicity. *Ann Neurol.* 1983;13:453-455.
9. Atack JR, Broughton HB, Pollack SJ. Structure and mechansim of inositol monophosphatase. *FEBS Lett.* 1995;361:1-7.
10. Atherton JC, Doyle A, Gee A, et al. Lithium clearance: modification by the loop of Henle in man. *J Physiol.* 1991;437:377-391.
11. Awad SS, Miskulin J, Thompson N. Parathyroid adenomas versus four-gland hyperplasia as the cause of primary hyperparathyroidism in patients with prolonged lithium therapy. *World J Surg.* 2003;27:486-488.
12. Baastrup PC, Hollnagel P, Sorensen R, et al. Adverse reactions in treatment with lithium carbonate and haloperidol. *JAMA.* 1976;236:2645-2646.
13. Baethge C, Blumentritt H, Berghofer A, et al. Long-term lithium treatment and thyroid antibodies: a controlled study. *J Psychiatry Neurosci.* 2005;30:423-427.
14. Bailey B, McGuigan M. Comparison of patients hemodialyzed for lithium poisoning and those for whom dialysis was recommended by PCC but not done: what lesson can we learn? *Clin Nephrol.* 2000;54:388-392.
15. Baldessarini RJ, Tondo L. Suicide risk and treatments for patients with bipolar disorder. *JAMA.* 2003;290:1157-1159.
16. Baldessarini RJ, Tondo L, Davis P, et al. Decreased risk of suicides and attempts during long-term lithium treatment: a meta-analytic review. *Bipolar Disord.* 2006;8:625-639.
17. Baldessarini RJ, Tondo L, Hennen J. Treating the suicidal patients with bipolar disorder: reducing suicidal risk with lithium. *Ann NY Acad Sci.* 2001;932:24-38.
18. Baraban JM, Worley PF, Snyder SH. Second messenger systems and psychoactive drug action: focus on the phosphoinositide system and lithium. *Am J Psychiatry.* 1989;146:1251-1260.
19. Barclay ML, Brownlie BE, Turner JG, et al. Lithium associated thyrotoxicosis: a report of 14 cases, with statistical analysis of incidence. *Clin Endocrinol (Oxf).* 1994;40:759-764.
20. Bartha L, Marksteiner J, Bauer G, et al. Persistent cognitive deficits associated with lithium intoxication: a neuropsychological case description. *Cortex.* 2002;38:743-752.
21. Batlle DC, von Riotte AB, Gaviria M, et al. Amelioration of polyuria by amiloride in patients receiving long-term lithium therapy. *N Engl J Med.* 1985;312:408-414.
22. Bauer M, Alda M, Priller J, et al. Implications of the neuroprotective effects of lithium for the treatment of bipolar and neurodegenerative disorders. *Pharmacopsychiatry.* 2003;36(suppl 3):S250-S254.
23. Baum L, Seger R, Woodgett JR, et al. Overexpressed tau protein in cultured cells is phosphorylated without formation of PHF: implication of phosphoprotein phosphatase involvement. *Brain Res Mol Brain Res.* 1995;34:1-17.
24. Baum M, Dwarakanath V, Alpern RJ, et al. Effects of thyroid hormone on the neonatal renal cortical Na+/H+ antiporter. *Kidney Int.* 1998;53:1254-1258.
25. Beaulieu JM. Not only lithium: regulation of glycogen synthase kinase-3 by antipsychotics and serotonergic drugs. *Int J Neuropsychopharmacol.* 2007;10:3-6.
26. Beaulieu JM, Caron MG. Looking at lithium: molecular moods and complex behaviour. *Mol Interv.* 2008;8:230-241.
27. Beaulieu JM, Gainetdinov RR, Caron MG. Akt/GSK3 signaling in the action of psychotropic drugs. *Annu Rev Pharmacol Toxicol.* 2009;49:327-347.
28. Beaulieu JM, Gainetdinov RR, Caron MG. The Akt-GSK-3 signaling cascade in the actions of dopamine. *Trends Pharmacol Sci.* 2007;28:166-172.
29. Beaulieu JM, Marion S, Rodriguiz RM, et al. A beta-arrestin 2 signaling complex mediates lithium action on behavior. *Cell.* 2008;132:125-136.
30. Beaulieu JM, Sotnikova TD, Marion S, et al. An Akt/beta-arrestin 2/PP2A signaling complex mediates dopaminergic neurotransmission and behavior. *Cell.* 2005;122:261-273.
31. Beaulieu JM, Sotnikova TD, Yao WD, et al. Lithium antagonizes dopamine-dependent behaviors mediated by an AKT/glycogen synthase kinase 3 signaling cascade. *Proc Natl Acad Sci U S A.* 2004;101:5099-5104.
32. Beaulieu JM, Tirotta E, Sotnikova TD, et al. Regulation of Akt signaling by D2 and D3 dopamine receptors in vivo. *J Neurosci.* 2007;27:881-885.
33. Beaulieu JM, Zhang X, Rodriguiz RM, et al. Role of GSK3 beta in behavioral abnormalities induced by serotonin deficiency. *Proc Natl Acad Sci U S A.* 2008;105:1333-1338.
34. Beckman U, Oakley PW, Dawson AH, et al. Efficacy of continuous venovenous hemodialysis in the treatment of severe lithium toxicity. *Clin Toxicol.* 2001;39:393-397.
35. Bell EC, Willson MC, Wilman AH, et al. Lithium and valproate attenuate dextroamphetamine-induced changes in brain activation. *Hum Psychopharmacol Clin Exp.* 2005;20:87-96.
36. Bellomo R, Kearly Y, Parkin G, et al. Treatment of life-threatening lithium toxicity with continuous arterio-venous hemodiafiltration. *Crit Care Med.* 1991;19:836-837.
37. Bendz H, Sjodin I, Toss G, et al. Hyperparathyroidism and long-term lithium therapy—a cross-sectional study and the effect of lithium withdrawal. *J Intern Med.* 1996;240:357-365.
38. Bocchetta A, Cocco F, Velluzzi F, et al. Fifteen-year follow-up of thyroid function in lithium patients. *J Endocrinol Invest.* 2007;30:363-366.
39. Bocchetta A, Loviselli A. Lithium treatment and thyroid abnormalities. *Clin Pract Epidemol Ment Health.* 2006;2:23.
40. Boer WH, Fransen R, Shirley DG, et al. Evaluation of the lithium clearance method: direct analysis of tubular lithium handling by micropuncture. *Kidney Int.* 1995;47:1023-1030.
41. Boer WH, Koomans HA, Dorhout Mees EJ. Lithium clearance in healthy humans suggesting lithium reabsorption beyond the proximal tubules. *Kidney Int Suppl.* 1990;28(suppl):S39-S44.
42. Boggs D, Joyce RA. The hematopoietic effects of lithium. *Semin Hematol.* 1983;20:129-138.
43. Bosinski T, Bailie GR, Eisele G. Massive and extended rebound of serum lithium concentrations following hemodialysis in two chronic overdose cases. *Am J Emerg Med.* 1998;16:98-100.
44. Brady HR, Horgan JH. Lithium and the heart. Unanswered questions. *Chest.* 1988;93:166-169.
45. Brunello N, Tascedda F. Cellular mechanisms and second messengers: relevance to the psychopharmacology of bipolar disorders. *Int J Neuropsychopharmacol.* 2003;6:181-189.
46. Brust JC, Hammer JS, Challenor Y, et al. Acute generalized polyneuropathy accompanying lithium poisoning. *Ann Neurol.* 1979;6:360-362.
47. Caccamo A, Oddo S, Tran LX, et al. Lithium reduces tau phosphorylation but not A beta or working memory deficits in a transgenic model with both plaques and tangles. *Am J Pathol.* 2007;170:1669-1675.
48. Cade JF. John Frederick Joseph Cade: family memories on the occasion of the 50th anniversary of his discovery of the use of lithium in mania. 1949. *Aust N Z J Psychiatry.* 1999;33:615-618.
49. Cade JF. Lithium salts in the treatment of psychotic excitement. 1949. *Bull World Health Organ.* 2000;78:518-520.
50. Camus M, Hennere G, Baron G, et al. Comparison of lithium concentrations in red blood cells and plasma in samples collected for TDM, acute toxicity, or acute-on-chronic toxicity. *Eur J Clin Pharmacol.* 2003;59:583-587.
51. Cantor C. The impact of lithium long-term medication on suicidal behavior and mortality of bipolar patients. *Arch Suicide Res.* 2006;10:303-304.
52. Carmichael J, Sugars KL, Bao YP, et al. Glycogen synthase kinase-3-beta inhibitors prevent cellular polyglutamine toxicity caused by the Huntington's disease mutation. *J Biol Chem.* 2002;277:33791-33798.
53. Chen G, Zeng WZ, Yuan PX, et al. The mood-stabilizing agents lithium and valproate robustly increase the levels of the neuroprotective protein bcl-2 in the CNS. *J Neurochem.* 1999;72:879-882.
54. Christensen S, Kusano E, Yusufi AN, et al. Pathogenesis of nephrogenic diabetes insipidus due to chronic administration of lithium in rats. *J Clin Invest.* 1985;75:1869-1879.
55. Chuang D. Neurotransmitter receptors and phosphoinositide turnover. *Annu Rev Pharmacol Toxicol.* 1989;29:71-110.
56. Chuang DM, Chen RW, Chelecka-Franaszek E, et al. Neuroprotective effects of lithium in culutured cells and animal models of diseases. *Bipolar Disord.* 2002;4:129-136.
57. Cipriani A, Smith K, Burgess S, et al. Lithium versus antidepressants in the long-term treatment of unipolar affective disorder. *Cochrane Database Syst Rev.* 2006:CD003492.

58. Cohen WJ, Cohen NH. Lithium carbonate, haloperidol, and irreversible brain damage. *JAMA*. 1974;230:1283-1287.
59. Connemann BJ. Lithium and suicidality revisited. *Am J Psychiatry*. 2006; 163:550.
60. Connolly DL, Shanahan CM, Weissberg PL. Water channels in health and disease. *Lancet*. 1996;347:210-212.
61. Corcoran AC, Taylor RD, Page IH. Lithium poisoning from the use of salt substitutes. *JAMA*. 1949;139:685-688.
62. Cross D, Culbert AA, Chalmers KA, et al. Selective small-molecule inhibitors of glycogen synthase kinase-3 activity protect primary neurones from death. *J Neurochem*. 2001;77:94-102.
63. Darbar D, Yang T, Churchwell K, et al. Unmasking of brugada syndrome by lithium. *Circulation*. 2005;112:1527-1531.
64. Dodd S, Berk M. The pharmacology of bipolar disorder during pregnancy and breastfeeding. *Expert Opin Drug Saf*. 2004;3:221-229.
65. Dorhout Mees EJ, Beutler JJ, Boer WH, et al. Does lithium clearance reflect distal delivery in humans? Analysis with furosemide infusion. *Am J Physiol*. 1990;258:F1100-1104.
66. Drevets WC. Functional anatomical abnormalities in limbic and prefrontal cortical structures in major depression. *Prog Brain Res*. 2000;126: 413-431.
67. Dupuis RE, Cooper AA, Rosamond LJ, et al. Multiple delayed peak lithium concentrations following acute intoxication with an extended-release product. *Ann Pharmacother*. 1996;30:356-360.
68. Dyson EH, Simpson D, Prescott LF, et al. Self-poisoning and therapeutic intoxication with lithium. *Hum Toxicol*. 1987;6:325-329.
69. Ehrlich BE, Diamond JM. Lithium, membranes, and manic-depressive illness. *J Membr Biol*. 1980;52:187-200.
70. Ehrlich BE, Wright EM. Choline and PAH transport across blood-CSF barriers: the effect of lithium. *Brain Res*. 1982;250:245-249.
71. El Balkhi S, Megarbane B, Poupon J, et al. Lithium poisoning: is determination of the red blood cell lithium concentration useful? *Clin Toxicol*. 2009;47:8-13.
72. Eyer F, Pfab R, Felgenhauer N, et al. Lithium poisoning: pharmacokinetics and clearance during different therapeutic measures. *J Clin Psychopharmacol*. 2006;26:325-330.
73. Facci L, Stevens DA, Skaper SD. Glycogen synthase kinase-3 inhibitors protect central neurons against excitotoxicity. *Neuroreport*. 2003;14: 1467-1470.
74. Finch CK, Kelley KW, Williams RB. Treatment of lithium-induced diabetes insipidus with amiloride. *Pharmacotherapy*. 2003;23:546-550.
75. Finley PR, O'Brien JG, Coleman RW. Lithium and angiotensin-converting enzyme inhibitors: evaluation of a potential interaction. *J Clin Psychopharmacol*. 1996;16:68-71.
76. Finley PR, Warner MD, Peabody CA. Clinical relevance of drug interactions with lithium. *Clin Pharmacokinet*. 1995;29:172-191.
77. Fornai F, Longone P, Cafaro L, et al. Lithium delays progression of amyotrophic lateral sclerosis. *Proc Natl Acad Sci U S A*. 2008;105: 2052-2057.
78. Fransen R, Boer WH, Boer P, et al. Amiloride-sensitive lithium reabsorption in rats: a micropuncture study. *J Pharmacol Exp Ther*. 1992;263: 646-650.
79. Fransen R, Boer WH, Boer P, et al. Effects of furosemide or acetazolamide infusion on renal handling of lithium: a micropuncture study in rats. *Am J Physiol*. 1993;264:R129-R134.
80. Friedrich MJ. Molecular studies probe bipolar disorder. *JAMA*. 2005;293: 535-536.
81. Frye MA, Yatham L, Ketter TA, et al. Depressive relapse during lithium treatment associated with increased serum thyroid-stimulating hormone: results from two placebo-controlled bipolar I maintenance studies. *Acta Psychiatr Scand*. 2009;120(1):10-13.
82. Gehrke JC, Watling SM, Gehrke CW, et al. In-vivo binding of lithium using the cation exchange resin sodium polystyrene sulfonate. *Am J Emerg Med*. 1996;14:37-38.
83. Gelenberg AJ, Carroll JA, Baudhuin MG, et al. The meaning of serum lithium levels in maintenance therapy of mood disorders: a review of the literature. *J Clin Psychiatry*. 1989;50(suppl):17-22.
84. Gelenberg AJ, Kane JM, Keller MB, et al. Comparison of standard and low serum levels of lithium for maintenance treatment of bipolar disorder. *N Engl J Med*. 1989;321:1489-1493.
85. Goldberger ZD. Sinoatrial block in lithium toxicity. *Am J Psychiatry*. 2007;164:831-832.
86. Gonzalez-Pinto A, Mosquera F, Alonso M, et al. Suicidal risk in bipolar I disorder patients and adherence to long-term lithium treatment. *Bipolar Disord*. 2006;8:618-624.
87. Goodwin FK, Fireman B, Simon GE, et al. Suicide risk in bipolar disorder during treatment with lithium and divalproex. *JAMA*. 2003;290: 1467-1473.
88. Gould E, Gross CG. Neurogenesis in adult mammals: some progress and problems. *J Neurosci*. 2002;22:619-623.
89. Grandjean EM, Aubry JM. Lithium: updated human knowledge using an evidence-based approach: part I: clinical efficacy in bipolar disorder. *CNS Drugs*. 2009;23:225-240.
90. Grignon S, Bruguerolle B. Cerebellar lithium toxicity: a review of recent literature and tentative pathophysiology. *Therapie*. 1996;51:101-106.
91. Hall AC, Lucas FR, Salinas PC. Axonal remodeling and synaptic differentiation in the cerebellum is regulated by Wnt-7a signaling. *Cell*. 2000;100: 525-535.
92. Hanlon LW, Romaine MI, Gilroy FJ, et al. Lithium chloride as a substitute for sodium chloride in the diet. *JAMA*. 1949;139:688-692.
93. Hansen HE, Amdisen A. Lithium intoxication. (Report of 23 cases and review of 100 cases from the literature). *Q J Med*. 1978;47:123-144.
94. Harvey NS, Merriman S. Review of clinically important drug interactions with lithium. *Drug Saf*. 1994;10:455-463.
95. Harwood AJ. Lithium and bipolar mood disorder: the inositol-depletion hypothesis revisited. *Mol. Psychiatry*. 2005;10:117-126.
96. Harwood AJ, Agam G. Search for a common mechanism of mood stabilizers. *Biochem Pharmacol*. 2003;66:179-189.
97. Hazouard E, Ferrandiere M, Rateau H, et al. Continuous veno-venous haemofiltration versus continuous veno-venous haemodialysis in severe lithium self-poisoning: a toxicokinetics study in an intensive care unit. *Nephrol Dial Transplant*. 1999;14:1605-1606.
98. Hetman M, Cavanaugh JE, Kimelman D, et al. Role of glycogen synthase kinase-3B in neuronal apoptosis induced by trophic withdrawal. *J Neurosci*. 2000;20:2567-2574.
99. Hollander E, Pallanti S, Allen A, et al. Does sustained-release lithium reduce impulsive gambling and affective instability versus placebo in pathological gamblers with bipolar spectrum disorders? *Am J Psychiatry*. 2005;162:137-145.
100. Holubek WJ, Hoffman RS, Goldfarb DS, et al. Use of hemodialysis and hemoperfusion in poisoned patients. *Kidney Int*. 2008;74:1327-1334.
101. Hsu CH, Liu PY, Chen JH, et al. Electrocardiographic abnormalities as predictors for over-range lithium levels. *Cardiology*. 2005;103:101-106.
102. Iqbal MM, Sohhan T, Mahmud SZ. The effects of lithium, valproic acid, and carbamazepine during pregnancy and lactation. *J Toxicol Clin Toxicol*. 2001;39:381-392.
103. Jacobsen D, Aasen G, Frederichsen P, et al. Lithium intoxication: pharmacokinetics during and after terminated hemodialysis in acute intoxications. *Clin Toxicol*. 1987;25:81-94.
104. Jaeger A, Sauder P, Kopferschmitt J, et al. Toxicokinetics of lithium intoxication treated by hemodialysis. *J Toxicol Clin Toxicol*. 1985;23:501-517.
105. Jaeger A, Sauder P, Kopferschmitt J, et al. When should dialysis be performed in lithium poisoning? A kinetic study in 14 cases of lithium poisoning. *J Toxicol Clin Toxicol*. 1993;31:429-447.
106. Jermain DM, Crismon ML, Martin ES 3rd. Population pharmacokinetics of lithium. *Clin Pharm*. 1991;10:376-381.
107. Jin N, Kovacs AD, Sui Z, et al. Opposite effects of lithium and valproic acid on trophic factor deprivation-induced glycogen synthase kinase-3 activation, c-Jun expression and neuronal cell death. *Neuropharmacology*. 2005;48:576-583.
108. Jope R. Lithium and GSK3: one inhibitor, two inhibitory actions, multiple outcomes. *Trends Pharmacol Sci*. 2003;24:441-443.
109. Jope RS, Johnson GV. The glamour and gloom of glycogen synthase kinase-3. *Trends Biochem Sci*. 2004;29:95-102.
110. Jorge RE, Robinson RG, Arndt S, et al. Mortality and poststroke depression: a placebo-controlled trial of antidepressants. *Am J Psychiatry*. 2003;160: 1823-1829.
111. Josephson IR, Lederer WJ, Hartmann HA. Letter regarding article by Darbar et al, "unmasking of Brugada syndrome by lithium." *Circulation*. 2006;113:e408.
112. Juul-Jensen P, Schou M.Permanent brain damage after lithium intoxication [letter]. *Br Med J*. 1973;4:673.
113. King LS, Agre P. Pathophysiology of the aquaporin water channels. *Annu Rev Physiol*. 1996;58:619-648.

114. Kofman O, Belmaker RH. Biochemical, behavioral, and clinical studies of the role of inositol in lithium treatment and depression. *Biol Psychiatry.* 1993;34:839-852.
115. Kores B, Lader MH. Irreversible lithium neurotoxicity: an overview. *Clin Neuropharmacol.* 1997;20:283-299.
116. Kosten TR, Forrest JN. Treatment of severe lithium-induced polyuria with amiloride. *Am J Psychiatry.* 1986;143:1563-1568.
117. Lang EJ, Davis SM. Lithium neurotoxicity: the development of irreversible neurological impairment despite standard monitoring of serum lithium levels. *J Clin Neurosci.* 2002;9:308-309.
118. Laroche M, Lamboley V, Amigues JM, et al. Hyperparathyroidism during lithium therapy. Two new cases. *Rev Rheum Engl Ed.* 1997;64:132-134.
119. Leblanc M, Raymond M, Bonnardeaux A, et al. Lithium poisoning treated by high-performance continuous arteriovenous and venovenous hemodiafiltration. *Am J Kidney Dis.* 1996;27:365-372.
120. Lenox RH, Hahn CG. Overview of the mechanism of action of lithium in the brain: fifty-year update. *J Clin Psychiatry.* 2000;61:5-15.
121. Lenox RH, McNamara RK, Papke RL, et al. Neurobiology of lithium: an update. *J Clin Psychiatry.* 1998;59:37-47.
122. Leyhe T, Eschweiler GW, Stransky E, et al. Increase of BDNF serum concentration in lithium treated patients with early Alzheimer's disease. *J Alzheimers Dis.* 2009;16:649-656.
123. Li X, Lu F, Tian Q, et al. Activation of glycogen synthase kinase-3 induces Alzheimer-like tau hyperphosphorylation in rat hippocampus slices in culture. *J Neural Transm.* 2006;113:93-102.
124. Li X, Rosborough KM, Friedman AB, et al. Regulation of mouse brain glycogen synthase kinase-3 by atypical antipsychotics. *Int J Neuropsychopharmacol.* 2007;10:7-19.
125. Li X, Zhu W, Roh MS, et al. In vivo regulation of glycogen synthase kinase-3beta (GSK3beta) by serotonergic activity in mouse brain. *Neuropsychopharmacology.* 2004;29:1426-1431.
126. Linakis JG, Eisenberg MS, Lacouture PG, et al. Multiple-dose sodium polystyrene sulfonate in lithium intoxication: an animal model. *Pharmacol Toxicol.* 1992;70:38-40.
127. Linakis JG, Hull KM, Lee CM, et al. Effect of delayed treatment with sodium polystyrene sulfonate on serum lithium concentrations in mice. *Acad Emerg Med.* 1995;2:681-685.
128. Linakis JG, Hull KM, Lacouture PG, et al. Enhancement of lithium elimination by multiple-dose sodium polystyrene sulfonate. *Acad Emerg Med.* 1997;4:175-178.
129. Linakis JG, Hull KM, Lacouture PG, et al. Sodium polystyrene sulfonate treatment for lithium toxicity: effects on serum potassium concentrations. *Acad Emerg Med.* 1996;3:333-337.
130. Linakis JG, Lacouture PG, Eisenberg MS, et al. Administration of activated charcoal or sodium polystyrene sulfonate (Kayexalate) as gastric decontamination for lithium intoxication: an animal model. *Pharmacol Toxicol.* 1989;65:387-389.
131. Linakis JG, Savitt DL, Lockhart GR, et al. In vitro binding of lithium using the cation exchange resin sodium polystyrene sulfonate. *Am J Emerg Med.* 1995;13:669-670.
132. Linakis JG, Savitt DL, Schuyler JE, et al. Lithium has no direct effect on cardiac function in the isolated, perfused rat heart. *Pharmacol Toxicol.* 2000;87:39-45.
133. Linakis JG, Savitt DL, Trainor BJ, et al. Potassium repletion fails to interfere with reduction of serum lithium by sodium polystyrene sulfonate in mice. *Acad Emerg Med.* 2001;8:956-960.
134. Linakis JG, Savitt DL, Wu TY, et al. Use of sodium polystyrene sulfonate for reduction of plasma lithium concentrations after chronic lithium dosing in mice. *J Toxicol Clin Toxicol.* 1998;36:309-313.
135. Macdonald A, Briggs K, Poppe M, et al. A feasibility and tolerability study of lithium in Alzheimer's disease. *Int J Geriatr Psychiatry.* 2008;23:704-711.
136. MacGregor DA, Baker AM, Appel RG, et al. Hyperosmolar coma due to lithium-induced diabetes insipidus. *Lancet.* 1995;346:413-417.
137. MacGregor DA, Dolinski SY. Hyperosmolar coma. *Lancet.* 1999;353:1189.
138. Mani J, Tandel SV, Shah PU, et al. Prolonged neurological sequelae after combination treatment with lithium and antipsychotic drugs. *J Neurol Neurosurg Psychiatry.* 1996;60:350-351.
139. Manji HK, Hsiao JK, Risby ED, et al. The mechanisms of action of lithium: I. Effects on serotonergic and noradrenergic systems in normal subjects. *Arch Gen Psychiatry.* 1991;48:505-512.
140. Manji HK, Lenox RH. Long-term action of lithium: a role for transcriptional and posttranscriptional factors regulated by protein kinase C. *Synapse.* 1994;16:11-28.
141. Manji HK, Moore GJ, Chen G. Lithium up-regulates the cytoprotective protein Bcl-2 in the CNS in vivo: a role for neurotrophic and neuroprotective effects in manic depressive illness. *J Clin Psychiatry.* 2000;61(suppl 9):82-96.
142. Manji HK, Potter WZ, Lenox RH. Signal transduction pathways: molecular targets for lithium's actions. *Arch Gen Psychiatry.* 1995;52:531-543.
143. Manto M, Godaux E, Jacquy J, et al. Analysis of cerebellar dysmetria associated with lithium intoxication. *Neurol Res.* 1996;18:416-424.
144. Markowitz GS, Radhakrishnan J, Kambham N, et al. Lithium nephrotoxicity: a progressive combined glomerular and tubulointerstitial nephropathy. *J Am Soc Nephrol.* 2000;11:1439-1448.
145. Marmol F. Lithium: bipolar disorder and neurodegenerative diseases: possible cellular mechanisms of the therapeutic effects of lithium. *Prog Neuropsychopharmacol Biol Psychiatry.* 2008;32:1761-1771.
146. Marples D. Water channels: who needs them anyway? *Lancet.* 2000;355:1571-1572.
147. Marx CE, Yuan P, Kilts JD, et al. Neuroactive steroids, mood stabilizers, and neuroplasticity: alterations following lithium and changes in Bcl-2 knockout mice. *Int J Neuropsychopharmacol.* 2008;11:547-552.
148. Mast BT, Neufeld S, MacNeill SE, et al. Longitudinal support for the relationship between vascular risk factors and late-life depressive symptoms. *Am J Geriatr Psychiatry.* 2004;12:93-101.
149. Mendes CT, Mury FB, de Sa Moreira E, et al. Lithium reduces Gsk3b mRNA levels: implications for Alzheimer disease. *Eur Arch Psychiatry Clin Neurosci.* 2009;259:16-22.
150. Meyer RJ, Flynn JT, Brophy PD, et al. Hemodialysis followed by continuous hemofiltration for treatment of lithium intoxication in children. *Am J Kidney Dis.* 2001;37:1044-1047.
151. Mignat C, Unger T. ACE inhibitors. Drug interactions of clinical significance. *Drug Saf.* 1995;12:334-347.
152. Mikoshiba K. Inositol 1,4,5-trisphosphate receptor. *Trends Pharmacol Sci.* 1993;14:86-89.
153. Moretti ME, Koren G, Verjee Z, et al. Monitoring lithium in breast milk: an individualized approach for breast-feeding mothers. *Ther Drug Monit.* 2003;25:364-366.
154. Nagamine M, Yoshino A, Ishii M, et al. Lithium-induced Hashimoto's encephalopathy: a case report. *Bipolar Disord.* 2008;10:846-848.
155. Nagaraja D, Taly AB, Sahu RN, et al. Permanent neurological sequelae due to lithium toxicity. *Clin Neurol Neurosurg.* 1987;89:31-34.
156. Newland KD, Mycyk MB. Hemodialysis reversal of lithium overdose cardiotoxicity. *Am J Emerg Med.* 2002;20:67-68.
157. Nishizuka Y. Membrane phospholipid degradation and protein kinase C for cell signaling. *Neurosci Res.* 1992;15:3-5.
158. Nunes PV, Forlenza OV, Gattaz WF. Lithium and risk for Alzheimer's disease in elderly patients with bipolar disorder. *Br J Psychiatry.* 2007;190:359-360.
159. O'Brien WT, Harper AD, Jove F, et al. Glycogen synthase kinase-3beta haploinsufficiency mimics the behavioral and molecular effects of lithium. *J Neurosci.* 2004;24:6791-6798.
160. O'Donnell T, Rotzinger S, Nakashima TT, et al. Chronic lithium and sodium valproate both decrease the concentration of myo-inositol and increase the concentration of inositol monophosphates in rat brain. *Brain Res.* 2000;880:84-91.
161. Oakley PW, Dawson AH, Whyte IM. Lithium: thyroid effects and altered renal handling. *J Toxicol Clin Toxicol.* 2000;38:333-337.
162. Odagaki Y, Koyama T, Matsubara S, et al. Effects of chronic lithium treatment on serotonin binding sites in rat brain. *J Psychiatr Res.* 1990;24:271-277.
163. Okusa MD, Crystal LJ. Clinical manifestations and management of acute lithium intoxication. *Am J Med.* 1994;97:383-389.
164. Omata N, Murata T, Omori M, et al. A patient with lithium intoxication developing at therapeutic serum lithium levels and persistent delirium after discontinuation of its administration. *Gen Hosp Psychiatry.* 2003;25:53-55.
165. Omata N, Murata T, Takamatsu S, et al. Neuroprotective effect of chronic lithium treatment against hypoxia in specific brain regions with upregulation of cAMP response element binding protein and brain-derived neurotrophic factor but not nerve growth factor: comparison with acute lithium treatment. *Bipolar Disord.* 2008;10:360-368.

166. Oudit GY, Korley V, Backx PH, et al. Lithium-induced sinus node disease at therapeutic concentrations: linking lithium-induced blockade of sodium channels to impaired pacemaker activity. *Can J Cardiol.* 2007;23:229-232.
167. Paclt I, Slavicek J, Dohnalova A, et al. Electrocardiographic dose-dependent changes in prophylactic doses of dosulepine, lithium and citalopram. *Physiol Res.* 2003;52:311-317.
168. Peces R, Pobes A. Effectiveness of haemodialysis with high-flux membranes in the extracorporeal therapy of life-threatening acute lithium intoxication. *Nephrol Dial Transplant.* 2001;16:1301-1303.
169. Phiel CJ, Klein PS. Molecular targets of lithium action. *Annu Rev Pharmacol.* Toxicol 2001;41:789-813.
170. Pomara N. Lithium treatment in Alzheimer's disease does not promote cognitive enhancement, but may exert long-term neuroprotective effects. *Psychopharmacology (Berl).* 2009, in press.
171. Porto FH, Leite MA, Fontenelle LF, et al. The syndrome of irreversible lithium-effectuated neurotoxicity (SILENT): one-year follow-up of a single case. *J Neurol Sci.* 2009;277:172-173.
172. Price LH, Heninger GR. Lithium in the treatment of mood disorders. *N Engl J Med.* 1994;331:591-598.
173. Pringuey D, Yzombard G, Charbit J, et al. Lithium kinetics during hemodialysis in a patient with lithium poisoning. *Am J Psychiatry.* 1981;138:249-251.
174. Rana RS, Hoken LE. Role of phosphoinositides in transmembrane signaling. *Physiol Rev.* 1990;70:115-164.
175. Rao R, Zhang MZ, Zhao M, et al. Lithium treatment inhibits renal GSK-3 activity and promotes cyclooxygenase 2-dependent polyuria. *Am J Physiol Renal Physiol.* 2005;288:F642-649.
176. Roberge RJ, Martin TG, Schneider SM. Use of sodium polystyrene sulfonate in a lithium overdose. *Ann Emerg Med.* 1993;22:1911-1915.
177. Roberts DE, Berman SM, Nakasato S, et al. Effect of lithium carbonate on zidovudine-associated neutropenia in the acquired immunodeficiency syndrome. *Am J Med.* 1988;85:428-431.
178. Roh MS, Eom TY, Zmijewska AA, et al. Hypoxia activates glycogen synthase kinase-3 in mouse brain in vivo: protection by mood stabilizers and imipramine. *Biol Psychiatry.* 2005;57:278-286.
179. Rowe MK, Chuang DM. Lithium neuroprotection: molecular mechanisms and clinical implications. *Expert Rev Mol Med.* 2004;6:1-18.
180. Ryves WJ, Harwood AJ. Lithium inhibits glycogen synthase kinase-3 by competition for magnesium. *Biochem Biophys Res Commun.* 2001;280:720-725.
181. Sachs GS, Renshaw PF, Lafer B, et al. Variability of brain lithium levels during maintenance treatment: a magnetic resonance spectroscopy study. *Biol Psychiatry.* 1995;38:422-428.
182. Sakae R, Ishikawa A, Niso T, et al. Decreased lithium disposition to cerebrospinal fluid in rats with glycerol-induced acute renal failure. *Pharm Res.* 2008;25:2243-2249.
183. Scharman EJ. Methods used to decrease lithium absorption or enhance elimination. *J Toxicol Clin Toxicol.* 1997;35:601-608.
184. Schieppati A, Remuzzi G. Nephrology. The year of the pores. *Lancet.* 1996;348(suppl 2):SII13.
185. Schneider JA, Mirra SS. Neuropathologic correlates of persistent neurologic deficit in lithium intoxication. *Ann Neurol.* 1994;36:928-931.
186. Schou M. Long-lasting neurological sequelae after lithium intoxication. *Acta Psychiatr Scand.* 1984;70:594-602.
187. Schou M. Clinical aspects of lithium in psychiatry. In: Birch NJ, ed. *Lithium and the Cell: Pharmacology and Biochemistry.* London: Academic Press; 1991:1-6.
188. Schou M. Forty years of lithium treatment. *Arch Gen Psychiatry.* 1997;54:9-13.
189. Schou M. Pharmacology and toxicology of lithium. *Annu Rev Pharmacol Toxicol.* 1976;16:231-243.
190. Senatorov VV, Ren M, Kanai H, et al. Short-term lithium treatment promotes neuronal survival and proliferation in rat striatum infused with quinolinic acid, an excitotoxic model of Huntington's disease. *Mol Psychiatry.* 2004;9:371-385.
191. Shaldubina A, Agam G, Belmaker RH. The mechanism of lithium action: state of the art, ten years later. *Prog Neuropsychopharmacol Biol Psych.* 2001;5:855-866.
192. Shastry BS. Bipolar disorder: an update. *Neurochem Int.* 2005;46:273-279.
193. Sheean GL. Lithium neurotoxicity. *Clin Exp Neurol.* 1991;28:112-127.
194. Shiraki T, Kohno K, Saito D, et al. Complete atrioventricular block secondary to lithium therapy. *Circ J.* 2008;72:847-849.
195. Silverstone PH, McGrath BM, Kim H. Bipolar disorder and myo-inositol: a review of the magnetic resonance spectroscopy findings. *Bipolar Disord.* 2005;7:1-10.
196. Simard M, Gumbiner B, Lee A, et al. Lithium carbonate intoxication. A case report and review of the literature. *Arch Intern Med.* 1989;149:36-46.
197. Singer I, Rotenberg D. Mechanisms of lithium action. *N Engl J Med.* 1973;289:254-260.
198. Singer I, Rotenberg D, Puschett JB. Lithium-induced nephrogenic diabetes insipidus: in vivo and in vitro studies. *J Clin Invest.* 1972;51:1081-1091.
199. Smith SW, Ling LJ, Halstenson CE. Whole-bowel irrigation as a treatment for acute lithium overdose. *Ann Emerg Med.* 1991;20:536-539.
200. Stein R, Beaman, C, Ali, MY, Hansen, R, Jenkins, DD, Jume'an, HG. Lithium carbonate attenuation of chemotherapy-induced neutropenia. *N Engl J Med.* 1977;297:430-431.
201. Strayhorn JM Jr, Nash JL. Severe neurotoxicity despite "therapeutic" serum lithium levels. *Dis Nerv Syst.* 1977;38:107-111.
202. Swartz CM, Dolinar LJ. Encephalopathy associated with rapid decrease of high levels of lithium. *Ann Clin Psychiatry.* 1995;7:207-209.
203. Swartz CM, Jones P. Hyperlithemia correction and persistent delirium. *J Clin Pharmacol.* 1994;34:865-870.
204. Szerlip HM, Heeger P, Feldman GM. Comparison between acetate and bicarbonate dialysis for the treatment of lithium intoxication. *Am J Nephrol.* 1992;12:116-120.
205. Talati SN, Aslam AF, Vasavada B. Sinus node dysfunction in association with chronic lithium therapy: a case teport and teview of literature. *Am J Ther.* 2009;16(3):274-278.
206. Terao T. Lithium for prevention of Alzheimer's disease. *Br J Psychiatry.* 2007;191:361.
207. Thompson CJ, France AJ, Baylis PH. Persistent nephrogenic diabetes insipidus following lithium therapy. *Scott Med J.* 1997;42:16-17.
208. Thomsen K, Bak M, Shirley DG. Chronic lithium treatment inhibits amiloride-sensitive sodium transport in the rat distal nephron. *J Pharmacol Exp Ther.* 1999;289:443-447.
209. Thomsen K, Schou M. Avoidance of lithium intoxication: advice based on knowledge about the renal lithium clearance under various circumstances. *Pharmacopsychiatry.* 1999;32:83-86.
210. Thomsen K, Schou M. Renal lithium excretion in man. *Am J Physiol.* 1968;215:823-827.
211. Tilkian AG, Schroeder JS, Kao JJ, et al. The cardiovascular effects of lithium in man. A review of the literature. *Am J Med.* 1976;61:665-670.
212. Timmer RT, Sands JM. Lithium intoxication. *J Am Soc Nephrol.* 1999;10:666-674.
213. Treiser SL, Cascio CS, O'Donohue TL, et al. Lithium increases serotonin release and decreases serotonin receptors in the hippocampus. *Science.* 1981;213:1529-1531.
214. van Bommel EF. Should continuous renal replacement therapy be used for "non-renal" indications in critically ill patients with shock? *Resuscitation.* 1997;33:257-270.
215. van Bommel EF, Kalmeijer MD, Ponssen HH. Treatment of life-threatening lithium toxicity with high-volume continuous venovenous hemofiltration. *Am J Nephrol.* 2000;20:408-411.
216. van Bommel EF, Leunissen KM, Weimar W. Continuous renal replacement therapy for critically ill patients: an update. *J Intensive Care Med.* 1994;9:265-280.
217. Von Hartitzsch B, Hoenich NA, Leigh RJ, et al. Permanent neurological sequelae despite haemodialysis for lithium intoxication. *Br Med J.* 1972;4:757-759.
218. Waise A, Fisken RA. Unsuspected nephrogenic diabetes insipidus. *Br Med J.* 2001;323:96-97.
219. Walcher J, Schoecklmann H, Renders L. Lithium acetate therapy in a maintenance hemodialysis patient. *Kidney Blood Press Res.* 2004;27:200-202.
220. Waldron AM. Lithium intoxication. *JAMA.* 1949;139:733.
221. Walker RJ, Weggery S, Bedford JJ, et al. Lithium-induced reduction in urinary concentrating ability and urinary aquaporin 2 (AQP2) excretion in healthy volunteers. *Kidney Int.* 2005;67:291-294.
222. Williams R, Ryves WJ, Dalton EC, et al. A molecular cell biology of lithium. *Biochem Soc Trans.* 2004;32:799-802.
223. Wilson R, McKillop JH, Crocket GT, et al. The effect of lithium therapy on parameters thought to be involved in the development of autoimmune thyroid disease. *Clin Endocrinol (Oxf).* 1991;34:357-361.
224. Wolfson M, Bersudsky Y, Zinger E, et al. Chronic treatment of human astrocytoma cells with lithium, carbamazepine or valproic acid decreases inositol uptake at high inositol concentrations but increases it at low inositol concentrations. *Brain Res.* 2000;855:158-161.
225. Woodgett JR. Judging a protein by more than its name: GSK-3. *Sci STKE.* 2001;2001:RE12.

226. Woodgett JR. Physiological roles of glycogen synthase kinase-3: potential as a therapeutic target for diabetes and other disorders. *Curr Drug Targets Immune Endocr Metabol Disord.* 2003;3:281-290.
227. Woosley RL. Lithium. In: *Therapeutics.* Tuscon, AZ: The University of Arizona Health Sciences Center; 2005. Retrieved October 4, 2009, from http://www.qtdrugs.org/medical-pros/drug-lists/browse-drug-list.cfm?alpha=L.
228. Xia Y, Wang CZ, Liu J, et al. Lithium protection of phencyclidine-induced neurotoxicity in developing brain: the role of phosphatidylinositol-3 kinase/Akt and mitogen-activated protein kinase kinase/extracellular signal-regulated kinase signaling pathways. *J Pharmacol Exp Ther.* 2008;326:838-848.
229. Yildiz A, Moore CM, Sachs GS, et al. Lithium-induced alterations in nucleoside triphosphate levels in human brain: a proton-decoupled 31P magnetic resonance spectroscopy study. *Psychiatry Res.* 2005;138:51-59.
230. Youdim MB, Arraf Z. Prevention of MPTP (N-methyl-4-phenyl-1,2,3,6-tetrahydropyridine) dopaminergic neurotoxicity in mice by chronic lithium: involvements of Bcl-2 and Bax. *Neuropharmacology.* 2004;46:1130-1140.
231. Zhang F, Phiel CJ, Spece L, et al. Inhibitory phosphorylation of glycogen synthase kinase-3 (GSK-3) in response to lithium. Evidence for autoregulation of GSK-3. *J Biol Chem.* 2003;278:33067-33077.

CHAPTER 71
MONOAMINE OXIDASE INHIBITORS

Alex F. Manini

Monoamine oxidase (MAO) inhibitors (MAOI) have a unique history, pharmacology, and toxic syndromes associated with their use. This drug class has fallen in and out of favor with scientists and clinicians over the past several decades. While toxicity from MAOI ingestion is becoming less common due to more limited clinical usage of the traditional nonselective MAOIs, an understanding of MAOI toxicity is fundamental to any clinician who takes care of patients with acute poisoning and xenobiotics overdoses. In this chapter, an overview of clinical manifestations from MAOI toxicity is presented along with an approach to management.

HISTORY

Monoamine oxidase was discovered in 1928 and named by Zeller when the enzyme was recognized to be capable of metabolizing primary, secondary, and tertiary amines such as tyramine and norepinephrine.[126] Subsequently, the monoamine hypothesis postulated depression as a monoamine deficiency state and MAOI drugs were used to target monoamine metabolism for therapeutic benefit. In the early 1950s iproniazid, a drug previously used to treat tuberculosis, was found to produce favorable behavioral side effects. By the mid-1950s, it was demonstrated that iproniazid inhibited MAO, and it then became the first antidepressant used clinically.[46]

Another crucial finding in the late 1960s was the existence of two MAO isoforms, each with their own substrate and inhibitor specificity. This paved the way for future development of selective MAOIs in attempts to minimize the many food and drug interactions that occur with the traditional nonselective MAOIs. Nonselective MAOIs proved to be potent and efficient antidepressants and at one point were utilized as first-line therapy for depression. In the 1970s, MAOIs were competing with alternative therapies for depression, such as tricyclic antidepressants, which were achieving good clinical results without as many food interactions.

EPIDEMIOLOGY

Intentional MAOI overdose is relatively uncommon and accounts for a dwindling number of annual exposures reported to the American Association of Poison Control Centers. In 2006, there were only 268 exposures reported[16] or 0.3% of all antidepressant exposures. Of the reported exposures in 2006, there were only three cases of "major toxic effect" (defined as life-threatening signs or symptoms) and no deaths were reported. Over the past two decades, annual reported MAOI exposures have decreased 34% since 1985 (see Chap. 135). Global MAOI exposure rates most likely mirror the decline occurring in the United States, with the possible exception of exposures to moclobemide, a drug which is not approved by the United States FDA.[33]

PHARMACOLOGY

CHEMISTRY

Monoamines, also known as biogenic amines, are a group of neurotransmitters including norepinephrine, dopamine, and serotonin that have in common the presence of a single amine group and the ability to be metabolized by MAO. Monoamine oxidase is a flavin-containing enzyme present on the outer mitochondrial membrane of central nervous system (CNS) neurons, hepatocytes, and platelets. In a two-step reaction, MAO catalyzes the oxidative deamination of its various substrates. Importantly, the reaction liberates H_2O_2, a reactive oxygen species. Deamination by MAO is one of two major routes of elimination of monoamines, the other being extracellular degradation by catechol-*O*-methyltransferase (COMT). Serotonin is the monoamine exception to this rule, as it is not metabolized by COMT.

MONOAMINE NEUROTRANSMITTER STORES

Monoamine neurotransmitter synthesis, vesicle transport, vesicle storage, uptake, and degradation are described in detail in Chap. 13 ("Neurotransmitters and Neuromodulators"). In the neuron, MAO functions as a "safety valve" to metabolize and inactivate any excess monoamine neurotransmitter molecules. Once monoamines undergo reuptake back into the cytoplasm from the synaptic cleft, they can either be transported back into vesicles for further storage and release, or can be quickly enzymatically degraded by MAO which is expressed on the outer mitochondrial membrane. Thus, under normal conditions, MAO degradation of monoamines helps regulate presynaptic neurotransmitter stores.

MAO ISOFORMS

There are two MAO isoforms, each with their own substrate and inhibitor specificity (Table 71–1). MAO-A preferentially metabolizes norepinephrine and serotonin, and MAO-B preferentially metabolizes benzylamine in vitro. Both isoforms metabolize tyramine and dopamine equally efficiently, but they are localized to differing regions of mammalian anatomy, with MAO-A more concentrated in intestine and liver whereas MAO-B is more concentrated in the basal ganglia region of the brain.[22]

MECHANISM OF ACTION

Monoamine oxidase inhibitors are transported into the neuron by the Na^+-dependent membrane norepinephrine-reuptake transporter.[73] Inhibition of MAO prevents presynaptic degradation of monoamines, thus increasing the concentration of monoamine neurotransmitters available for synaptic storage and subsequent release (Fig. 71–1). Inhibition of MAO also results in some indirect release of norepinephrine into the synapse, via displacement from presynaptic vesicles by raising pH in a manner similar to amphetamines.[112]

Elevated synaptic concentration of serotonin is most closely correlated with the antidepressant therapeutic effects of MAOIs. As with other antidepressants, the enzymatic inhibitions produced by MAOIs precede their clinical effects by as long as 2 weeks. This finding may relate to relatively slow downregulation of postsynaptic CNS serotonin receptors.[90]

Monoamine oxidase inhibitors impair norepinephrine synthesis due to dopamine-β-hydroxylase inhibition. Impaired norepinephrine synthesis leads to eventual depletion of norepinephrine stores. Additionally, indirect dopamine agonism occurs via elevated synaptic concentrations of dopamine. Dopamine agonism results in β-adrenergic stimulation, peripheral vasodilation, and direct α-adrenergic stimulation at high doses.

TABLE 71–1. Monoamine Oxidase (MAO) Isoforms: Substrate Affinities and Localization

	MAO Isoforms	
	MAO-A	MAO-B
Substrate Affinity		
Dopamine	Moderate	Moderate
Epinephrine	Moderate	Moderate
Norepinephrine	High	Low
Serotonin	High	Low
Tyramine	Moderate	Moderate
Localization		
Brain	Low	High
Intestine	Moderate	Low
Liver	Moderate	Moderate
Placenta	High	Absent
Platelets	Absent	High

The hydrazide MAOIs (eg, phenelzine, isocarboxazid) are thought to be cleaved to liberate pharmacologically active products (eg, hydrazines) which are cleared by acetylation in the liver (see Chap. 117).

FIRST-GENERATION MAOIs: NONSELECTIVE AND IRREVERSIBLE

Monoamine oxidase inhibitors are a chemically heterogeneous group of xenobiotics (Fig. 71–2). First-generation MAOIs (ie, irreversible and nonselective) in clinical use include the reactive hydrazine derivatives (phenelzine, isocarboxazid) and an amphetamine derivative (tranylcypromine).[45] First-generation MAOIs bind covalently to MAO and irreversibly inhibit the enzyme's function. Thus, patients taking these MAOIs are depleted of the enzyme until new MAO is synthesized, a process that typically takes up to 3 weeks. Patients taking first-generation MAOIs remain at risk for food and xenobiotic interactions during much of this period. Because nonselective MAOIs inhibit both isoforms of MAO (ie, MAO-A and MAO-B), inhibition of intestinal and hepatic degradation of biogenic amines occurs. As a result, patients taking these xenobiotics must be placed on a restrictive diet to prevent adverse events resulting from the absorption of undigested tyramine from the gut.

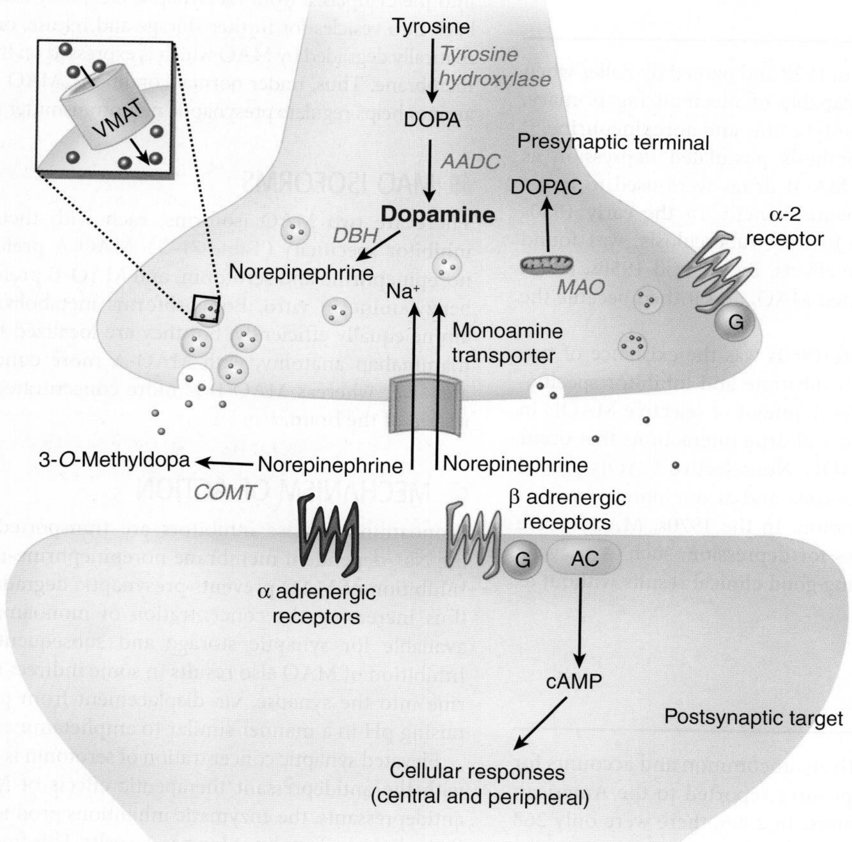

FIGURE 71–1. Sympathetic nerve terminal. Dopamine is synthesized in the sympathetic nerve cell and transported into vesicles where it is converted to norepinephrine (NE); and stored in vesicles ( ). An action potential causes the vesicles to migrate to and fuse with the presynaptic membrane. NE diffuses across the synaptic cleft and binds with and activates postsynaptic α- and β-adrenergic receptors. Neuronal NE reuptake occurs via the monoamine transporter. NE is transported back into vesicles by the vesicular monoamine transporter (VMAT; inset) or metabolized to 3, 4 dihydroxyphenyl acetic acid (DOPAC) by mitochondrial monoamine oxidase (MAO). NE that diffuses away from the synaptic cleft is inactivated by catechol-*O*-methyl transferase (COMT). AADC = aromatic L-amino acid decarboxylase; DBH = Dopamine beta-hydroxylase; HR= heart rate; NET = NE transporter.

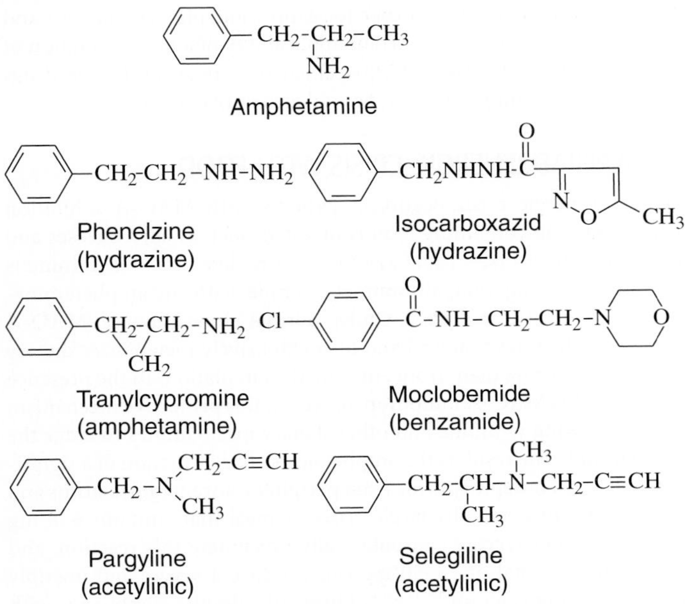

Amphetamine

Phenelzine (hydrazine)

Isocarboxazid (hydrazine)

Tranylcypromine (amphetamine)

Moclobemide (benzamide)

Pargyline (acetylinic)

Selegiline (acetylinic)

FIGURE 71–2. Structural similarities between amphetamine and the monoamine oxidase inhibitors. The words in parentheses are the chemical classes of the MAOI.

Phenelzine, isocarboxazid, and tranylcypromine are currently FDA approved for treatment of refractory depression.[58,77] Pargyline, previously approved for use as an antihypertensive due to chronic effects to generally decrease sympathetic outflow, is no longer routinely used.[122] Metabolites of amphetamine, such as phentermine, are also nonselective MAO inhibitors.[118]

Other enzyme systems inhibited by first generation MAOIs include amine oxidases such as diamine oxidase and semicarbazide-sensitive oxidases, arylamine *N*-acetyltransferase (by tranylcypromine), ceruloplasmin, alcohol dehydrogenase (by tranylcypromine), dopa decarboxylase, L-glutamic acid decarboxylase, γ-aminobutyric acid (GABA) and GABA transaminase (by hydrazide MAOIs), alanine decarboxylase and GABA transaminase (by hydrazide MAOIs), alanine aminotransferase (by phenelzine), and other pyridoxine (B_6)-containing enzyme systems.[49] The clinical implications of inhibiting these diverse enzyme systems, other than cytochrome P450,[99] are poorly understood.

SECOND-GENERATION MAOIs: SELECTIVE AND IRREVERSIBLE

Selective MAOIs preferentially inhibit one of the two MAO isoforms, although isoform selectivity is lost as the dose is increased.

MAO-A Inhibitors Clorgyline is an MAO-A inhibitor which is structurally related to pargyline. Once thought to be useful for treatment of depression, it has not found a widespread therapeutic niche.

MAO-B Inhibitors Selegiline is a selective MAO-B inhibitor that is FDA approved for the treatment of Parkinson disease,[58] although it does exhibit weak MAO-A inhibition at therapeutic doses.[68] Selegiline transdermal system is FDA approved for treatment of major depressive disorder in adults as an alternative to the traditional oral delivery system.[6,58,94] Rasagiline is another MAO-B selective MAOI that is FDA approved to treat Parkinson disease.[19]

THIRD-GENERATION MAOIs: SELECTIVE AND REVERSIBLE

Reversible inhibitors of monoamine oxidase (RIMA) are reversible and thus do not bind to MAO for the "lifetime" of the enzymes, such that high concentrations of substrate can displace the RIMA.[58] These drugs were developed in an effort to compensate for the limitations of first- and second-generation MAOIs (see Clinical Manifestations). RIMAs can be displaced by tyramine from the active site of the enzyme MAO-B, thereby enabling the amine to be metabolized peripherally. Because tyramine is not present in high concentrations in the brain, MAO-A continues to be inhibited and the antidepressant effects are achieved.[58] Moclobemide is the most widely studied RIMA and is approved as an antidepressant in Europe and other parts of the world but not currently in the United States.[33] Brofaromine and toloxatone are other RIMAs that were recently introduced but are less well studied.

NATURALLY OCCURRING MAOIs

The plant extract St. John's wort (*Hypericum perforatum*) is licensed in Germany for use as an antidepressant. Although hypericin or hyperforin have weak MAOI activity, it is debated whether this is responsible for its antidepressant effect. However, MAOI activity explains sporadic reports of hypertensive crises, cardiovascular collapse during anesthesia, and serotonin syndrome associated with use of this herbal product.[53,83]

Ayahuasca, a hallucinogenic beverage used by South American natives, uses an ethnobotanical mixture to circumvent gastrointestinal MAO. Dimethyltryptamine, which is derived from several local plant species, is a potent visual hallucinogen[27] that alone is not orally bioavailable because of its first-pass metabolism by MAO.[74] *Banisteriopsis caapi*, a plant containing the MAO-inhibiting harmala alkaloids, is mixed with dimethyltryptamine-containing plants to improve the bioavailability of this hallucinogenic amine.[74,75]

MAO-B activity in tobacco plants has prompted studies to find a link between the lower platelet MAO-B activity of smokers and their lower rate of Parkinson disease in this group.[18] This has led to interest in studying other MAO-B inhibitors for potential applications as neuroprotective xenobiotics.[125]

MISCELLANEOUS AND EXPERIMENTAL MAOIs

Some other xenobiotics with nonselective MAO inhibitory properties are used for purposes unrelated to MAO inhibition. Furazolidone is an antimicrobial used to treat protozoan-related diarrhea and bacterial enteritis. Procarbazine is a hydrazine derivative indicated as a chemotherapeutic agent for the treatment of Hodgkin lymphoma and some brain tumors. Linezolid is an antibiotic that produces weak, nonselective MAO inhibition.[30,108,116]

Research is active for novel MAO combination drugs that target multiple mechanistic approaches for the treatment of dementia and parkinsonism.[28] Ladostigil combines the cholinergic effects of a carbamate with the aminergic effects of MAO-B inhibition.[100] M30 is an actively researched drug that combines iron chelation and radical scavenger effects with irreversible, nonselective MAO inhibition.[35] Neither drug has been approved by the FDA.

PHARMACOKINETICS AND TOXICOKINETICS

Monoamine oxidase inhibitors are absorbed readily when given by mouth, and peak plasma concentrations are reached within 2–3 hours. Like other antidepressants, these xenobiotics are lipophilic and readily cross the blood–brain barrier. MAOIs are hepatically metabolized by both oxidation (various CYP450 isoenzymes including 2D6 and 2C19) and acetylation (*N*-acetyltransferase), and the metabolites are excreted in the urine.[8]

Phenelzine and isocarboxazid are hydrazides, as is the original MAOI, iproniazid. Hydrazides are metabolized to hydrazines.

The rate of metabolism of the hydrazide MAOIs is dependent on the *N*-acetyltransferase phenotype (ie, "acetylator status") of the patient (ie, fast or slow). About one-half of US populations are so-called slow-acetylators, which may contribute to exaggerated clinical effects despite standard therapeutic dosing or even mild overdose.

The clinical effects of MAOI inhibition occur rapidly and are usually maximal within a few days. First-generation (ie, irreversible) MAOIs have durations of effect that far surpass their pharmacologic half-lives, and recovery from their effects requires the synthesis of new enzyme over a period of up to 3 weeks ("washout period").[113] Thus, when switching from one serotonergic (ie, MAOI, SSRI, cyclic antidepressant), a sufficient washout must be allowed to prevent an adverse drug interaction.

PATHOPHYSIOLOGY

Increasing the concentration of norepinephrine, serotonin, and dopamine that are available for synaptic storage and release contributes to the majority of MAOI toxicity. Indirect release of monoamine neurotransmitters into the synapse as well as displacement of monoamine neurotransmitters (eg, norepinephrine) from vesicles (similar to amphetamines) also occurs.[112] These effects contribute to adrenergic stimulation that may lead to hyperadrenergic crisis. Furthermore, there is a synergistic effect on elevated presynaptic monoamine stores in the setting of coadministration with foods or xenobiotics that serve as substrates for, or enhancers of, monoamine formation, such as tyramine.[63]

Phenelzine and tranylcypromine are capable of stimulating the release of norepinephrine (and presumably other monoamines) from sympathetic nerve endings.[64] Norepinephrine release combined with MAO inhibition may result in so-called autopotentiation, or synergistic sympathomimetic effects. Autopotentiation may be responsible for paradoxical or hypertensive reactions sometimes observed following therapeutic doses of these xenobiotics.[5,23]

Hydrazide MAOIs, phenelzine and isocarboxazid are metabolized to hydrazines, which to some extent inactivate pyridoxal 5' phosphate, the cofactor necessary for neuronal decarboxylation of glutamic acid to the inhibitory neurotransmitter GABA. In addition, hydrazides may complex with pyridoxine, the precursor of pyridoxal 5' phosphate, thus enhancing its urinary elimination and further inhibiting the formation of neuronal GABA.[82] Decreased availability of neuronal GABA stores may lead to CNS excitation following overdose of hydrazide MAOIs (see Chap. 117 and Chap. 57).[61]

Impaired $GABA_A$ activity may contribute to symptoms of CNS excitation such as seizures which occur in MAOI overdose. In animal models, isocarboxazid and tranylcypromine directly inhibit GABA-mediated Cl^- influx at $GABA_A$ receptors.[109] The exact binding site of MAOIs on the $GABA_A$ receptor complex is unknown. Localization of GABA effects appears to be most pronounced in the caudate-putamen and nucleus accumbens areas in one animal model.[82] In addition, elevated neuronal glutamate concentrations due to MAOI effects may synergistically enhance CNS excitation.[102]

CLINICAL MANIFESTATIONS

The prescription of nonselective MAOIs is currently limited to resistant or atypical depression with prominent neurovegetative symptoms.[31] However, selective and reversible MAOIs are becoming the subject of renewed clinical applicability and basic science research interest. MAO-B selective drugs, such as selegiline, are used for the treatment of Parkinson disease. Reversible inhibitors of MAO, such as moclobemide, are used in Europe for depression, phobias, anxiety, and other select indications.[124] Current applicability of a new generation of experimental MAOIs is being investigated as neuroprotective drugs used in a broadening variety of neurodegenerative diseases.[125]

HYPERADRENERGIC CRISIS WITH FOOD

Hyperadrenergic crisis occurs in patients with MAO-A inhibition when tyramine-containing food is ingested, such as aged cheeses and fermented drinks (see Table 71–2 for a complete list).[125] Tyramine is an indirect-acting sympathomimetic amine with an amphetamine-like mechanism of action.[127] Under normal circumstances, MAO-A present in the intestinal wall and liver extensively metabolizes dietary amines preventing them from entering the circulation. In the presence of irreversible MAO-A inhibition, however, this protective mechanism is lost, allowing tyramine and other dietary monoamines to enter the circulation.[12] The result is the amphetamine-like induction of a significant release of norepinephrine from peripheral adrenergic neurons and provocation of hyperadrenergic crisis. A meal that contains 6–8 mg of tyramine per serving can potentially precipitate this reaction, and ingestion of a total of 25–50 mg can produce a severe and possibly life-threatening reaction.[29,114,120] Additionally, despite compliance with diet, chronically elevated cytoplasmic and synaptic concentrations of norepinephrine due to therapeutic MAOI administration can lead to occasional and unpredictable adrenergic crisis in some patients. Dietary restrictions and recommendations for patients prescribed first-generation MAOIs are summarized in Table 71-2.[29,114,120] A "washout" period of 3 weeks is sufficient to allow the inhibition caused by the irreversible MAOIs to end and a normal diet may then be resumed.[115]

The clinical syndrome of tyramine-related hyperadrenergic crisis is characterized by hypertension, headache, flushing, diaphoresis, mydriasis, neuromuscular excitation, and potential cardiac dysrhythmias.[117] This reaction is subjectively reported in up to 10% of patients taking MAOIs chronically,[88] and can occur up to 3 weeks following discontinuation of the drug.[123] Monoamine oxidase inhibitors specific for the MAO-B isoform are less likely to predispose to food or drug interactions by maintaining significant hepatic MAO-A activity, however isoform specificity is lost as dose is increased.

TABLE 71–2. Dietary Restrictions for Patients Taking MAOIs

LOW Tyramine Content (0–4 mg/serving)	MODERATE Tyramine Content (4–8 mg/serving)	HIGH Tyramine Content (>8 mg/serving)
Cottage cheese, cream cheese, yogurt, sour cream	Avocado/guacamole	Aged, mature cheeses
Chocolate	Meat extracts	Broad beans or fava beans
Distilled alcohol	Pasteurized light and pale beers	Red wines, selected beers
Non-overripe fruit	Overripe fruit/ figs	Smoked, pickled, aged, putrefying meats or fish, caviar
Soy sauce	Banana peels or stewed whole bananas	Yeast and meat extracts
		Fermented sausage
		Liver

Recommendation: Foods with *high* tyramine content should be avoided, those with *moderate* content should be consumed in restricted moderation, and those with *low* content may be cautiously consumed.

SEROTONIN SYNDROME

Any xenobiotic with serotonin-potentiating activity can interact with the MAOIs to produce serotonin syndrome. Combinations of xenobiotics commonly implicated in this reaction are involved with serotonin synthesis (eg, L-tryptophan), release (eg, amphetamines), agonism (eg, triptans that are metabolized by MAO), neuromodulation (eg, lithium), or reuptake inhibition (eg, selective serotonin reuptake inhibitors, meperidine, dextromethorphan). Animal studies have demonstrated that both meperidine[104] and dextromethorphan[105] administration can lead to fatal serotonin syndrome. Serotonin syndrome most commonly occurs in patients receiving combination therapy with two or more serotonergic agents; however, it may rarely occur with just one serotonergic agent.[81]

Clinically, this syndrome runs a spectrum of severity,[13] and is described in detail in Chap. 72. Minor findings can include akathisia, myoclonus, hyperreflexia, diaphoresis, penile erection, shivering, hyperactive bowel sounds, and tremor. Tremor and hyperreflexia are typically greater in the lower extremities. Shivering classically described with this syndrome is visually similar to "wet dog shakes," which may be analogous to serotonergic-mediated behavior in rodents,[43] and can occur at a range of body temperatures.[80] Severe signs and symptoms can include life-threatening autonomic instability, muscular rigidity, and hyperthermia.

Several diagnostic schemes for serotonin syndrome exist.[13,25,47,89,110] However, the key diagnostic criterion is exposure to a serotonergic. Because no diagnostic test is yet available, the diagnosis of serotonin syndrome must be established on clinical grounds. The onset of clinical symptoms may occur within minutes after a change in medication or self-poisoning.[69] The majority of patients with serotonin syndrome develop symptoms within 6 hours. Serotonin syndrome is not thought to resolve spontaneously if the serotonergic exposure is ongoing. Key clinical features of MAOI-induced serotonin syndrome are summarized in Table 71-3.

OVERDOSE

Monoamine oxidase inhibitor overdose may result in severe and life-threatening clinical manifestations, especially if the MAOI is a first-generation drug such as phenelzine. Classically, the clinical course involves a biphasic response characterized by initial CNS excitation and peripheral sympathetic stimulation which terminates in coma and cardiovascular collapse.[66] This biphasic model is hypothesized to result from an initial adrenergic crisis followed by inhibition of norepinephrine release,[127] and is supported by animal studies.[37,41] Additionally, depletion of norepinephrine stores may be partially or fully responsible for late hypotension observed in MAOI overdose. Toxic dose-response relationships in man are unclear, but overdose of 5 mg/kg of a first-generation MAOI is potentially life threatening.[11,66] Clinical manifestations of MAOI overdose are summarized in Table 71–3.

Patients with MAOI overdose are initially asymptomatic for several hours. Delays in clinical toxicity are well described.[70,72,92] Unstudied hypotheses that might explain this phenomenon include all of the following: initial reversible binding to MAO, cumulative effects, time-dependent alterations to MAO substrate stores, individual acetylator status, and hydrolysis of the hydrazide MAOIs. However, it must be highlighted that clinical toxicity should generally occur within the first 24 hours after overdose.[66]

Neurologic effects can be categorized as neuropsychiatric effects, neuromuscular effects, mental status effects, seizures, and chronic effects. *Neuropsychiatric* effects include agitation, akathisia, and hallucinations. *Neuromuscular* effects include flailing and tremor of the extremities, nystagmus, opsoclonus, fasciculation, myoclonus, hypertonia, hyperreflexia, muscular irritability, and muscular rigidity, the latter of which may lead to secondary effects such as hyperthermia and rhabdomyolysis. Effects on *mental status* include a variable spectrum from confusion to coma, the latter of which is a typically end-stage finding. Seizures may be either partial or generalized, and decorticate or decerebrate rigidity may alternate with periods of flaccid paralysis. Chronic use of phenelzine is also associated with and isoniazid-like peripheral neuropathy,[42] possibly explained by pyridoxine deficiency.[111]

Severe hyperthermia (40.5°C or 105°F)[103] due to MAOI toxicity may have a multifactorial etiology and is an ominous sign. Temperature dysregulation may be due to adrenergic crisis, muscular hypertonia, or CNS effects. Rigors may be present. Secondary effects from severe hyperthermia include disseminated intravascular coagulation and metabolic acidosis.[72]

Cardiovascular effects follow the previously described initial hyperadrenergic crisis followed by cardiovascular collapse. Thus, initially, hypertension, tachycardia, palpitations, and tachydysrhythmias are to be expected.[56] In severe poisoning, late toxicity can include development of hypotension, reflex tachycardia or bradycardia, bradydysrhythmias, and sudden death.[70,93] Alterations in myocardial supply/demand dynamics may lead to myocardial injury with elevations of serum cardiac biomarkers (eg, troponin I). Myonecrosis[84] and myocarditis[121] are also attributed to MAOI overdose.

TABLE 71–3. Comparison of Clinical Manifestations due to MAOI Toxicity

Clinical Category	Hyperadrenergic Crisis	Serotonin Syndrome	MAOI Overdose
Onset	Minutes–hours	Minutes–hours	Up to 24 hours
Duration	Hours	Hours	Days
Temperature	Normal	Elevated	Elevated
Neurological	Headache, hemorrhagic stroke Neuromuscular excitation	Akathisia, hyperreflexia, shivering, tremor, seizures, autonomic instability, coma Myoclonus, "wet dog shakes," muscular rigidity	Neuropsychiatric effects, neuromuscular effects, headache, seizures Myoclonus, muscular rigidity
Cardiovascular	Hypertension, dysrhythmias, myocardial injury	Hypertension, hypotension, tachycardia, palpitations, dysrhythmias	Hypertension (early), hypotension (late), tachycardia, palpitations, dysrhythmias, myocardial injury
Gastrointestinal	Nausea	Hyperactive bowel sounds	Nausea, vomiting, diarrhea
Dermatological	Flushing, diaphoresis	Diaphoresis	Flushing, piloerection, diaphoresis
Ophthalmologic	Mydriasis	Mydriasis	Mydriasis, ocular clonus

Electrocardiographic (ECG) abnormalities may include ischemic ECG changes (contiguous lead findings of T-wave inversion or ST-segment depression/elevation). Peaked T waves, in the presence[66] or absence[87] of hyperkalemia, are also noted. Myocardial manifestations associated with catastrophic CNS processes (eg, intracranial hemorrhage) can also lead to T wave inversions.

In addition to the effects mentioned above and listed in Table 71–3, reported complications of MAOI overdose include acute renal failure,[66,70,84,93] fetal demise,[93] and hemolysis.[66,72]

SELEGILINE OVERDOSE

Selegiline is metabolized to L-methamphetamine, which may result in hypertension and tachycardia, even at therapeutic doses.[1,7,97] Because selegiline overdose has not been reported in the routinely accessible medical literature, the clinical consequences of such an event are unknown.

MOCLOBEMIDE OVERDOSE

Moclobemide overdose typically produces mild to moderate CNS depression (drowsiness, disorientation), GI effects (nausea), and cardiovascular effects (tachycardia and mild hypertension).[33,76] Serotonin syndrome due to the ingestion of moclobemide, alone[51] and in combination with other serotonergics,[24,50,78,119] is well described. In massive overdose, fatalities attributed solely to the toxic effects of moclobemide have been reported.[17,34,40]

OTHER ADVERSE DRUG REACTIONS

Clinically significant drug interactions with MAOIs can be due to serotonergic effects (see Serotonin Syndrome earlier) as well as alterations to drug metabolism. Administration of opioids with serotonergic properties (eg, meperidine, dextromethorphan) is absolutely contraindicated due to risk of precipitating the serotonin syndrome.[13,39,96,104,105] Adverse drug reactions with other coadministered drugs that are metabolized by cytochrome P450 may be problematic, as first- generation MAOIs have an extensive inhibitory effect on hepatic cytochrome P450 enzymes 2C9, 2C19, and 2D6.[8,99] Thus, barbiturates (eg, phenobarbital) and benzodiazepines (eg, diazepam, lorazepam) that are metabolized by hepatic cytochrome P450 may produce prolonged sedation and respiratory depression. Table 71–4 summarizes analgesic safety in combination with MAOI drugs.[39]

TABLE 71–4. Adverse Drug Events Associated with Monamine Oxidase Inhibitors

Analgesic Class	Safe	Monitor Closely and Consider Alternative	Avoid Combination (*Contraindicated*)
Nonprescription	Acetaminophen Aspirin NSAIDs		Dextromethorphan
Opioids	Buprenorphine Codeine Morphine Oxycodone	Fentanyl Propoxyphene Remifentanil	Meperidine Methadone Pentazocine
Nonopioids	Inhalational anesthetics Nitroglycerin	Barbiturates† Benzodiazepines† Ethchlorvynol	Cyclobenzaprine Tramadol
Local anesthetics	Lidocaine		Cocaine

† Drugs that are metabolized by hepatic cytochrome P450 may produce prolonged sedation and respiratory depression when combined with MAOIs.

WITHDRAWAL REACTIONS

Monoamine oxidase inhibitor withdrawal may be severe, beginning 24–72 hours after discontinuation. Classically, MAOI withdrawal symptoms are the worst following discontinuation of high therapeutic doses of tranylcypromine and isocarboxazid.[9] Symptoms range from nausea, vomiting, and malaise, to CNS symptoms such as agitation, psychosis, and convulsions. Treatment is generally supportive and typically involves a benzodiazepine such as diazepam and restarting the medication if clinically indicated.

DIAGNOSTIC TESTING

The clinical utility of therapeutic drug monitoring in the routine use of MAOIs is limited. Evaluation of MAO activity is not routinely available, requires a fresh specimen (preferably jejunal biopsy),[65] and is therefore not recommended. Experimental evidence suggests that inhibition of human platelet MAO-B activity by at least 85% may be associated with a favorable clinical antidepressant response to phenelzine.[32,36]

Evaluation of MAOI toxicity remains a clinical diagnosis. Serum concentrations of MAOIs that correlate meaningfully with clinical effects are not well established. In addition, serum concentrations of any antidepressant, in general, can be misleading when obtained postmortem for forensic purposes.[86,95] Hyperglycemia and leukocytosis may be present. Elevations in serum lactate concentrations and metabolic acidosis may be present from seizures, muscular hypertonia, or hyperthermia.

Measurement of blood and urinary concentrations of MAO substrates may provide indirect evidence of MAOI effects. MAOIs may cause increase serum serotonin, increase or decrease serum norepinephrine, increase urinary epinephrine and norepinephrine, and decrease urinary serotonin metabolites. Due to the indirect nature of this testing and the fact that its interpretation is frought with confounding factors (eg, if the patient is receiving vasopressors), the routine measurement of plasma and urinary MAO substrates is not recommended in the assessment of MAOI toxicity. Of note, patients taking selegiline[101] and tranylcypromine[128] may test positive for amphetamines on drug screens due to their metabolites.

MANAGEMENT

OUT OF HOSPITAL

Decisions regarding referral to the emergency department (ED) must take into account factors such as patient age, intent of exposure, symptoms, as well as timing of exposure. All patients with MAOI exposures who display suicidal intent should be referred to an ED for evaluation. Children with exposure to even one adult formulation MAOI tablet or selegiline patch should be referred to the ED due to the potential for late-onset significant toxicity.[3] Patients who exhibit more than mild headache, minimal diaphoresis following an acute MAOI ingestion should be referred to an ED. Observation at home is warranted in patients who are asymptomatic and more than 24 hours have elapsed since the time of ingestion. Due to paucity of data at this time, patients with selegiline patch ingestions should be referred to the ED for observation, even if suicidal intent is absent.

PRE-HOSPITAL

Induction of emesis is not recommended.[3] Activated charcoal can be administered to asymptomatic patients who have ingested overdoses of MAOI if no contraindications are present.[2] Transportation to the hospital should not be delayed in order to administer activated charcoal. Use of intravenous benzodiazepines for seizures and external cooling measures for severe hyperthermia (40.5°C [105°F])[103] should be performed in consultation/authorization with EMS medical direction, by a written treatment protocol or policy, or with direct medical oversight.

INITIAL APPROACH IN THE EMERGENCY DEPARTMENT

As with any serious ingestion, initial stabilization must include rapid assessment of the airway, breathing, and circulation as well as establishment of intravenous access, supplemental oxygen, and cardiac monitoring. Evidence of hyperthermia or hemodynamic instability following MAOI ingestion may be a manifestation of significant toxicity. Intravenous volume repletion should begin while gastrointestinal decontamination is considered. In any patient with altered mental status who will likely deteriorate progressively, early orotracheal intubation may facilitate safe gastric decontamination measures. Subsequent management should focus on stabilization of hyperthermia, seizures, and muscular rigidity.

GASTRIC DECONTAMINATION

Patients who overdose with MAOIs are more likely to benefit from gastrointestinal decontamination than most other overdose patients because of their high potential for morbidity/mortality.[59,85] Orogastric lavage with a large bore orogastric tube (36-40 French) should be considered if a life-threatening ingestion is suspected to have occurred within several hours prior to presentation.[39,59,85] Single-dose activated charcoal should be orally administered for ingestions presenting within several hours, unless contraindications are present. Whole bowel irrigation with oral polyethylene glycol has limited utility unless there are co-ingestions with other sustained-release preparation medications. The lack of early clinical findings of poisoning should not dissuade the use of gastrointestinal decontamination given the potential for delayed clinical deterioration.

COOLING MEASURES

Severe hyperthermia must be treated aggressively. Use of ice baths (first choice for life-threatening hyperthermia),[106] cold water, and fans are the mainstay of treatment (see Chap. 15). Indications for ice bath immersion to treat MAOI toxicity include rectal temperature greater than 40.5°C (105°F),[103] rigidity, and altered mental status. If an ice bath is unavailable, ice packs should be placed in both the axillae and the groin. Benzodiazepines help control muscular rigidity, seizures, and agitation that may contribute to amelioration of hyperthermia and tachycardia. Patients with refractory hyperthermia despite the above measures may require neuromuscular blockade, using nondepolarizing paralytics, in conjunction with tracheal intubation and ventilation. The depolarizing paralytic succinylcholine should be avoided in severe MAOI toxicity due to the risk of precipitating lethal dysrhythmia due to hyperkalemia in the setting of rhabdomyolysis. Neuromuscular blockade eliminates hyperthermia that results from muscular rigidity, and can be employed if first-line treatments are unsuccessful. Antipyretics such as acetaminophen are unlikely to be efficacious because the hyperthermia is not due to alterations in the hypothalamic temperature set point.[103]

BLOOD PRESSURE CONTROL

Because there is characteristic fluctuation in vital signs associated with MAOI overdose, hemodynamic monitoring should be instituted even for patients who initially are stable. When supporting the patient's blood pressure, preference should be given to titratable drugs with a rapid onset and termination of action because of the potential for rapid hemodynamic changes. Use of β-adrenergic antagonists is relatively contraindicated for control of hypertension in MAOI-related toxicity because the action of monoamines (eg, norepinephrine) at the neuronal synapse in the autonomic nervous system could result in refractory hypertension due to unopposed α-adrenergic agonism.[91]

Patients who are normotensive at baseline and who experience MAOI-related severe *hypertension* can be treated with a short-acting α-adrenergic antagonist such as phentolamine (2–5 mg IV) for effective control.[12] Xenobiotics such as nitroprusside and nitroglycerin may be preferred because they allow for titratable blood pressure control.[21] Tyramine-related hypertensive crises can successfully be controlled with the dihydropyridine calcium channel blockers such as nifedipine and possibly the oral α-adrenergic antagonists such as terazosin but should be used with caution.[20,48] Particular caution must be exercised in patients with baseline hypertension because overly aggressive blood pressure lowering may reduce cerebral perfusion pressure sufficiently to cause cerebral ischemia.

Patients who are *hypotensive* may require aggressive support with intravenous fluid resuscitation and vasopressors. Direct-acting sympathetic agents (eg, epinephrine, norepinephrine) can be used safely in patients taking MAOIs.[14] Rather than causing release of a stored pool of norepinephrine, these xenobiotics bind directly with postsynaptic α- and β-adrenergic receptors.

Dopamine is relatively contraindicated in hypotensive patients who have overdosed on MAOIs for several reasons. The indirect action of dopamine administration may produce a synergistic effect with MAOI, resulting in excessive adrenergic activity and exaggerated rises in blood pressure. In addition, most of dopamine's α-adrenoceptor–mediated vasoconstriction is secondary to norepinephrine release; in the presence of MAOIs, norepinephrine synthesis may be impaired from concomitant dopamine-β-hydroxylase inhibition, and dopamine may not reliably raise blood pressure if cytoplasmic and vesicular neuronal stores have been depleted. Finally, in the presence of impaired norepinephrine release or α-adrenergic blockade by any cause, unopposed dopamine-induced vasodilation from action on peripheral dopamine and β-adrenoceptors may paradoxically lower blood pressure further.

DYSRHYTHMIAS

Due to the unique pharmacological and toxicokinetic considerations of MAOI toxicity, adherence to advance cardiac life support (ACLS) protocols may not provide optimal results.[4] In any stable patient, removal of the offending xenobiotic as well as correction of hypoxia, hypokalemia, and hypomagnesemia, if present, is a rational initial step.

Patients with immediately *life-threatening dysrhythmias* require rapid cardioversion. In the presence of the nonperfusing dysrhythmias such as ventricular fibrillation, pulseless ventricular tachycardia, and torsades de pointes unsynchronized electrical defibrillation is the treatment of choice.

Stable patients with *ventricular tachycardia* may benefit from a trial of antidysrhythmic drugs such as amiodarone or lidocaine. High-quality studies evaluating the use of these xenobiotics in the setting of MAOI overdose are not available.

Hemodynamically significant *supraventricular tachycardia* from MAOI toxicity should be corrected to prevent myocardial ischemia/infarction, ventricular dysrhythmia, and high-output heart failure. Benzodiazepines are safe and effective to treat sinus tachycardia, as long as respiratory status remains monitored. Adenosine and synchronized cardioversion are unlikely to be useful in the setting of ongoing presence of the MAOI, but may be considered in rare cases that are unresponsive to benzodiazepines. In patients with borderline hypotension, nondihydropyridine calcium-channel antagonists such as diltiazem and verapamil are relatively contraindicated because they may further lower blood pressure.

Hemodynamically significant *bradycardia* from MAOI toxicity may be refractory to standard ACLS protocols. An initial approach with intravenous atropine is a rational first-line therapy to temporize the patient with bradycardia and hypotension. Epinephrine and isoproterenol may also be considered. Multiple boluses of atropine in conjunction with intravenous fluid resuscitation may be necessary, while a pacemaker (transcutaneous or transvenous) is considered.

MANAGEMENT OF CNS MANIFESTATIONS

In acute altered mental status, hypoglycemia should be rapidly excluded.[15,98] Mild to moderate CNS excitation may be treated with small incremental doses of parenteral diazepam. Seizures should be treated with benzodiazepines such as lorazepam in standard incremental doses. Empiric administration of pyridoxine (vitamin B_6), intravenously at 70 mg/kg, up to 5 g in adults) should be considered in patients with status epilepticus, particularly following massive ingestions of hydrazine-derived MAOIs such as phenelzine which may deplete endogenous pyridoxine stores (see A-15 Pyridoxine).[111] Theoretically, phenytoin is not likely to be useful for treatment of MAOI-induced seizures because there is no distinct seizure focus, but rather generalized presence of MAOI (and metabolites) in the CNS.

CYPROHEPTADINE

Cyproheptadine is a nonselective serotonin antagonist that is recommended as third-line therapy (after benzodiazepine administration and cooling measures) for MAOI-induced serotonin syndrome.[13] Cyproheptadine prevents lethality in animal models of serotonin syndrome[79] and reportedly is beneficial in humans with serotonin syndrome although its efficacy has not been rigorously established.[38,44] It should be strongly considered when the diagnosis of serotonin syndrome is likely, especially if incomplete response has been achieved with aggressive cooling and benzodiazepine therapy.[62] In addition, its use to treat neuromuscular rigidity and hyperthermia associated with MAOI overdose has been reported.[10,26]

The recommended initial dose in adults is 12 mg orally, to be followed by 2 mg every 2 hours while symptoms continue.[13] Maintenance dosing involves the administration of 8 mg of cyproheptadine every 6 hours. A dose of 12–32 mg will bind 85%–95% of serotonin receptors.[55] The dose of cyproheptadine used to treat the serotonin syndrome may cause sedation, but this effect is a goal of therapy and should not deter clinicians from using the drug. Relative contraindications to its use include acute asthma exacerbation, GI obstruction, and age less than 2 years (due to lack of safety information for this age group).

DANTROLENE

Use of dantrolene in patients with serotonin syndrome is not recommended (see Antidote in Depth A22: Dantrolene Sodium). Case reports citing its utility probably involved a misdiagnosis of serotonin syndrome.[13,54] Dantrolene is indicated for treatment of malignant hyperthermia, a disease generally considered to be unrelated to serotonin syndrome. In animal models of serotonin syndrome, dantrolene administration has no effect on survival.[52,79] Use of dantrolene in one report of serotonin syndrome was implicated with causing fatality.[57]

EXTRACORPOREAL ELIMINATION

The utility of extracorporeal measures, such as hemodialysis, to treat MAOI toxicity remains to be demonstrated. The ability to dialyze a xenobiotic depends largely on its protein binding the volume of distribution. Unfortunately, data regarding protein-binding and volumes of distribution of the first generation MAOI drugs such as isocarboxazid are not well characterized. Use of peritoneal dialysis[67] and hemodialysis[71] to treat MAOI overdose has been reported in the literature. However, time to resolution of symptoms for all cases did not differ (~24 hours) from those in which hemodialysis was not employed. Therefore, extracorporeal elimination is not recommended in the management of MAOI overdose unless other indications are present such as severe acidemia or life-threatening hyperkalemia, or the need to eliminate dialyzable toxic co-ingestions.

DISPOSITION

Recommendations for the ideal time frame for observation of patients with suspected MAOI overdose are limited by a paucity of relevant studies in the clinical toxicology literature. Patients with presumed MAOI overdose should be observed with telemetry monitoring, preferably in an intensive care unit, for at least 24 hours regardless of the initial clinical findings. This recommendation takes into account the potential for delayed-onset of clinical toxicity as well as the potential for severe morbidity and mortality.[70,72,92] However, patients with MAOI–food or MAOI–xenobiotic interactions may not require hospital admission if the interaction is mild, resolution of symptoms is complete, and the patient has been observed for 4–8 hours.

SUMMARY

Toxicity from MAOI exposures is becoming less common due to more limited clinical usage of the traditional nonselective MAOIs; however, clinical and research use of selective MAOIs and RIMAs is increasing. Inhibition of MAO has effects on myriad neuronal neurotransmitters which are responsible for the majority of the therapeutic and toxic effects of MAOIs. The clinical effects of MAOI overdose may be life threatening and should be managed aggressively. Other consequential manifestations of MAOI toxicity may include hyperadrenergic crisis and the serotonin syndrome.

REFERENCES

1. Am OB, Amit T, Youdim MB. Contrasting neuroprotective and neurotoxic actions of respective metabolites of anti-Parkinson drugs rasagiline and selegiline. *Neurosci Lett.* 2004;355:169-172.
2. American Academy of Clinical Toxicology and European Association of Poisons Centres and Clinical Toxicologists. Position paper: single dose activated charcoal. *Clin Toxicol.* 2005;43:61-87.
3. American Academy of Pediatrics Committee on Injury, Violence, and Poison Prevention. Poison treatment in the home. *Pediatrics.* 2003;112:1182-1185.
4. American Heart Association (AHA). 2005 AHA Guidelines for Cardiopulmonary Resuscitation and Emergency Cardiovascular Care, Part 10.2: Toxicology in ECC. *Circulation.* 2005;112:IV-126-132.
5. American Medical Association Council on Drugs. Paradoxical hypertension from tranylcypromine sulfate. *JAMA.* 1963;254:94.
6. Amsterdam JD. A double-blind, placebo-controlled trial of the safety and efficacy of selegiline transdermal system without dietary restrictions in patients with major depressive disorder. *J Clin Psychiatry.* 2003;64:208-214.
7. Azzaro AJ, VanDenBerg CM, Ziemniak J, et al. Evaluation of the potential for pharmacodynamic and pharmacokinetic drug interactions between selegiline transdermal system and two sympathomimetic agents in healthy volunteers. *J Clin Pharmacol.* 2007;47:978-990.
8. Baker GB, Urichuk LJ, McKenna KF, et al. Metabolism of monoamine oxidase inhibitors. *Cell Mol Neurobiol.* 1999;19:411-426.
9. Baldessarini RJ, Tondo L, Viguera AC. Discontinuing psychotropic agents. *J Psychopharmacol.* 1999;13:292-293.
10. Beasley CM Jr, Masica DN, Heiligenstein JH, et al. Possible monoamine oxidase inhibitor-serotonin uptake inhibitor interaction: fluoxetine clinical data and preclinical findings. *J Clin Psychopharmacol.* 1993;13:312-320.

11. Bell DB, Scaff J. Fatal reaction to tranylcypromine (Parnate). *Hawaii Med J.* 1963;22:440-441.
12. Bieck PR, Antonin KH. Oral tyramine pressor test and the safety of monoamine oxidase inhibitor drugs: comparison of brofaromine and tranylcypromine in healthy subjects. *J Clin Psychopharmacol.* 1988;8:237-245.
13. Boyer EW, Shannon M. The serotonin syndrome. *N Engl J Med.* 2005;352: 1112-1120.
14. Braverman B, McCarthy RJ, Ivankovich AD. Vasopressor challenges during chronic MAOI or TCA treatment in anesthetized dogs. *Life Sci.* 1987;40:2587-2595.
15. Bressler R, Vargas-Cord M, Lebovitz HE. Tranylcypromine: a potent insulin secretagogue and hypoglycemic agent. *Diabetes.* 1968;17:617-624.
16. Bronstein AC, Spyker DA, Cantilena LR, et al. 2006 annual report of the American Association of Poison Control Centers' National Poison Data System (NPDS). *Clin Toxicol.* 2007;45:815-917.
17. Camaris C, Little D. A fatality due to moclobemide. *J Forensic Sci.* 1997;42: 954-955.
18. Castagnoli K, Murugesan T. Tobacco leaf, smoke and smoking, MAO inhibitors, Parkinson's disease and neuroprotection: are there links? *Neurotoxicology.* 2004;25:279-291.
19. Chen JJ, Swope DM, Dashtipour K. Comprehensive review of rasagiline, a second-generation monoamine oxidase inhibitor, for the treatment of Parkinson's disease. *Clin Ther.* 2007;29:1825-1849.
20. Clary C, Schweizer E. Treatment of MAOI hypertensive crisis with sublingual nifedipine. *J Clin Psychiatry.* 1987;48:249-250.
21. Cockhill LA, Remick RA. Blood pressure effects of monoamine oxidase inhibitors—the highs and lows. *Can J Psychiatry.* 1987;32:803-808.
22. Collins G, Sandler M, Williams E, et al. Mulitple forms of human brain monoamine oxidase. *Nature.* 1970;225:817-820.
23. Cooper AJ, Magnus RV, Rose MJ. Hypertensive syndrome with tranylcypromine medication. *Lancet.* 1964;1:527-529.
24. Dingemanse J, Wallnofer A, Gieschke R, et al. Pharmacokinetic and pharmacodynamic interactions between fluoxetine and moclobemide in the investigation of development of the "serotonin syndrome." *Clin Pharmacol Ther.* 1998;63:403-413.
25. Dunkley EJ, Isbister GK, Sibbritt D, et al. The Hunter Serotonin Toxicity Criteria: simple and accurate diagnostic decision rules for serotonin toxicity. *Q J Med.* 2003;96:635-642.
26. Erich JL, Shih RD, O'Connor RE. "Ping-pong" gaze in severe monoamine oxidase inhibitor toxicity. *J Emerg Med.* 1995;13:653-655.
27. Erowid, the Vaults of: N,N-DMT. Accessed online at: www.erowid.org/chemicals/dmt on September 19, 2008.
28. Fernandez HH, Chen JJ. Monoamine oxidase inhibitors: current and emerging agents for Parkinson disease. *Clin Neuropharmacol.* 2007;30: 150-168.
29. Folks DG. Monoamine oxidase inhibitors: reappraisal of dietary considerations. *J Clin Psychopharmacol.* 1983;3(4):249-252.
30. French G. Safety and tolerability of linezolid. *J Antimicrob Chemother.* 2003;51(Suppl 2):ii45-ii53.
31. Frieling H, Bleich S. Tranylcypromine: new perspectives on an "old" drug. *Eur Arch Psychiatry Clin Neuropsy.* 2006;256:268-273.
32. Fritz RR, Malek-Ahmadi P, Rose RM, et al. Tranylcypromine lowers human platelet MAO B activity but not concentration. *Biol Psychiatry.* 1983;18:685-694.
33. Fulton B, Benfield P. Moclobemide: an update of its pharmacological properties and therapeutic use. *Drugs.* 1996;52:450-474.
34. Gaillard Y, Pepin G. Moclobemide fatalities: report of two cases and analytical determinations by GC-MS and HPLC-PDA after solid-phase extraction. *Forensic Sci Int.* 1997;87:239-248.
35. Gal S, Fridkin M, Amit T, et al. M30, a novel multifunctional neuroprotective drug with potent iron chelating and brain selective monoamine oxidase-ab inhibitory activity for Parkinson disease. *J Neural Transm Suppl.* 2006;70:447-56.
36. Georgotas A, McCue RE, Friedman E, et al. Prediction of response to nortriptyline and phenelzine by platelet MAO activity. *Am J Psychiatry.* 1987;144:338-340.
37. Gessa GL, Cuenca E, Costa E. On the mechanism of hypotensive effects of MAO inhibitors. *Ann NY Acad Sci.* 1963;107:935-944.
38. Gillman PK. The serotonin syndrome and its treatment. *J Psychopharmacol.* 1999;13:100-109.
39. Gillman PK. Monoamine oxidase inhibitors, opioid analgesics, and serotonin toxicity. *Br J Anaesth.* 2005;95:434-41.
40. Giroud C, Horisberger B, Eap C, et al. Death following acute poisoning by moclobemide. *Forensic Sci Int.* 2004;140:101-107.
41. Goldberg ND, Shideman FE. Species differences in the cardiac effects of a monoamine oxidase inhibitor. *J Pharmacol Exp Ther.* 1963;136:142-151.
42. Goodheart RS, Dunne JW, Edis RH. Phenelzine associated peripheral neuropathy—clinical and electrophysiologic findings. *Aust N Z J Med.* 1991;21:339-340.
43. Gorzalka BB, Hanson LA. Sexual behavior and wet dog shakes in the male rat: regulation by corticosterone. *Behav Brain Res.* 1998;97:143-151.
44. Graudins A, Stearman A, Chan B. Treatment of the serotonin syndrome with cyproheptadine. *J Emerg Med.* 1998;16:615-619.
45. Haefely W, Burkard WP, Cesura AM, et al. Biochemistry and pharmacology of moclobemide, a prototype RIMA. *Psychopharmacology.* 1992;106:S6-S14.
46. Healy D. *The Antidepressant Era.* Cambridge, MA: Harvard University Press; 1997.
47. Hegerl U, Bottlender R, Gallinat J, et al. The serotonin syndrome scale: first results on validity. *Eur Arch Psychiatry Clin Neurosci.* 1998;248:96-103.
48. Hesselink JM. Safer use of MAOIs with nifedipine to counteract potential hypertensive crisis. *Am J Psychiatry.* 1991;148:1616.
49. Holt A, Berry MD, Boulton AA. On the binding of monoamine oxidase inhibitors to some sites distinct from the MAO active site, and effects thereby elicited. *Neurotoxicology.* 2004;25:251-266.
50. Ip A, Renouf T. Serotonin syndrome due to an overdose of moclobemide? *CJEM.* 2002;4:98-101.
51. Isbister GK, Hackett LP, Dawson AH, et al. Moclobemide poisoning: toxicokinetics and occurrence of serotonin toxicity. *Br J Clin Pharmacol.* 2003;56:441-450.
52. Isbister GK, Whyte IM. Serotonin toxicity and malignant hyperthermia: role of 5-HT2 receptors. *Br J Anaesth.* 2002;88:603-604.
53. Izzo AA. Drug interactions with St. John's wort (*Hypericum perforatum*): a review of the clinical evidence. *Int J Clin Pharmacol Ther.* 2004;42: 139-148.
54. Kaplan RF, Feinglass NG, Webster W, et al. Phenelzine overdose treated with dantrolene sodium. *JAMA.* 1986;255:642-644.
55. Kapur S, Zipursky RB, Jones C, et al. Cyproheptadine: a potent in vivo serotonin antagonist. *Am J Psychiatry.* 1997;154:884.
56. Keck PE Jr, Vuckovic A, Pope HG Jr, et al. Acute cardiovascular response to monoamine oxidase inhibitors: a prospective assessment. *J Clin Psychopharmacol.* 1989;9:203-206.
57. Kline SS, Mauro LS, Scala-Barnett DM, et al. Serotonin syndrome versus neuroleptic malignant syndrome as a cause of death. *Clin Pharm.* 1989;8:510-514.
58. Krishnan KR. Revisiting monoamine oxidase inhibitors. *J Clin Psychiatry.* 2007;68(Suppl 8):35-41.
59. Kulig K, Bar-Or D, Cantrill SV, et al. Management of acutely poisoned patients without gastric emptying. *Ann Emerg Med.* 1985;14:562-7.
60. Lancranjan I. The endocrine profile of bromocriptine: its application in endocrine diseases. *J Neural Transm.* 1981;51:61-82.
61. Landolt HP, Gillin JC. Different effects of phenelzine treatment on EEG topography in waking and sleep in depressed patients. *Neuropsychopharmacology.* 2002;27:462-469.
62. Lappin RI, Auchincloss EL. Treatment of the serotonin syndrome with cyproheptadine. *N Engl J Med.* 1994;331:1021-1022.
63. Lavin MR, Mendelowitz A, Kronig MH. Spontaneous hypertensive reactions with monoamine oxidase inhibitors. *Biol Psychiatry.* 1993;34:146-151.
64. Lee WC, Shin YH, Shideman FE. Cardiac activities of several monoamine oxidase inhihitors. *J Pharmacol Exp Ther.* 1961;133:180-185.
65. Levine RJ, Sjoerdsma A. Estimation of monoamine oxidase activity in man: techniques and applications. *Ann NY Acad Sci.* 1963;107:966-974.
66. Linden CH, Rumack BH, Strehlke C. Monoamine oxidase inhibitor overdose. *Ann Emerg Med.* 1984;13:1137-1144.
67. Lipkin D, Kuslmick T. Pargyline hydrochloride poisoning in a child. *JAMA.* 1967;201:135-136.
68. Mann JJ, Aarons SF, Frances AH, et al. Studies of selective and reversible monoamine oxidase inhibitors. *J Clin Psychiatry.* 1984;45:62-66.
69. Mason PJ, Morris VA, Balcezak PJ. Serotonin syndrome: presentation of 2 cases and a review of the literature. *Medicine (Baltimore).* 2000;79:201-209.
70. Matell G, Thorstrand C. A case of fatal nialamid poisoning. *Acta Med Scand.* 1967;181:79-82.
71. Matter BJ, Donat PE, Brill ML, et al. Tranylcypromine sulfate poisoning. Successful treatment by hemodialysis. *Arch Intern Med.* 1965;116:18-20.
72. Mawdsley JA. "Parstelin:" a case of fatal overdose. *Med J Aust.* 1968;2:292.

73. McDaniel KD. Clinical pharmacology of monoamine oxidase inhibitors. *Clin Neuropharmacol.* 1986;9:207-234.
74. McKenna DJ. Clinical investigations of the therapeutic potential of ayahuasca: rationale and regulatory challenges. *Pharmacol Ther.* 2004;102:111-129.
75. McKenna DJ, Towers GH, Abbott F. Monoamine oxidase inhibitors in South American hallucinogenic plants: tryptamine and beta-carboline constituents of ayahuasca. *J Ethnopharmacol.* 1984;10:195-223.
76. Myrenfors PG, Eriksson T, Sandsted CS, et al. Moclobemide overdose. *J Intern Med.* 1993;233:113-115.
77. Nelson SD, Mitchell JR, Timbrell JA, et al. Isoniazid and iproniazid: activation of metabolites to toxic intermediates in man and rat. *Science.* 1976;193:901-903.
78. Neuvonen PJ, Pohjola-Sintonen S, Tacke U, et al. Five fatal cases of serotonin syndrome after moclobemide-citalopram or moclobemide-clomipramine overdoses. *Lancet.* 1993;342:1419.
79. Nisijima K, Yoshino T, Yui K, et al. Potent serotonin (5-HT)(2A) receptor antagonists completely prevent the development of hyperthermia in an animal model of the 5-HT syndrome. *Brain Res.* 2001;890:23-31.
80. Okada F, Okajima K. Abnormalities of thermoregulation induced by fluvoxamine. *J Clin Psychopharmacol.* 2001;21(6):619-621.
81. Pan JJ, Shen WW. Serotonin syndrome induced by low-dose venlafaxine. *Ann Pharmacother.* 2003;37:209-211.
82. Parent MB, Master S, Kashlub S, et al. Effects of the antidepressant/antipanic drug phenelzine and its putative metabolite phenylethylidenehydrazine on extracellular gamma-aminobutyric acid levels in the striatum. *Biochem Pharmacol.* 2002;63:57-64.
83. Patel S, Robinson R, Burk M. Hypertensive crisis associated with St. John's wort. *Am J Med.* 2002;112:507-508.
84. Platts MM, Usher A, Stentiford NH. Phenelzine and trifluoperazine poisoning. *Lancet.* 1965;2:738.
85. Pond SM, Lewis-Driver DJ, Williams GM, et al. Gastric emptying in acute overdose: a prospective randomized controlled trial. *Med J Aust.* 1995;163:345-349.
86. Prouty RW, Anderson WH. The forensic science implications of site and temporal influences on postmortem blood-drug concentrations. *J Forensic Sci.* 1990;35:243-270.
87. Quill TE. Peaked T waves with tranylcypromine (Parnate) overdose. *Int J Psychiatr Med.* 1981;11:155-160.
88. Rabkin JG, Quitkin FM, McGrath P, et al. Adverse reactions to monoamine oxidase inhibitors, part II: treatment, correlates and clinical management. *J Clin Psychopharmacol.* 1985;5:2-9.
89. Radomski JW, Dursun SM, Reveley MA, et al. An exploratory approach to the serotonin syndrome: an update of clinical phenomenology and revised diagnostic criteria. *Med Hypotheses.* 2000;55:218-224.
90. Raft D, Davidson J, Wasik J, et al. Relationship between response to phenelzine and MAO inhibition in a clinical trial of phenelzine, amitriptyline and placebo. *Neuropsychobiology.* 1981;7:122-126.
91. Ramoska E, Sacchetti AD. Propranolol-induced hypertension in treatment of cocaine intoxication. *Ann Emerg Med.* 1985;14:1112-1113.
92. Reid DD, Kerr WC. Phenelzine poisoning responding to phanothiazine. *Med J Aust.* 1969;2:1214-1215.
93. Robertson JC. Recovery after massive MAOI overdose complicated by malignant hyperpyrexia, treated with chlorpromazine. *Postgrad Med J.* 1972;48:64-65.
94. Robinson DS, Amsterdam JD. The selegiline transdermal system in major depressive disorder: a systematic review of safety and tolerability. *J Affect Disord.* 2008;105:15-23.
95. Rogde S, Hilberg T, Teige B. Fatal combined intoxication with new antidepressants. Human cases and an experimental study of postmortem moclobemide redistribution. *Forensic Sci Int.* 1999;100:109-116.
96. Rogers KJ, Thornton JA. The interaction between monoamine oxidase inhibitors and narcotic analgesics in mice. *Br J Pharmacol.* 1969;36:470-480.
97. Rose LM, Ohlinger MJ, Mauro VF. A hypertensive reaction induced by concurrent use of selegiline and dopamine. *Ann Pharmacother.* 2000;34:1020-1024.
98. Rowland MJ, Bransome ED Jr, Hendry LB. Hypoglycemia caused by selegiline, an antiparkinsonian drug: can such side effects be predicted? *J Clin Pharmacol.* 1994;34:80-85.
99. Salsali M, Holt A, Baker GB. Inhibitory effects of the monoamine oxidase inhibitor tranylcypromine on the cytochrome P450 enzymes CYP2C19, CYP2C9, and CYP2D6. *Cell Molec Neurobiol.* 2004;24:63-76.
100. Sagi Y, Drigues N, Youdim MB. The neurochemical and behavioral effects of the novel cholinesterase-monoamine oxidase inhibitor, ladostigil, in response to L-dopa and L-tryptophan, in rats. *Br J Pharmacol.* 2005;146: 553-560.
101. Shin HS. Metabolism of selegiline in humans. *Drug Metab Dispos.* 1997;25:657-662.
102. Shioda K, Nisijima K, Yoshino T, et al. Extracellular serotonin, dopamine and glutamate levels are elevated in the hypothalamus in a serotonin syndrome animal model induced by tranylcypromine and fluoxetine. *Prog Neuropsychopharmacol Biol Psychiatry.* 2004;28:633-640.
103. Simon, HB. Hyperthermia. *N Engl J Med.* 1993;329:483-487.
104. Sinclair JG. The effects of meperidine and morphine in rabbits pretreated with phenelzine. *Toxicol Appl Pharmacol.* 1972;22:231-240.
105. Sinclair JG. Dextromethorphan-monoamine oxidase inhibitor interaction in rabbits. *J Pharm Pharmacol.* 1973;25:803-808.
106. Smith JE. Cooling methods used in the treatment of exertional heat illness. *Br J Sports Med.* 2005;39:503-507.
107. Snider [AU: please cite Rf. 107 in text]SR, Hutt C, Stein B, et al. Increase in brain serotonin produced by bromocriptine. *Neurosci Lett.* 1975;1: 237-241.
108. Sola CL, Bostwick M, Hart DA, et al. Anticipating potential linezolid-SSRI interactions in the general hospital setting: an MAOI in disguise. *Mayo Clin Proc.* 2006;81:330-334.
109. Squires RF, Saederup E. Antidepressants and metabolites that block $GABA_A$ receptors coupled to ^{35}S-*t*-butylbicyclophosphorothionate binding sites in rat brain. *Brain Res.* 1988;441:15-22.
110. Sternbach H. The serotonin syndrome. *Am J Psychiatry.* 1991;148:705-713.
111. Stewart J, Harrison W, Quitkin F, et al. Phenelzine-induced pyridoxine deficiency. *J Clin Psychopharmacol.* 1984;4:225-226.
112. Sulzer D, Rayport S. Amphetamine and other psychostimulants reduce pH gradients in midbrain dopaminergic beurons and chromaffin granules: a mechanism of action. *Neuron.* 1990;5:797-808.
113. Szuba MP, Hornig-Rohan M, Amsterdam JD. Rapid conversion from one monoamine oxidase inhibitor to another. *J Clin Psychiatry.* 1997;58: 307-310.
114. Tailor SA, Shulman KI, Walker SE, et al. Hypertensive episodes associated with phenelzine and tap beer – a reanalysis of the role of pressor amines in beer. *J Clin Psychopharmacol.* 1994;14:5-14.
115. Thase ME, Trivedi M, Rush AJ, et al. MAOIs in the contemporary treatment of depression. *Neuropsychopharmacology.* 1995;12:185-219.
116. Thomas CR, Rosenberg M, Blythe V, et al. Serotonin syndrome and linezolid. *J Am Acad Child Adolesc Psychiatry.* 2004;43:790.
117. Tollefson GD. Monoamine oxidase inhibitors: a review. *J Clin Psychiatry.* 1983;44:280-288.
118. Ulus IH, Maher TJ, Wurtman RJ. Characterization of phentermine and related compounds as monoamine oxidase (MAO) inhibitors. *Biochem Pharmacol.* 2000;59:1611-1621.
119. Vuori E, Henry JA, Ojanpera I, et al. Death following ingestion of MDMA (ecstasy) and moclobemide. *Addiction.* 2003;98:365-368.
120. Walker SE, Shulman KI, Tailor SA, et al. Tyramine content of previously restricted foods in monoamine oxidase inhibitor diets. *J Clin Psychopharmacol.* 1996;16:383-388.
121. Waring WS, Wallace WA. Acute myocarditis after massive phenelzine overdose. *Eur J Clin Pharmacol.* 2007;63:1007-1009.
122. Wells DG, Bjorksten AR. Monoamine oxidase inhibitors revisited. *Can J Anaesth.* 1989;36:64-74.
123. White K, Pistole T, Boyd J. Combined monoamine oxidase inhibitor-tricyclic antidepressant treatment: a pilot study. *Am J Psychiatry.* 1980;137: 1422-1425.
124. Yamada M, Yasuhara H. Clinical pharmacology of MAO inhibitors: safety and future. *Neurotoxicology.* 2004;25:215-221.
125. Youdim MB, Bakhle YS. Monoamine oxidase: isoforms and inhibitors in Parkinson's disease and depressive illness. *Br J Pharmacol.* 2006;147:S287-S296.
126. Youdim MB, Riederer PF. A review of the mechanisms and role of monoamine oxidase inhibitors in Parkinson's disease. *Neurology.* 2004;63:S32-S35.
127. Youdim MB, Weinstock M. Therapeutic applications of selective and nonselective inhibitors of monoamine oxidase A and B that do not cause significant tyramine potentiation. *Neurotoxicology.* 2004;25:243-250.
128. Youdim MBH, Aronson JK, Blau K, et al. Tranylcypromine concentrations and MAO inhibitory activity and identification of amphetamines in plasma. *Psychol Med.* 1997;9:377-382.

CHAPTER 72
SEROTONIN REUPTAKE INHIBITORS AND ATYPICAL ANTIDEPRESSANTS

Christine M. Stork

Antidepressants modulate the activity of serotonin and norepinephrine to achieve their effect. The class of selective serotonin reuptake inhibitors (SSRIs) includes citalopram, escitalopram (active enantiomer of citalopram), fluoxetine, fluvoxamine, paroxetine, and sertraline (Fig. 72–1). Atypical antidepressants expand the pharmacologic principles of SSRIs to achieve additional beneficial effects for patients with depression.

In a brief period of time these new xenobiotics have become the standard, with excellent profiles as compared to the monoamine oxidase inhibitors and the cyclic antidepressants. Like many new xenobiotics the appropriateness of their use and the associated morbidity and mortality have come into question as the patient population has aged and comorbidity profiles of those using the SSRIs have changed.

HISTORY AND EPIDEMIOLOGY

SSRIs initially were marketed in the United States in the early 1980s and still are considered a first-line therapy for treatment of depressive disorders in the United States and in Europe.[18,164,209] SSRIs are as effective as the cyclic antidepressants and monoamine oxidase inhibitors for treatment of major depression and have fewer significant side effects associated with therapeutic use and overdose (Chaps. 71 and 73).[67,135] SSRIs also are used to treat obsessive-compulsive disorders, panic disorders, alcoholism, obesity, and various medical and psychologic disorders such as migraine headache and chronic pain syndromes.[10,147,154]

An increased risk of suicidal behavior is reported with the use of many antidepressants compared with nondrug therapy or no therapy.[6,126] This is particularly true in children. The reason for this finding may be related to delayed onset of drug efficacy coupled with the increased energy associated with the initiation of drug therapy.

PHARMACOLOGY

Table 72–1 lists the pharmacology, therapeutic doses, and metabolism of the currently available SSRIs and the atypical antidepressants. Modulation of serotonin and norepinephrine neurotransmission has a significant role in the treatment of depression.[173] The selectivity of SSRIs for serotonin reuptake is structurally related to p-trifluoromethyl or p-fluoro substitution, which is present in many of these drugs.[218] Serotonin neurons are located almost exclusively in the median raphe nucleus of the brainstem, where they extend into and are in close proximity to norepinephrine neurons that are located primarily in the locus coeruleus (Fig. 72–2).[9] The interplay between norepinephrine and serotonin likely explains the effectiveness of other atypical antidepressants that do not directly modulate serotonin neurotransmission.

The exact etiology of depression and the mechanism by which increased serotonergic and norepinephrine neurotransmission modulates mood remain unclear. Some postulated causes of depression include decreased neuronal serotonin storage, decreased synaptic serotonin, increased serotonin receptor sensitivity, and serotonin overactivity resulting in depressed dopamine neurotransmission.[173,196,212,216] According to the first theory, desensitization and downregulation of serotonin of the somatodendritic and presynaptic inhibitory autoreceptors occur after extended use of SSRIs.[34] Ultimately these effects result in increased activity of raphe neurons, increased synthesis of serotonin, and increased release of serotonin. Unfortunately, no difference in the concentration of serotonin binding sites is reported between depressed patients who respond to SSRIs and those who do not respond.[182] In the second theory, SSRIs potentiate the activity of neuronally released serotonin at 5-HT_{2A} receptors and subsequently decrease the sensitivity of the serotonin receptor.[34] In depressed patients, these receptors are downregulated after treatment, but no overall difference in receptor activity is observed between depressed and nondepressed populations. Finally, increased serotonergic activity, particularly at 5-HT_{2A} receptors, is theorized to result in antidepressant activity through modulation of dopaminergic release.[216] Although the causes of depression are diverse and not well understood, recent data indicate that genetic polymorphisms of the serotonin transporter may play a role in individual response to SSRI therapy.[166]

Unlike cyclic antidepressants and other atypical antidepressants, SSRIs have little direct interaction with cholinergic receptors, γ-aminobutyric acid (GABA) receptors, sodium channels, or adrenergic reuptake (Table 72–2).

PHARMACOKINETICS AND TOXICOKINETICS

The SSRIs display diverse elimination patterns and have numerous active metabolites, which substantially increase both the duration of therapeutic effectiveness and the duration during which drug interactions and adverse drug effects can occur after the drug is discontinued (Table 72–1). Important pharmacokinetic and pharmacodynamic drug interactions are reported with therapeutic dosing (see Serotonin Syndrome). The SSRIs and their active metabolites are substrates for, and potent inhibitors of, CYP2D6 and other CYP enzymes.[89,174] For example, fluoxetine, fluvoxamine, citalopram, venlafaxine, mirtazapine, paroxetine, and sertraline are substrates for CYP2D6, whereas paroxetine, norfluoxetine, and fluoxetine inhibit the same enzyme (Table 72–1). Alternatively, mirtazapine induces CPY3A4 enzymes, while trazodone metabolism may be decreased after this same enzyme is inhibited.[191,197] The consequences of these interactions are manifest when the metabolism of xenobiotics that rely on these enzymes for metabolic transformation is altered (Chap. 12).

CLINICAL MANIFESTATIONS

ACUTE OVERDOSE

The majority of effects that occur following overdose are direct extensions of the pharmacologic activity of SSRIs in therapeutic doses. Excess serotonergic stimulation is prominent and nonselective. Acute signs and symptoms include nausea, vomiting, dizziness, blurred vision, and, less commonly, central nervous system (CNS) depression and sinus tachycardia.[28,30] Seizures and electrocardiographic changes including prolongation of the QRS complex and QT internal duration are reported, but rarely occur with most SSRIs, even after large overdoses (Table 72–3).[93,110,168]

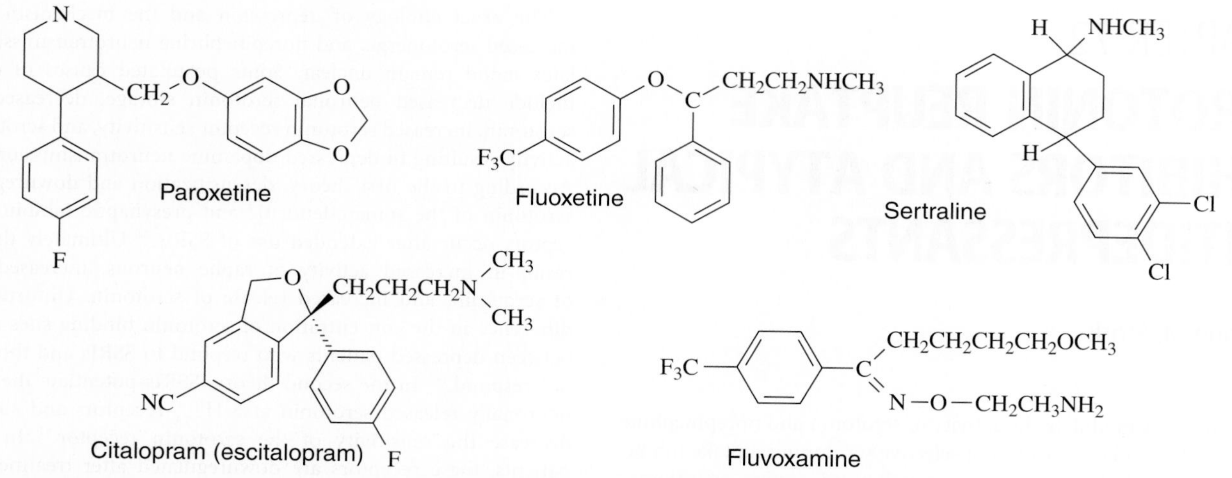

Paroxetine

Fluoxetine

Sertraline

Citalopram (escitalopram)

Fluvoxamine

FIGURE 72–1. Structures of common selective serotonin reuptake inhibitors. Citalopram is shown as the *S*-enantiomer (escitalopram).

Infrequently, SSRI overdose results in life-threatening effects. In two fatalities, the patients reportedly ingested 40–75 times the maximum daily dose of fluoxetine. Serum fluoxetine concentrations were 4500 and 6000 ng/mL, the latter with a measured norfluoxetine concentration of 5000 ng/mL—more than 10 times higher than therapeutic steady-state serum concentrations.[43,116]

Citalopram Citalopram and its enantiomer escitalopram cause QT interval prolongation and seizures in a dose-related manner. These effects are reported at doses as low as 400 mg for citalopram and 190 mg for escitalopram.[40,223] Larger case series found that these effects typically occur after exposure to doses exceeding 600 mg citalopram or in patients with serum concentrations more than 40 times the expected therapeutic concentrations.[90,160,161] In two large case series, seizures were an early finding, whereas the development of ECG abnormalities was delayed for as long as 24 hours following ingestion.[108,161] A recent case report documents prolongation of the QT interval and torsades de pointes occurring at 32.5 hours after ingestion with concentrations of citalopram and desmethylcitalopram of 477 mg/mL and 123.2 mg/mL, respectively.[205]

Although the mechanisms are unclear, experimental models suggest that the didesmethylcitalopram metabolite of citalopram prolongs the QT interval by blocking I_{Kr}, whereas high concentrations of both the parent drug and this metabolite result in seizures (Chaps. 22 and 23).[27,37] The elimination half-life of the *R*-enantiomer of citalopram appears to exceed that of the *S*-enantiomer.[213] The implications of this difference on the formation and effects of racemic forms of didesmethylcitalopram are unclear.

Management Treatment of patients with acute SSRI overdose is largely supportive. Dextrose and thiamine should be considered for patients who present with altered mental status when clinically warranted. Although cardiac manifestations after SSRI overdose are rare, a 12-lead ECG should be obtained to identify other cardiotoxic drugs such as cyclic antidepressants to which the patient may have access (Chaps. 22, 23 and 73). If overdose of citalopram or escitalopram is suspected, 24 hours of cardiac monitoring is recommended to exclude the possibility of QT prolongation and subsequent risk for ventricular dysrhythmias. In a single case, sodium bicarbonate was effective in reversing junctional bradycardia, and QT prolongation.[35]

After the patient is stabilized, oral activated charcoal (1 g/kg) may be useful to adsorb drug remaining in the gastrointestinal tract. In fact, pharmacokinetic lowering of blood concentrations and reduction in risk for QT prolongation is demonstrated when activated charcoal is given early after citalopram ingestion.[69,70] Because SSRI overdose is rarely life threatening, orogastric lavage is not generally indicated. Patients with small unintentional overdoses of SSRIs other than citalopram and escitalopram are not expected to develop significant signs and symptoms of poisoning. Fatalities resulting from SSRIs are rare and most commonly occur after multiple drug ingestions and manifestations of drug interactions resulting from excess serotonergic effects (see Serotonin Syndrome).[84] Forensic analysis suggests the minimum lethal concentrations of fluoxetine, paroxetine, and sertraline after isolated overdose are 0.63, 0.4, and 1.5 mg/L, respectively. Postmortem concentrations of citalopram include a heart blood concentration of 3.35 mg/L, a whole blood concentration of 11.6 mg/L, and urine concentrations of 32.43–149.67 mg/L.[105,131] When mono-n-desmethylcitalopram was measured, concentrations of 1.02 mg/L were found in the blood and 12.1 mg/L in the urine. A case of infant survival occurred with blood concentrations of 1.4 mg/L.[133]

Patients, frequently children, with well-defined small unintentional oral ingestions can be managed safely at home with close observation.[146]

ADVERSE EFFECTS AFTER THERAPEUTIC DOSES

Adverse effects commonly attributed to therapeutic doses of SSRIs that also may occur in overdose include gastrointestinal symptoms (anorexia, nausea, vomiting, diarrhea), sexual dysfunction in both men and women, headache, insomnia, jitteriness, dizziness, and fatigue.[220] Genetic polymorphism typing holds promise in identifying patients at highest risk for adverse drug events with therapeutic dosing.[23,98,195,222] However, pharmacokinetic polymorphisms do not appear to be important with fluoxetine.[80] Less common adverse effects include sedation, particularly following citalopram and paroxetine use as a result of their weak anticholinergic activity, and anxiety following fluoxetine treatment.[129]

Serotonin activity inhibits platelet secretory response, platelet aggregation, and platelet plug formation.[51] Although the effect increases in SSRIs with increased potency, clinical bleeding is rare and significant only in patients concurrently on other antiplatelet medications, most notably nonsteroidal antiinflammatory drugs such as aspirin.[51,137] This effect may be of potential benefit in patients at risk for cardiovascular events.[134] Other rarely reported adverse effects include new onset panic disorder, priapism, various cutaneous effects, bradycardia, hepatotoxicity, and urinary incontinence.[2,22,32,58,121,143,198] Movement disorders,

TABLE 72–1. Pharmacology of Currently Available SSRIs and Atypical Antidepressants

Drug	Typical Daily Dose Range (mg)	V_d (L/kg)	$t_{1/2}$ (h)	Major Metabolic Isoenzyme	Major Active Metabolites	Major Active Metabolite $t_{1/2}$	Drug (d) or Metabolite (m) Inhibits CYP
Selective serotonin reuptake inhibitors (SSRI)							
Citalopram (Celexa)	20–60	12–15	33–37	2C19, 3A4, 2D6	Monodesmethylcitalopram, didesmethylcitalopram	59 h	None/unknown
Escitalopram (Lexapro)	10–20	19	22–32	2C19, 3A4, 2D6,	S(+)-Desmethylcitalopram	59 h	None
Fluoxetine (Prozac)	10–80	14–100	24–144	2C9, 2D6	Norfluoxetine	4–16 d	2D6 (d,m), 2C19 (d,m), 2D6 (d,m), 3A4 (m)
Fluvoxamine (Luvox)	100–300	25	15–23	1A2, 2D6	None	N/A	1A2, 2C9, 2C19, 3A4
Paroxetine (Paxil)	10–50	8–28	2.9–44	2D6	None	N/A	2D6
Sertraline (Zoloft)	50–200	20	24	2C9, 2B6, 2C19, 2D6, 3A4	Desmethylsertraline	62–104 h	2C19 (d,m)
SSRI with α_1-adrenergic antagonism							
Trazodone (Desyrel)	50–600	0.47–1	3–9	2D6, 3A inhibitors may increase concentration	Metachlorophenylpiperazine	?	None/unknown
SSRI with inhibition of reuptake of norepinephrine							
Venlafaxine (Effexor)	75–375	6–7	3–4	2D6	*O*-desmethylvenlafaxine, depends on 3A4 and 2C19 for metabolism	10 h	None/unknown
Duloxetine (Cymbalta)	40–60	23	8–17	2D6, 1A2	None	N/A	2D6
SSRI with α_2-adrenergic antagonism: $5HT_2/5HT_3$ antagonism							
Mirtazapine (Remeron)	15–45	?	20–40	3A4	Desmethylmirtazapine	unknown	3A4 induction
Inhibition of reuptake of biogenic amines or dopamine							
Bupropion (Wellbutrin, Zyban)	150–450	20	9.6–20.9	2D6	Hydroxybupropion, erythrohydrobupropion, threohydrobupropion	24–37 h	None/unknown

NA = Not applicable

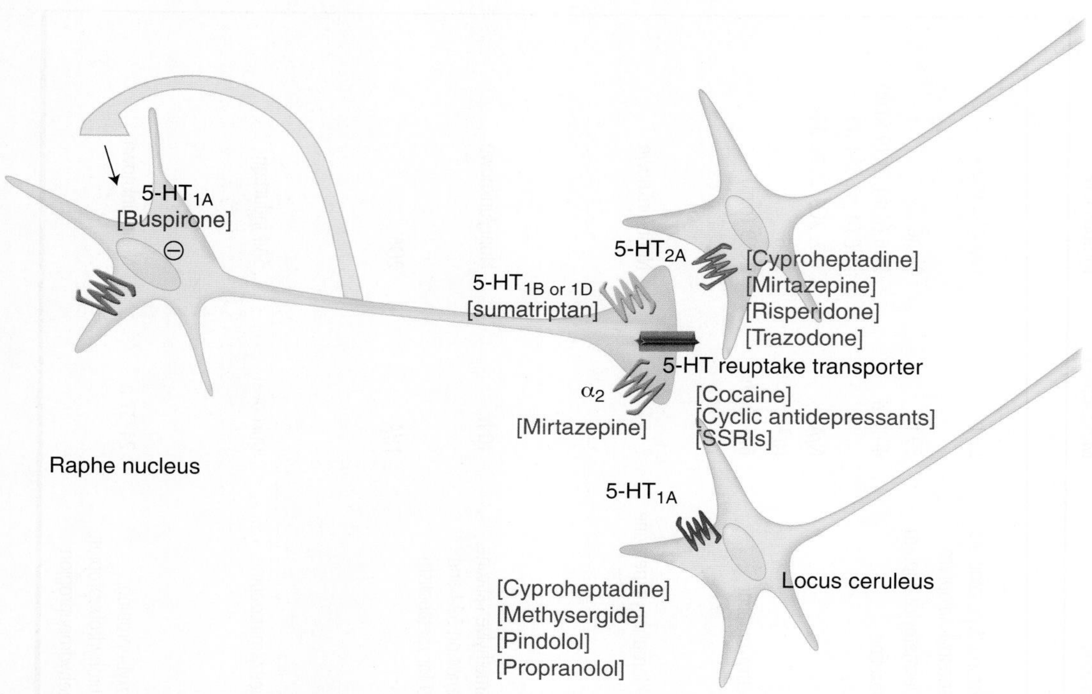

FIGURE 72–2. Neuroanatomy and effects of several common xenobiotics on serotonin neurotransmission in the brain. The 5-HT_{1A} autoreceptors decrease firing in the raphe nucleus when activated by 5-HT. The 5-HT_{1B} and 5-HT_{1D} autoreceptors reduce the release of serotonin.

TABLE 72–2. Receptor Activity of SSRIs and Related Antidepressants

Drug	Mechanism	Degree of Norepinephrine Reuptake Inhibition	Degree of Serotonin Reuptake Inhibition	Degree of Dopamine Reuptake Inhibition	Degree of Peripheral α-Adrenergic Agonism
SSRIs					
Citalopram (Celexa)	SSRI, antimuscarinic	0	++++	0	0
Escitalopram (Lexapro)	SSRI	0	++++	0	0
Fluoxetine (Prozac)	SSRI	0	++++	0	0
Fluvoxamine (Luvox)	SSRI	0	++++	0	0
Paroxetine (Paxil)	SSRI, antimuscarinic	+	++++	+	0
Sertraline (Zoloft)	SSRI	0	++++	+	+
Other					
Bupropion (Wellbutrin, Zyban)	Inhibits reuptake of biogenic amines	++	+	+	+++
Duloxetine (Cymbalta)	SRI, norepinephrine reuptake inhibitor	++	++++	0	++
Mirtazapine (Remeron)	α_2-adrenergic antagonism, $5HT_2/5HT_3$ antagonism	0	++++	0	+
Reboxetine (Edronax, Vestra)	Selective norepinephrine reuptake inhibitor	++++	0	0	++++
Trazodone (Desyrel)	SRI, α-adrenergic antagonist	0	++++	0	0 – +
Venlafaxine (Effexor)	SRI, norepinephrine reuptake inhibitor	++	++++	0	++

SSRI = selective serotonin reuptake inhibitor; SRI = serotonin reuptake inhibitor.

+ weak if any agonism; ++, weak agonism; +++, strong agonism; ++++, very strong agonism; 0, no effect.

TABLE 72–3. Predictive Analysis of the Relative Potential for Seizures and ECG Abnormalities of SSRIs and Atypical Antidepressants

Drug	Seizures	QT Prolongation	QRS Prolongation
Classic SSRIs			
Citalopram (Celexa)	+++	+++	0 – +
Escitalopram (Lexapro)	+++	+++	0 – +
Fluoxetine (Prozac)	+	0	0 – +
Fluvoxamine (Luvox)	+	0	0 – +
Paroxetine (Paxil)	+	0	0 – +
Sertraline (Zoloft)	+	0	0 – +
Atypical Antidepressants			
Bupropion (Wellbutrin, Zyban)	++++	0 – +	+
Duloxetine (Cymbalta)	++++	Unknown	Unknown
Mirtazapine (Remeron)	Unknown	Unknown	++
Reboxetine (Edronax, Vestra)	++++	Unknown	Unknown
Trazodone (Desyrel)	0 – +	0	0
Venlafaxine (Effexor)	+++	0 – +	+++

0 does not cause; + very rarely causes; ++ rarely causes; +++ causes; ++++ very commonly causes.

TABLE 72–4. Potential Xenobiotic Causes of Serotonin Syndrome

Inhibition of Serotonin Breakdown
- Linezolid[41,55]
- Methylene blue[79]
- Monoamine oxidase inhibitors (nonselective)
  - Phenelzine, moclobemide, clorgyline, isocarboxazid[31,38,42,68,82,87,99,113,163,175,189,193,194,203,206]
- Harmine and harmaline from Ayahuasca preparations, psychoactive beverage used for religious purposes in the Amazon and Orinoco River basins[38]

Blockade of Serotonin Reuptake
- Bupropion[145]
- Clomipramine[119,163,178,195]
- Cocaine[207]
- Dextromethorphan[148,176]
- Fentanyl[3]
- Meperidine[4,82]
- Pentazocine[95]
- SSRIs
  - Fluoxetine, citalopram, paroxetine, fluvoxamine, sertraline[3,4,11,17,20,31,41,44,55,57,64,68,75,78,79,87,88,95,127,144,145,155,163,170,179,189,192]
- Tramadol[118]
- Trazodone[75,85,150,169,170]
- Venlafaxine[47,99,120]

Serotonin Precursors or Agonists
- L-Tryptophan[195]
- Lysergic acid diethylamide (LSD)[188]

Enhancers of Serotonin Release
- Amphetamines, especially MDMA (ecstasy)[113,193]
- Buspirone[11,85]
- Cocaine[206]
- Lithium[119,144,151]
- Mirtazapine[20,55,57]

most commonly akathisia, parkinsonism, myoclonus, and dystonia, also occur after SSRI use.[7,185] These extrapyramidal side effects may be related to the complex interplay between serotonergic and dopaminergic activity. Predisposing factors for the development of movement disorders include concomitant use of dopamine antagonists such as the antipsychotics.[122]

The syndrome of inappropriate antidiuretic hormone (SIADH) (see Chap. 16), in which severe hyponatremia may occur rapidly, is associated with SSRI use. In an animal model, the effect appears to be serotonin mediated, with increased concentrations of serum cortisol, adrenocorticotropin (ACTH), and vasopressin.[72] Rat studies demonstrate that stimulation of $5HT_{1C}$ receptors increases antidiuretic hormone secretion.[159] However, human case control studies have not confirmed defects in osmoregulated release of vasopressin through normal water loading tests and measurement of vasopressin concentrations after 3–11 months of paroxetine use.[132] A review of the literature identified women older than 70 years who are concomitantly receiving diuretic therapy and have low baseline serum sodium concentrations to be at the greatest risk for developing SIADH.[24,112,117] Although reported to occur from 3 days to 4 months after initiation of therapy, a case-matched control study of 203 patients identified that SIADH occurs most frequently within the first 2 weeks of therapy.[142] Hyponatremia is demonstrated to occur when switching from one SSRI to another.[8] Efforts to predict risk through poor CYP2D6 genotype metabolizer status or high serum concentrations have not been successful.[200]

Patients older than 50 years of age using SSRIs may be at increased risk for bone fracture theorized due to a serotinergic effect on osteoblasts and osteocytes.[172] However, depression itself is also implicated in decreasing bone density in adults and children, and the implications of these findings are unknown.[214]

Serotonin Syndrome The most common severe adverse effect associated with SSRIs is the development of the serotonin syndrome. This syndrome, also referred to as the serotonin behavioral or hyperactivity syndrome, was first described in patients treated with MAOIs who were given other drugs that enhance serotonergic activity.[42,88,153,194] However, ingestion of an MAOI is not required for this syndrome to develop, and its development is unpredictable (Table 72–4).

Pathophysiology. The pathophysiologic mechanism of the serotonin syndrome is not completely understood but involves excessive selective stimulation of serotonin $5\text{-}HT_{2A}$ and perhaps $5\text{-}HT_{1A}$ receptors.[29] Animal models demonstrate that specific stimulation of $5\text{-}HT_{1A}$ receptors results in signs and symptoms of serotonin syndrome even when $5\text{-}HT_{2A}$ receptors were inactivated using a specific antagonist.[48] However, a subsequent animal study and a human retrospective case series showed that the potency of $5\text{-}HT_{2A}$ antagonist therapy was directly related to resolution of symptoms attributed to serotonin syndrome.[81] $5\text{-}HT_{1D}$ receptors are not implicated in cases of serotonin syndrome.

Clinical Manifestations. Symptoms of serotonin syndrome include altered mental status, agitation, myoclonus, hyperreflexia, diaphoresis, tremor, diarrhea, incoordination, muscle rigidity, and hyperthermia (Table 72–5). The clinical manifestations of serotonin syndrome are diverse, and minor manifestations are common after initiation of SSRI and atypical antidepressant therapy. In fact, a prospective study of depressed inpatients given clomipramine demonstrated that 16 of 38 patients experienced symptoms consistent with the serotonin syndrome, 14 of whom spontaneously recovered within 1 week without discontinuation of therapy.[125]

Life-threatening effects invariably result from hyperthermia caused by excessive muscle activity which may be more prominent in the lower extremities. Sustained severe hyperthermia can lead to death through denaturation of essential protein and enzymatic function that ultimately results in elevated lactate and metabolic acidosis, rhabdomyolysis, myoglobinuria, renal and hepatic dysfunction, disseminated intravascular coagulation, or adult respiratory distress syndrome (Chap. 15).[138,201]

Diagnosis. The serotonin syndrome occurs most frequently following use of combinations of serotonergic agents (Table 72–4). Xenobiotic interactions resulting in serotonin syndrome can occur while switching serotonergic pharmacologic agents when an insufficient time lag occurs before initiating the alternative therapy.[179,180] Residual pharmacologic effect, receptor downregulation or upregulation, and the presence of active metabolites may be causative in these circumstances. For example, fluoxetine metabolism results in the active metabolite norfluoxetine, which has comparable pharmacologic effects and a half-life substantially longer than that of the parent xenobiotic. The metabolite persists and may result in serotonin syndrome when another serotonergic agent, usually another antidepressant, is given prior to complete clearance of norfluoxetine, which takes approximately 2 weeks.[44]

This syndrome is reported in patients following a single dose, high therapeutic dosing, or overdoses of certain serotonergic agents in adults and children.[47,78,94,114,126,157,169] Although sporadic reports occur, selective MAO subtype B (MAO-B) inhibitor drug combinations are rarely reported to result in serotonin syndrome at therapeutic doses.[61,140]

Currently no diagnostic test capable of determining whether a patient is experiencing serotonin syndrome is available. A single case report demonstrated increased urinary serotonin concentrations after serotonin syndrome.[36] Although fulminant life-threatening cases are easy to recognize, mild cases are more difficult to distinguish from other causes. In an effort to determine diagnostic criteria, a study that included 38 cases of presumed serotonin syndrome was performed. This trial led to suggested diagnostic criteria for serotonin syndrome that include three of the following signs and symptoms—altered level of consciousness, agitation, myoclonus, hyperreflexia, diaphoresis, tremor, diarrhea, and incoordination—when other etiologies are excluded.[202] A modification, the Hunter Serotonin Toxicity Criteria, which included the variables myoclonus, agitation, diaphoresis, hyperreflexia, hypertonicity, and fever, was validated in 473 patients and found to correlate best with a clinical toxicologic diagnosis of the serotonin syndrome.[63,201] The most comprehensive review of signs and symptoms in a literature review found altered mental status, other neurologic signs and symptoms, vital signs, and autonomic manifestations most commonly associated with the development of serotonin syndrome. Diagnostic criteria based on these clinical findings are given in Table 72–5.[167]

TABLE 72–5. Diagnostic Criteria for Serotonin Syndrome

Major	Minor
Mental Status	
Consciousness altered	Insomnia
Elevated mood	Restlessness
Other Neurologic Signs and Symptoms	
Coma	Akathisia
Hyperreflexia	Incoordination
Myoclonus	Mydriasis
Rigidity	
Shivering	
Tremor	
Vital Signs and Autonomic Manifestations	
Fever (Hyperthermia)	Hypertension or hypotension
Sweating	Tachycardia
	Tachypnea or Dyspnea
	Diarrhea

Serotonin syndrome is diagnosed by the presence of at least four major symptoms or three major plus two minor symptoms following the addition or an increase in a known serotonergic agent. Underlying psychiatric disorder should be excluded. Other etiologies must be excluded, including initiation of a neuroleptic or other dopamine antagonist or withdrawal from a dopamine agonist.

Management. Treatment of patients with serotonin syndrome begins with supportive care and focuses on decreasing muscle rigidity. Because muscular rigidity is thought to be partly responsible for hyperthermia and death, rapid external cooling in conjunction with aggressive use of benzodiazepines should limit complications and mortality. In severe cases, neuromuscular blockade should be considered to achieve rapid muscle relaxation. The time course of the serotonin syndrome is variable and related to the time required to offending drug effects. In most patients, the serotonin syndrome resolves within 24 hours after the offending drug is removed. However, the serotonin syndrome can be prolonged when it is caused by drugs with long half-lives, protracted duration of effects, or active metabolites.

Animal models indicate that pretreatment with serotonin antagonists can prevent development of the serotonin syndrome.[77,103,199] Several case reports indicate the successful use of 4 mg oral or intravenous cyproheptadine, an antihistamine with nonspecific antagonist effects at 5-HT_{1A} and 5-HT_{2A} receptors.[88,123] Current recommendation allows doses at 8–16 mg. Patients who responded typically had mild to moderate symptoms of serotonin syndrome and were not hyperthermic evidence supports the use of cyproheptadine in this patient group. Further research is warranted to determine the success of higher doses given to gain sufficient 5-HT_{2A} antagonistic effects in more severely affected patients.[81] Other drugs that are anecdotally reported to be successful for treatment of symptoms caused by the serotonin syndrome include methysergide, chlorpromazine, atypical antipsychotics, and propranolol.[81,82,85,91,181] Because all of these drugs are of unproven utility and can be dangerous, aggressive cooling and sedation with a benzodiazepine remain the basis of therapy.

Differential Diagnosis of the Serotonin Syndrome from the Neuroleptic Malignant Syndrome Many features overlap between the serotonin syndrome and the neuroleptic malignant syndrome (NMS) (Chap. 68). Some authors call these "spectrum disorders" that can be caused by drugs with antidopaminergic and/or proserotonergic effects.[139,221] This position is supported by the finding that 5-HT_{2A} agonism results

TABLE 72–6. Comparison of Neuroleptic Malignant Syndrome (NMS) and Serotonin Syndrome (SS)

	NMS	SS
Historical Diagnostic Clue		
Inciting drug pharmacology	Dopamine antagonist	Serotonin agonist
Time course of initiation of symptoms after exposure	Days to weeks	Hours
Duration of symptoms	Days to 2 weeks	Usually 24 hours
Symptoms		
Autonomic instability	+++	+++
Fever	+++	+++
Altered level of consciousness (depressed/confusion)	+++	+++
Altered mental status (agitation/hyperactivity)	+	+++
Lead pipe rigidity	+++	+
Tremor, hyperreflexia, myoclonus	+	+++
Shivering	–	+++
Bradykinesia	+++	–

– not found; + rare finding; +++ common finding.

in an overall decrease in neuronal dopamine release. Some authors report NMS with use of serotonin-enhancing drugs. However, low concentrations of measured dopamine and normal concentrations of serotonin metabolites in the NMS patients reported support the hypothesis of central dopaminergic hypoactivity.[12,150] It now is clear that the implicated drugs, time course, pathophysiologic mechanism, and manifestations are distinct (Table 72–6).[81] Altered mental status, autonomic instability, and changes in neuromuscular tone that may result in hyperthermia are common to both syndromes. The development of NMS involves rapid blockade of dopaminergic neurons in the CNS, whereas the serotonin syndrome appears to result from acute overstimulation of serotonin receptors ($5\text{-}HT_{2A}$).

In addition to the associated medications, the time courses of the two syndromes are substantially different. Signs and symptoms of the serotonin syndrome develop within minutes to hours after exposure to the offending xenobiotics, whereas NMS typically develops days to weeks after daily exposure to the drug in question.[87] In addition, after symptoms develop and offending xenobiotics are discontinued, NMS can last for as long as 2 weeks, whereas the serotonin syndrome usually resolves quickly, directly correlated with the pharmacokinetic metabolic profile of the offending xenobiotic. A review of the literature indicates that patients presenting with serotonin syndrome were more likely to exhibit agitation, hyperactivity, clonus and myoclonus, ocular oscillations, (opsoclonus), shivering, tremors, and hyperreflexia, whereas patients presenting with NMS were more likely to exhibit bradykinesia and lead pipe rigidity.[81]

ATYPICAL ANTIDEPRESSANTS

Atypical antidepressants are defined as not belonging strictly to a set classification of antidepressants. They are not SSRIs, cyclic antidepressants, or MAOIs. In general, the atypical antidepressants are the newer antidepressants, most of which are derivatives of SSRIs and have additional pharmacologic effects that were selected in an attempt to decrease the undesirable side effects of traditional antidepressants.

SEROTONIN/NOREPINEPHRINE REUPTAKE INHIBITORS

Venlafaxine

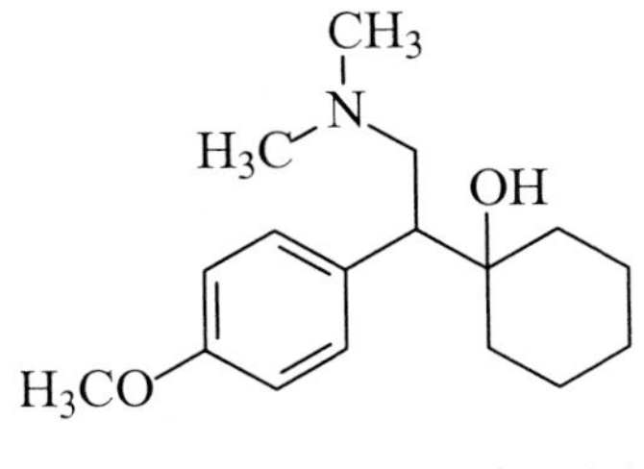

In addition to inhibiting serotonin reuptake, venlafaxine inhibits norepinephrine reuptake. Venlafaxine produces rapid downregulation of central β-adrenergic receptors, which may result in a faster onset of antidepressant effect.[187] Patients with acute venlafaxine overdose may present with nausea, vomiting, dizziness, tachycardia, CNS depression, hypotension, hyperthermia, hepatic toxicity that include zone 3 necrosis, rhabdomyolysis and seizures.[104,187,215,217,224] (see Chap. 26). Sodium and potassium channel blocking effects are rarely clinically apparent; however, QRS prolongation, QT prolongation, and ventricular tachycardia have resulted in death.[16,26,128,178,224] One report indicated a positive association of toxicity to serum venlafaxine concentration.[136] Although no clinical data regarding efficacy are available, sodium bicarbonate may be helpful in attenuating the sodium channel blocking effects leading to QRS prolongation (Antidotes in Depth A5: Sodium Bicarbonate). Chronic reported adverse effects after venlafaxine include alopecia, yawning, focal myositis facial flushing, and dose-related increases in blood pressure.[54,59,65,109,158]

Duloxetine, a drug similar to venlafaxine, has similar effects.[62]

OTHER ATYPICAL ANTIDEPRSSANTS WITH REUPTAKE INHIBITION AS PART OF THEIR MECHANISM

Bupropion

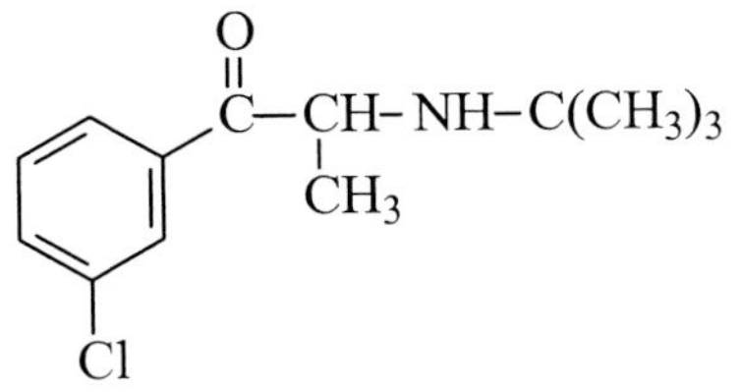

The pharmacologic mechanism of action of bupropion, a unicyclic antidepressant, is unclear, but both the parent xenobiotic and an active metabolite inhibit the reuptake of dopamine and, to a lesser extent, serotonin and norepinephrine.[173] Extended-release formulations of bupropion are frequently used as adjuncts in smoking cessation therapy.[107] Chronic doses greater than 450–500 mg/d place the patient at risk for seizures.[50,112]

Frequent effects after overdose include tachycardia, hypertension, gastrointestinal symptoms, and agitation.[15,19] Large acute overdoses may result in seizures and/or QRS prolongation.[46,83,97,141,156,190,202] In some cases, effects were delayed for up 10 hours, particularly after ingestion of sustained-release preparations.[96,190] Symptoms can continue for up to 48 hours.

Several studies suggest that seizures following either bupropion overdose or high therapeutic doses are caused by its metabolite hydroxybupropion.[71,162] Elevated hydroxybupropion concentrations are documented after seizures when bupropion concentrations were no longer detectable. The exact mechanism for the development of seizures caused by hydroxybupropion is unclear at this time.[50,71,176]

Treatment, when required for seizures, should be supportive and includes judicious use of benzodiazepines, followed by barbiturates if necessary. If QRS prolongation occurs, the patient should be treated with sodium bicarbonate (Antidotes in Depth A5: Sodium Bicarbonate). Intravenous fat emulsion therapy was used to successfully resuscitate a 17-year-old woman who ingested multiple drugs including bupropion after sodium bicarbonate and advanced life support failed and should be considered in similar cases (Antidotes in Depth A21: Intravenous Fat Emulsion).[190] Early after sustained-release bupropion overdose, activated charcoal should be considered, with use of multiple doses of activated charcoal or whole-bowel irrigation after large, potentially life-threatening ingestions.

Other serious adverse effects reported after bupropion use include cholestatic and hepatocellular hepatic dysfunction, and rhabdomyolysis, with isolated reports of chest pain, dystonia, trigeminal nerve dysfunction, mania, generalized erythrodermic psoriasis, erythema multiforme, dyskinesias, altered vestibular and sensory function, and serum sickness.[5,45,49,53,60,74,86,115,130,207,221]

Trazodone

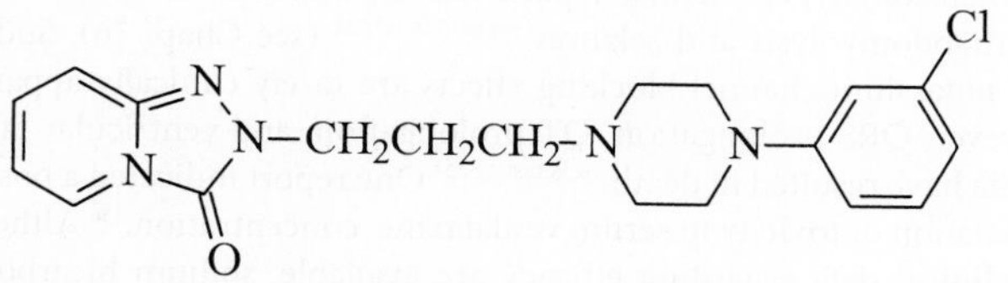

Trazodone is a serotonin agonist that acts through inhibition of serotonin reuptake. In addition, trazodone has peripheral α-adrenergic antagonist activity. CNS depression and orthostatic hypotension are the most common complications after acute overdose of trazodone.[73] Trazodone is rarely reported to cause SIADH. This effect may be responsible for seizures, which also may occur after acute overdose.[13,210] Priapism, reported with trazodone, may also occur occasionally after overdose.[39,73] Management of hypotension includes supportive care and administration of fluids and vasopressors, if necessary.

Mirtazapine

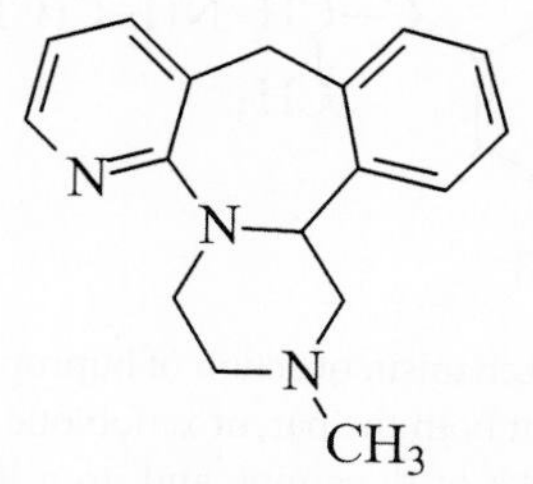

The mechanism of mirtazapine action is unique. In addition to serotonin reuptake inhibition, mirtazapine increases neuronal norepinephrine and serotonin through α_2-adrenergic antagonism.[52] Mirtazapine also blocks some subtypes of 5-HT receptors, including 5-HT_2 and 5-HT_3, which appear to have antidepressant effects.[152] The main effects that occur after acute mirtazapine overdoses include altered mental status, tachycardia, and hypothermia.[33,171,211] Large overdoses may cause respiratory depression and prolongation of the QT interval.[33,76,102,172] Because more overdose data are required before a precise constellation of symptoms can be attributed to this xenobiotic, careful clinical monitoring is advised. Therapeutic use of mirtazapine causing serotonin syndrome, hepatitis, hypertension, and reversible agranulocytosis is reported.[1,100,106,149,208]

DRUG DISCONTINUATION SYNDROME

The term *drug discontinuation syndrome* is used to describe the physiologic manifestations that occur after antidepressant withdrawal. The choice of terminology is unclear, but may relate to the manifestations occurring after therapeutic use versus misuse of the drug. Drug discontinuation syndromes are commonly reported after withdrawal of conventional antidepressants, including cyclic antidepressants and MAOIs (Chaps. 71 and 73).[124] SSRIs cause a discontinuation syndrome that typically begins within 5 days after drug discontinuation and may last up to 3 weeks.[92] The most frequently reported symptoms include dizziness, lethargy, paresthesias, nausea, vivid dreams, irritability, and depressed mood.[185] The risk factors associated with development of a discontinuation syndrome are not fully clarified. The syndrome is more common with SSRIs that have shorter elimination half-lives (paroxetine > fluvoxamine > sertraline > fluoxetine). In addition, SSRIs with high-potency serotonin reuptake inhibition are more frequently implicated (paroxetine > sertraline > clomipramine > fluoxetine > venlafaxine > trazodone). Of the SSRIs, paroxetine most often results in discontinuation syndrome, which results in mild to moderate symptoms in 20%–40% of patients, respectively, receiving 20 mg daily.[14] Several studies demonstrate that the vast majority of cases are attributed to paroxetine with an approximately 20% risk with sertraline, and escitalopram and 10% decrease in risk with fluvoxamine.[14,25] Fluoxetine discontinuation syndrome occurs less frequently, at only two cases per million prescriptions.[165] The long elimination half-life of fluoxetine and its active metabolite norfluoxetine probably decrease the incidence of discontinuation syndrome by providing a tapered effect after cessation.

Because of difficulty in distinguishing symptoms of discontinuation syndrome from underlying disease, many authors have proposed diagnostic criteria for the SSRI discontinuation syndrome.[25] All proposed criteria include discontinuation of the SSRI in concordance with CNS effects, gastrointestinal distress, or anxiety.[205]

The biochemical basis of the discontinuation syndrome appears to be similar to tryptophan depletion, both of which result in an acute decrease in synaptic serotonin.[56] In fact, abrupt discontinuation versus drug taper was a noted risk factor in paroxetine cases when compared with those who did not suffer discontinuation symptoms.[101] Although postulated, antimuscarinic withdrawal seems an unlikely cause because the antimuscarinic effects of desipramine failed to protect against paroxetine withdrawal in a human model.[66]

Treatment of patients exhibiting discontinuation symptoms should include supportive care and reinitiation of the discontinued drug or administration of another SSRI if reinitiation of the drug is contraindicated.[184] The drug then should be tapered at a rate that allows for improved patient tolerance.

Many of the other antidepressants discussed in this chapter also result in discontinuation reactions. Symptoms appear similar to those reported after discontinuation of SSRIs and are treated in a similar manner.[21,111]

SUMMARY

In acute overdose, SSRIs or atypical antidepressants usually are not life threatening, although a few drugs produce seizures or cardiac toxicity. Treatment is generally supportive for all of these drugs. In particular, patients with citalopram or escitalopram overdoses should be monitored for 24 h for QT prolongation. However, significant drug interactions and adverse drug effects are associated with serotonin reuptake inhibitors and may lead to acute life-threatening events including serotonin syndrome. In addition, the management of these patients frequently is complicated because they likely have concomitant access to more life-threatening antidepressants such as cyclic antidepressants and MAOIs.

REFERENCES

1. Abo-Zena RA, Bobek MB, Dweik RA. Hypertensive urgency induced by an interaction of mirtazapine and clonidine. *Pharmacotherapy.* 2000;20:476-478.
2. Aframian DJ. Oral adverse effects for escitalopram (Cipralex). *Br J Dermatol.* 2007;156:1046-1047.
3. Ailawadhi S, Sung KW, Carlson LA, Baer MR. Serotonin syndrome caused by interaction between citalopram and fentanyl. *J Clin Pharm Ther.* 2007;32(2):199-202.
4. Altman EM, Manos GH. Serotonin syndrome associated with citalopram and meperidine. *Psychosomatics.* 2007;48:361-363.
5. Amann B, Hummel B, Rall-Autenrieth H, Walden J, Grunze H. Bupropion-induced isolated impairment of sensory trigeminal nerve function. *Int Clin Psychopharmacol.* 2000;15:115-116.
6. Anonymous. Effexor (venlafaxine) warnings added for neonatal effects and suicidality risk, *Medwatch,* June 2004.
7. Anonymous. Extrapyramidal effects of SSRI antidepressants. *Prescrire Int.* 2001;10:118-119.
8. Arinzon ZH, Lehman YA, Fidelman ZG, Krasnyansky II. Delayed recurrent SIADH associated with SSRIs. *Ann Pharmacother.* 2002;36:1175-1177.
9. Asnis GM, Wetzler S, Sanderson WC, Kahn RS, van Praag HM. Functional interrelationship of serotonin and norepinephrine: cortisol response to MCPP and DMI in patients with panic disorder, patients with depression, and normal control subjects. *Psychiatry Res.* 1992;43:65-76.
10. Atkinson JH, Slater MA, Capparelli EV, et al. Efficacy of noradrenergic and serotonergic antidepressants in chronic back pain: a preliminary concentration-controlled trial. *J Clin Psychopharmacol.* 2007;27:135-142.
11. Baetz M, Malcolm D. Serotonin syndrome from fluvoxamine and buspirone. *Can J Psychiatry.* 1995;40:428-429.
12. Bakheit AM, Behan PO, Prach AT, Rittey CD, Scott AJ. A syndrome identical to the neuroleptic malignant syndrome induced by LSD and alcohol. *Br J Addict.* 1990;85:150-151.
13. Baldessarini RJ. Drugs and the treatment of psychiatric disorders. In: Hardman JG, Limbird LE, Molinoff PB, ed. *Goodman & Gillman's The Pharmacological Basis of Therapeutics.* 9th ed. New York: McGraw-Hill, 1996:431-459.
14. Baldwin DS, Montgomery SA, Nil R, Lader M. Discontinuation symptoms in depression and anxiety disorders. *Int J Neuropsychopharmacol.* 2007;10:73-84.
15. Balit CR, Lynch CN, Isbister GK. Bupropion poisoning: a case series. *Med J Aust.* 2003;178:61-63.
16. Banham ND. Fatal venlafaxine overdose. *Med J Aust.* 1998;169:445.
17. Bastani JB, Troester MM, Bastani AJ. Serotonin syndrome and fluvoxamine: a case study. *Nebr Med J.* 1996;81:107-109.
18. Bauer M, Monz BU, Montejo AL, et al. Prescribing patterns of antidepressants in Europe: results from the Factors Influencing Depression Endpoints Research (FINDER) study. *Eur Psychiatry.* 2008;23:66-73.
19. Belson MG, Kelley TR. Bupropion exposures: clinical manifestations and medical outcome. *J Emerg Med.* 2002;23:223-230.
20. Benazzi F. Serotonin syndrome with mirtazapine-fluoxetine combination. *Int J Geriatr Psychiatry* 1998;13:495-496.
21. Benazzi F. Mirtazapine withdrawal symptoms. *Can J Psychiatry.* 1998;43:525.
22. Beyenburg S, Schonegger K. Severe bradycardia in a stroke patient caused by a single low dose of escitalopram. *Eur Neurol.* 2007;57:50-51.
23. Bishop JR, Moline J, Ellingrod VL, Schultz SK, Clayton AH. Serotonin 2A-1438 G/A and G-protein Beta3 subunit C825T polymorphisms in patients with depression and SSRI-associated sexual side-effects. *Neuropsychopharmacology.* 2006;31:2281-2288.
24. Bissram M, Scott FD, Liu L, Rosner MH. Risk factors for symptomatic hyponatraemia: the role of pre-existing asymptomatic hyponatraemia. *Intern Med J.* 2007;37:149-155.
25. Black K, Shea C, Dursun S, Kutcher S. Selective serotonin reuptake inhibitor discontinuation syndrome: proposed diagnostic criteria. *J Psychiatry Neurosci.* 2000;25:255-2.
26. Blythe D, Hackett LP. Cardiovascular and neurological toxicity of venlafaxine. *Hum Exp Toxicol.* 1999;18:309-313.
27. Boeck V, Overo KF, Svendsen O. Studies on acute toxicity and drug levels of citalopram in the dog. *Acta Pharmacol Toxicol.* 1982;50:169-174.
28. Borys DJ, Setzer SC, Ling LJ, Reisdorf JJ, Day LC, Krenzelok EP. Acute fluoxetine overdose: a report of 234 cases. *Am J Emerg Med.* 1992;10:115-120.
29. Boyer EW, Shannon M. The serotonin syndrome. [see comment] [erratum appears in *N Engl J Med.* 2007 Jun 7;356(23):2437]. *N Engl J Med.* 2005;352:1112-1120.
30. Braitberg G, Curry SC. Seizure after isolated fluoxetine overdose. *Ann Emerg Med.* 1995;26:234-237.
31. Brannan SK, Talley BJ, Bowden CL. Sertraline and isocarboxazid cause a serotonin syndrome. *J Clin Psychopharmacol.* 1994;14:144-145.
32. Brauer HR, Nowicki PW, Catalano G, Catalano MC. Panic attacks associated with citalopram. *South Med J.* 2002;95:1088-1089.
33. Bremner JD, Wingard P, Walshe TA. Safety of mirtazapine in overdose. *J Clin Psychiatry.* 1998;59:233-235.
34. Briley M, Moret C. Neurobiological mechanisms involved in antidepressant therapies. *Clin Neuropharmacol.* 1993;16:387-400.
35. Brucculeri M, Kaplan J, Lande L. Reversal of citalopram-induced junctional bradycardia with intravenous sodium bicarbonate. *Pharmacotherapy.* 2005;25:119-122.
36. Brvar M, Stajer D, Kozelj G, Osredkar J, Mozina M, Bunc M. Urinary serotonin level is associated with serotonin syndrome after moclobemide, sertraline, and citalopram overdose. *Clin Toxicol.* 2007;45:458-460.
37. Burgh VDM. Citalopram product monograph. Copenhagen, Denmark. H. Lundbeck A/S: 1994.
38. Callaway JC, Grob CS. Ayahuasca preparations and serotonin reuptake inhibitors: a potential combination for severe adverse interactions. *J Psychoactive Drugs.* 1998;30:367-369.
39. Carson CC, 3rd, Mino RD. Priapism associated with trazodone therapy. *J Urol.* 1988;139:369-370.
40. Catalano G, Catalano MC, Epstein MA, Tsambiras PE. QTc interval prolongation associated with citalopram overdose: a case report and literature review. *Clin Neuropharmacol.* 2001;24:158-162.
41. Clark DB, Andrus MR, Byrd DC. Drug interactions between linezolid and selective serotonin reuptake inhibitors: case report involving sertraline and review of the literature. *Pharmacotherapy.* 2006;26:269-276.
42. Cohen RM, Pickar D, Murphy DL. Myoclonus-associated hypomania during MAO-inhibitor treatment. *Am J Psychiatry.* 1980;137:105-106.
43. Compton R, Spiller HA, Bosse GM. Fatal fluoxetine ingestion with postmortem blood concentrations. *Clin Toxicol.* 2005;43:277-279.
44. Coplan JD, Gorman JM. Detectable levels of fluoxetine metabolites after discontinuation: an unexpected serotonin syndrome. *Am J Psychiatry.* 1993;150:837.
45. Cox NH, Gordon PM, Dodd H. Generalized pustular and erythrodermic psoriasis associated with bupropion treatment. *Br J Dermatol.* 2002;146:1061-1063.
46. Curry SC, Kashani JS, LoVecchio F, Holubek W. Intraventricular conduction delay after bupropion overdose. *J Emerg Med.* 2005;29:299-305.
47. Daniels RJ. Serotonin syndrome due to venlafaxine overdose. *J Accid Emerg Med.* 1998;15:333-334.
48. Darmani NA, Zhao W. Production of serotonin syndrome by 8-OH DPAT in Cryptotis parva. *Physiol Behav.* 1998;65:327-331.
49. David D, Esquenazi J. Rhabdomyolysis associated with bupropion treatment. *J Clin Psychopharmacol.* 1999;19:185-186.
50. Davidson J. Seizures and bupropion: a review. [see comment]. *J Clin Psychiatry.* 1989;50:256-261.
51. de Abajo FJ, Montero D, Rodriguez LA, Madurga M. Antidepressants and risk of upper gastrointestinal bleeding. *Basic Clin Pharmacol Toxicol.* 2006;98:304-310.
52. de Boer T. The pharmacologic profile of mirtazapine. *J Clin Psychiatry.* 1996;57:19-25.
53. de Graaf L, Diemont WL. Chest pain during use of bupropion as an aid in smoking cessation. *Br J Clin Pharmacol.* 2003;56:451-452.
54. De Las Cuevas C, Sanz EJ. Duloxetine-induced excessive disturbing and disabling yawning. *J Clin Psychopharmacol.* 2007;27:106-107.
55. DeBellis RJ, Schaefer OP, Liquori M, Volturo GA. Linezolid-associated serotonin syndrome after concomitant treatment with citalopram and mirtazepine in a critically ill bone marrow transplant recipient. *J Intensive Care Med.* 2005;20:351-353.

56. Delgado PL. Monoamine depletion studies: implications for antidepressant discontinuation syndrome. *J Clin Psychiatry*. 2006;67:22-26.
57. Demers JC, Malone M. Serotonin syndrome induced by fluvoxamine and mirtazapine. *Ann Pharmacother*. 2001;35:1217-1220.
58. Dent LA, Brown WC, Murney JD. Citalopram-induced priapism. *Pharmacotherapy*. 2002;22:538-541.
59. Derby MA, Zhang L, Chappell JC, et al. The effects of supratherapeutic doses of duloxetine on blood pressure and pulse rate. *J Cardiovasc Pharmacol*. 2007;49:384-393.
60. Detweiler MB, Harpold GJ. Bupropion-induced acute dystonia. *Ann Pharmacother*. 2002;36:251-254.
61. Dingemanse J, Wallnofer A, Gieschke R, Guentert T, Amrein R. Pharmacokinetic and pharmacodynamic interactions between fluoxetine and moclobemide in the investigation of development of the "serotonin syndrome". *Clin Pharmacol Therapeutics*. 1998;63:403-413.
62. Dugan SE, Fuller MA. Duloxetine: a dual reuptake inhibitor. *Ann Pharmacother*. 2004;38:2078-2085.
63. Dunkley EJ, Isbister GK, Sibbritt D, Dawson AH, Whyte IM. The Hunter Serotonin Toxicity Criteria: simple and accurate diagnostic decision rules for serotonin toxicity. *QJM* 2003;96:635-642.
64. Dursun SM, Mathew VM, Reveley MA. Toxic serotonin syndrome after fluoxetine plus carbamazepine. *Lancet*. 1993;342:442-443.
65. Ezzo DC, Patel PN. Facial flushing associated with duloxetine use. *Am J Health-System Pharm* .2007;64:495-496.
66. Fava GA, Grandi S. Withdrawal syndromes after paroxetine and sertraline discontinuation. *J Clin Psychopharmacol*. 1995;15:374-375.
67. Finley PR. Selective serotonin reuptake inhibitors: pharmacologic profiles and potential therapeutic distinctions. *Ann Pharmacother*. 1994;28:1359-1369.
68. FitzSimmons CR, Metha S. Serotonin syndrome caused by overdose with paroxetine and moclobemide. *J Accid Emerg Med*. 1999;16:293-295.
69. Friberg LE, Isbister GK, Duffull SB. Pharmacokinetic-pharmacodynamic modelling of QT interval prolongation following citalopram overdoses. *Br J Clin Pharmacol*. 2006;61:177-190.
70. Friberg LE, Isbister GK, Hackett LP, Duffull SB. The population pharmacokinetics of citalopram after deliberate self-poisoning: a Bayesian approach. *J Pharmacokinet Pharmacodyn*. 2005;32:571-605.
71. Friel PN, Logan BK, Fligner CL. Three fatal drug overdoses involving bupropion. *J Anal Toxicol*. 1993;17:436-438.
72. Fuller RW. Serotonergic stimulation of pituitary-adrenocortical function in rats. *Neuroendocrinology*. 1981;32:118-127.
73. Gamble DE, Peterson LG. Trazodone overdose: four years of experience from voluntary reports. *J Clin Psychiatry*. 1986;47:544-546.
74. Gardos G. Reversible dyskinesia during bupropion therapy. *J Clin Psychiatry*. 1997;58:218.
75. George TP, Godleski LS. Possible serotonin syndrome with trazodone addition to fluoxetine. *Biol Psychiatry*. 1996;39:384-385.
76. Gerritsen AW. Safety in overdose of mirtazapine: a case report. *J Clin Psychiatry*. 1997;58:271.
77. Gerson SC, Baldessarini RJ. Motor effects of serotonin in the central nervous system. *Life Sci* .1980;27:1435-1451.
78. Gill M, LoVecchio F, Selden B. Serotonin syndrome in a child after a single dose of fluvoxamine. *Ann Emerg Med*. 1999;33:457-459.
79. Gillman PK. Methylene blue implicated in potentially fatal serotonin toxicity. *Anaesthesia*. 2006;61:1013-1014.
80. Gillman PK. Re: no evidence of increased adverse drug reactions in cytochrome P450 CYP2D6 poor metabolizers treated with fluoxetine or nortriptyline. *Human Psychopharmacol*. 2005;20:61-62.
81. Gillman PK. The serotonin syndrome and its treatment. [see comment]. *J Psychopharmacol*. 1999;13:100-109.
82. Gillman PK. Possible serotonin syndrome with moclobemide and pethidine. *Med J Aust*. 1995;162:554.
83. Givens ML, Gabrysch J. Cardiotoxicity associated with accidental bupropion ingestion in a child. *Pediatr Emerg Care*. 2007;23:234-237.
84. Goeringer KE, Raymon L, Christian GD, Logan BK. Postmortem forensic toxicology of selective serotonin reuptake inhibitors: a review of pharmacology and report of 168 cases. *J Forensic Sci*. 2000;45:633-648.
85. Goldberg RJ, Huk M. Serotonin syndrome from trazodone and buspirone. *Psychosomatics*. 1992;33:235-236.
86. Goren JL, Levin GM. Mania with bupropion: a dose-related phenomenon? *Ann Pharmacother*. 2000;34:619-621.
87. Graber MA, Hoehns TB, Perry PJ. Sertraline-phenelzine drug interaction: a serotonin syndrome reaction. *Ann Pharmacother*. 1994;28:732-735.
88. Graudins A, Stearman A, Chan B. Treatment of the serotonin syndrome with cyproheptadine. *J Emerg Med*. 1998;16:615-619.
89. Greenblatt DJ, von Moltke LL, Harmatz JS, Shader RI. Human cytochromes and some newer antidepressants: kinetics, metabolism, and drug interactions. *J Clin Psychopharmacol*. 1999;19:23S-35S.
90. Grundemar L, Wohlfart B, Lagerstedt C, Bengtsson F, Eklundh G. Symptoms and signs of severe citalopram overdose. *Lancet*. 1997;349:1602.
91. Guze BH, Baxter LR, Jr. The serotonin syndrome: case responsive to propranolol. *J Clin Psychopharmacol*. 1986;6:119-120.
92. Haddad P. Newer antidepressants and the discontinuation syndrome. *J Clin Psychiatry*. 1997;58:17-21.
93. Hancox JC, Mitcheson JS. Combined hERG channel inhibition and disruption of trafficking in drug-induced long QT syndrome by fluoxetine: a case-study in cardiac safety pharmacology. *Br J Pharmacol*. 2006;149:457-459.
94. Hanekamp BB, Zijlstra JG, Tulleken JE, Ligtenberg JJ, van der Werf TS, Hofstra LS. Serotonin syndrome and rhabdomyolysis in venlafaxine poisoning: a case report. *Neth J Med*. 2005;63:316-318.
95. Hansen TE, Dieter K, Keepers GA. Interaction of fluoxetine and pentazocine. *Am J Psychiatry*. 1990;147:949-950.
96. Harmon T, Jurta D, Krenzelok E. Delayed seizures from sustained-release bupropion overdose. *J Toxicol Clin Toxicol*, 1998;36:522.
97. Harris CR, Gualtieri J, Stark G. Fatal bupropion overdose. *J Toxicol Clin Toxicol*. 1997;35:321-324.
98. Hedenmalm K, Guzey C, Dahl ML, Yue QY, Spigset O. Risk factors for extrapyramidal symptoms during treatment with selective serotonin reuptake inhibitors, including cytochrome P-450 enzyme, and serotonin and dopamine transporter and receptor polymorphisms. *J Clin Psychopharmacol*. 2006;26:192-197.
99. Heisler MA, Guidry JR, Arnecke B. Serotonin syndrome induced by administration of venlafaxine and phenelzine. *Ann Pharmacother*. 1996;30:84.
100. Hernandez JL, Ramos FJ, Infante J, Rebollo M, Gonzalez-Macias J. Severe serotonin syndrome induced by mirtazapine monotherapy. *Ann Pharmacother*. 2002;36:641-643.
101. Himei A, Okamura T. Discontinuation syndrome associated with paroxetine in depressed patients: a retrospective analysis of factors involved in the occurrence of the syndrome. *CNS Drugs*. 2006;20:665-672.
102. Hoes MJ, Zeijpveld JH. First report of mirtazapine overdose. *Int Clin Psychopharmacol*. 1996;11:147.
103. Hoes MJ, Zeijpveld JH. Mirtazapine as treatment for serotonin syndrome. *Pharmacopsychiatry*. 1996;29:81.
104. Holliday SM, Benfield P. Venlafaxine. A review of its pharmacology and therapeutic potential in depression. *Drugs*. 1995;49:280-294.
105. Horak EL, Jenkins AJ. Postmortem tissue distribution of olanzapine and citalopram in a drug intoxication. *J Forensic Sci*. 2005;50:679-681.
106. Hui CK, Yuen MF, Wong WM, Lam SK, Lai CL. Mirtazapine-induced hepatotoxicity. *J Clin Gastroenterol*. 2002;35:270-271.
107. Hurt RD, Sachs DP, Glover ED, et al. A comparison of sustained-release bupropion and placebo for smoking cessation. *N Engl J Med*. 1997;337:1195-1202.
108. Isbister GK, Friberg LE, Stokes B, et al. Activated charcoal decreases the risk of QT prolongation after citalopram overdose. *Ann Emerg Med*. 2007;50:593; No-600.
109. Jewell DP, Thompson IW, Sullivan BA, Bondeson J. Reversible focal myositis in a patient taking venlafaxine. *Rheumatology*. 2004;43:1590-1593.
110. Johnsen CR, Hoejlyng N. Hyponatremia following acute overdose with paroxetine. *Int J Clin Pharmacol Ther*. 1998;36:333-335.
111. Johnson H, Bouman WP, Lawton J. Withdrawal reaction associated with venlafaxine. *BMJ*. 1998;317:787.
112. Johnston JA, Lineberry CG, Ascher JA, et al. A 102-center prospective study of seizure in association with bupropion. *J Clin Psychiatry*. 1991;52:450-456.
113. Kaskey GB. Possible interaction between an MAOI and "ecstasy". *Am J Psychiatry*. 1992;149:411-412.
114. Keltner NL, Hall S. Neonatal serotonin syndrome. *Perspect Psychiatr Care*. 2005;41:88-91.
115. Khoo AL, Tham LS, Lee KH, Lim GK. Acute liver failure with concurrent bupropion and carbimazole therapy. *Ann Pharmacother*. 2003;37:220-223.
116. Kincaid RL, McMullin MM, Crookham SB, Rieders F. Report of a fluoxetine fatality. *J Anal Toxicol*. 1990;14:327-329.
117. Kirchner V, Silver LE, Kelly CA. Selective serotonin reuptake inhibitors and hyponatraemia: review and proposed mechanisms in the elderly. *J Psychopharmacol*. 1998;12:396-400.

118. Kitson R, Carr B. Tramadol and severe serotonin syndrome. *Anaesthesia.* 2005;60:934-935.
119. Kojima H, Terao T, Yoshimura R. Serotonin syndrome during clomipramine and lithium treatment. *Am J Psychiatry.* 1993;150:1897.
120. Kolecki P. Isolated venlafaxine-induced serotonin syndrome. *J Emerg Med.* 1997;15:491-493.
121. Krasowska D, Szymanek M, Schwartz RA, Myliski W. Cutaneous effects of the most commonly used antidepressant medication, the selective serotonin reuptake inhibitors. *J Am Acad Dermatol.* 2007;56:848-853.
122. Lane RM. SSRI-induced extrapyramidal side-effects and akathisia: implications for treatment. *J Psychopharmacol.* 1998;12:192-214.
123. Lappin RI, Auchincloss EL. Treatment of the serotonin syndrome with cyproheptadine. *N Engl J Med.* 1994;331:1021-1022.
124. Lejoyeux M, Ades J. Antidepressant discontinuation: a review of the literature. *J Clin Psychiatry.* 1997;58:11-15.
125. Lejoyeux M, Rouillon F, Ades J. Prospective evaluation of the serotonin syndrome in depressed inpatients treated with clomipramine. *Acta Psychiatr Scand.* 1993;88:369-371.
126. Lenzer J. Secret US report surfaces on antidepressants in children. *BMJ.* 2004;329:307.
127. Lenzi A, Raffaelli S, Marazziti D. Serotonin syndrome-like symptoms in a patient with obsessive-compulsive disorder, following inappropriate increase in fluvoxamine dosage. *Pharmacopsychiatry.* 1993;26:100-101.
128. Letsas K, Korantzopoulos P, Pappas L, Evangelou D, Efremidis M, Kardaras F. QT interval prolongation associated with venlafaxine administration. *Int J Cardiol.* 2006;109:116-117.
129. Levinson ML, Lipsy RJ, Fuller DK. Adverse effects and drug interactions associated with fluoxetine therapy. [see comment]. *DICP.* 1991;25: 657-661.
130. Lineberry TW, Peters GE, Jr, Bostwick JM. Bupropion-induced erythema multiforme. *Mayo Clin Proc.* 2001;76:664-666.
131. Luchini D, Morabito G, Centini F. Case report of a fatal intoxication by citalopram. *Am J Forensic Med Pathol.* 2005;26:352-354.
132. Marar IE, Towers AL, Mulsant BH, Pollock BG, Amico JA. Effect of paroxetine on plasma vasopressin and water load testing in elderly individuals. *J Geriatr Psychiatry Neurol.* 2000;13:212-216.
133. Masullo LN, Miller MA, Baker SD, Bose S, Levsky M. Clinical course and toxicokinetic data following isolated citalopram overdose in an infant. *Clinical Toxicol.* 2006;44:165-168.
134. Maurer-Spurej E. Serotonin reuptake inhibitors and cardiovascular diseases: a platelet connection. *Cell Mol Life Sci.* 2005;62:159-170.
135. McKenzie MS, McFarland BH. Trends in antidepressant overdoses. *Pharmacoepidemiol Drug Saf.* 2007;16:513-523.
136. Megarbane B, Bloch V, Deye N, Baud FJ. Pharmacokinetic/pharmacodynamic modelling of cardiac toxicity in venlafaxine overdose. *Intensive Care Med.* 2007;33:195-196.
137. Meijer WE, Heerdink ER, Nolen WA, Herings RM, Leufkens HG, Egberts AC. Association of risk of abnormal bleeding with degree of serotonin reuptake inhibition by antidepressants. *Arch Intern Med.* 2004;164: 2367-2370.
138. Miller F, Friedman R, Tanenbaum J, Griffin A. Disseminated intravascular coagulation and acute myoglobinuric renal failure: a consequence of the serotonergic syndrome. *J Clin Psychopharmacol.* 1991;11:277-279.
139. Miyaoka H, Kamijima K. Encephalopathy during amitriptyline therapy: are neuroleptic malignant syndrome and serotonin syndrome spectrum disorders?. *Int Clin Psychopharmacol.* 1995;10:265-267.
140. Montastruc JL, Chamontin B, Senard JM, et al. Pseudophaeochromocytoma in parkinsonian patient treated with fluoxetine plus selegiline. *Lancet.* 1993;341:555.
141. Morazin F, Lumbroso A, Harry P, et al. Cardiogenic shock and status epilepticus after massive bupropion overdose. *Clinical Toxicol.* 2007;45:794-797.
142. Movig KL, Leufkens HG, Lenderink AW, Egberts AC. Serotonergic antidepressants associated with an increased risk for hyponatraemia in the elderly. *Eur J Clin Pharmacol.* 2002;58:143-148.
143. Movig KL, Leufkens HG, Belitser SV, Lenderink AW, Egberts AC. Selective serotonin reuptake inhibitor-induced urinary incontinence. *Pharmacoepidemiol Drug Saf.* 2002;11:271-279.
144. Muly EC, McDonald W, Steffens D, Book S. Serotonin syndrome produced by a combination of fluoxetine and lithium. *Am J Psychiatry.* 1993; 150:1565.
145. Munhoz RP. Serotonin syndrome induced by a combination of bupropion and SSRIs. *Clin Neuropharmacol.* 2004;27:219-222.
146. Myers LB, Krenzelok EP. Paroxetine (Paxil) overdose: a pediatric focus. *Vet Human Toxicol.* 1997;39:86-88.
147. Naranjo CA, Bremner KE. Clinical pharmacology of serotonin-altering medications for decreasing alcohol consumption. *Alcohol Alcohol.* 1993;221-229.
148. Navarro A, Perry C, Bobo WV. A case of serotonin syndrome precipitated by abuse of the anticough remedy dextromethorphan in a bipolar patient treated with fluoxetine and lithium. *Gen Hosp Psychiatry.* 2006;28:78-80.
149. Nelson JC. Safety and tolerability of the new antidepressants. *J Clin Psychiatry.* 1997;58:26-31.
150. Nisijima K, Ishiguro T. Cerebrospinal fluid levels of monoamine metabolites and gamma-aminobutyric acid in neuroleptic malignant syndrome. *J Psychiatr Res.* 1995;29:233-244.
151. Nisijima K, Shimizu M, Abe T, Ishiguro T. A case of serotonin syndrome induced by concomitant treatment with low-dose trazodone and amitriptyline and lithium. *Int Clin Psychopharmacol.* 1996;11:289-290.
152. Nutt D. Mirtazapine: pharmacology in relation to adverse effects. *Acta Psychiatr Scand.* 1997;31-73.
153. Oates JA, Sjoerdsma A. Neurologic effects of tryptophan in patients receiving a monoamine oxidase inhibitor. *Neurology.* 1960;10:1076-1078.
154. O'Reardon JP, Allison KC, Martino NS, Lundgren JD, Heo M, Stunkard AJ. A randomized, placebo-controlled trial of sertraline in the treatment of night eating syndrome. *Am J Psychiatry.* 2006;163:893-898.
155. Pao M, Tipnis T. Serotonin syndrome after sertraline overdose in a 5-year-old girl. *Arch Pediatr Adolesc Med.* 1997;151:1064-1067.
156. Paris PA, Saucier JR. ECG conduction delays associated with massive bupropion overdose. *J Toxicol Clinical Toxicol.* 1998;36:595-598.
157. Paruchuri P, Godkar D, Anandacoomarswamy D, Sheth K, Niranjan S. Rare case of serotonin syndrome with therapeutic doses of paroxetine. *Am J Ther.* 2006;13:550-552.
158. Pereira CE, Goldman-Levine JD. Extended-release venlafaxine-induced alopecia. *Ann Pharmacother.* 2007;41:1084.
159. Pergola PE, Sved AF, Voogt JL, Alper RH. Effect of serotonin on vasopressin release: a comparison to corticosterone, prolactin and renin. *Neuroendocrinology.* 1993;57:550-558.
160. Personne M, Persson H, Sjoberg E. Citalopram toxicity. *Lancet.* 1997;350:518-519.
161. Personne M, Sjoberg G, Persson H. Citalopram overdose—review of cases treated in Swedish hospitals. *J Toxicol Clin Toxicol.* 1997;35:237-240.
162. Popli AP, Tanquary J, Lamparella V, Masand PS. Bupropion and anticonvulsant drug interactions. *Ann Clin Psychiatry.* 1995;7:99-101.
163. Power BM, Pinder M, Hackett LP, Ilett KF. Fatal serotonin syndrome following a combined overdose of moclobemide, clomipramine and fluoxetine. *Anaesth Intensive Care.* 1995;23:499-502.
164. Preskorn SH, Burke M. Somatic therapy for major depressive disorder: selection of an antidepressant. [see comment]. *J Clin Psychiatry.* 1992;53:5-18.
165. Price JS, Waller PC, Wood SM, MacKay AV. A comparison of the post-marketing safety of four selective serotonin re-uptake inhibitors including the investigation of symptoms occurring on withdrawal. *Br J Clin Pharmacol.* 1996;42:757-763.
166. Putzhammer A, Schoeler A, Rohrmeier T, Sand P, Hajak G, Eichhammer P. Evidence of a role for the 5-HTTLPR genotype in the modulation of motor response to antidepressant treatment. *Psychopharmacology (Berl).* 2005;178:303-308.
167. Radomski JW, Dursun SM, Reveley MA, Kutcher SP. An exploratory approach to the serotonin syndrome: an update of clinical phenomenology and revised diagnostic criteria. *Med Hypotheses.* 2000;55:218-224.
168. Rajamani S, Eckhardt LL, Valdivia CR, et al. Drug-induced long QT syndrome: hERG K^+ channel block and disruption of protein trafficking by fluoxetine and norfluoxetine. *Br J Pharmacol.* 2006;149:481-489.
169. Rao R. Serotonin syndrome associated with trazodone. *Int J Geriatr Psychiatry.* 1997;12:129-130.
170. Reeves RR, Bullen JA. Serotonin syndrome produced by paroxetine and low-dose trazodone. *Psychosomatics.* 1995;36:159-160.
171. Retz W, Maier S, Maris F, Rosler M. Non-fatal mirtazapine overdose. *Int Clin Psychopharmacol.* 1998;13:277-279.
172. Richards JB, Papaioannou A, Adachi JD, et al. Effect of selective serotonin reuptake inhibitors on the risk of fracture. *Arch Intern Med.* 2007;167:188-194.
173. Richelson E. Pharmacology of antidepressants. *Mayo Clin Proc.* 2001;76:511-527.
174. Richelson E. Pharmacokinetic drug interactions of new antidepressants: a review of the effects on the metabolism of other drugs. *Mayo Clin Proc.* 1997;72:835-847.

175. Rivers N, Horner B. Possible lethanl interaction between Nardil and dextromethorphan. *Can Med Assoc J.* 1970;103:85.
176. Rohrig TP, Ray NG. Tissue distribution of bupropion in a fatal overdose. *J Anal Toxicol.* 1992;16:343-345.
177. Rosebush PI, Margetts P, Mazurek MF. Serotonin syndrome as a result of clomipramine monotherapy. *J Clin Psychopharmacol.* 1999;19:285-287.
178. Rudolph RL, Derivan AT. The safety and tolerability of venlafaxine hydrochloride: analysis of the clinical trials database. *J Clin Psychopharmacol.* 1996;16:54S-59S.
179. Ruiz F. Fluoxetine and the serotonin syndrome. *Ann Emerg Med.* 1994;24:983-985.
180. Safferman AZ, Masiar SJ. Central nervous system toxicity after abrupt monoamine oxidase inhibitor switch: a case report. *Ann Pharmacother.* 1992;26:337-338.
181. Sandyk R. L-dopa induced "serotonin syndrome" in a parkinsonian patient on bromocriptine. *J Clin Psychopharmacol.* 1986;6:194-195.
182. Sargent PA, Kjaer KH, Bench CJ, et al. Brain serotonin1A receptor binding measured by positron emission tomography with [11C]WAY-100635: effects of depression and antidepressant treatment. *Arch Gen Psychiatry.* 2000;57:174-180.
183. Schatzberg AF, Blier P, Delgado PL, Fava M, Haddad PM, Shelton RC. Antidepressant discontinuation syndrome: consensus panel recommendations for clinical management and additional research. *J Clin Psychiatry.* 2006;67:27-30.
184. Schatzberg AF, Haddad P, Kaplan EM, et al. Serotonin reuptake inhibitor discontinuation syndrome: a hypothetical definition. Discontinuation Consensus panel. [see comment]. *J Clin Psychiatry.* 1997;58:5-10.
185. Schillevoort I, van Puijenbroek EP, de Boer A, Roos RA, Jansen PA, Leufkens HG. Extrapyramidal syndromes associated with selective serotonin reuptake inhibitors: a case-control study using spontaneous reports. *Int Clin Psychopharmacol.* 2002;17:75-79.
186. Schweizer E, Weise C, Clary C, Fox I, Rickels K. Placebo-controlled trial of venlafaxine for the treatment of major depression. *J Clin Psychopharmacol.* 1991;11:233-236.
187. Shaw MW, Sheard JD. Fatal venlafaxine overdose with acinar zone 3 liver cell necrosis. *Am J Forensic Med Pathol.* 2005;26:367-368.
188. Silbergeld EK, Hruska RE. Lisuride and LSD: dopaminergic and serotonergic interactions in the "serotonin syndrome". *Psychopharmacology (Berl).* 1979;65:233-237.
189. Singer PP, Jones GR. An uncommon fatality due to moclobemide and paroxetine. *J Anal Toxicol.* 1997;21:518-520.
190. Sirianni AJ, Osterhoudt KC, Calello DP, et al. Use of lipid emulsion in the resuscitation of a patient with prolonged cardiovascular collapse after overdose of bupropion and lamotrigine. *Ann Emerg Med.* 2008;51:412; Ar-415.
191. Sitsen J, Maris F, Timmer C. Drug-drug interaction studies with mirtazapine and carbamazepine in healthy male subjects. *Eur J Drug Metab Pharmacokinet.* 2001;26:109-121.
192. Skop BP, Finkelstein JA, Mareth TR, Magoon MR, Brown TM. The serotonin syndrome associated with paroxetine, an over-the-counter cold remedy, and vascular disease. *Am J Emerg Med.* 1994;12:642-644.
193. Smilkstein MJ, Smolinske SC, Rumack BH. A case of MAO inhibitor/MDMA interaction: agony after ecstasy. *J Toxicol Clin Toxicol.* 1987;25:149-159.
194. Smith B, Prockop DJ. Central-nervous-system effects of ingestin of L-tryptophan by normal subjects. *N Engl J Med.* 1962;267:1338-1341.
195. Smits K, Smits L, Peeters F, et al. Serotonin transporter polymorphisms and the occurrence of adverse events during treatment with selective serotonin reuptake inhibitors. *Int Clin Psychopharmacol.* 2007;22:137-143.
196. Snyder SH, Peroutka SJ. A possible role of serotonin receptors in antidepressant drug action. *Pharmacopsychiatria.* 1982;15:131-134.
197. Spaans E, van den Heuvel MW, Schnabel PG, et al. Concomitant use of mirtazapine and phenytoin: a drug-drug interaction study in healthy male subjects. *Eur J Clin Pharmacol.* 2002;58:423-429.
198. Spigset O, Hagg S, Bate A. Hepatic injury and pancreatitis during treatment with serotonin reuptake inhibitors: data from the World Health Organization (WHO) database of adverse drug reactions. *Int Clin Psychopharmacol.* 2003;18:157-161.
199. Sprouse JS, Aghajanian GK. (–)-Propranolol blocks the inhibition of serotonergic dorsal raphe cell firing by 5-HT1A selective agonists. *Eur J Pharmacol.* 1986;128:295-298.
200. Stedman CA, Begg EJ, Kennedy MA, Roberts R, Wilkinson TJ. Cytochrome P450 2D6 genotype does not predict SSRI (fluoxetine or paroxetine) induced hyponatraemia. *Human Psychopharmacol.* 2002;17:187-190.
201. Sternbach H. The serotonin syndrome.[see comment]. *Am J Psychiatry.* 1991;148:705-713.
202. Storrow AB. Bupropion overdose and seizure. *Am J Emerg Med.* 1994;12:183-184.
203. Tackley RM, Tregaskis B. Fatal disseminated intravascular coagulation following a monoamine oxidase inhibitor/tricyclic interaction. *Anaesthesia.* 1987;42:760-763.
204. Tamam L, Ozpoyraz N. Selective serotonin reuptake inhibitor discontinuation syndrome: a review. *Adv Ther.* 2002;19:17-26.
205. Tarabar AF, Hoffman RS, Nelson L. Citalopram overdose: late presentation of torsades de pointes (TdP) with cardiac arrest. *J Med Toxicol.* 2008;4:101-105.
206. Tordoff SG, Stubbing JF, Linter SP. Delayed excitatory reaction following interaction of cocaine and monoamine oxidase inhibitor (phenelzine). *Br J Anaesth.* 1991;66:516-518.
207. Tripathi A, Greenberger PA. Bupropion hydrochloride induced serum sickness-like reaction. *Ann Allergy Asthma Immunol.* 1999;83:165-166.
208. Ubogu EE, Katirji B. Mirtazapine-induced serotonin syndrome. *Clin Neuropharmacol.* 2003;26:54-57.
209. Vaczek D. Top 200 prescription drugs of 2003. *Pharm Times.* 2004;46-69.
210. Vanpee D, Laloyaux P, Gillet JB. Seizure and hyponatraemia after overdose of trazadone. *Am J Emerg Med.* 1999;17:430-431.
211. Velazquez C, Carlson A, Stokes KA, Leikin JB. Relative safety of mirtazapine overdose. *Vet Human Toxicol.* 2001;43:342-344.
212. Vetulani J, Stawarz RJ, Dingell JV, Sulser F. A possible common mechanism of action of antidepressant treatments: reduction in the sensitivity of the noradrenergic cyclic AMP gererating system in the rat limbic forebrain. *Naunyn-Schmiedeberg's Arch Pharmacol.* 1976;293:109-114.
213. von Moltke LL, Greenblatt DJ, Giancarlo GM, Granda BW, Harmatz JS, Shader RI. Escitalopram (S-citalopram) and its metabolites in vitro: cytochromes mediating biotransformation, inhibitory effects, and comparison to R-citalopram. *Drug Metab Dispos.* 2001;29:1102-1109.
214. Weller EB, Weller RA, Kloos AL, Hitchcock S, Kim WJ, Zemel B. Impact of depression and its treatment on the bones of growing children. *Curr Psychiatry Rep.* 2007;9:94-98.
215. White CM, Gailey RA, Levin GM, Smith T. Seizure resulting from a venlafaxine overdose. *Ann Pharmacother.* 1997;31:178-180.
216. Willner P. Dopamine and depression: a review of recent evidence. I. Empirical studies. *Brain Res.* 1983;287:211-224.
217. Wilson AD, Howell C, Waring WS. Venlafaxine ingestion is associated with rhabdomyolysis in adults: a case series. *J Toxicol Sci.* 2007;32:97-101.
218. Wong DT, Bymaster FP, Horng JS, Molloy BB. A new selective inhibitor for uptake of serotonin into synaptosomes of rat brain: 3-(*p*-trifluoromethylphenoxy). N-methyl-3-phenylpropylamine. *J Pharmacol Exp Ther.* 1975;193:804-811.
219. Woodrum ST, Brown CS. Management of SSRI-induced sexual dysfunction. *Ann Pharmacother.* 1998;32:1209-1215.
220. Yamada J, Sugimoto Y, Wakita H, Horisaka K. The involvement of serotonergic and dopaminergic systems in hypothermia induced in mice by intracerebroventricular injection of serotonin. *Jpn J Pharmacol.* 1988;48:145-148.
221. Yolles JC, Armenta WA, Alao AO. Serum sickness induced by bupropion. *Ann Pharmacother.* 1999;33:931-933.
222. Yoshida K, Naito S, Takahashi H, et al. Monoamine oxidase A gene polymorphism, 5-HT 2A receptor gene polymorphism and incidence of nausea induced by fluvoxamine. *Neuropsychobiology.* 2003;48:10-13.
223. Yuksel FV, Tuzer V, Goka E. Escitalopram intoxication. *Eur Psychiatry.* 2005;20:82.
224. Zhalkovsky B, Walker D, Bourgeois JA. Seizure activity and enzyme elevations after venlafaxine overdose. *J Clin Psychopharmacol.* 1997;17:490-491.

CHAPTER 73
CYCLIC ANTIDEPRESSANTS

Erica L. Liebelt

The term *cyclic antidepressant* (CA) refers to a group of pharmacologically related xenobiotics used for treatment of depression, neuralgic pain, migraines, enuresis, and attention deficit hyperactivity disorder. Most CAs have at least three rings in their chemical structure. They include the traditional tricyclic antidepressants (TCAs) imipramine, desipramine, amitriptyline, nortriptyline, doxepin, trimipramine, protriptyline, and clomipramine, as well as other cyclic compounds such as maprotiline and amoxapine.

HISTORY AND EPIDEMIOLOGY

Imipramine was the first TCA used for treatment of depression in the late 1950s. However, the synthesis of iminodibenzyl, the "tricyclic" core of imipramine, and the description of its chemical characteristics date back to 1889. Structurally related to the phenothiazines, imipramine was originally developed as a hypnotic agent for agitated or psychotic patients and was serendipitously found to alleviate depression. From the 1960s until the late 1980s, the TCAs were the major pharmacologic treatment for depression in the United States. However, by the early 1960s, cardiovascular and central nervous system (CNS) toxicities were recognized as major complications of TCA overdoses.[99] The newer CAs developed in the 1980s and 1990s were designed to decrease some of the adverse effects of older TCAs, improve the therapeutic index, and reduce the incidence of serious toxicity. Other CAs include the tetracyclic drug maprotiline and the dibenzoxapine drug amoxapine.

The epidemiology of CA poisoning has evolved significantly in the last 20 years, resulting in great part from the introduction of the newer selective serotonin reuptake inhibitors (SSRIs) for the treatment of depression. Although the use of CAs for depression has decreased over the last 15 years, other medical indications, including chronic pain, obsessive-compulsive disorder, and, particularly in children, enuresis and attention deficit hyperactivity disorder have emerged, resulting in their continued use. The antidepressants are a leading cause of drug-related self-poisonings in the developed world, primarily because of their ready availability to people with depression who by virtue of the disease are at high risk for overdose. However, despite the increase in SSRI use and overdose, patients with TCA overdoses continue to have higher rates of hospitalization (78.7% versus 64.7%) and fatality (0.73% versus 0.14%) than do those with SSRI overdose.[73]

Children younger than 6 years have consistently accounted for approximately 12%–13% of all CA exposures reported to poison centers during each of the last 15 years (see Chap. 135). Despite the emergence of the SSRIs in the early 1990s, TCAs were still among the top five psychotropic drugs most frequently prescribed by pediatric office-based practices in 1995.[48] The use of TCAs has remained stable in adolescents but has declined in prepubertal children.[116] Thus CA poisoning likely will continue to be among the most lethal unintentional drug ingestions in younger children because only one or two adult-strength pills can produce serious clinical effects in young children.

PHARMACOLOGY

In general, the TCAs can be classified into tertiary and secondary amines based on the presence of a methyl group on the propylamine side chain (Table 73–1). The tertiary amines amitriptyline and imipramine are metabolized to the secondary amines nortriptyline and desipramine, respectively, which themselves are marketed as antidepressants. In therapeutic doses, the CAs produce similar pharmacologic effects on the autonomic system, CNS, and cardiovascular system. However, they can be distinguished from each other by their relative potencies.[118]

At therapeutic doses, CAs inhibit presynaptic reuptake of norepinephrine and/or serotonin, thus functionally increasing the amount of these neurotransmitters at CNS receptors. The tertiary amines, especially clomipramine, are more potent inhibitors of serotonin reuptake, whereas the secondary amines are more potent inhibitors of norepinephrine reuptake. Although these pharmacologic actions formed the basis of the monoamine hypothesis of depression in the 1960s, antidepressant actions of these drugs appear to be much more complex.

Extensive research has led to the "receptor sensitivity hypothesis of antidepressant drug action," which postulates that following chronic CA administration, alterations in the sensitivity of various receptors are responsible for antidepressant effects. Chronic TCA administration alters the number and/or function of central β-adrenergic and serotonin receptors. In addition, TCAs modulate glucocorticoid receptor gene expression and cause alterations at the genomic level of other receptors.[7,57] All of these actions likely play a role in the antidepressant effects of TCAs.

Additional pharmacologic mechanisms of CAs are responsible for their side effects with therapeutic dosing and clinical effects following overdose. All of the CAs are competitive antagonists of the muscarinic acetylcholine receptors, although they have different affinities. The CAs also antagonize peripheral α_1-adrenergic receptors. The most prominent effects of CA overdose result from binding to the cardiac sodium channels, which is also described as a membrane stabilizing effect (Fig. 73–1) (see Chap. 22). The tricyclic antidepressants are potent inhibitors of both peripheral and central postsynaptic histamine receptors. Finally, animal research demonstrates that the CAs interfere with chloride conductance by binding to the picrotoxin site on the GABA–chloride complex.[106]

Amoxapine is a dibenzoxapine CA derived from the active antipsychotic loxapine. Although it has a 3-ringed structure, this drug has little similarity to the other tricyclics. It is a potent norepinephrine reuptake inhibitor, has no effect on serotonin reuptake, and blocks dopamine receptors. Maprotiline is a tetracyclic antidepressant that predominantly blocks norepinephrine reuptake. Both of these CAs have a slightly different toxic profile than the traditional TCAs.[53,54,118]

PHARMACOKINETICS AND TOXICOKINETICS

The CAs are rapidly and almost completely absorbed from the gastrointestinal (GI) tract, with peak concentrations 2–8 hours after administration of a therapeutic dose. They are weak bases (high pK_a). In overdose, the decreased GI motility caused by anticholinergic effects and ionization in gastric acid delay CA absorption. Because of extensive first-pass metabolism by the liver, the oral bioavailability of CAs is low and variable, although metabolism may become saturated in overdose, increasing bioavailability.

The CAs are highly lipophilic and possess large and variable volumes of distribution (15–40 L/kg). They are rapidly distributed to the heart, brain, liver, and kidney, where the tissue-to-plasma ratio generally exceeds 10:1. Less than 2% of the ingested dose is present in blood several hours after overdose, and serum TCA concentrations decline biexponentially. The CAs are extensively bound to α_1-acid glycoprotein (AAG)

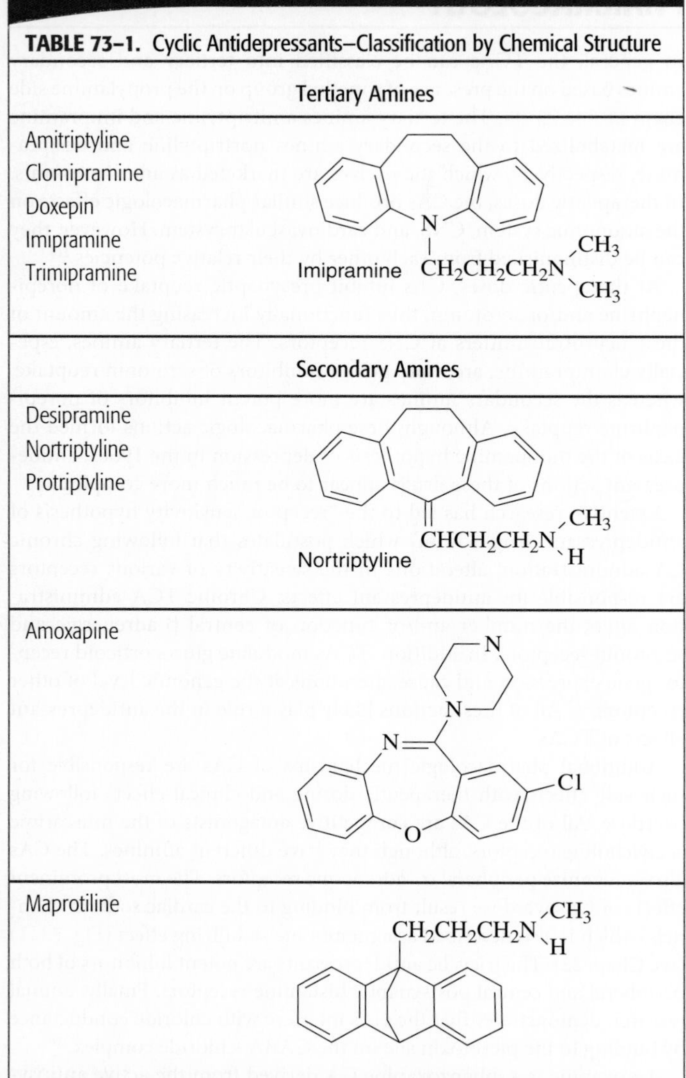

TABLE 73–1. Cyclic Antidepressants–Classification by Chemical Structure

Drug	Structure
Tertiary Amines	
Amitriptyline Clomipramine Doxepin Imipramine Trimipramine	Imipramine $CH_2CH_2CH_2N(CH_3)_2$
Secondary Amines	
Desipramine Nortriptyline Protriptyline	Nortriptyline $CHCH_2CH_2N(CH_3)H$
Amoxapine	N, Cl, O
Maprotiline	$CH_2CH_2CH_2N(CH_3)H$

in the plasma, although differential binding among the specific CAs is observed.[2] Changes in AAG concentration or pH can alter binding and the percentage of free or unbound drug.[87,98] Specifically, a low blood pH (which often occurs in a severely poisoned patient) may increase the amount of free drug, making it more available to exert its effects. This property serves as the basis for alkalinization therapy (see below).

The TCAs undergo demethylation, aromatic hydroxylation, and glucuronide conjugation of the hydroxy metabolites. The tertiary amines imipramine and amitriptyline are demethylated to desipramine and nortriptyline, respectively. The hydroxy metabolites of both tertiary and secondary amines are pharmacologically active and may contribute to toxicity. The glucuronide metabolites are inactive.

Genetically based differences in the activity of the CYP2D6 enzymes, which are responsible for hydroxylation of imipramine and desipramine, account for wide interindividual variability in metabolism and steady-state serum concentrations.[17] "Poor metabolizers" may recover more slowly from an overdose or demonstrate toxicity with therapeutic dosing.[110] The metabolism of CAs also may be influenced by concomitant ingestion of ethanol and other medications that induce or inhibit the CYP2D6 isoenzyme (see Chap. 12 Appendix).[16] Patient variables such as age and ethnicity also affect CA metabolism.

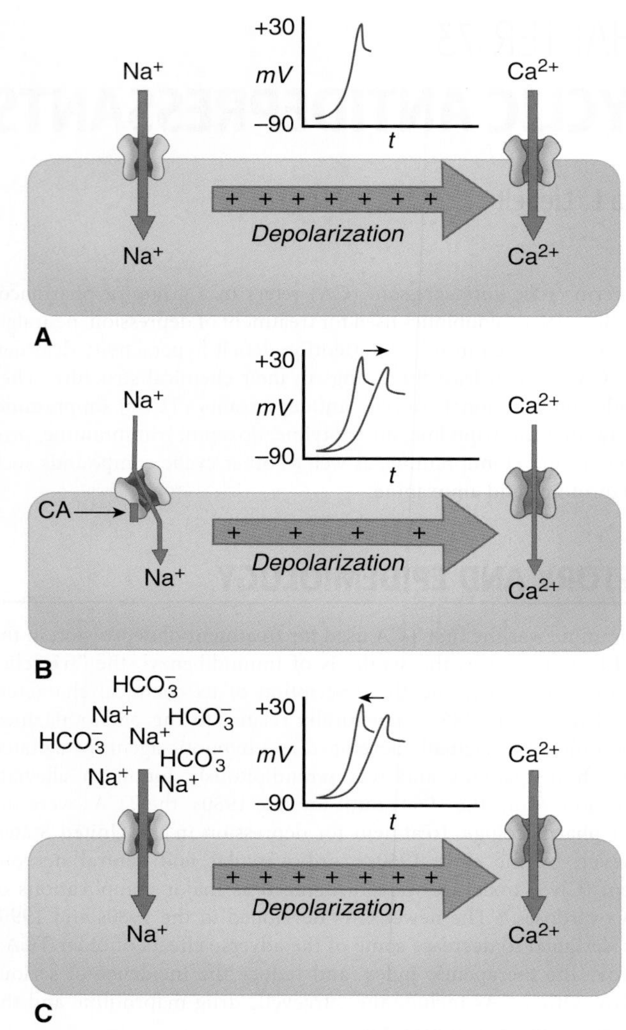

FIGURE 73–1. Effects of cyclic antidepressants on the fast sodium channel. **(A)** Sodium depolarizes the cell, which both propagates conduction; allowing complete cardiac depolarization; and opens voltage-dependent Ca^{2+} channels, producing contraction. **(B)** Cyclic antidepressants and other sodium channel blockers alter the conformation of the sodium channel, slowing the rate of rise of the action potential, which produces both negative dromotropic and inotropic effects. **(C)** Raising the Na^+ gradient across the affected sodium channel speeds the rate of rise of the action potential, counteracting the drug-induced effects. Raising the pH removes the CA from the binding site on the Na^+ channel. See Figure 73-3 for the effects noted on the ECG.

Elimination half-lives for therapeutic doses of CAs vary from 7–58 hours (54–92 hours for protriptyline), with even longer half-lives in the elderly. The half-lives may also be prolonged following overdose as a result of saturable metabolism. A small fraction (15%–30%) of CA elimination occurs through biliary and gastric secretion. The metabolites are then reabsorbed in the systemic circulation, resulting in enterohepatic and enterogastric recirculation and reducing their fecal excretion. Finally, less than 5% of CAs are excreted unchanged by the kidney.

PATHOPHYSIOLOGY

The CAs slow the recovery from inactivation of the fast sodium channel, slowing phase 0 depolarization of the action potential in the distal His-Purkinje system and the ventricular myocardium[117,119]

(Fig. 73–1 and Fig. 22-2; see Chaps. 22 and 23 (Hemodynamic Principles)). Impaired depolarization within the ventricular conduction system slows the propagation of ventricular depolarization, which manifests as prolongation of the QRS interval on the electrocardiogram (Fig. 73–1). The right bundle branch has a relatively longer refractory period, and it is affected disproportionately by xenobiotics that slow intraventricular conduction. This slowing of depolarization results in a rightward shift of the terminal 40-millisecond (T40-ms) of the QRS axis and the right bundle-branch block pattern that is noted on the electrocardiogram of patients who are exposed to, or overdose with, a CA.[121]

Because CAs are weakly basic, they are increasingly ionized as the ambient pH falls, and less ionized as the pH rises. Changing the ambient pH therefore likely alters their binding to the sodium channel. That is, since it is probable that 90% of the binding of TCA to the sodium channel occurs in the ionized state, alkalinizing the blood facilitates the movement of the TCA away from the hydrophilic sodium channel and into the lipid membrane.

Sinus tachycardia is due to the antimuscarinic, vasodilatory (reflex tachycardia), and sympathomimetic effects of the CAs. Wide-complex tachycardia most commonly represents aberrantly conducted sinus tachycardia rather than ventricular tachycardia. However, by prolonging anterograde conduction, nonuniform ventricular conduction may result, leading to reentrant ventricular dysrhythmias.[117]

Electrophysiologic studies in a canine model demonstrate that QRS prolongation is rate dependent, a characteristic effect of the type I antidysrhythmics (Chap. 63). In these studies, when the heart rate could not accelerate because of a crushed sinus node the dogs never developed QRS prolongation. Furthermore, pharmacologic induction of bradycardia prevents or narrows wide-complex tachycardia by allowing time for recovery of the sodium channel from inactivation.[4,97] However, since bradycardia adversely affects cardiac output, induction of bradycardia is not recommended.

A Brugada electrocardiographic pattern, specifically Type 1 or "coved" pattern, is rarely associated with CA overdose. The Brugada syndrome originates from a structural change in the myocardial sodium channel that results in functional sodium channel alterations similar to those caused by the CAs.[10,78] It is possible that this small cohort of patients may have had subclinical Brugada syndrome that was uncovered by the CA.

QT interval prolongation can occur in the setting of both therapeutic use and overdose of CAs. This apparent prolongation of repolarization results primarily from slowed depolarization (ie, QRS prolongation) rather than altered repolarization.[93] Although QT prolongation predisposes to the development of torsades de pointes, this dysrhythmia is uncommon in patients with CA poisoning due to the prominent tachycardia.

Hypotension is caused by direct myocardial depression secondary to altered sodium channel function, which disrupts the subsequent excitation-contraction coupling of myocytes and impairs cardiac contractility. Peripheral vasodilation from α-adrenergic blockade by CAs also contributes prominently to postural hypotension. In addition, downregulation of adrenergic receptors may cause a blunted physiologic response to catecholamines.[77]

Agitation, delirium, and depressed sensorium are primarily caused by the central anticholinergic and antihistaminic effects. Hemodynamic effects are likely to contribute in only the most severely poisoned patients. Details regarding the exact mechanism of CA-induced seizures remain elusive.[65] CA-induced seizures may result from a combination of an increased concentration of monoamines (particularly norepinephrine), muscarinic antagonism, neuronal sodium channel alteration, and GABA inhibition.[65,79]

Acute lung injury may occur in the setting of CA overdose. In one study, amitriptyline exposure caused dose-related vasoconstriction and bronchoconstriction in isolated rat lungs.[109] Many substances implicated in acute lung injury, such as platelet-activating factor and protein kinase activation, were important in mediating amitriptyline-induced lung function impairment in this experimental model. Another animal model demonstrated that acute amitriptyline poisoning causes dose-dependent rises in pulmonary artery pressure, pulmonary edema, and sustained vasoconstriction that could be attenuated by either calcium channel inhibition or a nitric oxide donor.[64]

CLINICAL MANIFESTATIONS OF TOXICITY

The toxic profile is qualitatively the same for all of the first-generation TCAs, but is slightly different for some of the other CAs.[118] The progression of clinical toxicity is unpredictable and may be rapid. Patients commonly present to the emergency department (ED) with minimal apparent clinical abnormalities only to develop life-threatening cardiovascular and CNS toxicity within hours.

The CAs have a low therapeutic index, meaning that a small increase in serum concentration over the therapeutic range may result in toxicity. Acute ingestion of 10–20 mg/kg of most CAs causes significant cardiovascular and CNS manifestations (therapeutic dose 2–4 mg/kg/d). Thus, in adults, ingestions of more than 1 gram of a CA is usually associated with life-threatening effects. As few as two 50-mg imipramine tablets may cause significant toxicity in a 10-kg toddler (ie, 10 mg/kg). In a series of children with unintentional TCA exposure, all patients with reported ingestions of more than 5 mg/kg manifested clinical toxicity.[72]

ACUTE TOXICITY

Most of the reported toxicity from CAs derives from patients with acute ingestions, especially in patients who are chronically taking the medication. Clinical manifestations of these two cohorts do not appear to be different, and most studies do not distinguish between them.

Acute Cardiovascular Toxicity Cardiovascular toxicity is primarily responsible for the morbidity and mortality attributed to CAs. Refractory hypotension due to myocardial depression probably is the most common cause of death from CA overdose.[19,108] Hypoxia, acidosis, volume depletion, seizures, or concomitant ingestion of other cardiodepressant or vasodilating drugs can exacerbate hypotension.

The most common dysrhythmia observed following CA overdose is sinus tachycardia (rate 120–160 beats/min in an adult) and this finding is present in most patients with clinically significant TCA poisoning. The electrocardiogram typically demonstrates intraventricular conduction delay that manifests as a rightward shift of the T40-ms QRS axis and a prolongation of the QRS complex duration. These findings can be used to identify and risk-stratify, respectively, patients with CA poisoning (see Diagnostic Testing). PR, QRS, and QT interval prolongation can occur in the setting of both therapeutic and toxic amounts of TCAs.[67]

Wide-complex tachycardia is the characteristic potentially life-threatening dysrhythmia observed in patients with severe toxicity (Fig. 73–2A–C). Ventricular tachycardia may be difficult to distinguish from aberrantly conducted sinus tachycardia which occurs more commonly. In the former cases, the preceding P wave may not be apparent because of prolonged AV conduction, widened QRS interval, or both. Ventricular tachycardia occurs most often in patients with prolonged QRS complex duration and/or hypotension.[62,112] Hypoxia, acidosis, hyperthermia, seizures, and β-adrenergic agonists may also predispose

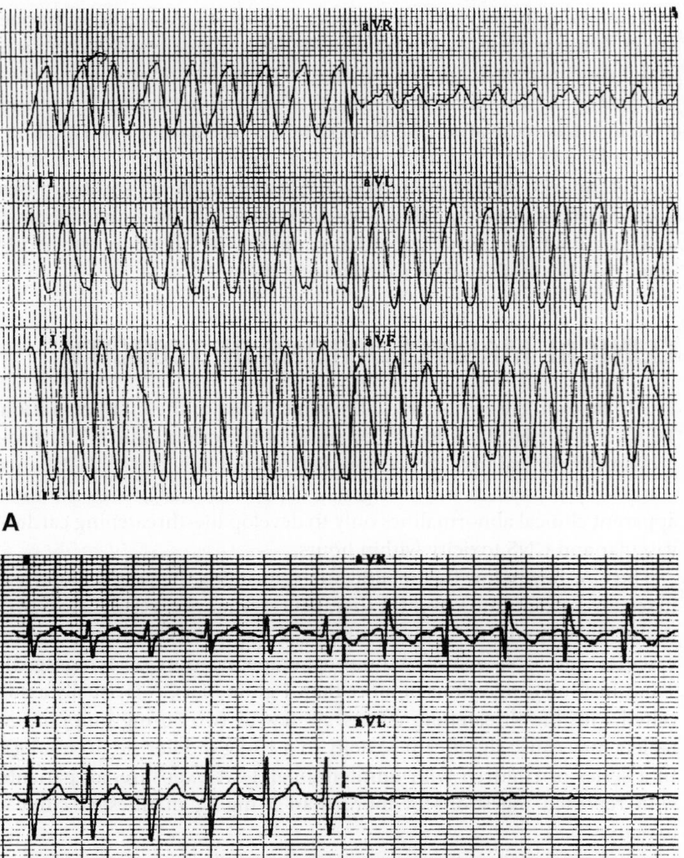

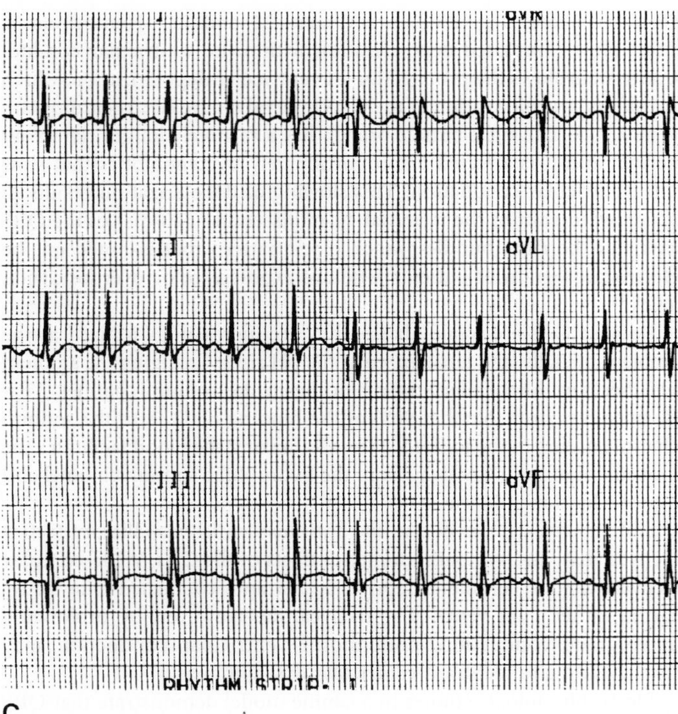

FIGURE 73–2. (**A**) ECG shows a wide-complex tachycardia with a variable QRS duration (minimum 220 ms). (**B**) ECG 30 minutes after presentation following sodium bicarbonate shows narrowing of the QRS interval to a duration of 140 ms and an amplitude of RaVR of 6.0 mm. (**C**) ECG 9 hours after presentation shows further narrowing of the QRS interval to 80 ms and decrease in the amplitude of RaVR to 4.5 mm. (Reproduced with permission from Liebelt EL, Targeted management strategies for cardiovascular toxicity from tricyclic antidepressant overdose: the pivotal role for alkalinization and sodium loading. *Pediatr Emerg Care* 1998;14:293–298.)

to ventricular tachycardia.[62,112] Fatal dysrhythmias are rare, as ventricular tachycardia and fibrillation occur in only approximately 4% of all cases.[39,90] Both the Brugada Type I electrocardiogram pattern and torsades de pointes are uncommon with acute TCA overdose.

Acute Central Nervous System Toxicity Altered mental status and seizures are the primary manifestations of CNS toxicity. Delirium, agitation, and/or psychotic behavior with hallucinations may be present and most likely result from antagonism of muscarinic and histaminergic receptors. These alterations in consciousness usually are followed by lethargy which is followed by rapid progression to coma. The duration of coma is variable and does not necessarily correlate or occur concomitantly with electrocardiographic abnormalities.[54]

Seizures usually are generalized and brief, most often occurring within 1–2 hours of ingestion.[26] The incidence of seizures is similar to ventricular tachycardia and occurs in an estimated 4% of patients presenting with overdose and 13% of fatal cases.[123] Status epilepticus is uncommon. Abrupt deterioration in hemodynamic status, namely, hypotension and ventricular dysrhythmias, may develop during or within minutes after a seizure.[26,62,112] This rapid cardiovascular deterioration likely results from seizure-induced acidosis that exacerbates cardiovascular toxicity. The risk of seizures with CA overdoses may be increased in patients undergoing long-term therapy or who have other risk factors such as history of seizures, head trauma, or concomitant drug withdrawal.[104] Myoclonus and extrapyramidal symptoms may also occur in CA-poisoned patients.

Discontinuation of CAs may produce a withdrawal syndrome in some patients. The syndrome is typified by gastrointestinal and somatic distress, sleep disturbances, movement disorders, and mania.[35]

Other Clinical Effects Anticholinergic effects can occur early or late in the course of CA toxicity. Pupils may be dilated and poorly reactive to light. Other anticholinergic effects include dry mouth, dry flushed skin, urinary retention, and ileus. Though prominent, these findings are typically clinically inconsequential.

Reported pulmonary complications include acute lung injury, aspiration pneumonitis, and multisystem organ failure. Acute lung injury may be the result of aspiration, hypotension, pulmonary infection, and excessive fluid administration, along with the primary toxic effects of CAs.[101,103] Bowel ischemia, pseudoobstruction, and pancreatitis are reported in patients with CA overdose.[75]

Death directly caused by CA toxicity usually occurs in the first several hours after presentation and is secondary to refractory hypotension in patients who reach healthcare facilities. Late deaths (>1–2 days after presentation) usually are secondary to other factors such as aspiration pneumonitis, adult respiratory distress syndrome from refractory hypotension, and/or infection.[19]

CHRONIC TOXICITY

Chronic CA toxicity usually manifests as exaggerated side effects, such as sedation and sinus tachycardia, or is identified by supratherapeutic drug concentrations in the blood in the absence of an acute overdose.[37] Unlike chronic theophylline and aspirin poisoning, chronic CA toxicity does not appear to cause life-threatening toxicity. A sparse literature describes the clinical course of this cohort.

Several reports describe sudden death in children taking therapeutic doses of CAs.[91,92,111] QT prolongation with resultant torsades de pointes, advanced atrioventricular conduction delays, blood pressure fluctuations, and ventricular tachycardia are postulated mechanisms, although whether any of these effects contributed to the deaths is unknown. Prospective studies using 12-lead ECG, 24-hour ECG recording, and Doppler echocardiography in children receiving therapeutic doses of CAs have failed to find any significant cardiac abnormalities when compared to children not taking CAs.[12,28] However, authors recommend that CAs not be initiated or continued in any child with a resting QT interval greater than 450 ms or with bundle-branch block.[31]

UNIQUE TOXICITY FROM "ATYPICAL" CYCLIC ANTIDEPRESSANTS

Although the incidence of serious cardiovascular toxicity is lower in patients with amoxapine overdoses, the incidence of seizures is significantly greater than with the traditional CAs.[54,63] Moreover, seizures may be more frequent or status epilepticus may develop.[78] Similarly, the incidences of seizures, cardiac dysrhythmias, and duration of coma are greater with maprotiline toxicity compared to the CAs.[53]

DIAGNOSTIC TESTING

Diagnostic testing for patients with CA poisoning primarily relies on indirect bedside tests (ECG) and other qualitative laboratory analyses. Quantification of CA concentration provides little help in the acute management of patients with CA overdose, but provides adjunctive information to support the diagnosis.

ELECTROCARDIOGRAPHY

The ECG can provide important diagnostic information and may predict clinical toxicity after a CA overdose. CA toxicity results in distinctive and diagnostic electrocardiographic changes that may allow early diagnosis and targeted therapy when the clinical history and physical examination are unreliable.

A T40-ms axis between 120° and 270° is associated with CA toxicity and in one study was a sensitive indicator of drug presence.[21,81,121] A terminal QRS vector of 130°–270° discriminated between 11 patients with positive toxicology screens for CAs and 14 patients with negative toxicology screens.[81] With further analyses, this report concluded that the positive and negative predictive values of this ECG parameter for CA ingestions were 66% and 100%, respectively, in a population of 299 general overdose patients. A retrospective study reported that a CA-poisoned patient was 8.6 times more likely to have a T40-ms axis greater than 120° than was a non–CA-poisoned patient.[121] This parameter was a more sensitive indicator of CA-induced altered mental status, but not necessarily of seizure or dysrhythmia. However, the T40-ms axis is not easily measured in the absence of specialized computer-assisted analysis, which limits its practical utility. An abnormal terminal rightward axis can be estimated by observing a negative deflection (terminal S wave) in leads I and aVL and a positive deflection (terminal R wave) in lead aVR (Fig. 73–3).

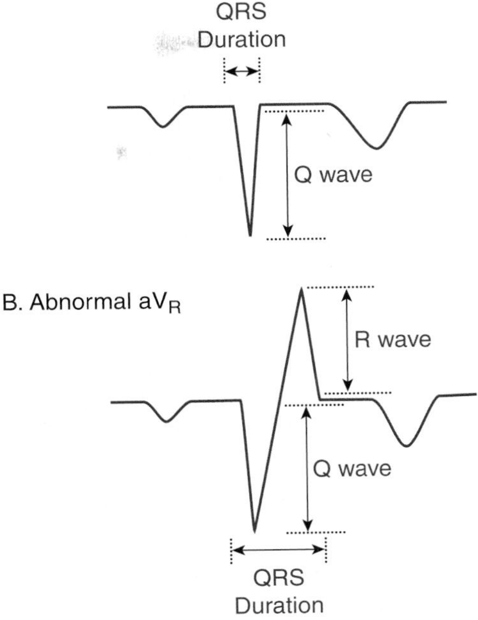

FIGURE 73–3. (A) Normal QRS complex in lead aVR. (B) Abnormal QRS complex in a patient with cyclic antidepressant (CA) poisoning. The R wave in lead aVR is measured as the maximal height in millimeters of the terminal upward deflection in the QRS complex. In this example, the QRS complex duration is prolonged, indicating significant CA poisoning.

The maximal limb lead QRS complex duration is an easily measured ECG parameter that is a sensitive indicator of toxicity. One investigation reported that 33% of patients with a limb lead QRS interval greater than or equal to 100 ms developed seizures and 14% developed ventricular dysrhythmias.[14] No seizures or dysrhythmias occurred in those patients whose QRS interval remained less than 100 ms. There was a 50% incidence of ventricular dysrhythmias among patients with a QRS duration greater than or equal to 160 ms. No ventricular dysrhythmias occurred in patients with a QRS duration less than 160 ms. Subsequent studies confirmed that a QRS duration greater than 100 ms is associated with an increased incidence of serious toxicity, including coma, need for intubation, hypotension, seizures, and dysrhythmias, making this ECG parameter a useful indicator of toxicity.[21,60]

Evaluation of lead aVR on a routine ECG may also predict toxicity (Figs. 73–2 and 73–3). When prospectively studied, 79 patients with acute CA overdoses demonstrated that the amplitude of the terminal R wave and R/S wave ratio in lead aVR (R_{aVR}, R/S_{aVR}) were significantly greater in patients who developed seizures and ventricular dysrhythmias.[60] The sensitivity of R_{aVR} = 3 mm and R/S_{aVR} = 0.7 in predicting seizures and dysrhythmias was comparable to the sensitivity of QRS = 100 ms.

The Type 1 Brugada pattern is similar to a right bundle branch block (rSR′), with downsloping ST elevations ("coved") in the right precordial leads (V1-V3).[10,78] This pattern is neither highly sensitive nor specific for CA toxicity, and it is reported in patients with cocaine and phenothiazine toxicity as well as those on Type IA antidysrhythmic therapy. In one series of over 400 pateints with CA overdose, a significant increase in adverse outcomes (ie, seizures, widened QRS interval, and hypotension) was identified in those patients with a Brugada ECG pattern compared to those who did not have the pattern.[10] However, there were no deaths or dysrhythmias in the nine patients with this pattern.

Serial ECGs should be obtained as the electrocardiographic changes can be dynamic. Electrocardiographic parameters should always be interpreted in conjunction with the patient's clinical presentation, history, and course during the first several hours to assist in decision making regarding interventions and disposition.[61]

LABORATORY TESTS

Determination of serum CA concentrations has limited utility in the immediate evaluation and management of patients with acute overdoses. In one study, serum drug concentrations failed to accurately predict the development of seizures or ventricular dysrhythmias.[14] The pharmacologic properties of CAs—namely, large volumes of distributions, prolonged absorption phase, long distribution half-lives, pH-dependent protein binding, and the wide interpatient variability of terminal elimination half-lives, explain the limited value of serum concentrations in this situation. Any concentration above the therapeutic range (50–300 ng/mL, including active metabolites) may be associated with adverse effects, and is an indication to decrease or discontinue the medication.

Although CA concentrations greater than 1000 ng/mL usually are associated with significant clinical toxicity such as coma, seizures, and dysrhythmias, life-threatening toxicity may be observed in patients with serum concentrations less than 1000 ng/mL.[14,56] Serious toxicity at lower concentrations probably results from a number of factors, including the timing of the specimen in relation to the ingestion and the limitations of measuring the concentration in blood and not the affected tissue. Quantitative concentrations usually cannot be readily obtained in most hospital laboratories. However, qualitative screens for CAs using an enzyme-multiplied immunoassay test are available at many hospitals. Unfortunately, false-positive results can occur with many drugs such as carbamazepine, cyclobenzaprine, thioridazine, diphenhydramine, quetiapine, and cyproheptadine (Chap. 6). Thus the presence of a CA on a qualitative assay should not be relied upon to confirm the diagnosis of CA poisoning in the absence of corroborating historical or clinical evidence.

Quantitative concentrations may be helpful in determining the cause of death in suspected overdose patients. CA concentrations reported in lethal overdoses typically range from 1100–21,800 ng/mL. CA concentrations may increase over 5-fold because of postmortem redistribution (Chap. 33).[5] Measurement of liver CA concentration or the parent-to-metabolite drug ratio may be useful in the postmortem setting.

TABLE 73–2. Treatment of Cyclic Antidepressant Toxicity

Toxic Effect	Treatment
Sinus rhythm with a QRS >100 ms	Sodium bicarbonate: 1--2 mEq/kg IV boluses at 3 to 5 min intervals to reverse the abnormality or to a target serum pH no greater than 7.55 Controlled ventilation (if clinically indicated for hypoventilation)
Wide-complex tachycardia/ ventricular tachycardia	Sodium bicarbonate: 1--2 mEq/kg IV boluses to reverse the dysrhythmias or to a target serum pH no greater than 7.55 Correct hypoxia, acidosis, hypotension Consider lidocaine: 1 mg/kg slow IV bolus, followed by infusion of 20--50 µg/kg/min Consider hypertonic saline (3% NaCl) Consider magnesium sulfate 25--50 mg/kg (maximum 2 g) IV over 2 min
Torsades de pointes	Magnesium sulfate Overdrive pacing (caution due to rate dependence of CA)
Hypotension	Isotonic saline (0.9% NaCl) boluses (up to 30 mL/kg) Correct hypoxia, acidosis Sodium bicarbonate: 1--2 mEq/kg IV boluses to a target serum pH of no greater than 7.50–7.55 Norepinephrine
Seizures	Benzodiazepines Secure airway with intubation if necessary Correct hypoxia, acidosis Barbiturates Continuous infusion of midazolam or propofol if barbiturates fail Consider neuromuscular paralysis/general anesthesia with EEG monitoring if all other measures fail
Refractory poisoning	Consider intravenous fat emulsion in moribund patients Consider extracorporeal mechanical circulation (extracorporeal membrane oxygenation, cardiopulmonary bypass)

MANAGEMENT

Any person with a suspected or known ingestion of a CA requires immediate evaluation and treatment (Table 73–2). The patient should be attached to a cardiac monitor and intravenous access should be secured. Early intubation is advised for patients with CNS depression and/or hemodynamic instability because of the potential for rapid clinical deterioration. A 12-lead ECG should be obtained for all patients. Laboratory tests including concentrations of glucose and electrolytes should be performed for all patients with altered mental status, as well as blood gas analysis to both assess the degree of acidemia and guide alkalinization therapy. Aggressive interventions for maintenance of blood pressure and peripheral perfusion must be performed early to avoid irreversible damage. Both children and adults receiving cardiopulmonary resuscitation have recovered successfully despite periods of asystole exceeding 90 minutes.[23,25,83,105] The options for GI decontamination discussed in the following section should then be considered.

GASTROINTESTINAL DECONTAMINATION

Induction of emesis is contraindicated, given the potential for precipitous neurologic and hemodynamic deterioration. Because of the potential lethality of large quantities of CAs, orogastric lavage should be considered in the symptomatic patient with an overdose. Although the benefits of orogastric lavage for CA toxicity are not substantiated by controlled trials, the potential benefits of removing significant quantities of a highly toxic drug must be weighed against the risks of the procedure (Chap. 7).[15] Because the anticholinergic actions of some CAs may decrease spontaneous gastric emptying, attempts at orogastric lavage up to 12 hours after ingestion may yield unabsorbed drug. Because of the potential for rapid deterioration of mental status and seizures, orogastric lavage should only be performed after endotracheal intubation has assured airway protection. Orogastric lavage in young children with unintentional ingestions of CAs may be associated with more risk and impracticalities, such as the inadequate hole size of pediatric tubes, and less benefit given the amount of drug usually ingested. Activated charcoal should be administered in nearly all cases. Irrespective of age, an additional dose of activated charcoal several hours later is reasonable in a seriously poisoned patient in whom unabsorbed drug may still be present in the GI tract, or in the case of desorption of CAs from activated charcoal. It is important to monitor for the development of an ileus to prevent abdominal complications from additional doses of activated charcoal.[75]

WIDE-COMPLEX DYSRHYTHMIAS, CONDUCTION DELAYS, AND HYPOTENSION

The mainstay therapy for treating wide-complex dysrhythmias and for reversing conduction delays and hypotension is the combination of serum alkalinization and sodium loading. Increasing the extracellular concentration of sodium, or sodium loading, may overwhelm the effective blockade of sodium channels presumably through gradient effects (Fig. 73–1). Controlled in vitro and in vivo studies in various animal models demonstrate that hypertonic sodium bicarbonate effectively reduces QRS complex prolongation, increases blood pressure, and reverses or suppresses ventricular dysrhythmias caused by CAs.[85,95–97] These studies showed a clear benefit of hypertonic sodium bicarbonate when compared to hyperventilation, hypertonic sodium chloride, or nonsodium buffer solutions. A systematic review of all animal and human studies published until 2001 revealed that alkalinization therapy was the most beneficial therapy for consequential dysrhythmias and shock[13] (see Antidote in Depth A5: Sodium Bicarbonate).

The optimal dosing and mode of administration of hypertonic sodium bicarbonate and the indications for initiating and terminating this treatment are unsupported by controlled clinical studies. Instead, the information is extrapolated from animal studies, clinical experience, and an understanding of the pathophysiologic mechanisms of CA toxicity. A bolus, or rapid infusion over several minutes, of hypertonic sodium bicarbonate (1–2 mEq/kg) should be administered initially.[69,102] Additional boluses every 3–5 minutes can be administered until the QRS interval narrows and the hypotension improves (Fig. 73–2). Blood pH should be carefully monitored after several bicarbonate boluses, aiming for a target pH of no greater than 7.50–7.55. Because CA may redistribute from the tissues into the blood over several hours, it may be reasonable to begin a continuous sodium bicarbonate infusion to maintain the pH in this range. Differences in outcomes between repetitive boluses versus bicarbonate infusions are not well studied. Although diluting sodium bicarbonate in 5% dextrose in water and infusing it slowly renders it less able to increase the sodium gradient across the cell, the beneficial effects of pH elevation still warrant its use once the patient is stabilized. No evidence supports prophylactic alkalinization in the absence of cardiovascular toxicity.

Hypertonic sodium chloride (3% NaCl) reverses cardiotoxicity in several animal studies,[45,70,85] and numerous reports and extensive clinical experience support its efficacy in humans.[13,46,47,74] However, the dose of hypertonic saline for CA poisoning has never been evaluated in humans for safety or efficacy, and the dose suggested by animal studies (up to 15 mEq/kg) exceeds the amount that most clinicians would consider safe (1–2 mEq/kg). Hypertonic sodium chloride is associated with a hyperchloremic metabolic acidosis, an undesired effect that highlights one benefit of hypertonic sodium bicarbonate. However, hypertonic saline could be considered in situations in which alkalinization with sodium bicarbonate is not possible.

Hyperventilation of an intubated patient is a more rapid and easily titratable method of serum alkalinization but is not as effective as $NaHCO_3$ in reversing cardiotoxicity.[49,69] Simultaneous hyperventilation and sodium bicarbonate administration may result in profound alkalemia and should be performed only with extreme caution and careful monitoring of pH.[122] Hyperventilation without bicarbonate administration may be indicated in patients with acute lung injury or congestive heart failure in whom administration of large quantities of sodium are contraindicated.

Alkalinization and sodium loading with hypertonic sodium bicarbonate and/or hypertonic saline along with controlled ventilation (if clinically indicated) should be administered to all CA overdose patients presenting with major cardiovascular toxicity and altered mental status. Indications include conduction delays (QRS > 100 ms) and hypotension. It is imperative to initiate treatment until CA toxicity can be excluded because of the risk for rapid and precipitous deterioration. Although commonly assumed, it is unclear whether the failure of the QRS complex to narrow with sodium bicarbonate treatment excludes CA toxicity.

It is unclear whether alkalinization and sodium loading is effective for reversing the Brugada pattern. The sparse available literature is equivocal.[9,78] It would seem prudent to administer sodium bicarbonate in the presence of a presumed TCA-induced Brugada pattern, especially with concomitant signs of other TCA toxicity.

Alkalinization may be continued for at least 12–24 hours after the ECG has normalized because of the redistribution of the drug from the tissue. However, the time observed for resolution or normalization of conduction abnormalities is extremely variable, ranging from several hours to several days, despite continuous bicarbonate infusion.[61] We recommend stopping alkalinization when the patient's mental status improves and there is improvement, but not necessarily normalization, of abnormal ECG findings.

ANTIDYSRHYTHMIC THERAPY

Lidocaine is the antidysrhythmic most commonly advocated for treatment of CA-induced dysrhythmias, although no controlled human studies demonstrate its efficacy.[86] Because lidocaine has sodium channel blocking properties, some investigators argue against its use in CA poisoning.[1] These theoretical concerns are not well supported in the literature, and the class IB antidysrhythmic channel binding kinetics may prove favorable. Although limited data also suggest that the IB antidysrhythmic phenytoin prevents or reverses conduction abnormalities,[41,68] these data were poorly controlled for other confounding factors, such as blood pH and sodium bicarbonate administration, they had very small numbers, and, in some, the cardiotoxicity was not severe. Since phenytoin exacerbates ventricular dysrhythmias in animals[20] and fails to protect against seizures,[8] its use is no longer recommended.

The use of class IA (quinidine, procainamide, disopyramide, and moricizine) and class IC (flecainide, propafenone) antidysrhythmics is absolutely contraindicated because they have similar pharmacologic actions to CAs and thus may worsen the sodium channel inhibition and exacerbate cardiotoxicity. Class III antidysrhythmics (amiodarone, bretylium, and sotalol) prolong the QT interval and, although unstudied, may be contraindicated as well (see Chap. 63).

Because magnesium sulfate has antidysrhythmic properties, it may be beneficial in the treatment of ventricular dysrhythmias. Animal studies of the effects of magnesium on CA-induced dysrhythmias yield conflicting results.[50,51] However, successful use of magnesium sulfate in the treatment of refractory ventricular fibrillation after TCA overdose is reported.[23,25,52,94] When dysrhythmias fail to reverse after alkalinization, sodium loading, and a trial of lidocaine, or magnesium sulfate may be warranted.

Slowing the heart rate in the presence of CAs may allow more time during diastole for CA unbinding from sodium channels and result in an improvement in ventricular conduction.[3,96] This may abolish the reentry mechanism for dysrhythmias and was one rationale for the past use of physostigmine and propranolol. Thus, decreasing the sinus rate may itself be effective in abolishing ventricular dysrhythmias by eliminating rate-dependent conduction slowing. Propranolol terminated ventricular tachycardia in an animal model but also caused significant hypotension and death.[97] In one case series, patients developed severe hypotension or had a cardiac arrest shortly after receiving a β-adrenergic antagonist.[33] Other animal studies suggest that preventing or abolishing tachycardia by sinus node destruction, or by using bradycardic agents that impede sinus node automaticity without affecting myocardial repolarization or contractility, may successfully prevent CA-induced ventricular dysrhythmias.[3,4] The combined negative inotropic effects of β-adrenergic antagonists and CAs, along with the significant cardiac and CNS effects reported with physostigmine use, do not support their routine use in the management of CA-induced tachydysrhythmias.

HYPOTENSION

Standard initial treatment for hypotension should include volume expansion with isotonic saline or sodium bicarbonate. Hypotension unresponsive to these therapeutic interventions necessitates the use of inotropic or vasopressor support and possibly extracorporeal cardiovascular support.

No controlled human trials are available to guide the use of vasopressor therapy. The pharmacologic properties of CAs complicate the choice of a specific agent. Specifically, CA blockade of neurotransmitter reuptake theoretically could result in depletion of intracellular catecholamines. This could blunt the effect of dopamine, which is dependent on the release of endogenous norepinephrine for its inotropic activity.[18] This suggests that a direct-acting vasopressor such as norepinephrine is more efficacious than an indirect-acting catecholamine such as dopamine.

In fact, limited clinical data suggest that norepinephrine is more efficacious than dopamine.[113] In a retrospective study of 26 adult hypotensive patients receiving nonstandardized therapy, response rates to norepinephrine (5–53 μg/min) were significantly better than response rates to dopamine (5–10 μg/kg/min).[114] Patients who did not respond to dopamine at vasopressor doses (10–50 μg/kg/min) responded to norepinephrine (5–74 μg/min). Animal data comparing various treatments are conflicting, and their direct applicability to clinical human poisoning is limited.[29,115] Both norepinephrine and epinephrine increased the survival rate in CA-poisoned rats. In addition, epinephrine was superior to norepinephrine when used both with and without sodium bicarbonate, and the most effective treatment regimen in this study was epinephrine plus sodium bicarbonate; neither precipitated dysrhythmias. The authors propose that epinephrine is more efficacious because it augments myocardial perfusion more than norepinephrine and improves the recovery of CA sodium channel blockade by hyperpolarization of the membrane potential through its stimulation of increased potassium intracellular transport.

Based on the available data, pharmacologic effects, theoretical concerns, and experience, norepinephrine (0.1–0.2 μg/kg/min) is recommended for hypotension that is unresponsive to volume expansion and hypertonic sodium bicarbonate therapy. Central venous pressure and/or pulmonary artery catheterization may be necessary to guide the choice of additional vasopressor or inotropic agents, especially in the presence of other cardiodepressant drugs.

If these measures fail to correct hypotension, extracorporeal life support measures should be considered. Extracorporeal membrane oxygenation, extracorporeal circulation, and cardiopulmonary bypass are successful adjuncts for refractory hypotension and life support when maximum therapeutic interventions fail.[40,55,105,120] These modalities can provide critical perfusion to the heart and brain and maintain metabolic function while giving the body time to metabolize and eliminate the CA by maintaining hepatorenal blood flow.

INVESTIGATIONAL THERAPY

Intravenous fat emulsion is reported to be effective in reversing cardiovascular toxicity due to several lipophilic drugs including clomipramine. Its use is currently reserved for moribund patients, though as more data emerges the indications may be expanded or its use eliminated[43] (see Antidotes in Depth: Intravenous Fat Emulsion).

CENTRAL NERVOUS SYSTEM TOXICITY

Seizures caused by CAs usually are brief and may stop before treatment can be initiated. Recurrent seizures, prolonged seizures (>2 minutes), and status epilepticus require prompt treatment to prevent worsening acidosis, hypoxia, and development of hyperthermia and rhabdomyolysis. Benzodiazepines are effective as first-line therapy for seizures. If this therapy fails, barbiturates or propofol should be administered. Propofol controlled refractory seizures resulting from amoxapine toxicity.[76] Failure to respond to barbiturates or propofol should lead to consideration of neuromuscular paralysis and general anesthesia with continuous EEG monitoring. Phenytoin is not recommended for seizures because data not only demonstrate a failure to terminate seizures, but also suggest enhanced cardiovascular toxicity.[8,20]

Use of flumazenil in the patient with known or suspected CA ingestion is contraindicated. Several case reports of patients with CA overdoses describe seizures following administration of flumazenil.[42,58,71] Physostigmine was used in the past to reverse the acute CNS toxicity of CAs (Antidotes in Depth A12: Physostigmine). However, physostigmine is not recommended because it may increase the risk of cardiac toxicity, cause bradycardia and asystole, and precipitate seizures in acutely CA-poisoned patients.[89]

ENHANCED ELIMINATION

No specific treatment modalities have demonstrated clinical significant efficacy in enhancing the elimination of CAs. Some investigators propose multiple doses of activated charcoal to enhance CA elimination because of their small enterohepatic and enterogastric circulation.[66] Human volunteer studies and case series of patients with CA overdoses suggest that the half-life of CAs may be decreased by multiple-dose activated charcoal (MDAC).[24,82,111]Activated charcoal reduced the apparent half-life of amitriptyline to 4–40 hours in overdose patients, compared to previously published values of 30 to more than 60 hours.[111] Changes in the severity or duration of clinical toxicity, however, were not reported. Other investigators showed that in human volunteers MDAC reduced the half-life of therapeutic doses of amitriptyline approximately 20% compared with no activated charcoal administration. However, the methodologic flaws and equivocal findings of these studies and the lack of any positive outcome data for this intervention from additional studies do not provide evidence supporting its use in this setting.[22,38] Pharmacokinetic properties of CAs (large volumes of distribution, high plasma-protein binding) weighed against the small increases in clearance and the potential complications of MDAC, such as impaction, intestinal infarction, and perforation, do not warrant its routine use.[22,75] One additional dose of activated charcoal may be given to decrease GI absorption in patients with evidence of significant CNS and cardiovascular toxicity if bowel sounds are present.

Measures to enhance urinary CA excretion have a minimal effect on total clearance. Urinary alkalinization does not enhance, and may reduce, urinary clearance due to passive reabsorption of the unionized CA from an alkaline urine. Hemodialysis is ineffective in enhancing the elimination of CAs because of their large volumes of distribution, high lipid solubility, and extensive protein binding.[44] Hemoperfusion overcomes some of the limitations of hemodialysis, but may not be effective because of the large volumes of distributions of CAs. Although several uncontrolled case reports and a case series described improvement in cardiotoxicity during hemoperfusion, this finding may be coincidental.[11,23,32]

HOSPITAL ADMISSION CRITERIA

All patients who present with known or suspected CA ingestion should undergo continuous cardiac monitoring and serial electrocardiography for a minimum of 6 hours. Recommendations in the older literature for 48–72 hours of ICU monitoring even for patients with minor CA ingestions stem from isolated case reports of late-onset dysrhythmias, CNS effects, and sudden deaths.[34,36,88] However, review of these cases shows inadequate gastric decontamination, inadequate therapeutic interventions, and significant ongoing complications of overdose. Several retrospective studies demonstrate that late, unexpected complications in CA overdoses such as seizures, dysrhythmias, and death did not occur in patients who had few or no major signs of toxicity at presentation or a normal level of consciousness and a normal ECG for 24 hours.[19,25,27,90] A disposition algorithm has been proposed based on clinical signs and symptoms.[6,24,112] If the patient is asymptomatic at presentation, undergoes GI decontamination, has normal ECGs, or has sinus tachycardia (with normal QRS complexes) that resolves, and the patient remains asymptomatic in the healthcare facility for a minimum of 6 hours without any treatment interventions, the patient may be medically cleared for psychiatric evaluation (if appropriate) or discharged home as appropriate.

A prospective study of 67 patients used the Antidepressant Overdose Risk Assessment (ADORA) criteria to identify patients who were at high risk for developing serious toxicity and proposed criteria for hospitalization.[30] In this study, the presence of QRS interval greater than 100 ms, cardiac dysrhythmias, altered mental status, seizures, respiratory depression, or hypotension on presentation to the ED (or within 6 hours of ingestion, if the time was known) was 100% sensitive in identifying patients with significant toxicity and subsequent complications. Criteria specific for ICU admission (other than patients requiring ventilatory and/or blood pressure support), versus an inpatient bed with continuous cardiac monitoring, are less clear and probably are institution dependent.[107]

The disposition of patients with persistent isolated sinus tachycardia, or prolonged QT interval with no concomitant altered mental status, or blood pressure changes, is not clearly defined. Previous studies demonstrate that these two parameters alone are not predictive of subsequent clinical toxicity or complications.[30,31] In addition, the sinus tachycardia may persist for up to 1 week following ingestion.[80,100] However, a study of isolated CA overdose patients reported that a heart rate greater than 120 beats/min and QT interval greater than 480 ms were associated with an increased likelihood of major toxicity.[21] These patients are candidates for observation units with continuous ECG monitoring and serial ECGs for 24 hours.

INPATIENT CARDIAC MONITORING

The duration of cardiac monitoring in any patient initially exhibiting signs of major clinical toxicity depends on many factors. Certainly the duration of CA cardiotoxicity and neurotoxicity may be prolonged, and using normalization of ECG abnormalities as an end point for therapy and discharge, is problematic. Some studies document the variable resolution and normalization of QRS prolongation and T40-ms axis rotation.[84,103] Based on the available literature, it is reasonable to recommend that after the mental status and blood pressure normalize, and the electrocardiogram improves, patients who exhibited significant poisoning should be monitored for another 24 hours off of all of therapy, including alkalinization, antidysrhythmics, and inotropics/vasopressors.

SUMMARY

Cyclic antidepressant poisoning continues to be a cause of serious morbidity and mortality worldwide. The distinctive characteristics of these drugs can cause significant CNS and cardiovascular toxicity, the latter being responsible for mortality as a result of overdose of these drugs. Cardiovascular toxicity ranges from mild conduction abnormalities and sinus tachycardia to wide-complex tachycardia, hypotension, and asystole. CNS toxicity includes delirium, lethargy, seizures, and coma. The ECG is a simple, readily available diagnostic test that can predict the development of significant toxicity, particularly seizures and/or dysrhythmias. Management strategies are based primarily on the pathophysiology of these drugs, namely, sodium channel blockade in the myocardium. Alkalinization and sodium loading with hypertonic sodium bicarbonate and isotonic saline are the principal modes of specific therapy for cardiovascular toxicity. Guidelines for observing or admitting patients to the hospital may be based on initial clinical presentation or development of clinical symptomatology and ECG changes.

REFERENCES

1. Ahmad S. Management of cardiac complications in tricyclic antidepressant poisoning. *J R Soc Med.* 1980;73:79.
2. Amitai Y, Kennedy EJ, De Sandre P, Frischer H. Distribution of amitriptyline and nortriptyline in blood: Role of α_1-glycoprotein. *Ther Drug Monit.* 1993;15:267-273.
3. Ansel GM, Coyne K, Arnold S, et al. Mechanisms of ventricular arrhythmia during amitriptyline toxicity. *J Cardiovasc Pharmacol.* 1993;22:798-803.
4. Ansel GM, Meimer JP, Nelson SD. Prevention of tricyclic antidepressant-induced ventricular tachyarrhythmia by a specific bradycardic agent in a canine model. *J Cardiovasc Pharmacol.* 1994;24:256-260.
5. Apple FS. Postmortem tricyclic antidepressant concentrations: assessing cause of death using parent drug to metabolite ratio. *J Anal Toxicol.* 1989;13:197-198.
6. Banahan B, Schelkum P. Tricyclic antidepressant overdose: conservative management in a community hospital with cost-saving implications. *J Emerg Med.* 1990;8:451-454.
7. Barden N. Modulation of glucocorticoid receptor gene expression by antidepressant drugs. *Pharmacopsychiatry.* 1996;29:12-22.
8. Beaubien AR, Carpenter DC, Mathieu, LF, MacConaill M, Hrdina PD. Antagonism of imipramine poisoning by anticonvulsants in the rat. *Toxicol Appl Pharmacol.* 1976;38:1-6.
9. Bebarta VS, Waksman JC. Amtriptyline-induced Brugada pattern fails to respond to sodium bicarbonate. *Clin Toxicol.* 2007;45:186-188.
10. Bebarta VS, Phillips S, Eberhardt A, et al. Incidence of Brugada electrocardiographic pattern and outcomes of these patients after intentional tricyclic antidepressant ingestion. *Am J Cardiol.* 2007;100:656-660.
11. Bek K, Ozkaya O, Mutlu B, et al. Charcoal haemoperfusion in amitriptyline poisoning: experience in 20 children. *Nephrology.* 2008;13:193-197.
12. Biederman J, Baldessarini RJ, Goldblatt A. A naturalistic study of 24-hour electrocardiographic recordings and echocardiographic findings in children and adolescents treated with desipramine. *J Am Acad Child Adolesc Psychiatry.* 1993;32:805-813.
13. Blackman K, Brown SF, Wilkes GJ. Plasma alkalinization for tricyclic antidepressant toxicity: a systematic review. *Emerg Med.* 2001;13:204-210.

14. Boehnert M, Lovejoy FH. Value of the QRS duration versus the serum drug level in predicting seizures and ventricular arrhythmias after an acute overdose of tricyclic antidepressants. *N Engl J Med.* 1985;313:474-479.
15. Bosse GM, Barefoot JA, Pfeifer MP, et al. Comparison of three methods of gut decontamination in tricyclic antidepressant overdose. *J Emerg Med.* 1995;13:203-209.
16. Brosen K, Skjelbo E. Fluoxetine and norfluoxetine are potent inhibitors of P450IID6—the source of the sparteine/debrisoquine oxidation polymorphism. *Br J Clin Pharmacol.* 1991;31:136-137.
17. Brosen Z, Zeugin T, Myer UA. Role of P450IID6, the target of the sparteine/debrisoquin oxidation polymorphism, in the metabolism of imipramine. *Clin Pharmacol Ther.* 1991;49:609-617.
18. Buchman AL, Dauer J, Geiderman J. The use of vasoactive agents in the treatment of refractory hypotension seen in tricyclic antidepressant overdose. *J Clin Psychopharmacol.* 1990;10:409-413.
19. Callaham M, Kassel D. Epidemiology of fatal tricyclic antidepressant ingestion: implications for management. *Ann Emerg Med.* 1985;14:1-9.
20. Callaham M, Schumaker H, Pentel P. Phenytoin prophylaxis of cardiotoxicity in experimental amitriptyline poisoning. *J Pharmacol Exp Ther.* 1988;245:216-220.
21. Caravati EM, Bossart PJ. Demographic and electrocardiographic factors associated with severe tricyclic antidepressant toxicity. *J Toxicol Clin Toxicol.* 1991;29:31-43.
22. Chyka P. Multiple-dose activated charcoal and enhancement of systemic drug clearance: summaries of studies in animals and human volunteers. *J Toxicol Clin Toxicol.* 1995;33:399-405.
23. Citak A, Soysal DD, Ucsel R, et al. Efficacy of long duration resuscitation and magnesium sulphate treatment in amitriptyline poisoning. *Eur J Emerg Med.* 2002;9:63-66.
24. Crome P, Dawling S, Braithwaite RA. Effect of activated charcoal on absorption of nortriptyline. *Lancet.* 1977;1:1203-1205.
25. Deegan C, O'Brien K. Amitriptyline poisoning in a 2 year old child. *Paediatr Anaesth.* 2006;16:174-177.
26. Ellison DW, Pentel PR. Clinical features and consequences of seizures due to cyclic antidepressant overdose. *Am J Emerg Med.* 1989;7:5-10.
27. Fasoli R, Glauser F. Cardiac arrhythmias and ECG abnormalities in TCA overdose. *J Toxicol Clin Toxicol.* 1981;18:155-163.
28. Fletcher SE, Case CL, Sallee FR, et al. Prospective study of the electrocardiographic effects of imipramine in children. *J Pediatr.* 1993;122:652-654.
29. Follmer CH, Lum BK. Protective action of diazepam and of sympathomimetic amines against amitriptyline-induced toxicity. *J Pharmacol Exp Ther.* 1982;222:424-429.
30. Foulke GE. Identifying toxicity risk early after antidepressant overdose. *Am J Emerg Med.* 1995;13:123-126.
31. Foulke GE, Albertson TE, Walby WF. Tricyclic antidepressant overdose: emergency department findings as predictors of clinical course. *Am J Emerg Med.* 1986;4:496-500.
32. Frank RD, Kierdorf HP. Is there a role for hemoperfusion/hemodialysis as a treatment option in severe tricyclic antidepressant intoxication? *Int J Artif Organs.* 2000;23:618-623.
33. Freeman JW, Loughhead MG. Beta blockade in the treatment of tricyclic antidepressant overdosage. *Med J Aust.* 1973;1:1233-1235.
34. Freeman JW, Mundy GR, Beattie RR, Ryan C. Cardiac abnormalities in poisoning with tricyclic antidepressants. *BMJ.* 1969;2:610-613.
35. Garner EM, Kelly MW, Thompson DF. Tricyclic antidepressant withdrawal syndrome. *Ann Pharmacother.* 1993;27:1068-1072.
36. Giles HM. Imipramine poisoning in childhood. *BMJ.* 1963;2:844-846.
37. Giller EL, Bialos DS, Docherty JP, et al. Chronic amitriptyline toxicity. *Am J Psychiatry.* 1979;136:458-459.
38. Goldberg MJ, Park GD, Spector R, et al. Lack of effect of oral activated charcoal on imipramine clearance. *Clin Pharmacol Ther.* 1985;38:350-353.
39. Goldberg RJ, Capone RJ, Hunt JD. Cardiac complications following tricyclic antidepressant overdose—issues for monitoring policy. *JAMA.* 1985;254:1772-1775
40. Goodwin DA, Lally KP, Null DM. Extracorporeal membrane oxygenation support for cardiac dysfunction from tricyclic antidepressant overdose. *Crit Care Med.* 1993;21:625-627.
41. Hagerman GA, Hanashiro PK. Reversal of tricyclic-antidepressant induced cardiac conduction abnormalities by phenytoin. *Ann Emerg Med.* 1981;10:82-86.
42. Haverkos GP, DiSalvo RP, Imhoff TE. Fatal seizures after flumazenil administration in a patient with mixed overdose. *Ann Pharmacother.* 1994;28:1347-1349.
43. Harvey M, Cave G. Intralipid outperforms sodium bicarbonate in a rabbit model of clomipramine toxicity. *Ann Emerg Med.* 2007;49:178-185.
44. Heath A, Wickstron I, Martensson E, et al. Treatment of antidepressant poisoning with resin hemoperfusion. *Hum Toxicol.* 1982;1:361-371.
45. Hoegholm A, Clementson P. Hypertonic sodium chloride in severe antidepressant overdosage. *J Toxicol Clin Toxicol.* 1991;29:297-298.
46. Hoffman JR, McElroy CR. Bicarbonate therapy for dysrhythmias and hypotension in tricyclic antidepressant overdose. *West J Med.* 1981;134:60-64.
47. Hoffman JR, Votey SR, Bayer M, et al. Effect of hypertonic sodium bicarbonate in the treatment of moderate-to-severe cyclic antidepressant overdose. *Am J Emerg Med.* 1993;11:336-341.
48. Jensen PS, Bhatara VS, Vitiello B, et al. Psychoactive medication prescribing practices for US children: gaps between research and clinical practice. *J Am Acad Child Adolesc Psychiatry.* 1999;38;557-565.
49. Kingston ME. Hyperventilation in tricyclic antidepressant poisoning. *Crit Care Med.* 1979;7:550-551.
50. Kline JA, DeStefano AA, Schroeder JD, et al. Magnesium potentiates imipramine toxicity in the isolated rat heart. *Ann Emerg Med.* 1994;24:224-232.
51. Knudsen K, Abrahamsson J. Effects of magnesium sulfate and lidocaine in the treatment of ventricular arrhythmias in experimental amitriptyline poisoning in the rat. *Crit Care Med.* 1994;22:494-498.
52. Knudsen K, Abrahamsson J. Magnesium sulphate in the treatment of ventricular fibrillation in amitriptyline poisoning. *Eur Heart J.* 1997;18:881-882.
53. Knudsen K, Heath A. Effects of self-poisoning with maprotiline. *BMJ.* 1984;288:601-603.
54. Kulig K, Rumack BH, Sullivan JB, et al. Amoxapine overdose: coma and seizures without cardiotoxic effects. *JAMA.* 1982;248: 1092-1094.
55. Larkin GL, Graeber GM, Hollingshed MJ. Experimental amitriptyline poisoning: treatment of severe cardiovascular toxicity with cardiopulmonary bypass. *Ann Emerg Med.* 1994;23:480-486.
56. Lavoie FW, Gansert GG, Weiss RE. Value of initial ECG findings and plasma drug levels in cyclic antidepressant overdose. *Ann Emerg Med.* 1990;19:696-700.
57. Lesch KP, Manji HK. Signal-transducing G proteins and antidepressant drugs: evidence for modulation of alpha subunit gene expression in rat brain. *Biol Psychiatr.* 1992;32:549-579.
58. Lheureux P, Vranckx M, Leduc D, et al. Flumazenil in mixed benzodiazepine/tricyclic antidepressant overdose: a placebo-controlled study in the dog. *Am J Emerg Med.* 1992;10:184-188.
59. Liebelt EL. Targeted management strategies for cardiovascular toxicity from tricyclic antidepressant overdose: the pivotal role for alkalinization and sodium loading. *Pediatr Emerg Care.* 1998;14:293-298.
60. Liebelt EL, Francis PD, Woolf AD. ECG lead aVR versus QRS interval in predicting seizures and arrhythmias in acute tricyclic antidepressant toxicity. *Ann Emerg Med.* 1995;26:195-201.
61. Liebelt EL, Ulrich A, Francis PD, et al. Serial electrocardiogram changes in acute tricyclic antidepressant overdoses. *Crit Care Med.* 1997;25:1721-1726.
62. Lipper B, Bell A, Gaynor B. Recurrent hypotension immediately after seizures in nortriptyline overdose. *Am J Emerg Med.* 1994;12:451-457.
63. Litovitz TL, Troutman WG. Amoxapine overdose: seizures and fatalities. *JAMA.* 1983;250:1069-1071.
64. Liu X, Emery CJ, Laude E, et al. Adverse pulmonary vascular effects of high dose tricyclic antidepressants: acute and chronic animal studies. *Eur Respir J.* 2002;20:344-352.
65. Malatynska E, Miller C, Schindler N, et al. Amitriptyline increases GABA-stimulated 36Cl-influx by recombinant (alpha 1 gamma) GABA A receptors. *Brain Res.* 1699;851:277-280.
66. Manoguerra AS, Weaver LC. Poisoning with tricyclic antidepressant drugs. *Clin Toxicol.* 1977;10:149-158.
67. Marshall JB, Forker AD. Cardiovascular effects of tricyclic antidepressant drugs: therapeutic usage, overdose, and management of complications. *Am Heart J.* 1982;103:401-414.
68. Mayron R, Ruiz E. Phenytoin: does it reverse tricyclic antidepressant-induced cardiac conduction abnormalities? *Ann Emerg Med.* 1986;15:876-880.
69. McCabe JL, Cobaugh DJ, Menegazzi JJ, et al. Experimental tricyclic antidepressant toxicity: a randomized, controlled comparison of hypertonic saline solution, sodium bicarbonate, and hyperventilation. *Ann Emerg Med.* 1998;32:329-333.
70. McCabe JL, Menegazzi JJ, Cobaugh DJ, et al. Recovery from severe cyclic antidepressant overdose with hypertonic saline/dextran in a swine model. *Acad Emerg Med.* 1994;1:111-115.

71. McDuffee AT, Tobias JD. Seizure after flumazenil administration in a pediatric patient. *Pediatr Emerg Care.* 1995;11:186-187.
72. McFee RB, Caraccio TR, Mofenson HC. Selected tricyclic antidepressant ingestions involving children 6 years old or less. *Acad Emerg Med.* 2001;8:139-144.
73. McKenzie MS, McFarland BH. Trends in antidepressant overdoses. *Pharmacoepidemiol Drug Saf.* 2007;16:513-523.
74. McKinney PE, Rasmussen R. Reversal of severe tricyclic antidepressant-induced cardiotoxicity with intravenous hypertonic saline solution. *Ann Emerg Med.* 2003;42:20-24.
75. McMahon AJ. Amitriptyline overdose complicated by intestinal pseudo-obstruction and caecal perforation. *Postgrad Med J.* 1989;65:948-949.
76. Merigian KS, Browning RG, Leeper KV. Successful treatment of amoxapine-induced refractory status epilepticus with propofol (Diprivan). *Acad Emerg Med.* 1995;2:128-133.
77. Merigian KS, Hedges JR, Kaplan LA, et al. Plasma catecholamine levels in cyclic antidepressant overdose. *J Toxicol Clin Toxicol.* 1991; 29:177-190.
78. Monteban-Kooistra WE, van den Berg MP, Tulleken JE. Brugada electrocardiographic pattern elicited by cyclic antidepressants overdose. *Intensive Care Med.* 2006;32:281-285.
79. Nakashita M, Sasaki K, Sakai N, et al. Effects of tricyclic and tetracyclic antidepressants on the three subtypes of GABA transporter. *Neurosci Res.* 1997;29:87-91.
80. Nicotra MB, Rivera M, Pool JL, et al. TCA overdose: clinical and pharmacologic observations. *J Toxicol Clin Toxicol.* 1981;18:599-613.
81. Niemann JT, Bessen HA, Rothstein RJ, et al. Electrocardiographic criteria for tricyclic antidepressant cardiotoxicity. *Am J Cardiol.* 1986;57:1154-1159.
82. Oppenheim RC, Stewart NF. Adsorption of tricyclic antidepressants by activated charcoal. I. Adsorption in low pH conditions. *Aust J Pharm Sci.* 1975;4:79-84.
83. Orr DAK, Bramble MG. Tricyclic antidepressant poisoning and prolonged external cardiac massage during asystole. *BMJ.* 1981;283:1107-1108.
84. Pellinen TJ, Färkkilä M, Heikkilä J, et al. Electrocardiographic and clinical features of tricyclic antidepressant intoxication. *Ann Clin Res.* 1987;19:12-17.
85. Pentel P, Benowitz N. Efficacy and mechanism of action of sodium bicarbonate in the treatment of desipramine toxicity in rats. *J Pharmacol Exp Ther.* 1984;230:12-19.
86. Pentel PR, Benowitz NL. Tricyclic antidepressant poisoning—management of arrhythmias. *Med Toxicol.* 1986;1:101-121.
87. Pentel PR, Keyler DE. Effects of high dose alpha-1-acid glycoprotein on desipramine toxicity in rats. *J Pharmacol Exp Ther.* 1988; 246:1061-1066.
88. Pentel P, Olson KR, Becker CE, et al. Late complications of tricyclic antidepressant overdose. *West J Med.* 1983;138:423-424.
89. Pentel P, Peterson CD. Asystole complicating physostigmine treatment of tricyclic antidepressant overdose. *Ann Emerg Med.* 1980;9:588-590.
90. Pentel P, Sioris L. Incidence of late arrhythmias following tricyclic antidepressant overdose. *Clin Toxicol.* 1981;18:543-548.
91. Popper CW, Ziminitzky B. Sudden death putatively related to desipramine treatment in youth: a fifth case and a review of speculative mechanisms. *J Child Adolesc Psychopharmacol.* 1995:5:283-300.
92. Riddle MA, Nelson JC, Kleinman CS, et al. Sudden death in children receiving Norpramin: a review of three reported cases and commentary. *J Am Acad Child Adolesc Psychiatry.* 1991;30:104-108.
93. Rodriguez S, Tomargo J. Electrophysiological effects of imipramine on bovine ventricular muscle and Purkinje fibres. *Br J Pharmacol.* 1980;70:15-23.
94. Sarisoy O, Babaoglu K, Tukay S, et al. Effect of magnesium sulfate for treatment of ventricular tachycardia in amitriptyline intoxication. *Pediatr Emerg Care.* 2007;23:646-648.
95. Sasyniuk BI, Jhamandas V. Mechanism of reversal of toxic effects of amitriptyline on cardiac Purkinje fibers by sodium bicarbonate. *J Pharmacol Exp Ther.* 1984;231:387-394.
96. Sasyniuk BI, Jhamandas V. Frequency-dependent effects of amitripty-line on V_{max} in canine Purkinje fibers and its alteration by alkalosis. *Proc West Pharmacol Soc.* 1986;29:73-75.
97. Sasyniuk BI, Jhamandas V, Valois M. Experimental amitriptyline intoxication: treatment of cardiac toxicity with sodium bicarbonate. *Ann Emerg Med.* 1986;15:1052-1059.
98. Seaberg DC, Weiss LD, Yeally DM, et al. Effects of alpha-1-acid glycoprotein on the cardiovascular toxicity of nortriptyline in a swine model. *Vet Hum Toxicol.* 1991;33:226-230.
99. Sedal L, Korman M, Williams P, et al. Overdosage of tricyclic antidepressants. *Med J Aust.* 1972;2:74-79.
100. Serafimovski N, Thorball N, Asmussen I, et al. Tricyclic antidepressive poisoning with special references to cardiac complications. *Acta Anaesthesiol Scand Suppl.* 1975;57:55-63.
101. Shannon M, Lovejoy FH. Pulmonary consequences of severe tricyclic antidepressant ingestion. *J Toxicol Clin Toxicol.* 1987;25: 443-461.
102. Shannon MW, Merola J, Lovejoy Jr FH. Hypotension in severe tricyclic antidepressant overdose. *Am J Emerg Med.* 1988;6:439-442.
103. Shannon MW. Duration of QRS disturbances after severe tricyclic antidepressant intoxication. *J Toxicol Clin Toxicol.* 1992;30:377-386.
104. Skowron DM, Stimmel GL. Antidepressants and the risk of seizures. *Pharmacotherapy.* 1992;12:18-22.
105. Southall DP, Kilpatrick SM. Imipramine poisoning: survival of a child after prolonged cardiac massage. *BMJ.* 1974;4:508.
106. Squires RF, Saederup E. Antidepressants and metabolites that block $GABA_A$ receptors coupled to 35S-t-butylbicyclophosphorothionate binding sites in rat brain. *Brain Res.* 1988;441:15-22.
107. Stern TA, O'Gara PT, Mulley AG. Complications after overdose with tricyclic antidepressants. *Crit Care Med.* 1985;13:672-674.
108. Strom J, Sloth-Madsen P, Nygaard-Nielsen N. Acute self-poisoning with TCA in 295 consecutive patients treated in an ICU. *Acta Anaesthesiol Scand.* 1984;28:666-670.
109. Svens K, Ryrfeldt A. A study of mechanisms underlying amitriptylineinduced acute lung function impairment. *Toxicol Appl Pharmacol.* 2001;177:179-187.
110. Swanson JR, Jones GR, Krasselt W, et al. Death of two subjects due to imipramine and desipramine metabolite accumulation during chronic therapy: a review of the literature and possible mechanisms. *J Forensic Sci.* 1997;42:335-339.
111. Swartz CM, Sherman A. The treatment of tricyclic antidepressant overdose with repeated charcoal. *J Clin Psychopharmacol.* 1984;4:336-340.
112. Taboulet P, Michard F, Muszynski J, et al. Cardiovascular repercussions of seizures during cyclic antidepressant poisoning. *J Toxicol Clin Toxicol.* 1995;33:205-211.
113. Teba L, Schiebel F, Dedhia HV, et al. Beneficial effect of norepinephrine in the treatment of circulatory shock caused by tricyclic antidepressant overdose. *Am J Emerg Med.* 1988;6:566-568.
114. Tran TP, Panacek EA, Rhee KJ, et al. Response to dopamine vs norepinephrine in tricyclic antidepressant-induced hypotension. *Acad Emerg Med.* 1997;4:864-868.
115. Vernon DD, Banner W, Garrett JS, et al. Efficacy of dopamine and norepinephrine for treatment of hemodynamic compromise in amitriptyline intoxication. *Crit Care Med.* 1991;19:544-549.
116. Vitiello B, Zuvekas SH, Norquist GS. National estimates of antidepressant medication use among U.S. children, 1997-2002. *J Am Acad Child Adolesc Psychiatry.* 2006;45:271-279.
117. Vohra J, Burrows G, Hunt D, et al. The effect of toxic and therapeutic doses of tricyclic antidepressant drugs on intracardiac conduction. *Eur J Cardiol.* 1975;3:219-227.
118. Wedin GP, Oderda GM, Klein-Schwartz W. Relative toxicity of cyclic antidepressants. *Ann Emerg Med.* 1986;15:797-804.
119. Weld FM, Bigger JT. Electrophysiological effects of imipramine on ovine cardiac Purkinje and ventricular muscle fibers. *Circ Res.* 1980;46: 167-174.
120. Williams JM, Hollingshed MJ, Vasilakis A, et al. Extracorporeal circulation in the management of severe tricyclic antidepressant overdose. *Am J Emerg Med.* 1994;12:456-458.
121. Wolfe TR, Caravati EM, Rollins DE, et al. Terminal 40-ms frontal plane QRS axis as a marker for tricyclic antidepressant overdose. *Ann Emerg Med.* 1989;18:348-351.
122. Wrenn K, Smith BA, Slovis CM. Profound alkalemia during treatment of tricyclic antidepressant overdose: A potential hazard of combined hyperventilation and intravenous bicarbonate. *Am J Emerg Med.* 1992;10:553-555.
123. Zaccara G, Muscas GC, Messori A. Clinical features, pathogenesis and management of drug-induced seizures. *Drug Saf.* 1990;5:109-151.

CHAPTER 74
SEDATIVE-HYPNOTICS

David C. Lee and Kathy Lynn Ferguson

Sedative-hypnotics are xenobiotics that limit excitability (sedation), and/or induce drowsiness and sleep (hypnosis). *Anxiolytics* (formerly known as *tranquilizers*) are medications prescribed for their sedative-hypnotic properties. There are many different types of medications used to induce anxiolysis or sleep. This chapter focuses primarily on pharmaceuticals prescribed for their sedative-hypnotic effects, many of which interact with the γ-aminobutyric acid-A ($GABA_A$) receptor (Table 74–1). Specific sedative-hypnotics such as ethanol and γ-hydroxybutyric acid are discussed in more depth in their respective chapters (Chaps. 77 and 80).

HISTORY AND EPIDEMIOLOGY

Mythology of ancient cultures is replete with stories of xenobiotics that cause sleep or unconsciousness (Chap. 1). Symptomatic overdoses of sedative-hypnotics were described in the medical literature soon after the commercial introduction of bromide preparations in 1853. Other commercial xenobiotics that subsequently were developed include chloral hydrate, paraldehyde, sulfonyl, and urethane.

The barbiturates were introduced in 1903 and quickly supplanted the older xenobiotics. This class of medications dominated the sedative-hypnotic market for the first half of the 20th century. Unfortunately, because they have a narrow therapeutic-to-toxic ratio and substantial potential for abuse, they quickly became a major health problem. By the 1950s, barbiturates were frequently implicated in overdoses and were responsible for the majority of drug-related suicides. As fatalities from barbiturates increased, attention shifted toward preventing their abuse and finding less toxic alternatives.[19] The "safer" drugs of that era included methyprylon, glutethimide, ethchlorvynol, bromides, and methaqualone. Unfortunately, many of these sedative hypnotics also had significant undesirable effects. After the introduction of benzodiazepines in the early 1960s, barbiturates and the other alternatives were quickly replaced as commonly used sedatives in the United States.

Intentional and unintentional overdoses with sedative-hypnotics occur frequently. According to the American Association of Poison Control Centers, sedative-hypnotics is consistently one of the top five classes of xenobiotics associated with overdose fatalities (see Chap. 135). With the ubiquitous worldwide use of sedative-hypnotics, they may be associated with a substantially higher number of overdoses and deaths than are officially reported. For example, a recent report described benzodiazepines as being increasingly used in drug-facilitated thefts outside the United States.[75]

Chlordiazepoxide, the first commercially available benzodiazepine, initially was marketed in 1960. Since then, more than 50 benzodiazepines have been marketed, and more are being developed. Compared with barbiturate overdoses, overdoses of benzodiazepines alone account for relatively few deaths.[37] Most deaths associated with benzodiazepines result from mixed overdoses with other centrally acting respiratory depressants.[46]

Benzodiazepines remain the most popular prescribed anxiolytics. However, the recently introduced hypnotics zolpidem, zaleplon, zopiclone, and eszopiclone have replaced benzodiazepines as the most commonly prescribed pharmaceutical sleep aids. Melatonin and ramelteon are emerging as popular sleep aids whose effects are mediated through melatonin receptor subtypes MT-1 and MT-2 specifically.[107,112,127] Dexmedetomidine, a central α_2-adrenergic agonist, is now increasingly used in the hospital setting for short-term sedation.[5,111]

PHARMACODYNAMICS/TOXICODYNAMICS

All sedative-hypnotics induce central nervous system (CNS) depression. Most clinically effective sedative-hypnotics produce their physiologic effects by enhancing the function of GABA-mediated chloride channels via agonism at the $GABA_A$ receptor. These receptors are the primary mediators of inhibitory neurotransmission in the brain (see Chap. 13). The $GABA_A$ receptor is a pentameric structure composed of varying polypeptide subunits associated with a chloride channel on the postsynaptic membrane. These subunits are classified into families (α, β, γ, etc.). Variations in the five subunits of the GABA receptor confer the potency of its sedative, anxiolytic, hypnotic, amnestic, and muscle relaxing properties. The most common $GABA_A$ receptor in the brain is composed of $\alpha_1\beta_2\gamma_2$ subunits. Almost all sedative-hypnotics bind to $GABA_A$ receptors containing the α_1 subunit. One exception may be etomidate, which has been shown to produce sedation at the β_2 unit and anesthesia at the β_3 subunit.[24,91,104,150] Low doses of benzodiazepines will be effective only at $GABA_A$ receptors with the γ_2 subunit. Even within classes of sedative-hypnotics, there will be varying affinities for differing subunits of the GABA receptor.[30,79]

Many sedative-hypnotics also act at receptors other than the $GABA_A$ receptor. Trichloroethanol and propofol, also inhibit glutamate-mediated *N*-methyl-D-aspartate (NMDA) receptors, thereby inhibiting excitatory neurotransmission.[26,99,116] Some benzodiazepines may also inhibit adenosine metabolism and reuptake, thereby potentiating both A_1-adenosine (negative dromotropy) and A_2-adenosine (coronary vasodilation) receptor-mediated effects.[87,124] Benzodiazepines also interact with specific benzodiazepine receptors that are not associated with the GABA receptor. These receptors have been labeled ω receptors. Benzodiazepines can also interact with serotonergic pathways. For example, diazepam modulates morphine analgesia via interactions with serotonin receptors. In addition, the anxiolytic effects of clonazepam can be partially explained by upregulation of serotonergic receptors, specifically $5\text{-}HT_1$ and $5\text{-}HT_2$.[8,88,157] Newer sleep aids, such as melatonin and ramelteon, do not appear to act at the $GABA_A$ receptor. Instead, they are agonists at melatonin receptor subtypes MT-1 and MT-2 in the suprachiasmatic nucleus of the brain.[127] Dexmedetomidine, a central α_2-adrenergic agonist similar to clonidine, induces a state of "cooperative sedation."[136]

PHARMACOKINETICS/TOXICOKINETICS

Most sedative-hypnotics are rapidly absorbed via the gastrointestinal (GI) tract, with the rate-limiting step consisting of dissolution and dispersion of the xenobiotic. Barbiturates and benzodiazepines are primarily absorbed in the small intestine. Clinical effects are determined by their relative ability to penetrate the blood–brain barrier. Drugs that are highly lipophilic penetrate most rapidly. The ultrashort-acting barbiturates are clinically active in the most vascular parts of the brain (gray matter first), with sleep occurring within 30 seconds of administration. Table 74–1 lists individual sedative-hypnotics and some of their pharmacokinetic properties.

TABLE 74–1. Pharmacology of Sedative-Hypnotics

	Equipotent Dosing Oral Dose (mg)[a]	$t_{1/2}$ (hours)	Protein Binding (%)	V_d (L/kg)	Active Metabolite Important
Benzodiazepines					
Agents with full agonist activity at the benzodiazepine site					
Alprazolam (Xanax)	1.0	10–14	80	0.8	No
Chlordiazepoxide (Librium)	50	5–15	96	0.3	Yes
Clorazepate (Tranxene)	15	97	0.9	Yes	
Clonazepam (Klonopin)	0.5	18–50	85.4	Unclear	Yes
Diazepam (Valium)	10	20–70	98.7	1.1	Yes
Estazolam (ProSom)	2.0	8–31	93	0.5	No
Flunitrazepam[b] (Rohypnol)	1.0	16–35	80	1.0–1.4	Yes
Flurazepam (Dalmane)	30	2.3	97.2	3.4	Yes
Lorazepam (Ativan)	2.0	9–19	90	1–1.3	None
Midazolam (Versed)	–	3–8	95	0.8–2	Yes
Oxazepam (Serax)	30	5–15	Unclear	Unclear	No
Temazepam (Restoril)	30	10–16	97	0.75–1.37	No
Triazolam (Halcion)	0.25	1.5–5.5	90	0.7–1.5	Yes
Nonbenzodiazepines active mainly at the type I (ω_1) benzodiazepine site					
Eszoplicone (Lunesta)	?	6	55	1.3	No
Zaleplon (Sonata)	20	1.0	92	0.54	No
Zolpidem (Ambien)	20	1.7	92	0.5	No
Barbiturates					
Amobarbital (Amytal)	–	8–42	Unclear	Unclear	Unclear
Aprobarbital[b] (Alurate)	–	14–34	Unclear	Unclear	Unclear
Butabarbital (Butisol)	–	34–42	Unclear	Unclear	Unclear
Barbital[b]	–	6–12	25	Unclear	Unclear
Mephobarbital (Mebaral)	–	5–6	40–60	Unclear	Yes
Methohexital (Brevital)	–	3–6	73	2.2	Unclear
Pentobarbital (Nembutal)	100	15–48	45–70	0.5–1.0	Unclear
Phenobarbital (Luminal)	30	80–120	50	0.5–0.6	No
Primidone (Mysoline)	–	3.3–22.4	19	Unclear	Yes
Secobarbital (Seconal)	–	15–40	52–57	Unclear	Unclear
Thiopental (Pentothal)	–	6–46	72–86	1.4–6.7	Unclear
Other					
Chloral hydrate (Aquachloral)	NA	4.0–9.5	35–40	0.6–1.6	Yes
Ethchlorvynol[b] (Placidyl)	NA	10–25	30–40	4	Unclear
Etomidate (Amidate)	NA	2.9–5.3	98	2.5–4.5	Unclear
Glutethimide[b] (Doriden)	NA	5–22	47–59	2.7	Unclear
Methyprylon[b] (Nodular)	NA	3–6	60	0.97	Unclear
Meprobamate[b] (Miltown)	NA	6–17	20	0.75	Unclear
Methaqualone[b] (Quaalude)	NA	19	80–90	5.8–6.0	Yes
Paraldehyde[b] (Paral)	NA	7	Unclear	0.9	Unclear
Propofol (Diprivan)	NA	4–23	98	2–10	No
Ramelteon (Rozerem)	NA	1–2.6	82	High	Yes
Dexmedetomidine (Precedex)	NA	2	94	1.5	No

NA = not applicable comparison.

[a]This table is an approximation of equipotent doses of xenobiotics affecting the benzodiazepine receptor and several barbiturates. All of the full agonist benzodiazepines have similar amnestic, anxiolytic, sedative, and hypnotic effects. These effects are a reflection of dose and serum concentration. There can be significant variation of these effects according to age and gender.

[b]Not presently available in the United States.

After initial distribution, many of the sedative-hypnotics undergo a redistribution phase as they are dispersed to other body tissues, specifically fat. Xenobiotics that are redistributed, such as the lipophilic (ultrashort-acting) barbiturates and some of the benzodiazepines (diazepam, midazolam), may have a brief clinical effect as the early peak concentrations in the brain rapidly decline. The clinical activity of many of them after single doses is determined by their rapid distribution and redistribution (alpha phase) and not by their elimination (beta phase) (see Chap. 8).

Many of the sedative-hypnotics are metabolized to pharmacologically active intermediates. This is particularly true for chloral hydrate and some of the benzodiazepines. Benzodiazepines can be demethylated, hydroxylated, or conjugated with glucuronide in the liver. Glucuronidation results in the production of inactive metabolites. Benzodiazepines, such as diazepam, are demethylated which produces active intermediates with a more prolonged therapeutic half-life than the parent compound. Because of the individual pharmacokinetics of sedative-hypnotics and the production of active metabolites, there is often little correlation between the therapeutic and biologic half-lives.

The majority of sedative-hypnotics, such as the highly lipid-soluble barbiturates and the benzodiazepines, are highly protein bound. These drugs are poorly filtered by the kidneys. Elimination occurs principally by hepatic metabolism. Chloral hydrate and meprobamate are notable exceptions. Xenobiotics with a low lipid-to-water partition coefficient, such as meprobamate and the longer-acting barbiturates, are poorly protein bound and more subject to renal excretion. Phenobarbital is a classic example of a drug whose elimination can be enhanced through alkalinization. Most other sedative-hypnotics are not amenable to urinary pH manipulation.

Overdoses of combinations of sedative-hypnotics enhance toxicity through synergistic effects. For example, both barbiturates and benzodiazepines act on the $GABA_A$ receptor, but barbiturates prolong the opening of the chloride ionophore, whereas benzodiazepines increase the frequency of ionophore opening.[128] Various sedative-hypnotics may increase the affinity of another xenobiotic at its respective binding site. For example, pentobarbital increases the affinity of γ-hydroxybutyrate (GHB) for its non-GABA binding site.[130] Propofol potentiates the effect of pentobarbital on chloride influx at the GABA receptor.[142] Propofol also increases the affinity and decreases the rate of dissociation of benzodiazepines from their site on the GABA receptor.[18,106] These actions increase the clinical effect of each xenobiotic and may lead to deeper CNS and respiratory depression.

Another mechanism of synergistic toxicity occurs via alteration of metabolism. The combination of ethanol and chloral hydrate, historically known as a "Mickey Finn," has additive CNS depressant effects. Chloral hydrate competes for alcohol and aldehyde dehydrogenases, thereby prolonging the half-life of ethanol. The metabolism of ethanol generates the reduced form of nicotinamide adenine dinucleotide (NADH), which is a cofactor for the metabolism of choral hydrate to trichloroethanol, an active metabolite. Finally, ethanol inhibits the conjugation of trichloroethanol, which in turn inhibits the oxidation of ethanol (Fig. 74–1).[16,80,121,122] The end result of these synergistic pharmacokinetic interactions is enhanced CNS depression.

Multiple drug–drug interactions can occur that may prolong the half-life of many sedative-hypnotics and significantly increase their potency or duration of action. The half-life of midazolam, which undergoes hepatic metabolism via cytochrome CYP3A4, can change dramatically in the presence of certain drugs that compete for its metabolism, or that induce or inhibit CYP3A4.[94,145] For example, the half-life of midazolam rises 400-fold when coadministered with itraconazole.[7] Various receptor and metabolic enzyme alterations resulting in upregulation or downregulation may occur in the setting of acute or chronic exposure to certain sedative-hypnotics.

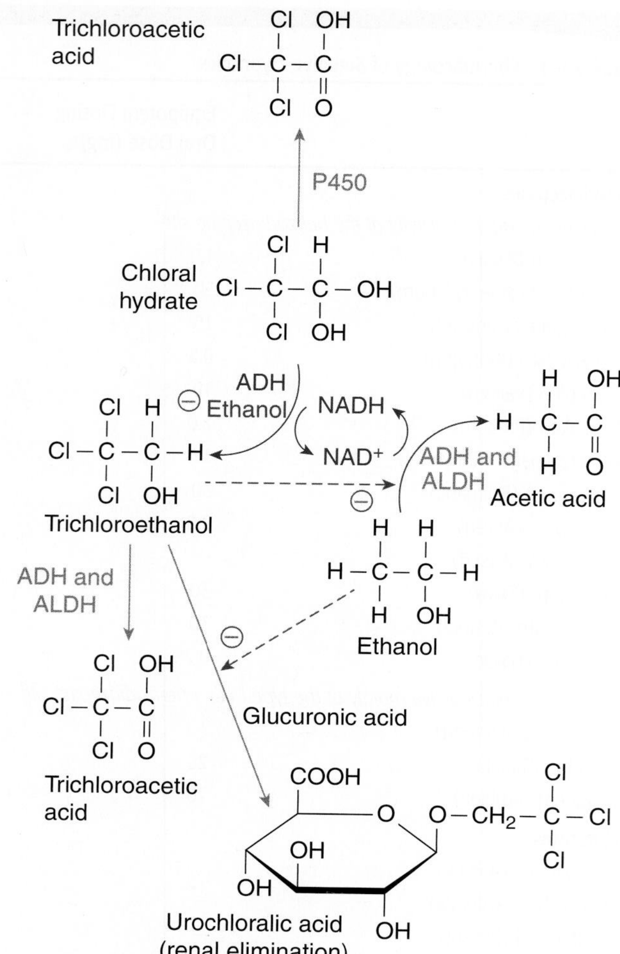

FIGURE 74–1. Metabolism of chloral hydrate and ethanol, demonstrating the interactions between chloral hydrate and ethanol metabolism. Note the inhibitory effects (dotted lines) of ethanol on trichloroethanol metabolism and the converse.

TOLERANCE/WITHDRAWAL

Ingestions of relatively large doses of sedative-hypnotics may not have predictable effects in patients who chronically use them. This is due to *tolerance*, defined as the progressive diminution of effect of a particular drug with repeated administrations that results in a need for greater doses to achieve the same effect. Tolerance occurs when adaptive neural and receptor changes (plasticity) occur after repeated exposures. These changes include a decrease in the number of receptors (downregulation), reduction of firing of receptors (receptor desensitization), structural changes in receptors (receptor shift), or reduction of coupling of sedative-hypnotics and their respective $GABA_A$ related receptor site (see Chap. 14). Tolerance can also be secondary to pharmacokinetic factors. However, in the majority of cases, tolerance to sedative-hypnotics is caused by pharmacodynamic changes such as receptor downregulation.[129]

Cross-tolerance readily exists among the sedative-hypnotics. For example, chronic use of benzodiazepines not only decreases the activity of the benzodiazepine site on the GABA receptor but also decreases the binding affinity of the barbiturate sites.[3,55] Many sedative-hypnotics are also associated with drug dependence after chronic exposure. Some of these, classically the barbiturates, benzodiazepines, and ethanol, are associated with characteristic potentially life-threatening withdrawal syndromes.

CLINICAL MANIFESTATIONS

Patients with sedative-hypnotic overdoses may exhibit slurred speech, ataxia, and incoordination. Larger doses result in stupor or coma. In most instances, respiratory depression parallels CNS depression. However, not all sedative-hypnotics cause significant hypoventilation. Oral overdoses of benzodiazepines alone may lead to sedation and hypnosis, but rarely life-threatening hypoventilation. Typically, the patient may appear comatose but have relatively normal vital signs. In contrast, large intravenous doses of benzodiazepines may lead to potentially life-threatening respiratory depression. Single overdoses of zolpidem and its congeners have not been shown to cause life-threatening respiratory depression in adults.[40]

Although the physical examination is rarely specific for a particular sedative-hypnotic, it can sometimes offer clues of exposure based on certain physical and clinical findings (Table 74–2). Hypothermia has been described with most of the sedative-hypnotics but may be more pronounced with barbiturates.[56,113] Barbiturates may cause fixed drug eruptions that often are bullous and appear over pressure-point areas. Although classically referred to as "barbiturate blisters," this phenomenon is not specific to barbiturates and has been documented with other CNS depressants, including carbon monoxide, methadone, imipramine, glutethimide, and benzodiazepines. Methaqualone can cause muscular rigidity and clonus.[1] Glutethimide can result in anticholinergic signs and symptoms.[47] Chloral hydrate use may result in vomiting, gastritis, and cardiac dysrhythmias.[45,71,92,149] Meprobamate overdoses may present with significant hypotension due to myocardial depression.[21]

Large or prolonged intravenous doses of sedative-hypnotics may also be associated with toxicities due to their diluents. Propylene glycol is a classic example of a diluent that may accumulate with prolonged infusions of certain medications such as lorazepam. Rapid infusions of propylene glycol may induce hypotension. Accumulated amounts of propylene glycol may lead to metabolic acidosis and a hyperosmolar state with elevated serum lactate concentrations.[68,72,78,105,146] In one study, two-thirds of critical care patients given high doses of lorazepam (0.16 mg/kg/h) for more than 48 hours had significant accumulations of propylene glycol as manifested by hyperosmolar anion gap metabolic acidosis[6] (see Chap. 55).

TABLE 74–2. Clinical Findings of Sedative-Hypnotic Overdose

Clinical Signs	Sedative-Hypnotics
Hypothermia	Barbiturates, bromides, ethchlorvynol
Unique odors	Chloral hydrate (*pear*), ethchlorvynol (*new vinyl shower curtain*)
Cardiotoxicity	
Myocardial depression	Meprobamate
Dysrhythmias	Chloral hydrate
Muscular twitching	GHB, methaqualone, propofol, etomidate
Acneiform rash	Bromides
Fluctuating coma	Glutethimide, meprobamate
GI hemorrhage	Chloral hydrate, methaqualone
Discolored urine	Propofol (green/pink)
Anticholinergic signs	Glutethimide

DIAGNOSTIC TESTING

When overdose is a primary concern in the undifferentiated comatose patient without a clear history laboratory testing, including electrolytes, liver enzymes, thyroid function tests, blood urea nitrogen (BUN), creatinine, glucose, venous or arterial blood gas analysis, and cerebrospinal fluid analysis, may be useful to exclude metabolic abnormalities. With any suspected intentional overdose, a serum acetaminophen concentration should be obtained. Diagnostic imaging studies, such as head CT scans, may be warranted on a case-by-case basis.

Routine laboratory screening for "drugs of abuse" generally is not helpful in the management of undifferentiated comatose adult patients, although screening may be useful for epidemiologic purposes in a particular community. These tests vary in type, sensitivity, and specificity. Furthermore, many sedative-hypnotics are not included on standard screening tests for drugs of abuse. For example, a typical benzodiazepine urine screen identifies metabolites of 1,4-benzodiazepines, such as oxazepam or desmethyldiazepam. Many benzodiazepines that are metabolized to alternative compounds remain undetected and thus may exhibit a false-negative result on the benzodiazepine screening assay. Benzodiazepines that are 7-amino analogs, such as clonazepam and flunitrazepam, may not be detected because they do not have a metabolite with a 1,4-benzodiazepine structure. Alprazolam and triazolam are not detected because they undergo minimal metabolism.[33]

Specific concentrations of xenobiotics such as ethanol or phenobarbital may be helpful to confirm or disprove exposure. However, specific concentrations of most other sedative-hypnotics are not routinely performed in hospital laboratories. Abdominal radiographs may detect chloral hydrate in the gastrointestinal tract because of its potential radiopacity (see Chap. 5). Although immediate identification of a particular sedative-hypnotic may be helpful in predicting the length of toxicity, it rarely affects the acute management of the patient. One exception is phenobarbital, for which urinary alkalinization and MDAC may enhance elimination.[39,102]

MANAGEMENT

Death secondary to sedative-hypnotic overdose usually results from cardiorespiratory collapse. Careful attention should focus on monitoring and maintaining adequate airway, oxygenation, and hemodynamic support. Supplemental oxygen, respiratory support, and prevention of aspiration are the cornerstones of treatment. Hemodynamic instability, although often a secondary or a delayed manifestation of sedative-hypnotic poisoning, should be treated initially with volume expansion. Historically, analeptics and other nonspecific arousal xenobiotics (see Chap. 1) were used, but their use is no longer recommended. With good supportive care and adequate early airway/respiratory support as needed, patients with sedative-hypnotic overdoses should eventually recover. Patients with meprobamate and chloral hydrate overdoses, however, may present with both respiratory depression and cardiac toxicity. Meprobamate toxicity may be associated with myocardial depression and significant hypotension, often resistant to standard intravenous fluid resuscitation.[21] Chloral hydrate cardiotoxic effects include lethal ventricular dysrhythmias, resulting from its active halogenated metabolite trichloroethanol. In the setting of cardiac dysrhythmias from chloral hydrate, judicious use of β-adrenergic antagonists is recommended.[15,45,158]

The use of gastrointestinal decontamination should be decided on a case-by-case basis. The benefits of activated charcoal (AC) must be balanced with the risks of its aspiration and subsequent potential for pulmonary toxicity. The use of AC should be determined judiciously based upon a patient's current mental status, potential for further deterioration, the xenobiotic(s) ingested if known, and the expected clinical course. Phenobarbital overdose is one particular scenario in which multiple-dose AC (MDAC) may be considered. MDAC increases phenobarbital elimination by 50%–80%.[9,10,14] However, in the only controlled study, no difference could be demonstrated in outcome measures (time to extubation and length of hospitalization) in intubated, phenobarbital-poisoned patients who were randomized to single-dose activated charcoal versus MDAC.[101] Although inconclusive, after ensuring an adequately protected airway, activated charcoal may have potential benefits in certain situations (Antidotes in Depth A2: Activated Charcoal).

Although the efficacy of delayed orogastric lavage is controversial, orogastric lavage may be considered in overdoses with xenobiotics that slow GI motility or that are known to develop concretions, specifically phenobarbital and meprobamate.[21,59,119] Orogastric lavage in the setting of oral benzodiazepine overdoses alone is not recommended, as the benefits of lavage are minimal compared to the significant risks of aspiration. The use of orogastric lavage in sedative-hypnotic overdose should always be done cautiously as outlined in Chap. 7. No antidote counteracts all sedative-hypnotic overdoses. Flumazenil, a competitive benzodiazepine antagonist, rapidly reverses the sedative effects of benzodiazepines as well as zolpidem and its congeners.[30,73,156] However, flumazenil has been documented to precipitate life-threatening benzodiazepine withdrawal in benzodiazepine-dependent patients and precipitate seizures, especially in patients who have overdosed on tricyclic antidepressants[41,132,133] (see Antidotes in Depth A23: Flumazenil).

Patients with sedative-hypnotic overdoses rarely require invasive therapy other than respiratory support. Hemodialysis may be considered in patients with chloral hydrate overdoses who develop life-threatening cardiac manifestations or in patients who ingest extremely large quantities of phenobarbital and meprobamate who might require prolonged intubation.

Because the lethality of sedative-hypnotics is associated with their ability to cause respiratory depression, asymptomatic patients can be downgraded to a lower level of care after a period of observation with no signs of respiratory depression. Patients with symptomatic overdoses of long-acting sedative hypnotics, such as meprobamate and clonazepam, or drugs that can have significant enterohepatic circulation, such as glutethimide, may require 24 hours of observation (see Chap. 10). Patients with mixed overdoses of various sedative-hypnotics and CNS depressants also warrant closer observation for respiratory depression due to synergistic respiratory depressant effects.

SPECIFIC SEDATIVE-HYPNOTICS

BARBITURATES

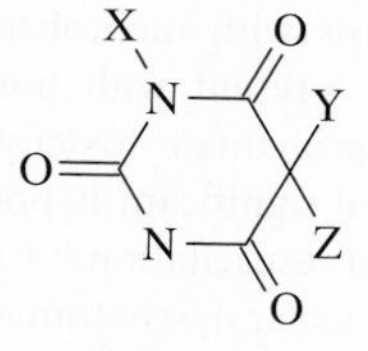

Barbital became the first commercially available barbiturate in 1903. Although many other barbiturates were subsequently developed, their popularity has greatly waned since the introduction of benzodiazepines. Barbiturates are derivatives of barbituric acid (2,4,6-trioxo-hexahydropyrimidine), which itself has no CNS depressant properties. The addition of various side chains influence pharmacologic properties. Barbiturates with long side chains tend to have increased lipophilicity, potency, and slower rates of elimination. However, the observed clinical effects also depend on absorption, redistribution, and the presence of active metabolites. For this reason, the duration of action of barbiturates (like those of benzodiazepines) does not correlate well with their biologic half-lives.

Oral barbiturates are preferentially absorbed in the small intestine and are eliminated by both hepatic and renal mechanisms. Longer-acting barbiturates tend to be more lipid soluble, more protein bound, have a high pK_a, and are metabolized almost completely by the liver. Renal excretion of unchanged drug is significant for phenobarbital, a long-acting barbiturate with a relatively low pK_a (7.24). Alkalinizing the urine with sodium bicarbonate to a urinary pH of 7.5–8.0 can increase the amount of phenobarbital excreted by 5- to 10-fold. This procedure is not effective for the short-acting barbiturates because they have higher pK_a values, are more protein bound, and are primarily metabolized by the liver with very little unchanged drug excreted by the kidneys (see Chap. 9).

Barbiturates (especially the shorter-acting barbiturates) can accelerate their own hepatic metabolism by cytochrome P450 enzyme autoinduction. Phenobarbital is a nonselective inducer of hepatic cytochromes, the greatest effects being on CYP2B1, CYP2B2, and CYP2B10, although CYP3A4 is also affected.[65,93,115,126,143] Not surprisingly, a variety of interactions are reported following the use of barbiturates. Clinically significant interactions as a result of enzyme induction lead to increased metabolism of β-adrenergic antagonists, corticosteroids, doxycycline, estrogens, phenothiazines, quinidine, theophylline, and many other xenobiotics.

Similar to other sedative-hypnotics, patients with significant barbiturate overdoses present with CNS and respiratory depression. Hypothermia and cutaneous bullae ("barb blisters") are often present. These two signs are also described for other patients with sedative-hypnotic overdoses, but they may be more pronounced with barbiturates.[11,32] Early deaths caused by barbiturate ingestions result from respiratory arrest and cardiovascular collapse. Delayed deaths result from acute renal failure, pneumonia, acute lung injury, cerebral edema, and multiorgan system failure as a result of prolonged cardiorespiratory depression.[2,48]

BENZODIAZEPINES

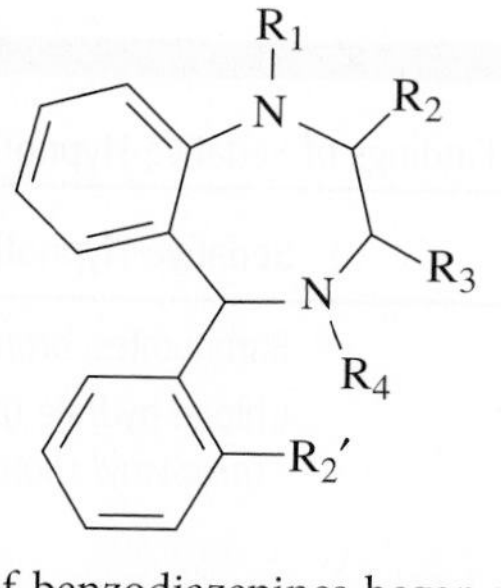

The commercial use of benzodiazepines began with the introduction of chlordiazepoxide for anxiety in 1961 and diazepam for seizures in 1963. Benzodiazepines are used principally as sedatives and anxiolytics. Clonazepam is the only benzodiazepine approved for use as a chronic anticonvulsant. Benzodiazepines may rarely cause paradoxical psychological effects, including nightmares, delirium, psychosis, and transient global amnesia.[12,13,34,86] The incidence and intensity of CNS adverse events increases with age.[81]

Similar to barbiturates, various benzodiazepine side chains influence potency, duration of action, metabolites, and rate of elimination. Most benzodiazepines are highly protein bound and lipophilic. They passively diffuse into the CNS, their main site of action. Because of their lipophilicity, benzodiazepines are extensively metabolized via oxidation and conjugation in the liver prior to their renal elimination.

Benzodiazepines bind nonselectively to "central" benzodiazepine receptors within the brain, termed ω_1 and ω_2. ω_1 receptors are located throughout the brain and contain the $GABA_A$ α_1 subunit.[30] They are hypothesized to affect anxiety, sleep, and amnesia. ω_2 receptors are concentrated predominantly in the hippocampus, striatum, and the spinal cord. They are hypothesized to affect muscle relaxation, cognition, memory, and dependence. Peripheral benzodiazepine receptors ω_3 are found throughout the body, with the greatest concentrations in steroid-producing cells in the adrenal gland, anterior pituitary gland, and reproductive organs (Antidote in Depth A24: Benzodiazepines).

One unique property of the benzodiazepines is their relative safety even after substantial ingestion, which probably results from their GABA receptor properties.[30,95] Unlike many other sedative-hypnotics, benzodiazepines do not open GABA channels independently at high concentrations. Benzodiazepines are not known to cause any specific systemic injury, and their long-term use is not associated with specific organ toxicity. Deaths resulting from benzodiazepine ingestions alone are extremely rare. Most often deaths are secondary to a combination of alcohol or other sedative-hypnotics.[46,123] Supportive care is the mainstay of treatment.

Tolerance to the sedative effects of benzodiazepines occurs more rapidly than does tolerance to the antianxiety effects.[74,110] Abrupt discontinuation following long-term use of benzodiazepines may precipitate benzodiazepine withdrawal, which is characterized by autonomic instability, changes in perception, paresthesias, headaches, tremors, and seizures. Withdrawal from benzodiazepines is common, manifested by almost one-third of long-term users.[66] Alprazolam and lorazepam are associated with more severe withdrawal syndromes compared with chlordiazepoxide and diazepam.[66,67] This is likely due to the fact that both chlordiazepoxide and diazepam have active metabolites. Withdrawal may also occur when a chronic user of a particular benzodiazepine is switched to another benzodiazepine with different receptor activity.[76]

CHLORAL HYDRATE

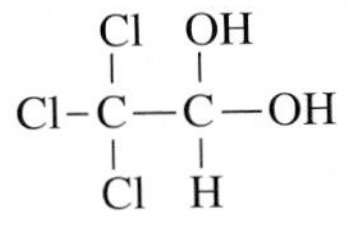

```
    Cl OH
    |  |
Cl-C--C-OH
    |  |
    Cl H
```

Chloral hydrate, first introduced in 1832, belongs to one of the oldest classes of pharmaceutical hypnotics, the chloral derivatives. Although still used fairly commonly in children, its use has substantially decreased. Chloral hydrate is well absorbed but is irritating to the GI tract. It has a wide tissue distribution, rapid onset of action, and rapid hepatic metabolism by alcohol and aldehyde dehydrogenases. Trichloroethanol is a lipid soluble, active metabolite that is responsible for the hypnotic effects of chloral hydrate. It has a plasma half-life of 4–12 hours and is metabolized to inactive trichloroacetic acid by alcohol dehydrogenases. It is also conjugated with glucuronide and excreted by the kidney as urochloralic acid. Less than 10% of trichloroethanol is excreted unchanged.

Metabolic rates in children vary widely because of variable development and function of hepatic enzymes, in particular glucuronidation.[16,80] The elimination half-life of chloral hydrate and triculoroethanol is markedly increased in children younger than 2 years. This may be especially of concern in neonates and in infants exposed to repetitive doses.

Acute chloral hydrate poisoning is unique compared with that of other sedative-hypnotics. Cardiac dysrhythmias are believed to be the major cause of death.[45] Chloral hydrate and its metabolites reduce myocardial contractility, shorten the refractory period, and increase myocardial sensitivity to catecholamines.[17,18,26,158] Persistent cardiac dysrhythmias (ventricular fibrillation, ventricular tachycardia, torsades de pointes) are common terminal events.[45] Standard antidysrhythmics often are ineffective, and β-adrenergic antagonists are considered the treatment of choice.[15,17,70,163] In addition to cardiotoxicity, chloral hydrate toxicity may cause vomiting, hemorrhagic gastritis, and rarely gastric and intestinal necrosis, leading to perforation and esophagitis with stricture formation.[71,92] Chloral hydrate is radiopaque and may be detected on radiographs; however, a negative radiograph should not be used to exclude chloral hydrate ingestion. Few hospital-based laboratories have the ability to rapidly detect chloral hydrate or its metabolites.

MEPROBAMATE/CARISOPRODOL

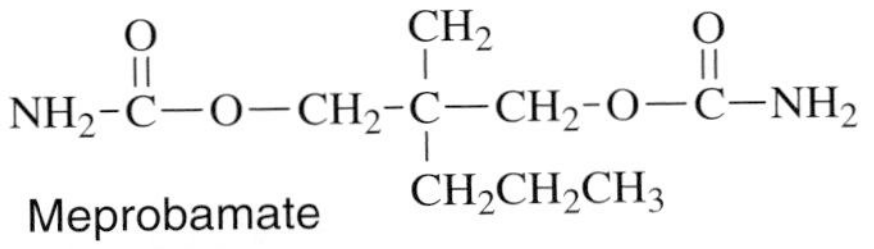

```
       O               CH2             O
       ||              |               ||
NH2-C--O--CH2-C--CH2-O--C--NH2
                       |
                 CH2CH2CH3
```

Meprobamate

Meprobamate was introduced in 1950 and was used for its muscle-relaxant and anxiolytic characteristics. Carisoprodol, which was introduced in 1955, is metabolized to meprobamate. Both drugs have pharmacologic effects on the $GABA_A$ receptor similar to those of the barbiturates. Like barbiturates, meprobamate can directly open the GABA-mediated chloride channel and may inhibit NMDA receptor currents.[108] Both are rapidly absorbed from the GI tract. Meprobamate is metabolized in the liver to inactive hydroxylated and glucuronidated metabolites that are excreted almost exclusively by the kidney. Of all the nonbarbiturate tranquilizers, meprobamate most likely will produce euphoria.[57,58] Unlike most sedative-hypnotics, meprobamate has been reported to cause profound hypotension from myocardial depression.[21] Large masses or bezoars of pills have been noted in the stomach at autopsy after large meprobamate ingestions.[119] Orogastric lavage with a large-bore tube and MDAC may be indicated for significant meprobamate ingestion; however, the potential benefits of orogastric lavage must be weighed against the risks of aspiration. Whole-bowel irrigation may be helpful if multiple pills or small concretions are noted. It is important to note that patients can experience recurrent toxic manifestations as a result of concretion formation with delayed drug release and absorption. Careful monitoring of the clinical course is essential even after the patient shows initial improvement because recurrent and cyclical CNS depression may occur.[119]

BROMIDES

Bromides have been used in the past as "nerve tonics," headache remedies, and anticonvulsants. Although medicinal bromides have largely disappeared from the US pharmaceutical market, bromide toxicity still occurs through the availability of bromide salts of common drugs, such as dextromethorphan.[89] Poisoning also may occur in immigrants and travelers from other countries where bromides are still therapeutically used.[38] An epidemic of more than 400 cases of mass bromide poisoning occurred in the Cacuaco municipality of Luanda Province, Angola in 2007. According to a World Health Organization report, the etiology of the bromide exposure in these cases was believed to be table salt contaminated with sodium bromide. Although the majority of persons affected were children, no actual deaths were attributed to bromide poisoning in this epidemic.[159]

Bromides tend to have long half-lives and toxicity typically occurs over time as concentrations accumulate in tissue. Bromide and chloride ions have a similar distribution pattern in the extracellular fluid. It is postulated that because the bromide ion moves across membranes slightly more rapidly than the chloride ion, it is more quickly reabsorbed in the tubules from the glomerular filtrate than the chloride ion. Although osmolar equilibrium persists, CNS function is progressively impaired by a poorly understood mechanism, with resulting inappropriateness of behavior, headache, apathy, irritability, confusion, muscle weakness, anorexia, weight loss, thickened speech, psychotic behavior, tremulousness, ataxia, and eventually coma.[20,164] Delusions and hallucinations can occur. Bromide can lead to hypertension, increased intracranial pressure, and papilledema. Chronic use of bromides can also lead to dermatologic changes, with the hallmark characteristic of a facial acneiform rash.[53,141] Toxicity with bromides during pregnancy may lead to accumulation of bromide in the fetus.[100] A spurious laboratory result of hyperchloremia with decreased anion gap may result from bromide's interference with the chloride assay on older analyzers[161] (Chap. 16). Thus an isolated elevated serum chloride concentration with neurologic symptoms should raise suspicion of possible bromide poisoning.

ZOLPIDEM/ZALEPLON/ZOPICLONE/ESZOPICLONE

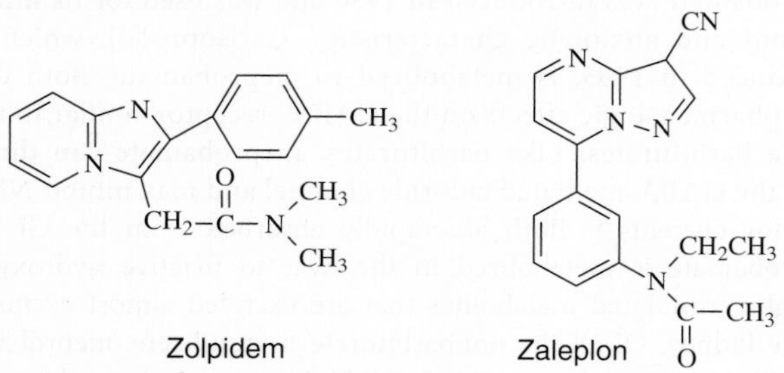

Zolpidem

Zaleplon

These oral xenobiotics have supplanted benzodiazepines as the most commonly prescribed sleep aid medications.[35] Although they are structurally unrelated to the benzodiazepines, they bind preferentially to the ω_1 benzodiazepine receptor subtype in the brain, specifically the $GABA_A$ α_1 subunit.[30] They have a lower affinity for ω_2 receptors than benzodiazepines, therefore they have potent hypnotic effects with less potential for dependence.[30,52] Each of these xenobiotics has a relatively short half-life (≤6 hours), with zaleplon exhibiting the shortest half-life (1 hour). Unlike benzodiazepines that prolong the first two stages of sleep and shorten stages 3 and 4 of rapid eye movement (REM) sleep, zolpidem and its congeners all decrease sleep latency with little effect on sleep architecture. Because of their receptor selectivity, they appear to have minimal effect at other sites on the GABA receptor that mediate anxiolytic, anticonvulsant, or muscle-relaxant effects.[69,151]

They are hepatically metabolized by various CYP450 enzymes. Zolpidem is mainly metabolized by CYP3A4. Zaleplon is primarily metabolized by aldehyde oxidase, but CYP3A4 is also involved in parent compound oxidation. Zopiclone is primarily metabolized by CYP3A4 and CYP2C8, whereas eszopiclone is metabolized mainly by CYP3A4 and CYP2E1. Various pharmacokinetic interactions with inhibitors or inducers of CYP450 enzymes and these medications have been reported.[51]

In isolated overdoses, drowsiness and CNS depression are common. However, prolonged coma with respiratory depression is exceptionally rare. Isolated overdoses usually manifest with depressed level of consciousness without respiratory depression. For example, even at 40 times the therapeutic dose of zolpidem, no biologic or electrocardiographic abnormalities were reported.[40] Tolerance to zolpidem and its congeners has also been described. Withdrawal has been reported after abrupt discontinuation following chronic use but typically is mild.[50,155] Flumazenil may reverse the hypnotic or cognitive effects of these agents.[73,156] Deaths have resulted when zolpidem was taken in large amounts with other CNS depressants (Antidote in Depth A23 Flumazenil).[40]

PROPOFOL

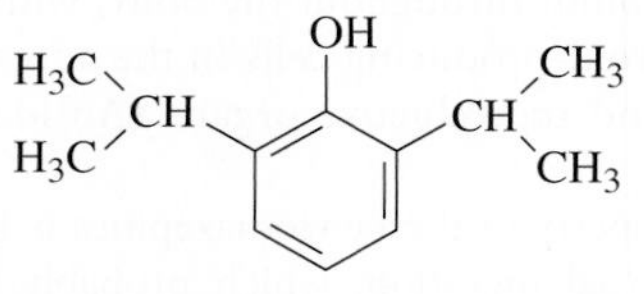

Propofol is a rapidly acting intravenous sedative-hypnotic that is a postsynaptic $GABA_A$ agonist and also induces presynaptic release of GABA.[117] Propofol is also an antagonist at NMDA receptors.[63,64,131] In addition, propofol also interacts with dopamine, promotes nigral dopamine release possibly via $GABA_B$ receptors,[96,120] and has partial agonist properties at dopamine (D_2) receptors.[118] Propofol is used for procedural sedation and either induction or maintenance of general anesthesia. It is highly lipid soluble, so it crosses the blood–brain barrier rapidly. The onset of anesthesia usually occurs in less than 1 minute. The duration of action after short-term dosing is usually less than 8 minutes due to its rapid redistribution from the CNS.

Propofol use is associated with various adverse effects. Acutely, propofol causes dose-related respiratory depression. Propofol may decrease systemic arterial pressure and cause myocardial depression. Although short-term use of propofol does not typically cause dysrhythmias or myocardial ischemia, atropine-sensitive bradydysrhythmias have been noted, specifically sinus bradycardia and Mobitz type I atrioventricular block.[140,154,162] Short-term use of propofol in the perioperative setting is associated with a myoclonic syndrome manifesting as opisthotonus, myoclonus, and sometimes myoclonic seizure like activity.[82,90]

Prolonged propofol infusions for more than 48 hours at rates of 4–5 mg/kg/h or greater are associated with a life-threatening *propofol-infusion syndrome* (PIS) involving metabolic acidosis, cardiac dysrthythmias, and skeletal muscle injury.[61] The clinical signs of PIS often begin with the development of a new right bundle branch block and ST segment convex elevations in the electrocardiogram precordial leads.[60] Predisposing factors to the development of PIS include young age, severe brain injury (especially in the setting of trauma), respiratory compromise, concurrent exogenous administration of catecholamines or glucocorticoids, inadequate carbohydrate intake, and undiagnosed mitochondrial myopathy. Some authors propose a "priming" and "triggering" mechanism for PIS with endogenous glucocorticoids, catecholamines, and possibly cytokines as "priming" agents, and exogenous catecholamines and glucocorticoids in the setting of high-dose propofol infusion as "triggering" stimuli.[147] Propofol is suggested to induce disruption of mitochondrial free fatty acid utilization and metabolism, causing a syndrome of energy imbalance and myonecrosis similar to other mitochondrial myopathies.[22,125,148] Case reports associate propofol with metabolic acidosis with elevated lactate concentration and fatal myocardial failure in children and young adults; however, it has been reported in older adults as well.[98] Cases of metabolic acidosis may be associated with an inborn disorder of acylcarnitine metabolism.[160] Caution is advised when prolonged propofol infusions are used in any patient, especially children, as they may have a previously undiagnosed myopathy that would cause them to be at increased risk for PIS. Despite the increasing number of reports of PIS in the literature, a direct cause-and-effect relationship remains to be fully elucidated.

The unique nature of propofol's carrier base, a milky soybean emulsion formulation, is associated with multiple adverse events. It is a fertile medium for many organisms, such as enterococcal, pseudomonal, staphylococcal, streptococcal, and candidal strains. In 1990, the Centers for Disease Control and Prevention (CDC) reported an outbreak of *Staphylococcus aureus* associated with contaminated propofol. This carrier base also impairs macrophage function,[22] causes hypertriglyceridemia[33,55,67,76] and histamine-mediated anaphylactoid reactions,[31,62,148] and impairs platelet and coagulation function.[4,29]

ETOMIDATE

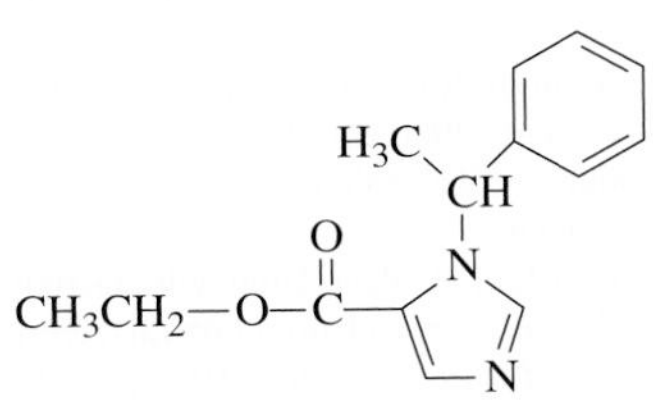

H_3C—CH (phenyl); CH_3CH_2—O—C(=O)— imidazole (N, N)

Etomidate is an intravenous nonbarbiturate, hypnotic primarily used as an anesthesia induction agent. It is active at the $GABA_A$ receptor, specifically the β_2 and β_3 subunits.[91,104] Only the intravenous formulation is available in the United States. The onset of action is less than 1 minute and its duration of action is less than 5 minutes.

Etomidate is commercially available as a 2 mg/mL solution in a 35% propylene glycol solution. Propylene glycol toxicity from prolonged etomidate infusions is implicated in the development of hyperosmolar metabolic acidosis.[78,144,146] Etomidate has minimal effect on cardiac function, but rare cases of hypotension are reported.[42–44,135] Etomidate has both proconvulsant and anticonvulsant properties.[25,103] Involuntary muscle movements are common during induction, and may be caused by etomidate interaction with glycine receptors at the spinal cord level.[27,84,85]

Etomidate depresses adrenal production of cortisol and aldosterone and has thus been associated with adrenocortical suppression, usually after prolonged infusions.[117,152,153] One prospective randomized trial demonstrated chemical adrenal suppression with decreased serum cortisol levels and decreased responses to ACTH stimulation in trauma patients even after receiving single-dose etomidate.[54] The authors postulate that this may have been associated with prolonged duration of hospital and ICU stays, as well as prolonged ventilator requirements. Other authors question the clinical significance of adrenal suppression from single-dose etomidate administration.[137]

DEXMEDETOMIDINE

Dexmedetomidine is a central α_2 adrenergic agonist that decreases central presynaptic catecholamine release, primarily in the locus coeruleus. It was approved by the FDA in 1999 for short-term use in the critical care setting. It has a terminal half-life of 1.8 hours and its volume of distribution is less than 1 L/kg. When dexmedetomidine is used to help wean patients from ventilators, a better level of desired sedation is achieved with less associated delirium.[97,136] It is also used for procedural sedation in certain settings such as interventional radiology procedures and awake fiberoptic intubations. In addition, other authors have described lesser opioid requirements in postoperative patients sedated with dexmedetomidine, compared with propofol. Individual case reports also document the use of dexmedetomidine in benzodiazepine, opioid, or ethanol withdrawal.[28,36,114,138,139]

Dexmedetomidine has no effect at the GABA receptor, and unlike other sedative-hypnotics, it is not associated with significant respiratory depression. Although mechanistically similar to clonidine, dexmedetomidine does not appear to cause as much respiratory depression as clonidine. Dexmedetomidine is said to induce a state of "cooperative sedation," in which a patient is sedated but yet able to interact with health-care providers. Dexmedetomidine may also have analgesic effects.[23]

Dexmedetomidine is currently approved for use only for less than 24 hours, as safety trials have not yet explored its use beyond 24 hours. Unlike clonidine, rebound hypertension and tachycardia have not been described upon cessation of dexmedetomidine. Because dexmedetomidine decreases central sympathetic outflow, its use should probably be avoided in patients whose clinical stability is dependent on high resting sympathetic tone. The most common adverse effects from its use are nausea, dry mouth, bradycardia, and varying effects on blood pressure (usually hypertension followed by hypotension). Slowing of the continuous infusion may help to prevent or lessen the hypotensive effects.[23]

RAMELTEON/MELATONIN

Ramelteon is a synthetic melatonin-analog that is FDA approved for the treatment of chronic insomnia. Ramelteon has been proposed to decrease both latency to sleep induction and length of persistent sleep.[127] Melatonin (*N*-acetyl-5-methoxytryptamine) and melatonin-containing products are sold as dietary supplements. Melatonin is naturally synthesized from tryptophan by the enzyme 5-hydroxyindole-*O*-methyltransferase, primarily within the pineal gland in humans. Melatonin and ramelteon both act as agonists at MT-1 and MT-2 receptors, which are G protein–coupled receptors mainly located in the suprachiasmatic nucleus of the brain.[127] Ramelteon is specific for MT-1 and MT-2 receptors, whereas melatonin is active at other melatonin receptors that are likely not involved in sleep. MT-1 receptors appear to be involved in sleep induction, whereas MT-2 receptors are involved in regulation of the circadian sleep-wake cycle in humans.[134]

Ramelteon is administered as an oral medication that is rapidly absorbed but undergoes significant first-pass metabolism. Ramelteon is metabolized primarily by CYP1A2 hepatic isoenzyme. The half-life of ramelteon with therapeutic use is roughly 1.5 hours.

Adverse effects of ramelteon are often mild, and usually include dizziness, fatigue, headache. The endocrine effects of long-term exposure to ramelteon seem to be limited to subclinical increases in serum prolactin concentration in women, and do not appear to affect adrenal or thyroid function.[109] In addition, ramelteon has a low abuse potential and does not appear to be associated with a withdrawal syndrome or with rebound insomnia.[49,77,83] As of yet, there are no reported cases of significant toxicity from ramelteon overdose.

SUMMARY

Sedative-hypnotics encompass a wide range of xenobiotics with varying mechanisms of action. Patients with sedative-hypnotic overdoses often present with the primary manifestation of CNS depression; however, death typically results from respiratory depression and subsequent cardiovascular collapse in the setting of concurrent co-ingestion of other CNS depressants. Careful monitoring, airway protection, and good supportive care are the cornerstones of treatment. Specific antidotes such as flumazenil and treatments such as hemodialysis are rarely indicated.

REFERENCES

1. Abboud RT, Freedman MT, Rogers RM, et al. Methaqualone poisoning with muscular hyperactivity necessitating the use of curare. *Chest.* 1974;65:204-205.
2. Afifi AA, Sacks ST, Liu VY, et al. Accumulative prognostic index for patients with barbiturate, glutethimide and meprobamate intoxication. *N Engl J Med.* 1971;285:1497-1502.
3. Allan AM, Zhang X, Baier LD. Barbiturate tolerance: effects on GABA-operated chloride channel function. *Brain Res.* 1992;588:255-260.
4. Aoki H, Mizobe T, Nozuchi S, et al. In vivo and in vitro studies of the inhibitory effect of propofol on human platelet aggregation. *Anesthesiology.* 1998;88:362-370.
5. Arpino PA, Kalafatas K, Thompson BT. Feasibility of dexmedetomidine in facilitating extubation in the intensive care unit. *J Clin Pharm Ther.* 2008;33:25-30.
6. Arroliga AC, Shehab N, McCarthy K, et al. Relationship of continuous infusion lorazepam to serum propylene glycol concentration in critically ill adults. *Crit Care Med.* 2004;32:1709-1714.
7. Backman JT, Kivisto KT, Olkkola KT, et al. The area under the plasma concentration-time curve for oral midazolam is 400-fold larger during treatment with itraconazole than with rifampicin. *Eur J Clin Pharmacol.* 1998;54:53-58.
8. Bailey SJ, Toth M. Variability in the benzodiazepine response of serotonin 5-HT1A receptor null mice displaying anxiety-like phenotype: evidence for genetic modifiers in the 5-HT-mediated regulation of GABA(A) receptors. *J Neurosci.* 2004;24:6343-6351.
9. Berg MJ, Berlinger WG, Goldberg MJ, et al. Acceleration of the body clearance of phenobarbital by oral activated charcoal. *N Engl J Med.* 1982; 307:642-644.
10. Berg MJ, Rose JQ, Wurster DE, et al. Effect of charcoal and sorbitol-charcoal suspension on the elimination of intravenous phenobarbital. *Ther Drug Monit.* 1987;9:41-47.
11. Beveridge GW. Bullous lesions in poisoning. *Br Med J.* 1971;4:116-117.
12. Bixler EO, Kales A, Brubaker BH, et al. Adverse reactions to benzodiazepine hypnotics: spontaneous reporting system. *Pharmacology.* 1987;35:286-300.
13. Boatwright DE. Triazolam, handwriting, and amnestic states: two cases. *J Forensic Sci.* 1987;32:1118-1124.
14. Boldy DA, Vale JA, Prescott LF. Treatment of phenobarbitone poisoning with repeated oral administration of activated charcoal. *Q J Med.* 1986;61:997-1002.
15. Bowyer K, Glasser SP. Chloral hydrate overdose and cardiac arrhythmias. *Chest.* 1980;77:232-235.
16. Bronley-DeLancey A, McMillan DC, McMillan JM, et al. Application of cryopreserved human hepatocytes in trichloroethylene risk assessment: relative disposition of chloral hydrate to trichloroacetate and trichloroethanol. *Environ Health Perspect.* 2006;114:1237-1242.
17. Brown AM, Cade JF. Cardiac arrhythmais after chloral hydrate overdose. *Med J Aust.* 1980;1:28-29.
18. Bruner KR, Reynolds JN. Propofol modulation of [3H]flunitrazepam binding to $GABA_A$ receptors in guinea pig cerebral cortex. *Brain Res.* 1998;806:122-125.
19. Buckley NA, Whyte IM, Dawson AH, et al. Correlations between prescriptions and drugs taken in self-poisoning. Implications for prescribers and drug regulation. *Med J Aust.* 1995;162:194-197.
20. Carney MW. Five cases of bromism. *Lancet.* 1971;2:523-524.
21. Charron C, Mekontso-Dessap A, Chergui K, et al. Incidence, causes and prognosis of hypotension related to meprobamate poisoning. *Intensive Care Med.* 2005;31:1582-1586.
22. Chen RM, Wu CH, Chang HC, et al. Propofol suppresses macrophage functions and modulates mitochondrial membrane potential and cellular adenosine triphosphate synthesis. *Anesthesiology.* 2003;98:1178-1185.
23. Chrysostomou C, Schmitt CG. Dexmedetomidine: sedation, analgesia and beyond. *Expert Opin Drug Metab Toxicol.* 2008;4:619-627.
24. Cirone J, Rosahl TW, Reynolds DS, et al. Gamma-aminobutyric acid type A receptor beta 2 subunit mediates the hypothermic effect of etomidate in mice. *Anesthesiology.* 2004;100:1438-1445.
25. Conca A, Germann R, Konig P. Etomidate vs. thiopentone in electroconvulsive therapy. An interdisciplinary challenge for anesthesiology and psychiatry. *Pharmacopsychiatry.* 2003;36:94-97.
26. Criswell HE, Ming Z, Pleasant N, et al. Macrokinetic analysis of blockade of NMDA-gated currents by substituted alcohols, alkanes and ethers. *Brain Res.* 2004;1015:107-113.
27. Daniels S, Roberts RJ. Post-synaptic inhibitory mechanisms of anaesthesia; glycine receptors. *Toxicol Lett.* 1998;100-101:71-76.
28. Darrouj J, Puri N, Prince E, et al. Dexmedetomidine infusion as adjunctive therapy to benzodiazepines for acute alcohol withdrawal. *Ann Pharmacother.* 2008;42:1703-1705.
29. De La Cruz JP, Paez MV, Carmona JA, et al. Antiplatelet effect of the anaesthetic drug propofol: influence of red blood cells and leucocytes. *Br J Pharmacol.* 1999;128:1538-1544.
30. Doble A. New insights into the mechanism of action of hypnotics. *J Psychopharmacol.* 1999;13(4):S11-20.
31. Ducart AR, Watremez C, Louagie YA, et al. Propofol-induced anaphylactoid reaction during anesthesia for cardiac surgery. *J Cardiothorac Vasc Anesth.* 2000;14:200-201.
32. Dunn C, Held JL, Spitz J, et al. Coma blisters: report and review. *Cutis.* 1990;45:423-426.
33. Dunn W. Various laboratory methods screen and confirm benzodiazepines. *Emerg Med News.* 2000:21-24.
34. Einarson TR, Yoder ES. Triazolam psychosis—a syndrome? *Drug Intell Clin Pharm.* 1982;16:330.
35. Elie R, Ruther E, Farr I, et al. Sleep latency is shortened during 4 weeks of treatment with zaleplon, a novel nonbenzodiazepine hypnotic. Zaleplon Clinical Study Group. *J Clin Psychiatry.* 1999;60:536-544.
36. Farag E, Chahlavi A, Argalious M, et al. Using dexmedetomidine to manage patients with cocaine and opioid withdrawal, who are undergoing cerebral angioplasty for cerebral vasospasm. *Anesth Analg.* 2006;103: 1618-1620.
37. Finkle BS, McCloskey KL, Goodman LS. Diazepam and drug-associated deaths. A survey in the United States and Canada. *JAMA.* 1979;242: 429-434.
38. Frances C, Hoizey G, Lamiable D, et al. Bromism from daily over intake of bromide salt. *J Toxicol Clin Toxicol.* 2003;41:181-183.
39. Fukunaga K, Saito M, Muto M, et al. Effects of urine pH modification on pharmacokinetics of phenobarbital in healthy dogs. *J Vet Pharmacol Ther.* 2008;31:431-436.
40. Garnier R, Guerault E, Muzard D, et al. Acute zolpidem poisoning—analysis of 344 cases. *J Toxicol Clin Toxicol.* 1994;32:391-404.
41. Geller E, Crome P, Schaller MD, et al. Risks and benefits of therapy with flumazenil (Anexate) in mixed drug intoxications. *Eur Neurol.* 1991;31: 241-250.
42. Gooding JM, Corssen G. Etomidate: an ultrashort-acting nonbarbiturate agent for anesthesia induction. *Anesth Analg.* 1976;55:286-289.
43. Gooding JM, Corssen G. Effect of etomidate on the cardiovascular system. *Anesth Analg.* 1977;56:717-719.
44. Gooding JM, Weng JT, Smith RA, et al. Cardiovascular and pulmonary responses following etomidate induction of anesthesia in patients with demonstrated cardiac disease. *Anesth Analg.* 1979;58:40-41.
45. Graham SR, Day RO, Lee R, et al. Overdose with chloral hydrate: a pharmacological and therapeutic review. *Med J Aust.* 1988;149:686-688.
46. Greenblatt DJ, Allen MD, Noel BJ, et al. Acute overdosage with benzodiazepine derivatives. *Clin Pharmacol Ther.* 1977;21:497-514.
47. Greenblatt DJ, Allen MD, Harmatz JS, et al. Correlates of outcome following acute glutethimide overdosage. *J Forensic Sci.* 1979;24:76-86.
48. Greenblatt DJ, Allen MD, Harmatz JS, et al. Overdosage with pentobarbital and secobarbital: assessment of factors related to outcome. *J Clin Pharmacol.* 1979;19:758-768.
49. Griffiths RR, Johnson MW. Relative abuse liability of hypnotic drugs: a conceptual framework and algorithm for differentiating among compounds. *J Clin Psychiatry.* 2005;66 Suppl 9:31-41.
50. Hajak G, Muller WE, Wittchen HU, et al. Abuse and dependence potential for the non-benzodiazepine hypnotics zolpidem and zopiclone: a review of case reports and epidemiological data. *Addiction.* 2003;98:1371-1378.
51. Hesse LM, von Moltke LL, Greenblatt DJ. Clinically important drug interactions with zopiclone, zolpidem and zaleplon. *CNS Drugs.* 2003;17:513-532.
52. Heydorn WE. Zaleplon—a review of a novel sedative hypnotic used in the treatment of insomnia [In Process Citation]. *Expert Opin Investig Drugs.* 2000;9:841-858.
53. Hezemans-Boer M, Toonstra J, Meulenbelt J, et al. Skin lesions due to exposure to methyl bromide. *Arch Dermatol.* 1988;124:917-921.

54. Hildreth AN, Mejia VA, Maxwell RA, et al. Adrenal suppression following a single dose of etomidate for rapid sequence induction: a prospective randomized study. *J Trauma.* 2008;65:573-579.
55. Hu XJ, Ticku MK. Chronic benzodiazepine agonist treatment produces functional uncoupling of the gamma-aminobutyric acid-benzodiazepine receptor ionophore complex in cortical neurons. *Mol Pharmacol.* 1994;45:618-625.
56. Ivnitsky JJ, Schafer TV, Malakhovsky VN, et al. Intermediates of Krebs cycle correct the depression of the whole body oxygen consumption and lethal cooling in barbiturate poisoning in rat. *Toxicology.* 2004;202:165-172.
57. Jacobsen D, Frederichsen PS, Knutsen KM, et al. Clinical course in acute self-poisonings: a prospective study of 1125 consecutively hospitalised adults. *Hum Toxicol.* 1984;3:107-116.
58. Jacobsen D, Frederichsen PS, Knutsen KM, et al. A prospective study of 1212 cases of acute poisoning: general epidemiology. *Hum Toxicol.* 1984;3:93-106.
59. Johanson WG, Jr. Massive phenobarbital ingestion with survival. *JAMA.* 1967;202:1106-1107.
60. Kam PC, Cardone D. Propofol infusion syndrome. *Anaesthesia.* 2007;62: 690-701.
61. Kang TM. Propofol infusion syndrome in critically ill patients. *Ann Pharmacother.* 2002;36:1453-1456.
62. Kimura K, Adachi M, Kubo K. Histamine release during the induction of anesthesia with propofol in allergic patients: a comparison with the induction of anesthesia using midazolam-ketamine. *Inflamm Res.* 1999;48: 582-587.
63. Kingston S, Mao L, Yang L, et al. Propofol inhibits phosphorylation of N-methyl-D-aspartate receptor NR1 subunits in neurons. *Anesthesiology.* 2006;104:763-769.
64. Kotani Y, Shimazawa M, Yoshimura S, et al. The experimental and clinical pharmacology of propofol, an anesthetic agent with neuroprotective properties. *CNS Neurosci Ther.* 2008;14:95-106.
65. Kozawa M, Honma M, Suzuki H. Quantitative prediction of in vivo profiles of CYP3A4 induction in humans from in vitro results with reporter gene assay. *Drug Metab Dispos.* 2009.
66. Lader M. Anxiolytic drugs: dependence, addiction and abuse. *Eur Neuropsychopharmacol.* 1994;4:85-91.
67. Lader M. Biological processes in benzodiazepine dependence. *Addiction.* 1994;89:1413-1418.
68. Laine GA, Hossain SM, Solis RT, et al. Polyethylene glycol nephrotoxicity secondary to prolonged high-dose intravenous lorazepam. *Ann Pharmacother.* 1995;29:1110-1114.
69. Langtry HD, Benfield P. Zolpidem. A review of its pharmacodynamic and pharmacokinetic properties and therapeutic potential. *Drugs.* 1990;40: 291-313.
70. Laurent Y, Wallemacq P, Haufroid V, et al. Electrocardiographic changes with segmental akinesia after chloral hydrate overdose. *J Emerg Med.* 2006;30:179-182.
71. Lee DC, Vassalluzzo C. Acute gastric perforation in a chloral hydrate overdose. *Am J Emerg Med.* 1998;16:545-546.
72. Levy ML, Aranda M, Zelman V, et al. Propylene glycol toxicity following continuous etomidate infusion for the control of refractory cerebral edema. *Neurosurgery.* 1995;37:363-369; discussion 369-371.
73. Lheureux P, Debailleul G, De Witte O, et al. Zolpidem intoxication mimicking narcotic overdose: response to flumazenil. *Hum Exp Toxicol.* 1990;9:105-107.
74. Lucki I, Rickels K. The effect of anxiolytic drugs on memory in anxious subjects. *Psychopharmacol Ser.* 1988;6:128-139.
75. Majumder MM, Basher A, Faiz MA, et al. Criminal poisoning of commuters in Bangladesh: prospective and retrospective study. *Forensic Sci Int.* 2008; 180:10-16.
76. Marks J. Techniques of benzodiazepine withdrawal in clinical practice. A consensus workshop report. *Med Toxicol Adverse Drug Exp.* 1988;3:324-333.
77. Mayer G, Wang-Weigand S, Roth-Schechter B, et al. Efficacy and safety of 6-month nightly ramelteon administration in adults with chronic primary insomnia. *Sleep.* 2009;32:351-360.
78. McConnel JR, Ong CS, McAllister JL, et al. Propylene glycol toxicity following continuous etomidate infusion for the control of refractory cerebral edema. *Neurosurgery.* 1996;38:232-233.
79. Mehta AK, Ticku MK. An update on GABAA receptors. *Brain Res Brain Res Rev.* 1999;29:196-217.
80. Merdink JL, Robison LM, Stevens DK, et al. Kinetics of chloral hydrate and its metabolites in male human volunteers. *Toxicology.* 2008;245:130-140.
81. Meyer BR. Benzodiazepines in the elderly. *Med Clin North Am.* 1982;66: 1017-1035.
82. Miner JR, Danahy M, Moch A, et al. Randomized clinical trial of etomidate versus propofol for procedural sedation in the emergency department. *Ann Emerg Med.* 2007;49:15-22.
83. Mini L, Wang-Weigand S, Zhang J. Ramelteon 8 mg/d versus placebo in patients with chronic insomnia: post hoc analysis of a 5-week trial using 50% or greater reduction in latency to persistent sleep as a measure of treatment effect. *Clin Ther.* 2008;30:1316-1323.
84. Modica PA, Tempelhoff R, White PF. Pro- and anticonvulsant effects of anesthetics (Part II). *Anesth Analg.* 1990;70:433-444.
85. Modica PA, Tempelhoff R, White PF. Pro- and anticonvulsant effects of anesthetics (Part I). *Anesth Analg.* 1990;70:303-315.
86. Morris HHd, Estes ML. Traveler's amnesia. Transient global amnesia secondary to triazolam. *JAMA.* 1987;258:945-946.
87. Narimatsu E, Aoki M. Involvement of the adenosine neuromodulatory system in the benzodiazepine-induced depression of excitatory synaptic transmissions in rat hippocampal neurons in vitro. *Neurosci Res.* 1999; 33:57-64.
88. Nemmani KV, Ramarao P. Role of benzodiazepine-GABAA receptor complex in attenuation of U-50,488H-induced analgesia and inhibition of tolerance to its analgesia by ginseng total saponin in mice. *Life Sci.* 2002;70:1727-1740.
89. Ng YY, Lin WL, Chen TW, et al. Spurious hyperchloremia and decreased anion gap in a patient with dextromethorphan bromide. *Am J Nephrol.* 1992;12:268-270.
90. Nimmaanrat S. Myoclonic movements following induction of anesthesia with propofol: a case report. *J Med Assoc Thai.* 2005;88:1955-1957.
91. O'Meara GF, Newman RJ, Fradley RL, et al. The GABA-A beta3 subunit mediates anaesthesia induced by etomidate. *Neuroreport.* 2004;15:1653-1656.
92. Ogino K, Hobara T, Kobayashi H, et al. Gastric mucosal injury induced by chloral hydrate. *Toxicol Lett.* 1990;52:129-133.
93. Olinga P, Elferink MG, Draaisma AL, et al. Coordinated induction of drug transporters and phase I and II metabolism in human liver slices. *Eur J Pharm Sci.* 2008;33:380-389.
94. Olkkola KT, Backman JT, Neuvonen PJ. Midazolam should be avoided in patients receiving the systemic antimycotics ketoconazole or itraconazole. *Clin Pharmacol Ther.* 1994;55:481-485.
95. Orser BA, McAdam LC, Roder S, et al. General anaesthetics and their effects on GABA(A) receptor desensitization. *Toxicol Lett.* 1998;100-101: 217-224.
96. Pain L, Gobaille S, Schleef C, et al. In vivo dopamine measurements in the nucleus accumbens after nonanesthetic and anesthetic doses of propofol in rats. *Anesth Analg.* 2002;95:915-919, table of contents.
97. Pandharipande PP, Pun BT, Herr DL, et al. Effect of sedation with dexmedetomidine vs lorazepam on acute brain dysfunction in mechanically ventilated patients: the MENDS randomized controlled trial. *JAMA.* 2007;298:2644-2653.
98. Parke TJ, Stevens JE, Rice AS, et al. Metabolic acidosis and fatal myocardial failure after propofol infusion in children: five case reports [see comments]. *BMJ.* 1992;305:613-616.
99. Peoples RW, Weight FF. Trichloroethanol potentiation of gamma-aminobutyric acid-activated chloride current in mouse hippocampal neurones. *Br J Pharmacol.* 1994;113:555-563.
100. Pleasure JR, Blackburn MG. Neonatal bromide intoxication: prenatal ingestion of a large quantity of bromides with transplacental accumulation in the fetus. *Pediatrics.* 1975;55:503-506.
101. Pond SM, Olson KR, Osterloh JD, et al. Randomized study of the treatment of phenobarbital overdose with repeated doses of activated charcoal. *JAMA.* 1984;251:3104-3108.
102. Proudfoot AT, Krenzelok EP, Vale JA. Position Paper on urine alkalinization. *J Toxicol Clin Toxicol.* 2004;42:1-26.
103. Reddy RV, Moorthy SS, Dierdorf SF, et al. Excitatory effects and electroencephalographic correlation of etomidate, thiopental, methohexital, and propofol. *Anesth Analg.* 1993;77:1008-1011.
104. Reynolds DS, Rosahl TW, Cirone J, et al. Sedation and anesthesia mediated by distinct GABA(A) receptor isoforms. *J Neurosci.* 2003;23: 8608-8617.

105. Reynolds HN, Teiken P, Regan ME, et al. Hyperlactatemia, increased osmolar gap, and renal dysfunction during continuous lorazepam infusion. *Crit Care Med*. 2000;28:1631-1634.
106. Reynolds JN, Maitra R. Propofol and flurazepam act synergistically to potentiate $GABA_A$ receptor activation in human recombinant receptors. *Eur J Pharmacol*. 1996;314:151-156.
107. Reynoldson JN, Elliott E, Sr., Nelson LA. Ramelteon: a novel approach in the treatment of insomnia. *Ann Pharmacother*. 2008;42:1262-1271.
108. Rho JM, Donevan SD, Rogawski MA. Barbiturate-like actions of the propanediol dicarbamates felbamate and meprobamate. *J Pharmacol Exp Ther*. 1997;280:1383-1391.
109. Richardson G, Wang-Weigand S. Effects of long-term exposure to ramelteon, a melatonin receptor agonist, on endocrine function in adults with chronic insomnia. *Hum Psychopharmacol*. 2009;24:103-111.
110. Rickels K, Schweizer E, Csanalosi I, et al. Long-term treatment of anxiety and risk of withdrawal. Prospective comparison of clorazepate and buspirone. *Arch Gen Psychiatry*. 1988;45:444-450.
111. Riker RR, Shehabi Y, Bokesch PM, et al. Dexmedetomidine vs midazolam for sedation of critically ill patients: a randomized trial. *JAMA*. 2009;301:489-499.
112. Rivara S, Mor M, Bedini A, et al. Melatonin receptor agonists: SAR and applications to the treatment of sleep-wake disorders. *Curr Top Med Chem*. 2008;8:954-968.
113. Rosenberg J, Benowitz NL, Pond S. Pharmacokinetics of drug overdose. *Clin Pharmacokinet*. 1981;6:161-192.
114. Rovasalo A, Tohmo H, Aantaa R, et al. Dexmedetomidine as an adjuvant in the treatment of alcohol withdrawal delirium: a case report. *Gen Hosp Psychiatry*. 2006;28:362-363.
115. Sahi J, Shord SS, Lindley C, et al. Regulation of cytochrome P450 2C9 expression in primary cultures of human hepatocytes. *J Biochem Mol Toxicol*. 2009;23:43-58.
116. Scheibler P, Kronfeld A, Illes P, et al. Trichloroethanol impairs NMDA receptor function in rat mesencephalic and cortical neurones. *Eur J Pharmacol*. 1999;366:R1-2.
117. Schenarts CL, Burton JH, Riker RR. Adrenocortical dysfunction following etomidate induction in emergency department patients. *Acad Emerg Med*. 2001;8:1-7.
118. Schulte D, Callado LF, Davidson C, et al. Propofol decreases stimulated dopamine release in the rat nucleus accumbens by a mechanism independent of dopamine D2, $GABA_A$ and NMDA receptors. *Br J Anaesth*. 2000; 84:250-253.
119. Schwartz HS. Acute meprobamate poisoning with gastrotomy and removal of a drug-containing mass. *N Engl J Med*. 1976;295:1177-1178.
120. Schwieler L, Delbro DS, Engberg G, et al. The anaesthetic agent propofol interacts with GABA(B)-receptors: an electrophysiological study in rat. *Life Sci*. 2003;72:2793-2801.
121. Sellers EM, Carr G, Bernstein JG, et al. Interaction of chloral hydrate and ethanol in man. II. Hemodynamics and performance. *Clin Pharmacol Ther*. 1972;13:50-58.
122. Sellers EM, Lang M, Koch-Weser J, et al. Interaction of chloral hydrate and ethanol in man. I. Metabolism. *Clin Pharmacol Ther*. 1972;13:37-49.
123. Serfaty M, Masterton G. Fatal poisonings attributed to benzodiazepines in Britain during the 1980s [see comments]. *Br J Psychiatry*. 1993;163:386-393.
124. Seubert CN, Morey TE, Martynyuk AE, et al. Midazolam selectively potentiates the A(2A)—but not A1—receptor-mediated effects of adenosine: role of nucleoside transport inhibition and clinical implications. *Anesthesiology*. 2000;92:567-577.
125. Short TG, Young Y. Toxicity of intravenous anaesthetics. *Best Pract Res Clin Anaesthesiol*. 2003;17:77-89.
126. Sills G, Brodie M. Pharmacokinetics and drug interactions with zonisamide. *Epilepsia*. 2007;48:435-441.
127. Simpson D, Curran MP. Ramelteon: a review of its use in insomnia. *Drugs*. 2008;68:1901-1919.
128. Sivilotti L, Nistri A. GABA receptor mechanisms in the central nervous system. *Prog Neurobiol*. 1991;36:35-92.
129. Smith PF, Darlington CL. The behavioural effects of long-term use of benzodiazepine sedative and hypnotic drugs: what can be learned from animal studies? *New Zealand J Psychol*. 1994;23:48-63.
130. Snead OC, Nichols AC, Liu CC. γ-Hydroxybutyric acid binding sites: interaction with the GABA-benzodiazepine-picrotoxin receptor complex. *Neurochem Res*. 1992;17:201-204.
131. Snyder GL, Galdi S, Hendrick JP, et al. General anesthetics selectively modulate glutamatergic and dopaminergic signaling via site-specific phosphorylation in vivo. *Neuropharmacology*. 2007;53:619-630.
132. Spivey WH. Flumazenil and seizures: analysis of 43 cases. *Clin Ther*. 1992;14: 292-305.
133. Spivey WH, Roberts JR, Derlet RW. A clinical trial of escalating doses of flumazenil for reversal of suspected benzodiazepine overdose in the emergency department. *Ann Emerg Med*. 1993;22:1813-1821.
134. Srinivasan V, Pandi-Perumal SR, Trahkt I, et al. Melatonin and melatonergic drugs on sleep: possible mechanisms of action. *Int J Neurosci*. 2009;119:821-846.
135. Stowe DF, Bosnjak ZJ, Kampine JP. Comparison of etomidate, ketamine, midazolam, propofol, and thiopental on function and metabolism of isolated hearts. *Anesth Analg*. 1992;74:547-558.
136. Szumita PM, Baroletti SA, Anger KE, et al. Sedation and analgesia in the intensive care unit: evaluating the role of dexmedetomidine. *Am J Health Syst Pharm*. 2007;64:37-44.
137. Tekwani KL, Watts HF, Rzechula KH, et al. A prospective observational study of the effect of etomidate on septic patient mortality and length of stay. *Acad Emerg Med*. 2009;16:11-14.
138. Tobias JD. Dexmedetomidine to treat opioid withdrawal in infants following prolonged sedation in the pediatric ICU. *J Opioid Manag*. 2006;2: 201-205.
139. Tobias JD. Subcutaneous dexmedetomidine infusions to treat or prevent drug withdrawal in infants and children. *J Opioid Manag*. 2008;4: 187-191.
140. Tramer MR, Moore RA, McQuay HJ. Propofol and bradycardia: causation, frequency and severity. *Br J Anaesth*. 1997;78:642-651.
141. Trump DL, Hochberg MC. Bromide intoxication. *Johns Hopkins Med J*. 1976;138:119-123.
142. Uchida I, Li L, Yang J. The role of the GABA(A) receptor alpha1 subunit N-terminal extracellular domain in propofol potentiation of chloride current. *Neuropharmacology*. 1997;36:1611-1621.
143. van de Kerkhof EG, de Graaf IA, Ungell AL, et al. Induction of metabolism and transport in human intestine: validation of precision-cut slices as a tool to study induction of drug metabolism in human intestine in vitro. *Drug Metab Dispos*. 2008;36:604-613.
144. Van de Wiele B, Rubinstein E, Peacock W, et al. Propylene glycol toxicity caused by prolonged infusion of etomidate. *J Neurosurg Anesthesiol*. 1995;7:259-262.
145. van Herwaarden AE, Smit JW, Sparidans RW, et al. Midazolam and cyclosporin a metabolism in transgenic mice with liver-specific expression of human CYP3A4. *Drug Metab Dispos*. 2005;33:892-895.
146. Varon J, Marik P. Etomidate and propylene glycol toxicity. *J Emerg Med*. 1998;16:485.
147. Vasile B, Rasulo F, Candiani A, et al. The pathophysiology of propofol infusion syndrome: a simple name for a complex syndrome. *Intensive Care Med*. 2003;29:1417-1425.
148. Vasileiou I, Xanthos T, Koudouna E, et al. Propofol: a review of its non-anaesthetic effects. *Eur J Pharmacol*. 2009;605:1-8.
149. Veller ID, Richardson JP, Doyle JC, et al. Gastric necrosis: a rare complication of chloral hydrate intoxication. *Br J Surg*. 1972;59:317-319.
150. Wafford KA, Macaulay AJ, Fradley R, et al. Differentiating the role of gamma-aminobutyric acid type A ($GABA_A$) receptor subtypes. *Biochem Soc Trans*. 2004;32:553-556.
151. Wagner J, Wagner ML, Hening WA. Beyond benzodiazepines: alternative pharmacologic agents for the treatment of insomnia. *Ann Pharmacother*. 1998;32:680-691.
152. Wagner RL, White PF. Etomidate inhibits adrenocortical function in surgical patients. *Anesthesiology*. 1984;61:647-651.
153. Wagner RL, White PF, Kan PB, et al. Inhibition of adrenal steroidogenesis by the anesthetic etomidate. *N Engl J Med*. 1984;310:1415-1421.
154. Warden JC, Pickford DR. Fatal cardiovascular collapse following propofol induction in high-risk patients and dilemmas in the selection of a short-acting induction agent [see comments]. *Anaesth Intensive Care*. 1995;23: 485-487.
155. Watsky E. Management of zolpidem withdrawal. *J Clin Psycho-pharmacol*. 1996;16:459.
156. Wesensten NJ, Balkin TJ, Davis HQ, et al. Reversal of triazolam- and zolpidem-induced memory impairment by flumazenil. *Psychopharmacology (Berl)*. 1995;121:242-249.

157. Wesolowska A, Paluchowska M, Chojnacka-Wojcik E. Involvement of presynaptic 5-HT(1A) and benzodiazepine receptors in the anticonflict activity of 5-HT(1A) receptor antagonists. *Eur J Pharmacol.* 2003;471:27-34.
158. White JF, Carlson GP. Epinephrine-induced cardiac arrhythmias in rabbits exposed to trichloroethylene: role of trichloroethylene metabolites. *Toxicol Appl Pharmacol.* 1981;60:458-465.
159. WHO. World Health Organization http://www.who.int/environmental_health_emergencies/events/Angola%20cause%20finding%20mission%20report%20Exeutive%20Summary%20for%20Web%20V190308.pdf.
160. Withington DE, Decell MK, Al Ayed T. A case of propofol toxicity: further evidence for a causal mechanism. *Paediatr Anaesth.* 2004;14:505-508.
161. Yamamoto K, Kobayashi H, Kobayashi T, et al. False hyperchloremia in bromism. *J Anesth.* 1991;5:88-91.
162. Zaballos M, Almendral J, Anadon MJ, et al. Comparative effects of thiopental and propofol on atrial vulnerability: electrophysiological study in a porcine model including acute alcoholic intoxication. *Br J Anaesth.* 2004;93:414-421. Epub 2004 Jul 2009.
163. Zahedi A, Grant MH, Wong DT. Successful treatment of chloral hydrate cardiac toxicity with propranolol. *Am J Emerg Med.* 1999;17:490-491.
164. Zatuchni J, Hong K. Methyl bromide poisoning seen initially as psychosis. *Arch Neurol.* 1981;38:529-530.

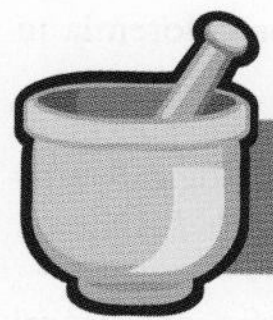

ANTIDOTES IN DEPTH (A23)

FLUMAZENIL

Mary Ann Howland

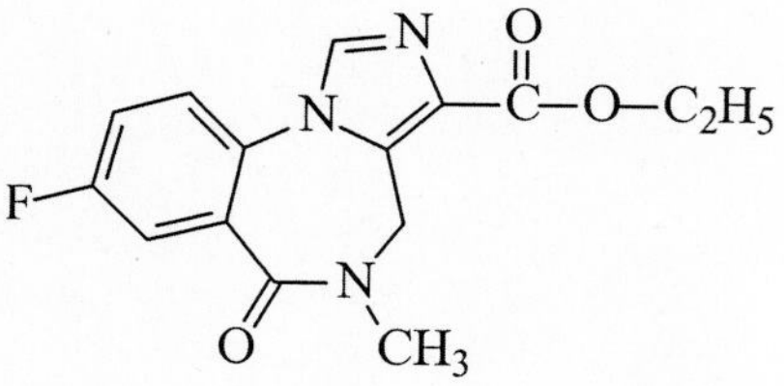

Flumazenil

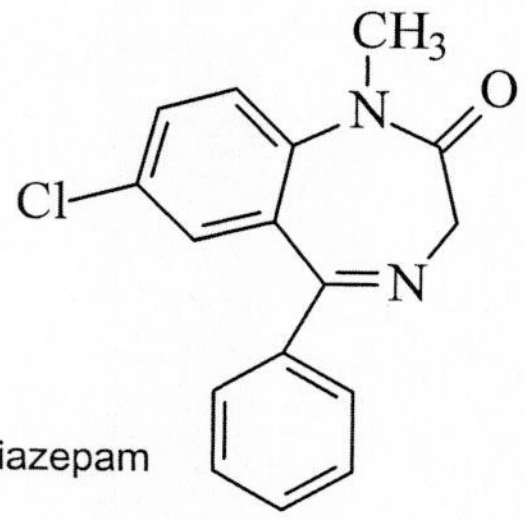

Diazepam

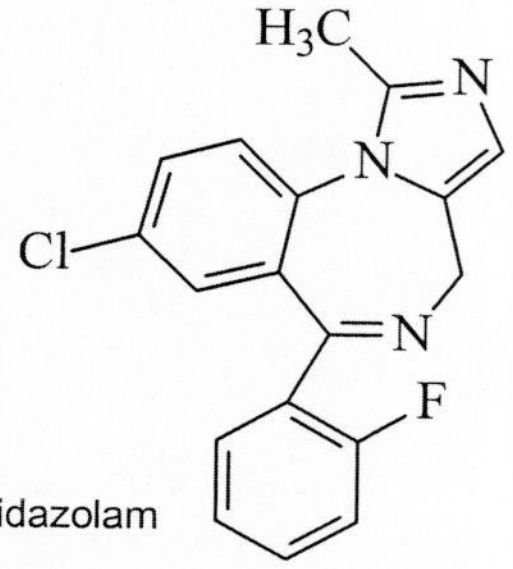

Midazolam

Flumazenil is a competitive benzodiazepine receptor antagonist. Its role in patients with unknown overdose is limited because seizures and dysrhythmias may develop when the effects of a benzodiazepine are reversed in a mixed overdose. Flumazenil also has the potential to induce benzodiazepine withdrawal symptoms, including seizures in patients who are benzodiazepine dependent. Flumazenil does not reliably reverse the respiratory depression induced by intravenous benzodiazepines.[57] Flumazenil is the ideal antidote for the relatively few patients who are both naïve to benzodiazepines and who overdose solely on a benzodiazepine as well as benzodiazepine-naïve patients whose benzodiazepine component must be reversed after procedural sedation. Because the duration of effect of flumazenil is shorter than that of most benzodiazepines, repeat doses may be necessary and vigilance is warranted. Flumazenil has no role in the management of ethanol intoxication but may be considered for patients with hepatic encephalopathy. However, further study is needed before its routine use can be recommended.[4] Case reports raise the possibility of a role for flumazenil in patients with paradoxical reactions to therapeutic doses of benzodiazepines.[75] Flumazenil is not expected to be effective in sedating overdoses such as baclofen in which a benzodiazepine receptor is not involved.[14] Flumazenil is effective for overdoses of zolpidem and zaleplon, nonbenzodiazepines that interact with ω_1 receptors, a subclass of central benzodiazepine receptors.[41,51,54]

HISTORY

Haefely and Hunkeler's initial work on chlordiazepoxide synthesis[69] led to an attempt to develop benzodiazepine derivatives that would act as antagonists.[32] This endeavor was initially unsuccessful but led to the promising γ-aminobutyric acid (GABA) hypothesis of benzodiazepine mechanism of action. In 1977, the then-new technique of radioligand binding identified specific high-affinity benzodiazepine binding sites. Other investigators simultaneously isolated a product produced by a *Streptomyces* species that had the basic 1,4-benzodiazepine structure. Synthetic compounds subsequently were derived from this molecule to act as potential tranquilizers. Further research attempted to produce benzodiazepines with potent anxiolytic and anticonvulsant activity and diminished sedative and muscle-relaxing properties. Testing revealed these derivatives had high in vitro binding affinities but lacked in vivo activity. An inability to enter the CNS was considered an explanation for the discordance. During an experiment that attempted to demonstrate CNS penetration of these derivatives, diazepam given to incapacitate the animals had a surprisingly weak effect. This lack of potency led to the discovery of a benzodiazepine antagonist. Further modifications led to the synthesis of flumazenil (Ro 15-1788).[20,55]

PHARMACOLOGY

The benzodiazepine receptor modulates the effect of GABA on the $GABA_A$ receptor by increasing the frequency of Cl^- channel opening, leading to hyperpolarization. Agonists such as diazepam stimulate the benzodiazepine receptor to produce anxiolytic, anticonvulsant, sedative, amnestic, and muscle relaxant effects at low doses, and hypnosis at high doses.[33] Flumazenil is a water-soluble benzodiazepine analog with a molecular weight of 303 Daltons. It is a competitive antagonist at the benzodiazepine receptor, with very weak agonist properties both in animal models and in humans.[50] Inverse agonists bind the benzodiazepine receptor and result in the opposite effects of anxiety, agitation, and seizures. Antagonists, such as flumazenil, competitively occupy the benzodiazepine receptor without causing any functional change and without allowing an agonist or inverse agonist access to the receptor. The zero set point of intrinsic activity may be influenced by the activity of the GABA system or by chronic treatment with benzodiazepines.[22] Positron emission tomography investigations reveal that 1.5 mg flumazenil leads to an initial receptor occupancy of 55%, whereas 15 mg causes almost total blockade of benzodiazepine receptor sites.[60]

The structures of flumazenil, diazepam, and midazolam are shown above. Table A23–1 summarizes the physiochemical and pharmacologic properties of flumazenil.[37]

VOLUNTEER STUDIES

Volunteer studies demonstrate that the ability of flumazenil to reverse the effects of sedating doses of intravenous (IV) benzodiazepines (such as 30 mg diazepam, 3 mg lorazepam, 10 mg midazolam) is dose dependent and begins within minutes.[18] Peak effects occur within 6 to 10 minutes.[57] Most individuals achieve complete reversal of benzodiazepine effect with

TABLE A23–1. Physicochemical and Pharmacologic Properties of Flumazenil

pK_a	Weak base
Partition coefficient at pH 7.4	14 (octanol/aqueous PO_4 buffer)
Volume of distribution	1.06 L/kg
Distribution half-life ($t_{1/2}\alpha$)	≤5 minutes
Metabolism	Hepatic: three inactive metabolites High clearance
Elimination	First order
Protein binding	54%–64%
Elimination half-life ($t_{1/2}\beta$)	53 minutes
Onset of action	1–2 minutes
Duration of action	Dependent on dose and elimination of benzodiazepine, time interval, dose of flumazenil, and hepatic function

a total IV dose of 1 mg, titrated in 0.2-mg aliquots.[5,13] A 3-mg IV dose produces similar effects that last approximately twice as long as the 1-mg dose.

CONSCIOUS SEDATION

A number of studies evaluated patients who received diazepam or midazolam as conscious sedation for endoscopy or cardioversion.[6,12,13,17,39,40] When a benzodiazepine is given for conscious sedation during a procedure, flumazenil appears safe and effective for reversal of sedation and partial reversal of amnesia and cognitive impairment.[25] Most patients respond to total doses of 0.4 to 1 mg. Administering flumazenil slowly at a rate of 0.1 mg/min minimizes the disconcerting symptoms associated with rapid arousal, such as confusion, agitation, and emotional lability. Residual sedation becomes evident within 20 to 120 minutes, depending on the dose and pharmacokinetics of the specific benzodiazepine and the dose of flumazenil.[25] For this reason, patients must be carefully monitored and subsequent doses of flumazenil titrated to clinical response. Because the amnestic effect of benzodiazepines and the cognitive and psychomotor effects are not fully reversed, posttreatment instructions should be reinforced in writing and given to a responsible caregiver accompanying the patient.[18,25] Because of the risk of resedation, many practitioners elect not to use flumazenil routinely.

Two patients undergoing endoscopy who developed seizures following benzodiazepine reversal are reported.[64] One patient had a history of seizures, and the other had no obvious etiology. Both patients recovered uneventfully.

USE FOR PARADOXICAL REACTION TO MIDAZOLAM AND OTHER BENZODIAZEPINES

Paradoxical reactions to benzodiazepines are unpredictable and documented in as many as 10% of adults and in 3.4% of children.[28,46] Common features include worsening restlessness, agitation, disorientation, flailing, and dysphoria.[24,26,52,75] The mechanism is unclear and has been attributed to a disinhibition reaction.[21] These reactions are reported to occur anywhere from several minutes to 210 minutes after sedation is begun.[26,75] Management strategies include administering higher doses of the benzodiazepines, adding other drugs such as opioids or droperidol, stopping the procedure, and using flumazenil.[24,36,52,56,65,66,75] Intravenous flumazenil was administered to six adults with paradoxical reactions to midazolam in 0.1-mg aliquots. Doses of 0.2 to 0.5 mg were effective in all the patients with a response occurring within 30 seconds.[75] Attention to other causes of unexpected behavior such as hypoxia or hypoglycemia must be addressed and corrected.

EFFECTS ON BENZODIAZEPINE-INDUCED RESPIRATORY DEPRESSION

Flumazenil has not consistently reversed benzodiazepine-induced respiratory depression and is not suggested as the initial intervention should respiratory depression occur.[15,29,44,48,57,62,70,73] It is likely that following oral overdose, benzodiazepine-induced respiratory insufficiency is related to smooth muscle relaxation resulting in a mechanical effect with an increase in upper airway resistance and obstructive apnea rather than a central effect.[31] Although flumazenil might improve the situation,[31,53] other standard procedures such as airway repositioning, supplemental oxygen, bag-valve-mask ventilation, and endotracheal intubation, if indicated, should be used either prior to or during reversal.

USE IN THE OVERDOSE SETTING

The role of flumazenil in the overdose setting is controversial.[71] The first argument against flumazenil use is the rare morbidity and mortality associated with benzodiazepine use. An analysis of 702 patients who had taken benzodiazepines alone or in combination with ethanol or other drugs and were subsequently admitted to a medical intensive care unit (ICU) over a 14-year period revealed a 0.7% fatality rate (five deaths) and 9.8% complication rate (69 patients).[35] In comparison, the fatality rate for patients with nonbenzodiazepine-related overdoses was 1.6% (55 of 3430 patients). In the pure benzodiazepine group, two patients died and 18 (12.5%) of 144 patients had complications, mostly aspiration pneumonitis and decubitus ulcers. Proponents of flumazenil therapy suggest that some of the 29 diagnostic procedures used in the patients were unnecessary, and some of the complications could have been prevented. Opponents of flumazenil therapy suggest that many of the cases of aspiration pneumonitis occurred prior to hospital admission and that the patients also suffered from trauma and infectious disease, making most diagnostic procedures necessary.

In an effort to develop indications for safe and effective use of flumazenil, overdosed comatose patients were retrospectively assigned to either a low-risk or non–low-risk group.[30] Low-risk patients had CNS depression with normal vital signs, no other neurologic findings, no evidence of ingestion of a tricyclic antidepressant by history or electrocardiogram (ECG), no seizure history, and absence of an available history of chronic benzodiazepine use. All other patients fell into the non–low-risk category. Of 35 consecutive comatose patients, four patients were assigned to the low-risk group. Flumazenil caused complete awakening in three patients and partial awakening in the fourth patient in the low-risk group, with no adverse effects. In the non–low-risk group of 31 patients, flumazenil caused complete awakening in four patients and partial awakening in five patients. Seizures occurred in five patients, of whom only one had a history of seizures, five were long-term benzodiazepine users, four had abnormal vital signs prior to reversal, and three had evidence of hyperreflexia or myoclonus. Therefore, although flumazenil use probably was safe and effective in the low-risk group, few patients met the criteria for inclusion in that risk group. The risk of seizures appears substantial in non–low-risk patients.

TABLE A23–2. Indications for Flumazenil Use in the Overdose Setting

Pure benzodiazepine overdose in a nontolerant individual who has
- CNS depression
- Normal vital signs, including SaO_2
- Normal ECG
- Otherwise normal neurologic examination

CNS, central nervous system; ECG, electrocardiogram.

In conclusion, the risks of flumazenil usually outweigh the benefits in overdose patients.[61] When non–benzodiazepine-dependent patients ingest benzodiazepines alone in overdose, as rarely occurs in adults but might be expected in children, the risks associated with flumazenil use may be limited.[77] Table A23–2 summarizes the indications for flumazenil use in the overdose setting.

ADVERSE EFFECTS AND SAFETY ISSUES

Flumazenil has been studied in more than 3500 patients worldwide, including healthy volunteers and overdosed patients, or patients who had undergone conscious sedation. The safety of flumazenil in healthy volunteers is well established, with no discernible objective or subjective effects. However, precipitation of seizures in benzodiazepine-dependent patients, unmasking of dysrhythmias in patients who coingest a benzodiazepine with a prodysrhythmic drug, and resedation within 20 to 120 minutes in patients receiving benzodiazepines for conscious sedation are recognized adverse effects associated with flumazenil administration.

The ability of flumazenil to precipitate acute benzodiazepine withdrawal seizures in a more controlled environment than the overdose setting was demonstrated by reversal of long-term benzodiazepine sedation in the ICU. A study of 1700 patients revealed that 14 patients developed adverse drug reactions, probably half related to abrupt arousal.[6] Two patients with a history of epilepsy developed tonic–clonic seizures, and one patient developed myoclonic seizures.[6] Dose-dependent induction of withdrawal reactions is therefore suggested. Small total doses (less than 1 mg) of titrated flumazenil may allow sufficient occupation of the benzodiazepine receptor sites by benzodiazepines so that abrupt withdrawal seizures are uncommon.

In a study of 12 patients receiving midazolam sedation for 4 ± 3 days, 0.5 mg flumazenil was administered as a rapid bolus. Serum norepinephrine and epinephrine concentrations rose within 10 minutes, returned to baseline within 30 minutes, and correlated with increased heart rate, blood pressure, and myocardial oxygen consumption.[38]

Flumazenil causes a significant overshoot in cerebral blood flow and may cause a large increase in intracranial pressure in patients who receive midazolam for severe head injury.[79]

In one review, 30 published case studies involving 758 patients with drug overdoses were reviewed.[23] In total, 387 patients participated in double-blind study protocols and 371 patients in open-label studies.[23] Fifty percent of cases were mixed overdoses. The doses of flumazenil ranged from 0.2 to 5 mg. Five cases of seizures were temporally related to flumazenil administration, all after large bolus doses. In three of the five patients, high concentrations of tricyclic antidepressants were present in the blood. The seizures resolved either without treatment or following administration of a small dose of a benzodiazepine. Dysrhythmias developed in two patients given small doses of flumazenil, both presumably associated with the presence of a tricyclic antidepressant. Of 497 patients enrolled in two clinical US studies sponsored by the manufacturer,[23] six patients developed seizures (five had coingested tricyclic antidepressants) and one patient who had taken a tricyclic antidepressant and carbamazepine had a junctional tachycardia, which normalized after several minutes. Thus, in reviewing 1255 patients, 11 patients had seizures and three developed dysrhythmias, for an incidence of approximately 0.9%. The consensus report was that (1) flumazenil is not a substitute for primary emergency care; (2) hypoxia and hypotension should be corrected before flumazenil is used; (3) when used small titrated doses of flumazenil should be used; (4) flumazenil should not be used in patients with a history of seizures, evidence of seizures or jerking movements, or evidence of a tricyclic antidepressant overdose; and (5) flumazenil should not be used by inexperienced clinicians.

An analysis of all seizures associated with flumazenil gathered from previously published cases or reports to the manufacturer was published.[64] Forty-three patients had seizures and 6 patients died, but the author believed that none of the deaths were attributable to flumazenil.[64] Four patients developed status epilepticus; two were presumed to be caused by concomitant tricyclic antidepressant exposure, and the other two patients had received benzodiazepines to treat status epilepticus prior to flumazenil therapy. In six of 43 seizure episodes, the relationship to flumazenil use was believed to be inadequately defined. The remaining 37 patients were stratified into five categories. In category 1, seven patients were given flumazenil after they had received a benzodiazepine for treatment of a seizure disorder. Six of these seven patients received greater than 1 mg flumazenil. In category 2, 20 patients received flumazenil for reversal of a benzodiazepine in a mixed-drug overdose. Many of these patients had coingested tricyclic antidepressants. Thirteen of these patients received greater than 1 mg flumazenil. Two of the patients in this group developed status epilepticus and died, possibly secondary to a severe tricyclic antidepressant overdose. Category 3 included five patients who received benzodiazepines for suppression of non–drug-induced seizures. Two of these five patients received greater than 1 mg flumazenil. Category 4 included three patients with acute benzodiazepine overdoses in the presence of chronic benzodiazepine dependence. Category 5 included two patients who received a benzodiazepine for conscious sedation. Therefore, flumazenil use may place the patient at risk for seizures by unmasking a toxic effect in mixed overdose, by removing the protective anticonvulsant effect in a patient with non–drug-induced seizures, or by precipitating acute benzodiazepine withdrawal. Table A23–3 summarizes the contraindications to flumazenil use.

TABLE A23–3. Contraindications to Flumazenil Use

History	Clinical
Seizure history or current treatment of seizures	Potential ECG evidence of cyclic antidepressant use: terminal rightward 40 ms axis, QRS or QT prolongation
Ingestion of a xenobiotic capable of provoking seizures or cardiac dysrhythmias	Hypoxia
Long-term use of benzodiazepines	Hypotension.

DOSING

Slow IV titration (0.1 mg/min) to a total dose less than or equal to 1 mg seems most reasonable. Resedation may occur at 20 to 120 minutes, and readministration of flumazenil may be necessary. Although not approved by the US Food and Drug Administration (FDA), continuous IV infusion of flumazenil 0.1 to 1.0 mg/h in 0.9% sodium chloride solution or 5% dextrose in water has been used following the loading dose.[41,76,78]

AVAILABILITY

Flumazenil is available as Romazicon and as a generic formulation by many manufacturers in a concentration of 0.1 mg/mL with parabens in 5-mL and 10-mL vials.

ROLE IN NONBENZODIAZEPINE TOXICITY

HEPATIC ENCEPHALOPATHY

Hepatic encephalopathy is considered a reversible metabolic encephalopathy characterized by a spectrum of CNS effects. Symptoms may progress from confusion and somnolence to coma. One current hypothesis implicates an increase in GABAergic tone in the development of encephalopathy.[7,63]

Animal studies of hepatic encephalopathy secondary to galactosamine or thioacetamide (hepatotoxins) demonstrate an increase in GABA effect, which is antagonized by flumazenil, bicuculline (a GABA-receptor antagonist), and isopropylbiclophosphate chloride (a calcium channel blocker).[7] Cerebrospinal fluid (CSF) from these animals contained a benzodiazepine receptor ligand with agonist activity. Rat studies involving hepatic encephalopathy resulting from acute liver ischemia showed only a slight response to flumazenil, but significant improvement after administration of a partial inverse agonist.[11,72]

Human studies have detected benzodiazepine-binding activity in the CSF, (but not in serum), of patients with hepatic encephalopathy. One group identified four to 19 peaks representing benzodiazepine-binding ligands from the frontal cortex of 11 patients who died of hepatic encephalopathy.[10] Two of the peaks were further characterized as diazepam and *N*-desmethyldiazepam. Brain concentrations of these substances were two to 10 times higher than normal in six of the patients and were normal in five patients. Patients with idiopathic recurring stupor who have measurable "endozepines" (endogenous benzodiazepine ligands) in serum and CSF are reported.[58,68]

Flumazenil improves the clinical and electrophysiologic responses of patients with hepatic encephalopathy and idiopathic recurring stupor.[4,8,19,58,68] Some patients with encephalopathy have improved from stage IV to stage II encephalopathy after intravenous flumazenil. Maximal improvement after flumazenil lasts approximately 1 to 2 hours and gradually dissipates within 6 hours. The response rate in a meta-analysis averaged approximately 30%.[27] The proposed explanations for the unresponsiveness include cerebral edema, hypoxia, other systemic diseases or complications, and irreversible CNS damage.

Animal and human data convincingly support the concept that increased GABAergic tone is responsible for hepatic encephalopathy. Evidence for endogenous benzodiazepine ligands that enhance GABA action also are demonstrated but controversial.[1,3] The source of these benzodiazepine receptor agonists is unclear, but diet and/or production by gut bacteria is postulated.[7] Most authorities believe endogenous de novo synthesis is unlikely and propose prior benzodiazepine exposure and persistence as an explanation. Neurosteroids and hemoglobin metabolites are also implicated in the pathophysiology of hepatic encephalopathy.[3,59]

Flumazenil can lead to short-term improvement of the clinical condition of a subgroup of patients with hepatic encephalopathy and may prove useful as an addition to conventional therapy.[2,4,9] Additional research is necessary to prospectively identify responders, provide dosing considerations, and evaluate adverse effects. There is no survival benefit.

ETHANOL INTOXICATION

Animal studies indicate that many of the actions of ethanol are mediated through GABA neurotransmission.[67] Acute ethanol administration appears to enhance GABA transmission and inhibit *N*-methyl-d-aspartate (NMDA) excitation. Chronic ethanol administration leads to downregulation of the GABA system. Ethanol enhances $GABA_A$-induced chloride influx in a dose-dependent fashion without a direct effect on chloride. Flumazenil does not influence this action of GABA. Chronic ethanol use selectively increases the sensitivity to inverse benzodiazepine agonists, invoking a change in coupling or conformation of the receptor. These changes may explain the development of tolerance and the kindling and production of seizures that occur on ethanol withdrawal.

Two double-blind studies in patients with benzodiazepine or ethanol overdose evaluated the response to flumazenil. In one study of 13 patients with suspected ethanol intoxication, six had no response to placebo when it was given first, whereas all 13 patients responded to 5 mg flumazenil.[47] Improved consciousness occurred after 15 minutes, and respiratory rates increased from 14 to 16 breaths/min. Heart rate and blood pressure were not affected. The 5-mg dose of flumazenil was selected because no improvement in mental status or vital signs was observed when 1 mg flumazenil was administered to four patients.

Another comparable study demonstrated similar results.[42] Flumazenil (1 mg) administered to nine ethanol-intoxicated patients produced the same effects as placebo. Subsequent administration of 2 to 5 mg flumazenil in the open part of the study produced a clear improvement in the modified Glasgow Coma Score scale in five of 11 patients. However, a closer inspection of phase 1 of the study reveals that an arousal reaction occurred in seven of nine patients after the flumazenil dose and in five of nine patients following placebo administration. It is conceivable that the improvement in phase 2 was a continuation of the arousal reaction.

One case report indicates that ethanol-induced respiratory depression was reversed by flumazenil,[45] but whether the actual data support the authors' conclusions is unclear.

A randomized, double-blind, crossover study of eight male volunteers given IV ethanol to achieve a constant serum ethanol concentration of 160 mg/dL was conducted.[16] Once stabilized, the volunteers were given either placebo or 5 mg flumazenil. Subjective and objective psychomotor tests were conducted, with no differences noted between volunteers given flumazenil and volunteers given placebo. Thus the probability of ethanol reversal at the suggested doses appears unlikely.

Based on this information, flumazenil likely does not have a significant effect on ethanol intoxication, and low doses of flumazenil (less than 1 mg) have no effect. The 5-mg doses reportedly produce favorable changes in sensorium, but these findings may be the result of confounding factors. Because we would not administer 5 mg flumazenil in the overdose setting to avoid the increased risk of adverse effects at this dose, flumazenil cannot be recommended for reversal of ethanol intoxication.

SUMMARY

The risks of flumazenil appear to greatly outweigh the potential benefits of reversal when benzodiazepines are used chronically or acutely to treat a seizure disorder. Flumazenil is best avoided in the overdose setting when evidence indicates coingestion of a drug capable of causing seizures or dysrhythmias. For example, any indication that theophylline, carbamazepine, chloral hydrate, chloroquine, and/or chlorinated hydrocarbons was ingested is a contraindication to flumazenil use.[74] Flumazenil should also not be used when involvement of a tricyclic antidepressant is strongly suggested based on history, clinical findings, or ECG findings (prolonged QRS complex).[34,43,49,74] In the event of flumazenil-induced seizure, a therapeutic dose of a benzodiazepine such as diazepam should be effective. Flumazenil is a competitive antagonist; higher doses of benzodiazepines will reverse higher doses of flumazenil.

REFERENCES

1. Ahboucha S, Butterworth RF. Pathophysiology of hepatic encephalopathy: a new look at GABA from the molecular standpoint. *Metab Brain Dis.* 2004;19:331-343.
2. Ahboucha S, Butterworth RF. Role of endogenous benzodiazepine ligands and their GABA-A associated receptors in hepatic encephalopathy. *Metab Brain Dis.* 2005;20:425-437.
3. Ahboucha S, Pomier-Layrargues G, Butterworth RF. Increased brain concentrations of endogenous (non-benzodiazepine) GABA-a receptor ligands in human hepatic encephalopathy. *Metab Brain Dis.* 2004;19:241-251.
4. Als-Nielsen B, Kjaergard LL, Gluud C. Benzodiazepine receptor antagonists for acute and chronic hepatic encephalopathy. *Cochrane Database Syst Rev.* 2004;2:CD002798.
5. Amrein R, Hetzel W, Hartmann D, Lorscheid T. Clinical pharmacology of flumazenil. *Eur J Anaesth.* 1988;2:65-80.
6. Amrein R, Leishman B, Bentzinger C, Roncari G. Flumazenil in benzodiazepine antagonism: actions and clinical use in intoxications and anaesthesiology. *Med Toxicol.* 1987;2:411-429.
7. Anonymous. Benzodiazepine compounds and hepatic encephalopathy. *N Engl J Med.* 1991;325:509-510.
8. Anonymous. Flumazenil in the treatment of hepatic encephalopathy. *Ann Pharmacother.* 1993;27:46-47.
9. Barbaro G, Di Lorenzo G, Soldini M, et al. Flumazenil for hepatic encephalopathy grade III and IVa in patients with cirrhosis: an Italian multicenter double-blind, placebo-controlled, cross-over study. *Hepatology.* 1998;28:374-378.
10. Basile AS, Hughes RD, Harrison PM, et al. Elevated brain concentrations of 1,4-benzodiazepines in fulminant hepatic failure. *N Engl J Med.* 1991;325:473-478.
11. Bosman DK, Van Den Buijs CACG, De Haan JC, et al. The effects of benzodiazepine-receptor antagonists and partial inverse agonists on acute hepatic encephalopathy in the rat. *Gastroenterology.* 1991;101:772-781.
12. Breheny FX. Reversal of midazolam sedation with flumazenil. *Crit Care Med.* 1991;20:736-739.
13. Brogden RN, Goa KL. Flumazenil: a reappraisal of its pharmacological properties and therapeutic efficacy as a benzodiazepine antagonist. *Drugs.* 1991;42:1061-1089.
14. Byrnes SMA, Watson GW, Hardy PAJ. Flumazenil: an unreliable antagonist in baclofen overdose. *Anaesthesiology.* 1996;51:481-482.
15. Carter AS, Bell GD, Coady T, et al. Speed of reversal of midazolam-induced respiratory depression by flumazenil: a study in patients undergoing upper GI endoscopy. *Acta Anaesth Scand.* 1990;34:59-64.
16. Clausen TG, Wolff J, Carl P, Theilgaard A. The effect of the benzodiazepine antagonist, flumazenil, on psychometric performance in acute ethanol intoxication in man. *Eur J Clin Pharmacol.* 1990;38:233-236.
17. Coll-Vincent B, Sala X, Fernandez C, et al. Sedation of cardioversion in the emergency department: analysis of effectiveness in four protocols. *Ann Emerg Med.* 2003;42:767-772.
18. Dunton AW, Schwam E, Pitman V, et al. Flumazenil: US clinical pharmacology studies. *Eur J Anaesth.* 1988;2:81-95; discussion *Eur J Anaest.* 1988;2(Suppl):233-235.
19. Ferenci P, Grimm G, Meryn S, Gangl A. Successful long-term treatment of portal-systemic encephalopathy by the benzodiazepine antagonist flumazenil. *Gastroenterology.* 1989;96:240-243.
20. File SE, Pellow S. Intrinsic actions of the benzodiazepine receptor antagonist Ro 15-1788. *Psychopharmacology.* 1986;88:1-11.
21. Fulton SA, Mullen KD. Completion of upper endoscopic procedures despite paradoxical reaction to midazolam: a role for flumazenil? *Arch J Gastroenterol.* 2000;95:809-811.
22. Gardner CR. Functional in vivo correlates of the benzodiazepine agonist-inverse agonist continuum. *Prog Neurobiol.* 1988;31:425-476.
23. Geller E, Crome P, Schaller MD, et al. Risks and benefits of therapy with flumazenil (Anexate) in mixed drug intoxications. *Eur Neurol.* 1991;31:241-250.
24. George M, Sury M. Reversal of paradoxical excitement to diazepam sedation. *Pediatr Anesth.* 2008;18:546-547.
25. Girdler NM, Fairbrother KJ, Lyne JP. A randomised crossover trial of post-operative cognitive and psychomotor recovery from benzodiazepine sedation: effects of reversal with flumazenil over a prolonged recovery period. *Br Dent J.* 2002;192:335-339.
26. Golparvar M, Saghaei M, Sajedi P, et al. Paradoxical reaction following intravenous midazolam premedication in pediatric patients—a randomized placebo controlled trial of ketamine for rapid tranquilization. *Pediatr Anesth.* 2004;14:924-930.
27. Goulenok C, Bernard B, Cadranel JF, et al. Flumazenil vs. placebo in hepatic encephalopathy in patients with cirrhosis: a meta-analysis. *Aliment Pharmacol Ther.* 2002;16:361-372.
28. Greenblatt DJ, Shader RI. Benzodiazepines (first of two parts). *N Engl J Med.* 1974;291:1011-1015.
29. Gross JB, Weller RS, Conard P. Flumazenil antagonism of midazolam-induced ventilatory depression. *Anesthesiology.* 1991;75:179-185.
30. Gueye PN, Hoffman JR, Taboulet P, et al. Empiric use of flumazenil in comatose patients: limited applicability of criteria to define low risk. *Ann Emerg Med.* 1996;27:730-735.
31. Gueye P, Lofaso F, Borron S, et al. Mechanism of respiratory insufficiency in pure or mixed drug induced coma involving benzodiazepines. *Clin Tox.* 2002;40:35-47.
32. Haefely W, Hunkeler W. The story of flumazenil. *Eur J Anaesth.* 1988;2:3-14.
33. Hart YM, Meinardi H, Sander JW, et al. The effect of intravenous flumazenil on interictal electroencephalographic epileptic activity: results of a placebo-controlled study. *J Neurol Neurosurg Psychiatry.* 1991;54:305-309.
34. Haverkos GP, DiSalvo RP, Imhoff TE. Fatal seizures after flumazenil administration in a patient with mixed overdose. *Ann Pharmacother.* 1994;28:1347-1349.
35. Höjer J, Baehrendtz S. The effect of flumazenil (Ro 15-1788) in the management of self-induced benzodiazepine poisoning: a double-blind controlled study. *Acta Med Scand.* 1988;224:357-365.
36. Honan VJ. Paradoxical reaction to midazolam and control with flumazenil. *Gastrointest Endosc.* 1994;40:86-88.
37. Hunkeler W. Preclinical research findings with flumazenil (Ro 15-1788, Anexate): chemistry. *Eur J Anaesth.* 1988;2(Suppl):37-62.
38. Kamijo Y, Masuda T, Nishikawa T, et al. Cardiovascular response and stress reaction to flumazenil injection in patients under infusion with midazolam. *Crit Care Med.* 2000;28:318-323.
39. Katz JA, Fragen RJ, Dunn KL. Flumazenil reversal of midazolam sedation of the elderly. *Reg Anesth Pain Med.* 1991;16:247-252.
40. Kirkegaard L, Knudsen L, Jensen S, Kruse A. Benzodiazepine antagonist Ro 15-1788. *Anaesthesia.* 1986;41:1184-1188.
41. L'heureux P. Continuous flumazenil for zolpidem toxicity—commentary. *J Toxicol Clin Toxicol.* 1998;36:745-746.
42. L'heureux P, Askenasi R. Efficacy of flumazenil in acute alcohol intoxication: double-blind placebo controlled evaluation. *Hum Exp Toxicol.* 1991;10:235-239.
43. L'heureux P, Vranckx M, Leduc D, Askenasi R. Flumazenil in mixed benzodiazepine/tricyclic antidepressant overdose: a placebo-controlled study in the dog. *Am J Emerg Med.* 1992;10:184-188.
44. Lim AG. Death after flumazenil. *BMJ.* 1989;299:858-859.
45. Linowiecki K, Paloucek F, Donnelly A, Leikin JB. Reversal of ethanol-induced respiratory depression by flumazenil. *Vet Hum Toxicol.* 1992; 34:417-419.
46. Litchfield NB. Complications of intravenous diazepam. Adverse psychological reactions. *Anesth Prog.* 1980;27:175-183.
47. Martens F, Köppel C, Ibe K, et al. Clinical experience with the benzodiazepine antagonist flumazenil in suspected benzodiazepine or ethanol poisoning. *J Toxicol Clin Toxicol.* 1990;28:341-356.
48. Mora CT, Torjman M, White PF. Effects of diazepam and flumazenil on sedation and hypoxic ventilatory response. *Anesth Analg.* 1989;68:473-478.

49. Mordel A, Winkler E, Almog S, et al. Seizures after flumazenil administration in a case of combined benzodiazepine and tricyclic antidepressant overdose. *Crit Care Med.* 1992;20:1733-1734.
50. Neave N, Reid C, Scholey AB, et al. Dose-dependent effects of flumazenil on cognition, mood, and cardio-respiratory physiology in healthy volunteers. *Br Dent J.* 2000;189:668-674.
51. Noguchi H, Kitazumi K, Mori M, Shiba T. Binding and neuropharmacological profile of zaleplon, a novel nonbenzodiazepine sedative/hypnotic. *Eur J Pharmacol.* 2002;434:21-28.
52. Olshaker J, Flanigan J. Flumazenil reversal of lorazepam induced acute delirium. *J Emerg Med.* 2003;24:181-183.
53. Oshima T, Masaki Y, Tpyooka H. Flumazenil antagonizes midazolam-induced airway narrowing during nasal breathing in humans. *Br J Anaesthesia.* 1999; 82:698-702.
54. Patat A, Naef MM, Van Gessel E, et al. Flumazenil antagonizes the central effects of zolpidem, an imidazopyridine hypnotic. *Clin Pharmacol Ther.* 1994;56:430-436.
55. Persson A, Pauli S, Halldin C, et al. Saturation analysis of specific ^{11}C Ro 15-1788 binding to the human neocortex using positron emission tomography. *Hum Psychopharmacol.* 1989;4:21-31.
56. Rodrigo CR. Flumazenil reverses paradoxical reaction with midazolam. *Anesth Prog.* 1991;38:65-68.
57. Romazicon [package insert]. Nutley, NJ: Roche Laboratories, Inc; September 2004.
58. Rothstein JD, Guidotti A, Tinuper P, et al. Endogenous benzodiazepine receptor ligands in idiopathic recurring stupor. *Lancet.* 1992;340:1002-1004.
59. Ruscito BJ, Harrison NL. Hemoglobin metabolites mimic benzodiazepines and are possible mediators of hepatic encephalopathy. *Blood.* 2003;102:1525-1528.
60. Savic I, Widen L, Stone-Eldaner S. Feasibility of reversing benzodiazepine tolerance with flumazenil. *Lancet.* 1991;337:133-137.
61. Seger DL. Flumazenil—treatment or toxin. *J Toxicol Clin Toxicol.* 2004;42:209-216.
62. Shalansky SJ, Naumann TL, Englander FA. Therapy update: effect of flumazenil on benzodiazepine-induced respiratory depression. *Clin Pharm.* 1993;12:483-487.
63. Skolnick P. The γ-aminobutyric acid A ($GABA_A$) receptor complex. In: Jones EA, moderator: the γ-aminobutyric acid A ($GABA_A$) receptor complex and hepatic encephalopathy: some recent advances. *Ann Intern Med.* 1989;100:532-546.
64. Spivey WH. Flumazenil and seizures: analysis of 43 cases. *Clin Ther.* 1992;14:292-305.
65. Thakker P, Gallagher TM. Flumazenil reverses paradoxical reaction to midazolam in a child. *Anaesth Intensive Care.* 1996;24:505-507.
66. Thurston TA, Williams CG, Foshee SL. Reversal of a paradoxical reaction to midazolam with flumazenil. *Anesth Analg.* 1996;83:192.
67. Ticku MK, Mhatre M, Mehta AK. Modulation of GABAergic transmission by ethanol. In: Biggio G, Costa E, eds. *GABAergic Synaptic Transmission.* New York: Raven; 1992:255-268.
68. Tinuper P, Montagna P, Cortelli P, et al. Idiopathic recurring stupor: a case with possible involvement of the gamma-aminobutyric acid (GABA)ergic system. *Ann Neurol.* 1992;31:503-506.
69. Tobin JM, Lewis N. New psychotherapeutic agent chlordiazepoxide. *JAMA.* 1960;174:1242-1249.
70. Tolksdorf W, Ney C, Ney R, Amberger M. The influence of flumazenil on respiration after midazolam and/or fentanyl [abstract]. *Anesth Analg.* 1990;70:S409.
71. Tote S, Mulleague L. The role of flumazenil in self-harm with benzodiazepines: to give or not to give? *Hosp Med.* 2005;66:308.
72. Van der Rijt CC, de Knegt RJ, Schalm SW, et al. Flumazenil does not improve hepatic encephalopathy associated with acute ischemic liver failure in the rabbit. *Metab Brain Dis.* 1990;3:131-141.
73. Weinbroum A, Geller E. The respiratory effects of reversing midazolam sedation with flumazenil in the presence or absence of narcotics. *Acta Anaesth Scand.* 1990;92:65-69.
74. Weinbroum A, Halpern P, Geller E. The use of flumazenil in the management of acute drug poisoning: a review. *Intensive Care Med.* 1991;17:S32-S38.
75. Weinbroum A, Szold O, Ogorek D, et al. The midazolam-induced paradox phenomenon is reversible by flumazenil. Epidemiology, patient characteristics and review of the literature. *Eur J Anaesthesiology.* 2001;18:789-797.
76. Weinbroum MD, Rudick V, Sorkine P, et al. Use of flumazenil in the treatment of drug overdose: a double-blind and open clinical study in 110 patients. *Crit Care Med.* 1996;24:199-206.
77. Wiley CC, Wiley JF 2nd. Pediatric benzodiazepine ingestion resulting in hospitalization. *J Toxicol Clin Toxicol.* 1998;36:227-231.
78. Winkler E, Shlomo A, Kriger D, et al. Use of flumazenil in the diagnosis and treatment of patients with coma of unknown etiology. *Crit Care Med.* 1993;21:538-542.
79. Whitwan G, Amrein R. Pharmacology of flumazenil. *Acta Anaesthesiol Scand.* 1995;39(Suppl 108):3-14.

H.

SUBSTANCES OF ABUSE

CHAPTER 75
AMPHETAMINES

William K. Chiang

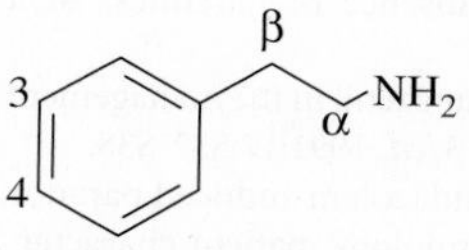

Phenylethylamine

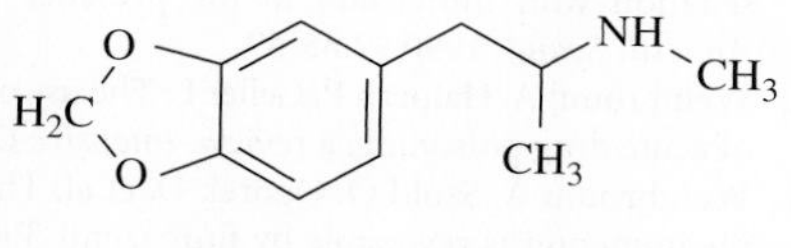

Methylenedioxymethamphetamine

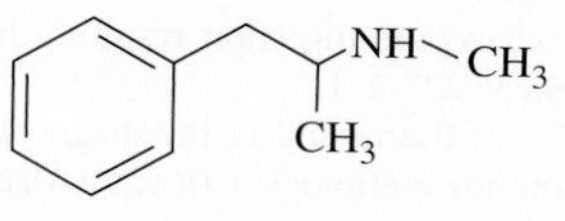

Methamphetamine

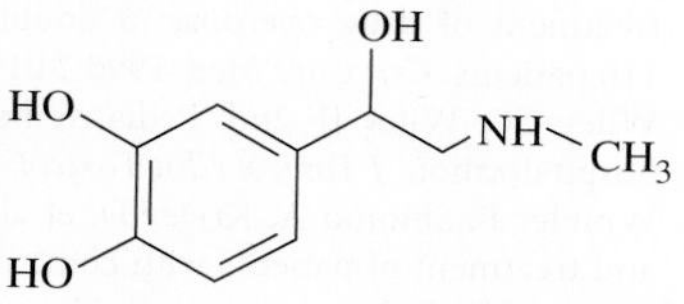

Epinephrine

Amphetamine is the trivial name and acronym for racemic β-phenylisopropylamine or α-methylphenylethylamine. Numerous substitutions of the phenylethylamine structure are possible, resulting in different amphetamine like compounds. Commonly, these compounds are referred to as amphetamines or amphetamine analogs, although phenylethylamine is the more precise term. For the purposes of this chapter, the term *amphetamines* refers to amphetamine analogs, and *amphetamine* specifically refers to β-phenylisopropylamine.

Since the initial marketing of amphetamines, continued abuse and misuse have been substantial.[18,103,184] Over the years amphetamines have been advocated by the medical communities for the treatment of depression, obesity, enuresis, postencephalitic parkinsonism, coma, ADHD, and even alcoholism.[103,139]

Currently, there are very few medical indications for amphetamines, which include narcolepsy, attention deficit hyperactivity disorder, and short-term weight reduction.[124] The prescriptive amphetamines include methylphenidate, pemoline, phentermine, phendimetrazine, amphetamine, dextroamphetamine, and methamphetamine. Due to their structural differences, some amphetamines can technically be marketed as nonamphetamine products. There continues to be a resurgence of amphetamine abuse, particularly with methamphetamine and methylenedioxymethamphetamine (MDMA).[49,101,208,210,268,275]

HISTORY AND EPIDEMIOLOGY

Edeleano first synthesized amphetamine (racemic β-phenylisopropylamine) in 1887.[103] However, it was not rediscovered until the 1920s, when there was significant concern about the supply of ephedrine for asthma therapy. In the search for the synthesis for ephedrine, Alles from UCLA rediscovered dextroamphetamine, and Ogata from Japan discovered methamphetamine (*d*-phenylisopropylmethylamine hydrochloride).[103] Amphetamine was marketed as Benzedrine inhaler, a nasal decongestant, by Smith, Kline, and French in 1932.[18] Amphetamine tablets were available in 1935 for the treatment of narcolepsy, and were advocated as anorexiants in 1938. The stimulant and euphoric effects of amphetamines were widely recognized, resulting in diverse forms of abuse and misuse. Amphetamine abuse was reported as early as 1936.[139] Benzedrine inhalers, each containing 250 mg of amphetamine, were widely abused, leading to a ban by the FDA in 1959. Propylhexedrine found in Benzedrex inhalers, a less-potent amphetamine like xenobiotic marketed in 1949, supplanted Benzedrine inhalers.[7] Propylhexedrine was also significantly misused.[7]

Both amphetamine and methamphetamine were supplied as stimulants for soldiers and prisoners of war in World War II.[18,185] Widespread methamphetamine abuse in Japan persisted for more than a decade after the war. From 1950 to the 1970s, there were sporadic periods of widespread amphetamine use and abuse in the United States. In the 1960s, various amphetamine derivatives such as methylenedioxyamphetamine (MDA) and *para*-methoxyamphetamine (PMA) were popularized as hallucinogens.[47] Until 1971, only a small proportion of the amphetamines produced by pharmaceutical companies was used for legitimate medical problems.[103,187] The Controlled Substance Act of 1970 placed amphetamines in Schedule II to prevent the diversion of pharmaceutical amphetamines for nonmedicinal uses.[54] Amphetamine abuse subsequently declined in the 1970s.[39,149,183,187]

In the 1980s, the so-called designer amphetamines (Table 75–1), mostly methylenedioxy derivatives of amphetamine and methamphetamine, came into vogue, as a mechanism of circumventing existing regulations. The most well-known xenobiotics were MDMA and 3,4-methylenedioxyethamphetamine (MDEA), but more than 200 different derivatives are known.[64,249] Before 1986, the Controlled Substances Act classified drugs as illegal only after they were synthesized and formally recognized by their structure, effects, or illegal usage. During this period, any analogs, such as these "designer drugs" not yet formally classified could be sold legally. In 1986, the standard became prospective for any xenobiotic that was used as a stimulant, hallucinogen, or depressant, and for any xenobiotic designed as such.[27] In effect, this amendment eliminated the legal loophole that allowed the designer drug industry to flourish. Although the meaning of the term "designer drugs" has changed and is no longer legally relevant, many of these analogs are still illicitly available.[119,131,177]

From the late 1980s until today, a dramatic resurgence of methamphetamine abuse spread throughout much of the United States. A high purity preparation of methamphetamine hydrochloride was marketed in a large crystalline form termed "ice" by abusers.[10,44,67,184] In fact, methamphetamine surpassed cocaine and became the primary substance of abuse among those seeking care in the drug treatment programs of San Diego and San Francisco counties in the 1990s.[101,116,188] From 1991 to

TABLE 75–1. Designer Amphetamines

Xenobiotic	Clinical Manifestations	Structure
4-Bromo-2,5-dimethoxyamphetamine (DOB)	Marked psychoactive effect potency > mescaline Delayed onset of action, peak 3–4 h Fantasy, mood altering for 10 h, resolution 12–24 h Agitation, sympathetic excess Sold as impregnated paper, like LSD	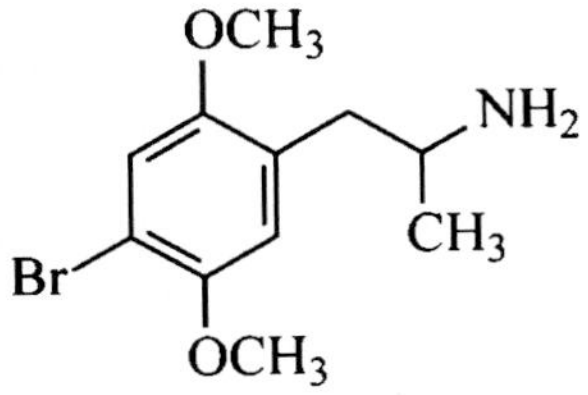 OCH_3, NH_2, CH_3, Br, OCH_3
4-Bromo-2,5-methoxyphenyl-ethylamine (2CB, MFT)	Relaxation Sensory distortion Agitation Hallucination Potency > mescaline	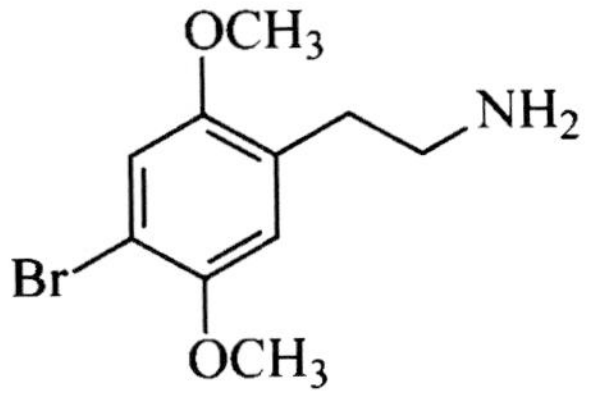 OCH_3, NH_2, Br, OCH_3
Methcathinone (cat, Jeff, Khat, ephedrone)	Hallucinations sympathetic excess	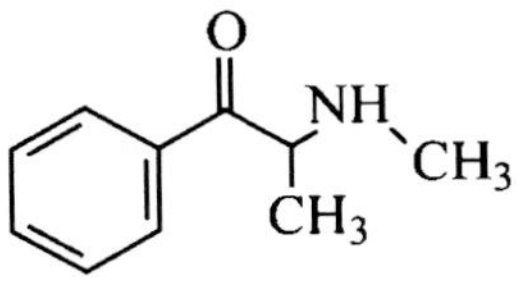 O, NH, CH_3, CH_3
4-Methyl-2,5-dimethoxyamphetamine (DOM/STP) (serenity, tranquility, peace)	Narrow therapeutic index Euphoria, perceptual distortion Hallucinations, sympathetic excess	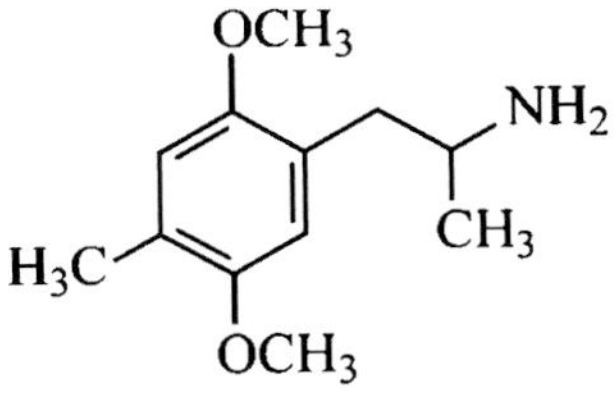 OCH_3, NH_2, CH_3, H_3C, OCH_3
3,4-Methylenedioxyamphetamine (MDA, love drug)	Empathy, euphoria Agitation, delirium, hallucinations, death associated with sympathetic excess	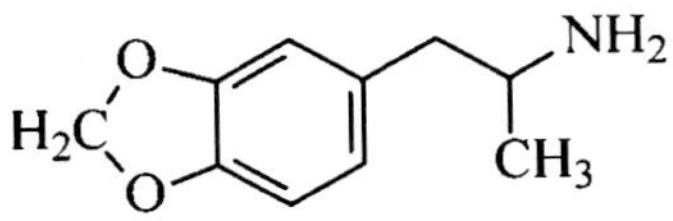 O, H_2C, O, NH_2, CH_3
3,4-Methylenedioxyethamphetamine (MDEA, Eve)	Comparable to MDMA Sympathetic excess	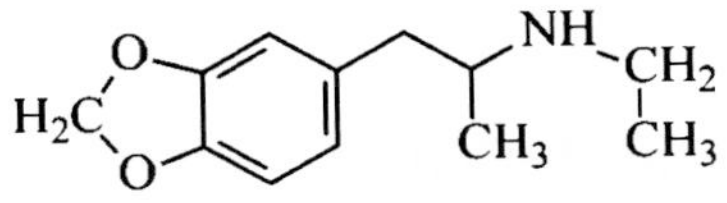 O, H_2C, O, NH, CH_2, CH_3, CH_3
3,4-Methylenedioxymethamphetamine (MDMA, Adam, ecstasy, XTC)	Psychotherapy "facilitator" Euphoria, empathy Nausea, anorexia Anxiety, insomnia Sympathetic excess	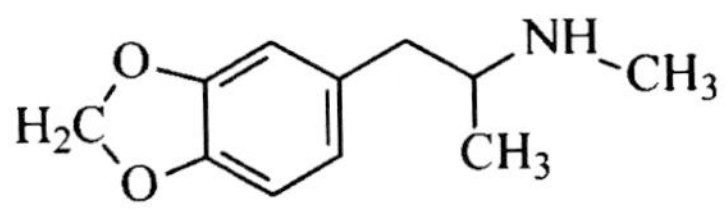 O, H_2C, O, NH, CH_3, CH_3
para-Methoxyamphetamine (PMA)	Potent hallucinogen Sympathetic excess	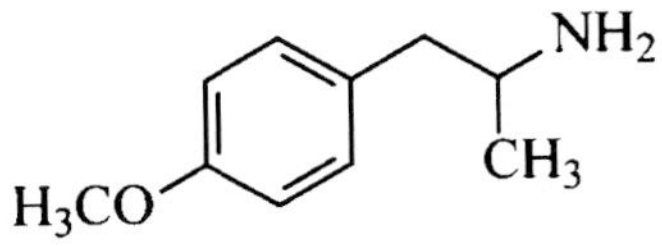 NH_2, CH_3, H_3CO
2,4,5-Trimethoxyamphetamine	Similar to mescaline	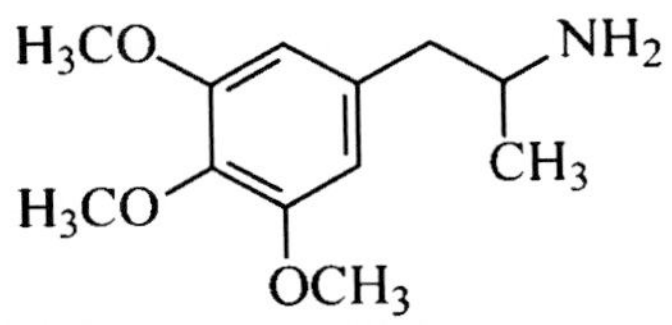 H_3CO, H_3CO, OCH_3, NH_2, CH_3

1994, the number of methamphetamine-related deaths in the United States reported by medical examiners tripled from 151 to 433, with a disproportional distribution from the Los Angeles, San Diego, San Francisco, and Phoenix metropolitan areas. The number of methamphetamine-related emergency department (ED) visits also increased from 4900 in 1991 to 17,400 in 1994.[101] The number of methamphetamine-related ED visits has remained stable since the mid-1990s despite significant local geographical changes.[73] The 2007 national survey on drug use and health demonstrated a stabilization or slight decline in methamphetamine use.[261] Recently, methamphetamine use has become particularly prevalent among men having sex with men in New York City.[108] Although the initial source of methamphetamine was from Pacific Rim countries such as Korea and Taiwan, currently the majority is produced in the United States.[45,80,268] Methamphetamine is the most common illicit drug produced by clandestine laboratories in the United States at this time. Because of the ease and low cost of methamphetamine synthesis and the local production, the end user cost of methamphetamine is less than one-third that of cocaine.[80] Methamphetamine production in the United States was primarily located in California and Oregon in the late 1990s, but it has spread through every state, although it remains particularly prevalent in the midwest and western United States.[268] The number of clandestine methamphetamine laboratory seizures nationally increased from 327 in 1995 to 15,994 in 2004. Both the cost and the prolonged duration of effect may contribute to the increased popularity of methamphetamine.[101,268]

Beginning in the mid-1990s, MDMA became and remains the amphetamine most widely used by college students and teenagers. MDMA is used by this population in large gatherings, known as "rave" or "techno" parties in England, Australia, and the United States.[215,216,275] MDMA use is prevalent in parties and clubs worldwide. Other MDMA-like analogs are often used or sold as MDMA in these gatherings.[11,275] Despite the popularity of MDMA, recent data in the United States demonstrate a decline in its past year use.[262]

Reports of methcathinone (a Khat-derived substance) use in the midwestern United States,[96,286] and a resurgence of 4-bromo-2,5-methoxyphenylethylamine (2CB) in dance clubs occurred in the 1990s.[77,90] Fortunately, the fear for the widespread use of these agents never materialized. Although the trend of a particular amphetamine analog waxes and wanes, use and abuse of amphetamines in general has continued unabated for the last quarter century.

PHARMACOLOGY

The pharmacologic effects of amphetamines are complex but the primary mechanism of action is the release of catecholamines, particularly dopamine and norepinephrine, from the presynaptic terminals. Although there are conflicting mechanistic models of amphetamine induction of catecholamine release, the variable results may be directly correlated with the different concentrations of amphetamines used in experimental models.[189] The best models to study the mechanism of action of amphetamines are based on dopaminergic neurons; similar mechanisms are invoked for norepinephrine and serotonin. Two storage pools exist for dopamine in the presynaptic terminals: the vesicular pool and the cytoplasmic pool. The vesicular storage of dopamine and other biogenic amines is maintained by the acidic environment within the vesicles and the persistence of a stabilizing electrical gradient with respect to the cytoplasm. This environment is maintained by an adenosine triphosphate (ATP)-dependent active proton transport system.[243] At low doses, amphetamines release dopamine from the cytoplasmic pool by exchange diffusion at the dopamine uptake transporter site in the membrane. At moderate doses, amphetamines diffuse through the presynaptic terminal membrane and interact with the neurotransmitter transporter on the vesicular membrane to cause exchange release of dopamine into the cytoplasm. Dopamine is subsequently released into the synapse by reverse transport at the dopamine uptake site.[243,264] At high doses, an additional mechanism is invoked as amphetamine diffuses through the cellular and vesicular membranes, alkalinizing the vesicles, and permitting dopamine release from the vesicles and delivery into the synapse by reverse transport.[264,265] Binding selectivity to the neurotransmitter transporters largely determines the range of pharmacologic effects for the particular amphetamine. The affinity of MDMA for serotonin transporters is 10 times greater than that for dopamine and norepinephrine transporters, hence it produces primarily serotonergic effects.[99]

Amphetamines may also block the reuptake of catecholamines by competitive inhibition.[104,124] However, the effects of this mechanism are considered to be minor. At higher doses, amphetamines can cause the release of serotonin (5-hydroxytryptamine [5-HT]) and affect central serotonin receptors. Certain amphetamines, such as MDMA and 4-bromo-2,5-dimethoxyamphetamine (DOB), have more significant serotonergic effects.[87,124] Amphetamines are structurally similar to nonhydrazine amine-derivative monoamine oxidase inhibitors such as phenelzine and tranylcypromine, and most amphetamines retain a weak monoamine oxidase-inhibiting activity, the clinical significance of which is unclear.[212]

The most identifiable effects of amphetamines are those caused by catecholamine release and the resultant stimulation of peripheral α- and β-adrenergic receptors. In the central nervous system, increased norepinephrine at the locus caeruleus mediates the anorectic and alerting effects, and also some locomotor stimulation.[103] The increase in central nervous system dopamine, particularly in the neostriatum, mediates stereotypical behavior and other locomotor activities.[53,94,104,141] The activity of dopamine in the neostriatum appears to be linked to glutamate release and inhibition of GABAergic efferent neurons.[94,140,141] Stimulation of the glutamatergic system contributes significantly to the stereotypical behavior, locomotor activity, and neurotoxicity of amphetamines.[19,25,140,141,257,258] The effects of serotonin and dopamine on the mesolimbic system alter perception and cause psychotic behavior.[94,123,263]

Because amphetamines directly interact with neurotransmitter transporters, minor modifications of the molecule may significantly alter its pharmacologic profile.[129] The α-methyl group in the amphetamine structure introduces chirality to the molecule. Except for MDMA and certain MDMA analogs, the *d*-enantiomers are typically 4–10 times more potent than the *l* forms of amphetamines. Substitutions at different positions of the phenylethylamine molecule alter the general clinical effects of amphetamines, as demonstrated by both animal and human observations. Xenobiotics with methyl substitution at the α carbon, such as amphetamine and methamphetamine, possess strong stimulant, cardiovascular, and anorectic properties.[93,196] Large group substitution at the α carbon reduces the stimulant and cardiovascular effects, but retains the anorectic properties (such as in phentermine).[13] Substitution at the *para* position of the phenyl ring enhances the hallucinogenic or serotonergic effects of amphetamines (such as in *para*-chloroamphetamine and MDMA).[13,84,181] Although some of these generalizations enable scientists to understand the effects of amphetamines, there are many exceptions, and such generalizations may not apply when large doses of a particular molecule are ingested.[74] In terms of the spectrum of activities, methamphetamine results in the most potent cardiovascular effects, and DOB results in the most consequential hallucinogenic and serotonergic effects.[93,196]

PHARMACOKINETICS AND TOXICOKINETICS

In general, amphetamines are relatively lipophilic and hence they can readily cross the blood–brain barrier. They have large volumes of distribution, varying from 3–5 L/kg for amphetamine and 3–4 L/kg for methamphetamine and phentermine, to 11–33 L/kg for methylphenidate. Pemoline is the exception as it has a small volume of distribution (0.2–0.6 L/kg).[12] Amphetamines differ from catecholamines in that they lack the catechol structure (hydroxyl groups at the 3 and 4 positions of the phenyl ring) and are resistant to metabolism by catechol-O-methyltransferase (COMT).[124] The addition of an α-methyl group in amphetamines confers resistance to metabolism by monoamine oxidase. These characteristics permit better oral bioavailability and a longer duration of effects.[196]

Amphetamines are eliminated via multiple pathways, including diverse routes of hepatic transformation, and by renal elimination. For MDMA and its analogs, *N*-dealkylation, hydroxylation, and demethylation are the dominant hepatic pathways.[45,46,172] Depending on the particular xenobiotic, active metabolites of secondary amphetamines and ephedrine derivatives may be formed.[12,45] *N*-demethylation of methamphetamine and MDMA result in the formation of amphetamine and MDA, respectively.[45] Dealkylation and demethylation are mainly performed by cytochrome P450 (CYP) isoenzymes, including CYP1A2, CYP2D6, and CYP3A4, but they are also performed by flavin monooxygenases.[172] Polymorphism of CYP2D6 in humans was discovered as a result of decreased *p*-hydroxylation of amphetamine in certain individuals. Since its discovery, CYP2D6 polymorphism has been implicated in drug toxicity, substance use and abuse, and lack of drug efficacy in predisposed individuals.[246] Increased amphetamine toxicity is a potential concern in patients with decreased CYP2D6 activity. Although animals with CYP2D6 deficiency are more susceptible to MDMA toxicity,[51] limited studies in humans do not demonstrate an association of mortality and CYP2D6 deficiency.[88,199] In general, because multiple enzymes and pathways, including renal are involved in amphetamine elimination, it is less likely that CYP2D6 polymorphism or drug interactions with CYP3A4 alone will significantly increase toxicity. However, it is unclear if toxicity is enhanced in the simultaneous presence of altered drug metabolism and renal dysfunction.

Renal elimination is substantial for amphetamine (30%), methamphetamine (40%–50%), MDMA (65%), and phentermine (80%). Amphetamines are relatively strong bases with a typical pK_a range from 9–10, and renal elimination varies depending on the urine pH.[12] The half-life of amphetamines varies significantly: amphetamine, 8–30 hours; methamphetamine, 12–34 hours; MDMA, 5–10 hours; methylphenidate, 2.5–4 hours; and phentermine, 19–24 hours.[12,45] Repetitive administration, which typically occurs during binge use, may lead to drug accumulation and prolongation of the apparent half-life and duration of effect.[133]

CLINICAL MANIFESTATIONS

The clinical effects of amphetamines are largely related to the stimulation of central and peripheral adrenergic receptors. These clinical manifestations and their associated complications are similar to those from cocaine use and may be indistinguishable except for the duration of effect of amphetamines, which tends to be longer (up to 24 hours).[67]

Compared to cocaine, amphetamines are less likely to cause seizures, dysrhythmias, and myocardial ischemia. This may be related to the sodium channel–blocking effects and to the thrombogenic effect of cocaine.[95] Psychosis appears to be more likely with amphetamines than cocaine, which may be related to the more prominent dopaminergic effects of amphetamines.[9,94] Tachycardia and hypertension are the most common manifestations of cardiovascular toxicity. Most patients present to the ED, however, because of the CNS manifestations.[67,130,279] These patients are anxious, volatile, aggressive, and may have life-threatening agitation. Visual and tactile hallucinations, as well as psychoses, are common.[22,68,69,114,164,226,239] Other sympathetic findings include mydriasis, diaphoresis, and hyperthermia (Table 75–2).[68,72]

TABLE 75–2. Clinical Manifestations of Amphetamine Toxicity

Acute	Mydriasis
Cardiovascular system	Tremor
Hypertension	Nausea
Tachycardia	**Other organ system manifestations**
Dysrhythmias	Rhabdomyolysis
Myocardial ischemia	Muscle rigidity
Aortic dissection	Acute lung injury
Vasospasm	Ischemic colitis
Central nervous system	**Laboratory abnormalities**
Hyperthermia	Leukocytosis
Agitation	Hyperglycemia
Seizures	Hyponatremia
Intracerebral hemorrhage	Elevated CPK
Headache	Elevated liver enzymes
Euphoria	Myoglobinuri
Anorexia	
Bruxism	**Chronic**
Choreoathetoid movements	Vasculitis
Hyperreflexia	Cardiomyopathy
Paranoid psychosis	Pulmonary hypertension
Other sympathetic symptoms	Aortic and mitral regurgitation
Diaphoresis	Permanent damage to dopaminergic
Tachypnea	and serotonergic neurons

Death from amphetamine toxicity most commonly results from hyperthermia, dysrhythmias, and intracerebral hemorrhage.[40,63,81,136,143,163,206,227] Direct CNS effects may result in seizures. Tachycardia, hypertension, and vasospasm may lead to cerebral infarction,[97,153,231] intraparenchymal and subarachnoid hemorrhage,[59,112,127,142,258,281] myocardial ischemia or infarction,[83,207,272] aortic dissection,[59,71] acute lung injury,[30,193,194] obstetrical complications, fetal death,[162] and ischemic colitis.[17,121,134] Dysrhythmias vary from premature ventricular complexes to ventricular tachycardia and ventricular fibrillation.[136,165] Agitation, increased muscular activity, and hyperthermia can result in metabolic acidosis, rhabdomyolysis,[56] acute tubular necrosis (acute renal failure), and coagulopathy.[72,89,135,144] Unless these systemic signs and symptoms are rapidly reversed, multiorgan failure and death may ensue.

Amphetamine users seeking intense "highs" may go on "speed runs" for days to weeks. Because of the development of acute CNS tolerance, they use increasing amounts of amphetamines during these periods, usually without much nutritional sustenance or sleep, attempting to achieve their desired euphoria.[18,54,155,253,266] Acute psychosis resembling paranoid schizophrenia may occur during these binges and has contributed to both amphetamine-related suicides and homicides.[75,151] Return to a normal sensorium occurs within a few days after discontinuation of the drug. Once an amphetamine user experiences psychosis, it is likely to be recurrent, even after prolonged abstinence, which may be related to a *kindling phenomenon*.[18,204,266] Amphetamine-induced psychosis has contributed to the understanding of the function of dopamine in schizophrenia. Typically after such binges, patients may sleep for prolonged periods of time, feeling hungry and depressed when awake. During this period of depression or withdrawal, the patient continues to crave amphetamines.[114,152,158]

There are some direct neurologic effects of amphetamines. Compulsive repetitive behavior patterns are reported in humans and animals. Individuals may constantly pick at their skin, grind their teeth (bruxism), or perform repetitive tasks, such as constantly cleaning their house or car.[18] MDMA users often carry pacifiers to relieve bruxism. Choreoathetoid movements, although uncommon, are reported with acute and chronic amphetamine usage.[150,167,171,219,238,252] The etiology of the choreoathetoid movements may be related to increased dopaminergic stimulation in the striatal area.

Necrotizing vasculitis is associated with amphetamine abuse.[20,48] Angiography typically demonstrates beading and narrowing of the small- and medium-sized arteries (see Fig. 5–25).[233,260] Progressive necrotizing arteritis[59] can involve multiple organ systems, including the central nervous, cardiovascular, gastrointestinal, and renal systems. Complications include cerebral infarction and hemorrhage, coronary artery disease, pancreatitis, and renal failure.[48,111,166,233,237,260,281,285] The etiology of the arteritis remains unclear. Although various contaminants associated with injection drug use were postulated as potential etiologies, oral and IV amphetamine use in animal models are also associated with vasculitis, suggesting that this is a direct amphetamine effect.[234,235,269] Cardiomyopathy is also reported with acute and chronic amphetamine abuse.[20,125,200,255] Excessive catecholamine exposure in patients with pheochromocytomas and chronic cocaine use may be responsible for their associated cardiomyopathies; amphetamine-induced cardiomyopathy may be produced by similar mechanisms.[103,138,278]

Valvular heart disease is also associated with the use of the appetite-suppressants fenfluramine, dexfenfluramine, and phentermine, particularly if the duration of therapy is greater than 4 months.[52,85,132,146,276] The initial reports, in 1997, implicated significant aortic and mitral regurgitation with the use of these drugs and the prevalence was as high as 32%.[38] These reports resulted in the withdrawal of fenfluramine and dexfenfluramine. Subsequent studies demonstrated mostly mild aortic regurgitation and possibly mitral regurgitation; the overall prevalence varies from study to study, ranging from 0.14% to 22.7%.[85,132,146,274,283] The highest risks appear to be in patients taking combination therapy with fenfluramine and phentermine, and those who used the drugs for prolonged periods (>4 months).[132] The dramatic differences in the overall prevalence rate in these studies may be related to differences in patient population, duration of therapy, and the timing of echocardiography (ie, during therapy or after the cessation of therapy). A meta-analysis demonstrated a 12% prevalence rate of valvular regurgitation (mostly aortic) with more than 90-day use of the appetite-suppressants, compared to 5.9% in the unexposed group. There was no difference when the appetite suppressants were used less than 90 days.[236] Echocardiographic findings of the valvular dysfunction typically improve following cessation of these drugs.[120] The exact etiology of the valvular disease is postulated to be related to increased serotonin or direct effects on 5-HT_{2B} receptors. Similar valvular disorders are recognized in patients exposed to persistently increased serotonin concentrations with conditions such as malignant carcinoid syndrome; it is unclear why the carcinoid syndrome predominantly affects right-sided valves, whereas these drugs primarily affect left-sided valves.[228]

Primary pulmonary hypertension, a rare and potentially fatal disease, is reported with chronic methamphetamine and propylhexedrine use.[7,43,70,156,241] However, substantial epidemiologic risk for primary pulmonary hypertension is demonstrated only with fenfluramine, aminorex (2-amino-5-phenyl-2-oxazoline), and methamphetamine.[24,105,250] One recent study also linked methampetamine use with pulmonary hypertension.[43] Pulmonary hypertension was associated with the use of Aminorex—as an anorectic agent in Europe from 1965 to 1968.[106] In 1996, a case-controlled study substantiated the increased risk of pulmonary hypertension with the use of amphetamine appetite-suppressant drugs, particularly with fenfluramine.[1] The risk of pulmonary hypertension was increased 23-fold when the cumulative use of anorectics totaled more than 3 months,[1] but may develop following exposure to anorectics that may be as brief as 3 weeks.[105] Increased serotonin or direct effects on 5-HT_{2B} receptors in the pulmonary vasculature is postulated to result in pulmonary vasoconstriction and endothelial proliferation.[122,193,229] Interestingly, although fenfluramine is a weak agonist for 5-HT_{2B} receptors, its metabolite norfenfluramine is a potent agonist for 5-HT_{2B} receptors and may be responsible for causing pulmonary hypertension.[126] Although MDMA use has not been associated with pulmonary hypertension, MDMA and its metabolite MDA have significant effects on 5-HT_{2B} receptor activity and can induce cardiac valvular interstitial cell proliferation in vitro.[230] With widespread MDMA use, both pulmonary hypertension and valvular diseases are potential public health concerns.[247] Pulmonary hypertension that develops following the use of anorectics may be partially reversible after withdrawal of the xenobiotic; however, the median survival of patients studied during the European Aminorex epidemic was 3.5 years from the time of diagnosis.[105] With current advances in therapy, improved survival is expected.[232]

Although the chronic administration of MDMA and its analogs are better publicized, chronic administration of various amphetamines, including amphetamine and methamphetamine, to animals alters dopamine and serotonin transporter functions, depletes dopamine and serotonin in the neuronal synapses, and produces irreversible destruction of those neurons.[16,87,222,223,225,242,281] The etiology of neuronal toxicity may be related to the generation of oxygen free radicals, resulting in the generation of toxic dopamine and serotonin metabolites and neuronal destruction.[87,157,244,281,282] Based on animal models, dose, frequency and duration of exposure, and ambient temperature can affect neurologic injuries. Intact dopamine or serotonin transporters are necessary to produce neurologic injury. Xenobiotics that inhibit transporter function may prevent neurologic injuries in animals.[99] Significant differences are also noted across species; mice are typically resistant to MDMA-induced neurologic injury.[175] Although not as well studied as MDMA, studies of former methamphetamine users demonstrated impaired memory and psychomotor functions, as well as corresponding dopamine transporter dysfunction and abnormal glucose metabolism on PET scans.[245,270,271] However, it is still not clear as to the difference in species susceptibility to neurologic injuries, the duration of effects in primates and humans, and functional consequences of neurotoxicity in humans. The potential for permanent neurologic effects associated with chronic amphetamine use in humans requires further study. Despite the first report of neurologic injuries from methamphetamine in animals in 1976, many questions remain unanswered.

Finally, multiple medical complications can result from injection drug use and from the associated contaminants. Contamination with microbials may result in HIV infection, hepatitis, and malaria. Bacterial and foreign-body contamination may result in endocarditis, tetanus, wound botulism, osteomyelitis, and pulmonary and soft-tissue abscesses.[42]

DIAGNOSTIC TESTING

Diagnosis by history is rarely reliable as patients often do not know the exact xenobiotic they have used.[149] Also, there is no readily available xenobiotic-specific serum analysis. Qualitative urine immunoassay testing for amphetamines is available, but it is not valuable in the acute overdose setting. Typically, the turnaround time for the test result is at least several hours, which is far too long to be clinically useful. Both false-positive and false-negative results are common. For example, many cold preparations contain structurally similar substances such as pseudoephedrine that may cross-react with the immunoassay.[50,57,82,213] Likewise, selegiline, a selective monoamine oxidase type B (MAO-B) inhibitor used for the treatment of parkinsonism, is metabolized to amphetamine and methamphetamine. Patients taking selegiline will have a positive screen with most amphetamine-testing techniques.[139] Even a true-positive result only means the patient has used an amphetamine analog within the last several days. In addition, most immunoassays do not react with all amphetamines, resulting in false-negative results. For example, MDMA frequently is unrecognized on standard urinary drug testing.[17,50] Although newer, rapid, serum qualitative drug screens are available, false-positive and false-negative results remain common and may be misleading. The gold standard for drug testing, gas chromatography–mass spectrometry analysis, can misidentify isomeric substances such as *l*-methamphetamine, which is present in nasal inhalers, with *d*-methamphetamine, if performed by inexperienced personnel.[254] In summary, the suspicion of amphetamine toxicity cannot be confirmed rapidly with a high degree of reliability by the laboratory.

The physical and psychological assessment is nonspecific, and polydrug use is quite common. As such, the prevalence of amphetamine use in the local geographic region should heighten the suspicion of amphetamine toxicity in patients with a suggestive presentation. Management decisions must be determined by the clinical manifestations and impressions.

Blood specimens should be sent for glucose, BUN, and electrolyte assays. Hyponatremia should be considered for any patient with an altered sensorium and suspected MDMA usage (Chap. 16).[173] An ECG should be obtained to exclude ischemia, hyperkalemia, and drug toxicity (cyclic antidepressant), and continuous cardiac monitoring should be initiated. A complete blood count, urinalysis, coagulation profile, chest radiograph, CT of the head, and lumbar puncture may be necessary, depending on the clinical presentation.

MANAGEMENT

Table 75–3 summarizes the therapeutic approach to a patient with amphetamine toxicity. The initial medical assessment of the agitated patient must include the vital signs and a rapid complete physical examination.

Hyperthermia, a frequent and rapidly fatal manifestation in patients with drug-induced delirium, requires immediate interventions to achieve cooling.[89,135,144] Some patients will require physical restraint to gain clinical control and prevent personal harm to themselves or others. Because agitation and resistance against physical restraint may lead to rhabdomyolysis and continued heat generation, intravenous chemical sedation should be instituted immediately. Intravenous (IV) glucose ($D_{50}W$, 0.5–1 g/kg) and thiamine 100 mg should be given as indicated.

Because the clinician cannot accurately distinguish the diverse etiologies of xenobiotic-induced delirium, the choice of chemical sedation should be safe and effective regardless of the etiology. The most appropriate choice of sedation is benzodiazepines because they have a high therapeutic index and good anticonvulsant activity. They are effective not only for the treatment of delirium induced by acute overdose of cocaine, amphetamines, and other xenobiotics but also the delirium associated with ethanol and sedative-hypnotic withdrawal (see A-24 Benzodiazepines).[65,68,95,205] The dose of the chosen benzodiazepine should be titrated rapidly intravenously until the patient is calm. In our clinical experience, cumulative benzodiazepine dosages required in the initial 30 minutes to achieve adequate sedation frequently exceed 100 mg of diazepam or its equivalent. Antipsychotics, particularly potent dopamine antagonists such as haloperidol and droperidol, are frequently recommended by others for amphetamine-induced delirium. Antipsychotics may actually antagonize some of the effects of amphetamines via dopamine blockade.[65,66,78] In animal models, haloperidol may be superior to diazepam in preventing mortality from amphetamine toxicity.[35,61,65,66] In clinical experience, however, the benzodiazepines appear to be as efficacious as the antipsychotics in the management of amphetamine toxicity.[68] Antipsychotics may lower the seizure threshold, alter temperature regulation, may cause acute dystonia and cardiac dysrhythmias, and do not interact with the benzodiazepine–γ-aminobutyric acid (GABA)–chloride channel receptor complex. All of these effects may worsen the clinical outcomes related to occult or concomitant cocaine toxicity and ethanol withdrawal.[95,100,205]

Rhabdomyolysis from amphetamine toxicity usually results from agitation and hyperthermia.[84,144] Sedation prevents further muscle contraction and heat production. External cooling should be instituted for significant hyperthermia. Adequate IV hydration and cardiovascular support should maintain urine output of 1–2 mL/kg/h. Although urinary acidification can significantly increase amphetamine elimination and decrease the half-lives of amphetamine and methamphetamine,[12,14,15,60] this pH manipulation does not decrease toxicity, and, in fact, may increase the risk of renal compromise and acute tubular necrosis from rhabdomyolysis by precipitating ferrihemate in the renal tubules.[56] Patients with acute renal failure, acidemia, and hyperkalemia will likely require urgent hemodialysis.

Amphetamine body packers should be treated similarly to those who transport cocaine (Chap. 76 and Special Considerations: SC-4 Internal Concealment of Xenobiotics). Any sympathomimetic symptom suggesting leakage of the packets requires surgical intervention.[273] Intravenous fluids, benzodiazepines, intubation, and external cooling may be necessary to stabilize these patients.

TABLE 75–3. Management of Patients with Amphetamine Toxicity

Agitation
Benzodiazepines (usually adequate for the cardiovascular manifestations)
Diazepam 10 mg (or equivalent) IV, repeat rapidly until the patient is calm (cumulative dose may be as high as 100 mg of diazepam)
Seizures
Benzodiazepines
Barbiturates
Propofol
Hyperthermia
External cooling
Control agitation rapidly
Gastric decontamination and elimination
Activated charcoal for recent oral ingestions
Hypertension
Control agitation first
α-Adrenergic receptor antagonist (phentolamine)
Vasodilator (nitroprusside, nitroglycerin or possibly nicardipine)
Delirium or hallucinations with abnormal vital signs
If agitated: benzodiazepines
Delirium or hallucinations with normal vital signs
Consider risk/benefit of haloperidol or droperidol

INDIVIDUAL XENOBIOTICS

METHAMPHETAMINE

From the 1950s to the 1970s, there were multiple epidemics of methamphetamine abuse in the United States.[18] Methamphetamine was and sometimes still is referred to as "crack," "speed," "yaba," and "go." The pharmacologic profile of methamphetamine is quite similar to amphetamine, although the effects on the central nervous system are more substantial.[44] "Ice," the common name for methamphetamine in the 1990s because of the crystal forms, does not differ pharmacologically from other forms of methamphetamine. Methamphetamine is readily absorbed by the oral, parenteral, and inhalational routes. Because of a prolonged half-life of 19–34 hours, the duration of its acute effects can be greater than 24 hours.[44,67,68]

Since the 1990s, the activity and purity of methamphetamine available on the street is substantially higher than previous epidemics because of the improved methods of synthesis.[160] Methamphetamine is now typically greater than 80%–90% pure and almost exclusively in the dextroisomer form, which is most active on the CNS.

Methamphetamine is easily synthesized with the proper chemicals and minimal equipment.[86] The primary ingredient of methamphetamine synthesis is ephedrine, which can be hydrogenated into methamphetamine. The ephedrine method, using pharmaceutical grade L-ephedrine, produces a product with few contaminants that is stereochemically pure.[67,214] The production of the large crystal is possible by creating a supersaturated solution of methamphetamine hydrochloride.[67] Nonprescription sales of ephedrine are now restricted and monitored in many states.[268] Phenyl-2-propanone (P2P), as an alternative ingredient, can be methylated into ephedrine and then into methamphetamine.[29] Because of the strict control of ephedrine and P2P, illicit chemists use phenylacetic acid to synthesize P2P.[29,58] Lead acetate, which is used as a substrate for the reaction, resulted in an epidemic of lead poisoning associated with methamphetamine abuse in Oregon.[3,41] Lead concentrations reported in drug users were as high as 513 μg/dL, and some samples of illicitly manufactured methamphetamine had lead contents as high as 60% by weight.[41] Mercury contamination was also documented, although clinical mercury toxicity has not been reported.[27] The number of potential chemicals involved in the methamphetamine manufacturing process is significant, and without any legal monitoring, contamination of the product and the environment is inevitable.[4,29,128,154,217] In fact, in certain periods 20%–30% of the illicit methamphetamine manufacturing sites discovered were discovered because of laboratory explosions.[80] In San Bernardino County, California alone in 1995, 360 methamphetamine laboratories were identified and closed by drug enforcement agents.[80] These makeshift methamphetamine laboratories pose a significant health risk to law enforcement officers and the general public, causing respiratory and ophthalmic irritation, headaches, and burns.[36,259] Methamphetamine laboratory–related burns were well reported from burn centers and associated with increased mortality. Currently, the sale of other potential amphetamine synthetic ingredients, such as hydrochloric acid, hydrogen chloride gas, anhydrous ammonia, red phosphorus, and iodine, are also monitored and restricted in the United States.[29,37,268]

3,4-METHYLENEDIOXYMETHAMPHETAMINE

MDMA was first synthesized in 1912, and was rediscovered in 1965 by Shulgin.[27] It is currently one of the most widely abused amphetamines by college students and teenagers.[49,208,275,279] It is commonly known as "ecstasy," "E," "Adam," "XTC," "M&M," and "MDM." Other structural relatives of MDMA, MDEA ("Eve") and MDA ("love drug"), are also used or distributed as MDMA in areas of MDMA use. These xenobiotics have similar clinical effects and acute and chronic toxicity. Other MDMA-related xenobiotics have been found at "rave" scenes, 2CB, 2,4-dimethoxy-4-(*n*)-propylthiophenylethylamine (2C-T7), and *N*-methyl-1-(3, 4-methylenedioxyphenyl)-2-butanamine (MBDB).[34,77,90,147] The term, "ecstasy" may be used for all of these xenobiotics. Typically, MDMA is available in colorful and branded tablets that vary from 50 mg to 200 mg. MDMA and similar analogs are so-called entactogens (meaning touching within), capable of producing euphoria, inner peace, and a desire to socialize.[177,256] In addition, some psychologists used MDMA to enhance psychotherapy until the Controlled Substances Act of 1986.[195] People who use MDMA report that it enhances pleasure, heightens sexuality, and expands consciousness without the loss of control.[27,102,177] Negative effects reported with acute use included ataxia, restlessness, confusion, poor concentration, and impaired memory.[256] MDMA has about one-tenth the CNS stimulant effect of amphetamine. Unlike amphetamine and methamphetamine, MDMA is a potent stimulus for the release of serotonin.[31,62,104] The concentration of MDMA required to stimulate the release of serotonin is 10 times less than that required for the release of dopamine or norepinephrine. In animal models, the stereotypic and discriminatory effects of MDMA and its congeners can be distinguished from those of other amphetamines.[32,195]

The sympathetic effects of MDMA are mild in low doses. However, when a large amount of MDMA is taken, the clinical presentation is similar to that of other amphetamines and deaths can result from abuse.[72,118,119,191,279] Those patients at greatest risk develop dysrhythmias, hyperthermia, rhabdomyolysis, and disseminated intravascular coagulation.[72,117,251] Significant hyponatremia is reported with MDMA use.[2,115,174,197] MDMA and its metabolites increase the release of vasopressin (antidiuretic hormone) and may be related to their serotonergic effects.[79,117] Furthermore, substantial free-water intake combined with sodium loss from physical exertion in dance clubs may be crucial to the development of hyponatremia.

A major concern with MDMA usage is its long-term effects on the brain. In numerous animal models, acute administration of MDMA leads to the decrease in serotonin reuptake transporter (SERT) function and numbers. Recovery of SERT function may take several weeks. Repetitive administration of MDMA ultimately leads to permanent damage to serotonergic neurons, typically causing injury to the axons and the terminals while sparing the cell bodies.[174,178,180,201,220,222] Some regeneration of synaptic terminals can occur even with neuronal damage, but functional recovery is incomplete. Intact SERT function is necessary for MDMA-induced neurotoxicity. Xenobiotics that inhibit the uptake of serotonin prevent MDMA-induced neurotoxicity in animals. Animal data suggest that MDMA induces hydroxyl free-radical generation and decreases antioxidants in serotonergic neurons.[224,248] MDMA does not directly cause neurotoxicity, but its metabolites 3-methyldopamine and *N*-methyl-α-methyldopamine do produce neurotoxicity in animals.[186] When antioxidants are depleted, neuronal damage may occur.

The evidence for these potential neurotoxic effects in humans is less clear.[148] Indirect evidence of serotonergic effects in humans includes lower concentrations of 5-hydroxyindoleacetic acid (5-HIAA) in the cerebral spinal fluid of MDMA users than in controls.[221] Case reports and studies of MDMA users demonstrate alteration in mood, sleep, anxiety, cognition, memory, and impulse control—all functions that are believed to be affected by serotonin.[5,176,179,181,185] Either single-photon emission tomography (SPECT) or positron emission tomography (PET) demonstrates decreased SERT function in MDMA users, even after prolonged abstinence.[28,202,218] Memory deficits appeared to persist even when MDMA users were abstinent.[98,190] A major deficit in human studies is finding appropriate control groups as people with psychiatric disease are also more likely to be or have been MDMA users.[182] MDMA users often are polydrug users. Currently, there are no available human postmortem histopathologic data for MDMA users.[147] Further studies are required to address the long-term neuropsychiatric effects of MDMA.

PROPYLHEXEDRINE

NH—CH_3
CH_3

Smith, Kline, and French introduced propylhexedrine in 1949 as the primary active ingredient in the Benzedrex nasal inhaler, which was to replace the widespread abuse of amphetamine nasal inhalers.[8,84] Propylhexedrine is an alicyclic aliphatic sympathomimetic amine that is structurally similar to amphetamine, with a local vasoconstrictive effect and approximately 10% of the CNS stimulatory effect of amphetamine.[8] Propylhexedrine abuse became prevalent after the removal of amphetamine from nasal inhalers. The abusers disassembled the inhaler and ingested the cotton pledget vehicle of propylhexedrine itself, diluted it in beverages, or reconstituted the drug for intravenous injection. Numerous effects were reported with propylhexedrine abuse, including sudden death, myocardial infarction, cardiomyopathy, pulmonary hypertension, and acute psychosis.[7,8,55,70,84,161,169,170,277] Although propylhexedrine in nasal inhalers has largely been replaced by safer sympathomimetics (Chap. 50), the drug is still readily available and is abused as an inexpensive, legal "high."

KHAT, CATHINONE, AND METHCATHINONE

Khat (also known as quat and gat), the fresh leaves and stems from the *Catha edulis* shrub, is a commonly used drug in eastern and central Africa, and in parts of the Arabian peninsula. Attention to khat was highlighted in the early 1990s by war media coverage in Somalia and Ethiopia. Khat is sold in small bundles of leaves in the local markets of these countries. The leaves and the tender stems are chewed or occasionally concocted into tea. Khat chewing has a significant role at social gatherings in these countries.[168] There is a trend of increasing khat consumption and binges among adolescents in these countries.[202] When the dried leaves and stems were studied, the primary active ingredient was thought to be cathine (norpseudoephedrine), present as 0.1%–0.2% of the dried material. Cathine has about one-tenth the stimulant effects of D-amphetamine and numerous other amphetamine-like compounds were also isolated, but occur in minute quantities.[137] When the fresh leaves are analyzed, however, cathinone (benzylketoamphetamine), a more potent psychoactive compound, was demonstrated to be the primary active agent.[91,107,137] As the leaves age, cathinone is degraded into cathine, which also explains why dried khat is neither popular nor widely distributed. Imported fresh khat must be consumed within a week, before it loses much of its potency. The primary effects of khat are increased alertness, insomnia, euphoria, anxiety, and hyperactivity. Increased khat consumption is linked to psychosis. Significant adrenergic complications are much less frequent than those associated with amphetamine abuse. Epidemiological studies demonstrated an association among khat chewing, psychosis, and myocardial infarction.[6,203]

Methcathinone, the methyl derivative of cathinone, chemically synthesized from ephedrine, has been abused in Russsia and other former countries of the Soviet Union, for many years. The potency of methcathinone is comparable to that of methamphetamine.[92,284] Methcathinone—also termed ephedrone, or sold under the street names of "cat" or "Jeff"—currently remains widely abused in Russia (see Chap. 95). Methcathinone abuse was first reported in Michigan[76] in the early 1990s and is now reported in other states as well.

EPHEDRINE OR MA-HUANG HERBAL PRODUCTS

OH
NH—CH_3
CH_3

Ephedrine is commonly found in nonprescription cold preparations. Ephedrine is also the active substance in the Chinese plant ma-huang, which has been used for centuries for the treatment of asthma. Although ephedrine is much less potent than amphetamine, when combined with other catecholamine stimulating xenobiotics, or when taken in large quantities, significant toxicity may occur.[26,33,209,240] In the United States, numerous ephedrine products, such as "go," "ultimate xphoria," "up your gas," and "herbal ecstasy," are marketed primarily to teenagers. Some of these products contain more than 500 mg of ephedrine, which may be combined with pseudoephedrine, phenylpropanolamine, and caffeine; other products contain the plant extract ma-huang.[159,209,211] Many of these products are marketed as legal stimulants or safe herbal stimulants for a natural "high." Similarly, ma-huang is also widely marketed as a "safe" herbal weight-reducing product. Sales appeared to increase when it was recognized that phenylpropanolamine was associated with intracerebral hemorrhage in women.[145] Unfortunately, these products are linked to numerous deaths and adverse reactions.[109,110,192,211,267,280,286] Because these products are sold as food supplements, they are not regulated by the FDA unless a product can be demonstrated to be unsafe (Chap. 43). In 2004, the FDA finally banned the use of ephedra products. In April 2005, a federal judge in Utah reversed the ban of ephedra sales in Utah, illustrating the difficulty of the FDA in the regulation of herbal products.[113] Herbal products with *Citrus aurantium* (bitter orange), contain a number of adrenergic amines, including synephrine and have now supplanted ephedra products. *Citrus aurantium* has similar pharmacologic effects and toxicity as ephedra.[21,198]

SUMMARY

Amphetamine usage continues to increase dramatically throughout the United States. Similarly, ED visits and morbidity and mortality related to amphetamines parallel amphetamine usage. Many of these complications are similar to those of cocaine, such as agitation, hyperthermia, rhabdomyolysis, myocardial ischemia, and cerebral infarction. Physicians, more than ever, must understand the pathophysiology of amphetamines and be prepared to diagnose and treat its toxicity. The chronic effects of amphetamines as demonstrated in animal models pose serious concerns for humans, particularly as amphetamine usage becomes more prevalent; further studies are required to achieve prevention and management.

REFERENCES

1. Abenhaim L, Moride Y, Brenot F, et al. Appetite-suppressant drugs and the risk of primary pulmonary hypertension. *N Engl J Med.* 1996;335:609-615.
2. Ajaelo I, Koenig K, Snoey E. Severe hyponatremia and inappropriate antidiuretic hormone secretion following ecstasy use. *Acad Emerg Med.* 1998;5:839-840.

3. Allcott JV, Barnhart RA, Mooney LA. Acute lead poisoning in two users of illicit methamphetamine. *JAMA*. 1987;258:510-511.
4. Allen A, Cantrell T. Synthetic reductions in clandestine amphetamine and methamphetamine labs. *J Forensic Sci*. 1989;42:183-199.
5. Allen RP, McCann UD, Ricaurte GA. Persistent effects of (+)3,4-methylenedioxymethamphetamine (MDMA, "ecstasy") on human sleep. *Sleep*. 1993;16:560-564.
6. Al-Motarreb A, Briancon S, Al-Jaber N, et al. Khat chewing is a risk factor for acute myocardial infarction: a case-control study. *Br J Clin Pharmacol*. 2005;59:574-581.
7. Anderson RJ, Garza HR, Garriott JC, et al. Intravenous propylhexedrine abuse and sudden death. *Am J Med*. 1979;67:15-20.
8. Anderson RJ, Reed WG, Hillis LD. History, epidemiology, and medical complications of nasal inhaler abuse. *Clin Toxicol*. 1982;19:95-107.
9. Angrist B: Amphetamine psychosis: clinical variation of the syndrome. In: Cho AK, Segal DS, eds. *Amphetamines and Its Analogs. Psychopharmacology, Toxicity, and Abuse*. San Diego, CA: Academic Press; 1994:387-414.
10. Baggott M, Heifets B, Jones RT, et al. Chemical analysis of ecstasy pills. *JAMA*. 2000;284:2190.
11. Bailey DN, Shaw RF. Cocaine and methamphetamine-related deaths in San Diego County (1987): homicides and accidental overdoses. *J Forensic Sci*. 1989;34:407-422.
12. Baselt RC, Cravey RH. *Disposition of Toxic Drugs and Chemicals in Man*, 3rd ed. Chicago: Year Book; 1989.
13. Battaglia G, DeSouza EB. Pharmacologic profile of amphetamine derivatives at various brain recognition sites: selective effects on serotonergic systems. *NIDA Res Monogr*. 1989;94:240-258.
14. Beckett AH, Rowland M, Turner P. Influence of urinary pH on excretion of amphetamine. *Lancet*. 1965;1:303.
15. Beckett AH, Rowland M. Urinary excretion kinetics of amphetamine in man. *J Pharm Pharmacol*. 1965;17:628-639.
16. Berger UV, Grzanna R, Molliver ME. Depletion of serotonin using *p*-chlorophenylalanine (PCPA) and reserpine protects against the neurotoxic effects of *p*-chloroamphetamine (PCA) in the brain. *Exp Neurol*. 1989;103:111-115.
17. Beyer KL, Bicker JT, Butt JH. Ischemic colitis associated with dextroamphetamine use. *J Clin Gastroenterol*. 1991;13:198-201.
18. Blum K. Central nervous system stimulants. In: Blum K, ed. *Handbook of Arousable Drugs*. New York: Gardner; 1984:305-347.
19. Borowski TB, Kirkby RD, Kokkinidis L. Amphetamine and antidepressant drug effects on GABA-and NMDA-related seizures. *Brain Res Bull*. 1993;30:607-610.
20. Boswick DG. Amphetamine-induced cerebral vasculitis. *Hum Pathol*. 1981;12:1031-1033.
21. Bouchard NC, Howland MA, Greller HA, et al. Ischemic stroke associated with use of an ephedra-free dietary supplement containing synephrine. *Mayo Clin Proc*. 2005;80:541-545.
22. Bowen JS, Davis GB, Kearney TE, Bardin J. Diffuse vascular spasm associated with 4-bromo-2,5-dimethoxyamphetamine ingestion. *JAMA*. 1983;249:1477-1479.
23. Boyer EW, Quang L, Woolf, et al. Dextromethorphan and ecstasy pills. *JAMA*. 2001;285:409-410.
24. Brenot F, Herve P, Petitpretz P, et al. Primary pulmonary hypertension and fenfluramine use. *Br Heart J*. 1993;70:537-541.
25. Bristow LJ, Thorn L, Tricklebank MD, et al. Competitive NMDA receptor antagonists attenuate the behavioural and neurochemical effects of amphetamine in mice. *Eur J Pharmacol*. 1994;264:353-359.
26. Bruno A, Nolte KB, Chapin J. Stroke associated with ephedrine use. *Neurology*. 1993;43:1313-1316.
27. Buchanan JF, Brown CR. "Designer drugs": a problem in clinical toxicology. *Med Toxicol*. 1988;3:1-17.
28. Buchert R, Thomasius R, Nebeling B, et al. Long-term effects of "ecstasy" use on serotonin transporters of the brain investigated by PET. *J Nucl Med*. 2003;44:375-384.
29. Burton BT. Heavy metal and organic contaminants associated with illicit methamphetamine production. *NIDA Res Monogr*. 1991;115: 47-59.
30. Call TD, Hartneck J, Dickinson WA, et al. Acute cardiomyopathy secondary to intravenous amphetamine abuse. *Ann Intern Med*. 1982; 97: 559-560.
31. Callaway CW, Johnson MP, Gold LH, et al. Amphetamine derivatives induce locomotor hyperactivity by acting as indirect serotonin agonists. *Psychopharmacology*. 1991;104:293-301.
32. Callaway CW, Wing LL, Geyer MA. Serotonin release contributes to the locomotor stimulant effects of 3,4-methylenedioxymethamphetamine in rats. *J Pharmacol Exp Ther*. 1990;254:456-464.
33. Capwell RR. Ephedrine-induced mania from an herbal diet supplement. *Am J Psychiatry*. 1995;152:647.
34. Carter N, Rutty GN, Milroy CM, et al. Deaths associated with MBDB misuse. *Int J Legal Med*. 2000;113:168-170.
35. Catravas JD, Waters IW, Davis WM, Hickenbottom JP. Haloperidol for acute amphetamine poisoning: a study in dogs. *JAMA*. 1975;231: 1340-1341.
36. Centers for Disease Control and Prevention (CDC). Acute public health consequences of methamphetamine laboratories—16 states, January 2000-June 2004. *MMWR Morb Mortal Wkly Rep*. 2005;54:356-359.
37. Centers for Disease Control and Prevention (CDC). Anhydrous ammonia thefts and releases associated with illicit methamphetamine production—16 states, January 2000-June 2004. *MMWR Morb Mortal Wely Rep*. 2005;54:359-361.
38. Centers for Disease Control and Prevention (CDC). Cardiac valvulopathy associated with exposure to fenfluramine or dexfenfluramine: US Department of Health and Human Services interim public health recommendations, November 1997. *MMWR Morb Mortal Wkly Rep*. 1997;46:1061-1066.
39. Chambers CD, The epidemiology of stimulant abuse: a focus on the amphetamine-related substances. In: Smith DE, Wesson DR, Buxton ME, et al, eds. *Amphetamine Use, Misuse, and Abuse*. Boston: GK Hall; 1979:92-103.
40. Chan P, Chen JH, Lee MH, et al. Fatal and nonfatal methamphetamine intoxication in the intensive care unit. *J Toxicol Clin Toxicol*. 1994;32:147-155.
41. Chandler DB, Norton RL, Kauffman J, et al. Lead poisoning associated with intravenous methamphetamine use—Oregon, 1988. *MMWR Morb Mortal Wkly Rep*. 1989;38:830-831.
42. Chiang WK, Goldfrank LG. Medical complications of drug abuse. *Med J Aust*. 1990;152:83-88.
43. Chin KM, Channick RN, Rubin LJ. Is methamphetamine use associated with idiopathic pulmonary arterial hypertension? *Chest*. 2006;130:1657-1663.
44. Cho AK, Kumagai Y. Metabolism of amphetamine and other arylisopropylamines. In: Cho AK, Segal DS, eds. *Amphetamines and Its Analogs. Psychopharmacology, Toxicity, and Abuse*. San Diego, CA: Academic Press; 1994:43-77.
45. Cho AK, Wright J. Pathways of metabolism of amphetamine. *Life Sci*. 1978;22:363-371.
46. Cho AK. Ice: a new dosage form of an old drug. *Science*. 1990;249:631-634.
47. Cimbura G. PMA deaths in Ontario. *Can Med Assoc J*. 1974;110:12631267.
48. Citron BP, Halpern M, McCarron M, et al. Necrotizing angitis associated with drug abuse. *N Engl J Med*. 1970;283:1003-1011.
49. Cloud J. It's all the rave. *Time Europe*. 2000;155:64-66.
50. Cody JT, Schwarzhoff R. Fluorescence polarization immunoassay of amphetamine, methamphetamine, and illicit amphetamine analogues. *J Anal Toxicol*. 1993;17:23-33.
51. Colado MI, Williams JL, Green AR. The hyperthermic and neurotoxic effects of "ecstasy" (MDMA) and 3,4-methylenedioxyamphetamine (MDA) in the Dark Agouti (DA) rat, a model of CYP2D6 poor metabolizer phenotype. *Br J Pharmacol*. 1995;115:1281-1289.
52. Connolly HM, Crary JL, McGoon MD, et al. Valvular heart disease associated with fenfluramine-phentermine. *N Engl J Med*. 1997;337:581-588.
53. Costall B, Naylor RJ. Extrapyramidal and mesolimbic involvement with the stereotypic activity of D- and L-amphetamine. *Eur J Pharmacol*. 1974;15:121-129.
54. Council on Scientific Affairs. Clinical aspects of amphetamine abuse. *JAMA*. 1978;240:2317-2319.
55. Croft CH, Firth BG, Hillis LD. Propylhexedrine-induced left ventricular dysfunction. *Ann Intern Med*. 1982;97:560-561.
56. Curry SC, Chang D, Connor D. Drug- and toxin-induced rhabdomyolysis. *Ann Emerg Med*. 1989;18:1068-1084.
57. D'Nicoula J, Jones R, Levine B, et al. Evaluation of six commercial amphetamine and methamphetamine immunoassays for cross-reactivity to phenylpropanolamine and ephedrine in urine. *J Anal Toxicol*. 1992;16:211-213.
58. Dal Carson TA, Angelos JA, Raney JK. A clandestine approach to the synthesis of phenyl-2-propanone from phenylpropenes. *J Forensic Sci*. 1984;29:1187-1208.
59. Davis GG, Swalwell CI. Acute aortic dissections and ruptured berry aneurysms associated with methamphetamine abuse. *J Forensic Sci*. 1994;39:1481-1485.

60. Davis JM, Kopin IJ, Lemberger L, et al. Effects of urinary pH on amphetamine metabolism. *Ann N Y Acad Sci.* 1971;179:493-501.
61. Davis MW, Logston DG, Hickenbottom JP. Antagonism of acute amphetamine intoxication by haloperidol and propranolol. *Toxicol Appl Pharmacol.* 1974;29:397-403.
62. De Souza EB, Battaglia G. Effects of MDMA and MDA on brain serotonin neurons: evidence from neurochemical and autoradiographic studies. *NIDA Res Monogr.* 1989;94:196-222.
63. Delaney P, Estes M. Intracranial hemorrhage with amphetamine abuse. *Neurology.* 1980;30:1125-1128.
64. Delliou D, Bromo DMA. New hallucinogenic drug. *Med J Aust.* 1980;1:83.
65. Derlet RW, Albertson TE, Rice P. Antagonism of cocaine, amphetamine, and methamphetamine toxicity. *Pharmacol Biochem Behav.* 1990;36:745-749.
66. Derlet RW, Albertson TE, Rice P. Protection against d-amphetamine toxicity. *Am J Emerg Med.* 1990;8:105-108.
67. Derlet RW, Heischober B. Methamphetamine. Stimulant of the 1990s? *West J Med.* 1990;153:625-628.
68. Derlet RW, Rice P, Horowitz BZ, Lord RV. Amphetamine toxicity: experience with 127 cases. *J Emerg Med.* 1989;7:157-161.
69. Devan GS. Phentermine and psychosis. *Br J Psychiatry.* 1990;156: 442-443.
70. Di Maio VJM, Garriott JC. Intravenous abuse of propylhexedrine. *J Forensic Sci.* 1977;22:152-158.
71. Doflou J, Mark A. Aortic dissection after ingestion of "ecstasy" (MDMA). *Am J Forensic Med Pathol.* 2000;21:261-263.
72. Dowling GP, McDonough ET, Bost RO. "Eve" and "ecstasy." A report of five deaths associated with the use of MDEA and MDMA. *JAMA.* 1987;257:1615-1617.
73. Drug Abuse Warning Network, 2002. National estimates of drug-related emergency department visits. U.S. Department of Health and Human Services, Substance Abuse and Mental Health Services Administration.
74. Edison GR. Amphetamines: a dangerous illusion. *Ann Intern Med.* 1971;74:605-610.
75. Ellinwood EH. Assault and homicide associated with amphetamine abuse. *Am J Psychiatry.* 1971;127:1170-1175.
76. Emerson TS, Cisek JE. Methcathinone ("cat"): a Russian designer amphetamine infiltrates the rural Midwest. *Ann Emerg Med.* 1993;22:1897-1903.
77. Erowid's psychoactive vaults. http://www.erowid.org/psychoactives/psychoactives.shtml. Last accessed April 8, 2009.
78. Espelin DE, Done AK. Amphetamine poisoning. Effectiveness of chlorpromazine. *N Engl J Med.* 1968;278:1361-1365.
79. Fallon JK, Shah D, Kicman AT, et al. Action of MDMA (ecstasy) and its metabolites on arginine vasopressin release. *Ann N Y Acad Sci.* 2002;965:399-409.
80. Feinstein D. The Methamphetamine Control Act of 1996. http://feinstein.senate.gov/methamphetamine_control.html. Last accessed April 8, 2009.
81. Felgate HE, Felgate PD, James RA, et al. Recent paramethoxyamphetamine deaths. *J Anal Toxicol.* 1998;22:169-172.
82. Fitzgerald RL, Ramos JM Jr, Bogema SC, et al. Resolution of methamphetamine stereoisomers in urine drug testing: urinary excretion of R(2)-methamphetamine following use of nasal inhalers. *J Anal Toxicol.* 1988;12:255-259.
83. Furst SR, Fallon SP, Reznik GN, et al. Myocardial infarction after inhalation of methamphetamine. *N Engl J Med.* 1990;323:1147-1148.
84. Gal J. Amphetamines in nasal inhalers. *Clin Toxicol.* 1982;19:577-578.
85. Gardin JM, Schumacher D, Constantine G, et al. Valvular abnormalities and cardiovascular status following exposure to dexfenfluramine or phentermine/fenfluramine. *JAMA.* 2000;283:1703-1709.
86. Gary NE, Saidi M. Methamphetamine intoxication. A speedy new treatment. *Am J Med.* 1978;64:537-540.
87. Gibb JW, Johnson M, Elayan I, et al. Neurotoxicity of amphetamines and their metabolites. *NIDA Res Monogr.* 1997;173:128-145.
88. Gilhooly TC, Daly AK. Cyp2D6 deficiency, a fact in ecstasy related death? *Br J Clin Pharmacol.* 2002;54:69-70.
89. Ginsberg MD, Hertzman M, Schmidt-Nowara W. Amphetamine intoxication with coagulopathy, hyperthermia, and reversible renal failure. A syndrome resembling heatstroke. *Ann Intern Med.* 1970;73:81-85.
90. Giroud C, Augsburger M, River L, et al. 2C-B: a new psychoactive phenylethylamine recently discovered in Ecstasy tablets sold on the Swiss black market. *J Anal Toxicol.* 1998;22:345-354.
91. Glennon RA, Showalter D. The effects of cathinone and several related derivatives on locomotor activity. *Res Commun Subst Abuse.* 1981;2:186-191.
92. Glennon RA, Yousif M, Naiman N, et al. Methcathinone: a new and potent amphetamine-like agent. *Pharmacol Biochem Behavior.* 1987;26:547-551.
93. Glennon RA. Stimulus properties of hallucinogenic phenalkylamines and related designer drugs: formulation of structure-activity relationship. *NIDA Res Monogr.* 1989;94:43-67.
94. Gold LHG, Geyer MA, Koob GF. Neurochemical mechanisms involved in behavioral effects of amphetamines and related designer drugs. *NIDA Res Monogr.* 1989;94:101-126.
95. Goldfrank LR, Hoffman RS. The cardiovascular effects of cocaine. *Ann Emerg Med.* 1991;20:165-175.
96. Goldstone MS. "Cat": methcathinone—a new drug of abuse. *JAMA.* 1993;269:2508.
97. Gospe SM Jr. Transient cortical blindness in an infant exposed to methamphetamine. *Ann Emerg Med.* 1995;26:380-382.
98. Gouzoulis-Mayfrank E, Daumann J, Tuchtenhagen F, et al. Impaired cognitive performance in drug-free users of recreational ecstasy (MDMA). *J Neurol Neurosurg Psychiatry.* 2000;68:719-725.
99. Green AR, Mechan AO, Elliott JM, et al. The pharmacology and clinical pharmacology of 3,4-methylenedioxymethamphetamine (MDMA, "ecstasy"). *Pharmacol Rev.* 2003;55:463-508.
100. Greenblatt DJ, Gross PL, Harris J, et al. Fatal hyperthermia following haloperidol therapy of sedative-hypnotic withdrawal. *J Clin Psychiatry.* 1978;39:673-675.
101. Greenblatt JC, Gfroerer JC, Melnick D. Increasing morbidity and mortality associated with abuse of methamphetamine—United States, 1991-1994. *MMWR Morb Mortal Wkly Rep.* 1995;44:882-886.
102. Greer G, Tolbert R. Subjective reports on the effects of MDMA in a clinical setting. *J Psychoactive Drugs.* 1986;18:319-327.
103. Grinspoon L, Bakalar JB. Amphetamines: medical and health hazards. In: Smith DE, Wesson DR, Buxton ME, et al, eds. *Amphetamine Use, Misuse, and Abuse.* Boston: GK Hall; 1979:18-34.
104. Groves PM, Ryan LJ, Diana M, et al. Neuronal actions of amphetamine in the rat brain. *NIDA Res Monogr.* 1989;94:127-145.
105. Gurtner HP, Gertsch M, Salzmann C, et al. Haufen sich die primar vascularen Formen des chronischen Cor pulmonale? *Schweiz Med Wochenschr.* 1968;98:1579-1589.
106. Gurtner HP. Aminorex and pulmonary hypertension. *Cor Vasa.* 1985; 27:160-171.
107. Halbach H. Medical aspects of the chewing of khat leaves. *Bull WHO.* 1972;27:21-29.
108. Halkitis PN, Green KA, Mourgues, P. Longitudinal investigation of methamphetamine use among gay and bisexual men in New York City: findings from project BUMPS. *J Urban Health.* 2005;82:18-25.
109. Haller CA, Benowitz NL. Adverse cardiovascular and central nervous system events associated with dietary supplements containing ephedra alkaloids. *N Engl J Med.* 2000;343:1833-1838.
110. Haller CA, Meier KH, Olson KR. Seizures reported in association with use of dietary supplements. *Clin Toxicol.* 2005;1:23-30.
111. Hamer R, Phelphs D. Inadvertent intra-arterial injection of phentermine: a complication of drug abuse. *Ann Emerg Med.* 1981;10:148-150.
112. Harrington H, Heller HA, Dawson D, et al. Intracerebral hemorrhage and oral amphetamine. *Arch Neurol.* 1983;40:503-507.
113. Harris G. Judge's decision lifts ban on sale of ephedra in Utah. *New York Times,* April 15, 2004, p. A12.
114. Hart JB, Wallace J. The adverse effects of amphetamines. *Clin Toxicol.* 1975;8:179-190.
115. Hartung TK, Schofield E, Short AI, et al. Hyponatraemic states following 3,4-methylenedioxymethamphetamine (MDMA, "ecstasy") ingestion. *Q J Med.* 2002;95:431-437.
116. Heischober B, Miller MA. Methamphetamine abuse in California. *NIDA Res Monogr.* 1991;115:60-71.
117. Henry JA, Fallon JK, Kicman AT, et al. Low-dose MDMA ("ecstasy") induces vasopressin secretion. *Lancet.* 1998;351:1784.
118. Henry JA, Hill IR. Fatal interaction between ritonavir and MDMA. *Lancet.* 1998;325:1751-1752.
119. Henry JA, Jeffrey KJ, Dawling S. Toxicity and deaths from 3,4-methylenedioxymethamphetamine ("ecstasy"). *Lancet.* 1992;340:384-387.
120. Hensrud DD, Connolly HM, Grogan M, et al. Echocardiographic improvement over time after cessation of use of fenfluramine and phentermine. *Mayo Clin Proc.* 1999;74:1191-1197.

121. Herr RD, Caravati EM. Acute transient ischemic colitis after oral methamphetamine ingestion. *Am J Emerg Med.* 1991;9:406-409.
122. Herve P, Launay J, Scrobohaci M, et al. Increased plasma serotonin in primary pulmonary hypertension. *Am J Med.* 1995;99:249-254.
123. Hirata H, Ladenheim B, Rothman RB, et al. Methamphetamine-induced serotonin neurotoxicity is mediated by superoxide radicals. *Brain Res.* 1995;677:345-347.
124. Hoffman BB, Lefkowitz RJ. Catecholamines, sympathomimetic drugs, and adrenergic receptor antagonists. In: Hardman JG, Limbird LE, Molinoff PB, et al, eds. *Goodman and Gilman's The Pharmacological Basis of Therapeutics*, 9th ed. New York, McGraw-Hill, 1996, pp. 199-227.
125. Hong R, Matsuyama E, Nur K. Cardiomyopathy associated with the smoking of crystal methamphetamine. *JAMA.* 1991;265:1152-1154.
126. Hong Z, Olshewski A, Reeve HL, et al. Nordexfenfluramine causes more severe pulmonary vasoconstriction than dexfenfluramine. *Am J Physiol Lung Cell Mol Physiol.* 2004;531-538.
127. Imanse J, Vanneste J. Intraventricular hemorrhage following amphetamine abuse. *Neurology.* 1990;40:1318-1319.
128. Irvine GD, Chin L. The environmental impact and adverse health effects of the clandestine manufacture of methamphetamine. *NIDA Res Monogr.* 1991;115:33-46.
129. Iversen L. Neurotransmitter transporters: fruitful targets for CNS drug discovery. *Mol Psychiatry.* 2000;5:357-362.
130. Jackson JG. Hazards of smokable methamphetamine. *N Engl J Med.* 1989;321:907.
131. Jerrard DA. "Designer drugs"—a current perspective. *J Emerg Med.* 1990;8:733-741.
132. Jick H, Vasilakis C, Weinrauch LA, et al. A population-based study of appetite-suppressant drugs and the risk of cardiac-valve regurgitation. *N Engl J Med.* 1998;339:719-724.
133. Johnson LE, Anggaro E, Gunne LM. Blockade of intravenous amphetamine euphoria in man. *Clin Pharmacol Ther.* 1971;12:889-896.
134. Johnson TD, Berenson MM. Methamphetamine-induced ischemic colitis. *J Clin Gastroenterol.* 1991;13:687-689.
135. Jordan SC, Hampson F. Amphetamine poisoning associated with hyperpyrexia. *Br J Med.* 1960;2:844.
136. Kalant H, Kalant OJ. Death in amphetamine users: causes and rates. *Can Med Assoc J.* 1975;112:299-304.
137. Kalix P. Pharmacological properties of the stimulant khat. *Pharmacol Ther.* 1990;48:397-416.
138. Karch SB, Billingham ME. The pathology and etiology of cocaine-induced heart disease. *Arch Pathol Lab Med.* 1988;112:225-230.
139. Karch SB. Synthetic stimulants. In: Karch SB: *The Pathology of Drug Abuse.* Boca Raton, FL: CRC Press; 1993:165-218.
140. Karler R, Calder LD, Thai LH, et al. A dopaminergic-glutamatergic basis for the action of amphetamine and cocaine. *Brain Res.* 1994;658: 8-14.
141. Karler R, Calder LD, Thai LH, et al. The dopaminergic, glutamatergic, GABAergic bases for the action of amphetamine and cocaine. *Brain Res.* 1995;671:100-104.
142. Kase CS, Foster TE, Reed JE, et al. Intracerebral hemorrhage and phenylpropanolamine use. *Neurology.* 1987;37:399-404.
143. Katsumata S, Sato K, Kashiwade H, et al. Sudden death due presumably to internal use of methamphetamine. *Forensic Sci Int.* 1993;62: 209-215.
144. Kendrick WC, Hull AR, Knochel JP. Rhabdomyolysis and shock after intravenous amphetamine administration. *Ann Intern Med.* 1977;86: 381-387.
145. Kernan WN, Viscoli CM, Brass LM, et al. Phenylpropanolamine and the risk of hemorrhagic stroke. *N Engl J Med.* 2000;343:1826-1832.
146. Khan MA, Herzog CA, St. Peter JV, et al. The prevalence of cardiac valvular insufficiency assessed by transthoracic echocardiography in obese patients treated with appetite-suppressants drugs. *N Engl J Med.* 1998;339:713-718.
147. Kintz P. Excretion of MBDB and BDB in urine, saliva, and sweat following single oral administration. *J Anal Toxicol.* 1997;21:570-575.
148. Kish SJ. How strong is the evidence that brain serotonin neurons are damaged in human users of ecstasy? *Pharmacol Biochem Behav.* 2002;71: 845-855.
149. Klatt EC, Montgomery S, Nemiki T, et al. Misrepresentation of stimulant street drugs: a decade of experience in analysis program. *J Toxicol Clin Toxicol.* 1986;24:441-450.
150. Klawans HL, Weiner WJ. The effects of d-amphetamine on choreiform movement disorder. *Neurology.* 1974;6:312-318.
151. Kojima T, Matsushima E, Iwama H, et al. Visual perception process in amphetamine psychosis and schizophrenia. *Psychopharmacol Bull.* 1986;22:768-773.
152. Kokkinidis L, Zacharko RM, Anisman H. Amphetamine withdrawal: a behavioral evaluation. *Life Sci.* 1968;38:1617-1623.
153. Kokkinos J, Levine SR. Possible association of ischemic stroke with phentermine. *Stroke.* 1993;24:310-313.
154. Kram TC, Kram BS, Kruegel AV. The identification of impurities in illicit methamphetamine exhibits by gas chromatography/mass spectrometry and nuclear magnetic resonance spectroscopy. *J Forensic Sci.* 1976;22:40-52.
155. Kramer JC, Fischman VS, Littlefield DC. Amphetamine abuse. Pattern and effects of high doses taken intravenously. *JAMA.* 1967;201:89-93.
156. Kringsholm B, Christoffersen P. Lung and heart pathology in fatal drug addiction. A consecutive autopsy study. *Forensic Sci Int.* 1987;34:39-51.
157. Kuhn DM, Geddes TJ. Molecular footprints of neurotoxic amphetamine action. *Ann N Y Acad Sci.* 2000;914:92S-103S.
158. Lago JA, Kosten TR. Stimulant withdrawal. *Addiction.* 1994;89:1477-1481.
159. Lake C, Quirk R. Stimulants and look-alike drugs. *Psychiatr Clin North Am.* 1984;7:689-701.
160. Lerner MA. The fire of ice. *Newsweek*, November 27, 1989, pp. 37-40.
161. Liggett SB. Propylhexedrine intoxication: clinical presentation and pharmacology. *South Med J.* 1982;76:250-251.
162. Little BB, Snell LM, Gilstrap LC. Methamphetamine abuse during pregnancy: outcome and fetal effects. *Obstet Gynecol.* 1988;72:541-544.
163. Logan BK, Fligner CL, Haddix T. Cause and manner of death in fatalities involving methamphetamine. *J Forensic Sci.* 1998;43:28-34.
164. Lucas AR, Weiss M. Methylphenidate hallucinosis. *JAMA.* 1971;217: 1079-1081.
165. Lucas BB, Gardner DL, Wolkowitz OM, et al. Methylphenidate-induced cardiac arrhythmias. *N Engl J Med.* 1986;315:1485.
166. Lukes SA. Intracerebral hemorrhage from an arteriovenous malformation after amphetamine injection. *Arch Neurol.* 1983;40:60-61.
167. Lundh H, Tunuing K. An extrapyramidal choreiform syndrome caused by amphetamine addiction. *J Neurol Neurosurg Psych.* 1981;44:728-730.
168. Luqman W, Danowski TS. The use of khat (Catha edulis) in Yemen social and medical observation. *Ann Intern Med.* 1976;85:246-249.
169. Mancusi-Ungaro HR, Decker WJ. Tissue injuries associated with parenteral propylhexedrine abuse. *J Toxicol Clin Toxicol.* 1983-1984; 21:359-372.
170. Marsden P, Sheldon J. Acute poisoning by propylhexedrine. *BMJ.* 1972;1:730.
171. Mattson RH, Calverley JR. Dextroamphetamine-sulfate-induced dyskinesis. *JAMA.* 1968;204:108-110.
172. Maurer HH, Bickeboeller-Friedrich J, Kraemer T, et al. Toxicokinetics and analytical toxicology of amphetamine-derived designer drugs ("ecstasy"). *Toxicol Lett.* 2000;112-113:133-142.
173. Maxwell DL, Polkey MI, Henry JA. Hyponatremia and catatonic stupor after taking "ecstasy." *BMJ.* 1993;307:1399.
174. McCann UD, Eligulashvilli V, Ricaurte GA. (+/-)3,4-Methylenedioxymethamphetamine ("ecstasy")-induced serotonin neurotoxicity: clinical studies. *Neuropsychology.* 2000;42:11-16.
175. McCann UD, Ricaurte GA. Amphetamine neurotoxicity: accomplishments and remaining challenges. *Neurosci Bio Rev.* 2004;27:821-826.
176. McCann UD, Ricaurte GA. Lasting neuropsychiatric sequelae of methylenedioxymethamphetamine ("ecstasy") in recreational users. *J Clin Psychopharamacology.* 1991;11:302-305.
177. McCann UD, Ricaurte GA. Use and abuse of ring-substituted amphetamines. In: Cho AK, Segal DS, eds. *Amphetamines and Its Analogs. Psychopharmacology, Toxicity, and Abuse.* San Diego, CA: Academic Press; 1994: 371-386.
178. McCann UD, Ridenour A, Shaham Y, et al. Serotonin neurotoxicity after 3,4-methylenedioxymethamphetamine (MDMA: "ecstasy"): a controlled study in humans. *Neuropsychopharmacology.* 1994;10: 129-138.
179. McCann UD, Slate SO, Ricaurte GA. Adverse reactions with 3,4-methylenedioxymethamphetamine (MDMA; "ecstasy"). *Drug Saf.* 1996;15:107-115.
180. McCann UD, Szabo Z, Scheffel U, et al. Positron emission tomographic evidence of toxic effect of MDMA ("ecstasy") on brain serotonin neurons in human beings. *Lancet.* 1998;352:1433-1437.
181. McGuire P. Long-term psychiatric and cognitive effects of MDMA use. *Toxicol Lett.* 2000;112-113:153-156.

182. McGuire PK, Cope HM, Fahy T, et al. Diverse psychiatric morbidity associated with use of 3,4-methylenedioxymethamphetamine ("ecstasy"). *Br J Psychiatry*. 1994;165:391-394.
183. Miller MA, Hughes AL. Epidemiology of amphetamine use in the United States. In: Cho AK, Segal DS, eds. *Amphetamines and Its Analogs. Psychopharmacology, Toxicity, and Abuse*. San Diego, CA: Academic Press; 1994:439-457.
184. Miller MA. Trends and patterns of methamphetamine smoking in Hawaii. *NIDA Res Monogr*. 1991;115:72-83.
185. Molliver ME, Berger UV, Mamounas LA, et al. Neurotoxicity of MDMA and related compounds: anatomic studies. *Ann N Y Acad Sci*. 1990;600:640-661.
186. Monks TJ, Jones DC, Bai F, Lau SS. The role of metabolism in 3,4-(±)-methylenedioxyamphetamine and 3,4-(±)-methylenedioxymethamphetamine (ecstasy) toxicity. *Ther Drug Monit*. 2004;26:132-136.
187. Morgan JP, Kagan D. Street amphetamine quality and the controlled substances act of 1970. In: Smith DE, Wesson DR, Buxton ME, et al, eds. *Amphetamine Use, Misuse, and Abuse*. Boston: GK Hall; 1979: 73-91.
188. Morgan JP. Amphetamine and methamphetamine during the 1990s. *Pediatr Rev*. 1992;13:330-333.
189. Morgan JP. The clinical pharmacology of amphetamine. In: Smith DE, Wesson DR, Buxton ME, et al, eds. *Amphetamine Use, Misuse, and Abuse*. Boston: GK Hall; 1979:3-10.
190. Morgan M. Memory deficits associated with recreational use of "ecstasy" (MDMA). *Psychopharmacology*. 1999;141:30-36.
191. Mueller PD, Korey WS. Death by "ecstasy": The serotonin syndrome? *Ann Emerg Med*. 1998;32:377-380.
192. Nadir A, Agrawal S, King PD, et al. Acute hepatitis associated with the use of a Chinese herbal product, ma-huang. *Am J Gastroenterol*. 1996;91:1436-1438.
193. Naeije R, Wauthy P, Maggiorini M, et al. Effects of dexfenfluramine on hypoxic pulmonary vasoconstriction and emboli pulmonary hypertension in dogs. *Am J Respir Crit Care Med*. 1995;151:692-697.
194. Nestor TA, Tamamoto WI, Kam TH. Acute pulmonary oedema caused by crystalline methamphetamine. *Lancet*. 1989;2:1277-1278.
195. Nichols DE, Oberlender R. Structure-activity relationships of MDMA-like substances. *NIDA Res Monogr*. 1989;94:1-29.
196. Nichols DE. Medicinal chemistry and structure-activity relationships. In: Cho AK, Segal DS, eds. *Amphetamines and Its Analogs. Psychopharmacology, Toxicity, and Abuse*. San Diego, CA: Academic Press; 1994:3-41.
197. Nuvials X, Masclans JR, Peracaula R, et al. Hyponatremic coma after ecstasy ingestion. *Intensive Care Med*. 1997;23:480.
198. Nykamp DL, Fackin MN, Compton AL. Possible association of acute lateral-wall myocardial infarction and bitter orange supplement. *Ann Pharmacother*. 2004;38:812-816.
199. O'Donohoe A, O'Flynn K, Shields K, et al. MDMA toxicity. No evidence for a major influence of metabolic genotype at CYP2D6. *Addict Biol*. 1998;3:309-314.
200. O'Neill ME, Arnolda LF, Coles DM, et al. Acute amphetamine cardiomyopathy in a drug addict. *Clin Cardiol*. 1983;6:189-191.
201. Obradovic T, Imel KM, White SR. Repeat exposure to methylenedioxymethamphetamine (MDMA) alters nucleus accumbens neuronal responses to dopamine and serotonin. *Brain Res*. 1998;785:1-9.
202. Obrocki J, Buchert R, Vaterlein O, et al. Ecstasy—Long-term effects on the human central nervous system revealed by positron emission tomography. *Br J Psych*. 1999;175:186-188.
203. Odenwald M, Neuner F, Schauer M, et al. Khat use as risk factor for psychotic disorders: a cross-sectional and case-control study in Somalia. *BMC Med*. 2005;3:5.
204. Ohmori T, Abekawa T, Muraki A, et al. Competitive and noncompetitive NMDA antagonists block sensitization to methamphetamine. *Pharmacol Biochem Behav*. 1994;48:587-591.
205. Olmedo R, Hoffman RS. Withdrawal syndromes. *Emerg Med Clin North Am*. 2000;18:273-288.
206. Ong BH. Hazards to health. Dextroamphetamine poisoning. *N Engl J Med*. 1962;266:1321-1322.
207. Packe GE, Garton MJ, Kennings K. Acute myocardial infarction caused by intravenous amphetamine abuse. *Br Heart J*. 1990;64:23-24.
208. Pedersen W, Skrondal A. Ecstasy and new patterns of drug use: a normal population study. *Addiction*. 1999;94:1695-1706.
209. Pentel P. Toxicity of over-the-counter stimulants. *JAMA*. 1984;252:1898-1903.
210. Peroutka SJ. Incidence of recreational use of MDMA "ecstasy" on an underground campus. *N Engl J Med*. 1987;317:1542-1543.
211. Perrotta DM, Coody G, Culmo C, et al. Adverse events associated with ephedrine-containing products—Texas, December 1993 to September 1995. *MMWR Morb Mortal Wkly Rep*. 1996;45:689-693.
212. Pitts DK, Marwah J. Cocaine and central monoaminergic neurotransmission: a review of electrophysiological studies and comparison to amphetamine and antidepressants. *Life Sci*. 1988;42:949-968.
213. Poklis A, Moore KA. Stereoselectivity of the TdxADx/FLx amphetamine/methamphetamine II amphetamine/methamphetamine immunoassay—response of urine specimens following nasal inhaler use. *J Toxicol Clin Toxicol*. 1995;33:35-41.
214. Puder KD, Kagan DV, Morgan JP. Illicit methamphetamine, analysis, synthesis, and availability. *Am J Drug Alcohol Abuse*. 1988;14:463-473.
215. Randall T. "Rave" scene, ecstasy use, leap Atlantic. *JAMA*. 1992;268:1506.
216. Randall T. Ecstasy-fueled "rave" parties become dances of death for English youths. *JAMA*. 1992;268:1505-1506.
217. Rasmussen S, Cole R, Spiehler V. Methamphetamine prevalence in sheriff's crime lab samples. *J Anal Toxicol*. 1989;12:263-267.
218. Reneman L, Booij J, Schmand B, et al. Memory disturbances in "ecstasy" users are correlated with an altered serotonin neurotransmission. *Psychopharmacology*. 2000;148:322-324.
219. Rhee KJ, Albertson TE, Douglas JC. Choreoathetoid disorder associated with amphetamine-like drugs. *Am J Emerg Med*. 1988;6:131-133.
220. Ricaurte GA, DeLanney LE, Irwin I, et al. Toxic effects of MDMA on central serotonergic neurons in the primate: importance of route and frequency of drug administration. *Brain Res*. 1988;446:165-168.
221. Ricaurte GA, Finnegan KF, Irwin I, et al. Aminergic metabolites in cerebrospinal fluid of humans previously exposed to MDMA: preliminary observations. *Ann N Y Acad Sci*. 1990;600:699-710.
222. Ricaurte GA, Finnegan KF, Nichols DE, et al. 3,4-Methylenedioxyethylamphetamine (MDE), a novel analogue of MDMA, produces long-lasting depletion of serotonin in the rat brain. *Eur J Pharmacol*. 1987;137:265-268.
223. Ricaurte GA, Guillery RW, Seiden LS, et al. Dopamine nerve terminal degeneration produced by high doses of methylamphetamine in the rat brain. *Brain Res*. 1982;235:93-103.
224. Ricaurte GA, McCann UD, Szabo Z, et al. Toxicodynamics and long-term toxicity of the recreational drug, 3,4-methylenedioxymethamphetamine (MDMA, "ecstasy"). *Toxicol Lett*. 2000;112-113:143-146.
225. Ricaurte GA, Seiden LS, Schuster CR. Further evidence that amphetamines produce long-lasting dopamine neurochemical deficits by destroying dopamine nerve fibers. *Brain Res*. 1984;303:359-364.
226. Richards KC, Borgstedt HH. Near fatal reaction to ingestion of the hallucinogenic drug MDA. *JAMA*. 1971;218:1826-1827.
227. Riley I, Corson J, Haider I, et al. Fenfluramine overdosage. *Lancet*. 1969;2:1162-1163.
228. Robiolio PA, Rigolin VH, Wilson JS, et al. Carcinoid heart disease: correlation of high serotonin levels with valvular abnormalities detected by cardiac catheterization and echocardiography. *Circulation*. 1995;92:790-795.
229. Rothman RB, Ayestas MA, Dersch CM, et al. Aminorex, fenfluramine, and chlorphentermine are serotonin transporter substrates. Implications for primary pulmonary hypertension. *Circulation*. 1999;100:869-875.
230. Rothman RB, Baumann MH, Savage JE, et al. Evidence for possible involvement of 5-HT2B receptors in the cardiac valvulopathy associated with fenfluramine and other serotonegic medications. *Circulation*. 2000;102:2836-2841.
231. Rothrock JF, Rubenstein R, Lyden PD. Ischemic stroke associated with methamphetamine inhalation. *Neurology*. 1988;38:589-592.
232. Rubin LJ. Primary pulmonary hypertension. *N Engl J Med*. 1997;336:111-117.
233. Rumbaugh CL, Bergeron RT, Fang HCH, et al. Cerebral angiographic changes in drug abuse patient. *Radiology*. 1971;101:335-344.
234. Rumbaugh CL, Bergeron RT, Scanlan RL, et al. Cerebral vascular changes secondary to amphetamine abuse in the experimental animal. *Radiology*. 1971;101:345-351.
235. Rumbaugh CL, Fang HCH, Higgins RE, et al. Cerebral microvascular injury in experimental drug abuse. *Invest Radiol*. 1976;11:282-294.
236. Sachdev M, Miller WC, Ryan T, et al. Effects of fenfluramine-derivative diet pills on cardiac valves: a meta-analysis of observational studies. *Am Heart J*. 2002;144:1065-1073.
237. Salanova V, Taubner R. Intracerebral haemorrhage and vasculitis secondary to amphetamine use. *Postgrad Med J*. 1984;60:429-430.
238. Sallee FR, Stiller RL, Perel JM, et al. Pemoline-induced abnormal involuntary movements. *J Clin Psychopharmacol*. 1989;9:125-129.

239. Sato M. Psychotoxic manifestations in amphetamine abuse. *Psychopharmacol Bull.* 1986;22:751-756.
240. Schaffer CB, Pauli MW. Psychotic reaction caused by proprietary oral diet agents. *Am J Psychiatry.* 1980;137:1256-1257.
241. Schaiberger PH, Kennedy TC, Miller FC, et al. Pulmonary hypertension associated with long-term inhalation of "crank" methamphetamine. *Chest.* 1993;104:614-616.
242. Seiden LS, Klever MS. Methamphetamine and related drugs: toxicity and resulting behavioral changes in response to pharmacological probes. *NIDA Res Monogr.* 1989;94:146-160.
243. Seiden LS, Sabol KE, Ricaurte GA. Amphetamine: effects on catecholamine systems and behavior. *Annu Rev Pharmacol Toxicol.* 1993;32:639-677.
244. Seiden LS. Neurotoxicity of methamphetamine: mechanisms of action and issues related to aging. *NIDA Res Monogr.* 1991;115:24-32.
245. Sekine Y, Iyo M, Ouchi Y, et al. Methamphetamine related psychiatric symptoms and reduced brain dopamine transporters studied with PET. *Am J Psychiatry.* 2001;158:1206-1214.
246. Sellers EM, Otton SV, Tyndale RF. The potential role of the cytochrome P-450 2D6 pharmacogenetic polymorphism of drug abuse. *NIDA Res Monogr* .1997;173:9-26.
247. Setola V, Hufeisen SJ, Grande-Allen J, et al. 3,4-Methylenedioxymethamphetamine (MDMA, "ecstasy") induces fenfluramine-like proliferative actions on human cardiac valvular interstitial cells in vivo. *Mol Pharmacol.* 2003;63:1223-1229.
248. Shankaran M, Yamamoto BK, Gudelsky GA. Ascorbic acid prevents 3,4-methylenedioxymethamphetamine (MDMA)-induced hydroxyl radical formation and the behavioral and neurochemical consequences of the depletion of brain 5-HT. *Synapse.* 2001;40:55-64.
249. Shulgin A, Shulgin A. *PIHKAL: A Chemical Love Story.* Berkeley, CA: Transform Press; 1991.
250. Simmonneau G, Fartoukh M, Sitbon O, et al. Primary pulmonary hypertension associated with the use of fenfluramine derivatives. *Chest.* 1998;114:195S-199S.
251. Simpson DL, Rumack BH. Methylenedioxyamphetamine. Clinical description of overdose, death, and review of pharmacology. *Arch Intern Med.* 1981;141:1507-1509.
252. Singh BK, Singh A, Chusid E. Chorea in long-term use of pemoline. *Ann Neurology.* 1983;13:218.
253. Smith DE, Fisher CM. An analysis of 310 cases of acute high-dose methamphetamine toxicity in Haight Ashbury. *Clin Toxicol.* 1970;3:117-124.
254. Smith FP, Kidwell DA. Isomeric amphetamines—a problem for urinalysis? *Forensic Sci Int.* 1991;50:153-165.
255. Smith HJ, Roche AHG, Herdson PB. Cardiomyopathy associated with amphetamine administration. *Am Heart J.* 1976;91:792-797.
256. Solowij N, Hall W, Lee N. Recreational MDMA use in Sidney: a profile of "ecstasy" users and their experiences with the drug. *Br J Addict.* 1992;87:1161-1172.
257. Sonsalla PK, Nicklas WJ, Heikkila RE. Role for excitatory amino acids in methamphetamine-induced nigrostriatal dopaminergic toxicity. *Science.* 1989;243:398-400.
258. Sonsalla PK. The role of *N*-methyl-D-aspartate receptors in dopaminergic neuropathology produced by the amphetamines. *Drug Alcohol Depend.* 1995;37:101-105.
259. Spann MD, McGwin Jr. G, Kerby JD, et al. Characteristics of burn patients injured in methamphetamine laboratory explosions. *J Burn Care Res.* 2006;27:496-501.
260. Stoessl AJ, Young GB, Feasby TE. Intracerebral haemorrhage and angiographic beading following ingestion of catecholaminergics. *Stroke.* 1985;16:734-736.
261. Substance Abuse and Mental Health Services Administration, Office of Applied Studies (2008). Results from the 2007 National Survey on Drug Use and Health: National Findings (NSDUH Series H-34, DHHS Publication No. SMA 08-4343). Rockville, MD.
262. Substance Abuse & Mental Health Services Administration (SAMHSA). 2003 National Survey on Drug Use & Health: Results. Rockville, MD, United States Department of Health and Human Services. 2004.
263. Sudilovsky A. Disruption of behavior in cats by chronic amphetamine intoxication. *Int J Neurol.* 1975;10:259-275.
264. Sulzer D, Chen TK, Lau YY, et al. Amphetamine redistributes dopamine from synaptic vesicles to the cytosol and promotes reverse transport. *J Neurosci.* 1995;15:4105-4108.
265. Sulzer D, Pothos E, Sung HM, et al. Weak base model of amphetamine action. *Ann N Y Acad Sci.* 1992;654:525-528.
266. Tadokoro S, Kuribara H. Reverse tolerance to the ambulation-increasing effect of methamphetamine in mice as an animal model of amphetamine-psychosis. *Psychopharmacol Bull.* 1986;22:757-762.
267. Traub SJ, Hoyek W, Hoffman RS. Dietary supplements containing ephedra alkaloids. *N Engl J Med.* 2001;344:1095-1097.
268. Trends Alert. Drug abuse in America—rural meth. Lexington, KY: The Council of State Governments; 2004.
269. Trugman JM. Cerebral arteritis and oral methylphenidate. *Lancet.* 1988;1:584-585.
270. Volkow ND, Chang L, Wang G, et al. Association of dopamine transporter reduction with psychomotor impairment in methamphetamine abusers. *Am J Psychiatry.* 2001;158:377-382.
271. Volkow ND, Chang L, Wang G, et al. Higher cortical and lower subcortical metabolism in detoxified methamphetamine abusers. *Am J Psychiatry.* 2001;158:383-389.
272. Waksman J, Taylor RN Jr, Bodor GS, et al. Acute myocardial infarction associated with amphetamine use. *Mayo Clin Proc.* 2001;76:323-326.
273. Watson CJ, Thomson HJ, Johnston PS. Body-packing with amphetamines—an indication for surgery. *J R Soc Med.* 1991;84:311-312.
274. Wee CC, Phillips RS, Aurigemma G. Risk for valvular heart disease among users of fenfluramine and dexfenfluramine who underwent echocardiography before use of medication. *Ann Intern Med.* 1998;129:870-874.
275. Weir E. Raves: a review of the culture, the drugs and the prevention of harm. *CMAJ.* 2000;162:1829-1830.
276. Weissman NJ, Tighe JF Jr, Gottdiener JS, et al. An assessment of heartvalve abnormalities in obese patients taking dexfenfluramine, sustained-release dexfenfluramine, or placebo. *N Engl J Med.* 1998;339:725-732.
277. White L, DiMaio VJM. Intravenous propylhexedrine and sudden death. *N Engl J Med.* 1977;297:1071.
278. Wiener RS, Lockhart JT, Schwartz RG. Dilated cardiomyopathy and cocaine abuse. Report of two cases. *Am J Med.* 1986;81:699-701.
279. William H, Dratcu L, Taylor R, et al. "Saturday night fever": Ecstasy-related problems in a London accident and emergency department. *J Accid Emerg Med.* 1998;15:322-326.
280. Wooten MR, Khangure MS, Murphy MJ. Intracerebral hemorrhage and vasculitis related to ephedrine use. *Ann Neurol.* 1983;13:337-340.
281. Wrona MZ, Yang Z, Zhang F, et al. Potential new insights into the molecular mechanism of methamphetamine-induced neurodegeneration. *NIDA Res Monogr.* 1997;173:146-174.
282. Yamamoto BK, Zhu W. The effects of methamphetamine on the production of free radical and oxidative stress. *J Pharmacol Exp Ther.* 1988;287:107-114.
283. Yoke YK, Derry S, Pritchard-copley A. Appetite suppressants and valvular heart disease – a systemic review. *BMC Clin Pharmacol.* 2002;23:6-15.
284. Young R, Glennon RA. Cocaine-stimulus generalization to two new designer drugs: Methcathinone and 4-methylaminorex. *Pharmacol Biochem Behav.* 1993;45:229-231.
285. Yu YJ, Cooper DR, Wellenstein DE, et al. Cerebral angiitis and intracerebral hemorrhage associated with methamphetamine abuse. *J Neurosurg.* 1983;58:109-111.
286. Zhinger KY, Dovensky W, Crossman A, et al. Ephedrone: 2-methylamino-1-phenylpropan-1-one (Jeff). *J Forensic Sci.* 1991;36:915-920.

CHAPTER 76
COCAINE

Jane M. Prosser and Robert S. Hoffman

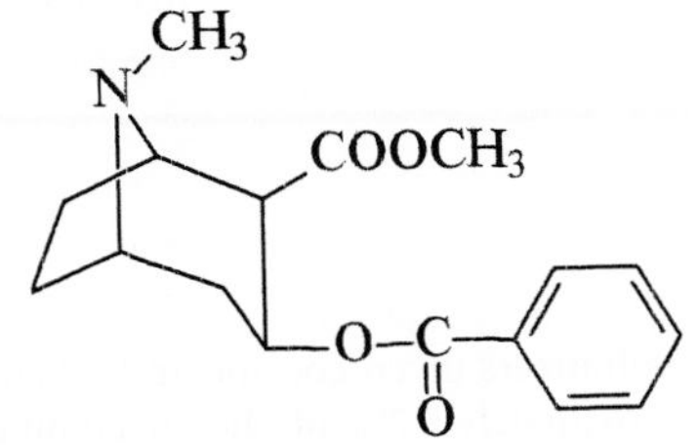

Cocaine is a naturally occurring alkaloid with unique local anesthetic and sympathomimetic activity, which served as the prototype for the synthesis of local anesthetics. Unlike other local anesthethics, cocaine has both anesthetic and vasoconstrictive properties, however many otolaryngologists no longer use cocaine because of its toxicity profile.[142] Cocaine is also a prevalent drug of abuse producing the characteristic sympathomimetic toxic syndrome that includes hypertension, tachycardia, tachypnea, hyperthermia, diaphoresis, mydriasis, and severe psychomotor agitation. The study of cocaine metabolism led early insights into pharmacogenetics, and the understanding of cocaine toxicity sheds light into the interactions of the control of the sympathetic nervous system.

HISTORY AND EPIDEMIOLOGY

Cocaine is contained in the leaves of *Erythroxylum coca*, a shrub that grows abundantly in Colombia, Peru, Bolivia, the West Indies, and Indonesia. As early as the 6th century, the inhabitants of Peru chewed or sucked on the leaves for social and religious reasons. In the 1100s, the Incas used cocaine-filled saliva as local anesthesia for ritual trephinations of the skull.[73]

In 1859, Albert Niemann isolated cocaine as the active ingredient of the plant. By 1879 Vassili von Anrep demonstrated that cocaine could numb the tongue.[120] However, Europeans knew little about cocaine until 1884, when the Austrian ophthalmologist Karl Koller introduced cocaine as an effective local anesthetic for eye surgery and Koller's colleague, Sigmund Freud, wrote extensively on the psychoactive properties of cocaine.[60] Following these revelations, Merck, Europe's main cocaine producer, increased production from less than 0.75 pounds in 1883 to more than 150,000 pounds in 1886.[114]

Simultaneously, reports of complications from the therapeutic use of cocaine began to appear. In 1886, a 25-year-old man had a "pulseless" syncopal event after cocaine was applied to his eye to remove a foreign body.[229] By 1887 more than 30 cases of severe toxicity were reported,[195] and by 1895 at least 8 fatalities resulting from a variety of doses and routes of administration were summarized in one article.[62] Recreational cocaine use was legal in the United States until 1914, when cocaine was restricted to medical use. It was not until 1982, however, that the first cocaine-associated myocardial infarction was reported in the United States.[29]

Currently, cocaine is an approved pharmaceutical. It is used primarily for topical anesthesia of cutaneous lacerations or during otolaryngology procedures as a vasoconstrictor and topical anesthetic. Although multiple factors have fostered a decline in the medicinal use of cocaine,[19,68,142] the recreational use of cocaine remains a significant problem. Recent estimates suggest that almost 34 million Americans have used cocaine at least once, with 1.7 million of those dependent or addicted.[43] European Union statistics estimate that cocaine has been used at least once by more than 12 million Europeans, representing almost 4% of all adults.[50]

PHARMACOLOGY

The alkaloid form of cocaine (benzoylmethylecgonine) is extracted from the leaf by mechanical degradation in the presence of a hydrocarbon. The resulting product is converted into a hydrochloride salt to yield a white powder (cocaine hydrochloride). Cocaine hydrochloride can be insufflated, applied topically to mucous membranes, dissolved in water and injected, or ingested; however, it degrades rapidly when pyrolyzed. Smokeable cocaine (crack) is formed by dissolving cocaine hydrochloride in water and adding a strong base. A hydrocarbon solvent is added, the cocaine base is extracted into the organic phase, and then evaporated. The term free-base refers to the use of cocaine base in solution.

Cocaine is rapidly absorbed following all routes of exposure; however, when applied to mucous membranes or ingested, its vasoconstrictive properties slow the rate of absorption and delay the peak effect. Bioavailability exceeds 90% with intravenous and smoked cocaine; it is approximately 80% following nasal application.[110] Data for ingested cocaine and application to other mucus membranes such as the urethra, vagina, or rectum are inadequately documented. Table 76–1 lists the typical onsets and durations of action for various uses of cocaine.

Following absorption cocaine is approximately 90% bound to plasma proteins, primarily α_1-acid glycoprotein.[182] Based on human volunteer studies, the volume of distribution is reported to be about 2.7 L/kg.[110] It is unclear if the volume of distribution changes with overdose.

The metabolism of cocaine is complex and dependent on both genetic and acquired factors. Three major pathways of cocaine metabolism are well described (Fig. 76–1). Cocaine undergoes *N*-demethylation in the liver to form norcocaine, a minor metabolite that rarely accounts for more than 5% of drug.[106,135,221,222] However, norcocaine readily crosses the blood–brain barrier and produces clinical effects in animals that are quite similar to cocaine.[13,35,113,159,160,166,206,209,245] Nearly half of a dose of cocaine is both nonenzymatically[222] and enzymatically hydrolyzed[41] to form benzoylecgonine (BE). When BE is injected into animals some reports suggest that it is virtually inactive,[115,159,160,206,217] while other studies demonstrate cerebral vasoconstriction[33] and seizures.[123,159] When either injected directly into the cerebral ventricles[160,209] or applied to the surface of cerebral arteries,[145] BE is a potent vasoconstrictor. Although BE traverses the blood–brain barrier poorly,[160] the potential effects are of concern as some BE is probably formed from cocaine that has already entered the CNS. In vitro, BE has little or no effect on cardiac sodium or potassium channels.[33,52] Finally, plasma cholinesterase (PChE) and other esterases metabolize cocaine to ecgonine methyl ester (EME). In normal individuals, between 32% and 49% of cocaine is metabolized to EME.[4,106] Like BE, EME crosses the blood–brain barrier poorly.[160] Although many authors state that EME has little or no pharmacologic activity,[35,52,159,160,206] diverse animal models demonstrate contradictory results, concluding that EME is a vasodilator,[145,180,207] sedative, anticonvulsant,[209] and protective metabolite against lethal doses of cocaine.[88]

TABLE 76–1. Pharmacology of Cocaine by Various Routes of Administration

Route of Exposure	Onset of Action (min)	Peak Action (min)	Duration of Action (min)	Relative Peak Concentrations (ng/mL)[111]
Intravenous	<1	3–5	30–60	180 ± 56
Nasal insufflation	1–5	20–30	60–120	220 ± 39
Smoking	<1	3–5	30–60	203 ± 88
Gastrointestinal	30–60	60–90	Unknown	Unknown

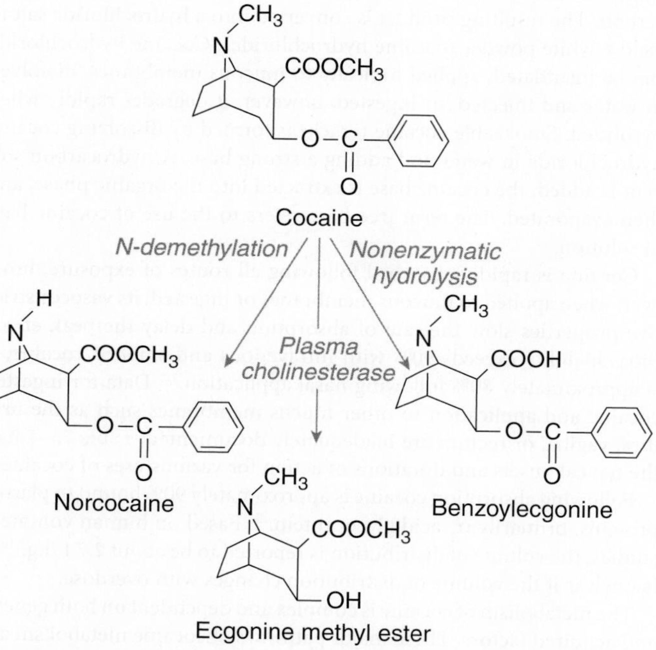

FIGURE 76–1. Metabolism of cocaine. The three principle metabolic pathways of cocaine are depicted.

The role of genetic or acquired alterations in PChE activity has been of interest for many years. Early in vitro studies showed that cocaine was poorly metabolized in serum from patients with succinylcholine sensitivity (low PChE activity). In subsequent studies and case series, patients with low PChE activity demonstrate increased sensitivity to cocaine,[45,86,175] findings that are corroborated in multiple animal models.[21,22,87,143,154,223,250]

Multiple other metabolites of cocaine are well characterized.[31] Several have clinical or diagnostic importance. In 1990, a unique metabolite was identified in patients who smoke cocaine, which has subsequently come to be known either as anhydroecgonine methyl ester (AEME) or methylecgonide.[108] The presence of this compound and its metabolite, ecgonidine, can be used to help determine the route of administration in cocaine users.[205] Additionally, AEME has demonstrable agonism at the muscarinic (M_2) receptors, which may have important clinical implications.[251]

Ethanol has a unique pharmacologic interaction with cocaine. A transesterification reaction between the two drugs produces benzoylethylecgonine which is also called "ethyl cocaine" or "cocaethylene" (CE).[14] In human volunteers given cocaine and ethanol, cocaethylene accounted for approximately 17% of the metabolites, producing a decrease in the amount of BE and an increase in the amount of EME formed.[77,78] Cocaethylene has a longer duration of action than cocaine and similar neurotoxic and cardiotoxic effects.

PATHOPHYSIOLOGY

NEUROTRANSMITTER EFFECTS

Cocaine blocks the reuptake of biogenic amines. Specifically, these effects are described on serotonin and the catecholamines dopamine, norepinephrine, and epinephrine. Several animal investigations have elucidated the particular roles of each neurotransmitter. Mice lacking the dopamine transporter are relatively insensitive to the locomotor effects of cocaine.[64] Tachycardia emanates from adrenally derived epinephrine, whereas hypertension results from neuronally derived norepinephrine.[227,228] Serotonin is an important modulator of dopamine and has a role in cocaine addiction and reward and seizures.[75,133,153,172]

Although much emphasis has been placed on the reuptake blockade of these biogenic amines, it is clear that this effect is insufficient to account for the clinical manifestations of cocaine toxicity. First, other xenobiotics that block the reuptake of biogenic amines, such as cyclic antidepressants, produce quite distinct clinical manifestations (Chap. 73).[230] Also, xenobiotics that block the effects of dopamine, epinephrine, and norepinephrine not only fail to protect against cocaine toxicity, they actually exacerbate it.[25,70,128,200] Although this may, in part, result from an unopposed α-adrenergic effect, hypertension and vasospasm fail to explain the increase in psychomotor agitation, seizures and hyperthermia that result.[25,70] These effects most likely result from an interaction between cocaine and excitatory amino acids. Cocaine increases excitatory amino acid concentrations in the brain,[216] and excitatory amino acid antagonists prevent both seizures and death in experimental animals.[15,192] Finally, because experimental evidence in animals[25,70,210] and clinical experience in humans demonstrate that sedation treats both the central effects of cocaine and the peripheral effects of biogenic amines, a newer model was proposed (Fig. 76–2). This model emphasizes the necessity of diffuse central nervous system excitation as a prerequisite for cocaine toxicity, explains experimental and clinical observations, and provides insight into the treatment of acute toxicity.

CARDIOVASCULAR EFFECTS

Cocaine use is associated with myocardial ischemia and myocardial infarction (MI). The increased risk of MI results from several different mechanisms. Hypertension and tachycardia increase myocardial

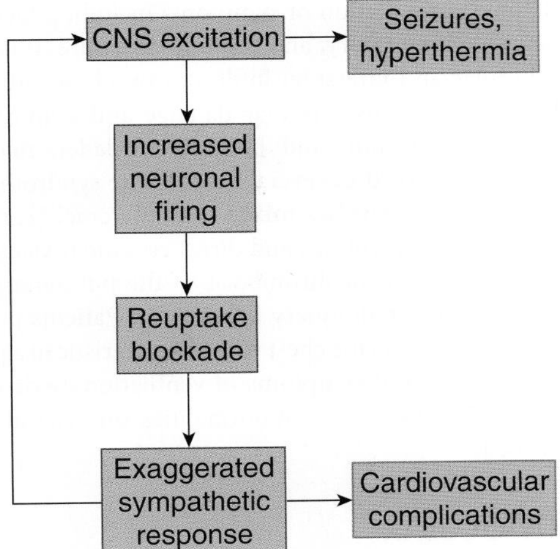

FIGURE 76–2. Cocaine-induced CNS effects modulate peripheral events.

oxygen demand. Cocaine use also leads to vasospasm, accelerated atherogenesis, and hypercoagulability.

Vasopasm Although increased myocardial oxygen demand may be sufficient to cause ischemia in some individuals, it is clear that cocaine also produces profound vasoconstriction. Evidence suggests that cocaine-induced vasoconstriction is mediated through both neuronal norepinephrine,[129,144] and benzoylecgonine (BE). BE has a direct effect on vessels that appears to be calcium mediated.[144] Additionally nicotine, which is simultaneously used by many substance users, has additive, if not synergistic, effects with cocaine.[165]

Atherogenesis Cocaine use accelerates atherosclerosis. Rabbits fed a normal diet supplemented with cholesterol do not develop atherosclerotic vascular disease. However, when that diet includes cocaine, rabbits develop classic atherosclerotic lesions.[121,131,132] Experiments with human endothelial cells demonstrate that cocaine directly increases the permeability to lipids by altering tight junctions.[122] This probably promotes the formation of subendothelial atherosclerotic plaques.

Dysrhythmias Like other local anesthetics (Chap. 66) cocaine blocks neuronal sodium channels, thereby preventing saltatory conduction. Because of homology between neuronal and cardiac sodium channels, cocaine also inhibits the rapid inward Na^+ current responsible for phase 0 depolarization of the cardiac action potential (Chaps. 5, 23, and 73). Experimental evidence suggests that cocaine enters the sodium channel and binds on the inner membrane.[35,120,187] Like many sodium channel blockers, binding is both pH and use dependent (ie, binding increases as pH falls or heart rate increases; Chap. 63).[36,239] Furthermore, although norcocaine has a greater affinity for inactivated sodium channels, it has a much more rapid offset of action than cocaine.[35] Consequently, cocaine can be characterized as a Vaughan-Williams type IC antidysrhythmic (Chap. 63).[249] Cocaine-induced QRS prolongation is exacerbated by Vaughan-Williams type IA antidysrhythmics,[246] and ameliorated by hypertonic sodium bicarbonate or lidocaine.[9,69,181] Another effect of sodium channel blockade, the Brugada pattern, is also associated with cocaine use.[141,177]

In addition to its sodium channel-blocking properties, cocaine also blocks cardiac potassium channels (Chaps. 22 and 23). This results in QT prolongation [185,226,239] and may produce torsades de pointes.[208] Cocaethylene also has dysrhythmogenic effects.[173] In vivo experiments demonstrated inhibition of the myocardial HERG potassium channels which may explain this phenomenon.[52] Cocaethylene, in animal studies, is associated with increased incidence of dysrhythmias, prolonged myocardial depression, and increased lethality.[115,244]

HEMATOLOGIC EFFECTS

Enhanced coagulation and impaired thrombolysis compound the effects of accelerated atherogenesis and vasospasm. Cocaine activates human platelets and causes α-granule release, resulting in platelet aggregation.[80,127] Thus even in the absence of endothelial injury, cocaine can initiate a thrombotic cascade while simultaneously enhancing the activity of plasminogen activator inhibitor type 1 (PAI-1), thereby impairing clot lysis.[164]

PULMONARY EFFECTS

Bronchospasm The association between cocaine use and asthma[195] was not recognized until smoked cocaine became prevalent.[49] Furthermore, experiments in human volunteers demonstrate that only smoked cocaine (not intravenous cocaine) produces bronchospasm.[225] Although it is possible that bronchospasm results from direct administration of cocaine to the airways, inhaled contaminants of cocaine, or thermal insult, and AEME (the unique pyrolytic metabolite of cocaine that acts as a muscarinic agonist) produces bronchospasm in experimental animals.[27]

CLINICAL MANIFESTATIONS

Many clinical manifestations of toxicity develop immediately following cocaine use. These are typically associated with the sympathetic overactivity, and their duration of effect is predictable based on the pharmacokinetics of cocaine use. Other manifestations, such as those associated with tissue ischemia, may present in a delayed fashion, with a clinical latency of hours to even days after last cocaine use. The reasons for this delay are not entirely apparent but may relate to the presence of an altered sensorium associated with acute cocaine use, anesthetic effects, changes in receptor regulation,[168] or affects on platelets, coagulation, and thrombolysis, which incite a slow cascade leading to thrombosis.

Vital sign abnormalities that develop during cocaine toxicity are characteristic of the sympathomimetic toxidrome. Thus, varying degrees of hypertension, tachycardia, tachypnea, and hyperthermia occur. Although any of these vital sign abnormalities can be life threatening, experimental and clinical evidence suggests that hyperthermia is the most critical.[25,70,150] Initially, with typically used doses, and at any time with a massive dose, apnea, hypotension, and bradycardia can result, all from direct suppression (anesthesia) of brainstem centers.[129,157] These effects are fleeting and rarely noted when patients present to healthcare as either the sympathetic overdrive rapidly ensues, or sudden death results. Additional sympathomimetic findings include mydriasis, diaphoresis, and neuropsychiatric manifestations.

Cocaine produces end-organ toxicity in virtually every organ system in the body. These events result from vasospasm, hemorrhage secondary to increased vascular sheer force (dP/dT), or enhanced coagulation. Each organ system is discussed separately in the following sections.

CENTRAL NERVOUS SYSTEM

Seizures, coma, headache, focal neurologic signs or symptoms, or behavioral abnormalities that persist longer than the predicted duration of effect of cocaine should alert the clinician to a potential catastrophic CNS event. Hemorrhage can occur at any anatomic site in the CNS. Subarachnoid, intraventricular, and intraparenchymal bleeding are all well described in association with cocaine use.[2,39,137,149,189,211] Early discussions suggested an underlying predisposition due to the presence of arteriovenous malformations or congenital aneurysms,[248] but subsequent larger studies failed to support this analysis, suggesting that effects can occur independently of preexisting disease.[2,170,237] Recent data suggests that ruptured intracerebral aneurysms in cocaine users are almost exclusively in the carotid artery circulation.[237] Presumably CNS bleeding is a manifestation of abnormal sheer force. Spontaneous extra-axial bleeding is also associated with cocaine use.[199]

Both vasospastic infarction and transient ischemic attack (TIA) are reported in association with cocaine use.[39,40,137] In one epidemiologic study, women younger than age 45 years who had strokes were seven times more likely to report cocaine use than controls.[186] Patients can present with any of the classic physical findings associated with thrombotic or embolic stroke. Vasospasm can injure the spinal cord, resulting in paralysis from an anterior spinal artery syndrome.[39,163]

Seizures are commonly provoked by cocaine use.[91,167] It is clear that cocaine use can serve as a trigger in patients with epilepsy, although an underlying focus is not necessary for seizures to occur.[124]

Headache is also well described in cocaine users. While the exact mechanism is unclear, hypertension, vasospasm, or dysregulated neurotransmitters may all be contributory. In addition to typical tension headache, classic migraine and cluster headaches are also reported.[184,201]

EYES, NOSE, AND THROAT

Sympathetic excess produces mydriasis through stimulation of the dilator fibers of the iris with characteristic retention of the ability to respond to light. Like other mydriatics, cocaine can produce acute angle closure glaucoma.[76] Vasospasm of the retinal vessels causes both unilateral and bilateral loss of vision.[89,139] Additionally, although cocaine produces excellent corneal anesthesia, it is highly toxic to the corneal epithelium. Following application of cocaine to the eye, the superficial corneal layer is shed, resulting in pain and decreased acuity.[190] The loss of eyebrow and eyelash hair from thermal injury associated with smoking crack cocaine is called *madarosis*.[224]

Chronic intranasal insufflation of cocaine can produce perforation of the nasal septum. This finding most likely results from repeated ischemic injury with resultant tissue loss. This ischemia is usually asymptomatic and necrotic tissue is sloughed. At least one reported case of wound botulism (Chap. 46) has been associated with intranasal insufflation. Presumably this resulted from accumulation of necrotic tissue in the nose, serving as a culture medium for *Clostridium botulinum*.[126]

Angioedema and oropharyngeal burns, located as far distally as the esophagus, are associated with smoking crack cocaine.[23,28,117,158] These effects are most likely the result of inhalation or ingestion of superheated fumes and hot liquid (from the smoking apparatus) rather than direct toxicity from cocaine.

PULMONARY

Pneumothorax, pneumomediastinum, and pneumopericardium are reported following both smoked and intranasal cocaine use.[146,203,230,234] These findings do not result directly from cocaine toxicity, but rather are epiphenomena related to the mechanism of drug use. Following insufflation or inhalation, the user commonly performs a Valsalva maneuver in an attempt to retain the drug. Bearing down against a closed epiglottis increases intrathoracic pressure and an alveolar bleb can rupture against the pleural, mediastinal or pericardial surfaces.

Cocaine use exacerbates reversible airway disease and it is common for patients to present with shortness of breath and wheezing.[49,136,178,194] Like so many manifestations of cocaine toxicity, it is unclear whether this is a direct effect of cocaine or related to inhalation of some contaminant of the drug. However, as discussed above, the muscarinic (M2) agonistic effects of the pyrolysis metabolite AEME might be contributory.

Crack lung is the term given to an acute pulmonary syndrome that occurs after inhalational use of crack cocaine. The pulmonary syndrome is a poorly defined constellation of symptoms including fever, hemoptysis, hypoxia, acute lung injury, and respiratory failure. It is associated with diffuse alveolar and interstital infiltrates on chest radiography.[191] Histopathology shows diffuse alveolar damage and hemorrhage with inflammatory cell infiltration and hemosiderin-laden macrophages. Eosinophilia has been noted in several cases.[58] The syndrome has been variously attributed to impurities mixed with the crack, carbonaceous material generated from pyrolysis, and direct cocaine toxicity.

Vasospasm and subsequent thrombosis of the pulmonary artery or its branches can produce pulmonary infarction.[42] Patients present with shortness of breath and pleuritic chest pain characteristic of a pulmonary embolus. Clinical signs and symptoms of ventilation–perfusion (V/Q) mismatch (Chap. 21), as well as abnormalities on arterial blood gas analysis, are noted.

CARDIOVASCULAR

Chest pain or discomfort is a common emergency department complaint in cocaine users.[17] Cocaine use is associated with cardiac ischemia and infarction in young people, and may account for as much as 25% of myocardial infarctions in patients younger than 45 years old.[188] Although myocardial infarction is of concern, only approximately 6% of patients with complaints referable to the heart will manifest biochemical evidence of myocardial injury.[96,240] Many others will have an ischemic cardiac event, but for the remainder the differential diagnosis is broad.[130] Entities to consider include the pulmonary and esophageal etiologies described previously, referred abdominal symptoms (see Abdominal below), chest wall injury,[67] aortic dissection,[37,104,138,140] coronary artery dissection,[202,220] and dysrhythmias. No single sign or symptom or combination of signs and symptoms reliably identifies cardiovascular injury from among the discussed differential diagnosis.[96]

Catecholamine-induced direct myocardial catecholamine toxicity contributes to both acute and chronic cardiac disease. *Takotsubo cardiomyopathy* is a reversible form of left ventricular apical ballooning associated with myocardial ischemia in the absence of atherosclerotic lesions. It is thought to result from catecholamine toxicity on the myocardium during high levels of stress and is also reported after cocaine use.[5] Chronic cocaine use is associated with a dilated cardiomyopathy,[82,130,176,243] the etiology of which is presumed to be the result of repeated subclinical ischemic events. Patients may present with signs and symptoms of congestive heart failure or pulmonary edema. The pathologic finding of contraction band necrosis also suggests that there may be some direct catecholamine toxicity as this finding only commonly occurs with cocaine and amphetamine use, pheochromocytoma, and in patients receiving high-dose vasopressors.[55,238]

ABDOMINAL

Abdominal pain, or other gastrointestinal complaints, suggests a broad differential diagnosis. Cocaine users have a disproportionate incidence of perforated ulcers.[134,183,214] The etiology has not been elucidated, but may be related to local ischemia of the gastrointestinal tract or increased acid production associated with sympathetic activity. Vasospasm produces ischemic colitis that can present with abdominal pain or bloody stools.[140,169] More severe vasospasm, with or without thrombosis, can lead to intestinal infarction[61,83,101,179] with attendant hypotension and metabolic acidosis. Signs and symptoms of bowel obstruction such as vomiting or distension might suggest body packing (gastrointestinal drug smuggling). Although less common, splenic[44,171] and renal infarctions,[46,161,198] may also occur. Spontaneous hemoperitoneum was also reported, although occult trauma could not be definitively excluded.[10]

Animals frequently develop hepatotoxicity following cocaine administration. In human cocaine users, minor elevations of liver enzyme concentrations are common and rarely associated with symptoms.[20,125] When more severe liver injury occurs, it is usually associated with multisystem organ dysfunction from hyperthermia or another type of hepatic injury.[6] Isolated hepatic injury from cocaine is distinctly uncommon and may result from differences in metabolic pathways, as animals are known to make a hepatotoxic metabolite of cocaine that has not been described in humans.[236]

MUSCULOSKELETAL

Rhabdomyolysis is common in all conditions that produce an agitated delirium and/or hyperthermia; cocaine is no exception.[32,103,196] Unlike most other toxicologic disorders, however, psychomotor agitation is not a prerequisite for cocaine-associated rhabdomyolysis.[252] Muscle injury may result from vasospasm or direct muscle toxicity; however, the mechanism remains unclear. Patients with cocaine toxicity present with a spectrum of illness that ranges from asymptomatic enzyme and electrolyte abnormalities characteristic of rhabdomyolysis, to localized or diffuse muscle pain, to frank compartment syndrome and renal failure.[47,56]

Limb ischemia associated with cocaine use has been reported.[71,155] Vasospasm, accelerated atherogenesis, and increased thrombogensis (see Pathophysiology) place users at increased risk.

Traumatic injury is also fairly common in the setting of cocaine use.[152] Clinicians should be aware of the possibilities of occult fractures or other injuries that may be masked by the anesthetic properties of cocaine.[142,151]

NEUROPSYCHIATRIC

The neuropsychiatric effects of cocaine are most likely dose dependent. Low-dose administration produces alertness, exhilaration, hypersexual behavior, and other "desired" effects. These effects rarely bring users to healthcare facilities. As the cocaine dose increases, agitation, aggressive behavior, confusion, disorientation, and hallucinations can develop.

Other possible manifestations include a variety of movement disorders that most likely result from depletion or dysregulation of dopamine. Patients may develop acute dystonias[24,53,235] or choreoathetoid movements that have been referred to as "crack-dancing."[38,72] Following binge use of cocaine, a "washed-out" syndrome occurs that is best described by dopamine depletion.[219,231] Patients complain of anhedonia, lethargy, and have trouble initiating and sustaining movement. However, they are arousable with minimal stimulation and usually remain cognitively intact.

OBSTETRICAL

The majority of obstetrical findings associated with cocaine use involve developmental problems in the fetus and neonate and are probably a result of a combination of chronic vascular insufficiency from cocaine-induced spasm of the uterine artery or distal vessels and other risk factors, such as poor maternal nutrition, cigarette smoking, and a lack of prenatal care. These events are extensively reviewed elsewhere.[26,51,213] Acute cocaine use during pregnancy is associated with abruptio placentae, causing patients to present with abdominal pain and vaginal bleeding.[1,57] The remaining maternal and fetal complications comprise every possible complication described in nonpregnant patients.

DIAGNOSTIC TESTING

Cocaine and benzoylecgonine, its principle metabolite, can be detected in blood, urine, saliva, hair, and meconium. Routine drug-of-abuse testing relies on urine testing using a variety of immunologic techniques (Chap. 6). Although cocaine is rapidly eliminated within just a few hours of use, benzoylecgonine is easily detected in the urine for 2–3 days following last use.[4] When more sophisticated testing methodology is applied to chronic users, cocaine metabolites can be identified for several weeks following last use.[243]

Urine testing, even using rapid point-of-care assays, offers little to clinicians managing patients with presumed cocaine toxicity because it cannot distinguish recent from remote cocaine use. In addition, false-negative testing can result when there is a large quantity of urine in the bladder with very recent cocaine use or when the urine is intentionally diluted by increased fluid intake[30] leading to a urine cocaine concentration below the cut-off value and interpretation of the test as negative. Under these circumstances, repeat testing is almost always positive. While false-positive tests do occur, they are more common with hair testing than urine or blood because of the increased risk of external contamination.[30,193] Because of the very low rate of false-positive results, confirmation of a positive urine is unnecessary for medical indications (Chap. 6).

The greatest benefit for cocaine testing is in cases of unintentional poisoning or suspected child abuse and neglect. Here confirmation of a clinical suspicion is essential to support a legal argument. In addition, there may be some usefulness for urine testing of body packers, especially when the concealed xenobiotic is unknown.[232] While many body packers will have negative urine throughout their hospitalization, a positive urine test is suggestive of the concealed drug but obviously not confirmatory. More importantly, a conversion from a negative study on admission to a positive study not only confirms the substance ingested, but also suggests packet leakage, which could be a harbinger of life-threatening toxicity (see SC4: Concealment). Another indication for urine testing for cocaine occurs in young patients with chest pain syndromes where the history of drug use, specifically cocaine, is not forthcoming.[92] Routine diagnostic tests such as a bedside rapid reagent glucose, electrolytes, renal function tests, and markers of muscle and cardiac muscle injury are more likely to be useful than urine drug screening. An ECG may show signs of ischemia or infarction, or dysrhythmias that require specific therapy. Unfortunately, in the setting of cocaine-associated chest pain, the ECG has neither the sensitivity nor the specificity necessary to permit exclusion or confirmation of cardiac injury.[99] Cardiac markers are therefore always required adjuncts when considering myocardial ischemia or infarction. Because cocaine use is associated with diffuse muscle injury, assays for troponin are preferred over myoglobin or myocardial band enzymes of creatine phosphokinase (CPK-MB).[98] Additionally, a chest radiograph may be useful to exclude certain etiologies in patients with chest discomfort, or to identify free air under the diaphragm when gastrointestinal perforation is suspected. Supplemental diagnostic studies, such as CT scans of the head, chest, or abdomen and functional cardiac imaging, should be guided by the clinical condition of the patient.[34,48,74]

MANAGEMENT

GENERAL SUPPORTIVE CARE

As in the case of all poisoned patients, the initial emphasis must be on stabilization and control of the patient's airway, breathing, and circulation. If tracheal intubation is required, it is important to recognize that cocaine toxicity may be a relative contraindication to the use of succinylcholine. Specifically, in the setting of rhabdomyolysis, hyperkalemia may be exacerbated by succinylcholine administration, and life-threatening dysrhythmias may result (Chap. 68). Additionally, it is essential to recognize that PChE metabolizes both cocaine and succinylcholine.[109] Thus their simultaneous use could either prolong cocaine toxicity or paralysis, or both. Human data are insufficient to predict which interaction is more likely to occur. If hypotension is present, the initial approach should be infusion of intravenous 0.9% sodium chloride solution as many patients are volume depleted as a result of poor oral intake and excessive fluid losses from uncontrolled agitation, diaphoresis, and hyperthermia.

In the setting of cocaine toxicity it is important to recognize that both animal[25,70] and human[150] experience suggests that elevated temperature represents the most critical vital sign abnormality. Determination of the core temperature is an essential element of the initial evaluation, even when patients are severely agitated. When hyperthermia is present, preferably rapid cooling with ice water immersion, or the combined use of mist and fanning, is required to achieve a rapid return to normal core body temperature (Chap. 15). Sedation or paralysis and intubation may be necessary to facilitate the rapid cooling process. Pharmacotherapy including antipyretics, drugs that prevent shivering (chlorpromazine or meperidine), and dantrolene[59] are not indicated as they are ineffective and have the potential for adverse drug interactions such as serotonin syndrome (meperidine) or seizures (chloropromazine).

Sedation remains the mainstay of therapy in patients with cocaine-associated agitation. It is important to remember that cocaine use is associated with hypoglycemia and that many of the peripheral findings of hypoglycemia are the result of a catecholamine discharge.[16,162] Consequently, a rapid reagent glucose test should be obtained, or hypertonic dextrose should be empirically administered if indicated, prior to or while simultaneously achieving sedation. Both animal models[25,70] and extensive clinical experience in humans support the central role of benzodiazepines. Although the choice among individual benzodiazepines is not well studied, an understanding of the pharmacology of these drugs allows for rational decision making. The goal is to use parenteral therapy with a drug that has a rapid onset and a rapid peak of action, making titration easy. Using this rationale, midazolam and diazepam are preferable to lorazepam, because significant delay to peak effect for lorazepam often results in oversedation when it is dosed rapidly, or in prolonged agitation when the appropriate dosing interval is used. Drugs should be administered in initial doses that are consistent with routine practices and increased incrementally based on an appropriate understanding of their pharmacology. For example, if using diazepam, the starting dose might be 5–10 mg, which can be repeated every 3–5 minutes and increased if necessary. Large doses of benzodiazepines may be necessary (on the order of 1 mg/kg of diazepam). This may result from cocaine-induced alterations in benzodiazepine receptor function.[65,66,112] (see Antidote in Depth A24)

On the rare occasion when benzodiazepines fail to achieve an adequate level of sedation, either a rapidly acting barbiturate or propofol should be administered. Controlled animal studies clearly show that the use of phenothiazines or butyrophenones is contraindicated.[25,70,247] In animal models, these drugs enhance toxicity (seizures), lethality, or both. Additional concerns about these drugs include interference with heat dissipation, exacerbation of tachycardia, prolongation of the QT interval, induction of torsade de pointes, and precipitation of dystonic reactions.

Once sedation is accomplished, often no additional therapy is required. Specifically, hypertension and tachycardia usually respond to sedation and volume resuscitation. In the uncommon event that hypertension and/or tachycardia persists, the use of a β-adrenergic antagonist or a mixed α- and β-adrenergic antagonist is contraindicated. Again, in both animal models and human reports, these drugs increase lethality and fail to treat the underlying problem.[12,25,70,200,231] The resultant unopposed α-adrenergic effect may produce severe and life-threatening hypertension or vasospasm. A direct-acting vasodilator like nitroglycerin, nitroprusside or possibly nicardipine or an α-adrenergic antagonist (such as phentolamine) may be considered. Other nonspecific therapies for rhabdomyolysis such as intravenous fluid should also be considered.

DECONTAMINATION

The majority of patients who present to the hospital following cocaine use will not require gastrointestinal decontamination as the most popular methods of cocaine use are smoking, intravenous and intranasal administration. If the nares contain residual white powder presumed to be cocaine, gentle irrigation with 0.9% sodium chloride solution will help remove adherent material. Less commonly, patients may ingest cocaine unintentionally or[19] in an attempt to conceal evidence during an arrest (body stuffing)[84,111,148,218] or transport large quantities of drug across international borders (body packing).[63] These patients may require intensive decontamination and possibly surgical removal[54,90,147,204,232,233,242] (see Special Considerations SC4: Body Stuffers and Body Packers).

SPECIFIC MANAGEMENT

End-organ manifestations of vasospasm that do not resolve with sedation, cooling, and volume resuscitation should be treated with vasodilatory agents (such as phentolamine). When possible, direct delivery via intra-arterial administration to the affected vascular bed is preferable. Because this approach is not always feasible, systemic therapy is typically indicated. Phentolamine can be dosed intravenously in increments of 1–2.5 mg, and repeated as necessary until symptoms resolve or systemic hypotension develops.

Acute Coronary Syndrome A significant amount of animal, in vitro, and in vivo human experimentation has been directed at defining the appropriate approach to a patient with presumed cardiac ischemia or infarction. In some instances an approach that is similar to the treatment of coronary artery disease (CAD) is indicated, although there are certain notable exceptions. An overall approach to care is available in the American Heart Association guidelines and a number of reviews.[3,100,130,156]

High-flow oxygen therapy is clearly indicated as it may help overcome some of the supply–demand mismatch that occurs with coronary insufficiency. Aspirin is safe in patients with cocaine-associated chest pain and is recommended for routine use.[156] In addition, administration of morphine is likely to be effective as it relieves cocaine-induced vasoconstriction.[197] Morphine also offers the same theoretical benefits of preload reduction and reduction of catecholamine release in response to pain that is thought to be responsible for its usefulness in patients with CAD.

After these interventions, the treatment of patients with cocaine-associated chest pain begins to deviate from the standard accepted approach to patients with CAD. Nitroglycerin is clearly beneficial as it reduces cocaine-associated coronary constriction of both normal and diseased vessels and relieves chest pain and associated symptoms.[18,95] Interestingly, in several clinical trials of cocaine-associated chest pain, benzodiazepines are at least as effective or superior to nitroglycerin.[8,102] Although the reasons for this are unclear, possible etiologies include blunting of central catecholamines or direct effects on cardiac benzodiazepine receptors. Either or both drugs can be used in standard dosing (See Antidotes in Depth A24: Benzodiazepines).

Over the last decade, the benefits of β-adrenergic antagonism have been demonstrated in patients with CAD. In contrast, β-adrenergic antagonism increases lethality in cocaine-toxic animals[25,70] and in humans, exacerbates cocaine-induced coronary vasoconstriction,[128] and produces severe paradoxical hypertension.[200] Similarly, with regard to treatment of coronary constriction, labetalol is no better than placebo.[12] Thus, in the setting of cocaine use, β-adrenergic antagonism is absolutely contraindicated. The 2008 American Heart Association Guidelines for the treatment of cocaine-associated chest pain and MI state that use of β-adrenergic antagonists should be avoided in the acute setting.[156] If, after the measures mentioned previously have been initiated, hypertension or vasospasm is still present and treatment is indicated, phentolamine is preferred based on its demonstrable experimental and clinical results.[94,129] If tachycardia does not respond to accepted therapies above, then diltiazem can be administered and titrated to effect.[11] Prior to the administation of any negative inotrope, it is essential to confirm that the tachycardia is not compensatory for a low cardiac output resulting from global myocardial dysfunction. Noninvasive methods of assessment of cardiac function have been used successfully in patients with cocaine-associated acute coronary syndromes.[7]

There are no data on the use of either unfractionated or low-molecular-weight heparins, glycoprotein IIb/IIIa inhibitors, or clopidogrel. The recent AHA guidelines recommend the administration of unfractionated heparin or low-molecular-weight heparin in patients with cocaine-associated MI.[156] The decision to use any of these medications should be based on a risk-to-benefit analysis. Consideration should be given to the possibility of underlying atherosclerotic heart disease. When acute thrombosis is likely, thrombolytic therapy should be considered. Mechanistically, cocaine inhibits endogenous thrombolysis through augmentation of the inhibitor of tissue plasminogen activator. Additionally, there is sufficient clinical evidence to support the safety of thrombolytic therapy in patients with cocaine-associated myocardial infarction.[85,93] Even though the number of patients treated with thrombolytic therapy is insufficient to demonstrate efficacy in terms of mortality, evidence of revascularization is encouraging. Similar to patients with ASHD, if available, cardiac catheterization with revascularization is preferable to thrombolysis.[212] Thrombolysis would not be expected to be useful in treating ischemia caused by vasospasm. Due to the high incidence of coexisting atherosclerotic disease and an increased hypercoaguable state in cocaine-associated MI, thrombolysis is an acceptable alternative when catheterization is unavailable. Standard contraindications such as persistent hypertension, aortic dissection, trauma, and altered mental status must be considered prior to thrombolysis.

Dysrhythmias Most patients present with sinus tachycardia that resolves following sedation, cooling, rehydration, and time to metabolize the drug. Other stable dysrhythmias should be treated similarly, and will often spontaneously revert because of the short duration of effect of cocaine. However, cocaine use is associated with atrial, supraventricular, and ventricular dysrhythmias including torsade de pointes.[107,130,208] Most notably, wide complex tachycardias result from sodium channel blockade. When approaching patients with cocaine-associated dysrhythmias, there are several important points to consider. The first is that β-adrenergic antagonism is contraindicated. Furthermore, classic types IA and IC antidysrhythmics are also contraindicated because of their ability to exacerbate cocaine-induced sodium and potassium channel blockade.[130,246] Additionally, although popular in many advanced cardiac life support dysrhythmia algorithms, the effects of amiodarone are largely unknown in the setting of cocaine toxicity. Because of the lack of data demonstrating a benefit for amiodarone, and because of concerns about its β-adrenergic antagonist effects, the use of this drug cannot be recommended. Finally, although adenosine and synchronized cardioversion may transiently help convert narrow complex tachycardias, if a substantial amount of cocaine is unmetabolized, the patient will likely revert back to the original dysrhythmia as these therapeutic interventions have short durations of effect. Thus for rapid atrial fibrillation and narrow complex reentrant tachycardias, a calcium channel blocker such as diltiazem is preferred. For wide-complex dysrhythmias, a trial of hypertonic sodium bicarbonate has demonstrable usefulness analogous to treating patients with cyclic antidepressant overdose (see Antidotes in Depth A5: Sodium Bicarbonate).[116,181,239,246] When the use of hypertonic sodium bicarbonate fails to treat the dysrhythmia, lidocaine can be used. Although lidocaine blocks sodium channels, its fast-on, fast-off properties allow it to antagonize the effects of cocaine. The benefits and safety of lidocaine were demonstrated in multiple animal models[69,81,246] and in humans with cocaine-associated myocardial infarction.[215]

DISPOSITION

Patients who present to healthcare facilities with classic sympathomimetic signs and symptoms that resolve spontaneously in the absence of signs of end-organ damage can be safely discharged after short periods of observation. Once hyperthermia, rhabdomyolysis, or other signs of end-organ damage are evident, hospital admission is usually required. Patients who use cocaine are at increased risk for sudden death likely related in part to dysrhythmias and myocardial ischemia. In one series, patients with cardiac arrest after smoking crack cocaine were younger, more likely to survive, and less likely to have neurologic sequelae than case controls.[105]

For patients with chest pain, a specific management algorithm has been derived based on substantial clinical experience. Those patients with clearly diagnostic or evolving ECGs suggestive of ischemia or infarction, positive cardiac markers, dysrhythmias other than sinus tachycardia, congestive heart failure, or persistent pain require admission. Patients who become pain free and whose ECGs are stable are candidates for discharge if a single cardiac marker obtained at least 8 hours after the onset of chest pain is normal.[241] The AHA guidelines recommend 9–12 hours of observation for low and intermediate risk patients with cocaine-associated chest pain. For all patients it is essential to provide a referral for detoxification, as repeated cocaine use is the greatest risk factor for future cardiovascular complications.[97,243]

SUMMARY

Cocaine is a unique drug that combines local anesthetic, vasoconstrictive, and neuropsychopharmacologic properties. Although its legitimate pharmaceutical use has diminished because of its high abuse potential, it remains a common recreational drug of abuse. Cocaine produces the prototypical agitated delirium that characterizes the sympathomimetic toxic syndrome. Most patients can be treated with sedation and cooling, but others require more intensive individualized care. The most essential and difficult aspect of care is providing access to programs that support cocaine detoxification.

REFERENCES

1. Addis A, Moretti ME, Ahmed Syed F, et al. Fetal effects of cocaine: an updated meta-analysis. *Reprod Toxicol.* 2001;15:341-369.
2. Aggarwal SK, Williams V, Levine SR, et al. Cocaine-associated intracranial hemorrhage: absence of vasculitis in 14 cases. *Neurology.* 1996;46:1741-1743.
3. Albertson TE, Dawson A, de Latorre F, et al. TOX-ACLS: toxico-logic-oriented advanced cardiac life support. *Ann Emerg Med.* 2001;37:S78-S90.
4. Ambre J, Fischman M, Ruo TI. Urinary excretion of ecgonine methyl ester, a major metabolite of cocaine in humans. *J Anal Toxicol.* 1984;8:23-25.
5. Arora S, Aflayoumi F, Srinivasan V. Transient left ventricular apical ballooning after cocaine use: is catecholamine cardiotoxicity the pathologic link? *Mayo Clin Proc.* 2006;81:829-832.
6. Balaguer F, Fernandez J, Lozano M, et al. Cocaine-induced acute hepatitis and thrombotic microangiopathy. *JAMA.* 2005;293:797-798.
7. Baumann BM, Perrone J, Hornig SE, et al. Cardiac and hemodynamic assessment of patients with cocaine-associated chest pain syndromes. *J Toxicol Clin Toxicol.* 2000;38:283-290.
8. Baumann BM, Perrone J, Hornig SE, et al. Randomized, double-blind, placebo-controlled trial of diazepam, nitroglycerin, or both for treatment of patients with potential cocaine-associated acute coronary syndromes. *Acad Emerg Med.* 2000;7:878-885.

9. Beckman KJ, Parker RB, Hariman RJ, et al. Hemodynamic and electrophysiological actions of cocaine: effects of sodium bicarbonate as an antidote in dogs. *Circulation.* 1991;83:1799-1807.
10. Bellows CF, Raafat AM. The surgical abdomen associated with cocaine abuse. *J Emerg Med.* 2002;23:383-386.
11. Billman GE. Effect of calcium channel antagonists on cocaine-induced malignant arrhythmias: protection against ventricular fibrillation. *J Pharmacol Exp Ther.* 1993;266:407-416.
12. Boehrer JD, Moliterno DJ, Willard JE, et al. Influence of labetalol on cocaine-induced coronary vasoconstriction in humans. *Am J Med.* 1993;94:608-610.
13. Borne RF, Bedford JA, Buelke JL, et al. Biological effects of cocaine derivatives I: improved synthesis and pharmacological evaluation of norcocaine. *J Pharm Sci.* 1977;66:119-120.
14. Bourland JA, Martin DK, Mayersohn M. In vitro transesterification of cocaethylene (ethylcocaine) in the presence of ethanol: esterase-mediated ethyl ester exchange. *Drug Metab Dispos.* 1998;26:203-206.
15. Brackett RL, Pouw B, Blyden JF, et al. Prevention of cocaine-induced convulsions and lethality in mice: effectiveness of targeting different sites on the NMDA receptor complex. *Neuropharmacology.* 2000;39:407-418.
16. Brady WJ Jr, Duncan CW. Hypoglycemia masquerading as acute psychosis and acute cocaine intoxication. *Am J Emerg Med.* 1999;17:318-319.
17. Brody SL, Slovis CM, Wrenn KD. Cocaine-related medical problems: consecutive series of 233 patients. *Am J Med.* 1990;88:325-331.
18. Brogan WE 3rd, Lange RA, Kim AS, et al. Alleviation of cocaine-induced coronary vasoconstriction by nitroglycerin. *J Am Coll Cardiol.* 1991;18:581-586.
19. Bush S. Is cocaine needed in topical anaesthesia? *Emerg Med J.* 2002;19:418-422.
20. Cantilena LR, Cherstniakova SA, Saviolakis G, et al. Prevalence of abnormal liver-associated enzymes in cocaine experienced adults versus health volunteers during phase 1 clinical trials. *Contemp Clin Trials.* 2007;28:695-704.
21. Carmona GN, Jufer RA, Goldberg SR, et al. Butyrylcholinesterase accelerates cocaine metabolism: in vitro and in vivo effects in non-human primates and humans. *Drug Metab Dispos.* 2000;28:367-371.
22. Carmona GN, Schindler CW, Shoaib M, et al. Attenuation of cocaine-induced locomotor activity by butyrylcholinesterase. *Exp Clin Psychopharmacol.* 1998;6:274-279.
23. Castro-Villamor MA, de las Heras P, Armentia A, Duenas-Laita A. Cocaine-induced severe angioedema and urticaria. *Ann Emerg Med.* 1999;34:296-297.
24. Catalano G, Catalano MC, Rodriguez R. Dystonia associated with crack cocaine use. *South Med J.* 1997;90:1050-1052.
25. Catravas JD, Waters IW. Acute cocaine intoxication in the conscious dog: studies on the mechanism of lethality. *J Pharmacol Exp Ther.* 1981;217:350-356.
26. Chasnoff IJ, Burns WJ, Schnoll SH, Burns KA. Cocaine use in pregnancy. *N Engl J Med.* 1985;313:666-669.
27. Chen LC, Graefe JF, Shojaie J, et al. Pulmonary effects of the cocaine pyrolysis product, methylecgonidine, in guinea pigs. *Life Sci.* 1995;56:P7-12.
28. Cohen ME, Kegel JG. Candy cocaine esophagus. *Chest.* 2002;121:1701-1703.
29. Coleman DL, Ross TF, Naughton JL. Myocardial ischemia and infarction related to recreational cocaine use. *West J Med.* 1982;136:444-446.
30. Cone EJ, Sampson-Cone AH, Darwin WD, et al. Urine testing for cocaine abuse: metabolic and excretion patterns following different routes of administration and methods for detection of false-negative results. *J Anal Toxicol.* 2003;27:386-401.
31. Cone EJ, Tsadik A, Oyler J, Darwin WD. Cocaine metabolism and urinary excretion after different routes of administration. *Ther Drug Monit.* 1998;20:556-560.
32. Counselman FL, McLaughlin EW, Kardon EM, Bhambhani-Bhavnani AS. Creatine phosphokinase elevation in patients presenting to the emergency department with cocaine-related complaints. *Am J Emerg Med.* 1997;15:221-223.
33. Covert RF, Schreiber MD, Tebbett IR, Torgerson LJ. Hemodynamic and cerebral blood flow effects of cocaine, cocaethylene and benzoylecgonine in conscious and anesthetized fetal lambs. *J Pharmacol Exp Ther.* 1994;270:118-126.
34. Cranston PE, Pollack CV Jr, Harrison RB. CT of crack cocaine ingestion. *J Comput Assist Tomogr.* 1992;16:560-563.
35. Crumb WJ Jr, Clarkson CW. Characterization of the sodium channel blocking properties of the major metabolites of cocaine in single cardiac myocytes. *J Pharmacol Exp Ther.* 1992;261:910-917.
36. Crumb WJ Jr, Clarkson CW. The pH dependence of cocaine interaction with cardiac sodium channels. *J Pharmacol Exp Ther.* 1995;274:1228-1237.
37. Daniel JC, Huynh TT, Zhou W, et al. Acute aortic dissection associated with use of cocaine. *J Vasc Surg.* 2007;46:427-433.
38. Daras M, Koppel BS, Atos-Radzion E. Cocaine-induced choreoathetoid movements ("crack dancing"). *Neurology.* 1994;44:751-752.
39. Daras M, Tuchman AJ, Marks S. Central nervous system infarction related to cocaine abuse. *Stroke.* 1991;22:1320-1325.
40. Daras MD, Orrego JJ, Akfirat GL, et al. Bilateral symmetrical basal ganglia infarction after intravenous use of cocaine and heroin. *Clin Imaging.* 2001;25:12-14.
41. Dean RA, Christian CD, Sample RH, Bosron WF. Human liver cocaine esterases: ethanol-mediated formation of ethylcocaine. *FASEB J.* 1991;5:2735-2739.
42. Delaney K, Hoffman RS. Pulmonary infarction associated with crack cocaine use in a previously healthy 23-year-old woman. *Am J Med.* 1991;91:92-94.
43. Department of Health and Human Services, Substance Abuse and Mental Health Services. Results Form the 2006 National Survey on Drug Abuse and Health. Available at: http://www.oas.samhsa.gov/latest.htm. Last accessed on May 22, 2008.
44. Dettmeyer R, Schlamann M, Madea B. Cocaine-associated abscesses with lethal sepsis after splenic infarction in a 17-year-old woman. *Forensic Sci Int.* 2004;140:21-23.
45. Devenyi P. Cocaine complications and pseudocholinesterase. *Ann Intern Med.* 1989;110:167-168.
46. Edmondson DA, Towne JB, Foley DW, et al. Cocaine-induced renal artery dissection and thrombosis leading to renal infarction. *WMJ.* 2004;103:66-69.
47. el-Hayek BM, Nogue S, Alonso D, Poch E. [Rhabdomyolysis, compartment syndrome and acute kidney failure related to cocaine consume.]. *Nefrologia.* 2003;23:469-470.
48. Eng JG, Aks SE, Waldron R, et al. False-negative abdominal CT scan in a cocaine body stuffer. *Am J Emerg Med.* 1999;17:702-704.
49. Ettinger NA, Albin RJ. A review of the respiratory effects of smoking cocaine. *Am J Med.* 1989;87:664-668.
50. European Monitoring Centre for Drugs and Addiction. State of the Drugs Problem in Europe. Annual Report. http://www.emcdda.europa.eu/publications/online/ar2007/en/cocaine. Last accessed 5/22/08.
51. Fajemirokun-Odudeyi O, Lindow SW. Obstetric implications of cocaine use in pregnancy: a literature review. *Eur J Obstet Gynecol Reprod Biol.* 2004;112:2-8.
52. Ferreira S, Crumb WJ Jr, Carlton CG, Clarkson CW. Effects of cocaine and its major metabolites on the HERG-encoded potassium channel. *J Pharmacol Exp Ther.* 2001;299:220-226.
53. Fines RE, Brady WJ, DeBehnke DJ. Cocaine-associated dystonic reaction. *Am J Emerg Med.* 1997;15:513-515.
54. Fineschi V, Centini F, Monciotti F, Turillazzi E. The cocaine "body stuffer" syndrome: a fatal case. *Forensic Sci Int.* 2002;126:7-10.
55. Fineschi V, Wetli CV, Di Paolo M, Baroldi G. Myocardial necrosis and cocaine. A quantitative morphologic study in 26 cocaine-associated deaths. *Int J Legal Med.* 1997;110:193-198.
56. Flaque-Coma J. Cocaine and rhabdomyolysis: report of a case and review of the literature. *Bol Asoc Med P R.* 1990;82:423-424.
57. Flowers D, Clark JF, Westney LS. Cocaine intoxication associated with abruptio placentae. *J Natl Med Assoc.* 1991;83:230-232.
58. Forrester JM, Steele AW, Waldron JA, Parsons PE. Crack lung: an acute pulmonary syndrome with a spectrum of clinical and histopathologic findings. *Am Rev Respir Dis.* 1990;142:462-467.
59. Fox AW. More on rhabdomyolysis associated with cocaine intoxication. *N Engl J Med.* 1989;321:1271.
60. Freud S. Uber coca. *Wien Centralbl Ther.* 1884;2:289-314.
61. Freudenberger RS, Cappell MS, Hutt DA. Intestinal infarction after intravenous cocaine administration. *Ann Intern Med.* 1990;113:715-716.
62. Garland OH. Fatal acute poisoning by cocaine. *Lancet.* 1895;1:1104-1105.
63. Gill JR, Graham SM. Ten years of "body packers" in New York City: 50 deaths. *J Forensic Sci.* 2002;47:843-846.
64. Giros B, Jaber M, Jones SR, et al. Hyperlocomotion and indifference to cocaine and amphetamine in mice lacking the dopamine transporter. *Nature.* 1996;379:606-612.
65. Goeders NE, Irby BD, Shuster CC, Guerin GF. Tolerance and sensitization to the behavioral effects of cocaine in rats: relationship to benzodiazepine receptors. *Pharmacol Biochem Behav.* 1997;57:43-56.

66. Goeders NE. Cocaine differentially affects benzodiazepine receptors in discrete regions of the rat brain: persistence and potential mechanisms mediating these effects. *J Pharmacol Exp Ther.* 1991;259:574-581.
67. Gotway MB, Marder SR, Hanks DK, et al. Thoracic complications of illicit drug use: an organ system approach. *Radiographics.* 2002;22:S119-35.
68. Grant SA, Hoffman RS, Goldfrank LR. Tetracaine protects against cocaine lethality in mice. *Ann Emerg Med.* 1993;22:1799-1803.
69. Grawe JJ, Hariman RJ, Winecoff AP, et al. Reversal of the electrocardiographic effects of cocaine by lidocaine. Part 2. Concentration-effect relationships. *Pharmacotherapy.* 1994;14:704-711.
70. Guinn MM, Bedford JA, Wilson MC. Antagonism of intravenous cocaine lethality in nonhuman primates. *Clin Toxicol.* 1980;16:499-508.
71. Gutierrez A, England JD, Krupski WC. Cocaine-induced peripheral vascular occlusive disease: a case report. *Angiology.* 1998;49:221-224.
72. Habal R, Sauter D, Olowe O, Daras M. Cocaine and chorea. *Am J Emerg Med.* 1991;9:618-620.
73. Haddad LM. 1978: Cocaine in perspective. *JACEP.* 1979;8:374-376.
74. Hahn IH, Hoffman RS, Nelson LS. Contrast CT scan fails to detect the last heroin packet. *J Emerg Med.* 2004;27:279-283.
75. Hall FS, Sora I, Drgonova J, et al. Molecular mechanisms underlying the rewarding effects of cocaine. *Ann N Y Acad Sci.* 2004;1025:47-56.
76. Hari CK, Roblin DG, Clayton MI, Nair RG. Acute angle closure glaucoma precipitated by intranasal application of cocaine. *J Laryngol Otol.* 1999;113:250-251.
77. Harris DS, Everhart ET, Mendelson J, Jones RT. The pharmacology of cocaethylene in humans following cocaine and ethanol administration. *Drug Alcohol Depend.* 2003;72:169-182.
78. Hart CL, Jatlow P, Sevarino KA, McCance-Katz EF. Comparison of intravenous cocaethylene and cocaine in humans. *Psychopharmacology (Berl).* 2000;149:153-162.
79. Havlik DM, Nolte KB. Fatal "crack" cocaine ingestion in an infant. *Am J Forensic Med Pathol.* 2000;21:245-248.
80. Heesch CM, Wilhelm CR, Ristich J, et al. Cocaine activates platelets and increases the formation of circulating platelet containing microaggregates in humans. *Heart.* 2000;83:688-695.
81. Heit J, Hoffman RS, Goldfrank LR. The effects of lidocaine pretreatment on cocaine neurotoxicity and lethality in mice. *Acad Emerg Med.* 1994;1:438-442.
82. Henzlova MJ, Smith SH, Prchal VM, Helmcke FR. Apparent reversibility of cocaine-induced congestive cardiomyopathy. *Am Heart J.* 1991;122: 577-579.
83. Hoang MP, Lee EL, Anand A. Histologic spectrum of arterial and arteriolar lesions in acute and chronic cocaine-induced mesenteric ischemia: report of three cases and literature review. *Am J Surg Pathol.* 1998;22: 1404-1410.
84. Hoffman RS, Chiang WK, Weisman RS, Goldfrank LR. Prospective evaluation of "crack-vial" ingestions. *Vet Hum Toxicol.* 1990;32:164-167.
85. Hoffman RS, Hollander JE. Thrombolytic therapy and cocaine-induced myocardial infarction. *Am J Emerg Med.* 1996;14:693-695.
86. Hoffman RS, Henry GC, Howland MA, et al. Association between life-threatening cocaine toxicity and plasma cholinesterase activity. *Ann Emerg Med.* 1992;21:247-253.
87. Hoffman RS, Henry GC, Wax PM, et al. Decreased plasma cholinesterase activity enhances cocaine toxicity in mice. *J Pharmacol Exp Ther.* 1992;263:698-702.
88. Hoffman RS, Kaplan JL, Hung OL, Goldfrank LR. Ecgonine methyl ester protects against cocaine lethality in mice. *J Toxicol Clin Toxicol.* 2004;42:349-354.
89. Hoffman RS, Reimer BI. "Crack" cocaine-induced bilateral amblyopia. *Am J Emerg Med.* 1993;11:35-37.
90. Hoffman RS, Smilkstein MJ, Goldfrank LR. Whole bowel irrigation and the cocaine body-packer: a new approach to a common problem. *Am J Emerg Med.* 1990;8:523-527.
91. Holland RW 3rd, Marx JA, Earnest MP, Ranniger S. Grand mal seizures temporally related to cocaine use: clinical and diagnostic features. *Ann Emerg Med.* 1992;21:772-776.
92. Hollander JE, Brooks DE, Valentine SM. Assessment of cocaine use in patients with chest pain syndromes. *Arch Intern Med.* 1998;158:62-66.
93. Hollander JE, Burstein JL, Hoffman RS, et al. Cocaine-associated myocardial infarction. Clinical safety of thrombolytic therapy. Cocaine-associated myocardial infarction (CAMI) study group. *Chest.* 1995;107: 1237-1241.
94. Hollander JE, Carter WA, Hoffman RS. Use of phentolamine for cocaine-induced myocardial ischemia. *N Engl J Med.* 1992;327: 361.
95. Hollander JE, Hoffman RS, Gennis P, et al. Nitroglycerin in the treatment of cocaine associated chest pain—clinical safety and efficacy. *J Toxicol Clin Toxicol.* 1994;32:243-256.
96. Hollander JE, Hoffman RS, Gennis P, et al. Prospective multicenter evaluation of cocaine-associated chest pain. Cocaine-associated chest pain (COCHPA) study group. *Acad Emerg Med.* 1994;1:330-339.
97. Hollander JE, Hoffman RS, Gennis P, et al. Cocaine-associated chest pain: one-year follow-up. *Acad Emerg Med.* 1995;2:179-184.
98. Hollander JE, Levitt MA, Young GP, et al. Effect of recent cocaine use on the specificity of cardiac markers for diagnosis of acute myocardial infarction. *Am Heart J.* 1998;135:245-252.
99. Hollander JE, Lozano M, Fairweather P, et al. "Abnormal" electrocardiograms in patients with cocaine-associated chest pain are due to "normal" variants. *J Emerg Med.* 1994;12:199-205.
100. Hollander JE. The management of cocaine-associated myocardial ischemia. *N Engl J Med.* 1995;333:1267-1272.
101. Hon DC, Salloum LJ, Hardy HW 3rd, Barone JE. Crack-induced enteric ischemia. *N J Med.* 1990;87:1001-1002.
102. Honderick T, Williams D, Seaberg D, Wears R. A prospective, randomized, controlled trial of benzodiazepines and nitroglycerine or nitroglycerine alone in the treatment of cocaine-associated acute coronary syndromes [see comment]. *Am J Emerg Med.* 2003;21:39-42.
103. Horowitz BZ, Panacek EA, Jouriles NJ. Severe rhabdomyolysis with renal failure after intranasal cocaine use. *J Emerg Med.* 1997;15:833-837.
104. Hsue PY, Salinas CL, Bolger AF, et al. Acute aortic dissection related to crack cocaine. *Circulation.* 2002;105:1592-1595.
105. Hsue PY, McManus D, Selby V, et al. Cardiac arrest in patients who smoke crack cocaine. *Am J Cardiol.* 2007;99:822-824.
106. Inaba T, Stewart DJ, Kalow W. Metabolism of cocaine in man. *Clin Pharmacol Ther.* 1978;23:547-552.
107. Isner JM, Estes NA 3rd, Thompson PD, et al. Acute cardiac events temporally related to cocaine abuse. *N Engl J Med.* 1986;315:1438-1443.
108. Jacob P 3rd, Jones RT, Benowitz NL, et al. Cocaine smokers excrete a pyrolysis product, anhydroecgonine methyl ester. *J Toxicol Clin Toxicol.* 1990;28:121-125.
109. Jatlow P, Barash PG, Van Dyke C, et al. Cocaine and succinylcholine sensitivity: a new caution. *Anesth Analg.* 1979;58:235-238.
110. Jeffcoat AR, Perez-Reyes M, Hill JM, et al. Cocaine disposition in humans after intravenous injection, nasal insufflation (snorting), or smoking. *Drug Metab Dispos.* 1989;17:153-159.
111. June R, Aks SE, Keys N, Wahl M. Medical outcome of cocaine body stuffers. *J Emerg Med.* 2000;18:221-224.
112. Jung ME, McNulty MA, Goeders NE. Cocaine increases benzodiazepine receptors labeled in the mouse brain in vivo with [3H]ro 15-1788. *NIDA Res Monogr.* 1989;95:512-513.
113. Just WW, Hoyer J. The local anesthetic potency of norcocaine, a metabolite of cocaine. *Experientia.* 1977;33:70-71.
114. Karch SB. Cocaine: history, use, abuse. *J R Soc Med.* 1999;92:393-397.
115. Katz JL, Terry P, Witkin JM. Comparative behavioral pharmacology and toxicology of cocaine and its ethanol-derived metabolite, cocaine ethyl-ester (cocaethylene). *Life Sci.* 1992;50:1351-1361.
116. Kerns W 2nd, Garvey L, Owens J. Cocaine-induced wide complex dysrhythmia. *J Emerg Med.* 1997;15:321-329.
117. Kestler A, Keyes L. Images in clinical medicine: uvular angioedema (Quincke's disease). *N Engl J Med.* 2003;349:867.
118. Kissner DG, Lawrence WD, Selis JE, Flint A. Crack lung: pulmonary disease caused by cocaine abuse. *Am Rev Respir Dis.* 1987;136:1250-1252.
119. Knuepfer MM, Branch CA. Cardiovascular responses to cocaine are initially mediated by the central nervous system in rats. *J Pharmacol Exp Ther.* 1992;263:734-741.
120. Knuepfer MM. Cardiovascular disorders associated with cocaine use: myths and truths. *Pharmacol Ther.* 2003;97:181-222.
121. Kolodgie FD, Wilson PS, Cornhill JF, et al. Increased prevalence of aortic fatty streaks in cholesterol-fed rabbits administered intravenous cocaine: the role of vascular endothelium. *Toxicol Pathol.* 1993;21:425-435.
122. Kolodgie FD, Wilson PS, Mergner WJ, Virmani R. Cocaine-induced increase in the permeability function of human vascular endothelial cell monolayers. *Exp Mol Pathol.* 1999;66:109-122.
123. Konkol RJ, Erickson BA, Doerr JK, et al. Seizures induced by the cocaine metabolite benzoylecgonine in rats. *Epilepsia.* 1992;33:420-427.

124. Koppel BS, Samkoff L, Daras M. Relation of cocaine use to seizures and epilepsy. *Epilepsia*. 1996;37:875-878.
125. Kothur R, Marsh F, Posner G. Liver function tests in nonparenteral cocaine users. *Arch Intern Med*. 1991;151:1126-1128.
126. Kudrow DB, Henry DA, Haake DA, et al. Botulism associated with clostridium botulinum sinusitis after intranasal cocaine abuse. *Ann Intern Med*. 1988;109:984-985.
127. Kugelmass AD, Oda A, Monahan K, et al. Activation of human platelets by cocaine. *Circulation*. 1993;88:876-883.
128. Lange RA, Cigarroa RG, Flores ED, et al. Potentiation of cocaine-induced coronary vasoconstriction by beta-adrenergic blockade. *Ann Intern Med*. 1990;112:897-903.
129. Lange RA, Cigarroa RG, Yancy CW Jr, et al. Cocaine-induced coronary-artery vasoconstriction. *N Engl J Med*. 1989;321:1557-1562.
130. Lange RA, Hillis LD. Cardiovascular complications of cocaine use. *N Engl J Med*. 2001;345:351-358.
131. Langner RO, Bement CL, Perry LE. Arteriosclerotic toxicity of cocaine. *NIDA Res Monogr*. 1988;88:325-336.
132. Langner RO, Bement CL. Cocaine-induced changes in the biochemistry and morphology of rabbit aorta. *NIDA Res Monogr*. 1991;108:154-166.
133. Lason W. Neurochemical and pharmacological aspects of cocaine-induced seizures. *Pol J Pharmacol*. 2001;53:57-60.
134. Lee HS, LaMaute HR, Pizzi WF, et al. Acute gastroduodenal perforations associated with use of crack. *Ann Surg*. 1990;211:15-17.
135. Leighty EG, Fentiman AF Jr. Metabolism of cocaine to norcocaine and benzoyl ecgonine by an in vitro microsomal enzyme system. *Res Commun Chem Pathol Pharmacol*. 1974;8:65-74.
136. Levine M, Iliescu ME, Margellos-Anast H, et al. The effects of cocaine and heroin use on intubation rates and hospital utilization in patients with acute asthma exacerbations. *Chest*. 2005;128:1951-1957.
137. Levine SR, Brust JC, Futrell N, et al. Cerebrovascular complications of the use of the "crack" form of alkaloidal cocaine. *N Engl J Med*. 1990;323: 699-704.
138. Li W, Su J, Sehgal S, et al. Cocaine-induced relaxation of isolated rat aortic rings and mechanisms of action: possible relation to cocaine-induced aortic dissection and hypotension. *Eur J Pharmacol*. 2004;496: 151-158.
139. Libman RB, Masters SR, de Paola A, Mohr JP. Transient monocular blindness associated with cocaine abuse. *Neurology*. 1993;43:228-229.
140. Linder JD, Monkemuller KE, Raijman I, et al. Cocaine-associated ischemic colitis. *South Med J*. 2000;93:909-913.
141. Littmann L, Monroe MH, Svenson RH. Brugada-type electrocardiographic pattern induced by cocaine. *Mayo Clin Proc*. 2000;75:845-849.
142. Long H, Greller H, Mercurio-Zappala M, et al. Medicinal use of cocaine: a shifting paradigm over 25 years. *Laryngoscope*. 2004;114:1625-1629.
143. Lynch TJ, Mattes CE, Singh A, et al. Cocaine detoxification by human plasma butyrylcholinesterase. *Toxicol Appl Pharmacol*. 1997; 145:363-371.
144. Madden JA, Konkol RJ, Keller PA, Alvarez TA. Cocaine and benzoylecgonine constrict cerebral arteries by different mechanisms. *Life Sci*. 1995;56:679-686.
145. Madden JA, Powers RH. Effect of cocaine and cocaine metabolites on cerebral arteries in vitro. *Life Sci*. 1990;47:1109-1114.
146. Maeder M, Ullmer E. Pneumomediastinum and bilateral pneumothorax as a complication of cocaine smoking. *Respiration*. 2003;70:407.
147. Makosiej FJ, Hoffman RS, Howland MA, Goldfrank LR. An in vitro evaluation of cocaine hydrochloride adsorption by activated charcoal and desorption upon addition of polyethylene glycol electrolyte lavage solution. *J Toxicol Clin Toxicol*. 1993;31:381-395.
148. Malbrain ML, Neels H, Vissers K, et al. A massive, near-fatal cocaine intoxication in a body-stuffer: case report and review of the literature. *Acta Clin Belg*. 1994;49:12-18.
149. Mangiardi JR, Daras M, Geller ME, et al. Cocaine-related intracranial hemorrhage. Report of nine cases and review. *Acta Neurol Scand*. 1988;77:177-180.
150. Marzuk PM, Tardiff K, Leon AC, et al. Ambient temperature and mortality from unintentional cocaine overdose. *JAMA*. 1998;279:1795-1800.
151. Marzuk PM, Tardiff K, Leon AC, et al. Fatal injuries after cocaine use as a leading cause of death among young adults in New York City. *N Engl J Med*. 1995;332:1753-1757.
152. Marzuk PM, Tardiff K, Leon AC, et al. Prevalence of recent cocaine use among motor vehicle fatalities in New York City. *JAMA*. 1990;263: 250-256.
153. Mateo Y, Budygin EA, John CE, Jones SR. Role of serotonin in cocaine effects in mice with reduced dopamine transporter function. *Proc Natl Acad Sci U S A*. 2004;101:372-377.
154. Mattes CE, Lynch TJ, Singh A, et al. Therapeutic use of butyrylcholinesterase for cocaine intoxication. *Toxicol Appl Pharmacol*. 1997;145: 372-380.
155. Mazzone A, Giani L, Faggioloi P et al. Cocaine-related peripheral vascular occlusive disease treated with iloprost in addition to anticoagulants and antibiotics. *Clin Toxicol*. 2007;45:65-66.
156. McCord J, Jneid H, Hollander JE, et al. Management of cocaine-associated chest pain and myocardial infarction. A scientific statement from the American Heart Assoication Acute Cardiac Care Committee of the Council on Clinical Cardiology. 2008;117;1897-1907.
157. Mehta A, Jain AC, Mehta MC. Electrocardiographic effects of intravenous cocaine: an experimental study in a canine model. *J Cardiovasc Pharmacol*. 2003;41:25-30.
158. Meleca RJ, Burgio DL, Carr RM, Lolachi CM. Mucosal injuries of the upper aerodigestive tract after smoking crack or freebase cocaine. *Laryngoscope*. 1997;107:620-625.
159. Mets B, Virag L. Lethal toxicity from equimolar infusions of cocaine and cocaine metabolites in conscious and anesthetized rats. *Anesth Analg*. 1995;81:1033-1038.
160. Misra AL, Nayak PK, Bloch R, Mule SJ. Estimation and disposition of [^{3}H] benzoylecgonine and pharmacological activity of some cocaine metabolites. *J Pharm Pharmacol*. 1975;27:784-786.
161. Mochizuki Y, Zhang M, Golestaneh L, et al. Acute aortic thrombosis and renal infarction in acute cocaine intoxication: a case report and review of literature. *Clin Nephrol*. 2003;60:130-133.
162. Mochson CM, Sharma AN, Hoffman RS. Hypoglycemia in cocaine-intoxicated mice. *Acad Emerg Med*. 2001;8:768.
163. Mody CK, Miller BL, McIntyre HB, et al. Neurologic complications of cocaine abuse. *Neurology*. 1988;38:1189-1193.
164. Moliterno DJ, Lange RA, Gerard RD, et al. Influence of intranasal cocaine on plasma constituents associated with endogenous thrombosis and thrombolysis. *Am J Med*. 1994;96:492-496.
165. Moliterno DJ, Willard JE, Lange RA, et al. Coronary-artery vasoconstriction induced by cocaine, cigarette smoking, or both. *N Engl J Med*. 1994;330:454-459.
166. Morishima HO, Whittington RA, Iso A, Cooper TB. The comparative toxicity of cocaine and its metabolites in conscious rats. *Anesthesiology*. 1999;90:1684-1690.
167. Mott SH, Packer RJ, Soldin SJ. Neurologic manifestations of cocaine exposure in childhood. *Pediatrics*. 1994;93:557-560.
168. Nademanee K, Gorelick DA, Josephson MA, et al. Myocardial ischemia during cocaine withdrawal. *Ann Intern Med*. 1989;111:876-880.
169. Niazi M, Kondru A, Levy J, Bloom AA. Spectrum of ischemic colitis in cocaine users. *Dig Dis Sci*. 1997;42:1537-1541.
170. Nolte KB, Brass LM, Fletterick CF. Intracranial hemorrhage associated with cocaine abuse: a prospective autopsy study. *Neurology*. 1996;46: 1291-1296.
171. Novielli KD, Chambers CV. Splenic infarction after cocaine use. *Ann Intern Med*. 1991;114:251-252.
172. O'Dell LE, Li R, George FR, Ritz MC. Molecular serotonergic mechanisms appear to mediate genetic sensitivity to cocaine-induced convulsions. *Brain Res*. 2000;863:213-224.
173. O'Leary ME. Inhibition of HERG potassium channels by cocaethylene: a metabolite of cocaine and ethanol. *Cardiovasc Res*. 2002;53:59-67.
174. O'Leary ME. Inhibition of human ether-a-go-go potassium channels by cocaine. *Mol Pharmacol*. 2001;59:269-277.
175. Om A, Ellahham S, Ornato JP, et al. Medical complications of cocaine: possible relationship to low plasma cholinesterase enzyme. *Am Heart J*. 1993;125:1114-1117.
176. Om A, Ellahham S, Ornato JP. Reversibility of cocaine-induced cardiomyopathy. *Am Heart J*. 1992;124:1639-1641.
177. Ortega-Carnicer J, Bertos-Polo J, Gutierrez-Tirado C. Aborted sudden death, transient Brugada pattern, and wide QRS dysrhythmias after massive cocaine ingestion. *J Electrocardiol*. 2001;34:345-349.
178. Osborn HH, Tang M, Bradley K, Duncan BR. New-onset bronchospasm or recrudescence of asthma associated with cocaine abuse. *Acad Emerg Med*. 1997;4:689-692.
179. Osorio J, Farreras N, Ortiz De Zarate L, Bachs E. Cocaine-induced mesenteric ischaemia. *Dig Surg*. 2000;17:648-651.

180. Pane MA, Traystman RJ, Gleason CA. Ecgonine methyl ester, a major cocaine metabolite, causes cerebral vasodilation in neonatal sheep. *Pediatr Res.* 1997;41:815-821.
181. Parker RB, Perry GY, Horan LG, Flowers NC. Comparative effects of sodium bicarbonate and sodium chloride on reversing cocaine-induced changes in the electrocardiogram. *J Cardiovasc Pharmacol.* 1999;34:864-869.
182. Parker RB, Williams CL, Laizure SC, Lima JJ. Factors affecting serum protein binding of cocaine in humans. *J Pharmacol Exp Ther.* 1995;275:605-610.
183. Pecha RE, Prindiville T, Pecha BS, et al. Association of cocaine and methamphetamine use with giant gastroduodenal ulcers. *Am J Gastroenterol.* 1996;91:2523-2527.
184. Penarrocha M, Bagan JV, Penarrocha MA, Silvestre FJ. Cluster headache and cocaine use. *Oral Surg Oral Med Oral Pathol Oral Radiol Endod.* 2000;90:271-274.
185. Perera R, Kraebber A, Schwartz MJ. Prolonged QT interval and cocaine use. *J Electrocardiol.* 1997;30:337-339.
186. Petitti DB, Sidney S, Quesenberry C, Bernstein A. Stroke and cocaine or amphetamine use. *Epidemiology.* 1998;9:596-600.
187. Przywara DA, Dambach GE. Direct actions of cocaine on cardiac cellular electrical activity. *Circ Res.* 1989;65:185-192.
188. Qureshi AI, Suri MF, Guterman LR, Hopkins LN. Cocaine use and the likelihood of nonfatal myocardial infarction and stroke: data from the third national health and nutrition examination survey. *Circulation.* 2001;103:502-506.
189. Ramadan NM, Levine SR, Welch KM. Pontine hemorrhage following "crack" cocaine use. *Neurology.* 1991;41:946-947.
190. Ravin JG, Ravin LC: Blindness due to illicit use of topical cocaine. *Ann Ophthalmol.* 1979;11:863-864.
191. Restrepo CS, Carrillo JA, Martinez S, et al. Pulmonary complications from cocaine and cocaine-based sustances: imaging manifestations. *Radiographics.* 2007;27:941-956.
192. Rockhold RW, Oden G, Ho IK, et al. Glutamate receptor antagonists block cocaine-induced convulsions and death. *Brain Res Bull.* 1991;27:721-723.
193. Romano G, Barbera N, Lombardo I. Hair testing for drugs of abuse: evaluation of external cocaine contamination and risk of false positives. *Forensic Sci Int.* 2001;123:119-129.
194. Rome LA, Lippmann ML, Dalsey WC, et al. Prevalence of cocaine use and its impact on asthma exacerbation in an urban population. *Chest.* 2000;117:1324-1329.
195. Ruetsch YA, Boni T, Borgeat A. From cocaine to ropivacaine: the history of local anesthetic drugs. *Curr Top Med Chem.* 2001;1:175-182.
196. Ruttenber AJ, McAnally HB, Wetli CV. Cocaine-associated rhabdomyolysis and excited delirium: different stages of the same syndrome. *Am J Forensic Med Pathol.* 1999;20:120-127.
197. Saland KE, Hillis LD, Lange RA, Cigarroa JE. Influence of morphine sulfate on cocaine-induced coronary vasoconstriction. *Am J Cardiol.* 2002;90:810-811.
198. Saleem TM, Singh M, Murtaza M, et al. Renal infarction: a rare complication of cocaine abuse. *Am J Emerg Med.* 2001;19:528-529.
199. Samkoff LM, Daras M, Kleiman AR, Koppel BS. Spontaneous spinal epidural hematoma: another neurologic complication of cocaine? *Arch Neurol.* 1996;53:819-821.
200. Sand IC, Brody SL, Wrenn KD, Slovis CM. Experience with esmolol for the treatment of cocaine-associated cardiovascular complications. *Am J Emerg Med.* 1991;9:161-163.
201. Satel SL, Gawin FH. Migraine-like headache and cocaine use. *JAMA.* 1989;261:2995-2996.
202. Satran A, Bart BA, Henry CR, et al. Increased prevalence of coronary artery aneurysms among cocaine users. *Circulation.* 2005;111:2424-2429.
203. Savader SJ, Omori M, Martinez CR. Pneumothorax, pneumomediastinum, and pneumopericardium: Complications of cocaine smoking. *J Fla Med Assoc.* 1988;75:151-152.
204. Schaper A, Hofmann R, Bargain P et al. Surgical treatment in cocaine body packers and body pushers. *Int J Colorectal Dis.* 2007;22:1531-1535.
205. Scheidweiler KB, Plessinger MA, Shojaie J, et al. Pharmacokinetics and pharmacodynamics of methylecgonidine, a crack cocaine pyrolyzate. *J Pharmacol Exp Ther.* 2003;307:1179-1187.
206. Schindler CW, Zheng JW, Goldberg SR. Effects of cocaine and cocaine metabolites on cardiovascular function in squirrel monkeys. *Eur J Pharmacol.* 2001;431:53-59.
207. Schreiber MD, Madden JA, Covert RF, Torgerson LJ. Effects of cocaine, benzoylecgonine, and cocaine metabolites in cannulated pressurized fetal sheep cerebral arteries. *J Appl Physiol.* 1994;77:834-839.
208. Schrem SS, Belsky P, Schwartzman D, Slater W. Cocaine-induced torsades de pointes in a patient with the idiopathic long QT syndrome. *Am Heart J.* 1990;120:980-984.
209. Schuelke GS, Konkol RJ, Terry LC, Madden JA. Effect of cocaine metabolites on behavior: possible neuroendocrine mechanisms. *Brain Res Bull.* 1996;39:43-48.
210. Schwartz AB, Janzen D, Jones RT, Boyle W. Electrocardiographic and hemodynamic effects of intravenous cocaine in awake and anesthetized dogs. *J Electrocardiol.* 1989;22:159-166.
211. Schwartz KA, Cohen JA. Subarachnoid hemorrhage precipitated by cocaine snorting. *Arch Neurol.* 1984;41:705.
212. Shah DM, Dy TC, Szto GY, Linnemeier TJ. Percutaneous transluminal coronary angioplasty and stenting for cocaine-induced acute myocardial infarction: a case report and review. *Catheter Cardiovasc Interv.* 2000;49:447-451.
213. Shankaran S, Lester BM, Das A, et al. Impact of maternal substance use during pregnancy on childhood outcome. *Semin Fetal Neonatal Med.* 2007;12:143-150.
214. Sharma R, Organ CH Jr, Hirvela ER, Henderson VJ. Clinical observation of the temporal association between crack cocaine and duodenal ulcer perforation. *Am J Surg.* 1997;174:629-632.
215. Shih RD, Hollander JE, Burstein JL, et al. Clinical safety of lidocaine in patients with cocaine-associated myocardial infarction. *Ann Emerg Med.* 1995;26:702-706.
216. Smith JA, Mo Q, Guo H, et al. Cocaine increases extraneuronal levels of aspartate and glutamate in the nucleus accumbens. *Brain Res.* 1995;683:264-269.
217. Spealman RD, Madras BK, Bergman J. Effects of cocaine and related drugs in nonhuman primates. II. Stimulant effects on schedule-controlled behavior. *J Pharmacol Exp Ther.* 1989;251:142-149.
218. Sporer KA, Firestone J. Clinical course of crack cocaine body stuffers. *Ann Emerg Med.* 1997;29:596-601.
219. Sporer KA, Lesser SH. Cocaine washed-out syndrome. *Ann Emerg Med.* 1992;21:112.
220. Steinhauer JR, Caulfield JB. Spontaneous coronary artery dissection associated with cocaine use: a case report and brief review. *Cardiovasc Pathol.* 2001;10:141-145.
221. Stewart DJ, Inaba T, Lucassen M, Kalow W. Cocaine metabolism: cocaine and norcocaine hydrolysis by liver and serum esterases. *Clin Pharmacol Ther.* 1979;25:464-468.
222. Stewart DJ, Inaba T, Tang BK, Kalow W. Hydrolysis of cocaine in human plasma by cholinesterase. *Life Sci.* 1977;20:1557-1563.
223. Sun H, Shen ML, Pang YP, et al. Cocaine metabolism accelerated by a re-engineered human butyrylcholinesterase. *J Pharmacol Exp Ther.* 2002;302:710-716.
224. Tames SM, Goldenring JM. Madarosis from cocaine use. *N Engl J Med.* 1986;314:1324.
225. Tashkin DP, Kleerup EC, Koyal SN, et al. Acute effects of inhaled and i.v. cocaine on airway dynamics. *Chest.* 1996;110:904-910.
226. Taylor D, Parish D, Thompson L, Cavaliere M. Cocaine induced prolongation of the QT interval. *Emerg Med J.* 2004;21:252-253.
227. Tella SR, Schindler CW, Goldberg SR. Cardiovascular effects of cocaine in conscious rats: relative significance of central sympathetic stimulation and peripheral neuronal monoamine uptake and release mechanisms. *J Pharmacol Exp Ther.* 1992;262:602-610.
228. Tella SR, Schindler CW, Goldberg SR. Cocaine: Cardiovascular effects in relation to inhibition of peripheral neuronal monoamine uptake and central stimulation of the sympathoadrenal system. *J Pharmacol Exp Ther.* 1993;267:153-162.
229. Thompson A. Toxic action of cocaine. *Br Med J.* 1886;1:67.
230. Torre M, Barberis M. Spontaneous pneumothorax in cocaine sniffers. *Am J Emerg Med.* 1998;16:546-549.
231. Trabulsy ME. Cocaine washed out syndrome in a patient with acute myocardial infarction. *Am J Emerg Med.* 1995;13:538-539.
232. Traub SJ, Hoffman RS, Nelson LS. Body packing—the internal concealment of illicit drugs. *N Engl J Med.* 2003;349:2519-2526.
233. Traub SJ, Su M, Hoffman RS, Nelson LS. Use of pharmaceutical promotility agents in the treatment of body packers. *Am J Emerg Med.* 2003;21:511-512.
234. Uva JL. Spontaneous pneumothoraces, pneumomediastinum, and pneumoperitoneum: consequences of smoking crack cocaine. *Pediatr Emerg Care.* 1997;13:24-26.
235. van Harten PN, van Trier JC, Horwitz EH, et al. Cocaine as a risk factor for neuroleptic-induced acute dystonia. *J Clin Psychiatry.* 1998;59:128-130.

236. Van Thiel DH, Perper JA. Hepatotoxicity associated with cocaine abuse. *Recent Dev Alcohol.* 1992;10:335-341.
237. Vannemreddy P, Caldito G, Willis B, Nanda A. Influence of cocaine on ruptured intracranial aneurysms: a case control study of poor prognostic indicators. *J Neurosurg.* 2008;108:470-476.
238. Virmani R. Cocaine-associated cardiovascular disease: clinical and pathological aspects. *NIDA Res Monogr.* 1991;108:220-229.
239. Wang RY. pH-dependent cocaine-induced cardiotoxicity. *Am J Emerg Med.* 1999;17:364-369.
240. Weber JE, Chudnofsky CR, Boczar M, et al. Cocaine-associated chest pain: how common is myocardial infarction? *Acad Emerg Med.* 2000;7:873-877.
241. Weber JE, Shofer FS, Larkin GL, et al. Validation of a brief observation period for patients with cocaine-associated chest pain. *N Engl J Med.* 2003;348:510-517.
242. Weiss RD, Gawin FH. Protracted elimination of cocaine metabolites in long-term high-dose cocaine abusers. *Am J Med.* 1988;85:879-880.
243. Willens HJ, Chakko SC, Kessler KM. Cardiovascular manifestations of cocaine abuse. A case of recurrent dilated cardiomyopathy. *Chest.* 1994;106:594-600.
244. Wilson LD, Jeromin J, Garvey L, Dorbandt A. Cocaine, ethanol, and cocaethylene cardiotoxicity in an animal model of cocaine and ethanol abuse. *Acad Emerg Med.* 2001;8:211-222.
245. Wilson MC, Bedford JA, Kibbe AH, Sam JA. Brief communication. Comparative pharmacology of norcocaine in *M. mulatta* and *M. fascicularis. Pharmacol Biochem Behav.* 1978;9:141-145.
246. Winecoff AP, Hariman RJ, Grawe JJ, et al. Reversal of the electrocardiographic effects of cocaine by lidocaine. Part 1. Comparison with sodium bicarbonate and quinidine. *Pharmacotherapy.* 1994;14:698-703.
247. Witkin JM, Goldberg SR, Katz JL. Lethal effects of cocaine are reduced by the dopamine-1 receptor antagonist SCH 23390 but not by haloperidol. *Life Sci.* 1989;44:1285-1291.
248. Wojak JC, Flamm ES. Intracranial hemorrhage and cocaine use. *Stroke.* 1987;18:712-715.
249. Wood DM, Dargan PI, Hoffman RS. Management of cocaine-induced cardiac arrhythmias due to cardiac ion channel dysfunction. *Clin Toxicol* (Phila). 2009;47:14-23.
250. Xie W, Altamirano CV, Bartels CF, et al. An improved cocaine hydrolase: the A328Y mutant of human butyrylcholinesterase is 4-fold more efficient. *Mol Pharmacol.* 1999;55:83-91.
251. Yang Y, Ke Q, Cai J, et al. Evidence for cocaine and methylecgonidine stimulation of M(2) muscarinic receptors in cultured human embryonic lung cells. *Br J Pharmacol.* 2001;132:451-460.
252. Zamora-Quezada JC, Dinerman H, Stadecker MJ, Kelly JJ. Muscle and skin infarction after free-basing cocaine (crack). *Ann Intern Med.* 1988;108:564-566.

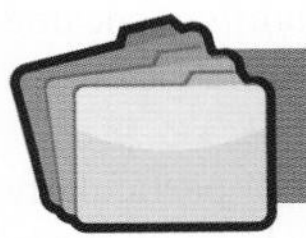

SPECIAL CONSIDERATIONS (SC4)

INTERNAL CONCEALMENT OF XENOBIOTICS

Jane M. Prosser

Internal concealment of illicit xenobiotics is a significant concern for local and international police efforts as well as medical, social, and public health practitioners. There are two distinct categories of concealment colloquially known as "body stuffers" and "body packers." The term body stuffer refers to individuals who hide drugs in a body cavity or ingest the drugs in an attempt to hide evidence from law enforcement officers. The xenobiotics are ingested in an unplanned manner and are often poorly wrapped. The term body packer refers to individuals who conceal xenobiotics, typically in large quantities, in a premeditated fashion almost exclusively for the purposes of international smuggling.

BODY PACKERS

Internal concealment of drugs for the purpose of smuggling was first reported in Canada in 1973. A 21-year-old man presented with a small bowel obstruction as a result of swallowing a condom filled with hashish. He had swallowed the condom in order to transport it into Canada after a trip to Lebanon.[13] Internal drug smuggling has become a worldwide problem as increased surveillance at international borders has made conventional transportation of illegal drugs more difficult. Improved detection of smugglers has increased the number of patients brought to the attention of healthcare providers. Pregnant women and children as young as 6 years of age have been used as body packers.[2,6,9]

Airline and airport personnel are trained to identify people who may be drug couriers. Suspicious behavior includes not eating or drinking on the airplane, abnormal behavior while going through customs, and overt signs of drug toxicity.[76,87]

COMPOSITION OF PACKAGES

Body packers typically swallow large numbers of well prepared packages, each filled with substantial amounts of drug. Packets may also be concealed by insertion into the vagina and rectum.[14,92] The most frequently smuggled cargo is either heroin or cocaine, but other drugs have been reported (Table SC4–1). Body packers often swallow 50 to 100 packages and ingestion of as many as 500 has been reported.[93] Each package typically contains from 0.5 to 10 g of drug. Therefore, one person may carry as much as 1.5 kg of drug.[84] Lethal doses of cocaine and heroin are difficult to determine based in part on sparse data and on widely variable purity. For reference, death from cocaine toxicity is reported after ingestion of as little as 2 to 3 g.[71] As such, each packet should be considered to contain a potentially lethal dose.

A number of materials have been used for drug packaging. Some, like latex, are used as wrappers. Others such as carbon paper and aluminum foil are used to change the radiodensity and decrease the likelihood of detection with diagnostic and forensic imaging studies. Packages have been made using plastic bags, plastic wrap, condoms, finger cots, balloons, cellophane, wax, tape, rubber gloves, surgical ligatures, paraffin, and fiberglass.[5,23,31,58,68]

Initial reports suggested a high rate of complications due to packaging failure.[58] More recently however, advances in constituents and technology of packet construction have decreased rates of rupture.[68] A typical packet in current use is composed of a core of compacted drug covered by several layers of latex and encased in an outer wax coat.[87]

Important historical details include the number and contents of packets, the constitution of the wrapping, time of ingestion, and any associated symptoms. Body packers often know exactly how many packets they are carrying in order to know when delivery is complete. However, they may be reluctant to give an accurate clinical history to the healthcare provider or legal authorities.

BIOAVAILABILITY

The oral bioavailability of cocaine hydrochloride is approximately 30% to 40%, which is similar to intranasal administration.[19,96] Rectal and vaginal bioavailability of cocaine hydrochloride and the oral, rectal and vaginal bioavailability of crack cocaine have not been studied.

Oral exposure to heroin results in rapid first pass metabolism to morphine[25] and can be considered a morphine prodrug.[19,39] The peak concentrations after 10 mg of oral heroin are similar to those expected from 10 mg of oral morphine.[3] The rectal bioavailability of morphine has a 1:1 ratio with oral administration. Although heroin is rectally bioavailable,[75] one study examining the bioavailability after rectal suppository administration in 2 opioid dependent patients found it to be approximately 50% less than the oral bioavailability.[27]

CLINICAL MANIFESTATIONS

Body packers undergoing medical examination may be asymptomatic or may have clinical manifestations consistent with either drug toxicity or mechanical obstruction. Physical examination should be thorough, with a focus on findings related to these problems (Chaps. 38 and 76).

The packets may be too large to pass and obstruction can occur at any point in the gastrointestinal tract. Couriers carrying packets containing opioids appear to be at higher risk of gastrointestinal obstruction even with intact packets.[24] The reason for this is unclear, but may be related to microperforation or contamination of the outside of the package during manufacture, resulting in opioid induced gastrointestinal stasis. Patients with a history of abdominal surgery may also be at increased risk of obstruction.[37,11] Gastrointestinal perforation and peritonitis can result if the obstruction is untreated.[11] Gastric ulcers,[62] gastric hemorrhage,[15] esophageal obstruction,[47] esophageal perforation and mediastinitis,[41] hematemesis,[37] hematochezia,[89] incarcerated hernias,[83] dysphagia,[7] uterine ischemia,[7] and septic shock[24] have resulted following packet rupture.

LABORATORY EVALUATION

Drug screening results may be difficult to interpret. Although generally, a positive result should raise concern for a ruptured packet, positive

TABLE SC4-1. Xenobiotics Associated with Internal Concealment

Substances reported in body stuffer ingestion
Cannabis[86]
Cocaine hydrochloride[72]
Crack cocaine[72]
Heroin[44]
Methamphetamine[32]
Prescription drugs[73]
Substances reported in body packer ingestion
Cannabis[54]
Cocaine[12]
Hashish [67] and hasish oil[59]
Heroin[23]
Methamphetamine[54]
Methylenedioxymethamphetamine (ecstasy)[85]
Oxycodone[2]

results may also be due to external contamination of the packet, from a microperforation or prior utilization. Thus, patients with packets that appear externally intact may have a positive urine drug screen.[24,59] The rate of positive drug screens in asymptomatic patients may be as great as 52% to 72%.[12,15] Screening typically correlates closely with the drug carried,[23] but may be misleading as patients transporting any product may ingest opioids for the purpose of slowing gastrointestinal transit time.[63] Additionally patients may be carrying a combination of drugs, known as "double breasting."[24]

A subsequent urine drug screen may be particularly useful in the setting of a patient with an initially negative screen. A screen that later becomes positive suggests a ruptured packet and is an indication for very close monitoring. This is of particular concern in the setting of a cocaine body packer when a change from a negative to a positive screen might indicate the potential for a precipitous decline.

RADIOGRAPHIC EVALUATION

All suspected body packers should undergo radiographic evaluation. Plain abdominal radiographs have a sensitivity of 75% to 95%, but this varies based on the number of packets and their methodology of construction.[5,58,91] Several authors suggest increased sensitivity with supine abdominal films.[56,93] Packets can be visualized as multiple radiodense foreign bodies. (Figs. 5-8 A–C) The "double condom sign" is a lucent ring surrounding the packet and results from air trapped in between layered wrappings.[69] The "rosette-like" sign results from the air trapped in the knot when the condom or balloon is tied.[80] Caution must be used when interpreting plain radiographic studies. In one series, 19% of patients had false negative radiographs, with one patient subsequently passing 135 packets.[58] False positives have also been reported from constipation,[46] intraabdominal calcifications[88] and bladder stones.[97] Contrast enhancement may increase the sensitivity of plain radiography.[22,35,56]

Several authors suggest that CT scanning has a higher sensitivity than plain radiographs,[30,49] but precise data on sensitivity is lacking. Although likely to identify patients with multiple packets, a false negative contrast CT scan following WBI was reported in a body packer who subsequently passed a single packet per rectum.[28] Retrospective review of the CT could not identify the packet. One study found a difference in Hounsfield units between packets containing cocaine (−219 HU) and heroin (−520 HU) suggesting that CT scanning can also potentially distinguish between package contents.[95]

Ultrasonography may be another useful screening tool particularly for evaluation of pregnant women. However, its utility has only been evaluated in a few small case series.[34,60] In one series of patients arrested on suspicion of body packing at an international airport, ultrasound examination correctly identified 40 of 42 body packers with positive plain radiographs. The 2 false negative results occurred when packets were located low in the rectum.[60] More investigation is needed to determine the sensitivity and specificity of ultrasound for use in these patients.

Magnetic resonance imaging (MRI) is not likely to provide any additional information when evaluating the gastrointestinal tract. The utility of MRI may be limited for examining the bowel because of the presence of air and normal peristalsis.[33]

Pregnant women may be targeted as body packers due to hesitation from customs officials and health care providers to obtain radiographs. However, the average radiation dose of 100 millirads from an abdominal radiograph is much less than the threshold thought to induce fetal malformations. Therefore, radiography should be obtained when medically indicated. Consideration should also be given to the use of ultrasonography in this situation.[9]

MANAGEMENT

Gastrointestinal decontamination is a vital element in the management of body packers. Initially, surgical intervention was thought to be necessary in all body packers secondary to perceived high rates of toxicity and death.[21,82] The incidence of life-threatening complications has decreased due in part to better packaging[58,68] and to increased rates of detection of asymptomatic carriers. Currently, a more conservative nonsurgical approach is suggested for asymptomatic patients[87] and is supported by a several large series.[4,5,12,58,76,91,93] (Fig. SC4–1)

Treatment with activated charcoal (AC) is frequently suggested on the basis that cocaine and heroin are both well adsorbed to activated charcoal.[55] There are no data showing an actual benefit, and the large doses needed to adsorb the many grams of drug released during packet rupture make AC impractical for use. Furthermore, AC may be detrimental if contamination of the peritoneal cavity occurs after gastrointestinal rupture or during surgery or if it obscures visualization during endoscopy. The risks and benefits must be weighed in each patient. Activated charcoal is of questionable value in cocaine packers given the higher risk of the need for surgical intervention. Activated charcoal is also not likely to improve the outcome of symptomatic heroin body packers, as these patients can be successfully managed with opioid antagonists and mechanical ventilation. Therefore, the administration of AC is not likely to be of benefit.

The utility of whole bowel irrigation (WBI) to enhance elimination is generally accepted, but has not been rigorously evaluated. There is a theoretical concern that polyethylene glycol could increase the water solubility of heroin should it leak,[91] and that it may decrease the adsorption of cocaine to AC if AC is given.[55] Given the lack of in vitro data to support these risks,[18] and its generally accepted benefit, WBI is recommended to decrease intestinal transit time (Antidotes in Depth A3: Whole Bowel Irrigation and other intestinal evacuants). Orogastric lavage is not indicated as packets are too large to fit though holes in the lavage tube.

Cathartics are sometimes recommended for gastrointestinal decontamination. Although oil based cathartics were frequently used in the past,[5,57] a non-oil based medication such as magnesium citrate is preferred. Paraffin oil may actually dissolve some packet wrappers

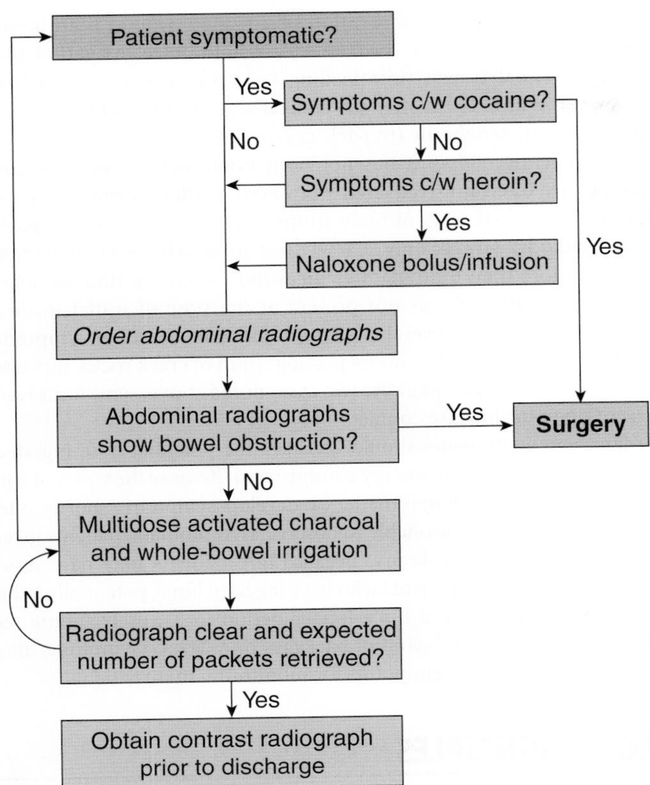

FIGURE SC4–1. Algorithm for managing cocaine or heroin body packers.

resulting in drug toxicity.[94] Safe use of promotility agents, such as metoclopramide and erythromycin, is also reported.[90] Enemas and manual disimpaction should be avoided or used with great caution as packet rupture may occur.[43,50]

Treatment for symptomatic patients depends on the nature of the drug ingested. Patients manifesting opioid toxicity should be treated with the opioid antagonist, naloxone and mechanical ventilation if necessary. Opioid antagonists also improve gastrointestinal motility (Antidotes in Depth A6: Opioid Antagonists). Surgical decontamination is generally not indicated for opioid poisoning, as optimal medical therapy should be adequate.

Rupture of a cocaine packet however, is a life-threatening emergency that requires aggressive medical and surgical therapy (Chap. 76). Benzodiazepines or other sedatives such as propofol may be used as a temporizing measure, but surgical decontamination should be performed emergently in body packers with *any* sign of cocaine toxicity. Indications for surgery include, but are not limited to, hypertension, tachycardia, agitation or other alteration in mental status, myocardial ischemia, bowel ischemia, seizures, respiratory distress and the transition of a urine drug screen from negative to positive.

Surgical removal of the packets is the therapy of choice in the case of cocaine toxicity or mechanical obstruction, but may not be definitive.[31,65,79] In one series, 6 of 70 patients were found to have retained packets postoperatively.[11] Also, emergent surgical removal is associated with a high rate of postoperative infection.[11,79] Endoscopy[74,78,91] and proctoscopy[26] have been used successfully for removal of packets in several cases. However, caution must be used as attempted endoscopic removal can cause packet rupture and resultant toxicity.[82]

It is essential to assure the passage of all packets prior to discharging a patient from medical care. Packets may remain even in patients with clear rectal effluent following WBI.[36] After negative plain radiographs are obtained, a confirmatory study should be done using contrast plain radiography or CT scan. However these modalities do not have 100% sensitivity and retained packets may be missed.[28] It is therefore recommended that patients be observed for twenty-four hours after the passage of 2 packet free stools[5] and a negative confirmatory radiograph or CT Scan (see Fig. SC4-1) (For more information see Antidotes In Depth A3: Whole Bowel Irrigation and Other Intestinal Evacuants and A6: Opioid Antagonists.). Complete GI decontamination must be assured before releasing the patient from close medical observation.

BODY STUFFERS

Body stuffers usually present to healthcare when they are taken into custody by law enforcement officers. Typically the person has hastily ingested the xenobiotic or inserted them into the rectum or vagina to hide the evidence from the police. Since the person was not planning to conceal the xenobiotic, they may be unwrapped, as in the case of crack cocaine "rocks,"[61] or poorly wrapped in materials intended for distribution. Although the overall incidence of toxicity is low, body stuffers are probably more likely to have symptoms, but are also probably less likely to have significant morbidity and mortality, as they typically ingest much smaller amounts of drug.

Pertinent historical information includes time of ingestion, xenobiotic, amount ingested, packaging and symptoms consistent with drug ingestion. Unfortunately, an accurate history is often difficult to obtain. Patients who are recent arrestees may anticipate a secondary gain of delayed incarceration by reporting the ingestion of drugs; alternatively the individuals may deny ingestion to avoid prosecution. Complicating the clinical picture is the possibility that law enforcement officers may assume internal concealment of illicit substances when they are unable to find the drugs after the arrest.

COMPOSITION OF PACKAGES

Since drugs are typically transported locally in plastic bags, condoms,[81] balloons,[8] glycine envelopes, aluminum foil[73] or crack vials,[35] these are the most frequently reported wrappers. Reported amounts vary from one dose to up to 30 packages of unspecified dose.[44] Cocaine, either in crack rocks or the hydrochloride salt form are most commonly ingested,[72] but other xenobiotics are also reported (see Table SC4-1). Typically, the drugs are ingested although other routes of exposure include the external auditory canal, rectum, and vagina.[48,53,86]

The importance of obtaining a precise history related to packaging material is highlighted by an in vitro study examining the effects of packet medium and pH on release of cocaine from drug packets. Cocaine was released almost immediately from paper packaging, and least readily from condoms. Cellophane packing led to intermediate concentrations; when double or triple wrapped in cellophane, decreased concentrations were noted. All packets released more drug in an acidic medium.[1]

CLINICAL MANIFESTATIONS

After oral ingestion of drug packets or crack rocks, toxicity is most frequently absent or mild.[44,45] However, although most case series report low rates of complications, both significant toxicity and death occur.[20,38,45,63] The time of onset of symptoms in body stuffers is typically within several hours.[44,45] Following the ingestion of cocaine in crack vials onset of symptoms may be delayed by 3 to 4 hours.[35]

Most patients with onset of symptoms greater than 6 hours have symptoms at the time of medical contact. Two exceptions are noted in the literature. A 50-year-old woman reported ingesting drugs at the time of incarceration. Seven hours later, a prison physician noted normal pulse and mental status and she was placed in her cell to be observed by staff members every half hour. Prison staff documentation noted that she was "correct" and sat up one-half hour before being found dead in the cell 11 hours after the time of ingestion. Postmortem examination revealed an open cocaine packet in the intestine.[64] A patient who placed methamphetamine in a plastic bag with a small hole in an attempt to create a sustained release mechanism presented for care of abdominal pain ten hours later. This patient remained without symptoms of methamphetamine intoxication until 42 hours after ingestion.[32]

LABORATORY EVALUATION

Laboratory drug testing may be difficult to interpret in body stuffers, as these patients are often habitual substance users. Thus a positive drug screen could be equally indicative of either prior use or current toxicity or both. Likewise, a negative result does not exclude recent ingestion or leaking packages. One study of 50 suspected body stuffers, found that urine drug screening correctly classified the presence or absence of packets only 57% of the time.[57] Several authors report drug toxicity or death occurring in the presence of a negative urine screen.[24,32] One explanation is that patients may die of drug toxicity before substantial urinary excretion occurs.

RADIOGRAPHIC EVALUATION

Although detection of stuffed xenobiotics may be possible by diagnostic imaging studies, the sensitivity is very poor.[16,44,57] Plastic bags, crack vials, and staples (enclosing plastic bags) are rarely visualized.[44] In one series of patients with crack vial ingestions, only 2 of 23 of abdominal radiographs were positive[35] in patients who subsequently passed vials. In two other series of cocaine body stuffers, all plain radiographs were negative.[45,81] Several authors suggest that radiographic detection can be increased with oral contrast though its utility has not been established.[10,45] Although CT scanning may identify some packets missed on plain radiographs, the sensitivity has not been investigated and missed packets have been reported with this modality as well.[16] Therefore, CT scanning is not likely to be clinically useful in these patients.

MANAGEMENT

Body stuffers who are exhibiting drug toxicity should be managed according to standard principles for managing that xenobiotic or suspected xenobiotic (Chaps. 38 and 76).

Patients with gastrointestinal complaints should be evaluated for ileus or obstruction. Removal of packets has been performed by endoscopy,[10,44,70] but is useful only for a small number of packets, as each package requires an additional passage of the endoscope. Endoscopy should be used with extreme caution as it may cause packet rupture with subsequent toxicity or aspiration of the packet with airway obstruction.[82] Bronchoscopic removal of pieces of a balloon wrapping in the airway was successful in one patient after attempted orogastric lavage led to balloon aspiration.[8] Use of colonoscopy[76] is also reported but carries a risk of rupture similar to that associated with upper endoscopy. The need for surgical intervention has been reported in only 1 case. This patient presented with complaint of epigastric pain 3 days after ingesting a large plastic bag filled with 15 to 20 smaller bags of cocaine. He showed no signs of cocaine toxicity, but required surgical removal, as the bag was still retained in the stomach 4 days postingestion.[16]

Management of asymptomatic body stuffers has not been rigorously evaluated. Treatment with AC and WBI was often advocated for high risk patients. Although these methods have not been proven to reduce morbidity or mortality, they offer theoretical benefits.[35,44,45,81] Activated charcoal may reduce the absorption of liberated drug as both heroin and cocaine are well adsorbed to AC. Whole bowel irrigation may reduce intestinal transit time leading to earlier passage of packets. However, it is unlikely to offer any clinical benefits, unless life threatening amounts of xenobiotic (in packages) are ingested.

A therapeutic endpoint has not been established in part because packages are often not recovered from body stuffers. Review of more than 600 published cases of body stuffers involving a variety of packaging methods, reveals only a few cases in which onset of toxicity occurred more than 6 hours after ingestion (when the time of ingestion is reported) and was not present at the time of initial medical evaluation. There are several cases reported when onset of symptoms occurred between 8 and 10 hours postingestion of crack rocks, however in all of these cases except in the two cases noted above, symptoms were present upon health care contact.[10,70]

Management strategies should consider the potential dose ingested, time since ingestion, and therapy administered. Because the vast majority of patients remain asymptomatic, or develop symptoms shortly after medical contact, it is reasonable to observe asymptomatic patients given activated charcoal for 6 hours. Because rare patients may have more delayed presentations, patients who have ingested large, potentially lethal doses should be observed for a longer period in a closely monitored setting. Multiple stools devoid of packages or a lack of symptoms after 24 hours are reasonable endpoints for monitoring these patients.

LEGAL PRINCIPLES

Because clinical errors have the potential for life-threatening consequences, it is essential to evaluate patients within the constructs of their unique social and legal settings. It is important to remember there may be significant motivation to deny ingestion altogether or secondary gain from over-reporting the dose in order to delay incarceration. Often, patients will refuse medical care either as an assertion of innocence, or over concerns that evidence produced might be incriminatory.

In the United States, patients may refuse care if they are competent to do so. This includes body stuffers and body packers who are under arrest. Patients with decisional capacity can not be forced to take AC, WBI, or any other form of therapy. If in police custody, they may however be kept in the hospital for an extended observation period. This strategy maintains patient's medical autonomy as well as assures clinical and legal stability. If signs of life-threatening toxicity subsequently develop, the patient will most likely have lost decisional capacity and therapy can proceed as medically necessary.

If a body packer who is not in legal custody presents for medical care, physicians may face an ethical dilemma. Calling the authorities is a violation of the patient's right to confidentiality. However, possession of large amounts of drugs may theoretically endanger the hospital staff as criminal elements expect drug delivery. Consultation with hospital legal counsel, risk management, and the ethics committee may be helpful in this situation (Chap. 140).

SUMMARY

Patients with intestinal concealment of drugs present a diagnostic and therapeutic challenge. History, laboratory and radiology studies must be interpreted with caution. Management strategies should focus on the drug ingested and be tailored to the needs of each individual patient. Gastrointestinal decontamination is the most important consideration in asymptomatic patients. A complex patient physician relation is common and must be effectively and rapidly developed to assure reliable and high quality care.

REFERENCES

1. Aks SE, Vander Hoek TL, Hryhorczuk DO, et al. Cocaine liberation from body packets in an in vitro model. *Ann Emerg Med.* 1992;21:1321-1325.
2. Beno S, Calello D, Baluffi A, Henretig FM. Pediatric body packing: Drug smuggling reaches a new low. *Pediatr Emerg Care.* 2005;21:744-146.
3. Brunton LL, Lazo JS, Parker KL, eds. *Goodman & Gilman's Pharmacological Basis of Therapeutics.* 11th ed. New York: McGraw-Hill; 2006.
4. Bulstrode N, Banks F, Shrotria S. The outcome of drug smuggling by 'body packers'—the British experience. *Ann R Coll Surg Engl.* 2002;84:35-38.
5. Caruana DS, Weinbach B, Goerg D, Gardner BL. Cocaine-packet ingestion: diagnosis, management and natural history. *Ann Intern Med.* 1984;100: 73-74.
6. Chakrabarty A, Hydros S, Puliyel JM. Smuggling contraband drugs using paediatric "body packers." *Arch Dis Child.* 2006;91:51.
7. Choudhary AM, Taubin H, Gupta T, Roberts I. Endoscopic removal of a cocaine packet from the stomach. *J Clin Gastroenterol.* 1998;27:155-156.
8. Cobaugh DJ, Schneider SM, Benitez JG, Donahoe MP. Cocaine balloon aspiration: successful removal with bronchoscopy. *Am J Emerg Med.* 1997;15:544-546.
9. Cordero DR, Medina C, Helfgott A. Cocaine body packing in pregnancy. *Ann Emerg Med.* 2006;48:323-325.
10. Cranston PE, Pollack Jr CV, Harrison BR. CT of crack cocaine ingestion. *J Comput Assist Tomogr.* 1992;16:560-563.
11. de Beer SA, Spiessens G, Mol W, Fa-Si-Oen PR. Surgery for body packing in the Caribbean: a retrospective study of 70 patients. *World J Surg.* 2008;32:281-285.
12. de Proust N, Lefebvre A, Questel F, et al. Prognosis of cocaine body packers. *Intensive Care Med.* 2005;31:955-958.
13. Deitel M, Syed AK. Intestinal obstruction by an unusual foreign body. *CMAJ.* 1973;109:211-212.
14. Diamant-Berger O, Gheradi R, Baud F, et al. Dissimulation intracorporelle de stupefiants: Experience des urgences medico-judiciaires de l'Hotel-Dieu de Paris: 100 cas. *Presse Med.* 1998;17:107-110.
15. Duenas-Laita A, Nogue S. Body parking. *NEJM.* 2004;350:1260.
16. Eng JGH, Aks SE, Waldron R, et al. False-negative abdominal CT scan in a cocaine body stuffer. *Am J Emerg Med.* 1999;17:702-704.
17. Expert Working Group of the European Association for Palliative Care. Morphine in cancer pain: modes of administration. *BMJ.* 1996;312: 823-826.
18. Farmer JW, Chan SB. Whole body irrigation for contraband bodypackers. *J Clin Gastroenterol.* 2003;37:147-150.
19. Fattinger K, Benowitz NL, Jones RT, Verotta D. Nasal mucosal versus gastrointestinal absorption of nasally administered cocaine. *Eur J Clin Pharmacol.* 2008;56:305-310.
20. Fineschi V, Centini F, Monciotti, Turillazzi E. The cocaine "body stuffer" syndrome: a fatal case. *Forensic Sci Int.* 2002;126:7-10.
21. Fishbain DA, Wetli CV. Cocaine intoxication, delirium and death in a body packer. *Ann Emerg Med.* 1981;10:531-532.
22. Gherardi R, Marc B, Alberti X, et al. A cocaine body packer with normal abdominal plain radiograms: Value of detection in urine and contrast study of the bowel. *Am J Forensic Med Pathol.* 1990;11:154-157.
23. Gherardi RK, Baud FJ, Leporc P, et al. Detection of drugs in the urine of body-packers. *Lancet.* 1988;1:1076-1077.
24. Gill JR, Graham SM: Ten years of "body packers" in New York City: 50 deaths. *J Forensic Sci.* 2002;47:843-846.
25. Girardin F, Rentsch KM, Schwab M, et al. Pharmacokinetics of high doses of intramuscular and oral heroin in narcotic addicts. *Clin Pharmacol Ther.* 2003;74:341-352.
26. Glass JM, Scott HJ. 'Surgical mules': The smuggling of drugs in the gastrointestinal tract. *J R Soc Med.* 1995;88:450-453.
27. Gyr E, Brenneise R, Bourquin D, et al. Pharmacodynamics and pharmacokinetics of intravenously, orally and rectally administered diacetylmorphine in opioid dependents, a two-patient pilot study within a heroin-assisted treatment program. *Int J Clin Pharmacol Ther.* 2000;38: 486-491.
28. Hahn IH, Hoffman RS, Nelson LS. Contrast CT scan fails to detect the last heroin packet. *J Emerg Med.* 2004;27:279-283.
29. Halbsguth U, Rentsch KM, Eich-Hochli D, et al. Oral diacetylmorphine (heroin) yields greater morphine bioavailability than oral morphine: bioavailability related to dosage and prior opioid exposure. *Br J Clin Pharmacol.* 2008;66:781-791.
30. Hartoko TJ, Demey HE, de Schepper AM, et al. The body packer syndrome—cocaine smuggling in the gastrointestinal tract. *Klin Wochenschr.* 1988;66:1116-1120.
31. Hassanian-Moghaddam H, Abolmasoumi Z: Consequence of body packing illicit drugs. *Arch Iran Med.* 2006;10:20-23.
32. Hendrickson RG, Horowitz BZ, Norton RL, Notenboom H. "Parachuting" meth: a novel delivery method for methamphetamine and delayed-onset toxicity from "body stuffing." *Clin Toxicol.* 2006;44:379-382.
33. Hergan K, Kofler K, Oser W. Drug smuggling by body packing: what radiologists should know about it. *Eur Radiol.* 2004;14:736-742.
34. Hierholzer J, Cordes M, Tantow H, et al. Drug smuggling by ingested cocaine-filled packages: conventional x-ray and ultrasound. *Abdom Imaging.* 1995;20:333-338.
35. Hoffman RS, Chiang WK. Prospective evaluation of "crack-vial" ingestions. *Vet Hum Toxicol.* 1990;32:164-167.
36. Hoffman RS, Smilkstein MJ, Goldfrank LR. Whole bowel irrigation and the cocaine body-packer: A new approach to a common problem. *Am J Emerg Med.* 1990;8:523-527.
37. Hutchins KD, Pierre-Louis PJB, Zaretski L, et al. Heroin body packing: Three fatal cases of intestinal perforation. *J Forensic Sci.* 2000;45:42-47.
38. Introna Jr F, Smialek JE. The "mini-packer" syndrome. *Am J Forensic Med Pathol.* 1989;10:21-24.
39. Inturrisi CE, Max MB, Foley KM, et al. The pharmacokinetics of heroin in patients with chronic pain. *JAMA.* 1984;310:1213-1217.
40. Jenkins AJ. Pharmacokinetics: Drug absorption, distribution and elimination. In: Karch SB, ed: *Drug Abuse Handbook.* 2nd ed. New York: CRC Press; 2007:195-196.
41. Johnson JA, Landreneau RJ. Esophageal obstruction and mediastinitis: a hard pill to swallow for drug smugglers. *Am Surg.* 1991;57:723-726.
42. Jones RT: pharmacology of cocaine. In: Grabowski J, ed. *Cocaine: Pharmacology, effects and treatment of abuse.* NIDA Reseach Monograph 50. 1984;50:34-53.
43. Jonsson S, O'Meara M, Young JB: Acute cocaine poisoning: importance of treating seizures and acidosis. *Am J Med.* 1983;75:1061-1064.
44. Jordan MT, Bryant SM, Aks SE, Wahl M. A five-year review of the medical outcome of heroin body stuffers. *J Emerg Med.* 2009;36:250-256.
45. June R, Aks SE, Keys N, Wahl M: Medical outcome of cocaine body stuffers. *J Emerg Med.* 2000;18:221-224.
46. Karhunen PJ. Suoranta H. Penttila A. Pitkaranta P. Pitfalls in the diagnosis of drug smuggler's abdomen. *J Foren Sci.* 1991;36:397-402.
47. Karkos PD, Cain AJ, White PS. An unusual foreign body in the oesophagus. The body packer syndrome. *Eur Arch Otorhinolaryngol.* 2005;262:154-156.
48. Kashani J, Ruha A. Methamphetamine toxicity secondary to intravaginal body stuffing. *J Toxicol Clin Toxicol.* 2004;42:987-989.
49. Kersschot EA, Beaucourt LE, Degryse HR, de Schepper AM. Roentgenographical detection of cocaine smuggling in the alimentary tract. *Rofo Fortschr Geb Rontgenstr Neuen Bildgeb Verfahr.* 1985;142:295-298.
50. Koehler SA, Ladham S, Rozin L, et al. The risk of body packing: a case of fatal cocaine overdose. *Forensic Sci Int.* 2005;151:81-84.
51. Lancashire MJR, Legg PK, Lowe M, et al. Surgical aspects of international drug smuggling. *BMJ.* 1988;296:1035-1037.
52. Litovitz TL, Holm KC, Bailey KM,Schmitz BF. 1991 annual report of the American Association of Poison Control Centers National Data Collection System. *Am J Emerg Med.* 1992;10:452-505.
53. Lopez HH, Goldman SM, Liberman II, Barnes DT. Cannabis—accidental peroral intoxication: the hashish smuggler roentgenographically unmasked. *JAMA.* 1974;227:1041-1042.
54. Low VHS, Dillon EK. Agony of the ecstasy: report of five cases of MDMA smuggling. *Australas Radiol.* 2005;49:400-403.
55. Makosiej FJ, Hoffman RS, Howland MA, Goldfrank LR. An in vitro evaluation of cocaine hydrochloride adsorption by activated charcoal and desorbption upon addition of polyethylene glycol electrolyte lavage solution. *J Toxicol Clin Toxicol.* 1993;31:381-395.
56. Marc B, Baud FJ, Aelion MJ, et al. The cocaine body-packer syndrome: Evaluation of a method of contrast study of the bowel. *J Forensic Sci.* 1990;35:345-355.
57. Marc B, Gherardi RK, Baud FJ, et al. Managing drug deals who swallow the evidence. *BMJ.* 1989;299:1082.
58. McCarron MM, Wood JD. The cocaine 'body packer' syndrome: diagnosis and treatment. *JAMA.* 1983;250:1417-1420.
59. Meatherall RC, Warren RJ. High urinary cannabinoids from a hashish body packer. *J Anal Toxicol.* 1993;17:439-440.
60. Meijer R, Bots ML. Detection of intestinal drug containers by ultrasound scanning: An airport screening tool?: *Eur Radiol.* 2003;13:1312-1315.

61. Merigan KS, Park LJ, Leeper KV, et al. Adrenergic crisis from crack cocaine ingestion: report of five cases. *J Emerg Med.* 1994;12:485-490.
62. Miller JS, Hendren SK, Liscum KR. Giant gastric ulcer in a body packer. *J Trauma.* 1998;45:617-619.
63. Nihira M, Hayashida M, Ohno Y, et al. Urinaysis of body hackers in Japan. *J Anal Toxicol.* 1998;22:61-65.
64. Norfolk GA. The fatal case of a cocaine body-stuffer and a literature review—towards evidence based management. *J Forensic Leg Med.* 2007;14:49-52.
65. Olmedo R, Nelson LS, Chu J, Hoffman RS. Is surgical decontamination definitive treatment of "body-packers"? *Am J Emerg Med.* 2001;19:593-596.
66. Paez A. Peru: poverty provides a growing number of 'drug mules.' Inter Press Service News Agency. August 14, 2008. http://ipsnews.net/news.asp?idnews=41264. Accessed October 2, 2008.
67. Pamilo M, Suoranta H, Suramo I. Narcotic smuggling and radiography of the gastrointestinal tract. *Acta Radiol Diagn.* 1986;27:213-216.
68. Pidoto RR, Aglita AM, Bertolini R, et al. A new method of packaging cocaine for international traffic and implications for the management of cocaine body packers. *J Emerg Med.* 2002;23:149-153.
69. Pinsky MF, Ducas J, Ruggere MD. Narcotic smuggling: the double condom sign. *Can Assoc Radiol J.* 1978;29:79-81.
70. Pollack Jr CV, Biggers DW, Carlton Jr FB, et al. Two crack cocaine body stuffers. *Ann Emerg Med.* 1992;21:1370-1380.
71. Price KR: Fatal cocaine poisoning. *J Forensic Sci Soc.* 1974;14:329-333.
72. Puschel K, Stein S, Stobbe S, Heinemann A. Analysis of 683 drug packages seized from "body stuffers." *Forensic Sci Int.* 2004;140:109-111.
73. Roberts JR, Price D, Goldfrank LR, Hartnett L. The bodystuffer syndrome: A clandestine form of drug overdose. *Am J Emerg Med.* 1986;4:24-27.
74. Robinson T, Birrer R, Mandava N, Pizzi WF. Body smuggling of illicit drugs: two cases requiring surgical intervention. *Surg.* 1993;113:709-711.
75. Rook EJ, Huitema ADR, van den Brink W, et al. Pharmacokinetics and pharmacokinetic variability of heroin and its metabolites: review of the literature. *Curr Clin Pharmacol.* 2006;1:109-118.
76. Schaper A, Hofmann R, Bargain R, et al. Surgical treatment in cocaine body packers and body pushers. *Int J Colorectal Dis.* 2007;22:1531-1535.
77. Schaper A, Hofmann R, Ebbecke M, et al. Kokain-body-packing: Seltene indikation zur laparotomie. *Chirug.* 2003;74:626-631.
78. Sherman A, Zinger BM. Successful endoscopic retrival of a cocaine body packer from the stomach. *Gastrointest Endosc.* 1990;36:152-154.
79. Silverberg D, Menes T, Kim U. Surgery for "body packers"—a 15-year experience. *World J Surg.* 2006;30:541-546.
80. Sinner W. The gastrointestinal tract as a vehicle for drug smuggling. *Gastrointest Radiol.* 1981;6:319-323.
81. Sporer KA, Firestone J. Clinical course of crack cocaine body stuffers. *Ann Emerg Med.* 1997;29:596-601.
82. Suarez CA, Arango A, Lester III JL: Cocaine-condom ingestion: surgical treatment. *JAMA.* 1977;238:1391-1392.
83. Swan MC, Byrom R, Nicolaou M, Paes T. Cocaine by internal mail: two surgical cases. *J R Soc Med.* 2003;96:188-189.
84. Taheri MS, Hassanian-Moghaddam H, Birang S, et al. Swallowed opium packets: CT diagnosis. *Abdom Imaging.* 2008;33:262-266.
85. Takekawa K, Ohmori T, Kido A, Oya M. Methamphetamine body packer: Acute poisoning death due to massive leaking of methamphetamine. *J Forensic Sci.* 2007;52:1219-1222.
86. Thompson AC, Terry RM. Cannabis-resin foreign body in the ear. *NEJM.* 1989;320:1758.
87. Traub SJ, Hoffman RS, Nelson LS: Body packing—the internal concealment of illicit drugs. *New Engl J Med.* 2003;349:2519-2526.
88. Traub SJ, Hoffman RS, Nelson LS: false-positive abdominal radiography in a body packer resulting from intraabdominal calcifications. *Am J Emerg Med.* 2003;21:607-608.
89. Traub SJ, Kohn GL, Hoffman RS, Nelson LS. Pediatric "body packing." *Arch Pediatr Adolesc Med.* 2003;157:174-177.
90. Traub SJ, Su M, Hoffman RS, Nelson LS. Use of pharmaceutical promotility agents in the treatment of body packers. *Am J Emerg Med.* 2003;21:511-512.
91. Utecht MJ, Stone AF, McCarron MM. Heroin body packers. *J Emerg Med.* 1993;11:33-40.
92. van der Vlies CH, Busch ORC: an intraabdominal cyst. *New Engl J Med.* 2007;357:e6.
93. van Geloven AAW, van Lienden KP, Gouma DJ. Bodypacking—an increasing problem in the Netherlands: conservative or surgical treatment? *Eur J Surg.* 2002;168:404-409.
94. Visser L, Stricker B, Hoogendoorn M, Vinks A. Do not give paraffin to packers. *Lancet.* 1998;352:1352.
95. Wackerle VB, Rupp N, von Clarmann M, et al. Nachweis von rauschgiftpackchen beim "body packer" durch bildgebende verfahren." *Fortschr Rontgenstr.* 1986;145:274-277.
96. Wilkinson P, Van Dyke C, Jatlow P, et al. Intranasal and oral cocaine kinetics. *Clin Pharmacol Ther.* 1980;27:386-394.
97. Wilogren J. Misdiagnosis leads to man's handcuffing, suit claims. *New York Times.* December 6, 1998;

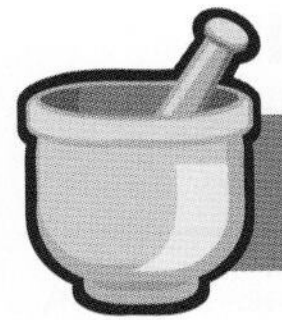

ANTIDOTES IN DEPTH (A24)

BENZODIAZEPINES

Robert S. Hoffman, Lewis S. Nelson, and Mary Ann Howland

Since the introduction of chlordiazepoxide in 1960,[53] benzodiazepines have gained acceptance as safe and effective drugs for a large variety of clinical indications. Specifically in medical toxicology, benzodiazepines are used as the first-line anticonvulsants for virtually all xenobiotic-induced seizures; as the sedatives of choice for most forms of xenobiotic-induced agitation; as muscle relaxants for diverse disorders such as serotonin syndrome, neuroleptic malignant syndrome, and poisoning from strychnine or black widow spider envenomation; and as sedative hypnotics for withdrawal from ethanol, γ-hydroxybutyric acid (GHB), and a variety of sedatives. Additional distinct indications for benzodiazepines can be found in overdose from chloroquine and possibly other quinine-derived antimalarials, and in patients with cocaine-associated myocardial ischemia and infarction.

This Antidotes in Depth provides a summary of the clinical pharmacology of benzodiazepines in order to provide the reader with the background necessary to administer these drugs as safely and effectively as possible.

CHEMISTRY

All benzodiazepines share a common chemical structure shown in Figure A24–1. This structure links a benzene ring with a diazepine ring and gives rise to the name used to describe the drug class. The additional phenyl ring is present in all clinically important benzodiazepines and serves as a site of substitution that modulates some pharmacologic characteristics. The pyrazolopyrimidines (zolpidem, zopiclone, and zaleplon) lack the typical benzodiazepine structure, but have similar pharmacologic effects.[20] Since these pharmaceuticals are largely unstudied for the antidotal indications described above, they are not discussed in depth here. A discussion of the manifestations and treatment of overdose of benzodiazepines and similar xenobiotics can be found in Chapter 74.

GABA RECEPTORS

Benzodiazepines target the γ-aminobutyric acid type A ($GABA_A$) receptor, which is a ligand-gated chloride channel (see Chap. 13, Fig. 13-10), but have no appreciable binding to $GABA_B$. In the absence of GABA, benzodiazepines have no effect on chloride conductance. However, when GABA is present on its $GABA_A$ receptor, benzodiazepines increase the frequency of channel opening resulting in enhanced flow of negatively charged chloride ions into the cell with resultant hyperpolarization.[56]

The $GABA_A$ receptor is assembled from five subunits that span the cell membrane in a circular fashion to create the chloride channel.[40] These subunits are coded as α, β, γ, δ, ε, Φ, π, or ρ, and at least 19 isoforms of these subunits (such as α_1, α_2, α_3, α_4, and α_5) are identified.[12] If the isoforms of the known subunits could assemble randomly, several hundred thousand possible configurations of the $GABA_A$ receptor would be possible.[58] However, it appears that a minimum of at least one α, one β, and either one γ or one δ subunit are required to form a functional chloride channel,[62] and as a result the actual number of configurations is limited. The most common configuration consists of one α, two β, and two γ isoforms.[58,62]

BENZODIAZEPINE RECEPTORS

Rapidly evolving neuroscience has resulted in an exponential expansion in the understanding of benzodiazepine receptors. As a result multiple, potentially confusing nomenclatures have developed.

CENTRAL

The term "central benzodiazepine receptors" is used to refer to benzodiazepine binding sites on GABAergic neurons of the nervous system. Although benzodiazepine binding to the $GABA_A$ receptor cannot occur unless at least one γ subunit is present,[15] the actual site of benzodiazepine binding is believed to be located at the interface of the α and γ subunits.[12] Since most receptors only contain a single α subunit, only one benzodiazepine binding site usually exists on each $GABA_A$ receptor. Anatomical variations in the α isoforms produce two common patterns of expression that account for some of the clinical variations between benzodiazepines and the pyrazolopyrimidines mentioned earlier.

Benzodiazepine type 1 (BZ1) receptors are also called ω_1 receptors. They have a predominance of the α_1 isoform, are located in the sensory and motor areas of the brain, and mediate sedative and hypnotic effects. Benzodiazepine type 2 (BZ2) receptors are also called ω_2 receptors. They have a predominance of the α_2, α_3, or α_5 isoforms; are located in the subcortical and limbic areas of the brain; and mediate anxiolytic and anticonvulsant effects.[39] Most typical benzodiazepines have substantial affinity for the α_1, α_2, α_3, and α_5 isoforms, which explains their combined sedative-hypnotic, anxiolytic, and anticonvulsant effects. In contrast, the pyrazolopyrimidines (such as zolpidem) have high affinity for α_1, intermediate affinity for α_2 and α_3, and low affinity for α_5 isoforms, which explains their lack of anticonvulsant effect.[20,41] The α_4 confers resistance to benzodiazepines.

PERIPHERAL

The term "peripheral benzodiazepine receptors" was originally used in the 1970s to define benzodiazepine binding sites outside of the nervous system.[10] Since peripheral benzodiazepines are now identified in most tissues including the central nervous system, the term best applies to binding sites not located on GABAergic neurons. These receptors have also been called BZ3 or ω_3 receptors to distinguish them from the "central receptors" described above.[31] However, numerous non-benzodiazepines have high-affinity binding for these receptors, and their structure and function are so dissimilar from $GABA_A$-associated benzodiazepine binding sites that other names such as translocator

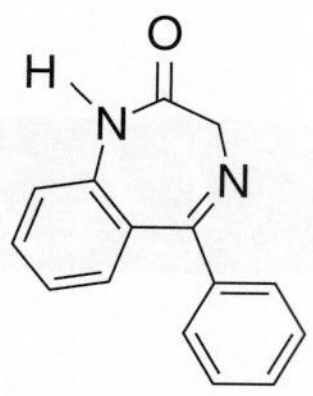

FIGURE A24–1. Generic structure of benzodiazepines.

protein (18 kDa), mitochondrial translocator protein (18 kDa), nuclear translocator protein (18 kDa), or simply translocator protein (18 kDa) may be more appropriate.[47,57,63] For simplicity and consistency they will be referred to as peripheral benzodiazepine receptors (PBRs) in the remainder of this discussion.

Peripheral benzodiazepine receptors are heterotrimers composed of an isoquinoline binding protein, which is the actual 18-kDa translocator protein or the actual receptor; a voltage-dependent anion channel (VDAC); and an adenine nucleotide transporter (ANT).[47] Although the actual function of each subunit is not well appreciated, the minimal functional unit of the PBR is the 18-kDa protein.[29] Sequencing of PBRs demonstrates that they are highly conserved in nature, with DNA from bacteria and fungi having a nearly 50% homology of the isoquinoline binding domain with human DNA.[19] Homology among mammals exceeds 75%.[19] These findings suggest that the PBRs perform a "housekeeping function," that is, they are involved in a process or processes that are essential for life. In higher life forms PBRs can be found primarily in the brain, adrenal glands, heart, and kidney. The translocator protein and the VDAC span the outer mitochondrial membrane, while the ANT bridges the outer and inner membranes (Fig. A24–2). PBRs are implicated in cholesterol and protoporphyrin transport required for the synthesis of steroids, heme, and bile salts; ischemia and reperfusion; regulation of calcium channels; mitochondrial respiration; apoptosis; microglial activation; and the immune response.[19,47,57]

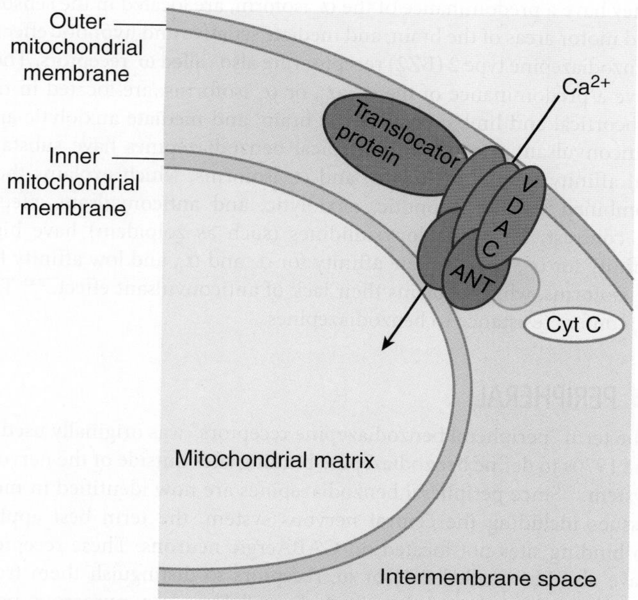

FIGURE A24–2. The peripheral benzodiazepine receptor has three main components: the 18-kDa translocator protein, a voltage-dependent anion channel (VDAC), and an adenine nucleotide transporter (ANT) which are shown on the mitochondrial membrane.

ROLE OF PERIPHERAL BENZODIAZEPINE RECEPTORS IN THE MANAGEMENT OF POISONING

Many chapters in this text discuss the use of benzodiazepines as $GABA_A$ agonists in the management of poisoned patients (see Chaps. 14, 18, 75, 76, and 78). In contrast to the highly evidence-based support for $GABA_A$ agonists in sympathomimetic overdose, xenobiotic-induced seizures, and sedative-hypnotic withdrawal, the use of benzodiazepines as modulators of PBRs for the treatment of poisoned patients is highly speculative. However, as this field is rapidly evolving, discussion of two xenobiotics, chloroquine (see Chap. 58) and cocaine (see Chap. 76) is warranted.

CHLOROQUINE

Although chloroquine overdose is uncommon, case fatality rates are extremely high, and ingestion of 5 g or more was once considered universally fatal. However, in 1988 a case series of patients with chloroquine overdose who survived with the use of an aggressive new regimen was described.[50] The protocol, consisting of early endotracheal intubation, high-dose epinephrine infusion, and intravenous diazepam (2 mg/kg over 30 minutes), resulted in the survival of 10 of 11 patients who ingested at least 5 g of chloroquine. This regimen was based on a controlled trial where diazepam improved the hemodynamic and electrocardiographic manifestations of chloroquine poisoning in pigs.[51] Although the study was not designed to determine the mechanism of effect of diazepam, there was no difference in the chloroquine concentrations between the treated and control groups, suggesting that diazepam did not change the distribution of chloroquine.

In isolated perfused hearts, high-dose diazepam has positive inotropic effects that are suppressed by a PBR antagonist.[34] Unfortunately, translation of these findings in an isolated rat heart to doses used in human poisoning is not necessarily valid. Also, benzodiazepines, chloroquine, and experimental PBR agonists share some structural elements (Fig. A24–3). Functional similarity is also suggested by evidence that both flurazepam and PK 11195 (a PBR agonist) have antimalarial

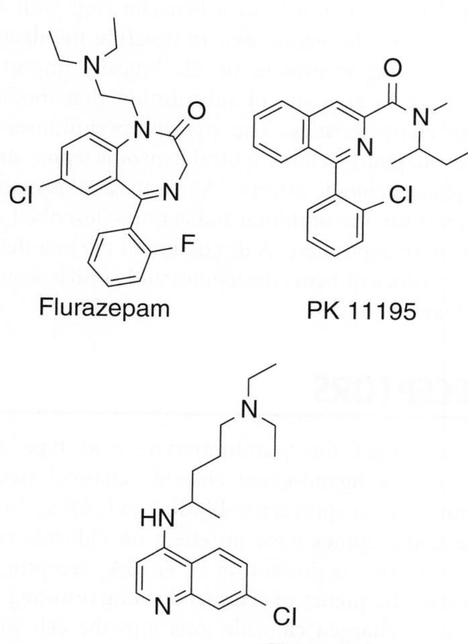

FIGURE A24–3. Comparative structures of flurazepam, PK 11195 (a PBR agonist) and chloroquine. Note the similarity and particularly the shared isoquinoline rings of chloroquine and PK 11195.

activity.[17] Thus, one could speculate that it is possible that the beneficial effects of high-dose diazepam result from competitive inhibition of an undefined interaction between chloroquine and PBRs.

COCAINE

Patients who use cocaine frequently present to emergency departments with either chest pain, or signs or symptoms that could represent myocardial ischemia or infarction.[11] Unlike most patients with acute cocaine toxicity, however, these patients often present hours after their last drug use and without the classic sympathomimetic findings of acute cocaine toxicity.[26] While the pathophysiology of cocaine-induced myocardial ischemia is complex and multifactorial (see Chap. 76), one component of delayed myocardial ischemia may result from the vasoconstrictive actions of benzoylecgonine, the principal metabolite of cocaine.[37] Benzoylecgonine is distinct from cocaine in that it has a much longer half-life,[3,4] does not produce central nervous system stimulation,[43,44] and directly vasoconstricts through modulation of calcium channels.[36]

Limited research suggests that chronic cocaine use is associated with an increased number of PBRs on human platelets.[14] Also in humans, cocaine withdrawal is associated with a decrease in PBRs on neutrophils. In the myocardium, PBRs are either present on mitochondria, or coupled to calcium channels.[42] Specifically, PBR ligands have demonstrable inhibitory effects on myocardial L-type calcium channels.[13] Also in a cardiac model of ischemia and reperfusion injury, an experimental PBR agonist limited myocardial infarction size following coronary artery occlusion.[32] This effect most likely occurs through inhibition of the opening of the mitochondrial permeability transition pore,[45] which is a common final mechanism of cell death. Additionally, although the exact mechanism is unclear, PBR agonists directly antagonize the vasoconstrictive effects of norepinephrine in rat aortic tissue.[21]

Benzodiazepines are commonly used to treat the agitation associated with sympathomimetic overdose (see Chaps. 75 and 76). While it is assumed that the normalization of vital signs results from a decrease in central nervous system stimulation and psychomotor agitation, effects on PBRs may be contributory. In the same isolated perfused hearts described above, low-dose diazepam has a negative inotropic effect that results from an interaction with calcium currents.[33] As noted above, interpreting the implications of varied benzodiazepine doses in an isolated rat model with regard to human beings may not be valid. More importantly, two randomized controlled studies evaluated the use of benzodiazepines in patients with cocaine-associated chest pain.[8,27] In the first study, patients were randomized to receive nitroglycerin, diazepam, or combined therapy.[8] Both drugs were associated with an improvement in chest pain, and combined therapy appeared to offer no additional benefit. The second study randomized patients to nitroglycerin or combined nitroglycerin with lorazepam therapy.[27] In this trial combined therapy was better than either therapy alone, possibly suggesting that benzodiazepines and nitroglycerin relieve chest pain by different mechanisms.

PHARMACOKINETICS AND PHARMACODYNAMICS

As mentioned above, in medical toxicology benzodiazepines are usually administered to treat seizures, psychomotor agitation, or sedative-hypnotic withdrawal. Since these disorders often represent life-threatening emergencies, the initial approach to treatment involves the use of parenteral drugs. Parenteral therapy provides guaranteed absorption with a relatively rapid onset of action. As such, this Antidotes in Depth: A24 focuses on the most commonly used parenteral benzodiazepines: diazepam, lorazepam, and midazolam. Clinically important pharmacologic parameters of these three drugs are listed in Table A24–1. Of note, since the existing literature is insufficient to

TABLE A24–1. Pharmacologic Properties of Select Benzodiazepines

Parameter	Diazepam	Midazolam	Lorazepam
Lipid solubility	++++	++++ (initially water soluble but becomes lipophilic at physiologic pH)	+++
Partition ratio (octanol/pH 6)	309	34	73
Volume of distribution (healthy adults) (L/kg)	0.89 ± 0.18	0.80 ± 0.19	1.28 ± 0.34
Protein binding (%)	97–99	96	85
Hepatic metabolism	Phase 1	Phase 1	Phase 2
Active metabolites	Yes (several)	Yes: Alpha hydroxymidazolam (10% of parent, but accumulates with chronic dosing)	No
Average dose (mg) in 70-kg adult[a]			
Sedation	10 mg over 2 min	2 mg over >2 min (not >1.5 mg in elderly or debilitated patients and over >>2 min) Wait 2 min before titrating	2 mg over 1 min (dilute with equal volume of NS or D_5W prior to injection) Wait 15 min before redosing
Status epilepticus (Initial dose)	10 mg	Not established	4 mg
Diluent	Alcohol 10% Benzyl alcohol 1.5% Propylene glycol 40%	Benzyl alcohol 1.0% Edetate Na_2 1%	Benzyl alcohol 2% Propylene glycol 80%
Available	5mg/mL Rectal gel 5 mg/mL	1 mg/mL 5 mg/mL	2 mg/mL 4 mg/mL

[a]Avoid intraarterial administration since severe spasm may occur with resulting ischemia or gangrene. Also avoid extravasation.

D_5W = 5% dextrose in water

NS = 0.9% NaCl.

absolutely differentiate individual roles for specific benzodiazepines in specific disorders, these three drugs are often used interchangeably for a variety of indications based on availability within the hospital and regional historic preferences. Only through an understanding of the pharmacology can the clinician select the optimal drug, dose, route, and interval to ensure adequate response and limit adverse reactions. As discussed below, it is important to note that the onset and peak effects of sedative and anticonvulsant activity are distinctly different for each drug and among drugs, so pharmacodynamic data are an important adjunct to the interpretation of pharmacokinetic data.

Intravenous administration guarantees complete and immediate absorption. When intravenous access is unavailable, intramuscular lorazepam or midazolam should be considered as they both have good absorptive profiles.[24,28,61] In contrast, the absorption following intramuscular diazepam is best described as slow, incomplete, erratic, and dependent on the site of administration.[16,28,59] Intramuscular injection of diazepam should therefore not be considered unless no other alternatives exist.

Other routes of administration are used for rapid drug delivery when intravenous access is not available. For example, and especially in children, intranasal and rectal administration can be considered. When rectal diazepam was compared with intravenous diazepam in children with seizures, the peak concentration was more variable and was delayed by about 20 minutes.[46] Additionally, failure rates are higher when rectal diazepam is compared with intravenous diazepam.[46,49] Similarly, although midazolam is more rapidly absorbed than diazepam following both nasal and rectal administration, the kinetic profile of nasal or rectal midazolam is still inferior than the intravenous administration or either diazepam or midazolam.[38,49]

Once absorbed, benzodiazepines must distribute into the central nervous system in order to produce their sedative and anticonvulsant effects. The differences among individual drugs can be evaluated in terms of their pharmacokinetics, such as cerebral drug concentrations, or pharmacodynamics, such as changes in either consciousness or electroencephalographic (EEG) findings. A cat model was used to compare cerebrospinal fluid (CSF) concentrations of benzodiazepines with EEG effects.[5] Following intravenous administration, diazepam, midazolam, and lorazepam all appeared rapidly in the CSF. However, the times to peak concentration, onset, and duration of EEG activities were remarkably different among the three drugs (Table A24–2).

In a similar study, human volunteers were given a 1-minute intravenous infusion of either diazepam (0.15 mg/kg) or midazolam (0.1 mg/kg) and EEG analysis was used as a surrogate for the pharmacodynamic effects of sedation. Peak EEG effects were present immediately at the end of the diazepam infusion, but were delayed for 5- to 10 minutes after the midazolam infusion.[23] These EEG effects lasted for 5 hours in diazepam-treated volunteers in comparison to only 2 hours in midazolam-treated volunteers. The same investigators compared the EEG effects of either intravenous lorazepam (low dose, 0.0225 mg/kg; high dose, 0.045 mg/kg) or diazepam (0.15 mg/kg) in human volunteers.[22] In comparison to diazepam, the EEG effects of lorazepam were slower in onset, delayed in peak (30 minutes), and prolonged in duration of effect. The relative effects of diazepam, lorazepam, and midazolam are shown in Table A24–3.

TABLE A24–2. Selected Pharmacokinetic and Pharmacodynamic Properties of Benzodiazepines in Animals[5]

Parameter	Diazepam	Midazolam	Lorazepam
Time to peak CSF concentration (min)	3.7 ± 1.3	3.7 ± 1.3	7.0 ± 4.2
Onset of EEG activity (min)	0.89 ± 0.31	0.29 ± 0.04	3.8 ± 3.1
Duration of EEG activity (min)	7.5 ± 1.4	6.3 ± 1.9	28.3 ± 10.1

CSF, cerebrospinal fluid; EEG, electroencephalographic.

TABLE A24–3. Relative Pharmacodynamic Properties of Benzodiazepines in Humans

	Diazepam	Midazolam	Lorazepam
Anticonvulsant			
Onset of action			
IV	Quick (min)	Quick (min)	Quick (min)
IM	Not advisable	2–10 min	9 min
Duration of action			
IV	1–2 h	30-80 min	Many hours
IM	Unpredictable	1–2 h	Many hours
Sedative			
Onset of action			
IV	Quick (min)	Quick (min)	5–20 min
IM	Unpredictable	5–10 min	20-30 min
Relative duration of action			
Single dose	Short	Short	Long
Repeated doses	Long (secondary to active metabolites)	Intermediate (secondary to active metabolites)	Long

IM, intravenous; IM, intramuscular.

DOSING AND ADMINISTRATION

In theory, an analysis of the pharmacokinetic and pharmacodynamic parameters presented in Tables A24–1 and A24–3 should allow clinicians to choose among the benzodiazepines based on the particular clinical situation. In reality, however, these choices may be difficult in patients with complex clinical presentations of uncertain etiologies. In addition, clinical studies seem to suggest less variability than might be predicted based on pharmacokinetic and pharmacodynamic modeling. For example, in an analysis of 28 studies of conscious sedation, 19 failed to demonstrate a significant difference in the times to recovery between diazepam and midazolam.[6] Likewise although multiple studies demonstrate that lorazepam is at least as effective and likely superior to diazepam in terminating status epilepticus, its onset of action does not appear to be delayed.[2,35,55]

Some of the observed inability to translate controlled pharmacologic analyses into clinical practice may result from imprecision in determining equivalent doses of these drugs. We offer the following guidance. Each of these three benzodiazepines discussed will likely have some efficacy in all clinical scenarios for which a benzodiazepine is indicated. It may therefore be preferable for many clinicians to understand and master the pharmacology and limitations of a single drug rather than attempt to use all three drugs selectively and run the risk of an improper dose or suboptimal therapeutic interval leading to an adverse effect. For those who wish to use these drugs selectively, three variables should be considered: onset of effect, peak effect, and duration of effect. For example, in patients with extreme psychomotor agitation intravenous diazepam or midazolam would be prefered both for their rapid onset and rapid peak effects. The relatively slow onset and delayed peak of lorazepam might lead to administration of multiple doses before the full effect of the first dose is appreciated, with resultant oversedation. When a short duration of sedation is anticipated, such as when treating a patient with toxicity following intravenous or inhaled use of cocaine, midazolam might be preferable over diazepam or lorazepam in that the duration of the effects of midazolam better matches the duration of effects of cocaine, thereby limiting oversedation after cocaine has been rapidly metabolized. For disorders where very long periods of agitation are expected, such as alcohol withdrawal, the choice of diazepam with its very active metabolites (desmethyldiazepam and oxazepam) may be preferable over lorazepam and midazolam in that less frequent dosing may be required and an auto-tapering effect may result at the end of therapy, because these metabolites persist longer than diazepam alone. When status epilepticus is present in the absence of substance use or withdrawal, lorazepam seems to offer a clear advantage. It is important to note that switching from one benzodiazepine to another is rarely indicated, and increases the risk of an adverse drug event from unpredictable peak effects, or improper therapeutic doses or dosing intervals. Specific recommendations can be found in Chapters 14, 18, 75, 76, and 78.

ADVERSE EFFECTS

The most common adverse effect of benzodiazepines is central nervous system depression. While this is unavoidable in some cases, it can generally be limited by selecting the optimal drug and the proper dose and dosing interval for the drug being used. Extra caution is advised in elderly patients as they appear to be more sensitive, particularly to the sedative and respiratory depressant effects of midazolam.[1] In contrast, paradoxical reactions may occur where patients become more agitated following benzodiazepine administration.[52,54,60] These infrequent reactions probably result from disinhibition and may respond to larger doses of benzodiazepines. Although paradoxical agitation also responds to flumazenil, reversal would be inappropriate following the antidotal use of benzodiazepines (see Antidotes in Depth A23–Flumazenil).

Intravenous benzodiazepines produce a mild reduction in heart rate and both systolic and diastolic blood pressure. The effects of midazolam may be greater than diazepam,[48] but this may merely be based on an inability to determine an equivalent dosing regimen. While these reductions result in part from diminished sympathetic tone, direct myocardial effects are rarely severe and are often considered desirable in the overdose setting.[48]

Whereas respiratory depression is generally not a concern with oral benzodiazepines, parenteral administration is documented to impair ventilation. Early investigations demonstrated that intramuscular diazepam (10 mg) blunted the hypoxic ventilatory drive in normal subjects.[30] Intravenous diazepam impaired the ventilatory response to a rising Pco_2 in normal volunteers.[7] The impaired response to a rising Pco_2 was evident almost immediately and lasted for at least 25 minutes following injection of 0.4 mg/kg of diazepam in healthy volunteers.[25] Studies with midazolam demonstrate similar alterations in respiratory physiology[18] that are comparable in magnitude to those reported with diazepam.[9] Apnea is reported following intravenous midazolam and appears to be dose and rate related, with doses greater than or equal to 0.15 mg/kg being of particular concern.[48] Individuals with preexisting pulmonary disorders, extremes of age, or other central nervous system or respiratory depressants may be more susceptible.

AVAILABILITY

Parenteral benzodiazepines are available from multiple manufacturers in varying concentrations. It is essential to recognize that some formulations contain several significant and varied excipients (see Table A24–1). Large doses or prolonged continuous infusions of benzodiazepines may result in toxicity from these excipients (see Chap. 55).

SUMMARY

Although benzodiazepines are commonly used in a variety of medical settings, subtle differences exist in their pharmacokinetics and pharmacodynamics. Optimal use of these drugs requires a thorough understanding of these differences. Clinicians should consider the desired onset of action, peak effect, and duration of action when choosing among different benzodiazepines. In general, intravenous administration is preferred in an emergency because of rapid and reliable absorption. Because of a rapid onset of action and short time to peak effect, sedation is best achieved with diazepam. When intravenous access is not available, pharmacokinetic and pharmacodynamic parameters favor the use of midazolam for sedation. A prolonged anticonvulsant effect is the major benefit of lorazepam. However, when used for sedation, the delayed peak effect of lorazepam (regardless of route of administration) is undesirable. Although the use of benzodiazepines as peripheral benzodiazepine receptor agonists may explain some unique therapeutic effects of these drugs, existing research is too limited to offer guidance with regard to choice of drug, dose, or dosing interval required to optimize peripheral benzodiazepine receptor response.

REFERENCES

1. Albrecht S, Ihmsen H, Hering W, et al. The effect of age on the pharmacokinetics and pharmacodynamics of midazolam. *Clin Pharmacol Ther.* 1999;65:630-639.
2. Alldredge BK, Gelb AM, Isaacs SM, et al. A comparison of lorazepam, diazepam, and placebo for the treatment of out-of-hospital status epilepticus. *N Engl J Med.* 2001;345:631-637.
3. Ambre J. The urinary excretion of cocaine and metabolites in humans: a kinetic analysis of published data. *J Anal Toxicol.* 1985;9:241-245.
4. Ambre J, Fischman M, Ruo TI. Urinary excretion of ecgonine methyl ester, a major metabolite of cocaine in humans. *J Anal Toxicol.* 1984;8:23-25.
5. Arendt RM, Greenblatt DJ, deJong RH, et al. In vitro correlates of benzodiazepine cerebrospinal fluid uptake, pharmacodynamic action and peripheral distribution. *J Pharmacol Exp Ther.* 1983;227:98-106.
6. Ariano RE, Kassum DA, Aronson KJ. Comparison of sedative recovery time after midazolam versus diazepam administration. *Crit Care Med.* 1994;22:1492-1496.
7. Bailey PL, Andriano KP, Goldman M, et al. Variability of the respiratory response to diazepam. *Anesthesiology.* 1986;64:460-465.
8. Baumann BM, Perrone J, Hornig SE, et al. Randomized, double-blind, placebo-controlled trial of diazepam, nitroglycerin, or both for treatment of patients with potential cocaine-associated acute coronary syndromes. *Acad Emerg Med.* 2000;7:878-885.
9. Berggren L, Eriksson I, Mollenholt P, Sunzel M. Changes in respiratory pattern after repeated doses of diazepam and midazolam in healthy subjects. *Acta Anaesthesiol Scand.* 1987;31:667-672.
10. Braestrup C, Squires RF. Specific benzodiazepine receptors in rat brain characterized by high-affinity (3H)diazepam binding. *Proc Natl Acad Sci U S A.* 1977;74:3805-3809.
11. Brody SL, Slovis CM, Wrenn KD. Cocaine-related medical problems: Consecutive series of 233 patients. *Am J Med.* 1990;88:325-331.
12. Burt DR. Reducing GABA receptors. *Life Sci.* 2003;73:1741-1758.
13. Campiani G, Fiorini I, De Filippis MP, et al. Cardiovascular characterization of pyrrolo[2,1-d][1,5]benzothiazepine derivatives binding selectively to the peripheral-type benzodiazepine receptor (PBR): from dual PBR

affinity and calcium antagonist activity to novel and selective calcium entry blockers. *J Med Chem.* 1996;39:2922-2938.
14. Chesley SF, Schatzki AD, DeUrrutia J, et al. Cocaine augments peripheral benzodiazepine binding in humans. *J Clin Psychiatry.* 1990;51:404-406.
15. Costa E, Guidotti A. Benzodiazepines on trial: a research strategy for their rehabilitation. *Trends Pharmacol Sci.* 1996;17:192-200.
16. Divoll M, Greenblatt DJ, Ochs HR, Shader RI. Absolute bioavailability of oral and intramuscular diazepam: effects of age and sex. *Anesth Analg.* 1983;62:1-8.
17. Dzierszinski F, Coppin A, Mortuaire M, et al. Ligands of the peripheral benzodiazepine receptor are potent inhibitors of plasmodium falciparum and toxoplasma gondii in vitro. *Antimicrob Agents Chemother.* 2002;46:3197-3207.
18. Forster A, Morel D, Bachmann M, Gemperle M. Respiratory depressant effects of different doses of midazolam and lack of reversal with naloxone—a double-blind randomized study. *Anesth Analg.* 1983;62:920-924.
19. Gavish M, Bachman I, Shoukrun R, et al. Enigma of the peripheral benzodiazepine receptor. *Pharmacol Rev.* 1999;51:629-650.
20. George CF. Pyrazolopyrimidines. *Lancet.* 2001;358:1623-1626.
21. Gimeno M, Pallas M, Newman AH, et al. The role of cyclic nucleotides in the action of peripheral-type benzodiazepine receptor ligands in rat aorta. *Gen Pharmacol.* 1994;25:1553-1561.
22. Greenblatt DJ, Ehrenberg BL, Gunderman J, et al. Kinetic and dynamic study of intravenous lorazepam: comparison with intravenous diazepam. *J Pharmacol Exp Ther.* 1989;250:134-140.
23. Greenblatt DJ, Ehrenberg BL, Gunderman J, et al. Pharmacokinetic and electroencephalographic study of intravenous diazepam, midazolam, and placebo. *Clin Pharmacol Ther.* 1989;45:356-365.
24. Greenblatt DJ, Joyce TH, Comer WH, et al. Clinical pharmacokinetics of lorazepam. II. Intramuscular injection. *Clin Pharmacol Ther.* 1977;21:222-230.
25. Gross JB, Smith L, Smith TC. Time course of ventilatory response to carbon dioxide after intravenous diazepam. *Anesthesiology.* 1982;57:18-21.
26. Hollander JE, Hoffman RS, Gennis P, et al. Prospective multicenter evaluation of cocaine-associated chest pain: cocaine associated chest pain (COCHPA) study group. *Acad Emerg Med.* 1994;1:330-339.
27. Honderick T, Williams D, Seaberg D, Wears R. A prospective, randomized, controlled trial of benzodiazepines and nitroglycerine or nitroglycerine alone in the treatment of cocaine-associated acute coronary syndromes. *Am J Emerg Med.* 2003;21:39-42.
28. Hung OR, Dyck JB, Varvel J, et al. Comparative absorption kinetics of intramuscular midazolam and diazepam. *Can J Anaesth.* 1996;43:450-455.
29. Lacapere JJ, Delavoie F, Li H, et al. Structural and functional study of reconstituted peripheral benzodiazepine receptor. *Biochem Biophys Res Commun.* 2001;284:536-541.
30. Lakshminarayan S, Sahn SA, Hudson LD, Weil JV. Effect of diazepam on ventilatory responses. *Clin Pharmacol Ther.* 1976;20:178-183.
31. Langer SZ, Arbilla S. Imidazopyridines as a tool for the characterization of benzodiazepine receptors: a proposal for a pharmacological classification as omega receptor subtypes. *Pharmacol Biochem Behav.* 1988;29:763-766.
32. Leducq N, Bono F, Sulpice T, et al. Role of peripheral benzodiazepine receptors in mitochondrial, cellular, and cardiac damage induced by oxidative stress and ischemia-reperfusion. *J Pharmacol Exp Ther.* 2003;306:828-837.
33. Leeuwin RS, Zeegers A, Van Wilgenburg H. Flunarizine but not theophylline modulates inotropic responses of the isolated rat heart to diazepam. *Eur J Pharmacol.* 1996;315:153-157.
34. Leeuwin RS, Zeegers A, Van Wilgenburg H. PK 11195 antagonizes the positive inotropic response of the isolated rat heart to diazepam but not the negative inotropic response. *Eur J Pharmacol.* 1996;299:149-152.
35. Leppik IE, Derivan AT, Homan RW, et al. Double-blind study of lorazepam and diazepam in status epilepticus. *JAMA.* 1983;249:1452-1454.
36. Madden JA, Konkol RJ, Keller PA, Alvarez TA. Cocaine and benzoylecgonine constrict cerebral arteries by different mechanisms. *Life Sci.* 1995;56:679-686.
37. Madden JA, Powers RH. Effect of cocaine and cocaine metabolites on cerebral arteries in vitro. *Life Sci.* 1990;47:1109-1114.
38. Malinovsky JM, Lejus C, Servin F, et al. Plasma concentrations of midazolam after i.v., nasal or rectal administration in children. *Br J Anaesth.* 1993;70:617-620.
39. McLeod M, Pralong D, Copolov D, Dean B. The heterogeneity of central benzodiazepine receptor subtypes in the human hippocampal formation, frontal cortex and cerebellum using [3H]flumazenil and zolpidem. *Brain Res Mol Brain Res.* 2002;104:203-209.
40. Mehta AK, Ticku MK. An update on GABAA receptors. *Brain Res Brain Res Rev.* 1999;29:196-217.
41. Meldrum BS, Chapman AG. Benzodiazepine receptors and their relationship to the treatment of epilepsy. *Epilepsia.* 1986;27(Suppl 1):S3-13.
42. Mestre M, Carriot T, Belin C, et al. Electrophysiological and pharmacological evidence that peripheral type benzodiazepine receptors are coupled to calcium channels in the heart. *Life Sci.* 1985;36:391-400.
43. Mets B, Virag L. Lethal toxicity from equimolar infusions of cocaine and cocaine metabolites in conscious and anesthetized rats. *Anesth Analg.* 1995;81:1033-1038.
44. Misra AL, Nayak PK, Bloch R, Mule SJ. Estimation and disposition of [3H] benzoylecgonine and pharmacological activity of some cocaine metabolites. *J Pharm Pharmacol.* 1975;27:784-786.
45. Obame FN, Zini R, Souktani R, et al. Peripheral benzodiazepine receptor-induced myocardial protection is mediated by inhibition of mitochondrial membrane permeabilization. *J Pharmacol Exp Ther.* 2007;323:336-345.
46. Ogutu BR, Newton CR, Crawley J, et al. Pharmacokinetics and anticonvulsant effects of diazepam in children with severe falciparum malaria and convulsions. *Br J Clin Pharmacol.* 2002;53:49-57.
47. Papadopoulos V, Baraldi M, Guilarte TR, et al. Translocator protein (18kDa): new nomenclature for the peripheral-type benzodiazepine receptor based on its structure and molecular function. *Trends Pharmacol Sci.* 2006;27:402-409.
48. Reves JG, Fragen RJ, Vinik HR, Greenblatt DJ. Midazolam: pharmacology and uses. *Anesthesiology.* 1985;62:310-324.
49. Rey E, Treluyer JM, Pons G. Pharmacokinetic optimization of benzodiazepine therapy for acute seizures: focus on delivery routes. *Clin Pharmacokinet.* 1999;36:409-424.
50. Riou B, Barriot P, Rimailho A, Baud FJ. Treatment of severe chloroquine poisoning. *N Engl J Med.* 1988;318:1-6.
51. Riou B, Rimailho A, Galliot M, et al. Protective cardiovascular effects of diazepam in experimental acute chloroquine poisoning. *Intensive Care Med.* 1988;14:610-616.
52. Schreiber S. Diazepam-induced disinhibition. *Harefuah.* 1993;124:681-682, 739.
53. Shader RI, Greenblatt DJ, Balter MB. Appropriate use and regulatory control of benzodiazepines. *J Clin Pharmacol.* 1991;31:781-784.
54. Smith VM. Paradoxical reactions to diazepam. *Gastrointest Endosc.* 1995; 41:182-183.
55. Treiman DM, Meyers PD, Walton NY, et al. A comparison of four treatments for generalized convulsive status epilepticus: Veterans Affairs Status Epilepticus Cooperative Study Group. *N Engl J Med.* 1998;339:792-798.
56. Twyman RE, Rogers CJ, Macdonald RL. Differential regulation of gamma-aminobutyric acid receptor channels by diazepam and phenobarbital. *Ann Neurol.* 1989;25:213-220.
57. Venneti S, Lopresti BJ, Wiley CA. The peripheral benzodiazepine receptor (translocator protein 18 kDa) in microglia. From pathology to imaging. *Prog Neurobiol.* 2006;80:308-322.
58. Wafford KA. GABAA receptor subtypes: any clues to the mechanism of benzodiazepine dependence? *Curr Opin Pharmacol.* 2005;5:47-52.
59. Watson DM, Uden DL. Promotion of intramuscular diazepam questioned. *Am J Hosp Pharm.* 1981;38:968, 970-971.
60. Weinbroum AA, Szold O, Ogorek D, Flaishon R. The midazolam-induced paradox phenomenon is reversible by flumazenil: epidemiology, patient characteristics and review of the literature. *Eur J Anaesthesiol.* 2001;18: 789-797.
61. Wermeling DP, Miller JL, Archer SM, et al. Bioavailability and pharmacokinetics of lorazepam after intranasal, intravenous, and intramuscular administration. *J Clin Pharmacol.* 2001;41:1225-1231.
62. Whiting PJ, McKernan RM, Wafford KA. Structure and pharmacology of vertebrate GABAA receptor subtypes. *Int Rev Neurobiol.* 1995;38:95-138.
63. Woods MJ, Williams DC. Multiple forms and locations for the peripheral-type benzodiazepine receptor. *Biochem Pharmacol.* 1996;52:1805-1814.

CHAPTER 77
ETHANOL

Luke Yip

Ethanol, or ethyl alcohol, is commonly referred to as "alcohol." This term is somewhat misleading since there are numerous other alcohols to which a patient may be exposed. However, ethanol is probably the most commonly used and abused xenobiotic in the world. Its use is pervasive among adolescents and adults of all ages and socioeconomic groups, and represents a tremendous financial and social cost.[3,209]

HISTORY AND EPIDEMIOLOGY

The ethanol content of alcoholic beverages is expressed by volume percent or by proof. Proof is a measure of the absolute ethanol content of distilled liquor, made by determining its specific gravity at an index temperature. In the United Kingdom, the Customs and Excise Act of 1952 declared proof spirits (100 proof) as those in which the weight of the spirits is 12/13 the weight of an equal volume of distilled water at 11°C (51°F). Thus, proof spirits are 48.24% ethanol by weight or 57.06% by volume. Other spirits are designated over or under proof, with the percentage of variance noted. In the United States, a proof spirit (100 proof) is one containing 50% ethanol by volume. The derivation of proof comes from the days when sailors in the British Navy suspected that the officers were diluting their rum (grog) ration and demanded "proof" that this was not the case. They achieved this by pouring a sample of grog on black granular gunpowder. If the gunpowder ignited by match or spark, the rum was up to standard, 100% proof that the liquor was 50% ethanol. This became shortened to 100 proof (Table 77–1). In addition to beverages, ethanol is present in hundreds of medicinal preparations used as a diluent or solvent in concentrations ranging from 0.3% to 75%.[28,44,52,106,164,208] Mouthwashes may have up to 75% ethanol (150 proof) and colognes typically contain 40% to 60% ethanol (80 to 120 proof).[16,104,164,177] These products occasionally cause intoxication, especially when unintentionally ingested by children.[31,49,88,210]

Veisalgia, "alcohol hangover," comes from the Norwegian *kveis*, "uneasiness following debauchery," and the Greek *algia*, pain. The "hangover" syndrome has been attributed to congeners, substances that appear in alcoholic beverages in addition to ethanol and water.[26,33,34] Congeners contribute to the special characteristics of taste, flavor, aroma, and color of a beverage. The combinations and exact amounts of congeners vary with the type of beverage, ranging from 33 mg/L in vodka, to averages of 500 mg/L in some whiskies and as much as 29,000 mg/L in specially aged whiskies or brandies.[26,33,34] The conventional listing of congeners includes fusel oil (a mixture containing amyl, buytyl, propyl, and methyl alcohol), aldehydes, furfural, esters, low-molecular-weight organic acids, phenols, and other carbonyl compounds, tannins, solids, and a relatively large number of additional organic and inorganic compounds, usually in trace amounts.[26,34]

Consumption of illicitly produced ethanol ("moonshine") has resulted in methanol, lead, or arsenic poisoning.[46,66,101,120,126,144,161] Incidental lead contamination is also reported in draught beers or wine contained in lead-capped bottles.[183,184] Of historic interest is that the addition of cobalt salts to beer to stabilize the "head" (foam) led to outbreaks of congestive cardiomyopathy among heavy beer drinkers in Canada and Belgium in the 1960s (see Chap. 92). The clinical-pathological pattern of this disease is distinct from the classical alcoholic cardiomyopathy.[136,138]

Alcoholism is the leading cause of morbidity and mortality in the United States. The prevalence of ethanol dependence in the United States has been relatively stable, at around 6% for men and 2% for women.[25] The overall estimated annual cost of health expenses related to ethanol is $185 billion.[151] More than 70% of the estimated costs were attributed to lost productivity, most of which resulted from ethanol-related illness or premature death. Most of the remaining estimated costs were expenditures for health care services to treat ethanol-induced disorders (14.3%), property and administrative costs of ethanol-related motor vehicle crashes (8.5%), and criminal justice system costs of ethanol-related crime (3.4%). More than 200,000 Americans die annually of alcoholism, far more than those who die of all illicit drugs of abuse combined. Ethanol is the leading cause of mortality in people 15 to 45 years of age. In 2007 there were 12,998 ethanol-related traffic fatalities in the United States that accounted for 31.7% of total traffic fatalities; 67% of ethanol-impaired driving fatalities were drivers with blood ethanol concentration 80 mg/dL or higher and 17% were passengers riding with the ethanol-impaired drivers.[149] Drivers age 21 to 34 accounted for 44% and drivers between 16 to 20 years accounted for 10% of all ethanol-impaired drivers in fatal crashes. Among 16- to 20-year-old male drivers, an increase of 20 mg/dL in blood ethanol concentration was estimated to more than double the relative risk of fatal single-vehicle crash injury compared with sober drivers of the same age and gender.[222,223] When the blood ethanol concentration was between 80 and 100 mg/dL (17–22 mmol/L), 100 and 150 mg/dL (22–33 mmol/L) and greater than 150 mg/dL (33 mmol/L), the relative risk of fatal single-vehicle crash injury was 52, 241, and 15,560 respectively.

The Global Burden of Disease Study identified three effects of ethanol: harmful effects in relation to injuries, harmful effects in relation to disease, and the protective effect in relation to ischemic heart disease.[151] Overall ethanol accounted for 3.5% of mortality and disability, 1.5% of all deaths, 2.1% of all life years lost, and 6% of all the years lived with disability.[151] In the United States, according to National Highway Traffic Safety Administration (NHTSA) information, all jurisdictions have enacted per se blood ethanol concentration for adults operating non-commercial motor vehicles.[150] The term *illegal per se* refers to state laws that make it a criminal offense to operate a motor vehicle at or above a specified ethanol (or drug) concentration in the blood, breath, or urine, which may or may not reflect clinical intoxication (Table 77–2). For example, while ethanol-tolerant patients may not exhibit impairment even at serum ethanol concentrations greater than 300 mg/dL (65 mmol/L), they are still considered impaired with regard to the laws that govern motor vehicle operation.[1]

There appears to be a dose–response relationship between ethanol consumption and risk of death in men aged 16–34 and in women aged 16–54. The level at which the risk is lowest increases with age, reaching 64–80 grams per week in men over 65 and 24–30 grams per week in women over 65. The level at which the risk is increased by 5% above this minimum is 40–50 grams per week in men aged 16–24 and 64–80 grams per week in women aged 16–24, increasing to 272–340 g and 160–200 g per week in men and women over 65, respectively.[214] Meta-analysis of aggregate data from epidemiologic dose–response ethanol and mortality cohort studies suggests that the level of ethanol consumption at which all-cause risk is lowest is approximately 5 g/d and that ethanol exerts a protective effect (J-shaped dose response curve) up to a daily intake of approximately 45 grams.[9] It is suggested that sensible drinking of ethanol for men is 8–10 g/d up to age 34, 16–20 g/d between 34 and 44 years of age, 24–30 g/d between 44 and 54 years of age, 32–40 g/d between 54 and 84 years of age, and 40–50 g/d over age 85. Women would be advised to limit their drinking to 8–10 g/d up to age 44, 16–20 g/d between 44 and

TABLE 77–1. Clinical Pharmacology and Pharmacokinetics of Ethanol

Ethanol MW: 46 daltons

$$\text{mmol} = \frac{\text{mg}}{\text{MW}} = \frac{\text{mg}}{46}$$

$$\text{mmol/L} = \frac{\text{mg/dL}}{4.6}$$

Specific gravity: 0.7939 (~0.8) g/mL

Volume of distribution (V_d): 0.6 L/kg

$$\text{Serum ethanol concentration (mg/dL)} = \frac{\text{dose (mg)}}{V_d\text{(L/kg)} \times \text{body weight (kg)} \times 10}$$

Average reduction in blood ethanol concentration (elimination phase):
- Nontolerant adult: 3.26–4.35 mmol/L/h (15–20 mg/dL/h, 100–125 mg/kg/h)
- Tolerant adult: 6.52–8.70 mmol/L/h (30–40 mg/dL/h, 175 mg/kg/h)

For a 70-kg individual:

Dose of ethanol	Serum ethanol concentration[a]
10 mL/kg of 10% (20 proof)	167 mg/dL (36.30 mmol/L)
3 mL/kg of 10% (20 proof)	50 mg/dL (10.87 mmol/L)
1.5 mL/kg of 10% (20 proof)	25 mg/dL (5.43 mmol/L)
150 mL (5 "shots") of 40% (80 proof)	143 mg/dL (31.09 mmol/L)
30 mL (1 "shot") of 40% (80 proof)	27 mg/dL (5.87 mmol/L)
A "standard drink" (15 g of ethanol), defined as 1 oz (30 mL) of 100 proof liquor, 4-oz (120 mL) glass of wine (12% ethanol), or 10-oz bottle (300 mL) of beer (5% ethanol)	43 mg/dL (9.35 mmol/L)

[a]This is the theoretical maximum concentration, based on instantaneous and complete ethanol absorption and no distribution or metabolism.

Blood concentration consistent with legal intoxication = 10.87–17.39 mmol/L (50–80 mg/dL or 0.05–0.08 g/dL [%]).

The legal breath ethanol concentration to blood ethanol concentration ratio has been set at 1:2100; the amount of ethanol in 1 mL of blood is the same amount in 2100 mL of exhaled air: Measured breath ethanol concentration (mmol/L) × 2100 = (calculated) blood ethanol concentration (mmol/L).

TABLE 77–2. Acute Ethanol Effects in Most Nontolerant Individuals

Serum Ethanol Concentration	Effects
20 mg/dL (4.35 mmol/L)[151,223]	Impairs driving-related skills
50 mg/dL (10.87 mmol/L)[142]	Gross motor control and orientation may be significantly affected
	Clinical ethanol intoxication is usually apparent

74 years of age, and 24–30 g/d over age 75.[214] However, no safe level of prenatal ethanol exposure has been established. The combination of a national tolerance of drinking and heavy advertising of ethanol makes it especially appealing to young people. In a society increasingly concerned with drug abuse, the excessive use of ethanol constitutes a serious and pervasive problem as well as a major health issue.

PHARMACOKINETICS/TOXICOKINETICS

Ethanol is rapidly absorbed from the gastrointestinal (GI) tract, with approximately 20% absorbed from the stomach and the remainder from the small intestine.[153] Factors that enhance absorption include rapid gastric emptying, ethanol intake without food, the absence of congeners, dilution of ethanol (maximum absorption occurs at a concentration of 20%), and carbonation. Under optimal conditions for absorption, 80% to 90% of an ingested dose is fully absorbed within 60 minutes. Factors that delay or decrease ethanol absorption include high concentrations of ethanol (by causing pylorospasm), presence of food, coexistence of GI disease, co-ingestion of drugs such as, aspirin,[102,158] time taken to ingest the drink, and individual variation. When any of these factors is present, absorption may be delayed for 2 to 6 hours. The relative amount of ethanol that is absorbed from the stomach is determined by the presence of alcohol dehydrogenase (ADH) in the gastric mucosa, which oxidizes a proportion of the ingested ethanol, thus reducing the amount available for absorption. This effect is more pronounced in men than in women and in nonalcoholics than in alcoholics.[11,58] Histamine$_2$ (H_2) receptor antagonists (ie, cimetidine and ranitidine) inhibit ADH activity in the gastric mucosa resulting in decreased first-pass metabolism and increase the bioavailability of imbibed ethanol.[7,22,24,40,51]

Following complete distribution, ethanol is present in body tissues in a concentration proportional to that of the tissue water content. Ethanol freely passes through the placenta, exposing the fetus to ethanol concentrations comparable to that achieved in the mother.

Ethanol is primarily eliminated by the liver, with 5%–10% excreted unchanged by the kidneys, lungs, and sweat. Ethanol is metabolized via at least three different pathways: the aforementioned alcohol dehydrogenase (ADH) pathway located in the cytosol of the hepatocytes, the microsomal ethanol oxidizing system (MEOS; CYP2E1), located on the endoplasmic reticulum, and the peroxidase-catalase system associated with the hepatic peroxisomes (Fig. 77–1.).[153]

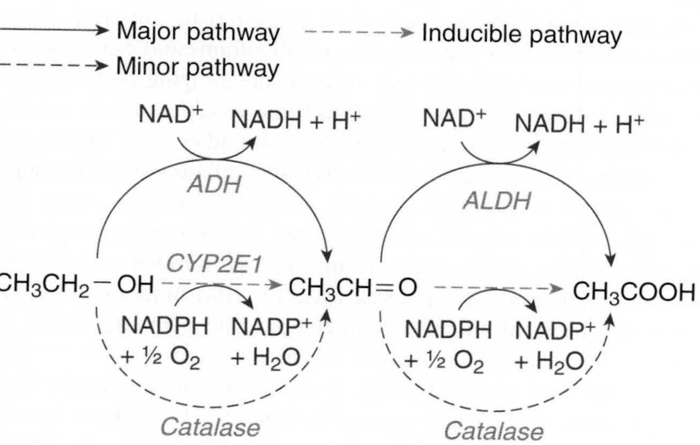

FIGURE 77–1. Ethanol (CH_3CH_2OH) is metabolized to acetaldehyde (CH_3CHO) and then to acetic acid (CH_3COOH) through major, minor and inducible pathways. ADH = alcohol dehydrogenase, ALDH = aldehyde dehydrogenase.

For a given ethanol dose 95%–98% is metabolized in the liver, first to acetaldehyde by ADH and then further to acetic acid by aldehyde dehydrogenase (ALDH).[94] The end products of ethanol oxidation are carbon dioxide and water. The remaining 2%–5% is excreted unchanged in urine, sweat, and expired air. In addition, less than 0.1% undergoes phase II conjugation reactions to produce ethyl glucuronide and ethyl sulfate, catalyzed by uridine diphosphate-glucuronosyltransferase and sulfotransferase, respectively.[32,56,78,179,180]

The ADH system is the main pathway for ethanol metabolism and is also the rate-limiting step. ADH is a zinc metalloenzyme that uses oxidized nicotinamide adenine dinucleotide (NAD^+) as a hydrogen ion acceptor to oxidize ethanol to acetaldehyde. In this process, hydrogen ion is transferred from ethanol to NAD^+, converting it to its reduced form, NADH. Subsequently, hydrogen ion is transferred from acetaldehyde to NAD^+. Under normal conditions acetate is converted to acetylcoenzyme A (acetyl-CoA), which enters the Krebs cycle and is metabolized to carbon dioxide and water. The entry of acetyl-CoA into the Krebs cycle is thiamine dependent (see Antidotes in Depth A25: Thiamine Hydrochloride).

The ADH gene family encodes enzymes that metabolize a wide variety of substrates. There are at least 7 genetic loci code for human ADH arising from the association of different subunits, and there are over 20 ADH isoenzymes.[2] These ADH forms have been divided into five major classes (I-V) according to their subunit, isoenzyme composition, and physicochemical properties.[97] Two of these gene loci exhibit polymorphism and they both involve Class I ADH genes; three alleles exist for ADH2 (ADH1B) ADH2*1 (ADH1B*1), ADH2*2 (ADH1B*2), and ADH2*3 (ADH1B*3)] and three for ADH3: (ADH1C) ADH3*1 (ADH1C*1), ADH3*2 (ADH1C*2), and ADH3*3 (ADH1C*3).[30] Class I enzymes are inducible intracellular hepatic enzymes and are believed to play a major role in ethanol metabolism.[123] Class IV ADH6 (σ-ADH) is the major ADH expressed in human gastric mucosa.[11,58] σ-ADH is usually present in non-Asians, whereas in a majority of Pacific Rim Asians the enzyme activity is either low or not detectable.[11,12,42] The ADH1B*2 allele is present in 90% of Pacific Rim Asians but occurs infrequently in most Caucasians, except for people of Jewish and perhaps Hispanic descent.[215] It appears to be responsible for the unusually rapid conversion of ethanol to acetaldehyde. People carrying ADH1B*2 alleles are about one-third as likely to be alcoholic compared with people without this allele.[215]

In the liver, ADH metabolizes ethanol to acetaldehyde, which is then converted to acetate by mitochondrial NAD-dependent ALDH. Human ALDH is divided into nine major gene families. There is a functional polymorphism of the mitochondrial ALDH2 gene and expression of an inactive form of the ALDH2, glutamate to lysine substitution at position 487 (E487K), results in impaired acetaldehyde metabolizing capacity. The variant allele ALDH2*2 encodes a protein subunit that confers low activity to the enzyme resulting in marked differences in the steady-state kinetic constants, which appears to be most prevalent in Pacific Rim Asians.[2,30,68,192,193] These metabolic polymorphisms contribute to differences in ethanol and acetaldehyde elimination rate; high-activity ADH variants are predicted to increase the rate of acetaldehyde generation, while the low-activity ALDH2 variant is associated with an inability to metabolize this compound, and may explain differences in ethanol-related behavior. Asians possessing an atypical ALDH2 gene are more sensitive to acute adverse responses to ethanol and tends to discourage ethanol consumption. Homozygous ALDH2*2 individuals are strikingly sensitive to small doses of ethanol (0.2 g/kg), as evidenced by the intense flushing, pronounced cardiovascular hemodynamic effects as well as subjective perception of general discomfort.[48,68,162,198,203] This effect may also be associated with the ADH2*2 and ADH3*1 allele, and is similar to that induced by disulfiram (see Chap. 79). The ethanol flushing response may involve prostaglandin and histamine release. Both prostaglandin antagonists (aspirin)[200] and anithistamines (H_1 and H_2)[139,188,195] may attenuate this response.

The MEOS (CYP2E1) is responsible for very little ethanol metabolism in the nontolerant drinker, but becomes more important as the ethanol concentration rises or as ethanol use becomes chronic (Fig. 77–1.). CYP2E1 uses oxidized nicotinamide adenine dinucleotide phosphate ($NADP^+$) as an electron acceptor to oxidize ethanol to acetaldehyde.[112] In this process, electrons are transferred from ethanol to $NADP^+$, converting it to its reduced form, NADPH. Subsequently, acetaldehyde is further oxidized to acetate as hydrogen ion is transferred from acetaldehyde to $NADP^+$. The ability of ethanol to induce the MEOS system forms the basis for the well-established interactions between ethanol and a host of other xenobiotics metabolized by this system.[41,57] In alcoholics and those with higher ethanol concentrations, cimetidine may also delay ethanol clearance by inhibiting the MEOS (CYP2E1).[74] However, the increase in blood ethanol concentration from such an interaction is of questionable clinical significance.[6,7,22,23]

ADH is saturated at relatively low blood ethanol concentrations. As the system is saturated, ethanol elimination changes from first-order to zero-order kinetics (see Chap. 8). In adults, the average rate of ethanol metabolism is 100 to 125 mg/kg/h in occasional drinkers and up to 175 mg/kg/h in habitual drinkers.[19,67] As a result, the average-sized adult metabolizes 7 to 10 g/h and the blood ethanol concentration falls 15 to 20 mg/dL/h (3.26–4.35 mmol/L/h). Tolerant drinkers, by recruiting CYP2E1, may increase their clearance of ethanol to 30 mg/dL/h (6.52 mmol/L/h).[19,67] Studies of ethanol intoxicated patients indicate that although the average ethanol clearance rate is about 20 mg/dL/h (4.35 mmol/L/h), there is considerable individual variation (standard deviation of about 6 mg/dL/h [1.30 mmol/L/h]).[19,67]

XENOBIOTIC INTERACTIONS

Ethanol interacts with a variety of xenobiotics (Table 77–3).[100,208] The most frequent ethanol–drug interactions occur as a result of ethanol-induced increase in hepatic xenobiotic-metabolizing enzyme activity. In contrast, acute ethanol use may inhibit metabolism of other xenobiotics and this may be due to competitive inhibition of hepatic enzyme activity or a reduction in hepatic blood flow. The interaction between ethanol and disulfiram (Antabuse) is well described and it can be rarely life threatening (see Chap. 79).

Concomitant use of cocaine and ethanol leads to the formation of an active metabolite, cocaethylene, through transesterification of cocaine by the liver.[169] Cocaethylene has a longer half-life than cocaine itself (2 hours versus 48 minutes), and this may explain some of the delayed cardiovascular effects attributed to cocaine use.[8,216] Both ethanol and cocaethylene inhibit the metabolism of cocaine, thereby prolonging the elimination of cocaine and enhancing its effect (see Chap. 76).[159]

Case reports and retrospective case series suggest that chronic ethanol consumption may predispose a person to acetaminophen (APAP) hepatotoxicity (see Chap. 34)[47,129,135,178,226] even when APAP has been taken according to the manufacturer's recommended dosage of not more than 4 grams daily.[225] Because ethanol induces cytochrome P450, the enzyme involved in the metabolism of acetaminophen to its hepatotoxic intermediate, NAPQI, a theoretical basis for this association exists. However, in a double-blind placebo control study where confirmed alcoholics were given acetaminophen 4 grams daily or placebo for three consecutive days there were no differences between the two groups with regard to liver enzymes or to their coagulation profile.[111] Recent fasting, common in alcoholics, was also associated with a predisposition

TABLE 77–3. Ethanol Xenobiotic Interactions

Xenobiotics	Adverse Effects
Antihistamines (H_1)	Additive sedative effect
Aspirin	Enhance antiplatelet effect
Carbamates	Disulfiram-like effect
Cephalosporins[a]	Disulfiram-like effect
Chloral hydrate	Additive sedative effect
Chloramphenicol	Disulfiram-like effect
Chlorpropamide	Disulfiram-like effect
Coprinus mushrooms	Disulfiram-like effect
Cyclic antidepressants	Additive sedative effect
Disulfiram (Antabuse)	Nausea, vomiting, abdominal pain, flushing, diaphoresis, chest pain, headache, vertigo, palpitations
Griseofulvin	Disulfiram-like effect
Isoniazid	Increased incidence of hepatitis; increased metabolism[b]
Methadone	Increased methadone metabolism[b]
Metronidazole	Disulfiram-like effect
Nitrofurantoin	Disulfiram-like effect
Opioids	Additive sedative effect
Oral hypoglycemics	Potentiates hypoglycemic effect
Phenothiazines	Additive sedative effect
Phenytoin	Increased phenytoin metabolism[b]
Ranitidine, cimetidine	Increased ethanol concentration
Sedative-hypnotics	Additive sedative effect
Thiram derivatives	Disulfiram-like effect
Vasodilators	Potentiates vasodilator effect
Warfarin	Increased warfarin metabolism[b]

[a] Those containing a *N*-methylthiotetrazole side chain.

[b] Effect possibly associated with chronic alcohol consumption.

to acetaminophen hepatotoxicity, likely due to depletion of glutathione (see Chap. 34).[213] However, in a retrospective study, heavy drinkers did not develop more severe hepatotoxicity following APAP overdose than nondrinkers.[130]

PATHOPHYSIOLOGY

Despite ethanol's long history of use and study, no specific receptor for ethanol has been identified, and the mechanism of action leading to intoxication remains the subject of debate.[163] Ethanol has been shown to affect a large number of membrane proteins that participate in signaling pathways, eg, neurotransmitter receptors, enzymes, and ion channels,[148,205] and there is extensive evidence that ethanol interacts with a variety of neurotransmitters.[50,201,202] The major actions of ethanol involve enhancing the inhibitory effects of gamma-aminobutyric acid (GABA) at $GABA_A$ receptors and blockade of the *N*-methyl-*D*-aspartate (NMDA) subtype of glutamate, an excitatory amino acid (EAA) receptor.[37,109,110,205] Animal studies indicate that the acute effects of ethanol result from competitive inhibition of glycine's binding to the NMDA receptor and disruption of glutamatergic neurotransmission by inhibiting the response of the NMDA receptor. Persistent glycine antagonism and attenuation of glutamatergic neurotransmission by chronic ethanol exposure results in tolerance to ethanol by enhancing EAA neurotransmission and NMDA receptor upregulation.[89,147,197,201,202] The latter appears to involve selective increases in NMDA R2B subunit expression and other molecular changes in specific brain loci.[4] The abrupt withdrawal of ethanol thus produces a hyperexcitable state that leads to the ethanol withdrawal syndrome and excitotoxic neuronal death.[17,37,202] GABA mediated inhibition, which normally acts to limit excitation is eliminated in the absence of ethanol during ethanol withdrawal syndrome, and further intensifies this excitation (see glutamate and NMDA receptors sections of Chaps. 13 and 78). In addition, NMDA receptors function to inhibit the release of dopamine in the nucleus accumbens and mesolimbic structures, which modulates the reinforcing action of addictive agents like ethanol.[20,21,187] By inhibiting NMDA receptor activity, ethanol could increase dopamine release from the nucleus accumbens and ventral tegmental area and could thus create dependence.[20] Chronic ethanol administration also results in tolerance, dependence, and an ethanol withdrawal syndrome, mediated, in part, by desensitization and/or downregulation of $GABA_A$ receptors.[191]

Chronic alcoholism has multiorgan system effects (Table 77–4), and the relationships between ethanol use, nutrition, and liver disease have been reviewed elsewhere.[122] In addition to the harmful effects of ethanol itself (eg, impairment of protein synthesis), its metabolite, acetaldehyde, is inherently toxic to biologic systems.[117,124,204,224] Acetaldehyde directly impairs cardiac contractile function, disrupts cardiac excitation-contractile coupling, inhibits myocardial protein synthesis, interferes with phosphorylation, causes structural and functional alterations in mitochondria and hepatocytes, and inactivates acetyl-coenzyme A. Acetaldehyde can also react with intracellular proteins to generate adducts. Acetaldehyde adducts are believed to play an important role in the early phase of alcoholic liver disease, and in advanced liver disease they contribute to the development of hepatic fibrosis.

Ethanol metabolism through the hepatic CYP2E1 pathway generates highly reactive oxygen radicals, including the hydroxyethyl radical (HER) molecule.[38] Elevated oxygen radical concentrations generate a state of oxidative stress, which leads to cell damage. Oxygen radicals can also initiate lipid peroxidation resulting in reactive molecules such as malondialdehyde (MDA) and 4-hydroxy-2-nonenal (HNE). These reactive molecules react with proteins or acetaldehyde to form adducts, which contribute to the development of alcoholic liver injury.

Oxidation of ethanol generates an excess of reducing potential in the cytosol in the form of NADH with the ratio of NADH to NAD^+ being dramatically increased. This ratio, also known as the redox potential, determines the ability of the cell to carry on various oxidative processes. The unfavorable change in redox potential due to ethanol metabolism contributes to the development of metabolic disorders (eg, impaired gluconeogenesis, alterations in fatty acid metabolism, fatty liver, hyperlipidemia, hypoglycemia, metabolic acidosis with evevated lactate concentration, hyperuricemia (gouty attacks), increased collagen and scar tissue formation associated with alcoholism, and a clinical syndrome of alcoholic ketoacidosis.

Recent studies in alcoholic liver disease have focused on Kupffer cell activation by endotoxin that is released by intestinal bacteria. When Kupffer cells are activated they produce regulatory nuclear factor kappa β (NFκβ) and generate significant amounts of superoxide radicals (O_2^-) and cytokines (tumor necrosis factor and interleukin-8), which has been shown to be an essential factor in the injury to hepatocytes associated with alcoholic liver disease.[134,212]

TABLE 77–4. Systemic Effects Associated With Alcoholism

- **Cardiovascular**
  - Cardiomyopathy
  - "Holiday heart" (dysrhythmias)
  - "Wet" beriberi (thiamine deficiency)
- **Endocrine and metabolic**
  - Hypoglycemia
  - Hypophosphatemia
  - Hypokalemia
  - Hypomagnesemia
  - Hypothermia
  - Hypertriglyceridemia
  - Hyperuricemia
  - Metabolic acidosis
  - Malnutrition
- **Gastrointestinal**
  - Mouth
    - Cancer of the mouth, pharynx, larynx
    - Cheilosis
    - Nutritional stomatitis
  - Esophagus
    - Boerhaave syndrome
    - Cancer of the esophagus
    - Diffuse esophageal spasm
    - Esophagitis
    - Mallory-Weiss tear
  - Stomach and duodenum
    - Gastritis
    - Chronic hypertrophic gastritis
    - Diarrhea
    - Hematemesis
    - Malabsorption
    - Peptic ulcer
  - Liver
    - Steatosis
    - Hepatitis
    - Cirrhosis
  - Pancreas
    - Pancreatitis (acute or chronic)
- **Genitourinary**
  - Hypogonadism
  - Impotence
  - Infertility
- **Hematologic**
  - Coagulopathy
  - Folate, B_{12}, iron deficiency anemias
  - Hemolysis (Zieve syndrome, stomatocytosis, spur cell anemia)
  - Leukopenia
  - Thrombocytopenia
- **Neurologic**
  - Alcohol amnestic syndrome
  - Alcoholic hallucinosis
  - Alcohol withdrawl
  - Central pontine myelinolysis
  - Cerebral atrophy (dementia)
  - Cerebellar degeneration
  - CVA (SAH, infarction)
  - Intoxication
  - Korsakoff psychosis
  - Wernicke encephalopathy
  - Marchiafava-Bignami disease
  - Myopathy
  - Polyneuropathy
  - Pellagra
- **Ophthalmic**
  - Tobacco–ethanol amblyopia
- **Psychiatric**
  - Animated behavior
  - Loss of self-restraint
  - Depression
  - Mania
  - Suicide
- **Respiratory**
  - Atelectasis
  - Pneumonia
  - Respiratory depression
  - Respiratory acidosis

ACUTE CLINICAL FEATURES

Ethanol is a selective central nervous system (CNS) depressant at low doses and a general depressant at high doses. Initially it depresses those areas of the brain involved with highly integrated functions. Cortical release leads to animated behavior and the loss of restraint. This paradoxical CNS stimulation is due to disinhibition. In cases of mild intoxication the signs of ethanol inebriation are quite variable. The patient may be energized and loquacious, expansive, emotionally labile, increasingly gregarious or may appear to have lost self-control, exhibit antisocial behavior, and be ill tempered. As the degree of intoxication increases, there is successive inhibition and impairment of neuronal activity.[142] The patient may become irritable, abusive, aggressive, violent, dysarthric, confused, disoriented, or lethargic. With severe intoxication, there is loss of airway protective reflexes, coma, and increasing risk of death from respiratory depression. An ethanol naïve adult with a blood ethanol concentration of greater than 250 mg/dL (54 mmol/L) is usually stuporous.[1]

The acute effects of ethanol ingestion also depend on the habituation of the drinker. This is mainly due to the development of tolerance, which has both a metabolic (pharmacokinetic) and a functional (pharmacodynamic) component.[191] Metabolic tolerance to ethanol is based on enhanced elimination by the ADH enzyme and CYP2E1 system. Functional tolerance (resistance to the effects of ethanol at the cellular level) is a more important determinant of habituation and may be mediated through alterations in $GABA_A$ and NMDA receptors as well as serotonergic and adrenergic neurons.[89,105,106,147,190,197,201,202] Acute ethanol tolerance may be demonstrated by the Mellanby effect, which involves the comparison of physiologic responses or behavioral effects at the same blood ethanol concentration on the ascending and descending limbs of the blood ethanol curve. Impairment is greater at a given blood ethanol concentration when it is increasing than for the same blood ethanol concentration when it is falling.[152,207] Although individuals who are acutely intoxicated move through a progressive sequence of events, the association of a particular aspect of intoxication with a specific blood ethanol concentration is not usually possible without knowing the pattern of ethanol use of the patient. Acute ethanol intoxication occurs in habitual drinkers when they raise their ethanol concentration an equivalent amount above baseline, and specific clinical manifestations of inebriation typically occur with significantly higher blood ethanol concentration than nontolerant individuals. Regardless, the absolute change above baseline may be important.

A patient may present with obvious signs and symptoms consistent with ethanol intoxication that include flushed facies, diaphoresis, tachycardia, hypotension, hypothermia, hypoventilation, mydriasis, nystagmus, vomiting, dysarthria, muscular incoordination, ataxia, altered consciousness, and coma. However, an ethanol-intoxicated patient may present to the ED with a broad range of diagnostic possibilities and should prompt a careful evaluation for a variety of covert clinical and metabolic disorders. A meticulous and systematic approach to the evaluation and management of an inebriated patient will help avoid the potential pitfalls in such a situation.[61] The presence or absence of an odor of ethanol on the breath is an unreliable means of ascertaining whether a person is intoxicated or whether ethanol was recently consumed.[146] Diplopia, visual disturbances, and nystagmus may be evident, which may be due to the toxic effects of ethanol or may represent Wernicke encephalopathy. Hypothermia may be exacerbated by environmental exposure, from malnutrition and loss of carbohydrate or energy substrate, and ethanol-induced vasodilation. Ethanol intoxication can impair cardiac output in patients with preexisting cardiac disease,[70] and dysrhythmias such as atrial fibrillation and nonsustained ventricular tachycardia as well as atrioventricular block are documented in binge drinkers.[45,71,72] The association between ethanol use and cardiac dysrhythmias, particularly supraventricular tachydysrhythmias in apparently healthy people, is called *holiday heart syndrome*.[107,113,137] The syndrome was first described in people with heavy ethanol consumption, who typically presented on weekends or after holidays, and it may also occur in patients who binge but who usually drink little ethanol. The most common dysrhythmia is atrial fibrillation, which usually reverts to normal sinus rhythm within 24 hours. Although the syndrome may recur, the clinical course is benign in patients without anatomic cardiac pathology and specific antidysrhythmic therapy is usually not warranted.[59,72] Acute heavy ethanol drinking may precipitate silent myocardial ischemia in patients with stable angina pectoris.[174] Variant angina is reported to occur in patients following ethanol ingestion at a time when the blood ethanol concentration has decreased almost to zero.[53,99,132,140,157,176,194] Ethanol induced seizures are reported in adults, but are more frequent in children with ethanol-induced hypoglycemia.[31,88] Patients presenting with acute ethanol intoxication commonly have decreased serum ionized magnesium concentrations while their total serum magnesium concentration is within the normal range.[221] However, total body magnesium may be depleted due to poor dietary intake, decreased GI absorption secondary to ethanol, and renal wasting due to the ethanol-related diuresis.[54,98,171,182,189]

DIAGNOSTIC TESTS

There are numerous qualitative and quantitative assays for ethanol in biological fluids and exhaled breath. Immunoassay or gas chromatography is commonly used for determination of ethanol in liquid specimens in most hospitals. Hospital laboratory analysis of blood samples for ethanol content is usually based on serum (liquid portion of whole blood after the cellular components and clotting factors have been removed), or rarely plasma (acellular liquid portion of whole blood). In contrast, forensic casework expresses ethanol concentration in whole blood. Serum contains slightly more water than does plasma and whole blood and will have a slightly higher ethanol concentration. In a study of ED patients the serum-to-whole blood ethanol concentration ratios range from 0.88 to 1.59 with the median ratio being 1.15.[168] As a result, a whole blood ethanol concentration of 100 mg/dL (22 mmol/L) might be equivalent to a serum ethanol concentration that ranges between 88 and 159 mg/dL (19–35 mmol/L). In patients receiving intravenous ethanol the mean ratio of plasma to whole blood ethanol concentration is 1.10, range 1.03:1 to 1.24:1.[96]

A fraction of ethanol is excreted by the lungs. Breath ethanol concentration measurement as a surrogate for blood ethanol concentration is popular with emergency departments and law-enforcement agencies because of the noninvasive nature and the ability to provide an immediate result. The use of breath to estimate blood ethanol concentration is based on respiratory physiology concepts and assumptions from the 1940s and 1950s, which are derived from initial exhaled air volume from the lungs and comes from the conducting airways and has little "alveolar air." Further exhalation results in air exhalation from the alveoli containing gas in equilibrium with pulmonary capillary blood. Extrapolation of data from low solubility gases (ie, nitrogen), and end tidal ethanol concentration is independent of exhaled volume after exhalation beyond anatomic dead space volume. Aveolar ethanol concentration is in thermodynamic equilibrium with the arterial blood ethanol concentration. Ethanol (gas phase) concentration remains constant throughout the respiratory tract; this relationship could be described by a partition coefficient—ratio between breath and blood ethanol concentration.[82] The mean breath-to-blood ratio is reported as 1:2300 during the postabosorptive phase of ethanol kinetics, and a ratio of 1:2100 is used in forensic casework, which is the programmed ratio used in breath analyzers.[153] There are significant individual and interindividual variations (±20%) in the breath-to-blood ethanol ratio.[91,95] Log-transformation of the normal breath-to-blood values has been used to calculate means and confidence intervals.[73,114] However, ethanol breath tests should be interpreted with caution. Breath ethanol concentration may not reflect the concentration of ethanol in blood. Confounding variables include recent use of ethanol containing products, belching or vomiting of gastric ethanol contents, breath holding or hyperventilation immediately prior to providing a breath sample, inadequate exhalation, prolonged expiration, obstructive pulmonary disease, mouth ethanol retained in the bridges or periodontal spaces, and poor technique.[5,92,93,118,199] Multidose inhalers (eg, Tornalate [bitolterol mesylate with 38% ethanol], Bronkometer [isoetharine mesylate with 30% ethanol], Primatene Mist [adrenaline with 34% ethanol], and salbutamol) and mouth washes (eg, Listerine [26.9% ethanol], Scope [18.9% ethanol], and Lavoris [6.0% ethanol]) may contain significant concentration of ethanol, and may cause elevations of breath ethanol above the legal criteria for intoxication.[13,69,127,141] However, these effects are transient and may be prevented by a 10- to 15-minute interval between the use of multidose inhaler or mouth wash and breath ethanol testing.[69,127,141]

Ethanol saliva testing is a promising alternative to breath ethanol analysis in the rapid assessment of blood ethanol concentrations in patients regardless of their mental status.[35,185] Fatty acid ethyl esters (FAEEs) may be a highly sensitive test for recent ethanol use.[15,43,186] Because FAEEs remain in the system for at least 24 hours they may have a role as a marker of recent ethanol use even after ethanol is completely metabolized. However, their availability is limited and their place in patient management is undefined.

Ethyl glucuronide and ethyl sulfate are nonoxidative direct ethanol metabolites and are excreted for a considerably longer time than ethanol.[18,32,77,175,179] Testing for these metabolites in urine has gained popularity as a sensitive method to detect recent ethanol intake and is favored over tests such as gamma glutamyl transferase (GGT) or carbohydrate-deficient transferrin (CDT) particularly by agencies concerned with monitoring an individual for recent ethanol consumption or relapse, confirming abstinence in treatment programs, workplaces, and schools, and providing legal proof of drinking.[76,166] The presence of ethyl glucuronide and ethyl sulfate provides a strong indication of recent drinking even when ethanol is no longer detectable.[77] However, caution should be applied in the interpretation of ethyl glucuronide testing results. Ethyl glucuronide may be sensitive to degradation or may be synthesized by bacteria (eg, *E coli*)-infected urine resulting in either a false-negative or false-positive test particularly when specimens have been improperly stored; ethyl sulfate degradation or formation has not been detected under similar conditions.[79,81] Detection windows for ethyl glucuronide and ethyl sulfate after drinking may be limited and dependent on the amount of ethanol consumed. For example, these metabolites are detectable in urine for less than or equal to 24 hours after intake of 0.25 g/kg ethanol and less than or equal to 48 hours after intake of 0.50 g/kg ethanol.[32,75,77,85,86,219] Depending on the analytical cut-off limit unintentional exposure to ethanol-based mouthwash and hand sanitizers may result in a urine positive for ethyl glucuronide or ethyl sulfate.[29,173] There appears to be a marked interindividual variation in the concentration-time profiles for both metabolites. In situations where the times for ethanol intake and urine specimen collection between drinking and sampling are uncertain, it would not be possible to link a single ethyl glucuronide and sulfate result to a specific ethanol dose taken at a specific time.[80] A common cut-off or reporting limit has yet to be determined for urinary ethyl glucuronide and ethyl sulfate when used as ethanol biomarkers.

Blood tests that should be considered for patients with ethanol intoxication include a rapid reagent glucose test, CBC, electrolytes, BUN, creatinine, ketones, acetone, lipase, liver enzymes, INR, ammonia, calcium, and magnesium. Patients with an anion gap metabolic acidosis should have urine ketones and a serum lactate concentration determined (see Chaps. 16 and 107). High serum acetone concentrations may be indicative of isopropanol intoxication whereas elevated serum or urinary ketones may be indicative of alcoholic ketoacidosis, starvation ketosis or diabetic ketoacidosis. Because the laboratory nitroprusside reaction detects only ketones (acetoacetate and acetone) and not β-hydroxybutyrate, the assay for urinary ketones in patients with alcoholic ketoacidosis may be only mildly positive.[60-64]

A blood ethanol concentration should be included in the initial laboratory studies.[87] If the blood ethanol concentration is inconsistent with the patient's clinical condition, prompt reevaluation of the patient is indicated to elucidate the etiology of the altered mental status including toxic-metabolic (eg, hypoglycemia, electrolyte or acid-base disorder, toxic alcohols, therapeutic or illicit drug overdose, ethanol withdrawal, hepatic encephalopathy, and Wernicke-Korsakoff syndrome), trauma-related, neurologic (eg, post-ictal condition), and infectious etiologies. Comatose patients with levels below 300 mg/dL (65 mmol/L) and those with values in excess of 300 mg/dL (65 mmol/L) who fail to improve clinically during a limited period of close observation should have a head CT scan, followed by a lumbar puncture if clinically indicated. Because chronically ethanol tolerant patients are prone to trauma and coagulopathies, both of which can cause intracerebral bleeding, the threshold for head CT scanning should be low.

MANAGEMENT OF THE INTOXICATED PATIENT

Ethanol is rapidly absorbed from the gastrointestinal tract. In situations where recent ingestion (within 1 hour of presentation), delayed absorption, and concomitant ingestions are under consideration gastrointestinal decontamination may be considered. Occasionally, the extremely intoxicated or comatose patient may have severe respiratory depression necessitating endotracheal intubation and ventilatory support.

Any patient with an acute altered mental status mandates immediate investigation and treatment of reversible etiologies such as hypoxia, hypoglycemia, and opioid intoxication. In addition, Wernicke encephalopathy should be considered. Supplemental oxygen should be administered if the patient is hypoxic; intravenous dextrose (0.5–1.0 g/kg), thiamine 100 mg, and naloxone should be administered as clinically indicated. Abnormal vital signs should be addressed and stabilized. Patients who are combative and violent should be both physically and then chemically (eg, benzodiazepine) restrained. Caution should be taken because of additive effects of ethanol and benzodiazepines on respiratory depression. Attempts by those who are clinically intoxicated to sign out against medical advice or attempt to leave should also be prevented (see Chap. 140). The patient's fluid and electrolyte status should be assessed and abnormalities corrected. Multivitamins with folate, thiamine, and magnesium may be added to the maintenance IV solution.

A variety of therapies have been advocated either to reverse the intoxicating effects of ethanol or to enhance its elimination. Those proven to be either ineffective or unreliable include coffee, caffeine, naloxone, flumazenil, and rapid intravenous saline loading.[55,121,154,155,172] Hemodialysis is an effective means of enhancing the systemic elimination of ethanol because of the small volume of distribution and low molecular weight of ethanol. In severe ethanol poisoning resulting in respiratory failure or coma, hemodialysis may be an adjunct treatment to supportive care. However, the risk–benefit of hemodialysis should be considered.

INDICATIONS FOR HOSPITALIZATION

A patient with uncomplicated ethanol intoxication can be safely discharged after a careful observation often with social service or psychiatric counseling. An individual should not be discharged while still clinically intoxicated. However, consideration may be given to a situation where the intoxicated patient is discharged to a protected environment under the supervision of a responsible non-intoxicated adult. In this case the clinical assessment of the patient is more important than the blood ethanol concentration. Indications for hospital admission include persistently abnormal vital signs, persistently abnormal mental status with or without an obvious cause, a mixed overdose with other concerning xenobiotics, concomitant serious trauma, consequential ethanol withdrawal, and those with an associated serious disease process such as pancreatitis or gastrointestinal hemorrhage.

Chronic alcoholism may result in an organic brain syndrome that is irreversible. The patient's socioeconomic condition and lack of ability to comply with a treatment plan are critical in making a disposition. Alcoholics requesting ethanol detoxification can be admitted for rehabilitation. Inpatient detoxification programs differ substantially from outpatient programs but their most consequential advantages may be that they enforce abstinence, provide more support and structure, and separate the patient from the social surroundings associated with drinking.[151,206] For patients who are not admitted, a referral should be offered to Alcoholics Anonymous or another suitable ethanol rehabilitation program.

ETHANOL-INDUCED HYPOGLYCEMIA

Hypoglycemia associated with ethanol consumption is believed to occur when ethanol metabolism increases the cellular redox ratio. The higher redox state favors the conversion of pyruvate to lactate, diverting pyruvate from gluconeogenesis (Fig. 77–2). Hypoglycemia typically occurs when there is a reduced caloric intake and only after the hepatic glycogen stores are depleted, as in an overnight fast. The mechanism by which hypoglycemia is associated with ethanol consumption in the well-nourished individual is less well defined.

Although the conditions that cause hypoglycemia in adults may also be present in infants and children, children with their smaller livers have less glycogen stores than adults and are more likely to develop hypoglycemia. Hypoglycemia associated with ethanol consumption usually occurs in malnourished chronic alcoholics and in children (see Chap. 48). It may also occur in binge drinkers who do not eat. A 22% incidence of hypoglycemia was reported in one retrospective study of children with documented ethanol ingestion.[119] In another retrospective study of children and adolescents there was a 3.4% incidence of hypoglycemia (serum glucose concentration less than 67 mg/dL [3.7 mmol/L]).[49] Ethanol-intoxicated children under 5 years of age have an increased risk of developing hypoglycemia and it is the most common reported clinical abnormality related to ethanol ingestion in this age group.[115,116]

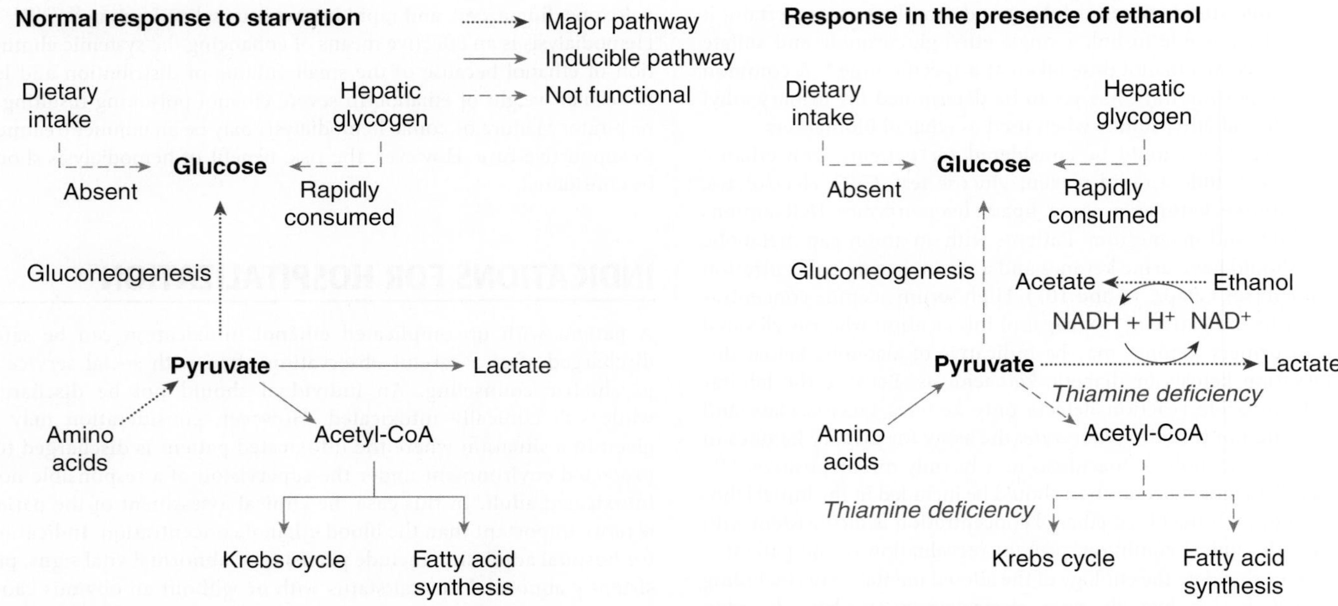

FIGURE 77–2. Central role of pyruvate in ethanol-induced hypoglycemia. Thiamine deficiency interrupts metabolism at the indicated steps.

CLINICAL FEATURES

Patients with ethanol associated hypoglycemia usually present with an altered consciousness 2 to 10 hours following ethanol ingestion. Other physical findings include hypothermia and tachypnea. Laboratory findings, in addition to hypoglycemia, usually include a positive blood ethanol concentration, ketonuria without glucosuria, and mild acidosis.

MANAGEMENT

Acute treatment of ethanol-induced hypoglycemia is similar to other causes of hypoglycemia (see Chap. 48), and should prompt a systematic evaluation for coexisting clinical and metabolic disorders. Hospital admission is indicated as this represents serious metabolic impairment.

ALCOHOLIC KETOACIDOSIS (AKA)

The development of AKA requires a combination of physical and physiologic events to occur. The normal response to starvation and depletion of hepatic glycogen stores is for amino acids to be converted to pyruvate. Pyruvate serves as a substrate for gluconeogenesis by being converted to acetyl-CoA, which enters the Krebs cycle, or undergoes conversion to fatty acids. As described earlier, ethanol metabolism generates NADH resulting in an excess of reducing potential. This high redox state favors the conversion of pyruvate to lactate, diverting pyruvate from being a substrate for gluconeogenesis. To compensate for the lack of normal metabolic substrates, the body mobilizes fat from adipose tissue and increases fatty acid metabolism as an alternative source of energy. This response is mediated by a decrease in insulin and an increased secretion of glucagon, catecholamines, growth hormone, and cortisol. Fatty acid metabolism results in the formation of acetyl-CoA and it combines with the excess acetate that is generated from ethanol metabolism to form acetoacetate (Fig. 77–3).[84] Most of the acetoacetate is reduced to β-hydroxybutyrate due to the excess reducing potential or high redox state of the cell. Volume depletion interferes with the renal elimination of acetoacetate and β-hydroxybutyrate and contributes to the acidosis. Metabolic acidosis with elevated lactate concentration due to hypoperfusion or infection may coexist with the underlying ketoacidosis.

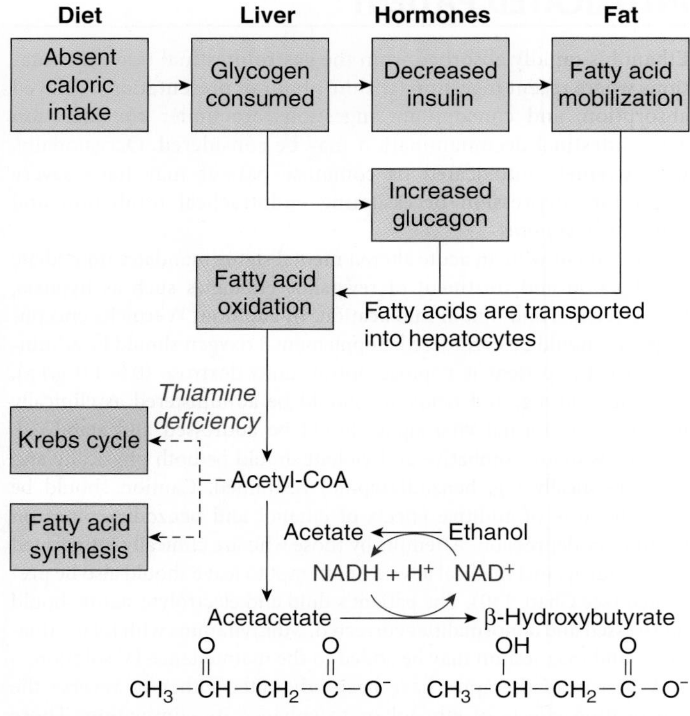

FIGURE 77–3. Mechanism of alcoholic ketoacidosis. Thiamine deficiency interrupts metabolism at the indicated steps.

CLINICAL FEATURES

Patients with AKA are typically chronic ethanol users, presenting after a few days of binge drinking, who become acutely starved because of cessation in oral intake due to binging itself or to nausea, vomiting, abdominal pain from gastritis, hepatitis, pancreatitis or a concurrent acute illness.[61,62,64] The patient may appear acutely ill with salt and water depletion, tachypnea, tachycardia, and hypotension. Underlying medical conditions such as sepsis, meningitis, pyelonephritis, or pneumonia may be present, and ethanol withdrawal may develop, all of which should be considered and systematically excluded. The diagnosis of AKA is a diagnosis of exclusion.

The blood ethanol concentration is usually low or undetectable because ethanol intake ceased substantially earlier in the clinical course. The hallmarks of AKA include an elevated anion gap metabolic acidosis with an elevated serum lactate concentration insufficient to account for the gap. However, some patients will have a normal arterial pH or be even alkalemic because of an associated primary metabolic alkalosis due to vomiting and a compensatory respiratory alkalosis (see Chap. 16).[60] When patients with AKA are compared with patients with diabetic ketoacidosis (DKA), those with AKA tended to have a higher blood pH, lower serum potassium and chloride concentrations, and a higher serum bicarbonate concentration.[60,63] The etiology of anion gaps in patients with AKA and DKA is very similar, with β-hydroxybutyrate being the primary anion contributor and lactate having a less consequential role.[63]

The nitroprusside test used to detect the presence of ketones in serum and urine may be negative or mildly positive in patients with AKA because the nitroprusside reaction detects only molecules containing ketone moieties. This includes acetone and acetoacetate but not β-hydroxybutyrate. Reliance on the nitroprusside test alone may underestimate the severity of ketosis. Specific assays for β-hydroxybutyrate may be performed in some hospital laboratories, and may be available as point of care testing at bedside. The blood glucose concentration may be low or mildly elevated. It is postulated that ethanol-induced hypoglycemia occurs first, causing increased levels of cortisol, growth hormone, glucagon, and epinephrine; this may correct the hypoglycemia and mobilize fatty acids, which are converted to ketones.[36] Therefore, alcoholic hypoglycemia and alcoholic ketoacidosis may be sequential events of the same process depending on the point in this process at which the patient is evaluated.

MANAGEMENT

Treatment should begin with adequate crystalloid fluid replacement, dextrose, and thiamine. Supplemental multivitamins, potassium, and magnesium should be instituted on an individual basis. The administration of dextrose will stimulate the release of insulin, decrease the release of glucagon, and reduce the oxidation of fatty acids. Exogenous glucose also facilitates the synthesis of adenosine triphosphate (ATP), which reverses the pyruvate-to-lactate and NADH/NAD$^+$ ratios. The provision of thiamine facilitates pyruvate entry into the Krebs cycle, thus increasing ATP production. Volume replacement restores glomerular flow and improves excretion of ketones and organic acids. Administration of either insulin or sodium bicarbonate in the management of AKA is usually unnecessary.[64]

During the recovery phase of AKA, β-hydroxybutyrate is converted to acetoacetate. As this process occurs, the nitroprusside test may become more positive because of higher concentrations of acetoacetate resulting in a transient hyperketonemia that actually represents improvement of the metabolic status.

Patients presenting with AKA are manifesting serious metabolic impairment and require hospital admission. They may succumb to other precipitating or coexisting medical or surgical disorders[61] such as occult trauma, pancreatitis, gastrointestinal hemorrhage or hepatorenal dysfunction, and infections. However, mortality is rare from ethanol-induced ketoacidosis.

ALCOHOLISM

Alcoholism is traditionally defined as a chronic, progressive disease characterized by tolerance and physical dependence to ethanol and pathologic organ changes. Alcoholism is a multifactorial, genetically influenced disorder.[30,83,151,162,170,181,196]

Concern for early detection and intervention led to attempts to create reliable diagnostic screening systems. The Brief Michigan Alcoholism Screening Test (MAST)[165] and the CAGE questions[133,211] represent two such tools (Tables 77–5 and 77–6). The presence of physical tolerance and/or dependence is not essential for a diagnosis of alcoholism.

TABLE 77–5. The Brief Michigan Alcoholism Screening Test

Question	Circle Correct Answer		Points
1. Do you feel you are a normal drinker?	Yes	No	N2
2. Do friends or relatives think you are a normal drinker?	Yes	No	N2
3. Have you ever attended a meeting of Alcoholics Anonymous?	Yes	No	Y5
4. Have you ever lost friends or girlfriends/boyfriends because of drinking?	Yes	No	Y2
5. Have you ever gotten into trouble at work because of drinking?	Yes	No	Y2
6. Have you ever neglected your obligations, your family, or your work for 2 or more days in a row because you were drinking?	Yes	No	Y2
7. Have you ever had delirium tremens (DTs) or severe shaking, or heard voices, or seen things that weren't there after heavy drinking?	Yes	No	Y2
8. Have you ever gone to anyone for help about your drinking?	Yes	No	Y5
9. Have you ever been in a hospital because of drinking?	Yes	No	Y5
10. Have you ever been arrested for drunk driving after drinking?	Yes	No	Y2
Score 6 = Probable diagnosis of alcoholism.			

Reprinted, with permission, from Pokorny AO, Miller BA, Kaplan HB. *Am J Psychiatry* 1972;129:342-345. Copyright 1972, American Psychiatric Association.

TABLE 77–6. The CAGE Questions

1. Have you ever felt you should **c**ut down on your drinking?
2. Have people **a**nnoyed you by criticizing your drinking?
3. Have you ever felt bad or **g**uilty about your drinking?
4. Have you ever had a drink first thing in the morning to steady your nerves or to get rid of a hangover (**e**ye-opener)?

Two or more affirmatives = probable diagnosis of alcoholism.

Reprinted, with permission, from West LJ, Maxwell DS, Noble EP, Soloman DH. Alcoholism. *Ann Intern Med* 1984;100:412-420.

Emphasis instead is placed on the social and behavioral concomitants of heavy drinking.[145] In the ED setting, questions concerning the patient's ability to function physically and psychologically are just as appropriate as quantifying the amount of ethanol consumed per day.

Alcoholism is commonly associated with affective disorders, especially depression.[143,167] There is a higher rate of alcoholism among patients with bipolar disorder than in the general population and there may be a genetic relationship between alcoholism and depression.[103,156,217,218] Ethanol affects mood, judgment, and self-control, creates a clinical condition conducive to violence directed at self and others, and is an important risk factor for suicide. Although many people drink in an attempt to ameliorate their depression, all available evidence suggests that alcoholism adversely affects mood and cognitive ability. Research indicates alcoholism may be partly under genetic control.[10,103,108,125] Chromosomal linkage analysis has implicated chromosomes 9, 15, and 16 in the genetic predisposition to alcoholism.[14,39,128] Polymorphism in ADH and ALDH genes appears to be a marker for risk of alcoholism.[27,30,48,196,198] The ADH1B*2, ADH1C*1, and ALDH2*2 alleles have been associated with reduced risk of alcoholism. Genetic epidemiologic studies strongly correlate Asians with homozygous ADH1B*2 and ALDH2*2 alleles with reduced ethanol consumption and incidence of alcoholism.[30,162,215] The incidence of both homozygous ADH1B*1 and ALDH2*1 alleles was significantly higher in patients with ethanol dependence and in patients with alcoholic liver disease.

Various strategies are employed to treat alcoholism including psychosocial interventions, pharmacological interventions, or both. Pharmacologic treatment of ethanol dependence that is of potential collateral toxicologic consequence include the opioid antagonists naltrexone and nalmefene and, disulfiram, serotonergic agents, and topiramate.[65,90]

Although it is a serious disease with important health and economic consequences, alcoholism remains underdiagnosed and remains a treatment challenge.[131,206,220]

SUMMARY

Ethanol is widely used in our society and ethanol use problems impose a staggering personal, social, and economic burden on our society. Most people are responsible drinkers of ethanol. However, some people drink ethanol in ways that are detrimental to themselves or others. Domestic violence, child abuse, fires, falls, rape, and other crimes such as robbery and assault, and medical consequences such as cancer, liver disease, and heart disease have all been associated with ethanol misuse. One interesting area in ethanol research has been the finding that genetics may be an important determinant in vulnerability to ethanol dependence. This finding suggests the biological basis of alcoholism.

Acute ethanol intoxication and chronic alcoholism are among the most common and complex toxicologic and societal problems. These patients may present with a diversity of clinical problems that challenge the clinician to be meticulous and systematic in their evaluation and management of these patients.

REFERENCES

1. Adinoff B, Gone GH, Linnoila M. Acute ethanol poisoning and the ethanol withdrawal syndrome. *Med Toxicol Adverse Drug Exp*. 1988;3:172-196.
2. Agarwal DP. Genetic polymorphisms of alcohol metabolizing enzymes. *Pathol Biol*. 2001;49:703-709.
3. Alcohol Epidemiologic Data Directory June 2008. [http://pubs.niaaa.nih.gov/publications/2008DataDirectory/2008DataDirectory.pdf]
4. Allgaier C. Ethanol sensitivity of NMDA receptors. *Neurochem Int*. 2002;41:377-382.
5. Alobaidi AA, Hill DW, Payne JP. Significance of variations in blood: breath partition coefficient of alcohol. *BMJ*. 1976; 2:1479-1481.
6. Amir I, Anwar N, Baraona E, et al. Ranitidine increases the bioavailability of imbibed alcohol by accelerating gastric emptying. *Life Sci*. 1996;58:511-518.
7. Arora S, Baraona E, Lieber CS. Alcohol levels are increased in social drinkers receiving ranitidine. *Am J Gastroenterol*. 2000;95:208-213.
8. Bailey DN, Bessler JB, Saucrey BA. Cocaine and cocaethylene-creatinine clearance ratios in humans. *J Anal Toxicol*. 1997;21:41-43.
9. Bagnardi V, Zambon A, Quatto P, et al. Flexible meta-regression functions for modeling aggregate dose-response data, with an application to alcohol and mortality. *Am J Epidemiol*. 2004;159:1077-1086.
10. Ball DM, Murray RM. Genetics of alcohol misuse. *Br Med J*. 1994;50:18-35.
11. Baraona E, Abittan CS, Dohmen K, et al. Gender differences in pharmacokinetics of alcohol. *Alcohol Clin Exp Res*. 2001;25:502-507.
12. Baraona E, Yokoyama A, Ishii H, et al. Lack of alcohol dehydrogenase isoenzyme activities in the stomach of Japanese subjects. *Life Sci*. 1991;49:1929-1934.
13. Barry PW, O'Callaghan C. New formulation metered dose inhaler increases breath alcohol levels. *Respir Med*. 1999;93:167-168.
14. Bergen AW, Yang XR, Bai Y, et al. Framingham Heart Study: genomic regions linked to alcohol consumption in the Framingham Heart Study. *BMC Genet*. 2003;4 Suppl 1:S101.
15. Best CA, Laposata M. Fatty acid ethyl esters: toxic non-oxidative metabolites of ethanol and markers of ethanol intake. *Front Biosci*. 2003;8:e202-217.
16. Bhatti SA, Walsh TF, Douglas CW. Ethanol and pH levels of proprietary mouthrinses. *Community Dent Health*. 1994;11:71-74.
17. Bleich S, Degner D, Sperling W, et al. Homocysteine as a neurotoxin in chronic alcoholism. *Prog Neuropsychopharmacol Biol Psychiatry*. 2004;28:453-464.
18. Borucki K, Schreiner R, Dierkes J et al. Detection of recent ethanol intake with new markers: comparison of fatty acid ethyl esters in serum and of ethyl glucuronide and the ratio of 5-hydroxytryptophol to 5-hydroxyindole acetic acid in urine. *Alcohol Clin Exp Res*. 2005;29:781-787.
19. Brennan DF, Betzelos S, Reed R, et al. Ethanol elimination rates in an ED population. *Am J Emerg Med*. 1995;13:276-280.
20. Brodie MS. Increased ethanol excitation of dopaminergic neurons of the ventral tegmental area after chronic ethanol treatment. *Alcohol Clin Exp Res*. 2002;26:1024-1030.
21. Brodie MS, Pesold C, Appel SB. Ethanol directly excites dopaminergic ventral tegmental area reward neurons. *Alcohol Clin Exp Res*. 1999;23:1848-1852.
22. Brown AS, James OF. Omeprazole, ranitidine, and cimetidine have no effect on peak blood ethanol concentrations, first pass metabolism or area under the time-ethanol curve under "real-life" drinking conditions. *Aliment Pharmacol Ther*. 1998;12:141-145.
23. Bye A, Lacey LF, Gupta S, et al. Effect of ranitidine hydrochloride (150 mg twice daily) on the pharmacokinetics of increasing doses of ethanol (0.15, 0.3, 0.6 g kg-1). *Br J Clin Pharmacol*. 1996;41:129-133.
24. Caballeria J, Barbona E, Podamilens M, et al. Effects of cimetidine on gastric alcohol dehydrogenase activity and blood ethanol levels. *Gastroenterology*. 1989;96:388-392.
25. Caetano R, Cunradi C. Alcohol dependence: a public health perspective. *Addiction*. 2002;97:633-45.

26. Chapman LF. Experimental induction of hangover. *Q J Stud Alcohol.* 1970;31:67-86.
27. Chen YC, Lu RB, Peng GS, et al. Alcohol metabolism and cardiovascular response in an alcoholic patient homozygous for the ALDH2*2 variant gene allele. *Alcohol Clin Exp Res.* 1999;23:1853-1860.
28. Committee on Drugs, 1983-1984, American Academy of Pediatrics: Ethanol in liquid preparations intended for children. *Pediatrics.* 1984;73:405-407.
29. Costantino A, Digregorio EJ, Korn W, et al. The effect of the use of mouthwash on ethylglucuronide concentrations in urine. *J Anal Toxicol.* 2006;30:659-662.
30. Crabb DW, Matsumoto M, Chang D, et al. Overview of the role of alcohol dehydrogenase and aldehyde dehydrogenase and their variants in the genesis of alcohol-related pathology. *Proc Nutr Soc.* 2004;63:49-63.
31. Cummins LH. Hypoglycemia and convulsions in children following alcohol ingestion. *J Pediatr.* 1961;58:23-26.
32. Dahl H, Stephanson N, Beck O, Helander A. Comparison of urinary excretion characteristics of ethanol and ethyl glucuronide. *J Anal Toxicol.* 2002;26:201-204.
33. Damrau F, Liddy E. Hangovers and whisky congeners: comparison of whisky with vodka. *J Nat Med Assoc.* 1960;52:262-264.
34. Damrau F, Goldberg AH. Adsorption of whisky congeners by activated charcoal. *Southwest Med.* 1971;53:175-182.
35. Degutis LC, Rabinovici R, Sabbaj A, et al. The saliva strip test is an accurate method to determine blood alcohol concentration in trauma patients. *Acad Emerg Med.* 2004;11:885-887.
36. Devenyi P. Alcoholic hypoglycemia and alcoholic ketoacidosis: sequential events of the same process? *Can Med Assoc J.* 1982;127:513.
37. De Witte P. Imbalance between neuroexcitatory and neuroinhibitory amino acids causing craving for ethanol. *Addict Behav.* 2004;29:1325-1339.
38. Dey A, Cederbaum AI. Alcohol and oxidative liver injury. *Hepatology.* 2006;43:S63-S74.
39. Dick DM, Edenberg HJ, Xuei X, et al. Association of GABRG3 with alcohol dependence. *Alcohol Clin Exp Res.* 2004;28:4-9.
40. Di Padova C, Poine R, Frezza M, et al. Effects of rantidine on blood alcohol levels after ethanol ingestion. *JAMA.* 1992;267:83-86.
41. Djordjevic D, Nikolic J, Stefanovic V. Ethanol interactions with other cytochrome P45 substrates including drugs, xenobiotics, and carcinogens. *Pathol Biol.* 1998;46:760-770.
42. Dohmen K, Baraona E, Ishibashi H, et al. Ethnic differences in gastric-alcohol dehydrogenase activity and ethanol first-pass metabolism. *Alcohol Clin Exp Res.* 1996;20:1569-1576.
43. Doyle KM, Cluette-Brown JE, Dube DM, et al. Fatty acid ethyl esters in the blood as markers of ethanol intake. *JAMA.* 1996;276:1152-1156.
44. Dukes GE, Kuhn JG, Evens RP. Alcohol in pharmaceutical products. *Am Fam Physician.* 1977;16:97-103.
45. Eilam O, Heyman SN. Wenckebach-type atrioventricular block in severe alcohol intoxication. *Am J Emerg Med.* 1991;9:1170.
46. Ellis T, Lacy R. Illicit alcohol (moonshine) consumption in West Alabama revisited. *South Med J.* 1998;91:858-860.
47. Embly DI, Fraser BN. Hepatotoxicity of paracetamol enhanced by ingestion of alcohol. *S Afr Med J.* 1977;51:208-209.
48. Eriksson CJ, Fukunaga T, Sarkola T, et al. Functional relevance of human ADH polymorphism. *Alcohol Clin Exp Res.* 2001;25(5 Suppl ISBRA): 157S-163S.
49. Ernst AA, Jones K, Nick TG, et al. Ethanol ingestion and related hypoglycemia in a pediatric and adolescent emergency department population. *Acad Emerg Med.* 1996;3:46-49.
50. Faingold CL, N'Gouemo P, Riaz A. Ethanol and neurotransmitter interactions—from molecular to integrative effects. *Prog Neurobiol.* 1998;55: 509-535.
51. Feely J, Wood AJ. Effects of cimetidine on the elimination and actions of ethanol. *JAMA.* 1982;247:2819-2821.
52. Feldstein TJ. Carbohydrate and alcohol content of 200 oral liquid medications for use in patients receiving ketogenic diets. *Pediatrics.* 1996;97:506-511.
53. Fernandez D, Rosenthal JE, Cohen LS, et al. Alcohol-induced Prinzmetal variant angina. *Am J Cardiol.* 1973;32:238-239.
54. Flink EB. Magnesium deficiency in alcoholism. *Alcohol Clin Exp Res.* 1986;10:590-594.
55. Fluckiger A, Hartmann D, Leishman B, et al. Lack of effect of the benzodiazepine antagonist flumazenil and the performance of healthy subjects during experimentally induced ethanol intoxication. *Eur J Clin Pharmacol.* 1988;34:273-276.
56. Foti RS, Fisher MB. Assessment of UDP-glucuronosyltransferase catalyzed formation of ethyl glucuronide in human liver microsomes and recombinant UGTs. *Forensic Sci Int.* 2005;153:109-116.
57. Fraser AG. Pharmacokinetic interactions between alcohol and other drugs. *Clin Pharmacokinet.* 1997;33:79-90.
58. Frezza M, DiRadova C, Pozzato G, et al. High blood alcohol levels in women: the role of decreased gastric alcohol dehydrogenase activity and first pass metabolism. *N Engl J Med.* 1990;322:95-110.
59. Fuenmayor AJ, Fuenmayor AM. Cardiac arrest following holiday heart syndrome. *Int J Cardiol.* 1997;59:101-103.
60. Fulop M. Alcoholic ketoacidosis. *Endocrinol Metab Clin North Am.* 1993;22: 209-219.
61. Fulop M. Alcoholism, ketoacidosis, and lactic acidosis. *Diabetes Metab Rev.* 1989;5:365-378.
62. Fulop M, Ben-Ezra J, Bock J. Alcoholic ketosis. *Alcohol Clin Exp Res.* 1986; 10:610-615.
63. Fulop M, Hoberman HD. Diabetic ketoacidosis and alcoholic ketosis. *Ann Intern Med.* 1979;91:796-797.
64. Fulop M, Hoberman HD. Alcoholic ketosis. *Diabetes.* 1975;24:785-790.
65. Garbutt JC, West SL, Carey TS, et al. Pharmacological treatment of alcohol dependence, a review of the evidence. *JAMA.* 1999;281:1318-1325.
66. Gerhardt RE, Crecelius EA, Hudson JB. Moonshine-related arsenic poisoning. *Arch Intern Med.* 1980;140:211-213.
67. Gershman H, Steper J. Rate of clearance of ethanol from the blood of intoxicated patients in the emergency department. *J Emerg Med.* 1991;9: 307-311.
68. Goedde HW, Agarwal DP, Fritze G, et al. Distribution of ADH2 and ALDH2 genotypes in different populations. *Hum Genet.* 1992;88:344-346.
69. Gomez HF, Moore L, McKinney P, et al. Elevation of breath ethanol measurements by metered-dose inhalers. *Ann Emerg Med.* 1995;25:608-611.
70. Gould L. Hemodynamic effects of ethanol in patients with cardiac disease. *Q J Stud Alcohol.* 1972;33:714-722.
71. Greenspon AJ. Provocation of ventricular tachycardia after consumption of alcohol. *N Engl J Med.* 1979;301:1049-1156.
72. Greenspon AJ, Schaal SF. The "holiday heart": electrophysiological studies of alcohol effects in alcoholics. *Ann Intern Med.* 1983;98:135-140.
73. Gullberg RG. Statistical evaluation and reporting of blood alcohol/breath ratio distribution data. *J Anal Toxicol.* 1991;15:343-344.
74. Haber PS, Gentry RT, Mak KM, et al. Metabolism of alcohol by human gastric cells: relation to first-pass metabolism. *Gastroenterology.* 1996;111:863-870.
75. Halter CC, Dresen S, Auwaerter V, et al. Kinetics in serum and urinary excretion of ethyl sulfate and ethyl glucuronide after medium dose ethanol intake. *Int J Legal Med.* 2008;122:123-128.
76. Helander A. Biological markers in alcoholism. *J Neural Transm Suppl.* 2003: 15-32.
77. Helander A, Beck O. Ethyl sulfate: a metabolite of ethanol in humans and a potential biomarker of acute alcohol intake. *J Anal Toxicol.* 2005;29:270-274.
78. Helander A, Beck O. Mass spectrometric identification of ethyl sulfate as an ethanol metabolite in humans. *Clin Chem.* 2004;50:936-937.
79. Helander A, Dahl H. Urinary tract infection: a risk factor for false-negative urinary ethyl glucuronide but not ethyl sulfate in the detection of recent alcohol consumption. *Clin Chem.* 2005;51:172817-30.
80. Helander A, Böttcher M, Fehr C, et al. Detection times for urinary ethyl glucuronide and ethyl sulfate in heavy drinkers during alcohol detoxification. *Alcohol Alcohol.* 2009;44:55-61.
81. Helander A, Olsson I, Dahl H. Postcollection synthesis of ethyl glucuronide by bacteria in urine may cause false indentification of alcohol consumption. *Clin Chem.* 2007;53:1855-1857.
82. Henry W. Experiments on the quantity of gases absorbed by water at different temperature and under different pressures. *Philos Trans R Soc Lond B Biol Sci.* 1803;93:29-42.
83. Higuchi S, Matsushita S, Muramatsu T, et al. Alcohol and aldehyde dehydrogenase genotypes and drinking behavior in Japanese. *Alcohol Clin Exp Res.* 1996;20:493-497.
84. Hoffman RS, Goldfrank LR. Ethanol-associated metabolic disorders. *Emerg Med Clin North Am.* 1989;7:943-961.
85. Høiseth G, Bernard JP, Karinen R, et al. A pharmacokinetic study of ethyl glucuronide in blood and urine: applications to forensic toxicology. *Forensic Sci Int.* 2007;172:119-124.
86. Høiseth G, Bernard JP, Stephanson N, et al. Comparison between the urinary alcohol markers EtG, EtS, and GTOL/5-HIAA in controlled drinking experiment. *Alcohol Alcohol.* 2008;43(2):187-191.

87. Holt S, Stewart IC, Dixon JM. Alcohol and the emergency service patient. *Br Med J.* 1980;281:638-640.
88. Hornfeldt CS. A report of acute ethanol poisoning in a child. *J Toxicol Clin Toxicol.* 1992;30:115-121.
89. Hu X-J, Ticku MK. Chronic ethanol treatment upregulates the NMDA receptor function and binding in mammalian cortical neurons. *Brain Res Mol Brain Res.* 1995;30:347-356.
90. Johnson RA. Progress in the development of topiramate for treating alcohol dependence: from a hypothesis to a proof-of-concept study. *Alcohol Clin Exp Res.* 2004;28:1137-1144.
91. Jones AW. Variability of the blood: breath alcohol ratio in vivo. *J Stud Alcohol.* 1978;39:1931-1939.
92. Jones AW. How breathing technique can influence the results of breath alcohol analysis. *Med Sci Law.* 1982;22:275-280.
93. Jones AW. Role of rebreathing in determination of the blood-breath ratio of expired ethanol. *J Appl Physiol.* 1983;55:1237-1241.
94. Jones AW. Excretion of alcohol in urine and diuresis in healthy men in relation to their age, the dose administered and the time after drinking. *Forensic Sci Int.* 1990;45:217-224.
95. Jones AW, Andersson L. Variability of the blood/breath alcohol ratio in drinking drivers. *J Forensic Sci.* 1996;41:916-921.
96. Jones AW, Hahn RG, Stalberg HP. Distribution of ethanol and water between plasma and whole blood: inter- and intra-individual variations after administration of ethanol by intravenous infusion. *Scand J Clin Lab Invest.* 1990;50:775-780.
97. Jornvall H, Hoog JO: Nomenclature of alcohol dehydrongenases. *Alcohol Alcohol.* 1995;30(2):153-161.
98. Kalbfleisch JM, Lindeman RD, Ginn HE, et al. Effects of ethanol administration on urinary excretion of magnesium and other electrolytes in alcoholic and normal subjects. *J Clin Invest.* 1963;42:1471-1475.
99. Kashima T, Tanaka H, Arikawa K, et al. Variant angina induced by alcohol ingestion. *Angiology.* 1982;33:137-139.
100. Kater RM, Roggin G, Tobon F, et al. Increased rate of clearance of drugs from the circulation of alcoholics. *Am J Med Sci.* 1969;258:35-39.
101. Kaufmann RB, Staes CJ, Matte TD. Deaths related to lead poisoning in the United States, 1979-1998. *Environ Res.* 2003;91:78-84.
102. Kechagias S, Jonsson KA, Norlander B, et al. Low-dose aspirin decreases blood alcohol concentrations by delaying gastric emptying. *Eur J Clin Pharmacol.* 1997;53:241-246.
103. Kendler KS, Heath AC, Neale MC, et al. Alcoholism and major depression in women. A twin study of the causes of comorbidity. *Arch Gen Psychiatry.* 1993;50:690-698.
104. Khan F, Alagappan K, Cardell K. Overlooked sources of ethanol. *J Emerg Med.* 1999;17:985-988.
105. Khanna JM, Kalant H, Le AD, et al. Role of serotonergic and adrenergic systems in alcohol tolerance. *Prog Neuropsychopharmacol.* 1981;5:459-465.
106. Khanna JM, Morato GS, Kalant H. Effect of NMDA antagonists, an NMDA agonist, and serotonin depletion on acute tolerance to ethanol. *Pharmacol Biochem Behav.* 2002;72:291-298.
107. Klatsky AL. Alcohol and cardiovascular diseases: a historical overview. *Novartis Found Symp.* 1998;216:2-12.
108. Koopmans JR, Boomsma DI. Familial resemblance in alcohol use: genetic or cultural transmission? *J Stud Alcohol.* 1996;57:19-28.
109. Krystal JH, Petrakis IL, Krupitsky E, et al. NMDA receptor antagonism and the ethanol intoxication signal: from alcoholism risk to pharmacotherapy. *Ann N Y Acad Sci.* 2003;1003:176-184.
110. Krystal JH, Petrakis IL, Mason G, et al. N-methyl-*D*-aspartate glutamate receptors and alcoholism: reward, dependence, treatment, and vulnerability. *Pharmacol Ther.* 2003;99:79-94.
111. Kuffner EK, Dart RC, Bogdan GM, et al. Effect of maximal daily doses of acetaminophen on the liver of alcoholic patients: a randomized, double-blind, placebo-controlled trial. *Arch Intern Med.* 2001;161:2247-2252.
112. Kunitoh S, Imaoka S, Hiroi T, et al. Acetaldehyde as well as ethanol is metabolized by human CYP2E1. *J Pharmacol Exp Ther.* 1997;280:527-532.
113. Kupari M, Koskinen P. Time of onset of supraventricular tachyarrhythmia in relation to alcohol consumption. *Am J Cardiol.* 1991;67:718-722.
114. Labianca DA, Simpson G. Statistical analysis of blood- to breath-alcohol ratio data in the logarithm-transformed and non-transformed modes. *Eur J Clin Chem Clin Biochem.* 1996;34:111-117.
115. Lamminpaa A. Alcohol intoxication in childhood and adolescence. *Alcohol Alcohol.* 1995;30:5-12.
116. Lamminpaa A, Vilska J. Acute alcohol intoxications in children treated in hospital. *Acta Paediatr Scand.* 1990;79:847-854.
117. Lang CH, Kimball SR, Frost RA, et al. Alcohol myopathy: impairment of protein synthesis and translation initiation. *Int J Biochem Cell Biol.* 2001;33:457-473.
118. Lester D. Breath tests for alcohol. *N Engl J Med.* 1971;284:1269-1270.
119. Leung AK. Ethyl alcohol ingestion in children. A 15-year review. *Clin Pediatr (Phila).* 1986;25:617-619.
120. Levy P, Hexdall A, Gordon P, et al. Methanol contamination of Romanian home-distilled alcohol. *J Toxicol Clin Toxicol.* 2003;41:23-28.
121. Li J, Mills T, Erato R. Intravenous saline has no effect on blood ethanol clearance. *J Emerg Med.* 1999;17:1-5.
122. Lieber CS. Relationships between nutrition, alcohol use, and liver disease. *Alcohol Res Health.* 2003;27:220-231.
123. Lieber CS. Ethnic and gender differences in ethanol metabolism. *Alcohol Clin Exp Res.* 2000;24:417-418.
124. Lieber CS. Biochemical and molecular basis of alcohol-induced injury to the liver and other tissues. *N Engl J Med.* 1988;319:1639-1644.
125. Liu IC, Blacker DL, Xu R, et al. Genetic and environmental contributions to the development of alcohol dependence in male twins. *Arch Gen Psychiatry.* 2004;61:897-903.
126. Liu JJ, Daya MR, Mann NC. Methanol-related deaths in Ontario. *J Toxicol Clin Toxicol.* 1999;37:69-73.
127. Logan BK, Distefano S, Case GA. Evaluation of the effect of asthma inhalers and nasal decongestant sprays on a breath alcohol test. *J Forensic Sci.* 1998;43:197-199.
128. Ma JZ, Zhang D, Dupont RT, et al. Mapping susceptibility loci for alcohol consumption using number of grams of alcohol consumed per day as a phenotype measure. *BMC Genet.* 2003;4 Suppl 1:S104.
129. Maddrey WC. Hepatic effects of acetaminophen—enhanced toxicity in alcoholics. *J Clin Gastroenterol.* 1987;9:180-185.
130. Makin A, Williams R. Paracetamol hepatotoxicity and alcohol consumption in deliberate and accidental overdose. *QJM.* 2000;93:341-349.
131. Mann K, Hermann D, Heinz A. One hundred years of alcoholism: the twentieth century. *Alcohol Alcohol.* 2000;35:10-15.
132. Matsuguchi T, Araki H, Anan T, et al. Provocation of variant angina by alcohol ingestion. *Eur Heart J.* 1984;5:906-912.
133. Mayfield D, McLeod G, Hall P. The CAGE questionnaire: validation of a new alcoholism screening instrument. *Am J Psychiatry.* 1974;131:1121-1126.
134. McClain CJ, Hill DB, Song Z, et al. Monocyte activation in alcoholic liver disease. *Alcohol.* 2002;27:53-61.
135. McClain CJ, Kromhout JP, Peterson FJ, et al. Potentiation of acetaminophen hepatotoxicity. *JAMA.* 1980;244:251-253.
136. McDermott PH, Delaney RL, Egon JD, et al. Myocarditis and cardiac failure in men. *JAMA.* 1966;198:253-256.
137. Menz V, Grimm W, Hoffmann J, et al. Alcohol and rhythm disturbance: the holiday heart syndrome. *Herz.* 1996;21:227-231.
138. Mercier G, Patry G. Quebec beer-drinkers' cardiomyopathy: clinical signs and symptoms. *Can Med Assoc J.* 1967;97:884-888.
139. Miller NS, Goodwin DW, Jones FC, et al. Antihistamine blockade of alcohol-induced flushing in orientals. *J Stud Alcohol.* 1988;49:16-20.
140. Miwa K, Igawa A, Miyagi Y. Importance of magnesium deficiency in alcohol-induced variant angina. *Am J Cardiol.* 1994;73:813-816.
141. Modell JG, Taylor JP, Lee JY. Breath alcohol values following mouthwash use. *JAMA.* 1993;270:2955-2956.
142. Modell JG. Behavioral, neurologic, and physiologic effects of acute ethanol ingestion. In Fassler D, ed. *The Alcoholic Patient: Emergency Medical Intervention.* New York: Gardner Press; 1990:25-34.
143. Modesto-Lowe V, Kranzler HR. Diagnosis and treatment of alcohol-dependent patients with comorbid psychiatric disorders. *Alcohol Res Health.* 1999;23:144-149.
144. Morgan BW, Parramore CS, Ethridge M. Lead contaminated moonshine: a report of Bureau of Alcohol, Tobacco and Firearms analyzed samples. *Vet Hum Toxicol.* 2004;46:89-90.
145. Morse RM, Flarin DK. The definition of alcoholism. *JAMA.* 1992;268:1012-1014.
146. Moskowitz H, Burns M, Ferguson S. Police officers' detection of breath odors from alcohol ingestion. *Accid Anal Prev.* 1999;31:175-180.
147. Nagy J. The NR2B subtype of NMDA receptor: a potential target for the treatment of alcohol dependence. *Curr Drug Targets CNS Neurol Disord.* 2004;3:169-179.

148. Narahashi T, Kuriyama K, Illes P, et al. Neuroreceptors and ion channels as targets of alcohol. *Alcohol Clin Exp Res*. 2001;25(5 Suppl ISBRA):182S-188S.
149. National Highway Traffic Safety Administration Traffic Safety Facts Research Note: 2007 traffic safety annual assessment – alcohol-impaired driving fatalities. August 2008 DOT HS 811 016. [http://www.nrd.nhtsa.dot.gov/Pubs/811016.PDF]
150. National Institute on Alcohol Abuse and Alcoholism. National Highway Traffic Safety Administration's *Digest of State Alcohol-Highway Safety Related legislation*. [http://www.alcoholpolicy.niaaa.nih.gov/index.asp?Type=B_BASIC&SEC={18705C0B-1B37-40E2-9FB6-E3AD00048B3C}]
151. National Institute on Alcohol Abuse and Alcoholism. Publications – Congressional Report to Congress. Tenth Special Report to the U.S. Congress on Alcohol and Health. [http://www.niaaa.nih.gov].
152. Nicholson ME, Wang M, Airhihenbuwa CO, et al. Variability in behavioral impairment involved in the rising and falling BAC curve. *J Stud Alcohol*. 1992;53:349-356.
153. Norberg A, Jones AW, Hahn RG, et al. Role of variability in explaining ethanol pharmacokinetics: research and forensic applications. *Clin Pharmacokinet*. 2003;42:1-31.
154. Nuotto E. Coffee and caffeine and alcohol effects on psychomotor function. *Clin Pharmacol Ther*. 1982;31:68-72.
155. Nuotto E, Palva ES. Naloxone fails to counteract heavy alcohol intoxication. *Lancet*. 1983;2:167-170.
156. Nurnberger JI Jr, Foroud T, Flury L, et al. Is there a genetic relationship between alcoholism and depression? *Alcohol Res Health*. 2002;26:233-240.
157. Oda H, Suzuki M, Oniki T, et al. Alcohol and coronary spasm. *Angiology*. 1994;45:187-197.
158. Oneta CM, Simanowski UA, Martinez M, et al. First pass metabolism of ethanol is strikingly influenced by the speed of gastric emptying. *Gut*. 1998;43:612-619.
159. Parker RB, Williams CL, Laizure SC, et al. Effects of ethanol and cocaethylene on cocaine pharmacokinetics in conscious dogs. *Drug Metab Dispos*. 1996;24:850-853.
160. Parker WA. Alcohol-containing pharmaceuticals. *Am J Drug Alcohol Abuse*. 1982-83;9:195-209.
161. Pegues DA, Hughes BJ, Woernle CH. Elevated blood lead levels associated with illegally distilled alcohol. *Arch Intern Med*. 1993;153:1501-1504.
162. Peng GS, Wang MF, Chen CY, et al. Involvement of acetaldehyde for full protection against alcoholism by homozygosity of the variant allele of mitochondrial aldehyde dehydrogenase gene in Asians. *Pharmacogenetics*. 1999;9:463-476.
163. Peoples RW, Li C, Weight FF. Lipid vs. protein theories of alcohol action in the nervous system. *Annu Rev Pharmacol Toxicol*. 1996;36:185-201.
164. Petroni NC, Cardoni AA. Alcohol content of liquid medicinals. *Clin Toxicol*. 1979;14:407-432.
165. Pokorny AD, Miller BA, Kaplan HB. The brief MAST. *Am J Psychiatry*. 1972;129:342-350.
166. Politi L, Leone F, Morini L, et al. Bioanalytical procedures for determination of conjugates or fatty acid esters of ethanol as markers of ethanol consumption: a review. *Anal Biochem*. 2007;368:1-16.
167. Raimo EB, Schuckit MA. Alcohol dependence and mood disorders. *Addict Behav*. 1998;23:933-946.
168. Rainey PM. Relation between serum and whole-blood ethanol concentrations. *Clin Chem*. 1993;39:2288-2292.
169. Randall T. Cocaine alcohol mix in body to form even longer lasting, more lethal drug. *JAMA*. 1992;267:1043-1044.
170. Reich T, Edenberg HJ, Goate A, et al. Genome-wide search for genes affecting the risk for alcohol dependence. *Am J Med Genet*. 1998;81:207-215.
171. Rivlin RS. Magnesium deficiency and alcohol intake: mechanisms, clinical significance and possible relation to cancer development. *J Am Coll Nutr*. 1994;13:416-423.
172. Roberts JR, Greenberg MI. Fluid loading: neither safe nor efficacious in the treatment of the alcohol-intoxicated patient in the ED. *Am J Emerg Med*. 2000;18(1):121.
173. Rohrig TP, Huber C, Goodson L, et al. Detection of ethylglucuronide in urine following the application of Germ-X. *J Anal Toxicol*. 2006;30:703-704.
174. Rossinen J, Partanen J, Koskinen P, et al. Acute heavy alcohol intake increases silent myocardial ischaemia in patients with stable angina pectoris. *Heart*. 1996;75:563-567.
175. Sarkola T, Dahl H, Eriksson CJ, et al. Urinary ethyl glucuronide and 5-hydroxytryptophol levels during repeated ethanol ingestion in healthy human subjects. *Alcohol Alcohol*. 2003;38:347-351.
176. Sato A, Taneichi Y, Sekine I, et al. Prinzmetal's variant angina induced only by alcohol ingestion. *Clin Cardiol*. 1981;4:193-195.
177. Scherger DL, Wruk KM, Kulig KW, et al. Ethyl alcohol (ethanol)-containing cologne, perfume, and after-shave ingestions in children. *Am J Dis Child*. 1988;142:630-632.
178. Schiodt FV, Rochling FA, Casey DL, et al. Acetaminophen toxicity in an urban county hospital. *N Engl J Med*. 1997;337:1112-1117.
179. Schmitt G, Aderjan R, Keller T, et al. Ethyl glucuronide: an unusual ethanol metabolite in humans. Synthesis, analytical data, and determination in serum and urine. *J Anal Toxicol*. 1995;19:91-94.
180. Schneider H, Glatt H. Sulpho-conjugation of ethanol in humans in vivo and by individual sulphotransferase forms in vitro. *Biochem J*. 2004;383:543-549.
181. Schuckit MA. Biological, psychological, and environmental predictors of alcoholism risk: a longitudinal study. *J Stud Alcohol*. 1998;59:485-494.
182. Shane SR, Flink EB. Magnesium deficiency in alcohol addiction and withdrawal. *Magnes Trace Elem*. 1991-1992;10(2-4):263-268.
183. Sherlock JC, Pickford CJ, White GF. Lead in alcoholic beverages. *Food Addit Contam*. 1986;3:347-354.
184. Smart GA, Pickford CJ, Sherlock JC. Lead in alcoholic beverages: a second survey. *Food Addit Contam*. 1990;7:93-99.
185. Smolle KH, Hofmann G, Kaufmann P, et al. Q.E.D. Alcohol test: a simple and quick method to detect ethanol in saliva of patients in emergency departments. Comparison with the conventional determination in blood. *Intensive Care Med*. 1999;25:492-495.
186. Soderberg BL, Salem RO, Best CA, et al. Fatty acid ethyl esters. Ethanol metabolites that reflect ethanol intake. *Am J Clin Pathol*. 2003;119 Suppl:S94-99.
187. Stobbs SH, Ohran AJ, Lassen MB, et al. Ethanol suppression of ventral tegmental area GABA neuron electrical transmission involves N-methyl-*D*-aspartate receptors. *J Pharmacol Exp Ther*. 2004;311:282-289.
188. Stowell A, Johnsen J, Ripel A, et al. Diphenhydramine and the calcium carbimide-ethanol reaction: a placebo-controlled clinical study. *Clin Pharmacol Ther*. 1986;39:521-525.
189. Sullivan JF, Wolpert PW, Williams R. Serum magnesium in chronic alcoholism. *Ann NY Acad Sci*. 1969;162:947-955.
190. Suwaki H, Kalant H, Higuchi S, et al. Recent research on alcohol tolerance and dependence. *Alcohol Clin Exp Res*. 2001;25(5 Suppl ISBRA):189S-196S.
191. Tabakoff B, Cornell N, Hoffman PL. Alcohol tolerance. *Ann Emerg Med*. 1986;15:1005-1012.
192. Takeshita T, Mao XQ, Morimoto K. The contribution of polymorphism in the alcohol dehydrogenase beta subunit to alcohol sensitivity in a Japanese population. *Hum Genet*. 1996;97:409-413.
193. Takeshita T, Morimoto K, Mao X, et al. Characterization of the three genotypes of low Km aldehyde dehydrogenase in a Japanese population. *Hum Genet*. 1994;94:217-223.
194. Takizawa A, Yasue H, Omote S, et al. Variant angina induced by alcohol ingestion. *Am Heart J*. 1984;107:25-27.
195. Tan OT, Stafford TJ, Sarkany I, et al. Suppression of alcohol-induced flushing by a combination of H1 and H2 histamine antagonists. *Br J Dermatol*. 1982;107:647-652.
196. Tanaka F, Shiratori Y, Yokosuka O, et al. High incidence of ADH2*1/ALDH2*1 genes among Japanese alcohol dependents and patients with alcoholic liver disease. *Hepatology*. 1996;23:234-239.
197. Thomas RJ. Excitatory amino acids in health and disease. *J Am Geriatr Soc*. 1995;43:1279-1289.
198. Thomasson HR, Crabb DW, Edenberg HJ, et al. Alcohol and aldehyde dehydrogenase polymorphisms and alcoholism. *Behav Genet*. 1993;23:131-136.
199. Trafford DJ, Makin HL. Breath-alcohol concentration may not always reflect the concentration of alcohol in blood. *J Anal Toxicol*. 1994;18:225-228.
200. Truitt EB Jr, Gaynor CR, Mehl DL. Aspirin attenuation of alcohol-induced flushing and intoxication in Oriental and Occidental subjects. *Alcohol Alcohol*. 1987;Suppl 1:595-599.
201. Tsai GE, Ragan P, Chang R, et al. Increased glutamatergic neurotransmission and oxidative stress after alcohol withdrawal. *Am J Psychiatry*. 1998;155:726-732.
202. Tsai GE, Coyle JT. The role of glutamatergic neurotransmission in the pathophysiology of alcoholism. *Annu Rev Med*. 1998;49:173-184.
203. Tsutaya S, Shoji M, Sito Y, et al. Analysis of aldehyde dehydrogenase 2 gene polymorphism and ethanol patch test as a screening method for alcohol sensitivity. *Tohoku J Exp Med*. 1999;187:305-310.

204. Tuma DJ, Casey CA. Dangerous byproducts of alcohol breakdown-focus on adducts. *Alcohol Res Health.* 2003;27:285-290.
205. Ueno S, Harris RA, Messing RO, et al. Alcohol actions on GABA(A) receptors: from protein structure to mouse behavior. *Alcohol Clin Exp Res.* 2001;25(5 Suppl ISBRA):76S-81S.
206. Walsh EC, Himpson RW, Merrigan DM. A randomized trial of treatment options for alcohol abusing workers. *N Engl J Med.* 1991;325:775-782.
207. Wang MQ, Nicholson ME, Mahoney BS, et al. Proprioceptive responses under rising and falling BACs: a test of the Mellanby effect. *Percept Mot Skills.* 1993;77:83-88.
208. Weathermon R, Crabb DW. Alcohol and medication interactions. *Alcohol Res Health.* 1999;23:40-45.
209. Welch C, Harrison D, Short A, et al. The increasing burden of alcoholic liver disease on United Kingdom critical care units: secondary analysis of a high quality clinical database. *J Health Serv Res Policy.* 2008;13 Suppl 2:40-44.
210. Weller-Fahy ER, Berger LR, Troutman WG. Mouthwash: a source of acute ethanol intoxication. *Pediatrics.* 1980;66:302-305.
211. West LJ, Maxwell DS, Noble EP, et al. Alcoholism. *Ann Intern Med.* 1984;100:405-406.
212. Wheeler MD. Endotoxin and Kupffer cell activation in alcoholic liver disease. *Alcohol Res Health.* 2003;27:300-306.
213. Whitcomb DC, Block GD. Association of acetaminophen hepatotoxicity with fasting and ethanol use. *JAMA.* 1994;272:1845-1850.
214. White IR, Altmann DR, Nanchahal K. Alcohol consumption and mortality: modelling risks for men and women at different ages. *BMJ.* 2002;325:191-197.
215. Whitfield JB. Meta-analysis of the effects of alcohol dehydrogenase genotype on alcohol dependence and alcoholic liver disease. *Alcohol Alcohol.* 1997;32(5):613-619.
216. Wilson LD, Hemming RJ, Suttheimer C, et al. Cocaethylene causes dose-dependent reductions in cardiac function in anesthetized dogs. *J Cardiovasc Pharmacol.* 1995;26:965-973.
217. Winokur G, Turvey C, Akiskal H, et al. Alcoholism and drug abuse in three groups—bipolar I, unipolars and their acquaintances. *J Affect Disord.* 1998;50:81-89.
218. Winokur G, Coryell W, Endicott J, et al. Familial alcoholism in manic-depressive (bipolar) disease. *Am J Med Genet.* 1996;67:197-201.
219. Wojcik MH, Hawthorne JS. Sensitivity of commercial ethyl glucuronide testing in screening for alcohol abstinence. *Alcohol Alcohol.* 2007;42(4): 317-320.
220. Wright C. Physician interventions in alcoholism—past and present. *Md Med J.* 1995;44:447-452.
221. Wu C, Kenny MA. Circulating total and ionized magnesium after ethanol ingestion. *Clin Chem.* 1996;42:625-629.
222. Zador PL, Krawchuk SA, Voas RB. Alcohol-related relative risk of driver fatalities and driver involvement in fatal crashes in relation to driver age and gender: an update using 1996 data. *J Stud Alcohol.* 2000;61:387-395.
223. Zador PL. Alcohol-related relative risk and fatal driver injuries in relation to driver age and sex. *J Stud Alcohol.* 1991;52:302-310.
224. Zhang X, Li SY, Brown RA, et al. Ethanol and acetaldehyde in alcoholic cardiomyopathy: from bad to ugly en route to oxidative stress. *Alcohol.* 2004;32:175-186.
225. Zimmerman HJ, Maddrey WC. Acetaminophen (paracetamol) hepatotoxicity with regular intake of alcohol: analysis of instances of therapeutic misadventure. *Hepatology.* 1995;22:767-773.
226. Zimmerman HJ. Effects of alcohol on other hepatotoxins. *Alcoholism.* 1986;10:3-15.

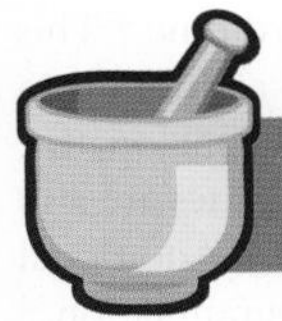

ANTIDOTES IN DEPTH (A25)

THIAMINE HYDROCHLORIDE

Robert S. Hoffman

$$\left[\ \text{Thiamine}\ \right]\ Cl^-$$

Thiamine (vitamin B_1) is a water-soluble vitamin found in organ meats, yeast, eggs, and green leafy vegetables that is essential in the creation and utilization of cellular energy. While there is no toxicity associated with thiamine excess, thiamine deficiency is responsible for "wet" beriberi (congestive heart failure) and "dry" beriberi (Wernicke encephalopathy and the Wernicke-Korsakoff syndrome). Patients at risk include those with poor oral intake (human immunodeficiency virus [HIV], chemotherapy, fad diets, hyperemesis gravidarum) and those with impaired absorption (alcoholism). Typical signs of Wernicke encephalopathy include ataxia, altered mental status, and ophthalmoplegia. Although administration of 100 mg of parenteral thiamine hydrochloride will protect against thiamine deficiency for more than 1 week, patients with clinical deficiencies may require larger doses.

BIOCHEMISTRY

As a coenzyme in the pyruvate dehydrogenase complex, thiamine diphosphate, the active form of thiamine, accelerates the conversion of pyruvate to acetylcoenzyme A (acetyl-CoA). This reaction occurs at the C2 atom of thiamine, which is located between the nitrogen and sulfur atoms on the thiazolium ring.[25] In the protein-rich environment of the enzyme complex, this C2 atom is deprotonated to form a carbanion that rapidly attaches to the carbonyl group of pyruvate, thereby stabilizing it for decarboxylation.[32] In a series of subsequent reactions, the hydroxyethyl group that remains bound to thiamine diphosphate is transferred to lipoamide, where an acetyl group is later broken off and attached to coenzyme A (CoA). This overall process links anaerobic glycolysis to the Krebs cycle, where subsequent aerobic metabolism produces the equivalent of 36 mol of adenosine triphosphate (ATP) from each mole of glucose (Fig. A25–1). When pyruvate cannot be converted to acetyl-CoA because of thiamine deficiency, for example, only 2 mol of ATP can be generated by anaerobic metabolism from each mole of glucose. Thiamine is also required as a cofactor for α-ketoglutarate dehydrogenase, a second enzyme in the Krebs cycle, and for transketolase, an enzyme in the pentose phosphate pathway, in which nicotinamide adenine dinucleotide phosphate (NADPH) is formed for subsequent use in reductive biosynthesis. In addition, thiamine is important in maintaining normal neuronal conduction.[67,84]

Naturally occurring thiamine is a base composed of a substituted pyrimidine ring and a substituted thiazole ring connected by a methylene bridge. This connection between the two rings is weak, and the molecule is unstable in an alkaline milieu and in a high temperature environment. In addition, thiamine is highly water soluble, allowing it to leach out of foods following prolonged washing or cooking in water. However, thiamine, which is synthesized as a hydrochloride salt, is usually quite stable. Thiamine requirements are determined by total caloric intake and energy demand, with a minimum daily requirement of 0.5 mg/1000 calories.[67]

PHARMACOLOGY

Thiamine is well absorbed from the human gastrointestinal tract by a complex process.[38,58] At low concentrations, thiamine absorption occurs through a saturable mechanism that is most effective in the duodenum, with absorption occurring to a lesser degree in the large bowel and stomach.[38] As thiamine concentrations increase, however, the majority of absorption occurs through simple passive diffusion. Although synthesized analogs such as thiamine propyl disulfide, benfotiamine, and fursultiamine have enhanced bioavailability, their use remains largely experimental.[25,76] Chronic liver disease, folate deficiency, steatorrhea, and other forms of malabsorption all significantly decrease the absorption of thiamine. Recently, bariatric surgery was recognized to predispose patients to thiamine deficiency.[2,23,63] Malabsorption has even greater clinical relevance in alcoholics.[5,75] In experimental studies, when healthy volunteers were given small amounts of ethanol, a 50% reduction in gastrointestinal thiamine absorption resulted.[75]

Thiamine is eliminated from the body largely by renal clearance, which consists of a combination of glomerular filtration, flow-dependent tubular secretion, and saturable tubular reabsorption.[82] In an animal model, furosemide, acetazolamide, chlorothiazide, amiloride, mannitol, and salt loading all significantly increased urinary elimination of thiamine.[43] This nonspecific flow-dependent elimination was confirmed in humans given small doses of furosemide.[57] Additionally, both furosemide and digoxin appear to inhibit thiamine uptake into myocardial cells.[87]

THIAMINE DEFICIENCY

PATHOPHYSIOLOGY

Mice develop signs of encephalopathy 10 days after being rendered thiamine deficient. Immunohistochemistry in these animals demonstrates destruction of the blood–brain barrier with resultant extravasation of albumin.[28] Similarly, rats develop symptoms after 10 days of thiamine deficiency, and subsequently demonstrate deterioration of the blood–brain barrier with hemorrhage into the mammillary bodies and other areas of the brain.[12] This pattern is similar to findings described in humans with Wernicke encephalopathy.[54]

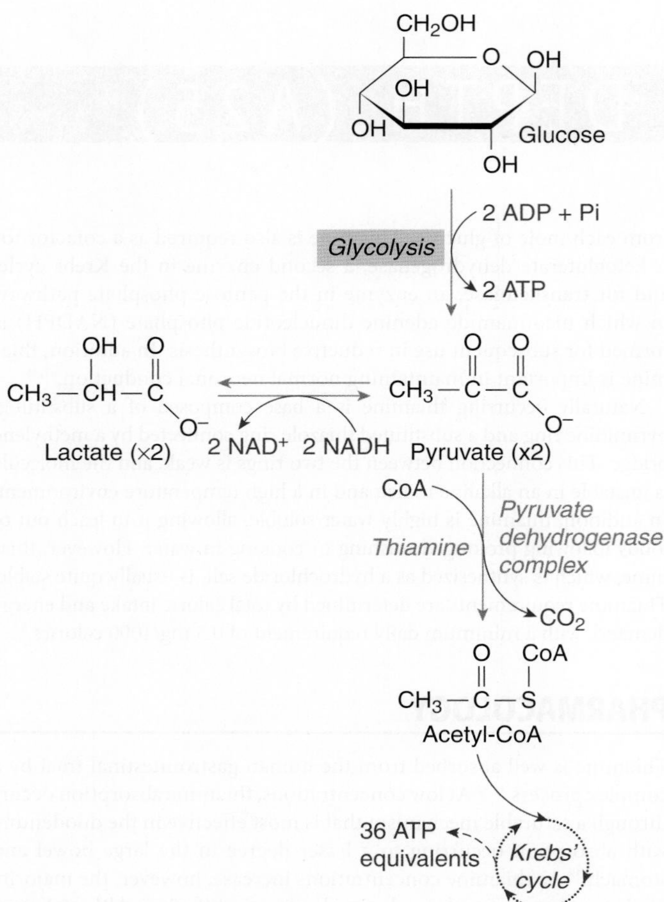

FIGURE A25–1. Thiamine links anaerobic glycolysis to the Krebs cycle. Anaerobic glycolysis only yields 2 mol of ATP as each mole of glucose is metabolized to 2 mol of pyruvate. To obtain the 36 additional ATP equivalents that can be derived as the Krebs cycle converts pyruvate to CO_2 and H_2O, pyruvate must first be combined with CoA to form acetyl-CoA and CO_2. This process is dependent on the thiamine-requiring enzyme system known as pyruvate dehydrogenase complex.

The exact cause of Wernicke encephalopathy is unclear. In human autopsy studies, brain samples from alcoholic patients with Wernicke-Korsakoff syndrome demonstrate decreased function of pyruvate dehydrogenase, α-ketoglutarate dehydrogenase, and transketolase when compared with controls.[11] However, a similar decrease in enzyme activity of neuronal tissue was demonstrated in alcoholics who died from hepatic coma without ever manifesting signs of Wernicke encephalopathy.[42] Likewise, the activity of thiamine-requiring Krebs cycle enzymes is reduced in thiamine-replete patients with neurodegenerative diseases.[8] Thus, while thiamine deficiency produces deficits in critical enzymes in humans, it is unclear whether these deficits are either necessary or sufficient to produce clinical disease.

Animal models offer insight into the mechanisms involved in developing thiamine-deficient neurologic injury. While the exact chain of events leading to these structural abnormalities is unclear, several models demonstrate key portions of the pathway. Thiamine deficiency in rats produces 200% to 640% increases in concentrations of glutamate,[41] which presumably results from blockade of α-ketoglutarate dehydrogenase. Excess α-ketoglutarate is shunted away from the Krebs cycle to form glutamate. Rats subsequently develop increases in lactate in vulnerable regions of the brain marked by the induction of the protooncogene c-fos. Both the histochemical lesions and the gene induction can be blocked by the administration of the calcium channel blocker nicardipine.[46] This suggests a strong role for excitatory amino acid–induced alterations in calcium transport in the genesis of thiamine-deficient encephalopathy. In other animal models of thiamine deficiency, neuronal tissues are also directly injured by oxidative stress and lipid peroxidation.[13] Additional investigations demonstrate roles for triggered mast cell degranulation,[22] histamine,[40] and nitric oxide[35] in the generation of neuronal injury. The final common pathway is localized cerebral edema, which may result from altered expression of aquaporin.[17]

CLINICAL MANIFESTATIONS

When thiamine is completely removed from the human diet, clinical manifestations of thiamine deficiency typically develop within 2 to 3 weeks, although tachycardia, the first sign of deficiency, may occur as early as 9 days after cessation of thiamine intake.[84] The clinical symptoms of thiamine deficiency present as two distinct patterns: "wet" beriberi or cardiovascular disease, and "dry" beriberi, the neurologic disease known as Wernicke-Korsakoff syndrome. Although some patients display symptoms consistent with both disorders, usually either the cardiovascular or the neurologic manifestations predominate. A genetic variant of transketolase activity, combined with low physical activity and low-carbohydrate diet, may predispose to neurologic symptoms, whereas high-carbohydrate diets and increased physical activity lead to cardiovascular symptoms.[7,84] Thus, cardiovascular disease is more common in the Asian population, and neurologic disease predominates in the northern European population.

Wet beriberi results from high-output cardiac failure induced by peripheral vasodilation and the formation of arteriovenous fistulae secondary to thiamine deficiency. These patients complain of fatigue, decreased exercise tolerance, shortness of breath, and peripheral edema. The classic triad of oculomotor abnormalities, ataxia, and global confusion defines dry beriberi or Wernicke encephalopathy. Other manifestations include hypothermia and the absence of deep-tendon reflexes.[81] Additionally, patients develop a peripheral neuropathy with paresthesias, hypesthesias, and an associated myopathy, all related to axonal degeneration.[67] Laboratory studies may reflect a metabolic acidosis with elevated lactate concentration brought on by excessive anaerobic glycolysis resulting from blocked entry of substrate into the Krebs cycle.[16,18,33,34,39,51,59,81] Interestingly, a primary respiratory alkalosis of unclear etiology seems to be simultaneously present.[20] Korsakoff psychosis, an irreversible disorder of learning and processing of new information characterized by a deficit in short-term memory and confabulation, often occurs together with Wernicke encephalopathy.[79] A 10% to 20% mortality rate is associated with Wernicke encephalopathy, with survivors having an 80% risk of developing Korsakoff psychosis.[56]

POPULATIONS AT RISK

In the United States, a healthy diet and mandatory thiamine supplementation of numerous food products protect most people from the manifestations of thiamine deficiency. This is, unfortunately, not true in other countries. A survey of the 17 major public hospitals in the Sydney, Australia, area identified more than 1000 cases of either acute Wernicke encephalopathy or Korsakoff psychosis between 1978 and 1993.[44] Similarly, a single Australian hospital identified 32 cases of Wernicke encephalopathy during a 33-month period.[85] In Australia, mandatory supplementation of flour with thiamine in 1991 resulted in a dramatic reduction in hospitalized cases during 1992 and 1993,[44] as well as of those subsequently identified by postmortem studies.[29] Current areas at risk include Ireland and New Zealand where lack of a mandatory supplementation program is correlated with a high prevalence of biochemical evidence of thiamine deficiency.[49]

Alcoholic patients, whose consumption of ethanol is their major source of calories, are the best described and most easily recognized patients at risk for thiamine deficiency.[56] Consequential thiamine deficiency is also described in incarcerated prisoners,[31] patients in drug rehabilitation,[24] patients receiving hemodialysis,[19] patients with hyperemesis gravidarum or anorexia nervosa,[74] patients receiving parenteral nutrition,[13,14,39,51,71,80] patients with acquired immunodeficiency syndrome (AIDS),[3,8,9,62] patients with malignancies,[6,36,60,71,78] the institutionalized elderly,[38,50,52] and patients with congestive heart failure on furosemide therapy.[37] Thus, despite routine dietary supplementation, many people are still at risk because of dietary limitations, alcohol abuse, or underlying medical conditions.

THIAMINE DOSING

Thiamine hydrochloride is included in the initial therapy for any patient with an altered mental status, potentially acting as both treatment and prevention of Wernicke encephalopathy. Many patients with altered levels of consciousness have had or will have a poor nutritional status, or will be hospitalized without oral intake for a number of days because of gastrointestinal disorders or altered mental status. Although thiamine concentrations can be either directly measured or functionally assessed by measuring erythrocyte transketolase activity at baseline and in response to thiamine diphosphate,[30] these determinations are unavailable for clinical use. Likewise, although clinical prediction models have been developed, they are cumbersome and unvalidated.[65] Glucose loading increases thiamine requirements, which can exacerbate marginal thiamine deficiencies, elevate lactate concentrations,[48] or even precipitate coma in the absence of parenteral thiamine supplementation.[56] Although it is commonly believed that acute glucose loading, in the form of a bolus of hypertonic dextrose, can precipitate Wernicke encephalopathy over several hours in normal individuals, there is only evidence to support this effect in patients who already have grave manifestations of thiamine deficiency.[81] Previously healthy patients require prolonged dextrose administration in order to develop Wernicke encephalopathy. Because the morbidity and mortality associated with Wernicke encephalopathy are so severe, and treatment is both benign and inexpensive, thiamine hydrochloride should be included in the initial therapy for all patients who receive dextrose, all patients with altered consciousness, and every potential alcoholic or nutritionally deprived individual who presents to the emergency department or other clinical setting.

Initial therapy consists of the immediate parenteral administration of 100 mg of thiamine hydrochloride. This can be given either intramuscularly or intravenously, but the oral route should be avoided because of its unpredictable absorption. In countries where thiamine propyl disulfide (a lipid-soluble thiamine preparation) is available, the oral route may be considered equally efficacious for the replacement of serious thiamine deficiencies.[5,75,76] In some patients, symptoms such as ophthalmoplegia are reported to respond rapidly to as little as 2 mg of thiamine; however, the other neurologic and cardiovascular manifestations of thiamine deprivation may necessitate higher doses and may respond more slowly, if at all. Although many sources recommend that daily doses of 100 mg of thiamine are sufficient as preventive therapy, others recommend initial doses as high as 200 or 250 mg,[1,77] based on limited data. Because of the safety of thiamine hydrochloride, and the urgency to correct the manifestations of thiamine deficiency, up to 1000 mg of thiamine hydrochloride can be used in the first 12 hours if a patient demonstrates persistent neurologic abnormalities.[47]

The practice of requiring the administration of parenteral thiamine prior to hypertonic dextrose in patients with altered consciousness is illogical.[26] Besides the fact that the first dose of dextrose is unlikely to cause thiamine deficiency, thiamine uptake into cells and activation of enzyme systems is slower than that of glucose uptake, which suggests that even pretreatment with thiamine offers little benefit over posttreatment.[73] Despite these limitations it is prudent to administer 100 mg of parenteral thiamine at the time of initial dextrose administration. The biochemical link between dextrose and thiamine is obvious, which demonstrates to the clinician the scientific basis for the administration of thiamine. Although thiamine is unlikely to offer immediate benefits for patients with altered consciousness, it will offer some long-term protection for these individuals at risk and initiate therapy for an uncommon, serious, insidious, and easily overlooked disorder.

A supplementary indication for the administration of thiamine hydrochloride occurs in patients with ethylene glycol poisoning. As shown in Fig. 107–2, a minor pathway for the elimination of glyoxylic acid involves its conversion to α-hydroxy-β-ketoadipate by α-ketoglutarate:glyoxylate carboligase, a thiamine and magnesium-requiring enzyme. There are no data to support an increase in α-hydroxy-β-ketoadipate formation following thiamine administration in ethylene glycol–poisoned animals or humans. However, animal models of primary hyperoxaluria show increases in urinary oxalate during thiamine deficiency, suggesting at least a potential importance of this pathway.[27,72] Because therapy is benign and inexpensive, it is prudent to administer standard doses of thiamine to patients with suspected or confirmed ethylene glycol poisoning.

Routine thiamine administration should also be considered in patients with congestive heart failure and long-term use of diuretics. Diuretics enhance renal thiamine elimination.[64] In one randomized trial, 200 mg of daily intravenous thiamine was able to increase cardiac ejection fraction by 22% at 7 weeks.[66] Unfortunately, although ejection fraction was not measured, another small study was unable to show a statistical benefit in a variety of clinical parameters.[68]

ADVERSE EVENTS

Very few complications are associated with the parenteral administration of thiamine. The older literature emphasized intramuscular administration because of numerous reports of anaphylactoid reactions associated with intravenous thiamine delivery.[21,55,61,70,83] It is generally believed that these reactions resulted from responses to the vehicle (chlorbutanol) or its contaminants rather than thiamine itself. Despite the availability of purer, aqueous preparations of thiamine, rare adverse reports still occur.[4,45,53,69] Although the intramuscular route is theoretically comparably efficacious in a healthy individual, many patients requiring thiamine may have diminished muscle mass or a coagulopathy, exacerbating the potential for pain and unpredictable absorption. The safety of thiamine use was evaluated in a large case series in which nearly 1000 patients received parenteral doses of up to 500 mg of thiamine without significant complications.[86] This study suggests that if anaphylaxis to thiamine exists, its occurrence is exceedingly rare, permitting the safe intravenous administration of thiamine to most patients.

PREGNANCY CATEGORY

Thiamine hydrochloride is listed in pregnancy category A and is also considered safe for use in lactating mothers.

AVAILABILITY

Multiple manufacturers formulate thiamine hydrochloride for intravenous or intramuscular administration. Typical concentrations are either 50 or 100 mg/mL. Although more concentrated solutions are available, their use is usually reserved for preparation of total parenteral nutrition solutions.

REFERENCES

1. Ambrose ML, Bowden SC, Whelan G. Thiamin treatment and working memory function of alcohol-dependent people: preliminary findings. *Alcohol Clin Exp Res.* 2001;25:112-116.
2. Angstadt JD, Bodziner RS. Peripheral polyneuropathy from thiamine deficiency following laparoscopic Roux-en-Y gastric bypass. *Obes Surg.* 2005;15:890-892.
3. Arici C, Tebaldi A, Quinzan GP, et al. Severe lactic acidosis and thiamine administration in an HIV-infected patient on HAART. *Int J Std AIDS.* 2001;12:407-409.
4. Assem ESK. Anaphylactic reaction to thiamine. *Practitioner.* 1973;322:565.
5. Baker H, Frank O. Absorption, utilization and clinical effectiveness of allithiamines compared to water-soluble thiamines. *J Nutri Sci Vitaminol.* 1976;22(Suppl):63-68.
6. Barbato M, Rodriguez PJ. Thiamine deficiency in patients admitted to a palliative care unit. *Palliat Med.* 1994;8:320-324.
7. Blass JP, Gibson GE. Abnormality of a thiamine-requiring enzyme in patients with Wernicke-Korsakoff syndrome. *N Engl J Med.* 1977;297:1367-1370.
8. Bubber P, Ke ZJ, Gibson GE. Tricarboxylic acid cycle enzymes following thiamine deficiency. *Neurochem Int.* 2004;45:1021-1028.
9. Butterworth RF, Gaudreau C, Vincelette J, et al. Thiamine deficiency and Wernicke's encephalopathy in AIDS. *Metab Brain Dis.* 1991;6:207-212.
10. Butterworth RF, Gaudreau C, Vincelette J, et al. Thiamine deficiency in AIDS. *Lancet.* 1991;338:1086.
11. Butterworth RF, Kril JJ, Harper CG. Thiamine-dependent enzyme changes in the brains of alcoholics: relationship to the Wernicke-Korsakoff syndrome. *Alcohol Clin Exp Res.* 1993;17:1084-1088.
12. Calingasan NY, Baker H, Sheu KF, Gibson GE. Blood–brain barrier abnormalities in vulnerable brain regions during thiamine deficiency. *Exp Neurol.* 1995;134:64-72.
13. Calingasan NY, Chun WJ, Park LC, Uchida K, Gibson GE. Oxidative stress is associated with region-specific neuronal death during thiamine deficiency. *J Neuropathol Exp Neurol.* 1999;58:946-958.
14. Centers For Disease Control. Deaths associated with thiamine-deficient total parenteral nutrition. *MMWR Morb Mortal Wkly Rep.* 1989;38:43-46.
15. Centers For Disease Control. Lactic acidosis traced to thiamine deficiency related to nationwide shortage of multivitamins for total parenteral nutrition—United States, 1997. *MMWR Morb Mortal Wkly Rep.* 1997;46:523-528.
16. Chadda K, Raynard B, Antoun S, et al. Acute lactic acidosis with Wernicke's encephalopathy due to acute thiamine deficiency. *Intensive Care Med.* 2002;28:1499.
17. Chan H, Butterworth RF, Hazell AS. Primary cultures of rat astrocytes respond to thiamine deficiency-induced swelling by downregulating aquaporin-4 levels. *Neurosci Lett.* 2004;366:231-234.
18. Cho YP, Kim K, Han MS, et al. Severe lactic acidosis and thiamine deficiency during total parenteral nutrition—case report. *Hepatogastroenterology.* 2004;51:253-255.
19. Descombes E, Dessibourg CA, Fellay G. Acute encephalopathy due to thiamine deficiency (Wernicke's encephalopathy) in a chronic hemodialyzed patient: a case report. *Clin Nephrol.* 1991;35:171-175.
20. Donnino MW, Miller J, Garcia AJ, McKee E, Walsh M. Distinctive acid-base pattern in Wernicke's encephalopathy. *Ann Emerg Med.* 2007;50:722-725.
21. Eisenstadt WS. Hypersensitivity to thiamine hydrochloride. *Minn Med.* 1942;85:861-863.
22. Ferguson M, Dalve-Endres AM, McRee RC, Langlais PJ. Increased mast cell degranulation within thalamus in early pre-lesion stages of an experimental model of Wernicke's encephalopathy. *J Neuropathol Exp Neurol.* 1999;58:773-783.
23. Foster D, Falah M, Kadom N, Mandler R. Wernicke encephalopathy after bariatric surgery: losing more than just weight. *Neurology.* 2005;65:1987.
24. Fozi K, Azmi H, Kamariah H, Azwa MS. Prevalence of thiamine deficiency at a drug rehabilitation centre in Malaysia. *Med J Malaysia.* 2006;61:519-525.
25. Greb A, Bitsch R. Comparative bioavailability of various thiamine derivatives after oral administration. *Int J Clin Pharmacol Ther.* 1998;36:216-221.
26. Hack JB, Hoffman RS. Thiamine before glucose to prevent Wernicke's encephalopathy: examining the conventional wisdom. *JAMA.* 1998;279:583-584.
27. Hannett B, Thomas DW, Chalmers AH, et al. Formation of oxalate in pyridoxine or thiamin deficient rats during intravenous xylitol infusions. *J Nutr.* 1977;107:458-465.
28. Harata N, Iwasaki Y. Evidence for early blood-brain barrier breakdown in experimental thiamine deficiency in the mouse. *Metab Brain Dis.* 1995;10:159-174.
29. Harper CG, Sheedy DL, Lara AI, et al. Prevalence of Wernicke-Korsakoff syndrome in Australia: has thiamine fortification made a difference? *Med J Aust.* 1998;168:542-545.
30. Herve C, Beyne P, Letteron P, Delacoux E. Comparison of erythrocyte transketolase activity with thiamine and thiamine phosphate ester levels in chronic alcoholic patients. *Clin Chim Acta.* 1995;234:91-100.
31. Jeyakumar D. Thiamine responsive ankle oedema in detention centre inmates. *Med J Malaysia.* 1995;50:17-20.
32. Kern D, Kern G, Neef H, et al. How thiamine diphosphate is activated in enzymes. *Science.* 1997;275:67-70.
33. Kitamura K, Takahashi T, Tanaka H, et al. Two cases of thiamine deficiency-induced lactic acidosis during total parenteral nutrition. *Tohoku J Exp Med.* 1993;171:129-133.
34. Klein M, Weksler N, Gurman GM. Fatal metabolic acidosis caused by thiamine deficiency. *J Emerg Med.* 2004;26:301-303.
35. Kruse M, Navarro D, Desjardins P, Butterworth RF. Increased brain endothelial nitric oxide synthase expression in thiamine deficiency: relationship to selective vulnerability. *Neurochem Int.* 2004;45:49-56.
36. Kuba H, Inamura T, Ikezaki K, et al. Thiamine-deficient lactic acidosis with brain tumor treatment: report of three cases. *J Neurosurg.* 1998; 89:1025-1028.
37. Kwok T, Falconer-Smith JF, Potter JF, Ives DR. Thiamine status of elderly patients with cardiac failure. *Age Ageing.* 1992;21:67-71.
38. Laforenza U, Patrini C, Alvisi C, et al. Thiamine uptake in human intestinal biopsy specimens, including observations from a patient with acute thiamine deficiency. *Am J Clin Nutr.* 1997;66:320-326.
39. Lange R, Erhard J, Eigler FW, Roll C. Lactic acidosis from thiamine deficiency during parenteral nutrition in a two-year-old boy. *Eur J Pediatr Surg.* 1992;2:241-244.
40. Langlais PJ, McRee RC, Nalwalk JA, Hough LB. Depletion of brain histamine produces regionally selective protection against thiamine deficiency-induced lesions in the rat. *Metab Brain Dis.* 2002;17:199-210.
41. Langlais PJ, Zhang SX. Extracellular glutamate is increased in thalamus during thiamine deficiency-induced lesions and is blocked by MK-801. *J Neurochem.* 1993;61:2175-2182.
42. Lavoie J, Butterworth RF. Reduced activities of thiamine-dependent enzymes in brains of alcoholics in the absence of Wernicke's encephalopathy. *Alcohol Clin Exp Res.* 1995;19:1073-1077.
43. Lubetsky A, Winaver J, Seligmann H, et al. Urinary thiamine excretion in the rat: effects of furosemide, other diuretics, and volume load. *J Lab Clin Med.* 1999;134:232-237.
44. Ma JJ, Truswell AS. Wernicke-Korsakoff syndrome in Sydney hospitals: before and after thiamine enrichment of flour. *Med J Aust.* 1995;163:531-534.
45. Morinville V, Jeannet-Peter N, Hauser C. Anaphylaxis to parenteral thiamine (vitamin B_1). *Schweiz Med Wochenschr.* 1998;128:1743-1744.
46. Munujos P, Vendrell M, Ferrer I. Proto-oncogene c-fos induction in thiamine-deficient encephalopathy. Protective effects of nicardipine on pyrithiamine-induced lesions. *J Neurol Sci.* 1993;118:175-180.
47. Nakada T, Knight RT. Alcohol and the central nervous system. *Med Clin North Am.* 1984;68:121-131.
48. Navarro D, Zwingmann C, Chatauret N, Butterworth RF. Glucose loading precipitates focal lactic acidosis in the vulnerable medial thalamus of thiamine-deficient rats. *Metab Brain Dis.* 2008;23:115-122.
49. O'Keeffe ST, Tormey WP, Glasgow R, Lavan JN. Thiamine deficiency in hospitalized elderly patients. *Gerontology.* 1994;40:18-24.
50. O'Keeffe ST. Thiamine deficiency in elderly people. *Age Ageing.* 2000;29:99-101.
51. Oriot D, Wood C, Gottesman R, Huault G. Severe lactic acidosis related to acute thiamine deficiency. *JPEN J Parenter Enteral Nutr.* 1991;15:105-109.
52. O'Rourke NP, Bunker VW, Thomas AJ, et al. Thiamine status of healthy and institutionalized elderly subjects: analysis of dietary in-take and biochemical indices. *Age Ageing.* 1990;19:325-329.
53. Proebstle TM, Gall H, Jugert FK, et al. Specific IgE and IgG serum antibodies to thiamine associated with anaphylactic reaction. *J Allergy Clin Immunol.* 1995;95:1059-1060.
54. Rao VL, Butterworth RF. Thiamine phosphatases in human brain: regional alterations in patients with alcoholic cirrhosis. *Alcohol Clin Exp Res.* 1995;19:523-526.
55. Reingold IM, Webb FR. Sudden death following intravenous injection of thiamine hydrochloride. *JAMA.* 1946;130:491-492.
56. Reuler JB, Girard DE, Cooney TG. Current concepts. Wernicke's encephalopathy. *N Engl J Med.* 1985;312:1035-1039.

57. Rieck J, Halkin H, Almog S, et al. Urinary loss of thiamine is increased by low doses of furosemide in healthy volunteers. *J Lab Clin Med.* 1999;134:238-243.
58. Rindi G, Laforenza U. Thiamine intestinal transport and related issues: recent aspects. *Proc Soc Exp Biol Med.* 2000;224:246-255.
59. Romanski SA, McMahon MM. Metabolic acidosis and thiamine deficiency. *Mayo Clin Proc.* 1999;74:259-263.
60. Rovelli A, Bonomi M, Murano A, et al. Severe lactic acidosis due to thiamine deficiency after bone marrow transplantation in a child with acute monocytic leukemia. *Haematologica.* 1990;75:579-581.
61. Schiff L. Collapse following parenteral administration of solution of thiamine hydrochloride. *JAMA.* 1941;117:609.
62. Schramm C, Wanitschke R, Galle PR. Thiamine for the treatment of nucleoside analogue-induced severe lactic acidosis. *Eur J Anaesthesiol.* 1999;16:733-735.
63. Sekiyama S, Takagi S, Kondo Y. Peripheral neuropathy due to thiamine deficiency after inappropriate diet and total gastrectomy. *Tokai J Exp Clin Med.* 2005;30:137-140.
64. Seligmann H, Halkin H, Rauchfleisch S, et al. Thiamine deficiency in patients with congestive heart failure receiving long-term furosemide therapy: a pilot study. *Am J Med.* 1991;91:151-155.
65. Sgouros X, Baines M, Bloor RN, et al. Evaluation of a clinical screening instrument to identify states of thiamine deficiency in inpatients with severe alcohol dependence syndrome. *Alcohol Alcohol.* 2004;39:227-232.
66. Shimon I, Almog S, Vered Z, et al. Improved left ventricular function after thiamine supplementation in patients with congestive heart failure receiving long-term furosemide therapy. *Am J Med.* 1995;98:485-490.
67. Skelton WP 3rd, Skelton NK. Thiamine deficiency neuropathy. It's still common today. *Postgrad Med.* 1989;85:301-306.
68. Smithline HA. Thiamine for the treatment of acute decompensated heart failure. *Am J Emerg Med.* 2007;25:124-126.
69. Stephen JM, Grant R, Yeh CS. Anaphylaxis from administration of intravenous thiamine. *Am J Emerg Med.* 1992;10:61-63.
70. Stiles MH. Hypersensitivity to thiamine chloride with a note on sensitivity to pyridoxine hydrochloride. *J Allergy.* 1941;12:507-509.
71. Svahn J, Schiaffino MC, Caruso U, et al. Severe lactic acidosis due to thiamine deficiency in a patient with B-cell leukemia/lymphoma on total parenteral nutrition during high-dose methotrexate therapy. *J Pediatr Hematol Oncol.* 2003;25:965-968.
72. Takasaki E. The urinary excretion of oxalic acid in vitamin B_1-deficient rats. *Invest Urol.* 1969;7:150-153.
73. Tate JR, Nixon PF. Measurement of Michaelis constant for human erythrocyte transketolase and thiamin diphosphate. *Anal Biochem.* 1987;160:78-87.
74. Tesfaye S, Achari V, Yang YC, et al. Pregnant, vomiting, and going blind. *Lancet.* 1998;352:1594.
75. Thomson AD, Baker H, Leevy CM. Patterns of 35S-thiamine hydrochloride absorption in the malnourished alcoholic patient. *J Lab Clin Med.* 1970;76:34-45.
76. Thomson AD, Frank O, Baker H, Leevy CM. Thiamine propyl disulfide: absorption and utilization. *Ann Intern Med.* 1971;74:529-534.
77. Thomson AD, Marshall EJ. The treatment of patients at risk of developing Wernicke's encephalopathy in the community. *Alcohol Alcohol.* 2006;41:159-167.
78. van Zaanen HC, van der Lelie J. Thiamine deficiency in hematologic malignant tumors. *Cancer.* 1992;69:1710-1713.
79. Victor M, Adams RD. The effect of alcohol on the nervous system. In: Meritt HH, Hare CC, eds. *Metabolic and Toxic Diseases of the Nervous System.* Baltimore: Williams & Wilkins; 1953:526-563.
80. Vortmeyer AO, Hagel C, Laas R. Haemorrhagic thiamine deficient encephalopathy following prolonged parenteral nutrition. *J Neurol Neurosurg Psych.* 1992;55:826-829.
81. Watson AJ, Walker JF, Tomkin GH, et al. Acute Wernicke's encephalopathy precipitated by glucose loading. *Ir J Med Sci.* 1981;150:301-303.
82. Weber W, Nitz M, Looby M. Nonlinear kinetics of the thiamine cation in humans: saturation of nonrenal clearance and tubular reabsorption. *J Pharmacokinet Biopharm.* 1990;18:501-523.
83. Weigand CG. Reactions attributed to administration of thiamine chloride. *Geriatrics.* 1950;5:274-279.
84. Wilson JD, Madison LL. Deficiency of thiamine (beriberi), pyridoxine, and riboflavin. In: Isselbacher KJ, Adams RD, Braunwald E, et al., eds. *Harrison's Principles of Internal Medicine*, 9th ed. New York: McGraw-Hill; 1980:425-429.
85. Wood B, Currie J. Presentation of acute Wernicke's encephalopathy and treatment with thiamine. *Metab Brain Dis.* 1995;10:57-72.
86. Wrenn KD, Murphy F, Slovis CM. A toxicity study of parenteral thiamine hydrochloride. *Ann Emerg Med.* 1989;18:867-870.
87. Zangen A, Botzer D, Zangen R, Shainberg A. Furosemide and digoxin inhibit thiamine uptake in cardiac cells. *Eur J Pharmacol.* 1998;361:151-155.

CHAPTER 78
ETHANOL WITHDRAWAL

Jeffrey A. Gold • Lewis S. Nelson

Alcohol withdrawal represents a major cause of morbidity in the alcoholic population and a substantial resource burden on certain medical centers and communities. Complicating management is that there is no diagnostic test for this clinical syndrome, and the diagnosis is established on the basis of the patient history and clinical findings. The impact on patient outcome and resource utilization can be enhanced through early recognition of risk factors and insight into the expected clinical course of these patients. This will allow for empiric initiation of therapy and targeted management. The underlying pathophysiology provides insight into the potential complications associated with alcohol withdrawal and the choice of therapy. It is important to seek alternative diagnoses and inciting factors for withdrawal, which may indeed be the same entity.

HISTORY AND EPIDEMIOLOGY

The medical problems associated with alcoholism and alcohol withdrawal were first described by Pliny the Elder in the 1st century B.C. In his work *Naturalis Historia*, the alcoholic and alcohol withdrawal were described as follows: "...drunkenness brings pallor and sagging cheeks, sore eyes, and trembling hands that spill a full cup, of which the immediate punishment is a haunted sleep and unrestful nights. ..."[80] Initial treatments as described by Osler were focused on supportive care, including confinement to bed, cold baths to reduce fever, and judicious use of potassium bromide, chloral hydrate, hyoscine, and possibly opium.[79]

Some of the initial large series of alcohol related complications in the early 20th century describe the alcohol withdrawal syndrome (AWS) as a major public health concern. At Bellevue Hospital in New York City, Jolliffe described 7000–10,000 admissions per year for alcohol-related problems from 1902–1935, with an estimated rate of 2.5–5 admissions per 1000 New York City residents.[54] Moore et al.[75] described similar numbers of admissions to Boston City Hospital, with up to 10% of alcoholics admitted with evidence of delirium tremens (DTs). The mortality at the beginning of their study among patients with DTs was 52% (1912), and DTs was the leading cause of death among admitted alcoholics. Over the ensuing 20 years, the mortality rate declined to approximately 10%–12%, a decrease believed to be secondary to improved supportive care and nursing.[75]

Though alcoholics were widely recognized to have a high incidence of delirium and psychomotor agitation, the etiology of these signs and symptoms was controversial and attributed to ethanol use, ethanol abstinence, or coexisting psychological disorders. Isbell and colleagues, in 1955, proved that abstinence from alcohol was the cause of this syndrome when they subjected nine male prisoners to chronic alcohol ingestion for a period of 6–12 weeks followed by 2 weeks of abstinence.[52] While they were ingesting alcohol daily none of these prisoners developed signs and symptoms of DTs but during the abstinence phase six of the nine men developed tremor, elevations in blood pressure and heart rate, diaphoresis, and varying degrees of either auditory or visual hallucinations, consistent with the diagnosis of DTs.[52] In addition, two of the nine abstinent men developed convulsions, further linking alcohol abstinence to seizures. However, it should be noted that the high rate of development of DTs (67%) in this study is atypical and does not represent the true prevalence found in later epidemiologic studies.[13]

Currently, alcoholism and alcohol withdrawal syndromes still represent a major problem in both the inpatient and outpatient setting. In a 10-year epidemiologic study, the prevalence of self-reported symptoms of alcohol withdrawal, including morning tremors and sweating, in the general population was quite low, with only 1%–3% of men describing one or more symptoms consistent with alcohol withdrawal; rates were even lower among women.[13] However, when the population in this study was enriched by those at risk for alcoholism, with at risk being defined as convicted for driving under the influence, nearly 19% met self-reported *Diagnostic and Statistical Manual of Mental Disorders* (DSM-IV) criteria for alcohol withdrawal. The prevalence was even higher among persons admitted for detoxification, with nearly 80% experiencing one or more withdrawal symptoms.[13]

Similar results have been obtained in the inpatient setting. Alcohol-related complications accounted for 21% of all medical ICU admissions in an inner city hospital, with alcohol withdrawal being the most common alcohol-related diagnosis.[72] In other studies, 8% of all general hospital admissions, 16% of all postsurgical patients, and 31% of all trauma patients developed AWS.[33,90] The development of AWS in postsurgical and trauma patients can increase the mortality in this population nearly 3-fold.[87,89] Furthermore, alcohol was involved in nearly 86% of homicides, 37% of assaults, and 25%–35% of nonfatal motor vehicle crashes.[15]

PATHOPHYSIOLOGY

Numerous studies over the past 2 decades have provided valuable insight into the mechanism of alcohol withdrawal, allowing for better understanding of both the clinical spectrum of the disorder and potential therapeutic interventions. Alcohol withdrawal is a neurologic disorder with a continuum of progressively worsening symptoms caused by the effects of chronic ethanol use on the central nervous system, and often exacerbated by the clinical manifestations of alcoholism which include nutritional depletion, impaired immunity, anemia, cirrhosis and head trauma.

The effects of chronic alcohol consumption on neurotransmitter function best explain the clinical findings. Persistent stimulation of the inhibitory γ-aminobutyric acid (GABA) receptor-chloride channel complex by ethanol leads to downregulation of GABA receptor–chloride channel complex.[12,57] This allows the alcohol user to maintain a relatively normal level of consciousness despite the presence of high and sedating concentrations of ethanol in the brain. A continued escalation of the steady-state ethanol concentration is required to achieve euphoria termed tolerance, which results in progressive desensitization of the GABA receptor–chloride channel complex.[28] The exact mechanism by which this adaptive change occurs is incompletely defined, but involves substitution of an α_4 for an α_1 receptor subunit on the $GABA_A$ receptor (Chap. 14).[14,66] A converse series of events occurs at the *N*-methyl-D-aspartate (NMDA) subtype of glutamate receptor. Binding by ethanol to the glycine binding site of this receptor inhibits the NMDA function, resulting in compensatory upregulation of these excitatory receptors.[42,50] Thus, withdrawal of alcohol is associated with both a decrease in GABAergic activity and an increase glutamatergic activity.[42] This phenomenon of a concomitant increased excitation and loss of inhibition results in the clinical manifestations of autonomic excitability and psychomotor agitation.

Repeated episodes of alcohol withdrawal may lead to poorly understood permanent alterations in neurotransmitters and their receptors. In rats, repeated episodes of alcohol withdrawal leads to persistent and progressive EEG abnormalities, with further episodes of withdrawal becoming increasingly resistant to benzodiazepines. Both clinical observation and in vitro data suggest that repeated episodes of alcohol withdrawal lead to permanent dysregulation of GABA receptors. This understanding may be an explanation for the "kindling phenomena," which is the clinical observation of increasing severity of alcohol withdrawal among individual subjects, and the development of benzodiazepine-resistant alcohol withdrawal.[11,37,104]

CLINICAL SYNDROMES

Alcohol withdrawal is defined in the DSM-IV as the cessation of substantial or prolonged alcohol use resulting, within a period of a few hours to several days, in the development of two or more of the clinical findings listed in Table 78–1.[32] Additionally, these symptoms must have no other organic etiology. Alcohol withdrawal syndromes can be classified both by timing (early vs. late) and severity (complicated vs. uncomplicated). However, there are no adequate or fully accepted criteria by which to define these categories. Furthermore, the clinical course of AWS can vary widely among patients, and progression of individual patients through these different stages is extremely variable. In fact, some substantial alcohol users experience no withdrawal syndromes following the cessation of alcohol consumption. Recognizing these limitations, this conceptual framework still proves helpful in the clinical management of patients with alcohol withdrawal.

EARLY UNCOMPLICATED WITHDRAWAL

Alcohol withdrawal begins as early as 6 hours after the cessation of drinking. Early withdrawal is characterized by autonomic hyperactivity including tachycardia, tremor, hypertension, and psychomotor agitation.[97] Although these symptoms are uncomfortable, they are not generally dangerous. Most patients who ultimately develop severe manifestations of AWS initially develop these findings, but this is not universal. Early in this "stage" of AWS, the symptoms are still readily amenable to treatment with ethanol, as is done daily by most chronic alcohol users.

TABLE 78–1. DSM-IV Criteria for Alcohol Withdrawal[32]

A. Cessation of (or reduction in) alcohol use that has been heavy and prolonged.
B. Two (or more) of the following, developing within several hours to a few days after criterion A:
   1. Autonomic hyperactivity (eg, sweating or pulse rate greater than 100)
   2. Increased hand tremor
   3. Insomnia
   4. Nausea or vomiting
   5. Transient visual, tactile, or auditory hallucinations or illusions
   6. Psychomotor agitation
   7. Anxiety
   8. Grand mal seizures
C. The symptoms in criterion B cause clinically significant distress or impairment in social, occupational, or other important areas of functioning.
D. The symptoms are not due to a general medical condition and are not better accounted for by another mental disorder.

ALCOHOLIC HALLUCINOSIS

Nearly 25% of patients with AWS will develop hallucinations, which are generally auditory and persecutory, and a subset of these patients will develop alcoholic hallucinosis, a syndrome of persistent hallucinations.[96,98] Although classically these persistent hallucinations are tactile or visual, other types of hallucinations are described. Tactile hallucinations include formication, or the sensation of ants crawling on the skin, which can result in repeated itching and excoriations. However, as opposed to DTs, alcoholic hallucinosis is associated with a clear sensorium. The presence of alcoholic hallucinosis is neither a positive nor a negative predictor of the subsequent development of DTs.[50]

ALCOHOL WITHDRAWAL SEIZURES

Approximately 10% of patients with AWS develop alcohol withdrawal seizures, or "rum fits." For many patients, a generalized alcohol withdrawal seizure may be the first manifestation of the AWS.[97] Approximately 40% of patients with alcohol withdrawal seizures have isolated seizures and 3% develop status epilepticus.[95,97] Alcohol withdrawal seizures may occur in the absence of other signs of alcohol withdrawal and are characteristically brief, generalized, tonic–clonic events with a short post-ictal period. Occasionally a flurry of seizures may occur over a short time period.[95] Regardless, rapid termination and normal post-ictal mental status belie the seriousness of an alcohol withdrawal seizure. For approximately one-third of patients with DTs, the sentinel event is an isolated alcohol withdrawal seizure. Alcohol withdrawal seizures occurring in the presence of an elevated ethanol concentration may be a poor prognostic indicator for the development of a more severe AWS because the relative protection against withdrawal of an elevated ethanol concentration will be lost as the concentration drops.[94] Finally, clinicians should be cognizant that anticonvulsants are prescribed for many alcoholics because they have a preexisting seizure disorder, often related to repetitive brain trauma.[35] Conversely, the use of anticonvulsants does not unequivocally indicate the presence of a preexisting seizure disorder because of the difficulty in differentiating these seizures from those of alcohol withdrawal.

DELIRIUM TREMENS

Delirium tremens is the most serious complication of the AWS, and generally occurs between 48 and 96 hours after the cessation of drinking.[97] Many of the clinical manifestations of DTs are similar to those of uncomplicated early alcohol withdrawal, differing only in severity, and include tremors, autonomic instability (hypertension and tachycardia), and psychomotor agitation. However, unlike AWS, DTs as defined in DSM-IV, is associated with either (1) disturbance of consciousness (such as reduced clarity of awareness of the environment) with reduced ability to focus, sustain, or shift attention, delirium, confusion, and frank psychosis, or (2) a change in cognition (such as memory deficit, disorientation, language disturbance) or the development of a perceptual disturbance that is not better accounted for by a preexisting, established, or evolving dementia.[32] Unlike the early manifestations of alcohol withdrawal, which typically last for 3–5 days, DT can last for up to 2 weeks (Table 78–2).[97]

TABLE 78–2. Diagnostic Criteria for Substance Withdrawal Delirium[32]

A. Disturbance of consciousness (ie, reduced clarity of awareness of the environment) with reduced ability to focus, sustain, or shift attention.
B. A change in cognition (such as memory deficit, disorientation, language disturbance) or the development of a perceptual disturbance that is not better accounted for by a preexisting, established, or evolving dementia.
C. The disturbance develops over a short period of time (usually hours to days) and tends to fluctuate during the course of the day.
D. There is evidence from the history, physical examination, or laboratory findings that the symptoms in criteria A and B developed during, or shortly after a withdrawal syndrome.

Note: This diagnosis should be made instead of a diagnosis of substance withdrawal only when the cognitive symptoms are in excess of those usually associated with the withdrawal syndrome and when the symptoms are sufficiently severe to warrant independent clinical attention.

RISK FACTORS FOR THE DEVELOPMENT OF ALCOHOL WITHDRAWAL

Factors determining whether an individual will develop AWS are not well identified. The strongest predictor for the development of AWS is a history of prior episodes of AWS/DTs and/or a family history.[31,62] The influence of family history on the development of AWS suggests a strong role for genetic factors. A growing number of studies have identified numerous polymorphisms associated with the development of AWS/DTs. These include genes involved in dopamine transmission, glutamate signaling, cannabinoid receptors and neuropeptide Y.[38,42,59,61,93] However, these findings must be interpreted with caution. First, whether or not they represent a predisposition to greater ethanol consumption because of an enhanced mesolimbic reward system, or some other underlying pathophysiologic effect, is unclear. In addition, they may be reflective of protective genetic alterations, as is noted with the GRK5 polymorphism of the β-adrenergic receptor.[67] Second, many of the studies do not systematically divide between AWS, withdrawal seizures, and DTs, all of which may be regulated by different pathways. Finally, almost uniformly these studies are small (less than 200 subjects) and are racially homogenous, making it imperative that they be replicated on a larger scale and in different racial groups.[59] Larger and more varied patient cohorts that include both women and nonwhite ethnic groups are required before any definitive conclusions can be drawn. Racial predisposition to the development or severity of AWS is not definitive, but the experience at our institution suggests that African American patients may be at lower risk of developing severe DTs than Caucasians.[17]

Because of the subjective nature of many of these findings, we discourage the use of pure clinical descriptors, such as DTs, tremors, rum fits, and the like, to classify the severity of alcohol withdrawal in any given patient. Furthermore, the necessity of having a standardized means of classification has enormous implications for epidemiologic, genetic, and treatment studies. One of the more commonly used means for accurately assessing alcohol withdrawal is the Clinical Institute Withdrawal Assessment of Alcohol Scale, Revised (CIWA-Ar) score (Fig. 78–1).[91] This scoring system contains 10 clinical categories and requires less than 5 minutes to complete. Scoring systems are not only essential for symptom-triggered therapy, but provide a basis for comparative analysis of clinical trials in ethanol withdrawal. Greater use of CIWA-Ar or a comparable validated scale will be essential for interpretation of both genetic and treatment trials in the future. The majority of scoring systems are validated only for patients with mild AWS who are in detoxification or rehabilitation environments and their direct applicability to patients with severe AWS is unclear.

CLINICAL AND BIOCHEMICAL PREDICTORS

Alcohol concentrations, homocysteine concentrations, and liver enzymes are often associated with the development of AWS in the results of some but not all studies.[8,94] Because many studies are based on small numbers of often highly selected subjects, their applicability to larger populations is extremely poor.

Numerous attempts have been made to develop biochemical predictors for the presence and/or severity of alcohol withdrawal. Although consistent abnormalities in readily obtained laboratory values are observed in patients with AWS (eg, aminotransferases, magnesium, erythrocyte parameters such as mean corpuscular volume), their role in predicting the severity of AWS is poorly described. In one study, an alanine aminotransferase (ALT) greater than 50 Units/L (odds ratio [OR] 9.0; 3.5–24), a serum chloride concentration less than 96 mEq/L (OR 61.5; 54.4–69.6), and a serum potassium concentration less than 3.6 mEq/L (OR 5.7; 2–16.4) were all associated with the development of alcohol withdrawal in patients admitted to a detoxification center.[102] However, the low specificity of these derangements makes it difficult to assess their predictive value, especially when accounting for other clinical characteristics such as prior history and admission CIWA-Ar score. In addition, there is a negative association between the presence of severe alcohol withdrawal and histopathologic cirrhosis, further clouding the usefulness of routine laboratory testing for prognostication.[3]

Other investigators have focused on admission ethanol concentration as a predictor for the severity of alcohol withdrawal in at risk subjects. In one study, an admission blood ethanol concentration of greater than 150 mg/dL had a 100% sensitivity and a 57% specificity for the need for treatment of alcohol withdrawal.[99] At a different treatment facility, an ethanol concentration of greater than 150 mg/dL had an 81% positive predictive value for the need to use more than a single dose of chlordiazepoxide for the treatment of AWS.[99] In addition, admission blood ethanol concentrations in patients with alcohol withdrawal seizures were 2-fold higher than in those without seizures, irrespective of whether or not they had a history of prior withdrawal seizures.[99] However, these results should be interpreted with caution, as other studies yield conflicting results. In one study, an admission ethanol concentration less than 100 mg/dL was associated with an increased risk of recurrent alcohol withdrawal seizures, and in another study, admission ethanol concentrations failed to predict the development of DTs.[21,81] There are many potential explanations for these disparate results, including differences in patient population, differences in cohort size, and the late onset of DTs, at a time when ethanol concentrations would be extremely low or nonexistent.[21]

More recently, investigators have looked at the prognostic usefulness of serum homocysteine concentrations. Numerous reports document hyperhomocysteinemia in patients with alcoholism, presumably caused by a deficiency of dietary folic acid.[25] Furthermore, homocysteine and its metabolites can act as excitatory neurotransmitters at the NMDA receptor and cause seizures and excitatory neuronal death.[69] In one study, serum homocysteine concentrations were predictive of alcohol withdrawal seizures. However, in this study, there was strong correlation ($r^2 = 0.7666$; $P < 0.001$) between admission blood ethanol concentrations and homocysteine concentrations, raising doubts as to whether this holds any advantage over blood ethanol concentrations.[8] Additionally, among men admitted for alcohol detoxification, those

Clinical Institute Withdrawal Assessment Of Alcohol Scale, Revised (CIWA-Ar)

The CIWA-Ar is *not* copyrighted and may be reproduced freely.

Patient:__________ Date:______ Time:______ (24 hour clock, midnight = 00:00)

Pulse or heart rate, taken for one minute:________ Blood pressure:________

NAUSEA AND VOMITING: Ask "Do you feel sick to your stomach? Have you vomited?" Observation.
0 No nausea and no vomiting
1 Mild nausea with no vomiting
2
3
4 Intermittent nausea with dry heaves
5
6
7 Constant nausea, frequent dry heaves and vomiting

TREMOR: Arms extended and fingers spread apart. Observation.
0 No tremor
1 Not visible, but can be felt fingertip to fingertip
2
3
4 Moderate, with patient's arms extended
5
6
7 Severe, even with arms not extended

PAROXYSMAL SWEATS: Observation.
0 No sweat visible
1 Barely perceptible sweating, palms moist
2
3
4 Beads of sweat obvious on forehead
5
6
7 Drenching sweats

ANXIETY: Ask "Do you feel nervous?" Observation.
0 No anxiety, at ease
1 Mild anxious
2
3
4 Moderately anxious, or guarded, so anxiety is inferred
5
6
7 Equivalent to acute panic states as seen in severe delirium or acute schizophrenic reactions

AGITATION: Observation.
0 Normal activity
1 Somewhat more than normal activity
2
3
4 Moderately fidgety and restless
5
6
7 Paces back and forth during most of the interview, or constantly thrashes about

TACTILE DISTURBANCES: Ask "Have you any itching, pins and needles sensations, any burning, any numbness, or do you feel bugs crawling on or under your skin?" Observation.
0 none
1 Very mild itching, pins and needles, burning or numbness
2 Mild itching, pins and needles, burning or numbness
3 Moderate itching, pins and needles, burning numbness
4 Moderately severe hallucinations
5 Severe hallucinations
6 Extremely severe hallucinations
7 Continuous hallucinations

AUDITORY DISTURBANCES: Ask " Are you more aware of sounds around you? Are they harsh? Do they frighten you? Are you hearing anything that is disturbing to you? Are you hearing things you know are not there?" Observation.
0 Not present
1 Very mild harshness or ability to frighten
2 Mild harshness or ability to frighten
3 Moderate harshness or ability to frighten
4 Moderately severe hallucinations
5 Severe hallucinations
6 Extremely severe hallucinations
7 Continuous hallucinations

VISUAL DISTURBANCES: Ask "Does the light appear to be too bright? Is its color different? Does it hurt your eyes? Are you seeing anything that is disturbing to you? Are you seeing things you know are not there?" Observation.
0 Not present
1 Very mild sensitivity
2 Mild sensitivity
3 Moderate sensitivity
4 Moderately severe hallucinations
5 Severe hallucinations
6 Extremely severe hallucinations
7 Continuous hallucinations

HEADACHE, FULLNESS IN HEAD: Ask "Does your head feel different? Does it feel like there is a band around your head?" Do not rate for dizziness or lightheadedness. Otherwise, rate severity.
0 No present
1 Very mild
2 Mild
3 Moderate
4 Moderately severe
5 Severe
6 Very severe
7 Extremely severe

ORIENTATION AND CLOUDING OF SENSORIUM: Ask "What day is this? Where are you? Who am I?"
0 Oriented and can do serial additions
1 Cannot do serial additions or is uncertain about date
2 Disoriented for date by no more than 2 calendar days
3 Disoriented for date by more than 2 calendar days
4 Disoriented for place/or person

Total CIWA-Ar score:______

Rater's initials:______

Maximum possible score 67

FIGURE 78–1. Clinical Institute Withdrawal Assessment. (Reproduced from Sullivan JT, Sykora K, Schneiderman J, et al. Assessment of alcohol withdrawal: the revised Clinical Institute Withdrawal Assessment of Alcohol Scale (CIWA-Ar). *Br J Addict* 1989;84:1353–1357.)

with a history of alcohol withdrawal seizures but no recent seizure had a significantly higher serum prolactin concentrations when compared to those without a prior alcohol withdrawal seizure ($P = 0.042$).[46] The robustness of an elevated prolactin or homocysteine concentration appears to be improved when combined, outperforming either individually and an elevated blood alcohol concentration in predicting the risk of alcohol withdrawal seizures.[47] However, additional study is needed before any definitive conclusions can be made.

In a recent study of 35 fatalities with an in-hospital diagnosis of DTs, restraint use and hyperthermia were both predictive of death.[58] Because this is likely a marker for undertreatment with appropriate doses of benzodiazepines (see next section), it highlights the need for aggressive early management.

MANAGEMENT

ALCOHOL WITHDRAWAL SEIZURES

Alcohol withdrawal seizures are perhaps the most rigorously studied complication of AWS. Although alcohol withdrawal seizures are generally self-limited, benzodiazepines are preferred for patients with persistent or recurrent alcohol withdrawal seizures. In a randomized, placebo-controlled trial of 229 subjects with alcohol withdrawal seizures, 2 mg of intramuscular lorazepam reduced the risk of recurrent seizure from 24% to 3% ($P < 0.001$) at 6 hours, and the need for hospital admission from 42% to 29% ($P = 0.0222$).[30] However, whether this interrupts the natural history of progression to DTs is not known. There is no role for phenytoin in either treatment or prevention of alcohol withdrawal seizures. In multiple trials, phenytoin was ineffective in preventing recurrence of alcohol withdrawal seizure.[1,18,82] The most likely explanation for the failure of phenytoin is its inability to regulate GABA or NMDA receptors, the principle mediators of the development of seizures in alcohol withdrawal. One exception to this lack of usefulness occurs in the alcoholic patient with a nonalcohol withdrawal-mediated seizure, or a history of underlying seizure disorders.

ALCOHOL WITHDRAWAL

In the early stages of alcohol withdrawal, many patients are able to self-medicate with additional alcohol consumption. Among those who seek medical attention, many patients with AWS can be safely managed as outpatients. Outpatient management has significant cost savings with little effect on treatment outcome when the patient is sufficiently stable to tolerate this option.[43] In one study, patients who exhibited a current lack of intoxication, no history of either DTs or alcohol withdrawal seizures, no comorbid psychiatric or medical disorders, and a CIWA-Ar score of less than 8 were safely managed as outpatients.[2] Patients not meeting these criteria were referred to inpatient detoxification centers or medical units, depending on the severity of withdrawal and other comorbid conditions.

For all patients with AWS, the initial stages of therapy remain the same, and should include a thorough assessment to identify coexisting medical, psychiatric, or toxicologic disorders. In particular, an assessment for central nervous system trauma and infection should include the appropriate use of computed tomography and lumbar puncture. Patients with altered cognition or an elevated body temperature should receive antibiotics as appropriate, pending the results of a lumbar puncture. In concert with this approach, adequate supportive care should be instituted, with attention to identifying treatable causes of abnormal vital signs and clinical findings.

Chronic alcohol consumption leads to severe vitamin and nutritional deficiencies and electrolytes disturbances that should be corrected.[25,49] Specifically, parenteral thiamine should be given to all patients to prevent the development of Wernicke encephalopathy. It is generally suggested that thiamine should be given prior to the administration of dextrose to prevent precipitation of Wernicke encephalopathy.[73,100] Although there is little evidence to support this approach, the administration of thiamine (see Antidote in Depth A25: Thiamine Hydrochloride) and dextrose together is a reasonable practice. Because there is typically a high incidence of intravascular volume depletion among alcoholics, all patients should receive adequate volume resuscitation. Of 39 deaths between 1915 and 1936 attributed to DTs in which volume status was recorded, all subjects were volume depleted.[75] Finally, for patients with AWS, particularly if severe, prevention of nosocomial complications is paramount for reducing hospital stay. Currently, in addition to adequate volume replacement, we recommend that all patients be kept with the head of the bed elevated to prevent pulmonary aspiration, and that deep vein thrombosis prophylaxis be given if the patient is bed bound for an extended period.

The association of severe alcohol withdrawal with severe psychomotor agitation led to early use of sedative-hypnotics. One of the first randomized trials compared chlorpromazine to paraldehyde. In both study arms there was a 0% mortality, suggesting equivalency of the two treatments.[34] Over the ensuing years, numerous trials documented similar efficacy between paraldehyde, benzodiazepines, and antipsychotics.[16,34,92] However, in a landmark study, 547 patients were randomized to 1 of 4 drugs (chlordiazepoxide, chlorpromazine, hydroxyzine, and thiamine) or to placebo for the treatment of alcohol withdrawal.[55] Patients receiving chlordiazepoxide had the lowest incidence of both DTs and alcohol withdrawal seizures, establishing benzodiazepines as a first-line agent for treatment of AWS. Of note, use of chlorpromazine, an antipsychotic, was associated with a significant increase in the incidence of seizures in both humans[55] and animal models.[10]

Since this study, numerous trials have compared different routes of administration among various sedative-hypnotics, both to each other and to placebo. Because of the historical use noted above, chlordiazepoxide remains widely used in outpatient and inpatient detoxification clinics. Oral benzodiazepine administration is generally effective in patients with early or mild AWS, although initial rapid titration with an intravenous regimen may be more efficient. Benzodiazepines administered intravenously have a rapid onset of action, and have long displaced paraldehyde as the sedative-hypnotic of choice for acute control. Among the benzodiazepines, diazepam offers the most rapid time to peak clinical effects, which limits oversedation that may occur following the administration of drugs with slower onset to the peak drug effect, such as lorazepam. Because of the delayed peak clinical effect of lorazepam of approximately 10–20 minutes, several doses may be administered in rapid succession with little clinical effect, followed by the appearance of oversedation from the cumulative doses. Midazolam may be administered intramuscularly if intravenous access is not available, but intramuscular injection significantly delays the time to both onset and peak clinical effect. Although no significant differences are observed between benzodiazepines and barbiturates in terms of mortality or the duration of delirium, the improved pharmacokinetic profile and ease of administration favor benzodiazepines as the preferred initial agent (see A24: Benzodiazepines).[2,63]

Other pharmacokinetic factors and experience confirm that diazepam is preferred for initial intravenous use in patients with moderate to severe AWS. Diazepam has a long half-life [43 ± 13 hours] and has active metabolites (desmethyldiazepam and oxazepam). The prolonged half-life (48–72 hours) of desmethyldiazepam further extends the effective duration of action of the initial dose of diazepam.[107] A retrospective review reported that the use of a single benzodiazepine rather than multiple benzodiazepines was a marker for treatment success in surgical patients experiencing alcohol withdrawal during surgical admission.[77] These data suggest that it is more important to rapidly sedate the patient with adequate doses of a single benzodiazepine than to use multiple benzodiazepines in hopes of finding an effective regimen. Finally, it should be noted that in patients with advanced liver disease, the use of diazepam may result in a very prolonged period of sedation because of impaired clearance of the parent compound and its metabolites. Consequently, in these patients, a benzodiazepine without active metabolites, such as lorazepam, may be a better drug.

The initial management of patients with AWS/DTs should include rapid titration with intravenous benzodiazepine to achieve sedation. The goal of therapy is to have the patient sedated but breathing spontaneously, with normal vital signs. Although normalization of vital signs is not a mandatory therapeutic endpoint, abnormal vital signs despite adequate sedation should prompt a search for comorbidities. In many patients, complete sedation with diazepam may allow for autotitration; that is, as the AWS resolves, the blood concentrations of diazepam and desmethyldiazepam decrease, allowing gradual recovery. In practicality, most patients need periodic redosing with diazepam to maintain adequate sedation. This is particularly important in patients with AWS with an elevated blood alcohol concentration.

Multiple studies now suggest that if additional doses are required, they should be administered based on symptoms ("symptom triggered"), as opposed to a fixed dosing schedule. In two randomized controlled trials, administration of benzodiazepine in a symptom-triggered fashion reduced both the total amount of benzodiazepine and the duration of treatment.[26,86] In these trials, benzodiazepines were administered every hour as long as the CIWA-Ar score remained greater than 8–10. In both trials, symptom-triggered therapy resulted in a 4- to 6-fold reduction in the duration of therapy and a 4- to 5-fold reduction in the total amount of benzodiazepine administered, with no increase in withdrawal seizures or adverse events.[26,86] Symptom-triggered doses in patients with moderate or severe AWS should be diazepam 10–20 mg IV or lorazepam 2–4 mg.[26,86] For less-symptomatic patients, oral chlordiazepoxide 50–100 mg should be administered. However, it is important to note that the decision to treat in the symptom-triggered group was made based on CIWA-Ar score (usually >8), which demonstrates the usefulness of standardized scoring and evaluation tools. It should also be noted that in both of these trials, patients had very mild withdrawal symptoms, with mean CIWA-Ar scores of 9–11. While experience suggests that this same regimen is also effective in patients with serious withdrawal and/or DTs it has not been validated in this population. Furthermore, it must be emphasized that protocolized use of the CIWA-Ar score is dependent on a significant history of recent heavy drinking and a communicative subject. A prospective analysis of complex medical/surgical patients enrolled in a CIWA-Ar protocol suggested more than 50% patients failed to meet these criteria, leading to unnecessary treatment.[44]

RESISTANT ALCOHOL WITHDRAWAL AND DELIRIUM TREMENS

There is a subgroup of patients with AWS who require very large doses of diazepam, or another comparable drug to achieve initial sedation.[40,68,78,105] This same group often has exceedingly high benzodiazepine requirements to maintain this level of sedation. Subjects with resistant AWS and DTs may have benzodiazepine requirements that exceed 2600 mg of diazepam within the first 24 hours, and generally require admission to an intensive care or stepdown unit.[105] Patients admitted to the Bellevue hospital medical ICU for resistant alcohol withdrawal had very high diazepam requirements, with a mean of 234 mg (range: 10–1490 mg) required in the first 24 hours, and individual doses of diazepam that often exceeded 100 mg, to control their agitation. At Bellevue, these patients comprise approximately 5% of all ICU admissions, with nearly 40% of patients requiring mechanical ventilation and a mean ICU length of stay of 5.7 days.[36]

The approach to the management of resistant AWS depends on several factors, including the availability of an intensive care unit bed. In the ICU, despite the perception of failure of high benzodiazepine requirements, we favor administration of benzodiazepines in a symptom-triggered fashion. This approach was confirmed in a study of patients who developed AWS postoperatively in the ICU.[88] In this study, a symptom-triggered strategy resulted in a shorter length of stay and a lower incidence of mechanical ventilation than did continuous infusion of midazolam.[88] Patients who receive this therapy generally respond to bolus doses of diazepam, which results in a brief period of sedation followed by recrudescence of their AWS. However, the dose range and drug required to achieve this may be dramatically different than what is observed in subjects with nonresistant AWS. In a recent study, use of escalating bolus doses of diazepam, up to 200 mg as an individual dose, combined with phenobarbital in subjects with continued benzodiazepine resistance (defined as the requirement for bolus doses more frequently than every hour), reduced the need for mechanical ventilation by nearly 50%.[36] In non-ICU settings, the ability to administer frequent intravenous doses of diazepam is limited, and the use of intravenous infusions with secondary sedative agents may be more practical.

In instances of extreme benzodiazepine resistance, patients often receive a second GABAergic drug because of "failure" of benzodiazepine therapy. Phenobarbital, given in combination with a benzodiazepine, in intravenous doses of up to 260 mg, is a reasonable choice.[36] Caution is required to avoid stacking doses of phenobarbital, as the onset of clinical effect takes approximately 20–40 minutes.[45,53] Alternatively, propofol in standard doses may be administered. Although propofol has a rapid onset, it is difficult to titrate, and high dose or long-term use is associated with profound metabolic consequences.[22,23,74] However, in a recent observational study, propofol was safely administered to 21 subjects intubated for severe benzodiazepine resistant DTs.[36] The main drawback to the use of these drugs is their narrow therapeutic–toxic index, with the potential for profound respiratory depression. This is especially true for propofol, which should generally only be used in the setting of mechanical ventilation. Both of these agents can act synergistically with benzodiazepines to enhance GABA-induced chloride channel opening. In addition, propofol uniquely antagonizes NMDA receptors, thus reducing the excitatory component of AWS.[27,41,51]

ETHANOL

Ethanol consumption is a common and effective means by which alcoholics can self-medicate to treat and/or prevent mild alcohol withdrawal. Consequently, some hospitals still administer ethanol for either prophylaxis and/or treatment of AWS. In one survey, 72% of 122 hospitals surveyed had administered either IV or oral ethanol for these indications.[9] Despite its widespread use, little randomized controlled data support its use. In one trial, 39 trauma patients without liver or CNS disease were successfully treated with 10% ethanol infusion for treatment of presumed AWS.[24] Conversely, IV ethanol was no more effective than flunitrazepam in one trial and inferior to diazepam in another in the prevention of AWS in postoperative surgical patients.[31,101] Although the authors did not report any adverse effects in these trials, the necessity for frequent blood alcohol monitoring, unpredictable elimination kinetics, potential for significant hepatic complications, the postulated adverse effects of ethanol on wound healing, and the difficulty in safely administering this therapy make it inappropriate to recommend this regimen.[29,48,73]

ADRENERGIC ANTAGONISTS

Numerous studies have investigated the use of sympatholytics to control the autonomic symptoms of alcohol withdrawal. Both β-adrenergic antagonists and clonidine reduced blood pressure and heart rate in randomized, placebo-controlled trials.[4,64,106] However, the inability of these xenobiotics to address the underlying pathophysiologic mechanism of AWS, and subsequently control the neurologic manifestations, makes them suboptimal as sole therapeutic xenobiotics. There are additional concerns that by altering the physiologic parameters that serve as classic markers for AWS severity, there is a risk of underadministering necessary amounts of benzodiazepines.[106] This was observed in a randomized controlled trial of the central α-agonist lofexidine.[56] Finally, while animal evidence suggests a potential role for dexmedetomidine for AWS, there are only scattered case reports documenting its use in humans.[84,85] Consequently, we do not recommend using these drugs for the treatment of AWS until it becomes clear that other standard therapies have failed.

MAGNESIUM

The theoretical benefits of magnesium supplementation are based both on the high prevalence of magnesium deficiency in alcoholics and its usefulness in preventing seizures in other disorders, including eclampsia.[5,49] Furthermore, magnesium deficiency has many clinical similarities to AWS, clouding the differential diagnosis. Numerous studies have evaluated the efficacy of magnesium supplementation. However, in a randomized, placebo-controlled trial, intravenous magnesium sulfate had no effect on either severity of alcohol withdrawal or incidence of withdrawal seizures.[103] Consequently, aside from repletion of electrolyte abnormalities, there is no indication for routine administration of magnesium for the treatment of AWS.

ANTICONVULSANTS

Carbamazepine has been used in multiple trials for treatment of mild AWS, more commonly in Europe where an intravenous preparation is available. In animal studies, carbamazepine increases both the central nervous system GABA concentrations and the seizure threshold in alcohol withdrawal models.[20] In humans, carbamazepine is superior to placebo and equally efficacious as benzodiazepines for treatment of mild to moderate AWS in both inpatients and outpatients.[7,70,71] Similar data have been obtained with valproic acid, which appears to have a benzodiazepine-sparing effect in patients with mild withdrawal.[83] In contrast, a recent randomized, placebo-controlled study of the newer anticonvulsant oxcarbazepine showed no difference between this xenobiotic and placebo in inpatient detoxification.[60] Consequently, while this class of drugs may be reasonably recommended as adjuncts, they should not be used as monotherapy for treatment of established AWS and DT.

NEWER XENOBIOTICS AND FUTURE DIRECTIONS

There is a constant search for newer xenobiotics to treat alcohol withdrawal, especially for agents that target NMDA receptors. In animal studies, NMDA antagonists have shown benefit in preventing AWS seizure, neurologic damage, and alcohol craving.[6,76] In humans, one NMDA receptor inhibitor, acamprosate, has undergone significant study in the prevention of relapse following alcohol detoxification.[19,39] Its effects on AWS are less clear, although in one study of patients capable of outpatient detoxification, it had no adverse effects on CIWA-Ar scores.[19] More recently, antiglutamanergic lamotrigine and topiramate were compared both to placebo and to diazepam for treatment of mild AWS.[65] All three demonstrated varying degrees of superiority compared to placebo, with no difference when compared to diazepam. However, the role of these xenobiotics in more severe withdrawal as either primary therapy or as adjuncts for use in combination with GABAergic agents remains unclear.

SUMMARY

Alcohol withdrawal is a complex physiologic process involving both enhanced neuronal excitation and reduced inhibition resulting in neuroexcitation. The manifestations of greatest concern are neurologic and include altered mental status and seizure, but the autonomic excess may be clinically consequential. Treatment includes supportive care and sedation with benzodiazepines in escalating doses. When benzodiazepines cannot produce adequate sedation, agents such as phenobarbital or propofol should be added.

REFERENCES

1. Alldredge BK, Lowenstein DH, Simon RP. Placebo-controlled trial of intravenous diphenylhydantoin for short-term treatment of alcohol withdrawal seizures. *Am J Med.* 1989;87:645-648.
2. Asplund CA, Aaronson JW, Aaronson HE. 3 regimens for alcohol withdrawal and detoxification. *J Fam Pract.* 2004;53:545-554.
3. Barrio E, Tome S, Rodriguez I, et al. Liver disease in heavy drinkers with and without alcohol withdrawal syndrome. *Alcohol Clin Exp Res.* 2004;28:131-136.
4. Baumgartner GR, Rowen RC. Clonidine vs chlordiazepoxide in the management of acute alcohol withdrawal syndrome. *Arch Intern Med.* 1987;147:1223-1226.
5. Belfort MA, Anthony J, Saade GR, Allen JC Jr. A comparison of magnesium sulfate and nimodipine for the prevention of eclampsia. *N Engl J Med.* 2003;348:304-311.
6. Bienkowski P, Krzascik P, Koros E, Kostowski W, Scinska A, Danysz W. Effects of a novel uncompetitive NMDA receptor antagonist, MRZ 2/579 on ethanol self-administration and ethanol withdrawal seizures in the rat. *Eur J Pharmacol.* 2001;413:81-89.
7. Bjorkqvist SE, Isohanni M, Makela R, Malinen L. Ambulant treatment of alcohol withdrawal symptoms with carbamazepine: a formal multicentre double-blind comparison with placebo. *Acta Psychiatr Scand.* 1976;53:333-342.
8. Bleich S, Degner D, Wiltfang J, et al. Elevated homocysteine levels in alcohol withdrawal. *Alcohol Alcohol.* 2000;35:351-354.
9. Blondell RD, Dodds HN, Blondell MN, et al. Ethanol in formularies of US teaching hospitals. *JAMA* 2003;289:552.
10. Blum K, Eubanks JD, Wallace JE, Hamilton H. Enhancement of alcohol withdrawal convulsions in mice by haloperidol. *Clin Toxicol.* 1976;9:427-434.
11. Booth BM, Blow FC. The kindling hypothesis: further evidence from a U.S. national study of alcoholic men. *Alcohol Alcohol.* 1993;28:593-598.
12. Buck KJ, Hahner L, Sikela J, Harris RA. Chronic ethanol treatment alters brain levels of gamma-aminobutyric acidA receptor subunit mRNAs: relationship to genetic differences in ethanol withdrawal seizure severity. *J Neurochem.* 1991;57:1452-1455.
13. Caetano R, Clark CL, Greenfield TK. Prevalence, trends, and incidence of alcohol withdrawal symptoms: analysis of general population and clinical samples. *Alcohol Health Res World.* 1998;22:73-79.
14. Cagetti E, Liang J, Spigelman I, Olsen RW. Withdrawal from chronic intermittent ethanol treatment changes subunit composition, reduces synaptic function, and decreases behavioral responses to positive allosteric modulators of $GABA_A$ receptors. *Mol Pharmacol.* 2003;63:53-64.
15. Centers for Disease Control and Prevention. Impaired Driving. 2008. http://www.cdc.gov/MotorVehicleSafety/Impaired_Driving/impaired-drv_factsheet.html.
16. Chambers JF, Schultz JD. Double-blind study of three drugs in the treatment of acute alcoholic states. *Q J Stud Alcohol.* 1965;26:10-18.
17. Chan GM, Hoffman RS, Gold JA, et al. Racial variations in the incidence of severe alcohol withdrawal. *J Med Toxicol.* 2009;5:8-14.

18. Chance JF. Emergency department treatment of alcohol withdrawal seizures with phenytoin. *Ann Emerg Med.* 1991;20:520-522.
19. Chick J, Howlett H, Morgan MY, Ritson B. United Kingdom Multicentre Acamprosate Study (UKMAS): a 6-month prospective study of acamprosate versus placebo in preventing relapse after withdrawal from alcohol. *Alcohol Alcohol.* 2000;35:176-187.
20. Chu NS. Carbamazepine: prevention of alcohol withdrawal seizures. *Neurology.* 1979;29:1397-1401.
21. Clothier J, Kelley JT, Reed K, Reilly EL. Varying rates of alcohol metabolism in relation to detoxification medication. *Alcohol.* 1985;2:443-445.
22. Coomes TR, Smith SW. Successful use of propofol in refractory delirium tremens. *Ann Emerg Med.* 1997;30:825-828.
23. Corbett SM, Montoya ID, Moore FA. Propofol-related infusion syndrome in intensive care patients. *Pharmacotherapy.* 2008;28:250-258.
24. Craft PP, Foil MB, Cunningham PR, Patselas PC, Long-Snyder BM, Collier MS. Intravenous ethanol for alcohol detoxification in trauma patients. *South Med J.* 1994;87:47-54.
25. Cravo ML, Gloria LM, Selhub J, et al. Hyperhomocysteinemia in chronic alcoholism: correlation with folate, vitamin B-12, and vitamin B-6 status. *Am J Clin Nutr.* 1996;63:220-24.
26. Daeppen JB, Gache P, Landry U, et al. Symptom-triggered vs fixed-schedule doses of benzodiazepine for alcohol withdrawal: a randomized treatment trial. *Arch Intern Med.* 2002;162:1117-1121.
27. Daniell LC. Effect of anesthetic and convulsant barbiturates on N-methyl-D-aspartate receptor-mediated calcium flux in brain membrane vesicles. *Pharmacology.* 1994;49:296-307.
28. Diamond I, Gordon AS. Cellular and molecular neuroscience of alcoholism. *Physiol Rev.* 1997;77:1-20.
29. DiPaula B, Tommasello A, Solounias B, McDuff D. An evaluation of intravenous ethanol in hospitalized patients. *J Subst Abuse Treat.* 1998;15:437-442.
30. D'Onofrio G, Rathlev NK, Ulrich AS, Fish SS, Freedland ES. Lorazepam for the prevention of recurrent seizures related to alcohol. *N Engl J Med.* 1999;340:915-919.
31. Eggers V, Tio J, Neumann T, et al. Blood alcohol concentration for monitoring ethanol treatment to prevent alcohol withdrawal in the intensive care unit. *Intensive Care Med.* 2002;28:1475-1482.
32. First MB. Diagnostic and Statistical Manual - Text Revision (DSM-IV-TR", 2000). Washington, DC: American Psychiatric Association; 2000.
33. Foy A, Kay J, Taylor A. The course of alcohol withdrawal in a general hospital. *QJM.* 1997;90:253-261.
34. Friedhoff AJ, Zitrin A. A comparison of the effects of paraldehyde and chlorpromazine in delirium tremens. *N Y State J Med.* 1959;59:1060-1063.
35. Gill JS, Shipley MJ, Tsementzis SA, et al. Alcohol consumption—a risk factor for hemorrhagic and non-hemorrhagic stroke. *Am J Med.* 1991;90:489-497.
36. Gold JA, Rimal B, Nolan A, Nelson LS. A strategy of escalating doses of benzodiazepines and phenobarbital administration reduces the need for mechanical ventilation in delirium tremens. *Crit Care Med.* 2007;35:724-730.
37. Gonzalez LP, Veatch LM, Ticku MK, Becker HC. Alcohol withdrawal kindling: mechanisms and implications for treatment. *Alcohol Clin Exp Res.* 2001;25:197S-201S.
38. Gorwood P, Limosin F, Batel P, Hamon M, Ades J, Boni C. The A9 allele of the dopamine transporter gene is associated with delirium tremens and alcohol-withdrawal seizure. *Biol Psychiatry.* 2003;53:85-92.
39. Gual A, Lehert P. Acamprosate during and after acute alcohol withdrawal: a double-blind placebo-controlled study in Spain. *Alcohol Alcohol.* 2001;36:413-418.
40. Hack JB, Hoffman RS, Nelson LS. Resistant alcohol withdrawal: does an unexpectedly large sedative requirement identify these patients early? *J Med Toxicol.* 2006;2:55-60.
41. Hans P, Bonhomme V, Collette J, Albert A, Moonen G. Propofol protects cultured rat hippocampal neurons against N-methyl-D-aspartate receptor-mediated glutamate toxicity. *J Neurosurg Anesthesiol.* 1994;6:249-253.
42. Haugbol SR, Ebert B, Ulrichsen J. Upregulation of glutamate receptor subtypes during alcohol withdrawal in rats. *Alcohol Alcohol.* 2005;40:89-95.
43. Hayashida M, Alterman AI, McLellan AT, et al. Comparative effectiveness and costs of inpatient and outpatient detoxification of patients with mild-to-moderate alcohol withdrawal syndrome. *N Engl J Med.* 1989;320:358-365.
44. Hecksel KA, Bostwick JM, Jaeger TM, Cha SS. Inappropriate use of symptom-triggered therapy for alcohol withdrawal in the general hospital. *Mayo Clin Proc.* 2008;83:274-279.
45. Hill A, Williams D. Hazards associated with the use of benzodiazepines in alcohol detoxification. *J Subst Abuse Treat.* 1993;10:449-451.
46. Hillemacher T, Bayerlein K, Frieling H, et al. Elevated prolactin serum levels and history of alcohol withdrawal seizures. *J Psychiatr Res.* 2007;41:702-706.
47. Hillemacher T, Frieling H, Bayerlein K, Wilhelm J, Kornhuber J, Bleich S. Biological markers to predict previous alcohol withdrawal seizures: a risk assessment. *J Neural Transm.* 2007;114:151-154.
48. Hodges B, Mazur JE. Intravenous ethanol for the treatment of alcohol withdrawal syndrome in critically ill patients. *Pharmacotherapy.* 2004;24:1578-1585.
49. Hoes MJ. Plasma concentrations of magnesium and vitamin B-1 in alcoholism and delirium tremens. Pathogenic and prognostic implications. *Acta Psychiatr Belg.* 1981;81:72-84.
50. Holloway HC, Hales RE, Watanabe HK. Recognition and treatment of acute alcohol withdrawal syndromes. *Psychiatr Clin North Am.* 1984;7:729-743.
51. Irifune M, Takarada T, Shimizu Y, et al. Propofol-induced anesthesia in mice is mediated by gamma-aminobutyric acid-A and excitatory amino acid receptors. *Anesth Analg.* 2003;97:424-429, table of contents.
52. Isbell H, Fraser HF, Wikler A. An experimental study of the etiology of "rum fits" and delerium tremens. *Q J Stud Alcohol.* 1955;16:1-33.
53. Ives TJ, Mooney AJ, 3rd, Gwyther RE. Pharmacokinetic dosing of phenobarbital in the treatment of alcohol withdrawal syndrome. *South Med J.* 1991;84:18-21.
54. Jolliffe N. Alcoholic admissions to Bellevue Hospital. *Science.* 1936;83:306-309.
55. Kaim SC, Klett CJ, Rothfeld B. Treatment of the acute alcohol withdrawal state: a comparison of four drugs. *Am J Psychiatry.* 1969;125:1640-1646.
56. Keaney F, Strang J, Gossop M, et al. A double-blind randomized placebo-controlled trial of lofexidine in alcohol withdrawal: lofexidine is not a useful adjunct to chlordiazepoxide. *Alcohol Alcohol.* 2001;36:426-430.
57. Keir WJ, Morrow AL. Differential expression of $GABA_A$ receptor subunit mRNAs in ethanol-naive withdrawal seizure resistant (WSR) vs. withdrawal seizure prone (WSP) mouse brain. *Brain Res Mol Brain Res.* 1994;25:200-208.
58. Khan A, Levy P, Dehorn S, Miller W, Compton S. Predictors of mortality in patients with delirium tremens. *Acad Emerg Med.* 2008;15:788-790.
59. Koehnke MD, Schick S, Lutz U, et al. Severity of alcohol withdrawal symptoms and the T1128C polymorphism of the neuropeptide Y gene. *J Neural Transm.* 2002;109:1423-1429.
60. Koethe D, Juelicher A, Nolden BM, et al. Oxcarbazepine—efficacy and tolerability during treatment of alcohol withdrawal: a double-blind, randomized, placebo-controlled multicenter pilot study. *Alcohol Clin Exp Res.* 2007;31:1188-1194.
61. Kohnke MD. Approach to the genetics of alcoholism: a review based on pathophysiology. *Biochem Pharmacol.* 2008;75:160-177.
62. Kraemer KL, Mayo-Smith MF, Calkins DR. Independent clinical correlates of severe alcohol withdrawal. *Subst Abuse.* 2003;24:197-209.
63. Kramp P, Rafaelsen OJ. Delirium tremens: a double-blind comparison of diazepam and barbital treatment. *Acta Psychiatr Scand.* 1978;58:174-190.
64. Kraus ML, Gottlieb LD, Horwitz RI, Anscher M. Randomized clinical trial of atenolol in patients with alcohol withdrawal. *N Engl J Med.* 1985;313:905-909.
65. Krupitsky EM, Rudenko AA, Burakov AM, et al. Antiglutamatergic strategies for ethanol detoxification: comparison with placebo and diazepam. *Alcohol Clin Exp Res.* 2007;31:604-611.
66. Kumar S, Fleming RL, Morrow AL. Ethanol regulation of gamma-aminobutyric acid A receptors: genomic and nongenomic mechanisms. *Pharmacol Ther.* 2004;101:211-226.
67. Liggett SB, Cresci S, Kelly RJ, et al. A GRK5 polymorphism that inhibits beta-adrenergic receptor signaling is protective in heart failure. *Nat Med.* 2008;14:510-517.
68. Lineaweaver WC, Anderson K, Hing DN. Massive doses of midazolam infusion for delirium tremens without respiratory depression. *Crit Care Med.* 1988;16:294-295.
69. Lipton SA, Kim WK, Choi YB, et al. Neurotoxicity associated with dual actions of homocysteine at the N-methyl-D-aspartate receptor. *Proc Natl Acad Sci U S A.* 1997;94:5923-5928.
70. Malcolm R, Myrick H, Roberts J, Wang W, Anton RF, Ballenger JC. The effects of carbamazepine and lorazepam on single versus multiple previous alcohol withdrawals in an outpatient randomized trial. *J Gen Intern Med.* 2002;17:349-355.
71. Malcolm R, Ballenger JC, Sturgis ET, Anton R. Double-blind controlled trial comparing carbamazepine to oxazepam treatment of alcohol withdrawal. *Am J Psychiatry.* 1989;146:617-621.

72. Marik P, Mohedin B. Alcohol-related admissions to an inner city hospital intensive care unit. *Alcohol Alcohol.* 1996;31:393-396.
73. Mayo-Smith MF, Beecher LH, Fischer TL, et al. Management of alcohol withdrawal delirium. An evidence-based practice guideline. *Arch Intern Med.* 2004;164:1405-1412.
74. McCowan C, Marik P. Refractory delirium tremens treated with propofol: a case series. *Crit Care Med.* 2000;28:1781-1784.
75. Moore M, Gray MG. Delerium tremens: a study of cases at the Boston City Hospital, 1915-1936. *N Engl J Med.* 1939;220:953-956.
76. Nagy J, Horvath C, Farkas S, Kolok S, Szombathelyi Z. NR2B subunit selective NMDA antagonists inhibit neurotoxic effect of alcohol-withdrawal in primary cultures of rat cortical neurones. *Neurochem Int.* 2004;44:17-23.
77. Newman JP, Terris DJ, Moore M. Trends in the management of alcohol withdrawal syndrome. *Laryngoscope.* 1995;105:1-7.
78. Nolop KB, Natow A. Unprecedented sedative requirements during delirium tremens. *Crit Care Med.* 1985;13:246-247.
79. Oldham AJ, Bott M. The management of excitement in a general hospital psychiatric ward by high dosage haloperidol. *Acta Psychiatr Scand.* 1971;47:369-376.
80. Picciotto MR. Common aspects of the action of nicotine and other drugs of abuse. *Drug Alcohol Depend.* 1998;51:165-72.
81. Rathlev NK, Ulrich A, Fish SS, D'Onofrio G. Clinical characteristics as predictors of recurrent alcohol-related seizures. *Acad Emerg Med.* 2000;7: 886-891.
82. Rathlev NK, D'Onofrio G, Fish SS, et al. The lack of efficacy of phenytoin in the prevention of recurrent alcohol-related seizures. *Ann Emerg Med.* 1994;23:513-518.
83. Reoux JP, Saxon AJ, Malte CA, Baer JS, Sloan KL. Divalproex sodium in alcohol withdrawal: a randomized double-blind placebo-controlled clinical trial. *Alcohol Clin Exp Res.* 2001;25:1324-1329.
84. Riihioja P, Jaatinen P, Oksanen H, Haapalinna A, Heinonen E, Hervonen A. Dexmedetomidine, diazepam, and propranolol in the treatment of ethanol withdrawal symptoms in the rat. *Alcohol Clin Exp Res.* 1997;21:804-808.
85. Rovasalo A, Tohmo H, Aantaa R, Kettunen E, Palojoki R. Dexmedetomidine as an adjuvant in the treatment of alcohol withdrawal delirium: a case report. *Gen Hosp Psychiatry.* 2006;28:362-363.
86. Saitz R, Mayo-Smith MF, Roberts MS, Redmond HA, Bernard DR, Calkins DR. Individualized treatment for alcohol withdrawal. A randomized double-blind controlled trial. *JAMA.* 1994;272:519-523.
87. Sonne NM, Tonnesen H. The influence of alcoholism on outcome after evacuation of subdural haematoma. *Br J Neurosurg.* 1992;6:125-130.
88. Spies CD, Otter HE, Huske B, et al. Alcohol withdrawal severity is decreased by symptom-orientated adjusted bolus therapy in the ICU. *Intensive Care Med.* 2003;29:2230-2238.
89. Spies CD, Dubisz N, Neumann T, et al. Therapy of alcohol withdrawal syndrome in intensive care unit patients following trauma: results of a prospective, randomized trial. *Crit Care Med.* 1996;24:414-422.
90. Spies CD, Nordmann A, Brummer G, et al. Intensive care unit stay is prolonged in chronic alcoholic men following tumor resection of the upper digestive tract. *Acta Anaesthesiol Scand.* 1996;40:649-656.
91. Sullivan JT, Sykora K, Schneiderman J, Naranjo CA, Sellers EM. Assessment of alcohol withdrawal: the revised clinical institute withdrawal assessment for alcohol scale (CIWA-Ar). *Br J Addict.* 1989;84:1353-1357.
92. Thomas DW, Freedman DX. Treatment of the alcohol withdrawal syndrome. Comparison of promazine and paraldehyde. *JAMA.* 1964;188: 316-318.
93. van Munster BC, Korevaar JC, de Rooij SE, Levi M, Zwinderman AH. Genetic polymorphisms related to delirium tremens: a systematic review. *Alcohol Clin Exp Res.* 2007;31:177-184.
94. Veatch LM, Gonzalez LP. Repeated ethanol withdrawal produces site-dependent increases in EEG spiking. *Alcohol Clin Exp Res.* 1996;20:262-267.
95. Victor M, Brausch C. The role of abstinence in the genesis of alcoholic epilepsy. *Epilepsia.* 1967;8:1-20.
96. Victor M. Treatment of the neurologic complications of alcoholism. *Mod Treat.* 1966;3:491-501.
97. Victor M, Adams RD. The effect of alcohol on the nervous system. *Res Publ Assoc Res Nerv Ment Dis.* 1953;32:526-573.
98. Victor M, Hope JM, Adams RD. Auditory hallucinations in the alcoholic patient. *Trans Am Neurol Assoc.* 1953;3:273-275.
99. Vinson DC, Menezes M. Admission alcohol level: a predictor of the course of alcohol withdrawal. *J Fam Pract.* 1991;33:161-167.
100. Watson AJ, Walker JF, Tomkin GH, Finn MM, Keogh JA. Acute Wernickes encephalopathy precipitated by glucose loading. *Ir J Med Sci.* 1981;150:301-303.
101. Weinberg JA, Magnotti LJ, Fischer PE, et al. Comparison of intravenous ethanol versus diazepam for alcohol withdrawal prophylaxis in the trauma ICU: results of a randomized trial. *J Trauma.* 2008;64:99-104.
102. Wetterling T, Kanitz RD, Veltrup C, Driessen M. Clinical predictors of alcohol withdrawal delirium. *Alcohol Clin Exp Res.* 1994;18:1100-1102.
103. Wilson A, Vulcano B. A double-blind, placebo-controlled trial of magnesium sulfate in the ethanol withdrawal syndrome. *Alcohol Clin Exp Res.* 1984;8:542-545.
104. Wojnar M, Bizon Z, Wasilewski D. Assessment of the role of kindling in the pathogenesis of alcohol withdrawal seizures and delirium tremens. *Alcohol Clin Exp Res.* 1999;23:204-208.
105. Wojnar M, Wasilewski D, Matsumoto H, Cedro A. Differences in the course of alcohol withdrawal in women and men: a Polish sample. *Alcohol Clin Exp Res.* 1997;21:1351-1355.
106. Worner TM. Propranolol versus diazepam in the management of the alcohol withdrawal syndrome: double-blind controlled trial. *Am J Drug Alcohol Abuse.* 1994;20:115-124.
107. Wretlind M, Pilbrant A, Sundwall A, Vessman J. Disposition of three benzodiazepines after single oral administration in man. *Acta Pharmacol Toxicol (Copenh).* 1977;40 Suppl 1:28-39.

CHAPTER 79
DISULFIRAM AND DISULFIRAM-LIKE REACTIONS

Edwin K. Kuffner

$$(C_2H_5)_2N{-}C({=}S){-}S{-}S{-}C({=}S){-}N(C_2H_5)_2$$

Disulfiram

Disulfiram continues to be prescribed as part of alcohol treatment programs and is being more widely studied for other drugs of abuse. Disulfiram toxicity associated with acute overdose, chronic therapy, and from disulfiram–ethanol reactions continues to be reported worldwide. Most of the adverse effects are from case reports and case series which are difficult to interpret because of complications and comorbidities associated with alcohol use and alcoholism, the potential effects of polypharmacy, use of other drugs of abuse, and difficulty in relating specific adverse effects to disulfiram, alcohol or a disulfiram–ethanol reaction. Although serious and life-threatening effects associated with disulfiram are rare, clinicians and toxicologists must remain vigilant in diagnosing and appropriately managing patients with disulfiram associated toxicity.

HISTORY AND EPIDEMIOLOGY

For over 200 years disulfiram (tetraethylthiuram disulfide) and related chemicals have been used in the rubber industry as catalytic accelerators for the vulcanization (stabilization) of rubber by the addition of sulfur.[117] In the early 1900s, workers exposed to disulfiram were observed to develop adverse reactions when exposed to ethanol. Williams, an American physician, suggested that disulfiram might be a useful adjunct in the treatment of alcoholism.[127] In the 1940s, two Danish physicians, Hald and Jacobsen, became ill after consuming alcohol while using disulfiram as an antihelmintic.[42] Subsequently, disulfiram was approved by the FDA for the the treatment for alcoholism in 1951. Although data supporting the benefit of using disulfiram in a comprehensive alcohol treatment program have been questioned, other pharmacologic therapies such as naltrexone and acamprosate have been approved for the treatment of alcohol dependence, and the potential benefits of disulfiram therapy continue to be evaluated in clinical trials disulfiram is still widely prescribed today.[38,47,70,95,115] Although the use of disulfiram for treating alcoholism is decreasing, its use in the management of addictions to other drugs of abuse such as cocaine is increasing.[92] Specific epidemiologic information about the three different forms of disulfiram toxicity is difficult to elucidate, even from an analysis of the American Association of Poison Control Centers (AAPCC) (Chap. 135).

Data from the AAPCC from 2003 to 2007 confirms that each year US poison centers are notified of between three and four hundred disulfiram exposures. Major adverse outcomes are rare. Since 1982 only 14 deaths associated with disulfiram have been reported to the AAPCC, most reported to involve a disulfiram-ethanol reaction.

Unlike many xenobiotics reported to the AAPCC, the majority of the disulfiram exposures were in adults. Serious adverse effects reported in the literature associated with both therapeutic use of disulfiram and with disulfiram overdose continue to be reported mostly in the form of case reports and case series. As such, these reports are difficult to interpret because of complications and comorbidities associated with alcohol use and alcoholism, the potential effects of polypharmacy, and the difficulty in relating the adverse effect to disulfiram, alcohol or a disulfiram–ethanol reaction.

PHARMACOLOGY AND PHARMACOKINETICS OF DISULFIRAM

Disulfiram does not produce central nervous system effects that alter an alcoholic's drinking behavior. The effectiveness of disulfiram in discouraging alcohol consumption is aversive in nature, as it is dependent on the patient's fear of developing a disulfiram–ethanol reaction. Therapeutic doses of disulfiram, used as part of a comprehensive alcohol treatment program, typically range from 125 to 500 mg/day.

ABSORPTION

Disulfiram is highly lipid soluble and very insoluble in water. Following ingestion, disulfiram is either absorbed as the parent compound or rapidly converted to diethyldithiocarbamic acid (diethyldithiocarbamate) in the acid environment of the stomach.[13] Diethyldithiocarbamic acid is also very unstable in this acid environment and either rapidly undergoes absorption and spontaneous decomposition to carbon disulfide and diethylamine, or chelates copper, forming a bis(diethyldithiocarbamate)-copper complex. The bis(diethyldithiocarbamate)-copper complex is more stable than diethyldithiocarbamic acid and also can be absorbed as it passes through the upper gastrointestinal tract. In fact, most disulfiram is absorbed from the small intestine as this bis(diethyldithiocarbamate)-copper complex. Approximately 70%–90% of an ingested therapeutic dose of disulfiram is absorbed. The bioavailability of disulfiram varies with different preparations. In one study, the mean serum disulfiram concentration in humans following a 250-mg dose was reported to be 0.38 ± 0.03 μg/mL.[29] Peak serum concentrations of disulfiram and its metabolites are achieved 8–10 hours following a 250-mg dose.[29]

DISTRIBUTION

Approximately 96% of disulfiram itself and approximately 80% of disulfiram metabolites are protein bound.[50] Following absorption, disulfiram and its metabolites are uniformly distributed throughout tissues. A specific volume of distribution for disulfiram is not recognized.

METABOLISM

Since absorbed disulfiram is rapidly converted to diethyldithiocarbamic acid by erythrocyte glutathione reductase and endogenous thiols, it may be difficult to detect parent drug in the bloodstream. Diethyldithiocarbamic acid in the blood also reversibly chelates copper, forming a bis(diethyldithiocarbamate)-copper complex. Diethyldithiocarbamic acid is metabolized by a number of different pathways, including glucuronidation, methylation, nonenzymatic degradation, and oxidation. Nonenzymatic degradation of diethyldithiocarbamic

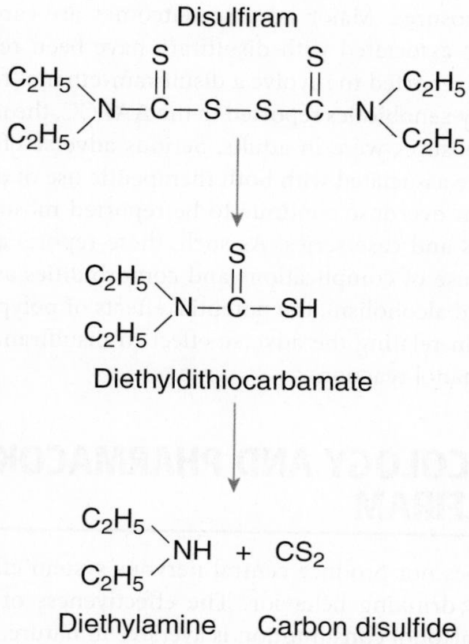

FIGURE 79–1. Disulfiram metabolism occurs in the liver and in the erythrocyte. The most consequential metabolites are diethyldithiocarbamate and carbon disulfide.

acid produces diethylamine and carbon disulfide. Carbon disulfide can be further oxidized to carbonyl sulfide, which, in turn, can be further oxidized to carbon dioxide. Phase II methylation of diethyldithiocarbamic acid, which is mediated by an *S*-methyltransferase, produces diethyldithiomethylcarbamic acid. Diethyldithiomethylcarbamic acid can be oxidized to diethylthiomethylcarbamic acid. Diethylthiomethylcarbamic acid is further oxidized to sulfoxide and sulfone metabolites and undergoes demethylation to form diethylthiocarbamic acid. Although diethyldithiocarbamic acid can be converted back to disulfiram, and carbon disulfide and diethylamine can be converted back to diethyldithiocarbamic acid, these reactions are not clinically significant[27] (Fig. 79–1). Significant interindividual variability exists in the metabolism of disulfiram resulting in varying concentrations of the different metabolites.[29]

ELIMINATION

Following a 250-mg dose, the half-lives of disulfiram, diethyldithiocarbamate, and carbon disulfide are 7.3 ± 1.5 hours, 15.5 ± 4.5 hours, and 8.9 ± 1.4 hours, respectively.[22] Approximately 20% of disulfiram is excreted unchanged in the feces and another 20% or more is excreted by the lungs as carbon disulfide. The majority of disulfiram is excreted in the urine as the glucuronidated metabolite of diethyldithiocarbamic acid.[50] At 48 hours after administration of a single 250-mg dose, there is a negligible amount of disulfiram and metabolites detectable in the serum.[29,48]

DISULFIRAM–ETHANOL REACTION

PHARMACOLOGY AND PHARMACOKINETICS OF DISULFIRAM–ETHANOL REACTION

Understanding the metabolism of ethanol is critical to understanding the mechanism of action of disulfiram as it relates to the disulfiram–ethanol reaction (Fig. 79–2). Disulfiram and its metabolites impair both cytosolic aldehyde dehydrogenase 1 (ALDH 1) and mitochondrial aldehyde dehydrogenase 2 (ALDH 2). A few days of treatment with disulfiram can reduce baseline aldehyde dehydrogenase activity

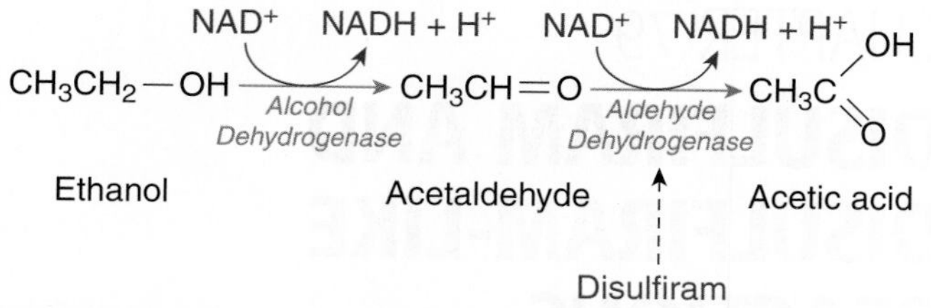

FIGURE 79–2. The site of action of disulfiram. The irreversible inactivation of aldehyde dehydrogenase results in an increased acetaldehyde concentration after ethanol is administered.

by 50%. Although aldehyde dehydrogenase is present throughout the body, inhibition of hepatic mitochondrial aldehyde dehydrogenase is most important in the disulfiram–ethanol reaction. This inhibition by disulfiram of ALDH 2 leads to a rise of acetaldehyde concentrations 5–10 times above baseline.

The exact mechanism by which disulfiram and its metabolites inhibit ALDH 1 and ALDH 2 is still unclear. Disulfiram may inactivate aldehyde dehydrogenase by oxidizing sulfhydryl groups and causing internal sulfur-sulfur bonds, or by competing for nicotinamide adenine dinucleotide.[99] The metabolites of disulfiram, including diethylthiomethylcarbamic acid and its sulfoxide and sulfone metabolites, may also inhibit aldehyde dehydrogenase.[42,50] Different metabolites possibly inactivate different isoenzymes of aldehyde dehydrogenase. Diethylthiocarbamic acid is believed to inactivate ALDH 2. Since aldehyde dehydrogenase inhibition is irreversible, new ALDH must be synthesized to metabolize acetaldehyde.[50] This explains why disulfiram has a longer duration of effect than would be predicted based on its half-life.

The duration of the inhibition of aldehyde dehydrogenase by disulfiram is partially dependent on the dose ingested and the route of administration. A 500-mg dose inhibits aldehyde dehydrogenase for up to 4 days, a 1000-mg dose for up to 6 days, and a 1500-mg dose up to 8 days.[42] Disulfiram-ethanol reaction has been reported up to 1–3 weeks following cessation of disulfiram therapy. There are also sustained-release and depot disulfiram preparations, but none are readily available in the United States. A patient reacted to oral ethanol 21 days following the subcutaneous injection of 2 g of disulfiram.[93] Although the severity of the disulfiram–ethanol reaction following subcutaneous disulfiram dosing is reported to be less than that following oral dosing, this has not been proven.

The accumulation of acetaldehyde, which would normally be metabolized rapidly by aldehyde dehydrogenase, is responsible for many of the symptoms produced by the disulfiram–ethanol reaction. In fact, intravenous administration of acetaldehyde to humans produces symptoms similar to those experienced by patients on disulfiram who consume ethanol.[1,122] Acetaldehyde may increase the release of histamine, which may also be responsible for some of the effects of the disulfiram–ethanol reaction.

Disulfiram–ethanol reactions are reported following exposure to disulfiram by the oral and subcutaneous routes, and to ethanol by any route. Disulfiram–ethanol reactions may follow exposure to the ethanol contained in many products other than alcoholic beverages. Table 79–1 lists some common household products containing ethanol.

OTHER ENZYMES INHIBITED BY DISULFIRAM

Disulfiram and its metabolites inhibit other enzymes besides ALDH 1 and ALDH 2, especially those that contain sulfhydryl groups and metalloproteins. Importantly, disulfiram inhibits dopamine β-hydroxylase (DBH), an enzyme necessary for norepinephrine synthesis.[39,83] The mechanism for this inhibition may be the chelation of copper by

TABLE 79–1. Common Household Products that Contain Ethanol and May Cause a Reaction with Disulfiram[59,91,93,95,99, and 112]

Adhesives
Alcohols: denatured alcohol, rubbing alcohol
Detergents
Foods: liquor-containing desserts, fermented vinegar, some sauces
Nonprescription xenobiotics: analgesics, antacids, antidiarrheals, cough and cold preparations, topical anesthetics, vitamins
Personal hygiene products: after-shave lotions, colognes, contact lens solutions, deodorants, liquid soaps, mouthwashes, perfumes, shampoos, skin liniments and lotions
Solvents

diethyldithiocarbamate, which is necessary for dopamine β-hydroxylase activity.[103] Inhibition of DBH leads to increased CNS concentrations of dopamine and decreased concentrations of epinephrine and norepinephrine. DBH inhibition may contribute to the therapeutic effects of disulfiram, especially in the management of cocaine addiction and may also explain some of the psychiatric effects following both acute disulfiram overdose and chronic disulfiram therapy. Although it has been theorized that some of the neurologic effects following both acute disulfiram overdose and chronic disulfiram therapy may be related to the metabolite carbon disulfide, this has not been confirmed in a well-controlled trial.[97] Decreased norepinephrine in the presence of acetaldehyde, a potential vasodilator, may also account for the hypotension associated with the disulfiram–ethanol reaction. This decrease is consistent with decreased urinary concentrations of vanillylmandelic acid in humans taking disulfiram.[43] Disulfiram and its metabolites may also inhibit microsomal carboxylesterases and plasma cholinesterases.[70]

DISULFIRAM AND THE CYTOCHROME P450 SYSTEM

Disulfiram and its metabolites are inhibitors of cytochrome P450 (CYP) 2E1.[52] Single doses of disulfiram administered to healthy humans result in 50% inhibition of baseline CYP2E1 activity for at least 3 days, with some inhibition for longer than 1 week.[26,28] Although animal studies suggest that disulfiram alters acetaminophen metabolism, a human study found that disulfiram did not significantly alter the metabolism of a therapeutic dose of acetaminophen, in either healthy patients or in patients with alcoholic liver disease.[94] Disulfiram may be an inducer of CYP2B1 and CYP2A1, but it does not appear to affect CYP2C9, CYP2C19, CYP2D6, or CYP3A4 activity.[36,50,52] The effects of disulfiram on CYP enzymes may be both dose and time dependent.

DISULFIRAM–XENOBIOTIC INTERACTIONS

Disulfiram may decrease the clearance of benzodiazepines (chlordiazepoxide, diazepam, and oxazepam),[68] phenytoin,[86] methylxanthines (theophylline[66] and caffeine[36] some tricyclic antidepressants (desipramine and imipramine)[21] and some monamine oxidase inhibitors (tranylcypromine[8]). Disulfiram increases the prothrombin time (international normalized ratio) in patients taking warfarin.[89,104] Combined therapy of disulfiram with omeprazole can cause catatonia.[41] Isoniazid,[126] metronidazole,[104] and methylphenidate[15] may potentiate the neuropsychiatric effects of disulfiram, producing confusion and psychosis.[104]

Patients taking disulfiram therapeutically may develop hypotension following the administration of anesthetic agents.[25] Disulfiram may also increase serum cocaine concentrations and potentiate the cardiovascular effects of cocaine.[75] There is a theoretical concern that disulfiram may decrease the metabolism of propylene glycol found in many liquid and parenteral drug formulations, but specific cases of toxicity have not been reported. Although animal studies suggest that disulfiram may increase the carcinogenicity of ethylene dibromide, this has not been substantiated in humans.[96,131]

DISULFIRAM AS AN ANTIDOTE

Case reports suggest that disulfiram may be useful for the treatment of nickel dermatitis.[20] However, a small double-blind, placebo-controlled study of patients with hand eczema and nickel allergy did not find a clinically significant difference between those treated with disulfiram and those treated with placebo.[51] The conditions of some patients have worsened with this therapy,[55] and because some patients treated for nickel dermatitis have developed hepatitis this therapy is not generally indicated.

Diethyldithiocarbamate, a disulfiram metabolite, is available as the chelator dithiocarb. Although animal data and human case series suggest that diethyldithiocarbamate may be an effective chelator for the treatment of nickel-carbonyl poisoning, no well-controlled human trial has evaluated this therapy.[116] Because disulfiram increases nickel absorption in humans, it is prudent to use disulfiram or diethyldithiocarbamate only for the treatment of nickel-carbonyl poisoning and not for the treatment of elemental or inorganic nickel poisoning. Although animal studies suggest that diethyldithiocarbamate may be effective for nickel-carbonyl poisoning there are no well-controlled human studies[10,93] (see Chap. 97).

CLINICAL MANIFESTATIONS

Data from clinical trails as well as clinical use suggest that there is considerable variation in the development and severity of disulfiram–ethanol reaction.[12,19,70] Symptoms of the disulfiram–ethanol reaction often begin within 15 minutes peak within 30 minutes to 1 hour, and then gradually subside over the next few hours.

Signs and symptoms of a disulfiram–ethanol reaction include nonallergic facial and generalized body warmth and flushing, conjunctival injection, pruritus, urticaria, diaphoresis, lightheadedness, vertigo, headache, nausea, vomiting, and abdominal pain. Cardiac effects include palpitations, chest pain, and dyspnea. Tachycardia and hypotension, including orthostatic hypotension, are common. Rare complications include altered mental status, electrocardiographic abnormalities, shock,[82] dysrhythmias, myocardial ischemia,[79] hypertension,[124,132] bronchospasm,[132] myoclonus,[118] and methemoglobinemia.[114] Esophageal rupture and intracranial hemorrhage secondary to profound vomiting may occur.[31] Deaths attributed to the disulfiram–ethanol reaction occur but are rare.[2,49,82] Many of the historical deaths were associated with doses of disulfiram in excess of current recommended doses.

DISULFIRAM–ETHANOL LIKE REACTIONS

The term *disulfiram like reaction* is commonly used to describe a presentation similar to the typical disulfiram–ethanol reaction when the patient has not been exposed to both disulfiram and ethanol. Most *disulfiram like* reactions involve an exposure to ethanol.[35,56,64,85]

Ingestion of ethanol following ingestion of various *Coprinus* species of mushrooms can cause symptoms of a disulfiram–ethanol reaction (Chap. 117).[102,111]

TABLE 79–2. Xenobiotics Reported to Cause a Disulfiram-like Reaction with Ethanol[6,14,44,56,57,81,85,95,105,111,121,131]

Antimicrobials
- Cephalosporins, especially those that contain a methylthiotetrazole (MTT) side chain, such as cefotetan, cefoperazone, cefamandole, and cefmenoxime.
- Metronidazole
- Moxalactam
- Trimethoprim-sulfamethoxazole
- Possible reactions with chloramphenicol, furazolidone, griseofulvin, nitrofurantoin, procarbazine quinacrine, sulfonamides

Calcium carbimide (citrated)

Carbon disulfide

Carbon tetrachloride

Chloral hydrate

Dimethylformamide

Mushrooms
- *Coprinus* mushrooms including *C. atramentarius, C. insignis, C. variegatus,* and *C. quadrifidus, Boletus luridus, Clitocybe clavipes, Polyporus sulphureus, Pholiota squarosa, Tricholoma aurantum, Verpa bohemica*

Nitrefazole

Phentolamine

Sulfonylurea oral hypoglycemics
- Chlorpropamide
- Tolbutamide

Tacrolimus

Thiram analogs (fungicides)
- Copper, mercuric, and sodium diethyldithiocarbamate
- Zinc and ferric dimethyldithiocarbamate
- Zinc and disodium ethylenebis [dithiocarbamate]

Thiuram analogs:
- Tetraethylthiuram monosulfide and disulfide (disulfiram)
- Tetramethylthiuram disulfide (thiram)

Tolazoline

Trichloroethylene

Many xenobiotics in combination with ethanol have been reported to produce symptoms of the disulfiram–ethanol reaction (Table 79–2). Unfortunately, the potential for disulfiram-like reactions with individual xenobiotics has rarely been studied systematically.[123] Alcohols other than ethanol and organic solvents, including mineral spirits, can also cause symptoms of a disulfiram–ethanol reaction.[109]

MANAGEMENT OF DISULFIRAM–ETHANOL REACTIONS

For most patients experiencing suspected disulfiram–ethanol reactions, it is frequently useful to confirm the presence of ethanol, either with an exhaled ethanol concentration or by obtaining a blood ethanol concentration. Because only small amounts of ethanol can precipitate a disulfiram–ethanol reaction, some patients, especially those with small ingestions or dermal exposures, may still manifest reactions in the absence of detectable ethanol concentrations at the time of evaluation. Elevated acetaldehyde concentrations in the blood will occur during a disulfiram–ethanol reaction, but acetaldehyde concentrations are not readily available, and thus are not clinically useful in managing most patients.

Symptomatic and supportive care is the mainstay of treatment. Gastrointestinal decontamination aimed at removing ethanol is unlikely to have any clinically significant effect on limiting the severity or duration of the disulfiram–ethanol reaction, because even small amounts of ethanol can cause toxicity in the presence of disulfiram. Additionally, because nausea and vomiting are common, patients often experience spontaneous gastric emptying. Antiemetics may improve nausea and vomiting, and histamine (H_1) receptor antagonists, such as diphenhydramine, may lessen cutaneous flushing.[113] Most patients with hypotension respond to intravenous crystalloid administration. Symptomatic hypotension refractory to these measures rarely occurs. If hypotension is refractory to crystalloid administration, a vasopressor should be administered. There is a theoretical benefit to administering a direct-acting vasopressor such as norepinephrine, because disulfiram inhibits dopamine β-hydroxylase, an enzyme necessary for norepinephrine synthesis. Indirect-acting vasopressors, such as dopamine, that require functioning dopamine β-hydroxylase to create a releasable pool of norepinephrine, may be less effective in the setting of disulfiram toxicity. Patients with cardiovascular instability should have an electrocardiogram performed.[62] Most patients with a typical disulfiram–ethanol reaction who have normal vital signs can be safely discharged following resolution of symptoms. More prolonged observation is essential for patients with persistent symptoms, ECG abnormalities, or any potentially life-threatening effect.

Fomepizole, an inhibitor of alcohol dehydrogenase, prevents the metabolism of ethanol to acetaldehyde.[9] Theoretically, by preventing the production of acetaldehyde, fomepizole could limit the effects of the disulfiram–ethanol reaction. A patient on disulfiram experiencing a disulfiram–ethanol reaction was given fomepizole experimentally, with an almost immediate decrease in the serum acetaldehyde concentration, and a rapid clinical improvement.[65] Fomepizole normalized blood acetaldehyde concentrations and relieved the symptoms of the disulfiram–ethanol reaction in four volunteers given calcium carbimide and ethanol.[65] Fomepizole should therefore be considered for patients with life-threatening signs or symptoms of a disulfiram–ethanol reaction who are unresponsive to standard treatment (see Antidotes in Depth A31: Fomepizole).

CLINICAL MANIFESTATIONS

ACUTE DISULFIRAM OVERDOSE

Acute overdose of disulfiram is uncommon and typically does not cause life-threatening toxicity. Most patients will develop symptoms within the first 12 hours following ingestion, with resolution of symptoms within 24 hours of ingestion.

Nausea, vomiting, and abdominal pain are common. A spectrum of central nervous system depression—from drowsiness to coma—may occur.[79] Metabolic acidosis is rare.[69] Dysarthria and movement disorders, including myoclonus, ataxia, dystonia, and akinesia, occur rarely. The movement disorders may be related to direct effects of carbon disulfide on the basal ganglia.[60,63,69] Sensorimotor neuropathy, subacute weakness, and psychosis are uncommon.[45,54] Hypotonia may be a prominent feature in children.[3,6] Persistent neurologic abnormalities, lasting for weeks to months, are reported in both children and adults, but are rare.[69,78,100,133]

CHRONIC DISULFIRAM THERAPY

In published clinical trials disulfiram at therapeutic doses for the treatment of alcoholism appears to be well tolerated.[17,18,24,37] Most of the serious adverse effects associated with disulfiram therapy are derived from case reports involving oral therapy. Toxicity associated with chronic disulfiram therapy correlates poorly with dose, and there is a wide variability in latency period between the time therapeutic dosing is initiated and when symptoms develop. Side effects associated with chronic disulfiram therapy, unsurprisingly, are obviously reported most commonly in alcoholic patients.

Adverse effects most typically involve the liver, the skin, or the central nervous system. Commonly reported effects include nausea, drowsiness, dizziness, irritability, anxiety, headache, a metallic taste in the mouth, halitosis, and skin odor described as having a sulfur or garlic smell, decreased libido, impotence, and hypertension.[43,71,121]

A spectrum of hepatic effects ranging from asymptomatic minor elevations of aminotransferase activity, to hepatic dysfunction, fulminant hepatic failure, and death are reported.[5] Hepatic effects most frequently occur at recommended doses with exposure durations that are extremely variable.[34] The true incidence of disulfiram-associated hepatic effects is unclear. Asymptomatic elevations in aminotransferase concentrations associated with disulfiram therapy have been reported to range from 6% to 30% in alcoholics.[40,119,129] The true incidence likely varies and is dependent on the frequency of sampling. The incidence of hepatic failure or death associated with disulfiram therapy is estimated at 1 in 25,000–30,000 patients treated per year[94] or 1 patient per 1.3 million daily doses distributed.[7] The mechanism of disulfiram-associated hepatotoxicity is poorly understood and may be caused by an immunologic or hypersensitivity reaction, by direct hepatotoxicity related to a metabolite, and possibly related to TNF-α.[22,67] Histologic patterns of toxicity are predominantly hepatocellular, involving eosinophilic leucocyte infiltration and centrilobular disappearance of hepatocytes due to necrosis or apoptosis.[7] Although it is reported that disulfiram-associated hepatotoxicity may be exacerbated by concurrent alcohol consumption and cirrhosis, nonalcoholic patients taking disulfiram as a treatment for nickel dermatitis and patients without biopsy-confirmed cirrhosis have also developed hepatotoxicity.[7,61,63] Although elevated aminotransferase concentrations has been suggested by some as a relative contraindication to initiating disulfiram therapy this has not been confirmed.[7,108] Aminotransferase concentration has not been shown to be different in alcoholics treated with disulfiram who had confirmed hepatitis compared to seronegative patients.[72] Although hepatic effects have most commonly been reported with oral dosage forms they have also been reported with implantable disulfiram.[76]

Dermatoses associated with disulfiram therapy include exfoliative dermatitis, contact dermatitis, urticaria, pruritus, acne, and yellow palms.[107,128] Localized skin reactions at the site of disulfiram implants as well as generalized reactions may occur.[53,120] Healthcare workers handling disulfiram medications may also develop dermatoses.[73] Interestingly, thiram and its analogs, which are found in rubber, are also potent skin sensitizers.[89] Some patients with rubber sensitivity develop localized and generalized dermatitis following ingestion of disulfiram, whereas other patients can be treated with disulfiram without dermatologic complications.[87,125] Disulfiram can also cause exacerbations of nickel and cobalt dermatitis.[55,77] Disulfiram may exacerbate nickel dermatitis because diethyldithiocarbamate complexes with nickel and increases its absorption.[46]

Reported neuropsychiatric side effects include headache, dizziness, confusion,[98] memory impairment,[71] ataxia, parkinsonian and extrapyramidal symptoms,[63] seizures,[23] optic neuropathy,[88] coma, peripheral neuropathy, psychosis including mania,[4,16] depression, catatonia,[32] punding,[30] and organic brain syndrome.[58,106] Confusion, memory impairment, peripheral neuropathy, and psychiatric diagnoses are common in alcoholic patients who are not taking disulfiram. Alcohol-induced and disulfiram-induced peripheral neuropathies are difficult to distinguish clinically. Disulfiram-induced peripheral neuropathy usually involves motor nerves more than sensory and autonomic nerves, is worse distally, and is usually bilateral. A small prospective study of alcoholics taking therapeutic doses of disulfiram revealed abnormalities of peripheral nerve function.[90] Neurologic symptoms may be related to both dose and duration of therapy, but these issues are not well studied.[28] Although case reports suggest an increased incidence of psychiatric complications, one prospective randomized study did not find an increased incidence of psychiatric complications in alcoholic patients taking disulfiram.[11]

Disulfiram therapy may increase serum cholesterol concentration.[74] Although patients with occupational exposures to carbon disulfide, a metabolite of disulfiram, have an increased risk of atherosclerosis and ischemic heart disease, this has not been proven for patients taking disulfiram.[117] One case report suggests that disulfiram may cause thrombocytopenia.[67] Disulfiram is not believed to be carcinogenic. Disulfiram is not routinely indicated for pregnant patients and is currently labeled as FDA pregnancy category C. Although case reports suggest potential teratogenic effects there are no adequate and well-controlled studies in pregnant women.[101]

DIAGNOSTIC TESTING

Serum disulfiram concentrations are not useful when managing most patients with suspected disulfiram toxicity following an acute overdose, chronic therapy, or a disulfiram–ethanol reaction. When interpreting a serum disulfiram concentration, it is important to note that because of rapid metabolism, only a small proportion of ingested disulfiram may appear in the blood as the parent compound.[50] Metabolites of disulfiram, including diethyldithiomethylcarbamic acid and diethylthiomethylcarbamic acid, can also be measured in the serum. Other markers of ingestion of disulfiram include carbon disulfide on the breath and diethylamine in the urine.[33] The activity of hepatic mitochondrial aldehyde dehydrogenase can be determined by liver biopsy, but this is impractical and dangerous. Leukocyte aldehyde dehydrogenase activity correlates most closely with hepatic mitochondrial aldehyde dehydrogenase activity. Decreased erythrocyte ALDH 1 activity and leukocyte ALDH 2 activity are markers of disulfiram exposure, although neither enzyme assay is commonly available.

CHRONIC DISULFIRAM THERAPY

Monitoring for evidence of drug-induced liver injury is recommended during the course of therapy. Unfortunately, for disulfiram specifically and for most other potentially hepatotoxic medications limited data are available on which to base monitoring recommendations.[110] Two common strategies employed for detecting and preventing severe hepatotoxicity include periodic monitoring of biomarkers including alanine aminotransferase (ALT), aspartate aminotransferase (AST), alkaline phosphatase, and total bilirubin as well as clinical monitoring for signs or symptoms of hepatic injury.[129,130] Given the lack of data to inform the most clinically effective and cost effective approach, clinicians should consider employing both strategies.

When monitoring biomarkers in patients on chronic disulfiram therapy, the most effective frequency or duration of testing or intervals between tests is unclear. Biomarker monitoring before initiation of disulfiram to establish a baseline and during the course of therapy is recommended.

Because isolated aminotransferase elevations, without other evidence of impaired hepatic function such as elevated total bilirubin or international normalized ratio (INR), are poor predictors of the development of hepatic dysfunction and hepatic failure, there is poor agreement on when disulfiram therapy should be modified or discontinued based on the finding of mildly elevated aminotransferase concentration.

There is much greater agreement that the development of an aminotransferase concentration greater than 3 times the upper limit of the reference range in combination with evidence of impaired hepatic synthetic function such as jaundice, elevated total bilirubin greater than 2 times the upper limit of the reference range or INR greater than 1.5 is suggestive of more severe drug-induced liver injury. In such situations mortality may be 16% or higher and should necessitate discontinuing disulfiram.[7,110]

As a method of determining compliance with chronic disulfiram therapy, some authors have advocated using ethanol patch testing to produce cutaneous vasodilation. Studies demonstrate that patch testing is not a reliable measure of compliance with disulfiram therapy. Measuring leukocyte aldehyde dehydrogenase activity, or serum concentrations of disulfiram and/or its metabolites, are better measures of compliance with disulfiram therapy.

MANAGEMENT OF DISULFIRAM TOXICITY

ACUTE DISULFIRAM OVERDOSE

Symptomatic and supportive care is the mainstay of treatment. There is no antidote for disulfiram toxicity. No studies have specifically addressed gastrointestinal decontamination in the setting of an acute disulfiram overdose. Unless otherwise contraindicated, activated charcoal, 1 g/kg of body weight, should be administered. It would be unusual for a patient with isolated disulfiram ingestion to require either orogastric lavage or whole-bowel irrigation. Emesis is not indicated, especially because some emetics contain ethanol, which could precipitate a disulfiram–ethanol reaction.

CHRONIC DISULFIRAM TOXICITY

There is indirect evidence that continued use of disulfiram in the face of elevated aminotransferase activity may increase the risk of developing life-threatening hepatotoxicity. Based on research with other medications, most patients on disulfiram who develop mild increased aminotransferase activity will likely adapt and their aminotransferases will normalize with continued disulfiram therapy.[110] Adaptation refers to the liver's ability to adjust to the presence of, and ongoing exposure to, medications such as disulfiram, such that serious hepatic injury or dysfunction does not develop.[84] Since isolated aminotransferase elevations, without other evidence of impaired hepatic function such as elevated total bilirubin or international normalized ratio (INR), are poor predictors of the development of hepatic dysfunction and hepatic failure, there is poor agreement on when disulfiram therapy should be modified or discontinued based on the finding of mildly elevated aminotransferase activity in otherwise asymptomatic patients. If the physician and patient determine that the risk benefit analysis favors continuing disulfiram therapy, enhanced periodic monitoring of aminotransferases and total bilirubin as well as vigilant clinical monitoring for signs and symptoms of hepatic injury such as anorexia, nausea, vomiting, abdominal pain, generalized weakness, malaise, fever, pruritus, scleral icterus, or jaundice is recommended.

Hepatotoxicity usually resolves following discontinuation of disulfiram therapy. Supportive care is the mainstay of treatment for disulfiram-associated hepatic failure. In severe cases, liver transplantation has been successfully performed for disulfiram-induced hepatic failure in both children and adults.[80,96]

SUMMARY

Because disulfiram is still used in comprehensive alcohol treatment programs, it is critical to understand the distinction between the different forms of disulfiram toxicity, including toxicity from an acute overdose, from chronic therapy, and from a disulfiram–ethanol reaction. Disulfiram toxicity following an acute overdose is unlikely to be life-threatening unless a massive amount is ingested, an event that is most likely to occur in suicidal adults. Although death is reported following disulfiram–ethanol reactions, most patients do not develop life-threatening toxicity.

Serious adverse effects associated with chronic disulfiram therapy continue to be reported and are associated with both therapeutic use of disulfiram and with disulfiram overdose. Most of the adverse effects are reported from case reports and case series which are difficult to interpret because of the complications and comorbidities associated with alcohol use and alcoholism, the potential effects of polypharmacy, and difficulty in relating the adverse effect to disulfiram, alcohol or a disulfiram–ethanol reaction. Although serious and life-threatening effects are associated with disulfiram the most significant is the disulfiram-associated hepatic failure which appears to be a very rare occurrence.

REFERENCES

1. Asmussen E, Hald J, Larsen V. The pharmacological action of acetaldehyde on the human organism. *Acta Pharmacol Toxicol*. 1948:4:311-320.
2. Becker MC, Sugarman G. Death following "test drink" of alcohol in patients receiving Antabuse. *JAMA*. 1952;149:568-571.
3. Benitz WE, Tatro DS. Disulfiram intoxication in a child. *J Pediatr*. 1984;105:487-489.
4. Bennett AE, McKeever LG, Turk RE. Psychotic reaction during tetraethylthiuram disulfide (Antabuse) therapy. *JAMA*. 1951;145:483-484.
5. Berlin RG. Disulfiram hepatotoxicity: a consideration of its mechanism and clinical spectrum. *Alcohol Alcohol*. 1989;24:241-246.
6. Billstein SA, Sudol TE. Disulfiram-like reactions rare with ceftriaxone. *Geriatrics*. 1992;47:70.
7. Björnsson E, Nordlinder H, Olsson R. Clinical characteristics and prognostic markers in disulfiram-induced liver injury. *J Hepatol*. 2006;44:791-797.
8. Blansjaar BA, Egberts T. Delirium in a patient treated with disulfiram and tranylcypromine. *Am J Psych*. 1995;152;2:296.
9. Blomstrand R, Theorell H. Inhibitory effect on ethanol oxidation in man after administration of 4-methylpyrazole. *Life Sci*. 1970;9:631-640.
10. Bradberry SM, Vale JA. Therapeutic review: do diethyldithiocarbamate and disulfiram have a role in acute nickel carbonyl poisoning? *J Toxicol Clin Toxicol*. 1999;37:259-264.
11. Branchey L, Davis W, Lee KK, et al. Psychiatric complications of disulfiram treatment. *Am J Psych*. 1987;144:1310-1312.
12. Brewer C. How effective is the standard dose of disulfiram? A review of the alcohol-disulfiram reaction in practice. *Br J Psychiatry*. 1984;144:202-204.
13. Brien JF, Loomis CW. Disposition and pharmacokinetics of disulfiram and calcium carbimide (calcium cyanamide). *Drug Metab Rev*. 1983;14:113-126.
14. Brown KR, Guglielmo BJ, Pons VG, et al. Theophylline elixir, moxalactam, and a disulfiram reaction. *Ann Intern Med*. 1982;97:621-622.
15. Caci H, Baylě F. A case of disulfiram-methylphenidate interaction: implications for treatment. *Am J Psych*. 2007;164:11
16. Ceylan ME, Turkcan A, Mutlu E, et al. Manic episode with psychotic symptoms associated with high dose of disulfiram. A case report. *J Clin Psychopharmacol*. 2007;27:224-225.
17. Chick J, Gough K, Falkowski W, et al. Disulfiram treatment of alcoholism. *Br J Psychiatry*. 1992;161:84-89

18. Christensen JK, Ronsted P, Vagg UH. Side effects after disulfiram. *Acta Psychiatr Scand*. 1984;69:265-273
19. Christensen JK, Moller IB, Ronsted P, et al. Dose-effect relationship of disulfiram in human volunteers. I. Clinical studies. *Pharmacol Toxicol*. 1991;68:163-165.
20. Christensen OB, Kristensen M. Treatment with disulfiram in chronic nickel hand dermatitis. *Contact Dermatitis*. 1982;8:59-63.
21. Ciraulo DA, Barnhill J, Boxenbaum H, et al. Pharmacokinetic interaction of disulfiram and antidepressants. *Am J Psychiatry*. 1985;142:1373-1374.
22. Cvek B. TNF-α could be responsible for disulfiram-mediated hepatotoxicity. *J Hepatol*. 2008;49:862-866.
23. Daniel DG, Swallows A, Wolff F. Capgras delusion and seizures in association with therapeutic dosages of disulfiram. *South Med J*. 1987;80:1577-1579.
24. DeSousa A, Desousa A. An open randomized study comparing disulfiram and acamprosate in the treatment of alcohol dependence. *Alcohol Alcohol*. 2006;40:545-548.
25. Diaz JH, Hill GE. Hypotension with anesthesia in disulfiram-treated patients. *Anesthesiology*. 1979;51:366-368.
26. Emery MG, Jubert C, Thymmel KE, et al. Duration of cytochrome P450 2E1 (CYP2E1) inhibition and estimation of functional CYP2E1 enzyme half-life after single-dose disulfiram administration in humans. *J Pharmacol Exp Ther*. 1999;291:213-219.
27. Eneanya DI, Bianchine JR, Duran DO, et al. The actions and metabolic fate of disulfiram. *Annu Rev Pharmacol Toxicol*. 1981;21:575-596.
28. Enghusen Poulsen H, Loft S, Andersen JR, et al. Disulfiram therapy-adverse drug reactions and interactions. *Acta Psychiatr Scand Suppl*. 1992;369:59-66.
29. Faiman MD, Jensen JC, La Coursiere R. Elimination of disulfiram and metabolites in alcoholics after single and repeated doses. *Clin Pharmacol Ther*. 1984;36:520-526.
30. Fan CC, Lin SK, Huang MC. Disulfiram-induced punding. *J Clin Psychopharmacol*. 2008;28:473-474.
31. Fernandez D. Another esophageal rupture after alcohol and disulfiram. *N Engl J Med*. 1972;286:610.
32. Fisher CM. “Catatonia” due to disulfiram toxicity. *Arch Neurol*. 1989;46:798-804.
33. Fletcher K, Stone E, Mohamad MW, et al. A breath test to assess compliance with disulfiram. *Addiction*. 2006;101:1705-1710.
34. Forns X, Caballeria J, Bruguera M, et al. Disulfiram-induced hepatitis. Report of four cases and review of the literature. *J Hepatol*. 1994;21:853-857.
35. Foster T, Raehl C, Wilson H. Disulfiram-like reactions associated with a parenteral cephalosporin. *Am J Hosp Pharm*. 1980;37:858-859.
36. Fry RF, Branch RA. Effect of chronic disulfiram administration on the activities of CYP1A2, CYP2C19, CYP2D6, CYP2E1 and N-acetyltransferase in healthy human subjects. *Br J Clin Pharmacol*. 2002;53:155-162.
37. Fuller RK, Brahchey L, Brightwell DR, et al. Disulfiram treatment of alcoholism: a Veterans Administration cooperative study *JAMA*. 1986;256:1449-1455.
38. Garbutt JC, West SL, Carey TS, et al. Pharmacological treatment of alcohol dependence. A review of the evidence. *JAMA*. 1999;281:1318-1325.
39. Goldstein M, Anagnoste B, Lauber E, et al. Inhibition of dopamine-β-hydroxylase by disulfiram. *Life Sci*. 1964;3:763-767.
40. Goyer PF, Major LF. Heptotoxicity in disulfiram treated patients. *J Stud Alcohol*. 1979;40:133-137.
41. Hajela R, Cunningham GM, Kapur BM, et al. Catatonic reaction to omeprazole and disulfiram in a patient with alcohol dependence. *CMAJ*. 1990;143:1207-1208.
42. Hald JE, Jacobsen E, Larsen V. The formation of acetaldehyde in the organism after ingestion of Antabuse (tetraethylthiuram disulfide) and alcohol. *Acta Pharmacol Toxicol*. 1948;4:285-310.
43. Heath RG, Nesselhof W, Bishop MP, et al. Behavioral and metabolic changes associated with administration of tetraethylthiuram disulfide (Antabuse). *Dis Nerv Sys*. 1965;26:99-104.
44. Heelon MW, White M. Disulfiram-cotrimoxazole reaction. *Pharmacotherapy*. 1998;18:869-870.
45. Hirschberg M, Ludolph A, Grotemeyer KH, et al. Development of a subacute tetraparesis after disulfiram intoxication. Case report. *Eur Neurol*. 1987;26:222-228.
46. Hopfer SM, Linden JV, Rezuke WN, et al. Increased nickel concentrations in body fluids of patients with chronic alcoholism during disulfiram therapy. *Res Commun Chem Pathol Pharmacol*. 1987;55:101-109.
47. Hughes JC, Cook CC. The efficacy of disulfiram: a review of outcome studies. *Addiction*. 1997;92:381-395.
48. Jensen JC, Faiman MD, Hurwitz A. Elimination characteristics of disulfiram in alcoholics after single and repeated doses. *Clin Pharmacol Ther*. 1984;36:500-506.
49. Jones RO. Death following ingestion of alcohol in Antabuse treated patient. *Can Med Assoc J*. 1949;60:609-612.
50. Johansson B. A review of the pharmacokinetics and pharmacodynamics of disulfiram and its metabolites. *Acta Psychiatr Scand Suppl*. 1992;369:15-26.
51. Kaaber K, Menne T, Veien N, et al. Treatment of nickel dermatitis with Antabuse: a double-blind study. *Contact Dermatitis*. 1983;9:297-299.
52. Kharasch ED, Hankins DC, Jubert C, et al. Lack of single-dose disulfiram effect on cytochrome P-450 2C9, 2C19, 2D6, and 3A4 activities: evidence for specificity toward P-450 2E1. *Drug Metab Dispos*. 1999;27:717-723.
53. Kieć-Świerczyńska M, Krecisz B, Fabicka B. Systemic contact dermatitis from implanted disulfiram. *Contact Dermatitis*. 2000;43:246-247.
54. Kirubakaran V, Liskow B, Mayfield D, et al. Case report of acute disulfiram overdose. *Am J Psychiatry*. 1983;140:1513-1514.
55. Klein LR, Fowler JF. Nickel dermatitis recall during disulfiram therapy for alcohol abuse. *J Am Acad Dermatol*. 1992;26:645-646.
56. Kline SS, Mauro VF, Forney RB, et al. Cefotetan-induced disulfiram-type reactions and hypoprothrombinemia. *Antimicrob Agents Chemother*. 1987;31:1328-1331.
57. Klink DD, Fritz RD, Franke GH. Disulfiram-like reaction to chlorpropamide. *Wis Med J*. 1969;68:134-136.
58. Knee ST, Razani J. Acute organic brain syndrome: a complication of disulfiram. *Am J Psychiatry*. 1974;131:1281-1282.
59. Koff RS, Papadimas I, Honig EG. Alcohol in cough mixture, a hazard to disulfiram user. *JAMA*. 1971;215:1988-1989.
60. Krauss JK, Mohadjer M, Wakhloo AK, et al. Dystonia and akinesia due to pallidoputaminal lesions after disulfiram intoxication. *Mov Disord*. 1992;6:166-170.
61. Kristensen ME. Toxic hepatitis induced by disulfiram in a non-alcoholic. *Acta Med Scand*. 1981;209:335-336.
62. Laaksonen E, Koski-Jannes A, Salaspuro M, et al. A randomized, multicentre, open label, comparative trial of disulfiram, naltrexone, and acamprosate in the treatment of alcohol dependence. *Alcohol Alcohol*. 2008;43:53-61.
63. Laplane D, Attal N, Sauron B, et al. Lesions of the basal ganglia due to disulfiram neurotoxicity. *J Neurol Neurosurg Psychiatry*. 1992;55:925-929.
64. Levy MS, Livingstone BL, Collins DM. A clinical comparison of disulfiram and calcium carbimide. *Am J Psychiatry*. 1967;123:1018-1022.
65. Lindros KO, Stowell A, Pikkarainen P, et al. The disulfiram (Antabuse)-alcohol reaction in male alcoholics: its efficient management by 4-methylpyrazole. *Alcohol Clin Exp Res*. 1981;5:528-530.
66. Loi CM, Day JD, Jue SG, et al. Dose-dependent inhibition of theophylline metabolism by disulfiram in recovering alcoholics. *Clin Pharmacol Ther*. 1989;45:476-486.
67. Lu JW, Wang H, Yan-Li J, et al. Differential effects of pyrrolidine dithiocarbamate on TNF-α-mediated liver injury in two different models of fulminant hepatitis. *J Hepatol*. 2008;48:442-552.
68. MacLeod SM, Sellers EM, Giles HG, et al. Interaction of disulfiram with benzodiazepines. *Clin Pharmacol Ther*. 1978;24:583-589.
69. Mahajan P, Lieh-Lai MW, Sarnaik A, et al. Basal ganglia infarction in a child with disulfiram poisoning. *Pediatrics*. 1997;99:605-608.
70. Malcolm R, Lechner, MFO, Lechner W. The safety of disulfiram for the treatment of alcohol and cocaine dependence in randomized clinical trials: guidance for clinical practice. *Expert Opin Drug Saf*. 2008;7:459-472.
71. Martensen-Larsen O. Five years experience with disulfiram in the treatment of alcoholics. *Q J Stud Alcohol*. 1953;14:406-418.
72. Martin B, Alfers J, Kulig C, et al. Disulfiram therapy in patients with hepatitis-C: a 12-month controlled study. *J Stud Alcohol*. 2004;65:651-657.
73. Mathelier-Fusade P, Leynadier F. Occupational allergic contact reaction to disulfiram. *Contact Dermatitis*. 1994;31:121-122.
74. Major LF, Goyer PF. Effects of disulfiram and pyridoxine on serum cholesterol. *Ann Intern Med*. 1978;88:53-56.
75. McCance-Katz EF, Kosten TR, Jatlow P. Disulfiram effects on acute cocaine administration. *Drug Alcohol Depend*. 1998;52:27-39.
76. Meier M, Woywodt A, Hoeper MM, et al. Acute liver failure: a message found under the skin. *Postgrad Med J*. 2005;81:269-270.
77. Menne T. Flare-up of cobalt dermatitis from Antabuse treatment. *Contact Dermatitis*. 1985;12:53.

78. Mesiwala AH, Loeser JD. Bilateral globus pallidus infarction secondary to disulfiram ingestion. *Pediatr Neurosurg.* 2001;34:224.
79. Milne HJ, Parke TRJ. Hypotension and ST depression as a result of disulfiram ethanol reaction. *Eur J Emerg Med.* 2007;14:228-229.
80. Mohanty SR, LaBrecque DR, Mitros FA, et al. Liver transplantation for disulfiram-induced fulminant hepatic failure. *J Clin Gastroenterol.* 2004;38:292-295.
81. Morales-Molina J, Mateu-de Antonio J, Grau S, et al. Alcohol ingestion and topical tacrolimus: a disulfiram-like interaction. *Ann Pharmacother.* 2005;39:772-773.
82. Motte S, Vincent JL, Gillet JB, et al. Refractory hyperdynamic shock associated with alcohol and disulfiram. *Am J Emerg Med.* 1986;4:323-325.
83. Musacchio JM, Goldstein M, Anagnoste B, et al. Inhibition of dopamine-β-hydroxylase by disulfiram in vivo. *J Pharmacol Exp Ther.* 1966;152:56-61.
84. Navarro VJ, Senior JR. Drug-related hepatotoxicity. *N Engl J Med.* 2006;354:731-739.
85. Neu HC, Prince AS. Interaction between moxalactam and alcohol. *Lancet.* 1980;1:1422.
86. Olesen OV. Disulfiram (Antabuse) as inhibitor of phenytoin metabolism. *Acta Pharmacol Toxicol.* 1966;24:317-322.
87. Olfson M. Disulfiram and allergy to rubber. *Am J Psych.* 1988;145:651-652.
88. Orakzai A, Guerin M, Beatty S. Disulfiram-induced transient optic and peripheral neuropathy: a case report. *Ir J Med Sci.* 2007;176:319-321.
89. O'Reilly RA. Interaction of sodium warfarin and disulfiram (Antabuse) in man. *Ann Intern Med.* 1973;78:73-76.
90. Palliyath SK, Schwartz BD, Gant L. Peripheral nerve functions in chronic alcoholic patients on disulfiram: a six-month follow-up. *J Neurol Neurosurg Psychiatry.* 1990;53:227-230.
91. Petroni NC, Cardoni AA. Alcohol content of liquid medicinals. *Clin Toxicol.* 1979;14:407-432.
92. Pettinati HM, Kampman KM, Lynch KG, et al. A double blind, placebo-controlled trial that combines disulfiram and naltrexone for treating co-occurring cocaine and alcohol dependence. *Addict Behav.* 2008;33:651-657.
93. Phillips M. Persistent sensitivity to ethanol following a single dose of parenteral sustained-release disulfiram. *Adv Alcohol Subst Abuse.* 1987;7:51-61.
94. Poulsen HE, Ranek L, Jorgensen L. The influence of disulfiram on acetaminophen metabolism in man. *Xenobiotica.* 1991;21:243-249.
95. Poulsen E, Loft H, Andersen JR, et al. Disulfiram therapy-adverse drug reactions and interactions. *Acta Psychaiatr Scand.* 1992;86:59-66.
96. Rabkin JM, Corless CL, Orloff SL, et al. Liver transplantation for disulfiram-induced hepatic failure. *Am J Gastroenterol.* 1998;93:830-831.
97. Rainey JM. Disulfiram toxicity and carbon disulfide poisoning. *Am J Psychiatry.* 1977;134:371-378.
98. Rathod NH. Toxic effects of disulfiram therapy, with two case reports. *Q J Study Alcohol.* 1958;19:418-427.
99. Refojo MF. Disulfiram-alcohol reaction caused by contact lens wetting solution. *Contact Intraocul Lens Med J.* 1981;7:172.
100. Reichelderfer TE. Acute disulfiram poisoning in a child. *Q J Study Alcohol.* 1969;30:724-728.
101. Reitnaurer P, Callanan NP, Farber RA, et al. Prenatal exposure to disulfiram implicated in the cause of malformations in discordant monozygotic twins. *Teratology.* 1997;56:358-362.
102. Reynolds WA, Lowe FH. Mushrooms and a toxic reaction to alcohol. *N Engl J Med.* 1965;272:630-631.
103. Rogers WK, Benowitz NL, Wilson KM, et al. Effect of disulfiram on adrenergic function. *Clin Pharmacol Ther.* 1979;25:469-477.
104. Rothstein E. Warfarin effect enhanced by disulfiram (Antabuse). *JAMA.* 1972;22:1052.
105. Rothstein E, Clancy DD. Toxicity of disulfiram combined with metronidazole. *N Engl J Med.* 1969;280:1006-1007.
106. Ryan TV, Sciara AD, Barth JT. Chronic neuropsychological impairment resulting from disulfiram overdose. *J Stud Alcohol.* 1993;54:389-392.
107. Santonastaso M, Cecchetti E, Pace M, et al. Yellow palms with disulfiram. *Lancet.* 1997;350:1176.
108. Saxon AJ, Sloan KL, Reoux J, et al. Disulfiram use in patients with abnormal liver function test results. *J Clin Psychiatry.* 1998;59:313-316.
109. Scott GE, Little FW. Disulfiram reaction to organic solvents other than ethanol. *N Engl J Med.* 1985;312:790.
110. Senior JR. Monitoring for hepatotoxicity: what is the predictive value of liver "function" tests. *Clin Pharmacol Therapeut.* 2009;85:331-334.
111. Spoerke DG, Rumack BH, eds. *Handbook of Mushroom Poisoning—Diagnosis and Treatment.* Boca Raton, FL: CRC Press; 1994.
112. Stoll D, King LE Jr. Disulfiram-alcohol skin reaction to beer-containing shampoo. *JAMA.* 1980;244:2045.
113. Stowell A, Johnson J, Ripel Å, et al. Diphenhydramine and the calcium carbimide-ethanol reaction: a placebo-controlled clinical trial. *Clin Pharmacol Ther.* 1986;39:521-525.
114. Stransky G, Lambing MK, Simmons GT, et al. Methemoglobinemia in a fatal case of disulfiram-ethanol reaction. *J Anal Toxicol.* 1997;21:178-179.
115. Suh JJ, Pettinati HM, Kampman KM, et al. The status of disulfiram: a half of a century later. *J Clin Psychopharmacol.* 2006;26:290-302.
116. Sunderman FW. Use of sodium diethyldithiocarbamate in the treatment of nickel carbonyl poisoning. *Ann Clin Lab Sci.* 1990;20:12-21.
117. Sweetnam PM, Taylor SWC, Elwood PC. Exposure to carbon disulphide and ischaemic heart disease in a viscose rayon factory. *Br J Indus Med.* 1987;44:220-227.
118. Syed J, Moarefi G. An unusual presentation of a disulfiram alcohol reaction. *Del Med J.* 1995;67:183.
119. Tamai H, Yokoyama A, Okuyama K, et al. Comparison of cyanamide and disulfiram in effects on liver function. *Alcohol Clin Exp Res.* 2000;24:97s-99s.
120. Thompson CC, Tacke RB, Woolley LH, et al. Purpuric oral and cutaneous lesions in a case of drug-induced thrombocytopenia. *J Am Dent Assoc.* 1982;105:465-467.
121. Truitt EB, Puritz G, Morgan AM, et al. Disulfiram-like actions produced by hypoglycemic sulfonylurea compounds. *Q J Stud Alcohol.* 1962;23:197-207.
122. Vallari RC, Pietruszko R. Human aldehyde dehydrogenase: mechanism of inhibition of disulfiram. *Science.* 1982;216:637-639.
123. Visapää JP, Tillonen JS, Kaihovaara PS. Lack of disulfiram-like reaction with metronidazonle and ethanol. *Ann Pharmacother.* 2002;36:971-974.
124. Volicer L, Nelson KL. Development of reversible hypertension during disulfiram therapy. *Arch Intern Med.* 1984;144:1294-1296.
125. Webb PK, Gibbs SC, Mathias CT, et al. Disulfiram hypersensitivity and rubber contact dermatitis. *JAMA.* 1979;241:2061.
126. Whittington HG, Grey L. Possible interaction between disulfiram and isoniazid. *Am J Psychiatry.* 1969;125:1725-1729.
127. Williams EE. Effects of alcohol on workers with carbon disulfide. *JAMA.* 1937;109:1472-1473.
128. Wilson H. Side effects of disulfiram. *BMJ.* 1962;2:1610.
129. Wright C, Vafier JA, Lake CR. Disulfiram-induced fulminating hepatitis: guidelines for liver-panel monitoring. *J Clin Psychiatry.* 1988;49:430-434.
130. Wright C, Moore R, Grodin DM, et al. Screening for disulfiram-induced liver test dysfunction in an in-patient alcoholism program. *Alcohol Clin Exp Res.* 1993;17:184-186.
131. Yodaiken RE. Ethylene dibromide and disulfiram—a lethal combination. *JAMA.* 1978;239:2783.
132. Zapata E, Orwin A. Severe hypertension and bronchospasm during disulfiram-ethanol test reaction. *BMJ.* 1992;305:870.
133. Zorzon M, Mase G, Biasutti E, et al. Acute encephalopathy and polyneuropathy after disulfiram intoxication. *Alcohol Alcohol.* 1995;30:629-631.

CHAPTER 80
γ-HYDROXYBUTYRIC ACID

Brenna M. Farmer

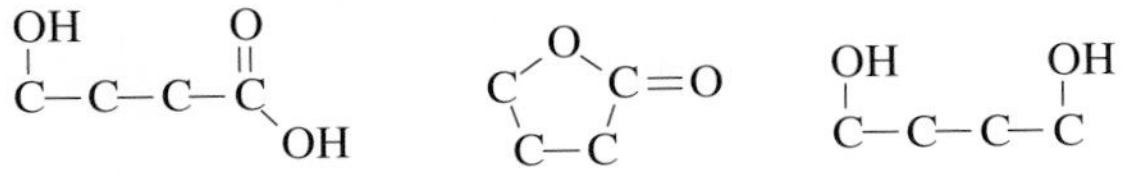

γ-Hydroxybutyric Acid [GHB] γ-Butyrolactone [GBL] Butanediol

Gamma-hydroxybutryic acid, or GHB, is an abused xenobiotic and a neurotransmitter and neuromodulator that is produced in the brain. It has also been synthesized and used and abused in this form. It has been used experimentally to treat absence seizures in animals,[63] as an adjunct to general anesthesia, as a sleep agent, as an anabolic nutritional supplement, and to treat alcohol dependence and alcohol withdrawal.[30,45,51,73] It is classified as a Schedule I drug due to its popularity as a drug of abuse and its association with drug facilitated sexual assault, and also as a Schedule III drug for the treatment of narcolepsy.[22] Two precursors of GHB, γ-butyrolactone (GBL) and 1,4-butanediol (1,4-BD)[64] have many industrial uses but are also used as recreational drugs and as drugs to achieve chemical submission (as "date rape" drugs). These two precursors exert their effects through conversion to GHB.[8,52] Numerous other analogs of GHB have industrial and commercial uses (see Table 80–1) and may result in GHB intoxication.

HISTORY AND EPIDEMIOLOGY

GHB was discovered in 1960 while searching for an analog for γ-aminobutyric acid (GABA).[33] Due to its CNS depressive and amnestic properties, GHB was used initially as an anesthetic adjunct, especially in Europe but never gained favor in the United States for this indication. During the 1970s, an FDA-investigational new drug protocol was submitted to test the use of GHB as a treatment for sleep disturbances. In the 1980s and 1990s, body builders popularized GHB as an anabolic dietary supplement due to its release of growth hormone. Its euphoric effects were recognized at this time, and it rapidly gained favor as a "club drug." Because it can cause coma and profound amnesia, GHB has been used in drug-facilitated sexual assault, and in 1990 the FDA banned all use of nonprescription GHB due to this concern.[61]

Following the FDA ban, the analogs GBL and 1,4-BD were quickly substituted for GHB in dietary supplements. After the Samantha Reid and Hillory J. Farias Date-Rape Prevention Act of 1999 was passed in 2000 the DEA classified GHB and its analogs as Schedule I substances claiming that GHB was a hazard to public safety.[19,61] Also in 2000, a new drug application was submitted to the FDA for GHB—under the generic name sodium oxybate and the trade name Xyrem®—to reduce the incidence of cataplexy and improve the symptoms of daytime sleepiness in patients with narcolepsy.[77] This latter indication was approved in 2002 and given a Schedule III designation by the DEA,[76] which was expanded, in 2005, to include the treatment of excessive daytime sleepiness in patients with narcolepsy.

In 2007, during an epidemic of toxicity from toy beads, marketed under the names Bindeez®or Aquadots®, 1,4-BD was identified in the sticky surface material that allowed the beads to reversibly adhere to one another. Multiple cases of toxicity were reported, largely in England and Australia.[26,56]

National statistics demonstrated a trend of escalating GHB abuse and poisoning throughout the 1990s. However, a decline has been seen in exposures reported to poison control centers and the Drug Abuse Warning Network in recent years. In 2002, there were 1386 exposures with GHB and its analogs and precursors reported to the American Association of Poison Control Centers (AAPCC)–Toxic Exposure Surveillance System, representing more than a 2-fold increase from approximately 600 GHB cases reported in 1996. Among these, 1181 exposures (85%) required treatment in a healthcare facility and resulted in 272 major outcomes and 3 deaths (see Chap. 135).[74] More recently there has been a further decline in the number of reported exposures to GHB and its analogs. From the 2006 AAPCC report, 485 cases mentioned exposure to GHB and its analogs. In 297 of those cases, GHB and or its analogs were listed as the single agent of exposure. Of the cases reported, 232 were treated in healthcare facilities with 145 of those cases resulting in "moderate" or "severe" findings according to the National Poison Center Database. One death was associated with confirmed GBL exposure when it was ingested with ethanol.[7] This trend in reduced use/abuse is also consistent with the Drug Abuse Warning Network's (DAWN) 2005 estimates which were 1861 emergency department (ED) visits for GHB exposures while their 2004 estimate was 2340 ED visits.[15]

The apparent trend of decreased GHB exposures in the United States after 2000 contrasts starkly with the increased use reported in some European countries (Denmark, Sweden, and Norway) and Australia.[11,14,32] In Melbourne, Australia, a recent retrospective study showed a 4% increase per month in the number of ambulance calls related to GHB and its analogs from March 2001 to October 2005.[11]

PHARMACOLOGY

GHB is both a precursor and degradation product of GABA.[64] It has a dual pharmacologic profile, with the neuropharmacology of endogenous GHB being distinct and divergent from that of exogenously administered GHB. The principal difference between their profiles is that the activity of endogenous GHB appears to be mediated by the GHB receptor, whereas the activity of exogenously administered GHB is most likely mediated by intrinsic activity at the $GABA_B$ receptor.

ENDOGENEOUS GHB

GHB is formed from GABA by the enzymes GABA transaminase and succinic semialdehyde reductase[41] (see Fig. 80–1). GHB is also endogeneously transformed from GBL by lactonases and from 1,4-BD by alcohol and aldehyde dehydrogenases. Endogeneous GHB acts as a putative neurotransmitter found in highest concentrations in the hippocampus, basal ganglia, hypothalamus, striatum, and substantia nigra.[41,43,71] It has subcellular systems for synthesis, vesicular uptake, and storage in presynaptic terminals. It is released in a Ca^{2+}-dependent manner following depolarization of neurons.

After release, GHB binds to GHB-specific receptors that modulate other neurotransmitter systems.

Endogeneous GHB acts predominantly on the GHB receptor, which is a G protein–linked receptor located presynaptically.[12,41,62] The GHB receptor is located in the synaptosomal membranes of neuronal cells most highly concentrated in the pons and hippocampus followed by the cerebral cortex and caudate. The GHB receptor has no affinity for typical $GABA_A$ or $GABA_B$ agonists such as GABA and baclofen,

TABLE 80–1. Common Synonyms for GHB and Analogs

GHB γ-Hydroxybutyrate	GBL γ-Butyrolactone	1,4-BD 1,4-bButanediol	GHV γ-Hydroxyvaleric Acid	GVL γ-Valerolactone	THF Tetrahydrofuran
γ-Hydroxybutyric acid 4-Hydroxybutyric acid sodium salt γ-Hydroxybutyric acid sodium salt Sodium oxybate Sodium 4-hydroxybutyrate 4-Hydroxybutanoic acid	2(3H)-Furanone dihydro Butyrolactone 4-Butyrolactone Dihydro-2(3H)-furanone 2(3H)-Furanone Tetrahydro-2-furanone 4-Deoxytetronic acid Butyryl lactone Butyric acid lactone Butyrolactone-gamma 4-Hydroxbutyric acid lactone γ-Hydroxybutyric acid lactone 4-Butanolide 1,4-Butanolide 1,4-Lactone	1,4-Butylene glycol 1,4-Dihydroxybutane 1,4-Tetramethylene glycol	γ-Methyl-GHB	4-Hydroxypentanoic acid lactone 4,5-Dihydro-5-methyl-2(3H)-furanone γ-Methyl-GHB	No other synonyms

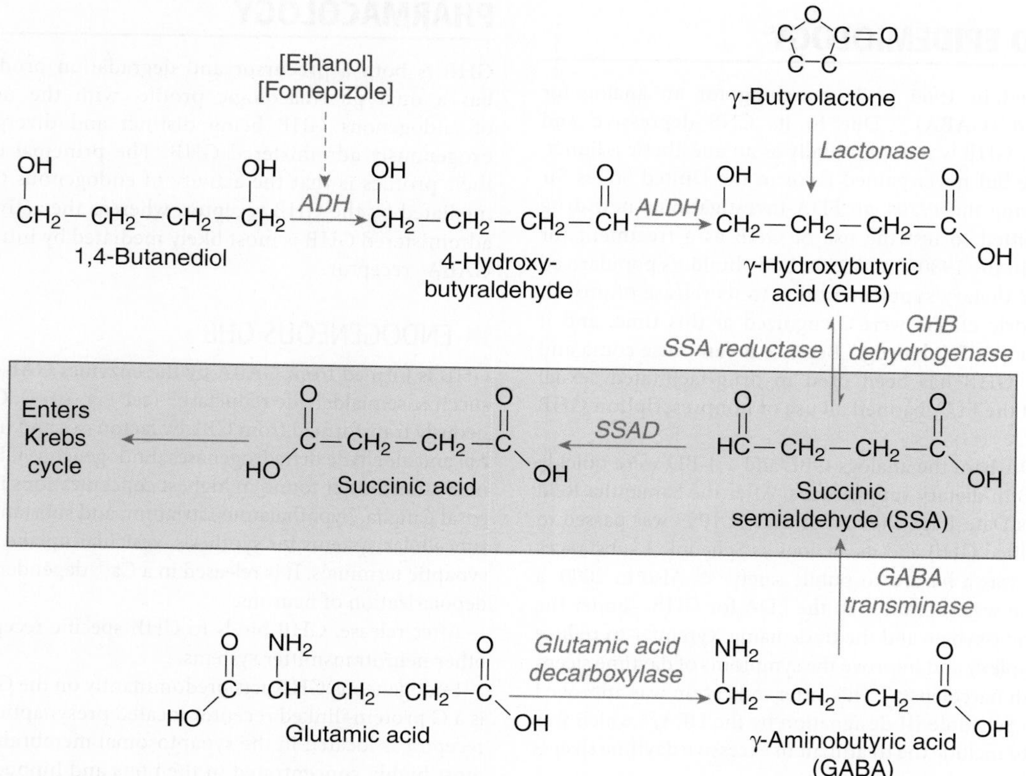

FIGURE 80–1. The synthesis and metabolism of γ-hydroxybutyric acid. ADH, alcohol dehydrogenase; ALDH, aldehyde dehydrogenase; SSA reductase, succinic semialdehyde reductase; SSAD, succinic semialdehyde dehydrogenase.

respectively. Localized application of GHB can produce a response that mimics the action of endogenous GHB released by nerve stimulation.[4,46]

GHB activity is terminated by active uptake from the synaptic cleft for metabolism by specific cytosolic and mitochondrial enzymes.

GHB receptors are highly associated with dopaminergic neurons and increase the concentration of dopamine by stimulating tyrosine hydroxylase to synthesize dopamine.[41,65,67] GHB is also a neuromodulator of dopamine, acetylcholine, endogeneous opioids, and glutamate.[41] It either increases (concentrations below 1 m*M*) or decreases (at higher concentrations) the release of dopamine throughout the mesolimbic system.[10] In contrast, GHB increases dopamine concentrations in the striatum and cortex in a dose-dependent manner by stimulating tyrosine hydroxylase to synthesize dopamine.[41,42,65] GHB also increases the turnover of serotonin in the brain by stimulating both serotonin synthesis and breakdown.[25,29] Furthermore, GHB decreases acetylcholine in the brainstem and corpus striatum, as well as in the hippocampus (via $GABA_B$ receptors).[47,65] GBL, but not GHB itself, increases total brain acetylcholine concentrations by decreasing firing of cholinergic neurons.[24,34,58]

Through an unclear mechanism, GHB increases the release of growth hormone by promoting slow wave sleep without effecting total sleep time and GHB release is enhanced.[69,72] Although GHB has no effect on total sleep time, it decreases latency to slow wave sleep while also decreasing the time spent in stage 1 and stage 2 of the sleep cycle.[35]

EXOGENEOUS GHB

Exogeneous GHB, which produces supraphysiologic GHB concentrations, acts predominantly on the $GABA_B$ receptor which is found throughout the cerebral cortex, cerebellum, and thalamus.[23,28,55,75] Presynaptically and postsynaptically, these receptors signal the adenylate cyclase system to activate calcium channels and G protein coupled inwardly rectifying potassium channels.[5] Through these $GABA_B$ receptor signaling pathways, both dopamine and acetylcholine pathways are altered leading to decreased dopamine release and decreased acetylcholine concentrations.[10,47] These effects of GHB are potentiated by baclofen, a $GABA_B$ receptor agonist. Further discussion of these receptors and pathways is found in Chapter 13.

GHB ANALOGS

GBL, like GHB, exists in the mammalian brain.[13] Its pharmacologic properties are only evident after conversion to its active metabolite, GHB. Like GBL, 1,4-BD occurs naturally in the brain and exerts its pharmacologic and toxicologic properties only when converted to GHB by alcohol dehydrogenase.[53]

Table 80–1 lists other GHB analogs known to result in similar toxicity and lists synonyms for GHB, GBL, and 1,4-BD that are often found on the labels of commercial and illicit products.

PHARMACOKINETICS AND TOXICOKINETICS

The endogeneous production and metabolism of GHB is shown in Figure 80–1. Exogeneous GHB is typically ingested in its sodium salt form. Oral bioavailability of exogeneous GHB is approximately 60% in rats.[36,38] It is rapidly absorbed from the GI tract in 15–45 minutes. GHB displays two-compartment distribution in animals with an initial volume of distribution of 0.4 L/kg and final volume of distribution 0.6 L/kg.[16,36–38] It is lipid soluble and crosses the blood–brain barrier rapidly. It does not bind significantly to any plasma proteins.[49] GHB is metabolized mainly by succinic semialdehyde reductase (also known as GHB dehydrogenase) to succinic semialdehyde, which is subsequently metabolized to succinate and enters the tricarboxylic acid cycle (see Fig. 80–1). GHB is also metabolized directly to succinate via beta oxidation in the liver.[51] GHB is subject to first-pass metabolism by the cytochrome P450 system.[36] In adult volunteers, the elimination half-life is 20–53 minutes. Less than 5% of GHB is excreted unchanged in the urine.[49]

Initial clinical effects of ingested GHB occur in 15–20 minutes and peak in 30–60 minutes.[6] The clinical manifestations of GHB follow a steep dose–response curve. Doses of 20–30 mg/kg create euphoria, memory loss, and drowsiness while doses of 40–60 mg/kg result in coma.[20,43] Doses of 25 mg/kg given to naïve healthy subjects result in mean serum GHB concentration of 39.4 + 25.2 μg/mL (range 4.7–76.3 μg/mL).[6]

GBL undergoes conversion to GHB by a lactonase.[53,54] In comparison to GHB, GBL is more rapidly absorbed from the gastrointestinal tract and has a longer duration of action, both of which result from higher lipid solubility. 1,4-BD exerts its effects after conversion to GHB by alcohol dehydrogenase (ADH).[8,52] Co-ingestion with ethanol can prolong the onset of clinical effects because of competitive inhibition of ADH.[48,57]

In HIV patients taking protease inhibitors, GHB first-pass metabolism is altered such that low doses of GHB can produce toxic manifestations. This results from the interactions of the protease inhibitors on the cytochrome P450 system.[1,27]

CLINICAL MANIFESTATIONS

The clinical manifestations of GHB are mainly due to its effects on the CNS. Vital sign changes include bradycardia, hypotension, bradypnea, and hypothermia. Pupils may be miotic and poorly responsive to light. Acute toxicity typically results in CNS depression/coma, respiratory depression, salivation, vomiting, and sometimes myoclonus.[16,40] Of these findings, the most concerning is respiratory depression, as death has resulted from apnea.[9,39,78] Salivation and vomiting can complicate the respiratory depression leading to pulmonary aspiration in an unconscious patient. Case series also report aggressive and combative behavior, which may become more prominent in the setting of assessing the gag reflex or trying to endotracheally intubate the unconscious patient.[16,79] Motor manifestations can be confusing. Although GHB induces seizure activity (EEG changes and convulsions) in animal models, this has never been demonstrated in humans. More commonly GHB induces myoclonus that can be confused with convulsions.[18] The sedative effects of GHB are synergistic with ethanol and other sedative-hypnotics or CNS depressants. When 1,4-BD is used simultaneously with ethanol, the effects of the 1,4-BD are prolonged as ethanol competitively inhibits alcohol dehydrogenase thus preventing the conversion of 1,4-BD to GHB.

Other findings reported in patients taking prescribed therapeutic doses for narcolepsy include confusion, abnormal thought processes, and depression.[77] The most common adverse effects reported in these patients using prescribed GHB include nausea, dizziness, headache, vomiting, and urinary incontinence.[77]

Electrocardiographic findings include sinus bradycardia and prominent U waves which may be related to the sinus bradycardia. Other standard laboratory tests are typically normal.[9]

Recovery from overdose occurs rapidly, typically in less than 6–8 hours, and patients often extubate themselves following rapid improvement of their level of consciousness. No sequelae should be expected if hypoxia or aspiration did not occur.

Frequent GHB users can develop both tolerance and dependence to GHB.[21,61] Such patients typically use GHB or one of its analogs every

2–4 hours over a prolonged period of time, with cumulative daily doses in the range of 10 grams or more.[44] In rats receiving doses of GHB every 3 hours for up to 6 days tolerance was observed.[2] Although the exact mechanism is unknown, tolerance may be the result of the induction of GHB metabolism and a decrease in CNS sensitivity.[70]

DIAGNOSTIC TESTING

Routine "screens" for drugs of abuse do not typically include analysis for GHB. Specific testing for GHB and its related substances usually is not requested unless there is suspicion of its use associated with drug-facilitated sexual assault. However, urine and serum testing can also be performed if needed for forensic purposes. Gas chromatography-mass spectrometry (GC/MS) is the test of choice for both urine and serum. GHB can be detected in the urine up to 12 hours after use.[6] Interpretation of these tests must include cutoff concentrations as GHB, GBL, and 1,4-BD also occur naturally. These cutoff concentrations must be able to distinguish endogenous production and therapeutic use (as in patients using prescribed GHB for narcolepsy) from abuse or misuse. Attempts to relate concentrations to clinical effects in any individual might not be valid, however, when used chronically and when tolerance develops. Due to rapid metabolism and elimination, concentrations return to baseline shortly after drug naïve patients become clinically normal. Endogeneous GHB urine concentrations are usually less than 5–10 μg/mL while endogeneous GHB serum concentrations are usually less than 5 μg/mL.[6] In patients receiving a 25 mg/kg dose of GHB, plasma GHB concentrations ranged from 4.7 μg/mL to 76.3 μg/mL 20–45 minutes after administration and urine concentrations from below the detection limit to 840 μg/mL. In general, loss of consciousness occurs when serum concentrations reach 50 μg/mL, and deep coma when concentrations rise above 260 μg/mL.[59]

Screening for GHB may also routinely be performed when specific genetic or metabolic disorders are of concern. In particular, elevated GHB concentrations on a urinary organic acid screen in a child may indicate a succinic semialdehyde dehydrogenase deficiency. These children have developmental delay, seizures, hypotonia and elevated GHB concentrations in the blood, urine, and CSF.[50] One case report reveals a child with a serum GHB concentration of 775 μg/mL, significantly higher than most patients with exogenous GHB poisoning.[31]

Other routine tests in patients with depressed levels of consciousness include a rapid evaluation of blood glucose, an ethanol concentration as clinically indicated, and an ECG. When intentional overdose or self-harm is suspected, a determination of serum acetaminophen concentration is also indicated. Other studies should be obtained based on the clinical condition of the patient.

MANAGEMENT

Supportive care is the mainstay of therapy for GHB toxicity. All patients presenting to the hospital should have their airway, breathing, and circulation assessed initially. Patients with GHB toxicity may require airway protection in the presence of profound coma and respiratory depression or apnea. However, many become combative during the intubation process. Supportive care with a nasal airway may suffice in the snoring patient who has an appropriate gag and respiratory function. The need for endotracheal intubation is a bedside clinical decision and should be based on the patient's ability to oxygenate and ventilate, especially when diagnosis is known or highly suspected as recovery is expected shortly. Atropine may be given as needed for severe bradycardia. However, in most instances, the bradycardia does not need to be treated in otherwise healthy patients. An IV catheter should be established and intravenous fluids infused as necessary for hypotension. Patients should be warmed if they are hypothermic.

There is no role for gastric decontamination in patients with GHB toxicity as GHB is rapidly absorbed from the gastrointestinal tract. The increased risk of vomiting and aspiration also limits any beneficial role of gastric decontamination. If a co-ingestant is present, appropriate decontamination methods may be employed if there are no contraindications to their use.

Other therapies such as dextrose and thiamine should be administered as clinically indicated. Some proposed antidotes include physostigmine, naloxone, and flumazenil. All of these antidotes lack a pharmacologic basis for use and may place the patient at increased risk as other drugs of abuse commonly used with GHB may interact with these medications. An animal model did not support the use of physostigmine in GHB intoxication,[3] nor did a systematic literature review.[68] Naloxone can be administered to the patient with respiratory and CNS depression in the setting of unknown or presumed overdose. In GHB-toxic patients, naloxone administration is largely unsuccessful at improving clinical status.[39]

Those patients whose symptoms resolve may be discharged from the hospital following appropriate psychosocial evaluation for abuse and dependency. All patients who do not follow the expected course of resolution of their clinical manifestations (in approximately 6 hours) should be admitted to the hospital and investigated for other potential etiologies.

GHB WITHDRAWAL

Patients who use GHB or its analogs daily in large quantities can develop dependence.[21] Such patients are prone to withdrawal if they abruptly cease or decrease their daily dose. In patients prescribed GHB for narcolepsy, withdrawal rarely develops when the GHB is used as prescribed as the recommended doses are low and given only at night.[66,77] The majority of patients with GHB withdrawal are body builders.

GHB withdrawal is similar to ethanol and benzodiazepine withdrawal. It can be severe and potentially life threatening. The onset of withdrawal typically occurs 1–6 hours after last use. Men appear to be more commonly affected than women.[44] Manifestations of withdrawal include tachycardia, hypertension, tremors, agitation, dysphoria, nausea/vomiting, auditory and visual hallucinations, and seizures.[17,21,44,66]

For acute withdrawal symptoms, benzodiazepines and supportive care are the mainstays of therapy.[44,66] Rapid cooling, intravenous fluids, and evaluation for other medical or traumatic illnesses should be performed. These patients may require large doses of benzodiazepines to control symptoms. In patients with withdrawal symptoms refractory to benzodiazepines, barbiturates and propofol can be considered.[44,60,66] In these refractory patients, endotracheal intubation may be required (see Chap. 14, Withdrawal Principles).

SUMMARY

GHB is a unique xenobiotic because it occurs naturally as an endogenous neurotransmitter, is a licensed pharmaceutical, as well as a drug of abuse. GHB, GBL, and 1,4-BD result in GHB toxicity through complex neuropharmacological effects. GHB toxicity rarely results in death when patients are treated with supportive care. A life-threatening withdrawal syndrome can occur with cessation or decreased use of the drug and its related analogs. This withdrawal syndrome should be treated in a manner similar to ethanol withdrawal or sedative-hypnotic withdrawal. With appropriate care of both acute intoxication and withdrawal, patients can recover without sequelae, but psychosocial care and referral for management of abuse or dependency is essential.

ACKNOWLEDGMENT

Lawrence S. Quang contributed to this chapter in a previous edition.

REFERENCES

1. Antoniou T, Tseng AL. Interactions between recreational drugs and antiretroviral agents. *Ann Pharmacother.* 2002;36:1598-1613.
2. Bania TC, Ashar T, Press G, et al. Gamma-hydroxybutyric acid tolerance and withdrawal in a rat model. *Acad Emerg Med.* 2003; 10:697-704.
3. Bania TC, Chu J. Physostigmine does not effect arousal but produces toxicity in an animal model of severe gamma-hydroxybutyrate intoxication. *Acad Emerg Med.* 2005;12:185-189.
4. Benavides J, Rumigny JF, Bourguignon JJ, et al. A high affinity, Na^+-dependent uptake system for gamma-hydroxybutyrate in membrane vesicles prepared from rat brain. *J Neurochem.* 1982;38:1570-1575.
5. Bettler B, Kaupman K, Mosbacher J, et al. Molecular structure and physiologic functions of $GABA_B$ receptors. *Physiol Rev.* 2004;84:835-867.
6. Brenneisen R, Elsohly MA, Murphy TP, et al. Pharmacokinetics and excretion of gamma-hydroxybutyrate (GHB) in healthy subjects. *J Anal Toxicol.* 2004;28:625-630.
7. Bronstein AC, Spyker DA, Cantilena Jr LR, et al. 2006 Annual Report of the American Association of Poison Control Centers' National Poison Data System (NPDS). *Clin Toxicol.* 2007;45:815-917.
8. Carai MA, Colombo G, Reali R, et al. Central effects of 1,4-butanediol are mediated by $GABA_B$ receptors via its conversion into gamma-hydroxybutyric acid. *Eur J Pharmacol.* 2002;441:157.
9. Chin RL, Sporer KA, Cullison B, et al. Clinical course of gamma-hydroxybutyrate overdose. *Ann Emerg Med.* 1998;31:716-722
10. Cruz HG, Ivanova T, Lunn ML, et al. Bi-directional effects of GABA(B) receptor agonists on the mesolimbic dopamine system. *Nat Neurosci.* 2004;7:153-159.
11. Dietze PM, Cvetkovski S, Barrat MJ, et al. Patterns and incidence of gamma-hydroxybutyrate (GHB)-related ambulance attendances in Melbourne, Victoria. *MJA.* 2008;188:709-711.
12. Doherty JD, Hattox SE, Snead OC, et al. Identification of endogeneous gamma-hydroxybutyrate in human and bovine brain and its regional distribution in human, guinea pig, and rhesus monkey brain. *J Pharmacol Exp Ther.* 1978;207:130-139.
13. Doberty JC, Snead OC, Roth RH. A sensitive method for quantitation of gamma-hydroxybutyric acid and gamma-butyrolactone in brain by electron capture gas chromatography. *Anal Biochem.* 1975;69:268-277.
14. Drasbek KR, Christensen J, Jensen K. Gamma-hydroxybutyrate – a drug of abuse. *Acta Neurol Scand.* 2006;114:145-156.
15. Drug Abuse Warning Network, 2005. National Estimates of Drug-Related Emergency Department Visits. DAWN Series D-29, DHHS Publication No. (SMA) 07-4256. March 2007.
16. Dyer JE. Gamma-hydroxybutyrate: a health-food product producing coma and seizurelike activity. Am J Emerg Med. 1991;9:321-324.
17. Dyer JE, Roth B, Hyma BA. Gamma-hydroxybutyrate withdrawal syndrome. *Ann Emerg Med.* 2001;37:147-153.
18. Entholzner E, Mielke, Pichlmeier R, et al. EEG changes during sedation with gamma-hydroxybutyric acid. *Anesthetist.* 1995;44:345-350.
19. *Federal Register.* March 13, 2000;65(49). Accessed online June 30, 2008 at http://www.deadiversion.usdoj.gov/fed_regs/sched_actions/2000/fr0313.htm.
20. Food and Drug Administration. Gamma hydroxybutyric acid. Press Release P90–53. Rockville, MD: 1990.
21. Freese TE, Miotto K, Reback CJ. The effects and consequences of selected club drugs. *J Subst Abuse Treat.* 2002;23:151-156.
22. Fuller DE, Hornfeldt CS. From club drug to orphan drug: sodium oxybate (Xyrem) for the treatment of cataplexy. *Pharmacotherapy.* 2003;23:1205-1209.
23. Gervasi N, Monnier Z, Vincent P, et al. Pathway-specific action of gamma-hydroxybutyric acid in sensory thalamus and its relevance to absence seizures. *J Neurosci.* 2003;23:11469-11478.
24. Giarman NJ, Schmidt KF. Some neurochemical aspects of the depressant action of gamma-butyrolactone on the central nervous system 1. *Br J Pharmacol.* 1963;20:563-568.
25. Gobaille S, Schleff C, Hechler V, et al. Gamma-hydroxybutyrate increases tryptophan availability and potentiates serotonin turnover in rat brain. *Life Sci.* 2002;70:2101-2112.
26. Gunja N, Doyle E, Carpenter K, et al. Gamma-hydroxybutyrate poisoning from toy beads. *Med J Aust.* 2008;188:54-55.
27. Harrington RD, Woodward JA, Hooton TM, et al. Life-threatening interactions between HIV-1 protease inhibitors and the illicit drugs MDMA and gamma-hydroxybutyrate. *Arch Intern Med.* 1999;159:2221-2224.
28. Hechler V, Ratomponirina C, Maitre M. Gamma-hydroxybutyrate conversion into GABA induces displacement of $GABA_B$ binding that is blocked by valproate and ethosuximide. *J Pharmacol Exp Ther.* 2003;281:753-760.
29. Hedner T, Ludnborg P. Effect of gammahydroxybutyric acid on serotonin synthesis, concentration, and metabolism in the developing rat brain. *J Neural Transm.* 1983;57:39-48.
30. Hunter AS, Long WJ, Ryrie CG. An evaluation of gamma-hydroxybutyric acid in paediatric practice. *Br J Anaesth.* 1971;43:620-628.
31. Ishiguro Y, Kajita M, Aoshima T, et al. The first case of 4-hydroxybutric aciduria in Japan. *Brain Dev.* 2001;23:128-130.
32. Knudsen K, Greeter J, Verdicchio M. High mortality rates among GHB abusers in Western Sweden. *Clin Toxicol.* 2008;46:187-192.
33. Laborit H. Sodium 4-hydroxybutyrate. *Int J Neuropharmacol.* 1964;32: 433-451.
34. Ladinsky H, Consolo S, Zatta A, et al. Mode of action of gamma-butyrolactone on the central cholinergic system. *Naunyn Schmiedebergs Arch Pharmacol.* 1983;322:42-48.
35. Lapierre O, Montplaisir J, Lamarre M, et al. The effect of gamma-hydroxybutyrate on nocturnal and diurnal sleep of normal subjects: further considerations on REM sleep-triggering mechanisms. *Sleep.* 1990; 13:24-30.
36. Lettieri JT, Fung HL. Absorption and first-pass metabolism of ^{12}C-gamma-hydroxybutyric acid. *Res Commun Chem Path Pharmacol.* 1976;13:425-437.
37. Lettieri JT, Fung HL. Dose-dependent pharmacokinetics and hypnotic effects of sodium gamma-hydroxybutyrate in the rat. *J Pharmacol Exp Ther.* 1979;208:7-11.
38. Lettieri JT, Fung HL. Improved pharmacological activity via pro-drug modification: comparative pharmacokinetics of sodium gamma-hydroxybutyrate and gamma-butyrolactone. *Res Commun Chem Path Pharmacol.* 1978;22:107-118.
39. Li J, Stokes SA, Woeckener A. A tale of novel intoxication: seven cases of gamma-hydroxybutyric acid overdose. *Ann Emerg Med.* 1998;31:723-728.
40. Liechti ME, Kunz I, Greminger P, et al. Clinical features of gamma-hydroxybutyrate and gamma-butyrolactone toxicity and concomitant drug and alcohol use. *Drug Alcohol Depend.* 2006;81:323-326.
41. Maitre M. The gamma-hydroxybutyrate signaling system in brain: organization and functional implications. *Proc Neurobiol.* 1997;51:337-361.
42. Mamelak M. Gamma-hydroxybutyrate: an endogeneous regulator of energy metabolism. *Neurosci Biobehav Rev.* 1989;13:187-198.
43. Mamelak M, Scharf MB, Woods M. Treatment of narcolepsy with gamma-hydroxybutyrate: a review of clinical and sleep laboratory findings. *Sleep.* 1993;16:216-220.
44. McDonough M, Kennedy N, Glasper A, et al. Clinical features and management of gamma-hydroxybutyrate (GHB) withdrawal: a review. *Drug Alcohol Depend.* 2004;75:3-9.
45. Meyer S, Gottschling S, Georg T, Lothschutz D, et al. Gamma-hydroxybutyrate versus chlorprothixene/phenobarbital sedation in children undergoing MRI studies. *Klin Padiatr.* 2003;215:69-73.
46. Muller C, Viry S, Miehe M, et al. Evidence of gamma-hydroxybutyrate (GHB) uptake by rat brain synaptic vesicles. *J Neurochem.* 2002;80:899-904.
47. Nava F, Carta G, Bortolato M, Gessa GL. Gamma-hydroxybutyric acid and baclofen decrease extracellular acetylcholine levels in the hippocampus via GABA(B) receptors. *Eur J Pharmacol.* 2001;430:261-263.
48. Nelson L. Butanediol and ethanol: a reverse Mickey Finn? *Int J Med Toxicol.* 2000;3:1-3.
49. Palatini P, Tedeschi L, Frison G, et al. Dose-dependent absorption and elimination of gamma-hydroxybutyric acid in healthy volunteers. *Eur J Clin Pharmacol.* 1993;45:353-356.
50. Pearl PL, Novotny EJ, Acosta MT, et al. Succinic semialdehyde dehydrogenase deficiency in children and adults. *Ann Neurol.* 2003;54:s73-s80.
51. Poldrugo F, Addolorato G. The role of gamma-hydroxybutyric acid in the treatment of alcoholism: from animal to clinical studies. *Alcohol Alcohol.* 1999;34:15-24.
52. Poldrugo F, Snead OC III. 1,4-Butanediol and ethanol compete for degradation in rat brain and liver in vitro. *Alcohol.* 1986;3:367-370.
53. Roth RH, Giarman NJ. Evidence that central nervous system depression by 1,4-butanediol is mediated through a metabolite, gamma-hydroxybutyrate. *Biochem Pharmacol.* 1968;17:735-739.

54. Roth RH, Levy R, Giarman NJ. Dependence of rat serum lactonase upon calcium. *Biochem Pharmacol.* 1967;16:596-598.
55. Rubin BA, Giarman NJ. The therapy of experimental influenza in mice with antibiotic lactones and related compounds. *Yale J Biol Med.* 1947;19:1017-1022.
56. Runnacles JLM, Stroobant J. Poisoning from toy beads. *BMJ.* 2008; 336:110.
57. Schneidereit T, Burkhart K, Donovan JW, et al. Butanediol toxicity delayed by preingestion of ethanol. *Int J Med Toxicol.* 2000;3:1-3
58. Sethy VH, Roth RH, Walters JR, et al. Effect of anesthetic doses of γ-hydroxybutyrate on the acetylcholine content of rat brain. *Naunyn Schmiedebergs Arch Pharmacol.* 1976;295:9-14.
59. Shannon M, Quang LS. Gamma-hydroxybutyrate, gamma-butyrolac-tone, and 1,4-butanediol: a case report and review of the literature. *Pediatr Emerg Care.* 2000;16:435-440.
60. Sivilotti ML, Burns MJ, Aaron CK, Greenberg MJ. Pentobarbital for severe gamma-butyrolactone withdrawal. *Ann Emerg Med.* 2001;38:660-665
61. Smith KM, Larive LL, Romanelli F. Club drugs: methylenedioxymethamphetamine, flunitrazepam, ketamine hydrochloride, and gamma-hydroxybutyrate. *Am J Health Syst Pharm.* 2002;59:1067-1076.
62. Snead OC III. Evidence for a G protein-coupled gamma-hydroxybutyric acid receptor. *J Neurochem.* 2000;75:1986-1996.
63. Snead OC III. γ-Hydroxybutyrate model of generalized absence seizures: further characterization and comparison with other absence models. *Epilepsia.* 1988;29:361-368.
64. Snead OC III, Furner R, Liu CC. In vivo conversion of gamma-aminobutyric acid and 1,4-butanediol to gamma-hydroxybutyric acid in rat brain: studies using stable isotopes. *Biochem Pharmacol.* 1989;38: 4375-4380.
65. Snead OC III, Liu C. Gamma-hydroxybutyric acid binding sites in rat and human brain synaptosomal membranes. *Biochem Pharmacol.* 1984;33: 2587-2590.
66. Tarabar AF, Nelson LS. The gamma-hydroxybutyrate withdrawal syndrome. *Toxicol Rev.* 2004;23:45-49.
67. Toide K, Kitazato K, Unemi N. Effects on 1,2-bis(tetrahydro-2-furanyl)-5-fluoro-2,4-pyrimidinedione(FD-1) on the central nervous system: 1. Effects of monoamines in the brain. *Arch Int Pharmacodyn Ther.* 1980;247: 243-256.
68. Traub SJ, Nelson LS, Hoffman RS. Physostigmine as a treatment for gamma-hydroxybutyrate toxicity: a review. *J Toxicol Clin Toxicol.* 2002;40:781-787.
69. Van Cauter E, Plat L, Scharf MB, et al. Simultaneous stimulation of slow-wave sleep and growth hormone secretion by gamma-hydroxybutyrate in normal young men. *J Clin Invest.* 1997;100:745-753.
70. van Sassenbroeck D, De Paepe P, Belpaire F, et al. Tolerance to gamma-hydroxybutyrate in the rat: pharmacokinetic and pharmacodynamic aspects. *Acad Emerg Med.* 2002;9:484-485.
71. Vayer P, Maitre M: Regional differences in depolarization-induced release of γ-hydroxybutyrate from rat brain slices. *Neurosci Lett.* 1988;87:99-103
72. Vescovi PP, Coirro V. Different control of GH secretions by gamma-amino-and gamma-hydroxy-butyric acid in 4-year abstinent alcoholics. *Drug Alcohol Depend.* 2001;61:217-221.
73. Vickers MD. Gammahydroxybutyric acid. *Int Anesthesiol Clin.* 1969;7:75-80.
74. Watson WA, Litovitz TL, Klein-Schwartz W, et al. 2003 Annual report of the American Association of Poison Control Centers Toxic Exposure Surveillance System. *Am J Emerg Med.* 2004;22:335-404.
75. Wu Y, Ali S, Ahmadian G, et al. Gamma-hydroxybutyric acid (GHB) receptor and the gamma-aminobutyric acid$_B$ receptor (GABA$_B$) binding sites are distinctive from one another: molecular evidence. *Neuropharmacology.* 2004;47:1146-1156.
76. The XYREM international study group. Further evidence supporting the use of sodium oxybate for the treatment of cataplexy: a double-blind, placebo-controlled study in 228 patients. *Sleep Med.* 2005;6:415-421.
77. XYREM (sodium oxybate) (prescribing information). Palo Alto, CA: Jazz Pharmaceuticals; 2005.
78. Zvosec DL, Smith SW, McCutcheon JR, et al. Adverse events, including death, associated with the use of 1,4-butanediol. *N Engl J Med.* 2001;344:87-94.
79. Zvosec DL, Smith SW. Agitation is common in gamma-hydroxybutyrate toxicity. *Am J Emerg Med.* 2005;23:316-320.

CHAPTER 81
INHALANTS

Heather Long

Inhalant abuse is defined as the deliberate inhalation of vapors for the purpose of changing one's consciousness or becoming "high." It is also referred to as volatile substance abuse and was first described in 1951.[32] Inhalants are appealing to adolescents because they are inexpensive, readily available, and sold legally. Initially, inhalant abuse was viewed as physically harmless, but reports of "sudden sniffing death" began to appear in the 1960s.[9] Shortly thereafter, evidence surfaced of other significant morbidities, including organic brain syndromes, peripheral neuropathy, and withdrawal.

EPIDEMIOLOGY

The demographics of inhalant abuse differ markedly from those of other traditional substances of abuse. The 2003 National Survey on Drug Use and Health found that more than 2.6 million youths between the ages of 12 and 17 years used inhalants at least once in their lifetime.[122] Inhalants were the most frequently reported illicit xenobiotics used in the past year by 12- and 13-year-old adolescents, and youths aged 12 to 17 years continued to report higher rates of past-year use than did adults aged 18 years and older. The lifetime prevalence of inhalant use peaked among 8th graders at 15.6%. The median age of first use is 13 years.[7] A worrisome trend reported by the 2007 Monitoring the Future Study is that perceived risk of even one-time use of an inhalant has fallen steadily since 2001.[89]

Although long considered to be a problem among boys, there has been a steady increase of inhalant abuse among girls, and their lifetime prevalence now equals that of boys.[11] In the United States, the problem is greatest among children of lower socioeconomic groups, and non-Hispanic white adolescents are the most likely and black adolescents the least likely to use inhalants.[85] Although inhalant use is a problem in both urban and rural communities, its prevalence is higher in rural settings.[116] This may relate to the easier access that teens in urban areas have to other drugs of abuse.

Inhalant abuse includes the practices of sniffing, huffing, and bagging. *Sniffing* entails the inhalation of a volatile substance directly from a container, as occurs with airplane glue or rubber cement. *Huffing* involves pouring a volatile liquid onto fabric, such as a rag or sock, and placing it over the mouth and/or nose while inhaling and is the method used by more than 60% of volatile-substance abusers.[85] *Bagging* refers to instilling a solvent into a plastic or paper bag and rebreathing from the bag several times; spray paint is among the xenobiotics commonly used with this method. A newly reported form of abuse, *"dusting,"* refers to the inhalation of compressed air cleaners containing halogenated hydrocarbons (eg, CRC Dust Off™), marketed for cleaning computers and electronics equipment. Reports of such exposures, including death and ventricular dysrhythmias, doubled in 2005 and tripled in 2006, yet dusting is not perceived to be harmful by users and, surprisingly, many users do not consider it a form of inhalant abuse.[84]

XENOBIOTICS COMMONLY USED

There are myriad xenobiotics abused as inhalants (Table 81–1), most of which are volatile hydrocarbons. Hydrocarbons are organic compounds comprised of carbon and hydrogen atoms and are divided into two basic categories: aliphatic (straight, branched, or cyclic chains) and aromatic. Most of the commercially available hydrocarbon products are mixtures of hydrocarbons; for example, gasoline is a mixture of aliphatic and aromatic hydrocarbons that may consist of more than 1500 compounds. Substituted hydrocarbons contain halogens or other functional groups such as hydroxyl or nitrite that are substituted for hydrogen atoms in the parent structure. Solvents are themselves a heterogeneous group of xenobiotics that are used to dissolve other chemical compounds or provide a vehicle for their delivery.

The most commonly inhaled volatile hydrocarbons are fuels, such as gasoline, and solvents, such as toluene.[116] Other commonly inhaled hydrocarbon-containing products include spray paints, lighter fluid, air fresheners, and glue. The choice of xenobiotic used likely reflects their availability: cases from the 1970s frequently reported abuse of antiperspirants and typewriter correction fluid. Now, abuse of computer and electronics cleaners is on the rise. In most reported cases of inhalant use, the inhalant is identified not by its chemical name (eg, butane, toluene) but rather by its form (eg, lighter fluid, paint thinner). Because exact components may vary between commercial products, this method is inaccurate and imprecise.

Although volatile alkyl nitrites are technically substituted hydrocarbons, they have pharmacologic and behavioral effects, as well as patterns of abuse, that are distinct from the other volatile hydrocarbons. For this reason, researchers usually classify them as a separate category among abused inhalants. Amyl nitrite is the prototypical volatile alkyl nitrite.[7] Amyl nitrite became popular in the 1960s with the appearance of "poppers," small glass capsules containing the chemical in a plastic sheath or gauze. When crushed, the ampules release the amyl nitrite. When nonprescription sales of amyl nitrite were restricted in 1968, sex and drug paraphernalia shops began selling small vials of butyl and isobutyl nitrites marketed as room deodorizers or liquid incense.[7,80] Because of further restrictions on sales of alkyl nitrites, most of these products now contain chemicals that are not technically alkyl nitrites, such as cyclohexyl nitrite.[7]

The most commonly used nonhydrocarbon inhalant is nitrous oxide. Nitrous oxide, or "laughing gas," is used medicinally as an inhalational anesthetic. It is the propellant in supermarket-bought whipped cream canisters, and cartridges of the compressed gas are sold for home use in whipped cream dispensers. These battery-sized metal containers of compressed gas may be used as "whippits," in which the container is punctured using a device known as a "cracker," and the escaping gas is either inhaled directly or collected in a balloon and then rebreathed.

PHARMACOLOGY

Although chemically heterogeneous, inhalants are generally highly lipophilic and gain rapid entrance into the central nervous system (CNS). Little is known about the cellular basis of the effects of inhalants. Evidence to date shows that the most commonly abused hydrocarbons have molecular mechanisms similar to those of other classic CNS depressants with frequently overlapping cellular sites of action. Their effects are probably best represented by the model for ethanol in which multiple different cellular mechanisms explain diverse pharmacologic and toxicologic effects.[7]

VOLATILE HYDROCARBONS

The clinical effects of the volatile hydrocarbons are likely mediated through stimulation of inhibitory neurotransmission within the CNS. Like ethanol, toluene, trichloroethane (TCE), and trichloroethylene enhance γ-aminobutyric acid type A ($GABA_A$) receptor–mediated synaptic currents as well as glycine receptor–activated ion function. Stimulation of

TABLE 81–1. Common Inhalants and the Constituent Xenobiotics

Inhalant	Chemical
Glues/adhesives	Toluene, *n*-hexane, benzene, xylene, trichloroethane, trichloroethylene, tetrachloroethylene, ethyl acetate, methylethyl ketone, methyl chloride
Spray paint	Toluene, butane, propane
VCR head cleaner	Ethyl chloride
Computer keyboard duster	Difluoroethane, tetrafluoroethane
Hair spray, deodorants, air fresheners	Butane, propane, fluorocarbons
Cigarette lighter fluid	Butane
Paint thinner	Toluene, methylene chloride, methanol
Gasoline	Aliphatic and aromatic hydrocarbons
Carburetor cleaner	Methanol, methylene chloride, toluene, propane
Dry cleaning agents, spot removers, degreasing agents	Tetrachloroethylene, trichloroethane, trichloroethylene
Typewriter correction fluid	Trichloroethane, trichloroethylene
Nail polish remover	Acetone
Paints, lacquers, varnishes	Trichloroethylene, toluene, *n*-hexane
"Poppers"	Amyl nitrite, isobutyl nitrite
Room deodorizers	Butyl nitrite, isobutyl nitrite, cyclohexyl nitrite
Whipped cream dispensers, "whippits"	Nitrous oxide

these receptors acts to increase chloride permeability, hyperpolarizing the neuronal cell membrane and inhibiting excitability.[13,62,118] Despite very different molecular structures, ethanol, enflurane, chloroform, toluene, and TCE compete for binding sites at α_1 glycine receptors.[12] Like ethanol, toluene, TCE, and benzene all also interfere with glutamate-mediated excitatory neurotransmission by inhibiting *N*-methyl-D-aspartate (NMDA) receptor–mediated currents in a concentration-dependent manner.[6,34,102] Furthermore, repeated toluene exposure increases NMDA receptors, suggesting that chronic exposure can lead to upregulation of NMDA receptors as occurs with alcohol.[6,138]

Toluene is the prototypical volatile hydrocarbon and the best studied. In animal models, differences in pharmacologic action are demonstrated between toluene and other alkylbenzenes, and halogenated hydrocarbons such as TCE, and acetone.[19,34,126] These differences may represent evidence that specific cellular sites for their actions exist. Additionally, these differences may explain the variation in their abuse potential or their clinical effects.[7] Despite these distinctions, there are marked similarities in the behavioral and pharmacologic effects of the volatile hydrocarbons. Moreover, the clinical effects profile shared by the volatile hydrocarbons, subanesthetic concentrations of general anesthetics, ethanol, and benzodiazepines suggests that they share cellular mechanisms. Shared clinical effects include anxiolytic effects,[23] anticonvulsant effects,[140] impaired motor coordination,[92] and evidence of physical dependence on withdrawal.[40,41]

Most research on inhalants has focused on the neural basis of their effects, yet it is the cardiotoxicity that is responsible for the majority of their lethal effects. In vivo, toluene reversibly inhibits myocardial voltage-activated sodium channels.[35] Similarly, it inhibits muscle sodium channels but with less potency.[48] Ethanol and toluene have opposite effects on potassium channels in vivo; ethanol potentiates the large conductance, calcium-activated potassium channels as well as certain G-protein-coupled inwardly rectifying potassium channels while toluene inhibits them.[37] This inhibition of the sodium channels and the inwardly rectifying potassium channels is postulated to play a role in cardiac dysrhythmias and sudden sniffing death associated with the aromatic and halogenated hydrocarbons. Animal studies show toluene and 1,1,1-trichloroethane produce biphasic dose–response curves for motor activity: low concentrations yield motor excitation while high concentrations produce sedation, motor impairment, and anesthesia.[20,133] Molecular mechanisms underlying both the neural and cardiac effects may optimize the conditions and explain the observed clinical phenomenon described in sudden sniffing deaths (see below).

There are scant data on the pharmacokinetics of the inhalants. Most data are derived from studies on occupational and environmental exposures and have limited applicability to intentional inhalation. More relevant to the understanding of inhalants are the similarities with the inhalational anesthetic agents, many of which are also halogenated hydrocarbons. Factors determining pharmacokinetic and pharmacodynamic effects of a given inhalational anesthetic include its concentration in inspired air; partition coefficient; interaction with other inhaled substances, alcohol, and drugs; the patient's respiratory rate and blood flow; their percent body fat; and individual variation in drug metabolism (Chap. 67).[52]

Partition coefficients measure the relative affinity of a gas for two different substances at equilibrium and are used to predict the rate and extent of uptake of an inhaled substance. The blood:gas partition coefficient is most commonly referenced. The higher the number, the more soluble the substance is in blood. Substances with a low blood:gas partition coefficient, like nitrous oxide, are rapidly taken up by the brain and, conversely, are rapidly eliminated from the brain once exposure is ended (Table 81–2).

In a rodent model of inhalation abuse of toluene and acetone, the rapidity of onset and the depth of CNS depression were dependent on the concentration of the solvent inhaled.[26] There was a parallel relationship between brain concentration and pharmacologic effect during induction (inhalation) and postexposure. Brain and liver concentrations dropped rapidly after exposure; concentration in blood decreased at the slowest rate. Elimination was biphasic: rapid elimination during the first step was a result of tissue redistribution, alveolar ventilation, and metabolic clearance. During the second phase there was a slow decrease in tissue concentrations as a result of the gradual mobilization from adipose tissue with subsequent exhalation or metabolism. Acetone, which is more water soluble than toluene, is less potent and more slow acting than toluene, but is eliminated much more slowly than toluene and has a much longer duration of action.[26] Positron emission tomography (PET) studies using (^{11}C) radiolabeled toluene, butane, and acetone in nonhuman primates showed rapid uptake of radioactivity in striatal and frontal regions of the cortex followed by rapid clearance from the brain.[49] Whole-body PET scans in mice showed excretion through the kidneys and liver.[50]

The inhalants are eliminated unchanged via respiration, undergo hepatic metabolism, or both (see Table 81–2). For some, the percentage that is metabolized versus eliminated unchanged varies with the exposure dose. Nitrous oxide and the aliphatic hydrocarbons are frequently eliminated unchanged in the expired air. The aromatic and halogenated hydrocarbons are metabolized extensively via the cytochrome P450 (CYP) system, particularly CYP2E1, which has a substrate spectrum that includes a number of aliphatic, aromatic, and halogenated hydrocarbons.[17,57,58,141] Extrahepatic expression of CYP2E1 occurs to

TABLE 81–2. Blood:Gas Partition Coefficients, Routes of Elimination, and Important Metabolites of Selected Inhalants

Xenobiotic	Blood:Gas Partition Coefficient (98.6°F/37°C)	Routes of Elimination	Important Metabolites
Acetone	243–300	Largely unchanged via exhalation 95% and urine 5%	None
n-Butane	0.019	Largely unchanged via exhalation	None
Carbon tetrachloride	1.6	50% unchanged via exhalation; 50% hepatic metabolism and urinary excretion	CYP2E1 to trichloromethyl radical, trichloromethyl peroxy radical, phosgene
n-Hexane	2	10%–20% exhaled unchanged; hepatic metabolism and urinary excretion	CYP2E1 to 2-hexanol, 2,5-hexanedione, γ-valerolactone
Methylene chloride	5–10	92% exhaled unchanged; hepatic metabolism and urinary excretion	(1) CYP2E1 to CO and CO_2 (2) Glutathione transferase to CO_2, formaldehyde, and formic acid
Nitrous oxide	0.47	>99% exhaled unchanged	None
Toluene	8–16	<20% exhaled unchanged; >80% hepatic metabolism and urinary excretion	CYP2E1 to benzoic acid, then (1) glycine conjugation to form hippuric acid (68%) (2) glucuronic acid conjugation to benzoyl glucuronide (insignificant pathway except following large exposure to toluene)
1,1,1-Trichloroethane	1–3	91% exhaled unchanged; hepatic metabolism and urinary excretion	CYP2E1 to trichloroethanol, then (1) conjugated with glucuronic acid (urochloralic acid) or (2) further oxidized to trichloracetic acid
Trichloroethylene	9	16% exhaled unchanged; 84% hepatic metabolism and urinary excretion	CYP2E1 to epoxide intermediate (transient); chloral hydrate (transient); trichloroethanol (45%), trichloroacetic acid (TCA) (32%). Urinary TCA peaks 2–3 days postexposure
1,2-dichloro-1,1-difluoroethane	NA	NA	CYP2E1 to 2-chloro-2,2-difluoroethyl glucuronide, 2-2chloro-2,2-difluoroethyl sulfate, chlorodifluoroacetic acid, chlorodifluoroacetaldehyde hydrate, chlorodifluoroacetaldehyde-urea adduct, and inorganic fluoride. No covalently bound metabolites to liver proteins

NA = Not available

a lesser extent but may be of toxicologic significance, particularly in the kidneys and the dopaminergic cells of the substantia nigra.[18,63,129] In humans, there appear to be no significant gender differences in CYP2E1; however, it is polymorphic and, as such, allelic distributions vary among different human populations.[18,114] Moreover, this polymorphism may explain the varying degrees of toxicity exhibited following inhalant abuse.

Reward and reinforcement effects of inhalants are readily demonstrated. While the mechanisms underlying their reinforcement behavior remain poorly studied, activation of the mesolimbic dopamine system is thought to play an important role in this as with more commonly studied drugs of abuse.[50,105]

VOLATILE ALKYL NITRITES

Unlike other volatile hydrocarbons, the volatile alkyl nitrites are not thought to have any direct effects on the CNS. Their effects are mediated through smooth muscle relaxation in the central and peripheral vasculature and they share a common cellular pathway with other nitric oxide (NO) donors similar to nitroglycerin and sodium nitroprusside.[71] A rat model of inhalation of isobutyl nitrite found a half-life of 1.4 minutes with almost 100% biotransformation to isobutyl alcohol. Bioavailability following inhalation was estimated to be 43%.[70]

NITROUS OXIDE

The pharmacokinetics and pharmacodynamics of nitrous oxide (N_2O) abuse are derived from its use as an inhalation anesthetic. Anesthetic uptake or induction, as well as emergence with N_2O, is rapid because of its low solubility in blood, muscle, and fat.[119] There is no appreciable metabolism of N_2O in human tissue. An animal study found N_2O significantly inhibited excitatory NMDA-activated currents and had no effect on GABA-activated currents.[64] N_2O also stimulates dopaminergic neurons, but the significance of this in mediating its anesthetic effects remains unclear.[68,93]

Animal studies suggest the analgesic effects (or more accurately the antinociceptive effects because it refers to animals) of N_2O appear to be mediated through opioid peptide release in the midbrain. These antinociceptive effects can be reversed by the opioid antagonist naloxone.[15] However, in humans the anesthetic effects are not attenuated by naloxone, and the subjective and psychomotor effects of N_2O are not extinguished by even high doses of naloxone.[115,142]

CLINICAL MANIFESTATIONS

Signs and symptoms of inhalant use may be subtle, tend to vary widely among individuals, and generally resolve within several hours of exposure. Following acute exposure, there may be a distinct odor of the abused inhalant on the patient's breath or clothing. Depending on the inhalant used and the method, there may be discoloration of skin around the nose and mouth. Mucous membrane irritation may cause sneezing, coughing, and tearing. Patients may complain of dyspnea and palpitations. Gastrointestinal complaints include nausea, vomiting, and abdominal pain. After an initial period of euphoria, patients may have residual headache and dizziness.

VOLATILE HYDROCARBONS

The CNS is the intended target of the inhalants and is most susceptible to its adverse effects. Initial CNS effects include euphoria and hallucinations, both visual and auditory, as well as headache and dizziness. As toxicity progresses, CNS depression worsens and patients may develop slurred speech, confusion, tremor, and weakness. Transient cranial nerve palsies are reported.[124] Further CNS depression is marked by ataxia, lethargy, seizures, coma, and respiratory depression. These acute encephalopathic effects generally resolve spontaneously and associated neuroimaging abnormalities are not reported.[43]

As can be expected, given the high lipophilicity of most inhalants, toxicity from chronic use is manifested most strikingly in the CNS. Toluene leukoencephalopathy, characterized by dementia, ataxia, eye movement disorders, and anosmia, is the prototypical manifestation of chronic inhalant neurotoxicity. Patients with toluene leukoencephalopathy display characteristic neurobehavioral deficits reflecting white matter involvement: inattention, apathy, and impaired memory and visuospatial skills with relative preservation of language.[43] Autopsy studies reveal white matter degeneration including cerebral and cerebellar atrophy and thinning of the corpus callosum.[72,106] On microscopy, there is diffuse demyelination with relative sparing of the axons. Abundant perivascular macrophages containing coarse or laminar myelin debris found in areas of the greatest myelin loss is a characteristic pathologic feature.[43] This targeting of myelin, which is 70% lipid, may be explained by toluene's lipophilicity.[43] As myelination continues at least through the second decade of life, the typical toluene abuser who begins inhaling during adolescence may be particularly susceptible to its toxic CNS effects.[42] Advances in magnetic resonance imaging (MRI) with gadolinium, which allow enhanced visualization of the cerebral white matter, demonstrate that the extent of white matter injury in the brain directly corresponds to the clinical severity of toluene leukoencephalopathy.[43] It is postulated that reactive oxygen species generated either by toluene or its metabolite benzaldehyde induce lipid peroxidation in the brain.[82,104] Genetic polymorphisms and host susceptibility among chronic abusers are also hypothesized to play a role.[54]

Acute cardiotoxicity associated with hydrocarbon inhalation is manifested most dramatically in "sudden sniffing death." In witnessed cases, sudden death frequently occurred when sniffing was followed by some physical activity. Examples include running or wrestling or a stressful situation like being caught sniffing by parents or police.[9] It is thought that the inhalant "sensitizes the myocardium" by blocking the potassium current (I_{KR}), thereby prolonging repolarization.[95] This produces a substrate for dysrhythmia propagation; the activity or stress then causes a catecholamine surge that initiates the dysrhythmia (Chap. 23).[95] Cardiac dysrhythmias following the inhalation of hydrocarbons were documented with the halogenated inhalational anesthetics in the early 1900s, and this association was subsequently confirmed in both animal and human studies.[44,125]

More typically, the clinical presentation of a patient with hydrocarbon cardiotoxicity may include palpitations, shortness of breath, syncope, and electrocardiographic (ECG) abnormalities, including atrial fibrillation, premature ventricular contractions, QT interval prolongation, and U waves.

Multiple case reports of ventricular fibrillation follow intentional inhalation of other hydrocarbons such as butane fuel,[56,137] Freon (Dupont trade name for fluorinated hydrocarbons), and Glade Air Freshener (SC Johnson), which contains a mixture of short-chain aliphatic hydrocarbons.[77] Among 44 patients with a history of inhalant abuse, specifically toluene exposure, the QT interval and corrected QT dispersion were significantly greater than in healthy controls. Furthermore, the QT interval and corrected QT dispersion were significantly greater in the 20 toluene abusers with a history of unexplained syncope than in asymptomatic abusers and controls.[2] Although cardiotoxic effects of inhalant abuse are generally acute, dilated cardiomyopathy is reported with chronic abuse of toluene and with trichloroethylene.[86,139] Microscopy reveals evidence of chronic myocarditis with fibrosis.[139]

The primary respiratory toxicity complication of inhalational abuse is hypoxia, which is either caused by rebreathing of exhaled air, as occurs with bagging, or displacement of inspired oxygen with the inhalant, reducing the fraction of inspired oxygen (FIO_2). Direct pulmonary toxicity associated with inhalants is most often a result of inadvertent aspiration of a liquid hydrocarbon (Chap. 106). Aspiration injury is associated with acute lung injury and the acute respiratory distress syndrome, a continuum of lung injury characterized by increased permeability of the alveolar–capillary barrier and the resulting influx of edema into the alveoli, neutrophilic inflammation, and an imbalance of cytokines and other inflammatory mediators.[132] Reports of asphyxiation initially ascribed to inhalant abuse were later found caused by suffocation by a plastic bag, mask, or container pressed firmly to the face, and not specifically by toxicity of the inhaled vapor.[9,29,131]

Irritant effects on the respiratory system are frequently transient, but patients may develop chemical pneumonitis. This syndrome is characterized by tachypnea, fever, tachycardia, crackles, rhonchi, leukocytosis, and radiographic abnormalities, including perihilar densities, bronchovascular markings, increased interstitial markings, infiltrates, and consolidation. Rebreathing of exhaled air, as occurs with bagging, may lead to hypercapnia and hypoxia. Acute eosinophilic pneumonia following abuse of a fabric protector containing 1,1,1-trichloroethane is also reported.[69] Barotrauma presents as pneumothorax, pneumomediastinum, or subcutaneous emphysema.[109]

Hepatoxicity is associated with exposure to halogenated hydrocarbons, particularly carbon tetrachloride, but also chloroform, trichloroethane, trichloroethylene, and toluene.[81] Intentional inhalation of carbon tetrachloride is rarely reported, but its toxic metabolite, the trichloromethyl radical, created by the cytochrome CYP2E1, can covalently bind to hepatocyte macromolecules and cause lipid peroxidation.[103] The resultant depletion of glutathione and the potentially fatal centrilobular necrosis mimic acetaminophen toxicity and have led to a postulated role for *N*-acetylcysteine (NAC) and its use is suggested. Animal studies on the efficacy of NAC in preventing carbon tetrachloride–induced hepatoxicity have yielded mixed results.[33,36] There are no clinical trials in humans, but case series suggest a protective role for NAC.[107] Two cases of centrilobular hepatic necrosis following inhalation of trichloroethylene are reported. In a case series of 34 serum-confirmed inhalant deaths, two of the three who died from trichloroethane and trichloroethylene inhalation had cirrhosis of the liver at autopsy. None of the victims of other inhalants had liver cirrhosis.[47] Inhalation of either toluene or one of the many halogenated hydrocarbons is associated with elevated liver enzymes and hepatomegaly that generally return to baseline within 2 weeks of abstinence.[5,61,66,76,94,97]

Most reported renal toxicity is associated with toluene inhalation. Traditionally, prolonged toluene inhalation was said to cause a distal renal tubular acidosis (RTA), resulting in hypokalemia. However, distal RTA is associated classically with a hyperchloremic metabolic acidosis and a normal anion gap, whereas toluene abuse may be associated with an increased anion gap. Production of hippuric acid, a toluene metabolite, plays an important role in the genesis of the metabolic acidosis.[30] Hippurate excretion, usually expressed as a ratio to creatinine, rises dramatically with toluene inhalation.[87] The excretion of abundant hippurate in the urine unmatched by ammonium mandates an enhanced rate of excretion of sodium and potassium cations. Continued loss of potassium in the urine leads to hypokalemia. Toluene is rapidly metabolized to hippuric acid, and the hippurate anion is swiftly cleared by the kidneys, leaving the hydrogen ion behind. This prevents the rise in the anion gap that would normally occur with an acid anion other than chloride, resulting in a normal anion gap. In some cases, the loss of sodium causes extracellular fluid volume contraction and a fall in the glomerular filtration rate, which may transform the metabolic acidosis with a normal anion gap into one with a high anion gap caused by the accumulation of hippurate and other anions.[30] Through unclear mechanisms, other renal abnormalities occur with toluene inhalation, including hematuria, albuminuria, and pyuria. Glomerulonephritis associated with hydrocarbon inhalation is also reported and is a result of antiglomerular basement membrane antibody-mediated immune complex deposition.[14,128,143]

Toluene-abusing patients may present with profound hypokalemic muscle weakness. In a study of 25 patients admitted to the hospital following inhalant abuse, nine presented with muscle weakness. The mean serum potassium concentration was 1.7 mEq/L and six of these patients also had manifestations of rhabdomyolysis. Four patients were quadriplegic on presentation and of these, two were initially diagnosed erroneously with Guillain-Barré syndrome. The patients had inhaled toluene 6 to 7 hours per day for 4 to 14 days prior to presentation.[120]

Acute dermatologic and upper airway toxicity is associated with the inhalation of fluorinated hydrocarbons. First- and second-degree burns of the face, neck, shoulder and chest are reported in a 12-year-old-girl inhaling difluoroethane from a computer cleaner.[90] Pyrolysis of difluoroethane may yield hydrofluoric acid burns.[45] Vesicular lesions resembling frostbite and massive, potentially life-threatening edema of the oropharyngeal, glottic, epiglottic, and paratracheal structures are also reported.[1,73,84] This is caused by the cooling of the gas associated with its rapid expansion once it is released from its pressurized container. With chronic abuse of volatile hydrocarbons, patients may develop severe drying and cracking around the mouth and nose as a consequence of a defatting dermatitis known as "huffer's eczema." Other manifestations of chronic irritation include recurrent epistaxis, chronic rhinitis, conjunctivitis, halitosis, and ulceration of the nasal and oral mucosa.[87]

Bone mineral density was significantly lower in 25 adolescent chronic glue sniffers compared with that of healthy controls.[39] In a mouse model, chronic exposure to toluene significantly reduced bone mineral density.[4]

Methylene chloride (dichloromethane), most commonly found in paint removers and degreasers, is unique among the halogenated hydrocarbons in that it undergoes metabolism in the liver by CYP2E1 to carbon monoxide.[98] In addition to acute CNS and cardiac manifestations, inhalation of methylene chloride is associated with delayed onset and prolonged duration of signs and symptoms of carbon monoxide (CO) poisoning. The CO metabolite is generated 4 to 8 hours after exposure and its apparent half-life is 13 hours, significantly longer than that of CO following inhalation (Chap. 125).[8,121] Methanol toxicity is reported following intentional inhalation of methanol-containing carburetor cleaners.[46,78,83] Significant findings may include hyperemic discs on funduscopic examination, metabolic acidosis, and CNS and respiratory depression (Chap. 107). Methanol-containing carburetor cleaners may also contain significant amounts of toluene (43.8%), methylene chloride (20.5%), and propane (12.5%). These xenobiotics may potentiate CNS depression and contribute to the toxicity associated with these products.

Chronic inhalation of the solvent *n*-hexane, a petroleum distillate and a simple aliphatic hydrocarbon found, for example, in rubber cement, can cause a sensorimotor peripheral neuropathy. Toxicity is mediated via a metabolite, 2,5-hexanedione, that interferes with glyceraldehyde-3-phosphate dehydrogenase–dependent axonal transport, resulting in axonal death.[38] Numbness and tingling of the fingers and toes is the most common initial complaint; progressive, ascending loss of motor function with frank quadriparesis may ensue.[31] Sural nerve biopsy shows axonal swelling and axonal loss, with secondary loss of myelin, probably as a result of retraction by axonal swelling, and accumulation of neurofilaments.[74] Nerve conduction studies show marked conduction slowing and conduction block (Chap. 18).[31,74]

Reports of polyneuropathy associated with chronic gasoline inhalation date to the 1960s and describe a symmetric, progressive, sensorimotor neuropathy with occasional superimposed mononeuropathies.[27,67] Initially these deficits were attributed to the presence of tetraethyl lead as an "antiknocking" agent in gasoline, but cases following abuse of unleaded gasoline are also reported.[27,110] *n*-Hexane is present in gasoline in concentrations of up to 3% and is thought to be the likely mediator of gasoline neuropathy.[134]

Teratogenicity Fetal solvent syndrome (FSS) was first reported in 1979.[127] The authors described a 20-year-old primigravida with a 14-year history of solvent abuse defined as "daily" and "heavy" who gave birth to an infant exhibiting facial dysmorphia, growth retardation, and microcephaly, a constellation of findings that resembles fetal alcohol syndrome (FAS). Since then a number of cases and case series have been reported.[3,60,108,136] A general limitation of these case series is their reliance on self-reporting of substance abuse. In a number of cases included for analysis of teratogenic effects, mothers admit to use during pregnancy of other potential teratogens, including ethanol, cocaine, heroin, and phenobarbital.[3,136] Cases purported to represent inhalant abuse in the absence of other drug abuse, particularly ethanol, are not verified by laboratory testing. A small study of infants born to mothers with a self-reported history of chronic solvent abuse found 16% had major anomalies, 12.5% had facial features resembling FAS, and 3.6% had cleft palate.[108] Craniofacial abnormalities common to both FAS and FSS include small palpebral fissures, thin upper lip, and midfacial hypoplasia. Features of FSS that distinguish it from FAS include micrognathia, low-set ears, abnormal scalp hair pattern, large anterior fontanelle, and downturned corners of the mouth.[127] Hypoplasia of the philtrum and nose are more characteristic of FAS.[100] Compared with matched controls, infants born to mothers who report inhalant abuse are more likely to be premature, have low birth weight, have smaller birth length, and have small head circumference.[3,136] Follow-up studies of these infants show developmental delay when compared with children matched for age, race, sex, and socioeconomic status.[3,60] A rat model of toluene-abuse embryopathy found a significant reduction in the number of neurons within each cortical layer, as well as abnormal neural migration.[53] In animal models of inhalant abuse, exposure to brief, repeated, high concentrations of toluene significantly increases rates of growth restriction, minor malformations, and impaired motor development.[21,65] In another rat model of maternal inhalant abuse, toluene levels in fetal brain tissue, the placenta, and amniotic fluid increased in a concentration-dependent manner.[22]

Withdrawal Observed similarities in the acute effects of inhalants compared with other CNS depressants have suggested similar patterns of tolerance and withdrawal. Rodent models of inhalant abuse with toluene and TCE show evidence of physical dependence that manifests as an increase in handling-induced seizures on cessation of inhalation.[41,135] Additionally, these studies demonstrate cross-tolerance of the benzodiazepine diazepam with the motor-stimulating effects of TCE and, to a lesser degree, with toluene. Inhalant abusers have themselves described tolerance with weekly usage in as little as 3 months.[55] Withdrawal symptoms, including irritability, insomnia, craving, nausea, tremor, and dry mouth lasting 2 to 5 days after last use, are described.[112]

VOLATILE ALKYL NITRITES

Methemoglobinemia caused by inhalation of amyl, butyl, and isobutyl nitrites is well reported.[24,79] Nitrites are strong oxidants that may induce hemoglobin oxidation from the ferrous (Fe^{2+}) to the ferric (Fe^{3+}) state. Patients may present with signs and symptoms of methemoglobinemia including shortness of breath, cyanosis, tachycardia, and tachypnea (Chap. 127). Eye pain and transient increased intraocular pressure are reported following use of amyl nitrite.[99]

NITROUS OXIDE

Reported deaths associated with abuse of nitrous oxide (N_2O) appear to be caused by secondary effects of N_2O, including asphyxiation and motor vehicle collisions while under the influence, and not to direct toxicity.[123,131] Investigations following deaths associated with N_2O have found many of the dead were discovered with plastic bags over their heads, in an apparent attempt to both prolong the duration of effect and increase the concentration to heighten the effect.[131] Autopsy findings in these cases were consistent with asphyxiation: acute lung injury, cardiac petechiae, and generalized visceral congestion.[123,131] Laboratory simulation of a reported death in which the victim was found with a plastic bag over his head with a belt fastened loosely around his neck and a spent whipped cream canister within the plastic bag showed N_2O displaces oxygen in a closed space.[131] Additionally, N_2O concentrations in this simulation were greater than 60%; at concentrations of nitrous oxide greater than 50%, the normal hypoxic response is diminished.[131] The combined effects of displaced oxygen and a blunted hypoxic drive may increase the risk of asphyxia.

Chronic abuse of N_2O is associated with neurologic toxicity mediated via irreversible oxidation of the cobalt ion of cyanocobalamin (vitamin B_{12}). Oxidation blocks formation of methylcobalamin, a coenzyme in the production of methionine and *S*-adenosylmethionine, required for methylation of the phospholipids of the myelin sheaths. Additionally, cobalamin oxidation inhibits the conversion of methylmalonyl to succinyl coenzyme A. The resultant accumulation of methylmalonate and propionate can result in synthesis of abnormal fatty acids and their subsequent incorporation into the myelin sheath (Chap. 67).[101] Case reports and small case series in humans following self-reported chronic, heavy abuse of N_2O found development of myeloneuropathy resembling the subacute combined degeneration of the dorsal columns of the spinal cord of classic vitamin B_{12} deficiency.[16,75,130] Presenting signs and symptoms reflect varying involvement of the posterior columns, the corticospinal tracts, and the peripheral nerves. Numbness and tingling of the distal extremities is the most common presenting complaint. Physical examination may reveal diminished sensation to pinprick and light touch, vibratory sensation and proprioception, gait disturbances, the Lhermitte sign (electric shock sensation from the back into the limbs with neck flexion), hyperreflexia, spasticity, urinary and fecal incontinence, and extensor plantar response.[28,101] Among reported patients with N_2O-associated neurotoxicity who had documented levels of vitamin B_{12}, approximately 50% had low serum vitamin B_{12} concentrations.[16,28,75,117,130] In the few patients who underwent Schilling tests, results were normal.[75,130] Nerve conduction studies and electromyography typically revealed a distal, axonal sensorimotor polyneuropathy.[28,75,130]

LABORATORY AND DIAGNOSTIC TESTING

Routine urine toxicology screens are unable to detect inhalants or their metabolites. Although most volatile inhalants can be detected using gas chromatography, the likelihood of detection is limited by the dose, time to sampling, and method of specimen storage. Blood is the preferred specimen, but urinalysis for metabolites and hippuric acid (for toluene) may extend the time until the limit of detection is reached.[25] Specimens should be stored at a temperature between 23°F (−5°C) and 39.2°F (4°C).[25] Testing is not readily available at most institutions and the need to send the specimen to a reference laboratory limits the clinical utility in most situations. A thorough history and physical examination and careful questioning of the patient's friends and family are probably more helpful in cases of suspected inhalant abuse.

TABLE 81–3. Inhalants With Unique Clinical Manifestations

Inhalant	Clinical Manifestations
Toluene	Hypokalemia; hepatotoxicity; leukoencephalopathy (chronic)
1,1,1-Trichloroethane, trichloroethylene	Hepatotoxicity
Methylene chloride	Carbon monoxide poisoning
Carburetor cleaner	Methanol poisoning
Alkyl nitrites (amyl, butyl, isobutyl)	Methemoglobinemia
n-Hexane	Peripheral neuropathy (chronic)
Nitrous oxide	Myeloneuropathy (chronic)

Depending on the patient's signs and symptoms, additional diagnostic testing may be indicated, including an ECG, chest radiograph, serum electrolytes, liver enzymes, and serum pH. Inhalation of some agents presents unique diagnostic considerations (Table 81–3). Routine laboratory testing, including cerebrospinal fluid analysis, is unremarkable in patients with inhalant-induced leukoencephalopathy. A computed tomography (CT) scan of the head is generally normal until late in the disease, when diffuse hypodensity of white matter becomes evident. T2-weighted MRI with its superior resolution of white matter is the diagnostic study of choice. Standard MRI does not detect initial changes caused by toluene leukoencephalopathy; measurement of *N*-acetyl aspartate (NAA), a marker of CNS axons, with magnetic resonance spectroscopy (MRS) may assist with earlier detection. A decrease in NAA concentration, usually expressed as the ratio of NAA to creatinine (NAA:Cr), may serve as a marker of axonal damage.[43]

MANAGEMENT

Management begins with assessment and stabilization of the patient's airway, breathing, and circulation (the "ABCs"). The patient should be attached to a pulse oximeter and cardiac monitor. Oxygen should be administered and the patient should be treated with nebulized β agonists if wheezing is present. Early consultation with a regional poison center or medical toxicologist may assist with identification of the xenobiotic and patient management.

Cardiac dysrhythmias associated with inhalant abuse carry a significantly poor prognosis. Sudden death following use is not limited to new users and there appears to be no premonitory signal to the user.[6,9,94] Life-threatening electrolyte abnormalities must be considered early and corrected in the patient presenting with dysrhythmia. Patients with nonperfusing rhythms should be managed following standard management with defibrillation. There are no evidence-based treatment guidelines for the management of inhalant-induced cardiac dysrhythmias, but β-adrenergic antagonists are thought to offer some cardioprotective effects to the sensitized myocardium.[95] Propranolol and esmolol have both been used successfully in treatment of ventricular dysrhythmias following inhalant abuse.[51,91]

Fluid and electrolyte abnormalities should be sought and corrected early. In the course of management other complications, including methemoglobinemia, elevated carboxyhemoglobin, and methanol toxicity, should be managed with the appropriate antidotal therapy. Patients with respiratory symptoms that persist beyond the initial complaints of gagging and choking should be evaluated for hydrocarbon pneumonitis and treated supportively (Chap. 106).

With abstinence, behavioral and neuroimaging changes associated with toluene-induced leukoencephalopathy may be partially reversible early on; beyond a poorly defined period, changes are irreversible.[43] Cessation of abuse is the most important therapeutic intervention in patients with *n*-hexane–induced neuropathy and N_2O-induced myeloneuropathy; limited anecdotal evidence supports the coadministration of vitamin B_{12} (1000 μg intramuscularly) and methionine (1 g orally) in cases of N_2O-induced myeloneuropathy.[28,111,117]

Agitation, either from acute effects of the inhalant or from withdrawal, is safely managed with a benzodiazepine. In the vast majority of patients, symptoms resolve quickly and hospitalization is not required. The potential toxicity of inhalants should be reinforced and patients should be referred for counseling. Subsets of users, meeting the criteria for inhalant dependence and inhalant-induced psychosis, require inpatient psychiatric care. Pharmacotherapy with carbamazepine or the antipsychotics haloperidol or risperidone appears beneficial to some patients with an inhalant-induced psychotic disorder.[59,88] Case reports describe successful treatment of inhalant dependence with lamotrigine, which inhibits excitatory glutamatergic tone, and with buspirone, an atypical anxiolytic.[96,113] Drug use treatment programs for inhalant abuse are scarce and few providers have special training in this area.[10]

SUMMARY

Inhalants are a heterogeneous group of xenobiotics that include the volatile hydrocarbons, the alkyl nitrates, and nitrous oxide. The incidence of abuse is greatest among adolescents. The central nervous system is the intended target for the inhalant users; early effects include euphoria, hallucinations, headache, and dizziness. Acute cardiotoxicity is manifested most dramatically in "sudden sniffing death." Unique considerations and toxicity are associated with specific agents (see Table 81–3). Diagnosis is largely clinical; further diagnostic testing should be guided by the patient's presenting complaint. Management begins with basic life support and care is generally supportive. Cessation of use is the only known treatment for many manifestations of chronic toxicity.

REFERENCES

1. Albright JT, Lebovitz BL, Lipson R, Luft J. Upper aerodigestive tract frostbite complicating volatile substance abuse. *Int J Pediatr Otorhinolaryngol.* 1999; 49:63-67.
2. Alper AT, Akyol A, Hasdemir H, et al. Glue (toluene) abuse: increased QT dispersion and relation with unexplained syncope. *Inhal Toxicol.* 2008;20:37-41.
3. Arnold GL, Kirby RS, Langendoerfer S, Wilkins-Haug L. Toluene embryopathy. clinical delineation and developmental follow-up. *Pediatrics.* 1994;93:216-220.
4. Atay AA, Kismet E, Turkbay T, et al. Bone mass toxicity associated with inhalation exposure to toluene. *Biol Trace Elem Res.* 2005;105:197-203.
5. Baerg RD, Kimberg DV. Centrilobular hepatic necrosis and acute renal failure in "solvent sniffers". *Ann Intern Med.* 1970;73:713-720.
6. Bale AS, Tu Y, Carpenter-Hyland EP, Chandler LJ, Woodward JJ. Alterations in glutamatergic and gabaergic ion channel activity in hippocampal neurons following exposure to the abused inhalant toluene. *Neuroscience.* 2005;130: 197-206.
7. Balster RL. Neural basis of inhalant abuse. *Drug Alcohol Depend.* 1998;51: 207-214.
8. Baselt RC. *Biological Monitoring Methods for Industrial Chemicals.* Davis, CA: Biomedical Publications; 1982.
9. Bass M. Sudden sniffing death. *JAMA.* 1970;212:2075-2079.
10. Beauvais F, Jumper-Thurman P, Plested B, Helm H. A survey of attitudes among drug user treatment providers toward the treatment of inhalant users. *Subst Use Misuse.* 2002;37:1391-1410.
11. Beauvais F, Wayman JC, Jumper-Thurman P, Plested B, Helm H. Inhalant abuse among American Indian, Mexican American, and non-Latino white adolescents. *Am J Drug Alcohol Abuse.* 2002;28:171-187.
12. Beckstead MJ, Phelan R, Mihic SJ. Antagonism of inhalant and volatile anesthetic enhancement of glycine receptor function. *J Biol Chem.* 2001;276:24959-24964.
13. Beckstead MJ, Weiner JL, Eger EI 2nd, Gong DH, Mihic SJ. Glycine and gamma-aminobutyric acid(A) receptor function is enhanced by inhaled drugs of abuse. *Mol Pharmacol.* 2000;57:1199-1205.
14. Beirne GJ, Brennan JT. Glomerulonephritis associated with hydrocarbon solvents: mediated by antiglomerular basement membrane antibody. *Arch Environ Health.* 1972;25:365-369.
15. Berkowitz BA, Ngai SH, Finck AD. Nitrous oxide "analgesia": resemblance to opiate action. *Science.* 1976;194:967-968.
16. Blanco G, Peters HA. Myeloneuropathy and macrocytosis associated with nitrous oxide abuse. *Arch Neurol.* 1983;40:416-418.
17. Bolt HM, Roos PH, Thier R. The cytochrome P-450 isoenzyme CYP2E1 in the biological processing of industrial chemicals: consequences for occupational and environmental medicine. *Int Arch Occup Environ Health.* 2003;76:174-185.
18. Botto F, Seree E, el Khyari S, et al. Tissue-specific expression and methylation of the human CYP2E1 gene. *Biochem Pharmacol.* 1994;48:1095-1103.
19. Bowen SE, Balster RL. A comparison of the acute behavioral effects of inhaled amyl, ethyl, and butyl acetate in mice. *Fundam Appl Toxicol.* 1997;35:189-196.
20. Bowen SE, Balster RL. A direct comparison of inhalant effects on locomotor activity and schedule-controlled behavior in mice. *Exp Clin Psychopharmacol.* 1998;6:235-247.
21. Bowen SE, Batis JC, Mohammadi MH, Hannigan JH. Abuse pattern of gestational toluene exposure and early postnatal development in rats. *Neurotoxicol Teratol.* 2005;27:105-116.
22. Bowen SE, Hannigan JH, Irtenkauf S. Maternal and fetal blood and organ toluene levels in rats following acute and repeated binge inhalation exposure. *Reprod Toxicol.* 2007;24:343-352.
23. Bowen SE, Wiley JL, Balster RL. The effects of abused inhalants on mouse behavior in an elevated plus-maze. *Eur J Pharmacol.* 1996;312:131-136.
24. Bradberry SM, Whittington RM, Parry DA, Vale JA. Fatal methemoglobinemia due to inhalation of isobutyl nitrite. *J Toxicol Clin Toxicol.* 1994;32:179-184.
25. Broussard LA. The role of the laboratory in detecting inhalant abuse. *Clin Lab Sci.* 2000;13:205-209.
26. Bruckner JV, Peterson RG. Evaluation of toluene and acetone inhalant abuse. I. Pharmacology and pharmacodynamics. *Toxicol Appl Pharmacol.* 1981;61:27-38.
27. Burns TM, Shneker BF, Juel VC. Gasoline sniffing multifocal neuropathy. *Pediatr Neurol.* 2001;25:419-421.
28. Butzkueven H, King JO. Nitrous oxide myelopathy in an abuser of whipped cream bulbs. *J Clin Neurosci.* 2000;7:73-75.
29. Byard RW, Chivell WC, Gilbert JD. Unusual facial markings and lethal mechanisms in a series of gasoline inhalation deaths. *Am J Forensic Med Pathol.* 2003;24:298-302.
30. Carlisle EJ, Donnelly SM, Vasuvattakul S, Kamel KS, Tobe S, Halperin ML. Glue-sniffing and distal renal tubular acidosis: sticking to the facts. *J Am Soc Nephrol.* 1991;1:1019-1027.
31. Chang AP, England JD, Garcia CA, Sumner AJ. Focal conduction block in *n*-hexane polyneuropathy. *Muscle Nerve.* 1998;21:964-969.
32. Clinger OW, Johnson NA. Purposeful inhalation of gasoline vapors. *Psychiatr Q.* 1951;25:557-567.
33. Corcoran GB, Racz WJ, Smith CV, Mitchell JR. Effects of *N*-acetylcysteine on acetaminophen covalent binding and hepatic necrosis in mice. *J Pharmacol Exp Ther.* 1985;232:864-872.

34. Cruz SL, Mirshahi T, Thomas B, Balster RL, Woodward JJ. Effects of the abused solvent toluene on recombinant *N*-methyl-D-aspartate and non-*N*-methyl-D-aspartate receptors expressed in Xenopus oocytes. *J Pharmacol Exp Ther.* 1998;286:334-340.
35. Cruz SL, Orta-Salazar G, Gauthereau MY, Millan-Perez Pena L, Salinas-Stefanon EM. Inhibition of cardiac sodium currents by toluene exposure. *Br J Pharmacol.* 2003;140:653-660.
36. De Ferreyra EC, Castro JA, Diaz Gomez MI, D'Acosta N, De Castro CR, De Fenos OM. Prevention and treatment of carbon tetrachloride hepatotoxicity by cysteine: studies about its mechanism. *Toxicol Appl Pharmacol.* 1974;27:558-568.
37. Del Re AM, Dopico AM, Woodward JJ. Effects of the abused inhalant toluene on ethanol-sensitive potassium channels expressed in oocytes. *Brain Res.* 2006;1087:75-82.
38. DiVincenzo GD, Kaplan CJ, Dedinas J. Characterization of the metabolites of methyl n-butyl ketone, methyl iso-butyl ketone, and methyl ethyl ketone in guinea pig serum and their clearance. *Toxicol Appl Pharmacol.* 1976;36:511-522.
39. Dundaroz MR, Sarici SU, Turkbay T, et al. Evaluation of bone mineral density in chronic glue sniffers. *Turk J Pediatr.* 2002;44:326-329.
40. Evans EB, Balster RL. CNS depressant effects of volatile organic solvents. *Neurosci Biobehav Rev.* 1991;15:233-241.
41. Evans EB, Balster RL. Inhaled 1,1,1-trichloroethane-produced physical dependence in mice: effects of drugs and vapors on withdrawal. *J Pharmacol Exp Ther.* 1993;264:726-733.
42. Filley CM. *The Behavioral Neurology of White Matter.* New York: Oxford Press; 2001.
43. Filley CM, Halliday W, Kleinschmidt-DeMasters BK. The effects of toluene on the central nervous system. *J Neuropathol Exp Neurol.* 2004;63:1-12.
44. Flowers NC, Horan LG. Nonanoxic aerosol arrhythmias. *JAMA.* 1972;219: 33-37.
45. Foster KN, Jones L, Caruso DM. Hydrofluoric acid burn resulting from ignition of gas from a compressed air duster. *J Burn Care Rehabil.* 2003;24:234-237; discussion 228.
46. Frenia ML, Schauben JL. Methanol inhalation toxicity. *Ann Emerg Med.* 1993;22:1919-1923.
47. Garriott J, Petty CS. Death from inhalant abuse: toxicological and pathological evaluation of 34 cases. *Clin Toxicol.* 1980;16:305-315.
48. Gauthereau MY, Salinas-Stefanon EM, Cruz SL. A mutation in the local anaesthetic binding site abolishes toluene effects in sodium channels. *Eur J Pharmacol.* 2005;528:17-26.
49. Gerasimov MR, Ferrieri RA, Pareto D, Logan J, Alexoff D, Ding YS. Synthesis and evaluation of inhaled [11C]butane and intravenously injected [11C]acetone as potential radiotracers for studying inhalant abuse. *Nucl Med Biol.* 2005;32:201-208.
50. Gerasimov MR, Schiffer WK, Marstellar D, Ferrieri R, Alexoff D, Dewey SL. Toluene inhalation produces regionally specific changes in extracellular dopamine. *Drug Alcohol Depend.* 2002;65:243-251.
51. Gindre G, Le Gall S, Condat P, Bazin JE. Late ventricular fibrillation after trichloroethylene poisoning. *Ann Fr Anesth Reanim.* 1997;16:202-203.
52. Gompertz D. Solvents—the relationship between biological monitoring strategies and metabolic handling. A review. *Ann Occup Hyg.* 1980;23: 405-410.
53. Gospe SM Jr, Zhou SS. Prenatal exposure to toluene results in abnormal neurogenesis and migration in rat somatosensory cortex. *Pediatr Res.* 2000;47:362-368.
54. Greenberg MM. The central nervous system and exposure to toluene: a risk characterization. *Environ Res.* 1997;72:1-7.
55. Grosse K, Grosse J. Propane abuse. Extreme dose increase due to development of tolerance. *Nervenarzt.* 2000;71:50-53.
56. Gunn J, Wilson J, Mackintosh AF. Butane sniffing causing ventricular fibrillation. *Lancet.* 1989;1:617.
57. Harris JW, Anders MW. Metabolism of the hydrochlorofluorocarbon 1,2-dichloro-1,1-difluoroethane. *Chem Res Toxicol.* 1991;4:180-186.
58. Herbst J, Koster U, Kerssebaum R, Dekant W. Role of P4502E1 in the metabolism of 1,1,2,2-tetrafluoro-1-(2,2,2-trifluoroethoxy)-ethane. *Xenobiotica.* 1994;24:507-516.
59. Hernandez-Avila CA, Ortega-Soto HA, Jasso A, Hasfura-Buenaga CA, Kranzler HR. Treatment of inhalant-induced psychotic disorder with carbamazepine versus haloperidol. *Psychiatr Serv.* 1998;49:812-815.
60. Hersh JH, Podruch PE, Rogers G, Weisskopf B. Toluene embryopathy. *J Pediatr.* 1985;106:922-927.
61. Hutchens KS, Kung M. "Experimentation" with chloroform. *Am J Med.* 1985;78:715-718.
62. Ikeuchi Y, Hirai H, Okada Y, Mio T, Matsuda T. Excitatory and inhibitory effects of toluene on neural activity in guinea pig hippocampal slices. *Neurosci Lett.* 1993;158:63-66.
63. Jenner P. Oxidative mechanisms in nigral cell death in Parkinson's disease. *Mov Disord.* 1998;13(Suppl 1):24-34.
64. Jevtovic-Todorovic V, Todorovic SM, Mennerick S, et al. Nitrous oxide (laughing gas) is an NMDA antagonist, neuroprotectant and neurotoxin. *Nat Med.* 1998;4:460-463.
65. Jones HE, Balster RL. Neurobehavioral consequences of intermittent prenatal exposure to high concentrations of toluene. *Neurotoxicol Teratol.* 1997;19:305-313.
66. Kaplan HG, Bakken J, Quadracci L, Schubach W. Hepatitis caused by halothane sniffing. *Ann Intern Med.* 1979;90:797-798.
67. Karani V. Peripheral neuritis after addiction to petrol. *Br Med J.* 1966;1:216.
68. Karuri AR, Kugel G, Engelking LR, Kumar MS. Alterations in catecholamine turnover in specific regions of the rat brain following acute exposure to nitrous oxide. *Brain Res Bull.* 1998;45:557-561.
69. Kelly KJ, Ruffing R. Acute eosinophilic pneumonia following intentional inhalation of Scotchguard. *Ann Allergy.* 1993;71:358-361.
70. Kielbasa W, Fung HL. Pharmacokinetics of a model organic nitrite inhalant and its alcohol metabolite in rats. *Drug Metab Dispos.* 2000;28:386-391.
71. Kielbasa W, Fung HL. Relationship between pharmacokinetics and hemodynamic effects of inhaled isobutyl nitrite in conscious rats. *AAPS PharmSci.* 2000;2:E11.
72. Kornfeld M, Moser AB, Moser HW, Kleinschmidt-DeMasters B, Nolte K, Phelps A. Solvent vapor abuse leukoencephalopathy. Comparison to adrenoleukodystrophy. *J Neuropathol Exp Neurol.* 1994;53:389-398.
73. Kurbat RS, Pollack CV Jr. Facial injury and airway threat from inhalant abuse: a case report. *J Emerg Med.* 1998;16:167-169.
74. Kuwabara S, Kai MR, Nagase H, Hattori T. *n*-Hexane neuropathy caused by addictive inhalation: clinical and electrophysiological features. *Eur Neurol.* 1999;41:163-167.
75. Layzer RB. Myeloneuropathy after prolonged exposure to nitrous oxide. *Lancet.* 1978;2:1227-1230.
76. Litt IF, Cohen MI. "Danger—vapor harmful": spot-remover sniffing. *N Engl J Med.* 1969;281:543-544.
77. LoVecchio F, Fulton SE. Ventricular fibrillation following inhalation of Glade Air Freshener. *Eur J Emerg Med.* 2001;8:153-154.
78. LoVecchio F, Sawyers B, Thole D, Beuler MC, Winchell J, Curry SC. Outcomes following abuse of methanol-containing carburetor cleaners. *Hum Exp Toxicol.* 2004;23:473-475.
79. Machabert R, Testud F, Descotes J. Methaemoglobinaemia due to amyl nitrite inhalation. a case report. *Hum Exp Toxicol.* 1994;13:313-314.
80. Maickel RP. The fate and toxicity of butyl nitrites. *NIDA Res Monogr.* 1988;83:15-27.
81. Marjot R, McLeod AA. Chronic non-neurological toxicity from volatile substance abuse. *Hum Toxicol.* 1989;8:301-306.
82. Mattia CJ, LeBel CP, Bondy SC. Effects of toluene and its metabolites on cerebral reactive oxygen species generation. *Biochem Pharmacol.* 1991;42:879-882.
83. McCormick MJ, Mogabgab E, Adams SL. Methanol poisoning as a result of inhalational solvent abuse. *Ann Emerg Med.* 1990;19:639-642.
84. McFee RB, Caraccio TR, McGuigan,M. "Dusting"—a new inhalant of abuse: office products containing difluoroethane. A case series including a fatality. *J Toxicol Clin Toxicol.* 2007;45:632.
85. McGarvey EL, Clavet GJ, Mason W, Waite D. Adolescent inhalant abuse: environments of use. *Am J Drug Alcohol Abuse.* 1999;25:731-741.
86. Mee AS, Wright PL. Congestive (dilated) cardiomyopathy in association with solvent abuse. *J R Soc Med.* 1980;73:671-672.
87. Meredith TJ, Ruprah M, Liddle A, Flanagan RJ. Diagnosis and treatment of acute poisoning with volatile substances. *Hum Toxicol.* 1989;8:277-286.
88. Misra LK, Kofoed L, Fuller W. Treatment of inhalant abuse with risperidone. *J Clin Psychiatry.* 1999;60:620.
89. Monitoring the future. 2007. http://www.monitoringthefuture.org/pub/monographs/overview2007.pdf.
90. Moreno C, Beierle EA. Hydrofluoric acid burn in a child from a compressed air duster. *J Burn Care Res.* 2007;28:909-912.
91. Mortiz F, de La Chapelle A, Bauer F, Leroy JP, Goulle JP, Bonmarchand G. Esmolol in the treatment of severe arrhythmia after acute trichloroethylene poisoning. *Intensive Care Med.* 2000;26:256.

92. Moser VC, Balster RL. Acute motor and lethal effects of inhaled toluene, 1,1,1-trichloroethane, halothane, and ethanol in mice: effects of exposure duration. *Toxicol Appl Pharmacol.* 1985;77:285-291.
93. Murakawa M, Adachi T, Nakao S, Seo N, Shingu K, Mori K. Activation of the cortical and medullary dopaminergic systems by nitrous oxide in rats: a possible neurochemical basis for psychotropic effects and postanesthetic nausea and vomiting. *Anesth Analg.* 1994;78:376-381.
94. Nathan AW, Toseland PA. Goodpasture's syndrome and trichloroethane intoxication. *Br J Clin Pharmacol.* 1979;8:284-286.
95. Nelson LS. Toxicologic myocardial sensitization. *J Toxicol Clin Toxicol.* 2002;40:867-879.
96. Niederhofer H. Treating inhalant abuse with buspirone. *Am J Addict.* 2007;16:69.
97. O'Brien ET, Yeoman WB, Hobby JA. Hepatorenal damage from toluene in a "glue sniffer". *Br Med J.* 1971;2:29-30.
98. Pankow D, Damme B, Schror K. Acetylsalicylic acid—inducer of cytochrome P-450 2E1? *Arch Toxicol.* 1994;68:261-265.
99. Pearlman JT, Adams GL. Amyl nitrite inhalation fad. *JAMA.* 1970; 212:160.
100. Pearson MA, Hoyme HE, Seaver LH, Rimsza ME. Toluene embryopathy: delineation of the phenotype and comparison with fetal alcohol syndrome. *Pediatrics.* 1994;93:211-215.
101. Pema PJ, Horak HA, Wyatt RH. Myelopathy caused by nitrous oxide toxicity. *AJNR Am J Neuroradiol.* 1998;19:894-896.
102. Raines DE, Gioia F, Claycomb RJ, Stevens RJ. The *N*-methyl-D-aspartate receptor inhibitory potencies of aromatic inhaled drugs of abuse: evidence for modulation by cation-pi interactions. *J Pharmacol Exp Ther.* 2004;311:14-21.
103. Reynolds ES, Treinen RJ, Farrish HH, Moslen MT. Metabolism of [14C]carbon tetrachloride to exhaled, excreted and bound metabolites. Dose-response, time-course and pharmacokinetics. *Biochem Pharmacol.* 1984;33:3363-3374.
104. Riegel AC, Ali SF, Torinese S, French ED. Repeated exposure to the abused inhalant toluene alters levels of neurotransmitters and generates peroxynitrite in nigrostriatal and mesolimbic nuclei in rat. *Ann N Y Acad Sci.* 2004;1025:543-551.
105. Riegel AC, Zapata A, Shippenberg TS, French ED. The abused inhalant toluene increases dopamine release in the nucleus accumbens by directly stimulating ventral tegmental area neurons. *Neuropsychopharmacology.* 2007;32:1558-1569.
106. Rosenberg NL, Kleinschmidt-DeMasters BK, Davis KA, Dreisbach JN, Hormes JT, Filley CM. Toluene abuse causes diffuse central nervous system white matter changes. *Ann Neurol.* 1988;23:611-614.
107. Ruprah M, Mant TG, Flanagan RJ. Acute carbon tetrachloride poisoning in 19 patients: implications for diagnosis and treatment. *Lancet.* 1985;1:1027-1029.
108. Scheeres JJ, Chudley AE. Solvent abuse in pregnancy: a perinatal perspective. *J Obstet Gynaecol Can.* 2002;24:22-26.
109. Seaman ME. Barotrauma related to inhalational drug abuse. *J Emerg Med.* 1990;8:141-149.
110. Seshia SS, Rjani KR, Boeckx RL, Chow PN. The neurological manifestations of chronic inhalation of leaded gasoline. *Dev Med Child Neurol.* 1978;20:323-334.
111. Sethi NK, Mullin P, Torgovnick J, Capasso G. Nitrous oxide "whippit" abuse presenting with cobalamin responsive psychosis. *J Med Toxicol.* 2006;2:71-74.
112. Shah R, Vankar GK, Upadhyaya HP. Phenomenology of gasoline intoxication and withdrawal symptoms among adolescents in India: a case series. *Am J Addict.* 1999;8:254-257.
113. Shen YC. Treatment of inhalant dependence with lamotrigine. *Prog Neuropsychopharmacol Biol Psychiatry.* 2007;31:769-771.
114. Shimada T, Yamazaki H, Mimura M, Inui Y, Guengerich FP. Interindividual variations in human liver cytochrome P-450 enzymes involved in the oxidation of drugs, carcinogens and toxic chemicals: studies with liver microsomes of 30 Japanese and 30 Caucasians. *J Pharmacol Exp Ther.* 1994;270:414-423.
115. Smith RA, Wilson M, Miller KW. Naloxone has no effect on nitrous oxide anesthesia. *Anesthesiology.* 1978;49:6-8.
116. Spiller HA, Krenzelok EP. Epidemiology of inhalant abuse reported to two regional poison centers. *J Toxicol Clin Toxicol.* 1997;35:167-173.
117. Stacy CB, Di Rocco A, Gould RJ. Methionine in the treatment of nitrous-oxide-induced neuropathy and myeloneuropathy. *J Neurol.* 1992;239: 401-403.
118. Stengard K, O'Connor WT. Acute toluene exposure decreases extracellular gamma-aminobutyric acid in the globus pallidus but not in striatum: a microdialysis study in awake, freely moving rats. *Eur J Pharmacol.* 1994;292:43-46.
119. Stenqvist O. Nitrous oxide kinetics. *Acta Anaesthesiol Scand.* 1994;38: 757-760.
120. Streicher HZ, Gabow PA, Moss AH, Kono D, Kaehny WD. Syndromes of toluene sniffing in adults. *Ann Intern Med.* 1981;94:758-762.
121. Sturmann K, Mofenson H, Caraccio T. Methylene chloride inhalation: an unusual form of drug abuse. *Ann Emerg Med.* 1985;14:903-905.
122. Substance Abuse and Mental Health Services Administration. http://oas.samhsa.gov/nhsda/2k3tabs/sect1pcTabs/to66.htm#tab1.24a.
123. Suruda AJ, McGlothlin JD. Fatal abuse of nitrous oxide in the workplace. *J Occup Med.* 1990;32:682-684.
124. Szlatenyi CS, Wang RY. Encephalopathy and cranial nerve palsies caused by intentional trichloroethylene inhalation. *Am J Emerg Med.* 1996;14: 464-466.
125. Taylor GJ 4th, Harris WS. Cardiac toxicity of aerosol propellants. *JAMA.* 1970;214:81-85.
126. Tegeris JS, Balster RL. A comparison of the acute behavioral effects of alkylbenzenes using a functional observational battery in mice. *Fundam Appl Toxicol.* 1994;22:240-250.
127. Toutant C, Lippmann S. Fetal solvents syndrome. *Lancet.* 1979;1:1356.
128. Venkataraman G. Renal damage and glue sniffing. *Br Med J (Clin Res Ed).* 1981;283:1467.
129. Vieira I, Sonnier M, Cresteil T. Developmental expression of CYP2E1 in the human liver. Hypermethylation control of gene expression during the neonatal period. *Eur J Biochem.* 1996;238:476-483.
130. Vishnubhakat SM, Beresford HR. Reversible myeloneuropathy of nitrous oxide abuse: serial electrophysiological studies. *Muscle Nerve.* 1991;14:22-26.
131. Wagner SA, Clark MA, Wesche DL, Doedens DJ, Lloyd AW. Asphyxial deaths from the recreational use of nitrous oxide. *J Forensic Sci.* 1992;37: 1008-1015.
132. Ware LB, Matthay MA. The acute respiratory distress syndrome. *N Engl J Med.* 2000;342:1334-1349.
133. Warren DA, Bowen SE, Jennings WB, Dallas CE, Balster RL. Biphasic effects of 1,1,1-trichloroethane on the locomotor activity of mice: relationship to blood and brain solvent concentrations. *Toxicol Sci.* 2000;56:365-373.
134. Weaver NK. *Gasoline.* Philadelphia: Williams & Wilkins; 1992.
135. Wiley JL, Bale AS, Balster RL. Evaluation of toluene dependence and cross-sensitization to diazepam. *Life Sci.* 2003;72:3023-3033.
136. Wilkins-Haug L, Gabow PA. Toluene abuse during pregnancy: obstetric complications and perinatal outcomes. *Obstet Gynecol.* 1991;77:504-509.
137. Williams DR, Cole SJ. Ventricular fibrillation following butane gas inhalation. *Resuscitation.* 1998;37:43-45.
138. Williams JM, Stafford D, Steketee JD. Effects of repeated inhalation of toluene on ionotropic $GABA_A$ and glutamate receptor subunit levels in rat brain. *Neurochem Int.* 2005;46:1-10.
139. Wiseman MN, Banim S. "Glue sniffer's" heart? *Br Med J (Clin Res Ed).* 1987; 294:739.
140. Wood RW, Coleman JB, Schuler R, Cox C. Anticonvulsant and antipunishment effects of toluene. *J Pharmacol Exp Ther.* 1984;230:407-412.
141. Yin H, Anders MW, Jones JP. Metabolism of 1,2-dichloro-1-fluoroethane and 1-fluoro-1,2,2-trichloroethane: electronic factors govern the regioselectivity of cytochrome P450-dependent oxidation. *Chem Res Toxicol.* 1996;9:50-57.
142. Zacny JP, Sparacino G, Hoffmann P, Martin R, Lichtor JL. The subjective, behavioral and cognitive effects of subanesthetic concentrations of isoflurane and nitrous oxide in healthy volunteers. *Psychopharmacology (Berl).* 1994;114:409-416.
143. Zimmerman SW, Groehler K, Beirne GJ. Hydrocarbon exposure and chronic glomerulonephritis. *Lancet.* 1975;2:199-201.

CHAPTER 82
HALLUCINOGENS

Kavita M. Babu

The term "hallucinogen" describes a diverse group of xenobiotics that alter and distort perception, thought, and mood without clouding the sensorium. Hallucinogens can be categorized by their chemical structures, and further divided into natural and synthetic members of each family. The major structural classes of hallucinogens include the lysergamides, tryptamines (indolealkylamines), amphetamines (phenylethylamines), arylhexamines, cannabinoids, harmine alkaloids, belladonna alkaloids, and the tropane alkaloids. In addition, there are several unique hallucinogens, such as *Salvia divinorum*, nutmeg, kratom, and kava kava. This chapter focuses on lysergamides, tryptamines, phenylethlyamines, and these unique hallucinogens. More on the other classes can be found in Chap. 71 (Monoamine oxidase inhibitors), Chap. 75 (Amphetamines), Chap. 83 (Cannabinoids), and Chap. 85 (Phencyclidine and Ketamine).

HISTORY

The term "hallucination" may be defined as false perception that has no basis in the external environment. The term is derived from the Latin alucinari, "to wander in mind." While the term "psychedelic" has been used for years to refer to the recreational and nonmedical effects of hallucinogens, other terms, like entheogen and entactogen, frequently appear in Internet discussions. Entheogens are "substances which generate the god or spirit within," while entactogens create an awareness of "the touch within."[41] These terms all refer to the same xenobiotics, used with differing intent or in varying settings. Hallucinations differ from illusions, which are distorted perceptions of objects based in reality.

Hallucinogens have been used for thousands of years by many different cultures, largely during religious ceremonies. The ancient Indian holy book, *Rig-Veda*, written over 3500 years ago, describes a sacramental xenobiotic called Soma both as a god and as an intoxicating xenobiotic. Although debated for many years, the source of Soma is now believed to be the juice of the mushroom *Amanita muscaria*.[98,105] The Aztecs used the psilocybin-containing teonanacatl (flesh of the gods), and *Ololiuqui* (morning glory species) in their religious ceremonies. To this day, the Native American Church in the United States uses peyote in religious ceremonies.

Synthetic hallucinogen use is often said to have begun with the discovery of lysergic acid diethylamide, or LSD. The synthesis of LSD resulted from extensive research on the medicinal uses of ergot alkaloids derived from the fungus, *Claviceps purpurea*. From medieval times through recent years, several large-scale epidemics of vasospastic ischemia, gangrene, and hallucinations (collectively called ergotism) have resulted from *C. purpurea* contamination of cereal crops.[136] The hallucinations from *Claviceps* ingestion have been attributed to the ergot alkaloid lysergic acid amide from which LSD was chemically synthesized. *Claviceps purpurea* has been suggested, but subsequently disproved, as the cause of the mass hysteria leading up to the Salem witch trials. Many of these adverse effects after ingestion of *C. purpurea* have been attributed to the serotonergic agonist effects of the ergot alkaloids (see Chap. 51).[38]

In 1938, Albert Hofmann, a Swiss chemist, synthesized LSD-25, the twenty-fifth substance in a series of lysergic acid derivatives being researched as new arousal, or analeptic, agents. These lysergic acid compounds were based on ergot extracts from *C. purpurea*. Five years later, LSD-25 was "tested" when Hofmann had an unintentional exposure in his laboratory, and subsequently developed hallucinations.[62,117] Soon thereafter, Sandoz laboratories began marketing LSD under the trademark Delysid as an adjunct for analytic psychotherapy. In the 1950s, a small number of psychiatrists began using LSD to release the repressed memories of patients, and as an experimental model for schizophrenia.[124] The Central Intelligence Agency reportedly experimented with the use of LSD as a tool for interrogating suspected communists and as a mind-control agent.[23,117]

In the 1960s, the concept of the "fifth freedom" emerged. As individuals explored this "right" to alter their consciousness as they saw fit, LSD (also called acid) became a fashionable recreational drug. In one of the most famous slogans of the 1960s, Dr. Timothy Leary popularized LSD as a way to "Tune in, Turn on, Drop out."[117] By 1966, federal law banned the use of LSD.[91] Initial reports of LSD-induced chromosomal damage appeared in the 1960s.[31,64,75] However, further studies of pregnant women who had taken LSD did not demonstrate an increased risk of abortions nor birth defects.[44,72]

LSD use diminished in the late 1970s and early 1980s, perhaps due to users' concerns regarding potential health risks of brain damage, "bad trips," and flashbacks.[97] In the meantime, there was a rise in the use of the "designer" hallucinogens. Exploiting a loophole in drug enforcement laws, these synthetic tryptamine and amphetamine hallucinogens were chemically similar to, but legally distinct from, their outlawed counterparts.

A resurgence in LSD use was reported among high school teens in the late 1990s, with more prevalent use in suburbs than in cities.[92,106] In 1997, two studies of adolescents showed a lifetime prevalence of LSD use at 13% and 14%.[66,97] In 2000, Drug Enforcement Administration (DEA) agents seized an LSD-production lab and apprehended two men involved in massive production of LSD in Kansas. Their incarceration resulted in a more than 90% decrease in LSD availability nationwide.[126]

All-night dance clubs host "rave parties," at which emerging hallucinogens are popular.[13] While the impact of these parties on the growth of hallucinogens in the United States is unclear, many of the newer hallucinogens have been christened "club drugs" because of this association.[53] The Internet has developed as a vehicle for the rapid and facile sharing of information on the synthesis of emerging drugs, user experiences, and adverse effects. Additionally, the Internet marketplace has made many "herbal" hallucinogens widely available via unregulated web sites.[35]

EPIDEMIOLOGY

The 2006 National Survey on Drug Use and Health (NSDUH) reported the following trends in hallucinogen use: more than 23 million Americans over the age of 12 reported LSD use during their lifetime, 6.6 million had used phencyclidine (PCP), and 12 million reported previous methylenedioxymethamphetamine (MDMA) use. Additionally, 2.3 million people reported prior use of ketamine, while only 700,000 reported use of α-methyltryptamine (AMT), dimethyltryptamine (DMT), or 5-methoxy-dimethyltryptamine (5-MeO-DMT). About 1.8 million people reported use of *S. divinorum* during their lifetime. In the reported results, the 18 to 25 age group was most likely to report use of any of these hallucinogens within the previous year.[119] Table 82–1 presents the structural classifications of hallucinogens.

TABLE 82–1. Structural Classifications of Hallucinogens

Classification
Lysergamides
d-Lysergic acid diethylamide (LSD)
Lysergic acid hydroxyethylamide
Ipomoea violacea (Morning glory)
Ololiuqui (South American Morning glory)
Ergine
Argyreia nervosa (Woodrose)
Indolealkylamines/Tryptamines
5-Methoxy-*N,N*-dimethyltryptamine
N,N-Dimethyltryptamine
Psilocin
Psilocybin
Phenylethylamines
Mescaline
MDMA (3,4-methylenedioxymethamphetamine)
2C-B
2C-T-7
Tetrahydrocannabinoids
Marijuana
Hashish
Belladonna alkaloids
Jimsonweed (*Datura stramonium*)
Henbane (*Hyoscyamus niger*)
Deadly nightshade (*Atropa belladonna*)
Brugmansia spp
Miscellaneous
Kava Kava
Ketamine
Kratom
Nutmeg
Phencyclidine (PCP)
Salvia divinorum

LYSERGAMIDES

Lysergamides are derivatives of lysergic acid, a substituted tetracyclic amine based on an indole nucleus (Fig. 82–1). Naturally occurring lysergamides are found in several species of morning glory (*Rivea corymbosa, Ipomoea violacea*) and Hawaiian baby woodrose (*Argyreia nervosa*).[58] Morning glory seeds contain multiple alkaloids, including lysergic acid hydroxyethylamide and ergonovine. The morning glory seeds were called ololiuqui in ancient Mexico, where Aztecs and other indigenous populations used them in religious rites.[121] However, in one volunteer study, ololiuqui use caused sedation rather than hallucinations.[63] Both morning glory and Hawaiian baby woodrose seeds can be legally purchased for planting in garden stores, and on the Internet.

The synthetic lysergamide, LSD, is derived from an ergot alkaloid of the fungus, *C. purpurea*. Although four LSD isomers exist, only the d-isomer is active. Lysergic acid diethylamide is a water-soluble, colorless, tasteless, and odorless powder. Currently, LSD is usually sold as liquid-impregnated blotter paper, microdots, tiny tablets, "window pane" gelatin squares, liquid, powder, or tablets.[106] LSD users typically experience heightened awareness of auditory and visual stimuli with size, shape, and color distortions. Auditory and visual hallucinations may occur, as well as synesthesia, a confusion of the senses, where users may report "hearing colors, or seeing sounds".[126] Other more complex perceptual effects may include depersonalization and a sensation of enhanced insight or awareness. A "bad trip" may occur with larger doses of LSD and produce anxiety, bizarre behaviors, and combativeness.[126]

LSD is classified by the DEA as a Schedule I drug, with high abuse potential, lack of established safety even under medical supervision, and no known use in medical treatment.[126]

INDOLEALKYLAMINES (TRYPTAMINES)

Indolealkylamines, or tryptamines, represent a class of natural and synthetic compounds that structurally share a substituted monoamine group (Fig. 82–2). Endogenous tryptamines include serotonin and melatonin. Naturally occurring exogenous tryptamines include psilocybin, bufotenine, and DMT. Psilocybin is found in three major genera of mushrooms: *Psilocyba, Panaelous,* and *Conocybe.*[105] Other psychoactive mushrooms include *Amanita muscaria* and *Amanita pantherina*, which contain ibotenic acid, muscimol, and muscazone, which are unrelated to the tryptamines.[58] Hallucinogenic mushrooms

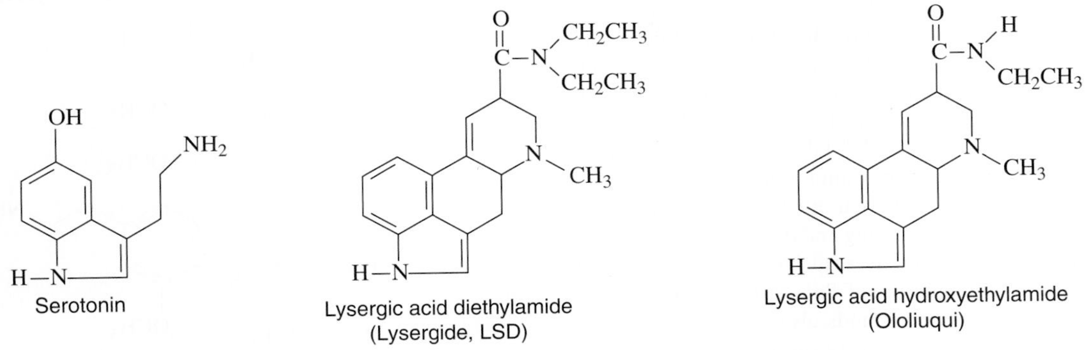

Serotonin

Lysergic acid diethylamide (Lysergide, LSD)

Lysergic acid hydroxyethylamide (Ololiuqui)

FIGURE 82–1. Hallucinogens of the lysergamide chemical class and their chemical similarity to serotonin.

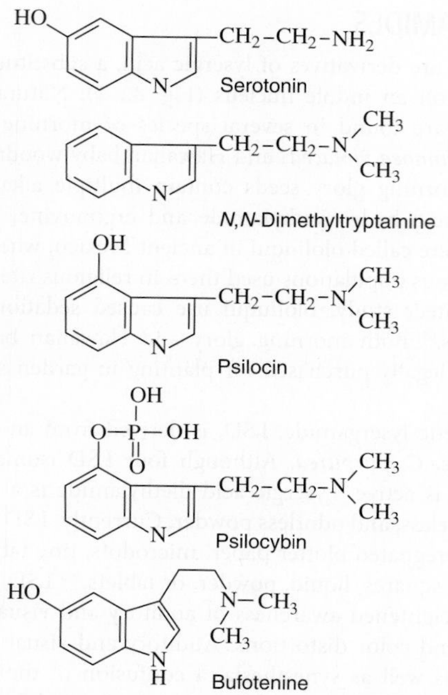

FIGURE 82–2. Hallucinogens of the indolealkylamine chemical class and their chemical similarity to serotonin.

are discussed in Chap. 117. Psilocybin-containing mushrooms, or "magic mushrooms," grow in the Pacific Northwest and southern United States, usually in cow pastures. The mushroom may be recognized by a green-blue color that it assumes after bruising, but misidentification is common.[11]

N,N-Dimethyltryptamine (DMT) is a potent, short-acting hallucinogen. It is found naturally in the bark of the Yakee plant (*Virola calophylla*), which grows in the Amazon Basin and is used by shamans as a hallucinogenic snuff to "communicate with the spirits."[105] DMT is also found in the hallucinogenic tea, ayahuasca, which is used by indigenous healers in the Amazon Basin. In ayahuasca, DMT-containing plants (e.g., *Psychotria viridis*) are combined with plants containing harmine alkaloids (e.g., *Banisteriopsis caapi*), which inhibit hepatic monoamine oxidases to increase the oral bioavailability of DMT (see Chap. 71).[84]

The use of toads in religious ceremonies and witchcraft dates back thousands of years. All species of the toad genus *Bufo* have parotid glands on their backs that produce a variety of substances, including dopamine, epinephrine, and serotonin.[77] Many of these toads produce bufotenine, a tryptamine, which causes hypertension, but does not cross the blood–brain barrier. Interest in bufotenine grew out of reports of a toad-licking fad in the 1980s, in which individuals would reportedly lick toads for recreational purposes.[76] However, further review suggests that bufotenine is not the hallucinogenic substance found in toad secretions. Instead, 5-MeO-DMT has been identified as the psychoactive substance.[135] 5-MeO-DMT is only found in one species of toad, *Bufo alvarius* (Sonoran Desert toad or Colorado River toad).[76] Although bufotenine is currently classified as a Schedule I drug by the DEA, 5-MeO-DMT is not scheduled.[88,128] Like DMT, 5-MeO-DMT is rapidly metabolized by intestinal monoamine oxidase enzymes; licking or ingesting toad skins would thus have limited potential as a route of recreational use.[21] Methods for extracting and drying *B. alvarius* secretions for smoking and insufflation are available and on the Internet. Death has resulted from wrongful use of *Bufo* secretions for purposes of aphrodisia.[29,55] The toad venom glands also produce cardioactive steroids, called bufodienolides, which may cause digoxin-like cardiac toxicity, and in some species can secrete tetrodotoxin.[86,139]

Two of the more important synthetic tryptamines include N,N-diisopropyl-5-methoxytryptamine (5-MeO-DiPT, Foxy Methoxy) and AMT (or IT-290). Since 2001, law enforcement authorities in more than 10 states have seized large amounts of 5-MeO-DiPT and AMT. These drugs are often sold surreptitiously as MDMA. 5-MeO-DiPT received Schedule I status in 2004.[129] AMT is a monoamine oxidase inhibitor that was sold as an antidepressant in the former Soviet Union.[111] AMT was given Schedule I status by the DEA in September 2004.[129]

PHENYLETHYLAMINES (AMPHETAMINES)

Endogenous phenylethylamines include dopamine, norepinephrine, and tyrosine. Exogenous phenylethylamines are known for their ability to stimulate catecholamine release and cause a variety of physiologic and psychiatric effects, including hallucinations. Substitution on the phenylalkylamine structure has important effects on both the hallucinogenic and stimulant potential. The presence of a methyl group in the side chain of the phenylethylamines is associated with a higher degree of hallucinogenic effect (Fig. 82–3).[68] MDMA, amphetamine, and methamphetamine are well-known members of this family and are discussed in detail in Chap. 75.

The best recognized of the naturally occurring phenylethylamines is mescaline. Mescaline is found in peyote (*Lophophora williamsii*), a small blue-green spineless cactus that grows in dry and rocky slopes throughout the southwestern United States and northern Mexico. Peyote buttons are the round, fleshy tops of the cactus that have been sliced off and dried. The legal use of peyote in the United States is restricted to the Native American Church where peyote buttons are used for both religious ceremonies and medical treatment for physical and psychological ailments.[24,27]

Other nonindigenous cactus species containing significant amounts of mescaline include the San Pedro cactus (*Trichocereus pachanoi*) and Peruvian torch cactus (*Trichocereus peruvianus*). These plants can be purchased for ornamental purposes in garden stores and on the Internet.[58]

The synthesis and effects of hundreds of other congeners of amphetamine have been described.[110] The most well-known of these synthetic

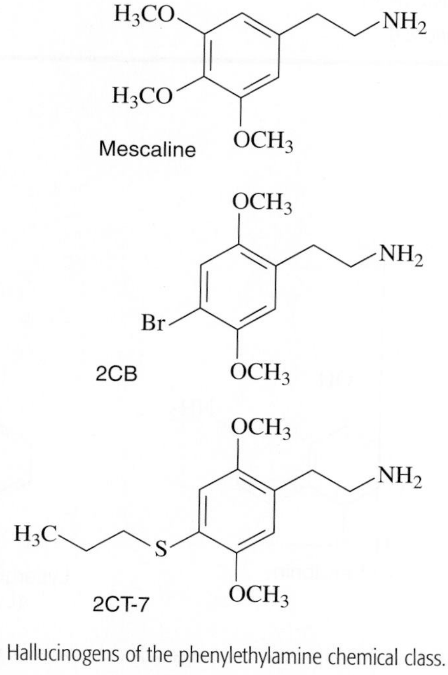

FIGURE 82–3. Hallucinogens of the phenylethylamine chemical class.

hallucinogenic amphetamines are 4-bromo-2,5-dimethoxyphenethylamine (2C-B, Nexus, Bromo, Spectrum) and 2,5-dimethoxy-4-N-propylthiopheneethylamine (2C-T-7, Blue Mystic). During the 1980s, 2C-B gained popularity as a legal alternative to MDMA. When 2C-B was given Schedule I status in 1995, 2C-T-7 emerged as another legal designer amphetamine.[9] In March 2004, 2C-T-7 also received Schedule I status.[33]

SALVIA DIVINORUM

Salvia divinorum is a perennial herbaceous member of the mint family. While there are more than 500 species of *Salvia*, *S. divinorum* is most recognized for its hallucinogenic properties. The plant is characterized by a height greater than 1 m, large green leaves, hollow square stems, and white flowers with purple calyces.[130] *Salvia divinorum* is native to areas of Oaxaca, Mexico, and grows well in sunny, temperate climates. Plants, leaves, and extracts may be purchased on the Internet, and tips for cultivation of plants are easily accessible.

Since the 16th century, the Mazatec Indians have employed *S. divinorum* as a hallucinogen in religious rites as a means of producing visions.[130] The Mazatecs continue to revere *S. divinorum* as an incarnation of the Virgin Mary, referring to the plant as "ska Maria." Currently, the Controlled Substances Act does not prohibit use of *S. divinorum* or extracts of its psychoactive agent, salvinorin A. Nationwide regulation of this substance exists in Australia, and there is local regulation in some municipalities where *S. divinorum* use among teenagers is rampant.[127] The possession and sale of *S. divinorum* is currently illegal in several states, including California, Delaware, Florida, and Georgia. There continues to be widespread marketing of this hallucinogen on the Internet as a "legal hallucinogen."[36]

KRATOM

Kratom, or *Mitragyna speciosa Korth*, is derived from the leaves of a tree native to Asia and Africa.[109] Kratom has dual properties as a stimulant and sedative, and was historically used in Southeast Asia by manual laborers to enhance productivity. Although hallucinogenic effects are uncommon, they have been reported in heavy use.[120] Kratom has been illegal in Thailand since 1946, and Australia since 2005. Kratom is currently legal to possess and use in the United States, where some patients who have chronic pain have adopted it to modulate opiate withdrawal symptoms.

NUTMEG

Nutmeg is derived from *Myristica fragrans*, an evergreen tree native to the Spice Islands. The fruits of the tree contain a central kernel called the nutmeg, while the surrounding red aril is used to produce a spice called mace.[96] While nutmeg is commonly available as a cooking spice, it has been used medicinally for centuries as an antidiarrheal and abortifacient.[57] It has also been used to produce euphoria and hallucinations, and is a low-cost and accessible recreational herbal that is frequently abused by adolescents.[34,96,102] There are currently no regulations affecting the recreational use of nutmeg.

BELLADONNA ALKALOIDS

The belladonna alkaloids, including the tropane alkaloids atropine, hyoscyamine, and scopolamine, can be isolated from a number of plants. Deadly nightshade (*Atropa belladonna*), a perennial plant, grows throughout the United States, and in areas of Europe and Africa. Belladonna alkaloids can be isolated from both the leaves and berries of this perennial plant. Jimson weed (*Datura stramonium*), also called loco weed, grows throughout warm and moist areas of the world. This bush contains pods full of small black seeds that are ingested for their hallucinogenic properties. The common name Angel's trumpet is used for plants of the Solanaceae family with large trumpet-shaped white flowers (*Brugmansia* or *Datura*). Given their wide availability, in the wild and over the Internet, these plants are frequently used as hallucinogens by adolescents.[54] Unfortunately, these plants can also produce significant morbidity from anticholinergic toxicity in unwary users. Moonflower, a common name given to several plants, including *Datura inoxia*, was responsible for anticholinergic poisoning of more than a dozen adolescents in one series.[30] Additionally, epidemics of unintentional poisoning have been reported among drug users who received heroin adulterated with scopolamine.[60]

TOXICOKINETICS

LSD is the most studied hallucinogen, and there is extensive information about its pharmacokinetics (Table 82–2). Ingestion is the most common route of exposure, and the gastrointestinal (GI) tract rapidly absorbs LSD. Other routes of administration include intranasal, parenteral, sublingual, smoking, and conjunctival instillation. Plasma protein binding is over 80% and volume of distribution is 0.28 L/kg. It is concentrated within the visual cortex, as well as the limbic and reticular activating systems. It is metabolized in the liver via hydroxylation and glucuronidation, and excreted predominantly as a pharmacologically inactive compound. LSD has an elimination half-life of about 2.5 hours. Only small amounts are eliminated unchanged in the urine.

While LSD use has been reported via intravenous and intramuscular routes, ingestion of blotter paper is the most common route of abuse. The minimum effective oral dose is 25 μg.[69] The onset of effects may occur 30 to 60 minutes after exposure, with a duration of 10 to 12 hours.

Ingestion of 200 to 300 morning glory seeds is required to achieve hallucinogenic effects. Hawaiian baby woodrose seeds contain ergine, and only five to 10 seeds are required to produce hallucinations. After ingestion of woodrose seeds, the effects typically last for 6 to 8 hours, and produce tranquility without marked euphoria.[4]

Peyote buttons are very bitter, and can be eaten whole or dried and crushed into a powder, which is reconstituted as tea.[58] Nausea, vomiting, and diaphoresis often precede the onset of hallucinations, which begin at 1 to 3 hours postingestion, and last for up to 12 hours.[96] Six to 12 peyote buttons, or 270 to 540 mg of mescaline, are commonly required to produce hallucinogenic effects.[104] Ingestion of up to 5 g of psilocybin-containing mushrooms may be required to produce hallucinogenic effects. After ingestion of psilocybe mushrooms, psilocybin is converted to psilocin, the active hallucinogen in the GI tract.[56] The effects of psilocin are similar to LSD, but with a shorter duration of action of about 4 hours.

For recreational purposes, DMT is typically smoked, snorted, or injected. Hallucinogenic effects peak in 5 to 20 minutes, with a duration of 30 to 60 minutes, which earned DMT the nickname the "businessman's trip." 5-MeO-DiPT is most commonly ingested, but may be smoked or insufflated. Effects begin 20 to 30 minutes after ingestion, and include disinhibition and relaxation. There is a dose-dependent response and at higher ranges, and symptoms include mydriasis, euphoria, auditory and visual hallucinations, nausea, diarrhea, and jaw clenching.[90,112] The hallucinogenic effects are reported to last from 3 to 6 hours.[85,112] Other substances may be used to heighten or prolong the hallucinogenic effects of 5-MeO-DiPT. These include sildenafil, γ-hydroxybutyrate, benzodiazepines, and marijuana. AMT is available as a white powder, which may be ingested, smoked, or insufflated. Hallucinations typically occur within 30 minutes, and may last from 12 to 16 hours.[74]

TABLE 82–2. Pharmacology of Selected Hallucinogens

Drug name or Source	Psychoactive Component (if Different)	Typical Oral Dose	Onset	Duration
Bufo species toads	5-MeO-DMT	5–15 mg (smoked)	Immediate (smoked)	5–20 min (smoked)
DMT	–	15–60 mg	5–20 min	30–60 min
"Foxy Methoxy"	5-MeO-DiPT	6–10 mg	20–30 min	3–6 h
Woodrose (*Argyreia nervosa)*	Ergine	5–10 seeds		6–8 h
Jimson weed (*Datura stramonium)*	Atropine, hyoscyamine, scopolamine	10 seeds	20–30 min	2–3 h
Kratom (*Mitragyna speciosa Korth)*	Mitragynine, 7-hydroxy-mitragynine	2–6 g (stimulant); >7 g (sedative)	10–15 min	4–6 h
LSD	Lysergic acid diethylamide	50–100 μg	30–60 min	10–12 h
"Magic mushrooms" (*Psilocybe* species)	Psilocybin, psilocin	5 g mushrooms	30 min–2 h	4 h
Nutmeg (*Myristica fragrans)*	Myristicin, elemicin	20 g	1 h	24 h
Peyote (*Lophophora williamsii)*	Mescaline	6–12 buttons, 270–540 mg mescaline	1–3 h	10–12 h
Salvia divinorum	Salvinorin A	–	30 min (inhaled); 1 h (po)	15–20 min (inhaled); 2 h (po)
2C-B	–	16–30 mg	1 h	6–10 h

Amphetamine, methamphetamine, and MDMA are well absorbed through the GI tract. The elimination half-life ranges from 8 to 30 hours for members of this class, and is dependent on urine pH.[12,32] Amphetamines are weak bases and undergo more rapid elimination in acidic urine.[107] The volume of distribution ranges from 3 to 5 L/kg for amphetamine, 3 to 4 L/kg for methamphetamine, and likely more than 5 L/kg for MDMA.[12,32,73,107] Elimination of other amphetamines occurs through multiple mechanisms including aromatic hydroxylation, aliphatic hydroxylation, and *N*-dealkylation.[73] Tolerance has been demonstrated in chronic amphetamine users.[70]

There is little information about 2C-B and 2C-T-7 in the medical literature. Both drugs may be used via oral, intranasal, and intrarectal routes. Both 2C-B and 2C-T-7 exert their hallucinogenic effects within 1 hour of use, and physiologic and psychologic effects may persist for 6 to 10 hours. Specific toxicokinetic data on 2C-B and 2C-T-7 are not available; however, the toxicokinetics of other phenylethylamines may be similar.

Salvia divinorum may be chewed, smoked, or ingested as tea. Hallucinations occur immediately after exposure to the drug and are typically quite vivid. Synesthesia is reported among Salvia users.[36] Hallucinogenic effects after *S. divinorum* use are typically brief, lasting only 1 to 2 hours. Pharmacokinetic data for *S. divinorum*, and its primary psychoactive, salvinorin A, have been described in one volunteer study.[113] Psychoactive effects were typically experienced 5 to 10 minutes after absorption of salvinorin A via the buccal mucosa, reaching a plateau during the first hour after exposure, and resolving within 2 hours. Vaporization and inhalation of salvinorin A led to more rapid effects at 30 seconds after exposure. These effects would plateau at 5 to 10 minutes, and typically subside after 20 to 30 minutes. In this study, ingestion of *S. divinorum* leaves did not produce the same effects as buccal or inhalational administration, leading to the theory that GI inactivation of salvinorin A occurs after ingestion.[113]

Kratom leaves can be decocted into tea, chewed, or smoked.[65] Kratom leaves contain approximately 0.8% mitragynine by weight, but this can vary by geographic origin of trees, as well as season.[108] Neuropsychiatric effects are dose dependent and occur within 5 to 10 minutes of exposure, with effects lasting 4 to 6 hours.[120] Stimulant effects predominate at doses of 2 to 6 g, while sedation becomes more pronounced at doses above 7 g.

Nutmeg is usually ingested as a paste, or mixed in a beverage; 15 to 20 g are required for clinical effects.[96] This dose is often unpalatable, and a case report of recreational use of encapsulated nutmeg has been described.[102] Clinical effects can begin 1 hour after nutmeg ingestion; nausea and vomiting precede the onset of hallucinations, and effects can persist for more than 24 hours after exposure.[96]

The belladonna alkaloids are most concentrated in the seeds of Jimson weed; each seed contains approximately 0.1 mg of atropine.[115] Ingestion of as few as 10 seeds can produce hallucinations within 20 to 30 minutes; these effects can last for 2 to 3 hours. While the roots and seeds of Angel's trumpet contain the highest alkaloid concentrations, users most often brew the blossom into a tea. Each blossom contains approximately 0.3 mg of atropine and 0.65 mg of scopolamine.[54] The elimination half-lives of atropine and hyoscyamine are 2.5 and 3.5 hours, respectively, while the elimination half-life of scopolamine is considerably longer, at 8 hours.[15]

PHARMACOLOGY

Although the lysergamide, indolealklylamine, and phenylethylamine hallucinogens are structurally distinct, the similarities in their effects on cognition support a common site of action on central serotonin receptors.[3,20,26,61,123] Serotonin modulates many psychological and physiologic processes, including mood, personality, affect, appetite, motor function, sexual activity, temperature regulation, pain perception, sleep induction, and antidiuretic hormone (ADH) release. There are more than 14 known 5-hydroxytryptamine, [serotonin (5-HT)] receptor subtypes (see Chap. 13); differing affinity for these subtypes occurs based on the structure of the hallucinogen, and may account for the subtle differences between their effects.

The lysergamide, indolealklylamine, and phenylethylamine hallucinogens all bind to the 5-HT_2 class of receptors. There is a good correlation between the affinity of both indolealkylamine and phenylethylamine hallucinogens for 5-HT_2 receptors in vitro and hallucinogenic potency in humans in vivo.[3,52,95,123] Of the multiple subtypes of 5-HT_2 receptors, 5-HT_{2A}, receptors are found with highest density in the cerebral cortex, making the 5-HT_{2A} receptor the most likely common site of hallucinogen action.[79] This theory is bolstered by an animal study that shows that a selective 5-HT_{2A} antagonist can inhibit the effects of LSD and a phenylethylamine, 2,5-dimethoxy-4-iodo-amphetamine (DOI). The response to high doses of LSD and DOI suggest that both lysergamides and phenylethylamines are partial agonists at cortical 5-HT_{2A} receptors.[51,79,101]

Although the majority of investigation has focused on the role of serotonin for drug-induced hallucinations, other neurotransmitters are involved. Stimulation of 5-HT_{2A} receptors enhances release of glutamate in the cortical layer V pyramidal cells.[3,8] LSD and other lysergamides stimulate both D_1 and D_2 dopamine receptors.[7,50,134] In animal models, LSD and phenylethylamine hallucinogens modulate *N*-methyl-D-aspartate (NMDA) receptor–mediated effects, and may have a protective effect against neurotoxicity secondary to PCP and ketamine.[8,43]

Another theory that incorporates these other neurotransmitters involves the concept of "thalamic filtering."[49] The thalamus receives input and output from the cortex and reticular activating system, and functions to filter relevant sensory input. This theory has been explored as an explanation for organic psychosis and the effects of hallucinogenic drugs. Multiple neurotransmitters, including dopamine, acetylcholine, γ-aminobutyric acid (GABA), and glutamate, exert their actions on the thalamus. Increased excitatory or decreased inhibitory neurotransmitter in this region of the brain may lead to "sensory overload," which manifests itself clinically as symptoms of psychosis.[49] Experimental evidence also demonstrates electroencephalographic (EEG) abnormalities after exposure to hallucinogens, confirming a cortical, rather the ophthalmologic, etiology for hallucinations.[42]

Salvinorin A, the psychoactive component of *S. divinorum*, is one of the most potent natural hallucinogens. The effect of salvinorin A occurs via binding at the κ-opioid receptor, making it structurally and mechanistically unique (Fig. 82–4).[138] The κ-opioid receptor is distinct from the μ-opioid receptor, stimulation of which generally causes euphoria and analgesia (see Chap. 38). Salvinorin A has not been demonstrated to have any serotonergic activity.[138]

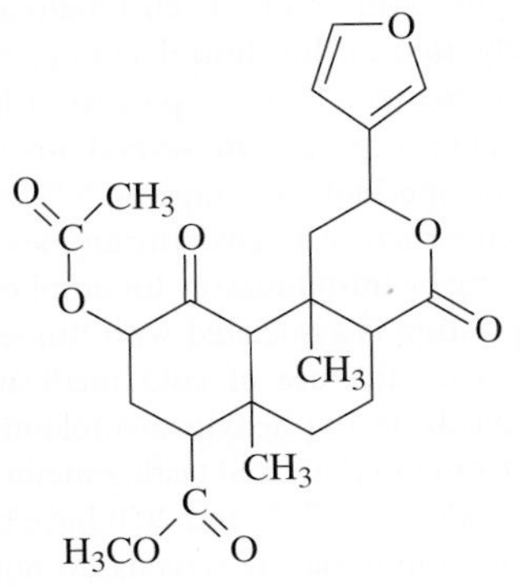

FIGURE 82–4. Structure of salvinorin A.

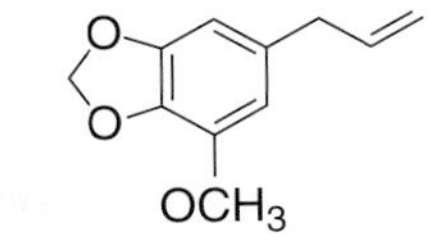

FIGURE 82–5. Structure of myristicin.

The opioid effects of Kratom have been attributed to mitragynine.[108,137] The most prevalent of the Kratom alkaloids, mitragynine shares a structural similarity with yohimbine.[10] In vitro, mitragynine is active at both supraspinal opioid δ and μ receptors.[122] This μ-receptor activity results in analgesia and efficacy in treating opioid withdrawal symptoms. Additionally, mitragynine activates noradrenergic and serotonergic pathways.[82] Another Kratom alkaloid, 7-hydroxymitragynine, also demonstrates antinociceptive effects and high affinity for opioid receptors.[83] In animal studies, 7-hydroxymitragynine has more analgesic potency than morphine, even after oral administration.[81]

Nutmeg contains a number of purportedly psychoactive compounds, including myristicin, elemicin, and safrole (Fig. 82–5). The psychoactive components of nutmeg include terpenes and alkyl benzyl derivatives (myristicin, elemicin, and safrole).[96]

It has been theorized that the aromatics found in nutmeg are metabolized to amphetaminelike compounds that create hallucinogenic effects.[96] However, this mechanism is unsupported by both theory and animal data.[102] Nutmeg contains myristicin and elemicin, both weak monoamine oxidase inhibitors, as well as other terpene compounds. Myristicin and elemicin both demonstrate serotonergic activity, which may account for nutmeg's clinical effects.[102]

The pharmacology of atropine, a competitive central and peripheral antimuscarinic agent and the most well-studied belladonna alkaloid, is discussed in detail (see Antidotes in Depth A34–Atropine). Like atropine, scopolamine and hyoscyamine are tertiary amines, which can cross the blood–brain barrier. Scopolomaine causes more sedation than atropine, and its transdermal availability has led to its use in motion sickness patches. Hyoscyamine is more potent than atropine; it has traditionally been used as an antispasmodic for GI conditions.

CLINICAL EFFECTS

Physiologic changes accompany and often precede the perceptual changes induced by lysergamides, tryptamines, and phenylethylamines. The physical effects may be caused by direct xenobiotic effect or by a response to the disturbing or enjoyable hallucinogenic experience. Sympathetic effects mediated by the locus coeruleus include mydriasis, tachycardia, hypertension, tachypnea, hyperthermia, and diaphoresis. They may occur shortly after ingestion and often precede the hallucinogenic effects. Other clinical findings that are reported include piloerection, dizziness, hyperactivity, muscle weakness, ataxia, altered mental status, coma, and rhythmic, pupillary dilation and constriction.[71] Nausea and vomiting often precede the psychedelic effects produced by psilocybin and mescaline. Potentially life-threatening complications, such as hyperthermia, coma, respiratory arrest, hypertension, tachycardia, and coagulopathy, were described in a report of eight patients with massive LSD overdoses.[67] Sympathomimetic effects are generally less prominent in LSD ingestion than in phenylethylamine toxicity. Similar sympathetic symptoms have been described after the use of 2C-B and 2C-T-7. Low doses of 2C-B and 2C-T-7 may produce hypertension, tachycardia, and visual hallucinations, while elevated doses are associated with shifts in color perception, and enhanced auditory and visual stimulation. An analog of 2C-B, called 2C-B-FLY, or BromoDragonFLY, has been implicated in finger amputations secondary to potent peripheral vasospastic activity, and sudden cardiac death.[93] Three deaths are associated with 2C-T-7 use; in one case death may have resulted from seizures or aspiration.[33,39,125]

The psychological effects of hallucinogens seem to represent a complex and elusive interaction between different neurotransmitters, including the serotonergic and dopaminergic systems. Based on this serotonergic mechanism, serotonin syndrome could theoretically occur after the use of any of the lysergamide, indolealkylamine, or phenylethylamine hallucinogens. Animal studies have documented LSD and tryptamine-induced serotonin syndrome.[114,131] Case reports have linked phenylethylamine use to fatal serotonin syndrome in recreational users.[89,133]

Tolerance to the psychological effects of LSD occurs within 2 or 3 days with daily dosing, but rapidly dissipates if the drug is withheld for 2 days. Psychological cross-tolerance among mescaline, psilocybin, and LSD is reported in humans.[14] There is no evidence for physiologic tolerance, physiologic dependence, or a withdrawal syndrome with LSD. Limited tolerance is demonstrated between psilocybin and cannabinoids such as marijuana.[22]

Salvia divinorum use results in vivid hallucinations and synesthesia.[113] Additionally, its use may cause dieresis, nausea, and dysphoria. These aversive effects may limit its long-term recurrent use.[10]

The dual stimulant and sedative properties of Kratom contributed to its traditional use among manual laborers. However, its opioidlike activity has led to a surge in contemporary use as an herbal treatment for opioid withdrawal among patients with chronic pain.[18,19] Anorexia, weight loss, and insomnia have been reported among Kratom addicts. Hyperpigmentation of the cheeks has also been described among chronic users.[120]

Recreational nutmeg use results in the desired effects of euphoria and hallucinations, as well as the adverse effects of nausea, vomiting, dizziness, flushing, tachycardia, and hypotension. Fatalities from nutmeg ingestion have been reported.[116]

The belladonna alkaloids produce classic symptoms of anticholinergic toxicity, including hyperthermia, tachycardia, mydriasis, flushing, anhidrosis, urinary retention, and ileus. The central effects can include restlessness, hallucinations, agitation, delirium, seizures, coma.[30] The psychosis produced by belladonna alkaloids can be profound; in one case, a young man auto-amputated his tongue and penis after ingestion of tea made from Angel's trumpet.[80]

The vast majority of morbidity from hallucinogen use stems from trauma. Hallucinogen users frequently report lacerations and bruises sustained during their "high." Additionally, dysphoric reactions may drive patients to react to stimuli with unpredictable, and occasionally aggressive, behaviors. Many Internet sites regarding hallucinogen use advise readers to take hallucinogens only while under the supervision of a "sitter."[40]

The psychological effects of hallucinogens are dose related and affect changes in arousal, emotion, perception, thought process, and self-image. The response to the xenobiotic is related to the person's mindset, emotions, or expectations at the time of exposure, and can be altered by the group or setting.[1] People experiencing the effects of a hallucinogen are usually fully alert, oriented, and aware that they are under the influence of a xenobiotic. Euphoria, dysphoria, and emotional lability may occur.

Illusions are common, typically involving distortion of body image and alteration in visual perceptions. Hallucinogen users may display acute attention to details with excessive attachment of meaning to ordinary objects and events. Usual thoughts seem novel and profound. Many people report an intensification of their sensory perceptions such as sound magnification and distortion. Colors often seem brighter with halolike lights around objects. Frequently, hallucinogen users relate a sense of depersonalization and separation from the environment, commonly called an "out-of-body" experience. Synesthesias, or sensory misperceptions, are frequent. Hallucinations may be visual, auditory, tactile, or olfactory.

Acute adverse psychiatric effects of hallucinogens include panic reactions, psychosis, and major depressive dysphoric reactions. Acute panic reactions, the most common adverse effect, present with frightening illusions, tremendous anxiety, apprehension, and a terrifying sense of loss of self-control.[46] These psychiatric effects may cause patients to seek care in the emergency department (ED).

DIFFERENTIAL DIAGNOSIS

Hallucinosis is the abnormal organic mental condition of persistent hallucinations. The major causes of hallucinosis can be divided by etiology into structural, infectious, functional, and toxic-metabolic. The diagnosis of hallucinogen exposure often must be established on the basis of history and physical examination alone. The person who has ingested hallucinogens typically is oriented and will often give a history of xenobiotic use. This stands in stark contrast to patients with xenobiotic-induced delirium, in whom orientation is, by definition, altered.

Xenobiotics such as amphetamine, cocaine, PCP, and anticholinergics produce delirium or psychosis at doses capable of producing hallucinations. Patients with psychiatric or "functional" causes of perceptual changes, such as schizophrenia, typically present with auditory hallucinations. Patients with central anticholinergic toxicity usually present with delirium, combative behavior, and incoherent mumbling, and may be unaware that the hallucinations are xenobiotic induced.[69] The presence of marked hyperthermia, uncontrollable behavior, or extreme agitation should suggest phenylethylamine use, or an alternative exposure, such as cocaine or PCP.

Evaluation for other causes of altered mental status and hallucinations should include early exclusion of hypoglycemia, encephalitis, meningitis, intracerebral hemorrhage, thyrotoxicosis, sepsis, decompensated psychiatric disease, withdrawal, and other toxic exposures. A computed tomography of the head and lumbar puncture are tests required in a patient where the history of hallucinogen exposure is not ascertained and the altered mental status is of unclear origin.

LABORATORY

Routine urine drug-of-abuse immunoassay screens do not detect LSD or other hallucinogens. Although LSD exposure can be detected by radioimmunoassay of the urine, confirmation by high-performance liquid chromatography (HPLC) or gas chromatography is necessary. These tests are rarely used in the clinical setting, but are much more common for forensic matters.[14,37] False-positive urine testing for LSD has been reported after exposure to several medications including fentanyl, sertraline, haloperidol, or verapamil.[47,99]

Depending on their structure, phenylethylamines may cause positive qualitative urine testing by immunoassay for amphetamines. However, amphetamine drug testing is associated with numerous false-positive results, particularly after the use of cold medications that contain ephedrine, pseudoephedrine, or phenylpropanolamine.[118] Gas chromatography-mass spectrometry (GC/MS) testing methods for detection of 5-MeO-DiPT, DMT, AMT, 2C-T-7, and 2CB have been described.[132]

Routine urine drug immunoassay screens do not detect salvinorin A, Kratom, or myrsiticin. HPLC and liquid chromatography-mass spectrometry (LC/MS) protocols have been applied to the quantitative analysis of salvinorin A and B in plant matter and in ex vivo animal studies. GC/MS identified salvinorin A in urine and saliva obtained after two human volunteers smoked *S. divinorum*.[94] Myristicin concentrations are not widely available, but have been obtained for confirmation of exposure after a fatality.[116]

TREATMENT

Most hallucinogen users rarely seek medical attention because they experience only the desired effect of the xenobiotic. For any hallucinogen user who does present to the ED, initial treatment must begin with attention to airway, breathing, circulation, level of consciousness, and abnormal vital signs. Even if an ingestion of a hallucinogen is suspected, the basic approach for altered mental status should include glucose, thiamine and oxygen therapy as indicated, as well as the vigorous search for other etiologies.

Hallucinogens rarely produce life-threatening toxicity. GI decontamination with activated charcoal may be considered for asymptomatic patients with recent ingestions, but is probably not helpful after clinical symptoms appear, and attempts may lead to further agitation. Sedation with benzodiazepines is usually sufficient to treat hypertension, tachycardia, and hyperthermia. The patient with a dysphoric reaction can be placed in a quiet location with minimal stimuli. A nonjudgmental advocate should attempt to reduce the patient's anxiety, provide reality testing, and remind the individual that a xenobiotic was ingested and the effect will wear off in a couple of hours. Excessive physical restraint (without chemical restraint) should be avoided to prevent hyperthermia and rhabdomyolysis. Benzodiazepines remain the cornerstone of therapy for both autonomic instability and dysphoria, as the sedating effect can diminish both endogenous and exogenous sympathetic effects.[87] Autonomic instability and hyperthermia may be a feature of phenylethylamine use, as well as tryptamine use or massive LSD overdose.[46,67,87] Hyperthermia resulting from agitation or muscle rigidity requires urgent sedation with benzodiazepines and rapid cooling. While central nervous system (CNS) depression is unlikely to be severe enough to require endotracheal intubation in a patient with a pure hallucinogen exposure, intubation and paralysis may be required in the patient with intractable hyperthermia.[16] Seizures may occur with tryptamine or phenylethylamine use, and can be initially treated with benzodiazepines. Seizures may also result from hyponatremia in MDMA users, and would necessitate treatment with 3% hypertonic saline (see Chap. 75).

The treatment of anticholinergic toxicity from the belladonna alkaloids involves several critical components: correction of abnormal vital signs, management of delirium, and rapid intervention for seizures or dysrhythmias. The mainstays of therapy are fluid resuscitation and benzodiazepines; however, physostigmine should be considered as antidotal therapy in cases of belladonna alkaloid poisoning. Conflicting data exist regarding the efficacy of physostigmine in decreasing morbidity and length of hospital stay when compared with benzodiazepines alone.[25,100] Based on the strength of this evidence, physostigmine should be considered in patients with evidence of anticholinergic delirium, or agitation refractory to treatment with benzodiazepines. More information on physostigmine can be found in Antidotes in Depth A12: Physostigmine Salicylate.

Morbidity and mortality typically result from the complications of hyperthermia including rhabdomyolysis and myoglobinuric renal failure, hepatic necrosis, and disseminated intravascular coagulopathy. For the most part, however, hydration, sedation, a quiet environment, and meticulous supportive care will prove adequate to prevent morbidity or mortality in recreational use or overdose.[28] Treatment of serotonin syndrome from phenylethylamine use is largely supportive, and includes the avoidance of further administration of serotonergic medications. Specific therapy with cyproheptadine may be warranted (see Chap. 72).[17]

The role of antipsychotics in controlling hallucinogen-induced agitation is unclear and should be avoided. Haloperidol, risperidone, and ziprasidone may have utility in controlling the acutely agitated patient. However, haloperidol and risperidone may worsen panic and visual symptoms, and increase the incidence of hallucinogen persisting perception disorder (HPPD; see below).[2] Ziprasidone safety in hallucinogen users has not yet been reported. While further study on these interventions is required, prolonged psychosis may require treatment with long-term antipsychotic therapy.

LONG-TERM EFFECTS

Long-term consequences of LSD use include prolonged psychotic reactions, severe depression, and exacerbation of preexisting psychiatric illness.[59,103] When LSD was initially popularized, some patients were noted to behave in a manner similar to schizophrenia and required admission to psychiatric facilities. In volunteer studies, panic reactions, HPPD, and extended psychoses were noted. When the drug was used for alleviation of anxiety and personality abnormalities, flashbacks and extended psychosis were reported.[45] It is suggested that these individuals had preexisting compensated psychological disturbances.[3,78]

Flashbacks have been reported in up to 15% to 80% of LSD users.[5] Anesthesia, alcohol intake, and medications may precipitate flashbacks.[48] These perceptions can be triggered during times of stress, illness, and exercise, and are often a virtual recurrence of the initial hallucinations. HPPD is a chronic disorder where flashbacks lead to impairment in social or occupational function. According to the Diagnostic and Statistical Manual IV, the diagnosis of HPPD requires the recurrence of perceptual symptoms that were experienced while intoxicated with the hallucinogen that causes functional impairment and is not due to a medical condition.[6] The etiology of HPPD is still unknown, and the reported incidence varies widely. Symptoms are primarily visual, and reality testing is typically intact in HPPD. Common perceptual and visual disturbances in HPPD include geometric forms; false, fleeting perceptions in the peripheral fields; flashes of color; intensified color; and halos around objects.[78] One finding described after LSD use is palinopsia, or "trailing," which refers to the continued visual perception of an object after it has left the field of vision. These visual perceptions have been associated with normal ophthalmologic examinations and abnormal EEG evaluations, suggesting a cortical etiology for the visual symptoms.

SUMMARY

Hallucinogens are a diverse group of xenobiotics that alter and distort perception, thought, and mood without clouding the sensorium. The lysergamide, phenylethylamine, and tryptamine hallucinogens share a serotonergic mechanism of action; however, other neurotransmitters may be responsible for the complex effects of these hallucinogens. Salvinorin A, a novel hallucinogen, exerts its effects via the opioid κ receptor. Acute adverse psychiatric effects of hallucinogens include panic reactions, true hallucinations, psychosis, and major depressive dysphoric reactions. Hallucinogens rarely produce life-threatening problems, but have been known to cause autonomic instability, seizures, and hyperthermia, particularly in overdose. Meticulous supportive care with attention to abnormal vital signs is often the only therapy required. Long-term consequence of LSD use may include prolonged psychotic reactions, severe depression, exacerbation of preexisting psychiatric illness, and HPPD.

ACKNOWLEDGMENT

Dr. Cynthia K. Aaron, Jeffrey R. Tucker, and Robert F. Ferm contributed to this chapter in previous editions.

REFERENCES

1. Abraham HD, Aldridge AM, Gogia P. The psychopharmacology of hallucinogens. *Neuropsychopharmacology.* 1996;14:285-298.
2. Abraham HD, Mamen A. LSD-like panic from risperidone in post-LSD visual disorder. *J Clin Psychopharmacol.* 1996;16:238-241.
3. Aghajanian GK, Marek GJ. Serotonin and hallucinogens. *Neuropsychopharmacology.* 1999;21:16S-23S.
4. Al-Assmar SE. The seeds of the Hawaiian baby woodrose are a powerful hallucinogen. *Arch Intern Med.* 1999;159:2090.
5. Aldurra G, Crayton JW. Improvement of hallucinogen persisting perception disorder by treatment with a combination of fluoxetine and olanzapine: case report. *J Clin Psychopharmacol.* 2001;21:343-344.
6. American Psychiatric Association. *Diagnostic and Statistical Manual of Mental Disorders*, 4th ed. Washington, DC: American Psychiatric Association; 1994.
7. Antkiewicz-Michaluk L, Romanska I, Vetulani J. Ca2+ channel blockade prevents lysergic acid diethylamide-induced changes in dopamine and serotonin metabolism. *Eur J Pharmacol.* 1997;332:9-14.
8. Arvanov VL, Liang X, Russo A, Wang RY. LSD and DOB: interaction with 5-HT_{2A} receptors to inhibit NMDA receptor-mediated transmission in the rat prefrontal cortex. *Eur J Neurosci.* 1999;11:3064-3072.
9. Babu K, Boyer EW, Hernon C, Brush DE. Emerging drugs of abuse. *Clin Pediatr Emerg Med.* 2005;6:81-84.
10. Babu KM, McCurdy CR, Boyer EW. Opioid receptors and legal highs: *Salvia divinorum* and Kratom. *Clin Toxicol (Phila).* 2008;46:146-152.
11. Badham ER. Ethnobotany of psilocybin mushrooms, especially *Psilocybe cubensis. J Ethnopharmacol.* 1984;10:249-254.
12. Baselt R, Cravey RH. *Amphetamine. Disposition of Toxic Drugs and Chemicals in Man*, 4th ed. Foster City: 1995; 44-47.
13. Bellis MA, Hughes K, Bennett A, Thomson R. The role of an international nightlife resort in the proliferation of recreational drugs. *Addiction.* 2003;98: 1713-1721.
14. Blaho K, Merigian K, Winbery S, Geraci SA, Smartt C. Clinical pharmacology of lysergic acid diethylamide: case reports and review of the treatment of intoxication. *Am J Ther.* 1997;4:211-221.
15. Bliss M. Datura poisoning. *Clin Toxicol Rev.* 2001;23:1-2.
16. Borowiak KS, Ciechanowski K, Waloszczyk P. Psilocybin mushroom (*Psilocybe semilanceata*) intoxication with myocardial infarction. *J Toxicol Clin Toxicol.* 1998;36:47-49.
17. Boyer E, Shannon M. Serotonin Syndrome. *N Engl J Med.* 2005; 352: 1112-1120.
18. Boyer EW, Babu KM, Adkins JE, McCurdy CR, Halpern JH. Self-treatment of opioid withdrawal using kratom (*Mitragynia speciosa Korth*). *Addiction.* 2008;103:1048-1050.
19. Boyer EW, Babu KM, Macalino GE. Self-treatment of opioid withdrawal with a dietary supplement, Kratom. *Am J Addict.* 2007;16:352-356.
20. Brubacher JR, Lachmanen D, Ravikumar PR, Hoffman RS. Efficacy of digoxin specific Fab fragments (Digibind) in the treatment of toad venom poisoning. *Toxicon.* 1999;37:931-942.
21. Brush DE, Bird SB, Boyer EW. Monoamine oxidase inhibitor poisoning resulting from Internet misinformation on illicit substances. *J Toxicol Clin Toxicol.* 2004;42:191-195.
22. Buckholtz NS, Zhou DF, Freedman DX. Serotonin2 agonist administration down-regulates rat brain serotonin2 receptors. *Life Sci.* 1988;42:2439-2445.
23. Buckman J. Brainwashing, LSD, and CIA: historical and ethical perspective. *Int J Soc Psychiatry.* 1977;23:8-19.
24. Bullis RK. Swallowing the scroll: legal implications of the recent Supreme Court peyote cases. *J Psychoactive Drugs.* 1990;22:325-332.
25. Burns MJ, Linden CH, Graudins A, Brown RM, Fletcher KE. A comparison of physostigmine and benzodiazepines for the treatment of anticholinergic poisoning. *Ann Emerg Med.* 2000;35:374-381.
26. Burris KD, Sanders-Bush E. Unsurmountable antagonism of brain 5-hydroxytryptamine2 receptors by (+)-lysergic acid diethylamide and bromo-lysergic acid diethylamide. *Mol Pharmacol.* 1992;42:826-830.
27. Calabrese JD. Spiritual healing and human development in the Native American Church: toward a cultural psychiatry of peyote. *Psychoanal Rev.* 1997;84:237-255.
28. Callaway CW, Clark RF. Hyperthermia in psychostimulant overdose. *Ann Emerg Med.* 1994;24:68-76.
29. Centers for Disease Control. Deaths associated with a purported aphrodisiac—New York City, February 1993–May 1995. *MMWR Morb Mortal Wkly Rep.* 1995;44:853-855, 861.
30. Centers for Disease Control. Suspected moonflower intoxication—Ohio, 2002. *MMWR Morb Mortal Wkly Rep.* 2003;52:788-791.
31. Cohen MM, Hirschhorn K, Frosch WA. In vivo and in vitro chromosomal damage induced by LSD-25. *N Engl J Med.* 1967;277:1043-1049.
32. de la Torre R, Farre M, Roset PN, et al. Human pharmacology of MDMA: pharmacokinetics, metabolism, and disposition. *Ther Drug Monit.* 2004;26:137-144.
33. DeBoer D, Gizjels M, Maes R. Data about the new psychoactive drug 2C-B. *J Anal Toxicol.* 1999;23:227.
34. Demetriades AK, Wallman PD, McGuiness A, Gavalas MC. Low cost, high risk: accidental nutmeg intoxication. *BMJ.* 2005;22:223-225.
35. Dennehy CE, Tsourounis C, Miller AE. Evaluation of herbal dietary supplements marketed on the internet for recreational use. *Ann Pharmacother.* 2005;39:1634-1639.
36. Drug Enforcement Administration. *Salvia divinorum.* http://www.deadiversion.usdoj.gov/drugs_concern/salvia_d/salvia_d.htm. Updated November 2008. Accessed March 2009.
37. Dupont R, Verebey K. The role of the laboratory in the diagnosis of LSD and ecstasy psychosis. *Psychiatr Annals.* 1994;24:142-144.
38. Eadie MJ. Convulsive ergotism: epidemics of the serotonin syndrome? *Lancet Neurol.* 2003;2:429-434.
39. Erowid. A Reported 2C-T-7 Death. http://www.erowid.org/chemicals/2ct7/2ct7_death1.shtml. Updated July 2003. Accessed March 2009.
40. Erowid. *Salvia divinorum* basics. http://www.erowid.org/plants/salvia/salvia_basics.shtml, Updated February 2009. Accessed March 2009.
41. Erowid. Terminology. http://www.erowid.org/psychoactives/psychoactives_def.shtml. Updated March 2009. Accessed March 2009.
42. Fairchild MD, Jenden DJ, Mickey MR, Yale C. EEG effects of hallucinogens and cannabinoids using sleep-waking behavior as baseline. *Pharmacol Biochem Behav.* 1980;12:99-105.
43. Farber NB, Hanslick J, Kirby C, McWilliams L, Olney JW. Serotonergic agents that activate $5HT_{2A}$ receptors prevent NMDA antagonist neurotoxicity. *Neuropsychopharmacology.* 1998;18:57-62.
44. Fody EP, Walker EM. Effects of drugs on the male and female reproductive systems. *Ann Clin Lab Sci.* 1985;15:451-458.
45. Frankel FH. The concept of flashbacks in historical perspective. *Int J Clin Exp Hypn.* 1994;42:321-336.
46. Friedman SA, Hirsch SE. Extreme hyperthermia after LSD ingestion. *JAMA.* 1971;217:1549-1550.
47. Gagajewski A, Davis GK, Kloss J, Poch GK, Anderson CJ, Apple FS. False-positive lysergic acid diethylamide immunoassay screen associated with fentanyl medication. *Clin Chem.* 2002;48:205-206.
48. Gaillard MC, Borruat FX. Persisting visual hallucinations and illusions in previously drug-addicted patients. *Klin Monatsbl Augenheilkd.* 2003;220: 176-178.
49. Gaudreau JD, Gagnon P. Psychotogenic drugs and delirium pathogenesis: the central role of the thalamus. *Med Hypotheses.* 2005;64:471-475.
50. Giacomelli S, Palmery M, Romanelli L, Cheng CY, Silvestrini B. Lysergic acid diethylamide (LSD) is a partial agonist of D2 dopaminergic receptors and it potentiates dopamine-mediated prolactin secretion in lactotrophs in vitro. *Life Sci.* 1998;63:215-222.
51. Glennon RA. Do classical hallucinogens act as 5-HT_2 agonists or antagonists? *Neuropsychopharmacology.* 1990;3:509-517.
52. Glennon RA, Titeler M, McKenney JD. Evidence for 5-HT_2 involvement in the mechanism of action of hallucinogenic agents. *Life Sci.* 1984;35:2505-2511.
53. Golub A, Johnson BD, Sifaneck SJ, Chesluk B, Parker H. Is the U.S. experiencing an incipient epidemic of hallucinogen use? *Subst Use Misuse.* 2001;36:1699-1729.

54. Gopel C, Laufer C, Marcus A. Three cases of angel's trumpet tea-induced psychosis in adolescent substance abusers. *Nord J Psychiatry.* 2002;56: 49-52.
55. Gowda RM, Cohen RA, Khan IA. Toad venom poisoning: resemblance to digoxin toxicity and therapeutic implications. *Heart.* 2003;89:e14.
56. Grieshaber AF, Moore KA, Levine B. The detection of psilocin in human urine. *J Forensic Sci.* 2001;46:627-630.
57. Hallstrom H, Thuvander A. Toxicological evaluation of myristicin. *Nat Toxins.* 1997;5:186-192.
58. Halpern JH. Hallucinogens and dissociative agents naturally growing in the United States. *Pharmacol Ther.* 2004;102:131-138.
59. Halpern JH, Pope HG, Jr. Do hallucinogens cause residual neuropsychological toxicity? *Drug Alcohol Depend.* 1999;53:247-256.
60. Hamilton RJ, Perrone J, Hoffman R, et al. A descriptive study of an epidemic of poisoning caused by heroin adulterated with scopolamine. *J Toxicol Clin Toxicol.* 2000;38:597-608.
61. Harrington MA, Zhong P, Garlow SJ, Ciaranello RD. Molecular biology of serotonin receptors. *J Clin Psychiatry.* 1992;53(Suppl):8-27.
62. Hofmann A. *History of the Discovery of LSD.* New York: Parthenon; 1994.
63. Isbell H, Gorodetzky CW. Effect of alkaloids of ololiuqui in man. *Psychopharmacologia.* 1966;8:331-339.
64. Jacobson CB, Berlin CM. Possible reproductive detriment in LSD users. *JAMA.* 1972;222:1367-1373.
65. Jansen KL, Prast CJ. Psychoactive properties of mitragynine (kratom). *J Psychoactive Drugs.* 1988;20:455-457.
66. Johnston L, O'Malley P, Bachman J. National Survey Results on Drug Abuse, the Monitoring the Future Study, 1975–1998. In: *NIoD Abuse.* NIH Publication No. 98-4346; 1999.
67. Klock JC, Boerner U, Becker CE. Coma, hyperthermia, and bleeding associated with massive LSD overdose, a report of eight cases. *Clin Toxicol.* 1975;8:191-203.
68. Kovar KA. Chemistry and pharmacology of hallucinogens, entactogens and stimulants. *Pharmacopsychiatry.* 1998;31(Suppl 2):69-72.
69. Kulig K. LSD. *Emerg Med Clin North Am.* 1990;8:551-558.
70. Lake CR, Quirk RS. CNS stimulants and the look-alike drugs. *Psychiatr Clin North Am.* 1984;7:689-701.
71. Leikin JB, Krantz AJ, Zell-Kanter M, Barkin RL, Hryhorczuk DO. Clinical features and management of intoxication due to hallucinogenic drugs. *Med Toxicol Adverse Drug Exp.* 1989;4:324-350.
72. Li JH, Lin LF. Genetic toxicology of abused drugs: a brief review. *Mutagenesis.* 1998;13:557-565.
73. Linden C, Kulig K, Rumack B. Amphetamines. *Top Emerg Med.* 1985;7:18-32.
74. Long H, Nelson LS, Hoffman RS. Alpha-methyltryptamine revisited via easy Internet access. *Vet Hum Toxicol.* 2003;45:149.
75. Louria DB. Lysergic acid diethylamide. *N Engl J Med.* 1968;278:435-438.
76. Lyttle T. Misuse and legend in the "toad licking" phenomenon. *Int J Addict.* 1993;28:521-538.
77. Lyttle T, Goldstein D, Gartz J. *Bufo* toads and bufotenine: fact and fiction surrounding an alleged psychedelic. *J Psychoactive Drugs.* 1996;28:267-290.
78. Madden JS. LSD and post-hallucinogen perceptual disorder. *Addiction.* 1994;89:762-763.
79. Marek GJ, Aghajanian GK. Indoleamine and the phenethylamine hallucinogens: mechanisms of psychotomimetic action. *Drug Alcohol Depend.* 1998;51:189-198.
80. Marneros A, Gutmann P, Uhlmann F. Self-amputation of penis and tongue after use of Angel's Trumpet. *Eur Arch Psychiatry Clin Neurosci.* 2006;256:458-459.
81. Matsumoto K, Horie S, Ishikawa H, et al. Antinociceptive effect of 7-hydroxymitragynine in mice: discovery of an orally active opioid analgesic from the Thai medicinal herb *Mitragyna speciosa. Life Sci.* 2004;74:2143-2155.
82. Matsumoto K, Suchitra T, Murakami Y, et al. Central antinociceptive effects of mitragynine in mice: contribution of descending noradrenergic and serotonergic systems. *Eur J Pharmacol.* 1996;317:75-81.
83. Matsumoto K, Yamamoto LT, Watanabe K, et al. Inhibitory effect of mitragynine, an analgesic alkaloid from Thai herbal medicine, on neurogenic contraction of the vas deferens. *Life Sci.* 2005;78:187-194.
84. McKenna DJ. Clinical investigations of the therapeutic potential of ayahuasca: rationale and regulatory challenges. *Pharmacol Ther.* 2004;102: 111-129.
85. Meatherall R, Sharma P. Foxy, a designer tryptamine hallucinogen. *J Anal Toxicol.* 2003;27:313-317.
86. Mebs D, Schmidt K. Occurrence of tetrodotoxin in the frog *Atelopus oxyrhynchus. Toxicon.* 1989;27:819-822.
87. Miller PL, Gay GR, Ferris KC, Anderson S. Treatment of acute, adverse psychedelic reactions. "I've tripped and I can't get down". *J Psychoactive Drugs.* 1992;24:277-279.
88. Most A. Bufo alvarius: *the Psychedelic Toad of the Sonoran Desert.* Denton: Venom Press; 1984.
89. Mueller PD, Korey WS. Death by "ecstasy": the serotonin syndrome? *Ann Emerg Med.* 1998;32:377-380.
90. National Drug Intelligence Center. Foxy Fast Facts. http://www.usdoj.gov/ndic/pubs6/6440/index.htm. Updated September 2003. Accessed March 2009.
91. Neill JR. "More than medical significance": LSD and American psychiatry 1953 to 1966. *J Psychoactive Drugs.* 1987;19:39-45.
92. O'Malley P, Johnston L, Bachman J. Adolescent substance use: epidemiology and implications for public policy. *Pediatr Clin North Am.* 1995;42:241-260.
93. Personne M, Hulten P. Bromo-Dragonfly, a life-threatening designer drug. *Clin Toxicol (Phila).* 2008;46:379.
94. Pichini S, Abanades S, Farre M, et al. Quantification of the plant-derived hallucinogen salvinorin A in conventional and non-conventional biological fluids by gas chromatography/mass spectrometry after *Salvia divinorum* smoking. *Rapid Commun Mass Spectrom.* 2005;19:1649-1656.
95. Rasmussen K, Glennon RA, Aghajanian GK. Phenethylamine hallucinogens in the locus coeruleus: potency of action correlates with rank order of 5-HT2 binding affinity. *Eur J Pharmacol.* 1986;132:79-82.
96. Richardson WH, Slone CM, Michels JE. Herbal drugs of abuse: an emerging problem. *Emerg Med Clinic North Am.* 2007;25:435-457.
97. Rickert VI, Siqueira LM, Dale T, Wiemann CM. Prevalence and risk factors for LSD use among young women. *J Pediatr Adolesc Gynecol.* 2003;16: 67-75.
98. Riedlinger TJ. Wasson's alternative candidates for soma. *J Psychoactive Drugs.* 1993;25:149-156.
99. Ritter D, Cortese CM, Edwards LC, Barr JL, Chung HD, Long C. Interference with testing for lysergic acid diethylamide. *Clin Chem.* 1997;43: 635-637.
100. Salen P, Shih R, Sierzenski P, Reed J. Effect of physostigmine and gastric lavage in a *Datura stramonium*-induced anticholinergic poisoning epidemic. *Am J Emerg Med.* 2003;21:316-317.
101. Sanders-Bush E, Burris KD, Knoth K. Lysergic acid diethylamide and 2,5-dimethoxy-4-methylamphetamine are partial agonists at serotonin receptors linked to phosphoinositide hydrolysis. *J Pharmacol Exp Ther.* 1988;246:924-928.
102. Sangalli B, Chiang W. Toxicology of nutmeg abuse. *J Toxicol Clin Toxicol.* 2000;38:671-678.
103. Schneier FR, Siris SG. A review of psychoactive substance use and abuse in schizophrenia. Patterns of drug choice. *J Nerv Ment Dis.* 1987;175: 641-652.
104. Schultes R, Hofmann A. *Plants of the Gods.* Rochester: Inner Traditions; 1992.
105. Schultes RE. Hallucinogens of plant origin. *Science.* 1969;163:245-254.
106. Schwartz RH. LSD. Its rise, fall, and renewed popularity among high school students. *Pediatr Clin North Am.* 1995;42:403-413.
107. Shannon M. Methylenedioxymethamphetamine (MDMA, "Ecstasy"). *Pediatr Emerg Care.* 2000;16:377-380.
108. Shellard E. The alkaloids of *Mitragyna* with special reference. *Bull Narc.* 1974;26:41-55.
109. Shellard EJ. Ethnopharmacology of Kratom and the *Mitragyna* alkaloids. *J Ethnopharmacol.* 1989;25:123-124.
110. Shulgin A. *Phenylethylamines I Have Known and Loved.* Berkley: Transform Press; 1991.
111. Shulgin A, Shulgin A. *TiHKAL: A Continuation.* Berkley: Transform Press; 1997.
112. Shulgin AT, Carter MF. N, N-Diisopropyltryptamine (DiPT) and 5-methoxy-N,N-diisopropyltryptamine (5-MeO-DIPT). Two orally active tryptamine analogs with CNS activity. *Commun Psychopharmacol.* 1980;4:363-369.
113. Siebert DJ. *Salvia divinorum* and salvinorin A: new pharmacologic findings. *J Ethnopharmacol.* 1994;43:53-56.
114. Silbergeld EK, Hruska RE. Lisuride and LSD: dopaminergic and serotonergic interactions in the "serotonin syndrome". *Psychopharmacology (Berl).* 1979;65:233-237.
115. Spina SP, Taddei A. Teenagers with Jimson weed (*Datura stramonium*) poisoning. *CJEM.* 2007;9:467-468.

116. Stein U, Greyer H, Hentschel H. Nutmeg (myristicin) poisoning—report on a fatal case and a series of cases recorded by a poison information centre. *Forensic Sci Int.* 2001;118:87-90.
117. Stevens J. *Storming Heaven.* New York: Harper and Row; 1987.
118. Stout PR, Klette KL, Horn CK. Evaluation of ephedrine, pseudoephedrine and phenylpropanolamine concentrations in human urine samples and a comparison of the specificity of DRI amphetamines and Abuscreen online (KIMS) amphetamines screening immunoassays. *J Forensic Sci.* 2004;49:160-164.
119. Substance Abuse and Mental Health Services Administration. The NSDUH Report. Use of Specific Hallucinogens. Rockville, MD: 2006.
120. Suwanlert S. A study of Kratom eaters in Thailand. *Bull Narc.* 1975; 27:21-27.
121. Taber WA, Heacock RA. Location of ergot alkaloid and fungi in the seed of *Rivea corymbosa. Can J Microbiol.* 1962;8:137-143.
122. Thongpradichote S, Matsumoto K, Tohda M, et al. Identification of opioid receptor subtypes in antinociceptive actions of supraspinally-administered mitragynine in mice. *Life Sci.* 1998;62:1371-1378.
123. Titeler M, Lyon RA, Glennon RA. Radioligand binding evidence implicates the brain 5-HT_2 receptor as a site of action for LSD and phenylisopropylamine hallucinogens. *Psychopharmacology (Berl).* 1988;94: 213-216.
124. Ulrich RF, Patten BM. The rise, decline, and fall of LSD. *Perspect Biol Med.* 1991;34:561-578.
125. US Department of Justice. 2,5-Dimethoxy-4-(n)-propylthiophenethylamine (2C-T-7). http://www.deadiversion.usdoj.gov/drugs_concern/2ct7.htm Updated July 2003. Accessed March 2009.
126. US Drug Enforcement Administration. Drugs and Chemicals of Concern. d-Lysergic Acid Diethylamide. http://www.deadiversion.usdoj.gov/drugs_concern/lsd/lsd.htm. Accessed March 2009.
127. US Drug Enforcement Administration. Information Bulletin. *Salvia Divinorum. Microgram Bull.* 2003;36:122-125.
128. US Drug Enforcement Administration. Psilocybin and Psilocyn and Other Tryptamines. http://www.usdoj.gov/dea/concern/psilocybin.html. Accessed March 2009.
129. US Drug Enforcement Administration. Schedules of controlled substances: placement of alpha-methyltryptamine and 5-methoxy-N,N-diisopropyltryptamine into Schedule I of the Controlled Substances Act. Final Rule. Federal Register, 2004; 69. 58950-58953.
130. Valdes LJ 3rd, Diaz JL, Paul AG. Ethnopharmacology of ska Maria Pastora (*Salvia divinorum*, Epling and Jativa-M.). *J Ethnopharmacol.* 1983;7:287-312.
131. Van Oekelen D, Megens A, Meert T, Luyten WH, Leysen JE. Role of 5-HT(2) receptors in the tryptamine-induced 5-HT syndrome in rats. *Behav Pharmacol.* 2002;13:313-318.
132. Vorce SP, Sklerov JH. A general screening and confirmation approach to the analysis of designer tryptamines and phenethylamines in blood and urine using GC-EI-MS and HPLC-electrospray-MS. *J Anal Toxicol.* 2004;28:407-410.
133. Vuori E, Henry JA, Ojanpera I, et al. Death following ingestion of MDMA (ecstasy) and moclobemide. *Addiction.* 2003;98:365-368.
134. Watts VJ, Lawler CP, Fox DR, Neve KA, Nichols DE, Mailman RB. LSD and structural analogs: pharmacological evaluation at D_1 dopamine receptors. *Psychopharmacology (Berl).* 1995;118:401-409.
135. Weil AT, Davis W. *Bufo alvarius*: a potent hallucinogen of animal origin. *J Ethnopharmacol.* 1994;41:1-8.
136. Woolf A. Witchcraft or mycotoxin? The Salem witch trials. *J Toxicol Clin Toxicol.* 2000;38:457-460.
137. Yamamoto LT, Horie S, Takayama H, et al. Opioid receptor agonistic characteristics of mitragynine pseudoindoxyl in comparison with mitragynine derived from Thai medicinal plant *Mitragyna speciosa. Gen Pharmacol.* 1999;33:73-81.
138. Yan F, Roth BL. Salvinorin A: a novel and highly selective kappa-opioid receptor agonist. *Life Sci.* 2004;75:2615-2619.
139. Yotsu-Yamashita M, Mebs D, Yasumoto T. Tetrodotoxin and its analogues in extracts from the toad *Atelopus oxyrhynchus* (family Bufonidae). *Toxicon.* 1992;30:1489-1492.

CHAPTER 83
CANNABINOIDS

Michael A. McGuigan

Cannabis is a collective term referring to the bioactive substances from *Cannabis sativa.* The *C. sativa* plant contains a group of more than 60 chemicals (C21 group) called cannabinoids. In this chapter, the term *cannabis* encompasses all cannabis products. The major cannabinoids are cannabinol, cannabidiol, and tetrahydrocannabinol. The principal psychoactive cannabinoid is Δ^9-tetrahydrocannabinol (THC). Marijuana is the common name for a mixture of dried leaves and flowers of the *C. sativa* plant. Hashish and hashish oil are the pressed resin and the oil expressed from the pressed resin, respectively. The concentration of THC varies from 1% in low-grade marijuana up to 50% in hash oil. Pure THC and a synthetic cannabinoid are available by prescription with the generic names of dronabinol and nabilone, respectively.

HISTORY AND EPIDEMIOLOGY

Cannabis has been used for more than 4000 years. The earliest documentation of the therapeutic use of marijuana is the 4th century BC in China.[82] Cannabis use spread from China to India to North Africa, reaching Europe around AD 500.[70] In colonial North America, cannabis was cultivated as a source of fiber.

Marijuana was used as an intoxicant from the 1850s until the 1930s when the US Federal Bureau of Narcotics began to portray marijuana as a powerful, addicting substance. Despite this, marijuana was listed in the *United States Pharmacopoeia* from 1850 to 1942. In 1970, The Controlled Substances Act classified marijuana as a Schedule I drug.

In all populations, cannabis use by males exceeds use by females. Currently, marijuana is the most commonly used illicit xenobiotic in the United States. A recent study by the Substance Abuse and Mental Health Services Administration[117] reported that in 2006 in the United States, 6.0% (14.8 million persons) ≥12 years used marijuana in the month prior to the survey; this prevalence is unchanged from previous years. The prevalence of past-month users aged 12 to 17 years was 6.7% (down from 8.2% in 2002). The number of first-time users was estimated to be 2.1 million, with 63.3% less than 18 years of age.

In 2004 in Europe, a mean of 20% (range 5%–31%) of people aged 15 to 64 years have used cannabis at least once in their lifetime; the general trend increased from the early 1990s to the early 2000s. Past-year use ranges from 1.7% to 10.4% and past-month use ranges from 0.5% to 6.2%; approximately 25% (range 19%–33%) of those who used at least once in the last month use it daily (~3 million daily users).[29]

In 2004 in Australia, 33.6% of people ≥14 years of age had used cannabis at least once in their life (unchanged from previous years) and 11.3% had used cannabis within the past year (down from a high of 17.9% in 1998).[4]

MEDICAL USES

Cannabinoids are proposed for use in the management of many clinical conditions (Table 83–1), but have generally only been approved for the control of chemotherapy-related nausea and vomiting that are resistant to conventional antiemetics, for breakthrough postoperative nausea and vomiting, and for appetite stimulation in human immunodeficiency virus (HIV) patients with anorexia-cachexia syndrome.[48] The claims of benefit in the other medical conditions in Table 83–1 are not supported by evidence.[6,41,63,131]

PHARMACOLOGY AND PATHOPHYSIOLOGY

Δ^9-THC (sometimes referred to in the literature as Δ^1-THC) was isolated in 1964. In the 1990s, two specific G protein–coupled cannabinoid-binding receptors were identified: CB1 (or *Cnr1)* and CB2 (or *Cnr2).* Subsequent research identified endogenous cannabinoid receptor ligands (anandamide, palmitoylethanolamide), as well as cannabinoid receptor agonists and antagonists.[30,47,118]

Both receptors inhibit adenylyl cyclase and stimulate potassium channel conductance.[98] CB1 receptors are distributed throughout the brain with high densities in the basal ganglia (particularly the globus pallidus), substantia nigra, cerebellum, hippocampus, and cerebral cortex (particularly the frontal regions). CB1 receptors are located presynaptically and their activation inhibits the release of acetylcholine, L-glutamate, γ-aminobutyric acid, noradrenaline, dopamine, and 5-hydroxytryptamine.[58,64,109] CB2 receptors are located peripherally in immune system tissues (splenic macrophages), B lymphocytes, peripheral nerve terminals, and the vas deferens. CB2 receptors are believed to participate in the regulation of immune responses and inflammatory reactions.

The neuropharmacologic mechanisms by which cannabinoids produce their psychoactive effects have not been fully elucidated.[49,58,98] Nevertheless, activity at the CB1 receptors is believed to be responsible for the clinical effects of cannabinoids,[12,30,58,118] including the regulation of cognition, memory, motor activities, nociception, and nausea and vomiting. Chronic administration of a cannabinoid agonist reduces CB1 receptor density in several regions of the rat brain.[13]

PHARMACOKINETICS AND TOXICOKINETICS

ABSORPTION

The pharmacokinetics of cannabinoids have been extensively reviewed.[40] The rate and completeness of absorption of cannabinoids depend on the route of administration and the type of cannabis product.

Inhalation of smoke containing THC results in the onset of psychoactive effects within minutes. From 10% to 35% of available THC is absorbed during smoking and peak serum THC concentrations occur an average of 8 (range: 3–10) minutes after the onset of smoking marijuana. Peak serum concentrations depend on the dose; a marijuana cigarette containing 1.75% THC produces a peak serum THC concentration of approximately 85 ng/mL.[52]

Ingestion of cannabis results in an unpredictable onset of psychoactive effects in 1 to 3 hours. Because of THC's instability in acidic gastric fluid and first-pass hepatic clearance,[95] 5% to 20% of available THC reaches the systemic circulation following ingestion. Peak serum THC concentrations usually occur 2 to 4 hours after ingestion but delays up to 6 hours are described.[35,71] The therapeutic serum THC concentration for the treatment of nausea and vomiting is greater than 10 ng/mL.[20]

Dronabinol has an oral bioavailability of approximately 10% with high interindividual variability.[37,90] THC is detectable in plasma 1.5 to 4.5 hours after ingestion of dronabinol; peak serum concentrations occur 6.5 to 107 hours after ingestion.[36] Nabilone has an oral bioavailability estimated to be greater than 90% and reaches peak serum concentrations 2 hours after ingestion.[108]

TABLE 83–1. Medical Conditions Proposed for Cannabinoid Use

Anorexia-cachexia syndrome secondary to HIV infection[a]
Anxiety
Asthma
Depression
Epilepsy
Glaucoma
Head injury
Insomnia
Migraine headaches
Multiple sclerosis
Muscle spasticity and spasms
Nausea and vomiting (resistant)[a]
Neurologic disorders
Pain
Parkinson disease
Tourette syndrome

[a] FDA approved use.

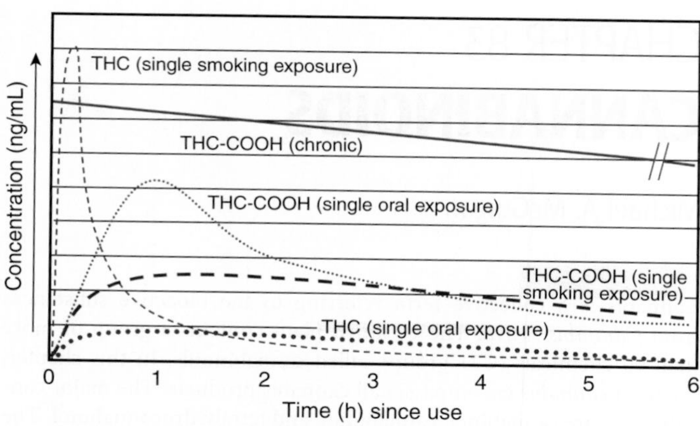

FIGURE 83–1. Estimated relative time course of THC and its major metabolite based on the route of exposure. THC = Δ^9 tetrahydrocannabinol; THC-COOH = Δ^9 THC carboxylic acid.

DISTRIBUTION

THC has a steady-state volume of distribution of approximately 2.5 to 3.5 L/kg.[40] Cannabinoids are lipid soluble and accumulate in fatty tissue in a biphasic pattern. Initially, THC is distributed to highly vascularized tissues such as the liver, kidneys, heart, and muscle. Following smoking or intravenous administration, the distribution half-life is less than 10 minutes.[52,95] After the initial distribution phase, THC accumulates more slowly in less vascularized tissues and body fat. Repeated administration of Δ^8-THC (an isomer of Δ^9-THC) to rats over 2 weeks resulted in steadily increasing concentrations of Δ^8-THC in body fat and liver, but not in brain tissue. Once administration of Δ^8-THC stopped, the cannabinoids were slowly released from fat stores as adipose tissue turned over.[94]

THC crosses the placenta and enters the breast milk. Concentrations in fetal serum are 10% to 30% of maternal concentrations. Daily marijuana smoking by a nursing mother resulted in concentrations of THC in breast milk that are eightfold higher than concomitant maternal serum concentrations; THC metabolites do not accumulate in breast milk.[100]

METABOLISM

THC is nearly completely metabolized by hepatic microsomal hydroxylation and oxidation by the cytochrome P450 system (primarily CYP2C9 and CYP3A4).[40] The primary metabolite (11-hydroxy-Δ^9-THC or 11-OH-THC) is active and is subsequently oxidized to the inactive 11-nor-Δ^9-THC carboxylic acid metabolite (THC-COOH) and many other metabolites.[1,3,103]

The serum concentrations of THC and its metabolites change over time. Smoking a marijuana cigarette results in peak serum THC concentrations before finishing the cigarette. In six volunteers, peak serum THC concentrations occurred at 8 (range: 6–10) minutes after onset of smoking, of 11-OH-THC at 13 (range: 9–23) minutes, and of THC-COOH at 120 (range: 48–240) minutes (Fig. 83–1).[52] Approximately 1 hour after beginning to smoke a marijuana cigarette, the THC-to-11-OH-THC ratio is 3:1 and the THC-to-THC-COOH ratio is 1:2; at approximately 2 hours the ratios are 2.5:1 and 1:8, respectively; at 3 hours the ratios are 2:1 and 1:16, respectively.[52]

Ingestion of cannabis results in much more variable concentrations and time courses of THC and metabolites (see Fig. 83–1). Nonetheless, at 2 to 3 hours postingestion the ratios are similar to those after smoking: THC-to-11-OH-THC is 2:1 and THC-to-THC-COOH ranges from 1:7 to 1:14.[35,127]

EXCRETION

Reported elimination half-lives of THC and its major metabolites vary considerably. Following intravenous doses of THC, the mean elimination half-life ranges from 1.6 to 57 hours.[40] Elimination half-lives are expected to be similar following inhalation.[40,52] The elimination half-life of 11-OH-THC is 12 to 36 hours and the elimination half-life of THC-COOH ranges from 1 to 6 days.[65,127]

THC and its metabolites are excreted in the urine and the feces. In the 72 hours following ingestion, approximately 15% of a THC dose is excreted in the urine and roughly 50% is excreted in the feces.[1,18,128] Following intravenous administration, approximately 15% of a THC dose is excreted in the urine and only 25% to 35% is excreted in the feces.[127] Inhalation is expected to produce results similar to intravenous administration.[40,52] In 5 days, 80% to 90% of a THC dose is excreted from the body.[45,56]

Cannabinoids were measured in the urine following smoking a marijuana cigarette containing 27 mg of THC (see Fig. 83–1).[78] THC urine concentrations peaked at 2 hours (mean: 21.5 ng/mL; range: 3.2–53.3 ng/mL) after smoking and were undetectable (less than 1.5 ng/mL) in five of the eight subjects by 6 hours after smoking. Urine concentrations of 11-OH-THC peaked at 3 hours (77.3 ± 29.7 ng/mL). The primary urinary metabolite is the glucuronide conjugate of THC-COOH.[130] THC-COOH urine concentrations peak at 4 hours (179.4 ± 146.9 ng/mL),[78] and it has an average urinary excretion half-life of 2 to 3 days (range: 0.9–9.8 days).[40] Both 11-OH-THC and THC-COOH remained detectable in the urine of all eight subjects for the 8 hours of the study.[78]

Following discontinuation of use, metabolites may be detected in the urine of chronic users for several weeks.[28,60] Factors such as age, weight, and frequency of use only partially explained the long excretion period.[28]

CLINICAL MANIFESTATIONS

The clinical effects of THC use, including time of onset and duration of effect, vary with the dose, the route of administration (ingestion is slower in onset than inhalation), the experience of the user, the user's vulnerability to psychoactive effects, and the setting in which the drug is used. The concomitant use of central nervous system depressants such as ethanol, or stimulants such as cocaine, alters the psychological and physiologic effects of cannabis.

PSYCHOLOGICAL EFFECTS

Use of cannabis produces variable psychological effects.[38] The variation, which occurs both between and within users, may be a result of drug tolerance, level or phase of clinical effects, physical and social settings, or user expectations or cognitive set. The most commonly self-reported effect is relaxation. Other commonly reported effects are perceptual alterations (heightened sensory awareness, slowing of time), a feeling of well-being (including giddiness or laughter), and increased appetite.[38]

PHYSIOLOGIC EFFECTS

Use of cannabis is associated with physiologic effects on cerebral blood flow, the heart, the lungs, and the eyes.

In a controlled, double-blind positron emission tomography study,[79] intravenous THC increased cerebral blood flow, particularly in the frontal cortex, insula, cingulate gyrus, and subcortical regions. These increases in cerebral blood flow occurred 30 to 60 minutes after use and were still elevated at 120 minutes.[80] Similar blood flow changes result from smoking marijuana.[97]

Common acute cardiovascular effects of cannabis use include increases in heart rate and decreases in vascular resistance.[62,114] Cannabis produces dose-dependent increases in heart rate within 15 minutes of starting a marijuana cigarette (from a baseline mean of 66 beats/min to a mean of 89 beats/min) that reach a maximum (mean: 92 beats/min) 10 to 15 minutes after peak plasma THC concentrations. These changes last for 2 to 3 hours.[8] Increases in blood pressure may occur with cannabis use. In a study of six subjects, an increase in blood pressure from a baseline mean of 119/74 mm Hg to a mean of 129/81 mm Hg occurred, but was not statistically significant.[8] In a double-blind, controlled study of men being investigated for angina pectoris, smoking a marijuana cigarette resulted in statistically significant changes in blood pressure from a baseline mean of 123/79 mm Hg to a peak mean of 132/84 mm Hg.[104] In contrast, repeated THC exposures resulted in significant slowing of heart rate (from a mean of 68 beats/min to a low of 62 beats/min) and lowering of blood pressure (from a mean of 116/62 mm Hg to a low of 108/53 mm Hg).[10] Decreased vascular tone may cause postural hypotension accompanied by dizziness and syncope.

Inhalation or ingestion of THC produces a dose-related short-term decrease in airway resistance and an increase in airway conductance in both normal and asthmatic individuals.[120] Smoking marijuana results in an immediate increase in airway conductance, which peaks at 15 minutes and lasts 60 minutes; ingestion of cannabis produces a significant increase in airway conductance at 30 minutes, which peaks at 3 hours and lasts 4 to 6 hours.[121,122,125] The mechanism for this effect is unclear.

The principal ocular effects of cannabis are conjunctival injection and decreased intraocular pressure. Cannabinoids, applied topically to a rabbit eye, resulted in hyperemia of the conjunctival blood vessels 2 hours after application.[86] Regardless of route of administration cannabis causes a fall in intraocular pressure in 60% of users[39] by acting on CB1 receptors in the ciliary body.[102] The mean reduction in intraocular pressure is 25% and lasts 3 to 4 hours.

ACUTE TOXICITY

In addition to the physiologic and psychological effects described above, acute toxicity may include decreases in coordination, muscle strength, and hand steadiness. Lethargy, sedation, postural hypotension, inability to concentrate, decreased psychomotor activity, slurred speech, and slow reaction time also may occur.[93,128]

In young children, the acute ingestion of cannabis is potentially life threatening.[61,81] Ingestion of estimated amounts of 250 to 1000 mg of hashish resulted in obtundation in 30 to 75 minutes. Tachycardia (>150 beats/min) was found in one-third of the children. Less commonly reported findings include apnea, cyanosis, bradycardia, hypotonia, and opisthotonus.

ACUTE ADVERSE REACTIONS

Cannabis users occasionally may experience distrust, dysphoria, fear, or panic reactions. Transient psychotic episodes are associated with cannabis use. Commonly reported adverse reactions at the prescribed dose of dronabinol or nabilone include postural hypotension, dizziness, sedation, xerostomia, abdominal discomfort, nausea, and vomiting.

One case of acute pancreatitis (serum amylase up to 3200 IU/mL) following a period of heavy cannabis use is reported, but the causal relationship is unclear.[37]

Life-threatening ventricular tachycardia (200 beats/min) has been reported.[105] In six individuals with acute cardiovascular deaths, postmortem whole-blood THC concentrations ranged from 2 to 22 ng/mL (mean: 7.2 ng/mL; median: 5 ng/mL).[5] While the temporal association is clear, causality is less clear because three of the six people had significant preexisting cardiac pathology. The risk of myocardial infarction is increased five times over baseline in the 60 minutes after marijuana use, but subsequently declines rapidly to baseline risk levels.[87] Atrial fibrillation with palpitations, nausea, and dizziness was temporally associated with smoking marijuana in four patients.[31,69,115]

CHRONIC USE ADVERSE EFFECTS

Long-term use of cannabis is associated with a number of adverse effects.

Immune System Cannabinoids affect host resistance to infection by modulating the secondary immune response (macrophages, T and B lymphocytes, acute phase and immune cytokines). However, an immune-mediated health risk from using cannabis has not been documented.[67]

Respiratory System Chronic use of marijuana is associated with clinical findings compatible with obstructive lung disease.[125] Smoking marijuana delivers more particulates to the lower respiratory tract than does smoking tobacco,[133] and marijuana smoke contains carcinogens similar to tobacco smoke. Case reports and a hospital-based case-control study suggest that cancers of the respiratory tract (mouth, larynx, sinuses, lung) are associated with daily or near-daily smoking of marijuana, although exposure to tobacco smoke and ethanol may be confounding factors.[19,120,123] A systematic review and a cohort study with 8 years of follow-up demonstrated no association between marijuana smoking and smoking-related cancers,[43,83] and a population-based case-control study found that marijuana use was not associated with an increased risk of developing oral squamous cell carcinoma.[107]

Cardiovascular System Marijuana use may be a risk for individuals with coronary artery disease. An exploratory prospective study of self-reported marijuana use among patients admitted for myocardial infarction found that patients who used marijuana were at significantly increased risk for cardiovascular and noncardiovascular mortality compared with nonusers.[87,90]

Reproductive System Reduced fertility in chronic users is a result of oligospermia, abnormal menstruation, and decreased ovulation.[15]

Cannabis is a class C drug in pregnancy[14] and affects birthweight and length but does not cause fetal malformations. Statistically significant reductions in birthweight (mean: 79 g less than nonusers) and length (mean: 0.5 cm shorter than nonusers) are reported in women who had urine assays positive for cannabis during pregnancy.[134] The results of three other studies are difficult to interpret because marijuana use in pregnancy was poorly documented.[44,47,134] Epidemiologic studies based on self-reporting of cannabis use do not support an association between the use of cannabis during pregnancy and teratogenesis.[68,74,132,134]

The effect of maternal use of cannabis during pregnancy on neurobehavioral development in the offspring has been studied. No detrimental effects are reported in children born to women who smoked marijuana daily (more than 21 cigarettes per week) in rural Jamaica.[26] Tremors and increased startling are reported in infants younger than 1 week of age whose mothers used cannabis during pregnancy.[33] These findings, which persisted beyond 3 days, were not associated with other signs of a withdrawal syndrome. There were no abnormalities in the children of parents who used greater than five cigarettes per week in Ottawa, Canada, at 12, 24, and 36 months of age, but lower scores in verbal and memory domains at 48 months of age are reported.[32,34,45] The results of studies evaluating the effect of in utero exposure to cannabis on postnatal neurobehavioral development are equivocal because of methodologic concerns regarding exposure assessment and control of covariates,[25] including the continued parental use of cannabis during the postnatal and early childhood periods. The role of secondhand exposure to cannabis on postnatal and early childhood development of neurobehavioral problems has not been evaluated.

Endocrine System In experimental animals, cannabis exposure is associated with suppression of gonadal steroids, growth hormone, prolactin, and thyroid hormone; in addition, cannabis alters the activity of the hypothalamic-pituitary-adrenal axis.[15] In human studies, the results are inconsistent, long-term effects have not been convincingly demonstrated, and clinical consequences are undefined.[15]

Neurobehavioral Effects There is a concern that chronic cannabis use results in deficits in cognition and learning that last well after cannabis use has stopped. Neuropsychological tests administered to 10 cannabis-dependent adolescents, eight adolescent noncannabis drug abusers, and nine nondrug users showed significant differences that persisted for the duration of the study (6 weeks of abstinence) between the cannabis group and the other groups in a visual retention test and a memory test.[112] In a study of three experienced marijuana smokers, cannabis impaired arithmetic and recall tasks up to 24 hours after smoking.[46] Adults who used cannabis more than seven times per week had impairments in math skills, verbal expression, and memory retrieval processes; people who used cannabis one to six times per week showed no impairments.[11] After 1 day of abstinence, 65 heavy marijuana users (median: use on 29 of past 30 days) showed greater impairment on neuropsychological tests of attention and executive functions than light marijuana users (median: use on 1 day of past 30 days).[101] The authors were uncertain whether this difference was caused by residual THC in the brain, a withdrawal effect from the drug, or a direct neurotoxic effect of cannabis.

There is little evidence that adverse cognitive effects persist after stopping the use of cannabis[59] or that cannabis use causes psychosocial harm to the user.[77] The hypothesis that there is a causal association between cannabis use and psychosis has not been proven unequivocally.[9]

An "amotivational syndrome" is attributed to cannabis use. The syndrome is a poorly defined complex of characteristics such as apathy, underachievement, and lack of energy.[22,111] The association of the syndrome with cannabis use is based primarily on anecdotal, uncontrolled observations.[49] Anthropologic field studies, evaluations of US college students, and controlled laboratory experiments have failed to identify a causal relationship between cannabis use and the amotivational syndrome.[49] A study evaluating the role of depression in the amotivational syndrome found significantly lower scores on "Need for Achievement" scales in heavy users (median: daily use for 6 years) with depressive symptoms compared with heavy users without depressive symptoms and light users (median: several times per month for 4.5 years) with or without depressive symptoms.[92] These data suggest that symptoms attributed to an amotivational syndrome are caused by depression, not cannabis. Another study found that behavior that could be interpreted as amotivation was inversely related to the perceived size of the reward.[22]

Abuse, Dependence, and Withdrawal The *Diagnostic and Statistical Manual of Mental Disorders*, 4th edition,[2] defines marijuana abuse as repeated instances of use under hazardous conditions; repeated, clinically meaningful impairment in social/occupational/educational functioning; or legal problems related to marijuana use. Marijuana dependence is defined as tolerance, compulsive use, impaired control, and continued use despite physical and psychological problems caused or exacerbated by use. In 2006, 4.2 million (1.7%) of the total population aged 12 or older were dependent on or abused marijuana or hashish.[117]

The amount, frequency, and duration of cannabis use required to develop dependence are not well established.[21,119] Much of the support for cannabis dependence is based on the existence of a withdrawal syndrome. In animals repeatedly given cannabis, the administration of a CB1 receptor antagonist produced signs of withdrawal.[73,116] In humans, chronic users experience unpleasant effects when abstaining from cannabis.[16] The time of onset of withdrawal symptoms is not well characterized.[15,116] The most reliably reported effects are irritability-restlessness-nervousness and appetite and sleep disturbances.[116] Other reported acute withdrawal manifestations include tremor, diaphoresis, fever, and nausea. These symptoms and signs are reversed by the oral administration of THC42.[9,42] The duration of withdrawal manifestations, without treatment, is not clearly established.[17,116]

CANNABIS AND DRIVING

The perceptual alterations caused by cannabis suggest that its recent use should be associated with automobile crashes. However, neither experimental nor epidemiologic studies have provided definitive answers about the effects cannabis use has on driving ability. The published analytical studies of the relationship between cannabis and driving behavior/motor vehicle crashes have been reviewed.[7] In experimental driving studies, cannabis impairs driving ability but cannabis-using drivers recognize their impairment and compensate for it by driving at slower speeds and increasing following distance. However, the slower reaction time caused by cannabis results in impaired emergency response behavior.

The epidemiologic studies evaluating the association of cannabis use and traffic crashes provide no evidence that cannabis alone increases the risk of causing fatal crashes or serious injuries.[7,96] Studies of 2500 drivers injured in multiple vehicle crashes found that those with blood tests positive for THC had no higher culpability rate than xenobiotic-free drivers.[75,76] A recent study comparing past driving records of subjects entering a drug treatment center with controls found that a self-reported history of cannabis use was associated with a statistically significant increase in adjusted relative risk for all crashes (relative risk 1.49, 95% confidence interval 1.17–1.89) and for "at fault" crashes (relative risk 1.68, 95% confidence interval 1.21–2.34).[23]

The results of studies evaluating the effect of a combination of cannabis and ethanol are contradictory.[7] One study supported potentiation of effects,[124] one could not evaluate the role of xenobiotics other than ethanol,[129] and one did not support potentiation.[57] Several issues were not addressed in these studies: the contribution of more than one central nervous system depressant, the concentrations of central nervous system depressants, and the effect of dependency or tolerance.

DIAGNOSTIC TESTING

Cannabinoids can be detected in plasma or urine. Enzyme-multiplied immunoassay technique (EMIT) and radioimmunoassay (RIA) are routinely available; gas chromatography-mass spectrometry (GC/MS) is the most specific assay and is used as the reference method.

EMIT is a qualitative urine test that is often used for screening purposes. EMIT identifies the metabolites of THC. In these tests, the concentrations of all metabolites present are additive. For the EMIT II Cannabinoid 20-ng Assay, the cutoff level for distinguishing positive from negative samples is 20 ng/mL. A positive test means that the total concentration of all the metabolites present in the urine was at least 20 ng/mL. A positive urine test for cannabis only indicates the presence of cannabinoids, it does not identify which metabolites are present or in what concentrations. Qualitative urine test results do not indicate or measure intoxication or degree of exposure. The National Institute on Drug Abuse guidelines for urine testing specify test cutoff concentrations of 50 ng/mL for screening and 15 ng/mL for confirmation.

Variables affecting the duration of detection of urinary metabolites include dose, duration of use, acute versus chronic use, route of exposure, and sensitivity of the method. In addition, factors affecting the quantitative values of urine THC and metabolites include urine volume, concentration, and pH. Using GC/MS, metabolites may be detected in the urine up to 7 days following a single marijuana cigarette.[54,55]

The length of time between stopping cannabis use and a negative EMIT urine test (<20 ng/mL) depends on the extent of use. Release of THC from adipose tissue is important in drug testing because chronic users may release cannabinoids in quantities sufficient to result in positive urine tests for several weeks. In addition, vigorous exercise may stimulate the release of cannabinoids from fat depots. In light users being tested daily under observed abstinence, the mean time to the first negative urine test is 8.5 days (range: 3–18 days) and the mean time to the last positive urine is 18.2 days (range: 7–34 days).[28] In heavy users (mean: 9 years of using at least once a day) being tested under the same conditions, the mean time to the first negative urine test result (EMIT assay less than 20 ng/mL) was 19.1 days (range: 3–46 days) and the mean time to the last positive urine sample was 31.5 days (range: 4–77 days).[28]

Standard laboratory analyses identify THC and its metabolites but cannot identify the source of the THC (eg, marijuana, hashish, dronabinol). EMIT will not identify nabilone because it is not THC; however, nabilone can be specifically identified using high-performance liquid chromatography-tandem mass spectrometry.[106]

Immunoassays may give false-negative and false-positive test results (Table 83–2). To help identify evidence tampering, negative urine immunoassays should be accompanied by examining the urine for clarity and measuring urinary specific gravity, pH, temperature, and creatinine.[113,126]

TABLE 83–2. Xenobiotics or Conditions Purported to Produce Inaccurate Screening Test Results for THC

False Negative[a]	False Positive
Bleach (NaOCl)	Dronabinol
Citric acid	Efavirenz
Detergent additives	Ethacrynic acid
Dettol[b]	Hemp seed oil
Dilution	NSAIDs
Glutaraldehyde	Promethazine
Lemon juice	Riboflavin
Potassium nitrite (KNO_2)	
Salt (NaCl)	
Tetrahydrozoline	
Vinegar (acetic acid)	
Water	

[a] Xenobiotics producing false-negative urine tests are usually added to a urine sample, not ingested.

[b] Dettol is an antiseptic containing isopropyl alcohol (8%–11%), pine oil (8.4%), and chloroxylenol (4.8%).

PASSIVE INHALATION

Studies of passive exposure to marijuana smoke and the urinary excretion of cannabinoids have used enclosed spaces with nonsmokers present during and after active smoking.[24,72,89,96,99]

In an unventilated 6.9 × 8.2 × 7.9-foot room (12,225.8 L of air), five adult volunteers were exposed to the sidestream smoke of four or 16 marijuana cigarettes (THC 25 mg/cigarette) smoked simultaneously over 1 hour on each of 6 consecutive days.[24] After being exposed to four marijuana cigarettes, four of the volunteers had at least one positive urine by EMIT assay (cutoff: 20 ng/mL) at some unspecified time during the 6 study days; exposure to 16 marijuana cigarettes resulted in positive EMIT assays only after the second day's exposure.

In a car (1650 L of air), three adult volunteers were exposed to the smoke from 12 marijuana cigarettes smoked by two people over 30 minutes.[89] EMIT analyses of urine samples from one passive inhaler were positive at time 0–4 hours and on days 2 and 3; a second passive inhaler had one positive urine test at time 4 to 24 hours after exposure.

Three adult volunteers in a 10 × 10 × 8-foot unventilated room (21,600 L of air) were exposed to the sidestream smoke of four marijuana cigarettes (THC 27 mg/cigarette) smoked simultaneously over 1 hour.[91] The concentrations of cannabinoids in urine samples taken 20 to 24 hours after exposure were less than 6 ng/mL when analyzed using RIA methodology.

Another study used an unventilated room (total volume of 27,950 L) containing three desks and a filing cabinet.[72] Over 10 to 34 minutes, each of six volunteers smoked a marijuana cigarette (THC 17.1 mg/cigarette) and left the room. Four nonsmoking adult males were in the study room for 3 hours from the start of smoking. The door was opened and closed 18 times during the study. The maximum urine cannabinoid concentration (measured by RIA) in the nonsmokers was 6.8 ng/mL at 6 hours after the start of smoking.

Another study used a closed 8 × 8 × 10-foot room (15,500 L of air) with each of four subjects smoking two marijuana cigarettes containing 2.5% THC on one occasion and 2.8% THC on a second occasion.[99] On each occasion, two nonsmoking subjects were in the room for 1 hour from the onset of smoking. None of the nonsmokers' urine samples (from 0–24 hours) from either exposure period tested positive on an EMIT assay with a cutoff of 20 ng/mL. An identical experiment in a closed car (approximately 3500 L of air) resulted in one of 23 urine specimens testing positive at 6 hours.

Therefore, passive inhalation of marijuana smoke is unlikely to result in positive urine test results unless the exposure has been extreme.

SALIVA

Saliva samples may be used to establish the presence of cannabinoids and time of cannabis consumption. Cannabinoids (THC, THC-COOH, 11-OH-THC) in saliva may be from the smoke of the marijuana or hashish, or from a preliminary metabolism in the mouth.[110] Saliva THC concentrations above 10 ng/mL are consistent with recent use and correlate with subjective intoxication and heart rate changes.[84]

HAIR

Hair sample analysis is not useful in identifying THC or its metabolites. Only small quantities of non-nitrogen-containing substances, such as cannabinoids, are found in hair pigments.[27,66,85]

SWEAT

The analysis of perspiration to test for cannabinoids is a recent development. Perspiration deposits drug metabolites on the skin and these are renewed even after the skin is washed. Detection threshold is reported to be 10 ng/mL but forensic confirmation by alternative means is required.[66]

ESTIMATING TIME OF EXPOSURE

A measurable serum concentration of THC is consistent with recent exposure and intoxication but there is poor correlation between serum THC concentrations and degree of intoxication.[50]

The ratio of THC to THC-COOH has been used to estimate time of smoking marijuana. Similar concentrations of each indicate cannabis use within 20 to 40 minutes and imply intoxication. In naïve users, a concentration of THC-COOH that is greater than THC indicates that use probably occurred more than 30 minutes ago. Serum THC-COOH concentrations greater than 40 ng/mL suggest chronic cannabis use.[88] The high background concentrations of THC-COOH in habitual users make estimations of time of exposure unreliable in this population.

Serum concentrations of THC and THC-COOH were used in a logarithmic equation to predict the time since smoking a marijuana cigarette.[78] The ratio provided acceptable results up to 3 hours after smoking (predicted time of exposure averaged 27 minutes longer than actual exposure time), but more than 3 hours after smoking the predicted exposure time was overestimated by 3 hours. Mean overestimations of predicted exposure time of 2.5 to 4.2 hours for smoking and of 1.6 hours for ingestions are reported when serum samples are taken more than 4 hours after exposure.[53]

Chronic use or oral administration of cannabis increases the concentration of 11-OH-THC relative to the concentrations of THC or THC-COOH. In these cases, estimating time of exposure based on relative concentrations is problematic.[51] In four subjects, ingestion of cannabis produced total serum metabolite concentrations less than 20 times the serum THC concentration for 3 hours after ingestion, suggesting that a ratio of this magnitude is consistent with recent oral consumption.[71]

MANAGEMENT

Gastrointestinal decontamination is not recommended for patients who ingest cannabis products, nabilone, or dronabinol because clinical toxicity is rarely serious and responds to supportive care. In addition, a patient with a significantly altered mental status, such as somnolence, agitation, or anxiety, has risks associated with gastrointestinal decontamination that outweigh the potential benefits of the intervention.

Agitation, anxiety, or transient psychotic episodes should be treated with quiet reassurance and benzodiazepines (lorazepam 1–2 mg intramuscularly or diazepam 5–10 mg intravenously) or antipsychotics (haloperidol, ziprasidone) as needed. There are no specific antidotes for cannabis. Coingestants, such as cocaine or ethanol, should be identified and their effects anticipated and treated as indicated.

SUMMARY

Cannabis is a commonly used and widely available xenobiotic. Common manifestations of acute cannabis toxicity include relaxation, perceptual alterations, sedation, tachycardia, postural hypotension, inability to concentrate, slurred speech, and slow reaction times. Feelings of distrust, fear, or panic may occur. Obtundation, apnea, bradycardia, hypotonia, and opisthotonus are reported in young children following ingestion of cannabis. THC or its metabolites can be identified in blood or urine, but treatment is not guided by drug concentrations. Treatment of an overdose, a high degree of toxicity, or an acute adverse reaction is symptomatic and supportive.

REFERENCES

1. Agurell S, Halldin M, Lindgren J. Pharmacokinetics and metabolism of delta-1-tetrahydrocannabinol and other cannabinoids with emphasis on man. *Pharmacol Rev.* 1986;38:21-43.
2. American Psychiatric Association. *Diagnostic and Statistical Manual of Mental Disorders*, 4th ed. Washington, DC: Author; 1994.
3. Anderson PO, McGuire GG. Delta-9-tetrahydrocannabinol as an anti-emetic. *Am J Hosp Pharm.* 1981;38:639-646.
4. Australian Institute of Health and Welfare 2005. 2004 National Drug Strategy Household Survey. First Results. AIHW cat. no. PHE 57. Canberra. AIHW (Drug Statistics Series No. 13). Accessed May 20, 2008.
5. Bachs L, Morland H. Acute cardiovascular fatalities following cannabis use. *Forensic Sci Int.* 2001;124:200-203.
6. Bagshaw SM, Hagen NA. Medical efficacy of cannabinoids and marijuana: a comprehensive review of the literature. *J Palliat Care.* 2002;18:111-122.
7. Bates MN, Blakely TA. Role of cannabis in motor vehicle crashes. *Epidemiol Rev.* 1999;21:222-232.
8. Beaconsfield P, Ginsburg J, Rainsbury R. Marijuana smoking. Cardiovascular effects in man and possible mechanisms. *N Engl J Med.* 1972;287:209-212.
9. Ben Amar M, Potvin S. Cannabis and psychosis: what is the link? *J Psychoactive Drugs.* 2007;39:131-142.
10. Benowitz NL, Jones RT. Cardiovascular effects of prolonged delta-9-tetrahydrocannabinol ingestion. *Clin Pharmacol Ther.* 1975;18:287-297.
11. Block RI, Ghoneim MM. Effects of chronic marijuana use on human cognition. *Psychopharmacology.* 1993;110:219-228.
12. Breivogel CS, Childers SR. The functional neuroanatomy of brain cannabinoid receptors. *Neurobiol Dis.* 1998;5:417-431.
13. Breivogel CS, Childers SR, Dedwyler SA, et al. Chronic delta 9-tetrahydrocannabinol treatment produces a time-dependent loss of cannabinoid receptors and cannabinoid receptor-activated G proteins in rat brain. *J Neurochem.* 1999;73:2447-2459.
14. Briggs GG, Freeman RK, Yaffe SJ. *Drugs in Pregnancy and Lactation*, 5th ed. Baltimore, MD: Williams & Wilkins; 1998.
15. Brown TT, Dobs AS. Endocrine effects of marijuana. *J Clin Pharmacol.* 2002;42:90S-96S.
16. Budney AJ, Hughes JR. The cannabis withdrawal syndrome. *Curr Opin Psychiatry.* 2006;19:233-238.
17. Budney AJ, Moore BA. Development and consequences of cannabis dependence. *J Clin Pharmacol.* 2002;42:28S-33S.
18. Busto U, Bendayan R, Sellers SM. Clinical pharmacokinetics of nonopiate abuse drugs. *Clin Pharmacokinet.* 1989;16:1-26.
19. Caplan GA. Marijuana and mouth cancer. *J R Soc Med.* 1991;84:386.
20. Chang AE, Shiling DJ, Stillman RC. Delta 9-tetrahydrocannabinol as an antiemetic in cancer patients receiving high dose methotrexate: a prospective randomized evaluation. *Ann Intern Med.* 1979;91:819-824.

21. Chen K, Kandel DB, Davies M. Relationships between frequency and quantity of marijuana use and last year proxy dependence among adolescents and adults in the United States. *Drug Alcohol Depend.* 1997;46:53-67.
22. Cherek DR, Lane SD, Bougherty DM. Possible amotivational effects following marijuana smoking under laboratory conditions. *Exp Clin Psychopharmacol.* 2002;10:26-38.
23. Chipman ML, Macdonald S, Mann RE. Being "at fault" in traffic crashes: does alcohol, cannabis, cocaine, or polydrug abuse make a difference? *Inj Prev.* 2003;9:343-348.
24. Cone EJ, Johnson RE, Darwin WD. Passive inhalation of marijuana smoke: urinalysis and room air levels of delta-9-tetrahydrocannabinol. *J Anal Toxicol.* 1987;11:89-96.
25. Day NL, Richardson GA. Prenatal marijuana use: epidemiology, methodologic issues, and infant outcomes. *Clin Perinatol.* 1991;18:77-91.
26. Dreher MC, Nugent K, Hudgins R. Prenatal marijuana exposure and neonatal outcomes in Jamaica: an ethnographic study. *Pediatrics.* 1994;93:254-260.
27. DuPont RL, Baumgartner WA. Drug testing by urine and hair analysis: complementary features and scientific issues. *Forensic Sci Int.* 1995;70:63-76.
28. Ellis GM Jr, Mann MA, Judson BA, et al. Excretion patterns of cannabinoid metabolites after last use in a group of chronic users. *Clin Pharmacol Ther.* 1985;38:572-578.
29. European Monitoring Centre for Drugs and Drug Addiction, *Statistical Bulletin 2006.* http://stats06.emcdda.europa.eu/en/home-en.html. Accessed May 18, 2008.
30. Felder CC, Glass M. Cannabinoid receptors and their endogenous agonists. *Ann Rev Pharmacol Toxicol.* 1998;38:179-200.
31. Fisher BAC, Ghuran A, Vadamalai V, et al. Cardiovascular complications induced by cannabis smoking. a case report and review of the literature. *Emerg Med J.* 2005;22:679-680.
32. Fried PA. Behavioral outcomes in preschool and school-age children exposed prenatally to marijuana: a review and speculative interpretation. *NIDA Res Monogr.* 1996;164:242-260.
33. Fried PA, Makin J. Neonatal behavioral correlates of prenatal exposure to marijuana, cigarettes and alcohol in a low risk population. *Neurotoxicol Teratol.* 1987;9:1-7.
34. Fried PA, Watkinson B. 36- and 48-month neurobehavioral follow-up of children prenatally exposed to marijuana, cigarettes, and alcohol. *J Dev Behav Pediatr.* 1990;11:49-58.
35. Frytak S, Moertel CG, Rubin J. Metabolic studies of delta-9-tetrahydrocannabinol in cancer patients. *Cancer Treat Rep.* 1984;68:1427-1431.
36. Goodwin RS, Gustafson RA, Barnes A, et al. Δ^9-tetrahydrocannabinol, 11-hydroxy-Δ^9-tetrahydrocannabinol and 11-nor-9-carboxy-Δ^9-tetrahydrocannabinol in human plasma after controlled oral administration of cannabinoids. *Ther Drug Monit.* 2006;28:545-551.
37. Grant P, Gandhi P. A case of cannabis-induced pancreatitis. *JOP.* 2004;5:41-43.
38. Green B, Kavanagh D, Young R. Being stoned: a review of self-reported cannabis effects. *Drug Alcohol Rev.* 2003;22:453-460.
39. Green K. Marijuana smoking vs cannabinoids for glaucoma therapy. *Arch Ophthalmol.* 1998;116:1433-1437.
40. Grotenhermen F. Pharmacokinetics and pharmacodynamics of cannabinoids. *Clin Pharmacokinet.* 2003;42:327-360.
41. Guy GW, Whittle BA, Robson PJ, eds. *The Medicinal Uses of Cannabis and Cannabinoids.* London: Pharmaceutical Press; 2004.
42. Haney M, Hart CL, Vosburg SK, et al. Marijuana withdrawal in humans: effects of oral THC or divalproex. *Neuropsychopharmacology.* 2004;29:158-170.
43. Hashibe M, Ford DE, Zhang AF. Marijuana smoking and head and neck cancer. *J Clin Pharmacol.* 2002;42:103S-107S.
44. Hatch EE, Bracken MB. Effect of marijuana use in pregnancy on fetal growth. *Am J Epidemiol.* 1986;124:986-993.
45. Hawks RL. The constituents of cannabis and the disposition and metabolism of cannabinoids. *NIDA Res Monogr.* 1982;42:125-137.
46. Heishman SJ, Huestis MA, Henningfield JE, et al. Acute and residual effects of marijuana: profiles of plasma THC levels, physiological, subjective, and performance measures. *Pharmacol Biochem Behav.* 1990;37:561-565.
47. Hingson R, Alpert JJ, Day N, et al. Effects of maternal drinking and marijuana use on fetal growth and development. *Pediatrics.* 1982;70:539-546.
48. Hirst RA, Lambert DG, Notcutt WG. Pharmacology and potential therapeutic uses of cannabis. *Br J Anaesth.* 1998;81:77-84.
49. Hollister LE. Health aspects of cannabis. *Pharmacol Rev.* 1986;38:1-20.
50. Hollister LE, Gillespie HK, Ohlsson A, et al. Do plasma concentrations of delta-9-tetrahydrocannabinol reflect the degree of intoxication? *J Clin Pharmacol.* 1981;21:171S-177S.
51. Huestis MA, ElSohly M, Nebro W, et al. Estimating time of last oral ingestion of cannabis from plasma THC and THCCOOH concentrations. *Ther Drug Monit.* 2006;28:540-544.
52. Huestis MA, Henningfield JE, Cone EJ. Blood cannabinoids. I. Absorption of THC and formation of 11-OH-THC and THCCOOH during and after smoking marijuana. *J Anal Toxicol.* 1992;16:276-282.
53. Huestis MA, Henningfield JE, Cone EJ. Blood cannabinoids. II. Models for the prediction of time of marijuana exposure from plasma concentrations of Δ^9-tetrahydrocannabinol (THC) and 11-nor-9-carboxy-Δ^9-tetrahydrocannabinol (THCCOOH). *J Anal Toxicol.* 1992;16:283-290.
54. Huestis MA, Mitchell JM, Cone EJ. Detection times of marijuana metabolites in urine by immunoassay and GC-MS. *J Anal Toxicol.* 1995;19:443-449.
55. Huestis MA, Mitchell JM, Cone EJ. Urinary excretion profiles of 11-Nor-9-carboxy-Δ^9-tetrahydrocannabinol in humans after single smoked doses of marijuana. *J Anal Toxicol.* 1996;20:441-452.
56. Hunt CA, Jones RT. Tolerance and disposition of tetrahydrocannabinol in man. *J Pharmacol Exp Ther.* 1980;215:35-44.
57. Hunter CE, Lokan RJ, Longo MC, et al. *The Prevalence and Role of Alcohol, Cannabinoids, Benzodiazepines and Stimulants in Nonfatal Crashes.* Adelaide, South Australia: Forensic Science, Department for Administrative and Information Services, South Australia; 1998.
58. Iverson L. Cannabis and the brain. *Brain.* 2003;126:1252-1270.
59. Iverson L. Long-term effects of exposure to cannabis. *Curr Opin Pharmacol.* 2005;5:69-72.
60. Johansson E, Halldin MM. Urinary excretion half-life of delta 1-tetrahydrocannabinol-7-oic acid in heavy marijuana users after smoking. *J Anal Toxicol.* 1989;13:218-223.
61. Johnson D, Convadi A, McGuigan M. Hashish ingestion in toddlers. *Vet Hum Toxicol.* 1991;33:393.
62. Jones RT. Cardiovascular system effects of marijuana. *J Clin Pharmacol.* 2002;42:58S-63S.
63. Joy JE, Watson SJ, Benson JA. *The Medical Value of Marijuana and Related Substances in Marijuana and Medicine: Assessing the Science Base.* Washington, DC: National Academy Press; 1999:137-192.
64. Katona I, Sperlagh B, Magloczky Z, et al. GABAergic interneurons are the targets of cannabinoid actions in human hippocampus. *Neuroscience.* 2000;100:797-804.
65. Kelly P, Jones RT. Metabolism of tetrahydrocannabinol in frequent and infrequent marijuana users. *J Anal Toxicol.* 1992;16:228-235.
66. Kidwell DA, Holland JS, Athanaselis S. Testing for drugs of abuse in saliva and sweat. *J Chromatogr B Biomed Sci Appl.* 1998;713:111-135.
67. Klein TW, Friedman H, Specter S. Marijuana, immunity and infection. *J Neuroimmunol.* 1998;83:102-115.
68. Kline J, Hutzler M, Levin B, et al. Marijuana and spontaneous abortion of known karyotype. *Paediatr Perinat Epidemiol.* 1991;5:320-332.
69. Kosior DA, Filipiak KJ, Stolarz P, et al. Paroxysmal atrial fibrillation following marijuana intoxication: a two-case report of possible association. *Int J Cardiol.* 2001:78:183-184.
70. Lagasse P, Goldman L, Hobson A, Norton SR, eds. *Columbia Encyclopedia,* 6th ed. New York: Columbia University Press; 2001.
71. Law B, Mason PS, Moffat AC, et al. Forensic aspects of the metabolism and excretion of cannabinoids following oral ingestion of cannabis resin. *J Pharm Pharmacol.* 1984;36:289-294.
72. Law B, Mason PA, Moffat AC, et al. Passive inhalation of cannabis smoke. *J Pharm Pharmacol.* 1984;36:578-581.
73. Lichtman AH, Martin BR. Marijuana withdrawal syndrome in the animal model. *J Clin Pharmacol.* 2002;42:20S-27S.
74. Linn S, Schoenbaum SC, Monson RR, et al. The association of marijuana use with outcome of pregnancy. *Am J Public Health.* 1983;73:1161-1164.
75. Longo MC, Hunter CE, Lokan RJ, et al. The prevalence of alcohol, cannabinoids, benzodiazepines and stimulants amongst injured drivers and their role in driver culpability. Part I. The prevalence of drug use in drivers, and characteristics of the drug-positive group. *Accid Anal Prev.* 2000;32:613-622.
76. Longo MC, Hunter CE, Lokan RJ, et al. The prevalence of alcohol, cannabinoids, benzodiazepines and stimulants amongst injured drivers and their role in driver culpability. Part II. The relationship between drug prevalence and drug concentration, and driver culpability. *Accid Anal Prev.* 2000;32:623-632.

77. Macleod J, Oakes R, Copello A, et al. Psychological and social sequelae of cannais and other illicit drug use by young people: a systematic review of logitundinal, general population studies. *Lancet.* 2004;363:1579-1588.
78. Manno JE, Manno BR, Kemp PM, et al. Temporal indication of marijuana use can be estimated from plasma and urine concentrations of Δ^9-tetrahydrocannabinol, ll-hydroxy-Δ^9-tetrahydrocannabinol, and ll-nor-Δ^9-tetrahydrocannabinol-9-carboxylic acid. *J Anal Toxicol.* 2001;25:538-549.
79. Mathew RJ, Wilson WH, Coleman RE, et al. Marijuana intoxication and brain activation in marijuana users. *Life Sci.* 1997;60:2075-2089.
80. Mathew RJ, Wilson WH, Turkington TG, et al. Time course of tetrahydrocannabinol-induced changes in regional cerebral blood flow measured with positron emission tomography. *Psychiatry Res.* 2002;116:173-185.
81. McNab A, Anderson E, Susak L. Ingestion of cannabis: a cause of coma in children. *Pediatr Emerg Care.* 1989;5:238-239.
82. Mechoulam R. *Cannabinoids as Therapeutic Agents.* Boca Raton, FL: CRC Press; 1986:1-19.
83. Mehra R, Moore BA, Crothers K, Tetrault J, Fiellin DA. The association between marijuana smoking and lung cancer: a systematic review. *Arch Intern Med.* 2006;166:1359-1367.
84. Menkes DB, Howard RC, Spears GFS, et al. Salivary THC following cannabis smoking correlates with subjective intoxication and heart rate. *Psychopharmacology.* 1991;103:277-279.
85. Mieczkowski T. A research note: the outcome of GC/MS/MS confirmation of hair assays on 93 cannabinoid (+) cases. *Forensic Sci Int.* 1995;70:83-91.
86. Mikawa Y, Matsuda S, Kanagawa T, et al. Ocular activity of topically administered anandamide in the rabbit. *Jpn J Ophthalmol.* 1997;41:217-220.
87. Mittleman MA, Lewis RA, Maclure M, et al. Triggering myocardial infarction by marijuana. *Circulation.* 2001;103:2805-2809.
88. Möller MR, Dörr G, Warth S. Simultaneous quantitation of delta-9-tetrahydrocannabinol (THC) and 11-Nor-9-carboxy-delta-9-tetrahydrocannabinol (THC-COOH) in serum by GC/MS using deuterated internal standards and its application to a smoking study and forensic cases. *J Forensic Sci.* 1992;37:969-983.
89. Mørland J, Bugge A, Skuterund B, Steen A, Wethe GH, Kjeldsen T. Cannabinoids in blood and urine after passive inhalation of *Cannabis* smoke. *J Forensic Sci.* 1985;30:997-1002.
90. Mukamal KJ, Maclure M, Muller JE, et al. An exploratory prospective study of marijuana mortality following acute myocardial infarction. *Am Heart J.* 2008;155:465-470.
91. Mule SJ, Lomax P, Gross SJ. Active and realistic passive marijuana exposure tested by three immunoassays and GC/MS in urine. *J Anal Toxicol.* 1988;12:113-116.
92. Musty RE, Kaback L. Relationships between motivation and depression in chronic marijuana users. *Life Sci.* 1995;56:151-158.
93. Nahas GG. Lethal cannabis intoxication. *N Engl J Med.* 1971;284:782.
94. Nahas G, Leger C, Tocque B, et al. The kinetics of cannabinoid distribution and storage with special reference to the brain and testis. *J Clin Pharmacol.* 1981;21:208S-214S.
95. Ohlsson A, Lingren JE, Wahlen A, et al. Plasma delta-9-tetrahydrocannabinol concentrations and clinical effects after oral and intravenous administration and smoking. *Clin Pharmacol Ther.* 1980;28:409-416.
96. O'Kane CJ, Tutt DC, Bauer L. Cannabis and driving: a new perspective. *Emerg Med (Fremantle).* 2002;14:296-303.
97. O'Leary DS, Block RI, Keoppel JA, et al. Effects of smoking marijuana on brain perfusion and cognition. *Neuropsychopharmacology.* 2002;26:802-816.
98. Onaivi ES, Leonard CM, Ishiguro H, et al. Endocannabinoids and cannabinoid receptor genetics. *Prog Neurobiol.* 2002;66:307-344.
99. Perez-Reyes M, Di Guiseppi S, Mason AP, et al. Passive inhalation of marihuana smoke and urinary excretion of cannabinoids. *Clin Pharmacol Ther.* 1983;34:36-41.
100. Perez-Reyes M, Wall ME. Presence of Δ^9-tetrahydrocannabinol in human milk. *N Engl J Med.* 1982;307:819-820.
101. Pope HG, Yurgelun-Todd D. The residual cognitive effects of heavy marijuana use in college students. *JAMA.* 1996;275:521-527.
102. Porcella A, Maxia C, Gessa GL, et al. The synthetic cannabinoid WIN55212-2 decreases the intraocular pressure in human glaucoma resistant to conventional therapies. *Eur J Neurosci.* 2001;13:409-412.
103. Poster DS, Penta JS, Bruno S, et al. Delta 9-tetrahydrocannabinol in clinical oncology. *JAMA.* 1981;245:2047-2051.
104. Prakash R, Aronow WS, Warren M, et al. Effects of marihuana and placebo marihuana smoking on hemodynamics in coronary disease. *Clin Pharmacol Ther.* 1975;118:90-95.
105. Rezkalla SH, Sharma P, Kloner RA. Coronary no-flow and ventricular tachycardia associated with habitual marijuana use. *Ann Emerg Med.* 2003;42:365-369.
106. Romolo FS, Perret D, Lopez A, et al. Determination of nabilone in bulk powders and capsules by high performance liquid chromatography/tandem mass spectrometry. *Rapid Commun Mass Spectrom.* 2004;18:128-130.
107. Rosenblatt KA, Daling JR, Chen C, et al. Marijuana use and risk of oral squamous cell carcinoma. *Cancer Res.* 2004;64:4049-4054.
108. Rubin A, Lemberger L, Warrick P, et al. Physiologic disposition of nabilone, a cannabinol derivative, in man. *Clin Pharmacol Ther.* 1977;22:85-91.
109. Schlicker E, Kathmann M. Modulation of transmitter release via presynaptic cannabinoid receptors. *Trends Pharmacol Sci.* 2001;22:565-572.
110. Schramm W, Smith RH, Craig PA, et al. Drugs of abuse in saliva: a review. *J Anal Toxicol.* 1992;16:1-9.
111. Schwartz RH. Marijuana: an overview. *Pediatr Clin North Am.* 1987;34:305-317.
112. Schwartz RH, Gruenewald PJ, Klitzner M, et al. Short-term memory impairment in cannabis-dependent adolescents. *Am J Dis Child.* 1989;143:1214-1219.
113. Schwartz RH, Hawks RL. Laboratory detection of marijuana use. *JAMA.* 1985;254:788-792.
114. Sidney S. Cardiovascular consequences of marijuana use. *J Clin Pharmacol.* 2002;42:64S-70S.
115. Singh GK. Atrial fibrillation associated with marijuana use. *Pediatr Cardiol.* 2000;21:284.
116. Smith NT. A review of the published literature into cannabis withdrawal symptoms in human users. *Addiction.* 2002;97:621-632.
117. Substance Abuse and Mental Health Services Administration, Office of Applied Studies. *National Survey on Drug Use and Health.* Washington, DC: US Department of Health and Human Services; 2006.
118. Sugiura T, Waku K. Cannabinoid receptors and their endogenous ligands. *J Biochem.* 2002;132:7-12.
119. Swift W, Hall W, Copeland J. One-year follow-up of cannabis dependence among long-term users in Sydney, Australia. *Drug Alcohol Depend.* 2000;59:309-318.
120. Tashkin DP. Airway effects of marijuana, cocaine, and other inhaled illicit agents. *Curr Opin Pulm Med.* 2001;7:43-61.
121. Tashkin DP, Shapiro BJ, Frank IM. Acute effects of smoked marijuana and oral Δ^9-tetrahydrocannabinol on specific airway conductance in asthmatic subjects. *Am Rev Respir Dis.* 1974;109:420-428.
122. Tashkin DP, Shapiro BJ, Frank IM. Acute pulmonary physiologic effects of smoked marijuana and oral Δ^9-tetrahydrocannabinol in healthy young men. *N Engl J Med.* 1973;289:336-341.
123. Taylor FM III. Marijuana as a potential respiratory tract carcinogen: a retrospective analysis of a community hospital population. *South Med J.* 1988;81:1213-1216.
124. Terhune KW, Ippolito CA, Hendricks DL, et al. The Incidence and Role of Drugs in Fatally Injured Drivers. Report no. DOT HS 808 065. Washington, DC: US Department of Transportation, National Highway Traffic Safety Administration; 1992.
125. Tetrault JM, Crothers K, Moore BA, et al. Effects of marijuana smoking on pulmonary function and respiratory complications: a systematic review. *Arch Intern Med.* 2007;167:221-228.
126. Uebel RA, Wium CA. Toxicological screening for drugs of abuse in samples adulterated with household chemical. *So Afr Med J.* 2002;92:547-549.
127. Wall ME, Sadler BM, Brine D, et al. Metabolism, disposition, and kinetics of delta-9-tetrahydrocannabinol in men and women. *Clin Pharmacol Ther.* 1983;34:352-363.
128. Weil AT. Adverse reactions to marijuana. *N Engl J Med.* 1970;282:997-1000.
129. Williams AF, Peat MA, Crouch DJ, et al. Drugs in fatally injured young male drivers. *Public Health Rep.* 1985;100:19-25.
130. Williams PL, Moffat AC. Identification in human urine of delta 9-tetrahydrocannabinol-11-oic acid glucuronide: a tetrahydrocannabinol metabolite. *J Pharm Pharmacol.* 1980;32:445-448.
131. Williamson EM, Evans FJ. Cannabinoids in clinical practice. *Drugs.* 2000;60:1303-1314.
132. Witter FR, Niebyl JR. Marijuana use in pregnancy and pregnancy outcome. *Am J Perinat.* 1990;7:36-38.
133. Wu T-C, Tashkin DP, Djahed B, et al. Pulmonary hazards of smoking marijuana as compared with tobacco. *N Engl J Med.* 1988;318:347-351.
134. Zuckerman B, Frank DA, Hingson R, et al. Effects of maternal marijuana and cocaine use on fetal growth. *N Engl J Med.* 1989;320:762-768.

CHAPTER 84
NICOTINE

Sari Soghoian

Nicotine

MW = 162 daltons

Nicotine is a highly addictive plant-derived alkaloid with stimulant properties, and the most widely used addictive xenobiotic in the world. It is related to coniine—the important alkaloid in poison hemlock—and to lobeline, which is found in *Lobalia inflata*, or Indian tobacco. Most nicotine is derived from members of the genus *Nicotiana*, collectively known as the tobacco plant, in the family Solanaceae. The most important species in human use today is *Nicotiana tabacum.*

The primary source of nicotine exposure is cigarette smoking, and there are over 3000 components to tobacco smoke. The health burden of cigarette smoking and use of other tobacco products is staggering. Epidemic tobacco abuse increases rates of chronic obstructive pulmonary disease (COPD), cardiovascular disease, pulmonary infections, macular degeneration, and cancers, and causes over five million deaths worldwide per year. Nicotine per se may not be the crucial factor in each of these health issues caused by tobacco products.

There are direct health effects of chronic nicotine exposure. Even in low doses, nicotine causes vasoconstriction and other cardiovascular effects related to catecholamine release, and promotes angiogenesis, neuroteratogenicity, and possibly some cancers.[41] Neither these nor the long-term effects of cigarette smoking and tobacco dependency are discussed further in this chapter. Instead, this chapter is concerned with the sources, effects, and management of acute toxicity referable to nicotinic receptor stimulation and cholinergic activation.

HISTORY AND EPIDEMIOLOGY

The tobacco plant is native to the Americas, and its use most likely predates the Mayan empire. In 1492 Christopher Columbus and his crew were given tobacco by the Arawaks, but threw it away not knowing any use for it. Ramon Pane, a monk who accompanied Columbus on his second voyage to America, is credited with introducing tobacco to Europe.[64]

Nicotine was isolated from tobacco in 1828. The principle source of nicotine today is still tobacco products including cigarettes, cigars, pipe tobacco, chewing tobacco, and snuff. Smoking cessation products containing nicotine are increasingly available and include gums, transdermal patches, lozenges, inhaler sprays, and pills. Exposure to tobacco plants during their harvest remains an important source of occupational nicotine toxicity known as green tobacco sickness. Nicotine insecticides are no longer in widespread use in the United States, but are used in other countries and can still be purchased from some online retailers. The neonicotinoids are the only major new class of insecticide developed in the past quarter century, and despite decreased affinity for mammalian compared to invertebrate nicotinic receptors they may still cause significant toxicity in humans. The nicotine receptor partial agonists, used to aid smoking cessation, are a new class of drug that mimics the physiologic effects of nicotine.

SOURCES AND USES OF NICOTINE

CIGARETTES

The amount of nicotine contained in a single cigarette is highly variable, and ranges from less than 10 mg in a "low nicotine" cigarette to 30 mg in some European cigarettes (Table 84–1). Since most nicotine is either lost in the sidestream (secondhand smoke) or left in the filter, the absorbed nicotine yield from a smoked cigarette is much less than this, on the order of 0.05 to 3 mg/cigarette.[25] Nicotine yield is determined by burning cigarettes on a smoke machine in a standardized manner. The amount of nicotine absorbed by a particular individual from a single smoked cigarette is highly variable among smokers, and depends on soufflé or "puff" rate, volume, the depth and duration of inhalation, and the size of the residual.[44]

The potential for nicotine toxicity from smoking is limited since peak effects by this route will occur within seconds and tend to limit further intake of drug. Most reports of acute nicotine toxicity referable to cigarette exposure are associated with cigarette and cigarette butt ingestion, usually by young children.[51,57,62]

CHEW

Smokeless or chewing tobacco is still widely used[18] despite a clear association with periodontal disease and dental cavities, and up to 48 times the risk of oropharyngeal cancers compared with people who do not use tobacco products.[19] The nicotine content of six major US brands of moist smokeless tobacco (dip) ranged from 3.37 to 11.04 mg/g in one study.[49] Because nicotine is a weak base, smokeless tobacco is buffered to facilitate buccal absorption. The pH of marketed products ranged from 5.24 to 8.35 in one survey.[49] Acute nicotine toxicity from smokeless tobacco is rarely reported in adults, however, a 14-month-old boy had muscle fasciculations and lethargy after ingesting material out of his father's spittoon but recovered within 24 hours with supportive care.[29]

GUM

Nicotine gum has been available without a prescription as an aide to smoking cessation in the United States since 1996. It is sold in 2-mg and 4-mg strengths. It is buffered to an alkaline pH to facilitate buccal absorption. The gum is supposed to be chewed until mouth and throat tingling and a peppery taste develops, signaling nicotine release. Approximately 53% to 72% of the nicotine in the gum is absorbed. The gum is then "parked" in the cheek until the sensation subsides, at which time it may be chewed again to release more drug.[52] If used correctly, serum nicotine concentrations rise gradually to a concentration slightly lower than normally achieved by cigarette smoking.[52] If the gum is swallowed whole, serum nicotine concentrations rise even more slowly since the acidic environment of the stomach delays absorption.[7] Conversely, if the gum is chewed vigorously and saliva is swallowed then nicotine concentrations may rise rapidly and adverse reactions may occur.[63]

TRANSDERMAL PATCHES

Nicotine patches have been US Food and Drug Administration (FDA) approved for purchase without prescription in the United States since 1996. Most nicotine transdermal delivery systems are designed to deliver 7, 14, or 21 mg of nicotine over 24 hours. Since many patch

TABLE 84–1. Sources of Nicotine

Source	Content (mg)	Delivered[a] (mg)
1 whole cigarette	10–30	0.05–3
1 cigarette butt	5–7	–
1 cigar	15–40	0.2–1
1 g snuff (wet)	12–16	2–3.5
1 g chewing tobacco	6–8	2–4
1 piece nicotine gum	2 or 4	1–2
1 nicotine patch	8.3–114	5–22 over 16 or 24 h
1 nicotine lozenge	2 or 4	2–4
1 nicotine nasal spray	0.5	0.2–0.4

[a] Delivered by intended use of standard dose.

users have difficulty sleeping, vivid dreams, or nightmares if they wear the patch overnight, systems designed for application for only 16 hours are now made. The patch reservoirs contain an estimated 36 to 114 mg of nicotine per patch.[53] For most children and many adults this exceeds the estimated LD_{50} for nicotine in humans of 1 mg/kg. With proper use only 7 to 21 mg is released into the skin[30] and absorbed. If the patch is punctured by biting or tearing, then delivery of the full content is possible, and severe toxicity may occur.

SPRAY/INHALER

A nicotine spray has been available since 1996 to aide efforts at smoking cessation. The most commonly reported adverse effects during initiation of therapy are due to local irritation and include rhinorrhea, lacrimation, sneezing, and nasal and throat irritation.[33] One spray delivers 0.5 mg of nicotine with the recommended dose of two sprays every 30 to 60 minutes as needed. The absorption is about 50% of the delivered dose and may be diminished or delayed by rhinitis or by α-adrenergic agonist decongestants.[40] No report of acute nicotine toxicity from nicotine inhalers has been published to date.

LOZENGES

Nicotine lozenges containing 2 and 4 mg of nicotine are available for purchase without prescription in the Unites States. The potential for rapid absorption of nicotine as a bolus dose from chewing the lozenge is a theoretical concern. No case of acute nicotine toxicity from nicotine lozenge misuse is published to date.

PLANTS/LEAVES

Green tobacco sickness is an occupational illness that affects workers who have direct contact with tobacco plants during cultivation and harvest. Residual moisture or dewdrops on tobacco leaves may contain as much as 9 mg of nicotine per 100 mL.[28] Sweat wrung out of the shirts worn by workers during tobacco harvest in one study contained up to 98 mg/mL of nicotine.[28] Green tobacco sickness is prevalent with an estimated 8.8% to 42% of tobacco harvesters affected each season.[2–4] Since farm workers are a medically underserved population in the United States, and many at-risk workers are undocumented immigrants, it is most likely underreported. Other risk factors for green tobacco sickness include younger age, working in wet tobacco, and a relative lack of work experience.[2,4,46,50] These factors may all be related to a lack of nicotine tolerance, although other aspects may be important for the development of toxicity. The use of rain suits or other barrier protection is the only protective factor consistently noted to be useful across multiple studies.[3,45,50]

SALTS (PESTICIDES)

Nicotine in the form of tobacco extracts was first reported as effective for pest control in 1690. In 1886 a mixture of tobacco and soapsuds was advocated for aphid control, but it was not until 1912 that the first commercial nicotine insecticides were developed. Crop dusting with nicotine sulfate began in 1917, though at the time this was mostly accomplished by horse-drawn carriage.[56]

The most widely known application of 40% nicotine sulfate, BlackLeaf 40, was discontinued in 1992. Nicotine is still available as a restricted-use pesticide for aphids and thrips, and a 14% preparation of nicotine is still marketed as a greenhouse smoke fumigator.[54] Since nicotine pesticides are highly concentrated, ingestion of even small amounts may produce serious toxicity including catastrophic brain injury[60] and death.[38]

NEONICOTINOIDS

The neonicotinoids are a new class of insecticides that have the theoretical advantage of decreased mammalian toxicity because of a lower affinity for the vertebrate, compared to the insect, nicotinic receptors.[65] Examples (and their year of patent) include the heterocyclics nithiazine (1977), imidacloprid (1985), thiacloprid (1985), and thiamethoxam (1989); and the acyclics nitenpyram (1988), acetamiprid (1989), clothianidin (1989), and dinotefuran (1994). Experience with human poisoning from neonicotinoid exposure is limited, and only a handful of case reports have been published to date.

NICOTINE RECEPTOR PARTIAL AGONISTS (VARENICLINE, CYTOSINE)

Nicotine receptor partial agonists have been developed to aide in smoking cessation by reducing smoking satisfaction (agonist antagonism effect) while helping to maintain moderate amounts of central dopamine release (partial agonist effect). Cytosine is a plant-derived insecticide with a chemical structure similar to nicotine that has been used in Eastern and Central Europe since the 1960s under the trade name Tabex® (Sopharma Pharmaceuticals) as a smoking cessation drug.[24] Despite widespread use it has not been well studied for its safety, efficacy, pharmacokinetics, and pharmacodynamics in humans.[24]

Varenicline (marketed as Chantix® in the United States, Champix® in Europe) is a xenobiotic developed by Pfizer Inc. as an analog of cytosine. It was FDA approved as a prescription-only aide to smoking cessation in 2006. Several randomized controlled trials have demonstrated efficacy in controlling nicotine cravings and evidence suggests that varenicline increases the probability of successful abstinence from smoking.[14] No reports of toxic manifestations (or lack thereof) after varenicline overdose have been published to date, but postmarketing experience suggests that there is an association with increased rates of suicide with therapeutic use.

PHARMACOLOGY/PHARMACOKINETICS

The pharmacologic characteristics of nicotine are listed in Table 84–2. Nicotine is well absorbed from mucosal surfaces, skin, the intestines, and the respiratory tract. Since nicotine is a weak base, more is nonionized—and will cross biologic membranes more easily—in an

TABLE 84–2. Pharmacologic Characteristics of Nicotine

Absorption	Lungs, oral mucosa, skin, intestinal tract; increased in more alkaline environment
Volume of distribution	Approximately 1 L/kg
Protein binding	5%–20%
Metabolism	80%–90% hepatic; remainder in lung, kidney; principal (inactive) metabolite is cotinine
Half-life	Nicotine: 1–4 h, decreases with repeated exposure; cotinine: 19–20 h
Elimination	2%–35% excreted unchanged in urine

alkaline environment. Cigar and pipe tobacco are air cured to achieve a pH of 8.5, and snuff, chewing tobacco, and nicotine gum are buffered in order to facilitate buccal absorption. Nicotine from cigarette smoke is carried on inhaled tar particles into the lungs where a large alveolar surface area allows rapid absorption into the pulmonary circulation.

Once absorbed, nicotine reaches the arterial circulation and diffuses almost immediately into the central nervous system (CNS). Nicotine readily crosses the placental barrier and is secreted in breast milk. Metabolism occurs primarily in the liver, and in the kidney and lung to a much lesser extent. About 70% of circulating nicotine is metabolized to cotinine, and much smaller amounts to nornicotine, nicotine-1-*N*-oxide, nicotine glucuronide, and 2'-hydroxynicotine. Hepatic transformation of nicotine is achieved by P450 cytochrome oxidases, aldehyde oxidase, flavin monooxygenase, and by glycosylation. Although multiple P450 enzymes are most likely involved, CYP2D6 and CYP2A6 are known to contribute to nicotine metabolism.

Renal excretion of unchanged nicotine accounts for 2% to 35% of total nicotine elimination,[13] and is pH dependent. Nicotine is reabsorbed in the proximal tubule where pH is relatively high. Acidification of the urine enhances elimination. The half-life of nicotine is 1 to 4 hours and decreases with repeated nicotine exposure as in habitual cigarette smoking. The elimination half-life of nicotine after transdermal patch removal is longer than that noted with nicotine exposure by other routes,[35] but this is most likely because a dermal reservoir of drug is established during patch use, from which absorption continues after removal. Cotinine and *trans*-3'-hydroxycotinine are eliminated in the urine as glucuronide esters independent of urine pH. The elimination half-life of cotinine is closer to 20 hours and urinary cotinine is therefore a more easily detected marker of nicotine exposure.

Serum concentrations of nicotine and cotinine are influenced most strongly by individual variations in clearance.[9,10] Nicotine metabolism is inducible and nicotine-dependent individuals metabolize the drug more rapidly than naïve ones.[32] Nicotine metabolism may also be linked to race and gender. Asians and African Americans metabolize nicotine more slowly than whites, and have prolonged cotinine clearance in the urine.[10,42,55] Women metabolize nicotine faster than men. This is further accelerated by oral contraceptive use and pregnancy, and is most likely mediated by an influence of estrogen on CYP2A6 activity.[32]

Cigarette smoking modulates the bioavailability and effectiveness of numerous medications through effects on drug absorption, metabolism, or pharmacodynamics. Cigarette smoking induces CYP1A2 and accelerates the metabolism of caffeine, clozapine, olanzapine, tacrine, theophylline, and erlotinib.[31,34] This effect may not involve nicotine, however, since nicotine administered intravenously does not affect theophylline metabolism.[7] Smokers also have diminished effectiveness of opioids, benzodiazepines, β-adrenergic antagonists, and nifedipine,[17] and are more likely to fail antacid and H_2-blocker therapy for peptic ulcer disease.[7] These interactions have not been clearly linked to an effect of nicotine per se, however.

The LD_{50} of nicotine has been estimated at 0.5 to 1 mg/kg in adults,[27,29,43] but severe toxicity has been reported with ingestion of less than 2 mg in a child[47,63] and this dose is sufficient to produce mild symptoms in an adult. Children under 6 years of age who ingest one or more cigarettes, or three or more cigarette butts, generally develop symptoms of nicotine toxicity.[63] A retrospective review of 10 children with cigarette ingestions found that the four patients with symptoms requiring medical evaluation and treatment had ingested at least two whole cigarettes.[43] The acute oral LD_{50} of imidacloprid in rats is 475 mg/kg, and the dermal LD_{50} is greater than 5 g/kg.[65]

Acute tolerance to nicotine develops in smokers who take in small doses of nicotine regularly throughout the day. Sensitization to the effects of nicotine is restored with overnight abstinence.[5,32] Tolerance may also develop in tobacco workers with regular exposure to tobacco plant leaves. The phenomenon of acute tolerance, however, along with considerable genetic variability in nicotine metabolism, implies a range of susceptibility to drug effect.

PATHOPHYSIOLOGY

Nicotine mimics the effects of acetylcholine release by binding to postsynaptic nicotinic receptors (nAchr) in the brain, spinal cord, autonomic ganglia, adrenal medulla, neuromuscular junctions, and chemoreceptors of the carotid and aortic bodies (Chap. 13). When nicotine binds to its receptor, the ion channel opens, allowing an influx of cations, mostly sodium and calcium. Voltage-gated calcium channels are then activated, leading to further influx of calcium and a variety of downstream effects including depolarization.

The clinical effects of nAchr stimulation are dose dependent. Low doses of nicotine and related compounds stimulate nicotinic receptors centrally and in autonomic and somatic motor nerve fibers. Prolonged stimulation at the receptor ultimately leads to receptor blockade (Chap. 68). Activation of nAchr in the CNS directly stimulates neurotransmitter release. At doses generally produced by cigarette smoking there is stimulation of the reticular activating system and an alerting pattern on electroencephalogram.[71] Release of dopamine most likely mediates the reinforcing effects of nicotine, and occurs in the mesolimbic area, the corpus striatum, the prefrontal cortex, and in the nucleus accumbens. Nicotine also stimulates glutaminergic activation and γ-aminobutyric acid (GABA)ergic inhibition of dopaminergic neurons in the ventral tegmental area of the midbrain.[6] These pathways are thought to be important neuromodulatory pathways for drug-induced reward and addiction. Norepinephrine, acetylcholine, GABA, serotonin, glutamate, and endorphins are also released by nicotine, and are associated with cognitive and mood enhancement as well as appetite suppression, increased basal energy expenditures, and anxiety reduction.[6]

At very high doses nicotine induces seizures. Nicotine-induced seizures can be blocked in mice by the nicotine-receptor antagonists mecamylamine, methyllycaconitine citrate (MLA), and hexamethonium.[20] Given to mice in slightly higher doses, however, these nicotine-receptor antagonists are themselves epileptogenic. The specific mechanisms by which nicotine produces seizures are unknown. A disinhibition model has been proposed, in which desensitization or antagonism of central nicotinic cholinergic neurons blocks excitatory input to GABAergic neurons, and a reduction of inhibitory GABAergic input to pyramidal cells then results in increased excitability and seizures.[1,15,23,26] An alternative hypothesis is that synchronous depolarization from activation of $\alpha 7^*$-subtype nicotinic receptors promotes kindling-induced seizures.[23]

CLINICAL MANIFESTATIONS

Nicotine is most rapidly absorbed in the lungs, and in decreasing order via the buccal mucosa, gastrointestinal tract, and skin. Time to onset of symptoms is within 5 to 60 seconds after inhalation of nicotine-containing smoke. Symptoms of nicotine toxicity are manifest within 15 to 30 minutes of chewing nicotine gum, but usually begin much sooner. Symptom onset is within 30 to 90 minutes after ingestion of tobacco products.

Exposure to nicotine in low doses comparable to cigarette smoking produces fine tremor, cutaneous vasoconstriction, increased gastrointestinal motility, nausea, and increases in heart rate, respiratory rate, and blood pressure. Low-dose nicotine also increases mental alertness and produces euphoria. Nicotine is rapidly metabolized, and patients who develop only mild symptoms are expected to recover quickly. An important exception to this rule is patients with symptoms of nicotine toxicity after transdermal nicotine patch application, since a reservoir of drug may persist in the skin after patch removal and can serve as a source of ongoing absorption.

Early symptoms of severe nicotine poisoning are referable to nicotinic cholinergic excess: increased salivation, nausea, vomiting, diaphoresis, and diarrhea may all occur within minutes of systemic absorption. Vomiting is the most common finding, and occurs in more than 50% of cases. Vasoconstriction may manifest with pallor and hypertension. Tachycardia may also occur. Neurologic signs and symptoms include headache, dizziness, ataxia, confusion, and perceptual distortions. Severe poisoning may include cardiac dysrhythmias, seizures, and muscle fasciculations early in the course of illness. Bradycardia, hypotension, coma, and neuromuscular blockade with respiratory failure from muscular paralysis may develop later on (Table 84–3). Nicotine is an irritant and ingestion of nicotine, including use of nicotine gum, may cause burning and pain in the mouth, and constriction of the throat muscles. Similarly, application of nicotine patches generally results in dermal irritation, which may be severe.

Data from poison centers in the United States suggests that most children with cigarette ingestions have a benign course. A series of 233 consecutive reports to poison centers of children under 6 years old who ingested cigarettes or butts found that 18% of patients developed symptoms, mostly vomiting (39%).[62] Twelve percent of the patients in this series were managed in an emergency department (ED), and none of them were admitted. Another series of 146 cases of cigarette ingestion by children less than 6 years old reported symptoms in 33.3% of the sample, again mostly vomiting (87%).[6] Follow-up was available for 90 patients, and all had recovered within 12 hours. The relative rarity of life-threatening symptoms after cigarette ingestion may be a result of auto-decontamination from vomiting, or because of limited exposure given the exploratory nature of most ingestions in children.

Cases of more severe toxicity from cigarette ingestion have been reported.[12,63] Severe toxicity including apnea and seizures is also reported in a 20-month-old child who had access to nicotine gum.[61] A retrospective review of nicotine exposures among children reported to one poison center in North America found that four out of five children aged 20 months to 9 years developed severe agitation after exposure to nicotine gum, and two of these patients developed tachycardia or hypotension.[63] The greater likelihood of becoming symptomatic after exposure to gum compared with tobacco products in this review was attributed to the rapid release of nicotine from the gum, rather than an absolute increase in dose. Atrial fibrillation is reported in adults who chew nicotine gum.[16,59]

Several reports have documented acute nicotine toxicity related to nicotine patch misuse. Toxicity from concurrent use of multiple patches as a means of attempted suicide is reported.[37,69] Children have developed symptoms after exploratory self-application of one or more patches to the skin,[66,68] and after biting, chewing, or swallowing all or part of a patch.[68] In a prospective case series of 36 exposures in children younger than 16 years, half were dermal and half oral exposures. Fourteen children (39%) developed symptoms (gastrointestinal distress, weakness, and dizziness), 10 children were evaluated in an ED and two were admitted for observation and supportive care.[68] Toxicity may also develop in people who continue to smoke cigarettes after beginning therapy with the nicotine patch.[67]

Acute nicotine toxicity including vomiting, bradycardia, and severe agitation was reported in an 8-year-old boy after application of a homemade remedy for eczema. The paste was made from a mixture of tobacco leaves, lime juice, and freeze-dried coffee after a recipe published in a book from Bangladesh and written in Bengali. The patient made a full recovery after 4 days with supportive care.[22] Severe poisoning after use of tobacco extract enema is also reported.[27] Tobacco extract and

TABLE 84–3. Signs and Symptoms of Acute Nicotine Poisoning

	Gastrointestinal	Respiratory	Cardiovascular	Neurologic
Early (0.25–1 h)	Nausea Vomiting Salivation Abdominal pain	Bronchorrhea Hyperpnea	Hypertension Tachycardia Pallor	Agitation Anxiety Dizziness Blurred vision Headache Hyperactivity Confusion Tremors Fasciculations Seizures
Late (0.5–4 h)	Diarrhea	Hypoventilation Apnea	Bradycardia Hypotension Dysrhythmias Shock	Lethargy Weakness Paralysis

tobacco smoke enemas were used in the pre-Columbian Americas by many tribes for both medicinal and spiritual purposes. They are still recommended by naturopaths and folk healers as a remedy for constipation, urinary retention, pinworm, and "hysterical convulsions."[36] Exposure to fresh tobacco leaves may produce green tobacco sickness. This syndrome has been likened to seasickness, and is characterized by dizziness, headache, nausea, weakness, vomiting, diarrhea, abdominal cramps, and chills. Signs of autonomic instability may be present in severe cases. Symptom onset is 3 to 17 hours after exposure and the duration of illness may be several days.[45]

Two suicide deaths are reported after ingestion of the neonicotinoid pesticide imidacloprid.[58] In both cases imidacloprid was implicated by postmortem liquid chromatography-mass spectrometry (LC/MS) analysis and no information was available regarding dosage or manner of death. Two other published case reports of intentional imidacloprid ingestions describe a more benign clinical course. In one of these cases symptoms included an initial period of drowsiness, disorientation, and dizziness that resolved within 12 to 15 hours, with subsequent development of fever and vomiting. Oral, esophageal, and gastric erosions were demonstrated by endoscopy.[70] Some of the clinical manifestations noted in this case may have been related to the solvent *N*-methyl pyrrolidone. Another patient who ingested a 17.8% imidacloprid solution also had initial altered level of consciousness followed by fever, bradycardia, and recurrent vomiting.[21] Both patients recovered with supportive care.

DIAGNOSTIC TESTING

Determination of serum or urinary concentrations of nicotine or its metabolites is unlikely to be helpful in the management of the acutely poisoned patient. The presence of measurable concentrations of nicotine or cotinine may reflect coincidental or chronic active or passive exposure, and does not necessarily imply acute intoxication. Cigarette smokers typically maintain serum nicotine concentrations around 30 to 50 ng/mL during the day, but may achieve concentrations as high as 100 ng/mL.[48]

Since urinary cotinine has a longer detection window, the absence of cotinine in the urine is often used to document abstinence from tobacco products. Conversely, urinary cotinine concentrations are used to document exposure to nicotine-containing products, including exposure to secondhand smoke, and to guide dosage adjustments in nicotine replacement therapy.[6,39,48]

MANAGEMENT

Most patients with unintentional or low-dose nicotine exposures will not require medical evaluation. Patients who ingest one or more cigarettes, three or more cigarette butts, any amount of nicotine or a neonicotinoid insecticide, or who have protracted vomiting or develop symptoms other than vomiting should be referred to an ED without delay. Patients with mild or no symptoms after exposure to low doses of nicotine can be observed for several hours and safely discharged home if no complicating circumstances are present such as significant comorbid cardiovascular illness, intent to self-harm, or the presence of clinical symptoms.

Vomiting is common and may limit absorption in some patients with nicotine toxicity. Induction of emesis with syrup of ipecac should be avoided since it is unlikely to be of added benefit and has the potential for harm. Orogastric lavage may be considered in patients who present immediately after large ingestions of nicotine-containing products. Activated charcoal adsorbs nicotine and can reduce absorption, but the risks of pulmonary aspiration from activated charcoal administration to patients with active vomiting seizing or a depressed level of consciousness outweigh the potential benefit.

Patients with dermal exposure to wet tobacco leaves or pesticides should be undressed completely, and the skin washed thoroughly with soap and copious amounts of water. Personal protective gear should be worn by medical staff charged with handling both clothes and patients prior to decontamination. Symptomatic patients should have any nicotine patches removed immediately and the skin washed with soap and water.

There is no specific antidote for nicotine toxicity. Treatment of acute nicotine toxicity is supportive. The first priority is to ensure airway protection and respiratory support. Seizures may be treated with a benzodiazepine. Hypotension should be treated with fluid boluses and an infusion 0.9% NaCl initially. Patients who fail to respond to volume infusion may require treatment with a vasopressor such as norepinephrine. Dysrhythmias should be treated according to standard protocols. Nicotine elimination is enhanced in acidic urine[8] but the potential risks outweigh the benefits of this elimination strategy.

SUMMARY

The primary source of nicotine is *Nicotiana* species and nicotine toxicity may occur after exposure to the fresh or dried leaves. An increasing number of nicotine-containing products are available today as alternate sources of drug that are intended to facilitate smoking cessation. Nicotine and the neonicotinoids are important pesticides that may also cause significant toxicity in humans. Nicotine is well absorbed after ingestion, inhalation, and dermal exposure. It is rapidly distributed to the brain, where it activates nicotinic acetylcholinergic receptors, stimulates the reticular activating system, and facilitates neurotransmitter release. Metabolism is via the hepatic cytochrome oxidase system, to inactive metabolites that are then slowly excreted in urine. The half-life of nicotine in the body is 1 to 4 hours, with more rapid clearance in individuals chronically exposed to the drug. Clinical manifestations of nicotine toxicity are those of nicotinic cholinergic excess, and most commonly include agitation and vomiting. Severe intoxication may cause seizures, cardiac dysrhythmias, hypotension, and neuromuscular blockade with respiratory failure from muscular paralysis. The clinical course in these cases is typically biphasic, with initial stimulation followed by inhibition. There are no antidotes for nicotine, and acute toxicity should be managed with symptom-directed, supportive care.

REFERENCES

1. Alkondon M, Pereira EF, Eisenberg HM, et al. Nicotine receptor activation in human cerebral cortical interneurons: a mechanism for inhibition and disinhibition of neuronal networks. *J Neurosci.* 2000;20:66-75.
2. Arcury TA, Quandt SA, Garcia DI, et al. A clinic-based, case-control comparison of green tobacco sickness among minority farmworkers: clues for prevention. *South Med J.* 2002;95:1008-1011.
3. Arcury TA, Quandt SA, Preisser JS. Predictors of incidence and prevalence of green tobacco sickness among Latino farmworkers in North Carolina, USA. *J Epidemiol Community Health.* 2001;55:818-824.
4. Ballard T, Ehler J, Freund E, et al. Green tobacco sickness: occupational poisoning in tobacco workers. *Arch Environ Health.* 1995;50:384-389.
5. Benowitz NL. Clinical pharmacology of nicotine: implications for understanding, preventing, and treating tobacco addiction. *Clin Pharmacol Ther.* 2008;83:531-541.
6. Benowitz NL. Neurobiology of nicotine addiction: implications for smoking cessation treatment. *Am J Med.* 2008;121:S3-10.
7. Benowitz NL. Pharmacologic aspects of cigarette smoking and nicotine addiction. *N Engl J Med.* 1988;319:1318-1330.
8. Benowitz NL, Jacob P III. Nicotine renal excretion rate influences nicotine intake during cigarette smoking. *J Pharmacol Exp Ther.* 1985;234:153-155.

9. Benowitz NL, Jacob P III, Perez-Stable E. CYP2D6 phenotype and the metabolism of nicotine and cotinine. *Pharmacogenetics.* 1996;6:239-242.
10. Benowitz N, Lessov-Schlaggar C, Swan G. Genetic influences in the variation in renal clearance of nicotine and cotinine. *Clin Pharmacol Ther.* 2008;84:243-247.
11. Benowitz N, Lessov-Schlaggar C, Swan GE, et al. Female sex and oral contraceptive use accelerate nicotine metabolism. *Clin Pharm Ther.* 2006;79:480-488.
12. Bonadio WA, Anderson Y. Tobacco ingestions in children. *Clin Pediatr.* 1989;28:592-593.
13. Byrd GD, Chang K-M, Greene JM, et al. Evidence for urinary excretion of glucuronide conjugates of nicotine, cotinine, and trans-3'-hydroxycotinine in smokers. *Drug Metab Dispos.* 1992;20:192-197.
14. Cahill K, Stead LF, Lancaster T. Nicotine receptor partial agonists for smoking cessation. *Cochrane Database of Syst Rev.* 2007;1:CD006103.
15. Chiodini FC, Tassonyi E, Hulo S, et al. Modulation of synaptic transmission by nicotine and nicotinic antagonists in the hippocampus. *Brain Res Bull.* 1999;48:623-628.
16. Choragudi NL, Aronow WS, DeLuca AJ. Nicotine gum-induced atrial fibrillation. *Heart Dis.* 2003;5:100-101.
17. Cone EJ, Fant RV, Henningfield JE. Chapter 13: nicotine and tobacco. In Mozayani A, Raymon LP, eds. *Handbook of Drug Interactions: A Clinical and Forensic Guide.* Humana Press; 2003:463-492.
18. Connolly GN, Orleans CT, Kogan M. Use of smokeless tobacco in major league baseball. *N Engl J Med.* 1988;318:1281-1284.
19. Consensus Conference: Health applications of smokeless tobacco use. *JAMA.* 1986;255:1045-1048.
20. Damaj MI, Glassco W, Dukat M, et al. Pharmacological characterization of nicotine-induced seizures in mice. *J Pharmacol Exp Ther.* 1999;291:1284-1291.
21. David D, George IA, Peter JV. Toxicology of the newer neonicotinoid insecticides: imidacloprid poisoning in a human. *Clin Toxicol.* 2007;45:485-486.
22. Davies P, Levy S, Pahari A, et al. Acute nicotine poisoning associated with a traditional remedy for eczema. *Arch Dis Child.* 2001;85:500-502.
23. Dobelis P, Hutton S, Lu Y, et al. GABAergic systems modulate nicotinic receptor-mediated seizures in mice. *J Pharmacol Exp Ther.* 2003;206:1159-1166.
24. Etter JF, Lukas RJ, Benowitz NL, et al. Cytisine for smoking cessation: a research agenda. *Drug Alcohol Depend.* 2008;92:3-8.
25. Federal Trade Comission Report. Tar, nicotine, and carbon monoxide of the smoke of 1,294 varieties of domestic cigarettes for the year 1998. http://www.ftc.gov/opa/2000/07/t&n2000.shtm (accessed May 20, 2008).
26. Freund RK, Jungschaffer DA, Collins AC, et al. Evidence for modulation of GABAergic neurotransmission by nicotine. *Brain Res.* 1988;453:215-220.
27. Garcia-Estrada H, Fischman C. An unusual case of nicotine poisoning. *Clin Toxicol.* 1977;10:391-393.
28. Gelbach SH, Perry LD, Williams WA, et al. Nicotine absorption by workers harvesting green tobacco. *Lancet.* 1975;1:478-480.
29. Goepferd SJ. Smokeless tobacco: a potential hazard to infants and children. *J Am Dent Assoc.* 1986;113:49-50.
30. Gupta SK, Benowitz NL, Jacob P III, et al. Bioavailability and absorption kinetics of nicotine following application of a transdermal system. *Br J Clin Parmacol.* 1993;36:221-227.
31. Hamilton M, Wolf JL, Rusk J, et al. Effects of smoking on the pharmacokinetics of erlotinib. *Clin Cancer Res.* 2006;12:2166-2171.
32. Hukkanen J, Jacob III P, Benowitz NL. Metabolism and disposition kinetics of nicotine. *Pharmacol Rev.* 2005;57:79-115.
33. Hurt RD, Dale LC, Croghan GA, et al. Nicotine nasal spray for smoking cessation: pattern of use, side effects, relief of withdrawal symptoms, and cotinine levels. *Mayo Clin Proc.* 1998;73:118-125.
34. Jusko WJ. Influence of cigarette smoking on drug metabolism in man. *Drug Metab Rev.* 1979;9:221-236.
35. Keller-Stanislawski B, Caspary S, Merz PG, et al. Transdermal nicotine substitution: pharmacokinetics of nicotine and cotinine. *Int J Clin Pharmacol Ther Toxicol.* 1993;31:417-421.
36. Kravetz RE. Tobacco enema. *Am J Gastroent.* 2002;97:2453.
37. LabelleA, Boulay LJ. An attempted suicide using transdermal nicotine patches. *Can J Psychiatry.* 1999;44:190.
38. Lavioe FW, Harris TM. Fatal nicotine ingestion. *J Emerg Med.* 1991;9:133-136.
39. Lawson GM, Hurt RD, Dale LC, et al. Application of urine nicotine and cotinine excretion rates to assessment of nicotine replacement in light, moderate, and heavy smokers undergoing transdermal therapy. *J Clin Pharmacol.* 1998;38:510-516.
40. Lunell E, Molander L, Leischow SJ, et al. Relative bioavailability of nicotine from a nasal spray in infectious rhinitis and after use of a topical decongestant. *Eur J Clin Pharmacol.* 1995;48:235-240.
41. Luo J, Ye W, Zendehdel K, et al. Oral use of Swedish moist snuff (snus) and risk for cancer of the mouth, lung, and pancreas in male construction workers: a retrospective cohort study. *Lancet.* 2007;369:2015-2020.
42. Malaiyandi V, Sellers AM, Tyndale RF. Implications of CYP2A6 genetic variation for smoking behaviors and nicotine dependence. *Clin Pharmacol Ther.* 2006;77:480-488.
43. Malizia E, Andreucci E, Alfani F, et al. Acute intoxication with nicotine alkaloids and cannabinoids in children from ingestion of cigarettes. *Hum Toxicol.* 1983;2:315-316.
44. Marion DJ, Fortmann SP. Nicotine yield and measures of cigarette smoke exposure in a large population. *Am J Public Health.* 1987;77:546-549.
45. McBride JS, Altman DG, Klein M, et al. Green tobacco sickness. *Tob Control.* 1998;7:294-298.
46. McKnight RH, Spiller HA. Green tobacco sickness in children and adolescents. *Public Health Rep.* 2005;120:602-605.
47. Mensch AR, Holden M. Nicotine overdose after a single piece of nicotine gum. *Chest.* 1984;86:801-802.
48. Moyer TP, Charlson JR, Enger RJ, et al. Simultaneous analysis of nicotine, nicotine metabolites, and tobacco alkaloids in serum or urine by tandem mass spectrometry, with clinically relevant metabolic profiles. *Clin Chem.* 2002;48:1460-1471.
49. MMWR. Determination of nicotine, pH, and moisture content of six commercial moist snuff products—Florida, January–February 1999. *MMWR.* 1999;48:398-401.
50. MMWR. Green tobacco sickness in tobacco harvesters—Kentucky, 1992. *MMWR.* 1993;42:237-240.
51. MMWR. Ingestion of cigarettes and cigarette butts by children—Rhode Island, January 1994–July 1996. *MMWR.* 1997;46:125-128.
52. Nicorette® [package insert]. Pfizer; 2002.
53. Nicoderm®CQ® [package insert]. GlaxoSmithKline Consumer Healthcare, L.P.; 2006.
54. Ohio Vegetable Production Guide. Ohio State University Bulletin 672-08. http://ohioline.osu.edu/b672/index.html (accessed September 6, 2008).
55. Perez-Stable EJ, Herrera B, Jacob P, et al. Nicotine metabolism and intake in black and white smokers. *JAMA.* 1998;280:152-156.
56. Pesticide Information Program, Clemson University. Fighting our insect enemies: achievements of Professional Entymology (1854–1954). http://entweb.clemson.edu/pesticid/history.htm (accessed September 6, 2008).
57. Petridou E, Polychronopoulou A, Kouri N, et al. Childhood poisonings from ingestion of cigarettes. *Lancet.* 1995;346:1296.
58. Proenca P, Teixeira H, Castanheira F, et al. Two fatal intoxication cases with imidacloprid: LC/MS analysis. *Forensic Sci Int.* 2005;153:75-80.
59. Rigotti NA, Eagle KA. Atrial fibrillation while chewing nicotine gum. *JAMA.* 1986;255:1018.
60. Rogers AJ, Denk LD, Wax PM. Catastrophic brain injury after nicotine insecticide ingestion. *J Emerg Med.* 2004;26:169-172.
61. Singer J, Janz T. Apnea and seizures caused by nicotine ingestion. *Pediatr Emerg Care.* 1990;6:135-137.
62. Sisselman SG, Mofenson HC, Caraccio TR. Childhood poisonings from ingestion of cigarettes. *Lancet.* 1996;347:200-201.
63. Smolinske SC, Spoerke DG, Spiller SK, et al. Cigarette and nicotine chewing gum toxicity in children. *Hum Toxicol.* 1988;7:27-31.
64. The tobacco timeline. http://www.tobacco.org/History/TobaccoHistory.html (accessed May 20, 2008).
65. Tomizzawa M, Casida JE. Neonicotinoid insecticide toxicology: mechanisms of selective action. *Ann Rev Toxicol.* 2005;45:247-268.
66. Wain AA, Martin J. Can transdermal nicotine patch cause acute intoxication in a child? A case report and review of the literature. *Ulster Med J.* 2004;73:65-66.
67. Weiss RD. Nicotine toxicity misdiagnosed as lithium toxicity. *Am J Psychiatry.* 1996;153:132.
68. Woolf A, Burkhart K, Caraccio T, Litovitz T. Childhood poisoning involving transdermal nicotine patches. *Pediatrics.* 1997;99:724.
69. Woolf A, Burkhart K, Caraccio T, Litovitz T. Self-poisoning among adults using multiple transdermal nicotine patches. *J Toxicol Clin Toxicol.* 1996;34:691-698.
70. Wu IW, Lin JL, Cheng ET. Acute poisoning with the neonicotinoid insecticide imidacloprid in *N*-methyl pyrrolidone. *J Toxicol Clin Toxicol.* 2001;39:617-621.
71. Zhang L, Samet J, Caffo B, et al. Power spectral analysis of EEG activity during sleep in cigarette smokers. *Chest.* 2008;133:427-432.

CHAPTER 85
PHENCYCLIDINE AND KETAMINE

Ruben E. Olmedo

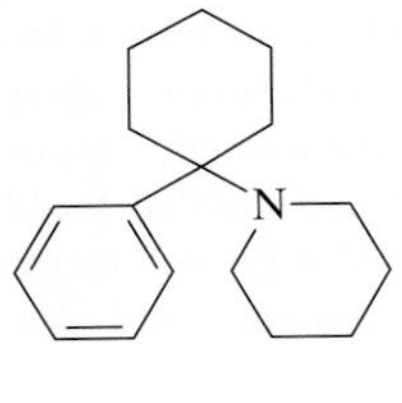

Phencyclidine (PCP)

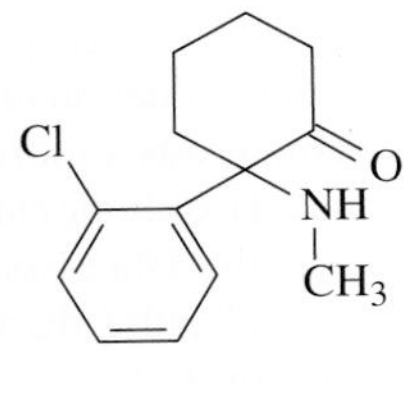

Ketamine

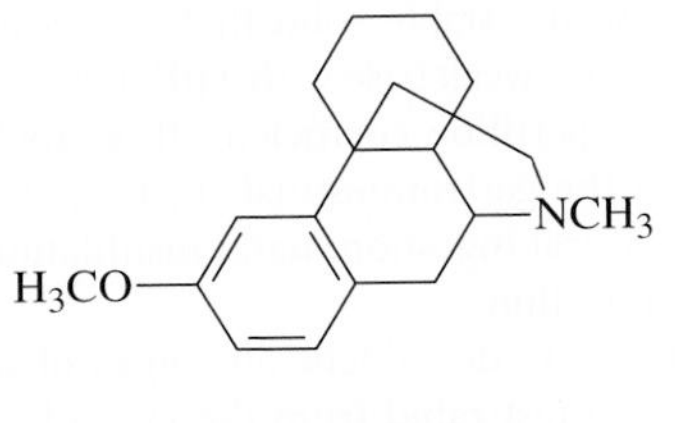

Dextromethorphan

Phencyclidine (PCP) and ketamine are dissociative anesthetics that are abused for their psychoactive effects, with ketamine having one-tenth the potency. PCP's popularity peaked during the 1970s. Ketamine gained popularity in the 1990s along with γ-hydroxybutyrate (GHB) and hallucinogenic amphetamines, which remain popular in nightclubs and "raves." Both xenobiotics affect the central nervous system (CNS), producing psychiatric and medical complications during an "out of body experience" and alteration in sensory perception. As a class of their own, they carry out these effects via inhibition of the *N*-methyl-D-aspartate (NMDA) receptor. The opioid, dextromethorphan, causes similar dissociative effects in high doses and has become popular among today's youth as it is easily obtained in cough suppressants. An understanding of the pharmacology and pathophysiology of PCP and ketamine is valuable in the diagnosis, management, and treatment of patients with toxicity from these agents.

HISTORY AND EPIDEMIOLOGY

PCP was discovered in 1926, but it was not developed as a general anesthetic until the 1950s. At the time, the Parke Davis drug company was searching for an ideal intravenous (IV) anesthetic that would rapidly achieve analgesia and anesthesia with minimal cardiovascular and respiratory depression.[36] It was marketed under the name Sernyl because it rendered an apparent state of serenity when administered to laboratory monkeys. Its surgical use began in 1963, but PCP was rapidly discontinued when a 10% to 30% incidence of postoperative psychoses and dysphoria was documented over the subsequent 2-year period.[81] By 1967 the use of PCP was limited exclusively to veterinary medicine as a tranquilizer marketed under the name Sernylan.

Simultaneously, in the 1960s, PCP was developing as a San Francisco street drug called "the PeaCe Pill."[66] Numerous street names have been given to phencyclidine: on the West Coast it was called "angel dust," PCP, "crystal," "crystal joints" (CJs); Chicago called it "THC" or "TAC"; the East Coast opted for "the sheets," "Hog," or "elephant tranquilizer."[121] Ironically, PCP was initially unpopular with drug users because of its dysphoric effects and unpredictable oral absorption.[157] With time, however, its use spread in a similar geographic pattern to that of marijuana and lysergic acid diethylamide (LSD), from the coastal United States to the Midwest region.[66]

Phencyclidine abuse became widespread during the 1970s.[25,182] The relatively easy and inexpensive synthesis coupled with the common masking of PCP as LSD, mescaline, psilocybin, cocaine, amphetamine, and/or "synthetic THC" (tetrahydrocannabinol) added to its allure and consumption.[121] By the late 1970s PCP abuse had reached epidemic proportions.[7] The Drug Abuse Warning Network (DAWN) reported that the number of PCP-related emergencies and deaths more than doubled in the 2 years from 1975 to 1977. In 1978 the National Institute of Drug Abuse reported that of young adults (18–25 years old), 13.9% had used PCP.[50] The manufacture of phencyclidine was ultimately prohibited in 1978 when it was added to the list of federally controlled substances. Classifying PCP as a Schedule II drug led to its decrease in availability and, consequently, a decrease in its use. Although the 1980s brought about a cocaine epidemic that eclipsed PCP, PCP has remained consistently available, primarily regionalized to large cities in the northeastern United States and in the Los Angeles area,[103] where PCP use continues to rise and fall with societal trends. Because many of the PCP congeners made during the manufacturing process were being abused in place of PCP, the Controlled Substance Act of 1986 made these derivatives illegal and established that the use of PCP's precursor, piperidine, necessitated mandatory reporting. With this new law in place, those possessing similar but not identical illegal substances could be prosecuted. This led to a further decline in the popularity of phencyclidine. Beginning in 1984, the overall use of PCP declined, reaching a nadir in 1994.[185] Since 1994, however, there has been an increase of reported PCP abuse. DAWN reported that the number of PCP-related emergencies increased 28% between 1995 and 2002, with the highest rate in 2002 encountered in Washington, DC; Philadelphia; Los Angeles; Chicago; and Newark.[186,189,190] According to the 2002 National Survey on Drug Use and Health (NSDUH), lifetime use of PCP was highest among those 26 years of age and older (3.5%) compared with people aged 18 to 25 years (2.7%) and those aged 12 to 17 years (0.9%).[185] In the 2003 NSDUH report, the number of PCP users remained stable at approximately 200,000.[187] It reported that in 2006 approximately 187,000 persons aged 12 or older used PCP in the past year and that 6.6 million persons had used PCP in their lifetime.[189] This number has not changed according to the NSDUH report of 2008.

Laboratory investigation of phencyclidine derivatives led to the discovery of ketamine, a chloroketone analog. Ketamine was introduced for general clinical practice in 1970 and was marketed as Ketalar, Ketaject and, for veterinary use, Ketavet. Because ketamine has approximately 5% to 10% of the potency of PCP and a much shorter duration of action, it provides greater control in clinical use. Thirty-five years of clinical experience have established that ketamine provides adequate surgical anesthesia, a rapid recovery, and less prominent emergence reactions than PCP.[56,78,160,201] Because of the simplicity and efficacy of its use it is regularly used in operating rooms, emergency departments (EDs), and throughout the developing world where little clinical monitoring is available during surgical and emergency procedures.[53,77,78,80,81,83,161,200]

Abuse of ketamine was first noted on the West Coast in 1971.[171] During the 1980s there were reports of its abuse internationally, as well as among physicians.[3,68] The nonmedical use of dissociative anesthetics has continued to increase throughout the 1990s and into the 2000s, in spite of the common complications associated with their use.[184] The same pharmacologic qualities that made ketamine more popular than PCP clinically are also responsible for its nonmedical popularity. Ketamine is regularly consumed at all-night "rave parties" and in nightclubs because of its "hallucinatory" and "out-of-body" effects, relatively inexpensive price, and short duration of effect: a single insufflation lasts between 15 and 20 minutes.[11,44,92,96,202]

The use of ketamine is not limited to the inner city. In the past decade, the media reported police arrests in affluent suburban communities for possession and sale of ketamine, as well as more in-depth and frequent reporting of the effects of its toxicity among users.[44,92,158,202] In contrast to PCP, ketamine is not manufactured illegally, but rather, it is diverted from legitimate medical, dental, and veterinary sources. Additionally, with the advent of the Internet, its availability has dangerously grown nationwide; a sham "biotech" Internet company was seized by New York City police in 2000 for selling so-called date-rape drugs, including ketamine.[133]

Adverse reactions do occur, although there are few reports of fatalities secondary to ketamine during this period of increased use.[72,112,116,138] Because of its abuse potential, ketamine was placed in Schedule III of the Controlled Substance Act in 1999.[160] In 2002, DAWN reported that there was a dramatic rise (more than 2000%) of ketamine-related ED visits between 1994 and 2001. Despite any clear reason, after peaking in 2001, there was a decline in ketamine-related ED visits in 2002.[187] The 2006 NSDUH estimated that 2.3 million persons aged 12 or older used ketamine in their lifetime, and 203,000 were past-year users.[188]

PHARMACOLOGY

CHEMISTRY

Phencyclidine's chemical name, 1-(1-phenylcyclohexyl)piperidine, provided the basis for its street acronym PCP. During its unlawful chemical synthesis, numerous analogs are made that have similar effects on the CNS and have been used as PCP substitutes. These "designer" arylcyclohexylamines are aliphatic- or aromatic-substituted amines, ketones, or halides, and appear similar to the parent compound. More than 60 psychoactive analogs are mentioned in the medical literature and the following salient points of the five most prevalent compounds are worth mentioning. TCP (1-[1-(2-thienyl)cyclohexyl] piperidine) and PCC (1-piperidino-cyclohexanecarbonitrile) are piperidine derivatives. Piperidine, the synthetic precursor, was formerly easily purchased for manufacturing PCP and its derivatives. TCP, a thiophene analog, produces even more intense effects than PCP. An intermediate of PCP synthesis, PCC was a constituent of up to 22% of illicit drug preparations analyzed for phencyclidine. This most likely resulted from a poor manufacturing process.[14,170] PCC degrades to piperidine, which is recognizable by its strong fishy odor. The presence of its carbonitrile group adds to its toxicity by generating cyanide when smoked.[12,14,177,178] The pyrrolidine derivative, PHP (phencycloclohexylpyrrolidine), is clinically comparable to PCP and is not detected by many of the available drug-screening methods.[27,89] More potent than PCP, PCE (1-phenyl-cyclohexylethylamine) was commonly available on the street as a white powder indistinguishable from PCP.[170]

Ketamine and tiletamine, two legal analogs of PCP, are used clinically for sedation and anesthesia. In larger quantities, both are also used in veterinary medicine for animal sedation. Ketamine (Ketaset and Ketalar) is the only dissociative anesthetic product manufactured for human use for the purpose of anesthesia, conscious sedation, and the treatment of bronchospasm. The development of a mechanistic approach to pain therapy in the last 15 years has brought a renewed interest in the use of ketamine as an adjuvant to multimodal pain treatment. Ketamine is used prophylactically and therapeutically in children and adults in the management of postoperative pain. For the treatment of pain ketamine is administered intravenously (median dose: 0.4 mg/kg; range: 0.1–1.6), orally, intramuscularly, rectally, subcutaneously, intraarticularly, caudally, epidurally, transdermally, intranasally, or added to a patient-controlled analgesia device.[61,82,90,107,163]

The molecular structure of ketamine [2-(ortho-chlorophenyl)-2-methylaminocyclohexanone] contains a chiral center, producing a racemic mixture of two resolvable optical isomers or enantiomers, the D(+)-isomer and L(−)-isomer. Commercially available preparations of ketamine contain equal concentrations of the two enantiomers. These two molecules differ in their pharmacodynamic effects. In a randomized, double-blind evaluation of patients undergoing surgery, the D(+)-isomer of ketamine was a more effective anesthetic, but manifested a higher incidence of psychotic emergence reactions than the L(−)-isomer. In other studies, the D(+)-isomer caused a greater increase in both blood pressure and pulse than the L(−)-isomer, and also had more bronchodilating effects.[161,201]

PHARMACOKINETICS AND TOXICOKINETICS

Phencyclidine is a white, stable solid that is readily soluble in both water and ethanol. It is a weak base with a pK_a between 8.6 and 9.4 with a high lipid-to-water-partition coefficient. It is rapidly absorbed from the respiratory and the gastrointestinal tracts; as such, it is typically self-administered by oral ingestion, nasal insufflation, smoking, or IV and subcutaneous injection.

The effects of PCP are dependent on routes of delivery and dose. Its onset of action is most rapid from the IV and inhalational routes (2–5 minutes) and slowest (30–60 minutes) following gastrointestinal absorption.[42,43] Sedation is commonly produced by doses of 0.25 mg intravenously, whereas oral ingestion typically requires 1 to 5 mg to produce similar sedation. Signs and symptoms of toxicity usually last 4 to 6 hours, and large overdoses generally resolve within 24 to 48 hours, but effects may persist in a chronic user.[16,54,57,120,144,157] However, in the PCP-poisoned patient, the relationships between dosage, clinical effects, and serum concentrations are not reliable or predictable.

There are several explanations for the protracted CNS effects of PCP. Its large volume of distribution of 6.2 L/kg[42,206] and high lipid solubility account for its entry and storage in adipose and brain tissue. Also, on reaching the acidic cerebrospinal fluid (CSF), PCP becomes ionized, producing CSF concentrations approximately six to nine times greater than those of serum.[135]

PCP undergoes first-order elimination over a wide range of doses. It has an apparent terminal half-life of 21 ± 3 hours under both control and overdose settings.[42,95] More prolonged toxicity has been reported in patients who "body-pack" PCP in plastic bags.[95,209] Ninety percent of PCP is metabolized in the liver and 10% is excreted in the urine unchanged. PCP undergoes hepatic oxidative hydroxylation into two monohydroxylated and one dihydroxylated metabolites.[43] All three compounds are conjugated to the more water-soluble glucuronide derivatives and then excreted in the urine.

Urine pH is an important determinant of renal elimination of PCP. In acidic urine, PCP becomes ionized and then cannot be reabsorbed. Acidification of the urine increased renal clearance of PCP from 1.98 ± 0.48 L/h to 2.4 ± 0.78 L/h.[42] Additional studies have found a much higher renal clearance (8.04 ± 1.56 L/h) if the urine pH was decreased to less than 5.0.[10] Although this may account for a 23% increase in the renal clearance, it only represents a 1.1% increase of the total clearance.

Similarly, ketamine is water soluble but also has a high lipid solubility that enables it to distribute to the CNS readily. It has a pK_a of

7.5 and a volume of distribution of 1.8 ± 0.7 L/kg. Ketamine has approximately 10% of the potency of PCP,[78,97] and human trials demonstrate that its clinical effects, similar to PCP, are both route and dose dependent.[46,49,56,179] Peak concentrations occur within 1 minute of IV administration and within 5 minutes of a 5-mg/kg intramuscular (IM) injection.[201,210] Ketamine distributes immediately into the CNS with the duration of its hypnotic and anesthetic effects being principally caused by its redistribution from the brain to other tissues.[201] Recovery time averages 15 minutes for IV administration, but it is prolonged to between 30 and 120 minutes for IM administration. Oral or rectal doses are not well absorbed and undergo substantial first-pass metabolism.[161,201] In contrast to oral administration of ketamine where symptoms last 4 to 8 hours, symptoms after nasal administration last for 45 to 90 minutes.

Ketamine is extensively metabolized in the liver by the cytochrome P450 (CYP) isoenzyme CYP2B6 and to a lesser extent by CYP3A4 and CYP2C9.[208] Its biotransformation is complex with numerous metabolites described.[2,161,201] The major pathway involves its *N*-demethylation to norketamine, a metabolite with one-third the anesthetic potency of ketamine. Norketamine is hydroxylated at different sites within its hexanone ring, producing varying second chiral centers. The majority of these diastereoisomers are glucuronidated to more water-soluble derivatives that are then excreted in the urine.[78,161] Ketamine also undergoes ring hydroxylation prior to *N*-demethylation as a minor metabolic pathway. The elimination half-life, which reflects both metabolic and excretory phases, is 2.3 ± 0.5 hours and is prolonged when xenobiotics requiring hepatic metabolism are coadministered.[118] Because of the enzymatic hepatic metabolism, both tolerance and enzyme induction are reported following chronic administration.[78,161]

AVAILABLE FORMS

PCP is available on the street in a variety of forms, including powder, liquid, tablets, leaf mixtures, and rock crystal. Because of its uncontrolled illegal manufacture, the contents of PCP vary considerably, with powder often the purest form, containing approximately 5 mg per dose.[156] Leaf mixtures are made by sprinkling approximately 1 to 10 mg of phencyclidine onto parsley, oregano, mint, tobacco, or marijuana. A typical PCP joint (known as "crystal joint," "KJ," or "supergrass") is developed for smoking and contains about 1 mg per 150 mg of plant product.[7] Mentholated cigarettes dipped into liquid PCP are known as "supercools."

Since PCP's inclusion in the federal Controlled Substance Act of 1970, it has been infrequently incorporated into marijuana cigarettes. There are reports of marijuana cigarettes being adulterated with PCP and sold on the street under varying names like "Illy" in Connecticut, "Hydro" in New York City, "Dip" in New Jersey, "Wet" in Philadelphia, and "Fry" in Texas.[91] The cigarettes are treated with embalming fluid, which allegedly enhances the drug's euphoric effects. Embalming fluid, which contains formalin (formaldehyde in methanol), is used as a medium to allow a uniform distribution of PCP in these cigarettes.[91] It is difficult to discern whether this "enhanced" mixture is purchased intentionally or is placed in these cigarettes surreptitiously.

On the street and on the Internet, ketamine is known as "vitamin K," "Special K," "Super K," "Ket," or simply "K." It is available in a liquid form that is dried into a pure-white crystalline powder and is typically self-administered by ingestion or insufflation in a fashion similar to PCP. It is rarely injected intravenously or intramuscularly in liquid form.

When used by injection there is an observed demographic and behavioral difference among those who initiate drug injection use with ketamine and those who initiate injection use with another xenobiotic and later transition into ketamine injection.[115]

Ketamine is primarily sold as tablets, capsules, or powder. These formulations are often adulterated with caffeine, methylenedioxymethamphetamine (MDMA), ephedrine, methamphetamine, heroin, and cocaine (a mixture known as CK or Calvin Klein).[59,164] In fact, in addition to alcohol, MDMA (39%), heroin (17%), and cocaine (14%) are the most frequently mentioned xenobiotics used with ketamine.[191] Exemplifying the commercial growth of ketamine, some of the tablets are even found to contain a "K" logo.[59] Common sedating doses are 75 to 300 mg orally (30–75 mg for insufflation). Higher doses, ranging between 300 and 450 mg orally (100–250 mg for insufflation), result in substantial CNS toxicity. These manifestations are similar to the clinical "emergence reactions" that patients experience ketamine anesthesia.

PATHOPHYSIOLOGY

The arylcyclohexylamines, of which PCP and ketamine are prototypes, are a group of anesthetics that functionally and electrophysiologically "dissociate" the somatosensory cortex from higher centers.[46,200] The precise mechanisms by which PCP and ketamine achieve these effects are complex and not fully understood; however, investigation of the nature of PCP-induced psychosis has led to a substantial identification of the various sites of PCP activity.

Most studies demonstrate that PCP and ketamine bind with high affinity to sites located in the cortex and limbic structures of the brain.[123] They block the NMDA receptors at serum concentrations encountered clinically.[195,211] Analogs of PCP (TCP, PCE, PHP, ketamine) and dizocilpine (MK-801) also interact with the NMDA receptor in a dose–response manner that corresponds appropriately to their neurobehavioral effect.[26,167,203] These xenobiotics bind to the NMDA receptor at a site independent of glutamate.[97,102,123,205] As such they antagonize glutamate's action on this channel and noncompetitively block Ca^{2+} influx (Fig. 13-14).

PCP and ketamine bind to the biogenic amine reuptake complex with 10% to 20% of the affinity to which they bind to the NMDA receptor. Binding occurs at physiologic concentrations that normally take place after subanesthetic doses.[4,152] This weak inhibition of the catecholamine reuptake accounts for the respective sympathomimetic and psychomotor effects. An increase in blood pressure and heart rate is induced. Rapid IV infusion produces a more pronounced effect than by IM injection, with the D(+)-isomer having a greater effect than the L(−)-isomer.[201]

In significant overdoses, PCP and ketamine also stimulate σ receptors at concentrations generally associated with coma, although with lower affinity than NMDA receptors.[180,204] Both D_2 and σ receptors have an inhibitory effect on the cholinergic receptor pathways.[204] At the higher concentrations typically associated with death, PCP and ketamine also bind to the nicotinic, opioid, and muscarinic cholinergic receptors.[194]

Data indicate that NMDA antagonists produce effects on behavior, sensation, and cognition that resemble aspects of endogenous psychoses, particularly schizophrenia.[98,149] The behavioral abnormalities were first observed in studies in the late 1950s when PCP, administered to healthy volunteers, generated a form of organic psychosis that mimicked schizophrenia. When PCP was administered to schizophrenic patients it uniformly intensified their primary symptoms of profound disorganization, and some of these symptoms lasted for weeks.[120] PCP psychosis is so similar to schizophrenia that many psychiatrists cannot distinguish them without a prior indication of drug abuse history.[176]

Current interest in the role of excitatory neurotransmitter systems in the pathophysiology of schizophrenia has led to similar observations in patients after ketamine administration. Subanesthetic doses of ketamine administered to both healthy and schizophrenic volunteers induced a mild, dose-related, short-lasting increase in psychotic symptoms. Although the normal and schizophrenic volunteers had different levels of baseline psychosis, the magnitude, time course, and dose–response changes in positive symptoms were similar across the two populations. Both groups experienced thought disorganization, such as concreteness and loose association, hallucinations, and delusions along a gradient of intensity.[110,112–114]

There is a connection between PCP psychosis and sensory processing. PCP and ketamine inhibit sensory perception in a dose-dependent manner. This processing in sensory information corresponds to their relative affinities to the NMDA receptor and not to the σ receptor.[6,152] Clinically, the impairment of sensory input produced by PCP resembles that of patients who are deprived of sensory stimulation.[134] When external stimulation was reduced by environmental sensory deprivation, the psychotomimetic effects of PCP were diminished,[40] giving credence to the theory that it may not be anxiety that causes perceptual dysfunction in schizophrenia, but the converse.

Many of the NMDA antagonists, including PCP and ketamine, have a negative effect on cognition and memory. There is substantial evidence in animal studies, including primates, where repeat administration of PCP and ketamine result in cognitive and memory impairement.[87,100] Both impair concentration, recall, learning, and retention of new information.[13,30,52,54,73,86–88,110,127,137,146] In human volunteers, ketamine selectively impairs explicit,[72] episodic,[51,141] and procedural memory,[141] and disrupts frontal cortical function, as measured by the Wisconsin Card Sorting Task and verbal fluency,[110,127] in a dose-dependent manner. Learning and memory impairments in volunteers who were administered subanesthetic doses of ketamine (0.65 mg/kg) are independent of the subject's attention and related psychosis.[127] Similar testing performed on chronic ketamine users produces similar results that are long lasting and have more marked effects on semantic and episodic memory.[51,52,142,143] Accordingly, it is presumed that the acute and repeated NMDA receptor antagonism interferes with those functions that integrate interoceptive and exteroceptive input in which goal-directed action becomes possible, similar to the organic psychosis in schizophrenia.

Hypofunction of the NMDA receptor causes neuroanatomical and neurobehavioral toxicologic effects. Animals exposed to NMDA antagonists such as PCP and dizocilpine transiently demonstrated neuronal vacuolar degeneration in the retrosplenial cortex and the posterior cingulate areas of the brain.[147,148] The major function of cingulate cortical neurons is to mediate affective responses to pain.[196] Single high doses or repeated exposure to NMDA receptor antagonists are associated with a higher incidence of cellular death.[45,62,63,147] This injury seems to be related to the induction of selective expression of individual heat shock proteins in this anatomical area.[169] Excitatory amino acids are neurotransmitters responsible for mediating seizure activity in the brain. As NMDA inhibitors, the anticonvulsant properties of PCP and ketamine are inconclusive. Animals administered PCP or PCP analogs progress through dose-related clonic activity followed by tonic–clonic convulsions, as is typical of classic convulsant compounds.[152] Animal research also demonstrates wide interspecies variability of the electroencephalographic (EEG) effects of PCP.[57] In a murine seizure model, ketamine possessed selective anticonvulsant properties.[31] In addition, ketamine preserves learning proficiency in rats when administered shortly after onset of status epilepticus, an effect that may prove useful in the clinical setting when combined with conventional antiepileptic medications.[181]

In humans, although these dissociative xenobiotics induce excitatory activity in the thalamus and limbic areas, they do not affect cortical regions.[48,49,56,69] Excitation, muscle twitching, posturing,[136] and tonic–clonic motor activity with or without EEG changes are reported with these subcortical EEG alterations.[34,47,69,136] In the clinical setting, many report ketamine to possess anticonvulsant properties at clinically relevant doses and may be explained by an NMDA inhibitory effect.[34,47]

The NMDA receptor is also responsible for the development of the neuronal organization of the central nervous system.[93,94,172,173] It is linked to hypoxic–ischemic brain injury by mediating calcium influx, a final pathway in cell death. The uninhibited firing of NMDA afferent neurons secondary to brain injury causes their death, as well as the death of efferent neurons downstream. In neonatal rats, ketamine increases the rate of neuronal apoptosis.[166] NMDA antagonists such as PCP block hypoxic brain injury from stroke and trauma.[17,119] In a rat model of ischemic stroke, PCP had a protective effect on the brain, demonstrated by a decreased rate of seizure activity.[17] This effect is transient and has not been studied in human subjects.

PCP induces modest tolerance in rats and squirrel monkeys. The development of tolerance is mostly secondary to PCP's pharmacologic effect rather than to biodispositional changes. Dependence was also observed in monkeys who self-administered PCP (10 mg/kg/d to serum concentrations of 100–300 ng/mL) over 1 month by the appearance of dramatic withdrawal signs when access was denied. Signs included vocalizations, bruxism, oculomotor hyperactivity, diarrhea, piloerection, difficulty remaining awake, tremors, and in one case convulsions.[15] These signs appeared within 8 hours of abstinence and were most severe at about 24 hours. When either PCP or ketamine (2.5 mg/kg/h) was readministered to the animals, PCP withdrawal symptoms were reversed, indicating cross-dependence from PCP to ketamine.[20,99,175]

Physiologic dependence in humans has not been formally studied. It is implied to occur by the observation that 68 chronic PCP users developed depression, anxiety, irritability, lack of energy, sleep disturbance, and disturbed thoughts after 1 day of abstinence from drug use.[159] Additionally, neonates whose mothers used PCP developed jitteriness, vomiting, and hypertonicity that lasted for at least 2 weeks.[183] These symptoms may represent PCP withdrawal or intrinsic teratogenic effects on neurologic development.[76,93] Although there are no controlled studies observing the physiologic symptoms of withdrawal in humans who chronically use PCP or ketamine, there is a definite psychological dependence on the sensations experienced during recreational use of the drugs.[171] There are few case reports of ketamine dependency in the medical literature where patients report a need to use an increased quantity of drug to get the same effect.[139,153] In addition, ketamine impairs response inhibition, which is found to be related to increases in subjective ratings of desire for the drug.[141]

CLINICAL MANIFESTATIONS

The reported signs and symptoms of patients presenting to the ED with PCP and ketamine toxicity are variable. The variations are a result of differences in dosage, the multiple routes of administration, concomitant xenobiotic use, and other associated medical conditions. In accordance with their pharmacologic effect, ketamine toxicity produces signs and symptoms similar to PCP with a shorter duration of action. Additionally, individual differences in xenobiotic susceptibility, the development of tolerance in chronic users, as well as contaminants in the drug manufacture, may account for erratic clinical findings.

VITAL SIGNS

Body temperature is rarely affected directly by PCP and ketamine. In one large series, only 2.6% of patients demonstrated hyperthermia (temperature greater than 101.8°F [38.8°C]).[130] In an experimental animal model, PCP failed to increase body temperature.[36,57] When hyperthermia does occur, all the known complications, including encephalopathy, rhabdomyolysis, myoglobinuria, acute renal failure, electrolyte abnormalities, and liver failure, occur (Chap. 15).[8,19,39,154]

Most PCP- and ketamine-toxic patients demonstrate mild sympathomimetic effects. PCP consistently increases both the systolic blood pressure (SBP) and diastolic blood pressure (DBP) in a dose-dependent fashion.[36,57] (Doses of 0.06 mg/kg of IV PCP increased the SBP and DBP by 8 mm Hg, whereas 0.25 mg/kg produce a 26 and 19 mm Hg increase in SBP and DBP, respectively.) PCP also increases the heart rate, although inconsistently.[84] Likewise, ketamine produces mild increases in blood pressure, heart rate, and cardiac output via this same mechanism.[49,122,179,192,201] In fact tachycardia was the most common finding on physical examination in a case series of ketamine abusers presenting to the ED.[199]

CARDIOPULMONARY

Rarely are cardiovascular catastrophes encountered in PCP toxicity.[60,131] These complications may result from direct vasospasm,[5,35] causing severe systemic hypertension[61] and cerebral hemorrhage.[22] Hypertension, along with abnormal behavior, miosis, and nystagmus in children, strongly suggest toxicity due to a dissociative anesthetic.[105]

The effect of PCP and ketamine on cardiac rhythm is controversial. Dysrhythmias are only observed in animals poisoned with very large doses of PCP. Ketamine both enhances and diminishes epinephrine-induced dysrhythmias in animals.[21,58,85,106] The considerable experience in the use of ketamine anesthesia on humans undergoing surgery or cardiac catheterization has not demonstrated prodysrhythmic effects.[65,145]

As these dissociative anesthetics were designed to retain normal ventilation, hypoventilation is uncommon. In clinical studies, PCP increased the minute ventilation, tidal volume, and respiratory rate of volunteers.[84] Clinically, in PCP-toxic patients, irregular respiratory patterns occur with tachypnea much more often than with bradypnea.[8,130] Hypoventilation, when present, is usually secondary to the use of particularly high doses of PCP. Acute lung injury secondary to respiratory depression is also a rare occurrence. Large doses of PCP (20 mg/kg) administered to laboratory animals produced respiratory depression.[36] Although respiratory depression in humans is an extremely rare event, it has been reported with fast or high-dose infusions of ketamine.[79,201] In fact, ketamine has been successfully used to prevent intubation in patients with refractory asthma. Ketamine relaxes bronchial smooth muscles, decreases mean airway pressure and $Paco_2$, and increases Pao_2.[71,162,184,201]

NEUROPSYCHIATRIC

The majority of patients with PCP and ketamine toxicity who are brought to medical attention manifest diverse psychomotor abnormalities.[12,18,28,68,100,199] As dissociative anesthetics, these xenobiotics impair response to external stimuli by separating various elements of the mind. Consciousness, memory, perception, and motor activity appear dissociated from each other. This dissociation prevents the user from attaining cognition and properly assembling all this information to construct a reality. Clinically the person may appear inebriated, either calm or agitated, and sometimes violent. In large overdoses, the anesthetic effect causes patients to develop stupor or coma. In recreational use, "dissociatives" are not taken for these effects, but rather for so-called out-of-body experiences. In addition patients often have disordered thought processes (including disorientation as to time, place, and person) or amnesia, paranoia, and dysphoria.[67]

The manifestations of PCP and ketamine toxicity are better illustrated by the results of their effects in controlled human studies. Volunteers who took oral PCP doses of up to 7.5 mg/d, or ketamine 0.1 mg/kg, exhibited inebriation, but higher doses (PCP greater than 10 mg/d; ketamine 0.5 mg/kg) generally caused a more severe impairment of mental function.[57,110] Intravenous doses of 0.1 mg/kg of PCP[16,54,120,144,165] or 0.5 mg/kg of ketamine[110,152] causes diminution in all sensory modalities (pain, touch, proprioception, hearing, taste, and visual acuity) in a dose-dependent fashion. Both drugs also cause feelings of apathy, depersonalization, hostility, isolation, and alterations in body image.[16,54,70,101,110,120,126,142,152] The deficits in sensory modalities are evident prior to the development of the psychological effects of PCP, with pain perception disappearing first. This alteration in analgesic perception is caused by a blocking action on the thalamus and midbrain (Fig. 85–1).[144]

Abnormal stereognosis and proprioception occur in a dose-dependent manner. This disturbed perception results in body image distortions described as "numbness," "sheer nothingness," and "depersonalization." The decrease of proprioceptive sensation to gravity probably gives the sensation of "tripping" or "flying." Because all sensory modalities are affected, visual, auditory, and tactile illusions and delusions are common. Hallucinations are typically auditory rather than visual, which are more common with LSD use. Ketamine's hallucinogenic effects on healthy human volunteers are linearly related to steady-state concentrations between 50 and 200 ng/mL.[23] The majority of ketamine users report experiencing a "k-hole," a slang term for the intense psychological and somatic state experienced while under the influence of ketamine. This experience varies with the individual, but can include buzzing, ringing or whistling sounds, traveling through a dark tunnel, intense visions, and out-of-body or near-death sensations.[55]

The reaction to the misperceived or disconnected reality may result in unintentional actions and violent behavior. The hallmark of PCP toxicity is the recurring delusion of superhuman strength and invulnerability resulting from both its anesthetic and dissociative properties. There are case reports of patients presenting with trauma either from

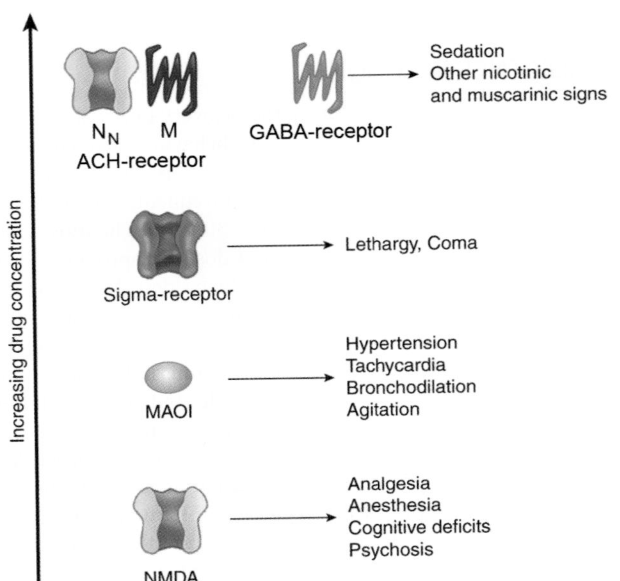

FIGURE 85–1. Clinical effects of phencyclidine and ketamine. Phencyclidine and ketamine bind to different receptors in the CNS with varying degrees of affinity; that is, an increasing concentration is necessary to achieve the various clinical effects. ACh, acetylcholine, GABA = δ amino butyric acid, N_N = nicotinic receptor, M = muscarinic receptor, NMDA = N-methyl-D-aspartate, MAOI = monoamine oxidase inhibitor.

jumping from high altitudes, fighting large crowds or the police, or self-mutilation. The true extent and incidence of violence is probably less than previously suggested.[24]

Typically, neurologic signs include horizontal, vertical, and/or rotatory nystagmus, ataxia, and altered gait. Initially, except for ataxia, motor movement is not impaired until the patient becomes unconscious. On physical examination, use of dissociative anesthetics typically produces relatively small pupils, nystagmus, and diplopia. In the largest case series reported to date, nystagmus and hypertension were noted in 57% of patients who had taken PCP.[130] Smaller and more limiting studies have found an incidence of nystagmus of 89% or higher.[18] In comparison, nystagmus was only found in 15% of patients with ketamine abuse.[199] Other cerebellar manifestations were also encountered, most notably dizziness, ataxia, dysarthria, and nausea. A pooled data compilation of 35 reports demonstrated that emesis occurred 8.5% of the time.[79] In fact, Internet chat groups devoted to substance abuse commonly direct users to "mix dissociatives with marijuana" for its antiemetic effect.

Larger doses of PCP produce loss of balance and confusion, the latter characterized by inability to repeat a set of objects, frequent loss of ideas, blocking, lack of concreteness, and disordered linguistic expression.[51,57,110,120,165] Similarly, ketamine users report a high incidence of incoordination, confusion, unusual thought content, and an inability to speak.[55] In general, dissociative anesthetics stimulate the CNS but seizures rarely occur, except at high doses. The largest case series of PCP-toxic patients detected a 3.1% incidence of seizures.[130]

Although PCP- and ketamine-toxic patients also present with motor disturbances, it is unclear to what extent PCP and ketamine are actually responsible for these manifestations. The most common of the reported disturbances are dystonic reactions: opisthotonos, torticollis, tortipelvis, and risus sardonicus (facial grimacing). Myoclonic movements, tremor, hyperactivity, athetosis, stereotypies, and catalepsy also occur.[12,29,68,130] A slight increase in muscle tone results from a dopaminergic effect.[120] Laryngospasm requiring intubation has been reported after the use of ketamine anesthesia. The incidence of this complication is less than 0.017%.[78] In comparison, the incidence of laryngospasm following traditional general anesthesia is 2%.[150]

EMERGENCE REACTION

The acute psychosis observed during the recovery phase of PCP anesthesia limits its clinical use. This bizarre behavior, characterized by confusion, vivid dreaming, and hallucinations, is termed an "emergence reaction." These reactions occur most frequently in middle-aged men, with a reported incidence of 17% to 30%.[84,104] The most violent emergence reactions follow an intravenous dose of approximately 0.25 mg/kg (total: 20 mg) of phencyclidine.[57] The mildest degrees of agitation produced by phencyclidine resemble the effects of ethanol intoxication. These same postanesthetic reactions also limit the clinical use of ketamine. The incidence of emergence reactions following ketamine administration may approximate 50% in adults and 10% in children.[78] Patients older than age 10 years, women, persons who normally dream frequently and/or have a prior personality disorder, premorbid denial of presence of illness or anosognosia, and paranoia incur the greatest risk.[78,132] The incidence of the occurrence of emergence reactions appears to be exacerbated when dissociative anesthetics are rapidly administered intravenously, and in those patients who are exposed to excessive stimuli during recovery. Although it has not been proved in a controlled study, reducing external stimuli during the recovery phase might reduce emergence reactions.

Both cholinergic and anticholinergic clinical manifestations occur in the PCP- or ketamine-toxic patient. Miosis or mydriasis, blurred vision, profuse diaphoresis, hypersalivation, bronchospasm, bronchorrhea, and urinary retention may occur.[12,18,117,129,130] Clinically, ketamine stimulates salivary and tracheobronchial secretions; both of which are equally and effectively inhibited by atropine and glycopyrolate.[139] Furthermore, in a randomized, double-blind trial, after infusion of 1.5 mg/kg of ketamine in healthy volunteers, physostigmine decreased nystagmus, blurred vision, and the time to recovery.[191]

Ironically, the very characteristics that were thought to make phencyclidine ideal for anesthesia—the preservation of muscle tone and cardiopulmonary function—magnify the difficulties in managing an individual who manifests dysphoria after an overdose. The course of delirium, stupor, and coma associated with PCP and ketamine is extremely variable, although the manifestations are much milder and shorter acting following ketamine use.

DIAGNOSTIC TESTING

If it is necessary to confirm the suspicion of PCP usage, urine is most commonly used for analysis, although serum, and possibly gastric contents, can be used. Rarely is it essential to make this determination. Most hospital laboratories do not perform quantitative analysis of PCP, but many can do a qualitative urine test for the presence of the drug. Qualitative testing is more important than a quantitative determination as serum concentrations do not correlate closely with the clinical effects. When a routine toxicologic screen is reported as negative this result should not lead to the erroneous conclusion that PCP exposure has been excluded. Routine toxicologic screening tests may not include PCP and it may be necessary to request a specific analysis if confirmation is required.

PCP is qualitatively detected by an enzyme immunoassay at a sensitivity of 10 ng/mL. High-affinity antibodies were once studied as specific PCP antagonists to reverse PCP-induced toxicity.[151,193] The detection of PCP is thus dependant on the concentration of PCP in the body fluid tested and the affinity of the antibody for the PCP molecule. As such, the immunoassay antibody binding to a molecule similar to PCP can produce false-positive reactions. Metabolites of PCP, such as PCE, PHP, TCP and its pyrrolizidine derivative TCPy, cross-react with the immunoassay at concentrations 30 times higher than those used to detect PCP. Because of its similar structure to PCP, dextromethorphan and its metabolite dextrorphan, also cross-react with Syva enzyme-multiplied immunoassay and fluorescence polarization PCP assays (Chap. 6).[92,198]

Although nonspecific, laboratory findings resulting from PCP use can include leukocytosis, hypoglycemia, and elevated concentrations of muscle enzymes, myoglobin, BUN, and creatinine.[130] The EEG reveals diffuse slowing with θ and δ waves, which may return to normal before the patient improves clinically.

There is no commercially available quantitative immunoassay for ketamine. When necessary, ketamine is detected by gas chromatography and mass spectroscopy. The increase in popularity in ketamine use in certain parts of the world has led to the development of rapid-detection urine assays that are sensitive, specific, and accurate.[37,197] There is anecdotal evidence that ketamine also cross-reacts with the urine PCP immunoassay because of their structural similarity.[168] Other authors, including the manufacturer who tests the reactivity of the commercially available PCP immunoassay with ketamine, do not find such results.[32,199]

MANAGEMENT

AGITATION

Conservative management is indicated for PCP and ketamine toxicity and includes maintaining adequate respiration, circulation, and thermoregulation. The psychobehavioral symptoms observed during acute dissociative reactions and during the emergence reaction are similar. To treat the symptoms of agitation and alteration of mental status of acutely toxic PCP patients, it is helpful to recognize that both pharmacologic[1,33,38,41,64,77,78,124,128] and behavioral[40,41,78,111] modalities have been used to diminish agitation and emergence phenomena during conscious sedation with ketamine. To prevent self-injury, a common form of PCP-induced morbidity and mortality, the patient must be safely restrained, initially physically, and then chemically. An IV line must be inserted and blood drawn for electrolytes, glucose, BUN, and creatinine concentrations. The use of 0.5 to 1.0 g/kg of body weight of dextrose and 100 mg of thiamine HCl intravenously should be considered if indicated.

Although body temperature is directly affected by PCP and ketamine, hyperthermia may occur secondary to psychomotor agitation and should be rapidly identified. Treatment should be accomplished immediately with adequate sedation to control motor activity. At presentation, placing the patient in a quiet room with low sensory stimuli will help achieve this goal. Physical restraint should only be used temporarily, if necessary, until chemical sedation is achieved. Rapid immersion in an ice water bath may be necessary because body temperatures greater than 106°F (41.1°C) place the patient at a great risk for end-organ injury. These patients will need volume repletion and electrolyte supplementation because hyperthermia increases fluid loss from sweat.

In the pharmacologic treatment of emergence reactions, benzodiazepines have been used with great success. A benzodiazepine such as diazepam, administered in titrated doses of up to 10 mg intravenously every 5 to 10 minutes until agitation is controlled, is usually safe and effective. Numerous studies demonstrate the benefits of benzodiazepines, although under certain conditions[38,78] they may prolong recovery time. Midazolam may be more effective than diazepam under certain circumstances.[33,128] Additionally, in a double-blind placebo-controlled study, lorazepam reduced the anxiety associated with ketamine without antagonizing ketamine's cognitive or psychotomimetic effects.[109] In contrast, phenothiazines may lower the seizure threshold, and both phenothiazines and butyrophenones may cause acute dystonic reactions. Phenothiazines may also cause significant hypotension due to their α-blocking effects on the vasculature, worsen hyperthermia, and exacerbate any anticholinergic effects from these drugs.

Some behavioral modalities have also been implemented in the treatment. Early studies demonstrated that the psychotomimetic effects of PCP were diminished when external stimulation was reduced by environmental sensory deprivation.[40] The practice of placing patients in a quiet room with minimal sensory stimulation is recommended by many, but has never been formally studied in a double-blind, controlled trial. Conversely, it is observed in patients undergoing ketamine anesthesia that emergence reactions are less violent when patients are talked to or when music is played.[111,174]

Although it is always important to ask the patient the names, quantities, times, and route of all xenobiotics taken, the information obtained from such a patient may be unreliable. Even when the patient is trying to cooperate and give an accurate history, many street psychoactive xenobiotics are mixtures whose contents are unknown to the patient. Consequently, pharmacologic management is complex and often sign or symptom dependent. Although some authors have attempted to define the appropriate therapy for specific PCP congeners and for ketamine-induced psychosis, no single approach has been consistently efficacious.[73,74,108,125]

DECONTAMINATION

Patients with a history of recent oral use of PCP are candidates for gastrointestinal decontamination. Although there is rarely, if ever, an indication, if coingestion is suspected, orogastric lavage may be initiated but the patient may need to be sedated. Activated charcoal, 1 g/kg, should be administered as soon as possible, and repeated every 4 hours for several doses. Activated charcoal will effectively adsorb PCP and increase its nonrenal clearance; even without prior gastric evacuation this approach is usually adequate.[158] Unless there are specific contraindications, a single dose of a cathartic, such as sorbitol, may be given.

Theoretically, xenobiotics that are weak bases, such as PCP, can be eliminated more rapidly if the urine is acidified. Although urinary acidification with ammonium chloride was previously recommended,[9] we do not recommend this approach. The risks associated with acidifying the urine—simultaneously inducing a systemic acidosis, thereby potentially increasing urinary myoglobin precipitation—outweigh any perceived benefits (Chap. 9).

As opposed to the problems in applying ion trapping to renal excretion, ion trapping results in the active mobilization of PCP into gastric secretions. Phencyclidine is in a substantially ionized (and therefore non–lipid-soluble) form in the acid of the stomach and can be absorbed only when it reaches the more alkaline intestine. As a result, gastric suction can remove a significant amount of the drug, as well as interrupt the gastroenteric circulation by which the xenobiotic is secreted into the acid environment of the stomach only to be reabsorbed again in the small intestine.[9] Continuous gastric suction, however, is unnecessary and can also be dangerous. It should be considered only in comatose patients. Continuous suction may result in trauma to the patient as well as in fluid and electrolyte loss, which can further complicate management and possibly interfere with the efficacy of activated charcoal. For these reasons the administration of multiple-dose activated charcoal rather than continuous nasogastric suction appears to be the safest and most effective way of removing ion-trapped drug from the stomach.

Most patients rapidly regain normal CNS function anywhere from 45 minutes to several hours after its use. However, those who have taken exceedingly high doses or who have an underlying psychiatric disorder may remain comatose or exhibit bizarre behavior for days, or even weeks, before returning to normal. Those who rapidly regain normal function should be monitored for several hours and then, after a psychiatric consultation, should receive drug counseling and any additional social support available. Patients whose recovery is delayed should be treated supportively and monitored carefully in an intensive care unit.

Many patients become depressed and anxious during the "post-high" period, and chronic users may manifest a variety of psychiatric disturbances.[207] These individuals typically present with repeated drug use, hospitalizations, and poor psychosocial functioning in the long term.

The major toxicity of PCP appears to be behaviorally related: self-inflicted injuries, injuries resulting from exceptional physical exertion, and injuries sustained as a result of resisting the application of physical restraints are frequent. Patients appear to be unaware of their surroundings and sometimes even oblivious to pain because of the dissociative anesthetic effects. In addition to major trauma, rhabdomyolysis and resultant myoglobinuric renal failure account in large measure for the high morbidity and mortality associated with PCP intoxication. If significant rhabdomyolysis[39,154] has occurred, myoglobinuria may be present. Early fluid therapy should be used to avoid deposition of myoglobin to the kidneys, leading to renal failure. Urinary alkalinization as part of the treatment regimen for rhabdomyolysis would potentially increase PCP reabsorption and deposition in fat stores, but this is only theoretical.

Although the clinical experience with recreational use of ketamine is limited, toxic manifestations appear to be similar, yet milder and shorter lived, when compared with PCP. In a study of 20 patients who presented with acute ketamine toxicity, all were treated conservatively and successfully with intravenous hydration, and sedation with benzodiazepines.[199]

SUMMARY

As "dissociative" anesthetics became clinically available, their abuse potential was also discovered. The popularity of PCP and ketamine results from their ability to produce an "out-of-body experience" with seemingly hallucinatory effects. The action of these drugs is largely mediated by the NMDA receptor. Their toxicity, in great part neuropsychiatric in nature, is managed by supportive care. The popularity of ketamine may be related to its lesser toxicity and milder distortion of the personality.

REFERENCES

1. Abajian JC, Page P, Morgan M. Effects of droperidol and nitrazepam on emergence reactions following ketamine anesthesia. *Anesth Analg.* 1973;52:385-389.
2. Adams JD, Baillie TA, Trevor AJ, et al. Studies on the biotransformation of ketamine—identification of metabolites produced in vitro from rat microsomal preparations. *Biomed Mass Spec.* 1981;8:527-538.
3. Ahmed SN, Petchkovsky L. Abuse of ketamine. *Br J Psychiatry.* 1980;137:303.
4. Akunne HC, Reid AA, Thurkuf A, et al. [^{3}H]1-[2-(2-thienyl) cyclohexyl]-piperidine labeled two high-affinity binding sites associated with the biogenic amine reuptake complex. *Synapse.* 1991;8:289-300.
5. Altura BT, Altura BM. Phencyclidine, lysergic acid diethylamide and mescaline: cerebral artery spasm and hallucinogenic activity. *Science.* 1981;212:1051-1052.
6. Anis NA, Berry SC, Burton NR, et al. The dissociative anaesthetics, ketamine and phencyclidine, selectively reduce excitation of central mammalian neurones by *N*-methyl-D-aspartate. *Br J Pharmacol.* 1983;79:565-575.
7. Anonymous. Phencyclidine: the new American street drug. *Br Med J.* 1980;281:1511-1512.
8. Armen R, Kanel G, Reynolds T. Phencyclidine-induced malignant hyperthermia causing submassive liver necrosis. *Am J Med.* 1984;77:167-172.
9. Aronow R, Done AK. Phencyclidine overdose: an emerging concept of management. *JACEP.* 1978;7:56-59.
10. Aronow R, Miceli JN, Done AK. Clinical observations during phencyclidine intoxication and treatment based on ion-trapping. *NIDA Res Monogr.* 1978;21:218-228.
11. Awuonda M. Swedes alarmed at ketamine misuse. *Lancet.* 1996; 348:122.
12. Bailey DN. Clinical findings and concentrations in biological fluids after non-fatal intoxication. *Am J Clin Pathol.* 1979;72:795-799.
13. Bakker CB, Amini FB. Observations on the psychotomimetic effects of Sernyl. *Compr Psychiatry.* 1961;2:269-280.
14. Ballinger JR, Chow AYK, Downie RH, et al. GLC quantitation of 1-piperidinocyclohexanecarbonitrile (PCC) in illicit phencyclidine (PCP). *J Anal Tox.* 1979;3:158-161.
15. Balster RL, Woolverton WL. Continuous access phencyclidine self-administration by rhesus monkeys leading to physical dependence. *Psychopharmacology.* 1980;70:5-10.
16. Ban TA, Lohrenz JJ, Lehmann HE. Observations on the action of Sernyl—a new psychotropic drug. *Can Psychiatr Assoc J.* 1961;6:150-156.
17. Barone FC, Price WJ, Jakobsen S, et al. Pharmacological profile of a novel neuronal calcium channel blocker includes cerebral damage and neurological deficits in rat focal ischemia. *Pharmacol Biochem Behav.* 1994;48:77-85.
18. Barton CH, Sterling ML, Vaziri ND. Phencyclidine intoxication: clinical experience with 27 cases confirmed by urine assay. *Ann Emerg Med.* 1981;10:243-246.
19. Barton CH, Sterling ML, Vaziri ND. Rhabdomyolysis and acute renal failure associated with phencyclidine intoxication. *Arch Intern Med.* 1980;140:568-569.
20. Beardsley PM, Balster RL. Behavioral dependence upon phencyclidine and ketamine in the rat. *J Pharmacol Exp Ther.* 1987;242:203-211.
21. Bednarski RM, Sams RA, Majors LJ, et al. Reduction of the ventricular arrhythmogenic dose of epinephrine by ketamine administration in halothane-anesthetized cats. *Am J Vet Res.* 1988;49:350-354.
22. Bessen HA. Intracranial hemorrhage associated with phencyclidine abuse. *JAMA.* 1982;248:585-587.
23. Bowdle TA, Radant A, Cowley DS, et al. Psychedelic effects of ketamine in healthy volunteers: relationship to steady-state plasma concentrations. *Anesthesiology.* 1998;88:82-88.
24. Brecher M, Wang BW, Wong H, Morgan JP. Phencyclidine and violence: clinical and legal issues. *J Clin Psychopharmacol.* 1988;8:397-401.
25. Brown JK, Malone HH. Street drug analysis: four years later. *Clin Toxicol Bull.* 1974;4:139-160.
26. Browne RG. Discriminative stimulus properties of PCP mimetics. In: Cloudet D, ed. *Phencyclidine: An Update.* NIDA Research Monograph 64. Rockville, MD: National Institute on Drug Abuse; 1986:134-147.
27. Budd RD. PHP, a new drug of abuse. *N Engl J Med.* 1980;303:588.
28. Burns RS, Lerner SE, eds. Phencyclidine: a symposium. *Clin Toxicol.* 1976;9:477-501.
29. Burrows FA, Seeman RG. Ketamine and myoclonic encephalopathy of infants (Kinsbourne syndrome). *Anesth Analg.* 1982;61:873-875.
30. Butelman ER. A novel NMDA antagonist, MK-801, impairs performance in a hippocampal-dependent spatial learning task. *Pharmacol Biochem Behav.* 1989;34:13-16.
31. Buterbaugh GG, Michelson HB. Anticonvulsant properties of phencyclidine and ketamine. In: Cloudet D, ed. *Phencyclidine: An Update.* NIDA Research Monograph 64. Rockville, MD: National Institute on Drug Abuse; 1986:67-79.
32. Caplan Y, Levine P. Abbott phencyclidine and barbiturates abused drug assays: evaluation and comparison of ADx, FPIA, TDx, FPIA, EMIT and GC/MS methods. *J Anal Toxicol.* 1989;13:289-292.
33. Cartwright PD, Pingel SM. Midazolam and diazepam in ketamine anesthesia. *Anesthesia.* 1984;39:439-442.
34. Celesia GG, Chen RC, Bamforth BJ. Effects of ketamine in epilepsy. *Neurology.* 1975;25:169-172.
35. Chen G, Ensor CR, Bohner B. An investigation on the sympathomimetic properties of phencyclidine by comparison with cocaine and desoxyephedrine. *J Pharmacol Exp Ther.* 1965;149:71-78.
36. Chen G, Ensor CR, Russell D, et al. The pharmacology of 1-(1-phenylcyclohexyl) piperidine-HCl. *J Pharmacol Exp Ther.* 1959;127:241-250.
37. Cheng JY, Mok VK. Rapid determination of ketamine in urine by liquid chromatography-tandem mass spectrometry for high throughput laboratory. *Forensic Sci Int.* 2004;142:9-15.
38. Chudnofsky CR, Weber JE, Stoyanoff PJ, et al. A combination of midazolam and ketamine for procedural sedation and analgesia in adult emergency department patients. *Acad Emerg Med.* 2000;7:228-235.
39. Cogen FC, Rigg G, Simmons JL, Domino EF. Phencyclidine associated acute rhabdomyolysis. *Ann Intern Med.* 1978;88:210-212.
40. Cohen BD, Luby ED, Rosenbaum G, et al. Combined Sernyl and sensory deprivation. *Comp Psychiatr.* 1960;1:345-348.
41. Cohen S. Angel dust. *JAMA.* 1977;238:515-516.
42. Cook CE, Brine DR, Jeffcoat AR, et al. Phencyclidine disposition after intravenous and oral doses. *Clin Pharmacol Ther.* 1982;31:625-634.
43. Cook CE, Brine DR, Quin GD, et al. Phencyclidine and phenylcyclohexene disposition after smoking phencyclidine. *Clin Pharmacol Ther.* 1982;31:635-641.
44. Cooper M. Special K. Rough catnip for clubgoers. *The New York Times.* January 28, 1996: sec 13, p. 4.
45. Corso TD, Sesma MA, Tenkova TI, et al. Multifocal brain damage induced by phencyclidine is augmented by pilocarpine. *Brain Res.* 1997;752:1-14.
46. Corssen G, Domino EF. Dissociative anesthesia: further pharmacologic studies and first clinical experience with the phencyclidine derivative CI-581. *Anesth Analg.* 1966;45:29-40.
47. Corssen G, Gutierez J, Reves J, et al. Ketamine in the anesthetic management of asthmatic patients. *Anesth Analg.* 1972;51:588-596.
48. Corssen G, Little SC, Tavakoli M. Ketamine and epilepsy. *Anesth Analg.* 1974;53:319-333.
49. Corssen G, Miyasaka M, Domino EF. Changing concepts in pain control during surgery: dissociative anesthesia with CI-581. A progress report. *Anesth Analg.* 1968;47:746-759.
50. Crider R. Phencyclidine: changing abuse patterns. In: Cloudet D, ed. *Phencyclidine: An Update.* NIDA Research Monograph 64. Rockville, MD: National Institute on Drug Abuse; 1986:163-173.
51. Curran HV, Monahan L. In and out of the K-hole: a comparison of the acute and residual effects of ketamine in frequent and infrequent ketamine users. *Addiction.* 2001;96:749-760.
52. Curran HV, Morgan C. Cognitive, dissociative and psychotogenic effects of ketamine in recreational users on the night of drug use and three days later. *Addiction.* 2000;95:575-590.
53. Dachs RJ, Innes GM. Intravenous ketamine sedation of pediatric patients in the emergency department. *Ann Emerg Med.* 1997;29:146-150.

54. Davies BM, Beech HR. The effect of 1-arylcyclohexylamine (Sernyl) on twelve normal volunteers. *J Ment Sci.* 1960;106:912-924.
55. Dillon P, Copeland J, Jansen K. Pattern of use and harms associated with non-medical ketamine use. *Drug Alcohol Depend.* 2003;69:23-28.
56. Domino EF, Chodoff P, Corssen G. Pharmacologic effects of CI-581, a new dissociative anesthetic in man. *Clin Pharmacol Ther.* 1965;6:279-291.
57. Domino EF. Neurobiology of phencyclidine (Sernyl), a drug with an unusual spectrum of pharmacological activity. *Int Rev Neurobiol.* 1964;6:303-347.
58. Dowdy EG, Kaya K. Studies of the mechanism of cardiovascular responses to CI-181. *Anesthesiology.* 1968;29:931.
59. Drug Enforcement Association. Unusual tablet combination (ephedrine, caffeine, ketamine, and phencyclidine). *Microgram Bulletin.* 2000;33:311.
60. Eastman JW, Cohen SN. Hypertensive crisis and death associated with phencyclidine poisoning. *JAMA.* 1975;231:1270-1271.
61. Elia N, Tramèr MR. Ketamine and postoperative pain—a quantitative systematic review of randomized trials. *Pain.* 2005;113(1-2):61-70.
62. Ellison G. Competitive and noncompetitive NMDA receptor antagonists induce similar limbic degeneration. *Neuroreport.* 1994;5:2688-2692.
63. Ellison G, Switzer RC. Dissimilar patterns of degeneration in brain following four different addictive stimulants. *Neuroreport.* 1993;5:17-20.
64. Erbguth PH, Reiman B, Klein RL. The influence of chlorpromazine, diazepam, and droperidol on emergence from ketamine. *Anesth Analg.* 1972;51:693-699.
65. Faithfull NS, Haider R. Ketamine for cardiac catheterization. *Anaesthesia.* 1971;26:318-323.
66. Fauman B, Aldinger G, Fauman M, et al. Psychiatric sequelae of phencyclidine abuse. *Clin Toxicol.* 1976;9:529-538.
67. Fauman B, Baker F, Coppleson LW. Psychosis induced by phencyclidine. *JACEP.* 1975;4:223-225.
68. Felser JM, Orban DJ. Dystonic reaction after ketamine abuse. *Ann Emerg Med.* 1892;11:673-675.
69. Ferrer-Allado T, Brechner V, Dymond A, et al. Ketamine-induced electroconvulsive phenomena in the human limbic and thalamic regions. *Anesthesiology.* 1973;38:333-344.
70. Fine J, Finestone SC. Sensory disturbances following ketamine anesthesia: recurrent hallucinations. *Anesth Analg.* 1973;52:428-430.
71. Fisher MM. Ketamine hydrochloride in severe bronchospasm. *Anesthesia.* 1977;32:771-772.
72. Ghoneim MM, Hinrichs JM, Mewaldt SP, et al. Ketamine: behavioral effects of subanaesthetics doses. *J Clin Psychopharmacol.* 1985;5:71-77.
73. Giannini AJ, Price WA, Loiselle RW, et al. Treatment of phenylcyclohexylpyrrolidine (PHP) psychosis with haloperidol. *J Toxicol Clin Toxicol.* 1985;23:185-189.
74. Giannini AJ, Underwood NA, Condon M. Acute ketamine intoxication treated by haloperidol: a preliminary study. *Am J Ther.* 2000;7:389-391.
75. Gill JR, Stajic M. Ketamine in non-hospital and hospital deaths in New York City. *J Forensic Sci.* 2000;45:655-658.
76. Golden NL, Sokol RJ, Rubin IL. Angel dust: possible effects on the fetus. *Pediatrics.* 1980;65:18-20.
77. Green SM. Ketamine sedation for pediatric therapy: part 1, a prospective series. *Ann Emerg Med.* 1990;19:1024-1032.
78. Green SM. Ketamine sedation for pediatric procedures: part 2, review and implications. *Ann Emerg Med.* 1990;19:1033-1046.
79. Green SM, Clark R, Hostetler MA, et al. Inadvertent ketamine overdose in children: clinical manifestations and outcome. *Ann Emerg Med.* 1999;34:492-497.
80. Green SM, Clem KJ, Rothrock SG. Ketamine safety profile in the developing world: survey of practitioners. *Acad Emerg Med.* 1996;3:598-604.
81. Green SM, Kuppermann N, Rothrock SG, et al. Predictors of adverse events with intramuscular ketamine sedation in children. *Ann Emerg Med.* 2000;35:35-42.
82. Green ST, Rothrock SG, Harris T, et al. Intravenous ketamine for pediatric sedation in the emergency department: safety profile with 156 cases. *Acad Emerg Med.* 1998;5:971-976.
83. Green SM, Rothrock SG, Lynch EL. Intramuscular ketamine for pediatric sedation in the emergency department: safety profile in 1,022 cases. *Ann Emerg Med.* 1998;31:688-697.
84. Greifenstein FE, DeVault M, Yoshitake J, et al. A study of a 1-aryl cyclohexylamine for anesthesia. *Anesth Analg.* 1958;37:283-294.
85. Hamilton IT, Bryson JS. The effect of ketamine on transmembrane potentials of Purkinje fibers of the pig heart. *Br J Anaesth.* 1974;46:636-642.
86. Harbourne GC, Watson FL, Healy DT, et al. The effects of subanesthetic doses of ketamine on memory, cognitive performance and subjective experience in healthy volunteers. *J Psychopharmacol.* 1996;10:134-140.
87. Harris EW, Ganong AH, Cotman CW. Long-term potentiation in the hippocampus involves activation of *N*-methyl-D-aspartate receptors. *Brain Res.* 1984;323:132-137.
88. Harris JA, Biersner RJ, Edwards D, et al. Attention, learning, and personality during ketamine emergence: a pilot study. *Anesth Analg.* 1975;54:169-172.
89. Heveran JE. Radioimmunoassay for phencyclidine. *J Forensic Sci.* 1980;25:79-87.
90. Himmelseher S, Durieux ME. Ketamine for perioperative pain management. *Anesthesiology.* 2005;102:211-220.
91. Holland JA, Nelson L, Ravikumar PR, et al. Embalming fluid-soaked marijuana. New high or new guise for PCP? *J Psychoactive Drugs.* 1998;30:215-219.
92. Hubel JA. Authorities cast a wary eye on raves. *The New York Times.* June 29, 1997: sec. 13LI, p. 15.
93. Ikonomidou C, Bosch F, Milsa M, et al. Blockade of NMDA receptors and apoptotic neurodegeneration in the developing brain. *Science.* 1999;283:70-74.
94. Ishimaru MJ, Ikonomidou C, Dikranian K, et al. Physiologic nervous system: NMDA (abstract). *Soc Neurosci.* 1997;895:23.
95. Jackson JE. Phencyclidine pharmacokinetics after a massive overdose. *Ann Intern Med.* 1989;111:613-615.
96. Jansen KL. Non-medical use of ketamine. *Br Med J.* 1993;306:601-602.
97. Javitt DC, Zukin SR. Recent advances in the phencyclidine model of schizophrenia. *Am J Psychiatry.* 1991;148:1301-1308.
98. Jentsch JD, Roth RH. The neuropsychopharmacology of phencyclidine: from NMDA receptor hypofunction to the dopamine hypothesis of schizophrenia. *Neuropsychopharmacology.* 1999;20:201-225.
99. Jentsch JD, Taylor JR, Elsworth JD, et al. Altered frontal cortical dopaminergic transmission in monkeys after subchronic phencyclidine exposure: involvement in frontostriatal cognitive deficits. *Neuroscience.* 1999;90:823-832.
100. Jentsch JD, Tran AN, Le D. Subchronic exposure to phencyclidine reduces mesofrontal dopamine utilization and impairs prefrontal cortical-dependent cognition in the rat. *Neuropharmacology.* 1997;17:92-99.
101. Johnson BD. Psychosis and ketamine. *Br Med J.* 1971;4:428.
102. Johnson KM, Snell LD, Sacaan AI, et al. Pharmacologic regulation of the NMDA receptor-ionophore complex. *NIDA Res Monogr.* 1993;133:14-40.
103. Johnston LD, O'Malley PM, Bachman JG. *National Survey Results on Drug Use From Monitoring the Future Survey, 1975-1993.* NIH publication no. 93-3597. Bethesda, MD: NIDA; 1994.
104. Johnstone M, Evans V. Sernyl (C1-395) in clinical anaesthesia. *Br J Anaesth.* 1959;31:433-439.
105. Karp HN, Kaufman ND, Anand SK. Phencyclidine poisoning in young children. *J Pediatr.* 1980;97:1006-1009.
106. Koehntop DE, Liao JC, Van Bergen FH. Effects of pharmacologic alterations of adrenergic mechanisms of cocaine, tropolone, aminophylline, and ketamine on epinephrine-induced arrhythmias during halothane-nitrous oxide anesthesia. *Anesthesiology.* 1977;46:83-93.
107. Kronenberg RH. Ketamine as an analgesic: parenteral, oral, rectal, subcutaneous, transdermal and intranasal administration. *J Pain Palliat Care Pharmacother.* 2002;16:27-35.
108. Krystal JH, D'Souza DC, Karper LP, et al. Interactive effects of subanesthetic ketamine and haloperidol in healthy humans. *Psychopharmacology.* 1999;145:193-204.
109. Krystal JH, Karper LP, Bennett A, et al. Interactive effects of subanesthetic ketamine and subhypnotic lorazepam in humans. *Psychopharmacology.* 135:213-299.
110. Krystal JH, Karper LP, Seibyl JP, et al. Subanesthetic effects of the noncompetitive NMDA antagonist, ketamine, in humans. *Arch Gen Psychiatry.* 1994;51:199-214.
111. Kumar A, Bajaj A, Sarkar P, et al. The effect of music on ketamine-induced emergence phenomena. *Anesthesia.* 1992;47:438-439.
112. Lahti AC, Holcomb HH, Gao XM, et al. NMDA-sensitive glutamate antagonism: a human model for psychosis. *Neuropsychopharmacology.* 1999;21:S158-S169.
113. Lahti AC, Koffel B, LaPorte D, et al. Subanesthetic doses of ketamine stimulate psychosis in schizophrenia. *Neuropsychopharmacology.* 1995;13:9-19.
114. Lahti AC, Weiler MA, Michaelidis T, et al. Effects of ketamine in normal and schizophrenic volunteers. *Neuropsychopharmacology.* 2001;25:455-467.

115. Lankenau SE, Clatts MC. Drug injection practices among high-risk youths: the first shot of ketamine. *J Urban Health.* 2004;81:232-248.
116. Licata M, Pierini G, Popoli G. A fatal ketamine poisoning. *J Forensic Sci.* 1994;39:1314-1320.
117. Liden CB, Lovejoy FH, Costello CE. Phencyclidine—nine cases of poisoning *JAMA.* 1975;234:513-516.
118. Lo JN, Cumming JF. Interaction between sedative premedicants and ketamine in man and isolated perfused rat livers. *Anesthesiology.* 1975;43:307-312.
119. Lu YF, Xing YZ, Pan BS, et al. Neuroprotective effects of phencyclidine in acute cerebral ischemia and reperfusion injury in rabbits. *Acta Pharmacol Sin.* 1992;13:218-222.
120. Luby EG, Cohen BD, Rosenbaum G, et al. Study of a new schizophrenomimetic drug—Sernyl. *AMA Arch Neurol Psychiatr.* 1959;129:363-369.
121. Lundberg GD, Gupta RC, Montgomery SH. Phencyclidine: patterns seen in street drug analysis. *Clin Toxicol.* 1976;9:503-511.
122. Lundy PM, Lockwood PA, Thompson G, et al. Differential effects of ketamine isomers on neuronal and extraneuronal catecholamine uptake mechanisms. *Anesthesiology.* 1986;64:359-363.
123. MacDonald JF, Barlett MC, Mody I, et al. The PCP site of the NMDA receptors complex. *Adv Exp Med Biol.* 1990;268:27-33.
124. Magbagbeola JAO, Thomas NA. Effect of thiopentone on emergence reaction to ketamine anaesthesia. *Can Anaesth Soc J.* 1974;21:321-324.
125. Malhotra AK, Adler CM, Kennison SD, et al. Clozapine blunts *N*-methyl-D-aspartate antagonist-induced psychosis: a study with ketamine. *Biol Psychiatry.* 1997;42:664-668.
126. Malhotra AK, Pinals DA, Adler CM, et al. Ketamine-induced exacerbation of psychotic symptoms and cognitive impairment in neuroleptic-free schizophrenics. *Neuropsychopharmacology.* 1997;17:141-150.
127. Maholtra AK, Pinals DA, Weingartner H, et al. NMDA receptor function and human cognition: the effects of ketamine in healthy volunteers. *Neuropsychopharmacology.* 1996;14:301-307.
128. Martinez-Aguirre E, Sansano C. Comparison of midazolam and diazepam as complement of ketamine-air anesthesia in children. *Acta Anesthesiol Belg.* 1986;37:15-22.
129. McCarron M, Schulze BW, Thompson GA, et al. Acute phencyclidine intoxication: clinical patterns, complications, and treatment. *Ann Emerg Med.* 1981;10:290-297.
130. McCarron M, Schulze BW, Thompson GA, et al. Acute phencyclidine intoxication: incidence of clinical findings in 1000 cases. *Ann Emerg Med.* 1981;10:237-242.
131. McMahon B, Ambre J, Ellis J. Hypertension during recovery from phencyclidine intoxication. *Clin Toxicol.* 1978;12:37-40.
132. Melkonian DL, Meshcheriakov AV. Possibility of predicting and preventing psychotic disorders during ketamine anesthesia. *Anesteziol Reanimatol.* 1989;3:15-18.
133. Metro News Briefs, New York. Police say web site was sham to sell drugs. *The New York Times.* February 25, 2000: sec. B, p. 6.
134. Meyer JS, Greifenstein F, Devault M. A new drug causing symptoms of sensory deprivation. Neurological, electroencephalographic and pharmacological effects of Sernyl. *J Nerv Ment Dis.* 1959;129:54-61.
135. Misra AL, Pontani RB, Bartolomeo J. Persistence of phencyclidine (PCP) and metabolites in brain and adipose tissue and implications for long-lasting behavioral effects. *Res Commun Chem Pathol Pharmacol.* 1979;24:431-445.
136. Modica P, Tempelhoff R, White P. Pro- and anticonvulsant effects of anesthetics (part II). *Anesth Analg.* 1990;70:433-444.
137. Moerschbaecher JM, Thompson DM. Differential effects of prototype opioid agonists on the acquisition of conditional discrimination in monkeys. *J Pharmacol Exp Ther.* 1983;226:738-748.
138. Moore KA, Kilbane EM, Jones R, et al. Tissue distribution of ketamine in a drug fatality. *J Forensic Sci.* 1997;2:1183-1185.
139. Moore NN, Bostwick JM. Ketamine dependence in anesthesia providers. *Psychosomatics.* 1999;40:356-359.
140. Morgan CJ, Curran HV. Acute and chronic effects of ketamine upon human memory: a review. *Psychopharmacology.* 2006;188:408-424.
141. Morgan CJ, Mofeez A, Brandner B, et al. Ketamine impairs response inhibition and is positive reinforcing in healthy volunteers: a dose–response study. *Psychopharmacology.* 2004;172:298-308.
142. Morgan CJ, Riccelli M, Maitland CH, et al. Long-term effects of ketamine: evidence for persisting impairment of source memory in recreational users. *Drug Alcohol Depend.* 2004;75:301-308.
143. Morgensen F, Muller D, Valentin N. Glycopyrrolate during ketamine/diazepam anaesthesia: a double-blind comparison with atropine. *Acta Anaesthesiol Scand.* 1986;30:332-336.
144. Morgenstern FS, Beech HR, Davies BM. An investigation of drug-induced sensory disturbances. *Psychopharmacologia.* 1962;3:193-201.
145. Morray JP, Lynn AM, Stamm SJ, et al. Hemodynamic effects of ketamine in children with congenital heart disease. *Anesth Analg.* 1984;63:895-899.
146. Newcomer JW, Farber NB, Jevtovic-Todorovic V, et al. Ketamine-induced NMDA receptor hypofunction as a model of memory impairment and psychosis. *Neuropsychopharmacology.* 1999;20:106-118.
147. Olney JW, Labruyere J, Price MT. Pathological changes induced in cerebrocortical neurons by phencyclidine and related drugs. *Science.* 1989;244:1360-1362.
148. Olney JW, Labruyere J, Wang G, et al. NMDA receptor antagonist neurotoxicity: mechanism and prevention. *Science.* 1991;254:1515-1518.
149. Olney JW, Newcomer JW, Farber NB. NMDA receptor hypofunction model of schizophrenia. *J Psychiatr Res.* 1999;33:523-533.
150. Olsson GL, Hallen B. Laryngospasm during anesthesia. A computer-aided incidence study in 136,929 patients. *Acta Anaesthesiol Scand.* 1984;28:567-575.
151. Owens SM, Mayersohn M. Phencyclidine-specific Fab fragments alter phencyclidine disposition in dogs. *Drug Metab Dispos.* 1986;14:52-58.
152. Oye I, Paulsen O, Maurset A. Effects of ketamine on sensory perception: evidence for a role of *N*-methyl-D-aspartate receptors. *J Pharmacol Exp Ther.* 1992;260:1209-1213.
153. Pal HR, Berry N, Kumar R, et al. Ketamine dependence. *Anaesth Intensive Care.* 2002;30:382-384.
154. Patel R, Connor G. A review of thirty cases of rhabdomyolysis associated acute renal failure among phencyclidine users. *J Toxicol Clin Toxicol.* 1985-1986;23:547-556.
155. Picchioni AC, Consroe PF. Activated charcoal: a phencyclidine antidote, or hog in dogs. *N Engl J Med.* 1979;300:202.
156. Pitts FN, Allen RE, Aniline O, et al. Occupational intoxication and long-term persistence of phencyclidine (PCP) in law enforcement personnel. *Clin Toxicol.* 1981;18:1015-1020.
157. Pradhan SN. Phencyclidine (PCP): some human studies. *Neurosci Biobehav Rev.* 1984;8:493-501.
158. Pristin T. New Jersey daily briefing. *The New York Times.* May 22, 1996: sec. B, p. 1.
159. Rawson RA, Tennant FS, McCann MA. Characteristics of 68 chronic phencyclidine abusers who sought treatment. *Drug Alcohol Depend.* 1981;8:223-227.
160. Rees DK, Wasem SE. The identification of ketamine hydrochloride. *Microgram Bulletin.* 2000;33:163-167.
161. Reich DL, Silvay G. Ketamine. An update on the first twenty-five years of clinical experience. *Can J Anaesth.* 1989;36:186-197.
162. Rock MJ, Reyes de la Rocha S, L'Hommedieu CS, et al. Use of ketamine in asthmatic children to treat respiratory failure refractory to conventional therapy. *Crit Care Med.* 1986;14:514-516.
163. Roelofse JA, Shipton EA, de la Harpe CJ, et al. Intranasal sufentanil/midazolam versus ketamine/midazolam for analgesia/sedation in the pediatric population prior to undergoing multiple dental extractions under general anesthesia: a prospective, double-blind, randomized comparison. *Anesth Prog.* 2004;51:114-21.
164. Rofael HZ, Turkall RM, Abdel-Raham MS. Effect of ketamine on cocaine-induced immunotoxicity. *Int J Toxicol.* 2003;22:343-358.
165. Rosenbaum G, Cohen BD, Luby ED, et al. Comparison of Sernyl with other drugs. *AMA Arch Gen Psychiatr.* 1959;1:651-657.
166. Scallet AC, Schmued LC, Slikker JR W, et al. Developmental neurotoxicity of ketamine: morphometric confirmation, exposure parameters, and multiple fluorescent labeling of apoptotic neurons. *Toxicol Sci.* 2004;81:364-370.
167. Shannon HE. Evaluation of phencyclidine analogues on the basis of discriminate stimulus properties in the rat. *J Pharmacol Exp Ther.* 1981;216:543-551.
168. Shannon M. Recent ketamine administration can produce a urine toxic screen which is falsely positive for phencyclidine. *Pediatr Emerg Care.* 1998;14:180.
169. Sharp FR, Jasper P, Hall J, et al. MK-801 and ketamine induce heat protein HSP72 in injured neurons in posterior cingulate and retrosplenial cortex. *Ann Neurol.* 1991;30:801-809.
170. Shulgin AT, Maclean DE. Illicit synthesis of phencyclidine (PCP) and several of its analogs. *Clin Toxicol.* 1976;9:553-560.
171. Siegel RK. Phencyclidine and ketamine intoxication: a study of four populations of recreational users. Phencyclidine (PCP) abuse: an appraisal. *NIDA Res Monogr.* 1978:119-147.

172. Singer W. Development and plasticity of cortical processing architecture. *Science.* 1995;270:758-764.
173. Sircar R, Li CS. PCP/NMDA receptor-channel complex and brain development. *Neurotoxicol Teratol.* 1994;16:369-373.
174. Sklar GS, Zukin SR, Reilly TA. Adverse reactions to ketamine anesthesia—abolition by a psychological technique. *Anesthesia.* 1981;36:183-187.
175. Slifer BL, Balster RL, Woolverton WL. Behavioral dependence produced by continuous phencyclidine infusion in rhesus monkeys. *J Pharmacol Exp Ther.* 1984;230:399-406.
176. Snyder SH. Phencyclidine. *Nature.* 1980;285:355-356.
177. Soine WH, Balster RL, Berglund KE, et al. Identification of a new phencyclidine analog, 1-(1-phenylcyclohexyl)-4-methylpiperidine, as a drug of abuse. *J Anal Toxicol.* 1982;6:41-43.
178. Soine WH, Vincek WC, Agee DT. Phencyclidine contaminant generates cyanide. *N Engl J Med.* 1979;301:438.
179. Stanley V, Hunt J, Willis KW, et al. Cardiovascular and respiratory function with CI-581. *Anesth Analg.* 1968;47:760-768.
180. Steinpreis RE. The behavioral and neurochemical effects of phencyclidine in humans and animals: some implications for modeling psychosis. *Behav Brain Res.* 1996;74:45-55.
181. Steward LS, Persinger MA. Ketamine prevents learning impairment when administered immediately after status epilepticus onset. *Epilepsy Behav.* 2001;2:585-591.
182. Stillman R, Petersen RC. The paradox of phencyclidine (PCP) abuse. *Ann Intern Med.* 1979;90:428-429.
183. Strauss AA, Modanlou HD, Bosu SK. Neonatal manifestations of maternal phencyclidine (PCP) abuse. *Pediatrics.* 1981;68:550-552.
184. Strube PJ, Hallam PL. Ketamine by continuous infusion in status asthmaticus. *Anesthesia.* 1986;41:1017-1019.
185. Substance Abuse and Mental Health Services Administration. National Household Survey on Drug Abuse. 1996. http:// www.samhsa.gov (accessed October 15, 2005).
186. Substance Abuse and Mental Health Service Administration, Office of Applied Studies. Emergency Department Trends From the Drug Abuse Warning Network, Final Estimates 1994-2001, DAWN Series D-21. Publication no. SMA 02-3635. Rockville, MD: DHHS; 2002.
187. Substance Abuse and Mental Health Services Administration, Office of Applied Studies. The DAWN Report, January. Trends in PCP-Related Emergency Department Visits. Rockville, MD; 2004.
188. Substance Abuse and Mental Health Services Administration, Office of Applied Studies. (February 14, 2008) The NSDUH Report. Use of Specific Hallucinogens. Rockville, MD: 2006.
189. Substance Abuse and Mental Health Services Administration, Office of Applied Studies. (March 27, 2008) The NSDUH Report. Substance Use and Dependence Following Initiation of Alcohol or Illicit Drug Use. Rockville, MD.
190. Substance Abuse and Mental Health Services Administration. Overview of Findings From the 2003 National Survey on Drug Use and Health. Office of Applied Studies, NSDUH Series H-24, Publication no. SMA 04-3963. Rockville, MD: DHHS; 2004.
191. Toro-Matos A, Rendon-Platas AM, Avila Valdez E, et al. Physostigmine antagonizes ketamine. *Anesth Analg.* 1980;59:764-767.
192. Tweed WA, Minuck M, Mymin D. Circulatory responses to ketamine anesthesia. *Anesthesiology.* 1972;37:613-619.
193. Valentine JL, Mayersohn M, Wessinger WD, et al. Antiphencyclidine monoclonal Fab fragment reverse phencyclidine-induced behavioral effects and ataxia in rats. *J Pharmacol Exp Ther.* 1996;278:709-716.
194. Vincent JP, Cavey D, Kamenka JM, et al. Interaction of phencyclidine with muscarinic and opiate receptors in the central nervous system. *Brain Res.* 1978;152:176-182.
195. Vincent JP, Kartalovski B, Geneste P, et al. Interaction of phencyclidine ("angel dust") with a specific receptor in rat brain membranes. *Proc Natl Acad Sci U S A.* 1979;76:4678-4682.
196. Vogt BA. Association and auditory cortices. In: Peters A, Jones EG, eds. *Cerebral Cortex, vol. 4.* New York: Plenum; 1985:89-149.
197. Wang KC, Shih TS, Cheng SG. Use of SPE and LC/TIS/MS/MS for rapid detection and quantitation of ketamine and its metabolite, norketamine, in urine. *Forensic Sci Int.* 2005;147:81-88.
198. Warner A. Dextromethorphan: analyte of the month. In: American Association of Clinical Chemistry. In Service Training and Continuing Education, Washington, DC. 1993;14:27-28. www. aacc.org (accessed October 15, 2005).
199. Weiner AL, Vieria L, McKay CA, et al. Ketamine abusers presenting to the emergency department. a case series. *J Emerg Med.* 2000;18:447-451.
200. Weingarten SM. Dissociation of limbic and neocortical EEG pattern in cats under ketamine anaesthesia. *J Neurosurg.* 1972;37:429-433.
201. White PF, Way WL, Trevor AJ. Ketamine—its pharmacology and therapeutic uses. *Anesthesiology.* 1982;56:119-136.
202. Wilgoren J. Police arrest 14 in drug raid at a nightclub in Manhattan. *The New York Times.* April 18, 1999: sec. 1, p. 41.
203. Willets J, Balster RL. Phencyclidine-like discriminate stimulus properties of MK-801 in rats. *Eur J Pharmacol.* 1988;146:167-169.
204. Wolfe SA, De Souza EB. Sigma and phencyclidine receptors in the brain-endocrine-immune axis. *NIDA Res Monogr.* 1993;133:95-123.
205. Wong EHF, Kemp JA. Sites for antagonism of *N*-methyl-D-aspartate receptor channel complex. *Annu Rev Pharmacol Toxicol.* 1991;31:401-425.
206. Woodworth JR, Owens SM, Mayersohn M. Phencyclidine (PCP) disposition kinetics in dogs as a function of dose and route of administration. *J Pharmacol Exp Ther.* 1985;234:654-661.
207. Wright HH, Cole EA, Batey SR, Hanna K. Phencyclidine-induced psychosis: eight-year follow-up of ten cases. *South Med J.* 1988;81:565-567.
208. Yanagihara Y, Kariya S, Ohtani M, et al. Involvement of CYP2B6 in *N*-demethylation of ketamine in human liver microsomes. *Drug Metab Dispos.* 2001;29:887-890.
209. Young JD, Crapo LM. Protracted phencyclidine coma from an intestinal deposit. *Arch Intern Med.* 1992;152:859-860.
210. Zsigmond EK, Domino EF. Ketamine. Clinical pharmacology, pharmacokinetics and current clinical uses. *Anesth Rev.* 1980;7:13-33.
211. Zukin SR, Zukin RS. Specific [^{3}H]phencyclidine binding in rat central nervous system. *Proc Natl Acad Sci U S A.* 1979;76:5372-5376.

I.

METALS

CHAPTER 86
ALUMINUM

Brenna M. Farmer

Aluminum (Al)		
Atomic number	=	113
Atomic weight	=	26.98 daltons
Normal concentrations		
Serum	≤	2 μg/L (< 0.074 μmol/L)
Whole blood concentration	<	12 μg/L (< 4.43 μmol/L)
Urine (24 hour)	=	4–12 μg/g creatinine (< 1.48–4.45 μmol/L)

Aluminum (Al) is the most abundant metal in the crust of the earth with ^{27}Al as the naturally occurring isotope. Aluminum is found in cookware, infant formula,[21] foil, vaccines as an adjuvant to boost immune response,[28] antiperspirants, antacids, and phosphate binders. It is also known to contaminate in hemodialysis (HD) fluids, intravenous (IV) fluids, total parenteral nutrition (TPN),[38] albumin,[39] and as alum solution (potassium aluminum sulfate or ammonium aluminum sulfate)—an astringent for bladder irrigation.[97] It has many industrial uses after extraction from bauxite. In the body, aluminum exists as a trivalent cation (Al^{3+}). In this chapter, aluminum metal is discussed as an occupational toxin with mainly lung manifestations. Aluminum salts, the more common form discussed for aluminum toxicity, primarily act as neurotoxins with both acute and chronic toxicity.

CHEMISTRY

Aluminum is a nonessential element and a trace metal with a single oxidation state, Al^{3+}. Aluminum is the most abundant metal in the earth's crust where it is found in many types of ores: bauxite, gibbite, boehmite, as alumina, and in gems like ruby, sapphire, and turquoise.

The aluminum industry is one of the world's largest industries. Aluminum ores are converted to alumina and then reduced to aluminum metal. The first step usually involves refining bauxite at high temperature and pressure in a caustic soda to form alumina (aluminum oxide, Al_2O_3). The second step occurs by a special method, the Hall-Heroult process, in potrooms and uses electrolytic reduction to form aluminum. Aluminum is then used alone or is processed into alloys to build a variety of products that are anticorrosive.[16]

HISTORY AND EPIDEMIOLOGY

The first case of aluminum toxicity with neurologic findings was reported in 1921. This patient had memory loss, tremor, and impaired coordination.[86] Subsequently, a case series described occupational asthma in Norwegian aluminum potroom workers ("potroom asthma"). These workers had a higher incidence of asthma than the general population.[22] In 1947, another report described German workers who developed pulmonary fibrosis after exposure to high concentrations of aluminum dust (also called "pyro powder") mixed with mineral oil–based lubricants. This pulmonary fibrosis, "aluminosis," was present in 26% of the workers.[24] Some potroom workers also developed neurologic findings described as a progressive encephalopathy and termed "potroom palsy."[45,51] Initially described in 1962, these patients had balance problems, impaired memory, an intention tremor, and decreased cognitive ability.[51,70]

In the 1970s, encephalopathy in patients with renal failure was attributed to using aluminum-salt-containing phosphate binders or, more rarely, to aluminum-contaminated dialysis fluid. This clinical syndrome known as "dialysis dementia" developed after years of HD. Manifestations included dyspraxia and multifocal seizures.[7] By 1976, elevated serum aluminum concentrations were reported in encephalopathic HD patients.[6] Both the relationship between aluminum and microcytic anemia and the connection between aluminum and osteomalacia in dialysis patients were recognized in 1978.[17,89] Treatment with the aluminum chelator deferoxamine to chelate the aluminum improved both symptoms. Since the recognition of chronic aluminum toxicity, phosphate binders rarely contain aluminum and dialysate is tested to ensure that very little aluminum is in the solution as a contaminant.

In 1982 alum (potassium aluminum sulfate or ammonium aluminum sulfate) was first used in the treatment of hemorrhagic cystitis.[64] Neurotoxicity can develop if patients absorb alum systemically, especially if renal insufficiency is present. This now appears to be the most common cause of acute aluminum toxicity.

Recently, aluminum has been linked to the spongioform leukoencephalopathy that rarely develops in heroin abusers "chasing the dragon." These patients inhale the pyrolysate of heroin heated on aluminum or tin foil. A 2007 study showed elevated urinary aluminum concentrations in patients abusing heroin in this way.[18] They then can develop bizarre behavior, and slowed speech and movements, as well as cognitive abnormalities.[44]

There is also a concern over the relationship between aluminum and Alzheimer disease. This linkage was studied because of the dialysis encephalopathy syndrome (dialysis dementia) and the association of aluminum with neuropsychiatric deficits and electroencephalographic (EEG) changes seen in welders of aluminum.[71] Although aluminum is a component of neurofibrillary tangles in senile plaques associated with AD, to date no studies have proven that aluminum is the cause of the disease.[57,66] Regardless, this association has led to several agencies in the United States and Canada to decrease the amount of aluminum contamination allowable in food and water products.[93]

ALUMINUM-CONTAINING XENOBIOTICS

ANTACIDS

Aluminum-containing products are rarely prescribed. However, patients may take antacids containing aluminum hydroxide for symptomatic control of dyspepsia and gastroesophageal reflux disease (GERD). Aluminum hydroxide is usually packaged with magnesium hydroxide to counteract the induced delay of gastric emptying and constipation caused by aluminum hydroxide. These antacids are poorly absorbed and are cleared from the stomach in about 30 minutes. The neutralizing effects of antacids last for 2 to 3 hours, especially in the presence of food.

SUCRALFATE

Sucralfate, an aluminum-containing salt with sucrose sulfate, is used for symptomatic control of ulcer disease, to accelerate healing of peptic ulcer disease, and as a protectant against stress ulcer formation. This sucrose aluminum complex is poorly absorbed from the gastrointestinal (GI) tract, and the little that is absorbed is excreted by the kidney without undergoing any metabolic changes. Although not approved by the US Food and Drug Administration (FDA) as a phosphate binder, it does have phosphate-binding properties.[14]

ALUM

Alum is usually a potassium aluminum sulfate salt [$KAl(SO_4)_2{}^*12H_2O$] or an ammonium aluminum sulfate salt [$NH_4Al(SO_4)_2{}^*12H_2O$], as a 1% solution, and is typically used as an astringent during bladder irrigation for hemorrhagic cystitis. It is rarely absorbed unless there is a defect in the bladder wall that allows for systemic absorption.

PHARMACOKINETICS AND TOXICOKINETICS

Aluminum is ubiquitous in the food we eat and water we drink.[65] The daily intake of aluminum in the United States is estimated to be 5 to 10 mg from food products alone.[93]

ABSORPTION

Gastrointestinal absorption mainly occurs in the proximal small intestine with uptake by the mucosal cells. Uptake is by both passive transport methods such as diffusion and active transport methods including active transferrin-mediated mechanisms.[25] Transferrin may also mediate methods leading to absorption into the blood.[25] Only approximately 0.3% of ingested aluminum is absorbed.[56,96] However, GI absorption increases in the presence of citrate, other small organic acids, and in uremia.[25,29,62,83] The GI absorption of aluminum is decreased in the presence of phosphorus and silicon.[29] There is negligible dermal absorption from the use of antiperspirants containing aluminum.[19] Pulmonary absorption is 1.5% to 2%, based on increased urinary aluminum excretion in workers exposed to aluminum-containing metal fumes.[58,81]

DISTRIBUTION

The initial distribution of aluminum appears to be consistent with blood volume 0.06 L/kg with equal distribution between plasma and cells in the blood.[90] Aluminum then becomes 90% bound to transferrin and approximately 10% bound to citrate.[87,92] From the blood, it distributes to many tissues including 50% to the bone, where it is concentrated at the mineralization front,[96] and approximately 1% to the brain, primarily in the gray matter.[6] The rest appears to variably distribute to the heart, liver, kidney, and other organ systems. The primary carrier in the cerebrospinal fluid (CSF) is citrate.[92] Intracellularly, aluminum appears to localize in the lysosomes of brain neurons, liver (not the Kupffer cells), spleen, kidney epithelial tubules and glomerular mesangium cells, cardiac myocytes,[5,74] and in the mitochondria of osteoblasts.[15]

METABOLISM/EXCRETION

Aluminum is not metabolized in the body, and is excreted unchanged in the urine (greater than 95% of the aluminum) with a daily urinary excretion of 4 to 12 μg.[61] Citrate in the blood may enhance the excretion of aluminum.[48] Less than 2% of aluminum is excreted by the bile.[40,68,94] Because of aluminum's primary renal excretion, patients with renal insufficiency or failure have decreased aluminum excretion. The elimination half-life for aluminum is approximately 85 days in dialysis patients.[75] Based on urinary excretion in workers (with preserved renal function) with prolonged occupational exposure, the apparent half-life is extended to years.[43] This prolonged half-life may be related to deposits of aluminum metal dust in the lungs of those workers (such as in those patients with pulmonary fibrosis from exposure to the aluminum dust). There is no normal reference point for elimination half-life.

PATHOPHYSIOLOGY

Little is known about the pathophysiology of aluminum toxicity. The information that follows is based on a summary of limited research. Some animal studies provide insight into mechanisms that may be responsible for the toxicity of aluminum, but the studies should not be considered to form a comprehensive understanding of aluminum toxicity as the basic science studies raise more questions. There remain many gaps in our knowledge of aluminum toxicity to different organ systems.

Pulmonary System In rats exposed to alumina and aluminum through intratracheal injection, fibrosis develops.[35,36] These animals develop epithelialization of alveoli with focal fibrosis occurring in the respiratory bronchioles and alveolar ducts with alveolar proteinosis.[27,67]

Central Nervous System Aluminum is associated with acute encephalopathy, dialysis dementia, seizures, and Alzheimer Disease.

The primary site of aluminum entry into the brain appears to be the cerebral microvasculature. Following IV administration in rats and rabbits, aluminum concentrations are higher in the frontal cortex than in the lateral ventricles. The cortex concentrations should result from blood supply while lateral ventricle concentration may represent blood supply or be CSF derived as the lateral ventricles are bathed in CSF.[95] The mechanisms of entry are postulated to be transferrin-mediated, endocytosis and other active processes.[2] Aluminum interacts with the acetylcholine pathways in the brain and decreases acetylcholine activity. Aluminum decreases the amount of high affinity choline uptake in the brains of rats and also decreases the activity of choline acetyltransferase in rabbit brains.[30,42] Aluminum-treated rabbits have significantly decreased acetylcholine outflow compared with controls that does not improve with potassium addition to the neurons. This finding suggests that aluminum may attenuate the response of neurons to potassium-induced depolarization.[95] Adult rabbits exposed to aluminum also have a significant reduction in conditioned responses compared with rabbits exposed in utero or in the first or second month postpartum.

Hematologic System Aluminum typically affects hematopoiesis prior to alterations on the central nervous system (CNS). A microcytic hypochromic anemia results. In rats, aluminum inhibits cell growth, while in humans hematopoietic cells are inhibited. In mice, aluminum decreases cell proliferation and hemoglobin synthesis.[3,55] It inhibits δ-aminolevulinic acid dehydrogenase in the heme synthesis pathway,[1,52] leading to the accumulation of erythrocyte protoporphyrins. Please see Fig. 24-3 for a diagram demonstrating this pathway. This effect is most noted in HD patients with aluminum overload.[9]

Musculoskeletal System Vitamin-D resistant osteomalacia and osteopathy occurs in patients with aluminum toxicity. It is characterized by hyperosteoidosis, minimal osteoblastic activity, and decreased mineralization. Calcium, magnesium, and phosphate metabolism/kinetics do not appear to be affected in these patients.[12] Aluminum concentrates in the mitochondria of the osteoblasts at the mineralization front.[15] It is theorized that aluminum competes and replaces other cations in the bone, leading to osteopathy.[26] The osteomalacia is not caused solely by chronic renal failure, but develops in the presence of aluminum exposure.[72] In rat studies exogeneous parathyroid hormone (PTH) enhanced aluminum deposition into bone, leading to osteopathy.[49,50]

MANIFESTATIONS

ACUTE TOXICITY

Regardless of etiology, patients with acute aluminum toxicity develop encephalopathy, myoclonus, and seizures. The encephalopathy manifests as disorientation, confusion, and coma. All symptoms appear to develop within days to a few weeks of receiving massive systemic aluminum exposure (usually to an aluminum salt). Serum concentrations range from barely elevated to extremely elevated. Most patients who manifest toxicity have systemically absorbed aluminum usually in the presence of renal insufficiency. In several case reports of acute aluminum toxicity, the initial exposure to aluminum is associated with alum bladder irrigations for hemorrhagic cystitis. In two patients, these symptoms developed after only weeks of exposure to aluminum containing phosphate binders in the presence of citrate,[37] and two neonates with uremia developed neurotoxicity after exposure to infant formula with high aluminum content over a 1 to 2 month period.[20] Recovery occurs in patients treated with deferoxamine and/or HD.[34,59] Patients in whom aluminum toxicity is not recognized and/or treated usually die (despite supportive care in the intensive care unit [ICU]), never recovering a normal mental status.[37,76,80]

CHRONIC TOXICITY

Two distinct types of chronic aluminum toxicity are reported: occupationally related lung problems, such as asthma and pulmonary fibrosis, and a multisystem syndrome most often noted in HD patients, which was initially described as dialysis encephalopathy syndrome or "dialysis dementia." As these names only describe one organ system involvement, they should not be used.

Pulmonary Potroom asthma consists of dyspnea, cough, wheezing, bronchitis, and chest tightness.[53] These symptoms may present after only a few months of exposure to the fumes and aluminum dust. The asthma may improve upon cessation of work in the potroom, although some workers never fully improve.[63] These symptoms may be a cause for high turnover in potroom workers and appears to have made long-term follow-up difficult.[33,85]

Pulmonary fibrosis from aluminum is very similar to the other pneumoconiosis, like silicosis, and appears to progress in a similar manner. This manifestation develops in workers exposed to aluminum metal dust. Patients experience cough, shortness of breath, dypsnea on exertion, and they eventually develop restrictive lung function.[41,54] Abnormal chest radiograph findings include decreased lung fields, distortion of pleura and diaphragms, and irregular opacities.[23,31,77,78] Recovery of lung function does not occur and several patients have died from complications of pulmonary disease such as pneumonia.

Multisystem Toxicity The other form of chronic aluminum toxicity has multisystem manifestations. It primarily affects three organ systems: hematopoietic, nervous, and musculoskeletal. In patients with renal insufficiency, the toxicity appears to occur after months to years of exposure to aluminum salt–contaminated dialysate and/or aluminum salt–containing phosphate binders such as aluminum hydroxide and sucralfate. A similar presentation has been reported in a patient using aluminum-coated cookware to boil methadone for intravenous abuse. The patient experienced 3 months of chronic aluminum toxicity (prior to presentation) after 4 years of processing his methadone this way.[21,97] Three industrial workers exposed to aluminum metal powder have also been reported to have encephalopathy. One of these workers was found to have a brain aluminum concentration 20 times normal.[45] One infant with renal insufficiency developed focal seizures, which eventually progressed to generalized seizures, hypotonia, poor head control, ataxia, and developmental delay in the presence of elevated serum aluminum concentration after 10 months of exposure to aluminum salt–containing phosphate binders.[69]

Microcytic hypochromic anemia is unresponsive to iron replacement therapy.[32] This clinical finding usually precedes encephalopathy and osteomalacia.[79] The encephalopathy of chronic aluminum toxicity was known as "dialysis dementia." Its features include speech disturbances, EEG abnormalities, myoclonic jerks, and dementia.[84] The characteristic speech disturbances include dyspraxia, dysphasia, stuttering, and possibly mutism.[46,73,84] EEG abnormalities include slowing of the normal rhythm and high voltage biphasic or triphasic spikes.[47,84] The myoclonic activity can include uncontrolled twitching movements, myoclonus, or seizures.[84] The osteopathy and osteomalacia can lead to bone pain and fractures.[13,93] Death is common in these patients when aluminum toxicity is not recognized and treated.

DIAGNOSTIC TESTS

Blood glucose status should also be tested in any patient with an altered mental status being evaluated for aluminum toxicity to ensure that hypo- or hyperglycemia is not a cause of this clinical manifestation.

Serum and urine concentrations of aluminum can estimate exposure. A serum aluminum concentration should be less than or equal to 2 µg/L[88] while a whole blood aluminum concentration should be less than 12 µg/L.[82] Daily urinary excretion of 4 to 12 µg aluminum is considered normal.[61] Toxicity has occurred in a wide range of serum and urine concentrations with patients dying who had severe manifestations and concentrations only slightly above normal.

Pulmonary function testing can be performed to evaluate for restrictive lung function, as occurs with aluminosis.

MANAGEMENT

Patients should be removed from their exposure once it has been identified. Exposure to aluminum in industry and exposure to antacids containing aluminum salts should also be limited. Patients with occupational asthma from aluminum exposure should be symptomatically treated with bronchodilators and steroids.

The only chelator with proven benefit is deferoxamine (DFO). Chelation therapy is recommended for both acute and chronic toxicity from aluminum salts. Chelation appears to limit and improve manifestations of neurotoxicity, anemia, and osteomalacia (see Antidotes in Depth A7–Deferoxamine). Other chelators such as *d*-penicillamine and 2,3-dimercapto-1-propanol have been tried in chronic HD patients without any improvement in their manifestations or aluminum concentrations.[11] A review of numerous chelator studies revealed that no other chelator has been found as an alternative to deferoxamine.[91]

ACUTE TOXICITY

A deferoxamine dose of 15 mg/kg/d intravenously is recommended. Adults have received doses ranging from 1 to 2 g for aluminum toxicity. Deferoxamine chelates the aluminum to form aluminoxamine, which is excreted in the urine or removed by HD.[92] Chelation mobilizes aluminum from its storage sites in blood and increases its renal elimination.

In patients with renal failure, chelation therapy is usually followed 6 to 8 hours later by HD with a high-flux membrane in order to clear the aluminoxamine (the aluminum-DFO product) in patients with renal insufficiency or failure.[59] Patients with normal kidney function may not require hemodialysis, as the aluminoxamine is excreted in the urine.

CHRONIC TOXICITY

Chelation therapy with DFO reverses dialysis dementia, osteomalacia, and anemia. Numerous case reports have demonstrated the reversal of the neurotoxicity, vitamin D–resistant bone disease, and iron-resistant anemia.[4,8,10] The National Kidney Foundation has issued complicated guidelines for the treatment of dialysis dementia. It consists of 4 months of once weekly DFO 5 mg/kg over 1 hour given 5 hours before a regularly scheduled HD session in patients with aluminum greater than 300 μg/L. In patients with aluminum concentrations between 50 and 300 μg/L, DFO 5 mg/kg is given the last hour of HD, once a week for 2 months. Serum aluminum concentrations are then monitored and this therapy is repeated as needed.[60]

SUMMARY

Both acute and chronic toxicity are associated with exposure to aluminum and aluminum salts. Aluminum metal causes pulmonary toxicity. Acutely, aluminum salts are neurotoxins with manifestations of encephalopathy and seizures. Chronically, aluminum salts affects at least three systems with manifestations of anemia, encephalopathy, dementia, and osteomalacia. Limiting or ending exposure, chelation, and HD have proven beneficial in the treatment of aluminum toxicity.

REFERENCES

1. Abdulla M, Svensson S, Haeger-Aronsen B. Antagonistic effects of zinc and aluminum on lead inhibition of delta-aminolevulinic acid dehydratase. *Arch Environ Health.* 1979;34:464-469.
2. Abreo K, Glass J. Cellular, biochemical, and molecular mechanisms of aluminium toxicity. *Nephrol Dial Transplant Suppl.* 1993;1:5-11.
3. Abreo K, Glass J, Sella M. Aluminum inhibits hemoglobin synthesis but enhances iron uptake in Friend erythroleukemia cells. *Kidney Int.* 1990;37:677-681.
4. Ackrill P, Ralston AJ, Day JP, et al. Successful removal of aluminum from patients with dialysis encephalopathy. *Lancet.* 1980;2:692-693.
5. Alfrey AC, Hegg A, Craswell P. Metabolism and toxicity of aluminum in renal failure. *Amer J Clin Nutr.* 1980;33:1509-1516.
6. Alfrey AC, LeGendre GR, Kaehny WD. The dialysis encephalopathy syndrome, possible aluminum intoxication. *N Engl J Med.* 1976;294:184-188.
7. Alfrey AC, Misholl JM, Burks J, et al. Syndrome of dyspraxia and multifocal seizures associated with chronic hemodialysis. *Trans Am Soc Artif Intern Organs.* 1972;18:257-261.
8. Arze RS, Parkinson IS, Cartlidge NEF, et al. Reversal of aluminum dialysis encephalopathy after deferrioxamine treatment. *Lancet.* 1981;ii:1116.
9. Bia MJ, Cooper K, Schnall S, et al. Aluminum induced anemia: pathogenesis and treatment in patients on chronic hemodialysis. *Kidney Int.* 1989;36(5):852-858.
10. Brown DJ, Ham KN, Dawborn JK, et al. Treatment of dialysis osteomalacia with desferrioxamine. *Lancet.* 1982;ii:343-345.
11. Burks JS, Alfrey AC, Huddlestone J, et al. A fatal encephalopathy in chronic hemodialysis patients. *Lancet.* 1976;I:764-768.
12. Burnatowska-Hledin MA, Kaiser L, Mayor GH. Aluminum, parathyroid hormone, and osteomalacia. *Spec Top Endocrinol Metab.* 1983;5:201-26.
13. Cannata-Andia JB, Fernadez-Martin JL. The clinical impact of aluminum overload in renal failure. *Nephrol Dial Transplant.* 2002;17(Suppl 2);9-12.
14. Carafate® Prescribing Information [package insert]. Axcan Scandipharm Inc; 2005.
15. Clarkson EM, Luck VA, Hynson WV, et al. The effect of aluminium hydroxide on calcium, phosphorus and aluminium balances, the serum parathyroid hormone concentration and the aluminium content of bone in patients with chronic renal failure. *Clin Sci.* 1972;43:519-31.
16. Dinman BD. Aluminum, alloys, and compounds. In: *Encyclopedia of Occupational Health and Safety, Vol. 1.* 1983;131-135.
17. Elliott HL, Dryburgh F, Fell GS, et al. Aluminum toxicity during regular dialysis. *BMJ.* 1978;1:1101-1103.
18. Exley C, Ahmed U, Polwart A, et al. Elevated urinary aluminum in current and past users of illicit heroin. *Addict Biol.* 2007;12:197-199.
19. Flarend R, Bin T, Elmore D, et al. A preliminary study of dermal absorption of aluminum from antiperspirants using aluminum-26. *Fd Chem Toxicol.* 2001;39:163-168.
20. Freundlich M, Zilleruelo G, Abitbol C, et al. Infant formula as a cause of aluminum toxicity in neonatal uraemia. *Lancet.* 1985;8454:527-529.
21. Friesen MS, Purssell RA, and Gair RD. Aluminum toxicity following IV use of oral methadone solution. *Clin Toxicol.* 2006;44:307-314.
22. Frostad EW. Fluoride intoxication in Norwegian aluminum plant workers. *Tidsskr Nor Laegeforen.* 1936;56:179-182.
23. Gaffuri E, Donna A, Pietra R. Pulmonary changes and aluminum levels following inhalation of alumina dust: a study on four exposed workers. *Med Lav.* 1985;76:246-250.
24. Goralewski G. Die aluminumlunge: ein neue gewerbeerkrankung. *Z Gestamte Inn Med.* 1947;2:665-673.
25. Greger JL, Sutherland JE. Aluminum exposure and metabolism. *Crit Rev Clin Lab Sci.* 1997;34:439-474.
26. Griswold WR, Reznik V, Mendoza SA, et al. Accumulation of aluminum in a nondialyzed uremic child receiving aluminum hydroxide. *Pediatrics.* 1983;71:56-58.
27. Gross P, Harley RA Jr, DeTreville RTP. Pulmonary reaction to metallic aluminum powders. *Arch Environ Health.* 1973;26:227-234.
28. Gupta RK, Relyveld EH. Adverse reactions after injection of adsorbed diphtheria-pertussis-tetanus (DPT) vaccine are not due only to pertussis organisms or pertussis components in the vaccine. *Vaccine.* 1991;9:699-702.
29. Health Canada, Environmental Health Directorate, Guidelines for Canadian Drinking Water Quality. Supporting Documentation. Part II. Aluminum. 1998:22.
30. Hofstetter JR, Vincent I, Bugiani O, et al. Aluminum induced decreases in choline acetyltransferase, tyrosine hydroxylase, and glutamate decarboxylase in selected regions of rabbit brain. *Neurochem Pathol.* 1987;6:177-193.
31. Jederlinic PJ, Abraham JL, Churg A, et al. Aluminum oxide workers: investigation of nine workers with pathology and microanalysis in three cases. *Am Rev Respir Dis.* 1990;142:1179-1184.
32. Jeffery EH, Abreo K, Burgess E, et al. Systemic aluminum toxicity: effects on bone, hematopoietic tissue, and kidney. *J Toxicol Environ Health.* 1996;48:649-665.
33. Kaltreider NL, Elder MJ, Cralley LV, et al. Health survey of aluminum workers with special reference to fluoride exposure. *J Occup Med.* 1972;14:531-541.
34. Kanwar VS, Jenkins III JJ, Mandrell BN, et al. Aluminum toxicity following intravesical alum irrigation for hemorrhagic cystitis. *Med Pediatr Oncol.* 1996;27:64-67.
35. King EJ, Harrison CV, Mohanty GP, Nagelschmidt G. The effect of various forms of alumina on the lungs of rats. *J Pathol Bracteriol.* 1955;69:81-93.
36. King EJ, Harrison CV, Mohanty GP, Yoganathan M. The effect of aluminum and of aluminum containing 5 percent of quartz in the lungs of rats. *J Pathol Bacteriol.* 1958;75:429-434.
37. Kirschbaum BB and Schoolwerth AC. Acute aluminum toxicity associated with oral citrate and aluminum-containing antacids. *J Med Sci.* 1989;297:9-11.
38. Klein GL, Alfrey AC, Miller NL, et al. Aluminum loading during total parenteral nutrition. *Am J Clin Nutr.* 1982;35:1425-1429.
39. Klein GL, Herndon DN, Rutan TC, et al. Elevated serum aluminum levels in severely burned patients who are receiving large quantities of albumin. *J Burn Care Rehabil.* 1990;11:526-30.
40. Kovalchik MT, Kaehny WD, Hegg AP, et al. Aluminum kinetics during hemodialysis. *J Lab Clin Med.* 1978;92:712-720.

41. Kraus T, Schaller KH, Angerer J, et al. Aluminum dust-induced lung disease in the pyro-powder-producing industry: detection by high-resolution computed tomography. *Int Arch Occup Environ Health.* 2000;73:61-64.
42. Lai JCK, Guest JF, Leung TKC, et al. The effects of cadmium, manganese, and aluminum on sodium-potassium activated and magnesium-activated adenosine triphosphatase activity and choline uptake in rat brain synaptosomes. *Biochem Pharmacol.* 1980;29:141-146.
43. Ljunggren KG, Lidums V, Sjogren B. Blood and urine concentrations of aluminum among workers exposed to aluminum flake powders. *Brit J Ind Med.* 1991;48:106-109.
44. Long H, Deore K, Hoffman RS, et al. A fatal case of spongioform leukoencephalopathy linked to chasing the dragon. *J Toxicol Clin Toxicol.* 2003;41:887-891.
45. Longstreth WT Jr, Rosenstock L, Heyer NJ. Potroom palsy? Neurologic disorder in three aluminum smelter workers. *Arch Intern Med.* 1985;145:1972-1975.
46. Madison DP, Baehr ET, Bazell M, et al. Communicative and cognitive deterioration in dialysis dementia: two case studies. *J Speech Hear Disord.* 1977;42:238-246.
47. Mahurkar SD, Meyers L, Cohen J, et al. Electroencephalographic and radionuclide studies in dialysis dementia. *Kidney Int.* 1978;13:306-315.
48. Maitani T, Kubota H, Hori N, et al. Distribution and urinary excretion of aluminum injected with several organic acids into mice: relationship with chemical state in serum studied by HPLC-ICP method. *J Appl Toxicol.* 1994;14:257-261.
49. Mayor GH, Sprague SM, Hourani MR, et al. Parathyroid hormone-mediated aluminum deposition and egress in the rat. *Kidney Int.* 1980;17;910-904.
50. McDermott JR, Smith AI, Iqbal K, et al. Aluminium and Alzheimer's disease. *Lancet.* 1977;2(8040):710-711.
51. McLaughlin AIB, Kazantzis G, King E, et al. Pulmonary fibrosis and encephalopathy associated with the inhalation of aluminum dust. *Br J Ind Med.* 1962;19:253-263.
52. Meredith PA, Elliott HL, Campbell BC, et al. Changes in serum aluminium, blood zinc, blood lead, and erythrocyte S-aminolaevulinic acid dehydratase activity during hemodialysis. *Toxicol Lett.* 1979;4:419.
53. Midttun O. Bronchial asthma in the aluminum industry. *Acta Allergol.* 1960;15:208-221.
54. Mitchell J, Manning GB, Molyneux M, et al. Pulmonary fibrosis in workers exposed to finely powdered aluminum. *Brit J Industr Med.* 1961;18:10-20.
55. Mladenovic J. Aluminum inhibits erythropoiesis in vitro. *J Clin Invest.* 1988;81(6):1661-1665.
56. Moore PB, Day JP, Taylor GA, et al. Absorption of aluminum-26 in Alzheimer's disease, measured using accelerator mass spectrometry. *Dement Geriatr Cogn Disord.* 2000;11:66-69.
57. Murray JC, Tanner CM, Sprague SM. Aluminum neurotoxicity: a re-evaluation. *Clin Neuropharmacol.* 1991;14:179-185.
58. Mussi I, Calzaferrri G, Buratti M, et al. Behavior of plasma aluminum levels in occupationally exposed subjects. *Int Arch Environ Health.* 1984;54:155-61.
59. Nakamura H, Mahieu P, Gersdorff M, et al. Encephalopathy with seizures after use of aluminum-containing bone cement. *Lancet.* 1994;344:1647.
60. National Kidney Foundation. K/DOQI clinical practice guidelines for bone metabolism and disease in chronic kidney disease. *Am J Kidney Dis.* 2003;42:S1-202.
61. Nieboer E, Gibson BL, Oxman AD, et al. Health effects of aluminum: a critical review with emphasis on aluminum in drinking water. *Environ Rev.* 1995;3:29-81.
62. Nolan Cr, DeGoes JJ, Alfrey AC. Aluminum and lead absorption from dietary sources in women ingesting calcium citrate. *South Med J.* 1994;87:894-898.
63. O'Connell TV, Welford B, Coleman ED. Potroom asthma: New Zealand experience and follow-up. *Am J Ind Med.* 1989;15:43-49.
64. Ostroff EB, Chenault OW. Alum irrigation for the control of massive bladder hemorrhage. *J Urol.* 1982;128:929-930.
65. Pennington JAT, Schoen SA. Estimates of dietary exposure to aluminum. *Fd Addit Contam.* 1995;12:119-128.
66. Perl DP, Brody AR. Alzheimer's disease: X-ray spectrometric evidence of aluminum accumulation in neurofibrillary tangle-bearing neurons. *Science.* 1980;208:297-299.
67. Pigott GH, Gaskell BA, Ishmael J. Effects of long-term inhalation of alumina fibres in rats. *Br J Exp Pathol.* 1981;62:323-331
68. Priest ND, Newton D, Day JP, et al. Human metabolism of aluminum-26 and gallium-67 injected as citrates. *Hum Exp Toxicol.* 1995;14:287-293.
69. Randall ME. Aluminum toxicity in an infant not on dialysis. *Lancet.* 1983;8337:1327-1328.
70. Rifat SL, Eastwood MR, McLachlan DRC, et al. Effect of exposure of miners to aluminum powder. *Lancet.* 1990;2:1162-1165.
71. Riihimaki V, Valkonen S, Engstrom B, et al. Behavior of aluminum in aluminum welders and manufacturers of aluminum sulfate-impact on biological monitoring. *Scand J Work Environ Health.* 2008;34:451-462.
72. Robertson JA, Felsenfeld AJ, Haygood CC, et al. Animal model of aluminum-induced osteomalacia: role of chronic renal failure. *Kidney Int.* 1983;23:327-335.
73. Rosenbek JC, McNeil MR, Lemme ML, et al. Speech and language findings in a chronic hemodialysis patient: a case report. *J Speech Hearing Dis.* 1975;40:245-252.
74. Roth A, Nogues C, Galle P, et al. Multiorgan aluminium deposits in a chronic haemodialysis patient. *Virchows Arch [Pathol Anat].* 1984;405:131-140.
75. Schulz W, Deuber HJ, Popperl G, et al. On the differential diagnosis and therapy of dialysis osteomalacia under special consideration to a therapy with oral phosphate binders. *Trace Elem Med.* 1984;1:120-127.
76. Seear MD, Dimmick JE, and Rogers PC. Acute aluminum toxicity after continuous intravesical alum irrigation for hemorrhagic cystitis. *Urology.* 1990;36;353-354.
77. Shaver C. Pulmonary changes encountered in employees engaged in the manufacture of alumina abrasives. *Occup Med.* 1948;5:718-128.
78. Shaver CG, Riddell AR. Lung changes associated with the manufacture of alumina abrasives. *J Ind Hyg Toxicol.* 1947;29:145-147.
79. Short AI, Winney RJ, Robson JS. Reversible microcytic hypochromic anaemia in dialysis patients due to aluminum intoxication. *Proc Eur Dial Transplant Assoc.* 1980;17:226-233.
80. Shoskes DA, Radzinski CA, Struthers NW, et al. Aluminum toxicity and death following intravesical alum irrigation in a patient with renal impairment. *J Urol.* 1992;147:697-699.
81. Sjorgren B, Lidums V, Haskansson M, et al. Exposure and urinary excretion of aluminum during welding. *Scand J Work Environ Health.* 1985;11:39-43.
82. Sjorgren B, Lundberg I, Lidums V. Aluminum in blood and urine of industrially exposed workers. *Br J Ind Med.* 1983;40:301-304.
83. Slanina P, Fech W, Esktrum LG, et al. Dietary citrate acid enhances absorption of aluminum in antacids. *Clin Chem.* 1986;32:539-541.
84. Smith EC, Mahurkar SD, Mamdani BH, et al. Diagnosing dialysis dementia. *Dial Transplant.* 1978;7:1264-1274.
85. Smith MM. The respiratory condition of potroom workers: the Australian experience. In: Hughes JP, ed. *Health Protection in Primary Aluminum Production.* London: International Primary Aluminum Institute; 1977:79-86.
86. Spofforth J. Case of aluminum poisoning. *Lancet.* 1921;1:1301.
87. Van Landeghem GF, De Broe MD, D'Haese PC. Al and Si: their speciation, distribution, and toxicity. *Clin Biochem.* 1998;31:385-397.
88. Wang ST, Pizzolato S, Demshar B et al. Aluminum levels in normal human serum and urine as determined by Zeeman atomic absorption spectrometry. *J Anal Toxicol.* 1991;15:66-70.
89. Ward MK, Feest TG, Ellis HA, et al. Osteomalacic dialysis osteodystrophy: evidence for a water-borne etiological agent, probably aluminum. *Lancet.* 1978;1:841-845.
90. Wilhelm M, Jager DE, Ohnesorge FK. Aluminum toxicokinetics. *Pharmacol Toxicol.* 1990;66:4-9.
91. Yokel RA. Aluminum chelation: chemistry, clinical, and experimental studies and the search for alternatives to desferrioxamine. *J Toxicol Environ Health.* 1994;41:131-174.
92. Yokel RA. Brain uptake, retention, and efflux of aluminum and manganese. *Environ Health Perspect.* 2002;110(Suppl 5):699-704.
93. Yokel RA. The toxicology of aluminum in the brain: a review. *Neurotoxicology.* 2000;21:813-828.
94. Yokel RA, Ackrill P, Burgess E, et al. Prevention and treatment of aluminum toxicity including chelation therapy: status and research needs. *J Toxicol Environ Health.* 1996;48:667-683.
95. Yokel RA, Allen DD, and Meyer JJ. Studies of aluminum neurobehavioral toxicity in the intact mammal. *Cell Mol Neurobiol.* 1994;14:791-808.
96. Yokel RA, McNamara PJ. Aluminum toxicokinetics: an updated minireview. *Pharmacol Toxicol.* 2001;88:159-167.
97. Yong RL, Holmes DT, Sreenivasan GM. Aluminum toxicity due to intravenous injection of boiled methadone. *N Engl J Med.* 2006;354:1210-1211.

CHAPTER 87
ANTIMONY

Asim F. Tarabar

Antimony (Sb)

Atomic number	=	51
Atomic weight	=	121.75 daltons
Normal concentrations:		
Serum	=	0.8–3 μg/L (6.6–24.6 nmol/L)
Urine (24 hour)	=	0.5–6.2 μg/L (4.1–50.1 nmol/L)
	<	3.5 μg/g creatinine (<28.7 nmol/g creatinine)

Antimony (Sb) and its compounds are among the oldest known remedies in the practice of medicine.[82,126] Because of a strong chemical similarity to arsenic, the features of antimony poisoning closely resemble arsenic poisoning (see Chap. 88), and antimony poisoning has many features in common with other metal poisonings. Although relatively uncommon, antimony poisoning still occurs, usually as a complication of the treatment of visceral leishmanias.[75] Acute overdose represents an even more rare but potentially lethal event.[112]

HISTORY AND EPIDEMIOLOGY

Objects discovered during exploration of ancient Mesopotamian life (third and fourth millennium BC) suggested that both the Sumerians and the Chaldeans were able to produce pure antimony.[82,126] The reference to eye paint in the Old Testament suggested the use of antimony.[82] For several thousand years, Asian and Middle Eastern countries used antimony sulfide in the production of cosmetics, including rouge and black paint for eyebrows, also known as kohl or surma.[78,83] Because of the scarcity of antimony sulfide, lead replaced antimony as a main component in more modern cosmetic preparations.

One of the first monographs on metals, written in the 16th century, included a description of antimony.[118] The medicinal use of antimony for the treatment of syphilis, whooping cough, and gout dates to the medieval period. Paracelsus was credited with establishing antimony compounds as therapeutic agents and increasing their popularity. In spite of being aware of its toxic potential, many of the disciples of Paracelsus enthusiastically continued the use of antimony.[82] Various antimony compounds were also used as topical preparations for the treatment of herpes, leprosy, mania, and epilepsy.[126] Orally administered tartar emetic (antimony potassium tartrate) was used for treatment of fever, pneumonia, inflammatory conditions, and as a decongestant, emetic, and sedative, but it was abandoned because of its significant toxicity.[18,38,54,66] The use of antimony as a homicidal agent[113] continued well into the 20th century (Chap. 1).

The current medical use of antimony is limited to the treatments of leishmaniasis and schistosomiasis, and to sporadic use as aversive therapy for substance abuse.[112] Pentavalent compounds are used because they are better tolerated. In the endemic regions of the world, generic pentavalent antimonials remain the mainstay of therapy because of their efficacy and low cost; however, the growing incidence of resistance may reduce future use.[87]

Some contemporary homeopathic[49] and anthroposophical[107] practices still recommend use of antimonial compounds as home remedies; however, these practices are rare.[82,126] In spite of its anticancer effects in vitro,[38] there is no current oncologic use of antimony.

The elemental form of antimony has very few industrial uses because of its physical limitations, particularly the fact that it is not malleable. In contrast, its alloys with copper, lead, and tin have important applications. Various antimony compounds can be used in the production of textiles, enamels, ceramics, fireworks, and pigments, and as catalysts in chemical reactions. Industrial and occupational exposure to antimony occurs mainly by the inhalation of dust or fumes during the processing or packaging of antimony compounds.[10] Smelter workers can also be occupationally exposed to antimony as it is often present arsenic-containing ore.[48] Antimony concentrations in cigarette smoke range from 10 to 60 mg/kg,[48,90] which may be responsible for a substantial percentage of antimony found in workers' lungs.[48]

In developed countries, antimony poisoning rarely occurs following intentional ingestion of antimony preparations.[126] Most recent descriptions of antimony toxicity result from parenteral exposures during the treatment of schistosomiasis and leishmaniasis. Oral exposures usually occur following the use of antimony potassium tartrate–containing compounds. Several cases were described after the use of old porcelain house ware or after use of antimony compounds as home remedies.[2,73,86,112]

CHEMISTRY

Antimony is located in the same group on the periodic table as arsenic (As), and as such it shares many chemical, physical, and toxicologic properties. Because it can react as both a metal and a nonmetal, antimony is classified as a metalloid (Chap. 11).[10,109] Pure antimony is a lustrous, silver-white, brittle, hard metal that is easily pulverized.[85,126] However, because elemental antimony is rapidly converted to either antimony oxide or antimony trioxide, it is extremely rare to find elemental antimony in nature.[10] It has been suggested that even its name originates from *anti monon* (enmity to solitude) because antimony is almost always found with some other metal.[82] Thus, for the purposes of this chapter, the term *antimony* refers to antimony ions.

In nature, antimony can be found in more than 100 different minerals,[68,82] including stibnite, cervantite, valentine, and kermesite.[43] The sulfide ore (stibnite) is the most abundant form,[82] and Bolivia and South Africa are among the leading producers.[126] Like arsenic, antimony forms both organic and inorganic compounds with trivalent (3^+) and pentavalent (5^+) oxidation states. Common inorganic trivalent antimony compounds include antimony potassium tartrate ($C_8H_4K_2O_{12}Sb_2$), antimony trichloride ($SbCl_3$), antimony trioxide (SbO_3), antimony trisulfide (SbS_3), and stibine (SbH_3). Antimony pentasulfide (Sb_2S_5) and pentoxide (Sb_2O_5) are inorganic compounds that can act as oxidizing agents.[55] Antimony pentachloride ($SbCl_5$) is used as a chemical reagent with acidic properties. It reacts with water, forming hydrochloric acid that causes a direct corrosive effect on skin and mucous membranes.[30]

From an industrial perspective, the most important application of antimony is the use of antimony oxychloride ($Sb_6O_6Cl_4$) as a flame retardant.[82]

Tartar emetic (antimony potassium tartrate) is an odorless trivalent antimony compound with a sweet metallic taste[56] and a potent emetic effect.[55] Antimony potassium tartrate is considered to be one of the most toxic antimony compounds, with minimal lethal doses reported between 200 mg[86] and 1200 mg.[82] There are large species variations of the LD_{50} in experimental animals, with a reported range of 115 mg/kg in rabbits and rats to 600 mg/kg in mice. In comparison, because of a low water solubility, antimony trioxide is considered to be nontoxic, with an LD_{50} greater than 20,000 mg/kg.[46]

PHARMACOLOGY

The antiparasitic mechanisms action of antimony may result from the inhibition of phosphofructokinase which is the rate-limiting step in the glycolytic pathway of schistosoma.[24] Trivalent antimony compounds inhibit phosphofructokinase, leading to energy failure from impaired adenosine triphosphate (ATP) synthesis.[21,126] It is speculated that antimonial preparations exert their antiparasitic effect through selective targeting of the guanosine diphosphate-mannose pryophosphorylase (GDP-MP), which interferes with nucleoside and mannose metabolism.[44] The result is that the parasites cannot synthesize purines and cannot survive without these mannose-containing glycoconjugates. Even less is known about the effects of antimony in humans. It has been proposed that, like other metals, antimony inactivates thiol-containing proteins and enzymes by binding to sulfhydryl groups.[35]

TOXICOKINETICS

ABSORPTION

Antimony may be absorbed by inhalation, ingestion, or transcutaneously. Absorption from the gastrointestinal tract begins immediately following ingestion, and the oral bioavailability of antimony ranges from 15% to 50%.[47,119] It is suggested that antimony absorption might be a saturable process, given that several studies failed to demonstrate a dose–response relationship for absorption.[1,110] In fact, after a lethal ingestion of antimony tartrate, the total body antimony burden was only 5% of the ingested dose.[77] This poor gastrointestinal absorption in humans, in addition to the concomitant emesis, necessitates parenteral administration of many antimony-based pharmaceuticals.

Pulmonary absorption of many inorganic antimony compounds is very slow and limited by low solubility.[82] In contrast, animal data suggest that inhaled trivalent antimony is well absorbed from the lung, distributed to various organs, and subsequently excreted in the feces and urine.[37]

Transcutaneous absorption of antimony trioxide and pentoxide was documented in studies with rabbits.[89] However, dermal absorption in humans of antimony trioxide is considered negligible.[103]

DISTRIBUTION

Distribution depends on the oxidation state of antimony. In animals, more than 95% of trivalent antimony is incorporated into the red blood cells within 2 hours of exposure, whereas in a similar time frame, 90% of pentavalent antimony remains in the serum.[39]

When administered intravenously or orally, antimony is predominantly distributed among highly vascular organs, including liver, kidneys, thyroid, and adrenals.[93,126] The antimony that was detected in the liver and spleen was predominantly in the pentavalent form whereas the thyroid accumulated trivalent forms.[9] Uptake by the liver occurs through the mechanisms of diffusion and saturable binding.[106] In a hamster model, following a single injection of organic antimonials, the greatest concentration of antimony was found in the liver.[47] After inhalation, antimony accumulates predominantly in red blood cells, and to a significantly lesser extent in liver and spleen.[37,39] It is possible that inhaled antimony is retained in the lungs for a prolonged period of time without significant systemic absorption and distribution.[48] Animal data also reported accumulation of antimony in the skeletal system and in fur.[40,41]

METABOLISM

Although antimony and arsenic share many toxicokinetic properties, unlike arsenic, inorganic trivalent antimony is not methylated in vivo.[5] Some microorganisms, however, are capable of biomethylation of antimony.[13] Rather, in humans antimony is converted by binding to macromolecules, by incorporation into lipids,[12] and by covalent interactions with sulfhydryl groups and phosphates. Pentavalent antimony may be converted to trivalent compounds in the liver.[126]

EXCRETION

Trivalent antimony is excreted in the bile after conjugation with glutathione. A significant proportion of excreted antimony undergoes enterohepatic recirculation.[5] The remainder is excreted in urine. The overall elimination is very slow, with only 10% of a given dose cleared in the first 24 hours, 30% in the first week,[7] and some urinary antimony is still detected in the urine 100 days after administration.[79,126] Pentavalent antimony is much more rapidly excreted by the kidneys than trivalent antimony (50%–60% versus 10% over the first 24 hours).[126] Urine and serum antimony concentrations remain elevated for several years following therapeutic use.[81] In actuality, renal excretion of sodium stibogluconate can be as high as 90% within 6 hours of an intramuscular administration.[100] In workers, urine concentrations of pentavalent antimony correlate well with the extent of exposure.[5]

The clearance of tartar emetic has a biphasic pattern, with 90% being excreted within 24 hours after acute exposure, followed by a second slower phase with an estimated half-life of approximately 16 days.[40]

The renal elimination half-life of inhaled stibine was estimated at approximately 4 days following occupational exposure.[74]

PATHOPHYSIOLOGY

Antimony has no known biological functions and is considered to be potentially toxic even at very low concentrations.[105] Like other toxic metals, antimony binds to sulfhydryl groups to inhibit a variety of metabolic functions.[25,35] Trivalent antimony compounds are more toxic than the pentavalent compounds because of their higher affinity for erythrocytes and sulfhydryl groups.[76] Tartar emetic and other antimony salts are also considered gastrointestinal irritants. One proposed mechanism for this local effect is the activation of enterochromaffin cells, which produce and secrete serotonin. Released serotonin acts on the 5-HT_3 receptors, stimulating vagal sensory fibers and activating the vomiting center.[53,121] In addition, there is apparent direct central medullary action, particularly after administration of higher doses of antimony.[126]

CLINICAL MANIFESTATIONS

Data on human toxicity of antimony are very limited, and are largely extrapolated from occupationally exposed patients and adverse effects that have occurred during treatment of leishmaniasis and schistosomiasis, and very few case reports of intentional antimony exposures.[86]

Workers with occupational exposures usually present with subtle clinical symptoms as chronic toxicity develops slowly over time. It is important to recognize that antimony ore contains a small concentration of arsenic, making it difficult to determine whether the effects on workers are caused by contaminants such as arsenic or by the antimony. Therapeutic side effects of antiparasitic treatment may have acute and subacute clinical manifestations, as some patients with leishmaniasis require prolonged antimonial treatment to achieve cure,[116] exposing them, over time, to very large cumulative doses.

Patients with ingestions present with acute symptoms mimicking the toxicity of arsenic and other metal and metalloid salts.

LOCAL IRRITATION

The most common manifestations of antimony toxicity involve local irritation. In sufficient concentration, antimony acts as an irritant to the eyes, skin, and mucosa. Chronic exposure can cause conjunctivitis.[15,43,101] Irritation of the upper respiratory tract can lead to pharyngitis and frequent nose bleeds.[124]

Antimony pentachloride is very irritating and can cause local dermal and mucosal burns. It reacts with water, releasing hydrochloric acid, heat, and antimony pentaoxide (Sb_2O_5). Following ingestion, contact with the water in saliva produces sufficient hydrochloric acid to potentially result in consequential gastrointestinal burns.

Ocular exposure to Sb_2O_5 can cause typical caustic injury resulting in blepharospasm, lacrimation, photophobia, and even corneal burns. Exposure to antimony trichloride fumes can cause similar ocular symptoms.[50]

Systemic ocular toxicity can manifest in optic atrophy, uveitis, and retinal hemorrhage with exudates resulting with diminished visual acuity.[27,72] Some of these changes can be permanent.[72]

Thrombophlebitis is common after intravenous (IV) use of antimony, but has been reported even when poisoning occurs orally.[77]

Gastrointestinal Following acute exposures, antimony can rapidly produce anorexia, nausea, vomiting, abdominal pain, and diarrhea.[77,122] Some patients may report a metallic taste in the mouth.[5,33] It is possible to sense a garlic odor on the breath, but this might be due to concomitant arsenic exposure. In severe overdose, gastrointestinal irritation can progress to hemorrhagic gastritis.[77] Workers chronically exposed to antimony dusts have a much higher incidence of gastrointestinal ulcers in comparison to controls (63 per 1000 versus 15 per 1000).[19] Many patients develop pancreatitis following treatment with pentavalent antimonial agents.[34,45,84] Because most cases improved despite continuation of treatment, a mechanism other than direct pancreatic toxicity is presumed. In another series, several patients with human immunodeficiency virus (HIV) who were treated with high doses of meglumine antimonate developed severe pancreatitis and died.[36]

Cardiovascular In animals, antimony decreases myocardial contraction, decreases coronary vasomotor tone producing decreased systolic pressure, and causes bradycardia.[32,126] The majority of reported human cardiac effects are related to the electrocardiographic (ECG) changes. Prolongation of the QT interval, inversion or flattening of T waves, and ST segment changes are frequently described during treatment of visceral leishmaniasis with pentavalent antimonial compounds (sodium stibogluconate and meglumine antimonate).[26,125] Torsades de pointes was described in the patients treated with pentavalent antimonial preparations.[92,115] In patients with underlying myocardial disease such as a cardiomyopathy, ECG changes can occur even at subtherapeutic antimony doses.[52] These changes are not necessarily associated with deterioration in cardiac function.[59] However, it is important to recognize that pentavalent antimonial drugs used for the treatment of leishmaniasis are associated with sudden deaths, probably as a result of the development of ventricular dysrhythmias.[23,111]

Respiratory Local irritation from antimony trioxide can produce laryngitis, tracheitis, and pneumonitis.[48,101,114] Pneumonitis is usually reversible after exposure ceases and can be followed radiologically.[101] Acute lung injury was reported after acute exposure to antimony pentachloride.[30,31]

Although antimony oxides are capable of causing metal fume fever,[4,42] this is much less common in comparison to exposure to zinc oxide (see Chap. 101).[4,42] Antimony metal fume fever is reported to occur even with air concentrations below 5 mg/m^3.[29]

Workers chronically exposed to antimony compounds for many years may develop "antimony pneumoconiosis."[28,83] Patients present with cough, wheezing, and exertional dyspnea that can progress to obstructive lung disease. Radiologically, antimony pneumoconiosis appears as diffuse, dense, punctate nonconfluent opacities with a predominant distribution in middle and lower lung lobes with or without pleural adhesions.[97]

Renal Patients treated with sodium stibogluconate can develop varied manifestations of renal toxicity ranging from renal cell casts, proteinuria, and increased blood urea nitrogen concentration[27] to renal failure.[6,99] Some patients can also develop renal tubular acidosis[65] and acute tubular necrosis.[98]

Hepatic Chronic therapeutic use of antimony compounds for the treatment of leishmaniasis can cause liver toxicity that can range from reversible elevations of aminotransferase concentrations to hepatic necrosis.[61,64,104,126]

Hematologic Severe anemia was reported in HIV-positive patients during treatment with sodium stibogluconate. Bone marrow biopsy documented transient severe marrow dyserythropoiesis, followed by complete recovery on discontinuation of the therapy.[63,80]

Patients treated with sodium stibogluconate for visceral leishmaniasis occasionally develop thrombocytopenia.[16,60,70] Rare cases of epistaxis are described during the treatment, and it is unclear if they are associated with thrombocytopenia.[71] Visceral leishmaniasis itself is known to be associated with pancytopenia, probably as a result of increased destruction of peripheral blood cells.[96] It may be difficult to determine whether this phenomenon is caused by disease itself or is secondary to the treatment, although some authors suggested a drug-induced immune thrombocytopenia.[96]

Leukopenia is frequently observed in patients treated with antimonial compounds.[36,126,127] Some authors speculate that antimony-induced lymphopenia is associated with an increased frequency of herpes zoster in HIV patients.[127]

Dermatologic Antimony spots[108] are papules and pustules that develop around sweat and sebaceous glands and may resemble varicella. Chronically exposed patients can develop areas of eczema and lichenification that typically occur in the summer and are usually found on the arms, legs, and in the joint creases with sparing of the face, hands, and feet.[83,101] A similar skin rash was described in the 18th century after external application of antimony tartrate for medicinal use.[82] Interestingly, these eruptions were usually interpreted as a sign of cure.[54] It is also suggested that antimony trioxide can cause contact dermatitis.[88]

Neurologic A patient with cutaneous leishmaniasis who was treated with sodium stibogluconate (pentavalent antimony) developed a reversible, peripheral sensory neuropathy in temporal association with treatment.[20]

Musculoskeletal Therapeutic use of parenteral antimonials can be associated with diffuse muscle and joint pain.[22,33,104,126]

Reproductive In animal studies, antimony exposure causes ovarian atrophy, uterine metaplasia, and impaired conception.[11] An association between spontaneous abortion and premature births is reported in women who were occupationally exposed to antimony salts. Antimony was found in the blood, urine, placenta, amniotic fluid, and breast milk of these women.[11]

Carcinogenicity Female rats developed lung tumors after inhalational exposure to antimony trioxide and antimony trisulfide.[14,51,120] A survey among antimony smelter workers suggested an excess of lung cancer, with a latency of 20 years, in comparison to a nonexposed population. However, concomitant exposure to arsenic and its effects could not be excluded and the data were poorly or inadequately controlled for workers' smoking habits.[69] Exposure to antimony oxide over 9 to 31 years did not suggest increased incidence of lung cancer in one group of workers.[97] Patients with schistosomiasis have an increased incidence of bladder tumors, and antimony compounds are considered to be one potential cause.[126]

Genotoxicity Both stibine and trimethylstibine are capable of damaging DNA, presumably by the generation of reactive oxygen species. No other forms of antimony tested including potassium antimony tartrate, potassium hexahydroxyantimonate, and trimethylantimony dichloride were found to be genotoxic.[3]

STIBINE

Antimony compounds can react with nascent hydrogen, forming an extremely toxic gas, stibine (SbH_3), which resembles arsine (AsH_3) (Chap. 88). Stibine is probably the most toxic antimony compound. It is a colorless gas with a very unpleasant smell that rapidly decomposes at temperatures above 302°F (150°C).[58,126] Historically, stibine release was reported during charging of lead storage batteries.[126] In addition to the onset of gastrointestinal symptoms that include nausea, vomiting, and abdominal pain, stibine has strong oxidative properties that may result in massive hemolysis (Chap. 24). Similar to arsine,[102] severe stibine exposure may result in hematuria, rhabdomyolysis, and death. Maintenance workers are advised to avoid use of drain cleaners containing sodium hydroxide, which is capable of releasing hydrogen in situations where antimony may be present.[94]

DIAGNOSTIC TESTING

Standard laboratory testing to help identify volume depletion and renal injury is indicated for patients with acute antimony toxicity. A complete blood count, electrolytes, renal function studies, and a urinalysis should be obtained. When there is a known or suspected exposure to stibine, additional studies should include tests for hemolysis, such as determinations of bilirubin and haptoglobin. Blood should also be obtained for a blood type and cross-match, as transfusions are likely to be required.

An ECG should be obtained to evaluate for QT prolongation and dysrhythimas. Patients with known myocardial disease should have frequent evaluations of cardiac function,[52] and continuous ECG monitoring is recommended for all patients with significant symptoms or abnormal cardiovascular status.

Antimony concentration in a 24-hour urine collection can be used for assessment of the intensity of exposure to either trivalent or pentavalent antimony.[5] A normal urinary antimony concentration in nonexposed patients is reported in the range of 0.5 to 6.2 µg/L.[95,123] A serum antimony concentration cannot be determined in a timely fashion. The normal serum concentration of antimony is 0.8 to 3 µg/L,[81] although some laboratories use higher values.[91]

TREATMENT

DECONTAMINATION

Following a significant acute ingestion, the majority of patients develop vomiting. Induction of emesis is unlikely to offer any additional benefit. In contrast, gastric lavage may be beneficial, especially if performed before the onset of spontaneous emesis. Although it is unknown whether antimony is adsorbed to activated charcoal, based on experience with salts of arsenic, thallium, and mercury, administration of activated charcoal is appropriate. Additionally, because antimony has a documented enterohepatic circulation, multiple-dose activated charcoal may be of value.[5] For patients exposed to stibine, decontamination involves removal from the exposure followed by the administration of high-flow oxygen. Theoretically, patients with severe stibine exposures may require exchange transfusion for removal of the stibine–hemoglobin complex.[102] Dermal exposures, particularly to antimony tri- or pentachloride, may require decontamination with soap and water. Prompt removal from the contaminated area is important for patients exposed to stibine. Rescuers need to take appropriate precautions to ensure their own safety (see Chap. 130).

SUPPORTIVE CARE

The mainstay of treatment for antimony poisoning is good supportive care. Clinicians should anticipate massive volume depletion and begin rehydration with isotonic crystalloid solutions. Electrolytes and urine output should be followed closely. A central venous pressure monitor may be required in patients with cardiovascular instability. Antiemetics are indicated both for patient comfort and to facilitate the administration of activated charcoal. Following stibine exposure, the hematocrit should be followed closely and blood should be transfused based on standard criteria.

CHELATION

Human experience with regard to chelation of antimony is rather limited because of the scarcity of serious toxicity and the rarity of instances when patients have received chelation. Most of the available data are based on animal experimentation. Dimercaprol, succimer, and dimercaptopropane-sulfonic acid (DMPS) all improve survival of experimental animals.[8,17,67,117] A group from Shanghai demonstrated the ability of the sodium salt of succimer to increase the murine LD_{50} of tartar emetic 16-fold.[128] One animal study that compared survival after treatment with multiple chelators concluded that the most effective antidotes were DMPS and succimer.[8]

A single case series documented survival in three of four patients exposed to tartar emetic who were treated with intramuscular dimercaprol at a dose of 200 to 600 mg/d. All four patients had increased urinary excretion of antimony.[77] In another case report, a patient survived after chelation with dimercaprol, but without evidence of enhanced urinary excretion of antimony.[5] Although specific recommendations are difficult to make, it is reasonable to begin therapy with intramuscular dimercaprol until it is certain that antimony is removed from the gastrointestinal tract, at which time the patient can be switched to oral succimer. Because chelation doses for antimony poisoning are not established, chelators should be administered in doses and regimens that are determined to be safe and effective for other metals (see Antidotes in Depth A26: Dimercaprol [British Anti-Lewisite or BAL] and Antidotes in Depth A27: Succimer [2,3-Dimercaptosuccinic Acid]).

SUMMARY

Antimony is an element whose physical, chemical, and toxicologic properties closely resemble arsenic. Although uncommon, antimony toxicity does occur. The hallmarks of toxicity are gastrointestinal manifestations leading to profound volume depletion and renal injury. ECG findings may assist in the identification of this xenobiotic. Treatment is largely supportive, although chelation may be indicated in life-threatening cases.

REFERENCES

1. Ainsworth N. Distribution and biological effects of antimony in contaminated grassland. Dissertation, 1988.
2. Andelman SL. Antimony poisoning—Illinois. *MMWR Mortal Morbid Wkly Rep*. 1964;13:250.

3. Andrewes P, Kitchin KT, Wallace K. Plasmid DNA damage caused by stibine and trimethylstibine. *Toxicol Appl Pharmacol.* 2004;194:41-48.
4. Anonymous. Metals and the lung. *Lancet.* 1984;2:903-904.
5. Bailly R, Lauwerys R, Buchet JP, et al. Experimental and human studies on antimony metabolism: their relevance for the biological monitoring of workers exposed to inorganic antimony. *Br J Ind Med.* 1991;48:93-97.
6. Balzan M, Fenech F. Acute renal failure in visceral leishmaniasis treated with sodium stibogluconate. *Trans R Soc Trop Med Hyg.* 1992;86: 515-516.
7. Barter FC, Cowie DB, Most H, et al. The fate of radioactive tartar emetic administered to human subjects. *J Trop Med Hyg.* 1947;27:403-416.
8. Basinger MA, Jones MM. Structural requirements for chelate antidotal efficacy in acute antimony (III) intoxication. *Res Commun Chem Pathol Pharmacol.* 1981;32:355-363.
9. Beliles, RP. The lesser metals. In: Oehme, FW, ed. *Toxicity of Heavy Metals in the Environment, Part II.* New York: Marcel Dekker; 1979:547-615.
10. Beliles RP. The metals: antimony. In: Clayton GD, Clayton FE, eds. *Patty's Industrial Hygiene and Toxicology, Vol. 2.* 11th ed. New York: John Wiley & Sons, Inc; 1994:1902-1913.
11. Belyaeva AP. The effect produced by antimony on the generative function. *Gig Tr Prof Zabol.* 1967;11:32-37.
12. Benson AA, Cooney RA. Antimony metabolites in marine algae. In: Craig PJ, Glockling F, eds. *Organometallic Compounds in the Environment. Principles and Reactions.* Harlow, UK: Longmans; 1988:135-37.
13. Bentley R, Chasteen TG. Microbial methylation of metalloids: arsenic, antimony, and bismuth. *Microbiol Mol Biol Rev.* 2002;66:250-271.
14. Beyersmann D, Hartwig A. Carcinogenic metal compounds: recent insight into molecular and cellular mechanisms. *Arch Toxicol.* 2008;82:493-512.
15. Bingham E, Cohrssen B, Powell CH. *Patty's Toxicology, Vol. 2.* 5th ed. New York: John Wiley & Sons; 1994:1902-1913.
16. Braconier JH, Miorner H. Recurrent episodes of thrombocytopenia during treatment with sodium stibogluconate. *J Antimicrob Chemother.* 1993;31:187-188.
17. Braun HA, Lusky LM, Calvery HO. The efficacy of 2,3-dimercaptopropanol (BAL) in the therapy of poisoning by compounds of antimony, bismuth, chromium, mercury and nickel. *J Pharmacol Exp Ther.* 1946;87:119-125.
18. Brieger GH. Therapeutic conflicts and the American medical profession in the 1860s. *Bull Hist Med.* 1967;41:215-222.
19. Brieger H, Semisch CW, Stasney J, Piatnek DA. Industrial antimony poisoning. *Indus Med Surg.* 1954;23:521-523.
20. Brummitt CF, Porter JA, Herwaldt BL. Reversible peripheral neuropathy associated with sodium stibogluconate therapy for American cutaneous leishmaniasis. *Clin Infect Dis.* 1996;22:878-879.
21. Bueding E, Fisher J. Factors affecting the inhibition of phosphofructokinase activity of *Schistosoma mansoni* by trivalent organic antimonials. *Biochem Pharmacol.* 1966;15:1197-1211.
22. Castro C, Sampaio RN, Marsden PD. Severe arthralgia, not related to dose, associated with pentavalent antimonial therapy for mucosal leishmaniasis. *Trans R Soc Trop Med Hyg.* 1990;84:362.
23. Cesur S, Bahar K, Erekul S. Death from cumulative sodium stibogluconate toxicity on Kala-Azar. *Clin Microbiol Infect.* 2002;8:606.
24. Chai Y, Yan S, Wong IL, Chow LM, Sun H. Complexation of antimony (Sb(V)) with guanosine 5′-monophosphate and guanosine 5′-diphospho-D-mannose: formation of both mono- and bis-adducts. *J Inorg Biochem.* 2005;99:2257-2263.
25. Chen G, Geiling EMK, Macuatton RM. Trypanocidal activity and toxicity of antimonials. *J Infect Dis.* 1945;76:144-151.
26. Chulay JD, Spencer HC, Mugambi M. Electrocardiographic changes during treatment of leishmaniasis with pentavalent antimony (sodium stibogluconate). *Am J Trop Med Hyg.* 1985;34:702-709.
27. Chunge CN, Gachihi G, Chulay JD, Spencer HC. Complications of kala azar and its treatment in Kenya. *East Afr Med J.* 1984;61:120-127.
28. Cooper DA, Pendergrass EP, Vorwald AJ, et al. Pneumoconiosis among workers in an antimony industry. *Am J Roentgenol Radium Ther Nucl Med.* 1968;103:495-508.
29. Cooper Hand Tools/Cheraw Plant. MSDS for lead-free solder. Revision date. August 4, 1999. http://www.cooperhandtools.com/MSDS/weller/LeadFreeSolderMSDSEnglish.pdf (accessed March 17, 2009).
30. Cordasco EM. Newer concepts in the management of environmental pulmonary edema. *Angiology.* 1974;25:590-601.
31. Cordasco EM, Stone FD. Pulmonary edema of environmental origin. *Chest.* 1973;64:182-185.
32. Cotton MD, Logan ME. Effects on antimony on the cardiovascular system and intestinal smooth muscle. *J Pharmacol Exp Ther.* 1966;151:7-22.
33. Davis A. Comparative trials of antimonial drugs in urinary schistosomiasis. *Bull World Health Organ.* 1968;38:197-227.
34. de Lalla F, Pellizzer G, Gradoni L, et al. Acute pancreatitis associated with the administration of meglumine antimonate for the treatment of visceral leishmaniasis (letter). *Clin Infect Dis.* 1993;16:730-731.
35. De Wolff FA. Antimony and health. *BMJ.* 1995;310:1216-1217.
36. Delgado J, Macias J, Pineda JA, et al. High frequency of serious side effects from meglumine antimonate given without an upper limit dose for the treatment of visceral leishmaniasis in human immunodeficiency virus type-1-infected patients. *Am J Trop Med Hyg.* 1999;61:766-769.
37. Djuric D, Thomas RG, Lie R. The distribution and excretion of trivalent antimony in the rat following inhalation. *Int Arch Gewerbepathol Gewerbehyg.* 1962;19:529-545.
38. Duffin J, Campling BG. Therapy and disease concepts: the history (and future?) of antimony in cancer. *J Hist Med Allied Sci.* 2002;57:61-78.
39. Edel J, Marafante E, Sabbioni E, et al. Metabolic behavior of inorganic forms of antimony in the rat. In: *Proceedings of Heavy Metal in the Environmental International Conference.* Heidelberg, Germany. 1983;1:1574-1577.
40. Felicetti SA, Thomas RG, McClellan RO. Metabolism of two valence states of inhaled antimony in hamsters. *Am Ind Hyg Assoc J.* 1974;355: 292-300.
41. Felicetti SW, Thomas RG, McClellan RO. Retention of inhaled antimony-124 in the beagle dog as a function of temperature of aerosol formation. *Health Phys.* 1974;26:525-531.
42. Finkel AJ. *Hamilton & Hardy's Industrial Toxicology.* Boston: John Wright PSG; 1983:13-16.
43. Friberg L, Nordberg GF, Vouk VB. *Handbook on the Toxicology of Metals.* 2nd ed. Amsterdam, NY: Elsevier; 1986:27-42.
44. Garami A, Ilg T. Disruption of mannose activation in Leishmania mexicana. GDP-mannose pyrophosphorylase is required for virulence, but not for viability. *EMBO J.* 2001;20:3657-3666.
45. Gasser RA Jr, Magill AJ, Oster CN, et al. Pancreatitis induced by pentavalent antimonial agents during treatment of leishmaniasis. *Clin Infect Dis.* 1994;18:83-90.
46. Gebel T. Arsenic and antimony: comparative approach on mechanistic toxicology. *Chemico-Biological Interactions.* 1997;107:131-144.
47. Gellhorn A, Tupikova NA, Van Dyke HB. The tissue distribution and excretion of four organic antimonials after single or repeated administration to normal hamsters. *J Pharmacol Exp Ther.* 1946;87:169-180.
48. Gerhardsson L, Brune D, Nordberg GF, Wester PO. Antimony in lung, liver and kidney tissue from deceased smelter workers. *Scand J Work Environ Health.* 1982;8:201-208.
49. Gibson S, Gibson R. *Homoeopathy for Everyone.* Harmondsworth, UK: Penguin Books; 1987.
50. Grant WM, Schuman JS. *Toxicology of the Eye.* 4th ed. Illinois: Charles C Thomas; 1993.
51. Groth DA, Stettler LE, Burg JR, et al. Carcinogenic effects of antimony trioxide and antimony ore concentrate in rats. *J Toxicol Environ Health.* 1986;18:607-626.
52. Gupta P. Electrocardiographic changes occurring after brief antimony administration in the presence of dilated cardiomyopathy. *Postgrad Med J.* 1990;66:1089.
53. Hain TC. Emesis. http://www.tchain.com/otoneurology/treatment/emesis.html (accessed May 12, 2003).
54. Haller JS. The use and abuse of tartar emetic in the 19th century materia medica. *Bull Hist Med.* 1975;49:235-257.
55. Harrison WN, Bradberry SM, Vale JA. UKPID Monograph. Antimony. IPCSINTOX databank. htpp://www/intox.org/databank/documents/pharm/anttart/ukpid37.htm (accessed on February 13, 2005).
56. Hawley GG. *The Condensed Chemical Dictionary.* 10th ed. New York: Van Nostrand Reinhold; 1981:79-82.
57. [AU: Refs. 57 and 62 are not cited.]Health and Safety Executive. Antimony—Health and Safety Precautions. Guidance Note EH 19. London: HMSO; 1978.
58. Health and Safety Executive. Stibine—Health and Safety Precautions. Guidance Note EH12. London: HMSO; 1978.
59. Henderson A, Jolliffe D. Cardiac effects of sodium stibogluconate. *Br J Clin Pharmacol.* 1985;19:73-77.
60. Hepburn NC. Thrombocytopenia complicating sodium stibogluconate therapy for cutaneous leishmaniasis. *Trans R Soc Trop Med Hyg.* 1993;87:691.

61. Hepburn NC, Nolan J, Fenn L, et al. Cardiac effects of sodium stibogluconate: myocardial, electrophysiological and biochemical studies. *QJM.* 1994;87:465-472.
62. Hepburn NC, Siddique I, Howie AF, et al. Hepatotoxicity of sodium stibogluconate in leishmaniasis. *Lancet.* 1993;342:238-239.
63. Hernandez JA, Navarro JT, Force L. Acute toxicity in erythroid bone marrow progenitors after antimonial therapy. *Haematologica.* 2001; 86:1319.
64. Herwaldt BL, Kaye ET, Lepore TJ, et al. Sodium stibogluconate (Pentostam) overdose during treatment of American cutaneous leishmaniasis. *J Infect Dis.* 1992;165:968-971.
65. Horber FF, Lerut J, Jaeger P. Renal tubular acidosis, a side effect of treatment with pentavalent antimony. *Clin Nephrol.* 1991;36:213.
66. Hoyt DM. *Practical Therapeutics.* St. Louis: AMA Mosby; 1914.
67. Hruby K, Donner A. 2,3-Dimercapto-1-propanesulphonate in heavy metal poisoning. *Med Toxicol.* 1987;2:317-323.
68. IRPTC. Antimony. In: *Scientific Reviews of Soviet Literature on Toxicity and Hazards of Chemicals.* Moscow, Russia: United Nations Environmental Program; 1984.
69. Jones RD. Survey of antimony workers. Mortality 1961-1992. *Occup Environ Med.* 1994;51:772-776.
70. Just G, Simader R, Helm EB, et al. Visceral leishmaniasis (kala-azar) in acquired immunodeficiency syndrome (AIDS). *Dtsch Med Wochenshr.* 1988;113:1920-1922.
71. Kager PA, Rees PH, Manguyu FM, et al. Clinical, haematological and parasitological response to treatment of visceral leishmaniasis in Kenya. A study of 64 patients. *Trop Geogr Med.* 1984;36:21-35.
72. Kassem A, Hussein HA, Abaza H, Sabry N. Optic atrophy following repeated courses of tartar emetic for the treatment of bilharziasis. *Bull Ophthalmol Soc Egypt.* 1976;69:459-463.
73. Kenley JB, Scheele AF, Skinner WF. Antimony poisoning—Virginia. *MMWR Mortal Morbid Wkly Rep.* 1965;14:27.
74. Kentner M, Leinemann M, Schaller KH, et al. External and internal antimony exposure in starter battery production. *Int Arch Occup Environ Health.* 1995;67:119-123.
75. Khalil EA, Ahmed AE, Musa AM, Hussein MH. Antimony-induced cerebellar ataxia. *Saudi Med J.* 2006;27:90-92.
76. Krachler M, Emons H. Speciations of antimony for the 21st century: promises and pitfalls. *Trends Anal Chem.* 2001;20:79-89.
77. Lauwers LF, Roelants A, Rosseel PM, et al. Oral antimony intoxications in man. *Crit Care Med.* 1990;18:324-326.
78. Leicester HM. *Discovery of the Elements.* Easton, PA: Mary Elvira Weeks; 1968:95-103.
79. Lippincott SW, Ellerbrook LD, Rhees M, Mason P. A study of the distribution and fate of antimony when used as tartar emetic and fouadin in the treatment of American soldiers with schistosomiasis japonica. *J Clin Invest.* 1947;26:370-378.
80. Mallick BK. Hypoplasia of bone marrow secondary to sodium antimony gluconate. *J Assoc Physicians India.* 1990;38:310-311.
81. Mansour MM, Rassoul AAA, Schulert RA. Anti-bilharzial antimony drugs. *Nature.* 1967;214:819-820.
82. McCallum RI. *Antimony in Medical History.* Edinburgh, Scotland: Pentland Press; 1999.
83. McCallum RI. The industrial toxicology of antimony. The Ernestine Henry Lecture 1987. *J R Coll Physicians Lond.* 1989;23:28-32.
84. McCarthy AE, Keystone JS, Kain KC. Pancreatitis occurring during therapy with stibogluconate: two case reports. *Clin Infect Dis.* 1993;17: 952-953.
85. McNally WD, ed. Antimony. In: *Toxicology.* Chicago: Industrial Medicine; 1937:285-290.
86. Miller JM. Poisoning by antimony: a case report. *South Med J.* 1982;75:592.
87. Mishra BB, Kale RR, Singh RK, Tiwari VK. Alkaloids: future prospective to combat leishmaniasis. *Fitoterapia.* 2009;80:81-90.
88. Motolese A, Truzzi M, Giannini A, Seidenari S. Contact dermatitis and contact sensitization among enamellers and decorators in the ceramics industry. *Contact Dermatitis.* 1993;28:59-62.
89. Myers R, Homan E, Well C, et al. Antimony Trioxide Range-Finding Toxicity Studies. Ots206062. Carnegie-Mellon Institute of Research, Carnegie-Mellon University, Pittsburgh, PA, 1978. Sponsored by Union Carbide. As cited in ATSDR 1990.
90. Nadkarni RA, Ehmann WD. Transference studies of trace elements from cigarette tobacco into smoke condensate, and their determination by neutron activation analysis. In: *Proceedings of the Tobacco Health Conference, Report 2.* Lexington: University of Kentucky; 1970:37-45.
91. National Medical Services. 24-Hour urine antimony reference value. In: Tietz NW, ed. *Textbook of Clinical Chemistry.* Philadelphia: WB Saunders; 1986:1814.
92. Ortega-Carnicer J, Alcazar R, De la Torre M, Benezet J. Pentavalent antimonial-induced torsade de pointes. *J Electrocardiol.* 1997;30:143-145.
93. Ozawa K. Studies on the therapy of schistosomiasis japonica. *Tohoku J Exp Med.* 1956;65:1-9.
94. Parish GG, Glass R, Kimbrough R. Acute arsine poisoning in two workers cleaning a clogged drain. *Arch Environ Health.* 1979;34:224-227.
95. Paschal DC, Ting BG, Morrow JC, et al. Trace metals in urine of United States residents: reference range concentrations. *Environ Res.* 1998;76:53-59.
96. Pollack S, Nagler A, Liberman D, et al. Immunological studies of pancytopenia in visceral leishmaniasis. *Isr J Med Sci.* 1988;24:70-74.
97. Potkonjak V, Pavlovich M. Antimoniosis: a particular form of pneumoconiosis. I. Etiology, clinical and x-ray findings. *Int Arch Occup Environ Health.* 1983;51:199-207.
98. Rai US, Kumar H, Kumar U, Amitabh V. Acute renal failure and 9th, 10th nerve palsy in patient of kala-azar treated with stibnite. *J Assoc Physicians India.* 1994;42:338.
99. Rai US, Kumar H, Kumar U. Renal dysfunction in patients of kala azar treated with sodium antimony gluconate. *J Assoc Physicians India.* 1994;42:383.
100. Rees PH, Keating MI, Kager PA, Hockmeyer WT. Renal clearance of pentavalent antimony (sodium stibogluconate). *Lancet.* 1980;2:226-229.
101. Renes LE. Antimony poisoning in industry. *AMA Arch Ind Hyg Occup Med.* 1953;7:99-108.
102. Romeo L, Apostoli P, Kovacic M, et al. Acute arsine intoxication as a consequence of metal burnishing operations. *Am J Ind Med.* 1997;32: 211-216.
103. Roper CS, Stupart L. The in vitro percutaneous absorption of diantimony trioxide through human skin, unpublished report on behalf of International Antimony Oxide Industry Association, Study Number 775440, report date 20.04.2006. Charles River Laboratories, Edinburgh, UK.
104. Saenz RE, de Rodriguez CG, Johnson CM, Berman JD. Efficacy and toxicity of pentostam against panamanian mucosal leishmaniasis. *Am J Trop Med Hyg.* 1991;44:394-398.
105. Smichowski P. Antimony in the environment as a global pollutant: a review on analytical methodologies for its determination in atmospheric aerosols. *Talanta.* 2008;75:2-14.
106. Smith SE. Uptake of antimony potassium tartrate by mouse liver slices. *Br J Pharmacol.* 1969;37:476-484.
107. Steiner R, Wegman I. *Fundamentals of Therapy: An Extension of the Art of Healing Through Spiritual Knowledge*, 4th ed. Chapters 14, 19, and 20. London: Rudolf Steiner Press; 1983.
108. Stevenson CJ. Antimony spots. *Trans St Johns Hosp Derm Soc.* 1965;51:40-45.
109. Sun H, Yan SC, Cheng WS. Interaction of antimony tartrate with the tripeptide glutathione: implication for its mode of action. *Eur J Biochem.* 2000;267:5450-5457.
110. Sunagawa S. Experimental studies on antimony poisoning. *Igaku Kenkyu.* 1981;51:129-142.
111. Sundar S, Sinha PR, Agrawal NK, et al. A cluster of cases of severe cardiotoxicity among kala-azar patients treated with a high-osmolarity lot of sodium antimony gluconate. *Am J Trop Med Hyg.* 1998;59:139-143.
112. Tarabar AF, Khan Y, Nelson LS, Hoffman RS. Antimony toxicity from the use of tartar emetic for the treatment of alcohol abuse. *Vet Hum Toxicol.* 2004;46:331-333.
113. Taylor AS. On poisoning by tartarized antimony; with medico-legal observations on the cases of Ann Palmer and others. In: Wilks S, Poland A, eds. *Guy's Hospital Reports, 3rd Series, Vol. III.* London: Levy's Hospital; 1857.
114. Taylor PJ. Acute intoxication from antimony trichloride. *Br J Ind Med.* 1966;23:318-321.
115. Temprano Vazquez S, Garcia Salazar MA, Jimenez Martin MJ, Lopez Martinez J. Torsade de pointes secondary to treatment with pentavalent antimonial drugs. *Med Clin (Barc).* 1998;110:717.
116. Thakur CP, Kumar M, Singh SK, et al. Comparison of regimens of treatment with sodium stibogluconate in kala-azar. *Br Med J.* 1984;288:895-897.

117. Thompson RHS, Whittaker VP. Antidotal activity of British anti-Lewisite against compounds of antimony, gold and mercury. *Biochem J.* 1947;41:342-346.
118. Van der Krogt P. Triumph-Wagen des Antimonij (Triumphal Chariot of Antimony). A monograph on Antimony: 1604 Basilius Valentinus (1565-1624). Elementymology and Elements Multidict—Stibium. Antimony; 2003. Last update. 02/10/2003 23:39. 34. http://www.vanderkrogt.net/elements/elem/sb.html (accessed October 15, 2005).
119. Waitz JA, Ober RE, Meisenhelder JE, Thompson PE. Physiological disposition of antimony after administration of ^{124}Sb-labelled tartar emetic to rats, mice and monkeys, and the effects of tris (*p*-aminophenyl) carbonium pamoate on this distribution. *Bull WHO.* 1965;33:537-546.
120. Watt WD. Chronic inhalation toxicity of antimony trioxide: validation of the threshold limit value [doctoral dissertation]. Detroit, MI: Wayne State University; 1983.
121. Weiss S, Hatcher RA. The mechanism of the vomiting induced by antimony and potassium tartrate (tartar emetic). *J Exp Med.* 1923;37:97-111.
122. Werrin M. Chemical food poisoning. *Q Bull Assoc Food Drug Office.* 1963;27:38-45.
123. Wester PO. Trace elements in serum and urine from hypertensive patients before and during treatment with chlorthalidone. *Acta Med Scand.* 1973;194:505-512.
124. White GP Jr, Mathias CG, Davin JS. Dermatitis in workers exposed to antimony in a melting process. *J Occup Med.* 1993;35:392-395.
125. WHO Expert Committee. The Leishmaniasis. Report of a. Technical Report Series 701. Geneva: World Health Organization; 1984.
126. Winship KA. Toxicity of antimony and its compounds. *Adverse Drug React Acute Poisoning Rev.* 1987;6:67-90.
127. Wortmann GW, Aronson NE, Byrd JC. Herpes zoster and lymphopenia associated with sodium stibogluconate therapy for cutaneous leishmaniasis. *Clin Infect Dis.* 1998;27:509-512.
128. Yu-I L, Chiao-Chen C, Yea-Lin T, Kuang-Sheng T. Studies on antibilharzial drugs VI: the antidotal effects of sodium dimercaptosuccinate and BAL-gludoside against tartar emetic. *Acta Physiol Sinica.* 1957;21:24-32.

CHAPTER 88
ARSENIC

Stephen W. Munday and Marsha D. Ford

Arsenic (As)		
Atomic number	=	33
Atomic weight	=	74.92 daltons
Normal concentrations		
Whole blood	<	5 μg/L (<0.067 μmol/L)
Urine (24 hour)	<	50 μg/L (< 0.67 μmol/L)
		1.33 μmol/g (<13.3 μmol/g creatinine)

The therapeutic use of arsenic (arsenic trioxide) for acute promyelocytic leukemia (APL), as well as its emergence as a significant environmental toxin, has renewed interest in its pharmacology and toxicology. The role of arsenic in our pharmacopeia may expand; its efficacy in treating various other leukemias, lymphomas, and multiple myeloma is being studied.[142] This chapter predominantly discusses the properties and toxicity of inorganic arsenic, the most prevalent toxic form.

HISTORY AND EPIDEMIOLOGY

Arsenic poisoning can be unintentional, suicidal, homicidal, occupational, environmental, or iatrogenic.[95,96,126,148] Mass poisonings have occurred. Nearly 400 residents of Hong Kong fell ill after eating contaminated bread from the Esing Bakery in 1857; two bakery foremen were thought to have tampered with the recipe.[79] The 1900 Staffordshire beer epidemic in England saw 6000 beer drinkers fall ill and 70 die from beer brewed with sugar made with arsenic-contaminated sulfuric acid.[95] In Wakayama, Japan, 67 people were poisoned by eating intentionally contaminated curry at a festival in 1998.[200] In 2003, the largest recent outbreak of arsenic poisoning in the United States occurred in New Sweden, Maine, when intentionally adulterated church coffee resulted in the death of one parishioner and the hospitalization of an additional 15 victims.[16] Arsenic trioxide reemerged as a treatment for acute promyelocytic leukemia in the 1990s after physicians in Harbin, China, found a high remission rate in patients given Ailing-1, a crude arsenic trioxide infusion.[111,236]

Contaminated soil, water, and food are the primary sources of arsenic for the general population. Pentavalent arsenic is the most common inorganic form in the environment.[49] Inorganic arsenic exposure from food is generally low and usually occurs from soil-derived foods such as rice and produce.[29,177,227,235] Exposure to organic arsenic compounds of low toxicity occurs from consumption of algae, fish, and shellfish. In the past 2 decades, consumption of contaminated water has emerged as the primary cause of large-scale outbreaks of chronic arsenic toxicity. Arsenic leaches from certain minerals and ores, as well as from industrial waste.[133] In Bangladesh, millions of people have been poisoned by drinking water from wells contaminated with arsenic leached from ground minerals.[151] Ironically, the wells were dug to obtain safer groundwater. Hydroarsenicism has also been reported in Chile, Taiwan, Brazil, India, Mexico, and Argentina.[32,43,49,89,133,151,216] In 2001, the US Environmental Protection Agency decreased the maximum contaminant level of arsenic in drinking water to 10 parts per billion (ppb), or 10 μg/L, after statistical modeling indicated an increased risk of lung and bladder cancer from water contaminated with arsenic at the formerly acceptable level of 50 ppb.[57] The World Health Organization also recommends a maximum concentration of 10 ppb.

CHEMISTRY

Arsenic is a metalloid that exists in multiple forms: elemental, gaseous (arsine), organic, and inorganic [(As^{3+} [trivalent, or arsenite] and As^{5+} [pentavalent, or arsenate])]. Tables 88–1 and 88–2 list sources of arsenic and regulatory standards about arsenic, respectively. Arsenic metal is considered nonpoisonous because of its insolubility in water and bodily fluids.[176] Arsine, which is highly toxic, is discussed in Chap. 24. Trivalent arsenicals include arsenic trioxide (As_2O_3), tetra-arsenic tetrasulfide (realgar; As_4S_4), and diarsenic trisulfide (orpiment; As_2S_3). Realgar and orpiment have been used by the Chinese to treat malignancies, diarrhea, and infections of the chest and liver.[124] Organic arsenicals vary in toxicity. Arsenobetaine, which is synthesized from inorganic arsenic by fish and crustaceans, and arsenosugars, which are synthesized by fish, crustaceans, and algae, have very low toxicity.[12,55,116] In contrast, the organoarsenical medication melarsoprol, used to treat the meningoencephalitic stage of African trypanosomiasis, has toxicity similar to inorganic arsenite.[24,165]

PHARMACOLOGY/PHYSIOLOGY

Arsenic trioxide (As_2O_3) is administered therapeutically for treating APL in doses of 0.15 to 0.16 mg/kg/d by either the intravenous or oral route.[109,111,183] At this dose its beneficial effects in APL occur predominantly by initiating cellular apoptosis when arsenic concentrations reach 0.5 to 2.0 μmol/L. Apoptosis is triggered by several mechanisms. The trivalent arsenic ion binds to mitochondrial membrane sulfhydryl (SH) groups, damaging mitochondrial membranes and collapsing membrane potentials. Cytochrome c is released from the damaged mitochondria with subsequent activation of caspases 9, 3, and 8, and initiation of apoptosis. Cells may be more susceptible if the intracellular concentrations of catalase and glutathione peroxidase (H_2O_2 scavenging enzymes) and glutathione-*S*-transferase (responsible for conjugating glutathione to xenobiotics) are reduced.[36,69,97,169] Arsenic trioxide also facilitates apoptosis by downregulating gene expression of BCL2, a prosurvival protein that protects against apoptosis.[33] Finally, arsenic trioxide can arrest cells early in mitosis, subsequently leading to apoptosis.[82]

Low-dose arsenic trioxide treatment (0.08 mg/kg/d) beneficially promotes cell differentiation of APL cells when arsenic concentrations reach 0.1 to 2.0 μmol/L. This differentiation is impaired by the promyelocytic leukemia-retinoic acid receptor α (PML-RARα) oncoprotein. This oncoprotein results from the APL-defining translocation of chromosomes 15 and 17. The PML portion of this oncoprotein plays a key role in leukemogenesis by interfering with RARα activity that is essential for normal myeloid cellular development. Trivalent arsenic degrades this PML portion, freeing RARα to facilitate cell differentiation.[36,137,144]

Melarsoprol is a trivalent organic arsenical compound used in Africa and parts of Europe to treat the meningoencephalitic stages of both species of African trypanosomes. It is ineffective against American trypanosomiasis and is available in the United States only directly from the Centers for Disease Control and Prevention (CDC) as it is not approved by the Food and Drug Administration (FDA). The mechanism of action is still poorly understood, but is believed to be related to inhibition of glycolysis and oxidation-reduction reactions.

TABLE 88–1. Sources of Exposure to Arsenic

Inorganic
- Occupational/manufacturing
  - Animal feed (additive)
  - Brass/bronze
  - Ceramics/glass
  - Computer chips (same as semiconductors)
  - Dyes/paints
  - Electron microscopy
  - Fireworks (Chinese)
  - Fossil fuel combustion—coal
  - Herbicides
  - Insecticides/pesticides
  - Metallurgy
  - Mining
  - Rodenticides
  - Semiconductors (gallium arsenide)
  - Smelting—copper, lead, zinc, sulfide minerals
  - Soldering
  - Wood preservatives
- Medicines/contaminated xenobiotics
  - Chemotherapy (acute promyelocytic leukemia)
  - Depilatory
  - Herbals/alternative medicines
  - Homeopathic remedies
  - Kelp
  - "Moonshine" ethanol
  - Opium
- Other
  - Contaminated well water
  - Contaminated foods/candies, eg, licorice

Organic
  - Melarsoprol (trypanocidal)
  - Thiacetarsamide (heartworm therapy in dogs)
  - Seafood (arsenobetaine)

The pharmaceutical compound also contains dimercaprol (BAL), which seems to reduce toxicity without diminishing effectiveness. The therapeutic use of melarsoprol can produce many of the toxic effects that occur with inorganic arsenic, including fever, encephalopathy, and acute cerebral edema with seizures and coma. Whether these effects are caused by drug toxicity or by an immune reaction elicited by trypanosomal antigens is unknown.[24,152] Other adverse effects include vomiting, abdominal pain, peripheral neuropathy with hypersensitivity reactions, hypertension, myocardial damage, and albuminuria. Hemolysis can occur in patients with glucose-6-phosphate dehydrogenase deficiency, and erythema nodosum in patients with leprosy.[24,152] In a study of the usefulness of melarsoprol as a treatment for refractory or advanced leukemia, efficacy was very limited, and reported adverse effects included fatigue, vomiting, diarrhea, vertigo, fever, seizures, headache, back pain, and injection site pain.[184]

TOXICOLOGY/PATHOPHYSIOLOGY

Investigations of the pathophysiologic effects induced by toxic doses of arsenic are discussed below. The apoptotic mechanisms[27] thought to be responsible for some therapeutic effects of arsenic trioxide have not been studied in toxicity models.

TRIVALENT ARSENIC

The primary biochemical lesion of As^{3+} is inhibition of the pyruvate dehydrogenase (PDH) complex (Fig. 88–1). Normally, dihydrolipoamide is recycled to lipoamide, a necessary cofactor in the conversion of pyruvate to acetylcoenzyme A (acetyl-CoA). As^{3+} binds the sulfhydryl groups of dihydrolipoamide, blocking lipoamide regeneration.[164] Acetyl-CoA is a central molecule in metabolism, and the resulting decrease leads to several deleterious effects:

- Decreased citric acid cycle activity and thus decreased adenosine triphosphate (ATP) production. Disruption of oxidative phosphorylation leads to production of hydrogen peroxide and oxygen radicals.
- Decreased gluconeogenesis that can worsen hypoglycemia. Pyruvate carboxylase catalyzes the conversion of pyruvate to oxaloacetate (initial step in gluconeogenesis), and this reaction requires the carboxylation of biotin, a CO_2 carrier attached to pyruvate carboxylase. Biotin cannot be carboxylated unless acetyl-CoA is attached to the enzyme.[165,188]

In the citric acid cycle, oxidation of α-ketoglutarate to succinyl-CoA uses an α-ketoglutarate dehydrogenase complex that contains the same cofactors as the PDH complex, including lipoamide. Succinyl-CoA is necessary for production of porphyrins and amino acids, and deficiency may contribute to the anemia and wasting seen with chronic arsenic poisoning. Arsenic inhibition of thiolase, the catalyst for the final step in fatty acid oxidation, also impairs ATP production. Diminished fatty acid oxidation results in decreased acetyl-CoA, in the loss of the reduced form of nicotinamide adenine dinucleotide (NADH) and the reduced form of flavin adenine dinucleotide ($FADH_2$) (electron carriers reduced during fatty acid breakdown whose subsequent oxidation yields ATP). Trivalent arsenic also inhibits glutathione synthetase, glucose-6-phosphate dehydrogenase (required to produce nicotinamide adenine dinucleotide phosphate [NADPH]), and glutathione reductase.[8] These inhibitions result in decreased levels of reduced glutathione, which is required to facilitate arsenic metabolism, protect red blood cells (RBCs) from oxidative damage, maintain hemoglobin in the ferrous state, and scavenge hydrogen peroxide and other organic peroxides.

Arsenic affects cardiac repolarization currents. When toxicity occurs, the result is ventricular dysrhythmias, including torsades de pointes. An in vitro study of cells exposed to As^{3+} demonstrated blockade of the delayed rectifier channels I_{Ks} and I_{Kr}. Interestingly, activation of $I_{K\text{-}ATP}$, a weak inward rectifier channel, also occurred; this activation could potentially counteract some of the effects of As^{3+} on the I_{Ks} and I_{Kr} channels.[52]

Animal experiments with phenylarsine oxide, a trivalent arsenical, demonstrate inhibition of insulin-induced glucose transport involving vicinal sulfhydryl groups, as well as β-cell damage in pancreatic islets attributed to inhibition of the α-ketoglutarate dehydrogenase complex.[22] The impaired glucose transport, plus the inhibited gluconeogenesis (discussed above), can lead to glycogen depletion and hypoglycemia.[166] Several animal experiments indicate improved central nervous system (CNS) glucose content[165] and increased in survival time with glucose treatment.[165]

TABLE 88–2. Regulations and Guidelines Applicable to Arsenic and Arsenic Compounds

Agency	Guideline Description	Concentration	Source
Air			
ACGIH	TLV (TWA) for arsenic and inorganic arsenic compounds	0.01 mg/m³	ACGIH 2004
NIOSH	REL (15-min ceiling limit) for arsenic and inorganic compounds	0.002 mg/m³	NIOSH 2005
	IDLH for arsenic and inorganic compounds	5 mg/m³	
OSHA	PEL (8-h TWA) for arsenic organic compounds (general industry, construction, and shipyard)	0.5 mg/m³	OSHA 2005 29 CFR 1910.1000; 1926.55; 1915.1000
	PEL (8-h TWA) for general industry for arsenic inorganic compounds	10 μg/m³	OSHA 2005 29 CFR 1910.1018
Water			
EPA	National primary drinking water standards for arsenic		EPA 2002
	MCL	10 μg/L (10 ppb)	
	MCLG	Zero	
FDA	Bottled drinking water	10 μg/L	FDA 2005 21 CFR 165.110
WHO	Drinking water quality guidelines for arsenic	10 μg/L	WHO 2004
ACGIH			ACGIH 2004
Confirmed human carcinogen			
EPA/NTP			IRIS 2007/ NTP 2005
IARC			IARC 2007

ACGIH, American Conference of Governmental Industrial Hygienists; CFR, Code of Federal Regulations; DWEL, drinking water equivalent level; EPA, Environmental Protection Agency; FDA, Food and Drug Administration; IARC, International Agency for Research on Cancer; IDLH, immediately dangerous to life or health; IRIS, Integrated Risk Information System; MCL, maximum contaminant level; MCLG, maximum contaminant level goal; MW, molecular weight; NIOSH, National Institute for Occupational Safety and Health; NTP, National Toxicology Program; OSHA, Occupational Safety and Health Administration; PEL, permissible exposure limit, REL, recommended exposure limit; TLV, threshold limit value; TWA, time-weighted average; WHO, World Health Organization.

Effects on RBCs include decreased membrane fluidity and ATP depletion.[223] Chronic arsenic exposure is associated with vascular disease; in vitro studies demonstrate inhibition of endothelial cell proliferation and glycoprotein synthesis in addition to lipid peroxidation.[34] A study on rodent and human platelets demonstrates increased platelet aggregation and arterial thrombosis.[118] Noncirrhotic hepatic portal fibrosis can develop. In a controlled study where mice chronically ingested water containing equal parts As^{3+} and As^{5+} for up to 15 months, the development of portal fibrosis was preceded by decreased hepatic glutathione (GSH), increased lipid peroxidation, and diminished levels or activities of numerous enzymes involved in regenerating GSH or scavenging free radicals.[174] Proposed mechanisms by which arsenic induces cancer include DNA damage induced by a dimethyl sulfide (DMS)-derived peroxyl radical, gene amplification, replacing phosphate in DNA during replication, increased cell proliferation, and decreased DNA repair efficiency.[14,102,226] Experimental evidence

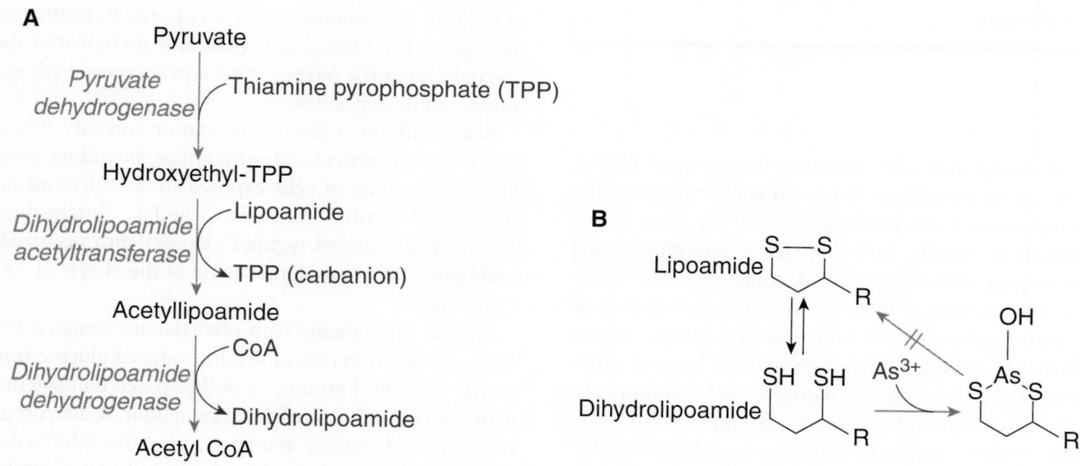

FIGURE 88–1. Effect of trivalent arsenicals (As^{3+}) on pyruvate dehydrogenase (PDH) complex. (A) The PDH complex is composed of the three enzymes, which use thiamine pyrophosphate (TPP) and lipoamide as cofactors to decarboxylate pyruvate and form acetyl CoA. (B) Arsenic interferes with the regeneration of lipoamide from dihydrolipoamide, thereby altering the function of the PDH complex.

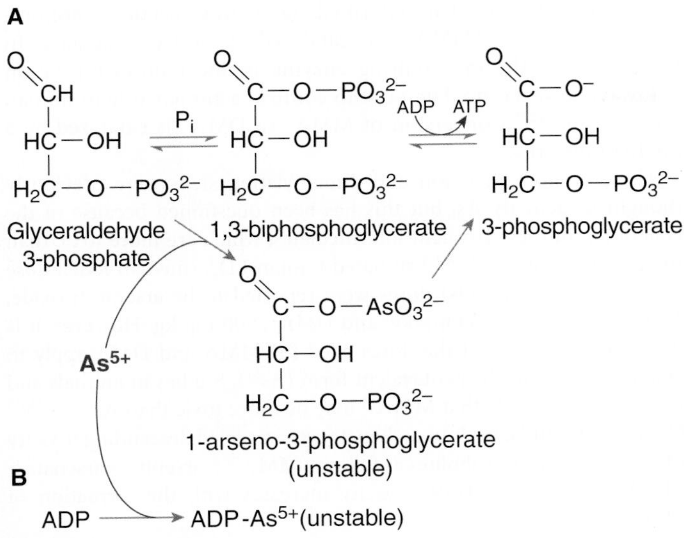

A

Glyceraldehyde 3-phosphate

1,3-biphosphoglycerate

3-phosphoglycerate

P_i

ADP ATP

As^{5+}

1-arseno-3-phosphoglycerate (unstable)

B

ADP → ADP-As^{5+}(unstable)

FIGURE 88–2. Pathophysiologic effects of pentavalent arsenic (As^{5+}; arsenate). **(A)** Arsenate (chemical formula AsO_4^{3-}) substitutes for inorganic phosphate (Pi; * indicates substitutions), bypassing the formation of 1,3-bisphosphoglycerate (1,3-BPG), and thus losing the ATP formation that occurs when 1,3-BPG is metabolized to 3-phosphoglycerate. **(B)** Energy loss also occurs if arsenate substitutes for Pi and blocks the formation of ATP from ADP. ADP, adenosine diphosphate; ATP, adenosine triphosphate.

and human studies support a number of etiologic or contributing factors for skin keratosis and cancer,[1] including chronic stimulation of keratinocyte-derived growth factors such as transforming growth factor-α (TGF-α), impaired methylation, mutation in the p53 tumor-suppressor gene, inhibition of poly(adenosine diphosphate [ADP]-ribose) polymerase vital for DNA repair, and interference with mitotic spindle and microtubular function.[7,71,92,122,225] Pigmentary changes also occur, and hyperpigmentation is attributed to increased melanin.

PENTAVALENT ARSENIC

Several mechanisms can cause toxicity from As^{5+}. Pentavalent arsenic can be reduced to As^{3+}.[93,208] Pentavalent arsenic also resembles phosphate chemically and structurally, may share a common transport system for cellular uptake with phosphate,[93] and can inhibit oxidative phosphorylation by substituting for inorganic phosphate (P_i) in the glycolysis reaction catalyzed by glyceraldehyde 3-phosphate dehydrogenase (Fig. 88–2)[31,167]. The resulting unstable product, 1-arseno-3-phosphoglycerate, spontaneously hydrolyzes to 3-phosphoglycerate, so glycolysis continues but the ATP normally produced during conversion of 1,3-bisphosphoglycerate to 3-phosphoglycerate is lost. Uncoupling may also occur if ADP forms ADP-arsenate, instead of ATP, in the presence of As^{5+}. The ADP-arsenate rapidly hydrolyzes, thus uncoupling oxidative phosphorylation.

PHARMACOKINETICS AND TOXICOKINETICS

ABSORPTION

Inorganic arsenic is tasteless and odorless and can be absorbed by the gastrointestinal (GI), respiratory, intravenous, and mucosal routes. *Gastrointestinal* absorption is facilitated by increased solubility and smaller particle size, and occurs predominantly in the small intestine, followed by the colon. Poorly soluble trivalent compounds such as arsenic trioxide (As_2O_3) are less well absorbed than more soluble trivalent and pentavalent compounds that, in aqueous solution, have an oral bioavailability greater than 90%. Therefore, when placed in an aqueous solution, As_2O_3 is more toxic than an identical dose of undissolved As_2O_3 eaten in food because of its failure to dissolve, thereby limiting absorption.[205] Organic arsenicals tend to be well absorbed; for example, a rodent study demonstrated approximately 70% GI absorption of the commonly used organic arsenical herbicide, dimethylarsinic acid (cacodylic acid).[186] Systemic absorption via the *respiratory* tract depends on the particulate size, as well as the arsenic compound and its solubility. Large, nonrespirable particles are cleared from the airways by ciliary action and swallowed, allowing GI absorption to occur. Respirable particles lodging in the lungs can be absorbed over days to weeks or remain unabsorbed for years.[25,220] *Dermal* penetration of arsenic through intact skin does not pose a risk for acute toxicity but potentially may be problematic with chronic application. Arsenic acid (H_3AsO_4) applied to intact skin in rhesus monkeys resulted in absorption of a mean of 2.0% to 6.4% of the applied dose.[221] Skin irritation and damage may increase systemic absorption.[68,168]

PHARMACOKINETICS OF ARSENIC TRIOXIDE

Intravenous administration of a single 10-mg dose of As_2O_3 to eight patients showed mean pharmacokinetic values as follows: maximum plasma concentration (Cp_{max}) of 6.85 μmol/L, α elimination half-life ($t_{1/2}$ α) of 0.89 ± 0.29 hours, and β elimination half-life ($t_{1/2}$ β) of 12.13 ± 3.31 hours.[180] In six patients, only 1% to 8% of the daily dose was eliminated in a 24-hour urine. Repeat pharmacokinetic studies on day 30 of treatment were not statistically different.[180] Another study of patients receiving a single dose of 5 mg of As_2O_3 intravenously demonstrated mean pharmacokinetic values as follows: Cp_{max} of 2.636 μmol/L, $t_{1/2}$ α of 1.413 hours, $t_{1/2}$ β of 9.411 hours, serum clearance of 1.987 L/h, and area under the plasma drug concentration versus time curve (AUC) of 12.706 μmol/L/h. A single dose of 10 mg intravenously showed a Cp_{max} of 6.799 ± 0.314 μmol/L.[179] Arsenic trioxide 10 mg given orally for APL demonstrated total plasma and blood AUC values that were 99% and 87%, respectively, of the corresponding values reported for a 10-mg intravenous dose administered in the same nine patients.[109]

A study in humans receiving intravenous radioarsenic isotope (^{74}As) showed arsenic clearing from the blood in three phases:

Phase 1 (2 to 3 hours)—Arsenic is rapidly cleared from the plasma with a $t_{1/2}$ of 1 to 2 hours; more than 90% may be cleared during this phase because of redistribution to tissue and renal elimination.

Phase 2 (3 hours to 7 days)—A more gradual plasma decline occurs, with an estimated $t_{1/2}$ of 30 hours.

Phase 3 (10 or more days)—Clearance continues from the plasma slowly with an estimated $t_{1/2}$ of 300 hours.[135]

The rapid clearance in phases 1 and 2 explains why blood testing for arsenic is unreliable, except early in acute poisoning.

Initial distribution is predominantly to liver, kidney, muscle, and skin. The skin is rich in sulfhydryl groups; the elimination $t_{1/2}$ of arsenic by the skin was estimated to be 1 month in a rabbit study.[53] Distribution to brain also occurs quickly. In the ^{74}As study, 0.30% of the administered dose was found in brain biopsy samples in the first hour postinfusion. This peak declined to 0.16% by day 7.[135] Ultimately, arsenic distributes to all tissues. In the single patient in this study who was followed for 18 days, 96.6% of the total injected arsenic dose was recovered in the urine. Fecal arsenic recovery was less than 1% of the total dose.[135] Other studies in humans demonstrate renal arsenic elimination of 46% to 68.9% within the first 5 days postingestion.[26,29,98,157] Approximately 30% is eliminated with a half-life of greater than 1 week, while the remainder is slowly excreted with a half-life of greater than 1 month.[26,134] Fecal elimination is considerably less, with reported amounts as much as 6.1% in humans.[190] Dog studies have revealed that the mechanisms of urinary elimination of unchanged arsenic and its methylated metabolites are via glomerular filtration and tubular secretion; active reabsorption also occurs.[198]

Arsenic crosses the placenta and accumulates in the fetus,[125] but two studies of breast milk excretion from women exposed to drinking water with arsenic levels of approximately 200 μg/L came to opposite conclusions. Breast milk arsenic levels were low in both studies, and only one of them demonstrated a correlation between maternal arsenic levels and levels in breast milk.[44,173]

Metabolism, by adding methyl groups, occurs primarily in the liver, as well as in the kidneys, testes, and lungs (Fig. 88–3). If the arsenic is pentavalent, approximately 50% to 70% will first be reduced to trivalent arsenic.[43,187,206] This bioactivation step requires the oxidation of glutathione[50] and can begin within 15 minutes of exposure.[206] *S*-adenosylmethionine (SAM) is the primary methyl donor. Nonenzymatic methylation has also been demonstrated in an in vitro study using human liver cytosol; here, methylcobalamin (methyl B_{12}) was the methyl donor.[232] Dietary and vitamin deficiencies, as well as high doses of inorganic arsenic, may diminish the ability to methylate arsenic, and folate supplementation has been shown to lower blood arsenic in a folate-deficient population.[65–67,84,85,156,207] However, a study in pregnant Bangladeshi women showed efficient arsenic methylation despite nutritional deficiencies.[121] Addition of one methyl group produces monomethylarsonic acid (MMA^{V}); adding a second methyl group produces dimethylarsinic acid (DMA^{V}).

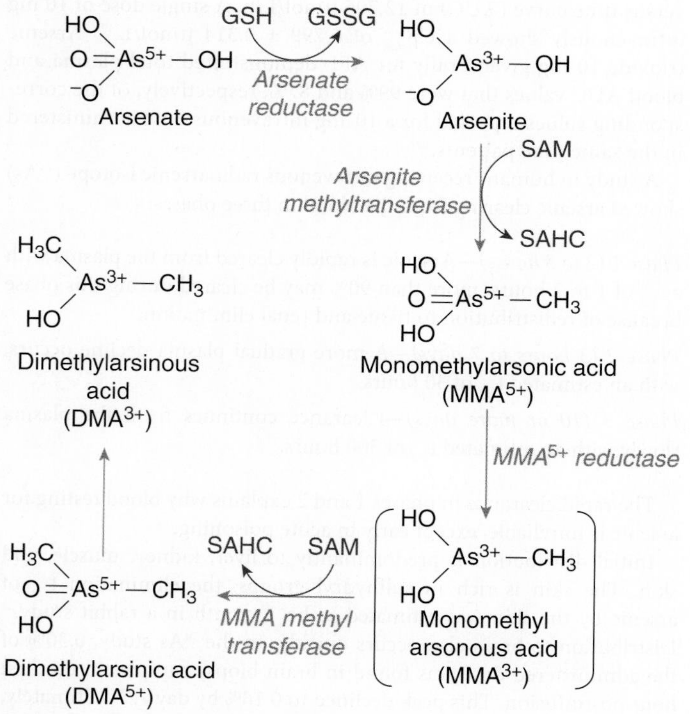

FIGURE 88–3. Metabolism of arsenate [As^{5+}] and arsenite [As^{3+}]. DMA, dimethylarsinic acid; GSH, glutathione; MMA, monomethylarsonic acid; SAHC, *S*-adenosylhomocysteine; SAM, *S*-adenosylmethionine. The asterisk (∗) denotes MMA^{V} reductase, the rate-limiting enzyme in rabbit studies of arsenic metabolism; the analogy to humans is unknown.

Production of a trivalent intermediate in this reaction, monomethylarsonous acid (MMA^{III}), is catalyzed by MMA^{V} reductase. In rabbits this is the rate-limiting enzyme in the biotransformation pathway; however, no data exist to confirm a similar role in human metabolism.[204,233] Conversion of MMA^{V} to DMA^{V} is catalyzed by a methyltransferase.

These monomethylation and dimethylation steps were previously thought to detoxify As, but this has been questioned because of the generation of these trivalent intermediates, which are more toxic than the parent compounds.[202] Estimated human LD_{50} (median lethal dose for 50% of test subjects) doses were reported to be arsenic trioxide, 1.43 mg/kg; MMA^{V}, 50 mg/kg; and DMA^{V}, 500 mg/kg. However, it is important to note that the doses cited for MMA and DMA apply to arsenic existing in the pentavalent form (As^{5+}). Studies in animals and cell cultures indicate that MMA^{III} may be more toxic than As^{3+}.[129,154,155] Cytotoxicity studies in human hepatocytes revealed descending toxicity of arsenic and its metabolites as follows: MMA^{III} > arsenite > arsenate > MMA^{V} = DMA^{V}.[154] Thus, toxicity increases with the formation of MMA^{III}.

There is some evidence that these findings have clinical relevance. In a study from a blackfoot disease–hyperendemic area of Taiwan, lower capacity to methylate inorganic arsenic to DMA^{V} was associated with increased risk of blackfoot disease. The capacity to methylate arsenic to DMA^{V} was measured as the ratio of DMA^{V} to MMA^{V} and the ratio of MMA^{V} to the sum of As^{III} and As^{V}.[196] In addition, a cohort study found that the odds of premalignant skin lesions increased with increasing urinary MMA^{V} and decreasing urinary DMA^{V}.[3] They also found that there was an increased risk of skin lesions associated with genetic polymorphisms of glutathaione S-transferase and borderline increased risk with polymorphisms of methylenetetrahydrofolate reductase. The authors suggested that the conversion of MMA^{V} to DMA^{V} may be saturable and that arsenic metabolism and toxicity are affected by genetics.[3]

Arsenobetaine (AsB) is also well absorbed and is excreted unchanged in the urine.[205] Elimination occurs more rapidly than with inorganic arsenic. In a study involving human volunteers, 25% was excreted within 2 to 4 hours, 50% by 20 hours, and 70% to 83.7% after 166 hours. A two-component exponential model shows nearly 50% of the AsB eliminated, with a first component $t_{1/2}$ of 6.9 to 11.0 hours and a second component $t_{1/2}$ of 75.7 hours.[98]

CLINICAL MANIFESTATIONS

INORGANIC ARSENICALS

Toxic manifestations vary, depending on the amount and form of arsenic ingested, as well as the chronicity of ingestion. Other influencing factors include individual variations in methylation and excretion. Larger doses of a potent compound, such as arsenic trioxide, will rapidly produce manifestations of acute toxicity, whereas chronic ingestion of substantially lower amounts of pentavalent arsenic in groundwater will result in a different clinical picture over time. Manifestations of subacute toxicity can develop in patients who survive acute poisoning, as well as in patients who are slowly poisoned environmentally.

Acute Toxicity Gastrointestinal signs and symptoms of nausea, vomiting, abdominal pain, and diarrhea, which occur 10 minutes to several hours following ingestion, are the earliest manifestations of acute poisoning by the oral route. The diarrhea has been compared to that seen with cholera and may resemble "rice water." Severe multisystem illness can ensue with extensive exposure. Cardiovascular signs, ranging from sinus tachycardia and orthostatic hypotension to shock, can develop. Reported cases have mimicked myocardial infarction or systemic inflammatory response syndrome, with intravascular volume depletion, capillary leak, myocardial dysfunction, and diminished systemic vascular resistance.[13,19,21,75,99,178] Acute encephalopathy can develop and progress over several days, with delirium, coma, and seizures attributed to cerebral edema and microhemorrhages.[61,178] Seizures may be secondary to dysrhythmias, and the underlying cardiac rhythm should be assessed. Seizures secondary to torsades de pointes associated with a prolonged QT interval developed 4 days to 5 weeks after acute arsenic ingestion.[19,73,185] Acute lung injury, acute respiratory distress syndrome and respiratory failure, hepatitis, hemolytic anemia, acute renal failure, rhabdomyolysis, other ventricular dysrhythmias, and death can occur.[21,59,78,139,189] Death may occur after suddenly developing bradycardia, followed by asystole.[21,99,126] Fever may develop, misleading the practitioner to diagnose sepsis.[54,99] Hepatitis can occur and may be a result of altered intrahepatic heme metabolism causing an increased synthesis of bilirubin or a result of altered protein transport between hepatocytes.[6] Acute renal failure may be secondary to ischemia caused by hypotension, tubular deposition of myoglobin or hemoglobin, renal cortical necrosis, and direct renal tubular toxicity.[23,70,175,199] Glutathione depletion may be contributory.[90] Unusual complications include phrenic nerve paralysis, unilateral facial nerve palsy, pancreatitis, pericarditis, and pleuritis.[15,234] Fetal demise has been reported, with toxic arsenic concentrations found in the fetal organs.[21,125]

Acutely poisoned patients with less severe illness may experience gastroenteritis and mild hypotension that persist despite antiemetic and intravenous crystalloid therapies. Hospitalization and continued intravenous fluids may be required for several days.[117] The prolonged character of the GI symptoms is atypical for most viral and bacterial enteric illnesses and should alert the physician to consider arsenic poisoning, especially if there is a history of repetitive GI illnesses. A metallic taste or oropharyngeal irritation, mimicking pharyngitis, can occur.[21,87] Gastrointestinal ulcerative lesions and hemorrhage have been reported.[61,75] Toxic erythroderma and exfoliative dermatitis result from a hypersensitivity reaction to arsenic.[191]

In the days and weeks following an acute exposure, prolonged or additional signs and symptoms in the nervous, GI, hematologic, dermatologic, pulmonary, and cardiovascular systems can occur. Encephalopathic symptoms of headache, confusion, decreased memory, personality change, irritability, hallucinations, delirium, and seizures may develop and persist.[54,64,170] Sixth cranial nerve palsy and bilateral sensorineural hearing loss are reported.[42,73] Peripheral neuropathy typically develops 1 to 3 weeks after acute poisoning, although in one series nine patients developed maximal neuropathy within 24 hours of exposure.[42,87,117,218] Sensory symptoms develop first, and diminished to absent vibratory sense may be present. Progressive signs and symptoms include numbness, tingling, and formication with physical findings of diminished to absent pain, touch, temperature, and deep-tendon reflexes in a stocking-glove distribution. Superficial touch of the extremities may elicit severe or deep aching pains, a finding that also occurs with thallium poisoning. Motor weakness may then develop. The most severely affected patients manifest an ascending flaccid paralysis that mimics Guillain-Barré syndrome.[42,87,117] Respiratory problems can include dry cough, rales, hemoptysis, chest pain, and patchy interstitial infiltrates.[87,153] These findings may be misinterpreted as viral or bronchitic disease. Leukopenia, and less commonly anemia and thrombocytopenia, occur from days to 3 weeks after an acute exposure, but resolve as bone marrow function returns.[95,120]

Dermatologic lesions can include patchy alopecia, oral herpetiform lesions, a diffuse pruritic macular rash, and a brawny nonpruritic desquamation (see Chap. 29). Diaphoresis and edema of the face and extremities can develop.[1] Mees lines (transverse striate leuconychia of the nails) are 1- to 2-mm-wide horizontal nail bands that represent disturbed nail matrix keratinization (see Fig. 88–4). They are uncommon in arsenic poisoning. A minimum of 30 days after exposure is required for the lines to extend visibly beyond the nail lunulae.[87,225] Contact dermatitis has been reported from topical exposure in an occupational setting. Other possible toxic manifestations of subacute inorganic arsenic toxicity include nephropathy, fatigue, anorexia with weight loss, torsades de pointes, and persistence of GI symptoms.[13,130]

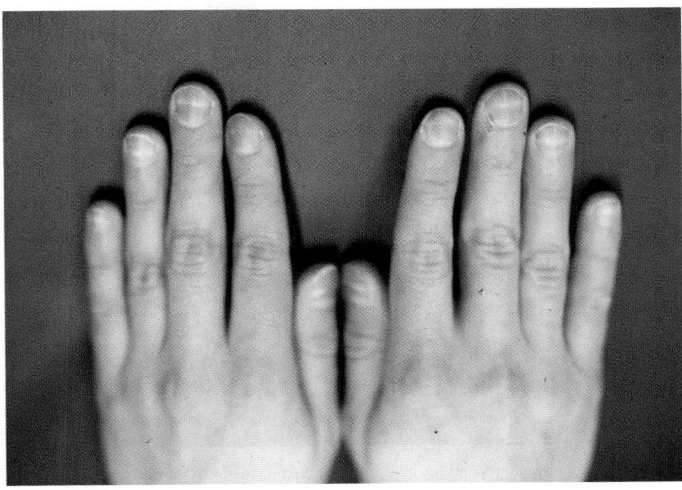

FIGURE 88–4. Mee's lines, parallel white bands across the nails result from exposures to metals, radiation, and chemotherapeutic agents, among others. *(Image contributed by the New York City Poison Center Toxicology Fellowship Program.)*

Chronic Toxicity Chronic low-level exposure to inorganic arsenicals typically occurs from occupational or environmental sources. Malignant and nonmalignant skin changes, hypertension, diabetes mellitus, peripheral vascular disease, and lung, bladder, and hepatic malignancies are associated with drinking water containing arsenic that is consumed by study populations.[136,151,158,229] The skin is very susceptible to the toxic effects of arsenic; multiple dermatologic lesions have been reported in populations suffering from hydroarsenicism.[133,229] Alterations in pigmentation occur first, with hyperpigmentation being the most common. Hypopigmentation ("raindrop" pattern) can also occur (see Fig. 88–5). Hyperkeratoses typically develop on the palms and soles, but can be diffuse (see Fig. 88–6). Squamous and basal cell

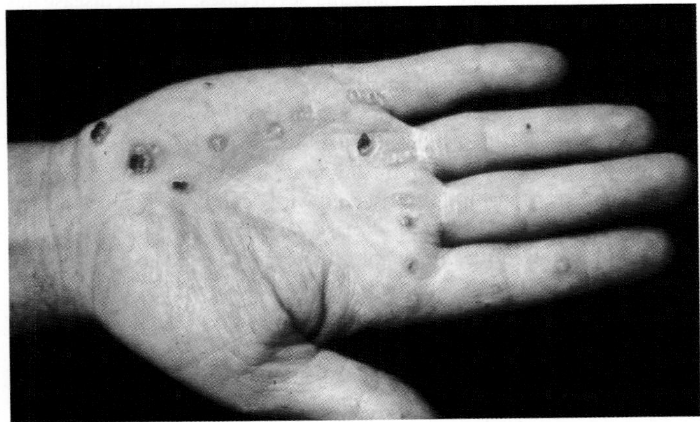

FIGURE 88–5. Characteristic hemorrhagic vesicles of arsenical dermatitis is shown. *(Image contributed by New York University Department of Dermatology.)*

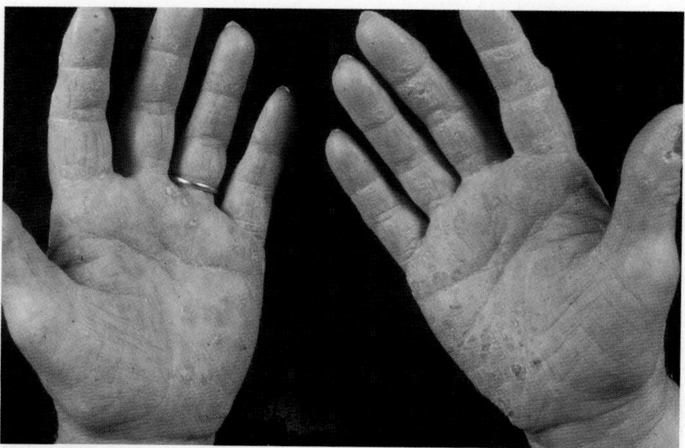

FIGURE 88–6. Characteristic vesicular xerotic arsenical dermatitis is shown. *(Image contributed by New York University Department of Dermatology.)*

carcinomas and Bowen disease (intraepidermal squamous cell carcinoma) may occur. Bowen disease usually proliferates in multiple sites, especially on the trunk, and is noted for developing on sun-protected areas. Latency periods for developing keratoses, Bowen disease, and squamous cell carcinoma were 28, 39, and 41 years, respectively, in 17 patients chronically exposed to environmental or medicinal arsenic.[48,224] Gastrointestinal symptoms of nausea, vomiting, and diarrhea are less likely but can occur. Hepatomegaly was present in 120 of 156 patients with hydroarsenicism; liver biopsy in 45 cases revealed a noncirrhotic portal fibrosis in 91.1%.[133] Rodent studies have also demonstrated hepatic fibrosis from inorganic arsenic exposure.[174] Portal hypertension and hypersplenism have occurred.[133,174] Hepatic angiosarcomas have been linked to arsenic exposure.[40,101,115]

Population studies in areas of Bangladesh and Taiwan with arsenic-contaminated water show an increased prevalence of diabetes mellitus (DM), pulmonary fibrosis, and other organ system effects.[160,161,197] A cross-sectional drinking water study from the United States revealed an odds ratio of 3.58 for prevalence of type 2 DM among those at the 80th percentile, as compared to those at the 20th percentile, despite a median total arsenic concentration of only 7.1 ppb.[114,143] The mechanism of this low-concentration arsenic effect is unclear. Animal studies have demonstrated that arsenic can decrease insulin-mediated uptake of glucose by cells and can also disrupt insulin transcription factor signal transduction.[150,213] In a study from West Bengal, restrictive lung disease was reported in nine of 17 patients, and a restrictive plus obstructive pattern occurred in another seven cases.[133] Lung disease has also been noted in other populations.[80] Proposed mechanisms include arsenic-induced inflammation and oxidative stress.[149] Aplastic anemia and agranulocytosis are documented in patients exposed to arsenic.[54] A dose–response relationship between arsenic exposure and vascular disease is reported in several populations.[215] After adjusting for age, sex, hypertension, DM, cigarette smoking, and alcohol consumption, a significant relationship was observed with cerebrovascular disease in a region of Taiwan.[39] Blackfoot disease, an obliterative arterial disease of the lower extremities, occurring in Taiwan, is linked to chronic arsenic exposure,[32,195] as is ischemic heart disease.[30] The incidence of Raynaud phenomenon and vasospasm was reported to be increased in smelter workers exposed to arsenic, compared with a control group.[113] Encephalopathy and peripheral neuropathy are the neurologic manifestations most commonly reported.[18,86] Electromyographic studies of 33 patients with chronic ingestion of arsenic-contaminated water revealed 10 patients with findings consistent with sensory neuropathy. The minimum duration of exposure was 2 years. Interestingly, three of these patients consumed water with an arsenic concentration that only slightly exceeded the contaminant concentration of 50 ppb previously permissible in the United States.[89]

Arsenic is classified as a definite carcinogen by the International Agency for Research on Cancer (IARC, Group 1) and the National Toxicology Program (NTP). Cancers known to develop include lung, skin, and bladder.[12,41,94,173,182] Transitional cell bladder carcinoma was the most common type in one large epidemiologic study.[38] A critical literature review of animal and human studies found that exposure to environmental arsenic was unlikely to cause reproductive or developmental toxicity.[51] However, a more recent rodent study revealed fetal growth retardation and neurotoxicity at doses relevant to human exposure and in the absence of maternal toxicity.[214] More concerning, two recent drinking water cohort studies from Bangladesh showed small but statistically significant increases in birth defects and fetal loss.[110,160,203] Moreover, in addition to possibly increasing the risk of birth defects there is also cross-sectional evidence that in utero or early childhood exposure may be associated with persistent neurocognitive effects in children.[28,46,194,211,216,217] Finally, there is evidence that in utero or early childhood exposure to arsenic in drinking water increases the risk of malignant and nonmalignant lung diseases in young adults.[182] In summary, there is accumulating evidence of persistent adverse effects from in utero or early childhood exposure, but prospective studies are needed to confirm these findings by decreasing the effects of confounding and bias that may explain the results.

Many of the questions regarding the chronic health effects of exposure to arsenic in drinking water are currently being investigated in the Health Effects of Arsenic Longitudinal Study (HEALS). This study was designed to evaluate the health effects of a full range of drinking water arsenic exposures including mortality, premalignant and malignant skin tumors, pregnancy outcomes, and children's cognitive development.[5]

This study is a prospective cohort study in Araihazar, Bangladesh. Participants were between the ages of 18 and 75 years and married, although both members of a couple were not required to enroll. A total of 11,764 subjects enrolled, 6704 women and 5042 men. The participation rate in the initial enrollment was 97.5% of those approached.[5]

Of those who agreed to participate 98% completed an extensive questionnaire that included demographic and lifestyle components and a validated food-frequency questionnaire. They also participated in a clinical examination with an extensive skin evaluation. Over 90% of this group also provided blood and spot urine arsenic samples.[5]

Approximately one-third of the participants consumed water in each of three groups: greater than 100 μg/L, 25 to 100 μg/L, and less than 25 μg/L. Average urinary concentrations of arsenic were approximately 140 μg/L.

Some findings from this cohort have been published. Studies of persons with arsenic-induced skin lesions have shown increasing risk of disease as exposure increases.[4] Modification of risk was noted in relationship to sunlight exposure, smoking, and some occupational exposures such as fertilizers and pesticides.[35] A dose–response relationship was also found for subclinical sensory neuropathy as measured by tactile thresholds.[81]

ADVERSE DRUG EFFECTS: ARSENIC TRIOXIDE

The most common adverse effects are *dermatologic* (skin dryness, pigmentary changes, maculopapular eruptions with or without pruritus); *GI* (nausea, vomiting, anorexia, diarrhea, and dyspepsia); *hematologic* (leukemoid reactions); *hepatic* (elevation of aminotransferase concentrations typically less than or equal to 10 times the upper limit of normal values, with a reported incidence of 20% with low-dose and 31.9% with conventional-dose therapy[179]); *cardiac* (prolonged QT interval in 40% to 63% of patients, first-degree atrioventricular block, ventricular ectopy, monomorphic nonsustained ventricular tachycardia, torsades de pointes, sudden asystole, and death);[172,179,183,201,222] *facial edema*; and *neurologic* (paresthesias, peripheral neuropathy, and headache). All of these effects occurred more commonly in one case series with conventional-dose therapy (0.16 mg/kg/d) when compared to low dose therapy. The majority are treated symptomatically without discontinuing As_2O_3 treatment. Leukemoid reactions, defined as white blood cell counts greater than 50×10^9/L, develop in nearly 50% of patients between 14 and 42 days of beginning treatment. Such patients are at risk for intracerebral hemorrhage or infarction and for the APL syndrome. This syndrome is similar to the differentiation syndrome (DS) that was formerly known as the retinoic acid syndrome.[138] The remission induction treatment phase is the period of greatest risk.[180] Common clinical findings in this syndrome include pulmonary interstitial infiltrates and/or pleural effusions, dyspnea, tachypnea, fluid retention, myalgias, arthralgias, fever, and weight gain; approximately 20% to 25% of patients treated with arsenic trioxide will develop one or more signs or symptoms of this syndrome.[131,142,172,179,180]

DIAGNOSTIC TESTING

Timing of testing for arsenic must be correlated with the clinical course of the patient and whether the poisoning is acute, subacute, chronic, or remote with residual clinical effects. To properly interpret laboratory measurements, confounding factors, such as food-derived organic arsenicals or accumulated arsenic (DMA and arsenobetaine) in patients with chronic renal failure, must be considered.[47,237,238] Failure to understand potential confounders, as well as the time course of arsenic metabolism, clearance, and effect on laboratory parameters, can cause erroneous assessment of possible arsenic poisoning.

URINE AND BLOOD

Diagnosis ultimately depends on finding an elevated urinary arsenic concentration. In an emergency, a spot urine may be sent prior to beginning chelation therapy. A markedly elevated arsenic concentration verifies the diagnosis in a patient with characteristic history and clinical findings, but a low concentration does not exclude arsenic toxicity.[212] In nine acutely symptomatic patients, initial spot urine arsenic concentrations ranged from 192 to 198,450 μg/L.[103] Definitive diagnosis of arsenic exposure hinges on finding a 24-hour urinary concentration equal to or greater than 50 μg/L, 100 μg/g creatinine, or 100 μg total arsenic. A study on arsenic exposure from drinking water showed excellent correlations between spot and 24-hour urine arsenic concentrations. There are not enough data to determine if this relationship holds true in acutely poisoned patients, so a 24-hour collection is still preferred.[29] Challenge testing with dimercaptopropane sulfonate (DMPS) has been performed in individuals exposed to arsenic in drinking water and clearly increases arsenic excretion; however, it also alters the percentages of the arsenic species recovered compared with controls and has not been correlated with clinical effects.[11] All urine should be collected in metal-free polyethylene containers; acid-rinsed containers are not recommended since the acid alters the arsenic species.[58] If testing is performed by an outside reference laboratory, specimens from acutely ill patients should be sent via express transportation with a request for a rapid result.

When interpreting slightly elevated urinary arsenic levels, laboratory findings must also be correlated with the history and clinical findings, because seafood ingestion is reported to transiently elevate urinary total arsenic excretion up to 1700 μg/L.[12] When seafood arsenic is a consideration, speciation of arsenic can be accomplished by high-performance liquid chromatography (HPLC) separation, followed by inductively coupled plasma-mass spectrometry (ICPMS), HPLC via ion-pair chromatography coupled with hydride-generation atomic-fluorescence spectrometry (HGAFS), or by hydride generation coupled with cold-trap gas chromatography-atomic absorption spectrometry. These techniques separate AsB, As^{3+}, As^{5+}, MMA, and DMA.[58] Arsenobetaine can also be directly measured by silica-based cation-exchange separation, followed by atomic absorption spectrometry.[145] Two other methods, selective hydride-generation atomic-absorption spectrometry (HGAAS) and resin-based ion-exchange chromatography, do not directly measure AsB; instead, they indirectly derive this value by subtracting the sum of all measured arsenic species from the total arsenic concentration.[145] If arsenic speciation cannot be done, the patient can be retested after a 1-week abstinence from fish, shellfish, and algae food products.

Conditions under which urine is stored can affect total arsenic recovery, as well as proportionality of the species. The various arsenic species—arsenate (As^{5+}), arsenite (As^{3+}), MMA, DMA, and AsB—remain stable for 2 months in urine stored without preservatives at either −4°F (−20°C; freezer) or 39.2°F (4°C; refrigerator); AsB is stable for 8 months under these conditions. Storage for longer than 2 months can alter the recovery of various species. Addition of 0.1% hydrochloric acid (HCl) facilitates reduction of arsenate to arsenite and also decreases MMA and DMA levels. Acid-washed collection containers should not be used if measurement of the various arsenic species is planned. Total arsenic recovery can be diminished by any of the following: specimen storage for greater than 2 months, acidification, or testing using HPLC-ICPMS and HPLC-HGAFS, since all these methods usually require that the samples be filtered prior to undergoing HPLC separation.[58]

Diagnostic evaluation of chronic toxicity should include laboratory parameters that may become abnormal within days to weeks following an acute exposure. Tests should include a complete blood count, renal and liver function tests, urinalysis, and 24-hour urinary arsenic determinations. Complete blood count findings can include a normocytic, normochromic, or megaloblastic anemia; an initial leukocytosis followed by development of leukopenia, with neutrophils depressed more than lymphocytes, and a relative eosinophilia; thrombocytopenia; and a rapidly declining hemoglobin, indicative of hemolysis or a GI hemorrhage.[112] Basophilic stippling of RBCs can be seen; this can occur in other toxic and clinical disorders. Karyorrhexis, a rupture of the RBC cell nucleus with chromatin disintegration into granules that are extruded from the cell, and dyserythropoiesis are reported in both lead- and arsenic-toxic patients. Both findings are caused by arsenic-induced inhibition of DNA synthesis and damage to the nuclear envelope.[56] The karyorrhexis can occur within 4 days and resolve by 2 weeks after poisoning, and may be an early indication of arsenic toxicity.[112] Elevated serum creatinine, aminotransferases, and bilirubin, as well as depressed haptoglobin concentrations, may develop. Urinalysis may reveal proteinuria, hematuria, and pyuria. Cerebrospinal fluid examination in patients with CNS findings can be normal or exhibit mild protein concentration elevation, measured at 26.5 mg/dL in one case.[87] Urinary arsenic excretion in subacute and chronic cases varies inversely with the postexposure time period, but low-level excretion can continue for months after exposure. In a study of 41 cases of arsenic-induced peripheral neuropathy, most patients with a neuropathy of 4 to 8 weeks duration had total 24-hour urinary arsenic measurements of 100 to 400 μg.[87]

HAIR AND NAIL TESTING

In cases of suspected arsenic toxicity, in which the urinary arsenic measurements fall below accepted toxic concentrations, analysis of hair and nails may yield the diagnosis. Arsenic can be detected in the proximal portions of hair within 30 hours of ingestion.[230] Inorganic arsenic is the form best absorbed by these tissues and the form most commonly found in human poisoning cases; small amounts of methylated metabolites may also be detected.[159] Arsenobetaine has not been found in hair and tissues in human and animal studies.[227,228] Hair grows at rates varying from 0.7 to 3.6 cm per month, with a mean rate of 1 cm per month.[219] The Society of Hair Testing has made the following recommendations for collection of hair specimens; however, these have only been validated for testing drugs of abuse: (1) collect approximately 200 mg of hair from the posterior vertex region of the scalp using scissors to cut as close to the scalp as possible, and (2) tie the hairs together, wrap in aluminum foil to protect from environmental contamination, and store at room temperature.[219] Nails grow approximately 0.1 mm per day. Total replacement of a fingernail requires 3 to 4 months, whereas toenails require 6 to 9 months of growth. These facts, plus the frequency of hair cutting, should be considered when estimating the usefulness of measuring arsenic levels in these tissues. The normal values of the testing laboratory should be used to determine whether arsenic concentrations are elevated. In cases of remote toxicity, hair and nail arsenic measurements may or may not be elevated, depending on the time elapsed since exposure. Sequential hair analysis to assess the time(s) of exposure can be performed by solid sampling graphite furnace atomic absorption spectrophotometry, or by X-ray fluorescence spectrometry.[104,192,193]

OTHER TESTS

Abdominal radiographs might demonstrate radiopaque material in the GI tract soon after an ingestion.[2,37,75,76,88] However, even after an acute ingestion the absence of radiopaque materials on abdominal radiographs is reported.[45] The incidence of positive radiographs after an ingestion is unknown, and a negative radiograph should not eliminate arsenic as a diagnostic consideration. Electrocardiographic changes reported include QRS widening, QT prolongation, ST segment depression, T-wave flattening, ventricular premature contractions, nonsustained monomorphic ventricular tachycardia, and torsades de pointes.[17,147,183,201] Nerve conduction studies (NCS) can confirm or diagnose clinical or subclinical axonopathy. Both the sensory nerve action potential (SNAP) and the motor compound muscle action potential (CMAP) measure the number of axons that can conduct impulses. However, the sensory studies are more sensitive than motor studies in detecting axonal degeneration and demyelination; decreased SNAP measurements can indicate subclinical neuropathy. In motor nerve studies, the amplitude (height of the CMAP) is a more sensitive measure of the number of axons that can conduct impulses than is the conduction velocity; this can be explained by the pattern of axonal destruction as opposed to myelin injury (which mainly affects conduction velocity). Nerve biopsies have confirmed disintegration of both axons and myelin in patients with arsenic-induced peripheral neuropathy; the axonal loss begins distally in the lower extremities and is initially scattered. Thus, conduction along the remaining functional axons can be sufficient to produce normal or only slightly decreased conduction measurements on NCS.[72,87,105,117,141,146]

MANAGEMENT

GENERAL

Acute arsenical toxicity is life threatening and mandates aggressive treatment. Advanced life support monitoring and therapies should be initiated when necessary, but with a few caveats. Careful attention to fluid balance is important because cerebral and pulmonary edema may be present. Xenobiotics that prolong the QT interval, such as the class IA, class IC, and class III antidysrhythmics, should be avoided (see Chap. 63). Potassium, magnesium, and calcium concentrations should be maintained within normal range to avoid exacerbating a prolonged QT interval. Glucose concentrations and glycogen stores should be maintained parenterally with dextrose and hyperalimentation solutions, or with enteral feedings, in view of their beneficial effects, in experimental models of arsenic poisoning.[123,165,166,188]

Gastrointestinal decontamination of patients acutely poisoned with arsenic is controversial. Arsenic poorly adsorbs to activated charcoal, cholestyramine, and bentonite.[163] Moreover, significantly poisoned patients usually have nausea and vomiting and may have altered mental status which make charcoal administration difficult. Despite these concerns, many medical toxicologists would give charcoal, in conjunction with airway protection if necessary, because of the relatively low likelihood of harming the patient and the hope that preventing even a small amount of absorption might prevent or lessen the potentially disastrous consequences of arsenic poisoning. If radiopaque material is visualized in the GI tract, whole-bowel irrigation can be administered until the radiopaque material is no longer visualized on repeat abdominal radiograph. Continuing nasogastric suction may be important in removing arsenic resecreted in the gastric or biliary tract. Arsenite was still detectable in the gastric aspirate in three patients 5 to 7 days following an ingestion.[128] There is no clinical experience with the use of *N*-acetylcysteine to increase glutathione levels; an animal experiment suggested a protective effect.[162]

In cases of chronic toxicity, patients should be removed from the arsenic source and gastric decontamination should be performed if there is evidence of arsenic in the GI tract. Arsenic can be readily removed from skin with soap, water, and vigorous scrubbing. In this situation, when homicidal intent is suspected, all hospital visitors should be closely monitored and outside nutritional products should be forbidden.

CHELATION THERAPY

Chelators Dimercaprol (BAL) and 2,3-dimercaptosuccinic acid (succimer) are the two chelators available in the United States. A third drug, DMPS, is distributed by Heyl, a German pharmaceutical company, as Dimaval, but it is not approved or marketed in the United States (see Antidotes in Depth, A26, A27). All contain vicinal dithiol moieties that bind arsenic to form stable 1,2,5-arsadithiolanes (Fig. 88–7), and all are most effective when administered in doses equimolar to the arsenic burden.[140] Dosing regimens and adverse effects are listed in Table 88–3.

The decision to initiate chelation therapy should depend on the clinical condition of the patient as well as the laboratory results for arsenic in urine, hair, or nails. A severely ill patient with known or suspected acute arsenic poisoning should be chelated immediately, prior to laboratory confirmation. In the United States, BAL remains the initial chelating drug for acute arsenical toxicity.[140] In a series of

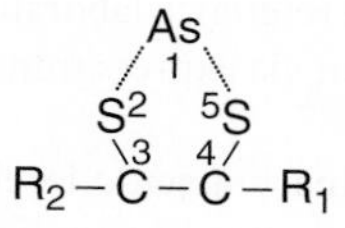

As
S2 5S
3 4
R_2–C–C–R_1

BAL adduct
R_1 = H, R_2 = CH_2OH

DMPS adduct
R_1 = H, R_2 = CH_2SO_2Na

Succimer adduct
R_1 = R_2 = COOH

FIGURE 88–7. 1,2,5-Arsadithiolane adducts with BAL, DMPS, and DMSA.

TABLE 88–3. Chelators for Arsenical Poisoning

Dosage	Adverse Effects
BAL 3–5 mg/kg every 4–6 h	Hypertension; febrile reaction; diaphoresis; nausea; vomiting; salivation; lacrimation; rhinorrhea; headache; painful injection; injection site sterile abscess; hemolysis in G6PD-deficient patients; chelation of essential metals (prolonged course)
SUCCIMER 10 mg/kg/dose every 8 h for 5 d, then 10 mg/kg/dose every 12 h	Nausea; vomiting; diarrhea; abdominal gas and pain; transient elevations of hepatic aminotransferases and alkaline phosphatase; ferases and alkaline phosphatase concentrations; rash; pruritus; sore throat; rhinorrhea; drowsiness; paresthesias; thrombocytosis; eosinophilia
DMPS (not FDA approved) Dose: 5 mg/kg/dose IM, administered as a 5% solution Day 1: q6–8h Day 2: q8–12h Day 3 and thereafter: q12–24h End point: for chelation is a 24 hour urinary arsenic concentration of <50 μg/L	Allergic reactions; increased copper and zinc excretion; nausea; pruritus; vertigo; weakness, toxic epidermal necrolysis

G6PD, glucose-6-phosphate dehydrogenase; IM, intramuscularly.

33 patients who had coma, seizures, or both, 24 patients were treated with BAL within 6 hours (mean: 1 hour) and 75% survived, compared with a survival rate of 45% of nine patients who were treated later (range: 9–72 hours; mean: 30 hours).[54] Cases of subacute and chronic toxicity can await rapid laboratory confirmation prior to beginning chelation, unless the clinical condition deteriorates.

In a cellular study of glucose uptake impaired by a lipophilic arsenical, BAL was superior to succimer and DMPS in restoring cellular equilibrium.[140] A human case series found increased survival with early use of BAL and improvement in encephalopathy within 24 hours of initiating therapy.[54] However, other acute cases treated promptly with BAL developed peripheral neuropathy.[117] In a study of subacute cases with peripheral neuropathy, BAL accelerated neurologic recovery but did not affect the overall recovery rate.[42] Despite starting BAL therapy 8 hours postexposure, a man who had ingested 2.15 g of arsenic developed severe toxicity and neurologic deficits.[60] Most concerning are the animal experiments indicating that BAL shifts arsenic into the brain and testes, two organs that have blood–organ barriers susceptible to this lipophilic drug.[10,91,107] It is clear that BAL has limitations, and that we need a safer, more effective intracellular/extracellular parenteral chelator.

Succimer is an oral hydrophilic analog of BAL and is the chelator of choice for subacute and chronic toxicity. It has proven effective in animal studies and in reported human cases.[10,106,119,127,181] In mice exposed to sodium arsenite, succimer was more effective than either DMPS or BAL in decreasing lethality, and more potent than BAL in restoring activity in the pyruvate dehydrogenase complex.[10] It is equal or superior to BAL in speeding arsenic elimination.[140] Liver function tests and essential metal concentrations should be monitored in patients requiring prolonged therapy.[63,77]

DMPS is also a water-soluble analog of BAL. It is not approved for use in the United States. It can be administered by the oral, intravenous, and intramuscular routes. It is eliminated from the body more slowly than succimer and has the advantage of intracellular as well as extracellular distribution.[7] It predominantly binds MMA^{3+} and possibly removes the MMA^{3+} from endogenous ligands. The DMPS–MMA^{3+} complex is eliminated in the urine.[9,11,74] It may also work by synergistically increasing the nonenzymatic methylation of As^{3+}.[232] Two brothers ingested nearly pure arsenic trioxide (1 and 4 g each) and were treated with intravenous and oral DMPS. The brother who ingested 4 g developed hypotension, renal failure, respiratory insufficiency, and asystolic cardiac arrest. DMPS was started 32 hours postingestion, and the patient survived with normal renal function and no neurologic dysfunction. His sibling had a milder course; DMPS was started 48 hours postingestion, and there were no neurologic sequelae on follow-up examination.[139] DMPS significantly increased biliary excretion of arsenic in a guinea pig model, but did not increase fecal excretion. The latter is most likely a result of enterohepatic recirculation of the DMPS–As complex.[163] However, in another guinea pig model, the addition of oral cholestyramine to either DMPS or DMSA increased fecal arsenic excretion; this effect cholestyranine was not seen with BAL.[140]

D-Penicillamine has not demonstrated efficacy in chelating or reversing the biochemical lesions of arsenic and should not be used. Its previous advantage of oral administration is no longer relevant with the availability of succimer.

Because of the limitations of currently available chelators, research is ongoing to find better chelators to treat arsenic toxicity. For example, some analogs of DMSA, especially its monoisoamyl ester, have increased intracellular penetration relative to the parent compound and have been shown to increase survival in arsenic-poisoned rats.[62,100] In addition to improved chelators, other treatments for arsenic toxicity are being investigated. Some rodent studies have suggested that certain micronutrients, such as zinc or selenium, can decrease arsenic toxicity.[62] However, early findings from the HEALS cohort are mixed. A cross-sectional substudy from this group revealed an inverse relationship between the severity of skin lesions and dietary intake of folate, pyridoxine, riboflavin, and vitamins A, C, and E.[231] In contrast, another study from the same cohort did not find a statistically significant relationship between the severity of skin lesions and supplementation with vitamin E, selenium, or both.[210] Until more data are available, nutritional supplementation, in the absence of dietary deficiency, remains controversial.

Hemodialysis Hemodialysis removes negligible amounts of arsenic, with or without concomitant BAL therapy, and is not indicated in patients with normal renal function.[20,83,132] In patients with renal failure, hemodialysis clearance rates have ranged from 76 to 87.5 mL/min, with or without concomitant BAL therapy.[209] In two acutely toxic patients with renal failure, total arsenic removed during a 4-hour dialysis measured 4.68 mg in one and 3.36 mg in the other. Concomitant 24-hour urinary arsenic excretions were 3.12 mg and 2.03 mg, respectively. When renal function returned, however, the 24-hour urinary excretion of arsenic far exceeded that recovered with dialysis, with reported levels of 18.99 mg in the first patient and 75 mg in the second patient.[209] There are no published rigorous data regarding hemodialysis removal of a water-soluble complex such as DMPS–As.[108]

SUMMARY

Environmental contamination of water sources has become a major health problem in many countries, including the United States. Arsenicals produce multisystem toxicity by a variety of pathophysiologic mechanisms. A thorough understanding of inorganic arsenic metabolism and excretion as well as the different clinical manifestations of acute, subacute, and chronic toxicity are necessary to avoid misdiagnosis. Chelation therapy with BAL in the United States, or with DMPS elsewhere, if available, should be started immediately in the severely ill patient. Treatment can await laboratory results for patients with subacute or chronic toxicity, unless clinical deterioration intervenes.

REFERENCES

1. Abernathy CO, Ohanian EV. Non-carcinogenic effects of inorganic arsenic. *Environ Geochem Health.* 1992;14:35-41.
2. Adelson L, George RA, Mandel A. Acute arsenic intoxication shown by roentgenograms. *Arch Intern Med.* 1961;107:401-404.
3. Ahsan H, Chen Y, Kibriya G, et al. Arsenic metabolism, genetic susceptibility and risk of premalignant skin lesions in Bangladesh. *Cancer Epidemiol Biomarkers Prev.* 2007;16:1270-1278.
4. Ahsan H, Chen Y, Parvez F, et al. Arsenic exposure from drinking water and risk of premalignant skin lesions in Bangladesh: baseline results from the health effects of arsenic longitudinal study. *Am J Epidemiol.* 2006;163:1138-1148.
5. Ahsan H, Chen Y, Parvez F, et al. Health effects of arsenic longitudinal Study (HEALS): description of a multidisciplinary epidemiologic investigation. *J Exp Sci Environ Epidemiology.* 2006;16:191-205.
6. Albores A, Cebrian ME, Bach PH, et al. Sodium arsenite induced alterations in bilirubin excretion and heme metabolism. *J Biochem Toxicol.* 1989;4:73-78.
7. Aposhian HV. Mobilization of mercury and arsenic in humans by sodium 2,3-dimercapto-1-propane sulfonate (DMPS). *Environ Health Perspect.* 1998;106(Suppl 4):1017-1025.
8. Aposhian HV, Aposhian MM. Newer developments in arsenic toxicity. *J Am Coll Toxicol.* 1989;8:1297-1305.
9. Aposhian HV, Arroyo A, Cebrian ME, et al. DMPS-arsenic challenge test. I: increased urinary excretion of monomethylarsonic acid in humans given dimercaptopropane sulfonate. *J Pharmacol Exp Ther.* 1997;282:192-200.
10. Aposhian HV, Carter DE, Hoover TD, et al. DMSA, DMPS, and DMPA-As arsenic antidotes. *Fundam Appl Toxicol.* 1984;4:S58-S70.
11. Aposhian HV, Zheng B, Aposhian MM, et al. DMPS-arsenic challenge test. II. Modulation of arsenic species, including monomethylarsonous acid (MMA^{III}), excreted in human urine. *Toxicol Appl Pharmacol.* 2000;165:74-83.
12. Arbouine MW, Wilson HK. The effect of seafood consumption on the assessment of occupational exposure to arsenic by urinary arsenic speciation measurements. *J Trace Elem.* 1992;6:153-160.
13. Armstrong CW, Stroube RB, Rubio T, et al. Outbreak of fatal arsenic poisoning caused by contaminated drinking water. *Arch Environ Health.* 1984;39:276-279.
14. Banerjee M, Sarma N, Biswas R, Roy J, et al. DNA repair deficiency leads to susceptibility to develop arsenic-induced premalignant skin lesions. *Int J Cancer.* 2008;123:283-287.
15. Bansal SK, Haldar N, Dhand UK, Chopra JS. Phrenic neuropathy in arsenic poisoning. *Chest.* 1991;100:878-880.
16. Banville B, Kesseli D. State closes New Sweden arsenic case. *Bangor Daily News*, Bangor, ME; April 19, 2006.
17. Barbey JT, Pezzullo JC, Soignet SL. Effect of arsenic trioxide on QT interval in patients with advanced malignancies. *J Clin Oncol.* 2003;21:3609-3615.
18. Beckett WS, Moore JL, Keogh JP, Bleecker ML. Acute encephalopathy due to occupational exposure to arsenic. *Br J Ind Med.* 1986;43:66-67.
19. Beckman KJ, Bauman JL, Pimental PA, et al. Arsenic-induced torsades de pointes. *Crit Care Med.* 1991;19:290-291.
20. Blythe D, Joyce DA. Clearance of arsenic by haemodialysis after acute poisoning with arsenic trioxide. *Intensive Care Med.* 2001;27:334.
21. Bolliger CT, van Zijl P, Louw JA. Multiple organ failure with the adult respiratory distress syndrome in homicidal arsenic poisoning. *Respiration.* 1992;59:57-61.
22. Boquist L, Boquist S, Ericsson I. Structural beta-cell changes and transient hyperglycemia in mice treated with compounds inducing inhibited citric acid cycle enzyme activity. *Diabetes.* 1988;37:89-98.
23. Bouletreau P, Ducluzeau R, Bui-Xuan B, et al. Acute renal complications of acute intoxications. *Acta Pharmacol Toxicol.* 1977;41(Suppl):49-63.
24. Bouteille B, Oukem O, Bisser S, Dumas M. Treatment perspectives for human African trypanosomiasis. *Fundam Clin Pharmacol.* 2003;17:171-181.
25. Brune D, Nordberg G, Wester PO. Distribution of 23 elements in the kidney, liver and lungs of workers from a smeltery and refinery in North Sweden exposed to a number of elements and of a control group. *Sci Total Environ.* 1980;16:13-35.
26. Buchet JP, Lauwerys R, Roels H. Comparison of the urinary excretion of arsenic metabolites after a single oral dose of sodium arsenite, monomethylarsonate or dimethylarsinate in man. *Int Arch Occup Environ Health.* 1981;48:71-79.
27. Bustamante J, Dock L, Vahter M, et al. The semiconductor elements arsenic and indium induce apoptosis in rat thymocytes. *Toxicology.* 1997;118:129-136.
28. Calderon J, Navarro ME, Jimenez-Capdeville ME, et al. Exposure to arsenic and lead and neuropsychological development in Mexican children. *Environ Res.* 2001;85:69-76.
29. Calderon RL, Hudgens E, Le XC, et al. Excretion of arsenic in urine as a function of exposure to arsenic in drinking water. *Environ Health Perspect.* 1999;107:663-667.
30. Chang CC, Ho SC, Tsai SS, Yang CY. Ischemic heart disease mortality reduction in an arseniasis-endemic area in southwestern Taiwan after a switch in the tap-water supply system. *J Toxicol Environ Health A.* 2004;67:1353-1361.
31. Chen B, Burt CT, Goering PL, et al. In vivo 31P nuclear magnetic resonance studies of arsenite induced changes in hepatic phosphate levels. *Biochem Biophys Res Commun.* 1986;139:228-234.
32. Chen C-J, Chuang Y-C, Lin T-M, Wu HY. Malignant neoplasms among residents of a blackfoot disease-endemic area in Taiwan: high-arsenic artesian well water and cancers. *Cancer Res.* 1985;45:5895-5899.
33. Chen GQ, Zhu J, Shi XG, et al. In vitro studies on cellular and molecular mechanisms of arsenic trioxide (As_2O_3) in the treatment of acute promyelocytic leukemia: As_2O_3 induces NB4 cell apoptosis with downregulation of Bcl-2 expression and modulation of PMLRAR alpha/PML proteins. *Blood.* 1996;88:1052-1061.
34. Chen GS, Asai T, Suzuki Y, et al. A possible pathogenesis for blackfoot disease: effects of trivalent arsenic (As_2O_3) on cultured human umbilical vein endothelial cells. *J Dermatol.* 1990;17:599-608.
35. Chen Y, Graziano JH, Parvez F, et al. Modification of risk of arsenic-induced skin lesions by sunlight exposure, smoking and occupational exposures in Bangladesh. *Epidemiology.* 2006;17:459-467.
36. Chen Z, Chen GQ, Shen ZX, et al. Treatment of acute promyelocytic leukemia with arsenic compounds: in vitro and in vivo studies. *Semin Hematol.* 2001;38:26-36.
37. Chernoff AI, Hartroft WS. Acute gastroenteritis. *Am J Med.* 1956;21:282-291.
38. Chiou HY, Chiou ST, Hsu YH, et al. Incidence of transitional cell carcinoma and arsenic in drinking water: a follow-up study of 8,102 residents in an arseniasis-endemic area in northeastern Taiwan. *Am J Epidemiol.* 2001;153:411-418.
39. Chiou HY, Huang WI, Su CL, et al. Dose–response relationship between prevalence of cerebrovascular disease and ingested inorganic arsenic. *Stroke.* 1997;28:1717-1723.
40. Chiu HF, Ho SC, Wang LY, et al. Does arsenic exposure increase the risk for liver cancer? *J Toxicol Environ Health A.* 2004;67:1491-1500.
41. Chu HA, Crawford-Brown DJ. Inorganic arsenic in drinking water and bladder cancer: a meta-analysis for dose-response assessment. *Int J Environ Res Public Health.* 2006;3(4):316-322.
42. Chuttani PN, Chawla LS, Sharma TD. Arsenical neuropathy. *Neurology.* 1967;17:269-274.
43. Concha G, Nermell B, Vahter MV. Metabolism of inorganic arsenic in children with chronic high arsenic exposure in northern Argentina. *Environ Health Perspect.* 1998;106:355-359.
44. Concha G, Vogler G, Nermell B, Vahter M. Low-level arsenic excretion in breast milk of native Andean women exposed to high levels of arsenic in the drinking water. *Int Arch Occup Environ Health.* 1998;71:42-46.
45. Cullen NM, Wolf LR, St. Clair D. Pediatric arsenic ingestion. *Am J Emerg Med.* 1995;13:432-435.
46. Dakeishi M, Murata K, Grandjean P. Long-term consequences of arsenic poisoning during infancy due to contaminated milk powder. *Environ Health.* 2006;5:31.

47. De Kimpe J, Cornelis R, Mees L, et al. More than tenfold increase of arsenic in serum and packed cells of chronic hemodialysis patients. *Am J Nephrol.* 1993;13:429-434.
48. DeChaudhuri S, Kundu M, Banerjee M, Das JK, et al. Arsenic-induced health effects and genetic damage in keratotic individuals: involvement of p53 arginine variant and chromosomal aberrations in arsenic susceptibility. *Mutat Res.* 2008 ;659:118-25.
49. Del Razo LM, Arellano MA, Cebrian ME. The oxidation states of arsenic in well-water from a chronic arsenicism area of northern Mexico. *Eviron Pollut.* 1990;64:143-153.
50. Delnomdedieu M, Basti MM, Otvos JD, Thomas DJ. Reduction and binding of arsenate and dimethylarsinate by glutathione: a magnetic resonance study. *Chem Biol Interact.* 1994;90:139-155.
51. DeSesso JM, Jacobson CF, Scialli AR, et al. An assessment of the developmental toxicity of inorganic arsenic. *Reprod Toxicol.* 1998;12:385-433.
52. Drolet B, Simard C, Roden DM. Unusual effects of a QT-prolonging drug, arsenic trioxide, on cardiac potassium currents. *Circulation.* 2004;109:26-29.
53. Du Pont O, Ariel I, Warren SL. The distribution of radioactive arsenic in the normal and tumor-bearing (Brown-Pearce) rabbit. *Am J Syph Gonorrhea Vener Dis.* 1941;26:96-118.
54. Eagle H, Magnuson HJ. The systemic treatment of 227 cases of arsenic poisoning (encephalitis, dermatitis, blood dyscrasias, jaundice, fever) with 2,3-dimercaptopropanol (BAL). *J Clin Invest.* 1946;25:420-441.
55. Edmonds JS, Shibata Y, Francesconi KA, et al. Arsenic transformations in short marine food chains studied by HPLC-ICP MS. *Appl Organometal Chem.* 1997;11:281-287.
56. Eichner ER. Erythroid karyorrhexis in the peripheral blood smear in severe arsenic poisoning: a comparison with lead poisoning. *Am J Clin Pathol.* 1984;81:533-537.
57. Environmental Protection Agency. National primary drinking water regulations; arsenic and clarifications to compliance and new source contaminants monitoring. Proposed rules. 40 CFR Parts 141 and 142. *Fed Reg.* 2000;65:63027-63035.
58. Feldmann J, Lai VW, Cullen WR, et al. Sample preparation and storage can change arsenic speciation in human urine. *Clin Chem.* 1999;45:1988-1997.
59. Fernandez-Sola J, Nogue S, Grau JM, et al. Acute arsenical myopathy: morphological description. *J Toxicol Clin Toxicol.* 1991;29:131-136.
60. Fesmire FM, Schauben JL, Roberge RJ. Survival following massive arsenic ingestion. *Am J Emerg Med.* 1988;6:602-606.
61. Fincher R-ME, Koerker RM. Long-term survival in acute arsenic encephalopathy: follow-up using newer measures of electrophysiologic parameters. *Am J Med.* 1987;82:549-552.
62. Flora SJS, Flora G, Saxena G, Mishra M. Arsenic and lead induced free radical generation and their reversibility following chelation. *Cell Mol Biol.* 2007;53(1):26-47.
63. Fournier L, Thomas G, Garnier R, et al. 2,3-Dimercaptosuccinic-acid treatment of heavy metal poisoning in humans. *Med Toxicol.* 1988;3:499-504.
64. Freeman JW, Crouch JR. Prolonged encephalopathy with arsenic poisoning. *Neurology.* 1978;28:853-855.
65. Gamble MV, Liu X, Ahsan H, et al. Folate and arsenic metabolism: a double-blind, placebo-controlled folic acid-supplementation trial in Bangladesh. *Am J Clin Nutr.* 2006;84:1093-1101.
66. Gamble MV, Liu X, Ahsan H, et al. Folate, homocysteine and arsenic metabolism in arsenic-exposed individuals in Bangladesh. *Environ Health Perspect.* 2005;113:1683-1688.
67. Gamble MV, Liu X, Slakovich V, Pilsner JR, et al. Folic acid supplementation lowers blood arsenic. *Am J Clin Nutr.* 2007;86:1202-1209.
68. Garb LG, Hine CH. Arsenical neuropathy: residual effects following acute industrial exposure. *J Occup Med.* 1977;19:567-568.
69. Gartenhaus RB, Prachand SN, Paniaqua M, et al. Arsenic trioxide cytotoxicity in steroid and chemotherapy-resistant myeloma cell lines: enhancement of apoptosis by manipulation of cellular redox state. *Clin Cancer Res.* 2002;8:566-572.
70. Gerhardt RE, Hudson JB, Rao RN, Sobel RE. Chronic renal insufficiency from cortical necrosis induced by arsenic poisoning. *Arch Intern Med.* 1978;138:1267-1269.
71. Germolec DR, Spalding J, Yu HS, et al. Arsenic enhancement of skin neoplasia by chronic stimulation of growth factors. *Am J Pathol.* 1998;153:1775-1785.
72. Goebel HH, Schmidt PF, Bohl J, et al. Polyneuropathy due to acute arsenic intoxication: biopsy studies. *J Neuropathol Exp Neurol.* 1990;49:137-149.
73. Goldsmith S, From AHL. Arsenic-induced atypical ventricular tachycardia. *N Engl J Med.* 1980;303:1096-1098.
74. Gong Z, Jiang G, Cullen WR, et al. Determination of arsenic metabolic complex excreted in human urine after administration of sodium 2,3-dimercapto-1-propane sulfonate. *Chem Res Toxicol.* 2002;15:1318-1323.
75. Gousios AG, Adelson L. Electrocardiographic and radiographic findings in acute arsenic poisoning. *Am J Med.* 1959;27:659-663.
76. Gray JR, Khalil A, Prior JC. Acute arsenic toxicity—an opaque poison. *Can Assoc Radiol J.* 1989;40:226-227.
77. Graziano JH, Cuccia D, Friedheim E. The pharmacology of 2,3-dimercaptosuccinic acid and its potential use in arsenic poisoning. *J Pharmacol Exp Ther.* 1978;207:1051-1055.
78. Greenberg C, Davies S, McGowan T, et al. Acute respiratory failure following severe arsenic poisoning. *Chest.* 1979;76:596-598.
79. Griffin JP. Famous names: the Esing Bakery, Hong Kong. *Adverse Drug React Toxicol Rev.* 1997;16:79-81.
80. Guha Mazumder DN. Arsenic and non-malignant lung disease. *J Environ Sci Health A Tox Hazard Subst Environ Eng.* 2007;42:1859-1867.
81. Hafeman DM, Ahsan H, Louis ED, et al. Association between arsenic exposure and a measure of subclinical sensory neuropathy in Bangladesh. *JOEN.* 2005;47:778-784.
82. Halicka HD, Smolewski P, Darzynkiewicz Z, et al. Arsenic trioxide arrests cells early in mitosis leading to apoptosis. *Cell Cycle.* 2002;1:201-209.
83. Hantson P, Haufroid V, Buchet JP, Mahieu P. Acute arsenic poisoning treated by intravenous dimercaptosuccinic acid (DMSA) and combined extrarenal epuration techniques. *J Toxicol Clin Toxicol.* 2003;41:1-6.
84. Heck JE, Gamble MV, Chen Y, et al. Consumption of folate-related nutrients and metabolism of arsenic in Bangladesh. *Am J Clin Nutr.* 2007;85:1367-1374.
85. Heck JE, Nievea JW, Chen Y, et al. Dietary intake of methionine, cycteine and protein and urinary arsenic excretion in Bangladesh. *Environ Health Perspect.* 2009;117:99-104.
86. Hessl SM, Berman E. Severe peripheral neuropathy after exposure to monosodium methylarsonate. *J Toxicol Clin Toxicol.* 1982;19:281-287.
87. Heyman A, Pfeiffer JB, Willett RW. Peripheral neuropathy caused by arsenical intoxication: a study of 41 cases with observations on the effects of BAL (2,3-dimercaptopropanol). *N Engl J Med.* 1956;254:401-409.
88. Hilfer RJ, Mandel A. Acute arsenic intoxication diagnosed by roentgenograms. *N Engl J Med.* 1962;266:663-664.
89. Hindmarsh JT, McLetchie OR, Heffernan LPM, et al. Electromyographic abnormalities in chronic environmental arsenicalism. *J Anal Toxicol.* 1977;1:270-276.
90. Hirata M, Tanaka A, Hisanaga A, Ishinishi N. Effects of glutathione depletion on the acute nephrotoxic potential of arsenite and on arsenic metabolism in hamsters. *Toxicol Appl Pharmacol.* 1990;106:469-481.
91. Hoover TD, Aposhian HV. BAL increases the arsenic-74 content of rabbit brain. *Toxicol Appl Pharmacol.* 1983;70:160-162.
92. Hsueh YM, Chiou HY, Huang YL, et al. Serum beta-carotene level, arsenic methylation capability, and incidence of skin cancer. *Cancer Epidemiol Biomarkers Prev.* 1997;6:589-596.
93. Huang R-N, Lee T-C. Cellular uptake of trivalent arsenite and pentavalent arsenate in KB cells cultured in phosphate-free medium. *Toxicol Appl Pharmacol.* 1996;136:243-249.
94. Huang Y, Zhang J, McHenry KT, Kim, MM, et al. Induction of cytoplasmic accumulation of p53: a mechanism for low levels of arsenic exposure to predispose cells for malignant transformation. *Cancer Res.* 2008;68:9131-9136.
95. Hunt E, Hader SL, Files D, Corey GR. Arsenic poisoning seen at Duke Hospital, 1965-1998. *N C Med J.* 1999;60:70-74.
96. Hutton JT, Christians BL, Dippel RL. Arsenic poisoning. *N Engl J Med.* 1982;307:1080.
97. Jing Y, Dai J, Chalmers-Redman RM, et al. Arsenic trioxide selectively induces acute promyelocytic leukemia cell apoptosis via a hydrogen peroxide-dependent pathway. *Blood.* 1999;94:2102-2111.
98. Johnson LR, Farmer JG. Use of human metabolic studies and urinary arsenic speciation in assessing arsenic exposure. *Bull Environ Contam Toxicol.* 1991;46:53-61.
99. Jolliffe DM, Budd AJ, Gwilt DJ. Massive acute arsenic poisoning. *Anaesthesia.* 1991;46:288-290.
100. Kalia K, Flora SJS. Strategies for safe and effective therapeutic measures for chronic arsenic and lead poisoning. *J Occup Health.* 2005;47:1-21.
101. Kasper ML, Schoenfield L, Strom RL, Theologides A. Hepatic angiosarcoma and bronchioloalveolar carcinoma induced by Fowler's solution. *JAMA.* 1984;252:3407-3408.

102. Kenyon EM, Hughes MF. A concise review of the toxicity and carcinogenicity of dimethylarsinic acid. *Toxicology*. 2001;160:227-236.
103. Kersjes MP, Maurer JR, Trestrail JH. An analysis of arsenic exposures referred to the Blodgett regional poison center. *Vet Hum Toxicol*. 1987;29:75-78.
104. Koons RD, Peters CA. Axial distribution of arsenic in individual human hairs by solid sampling graphite furnace AAS. *J Anal Toxicol*. 1994;18:36-40.
105. Kreiss K, Zack MM, Landrigan PJ, et al. Neurologic evaluation of a population exposed to arsenic in Alaskan well water. *Arch Environ Health*. 1983;38:116-121.
106. Kreppel H, Reichl FX, Kleine A, et al. Antidotal efficacy of newly synthesized dimercaptosuccinic acid (DMSA) monoesters in experimental arsenic poisoning in mice. *Fund Appl Toxicol*. 1995;26:239-245.
107. Kreppel H, Reichl FX, Szinicz L, et al. Efficacy of various dithiol compounds in acute As_2O_3 poisoning in mice. *Arch Toxicol*. 1990;64:387-392.
108. Kruszewska S, Wiese M, Kolacinski Z, Mielczarska J. The use of haemodialysis and 2,3-propanesulphonate (DMPS) to manage acute oral poisoning by lethal dose of arsenic trioxide. *Int J Occup Med Environ Health*. 1996;9:111-115.
109. Kumana CR, Au WY, Lee NS, et al. Systemic availability of arsenic from oral arsenic-trioxide used to treat patients with hematological malignancies. *Eur J Clin Pharmacol*. 2002;58:521-526.
110. Kwok RK, Kaufmann RB, Jakariya M. Arsenic in drinking water and reproductive health outcomes: a study of participants in the Bangladesh Integrated Nutrition Programme. *J Health Popul Nutr*. 2006;24:190-205.
111. Kwong YL. Arsenic trioxide in the treatment of haematological malignancies. *Expert Opin Drug Saf*. 2004;3:589-597.
112. Kyle RA, Pease GL. Hematologic aspects of arsenic intoxication. *N Engl J Med*. 1965;271:18-23.
113. Lagerkvist BE, Linderholm H, Nordberg GF. Arsenic and Raynaud's phenomenon. Vasospastic tendency and excretion of arsenic in smelter workers before and after the summer vacation. *Int Arch Occup Environ Health*. 1988;60:361-364.
114. Lai MS, Hsueh YM, Chen CJ, et al. Ingested inorganic arsenic and prevalence of diabetes mellitus. *Am J Epidemiol*. 1994;139:484-492.
115. Lander JJ, Stanley RJ, Sumner HW, et al. Angiosarcoma of the liver associated with Fowler's solution (potassium arsenite). *Gastroenterology*. 1975;68:1582-1586.
116. Le XC, Cullen WR, Reimer KJ. Human urinary arsenic excretion after one-time ingestion of seaweed, crab, and shrimp. *Clin Chem*. 1994;40:617-624.
117. Le Quesne PM, McLeod J. Peripheral neuropathy following a single exposure to arsenic: clinical course in four patients with electrophysiological and histological studies. *J Neurol Sci*. 1977;32:437-451.
118. Lee MY, Bae ON, Chung SM, et al. Enhancement of platelet aggregation and thrombus formation by arsenic in drinking water: a contributing factor to cardiovascular disease. *Toxicol Appl Pharmacol*. 2002;179:83-88.
119. Lenz K, Hruby K, Druml W, et al. 2,3-Dimercaptosuccinic acid in human arsenic poisoning. *Arch Toxicol*. 1981;47:241-243.
120. Lerman BB, Ali N, Green D. Megaloblastic, dyserythropoietic anemia following arsenic ingestion. *Ann Clin Lab Sci*. 1980;10:515-517.
121. Li L, Ekström EC, Goessler W, Lönnerdal B, et al. Nutritional status has marginal influence on the metabolism of inorganic arsenic in pregnant Bangladeshi women. *Environ Health Perspect*. 2008;116:315-321.
122. Li Y, Chen Y, Slavkovic V, et al. Serum levels of the extracellular domain of the epidermal growth factor receptor in individuals exposed to arsenic in drinking water in Bangladesh. *Biomarkers*. 2007;12:256-265.
123. Liebl B, Muckter H, Doklea E, et al. Influence of glucose on the toxicity of oxophenylarsine in MDCK cells. *Arch Toxicol*. 1995;69:421-424.
124. Lu DP, Wang Q. Current study of APL treatment in China. *Int J Hematol*. 2005;202(Suppl 01):316-318.
125. Lugo G, Cassady G, Palmisano P. Acute maternal arsenic intoxication with neonatal death. *Am J Dis Child*. 1969;117:328-330.
126. Mackell MA, Gantner GE, Poklis A, Graham M. An unsuspected arsenic poisoning murder disclosed by forensic autopsy. *Am J Forensic Med Pathol*. 1985;6:358-361.
127. Maehashi H, Murata Y. Arsenic excretion after treatment of arsenic poisoning with DMSA or DMPS in mice. *Jpn J Pharmacol*. 1986;40:188-190.
128. Mahieu P, Buchet JP, Roels HA, Lauwerys R. The metabolism of arsenic in humans acutely intoxicated by As_2O_3: its significance for the duration of BAL therapy. *Clin Toxicol*. 1981;18:1067-1075.
129. Mass MJ, Tennant A, Roop BC, et al. Methylated trivalent arsenic species are genotoxic. *Chem Res Toxicol*. 2001;14:355-361.
130. Massey EW, Wold D, Heyman A. Arsenic: homicidal intoxication. *South Med J*. 1984;77:848-851.
131. Mathews V, Balasubramanian P, Shaji RV, et al. Arsenic trioxide in the treatment of newly diagnosed acute promyelocytic leukemia: a single center experience. *Am J Hematol*. 2002;70:292-299.
132. Mathieu D, Mathieu-Nolf M, Germain-Alonso M, et al. Massive arsenic poisoning—effect of hemodialysis and dimercaprol on arsenic kinetics. *Intensive Care Med*. 1992;18:47-50.
133. Mazumder DN, Das GJ, Santra A, et al. Chronic arsenic toxicity in west Bengal—the worst calamity in the world. *J Indian Med Assoc*. 1998;96: 4-7:18.
134. McKinney JD. Metabolism and disposition of inorganic arsenic in laboratory animals and humans. *Environ Geochem Health*. 1992;14:43-48.
135. Mealey J, Brownell GL, Sweet WH. Radioarsenic in plasma, urine, normal tissues, and intracranial neoplasms. *Arch Neurol Psychiatry*. 1959;8: 310-320.
136. Meliker JR, Wahl RL, Cameron LL, Nriagu JO. Arsenic in drinking water and cerebrovascular disease, diabetes mellitus, and kidney disease in Michigan: a standardized mortality ratio analysis. *Environ Health*. 2007;6:4.
137. Melnick A, Licht JD. Deconstructing a disease: RARα, its fusion partners, and their roles in the pathogenesis of acute promyelocytic leukemia. *Blood*. 1999;93:3167-3215.
138. Montesinos P, Bergua JM, Vellenga E, et al. Differentiation syndrome in patients with acute promeylocytic leukemia treated with all-trans retinoic acid and anthracycline chemotherapy: characteristics, outcome, and prognostic factors. *Blood*. 2009;113:775-783.
139. Moore DF, O'Callaghan CA, Berlyne G, et al. Acute arsenic poisoning: absence of polyneuropathy after treatment with 2,3-dimercaptopropanesulphonate (DMPS). *J Neurol Neurosurg Psychiatry*. 1994;57: 1133-1135.
140. Muckter H, Liebl B, Reichl FX, et al. Are we ready to replace dimercaprol (BAL) as an arsenic antidote? *Hum Exp Toxicol*. 1997;16:460-465.
141. Mukherjee SC, Rahman MM, Chowdhury UK, et al. Neuropathy in arsenic toxicity from groundwater arsenic contamination in West Bengal, India. *J Environ Sci Health A Tox Hazard Subst Environ Eng*. 2003;38: 165-183.
142. Murgo AJ. Clinical trials of arsenic trioxide in hematologic and solid tumors: overview of the National Cancer Institute Cooperative Research and Development Studies. *Oncologist*. 2001;6(Suppl 2):22-28.
143. Navas-Acien A, Silbergeld EK, Pastor-Barriuso R, Guallar E. Arsenic exposure and prevalence of Type 2 diabetes in US adults. *JAMA*. 2008;300: 814-822.
144. Niu C, Yan H, Yu T, et al. Studies on treatment of acute promyelocytic leukemia with arsenic trioxide: remission induction, follow-up, and molecular monitoring in 11 newly diagnosed and 47 relapsed acute promyelocytic leukemia patients. *Blood*. 1999;94:3315-3324.
145. Nixon DE, Moyer TP. Arsenic analysis II. Rapid separation and quantification of inorganic arsenic plus metabolites and arsenobetaine from urine. *Clin Chem*. 1992;38:2479-2483.
146. Oh SJ. Electrophysiological profile in arsenic neuropathy. *J Neurol Neurosurg Psychiatry*. 1991;54:1103-1105.
147. Ohnishi K, Yoshida H, Shigeno K, et al. Prolongation of the QT interval and ventricular tachycardia in patients treated with arsenic trioxide for acute promyelocytic leukemia. *Ann Intern Med*. 2000;133:881-885.
148. Park MJ, Currier M. Arsenic exposures in Mississippi: a review of cases. *South Med J*. 1991;84:461-464.
149. Parvez F, Chen Y, Brand-Rauf PW, et al. Nonmalignant respiratory effects of chronic arsenic exposure from drinking water among never-smokers in Bangladesh. *Environ Health Perspect*. 2008;116:190-195.
150. Paul DS, Harmon AW, Devesa V, et al. Molecular mechanisms of the diabetogenic effects of arsenic: inhibition of insulin signaling by arsenite and methylarsonous acid. *Environ Health Perspect*. 2007;115:734-741.
151. Paul PC, Chattopadhyay A, Dutta SK, et al. Histopathology of skin lesions in chronic arsenic toxicity—grading of changes and study of proliferative markers. *Indian J Pathol Microbiol*. 2000;43:257-264.
152. Pepin J, Milord F. African trypanosomiasis and drug-induced encephalopathy: risk factors and pathogenesis. *Trans R Soc Trop Med Hyg*. 1991;85: 222-224.
153. Peters HA, Croft WA, Woolson EA, et al. Seasonal arsenic exposure from burning chromium-copper-arsenate treated wood. *JAMA*. 1984;251: 2393-2396.

154. Petrick JS, Ayala-Fierro F, Cullen WR, et al. Monomethylarsonous acid (MMA^{III}) is more toxic than arsenite in Chang human hepatocytes. *Toxicol Appl Pharmacol.* 2000;163:203-207.
155. Petrick JS, Jagadish B, Mash EA, Aposhian HV. Monomethylarsonous acid (MMA^{III}) and arsenite: LD_{50} in hamsters and in vitro inhibition of pyruvate dehydrogenase. *Chem Res Toxicol.* 2001;14:651-656.
156. Pilsner JR, Liu X, Ahsan H, et al. Genomic methylation of peripheral blood leukocyte DNA: influences of arsenic and folate in Bangladesh adults. *Am J Clin Nutr.* 2007;86:1179-1186.
157. Pomroy C, Charbonneau SM, McCullough RS, Tam GK. Human retention studies with ^{74}As. *Toxicol Appl Pharmacol.* 1980;53:550-556.
158. Pu YS, Uang SM, Huang YK, Chung CJ, et al. Urinary arsenic profile affects the risk of urothelial carcinoma even at low arsenic exposure. *Toxicol Appl Pharmacol.* 2007;218:99-106.
159. Raab A, Feldmann J. Arsenic speciation in hair extracts. *Anal Bioanal Chem.* 2005;381:332-338.
160. Rahman A, Vahter M, Ekstrom EC, et al. Association of arsenic exposure during pregnancy with fetal loss and infant death: a cohort study in Bangladesh. *Am J Epidemiol.* 2007;165:1389-1396.
161. Rahman M, Tondel M, Ahmad SA, Axelson O. Diabetes mellitus associated with arsenic exposure in Bangladesh. *Am J Epidemiol.* 1998;148: 198-203.
162. Ramos O, Carrizales L, Yanez L, et al. Arsenic increased lipid peroxidation in rat tissues by a mechanism independent of glutathione levels. *Environ Health Perspect.* 1995;103(Suppl 1):85-88.
163. Reichl F-X, Hunder G, Liebl B, et al. Effect of DMPS and various adsorbents on the arsenic excretion in guinea-pigs after injection with As_2O_3. *Arch Toxicol.* 1995;69:712-717.
164. Reichl F-X, Kreppel H, Forth W. Pyruvate and lactate metabolism in livers of guinea pigs perfused with chelation agents after repeated treatment with As_2O_3. *Arch Toxicol.* 1991;65:235-238.
165. Reichl F-X, Kreppel H, Szinicz L, et al. Effect of glucose treatment on carbohydrate content in various organs in mice after acute As_2O_3 poisoning. *Vet Hum Toxicol.* 1991;33:230-235.
166. Reichl F-X, Szinicz L, Kreppel H, Forth W. Effects of arsenic on carbohydrate metabolism after single or repeated injection in guinea pigs. *Arch Toxicol.* 1988;62:473-475.
167. Rein KA, Borrebaek B, Bremer J. Arsenite inhibits β-oxidation in isolated rat liver mitochondria. *Biochim Biophys Acta.* 1979;574:487-494.
168. Robinson TJ. Arsenical polyneuropathy due to caustic arsenical paste. *Br Med J.* 1975;3:139.
169. Rojewski MT, Korper S, Thiel E, Schrezenmeier H. Depolarization of mitochondria and activation of caspases are common features of arsenic(III)-induced apoptosis in myelogenic and lymphatic cell lines. *Chem Res Toxicol.* 2004;17:119-128.
170. Rosado JL, Ronquillo D, Kordas K, et al. Arsenic exposure and cognitive performance in Mexican schoolchildren. *Environ Health Perspect.* 2007;115:1371-1375.
171. Roses OE, Garcia Fernandez JC, Villaamil EC, et al. Mass poisoning by sodium arsenite. *J Toxicol Clin Toxicol.* 1991;29:209-213.
172. Rust DM, Soignet SL. Risk/benefit profile of arsenic trioxide. *Oncologist.* 2001;6(Suppl 2):29-32.
173. Samanta G, Das D, Manda BK, et al. Arsenic in the breast milk of lactating women in arsenic affected areas of West Bengal, India and its effect on infants. *J Environ Sci Health A Tox Hazard Subst Environ Enf.* 2007;42:1815-1825.
174. Santra A, Maiti A, Das S, et al. Hepatic damage caused by chronic arsenic toxicity in experimental animals. *J Toxicol Clin Toxicol.* 2000;38: 395-405.
175. Sanz P, Corbella J, Nogue S, et al. Rhabdomyolysis in fatal arsenic trioxide poisoning. *JAMA.* 1989;262:3271.
176. Savory J, Sedor FA. Arsenic poisoning. In: Brown SS, ed. *Clinical Chemistry and Chemical Toxicology of Metals.* New York: Elsevier/North Holland; 1977:271-286.
177. Schoof RA, Yost LJ, Eickhoff J, et al. A market basket survey of inorganic arsenic in food. *Food Chem Toxicol.* 1999;37:839-846.
178. Schoolmeester WL, White DR. Arsenic poisoning. *South Med J.* 1980;73: 198-208.
179. Shen Y, Shen ZX, Yan H, et al. Studies on the clinical efficacy and pharmacokinetics of low-dose arsenic trioxide in the treatment of relapsed acute promyelocytic leukemia: a comparison with conventional dosage. *Leukemia.* 2001;15:735-741.
180. Shen ZX, Chen GQ, Ni JH, et al. Use of arsenic trioxide (As_2O_3) in the treatment of acute promyelocytic leukemia (APL): II. Clinical efficacy and pharmacokinetics in relapsed patients. *Blood.* 1997;89: 3354-3360.
181. Shum S, Whitehead J, Vaughn L, Hale T. Chelation of organoarsenate with dimercaptosuccinic acid. *Vet Hum Toxicol.* 1995;37:239-242.
182. Smith AH, Marshal G, Yuan Y, et al. Increased mortality from lung cancer and bronchiectasis in young adults after exposure to arsenic in utero and in early childhood. *Environ Health Perspect.* 2006;114: 1293-1296.
183. Soignet SL, Frankel SR, Douer D, et al. United States multicenter study of arsenic trioxide in relapsed acute promyelocytic leukemia. *J Clin Oncol.* 2001;19:3852-3860.
184. Soignet SL, Tong WP, Hirschfeld S, Warrell RP Jr. Clinical study of an organic arsenical, melarsoprol, in patients with advanced leukemia. *Cancer Chemother Pharmacol.* 1999;44:417-421.
185. St. Petery J, Gross C, Victorica BE. Ventricular fibrillation caused by arsenic poisoning. *Am J Dis Child.* 1970;120:367-371.
186. Stevens JT, Hall LL, Farmer JD, et al. Disposition of ^{14}C and/or ^{74}As-cacodylic acid in rats after intravenous, intratracheal, or peroral administration. *Environ Health Perspect.* 1977;19:151-157.
187. Styblo M, Yamauchi H, Thomas DJ. Comparative in vitro methylation of trivalent and pentavalent arsenicals. *Toxicol Appl Pharmacol.* 1995;135:172-178.
188. Szinicz L, Forth W. Effect of As_2O_3 on gluconeogenesis. *Arch Toxicol.* 1988;61:444-449.
189. Szuler IM, Williams CN, Hindmarsh JT, Park-Dincsoy H. Massive variceal hemorrhage secondary to presinusoidal portal hypertension due to arsenic poisoning. *Can Med Assoc J.* 1979;120:168-171.
190. Tam GK, Charbonneau SM, Bryce F, et al. Metabolism of inorganic arsenic (^{74}As) in humans following oral ingestion. *Toxicol Appl Pharmacol.* 1979;50:319-322.
191. Tay CH, Seah CS. Arsenic poisoning from anti-asthmatic herbal preparations. *Med J Aust.* 1975;2:424-428.
192. Toribara TY. Analysis of single hair by XRF discloses mercury in-take. *Hum Exp Toxicol.* 2001;20:185-188.
193. Toribara TY, Jackson DA, French WR, et al. Nondestructive X-ray fluorescence spectrometry for determination of trace elements along a single strand of hair. *Anal Chem.* 1982;54:1844-1849.
194. Tsai SY, Chou HY, The HW, Chen CM, Chen CJ. The effects of chronic arsenic exposure from drinking water on the neurobehavioral development in adolescence. *Neurotoxicology.* 2003;24:747-753.
195. Tseng CH, Chong CK, Chen CJ, Tai TY. Dose–response relationship between peripheral vascular disease and ingested inorganic arsenic among residents in blackfoot disease endemic villages in Taiwan. *Atherosclerosis.* 1996;120:125-133.
196. Tseng CH, Huang YK, Huang YL, et al. Arsenic exposure, urinary arsenic speciation, and peripheral vascular disease in blackfoot disease-hyperendemic villages in Taiwan. *Toxicol Appl Pharmacol.* 2005;206: 299-308.
197. Tseng CH, Tai TY, Chong CK, et al. Long-term arsenic exposure and incidence of non-insulin-dependent diabetes mellitus: a cohort study in arseniasis-hyperendemic villages in Taiwan. *Environ Health Perspect.* 2000;108:847-851.
198. Tsukamoto H, Parker HR, Gribble DH. Metabolism and renal handling of sodium arsenate in dogs. *Am J Vet Res.* 1983;44:2331-2335.
199. Tsukamoto H, Parker HR, Gribble DH, et al. Nephrotoxicity of sodium arsenate in dogs. *Am J Vet Res.* 1983;44:2324-2330.
200. Uede K, Furukawa F. Skin manifestations in acute arsenic poisoning from the Wakayama curry-poisoning incident. *Brit J of Derm.* 2003;149: 757-762.
201. Unnikrishnan D, Dutcher JP, Varshneya N, et al. Torsades de pointes in 3 patients with leukemia treated with arsenic trioxide. *Blood.* 2001;97: 1514-1516.
202. Vahter M. Genetic polymorphism in the biotransformation of inorganic arsenic and its role in toxicity. *Toxicol Lett.* 2000;112-113:209-217.
203. Vahter M. Health effects of early life exposure to arsenic. *Basic Clin Pharmacol Toxicol.* 2008;102:204-211.
204. Vahter M. Mechanisms of arsenic biotransformation. *Toxicology.* 2002; 181-182:2111-2117.
205. Vahter M. Metabolism of arsenic. In: Fowler BA, ed. *Biological and Environmental Effects of Arsenic.* New York: Elsevier; 1983:171-198.

206. Vahter M. Methylation of inorganic arsenic in different mammalian species and population groups. *Sci Prog.* 1999;82(Pt 1):69-88.
207. Vahter M, Marafante E. Effects of low dietary intake of methionine, choline or proteins on the biotransformation of arsenite in the rabbit. *Toxicol Lett.* 1987;37:41-46.
208. Vahter M, Marafante E. Intracellular interaction and metabolic fate of arsenite and arsenate in mice and rabbits. *Chem Biol Interact.* 1983;47:29-44.
209. Vaziri ND, Upham T, Barton CH. Hemodialysis clearance of arsenic. *Clin Toxicol.* 1980;17:451-456.
210. Verret WJ, Chen Y, Ahmed A, et al. Effects of vitamin E and selenium on arsenic-induced skin lesions. *JOEM.* 2005;47:1026-1035.
211. Von Ehrenstein OS, Poddar S, Yuan Y, et al. Children's intellectual function in relation to arsenic exposure. *Epidemiology.* 2007;18:44-51.
212. Wagner SL, Weswig P. Arsenic in blood and urine of forest workers. *Arch Environ Health.* 1974;28:77-79.
213. Walton FS, Harmon AW, et al. Inhibition of insulin-dependent glucose uptake by trivalent arsenicals: possible mechanism of arsenic-induced diabetes. *Toxicol Appl Pharmacol.* 2004;198:424-433.
214. Wang A, Holladay SD, Wolf DC, Ahmed SA, Robertson JL. Reproductive and developmental toxicity of arsenic in rodents: a review. *Int J Toxicol.* 2006;25:319-331.
215. Wang CH, Hsiao CK, Chen CL Hsu LI, et al. A review of the epidemiologic literature on the role of the environmental arsenic exposure and cardiovascular diseases. *Toxicol Appl Pharmacol.* 2007;222:315-326.
216. Wasserman GA, Liu X, Parvez F, et al. Water arsenic exposure and children's intellectual function in Araihazar, Bangladesh. *Environ Health Perspect.* 2004;112:1329-1333.
217. Wasserman GA, Liu X, Parvez F, et al. Water arsenic exposure and intellectual function in 6-year-old children in Araihazar, Bangladesh. *Environ Health Perspect.* 2007;115:285-289.
218. Wax PM, Thornton CA. Recovery from severe arsenic-induced peripheral neuropathy with 2,3-dimercapto-1-propanesulphonic acid. *J Toxicol Clin Toxicol.* 2000;38:777-780.
219. Wennig R. Potential problems with the interpretation of hair analysis results. *Forensic Sci Int.* 2000;107:5-12.
220. Wester PO, Brune D, Nordberg G. Arsenic and selenium in lung, liver, and kidney tissue from dead smelter workers. *Br J Ind Med.* 1981;38:179-184.
221. Wester RC, Maibach HI, Sedik L, et al. In vivo and in vitro percutaneous absorption and skin decontamination of arsenic from water and soil. *Fundam Appl Toxicol.* 1993;20:336-340.
222. Westervelt P, Brown RA, Adkins DR, et al. Sudden death among patients with acute promyelocytic leukemia treated with arsenic trioxide. *Blood.* 2001;98:266-271.
223. Winski SL, Carter DE. Arsenate toxicity in human erythrocytes: characterization of morphologic changes and determination of the mechanism of damage. *J Toxicol Environ Health A.* 1998;53:345-355.
224. Wong SS, Tan KC, Goh CL. Cutaneous manifestations of chronic arsenicism: review of seventeen cases. *J Am Acad Dermatol.* 1998;38(2 Pt 1):179-185.
225. Woollons A, Russell-Jones R. Chronic endemic hydroarsenicism. *Br J Dermatol.* 1998;139:1092-1096.
226. Yamanaka K, Hasegawa A, Sawamura R, Okada S. Dimethylated arsenics induce DNA strand breaks in lung via the production of active oxygen in mice. *Biochem Biophys Res Commun.* 1989;165:43-50.
227. Yamato N. Concentrations and chemical species of arsenic in human urine and hair. *Bull Environ Contam Toxicol.* 1988;40:633-640.
228. Yamauchi H, Yamamura Y. Concentration and chemical species of arsenic in human tissue. *Bull Environ Contam Toxicol.* 1983;31:267-270.
229. Yoshida T, Yamauchi H, Fan SG. Chronic health effects in people exposed to arsenic via the drinking water: dose–response relationships in review. *Toxicol Appl Pharmacol.* 2004;198:243-252.
230. Young EG, Smith RP. Arsenic content of hair and bone in acute and chronic arsenical poisoning: review of 2 cases examined posthumously from medico-legal aspect. *Br Med J.* 1942;1:251-253.
231. Zablotska LB, Chen Y, Graziano JH, et al. Protective effects of B vitamins and antioxidants on the risk of arsenic-related skin lesions in Bangladesh. *Environ Health Perspect.* 2008;116:1056-1062.
232. Zakharyan RA, Aposhian HV. Arsenite methylation by methylvitamin B_{12} and glutathione does not require an enzyme. *Toxicol Appl Pharmacol.* 1999;154:287-291.
233. Zakharyan RA, Aposhian HV. Enzymatic reduction of arsenic compounds in mammalian systems: the rate-limiting enzyme of rabbit liver arsenic biotransformation is MMA^V reductase. *Chem Res Toxicol.* 1999;12: 1278-1283.
234. Zaloga GP, Deal J, Spurling T, et al. Case report: unusual manifestations of arsenic intoxication. *Am J Med Sci.* 1985;289:210-214.
235. Zavala YJ, Gerads R, Gorleyok H, Duxbury JM. Arsenic in rice: II. Arsenic speciation in USA grain and implications for human health. *Environ Sci Technol.* 2008;42:3861-3866.
236. Zhang P, Wang SY, Hu LH, et al. Treatment of 72 cases of acute promyelocytic leukemia by intravenous arsenic trioxide. *Chin J Hematol.* 1996;17: 58-62.
237. Zhang X, Cornelis R, De Kimpe J, et al. Accumulation of arsenic species in serum of patients with chronic renal disease. *Clin Chem.* 1996;42(8 Pt 1): 1231-1237.
238. Zhang X, Cornelis R, Mees L, et al. Chemical speciation of arsenic in serum of uraemic patients. *Analyst.* 1998;123:13-17.

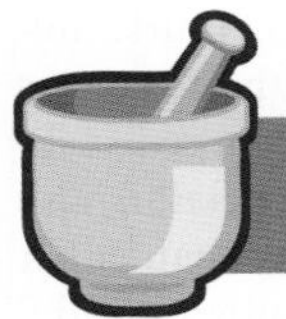

ANTIDOTES IN DEPTH (A26)

DIMERCAPROL (BRITISH ANTI-LEWISITE OR BAL)

Mary Ann Howland

```
     H
     |
 H—C—OH
     |
 H—C—SH
     |
 H—C—SH
     |
     H
```

BAL (2,3-Dimercaptopropanol; dimercaprol) is a metal chelator used clinically in conjunction with edetate calcium disodium ($CaNa_2EDTA$) for lead encephalopathy and severe lead toxicity.[22,29] In this instance BAL should precede the first dose of $CaNa_2EDTA$ by 4 hours to prevent redistribution of lead to the central nervous system (CNS). Because BAL has a narrow therapeutic index and must be given intramuscularly (IM), succimer is used for patients with less severe lead toxicity. Likewise, the roles of BAL in arsenic and mercury poisoning are being supplanted by succimer and the investigational agent 2,3-dimercaptopropane sulfonate (DMPS), unless the gastrointestinal tract is compromised and IM BAL is indicated.

HISTORY

Investigation into the use of sulfur donors as antidotes was precipitated by the World War II threat of chemical warfare with lewisite (dichloro[2-chlorovinyl]arsine) and mustard gas (dichlorodiethyl sulfide[$ClCH_2CH_2]_2S$).[1,30,31] Both are vesicant gases that cause tissue damage when combined with protein sulfhydryl (SH) groups (Chap. 131).[34] The investigations of Stocken and Thompson at Oxford led to the discovery of the dithiol 2,3-dimercaptopropanol, called British anti-Lewisite, which combines with lewisite to form a stable five-membered ring.[39,41]

CHEMISTRY

BAL has a molecular weight of 124.2 daltons and a specific gravity of 1.21.[32] Dimercaprol is an oily liquid with only 6% weight/volume water solubility, 5% weight/volume peanut oil solubility, and a disagreeable odor. Aqueous solutions are easily oxidized and therefore unstable. Peanut oil stabilizes BAL and benzyl benzoate (in the ratio of one part BAL to two parts of benzyl benzoate) renders the BAL miscible with peanut oil.[35]

PHARMACOKINETICS

There are no recent pharmacokinetic studies with BAL. The limited amount of information available dates back to the late 1940s.[1,23] Serum concentrations of BAL peak about 30 minutes after IM administration and distribution occurs quickly.[35,38] Within 2 hours after IM administration to rabbits, serum concentrations drop quickly. Urinary excretion of BAL metabolites, perhaps partially as glucuronic acid conjugates, accounted for nearly 45% of the dose within 6 hours and 81% of the dose within 24 hours.[35,37] Very little is excreted unchanged in the urine.[35] BAL is concentrated in the kidney, liver, and small intestine.[33] BAL can also be found in the feces, suggesting that enterohepatic circulation exists. Hemodialysis may be useful in removing the BAL–metal chelate in cases of renal failure.[22,28,40]

USE OF BAL FOR ARSENIC EXPOSURE

ANIMAL STUDIES

The fear of lewisite attack causing skin lesions, led researchers to investigate the potential for cutaneous application of BAL.[39] This was based on its limited water solubility and high lipid solubility. In a rodent model, low concentrations of topical BAL were very effective both in preventing lewisite-induced toxicity and in reversing toxicity when administered within 1 hour of skin exposure.[32,34] In rabbits, ocular application of BAL proved effective in preventing eye destruction if applied within 20 minutes of exposure.[22] Additionally, urinary arsenic concentrations were significantly increased after the application of BAL.[34]

The effectiveness of both parenteral single-dose and multiple-dose BAL against lewisite and other arsenicals was studied in rabbits. When begun within 2 hours of lewisite exposure, BAL injections of 4 mg/kg every 4 hours led to a 50% survival of exposed rabbits. This dosing regimen was demonstrated to be one-seventh of the maximum tolerated dose of BAL.[16]

The most recent animal studies demonstrate that although BAL increases the LD_{50} (median lethal dose for 50% of test subjects) of sodium arsenite, the therapeutic index of BAL is low and arsenic redistribution to the brain occurs.[4,6,7,19,36] In these same animal models, succimer and DMPS also increased the LD_{50}, but with a better therapeutic index and without causing redistribution to the brain.[3,4]

Ocular damage caused by lewisite is partly a result of the liberation of hydrochloric acid, which results in an acid injury causing localized superficial opacity of the cornea and deep penetration of lewisite into the cornea and aqueous humor with resultant rapid necrosis. In an experimental model, a 5% BAL ointment or solution applied within 2 minutes of exposure prevented the development of a significant reaction; application at 30 minutes lessened the reaction, but did not prevent permanent damage.[20]

HUMAN STUDIES

Earlier experiments in human volunteers who were given minute amounts of arsenic demonstrated that BAL increased urinary arsenic concentration by approximately 40%, with maximum excretion occurring 2 to 4 hours after BAL administration.[43] BAL was subsequently used in the treatment of arsenical dermatitis resulting from organic arsenicals used to treat syphilis. When applied to affected skin, topical BAL produced erythema, pruritus, and dysesthesias, but had no adverse effects on unaffected skin. Intramuscular BAL produced both subjective and objective improvement, limited the duration of the arsenical dermatitis, and increased urinary arsenic elimination.[12,26,27]

In a study of 227 patients with inorganic arsenic poisoning, maximal efficacy and minimal toxicity were achieved when 3 mg/kg of BAL was administered IM every 4 hours for 48 hours and then twice daily for 7 to 10 days. This regimen resulted in complete recovery in six of seven patients with severe arsenic-induced encephalopathy and demonstrated the importance of administering BAL as soon as possible after the exposure. Of 33 patients with severe arsenic-induced encephalopathy, 18 of 24 (75%) treated within 6 hours survived, versus only four of nine (44%) treated after a delay of at least 72 hours.[15] Furthermore, the effectiveness of BAL was also demonstrated in three patients who were treated successfully after mistakenly receiving 10 to 20 times the therapeutic dose of Mapharsen (oxophenarsine hydrochloride). A fourth patient, treated with inadequate doses of BAL, died.[15] These cases support the effectiveness of BAL in treating arsenic-induced agranulocytosis, encephalopathy, dermatitis, and probably arsenical fever.[15]

When BAL first became more widely available, 42 children who were treated following arsenic ingestions were compared with a historical group of 111 other children who had ingested arsenic and were not treated with BAL.[44] The percentage of children exhibiting symptoms on presentation were similar between groups (46%), but in the group of treated children the advantages were significant as there were fewer deaths (zero versus three), a shorter average hospital stay (1.6 versus 4.2 days), and fewer cases of persistent symptoms at 12 hours (0% versus 29.3%).

USE OF BAL FOR MERCURY EXPOSURE

Because mercury also reacts with sulfhydryl groups, animal studies were performed to assess the affinity and ability of thiols to competitively chelate inorganic mercury and prevent toxicity. As in the case of arsenic, the dithiols BAL and BAL glucoside were more effective than the monothiol 1-thiosorbitol in preventing mercury-induced death and uremia.[18] The clinical efficacy of BAL in treating inorganic mercury poisoning was substantiated in patients who ingested mercuric chloride.[24,25] Thirty-eight patients ingesting more than 1 g of mercuric chloride who were treated with BAL within 4 hours of exposure were compared with historical controls.[24] There were no deaths in the 38 patients treated with BAL as compared to 27 deaths in the 86 untreated patients. Death typically resulted from hemorrhagic gastritis and renal failure.[24] BAL is particularly useful for patients who have ingested a mercuric salt, as the associated gastrointestinal toxicity of the mercuric salt limits the potential of an orally administered antidote such as succimer.[42]

Animal models demonstrate that when BAL is administered following poisoning from elemental mercury vapor or exposure to short-chain organic mercury compounds, brain levels of mercury may increase.[9,11] As a result BAL therapy is not recommended in these circumstances.[2,5,22] Other therapies may have greater usefulness (Chap. 96).

USE OF BAL FOR LEAD EXPOSURE

BAL may be used in combination with $CaNa_2EDTA$ to treat patients with severe lead poisoning. In all other cases, succimer has become the chelator of choice. When administering BAL to patients with lead encephalopathy, it is essential to administer the BAL first, followed 4 hours later by $CaNa_2EDTA$, concomitantly with the second dose of BAL. This regimen prevents the $CaNa_2EDTA$ from redistributing lead into the brain.[13,14] Providing two different chelators also reduces the blood lead concentration significantly faster than either one alone, and maintains a better molar ratio of chelator to lead.[13] Once the mobilization of lead has begun, it is important to provide uninterrupted therapy to prevent redistribution of lead to the brain (see Chap. 94).[13]

ADVERSE EFFECTS AND SAFETY ISSUES

BAL has an LD_{50} in mice via intraperitoneal administration of 90 to 180 mg/kg, which is significantly lower than $CaNa_2EDTA$ at 4 to 6 g/kg, succimer at 2.48 g/kg, and DMPS at 1.1 to 1.4 g/kg.[2]

The toxicity of BAL is dose dependent and affected by urinary pH. Acidic urine allows dissociation of the BAL–metal chelate. Less than 1% of 700 IM injections resulted in minor reactions, such as pain at the injection site, among patients who received 2.5 mg/kg of BAL every 4 to 6 hours for 4 doses.[12] When doses of 4 mg/kg and 5 mg/kg were given, the incidence of adverse effects rose to 14% and 65%, respectively.[15] At these higher doses, the following symptoms were reported in decreasing order of frequency: nausea; vomiting; headache; burning sensation of lips, mouth, throat, and eyes; lacrimation; rhinorrhea; salivation; muscle aches; burning and tingling of extremities; tooth pain; diaphoresis; chest pain; anxiety; and agitation.[26] These effects were maximal within 10 to 30 minutes of exposure, and usually subsided within 30 to 50 minutes.[15] Elevations in systolic and diastolic blood pressure and tachycardia commonly occurred and correlated with increasing doses.[22,29] Thirty percent of children given BAL may develop a fever that can persist throughout the therapeutic period.[22] A transient reduction in the percentage of polymorphonuclear leukocytes may also occur.[22] Doses above 5 mg/kg should not be administered because of the high risk of adverse reactions. Doses above 25 mg/kg can be expected to produce a hypertensive encephalopathy with convulsions and coma.[44]

BAL is not very effective in the presence of arsenic-induced hepatotoxicity.[27] Moreover, in rats preexistent hepatotoxicity was exacerbated when BAL was used for treatment of arsenic poisoning. Therefore, unless the hepatotoxicity is considered to be arsenic induced, hepatic dysfunction is a contraindication to BAL use.[34] BAL should not be used for patients poisoned by methylmercury because animal studies demonstrate a redistribution of mercury to the brain.[5,22]

Because dissociation of the BAL–metal chelate will occur in acidic urine, the urine of patients receiving BAL should be alkalinized with hypertonic $NaHCO_3$ to a pH of 7.5 to 8.0 to prevent renal liberation of the metal.[22] BAL should be used with caution in patients with glucose-6-phosphate dehydrogenase (G6PD) deficiency, as it may cause hemolysis.[21] In these cases, a risk-to-benefit analysis must be made because G6PD-deficiency syndromes are variably expressed in young cells. In addition, chelators are relatively nonspecific and may bind metals other than those desired, thus causing deficiency of an essential metal. For example, BAL given to mice increased copper elimination to three times normal.[10] BAL is formulated in peanut oil; therefore, the patient should be questioned regarding any known peanut allergy. Limited evidence suggests that iron supplements should not be given to patients who are receiving BAL because the BAL–iron complex appears to cause severe vomiting and decreases metal chelation.[13,14,17]

Unintentional intravenous (IV) infusion of BAL could theoretically produce fat embolism, lipoid pneumonia, chylothorax, and associated hypoxia.[37]

DOSING

There has never been a clinical trial to identify the best dose of dimercaprol. The dosing for dimercaprol has been expressed in both mg/m^2 and mg/kg. Dimercaprol should only be administered by deep IM injection. The dose of BAL for lead encephalopathy is 75 mg/m^2 IM every 4 hours for 5 days in children.[13,14] As noted earlier, the first dose of dimercaprol should precede the first dose of $CaNa_2EDTA$ by 4 hours. Thereafter, IV $CaNa_2EDTA$, in a dose of 1500 mg/m^2/d (up to a maximum of 2–3 g) as a continuous infusion, or divided into two to four doses, should be administered. These daily doses are equimolar. For adults the dose of BAL is 4 mg/kg every 4 hours.[8]

The dose of BAL for severe inorganic arsenic poisoning has not been established. One regimen suggests the use of 3 mg/kg IM every 4 hours for 48 hours and then twice daily for 7 to 10 days.[15] Another regimen uses 3 to 5 mg/kg IM every 4 to 6 hours on the first day and then tapers the dose and frequency, depending on the patient's symptomatology. A third regimen reduces the number of injections by day 2 and terminates therapy within 5 to 7 days.[44]

The dose of BAL for patients exposed to inorganic mercury salts is 5 mg/kg IM initially, followed by 2.5 mg/kg every 12 to 24 hours until the patient appears clinically improved, up to a total of 10 days.[8]

Table 26–1

Calculations for average deep intramuscular (IM) BAL use when using body surface area (M^2)

Child	Avg. Height (in)	Avg. Weight (lbs)	M^2	75 mg/m^2* Every 4 h IM	50 mg/m^2** Every 4 h IM
2-year-old boy	36	30.5	0.593	44.5 mg	30 mg
2-year-old girl	35	29	0.57	43 mg	28.5 mg
4-year-old boy	42	39.75	0.73	55 mg	36.5 mg
4-year-old girl	41.75	38.75	0.72	54 mg	36 mg

*approximately 4 mg/kg
**approximately 3 mg/kg

AVAILABILITY

Commercially available BAL is a yellow, viscous liquid with a sulfur odor. It is available in 3-mL ampules containing 100 mg/mL of BAL, 200 mg/mL of benzyl benzoate, and 700 mg/mL of peanut oil.[8] BAL is for deep IM use only.

SUMMARY

BAL (dimercaprol) is a metal chelator used clinically in conjunction with $CaNa_2EDTA$ for lead encephalopathy and severe lead toxicity.[22,29] In this instance BAL should precede the first dose of $CaNa_2EDTA$ by 4 hours. The roles of BAL in arsenic and mercury poisoning are being supplanted by succimer and the investigational agent DMPS, unless the gastrointestinal tract is compromised and IM BAL is indicated.

REFERENCES

1. Aaseth J. Recent advances in the therapy of metal poisonings with chelating agents. *Hum Toxicol.* 1983;2:257-272.
2. Andersen O. Principles and recent developments in chelation treatment of metal intoxication. *Chem Rev.* 1999;99:2683-2710.
3. Aposhian HV, Aposhian MM. Arsenic toxicology: five questions. *Chem Res Toxicol.* 2006;19:1-15.
4. Aposhian HV, Carter DE, Hoover TD, et al. DMSA, DMPS, and DMPA as arsenic antidotes. *Fundam Appl Toxicol.* 1984;4:S58-S70.
5. Aposhian HV, Maiorino RM, Gonzalez-Ramirez D, et al. Mobilization of heavy metals by newer, therapeutically useful chelating agents. *Toxicology.* 1995;97:23-38.
6. Aposhian HV, Mershon MM, Brinkley FB, et al. Anti-Lewisite activity and stability of meso-dimercaptosuccinic acid and 2,3-dimercaptol-propane-sulfonic acid. *Life Sci.* 1982;31:2149-2156.
7. Aposhian HV, Tadlock CH, Moon TE. Protection of mice against the lethal effects of sodium arsenite—a quantitative comparison of a number of chelating agents. *Toxicol Appl Pharmacol.* 1981;61:385-392.
8. BAL in Oil Ampules (Dimercaprol Injection USP) [package insert]. Decatur, IL: Taylor Pharmaceuticals; 10/06.
9. Berlin M, Ullberg S. Increased uptake of mercury in mouse brain caused by 2,3-dimercaptopropanol. *Nature.* 1963;197:84-85.
10. Cantilena LR, Klaassen CD. The effect of chelating agents on the excretion of endogenous metals. *Toxicol Appl Pharmacol.* 1982;63:344-350.
11. Canty AJ, Kishimoto R. British anti-Lewisite and organ-mercury poisoning. *Nature.* 1972;253:123-125.
12. Carleton AB, Peters RA, Stocken LA, et al. Clinical uses of 2,3-dimercapto-propanol (BAL): VI. The treatment of complications of arseno-therapy with BAL. *J Clin Invest.* 1946;25:497-527.
13. Chisolm JJ Jr. The use of chelating agents in the treatment of acute and chronic lead intoxication in childhood. *J Pediatr.* 1968;73:1-38.
14. Committee on Drugs. Treatment guidelines for lead exposure in children. *Pediatrics.* 1995;96:155-160.
15. Eagle H, Magnuson HJ. The systemic treatment of 227 cases of arsenic poisoning (encephalitis, dermatitis, blood dyscrasias, jaundice, fever) with 2,3-dimercaptopropanol (BAL). *Am J Syph Gonorrhea Vener Dis.* 1946;30: 420-441.
16. Eagle H, Magnuson HJ, Fleischman R. Clinical uses of 2,3-dimercapto-propanol (BAL): I. The systemic treatment of experimental arsenic poisoning (Mapharsen, lewisite, phenyl arsenoxide) with BAL. *J Clin Invest.* 1946;25:451-466.
17. Edge WD, Somers GF. The effect of dimercaprol (BAL) in acute iron poisoning. *Q J Pharm Pharmacol.* 1948;21:364-369.
18. Gilman A, Allen RP, Philips FS, et al. Clinical uses of 2,3-dimercaptopropanol (BAL): X. The treatment of acute systemic mercury poisoning in experimental animals with BAL, thiosorbitol and BAL glucoside. *J Clin Invest.* 1946;25:549-556.
19. Hoover TD, Aposhian HV. BAL increases the arsenic-74 content of rabbit brain. *Toxicol Appl Pharmacol.* 1983;70:160-162.
20. Hughes WF. Clinical uses of 2,3-dimercaptopropanol (BAL): IX. The treatment of lewisite burns of the eye with BAL. *J Clin Invest.* 1946;25: 541-548.
21. Janakiraman N, Seeler RA, Royal JE, et al. Hemodialysis during BAL chelation therapy for high blood lead levels in two G6PD-deficient children. *Clin Pediatr.* 1978;17:485-487.
22. Klaassen CD. Heavy metals and heavy metal antagonists. In: Hardman JG, Limbird LE, eds. *The Pharmacological Basis of Therapeutics*, 10th ed. New York: Macmillan; 2001:1851-1875.
23. Kosnett MJ. Unanswered questions in metal chelation. *J Toxicol Clin Toxicol.* 1992;30:529-547.
24. Longcope WT, Luetscher JA. The use of BAL (British anti-Lewisite) in the treatment of the injurious effects of arsenic, mercury and other metallic poisons. *Ann Intern Med.* 1949;31:545-554.
25. Longcope WT, Luetscher JA, Calkins F, et al. Clinical uses of 2,3-dimercaptopropanol (BAL): XI. The treatment of acute mercury poisoning by BAL. *J Clin Invest.* 1946;25:557-567.
26. Longcope WT, Luetscher JA, Wintrobe MM, et al. Clinical uses of 2,3-dimercaptopropanol (BAL): VII. The treatment of arsenical dermatitis with preparations of BAL. *J Clin Invest.* 1946;25:528-533.
27. Luetscher JA, Eagle H, Longcope WT. Clinical uses of 2,3-dimercaptopropanol (BAL): VIII. The effect of BAL on the excretion of arsenic in arsenical intoxication. *J Clin Invest.* 1946;25:534-540.
28. Maher JF, Schreiner GE. The dialysis of mercury and mercury-BAL complex. *Clin Res.* 1959;7:298.
29. Mahieu P, Buchet JP, Roels HA, et al. The metabolism of arsenic in humans acutely intoxicated by As_2O_3: its significance for the duration of BAL therapy. *J Toxicol Clin Toxicol.* 1981;18:1067-1075.
30. Oehme FW. British anti-lewisite (BAL): the classic heavy metal antidote. *Clin Toxicol.* 1972;5:215-222.

31. Pearson RG. Hard and soft acids and bases; NSAB. Part II. Underlying theories. *J Chem Educ.* 1968;45:643-648.
32. Peters RA. Biochemistry of some toxic agents. *J Clin Invest.* 1955;34:1-20.
33. Peters RA, Spray GH, Stocken LA, et al. The use of British anti-Lewisite containing radioactive sulfur for metabolism investigations. *Biochem J.* 1947;41:370-373.
34. Peters RA, Stocken LA, Thompson RM. British anti-Lewisite (BAL). *Nature.* 1945;156:616-618.
35. Randall RV, Seeler AO. BAL. *N Engl J Med.* 1948;239:1004-1009, 1040-1048.
36. Schafer B, Kreppel H, Reichl FX, et al. Effect of oral treatment with BAL, DMPS or DMSA arsenic in organs of mice injected with arsenic trioxide. *Arch Toxicol.* 1991;14(Suppl):228-230.
37. Seifert SA, Dart RC, Kaplan EH. Accidental, intravenous infusion of a peanut oil-based medication. *J Toxicol Clin Toxicol.* 1998;36:733-736.
38. Spray GM, Stocken LA, Thompson RMS. Further investigations on the metabolism of 2,3-dimercaptopropanol. *Biochem J.* 1947;41:363-366.
39. Stocken LA, Thompson RM. Reactions of British anti-Lewisite with arsenic and other metals in living systems. *Physiol Rev.* 1949;29:168-194.
40. Vaziri ND, Upham T, Barton CM. Hemodialysis clearance of arsenic. *Clin Toxicol.* 1980;17:451-456.
41. Vilensky J, Redman K. British anti-Lewisite (dimercaprol): an amazing history. *Ann Emerg Med.* 2003;41:378-383.
42. Wang E, Mahajan N, Wills B, Leikin J. Successful treatment of potentially fatal heavy metal poisoning. *J Emerg Med.* 2007;32:289-294.
43. Wexler J, Eagle M, Tatum MJ, et al. Clinical uses of 2, 3-dimercaptopropanol (BAL): II. The effect of BAL on the excretion of arsenic in normal subjects after minimal exposure to arsenical smoke. *J Clin Invest.* 1946;25:467-473.
44. Woody NC, Kometani JT. BAL in the treatment of arsenic ingestion of children. *Pediatrics.* 1948;1:372-378.
45. Zimmer LJ, Carter DE. The effect of 2,3-dimercaptopropanol and D-penicillamine on methyl mercury-induced neurological signs and weight loss. *Life Sci.* 1978;23:1025-1034.

CHAPTER 89
BISMUTH

Rama B. Rao

Bismuth (Bi)

Atomic number	= 83
Atomic weight	= 208.98 daltons
Normal concentrations	
Blood	< 5 μg/dL (239.5 nmol/L)
Plasma	< 1 μg/dL (<47.9 nmol/L)
Urine	< 20 μg/L (<95.7 nmol/L)

Bismuth is a metal that is available either in its elemental form or compounded as a salt. Elemental bismuth is nontoxic. Bismuth salts have therapeutic uses and are responsible for the toxicities described in this chapter. Thus, the term "bismuth" in this chapter refers to bismuth salts. Bismuth is one of many xenobiotics commonly used in prescription and nonprescription oral preparations for treatment of traveler's diarrhea, nausea, and vomiting, as well as in bismuth-impregnated surgical packing paste for treatment of the flatus and odor associated with ileostomies and colostomies,[9,57] and as an adjunct in the treatment of ulcers.[14]

In the gastrointestinal (GI) tract, bismuth binds to sulfhydryl groups and decreases fecal odor through formation of bismuth sulfide.[50] Sulfhydryl binding is also the proposed mechanism of bismuth's antimicrobial effect, causing lysis of *Helicobacter pylori*, the causative bacteria in peptic ulcer formation. Bismuth may also inhibit bacterial enzyme function, as well as prevent adhesion of *H. pylori* to the gastric mucosa.[56]

HISTORY AND EPIDEMIOLOGY

Nearly 300 years ago, bismuth was recognized as medicinally valuable. It was included in topical salves and oral preparations for various GI disorders. Renal toxicity was described as early as 1802. In the early 20th century, renal failure was reported in children administered intramuscular bismuth salts for the treatment of gingivostomatitis.[7,25,47,48] Administration of bismuth thioglycollate and its related water-soluble compounds, triglycollamate and trithioglycollamate, was responsible for the renal failure.[8,12,29,55] Children with renal toxicity would typically present with abdominal pain, oliguria, anuria, malaise, depressed mental status, and vomiting. Renal failure occurred with as little as one or two treatments.[34,38,39] Alterations in consciousness usually abated with treatment or resolution of the uremia. As the use of intramuscular injections was abandoned, this form of bismuth-induced renal failure became uncommon. Syphilis was previously treated with intramuscular bismuth. A rash known as "erythema of the 9th day," consisting of a diffuse macular rash of the trunk and extremities, occasionally occurred and resolved without intervention.[16]

In patients administered "Analbis" antipyretic rectal suppositories, hepatic failure was described histopathologically as yellow atrophy with vacuolization.[3,22] An investigation of the suppositories suggested that diallylacetic acid, and not bismuth, was the hepatotoxin. This agent is no longer marketed in the United States. Enemas have been used.[54]

More recently, epidemics of bismuth-induced encephalopathy, particularly among patients with ileostomies or colostomies, were reported in France, Britain, and Australia. As a result, some countries banned or restricted bismuth preparations to prescription only. Bismuth subsalicylate, which is currently available in the United States as a nonprescription agent, is still periodically responsible for cases of encephalopathy.[15,17,30] Other reported causes of bismuth-induced encephalopathy include systemic absorption from bismuth-impregnated surgical packing paste and transdermal absorption from chronic application of a bismuth-containing skin cream.[24]

In 2006, the Food and Drug Administration (FDA) of the United States issued a warning on an alternative health product known as "bismacine"or "chromacine." This nonpharmaceutical product is not FDA approved, but has been used by some practitioners as an injectable treatment for Lyme disease, for which efficacy data are lacking. The product contains bismuth citrate and was associated with at least one death and other adverse events in patients administered this product.[2]

CHEMISTRY

Bismuth salts are divided into four groups based on their water or lipid solubility. The highly lipid-soluble compounds such as bismuth subsalicylate or bismuth subgallate are most commonly associated with neurotoxicity (Table 89–1). See Pathophsyiology section below.

TOXICOKINETICS

Bismuth is present in nature in both the trivalent and pentavalent forms. The trivalent form of bismuth is used for all medicinal uses, usually as the bismuthyl (BiO) moiety generated by hydrolysis of trivalent bismuth compounds to yield a low solubility alkaline salt. Most orally administered bismuth remains in the GI tract, being excreted in the feces, and only 0.2% is systemically absorbed.[19] Absorption of some bismuth preparations such as colloidal bismuth subcitrate may increase as gastric pH increases.[36] The time to peak absorption ranges between 15 and 60 minutes with high intra- and interindividual variation.[23,25] The serum-to-blood ratio of bismuth is 1.55.[4] The distribution and elimination of orally administered bismuth follows a complex, multicompartmental model. The volume of distribution in humans is unknown.[5,44]

Once in the circulation, bismuth binds to α_2-macroglobulin, IgM, β-lipoprotein, and haptoglobin. Bismuth rapidly enters liver, kidney, lungs, and bone.[51] Bismuth can cross the placenta and enter the amniotic fluid and fetal circulation.[53] It also readily crosses the blood–brain barrier.[35] Evidence in a rat model suggests that, when administered intramuscularly, bismuth can access the central nervous system (CNS) via retrograde axonal transport.[49] In both animal models and human reports bismuth is identified in the fenestrated membranes of synaptosomes,[38,41] localizing in the thalamus and cerebellum with diffuse cortical uptake as well.[25,35] Ninety percent of absorbed bismuth is eliminated through the kidneys, where it induces the production of its own metal-binding protein.[51]

Some authors propose three different half-lives to describe the pharmacokinetics of orally administered therapeutic doses of bismuth.[5,44] The first, a distribution half-life, is approximately 1 to 4 hours. The second, the apparent plasma half-life, lasts 5 to 11 days. The third is the apparent half-life of urinary excretion lasting between 21 and 72 days[4] with urinary bismuth detected as late as 5 months after the last oral dose.[23]

PATHOPHYSIOLOGY

Like other metals, bismuth toxicity involves multiple organ systems. The effect of different bismuth salts can be categorized into four groups based on solubility and GI absorption (see Table 89–1).[43]

TABLE 89–1. The Physiochemical Characteristics of Bismuth Salts

Group	Chemistry	Toxicity	Examples
I	Insoluble in water Inorganic	Minimal	Bismuth subnitrate Bismuth subcarbonate
II	Lipid soluble Organic	Neurologic	Bismuth subsalicylate Bismuth subgallate
III	Water soluble Organic	Renal	Bismuth triglycollamate
IV	Hydrolyzable Water soluble Organic	Minimal	Bismuth bicitropeptide

The mechanism of bismuth-induced encephalopathy is thought to be related to neuronal sulfhydryl binding. In patients who die of bismuth encephalopathy, the gray-matter concentration of bismuth is nearly twice that of white matter.[25] In a bismuth encephalopathic patient dying from concomitant sepsis, the autopsy revealed loss of cerebellar purkinje cells not expected from sepsis alone.[26] The factors predisposing some individuals to encephalopathy from group II bismuth salts, however, are not well defined. Age, gender, and duration of therapeutic use do not predict the likelihood of developing encephalopathy, but typically patients are on chronic bismuth therapy with a lipid soluble (group II) agent.

CLINICAL MANIFESTATIONS

ACUTE

Acutely, massive overdoses of bismuth may result in abdominal pain and oliguria or anuria. Acute renal failure can occur and is not limited to exposure to the water-soluble bismuth salts (group III).[34,39] In reported cases, overdoses of colloidal bismuth subsalicylate or tripotassium dicitratobismuthate (TDC) caused acute tubular necrosis.[1,18,20,48,52] Histopathologically, bismuth causes degeneration of the proximal tubule, similar to other heavy metals. While these substances are potentially neurotoxic, signs of encephalopathy are generally absent.[11,17] In one case, a patient with bismuth-induced renal failure was described as having diminished deep-tendon reflexes, muscle weakness, and myoclonus, without an alteration in consciousness.[18]

CHRONIC

The most common toxicologic finding associated with repeated therapeutic doses of oral bismuth compounds is a diffuse, progressive encephalopathy.[11,17] Affected patients exhibit neurobehavioral changes, such as apathy and irritability. With continued exposure, these patients may develop difficulty concentrating, diminished short-term memory, and occasionally, visual hallucinations.[27,28] A movement disorder characterized by muscle twitching, myoclonus, ataxia, and tremors may ensue.[11] This is often described as a myoclonic encephaloathy. Weakness and, rarely, seizures may advance to immobility.[30,32] With continued bismuth administration these patients can develop coma and die.

Rarely, patients recovering from severe encephalopathy may complain of scapular, humeral, or vertebral pain because of fractures caused by severe neuromuscular manifestations such as myoclonus.[13]

Like several other heavy metals, bismuth can cause a generalized pigmentation of skin. Deposition of bismuth sulfide into the mucosa causes a blue-black discoloration of gums.[58] This can occur in the absence of toxic effects. Formation of the same compound in the GI tract causes blackening of the stool. Liver failure is rarely reported, except in patients with multisystem organ failure from fatal neurotoxicity.

DIAGNOSIS

The clinician must have an index of suspicion based on the acute or chronic nature of the exposure. Patients with acute massive overdoses should be observed and evaluated for possible renal failure. The earliest findings suggestive of renal compromise may be hematuria and proteinuria on urinalysis. Formation of nuclear inclusion bodies can be identified on renal biopsy or on postmortem examination of the kidney.[12,40]

The diagnosis of bismuth-induced encephalopathy is based on a history of exposure coupled with diffuse neuropsychiatric and motor findings.[28] Other causes of encephalopathy should be entertained and excluded (Table 89–2). An abdominal radiograph will likely demonstrate radiopacities of bismuth in the intestines. Stool will be black and test negative for occult blood.

The presence of bismuth in the blood is confirmatory of exposure, but absolute concentrations correlate poorly with morbidity.[5] In a review of 310 patients with bismuth-induced encephalopathy, 288 patients (93%) had a blood concentration greater than 100 ng/mL, with the majority of these blood concentrations between 100 ng/mL and 1000 ng/mL.[27] Twenty-two patients suffered encephalopathy at blood concentrations below 100 ng/mL.[27] In another report, two patients with encephalopathy had blood concentrations of 900 ng/mL and 2500 ng/mL, both of whom recovered when the concentration fell below 500 ng/mL.[6] Just as blood concentrations do not reflect severity of illness, tissue concentrations may also poorly correlate with severity of illness. An example was noted in a patient who recovered from a severe encephalopathy. On discharge, he had low blood bismuth concentrations and died 3 months later of unrelated trauma. At autopsy he was found to have an elevated CNS bismuth burden but no reported symptoms at the time of the trauma.[10]

The electroencephalographic (EEG) findings of patients with bismuth encephalopathy generally demonstrate nonspecific slow wave changes.[15,18] In one study, the EEG findings were described in association with blood concentrations. At less than 50 ng/mL, the EEG was normal or demonstrated diffuse slowing. In patients with blood concentrations of less than 1500 ng/mL, the findings of sharp wave abnormalities were noted. At higher concentrations (greater than 2000 ng/mL), some patients with neurological events, such as myoclonic jerks, did not have corresponding EEG changes. The authors

TABLE 89–2. Differential Diagnosis of Bismuth Encephalopathy

Creutzfeld-Jacob disease
Ethanol withdrawal
Lithium toxicity
Neurodegenerative leukoencephalopathies
Nonketotic hyperosmolar coma
Postanoxic and posthypoglycemic encephalopathies
Progressive multifocal ataxia
Viral encephalopathies

proposed that an elevated body burden might have an inhibitory effect on the cerebral cortex.[10]

In encephalopathic patients with blood concentrations greater than 2000 ng/mL diagnostic imaging such as computed tomography may demonstrate a diffuse cortical hyperdensity of the gray matter. These findings tend to resolve with recovery. Magnetic resonance imaging was normal in another encephalopathic patient.[15]

TREATMENT

Typically, supportive care results in a complete recovery. Some authors suggest GI decontamination with activated charcoal and polyethylene glycol solution.[45] Although evidence for this approach is lacking, it appears to be a reasonable initial intervention, especially in patients with severe encephalopathy. In patients with renal toxicity, resolution is generally observed with supportive care and whole-bowel irrigation. The use of chelators in patients with acute overdose without neurotoxicity is probably not indicated.

It is uncertain whether different chelators affect the clinical course of encephalopathic patients. Withdrawal of the source of bismuth results in complete reversal of symptoms within days to weeks, even in severely ill patients. The precise timing, dosage, indications, and choice of chelator is not known; however, chelation with succimer has few side effects and may potentially limit the potentially fatal complications associated with prolonged immobilization. British anti-Lewisite (BAL), which has more side effects, can be considered in encephalopathic patients with renal failure in whom no neurological improvement is noted within 48 hours of whole-bowel irrigation and bismuth withdrawal (see Chelation section below).

Prevention is the most effective means of avoiding neurotoxicity. Blood concentrations of bismuth are not routinely performed, but a bismuth concentration above 100 ng/mL or symptoms at lower levels warrant withdrawal of bismuth therapy.

CHELATION

In general the data regarding chelation are limited and in vitro and animal models do not clearly predict in vivo human models. Chelation therapy with BAL is beneficial in experimental models,[45,48] reportedly beneficial in humans,[31] and often recommended, although clear evidence of efficacy is lacking. BAL undergoes biliary elimination, offering a major advantage over other chelators in patients who may develop renal insufficiency. One study advocated the addition of dimercaptopropane sulfonate (DMPS), as BAL with hemodialysis did not affect clearance, whereas the addition of DMPS to patients needing hemodialysis was effective in enhancing elimination.[48] It is uncertain whether the clinical course of the patients was improved. In human volunteers given colloidal bismuth subcitrate, succimer and DMPS, both at a dose of 30 mg/kg, increased urinary elimination of bismuth by 50-fold.[46]

In an animal model, D-penicillamine was most efficacious in enhancing elimination of bismuth. In a human volunteer model using therapeutic doses of tripotassium-dicitrato-bismuthate, however, a single dose of D-penicillamine did not enhance urinary excretion.[33]

BISMUTH DRUG INTERACTIONS AND REACTIONS

The coadministration of proton pump inhibitors (PPIs) may increase the absorption of some bismuth preparations. In a prospective evaluation of patients receiving different treatment regimens for *H. pylori*–induced dyspepsia or peptic ulcer disease, individuals taking PPIs had a statistically significant elevation in their blood bismuth concentrations with three patients exceeding 50 μg/L, compared with a similar group administered bismuth without PPIs. The authors suggest that the bismuth preparation used, colloidal bismuth subcitrate, is more soluble and absorbable at the higher gastric pH of patients on PPIs.[19] All of these patients received short courses of therapy (2 weeks). While the investigators did not attempt to follow neurobehavioral or neuropsychiatric changes, none of the patients had clinically evident bismuth toxicity.[36]

Based on this investigation, coadministration of PPIs with longer courses of colloidal bismuth subcitrate should be avoided or only offered with extreme caution. Ranitidine, which is frequently prescribed with a bismuth compound for dyspepsia or ulcer disease, does not affect the pharmacokinetics of bismuth absorption.[23]

In the United States, where bismuth subsalicylate is the most common oral bismuth-containing compound, up to 90% of the salicylate is absorbed.[37,42] Salicylate toxicity has been reported and salicylate concentrations should be determined in both acute and chronic exposures.[42,47] Methemoglobinemia from subnitrate salt of bismuth is uncommonly described.[21]

SUMMARY

The most likely manifestations of bismuth toxicity are either neuropsychiatric or renal, depending on the type of compound and whether the etiology is related to chronic therapy or acute overdose, respectively. The factors predisposing some individuals to neurotoxicity from therapeutic use of oral bismuth compounds are poorly understood. Thus, patients using therapeutic bismuth with new movement disorders or alterations in mental status should be assessed for possible bismuth-induced encephalopathy.

REFERENCES

1. Akpolat I, Kahraman H, Akpolat T, et al. Acute renal failure due to overdose of colloidal bismuth. *Nephrol Dial Transplant.* 1996;11:1890-1898.
2. Anonymous. Warning on bismacine. *FDA Consumer.* 2006;40:5.
3. Barnett RN. Reactions to a bismuth compound. Toxic manifestations following the use of the bismuth salt of heptadienecarboxylic acid in suppositories. *JAMA.* 1947;135:28-30.
4. Benet LZ. Safety and pharmacokinetics: colloidal bismuth subcitrate. *Scand J Gastroenterol.* 1991;25(Suppl 185):29-35.
5. Bennet JE, Wakefield JC, Lacey LF. Modeling trough plasma bismuth concentrations. *J Pharmacokinet Biopharm.* 1997;25:79-106.
6. Bes A, Caussanel JP, Geraud G, et al. Encephalopathie toxique par les sels de bismuth. *Rev Med Toulouse.* 1976;12:810-813.
7. Bierer DW. Bismuth subsalicylate: history chemistry, and safety. *Rev Infect Dis.* 1990;12:S3-S8.
8. Boyette DP, Ahiskie NC. Bismuth nephrosis with anuria in an infant. *J Pediatr.* 1946;28:493-497.
9. Bridgeman AM, Smith AC. Iatrogenic bismuth poisoning: case report. *Aust Dental J.* 1994;39:279-281.
10. Buge A, Supino-Viterbo V, Rancurel G, Pontes C. Epileptic phenomena in bismuth toxic encephalopathy. *J Neurol Neurosurg Psychiatr.* 1981;44:62-67.
11. Burns R, Thomas DW, Barron VJ. Reversible encephalopathy possibly associated with bismuth subgallate ingestion. *Br Med J.* 1974;1:220-223.
12. Czerwinski AW, Ginn HE. Bismuth nephrotoxicity. *Am J Med.* 1964;37:969-975.
13. Emile J, De Bray JM, Bernat M, et al. Osteoarticular complications in bismuth encephalopathy. *Clin Toxicol.* 1981;18:1285-1290.
14. Goldenberg MM, Honkomp LJ, Davis CS. Antinauseant and antiemetic properties of bismuth subsalicylate in dogs and humans. *J Pharmacol Sci.* 1976;65:1398-1400.

15. Gordon MF, Abrams RI, Rubin DB, et al. Bismuth subsalicylate toxicity as a cause of prolonged encephalopathy with myoclonus. *Mov Disord.* 1995;10:220-222.
16. Gryboski JD, Gotoff SP. Bismuth nephrotoxicity. *N Engl J Med.* 1961;265: 1289-1291.
17. Hasking GJ, Duggan JM. Encephalopathy from bismuth subsalicylate. *Med J Aust.* 1982;2:167.
18. Hudson M, Mowat NAG. Reversible toxicity in poisoning with colloidal bismuth subcitrate. *BMJ.* 1989;299:159.
19. Hundal O, Bergseth M, Gharehnia B, et al. Absorption of bismuth from two bismuth compounds before and after healing of peptic ulcers. *Hepatogastroenterology.* 1999;46:2882-2886.
20. Huwez F, Pall A, Lyons D, Stewart MJ. Acute renal failure after overdose of colloidal bismuth subcitrate. *Lancet.* 1992;340:1298.
21. Jacobsen JB, Huttel MS. Methemoglobin after excessive intake of a subnitrate containing antacid. *Ugeskr Laeger.* 1982;144:2340-2350.
22. Karelitz S, Freedman AD. Hepatitis and nephrosis due to soluble bismuth. *Pediatrics.* 1951;8:772-776.
23. Koch KM, Kerr BM, Gooding AE, Davis IM. Pharmacokinetics of bismuth and ranitidine following multiple doses of ranitidine bismuth citrate. *Br J Clin Pharmacol.* 1996:42:207-211.
24. Kruger G, Thomas DJ, Weinhardt F, Hoyer S. Disturbed oxidative metabolism in organic brain syndrome caused by bismuth in skin creams. *Lancet.* 1976;1:485-487.
25. Lambert JR. Pharmacology of bismuth-containing compounds. *Rev Infect Dis.* 1991;13:S691-S695.
26. Liessens JL, Monstrey J, Vanden Eeckhout E, Djudzman R, Martin JJ. Bismuth encephalopathy. *Act Neurol Belg.* 1978;78:301-309.
27. Martin-Bouyer G, Foulon G, Guerbois H, Barin C. Epidemiological study of encephalopathies following bismuth administration per os. Characteristics of intoxicated subjects: comparison with a control group. *Clin Toxicol.* 1981;18:1277-1283.
28. Martin-Bouyer G, Weller M. Neuropsychiatric symptoms following bismuth intoxication. *Postgrad Med J.* 1988;64:308-310.
29. McClendon SJ. Toxic effects with anuria from a single injection of a bismuth preparation. *Am J Dis Child.* 1941;61:339-341.
30. Mendelowitz PC, Hoffman RS, Weber S. Bismuth absorption and myoclonic encephalopathy during bismuth subsalicylate therapy. *Ann Intern Med.* 1990;112:140-141.
31. Molina JA, Calandre L, Bermego F. Myoclonic encephalopathy due to bismuth salts: treatment with dimercaprol and analysis of CSF transmitters. *Acta Neurol Scand.* 1989;79:200-203.
32. Monseu G, Struelens M, Roland M. Bismuth encephalopathy. *Acta Neurol Belg.* 1976;76:301-308.
33. Nwokolo CU, Pounder RE. D-Penicillamine does not increase urinary bismuth excretion in patients treated with tripotassium dicitrato bismuthate. *Br J Clin Pharmacol.* 1990;30:648-650.
34. O'Brien D. Anuria due to bismuth thioglycollate. *Am J Dis Child.* 1959;97:384-386.
35. Pamphlett R, Stoltenberg M, Rungby J, Danscher G. Uptake of bismuth in motor neurons of mice after single oral doses of bismuth compounds. *Neurotoxicol Teratol.* 2000;22:559-563.
36. Phillips RH, Whitehead MW, Diog LA, et al. Is eradication of *Helicobacter pylori* with colloidal bismuth subcitrate quadruple therapy safe? *Helicobacter.* 2001;6:151-156.
37. Pickering LK, Feldman S, Ericsson CD, Cleary TG. Absorption of salicylate and bismuth from a bismuth subsalicylate containing compound (Pepto-Bismol). *J Pediatr.* 1981;99:654-656.
38. Pollet S, Albouz S, Le Saux F, et al. Bismuth intoxication: bismuth level in pig brain lipids and in subcellular fractions. *Toxicol Eur Res.* 1979;2:123-125.
39. Randall RE, Osheroff RJ, Bakerman S, Setter JG. Bismuth nephrotoxicity. *Ann Intern Med.* 1972;77:481-482.
40. Rodilla V, Miles AT, Jenner W, Hawksworth GM. Exposure of human cultured proximal tubule cells to cadmium, mercury, zinc, and bismuth: toxicity and metallothionein induction. *Chem Biol Interact.* 1998;115: 71-83.
41. Ross JF, Broadwell RD, Poston MR, Lawhorn GT. Highest brain bismuth levels and neuropathology are adjacent to fenestrated blood vessels in mouse brain after intraperitoneal dosing of bismuth subnitrate. *Toxicol Appl Pharmacol.* 1994;124:191-200.
42. Sainsbury SJ. Fatal salicylate toxicity from bismuth subsalicylate. *West J Med.* 1991;155:637-639.
43. Serfontein WJ, Mekel R. Bismuth toxicity in man II. Review of bismuth blood and urine levels in patients after administration of therapeutic bismuth formulations in relation to the problem of bismuth toxicity in man. *Res Commun Chemical Pathol Pharmacol.* 1979;26:391-411.
44. Serfontein WJ, Mekel R, Bank S, et al. Bismuth toxicity in man I: bismuth blood and urine levels in patients after administration of a bismuth protein complex (bictropeptide). *Res Commun Chem Pathol Pharmacol.* 1979;26: 383-389.
45. Slikkerveer A, Jong HB, Helmich RB, de Wolff FA. Development of a therapeutic procedure for bismuth intoxication with chelating agents. *J Lab Clin Med.* 1992;119:529-537.
46. Slikkerveer A, Noach LA, Tytgat GN, et al. Comparison of enhanced elimination of bismuth in humans after treatment with meso-2,3 dimercaptosuccinic acid and d,l-2,3-dimercaptopropane-1-sulfonic acid. *Analyst.* 1998;123:91-92.
47. Stevens PE, Bierer DW. Bismuth subsalicylate: history chemistry, and safety. *Rev Infect Dis.* 1990;12:S3-S8.
48. Stevens PE, Moore DF, House IM, et al. Significant elimination of bismuth by haemodialysis with a new heavy metal chelating agent. *Nephrol Dial Transplant.* 1995;10:696-698.
49. Stoltenberg M, Schionning JD, Danscher G. Retrograde axonal transport of bismuth: an automettalographic study. *Acta Neuropathol.* 2001;101: 123-128.
50. Suarez FL, Furne JK, Springfield J, Levitt MD. Bismuth subsalicylate markedly decreases hydrogen sulfide release in the human colon. *Gastroenterology.* 1998;114:923-929.
51. Szymanska JA, Zelazowski AJ, Kawiorski S. Some aspects of bismuth metabolism. *Clin Toxicol.* 1981;18:1291-1298.
52. Taylor EG, Klenerman P. Acute renal failure after bismuth subcitrate overdose. *Lancet.* 1990;335:670-671.
53. Thompson HE, Steadman LT, Pommeranke WT. The transfer of bismuth into fetal circulation after maternal administration of sobisimol. *Am J Syp.* 1941;25:725-730.
54. Tremaine WJ, Sandborn WJ, Wolff BG, et al. Bismuth carbomer foam enemas for chronic pouchitis: a randomized, double-blind, placebo-controlled trial. *Aliment Pharmacol Ther.* 1997;11:1041-1046.
55. Urizar R, Vernier RL. Bismuth nephropathy. *JAMA.* 1966;198:207-209.
56. Walsh JH, Peterson WL. Drug therapy: the treatment of *Helicobacter pylori* infection in the management of peptic ulcer disease. *N Engl J Med.* 1995;333:984-991.
57. Wilson APR. The dangers of BIPP. *Lancet.* 1994;334:1313-1314.
58. Zala L, Hunziker T, Braathen LR. Pigmentation following long-term bismuth therapy for pneumatosis cystoides intestinalis. *Dermatology.* 1993;187:288-289.

CHAPTER 90
CADMIUM

Stephen J. Traub and Robert S. Hoffman

Cadmium (Cd)		
Atomic number	=	48
Atomic weight	=	112.40 daltons
Normal concentrations		
Whole blood	<	5 µg/L (<44.5 nmol/L)
Urine (24 hour)	<	3 µg/g creatinine
	<	26.7 nmol/g creatinine

Cadmium, which is currently used for a variety of industrial purposes, may cause both acute and chronic toxicological injury. After acute inhalation, patients may develop life-threatening pneumonitis; after acute ingestion, they may develop gastrointestinal (GI) necrosis. Chronic toxicity usually presents with renal impairment (proteinuria), although effects on bone and lung are also reported.

HISTORY AND EPIDEMIOLOGY

Cadmium, atomic number 48, is a transition metal in group IIB of the periodic table. In its pure atomic form, it is a bluish solid at room temperature. It is readily oxidized to a divalent ion, Cd^{2+}. Naturally occurring cadmium commonly exists as cadmium sulfide (CdS), a trace contaminant of zinc-containing ores.[36]

Cadmium sulfide, cadmium oxide, and other cadmium-containing compounds are refined to produce elemental cadmium, which is used for industrial purposes. When combined with other metals, cadmium forms alloys of relatively low melting points, which accounts for its extensive use in solders and brazing rods. Today, cadmium is principally used as a reagent in electroplating and in the production of nickel-cadmium batteries. Other uses of cadmium include as a pigment, as part of the phosphorescent system in black-and-white televisions, and as a neutron absorber in nuclear reactors. Cadmium salts have also been used as veterinary antihelminthics.[12]

As cadmium processing has increased, so has the incidence of cadmium toxicity. Cadmium exposure with resultant toxicity usually occurs in the environment, occupations, or hobby work.

ENVIRONMENTAL EXPOSURE

Environmental exposure to cadmium generally occurs by the consumption of foods grown in cadmium-contaminated areas. Because cadmium is fairly common as an impurity in ores, areas where mining or refining of ores takes place are the most likely to contain cadmium contamination.

In the 1950s, a mine near the Jinzu River basin discharged large amounts of cadmium into the environment, contaminating the rice that was a staple of the local food supply. An epidemic of painful osteomalacia followed, affecting hundreds of people, with postmenopausal multiparous women being most affected.[67] The afflicted were prone to develop pathologic fractures, and were reported to call out "itai-itai" (translated literally as "ouch-ouch") as they walked, because of the severity of their pain.[28] These symptoms were ultimately linked to the cadmium. Less consequential environmental cadmium exposures have also occurred in Sweden,[46] Belgium,[10] and China.[48] Environmental exposure also occurs in smokers, who have higher blood cadmium concentrations than nonsmokers,[88] probably as a result of soil contamination. This is noteworthy, in that cadmium and tobacco may be synergistic causes of chronic pulmonary disease.[62]

OCCUPATIONAL AND HOBBY EXPOSURE

Welders, solderers, and jewelry workers who use cadmium-containing alloys are at risk for developing acute cadmium toxicity due to inhalation of cadmium oxide fumes. Other workers who do not work with metals per se may develop significant chronic cadmium toxicity through exposure to cadmium-containing dust.

Hobbyists who work with cadmium solders have exposures similar to occupational metalworkers. Significant cadmium toxicity in this population invariably results from metalworking in a closed space with inadequate ventilation and/or improper respiratory precautions.

TOXICOKINETICS

There is no known biologic role for cadmium. The bioavailability of elemental cadmium is unknown. Orally ingested cadmium salts are poorly bioavailable (5%–20%). However, inhaled cadmium fumes (cadmium oxide) are readily bioavailable (up to 90%).[96] As the only data on cadmium toxicokinetics are derived from work with cadmium salts and oxides, "cadmium" in the following discussion refers to these species unless otherwise noted.

After exposure, cadmium is absorbed into the bloodstream, where it is bound to α_2-macroglobulin and albumin.[97] It is then quickly and preferentially redistributed to the liver and kidney. Although other organs, such as the pancreas, spleen, heart, lung, and testes, can take up part of an acute cadmium load, they do so much less avidly.[25] Cadmium enters target organs by three mechanisms: zinc and calcium transporters; uptake of cadmium–glutathione or cadmium–cysteine complexes by transport proteins; and endocytosis of cadmium–protein complexes.[102]

After incorporation into the liver and kidney, cadmium is complexed with metallothionein, an endogenous thiol-rich protein that is produced in both organs. Metallothionein binds and sequesters cadmium. Slowly, hepatic stores of the cadmium–metallothionein complex (Cd-MT) are released. Circulating Cd-MT is then filtered by the glomerulus. A significant amount is reabsorbed and concentrated in proximal tubular cells.[19,83,84] This in part explains why the kidney is the principal target organ in cadmium toxicity.

There is no evidence that cadmium ions are oxidized, reduced, methylated, or otherwise biotransformed in vivo. The volume of distribution (Vd) of cadmium is unknown, but is presumably quite large as a consequence of significant hepatic sequestration. Cadmium distribution and elimination are complex, and an eight-compartment kinetic model was proposed.[54] The slow release of cadmium from metallothionein-complexed hepatic stores accounts for its very long biologic half-life of 10 or more years.

PATHOPHYSIOLOGY

CELLULAR PATHOPHYSIOLOGY

Cadmium toxicity results from interaction of the free cation with target cells.[25,35,60,65,84] Complexation with metallothionein is cytoprotective,[22,60] and metallothionein functions as a natural chelator with a strong affinity for cadmium.[18,55] Although metallothionein may play a role in proximal tubular concentration of cadmium, renal damage is actually

TABLE 90–1. Chronic and Acute Organ System Effects of Cadmium

Organ	Acute	Chronic
Kidney		Proteinuria Nephrolithiasis
Bone		Osteomalacia
Lung	Pneumonitis	Cancer
Gastrointestinal system	Caustic injury	

attenuated by metallothionein, as metallothionein-deficient mice demonstrate more toxicity after cadmium exposure than controls.[60]

There are several mechanisms by which cadmium interferes with cellular function. Cadmium binds to sulfhydryl groups, denaturing proteins and/or inactivating enzymes. The mitochondria are severely affected by this process,[1] which may result in an increased susceptibility to oxidative stress.[47] Cadmium also interferes with E-cadherin, N-cadherin, and β-catenin–mediated cell–cell adhesion.[71–73] Finally, the demonstrated interference of cadmium with calcium transport mechanisms[93,94] might lead to intracellular hypercalcemia and, ultimately, apoptosis (Table 90–1).

SPECIFIC ORGAN SYSTEM INJURY

Kidney The renal damage caused by cadmium develops over years. Proteinuria is the most common clinical finding, and correlates with proximal tubular dysfunction, which manifests as urinary loss of low-molecular-weight proteins such as β_2-microglobulin and retinol-binding protein. Cadmium also produces hypercalciuria,[80] possibly also via damage to the proximal tubule.

Bone Cadmium-induced osteomalacia is a result of abnormalities in calcium and phosphate homeostasis, which, in turn, result from renal proximal tubular dysfunction. In one autopsy study, the severity of osteomalacia in cadmium-exposed subjects correlated with a decline in the serum calcium-phosphate product.[87]

Lung Acute cadmium pneumonitis is characterized by infiltrates on chest radiograph and hypoxia. Human autopsy studies[32,70,81,98] generally show degeneration and/or loss of bronchial and bronchiolar epithelial cells.

Gastrointestinal Tract Based on case reports,[11,99] ingested cadmium salts are caustic with the potential to induce significant nausea, vomiting, and abdominal pain, and result in GI hemorrhage, necrosis, and perforation. With respect to their effect on the GI mucosa, cadmium salts act similar to mercuric salts (Chap. 96).

CLINICAL MANIFESTATIONS

ACUTE POISONING

Pulmonary/Cadmium Fumes Cadmium pneumonitis results from inhalation of cadmium oxide fumes. The acute phase of cadmium pneumonitis may mimic metal fume fever (Chap. 124), but in fact, the two entities are distinctly different, with regard to both mechanism and clinical consequences. Whereas metal fume fever is benign and self-limited, acute cadmium pneumonitis can progress to hypoxia, respiratory insufficiency, and death.

Published case reports of patients who develop acute cadmium pneumonitis[4,5,32,70,81,90,98,101] are strikingly similar in their presentation. Within 6 to 12 hours of soldering or brazing with cadmium alloys in a closed space, patients typically develop constitutional symptoms, such as fever and chills, as well as a cough and respiratory distress.

On initial presentation these patients, rather than appear seriously ill, instead may have a normal physical examination, oxygenation, and chest radiograph. However, this relatively benign presentation may lead both to the misdiagnosis of metal fume fever and the underestimation of the severity of the patient's illness. As the pneumonitis progresses to acute lung injury (ALI) (Chap. 124), crackles and rhonchi develop, oxygenation becomes impaired, and the chest radiograph develops a pattern consistent with alveolar filling. Despite aggressive supportive care, death may occur, usually within 3 to 5 days.[32,70,81,98]

Patients who survive an episode of acute cadmium pneumonitis may develop chronic pulmonary ailments, including restrictive lung disease,[4,5] diffusion abnormalities,[4] and pulmonary fibrosis.[90] Recovery without sequelae is also reported.[101]

Oral/Cadmium Salts Most acute cadmium exposures are inhalational, and acute ingestions are rare. Based on case report data, GI injury is likely to be the most significant clinical finding after acute ingestion.

In one case,[11] a 17-year-old woman ingested approximately 150 g of cadmium chloride and presented to the emergency department with hypotension and edema of the face, pharynx, and neck. Her condition quickly deteriorated, and she suffered a respiratory arrest. She was intubated and underwent orogastric lavage, chelation with an unspecified agent, and charcoal hemoperfusion. Multisystem organ failure ensued, and she died within 30 hours of presentation. At autopsy, the most significant finding was hemorrhagic necrosis of the upper GI tract. Her blood cadmium concentration was more than 2000 times normal.

In a second reported case of oral ingestion a 23-year-old man ingested approximately 5 g of cadmium iodide in a suicide attempt and presented with acute hemorrhagic gastroenteritis.[99] His condition deteriorated, and despite treatment with ethylenediaminetetraacetic acid (EDTA) and supportive measures, he died on hospital day 7. Autopsy did not reveal a specific cause of death.

CHRONIC POISONING

Chronic cadmium poisoning generally occurs to individuals through occupational exposures, although instances of mass environmental exposure, such as occurred in Japan,[28,66] are reported. All studies of chronic cadmium poisoning in humans are retrospective; conclusions about clinical course and treatment are therefore neither randomized nor controlled. In addition, and especially in the industrial setting, cadmium exposure may serve simply as a marker for other exposures, such as toxic vapors, other metals, or solvents. These other xenobiotics may contribute to, or cause, the pathologic condition described.

Nephrotoxicity The most common finding in chronic cadmium poisoning is proteinuria. Low-molecular-weight proteinuria is usually more significant than, and generally precedes, glomerular dysfunction, although some cadmium-exposed workers manifest predominantly glomerular proteinuria.[7] There is a dose–response relationship between total body cadmium burden and renal dysfunction,[10,44,46,67,92] although this relationship may not be as strong at low doses.[39] Patients with diabetes mellitus may be particularly susceptible to the nephrotoxic effects of cadmium.[37] In most cases, proteinuria is generally considered to be irreversible even after removal from exposure,[38,52,76] but improvement is sometimes reported.[91] Less clear is the question of whether renal dysfunction progresses after removal from exposure, with studies showing both stable[38] and deteriorating[42,75,76] renal function in cadmium-exposed workers who are removed from exposure. The routes and duration of exposure, as well as blood and urine cadmium concentrations, differ markedly among these studies, limiting wider applicability of any analysis.

Occupational cadmium exposure is also associated with nephrolithiasis,[45,79] likely as a result of hypercalciuria.[80]

Pulmonary Toxicity Large studies of workers chronically exposed to cadmium fail to demonstrate consistent effects on the lung. In one study of 57 workers with sufficient exposure to cadmium oxide to produce renal dysfunction, there was no evidence of pulmonary dysfunction, even in those with the greatest cumulative cadmium exposure.[27] In contrast, other studies demonstrate both restrictive[17] and obstructive[21,78] changes on pulmonary function tests. Interestingly, a follow-up study of the group with restrictive lung disease showed improvements after cadmium exposure was reduced.[16] The discrepancies in these results may be partly a result of markedly different doses and durations of exposure among the various groups.

Cadmium is associated with pulmonary neoplasia; the carcinogenicity of cadmium is discussed separately (see Cancer section below).

Musculoskeletal Toxicity Cadmium-induced osteomalacia usually occurs in the setting of environmental exposure, as was true in Japan and Sweden.[43] Although mentioned in case reports,[8,52] osteomalacia is generally not a prominent feature of occupational exposure to cadmium. One possible reason for this apparent difference is, whereas victims of the original Itai-Itai epidemic were mostly women, occupational cadmium exposures typically occur in men. In addition, differences in cumulative dosing and in route of exposure (oral versus pulmonary) may partly account for the unique prominence of osteomalacia in environmental exposures.

Hepatotoxicity Although the liver stores as much cadmium as any other organ, hepatotoxicity is not a prominent feature in humans with cadmium exposure, probably because hepatic cadmium is usually complexed to metallothionein.[40] The liver can potentially be a target organ, however, and hepatotoxicity is easily inducible in animals.[1,25,26,74]

Neurologic Toxicity Cadmium exposure is linked to olfactory disturbances,[63,77,86] impaired higher cortical function,[95] and Parkinson syndrome.[68,95]

Other Organ Systems Cadmium induces hypertension in rats,[59] but human studies have only yielded unconvincing and conflicting results.[31,58,69,89] Although there is evidence that cadmium may cause immunosuppression affecting both humoral and cell-mediated immunity in animals,[24] a single human study showed no overt immunopathology in an occupationally exposed cohort.[51] The testes are clearly a target organ in animal exposures,[57] but they are not considered a major target organ in humans.

Cancer Cadmium induces tumors in multiple animal organs, an effect that is exacerbated by zinc deficiency.[96] In humans, cadmium exposure is associated with lung cancer, although the strength of this association has been questioned because most studies have methodologic problems, such as coexposure to arsenic, a known pulmonary carcinogen.[9,53] Despite these confounding coexposures, cadmium is officially designated as a human carcinogen by the International Agency for Research on Cancer.[41]

DIAGNOSTIC TESTING

Cadmium concentrations have limited usefulness in the management of the acutely exposed patient, other than to confirm exposure. Diagnosis and treatment are based on the patient's history, physical examination, and symptoms. In a patient exposed to cadmium oxide fumes, ancillary tests, such as pulse oximetry and chest radiography, are more useful than actual cadmium concentrations.

In the patient chronically exposed to cadmium, both cadmium concentrations and ancillary testing may prove helpful. Urinary cadmium concentrations, which reflect the slow, steady-state turnover and release of metallothionein-bound cadmium from the liver, are a better reflection of the total-body cadmium burden than are whole blood concentrations.

Workers at high risk for cadmium toxicity should routinely have blood and urine cadmium testing and urinary protein testing. Workers with a urinary cadmium concentration greater than 7 μg/g urinary creatinine or a blood cadium concentration greater than 10 μg Cd/L require immediate reassignment to a cadmium-free area. Workers with significant proteinuria (β_2-microglobulin concentrations of 750 μg/g urinary creatinine) should also be reassigned if additional testing confirms cadmium exposure (as defined by a urinary cadmium concentration greater than 3 μg/g urinary creatinine or a blood cadium concentration greater than 5 μg/L). These numbers are reasonable in light of the fact that renal dysfunction can occur at cadmium concentrations as low as 5 μg/g urinary creatinine,[20,44] a concentration significantly higher than that of the general US population, 95% of whom have concentrations that are less than 2 μg/g urinary creatinine.[15]

MANAGEMENT

ACUTE EXPOSURE

Oral Exposure/Cadmium Salts After the status of the patient's airway, breathing, and circulation are addressed, attention can be given to GI decontamination. Although large ingestions of soluble cadmium salts are rare, they frequently prove fatal.[11,99] The lowest reported human lethal dose is 5 g. In light of this, if a significant ingestion occurs but emesis has not occurred, gastric lavage is appropriate. In this situation, a small nasogastric tube should suffice, as inorganic cadmium salts are powders, not pills.

Given the relative lack of experience with acute oral cadmium poisoning, all patients with known exposures and/or abnormal findings consistent with cadmium toxicity or exposure should be admitted to the hospital for supportive care, monitoring of renal and hepatic function, and possibly evaluation of the GI tract for injury.

Although it seems logical to use chelation therapy in any patient with an acute life-threatening ingestion of a metal compound, the benefit of chelation in acute cadmium exposure is unproven. Multiple chelators have been used, all in animal models, with inconsistent results.

The ideal chelator for treatment of oral cadmium toxicity would be well tolerated, and would decrease GI absorption of cadmium and decrease the concentration of cadmium in organs such as the kidney and liver, while not increasing cadmium concentrations in other critical organs such as the brain. Of the chelators currently studied for cadmium toxicity, succimer comes closest to fulfilling these criteria. In models of acute oral cadmium toxicity, succimer decreases the GI absorption of cadmium,[3,6] without increasing cadmium burdens in target organs, and improves survival.[2,6,50]

In a patient thought to have ingested potentially lethal amounts of cadmium, treatment with succimer is reasonable. Succimer should be given as soon as possible after the ingestion, as the effectiveness of chelators decreases dramatically over time in experimental models of cadmium poisoning.[14]

It must be stressed, however, that supporting data for chelation are promising, but not definitive, and are only derived from animal models. Succimer dosing in human cadmium poisoning is unstudied. Doses that are well tolerated (10 mg/kg/dose tid) are appropriate (see Antidotes in Depth A27–Succimer [2,3-Dimercaptosuccinic Acid]).

Other chelators that may be beneficial, but for which further investigation is needed, include diethylenetriaminepentaacetic acid (DTPA)[6,13] and 2,3-dimercaptopropane sulfonate (DMPS),[13,50] both of which reduce tissue burdens and increase survival.

Most other chelators are either ineffective or detrimental, including 2,3-dimercaptopropanol (British anti-Lewisite, BAL),[13,19,49] penicillamine,[13,61] cyclic tetramines (such as cyclam and tACPD),[85] detergent formula chelators such as sodium tripolyphosphate (STPP) and nitrilotriacetic acid (NTA),[29,30] EDTA,[64] and dithiocarbamates.[3,33]

Pulmonary/Cadmium Fumes The patient who is ill after exposure to cadmium fumes (generally cadmium oxide) invariably presents with respiratory complaints and possibly also with constitutional symptoms. The airway should be assessed and appropriate oxygenation ensured, although hypoxia may not be a problem acutely. Steroids are used in most reported cases, but there are no studies to support their efficacy. Because cadmium inhalation injuries are neither benign nor self-limited, all patients with acute inhalational exposures to cadmium should be admitted to the hospital for observation and supportive care until respiratory symptoms have resolved. All such patients should have long-term follow-up arranged with a pulmonologist to assess the possibility of chronic lung injury, even following a single exposure.

Chelation should not be entertained as an option for patients with single acute exposures to cadmium fumes, as these patients do not appear to develop extrapulmonary injury.[4,5,90,101]

CHRONIC EXPOSURE

Patients chronically exposed to cadmium frequently come to attention during routine screening, as those who work with cadmium are under close medical surveillance. These patients may have developed proteinuria or, less commonly, chronic pulmonary complaints.

Management is challenging. Cessation of cadmium exposure is the first intervention. However, as mentioned earlier, chronic cadmium-induced renal and pulmonary changes are largely irreversible.

Chelation for chronic cadmium toxicity is not currently recommended. There is no evidence that chelation of chronically poisoned animals improves long-term outcomes, and one study in humans found no improvement in cadmium-induced renal dysfunction with periodic EDTA chelation.[100] Furthermore, in a chronically exposed patient, the majority of cadmium is bound to intracellular metallothionein, which greatly reduces its toxicity. Any attempt to remove cadmium from these deposits risks redistributing cadmium to other organs, possibly exacerbating toxicity, as is known to occur with BAL therapy.[23]

Of all the chelators tested thus far in animal models of chronic cadmium toxicity, the dithiocarbamates have shown the most success in reducing total body cadmium burdens. Unfortunately, these chelators tend to cause redistribution of cadmium to the brain as their lipophilicity not only allows them to cross cell membranes into hepatocytes (to access stored cadmium), but also promotes their uptake into the lipid-rich central nervous system (CNS).[34] Numerous dithiocarbamates have been synthesized and studied with regard to cadmium decorporation, however, and several species effectively reduce whole-body, renal, and hepatic cadmium concentrations without an increase in CNS cadmium.[56,82]

Further research into the subject of chelation for chronic cadmium poisoning is ongoing, and may produce an agent that is both safe and effective without exacerbating end organ toxicity. At present, there is insufficient evidence to justify the use of any chelator in the treatment of chronic cadmium toxicity.

SUMMARY

Cadmium is a toxic element that causes acute and chronic effects dependent on the total dose and route of exposure. After acute oral exposure, GI injury predominates. After acute inhalation, a severe chemical pneumonitis may ensue. With chronic environmental or occupational exposure, nephrotoxicity (usually manifested by proteinuria) is the most significant finding, although other organ systems, such as the lungs, can be affected. Treatment for all patients with suspected cadmium poisoning consists of removal from the source, decontamination if possible, and supportive care. In the rare instance of exposure from acute cadmium salt ingestion, treatment with succimer may be warranted. At this time there is insufficient evidence to recommend chelation in the patient who is chronically poisoned by cadmium.

REFERENCES

1. Al-Nasser IA. Cadmium hepatotoxicity and alterations of the mitochondrial function. *J Toxicol Clin Toxicol.* 2000;38:407-413.
2. Andersen O, Nielsen JB. Oral cadmium chloride intoxication in mice: effects of penicillamine, dimercaptosuccinic acid and related compounds. *Pharmacol Toxicol.* 1988;63:386-389.
3. Anderson O, Nielsen JB, Svendsen P. Oral cadmium chloride intoxication in mice: diethyldithiocarbamate enhances rather than alleviates acute toxicity. *Toxicology.* 1988;52:331-342.
4. Anthony JS, Zamel N, Aberman A. Abnormalities in pulmonary function after brief exposure to toxic metal fumes. *Can Med Assoc J.* 1978;119:586-588.
5. Barnhart S, Rosenstock L. Cadmium chemical pneumonitis. *Chest.* 1984;86:791.
6. Basinger MA, Jones MM, Hoscher MA, et al. Antagonists for acute oral cadmium chloride intoxication. *J Toxicol Environ Health.* 1988;23:77-89.
7. Bernard A, Roels H, Hubermont G, et al. Characterization of the proteinuria of cadmium-exposed workers. *Int Arch Occup Environ Health.* 1976;38:19-30.
8. Blainey JD, Adams RG, Brewer DB, et al. Cadmium-induced osteomalacia. *Br J Ind Med.* 1980;37:278-284.
9. Bofetta P. Methodological aspects of the epidemiological association between cadmium and cancer in humans. *IARC Sci Publ.* 1992;118:425-434.
10. Buchet JP, Lauwerys R, Roels H, et al. Renal effects of cadmium body burden of the general population. *Lancet.* 1990;336:699-702.
11. Buckler HM, Smith WD, Rees WD. Self-poisoning with oral cadmium chloride. *Br Med J.* 1986;292:1559-1560.
12. Budavari S, O'Neil MJ, Smith A, et al, eds. *The Merck Index.* Whitehouse Station, NJ: Merck & Company; 1996:1665.
13. Cantilena LR, Klaassen CD. Comparison of the effectiveness of several chelators after single administration on the toxicity, excretion, and distribution of cadmium. *Toxicol Appl Pharmacol.* 1981;58:452-460.
14. Cantilena LR, Klaassen CD. Decreased effectiveness of chelation therapy with time after acute cadmium poisoning. *Toxicol Appl Pharmacol.* 1982;63:173-180.
15. Centers for Disease Control and Prevention. Second national report on human exposure to environmental chemicals. NCEH Pub. No. 02-0716. March 2003:13-16. Atlanta.
16. Chan OY, Poh SC, Lee HS, et al. Respiratory function in cadmium battery workers—a follow-up study. *Ann Acad Med Singapore.* 1988;17:283-287.
17. Chan OY, Poh SC, Tan KT, Kwok SF. Respiratory function in cadmium battery workers. *Singapore Med J.* 1986;27:108-119.
18. Cherian MG, Goyer RA, Delaquerriere-Richardson L. Cadmium-metallothionein-induced nephropathy. *Toxicol Appl Pharmacol.* 1976;38:399-408.
19. Cherian MG, Rodgers K. Chelation of cadmium from metallothionein in vivo and its excretion in rats repeatedly injected with cadmium chloride. *J Pharmacol Exp Ther.* 1982;222:699-704.
20. Chia KS, Tan AL, Chia SE, et al. Renal tubular function of cadmium exposed workers. *Ann Acad Med Singapore.* 1992;21:756-759.
21. Cortona G, Apostoli P, Toffoletto F, et al. Occupational exposure to cadmium and lung function. *IARC Sci Publ.* 1992;118:205-210.
22. Coyle P, Niezing G, Shelton TL, et al. Tolerance to cadmium toxicity by metallothionein and zinc: in vivo and in vitro studies with MT-null mice. *Toxicology.* 2000;150:53-67.
23. Dalhamn T, Friberg L. Dimercaprol (2,3-dimercaptopropanol) in chronic cadmium poisoning. *Acta Pharmacol Toxicol.* 1955;11:68-71.
24. Dan G, Lall SB, Rao DN. Humoral and cell-mediated immune response to cadmium in mice. *Drug Chem Toxicol.* 2000;23:349-360.

25. Dudley RE, Gammal LM, Klaassen CD. Cadmium-induced hepatic and renal injury in chronically exposed rats: likely role of hepatic cadmium-metallothionein in nephrotoxicity. *Toxicol Appl Pharmacol.* 1985;77: 414-426.
26. Dudley RE, Svoboda DJ, Klaassen CD. Acute exposure to cadmium causes severe liver injury in rats. *Toxicol Appl Pharmacol.* 1982;65:302-313.
27. Edling C, Elinder CG, Randma E. Lung function in workers using cadmium containing solder. *Br J Ind Med.* 1986;43:657-662.
28. Emmerson BT. "Ouch-ouch" disease: the osteomalacia of cadmium nephropathy. *Ann Intern Med.* 1970;73:854-855.
29. Engstrom B. Influence of chelating agents on toxicity and distribution of cadmium among proteins of mouse liver and kidney following oral or subcutaneous exposure. *Acta Pharmacol Toxicol.* 1981;48:108-117.
30. Engstrom B, Nordberg GF. Effects of detergent formula chelating agents on the metabolism and toxicity of cadmium in mice. *Acta Pharmacol Toxicol.* 1978;43:387-397.
31. Engvall J, Perk J. Prevalence of hypertension among cadmium-exposed workers. *Arch Environ Health.* 1985;40:185-190.
32. Fuortes L, Leo A, Ellerbeck PG, Friell LA. Acute respiratory fatality associated with exposure to sheet metal and cadmium fumes. *J Toxicol Clin Toxicol.* 1991;29:279-283.
33. Gale GR, Atkins LM, Walker EM, et al. Comparative effects of diethyldithiocarbamate, dimercaptosuccinate, and diethylenetriaminepentaacetate on organ distribution and excretion of cadmium. *Ann Clin Lab Sci.* 1983;13:33-44.
34. Gale GR, Atkins LM, Walker EM, et al. Mechanism of diethyldithiocarbamate, dihydroxyethyldithiocarbamate, and dicarboxymethyldithiocarbamate action on distribution and excretion of cadmium. *Ann Clin Lab Sci.* 1983;13:474-481.
35. Goyer RA, Miller CR, Zhu SY, Victery W. Non-metallothioneinbound cadmium in the pathogenesis of cadmium nephrotoxicity in the rat. *Toxicol Appl Pharmacol.* 1989;101:232-244.
36. Hammond CR. Cadmium. In: Lide DR, ed. *CRC Handbook of Chemistry and Physics*, 80th ed. Boca Raton, FL: CRC Press; 1989:4-8.
37. Haswell-Elkins M, Satarug S, O'Rourke P, et al. Striking association between urinary cadmium level and albuminuria among Torres Strait Islander people with diabetes. *Environ Res.* 2008;106:379-383.
38. Hotz P, Buchet JP, Bernard A, et al. Renal effects of low-level environmental cadmium exposure: 5-year follow-up of a subcohort from the Cadmibel study. *Lancet.* 1999;354:1508-1513.
39. Ikeda M, Moon CS, Zhang ZW, et al. Urinary alpha$_1$-microglobulin, beta$_2$-microglobulin, and retinol-binding protein levels in general populations in Japan with references to cadmium in urine, blood, and 24-hour food duplicates. *Environ Res.* 1995;70:35-46.
40. Ikeda M, Watanabe T, Zhang Z-W, et al. The integrity of the liver among people environmentally exposed to cadmium at various levels. *Int Arch Occup Environ Health.* 1997;69:379-385.
41. International Agency for Research on Cancer. Cadmium. http://www-cie.iarc.fr/htdocs/monographs/vol58/mono58-2.htm (accessed January 5, 2005).
42. Iwata K, Saito H, Moriyama M, Nakano A. Renal tubular function after reduction of environmental cadmium exposure: a ten-year follow-up. *Arch Environ Health.* 1993;48:157-163.
43. Järup L, Alfvén T. Low level cadmium exposure, renal and bone effects—the OSCAR study. *Biometals.* 2004;17(5):505-509.
44. Järup L, Elinder CG. Dose-response relations between urinary cadmium and tubular proteinuria in cadmium-exposed workers. *Am J Ind Med.* 1994;26:759-769.
45. Järup L, Elinder CG. Incidence of renal stones among cadmium exposed battery workers. *Br J Ind Med.* 1993;50:598-602.
46. Järup L, Hellstrom L, Alfven T, et al. Low-level exposure to cadmium and early kidney damage: the OSCAR study. *Occup Environ Med.* 2000;57:668-672.
47. Jimi S, Uchiyama M, Takaki A, et al. Mechanisms of cell death induced by cadmium and arsenic. *Ann N Y Acad Sci.* 2004;1011:325-331.
48. Jin T, Nordberg G, Ye T, et al. Osteoporosis and renal dysfunction in a general population exposed to cadmium in China. *Environ Res.* 2004;96:353-359.
49. Jones MM, Cherian MG, Singh PK, et al. A comparative study on the influence of vicinal dithiols and a dithiocarbamate on the biliary excretion of cadmium in rat. *Toxicol Appl Pharmacol.* 1991;110:241-250.
50. Jones MM, Weater AD, Weller WL. The relative effectiveness of some chelating agents as antidotes in acute cadmium poisoning. *Res Commun Chem Pathol Pharmacol.* 1978;22:581-588.
51. Karakaya A, Yucesoy B, Sardas OS. An immunological study on workers occupationally exposed to cadmium. *Hum Exp Toxicol.* 1994;13:73-75.
52. Kazantis G. Renal tubular dysfunction and abnormalities of calcium metabolism in cadmium workers. *Environ Health Perspect.* 1979;28:155-159.
53. Kazantis G, Blanks RG, Sullivan KR. Is cadmium a human carcinogen? *IARC Sci Publ.* 1992;118:435-446.
54. Kjellstrom T, Nordberg GF. A kinetic model of cadmium metabolism in the human being. *Environ Res.* 1978;16:248-269.
55. Klaassen CD, Liu J, Choudhuri S. Metallothionein. An intracellular protein to protect against cadmium toxicity. *Annu Rev Pharmacol Toxicol.* 1999;39:267-294.
56. Kojima S, Ono H, Kiyozumi M, et al. Effect of *N*-benzyl-D-glucamine dithiocarbamate on the renal toxicity produced by subacute exposure to cadmium in rats. *Toxicol Appl Pharmacol.* 1989;98:39-48.
57. Kojima S, Sugimura Y, Hirukawa H, et al. Effects of dithiocarbamates on testicular toxicity in rats caused by acute exposure to cadmium. *Toxicol Appl Pharmacol.* 1992;116:24-29.
58. Kurihara I, Kobayashi E, Suwazono Y, et al. Association between exposure to cadmium and blood pressure in Japanese peoples. *Arch Environ Health.* 2004;59:711-716.
59. Lall SB, Das N, Rama R, et al. Cadmium-induced nephrotoxicity in rats. *Indian J Exp Biol.* 1997;35:151-154.
60. Liu J, Liu Y, Habeebu SS, Klaassen CD. Susceptibility of MT null mice to chronic $CdCl_2$-induced nephrotoxicity indicates that renal injury is not mediated by the CdMT complex. *Toxicol Sci.* 1998;46:197-203.
61. Lyle WH, Green JN, Gore V, et al. Enhancement of cadmium nephrotoxicity by penicillamine in the rat. *Postgrad Med J.* 1968;Suppl:18-21.
62. Mannino DM, Holguin F, Greves HM, et al. Urinary cadmium levels predict lower lung function in current and former smokers: data from the Third National Health and Nutrition Examination Survey. *Thorax.* 2004;59:194-198.
63. Mascagni P, Consonni D, Bregante G, et al. Olfactory function in workers exposed to moderate airborne cadmium levels. *Neurotoxicology.* 2003;24:717-724.
64. McGivern J, Mason J. The effect of chelation on the fate of intravenously administered cadmium in rats. *J Comp Pathol.* 1979;89:1-9.
65. Min K-S, Onosaka S, Tanaka K. Renal accumulation of cadmium and nephropathy following long-term administration of cadmiummetallothionein. *Toxicol Appl Pharmacol.* 1996;141:102-109.
66. Murata I, Hirono T, Saeki Y, et al. Cadmium enteropathy, renal osteomalacia ("Itai-Itai" disease in Japan). *Bull Soc Int Chir.* 1970;29:34-42.
67. Nogawa K, Kido T, Shaikh ZA. Dose-response relationship for renal dysfunction in a population environmentally exposed to cadmium. *IARC Sci Publ.* 1992;118:311-318.
68. Okuda B, Iwamoto Y, Tachibana H, Sugita M. Parkinsonism after acute cadmium poisoning. *Clin Neurol Neurosurg.* 1997;99:263-265.
69. Ostergaard K. Cadmium and hypertension. *Lancet.* 1977;8013:677-678.
70. Patwardhan JR, Finckh ES. Fatal cadmium-fume pneumonitis. *Med J Aust.* 1976;1:962-966.
71. Pearson CA, Lamar PC, Prozialeck WC. Effects of cadmium on E-cadherin and VE-cadherin in mouse lung. *Life Sci.* 2003;72:1303-1320.
72. Prozialeck WC. Evidence that E-cadherin may be a target for cadmium toxicity in epithelial cells. *Toxicol Appl Pharmacol.* 2000;164:231-249.
73. Prozialeck WC, Lamar PC, Lynch SM. Cadmium alters the localization of N-cadherin, E-cadherin, and beta-catenin in the proximal tubule epithelium. *Toxicol Appl Pharmacol.* 2003;189:180-195.
74. Rikans LE, Yamano T. Mechanisms of cadmium-mediated acute hepatotoxicity. *J Biochem Mol Toxicol.* 2000;14:110-117.
75. Roels H, Djubgang J, Buchet JT, et al. Evolution of cadmium-induced renal dysfunction in workers removed from exposure. *Scand J Work Environ Health.* 1982;8:191-200.
76. Roels HA, Lauwerys RR, Buchet JP, et al. Health significance of cadmium-induced renal dysfunction: a five-year follow-up. *Br J Ind Med.* 1989;46: 755-764.
77. Rose CS, Heywood PG, Costanzo RM. Olfactory impairment after chronic occupational cadmium exposure. *J Occup Med.* 1992;34:600-605.
78. Sakurai H, Omae K, Toyama T, et al. Cross-sectional study of pulmonary function in cadmium alloy workers. *Scand J Work Environ Health.* 1982;8(Suppl 1):122-130.
79. Scott R, Cunningham C, McLelland A, et al. The importance of cadmium as a factor in calcified upper urinary tract stone disease—a prospective 7-year study. *Br J Urol.* 1982;54:584-589.

80. Scott R, Patterson PJ, Burns R, et al. Hypercalciuria related to cadmium exposure. *Urology.* 1978;11:462-465.
81. Seidal K, Jorgensen N, Elinder CG, et al. Fatal cadmium-induced pneumonitis. *Scand J Work Environ Health.* 1993;19:429-431.
82. Singh PK, Jones SG, Gale GR, et al. Selective removal of cadmium from aged hepatic and renal deposits: N-substituted talooctamine dithiocarbamates as cadmium mobilizing agent. *Chem Biol Interact.* 1990;74:79-91.
83. Squibb KS, Pritchard JB, Fowler BA. Cadmium-metallothionein nephropathy. Relationships between ultrastructural/biochemical alterations and intracellular cadmium binding. *J Pharmacol Exp Ther.* 1984;229:311-321.
84. Squibb KS, Ridlington JW, Carmichael NG, Fowler BA. Early cellular effects of circulating cadmium-thionein on kidney proximal tubules. *Environ Health Perspect.* 1979;28:287-296.
85. Srivasta RC, Gupta S, Ahmad N, et al. Comparative evaluation of chelating agents on the mobilization of cadmium: a mechanistic approach. *J Toxicol Environ Health.* 1996;47:173-182.
86. Suruda AJ. Measuring olfactory dysfunction from cadmium in an occupational and environmental medicine office practice. *J Occup Environ Med.* 2000;42:337.
87. Takebayashi S, Jimi S, Segawaa M, Kiyoshi Y. Cadmium induces osteomalacia mediated by proximal tubular atrophy and disturbances of phosphate reabsorption. A study of 11 autopsies. *Pathol Res Pract.* 2000;196:653-663.
88. Telisman S, Jurasovic J, Pizent A, et al. Cadmium in the blood and seminal fluid of nonoccupationally exposed adult male subjects with regard to smoking habits. *Int Arch Occup Environ Health.* 1997;70:243-248.
89. Tellez-Plaza M, Navas-Acien A, Crainiceanu CM, Guallar E. Cadmium exposure and hypertension in the 1999-2004 National Health and Nutrition Examination Survey (NHANES). *Environ Health Perspect.* 2008;116:51-56.
90. Townshend RH. Acute cadmium pneumonitis: a 17-year follow up. *Br J Ind Med.* 1982;39:411-412.
91. Tsychya K. Proteinuria of cadmium workers. *J Occup Med.* 1976;18:463-466.
92. van Sittert NJ, Ribbens PH, Huisman B, Lugtengurg D. A nine-year follow-up study of renal effects in workers exposed to cadmium in a zinc ore refinery. *Br J Ind Med.* 1993;50:603-612.
93. Verbost PM, Filk G, Pang PKT, et al. Cadmium inhibition of the erythrocyte Ca^{2+} pump. *J Biol Chem.* 1989;264:5613-5615.
94. Verbost PM, Senden MHMN, van Os CH. Nanomolar concentrations of Cd^{2+} inhibit Ca^{2+} transport systems in plasma membranes and intracellular Ca^{2+} stores in intestinal epithelium. *Biochem Biophys Acta.* 1987;902:247-252.
95. Viaene, MK, Masschelein R, Leenders J, et al. Neurobehavioural effects of occupational exposure to cadmium: a cross-sectional epidemiological study. *Occup Environ Med.* 2000;57:19-27.
96. Waalkes MP. Cadmium carcinogenesis in review. *J Inorg Biochem.* 2000;79:241-244.
97. Watkins SR, Hodge RM, Cowman DC, Wickham PP. Cadmium-binding serum protein. *Biochem Biophys Res Commun.* 1977;74:1403-1410.
98. Winston RM. Cadmium fume poisoning. *Br Med J.* 1971;758:401.
99. Wisniewska-Knypl JM, Jablonska J, Myslak Z. Binding of cadmium on metallothionein in man: an analysis of a fatal poisoning by cadmium iodide. *Arch Toxicol.* 1971;28:46-55.
100. Wu X, Su S, Zhai R, et al. Lack of reversal effect of EDTA treatment on cadmium induced renal dysfunction. a fourteen-year follow-up. *Biometals.* 2004;17:435-441.
101. Yates DH, Goldman KP. Acute cadmium poisoning in a foreman plant welder. *Br J Ind Med.* 1990;47:429-431.
102. Zalups RK, Ahmad S. Molecular handling of cadmium in transporting epithelia. *Toxicol Appl Pharmacol.* 2003;186:163-188.

CHAPTER 91
CHROMIUM

Steven B. Bird

Chromium (Cr)		
Atomic number	=	24
Atomic weight	=	51.99 daltons
Normal concentrations		
Whole blood	=	20–30 µg/L (380–580 nmol/L)
Serum	=	0.05–2.86 µg/L (1–56 nmol/L)
Urine	<	1 µg/g creatinine (<19.2 nmol/g creatinine)

Chromium toxicity may result from occupational exposure, environmental exposure, or a combination of both routes. Similar to the case with many metals, the clinical manifestations of chromium toxicity depend on whether the exposure is acute or chronic and on the chemical form of chromium. Whereas acute toxicity is more likely to involve multiple organ failure, chronic exposure may lead to cancer.

HISTORY AND EPIDEMIOLOGY

Chromium (from the Greek word for color, *chroma*) is a naturally occurring element that may be found in oxidation states of −2 to +6 but primarily exists in the trivalent (Cr^{3+}) and hexavalent (Cr^{6+}) forms. It was first discovered in 1797 in the form of Siberian red lead (crocoite: $PbCrO_4$) and occurs only in combination with other elements, primarily as halides, oxides, or sulfides (Table 91–1). Chromium is found most abundantly in chromite ore ($FeCr_2O_4$).[9] Elemental chromium (Cr^0) does not occur naturally but is extracted commercially from ore.

Elemental chromium is a blue-white metal that is hard and brittle. It can be polished to a fine, shiny surface; affords significant protection against corrosion; and can be added to steel to form stainless steel (an alloy of chromium, nickel, and iron). One of the most important uses of chrome plating is to apply a hard, smooth surface to machine parts such as crankshafts, printing rollers, ball bearings, and cutting tools. This is known as "hard" chrome plating. Elemental chromium is also used in armor plating safes and is used in forming brick molds because of its high melting point and moderate thermal expansion.

The carcinogenic potential of hexavalent chromium was first recognized as a cause of nasal tumors in Scottish chrome pigment workers in the late 1800s. In the 1930s, the pulmonary carcinogenicity of hexavalent chromium was first described in German chromate workers.[12]

PHARMACOLOGY

Chromium is an essential element involved in glucose metabolism. This may be through facilitation of insulin binding to insulin receptors or by amplification of the effects of insulin on carbohydrate and lipid metabolism. Chromium deficiency may have a causal link to diabetes mellitus and atherosclerosis.

The chemical properties and health risks of chromium depend mostly on its oxidative state and on the solubility of the chromium compound. Chromium is found naturally in the hexavalent (Cr^{6+}) or in the trivalent (Cr^{3+}) valence states, and these are the species to which most human exposures occur. However, chromium in the Cr^{6+} and Cr^{3+} oxidation states has very different properties. The relationship between these oxidative states is described by the following equation:[14]

$$Cr_2O_7^{2-} + 14\ H^+ + 6\ \text{electrons} \rightarrow 2Cr^{3+} + 7H_2O + 1.33\ \text{eV}$$

This difference of 1.33 eV in electric potential between the Cr^{6+} (in $Cr_2O_7^{2-}$) and Cr^{3+} states reflects both the significant oxidizing potential of Cr^{6+} and the high energy required for the oxidation of Cr^{3+} to Cr^{6+}. Reduction of Cr^{6+} to Cr^{3+} occurs in vivo by abstraction of electrons from cellular constituents such as proteins, lipids, DNA, RNA, and plasma transferrin which accounts for the toxicity of Cr^{6+}.[34]

The rapidity and completeness of the reduction of Cr^{6+} has been the subject of considerable scientific debate. Hexavalent chromium is reduced to Cr^{3+} in saliva, the gastrointestinal (GI) tract, respiratory tract epithelium and pulmonary macrophages, and blood.[4,31] During this reduction, several other oxidative states transiently occur (namely Cr^{4+} and Cr^{5+}) and contribute to the cytotoxicity, genotoxicity, and carcinogenicity of Cr^{6+} chromium compounds.[43]

Although most Cr^{6+} is rapidly reduced on entering the GI tract, ingestion of Cr^{6+} in drinking water does lead to measurable chromium concentrations in serum, red blood cells (RBCs), and urine. Hexavalent chromium may accumulate in most body tissues, raising concerns that chromium-induced toxicity and carcinogenesis may be more widespread than is currently appreciated.[12]

ENVIRONMENTAL EXPOSURE

The processing of chromium ores primarily releases Cr^{3+} into the environment. However, some hexavalent chromium is released from chromate manufacturing and coal-based power plants. The most significant environmental sources of Cr^{6+} are chromate production, ferrochrome pigment manufacturing, chrome plating, and certain types of welding.

The general population may be exposed to chromium via drinking water, food and food supplements (eg, chromium picolinate), joint arthroplasty, coronary artery stents, and cigarettes. Chromium has been used extensively to prevent equipment and piping corrosion in industrial cooling towers and air conditioning (trivalent chromium). Dermal exposure may occur from use of tanned leather products or wood treated with CCA (copper, chromate, and arsenate), which contains hexavalent chromium that is reduced to trivalent chromium by organic compounds after it is inside wood. CCA-treated lumber was voluntarily removed from the U.S. consumer market in December 2003 because of possible health concerns as a result of exposure to the arsenic and chromium. No specific adverse health effects related to CCA-treated lumber were reported by the Environmental Protection Agency before the voluntary withdrawal. A recent reanalysis of cancer mortality and hexavalent chromium-contaminated drinking water from Liaoning Province, China, demonstrated an increase in stomach cancer rate in communities with chromium-contaminated drinking water.[7] Significant exposure from more than 160 chromate production waste sites within Hudson County, New Jersey, was discovered in the late 1980s.[18] A final report published by the Agency for Toxic Substances and Disease Registry in 2008 found an increased risk of lung cancer incidence in populations living in close proximity to historic chromium ore processing residue sites, although the increases were not statistically significant.[3]

OCCUPATIONAL EXPOSURE

Workers in industries that use chromium may be exposed to 100 times greater concentrations of chromium than the general population.

TABLE 91–1. Common Forms of Chromium

Name	Chemical Formula	Oxidation State	Uses
Barium chromate	$BaCrH_2O_4$	6+	Safety matches, anticorrosive, paint pigment
Calcium chromate	$CaCrO_4$	6+	Batteries, metallurgy
Chromic acid	H_2CrO_4	6+	Electroplating, oxidizer
Lead chromate	$PbCrO_4$	6+	Yellow pigment for paints and dyes
Potassium dichromate	$K_2Cr_2O_7$	6+	Oxidizer of organic compounds, leather tanning, porcelain painting
Chromic chloride	$CrCl_3$	3+	Supplement in total parenteral nutrition
Chromic fluoride	CrF_3	3+	Mordant in dye industry, moth-proofing agent for wool
Chromic oxide	Cr_2O_3	3+	Metal plating, wood treatment
Chromite ore	$FeCr_2O_4$	3+	Water tower treatment
Chromium picolinate	$C_{18}H_{12}CrN_3O_6$	3+	Nutritional

Whereas chromium pigmentation production and leather tanning use significantly more Cr^{6+} compounds, metal finishing, wood preservation, and cooling towers use Cr^{3+} compounds (Table 91–2).

Several studies have focused on the risk of chromium exposure in welders.[38,39] Stainless steel welding liberates significantly more hexavalent chromium than do other types of welding. Although the lung cancer rate of stainless steel (containing chromium) welders has not been found to be different than that in regular steel welders, in 2006, the Occupational Safety and Health Administration (OSHA) lowered the permissive exposure limit of hexavalent chromium by 10-fold for welders.

TABLE 91–2. Occupations at Risk for Chromium Exposure

Cement workers	Machinists
Chromite ore workers	Painters
Electroplaters	Photograph developers
Foundry workers	Tanners
Galvanized steel workers	Textile dyers
Glass polishers and glazers	Welders
Lithographers	Wood preservers

PHARMACOKINETICS AND TOXICOKINETICS

Because they possess significantly different properties, Cr^{3+} and Cr^{6+} must be evaluated separately.

ABSORPTION

Trivalent Chromium Compounds Oral absorption of Cr^{3+} salts is limited. Approximately 98% is recovered in the feces, just 0.1% is excreted in the bile, and 0.5% to 2.0% is excreted in the urine.[16,30] Human case reports and animal studies also corroborate the generally poor absorption of Cr^{3+} salts by the oral, inhalational, and dermal routes, except through burns and other disrupted mucosal or epithelial surfaces.[26]

Hexavalent Chromium Compounds Cr^{6+} is modestly absorbed after ingestion partly as a result of the structural similarity between hexavalent chromium compounds and phosphate and sulfate.[13] These three chemicals undergo facilitated diffusion through nonspecific anion channels as well as active transport. In human volunteers, approximately 10% of an orally ingested dose of sodium chromate was absorbed; duodenal administration increased this to roughly 50%.[16] This difference likely relates to the reduction of the hexavalent chromium to trivalent chromium in the acidic environment of the stomach. Similarly, 3 hours after a lethal ingestion of potassium dichromate (hexavalent), greater than 80% of the chromium was reduced to the trivalent state in the blood.[20] Hexavalent chromium compounds are generally not well absorbed after dermal exposure. Whatever the route of exposure, Cr^{6+} is absorbed much more readily than Cr^{3+}, but the Cr^{6+} is then rapidly reduced to Cr^{3+} after absorption.

Epidemiologically, inhalational of Cr^{6+} is the most consequential route of exposure. Furthermore, the greatest health consequences from Cr^{6+} exposure are from inhalation. The exact rate of absorption is unknown but is dependent on the solubility of the specific Cr^{6+} compound, the size of the particles, the phagocytic activity of the pulmonary macrophages, and the general health of the lungs. Animal studies suggest that roughly 50% to 85% of small (<5 μm) Cr^{6+} potassium dichromate particles are absorbed.[2]

DISTRIBUTION

Because most of the Cr^{6+} is rapidly reduced upon absorption by the GI tract and by RBCs, Cr^{3+} accounts for virtually the entire body burden of chromium. Trivalent chromium accumulates to the greatest extent in the kidneys, bone marrow, lungs, lymph nodes, liver, spleen, and testes. The kidneys and liver alone account for approximately 50% of the total body burden.[13]

ELIMINATION

Urinary excretion of trivalent chromium occurs rapidly. Roughly 80% of parenterally administered Cr^{6+} is excreted as Cr^{3+} in the urine and 2% to 20% in the feces.[30] The urinary excretion half-life of Cr^{6+} ranges from 15 to 41 hours.[21] Because Cr^{6+} undergoes reduction to Cr^{3+} after uptake by RBCs, an apparent slow compartment is created, with the elimination half-life dependent on the life span of erythrocytes. Small amounts of chromium are detectable in sweat, breast milk, nails, and hair.

PATHOPHYSIOLOGY

TRIVALENT CHROMIUM

Cr^{3+} is an essential trace metal required for the metabolism of glucose and fats. The complex nutritional interactions of trivalent chromium with numerous metabolic pathways are not understood and remain the subject of much debate among researchers. However, it is clear that dietary chromium deficiency leads to elevated insulin concentrations, hypercholesterolemia, hyperglycemia, increased body fat, and the attendant risks of these metabolic derangements. Cr^{3+} enhances insulin sensitivity and glucose disappearance concomitantly with lower insulin concentrations in a obese rat models, with no difference in lean controls.[11]

Chromium picolinate is a popular Cr^{3+} dietary supplement. There is a dearth of rigorous science concerning its efficacy and safety. However, it appears that organ deposition of Cr^{3+} occurs.[37] There is no strong evidence of any significant end-organ toxicity from exposure to Cr^{3+}, perhaps because Cr^{3+} is so poorly absorbed. There is little or no rigorous evidence that exposure to Cr^{3+} compounds increases cancer risk. Animal work and epidemiologic studies of workers exposed to Cr^{3+} compounds have failed to demonstrate a statistically significant increased incidence of cancer.[5]

HEXAVALENT CHROMIUM

Cr^{6+} is a powerful oxidizing agent that has corrosive and irritant effects. The greatest toxicity from Cr^{6+} lies in its ability to produce oxidative DNA damage. DNA strand breaks, DNA–DNA and DNA–protein cross-links, and nucleotide modifications all occur.[14] Although the exact mechanisms of how Cr^{6+} affects this genotoxicity are unknown, transient toxic chromium intermediates such as Cr^{4+} and Cr^{5+} are probably responsible.[36]

Inconsistent data suggest that either immunostimulation or immunosuppression results from chronic chromium exposure. At least one study suggests that chromium-induced immunosuppression may be responsible for implant-associated infections in patients after hip or knee arthroplasty.[44] Although human data are missing, adverse developmental effects, including cleft palate, hydrocephalus, and neural tube defects, have been demonstrated in animals.[15]

CLINICAL MANIFESTATIONS

The clinical manifestations of chromium poisoning depend on the valence, the source and route of exposure, and the duration of exposure. The clinical manifestations of chromium exposure are best divided into acute and chronic (low-level exposure) effects.

ACUTE

Manifestations of acute, massive Cr^{6+} ingestions are similar to other corrosive metal ingestions. GI hemorrhage, with or without bowel perforation, may occur acutely.[47] Because of the strong oxidative properties of Cr^{6+}, intravascular hemolysis with disseminated intravascular coagulation may also develop. Renal effects include acute tubular necrosis leading to renal failure.[46] Metabolic abnormalities after acute, massive exposure include metabolic acidosis with elevated lactate concentration, hyperkalemia, and uremia. Acute lung injury may develop up to 3 days after exposure. Although Cr^{6+} is generally not well absorbed after dermal exposure, it is a corrosive that causes skin inflammation and ulceration, which may lead to increased dermal absorption. Dermal chromic acid (H_2CrO_4) burns may lead to severe systemic toxicity with as little as 10% body surface area involvement.

CHRONIC

Because most chronic exposures are inhalational, the respiratory tract is the organ most affected after chronic chromium exposure. When inhaled, Cr^{6+} is a respiratory tract irritant that causes inflammation and, with continued exposure, ulceration (including nasal septum perforation).[22] Furthermore, the sensitizing effects of Cr^{6+} may lead to chronic cough, shortness of breath, occupational asthma, bronchospasm, and anaphylactoid-like reactions. Chronic deposition of chromium dust may also lead to pneumoconiosis.[35]

Epidemiologic studies of chromate workers in the 1980s indicated a significantly increased risk of lung cancer in individuals exposed to Cr^{6+} compounds.[23,32] Small cell and poorly differentiated carcinomas are the most common types, although nearly all pathologic types of lung cancer are associated with inhalational Cr^{6+} exposure.[1] The latency between exposure and development of lung cancer ranges from 13 to 30 years, although cases have been reported after as few as 2 years.[8]

Although conclusive evidence is missing, it appears that chronic exposure to Cr^{6+} via all routes may cause mild to moderate elevation in hepatic aminotransferases and abnormal liver architecture visible on histologic specimens.[47] Unlike acute exposures, low-dose chronic chromium exposure occasionally causes only transiently elevated urinary β_2-microglobulin concentrations, with no obvious lasting effects.[46]

Type IV (delayed-type) hypersensitivity reactions may occur after acute exposure to hexavalent chromium compounds. Chronic hexavalent chromium exposures also occur via dermal contact. Up to 24% of cement workers who have frequent contact with wet cement (which contains Cr^{6+}), automobile part handlers, and locksmiths develop skin sensitivity to chromium compounds.[25,27]

Occupational chromium exposure may also lead to contact dermatitis (dermatitis toxicosis) in as many as 10% to 20% of chromium workers.[41] There remains considerable debate over the relative sensitization abilities of Cr^{3+} and Cr^{6+}. Furthermore, what was initially thought to be sensitization to Cr^{3+} exposure may actually have been exposure to Cr^{6+} with subsequent in vivo reduction to Cr^{3+}. It appears, however, the Cr^{6+} is a more potent sensitizer than Cr^{3+} and that there may be limited cross-reactivity between the two forms of chromium.[17] Similarly, chromium-containing gaming table felt has led to hand dermatitis referred to as "blackjack disease," and virtually all occupations that involve exposure to chromium may lead to painless scarring and skin and nasal septum ulcerations referred to as "chrome holes."[24]

DIAGNOSTIC TESTING

Chromium may be detected in the blood, urine, and hair of exposed individuals. Because of the great difficulty in speciation, differentiation between Cr^{3+} and Cr^{6+} is generally not performed; instead, the total chromium concentration is usually reported. Needles used for phlebotomy and plastic containers used for sample storage may contain significant amounts of chromium. Unfortunately, there are no commercially available chromium-free needles. The use of modern, highly sensitive assay equipment, such as graphite furnace atomic absorption spectrometry, neutron activation analysis, and graphite spark atomic emission spectrometry, requires diligence in sample handling to ensure that biologic samples are not contaminated.

Because of the inherent difficulties in quantifying trace elements such as chromium and the lack of standard chromium reference materials, the reported normal serum and urine chromium concentrations in unexposed people have varied by more than 5000-fold over the past 50 years.[2] Consequently, older reference ranges should be interpreted with caution. Lastly, although cigarette smoke contains chromium, no studies have quantified the effect of smoking on serum, blood, or urinary chromium concentrations.

BLOOD OR SERUM

Chromium is distributed evenly between the serum and erythrocytes. Serum chromium concentrations are reflective of recent exposure to both Cr^{3+} and Cr^{6+}. Serum concentrations in people without occupational exposure to chromium have been reported to be from 0.05 μg/L (1 nmol/L)[10] up to more than 2.8 μg/L (56 nmol/L).[2] It is not certain whether concentrations above these values should be considered potentially toxic because no clear correlation has been found between serum or blood concentrations and physiologic effects.

URINE

Although urine chromium concentrations reflect the acute absorption of chromium over the previous 1 to 2 days, wide individual variation in metabolism and total body burden limit the value of urinary chromium monitoring. Urine should be collected over a 24-hour period because of diurnal variation in excretion. Data from the third National Health and Nutrition Examination Survey (NHANES III) demonstrated mean and median urinary chromium concentrations in approximately 500 individuals without known exposure to chromium of 0.22 μg/L (4.4 nmol/L) and 0.13 μg/L (2.6 nmol/L). When corrected for creatinine, the values were 0.21 and 0.12 μg/g creatinine, respectively.[29]

HAIR AND NAILS

Hair and nail samples are not reliable indicators of exposure to chromium because of the difficulty in distinguishing between chromium contamination of the hair sample from chromium incorporated into the hair during normal hair protein synthesis. Chromium found in hair is not caused by contamination or exposure to shampoo or tap water.[19] Chromium concentrations in hair may be up to 1000 times higher than those found in serum.

ANCILLARY TESTS

After confirmed or suspected acute chromium exposure, complete blood count, serum electrolytes, blood urea nitrogen, creatinine, urinalysis, and liver enzymes testing should be performed. If signs of systemic toxicity are evident, serial determination of coagulation function and disseminated intravascular coagulation may be useful to guide therapy.

MANAGEMENT

Acute chromium ingestions are infrequent but often severe, with significant morbidity and mortality. Consequently, after adequate airway, breathing, and circulatory support have been addressed, attention should be given to decontamination.

DECONTAMINATION

As a consequence of its serious but very limited toxicity, Cr^{3+} compounds should require limited decontamination measures. However, because coingestants may be present, standard gut decontamination with activated charcoal should be considered if a patient presents soon after exposure. Similar to most other dermal exposures, decontamination with soap and water should be performed after skin contact. No specific pulmonary decontamination is required.

Hexavalent chromium is corrosive, and profuse vomiting and hematemesis usually occur after acute ingestions. Nasogastric lavage may be beneficial after Cr^{6+} ingestions if the patient presents to the emergency department within 1 to 2 hours of exposure and no vomiting has occurred. There are no data regarding the use of activated charcoal in acute chromium ingestions. Endoscopic visualization may be difficult after administration of activated charcoal, and the relative benefits of these two modalities need to be considered. If there is a low likelihood of a coingestion, it is better to forego activated charcoal in order to obtain adequate endoscopic visualization. Known or suspected perforation is an absolute contraindication to activated charcoal.

Oral *N*-acetylcysteine increases the renal excretion of chromium in rats,[6] but there are no human data to support this therapy. Years of clinical experience using *N*-acetylcysteine for other indications and the very low incidence of adverse effects, however, favor the administration of oral *N*-acetylcysteine in the setting of acute chromium toxicity.

Although ascorbic acid facilitates reduction of Cr^{6+} to Cr^{3+} in vitro, no data are available to substantiate decreased absorption.[41] Some evidence suggests that topical ascorbic acid may reduce dermal Cr^{6+} exposure, but this has not been demonstrated in controlled trials.[36] Therefore, the routine use of ascorbic acid cannot be advocated at this time.

CHELATION THERAPY

The currently available chelators do not appear efficacious at either lowering serum or blood chromium concentrations or ameliorating chromium toxicity in experimental models. Specifically, ethylenediaminetetraacetic acid (EDTA) was found to have no effect on urinary chromium excretion in human subjects,[45] and dimercaprol (British anti-Lewsite, BAL) was not beneficial in an animal model of chromium poisoning.[28]

In a single study, dimercaptopropane sulfonate (DMPS) had no effect on urinary chromium excretion in humans.[42] D-penicillamine also failed to increase urinary excretion of chromium.[28] There have been no studies of chromium chelation with 2,3-dimercaptosuccinic acid (succimer). Therefore, at this time, there is no evidence to support the use of chelation therapy after acute Cr^{6+} or Cr^{3+} poisoning.

EXTRACORPOREAL ELIMINATION

Hemodialysis, hemofiltration, and peritoneal dialysis (PD) do not efficiently remove chromium. Studies in animals and human case reports indicate that as little as 1% of chromium is removed by hemodialysis or hemofiltration after acute dichromate (a hexavalent compound) exposure.[20,40] Exchange transfusions may rapidly reduce blood chromium concentrations, but no data are available to suggest that clinical outcomes are positively affected. Limited data in dialysis patients have demonstrated some ability of PD and hemodialysis to remove intravenously administered chromium.[33] Therefore, in the setting of normal renal function, extracorporeal means of eliminated chromium are not likely to be of benefit. In the setting of acute or chronic renal failure, PD or hemodialysis may be beneficial in reducing serum chromium concentrations, although no data are available showing that clinical outcomes are affected.

SUMMARY

Whereas hexavalent chromium remains an uncommon but serious cause of acute metal poisoning, trivalent chromium lacks toxicity. The acute exposure to Cr^{6+} salts by ingestion causes GI hemorrhage, hepatic necrosis, and renal failure. Toxicity after chronic Cr^{6+} exposure includes ulcerations of the skin and nasopharynx ("chrome holes") and, more significantly, lung and stomach cancer. Definitive data regarding other types of cancer resulting from chronic Cr^{6+} exposure are unavailable. Regardless of the time course of the poisoning, treatment for chromium exposure includes removal of the patient from the source of exposure, GI decontamination, and supportive care. There is insufficient evidence to support the use of chelating agents in either acute or chronic chromium poisoning.

REFERENCES

1. Abe S, Ohsaki Y, Kimura K, et al. Chromate lung cancer with special reference to its cell type and relation to the manufacturing process. *Cancer.* 1982;49:783-787.
2. Agency for Toxic Substances and Disease Registry. *Toxicologic Profile for Chromium Compounds.* Atlanta, GA. US Department of Health and Human Services: Agency for Toxic Substances and Disease Registry; 2000.
3. Agency for Toxic Substances and Disease Registry. *Analysis of Lung Cancer Incidence Near Chromium-Contaminated Sites in New Jersey (a/k/a Hudson County Chromium Sites).* Jersey City, Hudson County, NJ: US Department of Public Health, Agency for Toxic Substances and Disease Registry; 2008.
4. Aitio A, Jarvisalo J, Kiilunen M, et al. Urinary excretion of chromium as an indicator of exposure to trivalent chromium sulphate in leather tanning. *Int Arch Occup Environ Health.* 1984;54:241-249.
5. Axelsson G, Rylander R, Schmidt A. Mortality and incidence of tumours among ferrochromium workers. *Br J Ind Med.* 1980;37:121-127.
6. Banner W, Jr., Koch M, Capin DM, et al. Experimental chelation therapy in chromium, lead, and boron intoxication with N-acetylcysteine and other compounds. *Toxicol Appl Pharmacol.* 1986;83:142-147.
7. Beaumont JJ, Sedman RM, Reynolds SD, et al. Cancer mortality in a Chinese population exposed to hexavalent chromium in drinking water. *Epidemiology.* 2008;19:12-23.
8. Becker N. Cancer mortality among arc welders exposed to fumes containing chromium and nickel. Results of a third follow-up: 1989–1995. *J Occup Environ Med.* 1999;41:294-303.
9. Bencko V. Chromium: a review of environmental and occupational toxicology. *J Hyg Epidemiol Microbiol Immunol.* 1985;29:37-46.
10. Brune D, Aitio A, Nordberg G, et al. Normal concentrations of chromium in serum and urine—a TRACY project. *Scand J Work Environ Health.* 1993;19(suppl 1):39-44.
11. Cefalu WT, Wang ZQ, Zhang XH, et al. Oral chromium picolinate improves carbohydrate and lipid metabolism and enhances skeletal muscle glut-4 translocation in obese, hyperinsulinemic (JCR-LA corpulent) rats. *J Nutr.* 2002;132:1107-1114.
12. Cohen MD, Kargacin B, Klein CB, et al. Mechanisms of chromium carcinogenicity and toxicity. *Crit Rev Toxicol.* 1993;23:255-281.
13. Costa M. Toxicity and carcinogenicity of Cr(VI) in animal models and humans. *Crit Rev Toxicol.* 1997;27:431-442.
14. Dayan AD, Paine AJ. Mechanisms of chromium toxicity, carcinogenicity and allergenicity: review of the literature from 1985 to 2000. *Hum Exp Toxicol.* 2001;20:439-451.
15. Domingo JL. Metal-induced developmental toxicity in mammals: a review. *J Toxicol Environ Health.* 1994;42:123-141.
16. Donaldson RM, Jr., Barreras RF. Intestinal absorption of trace quantities of chromium. *J Lab Clin Med.* 1966;68:484-493.
17. Eisler R. *Handbook of Chemical Risk Assessment: Health Hazards to Humans, Plants, and Animals.* Boca Raton, Florida: CRC Press; 2000.
18. Freeman NC, Stern AH, Lioy PJ. Exposure to chromium dust from homes in a Chromium Surveillance Project. *Arch Environ Health.* 1997;52:213-219.
19. Hambidge KM, Franklin ML, Jacobs MA. Hair chromium concentration: effects of sample washing and external environment. *Am J Clin Nutr.* 1972;25:384-389.
20. Iserson KV, Banner W, Froede RC, et al. Failure of dialysis therapy in potassium dichromate poisoning. *J Emerg Med.* 1983;1:143-149.
21. Kerger BD, Finley BL, Corbett GE, et al. Ingestion of chromium(VI) in drinking water by human volunteers: absorption, distribution, and excretion of single and repeated doses. *J Toxicol Environ Health.* 1997;50:67-95.
22. Koutkia P, Wang RY. Electroplaters. In: Greenberg MI, Hamilton RJ, Phillips SD, McCluskey GJ, eds. *Occupational, Industrial, and Environmental Toxicology.* Boston: Mosby; 2003:126-139.
23. Langard S, Vigander T. Occurrence of lung cancer in workers producing chromium pigments. *Br J Ind Med.* 1983;40:71-74.
24. Lee HS, Goh CL. Occupational dermatosis among chrome platers. *Contact Dermatitis.* 1988;18:89-93.
25. Liden C, Skare L, Nise G, et al. Deposition of nickel, chromium, and cobalt on the skin in some occupations—assessment by acid wipe sampling. *Contact Dermatitis.* 2008;58:347-354.
26. Matey P, Allison KP, Sheehan TM, et al. Chromic acid burns: early aggressive excision is the best method to prevent systemic toxicity. *J Burn Care Rehabil.* 2000;21:241-245.
27. Newhouse ML. A cause of chromate dermatitis among assemblers in an automobile factory. *Br J Ind Med.* 1963;20:199-203.
28. Nowak-Wiaderek W. Influence of various drugs on excretion and distribution of chromium-51 in acute poisoning in rats. *Mater Med Pol.* 1975;7:308-310.
29. Paschal DC, Ting BG, Morrow JC, et al. Trace metals in urine of United States residents: reference range concentrations. *Environ Res.* 1998;76:53-59.
30. Paustenbach DJ, Hays SM, Brien BA, et al. Observation of steady state in blood and urine following human ingestion of hexavalent chromium in drinking water. *J Toxicol Environ Health.* 1996;49:453-461.
31. Proctor DM, Otani JM, Finley BL, et al. Is hexavalent chromium carcinogenic via ingestion? A weight-of-evidence review. *J Toxicol Environ Health A.* 2002;65:701-746.
32. Satoh K, Fukada Y, Torii K, et al. Epidemiological study of workers engaged in the manufacture of chromium compounds. *J Occup Med.* 1981;23:835-838.
33. Schiffl H, Weidmann P, Weiss M, et al. Dialysis treatment of acute chromium intoxication and comparative efficacy of peritoneal versus hemodialysis in chromium removal. *Miner Electrolyte Metab.* 1982;7:28-35.
34. Shrivastava R, Upreti RK, Seth PK, et al. Effects of chromium on the immune system. *FEMS Immunol Med Microbiol.* 2002;34:1-7.
35. Sluis-Cremer GK, Du Toit RS. Pneumoconiosis in chromite miners in South Africa. *Br J Ind Med.* 1968;25:63-67.
36. Stearns DM, Kennedy LJ, Courtney KD, et al. Reduction of chromium(VI) by ascorbate leads to chromium-DNA binding and DNA strand breaks in vitro. *Biochemistry.* 1995;34:910-919.
37. Stearns DM, Wise JP, Sr., Patierno SR, et al. Chromium(III) picolinate produces chromosome damage in Chinese hamster ovary cells. *FASEB J.* 1995;9:1643-1648.
38. Stern RM. In vitro assessment of equivalence of occupational health risk: welders. *Environ Health Perspect.* 1983;51:217-222.
39. Stern RM, Hansen K, Madsen AF, et al. In vitro toxicity of welding fumes and their constituents. *Environ Res.* 1988;46:168-180.
40. Stift A, Friedl J, Laengle F. Liver transplantation for potassium dichromate poisoning. *N Engl J Med.* 1998;338:766-767.
41. Suzuki Y. Reduction of hexavalent chromium by ascorbic acid in rat lung lavage fluid. *Arch Toxicol.* 1988;62:116-122.
42. Torres-Alanis O, Garza-Ocanas L, Bernal MA, et al. Urinary excretion of trace elements in humans after sodium 2,3-dimercaptopropane-1-sulfonate challenge test. *J Toxicol Clin Toxicol.* 2000;38:697-700.
43. Vasant C, Balamurugan K, Rajaram R, et al. Apoptosis of lymphocytes in the presence of Cr(V) complexes: role in Cr(VI)-induced toxicity. *Biochem Biophys Res Commun.* 2001;285:1354-1360.
44. Wang JY, Wicklund BH, Gustilo RB, et al. Prosthetic metals impair murine immune response and cytokine release in vivo and in vitro. *J Orthop Res.* 1997;15:688-699.
45. Waters MD, Gardner DE, Aranyi C, et al. Metal toxicity for rabbit alveolar macrophages in vitro. *Environ Res.* 1975;9:32-47.
46. Wedeen RP, Qian LF. Chromium-induced kidney disease. *Environ Health Perspect.* 1991;92:71-74.
47. Wood R, Mills PB, Knobel GJ, et al. Acute dichromate poisoning after use of traditional purgatives. A report of 7 cases. *S Afr Med J.* 1990;77:640-642.

CHAPTER 92
COBALT

Gar Ming Chan, MD

Cobalt (Co)		
Atomic number	=	27
Atomic weight	=	58.9 daltons
Normal concentrations		
Serum	=	0.1–1.2 μg/L (1.7–20.4 nmol/L)
Urine	=	0.1–2.2 μg/L (1.7–37.3 nmol/L)

Cobalt is extensively mined, has numerous industrial uses, and is an essential trace element in vitamin B_{12}. ^{60}Cobalt is remarkably important in radiotherapy, but an epidemic of cardiomyopathy ensued when cobalt was added to beer to improve the esthetics of the "foam." Toxicologic concerns today have diminished because of preventive respiratory measures in the mining industry. The ingestion of cobalt salts is quite uncommon.

HISTORY AND EPIDEMIOLOGY

The name cobalt (Co) originates from *kobold* German for "goblin," and was given to the cobalt-containing ore cobaltite (CoAsS) because it made exposed miners ill. However, the miners' illness was more likely a result from the arsenic exposure rather than exposure to cobalt. Brandt discovered cobalt in 1753 during an attempt to prove that an element other than bismuth gave glass a blue hue.

With an atomic number of 27 and a molecular weight of 58.93 daltons, Co is a light metal that has a melting point of 1768.2°K and a boiling point of 3373°K. These attributes make elemental cobalt a very useful industrial metal. The main industrial use of cobalt use is the formation of hard, high-speed, high-temperature cutting tools. When aluminum and nickel are blended with cobalt, an alloy (Alnico) with magnetic properties is formed. Other uses for cobalt include electroplating because of its resistance to oxidation and as an artist's pigment because of its bright blue color.

A Co^{3+} ion is at the center of cyanocobalamin (vitamin B_{12}), which is synthesized only by microorganisms and is not found in plants. Common dietary sources are fish, eggs, chicken, pork, and seafood. A diet deficient in cyanocobalamin results in pernicious anemia. Hydroxocobalamin, a Co^{3+}-containing precursor to cyanocobalamin, is used as an antidote for cyanide poisoning (see Antidotes in Depth A40: Hydroxocobalamin).

Historically, cobalt chloride was combined with iron salts and marketed in the 1950s as "Roncovite" for the medical treatment of anemia. As recently as 1976, physicians still used cobalt to reduce transfusion requirements in anemic patients despite concomitant adverse effects.[35] The other common medical use of cobalt is as a radioactive isotope, cobalt-60 (^{60}Co). This γ emitter was formerly used in the radiotherapy of cancers but has been largely replaced by linear accelerators in the Western world. It may also be targeted by terrorist groups as a source of radioactive material.

Epidemics of cardiomyopathy and goiter termed "beer drinker's cardiomyopathy"[12] and "cobalt-induced goiter"[59] occurred in the 1960s and 1970s. During this period, cobalt sulfate was added to beer as a foam stabilizer. In the 1970s, these epidemics were halted with the discontinued utilization of cobalt for this purely aesthetic purpose.[92]

Current sources of cobalt exposure include chemistry kits,[64] weather indicators,[64] antiquated anemia therapies,[64] cement,[71] fly ash,[71] mineral wool,[71] asbestos,[71] molds for ceramic tiles,[41] the production of Widia-steel (used in the wood industry),[126] mining,[65] porcelain paint,[110] orthopedic implants,[63] and dental hardware.[5]

The most clinically important source, however, arises through the formation of cemented tungsten carbide, a "hard metal." In tungsten carbide factories, powdered cobalt and tungsten are combined through an intense sintering process that exposes the metals to hydrogen heated to 1000°C. The first published investigation of these factories reported a 10-fold increase in workspace cobalt concentrations compared with atmospheric concentrations.[38] These respiratory exposures have resulted in pulmonary toxicity, known as "hard metal disease." As a result of this historic report, occupational studies and preventive respiratory measures have greatly reduced the acceptable cobalt exposure concentration in the workplace.

CHEMISTRY

Similar to other metals, cobalt occurs in elemental, inorganic, and organic forms. The clinical effects of each form are less well defined than more common metals such as lead, mercury, or arsenic. Elemental cobalt (Co^0) toxicity is reported through both inhalational[139] and oral exposures.[58,59] Inorganic Co salts most commonly occur in one of two oxidation states: cobaltous (Co^{2+}) or cobaltic (Co^{3+}). Inorganic Co salts, such as cobaltous chloride ($CoCl_2$) and cobaltous sulfate ($CoSO_4$), were historically used for the treatment of anemias[13,48,54,109,146] and were implicated in the "beer drinker's cardiomyopathy" case series.[1,88,94]

Organic cobalt exposure results from cyanocobalamin (vitamin B_{12}) ingestion but because of its limited oral absorption and its rapid renal elimination, it is considered of low toxicity.[106] Another organic form of cobalt (stearate) is toxic in rodents.[15] In animal models, the inorganic chloride, sulfate, and nitrate cobalt salts are more toxic than the organic forms such as cobalt stearate.[15]

TOXICOKINETICS

Based on animal studies, oral absorption of cobalt oxides, salts, and metal is highly variable, with a reported bioavailability of 5% to 45%.[72,82] In human studies, both iron deficiency and iron overload (hemochromatosis) enhance radiolabeled $^{57}CoCl_2$ absorption in the small bowel.[100] Inhaled cobalt oxide is about 30% bioavailable,[82] but the volume of distribution and elimination half-life are not well defined.

Most (50% to 88%) absorbed cobalt (organic and inorganic) is eliminated renally, and the remainder is eliminated in the feces.[124] Acutely, an increase in inorganic cobalt concentrations will result in an increased renal elimination.[69] However, this initial increased elimination decreases rapidly despite a large body burden.[2,100]

The elimination of cobalt correlates with the patterns of occupational exposure.[139] For example, a worker with a standard workweek will have much higher urine cobalt concentrations on Friday morning compared with Monday morning.[139] However, Monday afternoon urine cobalt concentrations may be higher than Friday morning concentrations, which is because of the rapid elimination that occurs after an initial exposure.[2,139] Based on these findings, the exposure over time must be considered when interpreting urinary cobalt levels in occupationally exposed individuals.[9]

PATHOPHYSIOLOGY

Similar to other metals, cobalt is a multiorgan toxin. Co^{2+} inhibits several key enzyme systems and interferes with initiation of protein synthesis.[10] First, polynucleotide phosphorylase, an essential enzyme in RNA synthesis, requires Mg^{2+} to function normally. The enzyme functions at 50% that of normal in the presence of Co^{2+}.[10] It is hypothesized that Co^{2+} is capable of displacing Mg^{2+} from this cofactor site of the enzyme.[10]

The second enzyme cobalt salts interfere with is α-ketoglutarate dehydrogenase, a mitochondrial Krebs cycle enzyme. Co^{2+} increases the rate of glycolysis and at the same time decreases oxygen consumption,[22] suggesting that Co^{2+} inhibits aerobic metabolism. In vitro studies demonstrate that other divalent cations, Zn^{2+}, Cd^{2+}, Cu^{2+}, and Ni^{2+}, inhibit α-ketogluturate dehydrogenase (see Chap. 12).[143] Compared with these divalent cations, Co^{2+}, is not as potent an inhibitor.[143] In an vitro model, Co^{2+} is capable of almost entirely inhibiting the reaction when nicotinamide adenine dinucleotide (NADH) is added to the reaction.[143] This model may suggest that NADH abundance, such as in chronic ethanol use, may potentiate the inhibition of α-ketogluturate dehydrogenase.[144]

Moreover, cobalt salts are capable of inhibiting α lipoic acid and dihydrolipoic acid by complexing with its sulfhydryl groups.[25,143] These reactions result in the inability to convert both pyruvate into acetyl-CoA and α-ketoglutarate into succinyl-CoA (see Chapter 12 and Antidotes in Depth A25: Thiamine). These toxic effects may help explain why the combination of chronic ethanol use and cobalt exposure results in cardiomyopathy (see Clinical Effects: Cardiac).[143]

In addition to enzyme inhibition, cobalt chloride induces oxidant-mediated pulmonary toxicity (see Clinical Effects: Pulmonary).[98] Xenobiotics implicated in free radical–mediated pulmonary injury are capable of accepting an electron from a reductant and subsequently transferring the electron to oxygen, forming a superoxide free radical (see Chap. 11). Cobalt is then capable of accepting another electron, which starts the cycle over again, a process known as redox cycling. This results in an accumulation of free radicals in the lung because of the abundance of oxygen ready to receive electrons and results in injury (see Chap. 124).

Within the endocrine system, $CoCl_2$ is capable of inhibiting tyrosine iodinase.[75] This enzyme is responsible for combining iodine (I_2) with tyrosine to form monoiodotyrosine and serves as the first step in the synthesis of thyroid hormone (see Chap. 49). Inhibition of tyrosine iodinase leads to a decrease of circulating triiodothyronine (T_3) and thyroxine (T_4), which may result in hypothyroidism (see Clinical Effects: Endocrine).

The hematopoietic system is also affected by Co salts. Multiple animal models demonstrate that $CoCl_2$ administration results in reticulocytosis, polycythemia, and erythropoeisis.[44,73,91,101,102,146] These events occur in both the bone marrow and extramedullary locations.[13,46] Although the pathogenesis remains largely unknown,[25] one theory is that cobalt binds to iron binding sites such as transferrin,[66] resulting in impaired oxygen transport to renal cells, which in turn induces erythropoietin production. A second theory in which cobalt is thought to stimulate erythropoiesis is through improving iron availability. In an animal model of anemia, a greater degree of gastrointestinal (GI) iron uptake occurs in cobalt-treated rats compared with rats with either hypoxia or nephrectomy.[46] A similar study in mice suggested that the increase in iron uptake exceeded that after exogenous erythropoietin.[3]

Finally, within the nervous system, $CoCl_2$ inhibits neuromuscular transmission by competing with Ca^{2+}, another divalent ion. Cobalt is 20 times more potent than magnesium with regard to its ability to compete with calcium for a site on the motor nerve terminal.[142]

TOXICITY

The single acute minimal toxic dose of cobalt salts is not well defined. In fact, varying effects have occurred at variable doses in different patients. Whereas patients with "beer drinker's cardiomyopathy" received an average daily dose of 6 to 8 mg of $CoSO_4$ (over weeks to months) and developed toxic effects of acidemia, cardiomyopathy, shock, and death,[70,94] infants being treated for anemia who received much higher daily cobalt doses of an iron–cobalt preparation (40 mg of $CoCl_2$ and 75 mg of $FeSO_4$) for 3 months did not develop toxicity.[115] The inconsistency of these findings suggests that multiple factors are responsible for the development of the clinical manifestations; in this case, the role of ethanol metabolism may be an important variable.[64]

CLINICAL MANIFESTATIONS

Organ systems affected by acute cobalt poisoning are the endocrine,[58] GI,[35,48] central[48,123] and peripheral nervous,[123] hematologic,[44,73,91,146] cardiovascular,[59] and metabolic[59] systems. Chronic inhalational exposures affect the pulmonary[18,23,38,77,78,112,131] and dermatologic systems.[42,118,145] Radioactive[60] Co used for radiation therapy has been associated with radiation burns (see Chap. 133). Unlike acute toxicity, chronic cobalt exposure is not associated with an increased mortality; a cohort study evaluating more than 1100 persons with pulmonary exposures to cobalt salts and oxides over a 30-year period was unable to show an increased mortality rate.[96]

ACUTE EXPOSURE

Cardiovascular ***"Beer Drinkers' Cardiomyopathy".*** In 1966, a Veterans Affairs Hospital in Nebraska cared for 28 white men with a history of beer drinking who presented with tachycardia, dyspnea, and metabolic acidosis with elevated lactate concentration but without any finding of congestive heart failure.[88] The mortality rate for these cases was 38% and death occurred rapidly within 72 hours of presentation because of severe acute metabolic acidosis and cardiac failure.[88] The survivors were successfully treated with supportive care and thiamine supplementation.[88] Of the survivors, most responded immediately to therapy, and a lack of response was found to be secondary to complications, most commonly, symptomatic pericardial effusions or embolic events.[88] Epidemiologic evaluation of this case series revealed that these men commonly drank large quantities of beer.

Ultimately, 64 cases and 30 fatalities were reported from Nebraska.[138] Of the reported 30 deaths, 26 decedents received autopsies. Common postmortem cardiac findings were dilated cardiomyopathy and cellular degeneration with vacuolization and edema with a lack of inflammation or fibrosis.[88] When cobalt was implicated in the pathogenesis of these deaths, the preserved cardiac tissue of eight decedents revealed cobalt concentrations 10 times greater than those of control subjects.[138]

Within 1 year of the Nebraska cases, reports began to emerge from Quebec.[94] Forty-eight beer drinkers (only two of whom were women) developed unexplained cardiomyopathy, with a mortality rate of 46%.[94] The only association between these patients was the common consumption of a given brand of beer.[94] The producers of this beer had factories in Quebec City and Montreal. The only difference between the two breweries was that the one in Quebec added 10 times the amount of $CoSO_4$ to the beer as a foam stabilizer.[92] Clinical findings in these cases included tachycardia, tachypnea, polycythemia, and low-voltage electrocardiograms (ECGs).[93] Cases began to appear 1 month after the beer with the excessive cobalt was released on the market, and no new cases were reported in Quebec after the beer with the excessive cobalt concentration was removed from the market.[92]

In 1972, 20 additional cases occurred in Minneapolis with similar findings of tachycardia, dyspnea, pericardial effusion, polycythemia, and metabolic acidosis with elevated lactate concentration; there was a mortality rate of 18% acutely and 43% over a 3-year period.[70]

Because the clinical findings resemble the cardiomyopathy associated with chronic alcoholism[40] and infantile malnutrition,[107] a debate persists as to whether cobalt is the sole cause of this syndrome. Cardiomyopathies caused by poor protein intake and vitamin deficiency both have similar histologic findings to cobalt cardiomyopathy. For example, myocardial biopsy of dogs with cobalt-induced cardiac failure revealed diffuse cytosolic vacuolization, loss of cross striations, and interstitial edema,[121] all of which are similar to findings of malnutrition.[40,107] However, some other findings may be specific to cobalt-associated cardiomyopathy. For example, a small retrospective analysis revealed myocyte atrophy and myofibril loss to be present in people with cobalt-associated cardiomyopathy significantly more often than in those with idiopathic dilated cardiomyopathy.[16]

Some animal models of cobalt cardiomyopathy were only able to reproduce pathologic and ECG findings if cobalt was combined with ethanol[7]; others required protein deficiency.[116] Contrary to these studies, several rat and canine models of cobalt poisoning and nutritional supplementation have demonstrated cardiac lesions,[52,120,121] cardiac failure[55,120,121] and ECG abnormalities.[53,120]

Despite the implication that cobalt-induced cardiomyopathy requires malnutrition or alcoholism, a case of cardiac toxicity after acute cobalt poisoning has been reported.[58,59] However, it is difficult to identify other cases reported outside of the aforementioned small epidemics in beer drinkers. In a controlled study of occupationally exposed subjects evaluated with echocardiograms, significantly more cobalt-exposed workers had diastolic dysfunction compared with control subjects.[80] However, none of these subjects under study developed congestive heart failure.[80] There have been rare reports of cardiomyopathy in chronically exposed workers,[11,21,68] which suggests that the cardiomyopathy reported in the "beer drinkers" cohort is multifactorial and not solely caused by cobalt.

Another source of criticism of the role of cobalt in the development of cardiomyopathy is the relatively low dose of cobalt needed to induce heart failure in these patients.[70] In patients receiving 20 to 75 mg/day of $CoCl_2$ for various red blood cell (RBC) dysplasias, there were no reports of heart failure,[70] but the "beer drinker's cardiomyopathy" group reportedly consumed only 6 to 8 mg/day of $CoSO_4$ from drinking 24 pints of cobalt-containing beer.[70,92] All patients who developed cardiomyopathies were malnourished, which supports the theory that a multifactorial nutritional deficiency in the presence of excessive cobalt may be necessary for the development of cardiomyopathy.[70]

Endocrine Both acute and chronic cobalt exposures are associated with thyroid hyperplasia and goiter. A series of patients with severe sickle cell anemia treated with cobalt therapy also developed goiter with varying degrees of thyroid dysfunction[54,74] including clinical hypothyroidism.[75] In one patient, the goiter was so severe that airway obstruction developed.[74]

More recent occupational data suggest that inhalational exposure to cobalt metals, salts, and oxides may result in abnormalities in thyroid function studies.[139] When 82 workers in a cobalt refinery were compared with gender- and age-matched control subjects, exposed workers had significantly lower T_3 concentrations.[139]

Within the previously mentioned beer drinker's cardiomyopathy cohort, 11 of 14 decedents had abnormal thyroid histology.[117] Among them, the most common findings were follicular cell abnormalities and colloid depletion, which did not exist on thyroid analysis from 11 randomly selected autopsies that served as control subjects.[117]

Hematologic Anemias of the newborn,[19,67,109] erythrocyte hypoplasia,[125] RBC aplasia,[141] renal failure,[48] and chronic infection[114] have all been successfully treated with cobalt salts. Patients undergoing $CoCl_2$ therapy for these diseases had increased hemoglobin,[48,109] hematocrit,[48,109] and RBC counts.[48] Furthermore, the effects did not persist after cessation of therapy.[48,109]

A published series of Peruvian cobalt miners working in an open pit at an elevation of 4300 m (2.7 miles) developed clinical effects, including headache, dizziness, weakness, mental fatigue, dyspnea, insomnia, tinnitus, anorexia, cyanosis, polycythemia, and conjunctival hyperemia consistent with acute mountain sickness.[65] When the study group was compared with age-, height-, and weight-matched high-altitude control subjects, the study group was noted to have higher chronic mountain sickness scores.[65] The only difference detected was elevated serum cobalt concentrations in the study group.[65]

In addition to effects on RBCs, recent work demonstrates transient hemolysis, methemoglobinemia, and methemoglobinuria from subcutaneous $CoCl_2$ exposure in mice.[60] These findings may explain reports of dark urine after cobalt exposure in other animal models.[50,133] Human cases have not been reported.

Other GI distress after the ingestion of "therapeutic" doses of cobalt salts[123] as well as elemental cobalt has been reported.[64] Decreased proprioception, impaired cranial nerve VIII function, and nonspecific peripheral nerve findings are reported with acute oral $CoCl_2$ exposures.[123]

CHRONIC

Pulmonary Two pulmonary diseases are associated with cobalt exposure: asthma and "hard metal disease." Occupational asthma is reported in hard metal workers with a prevalence of 2% to 5%[18,77,78] at exposure concentrations as low as 50 μg/m^3.[78] As is the case with most causes of occupational asthma, cobalt hypersensitivity–induced asthma is most likely immune mediated rather than toxicologic.[20,77,131] Most hard metal workers are exposed to other metals, such as tungsten (W) and nickel (Ni) in addition to Co, and these other metals may account for some cases of occupational asthma that are attributed to cobalt.[128,130] However, in a small but well-performed study in patients with cobalt-associated asthma, intradermal cobalt chloride ($CoCl_2$) resulted in a positive wheal response in all subjects, and 50% of patients had a positive radioallergosorbent test (RAST) scores, which correlated to the wheal size,[129] suggesting that Co salts independent of the other metals may illicit an immune response.

Cobalt-associated pulmonary toxicity was first noted in tungsten–carbide workers[38,56] and was subsequently referred to as "hard metal disease." Exposures result from the process by which tungsten–carbide is sintered with cobalt. Signs and symptoms of hard metal disease may include upper respiratory tract irritation, exertional dyspnea, severe dry cough, wheezing, and interstitial lung disease ranging from alveolitis to progressive fibrosis. The prevalence of hard metal disease is largely unknown. In one study, 11 of 290 (3.8%) exposed workers were diagnosed with interstitial infiltrates on chest radiographs but only two (0.7%) had a decreased predicted total lung capacity.[134]

Certain individuals who are exposed to large doses of hard metal for prolonged periods never develop disease, which suggests that a susceptible population exists. A glutamate substitution for lysine in position 69 of the β unit HLA-DP has a strong association with hard metal disease, similar to chronic beryllium disease.[108] Clinically, hard metal disease is difficult to distinguish from berylliosis, although an occupational history should be helpful.

Common findings of hard metal disease on histopathology are multinucleated giant cells and interstitial pneumonitis with bronchiolitis.[8] Elevated concentrations of cobalt in lung tissue can be detected,[113,132] even as long as 4 years after exposure.[113] Bronchioalveolar lavage (BAL) commonly reveals multinucleated giant cells, type II alveolar cells, and alveolar macrophages in patients with interstitial lung disease.[23] The finding of multinucleated giant cells from BAL washing is characteristic of hard metal disease.[20,26,27,89,140]

A cross-sectional study of more than 1000 tungsten carbide–exposed workers found an increased odds ratio of 2.1 for having a work-related wheeze when exposed to greater than 50 μg/m³ of Co.[135] In the same study, workers with exposures recorded at greater than 100 μg/m³ had higher odds (odds ratio [OR], 5.0) of having a chest radiograph profusion score of greater than or equal to 1/0.[135] This profusion score, established by the International Labor Organization (ILO) and most recently updated in 2000, is a grading system for pneumoconioses. When used to grade radiographs of asbestosis, this score correlates strongly with mortality risk,[87] reduced diffusing capacity, and decreased ventilatory capacity.[57,97] A score of 0/1 is suggestive but not diagnostic ("negative"), and a score of 1/0 is presumptively diagnostic but not unequivocal ("positive").[6] Additional studies have similarly concluded that pulmonary disease occurs when individuals are exposed to doses cobalt approach 100 μg/m³.[76] Thus, the current threshold limit value (TLV) is <50 μg/m³.

Until 1984, all reported cases of hard metal disease were associated with the combination of cobalt and other metals, such as nickel, cadmium, and tungsten.[8,56,78,135] Diamond polishers started to institute the use of high-speed grinding disks coated with abrasive microdiamonds embedded a matrix of cobalt powder.[79] Several case reports illustrate that cobalt-exposed diamond polishers develop similar clinical[79] and pathologic findings to hard metal disease, strengthening the link to cobalt.[20,26,99] Some authors still contend that the presence of other metals[8,56,78,135] and diamond dust[26,49,99] are confounding factors.[139] Similar to hard metal disease, most reported cases show resolution of symptoms upon removal from the exposure,[26] although this is not always sufficient.[99]

There are very few reports of isolated cobalt exposures. In an age- and gender-matched study of 82 workers with respiratory exposures to cobalt oxides, cobalt salts, cobalt metal, and no other metal, researchers were unable to detect a difference between exposed (mean, 8 years; TWA, 125 μg/m³, 25% >500 μg/m³) and unexposed workers with any objective measured pulmonary tests.[139] Neither group had any abnormality in chest radiography that would suggest pulmonary fibrosis.[139] The only significant pulmonary differences detected were a higher reported rate of dyspnea both on exertion and at rest and the presence of wheezing in the exposed group.[139] These authors concluded that cobalt contributes to the development of pulmonary disease but is not independently responsible for the development of pulmonary fibrosis.[139]

Despite the progressive and debilitating nature of hard metal disease, most signs and symptoms improve with cessation of exposure.[86,90,147] Moreover, the length and dose of exposure do not appear to correlate with the presence or severity of illness, suggesting that individual susceptibility is the most important risk factor for illness.[86,119]

Renal A single report associates reversible renal tubular necrosis with the chronic administration of $CoCl_2$ as treatment for anemia.[123] Some animal models of cobalt cardiomyopathy demonstrate cellular changes in renal tissue.[51] However, when 26 exposed hard metal workers were evaluated for urinary albumin, retinol binding protein (RBP), β_2-microglobulin, and tubular brush border antigens, no detectable difference could be found between the study group and control subjects.[45] Based on these few reports, it appears that acute and chronic exposure to cobalt has little effect on the kidneys.

Dermatologic In a study of 1782 construction workers, 23.6% developed dermatitis and 11.2% developed oil acne while using cobalt containing cement, fly ash, or asbestos.[71] As in hard metal disease, it is difficult to isolate cobalt as the sole contributor to the development of dermatitis. Nickel, the classic toxicant causing dermatitis, is commonly found in some of these preparations and may be implicated in the development of cutaneous sensitivity.[42,118]

Reproductive A pregnant woman with hard metal disease was able to bring the fetus to term and deliver without complications.[111] In pregnant rats, $CoCl_2$ exposure neither results in teratogenicity nor fetotoxicity.[104] Only doses that are toxic to the mother result in fetal toxicity.[34]

In mice, chronic exposure to cobalt results in impaired spermatogenesis and decreased fertility without affecting follicle-stimulating hormone (FSH) or luteinizing hormone (LH), but acute exposures did not demonstrate similar reproductive effects.[105] Additional murine studies discuss the possible interactions between cobalt with iron and zinc, which are both essential elements for spermatogenesis.[4] Despite these findings, there have been no reported human cases that associate cobalt exposure with teratogenicity or impaired fertility.

Carcinogenesis Based solely on animal experiments leading to the development of soft tissue sarcomas after the injection of $CoCl_2$ into soft tissue resulting in soft tissue sarcomas, the International Agency for Research on Cancer (IARC) considers cobalt and cobalt-containing compounds possibly carcinogenic to humans (group 2B).[14,24,36,136] There have been case reports and cohort studies suggesting that pulmonary exposure to Co^{2+} increases the risk for lung cancer. However, these studies were unable to control for other known carcinogens such as arsenic.[24] In the largest cohort study to date, which followed more than 1100 workers for more than 38 years, there was no increase in the prevalence of lung cancer.[95]

DIAGNOSTIC TESTING

Body fluid cobalt concentrations are not readily available and therefore cannot be used to direct emergent clinical care. Some adjunctive testing that may support a clinical diagnosis of cobalt toxicity should include complete blood count (CBC); reticulocyte count; erythropoietin (EPO) concentration; and T_3, T_4, and thyroid-stimulating hormone (TSH) concentrations. The results of these tests may reflect the level of exposure or potential toxicity discussed above.

CARDIAC STUDIES

ECG, echocardiography, and radionuclide angiocardiography with ^{99}Tc(RNA) are useful screening tests for detecting abnormalities associated with cobalt cardiomyopathy or pulmonary hypertension caused by hard metal disease.[21] It is important to remember that these cardiac tests are neither specific for nor diagnostic of cobalt-induced cardiomyopathy. Biopsy of myocardial tissue may show multinucleated giant cells, but testing of this nature is impractical.

PULMONARY TESTING

Patients with hard metal lung disease may demonstrate bilateral upper lobe interstitial lung disease on chest radiography. However, patients may have signs and symptoms of disease without specific radiographic findings.[111] Pulmonary function testing in occupationally exposed workers may show decreased vital capacity[111] and a decrease in diffusion capacity of lung for carbon monoxide (DLCO), both of which may be useful in identifying patients at risk for developing pulmonary fibrosis.[137] Some authors suggest an inversion of CD4/CD8 ratio in BAL washings as a useful tool for diagnosis and evaluation of progression of illness and that normalization is a marker for improvement.[112] Despite these available tests, a definitive diagnosis of hard metal disease requires a tissue sample with findings of multinucleated giant cells in the setting of interstitial pulmonary fibrosis.

COBALT TESTING

Cobalt is primarily eliminated in the urine and to a lesser extent in the feces, making urine cobalt evaluation most appropriate.[82] The difficulty lies in the interpretation of the result. Cobalt is detectable in the urine after inhalational exposure and reflects elimination kinetics that are rapid during an initial exposure but that slow after prolonged exposure.[82,122] Because of this variable elimination pattern, it is difficult to interpret both urine and blood concentrations unless the dose and length of exposure are precisely known. Furthermore, the defined patterns may be applicable only to shift workers using soluble forms of cobalt.[82]

Further complicating the interpretation of urinary cobalt concentrations is the abundance of organic cobalt in the form of vitamin B_{12}. A detailed vitamin supplementation history is required before the interpretation of a urine or blood cobalt concentration because a diet regimen high in vitamin B_{12} may increase urine cobalt concentrations. For this reason, speciation of cobalt has been investigated. The ratio of inorganic to organic cobalt is higher in occupationally exposed workers (2.3) compared with control subjects (1.01) independent of the wide variations of urinary cobalt concentrations.[47] This is a promising area of study for the evaluation of a cobalt-exposed worker.

Toxic concentrations of cobalt in serum and urine are poorly defined. Published literature on "normal levels" is fraught with variability, which may reflect differences in the population under study techniques for measurement. Normal serum concentrations of cobalt are frequently reported as 0.1 to 1.2 μg/L.[2,12,58,59,62,127] In comparison, a single acutely poisoned patient had a reported serum concentration of 41 μg/L.[58] Normal reference urine cobalt concentrations are between 0.1-2.2 μg/L.[2,12,58,59,62,103,127] In contrast, an acute elemental cobalt ingestion resulted in a concentration of 1700 μg/L on a spot urinalysis several days after the exposure.[59]

Patients with chronic exposures should be evaluated differently, as discussed above (see Toxicokinetics). Exposed workers without clinical disease have reported spot urine concentrations that range from 10 μg/L to several hundred μg/L.[61]

TREATMENT

ACUTE MANAGEMENT

Patients with acute cobalt poisoning require aggressive therapy. It is reasonable to conclude that the same decontamination principles used for other metals apply to cobalt. There have been no studies to date examining the benefits of gastric emptying, activated charcoal, or whole-bowel irrigation (WBI). An attempt at using WBI for radiopaque solid forms of cobalt should be made before endoscopic or surgical removal. Regardless of the decontamination procedure used, chelation therapy should not be initiated until the GI cobalt source has been removed. If there is a large stomach burden in a solid, endoscopic or surgical removal may be of benefit,[59] keeping in mind that the administration of activated charcoal before surgical removal may obscure visualization of the surgical field (see Antidote in Depth A2: Activated Charcoal). After decontamination, reduction of tissue burden and prevention of end-organ toxicity is the next crucial step.

Unfortunately, the data on chelation therapy are limited to animal models[28–34,83–85] and a single human case report.[59] The basis of chelation therapy originates from the mid 1900s when oral protein intake was found to result in a reduction of cobalt toxicity in calves[37] and rats.[52] Certain sulfur-containing proteins serve as good chelators for some metals.

In a series of animal models of acute cobalt toxicity, several treatments—N-acetylcysteine (NAC), succimer, ethylenediaminetetraacetic acid (EDTA), glutathione, and diethylenetriaminepentaacetic acid (DTPA)—were evaluated for their ability to enhance urinary and fecal elimination of cobalt.[84] Succimer and EDTA were able to enhance fecal elimination.[84] Glutathione and DTPA were able to enhance urinary elimination, and NAC was able to enhance elimination by both routes.[84]

In two separate animal studies, NAC reduced the tissue burden and injury caused by cobalt in the liver and spleen.[33,84] Glutathione, another sulfur-containing protein, also reduced tissue levels of cobalt but only in the spleen.[84]

The sulfur-containing proteins NAC,[29,33] L-cysteine,[29,29] L-methionine,[29] and L-histidine[31] were studied for their ability to reduce mortality in rats that were administered an LD_{50} of $CoCl_2$ orally and intraperitoneally. NAC, L-cysteine, and L-histidine[31] therapy are more effective than L-methionine in protecting against mortality, upwards of 100%. In a similar fashion, Na_2EDTA was effective in reducing mortality.[32] In all of these therapies, the successful reduction in mortality is predicated on its early administration.[28,29,31–33]

In a murine model, L-cysteine, NAC, glutathione, L-histidine, sodium salicylate, D,L-penicillamine, succimer, N-acetylpenicillamine (NAPA), diethyldithiocarbamate (DDC), BAL, 4,5-dihydroxy-1,3-benzene disulfonic acid, $Na_3CaDTPA$, $Na_2CaEDTA$, and deferoxamine mesylate were each evaluated for exposures to an LD_{50} and an LD_{99} of $CoCl_2$.[85] Agents that were ineffective at improving survival after an LD_{50} were sodium salicylate, NAPA, DOC, BAL, 4,5-dihydroxy-1,3-benzene disulfonic acid, and deferoxamine mesylate.[85] Chelators that were seemingly effective at LD_{50} and not at LD_{99} were L-histidine and D,L penicillamine.[83] NAC, L-cysteine, and succimer were able to improve survival by 40% to 50%.[85] The most effective chelators at LD_{99} were EDTA and DTPA.[83,85] An expanded analysis of these data revealed that EDTA and DTPA had a better therapeutic index compared with succimer.[85] In this study, BAL was ineffective as is suggested in an in vitro study in which BAL was unable to chelate Co^{2+} that is already bound to α-ketoglutarate.[143]

Human chelation data are available from a single pediatric case report involving the ingestion of multiple elemental cobalt–containing magnets yielding a serum cobalt concentration of 4.1 μg/dL.[59] Five days of 50 mg/kg/day of intravenous (IV) $CaNa_2EDTA$ enhanced renal elimination of cobalt, and the metabolic acidosis and the cardiac dysfunction also resolved simultaneously.[59]

In conclusion, based on a single human case report, several animal studies and safety profiles, $CaNa_2EDTA$ and NAC can be used as antidotal therapy. Indications for treatment should include patients who demonstrate end-organ manifestations of toxicity, including metabolic acidosis and cardiac failure. Patients with other manifestations of severe cobalt toxicity such as pericardial effusion, clinically significant goiter, and hyperviscosity syndrome should be treated aggressively with pericardiocentesis, airway protection, and phlebotomy, respectively. Based on years of experience with lead, $CaNa_2EDTA$ should be administered as doses of 1000 mg/m²/day by continuous infusion for 5 days. If the diagnosis is confirmed and signs of cardiac failure and metabolic acidosis persist after 5 days, an alternate chelator (ie, succimer or DTPA) can be started. Similarly, NAC dosing should be based on the acetaminophen experience. The 20-hour IV NAC protocol should be initiated and continued as in the case of fulminant hepatic failure (see Antidotes in Depth A4: N-acetylcysteine) for as long as the patient can tolerate therapy or continued if cardiac failure or acidemia persist.

If there are contraindications to IV NAC, oral NAC can be administered using one of the acetaminophen treatment regimens. Thiamine hydrochloride should be administered to all patients presenting with or without overt cardiomyopathy independent of whether the patient is alcoholic or malnourished. The dose of thiamine is not well defined but should be based on its safety and clinical experience with the treatment of Wernicke's encephalopathy. The daily administration of 100 mg of parenteral thiamine can be initiated with increasing doses to 100 mg every hour for life-threatening manifestations (ie, cardiac failure and metabolic acidosis) (see Antidotes in Depth A25: Thiamine Hydrochloride).

OCCUPATIONAL AND CHRONIC EXPOSURE

As is the case for occupational poisonings, prevention is of paramount importance. The use of skin protection and improvement of personal hygiene has reduced exposure and subsequently the amount of urinary cobalt in occupationally exposed workers.[81] Barrier and emollient creams cannot prevent the dermatitis associated with cobalt metal exposures.[43]

Large, statistically significant reductions in urinary cobalt were demonstrated after the implementation of aspirator systems over machines in the production of Widia steel.[17] These aspirators were found to reduce ambient cobalt concentrations by as much as a factor of six.[39]

SUMMARY

Acute cobalt toxicity results in multiorgan system toxicity, including the cardiac, endocrine, hematopoietic, GI, and neurologic systems. In contrast, chronic toxicity, dependent primarily on the route of exposure, mainly involves the pulmonary and dermal areas. The evaluation of the patient is determined by the cobalt source and type (ie, elemental, inorganic, or organic), route of poisoning, and time and duration of exposure. Cobalt measurements in blood and urine are possible, but toxic concentrations are poorly defined. Treatment of patients with chronic exposures is mainly symptomatic and often improved industrial hygiene is the most critical step. Acute poisoning with end-organ manifestations may require aggressive GI decontamination and chelation therapy using $CaNa_2EDTA$ and NAC and at times succimer.

REFERENCES

1. Alexander CS. Cobalt-beer cardiomyopathy. A clinical and pathologic study of twenty-eight cases. *Am J Med.* 1972;53:395-417.
2. Alexandersson R. Blood and urinary concentrations as estimators of cobalt exposure. *Arch Environ Health.* 1988;43:299-303.
3. Alippi RM, Boyer P, Leal T, et al. Higher erythropoietin secretion in response to cobaltous chloride in post-hypoxic than in hypertransfused polycythemic mice. *Haematologica.* 1992;77:446-449.
4. Anderson MB, Pedigo NG, Katz RP, et al. Histopathology of testes from mice chronically treated with cobalt. *Reprod Toxicol.* 1992;6:41-50.
5. Andreasen GF, Barrett RD. An evaluation of cobalt-substituted nitinol wire in orthodontics. *Am J Orthod.* 1973;63:462-470.
6. Anonymous. Diagnosis and initial management of nonmalignant diseases related to asbestos. *Am J Respir Crit Care Med.* 2004;170:691-715.
7. Anonymous. Synergism of cobalt and ethanol. *Nutr Rev.* 1971;29:43-45.
8. Anttila S, Sutinen S, Paananen M, et al. Hard metal lung disease: a clinical, histological, ultrastructural and X-ray microanalytical study. *Eur J Respir Dis.* 1986;69:83-94.
9. Apostoli P, Porru S, Alessio L. Urinary cobalt excretion in short time occupational exposure to cobalt powders. *Sci Total Environ.* 1994;150:129-132.
10. Babinet C, Roller A, Dubert JM, Thang MN, Grunberg-Manago M. Metal ions requirement of polynucleotide phosphorylase. *Biochem Biophys Res Commun.* 1965;19:95-101.
11. Barborik M, Dusek J. Cardiomyopathy accompanying industrial cobalt exposure. *Br Heart J.* 1972;34:113-116.
12. Barceloux DG. Cobalt. *J Toxicol Clin Toxicol.* 1999;37:201-206.
13. Berk L, Burchenal JH, Castle WB. Erythropoietic effect of cobalt in patients with or without anemia. *N Engl J Med.* 1949;240:754-761.
14. Beyersmann D, Hartwig A. The genetic toxicology of cobalt. *Toxicol Appl Pharmacol.* 1992;115:137-145.
15. Carson BL, Ellis HV III, McCann JL. *Toxicology and Biological Monitoring of Metals in Humans.* Chelsea (MI): Lewis Publishers, Inc. 1986. p. 21–46.
16. Centeno JA, Pestaner JP, Mullick FG, et al. An analytical comparison of cobalt cardiomyopathy and idiopathic dilated cardiomyopathy. *Biol Trace Elem Res.* 1996;55:21-30.
17. Cereda C, Redaelli ML, Canesi M, et al. Widia tool grinding: the importance of primary prevention measures in reducing occupational exposure to cobalt. *Sci Total Environ.* 1994;150:249-251.
18. Coates EO Jr, Sawyer HJ, Rebuck JW, et al. Hypersensitivity bronchitis in tungsten carbide workers. *Chest.* 1973;64:390.
19. Coles BL, James U. The effect of cobalt and iron salts on the anaemia of prematurity. *Arch Dis Child.* 1954;29:85-96.
20. Cugell DW, Morgan WK, Perkins DG, et al. The respiratory effects of cobalt. *Arch Intern Med.* 1990;150:177-183.
21. D'Adda F, Borleri D, Migliori M, et al. Cardiac function study in hard metal workers. *Sci Total Environ.* 1994;150:179-186.
22. Daniel M, Dingle JT, Weeb M, et al. The biological action of cobalt and other metals. I. The effect of cobalt on the morphology and metabolism of rat fibroblasts in vitro. *Br J Exp Pathol.* 1963;44:163-176.
23. Davison AG, Haslam PL, Corrin B, et al. Interstitial lung disease and asthma in hard-metal workers: bronchoalveolar lavage, ultrastructural, and analytical findings and results of bronchial provocation tests. *Thorax.* 1983;38:119-128.
24. De Boeck M, Kirsch-Volders M, Lison D. Cobalt and antimony: genotoxicity and carcinogenicity. *Mutat Res.* 2003;533:135-152.
25. de Moraes S, Mariano M. Biochemical aspects of cobalt intoxication. Cobalt ion action on oxygen uptake. *Med Pharmacol Exp Int J Exp Med.* 1967;16:441-447.
26. Demedts M, Gheysens B, Nagels J, et al. Cobalt lung in diamond polishers. *Am Rev Respir Dis.* 1984;130:130-135.
27. Demedts M, Gyselen A. [The cobalt lung in diamond cutters: a new disease]. *Verh K Acad Geneeskd Belg.* 1989;51:559-581.
28. Domingo JL, Llobet JM. The action of L-cysteine in acute cobalt chloride intoxication. *Rev Esp Fisiol.* 1984;40:231-236.
29. Domingo JL, Llobet JM. Treatment of acute cobalt intoxication in rats with L-methionine. *Rev Esp Fisiol.* 1984;40:443-448.
30. Domingo JL, Llobet JM, Bernat R. A study of the effects of cobalt administered orally to rats. *Arch Farmacol Toxicol.* 1984;10:13-20.
31. Domingo JL, Llobet JM, Corbella J. The effect of L-histidine on acute cobalt intoxication in rats. *Food Chem Toxicol.* 1985;23:130-131.
32. Domingo JL, Llobet JM, Corbella J. The effects of EDTA in acute cobalt intoxication in rats. *Toxicol Eur Res.* 1983;5:251-255.
33. Domingo JL, Llobet JM, Tomas JM. N-acetyl-L-cysteine in acute cobalt poisoning. *Arch Farmacol Toxicol.* 1985;11:55-62.
34. Domingo JL, Paternain JL, Llobet JM, et al. Effects of cobalt on postnatal development and late gestation in rats upon oral administration. *Rev Esp Fisiol.* 1985;41:293-298.
35. Duckham JM, Lee HA. The treatment of refractory anaemia of chronic renal failure with cobalt chloride. *Q J Med.* 1976;45:277-294.
36. Edel J, Pozzi G, Sabbioni E, et al. Metabolic and toxicological studies on cobalt. *Sci Total Environ.* 1994;150:233-244.
37. Ely R, Dunn K, Huffman C. Cobalt toxicity in calves resulting from high oral administration. *J Anim Sci.* 1948;7:239-243.
38. Fairhall LT, Keenan RG, Brinton HP. Cobalt and dust environment of the cemented tungsten carbide industry. *Pub Health Rep.* 1949;64:485-490.
39. Ferdenzi P, Giaroli C, Mori P, et al. Cobalt powdersintering industry (stone cutting diamond wheels): a study of environmental-biological monitoring, workplace improvement and health surveillance. *Sci Total Environ.* 1994;150:245-248.
40. Ferrans VJ. Alcoholic cardiomyopathy. *Am J Med Sci.* 1966;252:89-104.
41. Ferri F, Candela S, Bedogni L, et al. Exposure to cobalt in the welding process with stellite. *Sci Total Environ.* 1994;150:145-147.
42. Fischer T, Rystedt I. Cobalt allergy in hard metal workers. *Contact Dermatitis.* 1983;9:115-121.
43. Fischer T, Rystedt I. Skin protection against ionized cobalt and sodium lauryl sulphate with barrier creams. *Contact Dermatitis.* 1983;9:125-130.
44. Fisher JW, Langston JW. Effects of testosterone, cobalt and hypoxia on erythropoietin production in the isolated perfused dog kidney. *Ann N Y Acad Sci.* 1968;149:75-87.
45. Franchini I, Bocchi MC, Giaroli C, et al. Does occupational cobalt exposure determine early renal changes? *Sci Total Environ.* 1994;150: 149-152.
46. Fried W, Kilbridge T. Effect of testosterone and of cobalt on erythropoietin production by anephric rats. *J Lab Clin Med.* 1969;74:623-629.

47. Gallorini M, Edel J, Pietra R, et al. Cobalt speciation in urine of hard metal workers. A study carried out by nuclear and radioanalytical techniques. *Sci Total Environ.* 1994;150:153-160.
48. Gardner FH. The use of cobaltous chloride in the anemia associated with chronic renal disease. *J Lab Clin Med.* 1953;41:56-64.
49. Gennart JP, Lauwerys R. Ventilatory function of workers exposed to cobalt and diamond containing dust. *Int Arch Occup Environ Health.* 1990;62:333-336.
50. Giovannini E, Principato GB, Ambrosini MV, et al. Early effects of cobalt chloride treatment on certain blood parameters and on urine composition. *J Pharmacol Exp Ther.* 1978;206:398-404.
51. Greenberg SR. The beer drinker's kidney. *Nephron.* 1981;27:155.
52. Grice HC, Goodman T, Munro IC, et al. Myocardial toxicity of cobalt in the rat. *Ann N Y Acad Sci.* 1969;156:189-194.
53. Grice HC, Heggtveit HA, Wiberg GS, et al. Experimental cobalt cardiomyopathy: correlation between electrocardiography and pathology. *Cardiovasc Res.* 1970;4:452-456.
54. Gross RT, Kriss JP, Spaet TH. The hematopoletic and goltrogenic effects of cobaltous chloride in patients with sickle cell anemia. *Pediatrics.* 1955;15:284-290.
55. Haga Y, Hatori N, Hoffman-Bang C, et al. Impaired myocardial function following chronic cobalt exposure in an isolated rat heart model. *Trace Elements and Electrolytes.* 1996;13:69-74.
56. Harding HE. Notes on the toxicology of cobalt metal. *Br J Ind Med.* 1950;7:76-78.
57. Harkin TJ, McGuinness G, Goldring R, et al. Differentiation of the ILO boundary chest roentgenograph (0/1 to 1/0) in asbestosis by high-resolution computed tomography scan, alveolitis, and respiratory impairment. *J Occup Environ Med.* 1996;38:46-52.
58. Henretig F. Case presentation: an 11-year-old boy develops vomiting, weakness, weight loss, and a neck mass. *Internet J Med Toxicol.* 1998;1:13.
59. Henretig F. Further History: an 11-year-old boy develops vomiting, weakness, weight loss, and a neck mass. *Internet J Med Toxicol.* 1998;1:15.
60. Horiguchi H, Oguma E, Nomoto S, et al. Acute exposure to cobalt induces transient methemoglobinuria in rats. *Toxicol Lett.* 2004;151:459-466.
61. Ichikawa Y, Kusaka Y, Goto S. Biological monitoring of cobalt exposure, based on cobalt concentrations in blood and urine. *Int Arch Occup Environ Health.* 1985;55:269-276.
62. Iyengar V, Woittiez J. Trace elements in human clinical specimens: evaluation of literature data to identify reference values. *Clin Chem.* 1988;34:474-481.
63. Jacobs JJ, Skipor AK, Doorn PF, et al. Cobalt and chromium concentrations in patients with metal on metal total hip replacements. *Clin Orthop.* 1996:S256-263.
64. Jacobziner H, Raybin HW. Poison control: accidental cobalt poisoning. *Arch Pediatr.* 1961;78:200-205.
65. Jefferson JA, Escudero E, Hurtado ME, et al. Excessive erythrocytosis, chronic mountain sickness, and serum cobalt levels. *Lancet.* 2002;359:407-408.
66. Jones HD, Perkins DJ. Metal-ion binding of human transferrin. *Biochim Biophys Acta.* 1965;100:122-127.
67. Kato K. Iron-cobalt treatment of physiologic and nutritional anemia in infants. *J Pediatr.* 1937;11:385-396.
68. Kennedy A, Dornan JD, King R. Fatal myocardial disease associated with industrial exposure to cobalt. *Lancet.* 1981;1:412-414.
69. Kent NL, McCance RA. The absorption and excretion of "minor" elements by man. *Biochem J.* 1941;35.
70. Kesteloot H, Roelandt J, Willems J, et al. An enquiry into the role of cobalt in the heart disease of chronic beer drinkers. *Circulation.* 1968;37:854-864.
71. Kiec-Swierczynska M. Occupational dermatoses and allergy to metals in Polish construction workers manufacturing prefabricated building units. *Contact Dermatitis.* 1990;23:27-32.
72. Kirchgessner M, Reuber S, Kreuzer M. Endogenous excretion and true absorption of cobalt as affected by the oral supply of cobalt. *Biol Trace Elem Res.* 1994;41:175-189.
73. Kleinberg W, Gordon A, Charipper H. Effect of cobalt on erythropoiesis in anemic rabbits. *Proc Soc Exp Biol Med.* 1939;42:119-120.
74. Klinck GH. Thyroid hyperplasia in young children. *JAMA.* 1955;158:1347-1348.
75. Kriss JP, Carnes WH, Gross RT. Hypothyroidism and thyroid hyperplasia in patients treated with cobalt. *JAMA.*1955;157:117-121.
76. Kusaka Y, Ichikawa Y, Shirakawa T, et al. Effect of hard metal dust on ventilatory function. *Br J Ind Med.* 1986;43:486-489.
77. Kusaka Y, Iki M, Kumagai S, et al. Epidemiological study of hard metal asthma. Occup Environ Med 1996;53:188-193.
78. Kusaka Y, Yokoyama K, Sera Y, et al. Respiratory diseases in hard metal workers: an occupational hygiene study in a factory. *Br J Ind Med.* 1986;43:474-485.
79. Lahaye D, Demedts M, van den Oever R, et al. Lung diseases among diamond polishers due to cobalt? *Lancet.* 1984;1:156-157.
80. Linna A, Oksa P, Groundstroem K, et al. Exposure to cobalt in the production of cobalt and cobalt compounds and its effect on the heart. *Occup Environ Med.* 2004;61:877-885.
81. Linnainmaa M, Kiilunen M. Urinary cobalt as a measure of exposure in the wet sharpening of hard metal and stellite blades. *Int Arch Occup Environ Health.* 1997;69:193-200.
82. Lison D, Buchet JP, Swennen B, et al. Biological monitoring of workers exposed to cobalt metal, salt, oxides, and hard metal dust. *Occup Environ Med.* 1994;51:447-450.
83. Llobet JM, Domingo JL, Corbella J. Comparison of antidotal efficacy of chelating agents upon acute toxicity of Co(II) in mice. *Res Commun Chem Pathol Pharmacol.* 1985;50:305-308.
84. Llobet JM, Domingo JL, Corbella J. Comparative effects of repeated parenteral administration of several chelators on the distribution and excretion of cobalt. *Res Commun Chem Pathol Pharmacol.* 1988;60:225-233.
85. Llobet JM, Domingo JL, Corbella J. Comparison of the effectiveness of several chelators after single administration on the toxicity, excretion and distribution of cobalt. *Arch Toxicol.* 1986;58:278-281.
86. Mariano A, Sartorelli P, Innocenti A. Evolution of hard metal pulmonary fibrosis in two artisan grinders of woodworking tools. *Sci Total Environ.* 1994;150:219-221.
87. Markowitz SB, Morabia A, Lilis R, et al. Clinical predictors of mortality from asbestosis in the North American Insulator Cohort, 1981 to 1991. *Am J Respir Crit Care Med.* 1997;156:101-108.
88. McDermott PH, Delaney RL, Egan JD, et al. Myocardosis and cardiac failure in men. *JAMA.* 1966;198:253-256.
89. Migliori M, Mosconi G, Michetti G, et al. Hard metal disease: eight workers with interstitial lung fibrosis due to cobalt exposure. *Sci Total Environ.* 1994;150:187-196.
90. Miller CW, Davis MW, Goldman A, et al. Pneumoconiosis in the tungsten-carbide tool industry; report of three cases. *Arch Ind Hyg Occup Med.* 1953;8:453-465.
91. Morelli L, Di Giulio C, Iezzi M, et al. Effect of acute and chronic cobalt administration on carotid body chemoreceptors responses. *Sci Total Environ.* 1994;150:215-216.
92. Morin Y, Daniel P. Quebec beer-drinkers' cardiomyopathy: etiological considerations. *Can Med Assoc J.* 1967;97:926-928.
93. Morin Y, Tetu A, Mercier G. Cobalt cardiomyopathy: clinical aspects. *Br Heart J.* 1971;33(suppl):175-178.
94. Morin YL, Foley AR, Martineau G, et al. Quebec beer-drinkers' cardiomyopathy: forty-eight cases. *Can Med Assoc J.* 1967;97:881-883.
95. Moulin JJ, Wild P, Mur JM, et al. A mortality study of cobalt production workers: an extension of the follow-up. *Am J Ind Med.* 1993;23:281-288.
96. Mur JM, Moulin JJ, Charruyer-Seinerra MP, et al. A cohort mortality study among cobalt and sodium workers in an electrochemical plant. *Am J Ind Med.* 1987;11:75-81.
97. Murphy RL Jr, Gaensler EA, Holford SK, et al. Crackles in the early detection of asbestosis. *Am Rev Respir Dis.* 1984;129:375-379.
98. Nemery B, Lewis CP, Demedts M. Cobalt and possible oxidant-mediated toxicity. *Sci Total Environ.* 1994;150:57-64.
99. Nemery B, Nagels J, Verbeken E, et al. Rapidly fatal progression of cobalt lung in a diamond polisher. *Am Rev Respir Dis.* 1990;141:1373-1378.
100. Olatunbosun D, Corbett WE, Ludwig J, et al. Alteration of cobalt absorption in portal cirrhosis and idiopathic hemochromatosis. *J Lab Clin Med.* 1970;75:754-762.
101. Orten J. Blood volume studies in cobalt polycythemia. *J Am Biol Chem.* 1933;1936:457-463.
102. Orten J. On the mechanism of the hematopoietic action of cobalt. *Am J Physiol.* 1936;114:414-422.
103. Paschal DC, Ting BG, Morrow JC, et al. Trace metals in urine of United States residents: reference range concentrations. *Environ Res.* 1998;76:53-59.

104. Paternain JL, Domingo JL, Corbella J. Developmental toxicity of cobalt in the rat. J *Toxicol Environ Health*. 1988;24:193-200.
105. Pedigo NG, George WJ, Anderson MB. Effects of acute and chronic exposure to cobalt on male reproduction in mice. *Reprod Toxicol*. 1988;2:45-53.
106. Pitkin RM. *Dietary Reference Intakes: For Thiamin, Riboflavin, Niacin, Vitamin B6, Folate, Vitamin B12, Pantothenic Acid, Biotin, and Choline*; National Academy Press 2000, Washington, DC: Institute of Medicine; 1998.
107. Piza J, Troper L, Cespedes R, et al. Myocardial lesions and heart failure in infantile malnutrition. *Am J Trop Med Hyg*. 1971;20:343-355.
108. Potolicchio I, Mosconi G, Forni A, et al. Susceptibility to hard metal lung disease is strongly associated with the presence of glutamate 69 in HLA-DP beta chain. *Eur J Immunol*. 1997;27:2741-2743.
109. Quilligan JJ Jr. Effect of a cobalt-iron mixture on the anemia of prematurity. *Tex State J Med*. 1954;50:294-296.
110. Raffn E, Mikkelsen S, Altman DG, et al. Health effects due to occupational exposure to cobalt blue dye among plate painters in a porcelain factory in Denmark. *Scand J Work Environ Health*. 1988;14:378-384.
111. Ratto D, Balmes J, Boylen T, et al. Pregnancy in a woman with severe pulmonary fibrosis secondary to hard metal disease. *Chest*. 1988;93:663-665.
112. Rivolta G, Nicoli E, Ferretti G, et al. Hard metal lung disorders: analysis of a group of exposed workers. *Sci Total Environ*. 1994;150:161-165.
113. Rizzato G, Lo Cicero S, Barberis M, et al. Trace of metal exposure in hard metal lung disease. *Chest*. 1986;90:101-106.
114. Robinson JC, James GW, Kark RM. Effect of oral therapy with cobaltous chloride on blood of patients suffering with chronic suppurative infection. *N Engl J Med*. 1949;240:749-753.
115. Rohn RJ, Bond WH. Observations on some hematological effects of cobalt-iron mixtures. *Lancet*. 1953;73:317-324.
116. Rona G. Experimental aspects of cobalt cardiomyopathy. *Br Heart J*. 1971;33(suppl):171-174.
117. Roy PE, Bonenfant JL, Turcot L. Thyroid changes in cases of Quebec beer drinkers myocardosis. *Am J Clin Pathol*. 1968;50:234-239.
118. Rystedt I, Fischer T. Relationship between nickel and cobalt sensitization in hard metal workers. *Contact Dermatitis*. 1983;9:195-200.
119. Sabbioni E, Mosconi G, Minoia C, et al. The European Congress on Cobalt and Hard Metal Disease. Conclusions, highlights and need of future studies. *Sci Total Environ*. 1994;150:263-270.
120. Sandusky GE, Crawford MP, Roberts ED. Experimental cobalt cardiomyopathy in the dog: a model for cardiomyopathy in dogs and man. *Toxicol Appl Pharmacol*. 1981;60:263-278.
121. Sandusky GE, Henk WG, Roberts ED. Histochemistry and ultrastructure of the heart in experimental cobalt cardiomyopathy in the dog. *Toxicol Appl Pharmacol*. 1981;61:89-98.
122. Scansetti G, Lamon S, Talarico S, et al. Urinary cobalt as a measure of exposure in the hard metal industry. *Int Arch Occup Environ Health*. 1985;57:19-26.
123. Schirrmacher UO. Case of cobalt poisoning. *Br Med J*. 1967;1:544-545.
124. Schroeder HA, Nason AP. Trace-element analysis in clinical chemistry. *Clin Chem*. 1971;17:461-474.
125. Seaman AJ. Acquired erythrocyte hypoplasia: a recovery during cobalt therapy. *Acta Haematologica*. 1953;9:153-171.
126. Sesana G, Cortona G, Baj A, et al. Cobalt exposure in wet grinding of hard metal tools for wood manufacture. *Sci Total Environ*. 1994;150:117-119.
127. Shannon M. Differential diagnosis and evaluation: an 11-year-old boy develops vomiting, weakness, weight loss, and a neck mass. *Internet J Med Toxicol*. 1988;1:14.
128. Shirakawa T, Kusaka Y, Fujimura N, et al. Hard metal asthma: cross immunological and respiratory reactivity between cobalt and nickel? *Thorax*. 1990;45:267-271.
129. Shirakawa T, Kusaka Y, Fujimura N, et al. Occupational asthma from cobalt sensitivity in workers exposed to hard metal dust. *Chest*. 1989;95:29-37.
130. Shirakawa T, Kusaka Y, Morimoto K. Specific IgE antibodies to nickel in workers with known reactivity to cobalt. *Clin Exp Allergy*. 1992;22:213-218.
131. Sjogren I, Hillerdal G, Andersson A, et al. Hard metal lung disease: importance of cobalt in coolants. *Thorax*. 1980;35:653-659.
132. Skluis-Cremer GK, Glyn Thomas R, Solomon A. Hard-metal lung disease. A report of 4 cases. *S Afr Med J*. 1987;71:598-600.
133. Sobel H, Sideman M, Arce R. Effect of cobalt ion, nickel ion, an zinc ion on corticoid excretion by the guinea pig. *Proc Soc Exp Biol Med*. 1960;104:86-88.
134. Sprince NL, Chamberlin RI, Hales CA, et al. Respiratory disease in tungsten carbide production workers. *Chest*. 1984;86:549-557.
135. Sprince NL, Oliver LC, Eisen EA, et al. Cobalt exposure and lung disease in tungsten carbide production. A cross-sectional study of current workers. *Am Rev Respir Dis*. 1988;138:1220-1226.
136. Steinhoff D, Mohr U. On the question of a carcinogenic action of cobalt-containing compounds. *Exp Pathol*. 1991;41:169-174.
137. Suardi R, Belotti L, Ferrari MT, et al. Health survey of workers occupationally exposed to cobalt. *Sci Total Environ*. 1994;150:197-200.
138. Sullivan J, Parker M, Carson SB. Tissue cobalt content in "beer drinkers' myocardiopathy." *J Lab Clin Med*. 1968;71:893-911.
139. Swennen B, Buchet JP, Stanescu D, et al. Epidemiological survey of workers exposed to cobalt oxides, cobalt salts, and cobalt metal. *Br J Ind Med*. 1993;50:835-842.
140. van den Eeckhout AV, Verbeken E, Demedts M. [Pulmonary pathology due to cobalt and hard metals]. *Rev Mal Respir*. 1989;6:201-207.
141. Voyce MA. A case of pure red-cell aplasia successfully treated with cobalt. *Br J Haematol*. 1963;9:412-418.
142. Weakly JN. The action of cobalt ions on neuromuscular transmission in the frog. *J Physiol*. 1973;234:597-612.
143. Webb M. The biological action of cobalt and other metals. IV. Inhibition of alpha-oxoglutarate dehydrogenase. *Biochim Biophys Acta*. 1964;89:431-446.
144. Wiberg GS. The effect of cobalt ions on energy metabolism in the rat. *Can J Biochem*. 1968;46:549-554.
145. Wigren A. [Cobalt allergy reaction after knee arthroplasty with a Walldius prosthesis]. *Z Orthop Ihre Grenzgeb*. 1982;120:17.
146. Wintrobe M, Grinstein M, Dubash J, et al. The anemia of infection. VI. The influence of cobalt on the anemia associated with inflammation. *Blood*. 1947;2:323-331.
147. Zanelli R, Barbic F, Migliori M, et al. Uncommon evolution of fibrosing alveolitis in a hard metal grinder exposed to cobalt dusts. *Sci Total Environ*. 1994;150:225-229.

CHAPTER 93
COPPER

Lewis S. Nelson

Copper (Cu)

Atomic number	=	29
Atomic weight	=	63.5 daltons
Normal concentrations		
Whole blood	=	70–140 μg/dL (11–22 μmol/L)
Total serum	=	120–145 μg/dL (18.8–22.8 μmol/L)
Free serum	=	4–7 μg/dL (0.63–1.1 μmol/L)
Ceruloplasmin	=	25–50 μg/dL (3.9–7.8 μmol/L)
Urine	=	5–25 μg/24 h (.078–3.9 nmol/L)

Copper is a widely available metal that is associated with both acute and chronic poisoning. Although essential to life, acute overdose with copper salts produces severe gastrointestinal (GI) and systemic effects that may be life threatening. This clinical syndrome and the underlying mechanism is similar to that noted with iron poisoning. Regardless of the means of exposure, patients with acute copper poisoning require expeditious identification and empiric therapy.

HISTORY AND EPIDEMIOLOGY

Copper is available naturally, either as native copper (elemental copper) or as one of its sulfide or oxide ores. Important ores include malachite ($CuCO_3{\cdot}(OH)_2$), chalcocite (Cu_2S), cuprite (Cu_2O), and chalcopyrite ($CuFeS_2$ or $Cu_2S{\cdot}Fe_2S_3$). Chalcopyrite, a yellow sulfide ore, is the source of 80% of the world's copper production. The smelting, or separation, of copper ores began about 7000 years ago; copper gradually assumed its current level of importance at the start of the Bronze Age, around 3000 B.C. Smelting begins with roasting to dry the ore concentrate, which, in more modern times, is further purified by electrolysis to a 99.5% level of purity. The sulfide ores have a naturally high arsenic content, which is released during the extraction process, posing a risk to those who perform copper smelting.

Although acute copper poisoning is uncommon in the United States, the historical role of copper as a therapeutic agent remains noteworthy. Copper sulfate was used in burn wound debridement until cases of systemic copper poisoning were reported.[63] Interestingly, in one report, each wound debridement procedure was associated with an 8% to 10% decrease in the hematocrit. In the 1960s, copper sulfate (250-mg dose containing 100 mg copper ion) ironically was recommended as an emetic agent, typically for use in children after potentially toxic exposures.[70] It was recognized for its rapidity of onset and effectiveness, and it compared favorably with syrup of ipecac. However, copper-induced emesis was rapidly identified to be a highly dangerous practice, and this use was generally discontinued,[64,78,118] although fatal cases from this use still occur.[78] Copper salts are administered in religious rituals as a green-colored "spiritual water" containing 100 to 150 g/L of copper sulfate as an emetic to "expel one's sins."[7,117]

A growing body of knowledge links copper to the promotion of both physiologic and malignant angiogenesis.[59] In this latter case, copper may enable tumor expansion, invasion, and metastasis. Additionally, copper binding to amyloid fibers in the brain of patients with Alzheimer's disease may lead to local oxidative damage and cause the characteristic neurodegeneration.[25,39] Copper is also similarly implicated in the pathogenesis of both Parkinson's disease and autism.[28,131]

Acute or chronic copper poisoning may occur when the metal is leached from copper pipes or copper containers. This occurs frequently when carbon dioxide gas, used for postmix soft drink carbonation, backflows into the tubing transporting water to the soda dispensers, creating an acidic solution of carbonic acid that leaches copper from the equipment pipes.[127] Similarly, storage of acidic potable substances, such as orange or lemon juice, in copper vessels may cause copper poisoning. A particularly dangerous situation occurs when acidic water is inadvertently used for hemodialysis.[40,82] In this circumstance, the leached copper avoids the normal GI barrier and is delivered parenterally to the patient's circulation. In one reported series, the copper concentration in the dialysis water was 650 μg/L, causing several poisonings and the death of a patient with a whole-blood copper concentration of 2095 μg/L.[406] Similarly, stagnant water or hot water,[107] even if not highly acidic,[111] can accumulate copper ions from pipes and cause poisoning.[9,41]

Although most natural water contains a small quantity of copper (4–10 μg/L), it is tightly bound to organic matter and therefore not orally bioavailable. Copper pipes typically add about 1 mg of copper to the daily intake of an adult. The Environmental Protection Agency guidelines permit up to 1.3 mg/L of copper in drinking water,[34] although in some areas, intermittent concentrations may rise as high as 60 mg/L. Copper in water may be tasted at concentrations of 1 to 5 mg/L, and a blue-green discoloration is imparted when the concentrations are greater than 5 mg/L.[37] Acute GI symptoms occur when drinking water contains more than 25 mg/L,[65] although concentrations as low as 3 mg/L are associated with abdominal pain and vomiting in many, without an increase in the serum copper concentration.[100] In one blinded, randomized study comparing copper-adulterated water with pure water, women appeared more sensitive than men to copper, but both groups were symptomatic when the copper concentration in the water was 6 mg/L.[8]

Metallic copper is ideal for electrical wiring because it is highly malleable and can be drawn into fine wire. Its electrical conductivity is only exceeded by silver. Similarly, its excellent heat conductivity accounts for its widespread use in cookware. Although the metal is reactive with air, it forms a resistant layer of insoluble copper carbonate on its surface. It is this water- and air-resistant compound that accounts for the green coloration of ornamental roofing and statues. Because copper is a soft metal, it must be strengthened before use in structural applications or as a coinage metal. This is most commonly done by the creation of copper alloys. Brass is an alloy of copper compounded with as much as 35% zinc. Similarly, bronze contains copper combined with up to 14% tin. Gun metal is an alloy that contains 88% copper, 10% tin, and 2% zinc. Sterling silver and white gold also contain copper.

CHEMICAL PRINCIPLES

Metallic copper (Cu^0), although not in itself poisonous, may react in acidic environments to release copper ions. The metallic copper contraceptive intrauterine device (IUD) derives its efficacy from the local release of copper ions.[15] Metallic copper bracelets worn by patients with rheumatoid arthritis and other ailments purportedly derive their far-reaching antiinflammatory effect through dermal copper ion absorption and distribution to affected tissues.[125] Local copper ion release is responsible for the occasional case of dermatitis that occurs after skin exposure to copper metal.[64] Ingestion of large amounts of metallic copper—for example, as coins—may rarely produce acute copper poisoning.[103,130] Poisoning under these circumstances is a result of the release of large amounts of copper ion from copper alloy by the acidic gastric contents. Also, inhalation of finely divided metallic copper dust or bronze powder, which is used in industry and for gilding, may produce life-threatening bronchopulmonary irritation, presumably as a consequence of the local release of ions.[38,56]

The majority of patients with acute copper poisoning have been exposed to ionic copper. In copper sulfate, also known as cupric sulfate, the copper atom is in the +2 oxidation state. Copper sulfate is used as a fungicide and algicide and to eradicate tree roots that invade septic, sewage, and drinking water systems.[101] Copper sulfate is the most readily available form and is the form involved in the majority of nonindustrial copper salt exposures. Copper sulfate was a favorite ingredient in many home chemistry sets because of its brilliant blue color when dissolved in water. Although serious poisoning, particularly in children,[126] led regulatory agencies in the United States to restrict its use, it still accounts for the most consequential chemistry set–related toxic exposures reported in other countries.[88] Similarly, homegrown copper sulfate crystals from kits are occasionally responsible for fatal poisonings.[53]

Cuprous salts, containing copper in the +1 oxidation state, are unstable in water and readily oxidize to the cupric form. There are numerous copper salts with varying oxidation states used in industry and agriculture (Table 93–1), many of which are not poisonous. Because those salts that are water soluble are more likely to be toxic, it is important to determine the nature of the copper product implicated in an exposure. Analogously, when examining the medical literature, it is critical to discern which form of copper is involved in the scientific experiment or case report before applying the results to clinical practice.

PHARMACOLOGY AND PHYSIOLOGY

Copper is an essential metal that our body stores in milligram amounts (100–150 mg). Daily requirements of copper are approximately 50 μg/kg in infants and 30 μg/kg in adults. The average daily intake of copper in the United States noted in the Third National Health and Nutrition Examination Survey (NHANES III) is about 1.2 mg.[43]

The daily requirement of copper is satisfied by nuts, fish, and green vegetables such as legumes, although our largest source is generally from drinking water. Copper deficiency is exceedingly rare even in the poorest communities and is most frequently caused by excessive zinc intake[91] or by a genetic aberration such as Menkes "kinky-hair" syndrome, in which intestinal copper uptake is impaired. Menkes syndrome is characterized by mental retardation, thermoregulatory dysfunction, hypopigmentation, connective tissue abnormalities, and pili torti (kinky hair). Interestingly, with the increased focus on the role of copper in neurodegenerative disorders and cancer, some authors suggest intentionally depleting patients of their copper stores with tetrathiomolybdate, an experimental copper chelator.[50]

Copper is absorbed by an active process involving a copper adenosine triphosphatase (CuATPase) in the small intestinal mucosal cell membrane, also known as the Menkes ATPase (see below). The GI absorption varies with the copper intake and the food source[60] and is as low as 12% in patients with high copper intake. In the presence of damaged mucosa, such as after acute overdose, the fractional absorption is likely to be significantly higher.[79] After it has been absorbed, copper is rapidly bound to high-affinity carriers such as ceruloplasmin and low-affinity carriers such as albumin for transport to the liver and other tissues. The amount of unbound copper in the blood under

TABLE 93–1. Important Copper Products

Chemical Name	Chemical Structure	Common Name	Notes
Chalcopyrite	$CuFeS_2$	Copper iron sulfide	Copper ore; source of 80% of world's copper
Chromated cupric arsenate	35% CuO 20% CrO_3 45% As_2O_5	CCA	Wood preservative[a]
Copper octanoate	$Cu[CH_3(CH_2)_6COO]_2$	Copper soap	Fungicide in home garden products, paint, rot-proof rope and roofing
Copper triethanolamine complex	$Cu((HOCH_2CH_2)_3N)_2$	Chelated copper	Algicide
Cupric acetoarsenite	$Cu(C_2H_3O_2)_2 \cdot 3Cu(AsO_2)_2$	Paris or Vienna green	Insecticide, wood preservative, pigment[a]
Cupric arsenite	$CuHAsO_3$	Swedish or Scheele's green	Wood preservative, insecticide[a]
Cupric hydroxide	$Cu(OH)_2$	Copper hydroxide	Fungicide
Cupric chloride	$CuCl_2$		Catalyst in petrochemical industry
Cupric chloride, basic	$CuCl_2 \cdot 3Cu(OH)_2$	Basic copper chloride; copper oxychloride	Fungicide
Cupric oxide	CuO	Black copper oxide; tenorite	Glass pigment, flux, polishing agent
Cupric sulfate	$CuSO_4$	Roman vitriol, blue vitriol, bluestone, hydrocyanite	Fungicide, plant growth regulator, whitewash, homegrown crystals
Cupric sulfate, basic	$CuSO_4 \cdot 3Cu(OH)_2 \cdot 3CaSO_4$	Bordeaux solution	Fungicide
Cuprous cyanide	$CuCN$	Cupricin	Electroplating solutions
Cuprous oxide	Cu_2O	Red copper oxide, cuprite	Antifouling paint

[a]No longer used in the United States.

normal circumstances is well below 1%. After being released locally in the reduced form from its carrier, copper uptake by the hepatic cells occurs via a specific uptake pump.[104] This process, which is facilitated by the reducing agent ascorbic acid, provides a potential window, however brief, for detoxification of the ion by chelating agents. In acute overdose, a high fraction of the plasma copper remains bound to low-affinity proteins, such as albumin, and thus is biologically active.

In the hepatocyte, complex trafficking systems exist (involving ceruloplasmin, metallothionein, and other metallochaperones within the cytoplasm) to prevent copper toxicity and to aid delivery to the appropriate enzymes.[45,102] A distinct Cu-ATPase located on certain subcellular organelles such as the *trans*-Golgi network or pericanalicular lysosomes assists in the appropriate localization and elimination, respectively, of the metal.[26] By this mechanism, copper is either incorporated into enzymes or released, as a metallothionein–copper complex, directly into the biliary system for fecal elimination.

Some copper released from the liver is bound primarily to ceruloplasmin, an α_2-sialoglycoprotein with a molecular weight of 132,000 Daltons. Ceruloplasmin-bound copper accounts for approximately 90% to 95% of serum copper. Ceruloplasmin is a multifunctional protein that binds six atoms of copper per molecule. Copper bound to this carrier has a plasma half-life of approximately 24 hours. Ceruloplasmin is also involved in the mobilization of iron from its storage sites, and it serves an analogous role as a ferroxidase during the ferrous–ferric conversion. Cu^+ is oxidized directly by ceruloplasmin, thereby avoiding the generation of reactive oxygen species.

There are several important copper-containing enzymes in humans (Table 93–2). The common link among these enzymes is their participation in redox (reduction–oxidation) reactions in which a molecule, typically oxygen, donates or shares its electrons with another compound. In this respect, the physiology, chemistry, and toxicology of copper are most similar to those of iron. In fact, "blue-blooded" animals, such as octopi and spiders, use copper in hemocyanin, a blue pigment, in an analogous manner that "red-blooded" animals use iron in hemoglobin.

The volume of distribution of copper is 2 L/kg, and the half-life of erythrocyte copper is 26 days. The elimination of copper occurs predominantly through biliary excretion after complexation with ceruloplasmin. Biliary excretion approximates GI absorption and averages 2000 μg/24 h.[5,102,123] Renal elimination under normal conditions is trivial, accounting for approximately 5 to 25 μg/24 h.[5]

TABLE 93–2. Important Copper-Containing Enzymes and Proteins and Their Functions

Enzyme or Protein	Function
Alcohol dehydrogenase	Metabolism of alcohols
Catalase	Detoxifies peroxide
Ceruloplasmin enzymes	Copper transport, ferroxidase
Cytochrome C oxidase	Electron transport chain
Dopamine β-hydroxylase	Converts dopamine to norepinephrine
Factor V	Coagulation cascade
Lysyl oxidase	Cross-links collagen and elastin
Monoamine oxidase	Deamination of primary amines
Superoxide dismutase	Detoxifies free radicals
Tyrosinase	Melanin production

TOXICOLOGY AND PATHOPHYSIOLOGY

REDOX CHEMISTRY

Because copper is a transition metal, it is capable of assuming one of several different oxidation (or valence) states, and it is an active participant in redox reactions. In particular, participation in the Fenton reaction and Haber-Weiss cycle explains the toxicologic effects of copper as a generator of oxidative stress and inhibitor of several key metabolic enzymes (see Fig. 11-2).[42,47] In the presence of sulfhydryl-rich cell membranes, such as those on erythrocytes, cupric ions are reduced to cuprous ions, which are capable of generating superoxide radicals in the presence of oxygen.[74] This one-electron reduction of oxygen regenerates the cupric ion, allowing redox cycling and continuous generation of reactive oxygen species (Fig. 93–1). In particular, the mitochondrial electron transport chain and lipid membranes serve as ready sources of electrons for copper reduction, establishing a chain of events that ultimately leads to mitochondrial or membrane dysfunction, respectively.[90]

ERYTHROCYTES

Cupric ion inhibits sulfhydryl groups on enzymes in important antioxidant systems, including glucose-6-phosphate dehydrogenase and glutathione (GSH) reductase.[108] However, although support for these effects is only indirect, intraerythrocyte concentrations of reduced GSH decrease demonstrably after copper exposure.[86] This effect is presumably part of the protective role that GSH, a nucleophile or reducing agent, normally has on oxidants, such as either cupric ions or the reactive oxygen species they generate.[84,85] Thus, in the setting of copper poisoning, in which excessive quantities of oxidants are produced, the depletion of GSH presumably augments peroxidative membrane damage.

The importance of hemoglobin-derived reactive oxygen species is demonstrated by the lack of hemolysis in the presence of copper under anaerobic conditions or in an environment saturated with carbon monoxide.[12] The in vitro hemolytic activity of copper sulfate is reduced by albumin and several sulfhydryl-containing compounds, including

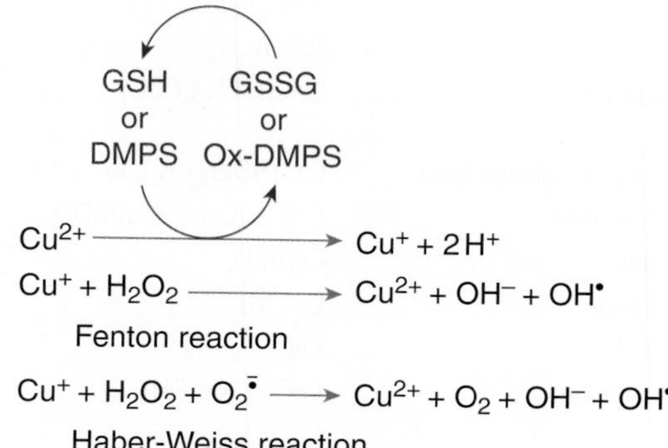

FIGURE 93–1. Copper in the cupric or Cu^{2+} state is reduced by sulfhydryl containing compounds such as glutathione (GSH) or dimercaptopropane sulfonate (DMPS) to its cuprous form (Cu^+), forming disulfide links in the process. Oxidized glutathione (GSSG) is subsequently enzymatically reduced by glutathione reductase to regenerate GSH. Superoxide anions, formed when molecular oxygen (O_2) acquires an additional electron, are continually generated by mitochondria. Both the Fenton and the Haber-Weiss reactions use the cuprous form of copper as a catalyst to convert hydrogen peroxide or superoxide radical into the more biologically consequential hydroxyl radical ($OH^\bullet$).[14,73]

D-penicillamine and succimer.[3] Interestingly, dimercaptopropane sulfonate (DMPS), another sulfhydryl-containing compound often used as a chelator, exacerbates copper-induced hemolysis. This paradoxic effect is variably attributed to concomitant inhibition of superoxide dismutase, an important antioxidant enzyme, or to the ability of DMPS to efficiently reduce either membrane dithiols or cupric ions, in either case increasing the generation of superoxide.[2]

Hemolysis frequently occurs within the first 24 hours after with acute copper poisoning.[32,117,129] This rapidity of hemolysis differs markedly from most other oxidant stressors, which may take several days, and is likely a result of the differing nature of the erythrocyte insult. That is, the hemolysis that occurs after most oxidant exposures is caused by precipitation of hemoglobin as Heinz bodies and subsequent erythrocyte destruction by the reticuloendothelial system. Hemoglobin precipitation may also occur in the setting of acute copper poisoning, particularly after less substantial exposure. Additionally, and accounting for the early hemolysis, copper also directly oxidizes the erythrocyte membrane, thereby initiating red cell lysis independently of the reticuloendothelial system.[4,106] Oxidant-induced disulfide cross-links in the erythrocyte membrane reduce its stability and flexibility, thereby predisposing to early cell rupture.[4]

Copper-induced oxidation of the heme iron within the erythrocyte produces methemoglobinemia.[89] Given the high incidence of hemolysis, the methemoglobin is commonly released within the plasma. In this situation, methylene blue may not reliably reduce the ferric iron.

LIVER

Although most of the accumulated copper in hepatocytes is rapidly complexed with metallothionein or otherwise used, failure to completely sequester copper ions allows their participation in redox reactions. Hepatic cells are protected from copper toxicity in vitro by induction of metallothionein with zinc or cadmium salts or by the infusion of metallothionein before exposure. These interventions demonstrate the toxicologic significance of free intracellular copper. These findings also explain the therapeutic use of zinc acetate in patients with Wilson disease because copper itself is not a good inducer of metallothionein in humans.

Copper ions also generate hydroxyl radicals, which are potent inducers of both lipid peroxidation, and other reactive oxygen species. The peroxidative effect on biologic membranes is more significant in animals deficient in vitamin E and is prevented by vitamin E replacement, presumably because of the role of vitamin E as a free radical scavenger.[69,116] These effects are most pronounced in mitochondria, perhaps as a consequence of the reduction of cupric to cuprous ion in these organelles.[52,115] Copper also accumulates in the cellular nuclei, where localized production of hydroxyl radicals may form DNA adducts and cause apoptosis.[105] Histologically, liver damage follows a centrilobular pattern of necrosis.

The sequelae of the potent hepatotoxic effects of copper are not isolated to the liver. After liver necrosis occurs, typically at liver copper concentrations greater than 50 mg/g dry weight, massive release of copper into the blood occurs, which may be of sufficient magnitude to cause hemolysis. This sequence of events is common during the crises of Wilson disease and may allow for an understanding of the delayed secondary episode of hemolysis that occurs in some copper-poisoned patients.

KIDNEYS

The kidneys bioaccumulate copper. Although primarily bound to metallothionein when available, copper is otherwise free to participate in oxidant-generating reactions in a manner analogous to that of iron. Thus, reactive oxygen species are probably also responsible for the nephrotoxic effects of copper. Pathologic analyses of the kidneys of oliguric or anuric patients typically reveal acute tubular necrosis that may demonstrate hemoglobin casts. These findings suggests that renal failure may result indirectly from the hemoglobinuria induced by the massive release of free extracellular hemoglobin. The urinary hemoglobin, similar to myoglobin, may undergo conversion to ferriheme or release its iron, either of which results in oxidative stress on the renal tubular epithelial cell. Additionally, free extracellular hemoglobin may cause renal vasoconstriction through the local scavenging of nitric oxide within the renal arterioles.

CENTRAL NERVOUS SYSTEM

Although charged entities such as copper ions do not readily cross the blood–brain barrier, elevated cerebrospinal fluid copper concentrations are characteristic of chronic copper overload conditions such as Wilson disease.[119] This accumulation is accomplished through carrier-mediated transport of albumin-bound, not ceruloplasmin-bound, copper into the central nervous system.

CLINICAL MANIFESTATIONS

ACUTE COPPER SALT POISONING

The acutely lethal dose of ingested copper sulfate is suggested to be 0.15 to 0.3 g/kg, but this is unverified. GI irritation is the most common initial manifestation of copper salt poisoning. This syndrome includes the rapid onset of emesis and abdominal pain, possibly followed by gastroduodenal hemorrhage, ulceration, or perforation.[8,33] Blue coloration of the vomitus may occur after the ingestion of certain copper salts, particularly copper sulfate.[53,112,126] Blue vomitus is not, however, pathognomonic for copper poisoning and also occurs in patients who ingest boric acid, methylene blue, or food dyes. Other common symptoms include retrosternal chest pain and a metallic taste.

Given its location within the GI tract, the liver receives the initial and most substantial exposure to any ingested copper. In patients with more severe acute copper sulfate poisoning, hepatotoxicity is a frequent, although rarely an isolated,[66] manifestation. Jaundice, although among the most common clinical and biochemical findings after overdose, can be hepatocellular or hemolytic.[10]

Hemolysis is more common than hepatotoxicity and occurs invariably in patients with liver damage.[86,114] As noted, copper-induced hemolysis often occurs rapidly after exposure and may be severe (see Pathophysiology above and Chap. 24). In most reported cases, the discovery of significant methemoglobinemia occurs early in the patient's clinical course and is rapidly followed by hemolysis.[31] Because free methemoglobin is filterable, methemoglobinuria may occur, although it cannot be differentiated from other heme forms in the urine without specialized testing.

Renal and pulmonary toxicity occur occasionally and represent extraerythrocytic manifestations of the oxidative effects of the copper ions. Despite massive intravascular hemolysis, hemoglobinuric renal failure is uncommon in patients who receive adequate volume-replacement therapy.[32]

Hypotension and cardiovascular collapse occur in patients with the most severe poisoning and is likely multifactorial in origin.[112] Undoubtedly, intravascular volume depletion from vomiting and diarrhea is involved. However, the severity and poor patient outcome despite appropriate volume repletion suggests that the direct effects of copper on vascular and cardiac cells are also involved. Sepsis, as a result of transmucosal bacterial invasion, may also be partially responsible.[79]

Depressed mental status, which ranges from lethargy to coma or seizures after acute poisoning, is likely an epiphenomenon related to damage to other organ systems. These findings are particularly common in patients with hepatic failure and are comparable to those of hepatic encephalopathy from other causes. In patients with chronic copper poisoning, such as Wilson disease, neurologic manifestations are prominent and typically involve movement disorders (see Chronic Copper Poisoning below).

Intravenous injection of copper sulfate reportedly produces a clinical syndrome identical to that that occurs after ingestion, although the GI findings may be less pronounced.[14,18,94] Subcutaneous administration of a veterinary copper glycinate solution produced skin necrosis in the area of the injection.[11,95]

Although not strictly a form of copper poisoning, inhalation of copper oxide fumes, generated during welding or other industrial processes, may produce metal fume fever, a syndrome historically called "brass chills" or "foundry workers' ague." Patients with this syndrome present with cough, chills, chest pain, or fever that are most likely immunologic, not toxicologic, in origin (see Chap. 124). However, copper oxide formation, unlike zinc oxide, only occurs at extremely high temperatures, accounting for the relative infrequency of copper-induced metal fume fever.

CHRONIC COPPER POISONING

Although hepatolenticular degeneration, known as Wilson disease, is a condition of chronic copper overload, there are qualitative similarities to acute copper poisoning. Wilson disease is an inherited autosomal recessive disorder of copper metabolism affecting approximately one in 40,000 persons. The gene implicated in this disease (*ATP7B*) codes for a hepatocyte membrane–bound, copper-binding protein that is required for the maturation of ceruloplasmin and the biliary excretion of copper. Transgenic replacement models, in which human *ATP7B* is expressed in deficient animals, demonstrate normalization of copper excretion.[83] The absence of this gene and the resultant increase in hepatic copper concentrations produce continuing oxidative stress on the hepatocyte and cellular necrosis with the inevitable development of cirrhosis. Patients undergo periodic fluctuations in the extent of their copper-induced hepatotoxicity, and episodes of severe hepatotoxicity are frequently associated with hemolysis as stored copper is released from dying hepatocytes.

The adverse effects of copper on the lenticular nucleus in the basal ganglia cause movement disorders such as ataxia, tremor, parkinsonism, dysphagia, and dystonia.[92] No other form of copper poisoning is associated with substantial or direct neurotoxicity. Psychiatric manifestations, such as behavioral changes or mood disorders, may also occur.[21] Accumulation of copper within the cornea accounts for the characteristic green-brown Kayser-Fleischer rings. Although patients' serum copper concentrations are decreased, they typically have a reduced ceruloplasmin concentration caused by the failure of copper incorporation into ceruloplasmin and release from the liver and an elevated urinary copper concentration. Treatment involves lifelong therapy with D-penicillamine, trientine (triethylene tetramine), or molybdenum salts if the patient is D-penicillamine sensitive. Zinc acetate, which has been approved by the Food and Drug Administration (FDA) as a maintenance therapy, induces the formation of intestinal metallothionein and thereby blocks copper absorption by enhancing intestinal mucosal cell sequestration.[22] Orthotopic liver transplantation results in improvement in nearly all aspects of the disease, including the central nervous system and ocular manifestations.[48]

Chronic exogenous copper poisoning is uncommon in adults but is reported after the use of copper-containing dietary supplements.[93] However, subacute or chronic exposure is common in children in some parts of the world. This condition, commonly called *childhood cirrhosis* in India or *idiopathic copper toxicosis* elsewhere, generally occurs in the setting of excessive dietary intake of copper because of copper-contaminated water from brass vessels used to store milk. These children may have a genetic predisposition to copper accumulation because signs of chronic liver disease develop by several months of age and progress rapidly.[110,113] Both serum copper and ceruloplasmin concentrations are markedly elevated, which differentiates this disease from Wilson disease. The incidence of the disease has decreased dramatically, probably as a result of improved nutrition and replacement of copper utensils and storage containers with those made of steel. One family of four developed abdominal pain, malaise, tachycardia, and anemia after approximately 1 month of eating homegrown vegetables treated with copper oxychloride pesticide.[54] Each patient had anemia and a slightly elevated (or upper limit of normal) serum copper concentration.

"Vineyard sprayer's lung," first described in 1969, refers to the occupational pulmonary disease that occurred among Portuguese vineyard workers applying Bordeaux solution, a 1% to 2% copper sulfate solution neutralized with hydrated lime ($Ca(OH)_2$).[97] The patients developed interstitial pulmonary fibrosis and histiocytic granulomas containing copper. Many of these workers also developed pulmonary adenocarcinoma, hepatic angiosarcoma, and micronodular cirrhosis, raising the possibility of a carcinogenic effect of chronic copper exposure.[98] There is also a suggestion of an increased incidence of pulmonary adenocarcinoma among smelters, who are, however, exposed to many other xenobiotics, including arsenic, a known carcinogen.[80] Copper is not on the list of suspected carcinogens compiled by the International Agency of Research on Cancer (IARC).

Ophthalmic effects of copper salts, primarily after occupational exposure, include irritation of the corneal, conjunctival, or adnexal structures. Chronic ophthalmic exposure to particulate elemental copper or one of its alloys may result in chalcosis lentis, from the Greek word *chalkos*, or copper. This chronic exposure manifests as a green-brown discoloration of the lens or cornea, similar to Kayser-Fleischer rings.

DIAGNOSTIC TESTING

Real-time testing for copper is impractical, and almost all management decisions must be based on clinical criteria. Copper concentrations are often obtained for confirmatory or investigative purposes. Although never adequately studied, whole-blood copper concentrations may correlate better with clinical findings than do serum copper concentrations.[33] The rapid movement of copper from serum into the erythrocyte presumably explains this finding. However, although there is a statistical relationship between the whole-blood copper concentrations and the severity of poisoning,[33,124] there is little correlation between clinical findings at any given copper concentration, regardless of which biologic tissue is measured. Similarly, other than at extremely high or low concentrations, there is no defined concentration at which the prognosis may be established with certainty. Reported serum copper concentrations in patients with hemolysis range from 96 to 747 μg/dL, and those after severe poisoning have values of 6600[53] to 8267 μg/dL.[31] Serum copper concentrations in 11 patients with copper-induced acute renal failure ranged from 115 to 390 μg/dL.[30] The normal urinary copper excretion per 24 hours is up to approximately 25 μg and is reportedly as high as 628 μg/24 h in patients with copper poisoning.[44]

Occasionally, serum copper concentrations reveal a secondary increase, likely as a consequence of release during hepatocellular necrosis. This secondary rise typically occurs only in patients with life-threatening poisoning, and clinical evaluation is far more important and relevant than serial copper concentrations.[114]

Elevated copper concentrations are also noted in patients with inflammatory conditions, biliary cirrhosis, pregnancy, and estrogenic oral contraceptive use.[24,62] These conditions are associated with an elevated ceruloplasmin level, and although the serum copper concentrations increase, the fraction of bound copper in the serum remains normal. Copper concentrations in the erythrocyte remain normal. Patients with Wilson disease have elevated hepatocyte copper content, but their serum copper concentrations are generally below normal unless hepatic necrosis is occurring.[81]

Although serum ceruloplasmin concentrations increase in patients with acute copper poisoning,[124] presumably reflecting increased hepatic synthesis, the ceruloplasmin concentration cannot be used to define the patient's prognosis. Tissue metallothionein concentrations may also increase after copper poisoning, but the implication of this finding, which is limited by the inability to rapidly obtain tissue samples, is unknown.[76] Ceruloplasmin concentrations are low in patients with Wilson disease, reflecting aberrant enzymatic activity.

Routine laboratory testing after acute copper salt poisoning should include an assessment for both hemolysis and hepatotoxicity. Differentiation of these causes as a cause for jaundice is made by standard methodology, such as comparison of the bilirubin fractions and an assessment of the hepatic enzymes and hemoglobin, that is, whereas indirect bilirubin is proportionally elevated in patients with hemolysis, the direct fraction increases in patients with hepatocellular necrosis. An assessment of the patient's electrolyte and hydration status is warranted. The prothrombin time may be prolonged in the absence of liver injury or disseminated intravascular coagulopathy and may be the result of a direct effect of free copper ions on the coagulation cascade.[89] In addition, many reports document abnormal glucose 6-phosphate dehydrogenase (G6PD) activity, suggesting for the cause of hemolysis. However, interpretation of this test result is difficult because copper poisoning interferes with the measurement of G6PD.

Although copper metal embedded in the skin is clearly visible, topically applied copper salts are not visualized.[16] The clinical usefulness of radiographs to identify ingested copper solutions has not been studied. Obtaining an abdominal radiograph, although probably of limited benefit, may be justified because it occasionally demonstrates the presence of radiopaque material in the GI tract.

MANAGEMENT

Supportive care is the cornerstone to the effective management of patients with acute copper poisoning, emphasizing antiemetic therapy, fluid and electrolyte correction, and normalization of vital signs before the consideration of chelation therapy. GI decontamination is of limited concern because the onset of emesis generally occurs within minutes of ingestion and is often protracted. In patients who present early after ingestion of a liquid copper solution and who have not yet vomited, aspiration with a nasogastric tube may remove copper ion. In one case, even after extensive vomiting, nasogastric aspiration still removed blue solution, but removing this remaining volume is unlikely to provide significant clinical benefit.[19] Although oral activated charcoal is unlikely to be harmful, it is of unproved benefit, and it may hinder the ability to perform GI endoscopy to evaluate the corrosive effects of a copper salt on the mucosal surface.[19] For this reason, even though activated charcoal may adsorb the remaining copper in the proximal GI tract, it is relatively contraindicated in most situations. Advanced therapy for patients with renal failure may include hemodialysis, and liver transplantation may be needed for patients with life-threatening hepatic failure.

CHELATION THERAPY

Chelation therapy should be initiated when hepatic or hematologic complications are present or there are other manifestations of severe poisoning. Studies on the efficacy of chelation therapy after acute copper salt poisoning are limited. Even when administered early and appropriately, organ damage and death still occur. Application of the data from the existing literature is complex because of the lack of controlled therapeutic studies of human copper poisoning. Although experimental animal models and uncontrolled human data exist, the results are frequently contradictory. Three chelators are clinically available, and most data regarding dosing and efficacy data are derived either from their use in the treatment of patients with Wilson disease or from their effects on copper elimination during chelation of patients manifesting toxicity from other metals.

Most patients with copper poisoning are initially treated with intramuscular British anti-Lewisite (BAL).[120,126] Although BAL may be less effective, its use is appropriate in patients in whom vomiting or GI injury prevents oral D-penicillamine administration. Furthermore, because the BAL–copper complex primarily undergoes biliary elimination, whereas D-penicillamine undergoes renal elimination, BAL proves useful in patients with renal failure. When tolerated, D-penicillamine therapy should be started simultaneously or shortly after the initiation of therapy with BAL (see Antidotes in Depth A26: Dimercaprol).

Calcium disodium ethylenediaminetetraacetate ($CaNa_2EDTA$) reduces the oxidative damage induced by copper ions in experimental models.[128] However, it does not greatly enhance the elimination of copper when used for the chelation of other metals.[109,121] In addition, short-term use of $CaNa_2EDTA$ inactivates dopamine β-hydroxylase in humans, presumably by chelating the copper moiety from its active site.[36] However, because the in vivo activity of this enzyme is restored on the addition of exogenous copper, the potential for inhibition of the formation of neuronal norepinephrine during the treatment of acute poisoning is unknown. Successful clinical use of $CaNa_2EDTA$ has been reported.[46,94,120] Interestingly, CuCaEDTA is used as a copper supplement in animals, and overdose of this formulation results in copper poisoning, suggesting that its chelating ability is limited[49] (see Antidotes in Depth A28: Edetate Calcium Disodium).

D-Penicillamine (Cuprimine), a structurally distinct metabolite of penicillin, is an orally bioavailable monothiol chelator. It is used in the treatment of lead, mercury, and copper toxicity, as well as in the management of rheumatoid arthritis and scleroderma. It has also recently been investigated for its antiangiogenesis effects in cancer therapy, which occur by chelation of copper that serves as a cofactor for certain growth factors, such as fibroblast growth factor.[55] D-Penicillamine is effective in preventing copper-induced hemolysis in patients with Wilson disease. Its protective mechanism is primarily mediated through chelation of unbound copper ions, rendering them unable to participate in redox reactions.[72] The D-penicillamine–copper complex undergoes rapid renal clearance in patients with competent kidneys. The use of D-penicillamine is not formally studied in the patients with acute copper salt poisoning, but case studies and animal models suggest that copper elimination is enhanced.[20,51,63] The recommended dose is 1.0 to 1.5 g/d given orally in four divided doses. D-Penicillamine is also indicated for the treatment of chronic exogenous copper poisoning, such as Indian childhood cirrhosis. Initiation early in the course of disease and discontinuation of the exposure are associated with hepatic recovery and dramatically improved survival rates.[13]

Although D-penicillamine appears to be effective, it is associated with several significant complications. In nearly 50% of patients treated with D-penicillamine for Wilson disease, there is worsening of the neurologic findings.[23] Subacute toxicities of D-penicillamine include aplastic anemia, agranulocytosis, and renal and pulmonary disease. Long-term use of D-penicillamine is also associated with the development of cutaneous lesions and immunologic dysfunction. However, in the brief treatment necessary for acutely poisoned patients, the major risk is the potential for hypersensitivity reactions that occur in 25% of patients who are allergic to penicillin. This hypersensitivity reaction is likely related to contamination of the pharmaceutical preparation with penicillin rather than immunologic cross-reactivity.[61,68] The use of D-penicillamine during pregnancy is associated with congenital abnormalities in fetuses, although all of the data are derived from women with Wilson disease who were receiving long-term therapy.[99]

Succimer is sometimes described as an ineffective copper chelator, although it is able to triple the baseline copper elimination in a murine model.[27] Given its ease of use, relative safety, and benefit in experimental models,[1] succimer may be used in lieu of D-penicillamine in patients with mild or moderate poisoning. Under these circumstances, the use of standard lead poisoning dosing regimens is warranted (see Chap. 93 and Antidote in Depth A27: Succimer [2,3-Dimercaptosuccinic Acid])

DMPS, an experimental chelator that is gaining popularity for the treatment of arsenic poisoning, prevents acute tubular necrosis in copper-poisoned mice.[87] DMPS also proved to be the most effective of a panel of chelators in a murine model of copper sulfate poisoning,[67] and it substantially increased urinary copper elimination in nonpoisoned individuals.[122] However, DMPS, unlike D-penicillamine, forms intramolecular disulfide bridges, which, in so doing, liberates an electron. This property, which accounts for its potency as a reducing agent, also probably explains its propensity to worsen copper-induced hemolysis in vitro.[2,3] Because an adequate analysis of risk versus benefit is unavailable, DMPS should not be used to chelate copper-poisoned patients at this time.

Trientine, an orally bioavailable xenobiotic, is the second-line chelator for patients with Wilson disease, but its use in patients with acute copper poisoning is unreported. This, too, is the case with zinc therapy to induce metallothionine synthesis, which is also of proven efficacy in Wilson disease but has an unknown role in the treatment of acute copper poisoning. The need for several weeks of zinc therapy before realizing full efficacy makes its therapeutic use in acutely poisoned patients questionable. Although large oral doses of zinc salts may limit the absorption of copper ion, the concomitant GI irritant effects of zinc ion make this therapy impractical.[58]

Tetrathiomolybdate, an FDA-recognized chelating agent with orphan drug status, although not marketed, may be available through compounding pharmacies, typically as ammonium tetrathiomolybdate. Tetrathiomolybdate is suggested to benefit copper-poisoned animals in uncontrolled studies,[96] but its use in acute copper poisoning in humans is unstudied. Tetrathiomolybdate depleted the copper stores in a patient with cancer who purchased the compound over the Internet as an "alternative" antiangiogenesis therapy.[77]

EXTRACORPOREAL ELIMINATION

There are limited data regarding the extent to which copper ion is eliminated by various extracorporeal means. Exchange transfusion is of undefined, but probably limited, benefit in acute copper sulfate poisoning.[31] Hemodialysis membranes undoubtedly allow copper ions to cross, based on the epidemics in which hemodialysis using copper-rich water inadvertently resulted in copper poisoning.[40] Although copper should be similarly cleared by hemodialysis, its relatively large volume of distribution limits the potential clinical usefulness of this technique. Furthermore, copper ions are highly protein bound, and the dialyzable concentration is typically less than 1 pmol/L, suggesting that hemodialysis would have little clinical usefulness. This fact is supported by case reports in which serum, tissue, or dialysate concentrations of copper are assessed.[6,94] Furthermore, given the propensity of hemodialysis to lyse erythrocytes, which may release stored copper and worsen toxicity, hemodialysis is not recommended.[57]

The molecular adsorbents recirculating system (MARS) and single-pass albumin dialysis (SPAD), which are modified forms of hemodialysis in which albumin is included in the dialysate, are reported to rapidly and substantially lower the serum copper concentrations in patients with fulminant Wilson disease, allowing a bridge to hepatic transplantation.[29,35] One patient was treated with albumin dialysis using a 44 g/L albumin-containing dialysate and a slow dialysate flow rate (1–2 L/h) in a manner similar to routine continuous venovenous hemodiafiltration reportedly removed 105 mg of copper and normalized the serum copper concentration.[17,73] The risk associated with hemolysis likely remains, and caution should be used when extrapolating therapy from Wilson disease to exogenous copper poisoning.

Plasma exchange enhanced the elimination of copper in patients with fulminant Wilson disease.[71,73] Copper removal ranged from 3 to 12 mg per treatment, but it is unclear if either of these removal techniques would be beneficial after an ingestion of gram quantities of copper sulfate. The same warning as above about inadvertent red cell lysis applies.

Peritoneal dialysis is not useful in patients with fulminant Wilson disease.[75] Peritoneal dialysis removed less than 700 μg in a copper sulfate-poisoned child whose copper concentration was 207 μg/dL.[57] However, in the same patient, the addition of albumin to the dialysate removed 9 mg of copper at a time when the child's serum copper concentration had already decreased substantially.

Management of hepatic toxicity requires little more than standard supportive care. The potential benefit of *N*-acetylcysteine has not been studied, although it is useful in many forms of fulminant hepatic failure. Liver transplantation should be considered, but specific criteria for transfer to a specialized liver unit or for transplant, other than those that are applicable for Wilson disease or other more common, noncopper etiologies, are undefined.

There are no controlled data on the treatment of acute copper poisoning in pregnancy. The available data on pregnant women with Wilson disease document that D-penicillamine is teratogenic and that zinc may be the preferred therapy.

SUMMARY

Acute copper poisoning is rare in the United States but is associated with dramatic toxicologic effects, primarily hemolysis and hepatotoxicity. The effects are primarily mediated by oxidative stress on the erythrocyte and hepatocyte, and this similarity to iron salt poisoning adds a framework for the conceptual understanding of the disease. The infrequency of acute copper poisoning severely limits our ability to perform controlled studies on its management. Chelation is most commonly performed with BAL and D-penicillamine. Succimer is more familiar to most clinicians and has fewer associated adverse effects and may therefore be an acceptable alternative. Extracorporeal elimination is unlikely to be of benefit. Fortunately, exhaustive research into diseases of copper metabolism, particularly Wilson disease, which has periodic exacerbations similar to acute copper poisoning, has provided insight into managing patients with acute copper salt poisoning.

REFERENCES

1. Aaseth J, Korkina LG, Afanas'ev IB. Hemolytic activity of copper sulfate as influenced by epinephrine and chelating thiols. *Zhongguo Yao Li Xue Bao.* 1998;19:203-206.
2. Aaseth J, Ribarov S, Bochev P. The interaction of copper (Cu^{++}) with the erythrocyte membrane and 2,3-dimercaptopropanesulphonate in vitro: a source of activated oxygen species. *Pharmacol Toxicol.* 1987;61:250-253.

3. Aaseth J, Skaug V, Alexander J. Haemolytic activity of copper as influenced by chelating agents, albumine and chromium. *Acta Pharmacol Toxicol (Copenh).* 1984;54:304-310.
4. Adams KF, Johnson G Jr, Hornowski KE, Lineberger TH. The effect of copper on erythrocyte deformability: a possible mechanism of hemolysis in acute copper intoxication. *Biochim Biophys Acta.* 1979;550:279-287.
5. Adelstein S, Vallee BL. Copper metabolism in man. *N Engl J Med.* 1961;265:892-897.
6. Agarwal BN, Bray SH, Bercz P, Plotzker R, Labovitz E. Ineffectiveness of hemodialysis in copper sulphate poisoning. *Nephron.* 1975;15:74-77.
7. Akintonwa A, Mabadeje AF, Odutola TA. Fatal poisonings by copper sulfate ingested from "spiritual water." *Vet Hum Toxicol.* 1989;31:453-454.
8. Araya M, Olivares M, Pizarro F, Llanos A, Figueroa G, Uauy R. Community-based randomized double-blind study of gastrointestinal effects and copper exposure in drinking water. *Environ Health Perspect.* 2004;112:1068-1073.
9. Arens P. Factors to be considered concerning the corrosion of copper tubes. *Eur J Med Res.* 1999;4:243-245.
10. Ashraf I. Hepatic derangements (biochemical) in acute copper sulphate poisoning. *J Ind Med Assoc.* 1970;55:341-342.
11. Atkinson D, Beasley M, Dryburgh P. Accidental subcutaneous copper salt injection: toxic effects and management. *N Z Med J.* 2004;117:U800.
12. Barnes G, Frieden E. Oxygen requirement for cupric ion induced hemolysis. *Biochem Biophys Res Commun.* 1983;115:680-684.
13. Bavdekar AR, Bhave SA, Pradhan AM, Pandit AN, Tanner MS. Long term survival in Indian childhood cirrhosis treated with D-penicillamine. *Arch Dis Child.* 1996;74:32-35.
14. Behera C, Rautji R, Dogra TD. An unusual suicide with parenteral copper sulphate poisoning: a case report. *Med Sci Law.* 2007;47:357-358.
15. Beltran-Garcia MJ, Espinosa A, Herrera N, Perez-Zapata AJ, Beltran-Garcia C, Ogura T. Formation of copper oxychloride and reactive oxygen species as causes of uterine injury during copper oxidation of Cu-IUD. *Contraception.* 2000;61:99-103.
16. Bentur Y, Koren G, McGuigan M, Spielberg SP. An unusual skin exposure to copper; clinical and pharmacokinetic evaluation. *J Toxicol Clin Toxicol.* 1988;26:371-380.
17. Berger MM, Shenkin A, Revelly JP, et al. Copper, selenium, zinc, and thiamine balances during continuous venovenous hemodiafiltration in critically ill patients. *Am J Clin Nutr.* 2004;80:410-416.
18. Bhowmik D, Mathur R, Bhargava Y, et al. Chronic interstitial nephritis following parenteral copper sulfate poisoning. *Ren Fail.* 2001;23:731-735.
19. Blundell S, Curtin J, Fitzgerald D. Blue lips, coma and haemolysis. *J Paediatr Child Health.* 2003;39:67-68.
20. Botha CJ, Naude TW, Swan GE, Dauth J, Dreyer MJ, Williams MC. The cupruretic effect of two chelators following copper loading in sheep. *Vet Hum Toxicol.* 1993;35:409-413.
21. Brewer GJ: Recognition, diagnosis, and management of Wilson's disease. *Proc Soc Exp Biol Med.* 2000;223:39-46.
22. Brewer GJ, Johnson VD, Dick RD, Hedera P, Fink JK, Kluin KJ. Treatment of Wilson's disease with zinc. XVII: treatment during pregnancy. *Hepatology.* 2000;31:364-370.
23. Brewer GJ, Turkay A, Yuzbaziyan-Gurkan V. Development of neurologic symptoms in a patient with asymptomatic Wilson's disease treated with penicillamine. *Arch Neurol.* 1994;51:304-305.
24. Buchwald A. Serum copper elevation from estrogen effect, masquerading as fungicide toxicity. *J Med Toxicol.* 2008;4:30-32.
25. Bush AI, Strozyk D. Serum copper: a biomarker for Alzheimer disease? *Arch Neurol.* 2004;61:631-632.
26. Camakaris J, Voskoboinik I, Mercer JF. Molecular mechanisms of copper homeostasis. *Biochem Biophys Res Commun.* 1999;261:225-232.
27. Cantilena LR Jr, Klaassen CD. The effect of chelating agents on the excretion of endogenous metals. *Toxicol Appl Pharmacol.* 1982;63:344-350.
28. Chauhan A, Chauhan V, Brown WT, Cohen I. Oxidative stress in autism: increased lipid peroxidation and reduced serum levels of ceruloplasmin and transferrin—the antioxidant proteins. *Life Sci.* 2004;75:2539-2549.
29. Chiu A, Tsoi NS, Fan ST. Use of the molecular adsorbents recirculating system as a treatment for acute decompensated Wilson disease. *Liver Transpl.* 2008;14:1512-1516.
30. Chugh KS, Sharma BK, Singhal PC, Das KC, Datta BN. Acute renal failure following copper sulphate intoxication. *Postgrad Med J.* 1977;53:18-23.
31. Chugh KS, Singhal PC, Sharma BK. Methemoglobinemia in acute copper sulfate poisoning [letter]. *Ann Intern Med.* 1975;82:226-227.
32. Chugh KS, Singhal PC, Sharma BK, et al. Acute renal failure due to intravascular hemolysis in the North Indian patients. *Am J Med Sci.* 1977;274:139-146.
33. Chuttani HK, Gupta PS, Gulati S, Gupta DN. Acute copper sulfate poisoning. *Am J Med.* 1965;39:849-854.
34. Cockell KA, Bertinato J, L'Abbe MR. Regulatory frameworks for copper considering chronic exposures of the population. *Am J Clin Nutr.* 2008;88 (suppl):863S-866S.
35. Collins KL, Roberts EA, Adeli K, Bohn D, Harvey EA. Single pass albumin dialysis (SPAD) in fulminant Wilsonian liver failure: a case report. *Pediatr Nephrol.* 2008;23:1013-1016.
36. De Paris P, Caroldi S. In vivo inhibition of serum dopamine-beta-hydroxylase by CaNa2 EDTA injection. *Hum Exp Toxicol.* 1994;13:253-256.
37. Dietrich AM, Glindemann D, Pizarro F, et al. Health and aesthetic impacts of copper corrosion on drinking water. *Water Sci Technol.* 2004;49:55-62.
38. Donoso A, Cruces P, Camacho J, Rios JC, Paris E, Mieres JJ. Acute respiratory distress syndrome resulting from inhalation of powdered copper. *Clin Toxicol (Phila).* 2007;45:714-716.
39. Doraiswamy PM, Finefrock AE. Metals in our minds: therapeutic implications for neurodegenerative disorders. *Lancet Neurol.* 2004;3:431-434.
40. Eastwood JB, Phillips ME, Minty P, Gower PE, Curtis JR. Heparin inactivation, acidosis and copper poisoning due to presumed acid contamination of water in a hemodialysis unit. *Clin Nephrol.* 1983;20:197-201.
41. Eife R, Weiss M, Muller-Hocker M, et al. Chronic poisoning by copper in tap water: II. Copper intoxications with predominantly systemic symptoms. *Eur J Med Res.* 1999;4:224-228.
42. Ercal N, Gurer-Orhan H, Aykin-Burns N. Toxic metals and oxidative stress part I: mechanisms involved in metal-induced oxidative damage. *Curr Top Med Chem.* 2001;1:529-539.
43. Ervin RB, Wang CY, Wright JD, Kennedy-Stephenson J. Dietary intake of selected minerals for the United States population: 1999–2000. *Adv Data.* 2004;(341):1-5.
44. Fairbanks VF. Copper sulfate-induced hemolytic anemia. Inhibition of glucose-6-phosphate dehydrogenase and other possible etiologic mechanisms. *Arch Intern Med.* 1967;120:428-432.
45. Florianczyk B. Copper in the organism—transport and storage in the cells. *Ann Univ Mariae Curie Sklodowska [Med].* 2003;58:85-88.
46. Franchitto N, Gandia-Mailly P, Georges B, et al. Acute copper sulphate poisoning: a case report and literature review. *Resuscitation.* 2008;78:92-96.
47. Gaetke LM, Chow CK. Copper toxicity, oxidative stress, and antioxidant nutrients. *Toxicology.* 2003;189:147-163.
48. Geissler I, Heinemann K, Rohm S, Hauss J, Lamesch P. Liver transplantation for hepatic and neurological Wilson's disease. *Transplant Proc.* 2003;35:1445-1446.
49. Giuliodori MJ, Ramirez CE, Ayala M. Acute copper intoxication after a Cu-Ca EDTA injection in rats. *Toxicology.* 1997;124:173-177.
50. Goodman VL, Brewer GJ, Merajver SD. Copper deficiency as an anticancer strategy. *Endocr Relat Cancer.* 2004;11:255-263.
51. Gooneratne SR, Christensen DA. Effect of chelating agents on the excretion of copper, zinc and iron in the bile and urine of sheep. *Vet J.* 1997;153:171-178.
52. Gu M, Cooper JM, Butler P, et al. Oxidative-phosphorylation defects in liver of patients with Wilson's disease. *Lancet.* 2000;356:469-474.
53. Gulliver JM. A fatal copper sulfate poisoning. *J Anal Toxicol.* 1991;15: 341-342.
54. Gunay N, Yildirim C, Karcioglu O, et al. A series of patients in the emergency department diagnosed with copper poisoning: recognition equals treatment. *Tohoku J Exp Med.* 2006;209:243-248.
55. Gupte A, Mumper RJ. Copper chelation by D-penicillamine generates reactive oxygen species that are cytotoxic to human leukemia and breast cancer cells. *Free Radic Biol Med.* 2007;43:1271-1278.
56. Haggerty RJ, Harris GB. Toxic hazards; bronze-powder inhalation. *N Engl J Med.* 1957;256:40-41.
57. Hamlyn AN, Gollan JL, Douglas AP, Sherlock S. Fulminant Wilson's disease with haemolysis and renal failure: copper studies and assessment of dialysis regimens. *Br Med J.* 1977;2:660-662.
58. Hantson P, Lievens M, Mahieu P. Accidental ingestion of a zinc and copper sulfate preparation. *J Toxicol Clin Toxicol.* 1996;34:725-730.
59. Harris ED. A requirement for copper in angiogenesis. *Nutr Rev.* 2004;62:60-64.
60. Harvey LJ, Dainty JR, Beattie JH, et al. Copper absorption from foods labelled intrinsically and extrinsically with Cu-65 stable isotope. *Eur J Clin Nutr.* 2005;59:363-368.

61. Herbst D. Detection of penicillin G and ampicillin as contaminants in tetracyclines and penicillamine. *J Pharm Sci.* 1977;66:1646-1648.
62. Hinks LJ, Clayton BE, Lloyd RS. Zinc and copper concentrations in leucocytes and erythrocytes in healthy adults and the effect of oral contraceptives. *J Clin Pathol.* 1983;36:1016-1021.
63. Holtzman NA, Elliott DA, Heller RH. Copper intoxication. Report of a case with observations on ceruloplasmin. *N Engl J Med.* 1966;275:347-352.
64. Hostynek JJ, Maibach HI. Copper hypersensitivity: dermatologic aspects. *Dermatol Ther.* 2004;17:328-333.
65. Hoveyda N, Yates B, Bond CR, Hunter PR. A cluster of cases of abdominal pain possibly associated with high copper levels in a private water supply. *J Environ Health.* 2003;66:29-32.
66. Jantsch W, Kulig K, Rumack BH. Massive copper sulfate ingestion resulting in hepatotoxicity. *J Toxicol Clin Toxicol.* 1984;22:585-588.
67. Jones MM, Basinger MA, Tarka MP. The relative effectiveness of some chelating agents in acute copper intoxication in the mouse. *Res Commun Chem Pathol Pharmacol.* 1980;27:571-577.
68. Juhlin L, Ahlstedt S, Andal L, Ekstrom B, Svard PO, Wide L. Antibody reactivity in penicillin-sensitive patients determined with different penicillin derivatives. *Int Arch Allergy Appl Immunol.* 1977;54:19-28.
69. Kadiiska MB, Mason RP. In vivo copper-mediated free radical production: an ESR spin-trapping study. *Spectrochim Acta A Mol Biomol Spectrosc.* 2002;58:1227-1239.
70. Karlsson B, Noren L. Ipecacuanha and copper sulphate as emetics in intoxications in children. *Acta Paediatr Scand.* 1965;54:331-335.
71. Kiss JE, Berman D, Van Thiel D. Effective removal of copper by plasma exchange in fulminant Wilson's disease. *Transfusion.* 1998;38:327-331.
72. Klein D, Lichtmannegger J, Heinzmann U, Summer KH. Dissolution of copper-rich granules in hepatic lysosomes by D-penicillamine prevents the development of fulminant hepatitis in Long-Evans cinnamon rats. *J Hepatol.* 2000;32:193-201.
73. Kreymann B, Seige M, Schweigart U, Kopp KF, Classen M. Albumin dialysis: effective removal of copper in a patient with fulminant Wilson disease and successful bridging to liver transplantation: a new possibility for the elimination of protein-bound toxins. *J Hepatol.* 1999;31:1080-1085.
74. Kumar KS, Rowse C, Hochstein P. Copper-induced generation of superoxide in human red cell membrane. *Biochem Biophys Res Commun.* 1978;83:587-592.
75. Kuno T, Hitomi T, Zaitu M, Sato T, Yoshida N, Miyazaki S. Severely decompensated abdominal Wilson disease treated with peritoneal dialysis: a case report. *Acta Paediatr Jpn.* 1998;40:85-87.
76. Kurisaki E, Kuroda Y, Sato M. Copper-binding protein in acute copper poisoning. *Forensic Sci Int.* 1988;38:3-11.
77. Lang TF, Glynne-Jones R, Blake S, Taylor A, Kay JD. Iatrogenic copper deficiency following information and drugs obtained over the Internet. *Ann Clin Biochem.* 2004;41:417-420.
78. Liu J, Kashimura S, Hara K, Zhang G. Death following cupric sulfate emesis. *J Toxicol Clin Toxicol.* 2001;39:161-163.
79. Liu Z, Chen B. Copper treatment alters the barrier functions of human intestinal Caco-2 cells: involving tight junctions and P-glycoprotein. *Hum Exp Toxicol.* 2004;23:369-377.
80. Lubin JH, Pottern LM, Stone BJ, Fraumeni JF Jr. Respiratory cancer in a cohort of copper smelter workers: results from more than 50 years of follow-up. *Am J Epidemiol.* 2000;151:554-565.
81. Mak CM, Lam CW. Diagnosis of Wilson's disease: a comprehensive review. *Crit Rev Clin Lab Sci.* 2008;45:263-290.
82. Manzler AD, Schreiner AW. Copper-induced acute hemolytic anemia. A new complication of hemodialysis. *Ann Intern Med.* 1970;73:409-412.
83. Meng Y, Miyoshi I, Hirabayashi M, et al. Restoration of copper metabolism and rescue of hepatic abnormalities in LEC rats, an animal model of Wilson disease, by expression of human ATP7B gene. *Biochim Biophys Acta.* 2004;1690:208-219.
84. Metz EN, Sagone AL Jr. The effect of copper on the erythrocyte hexose monophosphate shunt pathway. *J Lab Clin Med.* 1972;80:405-413.
85. Milne L, Nicotera P, Orrenius S, Burkitt MJ. Effects of glutathione and chelating agents on copper-mediated DNA oxidation: pro-oxidant and antioxidant properties of glutathione. *Arch Biochem Biophys.* 1993;304:102-109.
86. Mital VP, Wahal PK, Bansal OP. Study of erythrocytic glutathione in acute copper sulphate poisoning. *Ind J Pathol Bacteriol.* 1966;9:155-162.
87. Mitchell WM, Basinger MA, Jones MM. Antagonism of acute copper(II)-induced renal lesions by sodium 2,3-dimercaptopropanesulfonate. *Johns Hopkins Med J.* 1982;151:283-285.
88. Mucklow ES. Chemistry set poisoning. *Int J Clin Pract.* 1997;51:321-323.
89. Nagaraj MV, Rao PV, Susarala S. Copper sulphate poisoning, hemolysis and methaemoglobinemia. *J Assoc Phys. Ind.* 1985;33:308-309.
90. Nakatani T, Spolter L, Kobayashi K. Redox state in liver mitochondria in acute copper sulfate poisoning. *Life Sci.* 1994;54:967-974.
91. Nations SP, Boyer PJ, Love LA, et al. Denture cream: an unusual source of excess zinc, leading to hypocupremia and neurologic disease. *Neurology.* 2008;71:639-643.
92. Oder W, Prayer L, Grimm G, et al. Wilson's disease: evidence of subgroups derived from clinical findings and brain lesions. *Neurology.* 1993;43:120-124.
93. O'Donohue J, Reid M, Varghese A, Portmann B, Williams R. A case of adult chronic copper self-intoxication resulting in cirrhosis. *Eur J Med Res.* 1999;4:252.
94. Oldenquist G, Salem M. Parenteral copper sulfate poisoning causing acute renal failure. *Nephrol Dial Transplant.* 1999;14:441-443.
95. Oon S, Yap CH, Ihle BU. Acute copper toxicity following copper glycinate injection. *Intern Med J.* 2006;36:741-743.
96. Ortolani EL, Antonelli AC, de Souza Sarkis JE. Acute sheep poisoning from a copper sulfate footbath. *Vet Hum Toxicol.* 2004;46:315-318.
97. Pimentel JC, Marques F. "Vineyard sprayer's lung": a new occupational disease. *Thorax.* 1969;24:678-688.
98. Pimentel JC, Menezes AP. Liver disease in vineyard sprayers. *Gastroenterology.* 1977;72:275-283.
99. Pinter R, Hogge WA, McPherson E. Infant with severe penicillamine embryopathy born to a woman with Wilson disease. *Am J Med Genet A.* 2004;128A:294-298.
100. Pizarro F, Olivares M, Uauy R, Contreras P, Rebelo A, Gidi V. Acute gastrointestinal effects of graded levels of copper in drinking water. *Environ Health Perspect.* 1999;107:117-121.
101. Prociv P. Algal toxins or copper poisoning—revisiting the Palm Island "epidemic." *Med J Aust.* 2004;181:344.
102. Prohaska JR, Gybina AA. Intracellular copper transport in mammals. *J Nutr.* 2004;134:1003-1006.
103. Rebhandl W, Milassin A, Brunner L, et al. In vitro study of ingested coins: leave them or retrieve them? *J Pediatr Surg.* 2007;42:1729-1734.
104. Safaei R, Holzer AK, Katano K, Samimi G, Howell SB. The role of copper transporters in the development of resistance to Pt drugs. *J Inorg Biochem.* 2004;98:1607-1613.
105. Sagripanti JL, Goering PL, Lamanna A. Interaction of copper with DNA and antagonism by other metals. *Toxicol Appl Pharmacol.* 1991;110:477-485.
106. Salhany JM, Swanson JC, Cordes KA, Gaines SB, Gaines KC. Evidence suggesting direct oxidation of human erythrocyte membrane sulfhydryls by copper. *Biochem Biophys Res Commun.* 1978;82:1294-1299.
107. Salmon MA, Wright T. Chronic copper poisoning presenting as pink disease. *Arch Dis Child.* 1971;46:108-110.
108. Sansinanea AS, Cerone SI, Elperding A, Auza N. Glucose-6-phosphate dehydrogenase activity in erythrocytes from chronically copper-poisoned sheep. *Comp Biochem Physiol C Pharmacol Toxicol Endocrinol.*1996;114:197-200.
109. Sata F, Araki S, Murata K, Aono H. Behavior of heavy metals in human urine and blood following calcium disodium ethylenediamine tetraacetate injection: observations in metal workers. *J Toxicol Environ Health A.* 1998;54:167-178.
110. Scheinberg IH, Sternlieb I. Is non-Indian childhood cirrhosis caused by excess dietary copper? *Lancet.* 1994;344:1002-1004.
111. Schramel P, Muller-Hocker J, Meyer U, Weiss M, Eife R. Nutritional copper intoxication in three German infants with severe liver cell damage (features of Indian childhood cirrhosis). *J Trace Elem Electrolytes Health Dis.* 1988;2:85-89.
112. Schwartz E, Schmidt E. Refractory shock secondary to copper sulfate ingestion. *Ann Emerg Med.* 1986;15:952-954.
113. Sethi S, Grover S, Khodaskar MB. Role of copper in Indian childhood cirrhosis. *Ann Trop Paediatr.* 1993;13:3-5.
114. Singh MM, Singh G. Biochemical changes in blood in cases of acute copper sulphate poisoning. *J Ind Med Assoc.* 1968;50:549-554.
115. Sokol RJ, Devereaux MW, O'Brien K, Khandwala RA, Loehr JP. Abnormal hepatic mitochondrial respiration and cytochrome C oxidase activity in rats with long-term copper overload. *Gastroenterology.* 1993;105:178-187.
116. Sokol RJ, Devereaux M, Mierau GW, Hambidge KM, Shikes RH. Oxidant injury to hepatic mitochondrial lipids in rats with dietary copper overload. Modification by vitamin E deficiency. *Gastroenterology.* 1990;99:1061-1071.
117. Sontz E, Schwieger J. The "green water" syndrome: copper-induced hemolysis and subsequent acute renal failure as consequence of a religious ritual. *Am J Med.* 1995;98:311-315.

118. Stein RS, Jenkins D, Korns ME. Death after use of cupric sulfate as emetic [letter]. *JAMA*. 1976;235:801.
119. Stuerenburg HJ. CSF copper concentrations, blood-brain barrier function, and coeruloplasmin synthesis during the treatment of Wilson's disease. *J Neural Transm*. 2000;107:321-329.
120. Takeda T, Yukioka T, Shimazaki S. Cupric sulfate intoxication with rhabdomyolysis, treated with chelating agents and blood purification. *Intern Med*. 2000;39:253-255.
121. Thomas DJ, Chisolm J Jr. Lead, zinc and copper decorporation during calcium disodium ethylenediamine tetraacetate treatment of lead-poisoned children. *J Pharmacol Exp Ther*. 1986;239:829-835.
122. Torres-Alanis O, Garza-Ocanas L, Bernal MA, Pineyro-Lopez A. Urinary excretion of trace elements in humans after sodium 2,3-dimercaptopropane-1-sulfonate challenge test. *J Toxicol Clin Toxicol*. 2000;38:697-700.
123. Turnlund JR, Scott KC, Peiffer GL, et al. Copper status of young men consuming a low-copper diet. *Am J Clin Nutr*. 1997;65:72-78.
124. Wahal PK, Mehrotra MP, Kishore B, et al. Study of whole blood, red cell and plasma copper levels in acute copper sulphate poisoning and their relationship with complications and prognosis. *J Assoc Phys Ind*. 1976;24:153-158.
125. Walker WR, Keats DM. An investigation of the therapeutic value of the 'copper bracelet'-dermal assimilation of copper in arthritic/rheumatoid conditions. *Agents Actions*. 1976;6:454-459.
126. Walsh FM, Crosson FJ, Bayley M, McReynolds J, Pearson BJ. Acute copper intoxication. Pathophysiology and therapy with a case report. *Am J Dis Child*. 1977;131:149-151.
127. Witherell LE, Watson WN, Giguere GC. Outbreak of acute copper poisoning due to soft drink dispenser. *Am J Public Health*. 1980;70:1115.
128. Yamamoto H, Hirose K, Hayasaki Y, Masuda M, Kazusaka A, Fujita S. Mechanism of enhanced lipid peroxidation in the liver of Long-Evans cinnamon (LEC) rats. *Arch Toxicol*. 1999;73:457-464.
129. Yang CC, Wu ML, Deng JF. Prolonged hemolysis and methemoglobinemia following organic copper fungicide ingestion. *Vet Hum Toxicol*. 2004;46:321-323.
130. Yelin G, Taff ML, Sadowski GE. Copper toxicity following massive ingestion of coins. *Am J Forensic Med Pathol*. 1987;8:78-85.
131. Zecca L, Stroppolo A, Gatti A, et al. The role of iron and copper molecules in the neuronal vulnerability of locus coeruleus and substantia nigra during aging. *Proc Natl Acad Sci U S A*. 2004;101:9843-9848.

CHAPTER 94
LEAD

Fred M. Henretig

Lead (Pb)		
Atomic number	=	82
Atomic weight	=	207 daltons
Normal concentration		
Whole blood	<	10 µg/dL (<0.48 mmol/L)

Lead is a ubiquitous element in the earth's crust that has long been used by humans for a variety of purposes. Lead poisoning, or plumbism, has an equally long history, dating back to antiquity. Today, lead poisoning is primarily an important environmental health problem for young children exposed to deteriorated lead paint and an occupational illness of adults exposed via the workplace. There is no known physiologic role for lead, and thus any lead presence in human tissue represents toxic contamination.

PHYSICAL PROPERTIES

Lead is a silvery-gray, soft metal, with an atomic weight of 207.21 daltons and an atomic number of 82 Daltons. It has a low melting point, 621.3°F (327.4°C), and boils at 2948°F (1620°C) at atmospheric pressure.[159] It occurs principally as two isotopes, ^{206}Pb and ^{208}Pb. Metallic lead is relatively insoluble in water and dilute acids, but dissolves in nitric, acetic, and hot, concentrated sulfuric acids. In compounds, lead assumes valence states of +2 and +4. Inorganic lead compounds may be brightly colored and vary widely in water solubility; several are used extensively as pigments in paints such as lead chromate (yellow) and lead oxide (red). Lead also forms organic compounds, of which two, tetramethyl and tetraethyl lead (TEL), were used commercially as gasoline additives.[74] These are essentially insoluble in water but readily soluble in organic solvents.[135] Lead complexes with ligands containing sulfur, oxygen, or nitrogen as electron donors. It thus forms stable complexes with several ligands common to biologic molecules, including –OH, –SH, and $-NH_2$. Complexes with sulfhydryl (–SH) groups are thought to be of most toxicologic importance.

HISTORY AND EPIDEMIOLOGY

INDUSTRIAL APPLICATIONS

Lead's low melting point and high malleability made it one of the first metals smelted and used by humans. Ancient Egyptians and Hebrews used lead, and the Phoenicians established lead mines in Spain circa 2000 B.C. The Greeks and Romans released lead during the process of extracting silver from ore. Roman society found many uses for lead, including pipes, cooking utensils, and ceramic glazes, and a common practice was to use sapa, a grape syrup simmered down in lead vessels, as a sweetener and preservative.[109] Postindustrial lead use increased dramatically, and today lead is the most widely used nonferrous metal, with global extraction on the order of 9 million tons annually.[74] Lead is used widely for its waterproofing and electrical- and radiation-shielding properties. Use of both lead-based paint for house paint and leaded gasoline has been essentially eliminated by regulation in the United States since the 1980s, but is still a concern in many nations, and persistence of lead paint in older U.S. homes still constitutes an enormous environmental challenge.[3]

HISTORY OF LEAD-RELATED HEALTH EFFECTS

Dioscorides, a Greek physician in the 2nd century B.C., observed adverse cognitive effects, and Pliny cautioned the Romans of the danger of inhaled fumes from lead smelting.[105] Modern authors have suggested that extensive use of sapa in Roman aristocratic society contributed to the downfall of Roman dominance.[109] Lead poisoning was also recognized in American colonial times. Benjamin Franklin observed in 1763 the "dry gripes" (abdominal colic) and "dangles" (wristdrop) that afflicted tinkers, painters, and typesetters, as well as the "gripes" caused by rum distillation in leaden condensing coils.[96] Lead salts, particularly lead acetate (sugar of lead), were used medicinally in the early 19th century for control of bleeding and diarrhea. With the 19th-century Industrial Revolution, lead poisoning became a common occupational disease. The reproductive effects of lead poisoning were also noted by the turn of the 20th century, including the high rate of stillbirths, infertility, and abortions among women in the pottery industry or who were married to pottery workers.

The modern history of childhood plumbism can be traced to the recognition of lead-paint poisoning in Brisbane, Australia, in 1897.[105] Lead poisoning was reported in American children in 1917, and by 1943, it was established that children who recovered from clinical plumbism were frequently left with neurologic sequelae and intellectual impairment. Symptomatic childhood lead poisoning was a frequent occurrence in American pediatric medical centers throughout the 1950s and 1960s, a period during which research established effective chelation therapy protocols with British anti-Lewisite (BAL) and edetate calcium disodium ($CaNa_2EDTA$).[33] From the 1970s to the present, the research thrust in childhood lead poisoning has centered on the recognition and quantification of more subtle neurocognitive impairment caused by subclinical lead poisoning.[16,106] Over this time period, the Centers for Disease Control and Prevention (CDC) has steadily revised downward the definitions of a normal blood lead concentration (BLL) in children. The CDC definition of lead poisoning was 60 µg/dL in the early 1960s, but the current action concentration is 10 µg/dL.[22] Furthermore, considerable research in recent years has strongly suggested adverse cognitive effects in young children at BLLs below 10 µg/dL.[21]

SOURCES OF HUMAN EXPOSURE

Numerous sources of lead exposure exist and can be generally classified as environmental, occupational, or additional (somewhat "exotic") sources. *Environmental* exposures affect the entire population, particularly young children. These occur primarily by exposure to some form of lead paint derivative in most cases of childhood lead poisoning in the United States (Table 94–1). Because of its continuing, major impact in the United States today, lead paint exposure is further detailed here.

Lead pigments (typically lead carbonate) account for 50% by weight of many white house paints from the pre–World War II era. Since 1978, paint intended for interior or exterior residential surfaces, toys, or furniture in the United States may contain, by law, no more than 0.06% lead. However, an estimated 3 million tons of lead remain in 57 million U.S. homes built before 1980 and painted with lead-based paint. This aging housing stock has created an enormous environmental hazard of lead exposure to children and to adult homeowners, house painters, and construction workers who become involved in sanding, scraping, and restoration of painted surfaces in these homes. Furthermore, lead-based paint is still allowed for industrial; military; marine; and some outdoor uses, such as structural components of

TABLE 94–1. Environmental Lead Sources

Source	Comment
Paint	Especially pre-1978 homes
Dust	House dust from deteriorated lead paint
Soil	From yards contaminated by deteriorated lead paint, lead industry emissions, roadways with high leaded gasoline usage
Water	Leached from leaded plumbing (pipes, solder), cooking utensils, water coolers
Air	Leaded gasoline (pre-1976 United States; still prevalent worldwide), industrial emissions
Food	Lead solder in cans (pre-1991 United States; still prevalent in imported canned foods); "natural" dietary supplements; "moonshine" whiskey and lead foil–covered wines; contaminated flour, paprika, other imported foods and candy; lead leached from leaded crystal, ceramics, vinyl lunchboxes

bridges and highways; occasionally, some of this paint is inadvertently used in homes.[22] Attempts to abate lead-painted outdoor structures can pollute entire communities.[79]

Although paint-derived lead exposure may result from pica in some children, most lead paint exposure in childhood relates to the crumbling, peeling, flaking, or chalking of aging paint.[22] These fine paint particles are incorporated into household dust and yard soil, where ordinary childhood hand–mouth activity results in ingestion.[28] Seasonal variations in house dust contamination occur, with higher house dust lead levels and increased BLLs in exposed preschool children noted during the summer.

Adults with *occupational* exposures to lead constitute another large group of persons at risk. It is estimated that more than 1 million workers in the United States, employed in more than 100 occupations, are exposed to lead.[130] The most important route of absorption in occupational settings is inhalation of lead dust and fumes. In addition, workers may eat, drink, or smoke in lead-dust–contaminated areas, resulting in some ingestion. (Cigarettes use may provide a source of oral exposure.) However, the presence of lead in the workplace, per se, does not imply a significant risk of poisoning. The risk is correlated with several factors that contribute to the occurrence of respirable lead fumes or dust particles in the worksite atmosphere.[135] There are three general categories of such factors. The first relates to the degree of hazard inherent in the work process itself, including high temperatures; significant aerosol, dust, or fume production; and a less-mechanized workplace (with resulting greater "hands-on" employee exposure). Second, the adequacy of dust elimination, such as local and general ventilation, is critical. The third category is that of worksite and personal hygiene, including proper use of protective clothes and equipment, and thorough housekeeping. For example, lead smelting can be categorized as primary (from raw ore) and secondary (reclamation, such as from used car batteries). Secondary lead production workers may be at higher risk of poisoning because this job more typically involves small, sometimes "backyard" operations that are less likely to adhere to industry safety regulations than large, well-regulated primary smelters.[39] Despite the risk factors that may be specific to each worksite, some types of lead-related work are more hazardous than others. This ranking is based on actual surveys of BLLs and reported incidence of clinical poisoning (Table 94–2).[130,134]

For convenience, environmental and occupational or recreational lead exposures are discussed separately, although there is considerable overlap. For example, workers who fail to change lead dust–covered

TABLE 94–2. Occupational and Recreational Lead Sources

High-risk occupations
Automobile radiator repairers
Crystal glass makers
Firing range instructors, bullet salvagers
Lead smelters, refiners
Metal welders, cutters (includes bridge and highway reconstruction workers)
Painters, construction workers (sanding, scraping, or spraying of lead paint; demolition of lead-painted sites)
Polyvinyl chloride plastic manufacturers
Shipbreakers
Storage battery manufacturers, repairers, recyclers
Moderate-risk occupations
Automobile factory workers and mechanics
Enamelers
Glass blowers
Lead miners
Plumbers
Pottery glazers
Ship repairers
Shot makers
Solderers
Type founders
Varnish makers
Wire and cable workers
Possible increased-risk occupations
Electronics manufacturers
Jewelers
Pipefitters
Printers
Rubber product manufacturers
Traffic police officers, taxi drivers, garage workers, turnpike tollbooth operators, gas station attendants (exposed to leaded gasoline exhaust fumes; unlikely now in the United States but still a hazard in developing countries)
Recreational and hobby sources
Ceramic crafts
Furniture refinishing, restoring
Home remodeling, refinishing
Painting (fine artist's pigments)
Repair of automobiles, boats
Stained glass making
Target shooting, recasting lead for bullets
Additional sources
Complementary and alternative remedies; cosmetics; ingested lead foreign bodies and retained lead bullets; illicit substance abuse (heroin, methamphetamine, leaded gasoline "huffing"); burning batteries, leaded paper, or wood for fuel; use of lead-glazed ceramics; hand–mouth contact with pool cue chalk, glazes, leaded ink; vinyl mini-blinds; children's toys and jewelry (especially imported products)

work clothes or shoes may bring this occupational lead hazard home and secondarily contaminate their children's environment.[130]

Finally, numerous *additional sources* of lead exposure are also reported, including contaminated folk medications or cosmetics[20,80] ingested lead foreign bodies,[93,97,163] and retained bullets.[46,85,139]

Some potential exposures have raised considerable community concern and media coverage in recent years, for example, the discovery of lead contamination of some artificial turfs,[23] and imported toys coated with lead paint.[86] These, too, are highlighted separately in Table 94–2.

PREVALENCE

Several recent national and regional surveys have evaluated current U.S. population-based trends in BLLs and sociodemographic correlates. The CDC estimated in 2005 that BLLs are above 9 μg/dL (representing primarily excessive household exposure) in 310,000 children ages 1 to 5 years[18] and that approximately 10,000 adults are reported each year with BLLs above 24 μg/dL (typically reflecting excessive occupational exposure).[17] Although such numbers are impressive, they represent a considerable decrease from prevalence rates done in prior decades (eg, from 8.6% of children with elevated BLLs from 1988 to 1991 to 1.4% from 1999 to 2004)[70], and it is certainly the observed clinical experience that symptomatic pediatric plumbism, in particular, is far less common than it was a generation ago. Nevertheless, for young minority children and poor people who reside in our nation's deteriorating central cities, the battle is far from won. For example, the CDC reported in 2000 that children enrolled in Medicaid had a prevalence of elevated BLLs three times greater than those not enrolled.[25] Refugee, immigrant, and foreign-born adopted children remain at particularly high risk,[19,80] and remarkable cases of extremely elevated BLLs (>100 μg/dL) may still be detected on routine screening.[38]

TOXICOLOGY

PHARMACOKINETICS

Inorganic and Metallic Lead *Absorption.* Gastrointestinal (GI) absorption is less efficient than pulmonary absorption. Adults absorb an estimated 10% to 15% of ingested lead in food, and children have a higher GI absorption rate, averaging 40% to 50%,[1,53] although in animal studies, this varies by type of lead compound studied.[8] However, it should be noted that fasting and diets deficient in iron, calcium, and zinc—factors that are frequent among groups of young children—enhance GI absorption of lead.[53,88] The role of essential trace elements in decreasing lead absorption is assumed to be a consequence of competitive absorption processes. Metallic lead is absorbed as well, although less readily than most lead compounds.[8] The rate of absorption of metallic lead appears to be related to particle size, total surface area, and GI tract location (whereas gastric acidity favors dissolution, the small bowel is likely the site of maximal absorption).[93,97,163]

The overall absorption of inhaled lead averages 30% to 40%. Of note, both minute ventilation and the concentration of lead in air determine airborne lead exposure, so a worker engaged in vigorous physical activity will absorb considerably more lead than a person in the same atmosphere at rest. Likewise, children, with relatively greater volume of inhaled air per unit of body size because of higher metabolic rates, are proportionally at greater risk in a given degree of atmospheric lead pollution. It is estimated that children have a 2.7-fold higher lung deposition rate of lead than do adults.[1]

Cutaneous absorption of inorganic lead is low; one study found an average absorption of 0.06% through intact skin.[100] Soft tissue absorption of metallic lead follows exposure to retained bullets, and by analogy to GI lead foreign bodies, also depends on particle size, total surface area, and location (multiple small shot and location in which particles are bathed by synovial, serosal, or spinal fluid favor more a rapid increase in BLL).[46,85,139]

Transplacental lead transfer is critical in fetal and neonatal lead exposure, which has been under increasing scrutiny in recent years. Lead readily crosses the placental barrier throughout gestation, and lead uptake is cumulative until birth.[121]

Distribution. Absorbed lead enters the bloodstream, where at least 99% is bound to erythrocytes.[54] From blood, lead is distributed into both a relatively labile soft tissue pool and into a more stable bone compartment. This classic three-compartment model may be somewhat of an oversimplification. Currently, at least two bone compartments are recognized: a more labile pool in trabecular bone and a more stable pool in cortical bone. In adults, approximately 95% of the body lead burden is stored in bone versus only 70% for children. The remainder is distributed to the major soft tissue lead-storage sites, including the liver, kidney, bone marrow, and brain. Lead uptake into soft tissues occurs in a complex fashion that depends on numerous factors, including blood lead concentrations, external exposure factors, and specific tissue kinetics. Most of the toxicity associated with lead is a result of soft tissue uptake, so that the relative decrease in bone storage is another comparative disadvantage for lead-poisoned children.

Lead in the central nervous system (CNS) is of particular toxicologic importance, and studies have addressed specific storage sites. Lead preferentially concentrates in gray matter and certain nuclei.[54] Fetal brain uptake is relatively higher than with postnatal exposure in animal models. The highest brain concentrations are found in the hippocampus, cerebellum, cerebral cortex, and medulla.

Unlike soft tissue storage, bone lead accumulates throughout life. Bone storage begins in utero and occurs across all ranges of exposure, so that there is no threshold for bone lead uptake.[1] Total body accumulation of lead may range from 200 to 500 mg in workers with heavy occupational exposure.[54] Bone lead is thought to be relatively metabolically inert, but it can be mobilized from the more labile compartments and contributes as much as 50% of the blood lead content. This may be of particular importance during pregnancy and lactation, in elderly persons with osteoporosis,[147] and in children with immobilization.[94] Lead also accumulates in the teeth, particularly the dentine of children's teeth, a phenomenon that has been used to quantify cumulative lead exposure in young children.[106]

Excretion. Absorbed lead that is not retained is primarily excreted in urine (approximately 65%) and bile (approximately 35%).[1] A miniscule amount is lost via sweat, hair, and nails. Children excrete less of their daily uptake than adults, with an average retention of 33% versus 1% to 4%, respectively.[173] Biologic half-lives for lead are estimated as follows[1,90,122]: blood (adults, short-term experiments), 25 days; blood (children, natural exposure), 10 months; soft tissues (adults, short-term exposure), 40 days; bone (labile, trabecular pool), 90 days; and bone (cortical, stable pool), 10 to 20 years. Trace amounts of lead are also excreted in breast milk.[9]

Organic Lead Alkyl lead compounds are lipid soluble and have unique pharmacokinetics that are less well characterized than those of inorganic lead.[10] Animal studies and human clinical experience with acute ingestions and leaded gasoline sniffing demonstrate TEL absorption through ingestion, inhalation, and intact skin and subsequent distribution to lipophilic tissues, including the brain.[135,155,171] TEL is metabolized to triethyl lead, which is believed to be the major toxic compound. Alkyl leads may slowly release lead as the inorganic form, with subsequent kinetics as noted above.[10]

PATHOPHYSIOLOGY

GENERAL MECHANISMS

Similar to many metals, lead is a complex xenobiotic exerting numerous pathophysiologic effects in many organ systems.[54] Furthermore, genetic polymorphism may impact on individual susceptibility to lead.[110] Recently identified examples of such include the genes for apolipoprotein E, the vitamin D receptor, Na^+, K^+-ATPase, delta-aminolevulinic acid, and protein kinase C.[137] At the biomolecular level, lead functions in three general ways. First, its affinity for biologic electron-donor ligands, especially sulfhydryl groups, allows it to bind and impact numerous enzymatic, receptor, and structural proteins. Second, lead is chemically similar to the divalent cations calcium and zinc and interferes with numerous calcium- (and perhaps zinc-) mediated metabolic pathways, particularly in mitochondria and in second-messenger systems regulating cellular energy metabolism.[81] Lead-induced mitochondrial injury may result in apoptosis, a phenomenon particularly well studied in animal models of retinal cells.[81] Lead may function as an inhibitor or agonist of calcium-dependent processes. For example, lead inhibits neuronal voltage-sensitive calcium channels[8] and membrane-bound Na^+-K^+-ATPase (adenosine triphosphatase)[149] but activates calcium-dependent protein kinase C.[92] These effects adversely impact neurotransmitter function.[167] Third, lead exhibits mutagenic and mitogenic effects in mammalian cells in vitro and is carcinogenic in rats and mice.[42] There is mechanistic plausibility and some epidemiologic evidence for at least a facilitative role of lead in human carcinogenesis.[146]

NEUROTOXICITY

Lead's neurotoxicity involves several basic mechanisms, including apoptosis, excitotoxicity, adverse influence on neurotransmitter and second-messenger function, mitochondrial injury, cerebrovascular endothelial damage, neural cell adhesion molecule dysfunction, and impaired development and function of both oligodendroglia and astroglia, although particularly the former, with resultant abnormal myelin formation.[81,123,167] Lead-induced dysfunction is reported for several neurotransmitter systems and is linked to lead's calcium-mimetic properties. Lead blocks calcium influx through voltage-sensitive calcium channels, inhibiting evoked release of acetylcholine, dopamine, and amino acid neurotransmitters, but enhances spontaneous release.[35,54,81,167] This results in a decreased "signal to noise" ratio.[51] These effects are particularly important during early childhood, a period marked by rapid growth in brain synaptic connections followed by their "pruning." Because synapse persistence is likely modulated by motor and sensory stimulation, lead's adverse impact on neurotransmitter and synaptic function is believed to impair synaptic pruning, with resulting suboptimal cortical microarchitecture and function.[51] The hippocampus, an important locus of learning and memory, is believed to be a major site for this disturbance.[167] Lead also interferes with the 78-kDa chaperone glucose-regulated protein (GRP78) in astrocytes, which may result in adverse protein conformational effects that are thought to be associated with conditions such as Alzheimer's disease.[167] In severe cases, pathologic changes in cerebral microvasculature may result in cerebral edema and increased intracranial pressure, which are associated with the clinical syndrome of acute lead encephalopathy (Fig. 94–1). Peripheral neuropathy is a classic effect of lead poisoning in adults. The neuropathology in humans is poorly characterized. In animal models, it is associated with Schwann cell destruction, segmental demyelination, and axonal degeneration.[54] Sensory nerves are less affected than motor nerves.

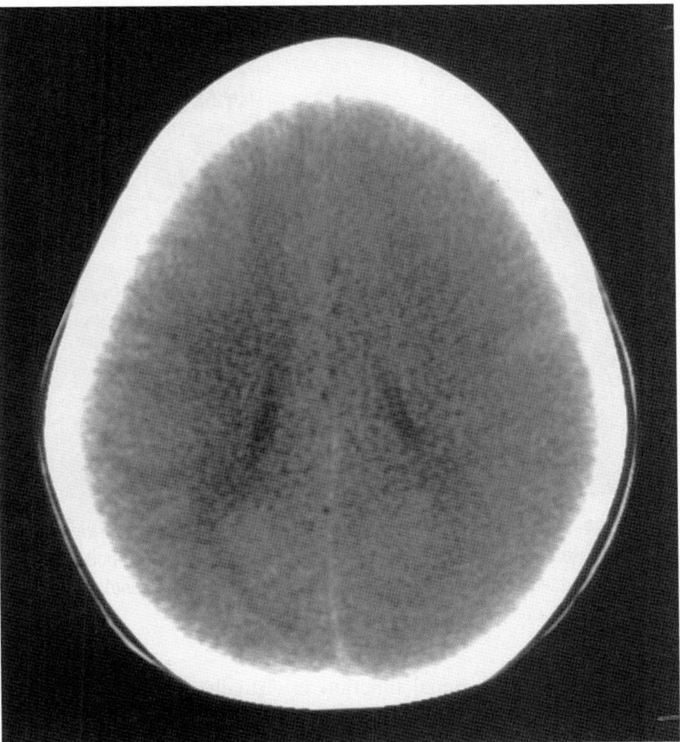

FIGURE 94–1. Computed tomography scan of the brain reveals diffuse cerebral edema and loss of gray-white matter differentiation on day 1 of hospitalization of a 3-year-old boy. He had presented with a brief prodrome of vomiting and altered mental status followed by status epilepticus, characteristic of acute lead encephalopathy. His blood lead concentration was 220 μg/dL. *(Image contributed by Department of Radiology, St. Christopher's Hospital for Children, Philadelphia, PA.)*

HEMATOLOGIC

Lead is hematotoxic in several ways, including via potent inhibition of several enzymes in the heme biosynthetic pathway (see Chap. 24 and Fig. 24–3). It also induces a defect in erythropoietin function secondary to associated renal damage.[59,129] A shortened erythrocyte life span is believed to be caused by increased membrane fragility. Inhibition of Na^+-K^+-ATPase and pyrimidine-5'-nucleotidase may impair erythrocyte membrane stability by altering energy metabolism. The inhibition of pyrimidine-5'-nucleotidase is also thought to underlie the appearance of basophilic stippling in erythrocytes, representing clumping of degraded RNA, which is normally eliminated by this enzyme.[111] (See Fig. 94–2.)

RENAL

Functional changes associated with acute lead nephropathy include decreased energy-dependent transport, resulting in a Fanconilike syndrome of aminoaciduria, glycosuria, and phosphaturia. These changes are related to disturbed mitochondrial respiration and phosphorylation and are reversible with discontinuation of exposure or treatment.[56] A pathologic finding is characteristic nuclear inclusion bodies in renal tubular cells composed of lead–protein complex. Chronic high-dose exposure may be associated with progressive interstitial fibrosis.[78] Lead is a renal carcinogen in rodent models, but its status in humans is uncertain.[42,54]

The association of plumbism with gout ("saturnine gout") was noted more than 100 years ago. Lead decreases renal uric acid excretion, with resulting elevated blood urate concentrations and urate crystal

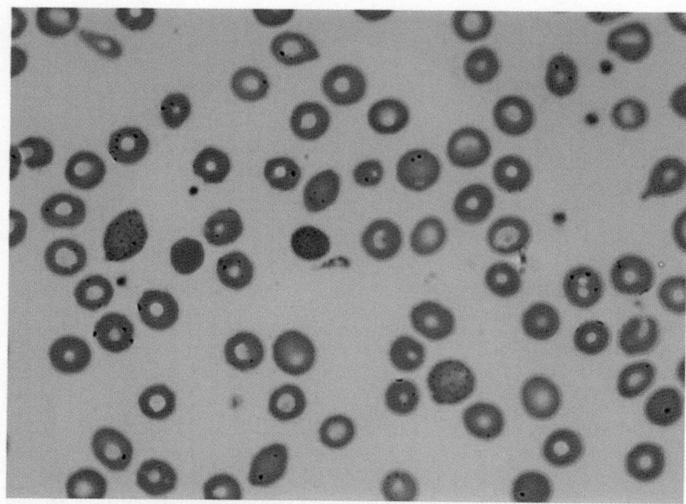

FIGURE 94–2. This peripheral smear of blood examined under high-power microscopy demonstrates the classic basophilic stippling associated with lead poisoning. The patient's blood lead concentration was over 100 mcg/dL. *(Image contributed by the New York City Poison Center Toxicology Fellowship Program).*

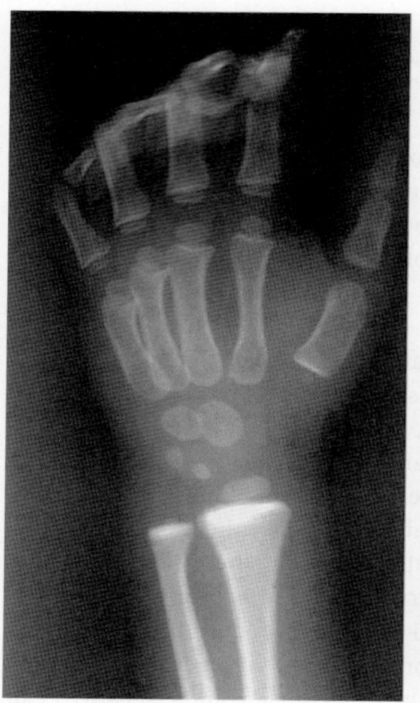

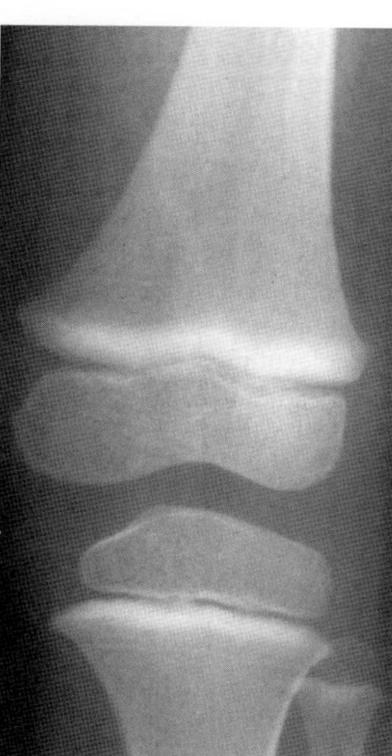

FIGURE 94–3. (**A**) Radiograph of the wrist reveals increased bands of calcification ("lead lines") in the same patient as in Figure 94-1. (**B**) Similar radiographic findings in another patient at the knee. *(Part A contributed by Department of Radiology, St. Christopher's Hospital for Children, Philadelphia, PA. Part B contributed by Richard Markowitz, MD, Department of Radiology, Children's Hospital of Philadelphia, Philadelphia, PA.)*

deposition in joints. Renal function is virtually always impaired in patients with gout.

CARDIOVASCULAR

The most important manifestation of lead toxicity on the cardiovascular system is hypertension. This is likely caused by altered calcium-activated changes in contractility of vascular smooth muscle cells secondary to decreased Na^+-K^+-ATPase activity and stimulation of the Na^+-Ca^{2+} exchange pump. Lead may also affect vessels by altering neuroendocrine input or sensitivity to such stimuli or by increasing reactive oxygen species that enhance nitric oxide inactivation.[84] Elevated plasma renin activity is found after periods of modest exposure, although activity may decrease to normal or lower in chronic severe exposure.[164] Rarely, direct cardiotoxicity is reported.[105,125,148] Animal models demonstrate increased sensitivity to norepinephrine-induced dysrhythmias and decreased myocardial contractility, protein phosphorylation, and high-energy phosphate generation.[75] Lead-induced impairment of intracellular calcium metabolism may impact on cardiac electrophysiology.

REPRODUCTIVE SYSTEM

Impairment of both male and female reproductive function is associated with overt plumbism. Gametotoxic effects in animals of both sexes and chromosomal abnormalities in workers with BLLs above 60 μg/dL are reported.[54] Testicular endocrine hypofunction occurs in smelter workers with BLLs in the 60-μg/dL range.[127]

ENDOCRINE

Reduced thyroid and adrenopituitary function are found in adult lead workers.[132,133] Children with elevated lead levels have a depressed secretion of human growth hormone and insulinlike growth factor.[66]

SKELETAL SYSTEM

In addition to the skeletal system's importance as the largest repository of lead body burden, studies suggest that bone metabolism also is adversely affected by lead.[54] Hormonal response is altered by reduced 1,25-dihydroxyvitamin D_3 concentrations and by inhibition of osteocalcin. Both new bone formation and coupling of normal osteoblast and osteoclast function may thus be impaired.[54] Bands of increased metaphyseal density on radiographs of long bones ("lead lines") in young children with heavy lead exposure represent increased calcium deposition (not primarily lead) in the zones of provisional calcification (Fig. 94–3). Impaired bone growth and shortened stature are associated with childhood lead poisoning. Impaired calcium or cyclic adenosine monophosphate (cAMP) messenger systems may underlie these cellular effects.

GASTROINTESTINAL

GI effects are partly explained by spasmodic contraction of intestinal wall smooth muscle, analogous to that believed to occur in vascular walls.[135]

CLINICAL PRESENTATION

INORGANIC LEAD

The numerous observed lead-induced pathophysiologic effects accurately predict that the clinical manifestations of lead poisoning are diverse. These manifestations of lead toxicity are often characterized as falling into distinct syndromes of acute and chronic symptomatology. In most cases, these distinctions really describe a continuum of dose- and time-related severity. Rarely, patients with massive acute exposure present with clinical findings that are somewhat unique but overlap considerably with the more severe cases of chronic lead exposure. These syndromes are sufficiently distinct in epidemiology, clinical manifestations, and current recommended management approaches that they are described separately (Tables 94–3 and 94–4). It should be first reemphasized that the occurrence of overt clinical

TABLE 94–3. Clinical Manifestations of Lead Poisoning in Children

Clinical Severity	Typical Blood Lead Concentrations (μg/dL)
Severe	>70–100
CNS: Encephalopathy (coma, altered sensorium, seizures, bizarre behavior, ataxia, apathy, incoordination, loss of developmental skills; papilledema, cranial nerve palsies, signs of increased ICP)	
GI: Persistent vomiting	
Hematologic: Pallor (anemia)	
Mild to moderate	50–70
CNS: Hyperirritable behavior, intermittent lethargy, decreased interest in play, "difficult" child	
GI: Intermittent vomiting, abdominal pain, anorexia	
Asymptomatic	≤49
CNS: Impaired cognition, behavior, balance, fine-motor coordination	
Miscellaneous: Impaired hearing, growth	

CNS, central nervous system; GI, gastrointestinal; ICP, intracranial pressure.

TABLE 94–4. Clinical Manifestations of Lead Poisoning in Adults

Clinical Severity	Typical Blood Lead Concentrations (μg/dL)
Severe	>100
CNS: Encephalopathy (coma, seizures, obtundation, delirium, focal motor disturbances, headaches, papilledema, optic neuritis, signs of increased ICP)	
PNS: Footdrop, wristdrop	
GI: Abdominal colic	
Hematologic: Pallor (anemia)	
Renal: Nephropathy	
Moderate	70–100
CNS: Headache, memory loss, decreased libido, insomnia	
PNS: peripheral neuropathy	
GI: Metallic taste, abdominal pain, anorexia, constipation	
Renal: Nephropathy with chronic exposure	
Miscellaneous: Mild anemia, myalgias, muscle weakness, arthralgias	
Mild	20–69 [a]
CNS: Tiredness, somnolence, moodiness, lessened interest in leisure activities	
Miscellaneous: Adverse effects on cognition, reproduction, renal function, or bone density; hypertension and cardiovascular disease; possible increased risk of cancer	

[a] Chronic lead exposure at lower blood lead concentrations may lead to cumulative body burdens of lead associated with these clinical findings.

CNS, central nervous system; GI, gastrointestinal; ICP, intracranial pressure; PNS, peripheral nervous system.

symptoms in lead-exposed persons is, in most cases, the culmination of a long history of lead exposure. As the total dose increases, these symptoms are almost always preceded first by measurable biochemical and physiologic impairment followed, in turn, by subtle prodromal clinical effects that may only become apparent in hindsight. In general, children are considered to be more susceptible than adults to toxicity for a given measured blood lead concentration; however, the data for this primarily concern effects on the CNS.

Symptomatic Children *Acute lead encephalopathy* is the most severe presentation of pediatric plumbism (see Table 94–3). It may be associated with cerebral edema and increased intracranial pressure (see Fig. 94–1). Encephalopathy is characterized by pernicious vomiting and apathy, bizarre behavior, loss of recently acquired developmental skills, ataxia, incoordination, seizures, altered sensorium, or coma. Physical examination may reveal papilledema, oculomotor or facial nerve palsy, diminished deep tendon reflexes, or other evidence of increased intracranial pressure.[20,169] Encephalopathy usually occurs in children ages 15 to 30 months; is associated with BLLs above 100 μg/dL, although it is reported with BLLs as low as 70 μg/dL; and tends to occur more commonly in summer months, when BLLs peak.[115] Milder but ominous symptoms that may portend incipient encephalopathy include anorexia, constipation, intermittent abdominal pain, sporadic vomiting, hyperirritable or aggressive behavior, periods of lethargy interspersed with lucid intervals, and decreased interest in play activities. Many such patients seek medical advice for vomiting and lethargy during the 2 to 7 days before onset of frank encephalopathy.[33,115] Physical examination of such children usually reveals no specific abnormalities.

Mortality caused by encephalopathy was 65% in the prechelation era, decreasing to below 5% with the advent of effective chelation. The incidence of permanent neurologic sequelae, including mental retardation, seizure disorder, blindness, and hemiparesis, is 25% to 30% in patients who develop encephalopathic symptoms before the onset of chelation (Fig. 94–4).[33]

Subencephalopathic symptomatic plumbism usually occurs in children 1 to 5 years old and is associated with BLLs above 70 μg/dL, but it may occur with concentrations as low as 50 μg/dL. Unfortunately, common complaints in well children of this age (eg, the "terrible twos," with functional constipation and who do not eat as much as parents expect) often overlap with the milder range of reported symptoms of lead poisoning. Frequently, parents of children diagnosed by routine blood screening recognize milder symptoms only in hindsight after chelation treatment results in clinical improvement ("it seemed as if the child was going through a phase").[49] This is especially true currently, when symptomatic plumbism is rarely reported.[20,22] Other uncommon clinical presentations are described, including isolated seizures without encephalopathy (indistinguishable from idiopathic epilepsy), chronic hyperactive behavior disorder, isolated developmental delay, progressive loss of cortical function simulating degenerative cerebral disease, peripheral neuropathy (reported particularly in children with sickle-cell hemoglobinopathy), and the occurrence of GI symptoms (colicky abdominal pain, vomiting, constipation) with myalgias of the trunk and proximal girdle muscles.[33,43]

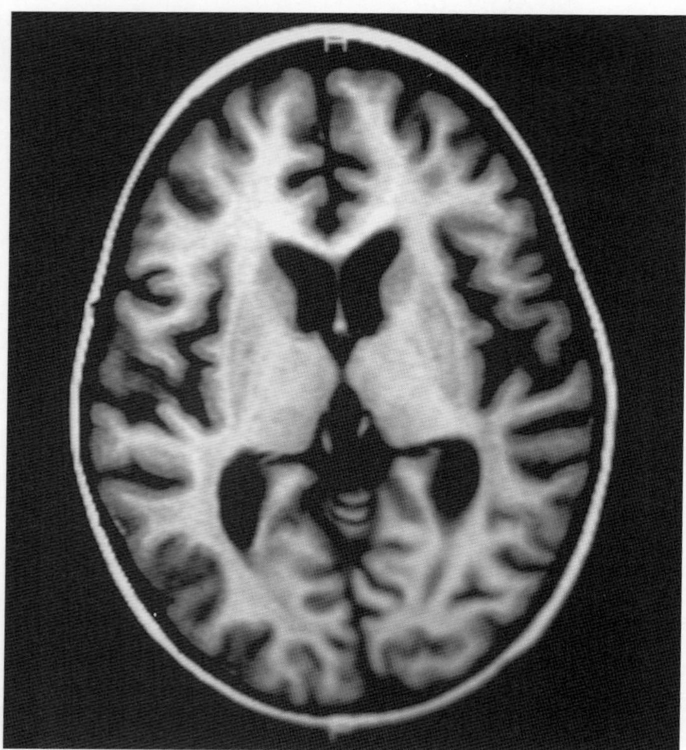

FIGURE 94–4. Magnetic resonance image of the brain reveals cortical atrophy and multiple areas of cerebral infarction in the same patient as in Figure 94–1, done on hospital day 22. At this time, the child's clinical status was notable for choreoathetoid movements and generalized hypotonia, inability to localize visual or auditory stimuli, and nonpurposeful movements of the extremities. *(Image contributed by Eric Faerber, MD, Department of Radiology, St. Christopher's Hospital for Children, Philadelphia, PA.)*

Asymptomatic Children Children with *elevated body lead burdens but without overt symptoms* represent the largest group of persons believed to be at risk for chronic lead toxicity. The subclinical toxicity of lead in this population centers around subtle effects on growth, hearing, and neurocognitive development. This last effect, in particular, is the subject of intense research interest and scrutiny. An effort to rigorously evaluate several modern (since 1979), carefully done studies of the association of low lead and reduced intelligence (cross-sectional studies with blood or tooth lead and prospective studies) and combine their results with a statistical meta-analysis technique have been reported.[117] The overall finding was that even though the majority of individual studies failed to achieve statistical significance when taken together, there was a significant inverse association between lead exposure and Intelligence Quotient (IQ), on the order of 1 to 2 IQ points for chronic BLL increases from 10 to 20 μg/dL. Since that publication, another study evaluated IQ in patients from 6 months to 5 years old and found that BLLs were inversely correlated with IQ at 3 and 5 years of age and that the magnitude of effect for all subjects was an average 4.6-point decrement in IQ for each 10-μg/dL increase in BLL. Of particular concern, this effect was even greater, with an estimated 7.4 point loss, for the subset of children in the 1 to 10 μg/dL BLL range.[16] The CDC recently compiled a number of studies confirming this association of adverse cognition and BLLs below 10 μg/dL.[21]

Adults Adults with occupational lead exposure may manifest numerous signs and symptoms representing disorders of several organ systems. Severity of symptoms correlates roughly with BLLs, although many conditions thought associated with low-dose chronic lead exposure are better correlated with markers of cumulative dose, such as bone lead or the cumulative blood lead index (area under the curve of BLLs versus time)[65,78] (see Table 94–4). True acute poisoning occurs rarely, after very high inhalational,[74] large oral,[107] or intravenous (IV) exposures.[108] Such patients may present with colic, hepatitis, pancreatitis, hemolytic anemia, and encephalopathy over days or weeks. Most adult plumbism is related to chronic respiratory exposure, although some authors have used the term *acute poisoning* to include patients with such exposure whose symptoms are severe and of relatively recent onset (within 6 weeks of presentation) and whose exposure is relatively brief (average, ≤1 year).[37]

The hallmark of severe toxicity is *acute encephalopathy*, which has been rarely reported in adults since the 1920s.[37] The majority of modern cases are actually not associated with occupational exposures but rather with more exotic exposures, such as ingestion of lead-contaminated illicit "moonshine" whiskey and ethnic alternative medications.[73,152] Encephalopathy in adults is usually associated with very high BLLs (typically >150 μg/dL) and is manifested by seizures (75% of cases), obtundation, confusion, focal motor disturbances, papilledema, headaches, and optic neuritis.[95,168] In addition, adult patients with severe plumbism often manifest attacks of abdominal colic, are virtually always anemic, and are at significant risk for severe peripheral nerve palsy such as wristdrop and footdrop and nephropathy. Rarely, cardiac dysfunction and electrocardiographic (ECG) abnormalities are reported.[125]

Moderate plumbism in adults typically involves CNS, peripheral nerve, hematologic, renal, GI, rheumatologic, endocrine or reproductive, and cardiovascular findings.[74,130,135] At BLLs above 70 μg/dL, such symptoms may include headache, memory loss, decreased libido, and insomnia. GI symptoms may include metallic taste, abdominal pain, decreased appetite, weight loss, and constipation. Musculoskeletal and rheumatologic complaints at this stage include muscle pain and joint tenderness. Peripheral neuropathy may occur, primarily motor, manifesting as muscle weakness, numbness of the legs, occasional paresthesias, tremor, and hyperreflexia. Many patients at this stage have mild anemia, and those with chronic exposure are at risk for nephropathy.

Mild plumbism may manifest as minor CNS findings, such as changes in mood and cognition. Subtle neurocognitive abnormalities demonstrable by neuropsychiatric testing are being found in both adults and children with modest elevations in blood lead concentration. Studies have documented abnormal psychometrics and nerve conduction in workers recently exposed to lead as BLLs increased to above 30 μg/dL.[89] Early symptoms, manifesting at BLLs of 40 to 70 μg/dL, may be subtle and include increased tiredness at the end of the day, disinterest in leisure-time pursuits, falling asleep easily, moodiness, and irritability. Effects on reproductive function and blood pressure may also be apparent in this range of exposure. Historically, infertility and stillbirths were common among heavily exposed female lead workers. More recent studies found reduced sperm counts, impaired sperm motility, and abnormal morphology in battery workers with BLLs above 40 μg/dL[6] and increased incidence of menstrual irregularity and spontaneous abortion in lead-exposed female workers in China[69] and Mexico.[11] Prematurity is more common in children of pregnancies associated with elevated maternal lead levels.[104]

Increased blood pressure is probably the most prevalent adverse health effect observed from lead exposure in adults. Epidemiologic studies document significant associations between hypertension and body lead burdens. The association is particularly strong for adult men ages 40 to 59 years, with an approximate 1.5- to 3.0-mm Hg increase in systolic pressure for every doubling of BLL beginning at 7 μg/dL.[116,158] Additional studies have correlated body lead burden with several other disorders of aging, including a decline in cognitive ability,[134,145] essential tremor,[41] cardiovascular and cerebrovascular events,[67,78,99] ECG abnormalities,[29] chronic renal dysfunction,[84,78] osteoporosis,[15] and cataract prevalence.[136]

Physical examination findings vary with the degree of severity. Mild and moderate symptoms usually occur in patients with normal examination findings.[39] In encephalopathic patients, typical changes of stupor, coma, posturing, and papilledema are noted. Milder abnormal neurologic findings include dominant wrist or hand weakness, paresthesia, and tremor. One author described grayish stippling of the retina circumferential to the optic disk,[151] but other authors dispute this finding.[112] A bluish-purple gingival lead line (Burton line) representing lead sulfide precipitation is described rarely in adult patients with poor oral hygiene. Abdominal guarding and tenderness are occasionally observed. Patients with saturnine gout may have typical joint findings of acute arthritis. Severely anemic patients may exhibit pallor. Careful neuropsychologic testing may reveal abnormalities of memory span, rapid motor tapping, visual motor coordination, and grip strength.[37]

ORGANIC LEAD

Clinical symptoms of TEL toxicity are usually nonspecific initially and include insomnia and emotional instability.[10,135] Nausea, vomiting, and anorexia may occur. The patient may exhibit tremor and increased deep tendon reflexes. In more severe cases, these symptoms progress to encephalopathy with delusions, hallucinations, and hyperactivity, which may resolve or deteriorate to coma and, occasionally, death. Severe cases may also develop hepatic and renal injury. Because many reported patients are exposed via intentional abuse of leaded gasoline, much of the literature reporting this syndrome may be confounded by accompanying volatile hydrocarbon toxicity.[155] Of note, in contrast to inorganic lead poisoning, patients with significant TEL toxicity do not consistently manifest hematologic abnormalities or elevations of heme synthesis pathway biomarkers. In addition, significant neurotoxicity may occur at BLLs considerably lower than those typically associated with inorganic lead poisoning.[61] A recent case report details the clinical course of a 13-year-old boy who unintentionally ingested a mouthful of fuel stabilizer containing 80% to 90% TEL. He developed progressive tremor, weakness, hallucinations, myoclonus, and hyperreflexia and required mechanical ventilation for 2 days and prolonged hospitalization for management of persistent hallucinations, weakness, dysphagia, and urinary and fecal incontinence. His peak BLL on the third day after ingestion was 62 μg/dL. [171]

ASSESSMENT

CLINICAL DIAGNOSIS IN SYMPTOMATIC PATIENTS

For all patients in whom plumbism is considered based on clinical manifestations, the medical evaluation should first include a comprehensive medical history. Further inquiry should elicit environmental, occupational, or recreational sources of exposure as detailed earlier (see Tables 94–1 and 94–2). Plumbism is more likely in a child between the ages of 1 and 5 years with prior plumbism or noted elevated BLLs, pica, including acute unintentional ingestions,[60] or aural, nasal, or esophageal foreign bodies[170], history of iron-deficiency anemia, residence in a pre-1960s–built home, especially with deteriorated paint, or one that has undergone recent remodeling; family history of lead poisoning, or foreign-born status.[3,31,172] Affected children may manifest persistent vomiting, lethargy, irritability, clumsiness, or loss of recently acquired developmental skills, afebrile seizures; or evidence of child abuse or neglect.[48,138] In adults, the history should focus on occupational and recreational activities that might involve lead exposure (see Table 94–2), a history of plumbism, and gunshot wounds with retained bullets.

The differential diagnosis of plumbism is broad. Adult patients may be misdiagnosed as having carpal tunnel syndrome, Guillain-Barré syndrome, sickle-cell crisis, acute appendicitis, renal colic, or infectious encephalitis. Children are often initially considered to have viral gastroenteritis or even to have insidious symptoms passed off as a difficult developmental phase.

A patient who presents to the ED with potential lead encephalopathy presents the physician with a dilemma: severe lead toxicity requires urgent diagnosis, but confirmatory blood lead assays are usually unavailable on an immediate basis.[63] For adults, a history of occupational exposure is often available from medical records or family members, and lead encephalopathy can be strongly considered with positive supportive laboratory findings (usually available on urgent basis) such as anemia, basophilic stippling, elevated erythrocyte protoporphyrin (especially >250 μg/dL), and abnormal urinalysis. In this context, it might be appropriate to institute presumptive chelation therapy while awaiting lead concentrations. In children, a similar indication for presumptive treatment would be suggested by a constellation of clinical features and ancillary studies, such as age 1 to 5 years, a prodromal illness of several days to weeks duration (suggestive of milder lead-related symptoms), history of pica and source of lead exposure, the laboratory features noted above, which are equally helpful in young children, radiologic findings of dense metaphyseal "lead lines" at wrists or knees (see Fig. 94–3), or evidence of recent pica for ingested foreign bodies or lead paint particles on abdominal radiographs (Figs. 94–5 and 94–6). Radiographic confirmation of retained bullets or shrapnel may be relevant in patients of any age (Fig. 94–7).[46,85,139,144] In both adults and children, the decision to institute empiric chelation treatment

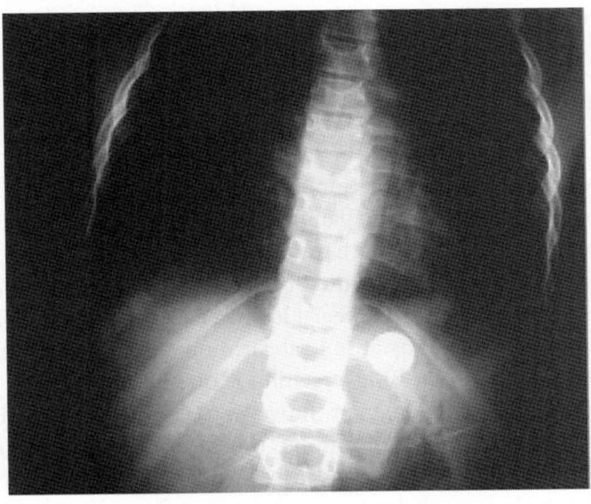

A

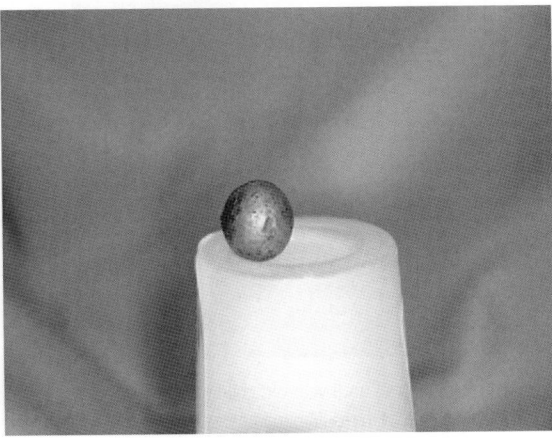

B

FIGURE 94–5. An unusual source of lead poisoning. (**A**) Radiograph of the abdomen reveals ingested metallic foreign body. (**B**) The ingested foreign body was a Civil War era musketball from the collection of the patient's father. *(Images contributed by Evaline Alessandrini, MD, Division of Emergency Medicine, Children's Hospital of Philadelphia, Philadelphia, PA.)*

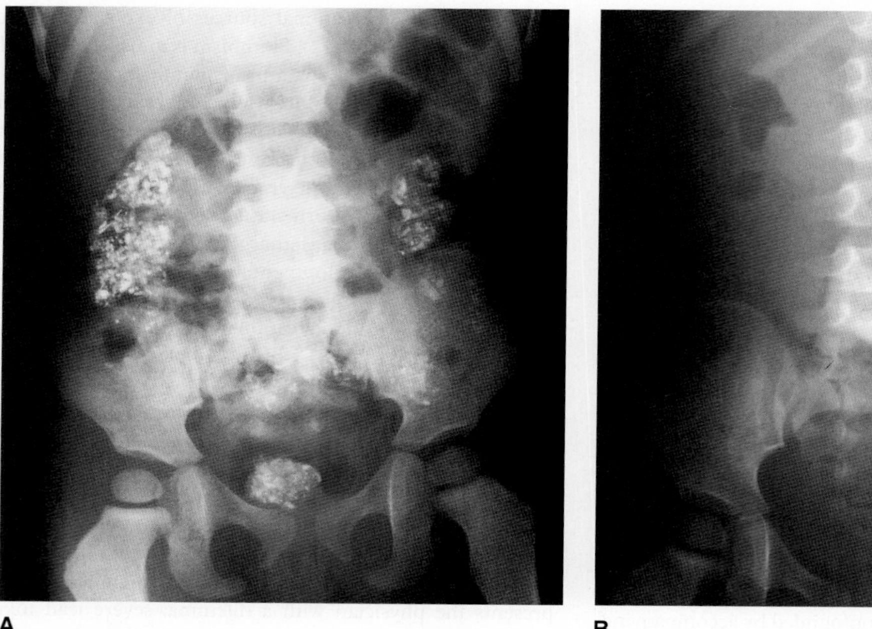

FIGURE 94–6. (A) Abdominal radiograph of a child who had massive paint chip ingestion. The dispersed radio dense (white) fragments are noted to follow the outline of the large intestine. (B) No remaining lead is seen on follow-up radiograph after whole-bowel irrigation. *(Images contributed by Department of Radiology, St. Christopher's Hospital for Children, Philadelphia, PA.)*

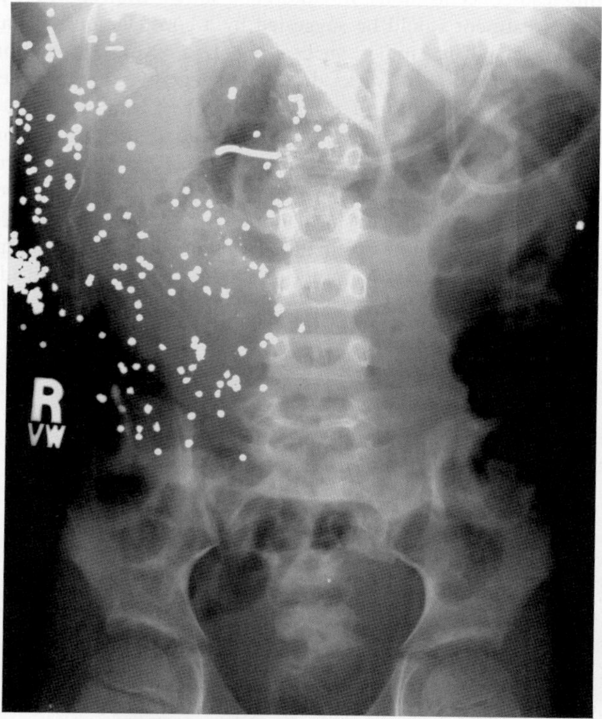

FIGURE 94–7. Abdominal radiograph of an 8-year-old child who sustained a shotgun wound to the right paraspinal area, with resultant paraplegia and multiple visceral injuries. The blood lead concentration was found to be 60 μg/dL at 11 weeks after injury, and chelation therapy was commenced. *(Reproduced with permission from Selbst SM, Henretig F, Fee MA, et al. Lead poisoning in a child with a gunshot wound.* Pediatrics. *1986;77:413-416.)*

should not deter additional emergent diagnostic efforts to exclude or to confirm other important entities while blood lead concentrations are pending. An important consideration in this context may be the suspicion of an acute, potentially treatable CNS infection (eg, bacterial meningitis or herpetic encephalitis). Lumbar puncture may be dangerous in patients with severe lead encephalopathy because of the risk of cerebral herniation.[34] If immediate lumbar puncture is thought to be highly desirable, a computed tomography scan would allow determination of severe cerebral edema, midline shift, or other evidence of an especially high risk for herniation. If performed, the minimal amount of fluid necessary for diagnosis (<1 mL) should be removed using a small-gauge needle. Alternatively, empiric treatment for infectious processes can be initiated while the lead concentration is pending, and delayed lumbar puncture can be performed if the blood lead concentration is normal.

LABORATORY EVALUATION

In patients suspected of having plumbism, laboratory testing is used to augment the evaluation of both lead exposure and lead toxicity. The *whole BLL* is the principal measure of lead exposure available in clinical practice, reflecting both recent and remote exposure. In any patient suspected of symptomatic plumbism, whole blood should be collected by venipuncture into special lead-free evacuated tubes. The BLL is typically determined by atomic absorption spectrophotometry. For asymptomatic children, BLL screening is often performed by capillary blood testing for convenience; however, venous confirmation of elevated capillary lead concentrations, unless extremely high (eg, >69 μg/dL) or unless the patient is clearly symptomatic, is still considered mandatory before chelation or other significant interventions. Hair and urine lead concentrations have little clinical utility. The *erythrocyte protoporphyrin concentration* reflects lead's inhibition of the heme synthesis pathway (see Chap. 24) and had been used as a screening tool in the past, but it is no longer considered sufficiently sensitive. The erythrocyte protoporphyrin concentration test may still be useful for tracking response to therapy and in distinguishing acute from chronic lead exposure; as an adjunct to the emergency diagnosis of symptomatic plumbism if emergent BLL determination is not available; and, rarely, in the evaluation of suspected factitious plumbism. Routine serum chemistries, renal function tests, liver function tests, urinalysis, and complete blood count are indicated in patients who are symptomatic or about to undergo chelation therapy. Radiographic studies may suggest retained bullets, as noted above (see Fig. 94–7), recent lead ingestion, or toxicity. Abdominal radiographs may reveal lead paint chips or other ingested lead foreign material (see Figs. 94–5 and 94–6). The finding of "lead lines," metaphyseal densities at the ends of long bones in young children, may substantiate a clinical diagnosis of plumbism before BLLs are available (see Fig. 94–2), although dense metaphyseal bands are rarely caused by other causes, including other heavy metals (arsenic, bismuth, and mercury), healing rickets, and recovery from scurvy.[120,171]

Finally, two measures of cumulative lead exposure are available. *X-ray fluorescence* technology measures bone lead, and thus indirectly estimates total body lead burden. The *cumulative blood lead index*, derived from several BLLs measured over the presumed course of lifetime lead exposure, calculated as an area under the concentration curve, has also been described.[65] Both techniques have been used in research studies of issues concerning past chronic lead exposure and a variety of current health outcomes.[64,77,166]

SCREENING

Although outside the scope of this discussion, screening is an essential public health practice for the prevention of severe plumbism in both children and adults from high-risk settings. Table 94–5 outlines the current CDC[21,26] pediatric recommendations, which also are endorsed by the American Academy of Pediatrics.[3] Likewise, the Occupational Safety and Health Administration (OSHA) maintains a lead standard for U.S. workers formulated to reduce workplace exposure to lead, decrease symptomatic lead poisoning, and provide quality medical care to workers with elevated blood lead levels.[159–161] Table 94–6A summarizes the OSHA-mandated action BLL values for worker notification, removal, and reinstatement.

TABLE 94–5. Pediatric Screening and Follow-up Guidelines[3,21,26]

Screening

1. The AAP and CDC recommend screening all children who are Medicaid eligible at age 1 and 2 years (and those ages 3–6 years who have not been screened previously). Children who may not be Medicaid eligible but whose families participate in any poverty assistance program should also be screened.
2. Certain local health departments (eg, New York, Chicago, and Philadelphia) recommend screening at younger ages or more frequently. Such recommendations include starting at age 6–9 months, testing every 6 months for children younger than 2 years, and provision of additional education and more rapid follow-up testing for children younger than 12 months old whose BLLs are 6–9 μg/dL.
3. In addition, children who are not Medicaid eligible but are designated high-risk by their state or local health departments should be screened as per these local policies.[a]
4. For children who are neither Medicaid eligible nor live in areas with locale-specific health department guidelines, recommendations are less clear. The AAP supports universal screening of such children as well.[b]
5. Recent immigrant, refugee, or international adoptee children should be screened on arrival to the United States.

Follow-up

BPb (μg/dL)	*Recommended Action*
≤9	Retest in 1 year
10–14	Retest in 3 months; education[20]
15–19	Retest in 2 months; education; if the level is 15–19 twice, refer for case management
20–44	Clinical evaluation; education; environmental investigation and lead hazard control
45–69	Clinical evaluation and case management within 48 hours; education; environmental investigation and lead hazard control; chelation therapy[3,22]
≥70	Hospitalize child; immediate chelation therapy; education; environmental investigation and lead hazard control

[a] Many relevant state and city health department contacts may be located at http://www.cdc.gov/nceh/lead/grants/contacts/CLPPP%20Map.htm.

[b] The 1997 CDC guidance[26] allowed for targeted screening of some children of low-risk geographic and demographic background based on a personal risk questionnaire. Subsequent studies have found that such survey-based targeted screening is not well validated.[3] Nevertheless, a listing of potential risk factors may be instructive and is summarized here. Screening was recommended if a child had any of the following high-risk factors:

Housing: Lives in or regularly visits a home built before 1950; lives in or regularly visits a home built before 1978 undergoing remodeling or renovation (or renovated within 6 months).

Medical history: Pica for paint chips or dirt; iron deficiency.

Personal, family, social history: Personal, family, or playmate history of lead poisoning; parental occupational, industrial, hobby exposures; live in proximity to major roadway; use of hot tap water for consumption; use of complementary remedies, cosmetics, ceramic food containers; trips or residence outside United States; parents are migrant farm workers, receive poverty assistance.

Educational interventions as per Table 94–7.

Chelation therapy as per Table 94–8.

AAP, American Academy of Pediatrics; BLL, blood lead concentration; BPb, venous blood lead; CDC, Centers for Disease Control and Prevention.

TABLE 94–6A. Occupational Safety and Health Administration General Industry[a] Standards for Various Blood Lead Concentrations (BLLs)

Number of Tests	BLL (μg/dL)	Action Required
1	≥40	Notification of worker in writing; medical examination of worker and consultation
3 (average)	≥50	Removal of worker from job with potential lead exposure
1	≥60	Removal of worker from job with potential lead exposure
2	<40	Reinstatement of worker in job with potential lead exposure

[a] The construction industry standard is similar for worker notification (at 40 μg/dL) and reinstatement (<40 μg/dL twice) but requires worker removal for a single value ≥50 μg/dL.

Adapted from U.S. Department of Labor, Occupational Safety and Health Administration. *Medical Surveillance Guidelines–1910.1025 App C.* Retrieved December 29, 2005, from http://www.osha.gov/pls/oshaweb/owadisp.show_document?p_table=STANDARDS&p_id=10033 and U.S. Department of Labor, Occupational Safety and Health Administration. *Medical Surveillance Guidelines. Lead–1926.62.* Retrieved December 29, 2005, from http://www.osha.gov/pls/oshaweb/owadisp.show_document?p_table=STANDARDS&p_id=10641. See also US Department of Labor.[160–162]

An expert panel convened by the Association of Occupational and Environmental Clinics recently published an alternative set of health-based management recommendations for lead-exposed workers. The authors propose that their recommendations are more reflective of recent research linking adverse health outcomes to chronic, low-dose lead exposure.[78] These guidelines are summarized in Table 94–6B.

TABLE 94–6B. Health-Based Occupational Surveillance Recommendations[a]

BLL (μg/dL)	Recommendation
<10	BLL every month for 3 months and then every 6 months (unless exposure increases); if BLL increases >4 μg/dL, exposure evaluation or reduction effort; exposure evaluation or reduction if BLL 5–9 μg/dL for women who are or may become pregnant
10–19	As for BLL <10 μg/dL and BLL every 3 months; exposure evaluation and reduction effort; consider removal if no improvement with exposure reduction or complicating medical condition[b]; resume BLL q 6 months if 3 BLLs <10 μg/dL
≥19	Remove from exposure if BLL >30 μg/dL or repeat BLL in 4 weeks; BLL every month; consider return to work after BLL <15 μg/dL twice

[a] All potentially lead-exposed workers warrant pre-employment clinical evaluation, baseline blood lead concentration (BLL), and serum creatinine level.

[b] Such conditions include chronic renal disease, hypertension, neurologic disorders, and cognitive dysfunction.

Adapted from Kosnett MJ, Wedeen RP, Rothenberg SJ, et al. Recommendations for medical management of adult lead exposure. *Environ Health Perspect.* 2007;115:463-471.

MANAGEMENT

There are several caveats about the management of patients with lead poisoning. First, the most important aspect of treatment is removal from further exposure to lead. Unfortunately, effective implementation of this therapy is often beyond the control of the clinician but rather depends on a complex interplay of public health, social, and political actions. Currently, the ability to control exposure is generally more applicable to adults with occupational exposures than to children exposed to residential hazards. Second, in children for whom some residual lead exposure potentially continues, optimization of nutritional status is vital in order to minimize absorption. Finally, pharmacologic therapy with chelators, although a mainstay of therapy for symptomatic patients, is an inexact science, with numerous unanswered questions despite almost 50 years of clinical use.[2,5,77] The rationale for chelation therapy of lead-poisoned patients is that chelators complex with lead, forming a chelate that is excreted in urine, feces, or both. Chelation therapy increases lead excretion, reduces blood concentrations, and reverses hematologic markers of toxicity during therapy. Reports from the 1950s found symptomatic improvement in adults chelated for lead colic.[165] The institution of effective combination chelation treatment of childhood lead encephalopathy in the 1960s contributed to the dramatic decline in mortality and morbidity of that devastating degree of plumbism.[33] However, the same era saw major advances in pediatric critical care in general and medical management of increased intracranial pressure in particular. The situation of chelation therapy for asymptomatic patients with mildly to moderately increased body burdens of lead is even less clear, and many questions regarding efficacy and safety remain.[31,55,77,114] To date, long-term reduction of target tissue lead content or reversal of toxicity is not demonstrated in human trials.[40,93,128]

DECREASING EXPOSURE

All patients with significantly elevated lead concentrations warrant identification of the lead exposure source and specific environmental and medical interventions or both (Table 94–7). In adults, this usually involves changes in their worksite.[39,78,135] Remedial actions might include improvements in ventilation, modification of personal hygiene habits, and optimal use of respiratory apparatus. It is vital to prohibit smoking, eating, and drinking in a lead-exposed work area. Work clothes should be changed after each shift and should not be lockered together with street clothes. In patients with plumbism caused by retained bullets, surgical removal of this lead source should be considered.[27,85,98] Table 94–7 also summarizes several specific educational guidelines that may be offered to parents of lead-exposed children.[3,14,22,] Overarching principles include home lead paint abatement (done preferably by professionals, with the family out of the home), home dust reduction techniques, decreasing soil lead exposure, and nutritional evaluation and counseling. Patients manifesting iron deficiency should be treated, and for others, a diet sufficient in trace nutrients, particularly iron and calcium (which may decrease lead absorption) and vitamin C (which may enhance renal lead excretion) is likely of value.[3] Clinicians who have primary responsibility for children with elevated lead levels should refer to the CDC's exhaustive monograph, which details such pediatric case mananagement.[22]

Occasionally, children may require urgent GI decontamination to reduce ongoing acute lead exposure. Patients with large burdens of lead paint chips may benefit from prompt institution of whole-bowel irrigation (WBI) (see Fig. 94–6). The presence of ingested lead foreign bodies is a unique situation that requires careful individualization of management. Several case reports document rapid absorption, with significantly elevated BLLs measured within 24 hours of ingestion in some cases. Such patients warrant baseline BLL determination

TABLE 94–7. Evaluation and Management of Patients with Lead Exposure

Workplace Efforts
Adults
Implement careful lead exposure monitoring (see Table 94-6B)
Improve ventilation
Use respiratory apparatus
Wear protective clothing; change from work clothes before leaving worksite
Modify personal hygiene habits
Prohibit eating, drinking, and smoking at the worksite
Evaluate possible sources beyond occupational setting (see Tables 94–1 and 94–2)
Children
Notify the local health department to initiate home inspection and abatement as needed
Home lead paint abatement (professional contractors if possible; use plastic sheeting, low dust-generating paint removal; replacement of lead-painted windows, floor treatment; final cleanup with high-efficiency particle air vacuum, wet-mopping)
Avoid most hazardous areas of the home and yard
Dust control: Wet mopping, sponging with high-phosphate detergent; frequent hand, toy, and pacifier washing
Soil lead exposure reduction by planting grass and shrubs around the house
Use only cold, flushed tap water for consumption
Optimize nutrition to reduce lead absorption: avoid fasting; iron, calcium, vitamin C sufficient diet; supplement iron and calcium as necessary
Avoid food storage in open cans
Avoid imported ceramic containers for food and beverage use
Evaluate parental occupations and hobbies and eliminate high-risk activity
Consider possible sources beyond lead paint exposure (see Tables 94–1 and 94–2)

and frequent repeat BLLs, with consideration for prompt endoscopic removal, particularly with gastric location and increasing BLLs.[97,103,163] Proton pump inhibitor and prokinetic therapy have also been recommended for gastric foreign bodies in an effort to decrease gastric acidity, retention time, and resultant lead dissolution.[47] WBI may be an adjunct for more distally located foreign bodies but has not been uniformly successful. Colonoscopy or surgery may be required in serious cases.[103,163] The issue of concomitant chelation therapy in patients with significant GI lead burdens is addressed in the following section.

CHELATION THERAPY

The indications for and specifics of chelation therapy are determined by the patient's age, blood lead concentration, and clinical symptomatology (Table 94–8). Three chelation agents are currently recommended as drugs of choice for the treatment of lead poisoning: (see Antidotes in Depth A26: Dimercaprol) BAL and $CaNa_2EDTA$ (see Antidotes in Depth A28: Edetate Calcium Disodium) are used parenterally for more severe cases, and succimer (see Antidotes in Depth A27: Succimer) is available for oral therapy. Pharmacologic profiles of these three chelators are detailed in the corresponding Antidotes in Depth. A fourth drug, D-penicillamine (see below), has been used orally for patients with mild to moderate excess lead burdens. Unfortunately, D-penicillamine has a toxicity profile that includes serious, life-threatening hematologic disorders and reversible, but serious, dermatologic and renal effects; consequently, since 1991, its role in lead poisoning treatment at most centers has been largely replaced by succimer. Currently, the American Academy of Pediatrics recommends D-penicillamine use only when unacceptable adverse reactions to both succimer and $CaNa_2EDTA$ occur, and it remains important to continue chelation.[2,3] Nevertheless, some authors still commend its use for mild lead intoxication, particularly at a reduced dose regimen.[143]

Chelation is not a panacea for lead poisoning. It is a relatively inefficient process, with a typical course of therapy decreasing body content of heavy metal by only 1% to 2%.[77,102] Furthermore, there is little evidence that chelating agents have significant access to critical sites in target organs, particularly in the brain.[36] Assumptions that reducing blood lead level will improve subtle neurocognitive dysfunction or other subclinical organ toxicity are appealing theoretically but are unproven.[40,128]

PEDIATRIC THERAPY

Lead encephalopathy is an acute life-threatening emergency and should be treated under the guidance of a multidisciplinary team in the intensive care unit of a hospital experienced in the management of critically ill children. Encephalopathy requires treatment by combination parenteral chelation therapy with maximum-dose BAL and $CaNa_2EDTA$ along with meticulous supportive care.[2,22,33] Such combination therapy has a dramatic effect on decreasing BLL—to 50% or less of baseline within 15 hours and to 75% to 80% of baseline by 48 to 72 hours. It is far superior to monotherapy with $CaNa_2EDTA$ in this regard.[33]

Chelation is instituted with 75 mg/m²/d (or 25 mg/kg/d) of intramuscular (IM) BAL in six divided doses.[2,22] The second dose of BAL is given 4 hours later followed immediately by IV $CaNa_2EDTA$, in maximum concentration of 0.5% solution, at 1500 mg/m²/d (or 50 mg/kg/d) as a continuous infusion over several hours or in divided-dose infusions.[2,22,115] The delay in initiating $CaNa_2EDTA$ infusion is based on past observations of clinical deterioration in encephalopathic patients treated with $CaNa_2EDTA$ alone.[2,33] Therapy is typically continued with both agents for 5 days, although in milder cases with prompt resolution of encephalopathy and decrease of BLL to below 50 μg/dL, BAL may be discontinued after 3 days, with continuation of $CaNa_2EDTA$ alone for 2 more days.

The presence of radiopaque material in the GI tract on radiography has raised concern that parenteral chelation might enhance absorption of residual gut lead. This issue is not settled fully,[31,71] but most experts advocate initiation of parenteral chelation without delay in seriously symptomatic patients. It seems reasonable to simultaneously attempt bowel decontamination,[2] as with a WBI solution. One case report described the successful use of chelation therapy begun with parenteral BAL and $CaNa_2EDTA$ and then enteral succimer (initiated after 3 days of WBI) for a child with lead encephalopathy and an extraordinarily high BLL of 550 μg/dL.[52] This issue applies as well to ingested lead foreign bodies, as noted above.[97,103,163] Generally, oral fluids, feedings, and medications are withheld for at least the first several days. Careful provision of adequate IV fluids optimizes renal function while avoiding overhydration and the risk of exacerbating cerebral edema. The occurrence of the syndrome of inappropriate secretion of antidiuretic hormone (SIADH) may be associated with lead encephalopathy,[33,154] so urine volume, specific gravity, and serum electrolytes should be closely monitored, especially as fluids are gradually liberalized with clinical improvement. In the context of lead encephalopathy, this approach would need to be tempered by the requirement for maintaining good urine output to optimize chelation efficacy.

Seizure control is usually accomplished with benzodiazepines. Ongoing anticonvulsant therapy is typically continued with phenytoin or phenobarbital. Rarely, continuous infusions of midazolam or high-dose pentobarbital therapy may be necessary.[169]

TABLE 94–8. Chelation Therapy Guidelines[2,3,22,74,115,118] for Initial Course of Treatment[a]

Condition, BLL (μg/dL)	Dose	Regimen/Comments
Adults		
Encephalopathy	BAL 450 mg/m²/d[a,b] and	75 mg/m² IM every 4 h for 5 d
	$CaNa_2EDTA$ 1000–1500 mg/m²/d[a]	Continuous infusion or two to four divided IV doses for 5 d (start 4 h after BAL)
Symptoms suggestive of encephalopathy or >100	BAL 300–450 mg/m²/d[a,b] and	50–75 mg/m² every 4 h for 3–5 d (base dose, duration on BPb, severity of symptoms; see text)
	$CaNa_2EDTA$ 1500 mg/m²/d[a]	Continuous infusion or two to four divided IV doses for 5 d (start 4 h after BAL)
		Lab: Baseline CT scan; CBC, Ca, BLL, BUN, Cr, LFTs, U/A; repeat CBC, Ca, BUN, Cr, LFTs, U/A daily; BLL on days 3 and 5
Mild symptoms or 70–100	Succimer 700–1050 mg/m²/d	350 mg/m² tid for 5 d, then bid for 14 d. Remove from exposure (Table 94–7)
		Lab: CBC, BLL, BUN, Cr, LFTs, U/A; repeat CBC, LFTs, BLL on days 7 and 21
Asymptomatic and <70	Usually not indicated	–
Children		
Encephalopathy	BAL 450 mg/m²/d[a] and	75 mg/m² IM every 4 h for 5 d
	$CaNa_2EDTA$ 1500 mg/m²/d[a]	Continuous infusion or two to four divided IV doses for 5 d (start 4 h after BAL)
		Lab: Baseline AXR, CT scan, CBC, Ca, BLL, BUN, Cr, LFTs, U/A; repeat CBC, Ca, BUN, Cr, LFTs, U/A daily; BLL on days 3 and 5
Symptomatic (without encephalopathy) or >69	BAL 300–450 mg/m²/d[a] and	50–75 mg/m² every 4 h for 3–5 d (base dose, duration on BPb, severity of symptoms; see text)
	$CaNa_2EDTA$ 1000–1500 mg/m²/d[a]	Continuous infusion or two to four divided IV doses for 5 d (start 4 h after BAL)
		Lab: Baseline AXR, CBC, Ca, BLL, BUN, Cr, LFTs, U/A; repeat CBC, Ca, BUN, Cr, LFTs, U/A on days 3 and 5 and BLL day 5
Asymptomatic: 45–69	Succimer 700–1050 mg/m²/d[a] or	350 mg/m² tid for 5 d and then bid for 14 d
		Lab: Baseline AXR, CBC, BLL, LFTs; repeat CBC, LFTs, BLL day 7 and 21
	$CaNa_2EDTA$, 1000 mg/m²/d[a]	Continuous infusion or two to four divided IV doses for 5 d (see text)
		Lab: Baseline AXR, CBC, Ca, BLL, BUN, Cr, LFTs, U/A; repeat Ca, BUN, Cr, LFTs, U/A on days 3 and 5 and BLL on day 5
	(*or rarely*, d-Penicillamine)	–
20–44	Routine chelation not indicated (see text)	If succimer used, same regimen as per above group
	Attempt exposure reduction	(see Table 94-7)
<20	Chelation not indicated	
	Attempt exposure reduction	(see Table 94-7)

[a] Subsequent treatment regimens should be based on postchelation BPb and clinical symptoms (see text).
Approximately equivalent doses are expressed in mg/kg: BAL 450 mg/m²/d (~24 mg/kg/d); 300 mg/m²/d (~18 g/kg/d)
$CaNa_2EDTA$ 1000 mg/m²/d (~25–50 mg/kg/d); 1500 mg/m²/d (~50–75 mg/kg/d); Adult maximum dose 2–3 g/d; Succimer 350 mg/m² (~10 mg/kg)
[b] Some clinicians recommend $CaNa_2EDTA$ alone in these contexts (see text).
AXR, abdominal radiography; BLL, blood lead level; BPb, venous blood lead; BUN, blood urea nitrogen; Ca, calcium; $CaNa_2EDTA$, edetate calcium disodium; CBC, complete blood count; Cr, creatinine, CT scan, computed tomography scan of the brain; IM, intramuscular; IV, intravenous; Lab = suggested laboratory and radiologic evaluation; LFTs, hepatic aminotransferases; U/A, urinalysis with microscopy (frequent monitoring of urine dipstick analysis for hematuria and proteinuria also advised during $CaNa_2EDTA$ therapy).

Modern approaches to the *management of cerebral edema and increased intracranial pressure (ICP)* have not as yet been critically evaluated in the currently rare context of lead encephalopathy. Lumbar puncture should probably be avoided if lead encephalopathy is highly suspected and acute infectious processes are not (of note, repeated lumbar puncture was used as an adjunct to the treatment of lead encephalopathy associated with increased ICP in the 1950s but was complicated by proximate death when signs of impending herniation were present[34]). It seems reasonable that noninvasive measures such as prevention of hypoxia and hypercarbia with tracheal intubation and controlled ventilation, seizure treatment and prophylaxis, maintenance of adequate cerebral perfusion pressure, mild hyperventilation with PCO_2 of 30 to 35 mm Hg, and neutral head positioning with elevation of the head of the bed to 30 degrees might have a salutary effect at minimal risk of increased iatrogenic morbidity.[2,153] Mannitol administration may prove beneficial in deteriorating patients and has been particularly suggested as an adjunctive therapy when cerebral edema is complicated by SIADH or impaired renal function.[33] Whether more aggressive measures, such acute hyperventilation for impending herniation, intracranial pressure monitoring, drainage of ventricular cerebrospinal fluid, induced hypothermia, or barbiturate coma would decrease mortality or morbidity further is unknown.

For children with *milder symptoms or who are asymptomatic with BLL > 70 μg/dL*, chelation with a two-drug regimen similar to that used for encephalopathy is recommended. It is likely that this group of patients will require only 2 to 3 days of BAL in addition to 5 days of $CaNa_2EDTA$. Some authors have suggested that asymptomatic patients in this group, particularly those with BLLs below 100, might also be adequately treated with $CaNa_2EDTA$ alone,[172] succimer plus $CaNa_2EDTA$, or even succimer alone, but these regimens have not been studied in such children. Intensive care monitoring may be prudent for such patients as well, at least during the initiation of chelation therapy.[102]

Chelation therapy is widely recommended for *asymptomatic children with BLLs between 45 and 70 μg/dL*.[2,5,22,102] Children without overt symptoms may be treated with succimer alone, which has documented efficacy in lowering BLLs and short-term safety since its approval by the Food and Drug Administration in 1991.[58,82] Succimer is initiated at 30 mg/kg/d (or 1050 mg/m^2/d) orally in three divided doses; this is continued for 5 days and then decreased to 20 mg/kg/d (or 700 mg/m^2/d) in two divided doses for 14 additional days.[2,57] The original data establishing this empiric dosing regimen were based on surface area rather than body weight.[57] For younger children, the alternative dosing by body weight results in suboptimal dosing.[126] Although the ability to chelate children orally with succimer makes it tempting to prescribe routinely for outpatient therapy and some animal evidence suggests succimer does not enhance enteral lead absorption,[72] clinical reports suggest that children must be protected from continued lead exposure during succimer chelation.[30,32] Home abatement and reinspection should be accomplished before initiation of ambulatory succimer therapy; if this is not feasible, hospitalization is still warranted. Alternative regimens (for rare patients with succimer intolerance or allergy or because of parental noncompliance) include inpatient parenteral chelation with $CaNa_2EDTA$ at 25 mg/kg/d for 5 days[2] or an outpatient oral course of D-penicillamine.

After initial chelation therapy, decisions to repeat treatment are based on clinical symptoms and follow-up BLLs. Patients with encephalopathy or any severe symptoms or with an initial BLL above 100 μg/dL often require repeated courses of treatment. It is suggested that at least 2 days elapse before restarting chelation. The precise regimen and dosing of chelating agents are determined by ongoing symptomatology and the repeat BLLs (see Table 94–8). A third course of chelation should rarely be necessary sooner than 5 to 7 days after the second course ends.[115] For patients with milder degrees of plumbism (eg, asymptomatic, initial BLL <70 μg/dL), it is reasonable to allow 10 to 14 days of reequilibration before restarting treatment.[2]

The management of *asymptomatic children with BLLs of 20 to 44 μg/dL* is controversial.[30,91,101,157] The National Institutes of Health–sponsored Treatment of Lead-exposed Children (TLC) trial found only modest efficacy of succimer in reducing BLL. Furthermore, at 3 years postenrollment, no benefit was noted in treated patients on measures of cognition, neuropsychiatric function, or behavior.[128] This large study enrolled 780 children in a multicenter, randomized, placebo-controlled, double-blind trial, but it still has been criticized, particularly for using a single chelating agent and having failed to lower BLL significantly over time between treated and control groups.[141] Of note, small but statistically significant decrements in growth velocity were noted in the treatment group, which might reflect trace mineral depletion.[114] Since its initial publication, the primary findings of the TLC trial on lack of cognitive improvement were confirmed in a 7-year follow-up study.[40] In addition, a reanalysis of the original data found that decreasing blood concentrations did correlate with improved cognitive scores over the initial 36-month trial period (~4 IQ points for each 10-μg/dL decrease in BLL), but only in the placebo group.[87] Nevertheless, there may still be potential indications for occasional chelation treatment in this group, including BLLs at the higher end of the range (eg, 35–44 μg/dL), especially if BLLs remain the same or increase over several months after rigorous environmental controls are instituted, in younger children (eg, younger than 2 years old), in children with evidence of biochemical toxicity (an elevated erythrocyte protoporphyrin concentration, after iron supplementation, if necessary), or any hint of subtle symptoms. Some clinicians suggest that a reduced dose regimen of D-penicillamine be considered for children with BLLs in this range. One retrospective study reviewed medical records for 55 children, with a mean BLL of 24 μg/dL, treated with 15 mg/kg/day of D-penicillamine in addition to lead hazard abatement. The treatment period averaged 77 days and achieved mean BLL of 16 μg/dL at the end of therapy, with few noted adverse effects.[143] Further study of such therapy on long-term BLLs and clinical outcomes is certainly warranted. Currently, the CDC[20] and the American Academy of Pediatrics[2,3] recommend aggressive environmental and nutritional interventions with close monitoring of blood lead concentrations, without routine chelation therapy, for such children.

BLLs of 10 to 19 μg/dL are defined by the CDC as representing excessive exposure to lead but do not require chelation therapy. Close monitoring (for the 10–14 μg/dL range) and careful environmental investigation and interventions as necessary (particularly for the 15–19 μg/dL range) are appropriate and sufficient.[2,3,22] The educational approaches outlined earlier should be included in the case management of all children with even modestly elevated lead levels (see Table 94–7).

ADULT THERAPY

General Considerations The first principle in the treatment of adults with lead poisoning is that chelation therapy may not substitute for adherence to OSHA lead standards at the worksite and should never be given prophylactically.[39,74] In addition to the guidelines for decreasing lead exposure noted earlier, chelation therapy is indicated for adults with significant symptoms (encephalopathy, abdominal colic, severe arthralgias, or myalgias), evidence of target organ damage (neuropathy or nephropathy), and possibly in asymptomatic workers with markedly elevated BLLs or evidence of biochemical toxicity or increased chelatable lead.[78,124,135,140] Table 94–8 outlines suggested chelation therapy regimens for adults. For encephalopathic adult patients, our practice is to recommend combined BAL and $CaNa_2EDTA$ therapy, just as for children, although some clinicians suggest that adults with severe lead poisoning may be successfully treated with $CaNa_2EDTA$ alone in doses of 2 to 4 g/day by continuous IV infusion.[76] Recent reports support the use of succimer in adult patients with mild to moderate plumbism after environmental and occupational remedies have been instituted.[83,118] Chelation therapy should also be considered in the perioperative period for patients undergoing surgical removal of retained bullets or debridement of adjacent lead-contaminated tissue.[85,98,139] Treatment of patients with acute TEL toxicity is largely supportive, with sedation as necessary. For patients seen soon after a large-volume ingestion, nasogastric suction, with airway protection as needed, may be warranted. In general, chelation therapy for TEL toxicity has been associated with enhanced lead excretion[12] but has not been found clinically efficacious.[135,155,171] However, for symptomatic, especially encephalopathic patients with very elevated BLLs (in whom there may be a significant component of metabolically derived inorganic lead toxicity), we strongly consider chelation therapy.

Pregnancy, Neonatal, and Lactation Issues An area of particular concern in the management of adult plumbism involves decisions regarding therapy during pregnancy. As noted previously, lead freely passes the placental barrier and accumulates in the fetus throughout gestation. Chelation therapy during early pregnancy poses theoretical problems of teratogenicity, particularly that caused by enhanced fetal excretion of potentially vital trace elements, or translocation of lead from mother to fetus (see also the relevant Antidotes in Depth A26, A27, A28). Symptomatic pregnant women with elevated BLLs certainly warrant chelation therapy, regardless of these concerns. Additionally, of some reassurance regarding fetal health, a recent case series and 25-year literature review of lead poisoning during pregnancy found no reports of chelation-associated birth defects in the handful of such published cases.[142] It should be noted that despite decreases in maternal BLL with chelation therapy, newborn BLLs may be considerably higher and, in some cases, may approximate the pretreatment maternal BLL, implying limited efficacy for in utero fetal chelation. However, in these cases, the newborn's hemoglobin level was generally much higher than the mother's, and thus some of the maternal–neonatal difference in lead concentrations may simply reflect this difference in hemoglobin concentration and hence total blood lead content. In general, there currently seems little support for routine chelation therapy in pregnant women who would not otherwise warrant treatment based on their own symptoms or degree of elevated BLL. Calcium carbonate supplementation may be considered because its use is associated with decreased bone resorption during pregnancy and thus possibly lessened fetal lead exposure.[68]

Postnatally, infant BLLs may decline over time without chelation, but this occurs very slowly.[131] In two reported neonates exposed to prenatal maternal chelation who were then monitored for 2 weeks postpartum, the BLL remained stable or increased until chelation therapy was instituted.[113,156] In two additional cases of neonates whose mothers were not treated prepartum, BLLs also remained stable or increased for 17 days to 3 weeks.[50,150] Thus, postpartum chelation therapy is warranted for neonates, depending on BLLs, as per the guidelines described above for older children. Exchange transfusion might be considered for neonates with extremely elevated BLLs.[13] Succimer chelation therapy has also been reported for one neonate whose exposure was presumably caused by organolead via maternal gasoline sniffing.[119]

Lastly, the issue of allowing mothers with elevated BLLs to breastfeed their infants may arise. Breast milk from heavily exposed mothers may be a potential source of lead exposure and may require lead concentration analysis before breastfeeding can be safely recommended.[9,44] One small case series found that breast milk from two women with BLLs of 34 and 29 μg/dL, respectively, had clinically insignificant lead content (<0.01 μg/mL).[9] Breast milk analysis may be warranted in some cases, particularly with BLLs of 35 μg/dL or greater, before safely advising continued nursing. Despite these considerations, the majority of women without excessive lead exposure should still be encouraged to breastfeed. Of note, one study has found that a relatively simple intervention, calcium supplementation (1200 mg/day of elemental calcium as calcium carbonate), reduces breast milk lead content by 5% to 10%.[45]

SUMMARY

Lead is a widely distributed element that has long been used by humans for a variety of purposes, including waterproofing; electrical and radiation shielding; and the production of ammunitions, paints, plastics, ceramics, glass, and explosives. Lead poisoning, or plumbism, has an equally long history, but today it primarily manifests as an important environmental health problem for young children exposed to deteriorated lead paint and as an occupational toxic exposure for adult workers, although numerous other exposure sources are continually reported.

Lead causes multiorgan toxicity, affecting especially the hematologic and neurologic systems in patients of all ages and renal injury with hypertension in adults. This may result in a broad spectrum of clinical effects ranging from subtle neurocognitive effects to vague constitutional symptoms without overt physical signs to acute encephalopathy with potentially fatal cerebral edema and increased intracranial pressure. Several techniques have been used to estimate increases in body lead burden, but currently, the measurement of whole-blood lead concentration is favored.

The mainstays of treatment are removal from exposure and chelation therapy for patients with symptoms or significantly elevated body lead burdens. Defining a group of asymptomatic patients that will benefit from chelation therapy has been difficult and controversial. Parenteral chelation with $CaNa_2EDTA$ and BAL is efficacious in lowering BLLs and reducing mortality and morbidity from severe lead poisoning. Succimer, an oral chelator, also has efficacy in reducing BLLs in asymptomatic children.

REFERENCES

1. Agency for Toxic Substances and Disease Registry. *The Nature and Extent of Lead Poisoning in Children in the United States: A Report to Congress.* Atlanta: Agency for Toxic Substances and Disease Registry; 1988.
2. American Academy of Pediatrics, Committee on Drugs. Treatment guidelines for lead exposure in children. *Pediatrics.* 1995;96:155-160.
3. American Academy of Pediatrics, Committee on Environmental Health. Lead exposure in children: prevention, detection and management. *Pediatrics.* 2005;116:1036-1046.
4. Amitai Y, Graef JW, Brown MJ, et al. Hazards of "deleading" homes of children with lead poisoning. *Am J Dis Child.* 1987;141:758-760.
5. Angle CR. Childhood lead poisoning and its treatment. *Annu Rev Pharmacol Toxicol.* 1993;32:409-434.
6. Assennato G, Paci C, Molinini R, et al. Sperm count suppression without endocrine dysfunction in lead-exposed men. *Annu Rev Pharmacol Toxicol.* 1986;41:387-390.
7. Audesirk G. Electrophysiology of lead intoxication: effects on voltage-sensitive ion channels. *Neurotoxicology.* 1993;14:137-147.
8. Barltrop D, Meek F. Absorption of different lead compounds. *Postgrad Med J.* 1975;51:805-809.
9. Baum CR, Shannon MW. Lead in breast milk. *Pediatrics.* 1996;97:932.
10. Bolanowska W, Piotrowski J, Garczynski H. Triethyl lead in the biologic material in cases of acute tetraethyl lead poisoning. *Arch Toxicol.* 1967;22:278-282.
11. Borja-Aburto VH, Hertz-Picciotto I, Lopez MR, et al. Blood lead levels measured prospectively and risk of spontaneous abortion. *Am J Epidemiol.* 1999;150:590-597.
12. Burns CB, Currie B. The efficacy of chelation therapy and factors influencing mortality in lead intoxicated petrol sniffers. *Aust N Z J Med.* 1995;25(3):197-203.
13. Calello DP, Chinnakaruppan N, Fleischer G, et al. Are we ready for prime time? Prenatal lead screening [abstract]. *Clin Toxicol.* 2008;46:608.
14. Campbell C, Osterhoudt KC. Prevention of childhood lead poisoning. *Curr Opin Pediatr.* 2000;12:428-437.
15. Campbell JR, Auginer P. The association between blood lead levels and osteoporosis among adults—results from the Third National Health and Nutrition Examination Survey (NHANES III). *Environ Health Perspect.* 2007;115:1018-1022.
16. Canfield RL, Henderson CR, Cory-Slechta DA, et al. Intellectual impairment in children with blood lead concentrations below 10 μg per deciliter. *N Engl J Med.* 2003;348:1517-1526.
17. Centers for Disease Control and Prevention. Adult blood lead epidemiology and surveillance—United States, 2002. *MMWR Morb Mortal Wkly Rep.* 2004;578-585.
18. Centers for Disease Control and Prevention. Blood lead levels in the United States, 1999–2002. *MMWR Morb Mortal Wkly Rep.* 2005;54:513-516.
19. Centers for Disease Control and Prevention. Elevated blood lead levels in refugee children—New Hampshire, 2003–2004. *MMWR Morb Mortal Wkly Rep.* 2005;54:42-46.
20. Centers for Disease Control and Prevention. Fatal pediatric poisoning from leaded paint—Wisconsin, 1990. *MMWR Morb Mortal Wkly Rep.* 1991;40:193-195.
21. Centers for Disease Control and Prevention. Interpreting and managing blood lead levels <10 μg/dL in children and reducing childhood exposures to lead. *MMWR Morb Mortal Wkly Rep.* 2007;56[RR-8]:1-14.

22. Centers for Disease Control and Prevention. *Managing Elevated Blood Lead Levels Among Young Children: Recommendations from the Advisory Committee on Childhood Lead Poisoning Prevention.* Atlanta: Centers for Disease Control and Prevention; 2002.
23. Centers for Disease Control and Prevention. Potential exposure to lead in artificial turf. *CDC Health Alert Network (HAN) Advisory*; June18, 2008. Retrieved Feb 24, 2009, from http://www2a.cdc.gov/HAN/ArchiveSys/ViewMsgV.asp?AlertNum=00275.
24. Centers for Disease Control and Prevention. *Preventing Lead Poisoning in Young Children.* Atlanta: US Department of Health and Human Services; 2005.
25. Centers for Disease Control and Prevention. Recommendations for blood lead screening of young children enrolled in Medicaid: targeting a group at high risk. *MMWR Morb Mortal Wkly Rep.* 2000;49:1-13.
26. Centers for Disease Control and Prevention. *Screening Young Children for Lead Poisoning: Guidance for State and Local Public Health Officials.* Atlanta: Centers for Disease Control and Prevention; 1997.
27. Chan GM, Hoffman RS, Nelson LS. Get the lead out. *Ann Emerg Med.* 2004;44:551-2.
28. Charney E, Sayre J, Coulter M. Increased lead absorption in inner-city children: where does it come from. *Pediatrics.* 1980;65:226-231.
29. Cheng Y, Schwartz J, Vokonas PS, et al. Electrocardiographic conduction disturbances in association with low-level lead exposure (the Normative Aging Study). *Am J Cardiol.* 1998;82:594-599.
30. Chisolm JJ Jr. BAL, EDTA, DMSA, and DMPS in the treatment of lead poisoning in children. *J Toxicol Clin Toxicol.* 1992;30:493-504.
31. Chisolm JJ Jr. Mobilization of lead by calcium disodium edetate: a reappraisal. *Am J Dis Child.* 1987;141:1256-1257.
32. Chisolm JJ Jr. Safety and efficacy of meso-2,3-dimercaptosuccinic acid (DMSA) in children with elevated blood lead concentrations. *J Toxicol Clin Toxicol.* 2000;38:365-375.
33. Chisolm JJ Jr. The use of chelating agents in the treatment of acute and chronic lead intoxication in childhood. *J Pediatr.* 1968;73:1-38.
34. Chisolm JJ Jr, Harrison HE. The treatment of acute lead encephalopathy in children. *Pediatrics.* 1957;19:2-20.
35. Corey-Slechta DA. Relationships between lead-induced learning impairments and changes in dopaminergic, cholinergic, and glutamatergic neurotransmitter system functions. *Annu Rev Pharmacol Toxicol.* 1995;35:391-415.
36. Cremin JJ, Luck M, Laughlin N, Smith DR. Efficacy of succimer chelation for reducing brain lead in a primate model of human lead exposure. *Toxicol Appl Pharmacol.* 1999;161:283-293.
37. Cullen MR, Robins JM, Eskenazi B. Adult inorganic lead intoxication: presentation of 31 new cases and a review of the literature. *Medicine (Baltimore).* 1983;62:221-247.
38. Davoli CT, Serwint JR, Chisolm JJ Jr. Asymptomatic children with venous lead levels >100 μg/dL. *Pediatrics.* 1996;98:965-968.
39. DeRoos FJ. Smelters and metal reclaimers. In: Greenberg MI, Hamilton R, Phillips S, McCluskey GJ, eds. *Occupational, Industrial and Environmental Toxicology*, 2nd ed. St. Louis: Mosby-Year Book; 2003:388-397.
40. Dietrich KN, Ware JH, Salganik M, et al. Effect of chelation therapy on the neuropsychological and behavioral development of lead-exposed children after school entry. *Pediatrics.* 2004;114:19-26.
41. Dogu O, Louis ED, Tamer L, et al. Elevated blood lead concentrations in essential tremor: a case-control study in Mersin, Turkey. *Environ Health Perspect.* 2007;115:1564-1568.
42. Environmental Protection Agency. *Evaluation of Potential Carcinogenicity of Lead and Lead Compounds. EPA/600/8–89/0454A.* Washington, DC: US Environmental Protection Agency, Office of Health and Environmental Assessment; 1989.
43. Erenberg G, Rinsler SS, Fish BG. Lead neuropathy and sickle cell disease. *Pediatrics.* 1974;54:438-441.
44. Ettinger AS, Tellez-Rojo MM, Amarasiriwardena C, et al. Levels of breast milk lead and their relation to maternal blood and bone lead levels at one-month postpartum. *Environ Health Perspect.* 2004;112:926-931.
45. Ettinger AS, Tellez-Rojo MM, Amarasiriwardena C, et al. Influence of maternal bone lead burden and calcium intake on levels of lead in breast milk over the course of lactation. *Am J Epidemiol.* 2006;163:48-56.
46. Farrell SE, Vandevander P, Schoffstall JM, Lee DC. Blood lead levels in emergency department patients with retained bullets and shrapnel. *Acad Emerg Med.* 1999;6:208-212.
47. Fergusson L, Malecky G, Simpson E. Lead foreign body ingestion in children. *J Paediatr Child Health.* 1997;33:542-544.
48. Flaherty EG. Risk of lead poisoning in abused and neglected children. *Clin Pediatr.* 1995;34:128-132.
49. Friedman JA, Weinberger HL. Six children with lead poisoning. *Am J Dis Child.* 1990;144:1039-1044.
50. Ghafour SY, Khuffash FA, Ibrahim HS, Reavey PC. Congenital lead intoxication with seizures due to prenatal exposure. *Clin Pediatr.* 1984;23:282-283.
51. Goldstein GW. Neurologic concepts of lead poisoning in children. *Pediatr Ann.* 1992;21:384-388.
52. Gordon RA, Roberts G, Amin Z, et al. Aggressive approach in the treatment of acute lead encephalopathy with an extraordinarily high concentration of lead. *Arch Pediatr Adolesc Med.* 1998;152:1100-1104.
53. Goyer RA. Lead toxicity: current concerns. *Environ Health Perspect.* 1993;100:177-187.
54. Goyer RA. Toxic effects of metals. In: Klaassen CD, ed. *Casarett and Doull's Toxicology: The Basic Science of Poisons*, 5th ed. New York: McGraw-Hill; 1996:691-709.
55. Goyer RA, Cherian MG, Jones MM, Reigart JR. Role of chelating agents for prevention, intervention and treatment of exposures to toxic metals. *Environ Health Perspect.* 1995;103:1048-1052.
56. Goyer RA, Rhyne B. Pathologic effects of lead. *Int Rev Exp Pathol.* 1973;12:1-77.
57. Graziano JH, Lolacono NJ, Meyer P. Dose–response study of oral 2,3-dimercaptosuccinic acid in children with elevated blood lead concentrations. *J Pediatr.* 1988;113:751-757.
58. Graziano JH, Lolacono LJ, Moulton T, et al. Controlled study of meso-2,3-dimercaptosuccinic acid for the management of childhood lead intoxication. *J Pediatr.* 1992;120:133-139.
59. Graziano JH, Slavkovic V, Factor-Litvak P, et al. Depressed serum erythropoietin in pregnant women with elevated blood lead. *Arch Environ Health.* 1991;46:347-350.
60. Hammer LD, Ludwig S, Henretig F. Increased lead absorption in children with accidental ingestions. *Am J Emerg Med.* 1985;3:301-304.
61. Hansen KS, Sharp FR. Gasoline sniffing, lead poisoning and myoclonus. *JAMA.* 1978;240:1375-1376.
62. Heard MJ, Chamberlain AC. Effect of minerals and food on uptake of lead from the gastrointestinal tract in humans. *Hum Toxicol.* 1982;1:411-415.
63. Henretig FM, Shannon MW. Toxicologic emergencies. In: Fleisher GR, Ludwig S, eds. *Textbook of Pediatric Emergency Medicine*, 3rd ed. Baltimore: Williams & Wilkins; 1993:779-781.
64. Hu H, Milder FL, Burger DE. The use of K x-ray fluorescence for measuring lead burden in epidemiological studies: high and low lead burdens and measurement uncertainty. *Environ Health Perspect.* 1991;94:107-110.
65. Hu H, Shih R, Rothenberg S, et al. The epidemiology of lead toxicity in adults: measuring dose and consideration of other methodologies. *Environ Health Perspect.* 2007;115:455-462.
66. Huseman CA, Varma MM, Angle CR. Neuroendocrine effects of toxic and low blood lead levels in children. *Pediatrics.* 1992;90:186-189.
67. Jain NB, Potula V, Schwartz J, et al. Lead levels and ischemic heart disease in a prospective study of middle-aged and elderly men: the VA normative aging study. *Environ Health Perspect.* 2007;115:871-875.
68. Jarakiraman V, Ettinger A, Mercado-Garcia A, et al. Calcium supplements and bone resorption in pregnancy: a randomized crossover trial. *Am J Prev Med.* 2003;24:260-264.
69. Jiang X, Liang Y, Wang Y. Studies of lead exposure on reproductive system: a review of work in China. *Biomed Environ Sci.* 1992;5:266-275.
70. Jones RL, Homa DM, Meyer PA, et al. Trends in blood lead levels and blood lead testing among US children aged 1 to 5 years, 1988–2004. *Pediatrics.* 2009;123:e376-e385.
71. Jugo S, Malikovic T, Kostial K. Influence of chelating agents on the gastrointestinal absorption of lead. *Toxicol Appl Pharmacol.* 1975;34:259-263.
72. Kapoor SC, Wielopolski L, Graziano JH, Lolacono NJ. Influence of 2,3-dimercaptosuccinic acid on gastrointestinal lead absorption and whole body lead retention. *Toxicol Appl Pharmacol.* 1989;97:525-529.
73. Kari SK, Saper RB, Kales SN. Lead encephalopathy due to traditional medicines. *Curr Drug Saf.* 2008;3:54-59.
74. Keogh JP. Lead. In: Sullivan JB Jr, Krieger GR, eds. *Hazardous Materials Toxicology: Clinical Principles of Environmental Health.* Baltimore: Williams & Wilkins; 1992:834-844.
75. Kopp SJ, Glonek T, Erlander M, et al. The influence of chronic low-level cadmium and/or lead feeding on myocardial contractility related to phosphorylation of cardiac myofibrillar proteins. *Toxicol Appl Pharmacol.* 1980;54:48-56.

76. Kosnett MJ. Lead. In: Brent J, Wallace KL, Burkhart KK, et al (eds). *Critical Care Toxicology: Diagnosis and Management of the Critically Poisoned Patient.* Philadelphia: Elsevier Mosby; 2005:821-832.
77. Kosnett MJ. Unanswered questions in metal chelation. *J Toxicol Clin Toxicol.* 1992;30:529-547.
78. Kosnett MJ, Wedeen RP, Rothenberg SJ, et al. Recommendations for medical management of adult lead exposure. *Environ Health Perspect.* 2007;115:463-471.
79. Landrigan PJ, Baker EL Jr, Himmelstein JS, et al. Exposure to lead from the Mystic River bridge: the dilemma of deleading. *N Engl J Med.* 1982;306:673-676.
80. Levin R, Brown MJ, Kashtock ME, et al. Lead exposures in U.S. children: implications for prevention. *Environ Health Perspect.* 2008;116:1285-1293.
81. Lidsky TI, Schneider JS. Lead neurotoxicity in children: basic mechanisms and clinical correlates. *Brain.* 2003;126:5-19.
82. Liebelt EL, Shannon M, Graef JW. Efficacy of oral meso-2,3 dimercaptosuccinic acid therapy for low-level childhood plumbism. *J Pediatr.* 1994;1214:313-317.
83. Lifshitz M, Hashkanazi R, Phillip M. The effect of 2,3-dimercaptosuccinic acid in the treatment of lead poisoning in adults. *Ann Med.* 1997;29:83-85.
84. Lin J-L, Lin-Tan D-T, Hsu K-H, Yu C-C. Environmental lead exposure and progression of chronic renal diseases in patients without diabetes. *N Engl J Med.* 2003;348:277-286.
85. Linden MA, Manton WI, Stewart RM, et al. Lead poisoning from retained bullets: pathogenesis, diagnosis and management. *Ann Surg.* 1982;195:305-313.
86. Lipton ES, Barboza D. As more toys are recalled, trail ends in China. *The New York Times*; June 19, 2007.
87. Liu X, Dietrich KN, Radcliffe J, et al. Do children with falling blood lead levels have improved cognition? *Pediatrics.* 2002;110:787-791.
88. Mahaffey KR. Nutrition and lead: strategies for public health. *Environ Health Perspect.* 1995;103:191-196.
89. Mantere P, Hanninen H, Hernberg S, Luukkonen R. A prospective follow-up study on psychological effects in workers exposed to low levels of lead. *Scand J Work Environ.* Health 1984;10:43-50.
90. Marcus AH. Multicompartment kinetic modules for lead: linear kinetics and variable absorption in humans without excessive lead exposures. *Environ Res.* 1985;36:459-472.
91. Marcus SM. Treatment of lead-exposed children. *Pediatrics.* 1996;98:161-162.
92. Markovac J, Goldstein GW. Picomolar concentrations of lead stimulate brain protein kinase C. *Nature.* 1988;334:71-73.
93. Markowitz ME, Bijur PE, Ruff H, Rosen JF. Effects of calcium disodium versenate ($CaNa_2EDTA$) chelation in moderate childhood lead poisoning. *Pediatrics.* 1993;92:265-271.
94. Markowitz ME, Weinberger HL. Immobilization-related lead toxicity in previously lead-poisoned children. *Pediatrics.* 1990;86:455-457.
95. Maslinski PG, Loeb JA. Pica-associated cerebral edema in an adult. *J Neurol Sci.* 2004;225:149-151.
96. McCord CP. Lead and lead poisoning in early America. Benjamin Franklin and lead poisoning. *Industr Med Surg.* 1953;22:394-399.
97. McKinney PE. Acute elevation of blood lead levels within hours of ingestion of large quantities of lead shot. *J Toxicol Clin Toxicol.* 2000;38:435-440.
98. Meggs WJ, Gerr F, Aly MH, et al. The treatment of lead poisoning from gunshot wounds with succimer (DMSA). *J Toxicol Clin Toxicol.* 1994;32:377-385.
99. Menke A, Muntner P, Batuman V, et al. Blood lead below 0.48 μmol/L (10 μg/dL) and mortality among US adults. *Circulation.* 2006:114:1388-1394.
100. Moore MR, Meredith PA, Watson WS, et al. The percutaneous absorption of lead-203 in humans from cosmetic preparations containing lead acetate, as assessed by whole-body counting and other techniques. *Food Cosmet Toxicol.* 1980;18:399-405.
101. Mortensen ME. Succimer chelation: what is known? *J Pediatr.* 1994;125:233-234.
102. Mortensen ME, Walson PD. Chelation therapy for childhood lead poisoning—the changing scene in the 1990s. *Clin Pediatr.* 1993;32:284-291.
103. Mowad E, Haddad I, Gemmel DJ. Management of lead poisoning from ingested fishing sinkers. *Arch Pediatr Adolesc Med.* 1998;152:485-488.
104. Mushak P, Davis JM, Crocewtti AF, Grant LD. Pre-natal and post-natal effects of low-level lead exposure: integrated summary of a report to the US Congress on childhood lead poisoning. *Environ Res.* 1989;50:11-36.
105. Needleman HL. The persistent threat of lead: medical and sociological issues. *Curr Probl Pediatr.* 1988;18:702-744.
106. Needleman HL, Gunnoe C, Leviton A, et al. Deficits in psychological and classroom performance of children with elevated dentine lead levels. *N Engl J Med.* 1979;300:689-695.
107. Nortier JWR, Sangster B, Van Kestern RG. Acute lead poisoning with hemolysis and liver toxicity after ingestion of red lead. *Vet Hum Toxicol.* 1980;22:145-147.
108. Norton RL, Weinstein L, Rafalski T, et al. Acute intravenous lead poisoning in a drug abuser: associated complications of hepatitis, pancreatitis, hemolysis and renal failure [abstract]. *Vet Hum Toxicol.* 1989;31:340.
109. Nriagu JO. Saturnine gout among Roman aristocrats. *N Engl J Med.* 1983;308:660-663.
110. Onalaja AO, Claudio L. Genetic susceptibility to lead poisoning. *Environ Health Perspect.* 2000;108(suppl 1):23-28.
111. Paglia DE, Valentine WN, Dahlgner JG. Effects of low level lead exposure on pyrimidine-5'-nucleotidase and other erythrocyte enzymes. *J Clin Invest.* 1976;56:1164-1169.
112. Pearce WG. More on retinal stippling. *N Engl J Med.* 1964;270:533-534.
113. Pearl M, Boxt LM. Radiographic findings in congenital lead poisoning. *Radiology.* 1980;136:83-84.
114. Peterson KE, Salganik M, Campbell C, et al. Effect of succimer on growth of preschool children with moderate blood lead levels. *Environ Health Perspect.* 2004;112:233-237.
115. Piomelli S, Rosen JF, Chisolm JJ Jr, Graef JW. Management of childhood lead poisoning. *J Pediatr.* 1984;105:523-532.
116. Pirkle JL, Schwartz J, Landis JR, Harlan WR. The relationship between blood lead levels and blood pressure and its cardiovascular risk implications. *Am J Epidemiol.* 1985;121:246-258.
117. Pocock SJ, Smith M, Baghurst P. Environmental lead and children's intelligence: a systematic review of the epidemiological evidence. *Br Med J.* 1994;309:1189-1197.
118. Porru S, Alessio L. The use of chelating agents in occupational lead poisoning. *Occup Med.* 1996;46:41-48.
119. Powell ST, Bolisetty S, Wheaton GR. Succimer therapy for congenital lead poisoning from maternal petrol sniffing. *Med J Aust.* 2006;184:84-85.
120. Raber SA. The dense metaphyseal band sign. *Radiology.* 1999;211:773-774.
121. Rabinowitz MB, Needleman HL. Temporal trends in the lead concentrations of umbilical cord blood. *Science.* 1982;216:1429-1431.
122. Rabinowitz MB, Wetherill GW, Kopple JD. Kinetic analysis of lead metabolism in healthy humans. *J Clin Invest.* 1976;58:260-270.
123. Regan CM. Neural cell adhesion molecules, neuronal development and lead toxicity. *Neurotoxicology.* 1993;14:69-74.
124. Rempel D. The lead-exposed worker. *JAMA.* 1989;262:532-534.
125. Restek-Samarzija N, Samarzija M, Momcilovic B. Ventricular arrhythmia in acute lead poisoning: a case report [abstract]. Presented at the EAPCCT XVI International Congress, Vienna, Austria; April 1994.
126. Rhoads GG, Rogan WJ. Treatment of lead-exposed children. *Pediatrics.* 1996;98:162-163.
127. Rodamilans M, Martinez-Osaba MJ, To-Figueras J, et al. Lead toxicity on endocrine testicular function in an occupationally exposed population. *Hum Toxicol.* 1988;7:125-128.
128. Rogan W, Dietrich K, Ware J, Dockery D, et al, for the Treatment of Lead-Exposed Children (TLC) Trial Group. The effect of chelation therapy with succimer on neuropsychological development in children exposed to lead. *N Engl J Med.* 2001;344:1421-1426.
129. Romeo R, Aprea C, Boccalon P, et al. Serum erythropoietin and blood lead concentrations. *Int Arch Occup Environ Health.* 1996;69:73-75.
130. Royce SE, Needleman HL. *Case Studies in Environmental Medicine. Lead Toxicity.* Atlanta: Agency for Toxic Substances and Disease Registry; 1992.
131. Ryu JE, Ziegler EE, Fomon SJ. Maternal lead exposure and blood lead concentration in infancy. *J Pediatr.* 1978;93:476-478.
132. Sandstead HH, Orth DN, Abe K, et al. Lead intoxication: effect on pituitary and adrenal function in man. *Clin Res.* 1970;18:76.
133. Sandstead HH, Stant EG, Brill AB, et al. Lead intoxication and the thyroid. *Arch Intern Med.* 1969;123:632-635.
134. Schwartz BS, Stewart WF, Bolla KI, et al. Past adult lead exposure is associated with longitudinal decline in cognitive function. *Neurology.* 2000;55:1144-1150.
135. Saryan LA, Zenz C. Lead and its compounds. In: Zenz C, Dickerson OB, Horvath EP Jr, eds. *Occupational Medicine*, 3rd ed. St. Louis: Mosby; 1994:506-541.

136. Schaumberg DA, Mendes F, Balaram M, et al. Accumulated lead exposure and risk of age-related cataract in men. *JAMA*. 2004;292:2750-2754.
137. Schwartz BS, Hu H. Adult lead exposure: time for change. *Environ Health Perspect*. 2007;115:451-4.
138. Selbst SM, Henretig FM, Pierce J. Lead encephalopathy in a child with sickle cell disease. *Clin Pediatr*. 1985;24:280-285.
139. Selbst SM, Henretig F, Fee MA, et al. Lead poisoning in a child with a gunshot wound. *Pediatrics*. 1986;77:413-416.
140. Seward JP. Occupational lead exposure and management. *West J Med*. 1996;165:222-224.
141. Shannon MW. Lead poisoning treatment—a continuing need. *J Toxicol Clin Toxicol*. 2001;39:661-663.
142. Shannon MW. Severe lead poisoning in pregnancy. *Ambul Pediatr*. 2003;3:37-39.
143. Shannon MW, Townsend MK. Adverse effects of reduced dose D-penicillamine in children with mild-moderate lead poisoning. *Ann Pharmacother*. 2000;34:15-18.
144. Shen J, Hirschtick R. Getting the lead out. *N Engl J Med*. 2004;351:1996.
145. Shih RA, Hu H, Weisskopf MG, et al. Cumulative lead dose and cognitive function in adults: a review of studies that measured both blood lead and bone lead. *Environ Health Perspect*. 2007;115:483-492.
146. Silbergeld EK. Facilitative mechanisms of lead as a carcinogen. *Mutat Res*. 2003;533:121-133.
147. Silbergeld EK, Scwartz J, Mahaffey K. Lead and osteoporosis: mobilization of lead from bone in post-menopausal women. *Environ Res*. 1988;47:79-94.
148. Silver W, Rodriguez-Torres R. Electrocardiographic studies in children with lead poisoning. *Pediatrics*. 1968;41:1124-1127.
149. Simons TJB. Cellular interactions between lead and calcium. *Br Med Bull*. 1986;42:431-434.
150. Singh N, Donovan CM, Hanshaw JB. Neonatal lead intoxication in a prenatally exposed infant. *J Pediatr*. 1978;93:1019-1021.
151. Sonkin N. Stippling of the retina—a new physical sign in the early diagnosis of lead poisoning. *N Engl J Med*. 1963;269:779-780.
152. Staes C, Matte T, Staeling N, et al. Lead poisoning deaths in the United States, 1979-1988. *JAMA*. 1995;273:847-848.
153. Steele D. Neurosurgical emergencies, nontraumatic. In: Fleisher GR, Ludwig S, Henretig FM (eds). *Textbook of Pediatric Emergency Medicine*, 5th edition. Philadelphia: Lippincott Williams & Wilkins; 2006:1717-1725.
154. Suarez CR, Black LE 3d, Hurley RM. Elevated lead levels in a patient with sickle cell disease and inappropriate secretion of antidiuretic hormone. *Pediatr Emerg Care*. 1992;8:88-90.
155. Tenenbein M. Leaded gasoline abuse: the role of tetraethyl lead. *Hum Exp Toxicol*. 1997;16:217-222.
156. Tinapu AE, Amin JS, Casalino MB, Yuceoglu AM. Congenital lead intoxication. *J Pediatr*. 1979;94:765-767.
157. Treatment of Lead-Exposed Children (TLC) Trial Group: Safety and efficacy of succimer in toddlers with blood lead levels of 20–44 μg/dL. *Pediatr Res*. 2000;48:593-599.
158. Tyroler HA. Epidemiology of hypertension as a public health problem: an overview as background for evaluation of blood lead-blood pressure relationship. *Environ Health Perspect*. 1988;78:3-8.
159. US Department of the Interior. *Minerals Yearbook for 1990*, vol 1. Washington, DC: Government Printing Office; 1991.
160. US Department of Labor, Occupational Safety and Health Administration: Lead *Exposure in Construction—Interim Final Rule* (29 CFR part 1926.62). *Fed Reg*. May 4, 1993.
161. US Department of Labor, Occupational Safety and Health Administration: Lead *Standard* (20 CFR 1910.1025; revised July 1, 1990). Washington, DC: US Government Printing Office; 1990.
162. US Department of Labor, Occupational Safety and Health Administration. *Occupational health and safety standard: occupational exposure to lead* (29 CFR 1910.1025). *Fed Reg*. 1978;42:52952-53014.
163. VanArsdale JL, Leiker RD, Kohn M, et al. Lead poisoning from a toy necklace. *Pediatrics*. 2004;114:1096-1099.
164. Vander AJ. Chronic effects of lead on renin-angiotensin system. *Environ Health Perspect*. 1988;78:77-83.
165. Wade JF, Burnum JF. Treatment of acute and chronic lead poisoning with disodium calcium versenate. *Ann Intern Med*. 1955;42:251-259.
166. Wedeen RP, Ty A, Udasin I, et al. Clinical application of in vivo tibial K-XRF for monitoring lead stores. *Arch Environ Health*. 1995;50:355-361.
167. White LD, Cory-Slechta DA, Gilbert ME, et al. New and evolving concepts in the *Neurotoxicology*. of lead. *Toxicol Appl Pharm*. 2007;225:1-27.
168. Whitfield CL, Ch'ien LT, Whitehead JD. Lead encephalopathy in adults. *Am J Med*. 1972;52:289-297.
169. Wiley J, Henretig F, Foster R. Status epilepticus and severe neurologic impairment from lead encephalopathy, November 1994 [abstract]. *J Toxicol Clin Toxicol*. 1995;33:529-530.
170. Wiley JF II, Henretig FM, Selbst SM. Blood lead levels in children with foreign bodies. *Pediatrics*. 1992;89:593-596.
171. Wills BK, Christensen J, Mazzoncini J, Miller M. Tetraethyl lead intoxication. *J Med Toxicol*. 2010 (March), in press.
172. Woolf AD, Goldman R, Bellinger DC. Update on the clinical management of childhood lead poisoning. *Pediatr Clin N Am*. 2007;54:271-294.
173. Ziegler EE, Edwards BB, Jensen RL, et al. Absorption and retention of lead by infants. *Pediatr Res*. 1978;12:29-34.

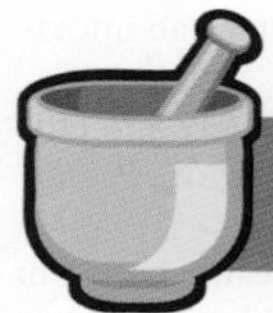

ANTIDOTES IN DEPTH (A27)

SUCCIMER (2,3-DIMERCAPTOSUCCINIC ACID)

Mary Ann Howland

Succimer
2,3-Dimercaptosuccinic acid

DMPS
2,3-Dimercapto-1-propanesulfonic acid

Succimer (meso-2,3-dimercaptosuccinic acid) is an orally active metal chelator that is approved by the Food and Drug Administration (FDA) for the treatment of lead poisoning in children with blood lead concentrations greater than 45 μg/dL. Succimer is also used to treat patients poisoned with arsenic and organic and inorganic mercury. Succimer has a wider therapeutic index and exhibits many advantages over dimercaprol and edetate calcium disodium ($CaNa_2EDTA$), the two other chelators used for the same clinical problems. Animal studies suggest that succimer does not redistribute lead or arsenic to the central nervous system (CNS). The role of succimer alone and in conjunction with other chelators to treat lead encephalopathy continues to be defined.[61,74]

HISTORY

Succimer was initially synthesized in 1949 in England.[72] In 1954, antimony-a,a′-dimercaptopotassium succinate (TWSb) was developed to treat schistosomiasis.[43] TWSb is antimony bound to the potassium salt of succimer in a 2:3 ratio, forming a water-soluble xenobiotic with 50 times less toxicity than the previously used antimony compound, tartar emetic. Several years later, a group from Shanghai demonstrated the ability of the sodium salt of succimer to increase the median lethal dose for 50% of test subjects (LD_{50}) of tartar emetic 16-fold in mice.[109] An early review of the Chinese experience with intravenous (IV) succimer in the treatment of occupational lead and mercury poisoning suggested efficacy similar to IV $CaNa_2EDTA$ in increasing urinary lead and to intramuscular (IM) DMPS (racemic-2,3-dimercapto-1-propanesulfonic acid, unithiol) for mercury, with little observed toxicity.[105] This experience, the subsequent widespread use in Asia[76,79,90,105,106,111] and Europe,[17,34,41,44,64,99] and the realization that succimer could be used orally,[7,50] led to US-based animal experiments, human trials, and FDA approval in 1991 for the treatment of lead-poisoned children.

PHARMACOLOGY AND PHARMACOKINETICS

Succimer is a white crystalline powder with a molecular weight of 182 daltons and a characteristic sulfur odor and taste.[6] Succimer is the meso form of 2,3-dimercaptosuccinic acid; the racemic form is being investigated.[38] Because it contains four ionizable hydrogen ions, succimer has four different pK_as—2.31, 3.69, 9.68, and 11.14—with the dissociation of the two lower values representing the carboxyl groups and the two higher values the sulfur groups.[4] Lead and cadmium bind to the adjoining sulfur and oxygen atoms, whereas arsenic and mercury bind to the two sulfur moieties, forming pH-dependent water-soluble complexes (see Fig. A27–1).[86] Succimer is highly protein bound to albumin through a disulfide bond. Subhuman primate studies of IV and oral ^{22}C succimer indicate that following an IV dose, radiolabel is eliminated almost exclusively via the kidney, with only trace amounts (less than 1%) excreted via feces or expired air.[72] Following the administration of a single oral dose of 10 mg/kg, succimer is rapidly and extensively metabolized.[69] Approximately 20% of the administered oral dose is recovered in the urine, presumably reflecting the low bioavailability of the drug.[10] Of the total drug eliminated in the urine, 89% is altered and in the form of disulfides of l-cysteine. The majority of the altered succimer is in the form of a mixed disulfide with two molecules of l-cysteine to one molecule of succimer.[8] The remaining 11% is excreted as unaltered free succimer.[69] Maximal excretion of succimer occurs in urine specimens collected between 2 and 4 hours after administration. Surprisingly, the blood only contains albumin-bound succimer and no evidence of the altered disulfide moieties, which suggests that the kidney may be involved in the biotransformation of succimer.

The pharmacokinetics of a single oral dose of succimer were determined in three children and three adults with lead poisoning, and in five healthy adult volunteers.[33] Children received 350 mg/m² of succimer, and adults received 10 mg/kg of succimer. The peak concentration and the time to peak blood concentration of total succimer (parent versus altered oxidized metabolites) were similar for all three groups. The half-life of total succimer was 1.5 times longer in the children than in either adult group. The renal clearance of total succimer was greater in healthy adults than in lead-poisoned patients. Distribution of succimer (parent and/or oxidized metabolites) into erythrocytes appeared greater in poisoned patients than in the healthy adults.[33]

The metabolism of succimer was studied in lead-poisoned children and in normal adults.[15] The results indicate that succimer undergoes an enterohepatic circulation facilitated by gastrointestinal (GI) microflora. Similar to the previous pharmacokinetic study, moderate lead exposure impaired the renal elimination of succimer.

USE FOR LEAD EXPOSURE

In addition to precise analysis of metal elimination kinetics, measures of clinical outcome are essential for an understanding of the utility of this chelator. The Treatment of Lead-Exposed Children (TLC) trial was a step in that direction.[102] The TLC trial was a randomized, multicenter, double-blind, placebo-controlled, ongoing study to examine the effects of succimer on cognitive development, behavior, stature, and blood pressure in children 1 to 3 years old with blood lead concentrations between

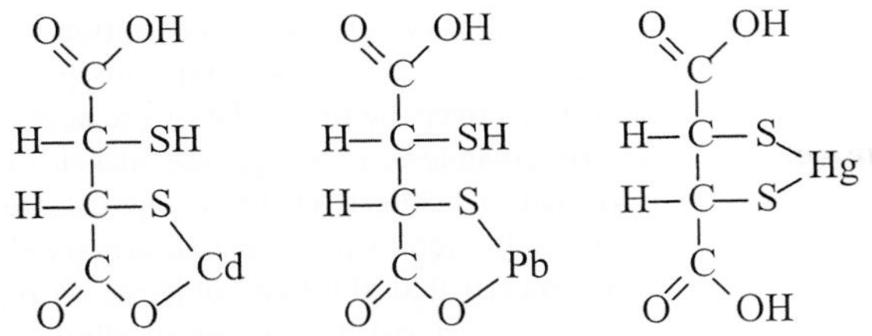

FIGURE A27–1. The chelation of cadmium, lead, and mercury with succimer.

20 and 44 μg/dL. In 2000 no beneficial effects on neuropsychological tests administered to those children was reported.[101] A follow-up study also demonstrated that although succimer lowered average blood lead concentrations, no beneficial effects on neuropsychological and behavioral development could be demonstrated in those children at 7 years old.[35] A case study showed similar results.[20] Similarly succimer showed no benefit on growth in children aged 12 to 33 months with blood lead concentrations of 20 to 44 μg/dL.[83]

Several groups are studying the efficacy of succimer in reducing blood, brain, and tissue lead by using rat and nonhuman primate models of childhood and adult lead poisoning.[91,92,94] Although monkeys most closely resemble humans in their lead-associated toxicity, using them in studies is costly[78]; the rat model is economical but limited because of species differences in lead and succimer metabolism and efficacy.

The validity of using blood lead concentrations as a marker of brain lead was studied in the adult rhesus monkey. Lead was administered orally for 5 weeks to achieve a target blood lead concentration of 35 to 40 μg/dL.[32] Five days after lead exposure ceased, succimer chelation was initiated in the currently approved dosage regimen. Two IV doses of radioactive lead tracer were administered prior to succimer chelation to study the kinetics of recent versus chronic lead uptake and distribution. Four areas of the brain, as well as blood and bone, were assayed for lead. Merely stopping further lead exposure significantly reduced blood lead concentrations by 63% and brain lead concentrations by 34% compared with pretreatment concentrations, and was not statistically different from succimer administration after halting exposure. However, when an integrated area under the serum lead concentration versus time curve (AUC) blood analysis was used over the 19-day succimer treatment course, instead of a single blood lead concentration, the differences between succimer and control were statistically significant. The clinical significance of these differences is unclear. Succimer-treated animals showed the greatest drop in blood lead concentrations over the first 5 days, while a similar end point was gradually achieved in the control. The lead from both the recent exposure (radioactive tracer lead) and chronic exposure declined to the same extent, independent of treatment with succimer. A better correlation was found between brain prefrontal cortex lead concentrations and an integrated blood lead analysis than with a single blood lead measurement.

Similarly, a study in neonatal rats demonstrated that increasing the duration of succimer chelation from 7 to 21 days decreased brain lead concentrations without a corresponding decrease in blood lead concentrations.[91] The authors proposed that a slow rate of egress of brain lead to the blood was responsible for the demonstrable benefit of prolonging therapy to 21 days. In this study, succimer decreased blood lead concentration by approximately 50% when compared to the vehicle as control, and this difference persisted for the 21 days of treatment. With succimer treatment, brain lead concentration decreased by 38% at 7 days and by 68% at 21 days. This same group also demonstrated that rats exposed to lead from postnatal day 1 to 30, then treated with succimer, demonstrated reductions in blood and brain lead concentrations and an improvement in cognitive deficits.[95]

revious animal studies demonstrated the ability of succimer to enhance urinary lead elimination[42,50,94] and to reduce blood,[16,30,39,40,55,81,92,94,96,98] brain,[16,30,81,97,98] liver,[94] and kidney lead concentrations,[16,30,39,55,81,98] while either reducing[16,55,81,98] or demonstrating no effect on bone lead concentrations.[30,94] These studies differ in the amounts and duration of lead administration prior to chelation, as well as in route, dose, and duration of chelation, but several months after a course of succimer chelation, tissue lead concentrations had returned to concentrations found in the pretreatment stage.[30] Given the limited absolute amount of lead that is actually eliminated by chelation in comparison to the total body burden, particularly bone, these transient effects are not surprising.

Under a variety of experimental conditions in animals, succimer prevents the deleterious effect of lead on heme synthesis,[16,50,81] blood pressure,[59] and behavior.[96]

Published studies of the use of succimer in both children and adults with chronic lead poisoning demonstrated consistent findings.[18,27,51–53,65,77] During the first 5 days of succimer chelation (1050 $mg/m^2/d$ in children, 30 mg/kg/d in adults both in 3 divided doses), the blood lead concentration dropped precipitously by approximately 60% to 70%. This blood lead concentration remained unchanged during the next 14 to 23 days of continued therapy. Increases in urinary lead excretion are concurrent with the drop in blood lead concentration, with maximal excretion occurring on day 1.[27,52] Calculations indicate that urinary lead excretion exceeds estimated blood content. This suggests that some lead is being removed from soft tissues as a concentration gradient is established from tissue to blood to urine.[27,53] Typically, 2 weeks after the completion of succimer, blood lead concentration rebounds to values 20% to 40% lower than pretreatment values. In the one randomized, double-blind, placebo-controlled trial of succimer use in children with pretreatment blood lead concentrations of 30 to 45 μg/dL, follow-up at 1 month and at 6 months showed no differences between succimer-treated children and controls.[77] Succimer restores red blood cell D-aminolevulinic acid dehydratase (ALA-D) activity, decreases erythrocyte protoporphyrin, and decreases urinary excretion of D-aminolevulinic acid and coproporphyrin.[18,27,52,53,77]

There is a large body of evidence reporting on the usage and safety profile of succimer in adults with chronic lead poisoning.[13,17,27,41,44,45,48,49,60,62,70,84,100,103] The published experience outside the United States with the use of oral succimer for metal poisoning includes nearly 100 adult cases and contributes considerably to the supporting evidence. At least 74 additional individuals have been successfully treated parenterally (IM or IV) with the sodium salt of succimer.[13,17,41,44]

USE FOR LEAD ENCEPHALOPATHY

The experience with the use of succimer in severely lead-poisoned subjects, including those with encephalopathy, is very limited.[41,44,52] Three children with mean blood lead concentrations of greater than 70 μg/dL who were treated with 5 days of succimer achieved comparable declines in blood lead concentration to two similar children who had been treated previously with a combination of British anti-Lewisite (BAL) for 3 days and $CaNa_2EDTA$ for 5 days.[52] Three adult patients with encephalopathy achieved significant improvement following succimer chelation.[41] A 3-year-old child with a massive lead exposure superimposed on chronic lead poisoning and a blood lead concentration of 550 μg/dL was given BAL and $CaNa_2EDTA$ for 5 days, with whole-bowel irrigation (WBI) performed on the first 3 days and succimer following WBI beginning on day 3 and continuing for 19 days. The blood lead concentration dropped from 550 μg/dL to 70 μg/dL on day 5, but rebounded to 99 μg/dL 2 days after BAL and $CaNa_2EDTA$, but not the succimer, were discontinued.[47]

USE OF SUCCIMER FOR ARSENIC EXPOSURE

Succimer has been used for arsenic toxicity in China and the Soviet Union since 1965.[7,13] Animal studies with sodium arsenite and lewisite demonstrate the ability of succimer to improve the LD_{50} with a good therapeutic index, lack of redistribution of arsenic to the brain as compared to BAL or control, and reduced kidney and liver arsenic concentrations.[7,13,63,82,87] A few case reports attest to the ability of succimer to enhance the urinary excretion of arsenic[31,88] and presumably normalize urinary arsenic concentrations following ingestion of arsenic trioxide ant bait by toddlers.[107] A randomized, placebo-controlled trial of succimer to treat 21 patients with chronic arsenic poisoning in India demonstrated improved clinical results and enhanced urinary excretion in both the treatment and placebo groups, but no statistical differences could be demonstrated.[71] A comparison of BAL, succimer, and DMPS as arsenic antidotes demonstrated higher therapeutic indices for succimer and DMPS over BAL in chronic arsenic poisoning.[75]

USE OF SUCCIMER FOR MERCURY EXPOSURE

Succimer enhances the elimination of mercury and has been used to treat patients poisoned with inorganic, elemental, and methylmercury. It improves survival, decreases renal damage, and enhances elimination of mercury in animals following exposure to inorganic mercury[4,22,55,58,66,85,110] and methylmercury.[1,2,9,67] However, one study in mice subjected to intraperitoneal mercuric chloride demonstrated an enhanced deposition of mercury in motor neurons following chelation with succimer or DMPS.[37] Of 53 construction workers who were exposed to mercury vapor, 11 received succimer and *N*-acetyl-*d*,*l*-penicillamine in a crossover study.[21] Mercury elimination was increased during the period of succimer administration compared with the period of *N*-acetyl-*d*,*l*-penicillamine administration. Because the chelators were administered for only 2 weeks and late in the clinical course, therapeutic benefit could not be evaluated. When succimer was given to victims of an extensive Iraqi methylmercury exposure, blood methylmercury half-life decreased from 63 days to 10 days.[7]

ADVERSE EFFECTS AND SAFETY ISSUES

Succimer is generally well tolerated with few serious adverse events reported.[27,28] Common adverse effects are gastrointestinal in nature, including nausea, vomiting, flatus, diarrhea, and a metallic taste in 10% to 20% of patients. Mild elevations in aspartate aminotransferase (AST) and alanine aminotransferase (ALT) are reported.[26,28,53,65,80] A single patient developed severe hyperthermia and hypotension reportedly related to succimer administration.[80] Rarely, chills, fever, urticaria, rash, reversible neutropenia, and eosinophilia are reported.[18,27,28,48] During the latest open-label prospective study in children, apparently unrelated adverse events included an elevation in bone-derived alkaline phosphatase, eosinophils, and elevated serum aminotransferases.[27]

The Chinese have reported a high incidence of more serious adverse effects (including dizziness and weakness) in response to IV or IM succimer.[106,111] This discrepancy is undoubtedly related to the substantially greater dose of succimer delivered from parenteral administration compared with the relatively low (approximately 20%)[72] oral bioavailability of succimer as a result of first-pass metabolism.

Incidental chelation of essential elements is always a concern with the use of chelators. A number of studies using succimer demonstrate no rise in urinary zinc, copper, iron, or calcium.[27,41,44,51–53] Urinary excretion of essential elements was the focus of a study in a primate model of childhood lead exposure.[92] Infant rhesus monkeys were exposed to lead for the first year of life to achieve blood lead concentrations of 40 to 50 μg/dL. Succimer was administered in the standard dosage regimen and complete urine collections over the first 5 days were analyzed for calcium, cobalt, copper, iron, magnesium, manganese, nickel, and zinc. Only when the data were analyzed collectively for all eight elements on all 5 days was there a statistically significant increased urinary elimination. These results raise concern that children subjected to repeated succimer chelation may also be at risk for enhanced elimination of essential elements.[27,92,94] An obvious concern regarding the safety of succimer is that there is still relatively limited clinical experience with the xenobiotic, particularly with regard to long-term administration.

One concern with administering succimer orally is that outpatient management might permit continued unintentional lead exposure and the possibility for succimer-facilitated lead absorption. Studies with D-penicillamine, dimercaprol,[56] and $CaNa_2EDTA$ demonstrate enhanced lead absorption and elevated blood lead concentrations.

Most blood lead concentrations are measured by graphite furnace atomic absorption spectrophotometry, in which case succimer does not interfere with the measurement. However, if blood lead concentrations were to be measured by anodic stripping voltammetry, succimer would affect the results by chelating the mercury in the electrode.[24] Succimer may cause a false-positive result for urinary ketones when tests using nitroprusside reagents (eg, Ketostix) are used, and a falsely decreased serum uric acid and creatine phosphokinase (CPK) may occur.[24]

Animal studies suggest that succimer does not promote lead retention in the setting of continued exposure unless lead exposure is overwhelming.[50,57,81] A radiolabeled lead tracer administered to adult volunteers suggested that succimer increased the net absorption of lead from the GI tract and may have distributed it to other tissues, as well as having enhanced urinary elimination.[93] Absorption is bimodal and consistent with an initial phase, followed by a delayed increase attributable to an enterohepatic effect. It may be that succimer-enhanced urinary lead elimination often exceeds enhanced lead absorption.[82] One study reported two children with environmental exposure and dramatic rises in blood lead concentration while receiving succimer.[27] In the event of unintentional exposure to a new lead source, decontamination of the GI tract should complement oral succimer.[73]

Although iron supplementation cannot be given concomitantly with BAL, because the BAL–iron complex may be a potent emetic, iron has been given concomitantly to patients receiving oral succimer without any adverse effects.[54] The prevalence of both iron deficiency and elevated blood lead concentrations is highest among poor, inner-city children.[68] Because heme is a constituent of all cells, including those of the brain, it appears clinically prudent to provide iron supplementation during chelation therapy, when the heme pathway is freed of the inhibitory effects of lead. The timing of administration of the iron should be separate from administration of the succimer.[27]

A case report describes a 3-year-old child who reportedly ingested 185 mg/kg of succimer and was asymptomatic.[89]

USE IN PREGNANCY

The use of succimer in pregnancy is restricted to women who warrant therapy based on their symptoms.[27] There was a dose-dependent effect of succimer on early and late fetal resorption and on fetal body weight and length when succimer was administered to pregnant mice during organogenesis. No observed teratogenic effects were noted when 410 mg/kg, or approximately 5% of the acute LD_{50}, of succimer was administered subcutaneously.[36] However, doses of 410 to 1640 mg/kg/d of succimer administered subcutaneously to pregnant mice during organogenesis is teratogenic and fetotoxic, and doses of more than 510 mg/kg/d to pregnant rats also showed problems with reflexes in the offspring.[24] Succimer 30 to 60 mg/kg/d was administered by gavage to lead-poisoned rats from day 6 to day 21 of gestation.[25] These doses of succimer decreased embryonic and fetal blood lead concentrations and normalized offspring body weight at 13 weeks. Although succimer was able to reverse some lead-induced immunotoxic effects, succimer itself caused problems with the immune system that persisted into adulthood.[25] Female mice exposed to lead in utero and then administered succimer from the fourth day of gestation to parturition demonstrated decreased blood lead concentrations; however, fetal liver and bone concentrations increased and worsened neural development in the offspring.[108]

COMBINED CHELATION THERAPY

Succimer can be combined with $CaNa_2EDTA$ to take advantage of the ability of succimer to remove lead from soft tissues, including the brain, while capitalizing on the ability of $CaNa_2EDTA$ to mobilize lead from bone.[30] A number of rodent models have examined this combination and found it to be superior in enhancing the elimination of lead, in reducing tissue concentrations of lead, and in restoring some lead-induced biochemical abnormalities.[39,40,97] Although the addition of succimer to $CaNa_2EDTA$ prevented the redistribution of lead to the brain caused by $CaNa_2EDTA$ alone, the combination also increased urinary excretion of zinc, calcium, and iron.[97,98] A retrospective review comparing dimercaprol plus $CaNa_2EDTA$ to succimer plus $CaNa_2EDTA$ in children with blood lead concentrations greater than 45 µg/mL, demonstrated a similar reduction in blood lead concentrations at the end of treatment and at 14 and 33 days following the termination of treatment.[19] Blood lead concentration reductions were approximately 75%, 40%, and 37% at the end of therapy, and at 14 and 33 days posttreatment, respectively. The succimer plus $CaNa_2EDTA$ combination was better tolerated.

DMPS

DMPS (racemic-2,3-dimercapto-1-propanesulfonic acid, Na salt) is a chelator that, like succimer, is a water-soluble analog of BAL.[7,9,23] A dose of 15 mg/kg of DMPS is equimolar to 12 mg/kg of succimer. DMPS was used in the Soviet Union since the late 1950s and continues to be used in Russia and other former Soviet countries. DMPS, which is an investigational drug in the United States, is marketed in both oral and parenteral forms in Germany as Dimaval. DMPS seems promising in mercury and arsenic poisoning.[3,5,7,9,11,14,23,46] DMPS is associated with an increase in the urinary excretion of copper and the development of Stevens-Johnson syndrome.[26,104] Like succimer, DMPS does not appear to redistribute mercury or lead to the brain. More research is needed to determine whether DMPS is more advantageous than succimer, given its lower LD_{50} in rodents (5.22 mmol/kg versus 16.5 mmol/kg for succimer).

DOSING AND AVAILABILITY

Succimer (Chemet) is available as 100-mg bead-filled capsules. For patients who cannot swallow the capsule whole, it can be separated immediately prior to use and the contents sprinkled into a small amount of juice or on apple sauce, ice cream, or soft food, or placed on a spoon and followed by a fruit drink. The dosage is 350 mg/m^2 in children, three times a day for 5 days, followed by 350 mg/m^2 twice a day for 14 days. In adults, the dosage is 10 mg/kg three times a day for 5 days followed by 10 mg/kg twice a day for 14 days. At approximately 5 years of age, dosing based on body surface area approximates the 10 mg/kg dose, while for children less than 5 years of age dosing by body surface area, as was done during the premarketing trials, gives higher doses and is recommended.[29,74]

Tables A27–1 A and B

Examples of dosing calculations

A. Succimer (available as 100-mg bead-filled capsules)

	Avg. Height (in.)	Avg. Weight (lbs.)	m^2	350 mg/m^2 [a]	10 mg/kg[a]
Child					
2-year-old boy	36	30.5	0.593	189 mg	
2-year-old girl	35	29	0.57	200 mg	
4-year-old boy	42	39.75	0.73	255 mg	
4-year-old girl	41.75	38.75	0.72	250 mg	
Adult					
50 kg					500 mg
70 kg					700 mg
90 kg					900 mg

B. Chemet (Succimer) Pediatric Dosing Chart

Pounds	Kilograms	Dose (mg)[a]	Number of Capsules[a]
18–35	8–15	100	1
36–55	16–23	200	2
56–75	24–34	300	3
76–100	35–44	400	4
>100	>45	500	5

[a] To be administered every 8 hours for 5 days, followed by dosing every 12 hours for 14 days.

SUMMARY

Succimer (meso-2,3-dimercaptosuccinic acid) is an orally active metal chelator that is FDA approved for the treatment of lead poisoning in children with blood lead concentrations greater than 45 µg/dL. There is no evidence at this time that succimer improves cognitive tests in patients with blood lead concentrations less than 45 µg/dL.[29]

Succimer is also used to treat patients poisoned with arsenic and organic and inorganic mercury. Succimer has many advantages over dimercaprol and $CaNa_2EDTA$, the two other chelators used for the same clinical problems. The advantages of succimer use include oral administration; limited effects on trace metals such as zinc; enhanced patient tolerance; limited toxicity; the ability to coadminister iron, if needed; and no contraindication in glucose-6-phosphate dehydrogenase–deficient individuals.[27] In contrast to $CaNa_2EDTA$, succimer does not redistribute lead to the brain of poisoned animals.[11,30] The role of succimer alone and in conjunction with other chelators to treat lead encephalopathy continues to be defined.[61,74]

REFERENCES

1. Aaseth J. Treatment of mercury and lead poisonings with dimercaptosuccinic acid and sodium dimercaptopropanesulfonate. *Analyst.* 1996;120:853-854.
2. Aaseth J, Friedheim EA. Treatment of methyl mercury poisoning in mice with 2,3-dimercaptosuccinic acid and other complexing thiols. *Acta Pharmacol Toxicol.* 1978;42:248-252.
3. Andersen O. Principles and recent developments in chelation treatment of metal intoxication. *Chem Rev.* 1999;99:2683-2710.
4. Aposhian HV. Succimer and DMPS—water-soluble antidotes for heavy metal poisoning. *Annu Rev Pharmacol Toxicol.* 1983;23:193-215.
5. Aposhian HV, Aposhian M. Aresenic toxicology: five questions. *Chem Res Toxicol.* 2006;19:1-15.

6. Aposhian HV, Aposhian MM. Meso-2,3-dimercaptosuccinic acid: chemical, pharmacological and toxicological properties of an orally effective metal chelating agent. *Annu Rev Pharmacol Toxicol.* 1990;30: 279-306.
7. Aposhian HV, Carter DE, Hoover TD, et al. Succimer, DMPS and DMPA as arsenic antidotes. *Fundam Applied Toxicol.* 1984;4:S58-S70.
8. Aposhian HV, Maiorino RM, Dart RC, et al. Urinary excretion of meso-2,3 dimercaptosuccinic acid in human subjects. *Clin Pharmacol Ther.* 1989;45:520-526.
9. Aposhian HV, Maiorino RM, Gonzalez-Ramirez D, et al. Mobilization of heavy metals by newer, therapeutically useful chelating agents. *Toxicology.* 1995;97:23-38.
10. Aposhian HV, Maiorino RM, Rivera M, et al. Human studies with the chelating agents, DMPS and succimer. *J Toxicol Clin Toxicol.* 1992;30: 505-528.
11. Aposhian M, Maiorano R, Xu Z, Aposhian HV. Sodium 2,3-dimercapto-1-propanesulfonate (DMPS) treatment does not redistribute lead or mercury to the brain of rats. *Toxicology.* 1996;109:49-55.
12. Aposhian HV, Mershon MM, Brinkley, Hsu CA. Anti-lewisite activity and stability of meso-dimercaptosuccinic acid and 2,3-dimercapto-1-propane-sulfonic acid. *Life Sci.* 1982;31:2149-2156.
13. Aposhian HV, Taklock CH, Moon TE. Protection of mice against the lethal effects of sodium arsenite: a quantitative comparison of a number of chelating agents. *Toxicol Appl Pharmacol.* 1981;61:385-392.
14. Aposhian HV, Zheng B, Aposhian M, et al. DMPS-arsenic challenge test. *Toxicol Appl Pharmacol.* 2000;165:74-83.
15. Asiedu P, Moulton T, Blum CB, et al. Metabolism of meso-2,3-dimercaptosuccinic acid in lead-poisoned children and normal adults. *Environ Health Perspect.* 1995;103:734-739.
16. Bankowska J, Hine C. Retention of lead in the rat. *Arch Environ Contam Toxicol.* 1985;14:621-629.
17. Bentur Y, Brook JG, Behar R, Taitelman U. Meso-2,3-dimercaptosuccinic acid in the diagnosis and treatment of lead poisoning. *J Toxicol Clin Toxicol.* 1987;25:39-51.
18. Besunder JB, Anderson RL, Super DM. Short-term efficacy of oral dimercaptosuccinic acid in children with low to moderate lead intoxication. *Pediatrics.* 1995;96:683-687.
19. Besunder JB, Super DM, Anderson R. Comparison of dimercaptosuccinic acid and calcium disodium ethylenediaminetetraacetic acid versus dimercaptopropanol and ethylenediaminetetraacetic acid in children with lead poisoning. *J Pediatr.* 1997;130:966-971.
20. Bhattacharya A, Smelser D, Berger O, et al. The effect of succimer therapy in lead intoxication using postural balance as a measure: a case study in a nine-year-old child. *Neurotoxicology.* 1998;19:57-64.
21. Bluhm RE, Bobbitt RG, Welch LW, et al. Elemental mercury vapour toxicity, treatment, and prognosis after acute, intensive exposure in chloralkali plant workers. I: history, neuropsychological findings and chelator effects. *Hum Exp Toxicol.* 1992;11:201-210.
22. Buchet JP, Lauwerys RR. Influence of 2,3 dimercaptopropane-1-sulfonate and dimercaptosuccinic acid on the mobilization of mercury from tissues of rats pretreated with mercuric chloride, phenylmercury acetate or mercury vapors. *Toxicology.* 1989;54:323-333.
23. Campbell JR, Clarkson TW, Omar MD. The therapeutic use of 2,3-dimercaptopropane-1-sulfonate in two cases of inorganic mercury poisoning. *JAMA.* 1986;256:3127-3130.
24. Chemet (succimer) [package insert]. Deerfield, IL: Manufactured by Schwartz Pharma Mfg Inc for Ovation Pharmaceuticals; 2007.
25. Chen S, Golemboski KA, Sanders FS, et al. Persistent effect of in utero meso-2,3-dimercaptosuccinic acid (succimer) on immune function and lead-induced immunotoxicity. *Toxicology.* 1999;132:67-69.
26. Chisolm JJ. BAL, EDTA, succimer and DMPS in the treatment of lead poisoning in children. *J Toxicol Clin Toxicol.* 1992;30:493-504.
27. Chisolm JJ. Safety and efficacy of meso-2,3-dimercaptosuccinic acid (succimer) in children with elevated blood lead concentrations. *J Toxicol Clin Toxicol.* 2000;38:365-375.
28. Committee on Drugs. Treatment guidelines for lead exposure in children. *Pediatrics.* 1995;96:155-160.
29. Committee on Environmental Health. Lead exposure in children: prevention, detection and management. *Peds.* 2005;116:1036-1046.
30. Cory-Slechta DA. Mobilization of lead over the course of succimer chelation therapy and long-term efficacy. *J Pharmacol Exp Ther.* 1988;246:84-91.
31. Cullen NA, Wolf LR, St. Clair D. Pediatric arsenic ingestion. *Am J Emerg Med.* 1995;13:432-435.
32. Cremin JD, Luck ML, Laughlin NK, Smith DR. Efficacy of succimer chelation for reducing brain lead in a primate model of human exposure. *Toxicol Appl Pharmacol.* 1999;161:283-293.
33. Dart RC, Hurlbut KM, Maiorino RM, et al. Pharmacokinetics of meso-2,3-dimercaptosuccinic acid in patients with lead poisoning and in healthy adults. *J Pediatr.* 1994;125:309-316.
34. Devars DuMayne JF, Prevost C, Gaudin B, et al. Lead poisoning treated with 2,3-dimercaptosuccinic acid. *Presse Med.* 1984;13:2209.
35. Dietrich K, Ware J, Salganik M et al. Effect of chelation therapy on the neuropsychological and behavioral development of lead exposed children after school entry. *Peds.* 2004;114:19-26.
36. Domingo JL, Paternain JL, Llobet JM, Corbella J. Developmental toxicity of subcutaneously administered meso-2,3-dimercaptosuccinic acid in mice. *Fundam Appl Toxicol.* 1986;11:715-722.
37. Ewan KB, Pamphlett R. Increased inorganic mercury in spinal motor neurons following chelating agents. *Neurotoxicology.* 1996;17:343-349.
38. Fang X, Fernando Q. Synthesis, structure, and properties of *rac*-2,3-dimercaptosuccinic acid, a potentially useful chelating agent for toxic metals. *Chem Res Toxicol.* 1994;7:148-156.
39. Flora GJS, Seth PK, Prakash AO, Mathur R. Therapeutic efficacy of combined meso-2,3-dimercaptosuccinic acid and calcium disodium edetate treatment during acute lead intoxication in rats. *Hum Exp Toxicol.* 1995;14:410-413.
40. Flora SJS, Bhattacharya R, Vijayaraghavan R. Combined therapeutic potential of meso-2,3-dimercaptosuccinic acid and calcium disodium versenate on the mobilization and distribution of lead in experimental lead intoxication in rats. *Fundam Appl Toxicol.* 1995;25:233-240.
41. Fournier L, Thomas G, Garnier R, et al. 2,3-Dimercaptosuccinic acid treatment of heavy metal poisoning in humans. *Med Toxicol.* 1988;3:499-504.
42. Friedheim E, Crovi C, Wakker CH. Meso-dimercaptosuccinic acid, a chelating agent for the treatment of mercury and lead poisoning. *J Pharm Pharmacol.* 1976;28:711-712.
43. Friedheim E, DaSilva JR. Treatment of schistosomiasis mansonii with antimony a, a′-dimercapto-potassium succinate (TWSb). *Am J Trop Med Hyg.* 1954;3:714-727.
44. Friedheim E, Graziano JH, Popovac D, et al. Treatment of lead poisoning by 2,3-dimercaptosuccinic acid. *Lancet.* 1978;2:1234-1235.
45. Glotzer DE. The current role of 2,3-dimercaptosuccinic acid (succimer) in the management of childhood lead poisoning. *Drug Saf.* 1993;9:85-92.
46. Gonzalez-Ramirez D, Zuniga-Charles M, Narro-Juarez A, et al. DMPS (2,3-dimercaptopropane-1-sulfonate, Dimaval) decreases the body burden of mercury in humans exposed to mercurous chloride. *J Pharm Exp Ther.* 1998;287:8-12.
47. Gordon R, Roberts G, Amin Z, et al. Aggressive approach in the treatment of acute lead encephalopathy with an extraordinarily high concentration of lead. *Arch Pediatr Adolesc Med.* 1998;152:1100-1104.
48. Grandjean P, Jacobsen IA, Jorgensen PJ. Chronic lead poisoning treated with dimercaptosuccinic acid. *Pharmacol Toxicol.* 1991;68:266-269.
49. Graziano JH. Role of 2,3-dimercaptosuccinic acid in the treatment of heavy metal poisoning. *Med Toxicol.* 1986;1:155-162.
50. Graziano JH, Leong JK, Friedheim E. 2,3-Dimercaptosuccinic acid: a new agent for the treatment of lead poisoning. *J Pharm Exp Ther.* 1978;206:696-700.
51. Graziano JH, LoIacono N, Meyer P. A dose–response study of oral 2,3-dimercaptosuccinic acid (succimer) in children with elevated blood lead concentrations. *J Pediatr.* 1988;113:751-757.
52. Graziano JH, LoIacono NJ, Moulton T, et al. Controlled study of meso-2,3-dimercaptosuccinic acid for the management of childhood lead intoxication. *J Pediatr.* 1992;120:133-139.
53. Graziano JH, Siris E, LoIacono N, et al. 2,3-Dimercaptosuccinic acid as an antidote for lead intoxication. *Clin Pharmacol Ther.* 1985;37:431-438.
54. Haust HL, Inwood M, Spence JD, et al. Intramuscular administration of iron during long-term chelation therapy with 3,2-dimercaptosuccinic acid in a man with severe lead poisoning. *Clin Biochem.* 1989;22:189-196.
55. Jones M, Basinger M, Gale G, Atkins L, Smith A, Stone A. Effect of chelate treatment on kidney, bone, and brain levels of lead-intoxicated mice. *Toxicology.* 1994;89:91-100.
56. Jugo S, Maljkovic T, Kostial K. Influence of chelating agents on the gastro-intestinal absorption of lead. *Toxicol Appl Pharmacol.* 1975;34:259-263.
57. Kapoor SC, Wielopolski L, Graziano JH, LoIacono NJ. Influence of 2,3-dimercaptosuccinic acid on gastrointestinal lead absorption and whole body lead retention. *Toxicol Appl Pharmacol.* 1989;97:525-529.
58. Keith RL, Setiarahardjo I, Fernando Q, et al. Utilization of renal slices to evaluate the efficacy of chelating agents for removing mercury from the kidney. *Toxicology.* 1997;116:67-75.

59. Khalil-Manesh F, Gonick HC, Weiler EW, et al. Effect of chelation treatment with dimercaptosuccinic acid (succimer) on lead-related blood pressure changes. *Environ Res.* 1994;65:86-99.
60. Klaassen CD. Heavy metals and heavy-metal antagonists. In: Gilman AG, Goodman LS, Rall TW, Murad F, eds. *Goodman and Gilman's the Pharmacological Basis of Therapeutics*, 7th ed. New York: Macmillan; 1985:1605-1627.
61. Kosnett MJ. Unanswered questions in metal chelation. *J Toxicol Clin Toxicol.* 1992;304:529-547.
62. Kosnett M, Wedeen R, Rothenberg S, et al. Recommendations for medical management of adult lead exposure. *Environ Health Perspec.* 2007;115:463-471.
63. Kreppel H, Paepcke U, Thiermann H, et al. Therapeutic efficacy of new dimercaptosuccinic acid (succimer) analogues in acute arsenic trioxide poisoning in mice. *Arch Toxicol.* 1993;67:580-585.
64. Lenz K, Hruby K, Druml W, et al. 2,3-Dimercaptosuccinic acid in human arsenic poisoning. *Arch Toxicol.* 1981;47:241-243.
65. Liebelt E, Shannon M. Oral chelators for childhood lead poisoning. *Pediatr Ann.* 1994;23:616-626.
66. Magos L. The effects of dimercaptosuccinic acid on the excretion and distribution of mercury in rats and mice treated with mercuric chloride and methylmercury chloride. *Br J Pharmacol.* 1976;56:479-484.
67. Magos L, Peristianis GC, Snowden RT. Postexposure preventive treatment of methylmercury intoxication in rats with dimercaptosuccinic acid. *Toxicol Appl Pharmacol.* 1978;45:463-475.
68. Mahaffey KR. Factors modifying susceptibility to lead. In: Mahaffey KR, ed. *Dietary and Environmental Lead: Human Health Effects*. New York: Elsevier; 1985:373-419.
69. Maiorino RM, Bruce DC, Aposhian HV. Determination and metabolism of dithiol chelating agents: VI. Isolation and identification of the mixed disulfides of meso-2,3-dimercaptosuccinic acid with l-cysteine in human urine. *Toxicol Appl Pharmacol.* 1989;97:338-349.
70. Mann KV, Travers JD. Succimer, an oral lead chelator. *Clin Pharm.* 1991;10:914-922.
71. Mazumder DN, Das Gupta J, Santra A, et al. Chronic arsenic toxicity in West Bengal—the worst calamity in the world. *J Indian Med Assoc.* 1998;96:4-7, 18.
72. McGown EL, Tillotson JA, Knudsen JJ, Dumlao CR. Biological behavior and metabolic fate of the BAL analogues succimer and DMPS. *Proc West Pharmacol Soc.* 1984;27:169-176.
73. McKinney PE. Acute elevation of blood lead levels within hours of ingestion of large quantities of lead shot. *J Toxicol Clin Toxicol.* 2000;38:435-440.
74. Mortensen ME. Succimer chelation: what is known? *J Pediatr.* 1994;125: 233-234.
75. Muckter H, Leibl B, Reichl FX. Are we ready to replace dimercaprol (BAL) as an arsenic antidote? *Hum Exp Toxicol.* 1997;16:460-465.
76. Ni W, Feng Y, Yu J, et al. A study of oral succimer in the treatment of lead poisoning. Personal communication, 1989.
77. O'Connor ME, Rich D. Children with moderately elevated lead levels: is chelation with succimer helpful? *Clin Pediatr (Phila).* 1999;38:325-331.
78. O'Flaherty EJ, Inskip MJ, Yagiminas AP, Franklin CA. Plasma and blood lead concentrations, lead absorption and lead excretion in sub-human primates. *Toxicol Appl Pharmacol.* 1996;138:121-130.
79. Okonishnokova IE, Rosenberg EE. Succimer as a means of chemoprophylaxis against occupational poisonings of workers handling mercury. *Gig Tr Prof Zabol.* 1971;15:29-32.
80. Okose P, Jennis T, Honcharuk L. Untoward effects of oral dimercaptosuccinic acid in the treatment of lead poisoning [abstract]. *Vet Hum Toxicol.* 1991;33:376.
81. Pappas JB, Ahlquist JT, Allen EM, Banner W. Oral dimercaptosuccinic acid and ongoing exposure to lead: effects on heme synthesis and lead distribution in a rat model. *Toxicol Appl Pharmacol.* 1995;133:121-129.
82. Pappas JB, Ahlquist T, Winn P, et al. The effect of oral succimer on ongoing exposure to lead [abstract]. *Vet Hum Toxicol.* 1992;34:361.
83. Peterson K, Salganik M, Campbell C, et al. Effect of succimer on growth of preschool children with moderate blood lead levels. *Environ Health Perspec.* 2004;112:233-237.
84. Piomelli S, Rosen JF, Chisolm JJ Jr, Graef JW. Management of childhood lead poisoning. *J Pediatr.* 1984;105:523-532.
85. Planas-Bohne F. The influence of chelating agents on the distribution and biotransformation of methylmercuric chloride in rats. *J Pharmacol Exp Ther.* 1981;217:500-504.
86. Rivera M, Zheng W, Aposhian HV, Fernando Q. Determination and metabolism of dithiol-containing agents VIII. Metal complexes of mesodimercaptosuccinic acid. *Toxicol Appl Pharmacol.* 1989;100:96-106.
87. Schafer B, Kreppel H, Reichl FX, et al. Effect of oral treatment with BAL, DMPS or succimer in organs of mice injected with arsenic tri-oxide. *Arch Toxicol.* 1991;14(Suppl):228-230.
88. Shum S, Whitehead J, Vaughn L. Chelation of organoarsenate with dimercaptosuccinic acid. *Vet Hum Toxicol.* 1995;37:239-242.
89. Sigg T, Burda A, Leikin JB, et al. A report of pediatric succimer overdose. *Vet Hum Toxicol.* 1998;40:90-91.
90. Singh PK, Jones MM, Xu Z, et al. Mobilization of lead by esters of meso-2,3-dimercaptosuccinic acid. *J Toxicol Environ Health.* 1989;27:423-434.
91. Smith D, Bayer L, Strupp B. Efficacy of succimer chelation for reducing brain Pb levels in a rodent model. *Environ Res.* 1998;78:168-176.
92. Smith DR, Calacsan C, Woodlard D, et al. Succimer and the urinary excretion of essential elements in a primate model of childhood lead exposure. *Toxicol Sci.* 2000;54:473-480.
93. Smith DR, Ilustre RP, Osterloh JD. Methodological considerations for the accurate determination of lead in human plasma and serum. *Am J Ind Med.* 1998;33:430-438.
94. Smith DR, Woolard D, Luck ML, et al. Succimer and the reduction of tissue lead in juvenile monkeys. *Toxicol Appl Pharmacol.* 2000;166:230-240.
95. Stangle D, Smith D, Besudin S, et al. Succimer chelation improves learning, attention, and arousal recognition in lead exposed rats but produces lasting cognitive impairment in the absence of lead exposure. *Environ Health Perspec.* 2007;115:201-209.
96. Stewart PW, Blaine C, Cohen M, et al. Acute and longer term effects of meso-2,3 dimercaptosuccinic acid (succimer) on the behavior of lead-exposed and control mice. *Physiol Behav.* 1996:59:849-855.
97. Tandon SK, Singh S, Jain V. Efficacy of combined chelation in lead intoxication. *Chem Res Toxicol.* 1994;7:585-589.
98. Tandon SK, Singh S, Prasad S, Mathur N. Mobilization of lead by calcium versenate and dimercaptosuccinate in the rat. *Clin Exp Pharmacol.* 1998;25:686-692.
99. Thomas G, Fournier L, Garnier R, Dally S. Nail dystrophy and dimercaptosuccinic acid. *J Toxicol Clin Exp.* 1987;7:285-287.
100. Thomas PS, Ashton C. An oral treatment for lead toxicity. *Postgrad Med J.* 1991;67:63-65.
101. Treatment of Lead Exposed Children (TLC) Trial Group. Safety and efficacy of succimer in toddlers with blood lead levels 20-44 μg/dL. *Pediatr Res.* 2000;48:593-599.
102. Treatment of Lead-Exposed Children (TLC) Trial Group. The Treatment of Lead-Exposed Children (TLC) trial: design and recruitment for a study of the effect of oral chelation on growth and development in toddlers. *Pediatr Perinatal Epidemiol.* 1998;12:313-333.
103. Tuntunji MF, al-Mahasneh QM. Disappearance of heme metabolites following chelation therapy with meso 2,3-dimercaptosuccinic acid (succimer). *J Toxicol Clin Toxicol.* 1994;32:267-276.
104. Van Der Linde A, Pillen S, Gerrits G, Bavinck J. Stevens-Johnson syndrome in a child with chronic mercury exposure and 2.3-dimercaptopropane-1-sulfate (DMPS) therapy. *Clin Toxicol.* 2008;46:479-481.
105. Wang SC, Ting KS, Wu CC. Chelating therapy with NaDMS in occupational lead and mercury intoxication. *Chin Med J.* 1965;84:437-439.
106. Xue H, Ni W, Xie Y, Cao T. Comparison of lead excretion of patients after injection of five chelating agents. *Chung Kuo Yao Li Hsuch Pao.* 1982;3:41-44.
107. Yarris J, Caravati M, Horowitz Z, et al. Acute arsenic trioxide ant bait ingestion by toddlers. *Clin Toxicol.* 2008;46:785-789.
108. Yu F, Liao Y, Jin Y, at al. Effects of in utero meso-2,3-dimercaptosuccinic acid with calcium and ascorbic acid on lead induced fetal development. *Arch Toxicol.* 2008;82:453-459.
109. Yu-I L, Chiao-Chen C, Yea-Lin T, Kuang-Sheng T. Studies on antibilharzial drugs VI: the antidotal effects of sodium dimercaptosuccinate and BAL-glucoside against tartar emetic. *Acta Physiol Sinica.* 1957;21: 24-32.
110. Zalups RK. Influence of 2,3-dimercaptopropoane-1-sulfonate (DMPS) and meso-2,3-dimercaptosuccinic acid (succimer) on the renal disposition of mercury in normal and uninephrectomized rats exposed to inorganic mercury. *J Pharmacol Exp Ther.* 1993;267:791-799.
111. Zhang J. Clinical observations in ethyl mercury chloride poisoning. *Am J Ind Med.* 1984;5:251-258.

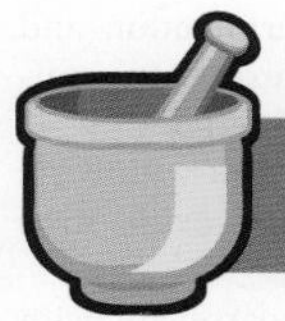

ANTIDOTES IN DEPTH (A28)

EDETATE CALCIUM DISODIUM ($CaNa_2EDTA$)

Mary Ann Howland

```
NaOOC—CH2          CH2—COONa
       |   CH2CH2   |
       N            N
  H2C                 CH2
   |                   |
  CH2       Ca        CH2
   |                   |
  COO                 OOC
```

Edetate calcium disodium ($CaNa_2EDTA$) is a chelating agent that is primarily used for the management of severe lead poisoning. Edetate calcium disodium has been replaced by succimer (2,3-dimercaptosuccinic acid) for the treatment of patients with lead concentrations between 45 and 70 μg/dL. Although, in conjunction with dimercaprol, $CaNa_2EDTA$ retains a critical role in the management of serious lead poisoning and lead encephalopathy.

CHEMISTRY

Edetate calcium disodium belongs to the family of polyaminocarboxylic acids. Although it is capable of chelating many metals, its current use is almost exclusively in the management of lead poisoning. The term *chelate* has its origin in the Greek word *chele*, which means "claw," implying an ability to tightly grasp the metal.[42] Implicit in chelation is the formation of a ring-structured complex. When $CaNa_2EDTA$ chelates lead, the calcium is displaced and the lead takes its place, forming a stable ring compound.[27]

PHARMACOKINETICS

Edetate calcium disodium is an ionic, water-soluble compound with a molecular weight of 374 daltons. The volume of distribution is small (0.05–0.23 L/kg), and due to its polar nature approximates that of the extracellular fluid compartment in normal individuals,[22,27] but is smaller in patients with renal dysfunction.[33] Edetate calcium disodium appears to penetrate erythrocytes poorly,[2,22] and less than 5% of $CaNa_2EDTA$ gains access to the spinal fluid.[22,27] Oral administration of $CaNa_2EDTA$ is not practical because of an oral bioavailability of less than 5%. The half-life is about 20 to 60 minutes.[4,22,27] Renal elimination approximates the glomerular filtration rate,[32] which correlates with creatinine clearance,[33] and results in the excretion of 50% of $CaNa_2EDTA$ in the urine within 1 hour, and more than 95% within 24 hours.[22,27] When $CaNa_2EDTA$ combines with lead, it forms a stable, soluble, nonionized compound that is subsequently excreted in the urine. Following $CaNa_2EDTA$ administration, urinary lead excretion is increased 20- to 50-fold.[9,34]

LEAD

ANIMALS

Animal studies demonstrate a decrease in tissue lead stores, including brain concentrations, when measurements are performed following $CaNa_2EDTA$ therapy.[25] A rat study examining the effect of a single dose of $CaNa_2EDTA$ on brain lead concentrations demonstrated a significant increase in brain lead concentrations,[17] suggesting that $CaNa_2EDTA$ may initially mobilize lead and facilitate redistribution to the brain. Additional doses enhance lead elimination, reduce blood lead concentrations, and subsequently reduce brain lead concentrations. The initial increase in brain lead may explain why some human case reports demonstrate worsening lead encephalopathy when $CaNa_2EDTA$ is used without concomitant dimercaprol (British anti-Lewisite [BAL]) therapy.

HUMANS

Edetate calcium disodium is capable of reducing blood lead concentrations, enhancing renal excretion of lead, and reversing the effects of lead on hemoglobin synthesis.[14] With chronic exposure, blood lead concentrations rebound considerably in the days to weeks following cessation of $CaNa_2EDTA$.[1,2,24] Although $CaNa_2EDTA$ has been used clinically since the 1970s, no rigorous clinical studies have ever been performed to evaluate whether $CaNa_2EDTA$ is capable of reversing the neurobehavioral effects of lead.[15,16] Chelators, including $CaNa_2EDTA$, are incapable of dramatically decreasing the body burden of lead, because only several milligrams of lead are eliminated during chelation.[9,11,35] A study of children with blood lead concentrations of 25 to 50 μg/dL who were given $CaNa_2EDTA$ for 5 days revealed very little difference in blood lead, bone lead, or erythrocyte protoporphyrin concentrations, when compared to pretreatment values.[28] Another study in children demonstrated no additional benefits of $CaNa_2EDTA$ on cognitive performance beyond that which was achieved by limiting further lead exposure and correcting an iron deficiency anemia.[34,36] A follow-up study in children with initial blood lead concentrations between 25 and 55 μg/dL also suggested an interaction between initial iron status, blood lead concentration and an improvement in perceptual motor performance over a 6-month period. Both correction of iron deficiency and a reduction in blood lead concentration (accomplished with limiting further exposure and or $CaNa_2EDTA$ chelation) contributed to the improvement, emphasizing the need to correct iron-deficiency anemia as well as limit lead exposure.[37]

$CaNa_2EDTA$ MOBILIZATION TEST

The $CaNa_2EDTA$ mobilization test was once widely recommended as a diagnostic aid for assessing the potential benefits of chelation therapy.[31,30] Currently,[10] it can only be considered obsolete.[10,14,17] Criticisms of the test include difficulties with administration of the antidote, unreliability as a predictor of total-body lead burden, expense, and the risk of worsening toxicity through redistribution of lead to either the kidney or brain.[14]

ADVERSE EFFECTS AND SAFETY ISSUES

The principal toxicity of $CaNa_2EDTA$ is related to the metal chelates it forms. In mice, the intraperitoneal (IP) LD_{50} (median lethal dose for 50% of test subjects) values of various $CaNa_2EDTA$ metal chelates are $CaNa_2EDTA$, 14.3 mmol/kg; lead EDTA, 3.1 mmol/kg; and mercury EDTA, 0.01 mmol/kg.

When $CaNa_2EDTA$ is given to patients with lead poisoning, the resultant sites of major renal toxicity are the proximal convoluted tubule, the distal convoluted tubule, and the glomeruli, possibly caused by the release of lead in the kidneys during excretion.[27] Of 130 children who received both dimercaprol and $CaNa_2EDTA$, 13% had biochemical evidence of nephrotoxicity, and 3% developed acute oliguric renal failure, which resolved over time without the need for hemodialysis.[31] Other studies failed to demonstrate any cases of renal failure in more than 1000 patient courses of therapy, when $CaNa_2EDTA$ was given in divided daily doses of 1000 mg/m^2 intravenously (IV) over 1 hour, every 6 hours.[29] Because lead toxicity causes renal damage independent of chelation, it is important to monitor renal function closely during $CaNa_2EDTA$ administration and to adjust the dose and schedule appropriately.[32,33] Nephrotoxicity may be minimized by limiting the total daily dose of $CaNa_2EDTA$ to 1 g in children or to 2 g in adults, although higher doses may be needed to treat lead encephalopathy. Continuous infusion while maintaining good hydration seems to increase efficacy and decrease toxicity.[32] Because the administration of disodium EDTA can lead to life-threatening hypocalcemia and death, $CaNa_2EDTA$ has become the preparation of choice and hypocalcemia is no longer a clinical concern.[5] Other adverse clinical effects of $CaNa_2EDTA$, most of which are uncommon, include malaise, fatigue, thirst, chills, fever, myalgias, dermatitis, headache, anorexia, urinary frequency and urgency, sneezing, nasal congestion, lacrimation, glycosuria, anemia, transient hypotension, increased prothrombin times, and inverted T waves.[27] Mild increases in alanine aminotransferase (ALT) and aspartate aminotransferase (AST) (usually reversible), and decreases in alkaline phosphatase are frequently reported. Extravasation may result in the development of painful calcinosis at the injection site.[34,38] Depletion of endogenous metals, particularly zinc, iron, and manganese, can result from chronic therapy.[8,41] A decrease in serum dopamine β-hydroxylase, a copper-dependent enzyme, occurred after a single injection of $CaNa_2EDTA$ in three adult lead welders, without any demonstrable decrease in serum copper.[18] Although the clinical relevance of this is unknown, it merits further investigation.[18]

An animal study suggests that gastrointestinal lead absorption may be enhanced by either IP or oral administration of $CaNa_2EDTA$[26]; consequently, removal of lead from the environment should always remain the first strategy in the management of lead toxicity. In the event of unintentional exposure to a new lead source, decontamination of the gastrointestinal tract must complement chelation.[30]

USES IN PREGNANCY

The safety of $CaNa_2EDTA$ has not been established in pregnancy, and a risk-to-benefit analysis must be made if its use is considered. In a model of lead poisoning in pregnant rats, fetal resorption decreased and the number of live fetuses increased when $CaNa_2EDTA$ was used, although the placental concentrations of lead were increased.[20] Zinc concentrations were not affected. Another study, however, found that when $CaNa_2EDTA$ was given to pregnant rats not poisoned with lead, increases in submucous clefts, cleft palate, adactyly/syndactyly, curly tail, and abnormal ribs and vertebrae resulted.[6] These teratogenic effects occurred with doses of $CaNa_2EDTA$ comparable to human doses and without causing noticeable changes in the mother except for weight gain. Use of zinc calcium EDTA and zinc EDTA preparations in pregnant rats caused no teratogenic effects at low doses, but resulted in the development of submucous cleft palates in 30% of the offspring receiving the higher dose of zinc calcium EDTA.[6]

DOSING AND ADMINISTRATION

There has never been a clinical trial to identify the best dose of $CaNa_2EDTA$. The most commonly recommended dose is determined by the patient's body surface area or weight (up to a maximum dose), the severity of the poisoning, and renal function (Chap. 94 and Table 94-8).[14,28,34] For patients with lead encephalopathy, the dose of $CaNa_2EDTA$ is 1500 mg/m^2/d approximately 50-75 mg/kg/d by continuous IV infusion, *starting 4 hours after the first dose of dimercaprol* and after an adequate urine flow is established.[13] The dose in obese patients has not been studied. A maximum dose of 3 g seems reasonable. Simultaneous dimercaprol and $CaNa_2EDTA$ therapy is administered for 5 days, followed by a rest period of at least 2 to 4 days, which permits lead redistribution. For adults with lead nephropathy, the following dosage regimen is recommended: 500 mg/m^2 every 24 hours for 5 days for patients with a serum creatinine of 2 to 3 mg/dL; every 48 hours for three doses for a serum creatinine of 3 to 4 mg/dL; and one dose for a serum creatinine greater than 4 mg/dL.[7] Previous recommendations were to limit the daily dose to 50 mg/kg when $CaNa_2EDTA$ is used in patients with renal dysfunction.[22,32,33] There is limited evidence to suggest that folic acid, pyridoxine, and thiamine increase the antidotal properties of $CaNa_2EDTA$.[39] There is inadequate data to recommend routine administration. A blood lead concentration should be measured 1 hour after the $CaNa_2EDTA$ infusion is discontinued, to avoid falsely elevated blood lead concentration determinations.

In symptomatic children without manifestations of lead encephalopathy, the dose of $CaNa_2EDTA$ is 1000 mg/m^2/d, approximately 25-50 mg/kg/d in addition to dimercaprol at 50 mg/m^2 every 4 hours. However, with Food and Drug Administration (FDA) approval of succimer, and the demonstrated ability to reduce brain lead concentrations in animals, succimer has essentially replaced $CaNa_2EDTA$ as the chelator of choice in lead-poisoned children without encephalopathy and lead concentration less than 70 μg/dL.[11,24]

Because of the pain associated with intramuscular (IM) administration, most clinicians recommend that $CaNa_2EDTA$ be administered at concentrations of approximately 0.5% by continuous IV infusion over 24 hours in 5% dextrose or 0.9% NaCl. Concentrations greater than 0.5% may lead to thrombophlebitis and should be avoided. Edetate calcium disodium is incompatible with other solutions. Careful attention to total fluid requirements in children and patients who have or who are at risk for, lead encephalopathy is paramount.[27,34] Rapid IV infusions in patients with lead encephalopathy may increase intracranial pressure and cerebral edema. In children with acute lead encephalopathy, starting BAL 4 hours prior to $CaNa_2EDTA$ appears to be more effective than starting $CaNa_2EDTA$ prior to and simultaneously with BAL.[12,15] In addition, treating with two chelators also reduces the blood lead concentration significantly faster than $CaNa_2EDTA$ alone, while maintaining a better molar ratio of chelator to lead.[12]

If $CaNa_2EDTA$ is to be administered IM to avoid the use of an IV and fluid overload, then either procaine or lidocaine is added to the $CaNa_2EDTA$ in a dose sufficient to produce a final concentration of 0.5% (5 mg/mL). This can be accomplished by mixing 1 mL of a 1% procaine or 1% lidocaine solution with each mL of chelator.[7,27] The procaine or lidocaine minimizes pain at the injection site.

Table A28–1. Calculations for Intravenous Edetate Calcium Disodium Infusion Over 24 hours

	Avg. Height (in.)	Avg. Weight (lbs.)	m^2	1000 mg/m^2 over 24 h IV	Dilute in D_5W or NS and Infuse over 24 h[a]	1500 mg/m^2 over 24 h IV	Dilute in D_5W or NS and Infuse over 24 h[a]
Child[b]							
2-year-old boy	36	30.5	0.593	593 mg	200 mL	890 mg	300 mL
2-year-old girl	35	29	0.57	570 mg	200 mL	855 mg	300
4-year-old boy	42	39.75	0.73	730 mg	250	1095 mg	400
4-year-old girl	41.75	38.75	0.72	720 mg	250	1080 mg	400
Adult[c,d]							
50 kg			1.5	1500 mg	500 mL	2250 mg	750 mL
70 kg			1.8	1800 mg	600 mL	2700 mg	1000 mL
90 kg			2.1	2100 mg	700 mL	3150 mg	1000 mL

Edetate calcium disodium comes in 5-mL ampules of 200 mg/mL.

D_5W, 5% dextrose in water; IV, intravenously; NS, 0.9% sodium chloride solution.

[a] Dilute in D_5W or 0.9% NaCl to concentrations of less than 0.5% to avoid thrombophlebitis with IV administration; be mindful of total fluid requirements if encephalopathic to avoid cerebral edema; if fluid is an issue consider intramuscular injection, otherwise infuse IV over 24 hours.

[b] Do not exceed adult dose.

[c] For adults with lead nephropathy, the following dosing regimen has been suggested: 500 mg/m^2 every 24 hours for 5 days for patients with serum creatinine levels of 2 to 3 mg/dL, every 48 hours for three doses for patients with creatinine concentrations of 3 to 4 mg/dL, and once weekly for patients with creatinine concentrations above 4 mg/dL.

[d] The dose in obese patients has not been studied. A maximum dose of 3 g seems reasonable.

COMBINATION THERAPY WITH SUCCIMER OR DMPS

The possible benefit of combining $CaNa_2EDTA$ with succimer or 2,3-dimercapto-1-propane-sulfonic acid (DMPS) is under investigation in animals.[19,21,40] The combination of $CaNa_2EDTA$ with succimer appears more potent than either individual agent in promoting urine and fecal lead excretion, and decreasing blood and liver lead concentrations. However, this approach might increase zinc depletion.[40]

A retrospective analysis compared the combination of BAL and $CaNa_2EDTA$ with succimer and $CaNa_2EDTA$ in children with blood lead concentrations of about 35 to 70 µg/dL (up to 90 µg/dL for the BAL group). They demonstrated equivalent reductions in blood lead concentrations with fewer side effects in the succimer group.[3] One case report of a child with lead encephalopathy and an extremely high blood concentration of 550 µg/dL used a combination of BAL and $CaNa_2EDTA$ initially followed by succimer, but a rebound increase in the lead concentration led to the addition of $CaNa_2EDTA$.[23] More data are needed to confirm this approach.

AVAILABILITY

Edetate calcium disodium is available as calcium disodium versenate in 5-mL ampules containing 200 mg of $CaNa_2EDTA$ per milliliter (1 g per ampule).[27] Disodium edetate (sodium EDTA) should not be considered an alternative to $CaNa_2EDTA$ because of the risk of life-threatening hypocalcemia associated with sodium EDTA use.

SUMMARY

Edetate calcium disodium reduces blood lead concentrations, enhances urinary lead excretion, and reverses lead-induced hematologic effects. Studies evaluating long-term effects in reversing lead-induced neurotoxicity have not been performed. Edetate calcium disodium remains the standard of care for patients with lead encephalopathy when used in conjunction with dimercaprol. A $CaNa_2EDTA$ challenge test is no longer recommended as a diagnostic gesture.[14,17] Recommended doses and dosage schedules should not be exceeded and should be reduced when the creatinine clearance is reduced. Patients should be well hydrated to achieve an adequate urine flow prior to and during $CaNa_2EDTA$ therapy.

REFERENCES

1. Angle CR. Childhood lead poisoning and its treatment. *Ann Rev Pharmacol Toxicol.* 1993;32:409-434.
2. Aposhian HV, Maiorinao RM, Gonzalez-Ramirez D, et al. Mobilization of heavy metals by newer, therapeutically useful chelating agents. *Toxicology.* 1995;97:23-38.
3. Besunder J, Super D, Anderson R. Comparison of dimercaptosuccinic acid and calcium disodium ethylenediaminetetraacetic acid versus dimercapto-propanol and ethylenediaminetetraacetic acid in children with lead poisoning. *J Peds.* 1997;130:966-971.
4. Bowazzi P, Lanzoni J, Marcussi F. Pharmacokinetic studies of EDTA in rats. *Eur J Drug Metab Pharmacokinet.* 1981;6:21-26.
5. Brown M, Willis T, Omalu B, et al. Deaths from hypocalcemia after administration of edetate disodium 2003-2205. *Peds.* 2006;118:e534-e536.

6. Brownie CF, Brownie C, Noden D, et al. Teratogenic effect of Ca EDTA in rats and the protective effect of zinc. *Toxicol Appl Pharmacol.* 1986;82: 426-443.
7. Calcium disodium versenate - edetate calcium disodium- injection [package insert]. Manufactured for 3M Pharmaceuticals, Northridge, CA, by Hospira Inc Lake Forest, IL; 2004.
8. Cantilena LR, Klaassen CD. The effect of chelating agents on the excretion of endogenous metals. *Toxicol Appl Pharmacol.* 1982;63:344-350.
9. Chisolm JJ Jr. The use of chelating agents in the treatment of acute and chronic lead intoxication in childhood. *J Pediatr.* 1968;73:1-38.
10. Chisolm JJ Jr. Mobilization of lead by calcium disodium edetate. *Am J Dis Child.* 1987;141:1256-1257.
11. Chisolm JJ Jr. BAL, EDTA, DMSA and DMPS in the treatment of lead poisoning in children. *J Toxicol Clin Toxicol.* 1992;30:493-504.
12. Chisolm JJ Jr. Safety and efficacy of meso-2,3-dimercaptosuccinic acid (DMSA) in children and elevated blood lead concentrations. *J Toxicol Clin Toxicol.* 2000;38:365-375.
13. Coffin R, Phillips LJ, Staples WL, et al. Treatment of lead encephalopathy in children. *J Pediatr.* 1966;69:198-206.
14. Committee on Drugs. Treatment guidelines for lead exposure in children. *Pediatrics.* 1995;96:155-160.
15. Corey-Slechta DA. Relationships between lead-induced learning impairments and changes in dopaminergic, cholinergic, and glutamatergic neurotransmitter system functions. *Annu Rev Pharmacol Toxicol.* 1995; 35:391-415.
16. Cory-Slechta DA, Weiss B. Efficacy of the chelating agent CaEDTA in reversing lead-induced changes in behavior. *Neurotoxicology.* 1989;10: 685-698.
17. Cory-Slechta DA, Weiss B, Cox C. Mobilization and redistribution of lead over the course of calcium disodium ethylenediamine tetraacetate chelation therapy. *J Pharmacol Exp Ther.* 1987;243:804-813.
18. Deparis P, Caroldi S. In vivo inhibition of serum dopamine B hydroxylase by $CaNa_2EDTA$ injection. *Hum Exp Ther.* 1994;13:253-256.
19. Flora GJS, Seth PK, Prakas A, et al. Therapeutic efficiency of combined meso-2,3-dimercaptosuccinic acid and calcium disodium ede-tate treatment during acute lead intoxication in rats. *Hum Exp Toxicol.* 1995;14: 410-413.
20. Flora SJ, Tandon SK. Influence of calcium disodium edetate on the toxic effects of lead administration in pregnant rats. *Indian J Physiol Pharmacol.* 1987;31:267-272.
21. Flora SJS, Bhattacharga R, Vijayaraghauan R. Combined therapeutic potential of meso-2,3-dimercaptosuccinic acid and calcium disodium edetate on the mobilization and distribution of lead in experimental lead intoxication in rats. *Fundam Appl Toxicol.* 1995;25:233-240.
22. Foreman H, Trujillo T. The metabolism of ^{14}C labeled ethylenediaminetetraacetic acid in human beings. *J Lab Clin Med.* 1954;43:566-571.
23. Gordon RA, Roberts G, Amin Z, et al. Aggressive approach in the treatment of acute lead encephalopathy with an extraordinarily high concentration of lead. *Arch Pediatr Adolesc Med.* 1998;152:1100-1104.
24. Graziano JH, Leong JK, Friedheim E. 2,3-Dimercaptosuccinic acid: a new agent for the treatment of lead poisoning. *J Pharmacol Exp Ther.* 1978;206:696-700.
25. Jones MM, Basinger MA, Gale GR, et al. Effect of chelate treatments on kidney, bone and brain lead levels of lead-intoxicated mice. *Toxicology.* 1994;89:91-100.
26. Jugo S, Maljkovic T, Kostial D. Influence of chelating agents on the gastrointestinal absorption of lead. *Toxicol Appl Pharmacol.* 1975;34:259-263.
27. Klaassen CD. Heavy metals and heavy metal antagonists. In: Gilman AG, Goodman LS, Rall TW, Murad F, eds. *Goodman and Gilman's the Pharmacological Basis of Therapeutics*, 11th ed. New York: McGraw-Hill; 1996:1753-1775.
28. Markowitz M, Bijur P, Ruff M, et al. Effects of calcium disodium versenate ($CaNa_2$-EDTA) chelation in moderate childhood lead poisoning. *Pediatrics.* 1993;92:265-271.
29. Markowitz M, Rosen J, Piomelli S, Weinberger H. Personal communication, 1995.
30. McKinney PE. Acute elevation of blood lead levels within hours of ingestion of large quantities of lead shot. *J Toxicol Clin Toxicol.* 2000;38:435-440.
31. Moel DI, Kumark, N. Reversible nephrotoxic reactions to a combined 2,3 dimercapto-1-propanol and calcium disodium ethylene diaminetetraacetic acid regimen in asymptomatic children with elevated blood lead levels. *Pediatrics.* 1982;70:259-262.
32. Morgan JW. Chelation therapy in lead nephropathy. *South Med J.* 1975;68: 1001-1006.
33. Osterloh J, Becker CE. Pharmacokinetics of $CaNa_2$-EDTA and chelation of lead in renal failure. *Clin Pharmacol Ther.* 1986;40:686-693.
34. Piomelli S, Rosen JF, Chisolm JJ Jr, Graef JW. Management of childhood lead poisoning. *J Pediatr.* 1984;105:523-532.
35. Rosen JF, Markowitz ME. Trends in the management of childhood lead poisonings. *Neurotoxicology.* 1993;14:211-217.
36. Ruff HA, Bijur PE, Markowitz M, et al. Declining blood levels and cognitive changes in moderately lead-poisoned children. *JAMA.* 1993;269: 1641-1646.
37. Ruff H, Markowitz M, Bijur P, Rosen J. Relationships among blood lead levels, iron deficiency, and cognitive development in two-year-old children. *Environ Health Perspect.* 1996;104:180-185.
38. Schumacher HR, Osterman AL, Choi SJ, et al. Calcinosis at the site of leakage from extravasation of calcium disodium edetate intravenous chelator therapy in a child with lead poisoning. *Clin Orthop.* 1987;219:221-225.
39. Tandon SK, Flora ST, Singh S. Chelation in metal intoxication: influence of various components of vitamin B complex on the therapeutic efficacy of CaEDTA in lead intoxication. *Pharmacol Toxicol.* 1987;60:62-65.
40. Tandon SK, Singh S, Jain VK. Efficiency at combined chelation in lead intoxication. *Chem Res Toxicol.* 1994;7:585-589.
41. Thomas DJ, Chisolm J. Lead, zinc, copper decorporation during Ca EDTA treatment of lead poisoned children. *J Pharmacol Exp Ther.* 1986;229:829-835.
42. Williams DR, Halstead BW. Chelating agents in medicine. *J Toxicol Clin Toxicol.* 1982-1983;19:1081-1115.

CHAPTER 95
MANGANESE

Sari Soghoian

Manganese (Mn)

Atomic number	=	25
Atomic weight	=	54.94 daltons
Normal concentrations:		
Whole blood	=	4–15 μg/L (73–273 nmol/L)
Serum	=	0.9–2.9 μg/L (16–52 nmol/L)
Urine (24h)	<	10 μg/L (182 nmol/L)

Manganese is an essential element of the diet and a known cofactor in many enzymatic processes. Most reported cases of manganese toxicity in humans have involved occupational exposure to inhaled manganese dusts and fumes. Toxicity has also occurred in patients receiving parenteral nutrition and recently in intravenous (IV) methcathinone users.

HISTORY AND EPIDEMIOLOGY

Manganese salts are brightly pigmented and were most likely first used to make paint. Manganese dioxide has been found in prehistoric paints and has been used as a decolorant in glass making since at least the Roman Empire. Manganese–iron alloys were found in Spartan weapons, but the combination was most likely fortuitous but unintentional. In the early 19th century, it was discovered that addition of manganese to iron produced a stronger metal alloy, and manganese became an important component of most steel. The largest industrial use of manganese today is in steelmaking, and more than 85% of manganese in production is used to make ferromanganese alloys.

Manganese, primarily in the form of oxides, is released during mining, and inhalational exposure to dusts from grinding manganese ore has been the most important source of manganese toxicity. Inhalation of inorganic manganese compounds may also occur during smelting, welding, or burning coal, oil, or fuel containing manganese compounds. Manganese was linked to the development of a characteristic neuropsychiatric syndrome since the 1800s when it was described in French pyrolusite mill workers.[17] A neuropsychiatric syndrome in welders is also attributed to inhalation of manganese oxide fumes[12,14,56]; however, many of the studies used to support this claim are methodologically flawed.[31,36]

Other industrial uses of manganese include: manganese chloride in dry-cell battery manufacture and as a catalyst for chlorination of organic compounds; manganese dioxide in batteries and glass production; and manganese sulfate to make ceramics, fungicides, and pesticides. Manganese toxicity from these professional applications has not been reported.

Permanganates were first discovered to be strong oxidizing agents in the 18th century. Weak solutions of potassium permanganate 0.01% are still used in medicine as topical drying and antiseptic skin preparations. Potassium, sodium, and barium permanganate also have uses in the pharmaceutical, chemical, and photographic industries. The toxicity of permanganates is mostly related to their oxidizing effects and is not discussed further here.

Manganese chloride and manganese sulfate are used as nutritional supplements.[10] Manganese toxicity is well documented in patients receiving total parenteral nutrition (TPN),[21,43,48] particularly infants and young children. An epidemic of manganese toxicity was recently reported from the use of IV methcathinone prepared using potassium permanganate as an oxidizing agent.[66] Manganese contamination of freebase cocaine may occur if manganese–carbonate is used as a reagent. The addition of methylcyclopentadienyl manganese tricarbonyl (MMT), a lead alternative, to gasoline has been allowed in Canada since 1976 and in the United States since 1995, but more research is needed to understand the contribution of MMT in gasoline to the environmental burden of manganese and to human health.

CHEMISTRY

Manganese is a transition metal atomic number 25, that is located between chromium and iron in the periodic table. It is dark grey, brittle, and paramagnetic. It is the 12th most abundant element in the earth's crust (0.106%) and occurs in several mineral forms. Most manganese in the environment is found complexed to oxygen, carbon, or chloride. The most economically important ore is pyrolusite, or manganese dioxide (MnO_2), from which metallic manganese was first isolated in 1774. Similar to magnetite and magnesium, the name *manganese* derives from *Magnesia*, a prefecture of Thessaly in ancient Greece. Ores from this region are abundant in manganese oxides and carbonates, among other elements.

Manganese can exist in several oxidation states from −3 to +7. Mn^{2+} is the most common, the most bioavailable, and the most physiologically important form.

PHARMACOLOGY AND PHYSIOLOGY

Divalent manganese ion (Mn^{2+}) is stable in aqueous solution at neutral pH and forms complexes with a variety of ligands in the body. Divalent manganese ion can substitute for Mg^{2+}, Ca^{2+}, and Fe^{2+} in complexes with proteins and enzymes.[45] Mn^{3+} is also biologically important and is, for example, the form of manganese in superoxide dismutase. Manganese is a cofactor in many other human enzyme systems, including hexokinase, xanthine oxidase, and glutamine synthase. It is also present in several metalloproteins.[10]

Manganese is considered an essential element in the diet. Although deficiency in humans is not reported, experimental manganese restriction produced a scaling, erythematous, pruritic rash; alterations in calcium homeostasis (eg, hypercalcemia, hyperphosphatemia); and increased alkaline phosphatase in healthy volunteers.[23] Manganese is present in human breast milk in its trivalent form bound to lactoferrin, which is readily absorbed via receptors in the small intestine. Divalent manganese salts—usually manganese sulfate or manganese chloride—that are typically added to infant formulas, processed foods, and dietary supplements are less well absorbed. Important dietary sources of manganese in adults are nuts, grains, legumes, fruits, and vegetables. Manganese salts in well water also contribute to dietary intake.[61] Most people consume 2 to 9 mg of manganese compounds per day, but vegetarians may consume more.

Normally, less than 5% of dietary manganese is absorbed throughout the length of the small intestine. However, enteral manganese absorption depends not only on the chemical form but also on the dietary needs of the host and the presence of similarly charged compounds. For example, because manganese can compete with iron for binding sites on transferrin, the percentage of absorbed manganese is increased in the presence of iron-deficiency anemia. Radioisotope studies demonstrate that absorption of dietary manganese is doubled in anemic subjects.[10,22] Manganese absorption from the gastrointestinal tract is also inversely proportional to the amount of calcium in the diet, most likely because of competition between divalent cations for transport.[10]

Divalent manganese can take the place of ferrous or ferric iron in hemoglobin. The incorporation of manganese into hemoglobin by substitution for iron accounts for the large difference between whole-blood manganese concentrations and the typically minute free serum manganese concentrations (<2.9 μg/L) that are measured in those with normal concentrations. Because about 85% of manganese in blood is bound up with hemoglobin in erythrocytes, normal measured whole-blood concentrations may be as much as five times higher than those measured in serum.[52] The remaining manganese in plasma is mostly bound to transferrin, β_1-globulin, and albumin.[6] Manganese is widely distributed to all tissues and crosses both the placental[10] and the blood–brain barrier.[5] Transport in the body is also facilitated by transport proteins and for Mn^{2+} by the divalent metal transporter (DMT-1).

The elimination half-life of manganese from the body is approximately 40 days[41] but is highly variable among subjects. Elimination of manganese may be prolonged in young women with high ferritin stores[22] or after the initiation of oral iron therapy for anemia.[41] This effect is most likely attributable to increased hepatic sequestration from increased production of iron transport and storage proteins. High concentrations of manganese are also found in patients with hemochromatosis, supporting the idea that increased or abnormal iron storage proteins also lead to increased hepatic manganese stores.[1]

Manganese is primarily eliminated via the bile in feces. It accumulates in bile against a concentration gradient, which suggests an active transport mechanism for its excretion.[33] Renal excretion is negligible; whereas 67% of a radiolabeled manganese dose injected IV is recovered in feces within 48 hours, less than 0.1% appears in the urine within 5 days of its administration.[33]

PATHOPHYSIOLOGY

Although manganese is widely distributed in the body, the most important clinical effects of manganese toxicity are related to its accumulation in brain. Increased brain manganese stores may be caused by overexposure or impaired elimination. Whereas normal liver function may protect against accumulation of manganese in the brain,[62] patients with hepatic disease have impaired manganese elimination and are also at risk for manganese toxicity from normal dietary intake.[53,58,62] Manganese concentrations are increased in the globus pallidum of cirrhotic patients compared with control subjects and in rats with either biliary cirrhosis or portacaval shunts.[58]

Manganese influx, but not efflux, into the central nervous system is tightly regulated by transferrin-dependent transport mechanisms.[5] Transferrin-receptor mediated endocytosis of bound Mn^{3+} is the major route of entry under normal conditions, but for unclear reasons, free manganese appears to cross the blood–brain barrier more quickly than protein-bound manganese.[47,55] Exposure to manganese in excess of blood ligand-binding capacity may therefore promote its distribution to the brain.

The exact mechanisms of manganese uptake into neuronal cells and its transport within the brain are still being elucidated. Transferrin may also play an important part in manganese accumulation in the basal ganglia, specifically because these are efferent to areas of high transferrin-receptor density.[6,19] The divalent-metal transporter is most likely also important, but more research is needed to understand its role.

Because of its low enteral absorption, ingestion of manganese in any form is unlikely to cause toxic manganese concentrations in the blood. This is more likely to occur with parenteral administration of nutrition or drugs containing manganese. Inhalation of manganese dusts or fumes during mining or welding may also cause acutely elevated blood concentrations or may create pulmonary manganese deposits that can prolong exposure even after the patient is removed from the environmental source.[49]

Manganese is cytotoxic, but the specific cellular mechanisms by which manganese leads to cell death are not well established. Similar to other transition metals, manganese probably causes some local damage by generating reactive oxygen species during redox cycling between the divalent and trivalent forms. The participation of manganese in Fenton reactions also occurs and results in oxidative tissue damage (see Chap. 11) Mn^{2+} concentrates in mitochondria and inhibits both mitochondrial F1-ATPase[6] and complex I[24] in the electron transport chain, thereby disrupting oxidative phosphorylation.[15,24,25,60,74,75] It may also impair glutamate synthesis and transport and alter the glycolytic enzyme glyceraldehyde-3-phosphate. Furthermore, the high-affinity binding of manganese-substituted hemoglobin to nitric oxide scavenges this vasodilatory compound.[37,50]

CLINICAL MANIFESTATIONS

The most characteristic clinical features of manganese toxicity are neuropsychiatric (Table 95–1). Early reports of manganism in German manganese workers[10] and Chilean miners[63] described a biphasic illness. The acute phase is characterized by psychiatric symptoms, or "manganese madness," that may also be progressive. Symptoms include visual hallucinations, behavioral changes, anxiety, impotence, and decreased libido.[10] This acute phase is followed by a late-developing movement disorder that includes tremor, impaired speech, loss of facial expression, and gait disturbances. This extrapyramidal movement disorder is similar to idiopathic Parkinson's disease but is more likely to present with only mild cognitive impairment or vestibular–auditory dysfunction rather than severe progressive dementia.[32] In addition, patients may lack tremors at rest, be more likely to have difficulty walking backward, have frequent falls, have a typical "cock walk" on the balls of

TABLE 95–1. Typical Features of Chronic Manganism

System	Early Manifestations	Late Manifestations
Constitutional	Asthenia, lethargy	—
Gastrointestinal	Anorexia	—
Neurologic	Fine intention tremor Headaches	Coarse intention tremor Visual hallucinations Cognitive impairment Loss of facial expression Dysphagia Micrographia Gait instability[a] Low-volume speech
Psychiatric	Apathy Irritability Emotional lability	Decreased libido or impotence Anxiety Additional behavioral changes
Musculoskeletal	Arthralgias	Muscle rigidity

[a] Decreased arm swing, toe walking, inability to turn or walk backward without falling.

the feet, and have low-volume speech. Furthermore, they may be less likely to improve with levodopa therapy compared with patients who have Parkinson's disease.[66]

Acute inhalational exposure to high concentrations of manganese oxides may also cause metal fume fever (see Chap. 124), with characteristic fever, child, nausea, headache, myalgias, and arthralgias.[10] Chronic exposure to manganese oxide fumes by factory workers is also associated with development of a persistent dry cough, bronchitis, chemical pneumonitis, and increased rates of pneumonia in factory workers but does not appear to cause pulmonary fibrosis.[38,57]

DIAGNOSTIC TESTING

Manganese concentrations in the blood are most commonly determined by flame or furnace atomic absorption spectrophotometry. Normal reference values for manganese in the blood and urine are published (see above), but toxic concentrations are not well defined. Elevated blood manganese concentrations are present in patients with acute toxicity, but this test is neither sensitive nor specific for chronic manganese toxicity. This occurs because manganese is rapidly cleared from the blood,[73] and elevated concentrations reflect only recent exposure. Symptoms of manganism are insidious and therefore likely to occur long after concentrations in the urine or blood have normalized. Increased urinary elimination of manganese after chelation challenge with edetate calcium disodium ($CaNa_2EDTA$) have been reported[59,66] but cannot be interpreted. In most situations, it is unclear whether the increased excretion signifies mobilization of physiologic manganese, an increased body burden of manganese, or toxicity.

Whole-blood manganese concentrations are the most reliable values for biomonitoring purposes, although they only correlate with group and not with individual exposure levels.[10] A cross-sectional study of workers from three different areas in a dry-cell battery plant found no significant differences in urinary manganese concentrations between workers with high, low, and no occupational exposure.[8] A large amount of background variation made it difficult to interpret axillary hair concentrations in this study. Whole-blood manganese concentrations revealed the least background variation and were positively correlated with group-based estimations of airborne manganese exposures.

Patients with manganese associated parkinsonism often have a pattern of magnetic resonance imaging (MRI) abnormalities that includes abnormal T1-weighted signal hyperintensity in the basal ganglia, particularly in the globus pallidus, with normal T2-weighted images.[4,31,32,51,66] This pattern is also reported in patients with iatrogenic manganism from long-term parenteral nutrition.[11,21,30,46,69] In patients without neurologic manifestations, manganese concentrations in TPN are positively correlated with the intensity of increased signal in the basal ganglia on T1-weighted MRI images,[11,69] and basal ganglia changes present on MRI during TPN therapy are reversible with its discontinuation.[46,68]

This MRI pattern also occurs in cirrhotic patients[54,65] and presumably represents an abnormal accumulation of dietary manganese caused by impaired hepatic excretion. The globus pallidi of cirrhotic patients who die with hepatic encephalopathy contain high concentrations of manganese compared with control subjects.[53] Increased T1-weighted signal in the basal ganglia occurs in individuals with many other conditions, however, and may also reflect iron, copper, or lipid deposition; hemorrhage; or neurofibromatosis.[10] MRI findings in patients with idiopathic Parkinson's disease more typically include a hypointense signal in the substantia nigra seen on T2-weighted images.[35,71,42] Positron emission tomography scans of patients with chronic manganese exposure and mild parkinsonism have failed to show abnormal nigrostriatal dopaminergic projections, although these are abnormal in patients with idiopathic parkinsonism.[51,72]

TREATMENT

The treatment of patients with acute or chronic manganese toxicity is primarily supportive. Removal from the source of exposure is paramount, although clinical manifestations of toxicity may progress even as body stores of manganese are decreasing.[29] Chelation therapy with $CaNa_2EDTA$ (A-28) or calcium diethylenetriamine pentaacetic acid (DTPA) (A-43) improves urinary excretion of manganese without affecting neurologic manifestations of toxicity.[59,66] Chelation of two workers with diemercaptosuccinic acid (DMSA) had no effect on manganese concentrations in the blood and urine or on clinical signs of manganism.[2]

Deferoxamine has not been studied as a potential therapy for manganese toxicity, and some evidence suggests that it might be counterproductive. In vitro studies with rat pheochromocytoma cells have demonstrated increased rates of apoptosis after coincubation with manganese and the iron chelator deferoxamine compared with incubation with manganese alone.[60] Because iron and manganese tend to compete for ligands, the increased cellular uptake of manganese in these experiments may have been caused by iron sequestration by deferoxamine leaving more transporters available to interact with manganese.

Although levodopa has reportedly improved parkinsonian signs in several manganese neurotoxic patients,[16,44,56] it did not improve the clinical course in double-blinded, randomized, placebo-controlled trials of manganese-associated parkinsonism.[34,39]

SUMMARY

Chronic exposure to high concentrations of manganese produces a characteristic neuropsychiatric disorder, manganism, that includes parkinsonian features, mild cognitive impairment, and possibly emotional instability. The clinical syndrome is associated with an increased signal in the globus pallidus on T1-weighted MRI. Elevated whole-blood manganese concentrations may also help differentiate the cause, but rapid clearance of manganese from the blood makes this a less sensitive test in cases in which exposure is remote from the onset of symptoms. Treatment is primarily supportive because no chelation regimen has been demonstrated to alter the clinical course.

REFERENCES

1. Altstatt LB, Pollack S, Feldman MH, Reba RC, Crosby WH. Liver manganese in hemochromatosis. *Proc Soc Exp Biol Med.* 1967;124:353-355.
2. Angle CR. Dimercaptosuccinic acid (DMSA): negligible effect on manganese in urine and blood. *Occup Environ Med.* 1995;52:846.
3. Aposhian HV, Ingersoll RT, Montgomery EB Jr. Transport and control of manganese ions in the central nervous system. *Environ Res.* 1999;80:96-98.
4. Arjona A, Mata M, Bonet M. Diagnosis of chronic manganese intoxication by magnetic resonance imaging. *N Engl J Med.* 1997;336:964-965.
5. Aschner M. Manganese homeostasis in the CNS. *Environ Res.* 1999;80:105-109.
6. Aschner M. Manganese. Transport and emerging research needs. *Environ Health Perspect.* 2000;108:429-432.
7. ATSDR. 2000. *Toxicological Profile for Manganese.* Atlanta: Agency for Toxic Substances and Disease Registry. Retrieved October 7, 2009, from http://www.atsdr.cdc.gov/toxprofiles/tp151.html.
8. Bader M, Dietz MC, Ihrig A, et al. Biomonitoring of manganese in blood, urine and axillary hair following low-dose exposure during the manufacture of dry cell batteries. *Int Arch Occup Environ Health.* 1999;72:521-527.
9. Barbeau A. Manganese and extrapyramidal disorder. *Neurotoxicology.* 1984;5:13-36.
10. Barceloux, DG. Manganese. *J Toxicol Clin Toxicol.* 1999;37:293-307.
11. Bertinet DB, Tinivella M, Balzola FA, et al. Brain manganese deposition and blood levels in patients undergoing home parenteral nutrition. *JPEN J Parenter Enteral Nutr.* 2000;24:223-227.

12. Bowler RM, Gysens S, Diamond E, et al. Neuropsychological sequelae of exposure to welding fumes in a group of occupationally exposed men. *Int J Hyg Environ Health.* 2003;206:517-529.
13. Calne DB, Chu NS, Huang CC, et al. Manganism and idiopathic parkinsonism: similarities and differences. *Neurology.* 1994:44:1583-1586.
14. Chandra SV, Shukla GS, Srivastava RS, et al. An exploratory study of manganese exposure to welders. *J Toxicol Clin Toxicol.* 1981;18:407-416.
15. Chen JY, Tsao GC, Zhao Q, et al. Differential cytotoxicity of Mn(II) and Mn(III): special reference to mitochondrial [Fe-S] containing enzymes. *Toxicol Appl Pharmacol.* 2001;175:160-168.
16. Cotzias GC, Papavasiliou PS, Ginos J, et al. Metabolic modification of Parkinson's disease and of chronic manganese poisoning. *Ann Rev Med.* 1971;22:305-326.
17. Couper J. On the effects of black oxide of manganese when inhaled into the lungs. *Br Ann Med Pharmacol.* 1837;1:41-42.
18. Crump KS. Manganese exposures in Toronto during use of the gasoline additive, methylcyclopentadienyl manganese tricarbonyl. *J Expo Anal Environ Epidemiol.* 2000;10:227-239.
19. Erikson KM, Thompson K, Aschner J, et al. Manganese neurotoxicity: a focus on the neonate. *Pharmacol Ther.* 2007;113:369-377.
20. Feldman RG. Manganese as a possible ecoetiologic factor in Parkinson's disease. *Ann NY Acad Sci.* 1992;648:266-267.
21. Fell JM, Reynolds AP, Meadows N, et al. Manganese toxicity in children receiving long-term parenteral nutrition. *Lancet.* 1996;347:1218-1221.
22. Finley JW. Manganese absorption and retention by young women is associated with serum ferritin concentration. *Am J Clin Nutr.* 1999;70:37-43.
23. Friedman BJ, Freeland-Graves J, Bales C, et al. Manganese balance and clinical observations in young men fed a manganese-deficient diet. *J Nutr.* 1987;117:133-143.
24. Galvani P, Fumagalli P, Sangostinono A. Vulnerability of the mitochondrial complex I in PC12 cells exposed to manganese. *Eur J Pharmacol Environ Toxicol.* 1995;293:377-383.
25. Gavin CE, Gunter KK, Gunter TE. Manganese and calcium efflux kinetics in brain mitochondria. Relevance to manganese toxicity. *Biochem J.* 1994;266:329-334.
26. Gavin CE, Gunter K, Gunter TE. Mn2+ sequestration by mitochondria and inhibition of oxidative phosphorylation. *Toxicol Appl Pharmacol.* 1992;115:1-5.
27. Gulson B, Mizon K, Taylor A, et al. Changes in manganese and lead in the environment and young children associated with the introduction of methylcyclopentadienyl manganese tricarbonyl in gasoline—preliminary results. *Environ Res.* 2006;100:100-114.
28. Hauser RA, Zesiewica TA, Martinez C, et al. Blood manganese correlates with brain magnetic resonance imaging changes in patients with liver disease. *Can J Neurol Sci.* 1996;23:95-98.
29. Huang CC, Chu NS, Lu CS, et al. Long-term progression in chronic manganism. *Neurology.* 1998;50:698-700.
30. Iinuma Y, Kubota M, Uchiyama M, et al. Whole-blood manganese levels and brain manganese accumulation in children receiving long-term home parenteral nutrition. *Pediatr Surg Int.* 2003;19:268-272.
31. Jankovic J. Searching for a relationship between manganese and welding and Parkinson's disease. *Neurology.* 2005;64:2021-2028.
32. Josephs KA, Ahlskog JE, Klos KJ, et al. Neurologic manifestations in welders with pallidal MRI T1 hyperintensity. *Neurology.* 2005;64:2033-2039.
33. Klaassen CD. Biliary excretion of manganese in rats, rabbits, and dogs. *Toxicol Appl Pharmacol.* 1974;29:458-468.
34. Koller WC, Lyons KE, Truly W. Effect of levodopa treatment for parkinsonism in welders. *Neurology.* 2004;62:730-733.
35. Kosta P, Argyropoulou MI, Markoula S, et al. MRI evaluation of the basal ganglia size and iron content in patients with Parkinson's disease. *J Neurol.* 2006;253:26-32.
36. Lees-Haley PR, Greiffenstein MF, Larrabee GJ, et al. Methodological problems in the neuropsychological assessment of effects of exposure to welding fumes and manganese. *Clin Neuropsychol.* 2004;18:449-464.
37. Liu X, Sullivan KA, Madl JE, et al. Manganese-induced neurotoxicity: the role of astroglial-derived nitric oxide in striatal interneuron degeneration. *Toxicol Sci.* 2006;91:521-531.
38. Lloyd Davies TA, Harding HE. Manganese pneumonitis: further clinical and experimental observations. *Br J Ind Med.* 1949;6:82-90.
39. Lu CS, Huang CC, Chu NS, et al. Levodopa failure in chronic manganism. *Neurology.* 1994;44:1600-1602.
40. Mahomedy MC, Mahomedy YH, Canham PAS, et al. Methaemoglobinemia following treatment by witch doctors. Two cases of potassium permanganate poisoning. *Anesthesia.* 1975;30:190-193.
41. Mahoney JP, Small WJ. The biological half-life of radiomanganese in man and factors which affect this half-life. *J Clin Invest.* 1968;47:643-653.
42. Martin WR, Wieler M, Gee M. Midbrain iron content in early Parkinson's disease: a potential biomarker of disease status. *Neurology.* 2008;70:1411-1417.
43. Masumoto K, Suita S, Taguchi T, et al. Manganese intoxication during intermittent parenteral nutrition: report of two cases. *J Parenter Enteral Nutr.* 2001;25:95-99.
44. Mena I, Court J, Fuenzalida S, et al. Modification of chronic manganese poisoning: treatment with L-dopa and 5-OH tryptophan. *N Engl J Med.* 1970;282:5-10.
45. Michalke B, Halbach S, Nischwitz V. Speciation and toxicological relevance of manganese in humans. *J Environ Monitor.* 2007;9:650-656.
46. Mirowitz SA, Westrich TJ. Basal ganglia signal intensity alterations: reversal after discontinuation of parenteral manganese administration. *Radiology.* 1992;185:535-536.
47. Murphy VA, Wadhwani KC, Smith QR, et al. Saturable transport of manganese (II) across the rat blood-brain barrier. *J Neurochem.* 1991;57:948-954.
48. Nagatomo S, Umehara F, Hanada K, et al. Manganese intoxication during total parenteral nutrition: report of two cases and review of the literature. *J Neurol Sci.* 1999;162:102-105.
49. Newland MC. Animal models of manganese's neurotoxicity. *Neurotoxicology.* 1999;20:415-432.
50. Normandin L, Hazell AS. Manganese neurotoxicity: an update of pathophysiologic mechanisms. *Metab Brain Dis.* 2002;17:375-387.
51. Olanow CW. Manganese-induced parkinsonism and Parkinson's disease. *Ann NY Acad Sci.* 2004;1012:209-223.
52. Pleban PA, Pearson KH. Determination of manganese in whole blood and serum. *Clin Chem.* 1979;23:95-98.
53. Pomier-Layrargues G, Spahr L, Butterworth RF. Increased manganese concentration in pallidum of cirrhotic patients. *Lancet.* 1995;345:735.
54. Pujol A, Pujol J, Graus F, et al. Hyperintense globus pallidus on T1-weighted MRI in cirrhotic patients is associated with severity of liver failure. *Neurology.* 1993;43:65-69.
55. Rabin O, Hegedus L, Bourre JM, et al. Rapid brain uptake of manganese (II) across the blood-brain barrier. *J Neurochem.* 1993;61:509-517.
56. Racette BA, McGee-Minnich, Moerlein SM, et al. Welding-related parkinsonism: clinical features, treatment, and pathophysiology. *Neurology.* 2001;56:8-13.
57. Roels H, Lauwerys R, Buchet JP, et al. Epidemiological survey among workers exposed to manganese: effects on lung, central nervous system, and some biological indices. *Am J Ind Med.* 1987;11:307-327.
58. Rose C, Butterworth RF, Zayed J, et al. Manganese deposition in basal ganglia structures results from both portal-systemic shunting and liver dysfunction. *Gastroenterology.* 1999;117:640-644.
59. Rosenstock HA, Simons DG, Meyer JS. Chronic manganism: neurologic and laboratory studies during treatment with levodopa. *JAMA.* 1971;217:1354-1358.
60. Roth JA, Feng L, Dolan KG, et al. Effect of the iron chelator desferrioxamine on manganese-induced toxicity of rat pheochromocytoma cells. *J Neurosci Res.* 2002;68:76-83.
61. Sahni V, Leger Y, Panaro M, et al. Case report: a metabolic disorder presenting as pediatric manganism. *Environ Health Persp.* 2007;115:1776-1779.
62. Schaumburg HH, Herskovitz S, Cassano VA. Occupational manganese neurotoxicity provoked by hepatitis C. *Neurology.* 2006;67:322-323.
63. Schuler P, Oyanguren H, Maturana V, et al. Manganese poisoning: environmental and medical study at a Chilean mine. *Ind Med Surg.* 1957;26:167-173.
64. Silbergeld EK. MMT: science and policy. *Environ Res.* 1999;80:93-95.
65. Spahr L, Butterworth RF, Fontaine S, et al. Increased blood manganese in cirrhotic patients: relationship to pallidal magnetic resonance signal hyperintensity and neurological symptoms. *Hepatology.* 1996;24:1116-1120.
66. Stepens A, Logina I, Liguts V, et al. A Parkinsonian syndrome in methcathinone users and the role of manganese. *N Engl J Med.* 2008;358:1009-1017.
67. Sumino K, Hayakawa K, Shibata T, et al. Heavy metals in normal Japanese tissues: amounts of 15 heavy metals in 30 subjects. *Arch Environ Health.* 1975;30:487-494.

68. Takagi Y, Okada A, Sando K, et al. Evaluation of indexes of in vivo manganese status and the optimal intravenous dose for adult patients undergoing home parenteral nutrition. *Am J Clin Nutr*. 2002;75:112-118.
69. Takagi Y, Okada A, Sando K, et al. On-off study of manganese administration to adult patients undergoing home parenteral nutrition: new indices of an in vivo manganese level. *JPEN J Parenter Enteral Nutr*. 2001;25:87-92.
70. Tanner CM, Goldman SM, Quinlan P, et al. Occupation and risk of Parkinson's disease (PD): a preliminary investigation of Standard Occupational Codes (SOC) in twins discordant for disease. *Neurology*. 2003;60:A415.
71. Tugrul AH, Oguz N, Tugba T, et al. T2-weighted MRI in Parkinson's disease: substantia nigra pars compacta hypointensity correlates with the clinical scores. *Neurol Ind*. 2004;52:332-337.
72. Wolters EC, Huang CC, Clark C, et al. Positron emission tomography in manganese intoxication. *Ann Neurol*. 1989;26:647-651.
73. Young RJ, Critchley JAJH, Young KK, et al. Fatal acute hepatorenal failure following potassium permanganate ingestion. *Human Exp Toxicol*. 1996;15:259-261.
74. Zwingmann C, Leibfritz D, Hazell AS. Brain energy metabolism in a subacute rat model of manganese neurotoxicity: an ex-vivo nuclear magnetic resonance study using [1-13C]glucose. *Neurotoxicology*. 2004;25:573-587.
75. Zwingmann C, Leibfritz D, Hazell AS. Energy metabolism in astrocytes and neurons treated with manganese: relation among cell-specific energy failure, glucose metabolism, and intracellular trafficking using multinuclear NMR-spectroscopic analysis. *J Cereb Blood Flow Metab*. 2003;23:756-771.

CHAPTER 96
MERCURY

Young-Jin Sue

Mercury (Hg)

Atomic number	=	80
Atomic weight	=	200.59
Normal concentrations		
Whole blood	<	10 µg/L (<50 nmol/L)
Urine	<	20 µg/L (<100 nmol/L)
	<	5 µg/g creatinine (<25 nmol/g creatinine)

Mercury is a naturally occurring metal that is widely toxic to multiple organ systems. Whereas elemental mercury produces pulmonary toxicity, inorganic mercury initially causes gastrointestinal (GI) symptoms followed by nephrotoxicity. A nearly pure neurologic toxicity results from organic (methylmercury) exposure.

HISTORY AND EPIDEMIOLOGY

The toxicologic manifestations of mercury are well known as a result of thousands of years of medicinal applications, industrial use, and environmental disasters.[58,92] Mercury occurs naturally in small amounts as the elemental silver-colored liquid (quicksilver); as inorganic salts such as mercuric sulfide (cinnabar), mercurous chloride (calomel), mercuric chloride (corrosive sublimate), and mercuric oxide; and as organic compounds (methylmercury and dimethylmercury). In recent centuries, mercury preparations were widely used to treat both syphilis and constipation. The musician Paganini was one of several famous persons whose gingivitis, dental decay, ptyalism (excessive salivation), and erethism (pathologic shyness) were attributed to mercury therapy.[67] In the 1800s, the United States witnessed an epidemic of "hatters' shakes" or "Danbury shakes" and "mercurial salivation" in hat industry workers.[103] Danbury, CT, was a U.S. center of felt hat manufacturing where mercuric nitrate was used to mat animal furs to make felt.[92,103]

In the early 1900s, acrodynia, or "pink disease," was described in children who received calomel for ascariasis or teething discomfort.[12] Vividly described in a series of 41 children, the development of acrodynia was more common in younger children, did not seem to correlate with mercury dose, and was not necessarily related to urine concentrations of mercury.[102]

One of the most devastating epidemics of mercury poisoning occurred as the result of a decade of contamination of Minamata Bay in Japan by a nearby vinyl chloride plant during the 1940s. Methylmercury accumulated in the bay's marine life and poisoned the inhabitants of the local fishing community. Although officially only 121 victims were initially counted, thousands more are believed to have been affected by what has subsequently been named Minamata disease.[72,94] The largest outbreak of methylmercury poisoning to date occurred in Iraq in late 1971. Approximately 95,000 tons of seed grain intended for planting and treated with methylmercury as a fungicide were baked into bread for direct consumption, resulting in widespread neurologic symptoms, 6530 hospital admissions, and more than 400 deaths.[4,18,77]

In 1990, the Environmental Protection Agency (EPA) banned mercury-containing compounds from interior paints.[2] However, mercury-containing paints manufactured before that ruling may still be on interior walls, and mercury-containing paint can still be sold for outdoor use. In 1997, a scientist succumbed to delayed, progressive neurologic deterioration after dermal exposure to a minute quantity of dimethylmercury.[64]

Contemporary exposures occur in the form of mercury-tainted seafood and mercury-based preservatives (thimerosal). However, a once widely feared source of potential poisoning, mercury-containing dental amalgam, does not result in clinically important poisoning. Occasionally, exposure to mercury from broken thermometers leads to poisoning in the home.

The recent movement to replace incandescent light bulbs with compact fluorescent bulbs has raised the concern of exposure to mercury in the home and environment. Promoted to reduce greenhouse gas emissions, each bulb contains 5 mg of elemental mercury. Recycling options are not yet widely available.[7] Tables 96–1 and 96–2 show the potential occupational and nonoccupational risks for mercury exposure.

FORMS OF MERCURY AND TOXICOKINETICS

The three important classes of mercury compounds—elemental, inorganic, and organic—differ with respect to their toxicodynamics and toxicokinetics (Table 96–3). Each class produces distinct clinical patterns of poisoning stemming in part from their unique kinetic features (Table 96–4). Within each class, the specific manifestations are determined by the route of exposure, rate of exposure, distribution, and biotransformation of mercury within the body and relative accumulation or elimination of mercury by the target organ systems.

ABSORPTION

Elemental Mercury Elemental mercury (Hg^0) is absorbed primarily via inhalation of vapor, although slow absorption after aspiration, subcutaneous deposition, and direct intravenous (IV) embolization occurs.[49,61,100,107] Volatility, moderate at room temperature, increases significantly with heating or aerosalization, both of which occur with vacuuming.[84] When inhaled by human volunteers, 75% to 80% of mercury vapor is absorbed.[35] However, elemental mercury is negligibly absorbed from a normally functioning gut, and it is usually considered nontoxic when ingested. Abnormal GI motility prolongs mucosal exposure to elemental mercury and increases subsequent ionization to more readily absorbed forms. Similarly, anatomic GI abnormalities such as fistulae or perforation may be associated with extravasation of mercury into the peritoneal space, where elemental mercury is oxidized to more readily absorbed inorganic forms.

Inorganic Mercury Salts The principal route of absorption for inorganic mercury salts is the GI tract. Approximately 10% of inorganic mercury salts are absorbed after dissociation of ingested soluble divalent mercuric salts such as mercuric chloride ($HgCl_2$).[55] Absorption of a relatively insoluble monovalent mercurous compound, such as calomel (HgCl), is thought to depend on its oxidation to the divalent form.[65] Inorganic mercury salts are also absorbed across the skin and mucous membranes, as evidenced by urinary excretion of mercury after dermal application of mercurial ointments and powders containing HgCl.[102] The degree of dermal absorption varies by the concentration of mercury, skin integrity, and lipid solubility of the vehicle. With substantial dermal exposures to inorganic mercury salts, skin absorption may be difficult to distinguish from concomitant absorption via other routes, such as ingestion.

TABLE 96–1. Potential Occupational Exposures to Mercury

Elemental	Salts	Organic
Amalgam	Disinfectants	Bactericide makers
Barometers	Dye makers	Drug makers
Bronzers	Explosives	Embalmers
Ceramic workers	Fireworks makers	Farmers
Chlorine workers	Fur processors	Fungicides
Dentists	Laboratory workers	Histology technicians
Electroplaters	Tannery workers	Pesticides
Jewelers	Taxidermists	Seed handlers
Mercury refiners	Vinyl chloride makers	Wood preservatives
Paint makers		
Paper pulp workers		
Photographers		
Thermometers		

TABLE 96–3. Classes of Mercury Compounds

	Chemical Formula	Example
Elemental mercury	Hg^0	Quicksilver
Inorganic mercury salts	Hg^+	Mercurous ion
	HgCl	Calomel, mercurous chlorine
	Hg^{2+}	Mercuric ion
	$HgCl_2$	Mercuric chloride
Organic mercury compounds	Short-chain alkyl–mercury compounds	Methylmercury, ethylmercury, dimethylmercury
	Long-chain aryl–mercury compounds	Methoxyethylmercury, phenylmercury

Organic Mercury Compounds As in the case of inorganic mercury salts, organic mercury compounds are primarily absorbed from the GI tract. Methylmercury, considered the prototype of the short-chain alkyl compounds, is approximately 90% absorbed from the gut.[65] Aryl and long-chain alkyl compounds have greater than 50% GI absorption.[65] Although both dermal and inhalational absorption of organic mercury compounds are reported, precise quantitation and exclusion of concomitant absorption by ingestion are difficult to determine.[22,28,104,105]

DISTRIBUTION AND BIOTRANSFORMATION

After it is absorbed, mercury distributes widely to all tissues, predominantly the kidneys, liver, spleen, and central nervous system (CNS). The initial distributive pattern into nervous tissue of elemental and organic mercury differs from that of the inorganic salts because of their greater lipid solubility.

Elemental Mercury Although peak concentrations of elemental mercury are delayed in the CNS as compared with other organs (2–3 days versus 1 day),[35] significant accumulation in the CNS may occur after an acute, intense exposure to elemental mercury vapor. Conversion of elemental mercury to the charged mercuric cation within the CNS favors retention and local accumulation of the metal. Because elemental mercury does not covalently bind to other compounds, its toxicity depends on its oxidation initially to the mercurous ion (Hg^+) and then to the mercuric ion (Hg^{2+}) by the enzyme catalase.[55] Because this oxidation–reduction reaction favors the mercuric cation at steady state, the distribution and late manifestations of metallic mercury toxicity eventually resemble those of inorganic mercury salt poisoning. Conversely, and to a lesser extent, inorganic mercuric ions are reduced to the elemental state, although the site and mechanism of this reaction are not well understood.[65]

TABLE 96–2. Nonoccupational Exposures to Mercury

Medicinal	Food	Other
Antiseptics	Fish	Button batteries
Calomel teething powders	Grains and seed, treated	Chemistry sets
Dental amalgam	Livestock fed treated grain	Home amalgam extraction
Diuretics		Lightbulbs (fluorescent)
Laxatives		Self-injection
Sphygmomanometers		Preservatives
Stool fixatives		Ritualistic use
Thermometers		
Weighted nasogastric tubes		

TABLE 96–4. Differential Characteristics of Mercury Exposure

	Elemental	Inorganic (Salt)	Organic (Alkyl)
Primary route of exposure	Inhalation	Oral	Oral
Primary tissue distribution	CNS, kidney	Kidney	CNS, kidney, liver
Clearance	Renal, GI	Renal, GI	Methyl: GI Aryl: Renal, GI
Clinical effects			
CNS	Tremor	Tremor, erethism	Paresthesias, ataxia, tremor, tunnel vision, dysarthria
Pulmonary	+++	–	–
Gastrointestinal	+	+++(caustic)	+
Renal	+	+++(ATN)	+
Acrodynia	+	++	–
Therapy	BAL, succimer	BAL, succimer	Succimer (early)

ATN, acute tubular necrosis; BAL, British anti-Lewisite.

Inorganic Mercury Salts The greatest concentration of mercuric ions is found in the kidneys, particularly within the renal tubules. Very little mercury is found as free mercuric ions. At least in animal studies, administration of mercury induces the renal synthesis of metallothionein, a compound that binds to and detoxifies mercuric ions.[9] In blood, mercuric ions are found within the red blood cells (RBCs) and are bound to plasma proteins in approximately equal proportions. Blood concentrations are greatest immediately after inorganic mercury exposure, with rapid waning as distribution to other tissues occurs. Although penetration of the blood–brain barrier is poor because of low lipid solubility, slow elimination and prolonged exposure contribute to consequential CNS accumulation of mercuric ions. Within the CNS, mercuric ions are concentrated in the cerebral and cerebellar cortices. Although inorganic mercurials undergo organification in marine life, as in the Minamata Bay disaster, the importance of this conversion in humans is unknown.[22] Animal studies demonstrate that the placenta functions as an effective barrier to mercuric ions.[65]

Organic Mercury Compounds Once absorbed, aryl and long-chain alkyl mercury compounds differ from the short-chain organic mercury compounds (ie, methylmercury) in an important way—the former possess a labile carbon-mercury bond, which is subsequently cleaved, releasing the inorganic mercuric ion. Thus, the distribution pattern and toxicologic manifestations produced by the aryl and long-chain alkyl compounds beyond the immediate postabsorptive phase are comparable to those of the inorganic mercury salts, but organification has facilitated absorption and reduced the caustic effects.[66] In contrast, short-chain alkyl mercury compounds possess relatively stable carbon–mercury bonds that survive the absorptive phase, although conversion to the inorganic mercuric cation at a rate of less than 1% per day may occur after absorption.[104] Because it is lipophilic, methylmercury readily distributes across all tissues, including the blood–brain barrier and placenta.[37] An important consequence of this property is the devastating neurologic degeneration that develops in prenatally exposed infants with Minamata disease.

After methylmercury is distributed to brain tissue, its fate is uncertain. Animal evidence indicates that methylmercury is converted to inorganic mercury in brain tissue.[52] Primates fed oral methylmercury daily for periods exceeding 1 year and then killed within a few days of the last exposure demonstrated an average brain inorganic mercury fraction of only 19%. When the postexposure period was extended to between 150 and 650 days, the inorganic mercury fraction increased to 88%. Similarly, long-term survivors of methylmercury poisoning had a higher ratio of inorganic mercury to total mercury in their brains.[25] In one patient who survived 22 years after methylmercury ingestion, autopsy revealed that the brain mercury was nearly completely in the inorganic form.

Methylmercury concentrates in RBCs to a much greater degree than do mercuric ions, with an RBC-to-plasma ratio of about 10:1 (in contrast to 1:1 RBC-to-plasma ratio for inorganic mercury).[46,65,104] However, despite this apparent affinity for nervous tissue and RBCs, the greatest methylmercury concentrations are found in the kidneys and liver. Also, because of the extensive sulfhydryl bonds in hair, methylmercury deposits in hair at concentrations approximately 250 times that found in whole blood.[45,93]

ELIMINATION

Elemental Mercury and Inorganic Mercury Salts Mercuric ions are excreted through the kidney by both glomerular filtration and tubular secretion and in the GI tract by transfer across gut mesenteric vessels into feces. Small amounts are reduced to elemental mercury vapor and volatilized from skin and lungs. The total-body half-life of elemental mercury and inorganic mercury salts is estimated at approximately 30 to 60 days.[17,55]

Organic Mercury Compounds In contrast to elemental mercury and inorganic mercury salts, the elimination of short-chain alkyl mercury compounds is predominantly fecal. Enterohepatic recirculation contributes to its somewhat longer half-life of about 70 days. Less than 10% of methylmercury is excreted in urine and feces as the mercuric cation.[104]

PATHOPHYSIOLOGY

The pervasive disruption of normal cell physiology by mercury is believed to arise from its avid covalent binding to sulfur, replacing the hydrogen ion in the body's ubiquitous sulfhydryl groups. Mercury also reacts with phosphoryl, carboxyl, and amide groups, resulting in widespread dysfunction of enzymes, transport mechanisms, membranes, and structural proteins. Mercury is being investigated in a variety of cellular alterations, including oxidant stress, microtubule disruption, protein and DNA synthesis, and cell membrane integrity.

Because mercury deposits in all tissues, the clinical manifestations of mercury toxicity involve multiple organ systems with variable features and intensity. Necrosis of the GI mucosa and proximal renal tubules, which occurs shortly after mercury salt poisoning, is thought to result from direct oxidative effect of mercuric ions. An immune mechanism is attributed to the membranous glomerulonephritis and acrodynia associated with the use of mercurial ointments.[10] Postmortem examination of the kidneys from two women who died after chronic abuse of mercurous chloride–containing laxatives revealed severe proximal tubular atrophy and mercury deposition within the cortical interstitium and renal macrophages.[101]

Neurologic manifestations of methylmercury poisoning correlate with pathologic findings in the brains of both adults and children who were prenatally exposed.[57,94] Grossly, atrophy of the brain is more severe in children who had prenatally or postnatally acquired methylmercury compared with the brains of those exposed as adults. In the adult brain, neuronal necrosis and glial proliferation are most prominent in the calcarine cortex of the cerebrum and in the cerebellar cortex. In fetal Minamata disease, similar lesions are present but in a more diffuse and severe form. Atrophy of the cerebellar hemispheres, postcentral gyri, and calcarine area of the brain demonstrated on magnetic resonance images in organic mercury–poisoned patients correlates with clinical findings of ataxia, sensory neuropathy, and visual field constriction, respectively.[48] Neuropathologic examination of the brain of a scientist who died after unintentional dermal exposure to dimethylmercury revealed lesions in the cerebellum, temporal lobe, and visual cortex.[87]

In rats, neuronal cytotoxicity of methylmercury may result partly from muscarinic receptor–mediated calcium release from smooth endoplasmic reticulum of cerebellar granule cells.[51] There is animal evidence that methylmercury may trigger reactive oxygen species production. In addition, methylmercury inhibits astrocyte uptake of cysteine, the rate-limiting step in the production of glutathione, a major antioxidant in mammalian cell systems.[86] Cultured astrocytes accumulated methylmercury and exhibited increased mitochondrial permeability and oxidative injury.[106]

CLINICAL MANIFESTATIONS

ELEMENTAL MERCURY

Symptoms of *acute elemental mercury inhalation* occur within hours of exposure and consist of cough, chills, fever, and shortness of breath.

GI complaints include nausea, vomiting, and diarrhea accompanied by a metallic taste, dysphagia, salivation, weakness, headaches, and visual disturbances. Chest radiography during the acute phase may reveal interstitial pneumonitis and both patchy atelectasis and emphysema. Symptoms may resolve or progress to acute lung injury, respiratory failure, and death. Survivors of severe pulmonary manifestations may develop interstitial fibrosis and residual restrictive pulmonary disease. The acute respiratory symptoms may occur concomitantly with or lead to the development of subacute inorganic mercury poisoning manifested by tremor, renal dysfunction, and gingivostomatitis.[13,44,75] Thrombocytopenia may also occur during the acute phase.[31]

Although acute exposure to elemental mercury vapor occurs most commonly in the occupational setting, poisonings caused by mishandling of the metal in the home are well reported.[16,40,59,89] In fact, attempts at home metallurgy using metallic mercury have resulted in fatalities with ambient air concentrations of mercury as high as 0.9 mg/m^3 (National Institute for Occupational Safety and Health recommended exposure level 8-hour time-weighted average 0.05 mg/m^3 for mercury vapor).[15] The lethal dose of inhaled elemental mercury has not been determined. As with other inhaled toxins, younger individuals may be more sensitive to the pulmonary toxicity of mercury vapor.[59] Although pulmonary toxicity from elemental mercury usually results from inhalation of vapor, massive endobronchial hemorrhage followed by death has occurred secondary to direct *aspiration of metallic mercury* into the tracheobronchial tree.[109]

Gradual volatilization of elemental mercury results in chronic toxicity from improper handling, such as vacuuming spilled mercury.[84]

The clinical importance of volatilized metallic mercury from dental amalgams for both the dentist and patient has been a point of contention. The preponderance of evidence refutes the idea that dental amalgam causes mercury poisoning. Several comprehensive reviews of the subject conclude that (1) occupational exposure to mercury from dental amalgam is acceptably low, provided that recommended preventive measures such as adequate ventilation are adhered to; (2) the quantity of mercury vaporized from dental amalgam by mechanical forces, such as chewing, is clinically insignificant; and (3) only in very rare cases will immunologic hypersensitivity to mercury amalgam (manifested as cutaneous signs and symptoms and confirmed by patch testing) necessitate removal of the amalgam.[27,29,30,50,88]

Unusual cases of chronic toxicity have resulted from intentional *subcutaneous or IV injection of elemental mercury* (see Figs. 5-6 and 96–1).[39,61] Aside from management of local and systemic mercury toxicity, local wound care and excision of deposits of mercury are additional therapeutic challenges presented by these cases. Serial or repeat radiographs are useful in guiding the removal of the radiopaque deposits.

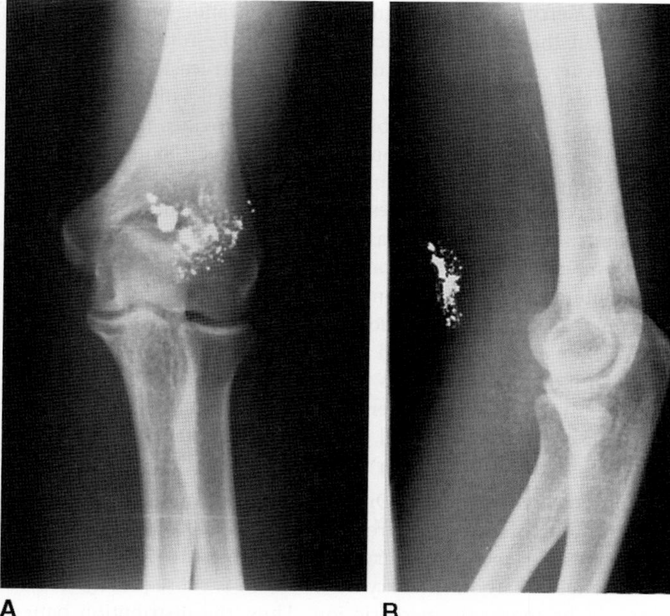

FIGURE 96–1. Anteroposterior (A) and lateral (B) views of the elbow after an unsuccessful suicidal gesture involving an attempted intravenous injection of mercury in the antecubital fossa. Note the extensive subcutaneous mercury deposition, which was partially removed by surgical intervention. *(Images contributed by Diane Sauter, MD.)*

INORGANIC MERCURY SALTS

Acute *ingestion of mercuric salts* produces a characteristic spectrum from severe irritant to caustic gastroenteritis. Immediately after the ingestion, a grayish discoloration of mucous membranes and metallic taste may accompany local oropharyngeal pain, nausea, vomiting, and diarrhea followed by abdominal pain, hematemesis, and hematochezia. The lethal dose of mercuric chloride is estimated to be 30 to 50 mg/kg.[96] The hallmarks of severe acute mercuric salt ingestion are hemorrhagic gastroenteritis, massive fluid loss resulting in shock, and acute tubular necrosis.[82]

Oropharyngeal injury, nausea, hematemesis, hematochezia, and abdominal pain were the most prominent symptoms in a series of 54 patients who presented after ingesting up to 4 g of mercuric chloride.[96] In this series, a fatal outcome was associated with the early development of oliguria (within 3 days). The development of anuria appeared to be related to the dose of mercuric chloride ingested. The histopathologic finding of proximal tubular necrosis after mercuric salt poisoning results from both direct toxicity to renal tubules by mercuric ions and renal hypoperfusion caused by shock. Consequently, aggressive fluid therapy is useful.[83]

Acute ingestion of mercuric salts is usually intentional, but unintentional ingestion occurs sporadically in both children and adults.[41] Although ingestion of button batteries containing mercuric oxide is associated with a greater incidence of fragmentation than with other batteries, clinically significant systemic mercury toxicity by this route has not been reported.[53,56]

Mercuric chloride–containing stool preservatives are another potential source of unintentional inorganic mercury poisoning. Ingestion of 10 to 20 mL of a polyvinyl alcohol preservative that contained 4.5% mercuric chloride resulted in bloody gastroenteritis and proteinuria.[85] Patent[39] and Ayurvedic[80,81] medicines are also associated with unintentional inorganic mercury poisoning.[43] Not subject to Food and Drug Administration (FDA) regulation and available without prescription, these xenobiotics are often inadequately labeled and of variable composition (see Chap. 43).

Subacute or chronic mercury poisoning occurs after inhalation, aspiration, or injection of elemental mercury; ingestion or application of inorganic mercury salts; or ingestion of aryl or long-chain alkyl mercury compounds. Slow in vivo oxidation of elemental mercury and dissociation of the carbon–mercury bond of aryl or long-chain alkyl mercury compounds result in the production of the inorganic mercurous and mercuric ions.

The predominant manifestations of subacute or chronic mercury toxicity include GI symptoms, neurologic abnormalities, and renal dysfunction. GI symptoms consist of a metallic taste and burning sensation in the mouth, loose teeth and gingivostomatitis, hypersalivation (ptyalism), and nausea.[102] The neurologic manifestations of chronic inorganic mercurialism include tremor, as well as the syndromes of neurasthenia and erethism. Neurasthenia is a symptom complex that includes fatigue, depression, headaches, hypersensitivity to stimuli, psychosomatic complaints, weakness, and loss of concentrating ability. Erethism, derived from the Greek word *red*, describes the easy blushing and extreme shyness of affected individuals. Other symptoms of erethism include anxiety, emotional lability, irritability, insomnia, anorexia, weight loss, and delirium. Mercury produces a characteristic central intention tremor (see Chap. 18) that is abolished during sleep. In the most severe forms of mercury-associated tremor, choreoathetosis and spasmodic ballismus may be present. Other neurologic manifestations of inorganic mercurialism include a mixed sensorimotor neuropathy, ataxia, concentric constriction of visual fields ("tunnel vision"), and anosmia.

Chronic poisoning with mercuric ions is associated with renal dysfunction, which ranges from asymptomatic, reversible proteinuria to nephrotic syndrome with edema and hypoproteinemia. An idiosyncratic hypersensitivity to mercury ions is thought to be responsible for acrodynia, or "pink disease," which is an erythematous, edematous, and hyperkeratotic induration of the palms, soles, and face, and a pink papular rash that was first described in a subset of children exposed to mercurous chloride powders.[102] The rash is described as morbilliform, urticarial, vesicular, and hemorrhagic. This symptom complex also includes excessive sweating, tachycardia, irritability, anorexia, photophobia, insomnia, tremors, paresthesias, decreased deep-tendon reflexes, and weakness. The acral rash may progress to desquamation and ulceration. The prognosis is favorable after withdrawal from mercury exposure. Childhood acrodynia has become uncommon since the abandonment of mercurial teething powders and diaper rinses. Occasional case reports are still noted, however, with fluorescent light bulbs and phenylmercuric acetate–containing paint implicated.[2,97]

Thimerosal is an example of an aryl or long-chain alkyl mercury compound that results in chronic inorganic mercury toxicity. It is a compound that was widely used as a preservative in the pharmaceutical industry (see Chap. 55). Although initial kinetics suggest a stable ethyl–mercury bond, the later elimination phase more closely resembles that of the inorganic mercury compounds. Thimerosal is approximately 50% mercury by weight. Generally considered safe, toxicity and death can nevertheless occur after both intentional overdose and excessive therapeutic application of Merthiolate (0.1% thimerosal or 600 μg/mL mercury).[71,76]

Concern that the cumulative dose of thimerosal in childhood immunizations may exceed federally recommended maximum mercury doses (EPA, 0.1 μg/kg/d; Agency for Toxic Substances and Disease Registry, 0.3 μg/kg/d; FDA, 0.4 μg/kg/d) led to a call by the American Academy of Pediatrics to reduce or eliminate thimerosal from vaccines.[3] In particular, controversy exists whether thimerosal causes autism. Although sensitization after use in vaccinations has been reported in atopic children,[70] clinical mercury toxicity has not been reported in appropriately immunized children. Moreover, a number of studies suggest that the incidence of autism is unrelated to the use of thimerosal-containing vaccines.[6,54,69,90] Similarly, no causal association with early thimerosal exposure and adverse neuropsychological outcomes was shown in children tested at 7 to 10 years of age.[95] At the present time, there is clearly more evidence for risk to child health from the diseases targeted for prevention by the vaccines than from thimerosal. Nevertheless, since 2001, routinely administered childhood vaccines in the United States, with the exception of injectable influenza vaccine, contain only trace amounts of thimerosal.[38]

ORGANIC MERCURY COMPOUNDS

In contrast to the inorganic mercurials, methylmercury produces an almost purely neurologic disease that is usually permanent except in the mildest of cases. Although the predominant syndrome associated with methylmercury is that of a delayed neurotoxicity, acute GI symptoms, tremor, respiratory distress, and dermatitis may occur.[22,104] In addition, electrocardiographic (ECG) abnormalities (ST segment changes) and renal tubular dysfunction are associated with this poisoning.[28,36]

The lipophilic property and slower elimination of methylmercury may contribute to its profound neurologic effects.[28] Characteristically, clinical manifestations occur after the initial poisoning by a latent period of weeks to months. Consequently, the lethal dose of methylmercury is difficult to determine. As noted previously, infants exposed prenatally to methylmercury were the most severely affected individuals in Minamata. Often born to mothers with little or no manifestation of methylmercury toxicity themselves, exposed infants exhibited decreased birth weight and muscle tone, profound developmental delay, seizure disorders, deafness, blindness, and severe spasticity. The development of neurologic symptoms in infants exclusively breastfed by women exposed to methylmercury after delivery and the detection of mercury in the milk of lactating women implies a risk for mercury poisoning via breast milk.[47] In one series of lactating women, mercury concentrations in milk were approximately 30% of the concentrations found in blood.[68] The rapid decline of blood mercury concentrations in both suckling rats and breastfeeding human infants is attributed to rapid growth of body volume combined with limited transport of mercury by milk.[63,78,79]

Several weeks after methylmercury-contaminated grain was ingested in Iraq, patients began to appear with paresthesias involving the lips, nose, and distal extremities. Symptomatic patients also noted headaches, fatigue, and tremor. More serious cases progressed to ataxia, dysarthria, visual field constriction, and blindness. Other neurologic deficits included hyperreflexia, hearing disturbances, movement disorders, salivation, and dementia. The most severely affected patients lay in a mute, rigid posture punctuated only by spontaneous crying, primitive reflexive movements, or feeding efforts.[77]

Although the outlook for methylmercury neurotoxicity is generally considered dismal, observations over the subsequent 2 years in 49 Iraqi children poisoned during the 1971 outbreak revealed complete resolution or partial improvement in all but the most severely affected.[4] Of 40 symptomatic children, 33 mildly to severely affected children showed partial to complete resolution of symptoms, but the seven children classified as "very severely poisoned" remained physically and mentally incapacitated.

The extreme toxicity of dimethylmercury was tragically demonstrated by the delayed fatal neurotoxicity that developed in a chemist who inadvertently spilled dimethylmercury on a break in the gloves on her hands. Over a period of several days, she developed progressive difficulty with speech, vision, and gait. Despite chelation and exchange transfusion, she died within several months of the exposure.[64]

An important route of organic mercury exposure is through seafood consumption. The safe level of methylmercury in seafood remains controversial. The FDA action concentration of 1 ppm for methylmercury in fish was set to limit consumption of methylmercury to less than one-tenth of levels found in cases of symptomatic poisoning. The EPA established a reference dose for methylmercury of 0.1 μg/kg/d.[73,98] Although elevated blood concentrations (19–53 μg/L) of mercury were found in one group of self-reported high consumers of seafood, increased incidence of cognitive and GI complaints were not.[42] Even so, concentrations at which fetuses experience adverse effects are unknown. Longitudinal studies of fish-eating populations are conflicting. No effect of a high prenatal fish diet was found on developmental markers in children followed to 11 years of age in the Seychelles Islands.[24] In the Faroe Island and New Zealand studies, however, a subtle but significant effect on neuropsychological development was seen.[21,33,91] In the Faroe Islands, this effect persisted when children were retested at 14 years of age.[26] One reason for the discrepancy that occurs between the two populations may be the different concentrations of methylmercury in the seafood consumed by each. The mean concentration of methylmercury in the whale meat consumed in the Faroe Islands was 1.6 μg/g, and the mean concentration of mercury found in New Zealand shark was 2.2 μg/g. In contrast, the mean methylmercury content of Seychellois fish was 0.3 μg/g.[62] The threshold concentration for neuropsychological effects may lie between these concentrations. The FDA recommends that at-risk populations (ie, pregnant women and women who may become pregnant, nursing mothers, and young children) avoid the large predator fish (eg, shark, swordfish, tilefish, and king mackerel) that contain concentrations of methylmercury approaching 1 ppm (1 μg/g).[99] The FDA has ruled that consumption advice is not indicated for the top 10 seafood species, which make up 80% of all seafood consumed: canned (nonalbacore) tuna, shrimp, pollock, salmon, cod, catfish, clams, flatfish, crabs, and scallops. These species contain concentrations of mercury less than 0.2 ppm and are rarely consumed in quantities in excess of the recommended weekly limit of 2.2 pounds. The recommendations are not as clear for albacore tuna, which may have concentrations of mercury as high as 0.34 ppm. The FDA-recommended limit of albacore tuna consumption by at-risk populations is less than 6 oz per week, but some consumer advocacy groups believe that the limit should be lower.[20] Others continue to believe that the benefits of modest fish ingestion, excepting a few select species, also outweigh the risks.[60]

DIAGNOSTIC TESTING

The dual findings of unexplained neuropsychiatric and renal abnormalities in an individual should alert the clinician to the possibility of mercurialism, as should an at-risk occupation or access by the patient to a mercurial product (see Tables 96–1 and 96–2).

Occupational or environmental exposure and a consistent clinical scenario may be suggestive of mercury poisoning, but demonstration of mercury in blood, urine, or tissues is necessary for confirmation of exposure. Of the many methods available to measure mercury, cold atomic absorption spectrometry is rapid, sensitive, and accurate but cannot distinguish the various forms of mercury. Thin-layer and gas chromatographic techniques can be used to distinguish organic from inorganic mercury.[22] Whole blood should be collected into a trace element collection tube obtained from the laboratory performing the assay. Urine should be collected for 24 hours into an acid-washed container obtained from a laboratory. Spot collections must be adjusted for creatinine concentration. Attempts to measure or otherwise handle the specimen should be avoided to prevent contamination.

There is considerable overlap among concentrations of mercury found in the normal population, asymptomatic exposed individuals, and patients with clinical evidence of poisoning. There is no definitive correlation between either whole blood or urine mercury concentrations and mercury toxicity. However, mercury serves no useful role in human physiology, and concentrations below 10 and 20 μg/L for whole blood and urine, respectively, are generally considered to reflect background exposure in nonpoisoned individuals. After long-term exposure to elemental mercury vapor, concentrations as low as 35 μg/L for whole blood and 150 μg/L for urine may be associated with nonspecific symptoms of mercury poisoning.[32]

For inorganic mercury poisoning, urine mercury concentrations may correlate roughly with exposure severity and neuropsychiatric symptoms,[74] but the relationship to total-body burden is probably poor. Urine mercury determinations have their greatest usefulness in confirming exposure and monitoring the efficacy of chelation therapy. Whole-blood mercury concentrations may reflect intense, acute inorganic mercury exposure but become less reliable as redistribution to tissues takes place.

Because organic mercury is eliminated via the fecal route, urine mercury concentrations are not useful in methylmercury poisoning. Because methylmercury concentrates in RBCs, the total-body methylmercury burden is best reflected acutely by whole blood concentrations.[22,46] As methylmercury distributes to and accumulates in brain, the severity of clinical manifestations probably more closely reflects the degree of the irreversible neuronal destruction that has taken place rather than the current body burden of mercury. Correlation of increasing whole-blood mercury concentrations with prevalence of paresthesias was suggested in a population of Iraqis studied early in the course of methylmercury poisoning.[19] However, in another group of patients, whole-blood concentrations did not correlate with severity of methylmercury poisoning.[77] This apparent discrepancy may have resulted from the finding that paresthesias are among the earliest reported symptoms of methylmercury poisoning.

Because mercury accumulates in the hair, hair analysis has been used as a tool for measuring mercury burden. However, because metal incorporation reflects past exposure and hair avidly binds mercury from the environment, the reliability of this method is questionable and is not recommended. In addition to mercury assays, neuropsychiatric testing, nerve conduction studies, and urine assays for *N*-acetyl-β-D-glucosaminidase and β_2-microglobulin are advocated for early detection of subclinical inorganic and organic mercury toxicity.[29,36,74]

GENERAL MANAGEMENT

After the initial assessment and stabilization, the early toxicologic management of a patient with mercury poisoning includes termination of exposure by removal from vapors; washing exposed skin; GI decontamination; supportive measures, such as hydration and humidified oxygen; baseline diagnostic studies, such as complete blood count, serum chemistries, arterial blood gas, radiographs, and ECG; specific analysis of whole blood and urine for mercury; consideration of possible cointoxicants; and meticulous monitoring.

ELEMENTAL MERCURY

Inhalation of mercury vapors or aspiration of metallic mercury may result in life-threatening respiratory failure; in this situation, stabilization of cardiorespiratory function is the initial priority. Postural drainage and endotracheal suction may be effective in removing aspirated metallic mercury. Parenteral deposition of subcutaneous or intramuscular (IM) mercury may be amenable to surgical excision, if well localized (see Fig. 96–1).

An adjunct to the initial management of patients with mercury poisoning is consideration for environmental decontamination. Elemental mercury that spills onto solid surfaces should be adsorbed to sand and the resulting mixture then swept into tightly sealed containers. Ideally, a mercury decontamination kit should be used. The kit consists of calcium polysulfide, which contains excess sulfur to convert mercury to water-insoluble mercuric sulfide (cinnabar). Absorbent surfaces, such as carpets, should be removed. Spilled mercury compounds should not be vacuumed because vacuuming could volatilize the mercury.[14] With respect to compact fluorescent bulbs, recommendations for decontamination after breakage include opening windows to release vapor, using adhesive tape to pick up visible fragments, and discarding in double-wrapped bags any remains after vacuuming. Guidance for decontamination of major spills and disposal of materials can be provided by local and federal hazardous materials agencies.

INORGANIC MERCURY SALTS

Ingestion of inorganic mercuric salts may lead to cardiovascular collapse caused by severe gastroenteritis and third-space fluid loss. Fluid resuscitation is a priority. GI decontamination of ingested inorganic salts of mercury is particularly problematic because of their causticity and risk for perforating injury. Nevertheless, one series of patients with mercuric chloride ingestion of up to 4 g reported recovery without long-term GI sequelae in patients who did not succumb to renal failure.[96] Therefore, unless there is high suspicion for penetrating GI mucosal injury, removal of mercury from absorptive surfaces should take priority over endoscopic evaluation. The prominence of vomiting makes gastric lavage unnecessary for most patients with inorganic mercury poisoning.

Metals are among the substances that are often considered to be poorly adsorbed to activated charcoal. Nevertheless, the serious nature of late sequelae after mercury absorption, the typically small quantities of mercury ingested, and evidence that inorganic mercuric salts actually have substantial adsorption to activated charcoal (800 mg mercuric chloride to 1 g activated charcoal in one in vitro study) justify routine administration of activated charcoal.[5] Whole-bowel irrigation with polyethylene glycol solution may also be useful in removing residual mercury and should be considered, with its progress followed with serial radiographs.

ORGANIC MERCURY COMPOUNDS

Organic mercury exposures do not typically present as single acute ingestions but rather as chronic or subacute ingestion of contaminated food. Therefore, GI decontamination is generally moot with respect to organic mercury poisoning. Nevertheless, its irreversible toxicity coupled with unsatisfactory treatments calls for aggressive decontamination when acute ingestions do occur.

CHELATION

After initial stabilization and decontamination, early institution of chelators may minimize or prevent the widespread effects of poisoning. A high degree of protein binding and distribution to the brain are responsible for the lack of efficacy of other measures to increase mercury clearance, such as peritoneal dialysis and hemodialysis.[82] In one report of the use of continuous venovenous hemodiafiltration in combination with a chelator in a patient with severe inorganic mercury poisoning, 12.7% of the ingested dose was recovered in the ultrafiltrate.[23] Hemodialysis may nevertheless ultimately be necessary because of the acute renal failure that often occurs after mercuric chloride poisoning.

Chelators have thiol groups that are believed to compete with endogenous sulfhydryl groups for the binding of mercury, thereby preventing inactivation of sulfhydryl-containing enzymes and other essential proteins (see Antidotes in Depth A26: Dimercaprol [British Anti-Lewisite or BAL] and Antidotes in Depth A27: Succimer [2,3-Dimercaptosuccinic Acid] for further discussion). A history of significant mercury exposure combined with the presence of typical symptoms of mercury poisoning is an appropriate indication for the institution of chelation therapy. Elevated whole-blood and urine mercury concentrations may help support the decision to begin chelation therapy in unclear cases and may also be used to guide the duration of therapy. Provocative chelation, in which urinary mercury excretion before and after a chelating dose is compared to determine the degree of mercury poisoning, is of no value.[42] Chelation tends to increase urinary elimination of mercury, regardless of exposure history and baseline excretion.

ELEMENTAL MERCURY AND INORGANIC MERCURY SALTS

For clinically significant acute inorganic mercury poisoning, dimercaprol (BAL) should be administered for 10 days in decreasing dosages of 5 mg/kg/dose every 4 hours IM for 48 hours, then 2.5 mg/kg every 6 hours for 48 hours, followed by 2.5 mg/kg every 12 hours for 7 days. This dosing regimen of BAL, derived from the use of BAL in lead poisoning, may be adjusted according to clinical response and the occurrence of adverse reactions.

When a patient is able to take oral medications, BAL therapy may be replaced with succimer (2,3-dimercaptosuccinic acid) at 10 mg/kg orally three times a day for 5 days, then twice a day for 14 days if the GI tract is clear. Because headache, nausea, vomiting, abdominal pain, and diaphoresis may result from BAL chelation therapy, oral succimer is recommended in patients who are not acutely ill or who have been chronically poisoned.

Either BAL or succimer is considered the treatment of choice for inorganic mercury poisoning in the United States, but a few other chelators deserve mention. DMPS (2,3-dimercapto-1-propanesulphonate) is a water-soluble dimercaprol derivative that is used in Europe. It may be administered both IV and orally. D-Penicillamine is an orally administered monothiol. Its adverse effects—GI distress, rashes, leukopenia, thrombocytopenia, and proteinuria—although uncommon in therapeutic doses, seriously limit the usefulness of the drug. *N*-acetyl-*d*,*l*-penicillamine (NAP), an investigational analog of D-penicillamine, is thought to be a more effective chelator of mercury than is D-penicillamine, perhaps because of its greater stability.[8,34]

ORGANIC MERCURY COMPOUNDS

The neurotoxicity of methylmercury and other organic mercury compounds is resistant to treatment, and therapeutic options are less than satisfactory. In rats, both BAL and D-penicillamine effectively reduced tissue mercury and prevented neurologic toxicity if administered within the first day of a methylmercury injection.[108] Neither treatment reversed neurologic toxicity when administered 12 days after methylmercury injection. DMPS, D-penicillamine, NAP, and a thiolated resin all led to a marked reduction of blood half-life of mercury (ie, 10, 24, 23, and 19 days, respectively, versus 60 days) during the outbreak of methylmercury poisoning in Iraq in 1971.[19] Clinical improvement was not observed in any treatment group, but it is reasonable to postulate that reducing the total-body burden of methylmercury may prevent or limit the progression of disease. When studied in mice poisoned with methylmercury,[1] succimer was superior to NAP, DMPS, and a thiolated resin in decreasing brain mercury and increasing urinary excretion. Brain mercury was decreased to 35% of control, and the total-body burden fell to 19%. Some animal evidence suggests that BAL may increase mercury mobilization into the brain.[11] For this reason and the lack of serious GI symptoms necessitating parenteral chelation, BAL should not be used for the treatment of patients with organic mercury poisoning.

Because the neurologic impairment associated with methylmercury is both profound and essentially irreversible, early recognition of poisoning and prevention of neurotoxicity are essential to a successful outcome. Although further investigation is necessary, succimer may prove to be the treatment of choice for methylmercury poisoning because of its apparently low toxicity and reported efficacy in animal trials.

SUMMARY

Mercury poisoning by any of the three major forms—elemental, inorganic, and organic—presents a complex toxicologic problem associated with a large variety of clinical presentations. An ever-present awareness of the problems coupled with the knowledge of the differing clinical forms is essential for both early recognition and effective treatment. Although some chelators do show promise in the treatment of mercury poisoning, neurologic sequelae, particularly those resulting from organic mercury exposures, remain largely irreversible. Promotion of public education regarding the dangers of mercury, its avoidance, and proper disposal may aid in the prevention of mercury poisoning.

REFERENCES

1. Aaseth J, Friedheim EAH. Treatment of methyl mercury poisoning in mice with 2,3-dimercaptosuccinic acid and other complexing thiols. *Acta Pharmacol Toxicol.* 1978;42:248-252.
2. Agocs MM, Etzel RA, Parrish G, et al. Mercury exposure from interior latex paint. *N Engl J Med.* 1990;323:1096-1100.
3. American Academy of Pediatrics, Committee on Infectious Diseases and Committee on Environmental Health: thimerosal in vaccines—an interim report to clinicians. *Pediatrics.* 1999;104(3 Pt 1):570-574.
4. Amin-Zaki L, Majeed MA, Clarkson TW, Greenwood MR. Methylmercury poisoning in Iraqi children: clinical observations over two years. *Br Med J.* 1978;1:613-616.
5. Andersen AH. Experimental studies on the pharmacology of activated charcoal. III: adsorption from gastrointestinal contents. *Acta Pharmacol.* 1948;4:275-284.
6. Andrews N, Miller E, Grant A, et al. Thimerosal exposure in infants and developmental disorders: a retrospective cohort study in the United Kingdom does not support a causal association. *Pediatrics.* 2004;114:584-591.
7. Appell D. Toxic bulbs. *Sci Am.* 2007;297:30-32.
8. Aronow R, Fleischmann LE. Mercury poisoning in children. *Clin Pediatr.* 1976;15;936-945.
9. Asano S, Eto K, Kurisaki E, et al. Acute inorganic mercury vapor inhalation poisoning. *Pathol Int.* 2000;50:169-174.
10. Becker CG, Becker EL, Maher JF, Schreiner GE. Nephrotic syndrome after contact with mercury. *Arch Intern Med.* 1962;110:178-186.
11. Berlin M, Rylander R. Increased brain uptake of mercury induced by 2,3-dimercaptopropanol (BAL) in mice exposed to phenylmercuric acetate. *J Pharmacol Exp Ther.* 1964;146:236-240.
12. Black J. The puzzle of pink disease. *J R Soc Med.* 1999;92:478-481.
13. Bluhm RE, Bobbitt RG, Welch LW, et al. Elemental mercury vapour toxicity, treatment, and prognosis after acute, intensive exposure in chloralkali plant workers: part I. History, neuropsychological findings and chelator effects. *Hum Exp Toxicol.* 1992;11:201-210.
14. Campbell D, Gonzales M, Sullivan JB. Mercury. In: Sullivan JB, Krieger GR, eds. *Hazardous Material Toxicology*. Baltimore: Williams & Wilkins; 1992:824-833.
15. Centers for Disease Control and Prevention. Acute, chronic poisoning, residential exposures to elemental mercury—Michigan, 1989–1990. *MMWR Morbid Mortal Wkly Rep.* 1991;40:393-395.
16. Centers for Disease Control and Prevention. Elemental mercury poisoning in a household. *MMWR Morbid Mortal Wkly Rep.* 1990;39:424-425.
17. Clarkson TE. Mercury. *J Am Coll Toxicol.* 1989;8:1291-1296.
18. Clarkson TW, Amin-Zaki L, Al-Tikriti SK. An outbreak of methylmercury poisoning due to consumption of contaminated grain. *Fed Proc.* 1976;35:2395-2399.
19. Clarkson TW, Magos L, Greenwood MR, et al. Tests of efficacy of antidotes for removal of methylmercury in human poisoning during the Iraq outbreak. *J Pharmacol Exp Ther.* 1981;218:74-83.
20. *Consumer Reports.* Is the government too lax in advice on tuna consumption? July 2004;69:8.
21. Crump KS, Kjellstrom T, Shipp AM, et al. Influence of prenatal mercury exposure upon scholastic and psychological test performance: benchmark analysis of a New Zealand cohort. *Risk Anal.* 1998;18:701-713.
22. Dales LG. The neurotoxicity of alkyl mercury compounds. *Am J Med.* 1972;53:219-232.
23. Dargan PI, Giles LJ, Wallace CI, et al. Case report: severe mercuric sulphate poisoning treated with 2,3-dimercaptopropane-1-sulphonate and haemodiafiltration. *Crit Care.* 2003;7:R1-R6.
24. Davidson PW, Myers GJ, Cox C, et al. Methylmercury and neurodevelopment: longitudinal analysis of the Seychelles child development cohort. *Neurotoxicol Teratol.* 2006;28:529-535.
25. Davis LE, Kornfeld M, Mooney HS, et al. Methylmercury poisoning: long-term clinical, radiological, toxicological, and pathological studies of an affected family. *Ann Neurol.* 1994;35:680-688.
26. Debes F, Budtz-Jorgensen E, Weihe P, et al. Impact of prenatal methylmercury exposure on neurobehavioral function at age 14 years. *Neurotoxicol Teratol.* 2006;28:536-547.
27. Eley BM, Cox SW. Mercury from dental amalgam fillings in patients. *Br Dent J.* 1987;163:221-225.
28. Elhassani SB. The many faces of methylmercury poisoning. *J Toxicol Clin Toxicol.* 1982–1983;19:875-906.
29. Eti S, Weisman RS, Hoffman RS, Reidenberg MM. Slight renal effect of mercury amalgam fillings. *Pharmacol Toxicol.* 1995;76:47-49.
30. Fung YK, Molvar MP. Toxicity of mercury from dental environment and from amalgam restorations. *J Toxicol Clin Toxicol.* 1992;30:49-61.
31. Fuortes LJ, Weismann DN, Graeff ML, et al. Immune thrombocytopenia and elemental mercury poisoning. *J Toxicol Clin Toxicol.* 1995; 33:449-455.
32. Goyer RA, Clarkson TW. Toxic effects of metals. In: Klaassen CD, ed. *Casarett and Doull's Toxicology: The Basic Science of Poisons*, 6th ed. New York: McGraw-Hill; 2001:811-867.
33. Grandjean P, Weihe P, White RF, et al. Cognitive deficit in 7-year-old children with prenatal exposure to methylmercury. *Neurotoxicol Teratol.* 1997;19:417-428.
34. Hryhorczuk DO, Meyers L, Chen G. Treatment of mercury intoxication in a dentist with N-acetyl-d,l-penicillamine. *Clin Toxicol.* 1982;19:401-408.
35. Hursh JB, Clarkson TW, Cherian MG, et al. Clearance of mercury (Hg-197, Hg-203) vapor inhaled by human subjects. *Arch Environ Health.* 1976;31:302-309.
36. Iesato K, Wakashin M, Wakashin Y, Tojo S. Renal tubular dysfunction in Minamata disease: detection of renal tubular antigen and beta-2-microglobulin in the urine. *Ann Intern Med.* 1977;86:731-737.
37. Inouye M, Kajiwara Y. Developmental disturbances of the fetal brain in guinea-pigs caused by methylmercury. *Arch Toxicol.* 1988;62:15-21.
38. Jacobson RM. Vaccine Safety. *Immunol Allergy Clin North Am.* 2003; 23:589-603.
39. Johnson HRM, Koumides O. Unusual case of mercury poisoning. *Br Med J.* 1967;1:340-341.
40. Jung RC, Aaronson J. Death following inhalation of mercury vapor at home. *West J Med.* 1980;132:539-543.
41. Kahn A, Denis R, Blum D. Accidental ingestion of mercuric sulphate in a 4-year-old child. *Clin Pediatr.* 1977;16:956-958.
42. Kales SN, Goldman, RH. Mercury exposure: current concepts, controversies, and a clinic's experience. *J Occup Environ Med.* 2002;44:143-154.
43. Kang-Yum E, Oransky SH. Chinese patent medicine as a potential source of mercury poisoning. *Vet Hum Toxicol.* 1992;34:235-238.
44. Kanluen S, Gottlieb CA. A clinical pathologic study of four adult cases of acute mercury inhalation toxicity. *Arch Pathol Lab Med.* 1991;115:56-60.
45. Katz SA, Katz RB. Use of hair analysis for evaluating mercury intoxication of the human body: a review. *J Appl Toxicol.* 1992;12:79-84.
46. Kershaw TG, Clarkson TW, Dhahir PH. The relationship between blood levels and dose of methylmercury in man. *Arch Environ Health.* 1980;35:28-36.
47. Koos BJ, Longo LD. Mercury toxicity in the pregnant woman, fetus, and newborn infant: a review. *Am J Obstet Gynecol.* 1976;126:390-409.
48. Korogi Y, Takahashi M, Shinzato J, Okajima T. MR findings in seven patients with organic mercury poisoning (Minamata disease). *Am J Neuroradiol.* 1994;15:1575-1578.
49. Krohn IT, Solof A, Mobini J, Wagner DK. Subcutaneous injection of metallic mercury. *JAMA.* 1980;243:548-549.
50. Langan DC, Fan PL, Hoos AA. The use of mercury in dentistry: critical review of the recent literature. *J Am Dent Assoc.* 1987;115:867-879.
51. Limke TL, Bearss JJ, Atchison WD. Acute exposure to methylmercury causes Ca2+ dysregulation and neuronal death in rat cerebellar granule cells through an M3 muscarinic receptor-linked pathway. *Toxicol Sci.* 2004;80:60-68.
52. Lind B, Friberg L, Nylander M. Preliminary studies on methylmercury biotransformation and clearance in the brain of primates: II. Demethylation of mercury in brain. *J Trace Elem Exp Med.* 1988;1:49-56.
53. Litovitz T, Schmitz BF. Ingestion of cylindrical and button batteries: an analysis of 2382 cases. *Pediatrics.* 1992;89:747-757.
54. Madsen KM, Lauritsen MB, Pedersen CB, et al. Thimerosal and the occurrence of autism: negative ecological evidence from Danish population-based data. *Pediatrics.* 2003;112:604-606.
55. Magos L. Mercury. In: Seiler HG, Sigel H, eds. *Handbook on Toxicity of Inorganic Compounds.* New York: Marcel Dekker; 1988:419-436.
56. Mant TGK, Lewis JL, Mattoo TK, et al. Mercury poisoning after disc-battery ingestion. *Hum Toxicol.* 1987;6:179-181.

57. Matsumoto H, Koya G, Takeuchi T. Fetal Minamata disease: a neuropathological study of two cases of intrauterine intoxication by a methyl mercury compound. *J Neuropathol Exp*. 1964;24:563-574.
58. Maurissen JPJ. History of mercury and mercurialism. *N Y State J Med*. 1981;81:1902-1909.
59. Moutinho ME, Tompkins AL, Rowland TW, et al. Acute mercury vapor poisoning. *Am J Dis Child*. 1981;135:42-44.
60. Mozaffarian D, Rimm EB. Fish intake, contaminants, and human health: evaluating the risks and the benefits. *JAMA*. 2006;296:1885-1899.
61. Murray KM, Hedgepeth JC. Intravenous self-administration of elemental mercury: efficacy of dimercaprol therapy. *Drug Intell Clin Pharm*. 1988;22:972-975.
62. Myers GJ. Prenatal methylmercury exposure from ocean fish consumption in the Seychelles child development study. *Lancet*. 2003;361:1686-1692.
63. Newland MC, Reile PA. Blood and brain mercury levels after chronic gestational exposure to methylmercury in rats. *Toxicol Sci*. 1999;50:106-116.
64. Nierenberg DW, Nordgren RE, Chang MB, et al. Delayed cerebellar disease and death after accidental exposure to dimethylmercury. *N Engl J Med*. 1998;338:1672-1676.
65. Nordberg GF, Skerfving S. Metabolism. In: Friberg L, Vostal J, eds. *Mercury in the Environment: An Epidemiological and Toxicological Appraisal*. Cleveland, OH: CRC Press; 1972:29-90.
66. Nordberg GF, ed. *Effects and Dose–Response of Toxic Metals*. New York: Elsevier; 1976:24-32.
67. O'Shea JG. Was Paganini poisoned with mercury? *J R Soc Med*. 1988;81: 594-597.
68. Oskarsson A, Palminger HI, Sundberg J. Exposure to toxic elements via breast milk. *Analyst*. 1995;120:765-770.
69. Parker SK, Schwartz B, Todd J, Pickering LK. Thimerosal-containing vaccines and autistic spectrum disorder: a critical review of published original data. *Pediatrics*. 2004;114:793-804.
70. Patrizi A, Rizzoli L, Vincenzi C, Trevisi P, Tosti A. Sensitization to thimerosal in atopic children. *Contact Dermatitis*. 1999;40:94-97.
71. Pfab R, Muckter H, Roider G, Zilker T. Clinical course of severe poisoning with thimerosal. *J Toxicol Clin Toxicol*. 1996;34:453-460.
72. Powell PP. Minamata disease: a story of mercury's malevolence. *South Med J*. 1991;84:1352-1358.
73. Rice DC. Methods and rationale for derivation of a reference dose for methylmercury by the US EPA. *Risk Anal*. 2003;23:107-115.
74. Rosenman KD, Valciukas JA, Glickman L, et al. Sensitive indicators of inorganic mercury toxicity. *Arch Environ Health*. 1986;41:208-215.
75. Rowens B, Guerrero-Betancourt D, Gottlieb CA, et al. Respiratory failure and death following acute inhalation of mercury vapor: a clinical and histologic perspective. *Chest*. 1991;99:185-190.
76. Royhans J, Walson PD, Wood GA, MacDonald WA. Mercury toxicity following Merthiolate ear irrigations. *J Pediatr*. 1984;104:311-313.
77. Rustam H, Hamdi T. Methyl mercury poisoning in Iraq. *Brain*. 1974;97: 499-510.
78. Sakamoto M, Kakita A, Wakabayashi K, et al. Evaluation of changes in methylmercury accumulation in the developing rat brain and its effects: a study with consecutive and moderate dose exposure throughout gestation and lactation periods. *Brain Res*. 2002;949:51-59.
79. Sakamoto M, Kubota M, Matsumoto S, et al. Declining risk of methylmercury exposure to infants during lactation. *Environ Res*. 2002;90: 185-189.
80. Saper RB, Kales SN, Paquin J, et al. Heavy metal content of ayurvedic herbal medicine products. *JAMA*. 2004;292:2868-2873.
81. Saper RB, Phillips RS, Sehgal A, et al. Lead, mercury, and arsenic in US- and Indian-manufactured Ayurvedic medicines sold via the Internet. *JAMA*. 2008;300:915-923.
82. Sauder PH, Livardjani F, Jaeger A, et al. Acute mercury chloride intoxication: effects of hemodialysis and plasma exchange on mercury kinetic. *J Toxicol Clin Toxicol*. 1988;26:189-197.
83. Schnellmann RG. Toxic responses of the kidney. In: Klaassen CD, ed. *Casarett and Doull's Toxicology: The Basic Science of Poisons*, 6th ed. New York: McGraw-Hill; 2001:491-514.
84. Schwartz JG, Snider TE, Montiel MM. Toxicity of a family from vacuumed mercury. *Am J Emerg Med*. 1992;10:258-261.
85. Seidel J. Acute mercury poisoning after polyvinyl alcohol preservative ingestion. *Pediatrics*. 1980;66:132-134.
86. Shanker G, Aschner M. Identification and characterization of uptake systems for cystine and cysteine in cultured astrocytes and neurons: evidence for methylmercury-targeted disruption of astrocyte transport. *J Neurosci Res*. 2001;66:998-1002.
87. Siegler RW, Nierenberg DW, Hickey WF. Fatal poisoning from liquid dimethylmercury: a neuropathologic study. *Hum Pathol*. 1999;30:720-723.
88. Snapp KR, Boyer DB, Peterson LC, Svare CW. The contribution of dental amalgam to mercury in blood. *J Dent Res*. 1989;68:780-785.
89. Snodgrass W, Sullivan JB, Rumack BH, Hashimoto C. Mercury poisoning from home gold ore processing. *JAMA*. 1981;246:1929-1931.
90. Stehr-Green P. Autism and thimerosal-containing vaccines: lack of consistent evidence for an association. *Am J Prev Med*. 2003;25:101-106.
91. Stern AH, Jacobsen JL, Ryan L, Burke TA. Do recent data from the Seychelles Islands alter the conclusions of the NRC report on the toxicologic effects of methylmercury? *Environ Health*. 2004;3:2.
92. Sunderman FW. Perils of mercury. *Ann Clin Lab Sci*. 1988;18:89-101.
93. Suzuki T, Hongo T, Yoshinaga J, et al. The hair-organ relationship in mercury concentration in contemporary Japanese. *Arch Environ Health*. 1993;48:221-229.
94. Takeuchi T. Pathology of Minamata disease. *Acta Pathol Jpn*. 1982; 32:73-99.
95. Thompson WW, Price C, Goodson B, et al. Early Thimerosal exposure and neuropsychological outcomes at 7-10 years. *New Engl J Med*. 2007;357:1281-1292.
96. Troen P, Kaufman SA, Katz KH. Mercuric bichloride poisoning. *N Engl J Med*. 1951;244:459-463.
97. Tunnessen WW, McMahon KJ, Baser M. Acrodynia: exposure to mercury from fluorescent light bulbs. *Pediatrics*. 1987;79:786-789.
98. US Environmental Protection Agency. *Mercury Report to Congress, Volume VI: Characterization of Human Health and Wildlife Risks from Anthropogenic Mercury Emissions in the United States*. EPA-452/R-97–001f. Washington, DC: Author; 1997.
99. US Food and Drug Administration. *Rationale for Issuance of Revised Advisory on Methylmercury and Fish Consumption*. Rockville, MD: Center for Food Safety and Applied Nutrition; February 2001.
100. Wallach L. Aspiration of elemental mercury—evidence of absorption without toxicity. *N Engl J Med*. 1972;287:178-179.
101. Wands JR, Weiss SH, Yardley JH, Maddrey WC. Chronic inorganic mercury poisoning due to laxative abuse. *Am J Med*. 1974;57:92-101.
102. Warkany J, Hubbard DM. Adverse mercurial reactions in the form of acrodynia and related conditions. *Am J Dis Child*. 1951;81:335-373.
103. Wedeen RP. Were the hatters of New Jersey "mad"? *Am J Ind Med*. 1989;16:225-233.
104. Winship KA. Organic mercury compounds and their toxicity. *Adverse Drug React Toxicol Rev*. 1986;3:141-180.
105. Yeh TF, Pildes RS, Firor HV. Mercury poisoning from mercurochrome treatment of an infected omphalocele. *Clin Toxicol*. 1978;13:463-467.
106. Yin Z, Milatovic D, Aschner JL, et al. Methylmercury induces oxidative injury, alterations in permeability and glutamine transport in cultured astrocytes. *Brain Res*. 2007;1131:1-10.
107. Yotsuyanagi T, Yokoi K, Sawada Y. Facial injury by mercury from a broken thermometer. *J Trauma*. 1996;40:847-849.
108. Zimmer LJ, Carter DE. The effect of 2,3-dimercaptopropanol and D-penicillamine on methyl mercury induced neurological signs and weight loss. *Life Sci*. 1978;23:1025-1034.
109. Zimmerman JE. Fatality following metallic mercury aspiration during removal of a long intestinal tube. *JAMA*. 1969;208:2158-2160.

CHAPTER 97
NICKEL

John A. Curtis and David A. Haggerty

Nickel (Ni)

Atomic number	=	28
Atomic weight	=	58.7 daltons
Normal concentrations		
Serum	<	1 μg/L (<17 nmol/L)
Urine	<	6 μg/L (<100 nmol/L)

Nickel is a ubiquitous metal commonly found in both the home and industry. It exists in a variety of chemical forms, from naturally occurring ores to synthetically produced nickel carbonyl. The toxicity of nickel is often overlooked outside of the occupational setting, yet it remains one of the most common causes of contact dermatitis worldwide. Nickel carbonyl in particular can produce significant morbidity and mortality, although fortunately such incidents are rare.

HISTORY AND EPIDEMIOLOGY

Nickel is a white, lustrous metal whose name is derived from the German word *kupfernickel* or "devil's copper." Swedish chemist Baron Axel Fredrik first identified nickel in 1751 in a mineral known as niccolite. Nickel comprises 0.008% of the earth's crust and is found in diverse locations, ranging from meteorites and soil to bodies of fresh- and saltwater.

First produced by the Chinese, nickel has been used as a component in a variety of metal alloys for more than 1700 years. The first malleable nickel was produced by Joseph Wharton after the American Civil War. Wharton went on to sell bulk quantities of nickel to the U.S. government for the minting of 3 cent coins and later donated the equivalent of 3.3 million of these coins to help fund what is today known as the Wharton School of Business.[90] The modern United States 5 cent piece, the "nickel," is actually only approximately 25% nickel by weight.[103]

Nickel ores typically consist of accumulations of nickel sulfide minerals of relatively low nickel content. Although a variety of technical methods for extracting nickel from ore have been developed, one method of special note was developed in 1890 by Ludwig Mond, who is credited with the discovery of nickel carbonyl. The Mond process for the extraction of nickel involves passing carbon monoxide over smelted ore. This creates nickel carbonyl, which then decomposes at high temperatures to produce purified nickel and carbon monoxide.[90] Nickel mining was stopped in the United States in 1993,[16] and despite an increasing worldwide demand, as of 2006, there were still no active domestic nickel mines.[49] Nickel is imported into the United States from other nickel-rich countries such as Canada, Russia, and Australia; domestic production of nickel in the United States is essentially limited to the recycling of nickel-containing metals.

Nickel is a siderophoric material that forms naturally occurring alloys with iron, a property that has made it useful for many centuries in the production of coins, tools, and weapons. Today, most nickel is used in the production of stainless steel, a highly corrosion-resistant alloy containing 8% to 15% nickel by weight.[114]

Occupational exposure to nickel and nickel-containing compounds occurs in a variety of industries, including nickel mining, refining, reclaiming, and smelting. Chemists, magnet makers, jewelry makers, oil hydrogenator workers, battery manufacturers, petroleum refinery workers, electroplaters, stainless steel and alloy workers, and welders are at increased risk for exposure to nickel and nickel-containing compounds.[61] The vast majority of nonindustrial human exposures to nickel are usually from dietary and environmental sources. Cigarette smoke contains nickel and elevates urinary nickel concentrations.[34,89] In the occupational setting, nickel carbonyl is responsible for the great majority of acute nickel toxicity; in clinical practice, the most common health issue related to nickel is the development of allergic dermatitis from jewelry and clothing. Nickel ranks behind *Toxicodendron* spp. exposure as the second most common cause of allergic contact dermatitis[31]; in a patch-testing study, more than 30% of adolescents demonstrated an allergy to nickel.[26]

TOXICOLOGY AND PHARMACOKINETICS

EXPOSURE

Nickel occurs naturally in soil, volcanic dust, and fresh- and saltwater but also enters the environment from the combustion of fuel oil, municipal incineration, nickel refining processes, and the production of steel and other nickel alloys that may allow aerosolized nickel to be disseminated into the environment.

The specific form of nickel emitted to the atmosphere depends on the source. Complex nickel oxides, nickel sulfate, and metallic nickel are associated with combustion and incineration, as well as smelting and refining processes. Consequently, ambient air concentrations of these forms of nickel tend to be higher in urban areas, and concentrations of nickel in urban household dust may be elevated under certain circumstances and thus may pose some variable exposure risk for young children who crawl or sit on floors.

Nickel carbonyl, $Ni(CO)_4$, deserves special mention. This highly volatile, highly useful, and very deadly liquid nickel compound is commonly used in nickel refining and petroleum processing and as a chemical reagent. Its high vapor pressure and high lipid solubility lead to rapid systemic absorption through the lungs. In the air and in the body, it decomposes into metallic nickel and carbon monoxide, and its toxicity has been compared to that of hydrogen cyanide.[50] Employees are commonly screened for low-level exposure to nickel carbonyl, but disasters such as the Gulf Oil Company refinery incident in 1953 and the Toa Gosei Chemical company incident in 1969 resulted in hundreds of inhalational exposures.[90]

Concentrations of metallic nickel in drinking water in the United States are generally below 20 μg/L.[62] Elevated concentrations of nickel in household and other potable and nonpotable water sources may result from corrosion and leaching of nickel alloys present in various plumbing fixtures, including valves and faucets.[3] Although many water suppliers in the United States monitor nickel concentrations in their water, there is currently no U.S. Environmental Protection Agency regulation regarding how much nickel is permissible in drinking water.

Dietary intake is a recognized source of nickel exposure for humans. Foods high in nickel include nuts, legumes, cereals, licorice, and chocolate. Recently, certain homeopathic medications, Ginseng products, Indian herbal teas, Nigerian herbal remedies, and Chinese herbal plants have been shown to have high nickel content, with some Nigerian herbal remedies containing up to 78 mg nickel/g substance.[23] Although evidence exists for uptake and accumulation of nickel in certain plants, nickel does not seem to bioaccumulate along the food chain.[114] Nickel is not considered an essential element for human health, and dietary recommendations for nickel have not been established. Normal consumption is between 0.3 to 0.6 mg per day, with the majority of this remaining unabsorbed by the gastrointestinal (GI) tract.[58] Although estimates vary widely, one author estimated that a 70-kg reference human contains 0.5 mg of nickel, giving an average body concentration of 7 ppb.[9] No clear biologic function has been determined for nickel in humans. However, it may serve as a cofactor for various enzymes, or it may facilitate iron absorption or metabolism in microorganisms, as in certain nickel-dependent blue-green algae.[109]

ABSORPTION

Nickel enters the body through the skin, lungs, and GI tract. The amount of absorption is dependent on the solubility of the nickel compound in water. Once in the body, nickel exists primarily as the divalent cation. Independent of the particular nickel compound available, elemental nickel, which typically exists as Ni^{+2} under normal conditions, is measured in the serum or urine.

After inhalational exposure, nickel accumulates in the lungs, but only 20% to 35% of nickel deposited in the human lung is systemically absorbed.[9,33] The remainder of the inhaled material is swallowed, expectorated, or deposited in the upper respiratory tract. Subsequent systemic absorption from the respiratory tract is dependent on the solubility of the specific nickel compound in question. The soluble nickel salts (nickel sulfate and nickel chloride) are more easily absorbed than the less soluble oxides and sulfides of nickel.

A man who died of adult respiratory distress syndrome 13 days after being exposed to fumes containing high concentrations of metallic nickel (~380 mg/m^3) had very high concentrations of nickel in his urine (700 μg/L).[73] This case report demonstrates that metallic nickel can be systemically absorbed from the lungs; however, many authorities believe that pulmonary concentrations must be high enough to result in direct pulmonary injury for systemic absorption to occur after inhalational exposure.

Because soluble nickel compounds tend to be more readily absorbed from the respiratory tract compared with nonsoluble or poorly soluble nickel,[102] exposure to the soluble nickel chloride or nickel sulfate results in higher urinary nickel concentrations than does exposure to less soluble nickel oxide or nickel subsulfide. The half-life of nickel in the lungs of rats exposed by inhalation is reported to be 32 hours for nickel sulfate,[37] 4.6 days for nickel subsulfide, and 120 days for green nickel oxide,[10] a fact that probably reflects slow dissolution and absorption from the lungs of less soluble nickel compounds.

After ingestion, approximately 27% of the total nickel in nickel sulfate given to humans in drinking water is absorbed, but only approximately 1% is absorbed when given in food.[95] Serum nickel concentrations peak between 1.5 and 3 hours after ingestion of nickel.[18,70,95] The bioavailability of nickel increased when nickel was administered in a soft drink but decreased when nickel was given with whole milk, coffee, tea, or orange juice.[85] The presence of food in the GI tract appears to reduce the absorption of nickel, and most ingested nickel remains in the gut and is excreted in the feces.

Human studies show that several nickel compounds are capable of penetrating the skin.[30,66] In one study, radioactive nickel sulfate was applied to occluded skin.[66] It was determined that 55% to 77% of the applied nickel was absorbed within 24 hours, with most of the nickel being absorbed in the first few hours. It could not be determined, however, if the nickel had been absorbed into the deep layers of the skin or into the bloodstream. In a study using excised human skin, whereas only 0.23% of an applied dose of nickel chloride permeated the skin after 144 hours when the skin was not occluded, 3.5% permeated occluded skin.[30]

DISTRIBUTION

In human serum, the exchangeable pool of primarily divalent nickel is bound to albumin, L-histidine, and α_2-macroglobulin.[65] A nonexchangeable pool of nickel that is tightly bound to a transport protein known as nickeloplasmin also exists in the serum. Nickel crosses the placenta[79] and may accumulate in breast milk, resulting in the potential for nickel exposure to offspring.[25]

Nickel also appears to be concentrated in various solid organs rather than in serum. An autopsy study of individuals not occupationally exposed to nickel reports the highest concentrations of nickel in the lungs followed by the thyroid, adrenal glands, kidneys, heart, liver, brain, spleen, and pancreas.[74] Nickel concentrations in the nasal mucosa are higher in workers exposed to less soluble nickel compounds relative to soluble nickel compounds,[102] indicating that after inhalation exposure, less soluble nickel compounds remain deposited on the nasal mucosa.

ELIMINATION

In humans, most ingested nickel is excreted in the feces; however, because more than 90% of ingested nickel does not leave the gut,[93] most of the nickel found in feces represents this unabsorbed fraction rather than the elimination of body nickel.[70,95] Absorbed nickel is primarily excreted in the urine and to a lesser degree in the saliva and sweat.[52]

Regardless of the route of exposure, workers occupationally exposed to nickel have increased urinary concentrations of nickel.[5,28,33,36,102] After inhalational exposure to green nickel oxide, nickel was only excreted in the feces, implying that the removal of nickel oxide from the lungs is macrophage mediated rather than through mechanisms dependent on dissolution and absorption.[10] After exposure to nickel subsulfide, nickel was excreted in both the urine and the feces, with greater amounts in the urine on days 6 to 14 after exposure. These results indicate that dissolution–absorption plays an important role in the removal of nickel subsulfide from the lungs; thus, in contrast to nickel oxide, nickel subsulfide behaves essentially like a soluble compound after inhalation.[10]

The elimination half-life of nickel depends on the source of exposure. It is important to note that prolonged elevation of serum and urine nickel concentrations after inhalational exposure to insoluble nickel represents continued slow absorption rather than delayed excretion.

In nickel workers, urinary excretion increased from the beginning to the end of the shift, indicating that a fraction of absorbed nickel is rapidly eliminated.[33,102] Similarly, urinary excretion increased as the workweek progresses, indicating the presence of a fraction that is excreted more slowly.[33]

Studies with radioactive nickel chloride injected into rats show that 68% of administered nickel is eliminated in the urine during the first day,[69] and the urine nickel concentration is commonly assumed to measure exposure over the past 2 to 3 days.[18]

In workers who unintentionally ingested water contaminated with nickel sulfate and nickel chloride, the mean serum half-life of nickel was 60 hours.[94] This half-life reportedly decreased substantially (to 27 hours) when the workers were treated with intravenous (IV) fluids.

No data exist regarding excretion of nickel in humans or animals after dermal exposure.

CLINICAL MANIFESTATIONS

ACUTE

The most important source of acute, nondermatologic nickel toxicity is nickel carbonyl. Exposure to this compound is associated with pulmonary, neurologic, and hepatic dysfunction[90] (Table 97–1.)

TABLE 97–1. Sequelae Associated with Nickel Carbonyl Poisoning

Acute lung injury or interstitial pneumonitis
Myocarditis
Altered mental status
Seizure
Profound weakness (sometimes requiring ventilatory support)
Prolonged neurasthenic syndrome (≤6 months after exposure)
Death (secondary to interstitial pneumonitis or cerebral edema)

The specific clinical manifestations associated with acute exposure to other forms of nickel depend on the specific compound and the route of exposure. Whereas inhalation of nickel-containing aerosolized particles tends to affect the lungs and upper airways directly, ingestion and IV administration may result in systemic toxicity, usually involving the neurologic system. By far the most common disorder associated with exposure to nickel is allergic dermatitis.

Nickel Dermatitis Nickel dermatitis was first reported in the late 1800s in nickel-plating workers and was recognized as an allergic reaction in 1925. Since then, nickel has been recognized as a common cause of allergic contact dermatitis. Nickel(2+) is not antigenic by itself. Instead, it acts as a hapten, binding larger proteins and inducing conformational changes such that these become recognized as non-self antigens.[42] One population survey reported that 3% of men and 15% of women demonstrated evidence of allergy to nickel.[57] The fivefold greater prevalence of nickel allergy in women is presumably a consequence of their higher rates of body piercing and more frequent wearing of jewelry, both of which are risk factors for nickel sensitization.[54,75]

Nickel dermatitis is classified into two types: primary and secondary. The more common primary dermatitis presents as a typical eczematous reaction in the area of skin that is in contact with nickel. It is characterized initially by erythematous papules that may proceed to lichenification because of pruritus and scratching. Areas typically involved are the wrists, as a result of wearing watches and bracelets; pierced ears; and periumbilical eruptions at the site of contact with nickel-containing buttons on jeans or nickel-containing belt buckles. (See Fig. 97–1)Approximately 50% of all belt buckles and 10% of buttons on blue jeans contain nickel.[17]

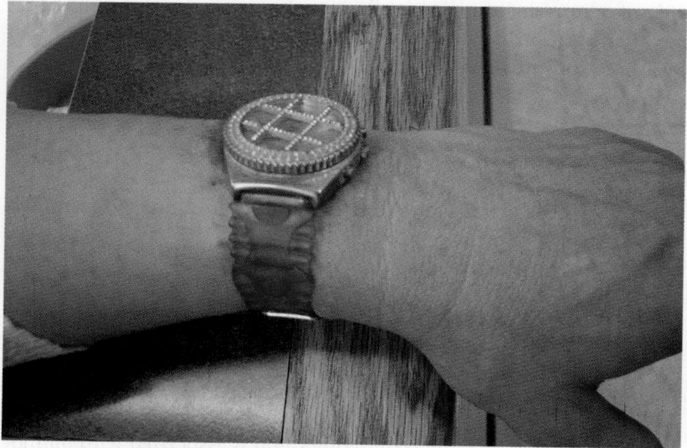

FIGURE 97–1. Nickel dermatitis from jewelry. *(Image contributed by Brian Wexler).*

The secondary form involves more widespread dermatitis as a result of other exposures, such as ingestion, transfusion, inhalation, and implantation of metal medical devices, and may be regarded as a systemic contact dermatitis elicited by nickel. Secondary eruptions are typically symmetrically distributed and may localize in the elbow flexure, on the eyelids, or on the sides of the neck and face, and they can become widespread. Nickel in foods, excessive skin contact, and certain orthodontic appliances with high nickel content are all linked to this eczematous eruption. Nonetheless, orthodontic exposure to nickel-containing alloys is unlikely to induce hypersensitivity reactions in patients without prior sensitization, and such reactions are still infrequent even in those sensitized.[32,41,71,72,81] In nickel-sensitive patients, these alloys do not seem to affect oral or gingival health.[8] Although patients wearing nickel-containing orthodontia have detectable nickel in their saliva, this is found in negligible concentrations (4–12 ppb) well below concentrations in the average daily dietary intake. Furthermore, these patients have no detectable difference between pre- and post-orthodontia serum nickel concentrations.[41]

Other types of medical devices containing nickel have the potential to induce either primary or local nickel dermatitis. Occlusion of a biliary stent caused by nickel allergy is reported.[47] Much debate has arisen over the past decade regarding metallic coronary stents and the potential for nickel allergy–induced restenosis. Several studies have suggested that inflammatory fibroproliferative restenosis occurs in nickel-sensitive patients, but others have failed to find such a correlation.[43,48,67] Stents containing immunosuppressant drugs such as sirolimus are currently being investigated as a possible solution to such proposed allergic reactions.[60]

The most common cause of nickel dermatitis in women is direct contact from jewelry, garments, or wristwatches and occupational contact in the metal, hairdressing, tailoring, hotel, and restaurant industries. In men, nickel dermatitis is often occupational but may also be related to jewelry, body piercing, and garments in some individuals. Recent case reports describe nickel dermatitis occurring in musicians through either direct contact with instruments or guitar strings.[84]

It is reported that the bimetallic core structure of the 1 and 2 Euro coins creates an electrical potential that results in the release of nickel when in contact with sweat.[64] Although studies report no increase in the prevalence of nickel sensitivity before and after the switch to the Euro in the general population,[54] positive patch tests to Euro coins[68] and cases of dermatitis in certain high-risk patients have been reported.[78]

Recently, reports have emerged involving cases of contact dermatitis in users of certain types of cellular phones.[11,53,113] Dimethylglyoxime spot testing has confirmed nickel release in such phones.[100] Nickel should be considered a potential cause in cases of facial contact dermatitis of unknown etiology.

One study showed that after skin application, nickel salts are retained in the skin for an extended period of time,[51] which could lead to prolonged antigen processing and consequent immune responses in dermal tissue. Additionally, when in contact with the skin, nickel is oxidized to form soluble, stratum corneum–diffusible compounds that may penetrate intact skin and have the potential to elicit allergic reactions.[39,40] A recent study showed that elicitation of nickel allergy is dependent on both the size and concentration of exposure.[29]

The allergic reaction caused by contact with nickel is a type IV delayed hypersensitivity immune response that typically occurs in two phases. In the first phase, sensitization occurs when nickel enters the body. The second phase occurs when the body is reexposed to nickel, at which time allergy manifests. The diagnosis of nickel allergy is suggested by specific historical findings listed in Table 97–2.

Nickel Carbonyl Nickel carbonyl is the most potentially harmful form of nickel, and the majority of acute occupational nickel exposures involve

TABLE 97–2. Findings Suggestive of Nickel Dermatitis

History of allergic response to jewelry
Multiple body piercings
Eruptions at the site of metal contact or flexural areas if generalized
Eruptions after placement of orthodontic appliances containing high concentrations of nickel (unusual)
Seasonal dermatitis in warm months (increased metal–skin contact and increased sweating)

nickel carbonyl. Once dissociated, nickel carbonyl can be oxidized in tissues to Ni^{2+}. Nickel carbonyl is described as having a "musty" or "sooty" odor, although thresholds for detection vary considerably, and potentially harmful exposures cannot be excluded simply by a reported lack of odor. Exposure to concentrations below 100 mg/m^3 is fatal in rats after 20 minutes.[91,96]

Nickel carbonyl exposure may cause symptoms rapidly, or symptoms may be delayed. In a series of 179 exposures, approximately 40% of patients reported symptoms within 1 hour of exposure. It is important to note, however, that symptoms were delayed for approximately 1 week in 20% of patients, and even patients with mild initial symptoms could develop severe delayed symptoms, although usually within the next 2 days.[82] In patients who developed symptoms shortly after exposure, the initial manifestations involved nonspecific complaints, including respiratory tract irritation, chest pain, cough, dyspnea, frontal headache, dizziness, weakness, and nausea. Cases manifesting only these initial signs are categorized as mild intoxication.[82]

Symptoms of severe acute nickel carbonyl poisoning generally develop over the course of several hours to days and may be associated with acute lung injury and interstitial pneumonitis. Myocarditis, marked by prolonged ECG changes, including ST- and T-wave changes, as well as QT interval prolongation, are reported.[82] Neurologic symptoms associated with severe poisoning include altered mental status, seizures, and extreme weakness that sometimes necessitates mechanical ventilation. Moderate leukocytosis (10,000–15,000 white blood cells/mm^3), nonspecific opacities on chest radiography, and elevation of aminotransferases may occur, but these tend to resolve over the course of several weeks. Deaths from nickel carbonyl are typically caused by interstitial pneumonitis and cerebral edema occurring within 2 weeks of initial exposure.[96] Survivors usually recover completely, although the development of a prolonged neurasthenic syndrome may occur and may last in some cases for up to 6 months.[82]

Parenteral Administration Acute parenteral toxicity from nickel-containing compounds occurred after the use of water for hemodialysis that had been heated in a nickel-plated tank.[111] The concentration of nickel in the delivered water was 0.25 mg/L, and serum concentrations were exceedingly elevated. These patients developed nonspecific symptoms, including headache, nausea, and vomiting, similar to the symptoms of nickel carbonyl poisoning, although no respiratory complaints were reported. The effects resolved after several hours, and the patients recovered without sequelae.[111]

Ingestion Acute ingestions of contaminated water containing 1.63 g Ni^{2+}/L caused nausea, vomiting, diarrhea, weakness, and headache, as well as pulmonary symptoms, including cough and dyspnea, lasting up to 48 hours.[94] Estimated ingested doses of nickel (as Ni^{2+}) were 0.5 to 2.5 g, and serum concentrations as high as 13.4 μg/L were reported. The death of a 2-year-old girl occurred after ingestion of 2.2 to 3.3 g Ni in the form of nickel sulfate crystals. After ingestion, this child reportedly developed depressed level of consciousness, nuchal rigidity, mydriasis, erythema, tachycardia, and acute lung injury.[27]

Inhalational Exposure A case report described seizure activity in two patients after occupational inhalational exposure to non-carbonyl nickel. Both patients exhibited elevated urinary nickel concentrations, with no recurrence of seizure activity upon removal from exposure.[24] This complication was documented previously in rats with nickel sulfate toxicity.[2,20] Although the mechanism for this is not quite clear, animal studies indicate that inhibition of the glutamate transporter may be involved.[55] Interstitial pneumonia is also associated with inhalational exposure while spray painting high-temperature nickel–chromium alloys.[38] As previously mentioned, inhalational exposure to metallic nickel may induce acute respiratory distress syndrome.[73]

Dermal Absorption Although transdermal absorption is typically of minor clinical significance, disruption of the normal integument may allow for more efficient systemic absorption. A metal refinery worker experienced a 40% body surface area partial-thickness chemical injury resulting from exposure to a chemical mixture that included nickel carbonate and nickel sulfate. Before the incident, this individual's measured serum nickel concentration was 1.33 μg/L (0.023 μmol/L). On the sixth day after the injury, the serum concentration was 28 μg/L (0.490 μmol/L). Two 5-day courses of chelation with edetate calcium disodium ($CaNa_2EDTA$) were begun for concomitant cobalt poisoning, and the patient's serum and urine nickel concentrations were within normal limits by 21 days after exposure. He subsequently recovered without manifesting signs of nickel toxicity.[63]

CHRONIC NICKEL EXPOSURE

Chronic inhalational exposure to nickel is associated with injury as well as specific histologic changes in the nasopharynx and upper respiratory tract, including atrophy of the olfactory epithelium,[35] rhinitis, sinusitis, nasal polyps, and septal damage.[14] Pulmonary effects may include asthma[56] and pulmonary fibrosis.[12,35]

Although evidence of the effects of chronic nickel exposure on reproduction remains limited, a study of Indian welders occupationally exposed to nickel and cadmium showed reduced sperm counts and quality, with a positive correlation between sperm tail defects and serum nickel concentrations.[22] Several epidemiologic studies investigating the effects of nickel exposure in female refinery workers have found no increased risk of spontaneous abortion, newborn genital malformation, or incidence of small-for-gestational-age newborns.[105–107]

The International Agency for Research on Cancer classifies nickel compounds as a group 1 carcinogen (carcinogenic to humans).[44] The potential for and mechanisms of carcinogenesis of nickel depend heavily on the specific compounds studied. Animal studies show a threshold dose–response curve for inflammation with soluble compounds (nickel sulfate), and similar curves describe the risks of pulmonary cancers with the less soluble nickel oxides and nickel subsulfide.[80] Although earlier studies of occupationally exposed workers, primarily electroplaters and refinery workers, also showed increased rates of nasal and pulmonary tumors, more recent studies of refinery workers in more modern environments with lower permissible limits of nickel exposure do not show an increased risk of cancer or any cause of mortality.[83,86,87]

Reactive oxygen species (ROS) formation occurs secondary to depletion of both glutathione and protein-bound sulfhydryl groups by nickel. Accumulation of ROS leads to lipid peroxidation and DNA damage.[88,108] Formation of ROS consequently causes depletion of ascorbic acid (vitamin C) as a free radical scavenger in conjunction with vitamin E. In vitro studies of human airway epithelial cells have shown that depletion of intracellular ascorbate from nickel causes the induction of hypoxic stress. Such nickel-induced stress leads to the activation of hypoxia-inducible factor (HIF-1) and upregulation of hypoxia-inducible genes.[76] Hypoxia is encountered in tumors as they outgrow their blood supply, thus selecting for cells with altered energy metabolism, changes in growth regulation, or resistance to apoptosis. HIF-1 activation and upregulation of hypoxia-inducible genes therefore mimics intracellular permanent hypoxia and may be related to nickel-induced carcinogenesis.[77]

Soluble compounds such as nickel sulfate cause a threshold-dependent inflammatory response and may act as promoters of malignancies without a directly genotoxic effect. Insoluble nickel oxides and nickel sulfide bind to chromatin and nucleic acids[19] and affect expression of various mRNAs.[110] Thus, under some conditions, these compounds may be carcinogenic through genetic or epigenetic mechanisms. The more potent carcinogenic effects of insoluble nickel compounds may be a consequence of their increased cellular uptake.[21]

DIAGNOSTIC TESTING

Although nickel is widely distributed to many body fluids and tissues, urine and blood are the most commonly analyzed samples. Urine collection should ideally use acid-washed, metal-free containers. Some authors recommend correcting urinary nickel concentration per gram of urine creatinine, but it is not clear that this offers any particular advantage in clinical decision making. The average nickel concentration in serum is 0.3 µg/L, and the value in urine ranges from 1 to 3 µg/L.[99] Concentrations among workers occupationally exposed to nickel may be substantially higher, and serum concentrations of more than 8 µg/L are indicative of excessive exposure.[59]

Nickel concentrations increase in urine, serum, and whole blood after oral administration. In these studies, serum concentrations were slightly higher than but correlated well with whole blood. Urine and blood concentrations primarily reflect exposure occurring within the previous 48 hours.[18]

Urine nickel concentrations are used more commonly than blood for monitoring of workplace exposures and for prognostic and therapeutic decision making in nickel carbonyl exposures (Table 97–3.) An 8-hour collection is typically performed, and the average urinary excretion of nickel (in these nickel workers) is 2 µg/L, with an upper limit of normal of 6 µg/L. In cases of nickel carbonyl poisoning, concentrations of below 100 µg/L in the initial 8-hour specimen may imply mild toxicity. Concentrations of 100 to 500 µg/L are classified as moderate, and concentrations above 500 µg/L are categorized as severe exposures.[96] These guidelines are often used in guiding treatment decisions. Urine nickel concentrations increase before the onset of symptoms in nickel carbonyl poisoning, making this determination a potentially useful screening tool for both workforce surveillance and the management of patients with acute exposures.

Testing metal surfaces for free nickel is possible and sometimes necessary in the evaluation and treatment of patients with nickel dermatitis. Patients with clinically important sensitivity or suspect medical histories can order an inexpensive, commercially packaged dimethylglyoxime spot test, allowing them to test metal objects for the presence of free nickel.[17]

TABLE 97–3. Regulatory Standards for Nickel Exposure

STANDARD	EXPOSURE LIMITS	
Elemental	1.5 mg/m³	
Soluble inorganic	0.1 mg/m³	
Insoluble inorganic	0.2 mg/m³	
Nickel subsulfide	0.1 mg/m³	
Nickel carbonyl	0.12 mg/m³	0.05 ppm
OSHA PEL-TWA		
Non-carbonyl nickel	1 mg/m³	
Nickel carbonyl	0.007 mg/m³	0.001 ppm
NIOSH REL-TWA		
Non-carbonyl nickel	0.015 mg/m³	
Nickel carbonyl	0.007 mg/m³	0.001 ppm

ACGIH, American Conference of Governmental Industrial Hygienists; NIOSH, National Institute for Occupational Safety and Health; OSHA, Occupational Safety and Health Administration; PEL, permissible exposure limits; REL, recommended exposure limits; TLV, threshold limit values; TWA, time-weighted average.

TREATMENT

The first step in treatment of nickel-related medical problems is eliminating the exposure, which includes detection and removal of the source. In the case of acute exposures to nickel carbonyl, removal of clothing to prevent continued exposure and thorough skin decontamination may be necessary.

Symptomatic treatment for pulmonary symptoms associated with hypoxia includes the administration of supplemental oxygen. The use of bronchodilators and corticosteroids may also be necessary for the treatment of concomitant bronchospasm. Mechanical ventilation may be required in the most severe cases.

The administration of IV fluids to promote diuresis reduces the half-life of orally ingested nickel chloride by approximately 50%.[94] It is important to note, however, that hemodialysis does not effectively remove nickel from the serum.[111]

CHELATION

Because there have been no controlled human trials, specific recommendations for the use of chelation to treat nickel toxicity are not currently supported by the literature. As a result, extrapolation from animal studies and case reports forms the basis for most treatment regimens. Most studies and reports involving treatment have focused on workers exposed to nickel carbonyl.

Several chelators are proposed as potential treatments for patients with nickel carbonyl exposures. Studies in rats with various chelators show some protection by administration of British anti-Lewisite (BAL) and D-penicillamine[112]; calcium EDTA had no protective effect.[92] Although BAL was been used in the past,[96] the most recent literature has focused on the use of diethyldithiocarbamate (DDC) (see Chaps. 79 and 99 and Antidotes in Depth A-26 and A-28).

DDC is a chelator formerly used as the color reagent for urine nickel measurements. Rats exposed to several times the LD_{50} (median lethal dose for 50% of test subjects) for nickel carbonyl had dramatically reduced mortality when pretreated with DDC; the antidotal efficacy, however, decreased with increasing delay to treatment.[7] A proposed treatment regimen for exposed workers focused on analysis both of the exposure and of the initial 8-hour urine collection.[96] Patients with suspected severe poisonings are typically given the first gram of DDC in divided oral doses. When less severe exposures are suspected, treatment decisions are based on the urinary nickel concentration (Table 97–4.) At concentrations below 100 µg/L, no initial therapy is recommended because delayed symptoms are unlikely to develop. At concentrations between 100–500 µg/L, an oral regimen consisting of

TABLE 97–4. Proposed Diethyldithiocarbamate (DDC) Treatment Regimen After Nickel Carbonyl Exposure[50,96]

Urine nickel	<10 μg/dL	No DDC therapy required
	≥10 mg/dL	1 g PO, then 0.8 g at 4 h, 0.6 g at 8 h, 0.4 g at 16 h, and then 0.4 g q8h
Critically ill		12.5 mg/kg IV (initial dose)
If DDC is unavailable	Disulfiram	750 mg PO q8h for 24 h and then 250 mg PO q8h

PO, orally.

1 g of DDC initially, 0.8 g at 4 hours, 0.6 g at 8 hours, and 0.4 g at 16 hours is used. DDC is continued at a dosage of 0.4 g every 8 hours until there is symptomatic improvement and urine nickel concentration is normal. Patients with severe exposures with urinary nickel concentrations above 500 μg/L may be treated using the same regimen, although they frequently require closer monitoring. Critically ill patients are given parenteral DDC starting at a dose of 12.5 mg/kg; however, given the animal data that the route and timing of administration are important to survival, some authors recommend that parenteral DDC be given as soon as possible after nickel carbonyl poisoning.[15] Although typically well tolerated, DDC is capable of inducing a disulfiram reaction (see Chap. 79) if taken with alcohol, and there are concerns about using DDC when there is concurrent cadmium exposure.[4]

Disulfiram is metabolized into two molecules of DDC. Given that DDC is not pharmaceutically available in the United States, there is some interest in the use of disulfiram as an antidote for nickel carbonyl. Although case reports describe successful treatment of nickel carbonyl toxicity with disulfiram,[50] concern exists because animal studies show that disulfiram increased nickel concentration in brain tissue.[6] One treatment regimen was 750 mg orally every 8 hours for 24 hours followed by 250 mg every 8 hours.[50]

Considering that the majority of the literature and almost all human case reports of nickel carbonyl refer to the use of DDC, it is considered the treatment of choice for nickel toxicity. Although commonly available as a reagent, pharmaceutical-grade DDC may be available commercially through a "complementary medicine pharmacy." It is recommended that the regional poison control center be contacted if necessary to assist with treatment decisions.

Treatments evaluated for divalent nickel exposure are D-penicillamine and *N*-benzyl-D-glucamine dithiocarbamate (NBG-DTC), which, although not commonly available, more effectively lowers brain nickel concentrations than does DDC, perhaps because of its lower lipid solubility.[97]

Patients with contact dermatitis from nickel are treated using standard measures, including avoidance, topical steroids, and oral antihistamines. Some patients have benefited from dietary alteration to reduce nickel intake. Although sometimes advised, there does not appear to be a role for avoiding stainless steel cookware to reduce the nickel content of food.[1]

SUMMARY

Nickel is an important metal that is ubiquitous in the human environment and vital to the functioning of an industrialized society. This constant exposure to nickel is reflected by high rates of nickel sensitivity and dermatitis in the public. Although systemic toxicity from nickel is rare, it is a potentially important cause of occupational illness. Acute toxicity from nickel carbonyl and the potential cancer risk posed by chronic inhalation of nickel-containing dusts and fumes remain important concerns in many industries.

ACKNOWLEDGMENT

Michael I. Greenberg contributed to this chapter in a previous edition.

REFERENCES

1. Accominotti M, Bost M, Haudrechy P, et al. Contribution to chromium and nickel enrichment during cooking of foods in stainless steel utensils. *Contact Dermatitis.* 1998;38:305-310.
2. Adler MW, Adler CH. Toxicity to heavy metals and relationship to seizure thresholds. *Clin Pharmacol Ther.* 1977;22:774-779.
3. Andersen KE, Nielsen GD, Flyvholm MA, et al. Nickel in tap water. *Contact Dermatitis.* 1983;9:140-143.
4. Andersen O, Nielsen JB, Svendsen P. Oral cadmium chloride intoxication in mice—DDC enhances rather than alleviates acute toxicity. *Toxicology.* 1998;52:331-342.
5. Angerer J, Lehnert G. Occupational chronic exposure to metals. II. Nickel exposure of stainless steel welders—biological monitoring. *Int Arch Occup Environ Health.* 1990;62:7-10.
6. Baselt RC, Hanson VW. Efficacy of orally-administered chelating agents for nickel carbonyl toxicity in rats. *Res Commun Chem Pathol Pharmacol.* 1982;38:113-124.
7. Baselt RC, Sunderman FW Jr, Mitchell J, et al. Comparisons of antidotal efficacy of sodium diethyldithiocarbamate, D-penicillamine and triethylenetetramine upon acute toxicity of nickel carbonyl in rats. *Res Commun Chem Pathol Pharmacol.* 1977;18:677-688.
8. Bass JK. Nickel hypersensitivity in the orthodontic patient. *Am J Orthod.* 1993;103:280-285.
9. Bennett BG. Environmental nickel pathways to man. In: Sunderman FW Jr, ed. *Nickel in the Human Environment.* Proceedings of a Joint Symposium, March 1983, Lyon, France (IARC Scientific Publication No. 53). Lyon, France: International Agency for Research on Cancer; 1984: 487-492.
10. Benson JM, Chang IY, Cheng YS, et al. Particle clearance and histopathology in lungs of F344/N rats and B6C3F1 mice inhaling nickel oxide or nickel sulfate. *Fundam Appl Toxicol.* 1995;28:232-244.
11. Bercovitch L, Luo J. Cellphone contact dermatitis with nickel allergy. *CMAJ.* 2008;178:23-24.
12. Berge SR, Skyberg K. Radiographic evidence of pulmonary fibrosis and possible etiologic factors at a nickel refinery in Norway. *J Environ Monit.* 2003;5:681-688.
13. Bernacki EJ, Parsons GE, Roy BR, et al. Urine nickel concentrations in nickel-exposed workers. *Ann Clin Lab Sci.* 1978;8:184-189.
14. Boysen M, Solberg LA, Andersen I, et al. Nasal histology and nickel concentration in plasma and urine after improvements in working environment at a nickel refinery in Norway. *Scand J Work Environ Health.* 1982;8:283-289.
15. Bradberry SM, Vale JA. Therapeutic review: do diethyldithiocarbamate and disulfiram have a role in acute nickel carbonyl poisoning? *J Toxicol Clin Toxicol.* 1999;37:259-264.
16. Bureau of Mines. *Chemical Industry Applications of Industrial Minerals and Metals. Bureau of Mines Special Publication.* Washington DC: Bureau of Mines; 1993:158.
17. Byer TT, Morrell DS. Periumbilical allergic contact dermatitis: blue-jeans or belt buckles. *Pediatr Dermatol.* 2004;21:223-226.
18. Christensen OB, Lagesson V. Nickel concentration of blood and urine after oral administration. *Ann Clin Lab Sci.* 1988;11:119-125.
19. Ciccarelli RB, Wetterhan KE. Nickel bound to chromatin, nucleic acids, and nuclear proteins from kidney and liver of rats treated with nickel carbonate in vivo. *Cancer Res.* 1984;44:3892-3897.
20. Cooper RM, Legare CE, Campbell Teskey G. Changes in (14)C-labeled 2-deoxyglucose brain uptake from nickel-induced epileptic activity. *Brain Res.* 2001;923:71-81.

21. Costa M, Mollenhauer HH. Carcinogenic activity of particulate nickel compounds is proportional to their cellular uptake. *Science.* 1980;209:515-517.
22. Danadevi K, Rozati R, Reddy PP, et al. Semen quality of Indian welders occupationally exposed to nickel and chromium. *Reprod Toxicol.* 2003;17:451-456.
23. De Medeiros LM, Fransway AF, Taylor JS, et al. Complementary and alternative remedies: an additional source of potential systemic nickel exposure. *Contact Dermatitis.* 2008;58:97-100.
24. Denays R, Kumba C, Lison D, et al. First epileptic seizure induced by occupational nickel poisoning. *Epilepsia.* 2005;46:961-962.
25. Dostal LA, Hopfer SM, Lin SM, et al. Effects of nickel chloride on lactating rats and their suckling pups, and the transfer of nickel through rat milk. *Toxicol Appl Pharmacol.* 1989;101:220-231.
26. Duarte I, Lazzarini R, Kobata CM: Contact dermatitis in adolescents. *Am J Contact Dermat.* 2003;14:200-204.
27. Daldrup T, Haarhoff K, Szathmary SC. Fatal nickel sulfate poisoning [German]. *Bericht Gerichtl Med.* 1983;41:141-144.
28. Elias Z, Mur JM, Pierre F, et al. Chromosome aberrations in peripheral blood lymphocytes of welders and characterization of their exposure by biological samples analysis. *J Occup Med.* 1989;31:477-483.
29. Fischer LA, Menne T, Johansen JD. Dose per unit area—a study of elicitation of nickel allergy. *Contact Dermatitis.* 2007;56:255-261.
30. Fullerton A, Andersen JR, Hoelgaard A, et al. Permeation of nickel salts through human skin in vitro. *Contact Dermatitis.* 1986;15:173-177.
31. Garner LA. Contact dermatitis to metals. *Dermatol Ther.* 2004;17:321-327.
32. Genelhu MC, Marigo M, Alves-Oliveira LF, et al. Characterization of nickel-induced allergic contact stomatitis associated with fixed orthodontic appliances. *Am J Orthod Dentofacial Orthop.* 2005;128:378-381.
33. Ghezzi I, Baldasseroni A, Sesana G, et al. Behaviour of urinary nickel in low-level occupational exposure. *Med Lav.* 1989;80:244-250.
34. Grandjean P. Human exposure to nickel. In: Sunderman FW Jr, ed. *Nickel in the Human Environment*, vol. 53. Lyon, France: International Agency for Research on Cancer; 1984:469-485.
35. Habor LT, Allen BC, Carole AK. Non-cancer risk assessment for nickel compounds: issues associated with dose–response modeling of inhalation and oral exposures. *Toxicol Sci.* 1998;43:213-229.
36. Hassler E, Lind B, Nilsson B, et al. Urinary and fecal elimination of nickel in relation to air-borne nickel in a battery factory. *Ann Clin Lab Sci.* 1983;13:217-224.
37. Hirano S, Shimada T, Osugi J, et al. Pulmonary clearance and inflammatory potency of intratracheally instilled or acutely inhaled nickel sulfate in rats. *Arch Toxicol.* 1994;68:548-554.
38. Hisatomi K, Ishii H, Hashiguchi K, et al. Interstitial pneumonia caused by inhalation of fumes of nickel and chrome. *Respirology.* 2006;11:814-817.
39. Hostynek JJ, Dreher F, Nakada T, et al. Human stratum corneum adsorption of nickel salts. Investigation of depth profiles by tape stripping in vivo. *Acta Derm Venereol Suppl (Stockh).* 2001;212:11-18.
40. Hostynek JJ, Dreher F, Pelosi A, et al. Human stratum corneum penetration by nickel. In vivo study after occlusive application of the metal as powder. *Acta Derm Venereol Suppl (Stockh).* 2001;212:5-10.
41. House K, Sernetz F, Dymock D, et al. Corrosion of orthodontic appliances—should we care? *Am J Orthod Dentofacial Orthop.* 2008;133:584-592.
42. Hostynek JJ. Sensitization to nickel: etiology, epidemiology, immune reactions, prevention, and therapy. *Rev Environ Health.* 2006;21:253-280.
43. Iijima R, Ikari Y, Amiya E, et al. The impact of metallic allergy on stent implantation: metal allergy and recurrence of in-stent restenosis. *Int J Cardiol.* 2005;104:319-325.
44. International Agency for Research on Cancer. *IARC Monographs on the Evaluation of carcinogenic Risks to Humans Overall Evaluations on Carcinogenicity: An updating on IARC Monographs Volumes 1 to 42.* Lyon, France: World Health Organization; 1987:264-269.
45. Jasim S, Tjalve H. Effects of sodium pyridinethione on the uptake and distribution of nickel, cadmium and zinc in pregnant and non-pregnant mice. *Toxicology.* 1986;38:327-350.
46. Kerosuo H, Moe G, Kleven E. In vitro release of nickel and chromium from different types of simulated orthodontic appliances. *Angle Orthod.* 1995;65:111-116.
47. Khan SF, Sherbondy MA, Ormsby A. Occlusion of metallic biliary stent related to nickel allergy. *Gastrointest Endosc.* 2007;66:413-414.
48. Koster R, Vieluf D, Kiehn M, et al. Nickel and molybdenum contact allergies in patients with coronary in-stent restenosis. *Lancet.* 2000;356: 1895-1897.
49. Kuck PH. *US Geological Survey Minerals Yearbook.* Washington DC: Minerals Yearbook; 2002:1-30.
50. Kurta DL, Dean BS, Krenzelok EP. Acute nickel carbonyl poisoning. *Am J Emerg Med.* 1993;11:64-66.
51. Lacy S A, Merritt K, Brown SA, et al. Distribution of nickel and cobalt following dermal and systemic administration with in vitro and in vivo studies. *J Biomed Mater Res.* 1996;32:279-283.
52. Leikin JB, Paloucek FP. *Poisoning and Toxicology Handbook.* Chicago: LexiComp; 1996.
53. Livideanu C, Giordano-Labadie F, Paul C. Cellular phone addiction and allergic contact dermatitis to nickel. *Contact Dermatitis.* 2007;57:130-131.
54. Lombardi C, Gargioni S, Dama A, et al. Euro coins and contact dermatitis. *Allergy.* 2004;59:669-670.
55. Mafra RA, Araujo DA, Beirao PS, et al. Glutamate transport in rat cerebellar granule cells is impaired by inorganic epileptogenic agents. *Neurosci Lett.* 2001;310:85-88.
56. Malo J-L, Cartier A, Doepner M, et al. Occupational asthma caused by nickel sulfate. *J Allergy Clin Immunol.* 1982;69:55-59.
57. Meding B, Liden C, Berglind N. Self-diagnosed dermatitis in adults. Results from a population survey in Stockholm. *Contact Dermatitis.* 2001;45: 341-345.
58. Menezes LM, Quintao CA, Bolognese AM. Urinary excretion levels of nickel in orthodontic patients. *Am J Orthod Dentofacial Orthop.* 2007;131:635-638.
59. Morgan LG, Rouge PJC. Biological monitoring in nickel refinery workers. In: Sunderman FW Jr, ed. *Nickel in the Human Environment.* Lyon, France: International Agency for Research on Cancer; 1984:507-520.
60. Nakazawa G, Tanabe K, Aoki J, et al. Sirolimus-eluting stents suppress neointimal formation irrespective of metallic allergy. *Circ J.* 2008;72: 893-896.
61. National Institute for Occupational Safety and Health. *Criteria for a Recommended Standard: Occupational Exposure to Inorganic Nickel* (DHEW-NIOSH Document No. 77-164). Washington, DC: US Government Printing Office; 1977.
62. National Research Council. *Medical and Biological Effects of Environmental Pollutants. Nickel.* Washington, DC: National Academy of Sciences; 1975.
63. Neligan PC. Transcutaneous metal absorption following chemical burn injury. *Burns.* 1996;22:232-233.
64. Nestle FO, Speidel H, Speidel MO. High nickel release from 1, 2 euro coins. *Nature.* 2002;419:432.
65. Nomoto S, Sunderman FW Jr. Presence of nickel in alpha-2-macroglobulin isolated from human serum by high-performance liquid chromatography. *Ann Clin Lab Sci.* 1988;18:78-84.
66. Norgaard O. Investigations with radioactive Ni57 into the resorption of nickel through the skin in normal and in nickel-hypersensitive persons. *Acta Derm Venereol.* 1955;35:111-117.
67. Norgaz T, Hobikoglu G, Serdar ZA, et al. Is there a link between nickel allergy and coronary stent restenosis? *Tohoku J Exp Med.* 2005;206: 243-246.
68. Nucera E, Schiavino D, Calandrelli A, et al. Positive patch tests to euro coins in nickel-sensitized patients. *Br J Dermatol.* 2004;150:500-503.
69. Onkelinx C, Becker J, Sunderman FW. Compartmental analysis of the metabolism of ^{63}Ni(II) in rats and rabbits. *Res Commun Chem Pathol Pharmacol.* 1973;6:663-676.
70. Patriarca M, Lyon TD, Fell GS. Nickel metabolism in humans investigated with an oral stable isotope. *Am J Clin Nutr.* 1997;66:616-621.
71. Pigatto PD, Guzzi G. Systemic contact dermatitis from nickel associated with orthodontic appliances. *Contact Dermatitis.* 2004;50:100-101.
72. Rahilly G, Price N. Current products and practice: nickel allergy in orthodontics. *J Orthod.* 2003;30:171-174.
73. Rendall REG, Phillips JI, Renton KA. Death following exposure to fine particulate nickel from a metal arc process. *Ann Occup Hyg.* 1994;38:921-930.
74. Rezuke WN, Knight JA, Sunderman FW Jr. Reference values for nickel concentrations in human tissue and bile. *Am J Ind Med.* 1987;11:419-426.
75. Rietschel RL, Fowler JF. *Fischer's Contact Dermatitis*, 4th ed. Baltimore: Williams & Wilkins; 1995:847-863.
76. Salnikow K, Donald SP, Bruick RK, et al. Depletion of intracellular ascorbate by the carcinogenic metal nickel and cobalt results in the induction of hypoxic stress. *J Biol Chem.* 2004;279:40337-40344.
77. Salnikow K, Zhitkovich A. Genetic and epigenetic mechanisms in metal carcinogenesis and cocarcinogenesis: nickel, arsenic, and chromium. *Chem Res Toxicol.* 2008;21:28-44.

78. Sanchez-Perez J, Ruiz-Genao D, Garcia Del Rio I, et al. Taxi driver's occupational allergic contact dermatitis from nickel in euro coins. *Contact Dermatitis.* 2003;48:340-341.
79. Schroeder HA, Balassa JJ, Vinton WH. Chromium, lead, cadmium, nickel and titanium in mice: effect on mortality, tumors and tissue levels. *J Nutr.* 1964;83:239-250.
80. Seilkop SK, Oller, AR. Respiratory cancer risks associated with low-level nickel exposure: an integrated assessment based on animal, epidemiological, and mechanistic data. *Regul Toxicol Pharmacol.* 2003;37:173-190.
81. Setcos JC, Babaei-Mahani A, Silvio LD, et al. The safety of nickel containing dental alloys. *Dent Mater.* 2006;22:1163-1168.
82. Shi ZC. Acute nickel carbonyl poisoning: a report of 179 cases. *Br J Ind Med.* 1986;43:422-424.
83. Sivulka DJ. Assessment of respiratory carcinogenicity associated with exposure to metallic nickel: a review. *Regul Toxicol Pharmacol.* 2005;43:117-133.
84. Smith VH, Charles-Holmes R, Bedlow A. Contact dermatitis in guitar players. *Clin Exp Dermatol.* 2006;31:143-145.
85. Solomons NW, Viteri F, Shuler TR, et al. Bioavailability of nickel in man: effects of foods and chemically-defined dietary constituents on the absorption of inorganic nickel. *J Nutr.* 1982;112:39-50.
86. Sorahan T. Mortality of workers at a plant manufacturing nickel alloys, 1958–2000. *Occup Med.* 2004;54:28-34.
87. Sorahan T, Williams SP. Mortality of workers at a nickel carbonyl refinery, 1958–2000. *Occup Environ Med.* 2005;62:80-85.
88. Stohs SJ, Bagchi D. Oxidative mechanism in the toxicity of metal ions. *Free Radic Biol Med.* 1995;18;321-336.
89. Stojanovic D, Nikic D, Lazarevic K. The level of nickel in smoker's blood and urine. *Cent Eur J Public Health.* 2004;12:187-189.
90. Sunderman FW. A pilgrimage into the archives of nickel toxicology. *Ann Clin Lab Sci.* 1989;19:1-16.
91. Sunderman FW. Nickel poisoning I. Experimental study of acute and subacute exposure to nickel carbonyl. *Arch Ind Hyg Occup Med.* 1953;8:48.
92. Sunderman FW. Nickel poisoning VI. A note concerning the ineffectiveness of edathamil calcium disodium (calcium disodium ethylenediaminetetraacetic acid). *Arch Ind Health.* 1958;18:480-482.
93. Sunderman FW Jr. A review of the metabolism and toxicology of nickel. *Ann Clin Lab Sci.* 1977;7:377-398.
94. Sunderman FW Jr, Dingle B, Hopfer SM, et al. Acute nickel toxicity in electroplating workers who accidentally ingested a solution of nickel sulfate and nickel chloride. *Am J Ind Med.* 1988;14:257-266.
95. Sunderman FW Jr, Hopfer SM, Swenney KR, et al. Nickel absorption and kinetics in human volunteers. *Proc Soc Exp Biol Med.* 1989;191:5-11.
96. Sunderman FW Sr. Use of sodium diethyldithiocarbamate in the treatment of nickel carbonyl poisoning. *Ann Clin Lab Sci.* 1990;20:12-21.
97. Tandon SK, Singh S, Jain VK, et al. Chelation in metal intoxication. XXXVIII: effect of structurally different chelating agents in treatment of nickel intoxication in rat. *Fundam Appl Toxicol.* 1996;31:141-148.
98. Tanojo H, Hostynek JJ, Mountford HS, et al. In vivo permeation of nickel salts through human stratum corneum. *Acta Derm Venereol Suppl (Stockh).* 2001;212:19-23.
99. Templeton DM, Sunderman FW Jr, Herber RF. Tentative reference values for nickel concentrations in human serum, plasma, blood, and urine: evaluation according to the TRACY protocol. *Sci Total Environ.* 1994;148: 243-251.
100. Thyssen JP, Johansen JD, Zachariae C, et al. The outcome of dimethylglyoxime testing in a sample of cell phone users. *Contact Dermatitis.* 2008;59:38-42.
101. Tola S, Kilpio J, Virtamo M. Urinary and plasma concentrations of nickel as indicators of exposure to nickel in an electroplating shop. *J Occup Med.* 1979;21:184-188.
102. Torjussen W, Andersen I. Nickel concentrations in nasal mucosa, plasma, and urine in active and retired nickel workers. *Ann Clin Lab Sci.* 1979;9: 289-298.
103. United States Code Title 31, Subtitle IV, Chapter 51, Subchapter II, § 5112. Denominations, specifications, and design of coins.
104. United States Environmental Protection Agency. *Consumer Fact Sheet on Nickel.* Washington, DC: Environmental Protection Agency. Retrieved October 5, 2009, from http://www.epa.gov/OGWDW/dwh/c-ioc/nickle.html
105. Vaktskjold A, Talykova LV, Chashchin VP, et al. Genital malformations of female nickel-refinery workers. *Scand J Work Environ Health.* 2006;32:41-50.
106. Vaktskjold A, Talykova LV, Chashchin VP, et al. Small-for-gestational-age newborns of female refinery workers exposed to nickel. *Int J Occup Med Environ Health.* 2007;20:327-338.
107. Vaktskjold A, Talykova LV, Chashchin VP, et al. Spontaneous abortions among nickel-exposed female refinery workers. *Int J Environ Health Res.* 2008;18:99-115.
108. Valko M, Morris H, Cronin MT. Metals, toxicity and oxidative stress. *Curr Med Chem.* 2005;12:1161-1208.
109. Van Baalen C, O'Donnell R. Isolation of a nickel-dependent blue-green algae. *J Gen Microbiol.* 1978;105:351-353.
110. Verma R, Ramnath J, Clemens F, et al. Molecular biology of nickel carcinogenesis: identification of differentially expressed genes in morphologically transformed C3H10T1/2 Cl 8 mouse embryo fibroblast cell lines induced by specific insoluble nickel compounds. *Mol Cell Biochem.* 2004;255:203-216.
111. Webster JD, Parker TF, Alfrey AC, et al. Acute nickel intoxication by dialysis. *Ann Intern Med.* 1980;92:631-633.
112. West B, Sunderman FW. Nickel poisoning. VII. The therapeutic effectiveness of alkyldithiocarbamates in experimental animals exposed to nickel carbonyl. *Am J Med Sci.* 1958;236:15-25.
113. Wohrl S, Jandl T, Stingl G, et al. Mobile telephone as new source for nickel dermatitis. *Contact Dermatitis.* 2007;56:113.
114. World Health Organization. *Environmental Health Criteria 108.* Geneva: World Health Organization; 1991:23.

CHAPTER 98
SELENIUM

Diane P. Calello

Selenium (Se)		
Atomic number	=	34
Atomic weight	=	78.96 daltons
Normal concentrations		
Whole blood	=	0.1–0.34 mg/L (1.27–4.32 μmol/L)
Serum	=	0.04–0.6 mg/L (0.51–7.6 μmol/L)
Urine	<	0.03 mg/L (<0.38 μmol/L)
Hair	<	0.4 μg/g (0.01 μmol/L)

Selenium was discovered by Jöns Berzelius in 1817 as a contaminant of sulfuric acid vats that caused illness in Swedish factory workers. He originally believed it to be the element tellurium (from the Latin *tellus*, "earth"), but on finding it to be an entirely new, yet similar, element, he named it from the Greek *selene*, "moon." Selenium has unusual light-sensitive electrical conductive properties, leading to its widespread use in industry. It is both an essential component of the human diet and a deadly poison.

HISTORY AND EPIDEMIOLOGY

Much of what is known about selenium centers around its role as an essential trace element required in the diet of most living things, not around its toxic properties. In the 1970s, it was discovered to be an essential cofactor of the enzyme glutathione peroxidase. Keshan disease, an endemic cardiomyopathy associated with multifocal myonecrosis, periacinar pancreatic fibrosis, and mitochondrial disruption, was described in 1979 in Chinese women and children who chronically consumed a selenium-poor diet.[9] Kashin-Beck disease, a disease causing shortened stature from chondrocyte necrosis, is described in young children in Russia, China, and Korea; although other factors are also likely involved, partial improvement results from with selenium supplementation.[2]

These observations prompted the establishment, in 1980, of the United States' recommended daily allowance (RDA) of selenium. Taking into account the level of supplementation required to achieve optimal glutathione peroxidase activity in selenium-deficient study populations, as well as the amounts required to cause toxicity, the recommendation calls for 55 μg/d. Deficiency occurs when daily intake falls below 20 μg/d.[9]

Chronic selenium toxicity, or selenosis, has occurred throughout history. Described first in animals, the acute syndrome of "blind staggers" and the more chronic "alkali disease" affected livestock eating highly seleniferous plants. Findings included blindness, walking in circles, anorexia, weight loss, ataxia, and dystrophic hooves. Humans in seleniferous areas of China and Venezuela develop similar integumentary symptoms (dermatitis, hair loss, and nail changes) at an intake of approximately 6000 μg/d, which is more than 100 times the RDA.[4,36] In recent years, there have been several outbreaks of chronic selenium toxicity related to improperly packaged dietary supplements.[14,35,42]

Selenium is widely distributed throughout the earth's crust, usually substituting for sulfur in sulfide ores such as marcasite (FeS_2), arsenopyrite (FeAsS), and chalcopyrite ($CuFeS_2$). It is found in the soil where it has leeched from bedrock, in groundwater, and in volcanic gas. The highest soil concentrations of selenium in the United States are in the Midwest and West. Dietary selenium is easily obtained through meats, grains, and cereals. Brazil nuts, grown in the foothills of the highly seleniferous Andes Mountains, contain the highest concentration measured in food, but chronic selenium toxicity from Brazil nuts has not been reported.[2]

In industry, selenium is generated primarily as a byproduct of electrolytic copper refining and in the combustion of rubber, paper, municipal waste, and fossil fuels. In general, selenium compounds are used in glass manufacture and coloring, photography and xerography, rubber vulcanization, and as insecticides and fungicides. Selenium sulfide is the active ingredient in many antidandruff shampoos. Gun bluing solution, used in the care of firearms to restore the natural color to the gun barrel, is composed of selenious acid in combination with cupric sulfate in hydrochloric acid, nitric acid, copper nitrate, or methanol. Tables 98–1 and 98–2 list features and regulatory standards of common selenium compounds.

CHEMICAL PRINCIPLES

Selenium is a nonmetal element of group VIA of the periodic table along with oxygen, sulfur, tellurium, and polonium. Selenium exists in elemental, organic, and inorganic forms, with four important oxidation states: selenide (Se^{2-}), elemental (Se^0), selenite (Se^{+4}), and selenate (Se^{+6}). Solubility in water generally increases with oxidation state. Selenium behaves similarly to sulfur in its tendency to form compounds and in biologic systems[2] and is both photovoltaic (able to convert light to electricity) and photoconductive (conducts electricity faster in bright light), which has led to its use in photography, xerography, and solar cells.

At least three solid allotropes of elemental selenium are described: "grey selenium," which predominates at room temperature; red crystalline selenium; and a red amorphous powder.[2] In general, toxicity from elemental selenium is rare and only occurs from long-term exposure. Hydrogen selenide (H_2Se) is formed from the reaction of water or acids with metal selenides or from the reaction of hydrogen with soluble selenium compounds; at room temperature, it exists in gaseous form and results in industrial inhalation exposures. The organic alkyl selenides (dimethylselenide, trimethylselenide) are the least toxic and are byproducts of endogenous selenium detoxification (methylation). Inorganic salts and acids are responsible for all cases of acute toxicity. Selenious acid (H_2SeO_3), generated from the reaction of selenium dioxide with water, is the most toxic form of selenium; ingestion of selenious acid is often fatal.

PHARMACOLOGY AND PATHOPHYSIOLOGY

Selenium exists in one of three forms in the body. First, *selenoproteins* contain selenocysteine residues and play specific selenium-dependent roles primarily in oxidation–reduction reactions. Second, nonspecific plasma proteins bind and may aid in transport of selenium; they may directly bind selenium (albumin, globulins) or contain it as selenocysteine or selenomethionine in place of cysteine and methionine, respectively. Third, there are several inorganic forms of selenium in transit throughout the body, such as selenate, alkyl selenides, and elemental selenium (Se°).

The known specific selenoproteins—glutathione peroxidase, iodothyronine 5-deiodinases, and thioredoxin reductase—each contain a selenocysteine residue at the active site. The most studied of these is glutathione peroxidase, which is responsible for detoxification of reactive oxygen species. Using reduced glutathione (GSH) as a substrate, glutathione

TABLE 98–1. Selenium Compounds

Name	Chemical Formula	Oxidation State	Uses
Selenium (elemental)	Se	0	Photography, catalyst, dietary supplement, xerography
Selenium sulfide	SeS_2	2⁻	Antidandruff shampoo, fungicide
Hydrogen selenide	H_2Se	2⁻	–
Dimethylselenide	CH_3SeCH_3	2⁻	Metabolite, garlic odor
Selenium dioxide	SeO_2	4⁺	Catalyst, photography, glass decolorizer, vulcanization of rubber, xerography
Selenium oxychloride	$SeOCl_2$	4⁺	Solvent, plasticizer
Selenious acid	H_2SeO_3	4⁺	Gun bluing solution
Sodium selenite	Na_2SeO_3	4⁺	Glass and porcelain manufacture
Selenium hexafluoride	SeF_6	6⁺	Gaseous electrical insulator
Sodium selenate	Na_2SeO_4	6⁺	Glass manufacture, insecticide

TABLE 98–2. Selenium Regulations and Advisories

Oral–Recommended Intake and Exposure Limits			
RDA (2000)		55 µg/d[a]	(0.8 µg/kg/d)
NAS-TUL		400 µg/d	(5.7 µg/kg/d)
ATSDR-chronic oral MRL[b]		5 µg/kg/d	
Water–Limits			
WHO	Drinking water	0.01 mg/L	
FDA	Bottled water	0.05 mg/L	
EPA	MCL, drinking	0.05 mg/L	
Air–Limits[c]			
NIOSH			
REL (TWA)		0.2 mg/m³	
IDLH		1.0 mg/m³	
OSHA			
PEL (TWA)		0.2 mg/m³	

[a] Values differ for pregnant and lactating women, children, and neonates.

[b] No acute or intermediate MRL has been established. Chronic ≥365 days.

[c] Ambient background air concentrations are usually in the ng/m³ range.

AHTSDR, American Toxic Surveillance and Disease Registry; EPA, Environmental Protection Agency; FDA, Food and Drug Administration; IDLH, Immediately Dangerous to Life or Health; MCL, maximum contaminant level; MRL, minimal risk level; NAS, National Academy of Sciences; NIOSH, National Institute for Occupational Safety and Health; OSHA, Occupational Safety and Health Administration; PEL, permissible exposure limit; RDA, recommended daily allowance; REL, recommended exposure limit; TUL, tolerable upper limit; TWA, time-weighted average; WHO, World Health Organization.

peroxidase catalyses the reduction of hydrogen peroxide to water and oxidized glutathione (GSSG, or glutathione disulfide); the reaction occurs by concomitant oxidation of the selenocysteine unit on the enzyme.[3,32] Other selenocysteine-containing proteins, such as thioredoxin reductase, also appear to have antioxidant properties. The selenocysteine-containing thyroid hormone deiodinases are responsible for the conversion of thyroxine (T_4) to the active triiodothyronine (T_3) form.

In selenium deficiency, glutathione peroxidase activity is decreased, and GSH and glutathione-S transferases are increased.[32] Consequently, selenium-deficient rats are more resistant to substances detoxified by glutathione-S transferase, such as acetaminophen and aflatoxin B[5], and less resistant to other prooxidants, such as nitrofurantoin, diquat, and paraquat.[5] In animal studies of metal toxicity, selenium also appears to modify the effects of silver, cadmium, arsenic, copper, zinc, mercury, and fluoride; conversely, vanadium, tellurium, and arsenic modify the effects of selenium deficiency or excess.[13,16,18,28,36] Although it is proposed that this is accomplished through the formation of insoluble selenium–metal complexes, these relationships are not entirely understood.[11]

Less is known about the biochemical mechanism of selenium toxicity, and what is known is from in vitro data. Paradoxically, excess selenium causes oxidative stress, presumably as a result of prooxidant selenide (R-Se⁻) anions. In addition, the replacement of selenium for sulfur in enzymes of cellular respiration may cause mitochondrial disruption, and the substitution of selenomethionine in place of methionine may interfere with protein synthesis. Integumentary effects are also most likely a result of selenium interpolation into disulfide bridges of structural proteins such as keratin.[40]

PHARMACOKINETICS AND TOXICOKINETICS

Gastrointestinal (GI) absorption varies with the species of selenium, and human data are limited. Elemental selenium is the least bioavailable (≤50%), followed by inorganic selenite and selenate salts (75%)[23]; selenious acid is quite well absorbed in the lungs and GI tract (~85% in animal studies[8]). Organic selenium compounds are the best absorbed at approximately 90% as determined by isotope tracers in human studies.[2,21]

Inhalational absorption was documented in a group of workers exposed to selenium dioxide and hydrogen selenide gas,[2,15] but quantitative inhalation studies in humans are not available. Dermal absorption appears to be limited. Selenium disulfide shampoos are not systemically absorbed as measured by urinary selenium levels[8] except in cases of repeated use on excoriated skin.[31]

The toxic dose of selenium varies widely between selenium compounds, as demonstrated by LD_{50} (median lethal dose for 50% of test subjects) animal studies,[36] making milligram per kilogram exposure estimates difficult to interpret. Elemental selenium has no reported adverse effects in acute overdose, although long-term exposure may be harmful. The selenium salts, particularly selenite, are more acutely toxic, as is selenium oxide (SeO_2) through its conversion to selenious acid in the presence of water. Selenious acid may be lethal with as little as a tablespoon of 4% solution in children.

Metabolic conversion of all forms of selenium to the selenide anion occurs through various means (Fig. 98–1), and the selenide ion undergoes one of three fates: (1) incorporation into selenoproteins such as glutathione peroxidase and triiodothyronine; (2) binding by nonspecific plasma proteins such as albumin or globulins; or (3) hepatic methylation into nontoxic, excretable metabolites. Trimethylselenide is the primary metabolite and is excreted by the kidneys, the major elimination pathway for selenium. Fecal elimination also occurs. Dimethylselenide production is usually minor but increases with exposure; this compound is volatilized through exhalation and sweat and is responsible for the garlic

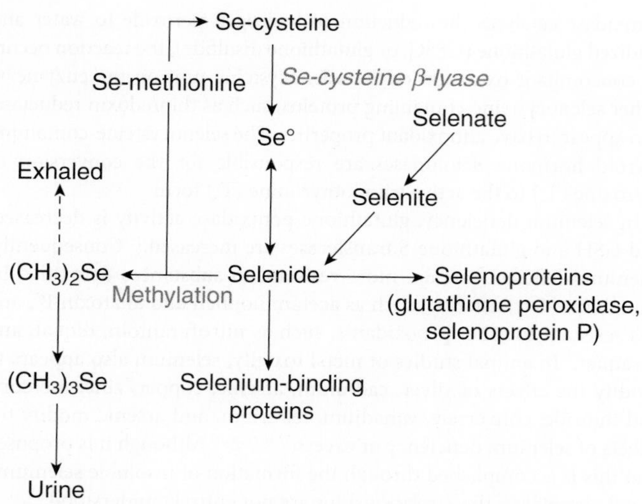

FIGURE 98–1. Metabolism of selenium. The selenide anion is central in selenium metabolism. Organic selenocysteine is converted via the β-lyase enzyme to elemental selenium and then to selenide. Selenomethionine may either undergo transsulfuration to selenocysteine or methylation to excretable metabolites. The selenate and selenite salts are reduced to selenide. Selenide then undergoes one of three processes: methylation, incorporation into selenoproteins, or binding by nonspecific plasma proteins.[1,13]

odor of patients exposed to excess selenium. The remaining selenium in the body is greater than 95% protein bound within 24 hours.[1,36] Toxicokinetic data are limited and vary by compound, and the significance of metabolism in acute selenium salt poisoning is unclear.

CLINICAL MANIFESTATIONS

ACUTE

Dermal and Ophthalmic Exposure Dermal exposure to selenious acid or to selenium dioxide (which is converted to selenious acid) and to selenium oxychloride (a vesicant that is hydrolyzed to hydrochloric acid) causes significantly painful caustic burns.[10] Excruciating pain may result from accumulation under fingernails. Corneal injury with severe pain, lacrimation, and conjunctival edema is reported after exposure to selenium dioxide sprayed unintentionally into the face.[24] In chronic exposures, "rose eye," a red discoloration of eyelids with palpebral conjunctivitis, is also described.

Inhalational Exposure When inhaled, all selenium compounds have the potential to be respiratory irritants. In general, inhaled elemental selenium dusts are less injurious than compounds converted to selenious acid. Hydrogen selenide inhalation toxicity is reported throughout the industrial literature.[6] Hydrogen selenide is oxidized to elemental selenium, so acutely, toxic exposures are limited to confined spaces where the hazardous gas may accumulate; however, similar to hydrogen sulfide (H_2S), its ability to cause olfactory fatigue, rendering the exposed persons anosmic to the toxic fumes, may prove very hazardous (see Chap. 20).[6] Acute exposure to high concentrations of hydrogen selenide gas produces throat and eye pain, rhinorrhea, wheezing, and pneumomediastinum, with residual restrictive and obstructive disease that may persist years later.[33]

In contrast, selenium dioxide and selenium oxide fumes form selenious acid in the presence of water in the respiratory tract. Twenty-eight workers in a selenium rectifier plant were inadvertently exposed to smoke and high concentrations of selenium oxide in an enclosed area. Initial symptoms included bronchospasm with upper respiratory irritation and burning. Some acutely developed hypotension, tachycardia, and tachypnea, which resolved over 2 hours. Patients went on to develop chemical pneumonitis, fever, chills, headache, vomiting, and diarrhea. Five patients required hospitalization for respiratory support, with fever, leukocytosis, and bilateral infiltrates. All patients recovered without sequelae.[44]

Selenium hexafluoride is a caustic gas used in industrial settings as an electrical insulator. Its caustic properties are derived from its conversion, in the presence of water, to elemental selenium and hydrofluoric acid. Severe pain and burning of the eyes, skin, and respiratory tract similar to that seen with hydrofluoric acid exposure can occur after inhalation of selenium hexafluoride (see Chap. 105).

Oral Exposure Acute selenium toxicity occurs after ingestion of inorganic selenium compounds, which include sodium selenite, sodium selenate, selenium dioxide, hydrogen selenide, selenic acid, and selenious acid. Selenious acid is the most toxic of these. Elemental selenium and organic selenium compounds do not cause acute toxicity.

Some authors have proposed a "triphasic" course of acute inorganic selenium toxicity, with GI, myopathic, and circulatory symptoms as the overdose progresses.[39] In reality, acute inorganic selenium poisoning is often rapid and fulminant, with onset of symptoms within minutes and, in some cases, death within 1 hour of ingestion. GI symptoms are the most commonly described and the first to occur and include abdominal pain, diarrhea, nausea, and vomiting. This may be partly caused by caustic esophageal and gastric burns but does not occur in all cases. Patients may have a garlic odor. The myopathic phase is characterized by weakness, hyporeflexia, myoclonus, fasciculations, and elevated creatine phosphokinase (CPK) concentrations with normal MB fraction. Renal insufficiency is also reported and presumably results from myoglobinuria and hemolysis. More severely poisoned patients may exhibit lethargy, delirium, and coma.

Circulatory failure is the hallmark of serious inorganic selenium toxicity. Patients present with dyspnea, chest pain, tachycardia, and hypotension. The initial electrocardiogram (ECG) may demonstrate ST elevation, a prolonged QT interval, and T-wave inversions. Refractory hypotension occurs as a combined product of decreased contractility from toxic cardiomyopathy and decreased peripheral vascular resistance. Pulmonary edema, ventricular dysrhythmias, myocardial and mesenteric infarction, and metabolic acidosis all contribute to poor outcome in these patients.[25,29,44] Death results from circulatory collapse in the setting of pump failure, hypotension, and ventricular dysrhythmias, often within 4 hours of ingestion.[7,17,19,30,38]

Other less frequent abnormalities include hypokalemia, hyperkalemia, coagulopathy, leukocytosis, hemolysis, thrombocytopenia, and metabolic acidosis with elevated lactate.[34,39]

The classic scenario of acute fatal inorganic selenium poisoning is in the context of selenious acid ingestion, usually as gun bluing solution. Similar toxicity may result from selenium oxide and dioxide, which are converted to selenious acid as well as sodium selenite and selenate. The underlying mechanism for this fulminant clinical syndrome is not well understood but may stem from a multifocal disruption of cellular oxidative processes and antioxidant defense mechanisms.

CHRONIC

Chronic elemental selenium toxicity, or selenosis, has received recent attention because of reports of improperly packaged nutritional supplements. In 2008, at least 200 people were affected by a manufacturing error in a selenium-containing dietary supplement and developed diarrhea, alopecia, fatigue, and nail deformities.[42] The manufacturer voluntarily recalled the product, and a Food and Drug Administration investigation revealed that the liquid supplement contained 800 μg/L instead of the 7.3 μg/L of selenium claimed on the packaging.[43] A similar outbreak occurred from a super-potent supplement in 1983, affecting at least 13 patients, all of whom recovered after discontinuation of the supplement.[14,35]

Selenosis is similar to arsenic toxicity, with the most consistent manifestations being nail and hair abnormalities. As with arsenic toxicity, nail or hair findings alone are unlikely to be the sole evidence of selenosis, but their absence makes the diagnosis unlikely. The hair becomes very brittle, breaking off easily at the scalp, with regrowth of discolored hair and the development of an intensely pruritic scalp rash. The nails also break easily, with white or red ridges that can be either transverse or longitudinal; the thumb is usually involved first, and paronychia and nail loss may develop.[27] The skin becomes erythematous, swollen, and blistered; slow to heal; and with a persistent red discoloration. Increased dental caries may occur.[12] Neurologic manifestations include hyperreflexia, peripheral paresthesia, anesthesia, and hemiplegia. Although cardiotoxicity is described with both selenium deficiency and acute poisoning, no such cases are reported with human selenosis. Aside from one case described in the Chinese population, in which there were insufficient postmortem data, there have been no reported deaths from intermediate or chronic exposure.

Selenosis is implicated in a number of long-term environmental exposures. Many descriptions come from inhabitants of the Hubei province of China from 1961 to 1964, the majority of whom developed clinical signs after an estimated average consumption of 5000 μg/d of selenium (but as little as 910 μg/d) derived from local crops and vegetation.[45] Inhabitants of a seleniferous area of Venezuela, consuming approximately 300 to 400 μg/d of selenium, also develop symptoms of selenium excess; however, the low socioeconomic and poor dietary status of the subjects may also contribute to their symptoms. In contrast, U.S. residents in a seleniferous area with a high selenium intake (724 μg/d) over 2 years who were compared with a control population and monitored for symptoms and laboratory abnormalities, remained asymptomatic, with only a clinically insignificant elevation of hepatic aminotransferases in the high-selenium group.[22] Average selenium concentrations were serum, 0.215 mg/L; whole blood, 0.322 mg/L; and urine, 0.17 mg/L.

Selenosis is also reported in the industrial setting. Copper refinery workers demonstrate garlic odor and GI and respiratory symptoms coincident with exposure to selenium dust and fumes.[15] Long before workplace biological monitoring took place, intense garlic odor of the breath and secretions was recognized as a reason to remove a worker from selenium until the odor subsided. Neuropsychiatric findings such as fatigue, irritability, and depression are reported throughout the industrial literature and are difficult to quantify. Early reports describe the selenium factory worker who "could not stand his children about him" at the end of the day.[10]

Although carcinogenicity is suggested by a number of animal studies, in humans, the data available suggest, if anything, an inverse correlation between selenium intake and cancer risk. The International Agency for Research on Cancer does not list selenium as a known or suspected carcinogen.[2]. Animal studies also suggest that selenium has embryotoxic and teratogenic properties.[11] A recent large randomized controlled trial of selenium supplementation suggested an increased the risk of diabetes mellitus with the ingestion of 200 μg/day of elemental selenium-fed baker's yeast compared with placebo.[41]

DIAGNOSTIC TESTING

Over time, selenium is incorporated into blood and erythrocyte proteins, making serum the best measure of acute toxicity and whole blood preferable for the assessment of patients with chronic exposure. Patients with acute poisoning generally demonstrate an initial serum concentration greater than 2 mg/L, which falls below 1 mg/L within 24 hours, reflecting redistribution.[27] Patients with long-term elemental exposures are reported to have serum concentrations of 0.5 to 1.0 mg/L. However, selenium concentrations do not demonstrate a predictable relationship with exposure, toxicity, or time course. Population-based studies suggest an average serum concentration of 0.126 mg/L in the United States.[26]

Urine concentrations reflect very recent exposure because urinary excretion of selenium is maximal within the first 4 hours. In addition, urine concentrations are an imperfect measure because they can be affected by the most recent meal and hydration status. However, in general, a normal urinary concentration is less than 0.03 mg/L. Freezing of urine specimens after collection is recommended to retard the enzymatic formation of difficult-to-detect volatile metabolites.[27]

Hair concentrations of selenium were measured in the Hubai Chinese populations of interest and may be a useful measure of exposure.[37,45] However, the usefulness of hair selenium is limited in countries such as the United States where the use of selenium sulfide shampoos is widespread.

Other ancillary tests to assess selenium toxicity include ECG, thyroid function, platelet counts, hepatic aminotransferases, creatinine, and serum creatine phosphokinase concentrations. These are abnormal in some patients (eg, in patients with selenious acid poisoning) and are not indicated in patients not expected to develop systemic toxicity.

MANAGEMENT

PAIN MANAGEMENT

Treating painful skin, nail bed burns, or ocular pain with 10% sodium thiosulfate solution or ointment may provide relief of symptoms as the result of a reduction of selenium dioxide to elemental selenium.[10] In one series, workers exposed to selenium dioxide fumes reported similar relief from inhalation of fumes from ammonium hydroxide–soaked sponges; the mechanism of this is unclear, and further study is required before this practice can be recommended.[44]

Workers exposed to selenium hexafluoride gas may be treated with calcium gluconate gel to the affected areas. This is the same treatment as in hydrofluoric acid exposures, which is discussed in Chapter 105.

DECONTAMINATION

As with any toxic exposure, prompt removal from the source is required if possible. Patients with dermal exposure should be irrigated immediately. There are limited data to support the use of aggressive GI decontamination after the ingestion of most elemental selenium–containing xenobiotics because there is little expected acute toxicity. However, in xenobiotics with the potential for producing systemic toxicity, such as the selenite salts, decontamination with gastric lavage or activated charcoal may be warranted. Although no charcoal adsorption data are available to guide this therapy, it should be considered in light of potential benefit until further information is available.

Special mention should be made of the ingestion of selenious acid, which is both a caustic with attendant decontamination difficulties and a serious systemic poison. The judicious use of nasogastric lavage may be indicated based on the time since ingestion, the amount and concentration ingested, the presence or absence of spontaneous emesis, and the clinical condition of the patient.

CHELATION AND ANTIDOTAL THERAPY

There are no proven antidotes for selenium toxicity. Animal studies and scant human data suggest that chelation with dimercaprol (BAL),[21] edetate calcium disodium ($CaNa_2EDTA$), or succimer form nephrotoxic complexes with selenium do not speed clinical recovery and may, in fact, worsen toxicity.[20,21,29] Arsenical compounds appear to ameliorate selenium toxicity through enhanced biliary excretion,[6,11,15,20] but there are no studies to guide this potentially toxic therapy. Vitamin C is hypothesized to limit oxidative damage but has not been studied. Bromobenzene may accelerate urinary excretion of selenium,[6] but its inherent toxicity limits its use, regardless of efficacy.

Extracorporeal removal techniques such as hemodialysis or hemofiltration decrease selenium concentrations in patients undergoing the procedure regularly for renal failure, so theoretically, this could be of use in lowering toxic serum selenium concentrations. However, because of extensive protein binding, this benefit may be only minor and only relevant to patients undergoing frequent dialysis. Although there are reports of using hemodialysis in patients with acute selenium poisoning, further study must occur before this can be recommended.[18,19]

SUPPORTIVE CARE

This is the mainstay of therapy in selenium poisoning. In particular, patients with selenious acid toxicity require intensive monitoring and multisystem support to survive.

SUMMARY

Selenium is an essential trace element and is required in the diet of both animals and humans. However, in overdose or with excessive chronic exposure, toxicity may result. In particular, ingestion of selenious acid is often fatal. Other selenium compounds cause variable toxicity, usually in the setting of occupational exposure. Topical and inhalational exposure causes burns and pulmonary irritation, respectively. Acute systemic exposure results in GI, myopathic, and circulatory symptoms. Long-term exposure to elemental selenium may cause selenosis, of which alopecia is the most consistent finding. Although it is possible to obtain blood, urine, and hair selenium concentrations to confirm exposure, there is no clear relationship between levels and clinical outcome. Supportive therapy remains the standard of care.

REFERENCES

1. Agency for Toxic Substances and Disease Registry (ATSDR). *Toxicological Profile for Selenium.* Atlanta: PHS U.S. Department of Health and Human Services; 2003.
2. Barceloux DG. Selenium. *J Toxicol Clin Toxicol.* 1999;37:146-172.
3. Berg JM, Tymoczko JL, Stryer L. *Biochemistry*, 5th ed. New York: WH Freeman; 2002.
4. Bratter P, Negretti de Bratter VE, Jaffe WG, et al. Selenium status of children living in seleniferous areas of Venezuela. *J Trace Elem Electrolytes Health Dis.* 1991;5:269-270.
5. Burk RF, Lane JM. Modification of chemical toxicity by selenium deficiency. *Fundam Appl Toxicol.* 1983;3:218-221.
6. Cerwenka EA, Cooper WC. Toxicology of selenium and tellurium and their compounds. *Arch Environ Health.* 1961;3:189-200.
7. Civil IDS, McDonald MJA. Acute selenium poisoning: case report. *N Z Med J.* 1978;87:354-356.
8. Cummins LM, Kimura ET. Safety evaluation of selenium sulfide antidandruff shampoos. *Toxicol Appl Pharmacol.* 1971;20:89-96.
9. Ge K, Xue A, Bai J, et al. Keshan disease-an endemic cardiomyopathy in China. *Virchows Arch.* 1983;401:1-15.
10. Glover JR. Selenium and its industrial toxicology. *Ind Med Surg.* 1970;39.
11. Goyer RA, Clarkson TW. Toxic effects of metals. In: Klassen CD, ed. *Casarett and Doul's Toxicology: The Basic Science of Poisons*, 6th ed. New York: McGraw-Hill; 2000:811-867.
12. Hadjimarkos DM. Selenium in relation to dental caries. *Food Cosmet Toxicol.* 1973;11:1083-1095.
13. Hadjimarkos DM. Selenium toxicity: effect of fluoride. *Experientia.* 1968;25:485-486.
14. Helzlsouer K, Jacobs R, Morris S. Acute selenium intoxication in the United States [abstract]. *Fed Proc.* 1985;44:1670.
15. Holness DL, Taraschuk IG, Nethercott JR. Health status of copper refinery workers with specific reference to selenium exposure. *Arch Environ Health.* 1989;44:291-297.
16. Huang Z, Pei Q, Sun G, et al. Low selenium status affects arsenic metabolites in an arsenic exposed population with skin lesions. *Clin Chim Acta.* 2008;387:139-144.
17. Hunsaker DM, Spiller HA, Williams D. Acute selenium poisoning: suicide by ingestion. *J Forensic Sci.* 2005;50:942-946.
18. Kise Y, Yoshimura S, Akieda K, et al. Acute oral selenium intoxication with ten times the lethal dose resulting in deep gastric ulcer. *J Emerg Med.* 2004;26:183-187.
19. Koppel C, Baudisch H, Veter KH, et al. Fatal poisoning with selenium dioxide. *J Toxicol Clin Toxicol.* 1986;24:21-35.
20. Levander OA. Metabolic interrelationships and adaptations in selenium toxicity. *Ann NY Acad Sci.* 1972;192:181-192.
21. Lombeck I, Menzel H, Frosch D. Acute selenium poisoning of a 2-year-old child. *Eur J Pediatr.* 1987;146:308-312.
22. Longnecker MP, Taylor PR, Levander OA, et al. Selenium in diet, blood, and toenails in relation to human health in a seleniferous area. *Am J Clin Nutr.* 1992;53:1288-1294.
23. McAdam PA, Lewis SA, Helzlsouer K, et al. Absorption of selenite and L-selenomethionine in healthy young men using a ^{74}selenium tracer [abstract]. *Fed Proc.* 1985;44:1670.
24. Middleton JM. Selenium burn of the eye. Review of a case with review of the literature. *Arch Ophthalmol.* 1947;38:806-811.
25. Nantel AJ, Brown M, Dery P, et al. Acute poisoning by selenious acid. *Vet Hum Toxicol.* 1985;27:531-533.
26. Niskar AS, Paschal DC, Kieszak SM, et al. Serum selenium levels in the US population: third National Health and Nutrition Examination Survey, 1988–1994. *Biol Trace Elem Res.* 2003;91:1-10.
27. Nuttall KL. Evaluating selenium poisoning. *Ann Clin Lab Sci.* 2006;36:406-420.
28. Parizek J, Kalouskova J, Benes J, et al. Interactions of selenium-mercury and selenium-selenium compounds. *Ann N Y Acad Sci.* 1980;355:347-359.
29. Pentel P, Fletcher D, Jentzen J. Fatal acute selenium toxicity. *J Forensic Sci.* 1985;30:556-562.
30. Quadrani DA, Spiller HA, Steinhorn D. A fatal case of gun blue ingestion in a toddler. *Vet Hum Toxicol.* 2000;42:96-98.
31. Ransone JW. Selenium sulfide intoxication. *N Engl J Med.* 1961;264:384-385.
32. Rotruck JT, Pope AL, Ganther HE, et al. Selenium: biochemical role as a component of glutathione peroxidase. *Science.* 1972;179:588-590.
33. Schecter A, Shanske W, Stenzler A, et al. Acute hydrogen selenide inhalation. *Chest.* 1980;77:554-555.
34. See KA, Lavercombe PA, Dillon J, et al. Accidental death from acute selenium poisoning. *Med J Aust.* 2006;185:388-389.
35. Selenium intoxication—New York. *MMWR Mortal Morbid Weekly Rep.* 1984;33:157-158.
36. Shamberger RJ. *Biochemistry of Selenium.* New York: Plenum Press; 1983.
37. Shamberger RJ. Validity of hair mineral testing. *Biol Trace Elem Res.* 2002;87:1-28.
38. Sioris LJ, Pentel PR. Acute selenium poisoning. *Vet Hum Toxicol.* 1980;22:364.
39. Spiller HA. Two fatal cases of selenium toxicity. *Forensic Sci Int.* 2007;171:67-72.
40. Stadtman T. Selenium biochemistry. *Science.* 1974;183:915-922.
41. Stranges S, Marshall JR, Natarajan R, et al. Effects of long-term selenium supplementation on the incidence of type 2 diabetes. *Ann Intern Med.* 2007;147:217-223.
42. Sutter ME, Thomas JD, Brown J, et al. Selenium toxicity: a case of selenosis caused by a nutritional supplement. *Ann Intern Med.* 2008;148:970-971.
43. U.S. Food and Drug Administration. *F.D.A. Completes Final Analysis of "Total Body Formula" and "Total Body Mega Formula" Products 2008.* Retrieved February 1, 2009, from http://www.fda.gov/bbs/topics/NEWS/2008/NEW01831.html.
44. Wilson HM. Selenium oxide poisoning. *N C Med J.* 1962;23:73-75.
45. Yang G, Wang S, Zhou R, et al. Endemic selenium intoxication of humans in China. *Am J Clin Nutr.* 1983;37:872-881.

CHAPTER 99
SILVER

Melisa W. Lai Becker and Michele Burns Ewald

Silver (Ag)

Atomic number	=	47
Atomic weight	=	107.9 daltons
Normal concentrations		
Serum	<	1 μg/L (<9 nmol/L)
Urine (24 hour)	<	2 μg/L (<18 nmol/L)

Silver, often referred to as a "precious metal," has been used for thousands of years in an impressive array of applications, including as coins and as a financial standard, instrument and tool material, chemical catalyst, electrical conductor, and medicinal ingredient and adjunct. It occurs throughout the earth's crust at an average concentration by weight of 80 ppb and in sea water at 0.1 ppb. Life-threatening toxicity of silver is uncommon, but chronic exposure may lead to permanent disability.

Silver has considerable strength and malleability, as well as excellent thermal and electrical conductivity, due to its weak interaction with oxygen (second only to gold). These properties are responsible for its widespread use throughout the health, science, and engineering industries, where it remains a key component of batteries, mechanical bearings, catalysts, coins, electroplating, mirrors, coatings, photography, medical bactericidal agents, and water purification.

This prevalence of silver notwithstanding, silver poisoning is rare and is often the result of occupational exposure or self-administration of silver-containing products for unproven medicinal purposes. Since the mid-20th century, the use of silver for medicinal purposes has infrequently resulted in iatrogenic overuse and subsequent *argyria*, which is a permanent bluish-gray discoloration of skin that is the primary manifestation of chronic silver overexposure.[5]

HISTORY

Although the symbol of silver, Ag, is derived from the Latin and Greek words for silver—*argentum* and *argyros*—the word we use in English is derived from Slavic and Germanic *Silubr* and *Sirebro* and Old English *Seolfor*. Even the alchemy symbol of silver (a crescent moon) and dalton symbol (a coinlike circumscribed letter S) etch the impression of silver as a valued and precious element.

In Asia Minor and on islands in the Aegean Sea, dumps of slag (scum formed by molten metal surface oxidation) demonstrate that silver may have been separated from lead as early as 4000 B.C. The use of silver as a precious metal with trade value appears to have begun around 600 B.C., when weighed pieces of silver were exchanged for goods. Silver coinage debuted circa 550 B.C. in the Mediterranean and was adopted by various empires, dynasties, and nation-states thereafter. Today, only Mexico uses silver in circulating coinage; the United States incorporates silver purely in commemorative and proof coins.

The Phoenicians and early Greeks knew to store water, wine, and vinegar in silver-lined vessels during long sea voyages, just as later American pioneers added silver coins to water barrels and jugs of milk to keep them fresh.[37] The phrase "born with a silver spoon in his mouth" referred originally to health rather than wealth because silver pacifiers and baby spoons were used to help ward off childhood illnesses.

A traded commodity on the world's markets, silver had been used as an abstract financial standard for various economies throughout modern banking history until the late 19th century.

Beyond the economic role of silver, the electrical and thermal conductive properties of the element make it an invaluable material for scientific instrument manufacture and engineering. Because silver contacts neither corrode nor overheat, silver is commonly used in electronic devices and appliances. Silver was a key component of early telecommunications—it was the choice for Morse's first telegraph contacts in 1844—and made the jet age possible because only silver-plated bearings have the adequate dry lubricity necessary for safe engine shutdown without volatile oil lubricants. Today, washing machines, cars, personal digital assistants, and consumer electronics all use small amounts of silver in their functional parts.

Silver is also used to "make rain"—silver iodide crystals, whose lattice structure is similar to ice, are released into "supercooled" (between 7° and 25°F) clouds, causing water droplets in clouds to attach and form ice crystals. Ice crystals that become large and heavy enough drop from the cloud and melt into raindrops en route to earth.

The medicinal value of silver has been greatly exaggerated, with the element being touted by some as a "cure-all." In the late nineteenth and early twentieth century claims were made that oral administration of colloidal silver proteins (CSPs) (gelatinous suspensions of finely divided elemental silver) would successfully treat diverse diseases, most without evidence.[16,51] However, in 1960, the United States Dispensary declared that "there is no justification for this internal use, either theoretically or practically," and silver was banned in all nonprescription drugs.[14] In 1999, the U.S. Food and Drug Administration issued a Final Rule declaring that all nonprescription drug products containing colloidal silver or silver salts are "not recognized as safe and effective and are misbranded."[15] However, CSPs and other silver-containing "natural" products have been reintroduced for use as health and dietary supplements.[16] After the anthrax terrorist acts of 2001, the mayor of Tampa, Florida, called for CSPs to be mixed into the town's water supply as a protective "elixir" without scientific justification.[2]

In 2002, the Associated Press reported on the reelection campaign of the Montana legislator known as the "blue" lawmaker who promoted the use of colloidal silver health supplements. Because silver-containing products continue to be marketed and sold online as "natural" health supplements with few warnings as to the possible development of argyria, there has been a small resurgence of case reports of argyria today.[19]

EPIDEMIOLOGY

Humans are exposed to minute but varying amounts of silver on a daily basis depending on the occupation. Silver is released into the environment during silver nitrate manufacture for use in photography (diminishing), mirrors, plating, inks and dyes, and porcelain, as well as for germicides, antiseptics, caustics, and analytical reagents. Silver-salt catalysts, used for oxidation–reduction and polymerization reactions, are another a source of silver exposure, as are silver powder pigments and paints.[27] Workplace exposure is often via transdermal, transmucosal, or inhalational routes as silver particles are liberated during various mining, refining, and manufacturing processes.

Additionally, industrial exposure of workers involved in silver mining and manufacturing increases the workplace risk of generalized argyria, although development of signs of argyria from uninterrupted occupational exposure takes a minimum of 24 years.[11] Employees are susceptible to localized argyria and corneal argyrosis from working with smaller amounts of silver in specific applications, as in the coating of metallic films on glass and china, manufacture of electroplating solutions and photographic processing, preparation of artificial pearls, and simple cutting and polishing of silver.

Today silver is used in water filtration cartridges and supermarket products for washing vegetables and to sterilize recycled drinking water on the MIR space station and NASA space shuttle.[44]

Both the National Institute for Occupational Safety and Health (NIOSH) and the Occupational and Safety Health Administration (OSHA) have established the safe occupational exposure limit to silver metal and soluble compounds as 10 μg/m^3 air per 8-hour work shift. The estimated oral intake of silver from average environmental exposure for humans not working in silver-related industries ranges from 10 to 88 μg/d.[13]

PHARMACOLOGY

Silver that is absorbed into the body is transported by globulins in blood and stored mainly in the skin and liver, with average daily intake excreted in the bile and eliminated in the feces (≤30–80 μg/d) and urine (≤10 μg/d).[11,12,14] Silver elimination through the feces occurs in two phases: phase one has a relatively short half-life ranging from 1 to 2.4 days, varying with route of administration (apparent oral half-life is 1 day, inhalational is 1.7 days, and intravenous (IV) is 2.4 days).[12,13,14,17,35] Phase two elimination has a half-life of 48–52 days, thought to represent liver deposition and clearance.[30,36]

Although one study on a single human subject showed 18% of a single dose of an orally administered silver acetate salt was retained after 30 weeks, animal studies show little silver absorption along the gastrointestinal (GI) tract, with 90% of ingested silver excreted within 2 days of ingestion.[12,13]

Humans retain only 0% to 10% of their daily silver exposure of 10 to 88 μg/d.[53] Minute amounts of silver can accumulate in humans throughout life, with a possible estimated lifetime accumulation of 230 to 480 mg by 50 years of age.[13]

Silver has a 1^+(Ag^+) valence when bonding with other elements and compounds to form complex ions and salts. Because of the microcidal effects of silver cations at low concentrations,[44] silver has been used as a simple medicinal and bactericidal agent.

The antibacterial activity of silver is related to both direct binding to biotic molecules and to disruption of hydrogen ions and thus pH balance. Silver ions bind to electron donor groups of proteins (sulfhydryl, amine, carboxyl, phosphate, and imidazole) to inhibit enzymatic activities and provoke protein denaturation and precipitation.[16] Silver also intercalates with DNA without destroying the double helix, thereby inhibiting fungal DNAse.[11,14] Silver ions induce proton leakage through a bacterial (*Vibrio cholerae*) membrane, leading to loss of the proton motive force in oxidative phosphorylation, with subsequent energy loss and cell death.[9] Bacterial resistance to silver was not reported until the mid-1970s followed shortly thereafter by the identification of the genes for silver resistance in bacteria.[44]

Although banned from routine administration via IV, intramuscular, and oral routes in the United States, silver salts are approved for use in topical medications, either as a caustic styptic or as a key component of burn care. Approved medicinal uses for silver in the United States apply only to silver salts and compounds and specifically preclude use of elemental silver (Table 99–1).

TABLE 99–1. Medicinal Silver-Containing Products

Product Name	Route of Administration	Applications
Silver nitrate (1% $AgNO_3$)	Ophthalmic	Prevention of gonorrheal ophthalmia neonatorum
Silver nitrate (10% $AgNO_3$)	Cutaneous	Chemical cautery of mucosa and exuberant granulations (Podiatry: corns, calluses; Dermatology: impetigo vulgaris, plantar warts, and papillomatous growths)
Silver sulfadiazine (0.2%, 1% micronized silver sulfadiazine)	Cutaneous	Antimicrobial adjunct for prevention and treatment of wound infection for patients with second- and third-degree burns

Silver sulfadiazine added to burn dressings kills bacteria and increases the rate of reepithelialization across partial-thickness wounds.[8] However, concerns of long-term toxicity may limit use by some clinicians.[7] Central venous catheters impregnated with silver sulfadiazine and silver-impregnated Foley catheters are used to lower rates of infection.[31] Recently, silver-lined endotracheal tubes have been shown to reduce the risk of ventilator-assisted pneumonia (VAP) by up to 51%, including specifically drug-resistant pathogens such as methicillin-resistant *Staphylococcus aureus*, *Pseudomonas aeruginosa*, and *Acinetobacter baumanii*.[43]

PATHOPHYSIOLOGY

In great enough quantities, silver manifests cardiovascular, hepatic, and hematopoietic toxicity. Acutely, administration of 50 mg or more of metallic silver IV in humans is fatal, leading to pulmonary edema; hemorrhage; and necrosis of bone marrow, liver, and kidneys.[1,14] The mechanism for this acute toxicity was studied only in the water flea (*Daphnia magna*) in which silver blocks Na^+-K^+-adenosine triphosphate (ATPase) activity.[3] Toxicity in animals is listed by system in Table 99–2.

Silver is neither classified as a human carcinogen nor found to be mutagenic, and no data link therapeutic use of silver to human cancer.[13] Although animal studies show that silver implanted subcutaneously may lead to local sarcoma formation, this reaction has been deemed uninterpretable in regard to carcinogenicity as implantation of other insoluble solids, such as plastic and smooth ivory, produce similar results.[13] Colloidal silver injected into rats induces growths at injection sites, but intramuscular injections of silver powder have not induced cancer.[18] Local inflammatory responses notwithstanding, silver is considered an inert substance and not a human carcinogen.

ARGYRIA

The most significant effect of silver overexposure in humans is argyria, a permanent bluish-gray discoloration of skin resulting from silver throughout the integument. (See Fig. 99–1)

Cases of argyria have been reported in the medical literature since at least the early 19th century. One of the most famous cases of argyria is that of the Barnum and Bailey Circus' "Blue Man" who died at New York's Bellevue hospital in 1923 and was described on autopsy as follows: "The color of the skin was of an unusually deep blue and from a distance appeared almost black. This deep color was almost uniform throughout the entire body, although it was more intense over the exposed skin areas."[21] An American woman who developed argyria

TABLE 99–2. Silver Toxicity: Systemic Manifestations

Cardiovascular	Rats given 0.1% silver nitrate in drinking water for 218 days developed cardiac ventricular hypertrophy that was not attributable to silver deposition in the heart despite advanced pigmentation in other body organs.[34]
Hepatic	Vitamin E and selenium deficient rats developed hepatic necrosis with ultrastructural changes after administration of silver salts.[7,10,48] Silver can induce selenium deficiency that consequently inhibits synthesis of the seleno-enzyme glutathione peroxidase.
Hematologic	Topical application of silver correlated with bone marrow depression and subsequent development of leukopenia or aplastic anemia.[7]
Renal	Tubular lesions are demonstrated in animals, and acute tubular necrosis is rarely identified in humans.[28]
Neurologic	Silver deposits in peripheral nerves, basal membranes, macrophages, and elastic fibers were found in one reported case of a 55-year-old woman with progressive vertigo, cutaneous hypoesthesia, and weakness after self-administration of silver salts to treat oral mycosis for 9 years.[50]
	Seizures were reported in a schizophrenic patient who ingested >20 mg silver daily for 40 years. Serum silver concentrations were elevated (12 μg/L). Seizures resolved concurrently with discontinuation of silver ingestion and a subsequent decrease in serum silver concentration (12 μg/L).[33]
Dermatologic	Generalized argyria, localized argyria, and argyrosis (silver deposition in the eyes) developed after chronic administration of silver.

as a teenager during the 1950s from use of a nasal CSP for allergies, has described her story on the Internet to warn others of the effects of prolonged contact with or ingestion of silver salts.[23] Her appearance was documented as an Image in Clinical Medicine in the *New England Journal of Medicine*.[5]

Generalized argyria may result from either simple mechanical impregnation of the skin by silver particles or inhalational and oral absorption of particulate silver. Local routes of silver absorption may be through the conjunctiva or oral mucous membranes after long-term topical treatment with silver salts. In 2002, a 42-year-old European man developed argyria after weekly application for 4 years of a topical nasal vasoconstrictor (Coldargan, manufactured by Siegfried, Sweden) available in Austria. The patient used this product to treat his rhinitis medicamentosa; each drop of medication contained 0.85 mg of silver protein.[46] More directly, colloidal silver protein ingestion for "health supplementation" leads to body burdens of silver that may produce argyria. Argyria was reported in a 33-year-old woman who had ingested 48 mg/d of elemental silver (from silver nitrate capsules) during alternating 2-week periods over 1 year to treat chronic GI symptoms.[4] Her serum silver concentrations remained at 500 μg/L for 3 months after discontinuation of the capsules, indicating significant silver deposition in tissues.

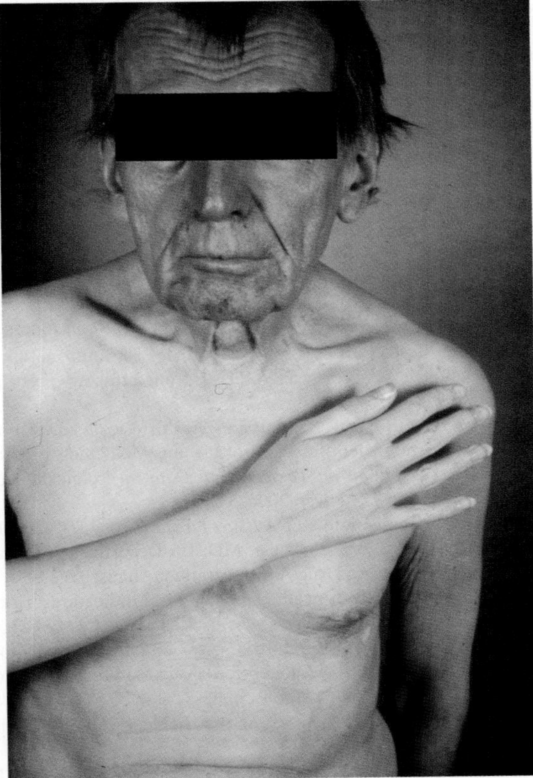

FIGURE 99–1. Long-term exposure to $AgNO_3$ in the workplace led to this patient's characteristic pigment changes of argyria. A normally pigmented arm is across the patient's chest. *(Image contributed by New York University Department of Dermatology).*

Mechanical impregnation of silver produces localized argyria or argyrosis (deposition into eyes) after repeated contact with metallic silver or silver salts.[25] Localized argyria is reported from both implanted acupuncture needles and short-contact acupuncture, when particle deposition may occur from silver needles used repeatedly during brief therapeutic sessions.[26] Silver sulfadiazine use produces localized argyria in and around wound scars.[17] Localized argyria of the tongue and gingiva is described in patients with silver dental amalgams.[24,39] These patients may also have elevated tissue concentrations of silver, but there are no known cases of significant absorption resulting in generalized argyria.[12] Even long-standing wearing of silver earrings has resulted in local contact argyria.[29,45,47] Corneal argyrosis was frequently reported from prolonged use of colloidal silver disinfectant eyedrops, but because these drops are no longer used, the condition has become an occupational disease caused by both inadequate eye protection and workers rubbing their eyes with hands contaminated by silver particles.[40,42,54]

Histopathology of Argyria There are no pathologic changes or inflammatory reactions visible at a histologic level from silver deposition or impregnation. Rather, the skin discoloration of argyria comes from the silver itself and from the induction of increased melanin production. Silver granules are initially found within fibroblasts and macrophages and then extracellularly along the basement membrane of blood vessels, sweat glands, and dermoepidermal junction and beside erector pili muscles (see Chap. 29). Patients with argyria commonly manifest increased pigmentation over sun-exposed skin. Although the mechanism for this process is not yet fully understood, it has been proposed that silver-complexed proteins are reduced to their elemental form via photoactivation from sunlight, similar to photographic image development. Silver plus light then further stimulates melanogenesis, increasing melanin in light-exposed areas and enhancing this cycle.

Argyria develops in stages, beginning with an initial gray-brown staining of gingiva, progressing to hyperpigmentation and bluish-gray discoloration in sun-exposed areas. Later, nail beds, sclerae and mucous membranes become hyperpigmented; on autopsy, viscera are noted to be blue. Confirmation of the diagnosis of argyria is through skin biopsy, showing brown-black clusters of silver granules.

Argyria occurs at exposure doses much lower than those associated with acutely toxic effects of silver; the degree of discoloration is directly proportional to the amount of silver absorbed or ingested.[20] The threshold dose for silver accumulation and retention resulting in generalized argyria varies considerably. Discoloration has been reported in some patients from as little as a cumulative 1 g of metallic silver administered IV (from 4 g of silver arsphenamine used to treat syphilis over a 2-year period in the early 1900s), but others have tolerated infusions containing up to 5 g of elemental silver over 9 months before a clinical change was noted.[20]

DIAGNOSTIC TESTING

Urine and serum concentrations of silver can be measured as indices of silver exposure. Hair is also tested for silver, but airborne silver particles may bind to hair and contaminate samples.

In individuals without a history of medicinal silver ingestion or occupational exposure, the normal serum silver concentration is 1 μg/L or below, and the normal urinary silver concentration is 2 μg/L or below (24-hour urine collection).[49] Workers who smelt and refine silver and who prepare silver salts for use in the photographic industry have mean serum concentrations of 11 μg/L and urine silver concentrations of 2.6 μg/L (in single "spot" urine samples).

TREATMENT OF ARGYRIA

Chelators are *ineffective* in treating both silver toxicity and argyria.[14] Dermatology conventional wisdom has suggested that topical hydroquinone 5% may reduce the number of silver granules in the upper dermis and around sweat glands, as well as diminish the number of melanocytes.[6] Sunscreens and opaque cosmetics can prevent further pigmentation darkening from sun exposure. Successful treatment of argyria using laser technology has only recently been reported.[38]

Because oxidant deficiencies may enhance silver toxicity, antioxidants, such as selenium and vitamin E, may play a role in reversing the effects of silver exposure. Selenium-dependent glutathione peroxidase synthesis is diminished when silver binds to, and thus reduces, intracellular selenium.[7,48] Supplemental vitamin E and selenium increase tolerance for silver in rats and chickens.[10] Selenium and sulfur are being considered as possible treatments for argyria. Selenium may act to precipitate or chelate silver: silver selenide is insoluble in vivo and should reduce the availability of monovalent silver to interfere with normal enzymatic activities.[1,32,41] Hence, increased selenium intake is theorized to bind silver for excretion rather than skin deposition. Silver–sulfur complexes may be investigated for similar effect, although the silver–sulfur complex is not as stable.[41]

EMERGENCY MANAGEMENT

Although systemic toxicity of silver is predominantly a result of chronic exposure, clinicians rarely encounter a patient who has ingested a colloidal silver product, a silver-containing medicinal product, or a silver salt. Burns from silver-salt cautery should be managed as chemical burns. Silver ingestion should be managed supportively. Silver-salt ingestion should be treated as a caustic ingestion (see Chap. 104).

SUMMARY

Silver toxicity—primarily argyria and burns—is still occasionally encountered[22,46,51,52]; the workplace environment and health supplementation products are the main sources of exposure. Despite frequent therapeutic use of silver and silver compounds, there is no evidence of silver acting as a mutagen or carcinogen. Significant toxicity is very rare, although argyria from chronic silver use is essentially a permanent manifestation. There are no proven effective means for removing accumulated silver and reversing argyria.

REFERENCES

1. Aaseth J, Halse J, Falch J. Chelation of silver in argyria. *Acta Pharmacol Toxicol.* 1986;59(suppl 7):471-474.
2. Associated Press. Silver-tongued mayor's anthrax "cure" rebutted. *St. Petersburg Times*; November 24, 2001.
3. Bianchini A, Wood CM. Mechanism of acute silver toxicity in Daphnia magna. *Environ Toxicol Chem.* 2003;22:1361-1367.
4. Blumberg H, Carey TN. Argyremia: detection of unsuspected and obscure argyria by the spectrographic demonstration of high blood silver. *JAMA.* 1934;103:1521-1524.
5. Bouts BA. Images in clinical medicine. Argyria. *N Engl J Med.* 1999;340:1554.
6. Browning JC, Levy ML. Argyria attributed to silvadene application in a patient with dystrophic epidermolysis bullosa. *Dermatol Online J.* 2008;14:9.
7. Caffee HH, Bingham HG. Leukopenia and silver sulfadiazine. *J Trauma.* 1982;22:586-587.
8. Demling RH, Leslie DeSanti MD. The rate of re-epithelialization across meshed skin grafts is increased with exposure to silver. *Burns.* 2002;28:264-266.
9. Dibrov P, Dzioba J, Gosink KK, Hase CC. Chemiosmotic mechanism of antimicrobial activity of Ag(+) in *Vibrio cholerae. Antimicrob Agents Chemother.* 2002;46:2668-2670.
10. Diplock AT, Green J, Bunyan J, et al. Vitamin E and stress. 3. The metabolism of D-alpha-tocopherol in the rat under dietary stress with silver. *Br J Nutr.* 1967;21:115-125.
11. DiVincenzo GD, Giordano CJ, Schriever LS. Biologic monitoring of workers exposed to silver. *Int Arch Occup Environ Health.* 1985;56:207-215.
12. Drasch G, Gath HJ, Heissler E, et al. Silver concentrations in human tissues. their dependence on dental amalgam and other factors. *J Trace Elem Med Biol.* 1995;9:82-87.
13. Environmental Protection Agency. *Silver* (CASRN 7440-22-4). US Environmental Protection Agency Integrated Risk Information System (IRIS); 2008. Retrieved February 28, 2009, from http://www.epa.gov/iris/subst/0099.htm.
14. European Union European Commission Health & Consumer Protection Directorate General Scientific Committee on Medicinal Products and Medical Devices. *Opinion on Toxicological Data on Colouring Agents for Medicinal Products: E 174 Silver*; 2000.
15. Food and Drug Administration. *FDA Issues Final Rule on OTC Drug Products Containing Colloidal Silver.* Rockville, MD: US Department of Health and Human Services, Food and Drug Administration; August 17, 1999.
16. Fung MC, Bowen DL. Silver products for medical indications: risk-benefit assessment. *J Toxicol Clin Toxicol.* 1996;34:119-126.
17. Furchner JE, Richmond CR, Drake GA. Comparative metabolism of radionuclides in mammals—IV. Retention of silver-110m in the mouse, rat, monkey, and dog. *Health Phys.* 1968;15:505-514.
18. Furst A, Schlauder MC. Inactivity of two noble metals as carcinogens. *J Environ Pathol Toxicol.* 1978;1:51-57.
19. Gaslin MT, Rubin C, Pribitkin EA. Silver nasal sprays: misleading Internet marketing. *Ear Nose Throat J.* 2008;87:217-220.
20. Gaul LE, Staud AH. Seventy cases of generalized argyrosis following organic and colloidal silver medication including a biospectrometric analysis of ten cases. *JAMA.* 1935;104:1387-1390.

21. Gettler AO, Rhoads CP, Weiss S. A contribution to the pathology of generalized argyria with a discussion of the fate of silver in the human body. *Am J Pathol.* 1927;3:631-652.
22. Hori K, Martin TG, Rainey P, Robertson WO. Believe it or not—silver still poisons! *Vet Hum Toxicol.* 2002;44:291-292.
23. Jacobs R. *Rosemary's Story—If My Doctor had Read the Medical Literature Instead of the Ads I Wouldn't Look Like this Today*; 1998. Retrieved January 31, 2009, from http://rosemaryjacobs.com.
24. Janner M, Marschelke I, Voigt H. Localized intramural silver impregnation of the tongue. Differential diagnosis from malignant melanoma [German]. *Hautarzt.* 1980;31:510-512.
25. Kapur N, Landon G, Yu RC. Localized argyria in an antique restorer. *Br J Dermatol.* 2001;144:191-192.
26. Legat FJ, Goessler W, Schlagenhaufen C, Soyer HP. Argyria after short-contact acupuncture. *Lancet.* 1998;352:241.
27. Mackison FW. *NIOSH/OSHA—Occupational Health Guidelines for Chemical Hazards.* Washington, DC: US Government Printing Office; 1981.
28. Maher JF. Toxic nephropathy. In: Brenner BM, Rector FC Jr, eds. *The Kidney.* Philadelphia: WB Saunders; 1976:1355-1395.
29. Morton CA, Fallowfield M, Kemmett D. Localized argyria caused by silver earrings. *Br J Dermatol.* 1996:484-485.
30. Newton D, Holmes A. A case of accidental inhalation of zinc-65 and silver-110m. *Radiat Res.* 1966;29:403-412.
31. Newton T, Still JM, Law E. A comparison of the effect of early insertion of standard latex and silver-impregnated latex Foley catheters on urinary tract infections in burn patients. *Infect Control Hosp Epidemiol.* 2002;23:217-218.
32. Nuttall KL. A model for metal selenide formation under biological conditions. *Med Hypotheses.* 1987;24:217-221.
33. Ohbo Y, Fukuzako H, Takeuchi K, Takigawa M. Argyria and convulsive seizures caused by ingestion of silver in a patient with schizophrenia. *Psychiatry Clin Neurosci.* 1996;50:89-90.
34. Olcott CT. Experimental argyrosis. V. Hypertrophy of the left ventricle of the heart in rats ingesting silver salts. *Arch Pathol.* 1950;49:138-149.
35. Phalen RF, Morrow PE. Experimental inhalation of metallic silver. *Health Phys.* 1973;24:509-518.
36. Polachek AA, Cope CB, Williard RF, Enns T. Metabolism of radioactive silver in a patient with carcinoid. *J Lab Clin Med.* 1960;56:499-505.
37. Powell J, Margarf H. Silver. Emerging as our mightiest germ fighter. *Sci Dig.* 1978;March:57-60.
38. Rhee DY, Chang SE, Lee MW, Choi JH, Moon KC, Koh JK. Treatment of argyria after colloidal silver protein ingestion using Q-switched 1,064-nm Nd:YAG laser. *Dermatol Surg.* 2008;34:1427-1430.
39. Rusch-Behrend GD, Gutmann JL. Management of diffuse tissue argyria subsequent to endodontic therapy: report of a case. *Quintessence Int.* 1995;26:553-557.
40. Sanchez-Huerta V, De Wit-Carter G, Hernandez-Quintela E, NaranjoTackman R. Occupational corneal argyrosis in art silver solderers. *Cornea.* 2003;22:604-611.
41. Sato S, Sueki H, Nishijima A. Two unusual cases of argyria: the application of an improved tissue processing method for X-ray microanalysis of selenium and sulphur in silver-laden granules. *Br J Dermatol.* 1999;140:158-163.
42. Scroggs MW, Lewis JS, Proia AD. Corneal argyrosis associated with silver soldering. *Cornea.* 1992;11:264-269.
43. Shorr AF. Impact of a silver-coated endotracheal tube on ventilator-associated pneumonia due to resistant pathogens. *Am J Respir Crit Care Med.* 2008;177:A530. As reported by Smith M. *American Thoracic Society (ATS): Silver Lining Prevents Ventilator Pneumonia.* Retrieved January 31, 2009, from http://www.medpagetoday.com/MeetingCoverage/ATS/9556.
44. Silver S. Bacterial silver resistance: molecular biology and uses and misuses of silver compounds. *FEMS Microbiol Rev.* 2003;27:341-353.
45. Sugden P, Azad S, Erdmann M. Argyria caused by an earring. *Br J Plast Surg.* 2001;54:252-253.
46. Tomi NS, Kranke B, Aberer W. A silver man. *Lancet.* 2004;363:532.
47. van den Nieuwenhuijsen IJ, Calame JJ, Bruynzeel DP. Localized argyria caused by silver earrings. *Dermatologica.* 1988;177:189-191.
48. Wagner PA, Hoekstra WG, Ganther HE. Alleviation of silver toxicity by selenite in the rat in relation to tissue glutathione peroxidase. *Proc Soc Exp Biol Med.* 1975;148:1106-1110.
49. Wan AT, Conyers RA, Coombs CJ, Masterton JP. Determination of silver in blood, urine, and tissues of volunteers and burn patients. *Clin Chem.* 1991;37:1683-1687.
50. Westhofen M, Schafer H. Generalized argyrosis in man: neurotological, ultrastructural and X-ray microanalytical findings. *Arch Otorhinolaryngol.* 1986;243:260-264.
51. White JM, Powell AM, Brady K, Russell-Jones R. Severe generalized argyria secondary to ingestion of colloidal silver protein. *Clin Exp Dermatol.* 2003;28:254-256.
52. Wickless SC, Shwayder TA, Baden LR. Medical mystery—the answer. *N Engl J Med.* 2004;351:2349-2350.
53. World Health Organization. 13. Inorganic constituents and physical parameters. In: WHO, ed. *Guidelines for Drinking-Water Quality*, vol. 2. *Health Criteria and Other Supporting Information*, 2nd ed. Geneva: World Health Organization; 1996:153-157.
54. Zografos L, Uffer S, Chamot L. Unilateral conjunctival-corneal argyrosis simulating conjunctival melanoma. *Arch Ophthalmol.* 2003;121:1483-1487.

CHAPTER 100
THALLIUM

Maria Mercurio-Zappala and Robert S. Hoffman

Thallium (Tl)

Atomic number	=	81
Atomic weight	=	204.37 daltons
Normal concentrations		
Whole blood	<	2 μg/L (<9.78 nmol/L)
Urine (24 hour)	<	5 μg/L (<24.5 nmol/L)

Thallium is a commonly found constituent of granite, shale, volcanic rock, and pyrites used to make sulfuric acid and is also recovered as flue dust from iron, lead, cadmium, and copper smelters.[23] It has been used in alloys as an anticorrosive, in optical lenses to increase the refractive index, in artists' paints, in lamps to improve tungsten filaments, in extreme cold thermometers, in imitation jewelry, as a catalyst, in fireworks, as a rodenticide, and as a medicinal. Diagnostically, small nontoxic amounts of thallium salts are used as radioactive contrast to image tumors and to permit the visualization of cardiac function.[65] Thallium toxicity presents as an uncommon constellation of signs and symptoms that most commonly include gastrointestinal (GI) distress, a painful ascending peripheral neuropathy, and alopecia.

HISTORY AND EPIDEMIOLOGY

Thallium, a metal with atomic number 81, is located between mercury and lead on the periodic table. Thallium is a soft, pliable metal that melts at 572°F (300°C), boils at 2699.6°F (1482°C), and is essentially nontoxic. Thallium forms univalent thallous and trivalent thallic salts, which are highly toxic.

In the early 1900s, thallium salts were used medicinally to treat syphilis, gonorrhea, tuberculosis, and ringworm of the scalp and as a depilatory.[6,65] Although the usual oral dose given for epilation in the treatment of ringworm of the scalp was 7 to 8 mg/kg, fatal doses ranged from 6 to 40 mg/kg.[13,54] Many cases of severe thallium poisoning (thallotoxicosis) resulted from the treatment of ringworm, with one author summarizing nearly 700 cases and 46 deaths.[67]

Because thallium sulfate is odorless and tasteless, it was also successfully used as a rodenticide. Commercially available as Thalgrain, Echol's Roach Powder, Mo-Go, Martin's Rat Stop liquid, and Senco Corn Mix, thallium sulfate was a very efficient rodenticide. As a consequence of numerous case reports of unintentional poisonings,[67,68,79] the use of thallium salts as a household rodenticide was restricted in the United States in 1965. Ultimately, even the commercial use of thallium salts as a rodenticide was banned in the United States in 1972 because of continued reports of human toxicity.

Life-threatening unintentional poisoning continues to occur in other countries where thallium salts are still commonly used as rodenticides.[12,77,85,100] Additional cases of thallium poisoning are reported in the United States and other countries as a result of the use of thallium as a homicidal agent[19,59,63,71,73,82,89] and through contamination of herbal products[86] and illicit drugs such as heroin[76] and cocaine.[41] Although occupational exposures to consequential amounts of thallium salts are uncommon, toxicity is well described in this setting.[35]

The following discussion of thallium toxicity refers to toxicity resulting from exposure to inorganic thallium salts, which represents virtually the entire literature on thallium poisoning. Although exceedingly rare, cases of poisoning with organic thallium compounds have been reported[2] and should be assessed and managed in a fashion similar to that used for patients with inorganic exposures.

TOXICOKINETICS

Exposures usually occur via one of three routes: *inhalation* of dust, *ingestion*, and *absorption* through intact skin. Thallium is rapidly absorbed following all routes of exposure. Bioavailability is greatest after ingestion and exceeds 90%.[37] Distribution follows three-compartment toxicokinetics[78] (see Chap. 8) into a final volume of distribution that is estimated to be about 3.6 L/kg.[17] Thallium can be found in all organs, but it is distributed unevenly, with the highest concentrations found in the large and small intestine, liver, kidney, heart, brain, and muscles.[6,49] In animals, the highest concentrations of thallium are found in the kidneys.[1,49]

The toxicokinetics of thallium can be described in the following three-phase model. The first phase occurs within the 4 hours after exposure during which thallium is distributed to a central compartment and to well-perfused peripheral organs such as the kidney, liver, and muscle. In the second phase, which may last between 4 and 48 hours, thallium is distributed into the central nervous system (CNS).[78] Whereas previous literature suggests that this distribution phase is generally completed within 24 hours of ingestion,[78] one human case suggests slower distribution into the CNS as evidenced by increasing cerebrospinal fluid (CSF) concentrations in the days after exposure when blood concentrations are declining.[89] The third or elimination phase usually begins within 24 hours after ingestion. The primary mechanism of thallium elimination is secretion into the intestine, but enteral reabsorption of thallium that is present in the bile subsequently reduces the fecal elimination.[17,63] Thallium is excreted primarily via the feces (51.4%) and the urine (26.4%).[53] It is filtered by the glomerulus, with approximately 50% being reabsorbed in the tubules. Thallium is also secreted into the tubular lumen in a manner similar to potassium.[3] The duration of the elimination phase depends on the route of exposure, dose, and treatment. Unlike many other metals, thallium does not have a major anatomic reservoir. For this reason, reported elimination half-lives are as short as 1.7 days in humans with thallium poisoning.[39]

PATHOPHYSIOLOGY

The mechanism of thallium toxicity is not well established. Thallium behaves biologically in a manner similar to potassium because both have similar ionic radii (0.147 nm for thallium and 0.133 nm for potassium). Because cell membranes cannot differentiate between thallium and potassium ions, thallous ions accumulate in areas with high potassium concentrations, such as the central and peripheral nervous system and hepatic and muscle tissue.[60,100] This accumulation is the fundamental principle that governs the use of radioactive thallium in cardiac imaging studies. Thallium replaces potassium in the activation of potassium-dependent enzymes.[60] In low concentrations, thallium stimulates these enzyme systems, but in high concentrations, it inhibits them.[7,62] Thallium also inhibits several potassium-dependent systems. Pyruvate kinase, a magnesium-dependent glycolytic enzyme that requires potassium to achieve maximum activity, has 50 times greater affinity for thallous ions than potassium ions.[45] Succinate dehydrogenase, an essential enzyme in the Krebs cycle, is inhibited by small doses of thallium in rats.[34] Sodium-potassium adenosine triphosphatase

(ATPase), which is responsible for active transport of monovalent ions across cell membranes, can use thallous ions at extremely low concentrations because of an affinity that is 10-fold greater than that of potassium ions[8,28] but is inhibited by thallium at higher concentrations.[42]

Thallium also impairs depolarization of muscle fibers.[65] Mitochondrial energy is decreased as a result of the inhibition of pyruvate kinase and succinate dehydrogenase, resulting in a decrease of adenosine triphosphate (ATP) generation via oxidative phosphorylation. Enzymatic destruction results in swelling and vacuolization of the mitochondria after exposure to thallium.[90] At low concentrations, thallium can activate other potassium-dependent enzymes such as phosphatase, homoserine dehydrogenase, vitamin B_{12}–dependent diol dehydrogenase, L-threonine dehydrogenase, and adenosine monophosphate (AMP) deaminase.[65] The net result of these processes is a failure of energy production.

Thallous ions have been used to isolate riboflavin from milk in the form of a reversible precipitate. Thallous ions may also form insoluble complexes and cause intracellular sequestration of riboflavin in vivo.[11] Riboflavin is the vitamin precursor of the flavin coenzyme flavin adenine dinucleotide (FAD). Because of a decrease in riboflavin, metabolic reactions dependent on flavoproteins decrease, causing disruption of the electron transport chain and a subsequent further decrease or impairment in the generation of cellular energy.[11] This decrease in cellular energy may lead to a decrease in mitotic activity and cessation of hair follicle formation, resulting in the clinical sign of alopecia. Subsequent hair loss is the result of combined arrested formation and local destruction of hair shaft cells in the hair bulb.[11,79] (see Chap. 29) Unfortunately, riboflavin supplementation was not beneficial in one animal model of thallium poisoning.[4] Data also demonstrate that the dermatologic, neurologic, and cardiovascular effects of thallium toxicity mirror the manifestations of thiamine deficiency (beriberi), highlighting the inhibitory effect of thallium on glycolytic enzymes.[11,65] It is unclear whether thiamine administration has any beneficial effect in patients with thallium poisoning.

Thallium has a high affinity for the sulfhydryl groups present in many other enzymes and other proteins. Keratin, a structural protein, consists of many cysteine residues that cross-link and form disulfide bonds. These disulfide bonds add strength to keratin. Thallium interferes with the formation of disulfide bonds, which may lead to the development of alopecia and defects in nail growth, resulting in Mees lines.[30,65,71,84,85] Additionally, the complexation of sulfhydryl groups with thallium results in a decrease in both the production of glutathione and the reduction of oxidized glutatione.[32,101] This results in oxidative damage[26] and the accumulation of lipid peroxides in the brain (which is most prominent in the cerebellum) and appears as dark, pigmented, lipofuscinlike areas.[33] The complexity and presumable multifactorial nature of thallium poisoning are again highlighted by the inability of *N*-acetylcysteine (NAC)–induced augmentation of glutathione stores to protect against toxicity in an animal model.[4]

Thallium also adversely affects protein synthesis in animals by damaging ribosomes, particularly the 60S subunit.[40] Although ribosomes are primarily dependent on potassium and magnesium, thallium will be used if present. In an experimental model, low concentrations of thallium are protective against hypokalemia-induced ribosomal inactivation. As thallium concentrations increase, the protective effects diminish, resulting in progressive destabilization and destruction of the ribosomes. Ribosomal destruction may also be produced by exposure to potassium concentrations of 4.5 to 20 times higher than the thallium concentrations necessary to achieve the same effect.[40]

Pathologic studies of the CNS in patients with thallium poisoning reveal localized areas of edema in the cerebral hemispheres and brainstem. Chromatolytic changes are prominent in neurons of the motor cortex, third nerve nuclei, substantia nigra, and pyramidal cells of the globus pallidus. In chronic exposures, there are signs of edema of the pial and arachnoidal membranes and chromatolysis, swelling, and fatty degeneration in the ganglion cells of the ventral and dorsal horns of the spinal cord.[6,79]

The peripheral nervous system, which is usually clinically affected before the CNS, develops a diffuse axonopathy in a classic dying back or Wallerian degeneration pattern.[5,6,15,21,61] (see Chap. 18) Fragmentation and degeneration of associated myelin sheaths are accompanied by activation of Schwann cells.[6,10,11] Because thallium affects the longer peripheral fibers—first sensory, then motor, and finally the shorter fibers—toxic effects occur initially in the lower extremities.[52,70,105]

CLINICAL MANIFESTATIONS

Many of the effects of thallium poisoning are somewhat nonspecific and occur over a variable time course.[50] When combined, however, a clear toxic syndrome can be defined (Table 100–1). Alopecia and a painful ascending peripheral neuropathy are the most characteristic findings.[5,25,63,70] Because of the delayed development of alopecia, the diagnosis of thallotoxicosis is often delayed. In fact, with acute exposures, a dose-dependent latent period of hours to days may precede initial symptoms.[50,65] When death occurs, it is usually the result of coma with loss of airway-protective reflexes, respiratory paralysis, and cardiac arrest.

Unlike most other metal salt poisonings, GI symptoms are usually modest or even absent in thallium toxicity.[13] The most common symptom is abdominal pain, which may be accompanied by vomiting and either diarrhea or constipation.[19,47,50,62,84,102,103] Constipation may be a result of decreased intestinal motility and peristalsis caused by direct involvement of the vagus nerve.[13,65] Rarely, severe symptoms, such as hematemesis, bloody diarrhea, or ulceration of the mucosal lining occur.

Pleuritic chest pain was described in a small series of poisoned patients.[59] Another patient was reported to have developed "chest tightness" shortly after drinking thallium-poisoned tea.[63] There is no known etiology for this finding, although it may also relate to involvement of the vagus nerve.

Tachycardia and hypertension frequently occur in patients with thallotoxicosis and usually develop during the first or second week after acute ingestion. A poor prognosis may be associated with a persistent and pronounced tachycardia. No exact mechanism has been determined for these cardiovascular effects of thallium toxicity. Some authors theorize that they result from autonomic neuropathic dysfunction directly related to involvement of the vagus nerve,[70] but others have noted early electrocardiographic (ECG) changes, such as prolongation of the QT interval, T-wave flattening or inversion, and nonspecific ST-segment abnormalities, which might suggest direct myocardial injury.[6,10,62,65,81] Another theory suggests that the stimulation of ATPase in the chromaffin cells by thallium may lead to increased output of catecholamines, resulting in sinus tachycardia.[3,63]

Neurologic symptoms usually appear 2 to 5 days after exposure. Patients may develop severely painful, rapidly progressive, ascending peripheral neuropathies.[5,6,21,59] Pain and paresthesias are present in the lower extremities (especially the soles of the feet), and although numbness is present in the fingers and toes, there is also decreased sensation to pinprick, touch, temperature, vibration, and proprioception.[5,86] The weight of bedsheets on the lower extremities may be sufficient to cause excruciating pain.[59,61] Motor weakness is always distal in distribution, with the lower limbs more affected than the upper limbs.[10,65]

Symptoms of confusion, delirium, psychosis, hallucinations, seizures, headache, insomnia, anxiety, tremor, ataxia, and choreoathetosis are common. Onset is variable and most likely dependent on dose. Ataxia

TABLE 100–1. Clinical Manifestations of Thallium Poisoning

Organ System	Onset of Effects			Residual Effects
	Immediate (<6 h)	Intermediate (Rarely in the First Few Days; within 2 wk)	Late (>2 wk)	
Gastrointestinal				
Nausea	†			
Vomiting	†			
Diarrhea	†			
Constipation	†	†		
Cardiovascular				
Nonspecific ECG changes	†	†		
Hypertension		†		
Tachycardia		†		
Respiratory				
Pleuritic chest pain	†	†		
Respiratory depression		†	†	
Renal				
Albuminuria		†		
Renal insufficiency		†		‡
Dermatologic				
Dry skin		†		
Alopecia		†		‡
Mees lines			†	‡
Neurologic				
Painful ascending sensory neuropathy		†	†	‡
Motor neuropathy		†	†	‡
Cranial nerve abnormalities		†		
Delirium, psychosis, coma		†		‡
Memory and cognitive deficits			†	‡
Optic neuritis	†	†		‡

† = Typical onset of symptoms. The time course outlined above may be accelerated with extremely large doses. When [a] appears in two adjacent columns, the time course is highly variable and may be dose dependent. With small ingestions, many of the effects listed above may not be evident.
‡ = Effects that may persist long after exposure, possibly permanently.

may develop within 48 hours after ingestion. Insomnia occurs in most patients and may progress to total reversal of sleep rhythm. Coma may occur, especially with larger exposures.[10,50,65,84] All cranial nerves can probably be affected by thallium, although abnormalities of cranial nerves I, V, and VIII have not been reported. Cranial nerve III involvement, as evidenced by ptosis, is common and may be asymmetric.[10] Nystagmus, another common finding, demonstrates involvement of cranial nerves IV and VI.[10] Cognitive abnormalities may persist for months after exposure.[56]

Thallium is toxic to both the retinal fibers and the neural retina.[87] In cases of a large, single ingestion of thallium, approximately 25% of patients may develop severe lesions of the optic nerve.[65,84] Optic neuropathy may lead to optic atrophy and a permanent decrease in visual acuity. In the early stages, the optic disk shows signs of neuritis, which is red and poorly defined, and later develops pallor from resultant optic nerve atrophy. In patients exposed to multiple small doses, nearly 100% suffer optic nerve injury.[62] Visual complaints may be delayed in comparison to other neurologic findings[87] and may include decreased acuity and central scotomata. Other described ophthalmic effects are noninflammatory keratitis, cataracts, and the color vision defect of tritanomaly (blue color defect).[93,94]

Renal function may remain normal in mild cases of thallium poisoning, even though the kidney has greater bioaccumulation than any other organ. Changes in renal function in patients with severe thallotoxicosis include oliguria, diminished creatinine clearance, elevated blood urea nitrogen, and albuminuria.[3,59,62,65] These findings correlate with morphologic studies in thallium-poisoned rats, demonstrating abnormalities in the renal medulla, mainly in the thick ascending limb of the loop of Henle, that occur by the second day after exposure and resolve by the tenth day.[3]

Alopecia is the most common and classic manifestation of thallium toxicity.[63,97] Typically occurring as the presenting symptom in patients

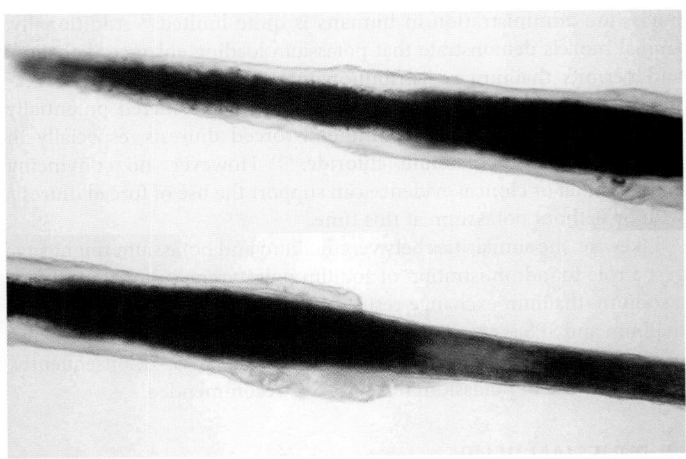

FIGURE 100–1. Hair from a patient with severe thallium poisoning (top) compared to a normal (bottom). Note the dark pigmented granules around the root of the poisoned patient. *(Image contributed by the New York City Poison Center Toxicology Fellowship Program).*

with chronic exposures after an acute exposure, epilation begins in approximately 10 days, and maximal hair loss usually occurs within 1 month.[25,63,67] Facial and axillary hair, especially the inner third of the eyebrows, may be spared, but in some cases, full beards, as well as all scalp hair, are lost.[79] Microscopic inspection of the hair reveals a diagnostic pattern of black pigmentation of the hair roots of the scalp in approximately 95% of poisoned patients,[9,63,84,97] which can be found within 3 to 5 days of initial exposure.[9,62] (See Fig. 100–1) In patients with recurrent exposures, several bands may be noted on the hair shaft, demonstrating multiple exposures. Initial hair regrowth is very fine and unpigmented but usually returns to normal after mild exposure.[62] In patients with severe exposures, alopecia may be permanent. Other dermatologic effects that are observed include acne, palmar erythema, and dry scaly skin that results from sebaceous gland damage.[97] Mees lines appear within 2 to 4 weeks after exposure.[63,71,84] (See Fig. 88–4)

Other less common findings include hepatotoxicity,[41] hypochloremic metabolic acidosis,[84] and anemia and thrombocytopenia.[51,84]

TERATOGENICITY

In animal models, thallium is teratogenic.[29,31] In humans, one study evaluated 297 children born in a region in which the population's urine thallium concentrations were higher than normal because of industrial contamination of their environment.[20] Urine thallium concentrations in the exposed children were as high as 76.5 μg/L. Although these children had a slightly higher than expected incidence of congenital abnormalities, no causal relationship could be established with regard to thallium exposure.[20]

There are few human reports of acute thallium poisoning during pregnancy. A comprehensive literature review demonstrated 25 cases, which included acute and chronic exposures that occurred during all trimesters.[36] Thallium slowly traverses the placenta and is able to cause characteristic fetal toxicity,[22,69] which manifests initially as decreased fetal movement, possibly as a consequence of fetal paralysis. The classic clinical signs and symptoms of thallium poisoning have been described both in the fetus after abortion and in neonate after viable delivery.[22,62,69,77] However, the outcome of the pregnancy may be normal despite significant maternal toxicity.[22,43] The only consistent finding is a trend toward prematurity and low birth weight, especially in children exposed during the first trimester.[36] One author recommends continuing the pregnancy as long as the mother is clinically improving.[22] It is reasonable to conclude that a fetus exposed to thallium during organogenesis has the potential for permanent injury. Those exposed later in pregnancy may recover without deficit if their exposures are limited and the mother recovers. If the exposure occurs closer to term, the child may be born with overt toxicity such as alopecia, dermatitis, nail growth disturbances, and permanent CNS injury.[62]

These few case reports and animal studies provide confusing and sometimes contradictory results. It seems that fetal outcome is determined both by the trimester of pregnancy and the extent of maternal toxicity. However, because there are insufficient data to predict the outcome of pregnancy complicated by maternal thallium poisoning, no specific course of action can be recommended other than extensive fetal monitoring and aggressive treatment for the mother. When a viable child is delivered, it is important to note that thallium is eliminated in breast milk, and a maternal toxicity reevaluation is essential because nursing may result in continued exposure.[34]

ASSESSMENT

Most patients with acute thallium toxicity seek healthcare soon after exposure because of alterations in their GI, cardiovascular, and neurologic function. Establishing the correct diagnosis at this early stage is essential to assure a satisfactory outcome. Unfortunately, many patients with either smaller acute exposures or chronic thallium poisoning first present days to weeks after their initial exposure, and diagnosis is often further delayed. In these instances, many valuable epidemiologic aspects of the exposure history may be difficult to obtain. GI symptoms may not have occurred or their consequence or etiology may have gone unrecognized because of their nonspecific, mild, and transient nature. Many patients with small acute or chronic exposures usually seek care because of alopecia or neuropathy.

The differential diagnosis of the neuropathy includes poisoning by arsenic, colchicine, and vinca alkaloids and disorders such as botulism, thiamine deficiency, and Guillain-Barré syndrome. Both the sensory neuropathy and the preservation of reflexes help differentiate thallium-induced neuropathy from Guillain-Barré syndrome and most other causes of acute neuropathy.[10] When GI symptoms are present in addition to a neuropathy and other end-organ effects, poisoning with metal salts such as arsenic and mercury should be considered (see Chaps. 88 and 96). The differential diagnosis of rapid onset alopecia is more restricted and includes arsenic, selenium, colchicine, and vinca alkaloid poisoning (see Chap. 29). When present, Mees lines indicate past exposure to metals, mitotic inhibitors, or antimetabolites and as such are nonspecific for thallium poisoning (see Chaps. 29, 88, and 96).

DIAGNOSTIC TESTING

Radiographs of tampered food products[59] or of the abdomen[30] can document the presence of a heavy metal such as thallium, which is radiopaque. Although abdominal radiography may be useful shortly after a suspected exposure, the sensitivity and specificity of this test is unknown. Similarly, the yield from other routine studies, such as the complete blood count, electrolytes, urinalysis, and ECG, is limited in that these other studies are often normal or at most, merely demonstrate nonspecific abnormalities. Although microscopic inspection of the hair is intriguing, this test is likely to be inconclusive for inexperienced observers.

The definitive clinical diagnosis of thallium poisoning can only be established by demonstrating elevated thallium concentrations in various body fluids or organs. Thallium can be recovered in the hair, nails, feces, saliva, CSF, blood, and urine, and standard assays and normal concentrations for most of these sources can be found.[65] Qualitative point of care urine spot tests notoriously give false-negative results and require the use of dangerous chemicals that are not routinely available (20% nitric acid) and therefore should be avoided.[84] The standard toxicologic testing method is to assay a 24-hour urine sample for thallium by atomic absorption spectroscopy.[14,104] Normal urine concentrations are below 5 μg/L. Some authors suggest a potassium mobilization test to enhance urinary elimination (similar to the ethylenediaminetetraacetic acid [EDTA] mobilization test) to assist in the diagnosis of thallium exposure.[9,41,84] We advise against this practice because of its lack of proven usefulness and its potential to exacerbate neurologic toxicity (see Potassium below).

MANAGEMENT

The treatment goals for a patient with thallium poisoning are initial stabilization, prevention of absorption, and enhanced elimination. After the initial assessment and stabilization of the patient's airway, breathing, and circulatory status, GI decontamination should be instituted in all patients with suspected thallium ingestions because of the morbidity and mortality associated with a significant exposure.

DECONTAMINATION

Patients who present within 1 to 2 hours after ingestion should be considered candidates for orogastric lavage (see Chap. 7). If the patient presents more than 2 hours after ingestion or has had considerable spontaneous emesis, gastric emptying is unnecessary.

Thallium salts are substantially adsorbed to activated charcoal in vitro.[38,47] Additionally, because thallium undergoes enterohepatic recirculation, activated charcoal may be useful both to prevent absorption after a recent ingestion and to enhance elimination of thallium in patients who present in the postabsorptive phase.[95] In fact, a rat model of thallium poisoning demonstrated that multiple-dose activated charcoal (given as 0.5 g/kg twice daily for 5 days) increased the fecal elimination of thallium by 82% and substantially improved survival.[53] Other data demonstrate that activated charcoal alone is superior to either forced diuresis or potassium chloride therapy.[48]

In patients with severe thallium toxicity, constipation is common, so the addition of mannitol[55,91,102] or another cathartic to the first dose of activated charcoal is appropriate. Although no studies address the efficacy of whole-bowel irrigation with polyethylene glycol electrolyte lavage solution, this technique may prove useful, especially when radiopaque material is demonstrated in the GI tract by abdominal radiography.

POTASSIUM

The similarities between the cellular handling of potassium ions and thallium ions led to the investigation of a possible role for potassium in the treatment of thallium poisoning. In humans, potassium administration is associated with an increase in urinary thallium elimination.[13,27,72] The magnitude of this increase is reported to be on the order of two- to threefold.[72] This is supported by animal models that demonstrate some benefit in terms of either enhanced thallium elimination or animal survival.[28,48,53] Potassium administration is believed to both block tubular reabsorption of thallium and mobilize thallium from tissue stores, thereby increasing thallium concentrations available for glomerular filtration.[66,84] However, the mobilization of the thallium is of concern. Many authors report either the development of acute neurologic toxicity or the significant exacerbation of neurologic symptoms during potassium administration.[5,27,59,72,81,98] Others cite data demonstrating that the augmentation of thallium elimination by potassium administration in humans is quite limited.[46] Additionally, animal models demonstrate that potassium loading enhances lethality[58] and permits thallium redistribution into the CNS.[34] For these reasons, the routine use of potassium should be considered potentially dangerous. Some authors recommend forced diuresis, especially in conjunction with potassium chloride.[18,95] However, no convincing experimental or clinical evidence can support the use of forced diuresis with or without potassium at this time.

Likewise, the similarities between thallium and potassium might suggest a role for administration of sodium polystyrene sulfonate (SPS) as a sodium–thallium exchange resin. Although in vitro binding between thallium and SPS is excellent, it is unlikely to be clinically useful because of preferential binding between potassium and SPS.[38] Consequently, neither the use of potassium nor of SPS is recommended.

PRUSSIAN BLUE

Prussian blue is a Food and Drug Administration–approved antidote for thallium toxicity (see Antidotes in Depth A29: Prussian Blue).[96] When given orally, Prussian blue acts as an ion exchanger for univalent cations, with its affinity increasing as the ionic radius of the cation increases. As such, Prussian blue interferes with the enterohepatic circulation of thallium by exchanging potassium ions from its lattice for thallium ions in the GI tract. This results in the formation of a concentration gradient, causing an increased movement of thallium into the GI tract.

Humans with thallium poisoning are routinely given Prussian blue, which appears to result in clinical benefits, enhanced fecal elimination, and decreasing thallium concentrations.[14,16,59,75,91,98,99,102,103] One series of 11 thallium-poisoned patients demonstrated both the safety of Prussian blue and its ability to substantially increase fecal thallium elimination.[91] Unfortunately, because there have been no controlled trials in humans that compare Prussian blue with other drugs and because many of the patients reported above received multiple therapies, the actual efficacy of Prussian blue is unknown.

The dose of Prussian blue is 250 mg/kg/d orally via a nasogastric tube in two to four divided doses.[91] For patients who are constipated, the Prussian blue may have greater benefit if dissolved in 50 mL of 15% mannitol.[95] Although any cathartic may be useful, most authors have used mannitol, possibly because of concerns regarding repeated use of magnesium-containing cathartics in patients with neurologic findings and the use of sorbitol in patients with poor GI mobility. (Other dosing regimens are discussed in Antidotes in Depth A29: Prussian Blue.)

EXTRACORPOREAL DRUG REMOVAL

Extracorporeal drug removal may have a limited beneficial role in patients with thallium toxicity, especially if it is begun shortly after the initial exposure while serum concentrations remain high before effective tissue distribution. Because a frequently quoted review attests to the benefits of hemodialysis,[62] many patients still receive this therapy.[61] The actual data, however, show that hemodialysis, at various stages of poisoning, is no better than forced diuresis.[16,74] Reported thallium removal rates by hemodialysis are trivial: 143 mg of thallium was removed by 120 hours,[75] 222.8 mg was removed by 121 hours,[16] and 128 mg was removed by 54 hours of hemodialysis.[16] These quantities can be placed in perspective knowing that the minimum lethal adult dose of thallium is estimated to be on the order of 1 g[65] and that many reported cases exceed that by a factor of 10. Data from a more recent hemodialysis experience suggest that by using high blood flow rates (300 mL/min), clearances as high as 90 to 150 mL/min could be obtained.[55] Although these clearances seem encouraging, they should be interpreted with an appreciation of the large volume of distribution of thallium.

TABLE 100–2. Treatment for Thallium Poisoning

Early (patients who present in the first 1–2 hours postexposure)

- Stabilize airway, breathing, and circulation if necessary.
- Consider orogastric lavage if the patient has not vomited.
- Consider whole-bowel irrigation with polyethylene glycol electrolyte lavage solution for patients with large ingestions or the presence of radiopaque material on abdominal radiographs.
- Begin multiple-dose activated charcoal therapy; add a cathartic to the first dose if the patient does not have diarrhea.
- Give 250 mg/kg/d of Prussian blue in two or four divided doses dissolved in water or 50 mL of 15% mannitol if the patient does not have diarrhea.
- Consider simultaneous charcoal hemoperfusion and hemodialysis, especially if the patient has renal insufficiency.

Late (patients who present more than 24 hours after exposure or with chronic toxicity)

- Stabilize airway, breathing, and circulation if necessary.
- Begin multiple-dose activated charcoal therapy; add a cathartic to the first dose if the patient does not have diarrhea.
- Give 250 mg/kg/d of Prussian blue in two or four divided doses dissolved in water or 50 mL of 15% mannitol if the patient does not have diarrhea.

With lower blood flow rates, charcoal hemoperfusion may be two to three times more efficient than hemodialysis, providing clearance rates as high as 139 mL/min.[16] Combined hemoperfusion and hemodialysis were used in several cases[2,16,17] and were reported to remove as much as 93 mg of thallium within 3 hours of therapy.[2] Although extracorporeal therapy alone is probably insufficient for patients with significant poisoning and unnecessary in those with small exposures, it may have some benefit when used in combination with other therapies, especially in patients with renal insufficiency and those with early massive, and presumed lethal, exposures. As is the case with other xenobiotics, thallium is probably not effectively removed by the use of peritoneal dialysis.[46] Table 100–2 summarizes the suggested therapy for thallium-poisoned patients.

CHELATION

Patients with thallium toxicity do not respond to traditional chelation therapy. Studies demonstrate that the use of EDTA and diethylenetriamine pentaacetic acid are without benefit.[65,84] Dimercaprol (British anti-Lewisite [BAL]) and D-penicillamine also fail to enhance thallium excretion in experimental models.[65,84] In one model in which D-penicillamine was able to enhance thallium elimination, it did so at the cost of substantial thallium redistribution into vital organs.[80] Similarly, sulfur-containing compounds such as cysteine and NAC have not been demonstrated to be beneficial.[53,57] Another chelator, diphenylthiocarbazone (dithizone), forms a minimally toxic complex with thallium, resulting in a 33% increase in fecal elimination of thallium in rats.[88] Unfortunately, dithizone is goitrogenic and diabetogenic in animal studies.[53,64,95] Dithiocarb (sodium diethyldithiocarbamate), an intermediate metabolite of tetraethylthiuram disulfide (disulfiram, or Antabuse) (see Chap. 79), also increases the urinary excretion of thallium.[88,92] Before thallium elimination, however, the formation of a lipophilic thallium–diethyldithiocarbamate complex may result in the redistribution of thallium into the CNS.[44,92] After decomposition of the chelate complex, thallium may remain in the CNS, potentially exacerbating neurologic symptoms.[44,82] Because of the significant adverse effects of dithizone and the redistribution of thallium after Dithiocarb use, neither agent is recommended in the treatment of patients with thallium poisoning.

Currently, there is renewed interest in the water-soluble analogs of BAL (DMPS [dimercaptopropane sulfonate] and succimer). However, in an animal model, DMPS failed to decrease tissues concentrations of thallium.[64] Similarly, in another animal model, although succimer improved survival over control subjects, the benefit was less than that achieved for Prussian blue and was at the cost of an increase in brain thallium concentrations.[83] One recent animal investigation demonstrated a significant reduction in serum thallium concentration after repeated administration of deferoxamine.[24] Although worthy of additional study, these results are too preliminary to recommend deferoxamine use in thallium-poisoned patients.

SUMMARY

The elimination of thallium salts from depilatories and rodenticides has substantially reduced the incidence of both intentional and unintentional thallium toxicity in the United States. Despite this, cases of significant poisoning still occur in countries where thallium-containing rodenticides remain in use, as well as in this country, from attempted homicide and by personal injury from contamination of foods and illicit drugs. Early recognition of the characteristic signs and symptoms of thallium poisoning and prompt initiation of safe and appropriate therapy will substantially improve the patient's prognosis. When recognition and subsequent treatment are delayed, morbidity and mortality may be consequential.

REFERENCES

1. Aoyama H. Distribution and excretion of thallium after oral and intraperitoneal administration of thallous malonate and thallous sulfate in hamsters. *Bull Environ Contam Toxicol.* 1989;42:456-463.
2. Aoyama H, Yoshida M, Yamamura Y. Acute poisoning by intentional ingestion of thallous malonate. *Hum Toxicol.* 1986;5:389-392.
3. Appenroth D, Gambaryan S, Winnefeld K, et al. Functional and morphological aspects of thallium-induced nephrotoxicity in rats. *Toxicology.* 1995;96:203-215.
4. Appenroth D, Winnefeld K. Is thallium-induced nephrotoxicity in rats connected with riboflavin and/or GSH? Reconsideration of hypotheses on the mechanism of thallium toxicity. *J Appl Toxicol.* 1999;19:61-66.
5. Bank WJ. Thallium. In: Spencer PS, Schaumburg HH, eds. *Experimental and Clinical Neurotoxicology.* Baltimore: Williams & Wilkins; 1980:570-577.
6. Bank WJ, Pleasure DE, Suzuki K, et al. Thallium poisoning. *Arch Neurol.* 1972;26:456-464.
7. Bostian K, Betts GF, Man WK, Hughes MN. Thallium activation and inhibition of yeast aldehyde dehydrogenase. *FEBS Lett.* 1975;59:88-91.
8. Britten JS, Blank M. Thallium activation of the (Na^+-K^+)-activated ATPase of rabbit kidney. *Biochim Biophys Acta.* 1968;159:160-166.
9. Burnett JW. Thallium poisoning. *Cutis.* 1990;46:112-113.
10. Cavanagh JB. What have we learnt from Graham Frederick Young? reflections on the mechanism of thallium neurotoxicity. *Neuropathol Appl Neurobiol.* 1991;17:3-9.
11. Cavanagh JB, Fuller NH, Johnson HR, Rudge P. The effects of thallium salts, with particular reference to the nervous system changes. A report of three cases. *Q J Med.* 1974;43:293-319.
12. Chakrabarti AK, Ghosh K, Chaudhuri AK. Thallium poisoning—a case report. *J Trop Med Hyg.* 1985;88:291-293.
13. Chamberlain PH, Stavinoha WB, Davis H, et al. Thallium poisoning. *Pediatrics.* 1958;22:1170-1182.
14. Chandler HA, Archbold GP, Gibson JM, et al. Excretion of a toxic dose of thallium. *Clin Chem.* 1990;36:1506-1509.

15. Davis LE, Standefer JC, Kornfeld M, et al. Acute thallium poisoning: toxicological and morphological studies of the nervous system. *Ann Neurol.* 1981;10:38-44.
16. De Backer W, Zachee P, Verpooten GA, et al. Thallium intoxication treated with combined hemoperfusion-hemodialysis. *J Toxicol Clin Toxicol.* 1982;19:259-264.
17. de Groot G, van Heijst AN. Toxicokinetic aspects of thallium poisoning. methods of treatment by toxin elimination. *Sci Total Environ.* 1988;71:411-418.
18. de Groot G, van Heijst AN, van Kesteren RG, Maes RA. An evaluation of the efficacy of charcoal haemoperfusion in the treatment of three cases of acute thallium poisoning. *Arch Toxicol.* 1985;57:61-66.
19. Desenclos JC, Wilder MH, Coppenger GW, et al. Thallium poisoning: an outbreak in Florida, 1988. *South Med J.* 1992;85:1203-1206.
20. Dolgner R, Brockhaus A, Ewers U, et al. Repeated surveillance of exposure to thallium in a population living in the vicinity of a cement plant emitting dust containing thallium. *Int Arch Occup Environ Health.* 1983;52:79-94.
21. Dumitru D, Kalantri A. Electrophysiologic investigation of thallium poisoning. *Muscle Nerve.* 1990;13:433-437.
22. English JC. A case of thallium poisoning complicating pregnancy. *Med J Aust.* 1954;41:780-782.
23. Ewers U. Environmental exposure to thallium. *Sci Total Environ.* 1988;71:285-292.
24. Fatemi SJ, Amiri A, Bazargan MH, Tubafard S, Fatemi SN. Clinical evaluation of desferrioxamine (DFO) for removal of thallium ions in rat. *Int J Artif Organs.* 2007;30:902-905.
25. Feldman J, Levisohn DR. Acute alopecia: clue to thallium toxicity. *Pediatr Dermatol.* 1993;10:29-31.
26. Galván-Arzate S, Pedraza-Chaverrí J, Medina-Campos ON, et al. Delayed effects of thallium in the rat brain: regional changes in lipid peroxidation and behavioral markers, but moderate alterations in antioxidants, after a single administration. *Food Chem Toxicol.* 2005;43:1037-1045.
27. Gastel B. Clinical conferences at the Johns Hopkins Hospital. Thallium poisoning. *Johns Hopkins Med J.* 1978;142:27-31.
28. Gehring PJ, Hammond PB. The interrelationship between thallium and potassium in animals. *J Pharmacol Exp Ther.* 1967;155:187-201.
29. Gibson JE, Becker BA. Placental transfer, embryotoxicity, and teratogenicity of thallium sulfate in normal and potassium-deficient rats. *Toxicol Appl Pharmacol.* 1970;16:120-132.
30. Grunfeld O, Hinostroza G. Thallium poisoning. *Arch Intern Med.* 1964;114:132-138.
31. Hall BK. Critical periods during development as assessed by thallium-induced inhibition of growth of embryonic chick tibiae in vitro. *Teratology.* 1985;31:353-361.
32. Hanzel CE, Villaverde MS, Verstraeten SV. Glutathione metabolism is impaired in vitro by thallium(III) hydroxide. *Toxicology.* 2005;207:501-510.
33. Hasan M, Ali SF. Effects of thallium, nickel, and cobalt administration of the lipid peroxidation in different regions of the rat brain. *Toxicol Appl Pharmacol.* 1981;57:8-13.
34. Hasan M, Chandra SV, Dua PR, et al. Biochemical and electrophysiologic effects of thallium poisoning on the rat corpus striatum. *Toxicol Appl Pharmacol.* 1977;41:353-359.
35. Hirata M, Taoda K, Ono-Ogasawara M, et al. A probable case of chronic occupational thallium poisoning in a glass factory. *Ind Health.* 1998;36:300-303.
36. Hoffman RS. Thallium poisoning during pregnancy: a case report and comprehensive literature review. *J Toxicol Clin Toxicol.* 2000;38:767-775.
37. Hoffman RS. Thallium toxicity and the role of Prussian blue in therapy. *Toxicol Rev.* 2003;22:29-40.
38. Hoffman RS, Stringer JA, Feinberg RS, Goldfrank LR. Comparative efficacy of thallium adsorption by activated charcoal, Prussian blue, and sodium polystyrene sulfonate. *J Toxicol Clin Toxicol.* 1999;37:833-837.
39. Hologgitas J, Ullucci P, Driscoll J, et al. Thallium elimination kinetics in acute thallotoxicosis. *J Anal Toxicol.* 1980;4:68-75.
40. Hultin T, Naslund PH. Effects of thallium (I) on the structure and functions of mammalian ribosomes. *Chem Biol Interact.* 1974;8:315-328.
41. Insley BM, Grufferman S, Ayliffe HE. Thallium poisoning in cocaine abusers. *Am J Emerg Med.* 1986;4:545-548.
42. Inturrisi CE. Thallium-induced dephosphorylation of a phosphorylated intermediate of the (sodium plus thallium-activated) ATPase. *Biochim Biophys Acta.* 1969;178:630-633.
43. Johnson W. A case of thallium poisoning during pregnancy. *Med J Aust.* 1960;47:540-542.
44. Kamerbeek HH, Rauws AG, ten Ham M, van Heijst AN. Dangerous redistribution of thallium by treatment with sodium diethyldithiocarbamate. *Acta Med Scand.* 1971;189:149-154.
45. Kayne FJ. Thallium (I) activation of pyruvate kinase. *Arch Biochem Biophys.* 1971;143:232-239.
46. Koshy KM, Lovejoy FH Jr. Thallium ingestion with survival: ineffectiveness of peritoneal dialysis and potassium chloride diuresis. *Clin Toxicol.* 1981;18:521-525.
47. Lehmann PA, Favari L. Parameters for the adsorption of thallium ions by activated charcoal and Prussian blue. *J Toxicol Clin Toxicol.* 1984;22:331-339.
48. Leloux MS, Nguyen PL, Claude JR. Experimental studies on thallium toxicity in rats. II—the influence of several antidotal treatments on the tissue distribution and elimination of thallium, after subacute intoxication. *J Toxicol Clin Exp.* 1990;10:147-156.
49. Leung KM, Ooi VE. Studies on thallium toxicity, its tissue distribution and histopathological effects in rats. *Chemosphere.* 2000;41:155-159.
50. Lovejoy FH. Thallium. *Clin Toxicol Rev.* 1982;4:1-2.
51. Luckit J, Mir N, Hargreaves M, et al. Thrombocytopenia associated with thallium poisoning. *Hum Exp Toxicol.* 1990;9:47-48.
52. Lukacs M. Thallium poisoning induced polyneuropathy—clinical and electrophysiological data [Hungarian]. *Ideggyogy Sz.* 2003;56:407-414.
53. Lund A. The effect of various substances on the excretion and the toxicity of thallium in the rat. *Acta Pharmacol Toxicol (Copenh).* 1956;12:260-268.
54. Lynche GR, Lond MB, Scovell JMS. The toxicology of thallium. *Lancet.* 1930;12:1340-1344.
55. Malbrain ML, Lambrecht GL, Zandijk E, et al. Treatment of severe thallium intoxication. *J Toxicol Clin Toxicol.* 1997;35:97-100.
56. McMillan TM, Jacobson RR, Gross M. Neuropsychology of thallium poisoning. *J Neurol Neurosurg Psychiatry.* 1997;63:247-250.
57. Meggs WJ, Cahill-Morasco R, Shih RD, et al. Effects of Prussian blue and *N*-acetylcysteine on thallium toxicity in mice. *J Toxicol Clin Toxicol.* 1997;35:163-166.
58. Meggs WJ, Goldfrank LR, Hoffman RS. Effects of potassium in a murine model of thallium poisoning [abstract]. *J Toxicol Clin Toxicol.* 1995;33:559.
59. Meggs WJ, Hoffman RS, Shih RD, et al. Thallium poisoning from maliciously contaminated food. *J Toxicol Clin Toxicol.* 1994;32:723-730.
60. Melnick RL, Monti LG, Motzkin SM. Uncoupling of mitochondrial oxidative phosphorylation by thallium. *Biochem Biophys Res Commun.* 1976;69:68-73.
61. Misra UK, Kalita J, Yadav RK, Ranjan P. Thallium poisoning: emphasis on early diagnosis and response to haemodialysis. *Postgrad Med J.* 2003;79:103-105.
62. Moeschlin S. Thallium poisoning. *Clin Toxicol.* 1980;17:133-146.
63. Moore D, House I, Dixon A. Thallium poisoning: diagnosis may be elusive but alopecia is the clue. *Br Med J.* 1993;306:1527-1529.
64. Mulkey JP, Oehme FW. Are 2,3-dimercapto-1-propanesulfonic acid or Prussian blue beneficial in acute thallotoxicosis in rats? *Vet Hum Toxicol.* 2000;42:325-329.
65. Mulkey JP, Oehme FW. A review of thallium toxicity. *Vet Hum Toxicol.* 1993;35:445-453.
66. Mullins LJ, Moore RD. The movement of thallium ions in muscle. *J Gen Physiol.* 1960;43:759-773.
67. Munch JC. Human thallotoxicosis. *JAMA.* 1934;102:1929-1933.
68. Munch JC, Ginsburg HM, Nixon C. The 1932 thallotoxicosis outbreak in California. *JAMA.* 1933;101:1315-1319.
69. Neal JB, Appelbaum E, Gaul LE, Masselink RJ. An unusual occurrence of thallium poisoning. *N Y State J Med.* 1935;35:657-659.
70. Nordentoft T, Andersen EB, Mogensen PH. Initial sensorimotor and delayed autonomic neuropathy in acute thallium poisoning. *Neurotoxicology.* 1998;19:421-426.
71. Pai V. Acute thallium poisoning. Prussian blue therapy in 9 cases. *West Ind Med J.* 1987;36:256-258.
72. Papp JP, Gay PC, Dodson VN, Pollard HM. Potassium chloride treatment in thallotoxicosis. *Ann Intern Med.* 1969;71:119-123.
73. Pau PW. Management of thallium poisoning. *Hong Kong Med J.* 2000;6:316-318.
74. Paulson G, Vergara G, Young J, Bird M. Thallium intoxication treated with dithizone and hemodialysis. *Arch Intern Med.* 1972;129:100-103.
75. Pedersen RS, Olesen AS, Freund LG, et al. Thallium intoxication treated with long-term hemodialysis, forced diuresis and Prussian blue. *Acta Med Scan.* 1978;204:429-432.

76. Questel F, Dugarin J, Dally S. Thallium-contaminated heroin. *Ann Intern Med.* 1996;124:616.
77. Rangel-Guerra R, Martinez HR, Villarreal HJ. Thallium poisoning: experience with 50 patients [Spanish]. *Gac Med Mex.* 1990;126:487-494.
78. Rauws AG. Thallium pharmacokinetics and its modification by Prussian blue. *Naunyn Schmiedebergs Arch Pharmacol.* 1974;284:294-306.
79. Reed D, Crawley J, Faro SN, et al. Thallotoxicosis. Acute manifestations and sequelae. *JAMA.* 1963;183:516-522.
80. Rios C, Monroy-Noyola A. D-Penicillamine and Prussian blue as antidotes against thallium intoxication in rats. *Toxicology.* 1992;74:69-76.
81. Roby DS, Fein AM, Bennett RH, et al. Cardiopulmonary effects of acute thallium poisoning. *Chest.* 1984;85:236-240.
82. Rusyniak DE, Furbee RB, Kirk MA. Thallium and arsenic poisoning in a small midwestern town. *Ann Emerg Med.* 2002;39:307-311.
83. Rusyniak DE, Kao LW, Nanagas KA, et al. Dimercaptosuccinic acid and Prussian blue in the treatment of acute thallium poisoning in rats. *J Toxicol Clin Toxicol.* 2003;41:137-142.
84. Saddique A, Peterson CD. Thallium poisoning: a review. *Vet Hum Toxicol.* 1983;25:16-22.
85. Saha A, Sadhu HG, Karnik AB, et al. Erosion of nails following thallium poisoning: a case report. *Occup Environ Med.* 2004;61:640-642.
86. Schaumburg HH, Berger A. Alopecia and sensory polyneuropathy from thallium in a Chinese herbal medication. *JAMA.* 1992;268:3430-3431.
87. Schmidt D, Bach M, Gerling J. A case of localized retinal damage in thallium poisoning. *Int Ophthalmol.* 1997;21:143-147.
88. Schwetz BA, O'Neil PV, Voelker FA, Jacobs DW. Effects of diphenylthiocarbazone and diethyldithiocarbamate on the excretion of thallium by rats. *Toxicol Appl Pharmacol.* 1967;10:79-88.
89. Sharma AN, Nelson LS, Hoffman RS. Cerebrospinal fluid analysis in fatal thallium poisoning: evidence for delayed distribution into the central nervous system. *Am J Forensic Med Pathol.* 2004;25:156-158.
90. Spencer PS, Peterson ER, Madrid R, Raine CS. Effects of thallium salts on neuronal mitochondria in organotypic cord-ganglia-muscle combination cultures. *J Cell Biol.* 1973;58:79-95.
91. Stevens W, van Peteghem C, Heyndrickx A, Barbier F. Eleven cases of thallium intoxication treated with Prussian blue. *Int J Clin Pharmacol Ther Toxicol.* 1974;10:1-22.
92. Sunderman FW. Diethyldithiocarbamate therapy of thallotoxicosis. *Am J Med Sci.* 1967;2:107-118.
93. Tabandeh H, Crowston JG, Thompson GM. Ophthalmologic features of thallium poisoning. *Am J Ophthalmol.* 1994;117:243-245.
94. Tabandeh H, Thompson GM. Visual function in thallium toxicity. *Br Med J.* 1993;307:324.
95. Thompson DF. Management of thallium poisoning. *Clin Toxicol.* 1981;18:979-990.
96. Thompson DF, Callen ED. Soluble or insoluble Prussian blue for radiocesium and thallium poisoning? *Ann Pharmacother.* 2004;38:1509-1514.
97. Tromme I, Van Neste D, Dobbelaere F, et al. Skin signs in the diagnosis of thallium poisoning. *Br J Dermatol.* 1998;138:321-325.
98. van der Merwe CF. The treatment of thallium poisoning. A report of 2 cases. *S Afr Med J.* 1972;46:560-561.
99. Vergauwe PL, Knockaert DC, Van Tittelboom TJ. Near fatal suba-cute thallium poisoning necessitating prolonged mechanical ventilation. *Am J Emerg Med.* 1990;8:548-550.
100. Villanueva E, Hernandez-Cueto C, Lachica E, et al. Poisoning by thallium. A study of five cases. *Drug Saf.* 1990;5:384-389.
101. Villaverde MS, Hanzel CE, Verstraeten SV. In vitro interactions of thallium with components of the glutathione-dependent antioxidant defence system. *Free Radic Res.* 2004;38:977-984.
102. Vrij AA, Cremers HM, Lustermans FA. Successful recovery of a patient with thallium poisoning. *Neth J Med.* 1995;47:121-126.
103. Wainwright AP, Kox WJ, House IM, et al. Clinical features and therapy of acute thallium poisoning. *Q J Med.* 1988;69:939-944.
104. Wakid NW, Cortas NK. Chemical and atomic absorption methods for thallium in urine compared. *Clin Chem.* 1984;30:587-588.
105. Yokoyama K, Araki S, Abe H. Distribution of nerve conduction velocities in acute thallium poisoning. *Muscle Nerve.* 1990;13:117-120.

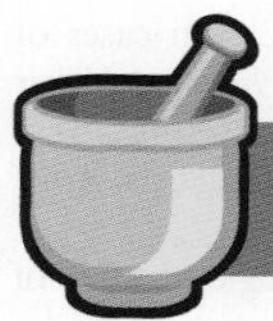

ANTIDOTES IN DEPTH (A29)

PRUSSIAN BLUE

Robert S. Hoffman

Prussian blue, the first artificially synthesized pigment, was discovered unintentionally by Diesbach in 1704 while he was attempting to make cochineal red lake. Although it immediately became popular in art and later in printing, it took approximately 250 years to recognize that Prussian blue was able to attract monovalent alkali metals into its crystal lattice. Subsequently, in 1963, Nigrovic was the first investigator to demonstrate that Prussian blue enhanced cesium elimination from the gut of rats.[33] In 2003, the US Food and Drug Administration (FDA) approved Prussian blue (Radiogardase®) for the treatment of thallium and radioactive cesium poisoning.

The literature associated with Prussian blue is complicated by many confusing chemical and physical terms. The product synthesized by Diesbach, $Fe_4[Fe(CN_6)]_3$, commonly known as insoluble Prussian blue, is assigned the Chemical Abstracts Service (CAS) number 14038-43-8, and is the FDA-approved product Radiogardase® (Fig. A29–1). Synonyms for Prussian blue include Berlin blue, Hamburg blue, mineral blue, Paris blue, and Pigment blue 27, among others.[51] These names are often used interchangeably to refer to both insoluble Prussian blue and a soluble (colloidal) Prussian blue that has the molecular formula either $KFe[Fe(CN)_6]_3$ or $K_3Fe[Fe(CN)_6]_3$. Thus "Prussian blue" also carries two additional CAS numbers: 25869-98-1 and 12240-15-2.[37] Compounds containing the same basic core structure, such as $NH_4Fe[Fe(CN)_6]_3$ (ammonium ferric ferrocyanide or Chinese blue) and sodium ferric ferrocyanide, may have similar efficacy in binding monovalent cations, and are also sometimes incorrectly called Prussian blue. For the purpose of clarity, general statements that follow use the term "Prussian blue." In many instances the terms "insoluble" and "soluble" are chosen to highlight differences between the compounds. Unfortunately, because many studies do not specify which Prussian blue is used, some inherent ambiguity persists.

PHARMACOLOGY

Typically, the crystal lattice of Prussian blue takes up cationic potassium ions from the surrounding environment. However, because its affinity increases as the ionic radius of the monovalent cation increases, Prussian blue preferentially binds cesium (ionic radius: 0.169 nm) and thallium (ionic radius: 0.147 nm) over potassium (ionic radius: 0.133 nm).[6,16] Additionally, binding for rubidium (ionic radius: 0.148 nm) has been demonstrated.[44] Thus, when given orally, Prussian blue binds unabsorbed thallium or cesium in the gastrointestinal tract, preventing absorption as well as reversing the concentration gradient to enhance elimination through gut dialysis. In addition, Prussian blue can interfere with enterohepatic circulation, causing a further reduction in tissue stores.

Insoluble Prussian blue is essentially not absorbed from the gastrointestinal tract and is eliminated in the feces at a rate determined by gastrointestinal transit time. In a radiolabeled study of healthy pigs, 99% of a single ingested dose was recovered unchanged in the stool.[30] In contrast, soluble Prussian blue is absorbed based on the clinical finding of a blue discoloration that develops in the sweat and tears of patients undergoing prolonged therapy.[12] This discoloration appears to be benign and resolves when therapy is stopped. No significant food or drug interactions are known to exist. Animal studies show no adverse effects of therapeutic doses,[39] and oral lethal doses are not known. The only significant adverse effects reported in humans receiving therapeutic doses are constipation and hypokalemia,[50] and the constipation may be related more to the thallium toxicity than to the Prussian blue.

Although there is some concern regarding the potential concentration of cyanide liberated from Prussian blue, this release appears to be quantitatively minimal. Cyanide release from soluble Prussian blue was less than 3 mg/24 h in simulated gastric fluid.[56] When three human volunteers were given 500 mg of radiolabeled soluble Prussian blue, only 2 mg of cyanide were absorbed.[31] Over the physiological range of potential gastrointestinal pH the maximal cyanide release of insoluble Prussian blue was determined to be 135 μg/g at pH 1.[59] When extrapolated, even repeated therapeutic doses would only deliver a trivial amount of cyanide.

IN VITRO ADSORPTION OF THALLIUM

In vitro and, presumably, in vivo binding of thallium to Prussian blue are influenced by its chemical formulation. An early investigation demonstrated that the soluble form more effectively adsorbs thallium than the insoluble form.[8] In a more rigorous study, the in vitro adsorptions of both forms were similar when thallium concentrations remained low.[15] However, as thallium concentrations increased, the colloidal (soluble) form demonstrated far greater adsorptive capacity. Although not proven, this difference may occur because the soluble form contains more potassium and can therefore exchange proportionally more cation. Furthermore, the actual size of the crystal lattice alters its efficacy. Laboratory synthesized Prussian blue (with a crystal size of 17.68 nm) was compared with a commercial preparation (with a crystal size of 31.19 nm). The laboratory synthesized product adsorbed more thallium in vitro, because its smaller size increased its surface area.[16] In vitro analysis of the FDA approved antidote demonstrated that pH and hydration state greatly influence binding with the maximal absorptive capacity (MAC) predicted to be as high as 1400 mg/g at pH 7.5.[60]

THALLIUM POISONING

A thorough analysis of the efficacy of Prussian blue in thallium poisoning is severely hampered by many factors. First, and most importantly, there are no controlled human trials. Second, although multiple patients have received Prussian blue in the setting of thallium poisoning, many were simultaneously treated with a variety of therapies, including forced potassium diuresis, single- or multiple-dose activated charcoal, and either hemodialysis or hemoperfusion. Thus, it is impossible to determine the specific effects of Prussian blue on mortality or other

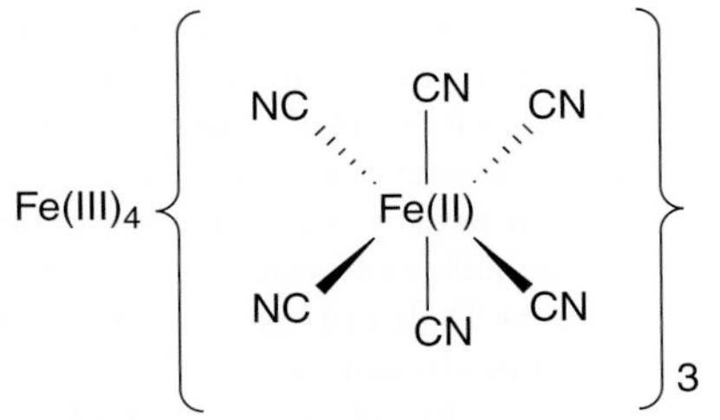

FIGURE A29–1. The chemical structure of insoluble Prussian blue. The Roman numerals II and III denote the valence state of iron. Although in the most current nomenclature this would be expressed as Fe^{2+} and Fe^{3+}, the figure is drawn this way to be consistent with most available references, which use the older nomenclature.

clinical outcomes, and even toxicokinetic data must be interpreted with caution. Third, many of the in vitro and animal investigations fail to specify the exact type of Prussian blue used. Those investigations that do specify the type of Prussian blue used typically used the soluble form, which is presently unavailable as a pharmaceutical preparation. Discussions of the available data in the following sections are limited by these considerations.

IN VITRO COMPARISON OF PRUSSIAN BLUE WITH ACTIVATED CHARCOAL

In one in vitro study, thallium was well adsorbed to Norit® brand activated charcoal.[15] Although numerical data are not supplied in the body of the paper, the 10% to 20% adsorption to activated charcoal demonstrated in a figure was far less than the results achieved with several different forms of Prussian blue tested simultaneously.[15] Two other binding studies showed different results from the Norit® activated charcoal study. An early investigation determined that the MAC of activated charcoal was 124 mg of thallium/g, whereas the MAC for Prussian blue was only 72 mg of thallium/g.[17] More recently, a MAC of only 59.7 mg of thallium/g was calculated for CharcoAid® activated charcoal, compared with a higher MAC for insoluble Prussian blue of 72.7 mg of thallium/g.[13] Although the MACs for Prussian blue in these two studies are nearly identical, they differ significantly from binding reported above, possibly as a result of different experimental conditions.[60] Similarly, the variable results for activated charcoal may also be a function of the study pH or the different types of activated charcoal used.

ANIMAL DATA: KINETICS, TISSUE CONCENTRATIONS, AND SURVIVAL

Sublethal doses of thallium were used to evaluate the effects of various antidotes in rats over an 8-day period.[17] Although the control group only eliminated 53% of the administered dose of thallium, 93% of the dose was eliminated in the activated charcoal and 82% was eliminated in the insoluble Prussian blue groups. In contrast, other investigators demonstrated only a modest increase in thallium elimination in rats treated with oral activated charcoal while a consistent benefit of Prussian blue was noted.[18]

Multiple studies clearly demonstrate that Prussian blue not only decreases the half-life of thallium in animals but also lowers thallium content in critical organs such as the brain and the heart.[11,27,28,43,45] Half-lives are typically reduced by approximately 50% when Prussian blue is given with or without a cathartic. The rationale for the cathartic is that constipation is invariably present in humans and animals with severe thallium poisoning.

Only a few studies evaluate the effects of Prussian blue on survival. In these studies, a statistically significant survival advantage is shown in thallium-poisoned rats[16,45] and mice[22] treated with Prussian blue. The experimental benefit is on the order of a 31% increase in the LD_{50} (median lethal dose for 50% of test subjects) in poisoned animals.[46]

RADIOACTIVE THALLIUM

There is no published experience describing human poisoning with radioactive thallium. Prussian blue has demonstrable efficacy in an animal model of radioactive thallium poisoning, as would be expected because the ionic radii of isotopes are generally similar. In one small study, insoluble Prussian blue decreased the biologic half-life of radioactive thallium in rats by approximately 40%.[2]

HUMAN DATA

Three patients, in 1971, were the first to receive Prussian blue as a treatment for thallium poisoning.[15] Although daily fecal thallium concentrations were not determined in two of the three patients because of severe constipation, an approximately sevenfold increase in fecal thallium elimination over baseline was attributed to Prussian blue therapy in the third patient. Subsequently, many humans with thallium poisoning have received Prussian blue, with or without a cathartic, as part of their therapy.[1,3,5,6,10,15,38,41,49,53,54,58] Unfortunately, other components of therapy that may have confounded the effects of Prussian blue in these cases include single- or multiple-dose activated charcoal, and the use of D-penicillamine, dimercaprol, ethylenediaminetetraacetic acid (EDTA), succimer, 2,3-dimercaptopropane-1-sulphate (DMPS), forced potassium diuresis, and either hemodialysis or hemoperfusion. There are no controlled trials of any of these modalities alone or in combination, and most of the data presented are based on single case reports or small case series.

One of the largest series was composed of 11 thallium-poisoned patients who were treated with soluble Prussian blue.[49] This report not only demonstrated the tolerability of Prussian blue, but also was the first to systematically evaluate its fecal elimination. In all individuals studied, fecal elimination remained high, even when urinary elimination fell, suggesting selective redistribution of thallium into the gut.[49] Although the authors commented on clinical improvement in these patients, the lack of controlled data makes these subjective observations difficult to interpret. Similarly, a substantial reduction in thallium half-life was demonstrated when Prussian blue was compared with no therapy at all in patients with thallium poisoning.[6]

DOSAGE AND ADMINISTRATION

The dosage of Prussian blue has never been investigated systematically in either humans or animals. In most of the case reports and series mentioned above, a total dose of 150 to 250 mg/kg/d was administered orally or via a nasogastric tube in two to four divided doses.[49] Because constipation or obstipation is often present or expected, Prussian blue is generally administered dissolved in 50 mL of 15% mannitol.[50] Although any cathartic may be appropriate, mannitol is used most frequently, possibly because of concerns over the risks associated with repeated doses of magnesium or sorbitol (see Antidotes in Depth A3–Whole-Bowel Irrigation and Other Intestinal Evacuants). The manufacturer of Radiogardase® recommends that adults and adolescents with thallium poisoning receive a total dose of 9 g divided daily (3 g every 8 hours) and that children receive a total dose of 3 g divided daily (1 g every 8 hours). Although the manufacturer does not recommend using a cathartic, a high-fiber diet is advocated when constipation is present. Because Prussian blue is well tolerated, the editors continue to favor the 150 to 250 mg/kg/d dosing because it provides more antidote. In addition, because many severely poisoned patients cannot eat, the use of a cathartic should be considered when constipation is consequential.

The end point of therapy is similarly poorly defined. By convention, Prussian blue is usually continued until urinary thallium concentrations fall below 0.5 mg/d. This end point may not be a meaningful measurement of thallium burden, as fecal elimination may continue, even when urinary elimination has diminished.[49] However, because most laboratories are not equipped to measure fecal thallium concentrations, the use of some urinary end point seems reasonable as the reported residual amounts of fecal elimination are small.

CESIUM POISONING

The radioactive isotope of cesium (^{137}Cs), a common byproduct of nuclear fission reactions, is a strong β and γ emitter with a physical half-life of more than 30 years and a biologic half-life of about 110 days. Another isotope (^{134}Cs) is only produced by neutron activation of the stable isotope (^{133}Cs) and has a physical half-life of about 2 years and a biologic half-life comparable to ^{137}Cs. Cesium is absorbed in the small bowel, distributes like potassium, and undergoes enteric recirculation in a manner comparable to thallium.[26] Approximately 80% of a given dose of cesium is eliminated in the urine, with 20% cleared in the feces.

The isotope ^{137}Cs is used clinically as a radiation source in nuclear medicine. Although uncommon, radiologic disasters such as Chernobyl and Goiânia (see Human Clinical Trials section below) have resulted in lethal incorporation exposures. Additionally, concerns over the use of ^{137}Cs in "dirty bombs" have increased the awareness of, and the potential need to treat, patients with radioactive cesium poisoning. Toxicity from nonradioactive cesium is also reported. Many cases of QT interval prolongation and torsades de pointes are reported in patients who take cesium chloride either as a dietary supplement or for its alleged antineoplastic effects.[4,20,36,42,47] To date, there have been no reports of Prussian blue therapy for nonradioactive cesium poisoning, but the following discussion is most likely applicable.

IN VITRO ADSORPTION OF CESIUM

Standard binding studies compared the ability of activated charcoal, sodium polystyrene sulfonate (SPS), and both soluble and insoluble Prussian blue to bind ^{137}Cs over a range of gastrointestinal pHs.[55] Unlike thallium, the adsorption of cesium to activated charcoal was negligible. Comparable to thallium, SPS offered no benefit, likely because of preferential effects on potassium. Although both forms of Prussian blue adsorbed cesium, the insoluble form was consistently superior. A pH of 7.5 was selected to represent the pH of the small bowel lumen, the location where most adsorption would occur. At this pH, a MAC of 238 mg of ^{137}Cs/g of insoluble Prussian blue was determined. In an interesting extension, when the same authors bound insoluble Prussian blue to a hemoperfusion column, they demonstrated a clearance of approximately 100 mL/min of ^{137}Cs from plasma, and projected that a 4-hour treatment would adsorb about 0.3 terabecquerel (TBq) of radioactive cesium.[57] When the FDA-approved antidote was analyzed, like thallium, pH and hydration introduced significant variations in binding, with a MAC of 715 mg/g noted at pH 7.5.[9]

ANIMAL DATA: KINETICS, TISSUE CONCENTRATIONS, AND SURVIVAL

Small animal investigations with either ^{134}Cs or ^{137}Cs consistently demonstrate that Prussian blue therapy reverses the urine-to-stool-elimination ratio from 8:1 to 0.3:1, and reduces the biologic half-life and the total body area under the curve by as much as 60%.[29,33,34,44,48] For example, rats given oral ^{134}Cs retained 84.7% of the ingested dose at 7 days. Treatment with insoluble and soluble Prussian blue, as well as Chinese blue, produced significant reductions in retained cesium (only 6.36%, 2.63%, and 2.43% of the dose was retained at 7 days, respectively).[7]

In addition to human toxicity, concern over radioactive cesium incorporation into cattle milk and meat has resulted in a number of large animal investigations. Daily Prussian blue therapy reduced radioactive cesium concentrations in sheep by as much as 42%.[14,40] Likewise, radioactive cesium transfer to milk was reduced by 85% in cows.[52] When dogs were contaminated with ^{137}Cs, Prussian blue reduced total-body burden by as much as 51%.[24] Similar efficacy in reducing the amount of cesium was demonstrated in meat from pigs fed ^{134}Cs-contaminated whey, with insoluble Prussian blue reducing activity from 359 Bq/kg to 11 Bq/kg.[7]

HUMAN VOLUNTEER STUDIES

Two human volunteers ingested meals contaminated with ^{134}Cs to compare the efficacy of both the soluble and insoluble forms of Prussian blue with controls.[7] At 14 days after loading and without therapy, the volunteers retained 94.7% of the ingested dose, compared with a retention of only 5.1% following therapy with insoluble Prussian blue and 4.9% following soluble Prussian blue. In another study, two volunteers demonstrated that Prussian blue decreased the biologic half-life of ingested radioactive cesium by approximately 33%.[21] Finally, in two volunteers, the effects of pretreatment were compared with simultaneous posttreatment Prussian blue. When a single dose of Prussian blue was administered 10 minutes before ^{134}Cs, absorption decreased from 100% (without therapy) to 3% to 10%. However, simultaneous administration of 0.5 or 1 g of Prussian blue with ^{134}Cs resulted in 38% to 63% absorption. Finally, when Prussian blue was given daily at a dose of 0.5 g every 8 hours in the postabsorptive phase, the biologic half-life of ^{134}Cs was reduced from 106 to 44 days.[32]

HUMAN CLINICAL TRIALS

There are no controlled trials of Prussian blue in radioactive cesium poisoning. Experience is derived exclusively from treating disaster victims. In 1987, a number of people in Goiânia, Brazil, were contaminated with radioactive cesium from a discarded radiotherapy unit.[35] Although the reported total number of individuals treated is uncertain because of multiple reports that probably include overlapping patients, one group describes 37 patients who were given insoluble Prussian blue in doses ranging from 3 g/d in children up to 10 g/d in adults. Untreated, elimination kinetics were first order and half-lives varied extensively from 39 to 106 days in adults (mean: 65.5 days in women and 83 days in men). Half-lives were shorter in children. Therapy with insoluble Prussian blue reduced half-lives by a mean of 32%[19] and reduced the retained cesium dose 51% to 84%.[23]

The nuclear disaster at Chernobyl, Ukraine, resulted in many cases of acute radiation exposure as well as incorporation into the population of radioactive iodine, cesium, and strontium. In one trial, insoluble Prussian blue was given to three victims of radioactive cesium incorporation many weeks after their exposure. The reported reduction in biologic half-life ranged from 12% to 52%.[25] The authors of this paper include data from the Chinese literature describing another six patients who demonstrated a similar reduction in the biologic half-life of cesium following Prussian blue therapy.

DOSAGE AND ADMINISTRATION

The manufacturer of Radiogardase® recommends that for radioactive cesium poisoning, adults receive a total daily dose of 9 g divided into

3 g, three times per day. Children should receive a total daily dose of 3 g divided into 1 g, three times per day. Although these are the same doses used for thallium poisoning, therapy for cesium poisoning should be continued for at least 30 days. Even though there are no recommendations of other criteria to determine the end point of therapy, quantitative and radiologic evaluations of cesium elimination should be performed.

PREGNANCY CATEGORY

Insoluble Prussian blue is listed as pregnancy category C. Because of the severe consequences of poisoning from radioactive cesium and thallium and the lack of systemic absorption of insoluble Prussian blue, a risk-to-benefit analysis favors the use of the antidote in all poisoned pregnant patients.

AVAILABILITY

Insoluble Prussian blue (Radiogardase®) is available as a 0.5-g blue powder in gelatin capsules for oral administration manufactured from Haupt Pharma Berlin GmbH for distribution by HEYL Chemisch-pharmazeutische Fabrik GmbH & Co. KG, Berlin.

ACKNOWLEDGMENT

Part of this chapter was adapted, with permission from the publisher, from Hoffman RS. Thallium toxicity and the role of Prussian blue in therapy. *Toxicol Rev.* 2003;22:29-40.

REFERENCES

1. Atsmon J, Taliansky E, Landau M, Neufeld MY. Thallium poisoning in Israel. *Am J Med Sci.* 2000;320:327-330.
2. Borisov VP, Seletskaia LI, Skomorokhova TN, Popov VA. Effectiveness of ferrocin in decreasing the resorption of radioactive thallium [Russian]. *Med Radiol.* 1984;29:15-18.
3. Chandler HA, Archbold GP, Gibson JM, et al. Excretion of a toxic dose of thallium. *Clin Chem.* 1990;36:1506-1509.
4. Dalal AK, Harding JD, Verdino RJ. Acquired long QT syndrome and monomorphic ventricular tachycardia after alternative treatment with cesium chloride for brain cancer. *Mayo Clin Proc.* 2004;79:1065-1069.
5. De Backer W, Zachee P, Verpooten GA, et al. Thallium intoxication treated with combined hemoperfusion-hemodialysis. *J Toxicol Clin Toxicol.* 1982;19:259-264.
6. de Groot G, van Heijst AN. Toxicokinetic aspects of thallium poisoning. Methods of treatment by toxin elimination. *Sci Tot Environ.* 1988;71:411-418.
7. Dresow B, Nielsen P, Fischer R, et al. In vivo binding of radiocesium by two forms of Prussian blue and by ammonium iron hexacyanofer-rate (II). *J Toxicol Clin Toxicol.* 1993;31:563-569.
8. Dvorak P. Colloidal hexacyanoferrates (II) as antidotes in thallium poisoning [German]. *Arzneimittelforschung.* 1969;151:89-92.
9. Faustino PJ, Yang Y, Progar JJ, et al. Quantitative determination of cesium binding to ferric hexacyanoferrate: Prussian blue. *J Pharm Biomed Anal.* 2008;47:114-125.
10. Ghezzi R, Bozza Marrubini M. Prussian blue in the treatment of thallium intoxication. *Vet Hum Toxicol.* 1979;21:64-66.
11. Heydlauf H. Ferric-cyanoferrate (II): an effective antidote in thallium poisoning. *Eur J Pharmacol.* 1969;6:340-344.
12. Hoffman RS. Thallium toxicity and the role of Prussian blue in therapy. *Toxicol Rev.* 2003;22:29-40.
13. Hoffman RS, Stringer JA, Feinberg RS, Goldfrank LR. Comparative efficacy of thallium adsorption by activated charcoal, Prussian blue, and sodium polystyrene sulfonate. *J Toxicol Clin Toxicol.* 1999;37:833-837.
14. Ioannides KG, Karamanis DT, Stamoulis KC, et al. Reduction of cesium concentration in ovine tissues following treatment with Prussian blue labeled with ^{59}Fe. *Health Phys.* 1996;71:713-718.
15. Kamerbeek HH, Rauws AG, ten Ham M, van Heijst AN. Prussian blue in therapy of thallotoxicosis. An experimental and clinical investigation. *Acta Med Scand.* 1971;189:321-324.
16. Kravzov J, Rios C, Altagracia M, et al. Relationship between physicochemical properties of Prussian blue and its efficacy as antidote against thallium poisoning. *J Appl Toxicol.* 1993;13:213-216.
17. Lehmann PA, Favari L. Parameters for the adsorption of thallium ions by activated charcoal and Prussian blue. *J Toxicol Clin Toxicol.* 1984;22:331-339.
18. Leloux MS, Nguyen PL, Claude JR. Experimental studies on thallium toxicity in rats. II—the influence of several antidotal treatments on the tissue distribution and elimination of thallium, after subacute intoxication. *J Toxicol Clin Exp.* 1990;10:147-156.
19. Lipsztein JL, Bertelli L, Oliveira CA, Dantas BM. Studies of cs retention in the human body related to body parameters and Prussian blue administration. *Health Phys.* 1991;60:57-61.
20. Lyon AW, Mayhew WJ. Cesium toxicity: a case of self-treatment by alternate therapy gone awry. *Ther Drug Monit.* 2003;25:114-116.
21. Madshus K, Stromme A. Increased excretion of ^{137}Cs in humans by Prussian blue. *Z Naturforsch B.* 1968;23:391-392.
22. Meggs WJ, Cahill-Morasco R, Shih RD, et al. Effects of Prussian blue and *N*-acetylcysteine on thallium toxicity in mice. *J Toxicol Clin Toxicol.* 1997;35:163-166.
23. Melo DR, Lipsztein JL, de Oliveira CA, Bertelli L. ^{137}Cs internal contamination involving a Brazilian accident, and the efficacy of Prussian blue treatment. *Health Phys.* 1994;66:245-252.
24. Melo DR, Lundgren DL, Muggenburg BA, Guilmette RA. Prussian blue decorporation of 137Cs in beagles of different ages. *Health Phys.* 1996;71:190-197.
25. Ming-Hua T, Yi-Fen G, Cheng-Yao S, et al. Measurement of internal contamination with radioactive caesium released from the Chernobyl accident and enhanced elimination by Prussian blue. *J Radiol Protect.* 1988;8:25-28.
26. Moore W Jr, Comar CL. Absorption of caesium 137 from the gastrointestinal tract of the rat. *Int J Radiat Biol.* 1962;5:247-254.
27. Mulkey JP, Oehme FW. A review of thallium toxicity. *Vet Hum Toxicol.* 1993;35:445-453.
28. Mulkey JP, Oehme FW. Are 2,3-dimercapto-1-propanesulfonic acid or Prussian blue beneficial in acute thallotoxicosis in rats? *Vet Hum Toxicol.* 2000;42:325-329.
29. Muller WH, Ducousso R, Causse A, Walter C. Long-term treatment of cesium 137 contamination with colloidal and a comparison with insoluble Prussian blue in rats. *Strahlentherapie.* 1974;147:319-322.
30. Nielsen P, Dresow B, Fischer R, et al. Intestinal absorption of iron from ^{59}Fe-labelled hexacyanoferrates(II) in piglets. *Arzneimittelforschung.* 1988;38:1469-1471.
31. Nielsen P, Dresow B, Fischer R, Heinrich HC. Bioavailability of iron and cyanide from oral potassium ferric hexacyanoferrate(II) in humans. *Arch Toxicol.* 1990;64:420-422.
32. Nielsen P, Dresow B, Fischer R, Heinrich HC. Inhibition of intestinal absorption and decorporation of radiocaesium in humans by hexacyanoferrates(II). *Arzneimittelforschung.* 1991;18:821-826.
33. Nigrovi'c V. Enhancement of the excretion of radiocaesium in rats by ferric cyanoferrate. II. *Int J Radiat Biol Relat Stud Phys Chem Med.* 1963;96:307-309.
34. Nigrovi'c V. Retention of radiocaesium by the rat as influenced by Prussian blue and other compounds. *Phys Med Biol.* 1965;10:81-92.
35. Oliveira AR, Hunt JG, Valverde NJ, et al. Medical and related aspects of the Goiania accident: an overview. *Health Phys.* 1991;60:17-24.
36. Olshansky B, Shivkumar K. Patient—heal thyself? Electrophysiology meets alternative medicine. *Pacing Clin Electrophysiol.* 2001;24:403-405.
37. O'Neil MJ, Smith A, Heckelman PE. *The Merck Index*, 13th ed. Whitehouse Station, NJ: Merck and Co, Inc; 2001:1650-1651.
38. Pai V. Acute thallium poisoning. Prussian blue therapy in 9 cases. *West Indian Med J.* 1987;36:256-258.
39. Pearce J. Studies of any toxicological effects of Prussian blue compounds in mammals—a review. *Food Chem Toxicol.* 1994;32:577-582.
40. Pearce J, Unsworth EF, McMurray CH, et al. The effects of Prussian blue provided by indwelling rumen boli on the tissue retention of dietary radiocaesium by sheep. *Sci Total Environ.* 1989;85:349-355.
41. Pedersen RS, Olesen AS, Freund LG, et al. Thallium intoxication treated with long-term hemodialysis, forced diuresis and Prussian blue. *Acta Med Scand.* 1978;204:429-432.

42. Pinter A, Dorian P, Newman D. Cesium-induced torsades de pointes. *N Engl J Med.* 2002;346:383-384.
43. Rauws AG. Thallium pharmacokinetics and its modification by Prussian blue. *Naunyn-Schmiedebergs Arch Pharmacol.* 1974;284:294-306.
44. Richmond CR, Bunde DE. Enhancement of cesium-137 excretion by rats maintained chronically on ferric ferrocyanide. *Proc Soc Exp Biol Med.* 1966;121:664-670.
45. Rios C, Kravsov J, Altagracia M, et al. Efficacy of Prussian blue against thallium poisoning: effect of particle size. *Proc West Pharmacol Soc.* 1991;34: 61-63.
46. Rios C, Monroy-Noyola A. D-Penicillamine and Prussian blue as antidotes against thallium intoxication in rats. *Toxicology.* 1992;74:69-76.
47. Saliba W, Erdogan O, Niebauer M. Polymorphic ventricular tachycardia in a woman taking cesium chloride. *Pacing Clin Electrophysiol.* 2001;24: 515-517.
48. Stather JW. Influence of Prussian blue on metabolism of ^{137}Cs and ^{86}Rb in rats. *Health Phys.* 1972;22:1-8.
49. Stevens W, van Peteghem C, Heyndrickx A, Barbier F. Eleven cases of thallium intoxication treated with Prussian blue. *Int J Clin Phamacol.* 1974;10:1-22.
50. Thompson DF. Management of thallium poisoning. *Pharmacotherapy.* 1981;18:979-990.
51. Thompson DF, Callen ED. Soluble or insoluble Prussian blue for radiocesium and thallium poisoning? *Ann Pharmacother.* 2004;38:1509-1514.
52. Unsworth EF, Pearce J, McMurray CH, et al. Investigations of the use of clay minerals and Prussian blue in reducing the transfer of dietary radiocaesium to milk. *Sci Total Environ.* 1989;85:339-347.
53. van der Merwe CF. The treatment of thallium poisoning. A report of 2 cases. *S Afr Med J.* 1972;46:560-561.
54. Vergauwe PL, Knockaert DC, Van Tittelboom TJ. Near fatal subacute thallium poisoning necessitating prolonged mechanical ventilation. *Am J Emerg Med.* 1990;8:548-550.
55. Verzijl JM, Joore JC, van Dijk A, et al. In vitro binding characteristics for cesium of two qualities of Prussian blue, activated charcoal and Resonium-A. *J Toxicol Clin Toxicol.* 1992;30:215-222.
56. Verzijl JM, Joore HC, van Dijk A, et al. In vitro cyanide release of four Prussian blue salts used for the treatment of cesium contaminated persons. *J Toxicol Clin Toxicol.* 1993;31:553-562.
57. Verzijl JM, Wierckx FC, van Dijk A, Glerum JH. In vitro binding of radiocesium to Prussian blue coated strips and Prussian blue containing hemoperfusion columns as a potential tool for the treatment of persons internally contaminated with radiocesium. *Artif Org.* 1995;19:86-93.
58. Wainwright AP, Kox WJ, House IM, et al. Clinical features and therapy of acute thallium poisoning. *Q J Med.* 1988;69:939-944.
59. Yang Y, Brownell C, Sadrieh N, May J, Del A. Quantitative measurement of cyanide released from Prussian blue. *Clin Toxicol.* 2007;45:776-781.
60. Yang Y, Faustino PJ, Progar JJ, et al. Quantitative determination of thallium binding to ferric hexacyanoferrate: Prussian blue. *Int J Pharm.* 2008;353:187-194.

CHAPTER 101
ZINC

Nima Majlesi

Zinc (Zn)

Atomic number	=	30
Atomic weight	=	65.37 daltons
Normal concentrations		
Blood	=	800 ± 200 μg/dL (122 ± 30 μmol/L)
Serum	=	109–130 μg/dL (16.7–20 μmol/L)
Urine (24 hour)	<	500 μg/d (<77 μmol/L)

Zinc is a ubiquitous element that is physiologically important to normal human function. However, zinc exposure can result in multiple consequential toxicities that are dependent on the dose and route. The typical systems affected are the respiratory, hematopoietic, and neurologic. Recent medical literature has contributed to the current knowledge of these effects.

HISTORY AND EPIDEMIOLOGY

The Babylonians used zinc alloys more than 5000 years ago,[1] and references to zinc oxide as a lotion to heal lesions around the eye can be found in the Ebers papyrus, written in 1500 B.C.[15] Zinc oxide and zinc sulfate were used in Western Europe during the late 1700s and early 1800s for gleet (urethral discharge), vaginal exudates, and convulsions. In the late 1800s, brass workers who inhaled zinc oxide fumes were noted to develop "zinc fever," "brass founders' ague," and "smelter shakes," all of which are now identified as metal fume fever (Chap. 124).[57]

Throughout history, humans have contaminated the environment with zinc. For example, release of zinc and other metals from mines produces elevated concentrations of zinc in the local water supply and vegetation, which may lead to elevated tissue zinc concentrations and clinical effects in the nearby population.[40,51]

The antiinflammatory effects of zinc sulfate were studied with mixed results in the late 1970s for acne vulgaris. However, a double-blinded controlled study found no difference between zinc and placebo.[63] The more recent use of zinc supplementation as an alternative preventive and treatment strategy is exposing large numbers of patients to undefined risks for unclear benefits.

CHEMISTRY

Zinc, a transition metal, has two common oxidation states, Zn^0 (elemental or metallic) and Zn^{2+}. Like other transition metals iron (Chap. 40) and copper (Chap. 93), zinc participates in reactions that result in the generation of reactive oxygen species. Such as superoxide radicals or hydroxyl radicals which can damage both local and remote tissues (Chapter 11).

The pure element exists as a blue to white shiny metal, but it also combines with other elements to form many compounds: zinc chloride ($ZnCl_2$), zinc oxide (ZnO), zinc sulfate ($ZnSO_4$), and zinc sulfide (ZnS). Once the metal is exposed to moisture, it becomes coated with zinc oxide or carbonate ($ZnCO_3$).[71]

PHARMACOLOGY AND PHYSIOLOGY

Zinc is an essential nutrient and found in more than 200 metalloenzymes, including acid phosphatase, alkaline phosphatase, alcohol dehydrogenase, carbonic anhydrase, superoxide dismutase, and DNA and RNA polymerases.[71] Zinc contributes to gene expression and chelates with either cysteine or histidine in a tetrahedral configuration, forming looped structures known as *zinc fingers*, which bind to specific DNA regions.[8,87] Other functions of zinc include membrane stabilization, vitamin A metabolism, and the development and maintenance of the nervous system. Zinc and copper concentrations generally have an inverse relationship in the serum with elevated zinc concentrations resulting in decreased copper concentrations (Chap. 93). Zinc accumulates in erythrocytes resulting in whole blood concentrations 6- to 7-fold higher than those in the serum.[59]

The average daily intake of zinc in the United States is 5.2–16.2 mg; foods that contain zinc include leafy vegetables (2 ppm), meats, fish, and poultry (29 ppm).[71] The recommended daily allowance is 11 mg/d for men and 8 mg/d for women. Pregnant and nursing women require 12 mg/d.

Zinc is important in maintaining olfactory and gustatory function (see Chap. 20). Serum, urine, and salivary zinc concentrations are lower in patients with dysfunctional senses of smell or taste. This is thought to be related to an abnormality in a salivary growth factor known as gustin/carbonic anhydrase VI.[30] Because this enzyme is zinc dependent, oral zinc may produce subjective improvement in taste and smell in patients with a known decrease in parotid gustin/carbonic anhydrase VI complex.[31] Oral zinc sulfate also improved subjective findings in a group of 25 patients with posttraumatic olfactory disorders.[4]

Zinc is also considered important for fetal growth. When 29 pregnant mothers who were at risk for small-for-gestational-age babies were given zinc citrate, zinc sulfate, or zinc aspartate, no intrauterine growth retardation was observed.[77] Subsequent studies have shown that zinc supplementation in women with low serum zinc concentrations in early pregnancy is associated with greater infant birth weights and head circumferences.[27] No adverse reproductive effects were observed in a rodent model exposed to inhalational zinc oxide.[54]

The role of zinc within the immune system is undefined. Zinc may be effective in the treatment of nonspecific infectious diarrhea, and specifically in the management of *Shigella* by improving the shigellacidal antibody response and increasing circulating B lymphocyte and plasma cells.[69,70]

Zinc – and zinc acetate–containing lozenges are sold as dietary supplements with conflicting evidence that they can shorten the duration of the "common cold."[36,53] One placebo-controlled study found that zinc nasal gel shortened the duration of viral syndromes when applied within 24 hours of the onset of symptoms.[32]

Zinc deficiency, or hypozincemia, is a well-described clinical entity. It can either be inherited as an autosomal recessive pattern known as acrodermatitis enteropathica, or develop due to a defect in zinc absorption in the GI tract.[64] Those patients at risk for acquiring the disorder include patients who receive total parenteral nutrition without adequate zinc supplementation, patients who have undergone intestinal bypass procedures, those with Crohn disease, and premature infants with low zinc storage. Physical findings that suggest the diagnosis of zinc deficiency, regardless of etiology, include the triad of dermatitis (acral and perioral), diarrhea, and alopecia. Zinc salts in initial doses of 5–10 mg/kg/d of elemental zinc followed by maintenance doses of 1–2 mg/kg/d are highly effective; in fact, skin lesions typically heal within 2–4 weeks and hair growth also restarts during this time frame.

The FDA approved zinc acetate in 1997 for maintenance therapy of Wilson disease, a disorder associated with copper overload.[9,49] Its use in this disorder is related to the ability of zinc to induce the formation of metallothionein, which assists in the elimination of copper from the blood and body tissues (Chap. 93)[5] (see next section for further discussion).

TOXICOKINETICS AND PATHOPHYSIOLOGY

When ingested the main site of zinc absorption is the jejunum, although absorption is reported to occur throughout the intestine by binding to metallothionein as a zinc–protein complex in the luminal cells.[86] Metallothionein is a family of specific metal-binding proteins with diverse and complex functions considered essential to metal homeostasis. Metallothioneins are of low molecular weight (3500–14000 Da) and are rich in thiol ligands; it is these ligands that allow high-affinity binding to metals such as zinc, copper, cadmium, mercury, and silver. Excess zinc absorption leads to upregulation of metallothioneins as a counterregulatory mechanism to prevent zinc overload. However, the affinity of other metals, especially copper, is higher for metallothionein, resulting is copper elimination. The primary route of excretion of the copper–metallothionein complex is fecal. The fecal loss of the zinc–metallothionein complex appears to also be the primary route of excretion with a small percentage excreted in the urine. Very little metallothionein is bound to zinc in the blood as it is primarily an intracellular cytosolic molecule. This appears to play a role in the peripheral utilization of zinc once it has been absorbed.[24] Albumin binds about two-thirds of zinc in the plasma and the remainder is bound to α_2-globulins.[71] Zinc concentrations in the body show a great variability by organ, with the prostate having the highest amount due to its high concentration of the zinc-containing enzyme acid phosphatase.[6]

The possibility of an inherited zinc overload syndrome has been proposed;[67,68,78] researchers believe the pattern of inheritance is either autosomal recessive or autosomal dominant with low penetrance or the development of new mutations. Whether the pathophysiology is analogous to the iron overload of hematochromatosis or to the copper overload with subsequent decreased zinc excretion of Wilson disease remains to be determined.

Zinc salts are used to enhance the solubility of pharmaceuticals such as insulin. Certain salts, such as zinc oxide, are used in baby powder, sun blocks, and topical burn preparations, and may be used on latex and latex-free gloves.

CLINICAL MANIFESTATIONS

The toxicity of zinc is dependent on the route of exposure. Each zinc compound has similar toxic manifestations following oral and dermal exposure; however, they have unique inhalational toxicities. The metallic form of zinc is not toxic per se, and only the salt forms are considered here unless otherwise specifically mentioned.

ACUTE

The hallmark of acute oral zinc (Zn^{2+}) toxicity is gastrointestinal (GI) distress, including nausea, vomiting, abdominal pain, and gastrointestinal bleeding.[6] In initial studies that evaluated the oral use of zinc sulfate ($ZnSO_4$) as an acne therapy, epigastric distress was noted in 33% of patients.[20,26] In a separate case report, a patient developed GI bleeding within a week of initiation of zinc sulfate at a therapeutic dose of 220 mg twice a day.[60] Zinc chloride solutions in concentrations greater than 20% are particularly corrosive when ingested. Partial- and full-thickness burns to the oral mucosa, pharynx, esophagus, and stomach, as well as to the laryngotracheal tree, can occur even following small unintentional ingestions of zinc chloride by children.[18,42,58] Delayed gastric stricture may occur after acute[58] or chronic zinc chloride consumption.[17] Pancreatitis was noted in a piglet model[25] and also in a 24-year-old man who inadvertently ingested liquid zinc chloride.[18] Hyperamylasemia, pulmonary edema, hypotension, vomiting, diarrhea, jaundice, anemia, thrombocytopenia, and subsequent death occurred following an unintentional intravenous infusion of 7.4 grams of zinc sulfate (via total parenteral nutrition) over 60 hours. The patient's serum zinc concentration was 4184 μg/dL.[10]

Inhalational toxicity will often depend on the type of zinc compound involved in the exposure. The water solubility of the various zinc salts plays an important role in the extent and time to onset of pulmonary toxicity. The solubility of zinc chloride in water at 25°C is 432 g/100 mL whereas that of zinc oxide at 29°C is 0.00016 g/100 mL.[71] Acute inhalation of zinc chloride aerosol from smoke bombs produces lacrimation, rhinitis, dyspnea, stridor, and retrosternal chest pain. Upper respiratory tract inflammation, acute lung injury (ALI), and acute respiratory distress syndrome (ARDS) may occur, generally with no manifestations of systemic absorption in the liver or kidneys.[33,35,55] Morbidity and mortality increase when the exposure to a zinc chloride aerosol occurs in an enclosed space.[74] Of 70 individuals exposed to a zinc chloride smoke bomb in a tunnel during World War II, 10 died within 4 days. Ambient zinc concentrations in the tunnel were measured at 33,000 mg/m^3.[21] Inhalation of zinc oxide, a far less water-soluble zinc salt, is associated with metal fume fever (see Chap. 124) and not pneumonitis despite similar ambient zinc concentrations[6] (see later for further discussion on metal fume fever).

Animal research suggests that intranasal zinc sulfate use can cause transient or persistent anosmia as a consequence of disruption of functional connections between the main olfactory bulb and the olfactory epithelium.[56] Topical zinc sulfate is used experimentally in both rat and mouse models to eliminate olfactory input.[84] Multiple patients, ages 31–55 years, who developed a burning sensation after intranasal zinc gluconate application to the olfactory epithelium later developed either a long-lasting or permanent anosmia and olfactory dysfunction.[39]

US pennies lodged in the distal esophagus release reactive zinc ions following exposure to gastric acids and can damage the local esophageal tissue.[14] The phenomenon of acid dissolution is demonstrated in animal[2] and in vitro models.[62]

Rare reports of renal complications exist. Hematuria was observed in a 24-year-old man who ingested liquid zinc chloride but whose renal function remained otherwise normal.[18] Intentional intravenous zinc sulfate administration can result in acute tubular necrosis and renal failure.[10]

Certain zinc salts, such as zinc oxide, found in baby powders and calamine lotion, are usually nonirritating for intact skin.[3] Although older studies suggested the possibility of pruritic, pustular rashes in workers who are exposed to zinc oxide, other causative factors, including personal hygiene, were not considered.[82] One case report describes urticaria and angioedema in a 34-year-old welder following contact with zinc oxides fumes at a smelting plant.[22] The patient was asymptomatic once he was removed from the environment and had no further difficulty during the welding process when personal protective equipment was employed.

CHRONIC

Chronic zinc toxicity following nutritional supplements and the ingestion of coins can produce a reversible sideroblastic anemia, as well as a reversible myelodysplastic syndrome.[11] Both anemia and granulocytopenia occur with the bone marrow showing vacuolated precursors and ringed sideroblasts; the mechanism appears to be zinc-induced copper deficiency.[23]

A 55-year-old schizophrenic patient with a 15-year history of pica (typically metal objects) presented with pancytopenia, including a hemoglobin of 3 g/dL and a white blood cell count of 1300/mm^3.[43]

A serum zinc concentration of 280 μg/mL and low serum copper concentration of <0.05 μg/mL reflected his ingestion of zinc-containing coins over many years. The patient refused surgery to remove the coins which formed a massive bezoar in his GI tract. Meat tenderizer and pancreatin were given in an unsuccessful to attempt to loosen the objects. Throughout his medical therapy the patient continued to ingest coins. Despite treatment efforts, he died of sepsis and multiorgan failure; an autopsy revealed a coin mass weighing 1870 g in his stomach and another bezoar at the site of a sigmoid volvulus. A 17-year-old boy who used megadoses of oral vitamins and mineral supplements containing zinc to treat acne over a 6–7 month period developed copper deficiency and anemia, leukopenia, and neutropenia.[73] A 28-month-old boy developed anemia, neutropenia, and developmental delay after 11 months of oral zinc gluconate. The parents were administering 314 mg/d of oral zinc gluconate (3.6 mg/kg/d of elemental zinc).[80] Hyperzincemia and hypocupremia were present and improved after discontinuation of zinc without copper supplementation.

It is suggested that zinc and other transition metals may be important in the pathogenesis of demyelinating diseases.[45,67] Clusters of cases of multiple sclerosis (MS) were described in northern New York in a factory where zinc was the primary occupational exposure. One hypothesis is that the allele frequency for transferrin (an iron- and zinc-binding protein) may differ in these MS patients.[75,79] Another cluster was found in Canada where excess metals, including zinc, were found in the soil and water.[28,38,37] A conclusive link to MS, however, has not been established.

Since the prostate contains the highest concentration of zinc in the human body, the role of zinc in the development of prostate cancer has been investigated. Specifically, American men participating in the Health Professionals Follow-Up Study were followed for 14 years, from 1986 to 2000. Of the 46,974 in the cohort, 2901 new cases of prostatic cancer were diagnosed, with 434 of them considered to be in an advanced stage.[50] Men who used zinc supplementation at a dose greater than 100 mg/d had a relative risk of 2.29 for advanced prostate cancer, and those using zinc for longer than 10 years had a relative risk of 2.37. To date, neither the International Agency for Research on Cancer (IARC) nor the Environmental Protection Agency (EPA) have classified zinc as a carcinogen.

A syndrome of progressive myeloneuropathy called *swayback* is defined by a spastic gait and a prominent sensory ataxia.[44,45,47,48] This neurologic syndrome may exist without the hematologic manifestations. These cases involve patients with copper deficiency, with a majority having a concomitant elevated serum zinc concentration. Though a history of excess zinc exposure could be obtained in some of the patients, many had no such history. The potential of an inherited zinc overload syndrome has been considered.[29] A 46-year-old man presented with evidence of bone marrow suppression followed by sensory ataxia and a progressive myelopathy. His neuroimaging evaluation was normal. His only remarkable laboratory studies included an elevated serum zinc concentration of 184 μg/dL (28.2 μmol/L) and a low copper concentration of less than 10 μg/dL (<2 μmol/L). There was no known exposure to or supplementation of zinc by history. Although his copper deficit improved with copper therapy, hyperzincemia persisted for more than 3 years that he was followed.

An unusual source of high concentration zinc that has recently been identified is denture creams, which may contain as much as 34 grams of zinc per gram of cream. Four patients with chronic exposure to excess denture cream were described to develop neurological abnormalities in the setting of hyperzincemia with associated hypocupremia.[61]

OCCUPATIONAL EXPOSURES

The United States penny currently contains 97.5% zinc and 2.5% copper.[83] Zinc is widely used in industry because it enhances the durability of iron and steel alloys; it also is commonly used in construction. Galvanization involves coating an iron product with metallic zinc to prevent it from oxidizing (rusting). Zinc is routinely encountered by electroplaters, smelters, jewelers, artists working on stained glass or sculpting metal, as well as aircraft manufacturing workers. Zinc chloride is commonly a component of flux which can be used for soldering galvanized iron.

Zinc is present in drinking water, and beverages stored in metal containers or that flow through pipes coated with zinc. Zinc concentrations in air are typically low; average zinc concentrations in the United States are less than 1 μg/m^3. Air concentrations near industrial areas can be higher, and may be substantially greater in certain occupational settings. The currently accepted occupational threshold limit value (TLV) time-weighted average (TWA) is 1 mg/m^3.[71]

METAL FUME FEVER

Metal fume fever (MFF) typically occurs within 12 hours after an exposure to zinc fumes. Patients develop fever, chills, cough, chest pain, dyspnea, dry throat, and a metallic taste in the mouth. Although exposure to zinc oxide fume is the most commonly associated exposure with this syndrome, other zinc compounds and other metal oxides may be implicated. The chest radiograph is often normal, but may show an infiltrate. Hypoxia and tachycardia are rare, but may occur. Overall, however, the syndrome is relatively benign, with tolerance developing within days. An immune mechanism is suggested, and chronic exposure is needed for sensitization (Chap. 124).

DIAGNOSTIC TESTING

Because zinc is ubiquitous in the environment and laboratory, great care must be taken to avoid contamination of any samples for investigation.[71] Since elevated zinc concentrations cause copper deficiency, a serum copper and ceruloplasmin concentration should be obtained in patients with zinc poisoning.

Urine zinc concentrations are not well defined. In a cohort of non-occupationally exposed patients, the mean urine concentrations were 450 μg/L, with a maximum concentration up to 1300 μg/L.[59] In the United States, normal urine values are generally accepted as less than 500 μg/day. The National Institute for Occupational Safety and Health states that the detection limits in urine and blood are as low as 0.1 μg per sample and 1 μg/100 g, respectively. Testing requires extraction of the metals from urine with polydithiocarbamate resin prior to digestion with concentrated acids and analysis.[71]

Errors can be caused by incorrect sample collection, equipment malfunction or miscalibration, inadequate reagent purity, and atmospheric deposition. Zinc oxide powder in some gloves can contaminate specimens, as can the rubber stoppers in certain blood collection tubes. Specific tubes are recommended with negligibly low concentrations of trace elements.[16] During sample analysis, laminar flow is recommended to prevent airborne particles from interfering.

Abdominal radiographs may play a role in determining the gastrointestinal burden of zinc, especially with ingestions of pennies. This may guide the decision to continue gastrointestinal decontamination in certain circumstances[13] (see Management).

Neuroimaging in patients with chronic zinc exposure leading to copper deficiency may reveal characteristic findings. MRI typically reveals increased T_2 signal in the dorsal columns of the cervical cord similar to that found in B_{12} deficiency.[46] These lesions are thought to represent Wallerian degeneration and demyelination of white matter. One case showed evidence of bilateral subcortical hyperintense T_2 abnormalities on an MRI of the brain.[61] These findings are likely the result of copper deficiency and not necessarily zinc toxicity.

MANAGEMENT

Treatment for acute oral zinc (Zn^{2+}) toxicity is primarily supportive. Efforts should be focused on hydration, as well as on antiemetic therapy. H_2 receptor antagonists or proton pump inhibitors may relieve abdominal discomfort when given for several days following the zinc salt ingestion.[6]

Gastrointestinal decontamination after zinc salt ingestion may include whole-bowel irrigation (WBI). A radiograph in a 16-year-old boy who ingested 50 zinc sulfate tablets each containing 500 mg noted no change in their position 4 hours after gastric evacuation. Within 1 hour of institution of WBI therapy, zinc tablets were present in the rectal effluent.[13]

Intravenous *N*-acetylcysteine (NAC) increased the urinary zinc excretion in a patient who had inhaled zinc chloride smoke.[65] Two individuals with inhalational zinc chloride–induced ARDS had simultaneous transient decreases in serum zinc concentrations and increases in urinary zinc excretion with intravenous and nebulized NAC.[33] However, they succumbed at days 25 and 32 after inhalation. Although an increase in urinary zinc excretion was noted in one rat model, ten healthy volunteers who were treated with oral NAC for 2 weeks had no significant change in either their serum or urine zinc concentrations.[34] This therapy requires further study and cannot be recommended at this time.

The data regarding the efficacy of chelation therapy for zinc are limited in humans. Edetate calcium disodium ($CaNa_2EDTA$) was used successfully in several cases, including in a child who was exposed to zinc chloride that was a component of soldering flux[66] and in a 24-year-old man exposed to liquid zinc chloride.[18] The combination of $CaNa_2EDTA$ and British anti-Lewisite (BAL) was used successfully in a 16-month-old toddler 74 hours after ingestion.[58] Both diethylenetriaminepentaacetic acid (DTPA) and ethylenediaminetetraacetic acid (EDTA) were effective in enhancing the urinary excretion of zinc in a rodent model of zinc acetate poisoning.[19] DTPA had its greatest antidotal efficacy when given within 30 minutes of the intraperitoneal injection of zinc acetate.[52] The urinary excretion of zinc increased 1.6- to 44-fold following a 3 mg/kg intravenous dose of sodium 2,3-dimercaptopropane-1-sulfonate (DMPS) in one human study where metal toxicity in patients with dental amalgams was the focus.[81] Two potential zinc-selective chelators, DPESA (4-{[2-(bis-pyridin-2-ylmethylamino)ethylamino]-methyl} phenylmethanesulfonic acid) sodium salt, as well as TPESA (4-{[2-(bis-pyridin-2-ylmethylamino) ethyl]pyridine-2-ylmethylamino}-methyl)phenyl] methanesulfonic acid) sodium salt, rapidly chelate zinc in vitro, but further detailed in vivo studies are needed before its clinical use can be considered.[41] Finally, an iron-chelator, deferiprone, was incidentally noted to cause decreased serum zinc concentrations in a transfusion overload study.[85] A subsequent prospective trial showed enhanced urinary excretion of zinc in children with thalassemia major who had received multiple blood transfusions.[7]

Many of the clinical and systemic manifestations of zinc toxicity are due to its ability to cause copper deficiency. In patients with zinc overload–related copper deficiency, the supplementation of oral copper alone was able to improve the hematopoeitic effects and prevent further neurological deterioration without chelation therapy.[72]

Though treatment with copper sulfate alone may be adequate for patients with neurological sequelae and mild hematopoietic effects, the addition of chelation may be required for patients with hemodynamic compromise or other consequential systemic manifestations. Limited experience exists in regard to treatment of these patients; however, 1000 mg/m^2/d IV $CaNa_2EDTA$ divided every 6 hours seems to be a reasonable choice based on case reports of successful use. The role of BAL is unclear; however, its ability to potentially increase copper elimination should deter its use.

Supportive care is used for patients with inhalational zinc exposures, including oxygen therapy and bronchodilators as clinically indicated, but these patients may necessitate ventilatory support in severe cases. Exposure to zinc oxide vapors by rescuers is minimal, although respiratory protective equipment should be worn.[76] In a case series of five soldiers exposed to zinc chloride during military training, the two individuals not wearing gas masks developed ARDS;[33] the others remained clinically well.

Metal fume fever is typically self-limited. Nonsteroidal antiinflammatory drugs should be sufficient to relieve the transient discomfort. Personal protection equipment and/or adequate engineering strategies may allow the individual to continue to work in this setting.

Dermal decontamination is paramount to prevent direct epidermal effects or systemic absorption of zinc salts.[12] However, water should not be used to perform dermal decontamination of patients exposed to metallic zinc because of concerns that zinc metal will ignite when wet. Treatment in these situations includes mechanical removal of any metallic particles with forceps and the application of mineral oil to the affected skin to protect the metal from ambient moisture.

SUMMARY

Zinc is a ubiquitous element. Exposures to humans occur as part of the diet, medicinal uses, nutritional supplements, and in occupational settings. Clinical manifestations include acute, life-threatening gastrointestinal and pulmonary effects, which are generally treated with supportive care. Copper supplementation alone often corrects systemic manifestations, but chelation therapy may be considered in acutely life-threatening circumstances.

REFERENCES

1. Abdel-Mageed AB, Oehme FW. A review of the biochemical roles, toxicity and interactions of zinc, copper and iron: I. Zinc. *Vet Hum Toxicol.* 1990;32:34-39.
2. Agnew DW, Barbiers RB, Poppenga RH, et al. Zinc toxicosis in a captive striped hyena (*Hyaena hyaena*). *J Zoo Wildl Med.* 1999;30:431-434.
3. Agren MS. Percutaneous absorption of zinc from zinc oxide applied topically to intact skin in man. *Dermatologica.* 1990;180:36-39.
4. Aiba T SM, Mori J, et al. Effect of zinc sulfate on sensorineural olfactory disorder. *Acta Otolaryngol Suppl.* 1998;538:202-204.
5. Askari FK GJ, Dick RD, et al. Treatment of Wilson's disease with zinc. XVIII. Initial treatment of the hepatic decompensation presentation with trientine and zinc. *J Lab Clin Med.* 2003;142:385-390.
6. Barceloux D. Zinc. *J Toxicol Clin Toxicol.* 1999;37:279-292.
7. Bartakke S BS, Kondurkar P, et al. Effect of deferiprone on urinary zinc excretion in multiply transfused children with thalassemia major. *Indian Pediatr.* 2005;42:150-154.
8. Berg JM SY. The galvanization of biology: a growing appreciation for the roles of zinc. *Science.* 1996;271:1081-1085.
9. Brewer G. Neurologically presenting Wilson's disease: epidemiology, pathophysiology, and treatment. *CNS Drugs.* 2005;19:185-192.
10. Brocks A, Reid H, Glazer G. Acute intravenous zinc poisoning. *BMJ.* 1977;1:1390-1391.
11. Broun ER, Greist A, Tricot G, et al. Excessive zinc ingestion. A reversible cause of sideroblastic anemia and bone marrow depression. *JAMA.* 1990;264:1441-1443.
12. Burgess JL, Kirk M, Borron SW, et al. Emergency department hazardous material protocol for contaminated patients. *Ann Emerg Med.* 1999;34:205-212.
13. Burkhart KK, Kulig KM, Rumack B. Whole bowel irrigation as treatment for zinc sulfate overdose. *Ann Emerg Med.* 1990;19:1167-1170.
14. Cantu S, Connors GP. The esophageal coin: is it a penny? *Am Surg.* 2002;68:417-420.

15. Cassel GH. Zinc: a review of current trends in therapy and our knowledge of its toxicity. *Del Med J.* 1978;50:323-328.
16. Chan S, Gerson B, Subramaniam S. The role of copper, molybdenum, selenium, and zinc in nutrition and health. *Clin Lab Med.* 1998;18:673-685.
17. Chew LS, Lim HS, Wong CY, et al. Gastric stricture following zinc chloride ingestion. *Singapore Med J.* 1986;27:163-166.
18. Chobanian S. Accidental ingestion of liquid zinc chloride: local and systemic effects. *Ann Emerg Med.* 1981;10:91-93.
19. Domingo JL, Llobet JM, Paternain JL, et al. Acute zinc intoxication: comparison of the antidotal efficacy of several chelating agents. *Vet Hum Toxicol.* 1988;30:224-228.
20. Dreno B, Moyse D, Alirezai M, et al. Multicenter randomized comparative double-blind controlled clinical trial of the safety and efficacy of zinc gluconate versus minocycline hydrochloride in the treatment of inflammatory acne vulgaris. *Dermatology.* 2001;203:135-140.
21. Evans EH. Casualties following exposure to zinc chloride smoke. *Lancet.* 1945;2:368-370.
22. Farrell FJ. Angioedema and urticaria as acute and late phase reactions to zinc fume exposure, with associated metal fume fever-like symptoms. *Am J Ind Med.* 1987;12:331-337.
23. Fiske DN, McCoy HE, Kitchens CS. Zinc-induced sideroblastic anemia: a report of a case, review of the literature, and description of the hematologic syndrome. *Am J Hematol.* 1994;46:147-150.
24. Fosmire GJ. Zinc toxicity. *Am J Clin Nutr.* 1990;51:225-227.
25. Gabrielson KL, Remillard RL, Huso DL. Zinc toxicity with pancreatic acinar necrosis in piglets receiving total parental nutrition. *Vet Pathol.* 1996;33:692-696.
26. Glover SC, White MI. Zinc again. *BMJ.* 1977;2:640-641.
27. Goldenberg RL, Tamura T, Neggers Y, et al. The effect of zinc supplementation on pregnancy outcome. *JAMA.* 1995;274:463-468.
28. Hader WJ, Irvine DG, Schiefer HB. A cluster-focus of multiple sclerosis at Henribourg, Saskatchewan. *Can J Neurol Sci.* 1990;17:391-394.
29. Hedera P, Fink JK, Bockenstedt PL, et al. Myelopolyneuropathy and pancytopenia due to copper deficiency and high zinc levels of unknown origin: further support for existence of a new zinc overload syndrome. *Arch Neurol.* 2003;60:1301-1306.
30. Henkin RI, Martin BM, Agarwal RP. Decreased parotid saliva gustin/carbonic anhydrase VI secretion: an enzyme disorder manifested by gustatory and olfactory dysfunction. *Am J Med Sci.* 1999;18:380-391.
31. Henkin RI, Martin BM, Agarwal RP. Efficacy of exogenous oral zinc in treatment of patients with carbonic anhydrase VI deficiency. *Am J Med Sci.* 1999;18:392-405.
32. Hirt M, Nobel S, Barron E. Zinc nasal gel for the treatment of common cold symptoms: a double-blind, placebo-controlled trial. *Ear Nose Throat J.* 2000;79:778-780.
33. Hjortso E, Qvist J, Bud MI, et al. ARDS after accidental inhalation of zinc chloride smoke. *Intensive Care Med.* 1988;14:17-24.
34. Hjortso E, Fomsgaard JS, Fogh-Andersen N. Does N-acetylcysteine increase the excretion of trace metals (calcium, magnesium, iron, zinc and copper) when given orally? *Eur J Clin Pharmacol.* 1990;39:29-31.
35. Homma S, Jones R, Qvist J, et al. Pulmonary vascular lesions in the adult respiratory distress syndrome caused by inhalation of zinc chlo-ride smoke: a morphometric study. *Hum Pathol.* 1992;23:45-50.
36. Hulisz D. Efficacy of zinc against common cold viruses: an overview. *J Am Pharm Assoc.* 2004;44:594-603.
37. Irvine DG, Schiefer HB, Hader WJ. Geotoxicology of multiple sclerosis: the Henribourg, Saskatchewan, cluster focus II: the soil. *Sci Total Environ.* 1988;77:175-188.
38. Irvine DG, Schiefer HB, Hader WJ. Geotoxicology of multiple sclerosis: the Henribourg, Saskatchewan, cluster focus I: the water. *Sci Total Environ.* 1989;84:45-59.
39. Jafek BW, Linschoten MR, Murrow BW. Anosmia after intranasal zinc gluconate use. *Am J Rhinol.* 2004;18:137-141.
40. Kachur AN, Arzhanova VS, Yelpatyevsky PV, et al. Environmental conditions in the Rudnaya River watershed–a compilation of Soviet and post-Soviet era sampling around a lead smelter in the Russian Far East. *Sci Total Environ.* 2003;303:171-185.
41. Kawabata E, Kikuchi K, Urano Y, et al. Design and synthesis of zinc-selective chelators for extracellular applications. *J Am Chem Soc.* 2005;127:818-819.
42. Knapp JF, Kennedy C, Wasserman GS, et al. A toddler with caustic ingestion. *Pediatr Emerg Care.* 1994;10:54-58.
43. Kumar A, Jazieh AR. Case report of sideroblastic anemia caused by ingestion of coins. *Am J Hematol.* 2001;66:126-129.
44. Kumar N. Copper deficiency myelopathy (human swayback). *Mayo Clin Proc.* 2006;81:1371-1384.
45. Kumar N, Ahlskog JE. Myelopolyneuropathy due to copper deficiency or zinc excess? *Arch Neurol.* 2004;61:604-605.
46. Kumar N, Ahlskog J, Klein CJ, Port JD. Imaging features of copper deficiency myelopathy: a study of 25 cases. *Neuroradiology.* 2006;48:78-83.
47. Kumar N, Crum B, Petersen RC, Vernino SA, Ahlskog JE. Copper deficiency myelopathy. *Arch Neurol.* 2004;61:762-766.
48. Kumar N, Gross JB Jr, Ahlskog JE. Myelopathy due to copper deficiency. *Neurology.* 2003;61:273-274.
49. Leggio L, Addolorato G, Abenavoli L, et al. Wilson's disease: clinical, genetic and pharmacological findings. *Int J Immunopathol Pharmacol.* 2005;18:7-14.
50. Leitzmann MF, Stampfer MJ, Wu K, et al. Zinc supplement use and risk of prostate cancer. *J Natl Cancer Inst.* 2003;95:1004-1007.
51. Liu H, Probst A, Liao B. Metal contamination of soils and crops affected by the Chenzhou lead/zinc mine spill (Hunan, China). *Sci Total Environ.* 2005;339:153-166.
52. Llobet JM, Colomina MT, Domingo JL, et al. Comparison of the antidotal efficacy of polyamincarboxylic acids (CDTA and DTPA) with time after acute zinc poisoning. *Vet Hum Toxicol.* 1989;31:25-28.
53. Macknin ML, Piedmonte M, Calendine C, et al. Zinc gluconate lozenges for treating the common cold in children: Aa randomized controlled trial. *JAMA.* 1998;279:1962-1967.
54. Marrs TC, Colgrave HF, Edginton JA, et al. The repeated dose toxicity of a zinc oxide/hexachloroethane smoke. *Arch Toxicol.* 1988;1988:123-132.
55. Matarese SL, Matthews JI. Zinc chloride (smoke bomb) inhalational lung injury. *Chest.* 1986;89:308-309.
56. McBride K, Slotnick B, Margolis FL. Does intranasal application of zinc sulfate produce anosmia in the mouse? An olfactometric and anatomical study. *Chem Senses.* 2003;28:659-670.
57. McCord CP, Friedlander A. An occupational syndrome among workers in zinc. *Am J Public Health (N Y).* 1926;16:274-280.
58. McKinney PE, Brent J, Kulig K. Acute zinc chloride ingestion in a child: local and systemic effects. *Ann Emerg Med.* 1994;23:1383-1387.
59. Minoia C, Sabbioni E, Apostoli P, et al. Trace element reference values in tissues from inhabitants of the European Community I. A study of 46 elements in urine, blood, and serum of Italian subjects. *Sci Total Environ.* 1990;95:89-105.
60. Moore R. Bleeding gastric erosion after oral zinc sulphate. *BMJ.* 1978;1:754.
61. Nations SP, Boyer PJ, Love LA, et al. Denture cream: an unusual source of excess zinc, leading to hypocupremia and neurologic disease. *Neurology.* 2008;71:639-643.
62. O'Hara SM, Donnelly LF, Chuang E, et al. Gastric retention of zinc-based pennies: radiographic appearance and hazards. *Radiology.* 1999;213:113-117.
63. Orris L, Shalita AR, Sibulkin D, et al. Oral zinc therapy of acne. Absorption and clinical effect. *Arch Dermatol.* 1978;114:1018-1020.
64. Perafán-Riveros C, Franca LF, Fortes AC, et al. Acrodermatitis enteropathica: case report and review of the literature. *Pediatr Dermatol.* 2002;19:426-431.
65. Pettila V, Takkunen O, Tukiainen P. Zinc chloride smoke inhalation: a rare cause of severe acute respiratory distress syndrome. *Intensive Care Med.* 2000;26:215-217.
66. Potter J. Acute zinc chloride ingestion in a young child. *Ann Emerg Med.* 1981;10:267-269.
67. Prodan CI, Holland NR. CNS demyelination from zinc toxicity? *Neurology.* 2000;54:1705-1706.
68. Prodan CI HN, Wisdom PJ, et al. CNS demyelination associated with copper deficiency and hyperzincemia. *Neurology.* 2002;59:1453-1456.
69. Rahman MJ, Sarker P, Roy SK, et al. Effects of zinc supplementation as adjunct therapy on the systemic immune responses in shigellosis. *Am J Clin Nutr.* 2005;81:495-502.
70. Raqib R, Roy SK, Rahman MJ, et al. Effect of zinc supplementation on immune and inflammatory responses in pediatric patients with shigellosis. *Am J Clin Nutr.* 2004;79:444-450.
71. Roney N, Osier M, Paikoff SJ, et al. ATSDR evaluation of potential for human exposure to zinc. *Toxicol Ind Health.* 2007;23:247-308.
72. Rowin J, Lewis SL. Copper deficiency myeloneuropathy and pancytopenia secondary to overuse of zinc supplementation. *J Neurol Neurosurg Psychiatry.* 2005;76:750-751.

73. Salzman MB, Smith EM, Koo C. Excessive oral zinc supplementation. *J Pediatr Hematol Oncol.* 2002;24:582-584.
74. Schenker MB, Speizer FE, Taylor JO. Acute upper respiratory symptoms resulting from exposure to zinc chloride aerosol. *Environ Res.* 1981;25:317-324.
75. Schiffer RB. Zinc and multiple sclerosis. *Neurology.* 1994;44:1987-1988.
76. Schultz M, Cisek J, Wabeke R. Simulated exposure of hospital emergency personnel to solvent vapors and respirable dust during decontamination of chemically exposed patents. *Ann Emerg Med.* 1995;26:324-329.
77. Simmer K, Lort-Phillips L, James C, et al. A double-blind trial of zinc supplementation in pregnancy. *Eur J Clin Nutr.* 1991;45:139-144.
78. Smith JC, Zeller JA, Brown ED, et al. Elevated plasma zinc: a heritable anomaly. *Science.* 1976;193:496-498.
79. Stein EC, Schiffer RB, Hall WJ, et al. Multiple sclerosis and the workplace: report of an industry-based cluster. *Neurology.* 1987;37:1672-1677.
80. Sugiura T, Goto K, Ito K, Ueta A, Fujimoto S, Togari H. Chronic zinc toxicity in an infant who received zinc therapy for atopic dermatitis. *Acta Paediatr.* 2005;94:1333-1335.
81. Torres-Alanis O, Garza-Ocanas L, Bernal MA, et al. Urinary excretion of trace elements after sodium 2,3-dimercaptoproprane-1-sulfonate challenge test. *J Toxicol Clin Toxicol.* 2000;38:697-700.
82. Turner JA. An occupational dermatoconiosis among zinc oxide workers. *Public Health Rep.* 1921;36:2727-2732.
83. United States Department of the Treasury USM. The Composition of the Cent. http://usmintgov/about_the_mint/fun_facts/indexcfm?flash=no&action=fun_facts2. 2004.
84. Van Denderen JCM, Van Wieringen GW, Hillen B, et al. Zinc sulphate-induced anosmia decreases the nerve fibre density in the anterior cerebral artery of the rat. *Auton Neurosci.* 2001;10:102-108.
85. Victor Hoffbrand A. Deferiprone therapy for transfusional iron overload. *Best Pract Res Clin Haematol.* 2005;18:299-317.
86. Walsh CT, Sandstead HH, Prasad H, et al. Zinc. Health effects and research priorities for the 1990s. *Environ Health Perspect.* 1994;102:5-46.
87. Wang R HD, Cukerman E, et al. Identification of genes encoding zinc finger motifs in the cardiovascular system. *J Mol Cell Cardiol.* 1997;86:281-287.

J.

HOUSEHOLD PRODUCTS

CHAPTER 102

ANTISEPTICS, DISINFECTANTS, AND STERILANTS

Paul M. Wax

INTRODUCTION

Antiseptics, disinfectants, and sterilants are a diverse group of antimicrobials used to prevent infection (Table 102–1). Although these terms are sometimes used interchangeably and some of these xenobiotics are used for both antisepsis and disinfection, the distinguishing characteristics between the groups are important to emphasize. An *antiseptic* is a chemical that is applied to living tissue to kill or inhibit microorganisms. Iodophors, chlorhexidine, and the alcohols (ethanol and isopropanol) are commonly used antiseptics. A *disinfectant* is a chemical or physical agent that is applied to inanimate objects to kill microorganisms. Bleach (sodium hypochlorite), phenolic compounds, and formaldehyde are examples of currently used disinfectants. Neither antiseptics nor disinfectants have complete sporicidal activity. A *sterilant* is a chemical or physical process that is applied to inanimate objects to kill all microorganisms as well as spores. Ethylene oxide and glutaraldehyde are examples of sterilants. Not unexpectedly many of the xenobiotics used to kill microorganisms also demonstrate considerable human toxicity.[17,60]

The use of these xenobiotics evolved during the 20th century as their toxicity and the principles of microbiology became better understood. Two of the more toxic antiseptics—iodine and phenol—were gradually replaced by the less toxic iodophors and substituted phenols. The use of mercuric chloride was superseded by the organic mercurials (eg, merbromin, thimerosal), which also proved toxic. In recent years, newer compounds, such as quaternary ammonium compounds, ethylene oxide, and glutaraldehyde, have become more extensively used.

ANTISEPTICS

CHLORHEXIDINE

This cationic biguanide has been in use as an antiseptic since the early 1950s. It is found in a variety of skin cleansers, usually as a 4% emulsion (eg, Hibiclens), and may also be found in mouthwash. Chlorhexidine is reported to have low toxicity.

Clinical Effects Few cases of deliberate ingestion of chlorhexidine are reported. Symptoms are usually mild and gastrointestinal irritation is the most likely effect after oral ingestion.[23] Chlorhexidine has poor enteral absorption. In one case, ingestion of 150 mL of a 20% chlorhexidine gluconate solution resulted in oral cavity edema and significant irritant injury of the esophagus.[111] In the same case, liver enzymes concentrations rose to 30 times normal on the fifth day after ingestion. Liver biopsy showed lobular necrosis and fatty degeneration. In another case, the ingestion of 30 mL of a 4% solution by an 89-year-old woman did not result in any GI injury.[44] An 80-year-old woman with dementia ingested 200 mL of a 5% chlorhexidine solution and subsequently aspirated.[70] She rapidly developed hypotension, respiratory distress, coma, and died 12 hours following ingestion.

Intravenous administration of chlorhexidine is associated with hemolysis, although this may be caused by the hypotonicity of the injected solution,[25] and acute respiratory distress syndrome.[80] Inhalation of vaporized chlorhexidine is reported to cause methemoglobinemia as a consequence of the conversion of chlorhexidine to *p*-chloraniline.[183] In one patient, the rectal administration of 4% chlorhexidine resulted in acute colitis with ulcerations.[59]

Topical absorption of chlorhexidine is negligible. Contact dermatitis is reported in up to 8% of patients who received repetitive topical applications of chlorhexidine.[60] More ominously, anaphylactic reactions, including shock, are associated with dermal application.[6,128] Some of these cases of chlorhexidine-related anaphylaxis occurred during surgery, appearing 15–45 minutes after application of the antiseptic.[12] Eye exposure may result in corneal damage.[177]

Management Treatment guidelines for chlorhexidine exposure are similar to those for other potential caustics. Patients with significant symptoms may require endoscopy, but the need for such extensive evaluation is quite uncommon.

HYDROGEN PEROXIDE

Hydrogen peroxide, an oxidizer with weak antiseptic properties, has been used for many years as an antiseptic and a disinfectant.[187] This oxidizer is generally available in two strengths: dilute hydrogen peroxide, with a concentration of 3%–9% by weight (usually 3%), sold for home use, and concentrated hydrogen peroxide, with a concentration greater than 10%, used primarily for industrial purposes. Commercial-strength hydrogen peroxide is commonly found in solutions varying from 27.5%–70%. Home uses for dilute hydrogen peroxide include ear cerumen removal, mouth gargle, vaginal douche, enema, and hair bleaching. Dilute hydrogen peroxide is also sometimes used as a veterinary emetic. Commercial uses of the more concentrated solutions include bleaching and cleansing textiles and wool, and producing foam rubber and rocket fuel. A 35% hydrogen peroxide solution is also available to the general public in health food stores and is sold as "hyperoxygenation therapy" and as a health food additive to aerate health food drinks.[76] This potentially dangerous therapy is touted as a treatment for a variety of conditions, including AIDS and cancer.

TABLE 102–1. Antiseptics, Disinfectants, Sterilants, and Related Xenobiotics

Xenobiotic	Commercial Product	Use	Toxic Effects	Therapeutics and Evaluation
Acids				
Boric acid	Borax Sodium perborate Dobell solution	Antiseptic Mouthwash Eyewash Roach powder	Blue-green emesis and diarrhea Boiled lobster appearance of skin CNS depression; renal failure	GI decontamination Hemodialysis (rare)
Alcohols (Chaps. 77 and 107)				
Ethanol	Rubbing alcohol (70% ethanol)	Antiseptic Disinfectant	CNS depression Respiratory depression Dermal irritant	Supportive
Isopropanol	Rubbing alcohol (70% isopropanol)	Antiseptic Disinfectant	CNS depression Respiratory depression Ketonemia, ketonuria GI irritation/bleeding Hemorrhagic tracheobronchitis	Supportive Hemodialysis (rare)
Aldehydes				
Formaldehyde	Formalin (37% formaldehyde, 12%–15% methanol)	Disinfectant Fixative Urea insulation	Caustic CNS depression Carcinogen	Gastric lavage Hemodialysis Sodium bicarbonate Endoscopy Folinic acid
Glutaraldehyde	Cidex (2% glutaraldehyde)	Sterilant	Mucosal and dermal irritant	Supportive
Chlorinated Compounds				
Chlorhexidine	Hibiclens	Antiseptic	GI irritation	Supportive
Chlorates	Sodium chlorate Potassium chlorate	Antiseptic Matches Herbicide	Hemolytic anemia Methemoglobinemia Renal failure	Exchange transfusion Hemodialysis
Chlorine		Disinfectant	Irritant	Supportive
Chlorophors (sodium hypochlorite)	Household bleach (5% NaOCl)	Disinfectant	Mild GI irritation	Endoscopy (rare)
	Dakin solution (1 part 5% NaOCl, 10 parts H_2O)	Decontaminating solution		
Ethylene Oxide		Sterilant Plasticizer	Irritant CNS depression Peripheral neuropathy Carcinogen?	Supportive
Mercurials (Chaps. 55 and 96)	Merbromin 2% (Mercurochrome)	Antiseptic (obsolete)	CNS	Gastric lavage, activated charcoal dimercaprol, succimer
	Thimerosal (Merthiolate)		Renal	
Iodinated Compounds				
Iodine	Tincture of iodine (2% iodine, 2% sodium iodide and 50% ethanol) Lugol solution (5% iodine)	Antiseptic	Caustic	Milk, starch, sodium thiosulfate Endoscopy
Iodophors	Povidone-iodine (Betadine) (0.01% iodine)	Antiseptic	Limited	Same as iodine

TABLE 102–1. Antiseptics, Disinfectants, Sterilants, and Related Xenobiotics (*Continued*)

Xenobiotic	Commercial Product	Use	Toxic Effects	Therapeutics and Evaluation
Oxidants				
Hydrogen peroxide	H_2O_2 3%–household H_2O_2 30%–industrial	Disinfectant	Oxygen emboli GI caustic	Gastric lavage Radiographic evaluation Endoscopy
Potassium permanganate	Crystals, solution	Antiseptic	Oxidizer, caustic, increased serum manganese	Decontamination Endoscopy as needed
Phenols				
Nonsubstituted	Phenol (carbolic acid)	Disinfectant	Caustic Dermal burns Cutaneous absorption CNS effects	Decontamination: polyethylene glycol or water Endoscopy as needed
Substituted	Hexachlorophene	Disinfectant	CNS effects	Supportive
Quaternary Ammonium Compounds				
Benzalkonium chloride	Zephiran	Disinfectant	GI caustic	Consider endoscopy

Toxicity from hydrogen peroxide may occur after ingestion or wound irrigation. Hydrogen peroxide has two main mechanisms of toxicity: local tissue injury and gas formation. The extent of local tissue injury and amount of gas formation is determined by the concentration of the hydrogen peroxide. Dilute hydrogen peroxide is an irritant and concentrated hydrogen peroxide is a caustic. Gas formation results when hydrogen peroxide interacts with tissue catalase, liberating molecular oxygen, and water. At standard temperature and pressure, 1 mL of 3% hydrogen peroxide liberates 10 mL of oxygen, whereas 1 mL of the more concentrated 35% hydrogen peroxide liberates more than 100 mL of oxygen. Gas formation can result in life-threatening embolization. Gas embolization may be a result of dissection of gas under pressure into the tissues or of liberation of gas in the tissue or blood following absorption. The use of hydrogen peroxide in partially closed spaces, such as operative wounds, or its use under pressure during wound irrigation increases the likelihood of embolization.

Clinical Effects Airway compromise manifested by stridor, drooling, apnea, and radiographic evidence of subepiglottic narrowing may occur.[39] The combination of local tissue injury and gas formation from the ingestion of concentrated hydrogen peroxide may cause abdominal bloating, abdominal pain, vomiting, and hematemesis.[77,105] Endoscopy may show esophageal edema and erythema and significant gastric mucosal erosions.[153]

Symptoms consistent with sudden oxygen embolization include rapid deterioration in mental status, cyanosis, respiratory failure, seizures, ischemic ECG changes, and acute paraplegia.[48,102] A 2-year-old boy died after ingesting 120–180 mL of 35% hydrogen peroxide.[27] Antemortem chest radiography showed gas in the right ventricle, mediastinum, and portal venous system. Portal vein gas is also a prominent feature in other cases.[76,105] Arterialization of oxygen gas embolization may result in cerebral infarction.[159] Encephalopathy with cortical visual impairment[21] and bilateral hemispheric infarctions detected by MRI imaging may occur after ingestion of concentrated hydrogen peroxide.[79] In a case of acute paraplegia after the ingestion of 50% hydrogen peroxide, MRI revealed discrete segmental embolic infacts of the cervical and thoracic spinal cord as well as both cerebral hemispheres and left cerebellar hemisphere.[102]

Death from intravenous injection of 35% hydrogen peroxide is also reported.[95] The use of a concentrated hydrogen peroxide solution as part of a hair highlighting procedure resulted in a severe scalp injury including necrosis of the galea aponeurotica.[154]

Clinical sequelae from the ingestion of dilute hydrogen peroxide are usually much more benign.[39,67] Nausea and vomiting are the most common symptoms.[39] A whitish discoloration may be noted in the oral cavity. Gastrointestinal injury is usually limited to superficial mucosal irritation, but multiple gastric and duodenal ulcers, accompanied by hematemesis, and diffuse hemorrhagic gastritis are reported.[67,117] Portal venous gas embolization may occur as a result of the ingestion of 3% hydrogen peroxide.[28,117,143]

The use of 3% hydrogen peroxide for wound irrigation may result in significant complications. Extensive subcutaneous emphysema occurred after a dog bite to a human's face was irrigated under pressure with 60 mL of 3% hydrogen peroxide.[162] Systemic oxygen embolism, causing hypotension, cardiac ischemia, and coma, resulted from the intraoperative irrigation of an infected herniorrhaphy wound.[11] Gas embolism, resulting in intestinal gangrene, was reported to occur following colonic lavage with 1% hydrogen peroxide during surgical treatment of meconium ileus.[157] Multiple cases of acute colitis are reported as a complication of administering 3% hydrogen peroxide enemas.[113] The use of 3% hydrogen peroxide as a mouth rinse is associated with the development of oral ulcerations.[145] Ophthalmic exposures may result in conjunctival injection, burning pain, and blurry vision.[39,112] Optic neuropathy including transient blindness (ability to visualize shadows only) and subsequent optic atrophy from possible inhalational of hydrogen peroxide has also been described.[40]

Diagnosis A careful examination should be performed to detect any evidence of gas formation. A chest radiograph might reveal gas in the cardiac chambers, mediastinum, or pleural space. An abdominal radiograph might show gas in the GI tract or portal system and define the extent of bowel distension. MRI and CT scan might be useful for detecting brain and spinal cord lesions secondary to gas embolism.[5,79,102] Endoscopic evaluation might be necessary in patients who ingest concentrated hydrogen peroxide to determine the extent of mucosal injury.

Management The treatment of patients with hydrogen peroxide ingestions depends, to a large degree, on whether the patient has ingested a diluted or concentrated solution. Those with ingestions of concentrated solutions require expeditious evaluation. Dilution with milk or water, although unstudied, is unlikely to be helpful. Nasogastric aspiration of hydrogen peroxide might be helpful if the patient presents immediately after ingestion. Induced emesis is contraindicated and activated charcoal offers no antidotal benefit. Patients with abdominal distension from gas formation should be treated with nasogastric suctioning. Those with clinical or radiographic evidence of gas in the heart should be placed in the Trendelenburg position to prevent gas from blocking the right ventricular outflow tract. Careful aspiration of intracardiac air through a central venous line may be attempted in patients in extremis.[27] Case reports suggest that hyperbaric therapy may be useful in cases of life-threatening gas embolization after hydrogen peroxide ingestion.[76,102,105,119,183] Asymptomatic patients who unintentionally ingest small amounts of 3% hydrogen peroxide can be safely observed at home.

IODINE AND IODOPHORS

Iodine is one of the oldest topical antiseptics.[155] Iodine usually refers to molecular iodine, also known as I_2, free iodine, and elemental iodine which is the active ingredient of iodine-based antiseptics. The use of ethanol as the solvent, such as tincture of iodine, allows substantially more concentrated forms of I_2 to be available. I_2 and tincture of iodine ingestions are much less common than in the past as a result of the change in antiseptic use from iodine to iodophor antiseptics.[41]

Iodophors have molecular iodine compounded to a high-molecular-weight carrier or to a solubilizing agent. Povidone-iodine (Betadine), a commonly used iodophor, consists of iodine linked to polyvinylpyrrolidone (povidone). Iodophors, which limit the release of molecular iodine and are generally less toxic, are the standard iodine-based antiseptic preparations. Iodophor preparations are formulated as solutions, ointments, foams, surgical scrubs, wound-packing gauze, and vaginal preparations. The most common preparation is a 10% povidone-iodine solution that contains 1% "available" iodine (referring to all oxidizing iodine species), but only 0.001% free iodine (referring only to molecular iodine).[17,60]

Iodine is used to disinfect medical equipment and drinking water. Iodine is an effective antiseptic against bacteria, viruses, protozoa, and fungi, and is used both prophylactically and therapeutically.[37] Iodine is cytotoxic and an oxidant. It is thought to work by binding amino and heterocyclic nitrogen groups, oxidizing sulfhydryl groups, and saturating double bonds. Iodine also iodinates tyrosine groups.[60]

There may be significant systemic absorption of iodine from topical iodine or iodophor preparations.[134] Markedly elevated iodine concentrations do occur in patients who receive topical iodophor treatments to areas of dermal breakdown, such as burn injuries.[93] Significant absorption occurs when iodophors are applied to the vagina, perianal fistulas, umbilical cords, and the skin of low-birth-weight neonates.[184] The mucosal application of povidone-iodine during a hysteroscopy procedure resulted in acute renal failure that transiently required hemodialysis.[13] A fatality following intraoperative irrigation of a hip wound with povidone-iodine is also reported.[32] In this latter case, the postmortem serum iodine concentration was 7000 μg/dL (normal: 5–8 μg/dL).

Clinical Effects Problems associated with the use of iodine include unpleasant odor, skin irritation, allergic reactions and clothes staining. Ingestion of iodine may cause abdominal pain, vomiting, diarrhea, GI bleeding, delirium, hypovolemia, anuria, and circulatory collapse. Severe caustic injury of the GI tract may occur. The ingestion of approximately 45 mL of a 10% iodine solution resulted in death from multisystem failure 67 hours after ingestion.[42]

Reports of adverse consequences from iodophor ingestions are rare. In one case report, a 9-week-old infant died within 3 hours of receiving povidone-iodine by mouth.[91] In this unusual case, the child was administered 15 mL of povidone-iodine mixed with 135 mL of polyethylene glycol by nasogastric tube over a 3-hour period for the treatment of infantile colic. Postmortem examination showed an ulcerated and necrotic intestinal tract. A blood iodine concentration of 14,600 μg/dL was recorded. Significant toxicity from intentional ingestions of iodophors in adults is not documented.

Acid–base disturbances are among the most significant abnormalities associated with iodine and iodophors. Metabolic acidosis occurred in several burn patients after receiving multiple applications of povidone-iodine ointment.[93,135] These patients had elevated serum iodine concentrations and normal lactate concentrations. The exact etiology of the acidosis remains unclear. Postulated mechanisms for the acidosis include the povidone-iodine itself (pH 2.43), bicarbonate consumption from the conversions of I_2 to NaI, and decreased renal elimination of H^+ as a consequence of iodine toxicity.[135] Metabolic acidosis associated with a high lactate level after iodine ingestion likely reflects tissue destruction.[37]

Electrolyte abnormalities also may occur following the absorption of iodine. A patient with decubitus ulcers who received prolonged wound care with povidone-iodine–soaked gauze developed hypernatremia, hyperchloremia, metabolic acidosis, and renal failure.[37] The hyperchloremia was thought to be caused by a spurious elevation of measured chloride ions as a consequence of iodine's interference with the chloride assay. This interference occurs on the Technicon STAT/ION autoanalyzer, but does not occur when the silver halide precipitation assay is used.[37] Spurious hyperchloremia from iodine (or iodide) may result in the calculation of a low or negative anion gap (Chap. 16).[22,46]

Other problems associated with topical absorption of iodine-containing preparations are hypothyroidism (particularly in neonates),[22,163] hyperthyroidism,[144,147] elevated liver enzyme concentrations, neutropenia anaphylaxis,[1] and hypoxemia.[37] Because of the lack of consistency between iodine concentrations and symptomatology, and because many of these patients had significant secondary medical problems that may have accounted for their symptoms, the exact relationship between iodine absorption and the development of a specific clinical syndrome remains speculative. However, a clinical controlled trial that compared preterm infants exposed to either topical iodinated antiseptics or to chlorhexidine-containing antiseptics showed that the infants exposed to topical iodine-containing antiseptics were more likely to have higher thyrotropin concentrations and elevated urine iodine concentrations than was the chlorhexidine group.[99]

Contact dermatitis can result from repetitive applications of iodophors.[108] A dermal burn may result from the trapping of an iodophor solution under the body of a patient in a pooled dependent position or under a tourniquet.[101,123]

Management The patient who ingests an iodine preparation requires expeditious evaluation, stabilization, and decontamination. Careful nasogastric aspiration and lavage may be performed to limit the caustic effect of the iodine if signs of perforation are absent. Irrigation with a starch solution will convert iodine to the much less toxic iodide and, in the process, turn the gastric effluent dark blue-purple. This change in color may serve as a useful guide in determining when lavage can be terminated. If starch is not available, milk may be a useful alternative. Instillation of 100 mL of a solution of 1%–3% sodium thiosulfate can also be used to convert any remaining iodine to iodide. Activated charcoal binds iodine and may be useful.[36] Early endoscopy may help assess the extent of the gastrointestinal injury.

Most patients with iodophor ingestion require only supportive management. The use of starch or sodium thiosulfate may be considered in symptomatic patients. Hemodialysis and continuous venovenous hemodiafiltration was used successfully to enhance elimination of iodine in patient with renal insufficiency who had become iodine toxic after undergoing continuous mediastinal irrigation with povidone-iodine.[87A] The benefit of hemodialysis or continuous venovenous hemodiafiltration is unknown in patients with normal renal function and therefore not recommended.

POTASSIUM PERMANGANATE

Potassium permanganate ($KMnO_4$) is a violet water-soluble xenobiotic that is usually sold as crystals or tablets or as a 0.01% dilute solution.[85] Historically, it was used as an abortifacient, urethral irrigant, lavage fluid for alkaloid poisoning, and snakebite remedy. Currently, potassium permanganate is most often used in baths and wet bandages as a dermal antiseptic, particularly for patients with eczema.

Potassium permanganate is a strong oxidizer and poisoning may result in local and systemic toxicity.[165] Upon contact with mucous membranes, potassium permanganate reacts with water to form manganese dioxide, potassium hydroxide, and molecular oxygen. Local tissue injury is the result of contact with the nascent oxygen, as well as the caustic effect of potassium hydroxide. A brown-black staining of the tissues occurs from the manganese dioxide. Systemic toxicity may occur from free radicals generated by absorbed permanganate ions.[193]

Clinical Effects Following ingestion, initial symptoms include nausea and vomiting. Laryngeal edema and ulceration of the mouth, esophagus, and, to a lesser extent, the stomach, may result from the caustic effects. Airway obstruction and fatal gastrointestinal perforation and hemorrhage may occur.[38,114,130] Esophageal strictures and pyloric stenosis are potential late complications.[89]

Although potassium permanganate is not well absorbed from the GI tract, systemic absorption may occur, resulting in life-threatening toxicity. Systemic effects include hepatotoxicity, renal damage, methemoglobinemia, hemolysis, hemorrhagic pancreatitis, airway obstruction, acute respiratory distress syndrome, disseminated intravascular coagulation, and cardiovascular collapse.[97,107,114,130] Elevation in blood or serum manganese concentration may also occur, confirming systemic absorption (normal concentrations blood manganese 3.9–15.0 μg/L; serum manganese 0.9–2.9 μg/L).

Chronic ingestion of potassium permanganate may result in classic manganese poisoning (manganism) characterized by behavioral changes, hallucinations, and delayed onset of parkinsonian-like symptoms. A 66-year-old man who mistakenly ingested 10 g of potassium permanganate over a 4-week period (because of medication mislabeling) developed impaired concentration and autonomic and visual symptoms. He also developed abdominal pain, gastric ulceration, and alopecia. Serum manganese concentration was elevated. Nine months later, the patient's neurologic examination displayed extrapyramidal signs consistent with parkinsonism (Chap. 95).[74]

Management Because the consequential effects of potassium permanganate ingestion are a result of its liberation of strong alkalis, the initial treatment of such a patient should include assessment for evidence of airway compromise. Dilution with milk or water may be useful. Patients with symptoms consistent with caustic injury should undergo early upper GI endoscopy. Corticosteroids along with antibiotics may be warranted if laryngeal edema is present. Analysis of liver enzymes, BUN, creatinine, lipase, serum manganese, and methemoglobin concentrations should be performed when systemic toxicity is suspected. Methemoglobinemia, if clinically significant, should be treated with methylene blue. Dermal irrigation with dilute oxalic acid may be successful in removing cutaneous staining.[165] The administration of *N*-acetylcysteine (see Antidotes in Depth A4: *N*-Acetylcysteine) to increase reduced glutathione production, thereby limiting free radical–mediated oxidative injury in cases of systemic potassium permanganate poisoning, has been suggested, but clinical trials have not been performed.[193]

OTHER ANTISEPTICS

ALCOHOLS

Isopropanol and ethanol are commonly used as skin antiseptics. Sold as rubbing alcohol, the standard concentration for these solutions is usually 70%. Their antiseptic action is thought to be a result of their ability to coagulate proteins. Isopropanol is slightly more germicidal than ethanol.[60] The alcohols have limited efficacy against viruses or spores. Isopropanol tends to be more irritating than ethanol and may cause more pronounced central nervous system depression.[185] The greater toxicity of isopropanol has caused some emergency departments to switch rubbing alcohol formulations from isopropanol to ethanol (Chaps. 77 and 107).

CHLORINE AND CHLOROPHORS

Chlorine, one of the first antiseptics, is still used in the treatment of the community water supply and in swimming pools. Chlorine is a potent pulmonary irritant that can cause severe bronchospasm and acute lung injury. Chapter 124 further discusses chlorine.

Sodium hypochlorite, found in household bleaches and in Dakin solution, remains a commonly used disinfectant. First used in the late 1700s to bleach clothes, its usefulness arises from its oxidizing capability, measured as "available chlorine," and its ability to release hypochlorous acid slowly. It is used to clean blood spills and to sterilize certain medical instruments. A 0.5% hypochlorite solution is sometimes recommended for dermal and soft-tissue wound decontamination after exposure to biologic and chemical warfare agents (Chaps. 131 and 132).[78] Toxicity from hypochlorite is mainly a result of its irritant effects. The ingestion of large amounts of household liquid bleach (5% sodium hypochlorite) on rare occasions can result in esophageal burns with subsequent stricture formation.[47] In a cat model of bleach ingestion, a high incidence of mucosal injury and stricture formation was noted.[188] However, the vast majority of household bleach ingestions in humans do not cause significant GI injuries.[136] Accordingly, endoscopic evaluation is usually not warranted when assessing most patients with household liquid bleach ingestions. The ingestion of a more concentrated "industrial strength" bleach preparation (eg, 35% sodium hypochlorite) increases the likelihood of local tissue injury and should be managed accordingly (Chap. 104).

MERCURIALS

Both inorganic mercurials, such as mercuric bichloride, and organic mercurials, such as merbromin (mercurochrome) and thimerosal (merthiolate), which both contain 49% mercury, were used in the past as topical antiseptic agents. The usefulness of mercurials is significantly limited because of their relatively weak bacteriostatic properties and the many problems associated with mercury toxicity (Chap. 96).

Repeated application of topical mercurials may result in significant absorption and systemic toxicity.[120,148] The use of high-dose hepatitis B immunoglobulin (HBIg) may cause mercury toxicity because of the use of thimerosal as a preservative in the HBIg preparation.[104] In one case, a 44-year-old male patient received 250 mL of HBIg (containing about 30 mg of thimerosal) over 9 days following liver transplantation.[104] He developed speech difficulties, tremor, and chorea. His whole blood mercury concentration was 104 μg/L (normal <10 μg/L). Increased mercury concentrations in both preterm and term infants, following immunizations with thimerosal-containing hepatitis B vaccine, have also generated much concern and led to the call to reduce or eliminate the mercury content of vaccines (Chap. 96).[57,167]

DISINFECTANTS

FORMALDEHYDE

Formaldehyde is a water-soluble, highly reactive gas at room temperature. Formalin consists of an aqueous solution of formaldehyde, usually containing approximately 37% formaldehyde and 12%–15% methanol. Formaldehyde is irritating to the upper airways, and its odor is readily detectable at low concentrations. Lethality in adults may follow ingestion of 30–60 mL of formalin.[43]

Formerly used as a disinfectant and fumigant, its role as a disinfectant is now largely confined to the disinfection of hemodialysis machines. Nonetheless, formaldehyde has many other applications. Healthcare workers are probably most familiar with the use of formaldehyde as a tissue fixative and embalming agent.

Exposure to formaldehyde, a potent caustic, may result in both local and systemic symptoms, causing coagulation necrosis, protein precipitation, and tissue fixation. Ingestions of formalin may result in significant gastric injury, including hemorrhage, diffuse necrosis, perforation, and stricture.[3,10] The most extensive damage appears in the stomach, with only occasional involvement of the small intestine and colon.[192] Chemical fixation of the stomach may occur. Esophageal involvement is not very prominent, and, if present, is usually limited to its distal segment.

The most striking and rapid systemic manifestation of formaldehyde poisoning is metabolic acidosis, resulting both from tissue injury and from the conversion of formaldehyde to formic acid. The patient may present with profound acidemia, accompanied by a large anion gap metabolic acidosis. Although the methanol component of the formalin solution is readily absorbed and has resulted in methanol concentrations as high as 40 mg/dL,[20,43] the rapid metabolism of formaldehyde to formic acid appears to be responsible for much of the acidosis (Chap. 107). Blindness as a consequence of the accumulation of formate, a retinal toxin, is not reported.

Clinical Effects Patients presenting after formaldehyde ingestions complain of the rapid onset of severe abdominal pain, which may be accompanied by vomiting and diarrhea. Altered mental status and coma usually follow rapidly. Physical examination may demonstrate epigastric tenderness, hematemesis, cyanosis, hypotension, and tachypnea. Hypotension may be profound with decreased myocardial contractility, as well as hypovolemic shock, contributing to the cardiovascular instability.[69,176] Early endoscopic findings include ulceration, necrosis, perforation, and hemorrhage of the stomach, with infrequent esophageal involvement. Chemical pneumonitis occurs after significant inhalational exposure.[138] Intravascular hemolysis is described in hemodialysis patients whose dialysis equipment contained residual formaldehyde after undergoing routine cleaning.[131,142]

Occupational and environmental exposure to formaldehyde receives considerable attention. In particular, there is concern over the potential off-gassing of formaldehyde from the widely used urea formaldehyde building insulation and particle boards.[129] Headache, nausea, skin rash, sore throat, nasal congestion, and eye irritation are associated with the use of these polymers.[34] Formaldehyde, at concentrations as low as 1 ppm, may cause significant irritation to mucous membranes of the upper respiratory tract and conjunctivae.[73,103] Formaldehyde is also a potential sensitizer for immune-mediated reversible bronchospasm.[66] The exact immunologic mechanism is not yet elucidated, although it is likely that formaldehyde acts as a hapten. In addition, formaldehyde is thought to be a dermal sensitizer.[164]

Recent concerns about the health effects from the off-gassing of formaldehyde in trailers used by the Federal Emergency Management Agency (FEMA) after Hurricane Katrina illustrates the potential public health issues related to low-level formaldehyde exposure.[106] Preliminary investigations from the Center for Disease Control (CDC) revealed that air formaldehyde concentrations in closed, unventilated trailers are, in fact, high enough to cause acute symptoms in some people.[4]

Both animal and human data suggest that formaldehyde exposure is associated with an increased incidence of nasopharyngeal carcinoma.[2,62,133,149] Although its role in the pathogenesis of cancer in humans is the subject of much debate,[30,109] in 2004 the International Agency for Research on Cancer (IARC) reclassified formaldehyde from a Group 2 *probable* to a Group 1 *known* carcinogen.

Management The immediate management of a patient who has ingested formaldehyde includes dilution with water. Although such an approach may be useful in reducing the caustic effect, strong evidence for a beneficial result is lacking. Gastric aspiration with a small-bore nasogastric tube may limit systemic absorption. The role of activated charcoal is not studied and it probably should not be used if endoscopy is considered likely. Significant acidemia should be treated with sodium bicarbonate and folinic acid (Chap. 107). Immediate hemodialysis may remove the accumulating formic acid as well as the parent molecules, formaldehyde, and methanol.[43] Independent treatment for methanol toxicity may be indicated (see Chap. 107). Early endoscopy is recommended for all patients with significant GI symptoms to assess the degree of burn injury. Surgical intervention may be required for those with suspected severe burns and/or perforation.[192] Emergent gastrectomy, as well as late surgical intervention to relieve formaldehyde-induced gastric outlet obstruction, is infrequently required.[63,90]

PHENOL

Phenol, also known as carbolic acid, is one of the oldest antiseptic agents. It is rarely used as an antiseptic today, secondary to its toxicity, and has been replaced by the many phenolic derivatives. Currently, phenol is used as a disinfectant, chemical intermediary, and nail cauterizer. The last application uses a highly concentrated 89% solution. Phenol is also a component (0.1%–4.5%) of various lotions, ointments, gels, gargles, lozenges, and throat sprays.[60] Campho-Phenique and Chloraseptic contain 4.7% and 1.4% phenol, respectively. Although many cases of phenol poisoning were reported in the past, acute oral overdoses of phenol-containing solutions are uncommon today.[53]

Phenol acts as a caustic causing cell wall disruption, protein denaturation, and coagulation necrosis. It also acts a central nervous system (CNS) stimulant. Intentional ingestion of concentrated phenol, ingestion of phenol-containing water, occupational exposure to aerosolized phenol, dermal contact, and parenteral administration may all result in symptomatic phenol poisoning. Phenol demonstrates excellent skin penetrance.[15] Severe dermal burns from phenol have resulted in systemic toxicity, even death within minutes to hours.[15,96] Parenteral administration of phenol has also resulted in death (see Chap. 135). The lethal oral dose may be as little as 1 g.[75]

Clinical Effects Clinical manifestations can be divided into local and systemic symptoms. Systemic symptoms from gastrointestinal (GI) or dermal absorption of phenol are usually more dangerous than the local effects. Manifestations of systemic toxicity include CNS and cardiac symptoms. CNS effects include central stimulation, seizures, lethargy, and coma.[56] In a study of patients who had ingested Creolin (26% phenol), CNS symptoms predominated.[166] Of the 52 patients who were evaluated at the hospital, 9 developed lethargy and 2 developed coma. Seizures were not reported. Cardiac symptoms from phenol include tachycardia, bradycardia, and hypotension.[56] Parenteral absorption of 10 mL concentrated 89% phenol resulted in hypoxemia, acute respiratory distress syndrome, pulmonary nodular opacities, and acute renal failure requiring intubation and hemodialysis.[55] This last case was associated with a phenol concentration of 87 mg/dL (normal <2 mg/dL).

Other systemic symptoms that may develop include hypothermia, metabolic acidosis, methemoglobinemia, and rabbit syndrome.[75,86] Rabbit syndrome is most commonly observed as a distinctive extrapyramidal effect from antipsychotic drugs and is characterized by fine rapid repetitive movements of the perioral musculature resembling a rabbit's chewing movements. Increased acetylcholine release and a relative dopaminergic hypofunction may explain the development of rabbit syndrome after phenol exposure.[86]

Local toxicity to the GI tract from the ingestion of phenol may result in nausea, painful oral lesions, vomiting, bloody diarrhea, dark urine, and severe abdominal pain.[7,84] Serious GI burns are uncommon, and strictures are rare. White patches in the oral cavity may be detected. In the Creolin study cited above, only 1 of 17 patients who underwent endoscopy had a significant esophageal burn.[166] Dermal exposures to phenol usually result in a light-brown staining of the skin. Excessive dermal absorption of phenol during chemical peeling procedures is associated with dysrhythmias and many of the other symptoms.[180,186]

Markedly elevated blood and urine concentrations of phenol may be detected after ingestion, or dermal absorption, of phenol and phenol-containing compounds (eg, Campho-Phenique).[15,75]

Management When phenol is mixed with water, a bilayer with unique properties is created that makes it difficult to remove from tissues. A variety of treatments have been suggested for dermal and gastric decontamination of phenol. A study employing a rat model showed that cutaneous decontamination with a low-molecular-weight polyethylene glycol solution decreased mortality, systemic effects, and dermal burns.[19] Although this study suggested that polyethylene glycol (PEG) was superior to water as a decontamination agent, a subsequent study using a swine model could not demonstrate a difference between these two therapies.[141] In another swine model, PEG 400 and 70% isopropanol were both superior to water washes and equally effective in decreasing dermal burn.[116] Given the lack of definitive efficacy data, either low-molecular-weight PEG, for example, PEG 300 or 400 (not to be confused with high-molecular-weight PEG that is used for whole-bowel irrigation), or high flow water is currently recommended for dermal irrigation and careful gastric decontamination. Isopropanol could also be considered as another treatment for dermal decontamination. Endoscopic evaluation, as needed to determine the extent of GI injury, and good supportive care are also recommended.

SUBSTITUTED PHENOLS AND OTHER RELATED COMPOUNDS

Hexachlorophene (pHisoHex), a trichlorinated *bis*-phenol, is one of the best known substituted phenols. Hexachlorophene, considered generally less tissue-toxic than phenol, was formerly used extensively as a disinfectant in hospitals. During the 1970s, an association was observed between repetitive whole-body washing of premature infants with 3% hexachlorophene and the development of vacuolar encephalopathy and cerebral edema.[110] There were also multiple reports of significant neurologic toxicity and death in children who became toxic after ingesting hexachlorophene.[68] In addition, fatalities also occurred after patients absorbed substantial amounts of hexachlorophene during the treatment of burn injuries.[26] The use of hexachlorophene has declined significantly.

Clinical Effects pHisoDerm contains sodium octylphenoxyethoxyethyl ether sulfonate and lanolin, and is a safe antiseptic. Irritative effects (nausea, vomiting, diarrhea) would be the main adverse effects with oral ingestions.

In a study of poisoning admissions to Hong Kong hospitals, the ingestion of Dettol liquid, a household disinfectant that contains 4.8% chloroxylenol, 9% pine oil, and 12% isopropanol, accounted for 10% of admissions.[24] Aspiration (perhaps, in part, because of the pine oil) occurred in 8% of these patients, resulting in upper airway obstruction, pneumonia, and acute respiratory distress syndrome. More common symptoms included nausea, vomiting, sore mouth, sore throat, drowsiness, abdominal pain, and fever. Dermal contact with Dettol may result in full-thickness chemical burns.[35]

Cresol, a mixture of three isomers of methylphenol, has better germicidal activity than phenol and is a commonly used disinfectant. Exposure to concentrated cresol may result in significant local tissue injury, hemolysis, renal injury, hepatic injury, and CNS and respiratory depression.[35,61,87,191] Phenol concentrations, as well as cresol concentrations, serve as markers of exposure.[191]

Management Treatment is mainly supportive.

QUATERNARY AMMONIUM COMPOUNDS

Quaternary ammonium compounds are a type of cationic surfactant (surface-active agent); they are used as disinfectants, detergents, and sanitizers. Chemically, the quaternary ammonium compounds are synthetic derivatives of ammonium chloride, and structurally similar to other quaternary ammonium derivatives, such as carbamate cholinesterase inhibitors and neuromuscular blockers. Other cationic surfactants include the pyridinium compounds and the quinolinium compounds. Benzalkonium chloride (Zephiran) was one of the most commonly employed quaternary ammonium compounds in the past. Many newer quaternary ammonium compounds have supplanted its use. However, nebulized solutions used for the treatment of asthma, including albuterol and ipratropium bromide, may contain small amounts of benzalkonium chloride.

Clinical Quaternary ammonium compounds are less toxic than phenol or formaldehyde. Most of the infrequent complications that are described result from ingestions of benzalkonium chloride. Complications of these ingestions include burns to the mouth and esophagus, CNS depression, elevated liver enzyme concentrations metabolic acidosis, and hypotension.[71,182,189] Paralysis is also occasionally described as a complication of these ingestions and is presumably a result of cholinesterase inhibition at the neuromuscular junction.[53] Chronic inhalational exposure is associated with occupational asthma.[16] Topical use of the quaternary ammonium compounds can cause contact dermatitis.[160] Few data are available on the toxicity of the newer quaternary ammonium compounds.

Ingestions of other cationic surfactants, such as the pyridinium agent cetrimonium bromide (Cetrimide), are associated with caustic burns to the mouth, lips, and tongue.[118] Peritoneal irrigation with cetrimonium bromide can produce metabolic abnormalities, hypotension, and methemoglobinemia.[8,115] Intravenous administration of cetrimide produced cardiac arrest, hemolysis, and muscle paralysis.[49]

Management Treatment recommendations following the ingestion of the quaternary ammonium compounds and other cationic surface-active agents are similar to those for other potentially caustic ingestions. Emergency department evaluation should be considered for all patients who ingest more than a taste of a dilute (less than 1%) solution. Therapy is mainly supportive. Endoscopy may be warranted if symptoms suggest the possibility of a burn injury.

STERILANTS

ETHYLENE OXIDE

Ethylene oxide is a gas that is commonly used to sterilize heat-sensitive material in healthcare facilities. Unlike antiseptics and disinfectants, which generally do not exhibit full sporicidal activity, sterilants, such as ethylene oxide, inactivate all organisms. Ethylene oxide is also used in the synthesis of many chemicals, including ethylene glycol, surfactants, rocket propellants, and petroleum demulsifiers, and has been used as a fumigant. Ethylene oxide has a cyclic ester structure that acts as an alkylating agent, reacting with most cellular components, including DNA and RNA.

Medical attention regarding ethylene oxide toxicity has centered on its mutagenic and possible carcinogenic effects.[92] Approximately 270,000 workers (including 96,000 hospital workers) in the United States are at risk for occupational exposure to ethylene oxide.[170] Retrospective studies suggest a possible excess incidence of leukemia and gastric cancer in ethylene oxide-exposed workers.[72,170] These studies are inconclusive, and the carcinogenicity of ethylene oxide remains subject to debate. It is also suggested that an increased incidence of spontaneous abortions may be associated with occupational exposure to ethylene oxide.[65]

Clinical Effects The acute toxicity of ethylene oxide is mainly the result of its irritant effects. Conjunctival, upper respiratory tract, GI, and dermal irritation may occur. Dermal burns from acute exposure to ethylene oxide are reported. Acute exposure to a broken ethylene oxide ampule by a 43-year-old recovery room nurse resulted in nausea, lightheadedness, malaise, syncope, and recurrent seizures.[152] There were no long-term complications. In another case of acute exposure, coma was followed by an irreversible parkinsonism.[9]

Chronic exposure to high concentrations of ethylene oxide may cause mild cognitive impairment and motor and sensory neuropathies.[18,54,127] The risk of cancer with occupational exposure is low.[29,169]

Management Treatment for patients with ethylene oxide exposure is supportive.

GLUTARALDEHYDE

Glutaraldehyde is a liquid solution used in the cold sterilization of nonautoclavable endoscopic, surgical, and dental equipment. It is also employed as a tissue fixative, embalming fluid, preservative, and tanning agent, in radiographic solutions, and in the treatment of warts.[51] Glutaraldehyde is a dialdehyde with two active carbonyl groups that is less volatile than formaldehyde. It kills all microorganisms, including viruses and spores. The germicidal ability of glutaraldehyde results from the alkylation of sulfhydryl, hydroxyl, carboxyl, and amino groups, within microbes interfering with RNA, DNA, and protein synthesis.[151] It is prepared as a 2% alkaline solution in 70% isopropanol (Cidex). Healthcare workers may be exposed to glutaraldehyde vapors when equipment is processed in poorly ventilated areas, or in open immersion baths or after spills. Under these circumstances, the evaporation of glutaraldehyde may result in the increase in ambient air concentrations that may easily exceed recommended limits. Approximately 35,000 workers are occupationally exposed to glutaraldehyde.[137] Patients may be exposed when diagnostic instruments are inadequately rinsed following cold sterilization with glutaraldehyde.

Clinical Clinical signs and symptoms are thought to be comparable to those of formaldehyde exposure although human toxicity data are limited. Animal studies show that glutaraldehyde's inhalational and dermal toxicity are comparable to formaldehyde at equivalent doses.[175]

Glutaraldehyde is a mucosal irritant. Coryza, epistaxis, headache, asthma, chest tightness, palpitations, tachycardia, and nausea are all associated with glutaraldehyde vapor exposure.[14,31,124,132] Contact dermatitis and ocular inflammation may also occur.[33,156] Colitis has been reported following the use of endoscopes contaminated with residual glutaraldehyde solution.[158] Patients with glutaraldehyde-induced colitis typically present with fever, chills, severe abdominal pain, bloody diarrhea, and an elevated white blood cell count blood within 48 hours after colonoscopy or sigmoidoscopy.

The IARC has not ranked the carcinogenic potential of glutaraldehyde.

Management Treatment recommendations are similar to those for patients with formaldehyde exposure. Prompt removal from the exposure is essential. Copious irrigation with water provides adequate dermal decontamination. Severe inhalational exposures may require hospital admission for observation, supportive care, and treatment of bronchospasm.

OTHER PRODUCTS

BORIC ACID

Boric acid is an odorless, transparent crystal, although it is most commonly available as a finely ground white powder. It is also commonly found as a 2.5%–5% aqueous solution. Boric acid (H_3BO_3), prepared from borax (sodium borate; $Na_2B_4O_7 \cdot 10\ H_2O$), was first used as an antiseptic by Lister in the late 19th century. Although used extensively over the years for antisepsis and irrigation, boric acid is only weakly bacteriostatic. As a result of its germicidal limitations and its inherent toxicity, boric acid is nearly obsolete in modern antiseptic therapy. Nonetheless, it continues to be used as an antimicrobial to treat such conditions as vulvovaginal candidiasis.[140] Boric acid is also employed in the treatment of cockroach infestation and as a soap, contact lens solution, toothpaste, and food preservative.[58]

Boric acid is readily absorbed through the GI tract, wounds, abraded skin, and serous cavities. Absorption does not occur through intact skin. Boric acid is predominantly eliminated unchanged by the kidney. Small amounts are also excreted into sweat, saliva, and feces.[50] Boric acid is concentrated in the brain and liver.

The exact mechanism of action of boric acid's toxicity remains unclear. Although it is an inorganic acid, it does not behave as a caustic. Local effects are limited to tissue irritation.

Over the years, boric acid has developed a reputation as an exceptionally potent toxin. This reputation was derived in great part from a series of reports involving neonatal exposures to boric acid resulting in high morbidity and mortality. Life-threatening toxicity resulted from the repetitive topical application of boric acid for the treatment of diaper rash or the use of infant formulas unintentionally contaminated with boric acid.[50,190] Fatality rates greater than 50% were reported in some series.[190] Although infants appear to be the most sensitive to the toxic effects of boric acid, many cases of significant adult toxicity are also reported. These cases date predominantly from the time when boric acid was widely used as an irrigant. Routes of exposure to boric acid, resulting in fatalities, include wound irrigation, pleural irrigation, rectal washing, bladder irrigation, and vaginal packing.[181]

Clinical Effects Classic boric acid poisoning usually involves multiple exposures over a period of days. Gastrointestinal, dermal, CNS, and renal manifestations predominate. The initial symptoms—nausea, vomiting, diarrhea, and occasionally crampy abdominal pain—may be confused with an acute gastroenteritis. At times, the emesis and diarrhea are greenish blue.[190] Following the onset of GI symptoms, the majority of patients develop a characteristic intense generalized erythroderma.[190] This rash, described as producing a "boiled lobster" appearance, may appear indistinguishable from toxic epidermal necrolysis or staphylococcal scalded skin syndrome in the neonate.[150] The rash may be especially noticeable on the palms, soles, and buttocks.[50] Typically, extensive desquamation takes place within 1–2 days. On occasion, prominent mucous membrane involvement of the oral cavity and conjunctivae is also apparent.[190] At about the time of the development of the erythroderma, patients, particularly young infants, may develop prominent signs of CNS irritability, resembling meningeal irritation. Seizures, delirium, and coma can occur.[50] Renal injury is common, both a result of the renal elimination of this compound and prerenal azotemia from GI losses.[50] Other complications of boric acid poisoning include hepatic injury, hyperthermia, and cardiovascular collapse. The abandonment of boric acid as an irrigant and particularly its removal from the nursery setting have led to a marked decrease in the incidence of significant boric acid poisoning.

Two retrospective studies on boric acid ingestions suggest that a single acute ingestion of boric acid is generally quite benign.[98,100] In these studies, 79–88% of patients remained asymptomatic. Symptoms, when present, primarily consist of GI irritative symptoms, such as nausea and vomiting. None of the 1184 patients in these two studies manifested the generalized erythroderma so commonly described in previous reports. Central nervous system manifestations of acute overdose were infrequent and limited to occasional lethargy and headache. Renal toxicity did not occur following single acute ingestions.

Several reports suggest, however, that significant toxicity from massive acute ingestion of boric acid can occur. Fatality resulted from a single ingestion of 2 cups (280 g) of boric acid crystals by a 45-year-old man.[146] Symptoms on presentation (2 days after ingestion) included nausea, vomiting, green diarrhea, lethargy, hypotension, renal failure, and a prominent "boiled lobster" rash on his trunk and extremities. In another case, the ingestion of 30 g of boric acid by a 77-year-old man resulted in similar symptoms and death 63 hours postingestion, despite hemodialysis.[81] The diagnosis of boric acid poisoning can be confirmed with the measurement of blood or serum boric acid concentrations (normal = 1.4 nmol/mL), but this test is not routinely available.

Long-term chronic exposure to boric acid results in alopecia in adults and seizures in children.[126] A 32-year-old woman who chronically ingested mouthwash containing boric acid over a 7-month period developed progressive hair loss.[174] The chronic application of a borax and honey mixture to pacifiers resulted in the development of recurrent seizures in nine infants, which resolved after the mixture was withheld.[52,126]

Management Treatment of boric acid toxicity is mainly supportive. Activated charcoal is not recommended because of its relatively poor adsorptive capacity for boric acid.[36] Since boric acid has a low molecular weight and relatively small volume of distribution, in cases of massive oral overdose or renal failure. Hemodialysis or perhaps exchange transfusion in infants, may be helpful in shortening the half-life of boric acid.[100,122,178,190] In patients with normal renal function, forced diuresis enhances renal elimination.[179]

CHLORATES

Sodium chlorate is a strong oxidizer. At one time, the chlorate salts, sodium chlorate and potassium chlorate, were used as medicinal to treat inflammatory and ulcerative lesions of the oral cavity and could be found in various mouthwash, toothpaste, and gargle preparations.[168] Although their use as local antiseptics is obsolete, chlorates are used as herbicides and in the manufacture of matches, explosives, and dyestuffs.[82] More recent cases of chlorate poisoning resulted from the ingestion of sodium chlorate–containing weed killers, or dispensing errors that confused sodium chlorate with sodium sulfate or sodium chloride.[82] Sodium chlorate in the form of white crystals has also been mistaken for table sugar.[64] A case of significant toxicity from the inhalation of atomized chlorates is also reported.[82]

Sodium chlorate is rapidly absorbed from the GI tract and eliminated predominantly unchanged from the kidneys.[83] Its systemic effects are chiefly hematologic and renal. Chlorate's major mechanism of toxicity is its ability to oxidize hemoglobin and increase red blood cell membrane rigidity.[161] Consequently, significant methemoglobinemia and hemolysis may result. Chlorates may also be directly toxic to the proximal renal tubule.[94] The hemolysis and the resultant hemoglobinuria may secondarily cause disseminated intravascular coagulation and potentiate renal toxicity. The worsening renal function is especially problematic because of its adverse effect on chlorate elimination. The methemoglobinemia may be severe and cause significant hypoxic stress. Methemoglobinemia may occur prior to or after the development of hemolysis.[125,171] Chlorates may also act locally as a GI irritant, and cause mild CNS depression after absorption.[53]

Clinical Clinical signs and symptoms of chlorate poisoning usually begin 1–4 hours after ingestion.[88] The earliest symptoms are GI, including nausea, vomiting, diarrhea, and crampy abdominal pain. Subsequently, the patient may exhibit cyanosis from the methemoglobinemia and black-brown urine from the hemoglobinuria. Obtundation and anuria may ensue. Laboratory studies may show methemoglobinemia, anemia, Heinz bodies, ghost cells, fragmented spherocytes, metabolic acidosis, decreased platelet count, and abnormal coagulation.[45] Hyperkalemia may be particularly problematic if the patient ingests potassium chlorate preparations.[121] In a recent case of chlorate poisoning from the ingestion of 120 potassium chlorate–containing matchsticks, an MRI revealed symmetric abnormal signal intensity within the deep gray matter and medial temporal lobes.[121] This finding can be explained by the basal ganglia's increased vulnerability to oxygen deprivation. Followup MRI two months later was normal.

Management Treatment of a patient with a significant chlorate ingestion should include orogastric lavage and the use of activated charcoal.[64] It has been suggested that administration of sodium thiosulfate may inactivate the chlorate ion by reducing it to the chloride ion,[64] but an in vitro study did not confirm this hypothesis.[173] Although methylene blue is used in the treatment of symptomatic methemoglobinemia, its efficacy in the treatment of chlorate-induced methemoglobinemia may be limited, as compared to its efficacy in the treatment of other oxidant-induced methemoglobinemias.[125,172] This may be a consequence of the inactivation by chlorates of glucose-6-phosphate dehydrogenase, an enzyme that is required for methylene blue to effectively reduce methemoglobin.[161] Exchange transfusion, peritoneal dialysis, and hemodialysis have all been advocated in the treatment of patients with severe chlorate poisoning.[125,172] Because the chlorate ion is easily dialyzable, hemodialysis is capable of removing this xenobiotic as well as treating any concomitant renal failure that may have developed.[82,88,94]

SUMMARY

A chemically diverse group of antiseptics, disinfectants, and sterilants exist. Many of the more toxic xenobiotics, such as iodine, phenol, and chlorates, are no longer commonly used as cleansers but may still be available in some settings. Formaldehyde exposures, although also uncommon, can also cause significant problems. Frequently employed antiseptics, such as chlorhexidine, pHisoDerm, and many of the currently used quaternary ammonium compounds, have a relatively limited toxicity. Ingestions of the iodophors do not usually cause significant toxicity, but absorption through other routes may produce significant adverse effects. Ingestions of hydrogen peroxide, particularly the more concentrated formulations, may result in life-threatening injuries.

REFERENCES

1. Adachi A, Fukunaga A, Hayashi K, Kunisada M, Horikawa T. Anaphylaxis to polyvinylpyrrolidone after vaginal application of povidone-iodine. *Contact Dermatitis.* 2003;48:133-136.
2. Albert RE, Sellakumar AR, Laskin S, Kuschner M, Nelson N, Snyder CA. Gaseous formaldehyde and hydrogen chloride induction of nasal cancer in the rat. *J Natl Cancer Inst.* 1982;68:597-603.
3. Allen RE, Thoshinsky MJ, Stallone RJ, Hunt TK. Corrosive injuries of the stomach. *Arch Surg* .1970;100:409-413.
4. Anonymous. An Update and Revision of ATSDR's February 2007 Health Consultation: Formaldehyde Sampling of FEMA Temporary-Housing TrailersBatonRouge,Louisiana,September-October,2006.Accessedat:http://wwwatsdrcdcgov/substances/formaldehyde/pdfs/revised_formaldehyde_report_1007pdf, 2007.
5. Ashdown BC, Stricof DD, May ML, Sherman SJ, Carmody RF. Hydrogen peroxide poisoning causing brain infarction: neuroimaging findings. *AJR Am J Roentgenol.* 1998;170:1653-1655.
6. Autegarden JE, Pecquet C, Huet S, Bayrou O, Leynadier F. Anaphylactic shock after application of chlorhexidine to unbroken skin. *Contact Dermatitis.* 1999;40:215.
7. Baker EL, Landrigan PJ, Bertozzi PE, Field PH, Basteyns BJ, Skinner HG. Phenol poisoning due to contaminated drinking water. *Arch Environ Health.* 1978;33:89-94.
8. Baraka A, Yamut F, Wakid N. Cetrimide-induced methaemoglobinaemia after surgical excision of hydatid cyst. *Lancet.* 1980;2:88-89.
9. Barbosa ER, Comerlatti LR, Haddad MS, Scaff M. Parkinsonism secondary to ethylene oxide exposure: case report. *Arq Neuropsiquiatr.* 1992;50:531-533.
10. Bartone NF, Grieco RV, Herr BS, Jr. Corrosive gastritis due to ingestion of formaldehyde: without esophageal impairment. *JAMA.* 1968;203:50-51.
11. Bassan MM, Dudai M, Shalev O. Near-fatal systemic oxygen embolism due to wound irrigation with hydrogen peroxide. *Postgrad Med J.* 1982;58:448-450.
12. Beaudouin E, Kanny G, Morisset M, et al. Immediate hypersensitivity to chlorhexidine: literature review. *Allerg Immunol (Paris).* 2004;36:123-126.
13. Beji S, Kaaroud H, Ben Moussa F, et al. [Acute renal failure following mucosal administration of povidone iodine]. *Presse Med.* 2006;35:61-63.
14. Benson WG. Exposure to glutaraldehyde. *J Soc Occup Med.* 1984;34:63-64.
15. Bentur Y, Shoshani O, Tabak A, et al. Prolonged elimination half-life of phenol after dermal exposure. *J Toxicol Clin Toxicol.* 1998;36:707-711.
16. Bernstein JA, Stauder T, Bernstein DI, Bernstein IL. A combined respiratory and cutaneous hypersensitivity syndrome induced by work exposure to quaternary amines. *J Allergy Clin Immunol.* 1994;94:257-259.
17. Block S. Definition of terms. In: Block S, ed. *Disinfection, Sterilization, and Preservation.* 4th ed. Philadelphia: Lea & Febiger; 1991:18-25.
18. Brashear A, Unverzagt FW, Farber MO, Bonnin JM, Garcia JG, Grober E. Ethylene oxide neurotoxicity: a cluster of 12 nurses with peripheral and central nervous system toxicity. *Neurology.* 1996;46:992-928.
19. Brown VK, Box VL, Simpson BJ. Decontamination procedures for skin exposed to phenolic substances. *Arch Environ Health.* 1975;30:1-6.
20. Burkhart KK, Kulig KW, McMartin KE. Formate levels following a formalin ingestion. *Vet Hum Toxicol.* 1990;32:135-137.
21. Cannon G, Caravati EM, Filloux FM. Hydrogen peroxide neurotoxicity in childhood: case report with unique magnetic resonance imaging features. *J Child Neurol.* 2003;18:805-808.
22. Chabrolle JP, Rossier A. Goitre and hypothyroidism in the newborn after cutaneous absorption of iodine. *Arch Dis Child.* 1978;53:495-498.
23. Chan TY. Poisoning due to Savlon (cetrimide) liquid. *Hum Exp Toxicol.* 1994;13:681-682.
24. Chan TY, Lau MS, Critchley JA. Serious complications associated with Dettol poisoning. *Q J Med.* 1993;86:735-738.
25. Cheung J, O'Leary JJ. Allergic reaction to chlorhexidine in an anaesthetised patient. *Anaesth Intensive Care.* 1985;13:429-430.
26. Chilcote R, Curley A, Loughlin HH, Jupin JA. Hexachlorophene storage in a burn patient associated with encephalopathy. *Pediatrics.* 1977;59:457-459.
27. Christensen DW, Faught WE, Black RE, Woodward GA, Timmons OD. Fatal oxygen embolization after hydrogen peroxide ingestion. *Crit Care Med.* 1992;20:543-544.
28. Cina SJ, Downs JC, Conradi SE. Hydrogen peroxide: a source of lethal oxygen embolism. Case report and review of the literature. *Am J Forensic Med Pathol.* 1994;15:44-50.
29. Coggon D, Harris EC, Poole J, Palmer KT. Mortality of workers exposed to ethylene oxide: extended follow up of a British cohort. *Occup Environ Med.* 2004;61:358-362.
30. Collins JJ, Acquavella JF, Esmen NA. An updated meta-analysis of formaldehyde exposure and upper respiratory tract cancers. *J Occup Environ Med.* 1997;39:639-651.
31. Connaughton P. Occupational exposure to glutaraldehyde associated with tachycardia and palpitations. *Med J Aust.* 1993;159:567.
32. D'Auria J, Lipson S, Garfield JM. Fatal iodine toxicity following surgical debridement of a hip wound: case report. *J Trauma.* 1990;30:353-355.
33. Dailey JR, Parnes RE, Aminlari A. Glutaraldehyde keratopathy. *Am J Ophthalmol.* 1993;115:256-258.
34. Dally KA, Hanrahan LP, Woodbury MA, Kanarek MS. Formaldehyde exposure in nonoccupational environments. *Arch Environ Health.* 1981;36:277-284.
35. DeBono R, Laitung G. Phenolic household disinfectants—further precautions required. *Burns.* 1997;23:182-185.
36. Decker WJ, Combs HF, Corby DG. Adsorption of drugs and poisons by activated charcoal. *Toxicol Appl Pharmacol.* 1968;13:454-460.
37. Dela Cruz F, Brown DH, Leikin JB, Franklin C, Hryhorczuk DO. Iodine absorption after topical administration. *West J Med.* 1987;146:43-45.
38. Dhamrait RS. Airway obstruction following potassium permanganate ingestion. *Anaesthesia.* 2003;58:606-607.
39. Dickson KF, Caravati EM. Hydrogen peroxide exposure—325 exposures reported to a regional poison control center. *J Toxicol Clin Toxicol.* 1994;32:705-714.
40. Domac FM, Kocer A, Tanidir R, Domac FM, Kocer A, Tanidir R. Optic neuropathy related to hydrogen peroxide inhalation. *Clin Neuropharmacol.* 2007;30:55-57.
41. Dyck RF, Bear RA, Goldstein MB, Halperin ML. Iodine/iodide toxic reaction: case report with emphasis on the nature of the metabolic acidosis. *Can Med Assoc J.* 1979;120:704-706.
42. Edwards NA, Quigley P, Hackett LP, et al. Death by oral ingestion of iodine. *Emerg Med Australas.* 2005;17:173-177.
43. Eells JT, McMartin KE, Black K, Virayotha V, Tisdell RH, Tephly TR. Formaldehyde poisoning. Rapid metabolism to formic acid. *JAMA.* 1981;246:1237-1238.
44. Emerson D, Pierce C. A case of a single ingestion of 4% Hibiclens. *Vet Hum Toxicol.* 1988;30:583.
45. Eysseric H, Vincent F, Peoc'h M, Marka C, Aitken Y, Barret L. A fatal case of chlorate poisoning: confirmation by ion chromatography of body fluids. *J Forensic Sci.* 2000;45:474-477.
46. Fischman RA, Fairclough GF, Cheigh JS. Iodide and negative anion gap. *N Engl J Med.* 1978;298:1035-1036.
47. French RJ, Tabb HG, Rutledge LJ. Esophageal stenosis produced by ingestion of bleach: report of two cases. *South Med J.* 1970;63:1140-1144.
48. Giberson TP, Kern JD, Pettigrew DW, 3rd, Eaves CC, Jr., Haynes JF, Jr. Near-fatal hydrogen peroxide ingestion. *Ann Emerg Med.* 1989;18:778-779.
49. Gode GR, Jayalakshmi TS, Kalla GN. Accidental intravenous injection of cetrimide. A case report. *Anaesthesia.* 1975;30:508-510.
50. Goldbloom R, Goldbloom A. Boric acid poisoning: a report of four cases and a review of 109 cases from the world literature. *J Pediatr.* 1953;43:631-643.
51. Goncalo S, Menezes Brandao F, Pecegueiro M, Moreno JA, Sousa I. Occupational contact dermatitis to glutaraldehyde. *Contact Dermatitis.* 1984;10:183-184.
52. Gordon AS, Prichard JS, Freedman MH. Seizure disorders and anemia associated with chronic borax intoxication. *Can Med Assoc J.* 1973;108:719-721.

53. Gosselin R, Smith R, Hodge H. *Clinical Toxicology of Commercial Products*. 5th ed. Baltimore: Williams & Wilkins; 1984.
54. Gross JA, Haas ML, Swift TR. Ethylene oxide neurotoxicity: report of four cases and review of the literature. *Neurology*. 1979;29:978-983.
55. Gupta S, Ashrith G, Chandra D, et al. Acute phenol poisoning: a life-threatening hazard of chronic pain relief. *Clin Toxicol (Phila)*. 2008;46: 250-253.
56. Haddad LM, Dimond KA, Schweistris JE. Phenol poisoning. *JACEP*. 1979;8:267-269.
57. Halsey NA. Limiting infant exposure to thimerosal in vaccines and other sources of mercury.[see comment][comment]. *JAMA*. 1999;282:1763-1766.
58. Hamilton RA, Wolf BC, Hamilton RA, Wolf BC. Accidental boric acid poisoning following the ingestion of household pesticide. *J Forensic Sci*. 2007;52:706-708.
59. Hardin RD, Tedesco FJ. Colitis after Hibiclens enema. *J Clin Gastroenterol*. 1986;8:572-575.
60. Harvey S. Antiseptics and disinfectants; fungicides; ectoparasiticides. In: Gilman A, Rall T, Nies A, Taylor P, eds. *Goodman and Gilman's The Pharmacological Basis of Therapeutics*. 7th ed. New York: Pergamon Press; 1985:959-979.
61. Hashimoto T, Iida H, Dohi S. Marked increases of aminotransferase levels after cresol ingestion. *Am J Emerg Med*. 1998;16:667-668.
62. Hauptmann M, Lubin JH, Stewart PA, Hayes RB, Blair A. Mortality from solid cancers among workers in formaldehyde industries. *Am J Epidemiol*. 2004;159:1117-1130.
63. Hawley CK, Harsch HH. Gastric outlet obstruction as a late complication of formaldehyde ingestion: a case report. *Am J Gastroenterol*. 1999;94: 2289-2291.
64. Helliwell M, Nunn J. Mortality in sodium chlorate poisoning. *BMJ*. 1979;1:1119.
65. Hemminki K, Mutanen P, Saloniemi I, Niemi ML, Vainio H. Spontaneous abortions in hospital staff engaged in sterilising instruments with chemical agents. *BMJ (Clin Res Ed)*. 1982;285:1461-1463.
66. Hendrick DJ, Lane DJ. Occupational formalin asthma. *Br J Ind Med*. 1977;34:11-18.
67. Henry MC, Wheeler J, Mofenson HC, et al. Hydrogen peroxide 3% exposures. *J Toxicol Clin Toxicol*. 1996;34:323-327.
68. Herskowitz J, Rosman NP. Acute hexachlorophene poisoning by mouth in a neonate. *J Pediatr*. 1979;94:495-496.
69. Hilbert G, Gruson D, Bedry R, Cardinaud JP. Circulatory shock in the course of fatal poisoning by ingestion of formalin. *Intensive Care Med*. 1997;23:708.
70. Hirata K, Kurokawa A. Chlorhexidine gluconate ingestion resulting in fatal respiratory distress syndrome. *Vet Hum Toxicol*. 2002;44:89-91.
71. Hitosugi M, Maruyama K, Takatsu A. A case of fatal benzalkonium chloride poisoning. *Int J Legal Med*. 1998;111:265-266.
72. Hogstedt C, Aringer L, Gustavsson A. Epidemiologic support for ethylene oxide as a cancer-causing agent. *JAMA*. 1986;255:1575-1578.
73. Holness DL, Nethercott JR. Health status of funeral service workers exposed to formaldehyde. *Arch Environ Health*. 1989;44:222-228.
74. Holzgraefe M, Poser W, Kijewski H, Beuche W. Chronic enteral poisoning caused by potassium permanganate: a case report. *J Toxicol Clin Toxicol*. 1986;24:235-244.
75. Horch R, Spilker G, Stark GB. Phenol burns and intoxications. *Burns*. 1994;20:45-50.
76. Horowitz BZ. Massive hepatic gas embolism from a health food additive. *J Emerg Med*. 2004;26:229-230.
77. Humberston CL, Dean BS, Krenzelok EP. Ingestion of 35% hydrogen peroxide. *J Toxicol Clin Toxicol*. 1990;28:95-100.
78. Hurst C. Decontamination. In: Sidell F, Takafuji E, Franz D, eds. *Medical Aspects of Chemical and Biological Warfare*. Washtington, DC: Office of the Surgeon General; 1997:351-359.
79. Ijichi T, Itoh T, Sakai R, et al. Multiple brain gas embolism after ingestion of concentrated hydrogen peroxide. *Neurology*. 1997;48:277-279.
80. Ishigami S, Hase S, Nakashima H, et al. Intravenous chlorhexidine gluconate causing acute respiratory distress syndrome. *J Toxicol Clin Toxicol*. 2001;39:77-80.
81. Ishii Y, Fujizuka N, Takahashi T, et al. A fatal case of acute boric acid poisoning. *J Toxicol Clin Toxicol*. 1993;31:345-352.
82. Jackson R, Elder W, McDonnell H. Sodium chlorate poisoning complicated by acute renal failure. *Lancet*. 1961;2:1381-1383.
83. Jansen H, Zeldenrust J. Homicidal chronic sodium chlorate poisoning. *Forensic Sci*. 1972;1:103-105.
84. Jarvis SN, Straube RC, Williams AL, Bartlett CL. Illness associated with contamination of drinking water supplies with phenol. *BMJ (Clin Res Ed)*. 1985;290:1800-1802.
85. Johnson TB, Cassidy DD. Unintentional ingestion of potassium permanganate. *Pediatr Emerg Care*. 2004;20:185-187.
86. Kamijo Y, Soma K, Fukuda M, Asari Y, Ohwada T. Rabbit syndrome following phenol ingestion. *J Toxicol Clin Toxicol*. 1999;37:509-511.
87. Kamijo Y, Soma K, Kokuto M, Ohbu M, Fuke C, Ohwada T. Hepatocellular injury with hyperaminotransferasemia after cresol ingestion. *Arch Pathol Lab Med*. 2003;127:364-366.
87a. Kanakiriya S, De Chazal I, Nath KA, et al: Iodine toxicity treated with hemodialysis and continuous venovenous hemodiafiltration. *Am J Kidney Dis* 2003;41:702-708.
88. Knight R, Trounce J, Cameron J. Suicidal chlorate poisoning treated with peritoneal dialysis. *BMJ*. 1967;3:601-602.
89. Kochar R, Das K, Mehta S. Potassium permanganate induced esophageal stricture. *Human Toxicol*. 1986;5:393-394.
90. Koppel C, Baudisch H, Schneider V, Ibe K. Suicidal ingestion of formalin with fatal complications. *Intensive Care Med*. 1990;16:212-214.
91. Kurt TL, Morgan ML, Hnilica V, Bost R, Petty CS. Fatal iatrogenic iodine toxicity in a nine-week old infant. *J Toxicol Clin Toxicol*. 1996;34:231-234.
92. Landrigan PJ, Meinhardt TJ, Gordon J, et al. Ethylene oxide: an overview of toxicologic and epidemiologic research. *Am J Ind Med*. 1984;6:103-115.
93. Lavelle KJ, Doedens DJ, Kleit SA, Forney RB. Iodine absorption in burn patients treated topically with povidone-iodine. *Clin Pharmacol Ther*. 1975;17:355-362.
94. Lee DB, Brown DL, Baker LR, Littlejohns DW, Roberts PD. Haematological complications of chlorate poisoning. *BMJ*. 1970;2:31-32.
95. Leiken J, Sing K, Woods K. Fatality from intravenous use of hydrogen peroxide for home "superoxygenation therapy" [abstract]. *Vet Hum Toxicol*. 1993;35:342.
96. Lewin JF, Cleary WT. An accidental death caused by the absorption of phenol through skin. A case report. *Forensic Sci Int*. 1982;19:177-179.
97. Lifshitz M, Shahak E, Sofer S. Fatal potassium permanganate intoxication in an infant. *J Toxicol Clin Toxicol*. 1999;37:801-802.
98. Linden CH, Hall AH, Kulig KW, Rumack BH. Acute ingestions of boric acid. *J Toxicol Clin Toxicol*. 1986;24:269-279.
99. Linder N, Davidovitch N, Reichman B, et al. Topical iodine-containing antiseptics and subclinical hypothyroidism in preterm infants. *J Pediatr*. 1997;131:434-439.
100. Litovitz TL, Klein-Schwartz W, Oderda GM, Schmitz BF. Clinical manifestations of toxicity in a series of 784 boric acid ingestions. *Am J Emerg Med*. 1988;6:209-213.
101. Liu FC, Liou JT, Hui YL, et al. Chemical burn caused by povidone-iodine alcohol solution—a case report. *Acta Anaesthesiol Sin*. 2003;41:93-96.
102. Liu TM, Wu KC, Niu KC, et al. Acute paraplegia caused by an accidental ingestion of hydrogen peroxide. *Am J Emerg Med*. 2007;25:90-92.
103. Loomis TA. Formaldehyde toxicity. *Arch Pathol Lab Med*. 1979;103: 321-324.
104. Lowell JA, Burgess S, Shenoy S, Curci JA, Peters M, Howard TK. Mercury poisoning associated with high-dose hepatitis-B immune globulin administration after liver transplantation for chronic hepatitis B. *Liver Transpl Surg*. 1996;2:475-478.
105. Luu TA, Kelley MT, Strauch JA, Avradopoulos K. Portal vein gas embolism from hydrogen peroxide ingestion. *Ann Emerg Med*. 1992;21: 1391-1393.
106. Madrid PA, Sinclair H, Bankston AQ, et al. Building integrated mental health and medical programs for vulnerable populations post-disaster: connecting children and families to a medical home. *Prehospital Disaster Med*. 2008;23:314-321.
107. Mahomedy MC, Mahomedy YH, Canham PA, Downing JW, Jeal DE. Methaemoglobinaemia following treatment dispensed by witch doctors. Two cases of potassium permanganate poisoning. *Anaesthesia*. 1975;30: 190-193.
108. Marks JG, Jr. Allergic contact dermatitis to povidone-iodine. *J Am Acad Dermatol*. 1982;6:473-475.
109. Marsh GM, Youk AO, Buchanich JM, et al. Pharyngeal cancer mortality among chemical plant workers exposed to formaldehyde. *Toxicol Ind Health*. 2002;18:257-268.
110. Martinez AJ, Boehm R, Hadfield MG. Acute hexachlorophene encephalopathy: clinico-neuropathological correlation. *Acta Neuropathol (Berl)*. 1974;28:93-103.

111. Massano G, Ciocatto E, Rosabianca C, Vercelli D, Actis GC, Verme G. Striking aminotransferase rise after chlorhexidine self-poisoning. *Lancet*. 1982;1:289.
112. Memarzadeh F, Shamie N, Gaster RN, Chuck RS. Corneal and conjunctival toxicity from hydrogen peroxide: a patient with chronic self-induced injury. *Ophthalmology*. 2004;111:1546-1549.
113. Meyer CT, Brand M, DeLuca VA, Spiro HM. Hydrogen peroxide colitis: a report of three patients. *J Clin Gastroenterol*. 1981;3:31-35.
114. Middleton SJ, Jacyna M, McClaren D, Robinson R, Thomas HC. Haemorrhagic pancreatitis—a cause of death in severe potassium permanganate poisoning. *Postgrad Med J*. 1990;66:657-658.
115. Momblano P, Pradere B, Jarrige N, Concina D, Bloom E. Metabolic acidosis induced by cetrimonium bromide. *Lancet*. 1984;2:1045.
116. Monteiro-Riviere NA, Inman AO, Jackson H, Dunn B, Dimond S. Efficacy of topical phenol decontamination strategies on severity of acute phenol chemical burns and dermal absorption: in vitro and in vivo studies in pig skin. *Toxicol Ind Health*. 2001;17:95-104.
117. Moon JM, Chun BJ, Min YI, Moon JM, Chun BJ, Min YI. Hemorrhagic gastritis and gas emboli after ingesting 3% hydrogen peroxide. *J Emerg Med*. 2006;30:403-406.
118. Mucklow ES. Accidental feeding of a dilute antiseptic solution (chlorhexidine 0.05% with cetrimide 1%) to five babies. *Hum Toxicol*. 1988;7:567-569.
119. Mullins ME, Beltran JT. Acute cerebral gas embolism from hydrogen peroxide ingestion successfully treated with hyperbaric oxygen. *J Toxicol Clin Toxicol*. 1998;36:253-256.
120. Mullins ME, Horowitz BZ. Iatrogenic neonatal mercury poisoning from Mercurochrome treatment of a large omphalocele. *Clin Pediatr (Phila)*. 1999;38:111-112.
121. Mutlu H, Silit E, Pekkafali Z, et al. Cranial MR imaging findings of potassium chlorate intoxication. *AJNR Am J Neuroradiol*. 2003;24:1396-1398.
122. Naderi AS, Palmer BF, Naderi ASA, Palmer BF. Successful treatment of a rare case of boric acid overdose with hemodialysis. *Am J Kidney Dis*. 2006;48:e95-97.
123. Nahlieli O, Baruchin AM, Levi D, Shapira Y, Yoffe B. Povidone-iodine related burns. *Burns*. 2001;27:185-188.
124. Norback D. Skin and respiratory symptoms from exposure to alkaline glutaraldehyde in medical services. *Scand J Work Environ Health*. 1988;14:366-371.
125. O'Grady J, Jarecsni E. Sodium chlorate poisoning. *Br J Clin Pract*. 1971;25:38-39.
126. O'Sullivan K, Taylor M. Chronic boric acid poisoning in infants. *Arch Dis Child*. 1983;58:737-739.
127. Ohnishi A, Murai Y. Polyneuropathy due to ethylene oxide, propylene oxide, and butylene oxide. *Environ Res*. 1993;60:242-247.
128. Okano M, Nomura M, Hata S, et al. Anaphylactic symptoms due to chlorhexidine gluconate. *Arch Dermatol*. 1989;125:50-52.
129. Olsen JH, Dossing M. Formaldehyde induced symptoms in day care centers. *Am Ind Hyg Assoc J*. 1982;43:366-370.
130. Ong KL, Tan TH, Cheung WL. Potassium permanganate poisoning—a rare cause of fatal self poisoning. *J Accid Emerg Med*. 1997;14:43-45.
131. Orringer EP, Mattern WD. Formaldehyde-induced hemolysis during chronic hemodialysis. *N Engl J Med*. 1976;294:1416-1420.
132. Palczynski C, Walusiak J, Ruta U, Gorski P. Occupational asthma and rhinitis due to glutaraldehyde: changes in nasal lavage fluid after specific inhalatory challenge test. *Allergy*. 2001;56:1186-1191.
133. Partanen T. Formaldehyde exposure and respiratory cancer—a meta-analysis of the epidemiologic evidence. *Scand J Work Environ Health*. 1993;19:8-15.
134. Pennington JA. A review of iodine toxicity reports. *J Am Diet Assoc*. 1990;90:1571-1581.
135. Pietsch J, Meakins JL. Complications of povidone-iodine absorption in topically treated burn patients. *Lancet*. 1976;1:280-282.
136. Pike D, Peabody J, Davis E, Lyons W. A reevaluation of the dangers of Clorox ingestion. *J Pediatr*. 1963;63:303-305.
137. Pinnas J, Meinke G. Other aldehydes. In: Sullivan J, Krieger GR, ed. *Hazardous Material Toxicology*. Baltimore: Williams & Wilkins; 1992:981-986.
138. Porter JA. Acute respiratory distress following formalin inhalation. *Lancet*. 1975;2:603-604.
139. Pritchett S, Green D, Rossos P, Pritchett S, Green D, Rossos P. Accidental ingestion of 35% hydrogen peroxide. *Can J Gastroenterol*. 2007;21:665-667.
140. Prutting SM, Cerveny JD. Boric acid vaginal suppositories: a brief review. *Infect Dis Obstet Gynecol*. 1998;6:191-194.
141. Pullin TG, Pinkerton MN, Johnston RV, Kilian DJ. Decontamination of the skin of swine following phenol exposure: a comparison of the relative efficacy of water versus polyethylene glycol/industrial methylated spirits. *Toxicol Appl Pharmacol*. 1978;43:199-206.
142. Pun KK, Yeung CK, Chan TK. Acute intravascular hemolysis due to accidental formalin intoxication during hemodialysis. *Clin Nephrol*. 1984;21:188-190.
143. Rackoff WR, Merton DF. Gas embolism after ingestion of hydrogen peroxide. *Pediatrics*. 1990;85:593-594.
144. Rath T, Meissl G. Induction of hyperthyroidism in burn patients treated topically with povidone-iodine. *Burns Incl Therm Inj*. 1988;14:320-322.
145. Rees TD, Orth CF. Oral ulcerations with use of hydrogen peroxide. *J Periodontol*. 1986;57:689-692.
146. Restuccio A, Mortensen ME, Kelley MT. Fatal ingestion of boric acid in an adult. *Am J Emerg Med*. 1992;10:545-547.
147. Robertson P, Fraser J, Sheild J, Weir P. Thyrotoxicosis related to iodine toxicity in a paediatric burn patient [letter]. *Intensive Care Med*. 2002;28:1369.
148. Rohyans J, Walson PD, Wood GA, MacDonald WA. Mercury toxicity following merthiolate ear irrigations. *J Pediatr*. 1984;104:311-313.
149. Roush GC, Walrath J, Stayner LT, Kaplan SA, Flannery JT, Blair A. Nasopharyngeal cancer, sinonasal cancer, and occupations related to formaldehyde: a case-control study. *J Natl Cancer Inst*. 1987;79:1221-1224.
150. Rubenstein AD, Musher DM. Epidemic boric acid poisoning simulating staphylococcal toxic epidermal necrolysis of the newborn infant: Ritter's disease. *J Pediatr*. 1970;77:884-887.
151. Russell AD. Glutaraldehyde: current status and uses. *Infect Control Hosp Epidemiol*. 1994;15:724-733.
152. Salinas E, Sasich L, Hall DH, Kennedy RM, Morriss H. Acute ethylene oxide intoxication. *Drug Intell Clin Pharm*. 1981;15:384-386.
153. Sansone J, Vidal N, Bigliardi R, Voitzuk A, Greco V, Costa K. Unintentional ingestion of 60% hydrogen peroxide by a six-year-old child. *J Toxicol Clin Toxicol*. 2004;42:197-199.
154. Schroder CM, Holler Obrigkeit D, Merk HF, Abuzahra F. [Necrotizing toxic contact dermatitis of the scalp from hydrogen peroxide]. *Hautarzt*. 2008;59:148-150.
155. Selvaggi G, Monstrey S, Van Landuyt K, Hamdi M, Blondeel P. The role of iodine in antisepsis and wound management: a reappraisal. *Acta Chir Belg*. 2003;103:241-247.
156. Shaffer MP, Belsito DV. Allergic contact dermatitis from glutaraldehyde in health-care workers. *Contact Dermatitis*. 2000;43:150-156.
157. Shaw A, Cooperman A, Fusco J. Gas embolism produced by hydrogen peroxide. *N Engl J Med*. 1967;277:238-241.
158. Sheibani S, Gerson LB, Sheibani S, Gerson LB. Chemical colitis. *J Clin Gastroenterol*. 2008;42:115-121.
159. Sherman SJ, Boyer LV, Sibley WA. Cerebral infarction immediately after ingestion of hydrogen peroxide solution. *Stroke*. 1994;25:1065-7106.
160. Shmunes E, Levy EJ. Quaternary ammonium compound contact dermatitis from a deodorant. *Arch Dermatol*. 1972;105:91-93.
161. Singelmann E, Steffen C. Increased erythrocyte rigidity in chlorate poisoning. *J Clin Pathol*. 1983;36:719.
162. Sleigh JW, Linter SP. Hazards of hydrogen peroxide. *BMJ (Clin Res Ed)*. 1985;291:1706.
163. Smerdely P, Lim A, Boyages SC, et al. Topical iodine-containing antiseptics and neonatal hypothyroidism in very-low-birthweight infants. *Lancet*. 1989;2:661-664.
164. Sneddon I. Dermatitis in an intermittent haemodialysis unit. *BMJ*. 1968;1:183-184.
165. Southwood T, Lamb CM, Freeman J. Ingestion of potassium permanganate crystals by a three-year-old boy. *Med J Aust*. 1987;146:639-640.
166. Spiller HA, Quadrani-Kushner DA, Cleveland P. A five year evaluation of acute exposures to phenol disinfectant (26%). *J Toxicol Clin Toxicol*. 1993;31:307-313.
167. Stajich GV, Lopez GP, Harry SW, Sexson WR. Iatrogenic exposure to mercury after hepatitis B vaccination in preterm infants. *J Pediatr*. 2000;136:679-681.
168. Stavrou A, Butcher R, Sakula A. Accidental self-poisoning by sodium chlorate weed-killer. *Practitioner*. 1978;221:397-399.
169. Steenland K, Stayner L, Deddens J. Mortality analyses in a cohort of 18 235 ethylene oxide exposed workers: follow up extended from 1987 to 1998. *Occup Environ Med*. 2004;61:2-7.

170. Steenland K, Stayner L, Greife A, et al. Mortality among workers exposed to ethylene oxide. *N Engl J Med.* 1991;324:1402-1407.
171. Steffen C, Seitz R. Severe chlorate poisoning: report of a case. *Arch Toxicol.* 1981;48:281-288.
172. Steffen C, Wetzel E. Chlorate poisoning: mechanism of toxicity. *Toxicology.* 1993;84:217-231.
173. Steffen C, Wetzel E. Pathophysiological aspects of chlorate poisoning. *Hum Toxicol.* 1984;4:541-542.
174. Stein KM, Odom RB, Justice GR, Martin GC. Toxic alopecia from ingestion of boric acid. *Arch Dermatol.* 1973;108:95-97.
175. Stonehill A, Krop S, Borick P. Buffered glutaraldehyde—a new chemical sterilization solution. *Am J Hosp Pharm.* 1963;20:458-465.
176. Strubelt O, Brasch H, Pentz R, Younes M. Experimental studies on the acute cardiovascular toxicity of formalin and its antidotal treatment. *J Toxicol Clin Toxicol.* 1990;28:221-233.
177. Tabor E, Bostwick DC, Evans CC. Corneal damage due to eye contact with chlorhexidine gluconate. *JAMA.* 1989;261:557-558.
178. Teshima D, Morishita K, Ueda Y, et al. Clinical management of boric acid ingestion: pharmacokinetic assessment of efficacy of hemodialysis for treatment of acute boric acid poisoning. *J Pharmacobiodyn.* 1992;15:287-294.
179. Teshima D, Taniyama T, Oishi R. Usefulness of forced diuresis for acute boric acid poisoning in an adult. *J Clin Pharm Ther.* 2001;26:387-390.
180. Unlu RE, Alagoz MS, Uysal AC, et al. Phenol intoxication in a child. *J Craniofac Surg.* 2004;15:1010-1013.
181. Valdes-Dapena M, Arey J. Boric acid poisoning: Three fatal cases with pancreatic inclusions and a review of the literature. *J Pediatr.* 1962;61:531-546.
182. van Berkel M, de Wolff FA. Survival after acute benzalkonium chloride poisoning. *Hum Toxicol.* 1988;7:191-193.
183. Vander Heide SJ, Seamon JP. Resolution of delayed altered mental status associated with hydrogen peroxide ingestion following hyperbaric oxygen therapy. *Acad Emerg Med.* 2003;10:998-1000.
184. Vorherr H, Vorherr U, Mehta P, et al. Vaginal absorption of povidone-iodine. *JAMA.* 1988;244:2628-2629.
185. Wallgren H. Relative intoxicating effects of ethyl, propyl and butyl alcohol. *Acta Pharmacol Toxicol.* 1960;16:217-220.
186. Warner MA, Harper JV. Cardiac dysrhythmias associated with chemical peeling with phenol. *Anesthesiology.* 1985;62:366-367.
187. Watt BE, Proudfoot AT, Vale JA, Watt BE, Proudfoot AT, Vale JA. Hydrogen peroxide poisoning. *Toxicol Rev.* 2004;23:51-57.
188. Weeks RS, Ravitch MM. Esophageal injury by liquid chlorine bleach: experimental study. *J Pediatr.* 1969;74:911-916.
189. Wilson JT, Burr IM. Benzalkonium chloride poisoning in infant twins. *Am J Dis Child.* 1975;129:1208-1209.
190. Wong L, Heimbach M, Truscott D, Duncan B. Boric acid poisoning: report of 11 cases. *Can Med Assoc J.* 1964;90:1018-1023.
191. Wu ML, Tsai WJ, Yang CC, Deng JF. Concentrated cresol intoxication. *Vet Hum Toxicol.* 1998;40:341-343.
192. Yanagawa Y, Kaneko N, Hatanaka K, et al. A case of attempted suicide from the ingestion of formalin. *Clin Toxicol (Phila).* 2007;45:72-76.
193. Young RJ, Critchley JA, Young KK, Freebairn RC, Reynolds AP, Lolin YI. Fatal acute hepatorenal failure following potassium permanganate ingestion. *Hum Exp Toxicol.* 1996;15:259-261.

CHAPTER 103
CAMPHOR AND MOTH REPELLENTS

Edwin K. Kuffner

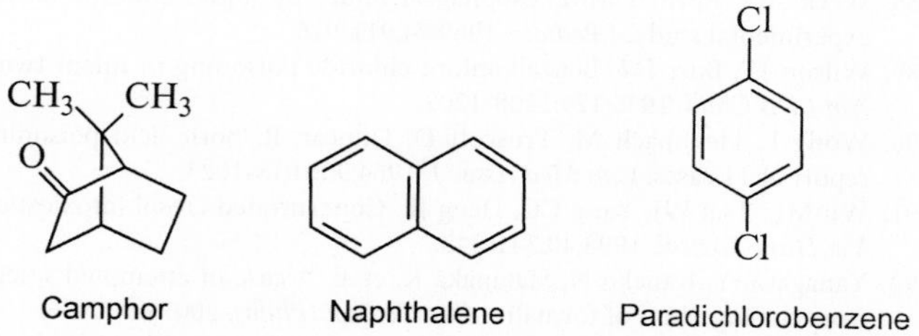

Camphor Naphthalene Paradichlorobenzene

Many different products have historically been used as moth repellents. In the United States, paradichlorobenzene has largely replaced both camphor and naphthalene as the most common active component of moth repellent and moth flakes because of its decreased toxicity. However, because paradichlorobenzene is widely available and because life-threatening camphor and naphthalene toxicity still occur, all of these xenobiotics need to be considered in evaluating possible exposure moth repellent.

CAMPHOR

HISTORY AND EPIDEMIOLOGY

Camphor (2-bormanone, 2-camphonone), a cyclic ketone of the terpene group, is an essential oil distilled from the bark of the camphor tree, *Cinnamomum camphora*. Today, most camphor is synthesized from the hydrocarbon pinene, a derivative of turpentine oil. Camphor has been used as an aphrodisiac, contraceptive, abortifacient, suppressor of lactation, analeptic, cardiac stimulant, antiseptic, cold remedy, muscle liniment, and drug of abuse.[27,34,40,45,50,60,71,72]

Camphorated oil and camphorated spirits contain varying concentrations of camphor. Historically, most camphorated oil was 20% weight (of solute) per weight (of solvent) (w/w) camphor with cottonseed oil, and most camphorated spirits contained 10% w/w camphor with isopropyl alcohol. Toxicity and death following ingestion of camphorated oil, which was confused with castor oil and cod liver oil, prompted the FDA to ban the nonprescription sale of camphorated oil in the United States in 1983.[3,21,40,64,81] Today, based on the 1983 FDA ruling, nonprescription camphor-containing products may not have greater than an 11% concentration of camphor. Camphorated oil is still used as an herbal remedy and muscle liniment, and products containing greater than 11% camphor can still be purchased outside of the United States.[78]

Common camphor-containing products include cold sore ointments (usually <1% camphor), muscle liniments, rubefacients (usually 4%–7% camphor), and camphor spirits (usually 10% camphor). Paregoric, camphorated tincture of opium, contains a combination of anhydrous morphine (0.4 mg/mL), alcohol (46%), and benzoic acid (4 mg/mL) but only a small amount of camphor.[43] Camphor for industrial use can be purchased legally in the United States and contains up to 100% camphor. Occupational exposures to camphor occur during the manufacture of plastic, celluloid, lacquer, varnish, explosives, embalming fluids, and numerous pharmaceuticals and cosmetics.[35]

Although products containing lower concentrations of camphor are implicitly safer, life-threatening toxicity and death may still result, usually from misuse or intentional overdose. Most reported cases of acute camphor poisoning are unintentional ingestions of camphor-containing liquids mistaken for other medications.[3,40,63,79] According to data obtained by the American Association of Poison Control Centers (AAPCC), each year there are approximately 10,000 exposures to camphor with very few reports of "major" toxicity. Over the past 20 years, according to the AAPCC, only six reported deaths were attributable to camphor, all in adults, at least two of which occurred in the setting of an intentional suicidal overdose. Chapter 135 contains complete references and discussion of the AAPCC data.

PHARMACOLOGY

Camphor is a colorless glassy solid. Camphor's pharmacologic activity is not well studied and its mechanism of action remains unclear. It is unlikely that camphor has therapeutic benefit as an expectorant or an antiinfective. Camphor may provide some local analgesic and antipruritic effects, but much safer xenobiotics are available for these indications. No therapeutic benefit of camphor has been proven in any well-controlled clinical trials.

PHARMACOKINETICS AND TOXICOKINETICS

There are limited data on the pharmacokinetics and toxicokinetics of camphor. Toxicity is reported following ingestion, inhalation, intranasal instillation, intraperitoneal administration, and transplacental transfer.[15,65,69,75,76,86] Dermal exposures have been reported to cause systemic toxicity.[30,61] Camphor from liquid preparations is rapidly absorbed from the gastrointestinal tract and camphor can be detected in the blood within 15–20 minutes postingestion.[65] Camphor is highly lipid soluble and is predominantly metabolized in the liver where it undergoes hydroxylation followed by conjugation with glucuronic acid. Inactive metabolites, including campherol, borneol, hydroxycamphor, and camphoglycuronic acid, are excreted by the kidneys.[66]

As with many xenobiotics, the toxic dose of camphor reported in the medical literature is highly variable.[31,40,74] As little as 1 teaspoon (approximately 5 gms) of 20% camphorated oil reportedly caused death in an infant.[74] Workplace standards include the Occupational Safety and Health Administration (OSHA) permissible exposure limit (PEL), which is 2 mg/m^3, the American Conference of Governmental Industrial Hygienists (ACGIH) threshold limit value (TLV), which is 12 mg/m^3 (2 ppm), and the ACGIH short-term exposure limit (STEL), which is 19 mg/m^3 (3 ppm); NIOSH Immediately Dangerous To Life or Health Concentration (IDLH) is 200 mg/m^3.[83]

PATHOPHYSIOLOGY

The mechanism of toxicity of camphor is unknown. Camphor is an irritant. Pathologic changes following ingestion include cerebral edema, neuronal degeneration, fatty changes, centrilobular congestion of the liver, and hemorrhagic lesions in the skin, gastrointestinal tract, and kidneys.[19,41,74,86]

CLINICAL MANIFESTATIONS

Exposure to camphor can often be detected by its characteristic aromatic odor (Chap. 20). Ingestion of camphor typically produces oropharyngeal irritation, nausea, vomiting, and abdominal pain. Generalized tonic–clonic seizures may be the first sign of camphor toxicity, usually occurring within 1–2 hours postingestion.[5,8] Most seizures are brief and self-limited, although some patients may have a more protracted course.[5,26,47,75] Delayed seizures, up to 9 hours following ingestion and up to 72 hours following dermal exposure, have been reported.[30,67] Central nervous system (CNS) depression is common, but rarely compromises respiratory function.[15,46] Other neurologic effects include headache, lightheadedness, transient visual changes, confusion, myoclonus, and hyperreflexia.[44,65,69] Psychiatric effects include agitation, anxiety, and hallucinations.[31,44,46] Dermal effects include flushing and petechial hemorrhages.[15,34,76] Camphor does not typically cause life-threatening cardiovascular effects although a case of myocarditis is reported.[9,34] Death is reported secondary to respiratory failure or seizures.[15]

Case reports suggest that acute ingestion of camphor can cause transient elevations of the hepatic aminotransferases.[3,41,65,69,74] Chronic administration of camphor to a child caused altered mental status and elevated hepatic aminotransferases concentrations suggestive of Reye syndrome.[41] When hepatotoxicity occurs, however, camphor does not typically produce morphologic changes of the liver characteristic of Reye syndrome. Albuminuria can also occur.[74]

Camphor crosses the placenta. Both fetal demise and delivery of healthy neonates are reported in mothers who develop camphor toxicity within 24 hours of term delivery.[10,65,86] Specific dose-related toxicity could not be determined from these case reports.

Inhalational and dermal exposure from camphor usually produces only mucous membrane and dermal irritation, respectively.[29]

DIAGNOSTIC TESTING

When managing most patients with camphor toxicity, no specific toxicologic diagnostic testing is indicated. Although camphor and its metabolites can be identified in blood and urine, concentrations are not useful in most cases of acute toxicity because they are not readily available and have not been proven to correlate with clinical toxicity.[34,45,66]

MANAGEMENT

The patients who should be evaluated in a healthcare facility after an acute ingestion include those who have signs or symptoms consistent with camphor toxicity, those who have ingested more than 1 g of camphor (1 teaspoon of 20% camphorated oil or approximately 2 teaspoons of 11% camphorated oil), suicidal patients, and any patient with a significant occupational exposure.

Gastric decontamination is not well studied in patients who have ingested camphor. If lavage is deemed necessary following recent ingestion of a camphor-containing solution, nasogastric suctioning and lavage are preferable to orogastric lavage. Because camphor-containing solutions are so rapidly absorbed, the benefit of gastrointestinal decontamination is expected to rapidly diminish as the time following ingestion increases. Emetics should not be administered because camphor-induced seizures can occur rapidly prior to the onset of emesis, raising the risk of pulmonary aspiration. There is no human evidence in support for or against the use of activated charcoal in camphor ingestions. A consensus panel has recommended against the use of activated charcoal in isolated camphor ingestions.[52] There is no antidote for camphor. Most patients survive with supportive care. Although the management of camphor-induced seizures is not well studied, patients should be treated with benzodiazepines. Repeat doses of benzodiazepines may be needed to control seizures. If benzodiazepines fail to control seizures, other sedative-hypnotic agents, including phenobarbital, pentobarbital, and propofol, should be administered. Case reports suggest that most patients who develop life-threatening camphor toxicity develop symptoms within a few hours postexposure. Based on this, an observation period of at least 2–4 hours following a potentially toxic ingestion of camphor is reasonable. Delayed seizures, up to 9 hours following ingestion and up to 72 hours following dermal exposure, have been reported.[30,67] In case reports, hemodialysis with a lipid dialysate and either hemoperfusion using an Amberlite resin or charcoal hemoperfusion successfully removed camphor.[3,25,46,47,53] Neither isolated lipid hemodialysis nor lipid dialysis in combination with hemoperfusion is routinely recommended or widely available.

NAPHTHALENE

HISTORY AND EPIDEMIOLOGY

Historically, naphthalene toxicity has resulted from its use as an antihelminthic and an antiseptic.[73] Toilet-bowl and diaper-pail deodorizers containing naphthalene have also caused toxicity.[14,91] Naphthalene is the single most abundant component of coal tar and is a component of petroleum. Occupational exposures to naphthalene may occur during the manufacture of dyes, synthetic resins, celluloid, solvents, and fuels. Naphthalene is a component of fuels and is also generated as a by-product of combustion.

Most unintentional exposures to naphthalene-containing moth repellents occur in children and do not cause life-threatening toxicity. According to data from the AAPCC, each year there are between 1500 and 2000 case mentions of naphthalene. Since 1998 there has not been a naphthalene-associated death reported to AAPCC, and reports of "major toxicity" are very unusual (see Chap. 135). Mothball vapors are also intentionally inhaled as a form of inhalant abuse.[49]

PHARMACOLOGY, PHARMACOKINETICS, AND TOXICOKINETICS

Naphthalene ($C_{10}H_8$), an aromatic bicyclic hydrocarbon, is a white, flakey crystalline solid with a noxious odor. Synonyms include white tar and tar camphor. Naphthalene toxicity is reported following ingestion, dermal application, and inhalation.[16,18,20,68,85] Although the absorption of naphthalene is not well studied, highly lipid-soluble compounds may increase both oral and dermal absorption. Naphthalene metabolism is complex and varies considerably among species and different anatomical regions.[11] Naphthalene is metabolized in the liver by CYP isoenzymes to naphthalene 1,2-oxide. Naphthalene 1,2-oxide can react with cellular components such as DNA and protein to form covalent adducts, can be spontaneously converted to 1-naphthol and 2-naphthol, the glucuronides and sulfates of which are renally eliminated, further metabolized to 1,4-naphthoquinone or detoxified by glutathione-*S*-transferase and excreted in the urine as mercaputuric acid metabolites.[11,64] These hepatic metabolites, primarily α-naphthol, but not the parent compound,[64,90] cause the oxidant stress responsible for naphthalene-induced hemolysis and methemoglobinemia. As with most xenobiotics, the toxic amount of naphthalene reported in the medical literature is highly variable. As little as one naphthalene mothball has resulted in toxicity, including hemolysis in an infant.[24,91] Workplace standards include the OSHA PEL, which is 50 mg/m^3 (10 ppm), ACGIH TLV, which is 52 mg/m^3 (10 ppm), and the ACGIH STEL, which is 79 mg/m^3 (15 ppm); NIOSH IDLH is 250 ppm (US Dept of Labor OSHA).[82]

PATHOPHYSIOLOGY

To understand naphthalene-induced hemolysis and methemoglobinemia, it is important to understand how oxidant stress affects erythrocytes and the normal mechanisms erythrocytes use to prevent and reverse the effects of oxidant stress.

Oxidant stressors can cause methemoglobinemia and/or hemolysis. When oxidant stress causes an iron atom from any of the four globin chains of hemoglobin to be oxidized from the ferrous state (Fe^{2+}) to the ferric state (Fe^{3+}) state, methemoglobin is formed (see Chap. 127). When oxidant stress causes hemoglobin denaturation, the heme groups and the globin chains dissociate and precipitate in the erythrocyte, forming Heinz bodies. An erythrocyte with denatured hemoglobin is more susceptible to hemolysis and removal by the reticuloendothelial system (see Chap. 24).

Hemolysis and methemoglobinemia can occur independently of each other or simultaneously in patients with either normal or deficient glucose-6-phosphate dehydrogenase (G6PD) activity.[24,39,85,91]

Theoretically, patients with G6PD deficiency are at increased risk for both hemolysis and methemoglobinemia following oxidant stress. In practice, however, patients with glucose-6-phosphate deficiency are at much greater risk of hemolysis than of methemoglobinemia.

Patients with G6PD deficiency are at increased risk for hemolysis because they have decreased glutathione stores.[85,90] Glucose-6-phosphate deficiency affects all races but is most prevalent in patients of African, Mediterranean and Asian descent. The gene that codes for G6PD is X-linked; consequently, men are affected more often than women.

Infants are also at increased risk of methemoglobinemia because fetal hemoglobin is more susceptible to the formation of methemoglobin and also because nicotinamide adenine dinucleotide (NADH) methemoglobin reductase activity is decreased, impairing the reduction of methemoglobin to hemoglobin.[42]

CLINICAL MANIFESTATIONS

Both acute and chronic exposures to naphthalene result in similar toxicity.[14,57,90] Ingestion and inhalational exposures to naphthalene commonly cause headache, nausea, vomiting, diarrhea, abdominal pain, fever, and altered mental status.[14,51,58] Dermal exposure results in dermatitis.[27]

Hemolysis or methemoglobinemia usually becomes clinically evident, as early as 24–48 hours postexposure, but more typically on the third day postexposure because of the time necessary for the metabolism of naphthalene.[18] Anemia secondary to hemolysis often does not reach its nadir until 3–5 days postexposure.[80]

Signs and symptoms of hemolysis and methemoglobinemia are nonspecific and include tachycardia, tachypnea, shortness of breath, generalized weakness, decreased exercise tolerance, and altered mental status. Methemoglobinemia may produce cyanosis, whereas hemolysis may produce pallor and jaundice (see Chap. 127). Renal failure as a complication of naphthalene-induced hemolysis and hemoglobinuria is reported. Naphthalene or its metabolites cross the placenta.[4] Naphthalene pica during pregnancy causes both maternal and fetal toxicity. Children born to mothers who were experiencing naphthalene toxicity at the time of delivery have developed hemolytic anemia believed to be related to the maternal naphthalene exposure.[90] Although cataracts have been reported in animals following naphthalene exposure, human data are limited.[55]

Although naphthalene is classified by the International Agency for Cancer Research (IARC) as a Group 2B carcinogen (possibly carcinogenic to humans), and by the EPA as a Group C possible human carcinogen, the data supporting human carcinogenicity of naphthalene are limited.[28,38]

DIAGNOSTIC TESTING

No specific diagnostic testing is indicated, although both naphthalene and its metabolites can be identified in blood and urine. Identification of 1-naphthol and 2-naphthol in the urine can confirm exposure to naphthalene;[59] qualitative or quantitative testing for naphthalene or its metabolites is rarely clinically indicated when managing a case of an acute overdose.

The presentation of naphthalene-induced hemolysis is similar to that of hemolysis from other causes. Reticulocytosis occurs as a response to restore a normal hemoglobin concentration. Hyperbilirubinemia from hemolysis is characterized by an elevation of the indirect bilirubin (unconjugated bilirubin) and a relatively normal direct (conjugated) fraction. Serum haptoglobin is usually low because the haptoglobin–hemoglobin complex is cleared by the kidneys. Both the direct and indirect Coombs tests are negative in naphthalene-induced hemolytic anemia. Lactate dehydrogenase is elevated because it is released from hemolyzed red blood cells. Gross or microscopic hemoglobinuria is confirmed by a urine dipstick that reacts strongly positive for hemoglobin with a paucity of red blood cells on microscopic examination of the urine sediment. This should be differentiated from myoglobinemia by measuring the serum creatine phosphokinase, which will be elevated in patients with rhabdomyolysis and myoglobinuria.

Examination of a peripheral blood smear can reveal evidence of hemolysis before a patient develops clinical or laboratory evidence of anemia. The peripheral smear may reveal red blood cell (RBC) fragmentation, anisocytosis, microspherocytosis, reticulocytosis, nucleated RBCs, Blister cells, and Heinz body formation (see Chap. 24). Peripheral smear abnormalities and anemia may occur within the first 24 hours following ingestion.[14,70,90,91] Testing for G6PD activity is not routinely recommended during an acute episode of hemolysis. Reticulocytes have higher G6PD activity than do older RBCs. If G6PD activity is measured during an episode of hemolysis when many of the older RBCs have already been destroyed, the G6PD activity may be falsely normal. It is best to delay testing for G6PD activity for a few months following an episode of hemolysis. Family members of patients with life-threatening G6PD deficiency should also be tested.

Naphthalene-induced methemoglobinemia is similar in presentation to methemoglobinemia from other xenobiotics. The percentage of methemoglobin can rapidly be determined using a cooximeter (see Chap. 127).

MANAGEMENT

Most patients with an unintentional exposure to all or part of one naphthalene-containing mothball do not require medical evaluation. Patients who should be evaluated in a healthcare facility following an acute ingestion include those who recently ingested more than one naphthalene-containing mothball equivalent, those with signs or symptoms of toxicity, especially hemolysis and/or methemoglobinemia, those with known or suspected G6PD deficiency, all intentional ingestions, and those patients with large inhalational exposures, especially after exposure occurs in an occupational setting.

Gastrointestinal decontamination is not well studied in patients who have ingested naphthalene. Most patients with unintentional exposures do not require gastrointestinal decontamination. Emesis may be useful following ingestion of multiple naphthalene-containing mothballs in children, provided it can be administered within 30–60 minutes postingestion. Administration of activated charcoal, 1 g/kg, although not of proven efficacy, is also reasonable because it is considered safe. Repeat doses of activated charcoal 0.5 g/kg and/or whole-bowel irrigation with polyethylene glycol electrolyte lavage solution would only be indicated for patients with large ingestions of naphthalene who are expected to have significant ongoing absorption of naphthalene within the gastrointestinal tract.

Diagnostic testing within the first 24–48 hours postexposure may detect the onset of methemoglobinemia and/or hemolysis before a patient becomes symptomatic. Most low-risk patients who are asymptomatic within the first 24–48 hours postexposure and who have no laboratory evidence of hemolysis or methemoglobinemia can be managed as outpatients if reevaluation within 24 hours can be arranged. Patients who are discharged should be instructed to return if they become symptomatic. High-risk patients, patients with laboratory evidence of hemolysis and/or methemoglobinemia, and patients who cannot reliably be managed as outpatients should be admitted.

Patients with life-threatening hemolysis and anemia should be transfused with packed red blood cells. However, most healthy patients will be able to compensate for the hemolysis and will not require a transfusion. Patients with symptomatic methemoglobinemia should receive methylene blue, 1–2 mg/kg (0.1–0.2 mL/kg of a 1% solution) intravenously. Repeat doses may be necessary (see Antidotes in Depth A41: Methylene Blue).

PARADICHLOROBENZENE

HISTORY AND EPIDEMIOLOGY

Paradichlorobenzene is widely used as a deodorizer, disinfectant, repellent, fumigant, insecticide, fungicide, and industrial solvent. Today, paradichlorobenzene is the most common component of moth repellents. Exposure to paradichlorobenzene in the United States is extremely common. A 1995 study suggested that 2,5-dichlorophenol, a metabolite of paradichlorobenzene, was detectable in the urine in 98% of the US population.[36]

Most unintentional exposures to paradichlorobenzene-containing moth repellents occur in children and do not cause toxicity. According to the AAPCC data there were no deaths and no reports of major toxicity associated with paradichlorobenzene between 1998 and 2007.

PHARMACOLOGY, PHARMACOKINETICS, TOXICOKINETICS, AND PATHOPHYSIOLOGY

Paradichlorobenzene ($C_6H_4Cl_2$) is a colorless solid with a noxious odor. It is available as pure white crystals, as a solid in combination with other chemicals, or as a liquid dissolved in volatile solvents or oil.[2] The mechanism for the effects and toxicology of paradichlorobenzene has not been studied. Although rare, paradichlorobenzene toxicity has been reported following ingestion and inhalation.[37,54] Inhalation toxicokinetics reveal that in humans there is rapid distribution to tissues, specifically adipose, and that the major route of elimination is urinary excretion followed by metabolism, not exhalation.[7,89] Workplace standards include the OSHA PEL, which is 450 mg/m^3 (75 ppm) TWA, ACGIH TLV, which is 60 mg/m^3 (10 ppm) TWA, and the ACGIH STEL, which is 675 mg/m^3 (110 ppm); NIOSH IDLH is 150 ppm.[84]

CLINICAL MANIFESTATIONS

Inhalation of paradichlorobenzene may cause nausea and vomiting, headache, and mucous membrane irritation.[17,37] Only a single case report links acute ingestion of a moth repellent, purportedly containing paradichlorobenzene with hemolysis. The demothing agent itself was not confirmed to be paradichlorobenzene.[32]

Case reports associate chronic exposure to paradichlorobenzene with weight loss, leukoencephalopathy, a spectrum of neuropsychiatric effects including weakness, ataxia and hypotonia, pulmonary granulomatosis, dyspnea, hepatotoxicity, anemia, and fixed drug eruptions.[12,13,17,22,33,36,54,56,77,87]

Paradicholorobenze is classified by IARC as a Group 2B, Possibly Carcinogenic to Humans.

DIAGNOSTIC TESTING

Both paradichlorobenzene and its metabolite, 2,5-dichlorophenol, can be identified in blood and urine following exposure.[7] Identification of 2,5-dichlorophenol can confirm exposure to paradichlorobenzene. Quantifying the amount of paradichlorobenzene in the urine of workers may be useful for monitoring occupational exposures.[23] Qualitative or quantitative testing for paradichlorobenzene or its metabolites is not generally indicated when managing a patient with an acute overdose. Structural CNS abnormalities including toxic leukoencephalopathy may be noted on imaging studies.[6]

MANAGEMENT

Referral to a Healthcare Facility Most unintentional exposures to paradichlorobenzene do not cause life-threatening toxicity. Thus most asymptomatic patients with unintentional exposures can be managed as outpatients. Patients who should be evaluated in a healthcare facility include those with clinical signs or symptoms, suicidal patients, and patients who have sustained a large exposure.

Gastrointestinal Decontamination Gastrointestinal decontamination has not been studied in patients who ingest paradichlorobenzene. Most patients with unintentional exposures do not require gastrointestinal decontamination. Administration of activated charcoal, 1 g/kg, although not studied, is reasonable for patients with large, intentional ingestions.

TABLE 103–1. Moth Repellents: Laboratory Differentiation[1,48,50,62,88]

Characteristic	Camphor	Naphthalene	Paradichlorobenzene
Water solubility (g/L)	1.2	0.03	0.08
Buoyancy in water	Floats	Sinks	Sinks
Buoyancy in water saturated with table salt	Floats	Floats	Sinks
Radiopacity	Radiolucent	Faintly radiopaque	Densely radiopaque
Melting point	350.6°F (177°C)	176°F (80°C)	127.4°F (53°C)
Placement in covered test tube in 140°F (60°C) water bath	Does not melt	Does not melt	Melts
Boiling point	399.2°F (204°C)	424.4°F (218°C)	345.2°F (174°C)
Addition of chloroform	Untested	Blue color	No reaction
Place on copper wire in a flame	Untested	Flame is yellow-orange	Initially flame is yellow-orange then bright green
Solubility in turpentine	Untested	Fast	Slow.

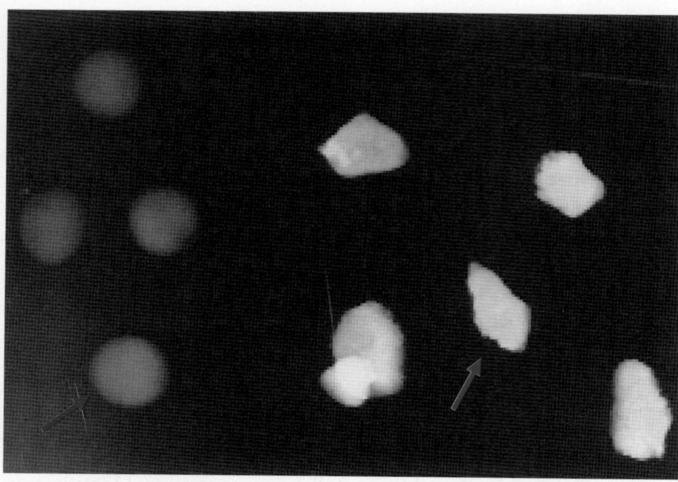

FIGURE 103–1. Radiograph of mothballs. Paradichlorobenzene (⟶) is densely radiopaque, whereas naphthalene (⟶) is faintly radiopaque.

MOTH REPELLENT RECOGNITION

Healthcare providers occasionally must determine whether a mothball is made of naphthalene, paradichlorobenzene, or camphor since management and prognosis differ. When the container is unavailable, as is often the case, mothballs are difficult to distinguish based on appearance, odor, texture, or size. Most mothballs are white, crystalline, and have a noxious odor.[88] Camphor moth repellents are more oily than both naphthalene and paradichlorobenzene mothballs. If controls are available, moth repellents can often be differentiated based on their odor and texture.[1] Although most new paradichlorobenzene moth repellents are slightly larger than most new naphthalene moth repellents, all moth repellents shrink over time when exposed to air, making size an unreliable differentiating characteristic. Identifying a moth repellent as paradichlorobenzene can often result in outpatient management, saving both money and undue worry. The tests described in Table 103–1 and shown in Figure 103–1 might allow rapid identification of the component of an unknown moth repellent. When performing these tests it is most helpful to have camphor, naphthalene, and paradichlorobenzene controls available for comparison.

SUMMARY

Historically, the most common components of moth repellents are camphor, naphthalene, and paradichlorobenzene. In the United States, paradichlorobenzene has largely replaced both camphor and naphthalene. If an unknown moth repellent can be identified as paradichlorobenzene, limited toxicity is expected following an acute exposure. It is important for clinicians to understand how to use simple tests to identify the component of an unknown mothball. Because life-threatening camphor and naphthalene toxicity are still reported, it is important for clinicians to understand how to manage patients exposed to both of these xenobiotics.

REFERENCES

1. Ambre J, Ruo TI, Smith-Coggins R. Mothball composition: three simple tests for distinguishing paradichlorobenzene from naphthalene. *Ann Emerg Med.* 1986;15:724-726.
2. Anonymous. Ortho, meta and para-dichlorobenzene. *Rev Environ Contam Toxicol.* 1988;106:51-68.
3. Antman E, Jacob G, Volpe B, et al. Camphor overdosage. Therapeutic considerations. *N Y Med J.* 1978;78:896-897.
4. Anziulewicz JA, Dick HJ, Chiarvili EE. Transplacental naphthalene poisoning. *Am J Obstet Gynecol.* 1959;78:519-521.
5. Aronow R, Spigiel RW. Implications of camphor poisoning. *Drug Intell Clin Pharm.* 1976;10:631-634.
6. Avila E, Schraeder P, Belliappa A, et al. Pica with paradichlorobenzene mothball ingestion associated with toxic leukoencephalopathy. *Am Soc Neuorimaging.* 2006;16:78-81.
7. Azouz WM, Parke DV, Williams RT. Studies in detoxification. The metabolism of halogenobenzenes. Ortho- and paradichlorobenzenes. *Biochem J.* 1955;59:410-415.
8. Benz RW. Camphorated oil poisoning with no mortality. Report of twenty cases. *JAMA.* 1919;72:1217-1218.
9. Bhaya M, Beniwal R. Camphor induced myocarditis. A case report. *Cardiovac Toxicol.* 2007;7:212-214.
10. Blackmon WP, Curry HB. Camphor poisoning: report of a case occurring during pregnancy. *J Fla Med Assoc.* 1957;43:999-1000.
11. Bogen KT, Benson JM, Yost GS, et al. Naphthalene metabolism in relation to target tissue anatomy, physiology, cytotoxicity and tumorigenic mechanism of action. *Reg Toxicol Pharmacol.* 2008;51:S27-S36.
12. Campbell DM, Davidson RJ. Toxic haemolytic anemia in pregnancy due to a pica for paradichlorobenzene. *J Obstet Gynaecol Br Commonw.* 1970;77:657-659.
13. Cheong R, Wilson RK, Cortese ICM, et al. Mothball withdrawal encephalopathy-case report and review of paradichlorobenzene neurotoxicity. *Subst Abus.* 2006;27:63-67.
14. Chusid E, Fried CT. Acute hemolytic anemia due to naphthalene ingestion. *Am J Dis Child.* 1955;89:612-614.
15. Clark TL. Fatal case of camphor poisoning. *BMJ.* 1924;1:467.
16. Cock TC. Acute hemolytic anemia in the neonatal period. *AMA J Dis Children.* 1957;94:77.
17. Cotter LH. Paradichlorobenzene poisoning from insecticides. *N Y State J Med.* 1953;53:1690-1699.
18. Dawson JP, Thayer WW, Desforges JF. Acute hemolytic anemia in the newborn infant due to naphthalene poisoning: A report of two cases with investigations into the mechanism of the disease. *Blood.* 1958;13:1113-1125.
19. Emery DP, Corban JG. Camphor toxicity. *J Paediatr Child Health.* 1999;35:105-106.
20. Fanburg SJ. Exfoliative dermatitis due to naphthalene. *Arch Derm Syph.* 1940;42:53-58.
21. Food and Drug Administration. Proposed rules: External analgesic drug products for over-the-counter human use; tentative final monograph. *Fed Reg.* 1983;48:5852-5869.
22. Frank SB, Cohen HJ. Fixed drug eruption due to paradichlorobenzene. *N Y State J Med.* 1961;61:4079.
23. Ghittori S, Imbriani M, Pezzagno G, et al. Urinary elimination of *p*-dichlorobenzene (*p* -DCB) and weighted exposure concentration. *G Ital Med Lav.* 1985;7:59-63.
24. Gidron E, Leurer J. Naphthalene poisoning. *Lancet.* 1956;1:228-233.
25. Ginn HE, Anderson KE, Mercier RK, et al. Camphor intoxication treated by lipid dialysis. *JAMA.* 1968;203:230-231.
26. Gouin S, Patel H. Unusual cause of seizure. *Pediatr Emerg Care.* 1996;12:298-300.
27. Greene RR, Ivy AC. The effect of camphor oil on lactation. *JAMA.* 1938;110:641-642.
28. Griego FY, Bogen KT, Price PS, et al. Exposure, epidemiology and human cancer incidence of naphthalene. *Reg Toxicol Pharmacol.* 2008;51:S22-S26.
29. Gronka PA, Bobkoskie RL, Tomchick GJ, et al. Camphor exposure in a packaging plant. *Am Ind Hyg Assoc J.* 1969;30:276-279.
30. Guilbert J, Flamant C, Hallalel F, et al. Anti-flatuence treatment and status epilepticus: a case of camphor intoxication. *Emerg Med J.* 2007;24:859-860.
31. Haft HH. Camphor liniment poisoning. *JAMA.* 1925;84:1571.
32. Hallowell M. Acute haemolytic anaemia following the ingestion of paradichlorobenzene. *Arch Dis Child.* 1959;34:74-75.
33. Harden RA, Baetjer MA. Aplastic anemia following exposure to paradichlorobenzene and naphthalene. *J Occup Med.* 1978;20:820-822.
34. Heard JD, Brooks RC. A clinical and experimental investigation of the therapeutic value of camphor. *Am J Med Sci.* 1913;145:238-253.
35. Herrmann AP Jr. Camphorated oil: Health, history and hazard. *Am Pharm.* 1978;18:15.

36. Hill RH, Ashley DL, Head SL, et al. *p* -Dichlorobenzene exposure among 1,000 adults in the United States. *Arch Environ Health*. 1995;50:277-280.
37. Hollingsworth RL, Rowe VK, Oyen F, et al. Toxicity of paradichlorobenzene: Determinations on experimental animals and human subjects. *Arch Indus Health*. 1956;14:138-147.
38. International Agency for Research on Cancer (IARC). Traditional herbal medicines, some mycotoxins, naphthalene and styrene. IARC monographs on the evaluation of carcinogenic risks to humans 2002;vol 82 IARC, Lyon, France.
39. Jacobziner H, Raybin HW. Accidental chemical poisonings. Naphthalene poisoning. *N Y State J Med*. 1964;1762-1766.
40. Jacobziner H, Raybin HW. Camphor poisoning. *Arch Pediatr*. 1962;79:28.
41. Jimenez JF, Brown AL, Arnold WC, et al. Chronic camphor ingestion mimicking Reye's syndrome. *Gastroenterology*. 1983;84:394-398.
42. Johnson CJ, Bonrud PA, Dosch TL, et al. Fatal outcome of methemoglobinemia in an infant. *JAMA*. 1987;257:2796-2797.
43. Kauffman RE, Banner W, Berlin CM, et al. Camphor revisited: Focus on toxicity. Committee on Drugs. American Academy of Pediatrics. *Pediatrics*. 1994;94:127-128.
44. Klingensmith WR. Poisoning by camphor. *JAMA*. 1934;102:2182-2183.
45. Köppel C, Tenczer J, Schirop T, et al. Camphor poisoning, abuse of camphor as a stimulant. *Arch Toxicol*. 1982;51:101-106.
46. Köppel C, Martens F, Schirop T, Ibe K. Hemoperfusion in acute camphor poisoning. *Intensive Care Med*. 1988;14:431-433.
47. Kopelman R, Miller S, Kelly R, et al. Camphor intoxication treated by resin hemoperfusion. *JAMA*. 1979;241:727-728.
48. Koyama K, Yamashita M, Ogura Y, et al. A simple test for mothball component differentiation using water and a saturated solution of table salt: Its utilization for poison information service. *Vet Hum Tox*. 1991; 33:425-427.
49. Kuczkowski K M. Mothballs and obstetric anesthesia. *Ann Fr Anesth Reanim*. 2006;25:464;465.
50. Lahoud CA, March JA, Proctor DD. Campho-Phenique ingestion: An intentional overdose. *South Med J*. 1997;90:647-648.
51. Linick M. Illness associated with exposure to naphthalene in mothballs. *MMWR Morb Mortal Wkly Rep*. 1983;32:34-35.
52. Manoguerra AS, Erdman AR, Wax PM, et al. Camphor poisoning: An evidence-based practice guideline for out-of-hospital management. *Clin Toxicol*. 2006;44:357-370.
53. Mascie-Taylor BH, Widop B, Davison AM. Camphor intoxication treated by charcoal hemoperfusion. *Postgrad Med J*. 1981;57:725-726.
54. Miyai I, Hirono N, Fujita M, et al. Reversible ataxia following chronic exposure to paradichlorobenzene. *J Neurol Neurosurg Psychiatry*. 1988; 51:453-454.
55. Molloy EJ, Boctor BA, Reed MD, et al. Perinatal/Neonatal case presentation. Perinatal toxicity of domestic naphthalaene exposure. *J Perinatol*. 2004;24:792-793.
56. Nalbandian RM, Pearce JF. Allergic purpura induced by exposure to *p*-dichlorobenzene. Confirmation by indirect basophil degranulation test. *JAMA*. 1965;194:238-239.
57. Nash FL. Naphthalene poisoning. *BMJ*. 1903;1:251-259.
58. Ostlere R, Amos R, Wass JAH. Haemolytic anaemia associated with ingestion of naphthalene-containing anointing oil. *J Toxicol Clin Toxicol*. 1988;64:444-446.
59. Owa JA, Izedonmwen OE, Ogundaini AO, et al. Quantitative analysis of 1-naphthol in urine of neonates exposed to mothballs: The value in infants with unexplained anaemia. *Afr J Med Sci*. 1993;22:71-76.
60. Rabl W, Katzgraber F, Steinlechner M. Camphor ingestion for abortion. *Forensic Sci Int*. 1997;89:137-140.
61. Rampini SK, Schneemann, Rentsch K, et al. Camphor intoxication after Cao Gio (coin rubbing) *JAMA*. 2002;288:45.
62. Reeves RR, Pendarvis RO. Mothball melting points. *Ann Emerg Med*. 1986;15:1377.
63. Reid FM. Accidental camphor ingestion. *JACEP*. 1979;8:339-340.
64. Rieders F, Brieger H: Hemolytic action of naphthalene and its oxidation products. *Pediatrics*. 1951;7:725-727.
65. Riggs J, Hamilton R, Homel S, et al. Camphorated oil intoxication in pregnancy: Report of a case. *Obstet Gynecol*. 1965;25:255-258.
66. Robertson JS, Mussain M. Metabolism of camphors and related compounds. *J Biochem*. 1969;113:57-64.
67. Ruha AM, Graeme KA, Field A. Late seizure following ingestion of Vicks VapoRub. *Acad Emerg Med*. 2003;10:691.
68. Schafer WB. Acute hemolytic anemia related to naphthalene. Report of a case in a newborn infant. *Pediatrics*. 1951;7:172-174.
69. Seife M, Leon JL. Camphor poisoning following ingestion of nose drops. *JAMA*. 1954;155:1059-1060.
70. Shannon K, Buchanan GR. Severe hemolytic anemia in black children with G-6-PD deficiency. *Pediatrics*. 1982;70:364-369.
71. Siegel E, Wason S. Camphor toxicity. *Pediatr Clin North Am*. 1986;33:375-379.
72. Siegel E, Wason S. Mothball toxicity. *Pediatr Clin North Am*. 1986;33: 369-374.
73. Smillie WG. Betanaphthol poisoning in the treatment of hookworm disease. *JAMA*. 1920;74:1503-1506.
74. Smith AG, Margolis G. Camphor poisoning, anatomical and pharmacologic study; report of a fatal case; experimental investigation of protective action of barbiturate. *Am J Pathol*. 1954;30:857-868.
75. Skoglund RR, Ware L, Schkanberger JE. Prolonged seizures due to contact and inhalation exposure to camphor. *Clin Pediatr*. 1977;16:901-902.
76. Summers GD. Case of camphor poisoning. *BMJ*. 1947;2:1009-1010.
77. Sumers J. Hepatitis with concomitant esophageal varices following exposure to mothball vapors. *N Y State J Med*. 1952;52:1048-1049.
78. Theis JG, Koren G. Camphorated oil: Still endangering the lives of Canadian children. *CMAJ*. 1995;152:1821-1824.
79. Tidcombe FS. Severe symptoms following the administration of a small teaspoonful of camphorated oil. *Lancet*. 1897;2:660.
80. Todisco V, Lamour J, Finberg L. Hemolysis from exposure to naphthalene mothballs. *N Engl J Med*. 1991;325:1660.
81. Trestrail JH, Spartz ME. Camphorated and castor oil confusion and its toxic results. *Clin Toxicol*. 1977;11:151-158.
82. United States Department of Labor Occupational Safety and Health Administration http://www.osha.gov/dts/chemicalsampling/data/CH_255800.html (accessed 3/21/2009) (naphthalene).
83. United States Department of Labor Occupational Safety and Health Administration http://www.osha.gov/dts/chemicalsampling/data/CH_224600.html (accessed 3/21/09) (camphor).
84. United States Department of Labor Occupational Safety and Health Administration http://www.osha.gov/dts/chemicalsampling/data/CH_232900.html (Accessed 3/21/09) (paradichlorobenzene).
85. Valaes T, Doxiadis SA, Fessas P. Acute hemolysis due to naphthalene inhalation. *J Pediatr*. 1963;63:904-915.
86. Weiss J, Catalano P. Camphorated oil intoxication during pregnancy. *Pediatrics*. 1973;52:713-716.
87. Weller RW, Crellin AJ. Pulmonary granulomatosis following extensive use of paradichlorobenzene. *AMA Arch Intern Med*. 1953;91:408-413.
88. Winkler JV, Kulig K, Rumack BH. Mothball differentiation: Naphthalene from paradichlorobenzene. *Ann Emerg Med*. 1985;14:30-32.
89. Yoshida T, Andoh K, Kosaka H, et al. Inhalation toxicokinetics of p-dichlorobenzene and daily absorption and internal accumulation in chronic low-level exposure to humans. *Toxicokinet Metab*. 2002;76:306-315.
90. Zinkham WJ, Childs B. A defect of glutathione metabolism in erythrocytes from patients with a naphthalene-induced hemolytic anemia. *Pediatrics*. 1958;22:461-471.
91. Zuelzer WW, Apt L. Acute hemolytic anemia due to naphthalene poisoning: Clinical and experimental study. *JAMA*. 1949;141:185-190.

CHAPTER 104
CAUSTICS

Jessica A. Fulton

Exposure to caustic agents may occur via the dermal, ocular, respiratory, and gastrointestinal routes with the most significant of these, by far, resulting from ingestion.

Morbidity and mortality from exposures to caustics is a worldwide problem. One study from India describing outcomes in patients following acid ingestions found that acute complications occurred in 39.1% of cases with death resulting in 12.2%.[131] In the United States, even though legislation limiting the concentration of caustic agents has existed since the early 20th century, exposures to both acids and alkalis continue to be significant. Data collected by the American Association of Poison Control Centers from 2002 through 2006 revealed 49,531 chemical acid exposures and 24,119 chemical alkali exposures. Of these, 7525 (15.2%) acid exposures and 4297 (17.8%) alkali exposures resulted in moderate to major outcomes and a total of 50 deaths occurred (see Chap. 135).

HISTORY AND EPIDEMIOLOGY

Caustics cause both histologic and clinical damage on contact with tissues. Table 104–1 lists common caustics and the commercial products that contain them. Many are available for home use, in both solid and liquid forms, with variations in viscosity, concentration, and pH.

As early as 1927, regulatory legislation in the United States governing the packaging of lye- and acid-containing products mandated that warning labels be placed on products containing these xenobiotics. In response to the recognition that caustic exposures were more frequent in children, in 1970 the Federal Hazardous Substances Act and Poison Prevention Packaging Act were passed, stating that all caustics with a concentration greater than 10% must be placed in child-resistant containers. By 1973, the household concentration for child-resistant packaging was lowered to 2%. In addition, the subsequent development of poison prevention education dramatically decreased the incidence of unintentional caustic injuries in children in the United States. The positive impact of both regulatory legislation and education is evident when observing the decrease of exposures in the United States compared to the number of exposures in developing nations that lack these policies.

Usually, children are unintentionally exposed to household products. Adults may be exposed to household or industrial products that result from occupational exposure or are suicide attempts.

Although less frequent, intentional exposures by adults are invariably more significant. One study noted that while children comprised 39% of admissions for caustic ingestions, adults comprised 81% of patients requiring treatment.[47] The severity of a caustic injury may not be immediately evident in patients who present shortly after exposure. Predicting which patients will require immediate interventions to prevent morbidity and mortality requires multiple clinical and laboratory parameters. This chapter reviews the pathophysiology and approach to patients with potentially serious exposures.

PATHOPHYSIOLOGY

A caustic is a xenobiotic that causes both functional and histologic damage on contact with tissue surfaces. Although there are many ways to categorize caustics, they are most typically classified as acids or alkalis. An acid is a proton donator[80] and causes significant injury, generally at a pH below 3. An alkali is a proton acceptor[80] and causes significant injury, generally at a pH above 11. Chapter 11 contains a more detailed discussion of the chemistry of acids and bases. The extent of injury is modulated by duration of contact; ability of the caustic to penetrate tissues; volume, pH, and concentration; the presence or absence of food in the stomach; and a property known as *titratable acid/alkaline reserve* (TAR). TAR quantifies the amount of neutralizing xenobiotic needed to bring the pH of a caustic to that of physiologic tissues. Neutralization of caustics takes place at the expense of the tissues, resulting in the release of thermal energy, producing burns. Generally, as the TAR of caustics increases, so does their ability to produce tissue damage.[6,11,30,44,50,95] Some xenobiotics, such as zinc chloride and phenol, have a high TAR and are capable of producing severe burns even though their pH is near physiologic.

ALKALIS

Following exposure to an alkaline xenobiotic, dissociated hydroxide (OH^-) ions penetrate tissue surfaces producing what is histologically described as liquefactive necrosis (see Figs. 104–1 and 104–2). This process includes protein dissolution, collagen destruction, fat saponification, cell membrane emulsification, transmural thrombosis, and cell death.[6,44] Animal studies following alkali exposure to the eye[49] demonstrate rapid formation of corneal epithelial defects with eventual deep penetration that may lead to perforation. Similarly, animal studies of the esophagus demonstrate that erythema and edema of the mucosa occur within seconds followed by an inflammatory reaction extending to the submucosa and muscular layers. The alkali, such as sodium hydroxide ("liquid lye"), then continues to penetrate until the OH^- concentration is sufficiently neutralized by the tissues.[6,63,67,116]

Although federal regulations have lowered the maximal available household concentration of many caustics, there are two industrial strength products that seem to be readily available and therefore warrant special mention: ammonium hydroxide and sodium hypochlorite. Ammonia (ammonium hydroxide) products are weak bases—partially dissociated in water—that can cause significant esophageal burns, depending on the concentration and volume ingested.[47,107,114,116] Household ammonium hydroxide ranges in concentration from 3% to 10%. Strictures have formed in patients who ingested 28% solutions.[89] Sodium hypochlorite is the major component in most industrial and household bleaches. Large case series and reports have found that severe injuries occur only in patients with large-volume ingestions of concentrated products[24] and that most other patients do well with supportive care.[17,47,113] A series of 393 patients with household bleach ingestions demonstrated no stricture formation.[66] Likewise, a canine model found that although vomiting was a common effect of bleach, no esophageal lesions were noted, and perforation occurred only following prolonged contact.[66]

Ingestion of button batteries were once considered a unique caustic exposure. Composed of metal salts and a variety of alkaline xenobiotics, such as sodium and potassium hydroxide, leakage of battery contents was a legitimate concern. In recent years, however, new techniques used in the production of button batteries that effectively prevent leakage have shifted the concern following their ingestion from caustic to foreign-body exposure. For a more in depth review of the management of button battery ingestion, the reader is referred to the previous editions of this text.

Household detergents, such as laundry powders and dishwasher detergents, contain silicates, carbonates, and phosphates, and have the

TABLE 104–1. Sources of Common Caustics

Xenobiotic	Applications
Acetic acid	Permanent wave neutralizers, photographic stop bath
Ammonia (ammonium hydroxide)	Toilet bowl cleaners, metal cleaners and polishes, hair dyes and tints, antirust products, jewelry cleaners, floor strippers, glass cleaners, wax removers
Benzalkonium chloride	Detergents
Boric acid	Roach powders, water softeners, germicide
Formaldehyde, formic acid	Deodorizing tablets, plastic menders, fumigant, embalming agent
Hydrochloric acid (muriatic acid)	Metal and toilet bowl cleaners
Hydrofluoric acid	Antirust products, glass etching, microchip etching
Iodine	Antiseptics
Mercuric chloride ($HgCl_2$)	Preservative
Methylethyl ketone peroxide	Industrial synthetic agent
Oxalic acid	Disinfectants, household bleach, metal polish, antirust products, furniture refinisher
Phenol (creosol, creosote)	Antiseptics, preservatives
Phosphoric acid	Toilet bowl cleaners
Phosphorus	Matches, fireworks, rodenticides, methamphetamine synthesis
Potassium permanganate	Illicit abortifacient, antiseptic solution
Selenious acid	Gun bluing agent
Sodium hydroxide	Detergents, paint removers, drain cleaners and openers, oven cleaners
Sodium borates, carbonates, phosphates, and silicates	Detergents, electric dishwasher preparations, water softeners
Sodium hypochlorite	Bleaches, cleansers
Sulfuric acid	Automobile batteries, drain cleaners
Zinc chloride	Soldering flux

potential to induce caustic burns and strictures even when ingested unintentionally.[18,114] Airway compromise also may occur,[18,27,73] but the majority of exposures result in only minor toxicity.

Cationic detergents include quinolinium compounds, pyridinium compounds, and quaternary ammonium salts. These are frequently found in products for industrial use, as well as household fabric softeners. A concentration greater than 7.5% can cause severe burns.[71]

ACIDS

In contrast to alkaline exposures, following exposure to an acid, hydrogen (H^+) ions desiccate epithelial cells, producing an eschar and

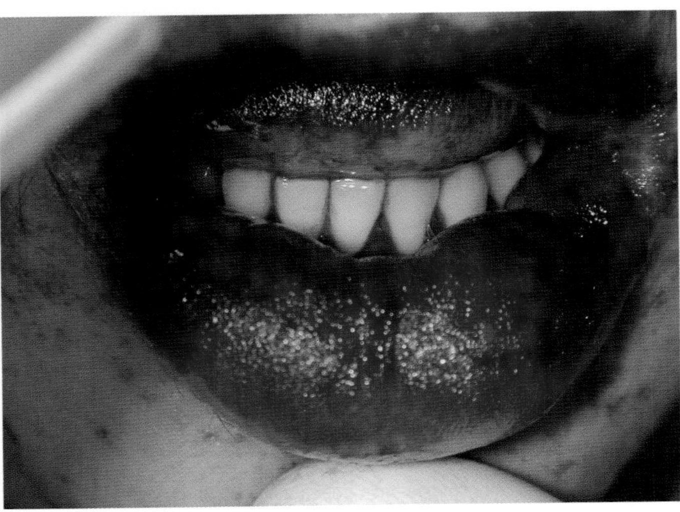

FIGURE 104–1. Photograph demonstrating burns to the lips and tongue of a 20-year-old man following ingestion of sodium hydroxide. *(Image contributed by the New York City Poison Center Toxicology Fellowship Program.)*

resulting in what is histologically referred to as *coagulation necrosis*. This process leads to edema, erythema, mucosal sloughing, ulceration, and necrosis of tissues. Dissociated anions of the acid (Cl^-, SO_4^{2-}, PO_4^{3-}) also act as reducing agents further injuring tissue.

Ophthalmic exposure to acids results in coagulative necrosis that tends to prevent further penetration into deeper layers of the eye.

In most series, following an acid ingestion, both the gastric and esophageal mucosa are equally affected.[25,56,131] On occasion, the esophagus may be spared damage while severe injury is noted in the stomach.[21,41,47,114] (See Fig. 104–3) This tends to be a rarer finding than concomitant injury to both stomach and esophagus, and is probably related to the rapid transit time of liquid acids through the upper gastrointestinal tract. Skip lesions from acid ingestions may be a function of viscosity and contact time.[47] Additionally, acid-induced pylorospasm may lead to gastric outlet obstruction, antral pooling, and perforation.[16,21,24,25,41,56,64,65,76,87,112,113,126,130] A cat model of the effects of sulfuric acid on the esophagus revealed a coagulative necrosis of the mucosa with whitish discoloration of the tissues and underlying smooth muscle spasm.[6] Other animal models demonstrate esophageal motility dysfunction and shortening.[110,111]

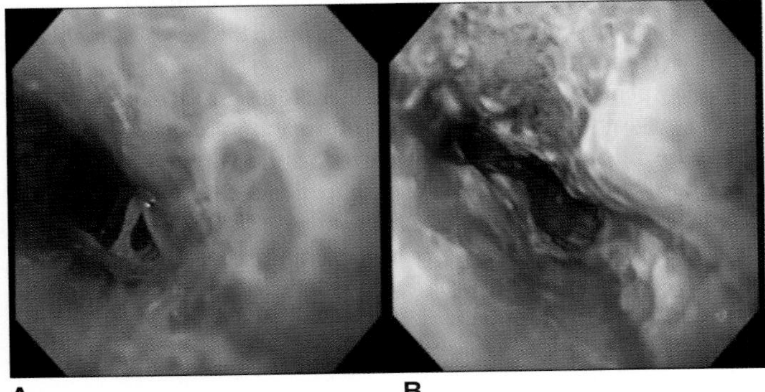

FIGURE 104–2. Endoscopy images of a 20-year-old man following ingestion of sodium hydroxide. **(A)** Grade IIa noncircumferential burn of the midesophagus. **(B)** Grade IIb circumferential burn of the distal esophagus. *(Image contributed by the New York City Poison Center Toxicology Fellowship Program.)*

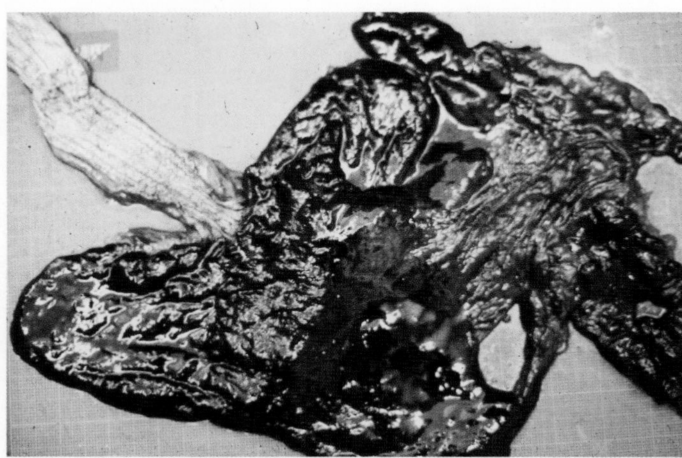

FIGURE 104–3. Postmortem specimen from a man with an intentional ingestion of a mixture of phosphoric and hydrochloric acid that was used as a brick cleaner. Note the relative sparing of the esophagus in contrast to full-thickness injury with perforation of the stomach. *(Image contributed by the New York City Poison Center Toxicology Fellowship Program.)*

Chapters 96 and 105 contain a more detailed discussion of mercury and hydrofluoric acid, respectively, each a uniquely caustic compound, and the management specific to their exposure.

CLASSIFICATION AND PROGRESSION OF CAUSTIC INJURY

Esophageal burns, secondary to both alkali and acid exposures, are classified based on endoscopic visualization that employs a grading system similar to that used with burns of the skin. Grade I burns are generally described as hyperemia or edema of the mucosa without evidence of ulcer formation.[20,62,130] Grade II burns include submucosal lesions, ulcerations, and exudates. Some authors further divide grade II lesions into grade IIa, noncircumferential lesions, and grade IIb, near-circumferential injuries.[17] Grade III burns are defined as deep ulcers and necrosis into the periesophageal tissues.[34,38,46,62]

Human case reports, postmortem studies, histologic inspection of surgical specimens, and experimental animal models reveal a consistent pattern of injury and repair following caustic injury.[1,32,39,74,82,104] As wound healing of gastrointestinal tract tissue occurs, neovascularization and fibroblast proliferation take place, laying down new collagen and replacing the damaged tissue with granulation tissue. A similar pattern of repair occurs following caustic injuries of the eye.

Burns of the esophagus may persist for up to 8 weeks as remodeling takes place, and may be followed by esophageal shortening.[124] If the initial injury penetrates deeply enough, there is progressive narrowing of the esophageal lumen. The dense scar formation presents clinically as a stricture.[22,44] Strictures can evolve over a period of weeks to months, leading to dysphagia and significant nutritional deficits.[100,105,124] Grade I burns carry no risk of stricture formation.[20,62,130] Grade II circumferential burns lead to stricture formation in approximately 75% of cases. Grade III burns invariably progress to stricture formation and are also at a high risk of perforation.[4,47,82]

CLINICAL PRESENTATION

The gastrointestinal tract, respiratory tract, eyes, and skin of a patient can be sites of caustic injury. Caustics may produce severe pain on contact with any of these tissues. By far, the majority of long-term morbidity and mortality from caustic exposure results from ingestion.

In general, patients who have ingested either alkaline or acid agents have similar initial presentations. Depending on the type, amount, and formulation (solid vs. liquid) of the substance, ingestion may lead to the development of severe pain of the lips, mouth, throat, chest, or abdomen. Oropharyngeal edema and burns may lead to drooling and rapid airway compromise. Symptoms of esophageal involvement include dysphagia and odynophagia, whereas epigastric pain and hematemesis may be symptoms of gastric involvement.

Respiratory tract damage may occur through direct inhalation or aspiration of vomitus leading to the clinical manifestations of hoarseness, stridor, and respiratory distress. Injury may result in epiglottitis, laryngeal edema and ulceration, pneumonitis, and impaired gas exchange. Patients may also be tachypneic or hyperpneic as a compensatory response to the metabolic acidosis with elevated lactate concentrations from necrotic tissue or hemodynamic compromise.

PREDICTORS OF INJURY

Many attempts have been made to define a method for clinical identification of patients with grade II or III esophageal injuries as these injuries typically progress to severe complications. Various studies, mostly involving alkaline xenobiotics, examine the predictive value of stridor, oropharyngeal burns, drooling, vomiting, and abdominal pain. A retrospective study of 378 children admitted for a caustic injury found that signs or symptoms could not be used to predict significant esophageal injury.[34] However, one prospective study of 79 children evaluated for vomiting, drooling, and stridor found that a combination of two or more of these signs were predictive of significant esophageal injury as visualized on endoscopy.[20] Another study found that drooling, buccal mucosal burns, and white blood cell count were significant independent predictors of severe gastrointestinal tract injury following acid ingestions.[45] Studies evaluating the presence or absence of oropharyngeal burns as a predictor of distal esophagogastric injury have repeatedly found this finding to be poorly predictive.[2,12,20,34,38,97,120] In one study esophageal injury was present 51.5% of the time in the absence of oropharyngeal lesions, and 22.2% of these were second- and third-degree burns.[97] A prospective study of alkali ingestions in both adults and children found that stridor was 100% specific for significant esophageal injury, but this was based on only three patients with this sign.[38]

Based on these findings, endoscopy, a standard diagnostic tool used in the management of caustic ingestions, is recommended in all patients with intentional ingestions. Endoscopy should also be performed in any patient with an unintentional ingestion in the presence of stridor, and in any patient with two or more of the following findings: pain, vomiting, and drooling.[20,99] Children with unintentional caustic ingestions who remain completely asymptomatic and tolerate liquids after a few hours of observation probably require no further medical care.

The abdominal examination is likewise an unreliable indicator of the severity of injury. The presence of abdominal pain suggests tissue injury, but the absence of pain or findings on abdominal examination do not preclude life-threatening gastrointestinal damage.[28,56,100,107,128] Esophageal perforations result in mediastinitis and are commonly associated with fever, dyspnea, chest pain, and subcutaneous emphysema of the neck and chest. Although indicative of viscus perforation, abdominal peritoneal signs are late findings.

In addition to the direct effects that occur with tissue contact, acids are systemically absorbed, resulting in damage to the spleen, liver, biliary tract, pancreas, and kidneys, as well as producing a metabolic acidosis, hemolysis, and, ultimately, death.[52,124]

Significant complications can occur at various stages of wound recovery. Most importantly, these include airway compromise, hemodynamic instability secondary to hemorrhage from vascular erosion or septic shock, perforations of the gastrointestinal tract with the development of mediastinitis or peritonitis, and other overwhelming infections from bacteria residing in the oropharynx. A patient who survives acute injury with an acid or an alkali may also subsequently develop stricture formation, gastric atony, decreased acid secretion, pseudodiverticula, and gastric outlet obstruction.[13,37,64,112,130]

Other complications include dysmotility of the pharynx and esophagus,[23] formation of aorto- and tracheoesophageal fistulas, delayed massive hemorrhage from erosion into a great vessel, and pulmonary thrombosis.[10,47,62,88,107,109]

Those patients surviving a few weeks after a grade II or III injury may subsequently present with dysphagia and vomiting from stricture formation. One study suggested that involvement of the entire length of the esophagus as well as hematemesis and increased serum lactic dehydrogenase are useful indicators for the development of strictures.[90] Strictures may also present with esophageal motility disorders caused by impaired smooth muscle reactivity.[119] The early assessment and long-term prognosis may be better defined by manometric studies of the esophagus which provide precise information on the severity of the initial injury and aid in long-term prognosis.[36]

Although the risk of carcinoma after caustic ingestions is inadequately studied, three patients developed squamous cell cancer of the stomach following acid ingestion[26] and 15 patients developed squamous cell cancer of the esophagus following lye ingestion many years after their initial injuries.[59] Long-term survivors of moderate and severe injury of the esophagus have a risk of esophageal carcinoma that is estimated to be 1000 times higher than that of the general population and appears to present with a latency of up to 40 years.[5]

DIAGNOSTIC TESTING

LABORATORY

All patients with presumed serious caustic exposure should have an evaluation of serum pH, blood type and cross-match, hemoglobin, coagulation parameters, electrolytes, and urinalysis. Elevated prothrombin time (PT) and partial thromboplastin times,[128] as well as an arterial pH lower than 7.22,[14] are associated with severe caustic injury.

Absorption of nonionized acid from the stomach mucosa may result in acidemia. Following ingestion of hydrochloric acid, hydrogen and chloride ions (both of which are accounted for in the measurement of the anion gap) dissociate in the serum resulting in a hyperchloremic normal anion gap metabolic acidosis. Other acids, such as sulfuric acid, result in an elevated anion gap metabolic acidosis because the sulfate anion (SO_4^{2-}) is not measured in the calculation of the anion gap. Although alkalis are not absorbed systemically, necrosis of tissue may result in a metabolic acidosis with an elevated lactate concentration.

A gastric pH greater than 7.30 correlated retrospectively with severe alkaline injury. The prospective usefulness of this information is limited, as obtaining gastric secretions without direct visualization is dangerous. One prospective study in children also found an increase in uric acid and decreases in phosphate and alkaline phosphatase concentrations to be useful in predicting the presence of esophageal injuries.[92]

RADIOLOGY

Chest and abdominal radiographs are useful in the initial stages of assessment to detect gross signs of esophageal or gastric perforation. Signs of alimentary tract perforation that may be present on plain radiographs include pneumomediastinum, pneumoperitoneum, and pleural effusion. However, these studies have a limited sensitivity, and an absence of findings does not preclude perforation.[128] Free intraperitoneal air is best visualized on an upright chest radiograph. Occasionally, free air may only be visible on the lateral view.[125] In patients too ill to obtain an upright chest radiograph, an abdominal radiograph obtained with the patient in a left-side-down position may reveal free intraperitoneal air adjacent to the liver. CT scanning is considerably more sensitive than radiography for detecting viscus perforation and should be obtained in patients with potentially serious caustic ingestions as soon as is feasible.[29,122]

A contrast esophagram is useful for defining the extent of esophageal injury (Fig. 104–4). Late after the ingestion, it can detect stricture formation. In patients for whom there is a high suspicion for esophageal perforation and in whom adequate visualization of the upper gastrointestinal tract by endoscopy is not possible (grade IIb circumferential burns or grade III burns), an enteric contrast study (esophagram and upper GI series) can be obtained 24 hours after the ingestion.[99,132] Extravasation of contrast outside of the gastrointestinal tract is diagnostic of perforation.[130] Water-soluble contrast should be used when perforation is suspected as it is less irritating to mediastinal and peritoneal tissues if extravasated.[32] However, barium contrast agents are more radiopaque than water-soluble agents and offer greater radiographic detail. Consequently, some authors recommend barium swallow if the water-soluble contrast study is nondiagnostic but demonstrates no leak.[42,70,115] In addition, if there is risk of aspiration, barium is preferred because water-soluble contrast material can cause a severe chemical pneumonitis. Significant necrosis with impending perforation may be suspected on enteric contrast studies when there is esophageal dilation, displacement of the pleural reflection, and widening of the pleuroesophageal line.[74] Enteric contrast studies may fail to detect perforation, and therefore must be interpreted within the context of the patient's clinical status.[10,19,43,56,74]

Although promising, a role for CT in caustic ingestions has not been formally investigated. CT has great sensitivity at detecting extraluminal air in the mediastinum or peritoneal cavity as a sign of perforation. In addition, CT can visualize the esophagus and stomach distal to severe caustic burns that cannot be safely seen using endoscopy or an esophagram. CT may therefore replace enteric contrast radiography for detection of perforation in the acute stage (within 24 hours) of a caustic ingestion. Other imaging modalities have been proposed. One study suggested a role for a technetium 99m-labeled sucralfate swallow for assessing esophageal injury after ingestion of caustic substances.[83] In another study, esophageal ultrasonography was helpful in determining the depth of injury.[86]

Another use of radiographic imaging is to noninvasively follow the patient after initial evaluation and stabilization. For example, contrast radiography is routinely used in the weeks or months following a caustic ingestion to detect esophageal narrowing representing stricture formation.[74,117] Chest CT may also be useful to determine the response of strictures to dilation procedures.[65]

ENDOSCOPY

Endoscopy should be performed within 12 hours and generally not later than 24 hours postingestion. Numerous case series demonstrate that the procedure is safe during this period. Early endoscopy serves multiple purposes in that it allows patients with minimal or no evidence of gastrointestinal injury to be discharged. It also offers a rapid means of obtaining diagnostic and prognostic information while shortening the period of time that patients forego nutritional support, permitting more precise treatment regimens.[17,22,24,28,44,47,69,81,99,107,108,121,125,130] The use of endoscopic assessment from the 2nd or 3rd day postingestion is discouraged and should be avoided between 5 days and 2 weeks postingestion as it is at this time that wound strength is least and the risk of perforation is greatest.

The choice of rigid versus flexible endoscopy is dependent on the comfort and experience of the endoscopist. The flexible endoscope has a smaller diameter but may require gentle insufflation of air to achieve or enhance visualization. A prospective evaluation of the role of fiberoptic endoscopy in the management of caustic ingestions

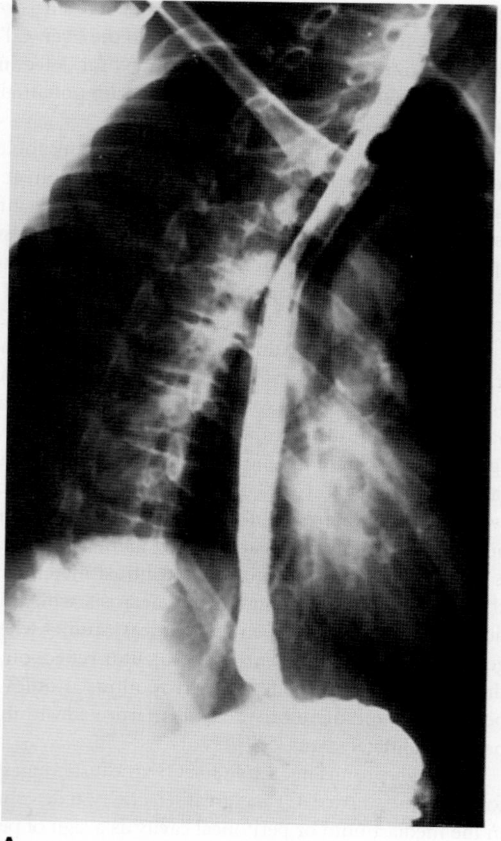

A

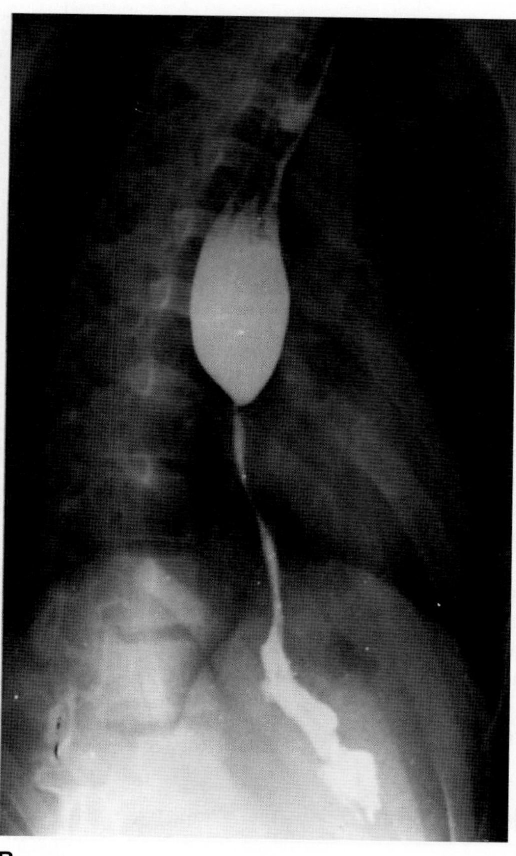

B

FIGURE 104–4. (A) Barium swallow several days after ingestion of liquid lye shows the esophagus to be atonic. There is poor coating of the esophagus, suggesting edema and intramural penetration. Note that the initial evaluation immediately following a caustic ingestion to assess the extent of injury is esophagoscopy, rather than a contrast esophagram. (B) Four months later, a repeat barium esophagram shows a severe stricture below the middle third of the esophagus. The barium barely passes the stricture, and the remainder of the esophagus is pencil thin. *(Images contributed by Emil J. Balthazar, MD, Professor of Radiology, New York University.)*

recommended the following guidelines: (1) direct visualization of the esophagus prior to advancing the instrument, (2) minimal insufflation of air, (3) passage into the stomach unless there is a severe (particularly circumferential) esophageal burn, and (4) avoidance of retroversion or retroflexion of the instrument within the esophagus. Provided that the patient is hemodynamically stable and endoscopy is indicated, every attempt should be made to visualize the esophagus, stomach, and duodenum after a caustic ingestion.

The absence of burns in the esophagus does not imply that severe necrosis and ulcerations do not exist in the stomach[81,114,120,130] and duodenum. In the case of termination of endoscopy because of grade IIb or grade III esophageal burns, barium studies,[99] CT scan, or consideration of surgical exploration should be undertaken to visualize remaining structures.

Endoscopy permits limited evaluation of gastrointestinal injury. For example, the endoscopist is able to appreciate only the mucosal surface of tissues, and not the serosal side. This is especially evident in stomach ulcerations, which may appear black and necrotic from a true burn through the layers of the stomach, or from the effect of stomach acid on the blood exposed from a shallow lesion. Some studies suggest that the use of endosonography during endoscopy may improve assessment of injury depth.[7,61] Often, though, only direct visualization of serosal and mucosal tissues with laparoscopy or laparotomy allows for definitive evaluation.

Most cases of perforation clearly linked to endoscopy have occurred when the endoscope was advanced through an esophagus with severe circumferential lesions—a violation of current endoscopic standards.[121] In addition, perforations are also more likely to occur when rigid instruments are used in children or in uncooperative patients. The use of the flexible endoscope has decreased the complications from endoscopic evaluation.[99] Some authors advocate the presence of a surgeon during endoscopy to assist in the assessment for potential surgical intervention.[105]

MANAGEMENT

ACUTE MANAGEMENT

As in the case of any patient presenting with a toxicologic emergency, the healthcare provider must adhere to universal precautions. Initial stabilization should include airway inspection and protection, basic resuscitation principles, and decontamination. Examination of the oropharynx for signs of injury, drooling, and vomitus, as well as careful auscultation of the neck and chest for stridor, may reveal signs of airway edema that should prompt immediate airway protection. Careful and constant attention to signs and symptoms of respiratory distress and airway edema, such as a change in voice, are essential and should prompt intubation as airway edema may rapidly progress over minutes to hours.

If airway involvement is significant enough to warrant intubation, it is best to mobilize a team of the most skilled physicians early in case of unforeseen complications. A delay in prophylactic airway protection may make subsequent attempts at intubation or bag-valve-mask ventilation difficult or impossible. Direct visual inspection of the vocal cords with a fiberoptic laryngoscope may also reveal signs of impending airway compromise. Patients necessitating intubation are best served by direct visualization of the airway either via direct laryngoscopy or fiberoptic endoscope, as perforation of edematous tissues of the pharynx and larynx is a grave complication that may occur during blind nasotracheal intubation attempts. Neuromuscular blockers should be avoided for induction of intubation as airway edema and bleeding may distort the ability to successfully ventilate via bag-valve-mask should intubation be unsuccessful.

Nonsurgical airway placement is recommended whenever possible as both cricothyrotomy and tracheostomy may interfere with the surgical field if esophageal repair is required.[128] Some patients with significant ingestions, however, may require emergent surgical airway intervention. The decision to perform the technique of a surgical airway is dependent on the status of the patient, the ability to orotracheally or nasotracheally intubate via a fiberoptic endoscope, and the comfort of the physician performing the procedure.

Following control of the airway, large-bore intravenous access should be secured and volume resuscitation initiated. Although not studied, most clinicians agree that patients with signs of caustic-induced airway edema benefit from dexamethasone 10 mg IV in adults and 0.6 mg/kg up to a total dose of 10 mg in children. Both acid and alkali ingestions cause "third spacing" of intravascular fluid to the interstitial space, which can result in hypotension. Empiric rehydration with clinical assessment of central venous pressures should be used to guide individual fluid requirements.

Serial physical examinations and constant monitoring of the vital signs and urine output may provide information on the severity of the exposure and the progression in clinical status.

DECONTAMINATION, DILUTION, AND NEUTRALIZATION

Decontamination should begin with careful, copious irrigation of the patient's skin and eyes when indicated to remove any residual caustic and to prevent contamination of other patients and staff.

Gastrointestinal decontamination is usually limited in patients with a caustic ingestion. Induced emesis is contraindicated, as it may cause reintroduction of the caustic to the upper gastrointestinal tract and airway. Activated charcoal is also contraindicated, as it will interfere with tissue evaluation by endoscopy and preclude a subsequent management plan. Additionally, most caustics are not adsorbed to activated charcoal.

Exceptions, such as cationic detergents, that do bind well to activated charcoal[71] have not been evaluated with a large series. For this reason, therapy with activated charcoal following any caustic ingestion cannot be recommended. Gastric emptying via cautious placement of a narrow nasogastric tube with gentle suction may be attempted to remove the remaining acid in the stomach only in patients with large life-threatening intentional ingestions of acid who present within 30 minutes.[95] Although this technique has never been studied and carries the risk of perforation, the outcome for these patients is often grave and options for treatment are limited. Therefore, preventing absorption of some portion of the ingested acid may have potential benefit in reducing systemic toxicity. Although the procedure has the potential to induce injury, a risk-to-benefit analysis favors gastric emptying following a presumed lethal ingestion.

In contrast, gastric emptying should be avoided with alkaline and unknown caustic ingestions as blind passage of a nasogastric tube carries the risk of perforation of damaged tissues; a risk that outweighs the benefit.

Exceptions to the general rules of gastrointestinal decontamination of caustic agents exist in the management of zinc chloride ($ZnCl_2$) and mercuric chloride ($HgCl_2$). Both are caustics with severe systemic toxicity.[15,77,78,96] Ingestion of these xenobiotics causes life-threatening illness from cationic metal exposure. The local caustic effects, though of great concern, are less consequential than the manifestations of systemic absorption. Therefore, prevention of systemic absorption should be addressed primarily, followed by the direct assessment and management of the local effects of these xenobiotics. Initial management to prevent systemic absorption includes aggressive decontamination with gentle nasogastric tube aspiration and administration of activated charcoal. In vitro data exist to suggest adequate charcoal adsorption of Hg^{2+}ion.[3]

The use of dilutional therapy has been examined using in vitro, ex vivo, and in vivo models in an attempt to assess its efficacy in caustic ingestions. An early in vitro model demonstrated a dramatic increase in temperature when either water or milk was added to crystal Drano.[106] Another in vitro model found less consequential increases in temperature despite large volumes of diluent. Results of both studies suggested that dilutional therapy was of limited benefit.[75] Dilutional therapy was also attended by an increase in temperature in an ex vivo study of harvested rat esophagi that examined the histopathologic effects of saline dilution after an alkali injury. Additionally, the usefulness of dilution appeared to be inversely related to the length of time from exposure, with minimal efficacy noted in as little as 30 minutes.[52,53] In contrast, an in vivo canine model of alkaline injury demonstrated that water dilution did not cause an increase in either temperature or intraluminal pressures.[55]

The extrapolation of these variable results to humans with caustic ingestions is limited, and suggests that histologic damage can only be attenuated by milk or water when administered within the first seconds to minutes following ingestion.[6,52,53,54,55,67,116] For solid, as opposed to liquid, substances (eg, crystal lye), there may be some value for delayed dilutional therapy, as tissue contact time is increased with solids and their concentration is usually 100% over a small surface area. Milk may be the best diluent to attenuate the heat generated by a caustic.[114]

Caution should be used in advising patients or family members about the use of dilutional agents. A child who refuses to swallow or take oral liquids should never be forced to do so. In general, dilutional therapy should be limited to patients within the first few minutes after ingestion who have no airway compromise, who are not complaining of significant pharyngeal, chest, or abdominal pain, who are not vomiting, and who are alert. Dilutional therapy should be avoided in patients with nausea, drooling, stridor, or abdominal distension as it may stimulate vomiting and result in reintroduction of the caustic into the upper gastrointestinal tract.[106]

Attempts at neutralization of ingested caustics should likewise be avoided. This technique has the potential to worsen tissue damage by forming gas and generating an exothermic reaction. In vitro and ex vivo models demonstrate that neutralization of caustics generates heat, requires a large volume to attain physiologic pH, and may have limited usefulness in preventing histologic damage if delayed beyond the first several minutes following caustic exposure.[51,76,106] In one in vivo canine model, orange juice was used to neutralize sodium hydroxide–induced gastric injury and demonstrated no change in temperature or intraluminal pressure.[55] Despite this study, neutralization is not recommended at this time as there are no other data demonstrating that clinical outcome is improved.

SURGICAL MANAGEMENT

The decision to perform surgery in patients with caustic ingestions is obvious in the presence of either endoscopic or diagnostic imaging evidence of perforation,[128] severe abdominal rigidity, or persistent hypotension. Hypotension is a grave finding and often indicates perforation or significant blood loss. Additionally, elevated prothrombin time (PT) and partial thromboplastin times,[128] as well as an arterial pH lower than 7.22,[14] are associated with severe caustic injury.

Many patients will not have an obvious indication for surgical intervention despite impending perforation, necrosis, sepsis, or delayed hemorrhage. Although more challenging to diagnose, all of these sequelae are potentially avoidable if surgery is performed early[91] as morbidity and mortality increase in patients whose surgery is delayed.[28,56,58,103,107] For this reason, some surgeons advocate surgery for all patients with grades II and III esophageal burns identified on endoscopy.[28,81] This aggressive approach allows for direct inspection of serosal surfaces and an opportunity for early surgical repair.

Multiple studies have attempted to codify the signs and symptoms necessary or sufficient to rapidly identify patients who would benefit from surgery, but who lack clear clinical indications. Several retrospective and prospective series of caustic ingestions found that patients with large ingestions (>150 mL), shock, acidemia, or coagulation disorders tended to have severe findings on surgical exploration. These studies also reinforce that the abdominal examination was frequently unreliable in predicting the need for surgery.[107,128,131] It should be noted, again, that patients with severe acid injuries may lack abdominal pain, abdominal tenderness, and have positive findings on diagnostic imaging.[25,56,131] One author used a stepwise approach of bronchoscopy, endoscopy, and abdominal ultrasonography to provide additional information regarding extent of injury prior to surgery. Respiratory distress, ascites, pleural fluid, and a serum pH less than 7.2 were used as indications for surgery.[128] A history of a large-volume caustic ingestion (between 40 and 200 mL) should also prompt consideration of early surgical intervention as delay is associated with increased mortality.[25,56,128]

Surgical intervention may include laparotomy for tissue visualization, resection, and repair of perforations. Laparoscopy may also be used, although it may not allow inspection of the posterior aspect of the stomach.

SUBACUTE MANAGEMENT

The extent of tissue injury dictates the subsequent management and disposition of patients with caustic ingestions.

Grade I Esophageal Injuries Patients with isolated grade I injuries of the esophagus do not develop strictures and are not at increased risk of carcinoma. Their diet can be resumed as tolerated. No further therapy is required. These patients can be discharged from the hospital as long as they are able to eat and drink and their psychiatric status is stable.

Grade IIa Esophageal Injuries If endoscopy reveals grade IIa lesions of the esophagus and sparing of the stomach, a soft diet can be resumed as tolerated, or a nasogastric tube can be passed under direct visualization. If oral intake is contraindicated because of the risk of perforation, feeding via gastrostomy, jejunostomy, or total parenteral nutrition should be instituted as rapidly as possible. Providing interim enteral support is imperative as metabolic demands are increased in any patient with a significant burn.

Grades IIb and III Esophageal Injuries Patients with grades IIb and III lesions must be followed for the complications of perforation, infection, and stricture development. Strictures are a debilitating complication of both acid and alkaline ingestions that can evolve over a period of weeks or months. They form as a result of the natural process by which the body repairs injured tissue through the production of collagen with resultant scar formation. Although steroid therapy is theorized to arrest the process of inflammatory repair and potentially prevent stricture formation, there is some evidence that grade III burns, in particular, will progress to stricture formation regardless of therapy.[4,47,82,121] In addition to stricture formation, patients with grade III burns are also at high risk for other complications, including fistula formation, infection, and perforation with associated mediastinitis and peritonitis. The use of corticosteroids in the management of grade III burns may mask infection and make the friable, necrotic esophageal tissue more prone to perforation.[94] For these reasons, steroid therapy is not a recommended therapy for grade III esophageal burns. When required in these patients for other indications such as caustic-induced airway inflammation, short-term steroids should be administered in conjunction with antibiotics.

Currently, some controversy exists regarding the use of steroid therapy in the management of grade IIb circumferential esophageal burns. A meta-analysis of studies completed from 1956–1991, with a total of 361 patients, evaluated the efficacy of corticosteroid therapy and found that in patients with grades II and III esophageal burns, strictures formed in 19% of the corticosteroid-treated group and in 41% of the untreated group.[57] The usefulness of the results of this study, however, are limited as no distinction was made between grades II and III burns. Another meta-analysis of studies from 1991 to 2003, with a total of 211 patients, was unable to find a benefit in treating patients with steroids with grades II and III esophageal burns.[94] However, no distinction was made between grades II and III burns. A systematic pooled analysis of studies from 1956 to 2006, with a total of 328 patients, attempted to reevaluate the usefulness of steroid therapy in grade II esophageal burns. Although methodologically limited, this study found no benefit in treating patients with steroids with grade II esophageal burns. A major limitation to the clinical usefulness of this study is that no distinction was made between grades IIa and IIb burns.[31] In addition, a multitude of case series also failed to clearly differentiate between grades IIa, IIb, and III lesions, making clinical application of their results difficult.[4,19,82,85,107,121]

Two prospective studies attempted to evaluate the efficacy of steroid therapy for caustic injuries to the esophagus. Both of these studies failed to show a benefit of steroid therapy and one even suggested harm.[3,4,60] It is imperative that the clinician understands that neither study clearly differentiates between grades IIb and III lesions.

Adequate human data demonstrating the efficacy of corticosteroids with or without antibiotics in the treatment of grade IIb circumferential lesions have yet to be generated. Because of the inherent risks involved in this therapy and the paucity of data supporting their use, steroid therapy in the management of grade IIb esophageal burns can no longer be routinely recommended.

No major outcome studies have investigated the use of antibiotics alone as prophylactic treatment for stricture prevention, but most clinicians would agree that it is probably best to reserve antibiotics for an identified source of infection.

A variety of other management strategies have been used in an attempt to prevent strictures and esophageal obstruction. In both animal models[102] and in human case series,[48,84,101] intraluminal stents and nasogastric tubes[84,125] made of silicone rubber tubing can successfully maintain the patency of the esophageal lumen. For nutritional support, the stents are usually attached to a feeding tube secured in the nasopharynx through which the patient can receive feedings without interfering with esophageal repair. These tubes are left in place for 3 weeks[101,102] and are often used with concomitant corticosteroid and antibiotic therapy. In animal models, the use of a stent for 3 weeks is superior in maintaining esophageal patency when compared to corticosteroids and antibiotics alone.[102]

Potential disadvantages of esophageal stents include mechanical trauma at the site and increased reflux, both of which may inhibit healing.[111] A feline model of esophageal exposure to sodium hydroxide used stents but reported deaths from aspiration and mediastinitis.[102] One series of 251 humans exposed to caustics who were managed with silicone rubber stents found that the procedure was successful in preventing stricture formation.[9]

Additionally, multiple therapies have been studied in various animal models in an attempt to identify agents that either inhibit synthesis or stimulate breakdown of collagen and thereby prevent stricture formation. β-Amino propionitrile (BAPN), penicillamine, *N*-acetylcysteine

(NAC), halofuginone, vitamin E, and colchicine are some of these agents.[118] BAPN was examined in a canine model in conjunction with dilation, and there was some suggestion that it was useful.[72] Both penicillamine and NAC were of some benefit in preventing strictures in rats and rabbits.[35,68,118] Halofuginone, a specific inhibitor of collagen type I synthesis, and vitamin E, a known antioxidant, significantly reduced esophageal stricture[93] and collagen synthesis,[40] respectively, in rats. In addition, epidermal growth factor and interferon-γ also decreased collagen synthesis and stenosis following sodium hydroxide burns in rats.[8] Colchicine, which decreases collagen synthesis, was found to delay wound healing and was associated with stricture formation in rabbits with sodium hydroxide-induced esophageal burns. Sphingosylphosphorylcholine, an intracellular second messenger, was shown to be effective in preventing caustic esophageal strictures via diminished collagen deposition in rats.[129] As none of these treatments have been adequately studied in humans, they cannot currently be recommended in the routine management of caustic ingestions.

CHRONIC TREATMENT OF STRICTURES

Commonly, the management of esophageal strictures includes early endoscopic dilation for which a variety of types of dilators are available. Contrast CT can be used to determine maximal esophageal wall thickness, which can then be used to predict response,[65] as well as the number of sessions required to achieve adequate dilation. Multiple dilations are often necessary. In one study, patients with a maximal esophageal wall thickness of 9 mm or greater required more than seven sessions to achieve adequate dilation. This was significantly higher than in patients with a lesser maximal wall thickness.[65] Measurement of maximal wall thickness may be also be useful in determining long-term followup, type of nutritional support, and the potential need for surgical repair as an alternative to dilations. It may also provide an indication for those who should undergo dilations under fluoroscopy to limit the risk of perforation.

The risk of perforation from esophageal dilation is decreased if the initial procedure is delayed beyond 4 weeks postingestion, when healing, remodeling, and potential stricture formation in the esophagus have already taken place. Several series report perforation secondary to esophageal dilation.[47,62,65,98,121] Following perforation, patients may complain of dyspnea or chest pain with associated subcutaneous emphysema or pneumomediastinum. Diagnostic imaging may identify the perforation and provide information for emergent surgical repair if the diagnosis is unclear.

Patients with stricture formation require long-term endoscopic followup for the presence of neoplastic changes of the esophagus that may occur with a delay of several decades.[5]

MANAGEMENT OF OPHTHALMIC EXPOSURES

Ophthalmic exposures frequently occur from splash injuries, and, more recently, from the alkaline byproducts of sodium azide released in automobile air bag deployment and rupture.[123] The mainstay of therapy for these patients is immediate irrigation of the eye for a minimum of 15 minutes with 0.9% sodium chloride, lactated Ringer solution, or tap water, if it is the only therapy immediately available. Several liters of irrigation fluid are recommended. The normal pH of ophthalmic secretions is close to 7.40. This can be tested colorimetrically by using a urine dipstick, which can test a range of pH from 5 to 9 using a color chart.[79] Litmus paper can be used in the same fashion. Another option is Nitrazine paper, which changes color from yellow to dark blue at a pH above 6.5,[33] and which may be useful in acid exposures. These different test strips can be applied to the ophthalmic secretions to test the baseline pH, and followed with intermittent evaluations after 15 minutes to determine the adequacy of irrigation. If these xenobiotics are not readily available, irrigation should not be delayed, as the depth of penetration of the caustic agent will determine outcome. Anterior chamber irrigation may be required; and should be performed emergently by an ophthalmologist. A thorough eye examination should be completed and followup should be arranged. Chapter 19 contains a more detailed description of the evaluation and management of toxicologic emergencies of the eye.

SUMMARY

Assessing the severity of injuries in patients with caustic exposures can be clinically challenging. For all patients with caustic exposures, the primary consideration is adherence to universal precautions by healthcare professionals in an effort to prevent further exposures. For patients with ingestions, this effort should be immediately followed by airway assessment and stabilization. Basic decontamination, and consideration of multiple bedside, laboratory, and diagnostic imaging factors to decide how best to inspect the affected tissues should then be considered. Ideally, early in the course of management of a caustic ingestion, gastroenterologists and surgeons are involved in the care of the patient, so that any surgical intervention deemed necessary can be performed promptly. Exposures to the skin and eyes require rapid decontamination with simple irrigants such as 0.9% sodium chloride solution.

Household and industrial exposures to caustics constitute a potentially life-threatening global health concern. Public health efforts, such as the successful implementation of child-proofing caustic substance containers and limiting the concentration in household items in the United States should be encouraged in developing nations as well.

ACKNOWLEDGMENT

Robert S. Hoffman and Rama B. Rao contributed to this chapter in previous editions.

REFERENCES

1. Aceto T, Terplan K, Firoe RR, Munschauer RW. Chemical burns of the esophagus in children and glucocorticoid therapy. *J Med.* 1970;1:101-109.
2. Alford BR, Harris HH. Chemical burns of the mouth, pharynx and esophagus. *Ann Otol Rhinol Laryngol.* 1959;68:122-128.
3. Andersen AH. Experimental studies on the pharmacology of activated charcoal. III. Adsorption of gastrointestinal contents. *Acta Pharmacol.* 1948;4:275-284.
4. Anderson KD, Rouse TM, Randolph JG. A controlled trial of corticosteroids in children with corrosive injury of the esophagus. *N Engl J Med.* 1990;323:637-640.
5. Appelqvist P, Salmo M. Lye corrosion carcinoma of the esophagus: a review of 63 cases. *Cancer.* 1980;45:2655-2658.
6. Ashcraft KW, Padula RT. The effect of dilute corrosives on the esophagus. *Pediatrics.* 1974;53:226-232.
7. Bernhardt J, Ptok H, Wilhelm L, Ludwig K. Caustic acid burn of the upper gastrointestinal tract: first use of endosonography to evaluate the severity of the injury. *Surg Endosc.* 2002;16:1004.
8. Berthet B, Di Costanzo J, Arnaud C, et al. Influence of epidermal growth factor and interferon gamma on healing of oesophageal corrosive burns in the rat. *Br J Surg.* 1994;81:395-398.
9. Berkovits RN, Bos CE, Wijburg FA, Holzki J. Caustic injury of the oesophagus. Sixteen years' experience and introduction of a new model oesophageal stent. *J Laryngol Otol.* 1996;110:1041-1045.
10. Borja AR, Ransdell HT, Thomas TV, Johnson W. Lye injuries of the esophagus: analysis of ninety cases of lye ingestion. *J Thorac Cardiovasc Surg.* 1969;57:533-538.
11. Cardona JC, Daly JF. Current management of corrosive esophagitis: an evaluation of results in 239 cases. *Ann Otol Rhinol Laryngol.* 1971;80:521-526.
12. Cello JP, Fogel RP, Boland CR. Liquid caustic ingestion—spectrum of injury. *Arch Intern Med.* 1980;140:501-504.

13. Chaudhary A, Puri AS, Dhar P, et al. Elective surgery for corrosive induced gastric injury. *World J Surg.* 1996;20:703-706.
14. Cheng YJ, Kao EL. Arterial blood gas analysis in acute caustic ingestion injuries. *Surg Today.* 2003;33:483-485.
15. Chobanian SJ. Accidental ingestion if liquid zinc chloride: local and systemic effects. *Ann Emerg Med.* 1981;10:91-93.
16. Chong SC, Beahrs OH, Payne WS. Management of corrosive gastritis due to ingested acid. *Mayo Clin Proc.* 1974;49:861-865.
17. Christensen BT. Prediction of complications following unintentional caustic ingestion in children. Is endoscopy always necessary? *Acta Paediatr.* 1995;84:1177-1182.
18. Clausen JO, Nielsen TLF, Fogh A. Admission to Danish hospitals after suspected ingestion of corrosives. *Dan Med Bull.* 1994;41:234-237.
19. Cleveland WW, Thornton N, Chesney JG, Lawson RB. The effect of prednisone in the prevention of esophageal stricture following the ingestion of lye. *South Med J.* 1958;51:861-864.
20. Crain EF, Gershel JC, Mezey AP. Caustic ingestions—symptoms as predictors of esophageal injury. *Am J Dis Child.* 1984;138:863-865.
21. Cullen ML, Klein MD. Spontaneous resolution of acid gastric injury. *J Pediatr Surg.* 1987;22:550-551.
22. Daly JF, Cardona JC. Acute corrosive esophagitis. *Arch Otolaryngol.* 1961;74:41-46.
23. Dantas RO, Mamede RCM. Esophageal motility in patients with esophageal caustic injury. *Am J Gastroenterol.* 1996;91:1157-1161.
24. Di Costanzo J, Noirclerc M, Jouglard J, et al. New therapeutic approach to corrosive burns of the upper gastrointestinal tract. *Gut.* 1980;21:370-375.
25. Dilawari JB, Singh S, Rao PN, Anand BS. Corrosive acid ingestion in man—a clinical and endoscopic study. *Gut.* 1984;25:183-187.
26. Eaton H, Tennekoon GE. Squamous carcinoma of the stomach following corrosive acid burns. *Br J Surg.* 1972;59:382-387.
27. Einhorn A, Horton L, Altieri M, et al. Serious respiratory consequences of detergent ingestions in children. *Pediatrics.* 1989;84:472-474.
28. Estera A, Taylor W, Mills LJ. Corrosive burns of the esophagus and stomach: a recommendation for an aggressive surgical approach. *Ann Thorac Surg.* 1986;41:276-283.
29. Fadoo F, Ruiz DE, Dawn SK, et al. Helical CT esophagography for the evaluation of suspected esophageal perforation or rupture. *AJR Am J Roentgenol.* 2004;182:1177-1179.
30. Friedman EM, Lovejoy FH Jr. The emergency management of caustic ingestions. *Emerg Med Clin North Am.* 1984;2:77-86.
31. Fulton JA, Hoffman RS. Steroids in second degree caustic burns of the esophagus: a systematic pooled analysis of fifty years of human data: 1956-2006. *Clin Tox.* 2007;45:402-408.
32. Gago O, Ritter FN, Martel W, et al. Aggressive surgical treatment for caustic injury of the esophagus and stomach. *Ann Thorac Surg.* 1972;13:243-250.
33. Garite TJ, Spellacy WN. Premature rupture of membranes. In: Scott JR, DiSaia PJ, Hammond CB, Spellacy WN, eds. *Danforth's Obstetrics and Gynecology*, 7th ed. Philadelphia: Lippincott; 1994:30.
34. Gaudreault P, Parent M, McGuigan MA, et al. Predictability of esophageal injury from signs and symptoms: a study of caustic ingestion in 378 children. *Pediatrics.* 1983;71:767-770.
35. Gehanno P, Geudon C. Inhibition of experimental esophageal lye strictures by penicillamine. *Arch Otolaryngol.* 1981;107:145-147.
36. Genc A, Mutaf O. Esophageal motility changes in acute and late periods of caustic esophageal burns and their relation to prognosis in children. *J Pediatr Surg.* 2002;37:1526-1528.
37. Gillis DA, Higgins G, Kennedy R. Gastric damage from ingested acid in children. *J Pediatr Surg.* 1985;20:494-496.
38. Gorman RL, Khin-Maung-Gyi MT, Klein-Schwartz W, et al. Initial symptoms as predictors of esophageal injury in alkaline corrosive ingestions. *Am J Emerg Med.* 1992;10:189-194.
39. Gossot D, Safarti E, Celerier M. Early blunt esophagectomy in severe caustic burns of the upper digestive tract: Report of 29 cases. *J Thorac Cardiovasc Surg.* 1987;94:188-191.
40. Gunel E, Caglayan F, Caglayan O, et al. Effect of antioxidant therapy on collagen synthesis in corrosive esophageal burns. *Pediatr Surg Int.* 2002;18:24-27.
41. Gupta S. A technique of repairing acid burns of the stomach. *Ann R Coll Surg Engl.* 1988;70:74-75.
42. Gupta S, Levine MS, Rubesin SE, et al. Usefulness of barium studies for differentiating benign and malignant strictures of the esophagus. *AJR Am J Roentgenol.* 2003;180:737-744.
43. Haller JA, Andrews HG, White JJ, et al. Pathophysiology and management of acute corrosive burns of the esophagus: results of treatment in 285 children. *J Pediatr Surg.* 1971;6:578-583.
44. Haller JA, Bachman K. The comparative effect of current therapy on experimental caustic burns of the esophagus. *Pediatrics.* 1964;34:236-245.
45. Havanond C, Havanond P. Initial signs and symptoms as prognostic indicators as severe gastrointestinal tract injury due to corrosive injury. *J Emerg Med.* 2007;33(4):349-353.
46. Hawkins DB. Dilatation and esophageal strictures: comparative morbidity of anterograde and retrograde methods. *Ann Otol Rhinol Laryngol.* 1988;97:460-465.
47. Hawkins DB, Demeter MJ, Barnett TE. Caustic ingestion: controversies in management. A review of 214 cases. *Laryngoscope.* 1980;90:98-109.
48. Hill JL, Norberg HP, Smith MD, et al. Clinical technique and success of the esophageal stent to prevent corrosive strictures. *J Pediatr Surg.* 1976;11:443-450.
49. Hirst LW, Summers PM, Griffiths, et al. Controlled trial of hyperbaric oxygen treatment for alkali corneal burn in the rabbit. *Clin Exp Ophthalmol.* 2004;32:67-70.
50. Hoffman RS, Howland MA, Kamerow HN, Goldfrank LR. Comparison of titratable acid/alkaline reserves and pH in potentially caustic household products. *J Toxicol Clin Toxicol.* 1989;27:241-261.
51. Homan CS, Maitra SR, Lane BP, et al. Effective treatment for acute alkali injury to the esophagus using weak acid neutralization therapy: an ex vivo study. *Acad Emerg Med.* 1995;2:952-958.
52. Homan CS, Maitra SR, Lane BP, et al. Histopathologic evaluation the therapeutic efficacy of water and milk dilution for esophageal acid injury. *Acad Emerg Med.* 1995;2:587-591.
53. Homan CS, Maitra SR, Lane BP, et al. Therapeutic effects of water and milk for acute alkali injury of the esophagus. *Ann Emerg Med.* 1994;24:14-19.
54. Homan CS, Maitra SR, Lane BP, Geller ER. Effective treatment of acute alkali injury of the rat esophagus with early saline dilution therapy. *Ann Emerg Med.* 1993;22:178-182.
55. Homan CS, Singer AJ, Henry MC, Thode HC. Thermal effects of neutralization therapy and water dilution for acute alkali exposure in canines. *Acad Emerg Med.* 1997;4:27-32.
56. Horvath OP, Olah T, Zentai G. Emergency esophagogastrectomy for the treatment of hydrochloric acid injury. *Ann Thorac Surg.* 1991;52:98-101.
57. Howell JM, Dalsey WC, Hartsell FW, Butzin CA. Steroids for the treatment of corrosive esophageal injury: a statistical analysis of past studies. *Am J Emerg Med.* 1992;10:421-425.
58. Hwang TL, Shen-Chen SM, Chen MF. Nonthoracotomy esophagectomy for corrosive esophagitis with gastric perforation. *Surg Gynecol Obstet.* 1987;164:537-540.
59. Isolauri J, Markkula H. Lye ingestion and carcinoma of the esophagus. *Acta Chir Scand.* 1989;155:269-271.
60. Jovic-Stosic J, Todorovic V, Doder R. Steroid treatment of corrosive injury. *J Toxicol Clin Toxicol.* 2004;42:417-418.
61. Kamijo Y, Kondo I, Soma K, et al. Alkaline esophagitis evaluated by endoscopic ultrasound. *J Toxicol Clin Toxicol.* 2001;39:623-625.
62. Kirsch MM, Peterson A, Brown JW, et al. Treatment of caustic injuries of the esophagus: a ten-year experience. *Ann Surg.* 1978;188:675-678.
63. Knox WG, Scott JR, Zintel HA, et al. Bougienage and steroids used singly or in combination in experimental corrosive esophagitis. *Ann Surg.* 1967;166:930-940.
64. Kocchar R, Mehta S, Nagi B, Goenka MK. Corrosive acid-induced esophageal intramural pseudodiverticulosis—a study of 14 patients. *J Clin Gastroenterol.* 1991;13:371-375.
65. Lahoti D, Broor SL, Basu P, et al. Corrosive esophageal strictures: predictors to response of endoscopic dilatation. *Gastrointest Endosc.* 1995;41:196-200.
66. Landau GD, Saunders WH. The effect of chlorine bleach on the esophagus. *Arch Otolaryngol.* 1964;80:174-176.
67. Leape LL, Ashcraft KW, Scarpelli DG, Holder TM. Hazard to health—liquid lye. *N Engl J Med.* 1971;284:578-581.
68. Liu A, Richardson M, Robertson WO. Effects of *N*-acetylcysteine on caustic burns. *Vet Hum Toxicol.* 1985;28:316.
69. Lowe JE, Graham DY, Boisaubin EV, Lanza FL. Corrosive injury to the stomach: the natural history and role of fiberoptic endoscopy. *Am J Surg.* 1979;137:803-806.
70. Luedtke P, Levine MS, Rubesin SE, et al. Radiologic diagnosis of benign esophageal strictures: a pattern approach. *Radiographics.* 2003;23:897-909.
71. Mack RB. Decant the wine, prune back your long-term hopes. *N C Med J.* 1987;48:593-595.

72. Madden JW, Davis WM, Butler C, Peacock EE. Experimental esophageal lye burns II: correcting established strictures with betaaminopropionitrile and bougienage. *Ann Surg.* 1973;178:277-284.
73. Mandarikan BA. Ingestion of dishwasher detergent by children. *Br J Clin Pract.* 1990;44:35-36.
74. Martel W. Radiologic features of esophagogastritis secondary to extremely caustic agents. *Diagn Radiol.* 1972;103:31-36.
75. Maull KI, Osmand AP, Maull CD. Liquid caustic ingestions: an in vitro study of the effects of buffer, neutralization, and dilution. *Ann Emerg Med.* 1985;14:1160-1162.
76. Maull KI, Scher LA, Greenfield LJ. Surgical implications of acid ingestion. *Surg Gynecol Obstet.* 1979;148:895-898.
77. McKinney PE. Zinc chloride ingestion in a child—exocrine pancreatic insufficiency. *Ann Emerg Med.* 1995;25:562.
78. McKinney PE, Brent J, Kulig K. Acute zinc chloride ingestion in a child—local and systemic effects. *Ann Emerg Med.* 1994;23:1383-1387.
79. McNeely MDD. Urinalysis. In: Sonnenwirth AC, Jarret L, eds: *Grad-wohl's Clinical Laboratory Methods and Diagnosis.* St. Louis: Mosby; 1980:483.
80. McQuarrie DA, Rock PA. Chemical reactivity. In: McQuarrie DA, Rock PA. *General Chemistry,* 3rd ed. New York: W H Freedman; 1991:100-137.
81. Meredith W, Kon ND, Thompson JN. Management of injuries from liquid lye ingestion. *J Trauma.* 1988;28:1173-1180.
82. Middlekamp JN, Ferguson TB, Roper CL, Hoffman FD. The management and problems of caustic burns in children. *J Thorac Cardiovasc Surg.* 1969;57:341-347.
83. Millar AJ, Numanoglu A, Mann M, et al. Detection of caustic oesophageal injury with technetium 99m-labelled sucralfate. *J Pediatr Surg.* 2001;36:262-265.
84. Mills LJ, Estrera AS, Platt MR. Avoidance of esophageal stricture following severe caustic burns by the use of an intraluminal stent. *Ann Thorac Surg.* 1979;28:63-65.
85. Mitani M, Hirata K, Fukuda M, Kaneko M. Endoscopic ultrasonography in corrosive injury of the upper gastrointestinal tract by hydrochloric acid. *J Clin Ultrasound.* 1996;24:40-42.
86. Mozingo DW, Smith AA, McManus WF, et al. Chemical burns. *J Trauma.* 1988;28:642-647.
87. Muhletaler CA, Gerlock AJ, de Soto L, Halter SA. Acid corrosive esophagitis: radiographic findings. *AJR Am J Roentgenol.* 1980;134:1137-1140.
88. Mutaf O, Avanoglu A, Ozok G. Management of tracheoesophageal fistula as a complication of esophageal dilatations in caustic esophageal burns. *J Pediatr Surg.* 1995;30:823-826.
89. Norton RA. Esophageal and antral strictures due to ingestion of household ammonia—report of two cases. *N Engl Med.* 1960;262:10-12.
90. Nunes AC, Romaozinho JM, Pontes JM, et al. Risk factors for stricture development after caustic ingestion. *Hepatogastroenterology.* 2002;49:1563-1566.
91. Ochi K, Ohashi T, Sato S, et al. Surgical treatment for caustic ingestion injury of the pharynx, larynx, and esophagus. *Acta Otolaryngol.* 1996;522 (Suppl):116-119.
92. Otcu S, Karnak I, Tanyel FC, et al. Biochemical indicators of caustic ingestion and/or accompanying esophageal injury in children. *Turk J Pediatr.* 2003;45:21-25.
93. Ozcelik MF, Pekmezci S, Saribeyoglu, et al. The effect of halofuginone, a specific inhibitor of collagen type 1 synthesis, in the prevention of esophageal strictures related to caustic injury. *Am J Surg.* 2004;187:257-260.
94. Pelclova D, Navratil T. Corrosive ingestion: the evidence base. Are steroids still indicated in second- and third-degree corrosive burns of the oesophagus? *J Toxicol Clin Toxicol.* 2004;42:414-416.
95. Penner GE. Acid ingestion—toxicology and treatment. *Ann Emerg Med.* 1980;9:374-379.
96. Potter JL. Acute zinc chloride ingestion in a young child. *Ann Emerg Med.* 1981;10:267-269.
97. Previterra C, Guisti F, Guglielmi M. Predictive value of visible lesions (cheeks, lips, oropharynx) in suspected caustic ingestion: may endoscopy reasonably be omitted in completely negative pediatric patients? *Pediatr Emerg Care.* 1990;6:176-178.
98. Ragheb MI, Ramadan AA, Khalia MA. Management of corrosive esophagitis. *Surgery.* 1976;79:494-498.
99. Ramasamy K, Gumaste VV. Corrosive ingestion in adults. *J Clin Gastroenterol.* 2003;37:119-124.
100. Ray JF III, Myers WO, Lawton BR, et al. The natural history of liquid lye ingestion—rationale for an aggressive surgical approach. *Arch Surg.* 1974;109:436-439.
101. Reyes HM, Hill JL. Modification of the experimental stent technique for esophageal burns. *J Surg Res.* 1976;20:65-70.
102. Reyes HM, Lin CY, Schlunk FF, Repogle RL. Experimental treatment of corrosive esophageal burns. *J Pediatr Surg.* 1974;9:317-327.
103. Ribet ME. Esophagogastrectomy for acid injury. *Ann Thorac Surg.* 1992;53:738-742.
104. Ritter FN, Newman MH, Newman DE. A clinical and experimental study of corrosive burns of the stomach. *Ann Otol Rhinol Laryngol.* 1968;77:830-842.
105. Rosenberg N, Kunderman PJ, Vroman L, Moolten SE. Prevention of experimental esophageal stricture by cortisone II. *Arch Surg.* 1953;66:593-598.
106. Rumack BH, Burrington JD. Caustic ingestions: a rational look at diluents. *Clin Toxicol.* 1977;11:27-34.
107. Safarti E, Gossot D, Assens P, Celerier M. Management of caustic ingestion in adults. *Br J Surg.* 1987;74:146-148.
108. Schild JA. Caustic ingestion in adult patients. *Laryngoscope.* 1985;95:1199-1201.
109. Scott JC, Jones B, Eisele DW, Ravich WJ. Caustic ingestion injuries of the upper aerodigestive tract. *Laryngoscope.* 1992;102:1-8.
110. Shirazi S, Schulze-Delrieu K, Custer-Hagen T, et al. Motility changes in opossum esophagus from experimental esophagitis. *Dig Dis Sci.* 1989;34:1668-1676.
111. Sinar DR, Fletcher JR, Cordova CC, et al. Acute acid-induced esophagitis impairs esophageal peristalsis in baboons. *Gastroenterology.* 1981;80:1286.
112. Subbarao KSVK, Kakar AK, Chandrasekhar V, et al. Cicatricial gastric stenosis caused by corrosive ingestion. *Aust N Z J Surg.* 1988;58:143-146.
113. Sugawa C, Lucas CE. Caustic injury of the upper gastrointestinal tract in adults: a clinical and endoscopic study. *Surgery.* 1989;106:802-807.
114. Sugawa C, Mullins RJ, Lucas CE, Leibold WC. The value of early endoscopy following caustic ingestion. *Surg Gynecol Obstet.* 1981;153:553-556.
115. Swanson JO, Levine MS, Redfern RO, Rubesin SE. Usefulness of high-density barium for detection of leaks after esophagogastrectomy, total gastrectomy, and total laryngectomy. *AJR Am J Roentgenol.* 2003;181:415-420.
116. Tewfik TL, Schloss MD. Ingestion of lye and other corrosive agents—a study of 86 infant and child cases. *J Otolaryngol.* 1980; 9:72-77.
117. Thompson JN. Corrosive esophageal injuries I: a study of nine cases of concurrent accidental caustic ingestions. *Laryngoscope.* 1987;97:1060-1066.
118. Thompson JN. Corrosive esophageal injuries II: an investigation of treatment methods and histochemical analysis of esophageal strictures in a new animal model. *Laryngoscope.* 1987;97:1191-1202.
119. Tugay M, Utkan T, Utkan Z. Effects of caustic lye injury to the esophageal smooth muscle reactivity: in vitro study. *J Surg Res.* 2003;113:128-132.
120. Viscomi GJ, Beekhuis GJ, Whitten CF. An evaluation of early esophagoscopy and corticosteroid therapy in the management of corrosive injury of the esophagus. *J Pediatr.* 1961;59:356-360.
121. Webb WR, Koutras P, Ecker RR, Sugg WL. An evaluation of steroids and antibiotics in caustic burns of the esophagus. *Ann Thorac Surg.* 1970;9:95-101.
122. White CS, Templeton PA, Attar S. Esophageal perforation: CT findings. *AJR Am J Roentgenol.* 1993;160:767-770.
123. White JE, McClafferty K, Orfon RB, et al. Ocular alkali burn associated with automobile air bag activation. *CMAJ.* 1995;153:933-934.
124. Wiesskopf A. Effects of cortisone on experimental lye burn of the esophagus. *Ann Otol Rhinol Laryngol.* 1952;61:681-691.
125. Wijburg FA, Beukers MM, Heymans HS, et al. Nasogastric intubation as a sole treatment of caustic esophageal lesions. *Ann Otol Rhinol Laryngol.* 1985;94:337-341.
126. Wilson DAB, Wormald PJ. Battery acid—an agent of attempted suicide in black South Africans. *S Afr Med.* 1994;84:529-531.
127. Woodring JH, Heiser MJ. Detection of pneumoperitoneum on chest radiographs: comparison of upright lateral and posteroanterior projections. *AJR Am J Roentgenol.* 1995;165:45-47.
128. Wu MH, Lai WW. Surgical management of extensive corrosive injuries of the alimentary tract. *Surg Gynecol Obstet.* 1993;177:12-16.
129. Yagmurlu A, Aksu B, Bingol-Kologlu M, et al. A novel approach for preventing esophageal stricture formation: sphingosylphosphorylcholine-enhanced tissue remodeling. *Pediatr Surg Int.* 2004;20(10):778-82.
130. Zargar SA, Kochlar R, Mehta S, Mehta SK. The role of fiberoptic endoscopy in the management of corrosive ingestion and modified endoscopic classification of burns. *Gastrointest Endosc.* 1991;37:165-169.
131. Zargar SA, Kochlar R, Nagi B, et al. Ingestion of corrosive acids: spectrum of injury to upper gastrointestinal tract and natural history. *Gastroenterology.* 1989;97:702-707.
132. Zwischenberger JB, Savage C, Bidani A. Surgical aspects of esophageal disease: perforation and caustic injury. *Am J Respir Crit Care Med.* 2002;165:1037-1040.

CHAPTER 105
HYDROFLUORIC ACID AND FLUORIDES

Mark Su

Hydrofluoric acid (HF) has multiple applications and is widely used throughout industry, especially in organofluorine chemistry. Organofluorine compounds (eg, Teflon, freon, etc.) are synthesized using HF as the source of fluorine. Since this widespread use of HF invariably leads to human exposures, it is essential for clinicians to recognize that HF and fluoride-containing compounds are protoplasmic poisons that may result in deleterious systemic effects.

HISTORY AND EPIDEMIOLOGY

Hydrofluoric acid has been known for centuries for its ability to dissolve silica. The Nuremberg artist Schwanhard is given credit for the first attempt (in 1670) to use HF vapors to etch glass.[42] Since then, HF has been developed for multiple uses in addition to glass etching, such as brick cleaning, etching microchips in the semiconductor industry, electroplating, leather tanning, rust removal, and the cleaning of porcelain.[23,42] From 2005 to 2007, the American Association of Poison Control Centers (AAPCC) reported more than 2500 exposures to HF and 5 deaths. Hands are by far the most common exposure location. Exposures to HF are often unintentional and they can be an occupationally related hazard. The actual number of work-related poisonings from HF appears difficult to quantitate because of limitations in ICD (*International Classification of Diseases*) medical coding and lack of notification of regional poison centers by worksites.[7]

Hydrofluoric acid is also the most common cause of fluoride poisoning, although other forms of fluoride, including sodium fluoride (NaF) and ammonium bifluoride (NH_4HF_2), may also produce significant toxicity. Historically, sodium fluoride has been used as an insecticide, rodenticide, antihelminthic agent in swine, and a delousing powder for poultry and cattle. Ammonium bifluoride is mainly used in industrial inorganic chemistry, especially in the processing of alloys and in glass etching. Other fluoride salts are widely used in, for example, the steel industry, drinking water, toothpaste additives, electroplating, lumber treatment, and the glass and enamel industries.

The widespread use of HF and fluoride-containing compounds has resulted in significant toxicity. In 1988, an oil refinery in Texas released a cloud of hydrogen fluoride gas that resulted in 36 people requiring hospital treatment.[42] The petroleum industry has since been plagued by similar HF incidents.[95] NaF was responsible for the poisoning of 263 people and 47 fatalities when it was mistaken for powdered milk and unintentionally combined with scrambled eggs.[52] These and other forms of fluoride salts can be converted to HF in vivo after ingestion. Consequently, many inorganic fluoride compounds can result in significant fluoride toxicity, especially when large exposures occur.

CHEMISTRY

Hydrofluoric acid has unique properties that can cause life-threatening complications following seemingly trivial exposure. Anhydrous HF is highly concentrated (>70%) and used almost exclusively for industrial purposes. The aqueous form of HF, which generally ranges in concentrations from 3% to 40%, is commonly used in both industrial and household products.

Hydrofluoric acid is synthesized as the product of gaseous sulfuric acid and calcium fluoride, which is subsequently cooled to a liquid.[53] Aqueous HF is a weak acid, with a pK_a of 3.5; as such, it is approximately 1000 times less dissociated than equimolar hydrochloric acid, a strong acid.

Sodium fluoride is commonly synthesized by the reaction of sodium hydroxide (NaOH) with HF, with subsequent purification by recrystallization. NaF is highly soluble and readily dissociates.[2]

To synthesize NH_4HF_2 ammonium fluoride (NH_4F) is first formed by the reaction of ammonium hydroxide (NH_4OH) and HF. Ammonium fluoride is then converted to bifluoride by dehydrating the aqueous solution.

Fluorine is the most electronegative element in the Periodic Table due to its relatively large number of protons in the nucleus compared to its molecular size, and the minimal amount of screening or shielding by inner electrons. Other halides also possess electronegative properties but to a lesser extent. Consequently, the corresponding anion of fluorine, the fluoride ion (F^-), is a weak base because of it is unwillingness to donate its electrons.

PATHOPHYSIOLOGY

Exposures to HF occur via dermal, ocular, inhalation, and oral routes with one reported case of toxicity from an HF enema.[15] A permeability coefficient of 1.4×10^{-4} cm/sec allows HF to penetrate deeply into tissues prior to dissociating into hydrogen ions and highly electronegative fluoride ions.[29] These fluoride ions avidly bind to extracellular and intracellular stores of calcium and magnesium, depleting them, and ultimately leading to cellular dysfunction and cell death.[8,51,60] The alteration in local calcium homeostasis causes neuroexcitation and accounts for the development of neuropathic pain. Furthermore, ischemia related to calcium dysregulation–mediated localized vasospasm is likely an additional contributory factor to the development of pain.[37,88]

Formation of insoluble calcium fluoride (CaF_2) is proposed as the etiology for both the precipitous fall in serum calcium concentration and the severe pain associated with tissue toxicity. There are several theories regarding the actual fate of calcium and fluoride ions in tissues. In vitro evidence suggests that fluorapatite is formed in the presence of phosphate and hydroxyapatite. This may be a more likely pathway for disposition of the fluoride ion.[8] Fluorapatite, like calcium fluoride, is insoluble and its formation may contribute to the clinical findings that occur with HF exposures.

Fluoride also binds magnesium and manganese and there is in vitro evidence that this interferes with many enzyme systems. In the anhydrous form, the high concentration of hydrogen ions in HF also produces a caustic burn similar to that caused by strong acids (see Chap. 104).

The minimal lethal dose in humans is approximated to be 1 mg/kg of fluoride ion.[42]

CLINICAL MANIFESTATIONS

LOCAL EFFECTS

Skin The extent of tissue injury following dermal exposures is determined by the volume, concentration, and contact time with the tissues. Following dermal exposure, concentration of HF is inversely related to the rapidity of onset of the excruciating pain at the contact site.[27,53,87] Concentrations of greater than 50% cause immediate pain with

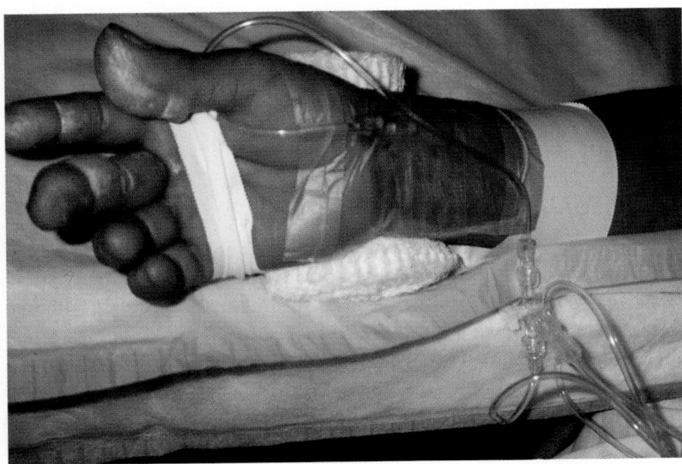

FIGURE 105–1. Severe injury to the fingers resulted from exposure to hydrofluoric acid. Note the arterial line in place for administration of calcium. *(Image contributed by the New York City Poison Center Toxicology Fellowship Program.)*

visible tissue damage.[81] Exposure to household rust-removal products (6% and 12% HF) is often associated with a delay of several hours before pain develops.[27,82,92,93] The initial site of injury may also appear relatively benign despite significant subjective complaints of pain. Over time, the tissue may become hyperemic, with subsequent blanching and coagulative necrosis. As calcium complexes precipitate, a white discoloration of the affected area may appear.[70] (See Fig 105–1) Ulcerations may form at a rate dependent on the concentration and duration of contact.[23,43,54] If more than 2% of the body surface area is burned with high-concentration HF, life-threatening systemic toxicity should be expected.[16,67,69,81,87] Small body surface area exposures to low concentrations typically do not result in life-threatening systemic toxicity, although fatalities have resulted with dermal exposures to concentrated HF covering less than 5% body surface area.[86]

Pulmonary Patients with inhalational exposures can present with a variety of signs and symptoms depending on the HF concentration and exposure time. Thirteen oil refinery workers exposed to a low-concentration HF mist experienced minor upper respiratory tract irritation.[49] In contrast, in a mass inhalational exposure to HF, throat burning and shortness of breath were among the more common chief complaints.[95] Some of these patients had altered pulmonary function tests and hypoxemia, and 16% developed hypocalcemia. Stridor, wheezing, rhonchi, and erythema and ulcers of the upper respiratory tract were described. Eye pain was also noted, reinforcing the fact that ophthalmic injury typically accompanies inhalational or dermal exposures.[49,58,76,95]

Gastrointestinal Intentional ingestion of concentrated HF (or other fluoride salts such as NaF) causes significant gastritis yet often spares the remainder of the gastrointestinal tract. Patients promptly develop vomiting and abdominal pain. Although systemic absorption is rapid and almost invariably fatal, there is at least one report of a patient with an ingestion of a low concentration of HF who suffered multiple episodes of ventricular fibrillation and was successfully resuscitated.[84] Following HF ingestion patients may present with an altered mental status, airway compromise, and dysrhythmias.[10,52,55,84]

Ophthalmic Hydrofluoric acid appears to result in more extensive injury to the eye than most other acids.[61] Ophthalmic exposures from liquid splashes or hydrogen fluoride gas denude the corneal and conjunctival epithelium, and lead to stromal corneal edema, conjunctival ischemia, sloughing, and chemosis.[42] Fluoride ions can penetrate deeply to affect the anterior chamber structures.[42] The effects are usually noted within one day.[42] Other possible findings include corneal revascularization, recurrent epithelial erosions, and, sometimes, keratoconjunctivitis sicca (dry eye) developing as a long-term complication.[4,61,77]

SYSTEMIC EFFECTS

Significant systemic toxicity can occur via any route of exposure because of the ability of HF to penetrate tissues. The potential for systemic toxicity is an important consideration in management as patients should be rapidly decontaminated and treated.[9,13,28,80,81,89,90] Fatal exposures to HF by any route share the similar features of hypocalcemia, hypomagnesemia, and, in many cases, hyperkalemia as preterminal events.[2,10,20,28,48,53,55,62,63,87] In some circumstances, the hypocalcemia severely disrupts the coagulation cascade, resulting in the inability of blood clotting, even on postmortem examination.[55,65,66]

Fatalities from HF may occur as a result of either sudden-onset myocardial conduction failure or ventricular fibrillation. Although the evidence regarding the mechanism of myocardial irritability is inconclusive, electrolyte disturbances that lead to ventricular dysrhythmias and fibrillation are thought to be the primary cause of death in patients with severe systemic fluoride poisoning.[16,67,81,87,98] Some postmortem cases reveal significant structural myocardial injury.[65] However, these findings are inconsistently encountered in humans and in animal cardiac arrest models that fail to demonstrate any histologic abnormalities of the myocardium.[22,59]

Although systemic fluoride toxicity results in systemic hypocalcemia, by mechanisms not fully elucidated, fluoride may induce intracellular hypercalcemia leading to an efflux of potassium ions into the extracellular space.[22,51,65] One in vitro study performed with human erythrocytes suggests that fluoride inhibition of Na^+-K^+ ATPase and Na^+-Ca^{2+} exchange leads to intracellular hypercalcemia.[64] The subsequent hyperkalemia may alter the automaticity and resting potential of the heart, leading to fatal dysrhythmias.[63] Dogs treated with quinidine, a potassium efflux blocker, are protected from lethal doses of intravenous sodium fluoride.[22] Likewise, amiodarone, which also possesses potassium efflux blockade properties, has demonstrable efficacy in both in vitro and in vivo models of fluoride toxicity.[18,85] However, efficacy in humans has not been studied or documented. Furthermore, the mechanism of toxicity may be much more complicated.[100] A child with systemic fluoride toxicity, who was appropriately repleted with calcium, and who had normal electrolytes still experienced nonfatal ventricular fibrillation.[9,100] Perhaps this is because serum potassium, calcium, and magnesium concentrations only partly represent tissue concentrations.[8,9,22,62,63] Furthermore, HF may directly impair myocardial function. Rabbits exposed to topical HF over 2% of their total body surface area developed focal necrosis of myocardial fibers, as well as significant elevations in cardiac enzymes that persisted for almost 5 days after injury.[99]

Assessing Severity of Clinical Exposures. Historical and clinical features of an exposure will determine which HF exposures are life-threatening. All oral and inhalational exposures should be considered potentially fatal, as should burns of the face and neck, regardless of HF concentration. Inhalational exposure should be assumed for all patients with skin burns of greater than 5% body surface area, any exposure to HF concentrations greater than 50%, and head and neck burns.[41] Patients presenting with altered mental status are critically ill and necessitate rapid therapy.

Hydrofluoric acid concentrations of greater than 20% have potential for significant toxicity in a patient even if only a small surface area has been exposed.[57] As a general rule, patients who experience severe pain within minutes of contact are most likely exposed to a very high concentration of HF and their condition can rapidly deteriorate. An otherwise well-appearing patient may have a precipitous demise without any clinical manifestations of hypocalcemia.

DIAGNOSTIC TESTING

Diagnostic testing for systemic fluoride poisoning is currently based on monitoring of serum electrolytes. Ionized calcium should be serially monitored along with magnesium and potassium.[28] Additional information may be obtained from a venous or arterial blood gas analysis. As systemic toxicity progresses, there is potential for development of metabolic acidosis.[8] Serum fluoride concentrations may be assessed but the results will not return in a clinically relevant timeframe. Although a serum fluoride concentration of 0.3 mg/dL has been reported as fatal, one patient survived with a serum fluoride concentration of 1.4 mg/dL.[87,100]

Electrocardiographic findings of both hypocalcemia (prolonged QT interval) and hyperkalemia (peaked T waves) may be reliable indicators of toxicity.[2,13,28,31,36,66,87] In fact, ECG findings of peaked T waves from hyperkalemia have preceded the onset of ventricular dysrhythmias, thus potentially serving as a marker of severe fluoride toxicity.[9,62]

MANAGEMENT

GENERAL

For patients with more than localized exposure to low concentration HF or exposures to high concentration HF, the mainstay of management is to prevent or limit systemic absorption, assess for systemic toxicity, and rapidly correct any electrolyte imbalances. Intravenous access should be obtained. An ECG should be examined for signs of hypocalcemia, hypomagnesemia, and hyperkalemia. The patient should be attached to continuous cardiac monitoring and have a rapid assessment of serum electrolyte concentrations. A Foley catheter should be placed as needed to follow urine output.

Rapid airway assessment and protection should occur early in patients with inhalation or ingestion, respiratory distress, ingestion with vomiting, or burns significant enough to cause a change in mental status or voice.

For patients with less-significant dermal exposures, recent studies have focused on alternatives to irrigation with water or saline as topical decontamination techniques. The compound "hexafluorine" has been promoted for dermal and ocular decontamination of HF splashes.[56,83] Hexafluorine is a proprietary name and not representative of a conventional chemical compound. Despite anecdotal supportive data, in a controlled and blinded experimental study hexafluorine treatment was less effective than irrigation with water followed by the application of topical calcium.[35] In a followup animal study, water irrigation was as effective as hexafluorine in preventing systemic toxicity from HF.[38] At this time, until further objective data are available, it is premature to recommend the routine use of hexafluorine for initial decontamination of HF exposures.

An iodine-containing preparation specifically formulated by the study authors was studied for HF-induced burns in guinea pigs.[96] Iodine has demonstrated protective effects against burns from various alkylating agents, including mustard gas, and is hypothesized to inhibit apoptosis.[96] Because experience with iodine treatment of human HF burns is lacking at this time, it cannot be recommended at this time.

To prevent absorption from dermal exposures, irrigation with copious amounts of water should be done. The most important therapy for skin exposures is rapid removal of clothing and irrigation of the affected area with copious amounts of water or saline, whichever is more readily available.[1,46,50,54]

One report describes a woman who was dying from severe HF toxicity who was treated by amputation of the affected limb, and survived. Although rarely considered, this may be an alternative measure for patients who are critically ill and demonstrating an inadequate response to all other therapeutic modalities.[12,45]

DERMAL TOXICITY

Several therapeutic options have been studied and described in animal models for treatment of topical HF burns. Unfortunately, many study designs use histologic or subjective wound inspection as outcome parameters,[14,72] some with unblinded inspection.[11,25,45,46,68] These animal models do not address the clinically important parameters of pain reduction, cosmesis, and functionality.

Topical calcium gel should be applied to the affected area. This is prepared by mixing 3.5 g of calcium gluconate powder in 150 mL of sterile water-soluble lubricant, or 25 mL of 10% calcium gluconate in 75 mL of sterile water-soluble lubricant.[1,14,41] If calcium gluconate is unavailable, calcium chloride or calcium carbonate can be used in a similar formulation.[17] Topical therapy for both severe and non–life-threatening exposures scavenges fluoride ions. An animal study examining the efficacy and mechanism of topical calcium gel therapy found that the fluoride ion concentration of the calcium gel was significantly higher than non–calcium-containing gel controls. Although this was a limited study, these animals also had a decrease in urinary fluoride ion concentration as compared to controls, suggesting less overall absorption of the HF into the tissues.[46] Delivery of calcium transcutaneously may be enhanced by various means. In a rodent study of HF burns, iontophoretic (facilitated transport using an electromotive force) delivery of calcium ions appeared to increase calcium concentrations in vitro and improve pathologic changes in vivo.[97] Significant limitations to this study are time to administration of therapy and feasibility in patients with complex burns.[78] Human data are lacking. Dimethyl sulfoxide (DMSO) mixed with topical calcium salts may also facilitate the transport of calcium ions through the skin to penetrate deeply into the tissues. It also is able to act as a scavenger of free radicals, thus limiting inflammation and ongoing injury.[31] Although one group of authors recently advocated the combined use of DMSO and calcium,[31] concerns remain over reported adverse effects of DMSO.[42] There is currently inadequate data to support the use of DMSO in the treatment of HF burns.

Four therapies have had variable success in human exposures: the application of calcium via topical, intradermal, intravenous, and intraarterial routes. After irrigation, a gel solution of calcium carbonate or gluconate can be applied directly to the affected area or mixed directly into a sterile surgical glove and then placed on the patient's hand for 30 minutes for hand burns. Two case series report limited success with this therapy.[1,17] Some patients describe prompt and dramatic relief of pain. Alternatively or simultaneously, analgesics can be administered orally or intravenously as needed, but preferably not to the point of sedation, because local pain response will guide therapy. Digital blocks with subcutaneous lidocaine or bupivacaine can be used for patients presenting 12–24 hours after the injury from a low concentration of HF and with no systemic signs of toxicity at which time topical calcium salts are unlikely to be effective.[24]

If topical gel therapy fails within the first few minutes of application, consideration should be given to intradermal therapy with dilute calcium gluconate, because the benefit in pain control often occurs immediately. This treatment may have limited usefulness, however, in nondistensible spaces such as fingertips. Histologic studies in animal models demonstrate that 10% calcium chloride solution can be damaging to the tissues and should be avoided.[24,30] The preferable method is to approach the wound from a distal point of injury and inject intradermally no more than 0.5 mL/cm^2 of 5% calcium gluconate. Although one author recommends a palmar fasciotomy whenever this method of treatment is used in the hand,[1] this practice is not currently recommended unless a compartment syndrome is present. The potential for iatrogenic injury exceeds the potential benefit of injections in the hand. The limits of intradermal injection include the potential to increase soft-tissue damage without adequate relief, infection, and inadequate space to safely inject without causing a compartment syndrome.

Effective pain relief is especially problematic for nail involvement, leading some authors to suggest removal of the nail. This approach has some advantages in accessing the affected area; however, it is a painful procedure that is often cosmetically undesirable and the outcome is not always significantly improved.

If the wound is large or on a section of the fingerpad or an area that is not amenable to intradermal injections, consideration should be given to the use of intraarterial calcium gluconate. This procedure delivers calcium directly to the affected tissue from a proximal artery. Placement should be ipsilateral and proximal to the affected area, usually in the radial or brachial artery. The method of obtaining access is somewhat debated. Because of the potential to damage the endothelial lining of the artery, and because extravasation can have potentially devastating consequences, angiographic confirmation or direct visualization of the vessel was formerly recommended. This practice is still prudent if cannulation of the artery is expected to be difficult because of prior surgery or if an anatomic deformity is suspected. If the arterial line is carefully placed in a single attempt, and a good confirmatory arterial tracing is obtained, the infusion can be started. The recommended protocol consists of 10 mL of 10% calcium gluconate added to either 40 mL of D_5W (dextrose 5% in water) or 0.9% sodium chloride solution infused continuously over 4 hours.[1,44,73,82,91,92] This results in a 2% calcium gluconate solution. An animal model examined the effect of undiluted 10% calcium gluconate intraaortically. Although the model did not involve exposure to HF, there was significant tissue injury in the vessel wall as compared to a 2% calcium gluconate solution.[24] Calcium chloride has also been used successfully, although the potential for vessel injury and extravasation are significant and there is no defined benefit over calcium gluconate.[91,101] The complications associated with the use of intraarterial calcium infusion in several case series were relatively benign, and include radial artery spasm, hematoma, inflammation at the puncture site, and a fall in serum magnesium.[79,92] After the infusion is initiated, patients typically experience significant pain relief. Patients requiring an arterial line for treatment should be admitted to the hospital, as the majority will require more than one treatment, and some patients may require as many as five separate infusions of calcium gluconate. Although wounds may require débridement,[1] some suggest that following intraarterial calcium infusion, tissue can be salvaged that initially would not have been considered viable.[93] There have been no reported cases of clinically significant hypercalcemia following infusion as the total dose infused is quite low, although serum calcium concentrations were not always routinely recorded.

Administration of magnesium salts is an alternative or adjunctive therapy to the administration of calcium for dermal HF burns. Magnesium hydroxide and magnesium gluconate gel used in rabbit models show some histologic evidence of efficacy in dermal HF burns.[14] Two other animal models of intravenous magnesium for the management of dermal HF burns also suggest efficacy in terms of wound healing.[21,94] Magnesium is suggested to be an antidote for fluoride poisoning because magnesium fluoride is more soluble than calcium fluoride and magnesium is readily excreted by the kidneys.[95] However, these magnesium models inadequately address the disadvantage of magnesium salt solubility, and both topical and intravenous magnesium therapy are insufficiently evaluated in humans.

Another reported therapy for localized HF poisoning is an intravenous Bier block technique that uses 25 mL of 2.5% calcium gluconate. In one case, the effects lasted 5 hours and there were no adverse events.[34] In two other cases of patients exposed to HF, a 6% calcium gluconate solution administered using this procedure resulted in rapid and complete analgesia and minimal tissue necrosis.[79] Although the intravenous Bier block technique is not reported as being used in a substantial number of patients, it may be particularly useful when intraarterial infusion is problematic.[79] Further data are required before this therapy is routinely recommended.

All patients with digital exposures should be observed over 4–6 hours, as the pain is likely to recur and reapplication of the gel or an alternative therapy may be necessary. Even if successful pain control is achieved, the patient will require specialized followup and wound care.

INHALATIONAL TOXICITY

Patients with symptomatic inhalational injuries can be treated with nebulized calcium gluconate. A report of patients exposed to a low concentration of HF and treated with 4 mL of a 2.5% nebulized calcium gluconate solution demonstrated a subjective decrease in irritation with no adverse effects.[49] Another report demonstrated a good outcome following nebulization of a 5% calcium gluconate solution in a patient with an inhalational exposure.[47] Because nebulized calcium gluconate appears to be a relatively benign therapy, a dilute solution should be given to all patients with symptomatic inhalational exposures to any concentration of HF.[26]

INGESTIONS

In patients with intentional ingestions of HF, gastrointestinal decontamination poses a dilemma. Induction of emesis is also potentially harmful. Although placement of a nasogastric tube to perform gastric lavage is clearly associated with risks to the patient, insertion of a nasogastric tube may be beneficial if done safely and in a timely manner. Consequently, gastric emptying via a nasogastric tube should be considered because these exposures are almost universally fatal.[2,10,55,66] Healthcare providers should exercise extreme caution during this procedure because dermal or inhalational exposures can occur in the absence of appropriate protection. Because aqueous HF is a weak acid, the risk of perforation by passage of a small nasogastric tube may be lower than the risk of death from systemic absorption.[2,55] In the acidic environment of the stomach, more of the weak acid solution remains unionized, thus penetrating the gastric mucosa and causing rapid systemic poisoning. Moreover, activated charcoal is unlikely to adsorb the relatively small fluoride ions.

If an oral exposure occurs, a solution of calcium or magnesium salt should be delivered to the stomach as soon as possible to prevent HF penetration and to provide an alternative source of cations for the damaging electronegative fluoride ions.

When considering the efficacy of calcium to magnesium salts, calcium may be better than magnesium in reducing the bioavailability of fluoride as described in a murine model.[33] Magnesium citrate in a standard cathartic dose, magnesium sulfate, or any of the calcium solutions can be administered orally to prevent absorption, (see Antidotes in Depth A30: Calcium). Although intuitive, evidence for the benefit of oral calcium or magnesium salts is limited. In a mouse model of oral HF toxicity, administration of calcium- or magnesium-containing solutions did not change average survival time.[32] The study results, however, were limited because the calcium and magnesium salts were premixed together with the HF during administration, thus being an atypical model of HF ingestion. In a more recent study, the survival rate of mice poisoned with NaF was significantly greater when treated with high doses of oral $CaCl_2$ or $MgSO_4$.[40]

OPHTHALMIC TOXICITY

Patients with ophthalmic exposures should have each eye irrigated with 1 L of 0.9% sodium chloride solution, lactated Ringer solution, or water.[61] Although there are limited data, repetitive or prolonged irrigation appears to worsen outcome.[61] A complete ophthalmic examination should be performed after the patient is deemed stable, and an ophthalmology consultation should be obtained (see Chap. 19). One case report demonstrated a good outcome following ocular HF exposure with the use of 1% calcium gluconate eyedrops.[4] Although two recent reviews also recommend the use of 1% calcium gluconate for this purpose,[26,31] calcium salts tend to be irritating to the eye and this therapy has not been adequately studied; consequently, routine use is not indicated at this time. There is no role for gel therapy or intraocular injection in these patients, because most calcium and magnesium salts are potentially toxic to ocular tissues and may actually worsen outcome.[3,61]

SYSTEMIC TOXICITY

If there is clinical suspicion of severe toxicity, the immediate intravenous administration of calcium and magnesium salts is recommended. In general, calcium gluconate is preferred over calcium chloride because of the risks associated with extravasation (see Antidotes in Depth A30: Calcium). Patients can require several grams of calcium to treat severe HF toxicity.[28,84] Intravenous magnesium can be administered to adults as 20 mL of a 20% solution (4 g) over 20 minutes. An approach that uses intravenous calcium or magnesium, and local calcium or magnesium gels to limit absorption may protect against life-threatening hypocalcemia and hyperkalemia. Due to the numerous adverse effects of systemic fluoride poisoning, administration of calcium and magnesium salts alone may be insufficient in improving survival from systemic fluoride poisoning.[19] Furthermore, an animal model of hydrogen fluoride toxicity found that maintaining a normal acid–base balance was protective against HF toxicity.[75] Moreover, in a study of patients receiving enflurane anesthesia, urine alkalinization improved the excretion of fluoride.[74] Thus, it may be beneficial to correct any significant acidemia with hydration and IV sodium bicarbonate (calcium salts and sodium bicarbonate cannot be mixed). Standard treatment for systemic fluoride toxicity includes administration of calcium salts and sodium bicarbonate, which may also improve the hyperkalemia.

Treatment with large quantities of calcium and magnesium has not generally resulted in significant hypercalcemia or hypermagnesemia.[26] Several explanations are proposed. First, in systemically HF poisoned patients total-body calcium and magnesium stores are severely decreased so that large doses are required for adequate repletion. Also, most patients who are exposed to HF are young and healthy, with intact renal function.[26] Administration of calcium also results in antidiuretic hormone antagonism on renal tubular reabsorption resulting in polyuria which facilitates the urinary excretion of calcium and magnesium.[26]

Because most of the fluoride ions are eliminated renally,[5,39,46,80] hemodialysis may be considered in patients with severe HF poisoning, particularly if renal function is compromised. There are several reported cases of successful clearance of fluoride ions via hemodialysis with one case also using continuous venovenous hemodialysis.[5,6] Because the reported clearance rate did not differ significantly from normally functioning kidneys, it is unclear whether hemodialysis alters outcome in patients with normal renal function.

Although the use of quinidine, a potassium channel blocker, is protective in dogs,[65] it has not been studied or used in humans, and at this time cannot be routinely recommended.

SUMMARY

Hydrofluoric acid and fluoride salts are extremely potent cellular toxins. Hydrofluoric acid exposure typically results in isolated local tissue damage but may also result in severe systemic toxicity and death especially in large exposures. Fluoride salts cause systemic toxicity only when ingested. Development of fluoride toxicity is dependent on many variables including form, concentration, route(s) of exposure, and immediacy and completeness of decontamination, as well as premorbid health conditions. Treatment consists of immediate decontamination, protection of staff, rapid administration of agents to detoxify fluoride ions, enhancement of elimination of fluoride ions, and, rarely, extracorporeal removal. It is imperative for clinicians to be aware of the potentially deceptive nature of fluoride, as well as the possible therapeutic modalities used to treat fluoride poisoned patients.

REFERENCES

1. Anderson WJ, Anderson JR. Hydrofluoric acid burns of the hand: mechanism of injury and treatment. *J Hand Surg*. 1988;13:52-57.
2. Baltazar RF, Mower MM, Reider R, et al. Acute fluoride poisoning leading to fatal hyperkalemia. *Chest*. 1980;78:660-663.
3. Beiran I, Miller B, Bentur Y. The efficacy of calcium gluconate in ocular hydrofluoric acid burns. *Hum Exp Toxicol*. 1997;16:223-228.
4. Bentur Y, Tannenbaum S, Yaffe Y, Halpert M. The role of calcium gluconate in the treatment of hydrofluoric acid eye burn. *Ann Emerg Med*. 1993;22:1488-1490.
5. Berman L, Taves D, Mitra S, Newmark K. Inorganic fluoride poisoning: treatment by hemodialysis. *N Engl J Med*. 1973;289:922.
6. Björnhagen V, Höjer J, Karlson-Stiber C, et al. Hydrofluoric acid-induced burns and life-threatening systemic poisoning-favorable outcome after hemodialysis. *J Toxicol Clin Toxicol*. 2003;41:855-860.
7. Blodgett DW, Suruda AJ, Crouch BI. Fatal unintentional occupational poisonings by hydrofluoric acid in the US. *Am J Ind Med*. 2001;40:215-220.
8. Boink AB, Wemer J, Meulenbelt J, et al. The mechanism of fluoride-induced hypocalcemia. *Hum Exp Toxicol*. 1994;13:149-155.
9. Bordelon BM, Saffle JR, Morris SE. Systemic fluoride toxicity in a child with hydrofluoric acid burns: case report. *J Trauma*. 1993;34: 437-439.
10. Bost RO, Springfield A. Fatal hydrofluoric acid ingestion: a suicide case report. *J Anal Toxicol*. 1995;19:535-536.
11. Bracken WM, Cuppage F, McLaury RL, et al. Comparative effectiveness of topical treatments for hydrofluoric acid burns. *J Occup Med*. 1985;27: 733-739.
12. Buckingham FM. Surgery: a radical approach to severe hydrofluoric acid burns—a case report. *J Occup Med*. 1988;30:873-874.
13. Burke WJ, Hoegg UR, Philips RE. Systemic fluoride poisoning resulting from a fluoride skin burn. *J Occup Med*. 1973;15:39-41.
14. Burkhart KK, Brent J, Kirk MA, et al. Comparison of topical magnesium and calcium treatment for dermal hydrofluoric acid burns. *Ann Emerg Med*. 1994;24:9-13.
15. Cappell MS, Simon T. Fulminant acute colitis following a self-administered enema. *Am J Gastroenterol*. 1993;88:122-126.
16. Chela A, Reig R, Sanz P, et al. Death due to hydrofluoric acid. *Am J Forensic Med Pathol*. 1989;10:47-48.
17. Chick LR, Borah G. Calcium carbonate gel therapy for hydrofluoric acid burns of the hand. *Plastic Reconstr Surg*. 1990;86:935-939.
18. Chu J, Su M, Bania TC, et al. Amiodarone improves survival in a murine model of fluoride toxicity. *Acad Emerg Med*. 2004;11:527b-528b.

19. Coffey JA, Brewer KL, Carroll R, et al. Limited efficacy of calcium and magnesium in a porcine model of hydrofluoric acid ingestion. *J Med Toxicol.* 2007;3:45-51.
20. Cordero SC, Goodhue WW, Splichal EM, et al. A fatality due to ingestion of hydrofluoric acid. *J Anal Toxicol.* 2004;28:211-213.
21. Cox RD, Osgood KA. Evaluation of intravenous magnesium sulfate for the treatment of hydrofluoric acid burns. *J Toxicol Clin Toxicol.* 1994;32: 123-136.
22. Cummings CC, McIvor ME. Fluoride-induced hyperkalemia—the role of calcium-dependent potassium channels. *Am J Emerg Med.* 1986;6:1-3.
23. Dibbell DG, Iverson RE, Jones W, et al. Hydrofluoric acid burns of the hand. *J Bone Joint Surg Am.* 1970;52:931-936.
24. Dowbak G, Rose K, Rohrich RJ. A biochemical and histological rationale for the treatment of hydrofluoric acid burns with calcium gluconate. *J Burn Care Rehabil.* 1994;15:323-327.
25. Dunn BJ, MacKinnon MA, Knowlden NF, et al. Hydrofluoric acid dermal burns—an assessment of treatment efficacy using an experimental pig model. *J Occup Med.* 1992;34:902-909.
26. Dünser MW, Öhlbauer M, Rider J, et al. Critical care management of major hydrofluoric acid burns: a case report, review of the literature, and recommendations for therapy. *Burns.* 2004;30:391-398.
27. El Saadi MS, Hall AH, Hall PK, et al. Hydrofluoric acid dermal exposure. *Vet Hum Toxicol.* 1989;31:243-247.
28. Greco RJ, Hartford CE, Haith LR, Patton ML. Hydrofluoric acid induced hypocalcemia. *J Trauma.* 1988;28:1593-1596.
29. Gutknecht J, Walter A. Hydrofluoric and nitric acid transport through lipid bilayer membranes. *Biochim Biophys Acta.* 1981;644:153-156.
30. Harris JC, Rumack BH, Bregman DJ. Comparative efficacy of injectable calcium and magnesium salts in the therapy of hydrofluoric acid burns. *Clin Toxicol.* 1981;18:1027-1032.
31. Hatzifotis M, Williams A, Muller M, Pegg S. Hydrofluoric acid burns. *Burns.* 2004;30:156-159.
32. Heard K, Delgado J. Oral decontamination with calcium or magnesium salts does not improve survival following hydrofluoric acid ingestion. *J Toxicol Clin Toxicol.* 2003;41:789-792.
33. Heard K, Hill RE, Cairns CB, et al. Calcium neutralizes fluoride bioavailability in a lethal model of fluoride poisoning. *J Toxicol Clin Toxicol.* 2001;39:349-53.
34. Henry JA, Hla KK. Intravenous regional calcium gluconate perfusion for hydrofluoric acid burns. *J Toxicol Clin Toxicol.* 1992;30: 203-207.
35. Höjer J, Personne M, Hultén P, et al. Topical treatments for hydrofluoric acid burns: a blind controlled experimental study. *J Toxicol Clin Toxicol.* 2002;40:861-866.
36. Holstege C, Baer A, Brady WJ. The electrocardiographic toxidrome: the ECG presentation of hydroflouric acid ingestion. *Am J Emerg Med.* 2005;23:171-176.
37. Huisman LC, Teijink JA, Overbosch EH, et al. An atypical chemical burn. *Lancet.* 2001 Nov 3;358(9292):1510.
38. Hultén P, Höjer J, Ludwigs U, et al. Hexafluorine vs. standard decontamination to reduce systemic toxicity after dermal exposure to hydrofluoric acid. *J Toxicol Clin Toxicol.* 2004;42:355-61.
39. Juncos LI, Donadio JV. Renal failure and fluorosis. *JAMA.* 1972;222:783-785.
40. Kao WF, Deng JF, Chiang SC, et al. A simple, safe, and efficient way to treat severe fluoride poisoning—oral calcium or magnesium. *J Toxicol Clin Toxicol.* 2004;42:33-40.
41. Kirkpatrick JJ, Burd DAR. An algorithmic approach to the treatment of hydrofluoric acid burns. *Burns.* 1995;21:495-499.
42. Kirkpatrick JJ, Enion DS, Burd DAR. Hydrofluoric acid burns: a review. *Burns.* 1995;21:483-493.
43. Klauder JV, Shelanski L, Gabriel K. Industrial uses of compounds of fluorine and oxalic acid. *Arch Environ Health.* 1955;12:412-419.
44. Kohnlein HE, Achinger R. A new method of treatment of the hydrofluoric acid burns of the extremities. *Chir Plast.* 1982;6:297-305.
45. Kohnlein HE, Merkle P, Springorum HW. Hydrogen fluoride burns: experiments and treatment. *Surg Forum.* 1973;24:50.
46. Kono K, Yoshida Y, Watanabe M, et al. An experimental study on the treatment of hydrofluoric acid burns. *Arch Environ Contam Toxicol.* 1992;22:414-418.
47. Kono K, Watanabe T, Dote T, et al. Successful treatments of lung injury and skin burn due to hydrofluoric acid exposure. *Int Arch Occup Environ Health.* 2000;73:S93-S97.
48. Kwok MC, Svancarek WP, Creer M. Fatality due to hydrofluoric acid exposure. *J Toxicol Clin Toxicol.* 1987;25:333-339.
49. Lee DC, Wiley JF, Snyder JW. Treatment of inhalational exposure to hydrofluoric acid with nebulized calcium gluconate. *J Occup Med.* 1993;35:470.
50. Leonard LG, Scheulen JJ, Munster AM. Chemical burns: effect of prompt first aid. *J Trauma.* 1982;22:420-423.
51. Lepke S, Paasow H. Effects of fluoride on potassium and sodium permeability of the erythrocyte membrane. *J Gen Physiol.* 1968;51: 365S-372S.
52. Lidbeck WL, Hill IB, Beeman JA. Acute sodium fluoride poisoning. *JAMA.* 1943;121:826-827.
53. MacKinnon MA. Hydrofluoric acid burns. *Dermatol Clin.* 1988;6:67-74.
54. MacKinnon MA. Treatment of hydrofluoric acid burns. *J Occup Med.* 1986;28:804.
55. Manoguerra AS, Neuman TS. Fatal poisoning from acute hydrofluoric acid ingestion. *Am J Emerg Med.* 1986;4:362-363.
56. Mathieu L, Nehles J, Blomet J, et al. Efficacy of hexafluorine for emergent decontamination of hydrofluoric acid eye and skin splashes. *Vet Hum Toxicol.* 2001;43:263-265.
57. Matsuno K. The treatment of hydrofluoric acid burns. *Occup Med* 1996;46:313-317.
58. Mayer L, Guelich J. Hydrogen fluoride (HF) inhalation and burns. *Arch Environ Health.* 1963;7:445-447.
59. Mayer TG, Gross PL. Fatal systemic fluorosis due to hydrofluoric acid burns. *Ann Emerg Med.* 1985;14:149-153.
60. McClure FJ. A review of fluorine and its physiologic effects. *Physiol Rev.* 1933;13:277-300.
61. McCulley JP, Whiting DW, Petitt MG, Lauber SE. Hydrofluoric acid burns of the eye. *J Occup Med.* 1983;25:447-450.
62. McIvor ME. Delayed fatal hyperkalemia in a patient with acute fluoride intoxication. *Ann Emerg Med.* 1987;16:1165-1167.
63. McIvor M, Baltazar RF, Beltran J, et al. Hyperkalemia and cardiac arrest from fluoride exposure during hemodialysis. *Am J Cardiol.* 1983; 51: 901-902.
64. McIvor ME, Cummings CC. *Sodium fluoride produces a K^+ efflux by increasing intracellular Ca^{2+} through Na^+-Ca^{2+} exchange. Toxicol Lett.* 1987;38(1-2):169-176.
65. McIvor ME, Cummings CE, Mower MM, et al. Sudden cardiac death from acute fluoride intoxication: the role of potassium. *Ann Emerg Med.* 1987;16:777-781.
66. Menchel SM, Dunn WA. Hydrofluoric acid poisoning. *Am J Forensic Med Pathol.* 1984;5:245-248.
67. Mullett T, Zoeller T, Bingham H, et al. Fatal hydrofluoric acid cutaneous exposure with refractory ventricular fibrillation. *J Burn Care Rehabil.* 1987;8:216-219.
68. Murao M. Studies on the treatment of hydrofluoric acid burn. *Bull Osaka Med Coll.* 1989;35:39-48.
69. Muriale L, Lee E, Genovese J, et al. Fatality due to acute fluoride poisoning following dermal contact with hydrofluoric acid in a palynology laboratory. *J Occup Med.* 1980;22:691-692.
70. Noonan T, Carter EJ, Edelman PA, Zawacki BE. Epidermal lipids and the natural history of hydrofluoric acid (HF) injury. *Burns.* 1994;20: 202-206.
71. O'Neil K. A fatal hydrogen fluoride exposure. *J Emerg Nurs.* 1994;20:451-453.
72. Paley A, Seifter J. Treatment of experimental hydrofluoric acid corrosion. *Proc Soc Exp Biol Med.* 1941;46:190-192.
73. Pegg SP, Siu S, Gillett G. Intra-arterial infusions in the treatment of hydrofluoric acid burns. *Burns.* 1985;11:440-443.
74. Proudfoot AT, Krenzelok EP, Vale JA. Position paper on urine alkalinization. *J Toxicol Clin Toxicol.* 2004;42:1-26.
75. Reynolds KE, Whitford GM, Pashley DH. Acute fluoride toxicity: the influence of acid-base status. *Toxicol Appl Pharmacol.* 1978;45:415-427.
76. Rose L. Further evaluation of hydrofluoric acid burns to the eye. *J Occup Med.* 1984;26:483.
77. Rubinfeld RS, Silbert DI, Arentsen JJ, Laibson PR. Ocular hydrofluoric acid burns. *Am J Ophthalmol.* 1992;114:420-423.
78. Rutan R, Rutan T, Deitch EA. Electricity and the treatment of hydrofluoric acid burns—the wave of the future or a jolt from the past? *Crit Care Med.* 2001;29:1646.
79. Ryan JM, McCarthy GM, Plunkett PJ. Regional intravenous calcium—an effective method of treating hydrofluoric acid burns to limb peripheries. *J Accid Emerg Med.* 1997;14:401-402.
80. Sadove R, Hainsworth D, Van Meter W. Total body immersion in hydrofluoric acid. *South Med J.* 1990;83:698-700.

81. Sheridan RL, Ryan CM, Quinby WC Jr, et al. Emergency management of major hydrofluoric acid exposures. *Burns*. 1995;21:62-64.
82. Siegel DC, Heard J. Intra-arterial calcium infusion for hydrofluoric acid burns. *Aviat Space Environ Med*. 1992;63:206-211.
83. Soderberg K, Kuusinen P, Mathieu L, et al. An improved method for emergent decontamination of ocular and dermal hydrofluoric acid splashes. *Vet Hum Toxicol*. 2004;46:216-218.
84. Stremski ES, Grande GA, Ling LJ. Survival following hydrofluoric acid ingestion. *Ann Emerg Med*. 1992;21:1396-1399.
85. Su M, Chu J, Howland MA, et al. Amiodarone attenuates fluoride-induced hyperkalemia in vitro. *Acad Emerg Med*. 2003;10:105-109.
86. Takase I, Kono K, Tamura A, et al. Fatality due to acute fluoride poisoning in the workplace. *Leg Med (Tokyo)*. 2004;6:197-200.
87. Tepperman PB. Fatality due to acute systemic fluoride poisoning following a hydrofluoric acid skin burn. *J Occup Med*. 1980;22:691-692.
88. Thomas D, Jaeger U, Sagoschen I, et al. Intra-arterial calcium gluconate treatment after hydrofluoric acid burn of the hand. Cardiovasc Intervent *Radiol*. 2009;32:155-158.
89. Trevino MA, Hermann GH, Sprout WL. Treatment of severe hydrofluoric acid exposures. *J Occup Med*. 1983;25:861-863.
90. Upfal M, Doyle C. Medical management of hydrofluoric acid exposure. *J Occup Med*. 1990;32:727-731.
91. Upton J, Mulliken JB, Murray JE. Major intravenous extravasation injuries. *Am J Surg*. 1979;137:497-506.
92. Vance MV, Curry SC, Kunkel DB, et al. Digital hydrofluoric acid burns: treatment with intraarterial calcium infusion. *Ann Emerg Med*. 1986;15:890-896.
93. Velvart J. Arterial perfusion for hydrofluoric acid burns. *Hum Toxicol*. 1983;2:233-238.
94. Williams JM, Hammad A, Cottington EC, Harchelroad FC. Intravenous magnesium in the treatment of hydrofluoric acid burns in rats. *Ann Emerg Med*. 1994;23:464-469.
95. Wing JS, Sanderson LM, Brender JD, et al. Acute health effects in a community after a release of hydrofluoric acid. *Arch Environ Health*. 1991;46:155-159.
96. Wormser U, Sintov A, Brodsky B, et al. Protective effect of topical iodine preparations upon head-induced and hydrofluoric acid-induced skin lesions. *Toxicol Pathol*. 2002;30:552-558.
97. Yamashita M, Yamashita M, Suzuki M, et al. Iontophoretic delivery of calcium for experimental hydrofluoric acid burns. *Crit Care Med*. 2001;29:1575-1578.
98. Yamaura K, Kao B, Iimori E, et al. Recurrent ventricular tachyarrhythmias associated with QT prolongation following hydrofluoric acid burns. *J Toxicol Clin Toxicol*. 1997;35:311-313.
99. Yan F, Ruan S, Li Y. An experimental study of myocardial injury by hydrofluoric acid in burned rabbits. *Zhonghua Shao Shang Za Zhi*. 2000;16:237-240.
100. Yolken R, Konecny P, McCarthy P. Acute fluoride poisoning. *Pediatrics*. 1976;58:90-93.
101. Yosowitz P, Ekland DA, Shah RC, Parsons RW. Peripheral intravenous infiltration necrosis. *Ann Surg*. 1975;182:553-556.

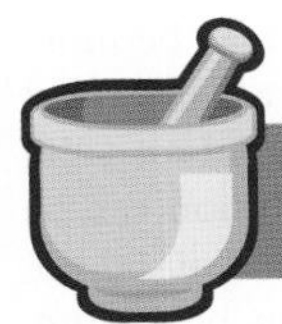

ANTIDOTES IN DEPTH (A30)

CALCIUM

Mary Ann Howland

Calcium is essential to maintaining the normal function of the heart, vascular smooth muscle, skeletal system, and nervous system. It is vital in enzymatic reactions, in neurohormonal transmission, and in the maintenance of cellular integrity.[25] The endocrine system maintains calcium homeostasis. Approximately half of the total serum calcium is ionized and active, and the remainder is primarily bound to albumin. Hypercalcemia raises the threshold for nerve and muscle excitation, resulting in muscle weakness, lethargy, cardiac conduction disturbances and coma.[25] Hypocalcemia can result in hyperreflexia, muscle spasms, tetany, and seizures (Chap. 16).[25]

CALCIUM CHANNEL BLOCKERS

Although calcium enters cells in numerous ways, only one of these, the voltage-dependent L-type channels in cardiac and smooth muscles, is inhibited by the calcium channel blockers (CCBs) available in the United States.[5,71] Calcium channel blocker overdoses (Chap. 60) may result in nausea, vomiting, hypotension, bradycardia, myocardial depression, sinus arrest, atrioventricular (AV) block, and metabolic acidosis with hyperglycemia, shock, pulmonary edema, altered mental status, and seizures.[58] Because CCBs do not alter either receptor-operated channels or the release of calcium from intracellular stores,[76] the serum calcium concentration remains normal in CCB overdose.

Intravenous (IV) administration of calcium to dogs poisoned with verapamil or diltiazem improves cardiac output secondary to increased inotropy.[29] The heart rate and cardiac conduction are affected minimally, if at all.[26,29,65] Case reports and reviews of the literature suggest similar findings in humans.[2,3,13,20,24,30,33,38,47,61,62,73]

Calcium should be administered to symptomatic patients with CCB overdoses.[34,43,46] Unfortunately, the most seriously ill patients respond inadequately, and other measures are often required. The dose of calcium needed to treat patients with CCB overdose is unknown. In animal experiments, there appears to be a dose-related improvement.[13,29] Since calcium chloride is extremely irritating to small vessels, subcutaneous tissue and muscle and may cause necrosis following extravasation, it is usually only administered through a central venous line. The customary approach is to administer an initial IV dose of 3 g of calcium gluconate (30 mL of 10% calcium gluconate) or 1 g of calcium chloride (10 mL of 10% calcium chloride) to adults.[58] Based on case reports, this dose may need to be repeated as clinically indicated. The hypothesis is that sufficient calcium must be present to compete with the CCB for binding to the L-type calcium channel. One author used a total of 10 g of calcium gluconate as 1 g boluses over 12 minutes after diltiazem-induced asystole and another 2.5 g of calcium gluconate minutes later for a second asystolic event, with a resultant serum calcium concentration of 3.36 mmol/L (normal: 2.2–2.6 mmol/L) about 1 hour after administration of the calcium gluconate.[36] Several authors have successfully treated patients with a total of 18 to 30 g of calcium gluconate or 13 g of calcium chloride over 2 to 12 hours, either by intermittent bolus dose or infusion, without apparent adverse effects.[13,34,35,43,46,47] Following the use of large doses of calcium, hypercalcemia can occur and is associated with severe consequences including myocardial depression and intense vasoconstriction leading to multiorgan ischemia.[70] Introduction of hyperinsulinemia euglycemia (see Antidotes in Depth A18: Insulin Euglycemia Therapy and A21: Intravenous Fat Emulsion) in the treatment of CCBs has diminished the need for excessive doses of calcium. This approach should be limited, and if used, meticulous monitoring of ionized calcium and blood glucose is advised to avoid hypercalcemia and hypoglycemia.

The administration of calcium to a patient with toxicity from cardioactive steroids such as digoxin could prove quite harmful.[28,81] In the event of concurrent overdose with both a cardioactive steroid and a CCB, the early use of digoxin-specific antibody fragments (A-20) should enable the subsequent safe use of calcium (see Chap. 64).

Therapy in children is based on even more limited data. The current pediatric guidelines of the American Heart Association[1] suggest an initial dose of 20 mg/kg of 10% calcium chloride (0.2 mL/kg) up to the adult dose. This is infused over 5 to 10 minutes, preferably into a central venous line. If a beneficial effect is observed an infusion of 20 to 50 mg/kg/h should follow. These guidelines preferentially suggest calcium chloride based on one study that compared the chloride to the gluconate salt in critically ill children with hypocalcemia.[12] However, since $CaCl_2$ may be irritating, calcium gluconate may be preferable, especially if central venous access is unavailable. A starting dose in children should be about 60 mg/kg of 10% calcium gluconate (0.6 mL/kg) titrating to the adult dose if needed.

β-ADRENERGIC ANTAGONISTS

In vitro studies suggest that the negative inotropic action of β-adrenergic antagonists are related to interference with both the forward and reverse transport of calcium in the sarcoplasmic reticulum and the inhibition of microsomal and mitochondrial calcium uptake (Chap. 61).[21,44,55] In a canine model of propranolol poisoning, the administration of calcium chloride improved mean arterial pressure, maximal left ventricular pressure change over time, and peripheral vascular resistance, but had no significant effect on bradycardia or QRS complex prolongation.[45] Several case reports attest to the beneficial effects of IV calcium in β-adrenergic antagonist overdose.[11,37,60,67] Because distinguishing an overdose of a CCB from that of a β-adrenergic antagonist may be difficult and the two may be taken simultaneously, a trial of IV calcium is appropriate for a presumed β-adrenergic antagonist overdose if cardioactive steroid toxicity which can produce similar effects can be excluded.

HYPOCALCEMIA SECONDARY TO ETHYLENE GLYCOL

Following ethylene glycol poisoning (Chap. 107) metabolism of the parent molecule generates oxalic acid, which complexes with calcium and subsequently precipitates in the kidneys, brain, and elsewhere, resulting in hypocalcemia.[2,35,57,71,74] After exposure to ethylene glycol, the ionized calcium concentration should always be monitored along with repeated examinations for such signs of hypocalcemia as prolongation of the QT interval on the electrocardiogram (ECG), hyperreflexia, muscle spasms, tetany, and seizures (Chap. 16). Intravenous calcium should be administered in the customary recommended doses (as above) to patients with these findings.

HYPOCALCEMIA SECONDARY TO HYDROFLUORIC ACID AND FLUORIDE-RELEASING XENOBIOTICS

Deaths from hypocalcemia secondary to dermal, gastrointestinal, and pulmonary hydrofluoric acid (HF) exposures are documented in the literature.[15,27,80] Any body contact with HF (Chap. 105) can result in severe burns and death, depending on concentration, area exposed, and duration of exposure. The pathophysiologic derangements noted result from (1) release of free hydrogen ions; (2) complexation of fluoride with calcium and magnesium to form insoluble salts, which causes cellular necrosis; (3) liberation of potassium ions; and (4) cellular dehydration.[8,9,14,23,48,50,52,77] Soluble salts of fluoride and bifluoride (eg, sodium, potassium, and ammonium) have all of the toxicity associated with HF and should be managed accordingly. Following HF exposure, the gluconate salt of calcium is used topically and subcutaneously to manage minor to moderate cutaneous burns, intravenously to treat systemic hypocalcemia, and intraarterially to manage significant burns.[2,8,9,14–16,19,23,27,48,50,54,59,64,66,69,77–79,84] Experimental studies demonstrate that when concentrated HF burns are immediately flushed with water and then treated with topical calcium there is a significant reduction in burn size.[10,77] A randomized clinical trial comparing the dimethyl sulfoxide (DMSO)/calcium gluconate combination to calcium gluconate alone is currently under way.[31] Although a DMSO preparation is not commercially available, a 2.5% calcium gluconate topical gel is marketed. In the event that the commercial preparation is inaccessible, a topical calcium gel can be prepared from calcium carbonate tablets, calcium gluconate powder or solution, and a water-soluble jelly such as K-Y Jelly® (mix 3.5 g calcium gluconate powder or 25 mL of calcium gluconate 10% solution or 10 g of calcium carbonate tablets with 5 ounces of K-Y Jelly®). An experimental study in rats demonstrated that iontophoretic delivery of calcium chloride appeared to enhance the delivery of calcium and to significantly reduce the burn area if applied within 30 minutes and may be a promising modality in the future.[65,83]

The chloride salt is also acceptable for topical therapy. However, calcium chloride should *never* be injected into tissues (subcutaneously, intramuscularly) since severe tissue necrosis can result.

In patients with severe topical HF exposures, aggressive administration of regional IV calcium using a Bier block technique (10 mL of 10% calcium gluconate plus heparin 5000 units in a total volume of 40 mL) or intraarterial calcium (10 mL of 10% calcium gluconate in 50 mL of 0.9% sodium chloride solution over 4 hours) may be required, along with frequent serum calcium determinations to titrate the dose.[31] One patient who was massively exposed to HF required a total of 267 mEq of calcium infused over a 24 hour period.[27]

In patients with life-threatening poisoning and particularly HF inhalation simultaneous administration of IV, oral, and nebulized 2.5% calcium gluconate can also be given to facilitate the availability of the maximum amount of calcium. To prepare nebulized calcium gluconate, mix 1.5 mL of 10% calcium gluconate solution with 4.5 mL of sterile water or saline to make a 2.5% solution. For moderate to severe burns (generally from HF concentrations greater than 10%) of the fingers and hands, an intraarterial calcium infusion may be more effective than local or IV therapy, although it is more invasive[59,69,75,78,79] and more hazardous.[69] A calcium gluconate solution (10 mL of 10%) mixed in 40 to 50 mL of 5% dextrose or 0.9% NaCl solution can be infused intraarterially over 4 hours followed by subsequent 40-50 mL infusions after 4 hours when pain persists.[78] Serum calcium, potassium, and serum magnesium concentrations should be carefully monitored in all severely poisoned patients.

HYPOCALCEMIA SECONDARY TO PHOSPHATES

Inappropriate use of oral and rectal phosphates as a laxative can result in hypocalcemia, hyperphosphatemia, and hyperkalemia with resultant morbidity and mortality.[4] Intravenous calcium may be needed for life-threatening hypocalcemia. However, since administration of calcium in the presence of hyperphosphatemia risks precipitation of calcium phosphate throughout the body, hemodialysis and other therapies should be considered in non–life-threatening cases.

HYPERMAGNESEMIA

Hypermagnesemia causes both direct and indirect depression of skeletal muscle, resulting in neuromuscular blockade, loss of reflexes, and profound muscular paralysis (Chap. 16).[42,53] Excess magnesium also causes prolongation of the PR interval and QRS complex on ECG, and depression of the sinoatrial (SA) node, leading to a bradycardic arrest. Intravenous calcium serves as a physiologic antagonist to these effects of magnesium (Table A30–1).

HYPERKALEMIA

Hyperkalemia causes significant myocardial depression. The resultant ECG changes are well defined: the height of the T wave increases and lengthening of the PR interval and QRS complex occur; ultimately, a sine wave pattern leading to cardiac arrest may occur if treatment is not initiated (Chaps. 16 and 22).[25] Calcium makes the membrane threshold potential less negative so that a larger stimulus is required to depolarize the cell. This stabilization antagonizes the hyperexcitability caused by modest hyperkalemia. However, when severe hyperkalemia exists, voltage-gated sodium channels are inactivated and cannot be depolarized, regardless of the strength of the impulse. Calcium may transform the voltage sensor of the sodium channel from inactive to closed, thus allowing the sodium channel to be opened with depolarization.[32] If hyperkalemia is secondary to the toxic effects of cardioactive steroids on the Na^+-K^+-adenosine triphosphatase (ATPase) pump, IV calcium can potentially exacerbate an already excessive intracellular calcium concentration, making IV calcium potentially harmful (see Chap. 64).[25]

BLACK WIDOW SPIDER ENVENOMATION (HISTORIC INDICATION)

Envenomation by the black widow spider (*Latrodectus* spp) (Chap. 119) leads to local and systemic symptoms. Most commonly, severe abdominal or back pain begins within several hours of envenomation.[17] The venom exerts its effects by opening sodium channels leading to calcium influx; the release of synaptic transmitters, including norepinephrine and acetylcholine, are believed to be involved.[63] Analgesics, benzodiazepines,

TABLE A30–1. Calcium Salts for Intravenous Use

	Calcium Gluconate[a]	Calcium Chloride ($CaCl_2$)[a,b]
10% Solution	10 mL = 1 g of Ca^{2+} gluconate 10 mL = 4.5 mEq elemental Ca^{2+}	10 mL = 1 g of $CaCl_2$ 10 mL = 13.6 mEq elemental Ca^{2+}
Adult dose	3 g (30 mL of 10% solution) over 10 min (unless in extremis–deliver over 30-60 sec) Repeat every several minutes as necessary[a]	1 g (10 mL of 10% solution) over 10 min (unless in extremis–deliver over 30-60 sec)[b] Repeat every several minutes as necessary[a]
Pediatric dose (not to exceed the adult dose)	60 mg/kg (0.6 mL/kg) of 10% solution infused over 5-10 minutes (unless in extremis–deliver over 30-60 sec)[b] Repeat every several minutes as necessary[b]	20 mg/kg (0.2 mL/kg) infused over 5-10 minutes (unless in extremis–deliver over 30-60 sec)[b] Repeat every several minutes as necessary[b]

[a] Monitor calcium after several doses and every 30 minutes during administration.

[b] Use of a central venous line is recommended to avoid extravasation.

and muscle relaxants are used to successfully relieve the pain and muscle spasms.[17,22,39,68] Rarely, antivenom may be indicated.

Intravenous calcium was previously recommended.[17,39] Animal studies suggested that the venom induces changes in the permeability of calcium that may be overcome by increasing the extracellular concentration of calcium.[40,56] In support, one prospective study noted improvement in six of 13 patients treated with calcium gluconate.[39] However, a large retrospective study of 163 patients cast doubt on the effectiveness of calcium.[17] Very few patients had adequate pain relief from calcium, and all but one patient also required opioids.[17] As a result, there is no longer a role for calcium in the management of black widow spider envenomation (see Chap. 119).

SAFETY ISSUES AND CALCIUM PREPARATIONS

Severe hypercalcemia is defined by a serum calcium concentration greater than 3.5 mmol/L (14.0 mg/dL) in a patient with a normal albumin concentration. The adverse effects of hypercalcemia (independent of the rate of administration) include nausea, vomiting, constipation, ileus, hypertension if intravascular volume is adequate, polyuria, polydipsia, cognitive difficulties, hyporeflexia, coma, and enhanced sensitivity to cardioactive steroids.[6] Significant hypercalcemia may lead to myocardial depression. The symptoms exhibited depend on the patient's age, rate of increase in the serum calcium concentration, and duration of the hypercalcemia.[6]

A variety of calcium salts are available for parenteral administration. The two most commonly used are calcium chloride and calcium gluconate (see Table A30-1). Neither salt should be combined and administered intravenously with sodium bicarbonate because calcium carbonate, a precipitate, is formed. Calcium chloride is an acidifying salt and is extremely irritating to tissue. It should *never* be given intramuscularly, subcutaneously, or perivascularly.[25,51] Calcium gluconate is less irritating, but care should also be taken to avoid extravasation. The best reason for choosing calcium gluconate in almost all clinical situations is that the tissue risk is far less. If extravasation should occur, subcutaneous injection of aliquots of hyaluronidase can be injected around the site (see Special Considerations SC3–Extravasation of xenobiotics). Equivalent molar doses of calcium found in calcium chloride (1 g $CaCl_2$ 10%) and calcium gluconate (3 g Ca gluconate 10%) produce similar serum ionized calcium concentrations, with peaks occurring within 30 seconds and accompanied by hemodynamic improvement.[49] These results support the idea that simple dissociation of calcium from gluconate is responsible for releasing calcium, rather than hepatic metabolism. Earlier evidence has been challenged that suggested that infusions of IV calcium chloride in hypocalcemic children[12] produce slightly larger increases in ionic calcium than infusions of calcium gluconate.[49,82] Intravenous calcium must be administered slowly, at a rate not exceeding 0.7 to 1.8 mEq/min or one 10-mL vial of calcium chloride or three 10 mL vials of calcium gluconate over 10 minutes in adults unless the patient is severely hypocalcemic. More rapid administration may lead to vasodilation, hypotension, bradycardia, dysrhythmias, syncope, and cardiac arrest.[7,18,41,51,72]

In cases of extreme life-threatening hypocalcemia or for a patient in extremis, a slow IV push may be required.

SUMMARY

Intravenous calcium infusion is an effective antidote for the hypocalcemia induced by either ethylene glycol, HF and fluoride–releasing xenobiotics. It serves as a physiologic antagonist to the cardiac and/or neurologic effects of hypermagnesemia and hyperkalemia and counteracts the effects of CCB overdoses. It may have some benefit in the treatment of β-adrenergic antagonist overdoses. Great care must be taken to avoid extravasation as calcium chloride in particular can cause tissue necrosis. Equivalent molar calcium doses found in appropriate volumes of calcium gluconate and calcium chloride deliver equal amounts of ionized calcium. Electrocardiographic monitoring and frequent ionized calcium concentration measurements are required to prevent iatrogenic toxicity. Although most clinical experience involves IV use, advances in intraarterial, topical, inhalational, and intraosseous calcium therapy may offer unique potential advantages.

REFERENCES

1. American Heart Association in collaboration with the International Liaison Committee on Resuscitation 2005. Guidelines for cardiopulmonary resuscitation and emergency cardiovascular care. Part 10: pediatric advanced life support. *Circulation.* 2005;112[Suppl I]:IV167-IV187.
2. Anderson WJ, Anderson JR. Hydrofluoric acid burns of the hand: mechanism of injury and treatment. *Am J Hand Surg.* 1988;13:52-57.

3. Ashraf M, Chaudry K, Nelson J, et al. Massive overdose of sustained release verapamil: a case report and review of the literature. *Am J Med Sci.* 1995;310:258-263.
4. Azzam I, Kovalev Y, Storch S, Elias N. Life threatening hyperphosphataemia after administration of sodium phosphate in preparation for colonoscopy. *Postgrad Med J.* 2004;80:487-488.
5. Bean BP. Classes of calcium channels in vertebrate cells. *Annu Rev Physiol.* 1989;51:367-384.
6. Belezekian JP. Management of acute hypercalcemia. *N Engl J Med.* 1992;326:1196-1215.
7. Berliner K. The effect of calcium injections on the human heart. *Am J Med Sci.* 1936;191:117-121.
8. Bertolini JC. Hydrofluoric acid: a review of toxicity. *J Emerg Med.* 1992;10:163-168.
9. Boink AB, Wemer J, Meulenbelt J, et al. The mechanism of fluoride-induced hypocalcemia. *Hum Exp Toxicol.* 1994;13:149-155.
10. Bracken WM, Cuppage F, McLaury RL, et al. Comparative effectiveness of topical treatments for hydrofluoric acid burns. *J Occup Med.* 1985;27:733-739.
11. Briacombe JR, Scully M, Swainston R. Propranolol overdose. A dramatic response to calcium chloride. *Med J Aust.* 1991;155:267-268.
12. Broner CW, Stidham GL, Westenkirchner DF, Watson DC. A prospective, randomized, double-blind comparison of calcium chloride and calcium gluconate therapies for hypocalcemia in critically ill children. *J Pediatr.* 1990;117:986-989.
13. Buckley N, Dawson AH, Howarth D, Whyte IM. Slow-release verapamil poisoning. *Med J Aust.* 1993;158:202-204.
14. Caravati EM. Acute hydrofluoric acid exposure. *Am J Emerg Med.* 1988;6:143-150.
15. Chan KM, Svancarek WP, Creer M. Fatality due to acute hydrofluoric acid exposure. *J Toxicol Clin Toxicol.* 1987;25:333-339.
16. Chick LR, Borah G. Calcium carbonate gel therapy of hydrofluoric acid burns of the hand. *Plast Reconstr Surg.* 1990;86:935-940.
17. Clark RF, Wethern-Kestner S, Vance MV, Gerkin R. Clinical presentation and treatment of black widow spider envenomation: a review of 163 cases. *Ann Emerg Med.* 1992;21:782-787.
18. Clarke NE. The action of calcium on the human electrocardiogram. *Am Heart J.* 1941;22:367-373.
19. Conway EE, Sockolow R. Hydrofluoric acid burn in a child. *Pediatr Emerg Care.* 1991;7:345-347.
20. DeWitt C, Waksman J. Pharmacology, pathophysiology and management of calcium channel blocker and beta blocker toxicity. *Toxicol Rev.* 2004;23:223-238.
21. Dhalla NS, Lee SL. Comparison of the actions of acebutolol, practolol, and propranolol on calcium transport by heart microsomes and mitochondria. *Br J Pharmacol.* 1976;57:215-221.
22. Diaz J, Leblanc K. Common spider bites. *Am Fam Physician.* 2007;75: 869-873.
23. Edinburg M, Swift R. Hydrofluoric acid burns of the hands: a case report and suggested management. *Aust N Z J Surg.* 1989;59:88-91.
24. Erickson F, Ling L, Grande G, et al. Diltiazem overdose? Case report and review. *J Emerg Med.* 1991;9:357-366.
25. Friedman P. Agents affecting mineral ion homeostasis and bone turnover. In: Brunton L, ed. *Goodman and Gilman's the Pharmacologic Basis of Therapeutics*, 11th ed. New York: McGraw-Hill; 2006:1647-1678.
26. Gay R, Algeo S, Lee R, et al. Treatment of verapamil toxicity in intact dogs. *J Clin Invest.* 1986;77:1805-1811.
27. Greco RJ, Hartford CE, Haith LR, Patton ML. Hydrofluoric acid-induced hypocalcemia. *J Trauma.* 1988;28:1593-1596.
28. Hack J, Woody J, Lewis D, et al. The effect of calcium chloride in treating hyperkalemia due to acute digoxin toxicity in a porcine model. *J Toxicol Clin Toxicol.* 2004;42:337-342.
29. Hariman RJ, Mangiardi LM, McAllister RG, et al. Reversal of the cardiovascular effects of verapamil by calcium and sodium: differences between electrophysiologic and hemodynamic responses. *Circulation.* 1979;59:797-804.
30. Harris NS. Case 24-2006. A 40-year-old woman with hypotension after an overdose of amlodipine. *N Engl J Med.* 2006;355:602-611.
31. Hatzifotis M, Williams A, Muller M, Pegg S. Hydrofluoric acid burns. *Burns.* 2004;30:156-159.
32. Hille B. *Ionic Channels of Excitable Membranes.* Sunderland, MA: Sinauer Associates; 1984.
33. Hofer CA, Smith JK, Tenholder MF. Verapamil intoxication: a literature review of overdoses and discussion of therapeutic options. *Am J Med.* 1993;95:431-438.
34. Hung Y, Olsen K. Acute amlodipine overdose treated by high dose intravenous calcium in a patient with severe renal insufficiency. *Clin Toxicol.* 2007;45:301-303.
35. Introna F Jr, Smialek JE. Antifreeze (ethylene glycol) intoxications in Baltimore: report of six cases. *Acta Morphol Hung.* 1989;37:245-263.
36. Isbister GK. Delayed asystolic cardiac arrest after diltiazem overdose: resuscitation with high dose intravenous calcium. *Emerg Med J.* 2002;19:355-357.
37. Jones JL. Metoprolol overdose. *Ann Emerg Med.* 1982;11:114-115.
38. Kerns W. Management of β-adrenergic blocker and calcium channel antagonist toxicity. *Emerg Med Clinics NA.* 2007;25:309-331.
39. Key GF. A comparison of calcium gluconate and methocarbamol (Robaxin) in the treatment of latrodectism (black widow spider envenomations). *Am J Trop Med Hyg.* 1981;30:273-277.
40. Kobernick M. Black widow spider bites. *Am Fam Physician.* 1984;29: 241-245.
41. Kuhn M. Severe bradyarrhythmias following calcium pretreatment. *Am Heart J.* 1991;121:1812-1813.
42. Kutsal E, Aydemir C, Eldes N. Severe hypermagnesemia as a result of excessive cathartic ingestion in a child without renal failure. *Pediatr Emerg Care.* 2007;23:570-572.
43. Lam YM, Tse HF, Lau CP. Continuous calcium chloride infusion for massive nifedipine overdose. *Chest.* 2001;119:1280-1282.
44. Langemeijer J, de Wildt D, de Groot G, Sangster B. Calcium interferes with the cardiodepressive effects of beta-blocker overdose in isolated rat hearts. *J Toxicol Clin Toxicol.* 1986;24:111-133.
45. Love J, Hanfling D, Howell J. Hemodynamic effects of calcium chloride in a canine model of acute propranolol intoxication. *Ann Emerg Med.* 1996;28:1-6.
46. Luscher TF, Noll G, Sturmer T, et al. Calcium gluconate in severe verapamil intoxication. *N Engl J Med.* 1994;330:718-719.
47. MacDonald D, Alguire P. Case reports: fatal overdose with sustained release verapamil. *Am J Med Sci.* 1992;303:115-117.
48. MacKinnon MA. Hydrofluoric acid burns. *Dermatol Clin.* 1988;6:67-74.
49. Martin T, Kang Y, Robertson K, et al. Ionization and hemodynamic effects of calcium chloride and calcium gluconate in the absence of hepatic function. *Anesthesiology.* 1990;73:62-65.
50. McCulley JP. Ocular hydrofluoric acid burns: animal model, mechanism of injury and therapy. *Am Ophthalmol Soc.* 1990;88:649-683.
51. McEvoy G, ed. *Calcium AHFS Drug Information.* Bethesda, MD: American Society of Health-System Pharmacists Inc; 2008:2722-2727.
52. Mistry DG, Wainwright DJ. Hydrofluoric acid burns. *Am Fam Physician.* 1992;45:1748-1754.
53. Moe S. Disorders of calcium, phosphorous and magnesium. *Prim Care Clin Office Pract.* 2008;35:215-237.
54. Nguyen LT, Mohr WJ 3rd, Ahrenholz DH, Solem LD. Treatment of hydrofluoric acid burn to the face by carotid artery infusion of calcium gluconate. *J Burn Care Rehabil.* 2004;25:421-424.
55. Noack E, Kurzmack M, Verjovski-Almeida S, Inesi G. The effect of propranolol and its analogs on Ca^{2+} transport by sarcoplasmic reticulum vesicles. *J Pharmacol Exp Ther.* 1978;206:281-288.
56. Pardel JF. Influence of calcium on ^{3}H-noradrenaline release by *Lactrodectus* venom gland extract on arterial tissue of the rat. *Toxicon.* 1979;17:455-465.
57. Parry MF, Wallach R. Ethylene glycol poisoning. *Am J Med.* 1974;57:143-150.
58. Pearigen PD, Benowitz NS. Poisoning due to calcium antagonists: experience with verapamil, diltiazem and nifedipine. *Drug Saf.* 1991;6:408-430.
59. Pegg SP, Siu S, Gillet G. Intra-arterial infusions in the treatment of hydrofluoric acid burns. *Burns.* 1985;11:440-443.
60. Pertoldi F, D'Orlando L, Mercanto W. Electromechanical dissociation 48 hours after atenolol overdose. Usefulness of calcium chloride. *Ann Emerg Med.* 1998;31:777-781.
61. Proano L, Chiang WK, Wang RY. Calcium channel blocker overdose. *Am J Emerg Med.* 1995;13:444-450.
62. Ramoska EA, Spiller HA, Winter M, Borys D. A one-year evaluation of calcium channel blocker overdoses: toxicity and treatment. *Ann Emerg Med.* 1993;22:196-200.
63. Rauber A. Black widow spider bites. *J Toxicol Clin Toxicol.* 1983-1984;21: 473-485.
64. Roberts JR, Merigian KS. Acute hydrofluoric acid exposure. *Am J Emerg Med.* 1989;7:125-126.
65. Rutan R, Rutan T. Electricity and the treatment of hydrofluoric acid burns—the wave of the future or a jolt from the past? *Crit Care Med.* 2001;29:1646-1647.

66. Sadove R, Hainsworth D, Van Meter W. Total body immersion in hydrofluoric acid. *South Med J.* 1990;83:698-700.
67. Sangster B, de Wildt D, van Dijk A. A case of acebutolol intoxication. *J Toxicol Clin Toxicol.* 1983;20:69-77.
68. Saucier J. Arachnid envenomation. *Emerg Clinics NA.* 2004;22:405-422.
69. Siegel DC, Heard JM. Intra-arterial calcium infusion for hydrofluoric acid burns. *Aviat Space Environ Med.* 1992;63:206-211.
70. Sim M, Stevenson F. A fatal case of iatrogenic hypercalcemia after calcium channel blocker overdose. *J Med Tox.* 2008;4:25-29.
71. Simpson E. Some aspects of calcium metabolism in a fatal case of ethylene glycol poisoning. *Ann Clin Biochem.* 1985;22:90-93.
72. Smallwood RA. Some effects of the intravenous administration of calcium in man. *Aust Acad Med.* 1967;16:126-131.
73. Spiller HA, Meyers A, Ziemba T, Riley M. Delayed onset of cardiac arrhythmias from sustained release verapamil. *Ann Emerg Med.* 1991;20:201-203.
74. Tarr BD, Winters LJ, Moore MP, et al. Low dose ethanol in the treatment of ethylene glycol poisoning. *J Vet Pharmacol Ther.* 1985;8:254-262.
75. Thomas D, Jaeger U, Sagoschen I, et al. Intra-arterial calcium gluconate treatment after hydrofluoric acid burn of the hand. *Cardiovasc Intervent Radiol.* 2009;32:155-158.
76. Triggle DJ. Calcium-channel antagonists: mechanisms of action, vascular selectivities, and clinical relevance. *Cleve Clin J Med.* 1992;59:617-626.
77. Upfal M, Doyle C. Medical management of hydrofluoric acid exposure. *J Occup Med.* 1990;32:726-731.
78. Vance MV, Curry SC, Kunkel DB, et al. Digital hydrofluoric acid burns: treatment with intraarterial calcium infusion. *Ann Emerg Med.* 1986;15:890-896.
79. Velvart J. Arterial perfusion for hydrofluoric acid burns. *Hum Toxicol.* 1983;2:233-238.
80. Vohra R, Velez L, Rivera W, et al. Recurrent life-threatening ventricular dysrhythmias associated with acute hydrofluoric acid ingestion: observations in one case and implications for mechanism of toxicity. *Clin Toxicol.* 2008;46:79-84.
81. Wagner J, Salzer WW. Calcium-dependent toxic effects of digoxin in isolated preparations. *Arch Int Pharmacodyn.* 1976;223:4-14.
82. White RD, Goldsmith RS, Rodriquez R, et al. Plasma ionic calcium levels following injection of chloride, gluconate, and gluceptate salts of calcium. *J Thorac Cardiovasc Surg.* 1976;71:609-613.
83. Yamashita M, Yamashita M, Suzuki M, et al. Iontophoretic delivery of calcium for experimental hydrofluoric acid burns. *Crit Care Med.* 2001;29:1575-1578.
84. Zachary LS, Reus W, Gottlieb J, et al. Treatment of experimental hydrofluoric acid burns. *J Burn Care.* 1986;7:35-39.

CHAPTER 106
HYDROCARBONS

David D. Gummin

Our present world could not exist without hydrocarbons. Nearly everything we touch today is either comprised of or coated with hydrocarbon products. In the practice of clinical toxicology, initial efforts usually entail precisely determining the specific xenobiotics that might be involved in a specific exposure, followed by defining the type and extent of the exposure. In this regard, hydrocarbon exposures are always clinically challenging. Despite significant chemical diversity, most classification schemes group hydrocarbons by specific uses or applications, rather than by chemical structure or physiologic properties. Most hydrocarbons in everyday use, such as gasoline, charcoal starter, and lamp oil, are actually mixtures of chemicals obtained from a common distillation fraction. The chemical diversity within a mixture makes it challenging to try to assess individual contribution to toxicity. As a result, generalities are often needed to describe the behavior of these complex mixtures. This chapter focuses primarily on toxicity of hydrocarbons present in such mixtures. Individual hydrocarbons are addressed only when they are commonly available in purified form, or when individual xenobiotics present unique toxicologic concerns.

HISTORY AND EPIDEMIOLOGY

Organic chemistry originated in the industrial revolution and evolved largely because of advances in coal tar technology. Coal liberates hydrocarbons in the coking process, when bituminous (soft) coal is heated to remove coal gas. The gas is then separated into a variety of natural gases. The viscous residue from the heating process forms coal tar, which can be further distilled into kerosene and other hydrocarbon mixtures.

Over the years, crude oil has replaced coal tar as the most common source for distillation of organic compounds. Crude oil distillation involves heating the oil to fixed temperatures in large-scale processors that separate hydrocarbons into fractions by vapor (boiling) point. Because of the relationship between boiling point and molecular weight, distillation roughly divides hydrocarbons into like-sized molecules. The most volatile fractions come off early, as gases. These are used primarily as heating fuels. The least volatile fractions (larger than about 10 carbons) are used chiefly for lubricants or as paraffins, petroleum jelly, or asphalt. The remaining volatile distillation fractions (C_5 to C_{10}) are the ones most commonly used in combustion fuels and as solvents. Petroleum distillates are also used as chemical feedstocks and as precursors or intermediates for production. The many contemporary applications of petroleum distillates in consumer and household products include paints and thinners, furniture polish, lamp oils, and lubricants (Table 106–1).

Mineral oil, castor oil, and glycerine are commonly used as laxatives. Hydrocarbon-based ointments, petroleum jelly, and camphor are used topically on skin and mucous membranes. Volatile oils (or essential oils) are fragrant hydrocarbon plant extracts. Examples include menthol, eucalyptus oil, clove oil, sassafras oil, and pennyroyal, among others. These oils have had a variety of medicinal uses over many centuries and are enjoying a resurgence with recent popularity of herbal products (Chap. 43). Phenol and substituted phenols are common medical disinfectants (Chap. 102). Diethyl ether and halogenated hydrocarbon compounds, like chloroform, were among the first general anesthetics used more than 150 years ago. Cyclopropane and trichloroethylene (TCE) were also widely used anesthetics.[135]

Three populations appear to be at particular risk for hydrocarbon-related illness, children who have unintentional exposures, often ingestions, workers with occupational exposures, often dermal and inhalational, and adolescents or young adults who intentionally abuse solvents through inhalation. Specific occupations at risk for exposure include petrochemical workers, plastics and rubber workers, printers, laboratory workers, painters, and hazardous waste workers. The Occupational Safety and Health Administration (OSHA) estimates that nearly 238,000 American workers are exposed annually to significant concentrations of benzene alone.[72] But the epidemiology of hydrocarbon exposure and hydrocarbon-related illness is difficult to assess. Most exposures do not involve ingestion, and most do not result in illness. Because a common property of hydrocarbons is high volatility, inhalation is extremely common. Lipid solubility facilitates dermal absorption when skin is exposed.[63] Exposures may range from self-pumping gasoline, to painting a spare bedroom, to applying or removing fingernail polish. Table 106-1 lists frequently encountered hydrocarbon compounds and properties.

During the years 2003 to 2007, American poison centers reported 52,398 average yearly human hydrocarbons exposures to the American Association of Poison Control Centers (AAPCC). These exposures accounted for 2.2% of total human exposures reported. The incidence of exposures has not changed appreciably in the AAPCC database since the first report in 1983. Over the most recent 5-year period, 34% of reported human exposures to hydrocarbons involved unintentional exposures in children younger than 6 years of age. Exposures in young children appear to be declining over the past decade of AAPCC reports, but this may be an artifact of the way in which cases are reported into the database. Within the AAPCC database, many thousands of hydrocarbon exposures are not listed as such, but are ascribed to chemicals, pesticides, personal care products, cleaning substances, paints, automotive products (see Chap. 135). The alarming rate of intentional misuse of volatile solvents by young people and the concomitant rate of death from volatile substance abuse is discussed in Chap. 81.

CHEMISTRY

A *hydrocarbon* is an organic compound made up primarily of carbon and hydrogen atoms, typically ranging from 1 to 60 carbon atoms in length. This definition includes products derived from plants (pine oil, vegetable oil), animal fats (cod liver oil), natural gas, petroleum, or coal tar. There are two basic types of hydrocarbon molecules, *aliphatic* (straight or branched chains) and *cyclic* (closed ring), each with its own subclasses. The aliphatic compounds include the *paraffins* (*alkanes*, with a generic formula C_nH_{2n+2}); the *olefins* (*alkenes* have one double bond and *alkadienes* have two double bonds); *acetylenes* (alkynes) with at least one triple bond; and the *acyclic terpenes* (polymers of isoprene, C_5H_8). Some aliphatic compounds have branches in which the subchain also contains carbon atoms; both the chain and branches are essentially straight.

The cyclic hydrocarbons include *alicyclic* (three or more carbon atoms in a ring structure, with properties similar to the aliphatics), and *aromatic* compounds, as well as the *cyclic terpenes.* The alicyclics are further divided into *cycloparaffins* (*naphthenes*) such as cyclohexane, and the *cycloolefins* (two or more double bonds) such as cyclopentadiene.

Saturated hydrocarbons contain carbon atoms that exist only in their most reduced state. This means that each carbon is bound to either hydrogen or to another carbon, with no double or triple bonds

TABLE 106–1. Classification and Viscosity of Common Hydrocarbons

Compound	Common Uses	Viscosity (SUS)[a]
Aliphatics		
Gasoline	Motor vehicle fuel	30
Naphtha	Charcoal lighter fluid	29
Kerosene	Heating fuel	35
Turpentine	Paint thinner	33
Mineral spirits	Paint and varnish thinner	30–35
Mineral seal oil	Furniture polish	30–35
Heavy fuel oil	Heating oil	>450
Aromatics		
Benzene	Solvent, reagent, gasoline additive	31
Toluene	Solvent, spray paint solvent	28
Xylene	Solvent, paint thinner, reagent	28
Halogenated		
Methylene chloride	Solvent, paint stripper, propellant	27
Carbon tetrachloride	Solvent, propellant, refrigerant	30
Trichloroethylene	Degreaser, spot remover	27
Tetrachloroethylene	Dry cleaning solvent, chemical intermediate	28

[a] Direct values for kinematic viscosity in Saybolt universal seconds (SUS) were not available for the following compounds: naphtha, xylene, methylene chloride, carbon tetrachloride, trichloroethylene, perchloroethylene, and toluene. SUS was calculated by converting from available measurements in centipoise viscosity and/or centistokes viscosity using the following conversions: the value in centistokes is estimated by dividing centipoise by density at 68°F (20°C); SUS is approximated from centistokes using $y = 3.2533x + 26.08$ ($R^2 = 0.9998$). Centipoise viscosity for naphtha was estimated from the value for butylbenzene. Centipoise viscosity for xylene is the average of *o*-, *m*-, and *p*-xylene.

present. Conversely, *unsaturated* compounds are those with hydrogens removed, in which double or triple bonds exist.

Solvents are a heterogenous class of xenobiotics used to dissolve and to provide a vehicle for delivery of other xenobiotics. The most common industrial solvent is water. The common solvents most familiar to toxicologists are *organic solvents* (containing one or more carbon atom), and most of these are hydrocarbons. Most are liquids in the conditions under which they are used. Specifically named solvents (Stoddard solvent, white naphtha, ligroin) represent mixtures of hydrocarbons emanating from a common petroleum distillation fraction.

Aromatic hydrocarbons are divided into the *benzene* group (one ring), *naphthalene* group (two rings), and the *anthracene* group (three rings). *Polycyclic aromatic hydrocarbons* (polynuclear aromatic hydrocarbons) have multiple, fused benzene-like rings. Aromatic organic compounds may also be *heterocyclic* (where oxygen or nitrogen substitutes for carbon in the ring). Structurally, all of these molecules are flat, with reactive electron clouds above and below the ring.

The *cyclic terpenes* are the principal components of the variety of plant-derived essential oils, often providing color, odor, and flavor. *Limonene* in lemon oil, *menthol* in mint oil, *pinene* in turpentine, and *camphor* are all terpenes (Chap. 42).[108]

Physical properties of hydrocarbons vary by the number of carbon atoms and by molecular structure. Unsubstituted, aliphatic hydrocarbons that contain up to 4 carbons are gaseous at room temperature, 5 to 19 carbon molecules are liquids, and longer-chain molecules tend to be tars or solids. Branching of chains tends to destabilize intermolecular forces, so that less energy is required to separate the molecules. The result is that, for a given molecular size, highly branched molecules have lower boiling points and tend to be more volatile.[104]

Gasoline is a mixture of alkanes, alkenes, naphthenes, and aromatic hydrocarbons, predominantly 5 to 10 carbon molecules in size. Gasoline is separated from crude oil in a common distillation fraction. However, most commercially available gasolines are actually blends of up to eight component fractions from refinery processors. More than 1500 individual xenobiotics may be present in commercial grades, but most analytical methods are only able to isolate 150 to 180 compounds from gasolines. Notably, *n*-hexane is present at up to 6%, and benzene is present between 1% and 6%, depending on the grade and the place of origin of the product. A number of additives may go into the final formulation: alkyl leads, ethylene dichloride, and ethylene dibromide in leaded gasoline, and oxygenates such as methyl *t*-butyl ether (MTBE), as well as methanol and ethanol.[170]

Organic halides contain one or more halogen atoms (fluorine, chlorine, bromine, iodine) usually substituted for a hydrogen atom in the parent structure. Examples include chloroform, trichloroethylene, and the freons.

Oxygenated hydrocarbons demonstrate toxicity specific to the oxidation state of the carbon, as well as to the atoms adjacent to it (the "R" groups). The *alcohols* are widely used as solvents in industry and in household products. Their toxicity is discussed in Chaps. 77 and 107. *Ethers* contain an oxygen bound on either side by a carbon atom. Acute toxicity from ethers tends to mirror that of the corresponding alcohols. *Aldehydes* and *ketones* contain a single carbon-oxygen double bond (C=O), the former at a terminal carbon, the latter somewhere in the middle. Organic *acids, esters, amides,* and *acyl halides* represent more oxidized states of carbon; human toxicity is agent-specific.

Phenols consist of benzene rings with an attached hydroxyl (alcohol) group. The parent compound, phenol, has only one hydroxyl group attached to benzene. The toxicity of phenol can be dramatically altered by addition of other functional groups to the benzene ring (Chap. 102). Cresols, catechols, and salicylate are examples of substituted phenols.

A variety of amines, amides, nitroso and nitro compounds, as well as phosphates, sulfites, and sulfates are used commercially and industrially. The addition of these functional groups to hydrocarbons dramatically alters the toxicity of the compound.

PHARMACOLOGY

Inhalation of hydrocarbon vapor depresses consciousness. Acute central nervous (CNS) toxicity from occupational overexposure or recreational abuse parallels the effect of administering an inhaled general anesthetic.[140] The concentration of volatile anesthetic that produces loss of nociception in 50% of patients defines the minimum alveolar concentration (MAC) required to induce anesthesia. Inhaled solvent vapor similarly produces unconsciousness in 50% of subjects when the partial pressure in the lung reaches its median effective dose (ED_{50}). The ED_{50} of occupational parlance is effectively the same as the MAC used in anesthesiology parlance (see Chap. 67). Virtually all patients will be anesthetized when the partial pressure is raised 30% above the MAC (MAC × 1.3), and death, if ventilation is not supported, typically occurs when the concentration reaches two to four times the MAC.[87] Dose–response curves suggest that essentially no individual will be rendered unconscious by an inhaled dose 30% below the MAC. However, impairment of cognitive and motor function may occur with much lower exposures.[18]

Occupational exposure to lipid-soluble solvents, such as aromatic, aliphatic, or chlorinated hydrocarbons, are more likely to cause acute and chronic CNS effects than exposure to water-soluble hydrocarbons such as alcohols, ketones, and esters.[94] The property of an inhaled anesthetic that correlates most closely with its ability to extinguish nociception is its lipid solubility. The Meyer-Overton hypothesis, proposed more than 100 years ago, implies that an anesthetic dissolves into some critical lipid compartment of the CNS, causing inhibition of neuronal transmission. In this construct, the target structure for general anesthetics is the neuronal lipid membrane itself.[64]

Inhaled hydrocarbons and other volatile anesthetic xenobiotics (Chap. 67) exhibit pharmacodynamic properties suggestive of a receptor-ligand interaction. The sigmoidal dose-response curves exhibit a near-linear midrange with a plateau effect at higher inhaled concentrations. Different xenobiotics produce curves whose linear segments parallel one another, implying that each xenobiotic produces the same physiologic effect at a particular concentration related to that xenobiotic's potency.[121] Thus, it has long been tempting to find the single, intangible "receptor" responsible for general anesthesia, and in doing so, to improve upon the Meyer-Overton hypothesis.

Unfortunately, a single mechanism remains elusive. Halothane, isoflurane, sevoflurane, enflurane, and desflurane inhibit fast sodium channels.[117] Toluene, trichloroethylene, perchloroethylene, and others inhibit neuronal calcium currents.[113,136] The halogenated hydrocarbons increase the outward potassium rectifying current.[137] Specific ligand-receptor interactions occur,[43] such as the inhibition of receptor function at nicotinic,[165] and at the glutamate receptors,[42] as well as enhancement of type-A γ-aminobutyric acid ($GABA_A$) and glycine receptor currents.[16] Independent of other mechanisms, halogenated hydrocarbons appear to decrease exocytosis of neuronal synaptic vesicles.[68] This growing body of research suggests that the Meyer-Overton hypothesis is too simplistic to explain the differences in pharmacologic profiles observed with this wide class of xenobiotics.

The effect of hydrocarbons on cardiac conduction remains an active arena of toxicologic research. Nearly all classes of hydrocarbons, to varying degrees, augment the dysrhythmogenic potential by "sensitizing" the myocardium. Sensitization occurs with both xenobiotic and class specificity. Ethylene and aliphatic ethers are very poor sensitizers. Aromatic, and even more so the halogenated hydrocarbons, are often potent sensitizers.[23]

Cardiac sensitization is incompletely understood.[43] Halothane and isoflurane inactivate sodium channels,[141] whereas chloroform and others attenuate potassium efflux through voltage-gated channels.[133] Sensitization may be mediated by slowed conduction velocity through membrane gap junctions. Dephosphorylation of connexin-43 results in a configurational change that increases gap junctional resistance. Halocarbons, in the presence of epinephrine, cause dephosporylation of this gap junction protein, thereby increasing gap junctional resistance and slowing conduction velocity in myocardial tissue.[77]

TOXICOKINETICS

Human toxicokinetic data are lacking for most hydrocarbons, and much of our understanding of the kinetics comes from animal studies. Hydrocarbons are variably absorbed through ingestion, inhalation, or dermal routes of exposure. Partition coefficients, in particular, are useful predictors of the rate and extent of the absorption and distribution of hydrocarbons into tissues as the higher the value the greater the potential for redistribution. A partition coefficient for a given chemical species is the ratio of concentrations achieved between two different media at equilibrium. The blood-to-air and tissue-to-air or tissue-to-blood coefficients directly relate to the pulmonary uptake and distribution of hydrocarbons. The tissue-to-blood partition coefficient is commonly determined by dividing the tissue-to-air coefficient by the blood-to-air coefficient.[53,120] Table 106–2 lists the partition coefficients for commonly encountered hydrocarbons. Where human data is limited, rat data is presented in the table, because human and rat data often correlate.[120]

Inhalation is a major route of exposure for most volatile hydrocarbons. The absorbed dose is determined by the air concentration, duration of exposure, minute ventilation, and the blood-to-air partition coefficient. Most hydrocarbons cross the alveolus through passive diffusion. The driving force for this is the difference in vapor concentration between the alveolus and the blood. Hydrocarbons that are highly soluble in blood and tissues are readily absorbed through inhalation, and blood concentrations rise rapidly following inhalation exposure. Aromatic hydrocarbons are generally well absorbed through inhalation, absorption of aliphatic hydrocarbons varies by molecular weight: aliphatic hydrocarbons with between 5 and 16 carbons are readily absorbed, through inhalation, whereas those with more than 16 carbons are less readily absorbed.[3]

Absorption of aliphatic hydrocarbons through the digestive tract is inversely related to molecular weight, ranging from complete absorption at lower molecular weights, to approximately 60% for C-14 hydrocarbons, 5% for C-28 hydrocarbons, and essentially no absorption for aliphatic hydrocarbons with more than 32 carbons.[3] Oral absorption of aromatic hydrocarbons with between 5 and 9 carbons ranges from 80% to 97%. Oral absorption data for aromatic hydrocarbons with more than 9 carbons are sparse.

While the skin is a common area of contact with solvents, for most hydrocarbons the dose received from dermal exposure is a small fraction of the dose received through other routes, such as inhalation. The skin is comprised of both hydrophilic (proteinaceous portion of cells) and lipophilic (cell membranes) regions. While many hydrocarbons can remove lipids from the stratum corneum, permeability is not simply the result of lipid removal; permeability also increases with hydration of the skin. When xenobiotics have near equality in the water-to-lipid partition coefficient, their rate of skin absorption is increased. Solvents that contain both hydrophobic and hydrophilic moieties (eg, glycol ethers, dimethylformamide, dimethylsulfoxide) are particularly well absorbed dermally.[94] Other factors, in addition to the partition coefficient and permeability constant, that determine penetration across the skin, include the thickness of the skin layer, the difference in concentration of the solvent on either side of the epithelium, the diffusion constant, and skin integrity (ie, normal versus cut or abraded).

The dose received via skin absorption will also depend on the surface area of the skin exposed and the duration of contact. Though highly volatile compounds may have a short duration of skin contact because of evaporation, skin absorption can also occur from contact with hydrocarbon vapor. In studies with human volunteers exposed to varying concentrations of hydrocarbon vapors, the dermal dose accounted for only 0.1%–2% of the inhalation dose. With massive exposure (eg, whole-body immersion), dermal absorption may contribute significantly to toxicity. Significant dermal absorption with resultant toxicity is described with carbon tetrachloride,[76] tetrachloroethylene,[63] and phenol.[93]

Once absorbed into the central compartment, hydrocarbons are distributed to target and storage organs based on their tissue-to-blood partition coefficients and on the rate of perfusion of the tissue with blood. During the onset of systemic exposure, hydrocarbons accumulate

TABLE 106–2. Kinetic Parameters of Selected Hydrocarbons

	Partition Coefficients		$t_{1/2}$			
	Blood/Air	Fat/Air	α	β	Elimination	Relevant Metabolites
Aliphatics						
n-Hexane	2.29[a]	159[a]	11 min	99 min	10%–20% exhaled; liver metabolism by CYP 2E1	2-Hexanol, 2,5-hexanedione, γ-valerolactone
Paraffin/tar	Not absorbed or metabolized					
Aromatics						
Benzene	8.19	499[a]	8 h	90 h	12% exhaled; liver metabolism to phenol	Phenol, catechol, hydroquinone, and conjugates
Toluene	18.0[a]	1021[a]	4–5 h	15–72 h	Extensive liver extraction and metabolism	80% metabolized to benzyl alcohol; 70% renally excreted as hippuric acid
o-Xylene	34.9	1877[a]	30–60 min	20–30 h	Liver CYP 2E1 oxidation	Toluic acid, methyl hippuric acid
Halogenated						
Methylene chloride	8.94	120[a]	Apparent $t_{1/2}$ of COHb 13 h	40 min	92% exhaled unchanged. Low doses metabolized; high doses exhaled. Two liver metabolic pathways	(a) CYP 2E1 to CO and CO_2 (b) Glutathione transferase to CO_2, formaldehyde, formic acid
Carbon tetrachloride	2.73	359[a]	84–91 min[a]	91–496 min[a]	Liver CYP 2E1, some lung exhalation (dose-dependent)	Trichloromethyl radical, trichloromethyl peroxy radical, phosgene
Trichloroethylene	8.11	554[a]	3 h	30 h	Liver CYP 2E1–epoxide intermediate; trichloroethanol is glucuronidated and excreted	Chloral hydrate, trichloroethanol, trichloroacetic acid
1,1,1- Trichloroethane	2.53	263[a]	44 min	53 h	91% exhaled; liver CYP 2E1	Trichloroacetic acid, trichloroethanol
Tetrachloroethylene	10.3	1638[a]	160 min	33 h	80% exhaled; liver CYP 2E1	Trichloroacetic acid, trichloroethanol

[a] Fat/blood partition coefficient is obtained by dividing the fat/air coefficient by the blood/air coefficient, as determined in rat models. All coefficients are determined at 98.6°F (37°C).

in tissues that have tissue/blood coefficients greater than 1 (eg, for toluene, the fat-to-blood partition coefficient is 60). Table 106-2 lists the distribution half-lives of selected hydrocarbons.

Hydrocarbons can be eliminated from the body unchanged, for example, through expired air, or can be metabolized to more polar compounds, which are then excreted in urine or bile. Table 106-2 lists the blood elimination half-lives (for first-order elimination processes) and metabolites of selected hydrocarbons. Some hydrocarbons are metabolized to toxic compounds (eg, methylene chloride, carbon tetrachloride, *n*-hexane, methyl-*n*-butyl ketone). The specific toxicities of these metabolites are discussed under Special Cases later in the chapter.

PATHOPHYSIOLOGY AND CLINICAL FINDINGS

RESPIRATORY

Several factors are classically associated with pulmonary toxicity after hydrocarbon ingestion. These include specific physical properties of the xenobiotics ingested, the volume ingested, and the occurrence of vomiting. Physical properties of viscosity, surface tension, and volatility are primary determinants of aspiration potential.

Dynamic (or absolute) viscosity is the measurement of the ability of a fluid to resist flow. This property is measured with a rheometer and is typically given in units of pascal-seconds. More frequently, engineers work with *kinematic viscosity,* measured in square millimeters per second, or centistokes. Dynamic viscosity is converted to kinematic viscosity by dividing the dynamic viscosity by the fluid's density. An older system for measuring viscosity was initially popularized by the petroleum industry and expresses kinematic viscosity in units of Saybolt Universal seconds (SUS). Unfortunately, many policy statements were developed in an era when SUS units were popular, so many still describe viscosity in SUS units. Various look-up tables and calculators are available to convert kinematic viscosity to SUS units. Table 106-1 shows kinematic viscosity of common hydrocarbons, measured in SUS. A unit conversion approximation is given in the table's footnote.

Hydrocarbons with low viscosities (less than 60 SUS; eg, turpentine, gasoline, naphtha) have a higher tendency for aspiration in animal models. The US Consumer Products Safety Commission issued a rule requiring child-resistant packaging for products that contain 10% or more hydrocarbon by weight and that have a viscosity less than 100 SUS.[160]

Surface tension is a cohesive force generated by attraction (ie, Van der Waals forces) between molecules.[118] This influences adherence of a liquid along a surface ("its ability to creep"). The lower the surface tension, the less well the liquid will creep and the higher the aspiration risk.[55]

Volatility is the tendency for a liquid to become a gas. Hydrocarbons with high volatility tend to vaporize, displace oxygen, and potentially lead to transient hypoxia.

It is not clear which physical property is most important in predicting toxicity. Early reports conflicted in attempting to relate risk of pulmonary toxicity to the amount of hydrocarbon ingested, or to the presence or absence of vomiting. One prospective study addressed both of these variables. The cooperative kerosene poisoning (COKP) study was a multicenter study that enrolled 760 cases of hydrocarbon ingestion. Of these, 409 could provide an estimate of the amount ingested. Patients who reportedly ingested more than 30 mL had a 52% chance of developing pulmonary complications, compared with 39% of those who ingested less than 10 mL. Risk of central nervous complications was 41%, compared with 24% using the same criterion. There was a 53% incidence of pulmonary toxicity when vomiting occurred, compared with 37% when there was no history of vomiting.[122] While this knowledge may help modify the index of suspicion regarding possible pulmonary toxicity, none of these parameters is completely predictive. Severe hydrocarbon pneumonitis may occur after ingestion of "low-risk" hydrocarbons.[131] Patients may develop severe lung injury after low-volume (less than 5 mL) ingestions, as well as after ingestions with no history of coughing, gagging, or vomiting.[9]

It is widely held that aspiration is the main route of injury from ingested simple hydrocarbons. The mechanism of pulmonary injury, however, is not fully understood. Intratracheal instillation of 0.2 mL/kg of kerosene causes physiologic abnormalities in lung mechanics (decreased compliance and total lung capacity) and pathologic changes such as interstitial inflammation, polymorphonuclear exudates, intraalveolar edema and hemorrhage, hyperemia, bronchial and bronchiolar necrosis, and vascular thrombosis.[11,61,156] These changes most likely reflect both direct toxicity to pulmonary tissue and disruption of the lipid surfactant layer.[173]

Most patients who go on to develop pulmonary toxicity after hydrocarbon ingestion will have an episode of coughing, gagging, or choking. This usually occurs within 30 minutes after ingestion and is presumptive evidence of aspiration. The majority of patients who have respiratory signs and symptoms beyond the initial history of gagging, choking, and coughing develop radiographic pneumonitis.[9] Absence of tachypnea on initial evaluation has 80% negative predictive value for pneumonitis.[168] Pulmonary toxicity may manifest as crackles, rhonchi, bronchospasm, tachypnea, hypoxemia, hemoptysis, acute lung injury (hemorrhagic or non-hemorrhagic), or respiratory distress.[156] Cyanosis develops in approximately 2% to 3% of patients.[99] This may result from simple asphyxiant effects from volatilized hydrocarbons, from ventilation–perfusion mismatch, or, rarely, from methemoglobinemia (aniline, nitrobenzene, or nitrite-containing hydrocarbons). Clinical findings often worsen over the first several days but typically resolve within a week. Death is rare (less than 2%), and typically occurs after a severe, progressive respiratory insult marked by hypoxia, ventilation–perfusion mismatch, and barotrauma.[14,180]

Intravenous (IV) and subcutaneous injection of hydrocarbons have been reported.[129,162] Severe hydrocarbon pneumonitis may occur following intravenous exposure. Animal experiments show that intravascular hydrocarbons injure the first capillary bed encountered. Intravenous injection thus causes pulmonary toxicity, and portal vein injection leads to direct hepatic injury.[127,175] The clinical course after IV hydrocarbon injection mirrors that of aspiration injury.

Radiographic evidence of pneumonitis develops in 40%–88% of admitted aspiration patients.[15,44,114,125] Findings can develop as early as 15 minutes or as late as 24 hours after exposure (Fig. 106–1).[36,51,122,163] Chest radiographs performed immediately on initial presentation are not useful in predicting infiltrates in either symptomatic or asymptomatic patients.[168] Ninety percent of patients who develop radiographic abnormalities do so by 4 hours postingestion.[36] Clinical signs of pneumonia (eg, crackles, rhonchi) are evident in 40%–50% of patients.[44] A small percentage (less than 5%) are completely asymptomatic after a period of observation, but still have radiographic findings.[9]

Specific radiologic findings include perihilar densities, bronchovascular markings, bibasilar infiltrates, and pneumonic consolidation.[56] Right-sided involvement occurs in 75% of cases and bilateral involvement in approximately 50%. Upper-lobe involvement is uncommon.[25] Pleural effusions develop in 3% of cases, with one-third appearing within 24 hours.[98] Pneumothorax, pneumomediastinum, and pneumatoceles occur uncommonly.[11,17,79] Initial radiographs after ingestion may reveal two liquid densities in the stomach, known as the "double-bubble" sign. This represents an air–fluid (hydrocarbon or water) and a hydrocarbon–water interface, as the hydrocarbon is not miscible with gastric fluids (primarily water) and may have a specific gravity less than that of water.[37]

Radiographic resolution does not correlate with clinical improvement, but rather lags behind by several days to weeks. There are few reports of long-term follow up on patients with hydrocarbon pneumonitis.[25,51,62,125,152] Frequent respiratory tract infections are described in individuals after hydrocarbon pneumonitis, but studies addressing this are poorly controlled.[51,156] Delayed formation of pneumatoceles may occur.[17,79] Bronchiectasis and pulmonary fibrosis are reported but appear to be uncommon.[59,125] In one study, 82% of patients examined 8–14 years after hydrocarbon-induced pneumonitis had asymptomatic minor pulmonary function abnormalities. The abnormalities were consistent with small-airway obstruction and loss of elastic recoil. The authors hypothesized that this group may be predisposed to chronic obstructive pulmonary disease.[62]

CARDIAC

The most concerning cardiac effect from hydrocarbon exposure is precipitation of a dysrhythmia by myocardial sensitization (see Pharmacology previously). These events are described with all classes of hydrocarbons, but halogenated compounds are most frequently implicated, followed by aromatic compounds.[13,126] Malignant dysrhythmias occur after exposure to high concentrations of volatile inhalants or inhaled anesthetics. Atrial fibrillation, ventricular tachycardia, junctional rhythm, ventricular fibrillation, and cardiac arrest are reported.[103,111,126] This is termed the "sudden sniffing death syndrome." Myocardial depression occurs by an unclear mechanism. Prolongation of the QT interval raises concern for torsades de pointes.[14,88,133]

Any route of exposure to hydrocarbons may result in cardiotoxicity. Classically, sudden death follows an episode of sudden exertion.[14] Tachydysrhythmias, cardiomegaly, and myocardial infarction are rarely reported after ingestion of hydrocarbons.[74,143] A retrospective followup cohort of exposed methylene chloride workers did not find evidence of excess long-term cardiac disease.[115]

CENTRAL NERVOUS SYSTEM

Transient CNS excitation may occur after acute hydrocarbon inhalation or ingestion.[88] More commonly, CNS depression or anesthesia occurs.[44] In cases of aspiration, hypoxemia from pulmonary damage may contribute to the CNS depression.[96,176] Coma and seizures are reported in 1%–3% of cases.[114,125,179] Chronic occupational exposure or volatile substance use may lead to a chronic neurobehavioral syndrome; the painter's syndrome, most notably described after toluene overexposure. The clinical features include ataxia, spasticity, dysarthria, and dementia, consistent with leukoencephalopathy.[49] Autopsy studies of the brains of chronic toluene abusers show atrophy and mottling of the white matter, as though the lipid-based myelin were dissolved away. Microscopic examination shows a consistent pattern of myelin and oligodendrocyte loss with relative preservation of axons.[86] Animal models of toluene poisoning reveal norepinephrine and dopamine depletion. The severity and reversibility of this syndrome depends on the intensity

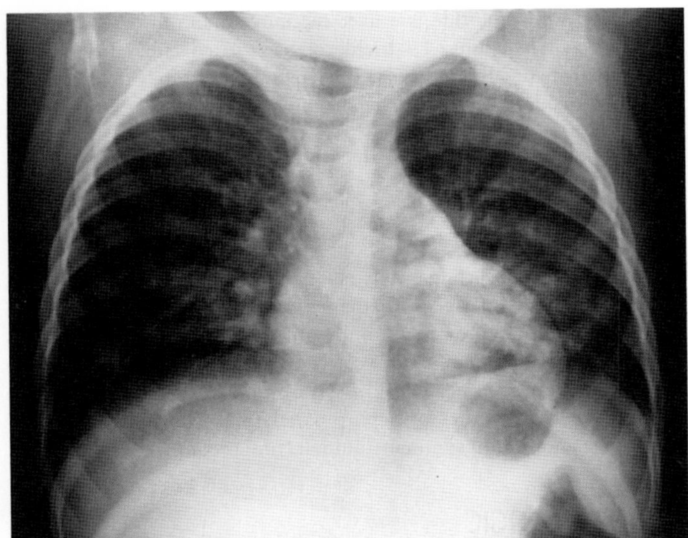

A

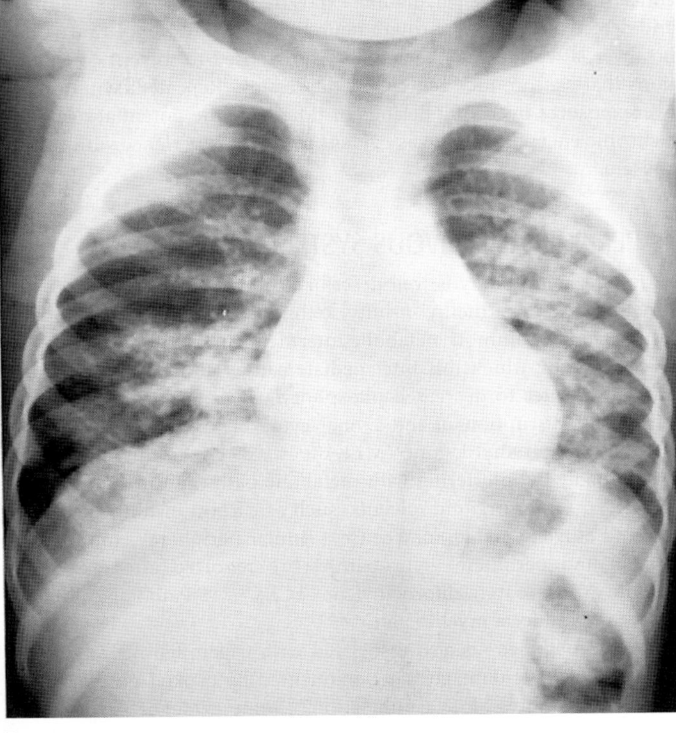

B

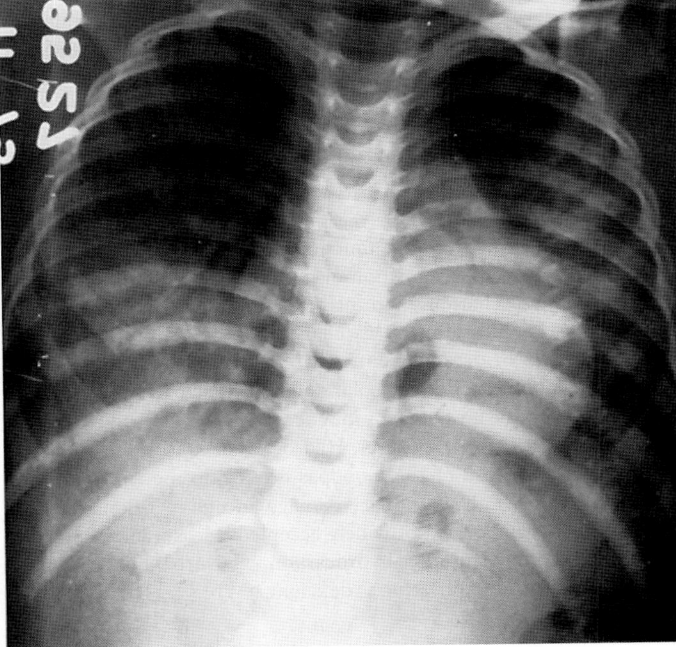

C

FIGURE 106–1. Three sequential radiographs of a young girl with severe hydrocarbon aspiration pneumonitis. **(A)** Initial: Patchy densities appear in basilar areas of both lung fields with increased interstitial markings and peribronchial thickening. **(B)** Day 2: More extensive diffuse alveolar infiltrates are apparent. **(C)** Day 6: Dense consolidation and atelectasis are evident in the right lower lobe. *(Images contributed by Nancy Genieser, MD, Professor of Radiology, New York University.)*

and duration of toluene exposure.[132] Infrequent exposure may produce no clinical neurologic signs, whereas heavy (eg, daily) use can lead to significant neurologic impairment after as little as one year, but more commonly after 2–4 years of ongoing exposure. The specific cognitive and neuropsychological findings in toluene-induced dementia are termed a white matter dementia.[46,52]

Initial findings of white matter dementia include behavioral changes, impaired sense of smell, impaired concentration, and mild unsteadiness of hand movements and gait. Further exposure leads to slurred speech, head tremor, poor vision, deafness, stiff-legged and staggering gait, and subsequent dementia. Physical findings may include nystagmus, ataxia, tremor, spasticity with hyperreflexia, abnormal Babinski reflexes, deafness, impaired vision, and a broad-based, staggering gait. An abnormal brainstem auditory-evoked response appears to be a sensitive indicator of toluene-induced CNS damage. The electroencephalogram can show mild, diffuse slowing. Computed tomography in severe cases shows mild-to-moderate cerebellar and cortical atrophy. MRI findings are consistent with white matter disease. Most cases show significant clinical improvement after 6 months of abstinence, although with moderate to severe abuse, improvement may be incomplete. Chronic toluene misuse is addicting and can produce withdrawal.[132]

In the occupational setting, exposures are rarely as extensive as those that occur with volatile substance misuse. Given the significantly lesser exposures, the findings among workers overexposed to solvent concentrations above permissible exposure limits are often subclinical, and detected primarily through neurobehavioral testing. In rare cases, however, a worker may be acutely overexposed to solvent concentrations that can produce acute CNS depression. Repeated, symptomatic overexposures over long periods of time have the potential to lead to a chronic encephalopathy, as evident from the experience with solvent abusers.[46]

PERIPHERAL NERVOUS SYSTEM

Peripheral neuropathy is well described following occupational exposure to *n*-hexane or methyl-*n*-butyl ketone (MnBK).[20] This axonopathy results from a common metabolic intermediate; 2,5-hexanedione. The mechanism by which this intermediate causes peripheral neuropathy probably relates to decreased phosphorylation of neurofilament proteins, with disruption of the axonal cytoskeleton (see Special Cases below). Methyl ethyl ketone (MEK) may exacerbate this neurotoxicity, probably by interfering with metabolic pathways of *n*-hexane and MnBK.[8,130] Other organic solvents, such as carbon disulfide, acrylamide, and ethylene oxide, may cause a similar peripheral axonopathy.[58] Cranial and peripheral neuropathies are reported after acute and chronic exposure to trichloroethylene (TCE).[78,92,149] Pathologically, TCE appears to induce a myelinopathy.[47,58]

Trichloroethylene is also associated with trigeminal neuralgia.[31,45,92] Trigeminal nerve damage was documented by evoked potentials following 15 minutes of TCE inhalation.[92] Some evidence suggests that decomposition products or impurities in TCE may be responsible for cranial neuropathy.[31,45]

Axonopathy from MnBK or *n*-hexane exposure typically begins in the distal extremities and progresses proximally (a classic, "dying-back" neuropathy) (see Chap. 18). Exposure to one of these hydrocarbons should be considered in the differential diagnosis of the patient with Guillain-Barré syndrome (GBS) although sensory findings are present with MnBK and absent in GBS.[139] The longest axons appear to be affected initially, so that the patient manifests a "length-dependent polyneuropathy." With discontinuation of exposure many of the effects reverse over weeks to months.[69,82,123,178] Alternatively, the phenomenon of "coasting" may occur, in which neuropathy progresses for a time (weeks to months) after discontinuation of the toxic insult.[139] A reversible peripheral neuropathy occurred in 40% of chronic toluene abusers and was characterized by severe motor weakness without sensory deficits or areflexia.[148] It is unclear whether the toluene in this series may have been contaminated by *n*-hexane or MnBK.[8,140]

GASTROINTESTINAL

Hydrocarbons irritate gastrointestinal mucous membranes. Nausea and vomiting are common after ingestion. As discussed earlier, vomiting may increase risk of pulmonary toxicity.[112,114,131] Hematemesis was reported in 5% of cases in one study.[112] Gastrointestinal ulcerations are seen in animal studies.[83]

HEPATIC

The chlorinated hydrocarbons (Table 106–1) and their metabolites are hepatotoxic. In most cases, activation occurs via a phase I reaction to form a reactive intermediate (Chap. 12). In the case of carbon tetrachloride, this intermediate is the trichloromethyl radical. This radical forms covalent bonds with hepatic macromolecules, and may initiate lipid peroxidation.[22] Carbon tetrachloride causes centrilobular necrosis after inhalational, oral ingestion, or dermal exposure.[101] Hepatotoxicity in animals has been ranked for common hydrocarbons as follows: carbon tetrachloride is greater than benzene, trichloroethylene is greater than pentane.[174] Vinyl chloride is a liver carcinogen, and trichloroethylene, tetrachloroethylene, and 1,1,1-trichloroethane are considered less acutely hepatotoxic than vinyl chloride.[101,154] Hepatotoxicity rarely follows ingestion of petroleum distillates.[75] Hepatic injury, manifested as aminotransferase elevation and hepatomegaly, is usually reversible except in massive overexposures (see Special Cases later in the chapter).

RENAL

Halogenated hydrocarbons such as chloroform, carbon tetrachloride, ethylene dichloride, tetrachloroethane, 1,1,1-trichloroethane, and TCE are nephrotoxic. Acute renal failure and distal renal tubular acidosis occur in some painters and volatile-substance abusers.[81] Toluene causes a renal tubular acidosis like syndrome (see Toluene later in the chapter). Human studies of nephrotoxicity are confounded by other exposures, and findings in many animal studies conflict.[2]

HEMATOLOGIC

Hemolysis has been sporadically reported to occur after hydrocarbon ingestion.[1,7,146] One retrospective study of 12 patients showed hemolysis in three individuals and disseminated intravascular coagulation in another.[7] Although one patient required transfusion, hemolysis is usually mild and does not require red blood cell transfusion (also see discussion of benzene's effects on bone marrow, under Benzene later in the chapter).

IMMUNOLOGIC

Hydrocarbons disturb the integrity of membrane lipid bilayers, causing swelling and increased permeability to protons and other ions. This alters the structural and functional integrity of the membrane. Changes in the lipid composition of the membrane occur, and membrane lipopolysaccharides and proteins are disturbed.[138] Resultant toxicity may directly destroy capillary endothelium.[21] Additionally, there appears to be derangement of basement membranes, and this is postulated to underlie both alveolar and glomerular toxicity of hydrocarbons.[144] Immune mechanisms may account for basement membrane dysfunction in chronic exposures. Hydrocarbon exposure is suggested as one possible cause of the Goodpasture syndrome (immune dysfunction causing both pulmonary damage and glomerulonephritis),[19] though the association is not widely accepted. Measurable changes in immune function occur after hydrocarbon exposure,[12] but our knowledge of any clinical implication is deficient.

DERMATOLOGIC

Most hydrocarbon solvents cause nonspecific irritation of skin and mucous membranes. Repeated, prolonged contact can dry and crack the skin. The mechanism of dermal injury appears to be defatting of the lipid layer of the stratum corneum. Up to 9% of workers may develop eczematous lesions from dermal contact.[177] Limonene and turpentine contain sensitizers that can rarely result in contact allergy (Chap. 29).

Contact dermatitis and blistering may progress to partial- and even full-thickness burns.[65] Severity is proportional to duration of exposure. Hydrocarbons are irritating to skin. Acute, prolonged exposure can cause dermatitis and even full-thickness dermal damage.[65] Chronic dermal exposure to kerosene or diesel fuel can cause oil folliculitis.[38,161] A specific skin lesion called chloracne is associated with exposure to chlorinated aromatic hydrocarbons with highly specific stereochemistry (eg, dioxins, polychlorobiphenyls).

Soft-tissue injection of hydrocarbon is locally toxic, leading to necrosis. Secondary cellulitis, abscess formation, and fasciitis can occur.

Infectious complications are treated by meticulous wound care, with surgical debridement as necessary. A particularly destructive injury involves high-pressure injection-gun injury. These injuries typically involve the extremities, with high-pressure injection of grease or paint into the fascial planes and tendon sheaths. Emergent surgical debridement is necessary in most of these cases.[48,106]

HYDROCARBONS WITH SPECIFIC AND UNIQUE TOXICITY

n-HEXANE

Hexane is a six-carbon simple aliphatic hydrocarbon. It is a constituent of some brake-cleaning fluids, rubber cement, glues, spray paints, coatings, and silicones. Outbreaks of *n*-hexane–related neurotoxicity have occurred in printing plants, sandal shops, furniture factories, and automotive repair shops.[32] Human exposure occurs primarily by inhalation. Both *n*-hexane and MnBK are well-known peripheral neurotoxins that cause a classic "dying-back" peripheral polyneuropathy, beginning in a "stocking-glove" distribution.[20,33] Neurotoxicity does not appear to be directly caused by the parent compounds, but results from a common metabolic intermediate—2,5-hexanedione. Toxicity appears related to the ability of this intermediate to form a ringed pyrrole structure, which causes decreased phosphorylation of neurofilament proteins, disrupting the axonal cytoskeleton.[58] Similar five- and seven-carbon species do not induce similar neurotoxicity, except those that are direct precursor intermediates in the metabolic pathway producing 2,5-hexanedione[58,150] (see Fig. 106–2).

METHYLENE CHLORIDE

Methylene chloride is commonly encountered in paint removers, as well as in cleaners and degreasers and in aerosol propellants. Like other halogenated hydrocarbons, it can rapidly induce general anesthesia by inhalation or ingestion. Unlike other hydrocarbon agents, methylene chloride and similar one carbon halomethanes (eg, methylene dibromide) are metabolized by liver P450 2E1 mixed-function oxidase to carbon monoxide. Significant, delayed, and prolonged carboxyhemoglobinemia can occur (Table 106–2 and Chap. 125).[4,124]

CARBON TETRACHLORIDE

Carbon tetrachloride (CCl_4), although not actually a hydrocarbon, has been used as an industrial solvent and reagent. Its use in the United States has declined dramatically since recognition of its toxicity caused the Environmental Protection Agency (EPA) to restrict its commercial use.[3] Absorption occurs by all routes, including dermal. CCl_4 is an irritant to skin and mucous membranes and is a potent gastric irritant when ingested. As with other halogenated hydrocarbons, aspiration can result in pneumonitis, and systemic absorption may result in ventricular dysrhythmias.

More unique to CCl_4 exposures are hepatotoxicity and nephrotoxicity. Both occur more commonly with repetitive exposure (eg, occupational exposures).[34,76,153] Toxicity follows phase-I dehalogenation of the parent compound, which produces free radicals, causes lipid peroxidation and the production of protein adducts.[22] Localization of specific phase-I hepatic enzymes in the centrilobular area of the liver results in regionalized (zone 3) centrilobular injury after CCl_4 exposure (Chap. 26). Hepatotoxicity is typically manifested as reversible aminotransferase concentration elevations with or without hepatomegaly. Cirrhosis is reported in both animal models and in humans with prolonged overexposures. Nephrotoxicity is less-well studied but may result from a similar mechanism. The proximal convoluted tubule and the loop of Henle appear to be specifically targeted.[50] Carbon tetrachloride is a suspected human carcinogen.[3]

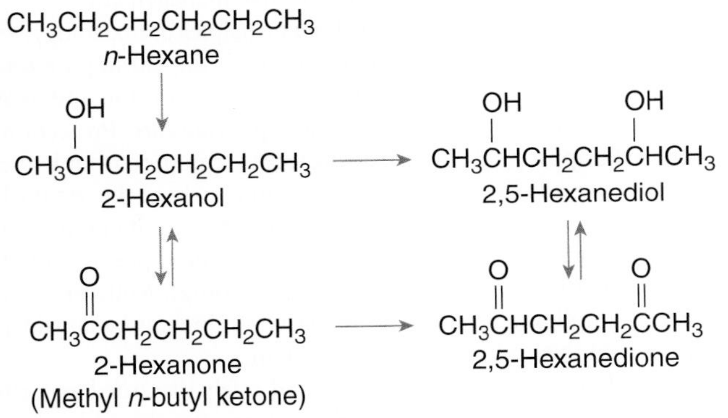

TRICHLOROETHYLENE

Trichloroethylene is a commonly used industrial solvent, cleanser, and degreaser. TCE was used for years as a general anesthetic agent, and hundreds of disposal sites in the United States. remain sources of ongoing human exposure. Its use as a general anesthetic was abandoned because of acute cardiotoxicity. TCE is also hepatotoxic, neurotoxic, and nephrotoxic in humans and animals. A recent report links TCE exposure to the development of neurodegenerative diseases, such as Parkinsonism.[54] This study has not been repeated or further validated.

An interagency group convened by the National Research Council recently assessed health risks associated with TCE. This group noted that compelling recent information implicates TCE as a human carcinogen. The final report calls upon federal agencies to finalize risk assessments so that informed risk management decisions about TCE can be made expeditiously.[107]

BENZENE

Benzene is hematotoxic and associated with acute hemolysis, or the delayed development of aplastic anemia and acute myelogenous leukemia.[5,57,89,100,119] Other aromatic hydrocarbons that are reported to cause similar hematologic effects most likely are contaminated with benzene. An excess risk of hematologic toxicity has not been demonstrated in groups with long-term exposure to toluene, xylene, or other aromatic hydrocarbons.[10,40,128,164,172] Other hematologic malignancies also may be linked to benzene, including chronic myelocytic leukemia, myelodysplastic syndromes, and lymphoma.[155] Chromosomal changes are believed to provide a marker for carcinogenicity.[159] Because of the carcinogenic risk, most benzene-based solvents have been unilaterally removed from the US market, and OSHA has limited the permissible worker exposure level to 1 ppm.[72]

TOLUENE

Toluene has essentially replaced benzene as the primary organic solvent in many commercial products. Many oil paints and stains contain primarily toluene as solvent. As such, it is readily available and readily abused as an inhalant. The CNS sequelae of chronic solvent inhalation are most frequently related to chronic toluene exposure.

Chronic toluene abuse can also cause a syndrome that resembles transient distal renal tubular acidosis (RTA).[151,166] Although the mechanism is incompletely understood, the acidosis results in great part from

$CH_3CH_2CH_2CH_2CH_2CH_3$ (*n*-Hexane) → $CH_3CH(OH)CH_2CH_2CH_2CH_3$ (2-Hexanol) ⇄ $CH_3C(=O)CH_2CH_2CH_2CH_3$ (2-Hexanone (Methyl *n*-butyl ketone))

2-Hexanol → $CH_3CH(OH)CH_2CH_2CH(OH)CH_3$ (2,5-Hexanediol)

2-Hexanone → $CH_3C(=O)CH_2CH_2C(=O)CH_3$ (2,5-Hexanedione)

2,5-Hexanediol ⇄ 2,5-Hexanedione

FIGURE 106–2. The metabolism of both organic solvents *n*-hexane and methyl *n*-butyl ketone produce the same common metabolite, 2,5-hexanedione.

the urinary excretion of hippuric acid (Table 106-2).[30,80] Renal potassium loss may be severe and can result in symptomatic hypokalemia.[80] Clinical findings are a hyperchloremic metabolic acidosis, hypokalemia, and aciduria. Typically an associated transient azotemia occurs, as well as proteinuria and an active urine sediment.[148,166] Some have reported a proximal RTA, or the Fanconi syndrome.[105,166] A metabolic acidosis resulting from the metabolism of toluene to benzyl alcohol through alcohol dehydrogenase to benzoic acid may be an adequate explanation for the serum and urine acid–base disturbances.

PINE OIL AND TERPENES

Pine oil is an active ingredient in many household cleaning products. It is a mixture of unsaturated hydrocarbons comprised of terpenes, camphenes, and pinenes. The major components are terpenes, which are found in plants and flowers. Wood distillates are products derived from pine trees and include pine oil and turpentine. Patients who ingest pine oil often emit a strong pine odor. Wood distillates are readily absorbed from the gastrointestinal tract and ingestion may cause CNS and pulmonary toxicity without aspiration.

The clinical features of pine oil ingestion can include CNS depression, respiratory failure, and gastrointestinal dysfunction and are rarely fatal.[85,171] Aspiration pneumonitis remains the primary clinical concern. Acute toxicity is similar to that of petroleum distillate ingestion, and management is similar. Rare reported complications of wood distillate ingestion include turpentine-associated thrombocytopenic purpura, acute renal failure, and hemorrhagic cystitis.[90,167]

TAR AND ASPHALT INJURY

Tar and asphalt injuries are common occupational hazards among construction workers. Asphalt workers are at risk for toxic gas exposure of hydrogen sulfide, carbon monoxide, propane, methane, and volatilized hydrocarbons.[70] In addition, cutaneous exposure to these hot hydrocarbon mixtures can cause severe burns. The material quickly hardens and is very difficult to remove. However immediate cooling with cold water is important to limit further thermal injury. Complete removal is essential to ensure proper burn management and to limit infectious complications. Attempts to mechanically remove hardened tar or asphalt often cause further damage. Dissolving the material with mineral oil, petroleum jelly, or antibacterial ointments are met with variable success. Surface-active agents combined with an ointment (De-Solv-it, Tween-80, Polysorbate 80) are more effective.[41,147,158]

DIAGNOSTIC TESTING

Laboratory and ancillary testing for hydrocarbon toxicity should be guided by available information regarding the specific xenobiotic, the route of exposure, and the best attempt at quantifying the exposure. Inhalation or ingestion of hydrocarbons associated with pulmonary aspiration is most likely to result in pulmonary toxicity. The use of pulse oximetry and arterial blood gas testing in this group of patients is warranted when clinically indicated. Early radiography is indicated in patients who are severely symptomatic; however, radiographs performed immediately after hydrocarbon ingestion demonstrate a low predictive value for the occurrence of aspiration pneumonitis. In the asymptomatic patient, early radiography is not cost-effective. Patients observed for 6 hours after an ingestion, who demonstrate no abnormal pulmonary findings, have adequate oxygenation, are not tachypneic, and have a normal chest radiograph after the 6-hour observation period, have a good medical prognosis with very low risk of subsequent deterioration.[9,168]

The choice of specific diagnostic laboratory tests to assess organ system toxicity or function following exposure to a hydrocarbon depends on the type, dose, and route of exposure, and on the assessment of the patient's clinical condition. Useful clinical tests may include pulse oximetry and an electrocardiogram (ECG).[116] Laboratory tests include serum or urine electrolytes, arterial blood gas, complete blood counts, and creatine phosphokinase. If a hydrocarbon has specific target organ toxicities (eg, benzene/bone marrow, carbon tetrachloride/liver, or *n*-hexane/peripheral nervous system), evaluating and monitoring target organ system function is indicated.

Specific diagnostic testing for hydrocarbon poisoning can include (1) bioassays for the specific hydrocarbon or its metabolites in blood, breath, or urine, or (2) assessment of toxicity. Bioassays for a hydrocarbon are seldom necessary for diagnosis or management of hydrocarbon poisoning in the emergency setting and rarely clinically available. Exceptions might include testing to assist in differential diagnosis (eg, testing for carbon tetrachloride in a comatose patient with unexplained hepatic and renal toxicity or a carboxyhemoglobin determination in a paint stripper with chest pain), testing for worker compensation purposes (eg, testing for urinary trichloroethanol and trichloroacetic acid in a worker exposed to trichloroethylene with unexplained bouts of dizziness), or for forensic purposes (eg, sudden death in a huffer).

When deciding whether to obtain a bioassay for a hydrocarbon, the clinician should determine the following: (1) What is the most informative biologic sample (blood, urine, breath) and how should it be collected, handled, and stored? (2) What are the kinetics of the hydrocarbon and the timing of exposure, and how should the results be interpreted in light of these kinetics? (3) What ranges of concentrations are associated with toxicity? Most hydrocarbon bioassays are performed by only a few, specialized clinical laboratories. The analytic toxicologist can often assist the clinician in determining the appropriate choice and timing of a bioassay. Table 106-2 provides useful information on the elimination kinetics of selected hydrocarbons and on their common metabolites.

Chronic overexposures to hydrocarbons, as occur with volatile substance use, can result in persistent damage to the central nervous system. Damage can be detected and quantified using neuroimaging methods such as magnetic resonance imaging (MRI) or positron emission tomography (PET). Major MRI findings in patients with chronic toluene abuse include atrophy, white matter T2 hyperintensity, and T2 hypointensity involving the basal ganglia and thalamus.[29] Neurobehavioral testing can be used to detect subtle central nervous system effects following chronic occupational overexposures.

MANAGEMENT

Identification of the specific type, route, and amount of hydrocarbon exposure is rarely essential to achieve effective management.

Decontamination is one of the cardinal principles of toxicology, with priority that is second only to stabilization of the cardiopulmonary status. Safe decontamination can avoid further absorption and avoids secondary casualties in those attempting to provide care. Protection of rescuers with appropriate personal protective equipment and rescue protocols is paramount, especially in situations where the victim has lost consciousness. The principle of removing the patient from the exposure (eg, vapor or gaseous hydrocarbon) or the exposure from the patient (eg, hydrocarbon liquid on skin or clothing), while protecting the rescuer, implies that personal protective equipment be considered at each level of the healthcare delivery system.

Exposed clothing should be removed and safely discarded as further absorption or inhalation of hydrocarbons from grossly contaminated clothing can worsen systemic toxicity.[145] Decontamination of the skin

TABLE 106–3. Orogastric Lavage for Hydrocarbon Ingestion

Contraindications
- Occurrence of spontaneous vomiting
- Asymptomatic initally and at initial medical evaluation

Indications
- Hydrocarbons with inherent systemic toxicity (CHAMP)
  - C: camphor
  - H: halogenated hydrocarbons
  - A: aromatic hydrocarbons
  - M: hydrocarbons containing metals
  - P: hydrocarbons containing pesticides

should have a high priority in massive hydrocarbon exposures, particularly those exposures involving highly toxic hydrocarbons (Table 106–3). Water alone may be ineffective in decontaminating most hydrocarbons, but early decontamination with soap and water may be adequate. The caregiver should remain aware that certain hydrocarbons are highly flammable and pose a fire risk to hospital staff (see Chap. 130).

Several studies have attempted to evaluate the role of gastric decontamination after hydrocarbon ingestion. Results were largely inconclusive and the level of evidence, poor. In the subset of patients who were randomized to receive gastric lavage, 44% had pulmonary complications, compared with 47% of those who were not lavaged. Available studies do not offer a conclusive answer to the question of gastric emptying after hydrocarbon ingestion.[122]

In the absence of a contraindication, gastric emptying is potentially useful only when the hydrocarbon has inherent severe toxicity or is co-ingested with a more potent xenobiotic (Table 106-3). Patients who have no symptoms at home or upon initial medical evaluation are unlikely to need gastric emptying.[9,95] For patients who do undergo gastric emptying, gastric lavage is likely the superior method.[109,110,122] If lavage is performed, a small nasogastric tube (18-French, not a large-bore tube) should be employed. If no gag reflex is present, an endotracheal tube should be placed prior to lavage (Chap. 7).

Activated charcoal (AC) has limited ability to decrease gastrointestinal absorption of hydrocarbons and may distend the stomach and predispose patients to vomiting and aspiration.[90,102,169] The use of AC may be justified in patients with mixed overdoses, but its role in isolated hydrocarbon ingestions appears very limited. The use of cathartics and promotility agents for hydrocarbon ingestions is also of limited importance in current management.

The use of olive oil or mineral oil was previously suggested as management for hydrocarbon ingestions.[15,51,179] Although these hydrocarbon oils have very high viscosities and low aspiration potential, they show no benefit in animal models,[102] can cause hydrocarbon pneumonitis and lipoid pneumonia themselves, and are therefore not indicated.[39]

Antibiotics are frequently administered in the setting of hydrocarbon pneumonitis to treat possible bacterial superinfection.[36,71,88,112,122,163] In experimental models, superinfection occurs as rapidly as 7 hours after aspiration.[71] Using radiolabeled *Staphylococcus aureus,* hydrocarbon-injured lungs were shown to have a decreased ability to clear bacteria by 4 hours after insult.[27]

Despite this, animal models, including guinea pigs, dogs, and baboons, did not demonstrate any efficacy of prophylactic antibiotics.[24,142,175] One study showed that administered antibiotic altered bacterial lung flora to predominantly Gram-negative organisms, compared to Gram-positive lung cultures in the controls.[24] These studies led to decreased use of prophylactic antibiotics, so that clinical evidence of infection dictated therapy for most clinicians.[44] This approach, however, is not without limitations. Abnormal lung auscultation, fever, leukocytosis, and abnormal radiographic findings are the initial manifestations of both bacterial pneumonia and hydrocarbon pneumonitis. Abnormal temperatures are reported to occur in 50%–90% of patients with hydrocarbon toxicity.[15,36,112,114] An elevated temperature is often initially noted, with the temperature reaching maximum at 8–12 hours, then declining over several days.[36,114] Leukocytosis is frequently reported, present in up to 60% of patients who aspirate hydrocarbons.[112,114,125]

Antibiotic administration may be justified in severely poisoned patients. Ideally, sputum cultures should direct antibiotic use. These, however, are often delayed and are not useful in critically ill patients. Most authorities do not recommend prophylactic antibiotics. Most recommend close observation of temperature and blood leukocyte count, as delayed elevation (24 hours after presentation) of temperature and/or leukocytes may signal bacterial superinfection. No human studies are available to support either approach, and this issue remains controversial.

Corticosteroids, like antibiotics, have been prophylactically administered in the setting of hydrocarbon pulmonary toxicity.[59,122] The rationale for their use is prevention and limitation of the inflammatory response in the lungs after hydrocarbon injury. Animal models do not show any benefit of corticosteroid administration.[6,24,142] In one study, corticosteroids increased the risk for bacterial superinfection with or without concomitant antibiotics.[24] Furthermore, two controlled human trials failed to show a benefit from corticosteroid administration.[66,97] It is clear that corticosteroid use does not improve the acute course of hydrocarbon pulmonary toxicity, although some authors suggest improved outcome with delayed corticosteroid therapy there is little supporting evidence.[79,84] Coupled with the possible increased risk of bacterial superinfection, corticosteroid administration in this setting is not recommended.

Patients with severe hydrocarbon toxicity pose unique problems for management. Respiratory distress requiring mechanical ventilation in this setting may be associated with a large ventilation–perfusion mismatch. The use of positive end-expiratory pressure (PEEP) in this setting is often beneficial. However, very high levels of PEEP may be required with subsequent increased risk of barotrauma.[131,180] High-frequency jet ventilation (HFJV), using very high respiratory rates (220–260) with small tidal volumes, has helped to decrease the need for PEEP.[28] Patients who continue to have severe ventilation–perfusion mismatch despite PEEP and HFJV have benefitted from extracorporeal membrane oxygenation (ECMO).[67,73,180] ECMO appears to be a useful option in severe pulmonary toxicity after other treatments have failed.

Cyanosis is uncommon after hydrocarbon toxicity. Although this is most often caused by severe hypoxia, methemoglobinemia associated with hydrocarbon exposure is reported.[35,91] The potential for methemoglobinemia should be investigated in patients who remain cyanotic following normalization of arterial oxygen tension.

Hypotension in severe hydrocarbon toxicity raises additional concerns. The etiology of hypotension in this setting is often compromise of cardiac output because of high levels of PEEP. Hydrocarbons do not have significant direct cardiovascular effects, and decreasing the PEEP may improve hemodynamics. The use of β-adrenergic agonists such as dopamine, epinephrine, isoproterenol, and norepinephrine should be avoided if possible, as certain hydrocarbons predispose to dysrhythmias.[14,126]

Management of dysrhythmias associated with hydrocarbon toxicity should include consideration of electrolyte and acid–base abnormalities such as hypokalemia and acidosis result from toluene, hypoxemia, hypotension, and hypothermia. Ventricular fibrillation poses a specific concern, as common resuscitation algorithms recommend epinephrine administration to treat this rhythm. If it is ascertained that the dysrhythmia emanates from myocardial sensitization by a hydrocarbon solvent, catecholamines should be avoided. In this setting, lidocaine has been used successfully, as have β-adrenergic antagonists.[103]

Hyperbaric oxygen (HBO) was studied in a rat model of severe kerosene-induced pneumonitis.[134] HBO at 4 ATA showed some benefit in 24-hour survival rates. No followup studies have been performed. Patients with carbon tetrachloride poisoning, however, may benefit from hyperbaric oxygen (see Antidotes in Depth A37: Hyperbaric Oxygen).[26,157]

In the past, hospital admission was routinely recommended for patients who had ingested hydrocarbons, because of concern over possible delayed symptom onset and progression of toxicity.[36,60] Several reports documented patients with relatively asymptomatic presentations who rapidly decompensated with respiratory compromise. However, progressive symptoms after hydrocarbon ingestion are rare.[9,95] In a retrospective study of 950 patients, only 14 (1.5%) had progression of pulmonary toxicity.[9] Of these 14, seven had persistence of symptoms for less than 24 hours. Eight hundred patients were asymptomatic on initial evaluation with normal chest radiographs, remained asymptomatic after 6–8 hours of observation, and had a normal repeat radiograph. No patient in this group of 800 had progressive symptoms, and all were discharged without clinical deterioration. Seventy-one of the 950 patients had initial respiratory symptoms but were asymptomatic at initial medical evaluation. Of the 71 patients, 36 had radiographic evidence of pneumonitis. Among these 36 patients, 2 (6%) developed progression of pulmonary symptoms during their 6-hour observation period. Of the 35 who had a normal radiograph, 2 (6%) developed pulmonary symptoms and radiographic pneumonitis during the 6-hour observation period. The four patients who were hospitalized for progression of symptoms became asymptomatic over the next 24 hours and had no complications.

A separate poison center-based study evaluated 120 asymptomatic patients for an 18-hour telephone followup period.[95] Sixty-two patients had initial pulmonary symptoms that quickly resolved. One of the 62 patients (1.6%) developed progressive pulmonary toxicity. This patient was hospitalized and had resolution of symptoms within 24 hours without complications.

A number of investigators have suggested protocols for determining which patients can be safely discharged.[9,83,95] None of these protocols has been prospectively validated. However, rational guidelines for hospitalization can be recommended. Those patients who have clinical evidence of toxicity, and most individuals with intentional ingestions, should be hospitalized. Patients who do not have any initial symptoms, have normal chest radiographs obtained at least 6 hours after ingestion, and who do not develop symptoms during the 6-hour observation period can be safely discharged. Care should be individualized for patients who are asymptomatic but who have radiographic evidence of hydrocarbon pneumonitis, and for patients who have initial respiratory symptoms but quickly become asymptomatic during medical evaluation. Reliable patients may be considered for possible discharge with next-day followup.

SUMMARY

Hydrocarbons are a diverse group of xenobiotics that can cause toxicity by inhalation, ingestion, or dermal absorption. Most hydrocarbons occur as mixtures of several to many chemicals. Ubiquitous use of hydrocarbons in our society means that exposures are extremely common. Populations at particular risk for toxicity include children who ingest hydrocarbon compounds, workers who are occupationally exposed by inhalation or dermal absorption, and youths who intentionally inhale volatile hydrocarbons.

Toxicity is largely determined by the route of exposure, and is xenobiotic-specific. Aspiration pneumonitis is the primary concern after hydrocarbon ingestion. Many hydrocarbons are poorly absorbed from the gastrointestinal tract and unlikely to produce systemic poisoning. Acute systemic toxicity is unlikely to occur in the absence of CNS effects such as excitation or sedation. Most hydrocarbons are capable of producing profound CNS depression, even general anesthesia if absorbed systemically.

Specific hydrocarbons may demonstrate specific organ toxicity: halogenated hydrocarbons are cardiotoxic, hepatotoxic, and nephrotoxic. Most are also acutely toxic to the CNS and some are peripheral neurotoxins. Diagnosis is predominantly clinical. Diagnostic studies are rarely specific, and hydrocarbon-specific studies are seldom helpful in the acute setting. Skin decontamination is important in massive dermal exposures. Gastrointestinal decontamination, as well as the use of prophylactic antibiotics or corticosteroids are rarely if ever indicated initially. Management is largely supportive, and no specific antidotes are available.

REFERENCES

1. Adler R, Robinson RG, Binkin NJ. Intravascular hemolysis: an unusual complication of hydrocarbon ingestion. *J Pediatr.* 1976;89:679-680.
2. Agency for Toxic Substances and Disease Registry (ATSDR). Toxicological Profile for Toluene. Washington, DC: US Public Health Service; 2000.
3. Agency for Toxic Substances and Disease Registry (ATSDR). Toxicological Profile for Total Petroleum Hydrocarbons. Washington, DC: US Public Health Service; 1999.
4. Ahmed AE, Kubic VL, Stevens JL, et al. Halogenated methanes: metabolism and toxicity. *Fed Proc.* 1980;39:3150-3155.
5. Aksoy M, Erdem S, Dincol G, et al. Aplastic anemia due to chemicals and drugs: a study of 108 patients. *Sex Transm Dis.* 1984;11(4 Suppl):347-350.
6. Albert WC. The efficacy of steroid therapy in the treatment of experimental kerosene pneumonitis. *Am Rev Respir Di.s* 1968;98:888-889.
7. Algren JT, Rodgers GC. Intravascular hemolysis associated with hydrocarbon poisoning. *Pediatr Emerg Care.* 1992;8:34-35.
8. Altenkirch H, Stoltenburg G, Wagner HM. Experimental studies on hydrocarbon neuropathies induced by methyl-ethyl-ketone (MEK). *J Neurol.* 1978;219:159-170.
9. Anas N, Namasonthi V, Ginsburg CM. Criteria for hospitalizing children who have ingested products containing hydrocarbon. *JAMA* 1981. 246:840-843.
10. Ashford NA. New scientific evidence and public health imperatives. *N Engl J Med.* 1987;316:1084-1085.
11. Baldachin BJ, Melmed RN. Clinical and therapeutic aspects of kerosene poisoning: a series of 200 cases. *Br Med J.* 1964;2:28-30.
12. Ban M, Hettich D, Bonnet P. Effect of inhaled industrial chemicals on systemic and local immune response. *Toxicology.* 2003;184:41-50.
13. Bass M. Death from sniffing gasoline. *N Engl J Med.* 1978;299:203.
14. Bass M. Sudden sniffing death. *JAMA.* 1970;212:2075-2079.
15. Beamon RF, Siegel CJ, Landers G, et al. Hydrocarbon ingestion in children: a six-year retrospective study. *JACEP.* 1976;5:771-775.
16. Beckstead MJ, Weiner JL, Eger EI, et al. Glycine and gamma-aminobutyric $acid_A$ receptor function is enhanced by inhaled drugs of abuse. *Mol Pharmacol.* 2000;57:1199-1205.
17. Bergeson PS, Hales SW, Lustgarten MD, Lipow HW. Pneumatoceles following hydrocarbon ingestion. Report of three cases and review of the literature. *Am J Dis Child.* 1975;129:49-54.
18. Bleecker ML; Bolla KI; Agnew J, et al. Dose-related subclinical neurobehavioral effects of chronic exposure to low levels of organic solvents. *Am J Ind Med.* 1991;19:715-728.
19. Bombassei GJ, Kaplan AA. The association between hydrocarbon exposure and anti-glomerular basement membrane antibody-mediated disease (Goodpasture's syndrome). *Am J Ind Med.* 1992;21:141-153.

20. Bos PM, de Mik G, Bragt PC. Critical review of the toxicity of methyl *n*-butyl ketone: risk from occupational exposure. *Am J Ind Med.* 1991;20:175-194.
21. Bratton L, Haddow JE. Ingestion of charcoal lighter fluid. *J Pediatr.* 1975;87:633-636.
22. Brent JA, Rumack BH. Role of free radicals in toxic hepatic injury: II. Are free radicals the cause of toxin-induced liver injury? *J Toxicol Clin Toxicol.* 1993;31:173-196.
23. Brock WJ, Rusch GM, Trochimowicz HJ. Cardiac sensitization: methodology and interpretation in risk assessment. *Regul Toxicol Pharmacol.* 2003;38:78-90.
24. Brown J III, Burke B, Dajani AS, et al. Experimental kerosene pneumonia: Evaluation of some therapeutic regimens. *J Pediatr.* 1974;84:396-401.
25. Brunner S, Rovsing H, Wulf H. Roentgenographic change in the lungs of children with kerosene poisoning. *Am Rev Respir Dis.*1964;89:250-254.
26. Burkhart KK, Hall AH, Gerace R, et al. Hyperbaric oxygen treatment for carbon tetrachloride poisoning. *Drug Saf.* 1991;6:332-338.
27. Burley S, Huber G. The effect of toxic agents commonly ingested by children on antibacterial defenses in the lung. *Proc Soc Pediatr Res.*1971;16:83.
28. Bysani GK, Rucoba RJ, Noah ZL. Treatment of hydrocarbon pneumonitis. High frequency jet ventilation as an alternative to extracorporeal membrane oxygenation. *Chest.* 1994;106:300-303.
29. Caldemeyer KS, Armstrong SW, George KK, et al. The spectrum of neuroimaging abnormalities in solvent abuse and their clinical correlation. *J Neuroimaging.* 1996;6:167-173.
30. Carlisle EJ, Donnelly SM, Vasuvattakul S, et al. Glue-sniffing and distal renal tubular acidosis: sticking to the facts. *J Am Soc Nephrol.* 1991;1:1019-1027.
31. Cavanagh JB, Buxton PH. Trichloroethylene cranial neuropathy: is it really a toxic neuropathy or does it activate latent herpes virus? *J Neurol Neurosurg Psychiatr.* 1989;52:297-303.
32. Centers for Disease Control and Prevention. *n*-Hexane–related peripheral neuropathy among automotive technicians—California, 1999–2000. *MMWR Morb Mortal Wkly Rep.* 2001;50:1011-1013.
33. Chang YC. Neurotoxic effects of *n*-hexane on the human central nervous system: evoked potential abnormalities in *n*-hexane polyneuropathy. *J Neurol Neurosurg Psychiatry.* 1987;50:269-274.
34. Clayton GD, Clayton FE, eds. *Patty's Industrial Hygiene and Toxicology, Vol. 2B: Toxicology,* 3rd ed. New York: John Wiley; 1981.
35. Curry S. Methemoglobinemia. *Ann Emerg Med.* 1982;11:214-221.
36. Daeschner CW, Blattner RJ, Collins VP. Hydrocarbon pneumonitis. *Pediatr Clin North Am.* 1957;4:243-253.
37. Daffner RH, Jimenez JP. The double gastric fluid level in kerosene poisoning. *Pediatr Radiol.* 1973;106:383-384.
38. Das M, Misra MP. Acne and folliculitis due to diesel oil. *Contact Dermatitis.* 1988;18:120-121.
39. De la Rocha SR, Cunningham JC, Fox E. Lipoid pneumonia secondary to baby oil aspiration: a case report and review of the literature. *Pediatr Emerg Care.* 1985;1:74-80.
40. Decoufle P, Blattner WA, Blair A. Mortality among chemical workers exposed to benzene and other agents. *Environ Res.* 1983;30:16-25.
41. Demling RH, Buerstatte WR, Perea A. Management of hot tar burns. *J Trauma.* 1980;20:242.
42. Dildy-Mayfield JE, Eger EI, Harris RA. Anesthetics produce subunit-selective actions on glutamate receptors. *J Pharmacol Exp Ther.* 1996;276: 1058-1065.
43. Dilger JP. The effects of general anaesthetics on ligand-gated ion channels. *Br J Anaesth.* 2002;89:41-51.
44. Eade NR, Taussig LM, Marks MI. Hydrocarbon pneumonitis. *Pediatrics.* 1974;54:351-357.
45. Feldman RG, Chirico-Post J, Proctor SP. Blink reflex latency after exposure to trichloroethylene in well water. *Arch Environ Health.* 1988;43:143-148.
46. Feldman RG, Ratner MH, Ptak T. Chronic toxic encephalopathy in a painter exposed to mixed solvents. *Environ Health Perspect.* 1999;107:417-422.
47. Feldman RG, White RF, Currie JN, et al. Long-term follow-up after single toxic exposure to trichloroethylene. *Am J Ind Med.* 1985;8:119-126.
48. Fialkov JA, Freiberg A. High pressure injection injuries: an overview. *J Emerg Med.* 1991;9:367-371.
49. Filley CM, Franklin GM, Heaton RK, Rosenberg NL. White matter dementia:clinical disorders and implications. *Neuropsychiatry Neuropsychol Behav Neurol.* 1988;1:239-254.
50. Finkel AJ, ed. *Hamilton and Hardy's Industrial Toxicology,* 4th ed. Boston: John Wright;1983.
51. Foley JC, Dreyer NB, Soule AB, et al. Kerosene poisoning in young children. *Radiology.* 1954;62:817-829.
52. Fornazzari L, Pollanen MS, Myers V, Wolf A. Solvent abuse-related toluene leukoencephalopathy. *J Clin Forensic Med.* 2003;10:93-95.
53. Gargas ML, Burgess RJ, Voisard DE, et al. Partition coefficients of low-molecular-weight volatile chemicals in various liquids and tissues. *Toxicol Appl Pharmacol.* 1989;98:87-99.
54. Gash DM, Rutland K, Hudson NL, et al. Trichloroethylene: parkinsonism and complex 1 mitochondrial neurotoxicity. *Ann Neurol.* 2008;63:184-92.
55. Gerarde HW. Toxicological studies on hydrocarbons: IX. The aspiration hazard and toxicity of hydrocarbons and hydrocarbon mixtures. *Arch Environ Health.* 1963;6:329-341.
56. Gershon-Cohen J, Bringhurst LS, Byrne RN. Roentgenography of kerosene poisoning. *Am J Roentgenol.* 1953;69:557.
57. Gosselin RE, Smith RP, Hodge HC, eds. *Clinical Toxicology of Commercial Products,* 5th ed. Baltimore: Williams & Wilkins; 1984.
58. Graham DG. Neurotoxicants and the cytoskeleton. *Curr Opin Neurol.* 1999;12:733-737.
59. Graham JR. Pneumonitis following aspiration of crude oil and its treatment by steroid hormones. *Trans Am Clin Climatol Assoc.* 1955–1956;67: 104-112.
60. Griffin JW, Daeschner CV, Collins VP, et al. Hydrocarbon pneumonitis following furniture polish ingestion. *J Pediatr.* 1954;13:13-26.
61. Gross P, McNerney JM, Babyak MA. Kerosene pneumonitis: an experimental study with small doses. *Am Rev Respir Dis.* 1963;88:656-663.
62. Gurwitz D, Katten M, Levison H, et al. Pulmonary function abnormalities in symptomatic children after hydrocarbon pneumonitis. *Pediatrics.*1978;62:789-794.
63. Hake CL, Stewart RD. Human exposure to tetrachloroethylene: inhalation and skin contact. *Environ Health Perspect.* 1977;21:231-238.
64. Halsey MJ. Physical chemistry applied to anaesthetic action. *Br J Anaesth.* 1974;46:172-180.
65. Hansbrough JF, Zapata-Sirvent R, Dominic W, et al. Hydrocarbon contact injuries. *J Trauma.* 1985;25:250-252.
66. Hardman G, Tolson R, Hadhdassarian O. Prednisone in the management of kerosene pneumonia. *Indian Pract.* 1960;13:615-620.
67. Hart LM, Cobaugh DJ, Dean BS, et al. Successful use of extracorpo-real membrane oxygenation (ECMO) in the treatment of refractory respiratory failure secondary to hydrocarbon aspiration. *Vet Hum Toxicol.* 1991;33:361.
68. Hemmings HC, Yan W, Westphalen RI, et al. The general anesthetic isoflurane depresses synaptic vesicle exocytosis. *Mol Pharmacol.* 2005;67:1591-9.
69. Herskowitz A, Ishii N, Schaumburg H. *n*-Hexane neuropathy: a syndrome occurring as a result of industrial exposure. *N Engl J Med.* 1971;285:82-85.
70. Hoidal CR, Hall AH, Robinson ND, et al. Hydrogen sulfide poisoning from toxic inhalations of roofing asphalt fumes. *Ann Emerg Med.* 1986;15:826-830.
71. Ikeda K. Oil aspiration pneumonia (lipoid pneumonia): clinical, pathologic and experimental consideration. *Am J Dis Child.* 1935;49:985-1006.
72. International Programme on Chemical Safety. Benzene: Environmental Health Criteria. Pub. 150. Geneva: World Health Organization; 199328-43.
73. Jaeger RW, Scalzo AS, Thompson MW. ECMO in hydrocarbon aspiration. *Vet Hum Toxicol.*1987;29:485.
74. James FW, Kaplan S, Bensing G. Cardiac complications following hydrocarbon ingestion. *Am J Dis Child.* 1971;121:431-433.
75. Janssen S, van der Geest S, Meijer S, et al. Impairment of organ function after oral ingestion of refined petrol. *Intensive Care Med.* 1988;14:238-240.
76. Javier Perez A, Courel M, Sobrado J, Gonzalez L. Acute renal failure after topical application of carbon tetrachloride. *Lancet.* 1987;1:515-516.
77. Jiao Z, De Jesús VR, Iravanian S, et al. A possible mechanism of halocarbon-induced cardiac sensitization arrhythmias. *J Mol Cell Cardiol.* 2006;41: 698-705.
78. Joron GE, Cameron DG, Halpenny GW. Massive necrosis of the liver due to trichloroethylene. *Can Med Assoc J.* 1955;73:890-891.
79. Kamijo Y, Soma K, Asari Y, Ohwada T. Pulse steroid therapy in adult respiratory distress syndrome following petroleum naphtha ingestion. *J Toxicol Clin Toxicol.* 2000;38:59-62.
80. Kao KC, Tsai YH, Lin MC, et al. Hypokalemic muscular paralysis causing acute respiratory failure due to rhabdomyolysis with renal tubular acidosis in a chronic glue sniffer. *J Toxicol Clin Toxicol.* 2000; 38:679-681.

81. Kaysen GA. Renal toxicology. In: La Dou J, ed. *Occupational Medicine.* Norwalk, CT: Appleton & Lange; 1994;259-260.
82. King PJ, Morris JG, Pollard JD. Glue sniffing neuropathy. *Aust N Z J Med.* 1985;15:293-299.
83. Klein BL, Simon JE. Hydrocarbon poisonings. *Pediatr Clin North Am.* 1986;33:411-419.
84. Kollef MH, Schuster DP. The acute respiratory distress syndrome. *N Engl J Med.* 1995;332:27-37.
85. Koppel C, Tenczer J, Tonnesmann U, et al. Acute poisoning with pine oil—metabolism of monoterpenes. *Arch Toxicol.* 1981;49:73-78.
86. Kornfeld M, Moser AB, Moser HW. Solvent vapor abuse leukoencephalopathy. Comparison to adrenoleukodystrophy. *J Neuropathol Exp Neurol.*1994;53:389-398.
87. Krasowski MD, Harrison NL. General anaesthetic actions on ligand-gated ion channels. *Cell Mol Life Sci.* 1999;55:1278-303.
88. Kulig K, Rumack B. Hydrocarbon ingestion. *Curr Top Emerg Med.* 1981;3:1-5.
89. Kwong YL, Chan TK. Toxic occupational exposures and paroxysmal nocturnal haemoglobinuria. *Lancet.* 1993;341:443.
90. Laass W. Therapy of acute oral poisonings by organic solvents: treatment by activated charcoal in combination with laxatives. *Arch Toxicol.*1980;4(Suppl):406-409.
91. Lareng L. Acute toxic methemoglobinemia from accidental ingestion of nitrobenzene. *Eur J Toxicol.* 1974;7:12-16.
92. Leandri M, Schizzi R, Scielzo C, et al. Electrophysiological evidence of trigeminal root damage after trichloroethylene exposure. *Muscle Nerve.* 1995;18:467-468.
93. Liao JT, Oehme FW. Literature reviews of phenolic compounds: I. Phenol. *Vet Hum Toxicol.* 1980;22:160-164.
94. Lundberg I, Hogstedt C, Liden C, Nise G. Organic solvents and related compounds. In: Rosenstock L, Cullen MR, eds. *Clinical Occupational and Environmental Medicine.* Philadelphia: WB Saunders; 1994:766-784.
95. Machado B, Cross K, Snodgrass WR, Accidental hydrocarbon ingestion cases telephoned to a regional poison center. *Ann Emerg Med.* 1988;17:804-807.
96. Mann MD, Pirie DJ, Wolfsdorf J. Kerosene absorption in primates. *J Pediatr.* 1977;91:495-498.
97. Marks MI, Chicoine L, Legere G, et al. Adrenocorticosteroid treatment of hydrocarbon pneumonia in children—a cooperative study. *J Pediatr.* 1972;81:366-369.
98. Matsumoto T, Koga M, Sata T, et al. The changes of gasoline compounds in blood in a case of gasoline intoxication. *J Toxicol Clin Toxicol.* 1992;30:653-662.
99. McNally WD. Kerosene poisoning in children. *J Pediatr.* 1956;48: 296-299.
100. Mehlman MA. Benzene health effects: unanswered questions still not addressed. *Am J Ind Med.* 1991;20:707-711.
101. Meredith TJ, Ruprah M, Liddle A, et al. Diagnosis and treatment of acute poisoning with volatile substances. *Hum Toxicol.* 1989;8:277-286.
102. Morgan DP. Effectiveness of activated charcoal, mineral oil, and castor oil in limiting gastrointestinal absorption of a chlorinated hydrocarbon pesticide. *Clin Toxicol.* 1977;11:61-70.
103. Moritz F, de La Chapelle A, Bauer F, et al. Esmolol in the treatment of severe arrhythmia after acute trichloroethylene poisoning. *Intensive Care Med.* 2000;26:256.
104. Morrison RT, Boyd RN. *Organic Chemistry,* 6th ed. Englewood Cliffs, NJ: Prentice Hall; 1992:.92-118.
105. Moss AH, Gabow PA, Kaehny WD, et al. Fanconi's syndrome and distal renal tubular acidosis after glue sniffing. *Ann Intern Med.* 1980;92:69-70.
106. Mrvos R, Dean BS, Krenzelok EP. High pressure injection injuries: a serious occupational hazard. *J Toxicol Clin Toxicol.*1987;25:297-304.
107. National Research Council. Assessing the Human Health Risks of Trichloroethylene. Washington, DC: National Academies Press; 2006. Available at http://www.nap.edu/catalog/11707.html, accessed April 12, 2009.
108. Nelson DL, Cox MM, eds. *Lehninger Principles of Biochemistry,* 3rd ed. New York: Worth Publishing; 2000.
109. Ng RC, Using syrup of ipecac for ingestion of petroleum distillates. *Pediatr Ann.* 1977;6:708-710.
110. Ng RC, Darwish H, Stewart DA. Emergency treatment of petroleum distillate and turpentine ingestion. *Can Med Assoc J.* 1974;3:537-538.
111. Nierenberg DW, Horowitz MB, Harris KM, et al. Mineral spirits inhalation associated with hemolysis, pulmonary edema, and ventricular fibrillation. *Arch Intern Med.* 1991;151:1437-1440.
112. Nouri L, Al-Rahim K. Kerosene poisoning in children. *Postgrad Med J.* 1970;46:71.
113. Okuda M, Kunitsugu I, Kobayakawa S, et al. Inhibitory effect of 1,1,1-trichloroethane on calcium channels of neurons. *J Toxicol Sci.* 2001;26:169-76.
114. Olstad RB, Lord RM Jr. Kerosene intoxication. *Am J Dis Child.* 1952;83: 446-453.
115. Ott MG, Skory LK, Holder BB, et al. Health evaluation of employees occupationally exposed to methylene chloride. *Scand J Work Environ Health.* 1983;9(Suppl 1):1-38.
116. Ottelio C, Giagheddu M, Marrosu F. Altered EEG pattern in aromatic hydrocarbon intoxication: a case report. *Acta Neurol.* 1993;15:357-362.
117. Ouyang W, Herold KF, Hemmings HC. Comparative effects of halogenated inhaled anesthetics on voltage-gated [sodium] channel function. *Anesthesiology.* 2009;110:582-90.
118. Padday JF. Theory of surface tension. In: Matijevic E, ed. *Surface and Colloid Science, Vol. 1.* New York: Wiley-Interscience; 1969;39-149.
119. Paustenbach DJ, Bass RD, Price P. Benzene toxicity and risk assessment, 1972–1992: implications for future regulation. *Environ Health Perspect.* 1993;101(Suppl 6):177-200.
120. Pierce CH, Dills RL, Silvey GW, et al. Partition coefficients between human blood or adipose tissue and air for aromatic solvents. *Scand J Work Environ Health.* 1996;22:112-118.
121. Pollard BJ. Sites of drug action. In Hugh C. Hemmings HC, Hopkins PM, eds. *Foundations of Anesthesia: Basic Sciences for Clinical Practice*, 2nd ed. Philadelphia: Elsevier; 2006:91-100.
122. Press E, Adams WC, Chittenden RF. Cooperative kerosene poisoning study: evaluation of gastric lavage and other factors in the treatment of accidental ingestion of petroleum distillate products. *Pediatrics.* 1962;29:648-674.
123. Prockop L. Neurotoxic volatile substances. *Neurology.* 1979;29:862-865.
124. Raphael M, Nadiras P, Flacke-Vordos N. Acute methylene chloride intoxication—a case report on domestic poisoning. *Eur J Emerg Med.* 2002;9:57-59.
125. Reed ES, Leikin S, Kerman HD. Kerosene intoxication. *Am J Dis Child.* 1950;79:623-632.
126. Reinhardt CF, Mullin LS, Maxfield ME. Epinephrine-induced cardiac arrhythmia potential of some common industrial solvents. *J Occup Med.* 1973;15:953-955.
127. Richardson JA, Pratt-Thomas HR. Toxic effects of varying doses of kerosene administered by different routes. *Am J Med Sci.* 1951;221: 531-536.
128. Rinsky RA, Smith AB, Hornung R, et al. Benzene and leukemia: an epidemiologic risk assessment. *N Engl J Med.* 1987;316:1044-1050.
129. Rush MD, Schoenfeld CN, Watson WA. Skin necrosis and venous thrombosis from subcutaneous injection of charcoal lighter fluid (naphtha). *Am J Emerg Med.* 1998;16:508-511.
130. Saida K, Mendell JR, Weiss HS. Peripheral nerve changes induced by methyl n-butyl ketone and potentiation by methyl ethyl ketone. *J Neuropathol Exp Neurol.* 1976;35:207-225.
131. Scalzo AJ, Weber TR, Jaeger RW, et al. Extracorporeal membrane oxygenation for hydrocarbon aspiration. *Am J Dis Child.* 1990;144:867-871.
132. Schaumburg HH. Toluene. In: Spencer PS, Schaumburg HH (eds.) *Experimental and Clinical Neurotoxicology,* 2nd ed. New York: Oxford University Press; 2000:1183-1189.
133. Scholz EP, Alter M, Zitron E, et al. In vitro modulation of HERG channels by organochlorine solvent trichlormethane as potential explanation for proarrhythmic effects of chloroform. *Toxicol Lett.* 2006;165:156-166.
134. Schwartz SI, Breslau RC, Kutner F, et al. Effects of drugs and hyper-baric oxygen environment on experimental kerosene pneumonitis. *Dis Chest.* 1965;47:353-359.
135. Secher O. Physical and chemical data on anaesthetics. *Acta Anaesthesiol Scand.* Suppl. 1971;42:1-95.
136. Shafer TJ, Bushnell PJ, Benignus VA, et al. Perturbation of voltage-sensitive [calcium] channel function by volatile organic solvents. *J Pharmacol Exp Ther.* 2005;315:1109-1118.
137. Shin WJ, Winegar BD. Modulation of noninactivating K+ channels in rat cerebellar granule neurons by halothane, isoflurane, and sevoflurane. *Anesth Analg.* 2003;96:1340-1344.
138. Sikkema J, de Bont JA, Poolman B. Mechanisms of membrane toxicity of hydrocarbons. *Microbiol Rev.* 1995;59:201-222.
139. Smith AG, Albers JW. *n*-Hexane neuropathy due to rubber cement sniffing. *Muscle Nerve.* 1997;20:1445-1450.

140. Snyder R, Andrews LS. Toxic effects of solvents and vapors. In Klaassen CD, ed. *Casarett and Doull's Toxicology: The Basic Science of Poisons,* 5th ed. New York: McGraw-Hill; 1996:737-771.
141. Stadnicka A, Kwok WM, Hartmann HA, et al. Effects of halothane and isoflurane on fast and slow inactivation of human heart hH1a sodium channels. *Anesthesiology.* 1999;90:1671-1683.
142. Steele RW, Conklin RH, Mark HM. Corticosteroids and antibiotics for the treatment of fulminant hydrocarbon aspiration. *JAMA.* 1972; 219:1434-1437.
143. Steiner MM. Syndromes of kerosene poisoning in children. *Am J Dis Child.* 1947;74:32-44.
144. Stevenson A, Yaqoob M, Mason H, et al. Biochemical markers of basement membrane disturbances and occupational exposure to hydrocarbons and mixed solvents. *QJM.* 1995;88:23-28.
145. Stewart RD, Dodd HC. Absorption of carbon tetrachloride, trichloroethylene, tetrachloroethylene, methylene chloride and 1,1,1-trichloroethane through human skin. *Am Ind Hyg Assoc J.* 1964;25:439-446.
146. Stockman JA. More on hydrocarbon-induced hemolysis. *J Pediatr.* 1977;90:848.
147. Strata RJ, Saffle JR, Kravitz M, et al. Management of tar and asphalt injuries. *Am J Surg.* 1983;146:766-769.
148. Streicher HZ, Gabow PA, Moss AH, et al. Syndromes of toluene sniffing in adults. *Ann Intern Med.* 1981;94:758-762.
149. Szlatenyi CS, Wang RY. Encephalopathy and cranial nerve palsies caused by intentional trichloroethylene inhalation. *Am J Emerg Med.* 1996;14: 464-466.
150. Takeuchi Y, Ono Y, Hisanaga N, et al. A comparative study on the neurotoxicity of *n*-pentane, *n*-hexane, and *n*-heptane in the rat. *Br J Ind Med.* 1980;37:241-247.
151. Tang HL, Chu KH, Cheuk A, et al. Renal tubular acidosis and severe hypophosphataemia due to toluene inhalation. *Hong Kong Med J.* 2005;11:50-53.
152. Taussig LM, Castro E, Landau LI, et al. Pulmonary function 8–10 years after hydrocarbon pneumonitis. *Clin Pediatr.* 1977;16:57-59.
153. Tomenson JA, Baron CE, O'Sullivan JJ, et al. Hepatic function in workers occupationally exposed to carbon tetrachloride. *Occup Environ Med.* 1995;52:508-514.
154. Torkelson TR. Halogenated aliphatic hydrocarbons. In Clayton GD, Clayton FE, eds. *Patty's Industrial Hygiene and Toxicology,* 4th ed. New York: John Wiley; 1994:4064-4068.
155. Travis LB, Li CY, Zhang ZN, et al. Hematopoietic malignancies and related disorders among benzene-exposed workers in China. *Leuk Lymphoma.* 1994;14:91-102.
156. Truemper E, Reyes de la Rocha SR, Atkinson SD. Clinical characteristics, pathophysiology, and management of hydrocarbon ingestion. *Pediatr Emerg Care.* 1987;3:187-193.
157. Truss CD, Killenberg PG. Treatment of carbon tetrachloride poisoning with hyperbaric oxygen. *Gastroenterology.* 1982;82;767-769.
158. Tsou TJ, Hutson HR, Bear M, et al. De-solv-it for hot paving asphalt burn: case report. *Acad Emerg Med.* 1996;3:88-89.
159. Turkel B, Egeli U. Analysis of chromosomal aberrations in shoe workers exposed long term to benzene. *Occup Environ Med.* 1994;51:50-53.
160. United States Code of Federal Regulations. 16 CFR 1700.14. Available at http://www.access.gpo.gov/nara/cfr/waisidx_02/16cfr1700_02.html Accessed April 20, 2009.
161. Upreti RK, Das M, Shanker R. Dermal exposure to kerosene. *Vet Hum Toxicol.* 1989;31:16-20.
162. Vaziri ND, Smith PJ, Wilson A. Toxicity with intravenous injection of naphtha in man. *Clin Toxicol.* 1980;16:335-343.
163. Victoria MS, Nangia BS. Hydrocarbon poisoning: a review. *Pediatr Emerg Care.* 1987;3:184-186.
164. Vigliano EC, Saita G. Benzene and leukemia. *N Engl J Med.* 1964;271: 872-876.
165. Violet JM, Downie DL, Nakisa RC, et al. Differential sensitivities of mammalian neuronal and muscle nicotinic acetylcholine receptors to general anesthetics. *Anesthesiology.* 1997;86:866-874.
166. Voights A, Kaufman CE. Acidosis and other metabolic abnormalities associated with paint sniffing. *South Med J.* 1983;76:443-452.
167. Wahlberg P, Nyman D. Turpentine and thrombocytopenic purpura. *Lancet.* 1969;2:215-216.
168. Wason S, Katona B. A review of symptoms, signs and laboratory findings predictive of hydrocarbon toxicity [abstract]. *Vet Hum Toxicol.* 1987;29:492.
169. Watson WA, Weinman SA, ACE Study Group.Activated charcoal (AC) dosing and the prevalence and predictors of emesis [abstract]. *J Toxicol Clin Toxicol.*1995;33:489-490.
170. Weaver NK. Gasoline. In Sullivan JB, Krieger GR, eds. *Hazardous Materials Toxicology: Clinical Principles of Environmental Health.* Philadelphia: Williams & Wilkins; 1992:807-817.
171. Welker JA, Zaloga GP. Pine oil ingestion: a common cause of poisoning. *Chest.* 1999;116:1822-1826.
172. White MC, Infante PF, Chu KC. A quantitative estimate of leukemia mortality associated with occupational exposure to benzene. *Risk Anal.* 1982;2:195-204.
173. Widmer LR, Goodwin SR, Berman LS, et al. Artificial surfactant for therapy in hydrocarbon-induced lung injury in sheep. *Crit Care Med.* 1996;24:1524-1529.
174. Wirtschafter ZT, Cronyn MW. Relative hepatotoxicity. *Arch Environ Health.* 1964;9:1980-1985.
175. Wolfsdorf J. Experimental kerosene pneumonitis in primates: relevance to the therapeutic management of childhood poisoning. *Clin Exp Pharmacol Physiol.* 1976;3:539-544.
176. Wolfsdorf J. Kerosene intoxication: an experimental approach to the etiology of the CNS manifestations in primates. *J Pediatr.* 1976;88:1037-1040.
177. Yakes B, Kelsey KT, Seitz T, et al. Occupational skin disease in newspaper pressroom workers. *J Occup Med.* 1991;33:711-717.
178. Yamamura Y. *n*-Hexane polyneuropathy. *Folia Psychiatr Neurol Jpn.* 1969;23:45-57.
179. Zieserl E. Hydrocarbon ingestion and poisoning. *Compr Ther.* 1979;5:35-42.
180. Zucker AR, Berger S, Wood LDH. Management of kerosene-induced pulmonary injury. *Crit Care Med.* 1986;14:303-304.

CHAPTER 107
TOXIC ALCOHOLS

Sage W. Wiener

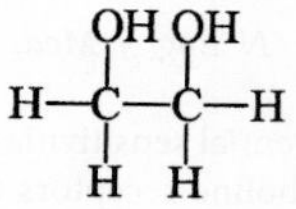

Ethylene glycol

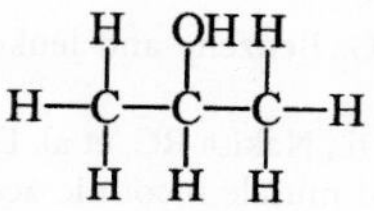

Isopropanol

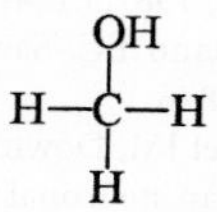

Methanol

Ethylene Glycol
MW = 62 Daltons
Isopropanol
MW = 60 Daltons
Methanol
MW = 32 Daltons

Toxic alcohols are important components of many household, automotive, and industrial products, and they are frequently implicated in suicidal, unintentional, and even epidemic poisoning. Consideration of toxic alcohols as a cause of illness is also often encountered clinically in the differential diagnosis of a metabolic acidosis with an elevated anion gap. Evaluation of these patients is complex, in part because serum concentrations are not readily available in many institutions. Treatment involves a choice between the antidotes fomepizole and ethanol in addition to multiple other therapeutic modalities including hemodialysis, bicarbonate, thiamine, pyridoxine, and folate. Further complicating matters, the role of hemodialysis remains controversial despite a long history of its effective use in treating patients poisoned by toxic alcohols.

HISTORY AND EPIDEMIOLOGY

Methanol was a component of the embalming fluid used in ancient Egypt. Robert Boyle first isolated the molecule in 1661 by distilling boxwood, calling it *spirit of box*.[23] The molecular composition was determined in 1834 by Dumas and Peligot, who coined the term *methylene* from the Greek roots for "wood wine."[145] Industrial production began in 1923, and today most methanol is used for the synthesis of other chemicals. Methanol-containing consumer products that are commonly encountered include model airplane fuel, windshield washer fluid, solid cooking fuel for camping and chafing dishes, photocopying fluid, perfumes, and gas line antifreeze ("dry gas"). Methanol is also used as a solvent by itself or as an adulterant in "denatured" alcohol.[95] Most reported cases of methanol poisoning in the United States involve ingestions of one of these products, with over 60% involving windshield washer fluid.[38] In a Tunisian series, ingested cologne was the most common etiology.[24] There have also been sporadic epidemics of mass methanol poisoning, most commonly involving tainted fermented beverages.[18,90] These epidemics are a continuing problem in many parts of the world.[12,105,133,173]

Ethylene glycol was first synthesized in 1859 by Charles-Adolphe Wurtz and first widely produced as an engine coolant during the second World War, when its precursor ethylene oxide became readily available.[47] Today its primary use remains as an engine coolant antifreeze used in car radiators. Antifreeze used in gas tanks generally contains methanol. Because of its sweet taste, it is unintentionally consumed by animals and children. Aversive bittering agents have been added to ethylene glycol-containing antifreeze to try to prevent ingestions by making the antifreeze unpalatable, an approach required by law in two states. However, no evidence suggest that this strategy is effective, and comparisons in poison center data between ethylene glycol ingestions where bittering agents were required and where they were not have revealed no significant differences in frequency or volume of ingestion, or any other outcome variable.[170]

Isopropanol is primarily available as rubbing alcohol. Typical household preparations contain 70% isopropanol. It is also a solvent used in many household, cosmetic, and topical pharmaceutical products. Perhaps because it is so ubiquitous, inexpensive, and its common name contains the word alcohol, isopropanol ingestions are the most common toxic alcohol exposure reported to poison centers in the United States,[29] typically in cases where it was used as an ethanol substitute (see Chap. 135).

CHEMISTRY

Alcohols are hydrocarbons that contain a *hydroxyl* (-OH) group. The term *toxic alcohols* traditionally refers to alcohols other than ethanol, those not intended for ingestion. In a sense, this is arbitrary, since all alcohols are toxic, causing inebriation and end-organ effects if taken in excess. The most common clinically relevant toxic alcohols are methanol and ethylene glycol (1,2-ethanediol). Ethylene glycol contains two hydroxyl groups; molecules with this characteristic are termed *diols* or *glycols* because of their sweet taste. Other common toxic alcohols include isopropanol (isopropyl alcohol or 2-propanol), benzyl alcohol (phenylmethanol), and propylene glycol (1,3-propanediol). *Primary* alcohols, such as methanol and ethanol, contain a hydroxyl group on the end of the molecule (the *terminal* carbon), whereas *secondary* alcohols, such as isopropanol, contain hydroxyl groups bound to middle carbons. Glycol ethers are glycols with a hydrocarbon chain bound to one or more of the hydroxyl groups (forming the basic structure $R^1O\text{-}CH_2\text{-}CH_2\text{-}O\text{-}R^2$ or $R^1O\text{-}CH_2\text{-}CH_2\text{-}CH_2\text{-}OR^2$). Poisoning with these compounds may clinically resemble toxic alcohol poisoning, and will be discussed in detail in Special Considerations: Diethylene Glycol. Glycol ethers commonly encountered include ethylene glycol butyl ether (also known as 2-butoxyethanol, ethylene glycol monobutyl ether, or butyl cellusolve), ethylene glycol methyl ether (2-methoxyethanol), and diethylene glycol (2,2'-dihydroxydiethyl ether).

TOXICOKINETICS/TOXICODYNAMICS

Alcohols are rapidly absorbed after ingestion[51,59] but not completely bioavailable because of metabolism by gastric alcohol dehydrogenase, as well as by first pass hepatic metabolism. Occasionally, delayed or prolonged absorption may occur.[45] Although methanol may also be absorbed in significant amounts by inhalation, poisoning by this route is uncommon. In workers exposed to methanol fumes from industrial processes for up to 6 hours at concentrations of 200 ppm (the Occupational Health and Safety Administration [OSHA] permissible exposure limit), there was no significant accumulation of methanol or its metabolite formate.[102] Another study showed that with methanol use in the semiconductor industry, ambient methanol concentrations generally do not approach this OSHA limit even in an a room with low ventilations rates and with no local exhaust ventilation.[57] Surprisingly, concentrations far in excess of the OSHA concentration limit can be present within the passenger compartment of a car when using the windshield wipers and methanol-containing windshield-washing fluid.[16] No cases of human poisoning have been reported from this type of exposure, probably because these concentrations are not sustained over a long time. However, cases of inhalational poisoning have been reported with intentional inhalation of methanol as a drug of abuse ("huffing") (see Chap. 81) and with massive exposures of rescue workers responding to the scene of an overturned rail car filled with methanol.[10,52,110,165] Two case series suggest that patients who present after chronic inhalation of methanol do well with folate and ADH blockade alone and without need for hemodialysis.[15,110] Ethylene glycol has low volatility and is not reported to cause poisoning by inhalation. In one study, human volunteers inhaled vaporized ethylene glycol at a concentration of 1340–1610 m*M* for 4 hours to simulate an industrial exposure. Afterward, the volunteers had detectable but not clinically significant concentrations of ethylene glycol and its metabolites.[164] Most alcohols have some dermal absorption, although isopropanol and methanol are able to penetrate the skin much better than ethylene glycol.[41,106,167] Most reported cases of toxic alcohol poisoning by this route involve infants,[37] because of their greater surface area to volume ratio, and likely also involved simultaneous inhalation. One reported case of transdermal methanol poisoning involved a 51-year-old woman, but details of the exposure were not reported.[156] Another case involved a 52-year-old woman who reportedly frequently massaged with methanol-containing cologne and spirit over the course of 3 days. That patient suffered significant visual and neurologic sequelae despite aggressive treatment with ethanol and hemodialysis.[1] One methanol fatality was deemed to be caused by transdermal absorption (in addition to blunt trauma) when high tissue methanol concentrations were measured in the absence of detectable methanol in the gastrointestinal tract,[11] but inhalational exposure could also conceivably have contributed. When human volunteers were exposed to 100% ethylene glycol applied to a 66 cm^2 area of skin under an occlusive dressing for 6 hours, detectable but not clinically significant amounts were absorbed.[164]

Once absorbed, alcohols are rapidly distributed to total body water. In human volunteers given an oral dose of methanol on an empty stomach, the measured Vd was 0.77 L/kg, with a distribution half-life of about 8 minutes.[59] This is only slightly longer than the absorption half-life, so serum concentrations typically peak soon after ingestion and then begin to fall.

Without intervention, toxic alcohols are metabolized through successive oxidation by alcohol dehydrogenase (ADH) and aldehyde dehydrogenase (ALDH), each of which is coupled to the reduction of NAD^+ to NADH and H^+. Methanol is metabolized to formaldehyde, then formic acid (Fig. 107–1). Ethylene glycol has two hydroxyl groups that are serially oxidized by ADH and ALDH, producing, in turn, glycoaldehyde, glycolic acid, glyoxylic acid, and finally oxalic acid (Fig. 107–2). Like ethanol, this metabolism follows zero-order kinetics, with a rate that is reported to be about 10 mg/dL/hr.[35,83,119] Additionally, this rate is apparently unchanged in chronic ethanol users.[65,66]

Alternate minor metabolic pathways such as catalase exist for methanol and ethylene glycol. After methanol ingestion, the formate metabolite is bound by tetrahydrofolate and then undergoes metabolism by 10-formyltetrahydrofolate dehydrogenase to carbon dioxide and water. Ethylene glycol is metabolized to ketoadipate and glycine using thiamine and pyridoxine as co-factors.[126] Because of the low toxicity of these ethylene glycol metabolites, these normally minor metabolic pathways are attractive targets for potential therapy.

Methanol and ethylene glycol may also be eliminated from the body as unchanged parent compounds. When renal function is normal, ethylene glycol is slowly cleared by the kidneys, with a half-life of approximately 11 to 18 hours.[22,33,154] Methanol does not have significant renal elimination and is cleared much more slowly than is ethylene glycol presumably as a vapor in expired air (half-life 30–54 hours).[26,134]

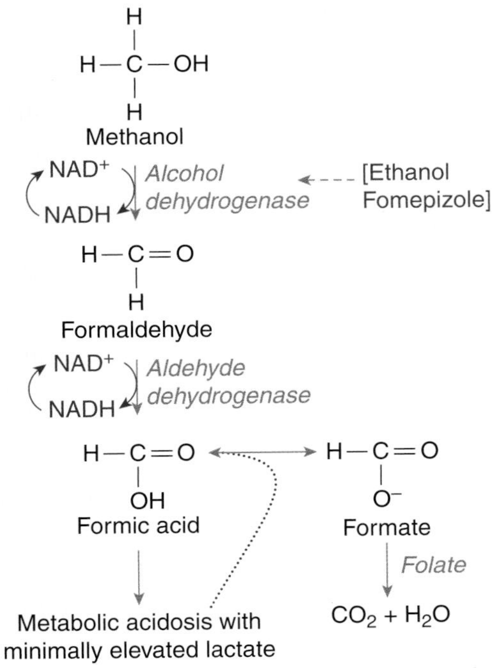

FIGURE 107–1. Major pathway of methanol metabolism.

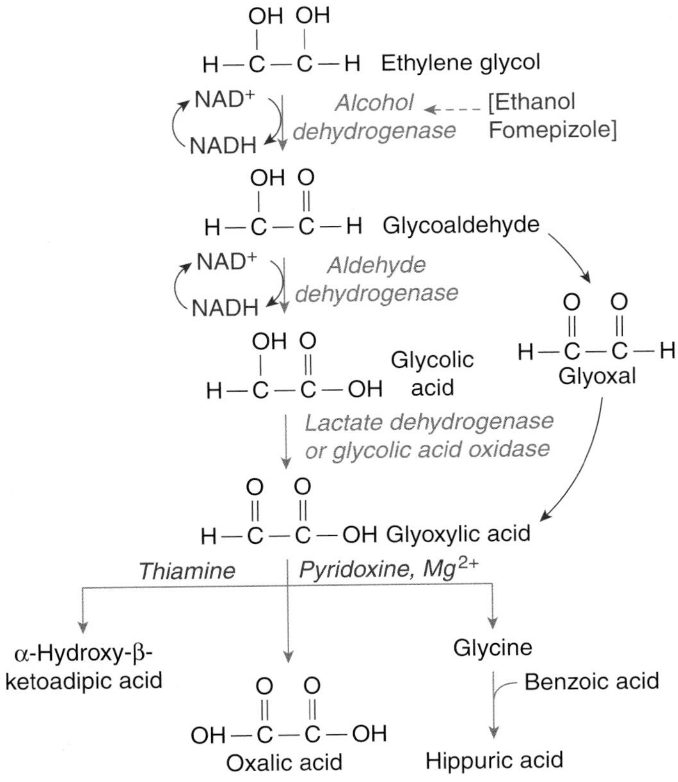

FIGURE 107–2. Pathways of ethylene glycol metabolism. Thiamine and pyridoxine enhance formation of nontoxic metabolites.

CLINICAL MANIFESTATIONS AND PATHOPHYSIOLOGY

CNS EFFECTS

All alcohols may cause inebriation, depending on the dose. Based on limited animal data, it appears that higher molecular weight alcohols are more intoxicating than lower molecular weight alcohols (therefore, isopropanol ≈ ethylene glycol > ethanol > methanol).[169] However, the absence of apparent inebriation does not exclude toxic alcohol ingestion, particularly if the patient chronically drinks ethanol and is thereby tolerant to its central nervous system (CNS) effects.[160] This is intuitively obvious; serum methanol concentrations of 25 to 50 mg/dL may potentially be associated with toxicity, whereas in most states one may legally drive a car with a blood alcohol concentration of 80 mg/dL.

The CNS manifestations of toxic alcohol poisoning are incompletely understood. It is assumed by analogy that inebriation is similar to that of ethanol, where effects are mediated through increased GABAergic tone both directly and through inhibition of presynaptic GABA, $GABA_A$ receptors as well as inhibition of the *N*-methyl-D-aspartic acid (NMDA) glutamate receptors.[6,31,60,72,121] Although the CNS effects of other alcohols are clinically similar, there is no direct evidence that they are mechanistically the same.

METABOLIC ACIDOSIS

Metabolic acidosis with an elevated anion gap is a hallmark of toxic alcohol poisoning. This is a consequence of the metabolism of these alcohols to toxic organic acids. The acids have no rapid natural metabolic pathway of elimination unlike acetic acid from ethanol metabolism, which can enter the Krebs cycle, and therefore they accumulate. In methanol poisoning, formic acid and lactic acid in the most seriously ill are responsible for the acidosis, whereas in ethylene glycol poisoning, glycolic acid is the primary acid responsible for the acidosis, with other metabolites making a minor contribution. An exception to the formation of an acid metabolite is isopropanol, which is metabolized to acetone. Acetone is a ketone, not an aldehyde, and therefore cannot be further metabolized by aldehyde dehydrogenase (ALDH) (Fig. 107–3). Thus it has no organic acid metabolite and does not cause metabolic acidosis. In fact, ketosis without acidosis is diagnostic of isopropanol poisoning. Occasionally, a non-anion gap metabolic acidosis may result from ethylene glycol poisoning (almost 18% in one series), often concurrently with anion gap acidosis.[155] The mechanism for this is unclear, but a similar pattern has been observed in the setting of diabetic ketoacidosis, lactic acidosis, alcoholic ketoacidosis, and toluene poisoning.

END-ORGAN MANIFESTATIONS

Additional end-organ effects depend on which alcohol is involved. Methanol causes visual impairment ranging from blurry or hazy vision or defects in color vision, to "snowfield vision" or total blindness in severe poisoning. On physical examination, central scotoma may be present on visual field testing, and both hyperemia and pallor of the optic disc, papilledema, and an afferent papillary defect are described as characteristic findings.[18,131,176] Electroretinography may demonstrate a diminished b-wave,[163] a marker of bipolar cell dysfunction, and optical coherence tomography (similar in principal to ultrasound, but using reflected light waves to image translucent tissues) may demonstrate peripapillary nerve fiber swelling and intraretinal fluid accumulation.[54] The formate metabolite of methanol is a mitochondrial toxin, inhibiting cytochrome oxidase and thereby interferes with oxidative phosphorylation.[46,127,128] Although it is unclear why this results in ocular toxicity while other tissues are relatively spared, retinal pigmented epithelial cells and optic nerve cells appear to be uniquely susceptible.[44,116,162,163]

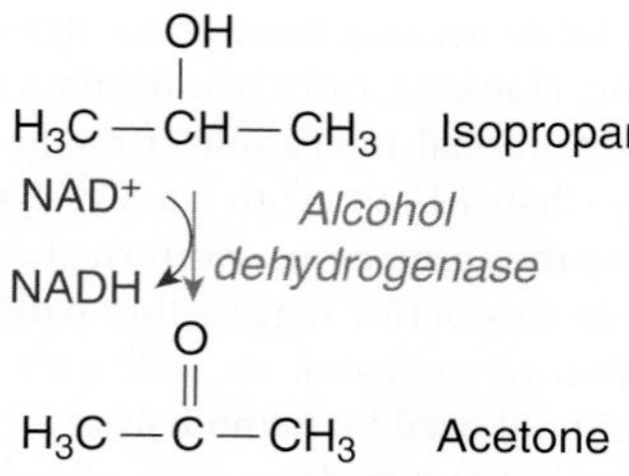

OH
$H_3C-CH-CH_3$ Isopropanol
NAD^+ → NADH *Alcohol dehydrogenase*
O
$H_3C-C-CH_3$ Acetone

FIGURE 107–3. Isopropanol metabolism.

Interestingly, neurons in the basal ganglia appear to be similarly susceptible to this toxicity; bilateral basal ganglia lesions, the putamen, and less commonly, caudate nucleus are characteristically abnormal visualized on cerebral computerized tomography or magnetic resonance imaging after methanol poisoning.[3,8,19,20,40,42,49,55,67,68,136,147,151] While lesions of this type are nonspecific, and may occur in other disease states, such as hypoxia, hypotension, and carbon monoxide exposure, they may occur in the absence of hypotension and hypoxia in methanol poisoning,[117] suggesting a direct toxic mechanism. In one series, typical radiological lesions were present in six of nine cases.[151] Other CNS lesions reported include necrosis of the corpus callosum[93] and intracranial hemorrhage.[9,150] Rarely, injury to other tissues may also occur; both renal failure and pancreatitis are reported after methanol poisoning.[70,96] For unclear reasons, one case series showed a much higher incidence of pancreatitis (50%)[70] and in another, 11 of 15 patients had pancreatitis[166] but this is not typical. Some of the renal failure that results from methanol poisoning may be due to myoglobinuria.[61] In one series of methanol-poisoned patients with renal failure, about half had associated myoglobinuria. Patients with renal failure were also more likely than a control group of patients to have severe poisoning, as manifested by low initial serum pH, high initial osmolality, and high peak formate concentration.[166]

The most prominent end organ effect of ethylene glycol is nephrotoxicity. The oxalic acid metabolite forms a complex with calcium to precipitate as calcium oxalate monohydrate crystals in the renal tubules, leading to acute renal failure.[50,62,64,118,141,159,161] The diagnosis of ethylene glycol poisoning has been made at autopsy by demonstrating this abnormality, including one homicide case;[7,104] in another case, the diagnosis was made by renal biopsy.[92] Although the intermediate products of ethylene glycol metabolism and possibly ethylene glycol itself were shown to be directly toxic to the renal tubules in some studies,[34,50,140,143] this appears not to occur at clinically relevant concentrations.[62] Currently no explanation exists for the presence of necrotic lesions to the glomerular basement membrane on some pathology specimens[50] as oxalic acid generally does not cause glomerular injury.[88]

Ethylene glycol can occasionally affect other organ systems. In severe poisoning, the oxalic acid metabolite may be present in sufficient amounts to cause systemic hypocalcemia by precipitation with calcium. This can result in prolongation of the QT interval on the electrocardiogram and ventricular dysrhythmias.[149] Cerebral edema was present on CT scan in two patients that died of ethylene glycol poisoning.[53,161] Precipitation of calcium oxalate crystals in the brain has also been found on autopsy after severe ethylene glycol poisoning[5,50,53] and may account for the multiple cranial nerve abnormalities that occasionally develop,[39,157] although there is as yet no direct evidence of causation. Peripheral polyradiculoneuropathy has been diagnosed by EMG in a case of ethylene glycol poisoning,[4] and intracranial hemorrhage involving the globus pallidus has also occurred.[30] A leukemoid reaction may also occur in the setting of severe ethylene glycol poisoning, but the mechanism remains unclear.[112,124] One pediatric case of hemophagocytic syndrome and liver failure in the setting of ethylene glycol poisoning resulted in fatality.[100] Finally, two patients developed parkinsonism after concomitant poisoning by methanol and ethylene glycol.[144]

Hemorrhagic gastritis has been reported in association with isopropyl alcohol intoxication. Although this has previously been assumed to be caused by a local irritant effect, one reported case of hemorrhagic gastritis after percutaneous isopropanol exposure suggests that this is not the only mechanism, and may in fact be a specific end-organ effect.[43] Hemorrhagic tracheobronchitis has occurred in fatal cases of isopropanol aspiration.[2]

DIAGNOSTIC TESTING

TOXIC ALCOHOL CONCENTRATIONS

Actual serum methanol, formate, ethylene glycol, oxalate, and isopropanol concentrations would be, in theory, the ideal tests to perform when toxic alcohol poisoning is suspected shortly after exposure. However, these concentrations are most commonly measured by gas chromatography with or without mass-spectrometry confirmation, methodologies that are not available in most hospital laboratories on a 24-hour basis, if at all. In fact, in many hospitals these are only available as "send-out" tests, so results arrive too late for early clinical decision-making.[91] Enzymatic assays for methanol, formic acid, ethylene glycol, and glycolic acid have been developed,[21,158,168] and these may lead to more readily-available clinical tests, but a commercial product is currently approved for veterinary use only. This veterinary test is effective for confirming the qualitative presence of ethylene glycol in human poisoning, although false-positives may occur with propylene glycol.[109] A group in Finland described a point-of-care breath test for methanol, using a portable Fourier transform infrared (FT-IR) analyzer similar to the "breathalyzers" used by law enforcement agents.[101] Although analyzers like this are used to check for methanol as a combustion product in industry, they are not yet approved for medical use in the United States. Once approved, they would be ideal for early clinical decision-making because they are easy to use and provide a rapid result. They also can provide continuous monitoring of concentrations, a feature that would be very helpful during hemodialysis. Unfortunately, this methodology could not be used to detect ethylene glycol because of its low volatility.

Patients presenting late after ingestion may already have metabolized all parent compound to toxic metabolites, and thus may have low or no measurable toxic alcohol concentrations. Fortuitously, the enzymatic assay for ethylene glycol is also capable of detecting glycolic acid, though as mentioned, this assay is only approved for veterinary use. Some authors have actually advocated for routine testing for glycolic acid in addition to testing for the parent compound when ethylene glycol poisoning is suspected.[143] Similarly, a formate concentration may be valuable when a patient presents late after methanol ingestion.[80,132] Formate has been detected in blood samples from 97% of patients who died of methanol poisoning in one series; all of these patients also had detectable blood or vitreous methanol.[89] Clearly, a low or undetectable toxic alcohol concentration must be interpreted within the context of the history and other clinical data, such as the presence of acidosis and end-organ toxicity, with glycolate and formate concentrations as potentially valuable additions.

Samples must be handled correctly for accurate toxic alcohol results. Particularly with the more volatile alcohols methanol and isopropanol, concentrations may be falsely low if the sample tubes are not airtight. This commonly results in low concentrations if alcohol concentrations are done as "add-on" tests to samples already opened for electrolyte or osmol determinations.

Other alcohols such as benzyl alcohol and propylene glycol are not routinely assessed for by gas chromatography. Thus these xenobiotics present a much greater diagnostic challenge than methanol and ethylene glycol. Enzymatic assays for methanol or ethylene glycol would also fail to detect these, although false-positive ethylene glycol tests may occur if propylene glycol is present. Thus a high index of suspicion is critical to establishing the diagnosis in these cases. If suspected on the basis of history, specific toxic alcohol testing should be performed.

Once alcohol concentrations are obtained, their interpretation represents a further point of controversy. Traditionally, a methanol or ethylene glycol concentration greater than 25 mg/dL has been considered toxic, but the evidence supporting this as a threshold is often questioned. In a case series of methanol-poisoned patients from the 1950s, a methanol concentration of 52 mg/dL was the lowest associated with vision loss.[18] This may have been the origin of the 25 mg/dL threshold, incorporating a 50% reduction as a margin of safety. However, the patient with the 52 mg/dL concentration presented 24 hours after his initial ingestion, and therefore was much more severely poisoned than suggested by his serum concentration at that point. In fact, almost all reported cases of methanol poisoning involve late presenters with metabolic acidosis.[97] The only reported patient who went untreated after presenting early with an elevated methanol concentration (45.6 mg/dL) and no acidosis never developed acidosis or end-organ toxicity.[25,97] A systematic review found that 126 mg/dL was the lowest methanol concentration resulting in an acidosis in a patient who arrived early after ingestion and met the authors' inclusion criteria. The authors concluded that the available data are currently insufficient to apply a 20 mg/dL treatment threshold in a patient presenting early after ingestion without acidosis.[97] However, until better data are available demonstrating the safe application of a higher concentration, it seems prudent to use a conservative concentration such as 25 mg/dL as a threshold for treatment.

Because of the problems with obtaining and interpreting actual serum concentrations, many surrogate markers have been used to assess the patient with suspected toxic alcohol poisoning. The initial laboratory evaluation should include: serum electrolytes including calcium, blood urea nitrogen, serum creatinine concentrations urinalysis, measured serum osmolality, and a serum ethanol concentration. Blood gas analysis with a lactate concentration is also helpful in the initial evaluation of ill-appearing patients.

ANION GAP AND OSMOL GAP

For a full discussion of the anion gap concept, refer to Chap. 16. As previously discussed, anion gap elevation is a hallmark of toxic alcohol poisoning. In fact, the possibility of methanol or ethylene glycol poisoning is often first considered when patients present with an anion gap acidosis of unknown etiology, frequently with no history of ingestion. Unless other clinical information suggests otherwise, it is important to exclude metabolic acidosis with elevated lactate concentration and ketoacidosis, which are the most common causes of anion gap acidosis, before pursuing toxic alcohols in these patients. This is because of the extensive evaluation and expensive, potentially invasive course of therapy to which they are otherwise committed. However, elevated lactate concentrations may be present in the setting of both methanol and ethylene glycol poisoning.

The unmeasured anions in toxic alcohol poisoning are the dissociated organic acid metabolites discussed above. The acidosis takes time to develop, sometimes up to 16–24 hours for methanol. Thus the absence of an anion gap elevation early after reported toxic alcohol ingestion does not exclude the diagnosis. If ethanol is present in the body, the development of acidosis will not begin to occur until the ratio of the ethanol to the toxic alcohol falls below a number that varies by alcohol.

A potential early surrogate marker of toxic alcohol poisoning is an elevated *osmol gap* (the principles and the calculations are discussed in detail in Chap. 16). However, it is important to recognize that osmol gap elevation is neither sensitive nor specific for toxic alcohol poisoning. Since a baseline osmol gap is generally not available when evaluating a patient, and a normal osmol gap ranges from −14 to +10 units, so-called "normal" osmol gaps cannot exclude toxic alcohol poisoning.[75] For example, in a patient with a baseline osmol gap of −10 units, a gap of +5 units represents a methanol concentration of 47 mg/dL or an ethylene glycol concentration of 93 mg/dL, values that might require hemodialysis. Inversely, a moderately elevated osmol gap (+10 to +20) is not necessarily diagnostic of toxic alcohol poisoning because other diseases such as alcoholic ketoacidosis and metabolic acidosis, with elevated lactate concentration, may raise the osmol gap.[148] Furthermore, mean osmol gaps vary within populations over time, further limiting their utility.[98] However, a markedly elevated osmol gap (>50) is difficult to explain by anything other than a toxic alcohol.

Further complicating matters, the anion gap and osmol gap have a reciprocal relationship over time. This is because soon after ingestion, the alcohols present in the serum raise the osmol gap, but do not affect the anion gap because metabolism to the organic acid anion has not yet occurred. As the alcohols are metabolized to organic acid anions, the anion gap rises while the osmol gap falls, because the metabolites are negatively charged particles that have already been accounted for in the calculated osmolarity by doubling of the sodium. Thus patients who present early after ingestion may have a high osmol gap and normal anion gap, while those who present later may have the reverse.[77,82] Figure 107–4 depicts a more intuitive visual representation of this process.

One retrospective and one prospective study have attempted to look at the performance characteristic of the osmol gap as a diagnostic test. Although in both cases, the osmol gap performed fairly well, the studies were small, 20 patients with toxic alcohol poisoning in the retrospective study and 28 patients with methanol poisoning in the prospective study, and the prospective study identified three patients with significant poisoning and acidosis but normal osmol gaps defined in the study as less than 25.[77,113] Therefore, these data do not eliminate the concern that someone with significant poisoning could be missed by relying on the osmol gap to exclude poisoning.

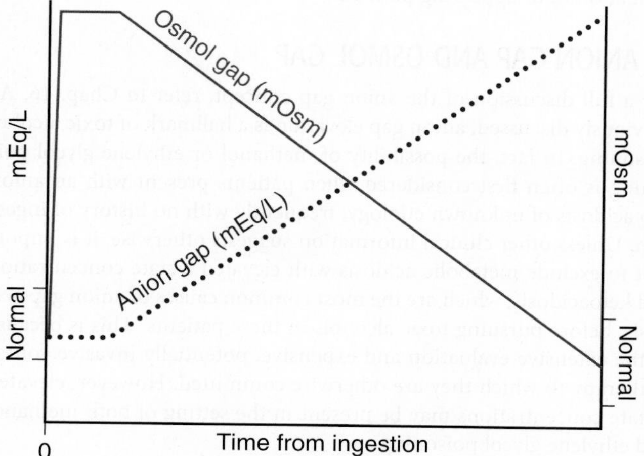

FIGURE 107–4. The reciprocal relationship of anion gap and osmol gap over time (hours). Note that patients presenting early may have a normal anion gap while patients who present late may have a normal osmol gap.

ETHANOL CONCENTRATION

A serum ethanol concentration is an important part of the assessment of the patient with suspected toxic alcohol poisoning. As discussed in Chap. 16, the ethanol concentration is necessary for the calculation of measured osmolarity. In addition, because ethanol is the preferred substrate of alcohol dehydrogenase (4:1 over methanol and 8:1 over ethylene glycol), a significant concentration would be protective if co-ingested with a toxic alcohol. In fact, ethanol concentrations near 100 mg/dL virtually preclude toxic alcohols as the cause of an unknown anion gap metabolic acidosis because the presence of such a concentration should have prevented metabolism to the organic acid. A possible exception would be ingestion of ethanol several hours after ingestion of a toxic alcohol.[73]

LACTATE CONCENTRATION

Both methanol and ethylene glycol can result in elevated lactate concentrations, for very different reasons. Formate, as an inhibitor of oxidative phosphorylation, can lead to anaerobic metabolism and resultant lactate elevation. Additionally, metabolism of all alcohols results in an increased $NADH/NAD^+$ ratio, which favors the conversion of pyruvate to lactate. Furthermore, hypotension and organ failure in severely poisoned patients can also result in elevated lactate concentrations. However, lactate production by these mechanisms tends to result in serum concentrations less than 5 mmol/L.

In ethylene glycol poisoning, the glycolate metabolite may also cause a false-positive lactate elevation when measured by some analyzers, particularly with whole blood arterial blood gas analyzers. Specific models implicated include: ABL 625, Radiometer ABL 700, Beckman LX 20, Chiron 865, Bayer (formerly Chiron) 860, Rapidlab (Bayer) 865, Integra and to a lesser extent, Hitachi 911 analyzers, but not the Vitros 950 or Vitros 250.[28,48,114,123,142,172] In such cases, the degree of lactate elevation directly correlates with the concentration of glycolate present,[114] and the artifact results from the lack of specificity of the lactate oxidase enzyme used in these machines,[123,142,172] although direct oxidation of glycolate at the analyzer anode has also been suggested as a possible mechanism.[152] It has been suggested that the presence of a "lactate gap" might also be used to diagnose ethylene glycol poisoning in hospitals where lactate assays are available with and without sensitivity to glycolate.[152]

OTHER DIAGNOSTICS

The urine may provide information in the assessment of the patient with suspected ethylene glycol poisoning. Calcium oxalate monohydrate (spindle-shaped) and dihydrate (envelope-shaped) crystals may be seen when the urine sediment is examined by microscopy, although this finding is neither sensitive nor specific.[56,83,122] In fact, calcium oxalate crystals were present in the urine of only 63% (12 of 19) of patients with proven ethylene glycol ingestion in one series.[27]

Some brands of antifreeze contain fluorescein to facilitate the detection of radiator leaks. If one of these products is ingested and the urine is examined with a Woods lamp within the first 6 hours, there may be urinary fluorescence.[171] False positive fluorescence may result from examining the urine in glass or plastic containers due to the inherent fluorescence of these materials, so if this test is performed, an aliquot of the urine should be poured onto a piece of white gauze or paper. Recent work has suggested a lack of utility of this test; almost all children had urinary fluorescence, and there was poor interrater agreement in determining fluorescence of specimens.[32,135]

The evaluation of patients with known or suspected ethylene glycol poisoning should also include a serum calcium and creatinine concentrations. Patients with methanol poisoning and abdominal pain also warrant an assessment of liver function tests and serum lipase and/or amylase because of the possibility of associated hepatitis and pancreatitis.

MANAGEMENT

As always, immediate resuscitation of critically ill patients starts with management of the airway, breathing, and circulation. Because alcohols may cause respiratory depression and coma, intubation and mechanical ventilation are commonly necessary for patients with severe poisoning. Alcohol-induced vasodilation combined with vomiting often lead to hypotension, and many patients will require fluid resuscitation with intravenous crystalloid. Gastrointestinal decontamination is rarely, if ever, indicated for toxic alcohols because of their rapid absorption and limited binding to activated charcoal. However, placement of a nasogastric tube and aspiration of any gastric contents is probably worthwhile in intubated patients, as absorption may sometimes be delayed after a large dose.[45]

ALCOHOL DEHYDROGENASE INHIBITION

The most important part of the initial management of patients with known or suspected toxic alcohol poisoning (after initial resuscitation) is blockade of ADH. This allows for the establishment of a definitive diagnosis and arrangement for hemodialysis while preventing the formation of toxic metabolites. Additionally, in some cases ADH blockade may itself serve as definitive therapy.

Teleologically, ADH exists for the purpose of metabolizing ethanol, so it is not surprising that the enzyme has a higher affinity for ethanol than for other alcohols. ADH metabolizes ethanol with a Km that is 15 times smaller in vitro than its Km for methanol metabolism and 67 times smaller than its Km for ethylene glycol metabolism.[137,138] Thus significant concentrations of ethanol prevent metabolism of other alcohols to their toxic products. Ethanol is the traditional method of ADH inhibition and may still be the only option in some institutions. A 10% solution is administered through a central venous catheter and titrated to maintain a serum concentration of 100 mg/dL (see Antidotes in Depth A32: Ethanol). Complications of the infusion, while uncommon,[146] include hypotension, respiratory depression (with supratherapeutic concentrations), flushing, hypoglycemia, hyponatremia, pancreatitis and gastritis, as well as inebriation, so patients getting intravenous ethanol require admission to an intensive care unit. Orally administered ethanol is also effective, and may be considered when intensive monitoring is unavailable, particularly in rural areas where there may be a significant delay in getting the patient to a hospital.

Fomepizole is a competitive antagonist of ADH that has many advantages over ethanol. It reliably inhibits ADH when administered as an intravenous bolus every 12 hours, and concentrations do not need to be monitored as with an ethanol infusion.[26,27] It does not cause inebriation and is associated with fewer adverse effects, so it does not require intensive care unit monitoring.[13,14,26,27] For these reasons, it has become the preferred method of ADH blockade, despite being significantly more expensive then ethanol. In fact, the savings in ICU monitoring and laboratory costs probably compensate for the higher drug cost of fomepizole, unless the patient requires intensive monitoring anyway based on the severity of illness.[22] The dose of fomepizole is 15 mg/kg intravenously as an initial loading dose followed by 10 mg/kg every 12 hours. Bradycardia and hypotension may occur after fomepizole infusion, so vital signs should be monitored closely during and after each dose.[103] After 48 hours of therapy, fomepizole induces its own metabolism, so the dose must be increased to 15 mg/kg every 12 hours. Pharmacokinetic data from a human volunteer study show that there is no significant difference in serum concentrations between oral and intravenous fomepizole.[115] However, there is currently no oral preparation of fomepizole on the market. (see Antidotes in Depth A31: Fomepizole)

Indications for fomepizole or ethanol therapy may be based on the history or on laboratory data. Any patient with a believable history of methanol or ethylene glycol ingestion should be treated until concentrations are available because as previously discussed, early symptoms and laboratory markers other than serum concentrations may be absent. In addition, any patient with an anion gap acidosis without another explanation or a markedly elevated osmol gap should also be treated. Once concentrations are available, therapy should be continued until the serum toxic alcohol concentration is predicted or measured to be below 20 mg/dL, although as discussed above, this value is based more on consensus opinion than on data.

HEMODIALYSIS

The definitive therapy for symptomatic patients poisoned by toxic alcohols is hemodialysis. Hemodialysis clears both the alcohols and their toxic metabolites from the blood, and corrects the acid-base disorder. The indications for hemodialysis have become more restricted with the advent of fomepizole because of its effectiveness combined with its low incidence of adverse effects. Particularly for ethylene glycol, which can generally be expected to be cleared within a few days once ADH is blocked if the GFR is normal, some have argued that the risks of an invasive procedure like hemodialysis are not warranted, in minimally symptomatic patients and in those whose symptoms are due to the parent toxic alcohol. However, patients with end-organ toxicity or severe acidosis have significant amounts of toxic metabolites, a problem not addressed by ADH blockade, and acidosis is associated with poor prognosis.[108] Additionally, although formate in normally cleared rapidly once ADH is blocked, the half-life increases with higher serum methanol concentrations and varies from 2.5 to 12.5 hours.[69,76] In one patient with severe poisoning, formate was eliminated at an extremely slow rate with a half-life of 49.5 hours until hemodialysis was initiated,[79] underscoring the importance of hemodialysis in patients with significant metabolic acidosis. In addition, patients with renal failure will not eliminate the parent compound once ADH is blocked, except very slowly in expired air in the case of methanol. Therefore, the consensus is that metabolic acidosis, signs of end-organ toxicity including coma and seizures and renal failure are indications for hemodialysis. A "toxic concentration" and possibly a very high osmol gap[139] are more relative indications for hemodialysis, and decisions must be based on the judgment of the clinician for the specific clinical scenario, considering the available resources. Some authors have advocated using toxic metabolite concentrations if available as additional criteria for hemodialysis. In data from case series, an elevated formate concentration appears to be a better predictor of clinically important toxicity than methanol concentrations.[132] Similarly, glycolate concentrations are a better predictor of death and renal failure than ethylene glycol concentrations.[143] However, although clearance of formate by hemodialysis is substantial,[86,87,94] the overall clearance in one case series did not appear to increase significantly above endogenous clearance in patients also treated with folate and bicarbonate.[94] Some have questioned the data quality in this series, pointing out: (1) that the pre-dialysis clearance in two patients was calculated using only two data points, and in the three others was calculated using three points, generally considered the minimum; (2) that several patients actually had decreased clearance during dialysis, contradicting all previous data; and (3) that two of the patients had variable blood flow during dialysis.[78,174]

The American Academy of Clinical Toxicology (AACT) practice guidelines are ambiguous with respect to a threshold methanol concentration for hemodialysis in the absence of acidosis, renal failure, end-organ effects or worsening clinical status.[13] However, until additional investigations are completed, a methanol concentration of 50 mg/dL remains a reasonable indication for consideration of hemodialysis in the absence of significant acidosis or end-organ effects. The AACT guidelines for ethylene glycol actually advise against hemodialysis for a concentration alone without any of these clinical indications.[14] Clearly, there are still insufficient data to establish threshold concentrations of alcohols or their metabolites where dialysis is absolutely indicated, and the decision is ultimately a subjective one based on the overall clinical scenario.[74]

Although hemodialysis effectively clears isopropanol and acetone from the blood, it is rarely if ever indicated for this purpose. Because isopropanol does not cause a metabolic acidosis and very rarely results in significant end-organ effects, the risks of hemodialysis likely outweigh the benefits.

Many patients will require multiple courses of hemodialysis to clear the toxin. Nephrologists may estimate the dialysis time required using the formula:

$$t = [-V \ln (5/A)/0.06\text{k}]$$

where t is the dialysis time required to reach a 5 mmol/L toxin concentration, V is the Watson estimate of total body water (liters), A is the initial toxin concentration (mmol/L) and k is 80% of the manufacturer-specified dialyzer urea clearance (mL/min) at the observed initial blood flow rate.[71,175] Additionally, the normalization of the osmol gap may guide the required duration of dialysis, but this has not been validated.[81] Regardless of how the duration of dialysis is determined, ADH blockade should be continued during and after hemodialysis until a subsequent concentration of the offending alcohol is confirmed to be nontoxic. Ethanol infusion rates must be increased during hemodialysis to maintain a therapeutic serum concentration as the ethanol is cleared (see Antidotes in Depth A32: Ethanol). Fomepizole should be redosed every 4 hours during hemodialysis to maintain therapeutic serum concentrations.[13,14]

ADJUNCTIVE THERAPY

There are several therapeutic adjuncts to ADH blockade with or (especially) without hemodialysis that should be considered for these patients. One of the differences that has been invoked to explain the absence of retinal toxicity from methanol in some species is the relative abundance of hepatic folate stores in these species such as the rat. Folate and leucovorin enhance the clearance of formate in animal models.[129,130] Thiamine enhances ethylene glycol's metabolism to ketoadipate, and pyridoxine enhances its metabolism to glycine and ultimately hippuiric acid (Fig. 107–2).[126] While all of these modalities offer theoretical advantages, they have yet to be proven to change outcome in humans. However, there is one human case report showing enhanced formate elimination with folinic acid therapy.[85] Additionally, some have suggested that the apparent lack of an increase in formate clearance by hemodialysis was because it was dwarfed by the effectiveness of folate supplementation in both the study group and the control group.[94] Because of the safety of vitamin supplementation, the potential benefit likely outweighs the risk of therapy (see Antidotes in Depth A25: Thiamine; Antidotes in Depth A13: Leucovorin (Folinic Acid) and Folic Acid; and Antidotes in Depth A15: Pyridoxine).

Formate (dissociated formic acid) is much less toxic than the undissociated formic acid, likely because undissociated formic acid has a much higher affinity for cytochrome oxidase in the mitochondria, the ultimate target site for toxicity.[107] In addition, the undissociated form is better able to diffuse into target tissues.[87] Alkalinization with a bicarbonate infusion shifts the equilibrium to favor the less toxic, dissociated form, in accordance with the Henderson-Hasselbach equation. This also enhances formate clearance in the urine by ion trapping.[87] Uncontrolled case series data exist showing that patients treated with bicarbonate alone had better than expected outcomes after severe methanol poisoning,[125] but the results are equivocal in patients also treated with ADH blockade and hemodialysis.[26,84,120] Additionally, the severity of the metabolic acidosis after methanol poisoning is a good predictor of severe neurological effects such as coma and seizures,[108] although it is not proven that alkalinization prevents these effects. However, in the absence of contraindications to a bicarbonate infusion (eg, hypokalemia, volume overload), alkalinization should be used in the patient with suspected methanol poisoning and a significant acidosis. A blood pH greater than 7.20 is a reasonable endpoint. Alkalinization should also be considered for patients with ethylene glycol poisoning and significant metabolic acidosis.

Aluminum citrate has potential promise as an adjunctive therapy for ethylene glycol poisoning. It interacts with the surface of calcium oxalate monohydrate crystals and prevents their aggregation. This decreases tissue damage from calcium oxalate monohydrate crystals in an *in vitro* model of human proximal tubule cells.[63] However, there are not yet any *in vivo* human studies or even case reports, so it cannot be recommended for clinical use.

One group has reported possible benefit of corticosteroids for retinal injury following methanol poisoning. This was an uncontrolled case series, but 13 of 15 patients showed improvement in their vision after treatment with 1 gram of methylprednisolone daily for 3 days, with one having worsening vision and one unchanged.[153] A patient in another case report had permanent vision loss despite steroid therapy using the same regimen.[54] Currently insufficient data exists to support the routine use of corticosteroids in methanol poisoning.

SPECIAL POPULATIONS

PREGNANT WOMEN AND PERINATAL EXPOSURE

There are very few reported cases of pregnant women with toxic alcohol poisoning, but some conclusions can be drawn from the available data. Toxic alcohols readily cross the placenta, and perinatal maternal methanol ingestion has resulted in death of a newborn.[17] One woman was initially misdiagnosed with eclampsia after ingesting ethylene glycol and presenting with seizures and metabolic acidosis in her 26th week of pregnancy. An emergency Caesarian section was performed, and she was later treated with hemodialysis and ethanol once the correct diagnosis was recognized. The child was severely ill, with an initial pH of 6.63 and an initial serum ethylene glycol concentration of 220 mg/dL. She was treated with exchange transfusion and ultimately survived without sequelae after a long hospital course.[99] In rat but not rabbit models of chronic high-dose ethylene glycol exposure, fetal axial skeletal malformations occur and are thought to be caused by glycolate.[36] No human case has yet been reported.

OTHER ALCOHOLS

PROPYLENE GLYCOL

Propylene glycol is commonly used as an alternative to ethylene glycol in "environmentally safe" antifreeze. It is also used as a diluent for many pharmaceuticals (such as phenytoin and lorazepam). This alcohol is successively metabolized by ADH and ALDH to lactate, so a metabolic acidosis results. This can result in extremely high lactic acid concentrations typically that would be incompatible with life if generated by any disease process. In other disease states associated with lactate accumulation and acidosis, the lactate is a reflection of underlying anaerobic metabolism, a marker of severe illness rather than part of the underlying pathophysiology. Lactic acidosis from propylene glycol is surprisingly well-tolerated because it represents nothing more sinister than its own metabolism, and it is rapidly cleared by oxidation to pyruvate, which then undergoes normal carbohydrate metabolism (see Chap. 55 for further discussion of propylene glycol).

BENZYL ALCOHOL

Benzyl alcohol is used as a preservative for intravenous solutions. Although it is no longer used in neonatal medicine, it has been responsible for "neonatal gasping syndrome," involving multiorgan system dysfunction, metabolic acidosis and death because of its metabolism to benzoic acid and hippuric acid[58,111] (see Chap. 55 for further discussion of benzyl alcohol).

SUMMARY

Toxic alcohol poisoning is complex and may result in consequential toxicity. Early symptoms may include inebriation, and subsequent toxicity results from metabolism to organic acid anions that cause metabolic acidosis and end-organ effects. The time required for this metabolism results in a delay before toxicity clinically manifests itself. Until serum concentrations are available, the serum anion gap and osmol gap may help with decision-making but do not exclude toxicity if the history is concerning. Therapy consists of ADH antagonism with fomepizole or ethanol, as well as adjunctive therapy with bicarbonate, folate or folinic acid, pyridoxine and thiamine. Hemodialysis is the definitive therapy for clinically ill patients as it removes the alcohol as well as toxic metabolites while correcting the metabolic acidosis and electrolyte abnormalities. However, hemodialysis may have a more limited role in the future, particularly for ethylene glycol poisoning (when renal function is normal) because of the safety and efficacy of fomepizole.

ACKNOWLEDGMENTS

Neal E. Flomenbaum, MD, Mary Ann Howland, PharmD, Neal A. Lewin, MD, and Adhi N. Sharma, MD, contributed to this chapter in previous editions.

REFERENCES

1. Adanir T, Ozkalkanli MY, Aksun M. Percutaneous methanol intoxication: a case report. European *J Anaesthesiology*. 2005;22:560-561.
2. Alexander CB, McBay AJ, Hudson RP. Isopropanol and isopropanol deaths: ten years' experience. *J Forensic Sci* 1982;27:541-548.
3. Almansori M, Ahmed SN. CT findings in methanol intoxication. *CMAJ*. 2007;176:620-623.
4. Alzouebi M, Sarrigiannis PG, Hadjivassilou M. Acute polyradiculoneuropthy with renal failure: mind the anion gap. *J Neurol Neurosurg Psychiatry*. 2008;79:842-844.
5. Anderson TJ, Shuaib A, Becker WJ. Neurologic sequelae of methanol poisoning. *Can Med Assoc J*. 1987;136:1177-1179.
6. Ariswodola OJ, Weiner JL. Ethanol potentiation of GABAergic synaptic transmission may be self-limiting: role of presynaptic $GABA_B$ receptors. *J Neurosci*. 2004;24:10679-10686.
7. Armstrong EJ, Engelhart DA, Jenkins A, Balraj EK. Homicidal ethylene glycol intoxication: a report of a case. *Am J Forensic Med Pathol*. 2006;27:151-155.
8. Arora V, Nijjar IB, Multani AS, et al. MRI findings in methanol intoxication: a report of two cases. *Br J Radiol*. 2007;80:e243-e246.
9. Askar A, Al-Suwaida A. Methanol intoxication with brain hemorrhage: catastrophic outcome of late presentation. *Saudi J Kidney Dis Transplant*. 2007;18:117-122.
10. Aufderheide TP, White SM, Brady WJ, Stueven HA. Inhalational and percutaneous methanol toxicity in two firefighters. *Ann Emerg Med*. 1993;22:1916-1918.
11. Avella J, Briglia E, Harleman G, Lehrer M. Case report: percutaeous absorption and distribution of methanol in a homicide. *J Anal Toxicol*. 2005;29:734-737.
12. Azmak D. Methanol related deaths in Edirne. *Legal Med*. 2006;8:39-42.
13. Barceloux DG, Bond GR, Krenzelok EP, et al. American Academy of Clinical Toxicology practice guidelines on the treatment of methanol poisoning. *J Toxicol Clin Toxicol*. 2002;40:415-446.
14. Barceloux DG, Krenzelok EP, Olson K, Watson W. American Academy of Clinical Toxicology practice guidelines on the treatment of ethylene glycol poisoning. *J Toxicol Clin Toxicol*. 1999;37:537-560.
15. Bebarta V, Heard K, Dart RC. Inhalational abuse of methanol products: elevated methanol and formate levels without vision loss. *Am J Emerg Med*. 2006;24:725-728.
16. Becalski A, Bartlett KH. Methanol exposure to car occupants from windshield washing fluid: a pilot study. *Indoor Air*. 2006;16:153-157.
17. Belson M, Morgan BW. Methanol toxicity in a newborn. *Clin Toxicol*. 2004;42:673-677.
18. Bennett IL, Cary FH, Mitchell GL, Cooper MN. Acute methyl alcohol poisoning: a review based on experiences in an outbreak of 323 cases. *Medicine*. 1953;32:432-463.
19. Bessell-Browne RJ, Bynevelt M. Two cases of methanol poisoning: CT and MRI features. *Australasian Radiol*. 2007;51:175-178.
20. Blanco M, Casado R, Vázquez F, Pumar JM. CT and MR imaging findings in methanol intoxication. *Am J Neuroradiol*. 2006;27:452-454.
21. Blomme B, Lheureux P, Gerlo E, Maes V. Cobas Mira" S Endpoint Enzymatic Assay for Plasma Formate. *J Anal Toxicol*. 2001;25:77-80.
22. Boyer EW, Mejia M, Woolf A, Shannon M. Severe ethylene glycol ingestion treated without hemodialysis. *Pediatrics*. 2001;107;172-173.
23. Boyle, R. *Sceptical Chymist*. London: F. Crooke; 1661;292.
24. Brahmi N, Blel Y, Abidi N, et al. Methanol poisoning in Tunisia: report of 16 cases. *Clin Toxicol*. 2007;45:717-720.
25. Brent J, Lucas M, Kulig K, Rumack B. Methanol poisoning in a 6-week-old infant. *J Pediatr*. 1991;118:644-666.
26. Brent J, McMartin K, Phillips S, et al. Fomepizole for the treatment of methanol poisoning. *N Engl J Med*. 2001;344:424-429.
27. Brent J, McMartin K, Phillips S, et al. Fomepizole for the treatment of ethylene glycol poisoning. *N Engl J Med*. 1999;340:832-838.
28. Brindley PG, Butler MS, Cembrowski G, Brindley DN. Falsely elevated point-of-care lactate measurement after ingestion of ethylene glycol. *CMAJ*. 2007;176:1097-1099.
29. Bronstein AC, Spyker DA, Cantilena LR Jr, et al. 2007 Annual Report of the American Association of Poison Control Centers' National Poison Data System (NPDS): 25th Annual Report. *Clin Toxicol*. 2008;46:927-1057.
30. Caparros-Lefebvre D, Policard J, Sengler C, et al. Bipallidal hemorrhage after ethylene glycol intoxication. *Neuroradiology*. 2005;47:105-107.
31. Carta M, Mameli M, Valenzuela CF. Alcohol enhances GABAergic transmission to cerebellar granule cells via an increase in Golgi cell excitability. *J Neurosci*. 2004;24:3746-3751.
32. Casavant MJ, Shah MN, Battels R. Does fluorescent urine indicate antifreeze ingestion by children? *Pediatrics*. 2001;107:113-114.
33. Cheng JT, Beysolow TD, Kaul B, et al. Clearance of ethylene glycol by kidneys and hemodialysis. *J Toxicol Clin Toxicol*. 1987;25:95-108.
34. Clay KL, Murphy RC. On the metabolic acidosis of ethylene glycol intoxication. *Toxicol Appl Pharmacol*. 1977;39:39-49.
35. Clay KL, Murphy RC, Watkins DW. Experimental methanol toxicity in the primate: analysis of metabolic acidosis. *Toxicol and Appl Pharmacol*. 1975;34:49-61.
36. Corley RA, Meek ME, Carney EW. Mode of action: Oxalate crystal-induced renal tubule degeneration and glycolic acid-induced dysmorphogenesis- Renal and developmental effects of ethylene glycol. *Crit Rev Toxicol*. 2005;35:691-702.

37. Darwish A, Roth CE, Duclos P, et al. Investigation into a cluster of infant deaths following immunization: evidence for methanol intoxication. *Vaccine.* 2002;20:3585-3589.
38. Davis LE, Hudson A, Benson BE, et al. Methanol poisoning exposures in the United States: 1993-1998. *J Toxicol Clin Toxicol.* 2002;40:499-505.
39. Delany C, Jay W. Papilledema and abducens nerve palsy following ethylene glycol ingestion. *Seminars in Opthalmology.* 2004;19:72-74.
40. Deniz S, Oppenheim C, Lehericy S, et al. Diffusion-weighted magnetic resonance imaging in a case of methanol intoxication. *NeuroToxicol.* 2000;21:405-408.
41. Driver J, Tardiff RG, Sedik L, et al. In vitro percutaneous absorption of [^{14}C] ethylene glycol by man. *J Exposure Anal Environ Epidemiol.* 1993;3:277-284.
42. Dujardin M, Peeters E, Ernst C, Stadnik T. Bilateral putaminal necrosis due to methanol abuse. *JBR-BTR.* 2006;89:315-317.
43. Dyer S, Mycyk MB, Ahrens WR, Zell-Kanter M. Hemorrhagic gastritis from topical isopropanol exposure. *Ann Pharmacother.* 2002;36:1733-1735.
44. Eells JT, Henry MM, Lewandowski MF, et al. Development and characterization of a rodent model of methanol-induced retinal and optic nerve toxicity. *NeuroToxicol.* 2000;21:321-330.
45. Elwell RJ, Darouian P, Bailie GR, et al. Delayed absorption and postdialysis rebound in a case of acute methanol poisoning. *Am J Emerg Med.* 2004;22:126-127.
46. Erecinska M, Wilson DF. Inhibitors of cytochrome c oxidase. *Pharmacol Ther.* 1980;8:1-10.
47. Ethylene Glycol. From Chemie.De information service. Available at: http://www.chemie.de/lexikon/e/Ethylene_glycol/ Accessed on 8/6/08.
48. Fijen J, Kemperman H, Ververs FFT, Meulenbelt J. False hyperlactatemia in ethylene glycol poisoning. *Intensive Care Med.* 2006;32:626-627.
49. Fontenat AP, Pelak VS. Development of neurologic symptoms in a 26-year-old woman following recovery from methanol intoxication. *Chest.* 2002;122:1436-1439.
50. Frang D, Csata S, Szemenyei K, Hamvasi G. [Kidney damage caused by ethylene glycol poisoning]. *Z Urol Nephrol.* 1967;60:465-471.
51. Frantz SW, Beskitt JL, Grosse CM, et al. Pharmacokinetics of ethylene glycol. I. Plasma disposition after single intravenous, peroral, or percutaneous doses in female Sprague-Dawley rats and CD-1 mice. *Drug Metab Dispos.* 1996;24:911-921.
52. Frenia ML, Schauben JL. Methanol inhalation toxicity. *Ann Emerg Med.* 1993;22:1919-1923.
53. Froberg K, Dorion RP, McMartin KE. The role of calcium oxalate crystal deposition in cerebral vessels during ethylene glycol poisoning. *Clin Toxicol.* 2006;44:315-318.
54. Fujihara M, Kikuchi M, Kurimoto Y. Methanol-induced retinal toxicity patient examined by optical coherence tomography. *Jpn J Ophthalmol.* 2006;50:239-241.
55. Fujita M, Tsuruta R, Wakatsuki J, et al. Methanol intoxication: differential diagnosis from anion gap-increased acidosis. *Intern Med.* 2004;43:750-754.
56. Gaines L, Waibel KH. Calcium oxalate crystalluria. *Emerg Med J.* 2007;24:310.
57. Gaffney S, Moody E, McKinley M, et al. Worker exposure to methanol vapors during cleaning of semiconductor wafers in a manufacturing setting. *J Occup Environ Hyg.* 2008;5:313-24.
58. Gershanik J, Boecler B, Ensley H, et al. The gasping syndrome and benzyl alcohol poisoning. *N Engl J Med.* 1982 25;307:1384-1388.
59. Graw M, Haffner HT, Althaus L, et al. Invasion and distribution of methanol. *Arch Toxicol.* 2000;74:313-321.
60. Grobin AC, Matthews DB, Devaud LL, Morrow AL. The role of $GABA_A$ receptors in the acute and chronic effects of ethanol. *Psychopharmacologia.* 1998;139:2-19.
61. Grufferman S, Morris D, Alvarez J. Methanol poisoning complicated by myoglobinuric renal failure. *Am J Emerg Med.* 1985;3:481-483.
62. Guo C, Cenac TA, Li Y, McMartin KE. Calcium oxalate, and not other metabolites, is responsible for the renal toxicity of ethylene glycol. *Toxicol Lett.* 2007;173:8-16.
63. Guo C, McMartin KE. Aluminum citrate inhibits cytotoxicity and aggregation of oxalate crystals. *Toxicology.* 2007;230:117-125.
64. Guo C, McMartin KE. The cytotoxicity of oxalate, metabolite of ethylene glycol, is due to calcium oxalate monohydrate formation. *Toxicology.* 2005;208:347-355.
65. Haffner HT, Banger M, Graw M, et al. The kinetics of methanol elimination in alcoholics and the influence of ethanol. *Forensic Sci Int.* 1997;89:129-136.
66. Haffner HT, Wehner HD, Scheytt KD, Besserer K. The elimination kinetics of methanol and the influence of ethanol. *Int J Legal Med.* 1992;105:111-114.
67. Halavaara J, Valanne L, Setala K. Neuroimaging supports the clinical diagnosis of methanol poisoning. *Neuroradiol.* 2002;44:924-928.
68. Hantson P, Duprez T, Mahieu P. Neurotoxicity to the basal ganglia shown by magnetic resonance imaging (MRI) following poisoning by methanol and other substances. *J Toxicol Clin Toxicol.* 1997;35:151-161.
69. Hantson P, Haufroid V, Wallemacq P. Formate kinetics in methanol poisoning. *Hum Exp Toxicol.* 2005;24:55-59.
70. Hantson P, Mahieu P. Pancreatic injury following acute methanol poisoning. *J Toxicol Clin Toxicol.* 2000;38:297-303.
71. Hirsch DJ, Jindal KK, Wong P, Fraser AD. A simple method to estimate the required dialysis time for cases of alcohol poisoning. *Kidney Int.* 2001;60:2021-2024.
72. Hoffman PL. NMDA receptors in alcoholism. *Int Rev Neurobiol.* 2003;56:35-82.
73. Hoffman RJ, Hoffman RS, Nelson LS. Ethylene glycol toxicity despite therapeutic ethanol level. *J Toxicol Clin Toxicol.* 2001;39:302.
74. Hoffman RS. Does consensus equal correctness? *J Toxicol Clin Toxicol.* 2000;38:689-690.
75. Hoffman RS, Smilkstein MJ, Howland MA, Goldfrank LR. Osmol gaps revisited: normal values and limitations. *J Toxicol Clin Toxicol.* 1993;31:81-93.
76. Hovda KE, Andersson KS, Urdal P, Jacobsen D. Methanol and formate kinetics during treatment with fomepizole. *Clin Toxicol.* 2005;43:221-227.
77. Hovda KE, Hunderi OH, Rudberg N, et al. Anion and osmolal gaps in the diagnosis of methanol poisoning: clinical study in 28 patients. *Intensive Care Med.* 2004;30:1842–1846.
78. Hovda KE, Jacobsen D. Expert opinion: fomipizole may ameliorate the need for hemodialysis in methanol poisoning. *Hum Exp Toxicol.* 2008;27:539-546.
79. Hovda KE, Mundal H, Urdal P, et al. Extremely slow formate elimination in severe methanol poisoning: a fatal case report. *Clin Toxicol.* 2007;45:516-521.
80. Hovda KE, Urdal P, Jacobsen D. Case report: increased serum formate in the diagnosis of methanol poisoning. *J Anal Toxicol.* 2005;29:586-588.
81. Hunderi OH, Hovda KE, Jacobsen D. Use of the osmolal gap to guide the start and duration of dialysis in methanol poisoning. *Scand J Urol Nephrol.* 2006;40:70-74.
82. Jacobsen D, Bredesen JE, Eide I, Ostborg J. Anion and osmolal gaps in the diagnosis of methanol and ethylene glycol poisoning. *Acta Med Scand.* 1982;212:17-20.
83. Jacobsen D, Hewlett TP, Webb R, et al. Ethylene glycol intoxication: evaluation of kinetics and crystalluria. *Am J Med.* 1988;84:145-152.
84. Jacobsen D, Jansen H, Wiik-Larsen E, et al. Studies on methanol poisoning. *Acta Med Scand.* 1982;212:5-10.
85. Jacobsen D, McMartin KE. Methanol and ethylene glycol poisonings: mechanism of toxicity, clinical course, diagnosis and treatment. *Med Toxicol.* 1986;1:309-334.
86. Jacobsen D, Ovrebo S, Sejersted OM. Toxicokinetics of formate during hemodialysis. *Acta Med Scand.* 1983;214:409-412.
87. Jacobsen D, Webb R, Collins TD, McMartin KE. Methanol and formate kinetics in late diagnosed methanol intoxication. *Med Toxicol Adverse Drug Exp.* 1988;3:418-423.
88. Jeghers H, Murphy R. Practical aspects of oxalate metabolism. *N Engl J Med.* 1945;233:208-215.
89. Jones GR, Singer PP, Rittenbach K. The relationship of methanol and formate concentrations in fatalities where methanol is detected. *J Forensic Sci.* 2007;52:1376-1382.
90. Kane RL, Talbert W, Harlan J, et al. A methanol poisoning outbreak in Kentucky. *Arch Environ Health.* 1968;17:119-129.
91. Kearney J, Rees S, Chiang WK. Availability of serum methanol and ethylene glycol levels: a national survey. *J Toxicol Clin Toxicol.* 1997;35:509.
92. Keiran S, Bhimani B, Dixit A. Ethylene glycol toxicity. *Am J Kidney Dis.* 2005;46:e31-3.
93. Keles GT, Orguc S, Toprak B, et al. Methanol poisoning with necrosis corpus callosum. *Clin Toxicol.* 2007;45:307-308.
94. Kerns W II, Tomaszewski C, McMartin K, et al. Formate kinetics in methanol poisoning. *J Toxicol Clin Toxicol.* 2002;40:137-143.
95. Kinoshita H, Nishiguchi M, Ouchi H, et al. Methanol: toxicity of the solvent in a commercial product should also be considered. *Hum Exp Toxicol.* 2005;24:663.
96. Korchanov LS, Lebedev FM, Lizanets MN, et al. [Treatment of patients with acute kidney insufficiency caused by methyl alcohol poisoning]. *Urol Nefrol (Mosk).* 1970;35:66-67.

97. Kostic MA, Dart RC. Rethinking the toxic methanol level. *J Toxicol Clin Toxicol. 2003*;41:793-800.
98. Krahn J, Khajuria A. Osmolality gaps: diagnostic accuracy and long-term variability. *Clin Chem.* 2006;52:737-739.
99. Kralova I, Stepanek Z, Dusek J. Ethylene glycol intoxication misdiagnosed as eclampsia. *Acta Anaesthesiol Scand.* 2006;50:385-387.
100. Kuskonmaz B, Duzova A, Kanbur NO, et al. Hemophagocytic syndrome and acute liver failure associated with ethylene glycol ingestion: a case report. *Pediatr Hematol Oncol.* 2006;23:427-432.
101. Laakso O, Haapala M, Jaakkola P, et al. FT-IR breath test in the diagnosis and control of treatment of methanol intoxications. *J Anal Toxicol.* 2001;25:26-30.
102. Leaf G, Zatman LJ. A study of the conditions under which methanol may exert a toxic hazard in industry. *Brit J Industr Med.* 1952;9:19-31.
103. Lepik KJ, Brubacher JR, DeWitt CR, et al. Bradycardia and hypotension associated with fomepizole infusion during hemodialysis. *Clin Toxicol.* 2008;46:570-573.
104. Leth PM, Gregersen M. Ethylene glycol poisoning. *Forensic Sci Int.* 2005;155:179-184.
105. Levy P, Hexdall A, Gordon P, et al. Methanol contamination of Romanian home-distilled alcohol. *J Toxicol Clin Toxicol.* 2003;41:23-28.
106. Lewin GA, Oppenheimer PR, Wingert WA. Coma from alcohol sponging. *JACEP.* 1977;6:165-167.
107. Liesivuori J, Savolainen H. Methanol and formic acid toxicity: biochemical mechanisms. *Pharmacol Toxicol.* 1991;69:157-163.
108. Liu JJ, Daya MR, Carrasquillo O, Kales SN. Prognostic factors in patients with methanol poisoning. *J Toxicol Clin Toxicol.* 1998;36:175-181.
109. Long H, Nelson LS, Hoffman RS. A rapid qualitative test for suspected ethylene glycol poisoning. *Acad Emerg Med.* 2008;15:688-690.
110. LoVecchio F, Sawyers B, Thole D, et al. Outcomes following abuse of methanol-containing carburetor cleaners. *Hum Exp Toxicol.* 2004;23:473-475.
111. Lovejoy FH Jr. Fatal benzyl alcohol poisoning in neonatal intensive care units. A new concern for pediatricians. *Am J Dis Child.* 1982;136:974-975.
112. Lovrić M, Granić P, Cubrilo-Turek M, et al. Ethylene glycol poisoning. *Forensic Sci Int.* 2007;170:213-215.
113. Lynd LD, Richardson KJ, Purssell RA, et al. An evaluation of the osmole gap as a screening test for toxic alcohol poisoning. *BMC Emerg Med.* 2008;8:1-10.
114. Manini AF, Hoffman RS, McMartin KE, Nelson LS. Relationship between serum glycolate and falsely elevated lactate in severe ethylene glycol poisoning. *J Anal Toxicol.* 2009;33:227-229.
115. Marraffa J, Forrest A, Grant W, et al. Oral administration of fomepizole produces similar blood levels as identical intravenous dose. *Clin Toxicol.* 2008;46:181-186.
116. Martin-Amat G, Tephly TR, McMartin KE, et al. Methyl alcohol poisoning II. Development of a model for ocular toxicity in methyl alcohol poisoning using the rhesus monkey. *Arch Ophthalmol.* 1977;95:1847-1850.
117. McLean DR, Jacobs H, Mielke BW. Methanol poisoning: a clinical and pathological study. *Ann Neurol.* 1980;8:161-167.
118. McMartin KE, Cenac TA. Toxicity of ethylene glycol metabolites in normal human kidney cells. *Ann N Y Acad Sci.* 2000;919:315-317.
119. McMartin KE, Makar AB, Martin-Amat G, et al. Methanol poisoning,I: the role of formic acid in the development of metabolic acidosis in the monkey and the reversal by 4-methylpyrazole. *Biochem Med.* 1975;13:319-333.
120. Meyer RJ, Beard MEJ, Ardagh MW, Henderson S. Methanol poisoning. *NZ Med J.* 2000;113:11-13.
121. Mihic SJ. Acute effects of ethanol on $GABA_A$ and glycine receptor function. *Neurochem Int.* 1999;35:115-123.
122. Morfin J, Chin A. Urinary calcium oxalate crystals in ethylene glycol intoxication. *N Engl J Med.* 2005;353:e21.
123. Morgan TJ, Clark C, Clague A. Artifactual elevation of measured plasma L-lactate concentration in the presence of glycolate. *Crit Care Med.* 1999;27:2177-2179.
124. Mycyk MB, Drendel A, Sigg T, Leikin JB. Leukemoid response in ethylene glycol intoxication. *Vet Human Toxicol.* 2002;44:304-306.
125. Naraqi S, Dethlefs RF, Slobodniuk RA, Sairere JS. An outbreak of acute methyl alcohol intoxication. *Aust NZ J Med.* 1979;9:65-68.
126. Nath R, Thind SK, Murthy MS, et al. Role of pyridoxine in oxalate metabolism. *Ann NY Acad Sci.* 1990;585:274-284.
127. Nicholls P. Formate as an inhibitor of cytochrome c oxidase. *Biochem Biophys Res Commun.* 1975;67:610-616.
128. Nicholls P. The effect of formate on cytochrome aa_3, and on electron transport in the intact respiratory chain. *Biochim Biophys Acta.* 1976;430:13-29.
129. Noker PE, Eells JT, Tephly TR. Methanol toxicity: treatment with folic acid and 5-formyl tetrahydrofolic acid. *Alcohol Clin Exp Res.* 1980;4:378-383.
130. Noker PE, Tephly TR. The role of folates in methanol toxicity. *Adv Exp Med Biol.* 1980;132:305-315.
131. Onder F, Ilker S, Kansu T, et al. Acute blindness and putaminal necrosis in methanol intoxication. *Int Ophthalmol.* 1999;22:81-84.
132. Osterloh JD, Pond SM, Grady S, Becker CE. Serum formate concentrations in methanol intoxication as a criterion for hemodialysis. *Ann Intern Med.* 1986;104:200-203.
133. Paasma R, Hovda KE, Tikkerberi A, Jacobsen D. Methanol mass poisoning in Estonia: outbreak in 154 patients. *Clin Toxicol.* 2007;45:152-157.
134. Palatnick W, Redman LW, Sitar DS, Tenenbein M. Methanol half life during ethanol administration: implications for management of methanol poisoning. *Ann Emerg Med.* 1995;26:202-207.
135. Parsa T, Cunningham SJ, Wall SJ, et al. The usefulness of urine fluorescence for suspected antifreeze ingestion in children. *Am J Emerg Med.* 2005;23:787-792.
136. Patankar T, Bichile L, Karnad D, et al. Methanol poisoning: brain computerized tomography scan findings in four patients. *Australasian Radiol.* 1999;43:526-528.
137. Pietruszko R. Human liver alcohol dehydrogenase inhibition of methanol activity by pyrazole, 4-methylpyrazole, 4-hydroxymethylpyrazole and 4-carbopyrazole. *Biochem Pharmacol.* 1975;24:1603-1607.
138. Pietruszko R, Voigtlander K, Lester D. Alcohol dehydrogenase from human and horse liver- substance specificity with diols. *Biochem Pharmacol.* 1978;27:1296-1297.
139. Pizon AF, Brooks DE. Hyperosmolality: another indication for hemodialysis following acute ethylene glycol poisoning. *Clin Toxicol.* 2206;44:181-183.
140. Poldelski V, Johnson A, Wright S, et al. Ethylene glycol-mediated tubular injury: identification of critical metabolites and injury pathways. *Am J Kidney Dis.* 2001;38:339-48.
141. Pomara C, Fiore C, D'Errico S, et al. Calcium oxalate crystals in acute ethylene glycol poisoning: a confocal laser scanning microscope study in a fatal case. *Clin Toxicol.* 2008;46:322-324.
142. Porter WH, Crellin M, Rutter PW, Oeltgen P. Interference by glycolic acid in the Beckman Synchron method for lactate: a useful clue for unsuspected ethylene glycol intoxication. *Clin Chem.* 2000;46:874-875.
143. Porter WH, Rutter PW, Bush BA, et al. Ethylene glycol toxicity: the role of serum glycolic acid in hemodialysis. *J Toxicol Clin Toxicol.* 2001;39:607-615.
144. Reddy NJ, Lewis LD, Gardner TB, et al. Two cases of rapid onset Parkinson's syndrome following toxic ingestion of ethylene glycol and methanol. *Clin Pharmacol Ther.* 2007;81:114-121.
145. Roscoe HE, Schorlemmer C. *A Treatise on Chemistry.* New York: D. Appleton and Co; 1884;200.
146. Roy M, Bailey B, Chalut D, et al. What are the adverse effects of ethanol used as an antidote in the treatment of suspected methanol poisoning in children? *J Toxicol Clin Toxicol* .2003;41:155-161.
147. Salzman M. Methanol neurotoxicity. *Clin Toxicol.* 2005;44:89-90.
148. Schelling JR, Howard RL, Winter SD, Linas SL. Increased osmolal gap in alcoholic ketoacidosis and lactic acidosis. *Ann Intern Med.* 1990;113:580-582.
149. Scully R, Galdabini J, McNealy B. Case records of the Massachusetts General Hospital. Weekly clinicopathological exercises. Case 38-1979. *N Engl J Med.* 1979;301:650-657.
150. Sebe A, Satar S, Uzun B, et al. Intracranial hemorrhage associated with methanol intoxication. *Mt. Sinai J Med.* 2006;73:1120-1122.
151. Sefibakht S, Rasekhi AR, Kamali K, et al. Methanol poisoning: acute MR and CT findings in nine patients. *Neuroradiology.* 2007;49:427-435.
152. Shirey T, Sivilotti M. Reaction of lactate electrodes to glycolate. *Crit Care Med.* 1999;27:2305-2307.
153. Shukla M, Shikoh I, Saleem A. Intravenous methylprednisolone could salvage vision in methyl alcohol poisoning. *Ind J Ophthalmol.* 2006;54:68-69.
154. Sivilotti MLA, Burns MJ, McMartin KE, Brent J. Toxicokinetics of ethylene glycol during fomepizole therapy: implications for management. *Ann Emerg Med.* 2000;36:114-124.
155. Soghoian S, Sinert R, Wiener SW, Hoffman RS. Ethylene Glycol Toxicity Presenting with Non-Anion Gap Metabolic Acidosis. *Basic Clin Pharmacol Toxicol.* 2009;104:22-26.
156. Soysal D, Kabayegit OY, Yilmaz S, et al. Transdermal methanol intoxication: a case report. *Acta Anaesthesiol Scand.* 2007;51:779-780.
157. Spillane L, Roberts JR, Meyer AE. Multiple cranial nerve deficits after ethylene glycol poisoning. *Ann Emerg Med.* 1991;20:137-169.

158. Standefer J, Blackwell W. Enzymatic method for measuring ethylene glycol with a centrifugal analyzer. *Clin Chem.* 1991;37:1734-1736.
159. Stokes MB. Acute oxalate nephropathy due to ethylene glycol ingestion. *Kidney International.* 2006;69:203.
160. Symington L, Jackson L, Klaassen. Toxic alcohol but not intoxicated—a case report. *Scott Med J.* 2005;50:129-130.
161. Takahashi S, Kanetake J, Kanawahu Y, Funayama M. Brain death with calcium oxalate deposition in the kidney: clue to the diagnosis of ethylene glycol poisoning. *Legal Med.* 2008;10:43-45.
162. Treichel JL, Henry MM, Skumatz CMB, et al. Formate, the toxic metabolite of methanol, in cultured ocular cells. *NeuroToxicol* .2003;24:825-834.
163. Treichel JL, Murray TG, Lewandowski MF, et al. Retinal toxicity in methanol poisoning. *Retina.* 2004;24:309-312.
164. Upadhyay S, Carstens J, Klein D, et al. Inhalation and epidermal exposure of volunteers to ethylene glycol: kinetics of absorption, urinary excretion, and metabolism to glycolate and oxalate. *Toxicol Lett.* 2008;178: 131-141.
165. Velez LI, Kulstad E, Shepherd G, Roth B. Inhalational methanol toxicity in pregnancy treated twice with fomepizole. *Vet Human Toxicol.* 2003;45:28-30.
166. Verhelst D, Moulin P, Haufroid V, et al. Acute renal injury following methanol poisoning: analysis of a case series. *Int J Toxicol.* 2004;23:267-273.
167. Vicas IM, Beck R. Fatal inhalational isopropyl alcohol poisoning in a neonate. *J Toxicol Clin Toxicol.* 1993;31:473-481.
168. Vinet B. An enzymic assay for the specific determination of methanol in serum. *Clin Chem.* 1987;33:2204-2208.
169. Wallgren H. Relative intoxicating effects on rats of ethyl, propyl and butyl alcohols. *Acta Pharmacol Toxicol Toxicol.* 1960;16:217-222.
170. White NC, Litovitz T, White MK, et al. The impact of bittering agents on suicidal ingestions of antifreeze. *Clin Toxicol.* 2008;46:507-514.
171. Winter ML, Ellis MD, Snodgrass WR. Urine fluorescence using a Wood's lamp to detect the antifreeze additive sodium fluorescein: a qualitative adjunctive test in suspected ethylene glycol ingestions. *Ann Emerg Med.* 1990;19:663-667.
172. Woo MY, Greenway DC, Nadler SP, Cardinal P. Artifactual elevation of lactate in ethylene glycol poisoning. *J Emerg Med.* 2003;25:289-293.
173. Yayci N, Agritmis H, Turla A, Koc S. Fatalities due to methyl alcohol intoxication in Turkey: an 8-year study. *Forensic Sci Int.* 2003;131:36-41.
174. Yip L, Jacobsen D. Endogenous formate elimination and total body clearance during hemodialysis. *J Toxicol Clin Toxicol.* 2003;41:257-258.
175. Youssef GM, Hirsch DJ. Validation of a method to predict required dialysis time for cases of methanol and ethylene glycol poisoning. *Am J Kidney Dis.* 2005;46:509-511.
176. Ziegler SL. The ocular menace of wood alcohol poisoning. *JAMA.* 1921;77:1160-1166.

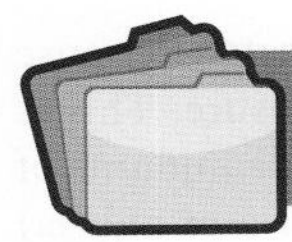

SPECIAL CONSIDERATIONS (SC5)

DIETHYLENE GLYCOL

Joshua G. Schier

$$HO—CH_2-CH_2-O—CH_2-CH_2-OH$$

Diethylene glycol is a common industrial solvent with physical and chemical properties similar to propylene glycol. (Chap. 55) Substitution of diethylene glycol for propylene glycol in oral elixirs has repeatedly caused epidemics of mass poisoning (Chap. 2). Patients develop neurologic symptoms and acute renal injury that often progresses to renal failure.

BRIEF HISTORY AND EPIDEMIOLOGY OF DIETHYLENE GLYCOL POISONING

Diethylene glycol (DEG) is produced by the condensation of two ethylene glycol molecules with an ether bond,[1] yielding a molecular weight of 106 Da. It was first isolated in 1869 and has been used in industry and manufacturing since 1928.[1] Since then it has found use as an antifreeze, as a finishing agent for wool, cotton, silk and other fabrics, and in dye manufacturing. DEG is chemically inert, does not ignite at normal temperatures, and has a higher boiling point than ethylene glycol (EG).[17,43] Its other physical properties are quite similar to EG, including a sweet taste.[17,43] It is often used as an intermediate in the production of polymers, higher glycols, morpholine, and dioxane.[26] Its physical properties enable it to serve as an excellent solvent for water-insoluble substances including drugs. This unfortunate use has accounted for the overwhelming majority of reported cases of illness.[4,6,7,9,11,12,14,15,21,23,29–33,36,38,43] In these recurring events, DEG was substituted for a safe and appropriate diluent such as glycerin or propylene glycol. Other causes of DEG-associated illness have resulted from the intentional addition of DEG to wine as a sweetening agent[40,41] and ingestion of radiator fluid or antifreeze,[27] brake fluid,[5] Sterno,[34] a "fog solution,"[16] cleaning solutions,[1] wallpaper stripper,[25] and as a substitute for ethanol.[44]

PHARMACOKINETICS/TOXICOKINETICS

Diethylene glycol is rapidly absorbed after ingestion and distributed primarily based on blood flow, with the kidneys receiving the most DEG, followed by the brain, the spleen, liver, and muscles.[17] The degree of protein binding and the volume of distribution (Vd) in humans is unknown but the Vd in the rat is approximately 1 L/kg.[17] Maximal DEG concentrations likely occur within 1 to 2 hours postingestion.[17,43] In both rats and dogs, as much as 30% of a given dose is converted to 2-(hydroxy) ethoxyacetic acid (HEAA).[10,26] In rats, there does not appear to be other metabolites although it is unclear if humans metabolize DEG by similar mechanisms.[17] Several early rat studies reported that oxaluria or calcium oxalate crystal formation occurred in renal tubules.[18,24,28] This limited evidence suggested that perhaps the ether bond joining the 2 ethylene glycol molecules was cleaved. This could then result in ethylene glycol-associated glycolate, glyoxylate and oxalate formation and the subsequent adverse health effects associated with ethylene glycol toxicity. (Chap. 107). Although this hypothesis for the pathophysiology of DEG induced renal toxicity remained popular for many years, more recent studies either failed to reproduce the oxaluria or found no difference in urinary oxalate concentrations when compared to control specimens.[24] In addition, during this previous work, there was no confirmation that the ingested DEG was the source of the oxalic acid production. In more recent work, rats given DEG with radiolabeled carbon had no subsequent radioactivity appear as ethylene glycol, glycoaldehyde, glycolate, glyxoylate, or exhaled carbon dioxide, indicating that there is no metabolism of DEG to any of these compounds.[42] The previous studies that found oxaluria all administered unlabeled DEG may have had unintentional contamination of their DEG with EG, because DEG is commercially prepared using EG.[42] Currently, it is believed that after ingestion, DEG undergoes oxidation by alcohol dehydrogenase to (2-hydroxyethoxy) acetaldehyde and then by aldehyde dehydrogenase to (2-hydroxyethoxy) acetic acid (HEAA). This was demonstrated when the formation of HEAA was decreased by 91% after administration of pyrazole (an alcohol dehydrogenase inhibitor) and by 66% after administration of diethyldithiocarbamate (an inhibitor of aldehyde dehydrogenase).[42] Further oxidation to diglycolic acid did not occur and is likely due to the subsequent formation of a cyclic compound that is not oxidized by alcohol or aldehyde dehydrogenase.[42] Rats pretreated with pyrazole and then administered the LD_{50} dose of DEG had decreased lethality.[42] However, pyrazole pretreatment did not confer a protective benefit in animals receiving greater than 25% above the LD_{50} dose.[42] This suggests that toxicity may be caused, in part, by another mechanism such as the parent compound, or another as of yet undiscovered metabolite. The possibility that higher doses of pyrazole were needed to protect against higher doses of DEG also exists.

Metabolism is saturable and as the dose increases, urinary elimination of the parent compound increases.[26] Carbon-14-labeled DEG is excreted primarily (~80%) in urine within 24 hours of ingestion.[26] Serum half-lives are dose-dependent with oral doses of 6 mL/kg and 12 mL/kg in rats producing biologic half-lives of 8 and 12 hours, respectively.[43] Another study found that urinary excretion half-lives for DEG in rats were dose dependent and ranged from 6 to 10 hours depending on doses ranging from 1–10 mL/kg.[17]At higher doses (≥5–10 mL/kg), DEG induces an osmotic diuresis, which accelerates elimination. This diuretic effect has a ceiling, as even greater doses of DEG (17.5 mL/kg) do not consistently trigger increased renal fluid losses.[17] At these greater doses, DEG elimination appears to follow first order kinetics with an elimination half-life of 3.6 hours.[17] However, increased doses are associated with lethargy, which limits oral intake and contributes to the development of oliguria and anuria.[17,26] This narcotic effect, triggered at doses of 5 and 10 mL/kg of DEG is strong evidence for DEG's ability to cross the blood brain barrier.[17]

TOXIC DOSE

Most available information on the pharmacokinetics and toxicokinetics of DEG is from studies in rats; however, limited data in humans are available. The median estimated toxic dose from the Haiti mass poisoning was determined to be 1.34 mL/kg (range, 0.22–4.42 mL/kg) or approximately 1–1.5 g/kg.[29] In the 1930s outbreak in the United States, the reported toxic doses in adults were similar.[6] Another study, examining postmortem DEG concentrations from a mass poisoning in Argentina in 1992, found a potentially lower lethal dose ranging from 0.014 to 0.170 mg/kg of body weight.[9,11] However, some questions remain concerning the validity and applicability of these calculations.[35] Furthermore, the analytical testing techniques used in this report may be subject to error due to cross-reactivity with other products formed as the result of normal postmortem processes.[13]

PATHOPHYSIOLOGY

The pathophysiology of DEG-induced nephrologic and neurologic illnesses are not well characterized. Limited evidence suggests that DEG may cause acute renal failure (ARF) through interruption of renal tubular transport processes.[22] This is consistent with observations made in the recent Panama poisonings.[37] In contrast, DEG-induced cortical necrosis is also reported.[25] The mechanism of DEG-induced neurologic toxicity remains unknown.[37] Furthermore, although HEAA is known to be a toxic metabolite, it is unclear if it is the only toxic compound. Questions remain about the possibility of inherent toxicity in the parent compound (DEG).

CLINICAL MANIFESTATIONS

The signs and symptoms of DEG poisoning are dependent on duration of exposure, dose, and other intrinsic host factors such as the presence of comorbidities. The presence of ARF remains the single unifying feature.[4,7,9,11,14,15,21,29–33,36,38] The permanence of DEG-induced ARF is unclear but it is not nearly or as readily reversible with either supportive or antidotal treatments (eg, fomepizole) as ethylene glycol-induced ARF. A spectrum of neurologic signs and symptoms can also occur and include unilateral or bilateral cranial VII (facial nerve) dysfunction, peripheral neuropathy, frank encephalopathy, and coma.[1,16,34,37]

In the Panama experience, the overwhelming majority of patients were adults who ingested small amounts of a product that was approximately 8% DEG concentration by volume.[33] The majority of patients presented with vague gastrointestinal or respiratory signs and symptoms and were found to be in ARF.[37] A significant number of these patients rapidly progressed to develop bilateral VII nerve paralysis and peripheral extremity weakness, often within several days. Finally, many also rapidly developed encephalopathy, coma, and death within 24 to 48 hours.[37] This incident was unique in that patients were mostly adults who received small amounts over an extended period of time in contrast to many other past incidents in which subjects were mostly children receiving relatively large doses of DEG.

DEG poisoning can also produce nausea, vomiting, abdominal pain, diarrhea, headache, metabolic acidosis, and confusion.[5] Some of the nonspecific symptoms may be attributable to ARF. Finally, patients may progress to develop multiple system organ failure and death.[5]

DIAGNOSTIC TESTING

Although specialized laboratory assays for DEG in blood and urine have been developed, they are not routinely available at most hospitals. The clinician will likely have to rely on a high index of suspicion and more commonly encountered "routine" testing methodologies including serum electrolytes and renal function tests. Nerve conduction studies may prove helpful in establishing the pattern of neuropathy if present. Use of an osmol gap has limitations[19] but may be helpful in patients with acute ingestions.

TREATMENT

Treatment of DEG poisoned individuals is complicated because they may not present until days after the initial exposure. This is especially true in individuals who have consumed small amounts of DEG over time as the first evidence of toxicity (oliguria or anuria) may be a delayed manifestation.[1,25,29,37] Following larger ingestions, symptoms such as confusion and altered mental status may present within hours of the ingestion.[3] Gastrointestinal decontamination including nasogastric lavage and activated charcoal administration should be strongly considered when the time to presentation to healthcare is minimal. Lavage is unlikely to be of any clinical benefit greater than 1 to 2 hours after ingestion as residual intragastric DEG beyond 2 hours is probably minimal or nonexistent. Although evidence supporting a clinical benefit with activated charcoal administration after 1 hour is lacking, little harm will result from giving a dose of activated charcoal when the patient has no contraindications to administration because DEG is potentially so toxic.[39] Unfortunately, however, gastrointestinal decontamination is unlikely to be of any benefit unless the patient presents within a few hours of the ingestion.

Fomepizole or other alcohol dehydrogenase inhibitors may be of some benefit in DEG poisoning.[42] However, the benefit appears to decrease or disappear as the dose increases, at least in animals.[42] This suggests that toxicity either may not be entirely caused by the primary metabolite (HEAA) or that larger doses of an inhibitor may be needed.[42] Fomepizole or ethanol was administered or coingested in at least four reports of DEG-associated illness.[1,3,5,34] In the first instance (and only case series), ethanol was administered to five of seven inmates who reportedly drank a DEG containing cleaning fluid and who presented to a tertiary healthcare facility for evaluation approximately 21 to 30 hours after the ingestion. Three of the 5 ill inmates had a severe metabolic acidosis (serum pH <7.1, or serum bicarbonate concentrations of 2.7 and 4 mEq/L) and elevated serum creatinine concentrations. All three were treated with ethanol and hemodialysis therapy but they either died or became hemodialysis dependent with persistent neurologic deficits. The remaining 2 ill inmates had evidence of milder toxicity including a milder metabolic acidosis (serum pH concentrations of 7.2 and 7.29 and serum bicarbonate concentrations of 16.4 and 12.1 mEq/L) and were treated with ethanol and hemodialysis, after which they had full recoveries.[1] The remaining two non-ill cases claimed a much milder exposure to the DEG containing fluid, were asymptomatic on hospital presentation and remained that way until discharge.[1]

There are limited conclusions that can be drawn from this information. The 2 patients who presented early (<10 hours)[3,5] and were treated aggressively (gastrointestinal decontamination, fomepizole, and hemodialysis) appeared to do much better than those who presented late (>10 hours).[1,16,34] Among the patients in the case series the three who died or had permanent neurologic and renal deficits, all presented late and with clinical manifestations of severe toxicity. Of the remaining four who reportedly drank DEG-containing brake fluid, all presented late but had full recoveries. As mentioned previously, of these four patients, two were asymptomatic on hospital presentation to begin with and remained that way. The remaining two patients had evidence of mild metabolic acidosis on presentation but no evidence of renal impairment. This strongly suggests that all four were exposed to a smaller dose than the first three and probably explains their lack of illness or recovery.[1]

In the Panama mass poisoning, the case-fatality rate was lower among patients who presented after the discovery of DEG as the etiology when compared to patients who presented before the etiology was discovered.[37] The reasons for this are unclear but may reflect a shorter time to critical therapies such as hemodialysis.[37] At least 1 report documented higher prehemodialysis and lower posthemodialysis concentrations of DEG suggesting that it is cleared by hemodialysis, although the gradient was relatively small (0–1.6 mg/dL).[5] Although the degree of DEG-protein binding is unknown, its molecular weight is 106.14 Da and its Vd is thought to be near 1 L/kg[17] (based on animal data), which suggest that hemodialysis would be effective in removing the compound.

At least one of the toxicants in DEG poisoning is the DEG metabolite HEAA.[42] If fomepizole or ethanol therapy is to be used in suspected or known cases of significant DEG poisoning, it should probably be administered in concert with hemodialysis, as the parent compound is most likely toxic as well.

SUMMARY

Patients with exposure to diethylene glycol present a diagnostic and therapeutic challenge. The repetitive epidemics of the use of this industrial solvent for human consumption has led to mass poisonings and critical nephrologic and neurologic illness. Early recognition of the epidemic and appropriate consideration of the antidotes fomepizole and ethanol as well as hemodialysis are indicated, although prevention of contamination of pharmaceuticals is truly most important.

DISCLAIMER

The findings and conclusions in this article are those of the authors and do not necessarily represent the views of the Centers for Disease Control and Prevention or the Agency for Toxic Substances and Disease Registry.

REFERENCES

1. Alfred S, Coleman P, Harris D, et al. Delayed neurologic sequelae resulting from epidemic diethylene glycol poisoning. *Clin Toxicol.* 2005;43:155-159.
2. Ballantyne B, Snellings WM. Developmental toxicity study with diethylene glycol dosed by gavage to CD rats and CD-1 mice. *Chem Toxicol.* 2005;43:1637-1646.
3. Borron SW, Baud FJ, Garnier R. Intravenous 4-methylpyrazole as an antidote for diethylene glycol and triethylene glycol poisoning: a case report. *Vet Hum Toxicol.* 1997;39:26-28.
4. Bowie MD, McKenzie D. Diethylene glycol poisoning in children. *South African Med J.* 1972; 931-934.
5. Brophy PD, Tenenbein M, Gardner J, et al. Childhood diethylene glycol poisoning treated with alcohol dehydrogenase inhibitor fomepizole and hemodialysis. *Am J Kidney Dis.* 2000;35:958-962.
6. Calvery HO, Klumpp TG. The toxicity for human beings of diethylene glycol with sulfanilamide. *SMJ.* 1939; 32:1105-1109.
7. Cantarell MC, Fort J, Camps J, et al. Acute intoxication due to topical application of diethylene glycol. *Ann Intern Med.* 1987;106:478-479.
8. Chyka PA, Seger D, Krenzelok EP, Vale JA. Position paper: single-dose activated charcoal. *J Toxicol Clin Toxicol.* 2004;42:843-854.
9. Drut R, Quijano G, Jones MC, Scanferla P. Hallazgos patologicos en la intoxicacion por dietilenglicol. *Medicina (Buenos Aires).* 1994;54:1-5.
10. Durand A, Auzépy P, Hébert JL, Trieu TC. A study of mortality and urinary excretion of oxalate in male rats following acute experimental intoxication with diethylene glycol. *Eur J Intens Care Med.* 1976;2:143-146.
11. Ferrari LA, Giannuzzi L. Clinical parameters, postmortem analysis and estimation of lethal dose in victims of a massive intoxication with diethylene glycol. *Forensic Sci Int.* 2005;153:45-51.
12. Geiling EMK, Coon JM, Schoeffel EW. Pathologic effects of elixir of sulfanilamide (diethylene glycol) poisoning. *JAMA.* 1938;111:919-926.
13. Gilliland MG, Bost RO. Alcohol in decomposed bodies: postmortem synthesis and distribution. *J Forensic Sci.* 1993;38:1266-1274.
14. Hanif M, Mobarak MR, Ronan A, et al. Fatal renal failure caused by diethylene glycol in paracetamol elixir: the Bangladesh epidemic. *BMJ.* 1995;311:88-91.
15. Hari P, Jain Y, Kabra SK. Fatal encephalopathy and renal failure caused by diethylene glycol poisoning. *J Trop Ped.* 2006:52:442-444.
16. Hasbani MJ, Sansing LH, Perrone J, et al. Encephalopathy and peripheral neuropathy following diethylene glycol ingestion. *Neurology.* 2005;64: 1273-1375.
17. Heilmair R, Lenk W, Lohr D. Toxicokinetics of diethylene glycol (DEG) in the rat. *Arch Toxicol.* 1993;67:655-666.
18. Herbert JL, Fabre M, Auzépy P, Paillas J. Acute experimental poisoning by diethylene glycol: acid base balance and histological data in male rats. *Toxicol Eur Res.* 1978;1:289-294.
19. Hoffman RS, Smilkstein MJ, Howland MA, Goldfrank LR. Osmol gaps revisited: normal values and limitations. *Clin Tox.* 1993;31:81-93.
20. Holland MG, Rosano TG. Osmolar gap method for detecting diethylene glycol. *J Tox Clin Tox.* 2007;6:221.
21. Junod SW. Diethylene Glycol Deaths in Haiti. *Public Health Reports.* 2000;115:78-86.
22. Kraul H, Jahn F, Braunlich H. Nephrotoxic effects of diethylene glycol (DEG) in rats. *Exp Pathol.* 1991;42:27-32.
23. Leech PN. Special article from the American Medical Association Chemical Laboratory. Elixir of sulfanilamide-massengill: chemical, pharmacologic, pathologic and necropsy reports; preliminary toxicity reports on diethylene glycol and sulfanilamide. *JAMA.* 1937;109:1531-1539.
24. Lenk W, Löhr D, Sonnenbichler J. Pharmacokinetics and biotransformation of diethylene glycol and ethylene glycol in the rat. *Xenobiotica.* 1989;19:961-979.
25. Marraffa JM, Holland MG, Stork CM, et al. Diethylene glycol: widely used solvent presents serious poisoning potential. *J Emerg Med.* 2008;35: 401-406.
26. Mathews JM, Parker MK, Matthews HB: Metabolism and disposition of diethylene glycol in rat and dog. *Drug Metab Disp.* 1991;19:1066-1070.
27. Milles G. Ethylene glycol poisoning. *Arch Pathol Lab Med.* 1946;41: 631-638.
28. Morris HG. Observations on the chronic toxicities of propylene glycol, ethylene glycol, diethylene glycol, ethylene glycol mono-ethyl-ether, and diethylene glycol mono-ethyl-ether. *J Phamacol Exp Ther.* 1942;74:266-273.
29. O'Brien KL, Selanikio JD, Hecdivert C, et al. Epidemic of pediatric deaths from acute renal failure caused by diethylene glycol poisoning. *JAMA.* 1995;279:1175-1180.
30. Okuonhghae HO, Ighogboja IS, Lawson JO, Nwana EJC. Diethylene glycol poisoning in Nigerian children. *AnnTrop Paed.* 1992;12:235-238.
31. Pandya SK. An unmitigated tragedy. *BMJ.* 1988;297:117-120.
32. Pilosuryl and severe diethylene glycol intoxication. *Prescrire Int.* 2004;13:59.
33. Rentz D, Lewis L, Mujica O, et al. Outbreak of acute renal failure syndrome due to diethylene glycol poisoning–Panama, 2006. Bulletin of the World Health Organization. http://www.who.int/bulletin/volumes/86/10/07-049965/en/index.html (accessed November 27, 2009).
34. Rollins YD, Filley CM, McNutt JT, et al. Fulminant ascending paralysis as a delayed sequela of diethylene glycol (Sterno) ingestion. *Neurology.* 2002;59:1460-1463.
35. Schep LJ, Slaughter RJ. Comments on diethylene glycol concentrations. *Forens Sci Int.* 2005;155:233.
36. Singh J, Dutta AK, Khare S, et al. Diethylene glycol poisoning in Gurgaon, India, 1998. Bulletin of the World Health Organization. 2001;79(2):88-95.
37. Sosa N, Rodriguez G. The clinical spectrum of DEG poisoning. *Clin Toxicol.* 2007;45:605–648. Lecture presentation at the North American Congress of Clinical Toxicology, September 2007, New Orleans, LA.
38. The CNA Corporation. After action report on HHS's response to the 2006 diethylene glycol poisonings in the Republic of Panama. IPR 12272/Draft. March 2007.
39. Vale JA, Kulig K: Position paper: gastric lavage. *J Toxicol Clin Toxicol.* 2004;42:933-943.
40. Van der Linden-Cremers PM, Sangster B: medical sequelae of the contamination of wine with diethylene glycol. *Ned Tijdschr Geneeskd.* 1985;129: 1890-1891.
41. Van Leusen R, Uges Dr: A patient with acute tubular necrosis as a consequence of drinking diethylene glycol-treated wine. *Ned Tijdschr Geneeskd.* 1987;131:768-771.
42. Weiner HL: Ethylene and diethylene glycol metabolism, toxicity and treatment. [dissertation]. Columbus, Ohio: Ohio State University; 1986.
43. Winek CL, Shingleton DP, Shanor SP. Ethylene and diethylene glycol toxicity. *Clin Toxicol.* 1978;13:297-324.
44. Wordley E. Diethylene glycol poisoning: report on two cases. *J Clin Pathol.* 1947;1:44-46.

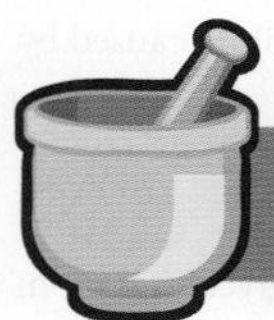

ANTIDOTES IN DEPTH (A31)

FOMEPIZOLE

Mary Ann Howland

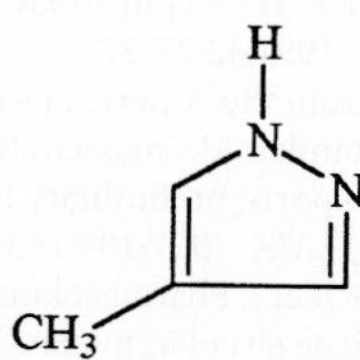

Fomepizole is a competitive inhibitor of alcohol dehydrogenase (ADH) that prevents the formation of toxic metabolites from ethylene glycol and methanol. It may also have a role in halting the disulfiram–ethanol reaction, and in limiting the toxicity from a variety of xenobiotics that rely on ADH for metabolism to toxic metabolites. In addition, as both an inducer and an inhibitor of certain cytochrome P450 (CYP) isoenzymes, the presence of fomepizole may lead to drug interactions.

HISTORY

In 1963, Theorell and associates described the inhibiting effect of pyrazole on the horse ADH-NAD^+ (nicotinamide adenine dinucleotide) enzyme–coenzyme system.[78] They noted that pyrazole blocked ADH by complexation, and that the administration of pyrazole to animals poisoned with methanol and ethylene glycol improved survival.[79] However, pyrazole also inhibited other liver enzymes, including catalase and the microsomal ethanol-oxidizing system.[55] Additional adverse effects of pyrazole administration resulted in bone marrow, liver, and renal toxicity, and these effects increased in the presence of ethanol and methanol.[66] These factors led to the search for less-toxic compounds with comparable mechanisms of action.

In 1969, Li and Theorell found that both pyrazole and 4-methylpyrazole (fomepizole) inhibited ADH in human liver preparations,[54] and studies in rodents found that fomepizole, unlike pyrazole, was relatively nontoxic regardless of the presence or absence of ethanol.[11] Subsequent studies of fomepizole in monkeys and humans poisoned with methanol and ethylene glycol confirmed both the inhibitory effect and relative safety of fomepizole.[16,17,66]

PHARMACOLOGY

Fomepizole has a molecular weight (MW) of 82 daltons, and a pKa of 2.91 at low concentrations and a pKa of 3.0 at high concentrations. The free base is used in the United States, whereas the salts are used in Europe. The free base is chemically equivalent to the chloride and sulfate salts at physiologic pH.[21]

Values for K_m (Michaelis-Menten dissociation constant; substrate concentration where the rate of metabolism is half the maximum) have been estimated for the toxic alcohols, along with the value for K_i (dissociation of enzyme-inhibitor complex inhibition constant) with fomepizole. The smaller the K_m, the higher the affinity of the substrate (alcohol) for the enzyme, and the lower the concentration of the substrate that is needed to half saturate the enzyme. Studies in monkey and human liver tissue demonstrate that fomepizole is a competitive inhibitor of alcohol dehydrogenase.[58,73] In monkey liver, fomepizole demonstrated very similar K_is for both ethanol and methanol at 7.5 and 9.1 μmol/L, respectively.[58] The affinity was 10 times higher when human liver was used.[72] Studies in monkeys demonstrate that a fomepizole concentration of 9 to 10 μmol/L (0.74–0.8 μg/mL) is needed to inhibit the metabolism of methanol to formate.[11,66] In human liver, the concentration needed to achieve inhibition is about 0.9 to 1 μmol/L.[54,72] The most recent trial using intravenous fomepizole attempted to maintain a serum fomepizole concentration above 10 μmol/L. Current dosing calls for a serum fomepizole concentration of 100 to 300 μmol/L to ensure a margin of safety.[1]

The CYP2E1 isoenzyme oxidizes to toxic metabolites ethanol and a number of other xenobiotics, including acetaminophen, carbon tetrachloride, nitrosamines, and benzene. Fomepizole, like ethanol and isoniazid, has the following effects on this isoenzyme: Fomepizole induces CYP2E1 in rat liver and kidney, but not in the lung, through a posttranscriptional mechanism not involving increased mRNA. However, when fomepizole is present, the isoenzyme is inhibited. It is not until after fomepizole is eliminated that the consequences of induction are manifest.[14,83,84] In hepatocyte culture, fomepizole stabilizes and maintains the induced metabolic activity of the isoenzyme for about 1 week.[85]

PHARMACOKINETICS

The volume of distribution of fomepizole is about 0.6 to 1 L/kg; it is metabolized to 4-carboxypyrazole, an inactive metabolite that accounts for 80% to 85% of the administered dose.[63] In healthy human volunteers, oral doses of fomepizole were rapidly absorbed and demonstrated saturation and nonlinear kinetics.[40,60] The K_m was estimated to be 75 μmol/L in two studies and 0.94 μmol/L in the most recent analysis, although the reason for the discrepancy is not known.[40,60,61] First-order kinetics were exhibited at concentrations below the K_m, whereas zero-order elimination occurred at concentrations 100% to 200% of the K_m.[40] Thus, elimination of fomepizole at doses of 10 mg/kg, 20 mg/kg, 50 mg/kg, and 100 mg/kg was 3.66, 5.05, 10.3, and 14.9 μmol/L/h, respectively.[40] Classical Michaelis-Menten kinetics would predict that the elimination rate should be the same at the two higher doses, but this is not the case. The authors speculate that multiple metabolic pathways with different affinities exist and predominate at different fomepizole concentrations. At a dose of 20 mg/kg, the half-life of fomepizole calculated from the linear portion of the curve was 5.2 hours and occurred when serum concentrations were less than 100 μmol/L. Peak concentrations after oral administration were achieved within 2 hours and were 132, 326, 759, and 1425 μmol/L following 10, 20, 50, and 100 mg/kg doses, respectively. Every increase of 10 mg/kg in the oral dose of fomepizole raised the serum concentration 130 to 160 μmol/L.[40] The renal clearance was low (0.016 mL/min/kg), and only 3% of the administered dose was excreted unchanged in the urine.[40]

In a pharmacokinetic study in healthy volunteers, oral administration produced similar serum concentrations to intravenous (IV) fomepizole.[60] The pharmacokinetics of IV fomepizole were studied in 14 patients being treated for ethylene glycol toxicity.[48] A mean peak concentration of 342 μmol/L (200–400 μmol/L) was achieved following a loading dose of 15 mg/kg (183 μmol/kg).[63,75] A significant weakness of the study involving toxicokinetic data is that the effect of simultaneous serum ethanol concentrations was not analyzed. The lowest serum fomepizole concentration of 105 μmol/L was present at 8 hours after the loading dose. The rate of elimination was determined to be zero order at 16 μmol/L/h compared with a first-order elimination half-life of 3 hours during hemodialysis. Other authors have reported similar fomepizole clearances (12.99 μmol/L/h).[18] A recent pharmacokinetic analysis in patients poisoned with methanol or ethylene glycol demonstrated a mean peak fomepizole concentration of 226 μmol/L (19 μg/mL), an apparent half-life of 14.5 hours (in the presence of methanol or ethylene glycol), and an apparent half-life of 40 hours in the presence of ethanol along with methanol or ethylene glycol. In the sole death, hepatic tissue contained 12 μg/g of fomepizole, even when the serum concentration was less than 1 μg/mL (12 μmol/L).[82]

The hemodialysis clearance of fomepizole ranges from 50 mL/min to 137 mL/min.[27,47] An analysis using determinations of dialysis fluid revealed an extraction ratio of approximately 75% and a dialysance of 117 mL/min, which was very similar to a simultaneous ethylene glycol determination.[27] The dialysance of fomepizole was similar to urea in a pig model and suggests no significant protein binding of fomepizole.[41]

The pharmacokinetic interactions between fomepizole and ethanol were studied in a double-blind crossover design in healthy human volunteers.[45] Fomepizole was given orally in doses of 10, 15, and 20 mg/kg one hour prior to oral ethanol at 0.5 to 0.7 g/kg as a 20% solution in orange juice. Fomepizole decreased the elimination rate of ethanol by approximately 40%, from 12 to 16 mg/dL/h to about 7 to 9.5 mg/dL/h. When IV fomepizole was administered at 5 mg/kg over 30 minutes and ethanol was administered orally at doses to achieve a concentration of 50 to 150 mg/dL for 6 hours beginning at the end of the fomepizole infusion, the elimination of fomepizole was decreased by approximately 50%.[45] This decrease occurred without a change in the amount or fraction of unchanged fomepizole appearing in the urine. The authors suggested that the ethanol probably inhibited the metabolism of fomepizole to 4-carboxypyrazole by the CYP system. A single low dose of fomepizole given to humans had a maximal effect on ethanol metabolism at 1.5 to 2 hours.[10] Thus, ethanol and fomepizole mutually inhibit the elimination of the other, prolonging their respective serum concentrations.[59,64] Methanol also decreases the elimination of fomepizole by approximately 25% in the monkey.[66]

METHANOL

IN VITRO AND ANIMAL STUDIES

Studies using human livers demonstrate the inhibitory effect of fomepizole on alcohol dehydrogenase.[72] Studies in monkeys, the animal species that most closely resembles humans in metabolizing methanol, also clearly demonstrate the inhibitory effect of fomepizole in preventing the accumulation of formate.[9,66,67]

HUMAN EXPERIENCE

The two largest fomepizole case series to date involved 11 and eight patients, respectively, who were given IV fomepizole in the approved US dosing regimen.[15,17,36] Following administration, formate concentrations in all patients fell and the arterial pH increased.[17] Case reports demonstrate similar findings.[18,29,32]

EFFECT OF FOMEPIZOLE ON METHANOL AND FORMATE CONCENTRATIONS

Methanol exhibits dose-dependent kinetics.[44] At low doses (0.08 g/kg), which achieve serum concentrations of about 10 mg/dL, methanol elimination is first order, with a half-life of about 2.5 to 3 hours.[48,51] In concentrations of about 100 to 200 mg/dL, methanol exhibits zero-order kinetics and is eliminated at about 8.5 to 9 mg/dL/h in untreated humans[46] and 4.4 to 7 mg/dL/h in untreated monkeys.[25,69] When monkeys were given 3 g/kg of methanol with resultant serum concentrations of about 500 mg/dL, the elimination of methanol exhibited apparent first-order kinetics. This alteration is likely caused by the greater contribution of other first-order pathways, such as pulmonary and urinary elimination, which may account for a greater fraction of the total body clearance under these circumstances.[44] Once fomepizole was administered, the elimination of methanol became first order in humans, and the half-life of methanol was about 54 hours.[17,36] When the metabolism of methanol to formate is blocked, formate is eliminated with a half-life dependent on dose and with an uncertain effect of folate and bicarbonate therapies. When formate was administered to monkeys in the absence of methanol, formate half-life was 30 to 50 minutes.[22] In monkeys given methanol followed by fomepizole, the formate concentrations decreased by more than 80% in 2 hours.[9] An analysis of formate concentrations in six patients with methanol poisoning treated with fomepizole, folate, and sodium bicarbonate revealed a formate half-life of 235 +/− 83 minutes.[49] A more recent analysis involving eight patients with methanol poisoning treated with fomepizole and sodium bicarbonate revealed a formate half-life of 156 minutes.[36]

ETHYLENE GLYCOL

IN VITRO AND ANIMAL STUDIES

Monkeys given 3 g/kg of ethylene glycol intraperitoneally recovered without treatment, whereas those given 4 g/kg died without therapy. All those given 4 g/kg of ethylene glycol with fomepizole survived.[22]

HUMAN EXPERIENCE

The first three patients treated with oral fomepizole improved clinically and tolerated the therapy.[4] Subsequent case reports and case series using fomepizole orally or IV, with or without hemodialysis, have also demonstrated effectiveness of fomepizole in preventing glycolate accumulation.[5,12,16,30,33,35,47,68,71,75]

EFFECT OF FOMEPIZOLE ON ETHYLENE GLYCOL AND GLYCOLATE CONCENTRATIONS IN HUMANS

Renal function is essential in the elimination of ethylene glycol. With normal renal function, the half-life of ethylene glycol is about 8.6 hours.[75] Based on pooled human data, the half-life of ethylene glycol after alcohol dehydrogenase is blocked by fomepizole is about 14 to 17 hours in patients with normal renal function, and about 49 hours in patients with impaired renal function.[4,33,75] Based on a limited number of determinations, the renal clearance of ethylene glycol averaged 31.5 mL/min during the first two days; the corresponding creatinine clearance was 112 mL/min, and estimated total body clearance during fomepizole therapy was 57 mL/min.[5] These calculations suggest that the renal clearance of ethylene glycol accounted for only 55% of estimated total body clearance. In a study where neither renal function was defined nor the amount of glycolate (MW = 76 daltons) excreted unchanged by the kidneys described, glycolate had a mean half-life of 10 ± 8 hours in patients treated with fomepizole before hemodialysis, and a mean half-life of less than three hours during hemodialysis.[42,50,68]

SAFETY AND ADVERSE EFFECTS

Retinol dehydrogenase, which is responsible for converting retinol to retinal in the eye, is an isoenzyme of ADH. As such, it was essential to study whether fomepizole would inhibit this enzyme and subsequently produce retinal damage.[66,67] Studies in several animal species demonstrate that fomepizole is relatively nontoxic, with no demonstrable signs of ophthalmic toxicity.[9] Two of the largest case series, and two recent case reports confirm the lack of retinal toxicity with fomepizole and demonstrate the reversibility of methanol-induced visual toxicity when patients are treated with fomepizole and hemodialysis before permanent ophthalmic toxicity developed.[16,17,26,77]

The LD_{50} (median lethal dose for 50% of test subjects) of fomepizole in mice and rats is 3.8 mmol/kg after IV administration, and 7.9 mmol/kg following oral administration.[57] An oral placebo-controlled, double-blind, single-dose, randomized, sequential, ascending-dose study was performed in healthy volunteers to determine fomepizole tolerance at 10 to 100 mg/kg.[44] There were no adverse effects in the 10 and 20 mg/kg groups, whereas at 50 mg/kg, three of four subjects experienced slight to moderate nausea and dizziness within 2.5 hours of fomepizole administration. All subjects reported comparable symptoms at 100 mg/kg, which lasted for 30 hours in one individual without vital sign or laboratory abnormalities noted. The most common adverse effects of the use of fomepizole reported by the manufacturer (in a total of 78 patients and 63 volunteers) were headache (14%), nausea (11%), and dizziness, increased drowsiness, and bad taste/metallic taste (6%).[1] Other less commonly observed adverse effects include phlebitis, rash, fever, and eosinophilia. A recent case report of a patient severely poisoned with ethylene glycol describes a temporal association between IV fomepizole administration during hemodialysis and the development of bradycardia and hypotension. However, this patient was severely acidotic, and when the patient received the fomepizole postdialysis no such adverse effects were noted.[52] Divided daily doses of fomepizole up to 20 mg/kg for 5 days have been administered without any demonstrable toxicity.[65] The most common laboratory abnormality after fomepizole administration is a transient elevation of aminotransferase levels, which was reported in six of 15 healthy volunteers.[43] In the two largest case series of patients treated with fomepizole for toxic alcohol poisoning, there were no adverse events classified as "definitely" or "probably" related to fomepizole.[16,17] Fomepizole is not approved for use in children, but has been used successfully in children who have ingested ethylene glycol and methanol.[6,13,19,23,24,34,82]

Fomepizole is pregnancy category C and thus should be used appropriately as indicated.

DISULFIRAM AND OTHER XENOBIOTICS

Fomepizole successfully terminated the adverse reactions resulting from the use of disulfiram administered to volunteers pretreated with a small dose of ethanol, and reactions occurring in a chronic alcoholic surreptitiously given disulfiram by his wife.[56] Pretreatment with oral fomepizole was also successful in preventing the facial flushing and tachycardia typically associated with ethanol administration in ethanol-sensitive Japanese subjects.[38,39]

Limited animal studies and a few case reports suggest that fomepizole may be effective in limiting the toxicity secondary to diethylene glycol, triethylene glycol, and 1,3-difluoro-2-propanol.[12,28,80] The role of fomepizole in overdoses secondary to 2-butoxyethanol (ethylene glycol monobutyl ether, butyl cellosolve) is unclear, but fomepizole may be useful if administered within several hours of ingestion and before rapid metabolism of butoxyethanol to butoxyacetic acid occurs.[62,70] Isopropanol is probably metabolized at least in part by alcohol dehydrogenase, but fomepizole therapy is not indicated, as this intervention would prolong the metabolism of isopropanol to acetone.[1]

COMPARISON TO ETHANOL

Ethanol has been used for many years to inhibit the metabolism of methanol and ethylene glycol to their respective toxic metabolites.[31,81] Although very inexpensive, ethanol has many disadvantages, compared to fomepizole. Ethanol causes central nervous system (CNS) depression that is at least additive to that of the methanol or ethylene glycol; dosing difficulties occur as a result of the rapid and often unpredictable rate of ethanol metabolism, and prolonged ethanol administration causes tolerance to ethanol to develop; an intravenous formulation of ethanol is no longer readily available[7]; the serum concentrations of ethanol must be closely monitored; a 5% or 10% IV preparation of ethanol is hyperosmolar[86]; and there is a great potential for hyponatremia and hypoglycemia or other ethanol-related adverse effects, such as pancreatitis and hepatitis. In contrast to all of these problems associated with ethanol administration, fomepizole has the advantage of being a very potent inhibitor of alcohol dehydrogenase without producing CNS depression. Fomepizole dosing is much easier without a need for serum concentration monitoring, thus allowing for every-12-hour dosing except during hemodialysis, when dosing should occur every 4 hours. Limited adverse effects of fomepizole include local reactions at the site of infusion when concentrations exceeding 25 mg/mL are used, nausea, dizziness, anxiety, headache, rash, transiently elevated aminotransferases, and eosinophilia.

Fomepizole is preferred to ethanol for all of the above reasons. Ethanol should only be used when fomepizole is not readily available. Hospitals should be encouraged to stock fomepizole.[53,76]

DOSING

The loading dose of fomepizole is 15 mg/kg IV, followed in 12 hours by 10 mg/kg every 12 hours for 4 doses. If therapy is necessary beyond 48 hours, the dose is then increased to 15 mg/kg every 12 hours, for as long as necessary. This increase is recommended because fomepizole stimulates its own metabolism. Patients undergoing hemodialysis require additional doses of fomepizole to replace the amount removed during hemodialysis.

The manufacturer recommends dosing fomepizole every 4 hours during hemodialysis.[1] Fomepizole should be administered at the beginning of hemodialysis if the last dose was more than 6 hours earlier. At the completion of hemodialysis, administer the next scheduled dose if more than 3 hours have transpired, or one-half of the dose if 1 to 3 hours have passed. Then continue with every-12-hour dosing.

The fomepizole dose must be diluted in 100 mL of 0.9% sodium chloride solution or dextrose 5% in water (D_5W) prior to IV administration, and then infused over 30 minutes to avoid venous irritation and phlebosclerosis. Once diluted, fomepizole remains stable for 24 hours when stored in the refrigerator or at room temperature.[1]

Fomepizole therapy should be continued until the methanol or ethylene glycol is no longer present in sufficient concentrations to produce toxicity. Although these concentrations are not precisely known, 25 to 50 mg/dL of either ethylene glycol or methanol is a conservative estimate that can be lowered in the presence of acid–base disturbances.[1–3]

The threshold concentrations for hemodialysis of methanol or ethylene glycol can be based on measurements when analyses can be done in a timely fashion. The duration of fomepizole therapy in the absence of hemodialysis can be estimated based on the assumption of half-life of the toxic alcohol when blocked with fomepizole. The half-life of methanol is approximately 54 hours in the presence of fomepizole.[12] The half-life of ethylene glycol in the presence of fomepizole is approximately 14 to 17 hours in patients with normal renal function, and 49 hours in patients with impaired renal function.[4,35,75]

The need for hemodialysis is based on the presence of toxic metabolites inferred by metabolic acidosis and presence of end-organ damage; the ability of the kidney to eliminate ethylene glycol and glycolic acid, and formate; the risk benefit of hemodialysis; and the length of time to remain hospitalized for elimination of the remaining methanol and ethylene glycol.[37,74]

AVAILABILITY

Fomepizole is marketed as Antizol injection by Jazz Pharmaceuticals (originally by Orphan Medical) in a tray pack containing four vials (1.5 mL vials of 1 g/mL). It is now also available generically by X-Gen Pharmaceuticals and Sandoz, both of whom allow the purchase of just one vial. Temperatures of less than 77°F (25°C) cause the contents of the fomepizole vials to solidify. Warming reliquifies the product without adversely affecting its potency.

SUMMARY

Fomepizole is a potent competitive inhibitor of alcohol dehydrogenase that is useful in inhibiting the metabolism of methanol, ethylene glycol, and other xenobiotics that use ADH in the formation of toxic metabolites. Once ADH is blocked, the decision to use hemodialysis depends on how much damage has occurred to the organs of elimination, and how well the body can eliminate both the parent compound and the toxic metabolites formed prior to fomepizole administration. Fomepizole appears to be safe and, although it has been used successfully orally, only an IV dosing regimen is approved and available. Fomepizole is more costly than ethanol, but its many advantages over ethanol, including the ability to often deliver care outside an intensive care unit, make fomepizole the preferred antidote. Hospitals should be encouraged to stock fomepizole.

REFERENCES

1. Antizol [package insert]. Minnetonka, MN: Orphan Medical; December 2000.
2. Barceloux DG, Bond GR, Krenzelok EP. American Academy of Clinical Toxicology practice guidelines on the treatment of methanol poisoning. *J Toxicol Clin Toxicol.* 2002;40:415-446.
3. Barceloux DG, Krenzelok EP, Olson K, Watson W. American Academy of Clinical Toxicology practice guidelines on the treatment of ethylene glycol poisoning. Ad Hoc Committee. *J Toxicol Clin Toxicol.* 1999;37:537-560.
4. Baud F, Bismuth C, Garnier R, et al. 4-Methylpyrazole may be an alternative to ethanol therapy for ethylene glycol intoxication in man. *J Toxicol Clin Toxicol.* 1986;24:463-483.
5. Baud F, Galliot M, Astier A, et al. Treatment of ethylene glycol poisoning with intravenous 4-methylpyrazole. *N Engl J Med.* 1988;319:97-110.
6. Baum CR, Langman CB, Oker EE, et al. Fomepizole treatment of ethylene glycol poisoning in an infant. *Pediatrics.* 2000;106:1489-1491.
7. Berberet B, Burda A, Breier C, Lodolce AE. Discontinuation of 5% alcohol in 5% dextrose injection: implications for antidote stocking. *Am J Health Sys Pharm.* 2008;65:2200, 2203.
8. Blair AH, Vallee BL. Some catalytic properties of human liver alcohol dehydrogenase. *Biochemistry.* 1966;5:2026-2034.
9. Blomstrand R, Ingelmansson S. Studies on the effect of 4-methylpyrazole on methanol poisoning using the monkey as an animal model: with particular reference to the ocular toxicity. *Drug Alcohol Depend.* 1984;13:343-355.
10. Blomstrand R, Theorell H. Inhibitory effect on ethanol oxidation in man after administration of 4-methylpyrazole. *Life Sci.* 1970;9:631-640.
11. Blomstrand R, Wintzell H, Lof A, et al. Pyrazoles as inhibitors of alcohol oxidation and as important tools in alcohol research: an approach to therapy against methanol poisoning. *Proc Natl Acad Sci U S A.* 1979;76:3499-3503.
12. Borron SW, Mégarbane B, Baud FJ. Fomepizole in treatment of uncomplicated ethylene glycol poisoning. *Lancet.* 1999;354:831.
13. Boyer EW, Mejia M, Woolf A, Shannon M. Severe ethylene glycol ingestion treated without hemodialysis. *Pediatrics.* 2001;107:172-173.
14. Brennan RJ, Mankes RF, Lefevre R, et al. 4-Methylpyrazole blocks acetaminophen hepatotoxicity in the rat. *Ann Emerg Med.* 1994,23:487-494.
15. Brent J, McMartin K, Phillips SP, et al. 4-Methylpyrazole (fomepizole) therapy of methanol poisoning: preliminary results of the META trial. *J Toxicol Clin Toxicol.* 1997;35:507.
16. Brent J, McMartin K, Phillips SP, et al. Fomepizole for the treatment of ethylene glycol poisoning. *N Engl J Med.* 1999;340:832-838.
17. Brent J, McMartin K, Phillips SP, et al. Fomepizole for the treatment of methanol poisoning. *N Engl J Med.* 2001;344:424-429.
18. Burns MJ, Graudins, Aaron CK, et al. Treatment of methanol poisoning with intravenous 4-methylpyrazole. *Ann Emerg Med.* 1997;30:829-832.
19. Caravati EM, Heileson HL, Jones M. Treatment of severe pediatric ethylene glycol intoxication without hemodialysis. *J Toxicol Clin Toxicol.* 2004;42:255-259.
20. Cheng JT, Beysolow TD, Kaul B, et al. Clearance of ethylene glycol by kidneys and hemodialysis. *J Toxicol Clin Toxicol.* 1987;25:95-108.
21. Chilukuri DM, Shah JC. pKa of 4MP and chemical equivalence in formulations of free base and salts of 4MP. *PDA J Pharm Sci Technol.* 1999;53:44-47.
22. Clay KL, Murphy RC, Watkins WD. Experimental methanol toxicity in the primate: analysis of metabolic acidosis. *Toxicol Appl Pharmacol.* 1975;13:319-333.
23. De Brabander N, Wojciechowski M, De Decker K, et al. Fomepizole as a therapeutic strategy in paediatric methanol poisoning. A case report and review of the literature. *Eur J Pediatr.* 2005;164:158-161.
24. Detaille T, Wallemacq P, Clement de Clety S, et al. Fomepizole alone for severe infant ethylene glycol poisoning. *Pediatr Crit Care Med.* 2004;5:490-491.
25. Eells JT, Makar AB, Noker PE, Tephly TR. Methanol poisoning and formate oxidation in nitrous oxide-treated rats. *J Pharmacol Exp Ther.* 1981;217:57-61.
26. Essama Mbia JJ, Guerit JM, Haufroid V, Hantson P. Fomepizole therapy for reversal of visual impairment after methanol poisoning: a case documented by visual evoked potentials investigation. *Am J Ophthalmol.* 2002;134:914-916.
27. Faessel H, Houze P, Baud FJ, Scherrmann JM. 4-Methylpyrazole monitoring during haemodialysis of ethylene glycol intoxicated patients. *Eur J Clin Pharmacol.* 1995;49:211-213.
28. Feldwick MS, Noakes PS, Prause U, et al. The biochemical toxicology of 1,3-difluoro-2-propanol, the major ingredient of the pesticide gliftor: the potential of 4-methylpyrazole as an antidote. *J Biochem Mol Toxicol.* 1998;12:41-52.
29. Girault C, Tamion F, Moritz F, et al. Fomepizole (4-methylpyrazole) in fatal methanol poisoning with early CT scan cerebral lesions. *J Toxicol Clin Toxicol.* 1999;35:777-780.
30. Goldfarb DS. Fomepizole for ethylene-glycol poisoning. *Lancet.* 1999;354:1646.
31. Grauer GF, Thrall MAH, Henre BA, Hjelle JJ. Comparison of the effects of ethanol and 4-methylpyrazole on the pharmacokinetics and toxicity of ethylene glycol in the dog. *Toxicol Lett.* 1987;35:307-314.
32. Hantson P, Wallemacq P, Brau M, et al. Two cases of acute methanol poisoning partially treated by oral 4-methylpyrazole. *Intensive Care Med.* 1999;25:528-531.

33. Hantson PH, Hassoun A, Mahieu P. Ethylene glycol poisoning treated by intravenous 4-methylpyrazole. *Intensive Care Med.* 1998;24:736-739.
34. Harry P, Jobard E, Briand M, et al. Ethylene glycol poisoning in a child treated with 4-methylpyrazole. *Pediatrics.* 1998;102:E31.
35. Harry P, Turcant A, Bouachour G, et al. Efficacy of 4-methylpyrazole in ethylene glycol poisoning. Clinical and toxicokinetic aspects. *Hum Exp Toxicol.* 1994;13:61-64.
36. Hovda KE, Andersson KS, Urdal P, Jacobsen D. Methanol and formate kinetics during treatment with fomepizole. *Clin Toxicol.* 2005;43:221-227.
37. Hovda KE, Jacobsen D. Expert opinion: fomepizole may ameliorate the need for hemodialysis in methanol poisoning. *Hum Exp Ther.* 2008;27:539-546.
38. Inoue K, Fukunaga M, Kiriyama T, Komura S. Accumulation of acetaldehyde in alcohol-sensitive Japanese: relation to ethanol and acetaldehyde oxidizing capacity. *Alcohol Clin Exp Res.* 1984;8:319-322.
39. Inoue K, Kera Y, Kiriyama T, Komura S. Suppression of acetaldehyde accumulation by 4-methylpyrazole in alcohol-hypersensitive Japanese. *Jpn J Pharmacol.* 1985;38:43-48.
40. Jacobsen D, Barron SK, Sebastian CS, et al. Nonlinear kinetics of 4-methylpyrazole in healthy human subjects. *Eur J Clin Pharmacol.* 1989;37:599-604.
41. Jacobsen D, Østensen J, Bredesen L, et al. 4-Methylpyrazole (4-MP) is effectively removed by hemodialysis in the pig model. *Vet Hum Toxicol.* 1992;34:362.
42. Jacobsen D, Øvrebo S, Østborg J, Sejersted OM. Glycolate causes the acidosis in ethylene glycol poisoning and is effectively removed by hemodialysis. *Acta Med Scand.* 1984:216:409-416.
43. Jacobsen D, Sebastian CS, Barron SK, et al. Effects of 4-methylpyrazole, methanol/ethylene glycol antidote, in healthy humans. *J Emerg Med.* 1990;8:455-461.
44. Jacobsen D, Sebastian CS, Blomstrand R, McMartin KE. 4-methylpyrazole: a controlled study of safety in healthy human subjects after single ascending doses. *Alcohol Clin Exp Res.* 1988;12:516-522.
45. Jacobsen D, Sebastian CS, Dies DF, et al. Kinetic interactions between 4-methylpyrazole and ethanol in healthy humans. *Alcohol Clin Exp Res.* 1996;20:804-809.
46. Jacobsen D, Webb R, Collins TD, McMartin KE. Methanol and formate kinetics in late diagnosed methanol intoxication. *Med Toxicol.* 1988;3:418-423.
47. Jobard E, Harry P, Turcant A, et al. 4-Methylpyrazole and hemodialysis in ethylene glycol poisoning. *J Toxicol Clin Toxicol.* 1996;34:373-377.
48. Jones AW. Elimination half-life of methanol during hangover. *Pharmacol Toxicol.* 1987;60:217-220.
49. Kerns W 2nd, Tomaszewski C, McMartin K, et al. META Study Group. Methylpyrazole for toxic alcohols. Formate kinetics in methanol poisoning. *J Toxicol Clin Toxicol.* 2002;40:137-143.
50. Knepshield JH, Shreiner GE, Lowenthal DT, et al. Dialysis of poisons and drugs: annual review. *Trans Am Soc Artif Intern Organs.* 1973;19:590-633.
51. Leaf G, Zatman LJ. A study of the conditions under which methanol may exert a toxic hazard in industry. *Br J Ind Med.* 1952;9:19-31.
52. Lepik KJ, Brubacher JR, Dewitt CR, et al. Bradycardia and hypotension associated with fomepizole infusion during hemodialysis. *Clin Toxicol.* 2008;46:570-573.
53. Lepik KJ, Levy AR, Sobolev BG, et al. Adverse drug events associated with the antidotes for methanol and ethylene glycol poisoning: a comparison of ethanol and fomepizole. *Ann Emerg Med.* 2009;53:451-453.
54. Li TK, Theorell H. Human liver alcohol dehydrogenase: inhibition by pyrazole and pyrazole analogs. *Acta Chem Scand.* 1969;23:892-902.
55. Lieber C, Rubin E, DeCarli L, et al. Effects of pyrazole on hepatic function and structure. *Lab Invest.* 1970;22:615-621.
56. Lindros KO, Stowell A, Pikkarainen P, Salaspuro M. The disulfiram (Antabuse)-alcohol reaction in male alcoholics: its efficient management by 4-methylpyrazole. *Alcohol Clin Exp Res.* 1981;5:528-530.
57. Magnusson G, Nyberg J-A, Bodin N-O, Hansson E. Toxicity of pyrazole and 4-methylpyrazole in mice and rats. *Experientia.* 1972;28:1198-1200.
58. Makar AB, Tephly TR. Inhibition of monkey liver alcohol dehydrogenase by 4-methylpyrazole. *Biochem Med.* 1975;13:334-342.
59. Makar AB, Tephly TR, Mannering GJ. Methanol metabolism in the monkey. *Mol Pharmacol.* 1968;4:471-483.
60. Marraffa J, Stork C, Howland MA, et al. Oral administration of fomepizole produces similar blood levels as identical intravenous dose. *Clin Toxicol.* 2008;46:181-186.
61. Mayersohn M, Owens, SM, Anaya AL, et al. 4-Methylpyrazole disposition in the dog: evidence for saturable elimination. *J Pharm Sci.* 1985;74:895-896.
62. McKinney PE, Palmer RB, Blackwell W, Benson BE. Butoxyethanol ingestion with prolonged hyperchloremic metabolic acidosis treated with ethanol therapy. *J Toxicol Clin Toxicol.* 2000;38:787-793.
63. McMartin KE, Brent J, META Study Group. Pharmacokinetics of fomepizole (4MP) in patients [abstract]. *J Toxicol Clin Toxicol.* 1998;36:450-451.
64. McMartin KE, Collins TD. Distribution of oral 4-methylpyrazole in the rat: inhibition of elimination by ethanol. *J Toxicol Clin Toxicol.* 1988;26:451-466.
65. McMartin KE, Heath A. The treatment of ethylene glycol poisoning with intravenous 4-methylpyrazole. *N Engl J Med.* 1989;320:125.
66. McMartin KE, Hedstrom K-G, Tolf B, et al. Studies on the metabolic interactions between 4-methylpyrazole and methanol using the monkey as an animal model. *Arch Biochem Biophys.* 1980;199:606-614.
67. McMartin KE, Makar AB, Martin A, et al. Methanol poisoning I. The role of formic acid in the development of metabolic acidosis in the monkey and the reversal by 4-methylpyrazole. *Biochem Med.* 1975;13:319-333.
68. Moreau CL, Kerns, W II, Tomaszewski CA, et al. Glycolate kinetics and hemodialysis clearance in ethylene glycol poisoning. *J Toxicol Clin Toxicol.* 1998;36:659-666.
69. Noker PE, Eells JT, Tephly TR. Methanol toxicity: treatment with folic acid and 5-formyl-tetrahydrofolic acid. *Alcohol Clin Exp Res.* 1980;4:378-383.
70. Osterhoudt KC. Fomepizole therapy for pediatric butoxyethanol intoxication. *J Toxicol Clin Toxicol.* 2002;40:929-930.
71. Parry MF, Wallach R. Ethylene glycol poisoning. *Am J Med.* 1974;57:143-150.
72. Pietruszko R. Human liver alcohol dehydrogenase inhibition of methanol activity by pyrazole, 4-methylpyrazole, 4-hydroxymethylpyrazole and 4-carboxypyrazole. *Biochem Pharmacol.* 1975;24:1603-1607.
73. Pietruszko R, Voigtlander K, Lester D. Alcohol dehydrogenase from human and horse liver—substrate specificity with diols. *Biochem Pharmacol.* 1978;27:1296-1297.
74. Rozenfeld RA, Leikin JB. Severe methanol ingestion treated successfully without hemodialysis. *Am J Ther.* 2007;14:502-503.
75. Sivilotti M, Burns M, McMartin K, et al. Toxicokinetics of ethylene glycol during fomepizole therapy: implications for management. *Ann Emerg Med.* 2000;36:114-125.
76. Sivilotti ML. Ethanol: tastes great! Fomepizole: less filling! *Ann Emerg Med.* 2009;53:451-453.
77. Sivilotti ML, Burns MJ, Aaron CK, et al. Reversal of severe methanol-induced visual impairment: no evidence of retinal toxicity due to fomepizole. *J Toxicol Clin Toxicol.* 2001;39:627-631.
78. Theorell H, Yonetani T, Sjoberg B. On the effects of some heterocyclic compounds on the enzymatic activity of liver alcohol dehydrogenase. *Acta Chem Scand.* 1969;23:255-260.
79. Van Stee E, Harris A, Horton M, et al. The treatment of ethylene glycol toxicosis with pyrazole. *J Pharmacol Exp Ther.* 1975;192:251-259.
80. Vassiliadis J, Graudins A, Dowsett RP. Triethylene glycol poisoning treated with intravenous ethanol infusion. *J Toxicol Clin Toxicol.* 1999;37:773-776.
81. Wacker WEC, Haynes H, Druyan R, et al. Treatment of ethylene glycol poisoning with ethyl alcohol. *JAMA.* 1965;194:1231-1233.
82. Wallemacq PE, Vanbinst R, Haufroid V, et al. Plasma and tissue determination of 4-methylpyrazole for pharmacokinetic analysis in acute adult and pediatric methanol/ethylene glycol poisoning. *Ther Drug Monit.* 2004;26:258-262.
83. Wu D, Cederbaum AI. Characterization of pyrazole and 4-methylpyrazole induction of cytochrome P4502E1 in rat kidney. *J Pharmacol Exp Ther.* 1994;270:407-413.
84. Wu D, Cederbaum AI. Induction of liver cytochrome P4502E1 by pyrazole and 4-methylpyrazole in neonatal rats. *J Pharmacol Exp Ther.* 1993;263:1468-1473.
85. Wu DF, Clejan L, Potter B, et al. Rapid decrease of cytochrome P45011E1 in primary hepatocyte culture and its maintenance by added 4-methylpyrazole. *Hepatology.* 1990;12:1379-1389.
86. Zahlten RN. Cyclic AMP and corticosteroids. *N Engl J Med.* 1974;290:743-744.

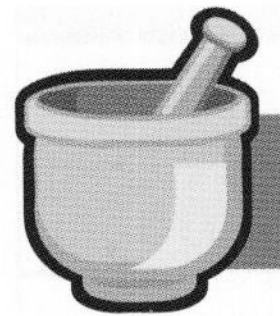

ANTIDOTES IN DEPTH (A32)

ETHANOL

Mary Ann Howland

```
    H   H
    |   |
H — C — C — OH
    |   |
    H   H
```

Ethanol is used therapeutically as a competitive substrate for xenobiotics metabolized by alcohol dehydrogenase, thus limiting the bioactivation of those xenobiotics to toxic metabolites. Methanol and ethylene glycol are potentially the two most lethal xenobiotics metabolized by this pathway.[8,9] Ethanol may also inhibit the metabolism of short-chain polyethylene glycols, such as di- and triethylene glycol,[50] as well as compete with monofluoroacetate and fluoroacetamide for binding to the tricarboxylic acid cycle via the formation of acetate. Ethanol also affects the cytochrome P450 (CYP) enzyme system, especially CYP2E1, for which it has biphasic properties as an inducer/inhibitor similar to fomepizole and isoniazid. The competitive relationship of ethanol with potentially toxic xenobiotics are used to therapeutic advantage, but the effect of ethanol on the CYP system often leads to unwanted drug interactions and pharmacokinetic tolerance after several days of administration.

AFFINITY FOR ALCOHOL DEHYDROGENASE

The dose of ethanol necessary to achieve competitive inhibition depends on the relative concentrations of the toxic alcohols and their affinity for the enzyme. An affinity constant, K_m, is used to express the degree of affinity: the lower the K_m value, the stronger the affinity. A summary of in vitro experiments using human liver cells demonstrated a K_m of 30 mM for ethylene glycol, 7 mM for methanol, and 0.45 mM for ethanol.[26,39,40] This means that the molar affinity of ethanol for alcohol dehydrogenase is 67 times that of ethylene glycol and 15.5 times that of methanol. Studies in methanol-poisoned monkeys revealed that when ethanol was administered at a molar ethanol-to-methanol ratio (E:M) of 1:4, the metabolism of methanol was reduced by 70%; at a 1:1 E:M ratio, metabolism was reduced by greater than 90%.[29] In these experiments, the dose of methanol was kept constant at about 1 g/kg (31 mmol/kg), whereas the dose of ethanol was varied. Although the serum methanol concentration was not measured, a calculation using this dose and a volume of distribution of 0.6 L/kg would predict a serum concentration of about 166 mg/dL. Even in molar ratios as high as 1:8, methanol did not inhibit ethanol metabolism. When ethylene glycol and methanol are administered together in a 0.5:1 molar ratio, ethylene glycol did not inhibit methanol metabolism.[29] When compared to methanol smaller amounts of ethanol are required to block the metabolism of ethylene glycol, as the affinity of ethylene glycol for alcohol dehydrogenase is less than that of methanol.[19,26,39,40,42,48]

Most authors[1,19,48] recommend either a serum ethanol concentration of 100 mg/dL, or at least a 1:4 molar ratio of ethanol to methanol or ethylene glycol, whichever is greater. Using this ratio, 100 mg/dL (~22 mmol/L) of ethanol protects against 88 mmol/L (286 mg/dL) of methanol or 88 mmol/L (546 mg/dL) of ethylene glycol. Inhibiting the metabolism of methanol and ethylene glycol impedes the formation of toxic metabolites and prevents the development of metabolic acidosis.[10,13,18,48] After this toxic metabolic pathway is blocked with ethanol, renal, pulmonary, and extracorporeal routes of toxic alcohol removal become the sole mechanisms for elimination.

Case reports attest to the efficacy of ethanol in preventing the sequelae of methanol and ethylene glycol poisoning when administered in a timely fashion after the toxic alcohol ingestion and before the accumulation of the toxic metabolites.[5,7,21,47,52] In the presence of sufficient blocking concentrations of ethanol, the half-life of ethylene glycol in two patients with normal kidney function was 17.5 hours, which was comparable to 17 hours in a case series of patients receiving fomepizole alone with normal kidney function.[5,46] A half-life of 46.5 hours for methanol was reported in a patient with methanol poisoning who had received a sufficient quantity of ethanol.[37] Again, this half-life for methanol in the presence of ethanol was quite similar to the 54 hours reported in a case series of methanol-poisoned patients treated only with fomepizole.[3,21]

PHARMACOKINETICS AND DOSING

Ethanol can be given either orally or intravenously (IV) (Tables A32–1 and A32–2). Concentrations of 20% to 30% orally and 5% to 10% IV are well tolerated. Intravenous administration has the advantages of complete absorption[23] and avoidance of most gastrointestinal symptoms, and it is a route that can be used in an unconscious or uncooperative patient. The disadvantages of IV ethanol include difficulty in obtaining and preparing an IV ethanol solution, the hyperosmolarity of a 5% ethanol solution (about 950 mOsm/L), and the possibilities of osmotic dehydration, hyponatremia, and venous irritation. Ethanol administered orally is rapidly absorbed and achieves peak concentrations in about 1 to 1.5 hours.[6,12,27,49] The amount of ethanol absorbed after oral administration is highly variable and dependent on a number of factors, such as ethanol dose, fasting, nutritional status, accelerated gastric emptying, gender, genetics, chronic alcohol use, lean body mass, and increasing age, as well as the presence of certain H_2 receptor antagonists.[4,7,12,22,24,34,51,53] Sufficient concentrations are generally achieved when 0.8 g/kg of ethanol is given orally over 20 minutes.[4,6,7,12,24,49]

Regardless of route, the objective is to rapidly achieve and maintain a serum concentration of at least 100 mg/dL of ethanol, which is adequate for enzyme inhibition in most cases. Inhibition is best achieved by administering a loading dose of ethanol, followed by a maintenance dose. Given that the volume of distribution for ethanol is approximately 0.6 L/kg,[54] the loading dose of ethanol is obtained by the following formula:

$$\begin{aligned}\text{Loading dose} &= C_p \times Vd\\ &= 1\text{ g/L (100 mg/dL)} \times 0.6\text{ L/kg}\\ &= 0.6\text{ g/kg}\\ C_p &= \text{plasma concentration which is comparable to the serum concentration}\end{aligned}$$

TABLE A32–1. Intravenous Administration of 10% Ethanol

Loading Dose[a]	Volume (mL)[b] (given over 1 h as tolerated)					
	10 kg	15 kg	30 kg	50 kg	70 kg	100 kg
0.8 g/kg of 10% ethanol (infused over 1 h as tolerated)	80	120	240	400	560	800

Maintenance Dose[c]	Infusion Rate[b] (mL/h for various weights)[d]					
	10 kg	15 kg	30 kg	50 kg	70 kg	100 kg
Ethanol Naive						
80 mg/kg/h	8	12	24	40	56	80
110 mg/kg/h	11	16	33	55	77	110
130 mg/kg/h	13	19	39	65	91	130
Ethanol Tolerant						
150 mg/kg/h	–	–	–	75	105	150
During hemodialysis						
250 mg/kg/h	25	38	75	125	175	250
300 mg/kg/h	30	45	90	150	210	300
350 mg/kg/h	35	53	105	175	245	350

[a] A 10% V/V concentration yields approximately 100 mg/mL.

[b] For a 5% concentration, multiply the amount by 2.

[c] Infusion to be started immediately following the loading dose. Concentrations above 10% are not recommended for IV administration. The dose schedule is based on the premise that the patient initially has a zero ethanol concentration. The aim of therapy is to maintain a serum ethanol concentration of 100 to 150 mg/dL, but constant monitoring of the ethanol concentration is required because of wide variations in endogenous metabolic capacity. Ethanol will be removed by hemodialysis, and the infusion rate of ethanol must be increased during hemodialysis. Prolonged ethanol administration may lead to hypoglycemia.

[d] Rounded to the nearest mL.

Adapted from Roberts JR, Hedges J, eds. *Clinical Procedures in Emergency Medicine*. Philadelphia: WB Saunders; 1985:1073-1074.

For a 70-kg person, the loading dose would be 42 g (70 kg × 0.6 g/kg) of ethanol, or 420 mL of 10% V/V (volume-to-volume) ethanol. However, a 0.8 g/kg or 8 mL/kg loading dose of a 10% ethanol solution is recommended in order to provide a margin of safety because of the inconsistencies in volume of distribution and the ongoing metabolism that occurs during administration.[23,41] The IV loading dose should be administered over 20 to 60 minutes, as tolerated by the patient. The 10% ethanol concentration is preferable to the 5% concentration in order to limit the volume of fluid administered. It is also preferred over the more concentrated solutions in order to limit local venous irritation and avoid postinfusion phlebitis. Because of the free water content and significant hypertonicity of the 10% solution, the patient should be closely observed for the development of hyponatremia.

To maintain an ethanol concentration of 100 mg/dL, enough ethanol has to be administered to replace the ethanol that is undergoing elimination (66–130 mg/kg/h). The average hourly dose for a 70-kg person is 4.6 g, but higher doses are required in ethanol tolerant patients (100–154 mg/kg/h) or others who may have induced enzymes, and in those undergoing hemodialysis (250–350 mg/kg/h) (Chap. 9).[9,19,30,37,38]

Because ethanol elimination varies in each individual, frequent serum ethanol determinations should be made to ensure adequate dosing while also monitoring blood glucose and fluid and electrolyte status. Also, any increase in the anion gap or decrease in bicarbonate concentration implies that the ethanol dose is inadequate to achieve blockade of alcohol dehydrogenase and the ethanol dosing should be increased.

Problems encountered with the administration of ethanol include further risk of central nervous system (CNS) depression;[11,15,31,35,36] behavioral disturbances or ethanol-related toxicities, such as hepatitis and pancreatitis, hypoglycemia, dehydration, and fluctuating serum concentrations, and potential drug interactions resulting in disulfiramlike reactions.[55]

AVAILABILITY

A more practical problem often involves preparing the ethanol to be given since commercial preparations of 5% ethanol in 5% dextrose are no longer available for IV administration.[2] Not having a commercially available preparation increases the delay to administration of IV ethanol and the potential for a medication error in preparation. Sterile ethanol USP (absolute ethanol) can be added to 5% dextrose to make a solution of approximately 10% ethanol concentration; 55 mL of absolute ethanol is then added to 500 mL of 5% dextrose to produce a total end volume of 555 mL (10% = 10 mL in 100 mL, in this case, 55 mL in 555 mL or 55/555). If oral administration is chosen, it is important to remember that in the United States the "proof" number on the label is double the concentration; that is, "100-proof" ethanol is 50% ethanol (50 g/100 mL). If there will be any delay in preparing ethanol for IV use and fomepizole is not available or used, oral therapy with ethanol should be initiated immediately.

TABLE A32–2. Oral Administration of 20% Ethanol

Loading Dose[a]	Volume (mL)					
	10 kg	15 kg	30 kg	50 kg	70 kg	100 kg
0.8 g/kg of 20% ethanol, diluted in juice (may be administered orally or via nasogastric tube)	40	60	120	200	280	400
Maintenance Dose[b]	**mL/h for various weights[c,d]**					
	10 kg	15 kg	30 kg	50 kg	70 kg	100 kg
Ethanol naive						
80 mg/kg/h	4	6	12	20	28	40
110 mg/kg/h	6	8	17	27	39	55
130 mg/kg/h	7	10	20	33	46	66
Ethanol tolerant						
150 mg/kg/h	8	11	22	38	53	75
During hemodialysis						
250 mg/kg/h	13	19	38	63	88	125
300 mg/kg/h	15	23	46	75	105	150
350 mg/kg/h	18	26	53	88	123	175

[a] A 20% V/V concentration yields approximately 200 mg/mL.

[b] Concentrations above 30% (60 proof) are not recommended for oral administration. The dose schedule is based on the premise that the patient initially has a zero ethanol concentration. The aim of therapy is to maintain a serum ethanol concentration of 100 to 150 mg/dL, but constant monitoring of the ethanol concentration is required because of wide variations in endogenous metabolic capacity. Ethanol will be removed by hemodialysis, and the dose of ethanol must be increased during hemodialysis. Prolonged ethanol administration may lead to hypoglycemia.

[c] Rounded to the nearest mL.

[d] For a 30% concentration, multiply the amount by 0.66.

Adapted from Roberts JR, Hedges J, eds. *Clinical Procedures in Emergency Medicine*. Philadelphia: WB Saunders; 1985:1073-1074.

COMPARISON TO FOMEPIZOLE

Although ethanol has been used as an antidote for toxic alcohols for many years in both adults and children[43] and has the advantages of easy access to oral ethanol and low acquisition cost, fomepizole is a very potent inhibitor of alcohol dehydrogenase with many important advantages.[14,16,20,28,32,33] Fomepizole does not produce CNS depression, is easier to dose, and does not require serum concentration monitoring. Although fomepizole is more costly than ethanol, its many advantages over ethanol make fomepizole the preferable antidote.[25,45] Hospitals should be strongly encouraged to stock fomepizole (see Antidotes in Depth A31: Fomepizole and Chap. 107).

SUMMARY

When administered appropriately, ethanol is an excellent first step in preventing further metabolism of methanol and ethylene glycol to their respective toxic metabolites. However, the disadvantages of ethanol compared with fomepizole (when available) now make ethanol an outmoded antidote. The only advantage that ethanol might have compared with fomepizole would be in a mass casualty situation until sufficient supplies of fomepizole could be procured.[35] It is important to remember, however, that neither fomepizole nor ethanol affect the toxic metabolites that are already present in the body. Once alcohol dehydrogenase is blocked, the decision whether to use hemodialysis depends on how much end-organ damage has occurred, how well the body can eliminate the parent compound without the benefit of hemodialysis, and how much toxic metabolite is already present. With the use of either ethanol or fomepizole alone (without subsequent hemodialysis), the increase in hospital length of stay in an intensive care unit or on a medical floor may be substantial for methanol-poisoned patients, and a risk-benefit analysis should be applied.[17,44]

REFERENCES

1. Agner K, Hook O, Von Porat B. The treatment of methanol poisoning with ethanol. *J Stud Alcohol.* 1949;9:515-522.
2. Berberet B, Burda A, Breier C, Lodolce A. Discontinuation of 5% alcohol in 5% dextrose injection: implications for antidote stocking. *Am J Health Sys Pharm.* 2008;65:2200-2203.
3. Brent J, McMartin K, Phillips SP, et al. Fomepizole for the treatment of methanol poisoning. *N Engl J Med.* 2001;344:424-429.
4. Caballeria L. First-pass metabolism of ethanol: its role as a determinant of blood alcohol levels after drinking. *Hepatogastroenterology.* 1992;39:62-66.
5. Cheng JT, Beysolow TD, Kaul B, et al. Clearance of ethylene glycol by kidneys and hemodialysis. *J Toxicol Clin Toxicol.* 1987;25:95-108.
6. Cobaugh DJ, Gibbs M, Shapiro DE, et al. A comparison of the bioavailabilities of oral and intravenous ethanol in healthy male volunteers. *Acad Emerg Med.* 1999;6:984-988.
7. Cole-Harding S, Wilson JR. Ethanol metabolism in men and women. *J Stud Alcohol.* 1987;48:380-387.

8. Davis DP, Bramwell KJ, Hamilton RS, Williams SR. Ethylene glycol poisoning: case report of a record-high level and a review. *J Emerg Med.* 1997;15:653-667.
9. Ekins BR, Rollins DE, Duffy DP, Gregory MC. Standardized treatment of severe methanol poisoning with ethanol and hemodialysis. *West J Med.* 1985;142:337-340.
10. Faci A, Plaa GL, Sharkawi M. Chloral hydrate enhances ethanol-induced inhibition of methanol oxidation in mice. *Toxicology.* 1998;131:1-7.
11. Fillmore MT, Vogel-Sprott M. Behavioral impairment under alcohol: cognitive and pharmacokinetic factors. *Alcohol Clin Exp Res.* 1998;22:1476-1482.
12. Fraser AG, Hudson M, Sawyer AM, et al. Ranitidine, cimetidine, famotidine have no effect on post-prandial absorption of ethanol (0.8 g/kg) taken after an evening meal. *Aliment Pharmacol Ther.* 1992;6:693-700.
13. Grauer G, Thrall MA, Henre B, et al. Comparison of the effects of ethanol on 4-methylpyrazole on the pharmacokinetics and toxicity of ethylene glycol in the dog. *Toxicol Lett.* 1987;35:307-314.
14. Hantson P, Wallemacq P, Brau M. Two cases of acute methanol poisoning partially treated by oral 4-methylpyrazole. *Intensive Care Med.* 1999;25:528-531.
15. Hantson P, Wittebole X, Haufroid V. Ethanol therapy for methanol poisoning: duration and problems. *Eur J Emerg Med.* 2002;9:278-279.
16. Hauser J, Szabo S. Extremely long protection by pyrazole derivatives against chemically induced gastric mucosal injury. *J Pharmacol Exper Ther.* 1991;256:592-598.
17. Hovda K, Jacobsen D. Expert opinion: fomepizole may ameliorate the need for hemodialysis in methanol poisoning. *Hum Exp Ther.* 2008;27:539-546.
18. Jacobsen D, Jansen H, Wiik-Larsen E, et al. Studies on methanol poisoning. *Acta Med Scand.* 1982;212:5-10.
19. Jacobsen D, McMartin KE. Methanol and ethylene glycol poisonings: mechanism of toxicity, clinical course, diagnosis and treatment. *Med Toxicol.* 1986;1:309-334.
20. Jacobsen D, Sebastian CS, Barron SK, et al. Effects of 4-methylpyrazole, methanol/ethylene glycol antidote, in healthy humans. *J Emerg Med.* 1990;8:455-461.
21. Jacobsen D, Webb R, Collins TD, McMartin KE. Methanol and formate kinetics in late diagnosed methanol intoxication. *Med Toxicol.* 1988;3:418-423.
22. Jones AW, Jönsson KA, Kechagias S. Effect of high-fat, high-protein, and high-carbohydrate meals on the pharmacokinetics of a small dose of ethanol. *Br J Clin Pharmacol.* 1997;44:521-526.
23. Julkunen RJ, Tannenbaum L, Baradna E, et al. First pass metabolism of ethanol: an important determinant of blood levels after alcohol consumption. *Alcohol.* 1985;2:437-441.
24. Korman MG, Bolin TD. Alcohol and H_2-receptor antagonists. *Med J Aust.* 1992;157:730-731.
25. Lepik KJ, Levy AR, Sobolev BG, et al. Adverse drug events associated with the antidotes for methanol and ethylene glycol poisoning: a comparison of ethanol and fomepizole. *Ann Emerg Med.* 2009;53:439-450.
26. Li TK, Theorell H. Human liver alcohol dehydrogenase: inhibition by pyrazole and pyrazole analogs. *Acta Chem Scand.* 1969;23:892-902.
27. Lieber CS. Gastric ethanol metabolism and gastritis: interactions with other drugs, *Helicobacter pylori*, and antibiotic therapy (1957-1997)—a review. *Alcohol Clin Exp Res.* 1997;21:1360-1366.
28. Makar AB, Tephly TR. Inhibition of monkey liver alcohol dehydrogenase by 4-methylpyrazole. *Biochem Med.* 1975;13:334-342.
29. Makar AB, Tephly TR, Mannering GJ. Methanol metabolism in the monkey. *Mol Pharmacol.* 1968;4:471-483.
30. McCoy HG, Cipolle RJ, Ehlers SM, et al. Severe methanol poisoning: application of a pharmacokinetic model for ethanol therapy and hemodialysis. *Am J Med.* 1979;67:804-807.
31. McKnight AJ, Langston EA, Marques PR, Tippetts AS. Estimating blood alcohol level from observable signs. *Accid Anal Prev.* 1997;29:247-255.
32. McMartin KE, Hedström K, Told B, et al. Studies on the metabolic interactions between 4-methylpyrazole and methanol using the monkey as an animal model. *Archiv Biochem Biophys.* 1980;199:606-614.
33. McMartin KE, Makar AB, Palese MA, Tephly TR. Methanol poisoning I. The role of formic acid in the development of metabolic acidosis in the monkey and the reversal by 4-methylpyrazole. *Biochem Med.* 1975;13:319-333.
34. Norberg A, Jones AW, Hahn R, Gabrielsson J. Role of variability in explaining ethanol pharmacokinetics research and forensic applications. *Clin Pharmacokinet.* 2003;42:1-31.
35. Paasma R, Hovda K, Jacobsen D. Methanol mass poisoning in Estonia: outbreak in 154 patients. *Clin Toxicol.* 2007;45:152-157.
36. Papineau KL, Roehrs TA, Petrucelli N, et al. Electrophysiological assessment (the multiple sleep latency test) of the biphasic effects of ethanol in humans. *Alcohol Clin Exp Res.* 1998;22:231-235.
37. Peterson C. Oral ethanol doses in patients with methanol poisoning. *Am J Hosp Pharm.* 1981;38:1024-1027.
38. Peterson CD, Collins AJ, Himes JM, et al. Ethylene glycol poisoning: pharmacokinetics during therapy with ethanol and hemodialysis. *N Engl J Med.* 1981;304:21-23.
39. Pietruszko R. Human liver alcohol dehydrogenase inhibition of methanol activity by pyrazole, 4-methylpyrazole, 4-hydroxymethylpyrazole and 4-carboxypyrazole. *Biochem Pharmacol.* 1975;24:1603-1607.
40. Pietruszko R, Voigtlander K, Lester D. Alcohol dehydrogenase from human and horse liver—substance specificity with diols. *Biochem Pharmacol.* 1978;27:1296-1297.
41. Rainey PM. Relation between serum and whole-blood ethanol concentrations. *Clin Chem.* 1993;39:2288-2292.
42. Roe O. Methanol poisoning: its clinical course, pathogenesis and treatment. *Acta Med Scand.* 1946;126(Suppl 182):1-253.
43. Roy M, Bailey B, Chalut D, et al. What are the adverse effects of ethanol used as an antidote in the treatment of suspected methanol poisoning in children? *J Toxicol Clin Toxicol.* 2003;44:155-161.
44. Rozenfeld R, Leikin J. Severe methanol ingestion treated successfully without hemodialysis. *Am J Ther.* 2007;14:502-503.
45. Sivilotti M. Ethanol: tastes great! Fomepizole: less filling! *Ann Emerg Med.* 2009;53:451-453.
46. Sivilotti ML, Burns MJ, McMartin KE, Brent J. Toxicokinetics of ethylene glycol during fomepizole therapy: implications for management. For the Methylpyrazole for Toxic Alcohols Study Group. *Ann Emerg Med.* 2000;36:114-125.
47. Sullivan M, Chen C, Madden JF. Absence of metabolic acidosis in toxic methanol ingestion: a case report and review. *Del Med J.* 1999;71:421-426.
48. Tarr B, Winters L, Moore M, et al. Low-dose ethanol in the treatment of ethylene glycol poisoning. *J Vet Pharm Ther.* 1985;8:254-262.
49. Tomaszewski C, Cline DM, Whitley TW, Grant T. Effect of acute ethanol ingestion on orthostatic vital signs. *Ann Emerg Med.* 1995;25:636-641.
50. Vassiliadis J, Graudins A, Dowsett RP. Triethylene glycol poisoning treated with intravenous ethanol infusion. *J Toxicol Clin Toxicol.* 1999;37:773-776.
51. Vestal RE, McGuire EA, Tobin JD, et al. Aging and ethanol metabolism. *Clin Pharmacol Ther.* 1975;21:343-353.
52. Wacker WE, Haynes H, Druyan R, et al. Treatment of ethylene glycol poisoning with ethyl alcohol. *JAMA.* 1965;194:173-175.
53. Whitfield JB. ADH and ALDH genotypes in relation to alcohol metabolic rate and sensitivity. *Alcohol Alcohol.* 1994;2:59-65.
54. Wilkinson P. Pharmacokinetics of ethanol: a review. *Alcohol Clin Exp Res.* 1980;4:6-21.
55. Williams CS, Woodcock KR. Do ethanol and metronidazole interact to produce a disulfiram-like reaction? *Ann Pharmacother.* 2000;34:255-257.

K.
PESTICIDES

CHAPTER 108
PESTICIDES: AN OVERVIEW OF RODENTICIDES AND A FOCUS ON PRINCIPLES

Neal E. Flomenbaum

Pesticides are defined by the US Federal Insecticide, Fungicide, and Rodenticide Act (FIFRA) as "any substance or mixture of substances intended for preventing, destroying, repelling, or mitigating any pest, and any substance or mixture of substances intended for use as a plant regulator, defoliant, or desiccant."[24,109] Pesticides are most commonly categorized into four major and several minor classes based on the intended targets. The four major classes are insecticides, herbicides (weeds), fungicides (fungi and molds), and rodenticides. Minor classes include acaricides and miticides (mites), molluscides (snails etc.), larvicides, pediculocides (lice), nematocides, and scabicides, as well as attractants (pheromones), defoliants, dessicants, plant regulators, and repellants.[23] Currently, the Annual Report of the American Association of Poison Control Centers, National Poison Data System (AAPCC-NPDS) lists six categories of pesticides: fumigants, fungicides, herbicides, insecticides, repellents, and rodenticides. In 2007, the total number of exposures mentioned was 95,657, of which 85,617 were described as unintentional and 43,469 were in children younger than 6 years of age. Remarkably, despite these large numbers, fewer than 20 annual deaths were attributed to all pesticides by AAPCC in 2006 and 2007 (Chap. 135).

REGULATION AND EPIDEMIOLOGY

Since 1947, the production, use, and distribution of pesticides in the United States have been regulated under FIFRA and its subsequent amendments in 1972, 1975, and 1978. In 1970, the Environmental Protection Agency (EPA) was given the authority to administer and enforce FIFRA regulations. Under FIFRA, all pesticides and their manufacturers must be registered with the EPA, and the pesticide must be classified for either general use or restricted use by licensed or certified applicators. Also, a pesticide must be sold exactly as formulated, registered, and labeled. Failure to comply with any of these regulations can result in civil and criminal penalties, and product recall, seizure, or ban from future sales.[109] The EPA and FDA together establish pesticide tolerance concentrations for agricultural products and foods, and the 1978 amendment to FIFRA allows individual states to enact and enforce pesticide regulations, resulting in some states establishing even more stringent requirements and lower acceptable concentrations than EPA itself.[109] However, the EPA retains the authority to act when states are unable or unwilling to do so.

In addition to its authority under FIFRA, the EPA regulates pesticides under several other acts: the Federal Environmental Pesticide Control Act; the Resource Conservation Recovery Act of 1972 (RCRA); the Comprehensive Environmental Response, Compensation and Liability Act (CERCLA, also called the "superfund" Act); the Toxic Substance Control Act (TSCA); the Clean Water Act and the Safe Drinking Water Act.

FIFRA is granted considerable authority to protect the health of the population. When evidence indicates that a pesticide may pose a significant hazard, one or more of the following actions may be taken: permissible workplace exposure limits may be issued, a product may be removed from sale or its registration canceled, restrictions on use or application of a product may be ordered and tolerance concentrations for pesticide residue on food stuffs or water contamination may be set.[109] However, since 1978, demonstration of efficacy may be waived, unless the pesticide actually affects public health. The Food Quality Protection Act of 1996 requires that EPA establish tolerances based in part on the higher vulnerability of children to pesticide residues, and on the aggregate exposures from residues from all sources and from all agents with the same mechanism of toxicity.[89] Table 108–1 summarizes the EPA toxicity classifications; the significance of oral median lethal doses for 50% of test subjects (LD_{50}) is discussed under rodenticides in the next section.

NEW RESTRICTIONS ON RODENTICIDES IN THE UNITED STATES

In an effort to reduce the risk of unintentional exposures to children, pets, and non-targeted wild life, in June 2008 the EPA announced significant new restrictions limiting the sale and use of 10 rodenticides. The 10 rodenticides covered by the new rules include the *nonanticoagulants* bromethalin, cholecalciferol, and zinc phosphide; the *"first-generation" anticoagulants* warfarin, chlorphacinone, and diphacinone; and the *"second-generation" anticoagulants* brodifacoum, bromadiolone, difenacoum, and difethialone. Under the new rules, use of all second-generation anticoagulants is restricted to use by professional applicators, and all other rodenticides available directly to consumers can only be sold in pre-loaded, tamper-resistant bait stations. Prohibited from sale are rodenticide baits in the form of meal, treated whole grain, loose pellets, and liquids, as are individual rodenticide "refills" sold without bait stations.

Insecticides are discussed in Chaps. 113 and 114, *herbicides* in Chap. 115, and *fumigants* including methyl bromide are discussed in Chapter 116. The remainder of this chapter explores the clinical problems posed by rodenticide poisoning. The specific rodenticides discussed

TABLE 108–1. EPA Toxicity Classifications

Category and Signal Word	Oral LD_{50} (mg/kg)	Dermal LD_{50} (mg/kg)	Inhalation LC_{50} (mg/L)	Eye Irritation	Skin Irritation
I Danger	0–50	0–200	0–0.05	Corrosive: corneal opacity not reversible within 21 d	Corrosive
II Warning	50–500	200–2000	0.05–0.5	Corneal opacity reversible within 8–21 d; irritation persisting for 7 d	Severe irritation at 72 h
III Caution	500–5000	2000–20,000	0.5–5.0	Corneal opacity; irritation reversible within 7 d	Moderate irritation at 72 h
IV None	>5000	>20,000	>5.0	Irritation cleared within 24 h	Mild or slight irritation at 72 h

here are α-naphthyl thiourea (ANTU), cholecaliciferol, norbormide, bromethalin, tetramethylene disulfotetramine (tetramine), α chloralose and salmonella-based rodenticides. Some of the oldest and most toxic rodenticides—including barium, sodium monofluoroacetate/fluoroacetamide, phosphorous, and strychnine—are individually discussed in Chaps. 109 to 112, and three highly toxic metallic rodenticides—arsenic, thallium and zinc phosphide—are considered in Chaps. 88, 100, and 101.

RODENTICIDES

INTRODUCTION

The prevention of rat-borne diseases and bites has been an important public health goal for centuries, and the use of chemical rodenticides—to achieve these goals has always been part of the efforts. Although the rodenticides legally available today in most of the industrialized world are far less toxic than those used a century ago, the "perfect rodenticide," one that effectively kills rodents but is not toxic to humans or pets, has yet to be discovered or synthesized. Instead, a wide variety of less-than-ideal rodenticides are commercially available, differing from one another in chemical composition, mechanism for killing rodents, and human toxicity.[43,60,61,73,84] Purportedly "effective and harmless" products are periodically introduced, only to be subsequently withdrawn when the true human toxicities become known.[50,53,58,69,90,91] Moreover, some of these products may remain in basements, on hardware store shelves, or in use by professional pest control operators long after they are officially withdrawn from sale.

EPIDEMIOLOGY

In 2007 and 2008, AAPCC-NPDS recorded about 15,000 rodenticide exposures in the United States each year, of which over 80% involved children younger than 6 years of age (Chap. 135). Despite the very large number of exposures, only one death from rodenticides was reported in 2006 and only two in 2007. The specific types of rodenticides tracked by AAPCC include anticoagulants of the long-acting/superwarfarin type, anticoagulants-warfarin type, α-naphthyl thiourea (ANTU), bromethalin, cholecalciferol, cyanide, monofluoroacetate, strychnine, vacor, zinc phosphide, and other/unknown.

Of the 11 rodenticide deaths reported by AAPCC between 2003 and 2007, second-generation long-acting anticoagulants accounted for three, strychnine accounted for two, bromethalin for two, zinc phosphide for one, and other/unknown accounted for three. However, in assessing the true human toll resulting from rodenticide exposures, it is important to recognize that the AAPCC database does not consider as a rodenticide exposure an encounter with a pesticide that is not labeled for use as a rodenticide, even when used by consumers for that purpose. An example of such product misuse is provided by a series of 35 cases referred to the New York City Poison Control Center from 1994 to 1997 involving an aldicarb insecticide illegally imported and sold as "Tres Pasitos" rodenticide.[74] Aldicarb, a carbamate cholinesterase inhibitor, can legally be used as an *insecticide* in some parts of the United States, but is not registered for use as a rodenticide, though it is sold that way in some neighborhood stores predominantly serving Dominican communities.

Children constitute the largest group of patients exposed to rodenticide; but the elderly; suicidal adults; potential homicide victims; intoxicated, psychiatric, or impaired persons; and pest control operators are also at substantial risk for intentional or unintentional exposures. The large number of unintentional ingestions of rodenticides placed in food containers or dishes, with or without added bait such as meal or peanut butter prompted EPA in 2008 to restrict the use of some rodenticides and require the use of tamper-resistant traps for all others.

DEFINITION AND CLASSIFICATION OF RODENTICIDES

A rodenticide is any product commercially marketed to kill rodents, mice, squirrels, gophers, and other small animals. Rodenticides are a heterogeneous group of chemicals bearing little or no relationship to one another, apart from their current or historic use as rodenticides. Rodenticides have been classified in several different ways: (1) as inorganic and organic compounds; (2) by animal selectivity; (3) by nature and onset of symptoms; and (4) according to their LD_{50} in rats.[5] Classification by LD_{50} is emphasized in this chapter and used to organize all of the rodenticides listed in Table 108–2.

INORGANIC AND ORGANIC COMPOUNDS

Inorganic compounds include the salts of arsenic (Chap. 88), thallium (Chap. 100), phosphorus (Chap. 111), barium (Chap. 109), and zinc (Chap. 101). Organic compounds include sodium monofluoroacetate (Chap. 110), ANTU, warfarin (Chap. 59), red squill[99,113] strychnine (Chap. 112), norbormide, and Vacor.[5,50,53,58,69,90,91]

TABLE 108–2. Management of Specific Rodenticide Ingestions

Rodenticide Name	Physical Characteristics	Toxic Mechanism	Estimated Fatal Dose	Signs and Symptoms	Onset	Antidote and/or Treatment*
Highly Toxic Signal Word: DANGER[a] (LD_{50} < 50 mg/kg)						
Thallium (Chap. 100)	White, crystalline, odorless, tasteless	Combines with mitochondrial sulfhydryl groups, interferes with oxidative phosphorylation	14 mg/kg	Anorexia, abdominal pain, diarrhea, painful neuropathy, delirium, coma, seizures, alopecia (late), Mees lines	GI symptoms acutely, other symptoms 12–14 h delay	Activated charcoal, Prussian blue
Sodium monofluoroacetate (SMFA, compound 1080)	White, crystalline, odorless, tasteless, water soluble	Fluoroacetate to fluorocitrate; interferes with Krebs cycle	3–7 mg/kg	Seizures, coma, tachycardia, PVCs, VT, VF, ST-T wave changes, rhabdomyolysis (hypocalcemia)	1/2–20 h	Experimental regimens: see text
Sodium fluoroacetamide (compound 1081) (Chap. 110)	Same as SMFA	Same as SMFA; fluoride toxicity	13–14 mg/kg	Same as SMFA	Same as SMFA	Same as SMFA
Strychnine (Chap. 112)	Bitter taste	Glycine receptor antagonist on spinal cord motor neurons	Children: 15 mg Adults: 1–2 mg/kg	Restlessness, anxiety, twitching, hyperextension alternating with relaxation, intense pain, trismus or facial grimacing ("risus sardonicus"), inability to swallow, opisthotonos	10–20 min	Quiet room, IV, benzodiazepines, neuromuscular blockade
Zinc phosphide (Chap. 101)	Heavy, gray, crystalline powder, water insoluble, "rotten fish" or "phosphorus" odor; normally used as 1% concentration	Releases phosphine on contact with water or acid or in GI tract	40 mg/kg in rats	"Rotten fish" breath odor, black vomitus, GI and cardiovascular toxicity, acute lung injury, agitation, coma, seizures, hepatic/renal toxicity	Within hours; inhalation may have delayed onset	Dilution with $NaHCO_3$ water or milk
Elemental phosphorus (yellow or white phosphorus) (Chap. 111)	Yellow, waxy paste, fat soluble, water insoluble	Local irritation and burns on contact followed by GI, liver, and renal damage, and interferes with clotting	1 mg/kg (more toxic if dissolved in alcohol, fats, oils)	Skin and GI burns, "smoking" luminescent vomitus and stools with garlic odor, jaundice, dysrhythmias, coma, delirium, seizures, cardiac arrest	1–2 h	Supportive care
Arsenic trioxide (Chap. 88)	White, crystalline powder	Combines with sulfhydryl groups and interferes with a variety of enzymatic reactions	1–4 mg/kg	Dysphagia, nausea and vomiting, bloody diarrhea, cardiovascular collapse, (VT, Torsades) garlic odor, altered mental status, late sensory/motor neuropathy	Symptoms: 1 h Death: 1–24 h	Succimer, dimercaprol until urine arsenic concentration <50 μg/L Hemodialysis to remove chelation compound if renal failure.
Barium (soluble forms: carbonate, chloride, hydroxide) (Chap. 109)	Yellow, white, slightly lustrous lump	Hypokalemia, neuromuscular blockade	20–30 mg/kg	Headache, paresthesias, peripheral weakness, paralysis, nausea, vomiting, diarrhea, abdominal pain, prolonged QT, dysrhythmias, cardiac and pulmonary failure	1–8 h	Orogastric lavage with Na_2SO_4, potassium replacement

(*Continued*)

TABLE 108–2. Management of Specific Rodenticide Ingestions (*Continued*)

Rodenticide Name	Physical Characteristics	Toxic Mechanism	Estimated Fatal Dose	Signs and Symptoms	Onset	Antidote and/or Treatment*
PNU (*N*-3-pyridylmethyl-*N'*-p-nitrophenyl urea, Vacor)	Yellow, resembling cornmeal or yellow green powder in bait; odor: peanuts	Interferes with nicotinamide metabolism in pancreas (destroying pancreatic beta cells), central and peripheral nervous system, and heart	5 mg/kg	Nausea and vomiting abdominal pain, severe orthostatic hypotension, hyperglycemia with or without ketoacidosis, GI perforation, pneumonia, neuropathy	4–48 h	Nicotinamide (Niacinamide) 500 mg IV or IM, manage diabetic ketoacidosis
Tetramine (tetramethylene disulfotetramine, TETS, TEM)	White powder	Non-competitive, GABA antagonism by direct blockade of chloride ionophore	5–10 mg/kg	Refractory status epilepticus, fainting, coma, coronary ischemia	1/2–13 h	Benzodiazepines Barbiturates, Neuromuscular blockers
Moderately Toxic Signal Word: WARNING[a] (LD_{50}, 50–500 mg/kg)						
α-Naphthylthiourea (ANTU)	Odorless, slightly bitter, fine, blue-gray powder, water-insoluble	Acute lung injury	>4 g/kg	Hypothermia, dyspnea, crackles, clear pulmonary froth, cyanosis	?	Supportive care
Cholecalciferol (vitamin D_3)	0.075% pellets, 364 pellets/oz; (1 pellet = 2308 U vitamin D)	Hypercalcemia	?	Headache, lethargy, weakness, fatigue, polyuria, renal injury and failure, hypertension, hypercalcemia	Hours to days	Fluids; if severe: furosemide, prednisone, calcitonin, bisphosphonates hemodialysis
Low Toxicity Signal Word: CAUTION[a] (LD_{50}, 500–5000 mg/kg)						
Red squill (Chap. 64)	Bitter taste	Cardioactive steroid poisoning	?	Myocardial irritability, blurred vision, hyperkalemia	30 min-6 h	Digoxin-specific Fab, atropine
Norbormide (dicarboximide)	Yellow cornmeal bait, peanut butter, 1% concentration	Vasoconstriction and ischemia in rats only via specific norbormide receptor in rat smooth muscle	Unknown, toxicity at <300mg	Transient hypothermia and hypotension	?	Supportive care
Bromethalin	7.5% concentrate, green pellets, with Bitrex (denatonium benzoate)	Uncouples oxidative phosphorylation; interrupts nerve impulse conduction	?	Muscle tremors, myoclonic jerks, flexion of major muscles, coma?, ataxia, focal motor seizures	Immediate	Supportive care
Anticogulants: Short Acting (Chap. 59)						
Warfarin	Yellow cornmeal, rolled oats (0.025%)	Anticoagulation via interference with clotting factors II, VII, IX, X	>5–20 mg/d for >5 d	Elevated INR; bleeding death from hemorrhage	12–48 h	Vitamin K_1, fresh frozen plasma (FFP) as indicated Activated factor VII Prothrombin complex concentrate
Prolin	Warfarin (0.025%) plus sulfaquinoxalin (0.025%)	Anticoagulant antibiotic combination eliminates intestinal vitamin K producing organisms	NA	Elevated INR; bleeding, death from hemorrhage		

Anticoagulants: Long Acting						
Hydroxycoumarins						
4-Hydroxycoumarin (brodifacoum, difenacoum)	0.005% grain-based bait	Anticoagulation via interference with clotting factors II, VII, IX, X	?	Elevated INR; bleeding death from hemorrhage	Delayed several days	Vitamin K_1, fresh frozen plasma (FFP) as indicated Activated factor VII Prothrombin complex concentrate
Warfacide (coumafuryl)	0.5% for dilution to 0.025% white powder, tasteless, odorless					
Indandiones						
Pindone (Pival)	Moldy, acrid odor, fluffy yellow powder, concentrations 0.005–2.5%	Anticoagulation via interference with clotting factors II, VII, IX, X	?	Chronic ingestion possibly produces cardiac and neurologic symptoms elevated INR; bleeding, death from hemorrhage	Delayed several days	Vitamin K_1, fresh frozen plasma (FFP) as indicated Activated factor VII Prothrombin complex concentrate
Pivalyn	0.5%					
Diphacinone	0.005–2.0%					
Chlorophacinone	0.005–2.5%					
Valone	0.005–2.5%					

[a]The LD_{50} values used in this table are derived from data on acute oral ingestions of the commercial product by rats. In some cases, the commercial product contains a very small percentage of active ingredient. The signal words that appear on labels of registered products may differ from the signal word assigned to the acute oral LD_{50} test because the label may also reflect another study (acute dermal or inhalational LD_{50}) requiring a more severe signal word. See Table 108-1 for the Consumer Product Safety Commission definitions and use of signal words as indicators of potential hazard of toxicity. Peacock D, Biologist, Registrations Division Office of Pesticide Programs, EPA, Washington, DC.

*Gastrointestinal decontamination should be provided as appropriate (Chap. 7); only unique or controversial aspects are discussed in this table.

ANIMAL SELECTIVITY

The cardioactive steroid *red squill* was promoted as a safe rodenticide because humans and other animals presumably would vomit the highly emetogenic xenobiotic prior to experiencing any cardiotoxic effects, whereas rats do not vomit and therefore would be expected to experience the cardiotoxic effects of red squill.[99,113] *Norbormide,* an irreversible smooth-muscle constrictor, causes widespread ischemic necrosis and death in rats, but does not appear to affect other animals or humans because it has been thought to act on a specific norbormide receptor found only in the smooth muscle of rats. ANTU, a relatively selective rodenticide, is a derivative of phenylthiourea, without the bitter taste characteristic of the thiourea. ANTU causes acute lung injury in rats that have not developed tolerance to it. ANTU, however, is only relatively selective: Although rats are more sensitive to it than other animals, large doses (greater than 4 g/kg) can also be lethal to primates.

All of the rodenticides classified as inorganic, and organic rodenticides such as strychnine and sodium fluoroacetate, are nonselective and of extreme concern when ingested by humans and domestic animals. Use of this entire group of rodenticides is restricted to commercial pest control operators and government agencies.

NATURE AND ONSET OF SYMPTOMS

Although a rodenticide classification system based purely on the nature and onset of symptoms would seem to be very appealing, such a system may be unreliable, may create a false sense of security, and may result in inappropriate management and/or inadequate followup. Many different rodenticides cause neurologic and/or gastrointestinal signs and symptoms, whereas characteristic or pathognomonic signs such as *risus sardonicus* from strychnine, or alopecia from thallium, may not be recognized, do not always occur consistently (especially after ingesting small amounts), or, as in the case of thallium-induced alopecia, would not occur until days after an acute ingestion. Classifying rodenticides by the time of onset of symptoms may similarly lump together within a late-onset group some of the least toxic (regular warfarin-type, cholecalciferol) and most toxic, (long-acting warfarin type, thallium) rodenticides.

LD_{50} IN RATS

Probably the most clinically useful way of classifying rodenticides at present is by toxicity based on LD_{50} data in rats. With a few noteworthy exceptions, the relative degree of toxicity per kilogram and the characteristic adverse effects generally hold among different mammals, allowing the healthcare provider the opportunity to consider a combination of historical and characteristic physical evidence to diagnose or exclude various rodenticides and to decide on an optimal management plan. The limitations of this classification system, however, must be understood to use it appropriately: (1) in rare cases, the LD_{50} may vary unpredictably among species as was the case with Vacor[50,53,58,69,90,91]; and (2) repeated ingestions of less toxic rodenticides (eg, short-acting anticoagulants, cholecalciferol) may, in fact, make them highly toxic (Table 108–2).

HIGHLY TOXIC RODENTICIDES (SIGNAL WORD: "DANGER")

According to FIFRA, highly toxic rodenticides are those substances with a single-dose LD_{50} of less than 50 mg/kg body weight. The label "Danger" is the strongest warning issued by the Consumer Product Safety Commission for a potential toxic hazard. Lower hazard levels are denoted by "Warning" and "Caution" (Table 108–1). The highly toxic "Danger" group includes thallium (Chap. 100), sodium monofluoroacetate (SMFA, compound 1080) and fluoroacetamide (compound 1081) (Chap. 110), strychnine (Chap. 112), zinc phosphide (Chap. 101), elemental phosphorus (Chap. 111), arsenic (Chap. 88), barium carbonate[57,70,87,97,104,105,117] (Chap. 109) and Vacor (N-3-pyridylmethyl-N′-p-nitrophenyl-urea)[3,50,53,58,69,90,91,101] (see Table 108–2 and the 7th edition of this text for an extensive discussion of Vacor).

MODERATELY TOXIC RODENTICIDES (SIGNAL WORD: "WARNING")

Moderately toxic rodenticides, those with an LD_{50} of 50 to 500 mg/kg body weight, include the "selective" rodenticide ANTU and *cholecalciferol (vitamin D_3),* one of the newer and increasingly popular rodenticides.

α-Naphthyl-Thiourea (ANTU) ANTU was first synthesized and tested in the United States during World War II in an effort to prevent rat-borne epidemics.[52] ANTU kills rats by causing acute lung injury (ALI) and pleural effusion, probably by damaging the lung capillaries, resulting in increased permeability.[11,96] Both morphine[23] and fructose-1,6-diphosphate (FDP)[64] appear to prevent or ameliorate ANTU-induced lung injury. Morphine modulates inducible nitric oxide synthetase and FDP inhibits activated neutrophils from producing oxygen free radicals that have been implicated in the pathogenesis of ALI and the resultant pulmonary edema. Young rats and rats exposed initially to small, nonlethal doses are relatively resistant to the lethal effects of ANTU, possibly by developing pulmonary cell hyperplasia.[9] The heart appears to be unaffected by ANTU.[11,96]

There are no well-documented human cases or series of human ANTU exposures from which human toxicity can be accurately determined. In several older series of combined ANTU plus chloralose ingestions, it appears that the respiratory symptoms are more severe from the combination than from chloralose alone, suggesting pulmonary effects of ANTU in humans. Of the 14 patients poisoned by the combination, 11 required intubation because of tracheobronchial hypersecretion.[36,43] Recommended treatment for ANTU ingestions is administration of activated charcoal (AC).[73] Supportive and symptomatic care should be provided, as there is no known antidote.

Cholecalciferol Cholecalciferol (vitamin D_3, Quintox®, Rampage®) was first registered and marketed in the United States in 1984 and can legally be purchased and applied by both pest control operators and consumers. Cholecalciferol mobilizes calcium from the bones of rodents and rabbits and in toxic doses produces hypercalcemia, osteomalacia, and metastatic calcification of the cardiovascular system, kidneys, stomach, and lungs; death typically occurs in 2 to 5 days.[66–68] Although all animals are susceptible to the effects of cholecalciferol, rats and mice succumb to much lower doses than do larger animals such as cats and dogs.[67,68] Cholecalciferol appears to be an effective rodenticide when either a large amount is consumed at one time, or smaller amounts consumed over a 2- to 3-day period.[67,68,92] Because death is not immediate and cholecalciferol does not impart unusual characteristics to the bait, the type of bait shyness that occurs with zinc phosphide, ANTU, strychnine, and other rodenticides typically does not occur.[66–68] Nevertheless, investigators in New Zealand hypothesized but failed to prove that dextromethorphan could prevent any acquired memory of sickness and cholecalciferol-induced anorexia by rats eating poisoned bait (resulting in poison shyness) though they claim that anorexia was reduced from 17 to 8 days.[41] The closely related vitamin D_2 (or ergocalciferol) has been used as a rodenticide in Europe and Canada since 1978, without the development of resistance reported to date.[66–68]

Although rats manifest signs of severe acute hypercalcemia, including lethargy and ultimately death from myocardial infarction in 2–5 days,[92] no serious human toxicity or deaths from the rodenticide form of cholecalciferol have been reported to date. It is important to note that all of the advice for managing human ingestions of cholecalciferol rodenticide is based on experience in the treatment of those poisoned from the therapeutic forms of vitamin D. One case of cholecalciferol poisoning in an industrial setting may be particularly relevant because, as might be the case of a child repeatedly ingesting small amounts of rodenticide, the exposure described was to small doses over a 32-day period resulting in prolonged hypercalcemia.[48]

Calciferol concentrations are not readily available, but a normal serum calcium concentration obtained 48 hours after an acute ingestion almost certainly will exclude any significant toxicity. Immediate intervention that may be considered after a large acute ingestion includes gastric emptying followed by gastric decontamination with AC, sorbitol, and multiple-dose activated charcoal (MDAC), but there is no data to confirm the effectiveness of this approach.

Treatment for moderate to severe degrees of hypercalcemia (greater than 11.5 mg/dL) includes IV fluid therapy with 0.9% sodium chloride solution, if the patient is hypovolemic and can tolerate a fluid load. Furosemide should be administered and potassium and magnesium concentrations monitored and maintained.

LOW-TOXICITY RODENTICIDES (SIGNAL WORD: "CAUTION")

The remaining rodenticides, with one exception, are of low toxicity (LD_{50}, 500 to 5000 mg/kg). This category includes red squill (*Urginea maritima*)[99,113] (Chap. 64), norbormide, bromethalin, and the anticoagulants (Chap. 59). The first-generation warfarin-based anticoagulant rodenticides and the second-generation long-acting superwarfarin forms together are responsible annually for more than 80% of the reported exposures, and the long-acting anticoagulants alone for 3 of the 11 deaths attributed to rodenticides between 2003 and 2007. Norbormide and bromethalin are discussed in the following sections.

Norbormide Norbormide, an irreversible smooth-muscle constrictor, appears to uniquely affect rats and has no known human toxicity. Rats die as a result of intense generalized vasoconstriction, resulting in tissue anoxia.[73] In vitro, norbormide promotes calcium entry into smooth muscle cells, inducing a myogenic contraction, selective for the small vessels in rats, whereas in the arteries of other mammals (and in the rat aorta), norbormide behaves like a calcium channel blocker.[12] Norboromide stimulates the opening of the rat mitochondrial permeability transition pore (mPTP) and induces changes in the fluidity of the lipid interior of the rat mitochondrial membranes, though the drug regulation of mPTP activity does not appear to be related to its lethal effects. The norbormide-sensitive mPTP target appears to be present in all species, and the selectivity may depend on unique properties of the system transporting norbormide to the internal matrix side of the rat mitochondria.[95,119] Following exposure, it is sufficient to achieve gastric decontamination with AC.

Bromethalin The commercial product formulation of bromethalin, is considered to be of low toxicity as defined previously. Bromethalin was registered with the EPA in 1982, became available in 1986.

From the time that bromethalin first became available, concern had been expressed about its potential toxicity.[66] However, the first possible bromethalin-induced case of human toxicity was not reported until 1996,[16] perhaps because as late as 1997, bromethalin had been registered in only six states. Two human deaths caused by bromethalin were reported by AAPCC in 2005, confirming fears of its potential lethality. From 2003 to 2007, AAPCC annually reported between 533 and 643 annual exposures, including 388 to 510 in children younger than 6 years of age. The outcome of the exposures has been almost entirely "none" to "moderate," except for the two deaths reported in 2005.

Bromethalin is considered a highly effective, single-feeding rodenticide with a mode of action reportedly involving the uncoupling of oxidative phosphorylation in the mitochondria, resulting in decreased adenosine triphosphate (ATP) production, increased fluid accumulation, and consequent increased pressure on nerve axons interrupting nerve impulse conduction.[67]

The pathologic changes resulting from a 1.5-mg/kg oral dose of bromethalin administered to cats, included spongy changes, hypertrophied fibrous astrocytes, and hypertrophied oligodendrocytes in the white matter of the cerebrum, cerebellum, brainstem, spinal cord, and optic nerve.[30,32] Prior to sacrifice of the animal, the clinical manifestations of bromethalin poisoning in these cats included ataxia, focal motor seizures, decerebrate posture, decreased proprioception, and depressed level of consciousness. Dogs given oral doses of 6.25 mg/kg of bromethalin developed hyperexcitability, tremors, seizures, depression, and death within 15 to 63 hours of exposure.[31] Death in animals is also usually preceded by paralysis and loss of tactile sensation.[114,115]

A 2006 report described the case of a 21-year-old man who presented with altered mental status a day after ingesting a bromethalin-based rodenticide. Over the next 7 days he developed obtundation, increased cerebrospinal fluid pressure, and cerebral edema, followed by death. Autopsy findings included diffuse histologic vacuolization in the CNS white matter on microscopic examination, and the presence of demethylated bromethalin in the liver and brain by gas chromatography-mass spectrometry. As predicted, clinical signs and microscopic pathology are clearly similar to that seen in animals poisoned with bromethalin.[81] Additional parallels to the clinical courses of exposed animals are the delay in appearance of clinical symptoms and signs, behavioral changes, anisocoria, cerebral edema, elevated CSF pressure, and subsequent death.[81]

Symptomatic and supportive care should be provided to patients exposed to bromethalin; there is no known antidote.

DANGEROUS OLD, NEW, AND UNUSUAL RODENTICIDES: THE GLOBAL PROBLEM

The confusion caused by nonrodenticide pesticides inappropriately used as rodenticides is compounded when a dangerous rodenticide favored in one part of the world is introduced and used in a different area, or when a highly toxic, previously abandoned rodenticide is "rediscovered." All three situations have become problematic in recent years. Widespread accessibility to products (including by the internet) and global travel probably contributes.

Tetramethylene Disulfotetramine (Tetramine, TETS, TEM) During the past decade, several reports have appeared in the medical literature describing the toxicity of the illegal Chinese rodenticide tetramine.[8,25] Patented as a rodenticide in the United States in 1953, tetramine was first used and then banned in China in 1984.[8] But this fast-acting, single-dose poison is still produced illegally in many parts of China and continues to be identified in unintentional or deliberate poisonings there and elsewhere. In China in September 2002, a deliberate adulteration of restaurant food with tetramine by a competing restaurant owner poisoned 300 people and caused 42 deaths, all in schoolchildren. In that same year, the first known case of tetramine poisoning in the United States resulted from a 15-month-old infant playing with the white powder brought back from China by her parents and applied to a kitchen corner.[8] The child developed convulsive status epilepticus refractory to lorazepam, phenobarbital, and pyridoxine and required intubation. She was left with multiple neurologic deficits that included persistent absence seizures, possible cortical blindness, multiple epileptogenic foci months later, and developmental delay 1 year later.[8]

Tetramine is an indirect-acting, γ-amino butyric acid (GABA) antagonist similar in some respects to picrotoxin and with an LD_{50} of 0.1–0.3 mg/kg.[35] Tetramine is more lethal than sodium fluoroacetate, the registered pesticide considered to be the most lethal by the World Health Organization (WHO). Tetramine may also be 100 times more toxic (on a g/kg basis)[8] to humans than potassium cyanide,[8] and as little as 5–10 mg/kg may be lethal.[25] Because of its high stability in water, tetramine is a relatively persistent environmental contaminant that theoretically could cause secondary poisonings.[25]

In addition to its most common manifestation of toxicity—refractory seizures[63]—tetramine also causes coma and possibly coronary ischemia. Symptoms begin from 30 minutes to 13 hours after exposure, and death may occur within 3 hours. A variety of methods have been used to treat tetramine poisoning in China, including AC, hemoperfusion, and hemodialysis, but none have proven to be uniformly successful and there are no proven antidotes for tetramine. Recently the use of sequential hemoperfusion (HP) and continous venovenous hemofiltration (CVVH) has been explored and in one study of 18 patients with severe tetramine poisoning treated this way, the 8 patients whose treatment was initiated within 24 hours of exposure had a higher cure rate than the 10 whose treatment began later.[27] Standard management includes gastrointestinal decontamination with AC, benzodiazepines for seizures, and effective airway protection.[118]

α-Chloralose (Glucochloral, Chloralosane) α-Chloralose is a crystalline powder (usually colored pink or blue) that is formed by the condensation of glucose with trichloroacetaldehyde (chloral). α-Chloralose is a central nervous system depressant, still used as a veterinary anesthetic.[100] Its effects in humans include sedation, anesthesia, spontaneous myoclonic movements, and generalized convulsions.[36,54] Most human exposures are nonfatal, and most current reports appear to emanate from France and Europe.[13,36,37,54] Management is supportive, with the use of airway protection and the administration of AC.

Salmonella-based Rodenticides *Salmonella enteritides*, a human pathogen, is an active ingredient in rodenticides still produced and used in Central America and Asia. The currently available formulation is made by coating rice grains with a combination of *S. enteritides* and warfarin. The strain of *Salmonella*—phage type 6a—is similar to the strain of *Salmonella* that was in a rodenticide used in Europe until the 1960s[79] and was responsible for human illness and deaths.[79] In 1954 and 1967, the WHO recommended against using *Salmonella*-based rodenticides because of the threat to human health. Since 1980, *S. enteritides* has been responsible for a global pandemic of foodborne illness associated with eggs and poultry.[79] In addition to inadvertent exposures, *Salmonella*-based rodenticides have been used intentionally to cause human illness.

MANAGING THE PATIENT EXPOSED TO AN UNKNOWN RODENTICIDE

For the patient exposed to an unknown rodenticide, the approach is more complicated than for a patient who ingests a known common commercial rodenticide, such as warfarin or cholecalciferol. First, as always, adequate breathing and circulation must be assured, as the patient is briefly examined. If the patient is initially stable, the next priority is to make every effort to fully identify the type and quantity of rodenticide ingested.

If the rodenticide and its package material do not accompany the patient, someone should be sent to retrieve them because identifying a harmless rodenticide ingestion early on is more cost-effective and less traumatic to the patient than treating for an unknown ingestion. If the rodenticide container is labeled, and the information is telephoned back to the health care provider, care should be taken to obtain the full name and not just the brand name. Rodenticide product and brand names are frequently used interchangeably by manufacturers. For example, until 1986, a line of rodenticides all carried the "Pied Piper" name on a variety of very different products: Pied Piper for Rats and Mice contained ANTU and warfarin; whereas Pied Piper Kwik-Kill Mouse Seed contained strychnine; and Pied Piper Rodenticide contained red squill. Many manufacturers still use similar names for dissimilar poisons.

Although full identification of the rodenticide is important, a careful physical examination should always be performed in all cases, searching for toxic signs that indicate specific rodenticides:

- Gastrointestinal symptomatology, paresthesias, and the late onset of hair loss are characteristic of thallium poisoning (Chap. 100).[10,26,28,44,49,62,72,75,83]
- Irritability or "apprehension" followed by seizures, coma, and death from respiratory failure or ventricular tachycardia and fibrillation are produced by SMFA, fluoroacetamide[18,19,20,21,40,78,86,93,107,110] (Chap. 110), and tetramine.
- Central nervous system stimulation, opisthotonos, prolonged recurrent motor seizures, and medullary paralysis followed by death suggest strychnine poisoning (Chap. 112).[6,15,33,46,51,56,59,76,77,80,85,94,102,108,112,116]
- Hypotension, vomitus with a rotten or "fishy" odor, cardiopulmonary collapse, coma, renal damage, and leukopenia suggest various metal phosphide exposures (Chap. 101).[1,2,4,17,22,39]
- Oral and skin burns, luminescent "smoking" vomitus, stools with a garlic odor, and gastrointestinal and biliary damage characterize yellow phosphorus (Chap. 111).[29,65,88,98,106,111]
- Dysphagia, muscle cramps, seizures, hematemesis, and bloody diarrhea followed by cardiovascular collapse suggest arsenic (Chap. 88).[55,103]
- The combination of striking hyperglycemia with or without ketoacidosis, severe postural hypotension, autonomic and peripheral neuropathies, and ileus and esophageal or GI perforation characterize Vacor poisoning (see Goldfrank's Toxicologic Emergencies, 7th ed., Chap. 90)[3,34,38,42,45,47,50,53,58,69,71,90,91,101]
- Muscle tremors, myoclonic jerks with flexion of major muscle groups, and unresponsiveness may be the human manifestations of bromethalin poisoning.
- Dyspnea, crackles, acute lung injury, pleural effusions, and hypothermia are seen with massive ingestions of ANTU.
- Nausea, vomiting, diarrhea, and abdominal pain will probably be the only effects of ingesting red squill, but when combined with signs of ventricular irritability (premature ventricular contractions and ventricular fibrillation), these signs and symptoms suggest exposure to this potent cardioactive steroid (Chap. 64).[82,99,113]
- Evidence of a bleeding disorder and abnormal coagulation or international normalized ratio (INR), or low concentrations of coagulation factors, point to either a large acute ingestion of a second-generation superwarfarin rodenticide, such as brodifacoum, or repeated (chronic) ingestion of a first-generation regular warfarin-type rodenticide (Chap. 59).[14]
- Signs and symptoms of hypercalcemia following (massive or chronic) rodenticide ingestion(s) suggests cholecalciferol (vitamin D_3).

If a toxic syndrome is identified, aggressive management, including the use of specific antidotes, may be indicated or necessary (see Table 108–2). Immediately following an ingestion and prior to the development of signs and symptoms of toxicity, there is no rodenticide currently in use for which orogastric lavage followed by AC (and possibly even an intestinal evacuant cathartic) is contraindicated—although they may be unnecessary. Once the patient is symptomatic however, orogastric lavage, AC, and catharsis must be individualized according to the specific toxin and the patient's clinical condition.

If every effort to identify the rodenticide fails, the following diagnostic evaluation may be indicated: A complete blood cell count and INR will help diagnose and manage repetitive ingestions of first-generation warfarin-type anticoagulant rodenticides, chronic ingestions of second-generation superwarfarin anticoagulant rodenticides, and a large single ingestion of a second-generation anticoagulant a few days later. Following acute ingestions, the CBC and INR will not be useful for at least 48 hours. Repetitive ingestions of the otherwise harmless first-generation warfarins is an important consideration for children who have pica, and for institutionalized, emotionally disturbed adults who may try to nibble rodenticides repeatedly. Tamper-resistant bait traps now mandated in the United States will hopefully reduce these risks further. Serum glucose, potassium, and bicarbonate concentrations will identify hyperglycemia and ketoacidosis caused by Vacor, and an elevated serum calcium concentration suggests cholecalciferol (vitamin D_3) ingestion. Liver enzyme, BUN, and creatinine concentrations are useful baseline determinations for rodenticides that cause hepatic or renal damage, respectively (eg, zinc phosphide, yellow phosphorus, cholecalciferol). A serum sample and 50 mL of urine should be obtained and sent to the toxicology laboratory with the request to hold it for possible heavy metals screening, especially if the patient is vomiting. Finally, if indicated by history or symptomatology, additional specimens may be collected for specific rodenticide determinations (eg, thallium, strychnine), and a digoxin concentration may point to red squill ingestion. Chest and abdominal radiographs may be useful because of the radiopaque nature of some of the uncommonly used rodenticides (Chap. 5).

If there is any doubt about the reliability of the patient (or parents) after the diagnostic evaluation, the patient should be admitted for observation. No matter what type of rodenticide was ingested, a determination should be made regarding the cause of the exposure, whether the ingestion was unintentional, a suicide gesture or attempt, or a manifestation of abuse or neglect.[7] A psychiatric assessment is, of course, indicated for any possible suicide attempt.

SUMMARY

As both the industrialized and underdeveloped parts of the world continue to experiment with and use exotic and sometimes lethal rodenticides, it will be even more important to be able to discriminate between the expected sequelae of known or suspected rodenticides and unexpected sequelae from other pesticides or xenobiotics used inappropriately for that purpose. The key to managing a patient who has ingested a rodenticide is to identify the rodenticide and the quantity ingested, its potential toxicity, and any available specific antidote. Toxic ingestions should be excluded or treated immediately; conversely, patients exposed to the most common commercial product acute anticoagulants, bromethalin, or cholecalciferol rodenticides should not be overtreated.

ACKNOWLEDGMENTS

Mary Ann Howland and Richard S. Weisman contributed to this chapter in a previous edition. Rebecca Tominack and Susan M. Pond contributed parts of the FIFRA discussion and Table 108–1.

REFERENCES

1. Abder-Rahman H. Effect of aluminum phosphide on blood glucose level. *Vet Hum Toxicol.* 1999;4:31-32.
2. Abder-Rahman HA, Baltah AH, Ibraheem YM et al. Aluminum phosphide fatalities, new local experience. *Med Sci Law.* 2000;40:164-168.
3. Ahn JS, Lee TH, Lee MC. Ultrastructure of neuromuscular junction in Vacor-induced diabetic rats. *Korean J Intern Med.* 1998;13:47-50.
4. Amr MM, Abbas EZ, El-Samra M, et al. Neuropsychiatric syndromes and occupational exposure to zinc phosphide in Egypt. *Environ Res.* 1997;73:200-206.
5. Arena JM, Drew RH. Rodenticides, fungicides, herbicides, fumigants and repellents. In Arena JM, Drew RH, eds. *Poisoning: Toxicology, Symptoms, Treatment*, 5th ed. Springfield, IL: Charles C Thomas; 1986:222-251.
6. Arneson D, Chi'en LT, Chance P, Wilroy RS. Strychnine therapy in nonketotic hyperglycinemia. *Pediatrics.* 1979;63:369-373.
7. Babcock J, Hartman K, Pedersen A, et al. Rodenticide-induced coagulopathy in a young child. A case of MÜnchausen syndrome by proxy. *Am J Pediatr Hematol Oncol.* 1993;15:126-130.
8. Barrueto F Jr, Furdyna PM, Hoffman RS, et al. Status epilepticus from an illegally imported Chinese rodenticide "tetramine." *J Toxicol Clin Toxicol.* 2003;41:991-994.
9. Barton CC, Bucci TJ, Lomax LG, et al. Stimulated pulmonary cell hyperplasia underlies resistance to alpha-naphthylthiourea. *Toxicology.* 2000;143:167-181.
10. Ben-Assa B: Indirect thallium poisoning in a Bedouin Family. *Harefuah.* 1962;62:378-380.
11. Bohm GM. Changes in lung arterioles in pulmonary oedema induced in rats by alpha-naphthyl-thiourea. *J Pathol.* 1973;110:343-345.
12. Bova S, Travis L, Debetto P, et al. Vasorelaxant properties of norbormide, a selective vasoconstrictor agent for the rat microvasculature. *Br J Pharmacol.* 1996;117:1041-1046.
13. Boyez E, Malherbe P. Curarization for contributing symptomatic treatment of myoclonic jerks induced by chloralose poisoning. *Ann Fr Anesth Reanim.* 2004;23:361-363.
14. Bruno CR, Howland MA, McMeeking A, Hoffman RS. Long-acting anticoagulant overdose: brodifacoum kinetics and optimal vitamin K dosing. *Ann Emerg Med.* 2000;36:262-267.
15. Boyd RE, Brennan PT, Deng JF, et al. Strychnine poisoning: recovery from profound lactic acidosis, hyperthermia, and rhabdomyolysis. *Am J Med.* 1983;74:507-512.
16. Buller G, Heard J, Gorman S. Possible bromethalin-induced toxicity in a human [abstract]. A case report. *J Toxicol Clin Toxicol.* 1996;34:572.
17. Chefurka W, Kashi KP, Bond EJ. The effect of phosphine on electron transport in mitochondria. *Pestic Biochem Physiol.* 1976;6:65-82.
18. Chenoweth MB. Monofluoroacetic acid and related compounds. *Pharm Rev.* 1949;1:383-424.
19. Chenoweth MB, Kandel A, Johnson LB, Bennett DR. Factors influencing fluoroacetate poisoning: practice treatment with glycerol monoacetate. *J Pharmacol Exp Ther.* 1951;102:31-49.
20. Chi CH, Chen KW, Chan SH, et al. Clinical presentation and prognostic factors in sodium monofluoroacetate intoxication. *J Toxicol Clin Toxicol.* 1996;34:707-712.
21. Chi CH, Lin TK, Chen KW. Hemodynamic abnormalities in sodium monofluoroacetate intoxication. *Hum Exp Toxicol.* 1999;18:351-353.
22. Chugh SN, Aggarwal HK, Mahajan SK. Zinc phosphide intoxication symptoms: analysis of 20 cases. *Int J Clin Pharmacol Ther.* 1998;36:406-407.
23. Comert M, Sipahl EY, Uston H, et al. Morphine modulates inducible nitric oxide synthetase expression and reduces pulmonary oedema induced by alpha-naphthylthiourea. *Eur J Pharmacol.* 2005; 511:183-189.
24. Costa LG. Toxic effects of pesticides. In Klaassen CD, ed. *Casarett & Doull's Toxicology: The Basic Science of Poisons*, 7th ed. New York: McGraw-Hill; 2008:883-884.
25. Croddy E. Rat poison and food security in the People's Republic of China: focus on tetramethylene disulfotetramine (tetramine). *Arch Toxicol.* 2004;78:1-6.
26. DeBacker W, Zachee P, Verpooten GA, Majelyne W. Thallium intoxication treated with combined hemoperfusion-hemodialysis. *J Toxicol Clin Toxicol.* 1982;19:259-264.
27. Dehua G, Daxi J, Honglang X et al. Sequential hemoperfusion and continuous venovenous hemofiltration in treatment of severe tetramine poisoning. *Blood Purif.* 2006;24:524-530.

28. Desenclos JC, Wilder MH, Coppenger GW, et al. Thallium poisoning: an outbreak in Florida, 1988. *South Med J.* 1992;85: 1203-1206.
29. Diaz-Rivera RS, Collazo PJ, Pons ER, et al. Acute phosphorus poisoning in man: a study of 56 cases. *Medicine.* 1950;29:269-298.
30. Dorman DC, Cote LM, Buck WB. Effects of an extract of Gingko biloba on bromethalin-induced cerebral lipid peroxidation and edema in rats. *Am J Vet Res.* 1992;53:138-142.
31. Dorman DC, Simon J, Harlin KA, Buck WB. Diagnosis of bromethalin toxicosis in the dog. *J Vet Diagn Invest.* 1990;2:123-128.
32. Dorman DC, Zachary JF, Buck WB. Neuropathologic findings of bromethalin toxicosis in the cat. *Vet Pathol.* 1992;29:138-144.
33. Edmunds M, Sheehan TMT, Van't Hoff W. Strychnine poisoning: clinical and toxicological observations on a non-fatal case. *J Toxicol Clin Toxicol.* 1986;24:245-255.
34. Esposti MD, Ngo A, Myers MA. Inhibition of mitochondrial complex I may account for IDDM-induced by intoxication with the rodenticide Vacor. *Diabetes.* 1996;45:1531-1534.
35. Esser T, Karu AE, Toia RF, Casida JE. Recognition of tetramethylene disulfotetramine and related sulfamides by the brain GABA-gated chloride channel and a cyclodiene-sensitive monoclonal antibody. *Chem Res Toxicol.* 1991;4:162-167.
36. Favarel-Garrigues JC, Boget JC. Intoxications aigues parles raticides a' base de chloralose et d'ANTU. *Concours Med.* 1968;90:2289-2298.
37. Federici S, Claudet I, Laporte-Turpin E et al. Severe chloralose intoxication in a toddler. *Arch Pediatr.* 2006;13:364-366.
38. Feingold KR, Lee TH, Chung MY, Siperstein MD. Muscle capillary basement membrane width in patients with Vacor-induced diabetes mellitus. *J Clin Invest.* 1986;78:102-107.
39. Frangides CY, Pneumatikos IA. Persistent severe hypoglycemia in acute toxic zinc phosphide poisoning. *Intensive Care Med.* 2002;28:223.
40. Gajdusek DC, Luther G. Fluoroacetate poisoning: a review and report of a case. *Am J Dis Child.* 1950;79:310-320.
41. Gould EM, Holmes SJ. The effect of dextromethorphan in preventing cholecalciferol-induced poison shyness and sickness-induced anorexia in the laboratory Norway rat. *Pest Manag Sci.* 2008; 64:197-202.
42. Hauser L, Sheehan P, Simpkins H. Pancreatic pathology in pentamidine induced diabetes in acquired immunodeficiency syndrome patients. *Hum Pathol.* 1991;22:926-929.
43. Hayes WJ. *Pesticides Studied in Man.* Baltimore, MD: Williams & Wilkins; 1982. pp. 473–478.
44. Heath A, Ahlmen J, Branegard B, et al. Thallium poisoning: toxin elimination and therapy in three cases. *J Toxicol Clin Toxicol.* 1983;20: 451-463.
45. Herken H. Antimetabolic action of 6-amino-nicotinamide on the pentose phosphate pathway in the brain. In Aldridge N, ed. *Mechanism of Toxicity.* London: St. Martin's; 1970:189.
46. Heiser JM, Daya MR, Magnussen AR, Norton RL. Massive strychnine intoxication: serial blood levels in a fatal case. *J Toxicol Clin Toxicol.* 1992;30:269-283.
47. Howland MA, Weisman R, Sauter D, Goldfrank L. Nonavailability of poison antidotes. *N Engl J Med.* 1986;314:927-928.
48. Jibani M, Hodges NH. Prolonged hypercalcemia after industrial exposure to vitamin D3. *Br Med J.* 1985;290:748-749.
49. Kamerbeek HH, Rauws AG, Ham MT, et al. Dangerous redistribution of thallium by treatment with sodium diethyldithiocarbamate. *Acta Med Scand.* 1971;189:149-154.
50. Karam JH, LeWitt PA, Young CH, et al. Insulinopenic diabetes after rodenticide (Vacor) ingestion: a unique model of acquired diabetes in man. *Diabetes.* 1980;29:971-978.
51. Katz J, Prescott K, Woolf AD. Strychnine poisoning from a Cambodian traditional remedy. *Am J Emerg Med.* 1996;14:475-477.
52. Keiner C. Wartime rate control, rodent ecology, and the rise and fall of chemical rodenticides. *Endeavour.* 2005; 29:119-125.
53. Kenney RM, Michaels IAL, Flomenbaum NE, Yu GSM. Poisoning with *N*-3-pyridylmethyl-*N*′-*p*-nitrophenyl-urea (Vacor). *Arch Pathol Lab Med.* 1981;105:367-370.
54. Kintz P, Doray S, Cirimele V, Ludes B. Testing for alpha-chloralose by headspace-GC/MS. A case report. *Forensic Sci Int.* 1999;104:59-63.
55. Kosnett MJ, Becker CE. Dimercaptosuccinic acid: utility in acute and chronic arsenic poisoning [abstract]. *Vet Hum Toxicol.* 1988;30:369.
56. Kuno M, Weakly JN. Quantal components of the inhibitory synaptic potential in spinal mononeurones of the cat. *J Physiol (Lond).* 1972; 224: 287-303.
57. Layzer RB. Periodic paralysis and the sodium-potassium pump. *Ann Neurol.* 1982;11:547-552.
58. LeWitt PA. The neurotoxicity of the rat poison Vacor: a clinical study of 12 cases. *N Engl J Med.* 1980;302:73-77.
59. Libenson MH, Yang JM. Weekly clinicopathological exercises: case 12-2001: a 16-year-old boy with an altered mental status and muscle rigidity. *N Eng J Med.* 2001;344:1232-1239.
60. Lisella FS, Long KR, Scott HG. Toxicology of rodenticides and their relation to human health. *J Environ Health.* 1970;33:231-237.
61. Lisella FS, Long KR, Scott HG. Toxicology of rodenticides and their relation to human health. *J Environ Health.* 1970;33:361-365.
62. Lovejoy FH. Thallium. *Clin Toxicol Rev.* 1982;5:1-2.
63. Lu Y, Wang X, Yan Y et al. Nongenetic cause of epileptic seizures in 2 otherwise healthy Chinese families: tetramine—case presentation and literature survey. *Clin Neuropharmacol.* 2008; 31:57-61.
64. Markov AK, Causey AL, Didlake RH, Lemos LB. Prevention of alpha-naphthylthiourea induced pulmonary edema with fructose-1,6-diphosphate. *Exp Lung Res.* 2002; 28:285-299.
65. Marin GA, Mantoya CA, Sierra JL, Senior JR. Evaluation of corticosteroid and exchange transfusion treatment of acute yellow phosphorous intoxication. *N Engl J Med.*1961;284:125-128.
66. Marsh R. Personal communication, June 29, 1993.
67. Marsh RE. Currrent (1987) and future rodenticides for commensal rodent control. *Bull Soc Vector Ecol.* 1988;13:102-107.
68. Marsh R, Tunberg A. Characteristics of cholecalciferol: rodent control—other options. *Pest Control Technol.* 1986;14:43-45.
69. Miller LV, Stokes JD, Silpipat C. Diabetes mellitus and autonomic dysfunction after Vacor rodenticide ingestion. *Diabetes Care.* 1978;1: 73-76.
70. Mills K, Kunkel D. Prevention of severe barium carbonate toxicity with oral magnesium sulfate [abstract]. *Vet Hum Toxicol.* 1993;35:342.
71. Molner GD, Berge KG, Rosenveas JW, et al. The effect of nicotinic acid in diabetes mellitus. *Metabolism.* 1974;13:181-189.
72. Moore D, House I, Dixon A, et al. Grand rounds, Guy's Hospital—thallium poisoning. *Br Med J.* 1993;306:1527-1529.
73. Morgan DP. *Recognition and Management of Pesticide Poisonings*, 4th ed. Washington, DC: United States Environmental Protection Agency;1989.
74. Nelson LS, Perrone J, DeRoos F, et al. Aldicarb poisoning by an illicit rodenticide imported into the United States: *Tres Pasitos. J Toxicol Clin Toxicol.* 2001;39:447-452.
75. Nogué S, Mas A, Parés A, et al. Acute thallium poisoning: an evaluation of different forms of treatment. *J Toxicol.* 1982;19: 1015-1021.
76. Oberpaur B, Donoso A, Claveria C, et al. Strychnine poisoning: an uncommon intoxication in children. *Pediatr Emerg Care.* 1999;15:264-265.
77. O'Callaghan WA, Joyce N, Counihan HE, et al. Unusual strychnine poisoning and its treatment: report of 8 cases. *Br Med J.* 1982;285:478.
78. Omara F, Sisodia CS. Evaluation of potential antidotes for sodium fluoroacetate in mice. *Vet Hum Toxicol.* 1990;32:427-431.
79. Painter JA, Molbak K, Sonne-Hansen J et al. Salmonella-based rodenticides and public health. *Emerg Infect Dis.* 2004;10:985-987.
80. Palatnick W, Meatherall R, Sitar D, Tenenbein M. Toxicokinetics of acute strychnine poisoning. *J Toxicol Clin Toxicol.* 1997;35:617-620.
81. Pasquale-Style MA, Sochaski MA, Dorman DC, et al. Fatal bromethalin poisoning. *J Forensic Sci.* 2006;51:1154-1157.
82. *PDR for Herbal Medicines,* 2nd ed. Montvale, NJ: Medical Economics; 2000.
83. Pedersen RS, Olesen AS, Freund LG, et al. Thallium intoxication treated with long-term hemodialysis, forced diuresis and Prussian blue. *Acta Med Scand.* 1978;204:429-432.
84. Pelfrene AF. Synthetic rodenticides. In Hayes WJ, Laws ER, eds. *Handbook of Pesticide Toxicology.* San Diego: Academic Press; 1991:1271-1316.
85. Perper JA. Fatal strychnine poisoning—a case report and review of the literature. *J Forensic Sci.* 1985;30:1248-1255.
86. Peters RA. Lethal synthesis. *Proc Roy Soc Lond.* 1952;13:139-143.
87. Phelan DM, Hagley SR, Guerin MD. Is hypokalaemia the cause of paralysis in barium poisoning? *Br Med J.* 1984;289:882.
88. Pietras RJ, Stavrakos C, Gunnar RM, Tobin JR. Phosphorus poisoning stimulating acute myocardial infarction. *Arch Intern Med.* 1968;122: 430-434.
89. Plunkett LM. Do current FIFRA testing guidelines protect infants and children? Lead as a case study. Federal Insecticide, Fungicide, and Rodenticide Act. *Regul Toxicol Pharmacol.* 1999;29:80-87.
90. Pont A, Rubino JM, Bishop D, Peal R. Diabetes mellitus and neuropathy following Vacor ingestion in man. *Arch Intern Med.* 1979;139:185-187.

91. Prosser PR, Karm JH. Diabetes mellitus following rodenticide ingestion in man. *JAMA.*1978;239:1148-1150.
92. Quintox. Product Information Sheet. Madison, WI: Bell Laboratories, 1985.
93. Reigart JR, Brueggeman JL, Keil JE. Sodium fluoroacetate poisoning. *Am J Dis Child.* 1975;129:1224-1226.
94. Reigart JR, Roberts JR. *Recognition and Management of Pesticide Poisonings,* 5th ed. Washington, DC: United States Environmental Protection Agency, 1999.
95. Ricchelli F, Dabbeni-Sala F, Petronilli V et al. Species-specific modulation of the mitochondrial permeability transition by norbormide. *Biochim Biophys Acta.* 2005;1708:178-186.
96. Richter CP. The development and use of alpha-naphthyl-thiourea (ANTU) as a rat poison. *JAMA.* 1945;129:927-931.
97. Roza O, Berman LB. The pathophysiology of barium, hypokalemia and cardiovascular effects. *J Pharmacol Exp Ther.* 1971;177: 433-439.
98. Rubitsky HJ, Myerson RM. Acute phosphorus poisoning. *Arch Intern Med.* 1949;83:164-178.
99. Sabouraud AE, Ortizberea M, Cano N, et al. Specific anti-digoxin Fab fragments: an available antidote for proscillaridin and scilliroside poisoning. *Hum Exp Toxicol.* 1990;9:191-193.
100. Segev G, Yas-Natan E, Shlosberg A, Aroch I. Alpha-chloralose poisoning in dogs and cats: a retrospective study of 33 canine and 13 feline confirmed cases. *Vet J.* 2006;172:109-113.
101. Seon YD, Lee TH, Lee MC. Changes of glomerular basement membrane components in Vacor-induced diabetic nephropathy. *Korean J Intern Med.* 1999;14:77-84.
102. Sgaragli GP, Mannaioni PF. Pharmacokinetic observations on a case of massive strychnine poisoning. *Clin Toxicol.* 1973;6: 533-540.
103. Shum S, Whitshead J, Vaughan L, et al. Chelation of organoarsonate with dimercapton succinic acid. *Vet Hum Toxicol.* 1995;37: 239-242.
104. Sigue G, Gamble L, Pelitere M, et al. From profound hypokalemia to life-threatening hyperkalemia. A case of barium sulfide poisoning. *Arch Intern Med.* 2000;160:548-551.
105. Silinsky EM. On the role of barium in supporting the asynchronous release of acetylcholine quanta by motor nerve impulses. *J Physiol.* 1978;274: 157-171.
106. Simon FA, Pickering LK. Acute yellow phosphorus poisoning. *JAMA.* 1976;235:1343-1366.
107. Singh M, Vijayaraghavan R, Pant SC, et al. Acute inhalation toxicity study of 2-fluoroacetamide in rats. *Biomed Environ Sci.* 2000;13:90-96.
108. Smith BA. Strychnine poisoning. *J Emerg Med.* 1990;8:321-325.
109. Sullivan JB, Krieger GR, eds. *Clinical Environmental Health and Toxic Exposures,* 2nd ed. Philadelphia, PA: Lippincott Williams & Wilkins; 2001:1056.
110. Taitelman U, Roy A, Hoffer E. Fluoroacetamide poisoning in man: the role of ionized calcium. *Arch Toxicol Suppl.* 1983;6:228-231.
111. Talley RC, Linhart JW, Trevino AJ, Moore L. Acute elemental phosphorous poisoning in man: cardiovascular toxicity. *Am Heart J.* 1972; 84:139-140.
112. Teitelbaum DT, Ott JE. Acute strychnine intoxication. *Clin Toxicol.* 1970;2:267-273.
113. Tuncok Y, Kozan O, Caudar C, et al. Urginea maritima (squill) toxicity. *J Toxicol Clin Toxicol.* 1995;33:83-86.
114. Van Lier RBL, Ottosen D. Studies on the mechanism of toxicity of bromethalin: a new rodenticide. *Theoret Toxicol.* 1981;1:114.
115. *Vengeance Rodenticide Technical Manual.* St. Louis City, MI: Velsicol Chemical Corp;1986:19.
116. Weiss S, Hatcher RA. Studies on strychnine. *J Pharm Exp Therap.* 1922;14: 419-482.
117. Wetherill SF, Guarino MJ, Cox RW. Acute renal failure associated with barium chloride poisoning. *Ann Intern Med.* 1981;95:187-188.
118. Whitlow KS, Belson M, Barrueto F et al. Tetramethylenedisulfotetramine: old agent and new terror. *Ann Emerg Med.* 2005; 45:609-613.
119. Zulian A, Petronilli V, Bovas S et al. Assessing the molecular basis for rat-selective induction of the mitochondrial permeability transition by norbormide. *Biochim Biophys Acta.* 2007;1767:980-988.

CHAPTER 109
BARIUM

Andrew Dawson

Barium (Ba)

Atomic number	=	56
Atomic weight	=	137.33 daltons
Normal concentrations		
Serum	=	0.2 mg/L (1.46 μmol/L)

Barium is commonly utilized as a pesticide, a depilatory, and a radiographic contrast material. Acute exposures following ingestion or inhalation are most common outside the hospital setting. Exposures during radiologic procedures are associated with aspiration during oral studies, intravasation during rectal procedures, and iatrogenic intravenous administration. Rapid recognition is essential to address these potentially life-threatening exposures.

HISTORY AND EPIDEMIOLOGY

Barium poisoning is a rare cause of exposure or poisoning as far fewer than 100 cases were reported to the AAPCC database in recent years (see Chap. 135). Toxicity is most commonly reported following the intentional ingestion of soluble salts found in rodenticides,[9] insecticides, or depilatories.[10] Barium carbonate has an appearance that is similar to flour and has been responsible for most unintentional barium poisonings.

Barium salts and barium hydroxide are extensively employed in industry particularly in thermoplastics and the manufacture of synthetic fibers, soap manufacture, and in lubricants (see Table 109–1). Toxicity has also followed occupational exposure to barium salts through ingestion or inhalation. An explosion of the propellant barium styphnate caused extensive burns and trauma in a 50-year-old man. The individual also developed significant barium toxicity within 2 hours of exposure that persisted for at least 4 days.[13] Despite the fact that barium sulfate is insoluble, rare cases of unintentional toxicity have been reported during radiographic procedures and include complications associated with oral[20] and rectal administration.[12,17,19,22] Toxicity and death occurred when soluble barium salts unintentionally contaminated contrast solution[24] and flour.[8]

CHEMISTRY

Barium is a soft metallic element that was first isolated by Sir Humphry Davey in 1808. With an atomic weight of 137.3 barium is located at number 56 in the periodic table (between cesium and lanthanum). The metal oxidizes easily when exposed to water or alcohol, has a melting point of 727°C (1341°F) and a boiling point of 1870°C (3398°F). Elemental barium is not found in nature; it normally occurs as an oxide, dioxide, sulphate (barite), or carbonate (witherite). Chemically, barium resembles calcium more than any other element. While some barium salts are naturally occurring, most used commercially are produced from the more commonly found carbonate or oxides. Barium salts are typically classified as either water soluble or insoluble, but the solubility of all barium salts increases as the milieu becomes more acidic. The soluble salts acetate, chloride, hydroxide, oxide, nitrate, and (poly)sulfide are the most commonly associated with toxicity (Table 109–1). Barium (poly)sulfide also produces toxicity through the formation of hydrogen sulfide when ingested and exposed to gastric hydrochloric acid.

The solubility of barium carbonate is low at physiological pH, but increases significantly as the pH is lowered. In addition, in gastric acid conversion to barium chloride occurs, which is highly soluble. The other insoluble barium salts such as arsenate, chromate, fluoride, oxalate, and sulfate are rarely associated with toxicity. However, toxicity has occurred in the unusual situation of intravasation of barium sulfate (see Toxicokinetics).

TOXICOKINETICS

Toxicity can result from ingestion of as little as 200 mg of a barium salt. Oral lethal doses are reported to range from 1 to 30 g of a barium salt. In ambient air, inhaled concentrations greater than 250 mg/m^3 are considered dangerous.[32]

Following ingestion, 5%–10% of soluble barium salts are absorbed,[14] with the rate of absorption dependent on the degree of water solubility of the salt. The time to peak serum concentration is 2 hours.[14]

The toxicokinetics are characterized by a rapid redistribution phase, followed by a slow decrease of serum barium concentrations with a reported half-life ranging between 18 and 85 hours.[14,23] Renal elimination of the absorbed dose accounts for 10%–28% of total barium excretion, with the predominant route of elimination through the gastrointestinal tract in the feces.

Death is uncommon following exposure but occurs most commonly following ingestion, and rarely following inhalation.[15] Death from an ingestion with barium chloride was associated with the following barium concentrations at autopsy: blood, 9.9 mg/L; bile, 8.8 mg/L; urine, 6.3 mg/L; and gastric contents, 10 g/L.[15]

Intravasation is a rare but serious complication of radiologic studies that administer barium sulfate under pressure, such as a barium enema. Following a small perforation, barium sulfate leaks into the peritoneal cavity or portal venous system.[19] Although sudden cardiovascular collapse may occur, it is unclear whether this is the result of venous occlusion (pulmonary embolism), overwhelming sepsis, or barium toxicity.[6,27,31] In at least one case report of intravasation, signs and symptoms were consistent with barium toxicity and elevated concentrations were confirmed.[20] If hypokalemia is present, then barium toxicity should be assumed.

Additionally, intravenous administration of barium sulfate has occurred as the result of iatrogenic error. Rapid recognition followed by aspiration through a central venous catheter was associated with a good outcome.[25]

PATHOPHYSIOLOGY

At a cellular level barium induces hypokalemia by two synergistic mechanisms. Barium is a competitive blocker of the potassium rectifier channel which is responsible for the efflux of intracellular potassium out of the cell. It may also directly increase cell membrane permeability to sodium. This causes a secondary increase Na^+-K^+ pump electrogenesis leading to a shift of extracellular potassium into the cell.

Intracellular trapping of potassium leads to depolarization and paralysis.[16] Additionally, the inhibition of potassium channels increases vascular resistance and reduces blood flow[3,5] and is the likely mechanism for hypertension and metabolic acidosis with elevated lactate concentration.

TABLE 109–1. Barium Salts: Solubility and Common Usages

Barium Salt	Solubility[a]	Common Uses
Acetate	58.8	Textile dyes
Carbonate	0.02 g/L increases in an acid pH; also, can be converted to barium chloride by gastric acid (HCl)	Rodenticide, welding fluxes, pigments, glass, ceramics, pyrotechnics, electronic devices, welding rods, ferrite magnet materials, optical glass, manufacture of caustic soda and other barium salts
Chloride	375	Textile dyes, barium salts, pigments, boiler detergents, in purifying sugar, as mordant in dyeing and printing textiles, as water softener, in manufacture of caustic soda and chlorine, polymers, stabilizers
Fluoride	1.2	Welding fluxes
Nitrate	87	Optical glass, ceramic glazes, pyrotechnics (green light), explosives, antiseptic preparation
Oxide	34.8	In glass, ceramics, refining oils and sugar, as an additive in petroleum products and also as materials of plastics, pharmaceuticals, polymers, glass and enamel industries
Styphenate	–	Propellent used in manufacture of explosive detonators
Sulfate	0.002	Radiopaque contrast media, manufacture of white pigments, paper making
Sulfide	Slightly soluble in H_2O	Depilatories, manufacture of fluorescent tubes

While severe hypokalemia is a major contributor to paralysis, some authors have found that muscle weakness correlates better with barium concentrations than with potassium concentrations.[21,28] This suggests a possible direct effect of barium on either skeletal muscle or neuromuscular transmission.

CLINICAL MANIFESTATION

Abdominal pain, nausea, vomiting, and diarrhea commonly occur within 1 hour of ingestion. Esophageal injury[1] and hemorrhagic gastritis are also reported.[15]

Severe hypokalemia is the cardinal feature of barium toxicity and can occur within 2 hours following oral or parenteral exposure. Hypokalemia may be exacerbated by blood transfusions, suggesting that fresh red blood cells provide a new reservoir for K^+ sequestration.[13] Progressive hypokalemia is associated with severe ventricular dysrhythmias, hypotension, profound flaccid muscle weakness, and respiratory failure (see Chap. 16).

Other effects less commonly reported include metabolic acidosis with elevated lactate concentration, hypophosphatemia, and rhabdomyolysis.[14] Altered level of consciousness, seizures,[7] and parkinsonism with MRI findings of bilateral hyperintensity of the basal ganglia are reported.[11] It is unclear whether these later findings are due to direct toxicity, deposition of barium or secondary to tissue ischemia.

DIAGNOSTIC TESTING

Barium can be measured by a variety of techniques. Mass spectrometry and graphite furnace atomic absorption spectrometry (GF-AAS) can quantitate barium in blood and urine.[16] Serum barium concentrations are not readily available, but values greater than 0.2 mg/L are considered abnormal.[4]

Following acute exposures, patients should have serum electrolytes (particularly potassium and phosphate) measured hourly while performing continuous ECG monitoring. CPK and acid base status and renal function should also be measured. A plain abdominal radiograph may show barium, but the sensitivity and specificity of radiography has never been determined for barium poisoning.[16]

DIFFERENTIAL DIAGNOSIS

Other causes of acute hypokalemia (see Chap. 16) associated with paralysis such as periodic hypokalemic paralysis, toluene toxicity, and diuretic use should be considered if there is no history or laboratory confirmation of barium exposure. Other toxicologic etiologies for flaccid paralysis such as hypermagnesemia, botulism, and the administration of neuromuscular blockers should also be considered.

MANAGEMENT

Patients should be admitted to an intensive care unit with expectant management of respiratory compromise support. Patients who are asymptomatic at 6 hours following ingestion with normal potassium concentrations can be discharged.

DECONTAMINATION

Activated charcoal is unlikely to be effective. Orogastric lavage should be considered in patients who present early after ingestion, but lavage is unlikely to provide substantial benefit in patients who are already symptomatic or who have had spontaneous emesis. Oral sodium sulfate administration may prevent absorption by precipitating unabsorbed barium ions as insoluble, nontoxic barium sulfate. Oral magnesium sulfate has had similar efficacy.[18] The oral dose of magnesium sulfate is 250 mg/kg for children and 30 g for adults. Intravenous magnesium sulfate or sodium sulfate is not advised as it may lead to renal failure due to precipitation of barium in the renal tubules.[21,30]

Patients in respiratory failure should receive assisted ventilation. Aggressive correction of hypokalemia is important to minimize the risk or to treat cardiac dysrhythmias. Large doses of potassium replacement (400 mEq in 24 hours) may be required to correct serum potassium although repletion may be inadequate to improve the resting membrane potential or muscle strength[16] (see Chap. 16). As hypokalemia is due to intracellular sequestration of potassium, potassium supplementation increases the total body potassium load. In this situation, rebound hyperkalemia may occur when barium is eliminated, especially in patients with impaired renal function. Observation for this clinical complication is essential.

Elimination Enhancement If the correction of hypokalemia does not restore normal motor function and muscle strength, hemodialysis can be considered. Hemodialysis for the management of severe barium toxicity is associated with rapid clinical improvement.[2,23,26,29] Additionally, in a case report, CVVHDF tripled the measured barium elimination, reduced serum barium half-life by a factor of three, stabilized serum potassium concentrations, and rapidly improved motor strength, with complete neurological recovery within 24 h.[16] Either method of enhanced elimination should be considered in any severely symptomatic patient who does not respond to correction of hypokalemia.

Management of Intravasation Following intravasation, patients should be admitted to an intensive care unit. Expectant management should include considerations of intraabdominal sepsis, hemorrhage and trauma, pulmonary embolus, and barium toxicity.[19] Prophylactic antibiotics seem reasonable and serial determinations of serum potassium concentrations are warranted. CT scanning of the chest and abdomen can demonstrate both the location and extent of the barium sulfate administered.[27]

SUMMARY

Although poisoning by barium salts is rare these salts are widely used in industry and therefore represent a substantial risk for human exposure. Barium salts typically produces a rapid onset of symptoms and can produce life-threatening toxicity. In addition to good supportive care the mainstay of treatment is rapid correction of hypokalemia.

REFERENCES

1. Aks SE, Mansour M, Hryhorczuk DO, Raba J, Vanden Hoek TL. Barium sulfide ingestions in an urban correctional facility population. *J Prison Jail Health.* 1993;12:3-12.
2. Bahlmann H, Lindwall R, Persson H. Acute barium nitrate intoxication treated by hemodialysis. *Acta Anaesthesiol Scand.* 2005:49:110-112.
3. Chilton L, Loutzenhiser R. Functional evidence for an inward rectifier potassium current in rat renal afferent arterioles. *Circulation Res.* 2001;88:152-158.
4. Crafoord B and Ekwall B. Time-related Lethal Blood Concentrations from Acute Human Poisoning of Chemicals. Part 2: The Monographs. No. 37 Barium. http://www.ctlu.se. 1998.
5. Dawes M, Sieniawska C, Delves T, Dwivedi R, Chowienczyk PJ, Ritter JM. Barium reduces resting blood flow and inhibits potassium-induced vasodilation in the human forearm. *Circulation.* 2002;105:1323-1328.
6. de Feiter PW, Soeters PB, Dejong CH. Rectal perforations after barium enema: a review. *Dis Colon Rectum.* 2006;49:261-271.
7. Deixonne B, Baumel H, Mauras Y, Allain P, Robert C, Raffanel C. [A case of barium-peritoneum with neurological involvement. Importance of barium determination in biological fluids]. *J Chir (Paris).* 1983;120:611-613.
8. Deng JF, Jan IS, Cheng HS. The essential role of a poison center in handling an outbreak of barium carbonate poisoning. *Vet Human Toxicol.* 1991;33:173-175.
9. Dhamija RM, Koley KC, Venkataraman S, Sanchetee PC. Acute paralysis due to barium carbonate. *J Assoc Physicians India.* 1990;38:948-949.
10. Downs JC, Milling D, Nichols CA. Suicidal ingestion of barium-sulfide-containing shaving powder. *Am J Forensic Med Pathol.* 1995;16:56-61.
11. Fogliani J, Giraud E, Henriquet D, Maitrasse B. [Voluntary barium poisoning]. *Ann Fr Anesth Reanim.* 1993;12:508-511.
12. Gross GF, Howard MA. Perforations of the colon from barium enema. *Am Surg.* 1972;38:583-585.
13. Jacobs IA, Taddeo J, Kelly K, Valenziano C. Poisoning as a result of barium styphnate explosion. *Am J Ind Med.* 2002;41:285-288.
14. Johnson CH, VanTassell VJ. Acute barium poisoning with respiratory failure and rhabdomyolysis. *Ann Emerg Med.* 1991;20:1138-1142.
15. Jourdan S, Bertoni M, Sergio P, Michele P, Rossi M. Suicidal poisoning with barium chloride. *Forensic Sci Int.* 2001;119:263-265.
16. Koch M, Appoloni O, Haufroid V, Vincent JL, Lheureux P. Acute barium intoxication and hemodiafiltration. *J Toxicol Clin Toxicol.* 2003;41:363-367.
17. Lewis JW, Jr., Kerstein MD, Koss N. Barium granuloma of the rectum: an uncommon complication of barium enema. *Ann.Surg.* 1975;181:418-423.
18. Mills K, Kunkel D. Prevention of severe barium carbonate toxicity with oral magnesium sulfate. *Vet Human Toxicol.* 1993;35:342.
19. O'Hara DE, Krakovitz EK, Wolferth CC. Barium intravasation during an upper gastrointestinal examination: a case report and literature review. *Am Surg.* 1995;61:330-333.
20. Pelissier-Alicot AL, Leonetti G, Champsaur P, Allain P, Mauras Y, Botta A. Fatal poisoning due to intravasation after oral administration of barium sulfate for contrast radiography. *Forensic Sci Int.* 1999;106:109-113.
21. Phelan DM, Hagley SR, Guerin MD. Is hypokalaemia the cause of paralysis in barium poisoning? *BMJ (Clin Res Ed).* 1984;289:882.
22. Salvo AF, Capron CW, Leigh KE, Dillihunt RC. Barium intravasation into portal venous system during barium enema examination. *JAMA.* 1976;235:749-751.
23. Schorn TF, Olbricht C, Schuler A, Franz A, Wittek K, Balks HJ, et al. Barium carbonate intoxication. *Intensive Care Med.* 1991;17:60-62.
24. Silva RF. CDC. Barium toxicity after exposure to contaminated contrast solution—Goias State, Brazil, 2003. *MMWR Morb Mortal Wkly Rep.* 2003;52: 1047-1048.
25. Soghoian S, Hoffman RS, Nelson L. Unintentional intravenous injection of barium sulfate in a child. *Clin Toxicol.* 2008;46:387.
26. Szajewski J. High-potassium haemodialysis in barium poisoning. *J Toxicol Clin Toxicol.* 2004:42:117.
27. Takahashi M, Fukuda K, Ohkubo Y, et al. Nonfatal barium intravasation into the portal venous system during barium enema examination. *Intern Med.* 2004;43:1145-1150.
28. Thomas M, Bowie D, Walker R. Acute barium intoxication following ingestion of ceramic glaze. *Postgrad Med J.* 1998;74:545-546.
29. Wells JA, Wood KE. Acute barium poisoning treated with hemodialysis. *Am J Emerg Med.* 2001;19:175-177.
30. Wetherill SF, Guarino MJ, Cox RW. Acute renal failure associated with barium chloride poisoning. *Ann Intern Med.* 1981;95:187-188.
31. White JS, Skelly RT, Gardiner KR, Laird J, Regan MC. Intravasation of barium sulphate at barium enema examination. *Br J Radiol.* 2006;79:e32-e35.
32. WHO. Environmental Health Criteria 107: Barium. IPCS INCHEM . 1-1-1990. 7-2-2005.

CHAPTER 110
SODIUM MONOFLUOROACETATE AND FLUOROACETAMIDE

Fermin Barrueto, Jr.

Sodium monofluoroacetate (SMFA) occurs naturally in plants native to Brazil, Australia, and South and West Africa, in the gifblaar (*Dichapetalum cymosum*).[11] The highest concentration (8.0 mg/g) is found in the seeds of a South African plant, *Dichapetalum braunii*.[11] In the 1940s, SMFA was released as a rodenticide (CAS No. 62-74-8) and assigned the compound number 1080, which was registered as its trade name. Fluoroacetamide, a similar pesticide, is known as Compound 1081. These compounds are used as poisons against most mammals and some amphibians.[23] Both products were banned in the United States in 1972, except in the form of collars intended to protect sheep and cattle from coyotes. Collars embedded with SMFA are placed around the neck of livestock, the typical point of attack for coyotes.

Sodium monofluoroacetate is used extensively in New Zealand and Australia to control the possum population and other animal species considered pests that have no natural predators. Its continued use is extremely controversial, but, following a recent review of the ramifications of the use of the compound, the government of New Zealand has retained both the aerosolized and collar applications.

PHARMACOKINETICS AND TOXICODYNAMICS

Sodium monofluoroacetate is an odorless and tasteless white powder with the consistency of flour. When it is dissolved in water, it is said to have a vinegar-like taste. Sodium monofluoroacetate and fluoroacetamide (CAS No. 640-19-7) are well absorbed by the oral and inhalational routes.[10,11,12,24] Detailed toxicokinetic data are lacking in humans, but in sheep, up to 33% can be excreted unchanged in the urine over 48 hours. Glucuronide and glutathione conjugates have also been isolated.[11] Substantial defluorination is not thought to occur in vivo. The serum half-life is estimated to be 6.6 to 13.3 hours in sheep.[10] Sodium monofluoroacetate has an LD_{50} of 0.07 mg/kg in dogs.[17] The oral dose thought to be lethal to humans is 2 to 10 mg/kg.[3]

PATHOPHYSIOLOGY

Sodium monofluoroacetate, a structural analog of acetic acid (Fig. 110–1), is an irreversible inhibitor of the tricarboxylic acid cycle (Fig. 12-3). Monofluoroacetic acid enters the mitochondria, where it is converted to monofluoroacetyl-coenzyme A (CoA) by acetate thiokinase. Once inside the mitochondria, citrate synthase joins the monofluoroacetyl-CoA complex with oxaloacetate to form fluorocitrate. Fluorocitrate then covalently binds aconitase, preventing the enzyme from any further interaction in the tricarboxylic acid cycle.[15] Thus, fluorocitrate acts as a "suicide inhibitor" of aconitase, producing a biochemical dead end. The presence of fluorocitrate and the subsequent increase in citrate, which chelates divalent cations, causes hypocalcemia. The toxicity caused by fluorocitrate results from the increase in substrate prior to inhibition of aconitase and the depletion of substrate after the step catalyzed by aconitase.

This inhibition of aconitase impairs energy production, leading to anaerobic metabolism and metabolic acidosis with an elevated lactate concentration. Additionally, other tricarboxylic acid cycle intermediates increase in concentration, contributing to the toxicity. α-Ketoglutarate depletion, caused by the lack of isocitrate, leads to glutamate depletion since α-ketoglutarate is a precursor of glutamate synthesis. Glutamate depletion leads to urea cycle disruption and ammonia accumulation. Impaired fatty acid oxidation leads to ketosis.

Disruption of the tricarboxylic acid and urea cycles affects every system in the human body, but the most consequential effects occur in the central nervous system (CNS) and the cardiovascular system. Fluoride toxicity from enzymatic defluorination of sodium monofluoroacetate and fluoracetamide does not occur substantially in vivo and is of minor significance.

CLINICAL MANIFESTATIONS

The majority of the clinical experience with SMFA is associated with intentional self-poisoning; fluoroacetamide poisoning is presumed to have a similar presentation.[9,14,16,26] Most patients develop symptoms within 6 hours after exposure. In the largest case series of 38 Taiwanese patients who ingested SMFA, 7 died.[6] The most common clinical findings recorded at the time of emergency department (ED) presentation were nausea and vomiting (74%), diarrhea (29%), agitation (29%), and abdominal pain (26%).[6] The mean time to presentation to the hospital was 10.9 ± 5.7 hours for those who died and 3.4 ± 0.6 hours for the survivors. All deaths occurred within 72 hours of admission to the hospital. The presence of respiratory distress and/or seizures was a poor prognostic indicator of death. All seven patients who died had systolic blood pressures less than 90 mm Hg on presentation to the ED, a finding noted in only 16% of the survivors.[6]

In a case series involving two patients, invasive hemodynamic monitoring revealed persistent low systemic vascular resistance and increased cardiac output despite adequate fluid resuscitation.[7] The authors theorized that the cardiovascular response may have been triggered by ATP depletion and inhibition of gluconeogenesis.[7] Anaerobic metabolism, mitochondrial inhibition, and sensitivity of the vasculature to SMFA are all also confounding factors.

The initial neurologic manifestations are agitation and confusion with progression to seizures. Neurologic sequelae such as cerebellar dysfunction may be permanent.[27] One case report describes a 15-year-old girl who survived an initial exposure to SMFA, but later developed cerebellar dysfunction and cerebral atrophy, demonstrated by brain computed tomography.[27] QT interval prolongation, premature ventricular contractions, ventricular fibrillation, ventricular tachycardia, and other dysrhythmias have been documented.[6] SMFA has negative inotropic effects, except in one case report that described episodic hypertension.[22] Signs and symptoms associated with severe poisoning are seizures, respiratory distress, and hypotension.

DIAGNOSTIC TESTING

The presence of SMFA and fluoroacetamide in the blood and urine can be confirmed with gas chromatography-mass spectrometry and thin-layer chromatography.[1,5,18] Simultaneous analysis for other rodenticides that can induce seizures, for example, fluoroacetamide and "tetramine," has been performed by gas chromatography in China, where exposure to these xenobiotics is more probable.[2,4,28] An elevated serum citrate concentration has been proposed as a useful marker for exposure to

```
   H  O
   |  ||
F—C—C—O⁻Na⁺     Sodium monofluoroacetate
   |
   H

   H  O
   |  ||
F—C—C—NH₂       Fluoroacetamide
   |
   H

   H  O
   |  ||
H—C—C—CoA       Acetyl CoA
   |
   H
```

FIGURE 110–1. Structural similarities among acetyl-CoA, sodium monofluoroacetate, and fluoroacetamide.

SMFA.[4] However, none of these studies can be performed in a clinically relevant period. A combination of history, signs, symptoms, and common laboratory tests can assist with the diagnosis.

Hypokalemia, anion gap metabolic acidosis, and an elevated creatinine concentration[8] are associated with severe poisoning but are very nonspecific.[6] The predominant electrolyte abnormality will be hypocalcemia, though hypokalemia can result from renal insufficiency and gastrointestinal losses. Creatinine, liver enzyme, and bilirubin concentrations may also be elevated as a result of multisystem organ toxicity. Ketones may be present in urine and serum. A complete blood cell count may reveal leukocytosis due to demargination. An electrocardiogram is valuable in the diagnosis of SMFA exposure; a prolonged QT interval, atrial fibrillation with a rapid ventricular response, ventricular tachycardia, and other dysrhythmias may be present. An initial brain computed tomography scan of the brain may be normal, but subsequent scans may reveal cerebral atrophy.[27]

TREATMENT

Initial decontamination should include removal of clothes and cleansing of skin with soap and water. Because there is no antidote for SMFA or fluoroacetamide poisoning, orogastric lavage should be considered for exposed patients who present to the ED prior to significant emesis. Appropriate patients should receive 1 g/kg of activated charcoal (AC) orally. A rat study showed that colestipol is more effective in binding SMFA than activated charcoal.[19] By extension, it seems reasonable to consider the use of colestipol, if available, for the treatment of life-threatening exposures in humans, although there are no data to support this statement. A typical oral starting dose would be 5 grams.

In animal models, ethanol and glycerol monoacetate (monacetin) are suggested to be antidotal. In this context, they function as acetate donors for ultimate incorporation into citrate in place of fluoroacetate.[26] Both ethanol and glycerol monacetate are converted to acetyl-CoA and compete with monofluoroacetyl-CoA for binding of citrate synthase. This may prevent the "suicide-inhibition" of aconitase, subsequent increase in citrate, and the formation of the toxic metabolite fluorocitrate.[26]

Ethanol has been used in human cases, although the appropriate dose is unknown and there is not enough evidence to support its use as a single antidote.[6,7,21] A reasonable therapeutic dose is the amount of ethanol required to obtain and sustain an ethanol serum concentration of 100 mg/dL (Antidotes in Depth A32: Ethanol) One intriguing case report involves a patient who ingested 240 mg of SMFA (typically a lethal dose) mixed with a Taiwanese wine (30% ethanol) and survived.[6] It is possible that the ethanol decreased or delayed the toxicity of SMFA.

In a mouse model,[20] use of a combination of calcium salts, sodium succinate, and α-ketoglutarate improved survival. The rationale of using these antidotes is to provide tricarboxylic acid cycle intermediates distal to the inhibited aconitase in an attempt to improve energy production. These antidotes were not effective unless calcium was coadministered, emphasizing the importance of replenishing electrolytes, particularly the divalent cations that are chelated by citrate.[13,25]

If a patient develops hypotension and shock, rapid administration of intravenous fluids should be followed by a vasopressor, such as norepinephrine, and/or vasopressin. Supportive care, correction of electrolyte abnormalities (calcium and potassium), ethanol infusion, and monitoring for dysrhythmias (prolonged QT interval) and seizures are the practical mainstays of treatment.

SUMMARY

Sodium monofluoroacetate and fluoroacetamide are potent pesticides that inhibit the tricarboxylic acid cycle, resulting in disrupted cellular energy production. Patients who are exposed to SMFA typically present with nausea, vomiting, agitation, and abdominal pain, which may be followed by hypotension, respiratory distress, shock, seizures, and death. Lactate accumulation, hypokalemia, hypocalcemia, metabolic acidosis, and elevation of serum creatinine also occur. Treatment of SMFA and fluoroacetamide poisoning involves replenishing electrolytes, correcting hypotension with intravenous fluids and vasopressors if necessary, monitoring for dysrhythmias, and treating seizures. Ethanol, although not a perfect antidote, is relatively familiar, is readily available, and can be administered safely. The efficacies of other experimental antidotes are unknown.

REFERENCES

1. Allender WJ. Determination of sodium fluoroacetate (Compound 1080) in biological tissues. *J Anal Toxicol.* 1990;14:45-49.
2. Barrueto F Jr, Furdyna PM, Hoffman RS, et al. Status epilepticus from an illegally imported Chinese rodenticide: "tetramine." *J Toxicol Clin Toxicol.* 2003;41:991-994.
3. Beasley M. Guidelines for the safe use of sodium fluoroacetate (1080). New Zealand Occupational Safety & Health Service, August 2002.
4. Bosakowski T, Levin AA. Serum citrate as a peripheral indicator of fluoroacetate and fluorocitrate toxicity in rats and dogs. *Toxicol Appl Pharmacol.* 1986;85:428-436.
5. Cai X, Zhang D, Ju H, et al. Fast detection of fluoroacetamide in body fluid using gas chromatography-mass spectrometry after solid-phase microextraction. *J Chromatogr B Analyt Technol Biomed Life Sci.* 2004;802:239-245.
6. Chi CH, Chen KW, Chan SH, et al. Clinical presentation and prognostic factors in sodium monofluoroacetate intoxication. *J Toxicol Clin Toxicol.* 1996;34:707-712.
7. Chi CH, Lin TK, Chen KW. Hemodynamic abnormalities in sodium monofluoroacetate intoxication. *Hum Exp Toxicol.* 1999;18:351-353.
8. Chung HM. Acute renal failure caused by acute monofluoroacetate poisoning. *Vet Hum Toxicol.* 1984;26(Suppl 2):29-32.
9. Deng HY, Gao Y, Li YJ. [Management of severe fluoroacetamide poisoning with hemoperfusion in children]. *Zhongguo Dang Dai Er Ke Za Zhi.* 2007;9:253-254. Chinese.
10. Eason CT, Gooneratne R, Fitzgerald H, et al. Persistence of sodium monofluoroacetate in livestock animals and risk to humans. *Hum Exp Toxicol.* 1994;13:119-122.
11. Eason C. Sodium monofluoroacetate (1080) risk assessment and risk communication. *Toxicology.* 2002;181-182:523-530.

12. Eason CT, Turck P. A 90-day toxicological evaluation of Compound 1080 (Sodium monofluoroacetate) in Sprague-Dawley rats. *Toxicol Sci.* 2002;69: 439-447.
13. Hornfeldt CS, Larson AA. Seizures induced by fluoroacetic acid and fluorocitric acid may involve chelation of divalent cations in the spinal cord. *Eur J Pharmacol.* 1990;179:307-313.
14. Jones K. Two outbreaks of fluoroacetate and fluroacetamide poisoning. *J Forensic Sci Soc.* 1965;12:76-79.
15. Liebecq C, Peters RA. The toxicity of fluoroacetate and the tricaraboxylic acid cycle 1949. *Biochim Biophys Acta.* 1989;1000:254-269.
16. Lin J, Jiang C, Ou J, Xia G. [Acute fluoroacetamide poisoning with main damage to the heart.] *Zhonghua Lao Dong Wei Sheng Zhi Ye Bing Za Zhi.* 2002;20:344-346. Chinese.
17. Meenken D, Booth LH. The risk to dogs of poisoning from sodium monofluoroacetate (1080) residues in possum (Trichosurus vulpecula). *New Zealand J Agric Res.* 1997;40:573-576.
18. Minnaar PP, Swan GE, McCrindle RI, et al. A high-performance liquid chromatographic method for the determination of monofluoroacetate. *J Chromatogr Sci.* 2000;38:16-20.
19. Norris WR, Temple WA, Eason CT, et al. Sorption of fluoroacetate (compound 1080) by colestipol, activated charcoal and anion-exchange in resins in vitro and gastrointestinal decontamination in rats. *Vet Hum Toxicol.* 2000;42:269-275.
20. Omara F, Sisodia CS. Evaluation of potential antidotes for sodium fluoroacetate in mice. *Vet Hum Toxicol.* 1990;32:427-431.
21. Ramirez M. Inebriation with pyridoxine and fluoroacetate: a case report. *Vet Hum Toxicol.* 1986;28:154.
22. Robinson RF, Griffith JR, Wolowich WR, et al. Intoxication with sodium monofluoroacetate (compound 1080). *Vet Hum Toxicol.* 2002;44:93-95.
23. Sherley M. The traditional categories of fluoroacetate poisoning signs and symptoms belie substantial underlying similarities. *Toxicol Lett.* 2004;151:399-406.
24. Singh M, Vijayaraghavan R, Pant SC, et al. Acute inhalation toxicity study of 2-fluoroacetamide in rats. *Biomed Environ Sci.* 2000;13:90-96.
25. Taitelman U, Roy A, Hoffer E. Fluoroacetamide poisoning in man: The role of ionized calcium. *Arch Toxicol Suppl.* 1983;6:228-231.
26. Taitelman U, Roy A, Raikhlin-Eisenkraft B, et al. The effect of monoacetin and calcium chloride on acid-base balance and survival in experimental sodium fluoroacetate poisoning. *Arch Toxicol Suppl.* 1983;6:222-227.
27. Trabes J, Rason N, Avrahami E. Computed tomography demonstration of brain damage due to acute sodium monofluoroacetate poisoning. *J Toxicol Clin Toxicol.* 1983;20:85-92.
28. Wu Q, Zhang MS, Lan ZR. Simultaneous determination of fluoroacetamide and tetramine by gas chromatography. *Se Pu.* 2002;20:381-382.

CHAPTER 111
PHOSPHORUS

Michael C. Beuhler

Phosphorus (P)		
Atomic number	=	15
Atomic weight	=	30.97 daltons
Normal concentrations		
Serum		3–4.5 mg/dL (1–1.4 mmol/L)

Elemental phosphorus is used for the production of matches, fireworks, rodenticides, and munitions. The more toxic form, white phosphorus, spontaneously combusts in air and has significant hepatic and renal toxicity when taken internally. The other common form, red phosphorus, has limited human toxicity. Although in many areas the prevalence of poisonings from phosphorus has markedly decreased, morbidity is high and treatment options remain limited.

HISTORY AND EPIDEMIOLOGY

Phosphorus is a nonmetallic element not naturally found in its elemental form; it was isolated from distilled urine by Hennig Brandt in 1669. White phosphorus has been used in munitions (mortar rounds, grenades, artillery shells, bombs) since World War I for its antipersonnel effect as well as its warning, incendiary, and smoke-producing properties. It is also used in fireworks made in countries other than the United States and China, in the production of matches, and for selected chemical synthetic processes (including some pesticides). White phosphorus was used extensively in the past as a rodenticide, but is no longer employed for this purpose in the United States. Because of its potential use for illicit drug manufacture, its sale is carefully monitored by the US Drug Enforcement Administration (DEA), which limits its availability in the United States. Before modern regulation, it was used in scientifically unfounded remedies primarily because its phosphorescent and reactive qualities suggested potency. Its occasional use as a homicidal agent was limited by its glowing, smoking qualities leaving obvious clues. It remains a common method of suicide in some countries.

Phosphorus was used extensively at the beginning of the 20th century in millions of "strike anywhere" matches (lucifers). However, safety concerns with the matches and illnesses in the workers producing the matches prompted a shift from using the more dangerous white phosphorus in the match heads to substituting the safer red phosphorus in the strikers. Workers chronically exposed to white phosphorus developed "phossy jaw," an illness characterized by disfiguring osteonecrosis of the mandible along with multiple draining abscesses.

CHEMISTRY

Phosphorus, atomic number 15, is a group 5A nonmetallic element sharing chemical properties with nitrogen (above) and arsenic (below) in the same periodic group. Elemental phosphorus can exist in several different allotropes (polymorphs); the two common forms considered here are red phosphorus and the highly reactive white phosphorus. The relatively nontoxic and nonreactive black form will not be considered further.

White phosphorus is a waxy whitish to yellow solid with a melting point of 44.1°C.[26] Often a small amount of red phosphorus being present results in discoloration, explaining its other name, "yellow" phosphorus. The word *phosphorus* means light-bearer, which originates from its property of glowing when exposed to air, likely due to the formation of reactive luminescent phosphorus oxide species on its surface. It is insoluble in water and often stored under it; it will dissolve in carbon disulfide and other organic solvents.[26] White phosphorus is very reactive, igniting spontaneously in air at approximately 34°C and oxidizing to form phosphorus pentoxide (P_4O_{10}), which has a cage-shaped molecular structure and usually appears as a white fume having a garliclike smell. Phosphorus pentoxide is hydroscopic and reacts with water to form phosphoric acid (H_3PO_4); it also reacts with organic molecules in dehydrating reactions and is irritating to biological membranes.

Red phosphorus is a red powdery compound of limited toxicologic significance. It is not luminescent, it does not combust in air, and its toxicity is orders of magnitude less than that of white phosphorus.

PHARMACOKINETICS AND TOXICOKINETICS

White phosphorus is insoluble in water, but it is soluble in lipids and lipophilic solvents. It is well absorbed from the intestinal tract and coingestion with fats, alcohol, and liquids has been associated with increased toxicity, probably from increased absorption.[8,9] White phosphorus is also well absorbed through skin, with dermal burns contributing to the absorption and significant morbidity and mortality arising from large surface areas burns. White phosphorus can also be absorbed by inhalation, but this route is rare with modern industrial hygiene. After ingestion, phosphorus is found in high concentrations in the blood, liver, and kidneys within 3 hours.[5,14]

Internally absorbed white phosphorus has significant toxicity. A dose of only about 1 mg/kg of white phosphorus in adults is likely to cause significant morbidity, but a lethal dose of 3 mg in a child is reported.[3] The mortality from white phosphorus ingestion is difficult to estimate since the majority of reported cases occurred before critical care was as advanced as it is now, but one can estimate a 25% mortality rate from a significant ingestion.[12]

PATHOPHYSIOLOGY

The mechanism of *dermal* injury from white phosphorus differs significantly from that of *ingested* white phosphorus. Externally, white phosphorus reacts with oxygen to form phosphorus pentoxide and other phosphorus oxides. Phosphorus pentoxide readily reacts with water in an exothermic reaction producing corrosive phosphoric acid.[17] Additionally, phosphorus pentoxide chemically reacts with (dehydrates) some organic molecules. These three mechanisms (exothermic, acid-producing, and dehydrating reactions) all contribute to the tissue injury observed, although the most damaging mechanism is the thermal injury from the heat of the reaction, as evidenced by the relatively short distance of tissue penetration by the acid and the relatively large amount of available water.[7,25] The evidence for describing white phosphorus as a cytoplasmic toxin is mostly derived from electron microscopy, which demonstrates an initial cytoplasmic injury of the rough endoplasmic reticulum rather than initial nuclear or mitochondrial changes.[13]

Red phosphorus has limited direct toxicological significance. It can cause gastrointestinal (GI) distress when ingested in significant amounts, but it is orders of magnitude less toxic than white phosphorus.

A resurgence of toxicity and human injury indirectly related to red phosphorus has resulted from the recent increase in North American domestic methamphetamine production. Red phosphorus is used in conjunction with elemental iodine to produce hydroiodic acid, the ultimate reducing agent required to convert ephedrine to methamphetamine. In this situation, red phosphorus contributes to human injury by causing fire because of its unintentional conversion to highly flammable white phosphorus. Additional pathology occurs because during heating, the reaction products of iodine and red phosphorus often generate phosphine (PH_3) a pulmonary irritant gas (see Chap. 124). Phosphine is only produced in significant amounts during an active methamphetamine "cook" using the red phosphorus method. This gas most likely contributes to some of the pulmonary symptoms occurring with chronic methamphetamine laboratory exposure, as well as several of the deaths resulting from performing the synthesis in an area with limited ventilation in order to hide the methamphetamine laboratory characteristic odors.[27] Unless specifically stated, all further references to phosphorus in this chapter refer to white phosphorus.

CLINICAL MANIFESTATIONS

GENERAL

Oral phosphorus poisoning was previously classified in three clinical stages. The initial symptoms may be delayed for a few hours, and the presence of a delay depends on the dose. During the first phase, patients experience vomiting, hematemesis, and abdominal pain, with hypotension and death occurring within 24 hours after large ingestions.[9,15] During the second stage, there is transient resolution of symptoms. During the third stage the patient develops hepatic injury with coagulopathy and jaundice as well as renal failure with oliguria and uremia. However, several case series demonstrate that three distinct phases is the exception rather than the rule, with significant overlap or absence of the "quiescent" second stage and death potentially occurring within hours of ingestion.[4,8,19,22,28] In the first 6 hours postexposure poor prognostic signs include altered sensorium, cyanosis, hypotension, metabolic acidosis, elevated prothrombin time, and hypoglycemia.[8,22] Survival to 3 days serves as a good prognostic sign; however, deaths delayed after several days have been reported.[9] Recovery usually occurs over 1 to 2 weeks.

GASTROINTESTINAL

Initial symptoms after ingestion of phosphorus include nausea, vomiting, and abdominal pain. Diarrhea, as well as constipation are reported, but are much less common. The breath and vomitus are sometimes described as having a garlic or musty sweet odor. The vomitus and diarrhea are sometimes luminescent and smoking, but this specific finding occurs in the minority of patients.[4,6,16] The smoking material is caused by the combustion of phosphorus upon its reexposure to air after being eliminated from the GI tract. Phosphorus causes an inflammatory injury to the GI tract characterized by local hemorrhage and hematemesis, but generally perforations do not occur. Massive GI bleeding later in the clinical course leading to mortality is occasionally reported, particularly when hepatic failure and coagulopathy occur.[12]

RENAL/ELECTROLYTES

In a rat model of dermal burns from phosphorus an initial diuresis occurs followed by renal failure manifested by hyperkalemia, hyponatremia, and hyperphosphatemia.[1] Renal cell swelling and necrosis with vacuolar degeneration of proximal convoluted tubules was also observed.[1] Poisoned patients demonstrated an increase in urinary white blood cells (WBC) and red blood cells (RBC) as well as casts and proteinuria.[3,15] Renal injury from phosphorus in humans is most likely acute tubular necrosis resulting from hypotension and salt and water depletion as well as a direct toxic effect.[9]

Significant electrolyte disturbances may result from both ingestion and dermal absorption of phosphorus. Hypocalcemia is common, but hypercalcemia is also occasionally reported.[17] Hyperphosphatemia may accompany the hypocalcemia but is not universal and can occur at any time in the clinical course.[3] The hyperphosphatemia is partially due to the conversion of absorbed phosphorus to phosphate; in an animal model those that died had increased concentrations of phosphorus, decreased concentrations of calcium, and hyperkalemia as early as 1 hour postexposure.[2] Hyperkalemia is occasionally reported in humans and may be secondary to tissue injury and renal failure.[1] The electrolyte disturbances are likely a leading cause of early mortality from phosphorus.

CARDIOVASCULAR

Death within 24 hours of the ingestion is likely the result of cardiovascular collapse. One human series of 41 suicide attempts demonstrated a variety of initial electrocardiogram (ECG) abnormalities. T-wave changes predominated in 24 patients but the series also had two cases of ventricular fibrillation. An increasing number of abnormalities occurred in those with larger ingestions, although the electrolyte abnormalities were not described in many patients.[9] An animal model of phosphorus exposure demonstrated prolonged QT interval and ST segment changes along with electrolyte abnormalities suggesting that many of the ECG changes might be due to these electrolyte abnormalities.[2] A small study of phosphorus exposure of rats observed a decrease in amino acid uptake in myocytes suggesting a direct effect beyond secondary effects due to electrolyte changes (hypocalcemia and hyperkalemia). Human autopsies have demonstrated fatty degeneration of the myocardium and vacuolated cytoplasm in a few patients many hours postingestion.[24]

HEPATIC

White phosphorus is a potent hepatoxin. Increase in prothrombin time, hyperbilirubinemia, and hypoglycemia usually occur within 3 days, with earlier signs of hepatic failure such as jaundice and coagulopathy indicative of a poor prognosis.[9,15,18] The increase in hepatic aminotransferases occurs over several days usually peaking at or below 1000 IU/L and almost always less than 3000 IU/L.[12] Other biochemical effects demonstrated by experimental phosphorus toxicity include an increase in glucose-6-phosphate activity and impairment of triglyceride metabolism. When death occurs after several days (as opposed to within 24 hours), hepatic injury is usually implicated. If survival occurs the hepatic damage usually resolves over several months, although persistent periportal fibrosis has been reported.[18]

With absorption of sufficient quantities, phosphorus causes a dose-related zone 1 or periportal hepatic injury, in contrast to the centrilobular pattern (zone 3) that occurs with other hepatotoxins (such as acetaminophen and carbon tetrachloride; see Chap. 26). Fatty degenerative changes and fatty infiltrates are also observed within 6 hours of ingestion.[8] Other histological changes include acute necrosis with large vacuoles and inflammatory changes. Electron microscopy in a rat model demonstrated an increase in the rough endoplasmic reticulum and an increase in the cytoplasmic fat without initial mitochondrial or nuclear injury.[13] Although the early pathological effects appear to be predominantly cytoplasmic, the formation of nuclear vacuoles can occur as well.[18]

NERVOUS SYSTEM

CNS effects include headache, altered mental status, coma, and rarely seizures. The altered mental status is probably due mostly to the presence of other organ dysfunction and shock; one example of the former is the encephalopathy secondary to hepatic injury. Patients with initial alterations in mental status or coma have an increased mortality rate independent of the presence of any electrolyte abnormalities.[19]

DERMAL/MUCOUS MEMBRANES

Dermal phosphorus exposure causes extensive burns, frequently in the military setting. Depending on the release conditions, white phosphorus can be a solid or liquid. Liquid white phosphorus splatters and can penetrate clothing; burning clothing commonly exacerbates the burn area.[17,20] Dermal penetration may be partially due to its lipophilicity as well as the compromise of the dermal barrier caused by the burn injury. The smoke produced by burning white phosphorus contains phosphorus pentoxide and is irritating to the conjunctiva and mucosa of the oropharynx and lungs.

Following a large burn, systemic illness manifested by electrolyte, cardiovascular, and hepatic abnormalities may result from absorbed phosphorus.[1,2] A 12% to 15% body surface area burn in a rat was lethal 50% of the time due to cardiovascular effects; human morbidity from large skin burns is similarly high. Rats with dermal burns from phosphorus also developed renal and hepatic injury. Healing time from phosphorus-induced burns is prolonged compared with thermal burns.[7]

DIAGNOSTIC TESTING

Serum elemental phosphorus concentrations are not clinically available and a serum phosphorus concentration does not reflect the serum elemental phosphorus concentration. Diagnosis of phosphorus poisoning must rely on history and physical examination. However, for optimal supportive care of the patient, many laboratory factors must be monitored such as electrolytes, serum pH, hepatic function, glucose, renal function, and coagulation parameters (see Management section).

MANAGEMENT

PROTECTION OF HEALTHCARE WORKERS

Caution should be exercised in decontamination and subsequent storage of contaminated clothing. After phosphorus ingestion, the patient's vomitus and diarrhea must be considered potentially hazardous and carefully handled. Any phosphorus fragments removed from the patient as well as all potentially contaminated clothing items should be kept under water. Fires and explosions are reported during GI decontamination efforts.[21]

GENERAL

General supportive care is the mainstay of treatment. Cardiac monitoring, frequent electrolyte analysis of calcium, phosphorus and potassium concentrations, and serial ECGs are essential for patients with a history of significant ingestions and/or overt toxicity, as dysrhythmias may occur rapidly.[9] Electrolyte disturbances such as hyperkalemia, hypocalcemia, and hypercalcemia should be corrected. With significant exposure to phosphorus, hepatic injury will occur and thus directed supportive care should be provided such as fresh frozen plasma, vitamin K, and lactulose when indicated. Adequate serum glucose concentrations are required to provide reducing equivalents (reduced form of nicotinamide adenine dinucleotide [NADH] and nicotinamide adenine dinucleotide phosphate [NADPH]) through glycolysis and the glucose-6-phosphate dehydrogenase (G6PD) pathways. Increased glucose concentrations may also theoretically offer protection by competing with phosphorus reuptake in the kidney, but the contribution to human morbidity is unclear. Steroids have not been shown to improve outcome following ingestions of white phosphorus.[18] Direct contact of phosphorus with the eye can result in serious ocular injury. Immediate copious ocular decontamination with water but not with copper sulfate is recommended.[23] A careful opthalmologic examination should be conducted by an ophthalmologist whenever possible.

DERMAL EXPOSURE

Initial treatment is to halt continuing injury by extinguishing combustion of the phosphorus. This is performed by submerging the affected area in cool water or, more practically, covering any areas with clean materials soaked in water or 0.9% sodium chloride solution to limit the white phosphorus contact with atmospheric oxygen. Decontamination is undertaken by removing the patient's clothing and using large amounts of cool water to remove any phosphorus fragments. In the past, sodium bicarbonate decontamination solution was recommended, but because the tissue injury is not due to the production of acid and because no clinical benefit was demonstrated, there is no role for specific neutralization fluids.[7,25] Water dilutes any phosphoric acid present and reacts with the phosphorus pentoxide to limit the dehydrating reactions.

Careful débridement is the next critical step as wounds that have not undergone adequate decontamination heal poorly, requiring additional débridement. Smoking pieces of phosphorus are not necessarily hot enough to cause thermal burns, but the oxidation process must be arrested. Fragments from the wound should be placed under water to prevent a fire hazard. Particles of phosphorus can be visualized by using a woods lamp as the chemical burns have a yellowish fluorescence. One author recommends turning off the lights to look for the glow of the phosphorescent particles; presumably this will only work if there has not been any copper metal wash solution used (see following paragraphs).[10] Because of the increased solubility of phosphorus in hydrophobic solvents, it is important not to use ointments until the wound is completely decontaminated.

A copper (II) sulfate solution was previously recommended for decontamination. Copper sulfate reacts with phosphorus to produce copper phosphide, a dark compound that is much more easily visualized in the tissues. This dark material coats the particle but the entire particle is not converted to copper phosphide. The use of high concentrations of copper sulfate solutions on exposed human flesh is no longer recommended because of potential systemic toxicity such as hemolysis caused by the copper (see Chap. 93).[23] This is especially concerning in patients at increased risk for oxidant injury, such as those with G6PD deficiency. The solutions of copper sulfate historically used ranged around 2% to 5% and were applied for several hours to the wounds, resulting in substantial amounts of copper absorption and morbidity.

However, copper sulfate solutions may have a role in the complete approach to the treatment of phosphorus wounds. A dilute copper sulfate solution 0.5% to less than or equal to 1.0% applied once to the wound and then rinsed off with water may not result in the morbidity that occurs with the more concentrated rinses and may provide temporary neutralization of the outer surface of the phosphorus. This approach may assist in identification of the small pieces of phosphorus that are difficult or impossible to visualize, especially in those with less experience débriding these wounds. The use of pads soaked in copper sulfate is *not* recommended. Wounds that are not treated with a copper solution may be at greater risk of requiring repeat débridement because of the persistence of small phosphorus particles missed during the initial decontamination efforts. Animal models have suggested improved healing from the initial treatment with a dilute copper solution, but a relatively large human case series did not find a difference in those who were treated with copper sulfate compared with those who were not.[7] The copper phosphide–coated particles must be removed as they still react slowly and can potentially cause toxicity. It is important to remember that the dilute copper sulfate solution is not a decontamination therapy, but a temporizing treatment that allows for better visualization for physical débridement and must be rinsed away immediately after application.[10]

Silver nitrate is suggested as a potential solution to replace the use of copper sulfate. It forms an insoluble, minimally reactive silver phosphide as well. Its use and preparation is similar to that described above; silver nitrate should be considered as a temporary neutralization tool and not a decontamination therapy. However, there is very limited experience with this approach in the literature and no detailed human data. Silver forms an insoluble precipitate with chloride and cannot be combined with 0.9% sodium chloride solutions; therefore, the amount of soluble silver ion that reaches the imbedded phosphorus may be more limited than with copper because of the presence of relatively large amounts of chloride ion in living tissues.[29]

After decontamination, good wound care and burn management is required as these burns (like other chemical burns) can require an extended period of time to heal. As mentioned, incomplete decontamination is a common reason for delayed wound healing. For significant burns, the patient should be admitted to a burn unit intensive care unit (ICU) for close monitoring of cardiovascular, renal, and electrolyte status. Because of the potential instability of these patients, it is important to weigh the risk-benefit ratio of transfer to a specialized center. The experience of the receiving center with phosphorus burns along with the acuity of the injury are important factors in making this decision.

GASTROINTESTINAL EXPOSURE

There is no evidence that GI decontamination or antidotal therapy following phosphorus ingestion is efficacious. In the past, several different lavage fluids were recommended in the past, ranging from the mostly benign (sodium bicarbonate) to the potentially dangerous (potassium permanganate). Milk might also be potentially harmful because of its lipophilic components. Some authors postulate better outcome with earlier GI decontamination, but there are no reliable studies available.[18] Activated charcoal may bind to white phosphorus and could be considered, although there are no data to support its use either. However, despite the lack of data of efficacy, given the poor outcome with large ingestions of phosphorus, decontamination efforts should be strongly considered. If lavage is considered, a nasogastric tube would not be expected to remove much because of the insoluble, solid nature of phosphorus. The tissue injury caused by phosphorus is not expected to cause early esophageal perforation and the use of an orogastric (OG) tube is therefore best. Caution to protect caregivers should be exercised with any lavaged material. After a fire and explosion, one author recommends keeping the free end of the OG tube under water while inserting and instilling small amounts of water (not air) to check for proper placement.[21]

N-acetylcysteine (NAC) is suggested as a potential adjunct in the treatment of phosphorus toxicity. Although NAC was used in a limited human series, the numbers were not great enough to demonstrate any benefit.[12] The use of superoxide dismutase (SOD) in an animal model suggested benefit but did not limit morbidity, suggesting that limiting oxidant injury may play a role in treatment.[11] There is no theoretical harm in using NAC for phosphorus toxicity and so it might reasonably be added to the treatment regimen. Methionine was used many years ago in the treatment of a few patients, but the number of treated patients was too few to draw any conclusions.[8]

SUMMARY

White phosphorus has been used in recent times in warfare, causing morbidity through dermal burns. These burns require large amounts of water irrigation and adequate débridement while protecting the health-care workers. Following ingestion, typically following suicide attempts, morbidity remains quite high and treatment options are limited to unproven decontamination therapies. Signs and symptoms of white phosphorus toxicity include vomiting, abdominal pain, confusion, dysrhythmias, hepatic injury, and renal failure. As early mortality is believed to be due to electrolyte abnormities and cardiac dysrhythmias, vigilant critical care is the mainstay of therapy. *N*-acetylcysteine may be used, but it has not been shown to alter human outcomes.

ACKNOWLEDGMENT

Heikki E. Nikkanen and Michele Burns Ewald contributed to this chapter in a previous edition.

REFERENCES

1. Ben-Hur N, Giladi A, Neuman Z, et al. Phosphorus burns—a pathophysiological study. *Br J Plastic Surg.* 1972;25:238-244.
2. Bowen TE, Whelan TJ, Nelson TG. Sudden death after phosphorus burns: experimental observations of hypocalcemia, hyperphosphatemia and electrocardiographic abnormalities following production of a standard white phosphorus burn. *Ann Surg.* 1971;174:779-784.
3. Brewer E, Haggerty RJ. Toxic hazards rat poisons II—phosphorus. *New Engl J Med.* 1958;258:147-148.
4. Brown CA, Halpert B. Poisoning with yellow phosphorus. *South Med J.* 1957;50:740-742.
5. Cameron JM, Patrick RS. Acute phosphorus poisoning—the distribution of toxic doses of yellow phosphorus in the tissues of experimental animals. *Med Sci Law.* 1966;6:209-214.
6. Chretien TE. Acute phosphorus poisoning report of a case with recovery. *N Engl J Med.* 1945;232:247-249.
7. Curreri PW, Asch MJ, Pruitt BA. The treatment of chemical burns: specialized diagnostic, therapeutic and prognostic considerations. *J Trauma.* 1970;10:634-642.
8. Diaz-Rivera RS, Collazo PJ, Pons ER, Torregrosa MV. Acute phosphorus poisoning in man: a study of 56 cases. *Medicine.* 1950;29:269-298.
9. Diaz-Rivera RS, Ramos-Morales F, Garcia-Palmieri MR, Ramirez EA. The electrocardiographic changes in acute phosphorus poisoning in man. *Am J Med Sci.* 1961;241:758-765.
10. Eldad A, Simon GA. The phosphorus burn—a preliminary comparative experimental study of various forms of treatment. *Burns.* 1991;17:198-200.
11. Eldad A, Wisoki M, Cohen H, et al. Phosphorus burns: evaluation of various modalities for primary treatment. *J Burn Care Rehabil.* 1995;16:49-55.
12. Fernandez OUB, Canizares LL. Acute hepatotoxicity from ingestion of yellow phosphorus-containing fireworks. *J Clin Gastroenterol.* 1995;21:139-142.
13. Ganote CE, Otis JB. Characteristic lesions of yellow phosphorus-induced liver damage. *Lab Invest.* 1969;21:207-213.
14. Ghoshal AK, Porta EA, Hartroft WS. Isotopic studies on the absorption and tissue distribution of white phosphorus in rats. *Exp Mol Path.* 1971;14:212-219.
15. Jacobziner H, Raybin HW. Activities of the Poison Control Center … phosphorus poisoning including two fatal case reports. *Arch Pediatrics.* 1961;78:396-402.
16. Jacobziner H, Raybin HW. Accidental chemical poisonings. Phosphorus and acute dextropropoxyphen intoxications. 1963;63:2126-2128. *N Y State J Med.* 1960;Sept:2742-2746.
17. Konjoyan TR. White phosphorus burns: case report and literature review. *Mil Med.* 1983;148:881-884.
18. Martin GA, Montoya CA, Sierra JL, Senior JR. Evaluation of corticosteroid and exchange transfusion treatment of acute yellow-phosphorus intoxication. *N Engl J Med.* 1971;284:125-128.
19. McCarron MM, Gaddis GP, Trotter AT. Acute yellow phosphorus poisoning from pesticide pastes. *Clin Toxicol.* 1981;18:693-711.

20. Mozingo DW, Smith AA, McManus WF, et al. Chemical burns. *J Trauma.* 1988;28:642-647.
21. Pande TK, Pandey S. White phosphorus poisoning—explosive encounter. *JAPI.* 2004;52:249-250.
22. Simon FA, Pickering LK. Acute yellow phosphorus poisoning: "smoking stool syndrome." *JAMA.* 1976;235:1343-1344.
23. Summerlin WT, Walder AI, Moncrief JA. White phosphorus burns and massive hemolysis. *J Trauma.* 1967;7:476-484.
24. Talley RC, Linhart JW, Trevino AJ, et al. Acute elemental phosphorus poisoning in man: cardiovascular toxicity. *Am Heart J.* 1972;84:139-140.
25. Walker J, Wexler J, Hill ML. Quantitative analysis of phosphorus-containing compounds formed in WP burns. Edgewood Arsenal Special Publication 100-49, Department of the Army. Maryland: Edgewood Arsenal Research Laboratories; 1969.
26. Weast RC, Astle MJ, Beyer WH, eds. *CRC Handbook of Chemistry and Physics*, 69th ed. Boca Raton, FL: CRC Press; 1988:B-27.
27. Willers-Russo LJ. Three fatalities involving phosphine gas, produced as a result of methamphetamine manufacturing. *J Forensic Sci.* 1999;44: 647-652.
28. Winek CL, Collom WD, Fusia EP. Yellow phosphorus ingestion—three fatal poisonings. *Clin Toxicol.* 1973;6:541-545.
29. Zong-yue S, Yao-ping L, Xue-qi G. Treatment of yellow phosphorus skin burns with silver nitrate instead of copper sulfate. *Scand J Work Environ Health.* 1985;11(Suppl 4):33.

CHAPTER 112
STRYCHNINE

Yiu-cheung Chan

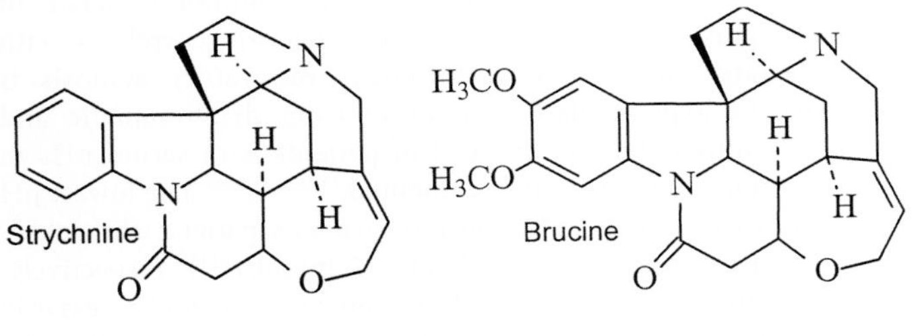

Strychnine Brucine

Strychnine alkaloid can be found naturally in *Strychnos nux-vomica*, a tree native to tropical Asia and North Australia, and in *Strychnos ignatii* and *Strychnos tiente*, trees native to South Asia. The alkaloid was first isolated in 1818 by Pelletier and Caventou.[5,17] It is an odorless and colorless crystalline powder that has a bitter taste when dissolved in water. Besides strychnine, the dried seeds of *S. nux-vomica* contain brucine, a structurally similar, although less potent, alkaloid.[89] In addition to the naturally occurring alkaloidal form, strychnine is available from commercial sources in its salt form, usually as nitrate, sulfate, or phosphate. In the past, strychnine poisoning was responsible for significant mortality, especially in children. Meticulous, supportive care remains the most important component of the management of the strychnine-poisoned patient.

HISTORY

Strychnine was first introduced as a rodenticide in 1540, and in subsequent centuries was used medically as a cardiac, respiratory, and digestive stimulant,[49] as an analeptic,[93] and as an antidote to barbiturate[92] and opioid overdoses.[60] Nonketotic hyperglycemia,[9,39,81] sleep apnea,[77] and snake bites[17] were also once considered indications for strychnine use. In 1982, at least 172 commercial products were found to contain strychnine, including 77 rodenticides, 25 veterinary products, and 41 products made for human use.[84] Currently, strychnine is used mainly as a pesticide and rodenticide (for moles, gophers, and pigeons),[84] and a research tool for the study of glycine receptors. Most commercially available strychnine-containing products contain about 0.25% to 0.5% strychnine by weight.[84]

EPIDEMIOLOGY

Between 1926 and 1928, strychnine killed more than three Americans every week.[5,30] In 1932, it was the most common cause of lethal poisoning in children,[5,84,99] and one-third of the unintentional poison-related deaths in children younger than 5 years were attributed to strychnine.[61] Currently, strychnine poisoning is rare and continues to decrease in the United States, although deaths are still reported. The Toxic Exposure Surveillance System (TESS) and National Poison Data System (NPDS) data of the American Association of Poison Control Centers (AAPCC) reports 1309 strychnine exposures during the past 10 years with only nine deaths (Chap. 135).

Strychnine poisoning has resulted from deliberate exposure with suicidal and homicidal intent,[12,30] from unintentional poisoning by a Chinese herbal medicine (Maqianzi),[18] a Cambodian traditional remedy (slang nut),[52,54,87] and adulteration of street drugs.[14] Maqianzi is used to treat limb paralysis, severe rheumatism, and inflammatory disease, whereas slang nut is used to treat gastrointestinal illness. The bitter taste and lethality of strychnine allow it to be substituted for heroin[46] and cocaine.[14,25,65] There are also reports of strychnine poisoning from adulterated amphetamines,[25] ecstasy (3,4-methylenedioxymethamphetamine [MDMA]),[28] Spanish fly,[13] and from the ingestion of gopher bait.[55]

TOXICOKINETICS

Standard references list the lethal dose of strychnine as approximately 50 to 100 mg[20,36,37,71,95] (1–2 mg/kg). However, mortality resulting from doses as low as 5 to 10 mg and, alternatively, survival following ingestions of 1 to 15 g of strychnine are reported.[6,20,98,83] Some of this variation may be attributed to the route of administration, with parenteral administration being more toxic than oral, and the limitations of self-reports of exposure quantities.

Strychnine is rapidly absorbed from the gastrointestinal tract and mucous membranes. There is also one case report of poisoning as a result of dermal absorption of strychnine from an alkaline solution, in which strychnine exists in the nonionized, alkaloid form.[38] Protein binding is minimal and strychnine is rapidly distributed to peripheral tissues[94] with a large volume of distribution (13 L/kg).[43] Based on postmortem findings, the highest concentrations of strychnine are found in the liver,[58,71,79] bile,[71] blood,[71] and gastric contents.[71,79] Relatively less strychnine is identified in kidney, urine, and brain.[79]

Strychnine is metabolized by hepatic P450 microsomes[1,62] producing strychnine-*N*-oxide as the major metabolite,[1] and this metabolism is increased by P450 induction.[47,51] Several urinary metabolites are identified,[66] and 1% to 30% of strychnine is excreted unchanged in urine,[10,42,70] in decreasing proportions when larger amounts are ingested.[82,94] In human case reports, strychnine follows first-order kinetics with an elimination half-life of 10 to 16 hours.[29,70,96]

PATHOPHYSIOLOGY

Glycine, one of the major inhibitory neurotransmitters in the spinal cord, opens a ligand-gated chloride channel, thus allowing the inward flow of Cl^- (see Fig. 13–12).[21] As Cl^- moves inward the cell becomes hyperpolarized or inhibited. Strychnine competitively inhibits the binding of glycine to the α-subunit of the glycinergic chloride channel.[14,22,97,99] Although strychnine affects all parts of the central nervous system in which glycine receptors are found, the most significant effect is in the spinal cord. With loss of the glycine inhibition to the motor neurons in the ventral horn, there is a loss of inhibitory influence on the normally suppressed reflex arc. The result is increased impulse transmission to the muscles, producing generalized muscular contraction. Rabbits pretreated with glycine were found to have a 40% increase in the strychnine "seizure" threshold, illustrating the competitive nature of strychnine and glycine activity on the glycinergic chloride channel.[19,78] Tetanus toxin (tetanospasmin) causes an identical clinical syndrome of muscular contractions, but does so by preventing the release of presynaptic glycine and does not function as a competitive antagonist. In dogs, strychnine also has positive chronotropic and inotropic effects on the heart,[85] but this effect is unlikely to exert a major effect in human poisoning.

CLINICAL MANIFESTATIONS

Strychnine poisoning is characterized by a rapid onset of signs and symptoms beginning within 15 to 60 minutes of ingestion[35] and, although less well documented, even sooner after parenteral or nasal administration. Delayed onset of clinical effects are rarely reported.[26,37] The typical symptoms of poisoning are involuntary, generalized muscular contractions resulting in neck, back, and limb pain. The contractions are easily triggered by trivial stimuli (such as turning on a light) and each episode usually lasts for 30 seconds to 2 minutes.[84] Recurrent episodes may last as long as 12 to 24 hours. Differences in the strength of various opposing muscle groups result in the classic signs of opisthotonus, facial trismus, and risus sardonicus, with flexion of the upper limbs and extensions of lower limbs predominating. Hyperreflexia, clonus, and nystagmus[11,63] are also evident on examination. Because strychnine affects glycine inhibition mainly in the spinal cord, the patient typically remains fully alert until metabolic complications arise. The combination of convulsive motor activity involving both sides of the body in the conscious patient has often resulted in imprecise descriptions such as "conscious seizure" or "spinal seizure." Hemodynamically, both hypotension,[27,29,65] or hypertension[14,32,64] in the presence of bradycardia[16,27,29,65] or tachycardia[14,16] are reported. Hyperthermia, presumably from increased muscular activity, is typical, and temperatures as high as 109.4°F (43°C) are reported.[14] Other nonspecific signs and symptoms include dizziness, vomiting, and chest and abdominal pain.[63]

Early in the course of strychnine poisoning, mortality is mainly due to hypoventilation and hypoxia secondary to muscular contractions.[32] Later, life-threatening complications include rhabdomyolysis with subsequent myoglobinuria and acute renal failure,[16] hypoxia or hyperthermia-induced multiorgan failure, aspiration pneumonitis,[86] anoxic brain injury, and pancreatitis.[45] Rarely, local neuromuscular sequelae such as weakness, myalgia, and anterior tibial compartment syndrome are reported.[14] As might be expected, the prognosis is related to the duration and extent of the episodes of muscle contractions.[34]

DIFFERENTIAL DIAGNOSIS

The diagnosis of strychnine poisoning is mainly established on clinical grounds, based on exposure history and compatible clinical manifestations, but can be confirmed by detection of strychnine in biological specimens. Several diagnoses need to be considered, the most important of which is tetanus because it produces similar muscular hyperactivity. With tetanus, however, the onset of symptoms is more gradual and the duration much longer than in the case of strychnine poisoning. Frequently, the diagnosis of tetanus is suggested by a history of recent injury, or the finding of an obvious wound. In general, patients with tetanus have either undocumented or incomplete tetanus immunization.

Strychnine poisoning can be differentiated from generalized seizures by the presence of a normal sensorium during the period of diffuse convulsions. That is, most patients with bilateral convulsions are having generalized seizures, which by definition involve the reticular activating system, producing unconsciousness. It is conceivable, although extraordinarily rare, to have bilateral focal seizures producing apparent "generalized" convulsions; in this case, because the reticular activating system may not be involved, the patient's mental status may be preserved. The diagnostic utility of the presence of consciousness in a patient with a generalized convulsion to establish the diagnosis of strychnine poisoning or tetanus is true at least in the early phase of the clinical course. At later times this finding may be obscured by metabolically induced alterations in sensorium.[19] When there is an alteration in the level of consciousness an electroencephalogram may be helpful, if it documents an absence of focal neurological deficits. A computed tomography (CT) scan can help to exclude structural brain lesions, and a lumbar puncture is helpful to exclude meningitis or encephalitis. Hypocalcemia, hyperventilation, and myoclonus secondary to renal or hepatic failure are evaluated by appropriate routine laboratory testing.

Although a drug-induced dystonic reaction should be considered when there is a relevant drug history, dystonic reactions are usually static, whereas strychnine poisoning results in dynamic muscular activity. Serotonin syndrome, malignant hyperthermia, neuroleptic malignant syndrome, and stimulant use should be considered, if the medical history is supportive.

DIAGNOSTIC TESTING

Respiratory and metabolic acidosis both commonly occur in strychnine-poisoned patients. Metabolic acidosis correlates with serum lactate concentrations,[14] whereas respiratory acidosis is secondary to hypoventilation resulting from diaphragmatic and respiratory muscle failure. Survival of patients with serum pHs in the range of 6.5 to 6.6 is well documented.[14,32,33,35,56,96] The lowest pH and highest lactate concentration reported in a patient who subsequently had full recovery was 6.5 and 32 mmol/L,[14,96] respectively. Thus, profound acidemia in strychnine poisoning is not necessarily associated with a poor prognosis. One proposed reason is that the serum pH does not correlate with the intracellular pH in the vital organs, namely the brain and heart.[7,8,14,74] In contrast to the metabolic acidosis with elevated lactate concentration that occurs in shock, the elevated lactate concentration of strychnine poisoning results from overactivity of the muscle instead of undersupply or underutilization of oxygen and nutrients.

Besides acidosis, other laboratory abnormalities expected from prolonged muscular activity include hyperkalemia and those associated with rhabdomyolysis, and acute renal failure.[14] There is also stress-induced leukocytosis,[14,45] elevated liver enzymes concentrations[45,63,91] hypocalcemia,[14,43] hypernatremia,[35] and hypokalemia.[31,63,86] The electrocardiogram is expected to remain normal or reflect changes consistent with the above electrolyte disturbances.[43] Chest radiography may show evidence of aspiration pneumonia or acute lung injury.

Strychnine can be detected by a variety of methods such as thin-layer chromatography,[48,67,90] high-performance liquid chromatography,[2,23] ultraviolet spectrometry,[67] a simple colorimetric reaction,[67] gas chromatography–mass spectrometry,[15,16,58,70,79] gas chromatography–flame ionization detector,[95] and capillary electrophoresis.[100] With the exception of the bedside colorimetric reaction, none of these tests are routinely available in a time frame useful to assist in clinical decisions. Strychnine is also detectable in amounts as low as 0.01 ppm in tissue,[2,24,59,73] and strychnine resists postmortem putrefaction. Additionally, even when available, quantitative concentrations do not correlate with clinical toxicity. Reported blood strychnine concentrations in fatal poisoning ranged from 0.5 to 61 mg/L.[95] Conversely, the highest initial blood concentration associated with survival was 4.73 mg/L from blood drawn 1.5 hours postingestion[96]; a concentration as low as 0.06 mg/L was found in a patient who solely had muscular irritability.[29]

MANAGEMENT

In strychnine poisoning, induced vomiting is absolutely contraindicated because of the risk of aspiration and loss of airway control following rapid onset of muscle contractions. Orogastric lavage should be considered on an individual basis after evaluating potential benefits and risks.[3] When orogastric lavage is thought to be indicated, it may be important to protect and secure the airway with an endotracheal tube before attempting lavage. Activated charcoal (AC) binds strychnine effectively at a ratio of approximately 1:1; 1 g of AC will bind 950 mg of strychnine.[4,89] In animal models, pretreatment[68] and posttreatment[72] with AC increase the median lethal dose in 50% of test subjects (LD_{50}) for strychnine. Clinical evidence of the effectiveness of AC for strychnine ingestion was first demonstrated in 1831, when Professor Touery survived the ingestion of a lethal dose of strychnine and AC in front of the French Academy of Medicine.

Currently, there is no evidence to recommend the use of multiple-dose AC or whole-bowel irrigation for strychnine poisoning. Although forced diuresis was once suggested as an effective means of enhancing the elimination of strychnine,[89] subsequent data failed to demonstrate an increase in clearance[82] and it is therefore no longer recommended. Peritoneal dialysis, hemodialysis, and hemoperfusion have not been extensively studied. Because strychnine is rapidly distributed to the tissues[94] with a large volume of distribution (13 L/kg), extracorporeal drug elimination procedures are unlikely to be useful and therefore not justified given their risks.

Supportive treatment remains the most important aspect of management in the majority of cases. The focus of care is to stop the muscular hyperactivity as soon as possible to prevent the metabolic and respiratory complications. At all times, unnecessary stimuli and manipulation of the patient should be avoided, as these activities trigger muscle contractions. Benzodiazepines remain the first-line treatment for strychnine-induced muscular hyperactivity.[84,96] Although much of the evidence concerning the efficacy of benzodiazepines is based on diazepam,[41,50,53,65] any of the other commonly used benzodiazepines (midazolam or lorazepam) would likely have similar effects. The initial dose of the benzodiazepine chosen should be the standard dose used for other indications, although doses of more than 1 mg/kg diazepam or its equivalent may be needed.[44,57] In case of failed intravenous access, lorazepam or midazolam can be given intramuscularly. Dosing should be repeated until the patient demonstrates muscle relaxation and the contractions cease. In addition to benzodiazepines, barbiturates and propofol are also effective, although considered secondary therapies, in stopping the strychnine-induced hyperactivity[40,54,75,88] Benzodiazepines and barbiturates both work through agonism of γ-aminobutyric acid (GABA) receptor chloride complexes to increase the inhibitory neurotransmission to the spinal cord from the brain, and thus raise the reflex arc threshold.[80] If these measures fail to control the muscular hyperactivity, a nondepolarizing neuromuscular blocker (NMB) should be administered. Only nondepolarizing NMBs should be used, as succinylcholine itself, a depolarizing NMB, induces muscle contractions.[14,29,54,65,82] It is important to remember that strychnine has no direct effects on consciousness, so that sedation must always accompany neuromuscular blockade. Generally, therapy is continued for about 24 hours, at which time the medications are slowly withdrawn, as tolerated.

The most important therapy for the metabolic complications of strychnine poisoning is to stop the further production of metabolic byproducts by terminating the muscular hyperactivity as soon as possible. Hyperthermia should be treated aggressively by active cooling with ice water immersion, cooling blanket, or mist and fan, depending on the magnitude of temperature elevation. Means to prevent rhabdomyolysis-induced acute renal failure include adequate fluid administration to ensure good urine output (greater than 1 mL/kg/h), the potential use of urinary alkalinization with sodium bicarbonate,[76] and temporary renal replacement therapy, if acute renal failure occurs. Metabolic acidosis rapidly resolves when muscular activity is controlled.[14,69]

Effective management in the first few hours of strychnine poisoning is crucial for survival. If the patient can be supported adequately for the first 6 hours, this may be considered a good prognostic sign.[14,37] All significantly poisoned patients should be managed in an intensive care unit with the help of a regional poison center or medical toxicologist. For patients unintentionally exposed to strychnine who remain asymptomatic, an observation period of 12 hours is sufficient to exclude significant risk.

SUMMARY

Strychnine is a lethal poison no longer frequently encountered, except in areas where it is used to exterminate small animals. A "conscious seizure" is the characteristic presentation of strychnine toxicity, and is rapidly followed by life-threatening metabolic and respiratory consequences. The mainstay of treatment is supportive care with the goal of rapidly terminating muscular contractions, providing adequate airway management, and rapidly treating hyperthermia and/or metabolic abnormalities. Although benzodiazepines are generally sufficient, neuromuscular paralysis with a nondepolarizing NMB may be required. Generally, the prognosis of strychnine poisoning is good, if the patient can be adequately supported and survives the first few hours of toxicity.

REFERENCES

1. Adamson RH, Fouts JR. Enzymatic metabolism of strychnine. *J Pharmacol Exp Ther*. 1959;127:87-91.
2. Alliot A, Bryant G, Guth PS. Measurement of strychnine by high performance liquid chromatography. *J Chromatogr*. 1982;232:440-442.
3. American Academy of Clinical Toxicology; European Association of Poisons Centres and Clinical Toxicologists. Position statement: gastric lavage. *J Toxicol Clin Toxicol*. 2004;42:933-943.
4. Anderson AH. Experimental studies on the pharmacology of activated charcoal. *Acta Pharmacol*. 1946;2:69-78.
5. Anonymous. The treatment of strychnine poisoning. *JAMA*. 1932;98: 1992-1994.
6. Arena JM. Report from the Duke University Poison Control Center. *N C Med J*. 1962:10:480-481.
7. Arieff AI, Kerian A, Massry SG, DeLima J. Intracellular pH of brain: alterations in acute respiratory acidosis and alkalosis. *Am J Physiol*. 1976:230:804-812.
8. Arieff AI, Park R, Leach WJ, Lazarowitz VC. Pathophysiology of experimental lactic acidosis in dogs. *Am J Physiol Renal Physiol*. 1980;239:135-142.
9. Arneson D, Chien L, Chance P, Wilriy R. Strychnine therapy in nonketotic hyperglycemia. *Pediatrics*. 1979;3:369-373.
10. Baselt, RC. *Disposition of Toxic Drugs and Chemicals in Man*, 5th ed. Foster City, CA: Chemical Toxicology Institute; 2000.
11. Blain PG, Nightingale S, Stoddart JC. Strychnine poisoning: abnormal eye movements. *J Toxicol Clin Toxicol*. 1982;19:215-217.
12. Bogan J, Rentoul E, Smith H, Weir WP. Homicidal poisoning by strychnine. *J Forensic Sci Soc*. 1966;6:166-169.
13. Boston Globe. Warning is issued on Spanish fly. Anita Manning. August 26, 1991.
14. Boyd RE, Brennan PT, Deng JF, Rochester DF, Spyker DA. Strychnine poisoning. Recovery from profound lactic acidosis, hyperthermia, and rhabdomyolysis. *Am J Med*. 1983;74:507-512.
15. Braselton WE, Johnson M. Thin-layer chromatography convulsant screen extended by gas chromatography–mass spectrometry. *J Vet Diagn Invest*. 2003;15:42-45.
16. Burn DJ, Tomson CR, Seviour J, Dale G. Strychnine poisoning as an unusual cause of convulsions. *Postgrad Med J*. 1989;65:563-564.
17. Campbell CH. Dr Mueller's strychnine cure of snakebite. *Med J Aust*. 1968;2:1-8.
18. Chan TY. Herbal medicine causing likely strychnine poisoning. *Hum Exp Toxicol*. 2002;21:467-468.
19. Ch'ien LT, Chance P, Arneson D. Glycine encephalopathy. *N Engl J Med*. 1978;298:687.
20. Cotton MS, Lane DH. Massive strychnine poisoning: a successful treatment. *J Miss State Med Assoc*. 1966;7:466-468.
21. Curtis DR, Hosli L, Johnston GAR. A pharmacological study of the depression of spinal neurons by glycine and related amino acids. *Exp Brain Res*. 1968;6:1-18.
22. Curtis DR, Duggan AW, Johnston GA. The specificity of strychnine as a glycine antagonist in the mammalian spinal cord. Exp Brain Res. 1971;12:547-565.
23. De Saqui-Sannes P, Nups P, Le Bars P, Burgat V. Evaluation of an HPTLC method for the determination of strychnine and crimidine in biological samples. *J Anal Toxicol*. 1986;20:185-188.

24. Decker W, Treuting J. Spot tests for rapid diagnosis of poisoning. *Clin Toxicol.* 1971;4:89-97.
25. Decker WJ, Baker HE, Tamulinas SH, Korndorffer WE. Two deaths resulting from apparent parenteral injection of strychnine. *Vet Hum Toxicol.* 1982;24:161-162.
26. Dickson E, Hawkins RC, Reynolds R. Strychnine poisoning: an uncommon cause of convulsions. *Aust NZJ Med.* 1992;22:500-501.
27. Dittrich K, Bayer MJ, Wanke LA. A case of fatal strychnine poisoning. *J Emerg Med.* 1984;1:327-330.
28. Drugscope. Contaminated ecstasy. May 1, 2001. www.drugscope.org.uk/news_item.asp?a=1&intID=234 (accessed November 10, 2004).
29. Edmunds M, Sheehan TM, Van't Hoff W. Strychnine poisoning: clinical and toxicological observations on a non-fatal case. *J Toxicol Clin Toxicol.* 1986;24:245-255.
30. Ferguson MB, Vance MA. Payment deferred: strychnine poisoning in Nicaragua 65 years ago. *J Toxicol Clin Toxicol.* 2000;38:71-77.
31. Fernandez X, Fernandez MC, Schumaker A. Hypokalemia related to strychnine ingestion. *J Toxicol Clin Toxicol.* 2000;38:524.
32. Flood RG. Strychnine poisoning. *Pediatr Emerg Care.* 1999;15:286-287.
33. Goldstein MR. Recovery from severe metabolic acidosis. *JAMA.* 1975;234:1119.
34. Goodman LS, Gilman A. *The Pharmacological Basis of Therapeutics*, 3rd ed. New York: Macmillan; 1965:345-348.
35. Gordon AM, Richards DW. Strychnine intoxication. *JACEP.* 1979;8: 520-522.
36. Gosselin RE, Hodge HC, Smith RP, Gleason MN. *Clinical Toxicology of Commercial Products*, 4th ed. Baltimore, MD: Williams & Wilkins Co; 1974:2.
37. Gosselin RE, Hodge HC, Smith RP, Gleason MN. *Clinical Toxicology of Commercial Products*, 5th ed. Baltimore, MD: Williams & Wilkins Co; 1984:375-379.
38. Greene R, Meatherall R. Dermal exposure to strychnine. *J Anal Toxicol.* 2001;25:344-347.
39. Haan EA, Kirby DM, Tada K. Difficulties in assessing the effect of strychnine on the outcome of non-ketotic hyperglycinemia. *Eur J Pediatr.* 1986;145:267-270.
40. Haggard H, Greenberg L. Antidotes for strychnine poisoning. *JAMA.* 1983;98:1133-1136.
41. Hardin JA, Griggs RC. Diazepam treatment in a case of strychnine poisoning. *Lancet.* 1971;2:372-373.
42. Hatcher RA, Smith MI. The Elimination of Strychnine by the Kidneys. *J Pharm Exptl Therap* 1916-1917;9:27-41.
43. Heiser JM, Daya MR, Magnussen AR, et al. Massive strychnine intoxication: serial blood levels in a fatal case. *J Toxicol Clin Toxicol.* 1992;30:269-283.
44. Herishanu Y Landau H. Diazepam in the treatment of strychnine poisoning. *Br J Anaesth.* 1972;44:747-748.
45. Hernandez AF, Pomares J, Schiaffino S, Pla A, Villanueva E. Acute chemical pancreatitis associated with nonfatal strychnine poisoning. *J Toxicol Clin Toxicol.* 1998;36:67-71.
46. Hoffman RS. The toxic emergency—strychnine. *Emerg Med.* 1994;Feb: 111-113.
47. Howes JF, Hunter WH. The stimulation of strychnine metabolism in rats by some anticonvulsant compounds. *J Pharm Pharmacol.* 1966;18: 52S-57S.
48. Hunter RT, Creekmur RE Jr. Liquid chromatographic determination of strychnine as poison in domestic animals. *J Assoc Off Anal Chem.* 1984;67:542-545.
49. Jackson G, Diggle G. Strychnine-containing tonics. *Br Med J.* 1973;2: 176-177.
50. Jackson G, Ng SH, Diggle GE, Bourke IG. Strychnine poisoning treated successfully with diazepam. *Br Med J.* 1971;3:519-520.
51. Kato R, Chiesara E, Vassanelli P. Increased activity of microsomal strychnine-metabolizing enzyme induced by phenobarbital and other drugs. *Biochem Pharmacol.* 1962;11:913-922.
52. Katz J, Prescott K, Woolf AD. Strychnine poisoning from a Cambodian traditional remedy. *Am J Emerg Med.* 1996;14:475-477.
53. Kempf GF, McCallum JTC, Zerfas LG. A successful treatment for strychnine poisoning: report of eleven cases. *JAMA.* 1933;100:548-551.
54. Libenson MH, Yang JM. Case 12-2001: a 16-year-old boy with altered mental status and muscle rigidity. *N Engl J Med.* 2001;344:1232-1239.
55. Lindsey T, O'Hara J, Irvine R, Kerrigan S. Strychnine overdose following ingestion of gopher bait. *J Anal Toxicol.* 2004;28:135.
56. Loughhead M, Braithwaite J, Denton M. Life at pH 6.6. *Lancet.* 1978;2:952.
57. Maron BJ, Krupp JR, Tune B. Strychnine poisoning successfully treated with diazepam. *J Pediatr.* 1971;78:697-699.
58. Marques EP, Gil F, Proenca P, et al. Analytical method for the determination of strychnine in tissues by gas chromatography/mass spectrometry: two case reports. *Forensic Sci Int.* 2000;110:145-152.
59. McConnell E, Van Rensburg I, Minne J. A rapid test for the diagnosis of strychnine poisoning. *JS Afr Vet Med Assn.* 1971;42:81-84.
60. McGarry RC, McGarry P. Please pass the strychnine: the art of Victorian pharmacy. *CMAJ.* 1999;161:1556-1558.
61. Metropolitan Life Insurance Company. *Statistical Bull.* 1930;11:11.
62. Mishima M, Tanimoto Y, Oguri Z, Yoshimura H. Metabolism of strychnine in vitro. *Drug Metab Dispos.* 1985;13:716-721.
63. Nishiyama T, Nagase M. Strychnine poisoning: natural course of a nonfatal case. *Am J Emerg Med.* 1995;13:172-173.
64. Oberpaur B, Donoso A, Claveria C, Valverde C, Azocar M. Strychnine poisoning: an uncommon intoxication in children. *Pediatr Emerg Care.* 1999;1:264-265.
65. O'Callaghan WG, Joyce N, Counihan HE, et al. Unusual strychnine poisoning and its treatment: report of eight cases. *Br Med J (Clin Res Ed).* 1982;285:478.
66. Oguri K, Tarimoto Y, Mishima M, Yoshimura H. Metabolic fate of strychnine in rats. *Xenobiotica.* 1989;19:171-178.
67. Oliver JS, Smith H, Watson AA. Poisoning by strychnine. *Med Sci Law.* 1979;19:134-137.
68. Olkkola KT. Does ethanol modify antidotal efficacy of oral activated charcoal: studies in vitro and in experimental animals. *J Toxicol Clin Toxicol.* 1984;22:425-432.
69. Orringer C, Eustace J, Wunsch, Gardner L. Natural history of lactic acidosis after grand mal seizures. *N Engl J Med.* 1977;297:697-699.
70. Palatnick W, Meatherall R, Sitar D, Tenenbein M. Toxicokinetics of acute strychnine poisoning. *J Toxicol Clin Toxicol.* 1997;35:617-620.
71. Perper JA. Fatal strychnine poisoning—a case report and review of the literature. *J Forensic Sci.* 1985;30:1248-1255.
72. Picchioni AL, Chin L, Verhulst HL. Activated charcoal vs "Universal Antidote" as an antidote for poisons. *Toxicol Appl Pharmacol.* 1966;8:447-454.
73. Platonow N, Funnell H, Oliver W. Determination of strychnine in biological materials by gas chromatography. *J Forensic Sci.* 1970;15: 433-446.
74. Posner JB, Plum F. Spinal fluid pH and neurologic symptoms in systemic acidosis. *N Engl J Med.* 1967;277:605-613.
75. Priest RE, Minn W. Strychnine poisoning successfully treated with sodium amytal. *JAMA.* 1938;110:1440.
76. Ralph D. Rhabdomyolysis and acute renal failure. *JACEP.* 1978;7:103-106.
77. Remmers JE, Anch AM, deGroot WJ. Oropharyngeal muscle tone in obstructive sleep apnea before and after strychnine. *Sleep.* 1980;3:447-453.
78. Roches JC, Zumstein HR, Fassler A, Scollo-Lavizzari G, Hosli L. Effects of taurine, glycine and GABA on convulsions produced by strychnine in the rabbit. *Eur Neurol.* 1979;18:26-32.
79. Rosano TG, Hubbard JD, Meola JM, Swift TA. Fatal strychnine poisoning: application of gas chromatography and tandem mass spectrometry. *J Anal Toxicol.* 2000;24:642-647.
80. Sangiah S. Effects of glycine and other inhibitory amino acid neurotransmitters on strychnine convulsive threshold in mice. *Vet Hum Toxicol.* 1985;27:97-99.
81. Sankaran K, Casey RE, Zaleski WA, Mendelson IM. Glycine encephalopathy in a neonate: treatment with intravenous strychnine and sodium benzoate. *Clin Pediatr.* 1982;21:636-637.
82. Sgaragli GP, Mannaioni PF. Pharmacokinetic observations on a case of massive strychnine poisoning. *Clin Toxicol.* 1973;6:533-540.
83. Shadnia S, Moiensadat M, Abdollahi M. A case of acute strychnine poisoning. *Vet Hum Toxicol.* 2004;46:76-79.
84. Smith BA. Strychnine poisoning. *J Emerg Med.* 1990;8:321-325.
85. Sofola OA, Odusote KA. Sympathetic cardiovascular effects of experimental strychnine poisoning in dogs. *J Pharmacol Exp Ther.* 1976;1:29-34.
86. Starretz-Hacham O, Sofer S, Lifshitz M. Strychnine intoxication in a child. *Isr Med Assoc J.* 2003;5:531-532.
87. Stewart MJ, Steenkamp V, Zuckerman M. The toxicology of African herbal remedies. *Ther Drug Monit.* 1988;20:510-516.
88. Swanson E. The antidotal effect of sodium amytal in strychnine poisoning. *J Lab Clin Med.* 1933;18:933-934.

89. Teitelbaum DT, Ott JE. Acute strychnine intoxication. *Clin Toxicol.* 1970;3:267-273.
90. Van den Heede M, Wauters A, Cordonnier J, Heyndrickx A, Timperman J. The toxicological investigation of two unexpected deaths due to poisoning by strychnine. In: Brandeberger H, R Brandnberger, eds. *Proceedings of the International Meeting of TIAFT.* Switzerland: Rigi-Kaltbaad; 1985:273-291.
91. Van Heerden PV, Edibam C, Augustson B, Thompson WR, Power BM. Strychnine poisoning—alive and well in Australia! *Anaesth Intensive Care.* 1993;21:876-877.
92. Volynskaia EL. Use of large doses of strychnine and bemegride in barbiturate coma. *Klin Med (Mosk).* 1970;48:139-140.
93. Wax PM. Analeptic use in clinical toxicology: a historical appraisal. *J Toxicol Clin Toxicol.* 1997;35:203-209.
94. Weiss S, Hatcher RA. Studies on strychnine. *J Pharmacol Exp Ther.* 1922;14:419-482.
95. Winek CL, Wahba WW, Esposito FM, Collom WD. Fatal strychnine ingestion. *J Anal Toxicol.* 1986;10:120-121.
96. Wood D, Webster E, Martinez D, Dargan P, Jones A. Case report: survival after deliberate strychnine self-poisoning, with toxicokinetic data. *Crit Care.* 2002;6:456-459.
97. Woodbury DM. Convulsant drugs: mechanism of action. *Adv Neurol.* 1980;27:249-303.
98. Yamarick W, Walson P, DiTraglia J. Strychnine poisoning in an adolescent. *J Toxicol Clin Toxicol.* 1992;30:141-148.
99. Young AB, Snyder SH. The glycine synaptic receptor: evidence that strychnine binding is associated with the ionic conductance mechanism. *Proc Natl Acad Sci USA.* 1974;71:4002-4005.
100. Zhang J, Wang S, Chen X, Hu Z, Ma X. Capillary electrophoresis with field-enhanced stacking for rapid and sensitive determination of strychnine and brucine. *Anal Bioanal Chem.* 2003;376:210-213.

CHAPTER 113
INSECTICIDES: ORGANIC PHOSPHORUS COMPOUNDS AND CARBAMATES

Michael Eddleston and Richard Franklin Clark

Globally, anticholinesterase insecticides likely kill more people each year than acute poisoning by any other xenobiotic. An estimated 200,000 die in rural Asia where intentional self-harm is common and extremely toxic organic phosphorus insecticides are widely used in agriculture.[53,84] An estimated 3000 to 6000 ventilators are constantly required in Asia alone to provide mechanical ventilation to poisoned patients.[84] Banning of the most toxic organic phosphorus insecticides has resulted in a 50% decrease in total suicides in Sri Lanka, showing that governmental regulation can be effective.[85] Severe occupational or unintentional poisoning also happens where such insecticides are used[199] but deaths are generally less common. Anticholinesterase poisoning is less important in industrialized countries where access to toxic insecticides is controlled. However, when anticholinesterase poisoning does occur, patients often require intensive care with long hospital stays.[65,155] A further threat is the terrorist use of organic phosphorus insecticides such as parathion to poison a water supply or flour used in bread baking. Such an event may result in many hundreds of casualties being treated by clinicians with limited experience of this potentially lethal toxic syndrome.

HISTORY AND EPIDEMIOLOGY

The first potent synthetic organic phosphorus anticholinesterase, tetraethylpyrophosphate (TEPP), was synthesized by Clermont in 1854. Clermont's report described the taste of the compound, a remarkable achievement because a few drops should be rapidly fatal.[94] In 1932, Lange and Krueger wrote of choking and blurred vision following inhalation of dimethyl and diethyl phosphorofluoridates. This account inspired Schrader in Germany to begin investigating these xenobiotics, initially as insecticides, and later for use in warfare (Chap. 131). During this research, Schrader's group synthesized hundreds of compounds, including the popular insecticide parathion and the chemical warfare agents, sarin, soman, and tabun. Allied scientists were also motivated during the same period by the work, and independently discovered other extremely toxic compounds such as diisopropylphosphofluoridate (DFP).[187] Since that time, it is estimated that more than 50,000 organic phosphorus compounds have been synthesized and screened for insecticidal activity, with dozens being produced commercially.[34]

The history of carbamates was first recorded by Westerners in the 19th century when they observed that the Calabar bean (*Physostigma venenosum* Balfour) was used in tribal cultural practice in West Africa.[95] These beans were imported to Great Britain in 1840, and in 1864 Jobst and Hesse isolated an active alkaloid component they named "physostigmine." Vée and Leven (1865) claimed to have obtained physostigmine in crystallized form, and named it *eserine*, from ésére, the African term for the "ordeal bean". Physostigmine was first used medicinally to treat glaucoma in 1877.[95] In the 1930s, the synthesis of aliphatic esters of carbamic acid led to the development and introduction of carbamate insecticides, marketed initially as fungicides. In 1953 the Union Carbide Corporation developed and first marketed carbaryl, the insecticide being prepared at the plant in Bhopal, India, during the catastrophic release of methyl isocyanate in 1984 (Chap. 2).[4,167]

Organic phosphorus compounds (OPs) and carbamates are the two groups of cholinesterase-inhibiting insecticides that commonly produce human toxicity. Although the term "organophosphate" is often used in clinical practice and in the literature to refer to all phosphorus-containing insecticides that inhibit cholinesterase, phosphates are compounds in which the P atom is surrounded by four O atoms, and there are other derivatives of phosphoric and phosphonic acids such as phosphonates that can exhibit cholinesterase inhibition. Some chemicals, such as parathion, contain thioesters, whereas others are vinyl esters. Those cholinesterase-inhibitors (anticholinesterases) that contain phosphorus will be collectively termed organic phosphorus compounds in this chapter. Those that contain the OC=ON linkage will be termed carbamates.

Anticholinesterases are broadly grouped according to their toxicity by the World Health Organization's Classification of Insecticides into five groups: Class Ia "Extremely hazardous," Class Ib "Highly hazardous," Class II "Moderately hazardous," Class III "Slightly hazardous," and "Active ingredients unlikely to present acute hazard in normal use."[204] This classification is based on comparative rat oral LD_{50} (median lethal dose in 50% of test subjects) data of the active ingredient. It seems useful to distinguish very toxic OPs (such as parathion, rat oral LD_{50} 13 mg/kg) that have killed many thousands of people from relatively safe OPs (such as temephos, rat oral LD_{50} 8600 mg/kg) that have not been reported to cause harm. The rat LD_{50} seems to be less useful to distinguish between insecticides within the same class. Here, the differential toxicity may be a result of differences in response to treatment, speed of onset, or coformulants.[58]

The case fatality ratio for OP and carbamate poisoning will vary according to which insecticides are used in local agriculture and the prehospital, healthcare, and hospital facilities available. Where fast acting, highly toxic insecticides are used in agriculture and for self-harm (as in much of the rural developing world), deaths will occur before patients present to a hospital. Hospital-based data therefore have a falsely low case fatality, although it is often still quite high at 10% to 30%.[53]

Before the recent ban of parathion in Germany, case fatality in the Munich toxicology intensive care unit was approximately 40%.[65,208] This was likely because the ambulance services in Germany were able to resuscitate and transport patients, before death but after they had become symptomatic with this fast-acting OP. Some had already aspirated or suffered hypoxic brain injury prior to arrival of the ambulance. Despite resuscitation at the scene, many of these patients subsequently died from their complications. Few of these patients would have survived to hospital admission in the developing world.

During the 5-year period from 2002 to 2006, the American Association of Poison Control Centers (AAPCC) recorded almost 30,000 exposures to organic phosphorus compounds and more than 14,000 exposures to carbamates. Although these totals are large, the number of reported exposures to both classes of insecticide have each dropped annually since 2002, likely due in part to a phase-out of their residential use during this period.[175] However, the number of fatalities reported to the AAPCC remained constant during this time, averaging about five per year. These insecticides still rank as the most lethal insecticides in use in the United States, and among the most lethal poisonings (see Chap. 135).

Since the overall case fatality ratio for OP and carbamate insecticide poisoning is approximately 10% to 20%, the 200,000 deaths a year in rural Asia must represent one million to two million poisonings. Respiratory failure is a major problem with OP and carbamate poisoning. Modeling suggests that the 20% to 30% of patients who develop respiratory failure will receive 1.1-2.3 million days of ventilation every year.[84] This will require constant use of 3140 to 6280 ventilators worldwide solely for managing self-poisoning with these insecticides.[84]

Patients typically present following unintentional or suicidal ingestion, or after working in areas recently treated. Children and adults can develop toxicity while playing in or inhabiting a residence recently sprayed or fogged by an insecticide applicator.[209] Direct dermal contact with certain types of these insecticides may be rapidly poisonous.[126] Outbreaks of mass poisoning regularly occur in the developing world, and less commonly in the United States, from contamination of crops or food.[26,35,47,48,64,156,190] Epidemics of cholinergic toxicity have also been reported among groups illegally importing and using the potent carbamate aldicarb.[140,152] Organic phosphorus compounds and carbamates have also been used for committing homicide.[22,46,158,179,192]

PHARMACOLOGY

ORGANIC PHOSPHORUS COMPOUNDS

Poisoning from OPs results in a rise in the concentration of acetylcholine (ACh) at muscarinic and nicotinic cholinergic receptors, which, in turn, leads to a syndrome of cholinergic excess. Figure 113–1 shows the basic formula for cholinesterase-inhibiting OPs.[72,181] The "X" or "leaving group" determines many of the characteristics of the OP and provides a means of classifying OPs into four main groups (Table 113–1). Group 1 OPs contain a quaternary nitrogen at the X position, and are collectively termed phosphorylcholines. Originally developed as weapons of war, these powerful cholinesterase inhibitors can also directly stimulate cholinergic receptors, presumably because of their structural resemblance to ACh. Group 2 OPs are called fluorophosphates because they possess a fluorine molecule as the leaving group. Like group 1 compounds, these OPs are volatile and highly toxic, making them well suited for chemical warfare. The leaving group of group 3 OPs is a cyanide molecule or a halogen other than fluorine. The most well-known members in this group are cyanophosphates such as tabun.

The fourth group is the broadest and comprises various subgroups based on the configuration of the R_1 and R_2 groups, with the majority falling into the category of either a dimethoxy or diethoxy compound. Most of the OPs in use today fall into this last class.[72]

"Direct-acting" OPs ("oxons") inhibit acetylcholinesterase (AChE) without first being metabolized in the body. However, many OPs, such as parathion and malathion, are "indirect" inhibitors (prodrugs or "thions") requiring partial metabolism (to paraoxon and malaoxon, respectively) within the body to become active. Desulfuration to the oxon occurs in the intestinal mucosa and liver following absorption.[111,176]

The OPs bind to a hydroxyl group at the active site of the AChE enzyme. As the leaving group of the OPs is split off by AChE, a stable but reversible bond results between the remaining substituted phosphate of the OP and AChE, effectively inactivating the enzyme (Fig. 113–2, normal metabolism; Fig. 113–3, inactivation; see Fig. 11–6 for a more detailed analysis).

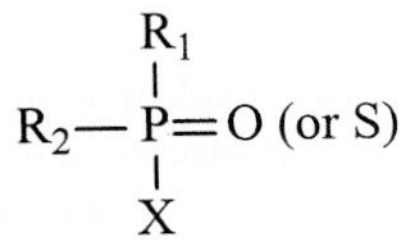

Although splitting of the choline–enzyme bond in normal ACh metabolism is completed within microseconds, the severing of the OP–enzyme bond is prolonged. The half-life of this reaction depends on the chemistry of the substituted phosphate. The in vitro half-life for spontaneous reactivation of human AChE inhibited by dimethoxy OPs is 0.7 to 0.86 hour; that of diethoxy inhibition is 31 to 57 hours.[67] Spontaneous reactivation is therefore far quicker with dimethoxy OPs.

Oximes, such as pralidoxime or obidoxime, markedly speed up the rate of reactivation.[67] However, if the phosphorus is allowed to remain bound to the AChE, because of late or inadequate administration of oximes, an alkyl group is nonenzymatically lost (see Fig. 113–2)—a process called "aging." Once aging has occurred, the AChE can no longer be reactivated by oximes. Again, the half-life of this reaction is determined by the substituted phosphorus. The in vitro half-life of aging of human AChE after poisoning with dimethoxy OPs is 3.7 hours; after diethoxy poisoning it is 31 hours.[67] Clinically, this means that patients who present to a hospital 4 hours after poisoning with a dimethoxy OP may already have as much as 50% of their AChE irreversibly inhibited; after 14 hours, the patients will be completely refractory to oxime therapy. In contrast, patients poisoned by diethoxy OPs presenting within 14 hours will have very little aged AChE and be responsive to oximes. De novo synthesis of AChE is required to replenish its supply once aging has occurred.[181]

OPs also vary by lipid solubility,[17] rate of activation (conversion from thion to oxon), rate of AChE inhibition,[67] and relative inhibition of the plasma butyrylcholinesterase. Some OPs do not fulfill the usual dimethoxy or diethoxy classification and have one of the alkyl groups linked to the phosphorus by a sulfur molecule, rather than oxygen (eg, profenofos, methamidophos). Aging seems to be particularly rapid for these OPs.[55] Spontaneous reactivation, aging, metabolism, and elimination are competing processes. The exact kinetics of these processes are poorly defined, making predictions about the course of any particular organic phosphorus compound in a particular individual quite difficult to predict (Tables 113–2 and 113–3).

CARBAMATES

Carbamate insecticides are *N*-methyl carbamates derived from carbamic acid (Fig. 113–4).[15] Medicinal carbamate compounds include physostigmine, pyridostigmine, and neostigmine.[181] Xenobiotics such as meprobamate and various urethanes are carbamate derivatives, but do not inhibit cholinesterase. Thiocarbamate fungicides and herbicides (eg, maneb, zineb, nabam, and mancozeb) also do not inhibit AChE and do not produce the cholinergic toxic syndrome (Chap. 115).

When exposed to carbamate compounds, AChE undergoes carbamylation in a manner similar to phosphorylation by OPs,[202] allowing ACh to accumulate in synapses. Aging cannot occur and the carbamate–AChE bond hydrolyzes spontaneously, reactivating the enzyme. As such, the duration of cholinergic symptoms in carbamate poisoning is generally less than 24 hours. However, severe complications from the cholinergic syndrome, in particular aspiration, can persist.

$$\begin{array}{c} R_1 \\ | \\ R_2\text{—}P\text{=O (or S)} \\ | \\ X \end{array}$$

FIGURE 113–1. General structure of organic phosphorus insecticides. X represents the leaving group. R_1 and R_2 may be aromatic or aliphatic groups that can be identical.

PHARMACOKINETICS AND TOXICOKINETICS

ORGANIC PHOSPHORUS COMPOUNDS

Organic phosphorus compounds are well absorbed from the lungs, gastrointestinal tract, mucous membranes, and conjunctiva following

TABLE 113–1. The Classification of Organic Phosphorus Compounds by Groups. Leaving Groups and Examples of Each Group Are Included

Group 1–phosphorylcholines
- Leaving group: substituted quarternary nitrogen
  - Echothiophate iodide

Group 2–fluorophosphates
- Leaving group: fluoride
  - Dimefox, sarin, mipafox

Group 3–cyanophosphates, other halophosphates
- Leaving group: CN^-, SCN^-, OCN^-, halogen other than fluoride
  - Tabun

Group 4–multiple constituents
- Leaving group:
  - Dimethoxy
    - Azinphos-menthyl, bromophos, chlorothion, crotoxyphos, dicapthon, dichlorvos, dicrotophos, dimethoate, fenthion, malathion, mevinphos, parathion-methyl, phosphamidon, temephos, trichlorfon
  - Diethoxy
    - Carbophenothion, chlorfenvinphos, chlorpyriphos, coumaphos, demeton, diazinon, dioxathion, disulfoton, ethion, methosfolan, parathion, phorate, phosfolan, TEPP
  - Other dialkoxy
    - Isopropyl paraoxon, isopropyl parathion
  - Diamino
    - Schradan
  - Chlorinated and other substituted dialkoxy
    - Haloxon
  - Trithioalkyl
    - Merphos
  - Triphenyl and substituted triphenyl
    - Triorthocresyl phosphate (TOCP)
  - Mixed substituent
    - Crufomate, cyanofenphos

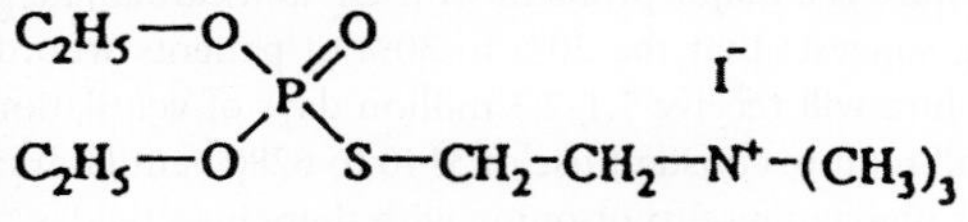

Echothiophate iodide

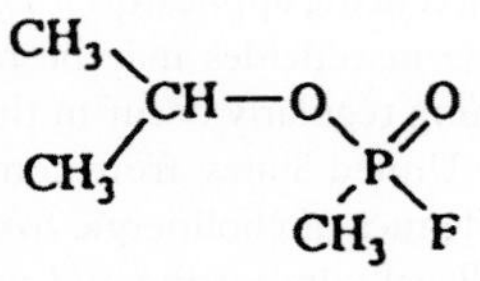

Sarin

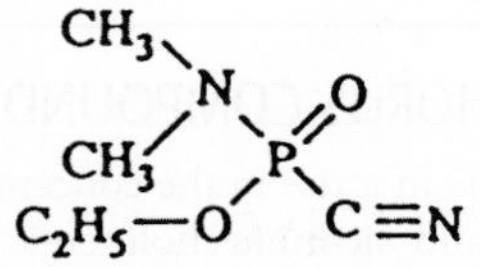

Tabun

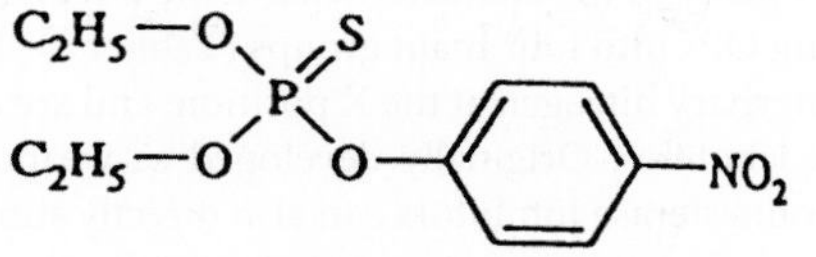

Parathion

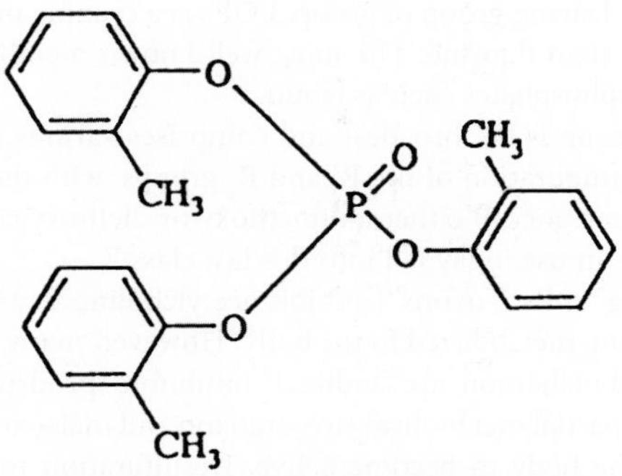

Triorthocresyl phosphate (TOCP)

inhalation, ingestion, or topical contact.[72] Although absorption through intact skin appears to be limited,[78] percutaneous exposure to highly toxic compounds can cause severe toxicity.[36,38,126,198] The presence of any dermatitis or skin damage and of higher environmental temperatures will enhance cutaneous absorption.[72]

Poisonings can be chronic or acute, although the differentiation has little clinical relevance. The difficulty in removing these compounds from the skin and clothing may explain some chronic poisonings, and inadequate skin and respiratory protection during insecticide application is responsible for most of the remainder of occupational exposures.

The time to peak serum concentration after self-poisoning is unknown. Human volunteer studies, using very low doses of chlorpyrifos, found C_{max} to be around 6 hours after oral ingestion.[141] However, patients ingesting large amounts of oxon or fast-acting thion OPs can

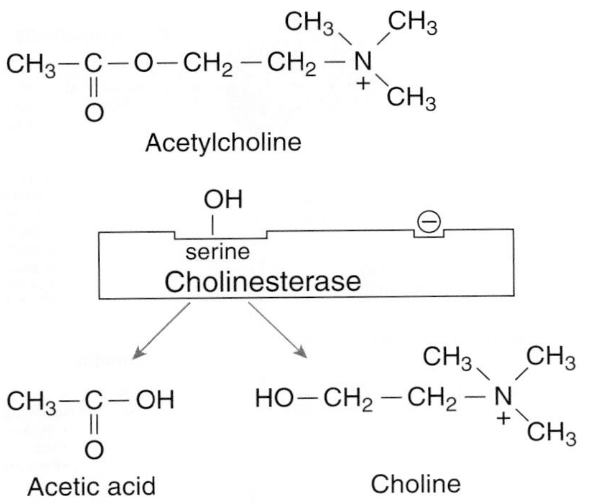

FIGURE 113–2. Normal metabolism of acetylcholine by acetylcholinesterase to choline and acetic acid.

become symptomatic within minutes,[65,118] suggesting that absorption can be rapid.

Most OPs are lipophilic[17] and are therefore predicted to have a large volume of distribution and to rapidly distribute into tissue and fat where they are protected from metabolism. Radiolabeled parathion injected into mice distributes most rapidly into the cervical brown fat and salivary glands, with high concentrations also measured in the liver, kidneys, and other adipose tissue.[70] Adipose tissue gradually accumulates the highest concentrations. Redistribution from these stores

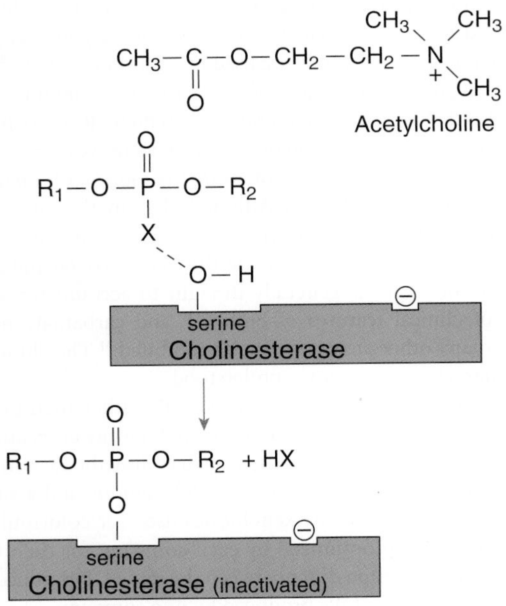

FIGURE 113–3. Mechanism of inhibition of acetylcholinesterase by an organic phosphorus compound. The X is the leaving group. A serine residue at the active site of the enzyme gives up a hydrogen atom to combine with the leaving group while the active site undergoes phosphorylation and inhibition. This initial inhibition is reversible with pralidoxime. However, as the inhibited phosphorylated enzyme "ages," one of the R groups is lost. The aged phosphorylated enzyme is unable to be rejuvenated by pralidoxime.

TABLE 113–2. Pharmacologic Properties of Dimethoxy Organic Phosphorus Insecticides

Compound	Bioactivation	Relative Lipophilicity[a]	Comments
Acephate	Liver	+	Hepatic metabolism
Azinphos-methyl	Yes (liver?)	+++	
Dimethoate	Liver	+	Hepatic metabolism
Fenthion	Liver	++++	
Malathion	Low C = 1A2/2B6 High C = 3A4	++	Inhibits BuChE > AChE Metabolism by CYP1A2
Methyl Parathion	Low C = 1A2/2B6 High C = 3A4	++	
Phosmet	Yes (liver?)	++	

For all dimethoxy compounds in this table, the half-life of spontaneous reactivation is about one hour, and the half-life of aging is about 4 hours.

[a]Derived from log P = octanol/water coefficient; C = concentration.

may allow for measurement of circulating OP concentrations for up to 48 days postingestion.[42,74,161]

Cholinergic crisis may recur in patients when unmetabolized OPs are mobilized from fat stores.[72] The more lipophilic compounds such as fenthion and dichlofenthion are particularly likely to cause this phenomenon.[42,58,129] Dimethoate, methamidophos, and oxydemeton methyl are three common OPs that are not lipophilic, with predicted small volumes of distribution and high serum OP concentrations.[43]

The distribution of OPs into fat will likely include both activated and unactivated compound. When released from the fat hours to days

TABLE 113–3. Pharmacologic Properties of Diethoxy Organic Phosphorus Insecticides

Compound	Bioactivation	Relative Lipophilicity[a]	Comments
Chlorpyrifos	Low C = 1A2/2B6 High C = 3A4	++++	Inhibits BuChE = AChE Metabolism by CYP1A2
Diazinon	Low C = 1A2/2B6 High C = 3A4	+++	Metabolism by CYP1A2
Parathion	3A4/5 and 2C8	+++	Hepatic metabolism
Phorate	Liver	+++	Inhibits BuChE > AChE Hepatic metabolism
Terbufos	Liver	++++	Hepatic metabolism

For all diethoxy compounds in this table, the half-life of spontaneous reactivation is 31-57 hours, and the half-life of aging is 31 to 94 hours.

[a]Derived from log P = octanol/water coefficient; C = concentration.

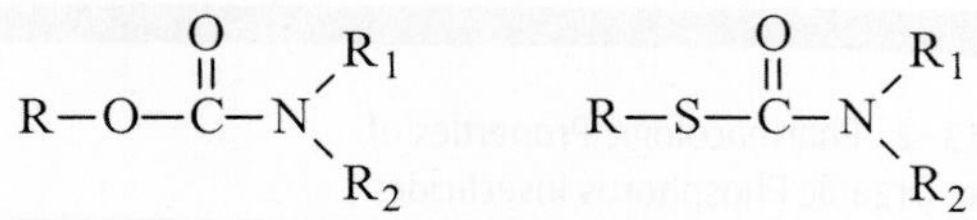

$$R{-}O{-}C({=}O){-}N(R_1)(R_2) \qquad R{-}S{-}C({=}O){-}N(R_1)(R_2)$$

FIGURE 113–4. General structure of carbamate insecticides.

later, the unactivated thion will require activation to cause clinical manifestations.

Thion OPs are activated by cytochrome P450 (CYP) enzymes in the liver and intestinal mucosa. The precise CYP enzymes responsible appear to vary according to the concentration of the OP. For example, chlorpyrifos, diazinon, parathion, and malathion are all activated by CYP1A2 and CYP2B6 at low concentrations.[27,28] However, at the higher concentrations more likely after self-poisoning, CYP3A4 becomes dominant. The particular enzymes involved in metabolism of the active oxon to inactive metabolites are less clear.

Studies have investigated possible relationships between human serum paraoxonase (PON) activity and susceptibility to acute and chronic effects of organic phosphorus poisoning.[37,168,170] PON can hydrolyze the active (oxon) metabolites of some OPs. Activity differs significantly among animal species. Some animal models of organic phosphorus poisoning demonstrate protection from toxicity when exogenous PON is administered, and greater susceptibility to poisoning when enzyme-deficient animals (such as genetically engineered knockout mice) are exposed.[168] Some authors have postulated that genetic polymorphisms in human PON activity may lead to variations in interindividual susceptibility to some OPs.[37]

CARBAMATES

Carbamates are absorbed across skin and mucous membranes, and by inhalation and ingestion. Peak blood cholinesterase inhibition occurs within 30 minutes of oral administration in rats.[143] Most carbamates undergo hydrolysis, hydroxylation, and conjugation in the liver and intestinal wall, with 90% excreted as metabolites in the urine within 3 to 4 days.[15]

There is a view that carbamates, unlike OPs, do not easily enter the brain. However, carbamates cause central nervous system (CNS) depression in humans[152] and are lipophilic,[17] and rat studies show inhibition of brain cholinesterases with multiple carbamates.[143] Furthermore, postmortem studies have shown high concentrations of carbamates in cerebrospinal fluid (CSF) and brain.[92,131,132] The evidence at present therefore suggests that they do not differ from OPs other than with regard to aging.

PATHOPHYSIOLOGY

Acetylcholine is a neurotransmitter found at both parasympathetic and sympathetic ganglia, skeletal neuromuscular junctions (NMJs), terminal junctions of all postganglionic parasympathetic nerves, postganglionic sympathetic fibers to most sweat glands, and at some nerve endings within the CNS (Fig. 113–5).[200] As the axon terminal is depolarized, vesicles containing ACh fuse with the nerve terminal, releasing ACh into the synapse or NMJ. ACh then binds postsynaptic receptors leading to activation (G proteins for muscarinic receptors and ligand-linked ion channels for the nicotinic receptors). Activation alters the flow of K^+, Na^+, and Ca^{2+} ionic currents on nerve cells, and alters membrane potential of the postsynaptic membrane, resulting in propagation of the action potential.

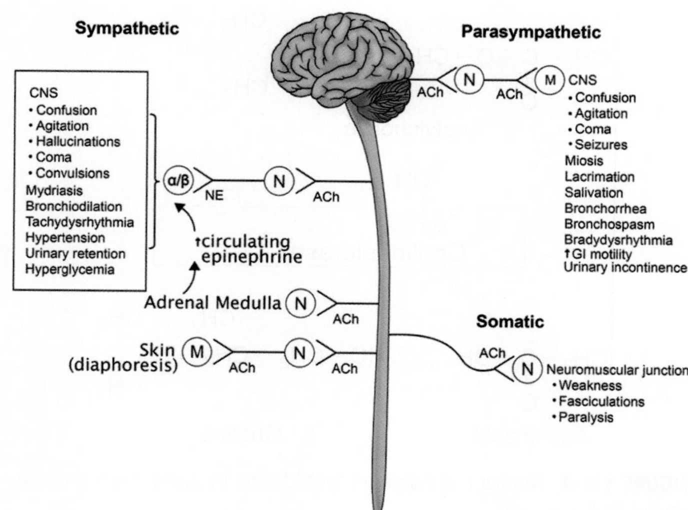

FIGURE 113–5. Pathophysiology of cholinergic syndrome as it affects the autonomic and somatic nervous systems.

Organic phosphorus insecticides and carbamates are inhibitors of carboxylic ester hydrolases within the body, including variably AChE (Enzyme Commission [EC] number 3.1.1.7), butyrylcholinesterase (plasma or pseudocholinesterase; BuChE; EC number 3.1.1.8), plasma and hepatic carboxylesterases (aliesterases), paraoxonases (A-esterases), chymotrypsin, and other nonspecific proteases.[31]

AChE hydrolyzes ACh into two inert fragments: acetic acid and choline. Under normal circumstances, virtually all ACh released by the axon is hydrolyzed almost immediately, with choline undergoing reuptake into the presynaptic terminal and being used to resynthesize ACh.[200] AChE is found in human nervous tissue and skeletal muscle, and on erythrocyte (red blood cell [RBC]) cell membranes.[123] Acutely, RBC AChE activity correlates well with the function of nervous system AChE.[185]

BuChE is a hepatic-derived protein that is found in human plasma, liver, heart, pancreas, and brain. Although the function of this enzyme is not well understood, its activity can be easily measured and has important clinical implications in anesthesia (Chaps. 66 and 68).

Inhibition of AChE is generally thought to account for all, or the majority, of clinical features of both OP and carbamate poisoning. However, many other enzymes are also inhibited.[31] The clinical effects of these interactions are not yet understood.

In addition, people ingest formulated OPs rather than pure active ingredient. OPs sold for agricultural use are typically emulsifiable concentrates in which an active ingredient such as dimethoate is mixed with an organic solvent such as xylene or cyclohexanone and a surfactant/emulsifier. Unfortunately, the xenobiotics used for coformulation are highly variable, being optimized by each company for each OP. As a result, coformulants often differ between the same OP produced by two companies, and for two OPs produced by one company.

The clinical effect of poisoning with these coformulants, in addition to the carbamate or OP, is poorly studied and uncertain. Complications of surfactant poisoning have been well described in glyphosate poisoning[24] but not with OPs. The acute toxicity of the solvents appears to be low—for example, the rat oral LD_{50}s for xylene and cyclohexanone are 4000-5000 and 1620 mg/kg, respectively. However, early respiratory arrest occurred in minipigs poisoned by dimethoate formulated with cyclohexanone at a point when red cell AChE was less than 30% inhibited, suggesting a non-AChE mechanism (Eddleston and Clutton, unpublished). Early work showed that dimethoate toxicity could be increased markedly by changing its solvent[32]; more recent work with chlorpyrifos has shown a modest change in toxicity after changing the solvent.[189] While potentially important, the major differences in clinical syndromes noted in Sri Lanka between dimethoate EC40, chlorpyrifos EC40, and fenthion EC50 cannot be attributed to the solvent since most Sri Lankan insecticides are generic, using 40% xylene as the solvent.[58]

A further effect of the solvents and surfactants occurs after aspiration. Ingestion of both OPs and carbamates can cause rapid loss of consciousness and respiratory arrest, increasing the risk of aspiration with the OP, solvent, and surfactant. Aspiration pneumonia is a major clinical problem in OP poisoning and cannot be effectively treated with oximes and atropine.

CLINICAL MANIFESTATIONS

ACUTE TOXICITY—ORGANIC PHOSPHORUS COMPOUNDS

Clinical findings of acute toxicity derive from excessive stimulation of muscarinic and nicotinic cholinergic receptors by ACh in the central and autonomic nervous systems, and at skeletal NMJs (see Fig. 113–5). The classically described patient with severe OP poisoning is one who is unresponsive, with pinpoint pupils, muscle fasciculations, diaphoresis, emesis, diarrhea, salivation, lacrimation, urinary incontinence, and an odor of garlic or solvents. Less severe poisoning is often not so typical.

The onset of symptoms varies according to the route, the degree of exposure, and particularly the OP. This is important since a more rapid onset of poisoning will reduce the likelihood of the patient reaching healthcare safely, before the need for intubation and ventilation, or the onset of complications such as aspiration. Onset of respiratory failure outside of a hospital in many parts of the world will result in the patient's death.

Patients ingesting large amounts can become symptomatic as quickly as 5 minutes following ingestion. Most patients with acute poisoning become symptomatic within a few hours of exposure, and practically all who will become ill show some features within 24 hours.

Oxon OPs (such as mevinphos and monocrotophos) are already active on exposure and patients become symptomatic very soon after ingestion. One man was reported to have died within 15 minutes of mevinphos ingestion.[118] Some thion OPs are very rapidly converted to oxons and can similarly produce symptoms rapidly, with patients ingesting parathion becoming unconscious within minutes.[65] In contrast, patients ingesting thions that are slowly converted to active oxons may not develop symptoms for hours.

The speed of onset will also be affected by the quantity ingested and the toxicity[67] of the individual OP. Patients ingesting very large doses or highly toxic compounds will more rapidly inhibit a clinically significant proportion of their AChE and exhibit features earlier.

Lipid solubility also likely affects time to onset—fat-soluble OPs such as fenthion will rapidly distribute to fat stores, in the process reducing their concentration in extracellular fluid where they impart their clinical effect.[58] Significant poisoning with such OPs is commonly delayed—respiratory failure with fenthion, for example, typically occurs after 24 hours, in contrast to the more rapid time course for less fat-soluble OPs.[61]

Symptoms following OP exposure may last for variable lengths of time, again based on the OP and the circumstances of the poisoning. For example, the more lipophilic compounds, such as dichlofenthion or fenthion, can cause recurrent cholinergic effects for many days following ingestion as they are released from fat stores.[42,129,150]

A variety of CNS findings are reported after OP exposure. Many patients present awake and alert, complaining of anxiety, restlessness, insomnia, headache, dizziness, blurred vision, depression, tremors, or other nonspecific symptoms.[13,138] The level of consciousness may deteriorate rapidly to confusion, lethargy, and coma, and patients may display inappropriate behavior. Where careful observational studies have been done, convulsions appear to be uncommonly associated with OP insecticide exposure compared with OP nerve agent poisoning.[58,194] The convulsions occurring with OPs may be due to hypoxia secondary to acute cholinergic toxicity.

The effects of excessive ACh on the autonomic nervous system may be variable because cholinergic receptors are found in both the sympathetic and parasympathetic nervous systems (see Fig. 113-5). Excessive muscarinic activity can be characterized by several mnemonics, including "SLUD" (salivation, lacrimation, urination, defecation) and "DUMBBELS" (defecation, urination, miosis, bronchospasm or bronchorrhea, emesis, lacrimation, salivation). Of these, miosis may be the most consistently encountered sign. Bronchorrhea can be so profuse that it mimics pulmonary edema.[138]

Although muscarinic findings are emphasized in these mnemonics, muscarinic signs may not always be clinically dramatic or initially predominant. Parasympathetic effects can be offset by excessive autonomic activity from stimulation of nicotinic adrenal receptors (resulting in catecholamine release) and postganglionic sympathetic fibers.[181] Mydriasis, bronchodilation, and urinary retention can occur as a result of sympathetic activity. Increased sympathetic activity usually induces white blood cell demargination, resulting in leukocytosis.[136,138]

Excessive adrenergic influences on metabolism cause glycogenolysis[182] with resultant hyperglycemia and ketosis simulating ketoacidosis.[127,206] Hypoglycemia can also occur, although the mechanism is unclear.[97] Disturbances of glucose metabolism do not seem to be common. A recent study of 79 patients with OP or carbamate poisoning showed hyperglycemia in only six patients[169]; an older study demonstrated it in seven of 105 patients.[88] It is possible that effects on glucose metabolism may be associated with specific OPs, such as malathion[97] and diazinon,[162] rather than all OPs. Larger cohorts of patients exposed to a single OP are required to determine whether such associations exist.

Hyperamylasemia appears to be relatively common in OP poisoning, occurring in four of 47 (9%) adult cases in one series[160] and five of 17 (29%) pediatric cases in a second series.[197] However, both included various anticholinesterases; a case series of only malathion poisoning reported 47 of 75 (63%) cases with hyperamylasemia.[39] The amylase likely comes from the pancreas since animal studies show OP-induced damage[98] and human poisoning cases show associated pancreatic edema and/or necrotizing pancreatitis.[25,87,144] The incidence of subclinical and clinical pancreatitis probably varies according to the OP ingested, and possibly the coformulants. Elevations of hepatic enzymes can also occur following OP exposures.[142,151,207]

Cardiovascular manifestations reflect mixed effects on the autonomic nervous system (including increased sympathetic tone), together with the consequences of OP-induced hypoxia and hypovolemia. The heart rate on admission is usually normal, with relatively few patients expressing a tachycardia or bradycardia. Patients who have received atropine before admission may be tachycardic. The literature is filled with reports of OP-associated QT interval prolongation and ventricular dysrhythmias.[14,79,109,157,159] However, most patients included had an electrocardiogram (ECG) done before they received any atropine or were so ill that atropine was ineffective. The first report described 46 patients with OP or carbamate poisoning in which ECG recordings taken on arrival were selected for analysis before the start of atropine treatment.[159] These cardiac rhythms are strongly confounded by the hypoxia and hypovolemia that characterizes the cholinergic syndrome. In a second study, 29 of the 35 patients with such dysrhythmias died.[120]

Hypotension may occur because of stimulation of vascular receptors by excessive circulating ACh.[9,105] Severe hypotension is a particularly significant problem in poisoning with the unusually fat-insoluble OP dimethoate.[43,58] Fatal poisoning is characterized by early respiratory failure followed by hypotension that can be treated only transiently with vasopressors. Such a syndrome was not found in poisoning with other fat-soluble OPs such as chlorpyrifos and fenthion.[58] The exact role of direct cardiotoxicity and peripheral vasodilatation is not yet clear, and whether this syndrome occurs with other fat-insoluble OPs, such as methamidophos and oxydemeton methyl, is also uncertain.[43]

Respiratory complications of OP poisoning include the direct pulmonary effects of bronchorrhea and bronchoconstriction, muscular junction failure of the diaphragm and intercostal muscles, and loss of central respiratory drive.[45] If severe and occurring before patients reach medical care, these effects can lead to hypoxemia and respiratory arrest, the most common cause of death after OP poisoning.[72] Both bronchorrhea and bronchoconstriction respond to adequate atropine therapy. Unfortunately, neither NMJ failure nor loss of central respiratory drive responds to atropine, and patients must be intubated and ventilated until respiratory function returns. An additional early respiratory complication is hydrocarbon aspiration that may occur after ingestion of formulated insecticides. The incidence of aspiration and the consequences of aspiration—whether pneumonia, chemical pneumonitis, or acute respiratory distress syndrome—are not yet known and likely differ according to the particular OP ingested.

Acetylcholine stimulation of nicotinic receptors governs skeletal muscle activity. The effects of excessive cholinergic stimulation at these sites are similar to that of a depolarizing neuromuscular blocking agent (succinylcholine) and initially result in fasciculations or weakness. This effect is considered to be the most reliable sign of parathion toxicity[138]; however, many severely poisoned patients lack this feature. Acute cranial nerve abnormalities are uncommon. Severe poisoning results in paralysis.[195] Rarely, patients may present only with paralysis from nicotinic effects without any other initial signs and symptoms suggestive of OP toxicity.[68,76] Extrapyramidal effects such as rigidity and choreoathetosis occur uncommonly after severe poisoning, but can persist for several days after cholinergic features have resolved.[7,21,114,134]

ACUTE TOXICITY—CARBAMATES

The effects of poisoning from carbamate insecticides appear identical to those of OPs except for the relative short duration of cholinergic features due to rapid hydroxylation of the carbamate–AChE bond. Persistent cholinergic features are not reported for carbamate poisoning.

DELAYED SYNDROMES

Intermediate Syndrome A syndrome of delayed muscle weakness resulting in respiratory failure without cholinergic features or fasciculations was first reported in 1974[195] and further refined in 1987.[164] This "intermediate syndrome" was defined as occurring 24 to 96 hours after acute OP poisoning, and following resolution of the cholinergic crisis.[106,164,195] Patients typically develop proximal muscle weakness, especially of the neck flexors, cranial nerve palsies, and progress to respiratory failure that may last for up to several weeks.[106] Consciousness is preserved unless complicated by hypoxia or pneumonia. The syndrome is important since apparently well patients can suddenly develop a respiratory arrest; therefore, an evaluation must occur in all poisoned patients if deaths are to be prevented.[16,145] The first sign is often weakness of neck flexion such that patients cannot lift their heads off the bed.

The exact pathophysiology of the syndrome is unknown. It is clearly due to dysfunction of the NMJ, with respiratory failure resulting from weakness affecting the diaphragm and intercostal muscles. Preservation of consciousness suggests that the central respiratory drive is unlikely to be involved. Clinicians have proposed that overwhelming NMJ stimulation causes downregulation of the NMJ synaptic mechanisms.[44,164] This dysfunction will require time to be repaired, even after the insecticide has been removed from the body, explaining the long periods of time that many patients require assisted ventilation.[61]

Case reports and small case series have been reported from around the world, with resulting comments that the intermediate syndrome is more common with certain OPs, such as parathion, methylparathion, malathion, and fenthion. Unfortunately, large cohorts of poisoning with specific OPs receiving standardized treatments have been rarely reported, making comparisons of incidence between OPs difficult. However, two cohorts have shown that the intermediate syndrome causing respiratory failure is much more common in fenthion poisoning than chlorpyrifos, malathion, or fenitrothion poisoning.[61,194]

Clinical examination remains the most reliable means of identifying the occurrence of intermediate syndrome.[106] Electromyograms (EMGs) will often show tetanic fade in these patients, and suggest both pre- and postsynaptic involvement.[106] Recent work has noted characteristic electrophysiological features, in particular the decrement-increment phenomenon, that can be identified before onset of neurological features and respiratory paralysis.[100] The majority of patients developing weakness in this series did not progress to respiratory failure, indicating that the intermediate syndrome is a spectrum disorder.

A study of severely poisoned patients suggested that the occurrence of intermediate syndrome strongly correlated with the initial degree of cholinergic crisis, and seemed to be a continuum with the neuromuscular paralysis resulting from the early stages of poisoning.[101] This view is supported by an earlier work[44] and a more recent study of dimethoate poisoning, which showed that peripheral NMJ dysfunction can occur simultaneously with the cholinergic syndrome.[61] Patients with moderate to severe dimethoate poisoning typically require intubation for respiratory failure soon after ingestion, during the acute cholinergic syndrome. However, this is relatively short lived and patients recover consciousness after a few days. As the cholinergic syndrome diminishes and patients regain consciousness, with recovery of the central respiratory drive, they still require ventilator support. Similar to patients with classical intermediate syndrome, they require ventilatory support for several weeks until their NMJ recovers function. In addition, this case series demonstrated that the classic intermediate syndrome—respiratory failure after resolution of the cholinergic syndrome—can occur before 24 hours and after 96 hours.[61]

These studies suggest that the original intermediate syndrome is just one important aspect of OP-induced peripheral NMJ dysfunction. It seems likely that the relative incidence and timing of the intermediate syndrome or delayed NMJ dysfunction for different OPs is determined by the rapidity and quantity of AChE inhibition. Where inhibition is intense, with fat-insoluble OPs like dimethoate that have very high blood concentrations, NMJ dysfunction develops at an early stage, before recovery from the cholinergic crisis. Fat-soluble OPs, such as fenthion, cause a more protracted AChE inhibition, likely explaining why fenthion-induced NMJ dysfunction and respiratory failure occur later.[61]

Some authors have suggested that insufficient oxime therapy explains the intermediate syndrome.[18] Of note, both dimethoate- and fenthion-inhibited AChE respond poorly to oximes, in contrast to chlorpyrifos, which responds well to oximes and has a much lower incidence of intermediate syndrome.[58,61] The occurrence of NMJ dysfunction in chlorpyrifos poisoning may well be due to inadequate oxime therapy. However, adequate oxime therapy after, for example, malathion poisoning[174] may be irrelevant since this dimethyl OP responds poorly to oximes. Overall, delayed NMJ dysfunction may be caused by ineffective

AChE reactivation, whether due to inadequate oxime therapy or to poisoning with OPs that do not respond to oxime therapy.

The treatment of intermediate syndrome is supportive with airway protection and mechanical ventilation. There are no substantial data demonstrating that pralidoxime or atropine is effective in the treatment of this disorder, although patients may require these medications to control concurrent cholinergic symptoms. Pralidoxime may be able to reverse the intermediate syndrome if given early in its development. Administration after the NMJ failure occurs is unlikely to be effective. The weakness and paralysis commonly resolve in 5 to 18 days.[61,89,100,101]

Organic Phosphorus–Induced Delayed Neuropathy Peripheral neuropathies can occur with chronic OP exposures or days to weeks following acute exposures. Organic phosphorus–induced delayed neuropathy (OPIDN) results from inhibition by phosphorylation of the enzyme neuropathy target esterase (NTE, now identified as a lysophospholipase [lysoPLA]) within nervous tissue.[30,75,102,103] This enzyme catalyzes breakdown of endoplasmic reticulum–membrane phosphatidylcholine, the major phospholipid of eukaryotic cell membranes. Neuropathic OPs cause a transient loss of NTE-lysoPLA activity, putatively disrupting membrane phospholipid homeostasis, axonal transport, and glial–axonal interactions.[75]

Such neuropathies may result from exposure to OPs that neither inhibit red blood cell cholinesterase nor produce clinical cholinergic toxicity.[33] The more commonly implicated chemicals include triaryl phosphates, such as triorthocresyl phosphate (TOCP), and dialkyl phosphates, such as mephosfolan, mipafox, and chlorpyrifos.[102] Pathologic findings demonstrate effects primarily on large distal neurons, with axonal degeneration preceding demyelination (see Chaps. 2 and 18).

Contaminated foods and beverages were responsible for epidemics of OP-induced delayed polyneuropathies and encephalopathy. In the 1930s, thousands of individuals in the United States became weak or paralyzed after drinking a supplement containing TOCP—an outbreak nicknamed "Ginger Jake paralysis" (see Chap. 2).[8,130] Contaminated cooking and mineral oils were responsible for outbreaks of delayed polyneuropathies in Vietnam and Sri Lanka.[47,163] Vague distal muscle weakness and pain are often the presenting symptoms and may progress to paralysis.[82] The administration of atropine or pralidoxime does not alter the onset and clinical course of these symptoms.[193] Pyramidal tract signs can appear weeks to months after acute exposures. EMGs and nerve conduction studies may be helpful in diagnosing this disorder by identifying the type of neuropathy (such as axonopathy, myelinopathy, or transmission neuropathy) and differentiating it from similar presentations such as Guillain-Barré syndrome.[1] The recovery of these patients is variable, commonly with residual deficits, and occurs over months to years.[130,163]

Delayed neuropathies are not usually associated with carbamate insecticides. One reason for this difference is presumed to be that aging of the neuropathy target esterase insecticide complex is a requirement for neuronal degeneration. Paradoxically, one study suggested that subgroups of carbamates may actually bind neuropathy target esterase and exert a protective effect against more toxic OPs.[3] However, several cases of delayed neuropathy associated with carbamates have been reported.[50,191,205] These cases involved ingestions of carbaryl, *m*-tolyl methyl carbamate, and carbofuran; included both sensory and motor tracts; and tended to resolve over 3 to 9 months.

CHRONIC TOXICITY–ORGANIC PHOSPHOROUS COMPOUNDS

Illness may also result from chronic exposure to excessive amounts of OPs. Chronic exposure most commonly occurs in workers who have regular contact with these xenobiotics, but may also occur in individuals who have repeated contact with excessive amounts of insecticides in their living environments. Chronic exposure to cholinergic ophthalmic preparations can also result in toxicity.[121] Although tolerance to acute cholinergic systemic effects of OPs (including death in rats) may be observed with long-term exposures,[72] persons who have long-term exposures begin to describe symptoms after a substantial length of time. These effects can range from vague neurological complaints, such as weakness and blurred vision, to miosis, nausea, vomiting, diarrhea, diaphoresis, and other cholinergic effects.[5,6,121,172] BuChE activity is usually the most sensitive measure of exposure, and workers in contact with these chemicals should have baseline BuChE testing for comparison and monitoring.[72,93]

Recent literature has linked Parkinson disease with chronic exposure to insecticides including OPs.[49,173] Some individuals may have a genetic susceptibility.[21] Additionally, significant acute exposures to OPs can lead to self-limited movement disorders resembling parkinsonism that resolve over weeks to months (see above). Although statistics derived from some epidemiologic studies suggest the connection,[63,91] other studies have failed to a find an association between OPs and parkinsonism.[180]

BEHAVIORAL TOXICITY

Behavioral changes may also occur after acute or chronic exposure to OPs.[66] Signs and symptoms include confusion, psychosis, anxiety, drowsiness, depression, fatigue, and irritability. Electroencephalographic changes may be noted and can last for weeks.[80] Single photon emission computed tomography (SPECT) scanning revealed morphologic changes in the basal ganglia of one child following poisoning.[23] Recent studies have shown a deficit in cognitive processing after acute OP self-poisoning lasting for at least 6 months and not found in matched patients who had poisoned themselves with paracetamol.[40,41] Thus far there appears to be no clear evidence for neuropsychiatric deficits resulting from subclinical exposure to OPs.[66]

DIAGNOSTIC TESTING

ORGANIC PHOSPHORUS COMPOUNDS

When confronted with a patient in cholinergic crisis who presents with a history of acute exposure to an OP, the diagnosis is straightforward. Although textbooks list a variety of clinical signs for the cholinergic crisis (DUMBELS, SLUD—see above), most patients with significant poisoning can be identified by the presence of pinpoint pupils, excessive sweat, and breathing difficulty.[56] However, when the history is unreliable or does not suggest poisoning, the clinician must turn to other means to confirm the diagnosis of OP or carbamate poisoning. Treatment of an ill patient with a cholinergic syndrome should not await confirmation of the diagnosis.

The most appropriate laboratory tests for confirming cholinesterase inhibition by insecticides are tests that measure (1) specific OPs and active metabolites in biologic tissues and (2) cholinesterase activity in plasma or blood. Unfortunately, although urine and serum assays for OPs and their metabolites are available,[2,86,99,112] such testing is rarely obtainable within hours. Moreover "normal" ranges and toxic concentrations are not established for most. Currently, therefore, verifying cholinesterase inhibitor poisoning relies on measurement of cholinesterase activity.[55,72]

Cholinesterase Activity The two cholinesterases commonly measured are butyrylcholinesterase (BuChE, plasma cholinesterase, EC 3.1.1.8) and red cell acetylcholinesterase (AChE, EC 3.1.1.7). The former is produced by the liver and then secreted into the blood, where it metabolizes xenobiotics, including succinylcholine and cocaine. Red cell AChE is expressed from the same gene as the enzyme found in neuronal synapses. The main difference is in their mechanism of membrane attachment which is due to posttranslational modification (red cell AChE is glycosylphosphatidyliositol anchor [GPI]-linked to the red cell while neuronal AChE is secreted and forms dimers and tetramers that are attached to the postsynaptic membrane by other proteins[123]). Inhibition of red cell AChE or BuChE only serves as a marker for cholinesterase inhibitor poisoning, since inhibition of these enzymes does not contribute to signs and symptoms of poisoning. However, red cell AChE activity seems to accurately reflect AChE activity in the NMJ soon after poisoning.[185]

There is tremendous interindividual and interchemical variability in the degree and duration with which the OPs affect particular cholinesterases. After a significant exposure, BuChE activity usually falls first, followed by a decrease in red cell AChE activity. The sequence may be highly variable, but by the time patients present with acute symptoms, both cholinesterase activities have usually fallen well below baseline values.[138] Of note, the presence of BuChE, AChE, and other esterases varies markedly between species,[115] complicating the interpretation of animal studies. Furthermore, AChE occurs at very low concentrations in human plasma or serum; therefore, papers citing human serum AChE activity (eg, [11,188]) are likely measuring serum BuChE.

Butyrylcholinesterase BuChE activity usually recovers before red cell AChE activity, returning to normal within a few days after a mild exposure in the absence of a repeat exposure to the inciting OP.[38] However, BuChE activity is less specific for exposure than red cell AChE activity.[72] Low BuChE activity can be found in patients with a number of disorders, including hereditary deficiency of the enzyme, malnutrition, hepatic parenchymal disease, chronic debilitating illnesses, and iron deficiency anemia.[107]

The wide normal range of BuChE activity allows for patients with high normal activity to suffer significant falls in activity, yet still register near normal BuChE activity on laboratory assay.[38] Additionally, day-to-day variation in the activity of this enzyme in healthy individuals may be as high as 20%.[72] Since BuChE inhibition varies between OPs and does not cause clinical effects, an admission activity by itself is of little value in predicting outcome. An admission activity can only be used to predict outcome if the ingested OP is known and its clinical usefulness has been studied specifically for that OP.[59]

Red Cell Acetylcholinesterase Red cell AChE activity is thought to more accurately reflect nervous tissue AChE activity because the AChE in red blood cells is true AChE. Some authors suggest that clinical OP poisoning occurs when red blood cell cholinesterase activity falls to below 50% of baseline.[138] Neuromuscular dysfunction is associated with a value of 30% of normal or less.[185] A major advantage of AChE is that its activity can be related to hemoglobin (Hb) concentration, reducing variation due to varying hematocrit.[203] Most people have a normal concentration of 600 to 700 mU/μmol Hb; a small study of Caucasians reported a mean of 651 ± 18 mU/μmol Hb.[203]

After poisoning, in the absence of oximes, red cell AChE may take many weeks to recover since erythrocytes in circulation at the time of OP exposure must be replaced. An average of 66 days may be necessary for red cell AChE activity to recover following severe inhibition (assuming no treatment with oxime). Rat studies suggest that neuronal AChE activity may return to normal more rapidly than red cell AChE.[83] Patients have been reported to have normal NMJ activity and no cholinergic features, yet low red cell AChE activity. For this reason, in subacute poisoning with OPs, it is difficult to accurately predict the actual time of onset or duration of exposure when only the red cell AChE activity is known.

Depressed red cell AChE activity may be the result of exposures or conditions other than OP or carbamate poisoning, for example, in pernicious anemia and during therapy with antimalarials or antidepressants (Table 113–4).[108,133]

TABLE 113–4. Interpreting Cholinesterase Concentrations

	Red Cell Cholinesterase	Butyrylcholinesterase
Advantage	Better reflection of synaptic inhibition	Easier to assay, declines faster
Site	RBC (reflects CNS gray matter, motor end plate)	CNS white matter, plasma, liver, pancreas, heart
Regeneration (untreated)	1%/day	25%–30% in first 7–10 days
Normalization (untreated)	35–49 days	28–42 days
Use	Unsuspected prior exposure with normal butyryl cholinesterase	Acute exposure
False depression in concentration	Pernicious anemia, hemoglobinopathies, antimalarial treatment, oxalate blood tubes	Liver dysfunction, malnutrition, hypersensitivity reactions, xenobiotics (succinylcholine, codeine, morphine), pregnancy, genetic deficiency

CNS, central nervous system; RBC, red blood cell.

Blood samples for cholinesterase activity must be obtained in the appropriate blood collecting tubes. Tubes containing fluoride will permanently inactivate the enzymes, yielding falsely low activity, and should not be used. Specimens for red cell AChE are usually drawn into tubes containing a chelating anticoagulant such as ethylenediaminetetraacetic acid (EDTA) to prevent clot formation. BuChE does not require an anticoagulant and can be drawn into a tube without chelators or anticoagulants. Of note, OPs and oximes in collected blood samples will continue to interact with red cell AChE; small differences in time between sampling and assay can result in marked artificial variation in results. The safest way to take blood for AChE is to immediately dilute it 1:20 or 1:100 into saline or water cooled to 4°C at the bedside, before rapidly freezing the sample. This process slows down both inhibitory and reactivating reactions in the tube, allowing more uniform results.[55,203] Such rapid reactions do not occur with BuChE, and bedside dilution and cooling are therefore not required.

Protein Adducts Current research is addressing means of detecting OP exposure many weeks after the event. New techniques using mass spectrometry are being developed to identify phosphorylated proteins, such as albumin or BuChE, in blood samples.[147,177]

CARBAMATES

Carbamates inhibit neuronal and red cell AChE, and BuChE. The relative ease with which spontaneous decarbamylation of cholinesterases takes place may result in the measurement of relatively normal red cell AChE activity despite severe cholinergic symptoms if the assay is not performed within several hours of sampling.[140] This emphasizes the importance of cooling and then freezing the blood sample within minutes of collection (see above). As in the case of OP poisoning, the wide "normal" range of BuChE activity makes interpretation of BuChE activity difficult at times when the patient's baseline concentrations are unknown. Unlike OPs, carbamates generally do not produce persistently depressed red cell AChE and BuChE activities.

ATROPINE CHALLENGE

An atropine challenge may be helpful in diagnosing cholinergic poisoning in a patient who presents with findings suggestive of this disorder, but in whom no history is available to suggest excessive exposure to an OP or carbamate. In an individual not exposed to significant amounts of insecticide a test dose of 1 mg of atropine in adolescents or adults, or 0.05 mg/kg in children up to an adult dose with a minimum of 0.1 mg, should produce classic antimuscarinic findings, in particular a tachycardia as well as mydriasis and dry mucous membranes. Conversely, the persistence of cholinergic signs and symptoms after an atropine challenge strongly suggests the presence of anticholinesterase poisoning.[138] However, some patients suffering from mild anticholinesterase poisoning may respond to this dose of atropine. Therefore, the reversal of cholinergic findings does not completely exclude cholinergic poisoning by one of these compounds.

ELECTROMYOGRAM STUDIES

Although measuring cholinesterase activity is the test most often used to estimate tissue and neuronal AChE activity, studies support the use of repetitive nerve stimulation testing as an accurate method of quantifying AChE inhibition at the NMJ.[10,19,100] Spontaneous repetitive potentials or fasciculations following single-nerve stimulation resulting from persistent acetylcholine at nerve terminals can be a sensitive indicator of AChE inhibition at the motor end plate, and may be useful in the early diagnosis of anticholinesterase poisoning.[19] This type of evaluation may also be of benefit in early detection of rebound cholinergic crisis caused by continued absorption or redistribution from adipose tissue or the onset of an intermediate syndrome.[10,19,100]

DIFFERENTIAL DIAGNOSIS

The differential diagnosis for cholinergic poisoning includes three main categories (Table 113–5). The first comprises insecticides and other noninsecticidal cholinesterase inhibitors including the medicinal anticholinesterases neostigmine, pyridostigmine, physostigmine, and echothiophate iodide. The patients who most commonly suffer cholinergic poisoning syndrome from medicinal cholinesterase inhibitors are those with myasthenia gravis who are given excessive doses of pyridostigmine. This entire group of xenobiotics should produce low BuChE and low red cell AChE activity.

TABLE 113–5. Categories of Cholinergic Poisoning

Cholinesterase Inhibitors	Cholinomimetics	Nicotine Alkaloids
Organic phosphorus insecticides	Pilocarpine Carbachol	Coniine Lobeline
Organic phosphorus ophthalmic medications	Aceclidine Methacholine	Nicotine
Carbamate insecticides	Bethanechol	
Carbamate medications	Muscarine-containing mushrooms	

The second category of compounds that produce a syndrome of cholinergic poisoning include those with cholinomimetic activity. These compounds directly stimulate muscarinic or nicotinic cholinergic receptors, but do not inhibit AChE. In individuals exposed to these compounds, BuChE and red cell AChE activity should be normal. Cholinomimetic medications include preparations of carbachol, methacholine, pilocarpine, and bethanechol. Nonpharmaceuticals such as muscarine-containing mushrooms can be cholinomimetic (Chap. 117). Finally, a third group of xenobiotics, the nicotine alkaloids (eg, nicotine, lobeline, and coniine) cause CNS, autonomic, and skeletal muscle symptoms similar to those occurring in OP and carbamate toxicity (Chap. 84).

MANAGEMENT

ORGANIC PHOSPHORUS INSECTICIDES

The primary cause of death after anticholinesterase poisoning is respiratory failure with subsequent hypoxemia. This results from muscarinic effects on the cardiovascular and pulmonary systems (bronchospasm, bronchorrhea, aspiration, bradydysrhythmias, or hypotension), nicotinic effects on skeletal muscles (weakness and paralysis), loss of central respiratory drive, and rarely seizures. Therefore, initial treatment for a patient exposed to OPs is directed at ensuring an adequate airway and ventilation, and at stabilizing cardiorespiratory function by reversing excessive muscarinic effects.[55,56] Seizures not secondary to hypoxemia are treated with standard anticonvulsants such as benzodiazepines.

Maintenance of the patient's airway is best assured by early endotracheal intubation and positive pressure ventilation in patients who are comatose, have significant weakness, or who are unable to handle copious secretions that may accompany the poisoning. Only a neuromuscular blocker that is not primarily metabolized by cholinesterases should be used to induce pharmacologic paralysis. The duration of action of the depolarizing agent succinylcholine and the nondepolarizing agent mivacurium, for example, will be extended in the presence of low BuChE activity, resulting in paralysis that can be prolonged for several hours.[148,165,166]

Antimuscarinic Therapy Simultaneously, with airway stabilization excessive muscarinic activity should be controlled since this will aid respiration and oxygenation. Atropine competitively antagonizes ACh at muscarinic receptors to reverse excessive secretions, miosis, bronchospasm, vomiting, diarrhea, diaphoresis, and urinary incontinence.[71,90,138] For adolescents and adults, intravenous doses should begin with boluses of 1 to 3 mg depending on the severity of symptoms; doses for children should start at 0.05 mg/kg up to adult doses with a minimum of 0.1 mg dose. Although many authors state that repeat doses of 1 to 5 mg should be given every 2 to 20 minutes until "atropinization" occurs, the most rapid method of obtaining control in severe cases is to give doubling doses every 5 minutes if the response to the previous dose has been inadequate.[54,56]

"Atropinization" is classically said to occur when patients exhibit dry skin and mucous membranes, decreased or absent bowel sounds, tachycardia, reduced secretions, no bronchospasm (in absence of other causes such as aspiration), and usually mydriasis.[54] However, patients die from cardiorespiratory compromise, not wet skin or miosis. Therefore, cardiorespiratory parameters, not pupil size or the presence of sweating, should guide administration of atropine. Atropine dosing should aim to reverse bronchorrhea and bronchospasm, and to provide adequate blood pressure and heart rate for tissue oxygenation (for example, systolic BP greater than 90 mm Hg and heart rate greater than 80 bpm). All can be easily and rapidly assessed.

Once atropinization occurs, it can be maintained by a constant infusion of atropine, typically initially giving 10% to 20% of the total loading dose per hour (usually maximum 2 mg/h). Regular assessment for signs of under- or overatropinization should guide the use of a further bolus or halting the infusion, followed by changes in the infusion rate.[56] Children have been managed with continuous infusions of atropine starting at 0.025 mg/kg/h.[23] Continuous infusions will be needed for patients severely poisoned by very fat-soluble OPs that continue to redistribute from the fat and freshly inhibit AChE. Such infusions have been used for as long as 32 days.[74]

Absent bowel sounds, marked tachycardia (greater than 120 bpm in a well-hydrated patient not withdrawing from alcohol), mydriasis, and urinary retention may indicate overatropinization or atropine toxicity. This is unnecessary and possibly dangerous because of associated hyperthermia, confusion, and agitation.[56] Tachycardia is not, however, an absolute contraindication to atropine therapy since it can result from hypovolemia, aspiration pneumonitis, or agitation. Isolated pulmonary manifestations may respond to administration of nebulized atropine or ipratropium, and this treatment can accompany parenteral administration of these medications. However, the risk/benefit of this pulmonary-specific treatment has not yet been assessed.

Large doses of atropine may be needed to reverse the bronchospasm, bronchorrhea, and bradycardia associated with severe OP toxicity.[138] Some patients with mild symptoms need only 1 or 2 mg of atropine to reverse cholinergic toxicity, but a moderately poisoned adolescent or adult commonly requires total doses as large as 40 mg.[52,54] Severe poisonings may necessitate even higher doses. Some adults have received over 1000 mg of atropine in 24 hours (with adequate pralidoxime dosing) without demonstrating antimuscarinic effects,[52,196] and total doses as high as 11,000 mg during the course of treatment have been reported.[96] However, the additional benefit of such extreme doses over more modest doses is unclear. One study reported that much smaller doses of around 1 mg/h were associated with adequate control of muscarinic features after initial atropinization.[186]

Atropine does not reverse nicotinic effects. Therefore, patients who improve after receiving atropine must still be closely monitored in an intensive care setting for impending respiratory failure from delayed NMJ dysfunction. Patients should be regularly clinically examined for proximal muscle weakness (in particular neck flexor weakness); once noted, tidal volume measurements should be made at least every 6 hours to detect impending respiratory failure and allow early initiation of ventilatory support.

When antimuscarinic CNS toxicity becomes evident, yet peripheral cholinergic findings such as bradycardia, bronchorrhea, or vomiting necessitate the administration of more atropine, glycopyrrolate can be substituted for atropine because its quaternary ammonium structure limits CNS penetration.[154] One randomized clinical trial compared atropine with glycopyrrolate in intensive care unit (ICU) management of OP poisoning but was too small to detect any difference between regimens.[12] The initial intravenous dose of glycopyrrolate for adults and adolescents is 1 to 2 mg, repeated as needed, or in children 0.025 mg/kg up to adult doses. As with atropine, much higher doses of glycopyrrolate may be required to stabilize patients with severe poisonings. Although scopolamine (hyoscine) has been used in place of atropine,[114,154] it may cause more pronounced CNS effects. If standard atropine supplies are exhausted during therapy, atropine ophthalmic preparations and other antimuscarinic agents such as diphenhydramine may be used.

However, in a large case series of Sri Lankan patients treated by necessity outside of an ICU, patients were safely atropinized without CNS toxicity by slowing atropine infusions whenever absent bowel sounds, confusion, or hyperthermia were detected.[56,58] It is therefore unclear whether glycopyrrolate or scopolamine is required for OP poisoning as long as the atropine regimen is adjusted and there is an adequate quantity for each patient.

OXIMES

Although phosphorylated AChE undergoes hydrolytic regeneration at a very slow rate, this process can be enhanced by using an oxime such as pralidoxime chloride (2-PAM) or obidoxime (Fig. 113–6).[67] Regeneration of AChE lowers ACh concentrations, improving both muscarinic and nicotinic effects. An immediate rise in red cell AChE activity, presumably paralleling a rise in neuronal AChE activity, can occur after effective administration of pralidoxime.[58,184]

As discussed above, phosphorylated AChE becomes aged, and therefore unresponsive to oximes at different rates according to the chemistry of the OP.[67] Oximes therefore have to be given early, within a few hours of exposure, after dimethoxy OP poisoning. In contrast, they can still be highly efficacious 48 hours after diethoxy poisoning, with some effects even when given several days after exposure. Oximes can also be efficacious weeks after poisoning with a fat-soluble OP. Therefore, some AChE may still be undergoing new inhibition for days or weeks after exposure in symptomatic patients, and such inhibition may be reversible by pralidoxime.[201] Case reports support this reasoning by noting dramatic effects in reversing paralysis, weakness, and cholinergic symptoms even after late administration of pralidoxime.[129,137]

However, the clinical effectiveness of oximes in significant OP poisoning is debated. The first clinical experience with pralidoxime was reported in the late 1950s when five patients with occupational parathion poisoning were treated.[137] All patients responded well to around 1 g of pralidoxime intravenously. As expected from occupational inhalational exposure, none of the patients were very ill. The use of much higher doses of pralidoxime, of 1 to 2 g infused over 20 to 30 minutes followed by 0.5 g/h, in patients with severe parathion poisoning was subsequently reported.[139] It was also noted that some OPs, including malathion, did not respond well to pralidoxime.[136]

Clinical experience of various intravenous pralidoxime regimens in Asia has led to debate about the efficacy of oximes.[62,104,149,153,178] However, a recent Indian clinical trial showed that very high doses of pralidoxime iodide, a 2-g loading dose followed by 1 g/h, reduced death and length

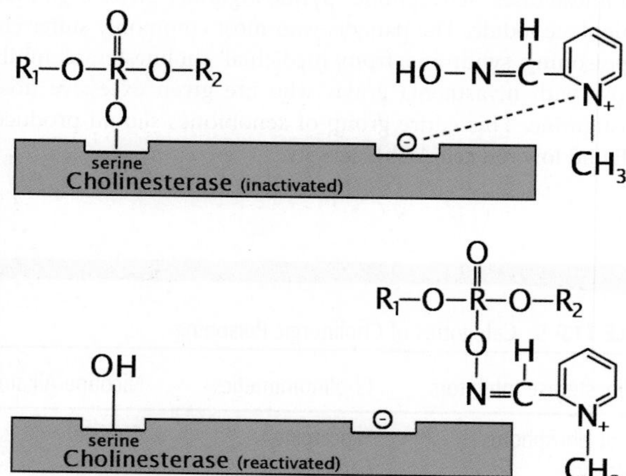

FIGURE 113–6. Mechanism of reactivation of acetylcholinesterase by pralidoxime. The positively charged aromatic nitrogen of pralidoxime is "attracted" to the anionic site of acetylcholinesterase, allowing the reactive oxime portion of the molecule to position itself over the phosphorylated active site of the enzyme. Pralidoxime then becomes phosphorylated, reactivating acetylcholinesterase.

of ventilation in moderately poisoned patients who presented early and were treated in an ICU.[146] However, we have found that similar doses of pralidoxime chloride did not reactivate AChE in severe poisoning with dimethoate and other dimethoxy insecticides.[58] Furthermore, analysis of a Sri Lankan cohort including 235 symptomatic OP insecticide poisoned patients was unable to find benefit from traditional doses of pralidoxime.[57] The exact role of oximes is currently unclear; however, the best quality evidence at present suggests that oximes should be given as soon as possible after exposure to increase the chance of benefit. The dosing regimens and length of pralidoxime therapy remain controversial for various OPs and clinical presentations.

Side effects of oximes are usually minimal at normal doses.[67,81,125] Rapid infusion causes emesis, hypertension (particularly diastolic), and possibly mild cholinergic effects because of transient blockade of AChE, and is said to cause neuromuscular blockade.[181] Occasional visual complaints are also reported in patients receiving pralidoxime. However, the recent Sri Lankan randomized, controlled trial suggests that sustained use of oximes at high concentrations may increase the risk of significant adverse effects.[57]

Some effects of oximes are not well understood. Their quaternary ammonium compound structures are thought to reduce their passage across the blood–brain barrier and prevent CNS effects.[181] However, obidoxime has been detected in CSF[67] and at least one case report describes pralidoxime-induced improvements in mental status and electroencephalograms not attributable to improved ventilation or perfusion.[119]

DIAZEPAM

Animal studies demonstrate that administering diazepam along with oximes in the treatment of poisoning with OP nerve agents or the insecticide dichlorvos can increase survival and decrease the incidence of seizures and neuropathy.[51,135] Diazepam can also decrease cerebral morphologic damage resulting from OP-related seizures.[20,124] One study suggests that diazepam may help attenuate OP-induced respiratory depression,[51] postulating that the benzodiazepines attenuate the overstimulation of central respiratory centers caused by OPs. However, seizures have been uncommon in large case series of patients poisoned by OPs,[58,194] and no clinical studies have yet been performed to determine whether benzodiazepines offer benefit to humans.[122] In the absence of this evidence, diazepam should be used to treat OP-related seizures and agitation and aid intubation, but not be given routinely to all cases (see Antidotes in Depth A24: Benzodiazepines).[122]

DECONTAMINATION

Cutaneous absorption of OPs and carbamates necessitates removal of all clothing as soon as possible. Medical personnel should avoid self-contamination by wearing neoprene or nitrile gloves. Double gloving with standard vinyl gloves may be protective. Skin should be triple washed with water, soap, and water, and rinsed again with water. Although alcohol-based soaps are sometimes recommended to dissolve hydrocarbons,[69] these products can be difficult to find, and expeditious skin cleansing should be the primary goal. Cutaneous absorption can also result from contact with OP and carbamate compounds in vomitus and diarrhea if the initial exposure was by ingestion. Oily insecticides may be difficult to remove from thick or long hair, even with repeated shampooing, and shaving scalp hair may be necessary. Exposed leather clothing or products should be discarded because decontamination is very difficult once impregnation has occurred.

Military institutions are now experimenting with cholinesterase sponges for cutaneous organic phosphorus decontamination.[77] The sponge consists of a cholinesterase enzyme covalently linked and immobilized in a polyurethane matrix. The sponge reportedly is effective in removing OPs from skin and surfaces.[77]

In substantial acute ingestions, if emesis has not occurred and the patient presents within several hours after ingestion, evacuation of stomach contents by lavage using a nasogastric tube can be done. Because the onset of coma, seizures, and paralysis can be rapid, airway protection is necessary to perform the procedure safely. Although there are data suggesting that activated charcoal (AC) may adsorb some OPs, a study of 1310 patients with OP or carbamate poisoning found no benefit from the use of multiple-dose activated charcoal.[60] Thus, the current recommendation is that patients with anticholinesterase poisoning receive only a single dose of 1 g/kg AC if the patient's airway is stable.

Healthcare providers must always maintain caution when coming into contact with stomach contents or other body fluids when managing these cases.[117] Bystanders have been poisoned by providing mouth-to-mouth resuscitation to a victim of an intentional ingestion of diazinon.[110] There have also been reports of nosocomial poisoning in emergency department (ED) staff.[29,73,117,171] A consensus statement on nosocomial poisoning has been developed.[117]

DISPOSITION

After atropinization, patients with cholinesterase-inhibitor poisoning should be continuously observed for evidence of (1) deteriorating neurologic function and potential paralysis, and (2) need for increases or reductions in atropine dosing.

Red cell AChE and BuChE activities can be measured intermittently after the institution of pralidoxime therapy.[65,67,183,201] Effective oxime therapy will normalize AChE activity but usually does not affect BuChE activity. In the absence of effective oxime therapy, red cell AChE activity may be markedly depressed long after neuronal AChE activity has returned to normal. Therefore, an individual who remains asymptomatic may be discharged home with subnormal cholinesterase activity. BuChE begins to rise when no more OP is left in the body.[55] A sudden fall in BuChE activity suggests that OP is being redistributed from fat stores. The relevance of a fall in BuChE activity that is not clinically apparent is uncertain. Overall, there is little evidence at present that repeated testing of AChE or BuChE activity improves management and outcome over clinical monitoring alone. Such testing is, however, important for research assessing new interventions.

When available, EMG studies to detect signs of motor end plate dysfunction and early AChE inhibition may be a more sensitive method for identifying recurrent cholinergic toxicity.[19] Again, the clinical usefulness of this approach has not yet been studied.

A patient who becomes asymptomatic, not requiring pralidoxime or atropine for 1 to 2 days, may be discharged. Although recurrent cholinergic crises and/or respiratory failure can occur after several days, such patients have usually previously shown clinical signs of some form. Patients should not be allowed to go home wearing clothing that was worn when the poisoning occurred. The clothing should be disposed of as medical waste and destroyed.

CARBAMATES

The treatment of patients with carbamate poisoning is identical to that of OP poisoning with two exceptions. First, the use of oximes in carbamate exposure is controversial and many providers will not administer them. Historical animal data had implied that pralidoxime might increase AChE inactivation in carbaryl poisoning.[113,116] Recent reports suggest aldicarb poisoning may also benefit from oxime therapy[152] and that the dose of pralidoxime may be important in carbaryl poisoning.[128] Comparative human data investigating the use of pralidoxime in carbamate poisonings are currently lacking. Fortunately, because of the rapid hydrolysis of the carbamate–AChE complex, symptoms, including weakness and paralysis, usually resolve within 24 to 48 hours without pralidoxime therapy. However, administering pralidoxime to a poisoned patient in a cholinergic crisis is appropriate when it is not known whether the patient is suffering from OP or carbamate insecticide poisoning. If the poisoning is from a carbamate insecticide, pralidoxime therapy may not be necessary, but if used will likely not prove detrimental.

Second, significant inhibition of red cell AChE and BuChE by carbamates generally does not last for more than 1 to 2 days, assuming absorption is complete. Patients exposed to carbamates usually have normal cholinesterase values by the time of discharge. There are no reported cases of recurrent or delayed poisonings following carbamate insecticide poisoning. Therefore, repeating cholinesterase activities after patients are asymptomatic is usually unnecessary. However, of note, complications of poisoning with carbamates—such as aspiration and hypoxic brain injury—can last many days.

SUMMARY

Organic phosphorus and carbamate insecticides kill hundreds of thousands of people each year. However, poisoning with these insecticides is not uniform; they differ markedly in their human toxicity, pharmacokinetics, clinical syndrome, and response to therapy. Symptoms result from inhibition of AChE and overstimulation of muscarinic and nicotinic receptors in synapses of the autonomic and central nervous systems and at the NMJ. Patients with substantial poisoning present with the cholinergic crisis and respiratory failure due to bronchospasm, bronchorrhea, loss of central respiratory drive, and dysfunction of NMJ. Resuscitation requires preservation of the airway, oxygen provision and ventilatory support as necessary, together with rapid administration of intravenous fluids and, for severe poisoning, doubling doses of atropine. Once stabilized, atropine should be administered as an infusion to sustain cardiorespiratory function. The clinical effectiveness of oximes for OP poisoning is still debated, but current evidence suggests that they are most effective if given soon after exposure and are more effective for poisoning with diethoxy compounds. Patients may develop NMJ dysfunction that progresses to respiratory failure; such patients often require ventilatory support for weeks. This respiratory failure can develop after several days and after the cholinergic features have settled; conscious patients in the days after exposure especially neck flexors have to be closely monitored for onset of proximal muscle weakness and reductions in tidal volume. Cholinergic features can recur many days after ingestion of very fat-soluble compounds such as fenthion because of redistribution from fat stores. Poisoning after ingestion of extremely toxic OPs such as parathion can develop within minutes, so that severely ill patients die before reaching medical care. Others become unconscious rapidly and aspirate the insecticide and stomach contents, so that a common cause of death is aspiration pneumonia. Regulation to withdraw the most toxic OPs and carbamates from agricultural practice may be the only way to rapidly reduce the number of deaths globally.

REFERENCES

1. Abou-Donia MB, Lapadula DM. Mechanisms of organophosphorus ester-induced delayed neurotoxicity: type I and type II. *Annu Rev Pharmacol Toxicol.* 1990;30:405-440.
2. Ageda S, Fuke C, Ihama Y, Miyazaki T. The stability of organophosphorus insecticides in fresh blood. *Leg Med (Tokyo).* 2006;8:144-149.
3. Ahmed MM, Glees P. Neurotoxicity of tricresylphosphate (TCP) in slow loris (Nycticebus coucang coucang). *Acta Neuropathol.* 1971;19:94-98.
4. Anon. Calamity at Bhopal. *Lancet.* 1984;2:1378-1379.
5. Anon. Neurological findings among workers exposed to fenthion in a veterinary hospital: Georgia. *MMWR.* 1985;34:402-403.
6. Anon. Organophosphate toxicity associated with flea-dip products: California. *MMWR.* 1988;37:329-336.
7. Arima H, Sobue K, So M, Morishima T, Ando H, Katsuya H. Transient and reversible parkinsonism after acute organophosphate poisoning. *J Toxicol Clin Toxicol.* 2003;41:67-70.
8. Aring CD. The systemic nervous affinity of triorthocresyl phosphate (Jamaica ginger palsy). *Brain.* 1942;65:34-47.
9. Asari Y, Kamijyo Y, Soma K. Changes in the hemodynamic state of patients with acute lethal organophosphate poisoning. *Vet Hum Toxicol.* 2004;46:5-9.
10. Avasthi G, Singh G. Serial neuro-electrophysiological studies in acute organophosphate poisoning—correlation with clinical findings, serum cholinesterase levels and atropine dosages. *J Assoc Physicians India.* 2000;48:794-799.
11. Aygun D, Doganay Z, Altintop L, et al. Serum acetylcholinesterase and prognosis of acute organophosphate poisoning. *J Toxicol Clin Toxicol.* 2002;40:903-910.
12. Bardin PG, van Eeden SF. Organophosphate poisoning: grading the severity and comparing treatment between atropine and glycopyrrolate. *Crit Care Med.* 1990;18:956-960.
13. Bardin PG, van Eeden SF, Moolman JA, Foden AP, Joubert JR. Organophosphate and carbamate poisoning. *Arch Intern Med.* 1994;154:1433-1441.
14. Bar-Meir E, Schein O, Eisenkraft A, et al. Guidelines for treating cardiac manifestations of organophosphate poisoning with special emphasis on long QT and Torsades de Pointes. *Crit Rev Toxicol.* 2007;37:279-285.
15. Baron RL. Carbamate insecticides. In: Hayes WJ, Laws ER, eds. *Handbook of Pesticide Toxicology*. San Diego, CA: Academic Press; 1991:1125-1189.
16. Basnyat B. Organophosphate poisoning: the importance of the intermediate syndrome. *J Inst Med.* 2000;22:248-250.
17. Benfenati E, Gini G, Piclin N, Roncaglioni A, Vari MR. Predicting log P of pesticides using different software. *Chemosphere.* 2003;53:1155-1164.
18. Benson B, Tolo D, McIntire M. Is the intermediate syndrome in organophosphate poisoning the result of insufficient oxime therapy? *J Toxicol Clin Toxicol.* 1992;30:347.
19. Besser R, Gutmann L, Dillmann U, Weilemann LS, Hopf HC. End-plate dysfunction in acute organophosphate intoxication. *Neurology.* 1989;39:561-567.
20. Bhagat YA, Obenaus A, Hamilton MG, Mikler J, Kendall EJ. Neuroprotection from soman-induced seizures in the rodent: evaluation with diffusion- and T2-weighted magnetic resonance imaging. *Neurotoxicology.* 2005;26:1001-1013.
21. Bhatt MH, Elias MA, Mankodi AK. Acute and reversible parkinsonism due to organophosphate pesticide intoxication. Five cases. *Neurology.* 1999;52:1467-1471.
22. Bohn G, Rucker G, Luckas KH. [Mass spectrometric and gaschromatographic detection of parathione in autopsy material after murder by poisoning]. *Z Rechtsmed.* 1971;68:45-52.
23. Borowitz SM. Prolonged organophosphate toxicity in a twenty-six-month-old child. *J Pediatr.* 1988;112:302-304.
24. Bradberry SM, Proudfoot AT, Vale JA. Glyphosate poisoning. *Toxicol Rev.* 2004;23:159-167.
25. Brahmi N, Blel Y, Kouraichi N, Abidi N, Thabet H, Amamou M. Acute pancreatitis subsequent to voluntary methomyl and dichlorvos intoxication. *Pancreas.* 2006;31:424-427.
26. Buchholz U, Mermin J, Rios R, et al. An outbreak of food-borne illness associated with methomyl-contaminated salt. *JAMA.* 2002;288:604-610.
27. Buratti FM, D'Aniello A, Volpe MT, Meneguz A, Testai E. Malathion bioactivation in the human liver: the contribution of different cytochrome P450 isoforms. *Drug Metab Dispo.* 2005;33:295-302.
28. Buratti FM, Volpe MT, Meneguz A, Vittozzi L, Testai E. CYP-specific bioactivation of four organophosphorothioate pesticides by human liver microsomes. *Toxicol Appl Pharmacol.* 2003;186:143-154.
29. Calvert GM, Barnett M, Mehler LN, et al. Acute pesticide-related illness among emergency responders, 1993–2002. *Am J Ind Med.* 2006;49:383-393.
30. Casida JE, Nomura DK, Vose SC, Fujioka K. Organophosphate-sensitive lipases modulate brain lysophospholipids, ether lipids and endocannabinoids. *Chem Biol Interact.* 2008;175(1-3):355-364.

31. Casida JE, Quistad GB. Organophosphate toxicology: safety aspects of non-acetylcholinesterase secondary targets. *Chem Res Toxicol.* 2004;17:983-998.
32. Casida JE, Sanderson DM. Toxic hazard from formulating the insecticide dimethoate in methyl 'Cellosolve'. *Nature.* 1961;189:507-508.
33. Cavanagh JB, Davies DR, Holland P, Lancaster M. Comparison of the functional effects of dyflos, tri-o-cresyl phosphate and tri-pethylphenyl phosphate in chickens. *Brit J Pharmacol.* 1961;17:21-27.
34. Chadwick JA, Oosterbaan RA. Actions on insects and other invertebrates. In: Koelle GB, ed. *Cholinesterases and Anticholinesterase Agents. Handbook Experimental Pharmak, Vol 15.* Berlin: Springer-Verlag; 1963:299-373.
35. Chaudhry R, Lall SB, Mishra B, Dhawan B. A foodborne outbreak of organophosphate poisoning. *BMJ.* 1998;317:268-269.
36. Clifford NJ, Bies AS. Organophosphate poisoning from wearing a laundered uniform previously contaminated with parathion. *JAMA.* 1989;262:3035-3036.
37. Costa LG, Cole TB, Vitalone A, Furlong CE. Measurement of paraoxonase (PON1) status as a potential biomarker of susceptibility to organophosphate toxicity. *Clin Chim Acta.* 2005;352:37-47.
38. Coye MJ, Barnett PG, Midtling JE, et al. Clinical confirmation of organophosphate poisoning by serial cholinesterase analyses. *Arch Intern Med.* 1987;147:438-442.
39. Dagli AJ, Shaikh WA. Pancreatic involvement in malathion anticholinesterase insecticide intoxication—a study of 75 cases. *Br J Clin Prac.* 1983;37:270-272.
40. Dassanayake T, Weerasinghe V, Dangahadeniya U, et al. Cognitive processing of visual stimuli in patients with organophosphate insecticide poisoning. *Neurology.* 2007;68:2027-2030.
41. Dassanayake T, Weerasinghe V, Dangahadeniya U, et al. Long-term event-related potential changes following organophosphorus insecticide poisoning. *Clin Neurophysiol.* 2008;119:144-150.
42. Davies JE, Barquet A, Freed VH, et al. Human pesticide poisonings by a fat soluble organophosphate pesticide. *Arch Environ Health.* 1975;30:608-613.
43. Davies JOJ, Roberts DM, Eyer P, Buckley NA, Eddleston M. Hypotension in severe dimethoate self-poisoning. *Clin Toxicol (Phila).* 2008;46:880-884.
44. de Bleecker JL. The intermediate syndrome in organophosphate poisoning: an overview of experimental and clinical observations. *J Toxicol Clin Toxicol.* 1995;33:683.
45. de Candole CA, Douglas WW, Lovatt Evans C, et al. The failure of respiration in death by anticholinesterase poisoning. *Brit J Pharmacol.* 1953;8:466-475.
46. De Letter EA, Cordonnier JA, Piette MH. An unusual case of homicide by use of repeated administration of organophosphate insecticides. *J Clin Forensic Med.* 2002;9:15-21.
47. Dennis DT. Jake walk in Vietnam. *Ann Intern Med.* 1977;86:665-666.
48. Dewan A, Patel AB, Pal RR, Jani UJ, Singel VC, Panchal MD. Mass ethion poisoning with high mortality. *Clin Toxicol.* 2008;46:85-88.
49. Dick FD. Parkinson's disease and pesticide exposures. *Br Med Bull.* 2006;79-80:219-231.
50. Dickoff DJ, Gerber O, Turovsky Z. Delayed neurotoxicity after ingestion of carbamate pesticide. *Neurology.* 1987;37:1229-1231.
51. Dickson EW, Bird SB, Gaspari RJ, Boyer EW, Ferris CF. Diazepam inhibits organophosphate-induced central respiratory depression. *Acad Emerg Med.* 2003;10:1303-1306.
52. du Toit PW, Muller FO, van Tonder WM, Ungerer MJ. Experience with the intensive care management of organophosphate insecticide poisoning. *S Afr Med J.* 1981;60:227-229.
53. Eddleston M. Patterns and problems of deliberate self-poisoning in the developing world. *Q J Med.* 2000;93:715-731.
54. Eddleston M, Buckley NA, Checketts H, et al. Speed of initial atropinisation in significant organophosphorus pesticide poisoning—a systematic comparison of recommended regimens. *J Toxicol Clin Toxicol.* 2004;42:865-875.
55. Eddleston M, Buckley NA, Eyer P, Dawson AH. Medical management of acute organophosphorus pesticide poisoning. *Lancet.* 2008;371:597-607.
56. Eddleston M, Dawson A, Karalliedde L, et al. Early management after self-poisoning with an organophosphorus or carbamate pesticide—a treatment protocol for junior doctors. *Crit Care.* 2004;8:R391-R397.
57. Eddleston M, Eyer P, Worek F, et al. Pralidoxime chloride in acute organophosphorus insecticide self-poisoning—a randomised placebo-controlled trial. *PLoS Med.* 2009;6:e1000104.
58. Eddleston M, Eyer P, Worek F, et al. Differences between organophosphorus insecticides in human self-poisoning: a prospective cohort study. *Lancet.* 2005;366:1452-1459.
59. Eddleston M, Eyer P, Worek F, Sheriff MHR, Buckley NA. Predicting outcome using butyrylcholinesterase activity in organophosphorus pesticide self-poisoning. *Q J Med.* 2008;101:467-474.
60. Eddleston M, Juszczak E, Buckley NA, et al. Multiple-dose activated charcoal in acute self-poisoning: a randomised controlled trial. *Lancet.* 2008;371:579-586.
61. Eddleston M, Mohamed F, Davies JOJ, et al. Respiratory failure in acute organophosphorus pesticide self-poisoning. *Q J Med.* 2006;99:513-522.
62. Eddleston M, Szinicz L, Eyer P, Buckley N. Oximes in acute organophosphorus pesticide poisoning: a systematic review of clinical trials. *Q J Med.* 2002;95:275-283.
63. Engel LS, Checkoway H, Keifer MC, et al. Parkinsonism and occupational exposure to pesticides. *Occup Environ Med.* 2001;58:582-589.
64. Etzel RA, Forthal DN, Hill RH, Demby A. Fatal parathion poisoning in Sierra Leone. *Bull World Health Organ.* 1987;65:645-649.
65. Eyer F, Meischner V, Kiderlen D, et al. Human parathion poisoning. A toxicokinetic analysis. *Toxicol Rev.* 2003;22:143-163.
66. Eyer P. Neuropsychopathological changes by organophosphorus compounds—a review. *Hum Exp Toxicol.* 1995;14:857-864.
67. Eyer P. The role of oximes in the management of organophosphorus pesticide poisoning. *Toxicol Rev.* 2003;22:165-190.
68. Fisher JR. Guillain-Barre syndrome following organophosphate poisoning. *JAMA.* 1977;238:1950-1951.
69. Fredriksson T. Percutaneous absorption of parathion and paraoxon. IV. Decontamination of human skin from parathion. *Arch Environ Health.* 1961;3:185-188.
70. Fredriksson T, Bigelow JK. Tissue distribution of P32-labeled parathion. Autoradiographic technique. *Arch Environ Health.* 1961;2:663-667.
71. Freeman G, Epstein MA. Therapeutic factors in survival after lethal cholinesterase inhibition by phosphorus pesticides. *N Engl J Med.* 1955;253:266-271.
72. Gallo MA, Lawryk NJ. Organic phosphorus pesticides. In: Hayes WJ, Laws ER, eds. *Handbook of Pesticide Toxicology.* San Diego, CA: Academic Press; 1991:917-1123.
73. Geller RJ, Singleton KL, Tarantino ML. Nosocomial poisoning associated with emergency department treatment of organophosphate toxicity—Georgia, 2000. *MMWR.* 2001;49:1156-1158.
74. Gerkin R, Curry SC. Persistently elevated plasma insecticide levels in severe methylparathion poisoning. *Vet Hum Toxicol.* 1987;29:483-484.
75. Glynn P. A mechanism for organophosphate-induced delayed neuropathy. *Toxicol Lett.* 2006;162:94-97.
76. Goldman H, Teitel M. Malathion poisoning in a 34-month-old child following accidental ingestion. *J Pediatr.* 1958;52:76-81.
77. Gordon RK, Feaster SR, Russell AJ, et al. Organophosphate skin decontamination using immobilized enzymes. *Chem Biol Interact.* 1999;119-120:463-470.
78. Griffin P, Mason H, Heywood K, Cocker J. Oral and dermal absorption of chlorpyrifos: a human volunteer study. *Occup Environ Med.* 1999;56:10-13.
79. Grmec S, Mally S, Klemen P. Glasgow Coma Scale score and QTc interval in the prognosis of organophosphate poisoning. *Acad Emerg Med.* 2004;11:925-930.
80. Grob D, Harvey AM, Langworthy OR, Lilienthal JL. The administration of diisopropyl fluorophosphate (DFP) to man. Effect on the central nervous system with special reference to the electrical activity of the brain. *Bull Johns Hopkins Hosp.* 1947;81:257.
81. Grob D, Johns RJ. Use of oximes in the treatment of intoxication by anticholinesterase compounds in normal subjects. *Am J Med.* 1958;24:497-511.
82. Gross D. Clinical aspects: diagnosis and symptomatology. In: Albertini AV, Gross D, Zinn WM, eds. *Triaryl-Phosphate Poisoning in Morocco 1959.* Stuttgart: George Thieme; 1968:53-81.
83. Grubic Z, Sketelj J, Klinar B, Brzin M. Recovery of acetylcholinesterase in the diaphragm, brain, and plasma of the rat after irreversible inhibition by soman: a study of cytochemical localization and molecular forms of the enzyme in the motor end plate. *J Neurochem.* 1981;37:909-916.
84. Gunnell D, Eddleston M, Phillips MR, Konradsen F. The global distribution of fatal pesticide self-poisoning: systematic review. *BMC Public Health.* 2007;7:357.
85. Gunnell D, Fernando R, Hewagama M, Priyangika WDD, Konradsen F, Eddleston M. The impact of pesticide regulations on suicide in Sri Lanka. *Int J Epidemiol.* 2007;36:1235-1242.
86. Hardt J, Angerer J. Determination of dialkyl phosphates in human urine using gas chromatography-mass spectrometry. *J Anal Toxicol.* 2000;24:678-684.

87. Harputluoglu MMM, Kantarceken B, Karincaoglu M, et al. Acute pancreatitis: an obscure complication of organophosphate intoxication. *Hum Exp Toxicol.* 2003;22:341-343.
88. Hayes MM, van der Westhuizen NG, Gelfand M. Organophosphate poisoning in Rhodesia. A study of the clinical features and management of 105 patients. *S Afr Med J.* 1978;54:230-234.
89. He F, Xu H, Qin F, Xu L, Huang J, He X. Intermediate myasthenia syndrome following acute organophosphate poisoning—an analysis of 21 cases. *Hum Exp Toxicol.* 1998;17:40-45.
90. Heath AJW, Meredith T. Atropine in the management of anticholinesterase poisoning. In: Ballantyne B, Marrs T, eds. *Clinical and Experimental Toxicology of Organophosphates and Carbamates.* Oxford: Butterworth Heinemann; 1992:543-554.
91. Herishanu YO, Medvedovski M, Goldsmith JR, Kordysh E. A case-control study of Parkinson's disease in urban population of southern Israel. *Can J Neurol Sci.* 2001;28:144-147.
92. Hoizey G, Canas F, Binet L, et al. Thiodicarb and methomyl tissue distribution in a fatal multiple compounds poisoning. *J Forensic Sci.* 2008;53:499-502.
93. Holmes JH. Organophosphorus insecticides in Colorado. *Arch Environ Health.* 1964;9:445-453.
94. Holmstedt B. Structure-activity relationship of the organophosphorus anticholinesterase agents. In: Koelle GB, ed. *Handbuch der Experimentellen Pharmakologie.* Berlin: Springer-Verlag; 1963:428-485.
95. Holmstedt B. The ordeal bean of Old Calabar: the pageant of Physostigma venenosum in medicine. In: Swain T, ed. *Plants in the Development of Modern Medicine.* Cambridge, MA: Harvard University Press; 1972:303-360.
96. Hopmann G, Wanke H. [Maximum dose atropine treatment in severe organophosphate poisoning]. *Dtsch Med Wochenschr.* 1974;99:2106-2108.
97. Hruban Z, Schulman S, Warner NE, Du Bois KP, Bunnag S, Bunnag SC. Hypoglycemia resulting from insecticide poisoning. Report of a case. *JAMA.* 1963;184:590-593.
98. Ikizceli I, Yurumez Y, Avsarofullari L, et al. Effect of interleukin-10 on pancreatic damage caused by organophosphate poisoning. *Regul Toxicol Pharmacol.* 2005;42:260-264.
99. Inoue S, Saito T, Mase H, et al. Rapid simultaneous determination for organophosphorus pesticides in human serum by LC–MS. *J Pharm Biomed Anal.* 2007;44:258-264.
100. Jayawardane P, Dawson AH, Weerasinghe V, Karalliedde L, Buckley NA, Senanayake N. The spectrum of intermediate syndrome following acute organophosphate poisoning: a prospective cohort study from Sri Lanka. *PLoS Med.* 2008;5:e147.
101. John M, Oommen A, Zachariah A. Muscle injury in organophosphorous poisoning and its role in the development of intermediate syndrome. *Neurotoxicology.* 2003;24:43-53.
102. Johnson MK. Organophosphates and delayed neuropathy—is NTE alive and well? *Toxicol Appl Pharmacol.* 1990;102:385-399.
103. Johnson MK. The delayed neurotoxic effect of some organophosphorus compounds. Identification of the phosphorylation site as an esterase. *Biochem J.* 1969;114:711-717.
104. Johnson MK, Jacobsen D, Meredith TJ, et al. Evaluation of antidotes for poisoning by organophosphorus pesticides. *Emerg Med.* 2000;12:22-37.
105. Kamijo Y, Soma K, Uchimiya H, Asari Y, Ohwada T. A case of serious organophosphate poisoning treated by percutaneus cardiopulmonary support. *Vet Hum Toxicol.* 1999;41:326-328.
106. Karalliedde L, Baker D, Marrs TC. Organophosphate-induced intermediate syndrome: aetiology and relationships with myopathy. *Toxicol Rev.* 2006;25:1-14.
107. Karalliedde L, Edwards P, Marrs TC. Variables influencing the toxic response to organophosphates in humans. *Food Chem Toxicol.* 2003;41:1-13.
108. Katewa SD, Katyare SS. Antimalarials inhibit human erythrocyte membrane acetylcholinesterase. *Drug Chem Toxicol.* 2005;28:467-482.
109. Kiss Z, Fazekas T. Arrhythmias in organophosphate poisoning. *Acta Cardiol.* 1979;34:323-330.
110. Koksal N, Buyukbese MA, Guven A, Cetinkaya A, Hasanoglu HC. Organophosphate intoxication as a consequence of mouth-to-mouth breathing from an affected case. *Chest.* 2002;122:740-741.
111. Kubistova J. Parathion metabolism in female rat. *Arch Int Pharmacodyn Ther.* 1959;118:308-316.
112. Kupfermann N, Schmoldt A, Steinhart H. Rapid and sensitive quantitative analysis of alkyl phosphates in urine after organophosphate poisoning. *J Anal Toxicol.* 2004;28:242-248.
113. Kurtz PH. Pralidoxime in the treatment of carbamate intoxication. *Am J Emerg Med.* 1990;8:68-70.
114. Kventsel I, Berkovitch M, Reiss A, Bulkowstein M, Kozer E. Scopolamine treatment for severe extra-pyramidal signs following organophosphate (chlorpyrifos) ingestion. *Clin Toxicol.* 2005;43:877-879.
115. Li B, Sedlacek M, Manoharan I, et al. Butyrylcholinesterase, paraoxonase, and albumin esterase, but not carboxylesterase, are present in human plasma. *Biochem Pharmacol.* 2005;70:1673-1684.
116. Lieske CN, Clark JH, Maxwell DM, Zoeffel LD, Sultan WE. Studies of the amplification of carbaryl toxicity by various oximes. *Toxicol Lett.* 1992;62:127-137.
117. Little M, Murray L. Consensus statement: risk of nosocomial organophosphate poisoning in emergency departments. *Emerg Med Australasia.* 2004;16:456-458.
118. Lokan R, James R. Rapid death by mevinphos poisoning while under observation. *Forensic Sci Int.* 1983;22:179-182.
119. Lotti M, Becker CE. Treatment of acute organophosphate poisoning: evidence of a direct effect on central nervous system by 2-PAM (pyridine-2-aldoxime methyl chloride). *J Toxicol Clin Toxicol.* 1982;19:121-127.
120. Lyzhnikov EA, Savina AS, Shepelev VM. Pathogenesis of disorders of cardiac rhythm and conductivity in acute organophasphate insecticide poisoning [Article in Russian]. *Kardiologiia.* 1975;15:126-129.
121. Manoguerra A, Whitney C, Clark RF, Anderson B, Turchen S. Cholinergic toxicity resulting from ocular instillation of echothiophate iodide eye drops. *J Toxicol Clin Toxicol.* 1995;33:463-465.
122. Marrs TC. Diazepam in the treatment of organophosphorus ester pesticide poisoning. *Toxicol Rev.* 2003;22:75-81.
123. Massoulie J, Anselmet A, Bon S, et al. Acetylcholinesterase: C-terminal domains, molecular forms and functional localization. *J Physiol (Paris).* 1998;92:183-190.
124. McDonough JH Jr, Jaax NK, Crowley RA, Mays MZ, Modrow HE. Atropine and/or diazepam therapy protects against soman-induced neural and cardiac pathology. *Fundam Appl Toxicol.* 1989;13:256-276.
125. Medicis JJ, Stork CM, Howland MA, Hoffman RS, Goldfrank LR. Pharmacokinetics following a loading plus a continuous infusion of pralidoxime compared with the traditional short infusion regimen in human volunteers. *Clin Toxicol.* 1996;34:289-295.
126. Meggs WJ. Permanent paralysis at sites of dermal exposure to chlorpyrifos. *J Toxicol Clin Toxicol.* 2003;41:883-886.
127. Meller D, Fraser I, Kryger M. Hyperglycemia in anticholinergic poisoning. *Can Med Assoc J.* 1981;124:745-748.
128. Mercurio-Zappala M, Hack JB, Salvador A, Hoffman RS. Pralidoxime in carbaryl poisoning: an animal model. *Hum Exp Toxicol.* 2007;26:125-129.
129. Merrill DG, Mihm FG. Prolonged toxicity of organophosphate poisoning. *Crit Care Med.* 1982;10:550-551.
130. Morgan JP, Penovich P. Jamaica ginger paralysis: Forty-seven-year follow-up. *Arch Neurol.* 1978;35:530-532.
131. Moriya F, Hashimoto Y. A fatal poisoning caused by methomyl and nicotine. *Forensic Sci Int.* 2005;149:167-170.
132. Moriya F, Hashimoto Y. Comparative studies on tissue distributions of organophosphorus, carbamate and organochlorine pesticides in decedents intoxicated with these chemicals. *J Forensic Sci.* 1999;44:1131-1135.
133. Muller TC, Rocha JB, Morsch VM, Neis RT, Schetinger MR. Antidepressants inhibit human acetylcholinesterase and butyrylcholinesterase activity. *Biochim Biophys Acta.* 2002;1587:92-98.
134. Muller-Vahl KR, Kolbe H, Dengler R. Transient severe parkinsonism after acute organophosphate poisoning. *J Neurol Neurosurg Psychiatry.* 1999;66:253-254.
135. Murphy MR, Blick DW, Dunn MA. Diazepam as a treatment for nerve agent poisoning in primates. *Aviat Space Environ Med.* 1993;64:110-115.
136. Namba T, Greenfield M, Grob D. Malathion poisoning. A fatal case with cardiac manifestations. *Arch Environ Health.* 1970;21:533-541.
137. Namba T, Hiraki K. PAM (pyridine-2-aldoxime methiodide) therapy of alkylphosphate poisoning. *JAMA.* 1958;166:1834-1839.
138. Namba T, Nolte C, Jackrel J, Grob D. Poisoning due to organophosphate insecticides. *Am J Med.* 1971;50:475-492.
139. Namba T, Taniguchi Y, Okazaki S, et al. Treatment of severe organophosphorus poisoning by large doses of PAM. *Naika no Ryoiki [Domain of Internal Medicine].* 1959;7:709-713.
140. Nelson LS, Perrone J, DeRoos F, Stork C, Hoffman RS. Aldicarb poisoning by an illicit rodenticide imported into the United States: Tres Pasitos. *J Toxicol Clin Toxicol.* 2001;39:447-452.

141. Nolan CM, Elarth AM, Barr HW. Intentional isoniazid overdosage in young Southeast Asian refugee women. *Chest.* 1988;93:803-806.
142. Pach D. The usefulness of scintigraphic examination for the evaluation of hepatotoxic impact of cholinesterase inhibitors. *Przegl Lek.* 1996;53: 313-323.
143. Padilla S, Marshall RS, Hunter DL, Lowit A. Time course of cholinesterase inhibition in adult rats treated acutely with carbaryl, carbofuran, formetanate, methomyl, methiocarb, oxamyl or propoxur. *Toxicol Appl Pharmacol.* 2007;219:202-209.
144. Panieri E, Krige JE, Bornman PC, Linton DM. Severe necrotizing pancreatitis caused by organophosphate poisoning. *J Clin Gastroenterol.* 1997;25:463-465.
145. Parker PE, Brown FW. Organophosphate intoxication: hidden hazards. *South Med J.* 1989;82:1408-1410.
146. Pawar KS, Bhoite RR, Pillay CP, Chavan SC, Malshikare DS, Garad SG. Continuous pralidoxime infusion versus repeated bolus injection to treat organophosphorus pesticide poisoning: a randomised controlled trial. *Lancet.* 2006;368:2136-2141.
147. Peeples ES, Schopfer LM, Duysen EG, et al. Albumin, a new biomarker of organophosphorus toxicant exposure, identified by mass spectrometry. *Toxicol Sci.* 2005;83:303-312.
148. Perez GF, Martinez Pretel CM, Tarin RF, et al. Prolonged suxamethonium-induced neuromuscular blockade associated with organophosphate poisoning. *Br J Anaesth.* 1988;61:233-236.
149. Peter JV, Moran JL, Graham P. Oxime therapy and outcomes in human organophosphate poisoning: an evaluation using meta-analytic techniques. *Crit Care Med.* 2006;34:502-510.
150. Peter JV, Prabhakar AT, Pichamuthu K. In-laws, insecticide—and a mimic of brain death. *Lancet.* 2008;371:622.
151. Prellwitz W, Schuster HP, Schylla G, et al. [Differential diagnosis of organ involvement in exogenous poisoning by means of clinical and clinicochemical studies]. *Klin Wochenschr.* 1970;48:51-53.
152. Ragoucy-Sengler C, Tracqui A, Chavonnet A, et al. Aldicarb poisoning. *Hum Exp Toxicol.* 2000;19:657-662.
153. Rahimi R, Nikfar S, Abdollahi M. Increased morbidity and mortality in acute human organophosphate-poisoned patients treated by oximes: a meta-analysis of clinical trials. *Hum Exp Toxicol.* 2006;25:157-162.
154. Robenshtok E, Luria S, Tashma Z, Hourvitz A. Adverse reaction to atropine and the treatment of organophosphate intoxication. *Isr Med Assoc J.* 2002;4:535-539.
155. Roberts DM, Fraser JF, Buckley NA, Venkatesh B. Experiences of anticholinesterase pesticide poisonings in an Australian tertiary hospital. *Anaesth Intens Care.* 2005;33:469-476.
156. Rosenthal E. The tragedy of Tauccamarca: a human rights perspective on the pesticide poisoning deaths of 4 children in the Peruvian Andes. *Int J Occup Environ Health.* 2003;9:53-58.
157. Roth A, Zellinger I, Arad M, Atsmon J. Organophosphates and the heart. *Chest.* 1993;103:576-582.
158. Ruangyuttikarn W, Phakdeewut T, Sainumtan W, Sribanditmongkol P. Children's plasma cholinesterase activity and fatal methomyl poisoning. *J Med Assoc Thai.* 2001;84:1344-1350.
159. Saadeh AM, Farsakh NA, al Ali MK. Cardiac manifestations of acute carbamate and organophosphate poisoning. *Heart.* 1997;77:461-464.
160. Sahin I, Onbasi K, Sahin H, Karakaya C, Ustun Y, Noyan T. The prevalence of pancreatitis in organophosphate poisonings. *Hum Exp Toxicol.* 2002;21:175-177.
161. Sakamoto T, Sawada Y, Nishide K, et al. Delayed neurotoxicity produced by an organophosphorus compound (Sumithion). A case report. *Arch Toxicol.* 1984;56:136-138.
162. Seifert J. Toxicologic significance of the hyperglycemia caused by organophosphorous insecticides. *Bull Environ Contam Toxicol.* 2001;67:463-469.
163. Senanayake N, Jeyaratnam J. Toxic polyneuropathy due to ginger oil contaminated with tri-cresyl phosphate affecting adolescent girls in Sri Lanka. *Lancet.* 1981;i:88-89.
164. Senanayake N, Karalliedde L. Neurotoxic effects of organophosphate insecticides: an intermediate syndrome. *N Engl J Med.* 1987;316:761-763.
165. Sener EB, Ustun E, Kocamanoglu S, Tur A. Prolonged apnea following succinylcholine administration in undiagnosed acute organophosphate poisoning. *Acta Anaesthesiol Scand.* 2002;46:1046-1048.
166. Seybold R, Brautigam KH. Prolonged suxamethonium-induced apnoea as a sign of organophosphate poisoning. *Ger Med Mon.* 1969;14:12-13.
167. Sharma DC. Bhopal: 20 years on. *Lancet.* 2005;365:111-112.
168. Shih DM, Gu L, Xia YR, et al. Mice lacking serum paraoxanase are susceptible to organophosphate toxicity and atherosclerosis. *Nature.* 1998;394:284-287.
169. Singh S, Bhardwaj U, Verma SK, Bhalla A, Gill K. Hyperamylasemia and pancreatitis following anticholinesterase poisoning. *Hum Exp Toxicol.* 2007;26:467-471.
170. Sozmen EY, Mackness B, Sozmen B, et al. Effect of organophosphate intoxication on human serum paraoxonase. *Hum Exp Toxicol.* 2002;21:247-252.
171. Stacey R, Morfey D, Payne S. Secondary contamination in organophosphate poisoning: analysis of an incident. *Q J Med.* 2004;97:75-80.
172. Steenland K, Dick RB, Howell RJ, et al. Neurologic function among termiticide applicators exposed to chlorpyrifos. *Environ Health Perspect.* 2000;108:293-300.
173. Stephenson J. Exposure to home pesticides linked to Parkinson disease. *JAMA.* 2000;283:3055-3056.
174. Sudakin DL, Mullins ME, Horowitz BZ, Abshier V, Letzig L. Intermediate syndrome after malathion ingestion despite continuous infusion of pralidoxime. *J Toxicol Clin Toxicol.* 2000;38:47-50.
175. Sudakin DL, Power LE. Organophosphate exposures in the United States: a longitudinal analysis of incidents reported to poison centers. *J Toxicol Environ Health A.* 2007;70:141-147.
176. Sultatos LG. Mammalian toxicology of organophosphorus pesticides. *J Toxicol Environ Health.* 1994;43:271-289.
177. Sun J, Lynn BC. Development of a MALDI-TOF-MS method to identify and quantify butyrylcholinesterase inhibition resulting from exposure to organophosphate and carbamate pesticides. *J Am Soc Mass Spectrom.* 2007;18:698-706.
178. Sundwall A. Minimum concentrations of N-methylpyridinium-2-aldoxime methane sulphonate (P2S) which reverse neuromuscular block. *Biochem Pharmacol.* 1961;8:413-417.
179. Svraka L, Sovljanski R, Sovljanski M. [4 cases of murder with organophosphorous compound]. *Arh Hig Rada Toksikol.* 1966;17:447-453.
180. Taylor CA, Saint-Hilaire MH, Cupples LA, et al. Environmental, medical, and family history risk factors for Parkinson's disease: a New England-based case control study. *Am J Med Genet.* 1999;88:742-749.
181. Taylor P. Anticholinesterase agents. In: Brunton LL, Lazo JS, Parker KL, eds. *Goodman and Gilman's the Pharmacological Basis of Therapeutics.* New York: McGraw-Hill; 2006:201-216.
182. Teimouri F, Amirkabirian N, Esmaily H, Mohammadirad A, Aliahmadi A, Abdollahi M. Alteration of hepatic cells glucose metabolism as a non-cholinergic detoxication mechanism in counteracting diazinon-induced oxidative stress. *Hum Exp Toxicol.* 2006;25:696-703.
183. Thiermann H, Kehe K, Steinritz D, et al. Red blood cell acetylcholinesterase and plasma butyrylcholinesterase status: important indicators for the treatment of patients poisoned by organophosphorus compounds. *Arh Hig Rada Toksikol.* 2007;58:359-366.
184. Thiermann H, Szinicz L, Eyer F, et al. Modern strategies in therapy of organophosphate poisoning. *Toxicol Lett.* 1999;107:233-239.
185. Thiermann H, Szinicz L, Eyer P, Zilker T, Worek F. Correlation between red blood cell acetylcholinesterase activity and neuromuscular transmission in organophosphate poisoning. *Chem Biol Interact.* 2005;157-8:345-347.
186. Thiermann H, Worek F, Szinicz L, et al. On the atropine demand in organophosphate poisoned patients. *J Toxicol Clin Toxicol.* 2003;41:457.
187. Tisdale WH, Flenver AL. Derivatives of dithiocarbamic acid as pesticides. *Ind Eng Chem.* 1942;34:506.
188. Tsai JR, Sheu CC, Cheng MH, et al. Organophosphate poisoning: 10 years of experience in southern Taiwan. *Kaohsiung J Med Sci.* 2007;23:112-119.
189. Tsai MC, Hwang JS, Chen CC, Wang SC, Liao JW. Safety evaluation in rats of alternative solvents for pesticides formulated with emulsifiable concentrate. *Plant Prot Bull.* 2004;46:267-280.
190. Tsai MJ, Wu SN, Cheng HA, Wang SH, Chiang HT. An outbreak of food-borne illness due to methomyl contamination. *J Toxicol Clin Toxicol.* 2003;41:969-973.
191. Umehara F, Izumo S, Arimura K, Osame M. Polyneuropathy induced by m-tolyl methyl carbamate intoxication. *J Neurol.* 1991;238:47-48.
192. van Hecke W. A case of murder by parathion (E605) which nearly escaped detection. *Med Sci Law.* 1964;4:197-199.
193. Vasilescu C, Alexianu M, Dan A. Delayed neuropathy after organophosphorus insecticide (Dipterex) poisoning: a clinical, electrophysiological, and nerve biopsy study. *J Neurol Neurosurg Psychiatry.* 1984;47:543-548.
194. Wadia RS, Bhirud RH, Gulavani AV, Amin RB. Neurological manifestations of three organophosphate poisons. *Indian J Med Res.* 1977;66: 460-468.

195. Wadia RS, Sadagopan C, Amin RB, Sardesai HV. Neurological manifestations of organophosphate insecticide poisoning. *J Neurol Neurosurg Psychiatry.* 1974;37:841-847.
196. Warriner RA, III, Nies AS, Hayes WJ Jr. Severe organophosphate poisoning complicated by alcohol and turpentine ingestion. *Arch Environ Health.* 1977;32:203-205.
197. Weizman Z, Sofer S. Acute pancreatitis in children with anticholinesterase insecticide intoxication. *Pediatrics.* 1992;90:204-206.
198. Wesseling C, Castillo L, Elinder CG. Pesticide poisonings in Costa Rica. *Scand J Work Environ Health.* 1993;19:227-235.
199. Wesseling C, McConnell R, Partanen T, Hogstedt C. Agricultural pesticide use in developing countries: health effects and research needs. *Int J Health Services.* 1997;27:273-308.
200. Westfall TC, Westfall DP. Neurotransmission: the autonomic and somatic motor nervous systems. In Brunton LL, Lazo JS, Parker KL, eds. *Goodman and Gilman's the Pharmacological Basis of Therapeutics.* New York: McGraw-Hill; 2006:137-181.
201. Willems JL, de Bisschop HC, Verstraete AG, et al. Cholinesterase reactivation in organophosphorus poisoned patients depends on the plasma concentrations of the oxime pralidoxime methylsulphate and of the organophosphate. *Arch Toxicol.* 1993;67:79-84.
202. Wislon IB, Hatch MA, Ginsburg S. Carbamylation of acetvlcholinesterase. *J Biol Chem.* 1960;235:2312-2315.
203. Worek F, Mast U, Kiderlen D, Diepold C, Eyer P. Improved determination of acetylcholinesterase activity in human whole blood. *Clin Chim Acta.* 1999;288:73-90.
204. World Health Organization. *The WHO Recommended Classification of Pesticides by Hazard and Guidelines to Classification: 2004.*, 0 edn. Geneva: WHO; 2005.
205. Yang PY, Tsao TCY, Lin JL, Lyu RK, Chaing PC. Carbofuran-induced delayed neuropathy. *J Toxicol Clin Toxicol.* 2000;38:43-46.
206. Zadik Z, Blachar Y, Barak Y, Levin S. Organophosphate poisoning presenting as diabetic ketoacidosis. *J Toxicol Clin Toxicol.* 1983;20:381-385.
207. Zhang J, Zhao J, Sun S, et al. [A clinical analysis of 104 cases of acute pure and mixed organophosphate poisoning]. *Zhonghua Nei Ke Za Zhi.* 2002;41:544-546.
208. Zilker T, Hibler A. Treatment of severe parathion poisoning. In Szinicz L, Eyer P, Klimmek R. *Role of Oximes in the Treatment of Anticholinesterase Agent Poisoning.* Heidelberg: Spektrum, Akademischer Verlag; 1996:9-17.
209. Zwiener RJ, Ginsburg CM. Organophosphate and carbamate poisoning in infants and children. *Pediatrics.* 1988;81:121-126.

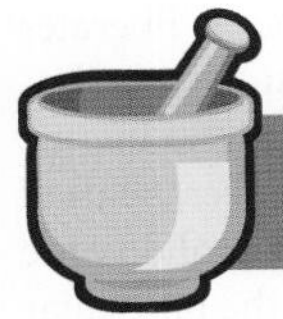

ANTIDOTES IN DEPTH (A33)

PRALIDOXIME

Mary Ann Howland

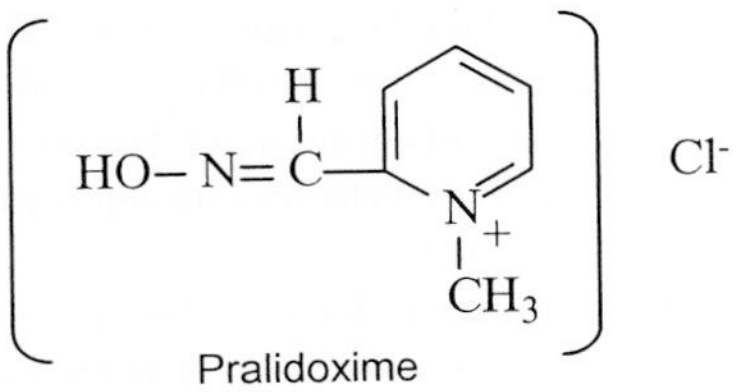

Cl^-

Pralidoxime

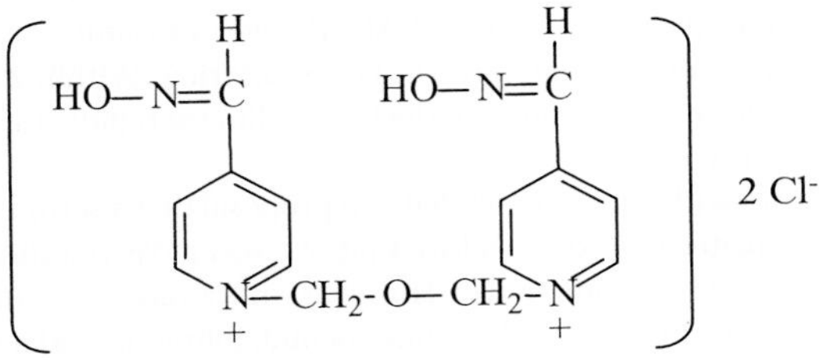

2 Cl^-

Obidoxime

2 Cl^-

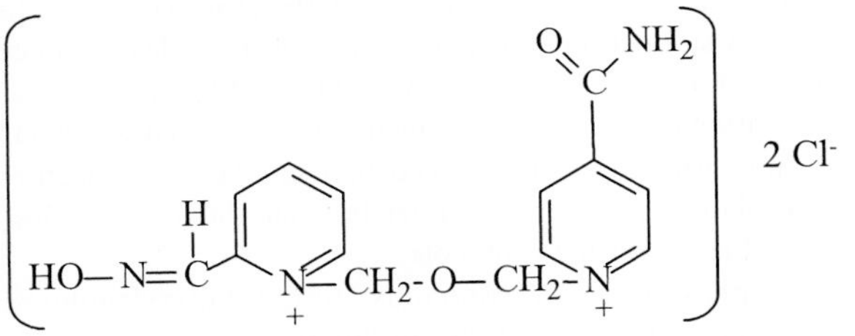

Asoxime (HI6)

Pralidoxime chloride (2-PAM) is the only cholinesterase-reactivating xenobiotic currently available in the United States.[55] It is used concomitantly with atropine in the management of patients poisoned by organic phosphorus (OP) compounds. Administration should be initiated as soon as possible after exposure, but could be effective even days after an exposure and therefore should be administered to all symptomatic patients independent of delay. Continuous infusion is preferable to intermittent administration for patients with serious toxicity, and a prolonged therapeutic course may be required.

CHEMISTRY

Pralidoxime chloride is a quaternary pyridinium oxime with a molecular weight of 173 daltons. The chloride salt exhibits excellent water solubility and physiologic compatibility. Another salt, pralidoxime iodide, with a molecular weight of 264 daltons, is less water soluble and can potentiallly induce iodism.[3]

REACTIVATION OF CHOLINESTERASES FOLLOWING ORGANIC PHOSPHORUS POISONING

Organic phosphorus compounds are powerful inhibitors of carboxylic esterase enzymes, including acetylcholinesterase (AChE; true cholinesterase, found in red blood cells, nervous tissue, and skeletal muscle) and plasma cholinesterase or butyrylcholinesterase (found in plasma, liver, heart, pancreas, and brain).[49] The OP binds firmly to the serine-containing esteratic site on the enzyme, inactivating it by phosphorylation (Fig. 113–3).[32,50,73] This reaction results in the accumulation of acetylcholine at muscarinic and nicotinic synapses in the peripheral and central nervous systems, leading to the clinical manifestations of OP poisoning. After phosphorylation, the enzyme is inactivated and can undergo one of three processes: endogenous hydrolysis of the phosphorylated enzyme; reactivation by a strong nucleophile, such as pralidoxime; and aging, which involves biochemical changes that stabilize the inactivated phosphorylated molecule.

Endogenous hydrolysis of the bond between the enzyme and the OP is generally extremely slow and is considered insignificant. This is in contrast to the rapid hydrolysis of the related bond between the enzyme and many carbamates. Studies in the 1950s demonstrated the ability of oximes to reactivate cholinesterase bound to OP compounds.[81,83,84] The positively charged quaternary nitrogen of pralidoxime is attracted to the negatively charged anionic site on the phosphorylated enzyme, bringing it in close proximity to the phosphorous moiety (Fig. 113–6). Pralidoxime then exerts a nucleophilic attack on the phosphate moiety, successfully releasing it from the AChE enzyme.[80] This action liberates the enzyme to a variable extent depending on the OP in question and restores enzymatic function.[40] It was previously believed that OP compounds with small substituted side chains were more easily reversed by oximes because of better steric positioning, allowing easier access for the oximes.[83] However, available data now refute that theory, but continue to emphasize the importance of spatial and steric considerations.[86]

In contrast to the usefulness of pralidoxime in the management of the cholinergic syndrome, current understanding of the pathophysiology of the intermediate syndrome is inadequate to determine whether pralidoxime can prevent the development of the syndrome.[71] However, if cholinergic receptor desensitization is responsible for the cause of the muscle weakness, then pralidoxime would be unlikely to prevent the syndrome, especially after large intentional ingestions.[12] Additionally, certain OP pesticides may lead to the development of delayed onset neurotoxicity, which involves inhibition of neurotoxic esterases that cannot be prevented or treated by pralidoxime.[18,43]

EFFICACY RELATED TO TIME OF ADMINISTRATION AFTER POISONING

Early in vitro evidence suggested that the successful use of cholinesterase reactivators depended on administration within 24 to 48 hours of exposure to the OPs; afterwards, the acetylcholinesterases would be irreversibly inactivated.[4,14,28,29,64] However, according to currently available information there is no absolute time limitation on reactivator function. The 48-hour limit was derived from in vitro experiments using a small number of tightly bound compounds and reactivators and data from plasma cholinesterase enzyme activity, which is now recognized to be relatively resistant to oxime-nucleophilic attack. These early data were accepted without consideration of their relevance to human systems, the use of newer and less tightly bound OP compounds, temperature and pH variation, blood flow, fat solubility, active metabolites, and species specificity. Fat-soluble OP compounds redistribute from fat stores over time, acting similarly to sustained-release products. Even if they have not aged, they continue to reinhibit AChE for days.

An in vitro experiment assessed the effect of aging on the ability of pralidoxime to regenerate rat erythrocyte and brain cholinesterases using three different OP compounds.[77] The rate of reactivation of erythrocyte and brain cholinesterases was significantly decreased over time for fenitrothion and methyl parathion, with no reactivation occurring at 48 hours. This is partly because dimethylated (dimethyl, dimethoxy) OP pesticides age more quickly than diethylphosphorylated agents.[18] In contrast, a very high reactivation rate for ethyl parathion was still apparent at 48 hours. Thus the structure of the OP compound is important in the rates of aging and reactivation with pralidoxime. Fenitrothion and methyl parathion are both O'O dimethyl OP compounds as is dimethoate, whereas ethyl parathion is an O'O diethyl OP compound.[77] Other studies also suggest that pralidoxime is effective long after the previously suggested 48-hour window of therapy.[2,5,8,13,16,18,19,47,79]

CARBAMATES

Acetylcholinesterases inactivated by most carbamates spontaneously reactivate with half-lives of 1 to 2 hours, and typical clinical recovery occurs in several hours. However, in severe cases, cholinergic findings may persist for 24 hours.[10,25] Pralidoxime is rarely indicated for carbamate poisoning, but it is not generally contraindicated as was previously suggested. This erroneous conclusion was based solely on data regarding a single carbamate, carbaryl, and inappropriately applied to all carbamates. Pralidoxime decreased the rate of carbamylation of 16 insecticidal carbamates, though it modestly increased the rates for three, one of which was carbaryl.[15] In vitro experiments demonstrated that pralidoxime had no effect on the reactivation of erythrocyte AChE carbamylated by aldicarb, methomyl, and carbaryl.[37] Furthermore, animal studies demonstrated the beneficial effects of pralidoxime in decreasing the lethality of several carbamate insecticides,[51,70] though it worsened the toxicity of carbaryl. It was suggested that this is possibly because the carbamate-oxime complex may actually be a more potent cholinesterase inhibitor than carbaryl alone.[25,51,70] However, even in the presence of carbaryl, the combination of atropine plus an oxime, a more clinically relevant situation, resulted in survival data comparable to that of atropine alone.[25] Previous animal data may also be confounded by using inappropriately high doses and potential overdoses of pralidoxime.[45] This evidence suggests that although pralidoxime is not usually a necessary adjunct to atropine for a patient with a pure carbamate overdose, it may nevertheless occasionally improve morbidity and mortality.[10] Thus pralidoxime should never be withheld in a seriously poisoned patient out of concern that a cholinergic xenobiotic may be a carbamate.[37] However, pralidoxime should be used in conjunction with atropine and never as the sole therapeutic agent.

PHARMACOLOGY

Pralidoxime is important at nicotinic sites where atropine is ineffective, most often improving muscle strength within 10 to 40 minutes after administration.[50,73] This effect is vital to maintaining the muscles of respiration. Pralidoxime is also synergistic with atropine, it liberates cholinesterase enzyme so that additional acetylcholine can be metabolized while atropine inhibits the effects of acetylcholine at cholinergic receptors. This suggests that pralidoxime should rarely, if ever, be used alone.[22,50] Some OP compounds respond much better to pralidoxime than others, depending on the affinity of pralidoxime for the particular type of phosphorylated enzyme, its reactivating ability, concentrations of both the oxime and the OP, aging, and OP redistribution from a depot site such as fat.[21,84]

The central nervous system (CNS) benefits of pralidoxime are controversial, as the molecule is a quaternary nitrogen compound and not expected to cross the blood–brain barrier.[42,50] Animal studies suggest conflicting results.[46] Rat studies using radiolabeled pralidoxime demonstrated a lack of any radioactivity in the CNS after intravenous (IV) administration.[76] Following exposure to IV fenitrothion, IV administration of pralidoxime in rats failed to improve survival or to reactivate brain cholinesterase, whereas intramedullary pralidoxime partially restored brain cholinesterase and eliminated fatalities.[76] A more recent rat experiment using a microdialysis technique demonstrated only 10% CNS penetration of pralidoxime.[63]

Clinical observations, however, have certainly suggested a CNS action of pralidoxime with a prompt return of consciousness reported in some cases.[49,50,58,80] A 3-year-old child who was comatose from parathion was given 500 mg of 2-PAM IV over 15 minutes with continuous electroencephalographic (EEG) monitoring. Within 2 minutes there was a dramatic response on the EEG, followed rapidly by normalization of consciousness.[31]

Early work with feline models led to a proposal that a serum concentration of greater than or equal to 4 μg/mL was a desired therapeutic concentration for pralidoxime.[72] However, more recent in vitro work with human erythrocytes and a mouse hemidiaphragm model suggests that higher serum concentrations are actually needed.[84] Twenty percent reactivation was achieved in 5 minutes with serum concentrations of 10 μg/mL.[84] A simulation and analysis suggests that plasma concentrations between 10 and 15 μg/mL (50–100 μmol/L) are necessary for optimal treatment of severely poisoned patients.[19,86] These recommendations await validation in poisoned patients. Serum concentrations are not available in a timely manner but may help in the design of future pralidoxime dosing protocols.

Organic phosphorous compounds inhibit butyrylcholinesterase (plasma cholinesterase) and AChE to different extents.[17] If performed correctly, butyrylcholinesterase may act as a surrogate marker for OP or carbamate elimination from the body.[34] Likewise, the reactivation of butyrylcholinesterase by pralidoxime is dependent on the concentration of pralidoxime and often has a flat dose response. For example, in an in vitro model of human blood taken from healthy volunteers and treated with paraoxon, pralidoxime was able to reactivate 1.3% and 18.1% of AChE at pralidoxime concentrations of 10 μM and 100 μM, respectively, compared with 1% and 5.5% of butyrylcholinesterase with 10 and 100 μM concentrations of pralidoxime.[31] Unless the effect of the specific OP on butyrylcholinesterase is known, there is no role for following serial butyrylcholinesterase concentrations.

PHARMACOKINETICS AND PHARMACODYNAMICS

Pralidoxime chloride pharmacokinetics are characterized by a two-compartment model. Pharmacokinetics values vary depending on whether calculations are determined in healthy volunteers or poisoned patients. The volume of distribution is larger in poisoned patients and most likely accounts for the prolonged elimination phase.[19]

In volunteers, the volume of distribution is about 0.8 L/kg and the half-life is 75 minutes.[30,56,69] Pralidoxime is renally excreted, and within 12 hours, 80% of the dose is recovered unchanged in the urine.[68]

A dose of 10 mg/kg of pralidoxime administered intramuscularly (IM) to volunteers results in peak serum concentrations of 6 μg/mL (reached 5–15 minutes after IM injection) and a half-life of approximately 75 minutes.[68] Following a standard IV 30-minute infusion dose of 1 g of pralidoxime in a 70-kg man, the serum concentration fell to less than 4 μg/mL (no longer thought to be a goal serum concentration) at 1.5 hours. In a simulated model, a continuous infusion of 500 mg/h of pralidoxime led to a concentration greater than 4 μg/mL after 15 minutes, which could be maintained throughout the infusion.[74] In a human volunteer study, an IV loading dose of 4 mg/kg over 15 minutes followed by 3.2 mg/kg/h for a total of 4 hours maintained serum pralidoxime concentrations greater than 4 μg/mL for 4 hours. The same total dose, 16 mg/kg, administered over 30 minutes only maintained those concentrations for 2 hours.[44] In poisoned patients receiving continuous infusions of pralidoxime as opposed to intermittent infusions, both the volume of distribution and the half-life are increased.[75] A volume of distribution of 2.77 L/kg, an elimination half-life of 3.44 hours, and a clearance of 0.57 L/kg/h were reported in poisoned adults given a mean loading dose of 4.4 mg/kg followed by an infusion of 2.14 mg/kg/h.[80] In poisoned children and adolescents, the volume of distribution varied with severity of poisoning from 8.8 L/kg in the severely poisoned patients to 2.8 L/kg in moderately poisoned patients.[65] After a mean loading dose of 29 mg/kg followed by a continuous infusion of about 14 mg/kg/h, a steady-state serum concentration of 22 μg/mL, a half-life of 3.6 hours, and a clearance of 0.88 L/kg/h were calculated.[65]

Oral administration of salts of pralidoxime (not used clinically because of OP poisoning–induced vomiting) demonstrated a peak concentration at 2 to 3 hours, a half-life of 1.7 hours, and an average urine recovery of 27% of unchanged pralidoxime in humans, and clinical efficacy in a mice model.[9,35] Autoinjector administration of 600 mg of pralidoxime chloride in an adult man (9 mg/kg) produced a concentration above 4 μg/mL at 7 to 16 minutes, a maximum serum concentration of 6.5 μg/mL at about 28 minutes, and a half-life of 2 hours.[56,67] Using traditional needle and syringe IM administration requires a longer time to achieve comparable serum concentrations. The autoinjectors more widely disperse the medication in the tissues resulting in faster absorption.[60,69]

OTHER REVERSAL AGENTS

The dihydropyridine derivative of pralidoxime, known as pro-2-PAM,[6] acts as a "prodrug" that allows passage through membranes such as the blood–brain barrier. Once across the membranes, spontaneous in vivo oxidation converts pro-2-PAM to the active form, demonstrating a 13-fold higher concentration of 2-PAM in the brain than when 2-PAM itself is administered under similar conditions. Further experiments support the significantly increased CNS effects of pro-2-PAM.[62] The toxicity of this compound has decreased enthusiasm for further investigation. The use of sugar oximes (the molecular combination of glucose with 2-PAM derivatives) to promote CNS penetration also appears promising.[38,59]

Obidoxime (Toxogonin) is an oxime used outside the United States that contains two active sites per molecule and is considered by some to be more effective than pralidoxime.[21,22,84] An in vitro study using human erythrocyte AChE supported the superiority of obidoxime to pralidoxime in reactivating AChE inhibited by the dimethyl phosphoryl (malaoxon, mevinphos) and diethyl phosphoryl OP compounds (paraoxon). On a molar basis, obidoxime is approximately 10 to 20 times more effective in reactivating AChE than pralidoxime.[84] A potential disadvantage is the concern that the phosphoryloxime generated from the reactivation of AChE by obidoxime could reinhibit AChE if not metabolized by a plasma enzyme similar or identical to human paraoxonase 1 (PON1). PON1 exhibits polymorphism[19] and one in 20 patients may not be able to metabolize this phosphorylobidoxime compound. Phosphorylpralidoxime is unstable and does not accumulate. The H series of oximes (named after Hagedorn; HI-6, HIo-7) were developed to act against the chemical warfare nerve agents.[7] These oximes have superior effectiveness against sarin, VX, and certain types of newer pesticides (eg, methyl-fluorophosphonylcholines).[3,11,33,36,39,61,84,85] Unfortunately, they are less efficacious for traditional OP insecticide poisoning, and their toxicity profile is inadequately defined.[11,33,36,39,61,84,85] In addition to reactivating AChEs, the Hagedorn oximes demonstrate direct central and peripheral anticholinergic effects at supratherapeutic concentrations.[61]

HUMAN TRIALS

There are four randomized clinical trials examining the efficacy of pralidoxime for the management of OP poisoning. Two of these trials were done in the 1990s in India using doses of pralidoxime now considered to be inadequate.[18] Neither study demonstrated a benefit for pralidoxime and, in fact, suggested an increase in mortality in patients receiving the higher but still inadequate dose of pralidoxime. Other criticisms include a delay in administration and too short a duration of treatment. The third clinical trial included 200 patients in India who were moderately to severely poisoned with an OP pesticide.[52] All patients received a 2-g loading dose of pralidoxime iodide over 30 minutes before being randomized to receive 1 g over 1 hour every 4 hours for 48 hours or a continuous infusion of 1 g/h for 48 hours. Beyond 48 hours all patients received 1 g every 4 hours until no longer ventilator dependent. In the continuous pralidoxime infusion arm the authors demonstrated reduced atropine requirements, a smaller number of patients requiring intubation, fewer intubated days, and a reduction in mortality from 8% to 1%. It should be noted that the iodide salt of pralidoxime was used and would equate to about 650 mg/h of the chloride salt.[20] Even though the majority of the patients by history ingested dimethoate, a dimethoxy compound with high lethality and rapid aging, the time to admission and administration of pralidoxime was very short with a median time of 2 hours. Criticisms of the study include a lack of blinding, no measurement of AChE or pesticide concentrations, and no objective monitoring of neuromuscular function.[20] In contrast, the most recent trial performed in Sri Lanka was unable to demonstrate a beneficial effect of pralidoxime in 121 patients compared to 114 patients treated with placebo.[18a] There was no difference in mortality between groups although pralidoxime effectively reactivated red cell AchE inhibited by diethyl OP insecticides. It also reactivated red cell AchE inhibited by dimethyl OP insecticides, but less so, as expected. In comparison to the third study[52] these patients arrived later (4.4 vs 2h), and the extent of supportive care was inferior. The exact reasons for these disparate results are unclear.

DURATION OF TREATMENT

The signs and symptoms of OP poisoning usually manifest within minutes but may be delayed up to 24 hours.[50] Delayed manifestations occur with the fat-soluble compounds, such as fenthion or chlorfenthion. The route of exposure may also influence the onset of systemic symptoms; for example, there may be a delay following dermal contact, which does not occur following ingestion or inhalation. When symptoms are either delayed or prolonged, or when treatment is delayed, extended therapy with pralidoxime may be indicated.[1,8,47] In one case of poisoning with the fat-soluble compound fenthion, 5 days elapsed before cholinergic symptoms appeared, and some symptoms then persisted for 30 days.[47] Pralidoxime and atropine were administered continuously in varying doses for the time that the patient was symptomatic. Ordinarily the recommendation is to continue the pralidoxime until atropine has not been needed for 12 to 24 hours.[17] Other proposals for estimating the duration of pralidoxime therapy include (1) measuring the serum or urinary concentration of the OP compound; (2) measuring serial determinations of plasma cholinesterase (increasing concentrations suggests the elimination of the OP compound); (3) incubating the patient's serum with an exogenous source of AChE or butyrylcholinesterase to look for inhibition; (4) incubating the patient's inhibited red blood cell cholinesterase with a high concentration of oxime in vitro, checking for reactivation.[19] In all cases, patients should be observed for recrudescent toxicity after termination of pralidoxime. If symptoms return, therapy should be continued for at least 24 hours.

ADVERSE EFFECTS

At therapeutic doses of pralidoxime in humans, adverse effects are minimal.[23,24,48-50,58,74] Transient dizziness, blurred vision, and elevations in diastolic blood pressure may be related to the rate of administration.[30,44] Doses of 45 mg/kg produce blood pressure elevations that may persist for several hours, but may be reversed with IV phentolamine.[67] The most recent randomized clinical trial revealed a higher percentage of patients with tachycardia and hypertension associated with pralidoxime compared to placebo after both the loading dose and the continuous infusion (75% vs 49% and 30% vs 14%). Rapid IV administration has produced sudden cardiac and respiratory arrest due to laryngospasm and muscle rigidity.[53,66,82] Other adverse effects reported following IM administration in normal volunteers include diplopia, dizziness, headache, drowsiness, nausea, tachycardia, increased systolic blood pressure, hyperventilation, decreased renal function, muscular weakness, and pain at the injection site.[56] Elevations in liver enzymes concentrations were observed in volunteers administered autoinjector doses of 1200 to 1800 mg; these enzyme concentrations returned to normal in 2 weeks.[56]

Pralidoxime is pregnancy category C and should be used as clinically indicated to protect the maternal fetal dyad.

DOSING AND ADMINISTRATION

The optimal dosage regimen for pralidoxime is unknown. A maintainence dose in adults of 1 g/h of the iodide salt of pralidoxime was used in the study from India and is approximally equal to 650 mg of pralidoxime chloride.[52] The package insert, last updated in 2004, recommends an adult dose of 1 to 2 g in 100 mL of 0.9% sodium chloride given intravenously over 15 to 30 minutes, with additional doses given every 3 to 8 hours as long as signs of poisoning recur. Difficulties arise because a target plasma concentration in humans has not been established, although in vitro studies suggest a target concentration closer to 17 μg/mL compared with the 4 μg/mL previously suggested.[19,21,31] This is complicated by the possibility that there is a ceiling dose and that some OP compounds are likely to be more easily reactivated than others. In addition, pharmacokinetic studies in volunteers suggest that a continuous infusion maintains a target concentration with less variation compared with intermittent boluses. Based on all of the above, we recommend a loading dose of pralidoxime chloride of 30 mg/kg (up to 2 grams) over 30 minutes followed by a maintenance infusion of 8 to 10 mg/kg/h (up to 650 mg/h).

Although IV administration is preferred, IM administration is acceptable using a 1-g vial of pralidoxime reconstituted with 3 mL of sterile water or 0.9% sodium chloride for injection to provide a solution containing 300 mg/mL (concentrations above 35% weight/volume produce muscle necrosis in animals).[55,68] This could be used until an IV site is established. Patients with reduced renal function may require dosage adjustment, but there are no specific recommendations on how to accomplish this.[55] In patients with acute lung injury the dose can be given as a 5% solution by a slow IV injection over at least 15 to 30 minutes.[55,68]

Depending on the severity of a nerve agent exposure, one to three injections with a pair of autoinjectors containing atropine and pralidoxime should be administered. The number of autoinjector doses administered to a child depends on the child's age and weight.[26,41] For children aged 3 to 7 (13–25 kg), one autoinjector of atropine and one autoinjector of pralidoxime should be administered, which should result in a projected pralidoxime dose of 24 to 46 mg/kg. For children aged 8 to 14, two autoinjectors of atropine and two autoinjectors of pralidoxime should be administered. These injections should result in a projected pralidoxime dose of 24 to 46 mg/kg. For anyone older than 14 years of age, three autoinjectors of atropine and pralidoxine should be administered. This results in a projected dose of pralidoxime of less than 35 mg/kg. For children younger than 3 years, during an emergency, one autoinjector of atropine and one of pralidoxime may be administered in accordance with a risk-benefit analysis. If time permits and only autoinjector doses are available, its contents may be transferred to a small sterile vial for traditional IM administration with a needle and syringe.[27]

In most cases, pralidoxime is continued for a minimum of 24 hours after symptoms have resolved and atropine is no longer required. Extended dosing may be necessary, depending on the patient's clinical condition and the nature of the OP.[78]

AVAILABILITY

Pralidoxime chloride (Protopam) is supplied in 20-mL vials containing 1 g of powder, ready for reconstitution with sterile water or 0.9% sodium chloride for injection.[54,55,57]

The addition of 20 mL of sterile water for injection to the 1-g vial of 2-PAM results in a 5% solution (50 mg/mL). Following reconstitution, the 2-PAM should be used within several hours. This solution can be further diluted to a volume of 100 mL of normal saline for IV infusion.

As noted above, pralidoxime chloride is also available for IM administration by an autoinjector containing 600 mg of pralidoxime in 2 mL of sterile water for injection with 20 mg benzyl alcohol and 11.26 mg glycine. The 2-PAM autoinjector is also packaged in a kit containing 600 mg of pralidoxime in 2 mL of sterile water for injection with 40 mg benzyl alcohol and 22.5 mg glycine, accompanied by an autoinjector containing 2.1 mg of atropine in 0.7 mL of a sterile solution containing 12.47 mg glycerin and not more than 2.8 mg phenol. This kit is called a "Mark 1 Nerve Agent Antidote Kit (NAAK)" and is designed to be used IM by first responders in case of a nerve agent attack. The needles extend 0.8 inch in length. The Mark 1 NAAK has recently been replaced by the DuoDote Autoinjector System, which uses technology that sequentially administers 2.1 mg in 0.7 mL atropine followed by 600 mg in 2 mL pralidoxime chloride IM through the same syringe. The 23-gauge needle is 0.8 inches in length.

SUMMARY

Pralidoxime is an effective reactivator of AChE in many OP compound poisonings. It primarily reverses neuromuscular manifestations but also has some CNS effects. New oximes may improve CNS penetration and efficacy. Pralidoxime and atropine are synergistic and should be used together in the management of patients with OP poisonings. If a patient requires multiple doses of atropine for muscarinic symptoms, then the use of 2-PAM is indicated. In symptomatic patients, AChE is partially inactivated and will remain so until new enzyme is synthesized or inactivated enzyme is reactivated. The resolution of all signs or symptoms with atropine alone indicates only that AChE inactivation is less than 50% and that endogenous hydrolysis by nonphosphorylated enzyme is sufficient to eliminate symptoms. This clinical response by no means indicates, however, that the enzyme systems are fully active; patients may still benefit from enzyme regeneration with the safe and effective antidote pralidoxime.

Finally, because newer fat-soluble OP pesticides are currently available, it may be necessary to administer atropine and 2-PAM for more prolonged periods of time than previously indicated based on the clinical manifestations and the predicted kinetics of the highly fat-soluble pesticides.[8]

ACKNOWLEDGMENT

Cynthia K. Aaron, MD contributed to this discussion in a previous edition.

REFERENCES

1. Aaron CK, Smilkstein M. Intermediate syndrome or inadequate therapy [abstract]. *Vet Human Toxicol.* 1988;30:370.
2. Amos WC Jr, Hall A. Malathion poisoning treated with Protopam. *Ann Intern Med.* 1965;62:1013-1016.
3. Antonijevic B, Stojiljkovic M. Unequal efficacy of pyridinium oximes in acute organophosphate poisoning. *Clin Med Res.* 2006;5:71-82.
4. Blaber LC, Creasey NH. The mode of recovery of cholinesterase activity in vivo after organophosphorus poisoning: I. Erythrocyte cholinesterase. *Biochem J.* 1960;77:591-596.
5. Blaber LC, Creasey NH. The mode of recovery of cholinesterase activity in vivo after organophosphorus poisoning: II. Brain cholinesterase. *Biochem J.* 1960;77:597-604.
6. Bodor N, Shek E, Higuchi T. Delivery of a quaternary pyridinium salt across the blood-brain barrier by its dihydropyridine derivative. *Science.* 1975;190:155-156.
7. Bokowjic D, Jovanovic D, Jokanovic M, et al. Protective effects of oximes HI-6, and PAM 2, applied by osmotic minipumps in quinalphos poisoned rats. *Arch Int Pharmacodyn Ther.* 1987;288:309-318.
8. Borowitz SM. Prolonged organophosphate toxicity in a twenty-six-month-old child. *J Pediatr.* 1988;112:303-304.
9. Bowls BJ, Freeman JM Jr, Luna JA, Meggs WJ. Oral treatment of organophosphate poisoning in mice. *Acad Emerg Med.* 2003;10:286-288.
10. Burgess JL, Bernstein JN, Hurlbut K. Aldicarb poisoning-A case report with prolonged cholinesterase inhibition and improvement after pralidoxime therapy. *Arch Intern Med.* 1994;154:221-224.
11. Clement JG, Bailey DG, Madill HD, et al. The acetylcholinesterase oxime reactivator HI-6, in man: pharmacokinetics and tolerability in combination with atropine. *Biopharm Drug Dispos.* 1995;16:415-425.
12. Costa L. Current issues in organophosphate toxicology. *Clinica Chimica Acta.* 2006;366:1-13.
13. Davies DR, Green AL. The kinetics of reactivation, by oximes, of cholinesterase inhibited by organophosphorus compounds. *Biochemistry.* 1956;63:529-535.
14. Davison AN. Return of cholinesterase activity in the rat after inhibition by organophosphorus compounds: I. Diethyl p-nitrophenyl phosphate (E600 Paraoxon). *Biochem J.* 1953;54:583-590.
15. Dawson RM. Oximes in treatment of carbamate poisoning. *Vet Rec.* 1994;134:687.
16. Durham WF, Hayes WJ Jr. Organic phosphorus poisoning and its therapy. *Arch Environ Health.* 1962;5:21-47.
17. Eddelson M, Buckley N, Eyer P, Dawson A. Management of acute organophosphorous pesticide poisoning. *Lancet.* 2008;371:597-607.
18. Eddleston M, Szinicz L, Eyer P, et al. Oximes in acute organophosphorous pesticide poisoning: a systematic review of clinical trials. *QJ Med.* 2002;95:275-283.

18a. Eddleston M, Eyer P, Worek F, et al. Pralidoxime in acute organophosphorus insecticide poisoning—a randomized controlled trial. *PLoS Medicine.* 2009;6:1-12.

19. Eyer P. The role of oximes in the management of organophosphorus pesticide poisoning. *Toxicol Rev.* 2003;22:166-190.
20. Eyer P, Buckley N. Pralidoxime for organophosphosphate poisoning. *Lancet.* 2006;368:2110-2111.
21. Eyer P, Szinicz L, Thiermann H, et al. Testing of antidotes for organophosphorous compounds: experimental procedures and clinical reality. *Toxicology.* 2007;233:108-119.
22. Finkelstein Y, Taitelman U, Biegon A. CNS involvement in acute organophosphate poisoning: specific pattern of toxicity, clinical correlates and antidotal treatment. *Ital J Neurol Sci.* 1988;9:437-446.
23. Grob D, Jones RJ. Use of oximes in the treatment of intoxication by anticholinesterase compounds in normal subjects. *Am J Med.* 1958;24:497-511.
24. Hagerstrom-Portnoy G, Jones R, Adams AJ, Jampolsky A. Effects of atropine and 2-PAM chloride on vision and performance in humans. *Aviat Space Environ Med.* 1987;10:47-53.
25. Harris LW, Talbot BG, Lennox WJ, et al. The relationship between oxime-induced reactivation of carbamylated acetylcholinesterase and antidotal efficacy against carbamate intoxication. *Toxicol Appl Pharmacol.* 1989;98:128-133.
26. Henretig FM, Cieslak TJ, Eitzen EM Jr. Biological and chemical terrorism. *J Pediatr.* 2002;141:311-326.
27. Henretig FM, Mechem C, Jew R. Potential use of autoinjector-packaged antidotes for treatment of pediatric nerve agent toxicity. *Ann Emerg Med.* 2002;40:405-408.
28. Hobbiger F. Chemical reactivation of phosphorylated human and bovine true cholinesterase. *Br J Pharmacol.* 1956;11:295-303.
29. Hobbiger F. Effect of nicotinehydroxamic acid methiodide on human plasma cholinesterase inhibited by organophosphates containing dialkylphosphate groups. *Br J Pharmacol.* 1955;10:356-362.
30. Jager BV, Staff GN. Toxicity of diacetyl monoxime and of pyridine-2-aldoxime methiodide in man. *Bull Johns Hopkins Hosp.* 1958;102:203-211.
31. Jun D, Musilova L, Kuca K, et al. Potency of several oximes to reactivate human acetylcholinesterase and butyrylcholinesterase inhibited by paraoxon in vitro. *Chem Biol Interact.* 2008;175:421-424.
32. Karczmar A. Invited review. Anticholinesterases: dramatic aspects of their use and misuse. *Neurochem Int.* 1998;32:401-411.
33. Kassa J, Cabal J. A comparison of the efficacy of a new asymmetric bispyridinium oxime BI-6, with currently available oximes and H oximes against soman in in vitro and in vivo methods. *Toxicology.* 1999;132:111-118.
34. Khan S, Hemalatha R, Jeyaseelan L, et al. Neuroparalysis and oxime efficacy in organophosphate poisoning: a study of butyrylcholinesterase. *Hum Exp Toxicol.* 2001;20:169-174.
35. Kondritzer A, Zvirblis P, Goodman A, Paplanus S. Blood plasma levels and elimination of salts of 2-PAM in man after oral administration. *J Pharm Sci.* 1968;57:1142-1145.
36. Kusic R, Jovanovic D, Randjelovic A, et al. HI-6, in man: efficacy of the oxime in poisoning by organophosphorus insecticides. *Hum Exp Toxicol.* 1991;10:113-118.
37. Lifshitz M, Rotenberg M, Sofer S, et al. Carbamate poisoning and oxime treatment in children: a clinical and laboratory study. *Pediatrics.* 1994;93:652-655.
38. Lotti M, Becker C. Treatment of acute organophosphate-poisoning: evidence of a direct effect on central nervous system by 2-PAM (pyridine-2-aldoxime methyl chloride). *J Toxicol Clin Toxicol.* 1982;19:121-127.
39. Lundy PM, Hansen AS, Hand BT, Boulet CA. Comparison of several oximes against poisoning by soman, tabun and GF. *Toxicology.* 1992;72:99-105.
40. Luo C, Saxena A, Smith M, et al. Phosphoryl oxime inhibition of acetylcholinesterase during oxime reactivation is prevented by edrophonium. *Biochemistry.* 1999;38:9937-9947.
41. Markenson D, Redlener I. Pediatric terrorism preparedness national guidelines and recommendations: findings of an evidenced-based consensus process. *Biosecur Bioterror.* 2004;2:301-319.
42. Matin M, Siddiqui R. Modification of the level of acetylcholinesterase activity by two oximes in certain brain regions and peripheral tissues of paraoxon treated rats. *Pharmacol Res Commun.* 1982;4:241-246.

43. Mattingly JE, Sullivan JE, Spiller HA, Bosse GM. Intermediate syndrome after exposure to chlorpyrifos in a 16-month-old girl. *J Emerg Med.* 2003;25: 379-381.
44. Medicis JJ, Stork CM, Howland MA, et al. Pharmacokinetics following a loading plus a continuous infusion of pralidoxime compared with the traditional short infusion regimen in human volunteers. *J Toxicol Clin Toxicol.* 1996;34:289-295.
45. Mercurio-Zappala M, Hack J, Salvador A, Hoffman R. Pralidoxime in carbaryl poisoning: an animal model. *Hum Exp Toxicol.* 2007;26:125-129.
46. Milosevic MP, Andjelkovic D. Reactivation of paraoxon-inactivated cholinesterase in the rat cerebral cortex by pralidoxime chloride. *Nature.* 1966;210:206.
47. Merrill D, Mihm F. Prolonged toxicity of organophosphate poisoning. *Crit Care Med.* 1982;10:550-551.
48. Namba T. Diagnosis and treatment of organophosphate insecticide poisoning. *Med Times.* 1972;100:100-126.
49. Namba T, Hiraki K. PAM (pyridine-2-aldoxime methiodide) therapy for alkyl-phosphate poisoning. *JAMA.* 1958;166:1834-1839.
50. Namba T, Nolte C, Jackrel J, Grob D. Poisoning due to organophosphate insecticides: acute and chronic manifestations. *Am J Med.* 1971;50:475-492.
51. Natoff IL, Reiff B. Effect of oximes on the acute toxicology of acetylcholinesterase carbamates. *Toxicol Appl Pharmacol.* 1973;25:569-575.
52. Pawar K, Pillay C, Chavan S, et al. Continuous pralidoxime infusion versus repeated bolus injection to treat organophosphorpus pesticide poisoning. a randomized trial. *Lancet.* 2006;368:2136-2141.
53. Pickering EN. Organic phosphate insecticide poisoning. *Can J Med Technol.* 1966;28:174-179.
54. Pralidoxime. In: Kastrup E, ed. *Facts and Comparisons.* Philadelphia: JB Lippincott; 1983.
55. Pralidoxime. In: McEvoy GK, Miller J, Litvak K, eds. *AHFS Drug Information 2004.* Bethesda, MD: American Society of Health-System Pharmacists; 2004:3541-3543.
56. Pralidoxime Chloride injection (Auto-Injector) [package insert]. The antidote treatment–nerve agent, auto-injector (ATNAA) package insert. Columbia, MD: Meridian Medical Technologies, Inc; 2002 Jan; and Columbia, MD: Meridian Medical Technologies; Inc, 2002 May.
57. Protopam Chloride (pralidoxime chloride) for injection [package insert]. Deerfield, IL: Baxter Healthcare Corporation; 2004.
58. Quimby G. Further therapeutic experience with pralidoximes in organic phosphorus poisoning. *JAMA.* 1963;187:202-206.
59. Rachaman E, Ashani Y, Leader H, et al. Sugaroximes, new potential antidotes against organophosphorus poisoning. *Arzneimittelforschung.* 1979;29:875-876.
60. Rotenberg J, Newmark J. Nerve agent attacks on children: diagnosis and management. *Peds.* 2003;112:648-658.
61. Rousseaux CG, Du AK. Pharmacology of HI-6, an H-series oxime. *Can J Physiol Pharmacol.* 1989;67:1183-1189.
62. Rump S, Faff J, Borkowska G, et al. Central therapeutic effects of dihydroderivative of pralidoxime (pro-2-PAM) in organophosphate intoxication. *Arch Int Pharmacodyn Ther.* 1978;232:321-331.
63. Sakurada K, Matsubara K, Shimizu K. Pralidoxime iodide (2-PAM) penetrates across the blood–brain barrier. *Neurochem Res.* 2003;28: 1401-1407.
64. Sanderson DM. Treatment of poisoning by anticholinesterase insecticides in the rat. *J Pharm Pharmacol.* 1961;13:435-442.
65. Schexnayder S, James L, Kearns G, Farrar H. The pharmacokinetics of continuous infusion pralidoxime in children with organophosphate poisoning. *J Toxicol Clin Toxicol.* 1998;36:549-555.
66. Scott RJ. Repeated asystole following PAM in organophosphate self-poisoning. *Anesth Intensive Care.* 1986;4:458-460.
67. Sidell FR. Nerve agents. In: Zajtchuk R, ed. *Textbook of Military Medicine: Medical Aspects of Chemical and Biological Warfare, Part I.* Office of the Surgeon General Department of the Army, United States of America; 1997:129-179.
68. Sidell FR, Groff WA. Intramuscular and intravenous administration of small doses of 2-pyridinium aldoxime methylchloride to man. *J Pharm Sci.* 1971;60:1224-1228.
69. Sidell FR, Markis J, Groff W, Kaminskis A. Enhancement of drug absorption after administration by an automatic injector. *J Pharm Sci.* 1974;2: 197-210.
70. Sterri S, Rognerud B, Fiskum S, Lyngaas S. Effect of toxogenin and P2S on the toxicity of carbamates and organophosphorus compounds. *Acta Pharmacol Toxicol.* 1979;45:9-15.
71. Sudakin D, Mullins M, Horowitz Z, et al. Intermediate syndrome after malathion ingestion despite continuous infusion of pralidoxime. *J Toxicol Clin Toxicol.* 2000;38:47-50.
72. Sundwall A. Minimum concentrations of n-methyl pyridinium-2-aldoxime methane sulphonate (PS2) which reverse neuromuscular block. *Biochem Pharmacol.* 1961;8:413-417.
73. Taylor P. Anticholinesterase agents. In: Hardman JG, Limbird LE, Molinoff PB, Ruddoev RW, eds. *Goodman and Gilman's the Pharmacological Basis of Therapeutics*, 9th ed. New York: Macmillan; 1996:100-119.
74. Thompson DF, Thompson GD, Greenwood RB, Trammel HL. Therapeutic dosing of pralidoxime chloride. *Drug Intell Clin Pharm.* 1987;21:1590-1593.
75. Tush G, Anstead M. Pralidoxime continuous infusion ion the treatment of organophosphate poisoning. *Ann Pharmacother.* 1997;31:441-444.
76. Uehara S, Hiromori T, Isobe N, et al. Studies on the therapeutic effect of 2-pyridine aldoxime methiodide (2-PAM) in mammals following organophosphorous compound (OP)-poisoning (report III): distribution and antidotal effect of 2-PAM in rats. *J Toxicol.* 1993;18:265-275.
77. Uehara S, Hiromori T, Suzuki T, et al. Studies on the therapeutic effect of 2-pyridine aldoxime methiodide (2-PAM) in mammals following organophosphorous compound (OP)-poisoning (report II): aging of OP-inhibited mammalian cholinesterase. *J Toxicol.* 1993;18:179-183.
78. Wiener SW, Hoffman RS. Nerve agents: a comprehensive review. *J Intensive Care Med.* 2004;19:22-37.
79. Willems JL, BeBisschop HC, Verstraete AG, et al. Cholinesterase reactivation in organophosphorus poisoned patients depends on the plasma concentrations of the oxime pralidoxime methylsulfate and of the organophosphate. *Arch Toxicol.* 1993;97:79-84.
80. Willems JL, Langenberg JP, Verstraete AC, et al. Plasma concentrations of pralidoxime methyl sulfate in organophosphorus poisoned patients. *Arch Toxicol.* 1992;66:260-266.
81. Wilson IB. Molecular complementarity and antidotes for alkylphosphate poisoning. *Fed Proc.* 1959;18(2 Part 1):752-758.
82. Wislicki L. Differences in the effect of oximes on striated muscle and respiratory centre. *Arch Int Pharmacodyn Ther.* 1960;120:1-19.
83. Wong L, Radic Z, Bruggemann RJ, et al. Mechanism of oxime reactivation of acetylcholinesterase analyzed by chirality and mutagenesis. *Biochemistry.* 2000;39:5750-5757.
84. Worek F, Backer M, Thiermann H, et al. Reappraisal of indications and limitations of oxime therapy in organophosphate poisoning. *Hum Exp Toxicol.* 1997;16:466-472.
85. Worek F, Thiermann H, Szinicz L. Reactivation and aging kinetics of human acetylcholinesterase inhibited by organophosphonylcholines. *Arch Toxicol.* 2004;78:212-217.
86. Worek F, Thiermann H, Szinicz L, Eyer P. Kinetic analysis of interactions between human acetylcholinesterase, structurally different organophosphorous compounds and oximes. *Biochem Pharmacol.* 2004;68: 2237-2248.

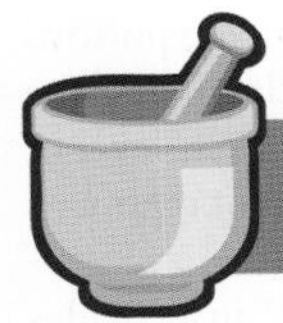

ANTIDOTES IN DEPTH (A34)

ATROPINE

Mary Ann Howland

Atropine is the prototypical antimuscarinic xenobiotic. It is a competitive antagonist at both central and peripheral muscarinic receptors, used to treat patients with symptoms following exposures to muscarinic agonists such as pilocarpine, and acetylcholinesterase inhibitors and *Clitocybe* mushrooms. The latter group includes pesticides, such as carbamate and organic phosphorous (OP) compounds, OP chemical warfare nerve agents, and some xenobiotics used to treat patients with Alzheimer disease (eg, donepezil, rivastigmine).

HISTORY

Many plants contain the alkaloids atropine and/or scopolamine. One notable example is *Atropa belladonna*, named by Linnaeus after Atropos, the goddess of fate in Greek mythology who could cut short a person's life. Belladonna means beautiful woman in Italian and comes from the practice by Italian women of placing belladonna extract in their eyes to produce aesthetically pleasing dilated pupils.[8] In the early 1800s, atropine was isolated and purified from plants. In the 1860s Fraser experimented with the dose–response relationship between atropine and physostigmine involving various organs such as the heart and the eye.[16] Experiments in the 1940s with cholinesterase inhibitors demonstrated that atropine reversed many of the effects of these xenobiotics and protected against doses two to three times the LD_{50} (median lethal dose in 50% of test subjects) in animals.[43]

CHEMISTRY

Atropine (dl-hyoscyamine), like scopolamine (l-hyoscine), is a tropane alkaloid with a tertiary amine structure that allows central nervous system (CNS) penetration. Tropane alkaloids are bicyclic nitrogen-containing compounds that are naturally found in the plants of the families Solanaceae (eg, deadly nightshade, datura) and Erythroxylaceae (eg, coca) and have a long history of use as poisons and therapeutic agents. Only l-hyoscyamine is active and found in nature. The process of isolation results in racemization and forms dl-hyoscyamine. Quaternary amine antimuscarinic agents such as glycopyrrolate, ipratropium, tiotropium, methylhomatropine bromide, and methylatropine bromide do not cross the blood–brain barrier into the CNS.

PHARMACOLOGY

Cholinergic receptors consist of muscarinic and nicotinic subtypes. Muscarinic receptors are coupled to G proteins and either inhibit adenylyl cyclase (M_2, M_4) or increase phospholipase C (M_1, M_3, M_5). Muscarinic receptors are widely distributed throughout the peripheral and central nervous systems.[19]

The competitive blockade of muscarinic receptors in normal individuals results in dose-dependent clinical effects that vary by organ system based on the degree of endogenous parasympathetic tone.[8,19] In adults, low doses (0.5 mg) of atropine cause a paradoxical bradycardia, and some drying of the mouth and sweat glands. Higher doses of atropine (2 mg) produce noticeable dryness; subjective feeling of warmth; slight flushing; slight tachycardia; reactive, slightly dilated pupils; blurred near vision; mild drowsiness; some postural hypotension; and urinary hesitation. At higher doses of 3 to 5 mg of atropine all the aforementioned symptoms are exaggerated, with escalating degrees of hyperthermia, tachycardia, drowsiness, difficulty voiding, prolonged gastrointestinal (GI) transit time, and decreased GI tone. Doses of greater than or equal to 10 mg of atropine produce incapacitation with hot, dry, flushed skin; dilated pupils; blurred vision; very dry mouth; tachycardia; urinary retention; constipation; increased drowsiness or disorientation; hallucinations; stereotypical movements; bursts of laughter; delirium; and finally, coma, and rarely death.[8,18]

This paradoxical bradycardia produced at low doses of atropine is thought to be a consequence of the inhibition of peripheral M_1 presynaptic postganglionic parasympathetic neurons; stimulation of these receptors by acetylcholine inhibits the further release of acetylcholine, and atropine interferes with this negative feedback.[8,41]

Centrally acting muscarinic antagonists include atropine, scopolamine, and homatropine. Glycopyrrolate, ipratropium, and tiotropium act peripherally. Scopolamine is about 10 times more potent than atropine.[25] Homatropine is at least one-tenth as potent as atropine depending on the measured outcome and route of administration.[24]

Cholinesterase inhibitors prevent the breakdown of acetylcholine by acetylcholinesterase, thereby increasing the amount of acetylcholine available to stimulate cholinergic receptors at both muscarinic and nicotinic subtypes, though the degree of effect varies widely among the class. Muscarinic agonists (eg, muscarine, methacholine, and pilocarpine) typically only stimulate muscarinic receptors. Atropine is a competitive antagonist of acetylcholine only at muscarinic receptors and not nicotinic receptors.[10]

Miosis from the topical instillation of a cholinesterase inhibitor into the eye will not be reversed by the systemic administration of atropine.[18] The systemic administration of 354 mg of atropine made one patient floridly anticholinergic but did not counteract the ophthalmic effects of a previously instilled topical cholinesterase inhibitor.[18]

PHARMACOKINETICS AND PHARMACODYNAMICS

Atropine is absorbed rapidly from most routes of administration including inhalation, oral, and intramuscular (IM).[3] Oral ingestion of 1 mg of atropine produces maximal effects on heart rate and on salivary secretions in 1 and 3 hours, respectively. The duration of action may last from 12 to 24 hours depending on the dose.

The distribution half-life of atropine following intravenous (IV) administration is approximately 1 minute. The apparent volume of distribution (Vd) is about 2 to 2.6 L/kg.[24] As a result of the rapid distribution, 10 minutes after IV administration less than 5% of the dose remains in the serum. The serum concentrations of atropine are similar at 1 hour following either 1 mg IV or IM in adults.[3,6] The elimination half-life is 6.5 hours.[34]

Following IM administration of 0.02 mg/kg in adults the absorption rate and elimination rates are comparable for the racemic dl-hyoscyamine and the active l-hyoscyamine at 8 minutes and 2.5 hours, respectively. The mean peak serum concentration and the area under the curve (AUC) are higher for the racemic mixture indicating a stereochemical difference in pharmacokinetics.[24] Renal elimination accounts for 34% to 57% of the excretion of the dose, and the majority of renal elimination occurs within 6 hours.[3] Serum concentrations of l-hyoscyamine correlate with effects on heart rate and the antisialagogue effects. Serum concentrations below 0.5 μg/L cause bradycardia, whereas higher concentrations cause tachycardia.[24]

Atropine autoinjectors are now given to first responders for use during chemical terrorist attacks. The administration of 2 mg of atropine by autoinjector was compared with 2 mg administered by conventional needle and syringe into the deltoid of six adult subjects.[39] The onset of tachycardia and the time to maximal increase in heart rate occurred sooner with the autoinjector (16 minutes versus 23 minutes, and 34 minutes versus 41 minutes, respectively). An analysis of radiographs of contrast material injected by autoinjector or conventional IM administration into a dog's leg demonstrated that the autoinjector appeared to "spray" the material into a larger tissue area accounting for a faster rate of absorption.[39]

Ophthalmic instillation of atropine causes cyclopegia and mydriasis by blocking the M_3 muscarinic receptor on the iris sphincter muscle.[28] The peak mydriatic effect occurs within 30 to 40 minutes and persists for 7 to 10 days. In contrast, the effects of topical homatropine on the eye occur sooner than topical atropine (10–30 minutes for mydriasis and 30–90 minutes for cycloplegia) and are shorter in duration (6–48 hours).

An investigation of the bioavailability of atropine eye drops in healthy adults revealed on average 65% systemic absorption, but with a wide individual variability.[23] The time to maximum serum concentration was 30 minutes and the elimination half-life was 2.5 hours.

The pharmacokinetics of three inhaled doses of atropine from a metered-dose nebulizer was compared with 2 mg of IM atropine in healthy adults.[20] Peak concentrations were comparable for the 2-mg inhaled and 2-mg IM atropine doses. The time to peak concentration following inhalation averaged 1.3 hours. A novel nanoatropine dry powder inhaler is being developed to rapidly achieve blood concentrations of atropine in the hopes of circumventing IM administration.[2]

CLINICAL USE

One of earliest descriptions of the effectiveness of atropine in parathion and tetraethylpyrophosphate insecticide poisoning was published in 1955.[17] The report emphasized improved survival when atropine was administered early and continued with adequate maintenance doses in conjunction with intubation and ventilation. The report also found that after parathion and tetraethylpyrophosphate insecticide exposure, dogs were more likely to develop heart block and bronchoconstriction, whereas humans were more likely to develop a relative rather than absolute bradycardia. Additionally, humans were more likely to die from respiratory causes stemming from central apnea, diaphragmatic weakness, and bronchorrhea.

In 1971, a landmark case series and review of OP insecticide poisonings was published. Included in this report was a table classifying the severity of poisoning along with treatment protocols for each level of severity.[29] This regimen served as the foundation of treatment regimens (atropine and pralidoxime) for many years.

In the 1930s and 1940s, the Germans synthesized OP insecticides (acetylcholinesterase inhibitors) that were further developed as chemical warfare nerve agents (Chap. 131).[38] Although these agents inhibit acetylcholinesterase in a manner similar to traditional OP insecticides, these so-called "nerve agents" also affect other cholinesterases, and at high doses, directly affect nicotinic and muscarinic receptors. Atropine was chosen in the late 1940s as the standard antidote for these nerve agents. The dose of atropine needed to antagonize these nerve agents is much less than that needed to effectively antagonize traditional OP insecticides, largely because of differences in pharmacokinetics. The benefits of adding pralidoxime to atropine were noted in the 1950s, and in the 1960s, pralidoxime was established as a standard antidote in addition to atropine for these agents (see Antidotes in Depth A33: Pralidoxime).

ADVERSE EFFECTS AND TOXICITY

When atropine is used in the absence of a xenobiotic that increases or mimics acetylcholine, adverse effects begin at 0.5 mg IV in the adult and include dry mouth and decreased sweat. However, in the presence of a muscarinic agonist or an anticholinesterase, these effects may not occur until many milligrams of atropine are administered.

Intravenous doses of greater than 10 mg of atropine and oral doses of 500 to 1000 mg have been administered with full recovery. Deaths from atropine use are usually correlated with hyperthermia.

An unintentional atropine dose of 1 g orally resulted in typical manifestations of anticholinergic poisoning that began within a short time and lasted 4 days.[1] In 2 hours the patient went from feeling hot and flushed with blurred vision to stuporous. Over the ensuing 24 hours he became tachycardic, hyperthermic, and comatose with dilated, nonreactive pupils and shallow respirations. By 40 hours he started to respond to his name and his temperature had normalized, but he remained dry with dilated and nonreactive pupils. He went from comatose to restless, hallucinating, and paranoid. At 4 days he regained a normal mental status with amnesia for the previous 4 days.

A survey of pediatric emergency departments in Israel reported on 240 children who were unintentionally injected with atropine autoinjectors during the Persian Gulf crisis.[4] Half of the children developed systemic effects that correlated with the doses of atropine administered. Eight percent of effects were serious but there were no seizures or deaths.

Systemic atropine toxicity may even occur when too large a dose of atropine, scopolamine or homatropine are instilled in the eye, especially in children.[31] Excessive absorption from other routes of administration (eg, rectal, inhaled) would also be expected to result in toxicity.[37] In the event of an atropine overdose, physostigmine, a reversible, CNS active, cholinesterase inhibitor, is the antidote of choice[30] (see Antidotes in Depth A12–Physostigmine Salicylate). Psychiatric patients in the 1950s were often given atropine as a remedy. Within 15 to 20 minutes of getting 32 to 212 mg of IM atropine, patients become restless and often confused. This progressed to muscular incoordination, ataxia, weakness, and garbled speech.[15] The patients then progressed to disorientation with illusions, visual hallucinations, and delirium, to coma. The coma often lasted for 4 to 6 hours and then patients recovered in a manner that in some respects is the reverse of intoxication. Regardless of the dose of atropine required to induce the coma, physostigmine 4 mg IM completely reversed it within 20 minutes, but the reversal only lasted for 30 to 45 minutes.[15,30]

Other precautions or contraindications to consider when administering atropine include those associated with all antimuscarinics and include narrow angle closure glaucoma, obstructive uropathy, gastroparesis, emptying, relaxation of the lower esophageal sphincter, and myasthenia gravis. Of course these issues must be weighed in light of the possible life-threatening nature of OP, carbamate, and chemical nerve agent poisoning.

Atropine is classified by the Food and Drug Administration (FDA) as pregnancy category C. Atropine crosses the placenta and may cause tachycardia in the fetus near term.[40]

DOSING AND ADMINISTRATION

The dosage regimen of atropine for an OP pesticide poisoning in adults has never been studied in a randomized, controlled trial, and there is considerable variation in textbook recommendations.[12] A recent prospective, observational study suggests that a dose doubling, titrated protocol provided equal efficacy with less atropine toxicity compared with a less-preplanned ad hoc dosing protocol.[33] Experience suggests that atropine should be initiated in adults in doses of 1 to 2 mg IV for mild to moderate poisoning and 3 to 5 mg IV for severe poisoning with unconsciousness.[29] This dose can be doubled every 3 to 5 minutes until improvement has begun, at which time dose doubling can stop and similar or smaller doses can be used.[13,35] We believe that the most important end point for adequate atropinization is clear lungs, and the reversal of the muscarinic toxic syndrome. It is, however, important not to confuse abnormal focal ausculatory sounds associated with pulmonary aspiration with those of extensive bronchorrhea.[13,35] Some authors suggest clear lungs, heart rate greater than or equal to 80 beats/min, and systolic blood pressure greater than or equal to 80 mm Hg as most important, and dry axillae and wider than pinpoint pupils as additional goals.[14] Once these end points have been achieved, a maintenance dose of atropine needs to be started. One group suggests administering 10% to 20% of the loading dose as an IV infusion every hour as a starting point with meticulous frequent reevaluation and titration.[12,13] The atropine can be diluted in 0.9% sodium chloride with rates of 0.5 to 1.5 mg/h of atropine commonly used.[33] For example, if a patient received atropine IV 2 mg, then 4 mg in 5 minutes, and 8 mg in 5 minutes when improvement in bronchorrhea is noticeable, the total loading dose to initial control would be 14 mg in 10 minutes. The initial IV infusion dose of atropine would be 1.4 mg/h. This could be prepared by mixing 10 mg of atropine in 100 mL of 0.9% sodium chloride to make a concentration of 0.1 mg/mL and infuse it at 14 mL (14 mg)/h. If too much atropine is administered, the patient demonstrates classic signs of peripheral and central anticholinergic toxicity as described above. The IV starting dose of atropine in children is 0.02 mg/kg up to the adult dose.[35,42] A continuous infusion of 0.025 mg/kg/h has been successfully used in a 2 year old following a fenthion poisoning.[7]

In the event that a person is exposed to a chemical warfare nerve agent, atropine should be administered in a dosage suitable for both the severity of the poisoning and the age of the patient. In a conscious adult with mild to moderate cholinergic effects, 2 mg of atropine IV or IM should be administered every 5 to 10 minutes until shortness of breath improves and drying of secretions occurs.[38] One adult autoinjector of atropine for IM administration, Mark 1 Nerve Agent Antidote Kit (NAAK), contains 2 mg of atropine, and therefore multiple injectors may be required. Total doses of 2 to 4 mg of atropine are usually all that is needed, which is much lower than the dose for most OP pesticide exposures. Patients who are unconscious or apneic require higher total doses with 5 to 15 mg usually sufficing.[38]

The appropriate total Mark 1 autoinjector doses of atropine for children depend on age and weight.[21,26] For ages 3 to 7 (13–25 kg), one autoinjector (2 mg) of atropine and one autoinjector of pralidoxime (600 mg) should be administered resulting in a projected atropine dose of 0.08 to 0.15 mg/kg. For ages 8 to 14, two autoinjectors of atropine and two autoinjectors of pralidoxime should be administered resulting in a projected atropine dose of 0.08 to 0.15 mg/kg. For patients older than 14 years of age, three autoinjectors of atropine and pralidoxime should be administered resulting in a projected dose of atropine of less than 0.11 mg/kg. In an emergency for children younger than 3 years of age a risk-benefit analysis would suggest injecting one autoinjector of atropine and one of pralidoxime. If time permits and only one autoinjector is available for use, its contents may be transferred to a small sterile vial for traditional IM administration with a needle and syringe.[22] Some experts recommend that children under the age of 1 be administered one pediatric atropine autoinjector (0.5 mg), AtroPen (Meridian Medical Technologies) if available, and children over the age of 1 be administered the Mark 1 autoinjector as described above.

When IV administration is not feasible, atropine may also be administered intraosseously at the standard IV dose. However, the dose for endotracheal administration in adults should be two to two-and-a-half times the IV dose, diluted in 5 to 10 mL of normal saline or sterile water. For children the 2005 American Heart Association guidelines for pediatric advanced life support recommend 0.03 mg/kg with a minimum dose of 0.1 mg in a child endotracheally followed by a flush of 5 mL of normal saline and then five manual ventilations to enhance absorption.[32]

AVAILABILITY

Atropine sulfate injection is available in many different strengths, with the following concentrations in each 1 mL vial or ampule: 50 μg, 300 μg, 400 μg, 500 μg, 800 μg, and 1 mg. Atropine sulfate is also available in prefilled 5-mL or 10-mL syringes with a concentration of 0.1 mg/mL for adults and in 5-mL syringes with a concentration of 0.05 mg/mL for pediatrics.

The AtroPen Auto-Injector is a prefilled syringe designed for IM injection by an autoinjector into the outer thigh.[5] It is available in four strengths: 0.25 mg, 0.5 mg (blue label), 1 mg (dark red label), and 2 mg (green label).

Atropine is also packaged in a kit designed for IM injection with a second autoinjector containing 600 mg of pralidoxime in 2 mL of sterile water for injection with 40 mg benzyl alcohol and 22.5 mg glycine. The pralidoxime injector is accompanied by an atropine autoinjector containing 2.1 mg of atropine in 0.7 mL of a sterile solution containing 12.47 mg glycerin and not more than 2.8 mg phenol. This particular combination kit is called a "Mark 1 Nerve Agent Antidote Kit" and is designed for IM use in case of a nerve agent attack. The needles are 0.8 inches in length.[27] The Mark 1 NAAK has recently been replaced by the DuoDote Autoinjector System, which uses technology that sequentially administers 2.1 mg in 0.7 mL atropine followed by 600 mg in 2 mL pralidoxime chloride IM through the same syringe. The 23-gauge needle is 0.8 inches in length.

Atropine is available orally in 300 μg, 400 μg, and 600 μg tablets.

In case of a shortage during an emergency, in vitro evidence suggests that outdated atropine retains its potency and that an extemporaneously prepared atropine solution from powder is stable for at least 3 days.[11,36] Other sources of atropine to consider in an emergency during a shortage would be atropine eye drops, which come as a 1% concentration (10 mg/mL). Homatropine, available as eye drops in a 2% or 5% concentration, compared favorably with atropine in preventing lethality when administered IM in a pretreatment rodent model using dichlorvos. In this experimental model, homatropine appeared to be half as potent as atropine.[9]

SUMMARY

Atropine has many clinical uses as a competitive antagonist at both central and peripheral muscarinic receptor sites. The use of atropine is extensive for patients with bradycardias, in advanced cardiac life support, and in those exposed to acetylcholinesterase inhibitors in the workplace, in the home, and potentially on the battlefield.

REFERENCES

1. Alexander E, Morris DP, Eslick RL. Atropine poisoning: report of a case with recovery after ingestion of one gram. *N Engl J Med.* 1946;234:258-259.
2. Ali R, Jain G, Iqbal Z, et al. Development and clinical trial of nano-atropine sulfate dry powder inhaler as a novel organophosphorous poisoning antidote. *Nanomedicine.* 2009;5:55-63.
3. Ali-Melkkila T, Kanto J, Iisalo E. Pharmacokinetics and related pharmacodynamics of anticholinergic drugs. *Acta Anaesthesiol Scand.* 1993;37:633-642.
4. Amitai Y, Almog S, Singer R, et al. Atropine poisoning in children during the Persian Gulf crisis: a national survey in Israel. *JAMA.* 1992;268:630-632.
5. AtroPen [package insert]. Columbia, MD: Meridian Medical Technologies, Inc; 2003 Sept.
6. Berghem L, Bergman U, Schildt B, et al. Plasma atropine concentrations determined by radioimmunoassay after single-dose I.V. and I.M. administration. *Br J Anaesth.* 1980;52:597-601.
7. Borowitz SM. Prolonged organophosphate toxicity in a twenty six month old child. *J Peds.* 1988;112:302-302.
8. Brown JH, Taylor P. Muscarinic receptor agonists and antagonists. In: Brunton L, Lazo J, Parker K, eds. *Goodman and Gilman's the Pharmacologic Basis of Therapeutics*, 11th ed. New York: McGraw-Hill; 2006:183-200.
9. Bryant S, Wills B, Rhee J, et al. Intramuscular ophthalmic homatropine versus atropine to prevent lethality in rats with dichlorvos poisoning. *J Med Tox.* 2006;2:156-159.
10. Caulfield MP, Birdsall NJ. International Union of Pharmacology: XVII. Classification of muscarinic acetylcholine receptors. *Pharmacol Rev.* 1998;50:279-290.
11. Dix J, Weber RJ, Frye RF, et al. Stability of atropine sulfate prepared for mass chemical terrorism. *J Toxicol Clin Toxicol.* 2003;41:771-775.
12. Eddleston M, Buckley NA, Checketts H, et al. Speed of initial atropinisation in significant organophosphorus pesticide poisoning—a systematic comparison of recommended regimens. *J Toxicol Clin Toxicol.* 2004;42:865-875.
13. Eddleston M, Buckley NA, Eyer P, et al. Management of acute organophosphorous pesticide poisoning. *Lancet.* 2008;371:597-607.
14. Eddleston M, Dawson A, Karalliedde L, et al. Early management after self-poisoning with an organophosphorus or carbamate pesticide—a treatment protocol for junior doctors. *Crit Care.* 2004;8:R391-R397.
15. Forrer GR, Miller JJ. Atropine coma: a somatic therapy in psychiatry. *Am J Psychiatry.* 1958;115:455-458.
16. Fraser TR. On the characters, action and therapeutic uses of the bean of Calabar. *Edinburgh Med J.* 1863;9:235-245.
17. Freeman G, Epstein MA. Therapeutic factors in survival after lethal cholinesterase inhibition by phosphorus insecticides. *N Engl J Med.* 1955;18;253:266-271.
18. Grob D. Anticholinesterase intoxication in man and its treatment. In: Koelle GB, ed. *Handbuch der Experimentellen Pharmakologie 15*, Suppl., Ch 22. New York: Springer-Verlag; 1963:989-1027.
19. Gyermek L. *Pharmacology of Antimuscarinic Agents.* Boca Raton, FL: CRC Press; 1997.
20. Harrison LI, Smallridge RC, Lasseter KC, et al. Comparative absorption of inhaled and intramuscularly administered atropine. *Am Rev Respir Dis.* 1986;134:254-257.
21. Henretig FM, Cieslak TJ, Eitzen EM Jr. Biological and chemical terrorism. *J Pediatr.* 2002;141:311-326.
22. Henretig FM, Mechem C, Jew R. Potential use of autoinjector-packaged antidotes for treatment of pediatric nerve agent toxicity. *Ann Emerg Med.* 2002;40:405-408.
23. Kaila T, Korte JM, Saari KM. Systemic bioavailability of ocularly applied 1% atropine eyedrops. *Acta Ophthalmol Scand.* 1999;77:193-196.
24. Kentala E, Kaila T, Iisalo E, et al. Intramuscular atropine in healthy volunteers: a pharmacokinetic and pharmacodynamic study. *Int J Clin Pharmacol Ther Toxicol.* 1990;28:399-404.
25. Longo VG. Behavioral and electroencephalographic effects of atropine and related compounds. *Pharmacol Rev.* 1966;18:965-996.
26. Mark I. *Nerve Agent Antidote Kit (NAAK).* Columbia, MD: Meridian Medical Technologies, Inc; 2002 Jan.
27. Markenson D, Redlener I. Pediatric terrorism preparedness national guidelines and recommendations: findings of an evidenced-based consensus process. *Biosecur Bioterror.* 2004;2:301-319.
28. Moroi SE, Lichter PR. Ocular pharmacology. In: Hardman JG, Limbird LE, Gilman AG, eds. *Goodman and Gilman's the Pharmacologic Basis of Therapeutics*, 10th ed. New York: McGraw-Hill; 2001:1821-1848.
29. Namba T, Nolte CT, Jackrel J, et al. Poisoning due to organophosphate insecticides. Acute and chronic manifestations. *Am J Med.* 1971;50:475-492.
30. Nickalls RWD, Nickalls EA. The first use of physostigmine in the treatment of atropine poisoning. *Anaesthesia.* 1988;43:776-779.
31. Palmer EA. How safe are ocular drugs in pediatrics? *Ophthalmology.* 1986;93:1038-1040.
32. Pediatric Advanced Life Support, Part 12. *Circulation.* 2005;112(Suppl 4) 167-187.
33. Perera P, Shahmy S, Gawarammana I, et al. Comparison of two commonly practiced atropinization regimens in acute organophosphorous and carbamate poisoning, doubling doses versus ad hoc: a prospective observational study. *Hum Exp Toxicol.* 2008;27:513-518.
34. Pihlajamaki K, Kanto J, Aaltonen L, et al. Pharmacokinetics of atropine in children. *Int J Clin Pharmacol Ther Toxicol.* 1986;24:236-239.
35. Roberts D, Aaron C. Management of acute organophosphorous pesticide poisoning. *BMJ.* 2007;334:629-634.
36. Schier JG, Ravikumar PR, Nelson LS, et al. Preparing for chemical terrorism: stability of injectable atropine sulfate. *Acad Emerg Med.* 2004;11:329-334.
37. Sharony R, Schwaber MJ, Bar-am I, et al. Atropinism following rectal administration of a therapeutic atropine dose. *J Toxicol Clin Toxicol.* 1998;36:41-42.
38. Sidell FR. Nerve agents. In: Zajtchuk R, ed. *Textbook of Military Medicine: Medical Aspects of Chemical and Biological Warfare. Part I.* Office of the Surgeon General Department of the Army, United States of America; 1997:129-177.
39. Sidell FR, Markis JE, Groff W, et al. Enhancement of drug absorption after administration by an automatic injector. *J Pharmacokinet Biopharm.* 1974;2:197-210.
40. *USP DI Volume I. Drug Information for the Health Care Professional. Atropine.* Thomson Healthcare, Inc; 2004:3.
41. Wellstein A, Pitschner HF. Complex dose–response curves of atropine in man explained by different functions of M_1- and M_2-cholinoceptors. *Naunyn Schmiedebergs Arch Pharmacol.* 1988;338:19-27.
42. WHO essential medicines list. http://www.who.int/selection_medicines/list/WMF2008.pdf (accessed Nov 29, 2008).
43. Wills JH. Pharmacological antagonists of the anticholinesterase agents. In: Koelle GB, ed. *Handbuch der Experimenteller Pharmakologie.* New York: Springer-Verlag; 1963:883-920.

CHAPTER 114

INSECTICIDES: ORGANIC CHLORINES, PYRETHRINS/PYRETHROIDS, AND INSECT REPELLENTS

Michael G. Holland

Organic chlorine pesticides are complex, cyclic, polychlorinated hydrocarbons having molecular weights generally in the range of 300 to 550 daltons. They are nonvolatile solids at room temperature. Most act as central nervous system (CNS) stimulants. In contrast, chlorinated hydrocarbon solvents and fumigants are low-molecular-weight, alkyl compounds that are volatile liquids or gases, and generally have CNS-depressant effects (Chap. 106). The pyrethrins, which are extracted from chrysanthemum flowers, are highly effective contact poisons. When properly used they have almost no mammalian systemic toxicity. These molecules are rapidly hydrolyzed and broken down by light with no environmental persistence or bioaccumulation.

ORGANIC CHLORINES

HISTORY AND EPIDEMIOLOGY

Until the 1940s, commonly available pesticides included highly toxic arsenicals, mercurials, lead, sulfur, and nicotine. When Nobel Prize–winning chemist Paul Müller demonstrated the insecticidal properties of dichlorodiphenyltrichloroethane (DDT) in the early 1940s, a whole new class of pesticides was introduced.[51] The organic chlorine insecticides were inexpensive to produce, nonvolatile, environmentally stable, and had relatively low acute toxicity when compared to previously available insecticides. Most organic chlorines have a negative temperature coefficient, making them more insecticidal at lower temperatures, and less toxic to warm-blooded organisms (Table 114–1).[172] Widespread use of these xenobiotics occurred from the 1940s until the mid-1970s. They were highly effective and revolutionized modern agriculture, allowing unprecedented crop output from each acre of arable land. Because of their stability, organic chlorines were used extensively in structural protection (from termites, carpenter ants) and soil treatments. Medical and public health applications of DDT and its analogues were also found in the control of typhus and eradication of malaria by eliminating the mosquito vector.[41] By 1953, DDT alone was credited for saving an estimated 50 million lives, and for averting one billion cases of human disease. It is suggested that because of this consequential impact on human health, DDT is the single most important factor in the population explosion that occurred between 1950 and 1970.[52]

However, the properties that made these chemicals such effective insecticides also made them environmental hazards: they are slowly metabolized, lipid soluble, chemically stable, and environmentally persistent. In her 1962 book, *Silent Spring*, Rachel Carson, a biologist with the US Fish and Wildlife Service, demonstrated that organic chlorines are bioconcentrated and biomagnified up the food chain.[19] She alleged that this persistence could eventually lead to future increases in cancer. Numerous publications since then have shown that organic chlorine residues in predatory birds, most notably grebes, peregrine falcons, bald eagles, and pelicans, caused eggshell thinning and decreased reproductive success.[51] However, conflicting results occurred when DDT-laced feedstuffs were administered in high concentrations to experimental birds. Testing on domesticated birds such as Japanese quail,[21,27,131] and chickens,[170] showed little or no eggshell thinning, whereas testing in mallard ducks showed thinning.[47,48] Hearings before the Environmental Protection Agency (EPA) regarding DDT registration also focused on the unproven fear of placing future generations at risk for cancer. This and the demonstration of persistent DDT residues in all humans, even those living in areas where DDT was never used such as Inuits, led to the severe restriction or total ban of DDT and most other organic chlorines in North America and Europe.[41] There is considerable evidence that since DDT was banned, the limited efficacy of the available alternative pesticides has placed many millions at risk for malaria and is responsible, at least in part, for millions of deaths from this disease.[104,128,129] Not surprisingly, DDT is still considered a highly effective mosquito control agent with a low order of acute toxicity, and is very inexpensive compared with newer replacement insecticides. For these reasons, the World Health Organization (WHO) exempted DDT from its list of banned pesticides, and it is still widely used for malaria control programs in many countries, since alternatives are more expensive and must be applied more often. Current use of DDT for indoor residual spraying is ongoing in endemic areas in Africa, and has been shown to be safe and effective as a public health initiative to control malaria, even in areas with resistant strains.[138] More recently, in the United States another organic chlorine was banned: in 2006, the EPA officially cancelled lindane's registration, and all use in agriculture will cease in 2009.[8]

The organic chlorine pesticides can be grouped into four categories based on their chemical structures and similar toxicities: (1) DDT and related analogues; (2) cyclodienes (the related isomers aldrin, dieldrin, and endrin; and heptachlor, endosulfan), and related compounds (toxaphene, dienochlor); (3) hexachlorocyclohexane, the primary organochlorine pesticide still in clinical use (more commonly termed lindane, the γ isomer, also referred to by the misnomer γ-benzene hexachloride). Isomerism is important, because the β and δ isomers are CNS depressants and have no insecticidal properties[3,32,117]; and (4) mirex and chlordecone (see Table 114–1; Fig. 114–1). These organic chlorine insecticides differ substantially, both between and within groups, with respect to toxic doses, skin absorption, fat storage, metabolism, and elimination.[41] The signs and symptoms of toxicity in humans, however, are remarkably similar within each group.

TOXICOKINETICS

Absorption All of the organic chlorine pesticides are well absorbed orally and by inhalation; dermal absorption is variable, depending on the particular compound. Absorption by any route may be affected by the vehicle and the physical state (solid or liquid) of the pesticide. None of the organic chlorines are water soluble, and are usually either dissolved in organic solvents or manufactured as powders for dusting.

DDT and its analogues are very poorly absorbed dermally, unless dissolved in a suitable hydrocarbon solvent.[126] DDT has limited volatility, so that air concentrations are usually low and toxicity by the respiratory route is unlikely.

All of the cyclodienes have significant dermal absorption rates. Cutaneous absorption of dieldrin is approximately 50% that of the oral route. Oral absorption of the cyclodienes is also high, and significant poisonings have occurred when foodstuffs were contaminated with these pesticides.[17,22] Although toxaphene is poorly absorbed through the skin, acute and chronic exposures occur.[143]

TABLE 114–1. Classification of Organic Chlorine Insecticides

Class	CAS[a] Registry #	Brand Name(s)	Current EPA Registration (US)	Acute Oral Toxicity (Man)	Dermal Absorption	Lipid Storage	Specific Characteristics
Hexachloro-cyclohexanes	Lindane (gamma isomer) 58–89–9	Kwell; Gustafson Flowable; Sorghum Guard	Topical scabicide; agricultural use cancelled 2006	Moderate	High	Low	Topical scabicide: seizures, CNS excitation; musty odor
DDT and Analogues	DDT (dichlorodiphenyltrichloroethane) 50–29–3	Neocid, Ixodex, Anofex, others	Cancelled 1972	Low to moderate	Low	Highest	Tremors, CNS excitation; odorless
	Methoxychlor 72–43–5	Marlate	Cancelled 2003	Low	Low	Moderate	Less toxic DDT substitute
	Dicofol 115–32–2	Kelthane	Residential use banned 1998; cotton, citrus, apple	Low	Low	Low	
	Chlorobenzilate 510–15–6	Benzilan, BenzoChlor	Cancelled 1983	Low	Low	Low	Much less environmental persistence than DDT
Cyclodienes and Related Compounds	Aldrin 309–00–2	Aldrex, Octalene, Toxadrin	Cancelled 1974	High	High	High	Rapidly metabolized to dieldrin; mild "chemical" odor
	Dieldrin 60–57–1	Dieldrite, Octalox, Quintox	Cancelled 1974	High	High	High	Stereoisomer of endrin; early and late seizures; odorless
	Endrin 72–20–8	Hexadrin	Cancelled 1974	Highest	High	None	Most toxic organic chlorine; rapid onset seizures, status epilepticus
	Chlordane 57–74–9	Octachlor, Toxichlor, others	Cancelled 1988	Moderate	High	High	Early and late seizures
	Endosulfan 115–29–7	Thiodan, Cyclodan, others	RED[b] 2002	High	High	Low	Strong sulfur odor
	Heptachlor 76–44–8	Drinox	Restricted: fire ant control soil treatment	Moderate	High	High	Toxic metabolite heptachlor epoxide; camphor odor
	Isobenzan 297–78–9	Telodrin	Never registered	High	Moderate	High	Also inhibits Mg^{++}-ATPase; mild "chemical" odor
	Dienochlor 2227–17–0	Pentac	Cancelled	NA	Low	Low	Toxic metabolite binds to GSH
	Toxaphene (polychlorinated camphene) 800–35–2	Alltox, Chemphene, Toxakil, others	Cancelled 1982	Moderate to high	Low	Low	Seizures; turpentinelike odor, often mixed with parathion
Chlordecone and Mirex	Chlordecone 143–50–0	Kepone	Cancelled 1977	Moderate	High	High	"Kepone shakes"; structurally similar to mirex
	Mirex 2385–85–5	Dechlorane	Cancelled 1976	Low	High	High	Metabolized to chlordecone, similar toxicity.

[a] CAS = Chemical Abstracts Service #—provided here to facilitate Toxline, Medline database searches.
[b] RED, Re-registration Eligibility Decision.
CNS, central nervous system; GSH, glutathione.

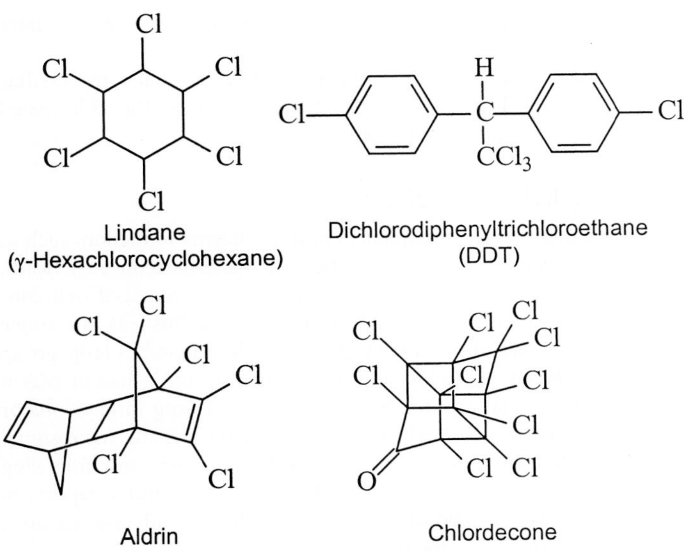

Lindane
(γ-Hexachlorocyclohexane)

Dichlorodiphenyltrichloroethane
(DDT)

Aldrin

Chlordecone

FIGURE 114–1. Structures of various organic chlorine insecticides.

In adults, lindane is well absorbed following topical application; the forearm skin absorption rate is 9.3% after 24 hours.[61] Anatomic sites vary in their absorptive capacities: axillary rates are 3.6 times greater and scrotal absorption is 42 times greater than forearm rates.[16,66,81,151] Animal studies and case reports suggest that the young, the malnourished, and those who receive repeated topical doses may have increased accumulation and toxicity.[118] Hot baths, occlusive clothing, or bandages, the vehicle for the lindane, and a disturbed cutaneous integrity, such as eczema, fissures, and other violations of the skin, all enhance dermal penetration.[150,151] The state of hydration of the skin also affects the amounts absorbed, so that bathing just prior to application can enhance absorption and increase the likelihood of toxicity.[102,151] Lindane is a stable compound and volatilizes easily when heated. It was used extensively in the past in home vaporizers, and toxicity was common via inhalation, or when vaporizer tablets were unintentionally ingested by children. Review of data following oral use of lindane as an antihelmintic demonstrates that 40 mg/d for 3 to 14 days generally produced no symptoms.[41]

Mirex and chlordecone are efficiently absorbed via skin, by inhalation, and orally.[60]

Distribution All organic chlorines are lipophilic, a property that facilitates penetration to many sites.[29] The fat-to-serum ratios at equilibrium are high, in the range of 660:1 for chlordane,[71] 220:1 for lindane,[144] and 150:1 for dieldrin.[42] Central nervous system redistribution to the blood and then to fat may account for the apparent rapid CNS recovery despite a persistent substantial total body burden. In the rat model, there is a direct correlation between the concentration of DDT or dieldrin in the brain and the clinical signs produced after a single dose of the insecticide.[41,45]

Serum lindane concentrations peak at 6 hours and have a half-life of 18 hours after topical application.[62]

Metabolism The high lipid solubility and very slow metabolic disposition of DDT, DDE (dichlorodiphenyl dichloroethylene, metabolite of DDT), dieldrin, heptachlor, chlordane, mirex, and chlordecone causes significant adipose tissue storage and increasing body burdens in chronically exposed populations.[60] Organic chlorines that are rapidly metabolized and eliminated, such as endrin (an isomer of dieldrin), endosulfan, lindane, methoxychlor, dienochlor, chlorobenzilate, dicofol, and toxaphene, tend to have less persistence in body tissues, despite being highly lipid soluble.[126]

Most organic chlorines are metabolized by the hepatic cytochrome P450 (CYP) enzyme systems by dechlorination and oxidation, with subsequent conjugation. However, metabolism may result in the production of a metabolite with more toxicity than the parent compound, such as heptachlor to heptachlor epoxide, chlordane to oxychlordane, and aldrin to dieldrin.

In animals, most organic chlorine pesticides are capable of inducing the hepatic microsomal enzyme systems.[40,174] Enzyme induction changes the biodegradation of the pesticide in rodents,[157] and in certain animal models the acute toxicity of organic phosphorus (OP) compounds and carbamates may be reduced by the administration of organic chlorines. Since this protective effect does not occur when the cytochrome P450 (CYP) inhibitor piperonyl butoxide is administered, it shows that hepatic microsomal enzyme induction by the organic chlorine and subsequent increased metabolism of the OP compound is responsible for this reduced toxicity of the OP in this rodent model.[41,174] However, induction of hepatic enzymes is rarely described in man.[60,71]

Elimination The half-lives of fat-stored compounds and poorly metabolized organic chlorines such as DDT and chlordecone are measured in months or years. The elimination half-life of lindane is 21 hours in adults.[103] The primary route of excretion of the organic chlorines is in the bile, but most also have detectable urinary metabolites. However, as with other compounds excreted in bile, most of the organic chlorines such as mirex and chlordecone have significant enterohepatic or enteroenteric recirculation.[14,31,60] All of the lipophilic compounds are excreted in maternal milk.[132]

MECHANISMS OF TOXICITY

The same neurotoxic properties that make the organic chlorines lethal to the target insects make them potentially toxic to higher forms of life. The organic chlorines exert their most important effects in the CNS. Electrophysiologic studies demonstrate that the organic chlorine insecticides affect the neuronal membrane by either interfering with repolarization, prolonging depolarization, or impairing the maintenance of the polarized state of the neuron. The end result is hyperexcitability of the nervous system and repetitive neuronal discharges.[52]

The voltage-gated sodium channel is a common site of action for natural and synthetic neurotoxins. There are at least 10 separate binding sites on the sodium channel, including those for local anesthetics and anticonvulsants. DDT, as well as the pyrethroids, bind at the same site on these channels. They preferentially bind when the channel is in the open state, allowing prolonged inward sodium conductance, repetitive action potentials, and extended tail currents. Prolonged axonal firing and repetitive stimuli eventually lead to nerve paralysis and death in target insects, whose sodium channels have much greater affinity for these insecticides than those of mammals.[108,109,111,152] In mammals, low-level stimuli cause exaggerated responses, manifested clinically as prominent tremors and abnormal startle reflexes observed in test animals.[79,166] This primary mechanism of action is demonstrated by the amelioration of DDT-induced tremor by pretreatment with phenytoin, a sodium channel blocker, which reduces the ability of voltage-dependent Na channels to recover from inactivation.[79,165]

The cyclodienes and lindane act as γ-aminobutyric acid (GABA) antagonists. They inhibit GABA binding at the $GABA_A$ receptor–chloride ionophore complex in the CNS, by interacting at the picrotoxin binding site.[3,11,32,70,74,110,117] In fact, the degree of binding at this site correlates well with the amount of Cl^- influx inhibited and the relative neurotoxicity of each insecticide (Figs. 13–9, 13–10, and 114–2).[11,70] Indeed, development of cyclodiene resistance seems to be related to alterations of the $GABA_A$ receptor–chloride ionophore complex in

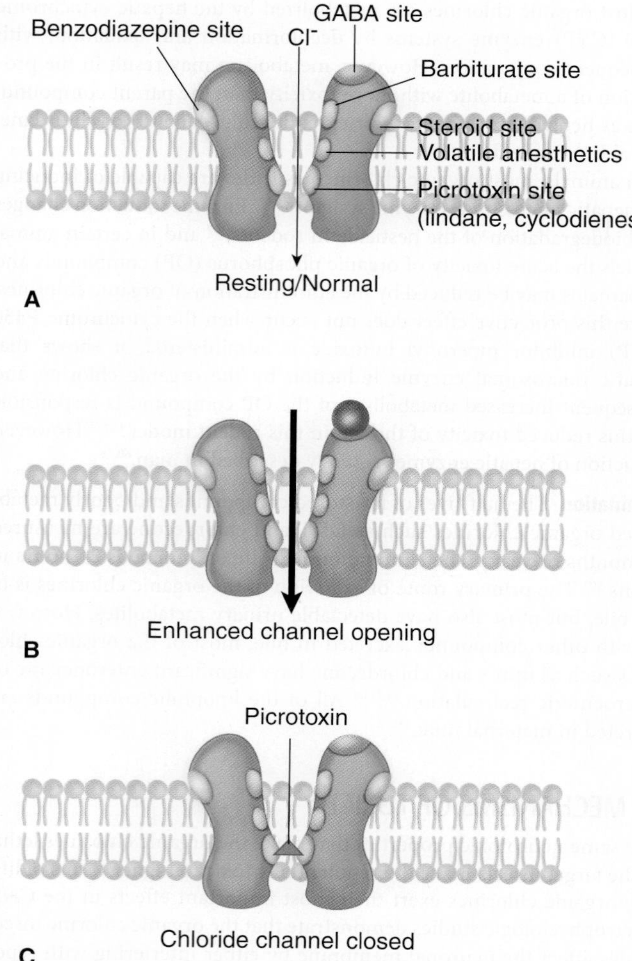

FIGURE 114–2. Chloride channel. (A) Under resting conditions, a tonic influx of chloride maintains the nerve cell in a polarized state. (B) Binding of GABA (●) or an indirect-acting GABA agonist (benzodiazepine, barbiturate, volatile anesthetic) opens the chloride channel. The subsequent chloride influx hyperpolarizes the cell membrane, making the neuron less likely to propagate an action potential in response to a stimulus. (C) GABA antagonists, such as picrotoxin, close the chloride channel, reducing chloride influx. The resulting decreased membrane polarity causes the neuron to become hyperexcitable to even those stimuli that are normally subthreshold in nature (Chap. 13).

these affected insects.[12,109] This also explains the efficacy of GABA agonists, such as benzodiazepines and phenobarbital, in treating seizures and neurotoxicity that result from the cyclodienes[75] and lindane.[178] Toxaphene also inhibits GABA binding at the $GABA_A$ receptor–chloride ionophore complex.[143]

The mechanisms of action of mirex and chlordecone are not as well understood. They inhibit Na^+–K^+-ATPase, and Ca^{2+}-ATPase. However, lindane, DDT, and the cyclodienes also inhibit these enzymes yet produce very different symptoms of toxicity, suggesting that these effects are not responsible for the clinical manifestations associated with mirex and chlordecone toxicity. Phenytoin and serotonin agonists exacerbate the prominent tremor associated with chlordecone poisoning, but conversely attenuate the tremors occurring with DDT poisoning, which further supports differing mechanisms of toxicity for the two compounds.[52] Mirex and chlordecone are poor inhibitors of GABA binding at the $GABA_A$ receptor–chloride ionophore complex; therefore, their mechanism of action is also likely not at this site,[60] and seizures have not been described with mirex or chlordecone.

Organic chlorines can predispose test animals to cardiac dysrhythmias,[126] likely via the same mechanism as the chlorinated hydrocarbon solvents (Chap. 106).

DRUG INTERACTIONS

There are theoretical consequences of liver enzyme induction, such as enhanced metabolism of therapeutic drugs and/or reduced efficacy. Dysfunctional uterine bleeding was attributed to enhanced oral contraceptive metabolism induced by chlordane, but this was in a single patient with weeks of excessive exposure to chlordane.[71] A large group of workers poisoned by chlordecone over many months had increased hepatic microsomal activity, but no evidence of drug interactions or adverse clinical effects.[60] Thus, induction of the hepatic microsomal enzyme system by organic chlorines probably occurs only following extended, substantial exposures.[126] There are no definitive reports of human enhanced metabolism of therapeutic drugs or adverse reactions due to microsomal enzyme induction.

CLINICAL MANIFESTATIONS

Acute Exposure In sufficient doses, organic chlorines lower the seizure threshold (DDT and related sodium channel agents) or remove inhibitory influences (antagonism to GABA effects) and produce CNS stimulation, with resultant seizures, respiratory failure, and death.[20,22,30,74,75,87,88,135,137] After DDT exposure, tremor may be the only initial manifestation. Nausea; vomiting; hyperesthesia of the mouth and face; paresthesias of face, tongue, and extremities; headache; dizziness; myoclonus; leg weakness; agitation; and confusion may subsequently occur. Seizures only occur after massive exposures, typically following the ingestion of large amounts.[52,75] DDT has a relatively low order of acute toxicity, and high doses of DDT (10 mg/kg or more) are usually necessary to produce symptoms.[75] There often are no prodromal signs or symptoms, and more often than not, the first manifestation of toxicity following exposure to lindane, the cyclodienes, and toxaphene is a generalized seizure.[20,22,51,52,75,88,135,154] If seizures develop, they often occur within 1 to 2 hours of ingestion when the stomach is empty, but may be delayed as much as 5 to 6 hours when the ingestion follows a substantial meal.[75]

Seizures related to dermal application of 1% lindane for treatment of ectoparasitic diseases may occur following a single inappropriate application,[95,118,162] or, more commonly, after repetitive prolonged exposures.[90,122] The time from application to seizure onset can vary from hours to days. The seizures are often self-limited, but may recur or result in status epilepticus. An epidemic of lindane poisoning related to the unintentional substitution of lindane powder for sugar in coffee demonstrated a delay of 20 minutes to 3 hours before the onset of nausea, vomiting, dizziness, facial pallor, severe cyanosis of the face and extremities, collapse, convulsions, and hyperthermia. Affected patients ingested an average of 86 mg/kg of lindane in a single time.[41]

The cyclodienes are also notable for their propensity to cause seizures that may recur for several days following an acute exposure. If the seizures are brief and hypoxia has not occurred, recovery is usually complete. Electroencephalographic (EEG) abnormalities are noted before, during, and following seizures.[88] Hyperthermia secondary to central mechanisms, increased muscle activity, and/or aspiration pneumonitis is common.[52]

The ingestion of combinations of xenobiotics such as for DDT and lindane may result in significantly increased toxicity because of synergy.[75]

Lindane: Specific Risks Patients are at risk for developing CNS toxicity from improper topical therapeutic use such as exceeding recommended application times or amounts, repeated applications, application following hot baths, and use of occlusive dressings or clothing shortly after application. Toxicity also occurs after unintentional ingestion of topical preparations. Young children appear at greatest risk, possibly because of greater skin permeability, increased ratio of body surface area to mass, or immature liver enzymes.[122,161,162] The elderly may also be at increased risk because of impaired hepatic metabolism, atrophic skin, and perhaps age-related increased sensitivity. Preexisting conditions causing increased risk of seizures include chlorpromazine treatment, CNS disease, or skin absorption changes.[5,43,62,90,95,112,118,122,150,151,161,162]

Despite the availability of safer and equally or more effective treatments such as permethrin, lindane continues to be used because of its low cost and generally good safety profile, when used according to directions. An evaluation of published English-language case reports and those submitted to the FDA divided toxicity into those associated with concentrations of lindane greater than or less than 1%.[90] Only six of 26 cases could be considered probably related to 1% lindane; six others were the result of ingestion or inappropriate skin application.[5] The sale of lindane-containing products for use in humans was recently banned in California because of its toxicity and environmental concerns.[17] In 1995, the FDA changed the labeling requirements for lindane adding a black-box warning, and relegating it to second-line therapy for ectoparasitic skin infections, because of its toxicity and the superior safety and efficacy of other products.[7]

Chronic Exposure Chlordecone (Kepone), unlike the other organic chlorines, produces an insidious picture of chronic toxicity related to its extremely long persistence in the body. Because of poor industrial hygiene practices in a makeshift chlordecone factory in Hopewell, Virginia, 133 workers were heavily exposed for 17 months from 1974 to 1975. They developed a clinical syndrome known as the "Hopewell epidemic," which consisted of a prominent tremor of the hands, a fine tremor of the head, and trembling of the entire body, known as the "Kepone shakes." Other findings included weakness, opsoclonus (rapid, irregular, dysrhythmic ocular movements), ataxia, mental status changes, rash, weight loss, and elevated liver enzyme concentrations. Idiopathic intracranial hypertension, oligospermia, and decreased sperm motility were also found in some of these workers. Severely affected workers even exhibited an exaggerated startle response, remarkably similar to that seen in animal studies. The exposures were so intense that some workers went home covered with chlordecone, and several workers' wives developed neurological symptoms, presumably from exposures while laundering their husbands' work clothes.[31,60]

This event led to substantial concern in environmental health centers with regard to persistent organic chemicals, such as the organic chlorine residues and polychlorinated biphenyls (PCBs). A recent review of the world literature reveals that since many of the organic chlorines are outlawed in many processes and countries, human burden appears to be decreasing.[98]

Carcinogenicity. DDT and other organic chlorine insecticides have estrogenic effects.[44,153] These estrogenic compounds adversely affect birds because differentiation of the avian reproductive system is estrogen dependent.[68] Breast cancer incidence rates in the United States have climbed 1% per year since the 1940s, coinciding with, among many other factors, the worldwide use of DDT. Because lifetime exposure to excess estrogen is a known risk factor for human breast cancer, it has been postulated that women who have higher concentrations of estrogenic organic chlorine compounds such as DDT and PCBs may be at greater risk for developing breast cancer.[139,176]

Several small case-control studies of women with breast cancer showed that women with the disease had higher average body burdens of DDT, DDE, and PCBs than their age-matched controls. These studies implicated the organic chlorines as a possible cause of human breast cancer. However, more recently, larger studies have shown no increased risk of breast cancer because of exposure to organic chlorines,[18] and that currently accepted hereditary and lifestyle risk factors were present in the patients with cancer.[80,91,139–141] In fact, other natural dietary estrogens such as flavonoids, lignans, sterols, and fungal metabolites are present in the human diet, and have much higher estrogenic potency; the organic chlorine contribution is probably minimal by comparison.[69] A recent meta-analysis of 22 studies found strong evidence to discard the putative relationship between p,p'-DDE (dichlorodiphenyldichloroethane) and breast cancer risk.[97]

The organic chlorines can induce liver tumors in mice, but have not been shown to do so in rats or hamsters.[76] Some reports suggest an association between long-term exposure to organic chlorine insecticides and hematologic disorders such as aplastic anemia, leukemia, and drug-induced thrombocytopenic purpura.[75,123,136] However, there is no convincing evidence that any of these xenobiotics are carcinogenic in humans. Workers heavily exposed to DDT and dieldrin do not have an increased incidence of neoplasms.[76] Epidemiologic evidence suggests that the incidence of deaths from liver cancer has steadily decreased since 1930, which includes the more than 50 years since the introduction of the organic chlorines.[75,76] There is some evidence that DDT can be a facilitator of carcinogenesis induced by other xenobiotics, such as aflatoxin, and that chlordane may have the same facilitative character regarding diethylnitrosamine.[75] A comprehensive review found no evidence of human cancer risk from exposure to aldrin or dieldrin.[156]

DIAGNOSTIC INFORMATION

The history of exposure to an organic chlorine insecticide is the most critical piece of information, because exposure is otherwise rare. By US law, the package label of these products must list the ingredients, the concentrations, and the vehicle. The EPA-registered use of the insecticide may be helpful in determining which agent is involved (Table 114–2). The presence of an unusual odor in the mouth, in the

TABLE 114–2. Common Household Insecticides

Pest	Typical Recommendation
Ants	Baygon, bendiocarb, chlorpyrifos, diazinon, permethrin, resmethrin, silica gel pyrethrum, boric acid
Bedbugs	Permethrin
Cockroaches	Baygon, bendiocarb, chlorpyrifos, diazinon, permethrin, resmethrin, silica gel pyrethrum, tetramethrin, boric acid
Fleas	Baygon, bendiocarb, chlorpyrifos, d-limonene, permethrin, pyrethrins, silica gel pyrethrum, resmethrin, tetramethrin
Flies (house)	Allethrin, pyrethrum, resmethrin, tetramethrin
Mosquitoes	Allethrin, pyrethrum, pyrethrins, resmethrin, tetramethrin
Silverfish	Baygon, bendiocarb, boric acid, chlorpyrifos, diazinon, silca gel pyrethrum
Spiders	Baygon, bendiocarb, chlorpyrifos, diazinon, permethrin, pyrethrins, resmethrin, tetramethrin
Termites	Restricted in use for application by certified applicators
Ticks	Baygon, chlorpyrifos, diazinon, malathion, tetramethrin

Reproduced, with permission, from Guide to Safe Pest Management Around the Home. New York State College of Agriculture and Life Sciences of Cornell University, 1997/1998, Misc Bull 74 Media Services at Cornell University.

vomitus, or on the skin may be helpful. Toxaphene, a chlorinated pinene, has a mild turpentine-like odor, and endosulfan has "rotten egg" sulfur odor (see Table 114–1). Following ingestion, an abdominal radiograph may reveal the presence of a radiopaque chlorinated insecticide, since chlorine increases the radiopacity of the xenobiotics (Chap. 5). A large number of other xenobiotics lead to seizures as the first manifestation of toxicity, and must be considered in the differential of an unknown exposure (Chaps. 13 and 18).

LABORATORY TESTING

Gas chromatography can detect organic chlorine insecticides in serum, adipose tissue, and urine.[42,80] If confirmation is indicated for purposes of documentation of source, it may be necessary to measure concentrations of organic chlorines. If the patient's history and toxidrome are obvious, then laboratory evaluation is unnecessary, as this determination will not alter the course of management, and these blood tests are not available on an emergent basis. At present, there are no data correlating health effects and tissue concentrations. Routine surveillance of serum concentrations in the occupationally exposed is not currently performed.[42]

Most humans studied have measurable concentrations of DDT in adipose tissue. In a study of a community with a very large exposure to DDT, serum DDT concentrations increased proportionally with age. These increasing concentrations were not associated with any apparent adverse health effects, but there was an association with increasing concentrations of the liver enzyme γ-glutamyltransferase (GGT), but significant hepatotoxicity did not occur. The Centers for Disease Control and Prevention's (CDC's) Third National Report on Human Exposure to Environmental Chemicals has demonstrated the presence of numerous organic chlorine insecticide residues in the lipid fraction of serum of US residents. These levels tend to increase with patient age, consistent with the bioaccumulation and fat-storing properties of the chemicals.[24] More recently, studies of occupationally exposed pesticide applicators and persons living in targeted regions confirmed higher serum concentrations over those not exposed, but no ill health effects are documented.[138]

Serum lindane concentrations document exposure, and most laboratories report toxic ranges. Lindane-exposed workers with chronic neurologic symptoms showed a blood lindane concentration of 0.02 mg/L.[5,75] A limited series of patients with acute lindane ingestion suggests that a serum concentration of 0.12 mg/L correlates with sedation, and that 0.20 mg/L is associated with seizures and coma.[5] After cutaneous application, lindane concentrations in the CNS are three to 12 times higher than serum concentrations.[31,46,151] In a group of factory workers with a prolonged exposure to chlordecone, clinical signs and symptoms of toxicity correlated with blood concentrations.[31]

MANAGEMENT

As in the care of any patient who presents with an altered mental status, the administration of dextrose and thiamine (in an adult) should be considered. Skin decontamination is essential, especially in the case of topical lindane exposure. Clothing should be removed and placed in a plastic bag that should be disposed of appropriately as biohazardous waste, and the skin washed with soap and water. Healthcare providers should be protected with rubber gloves and aprons. Because these insecticides are almost invariably liquids, a nasogastric tube can be used to suction and lavage gastric contents, if clinically indicated. This is most appropriate only with a very recent ingestion (Chap. 7). Activated charcoal (AC) can be used after or instead of gastric lavage, when lavage is not indicated.[75,101] However, the ability of AC to adsorb the various organic chlorines has not been adequately studied, and mixtures containing petroleum distillates would obviously preclude the use of AC (see Chap. 7). Because the organic chlorines are all neurotoxins, the risk of complications associated with seizures probably outweighs the risk of any of the gastrointestinal (GI) decontamination strategies in most acute settings. A murine model of lindane toxicity following intragastric administration showed a trend, but not a statistically significant benefit, of AC.[85] The use of cholestyramine, a nonabsorbable, bile acid–binding anion exchange resin, in the same murine model did show a statistically significant benefit by raising both the convulsive dose and the lethal dose.[85] Cholestyramine should be administered to all patients symptomatic from chlordecone, and possibly other organic chlorine exposures. Chlordecone undergoes both enterohepatic and enteroenteric recirculation, which can be interrupted by cholestyramine at a dosage of 16 g/d. Cholestyramine increased the fecal elimination of chlordecone three- to 18-fold in industrial workers exposed during the Hopewell epidemic, resulting in clinical improvement.[31]

Oil-based cathartics should never be used, as they may facilitate absorption. There is some evidence that sucrose polyester (olestra, a nonabsorbed synthetic dietary oil substitute) can increase excretion of a wide variety of fat-soluble organic chlorine chemicals.[82,106] It is useful for dioxin-poisoned patients when administered in potato chips.[72] This was most recently successfully used in treating Ukrainian President Viktor Yushenko.[155] This would be an inexpensive and more palatable alternative to cholestyramine in the effort to diminish toxicity by increasing excretion in patients with significant body burdens following chronic organic chlorine exposure.

Seizures should be controlled with a benzodiazepine followed by pentobarbital or a propofol infusion and, if necessary, neuromuscular blockade to control the peripheral manifestations of seizures, thereby preventing metabolic acidosis and rhabdomyolysis. As has been shown in other toxic exposures, phenytoin is much less effective in these cases, particularly with the GABA-chloride ionophore antagonists lindane, toxaphene, and the cyclodienes.[126] Hyperthermia should be managed with external cooling.

PYRETHRINS AND PYRETHROIDS

The pyrethrins are the active extracts from the flower *Chrysanthemum cinerariaefolium*. These insecticides are important historically, having been used in China since the first century AD[41] and developed for commercial application by the 1800s. They are produced by organic solvent extraction from ground Chrysanthemum flowers. The resulting concentrates have greater than 90% purity. Pyrethrum, the first pyrethrin identified, consists of six esters derived from chrysanthemic acid and pyrethric acid. These insecticides are highly effective contact poisons, and their lipophilic nature allows them to readily penetrate insect chitin (exoskeleton) and paralyze their nervous systems through Na^+ channel blockade.[29,107,126,152] When applied properly, they have essentially no systemic mammalian toxicity because of their rapid hydrolysis. Pyrethrins break down rapidly in light and in water, and therefore have no environmental persistence or bioaccumulation. This fact makes them extremely safe after human exposures, but unsuitable for commercial agriculture, since the constant reapplication would be cost prohibitive.

The pyrethroids are the synthetic derivatives of the natural pyrethrins (Table 114–3 and Fig. 114–3). They were developed in an effort to produce more environmentally stable products for use in agriculture. Originally, the pyrethroids were divided into two groups based on the poison syndromes they elicited in test animals. The

TABLE 114–3. Synthetic Pyrethroids in Common Use

Class	Generic Name, CAS #	Trademark Brand Names	Generation of Pyrethrold, Dates Introduced (if Available)
Type I	Allethrin 584–79–2	Pynamin	1st generation; first synthetic pyrethroid, 1949
	Bioallethrin 584–79–2	D-trans	2nd generation, 1969: trans isomer of allethrin
	Dimethrin 70–38–2	Dimetrin	2nd generation
	Phenothrin 26002–80–2	Fenothrin, Forte, Sumithrin	2nd generation, 1973
	Resmethrin 10453–86–8	Benzofluroline, Chrysron, Crossfire, pyrethrum Premgard, Pynosect, Pyretherm, Synthrin	2nd generation, 1967; 20× strength of pyrethrum
	Bioresmethrin 28434–01–7		2nd generation, 1967; 50× strength of pyrethrum, isomer of resmethrin
	Tetramethrin 7696–12–0	Neo-Pynamin	2nd generation, 1965
	Permethrin 52645–53–1	Ambush, Biomist, Dragnet, Ectiban, Elimite, Ipitox, Ketokill, Nix, Outflank, Perigen, Permasect, Persect, Pertox, Pounce, Pramex, etc.	3rd generation, 1972; effective topical scabicide and miticide, low toxicity
	Bifenthrin 82657–04–3	Capture, Talstar	4th generation
	Prallethrin 23031–36–9	SF, Etoc	4th generation
	Imiprothrin 72963–72–5	Multicide, Pralle, Raid Ant and Roach	3rd generation, 1998
Type II	Fenvalerate 51630–58–1	Belmark, Evercide, Extrin, Fenkill, Sanmarton, Sumicidin, Sumifly, Sumipower, Sumitox, Tribute	3rd generation, 1973
	Acrinathrin 103833–18–7	Rufast	4th generation
	Cyfluthrin 68359–37–5	Baythroid, Countdown, Cylense, Laser, Tempo, Bulldock, Cyfoxylate, Eulan SP, Solfac	4th generation
	Cyhalothrin 91465–08–6	Demand, Karate, Ninja 10WP , Scimitar, Warrior	4th generation
	Cypermethrin 52315–07–8	Ammo, Barricade, CCN52, Cymbush, Cymperator, Cynoff, Cypercopal; Cyperkill, Cyrux, Demon, Flectron, KafilSuper, Ripcord, Siperin, Mustang, and Fury	4th generation
	Deltamethrin 52918–63–5	Butoflin, Butox, Crackdown, Decis, DeltaDust, DeltaGard, Deltex, K-Othrine, Striker, Suspend	4th generation
	Esfenvalerate 66230–04–4	Asana, Asana-XL, Hallmark, Sumi-alpha	4th generation
	Fenpropathrin 39515–41–8	Danitol, Herald, Meothrin, Rody	4th generation, 1989
	Flucythrinate 70124–77–5	AASTAR, Cybolt, Fluent, Payoff, Guardian, Cythrin, StockGuard	4th generation
	Fluvalinate 102851–06–9	Apistan, Klartan, Mavrik, Mavrik Aqua Flow, Spur, Taufluvalinate, and Yardex	4th generation
	Imiprothrin 72963-72-5	Pralle; Multicide (mixture with d-phenothrin)	4th generation,1998
	Tefluthrin 79538–32–2	Demand, Force, Karate, Scimitar, Evict, Fireban, Force, and Raze	4th generation
	Tralomethrin 66841–25–6	Dethmor, SAGA, Scout, Scout X-TRA, Tralex	4th generation

T syndrome (for *t*remor seen in rats) was produced by intravenous administration of pyrethrin and most (15 of 18) of the pyrethroids that did not contain a cyano group at the central ester linkage. The CS syndrome (for *c*horeoathetosis and *s*alivation) was produced by 12 of the 17 pyrethroids that had an α-cyano group at the ester linkage. The original studies delineating the T or CS method of classification did not test several new currently registered pyrethroid pesticides, and the testing methods involved intravenous or intracerebral administration, which are not relevant to human exposures.[149]

The predominant classification scheme used today is based on the structure of the pyrethroid (see Fig. 114–3), its clinical manifestations in mammalian intoxication, its actions on insect nerve preparations, and its insecticidal activity. Type I pyrethroids have a simple ester bond at the central linkage without a cyano group. Commonly used type I pyrethroids include permethrin, allethrin, tetramethrin, and fenothrin. The type II pyrethroids have a cyano group at the carbon of this ester linkage. Type II pyrethroids in common use include cypermethrin, deltamethrin, fenpropathrin, fluvalinate, and fenvalerate. The cyano group greatly enhances neurotoxicity of the type II pyrethroids in both

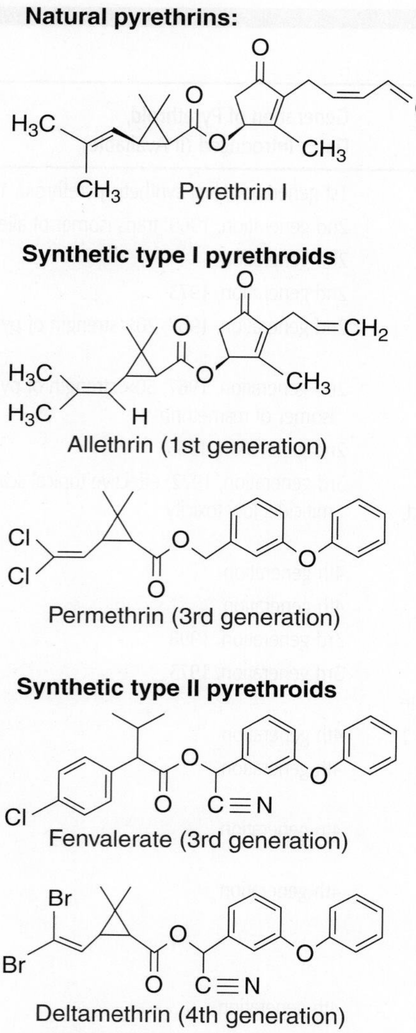

Natural pyrethrins:

Pyrethrin I

Synthetic type I pyrethroids

Allethrin (1st generation)

Permethrin (3rd generation)

Synthetic type II pyrethroids

Fenvalerate (3rd generation)

Deltamethrin (4th generation)

FIGURE 114–3. Representative structures of pyrethrin and pyrethroids.

mammals and insects, and type II agents tend to produce the CS syndrome in test animals and are generally considered more potent and toxic than the type I pyrethroids.[51,100,124,126,149]

The development of the pyrethroids can be divided into "generations," based on efficacy and dates of introduction.[172] The first generation began in 1949, with the development of allethrin. The second generation began in 1965, with the introduction of tetramethrin. The major advance of the second generation was a dramatic increase in potency compared with the pyrethrins. The third generation, introduced in the 1970s and including fenvalerate and permethrin, were the first pyrethroids with practical agricultural use. They are more potent and more environmentally stable, with efficacious crop residues lasting 4 to 7 days. The current fourth generation includes mostly type II pyrethroids, which have even greater insecticidal activity, are photostable (do not undergo photolysis "splitting" in sunlight), have minimal volatility, and provide extended residual effectiveness for up to 10 days under optimum conditions.[100,172]

There are more than 1000 pyrethroids, of which 16 to 20 are in widespread use today.[15,41] Pyrethrins and pyrethroids are found in more than 2000 commercially available products. These insecticides have a rapid paralytic effect ("knock down") on insects. On the other hand, most mammalian species are relatively resistant, because the pyrethrins can be rapidly detoxified by ester cleavage and oxidation.[116] Toxicity of the pyrethrins and pyrethroids is enhanced in insects by combination with microsomal enzyme inhibitors such as piperonyl butoxide (a synthetic analogue of sesamin, the methylenedioxyphenyl component of sesame oil) or *N*-octyl bicycloheptene dicarboximide [10,120]

Permethrin, a type I pyrethroid, is used medicinally as a topical treatment for ectoparasitic conditions in humans, and when impregnated in clothing and mosquito netting as an insect repellant. It has an excellent safety profile, with less than or equal to 2% being dermally absorbed.[102] Recent comprehensive reviews have confirmed that 5% permethrin is the drug of choice for scabies treatment, with the best efficacy versus safety profile of topical treatments for scabies and lice.[133,171] There are concerns of pediculosis resistance to the 1% over-the-counter product, but comparison trials still demonstrate clinical superiority as well as safety advantage compared with lindane.[17]

West Nile virus (WNV) was first identified in the United States in 1999, and rapidly spread to most U.S. states by 2006. Outbreaks of encephalitis caused by WNV occur in the late summer and early autumn months in the United States. Although birds are the reservoirs for WNV, transmission to humans occurs via mosquito bites, and hence many states and municipalities have increased their aerial spraying in an effort to control mosquito vectors of this disease. Most spraying programs use pyrethroid insecticides because of their favorable safety profile, and their efficacy against the adult mosquito. The widespread spraying programs have increased the potential for human exposures to these xenobiotics. A CDC study of pyrethroid spraying did not reveal an increase in detectable pyrethroid metabolites in the general public living in the sprayed areas.[9] Another study of asthma surveillance showed no increases in emergency department (ED) visits because of asthma-related conditions for the periods after pyrethroid spraying.[83]

TOXICOKINETICS

Absorption Pyrethrins are well absorbed orally and via inhalation, but skin absorption is poor. Piperonyl butoxide is also well absorbed orally, but likewise has poor dermal penetration.[120] The oral toxicity of pyrethrins in mammals is extremely low, because they are so readily hydrolyzed into inactive compounds. Dermal toxicity is even lower, due to slow penetration and rapid metabolism.[52,116]

The pyrethroids are more stable than the natural pyrethrins, and significant systemic toxicity has occurred following ingestion.[77] An average of 35% (range 27%–57%) of orally administered cypermethrin was absorbed in human volunteers.[177] Most exposures are from dermal absorption, the rate of which varies depending on the solvent vehicle. In the same volunteer study noted above, a mean of 1.2% (range 0.85%–1.8%) of dermally applied cypermethrin in soybean oil vehicle was absorbed systemically.[177] Intradermal metabolism of pyrethroids occurs in test animals, and likely further limits systemic absorption.[15] Direct absorption of pyrethroids through the skin to the peripheral sensory nerves probably accounts for the facial paresthesias that occur in these cases, as symptoms were prominent in areas of direct contact.[28,94] Absorption probably also occurs through the oral mucosa, as noted by a large study of Chinese insecticide sprayers who frequently used their mouths to clear clogged spray nozzles. The pyrethroids are also absorbed via inhalation; however, in these same sprayers, inhalation was not found to be a clinically significant route of exposure as analyzed by breathing zone assays.[28] The pyrethroids are not volatile compounds, so inhalation is always due to powders or sprayed mists, and mucosal and pulmonary toxicity may be because of hydrocarbon solvent vehicles. Systemic absorption and resultant effects may follow massive exposures, such as occurs in enclosed spraying or other extreme conditions.

Distribution The pyrethroids and pyrethrins are lipophilic and as such are rapidly distributed to the CNS. Because they are rapidly metabolized, there is no storage or bioaccumulation, which limits chronic toxicity.[51,52]

Metabolism Natural pyrethrins are readily metabolized by mammalian microsomal enzymes, and hence are essentially nontoxic to humans. They can induce CYP3A and CYP2B isoforms in vitro in human cultured hepatocytes, but clinical significance is doubtful.[119]

The synthetic pyrethroids are readily metabolized in animals and man by hydrolases and the CYP microsomal system. The metabolites are of lower toxicity than the parent compounds.[149] Piperonyl butoxide, a P450 inhibitor, enhances the potency of pyrethrins and pyrethroids 10- to 300-fold to target insects. It is often added to insecticide preparations to ensure lethality, as the initial "knock down" effect of a pyrethroid alone is not always lethal to the insect.[51] Testing of piperonyl butoxide on antipyrine metabolism (measure of CYP enzyme function) in humans at a dose exceeding 50 times that received in all-day confined-space pesticide spraying revealed no effect on this enzyme system.[120]

Elimination There is no evidence that the pyrethroids undergo enterohepatic recirculation. Deltamethrin disappeared from the urine of exposed workers within 12 hours, and fenvalerate disappeared within 24 hours.[28] Parent compounds and metabolites of the pyrethroids are found in the urine.[126] The most commonly assayed metabolites are 3-PBA (3-phenoxybenzoic acid, a nonspecific metabolite of multiple pyrethroids), cis-DCCA (cis-3-[2,2-dichloroethenyl]-dimethyl cyclopropane carboxylic acid, a metabolite of cis-permethrin, cypermethrin, and cyfluthrin), trans-DCCA (trans-3-[2,2-dichloroethenyl]-dimethyl cyclopropane carboxylic acid, a metabolite of trans-permethrin, cypermethrin, cyfluthrin), and Br2CA (3-[2,2-dibromovinyl]-2,2-dimethylcyclopropanecarboxlic acid, a metabolite of deltamethrin). The metabolite CDCA (chrysanthemumdicarboxylic acid) is also a nonspecific metabolite of natural pyrethrin I and the synthetic pyrethroids allethrin, resmethrin, and tetramethrin.[96,158] Monitoring of these metabolites is used in population-based studies for pesticide exposures. However, a recent review revealed that commonly assayed pyrethroid metabolites also occur in the environment from natural degradation. Therefore, the detection of these metabolites in the urine may be from a subject's exposure to the parent compound or from its metabolite in the environment.

PATHOPHYSIOLOGY

Like DDT, pyrethrins and pyrethroids prolong the activation of the neuronal voltage-dependent Na^+ channel by binding to it in the open state, causing a prolonged depolarization, as evidenced by an extended tail current associated with squid axon voltage clamp experiments (Chaps. 8 and 22).[108,109] Indeed, DDT and pyrethrin/pyrethroids bind to the same site on insect Na^+ channels, and resistance to one class causes cross-resistance to the other class as well.[111] The voltage-sensitive sodium channel binding is responsible for the insecticidal activity, and the toxicity of the pyrethroids to nontarget species. Natural pyrethrins and type I synthetic pyrethroids induce repetitive or "burst discharges" following a single stimulus, because they hold the Na^+ channel in its open state for shorter periods. The actual amplitude of the tail current is determined by the concentration of the pyrethroids, regardless of type. Type II pyrethroids cause the Na^+ channel to remain open longer, and allow a prolonged period of depolarization of the resting membrane potential, causing a longer duration of the tail current.[152,169] Type II pyrethroids are thus more potent, and lead to significant after-potentials and eventual nerve conduction block. The mammalian voltage-dependent sodium channel, unlike the insect, has many isoforms, and may help explain the relative resistance in mammalian species. Different pyrethroids have varied effects on mammal Na^+ channels; the effects are not additive and, in fact, may be antagonistic. Structure-activity relationship is important as well, because some pyrethroid trans isomers at the ester linkage are not insecticidal, but the cis isomers are, and some isomers are insecticidal but lack mammalian toxicity because of this isomerism.[149]

Pyrethroids also have activity at certain isoforms of the voltage-sensitive neuronal calcium channel, which may explain the neurotransmitter release that occurs in pyrethroid poisoning. Additionally, pyrethroids block voltage-sensitive chloride channels in test animals, producing the salivation seen in the CS syndrome. These effects may contribute to enhanced CNS toxicity,[149] and is likely responsible for the choreoathetosis that occurs in animal models of severe type II poisonings.[125] Some studies show some interference of the type II pyrethroids with the $GABA_A$-mediated inhibitory chloride channels, but only in high concentrations.[29,107] Antagonism of the $GABA_A$-chloride channels likely has a significant role in human pyrethroid exposures, and probably contributes to the seizures seen after severe poisoning by type II agents.[107,125] The pyrethroids may also act at the peripheral benzodiazepine receptor, as evidenced by decreased salivation in test animals when this receptor is blocked. The clinical significance of this is currently unknown.[15]

Natural pyrethrins and type I pyrethroids have a negative temperature coefficient, similar to DDT, and are more selectively toxic to non–warm-blooded target species. Type II pyrethroids have a positive temperature coefficient, which makes them more insecticidal at higher ambient temperatures, and thus more useful in agricultural applications.[172] However, this may also at least partly explain the greater mammalian toxicity of type II pyrethroids as compared to type I.[107]

CLINICAL MANIFESTATIONS

Pyrethrum probably has an LD_{50} (median lethal dose in 50% of test subjects) of well over 1 g/kg in man, as extrapolated from animal data. Most cases of toxicity associated with the pyrethrins are the result of allergic reactions.[116,173] Theoretically, those at highest risk for allergic reactions would be patients who are sensitive to ragweed pollen, 50% of whom may cross-react with chrysanthemums (ragweed and chrysanthemum are in the same botanical family). These allergic reactions have been postulated to be due to residual natural components present in the extracts.[126] However, recent reviews have cast some doubt on this explanation. First, there have been only four cases of life-threatening respiratory reactions reported in the literature, three of which were in known asthmatics.[120] Second, the presence of residual natural proteins is unlikely, as the purification procedures would allow little, if any, residuals. Third, most reported cases of contact urticaria have been erroneously classified as type I hypersensitivity reactions.[67] The synthetic pyrethroids can cause histamine release in vitro,[49] but generally do not induce IgE-mediated allergic reactions.[17]

In animals, type I pyrethroid poisoning most closely resembles that of DDT, with extensive tremors, twitching, increased metabolic rate, and hyperthermia. Excluding the rare possibility of skin irritation or allergy, the type I pyrethroids are unlikely to cause systemic toxicity in humans. Experimentally, pyrethroids have greater than 1000-fold more affinity for insect Na^+ channels than for mammals, explaining their low toxicity in higher life forms. This selectivity, along with the negative temperature coefficient and slower insect metabolism, combines to make the type I pyrethroids approximately 15,000 times more toxic in insects than in humans.[109] The type II pyrethroids are generally more potent and cause profuse salivation, ataxia, coarse tremor, choreoathetosis, and seizures in animals. In humans, type II pyrethroids cause paresthesias (secondary to sodium channel effects in cutaneous sensory nerves after topical exposure),[94] salivation, nausea, vomiting, dizziness, fasciculations, altered mental status, coma, seizures, and acute lung injury.[77] A review of more than 500 cases of acute pyrethroid poisoning from China highlights some similar manifestations between a massive acute type II pyrethroid overdose and an OP compound overdose. However, serious atropine toxicity and death have resulted when poisoning from a type II pyrethroid was mistaken for an OP compound, and treatment was directed at these seemingly cholinergic signs.[77] Features such as acute lung injury may be because of solvents and surfactants present in the agricultural products.[10] Although the type II pyrethroids contain a cyanide moiety, cyanide poisoning does not occur, and cyanide antidotal therapy is not indicated.

Most significant unintentional exposures are dermal, especially in occupational settings, and local symptoms predominate in the majority of these cases. Systemic effects from insecticidal sprayings have been reported from wind drift or inappropriate handling, and the more potent type II pyrethroids predominate in both case reports. An exposure of workers possibly affected by wind drift from a mixture of 32 oz of the type II pyrethroid cyfluthrin mixed with 18.5 gal of petroleum oil and 1800 gal water was reported in California in 2006. Spraying occurred in a citrus grove, and 23 female workers in an adjacent vineyard were possibly exposed. These workers complained of a "chemical" odor, and felt ill with headaches, nausea, eye irritation, weakness, anxiety, and shortness of breath. They were all evaluated in local EDs and discharged home. Despite the fact that no cyfluthrin was detected on these workers' clothing or on foliage in the field where they were alleged to have been exposed, the report concluded that cyfluthrin was the cause; no estimate of the contribution of the petroleum vehicle to the symptoms was posited.[25] The predominant feature after significant cutaneous exposures is local paresthesias in the areas of skin contact, due to Na^+-channel effects on cutaneous sensory nerves. Local skin irritation occurs in up to 10% of workers spraying pyrethroid insecticides, but rarely occurs after medicinal use of the pyrethroid creams and shampoos. Ocular contact causes more severe symptoms, including immediate pain, lacrimation, photophobia, and conjunctivitis.[15]

Intentional ingestions represent the most serious exposures, because of the higher doses involved and the greater exposures to vehicles and solvents. However, a study of 48 cases of permethrin/xylene/surfactant mixtures (38 were suicidal ingestions) revealed that mild GI signs and symptoms predominated (73%: sore throat, mouth ulcerations, dysphagia, epigastric pain, vomiting). Pulmonary signs and symptoms were documented in 29%, and eight patients (including one death) had aspiration pneumonitis. Thirty-three percent had CNS symptoms including confusion, coma, and seizures. The involvement of the CNS and lungs were less common, but clinically more significant.[180] The relative contributions of the xylene and surfactant were likely responsible for much of the GI and pulmonary effects, though they were not discussed in the report.

CHRONIC EXPOSURES

Since the pyrethroids are rapidly metabolized and are not biopersistent, they have not been shown to cause cumulative toxicity. A single case of motor neuron disease resulted from heavy daily inhalation exposure to pyrethroid mixtures in a confined space for 3 years, which resolved after exposure ceased.[50] Some investigators have expressed concerns regarding possible neurotoxicity of the pyrethroids. However, a recent review noted that regulatory studies in multiple species have shown no evidence supporting gross neurodevelopmental toxicity or adult neuronal loss in man.[125] In Germany, numerous civil lawsuits allege multiple chemical sensitivity (MCS) is caused by pyrethroid exposures. Scientific study of this phenomenon yields no scientific data to support this contention,[13] but the controversy is fueled by civil litigation and sensationalized by popular media, subsequently causing public fear,[6] not unlike the "toxic mold" concerns in the United States.[26,181]

TREATMENT

Initial treatment should be directed toward skin decontamination, as most poisonings occur from exposures by this route. Patients with large oral ingestions of a type II pyrethroid should be treated with a single standard dose of AC, provided the diluent of the pyrethroid does not contain a petroleum solvent. Contact dermatitis and acute systemic allergic reactions should be treated in the usual manner, using histamine blockers, corticosteroids, and β-adrenergic agonists as clinically indicated.

Treatment of systemic toxicity is entirely supportive and symptomatic, because there is no specific antidote. Benzodiazepines should be used for tremor and seizures. Topical vitamin E oil (dl-α-tocopherol) is especially effective in preventing and treating the cutaneous paresthesias due to topical pyrethroid exposures.[15,126]

INSECT REPELLENTS

Mosquitoes transmit more diseases to humans than any other biting insect. Worldwide, more than 700 million people are infected yearly by mosquito bites that transmit such diseases as viral encephalitis, yellow fever, dengue fever, bancroftian filariasis, and epidemic polyarthritis. Malaria alone is responsible for three million deaths annually.[63] In the United States, eight people died from WNV in New York City in 1999, and by January 2005 the virus, carried by mosquitoes from infected birds, had spread to all lower 48 states. By 2006, over 3000 cases of WNV infection were reported to the CDC. Since then, reducing the incidence of mosquito bites has become a major public health concern, not just control of an annoying insect, although utilization rates remain low in the US population.[92] Mosquito repellants are important public health tools, and DEET has been the time-tested primary tool for the past 5 decades. However, much controversy continues to surround DEET despite a remarkable safety profile with over a half-century of global use by billions of people. A growing trend in the United States and many Western cultures has been a chemophobia against synthetic products like DEET. Many people favor plant-based "natural" or "organic" repellents, paralleling the increasing consumer preference for natural or organic foods. Several xenobiotics have been proposed, but thus far few have been shown by objective blinded studies to even approach the efficacy of DEET, much less surpass it. Numerous comprehensive reviews of the subject have demonstrated the clear superiority of DEET in most cases, and DEET remains the insect repellent standard by which all others are measured (Table 114–4).

DEET

The topical insect repellent, *N,N*-diethyl-3-methylbenzamide (DEET, former nomenclature *N,N*-diethyl-*meta*-toluamide), was patented by the US Army in 1946, and commercially marketed in the United States since 1956. Currently, it is used worldwide by more than 200 million persons annually. The EPA estimates that 38% of the US population uses DEET each year. Despite the current search for alternatives, DEET is still the most effective insect repellant available, and that with the most clinical toxicity information.[64,65]

DEET can be purchased without prescription in concentrations ranging from 5% to 100%, and in multiple formulations of solutions, creams, lotions, gels, and aerosol sprays. DEET formulations can feel greasy or sticky, and can dissolve or damage some plastics (eyeglass frames, watches) and synthetic fabrics.

TABLE 114–4. Comparative Efficacy and Toxicity of Commonly Available Insect Repellents

Insect Repellent	EPA Approval	EPA Toxicity Rating[a]	Efficacy in Laboratory and Field Studies[b]	Notes
DEET	1957 (1980)	III	Most efficacious in laboratory and field studies; protective against ticks and mosquitoes	>50 years of experience, billions of users 10%–30% soln: safe, effective when used as directed
Picaridin	2001	IV	20% solution: Laboratory: Equivalent to DEET Field: Equivalent to DEET	All studies done on 20% picaridin; no studies done with 7% or 15 % (US formulas) Recommended by CDC as a DEET alternative[65]
IR3535	1999	IV	Laboratory: Inferior to DEET[65] Field: None available	Recommended by CDC as a DEET alternative[65]
Oil of lemon eucalyptus (p-menthane diol)	2000	IV (I, ocular)	Equivalent to DEET for mosquitoes; not tested for tick bite prevention	Recommended by CDC as a DEET alternative[65]
BioUD	2007	IV	Laboratory: Equivalent to 7% DEET Field: Equal to 25% and 30% DEET	Studies performed by patent holders and developers IR, no impartial evidence
Citronella oil	1948	IV	Laboratory: ineffective[56]	Candles only provide some repellency when within 1 meter

[a] EPA Acute Toxicity Ratings: Category I = very highly or highly toxic; Category II = moderately toxic; Category III = slightly toxic; Category IV = practically nontoxic.

[b] Lab tests: arm in cage studies for mosquito repellency; field studies: actual biting or tick attachment assays in natural conditions.

Mosquitoes are attracted to their hosts by temperature and chemical attractants, principally CO_2 and lactate. The mechanism by which DEET repels insects was thought to be because of some interference with the mosquito's chemoreceptors, rendering them unable to detect lactic acid and CO_2.[65,121] However, recent novel work has demonstrated that DEET does not simply "jam the signal"; rather, DEET is actually detected by mosquitoes' olfactory receptors and repels them independently of whether the normal physical or chemical attractants are present.[160]

Toxicokinetics DEET is extensively absorbed via the GI tract. Skin absorption is significant, depending on the vehicle and the concentration. It does not bind to stratum corneum, and only 0.08% or less of a dose remains in the skin 8 hours after application.[121] DEET is lipophilic, and skin absorption usually occurs within 2 hours, although it is eliminated from serum within 4 hours. The volume of distribution is large, in the range of 2.7 to 6.21 L/kg in animal studies. DEET is extensively metabolized by oxidation and hydroxylation by the hepatic microsomal enzymes, primarily by the isozymes CYP2B6, -3A4, -2C19, and -2A6.[167] DEET is excreted in the urine within 12 hours, mainly as metabolites, with 15% or less appearing as the parent compound.[64,121]

DEET has been extensively reviewed in terms of acute and chronic toxicity. It has been found safe for use in pregnant and lactating women[89]; it was found to have no specific target organ toxicity or oncogenicity in any observed rat, mouse, or dog studies[147]; and chronic DEET exposure together with other insecticides showed no increased cancer risks.[115]

Pathophysiology The exact mechanism of DEET toxicity is unknown. Recent reviews of adverse reactions to DEET have noted a total 26 reported cases with major morbidity including encephalopathy, ataxia, convulsions, respiratory failure, hypotension, anaphylaxis, or death, particularly after ingestion or dermal exposure to large amounts.[23,64,113,114,163,168] These primarily neurologic adverse reactions occurred mainly in children, and most involved prolonged use and excessive dosing beyond what is currently recommended. One fatal case involved a child who was known to be heterozygous for ornithine carbamoyl transferase (OCT) deficiency, and death was because of a Reyelike syndrome with hyperammonemia. This child had experienced prior episodes of hyperammonemia unrelated to DEET use, and DEET does not appear to affect, or be affected by, OCT activity in humans.[114] There is currently no evidence that enzyme polymorphism affects DEET metabolism or influences individual susceptibility to toxicity.

Although single, large, acute oral doses (1–3 g/kg) in rats produced seizures and CNS damage,[145] smaller, acute doses (500 mg/kg and less) and chronic multigenerational dosing in another rat study produced no obvious toxicity.[146] Teratogenicity studies in rats and rabbits failed to demonstrate toxicity except at the highest doses,[147,179] and DEET was not found to be carcinogenic.[121,147] In view of the billions of applications, the number of reports of toxicity appears exceedingly small, and suggests a remarkably wide margin of safety.[64,73,113,114,130,159]

Clinical Manifestations Most calls to poison centers regarding DEET exposures involve minor or no symptoms, and symptomatic exposures occur primarily when DEET is sprayed in the eyes or inhaled.[168] Except for suicidal ingestions, most serious reactions consist of seizures in children overexposed via the dermal route; in fact, some of these cannot be definitely attributed to DEET.[73,114] Most symptoms resolve without treatment and the majority of patients with serious toxicity recover fully with supportive care.

Treatment DEET exposures are treated with supportive care aimed at the primarily neurologic symptoms. In cases of dermal exposures skin decontamination should be a priority to prevent further absorption. Patients with intentional oral ingestions should receive a single dose of AC if clinically indicated.

An extensive review of the safety risk of DEET repellent use confirms its safe use for all populations when used according to labeling guidelines.[159] Despite its good safety profile, overuse of DEET must be avoided. The American Academy of Pediatrics (AAP) recently revised its recommendations for insect repellent use because of the emergence of WNV infections (prior recommendations were for use of products with DEET less than 10%).[148] They found that DEET-containing products are the most effective mosquito repellents available, and are also effective against a variety of other insects, including ticks. Insect repellants with a DEET concentration from 10% to 30% (the maximum recommended for children) appear to be equally safe when used according to the directions on the product labels. The safety of DEET does not appear to relate to differences in these concentrations, and higher concentrations have longer durations of effect.[1] As indicated in the AAP handbook, repellents are not recommended for children younger than 2 months of age.[2]

The higher concentrations prolong the repellency period, but there is a plateau at about 50% DEET concentration, and about 6 hours may be the maximum protection time from any single application. Newer longer-acting DEET formulations in lipids or polymers cause the DEET to evaporate more slowly, which affords protection for greater than 6 hours and also less systemic absorption.[86,142] Since mosquitoes are most active for a few hours preceding and following dusk, DEET should be promptly washed off the child's skin when protection is no longer needed. Soaking the skin is not more effective and may contribute to toxicity. DEET should be applied only to exposed skin. Use on abraded skin or skin with rashes should be avoided. Care should be taken to avoid exposure to eyes and sensitive skin areas. Avoid use on children's hands, so that the child does not wipe on eyes, mouth, genitalia, and so on. Adults should apply DEET to their own hands and then wipe onto the child's face, rather than spraying onto a child's face.

DEET combination products that include sunscreen should not be used, since it has been shown that these combination products mutually enhance the percutaneous absorption of each component in both a porcine in vivo study[84] and an in vitro mouse skin model.[134] Since mosquitoes are most active near dusk, there is clearly no need for the sunscreen component. Other options for protection include mechanical means, such as mosquito netting, as well as permethrin-impregnated clothing for tick prevention.

NEWER INSECT REPELLENTS

The efficacy of any xenobiotic, treatment, or repellent is directly related to compliance with the treatment. Despite its demonstrated efficacy and safety, many people view chemical insect repellents such as DEET as potentially harmful and avoid their use. Several survey results in the United States and Canada revealed that 56% of people believe repellents are likely to be harmful to children, and 45% believed insect repellents are likely to sicken adults.[175] This has led to an intense search for effective alternatives to DEET-based repellents.

Picaridin Picaridin (chemical name 2-(2-hydroxyethyl)-1-piperidinecarboxylic acid 1-methylpropyl ester) is a piperidine derivative and has low acute oral, dermal, and inhalation toxicity. The EPA classifies it as Toxicity Category IV for acute inhalation toxicity and primary dermal irritation, the lowest rating available, but category III for oral ingestion. It is not a dermal sensitizer, and no developmental toxicity was observed in chronic animal feeding studies. It was also not shown to be mutagenic in a battery of tests, and is not considered carcinogenic.[58] Picaridin is nearly as efficacious as DEET in comparison studies of the 20% solution used in Australia and Europe, but unfortunately no studies have compared the 7% formulation marketed in the United States (Cutter Advanced™; Avon Skin So Soft with Picaridin™). Since duration of protection is generally related to concentrations of the repellent (clearly shown with DEET), it would be reasonable to assume the 7% United States formula would not have as long a duration of effect.

Oil of Lemon Eucalyptus Oil of lemon eucalyptus occurs naturally in the lemon eucalyptus plant (*Eucalyptus citriodora*, also known as *Corymbia citriodor*). The natural oil can be extracted from the eucalyptus leaves and twigs; commercially the active ingredient, *p*-menthane-3,8-diol (PMD), is chemically synthesized, and is structurally similar to menthol. In its pure form, it is a solid at room temperature, and has a faint mintlike odor. PMD is placed into Toxicity Category IV for acute oral toxicity, dermal toxicity, and skin irritation, and Toxicity Category II for the end-use product for eye irritation. It is not a skin sensitizer. The EPA has determined that there is reasonable certainty of no harm to the general population or subpopulations, including infants and children, as the result of the use of PMD to formulate insect repellents.[59]

IR3535™ (CAS #52304-36-6) IR3535 (3-[N-butyl-N-acetyl]-aminopropionic acid, ethyl ester) is a substituted β amino acid structurally similar to naturally occurring β-alanine. The US EPA has classified IR3535 as a biochemical, based on the fact that it is functionally identical to naturally occurring β-alanine, and both repel insects, the basic molecular structure is identical, the end groups are not likely to contribute to toxicity, and it acts to control the target pest via a nontoxic mode of action. It is a liquid that contains 98% active ingredient and 2% inert ingredients. It has been used as an insect repellent in Europe for over 20 years with no substantial adverse effects. Toxicity tests show that IR3535 is not harmful when ingested, inhaled, or used on skin.[54,55]

2-Undecanone A newly formulated natural repellent, 2-undecanone, was approved for use as an insect repellant by the EPA in 2007, and is known by the brand name of BioUD™. Its active ingredient is derived from the wild tomato plant, *Lycopersicon hirsutum* Dunal f. *glabratum* C. H. Mull.[175] 2-Undecanone (also known as methyl nonyl ketone) was originally registered in 1966 as a dog and cat repellent/training aid and an iris borer deterrent. It received EPA approval as a topical insect repellent in 2007. The EPA Reregistration Eligibility Decision (RED) documents that in studies using laboratory animals, methyl nonyl ketone exhibited no toxicity via the oral and inhalation routes and was placed in Toxicity Category IV. Methyl nonyl ketone has slight dermal toxicity (Toxicity Category III) resulting in eye and dermal irritation as well as skin sensitization. Since it has a long history of safe use, is from a natural source, and is an approved food additive, it is considered nontoxic. Methyl nonyl ketone is currently found in only one insect repellent in the form of both a lotion and a spray.[57] The manufacturer lists an unpublished study on its website of a field test showing protection from mosquito bites that surpassed that of a 30% DEET product at 6 hours, and was equivalent at 4 hours.[78] A recent study done by the inventors and patent holders showed it was only as efficacious as lower DEET concentration products in laboratory arm-in-cage trials, but field trials revealed efficacy equivalent to 25% to 30% DEET formulations.[175]

Oil of Citronella Oil of citronella has been used for over 50 years as an insect repellent and as an animal repellent in candles and topical skin products. These products, which have little efficacy, are not expected to cause harm to humans, pets, or the environment when used according to the label.[56]

INSECTICIDES, DEET, AND THE GULF WAR SYNDROME

During operations Desert Shield/Desert Storm in 1991, nearly 700,000 Americans served in the Persian Gulf. Some returning troops began reporting a variety of symptoms and illnesses they attributed initially to exposure to burning oil well fires in Kuwait. Approximately 10% of these veterans have registered with the Persian Gulf Registry Health Examination Program. This program was initiated to study whether veterans were experiencing adverse health effects related to exposures encountered in the Persian Gulf War. The most common symptoms are largely nonspecific and multiorgan and include fatigue, rashes, headache, muscle aches, memory problems, dyspnea, insomnia, and GI symptoms. Multiple studies and expert panels have studied these veterans in an attempt to identify a causative xenobiotic responsible for this "Persian Gulf syndrome," now more accurately termed "Gulf War illness"(GWI).

Some investigators have suggested that combinations of DEET, permethrin, and pyridostigmine have additive neurotoxic effects and could be a cause of the symptoms.[93] Although there is laboratory evidence of synergistic neurotoxicity when large doses of these xenobiotics are gavaged or injected in test animals,[4,99] it is difficult to apply this methodology to human experience in the Gulf War. The exposures in the veterans were primarily dermal, and concomitant use at toxic dosages for any sustained time period was thought to be unlikely or a rare occurrence. Given the diversity and multisystem nature of symptoms experienced by these veterans, it has generally been felt that it was unlikely that use of these xenobiotics is responsible for the symptom complexes reported.[105] The newest report by the Research Advisory Committee (discussed below) chronicled many interviews with exposed soldiers, revealing that insecticide use and exposures were more intense than originally imagined, and in many ground troops were clearly excessive.

The Institute of Medicine Gulf War Committee initially evaluated the association of this GWI and multiple exposures. Six comprehensive review volumes have been authored by the Institute of Medicine (IOM) and published by the National Academy of Science from 2000 to 2008, along with three updates; the two most recent were published in July 2008. The committee found that although veterans of the first Gulf War report significantly more symptoms of illness than soldiers of the same period who were not deployed, studies have found no cluster of symptoms that constitute a syndrome unique to Gulf War veterans.[38,164] Moreover, there was evidence of an association with stress and many of the disorders and symptom complexes experienced by these veterans.[39] Earlier reports revealed that there was inadequate/insufficient evidence to link exposure to pyridostigmine and long-term health effects.[35] Extensive review has consistently shown that there is not enough evidence to link long-term health problems with exposure to depleted uranium,[33] or with exposure to low doses of sarin.[34] There was an association of exposure to combustion products and certain cancers such as lung, laryngeal, and bladder.[37] One volume found some limited evidence to link neurobehavioral effects with exposure to certain solvents and OP insecticides, but in the majority of cases, there was not enough evidence to determine whether there is an association between exposure and certain health effects.[36]

In November 2008, the Veteran's Administration's Research Advisory Committee on Gulf War Veterans' Illnesses published a comprehensive review of all of the research and epidemiology to date. This committee concluded that (1) the GWI was a complex syndrome, and that the inability to define a conventional diagnostic category or disease was the reason this disorder has heretofore *not* been recognized as a true illness; (2) despite a long safety history of pyridostigmine in myasthenia gravis treatment, use of the drug was associated with development of GWI; concomitant exposures to certain OP and carbamate insecticides was also causally linked; (3) a strong case can be made for a causal relationship between these two exposure types and GWI; and (4) the symptoms were not due to posttraumatic stress disorder (PTSD). The committee sent their report along to the IOM for expert review and analysis in November 2008.[127] Such a divergent conclusion made 17 years later and based largely on epidemiologic studies of exposure intensities raises the question of recall bias in those most affected. The controversy over this symptom complex will likely continue.

Despite the continued controversy, the prevalence of GWI complex among the veterans of that conflict is staggering. Estimates range that from one in seven to greater than 25% of US veterans of the war have some symptoms, and in the United Kingdom, 17% of Gulf War veterans have symptoms of "Gulf War syndrome." Similar postwar syndromes consisting of chronic pain, fatigue, depression, and other symptoms have plagued returning soldiers after every war in the 20th century. These syndromes have gone by a variety of names such as Da Costa syndrome, irritable heart, shell shock, neurocirculatory asthenia, and battle fatigue. After more than a decade of study, using more than $340 million of federally funded medical research, the cause of this medically unexplained syndrome continues to be investigated, and remains in dispute. Although Gulf War veterans have been shown to have an increased incidence of multisystem complaints such as multiple chemical sensitivity, chronic fatigue syndrome, and fibromyalgia, many investigators continue to feel that GWI likely represents, at least in part, a manifestation of PTSD.[53]

LEGAL STANDARDS FOR AN INSECTICIDE LABEL

The Federal Insecticide, Fungicide, and Rodenticide Act of 1962 (Table 108–1) established criteria for a "signal word" on an insecticide label, which implies the degree of toxicity based on an oral LD_{50}. Also, the label on the original container of these products is usually instructive and should always be brought to the medical facility (Chap. 108).

SUMMARY

The ideal insecticide is one that has low acute toxicity to humans and nontarget species (pyrethroids, DDT), is inexpensive to apply and produce (OP compounds, DDT), and would have no environmental persistence or bioaccumulation (OP compounds, pyrethroids). With research and development coupled with mass production techniques, some of the newer pyrethroids may come closer to this ideal than those most commonly used today. Until that goal is achieved, however, the neurotoxic organic chlorines will continue to be used. In January 2000, the Associated Press reported that 21 people in Iran were poisoned, and three died when DDT powder was inadvertently used in food preparation instead of flour, underscoring the continued clinical importance of organochlorine exposures in some areas of the world. Although organic chlorine pesticides are banned in North America and Europe, they are still widely used elsewhere, and will have important implications for toxicologists for some time to come.

REFERENCES

1. AAP Committee on Environmental Health. Follow Safety Precautions When Using DEET on Children, 2003. http://aapnews.aappublications.org/cgi/content/full/e200399v1 (accessed November 27, 2009).
2. AAP Committee on Environmental Health. Pesticides. In: Etzel RA, ed. *Pediatric Environmental Health*, 2nd ed. Elk Grove Village, IL: American Academy of Pediatrics; 2003.
3. Abalis IM, Eldefrawi ME, Eldefrawi AT. Effects of insecticides on GABA-induced chloride influx into rat brain microsacs. *J Toxicol Environ Health.* 1986;18:13-23.
4. Abou-Donia MB, Wilmarth KR, Jensen KF, et al. Neurotoxicity resulting from coexposure to pyridostigmine bromide, deet, and permethrin: implications of Gulf War chemical exposures. *J Toxicol Environ Health.* 1996;48:35-56.

5. Aks SE, Krantz A, Hryhrczuk DO, et al. Acute accidental lindane ingestion in toddlers. *Ann Emerg Med.* 1995;26:647-651.
6. Altenkirch H. Multiple chemical sensitivity (MCS)—differential diagnosis in clinical neurotoxicology: a German perspective. *Neurotoxicology.* 2000;21:589-597.
7. Anonymous. FDA Issues Health Advisory Regarding Labeling Changes for Lindane Products. US Food and Drug Administration, March 28, 2003. http://www.fda.gov/bbs/topics/ANSWERS/2003/ANS01205.html (accessed May 26, 2009).
8. Anonymous. Lindane Reregistration Eligibility Decision (RED); Notice of Availability Comment. Environmental Protection Agency (EPA). http://www.epa.gov/EPA-PEST/2002/September/Day-23/p24096.htm (accessed May 26, 2009).
9. Azziz-Baumgartner E. Mosquito Control and Exposure to Pesticides, Virginia and North Carolina 2003. CDC Lecture Series 2003. http://www.cdc.gov/ncidod/dvbid/westnile/conf/pdf/Azziz_Baumgartner_6_04.pdf.
10. Bateman DN. Management of pyrethroid exposure. *J Toxicol Clin Toxicol.* 2000;38:107-109.
11. Bloomquist JR. Intrinsic lethality of chloride-channel-directed insecticides and convulsants in mammals. *Toxicol Lett.* 1992;60:289-298.
12. Bloomquist JR, Roush RT, French-Constant RH. Reduced neuronal sensitivity to dieldrin and picrotoxinin in a cyclodiene-resistant strain of *Drosophila melanogaster* (Meigen). *Arch Insect Biochem Physiol.* 1992;19:17-25.
13. Bornschein S, Hausteiner C, Pohl C, et al. Pest controllers: a high-risk group for multiple chemical sensitivity (MCS)? *Clin Toxicol (Phila).* 2008;46:193-200.
14. Boylan JJ, Cohn WJ, Egle JL Jr, et al. Excretion of chlordecone by the gastrointestinal tract: evidence for a nonbiliary mechanism. *Clin Pharmacol Ther.* 1979;25:579-585.
15. Bradberry SM, Cage SA, Proudfoot AT, Vale JA. Poisoning due to pyrethroids. *Toxicol Rev.* 2005;24:93-106.
16. Brisson P. Percutaneous absorption. *Can Med Assoc J.* 1974;110:1182-1185.
17. Burkhart CG. Relationship of treatment-resistant head lice to the safety and efficacy of pediculicides. *Mayo Clin Proc.* 2004;79:661-666.
18. Calle EE, Frumkin H, Henley SJ, et al. Organochlorines and breast cancer risk. *CA Cancer J Clin.* 2002;52:301-309.
19. Carson R. *Silent Spring.* Boston: Houghton Mifflin Company; 1962.
20. Carvalho WA, Matos GB, Cruz SL, Rodrigues DS. Human aldrin poisoning. *Braz J Med Biol Res.* 1991;24:883-887.
21. Cecil HC, Fries GF, Bitman J, et al. Dietary p,p'-DDT, o,p'-DDT or p,p'-DDE and changes in egg shell characteristics and pesticide accumulation in egg contents and body fat of caged White Leghorns. *Poult Sci.* 1972;51:130-139.
22. Centers for Disease Control and Prevention (CDC). Acute convulsions associated with endrin poisoning—Pakistan. *MMWR Morb Mortal Wkly Rep.* 1984;33:687-688, 693.
23. Centers for Disease Control and Prevention (CDC). Seizures temporally associated with use of DEET insect repellent—New York and Connecticut. *MMWR Morb Mortal Wkly Rep.* 1989;38:678-680.
24. Centers for Disease Control and Prevention. Third National Report on Human Exposure to Environmental Chemicals. Atlanta, GA; 2005.
25. Centers for Disease Control and Prevention (CDC). Worker illness related to ground application of pesticide—Kern County, California, 2005. *MMWR Morb Mortal Wkly Rep.* 2006;55:486-488.
26. Chang C, Gershwin ME. Mold hysteria: origin of the hoax. *Clin Dev Immunol.* 2005;12:151-158.
27. Chang ES, Stokstad EL. Effect of chlorinated hydrocarbons on shell gland carbonic anhydrase and egg shell thickness in Japanese quail. *Poult Sci.* 1975;54:3-10.
28. Chen SY, Zhang ZW, He FS, et al. An epidemiological study on occupational acute pyrethroid poisoning in cotton farmers. *Br J Ind Med.* 1991;48:77-81.
29. Coats JR. Mechanisms of toxic action and structure-activity relationships for organochlorine and synthetic pyrethroid insecticides. *Environ Health Perspect.* 1990;87:255-62.
30. Coble Y, Hildebrandt P, Davis J, et al. Acute endrin poisoning. *JAMA.* 1967;202:489-493.
31. Cohn WJ, Boylan JJ, Blanke RV, et al. Treatment of chlordecone (Kepone) toxicity with cholestyramine. Results of a controlled clinical trial. *N Engl J Med.* 1978;298:243-248.
32. Cole LM, Casida JE. Polychlorocycloalkane insecticide-induced convulsions in mice in relation to disruption of the GABA-regulated chloride ionophore. *Life Sci.* 1986;39:1855-1862.
33. Committee on Gulf War and Health. *Gulf War and Health: Updated Literature Review of Depleted Uranium.* 2008.
34. Committee on Gulf War and Health. *Gulf War and Health: Updated Literature Review of Sarin.* 2004.
35. Committee on Gulf War and Health. *Gulf War and Health, Volume 1: Depleted Uranium, Sarin, Pyridostigmine Bromide, and Vaccines.* 2000.
36. Committee on Gulf War and Health. *Gulf War and Health, Volume 2: Insecticides and Solvents.* 2003.
37. Committee on Gulf War and Health. *Gulf War and Health, Volume 3: Fuels, Combustion Products, and Propellants.* 2005.
38. Committee on Gulf War and Health. *Gulf War and Health, Volume 4: Health Effects of Serving in the Gulf War.* 2006.
39. Committee on Gulf War and Health. *Gulf War and Health, Volume 6: Physiologic, Psychologic, and Psychosocial Effects of Deployment-Related Stress.* 2007.
40. Conney AH, Welch RM, Kuntzman R, Burns JJ. Effects of pesticides on drug and steroid metabolism. *Clin Pharmacol Ther.* 1967;8:2-10.
41. Costa LG. Basic toxicology of pesticides. *Occup Med.* 1997;12:251-268.
42. Coye MJ, Lowe JA, Maddy KJ. Biological monitoring of agricultural workers exposed to pesticides: II. Monitoring of intact pesticides and their metabolites. *J Occup Med.* 1986;28:628-636.
43. Crosby AD, D'Andrea GH, Geller RJ. Human effects of veterinary biological products. *Vet Hum Toxicol.* 1986;28:552-553.
44. Cummings AM. Methoxychlor as a model for environmental estrogens. *Crit Rev Toxicol.* 1997;27:367.
45. Dale WE, Gaines TB, Hayes WJ, Pearce GW. Poisoning by DDT: relation between clinical signs and concentration in rat brain. *Science.* 1963;142:1474-1476.
46. Davies JE, Dedhia HV, Morgade C, et al. Lindane poisonings. *Arch Dermatol.* 1983;119:142-144.
47. Davison KL. Calcium-45 uptake by shell gland, oviduct, plasma and eggshell of DDT-dosed ducks and chickens. *Arch Environ Contam Toxicol.* 1978;7:359-367.
48. Davison KL, Sell JL. DDT thins shells of eggs from mallard ducks maintained on ad libitum or controlled-feeding regimens. *Arch Environ Contam Toxicol.* 1974;2:222-232.
49. Diel F, Detscher M, Schock B, Ennis M. In vitro effects of the pyrethroid S-bioallethrin on lymphocytes and basophils from atopic and nonatopic subjects. *Allergy.* 1998;53:1052-1059.
50. Doi H, Kikuchi H, Murai H, et al. Motor neuron disorder simulating ALS induced by chronic inhalation of pyrethroid insecticides. *Neurology.* 2006;67:1894-1895.
51. Echobichon DJ. Toxic effects of pesticides. In: Klaassen CD, ed. *Casarett and Doull's Toxicology: The Basic Science of Poisons*, 5th ed. New York: MacMillan; 1996:643-669.
52. Echobichon DJ, Joy RM. *Pesticides and Neurological Diseases.* Boca Raton, FL: CRC Press; 1994.
53. Engel CC, Jaffer A, Adkins J, et al. Can we prevent a second 'Gulf War syndrome'? Population-based healthcare for chronic idiopathic pain and fatigue after war. *Adv Psychosom Med.* 2004;25:102-122.
54. Environmental Protection Agency. 3-[N-butyl-N-acetyl]-aminopropionic acid, ethyl ester (IR3535) Fact Sheet. US EPA, 2000.
55. Environmental Protection Agency. 3-[N-butyl-N-acetyl]-aminopropionic acid, ethyl ester (IR3535) Techical Document. US EPA, 1997.
56. Environmental Protection Agency. Citronella (Oil of Citronella) (021901) Fact Sheet. US EPA, November 1999. http://www.epa.gov/pesticides/biopesticides/ingredients/factsheets/factsheet_021901.htm (accessed November 27, 2009).
57. Environmental Protection Agency. Pesticide Re-registration Eligibility Decision. Methyl Nonyl Ketone (2-Undecanone). US EPA, 1995.
58. Environmental Protection Agency. Picaridin New Pesticide Fact Sheet. US EPA, 2005.
59. Environmental Protection Agency. Registration Eligibility Document for p-menthane-3,8-diol (oil of lemon eucalyptus). US EPA, 2000.
60. Faroon O, Kueberuwa S, Smith L, DeRosa C. ATSDR evaluation of health effects of chemicals. II. Mirex and chlordecone: health effects, toxicokinetics, human exposure, and environmental fate. *Toxicol Ind Health.* 1995; 11:1-203.
61. Feldmann RJ, Maibach HI. Percutaneous penetration of some pesticides and herbicides in man. *Toxicol Appl Pharmacol.* 1974;28:126-132.
62. Fischer TF. Lindane toxicity in a 24-year-old woman. *Ann Emerg Med.* 1994;24:972-974.

63. Fradin MS. Insect Repellents. emedicine, 2007.
64. Fradin MS. Mosquitoes and mosquito repellents: a clinician's guide. *Ann Intern Med.* 1998;128:931-940.
65. Fradin MS, Day JF. Comparative efficacy of insect repellents against mosquito bites. *N Engl J Med.* 2002;347:13-18.
66. Franz TJ. Kinetics of cutaneous drug penetration. *Int J Dermatol.* 1983;22:499-505.
67. Franzosa JA, Osimitz TG, Maibach HI. Cutaneous contact urticaria to pyrethrum-real?, common?, or not documented?: an evidence-based approach. *Cutan Ocul Toxicol.* 2007;26:57-72.
68. Fry DM. Reproductive effects in birds exposed to pesticides and industrial chemicals. *Environ Health Perspect.* 1995;103(Suppl 7):165-171.
69. Gaido K, Dohme L, Wang F, et al. Comparative estrogenic activity of wine extracts and organochlorine pesticide residues in food. *Environ Health Perspect.* 1998;106 (Suppl 6):1347-1351.
70. Gant DB, Eldefrawi ME, Eldefrawi AT. Cyclodiene insecticides inhibit $GABA_A$ receptor-regulated chloride transport. *Toxicol Appl Pharmacol.* 1987;88:313-321.
71. Garrettson LK, Guzelian PS, Blanke RV. Subacute chlordane poisoning. *J Toxicol Clin Toxicol.* 1984;22:565-571.
72. Geusau A, Schmaldienst S, Derfler K, et al. Severe 2,3,7,8-tetrachlorodibenzo- p-dioxin (TCDD) intoxication: kinetics and trials to enhance elimination in two patients. *Arch Toxicol.* 2002;76:316-235.
73. Goodyer L, Behrens RH. Short report: the safety and toxicity of insect repellents. *Am J Trop Med Hyg.* 1998;59:323-324.
74. Grutsch JF, Khasawinah A. Signs and mechanisms of chlordane intoxication. *Biomed Environ Sci.* 1991;4:317-326.
75. Hayes WJ. Chlorinated hydrocarbon insecticides. In: Hayes WJ, Lawes ER, eds. *Pesticides Studied in Man.* San Diego: Academic Press; 1991:731-868.
76. Hayes WJ, Lawes ER. *Handbook of Pesticide Toxicology.* San Diego: Academic Press; 1991.
77. He F, Wang S, Liu L, et al. Clinical manifestations and diagnosis of acute pyrethroid poisoning. *Arch Toxicol.* 1989;63:54-58.
78. Heal JD, Jones A. Field Evaluation of Two HOMS Mosquito Repellents to Repel Mosquitoes in Southern Ontario, 2006. http://www.bioud.com/Documents/HOMSfinalreport2006.pdf (accessed November 27, 2009)
79. Herr DW, Gallus JA, Tilson HA. Pharmacological modification of tremor and enhanced acoustic startle by chlordecone and p,p'-DDT. *Psychopharmacology (Berl).* 1987;91:320-325.
80. Hunter DJ, Hankinson SE, Laden F, et al. Plasma organochlorine levels and the risk of breast cancer. *N Engl J Med.* 1997;337:1253-1258.
81. Idson B. Vehicle effects in percutaneous absorption. *Drug Metab Rev.* 1983;14:207-222.
82. Jandacek RJ, Anderson N, Liu M, et al. Effects of yo-yo diet, caloric restriction, and olestra on tissue distribution of hexachlorobenzene. *Am J Physiol Gastrointest Liver Physiol.* 2005;288:G292-G299.
83. Karpati AM, Perrin MC, Matte T, et al. Pesticide spraying for West Nile virus control and emergency department asthma visits in New York City, 2000. *Environ Health Perspect.* 2004;112:1183-1187.
84. Kasichayanula S, House JD, Wang T, Gu X. Percutaneous characterization of the insect repellent DEET and the sunscreen oxybenzone from topical skin application. *Toxicol Appl Pharmacol.* 2007;223:187-194.
85. Kassner JT, Maher TJ, Hull KM, Woolf AD. Cholestyramine as an adsorbent in acute lindane poisoning: a murine model. *Ann Emerg Med.* 1993;22:1392-1397.
86. Katz TM, Miller JH, Hebert AA. Insect repellents: historical perspectives and new developments. *J Am Acad Dermatol.* 2008;58:865-781.
87. Kintz P, Baron L, Tracqui A, et al. A high endrin concentration in a fatal case. *Forensic Sci Int.* 1992;54:177-180.
88. Klaassen CD. Nonmetallic environmental toxicants. In: Hardman JG, Limbird LE, Molinoff PB, Ruddon RW, eds. *Goodman and Gilman's the Pharmacologic Basis of Therapeutics*, 9th ed. New York: McGraw-Hill; 1996:1684-1699.
89. Koren G, Matsui D, Bailey B. DEET-based insect repellents: safety implications for children and pregnant and lactating women. *CMAJ.* 2003;169: 209-212.
90. Kramer MS, Hutchinson TA, Rudnick SA, et al. Operational criteria for adverse drug reactions in evaluating suspected toxicity of a popular scabicide. *Clin Pharmacol Ther.* 1980;27:149-155.
91. Krieger N, Wolff MS, Hiatt RA, et al. Breast cancer and serum organochlorines: a prospective study among white, black, and Asian women. *J Natl Cancer Inst.* 1994;86:589-599.
92. Kuehn BM. CDC: new repellents for West Nile fight. *JAMA.* 2005;293:2583.
93. Kurt TL. Epidemiological association in US veterans between Gulf War illness and exposures to anticholinesterases. *Toxicol Lett.* 1998;102-103: 523-526.
94. Le Quesne PM, Maxwell IC, Butterworth ST. Transient facial sensory symptoms following exposure to synthetic pyrethroids: a clinical and electrophysiological assessment. *Neurotoxicology.* 1981;2:1-11.
95. Lee B, Groth P. Scabies: transcutaneous poisoning during treatment. *Pediatrics.* 1977;59:643.
96. Leng G, Gries W, Selim S. Biomarker of pyrethrum exposure. *Toxicol Lett.* 2006;162:195-201.
97. Lopez-Cervantes M, Torres-Sanchez L, Tobias A, Lopez-Carrillo L. Dichlorodiphenyldichloroethane burden and breast cancer risk: a meta-analysis of the epidemiologic evidence. *Environ Health Perspect.* 2004;112: 207-214.
98. Lucena RA, Allam MF, Jimenez SS, Villarejo ML. A review of environmental exposure to persistent organochlorine residuals during the last fifty years. *Curr Drug Saf.* 2007;2:163-172.
99. McCain WC, Lee R, Johnson MS, et al. Acute oral toxicity study of pyridostigmine bromide, permethrin, and DEET in the laboratory rat. *J Toxicol Environ Health.* 1997;50:113-124.
100. Mestres R, Mestres G. Deltamethrin: uses and environmental safety. *Rev Environ Contam Toxicol.* 1992;124:1-18.
101. Morgan DP, Dotson TB, Lin LI. Effectiveness of activated charcoal, mineral oil, and castor oil in limiting gastrointestinal absorption of a chlorinated hydrocarbon pesticide. *Clin Toxicol.* 1977;11:61-70.
102. Morgan-Glenn PD. Scabies. *Pediatr Rev.* 2001;22:322-323.
103. Mortensen ML. Management of acute childhood poisonings caused by selected insecticides and herbicides. *Pediatr Clin North Am.* 1986;33: 421-445.
104. Mouchet J, Manguin S, Sircoulon J, et al. Evolution of malaria in Africa for the past 40 years: impact of climatic and human factors. *J Am Mosq Control Assoc.* 1998;14:121-130.
105. Murphy FM. *A Guide to Gulf War Veterans' Health.* St. Louis, MO: Department of Veterans Affairs, Continuing Medical Education Program; 1998.
106. Mutter LC, Blanke RV, Jandacek RJ, Guzelian PS. Reduction in the body content of DDE in the Mongolian gerbil treated with sucrose polyester and caloric restriction. *Toxicol Appl Pharmacol.* 1988;92:428-435.
107. Narahashi T. Nerve membrane Na+ channels as targets of insecticides. *Trends Pharmacol Sci.* 1992;13:236-241.
108. Narahashi T, Frey JM, Ginsburg KS, Roy ML. Sodium and GABA-activated channels as the targets of pyrethroids and cyclodienes. *Toxicol Lett.* 1992;64-65:429-436.
109. Narahashi T, Zhao X, Ikeda T, et al. Differential actions of insecticides on target sites: basis for selective toxicity. *Hum Exp Toxicol.* 2007;26: 361-366.
110. Obata T, Yamamura HI, Malatynska E, et al. Modulation of γ-aminobutyric acid-stimulated chloride influx by bicycloorthocarboxylates, bicyclophosphorus esters, polychlorocycloalkanes and other cage convulsants. *J Pharmacol Exp Ther.* 1988;244:802-806.
111. O'Reilly AO, Khambay BP, Williamson MS, et al. Modeling insecticide-binding sites in the voltage-gated sodium channel. *Biochem J.* 2006;396: 255-263.
112. Ortiz Martinez A, Martinez-Conde E. The neurotoxic effects of lindane at acute and subchronic dosages. *Ecotoxicol Environ Saf.* 1995;30:101-105.
113. Osimitz TG, Grothaus RH. The present safety assessment of deet. *J Am Mosq Control Assoc.* 1995;11:274-278.
114. Osimitz TG, Murphy JV. Neurological effects associated with use of the insect repellent N,N-diethyl-m-toluamide (DEET). *J Toxicol Clin Toxicol.* 1997;35:435-441.
115. Pahwa P, McDuffie HH, Dosman JA, et al. Hodgkin lymphoma, multiple myeloma, soft tissue sarcomas, insect repellents, and phenoxyherbicides. *J Occup Environ Med.* 2006;48:264-274.
116. Paton DL, Walker JS. Pyrethrin poisoning from commercial-strength flea and tick spray. *Am J Emerg Med.* 1988;6:232-235.
117. Pomes A, Rodriguez-Farre E, Sunol C. Disruption of GABA-dependent chloride flux by cyclodienes and hexachlorocyclohexanes in primary cultures of cortical neurons. *J Pharmacol Exp Ther.* 1994;271:1616-1623.
118. Pramanik AK, Hansen RC. Transcutaneous gamma benzene hexachloride absorption and toxicity in infants and children. *Arch Dermatol.* 1979;115:1224-1225.

119. Price RJ, Giddings AM, Scott MP, et al. Effect of pyrethrins on cytochrome P450 forms in cultured rat and human hepatocytes. *Toxicology.* 2008;243:84-95.
120. Proudfoot AT. Poisoning due to pyrethrins. *Toxicol Rev.* 2005;24:107-113.
121. Qiu H, Jun HW, McCall JW. Pharmacokinetics, formulation, and safety of insect repellent N,N-diethyl-3-methylbenzamide (DEET): a review. *J Am Mosq Control Assoc.* 1998;14:12-27.
122. Rasmussen JE. The problem of lindane. *J Am Acad Dermatol.* 1981;5:507-516.
123. Rauch AE, Kowalsky SF, Lesar TS, et al. Lindane (Kwell)-induced aplastic anemia. *Arch Intern Med.* 1990;150:2393-2395.
124. Ray DE, Forshaw PJ. Pyrethroid insecticides: poisoning syndromes, synergies, and therapy. *J Toxicol Clin Toxicol.* 2000;38:95-101.
125. Ray DE, Fry JR. A reassessment of the neurotoxicity of pyrethroid insecticides. *Pharmacol Ther.* 2006;111:174-193.
126. Reigart JR, Roberts JR. *Recognition and Management of Pesticide Poisonings.* Washington, DC: Environmental Protection Agency; 1999.
127. Research Advisory Committee on Gulf War Veterans' Illnesses. *Gulf War Illness and the Health of Gulf War Veterans: Scientific Findings and Recommendations.* Washington, DC: US Government Printing Office; 2008.
128. Roberts DR, Laughlin LL, Hsheih P, Legters LJ. DDT, global strategies, and a malaria control crisis in South America. *Emerg Infect Dis.* 1997;3:295-302.
129. Roberts DR, Manguin S, Mouchet J. DDT house spraying and re-emerging malaria. *Lancet.* 2000;356:330-332.
130. Roberts JR, Reigart JR. Does anything beat DEET? *Pediatr Ann.* 2004;33:443-453.
131. Robson WA, Arscott GH, Tinsley IJ. Effect of DDE, DDT and calcium on the performance of adult Japanese quail (*Coturnix coturnix japonica*). *Poult Sci.* 1976;55:2222-2227.
132. Rogan WJ. Pollutants in breast milk. *Arch Pediatr Adolesc Med.* 1996;150:981-990.
133. Roos TC, Alam M, Roos S, et al. Pharmacotherapy of ectoparasitic infections. *Drugs.* 2001;61:1067-1088.
134. Ross EA, Savage KA, Utley LJ, et al. Insect repellent. *Drug Metab Dispos.* 2004;32:783-785.
135. Rowley DL, Rab MA, Hardjotanojo W, et al. Convulsions caused by endrin poisoning in Pakistan. *Pediatrics.* 1987;79:928-934.
136. Rugman FP, Cosstick R. Aplastic anaemia associated with organochlorine pesticide: case reports and review of evidence. *J Clin Pathol.* 1990;43:98-101.
137. Runhaar EA, Sangster B, Greve PA, Voortman M. A case of fatal endrin poisoning. *Hum Toxicol.* 1985;4:241-247.
138. Sadasivaiah S, Tozan Y, Breman JG. Dichlorodiphenyltrichloroethane (DDT) for indoor residual spraying in Africa: how can it be used for malaria control? *Am J Trop Med Hyg.* 2007;77:249-263.
139. Safe SH. Environmental and dietary estrogens and human health: is there a problem? *Environ Health Perspect.* 1995;103:346-351.
140. Safe SH. Is there an association between exposure to environmental estrogens and breast cancer? *Environ Health Perspect.* 1997;105:675-678.
141. Safe SH. Xenoestrogens and breast cancer. *N Engl J Med.* 1997;337:1303-1304.
142. Salafsky B, He YX, Li J, et al. Short report: study on the efficacy of a new long-acting formulation of N, N-diethyl-m-toluamide (DEET) for the prevention of tick attachment. *Am J Trop Med Hyg.* 2000;62:169-172.
143. Saleh MA. Toxaphene: chemistry, biochemistry, toxicity and environmental fate. *Rev Environ Contam Toxicol.* 1991;118:1-85.
144. Schenker MB, Louie S, Mehler LN, Albertson TE. Pesticides. In: Rom WN, ed. *Environmental and Occupational Medicine,* 3rd ed. Philadelphia: Lippincott-Raven; 1998:1157-1172.
145. Schoenig GP, Hartnagel RE, Jr, Schardein JL, Vorhees CV. Neurotoxicity evaluation of N,N-diethyl-m-toluamide (DEET) in rats. *Fundam Appl Toxicol.* 1993;21:355-365.
146. Schoenig GP, Neeper-Bradley TL, Fisher LC, Hartnagel RE Jr. Teratologic evaluations of N,N-diethyl-m-toluamide (DEET) in rats and rabbits. *Fundam Appl Toxicol.* 1994;23:63-69.
147. Schoenig GP, Osimitz TG, Gabriel KL, et al. Evaluation of the chronic toxicity and oncogenicity of N,N-diethyl-m-toluamide (DEET). *Toxicol Sci.* 1999;47:99-109.
148. Shelov SP. *Caring for Your Baby and Young Child: Birth to Age 5.* New York: Bantam Books; 1994.
149. Soderlund DM, Clark JM, Sheets LP, et al. Mechanisms of pyrethroid neurotoxicity: implications for cumulative risk assessment. *Toxicology.* 2002;171:3-59.
150. Solomon BA, Haut SR, Carr EM, Shalita AR. Neurotoxic reaction to lindane in an HIV-seropositive patient. An old medication's new problem. *J Fam Pract.* 1995;40:291-296.
151. Solomon LM, Fahrner L, West DP. Gamma benzene hexachloride toxicity: a review. *Arch Dermatol.* 1977;113:353-357.
152. Song JH, Nagata K, Tatebayashi H, Narahashi T. Interactions of tetramethrin, fenvalerate and DDT at the sodium channel in rat dorsal root ganglion neurons. *Brain Res.* 1996;708:29-37.
153. Soto AM, Chung KL, Sonnenschein C. The pesticides endosulfan, toxaphene, and dieldrin have estrogenic effects on human estrogen-sensitive cells. *Environ Health Perspect.* 1994;102:380-383.
154. Starr HG Jr, Clifford NJ. Acute lindane intoxication: a case study. *Arch Environ Health.* 1972;25:374-375.
155. Sterling JB, Hanke CW. Dioxin toxicity and chloracne in the Ukraine. *J Drugs Dermatol.* 2005;4:148-150.
156. Stevenson DE, Walborg EF Jr, North DW, et al. Monograph: reassessment of human cancer risk of aldrin/dieldrin. *Toxicol Lett.* 1999;109:123-186.
157. Street JC, Chadwick RW. Ascorbic acid requirements and metabolism in relation to organochlorine pesticides. *Ann N Y Acad Sci.* 1975;258:132-143.
158. Sudakin DL. Pyrethroid insecticides: advances and challenges in biomonitoring. *Clin Toxicol (Phila).* 2006;44:31-37.
159. Sudakin DL, Trevathan WR. DEET: a review and update of safety and risk in the general population. *J Toxicol Clin Toxicol.* 2003;41:831-839.
160. Syed Z, Leal WS. Mosquitoes smell and avoid the insect repellent DEET. *Proc Natl Acad Sci U S A.* 2008;105:13598-13603.
161. Telch J, Jarvis DA. Acute intoxication with lindane. *Can Med Assoc J.* 1982;127:821.
162. Tenenbein M. Seizures after lindane therapy. *J Am Geriatr Soc.* 1991;39:394-395.
163. Tenenbein M. Severe toxic reactions and death following the ingestion of diethyltoluamide-containing insect repellents. *JAMA.* 1987;258:1509-1511.
164. Thomas HV, Stimpson NJ, Weightman AL, et al. Systematic review of multi-symptom conditions in Gulf War veterans. *Psychol Med.* 2006;36:735-747.
165. Tilson HA, Hong JS, Mactutus CF. Effects of 5,5-diphenylhydantoin (phenytoin) on neurobehavioral toxicity of organochlorine insecticides and permethrin. *J Pharmacol Exp Ther.* 1985;233:285-289.
166. Tilson HA, Shaw S, McLamb RL. The effects of lindane, DDT, and chlordecone on avoidance responding and seizure activity. *Toxicol Appl Pharmacol.* 1987;88:57-65.
167. Usmani KA, Rose RL, Goldstein JA, et al. In vitro human metabolism and interactions of repellent N,N-diethyl-m-toluamide. *Drug Metab Dispos.* 2002;30:289-294.
168. Veltri JC, Osimitz TG, Bradford DC, Page BC. Retrospective analysis of calls to poison control centers resulting from exposure to the insect repellent N,N-diethyl-m-toluamide (DEET) from 1985-1989. *J Toxicol Clin Toxicol.* 1994;32:1-16.
169. Vijverberg HP, van den Bercken J. Neurotoxicological effects and the mode of action of pyrethroid insecticides. *Crit Rev Toxicol.* 1990;21:105-126.
170. Waibel GP, Speers GM, Waibel PE. Effects of DDT and charcoal on performance of White Leghorn hens. *Poult Sci.* 1972;51:1963-1967.
171. Walker GJ, Johnstone PW. Interventions for treating scabies [update in Cochrane Database Syst Rev. 2007;(3):CD000320; PMID. 17636630.
172. Ware GW, Whitacre DM. *An Introduction to Insecticides*, 4th ed. (Extracted from *The Pesticide Book,* 6th ed. Willoughby, OH: Meister Media Worldwide; 2004.)
173. Wax PM, Hoffman RS. Fatality associated with inhalation of a pyrethrin shampoo. *J Toxicol Clin Toxicol.* 1994;32:457-460.
174. Williams CH, Casterline JL Jr. Effects of toxicity and on enzyme activity of the interactions between aldrin, chlordane, piperonyl butoxide, and banol in rats. *Proc Soc Exp Biol Med.* 1970;135:46-50.
175. Witting-Bissinger BE, Stumpf CF, Donohue KV, et al. Novel arthropod repellent, BioUD, is an efficacious alternative to deet. *J Med Entomol.* 2008;45:891-898.

176. Wolff MS, Toniolo PG, Lee EW, Rivera M, Dubin N. Blood levels of organochlorine residues and risk of breast cancer. *J Natl Cancer Inst.* 1993;85:648-652.
177. Woollen BH, Marsh JR, Laird WJ, Lesser JE. The metabolism of cypermethrin in man: differences in urinary metabolite profiles following oral and dermal administration. *Xenobiotica.* 1992;22:983-991.
178. Woolley DE. Differential effects of benzodiazepines, including diazepam, clonazepam, Ro 5-4864 and devazepide, on lindane-induced toxicity. *Proc West Pharmacol Soc.* 1994;37:131-134.
179. Wright DM, Hardin BD, Goad PW, Chrislip DW. Reproductive and developmental toxicity of N,N-diethyl-m-toluamide in rats. *Fundam Appl Toxicol.* 1992;19:33-42.
180. Yang PY, Lin JL, Hall AH, et al. Acute ingestion poisoning with insecticide formulations containing the pyrethroid permethrin, xylene, and surfactant: a review of 48 cases. *J Toxicol Clin Toxicol.* 2002;40:107-113.
181. Zacharisen MC, Fink JN. Is indoor "mold madness" upon us? *Ann Allergy Asthma Immunol.* 2005;94:12-13.

CHAPTER 115
HERBICIDES

Darren M. Roberts

An herbicide is any chemical that regulates the growth of a plant, which encompasses a large number of xenobiotics of varying characteristics. Herbicides are used around the world for the destruction of plants in the home environment and also in agriculture where weeds are particularly targeted. Poisoning may occur following acute (intentional or unintentional poisoning) or chronic (such as occupational) exposures. Depending on the herbicide and the characteristics of the exposure, this may lead to clinically significant poisoning, including death.

Not all herbicide exposures are clinically significant. In developed countries, most acute herbicide exposures are unintentional and the majority of patients do not require admission to hospital. The National Poisoning and Exposure Database of the American Association of Poison Control Centers describes approximately 10,000 herbicide exposures each year. Over the last 12 years, there were only approximately five deaths per year and 20 patients per year with clinical outcomes categorized as "major" that were attributed to herbicide poisoning (see Chap. 135). Most deaths were due to paraquat and diquat, although more recently glyphosate and phenoxy acid compounds are more commonly implicated. Cases of severe poisoning that required hospitalization usually occurred following intentional self-poisoning. Significant toxicity may also occur with unintentional (eg, storage of a pesticide in food or drink containers) or criminal exposures.

This chapter focuses on the most widely used herbicides and also those associated with significant clinical toxicity. In particular, it discusses risk assessment and the management of patients with a history of acute herbicide poisoning.

HISTORY, CLASSIFICATION, AND EPIDEMIOLOGY

HISTORY

Prior to the 1940s, the main method of weed control and field clearance was manual labor, which was time consuming and expensive. A range of xenobiotics was tested including metals and inorganic compounds; however, their efficacy was limited. The first herbicide marketed was 2,4-dichlorphenoxyacetic acid during the 1940s, followed by other phenoxy acid compounds. Paraquat was initially marketed in the early 1960s and was followed by the benzoic acid compound dicamba later that decade. Since then there has been a progressive increase in the use and development of herbicides, which remains an active area of research. Increasing numbers of herbicide formulations are marketed every year including a number of novel structural compounds for which clinical toxicology data are unavailable. Hundreds of xenobiotics are classified as herbicides and a much larger number of commercial preparations are marketed. Some commercial preparations contain more than one herbicide to improve plant destruction. From another perspective, crops are being developed that are resistant to particular herbicides to maximize the selective destruction of weeds without reducing crop production.

Herbicides are the most widely sold pesticides in the world, accounting for more than 35% of the total world pesticide market and for more than 45% of the pesticide market in the United States. Home and garden domestic use accounts for 13% of the overall herbicide use in the United States, while the remainder is consumed by agriculture, government (for example, vegetation control on highways and railways), and industry. Sixteen herbicides are among the top 25 used pesticides in the United States and four herbicides are ranked in the top five: glyphosate is most widely used, followed by atrazine, acetochlor, and 2,4-dichlorophenoxyacetic acid. There was a decline in the overall total quantity of herbicides used worldwide between 1982 and 1987, which has since stabilized. In contrast, the domestic use of herbicides consistently increased between 1997 and 2001.[60]

CLASSIFICATION

Hundreds of xenobiotics are known to have herbicidal activity and they may be subclassified by a number of methods. Most commonly they are categorized in terms of their spectrum of activity (selective or nonselective), chemical structure, mechanism of action (contact herbicides or hormone dysregulators), use (preemergence or postemergence), or their toxicity to rats. Sometimes xenobiotics are classified as plant growth regulators rather than herbicides, but in this chapter all are considered to be herbicides.

Table 115–1 lists the extensive range of herbicides in current use.[56] By convention, they are subclassified according to their chemical class and their World Health Organization (WHO) hazard classification. Unfortunately, the utility of these (or any other) methods of classification has not been proven for predicting the hazard to humans with self-poisoning.

The WHO categorizes pesticides by their LD_{50}, which is the dose of pesticide required to kill 50% of test animals, usually rats, within a certain number of days in the absence of treatment. The WHO does not address morbidity or the effect of treatments. Further, the LD_{50} varies among studies in the same type of animal, and in particular among different species. For example, in the case of paraquat the LD_{50} in rats, monkeys, and guinea pigs was observed to be approximately 125 mg/kg, 50 mg/kg, and 25 mg/kg, respectively.[21,84] Therefore, extrapolation of the rat LD_{50} to estimate the toxicity in humans appears to be an imprecise approach to risk assessment. This variability was confirmed in preliminary studies with pesticide self-poisoning.[31,102] It should be emphasized that the intended application of this hazard classification is to achieve risk assessment for occupational exposures to operators who use the product as intended. Furthermore, the LD_{50} is determined by using pure herbicides, whereas proprietary formulations that result in poisoning also contain coformulants, which may have a significant influence on toxicity.

Herbicides within a single chemical class can manifest different clinical toxicity; for example, glyphosate is an organic phosphorus compound that does not inhibit acetyl cholinesterase. The mechanism of action of herbicides in plants usually differs from the mechanism of toxicity in humans; indeed, for some herbicides the mechanism of human toxicity is poorly described.

CONTRIBUTION OF COFORMULANTS

Commercial herbicides are generally identified by their active ingredients, but proprietary formulations almost always contain coformulants that may contribute to clinical toxicity. Hydrocarbon-based solvents and surfactants improve the contact of the herbicide with the plant and enhance penetration. Coformulants are generally considered "inactive" or "inert" because they lack herbicidal activity; however, increasingly their contribution to the toxicity is being realized.

The most widely discussed example of a coformulant dominating the toxicity of an herbicide product is that of glyphosate-containing

TABLE 115–1. Characteristics of the Major Herbicides, Categorized By Chemical Class and WHO Hazard Classification

Chemical Class[a]	Applications, Usage Data, and Mechanism of Action in Plants, If Known[b]	WHO Hazard Class[c]	Compounds Included	Clinical Effects, Potential Specific Treatments and Supportive Care
Alcohol and aldehyde	Broad-spectrum contact herbicide	Ib	Allyl alcohol (2-propen-1-ol) and acrolein (the metabolite of allyl alcohol)	Local irritation, cardiotoxicity, pulmonary edema, and death. Administer sulfhydryl-donors such as acetylcysteine or mesna.
Amide Fig. 115–1	Selective for grasses pre- or postemergence In 2001, acetochlor, propanil, alachlor, metolachlor, and dimethenamid are listed in the top 25 pesticides used in the United States. Propanil was among the top 10 pesticides used in the domestic sector Multiple mechanisms of action, including inhibition of photosynthesis at photosystem II and/or inhibition of dihydropteroate synthase and/or inhibition of cell division through inhibition of the synthesis of very-long-chain fatty acids and/or inhibition of acetolactate synthase (interferes with branched amino acid synthesis) and/or inhibition of microtubule assembly Some compounds may also be included in other chemical classes, including asulam (carbamate); oryzalin (dinitroaniline); clomeprop (phenoxy); diclosulam, flumetsulam, and metosulam (triazolopyrimidines)	III U	*Anilide derivatives*: Acetochlor, alachlor, dimethachlor, flufenacet, mefluidide, metolachlor, propachlor, propanil (DCPA) *Nonanilide derivatives*: Chlorthiamid, diphenamid *Anilide derivatives*: Butachlor, clomeprop, diclosulam, flamprop, flumetsulam, metosulam, mefenacet, metazachlor, pentanochlor, pretilachlor *Nonanilide derivatives*: Asulam, bromobutide, dimethenamid, isoxaben, napropamide,oryzalin, propyzamide, tebutam	See text for anilide derivatives. There are limited human data about the nonanilide derivatives. Lethargy or sedation preceded death in animals exposed to chlorthiamid. Behavioral changes, ataxia, and prostration were noted in animals exposed to diphenamid. Drowsiness and tachypnea were noted in goats following acute poisoning with napropamide
Aromatic acid	In 2001, dicamba was one of the top 25 pesticides used in the United States and the 7th most used in the domestic sector Dicamba is commonly coformulated with phenoxyacetic acid compounds Inhibits acetolactate synthase /or inhibition of microtubule assembly and/or indole acetic acid-like (synthetic auxins)	III U	Dicamba, 2,3,6-trichlorobenzoic acid (2,3,6-TBA) Bispyribac, chloramben (amiben), chlorthal, clopyralid, pyriminobac, pyrithiobac, quinclorac, quinmerac	Bispyribac causes gastrointestinal irritation, sedation, mortality (2.7%). Human data are limited for all other compounds, particularly single-agent exposures. In animals, myotonia, dyspnea, and death are reported with dicamba and 2,3,6-TBA poisoning
Arsenical	Unknown	III	Dimethylarsinic acid (cacodylic acid), methylarsonic acid (MAA)	See Chap. 88
Benzothiazole	Indole acetic acid-like (synthetic auxins) and/or inhibits photosynthesis at photosystem II	U	Benazolin, methabenzthiazuron	Limited human data
Bipyridyl	Nonselective, postemergence, contact herbicide Photosystem-I-electron diversion These compounds are part of a larger group of quaternary ammonium herbicides, including difenzoquat, which is also a pyrazole compounds (see below)	II	Paraquat, diquat	See text for paraquat and diquat

(*Continued*)

TABLE 115–1. Characteristics of the Major Herbicides, Categorized By Chemical Class and WHO Hazard Classification (*Continued*)

Chemical Class[a]	Applications, Usage Data, and Mechanism of Action in Plants, If Known[b]	WHO Hazard Class[c]	Compounds Included	Clinical Effects, Potential Specific Treatments and Supportive Care
Carbanilate	Inhibits photosynthesis at photosystem II and/or inhibits mitosis or microtubule organization	U	Carbetamide, desmedipham, phenmedipham, propham	Limited human data
Cyclohexane oxime	Postemergence, selective for grasses	III	Butroxydim, sethoxydim, tralkoxydim	Limited human data
	Inhibits acetyl-CoA carboxylase (lipid biosynthesis inhibitors)	U	Alloxydim, cycloxydim, cyhalofop	
Dinitroaniline	Preemergence, selective for grasses	III	Fluchloralin, pendimethalin	Pendimethalin induces mild clinical toxicity in most cases, but seizures and death due to respiratory failure are reported. Limited human data for the others
	In 2001, trifluralin and pendimethalin were among the top 25 pesticides used in the United States overall, while benfluralin and pendimethalin were among the top 10 used in the domestic sector Inhibits microtubule assembly	U	Benfluralin (benefin), butralin, dinitramine, ethalfluralin, oryzalin, prodiamine, trifluralin	Aniline metabolites are reported from trifluralin and oryzalin, which may induce methemoglobinemia and hemolysis with prolonged exposures. In rats, fluchloralin induces hyperexcitability, tremors, and convulsions prior to death. Many of these compounds are poorly absorbed and may be subject to enterohepatic recycling. Agitation, trembling, and fatigue occur in rats following lethal doses of trifluralin
Diphenyl ether	Postemergence (particularly broad leaves)	III	Acifluorfen, fluoroglycofen	Limited human data
	Contact herbicide, inhibits protoporphyrinogen oxidase, and/or inhibits carotenoid biosynthesis Aclonifen is also an amine compound	U	Aclonifen, bifenox, chlomethoxyfen, oxyfluorfen	
Halogenated aliphatic	Inhibit lipid synthesis	U	Dalapon, fluopropanate	Limited human data
Imidazolinone	Inhibit acetolactate synthase, interfering with branched amino acid synthesis	U	Imazamethabenz, imazapyr, imazaquin Imazethapyr	Limited human data. In a small case series, imazapyr induced sedation, respiratory distress, metabolic acidosis, hypotension, and hepatorenal dysfunction
Inorganic	Nonselective	III	Sodium chlorate	Nausea, vomiting, diarrhea, metabolic acidosis, renal failure, hemolysis, methemoglobinemia, rhabdomyolysis, and disseminated intravascular coagulation. Treatment includes hemodialysis, erythrocyte, and plasma transfusion. Methemoglobinemia is unresponsive to methylene blue, but sodium thiosulphate has been trialed
Nitrile	Pre-emergence, selective for grasses.	U	Ammonium sulfamate	Limited human data
	Inhibits photosynthesis at photosystem II &/or inhibition of cell wall (cellulose) synthesis	II	Bromoxynil, ioxynil	Limited human data; uncouples oxidative phosphorylation in animals.
	Commonly co-formulated with phenoxyacetic acid compounds	U	Dichlobenil	

Dinitrophenol	Uncoupling (membrane disruption)	Ib	Dinoterb, DNOC (4,6-dinitro-o-cresol)	Limited human data; methemoglobinemia is reported in animals. Dinitrophenol uncouples oxidative phosphorylation
Organic phosphorus	Bensulide: preemergence selective for grasses. Glyphosate and glufosinate and nonselective postemergence herbicides In 2001, glyphosate was the most used pesticide in the United States and the second most used in the domestic sector	II	Butamifos, bialaphos (bilanafos), anilofos, bensulide, piperophos	Limited human data. Bialaphos is metabolized to glufosinate in plants, but in humans only the metabolite L-amino-4-hydroxymethyl-phosphonoyl-butyric acid (L-AMPB) has been found. Clinical effects of poisoning include apnea, amnesia, and metabolic acidosis. Anilofos and bensulide are shown to inhibit acetyl cholinesterase
	Bialaphos and glufosinate inhibit glutamine synthetase, bensulide inhibits lipid synthesis, and glyphosate inhibits EPSP synthase, which interferes with aromatic amino acid synthesis	III	Glufosinate	See text for glufosinate, Fig. 115–5
		U	Fosamine, glyphosate	See text for glyphosate, Fig. 115–7. Limited human data for fosamine
Phenoxy Fig. 115–5	Postemergence, selective for grasses In 2001 2,4-D was the 5th most used pesticide in the United States but the most used in the domestic sector (mecoprop was 5th)	II	*Phenoxyacetic derivatives*: 2,4-D *Nonphenoxyacetic derivatives*: haloxyfop, quizalofop-P	See text for phenoxyacetic derivatives; similar clinical features of toxicity are noted for the chlorinated nonphenoxyacetic acid compounds. Mild clinical toxicity from fenoxaprop-ethyl. Limited human data on poisoning for others. Fluazifop 0.07 mg/kg was safely administered to humans in a volunteer study
	Inhibits acetyl-CoA carboxylase (lipid biosynthesis inhibitors; 'fops) or indole acetic acid-like (auxin growth regulators; chlorinated compounds) Clomeprop is also an amide compound	III	*Phenoxyacetic derivatives*: MCPA, 2,4,5-T *Nonphenoxyacetic derivatives*: Bromofenoxim, 2,4-DB, dichlorprop, diclofop, fluazifop, MCPB, mecoprop (MCPP), quizalofop, propaquizafop	
		U	*Nonphenoxyacetic derivatives*: Clomeprop, fenoxaprop-ethyl	
Pyrazole	May relate to inhibition of 4-hydroxyphenyl-pyruvate-dioxygenase or photosystem-I-electron diversion (difenzoquat is also a quaternary ammonium compound)	II	Difenzoquat	Limited human data
		III	Pyrazoxyfen, pyrazolynate	
		U	Azimsulfuron	
Pyridazine	Preemergence application. Inhibits photosynthesis at photosystem II	III	Pyridate	Limited human data
Pyridazinone	Inhibits photosynthesis at photosystem II or inhibits carotenoid biosynthesis at the phytoene desaturase step	U	Chloridazon, norflurazon	Limited human data. In animals, chloridazon appears to interfere with mitochondrial function. Respiratory distress, seizures and paralysis precede death
Pyridine	Inhibits carotenoid biosynthesis at the phytoene desaturase step and/or inhibits microtubule assembly and/or indole acetic acid-like (synthetic auxins)	III	Triclopyr	Limited human data on poisoning; triclopyr 0.5 mg/kg was safely administered to humans in a volunteer study. Picloram 5 mg/kg was safely administered to humans in a volunteer study
		U	Diflufenican, dithiopyr, fluroxypyr, fluthiacet, picloram	
Thiocarbamate	Preemergence, selective for grasses In 2001 EPTC was one of the top 25 pesticides used in the United States	II	EPTC, molinate, pebulate, prosulfocarb, thiobencarb, vernolate	Limited human data, including effects on cholinesterase. Some compounds display variable inhibition of nicotinic receptors, esterases, and aldehyde dehydrogenase in animals. Cycloate induces neurotoxicity in rats
		III	Cycloate, esprocarb, tri-allate	
	Inhibits lipid synthesis	U	Tiocarbazil	
Triazine Fig. 115–6	Mostly preemergence and nonselective	II	Cyanazine, terbumeton	See text
	In 2001 atrazine was the 2nd most used pesticide in the United States and simazine was in the top 25	III	Ametryn, desmetryn, dimethametryn, simetryn	
	Inhibits photosynthesis at photosystem II	U	Atrazine, prometon, prometryn, propazine, simazine, terbuthylazine, terbutryn, trietazine	

(Continued)

TABLE 115–1. Characteristics of the Major Herbicides, Categorized By Chemical Class and WHO Hazard Classification (*Continued*)

Chemical Class[a]	Applications, Usage Data, and Mechanism of Action in Plants, If Known[b]	WHO Hazard Class[c]	Compounds Included	Clinical Effects, Potential Specific Treatments and Supportive Care
Triazinone	Inhibits photosynthesis at photosystem II	II	Metribuzin, hexazinone	Limited human data. With hexazinone, rats and guinea pigs experience lethargy and ataxia, progressing to clonic seizures prior to death, while dogs were not particularly sensitive. Goats experience sedation, lethargy, and impaired respiration with metamitron poisoning
		III	Metamitron	
Triazole	Postemergent, nonselective Commonly coformulated with ammonium thiocyanate Inhibits lycopene cyclase; chlorophyll or carotenoid pigment inhibitor	U	Amitrole (aminotriazole)	Limited human data on single-agent exposures. Ingestion of 20 mg/kg in a human and >4000 mg/kg in rats did not induce symptoms
Triazolone	Inhibits acetolactate synthase	U	Flucarbazone	Limited human data
Triazolopy-rimidine	Inhibits acetolactate synthase. These herbicides are also amide compounds	U	Diclosulam, flumetsulam, metosulam	Limited human data. Asthma is reported from occupational exposures to flumetsulam
Uracil	Mostly preemergence. Inhibit photosynthesis at photosystem II	U	Bromacil, lenacil, terbacil	Limited human data
Urea	Both pre- and postemergence	III	Isoproturon, isouron, tebuthiuron	Limited human data. Some urea herbicides are metabolized to aniline compounds, which induce methemoglobinemia and hemolysis (similar to propanil, see text). Given the limited experience in treating poisonings with urea herbicides, it is reasonable to apply treatments described for amide herbicide poisoning (see text). Methemoglobinemia has been reported in products containing both metobromuron and metolachlor, which resolved with methylene blue. Wheeze is reported from occupational exposures to chlorimuron
	Inhibits acetolactate synthase (interferes with branched amino acid synthesis) and/or inhibits photosynthesis at photosystem II and/or inhibition of carotenoid biosynthesis	U	Bensulfuron, chlorbromuron, chlorimuron, chlorotoluron, cinosulfuron, cyclosulfa muron, daimuron, dimefuron, diuron, fenuron, fluometuron, linuron, methyldymron, metobromuron, metoxuron, metsulfuron, monolinuron, neburon, nicosulfuron, primisulfuron, pyrazosulfuron, rimsulfuron, siduron, sulfometuron, thifensulfuron, triasulfuron, tribenuron, triflusulfuron	Animal studies suggest that isoproturon causes CNS depression and tebuthiuron causes lethargy, ataxia, and anorexia
Miscellaneous	Clomazone may be coformulated with propanil Clomazone and fluridone: chlorophyll or carotenoid pigment inhibitor	II	Clomazone, endothal	Limited human data; in one case vomiting and gastric and pulmonary hemorrhage preceded death. Animal studies suggest that clomazone inhibits acetylcholinesterase and endothal induces lethargy, respiratory, and hepatic dysfunction
	Bentazone: pre- and postemergence for control of broadleaf plants. Inhibit photosynthesis	III	Bentazone, quinoclamine	Bentazone: gastrointestinal irritation, hepatic and renal failure, dyspnea, muscle rigidity, confusion, death
	Fluridone: chlorophyll or carotenoid pigment inhibitor	U	Benfuresate, cinmethylin, ethofumesate, fluridone, flurochloridone, oxadiazon	Limited human data

[a] Many of these classes can be further subclassified on the basis of chemical structure; however, the relationship between structure and clinical effects is not adequately described. The classification listed here is adapted from http://www.alanwood.net/pesticides/class_herbicides.html (accessed April 9, 2008).

[b] The mechanism by which a number of herbicides regulate plant growth is not fully described. The mechanisms listed here are adapted from http://www.plantprotection.org/HRAC/MOA.html (accessed April 9, 2008) and http://www.ces.purdue.edu/extmedia/WS/WS-23-W.html (accessed September 27, 2008).

[c] WHO Hazard Classification scale for oral liquid exposures of the technical grade ingredient based on rat LD_{50} (mg/kg body weight): Ia, "extremely hazardous," less than 20 mg/kg; Ib, "highly hazardous," 20 to 200 mg/kg; II, "moderately hazardous," 200 to 2000 mg/kg; III, "slightly hazardous," greater than 2000 mg/kg; and U, "technical grade active ingredients of pesticides unlikely to present acute hazard in normal use."

products, which is discussed below. Another example is imazapyr, which has an LD_{50} in rats of 1500 mg/kg intraperitoneally (IP), compared with 262 mg/kg IP when administered as the product ARSENAL®. This difference is attributed to the surfactant nonylphenol ethoxylate used in this product, which has an LD_{50} of 75 mg/kg IP.[40] In vitro studies with a number of formulations demonstrate increased cardiovascular toxicity compared with the technical herbicides.[18] Similarly, coformulants increase in vitro toxicity from phenoxyacetic acid derivatives and glufosinate.

Impurities may also be generated during manufacture or storage of the herbicide formulation, which contributes to toxicity. For example, phenolic byproducts from the manufacture of phenoxyacetic acid herbicides may be found as impurities in commercial formulations.

Some proprietary products contain a combination of herbicidal compounds that probably have additive effects, further complicating the risk assessment.

EPIDEMIOLOGY

The majority of herbicide exposures leading to severe poisoning or death are due to intentional self-harm and the specific herbicide taken, depending on local availability. Trends in herbicide poisoning usually reflect those of sales in the domestic sector because these products are most readily accessible to people with thoughts of self-harm.

Herbicide poisoning is a major issue in developing countries of the Asia-Pacific region where subsistence farming is common. In comparison, more recently the incidence of severe herbicide poisoning has decreased in developed countries because of restricted availability of highly toxic or concentrated solutions. In rural areas, the incidence of severe pesticide poisoning may be higher compared with urban regions because of easier access (see Chaps. 113 and 136).

Regulatory restrictions influence the herbicide exposures that are reported. For example, paraquat poisonings are now rare in the United States, while glyphosate poisonings are increasing. Similarly, paraquat was banned in Japan in the late 1980s and since then there has been an increase in the number of glufosinate poisonings.

REGULATORY CONSIDERATIONS

When properly used, the majority of herbicide formulations have a low potential toxicity for applicators because of their poor absorption across the skin and respiratory membranes. When inappropriately used, their toxicity is pronounced through enteral (or rarely parenteral) exposures.

The toxicity of herbicides varies among individual xenobiotics, but as a group, they appear to be intrinsically more toxic than medications when ingested with suicidal intent. Restrictions to the availability and formulation of toxic herbicides by regulatory authorities may improve outcomes from herbicide poisoning. For example, in the context of self-poisoning, the replacement of highly toxic pesticides with less toxic compounds may decrease the overall mortality[102] without altering agricultural outputs.[76] Prospective cohort studies have been useful for estimating the case fatality of individual herbicides so that the relative human toxicities were determined, as follows: fenoxaprop-P-ethyl 0%,[111] bispyribac 2.7%,[3] glyphosate 3.5%,[99] MCPA (4-chloro-2-methylphenoxyacetic acid) 4.4%,[103] propanil 10.7%,[101] and paraquat 50% to 90%.[33]

Regulatory bodies must also consider other factors, including the cost and efficacy of herbicides and their fate in the environment. An ideal herbicide is one that is selective for the target plant and does not migrate far from the site of application. Selective targeting may occur as a result of rapid inactivation or strong binding to soil components. For example, paraquat and glyphosate are inactivated when they come in contact with soil, which is favorable because they will remain in the region of application. In contrast, atrazine is more mobile, allowing it to leach into groundwater and migrate many kilometers. While the concentration at distant sites is low, there is concern that atrazine may have the potential to disrupt the growth and development of nontarget organisms.

GENERAL COMMENTS FOR THE MANAGEMENT OF ACUTE HERBICIDE POISONING

DIAGNOSIS

Herbicide poisoning is diagnosed following a specific history or other evidence of exposure (such as an empty bottle) and associated clinical symptoms. A detailed history, including the type of herbicide, amount, time since poisoning, and symptoms, is essential. Depending on local laboratory resources it may be possible to confirm the diagnosis with a specific assay, such as paraquat and glufosinate.

Because the principal criterion for diagnosis of acute herbicide poisoning is a history of exposure, a high index of suspicion is necessary. Because of the low incidence of herbicide poisoning in some regions it may not be considered in the differential diagnosis of patients presenting to hospital who are unable to provide a history. Therefore, clinicians should be familiar with the features of herbicide poisoning.

The pathophysiology of acute herbicide poisoning, and therefore the clinical manifestations, varies widely among individual compounds. Some herbicides induce multisystem toxicity due to interactions with a number of physiological systems. The mechanism of toxicity and pathophysiological changes in humans are discussed below for each herbicide individually.

INITIAL MANAGEMENT

An accurate risk assessment is necessary for the proper triage and subsequent management of patients with acute herbicide poisoning. Risk assessment involves consideration of the dose ingested, time since ingestion, clinical features, patient factors, and availability of medical facilities. All intentional exposures should be considered significant. If a patient presents to a facility that is unable to provide sufficient medical and nursing care or does not have ready access to necessary antidotes, then arrangements should be made to rapidly and safely transport the patient to a healthcare facility where these are available.

For many herbicides the initial management of an acute poisoning is empiric. All patients should receive prompt resuscitation paying close attention to airway, breathing, and circulation. Gastrointestinal toxicity, such as nausea, vomiting, and diarrhea, is common, leading to dehydration requiring administration of antiemetics and intravenous fluids to the patient.

Gastrointestinal decontamination may decrease absorption of the herbicide from the gut, decreasing systemic exposure. Gastric lavage is generally not recommended in acute poisoning because patients usually present too late or have self-decontaminated from vomiting and diarrhea. Lavage has been used by some practitioners for patients presenting shortly after an ingestion of a liquid formulation for which treatment options are limited. Depending on the procedure used, this treatment may cause harm and should only be conducted by an experienced clinician when the airway is protected. Oral activated charcoal may be given if the patient presents within 1 to 2 hours of ingestion.

Specific antidotes are available for only a few herbicides, which is in part because of their ill-defined mechanisms of toxicity.

Extracorporeal techniques, including hemoperfusion and hemodialysis, may decrease the systemic exposure by increasing the rate of elimination. The role of these treatments is discussed below for each pesticide.

Dermal decontamination is necessary if the patient has incurred clothing and cutaneous exposure. The patient should be washed with soap and water and contaminated clothes, shoes, and other leather materials should be removed and safely discarded in plastic bags.

Laboratory investigations may be useful for determining the evolution of organ toxicity, including serial measurement of biomarkers of liver and renal function, electrolytes, and acid–base status. Abnormalities should be corrected where possible. Respiratory distress and hypoxia with focal respiratory crackles soon after presentation are likely to result from aspiration pneumonitis, which can be confirmed on chest X-ray.

Patients with a history of acute ingestion should be observed for a minimum of 6 hours. Patients with a history of intentional ingestion and gastrointestinal symptoms should be observed for at least 24 hours given that clinical toxicity may progress or be delayed in some cases.

OCCUPATIONAL AND SECONDARY EXPOSURES (INCLUDING NOSOCOMIAL POISONING)

There is much concern regarding the risk of nosocomial poisoning to staff and family members who are exposed to patients with acute pesticide poisoning. The risk of nosocomial poisoning for health staff providing clinical care is low compared with other occupations, such as agricultural workers in whom toxicity is rarely observed. Universal precautions using nitrile gloves are most likely to provide sufficient protection for staff members.[73]

Few cases of secondary poisoning, if any, have been confirmed, and symptoms in these individuals were generally mild, such as nausea, dizziness, weakness, and headaches, probably relating to inhalation of the hydrocarbon solvent. These symptoms usually resolve after exposure to fresh air. Biomarkers for monitoring occupational exposures, as in the case of pesticide applicators, are outside the scope of this chapter.

AMIDE COMPOUNDS, IN PARTICULAR ANILIDE DERIVATIVES

Anilide compounds are the most widely used amide herbicides, of which propanil (3',4'-dichloropropionanilide, also known as DCPA), alachlor (2-chloro-2',6'-diethyl-*N*-methoxymethylacetanilide), and butachlor (*N*-butoxymethyl-2-chloro-2',6'-diethylacetanilide) are particularly common. Other amide herbicides and available toxicity data are listed in Table 115–1. In 2001, acetochlor, propanil, alachlor, metolachlor, and dimethenamid were each listed in the top 25 pesticides used in the United States, while propanil was among the top 10 pesticides in domestic use.[60] Anilide compounds are selective herbicides used mostly in rice cultivation in many parts of the world. Acute self-poisoning is reported particularly in Asia where subsistence farming is common. Data are limited for most compounds except propanil, butachlor, and alachlor. The case fatality of propanil is 10.9% compared with a combined mortality of 2.7% for butachlor and alachlor. Poor outcomes may reflect the inadequacies of current treatment regimens.

PHARMACOLOGY

Most of the clinical manifestations of propanil poisoning are mediated by its metabolites. 3,4-dichlorophenylhydroxylamine appears to be the most toxic metabolite because it directly induces methemoglobinemia and hemolysis in a dose-related manner.[78,80,112] 3,4-dichlorophenylhydroxylamine is cooxidized with oxyhemoglobin (Fe^{2+}) in erythrocytes to produce methemoglobin (Fe^{3+}) (see Chap. 127).[80,112]

However, toxicity may not be solely attributed to methemoglobinemia. Usually methemoglobin greater than 50% is required for severe poisoning and death, but fatal propanil poisoning is reported with methemoglobin as low as 40%.[22,87,127,128] Therefore, it seems likely that other toxic mechanisms contribute to clinical outcomes. Rats show signs of toxicity despite inhibition of hydrolytic enzymes and in the absence of methemoglobinemia, which may reflect direct toxicity from propanil itself.[112] Coformulants may also contribute.

The hydroxylamine metabolite has been shown to deplete glutathione, which may induce toxicity, although this is not consistently reported. Other possible toxicities from the metabolism of propanil include nephrotoxicity, lipoperoxidation, myelotoxicity, and immune dysfunction; the significance of these is not determined.

Para-hydroxylated aniline and other compounds are products of alachlor, butachlor, and acetochlor (2-chloro-*N*-ethoxymethyl-6'-ethylacet-*o*-toluidide) metabolism and may reduce glutathione and induce hepatotoxicity or cancer, particularly in rats.

PHARMACOKINETICS AND TOXICOKINETICS

Absorption is rapid in animals, with a peak concentration 1 hour postingestion. The volume of distribution (Vd) of propanil has not been determined, but is expected to be large given that both propanil and 3,4-dichloroaniline are highly lipid soluble. This Vd is consistent with data in the channel catfish where uptake and distribution of propanil was noted to be extensive. Anilide compounds interact with adenosine triphosphate (ATP)-binding cassette transporters, which may also influence the kinetics.

Anilide compounds undergo sequential metabolic reactions that produce toxic xenobiotics (Fig. 115–1). The first reaction is hydrolysis of the anilide to an aniline compound. This reaction is catalyzed by an esterase known as arylamidase, which has a high capacity in humans compared to rats (K_m = 473 μM and 271 μM, respectively) and sometimes by the cytochrome P450 system.[20] Examples include the bioconversion of propanil to 3,4-dichloroaniline[78,80,112] and also conversion of alachlor and butachlor to 2,6-diethylaniline.[20] These aniline intermediates are then oxidized by cytochrome P450, although the responsible isoenzyme has not been determined. N-hydroxylation of 3,4-dichloroaniline produces the hydroxylamine compound that

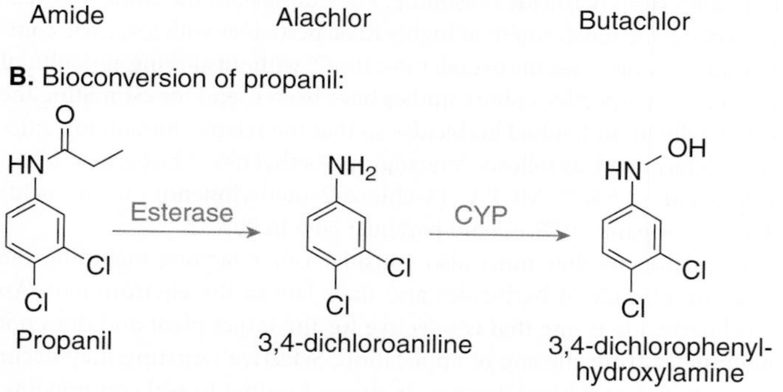

A. Common Anilide Xenobiotics

Amide — Alachlor — Butachlor

B. Bioconversion of propanil:

Propanil —Esterase→ 3,4-dichloroaniline —CYP→ 3,4-dichlorophenylhydroxylamine

FIGURE 115–1. Structure of common anilide compounds and the bioconversion of propanil.

induces hemolysis and methemoglobinemia, which are the obvious manifestations of propanil poisoning.[78,80,112]

These bioactivation reactions appear to be fairly rapid, where 3,4-dichloroaniline and methemoglobin are formed within 2 to 3 hours of parenteral administration of propanil to animals.[80] The hydroxylation of 3,4-dichloroaniline may be saturable (K_m = 120 μM in rats)[79] and slower than arylamidase, leading to a prolonged elimination of 3,4-dichloroaniline following large exposures.

In the case of alachlor, butachlor, and acetochlor, para-hydroxylated aniline compounds are produced, which appear to be carcinogens, particularly in rats.

These metabolic reactions are similar to those of dapsone, which are well characterized: the severity of methemoglobinemia relates to the amount of the dapsone metabolite; hydroxylamine, which varies with dose, and cytochrome P450 activity (see Chap. 127).

Propanil displays nonlinear toxicokinetics in humans with prolonged absorption continuing for approximately 10 hours following ingestion. Bioconversion to 3,4-dichloroaniline occurs largely within 6 hours, although it is particularly variable, which may reflect interindividual differences in esterase activity, dose, or coexposure to other pesticides. The median apparent elimination half-life of propanil is 3.2 hours compared with 3,4-dichloroaniline, which has a highly variable elimination profile. In general, the concentration of 3,4-dichloroaniline exceeds that of propanil and remains elevated for a longer period. In a case of coingestion of carbaryl the peak 3,4-dichloroaniline concentration was observed at 24 hours,[50] while in a fatal case the concentration of 3,4-dichloroaniline continued to increase until at least 30 hours postingestion.[101]

By 36 hours postingestion the concentration of 3,4-dichloroaniline is low in survivors, so clinical toxicity is unlikely to increase beyond this time.

PATHOPHYSIOLOGY

The predominant clinical manifestation in acute poisoning is methemoglobinemia. Methemoglobin is unable to bind and transport oxygen, inducing a relative hypoxia at the cellular level despite adequate arterial oxygenation. This leads to end-organ dysfunction, including central nervous system depression, hypotension, and acidosis. Because the serum concentration of 3,4-dichloroaniline remains elevated, methemoglobinemia persists for a similar time.[50,87,127] Sedation due to the direct effect of propanil or a hydrocarbon coformulant solvent may cause hypoventilation, which contributes to cellular hypoxia. Failure to correct these abnormalities may lead to irreversible cellular toxicity and death.

CLINICAL MANIFESTATIONS

Methemoglobinemia, hemolysis and anemia, coma, and death have also been reported following acute propanil poisoning. These manifestations occur in the clinical context of cyanosis, acidosis, and progressive end-organ dysfunction, which are consistent with severe and prolonged methemoglobinemia. A case fatality as high as 10.7% is reported and the median time to death was 36 hours. Patients who died were older with a depressed Glasgow coma scale (GCS) score and elevated concentration of propanil. Nausea, vomiting, diarrhea, tachycardia, dizziness, and confusion are also reported in patients who do not develop severe poisoning.[101]

Alachlor and butachlor appear to be less toxic than propanil, with a case fatality of 2.9% with self-poisoning. Hypotension and coma preceded death and other major symptoms included seizures, rhabdomyolysis, acidosis, renal failure, and cardiac dysrhythmias. Markers of milder clinical toxicity included gastrointestinal symptoms, agitation, dyspnea, and abnormal liver enzymes.[75] Methemoglobinemia was not reported, although it is unclear whether it was investigated for. Hepatic dysfunction has also occurred following dermal occupational exposure to butachlor.

Cyanosis was reported following acute ingestion of mefenacet (2-benzothiazol-2-yloxy-*N*-methylacetanilide) and imazosulfuron (1-[2-chloroimidazo(1,2-*a*)pyridin-3-ylsulfonyl]-3-[4,6-dimethoxypyrimidin-2-yl]urea) in the context of normal cooximetry, which was attributed to formation of a green pigment; green-colored urine was also reported. No other symptoms of toxicity were observed.[110]

Acute metolachlor (2-chloro-*N*-[6-ethyl-*o*-tolyl]-*N*-[(1*RS*)-2-methoxy-1-methylethyl]acetamide) poisoning in goats induced predominantly neuromuscular symptoms, including tremors, ataxia, and myoclonus, which progressed rapidly to death. Renal and hepatocellular toxicity were also noted. Acute acetochlor exposures in rats induced methemoglobinemia and hepatocellular toxicity.

DIAGNOSTIC TESTING

Specific investigations for the diagnosis of acute anilide herbicide poisoning are not widely available.

Patients with a history of propanil poisoning should be investigated for the presence of methemoglobinemia (see Chap. 127).

While the concentrations of propanil and 3,4-dichloroaniline appear to reflect clinical outcomes, this relationship is less marked for 3,4-dichloroaniline during the first 6 hours, which probably relates to the time for bioconversion from propanil.[101] However, propanil and 3,4-dichloroaniline assays are not commercially available and this observation has not been validated. Further, the relationship between concentration and outcomes varies with the time since ingestion and may depend on patient comorbidities.

MANAGEMENT

The minimum toxic dose has not been determined and the potential for severe poisoning and death is high, so all oral ingestions should be treated as significant and these patients should be monitored for a minimum of 12 hours. Symptomatic ingestions should be treated cautiously, including continuous monitoring for 24 to 48 hours, preferably in an intensive care unit.

Routine clinical observations are sufficient to detect the presence of poisoning, in particular, sedation and clinical cyanosis. Until more data are available it seems reasonable to focus treatment on reversal of methemoglobinemia. There is sufficient time to initiate specific treatments in propanil poisoning given that clinical signs of poisoning are noted early postingestion, yet the time to death is usually greater than 24 hours. There are no controlled clinical or laboratory data available on the effect of any specific treatment in acute symptomatic propanil poisoning, so management is largely empirical.

Resuscitation and Supportive Care Prompt resuscitation and close observation are required in all patients. Patients should be monitored clinically including pulse oximetry, and receive supportive care including supplemental oxygen, intravenous fluids, and ventilatory and hemodynamic support as required. In the absence of cooximetry analysis, significant methemoglobinemia is suspected when cyanosis does not correct with high-flow oxygen and ventilatory support. Euglycemia should be ensured since adequate glucose concentrations are required for endogenous reduction and maximizing the efficacy of methylene blue.

Hemoglobin concentrations should be monitored to detect hemolysis, and folate supplementation may be necessary during the recovery phase if anemia is significant.

Gastrointestinal Decontamination Toxicokinetic studies of propanil have demonstrated a prolonged absorption phase, so it is reasonable to administer activated charcoal to the patient a number of hours postingestion. Although a recent trial that did not demonstrate clinical benefits from activated charcoal in patients with pesticide poisoning included patients with propanil poisoning, subgroup analyses were not conducted.[32]

Extracorporeal Removal Treatment with combined hemodialysis and hemoperfusion was associated with a propanil elimination half-life of 1 hour, although clearance was not directly measured.[87] However, half-lives as short as 1 hour have been reported in patients who have not received this treatment[101] so its efficacy remains unknown. Exchange transfusion has the potential to decrease the concentration of propanil and free hemoglobin while replacing reduced hemoglobin and hemolyzed erythrocytes. But the function of transfused erythrocytes is temporarily impaired posttransfusion because of depletion of 2,3-bisphosphoglycerate (BPG) during storage. Further, transfusion reactions such as acute lung injury may occur, which is of concern when oxygenation is already impaired. In the absence of controlled studies, the role of such treatments in the routine management of acute propanil poisoning is poorly defined (see Chap. 9).

Antidotes Antidotes are largely used for the treatment of methemoglobinemia. Methylene blue (see Antidotes in Depth A41: Methylene Blue) is considered the first-line treatment for methemoglobinemia. Methylene blue has a half-life of 5 hours, which is commonly shorter than that of 3,4-dichloroaniline, so rebound poisoning (ie, an increase in methemoglobin following an initial recovery postadministration of methylene blue) is likely when a bolus regimen is used. This occurred in a previous case of propanil poisoning[127] and may be prevented by administration of methylene blue to the patient as a constant infusion.

Other potential treatments include toluidine blue, *N*-acetylcysteine, ascorbic acid, and cimetidine, but no clinical studies have assessed the role of these potential antidotes in the management of propanil poisoning.

BIPYRIDYL COMPOUNDS, PARAQUAT, AND DIQUAT

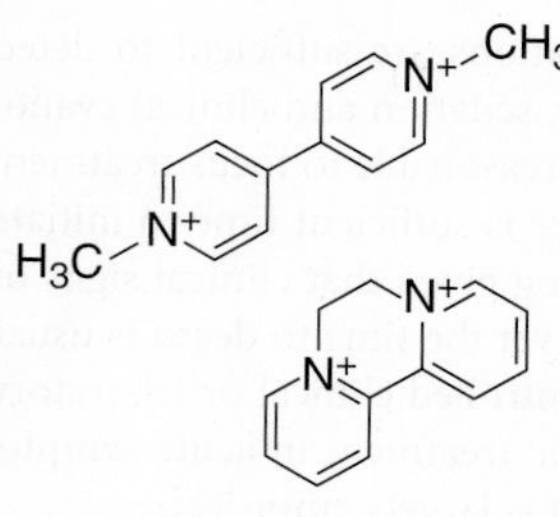

Paraquat

Diquat

Bipyridyl compounds are nonselective contact herbicides. The most widely used is paraquat (1,1'-dimethyl-4,4'-bipyridinium), but diquat (1,1'-ethylene-2,2'-bipyridyldiylium) is commonly used also. Paraquat is one of the most toxic pesticides available, as ingestion of as little as 10 to 20 mL of the 20% wt/vol solution is sufficient to cause death. Overall, the mortality varies between 50% and 90%, but in cases of intentional self-poisoning with concentrated formulations, mortality approaches 100%. Diquat is less toxic than paraquat so it may be coformulated with paraquat (allowing a lower concentration of paraquat) or used as an alternative in countries where paraquat is severely restricted. Because more data are available on paraquat than diquat, much of the following discussion and information relates particularly to paraquat.

PHARMACOLOGY

Paraquat and diquat formulations are highly irritating and often corrosive, causing direct toxicity. Paraquat induces intracellular toxicity by the generation of reactive oxygen species that nonspecifically damage the lipid membrane of cells, inducing cellular toxicity and death. Once paraquat enters the intracellular space it is oxidized to the paraquat radical. This radical is subsequently reduced by diaphorase in the presence of nicotinamide adenine dinucleotide phosphate (NADPH) to reform the parent paraquat compound and superoxide radical, a reactive oxygen species. This process is known as redox cycling (Fig. 115–2). The superoxide radical is susceptible to further reactions by other intracellular processes, leading to formation of other reactive oxygen species, including hydroxyl radicals and peroxynitrite. Reactive oxygen species are potent inducers of cytotoxicity. Paraquat redox cycling continues as long as NADPH and oxygen are available. Depletion of NADPH prevents recycling of glutathione and interferes with other intracellular processes, including energy production and active transporters, exacerbating toxicity. Intracellular protective mechanisms such as glutathione, superoxide dismutase, and catalase are overwhelmed or depleted following large exposures. Taken together, these cytotoxic reactions induce cellular necrosis, which is followed by an influx of neutrophils and macrophages. The reactions contribute to the inflammatory response and promote fibrosis and destruction of normal tissue architecture over a number of days.[23,27]

The lung is particularly susceptible to the effects of paraquat. Acute pneumonitis and hemorrhage occur, followed by ongoing inflammation and progressive pulmonary fibrosis.[27,109] Supplemental oxygen probably increases the generation of reactive oxygen species.

The highest concentration of paraquat is in the kidneys. Renal toxicity is commonly observed in acute paraquat and diquat poisoning, which is important since both are eliminated by the kidneys. Paraquat induces acute tubular necrosis due to direct toxicity to the proximal tubule in particular, and to a lesser degree distal structures. Other factors influencing the development of acute renal impairment include hypoperfusion from hypovolemia and/or hypotension and direct glomerular injury. Varying degrees of oliguria, proteinuria, hematuria, and glycosuria are reported.[17]

PHARMACOKINETICS AND TOXICOKINETICS

Absorption is limited following dermal exposures, although prolonged exposures (at least several hours) to concentrated formulations may degrade the epithelial barrier, allowing some systemic absorption. Absorption across the respiratory epithelium is also limited because of large droplets that impact the oropharynx or larger proximal airways rather than more permeable distal airways.

The oral bioavailability of paraquat varies among animal species, but it is overall quite low.[21,85,109] The bioavailability of paraquat in humans is estimated to be less than 5%,[21] yet an oral exposure of as little as 10 mL allows sufficient paraquat to be absorbed for significant clinical toxicity to occur. Absorption is rapid and the peak concentration occurs within 1 hour.[85] Coingestion of food may decrease the absorption of paraquat. Recently, paraquat was reformulated with an increased emetic concentration along with an alginate that formed a gelatinous mixture on contact with gastric acid, limiting release of the paraquat into the stomach. This formulation led to a decrease in paraquat absorption in animals[44] and improved outcomes from self-poisoning in humans (mortality of 64% compared to 74% with the standard preparation).[124]

Paraquat binds minimally to serum proteins. Paraquat and diquat rapidly distribute to all tissues where they accumulate but may redistribute

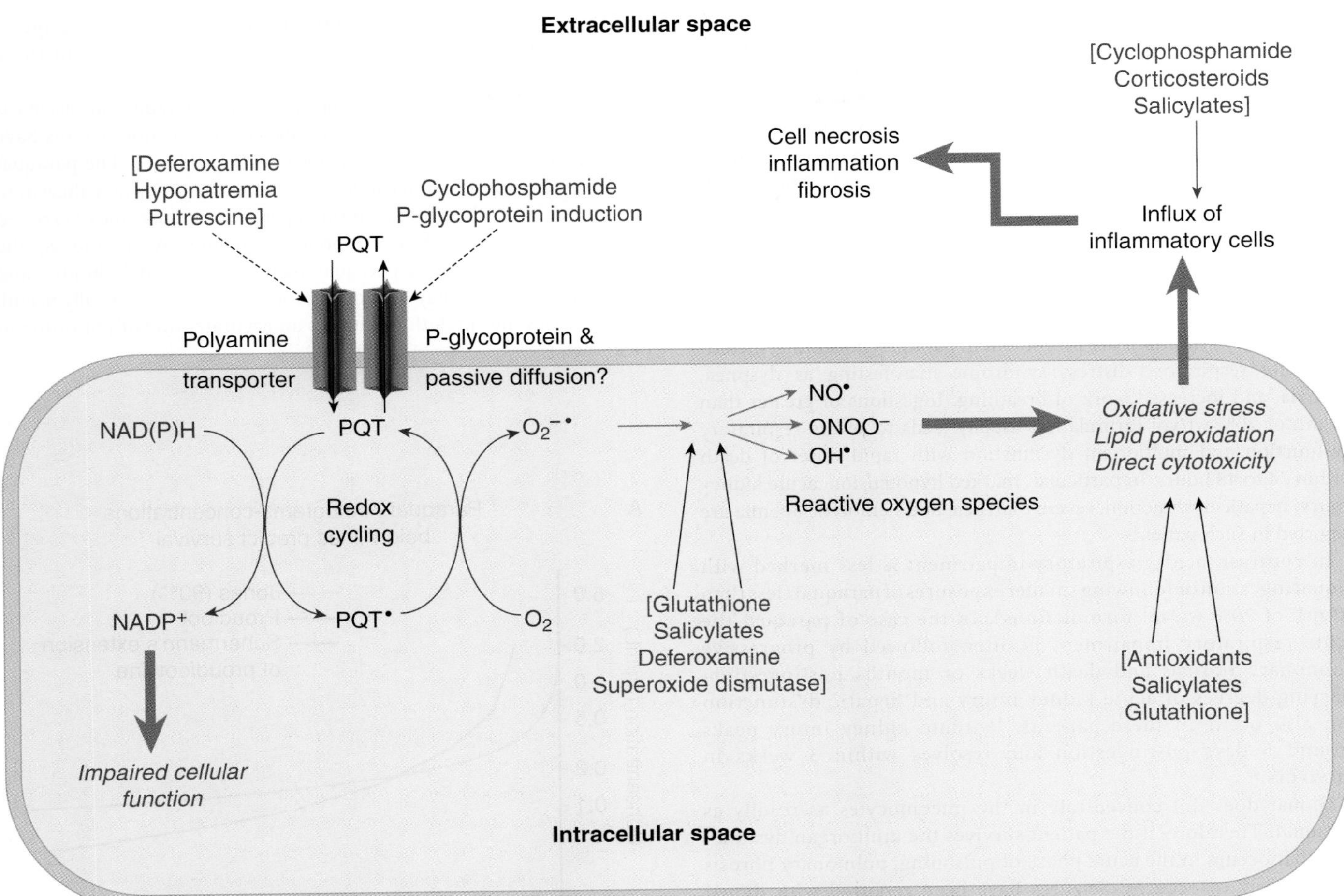

FIGURE 115–2. Toxicology of paraquat (PQT) and proposed mechanisms of action of potential treatments. PQT• = paraquat radical; NO• = Nitric oxide; ONOO− = peroxynitrite; OH• = hydroxyl radical.

back to the central circulation.[85] In humans the distribution half-life is approximately 5 hours.[52] Paraquat accumulates in alveolar cells so the concentration exceeds that of the blood,[85,104] with a peak occurring at around 6 hours postingestion in patients with normal renal function and a delay being recognized with renal impairment.[10] However, this accumulation appears to be a reversible process given that paraquat redistributes back to the systemic circulation as its concentration falls. This is possibly due to impaired function of the pneumocytes from acute lung injury.[5] The uptake of paraquat is an energy-dependent process that continues as long as the blood concentration of paraquat remains elevated.[104] This transporter also facilitates the uptake of endogenous polyamine compounds. In contrast, while there is some uptake of diquat this occurs to a limited extent.[104]

Paraquat is not metabolized and elimination is primarily renal[85] with more than 90% of a dose being excreted within the first 24 hours of poisoning if renal function is maintained.[52] Its clearance initially exceeds that of creatinine mostly because of active secretion, but also to a lesser degree through increased renal blood flow.[17] Renal clearance may be reduced by exogenous compounds or an acidic urine pH.[17] Renal impairment is commonly reported with paraquat and diquat poisoning, which decreases excretion and exacerbates clinical toxicity.[10] Elimination is prolonged with a terminal half-life of around 80 hours in humans.[52] Paraquat is detected in the urine of surviving patients beyond 30 days despite serum concentrations being quite low 48 hours postingestion.[7,109] In animals, the terminal elimination half-life of paraquat is more than 50 hours.[85]

PATHOPHYSIOLOGY

Paraquat induces nonspecific cellular necrosis. Pulmonary and renal toxicity is prominent in acute paraquat poisoning because of the high concentrations found in these cells. Acute pneumonitis reduces oxygen diffusion and induces dyspnea and hypoxia, which interfere with normal cellular function. Acute renal impairment interferes with normal fluid and electrolyte homeostasis, as well as interfering with paraquat elimination, which promotes systemic toxicity. Necrosis of the gut limits intake and causes fluid shifts that contribute to hypotension induced by direct vascular toxicity. Hypotension impairs tissue perfusion and if uncorrected progresses to irreversible shock. Failure to correct these abnormalities may lead to irreversible cellular toxicity and death.

CLINICAL MANIFESTATIONS

Topical exposures may induce painful irritation to the eyes and skin, progressing to ulceration or desquamation depending on the concentration of the solution, duration of exposure, and adequacy of decontamination. Intravenous administration induces severe poisoning from small exposures.

Most oral exposures to bipyridyl compounds induce clinical toxicity. Gastrointestinal toxicity occurs early, including nausea, vomiting, and abdominal and oral pain. Diarrhea and ileus are also reported. Necrosis of mucous membranes (occasionally referred to as pseudodiphtheria)[114] and ulceration are prominent and painful symptoms that generally occur within 12 hours. Injury has even been observed in cases where exposure to paraquat solution occurred without swallowing, despite the brief contact time as a result of immediate spitting and removal from the mouth. Dysphagia and odynophagia follow large exposures and may progress to esophageal rupture, mediastinitis, subcutaneous emphysema, and pneumothorax, which are preterminal events.

Respiratory symptoms are prominent in paraquat poisoning, including acute respiratory distress syndrome manifesting as dyspnea, hypoxia, and increased work of breathing. Ingestions of greater than 20 mL of 20% wt/vol formulation usually leads to severe respiratory dysfunction and multiorgan dysfunction with rapid onset of death within 24 to 48 hours. In particular, marked hypotension, acute kidney injury, hepatic dysfunction, severe diarrhea, and hemolytic anemia are reported in such patients.

In contrast, acute respiratory impairment is less marked with diquat ingestion or following smaller exposures of paraquat (less than 20 mL of 20% wt/vol formulations). In the case of paraquat the acute respiratory impairment is often followed by progressive pulmonary fibrosis and death weeks or months postingestion. Varying degrees of acute kidney injury and hepatic dysfunction can also occur in these patients.[9,55] Acute kidney injury peaks around 5 days postingestion and resolves within 3 weeks in survivors.[61]

Diquat does not concentrate in the pneumocytes as readily as paraquat. Therefore, if the patient survives the multiorgan dysfunction that occurs in the acute phase of poisoning, pulmonary fibrosis is less likely to occur.[129] Seizures have been reported with diquat poisoning.

DIAGNOSTIC TESTING

A diagnosis of paraquat poisoning is made on the basis of a history of exposure and the clinical symptoms, so a high index of clinical suspicion is required. Differential diagnoses include other corrosive exposures, sepsis, or other cellular poisons such as phosphine, colchicine, or iron.

Determination of the presence of a bipyridyl compound in blood confirms exposure, although such assays are increasingly of limited availability. The urinary dithionite test is a simple and quick method for confirming (or excluding) paraquat and diquat poisoning. Various methods are reported, including the addition of 1 g of sodium bicarbonate and 1 g of sodium dithionite, or 1% sodium dithionite in 1 M sodium hydroxide, to 10 mL of urine. A color change (blue for paraquat and green for diquat) confirms ingestion—the darker the color the higher the concentration.[7,105] If the test is negative on urine beyond 6 hours after ingestion, a large exposure is unlikely, but repeat testing should be conducted over 24 hours.

Given that outcomes from paraquat poisoning are generally poor, diagnostic tests may help differentiate patients who may survive from those in whom death is almost certain. The dose of paraquat is a well-established predictor of death, although this information may not be accurately known at the time of admission.[33] A range of investigations in patients with acute paraquat poisoning have attempted to determine the severity of poisoning and better define prognosis. Unfortunately, few have been validated so their predictive ability is unconfirmed. The range of prognostic tests were recently reviewed[33] and a selection of these are discussed below.

Quantitative analysis of the concentration of paraquat in plasma is useful for prognostication, and a number of similar nomograms have been developed to assist with this process (Fig. 115–3). The paraquat concentration must be interpreted relative to the time since ingestion. Determination of the concentration of paraquat in the urine of exposed patients has also been shown to predict outcomes. As mentioned, the availability of quantitative paraquat assays is increasingly limited and the turnaround time may be too long for the test to be clinically useful; in most cases interpretation requires an accurate time of poisoning to be known.[33]

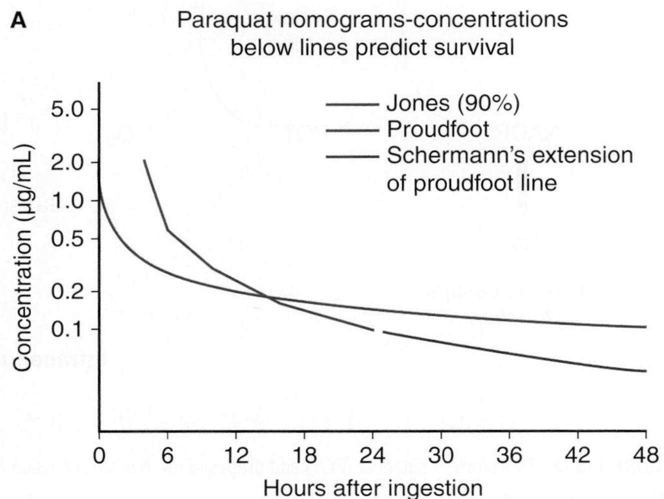

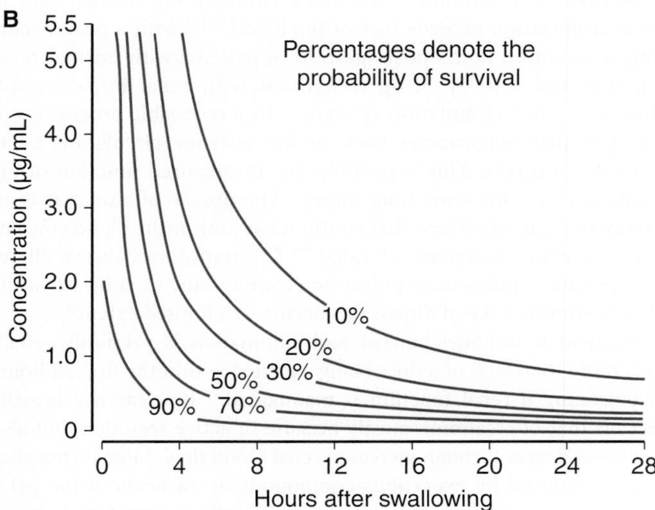

FIGURE 115–3. Nomograms for serum paraquat concentrations. **A.** Compilation of three nomograms proposed by: Proudfoot et al.[96a] Scherrmann et al.[107a] and Jones et al.[58a] **B.** Hart paraquat nomogram. Hart et al.[43a] In A, concentrations below lines predict survival. In B, lines link concentrations of equal probability of survival. (Derived from Eddleston, et al.[33] by permission of Oxford University Press.)

Other methods for predicting outcomes from paraquat poisoning have used various combinations of simple laboratory tests including blood gas analysis, complete blood count, electrolytes, renal function, and liver function tests.[33] A raised admission creatinine concentration predicts death (86% versus 40% if the concentration is normal), but is neither sensitive nor specific, which probably relates to differences in time to presentation. The higher the creatinine concentration, the higher the odds ratio of death.[61] The rate of increase in creatinine concentration is a simple test that may be a better predictor of prognosis. An increase less than 3 μmol/L/h over 5 hours predicts survival,[97] or greater than 5.4 μmol/L/h predicts death.[100] With such calculations, serial samples can be collected and the rate of increase determined irrespective of the time of poisoning. Paraquat and diquat interfere with creatinine assays using the Jaffe method causing a false elevation, although this largely occurs at concentrations exceeding 100 mg/L, which is rarely observed and likely to be associated with severe clinical toxicity.[95]

Other biomarkers that may inform prognosis include pulmonary surfactant protein-A and -B (but not -D), type IV collagen, and tissue inhibitor of metalloproteinase-1 (TIMP-1), but further research is required.

MANAGEMENT

Because death can occur following ingestion of as little as 10 to 20 mL of paraquat, all exposures should be treated as potentially life threatening. Patients suspected of ingesting paraquat should be observed in hospital for at least 6 hours postingestion or until a urinary dithionite test can be conducted.

Many medical interventions have been proposed for the treatment of patients with acute paraquat poisoning and these are described below. Unfortunately, data supporting the efficacy of any of these are lacking, largely because of the inadequacy of the clinical studies. Dose–response studies to determine the optimal dose are also lacking for most of the therapeutic interventions. The literature is complicated by case reports describing survival in patients who were administered one or a combination of therapies.

In countries where paraquat poisoning is relatively common, many clinicians elect to administer a number of therapies to patients concurrently in the hope of a benefit because of the high likelihood of death in patients with acute paraquat poisoning. Administration of activated charcoal, *N*-acetylcysteine, vitamins C and E, immunosuppressants, and hemodialysis and/or hemoperfusion to a patient is not uncommon.

The choice of which interventions should be administered to a patient is best made on a case-by-case basis by the treating physician in consultation with relevant resources. Detailed discussion with the patient and relatives early in the presentation is recommended to determine their preference for treatment modalities. In general, a comprehensive treatment regimen is reasonable in patients who present very early (within 2 hours of poisoning) or those with a faintly positive dithionite urinary test. Treatments that reduce the exposure to paraquat by either reducing absorption or increasing clearance should be initiated promptly. Immunosuppression with cyclophosphamide and corticosteroids, and probably administration of salicylates, is also reasonable even though the risk-benefit in such patients has not been determined. In contrast, these treatments seem unlikely to be of assistance to patients in whom this test is strongly positive, or those with evolving multiorgan dysfunction. Instead, palliation should be the priority, including oxygen for hypoxia and morphine for dyspnea and oropharyngeal and abdominal pain.

Serial pulse oximetry measurements and chest radiographs will demonstrate progression of the pneumonitis and pulmonary fibrosis. Lung transplantation has been trialed in patients who develop pulmonary fibrosis, but it was largely unsuccessful because of the prolonged elimination half-life of paraquat.[9,59] Patients developing acute kidney injury should receive hemodialysis or hemofiltration per usual guidelines if active treatment is to be pursued, and these treatments may also enhance elimination of herbicide.

A range of tests has been proposed for prognostication in acute paraquat poisoning, as discussed above. Where available, these might assist with decisions regarding whether patients should be actively treated, palliated, or discharged with confidence that harm will not occur.

Resuscitation and Supportive Care All patients should receive prompt routine resuscitation and close observation. Oxygen should be administered to patients for palliation only when there is confirmed hypoxia and the clinical assessment suggests that death is likely. Although controlled hypoxia does not prevent the development of pulmonary injury,[9] unnecessary supplemental oxygen can theoretically hasten the progression of injury. Intravenous fluids should be administered to patients who are volume depleted from poor intake, diarrhea, or third-space shifts, as this may reduce the extent of acute kidney injury and promote renal clearance of paraquat. Electrolyte abnormalities may also occur and these should be corrected as required.

Analgesia for oral and abdominal pain should be administered to patients, including intravenous opioids such as morphine and possibly topical anesthetics such as lidocaine.

Gastrointestinal Decontamination Paraquat is coformulated with an emetic so self-decontamination may have occurred by the time of presentation to hospital. Fuller's Earth and activated charcoal have been advocated to decrease absorption of paraquat. Data demonstrating the clinical superiority of Fuller's Earth over activated charcoal are not available. Fuller's Earth is now of limited supply, but activated charcoal appears to adsorb paraquat to a similar extent as Fuller's Earth.[8] However, given that paraquat is rapidly absorbed if activated charcoal is to be administered to a patient who has ingested paraquat, this should occur within 1 hour of ingestion. Gastric lavage has not been shown to improve outcomes and may even be harmful if administered to patients ingesting less than 30 mL.[125]

Extracorporeal Removal Extracorporeal techniques, including charcoal hemoperfusion and hemodialysis, aim to decrease the systemic exposure by increasing the rate of elimination. Hemoperfusion is more efficient than hemodialysis, and clearance is maximized when treatment is initiated within the first couple of hours because the plasma concentration is high.[46] Further, given that paraquat rapidly distributes from the circulation, prompt treatment is necessary to limit the uptake into pulmonary and other tissues. Experimentally, hemoperfusion reduces mortality in dogs only when it is commenced within a few hours of poisoning, and repeated treatments do not increase clearance to a large extent.[92]

Unfortunately, current experience suggests that these treatments do not sufficiently improve mortality in humans, particularly when the concentration is greater than 3 mg/L.[43] In some cases there may be a rebound in serum paraquat concentrations with intermittent regimens that may be minimized using continuous techniques. Hemoperfusion followed by continuous venovenous hemofiltration may prolong the time to death compared with hemoperfusion alone without changing the overall mortality in a randomized, controlled trial. All patients in this study also received high-dose dexamethasone and ascorbic acid.[63]

Extracorporeal techniques may also induce harm because of the requirement for central venous access, metabolic disequilibrium, or increased clearance of antidotes. Therefore, the use of extracorporeal techniques requires careful consideration.

Antidotes A large number of potential antidotes have been trialed in the treatment of acute paraquat poisoning. They attempt to counteract the effects of paraquat by targeting various steps in the pathogenesis of organ dysfunction or to alter cellular uptake (see Fig. 115–3). Unfortunately, none of these antidotes are proven to reduce mortality. However, two interventions that decrease paraquat exposure (either decreasing absorption[124] or increasing elimination[63]) prolonged the time to death, suggesting a beneficial effect. Combining these treatments with effective antidotes in a multimodal approach to treatment may reduce mortality. More research is required to support the use of such treatments in routine clinical care.

Immunosuppression with corticosteroids (dexamethasone or methylprednisolone) and cyclophosphamide are the most extensively trialed antidotes, including human randomized, controlled trials. These medicines aim to reduce inflammation, and initial studies were promising but not conclusive[33,72] because of serious concerns with the study design.[16,41] Regimens vary, including cyclophosphamide 10 to 15 mg/kg/d for 2 days, and methylprednisolone 15 mg/kg/d (up to 1 g) for 3 days, which is followed by dexamethasone 4 to 10 mg every 6 to 8 hours until recovery. In some reports cyclophosphamide was repeated if leukopenia did not develop, and pulse doses of methylprednisolone may also be repeated if deterioration is observed. Mesna was coadministered to patients in some series, and sirolimus has been trialed as an alternative immunosuppressant.

Generation of reactive oxygen species is an important step in the pathogenesis of paraquat poisoning (see Fig. 115–3). This leads to cytotoxicity, the extent of which depends on the concentration of paraquat at the cellular level and the efficiency of protective mechanisms. Endogenous scavenger defense mechanisms against reactive oxygen species include antioxidants such as vitamin C (ascorbic acid), vitamin E (alpha-tocopherol), and glutathione. Administration of these vitamins and/or a glutathione donator (such as acetylcysteine, S-carboxymethylcysteine, or captopril) to patients did not improve outcomes in every human or animal study. Poor intracellular penetration to the site of redox cycling may limit the effect of some compounds.[115] Potentially, vitamin C might increase oxidative toxicity.[27] These interventions have also been used in patients with acute poisoning. Typical doses include vitamin E 300 mg orally twice daily, vitamin C 25 mg/kg/d or 3 g/d for 7 days, and *N*-acetylcysteine 150 mg/kg over 3 hours as a loading dose followed by 500 mg/kg/d by continuous infusion. The scavenging agents superoxide dismutase and amifostine and the iron chelator desferrioxamine have also been trialed, but results were not encouraging.

Some treatments may influence the toxicokinetics of paraquat at the cellular level. Agents that decrease the uptake of paraquat by pneumocytes have been trialed such as putrescine, spermidine, and desferrioxamine, but their effect is limited and they do not alter efflux. Induction of P-glycoprotein with dexamethasone (100 mg/kg) increased cellular efflux and excretion of paraquat in rats, which is also promising.[26] Cyclophosphamide has also been shown to increase the efflux of paraquat from pneumocytes.[9]

Salicylates are proposed to inhibit multiple steps in the pathogenesis of paraquat poisoning, including decreasing production of reactive oxygen species, inhibition of NF-κB, antithrombotic effects, and chelation of paraquat.[25,29] Sodium salicylate 200 mg/kg decreased reactive oxygen species production and inflammation and improved survival in rats.[29] Similarly, lysine acetylsalicylate 200 mg/kg was noted to be the optimum dose to improve survival and minimize toxicity in rats.[28] A clinical study assessing the effect of intravenous acetylsalicylic acid in acute paraquat poisoning is currently under way in Sri Lanka.

Other antidotes and treatments have also been proposed, but less information regarding their effect is available and it is outside of the scope of this chapter to discuss every possible treatment.

GLUFOSINATE

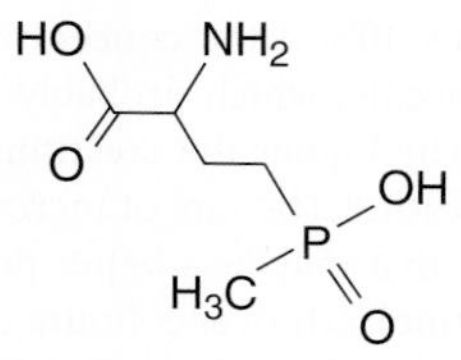

Glufosinate ([2*RS*]-2-amino-4-[hydroxy(methyl)phosphinoyl]butyric acid) is a nonselective herbicide used predominantly in Japan, which is where most cases of acute poisoning are reported. Commercial preparations contain 14% to 30% glufosinate as the ammonium salt and anionic surfactants. A case fatality as high as 17.7% has been reported from glufosinate poisoning.

PHARMACOLOGY

Glufosinate is neurotoxic, although the specific mechanism is incompletely described. Since it is structurally similar to glutamate, studies have explored whether it interferes with glutamate in the central nervous system. Rat studies have demonstrated both agonism[77,86] and antagonism[36] to glutamate receptors and no effect on other receptors in the brain.[42] Although glufosinate also interferes with glutamine synthetase activity,[30] this effect is unlikely to be significant given the limited alterations in the concentrations of ammonia or glutamate that result.[42]

Glufosinate was not found to inhibit cholinesterase enzymes in rat studies,[42] although it has been reported in humans on occasion, including one case where it decreased to around 40% of the lower limit of normal with subsequent recovery.[122] Ammonia concentrations were not markedly altered in rats[42]; however, serum ammonia was elevated in some patients with self-poisoning, which might contribute to clinical toxicity.[122]

The extent to which the surfactant contributes to clinical toxicity has not been confirmed. Rat studies suggest that hemodynamic changes due to glufosinate ammonium formulations are entirely caused by the surfactant component rather than glufosinate itself.[65] Surfactants may also cause uncoupling of oxidative phosphorylation, although this was not observed in a single case report of glufosinate ammonium poisoning.[74]

PHARMACOKINETICS AND TOXICOKINETICS

Kinetic analysis of glufosinate is limited to animal studies and a few human case reports. Minor differences in kinetics of the D- and L-glufosinate enantiomers are observed between patients, the clinical implications of which are not known.

The rate of absorption of glufosinate is slower in rats than mice, although this corrected when administered to the animals as the formulated product, and the concentration peaks at 1 hour postingestion. Less than 15% of a dose is absorbed by rats.

Glufosinate does not appear to bind to serum proteins to a significant extent. The Vd was calculated to be 1.44 L/kg in a case of acute poisoning by assuming that the renal excretion of glufosinate is similar to animals.[45] Glufosinate distributes to the central nervous system, and in a case of acute poisoning the cerebrospinal fluid concentration was one-third the serum concentration 27 hours postingestion. The rate of distribution to the cerebrospinal fluid has not been characterized, but it is theorized that glufosinate might distribute to the central nervous system slowly (perhaps due to active transporters) where it accumulates, which is why the onset of respiratory depression is delayed.[51] This theory was not supported in a case where glufosinate was not detected in the cerebrospinal fluid 6 hours after a seizure that occurred 30 hours postingestion.[118] Indeed, seizures have occurred in some patients after glufosinate was no longer detectable in the blood.[122] Seizures occur 3 hours postadministration of intracerebral glufosinate in rats, which further challenges the theory that distribution kinetics influence the delayed onset of seizures in humans.[42]

Glufosinate is subject to minimal metabolism and the majority of the bioavailable dose of glufosinate is excreted unchanged in urine.[37]

The elimination half-life in rats is 4 hours,[30] while in rabbits elimination is biphasic with a terminal elimination half-life of 1.9 hours, which was not dose dependent.[64] Kinetic data in humans are limited to a small number of cases of acute intentional poisoning where the elimination profile appeared biphasic with a distribution half-life of 2 to 4 hours and a terminal elimination of 10 to 18 hours.[45,49,116]

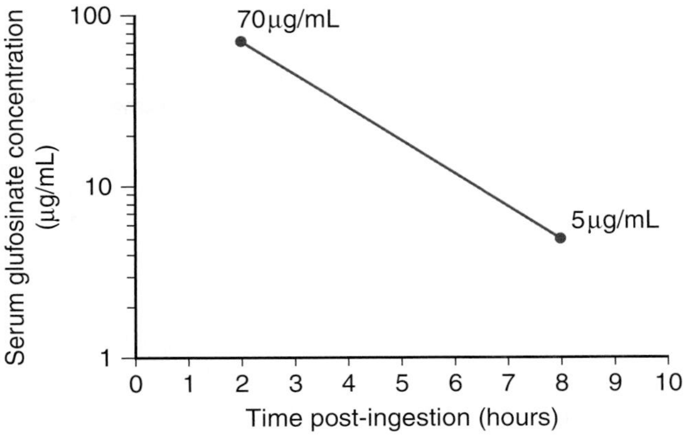

FIGURE 115–4. Glufosinate nomogram as described by Hori et al.[47] Concentrations above the line represent patients experiencing a greater degree of severity.

PATHOPHYSIOLOGY

It is not known whether the manifestations of glufosinate poisoning represent a primary (toxic) or secondary (downstream) effect. The most important manifestations are neurological, which interfere with respiration and subsequent oxygen delivery to vital organs, compromising normal cellular function. Hypotension also impairs tissue perfusion and if uncorrected progresses to shock. Failure to correct these abnormalities may lead to irreversible cellular toxicity and death.

CLINICAL MANIFESTATIONS

Nausea and vomiting are early features of acute poisoning. Altered level of consciousness may precede severe neurotoxicity, which occurs between 4 and 30 hours postingestion in the available reports, and includes seizures and central respiratory failure requiring ventilatory support. These symptoms may persist for a number of days. In rats, the onset of seizures is also delayed by a number of hours; however, the time to onset of the seizures decreases in a dose-dependent manner following the intraperitoneal administration of glufosinate.[77]

Other symptoms are reported including cardiac dysrhythmias, fever, amnesia, diabetes insipidus, and rhabdomyolysis. Refractory hypotension may be preterminal.

DIAGNOSTIC TESTING

Glufosinate poisoning is diagnosed clinically in the context of a history of exposure. Japanese clinicians and scientists have developed glufosinate assays for clinical use and a nomogram was developed for predicting clinical outcomes (Fig. 115–4).[47] Clinical chemistry assays including renal function, arterial blood gases, electrolytes, creatine kinase, and ammonia concentrations may support clinical management.

MANAGEMENT

Severe symptoms have been reported following unintentional ingestion, so all patients with oral exposures should be carefully monitored. Patients with confirmed exposures should be monitored for a minimum of 48 hours because of the possibility of delayed onset in clinical toxicity.

Resuscitation and Supportive Care Routine resuscitation, close observation, and supportive care are required. Careful monitoring for the onset of respiratory failure is necessary and early intubation and ventilation is recommended. Given that glufosinate and metabolites are primarily renally cleared, intravenous fluids to maintain a consistent urine output is suggested. Seizures should be treated along standard lines, including benzodiazepines as first-line and possibly barbiturates if required. This approach is suggested to be effective on the basis of animal studies. Biochemical and acid–base abnormalities should be corrected where possible.

Gastrointestinal Decontamination In most reports of glufosinate poisoning gastric lavage and activated charcoal were administered, but it is not possible to determine whether these interventions improved clinical outcomes. The high incidence of seizures and respiratory failure from glufosinate poisoning is a relative contraindication to the administration of activated charcoal to patients. However, if the airway is secured then activated charcoal could potentially be administered to the patient per usual recommendations, although there are insufficient data confirming that this is effective.

Extracorporeal Removal Hemodialysis and hemoperfusion have been used in the management of acute glufosinate poisoning. Hemodialysis appears to be superior to hemoperfusion in terms of extraction from whole blood in vitro,[119] with an extraction ratio of 80%.[118] However, the clearance by hemodialysis is less than 60% of renal clearance.[45] Although prompt hemodialysis in patients on admission to hospital decreased the concentration of glufosinate, this may not prevent the development of seizures a number of hours later. Thus, while hemodialysis appears to decrease the serum concentration, there is insufficient data to confirm its role in routine management. It is reasonable to attempt such treatments if the patient presents with renal impairment.

Antidotes Specific antidotes are not available. Rat studies did not demonstrate benefit with the use of atropine and pralidoxime.

GLYPHOSATE

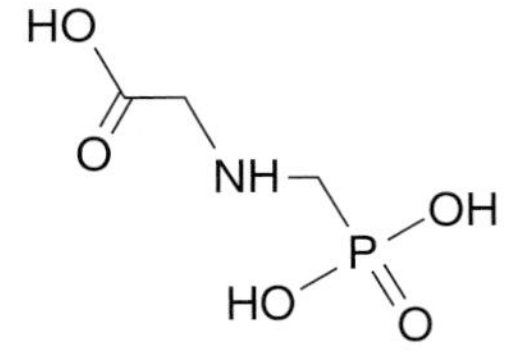

Glyphosate (*N*-[phosphonomethyl]glycine; Fig. 115–7) is a nonselective postemergence herbicide. It is used extensively worldwide, most commonly as the isopropylamine salt. Glyphosate-containing herbicides are available in various formulations, approximately 1% to 5% glyphosate (ready to use) or approximately 30% to 50% (concentrate requiring dilution before use). In 2001, glyphosate was the most frequently used pesticide in the United States and the second most commonly used pesticide in the domestic sector.[60] Products containing glyphosate trimesium are less widely used and may differ with respect to their toxicity profile.

PHARMACOLOGY

Glyphosate inhibits 5-enolpyruvylshikimate-3-phosphate synthase in plants, which interferes with their aromatic amino acid synthesis. Because this enzyme is not present in humans glyphosate appears to be relatively selective for plants.

The mechanism of toxicity of glyphosate-containing herbicides to humans has not been adequately described. The formulation is irritating, particularly high concentrations which are corrosive, causing direct toxicity to the gastrointestinal tract. Despite being an organic phosphorus compound, glyphosate is not considered to inhibit acetylcholinesterase. Patients with severe poisoning manifest multisystem effects, suggesting that the formulation is either nonspecific in its action or that it interferes with a physiological process common to a number of systems. Proposed mechanisms include disruption of cellular membranes and uncoupling of oxidative phosphorylation, although these may be interrelated.[11,88,90] Indeed, the mechanism of toxicity may vary between different formulations of glyphosate. In two cases of glyphosate trimesium poisoning cardiopulmonary arrest occurred within minutes of ingestion.[82,113] Since this is not reported from glyphosate isopropylamine, it is possible that these products differ in the mechanism of toxicity.

Experimentally, there appears to be minimal (if any) mammalian toxicity from glyphosate itself. Glyphosate is categorized as WHO class "U" (Unlikely to present acute hazard in normal use; LD_{50} greater than 4000 mg/kg).[56] Surfactant coformulants are considered the more toxic component in glyphosate-containing herbicides.[11,18,53,126] Polyoxyethyleneamine (POEA; tallow amine; LD_{50} equal to 1200 mg/kg) is the most common surfactant formulated in these products, but others are also used. Systemic exposure to surfactants induces hypotension, which is primarily due to direct effects on the heart and blood vessels.[18] Surfactants disrupt cellular and subcellular membranes by direct toxicity, including those of mitochondria, which has the potential to lead to systemic symptoms.[39] Coformulated potassium and isopropylamine may also contribute to toxicity. Isopropylamine has a rat LD_{50} of 111 to 820 mg/kg, decreases vascular resistance, and may either increase or decrease cardiac contractility and rate.[57,96]

PHARMACOKINETICS AND TOXICOKINETICS

The kinetics of the surfactant has not been described. Data about the kinetics of glyphosate are available but the importance of this is debated given that glyphosate is not considered very toxic to humans. However, the role of plasma concentrations for predicting outcomes in acute poisoning (as a surrogate marker of exposure) is currently being explored and will require kinetic data for proper interpretation. Ingestion is the most significant route of exposure of glyphosate-containing herbicides because they do not penetrate the skin to a significant extent. Up to 40% of an oral dose is absorbed in rats, although this could increase following exposure to concentrated solutions due to direct toxicity to the gastrointestinal epithelium. The peak glyphosate concentration occurs within 2 hours, distribution is limited, and there is minimal metabolism. Glyphosate is predominantly eliminated unchanged in the urine within 24 hours.[11,13,123] Glyphosate does not appear to readily cross the placenta on the basis of an ex vivo model.[83]

Human toxicokinetic data are limited to a few cases. These confirmed rapid elimination of glyphosate (undetectable in plasma within 12 hours because of a half-life of less than 4 hours) and minimal metabolism.[11,48]

PATHOPHYSIOLOGY

It is not known whether the manifestations of glyphosate poisoning represent a primary (toxic) or secondary (downstream) effect. Disruptions of oxidative phosphorylation globally impair normal cellular function as a result of limited energy supply (discussed further with the pathophysiology of phenoxy herbicides). Similarly, direct toxicity to cell membranes (including those of the mitochondria) interferes with normal cellular processes such as ion channels. Both disruptions induce multiorgan toxicity. Hypotension and dysrhythmias impair tissue perfusion, and hepatic and renal toxicity induce metabolic disequilibria and acidosis, which impairs normal physiological processes. Pulmonary toxicity may lead to hypoxia, which further compromises normal cellular functioning. Failure to correct these abnormalities may lead to irreversible cellular toxicity and death.

CLINICAL MANIFESTATIONS

Abdominal pain with nausea, vomiting, and/or diarrhea are the most common manifestations of acute poisoning. These may be mild and self-resolving, but in severe poisoning there may be inflammation, ulceration, or infarction. Severe diarrhea and recurrent vomiting may induce dehydration. Gastrointestinal burns and necrosis occurs with high doses of concentrated formulations and may be associated with hemorrhage. Extensive erosions of the upper gastrointestinal tract is associated with more severe systemic poisoning and a prolonged hospitalization.[19,54]

Severe poisoning manifests as hypotension, cardiac dysrhythmias, renal and hepatic dysfunction, hyperkalemia, pancreatitis, pulmonary edema or pneumonitis, altered level of consciousness, and metabolic acidosis. These effects may be transient or severe, progressing over 12 to 72 hours to shock and death. The mechanism of hypotension may relate to both hypovolemia (fluids shifts and increased losses) and direct cardiotoxicity.[11,71,117]

Intravenous self-administration of glyphosate-containing herbicide caused hemolysis in one patient, and intramuscular self-administration caused rhabdomyolysis in another.

In a recent review of the literature,[11] death occurred in 10.1% of all published cases of acute poisoning with this herbicide (38 of 377; largely retrospective case series), but more cases have since been reported. A subsequent prospective study reported a case fatality of 3.5% (10 of 286 patients) in patients presenting to rural hospitals in Asia where resources are limited.[99] It is possible that improved availability of intensive care facilities may improve outcomes.

Respiratory, ocular, and dermal symptoms may occur following occupational use of these preparations but are usually of minor severity. Significant skin reactions from topical exposure are also reported.

DIAGNOSTIC TESTING

Acute poisoning with a glyphosate-containing herbicide is diagnosed on the basis of a history of exposure and clinical symptomatology.

Quantitative glyphosate or surfactant assays are not routinely available for clinical use, and other specific diagnostic tests are not available. The differential diagnoses are wide, including any xenobiotic or medical condition associated with gastrointestinal symptomatology and progressive multisystem toxicity.

A number of clinical criteria for the classification of severity have been suggested, but none have been validated.[11,99,117,120] There are no clinical investigations to guide management, including specific biomarkers or tools to estimate prognosis in acute poisoning. Patients who develop marked nonspecific organ toxicity (eg, renal failure, pulmonary edema, sedation, dysrhythmias) appear more likely to die.[67,68]

Targeted laboratory and radiological investigations should be conducted in patients demonstrating anything more than mild gastrointestinal symptoms. Pulse oximetry and blood gas measurements may be useful for detection of metabolic disequilibria and respiratory impairment. Endoscopy can diagnose erosions or ulceration following exposures to the concentrated formulation. However, this procedure may be complicated by perforation, and therefore its use requires careful consideration.

Glyphosate serum concentration greater than 1000 mg/L is associated with severe poisoning, although the relevance of this is debated since glyphosate is not thought to induce clinical toxicity itself.[11] It might, however, be a reasonable biomarker of exposure to the product, but more research is required to explore this relationship.

MANAGEMENT

Retrospective studies suggest a correlation between dose, severity of poisoning, and death.[68,107,120] All patients except for those with trivial exposures should be observed for a minimum of 6 hours. In particular, patients presenting with intentional self-poisoning or ingestion of concentrated formulation must be carefully monitored. If gastrointestinal symptoms are noted then the patient should be observed for a minimum of 24 hours given that clinical toxicity may progress. Because the toxicity of individual surfactants has not been determined, treatment does not vary depending on specific coformulants.

Resuscitation and Supportive Care All patients should receive prompt resuscitation, close observation, and routine supportive care; other treatments are largely empiric. The airway is usually maintained but respiratory failure and respiratory distress occur, which require supplemental oxygen and possibly mechanical ventilation. The optimum management of hypotension is complicated because its etiology is potentially related to hypovolemia, negative inotropism, and reduced vascular resistance. A detailed clinical review is required, followed by cautious administration of intravenous fluids to the patient. If the response to prompt administration of 20 to 30 mL/kg intravenous fluid to the patient is insufficient or there is increasing pulmonary congestion, vasopressors should be used. Cardiac investigations such as echocardiography, central venous pressure, or pulmonary artery catheter may also guide management, if available.

Biochemical and acid–base abnormalities, such as hyperkalemia, should be corrected where possible. The contribution of uncoupling of oxidative phosphorylation to clinical toxicity and death has been proposed, but no specific treatment is available if this develops. In the context of acute poisoning with glyphosate-containing herbicides, signs suggestive of uncoupling of oxidative phosphorylation such as hyperthermia, metabolic acidosis with elevated lactate concentration and hypoglycemia may be a preterminal event (see Chap. 15).

Hemodialysis or hemofiltration should be administered to patients developing acute kidney injury per usual guidelines if active treatment is to be pursued.

Gastrointestinal Decontamination No data exist to support the role of gastrointestinal decontamination in acute poisoning with glyphosate-containing herbicides beyond the usual recommendations discussed above.

Extracorporeal Removal Patients have survived severe poisoning and received hemodialysis; however, other patients have died despite this treatment. Plasmapheresis has also been trialed but clearances were not determined. Early initiation of any of these treatments may be required for best results. The role of extracorporeal removal in routine care is not known given that there are limited quantitative data reporting direct clearances.

Antidotes No specific antidote has been proposed or tested for the treatment of acute poisoning with glyphosate-containing herbicides, which probably relates to the unknown mechanism of toxicity of these products.

PHENOXY HERBICIDES (PHENOXYACETIC DERIVATIVES), INCLUDING 2,4-D AND MCPA

Phenoxy compounds are selective herbicides that are widely used in both developing and developed countries. A large number of compounds are included in this category; however, the most widely used are the phenoxyacetic derivatives. This includes 2,4-dichlorophenoxyacetic acid (2,4-D), 4-chloro-2-methylphenoxyacetic acid (MCPA), 2,4,5-trichlorophenoxyacetic acid (2,4,5-T; no longer available), and mecoprop (MCPP; 2-[4-chloro-2-methylphenoxy]propionic acid; Fig. 115–5). Other phenoxy herbicides and available toxicity data are listed in Table 115-1. In 2001, 2,4-D was the fifth most commonly used pesticide in the United States but the most commonly used pesticide in the domestic sector (MCPP was fifth most commonly used in the domestic sector).[60]

Agent orange, a defoliant popularly used during the Vietnam War, was composed of an equal mixture of 2,4-D and 2,4,5-T. This product also contained the contaminant dioxin (2,3,7,8-tetrachlorodibenzo-dioxin; TCDD), which was a byproduct of the manufacture of phenoxy herbicides. Dioxin is a persistent organic pollutant that is alleged to induce chronic health conditions and cancer, although this has been debated. This chapter discusses only the outcomes of acute exposures to phenoxy herbicides.

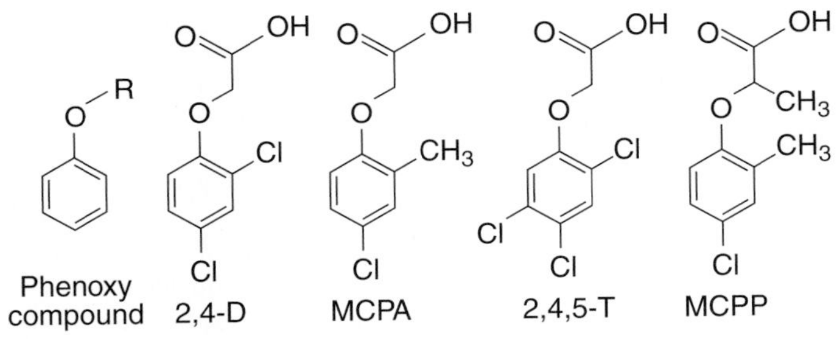

FIGURE 115–5. Structure of common phenoxy herbicides.

PHARMACOLOGY

The mechanism of toxicity of phenoxy compounds is not well described. As with other herbicide products, the formulation is irritating or corrosive, causing direct toxicity to the gastrointestinal tract. Patients with severe poisoning manifest multisystem effects, suggesting that the formulation is either nonspecific in its action or that it interferes with a physiological process common to a number of systems. As with other herbicide preparations, this may reflect the contribution of coformulants such as surfactants.

In rats, high serum concentrations of MCPA damage cell membranes and induce toxicity, but the correlation between serum concentrations, membrane damage, and toxicity is poor.

Uncoupling of oxidative phosphorylation also may contribute to the development of severe clinical toxicity. Phenoxyacetic derivatives demonstrate concentration-dependent uncoupling of rat mitochondria in vitro, although the specific process that is disrupted is not sufficiently described.[14,130] Features of uncoupling of oxidative phosphorylation were observed antemortem in clinical studies of patients with large phenoxy herbicide exposures.[103]

Phenoxy acid compounds inhibit the voltage-gated chloride channel CLC-1 in skeletal muscles, which is thought to contribute to the neuromuscular toxicity of these compounds. Dysfunction of CLC-1 induces myotonia due to hyperpolarization of the cell membrane. Other CLC channels are important for normal renal physiology. There are differences in the degree of inhibition between individual phenoxy acid compounds, which may contribute to the variability in animal LD_{50} and possibly clinical features.[2,69,70]

Other possible mechanisms of toxicity relate to their similarity to acetic acid, interfering with the utilization of acetylcoenzyme A (acetyl-CoA), or action as a false messenger at cholinergic receptors.[12]

PHARMACOKINETICS AND TOXICOKINETICS

Animal studies and human case reports have shown nonlinear kinetics for the phenoxy herbicide compounds. Dose-dependent changes in absorption, protein binding, and clearance all occur, and each will influence the concentration-time profile.

Absorption is usually first order[1]; however, the time to peak concentration may be delayed with increasing doses, which may suggest saturable absorption.[66,121]

As the dose of MCPA increases there is a change in the semilogarithmic serum concentration-time profile from linear to a biphasic convex profile. The inflection of this elimination curve in rats is approximately 200 mg/L,[34,35,121] which may reflect saturation of albumin binding. As the serum concentration exceeds this point the proportion of herbicide that is free (unbound) increases. This may increase the Vd and prolong the apparent plasma elimination half-life.

Another contributing mechanism to the observed biphasic convex concentration-time profile is saturation of renal clearance for which there is some interspecies variability. Dose-dependent renal clearance is attributed to saturation of an active transport process or direct nephrotoxicity. Renal clearance also varies with urine flow because of reabsorption from the distal tubule.

Similar to data from animal studies, the semilogarithmic serum concentration-time curve of phenoxy herbicides in humans with acute poisoning is generally convex, with an apparent inflection from a longer to shorter elimination half-life between 150 and 300 mg/L. The elimination half-lives are prolonged, which may explain the persistence of clinical toxicity and why death may occur a number of days postingestion of a phenoxyacetic herbicide.

Alterations in blood pH may also change tissue distribution because phenoxyacetic herbicides are weak acids (pKa approximately 3). Here, acidosis increases the proportion that is nonionized, and therefore lipophilic, which increases tissue binding and distribution. This has been observed in vitro and is similar to that observed for salicylates (see Chap. 35). Similarly, an alkaline plasma pH is expected to decrease tissue (and probably receptor) binding and increase plasma concentrations.

Experience with acute human poisonings noted a poor correlation between serum herbicide concentrations and peak toxicity.[103] This may reflect a discordance between serum (measured) and intracellular (eg, mitochondrial) concentrations.

PATHOPHYSIOLOGY

Direct toxicity to the gastrointestinal tract may cause vomiting and diarrhea, which induces hypovolemia and electrolyte abnormalities.[12] Nonspecific cellular toxicity and uncoupling of oxidative phosphorylation interfere with normal function of ion channels and other cellular functions, preventing normal physiological processes.

Uncoupling of oxidative phosphorylation may be caused by chemicals that disrupt mitochondrial function, and causes inefficiency in energy production. At a cellular level it describes an increase in oxygen consumption and heat production out of proportion to the generation of ATP due to mitochondrial dysfunction. Varying degrees of uncoupling of oxidative phosphorylation may occur. The initial physiological response to uncoupling is to increase mitochondrial respiration to maintain the supply of ATP, which increases heat production and respiratory rate. As ATP falls there is an increase in glycolysis, causing lactic acidosis and hypoglycemia. If the mitochondrial defect persists then there will be hyperthermia and insufficient ATP for essential cellular functions including active transport pumps such as Na^+,K^+-ATPase. This is followed by a loss of cellular ionic and volume regulation, which, if persistent, is irreversible and cell death occurs. Because mitochondria are the primary supplier of ATP for most physiological systems, uncoupling of oxidative phosphorylation is expected to induce multisystem toxicity.

CLINICAL MANIFESTATIONS

Vomiting, myotonia (confirmed on electromyography), and miosis are prominent features of 2,4-D poisoning in dogs. Severity varies in a dose-dependent manner, peaking 12 to 24 hours postingestion and persisting for a number of days.[6]

Gastrointestinal toxicity including nausea, vomiting, abdominal or throat pain, and diarrhea are common. Other clinical features include neuromuscular features (myalgia, rhabdomyolysis, weakness, myopathy, myotonia, and fasciculations), central nervous system features (agitation, sedation, confusion, miosis), tachycardia, hypotension, renal toxicity, hypocalcemia, and hypokalemia. In some patients, these effects persist for a number of days.

Tachypnea with respiratory alkalosis occurs in patients with phenoxy herbicide poisoning, some of who died, which may be consistent with increased mitochondrial respiration from mild uncoupling. More severe poisoning may be characterized by metabolic acidosis, hyperventilation, hyperkalemia, hyperthermia, elevated creatine kinase, generalized muscle rigidity, hypotension, pulseless electrical activity, or asystole.[12,24,89,103]

The mortality from acute phenoxy herbicide poisoning is potentially high. A systematic review of all acute phenoxy herbicide poisoning described severe clinical toxicity in most patients, including death in one-third of the cases.[12] Subsequently, a prospective study of MCPA exposures in Sri Lanka demonstrated minor toxicity in greater than

80% of patients and a mortality of 4.4% (eight of 181 patients).[103] When death occurs, it is usually delayed by 24 to 48 hours postingestion and results from cardiorespiratory arrest. The exact mechanism of death is inadequately described, but it may relate to uncoupling of oxidative phosphorylation or other metabolic dysfunction including renal toxicity, as discussed above.

DIAGNOSTIC TESTING

Commercial assays for the specific measurement of phenoxy herbicides are not available to assist in the diagnosis of acute poisoning. Further, their role in the management of acute poisoning is not confirmed because the relationship between serum phenoxy herbicide concentration and clinical toxicity is not adequately defined. Sedation is reported with a serum phenoxy concentration above 80 mg/L,[98] while concentrations more than 500 mg/L are associated with severe toxicity.[38] A patient survived severe MCPA poisoning (hypotension and limb myotonia) with a serum concentration of 546 mg/L. The myotonia persisted for a number of days and resolved when the MCPA serum concentration was less than 100 mg/L.[108] In contrast, death has been reported following MCPA poisoning at serum concentrations as low as 107 mg/L to 230 mg/L.[58,93,103]

Monitoring of electrolytes, renal function, pulse oximetry, and blood gases is recommended to detect progression of organ toxicity. Creatine kinase should also be determined since rhabdomyolysis may occur following acute poisoning. Urinalysis might be useful for identifying myoglobinuria. There are insufficient data describing the role of these measurements for prognostication.

MANAGEMENT

All significant poisonings, particularly symptomatic oral ingestions, should be treated cautiously, including continuous monitoring for 24 to 48 hours preferably in an intensive care unit. Initial mild toxicity (for example, gastrointestinal symptoms but normal vital signs and level of consciousness at presentation) does not preclude subsequent severe toxicity and death.[103]

Animal studies suggest that phenoxy herbicide toxicity increases when elimination is impaired. Empirically, this supports the use of treatments that decrease exposure either by decreasing absorption or increasing elimination. Unfortunately, there is insufficient evidence to recommend specific interventions in patients with acute phenoxy herbicide poisoning. However, an adequate urine output (greater than 1 mL/kg/h) may optimize the renal excretion of phenoxy herbicides as well as decreasing renal toxicity from rhabdomyolysis. Since signs consistent with uncoupling of oxidative phosphorylation are likely to be associated with a poor outcome, more advanced treatments such as hemodialysis can be considered in these patients.[12,103]

Resuscitation and Supportive Care All patients should receive routine resuscitation, close observation, and supportive care. It is reasonable to correct electrolyte abnormalities and acidosis given that this may promote the distribution of weak acids and increase the intracellular concentration.

Gastrointestinal Decontamination Gastrointestinal decontamination can be administered to patients per the guidelines listed above (see also Chap. 7). Delayed administration of activated charcoal to patients is reasonable given that absorption appears to be saturable, although clinical data supporting this are not available.

Extracorporeal Removal Because phenoxy compounds are small and water soluble, and subject to saturable protein binding with large exposures (increasing the free concentration), they are likely to be cleared by extracorporeal techniques. Extracorporeal elimination using resin hemoperfusion, hemodialysis, or plasmapheresis has been trialed in a few cases, with clearances approaching 75 mL/min. Hemodialysis should be considered in patients with severe toxicity if facilities are available.

Antidotes There are no specific antidotes for phenoxy herbicides, but sodium bicarbonate or other alkalinizing agents may have a role in management by altering the kinetics of phenoxy herbicides.

Data from animal studies and case reports suggest that urinary alkalinization increases the elimination of phenoxy herbicides. Increases in urinary pH increase clearance due to "ion trapping" of the phenoxy herbicide. For example, renal 2,4-D clearance was increased from 5.1 mL/min to 63 mL/min when urine pH increased from 5.0 to 8.0.[94] Compared with a total clearance of approximately 30 mL/min or less in volunteer studies,[62,106] this increase in renal clearance has the potential to be clinically significant. Prospective, randomized studies are required to confirm the efficacy of urinary alkalinization in humans.

Plasma alkalinization may also limit the distribution of phenoxy compounds from the central circulation by "ion trapping."

It is reasonable to consider plasma and urinary (urine pH greater than 7.5) alkalinization in patients who are symptomatic, particularly if there are features of uncoupling of oxidative phosphorylation or metabolic acidosis. Alkalinization is rarely associated with adverse effects when administered to patients with care and close observation (see Antidotes in Depth A5: Sodium Bicarbonate).

TRIAZINE COMPOUNDS, INCLUDING ATRAZINE

The 1,3,5-triazine or s-triazine compound (Fig. 115–9) is central to a large number of compounds, including herbicides, other pesticides (eg, cyromazine), resins (eg, melamine), explosives (RDX or C-4) and antiinfectives. Triazine herbicides are widely used, and in 2001 atrazine and simazine were among the 25 most used pesticides in the United States.[60] However, cases of acute poisoning are infrequent. Other herbicides included in this group are listed in Table 115–1. These selective herbicides may be used pre- or postemergence for weed control.

The safety of atrazine from an environmental health perspective is debated because of its persistence and propensity to spread across water systems and potential toxicity from chronic exposure. This led to restrictions on the use of triazine compounds recently in the European Union, but not elsewhere.

PHARMACOLOGY

Mechanism of toxicity is not fully determined, although it might relate to uncoupling of oxidative phosphorylation.[15] Atrazine is a direct arteriolar vasodilator.[18] Some metabolites of atrazine, particularly those remaining chlorinated, are thought to retain some biological activity.[4] Similarly, clinical features of prometryn poisoning resolved posthemodialysis despite persistence of the parent herbicide, suggesting that toxic metabolites were eliminated.[15]

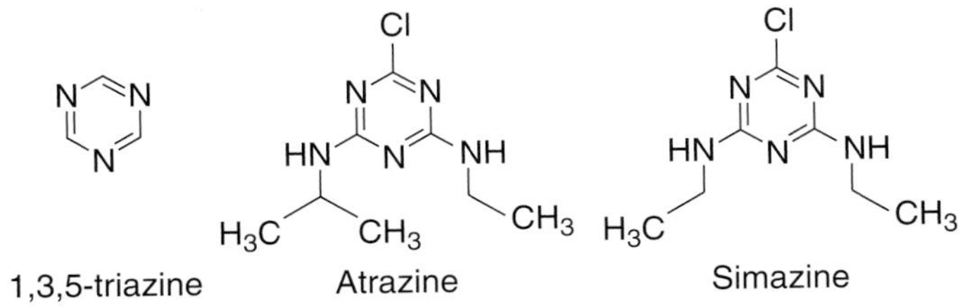

1,3,5-triazine Atrazine Simazine

FIGURE 115–9. Structure of common triazine herbicides.

PHARMACOKINETICS AND TOXICOKINETICS

Approximately 60% of an oral atrazine dose is absorbed in rats. The absorption phase of triazine compounds appears to be prolonged in humans where the serum concentration continues to increase during treatment with hemodialysis.[15,91] This is consistent with atrazine data in rats where the concentration peaks beyond 3 hours.[81] Atrazine is rapidly dealkylated to a metabolite that binds strongly to hemoglobin and serum proteins, allowing it to be detected in the blood for months. Metabolites are excreted in the urine and around 25% of them are conjugated to glutathione.[81]

The metabolism of atrazine has been studied in humans following occupational exposures, and animals, and a range of metabolites are described, in particular those derived from glutathione conjugation. Other metabolic products as a result of dealkylation and oxidation are also present.

Dermal absorption of atrazine is incomplete but increases with exposure to the proprietary formulation. Atrazine metabolites are readily measured in the urine of atrazine applicators.

CLINICAL MANIFESTATIONS

There are limited cases of triazine herbicide poisoning. Vomiting, depressed level of consciousness, tachycardia, hypertension, acute kidney injury, and lactic acidosis were described in a patient with acute prometryn and ethanol poisoning.[15] Similar clinical signs, in addition to hypotension with a low peripheral vascular resistance, were noted in a case of poisoning with atrazine, amitrole (see Table 115–1), and other toxic compounds. This was followed by progressive multiorgan dysfunction and death due to refractory shock 3 days later.[91]

DIAGNOSTIC TESTING

In a single case report, clinical toxicity did not directly relate to the concentration of prometryn, but the relationship to the concentration of metabolites has not been determined.[15] Routine biochemistry and arterial blood gases are useful for monitoring for the development of systemic toxicity.

MANAGEMENT

Few publications of triazine herbicide poisoning are available to guide management of patients with acute triazine poisoning.

Resuscitation and Supportive Care Routine resuscitation, close observation, and supportive care should be provided to all patients. Ventilatory support and correction of hypotension and metabolic disequilibria is reasonable.

Gastrointestinal Decontamination It is reasonable to administer activated charcoal to patients beyond 1 hour because of the slow absorption of these compounds.

Extracorporeal Removal Hemodialysis corrected metabolic acidosis in a case of prometryn poisoning without decreasing the serum concentration of prometryn, which might reflect ongoing absorption. In the absence of direct measurements of clearance, the efficacy of hemodialysis in removing prometryn cannot be determined but is probably limited.[15] Hemodialysis clearance of atrazine was 250 mL/min (extraction ratio 76%), but only 0.1% of the dose was removed after 4 hours of treatment. Further, similar to the previous case, atrazine concentrations continued to increase during the treatment.[91]

Antidotes No antidotes are available for the treatment of triazine herbicide poisoning.

SUMMARY

A large number of heterogeneous xenobiotics are classified as herbicides, and for many their toxicity in humans is incompletely described. Coformulants such as surfactants and solvents probably contribute to clinical toxicity in commercial preparations. Many herbicides induce multisystem toxicity for which treatments are often unsatisfactory, although some compounds induce organ-specific toxicity. All patients with acute intentional poisoning should be carefully observed for the development of poisoning. The priorities of treatment include a prompt resuscitation, a detailed history, ongoing monitoring, and supportive care. More research is required to better define the clinical syndromes associated with herbicide poisoning, the toxicokinetics of relevant compounds, and the efficacy of treatments including antidotes.

ACKNOWLEDGMENT

Rebecca L. Tominack and Susan M. Pond contributed to this chapter in previous editions.

REFERENCES

1. Arnold EK, Beasley VR. The pharmacokinetics of chlorinated phenoxy acid herbicides: a literature review. *Vet Hum Toxicol.* 1989;31:121-125.
2. Aromataris EC, Astill DS, Rychkov GY, et al. Modulation of the gating of ClC-1 by S-(-) 2-(4-chlorophenoxy) propionic acid. *Br J Pharmacol.* 1999;126:1375-1382.
3. Ashrafdeen M, Shukry M, Dawson A, et al. Acute intentional self-poisoning with a selective herbicide bispyribac sodium (BPS): a prospective observational study. Thailand: *Proceedings of the 6th Annual Congress of the Asia Pacific Association of Medical Toxicology*; 2007:131.
4. Barr DB, Panuwet P, Nguyen JV, et al. Assessing exposure to atrazine and its metabolites using biomonitoring. *Environ Health Perspect.* 2007;115:1474-1478.
5. Baud FJ, Houze P, Bismuth C, et al. Toxicokinetics of paraquat through the heart-lung block. Six cases of acute human poisoning. *J Toxicol Clin Toxicol.* 1988;26:35-50.
6. Beasley VR, Arnold EK, Lovell RA, et al. 2,4-D toxicosis. I: a pilot study of 2,4-dichlorophenoxyacetic acid- and dicamba-induced myotonia in experimental dogs. *Vet Hum Toxicol.* 1991;33:435-440.
7. Berry DJ, Grove J. The determination of paraquat (I,I′-dimethyl-4,4′-bipyridylium cation) in urine. *Clin Chim Acta.* 1971;34:5-11.
8. Berry DJ, Woollen BH, Wilks MF. Adsorptive properties of activated charcoal and Fuller's Earth used for treatment of paraquat ingestion. Thailand: *Proceedings of the 6th Annual Congress of the Asia Pacific Association of Medical Toxicology*; 2007:130.
9. Bismuth C, Garnier R, Baud FJ, et al. Paraquat poisoning. An overview of the current status. *Drug Saf.* 1990;5:243-251.
10. Bismuth C, Scherrmann JM, Garnier R, et al. Elimination of paraquat. *Hum Toxicol.* 1987;6:63-67.
11. Bradberry SM, Proudfoot AT, Vale JA. Glyphosate poisoning. *Toxicol Rev.* 2004;23:159-167.
12. Bradberry SM, Proudfoot AT, Vale JA. Poisoning due to chlorophenoxy herbicides. *Toxicol Rev.* 2004;23:65-73.
13. Brewster DW, Warren J, Hopkins WE. Metabolism of glyphosate in Sprague-Dawley rats: tissue distribution, identification, and quantitation of glyphosate-derived materials following a single oral dose. *Fundam Appl Toxicol.* 1991;17:43-51.
14. Brody TM. Effect of certain plant growth substances on oxidative phosphorylation in rat liver mitochondria. *Proc Soc Exp Biol Med.* 1952;80:533-536.
15. Brvar M, Okrajsek R, Kosmina P, et al. Metabolic acidosis in prometryn (triazine herbicide) self-poisoning. *Clin Toxicol (Phila).* 2008;46:270-273.
16. Buckley NA. Pulse corticosteroids and cyclophosphamide in paraquat poisoning. *Am J Respir Crit Care Med.* 2001;163:585.

17. Chan BSH, Lazzaro VA, Seale JP, et al. The renal excretory mechanisms and the role of organic cations in modulating the renal handling of paraquat. *Pharmacol Ther.* 1998;79:193-203.
18. Chan YC, Chang SC, Hsuan SL, et al. Cardiovascular effects of herbicides and formulated adjuvants on isolated rat aorta and heart. *Toxicol In Vitro.* 2007;21:595-603.
19. Chang C-Y, Peng Y-C, Hung D-Z, et al. Clinical impact of upper gastrointestinal tract injuries in glyphosate-surfactant oral intoxication. *Hum Exp Toxicol.* 1999;18:475-478.
20. Coleman S, Linderman R, Hodgson E, et al. Comparative metabolism of chloroacetamide herbicides and selected metabolites in human and rat liver microsomes. *Environ Health Perspect.* 2000;108:1151-1157.
21. Conning DM, Fletcher K, Swan AA. Paraquat and related bipyridyls. *Br Med Bull.* 1969;25:245-249.
22. De Silva WA, Bodinayake CK. Propanil poisoning. *Ceylon Med J.* 1997;42:81-84.
23. Denicola A, Radi R. Peroxynitrite and drug-dependent toxicity. *Toxicology.* 2005;208:273-288.
24. Dickey W, McAleer JJA, Callender ME. Delayed sudden death after ingestion of MCPP and ioxynil: an unusual presentation of hormonal weedkiller intoxication. *Postgrad Med J.* 1988;64:681-682.
25. Dinis-Oliveira RJ, de Pinho PG, Ferreira ACS, et al. Reactivity of paraquat with sodium salicylate: formation of stable complexes. *Toxicology.* 2008;249:130-139.
26. Dinis-Oliveira RJ, Duarte JA, Remiao F, et al. Single high dose dexamethasone treatment decreases the pathological score and increases the survival rate of paraquat-intoxicated rats. *Toxicology.* 2006;227:73-85.
27. Dinis-Oliveira RJ, Duarte JA, Sánchez-Navarro A, et al. Paraquat poisonings: mechanisms of lung toxicity, clinical features, and treatment. *Crit Rev Toxicol.* 2008;38:13-71.
28. Dinis-Oliveira RJ, Pontes H, Bastos ML, et al. An effective antidote for paraquat poisonings: the treatment with lysine acetylsalicylate. *Toxicology.* 2009;255:187-193.
29. Dinis-Oliveira RJ, Sousa C, Remião F, et al. Full survival of paraquat-exposed rats after treatment with sodium salicylate. *Free Radic Biol Med.* 2007;42:1017-1028.
30. Ebert E, Leist KH, Mayer D. Summary of safety evaluation toxicity studies of glufosinate ammonium. *Food Chem Toxicol.* 1990;28:339-349.
31. Eddleston M, Dawson AH, Buckley NA. Human toxicity of pesticides in self-poisoning. *Clin Toxicol.* 2006;44:415.
32. Eddleston M, Juszczak E, Buckley NA, et al. Multiple-dose activated charcoal in acute self-poisoning: a randomised controlled trial. *Lancet.* 2008;371:579-587.
33. Eddleston M, Wilks MF, Buckley NA. Prospects for treatment of paraquat-induced lung fibrosis with immunosuppressive drugs and the need for better prediction of outcome: a systematic review. *QJM.* 2003;96:809-824.
34. Elo H. Distribution and elimination of 2-methyl-4-chlorophenoxyacetic acid (MCPA) in male rats. *Acta Pharmacol Toxicol (Copenh).* 1976;39:58-64.
35. Elo HA, Ylitalo P. Distribution of 2-methyl-4-chlorophenoxyacetic acid and 2,4-dichlorophenoxyacetic acid in male rats: evidence for the involvement of the central nervous system in their toxicity. *Toxicol Appl Pharmacol.* 1979;51:439-446.
36. Fagg GE, Lanthorn TH. Cl-/Ca2+-dependent L-glutamate binding sites do not correspond to 2-amino-4-phosphonobutanoate-sensitive excitatory amino acid receptors. *Br J Pharmacol.* 1985;86:743-751.
37. FAO/WHO. *Pesticide residues in food—evaluations 1999. Part II—toxicological.* Geneva: WHO/PCS; 2000.
38. Flanagan RJ, Meredith TJ, Ruprah M et al. Alkaline diuresis for acute poisoning with chlorophenoxy herbicides and ioxynil. Lancet 1990;335:454-458.
39. Goldstein DA, Farmer DL, Levine SL, et al. Mechanism of toxicity of commercial glyphosate formulations: how important is the surfactant? *Clin Toxicol.* 2005;43:423-424.
40. Grisolia CK, Bilich MR, Formigli LM. A comparative toxicologic and genotoxic study of the herbicide arsenal, its active ingredient imazapyr, and the surfactant nonylphenol ethoxylate. *Ecotoxicol Environ Saf.* 2004;59:123-126.
41. Gunawardena G, Roberts DM, Buckley NA. Randomized control trial of immunosuppression in paraquat poisoning. *Crit Care Med.* 2007;35:330-331.
42. Hack R, Ebert E, Ehling G, et al. Glufosinate ammonium—some aspects of its mode of action in mammals. *Food Chem Toxicol.* 1994;32:461-470.
43. Hampson EC, Pond SM. Failure of haemoperfusion and haemodialysis to prevent death in paraquat poisoning. A retrospective review of 42 patients. *Med Toxicol Adverse Drug Exp.* 1988;3:64-71.
43a. Hart TB, Nevitt A, Whitehead A. A new statistical approach to the prognostic significance of serum paraquat concentrations. *Lancet.* 1984;2(8413):1222-1223).
44. Heylings JR, Farnworth MJ, Swain CM, et al. Identification of an alginate-based formulation of paraquat to reduce the exposure of the herbicide following oral ingestion. *Toxicology.* 2007;241:1-10.
45. Hirose Y, Kobayashi M, Koyama K, et al. A toxicokinetic analysis in a patient with acute glufosinate poisoning. *Hum Exp Toxicol.* 1999;18:305-308.
46. Hong SY, Yang JO, Lee EY, et al. Effect of haemoperfusion on plasma paraquat concentration in vitro and in vivo. *Toxicol Ind Health.* 2003;19:17-23.
47. Hori Y, Fujisawa M, Shimada K, et al. Determination of glufosinate ammonium and its metabolite, 3-methylphosphinicopropionic acid, in human serum by gas chromatography-mass spectrometry following mixed-mode solid-phase extraction and t-BDMS derivatization. *J Anal Toxicol.* 2001;25:680-684.
48. Hori Y, Fujisawa M, Shimada K, et al. Determination of the herbicide glyphosate and its metabolite in biological specimens by gas chromatography-mass spectrometry. A case of poisoning by Roundup(r) herbicide. *J Anal Toxicol.* 2003;27:162-166.
49. Hori Y, Fujisawa M, Shimada K, et al. Enantioselective analysis of glufosinate using precolumn derivatization with (+)-1-(9-fluorenyl)ethyl chloroformate and reversed-phase liquid chromatography. *J Chromatogr B Analyt Technol Biomed Life Sci.* 2002;776:191-198.
50. Hori Y, Nakajima M, Fujisawa M, et al. [Simultaneous determination of propanil, carbaryl and 3,4-dichloroaniline in human serum by HPLC with UV detector following solid phase extraction]. *Yakugaku Zasshi.* 2002;122:247-251.
51. Hori Y, Tanaka T, Fujisawa M, et al. Toxicokinetics of DL-glufosinate enantiomer in human BASTA poisoning. *Biol Pharm Bull.* 2003;26:540-543.
52. Houze P, Baud FJ, Mouy R, et al. Toxicokinetics of paraquat in humans. *Hum Exp Toxicol.* 1990;9:5-12.
53. Howe CM, Berrill M, Pauli BD, et al. Toxicity of glyphosate-based pesticides to four North American frog species. *Environ Toxicol Chem.* 2004;23:1928-1938.
54. Hung D-Z, Deng J-F, Wu T-C. Laryngeal survey in glyphosate intoxication: a pathophysiological investigation. *Hum Exp Toxicol.* 1997;16:596-599.
55. Hunt K, Thomas SHL. Renal impairment following low dose intravenous and oral diquat administration. *Clin Toxicol.* 2006;44:572-573.
56. IPCS. *The WHO recommended classification of pesticides by hazard and guidelines to classification 2000-2002.* World Health Organization; 2002.
57. Ishizaki T, Privitera PJ, Walle T, et al. Cardiovascular actions of a new metabolite of propranolol: isopropylamine. *J Pharmacol Exp Ther.* 1974;189:626-632.
58. Johnson HR, Koumides O. A further case of MCPA poisoning. *Br Med J.* 1965;629-630.
58a. Jones AL, Elton R, Flanagan R. Multiple logistic regression analysis of plasma paraquat concentrations as a predictor of outcome in 375 cases of paraquat poisoning. *QJM Mon J Assoc Physicians.* 1999;92(10):573-578.
59. Kamholz S, Veith FJ, Mollenkopf F, et al. Single lung transplantation in paraquat intoxication. *N Y State J Med.* 1984;84:82-84.
60. Kiely T, Donaldson D, Grube A. Pesticides industry sales and usage—2000 and 2001 market estimates. Washington, DC: US Environmental Protection Agency; 2004.
61. Kim SJ, Gil HW, Yang JO, et al. The clinical features of acute kidney injury in patients with acute paraquat intoxication. *Nephrol Dial Transplant.* 2009;24:1226-1232.
62. Kohli JD, Khanna RN, Gupta BN, et al. Absorption and excretion of 2,4,5-trichlorophenoxy acetic acid in man. *Arch Int Pharmacodyn Ther.* 1974;210:250-255.
63. Koo J-R, Kim J-C, Yoon J-W, et al. Failure of continuous venovenous hemofiltration to prevent death in paraquat poisoning. *Am J Kidney Dis.* 2002;39:55-59.

64. Koyama K, Kohda Y, Hisashi H, et al. Toxicokinetics of glufosinate, an herbicide structurally analogous to glutamic acid, that causes severe CNS disorders in human acute oral poisoning. *Toxicol Lett.* 1998;95:140.
65. Koyama K, Koyama Ky, Goto K. Cardiovascular effects of a herbicide containing glufosinate and an anionic surfactant: in vitro and in vivo analyses in rats. *Toxicol Appl Pharmacol.* 1997;145:409-414.
66. Lappin GJ, Hardwick TD, Stow R, et al. Absorption, metabolism and excretion of 4-chloro-2-methylphenoxyacetic acid (MCPA) in rat and dog. *Xenobiotica.* 2002;32:153-163.
67. Lee CH, Shih CP, Hsu KH, et al. The early prognostic factors of glyphosate-surfactant intoxication. *Am J Emerg Med.* 2008;26:275-281.
68. Lee H-L, Chen K-W, Chi C-H, et al. Clinical presentations and prognostic factors of a glyphosate-surfactant herbicide intoxication: a review of 131 cases. *Acad Emerg Med.* 2000;7:906-910.
69. Liantonio A, Accardi A, Carbonara G, et al. Molecular requisites for drug binding to muscle CLC-1 and renal CLC-K channel revealed by the use of phenoxy-alkyl derivatives of 2-(p-chlorophenoxy)propionic acid. *Mol Pharmacol.* 2002;62:265-271.
70. Liantonio A, De Luca A, Pierno S, et al. Structural requisites of 2-(p-chlorophenoxy)propionic acid analogues for activity on native rat skeletal muscle chloride conductance and on heterologously expressed CLC-1. *Br J Pharmacol.* 2003;139:1255-1264.
71. Lin C-M, Lai C-P, Fang T-C, et al. Cardiogenic shock in a patient with glyphosate-surfactant poisoning. *J Formos Med Assoc.* 1999;98:698-700.
72. Lin JL, Lin-Tan DT, Chen KH, et al. Repeated pulse of methylprednisolone and cyclophosphamide with continuous dexamethasone therapy for patients with severe paraquat poisoning. *Crit Care Med.* 2006;34:368-373.
73. Little M, Murray L. Consensus statement: risk of nosocomial organophosphate poisoning in emergency departments. *Emerg Med Australas.* 2004;16:456-458.
74. Lluis M, Nogue S, Miro O. Severe acute poisoning due to a glufosinate-containing preparation without mitochondrial involvement. *Hum Exp Toxicol.* 2008;27:519-524.
75. Lo YC, Yang CC, Deng JF. Acute alachlor and butachlor herbicide poisoning. *Clin Toxicol (Phila).* 2008;46:716-721.
76. Manuweera G, Eddleston M, Egodage S, et al. Do targeted bans of insecticides to prevent deaths from self-poisoning result in reduced agricultural output? *Environ Health Perspect.* 2008;116:492-495.
77. Matsumura N, Takeuchi C, Hishikawa K, et al. Glufosinate ammonium induces convulsion through N-methyl-D-aspartate receptors in mice. *Neurosci Lett.* 2001;304:123-125.
78. McMillan DC, Bradshaw TP, Hinson JA, et al. Role of metabolites in propanil-induced hemolytic anemia. *Toxicol Appl Pharmacol.* 1991;110:70-78.
79. McMillan DC, Freeman JP, Hinson JA. Metabolism of the arylamide herbicide propanil. I. Microsomal metabolism and in vitro methemoglobinemia. *Toxicol Appl Pharmacol.* 1990;103:90-101.
80. McMillan DC, McRae TA, Hinson JA. Propanil-induced methemoglobinemia and hemoglobin binding in the rat. *Toxicol Appl Pharmacol.* 1990;105:503-507.
81. McMullin TS, Brzezicki JM, Cranmer BK, et al. Pharmacokinetic modeling of disposition and time-course studies with [^{14}C]atrazine. *J Toxicol Environ Health A.* 2003;66:941-964.
82. Mortensen OS, SΦrensen FW, Gregersen M, et al. Forgiftninger med ukrudtsbekæmpelsesmidlerne glyphosat og glyphosat-trimesium. *Ugeskr Laeger.* 2000;162:4656-4659.
83. Mose T, Kjaerstad MB, Mathiesen L, et al. Placental passage of benzoic acid, caffeine, and glyphosate in an ex vivo human perfusion system. *J Toxicol Environ Health A.* 2008;71:984-991.
84. Murray RE, Gibson JE. A comparative study of paraquat intoxication in rats, guinea pigs and monkeys. *Exp Mol Pathol.* 1972;17:317-325.
85. Murray RE, Gibson JE. Paraquat disposition in rats, guinea pigs and monkeys. *Toxicol Appl Pharmacol.* 1974;27:283-291.
86. Nakaki T, Mishima A, Suzuki E, et al. Glufosinate ammonium stimulates nitric oxide production through N-methyl D-aspartate receptors in rat cerebellum. *Neurosci Lett.* 2000;290:209-212.
87. Ohashi N, Ishizawa J, Tsujikawa A. [DCPA [propanil] and NAC [carbaryl] herbicide poisoning]. *Jpn J Toxicol.* 1996;9:437-440.
88. Olorunsogo OO. Modification of the transport of protons and Ca2+ ions across mitochondrial coupling membrane by N-(phosphonomethyl) glycine. *Toxicology.* 1990;61:205-209.
89. O'Reilly JF. Prolonged coma anddelayed peripheral neuropathy after ingestion of phenoxyacetic acid weedkillers. *Postgrad Med J.* 1984;60:76-77.
90. Peixoto F. Comparative effects of the Roundup and glyphosate on mitochondrial oxidative phosphorylation. *Chemosphere.* 2005;61:1115-1122.
91. Pommery J, Mathieu M, Mathieu D, et al. Atrazine in plasma and tissue following atrazine-aminotriazole-ethylene glycol-formaldehyde poisoning. *J Toxicol Clin Toxicol.* 1993;31:323-331.
92. Pond SM, Rivory LP, Hampson EC, et al. Kinetics of toxic doses of paraquat and the effects of hemoperfusion in the dog. *J Toxicol Clin Toxicol.* 1993;31:229-246.
93. Popham RD, Davies DM. A case of MCPA poisoning. *BMJ.* 1964;1:677-678.
94. Prescott LF, Park J, Darrien I. Treatment of severe 2,4-D and mecoprop intoxication with alkaline diuresis. *Br J Clin Pharmacol.* 1979;7:111-116.
95. Price LA, Newman KJ, Clague AE, et al. Paraquat and diquat interference in the analysis of creatinine by the Jaffe reaction. *Pathology.* 1995;27:154-156.
96. Privitera PJ, Walle T, Gaffney TE. Nicotinic-like effects and tissue disposition of isopropylamine. *J Pharmacol Exp Ther.* 1982;222:116-121.
96a. Proudfoot AT, Stewart MS, Levitt T, Widdop B. Paraquat poisoning: significance of serum-paraquat concentrations. *Lancet.* 1979;2(8138):330-332.
97. Ragoucy-Sengler C, Pileire B. A biological index to predict patient outcome in paraquat poisoning. *Hum Exp Toxicol.* 1996;15:265-268.
98. Reingart JR, Roberts JR. Chlorophenoxy herbicides. In: *Recognition and Management of Pesticide Poisonings*, 5th ed. Washington: United States Environmental Protection Agency; 1999:94-98.
99. Roberts DM, Buckley NA. Acute intentional self-poisoning with glyphosate-containing herbicides. *Clin Toxicol.* 2006;44:414.
100. Roberts DM, Buckley NA. Changes in the concentrations of creatinine and cystatin C in patients with acute paraquat self-poisoning. Chandigarh, India: *Proceedings of the 7th Annual Scientific Meeting of the Asia Pacific Association of Medical Toxicology*; 2008.
101. Roberts DM, Heilmair R, Buckley NA, et al. Clinical outcomes and kinetics of propanil following acute self-poisoning: a prospective case series. *BMC Clin Pharmacol.* 2009;9:3.
102. Roberts DM, Karunarathna A, Buckley NA, et al. Influence of pesticide regulation on acute poisoning deaths in Sri Lanka. *Bull World Health Organ.* 2003;81:789-798.
103. Roberts DM, Seneviratne R, Mohammed F, et al. Intentional self-poisoning with the chlorophenoxy herbicide 4-chloro-2-methylphenoxyacetic acid (MCPA). *Ann Emerg Med.* 2005;46:275-284.
104. Rose MS, Smith LL, Wyatt I. Evidence for energy-dependent accumulation of paraquat into rat lung. *Nature.* 1974;252:314-315.
105. Salazar A, Vohra R, Cantrell FL, et al. Colorimetric detection of urinary diquat: in vitro demonstration. *Clin Toxicol.* 2007;45:381-382.
106. Sauerhoff MW, Braun WH, Blau GE, et al. The dose-dependent pharmacokinetic profile of 2,4,5-trichlorophenoxy acetic acid following intravenous administration to rats. *Toxicol Appl Pharmacol.* 1976;36:491-501.
107. Sawada Y, Nagai Y, Ueyama M, et al. Probable toxicity of surface-active agent in commercial herbicide containing glyphosate. *Lancet.* 1988;1:299.
107a. Scherrmann JM, Houze P, Bismuth C, Bourdon R. Prognostic value of serum and urine paraquat concentration. *Hum Toxicol.* 1987;6(1):91-93.
108. Schmoldt A, Iwersen S, Schlüter W. Massive ingestion of the herbicide 2-methyl-4-chlorophenoxyacetic acid (MCPA). *J Toxicol Clin Toxicol.* 1997;35:405-408.
109. Sharp CW, Ottolenghi A, Posner HS. Correlation of paraquat toxicity with tissue concentrations and weight loss of the rat. *Toxicol Appl Pharmacol.* 1972;22:241-251.
110. Shim YS, Gil HW, Yang JO, et al. A case of green urine after ingestion of herbicides. *Korean J Intern Med.* 2008;23:42-44.
111. Shukry M, Ashrafdeen M, Palasinghe C, et al. Acute intentional self-poisoning with a selective herbicide fenoxaprop-P-ethyl (FPPE): a prospective observational study. Thailand: *Proceedings of the 6th Annual Congress of the Asia Pacific Association of Medical Toxicology*; 2007:131.
112. Singleton SD, Murphy SD. Propanil (3,4-dichloropropionanilide)-induced methemoglobin formation in mice in relation to acylamidase activity. *Toxicol Appl Pharmacol.* 1973;25:20-29.
113. SΦrensen FW, Gregersen M. Rapid lethal intoxication caused by the herbicide glyphosate-trimesium (Touchdown). *Hum Exp Toxicol.* 1999;18:735-737.
114. Stephens DS, Walker DH, Schaffner W, et al. Pseudodiphtheria: prominent pharyngeal membrane associated with fatal paraquat ingestion. *Ann Intern Med.* 1981;94:202-204.

115. Suntres ZE. Role of antioxidants in paraquat toxicity. *Toxicology.* 2002;180:65-77.
116. Takahashi H, Toya T, Matsumiya N, et al. A case of transient diabetes insipidus associated with poisoning by a herbicide containing glufosinate. *J Toxicol Clin Toxicol.* 2000;38:153-156.
117. Talbot AR, Shiaw MH, Huang JS, et al. Acute poisoning with a glyphosate-surfactant herbicide ('Roundup'): a review of 93 cases. *Hum Exp Toxicol.* 1991;10:1-8.
118. Tanaka J, Matsuo H, Yamamoto T. Two cases of glufosinate poisoning with late onset convulsions. *Vet Hum Toxicol.* 1998;40:219-222.
119. Tanaka J, Yamashita M, Yamamoto T. A comparative study of direct hemoperfusion and hemodialysis for the removal of glufosinate ammonium. *J Toxicol Clin Toxicol.* 1995;33:691-694.
120. Tominack RL, Yang GY, Tsai WJ, et al. Taiwan National Poison Center survey of glyphosate—surfactant herbicide ingestions. *J Toxicol Clin Toxicol.* 1991;29:91-109.
121. van Ravenzwaay B, Pigott G, Leibold E. Absorption, distribution, metabolism and excretion of 4-chloro-2-methylphenoxyacetic acid (MCPA) in rats. *Food Chem Toxicol.* 2004;42:115-125.
122. Watanabe T, Sano T. Neurological effects of glufosinate poisoning with a brief review. *Hum Exp Toxicol.* 1998;17:35-39.
123. Wester RC, Melendres J, Sarason R, et al. Glyphosate skin binding, absorption, residual tissue distribution, and skin decontamination. *Fundam Appl Toxicol.* 1991;16:725-732.
124. Wilks MF, Fernando R, Ariyananda PL, et al. Improvement in survival after paraquat ingestion following introduction of a new formulation in Sri Lanka. *PLoS Med.* 2008;5:250-259.
125. Wilks MF, Tomenson JA, Buckley NA, et al. Influence of gastric decontamination on patient outcome after paraquat ingestion. *J Med Toxicol.* 2008;4:212-213.
126. Williams GM, Kroes R, Munro IC. Safety evaluation and risk assessment of the herbicide Roundup and its active ingredient, glyphosate, for humans. *Regul Toxicol Pharmacol.* 2000;31:117-165.
127. Yamashita M, Hukuda T. [The pitfall of the general treatment in acute poisoning]. *Kyukyu Igaku.* 1985;9:65-71.
128. Yamazaki M, Terada M, Kuroki H, et al. Pesticide poisoning initially suspected as a natural death. *J Forensic Sci.* 2001;46:165-170.
129. Yoshioka T, Sugimoto T, Kinoshita N, et al. Effects of concentration reduction and partial replacement of paraquat by diquat on human toxicity: a clinical survey. *Hum Exp Toxicol.* 1992;11:241-245.
130. Zychlinski L, Zolnierowicz S. Comparison of uncoupling activities of chlorophenoxyherbicides in rat liver mitochondria. *Toxicol Lett.* 1990;52:25-34.

CHAPTER 116
METHYL BROMIDE AND OTHER FUMIGANTS

Keith K. Burkhart

Fumigants are applied to control rodents, nematodes, insects, weed seeds, and fungi anywhere in soil, or on structures, crops, grains, and commodities.[20] Although many different chemical classes were used as fumigants, only a few remain in use today in the United States. Many fumigants, especially halogenated solvents, were abandoned because of their toxicity. In the 1987 Montreal Protocol an international agreement was adapted to phase out ozone-depleting chemicals such as methyl bromide, which was scheduled to be discontinued in 2005. Unfortunately many agricultural companies received exemptions, as satisfactory substitutes for some of its uses have not emerged.

Although fumigants exist as solids, liquids, or gases, they are most commonly used in the gaseous form or as volatile liquids, explaining why inhalation is the most common route of exposure (Table 116–1). Because of their gaseous forms, fumigants are generally heavier than air. Therefore, they will stay concentrated above the ground surface and lower floors of buildings. In addition, many do not have good warning properties. Several, such as methyl bromide and sulfuryl fluoride, are colorless and the toxic concentrations are below the odor threshold, making them particularly dangerous. While phosphides have a "rotten fish" or garliclike odor, toxic exposures are often debilitating, not allowing for escape.

METHYL BROMIDE

HISTORY AND EPIDEMIOLOGY

Methyl bromide (CH_3Br) was used as an anesthetic in the early 1900s, but fatalities halted this practice. It was used as a fire retardant during World War II, a role that persisted into the 1960s in Europe. Like many other halogenated hydrocarbons, methyl bromide was also used as a refrigerant, methylating agent, chemical precursor, and as a fumigant in fruit packaging. Industrial use and its naturally occurring environmental production in oceans have led to low concentrations of methyl bromide in ambient air, water, and food.[27] Diets that are high in marine products and fruits may increase environmental exposure to methyl bromide.[27]

Occupational and environmental exposures to methyl bromide as a fumigant are most common. Hazardous materials incidents are reported for methyl bromide, both during use and transport,[9,39] but they are relatively uncommon in residents and plant employees, living or working adjacent to agricultural fields where methyl bromide is applied.[8,9,20,39] Methyl bromide and other fumigants can also escape from fumigated structures into adjoining rooms, and adjacent or conjoined buildings, resulting in severe illness and fatalities.[33,50] For example, pipes adjoining sections of a greenhouse have led to exposures.[24] Fatalities have occurred when workers entered tanks containing fumigant residues.[30] Workers who repeatedly transfer methyl bromide between containers have developed severe neuropsychiatric sequelae. Defective or leaking canisters of methyl bromide are another source of exposure. In Europe, indoor and outdoor exposures to the contents of old fire extinguishers have caused severe poisoning and fatalities. Most symptoms reported by unintentionally exposed individuals are related to chloropicrin, which is usually formulated as 2% of the methyl bromide concentration. The overlap of the irritant and nonspecific symptoms of methyl bromide and chloropicrin make it difficult to absolutely differentiate between the two at the time of the exposure.[20] Rarely, fumigants are inhaled or ingested with suicidal intent.

OCCUPATIONAL EXPOSURE

Methyl bromide fumigation may expose workers to high concentrations at many steps in the process.[49] The Occupational Safety and Health Administration (OSHA) permissible exposure limit (PEL) is 20 parts per million (ppm). The American Conference of Governmental Industrial Hygienists (ACGIH) has recommended an 8-hour TWA (time-weighted average) of 3.9 mg/m^3 for methyl bromide; 1 mg/m^3 is 3.88 ppm.

Work clothes concentrations of 50 ppm have been recorded. Depending on ventilation conditions, concentrations up to 55 ppm occurred when the plastic sheets were removed 7 days after a soil application. Dermal and ocular exposures may occur during application secondary to employee error or equipment failure.[9] Leather and rubber gloves enhance skin contact with methyl bromide, and tight-fitting clothing may trap gas close to the skin.[9] Because of these properties, leather and rubber should be avoided for all applications, and work clothes should be changed after the application.

Methyl bromide is listed in the International Agency for Research on Cancers (IARC) as Group 3, or not classifiable as to its carcinogenicity in humans secondary to inadequate animal and human evidence.

TOXICOKINETICS

Methyl bromide is rapidly absorbed by oral, inhalational, and dermal routes. Life-threatening toxicity has been reported within the first hour of exposure. After absorption, bioactivation by oxidative metabolism by the cytochrome P450 enzymes occurs. These reactive metabolites can form protein adducts with albumin and hemoglobin.

There is significant individual variability for cytochrome P450 oxidative metabolism and patients exposed to methyl bromide demonstrate this variability. Three of seven methyl bromide workers had high hemoglobin adduct concentrations despite performing the same job as the other four.[46] S-methylcysteine albumin and hemoglobin adducts may persist for weeks.[7] Cysteine residues, at number 104 of the α chain and 93 of the β chain, appear to be preferentially methylated,[19] although it is unknown what role methylation plays in the toxic manifestations that follow methyl bromide metabolism.

PATHOLOGY/PATHOPHYSIOLOGY

Energy deprivation secondary to methylation of the sulfhydryl groups of metabolic enzymes is proposed as a common mechanistic pathway.[46] Pathologic examinations demonstrate the neurotoxicity of methyl bromide. Symmetric neuronal loss and gliosis have been described in both the central and peripheral nervous systems. The associated neurologic deficits have sometimes been irreversible. The cerebral lesions are reportedly similar to thiamine deficiency and Wernicke encephalopathy.

CLINICAL MANIFESTATIONS

Exposure to methyl bromide may lead to immediate life-threatening toxicity including a rapid loss of consciousness followed by seizures, dysrhythmias, and death. In contrast, symptoms may be delayed for days following low-level exposure. Cardiac, pulmonary, hepatic, neurologic, and renal toxicity may also develop following toxicity from methyl bromide exposure (Table 116–2). Some individuals may initially manifest irritant symptoms of the eye, nasopharynx, and oropharynx. These irritant symptoms may help differentiate upper

TABLE 116–1. Physical Properties and Industrial Use of Fumigants

	Chloropicrin	Dichloropropene	Ethylene Dibromide[a]	Metam Sodium	Methyl Bromide	Phosphine	Sulfuryl Fluoride	Methyl Iodide
MW (daltons)	164	111	188	129	95	34	102	142
Color	Colorless yellow-green	Yellow	Colorless	White	Colorless	Colorless	Colorless	Colorless
State	Liquid	Liquid	Liquid	Powder turns yellow-green liquid	Gas	Solid→gas	Gas	Liquid
Flammable	No	No	Low	No	No	High	No	No
Odor	Intense	Garlic	Sweet/chloroform	Sulfur	None	Rotten fish, garlic	None	Pungent
Use	Soil[b]	Soil	Soil, crop[b]	Soil	Soil, structural, crop[b]	Rodenticide[b]	Structural	Soil
Historical use			Fire extinguisher		Fire extinguisher			

[a] Ethylene dibromide has been banned and is no longer in use, but it is included for historical reference.

[b] Commodity fumigant, which is a class term used by the Environmental Protection Agency to refer to fumigation of a food or agricultural product.

respiratory and gastrointestinal viral syndromes from methyl bromide exposure. In some cases, the initial symptoms of methyl bromide poisoning are misdiagnosed as influenza or a viral like illness such as gastroenteritis.[33] In more severe poisonings pulmonary symptoms begin with cough or shortness of breath that may rapidly progress to bronchitis, pneumonitis, acute lung injury (ALI), and hemorrhage.

The neurologic effects of methyl bromide poisoning are the most consequential and may occur without antecedent irritant effects. Initial central nervous system signs and symptoms that may manifest in the first few hours after exposure include headache, vomiting, dizziness, drowsiness, euphoria, confusion, diplopia, dysmetria, dysarthria, and mood disorders or inappropriate affect. Those that may progress rapidly in the first day or manifest over the next few days include ataxia, psychotic delirium, intention tremor, fasciculations, myoclonus, seizures, and coma.

Many patients develop skin lesions such as erythema, vesicles, and bullae predominantly in moist areas or pressure points, including the

TABLE 116–2. Comparison of Clinical Effects of Fumigants

Clinical Effect	Chloropicrin	Dichloropropene	Ethylene Dibromide	Metam Sodium	Methyl Bromide	Phosphine	Sulfuryl Fluoride
Mucus membrane irritation	+ +	+	+ +	+ +	± High concentration	+ +	± High concentration
Dermatitis	–	+	+	+	+	–	+
Burns (frostbite)	+	–	–	+	+	–	+
Gastrointestinal:							
Nausea, vomiting, abdominal pain	+	+	+	+	+	+	+
Hepatic dysfunction	+	+	+ +	–	+	+	–
Chest pain	+	+	+	–		+	–
Acute lung injury		+	+	–	+	+	+
Cardiovascular:							
Hypotension	+	+	+	–	+	+	+
Dysrhythmias		+	Late	–	+	+ +	+ +
Nephrotoxicity	+	+	+ +	–	+	+	–
Mental status changes	+	+	+	+	+	+	+

+ = presence; – = absence; ± = variable; + + = very substantial.

groin, axilla, and wrist.[52] In one report, erythema and multiple vesicles developed on all four limbs of a fumigator who used protective respiratory gear.[31] This patient's skin lesions healed after 5 weeks, but he had a persistent peripheral neuropathy.

Patients chronically exposed may present with varied neurologic features including optic atrophy, nystagmus, paresthesias, dysesthesias, hypesthesia, hyporeflexia, and hyperreflexia. Visual loss associated with optic nerve degeneration may be permanent.[11] One chronically exposed worker had multiple presentations for psychosis before the underlying etiology of methyl bromide poisoning was determined.[51] Chronic exposure to methyl bromide is also associated with hepatotoxicity and nephrotoxicity. It is likely that acute poisoning produces similar effects and that critically ill patients simply may not survive to manifest fulminant hepatic failure. Autopsy findings have included acute tubular necrosis and degenerative nephritis.[33] Recovery of renal function is typical in survivors.

DIAGNOSTIC TESTING

Standard baseline laboratory tests should be obtained after an acute exposure, although they usually will be normal initially. Hepatic dysfunction should be assessed with hepatic aminotransferases and ammonia concentrations. Serum bromide concentrations are not readily available in most laboratories. Although a serum bromide concentration does not facilitate the clinical management of a methyl bromide–poisoned patient, the concentration may help confirm the diagnosis. Serum bromide concentrations may remain elevated for a week or more following an acute exposure. The elevation of the serum bromide, however, does not always correlate with the severity of the exposure.[24] An elevated serum bromide concentration may also cause a false elevation in serum chloride, when assayed using an ion selective electrode meter (see Chap. 16). Alternatively, in the setting of known methyl bromide exposure, the residual air concentration of methyl bromide can be measured.

TREATMENT

Treatment for methyl bromide poisoning relies on general and supportive care, and may require intensive care unit (ICU) management of coma, seizures, ALI, and hepatic and renal failure. Seizures are common and difficult to control with traditional anticonvulsants such as benzodiazepines and phenytoin. Pentobarbital coma and propofol have been required for many cases.[24] Decontamination should include the removal of clothing, as methyl bromide may bind to clothing, including rubber and leather. Clinical staff should exercise standard precautions using personal protective equipment. Irrigation of the eyes with saline and skin decontamination with soap and water should be performed by healthcare professionals using personal protective equipment. It is also reasonable to administer at least one dose of oral activated charcoal (AC) following ingestion.

Although hemodialysis can rapidly clear serum bromide, methyl bromide is probably completely metabolized by the time dialysis is considered. When dialysis is provided postdialysis neurological improvement was reported, but severe disabilities may remain. There is little evidence to support routine hemodialysis. Tissue injury following fumigant exposure occurs as the bromide is released into the serum, suggesting that the methylation of neuronal proteins has already occurred and the neurologic injury occurs so early that hemodialysis is unlikely to affect outcome.

PROGNOSIS

Most patients who develop seizures and coma will not survive and the few survivors of methyl bromide exposure who are described in the literature, with rare exception, had neuropsychiatric sequelae. These sequelae may or may not be permanent and have included myoclonus, cognitive deficits, paranoid delusions, depression, anxiety, mood disorders with rapid behavioral swings, and suicidal and homicidal thoughts.[7,48]

METHYL IODIDE

Iodomethane or methyl iodide (CH_3I) is currently under review by the Environmental Protection Agency (EPA). It is proposed fumigant to replace methyl bromide. However, a few reports from Europe suggest that the toxicity of methyl iodide may be similar to that of methyl bromide.[22,41] A recent report describes dermal exposure with severe burns and delayed neuropsychiatric sequelae, again similar to methyl bromide exposures.[43] This case of occupational exposure resulted from a breach in a protective suit.

DICHLOROPROPENE

$$\mathrm{Cl(H)C{=}CH{-}CH_2{-}Cl}$$

HISTORY AND EPIDEMIOLOGY

Dichloropropene was introduced in 1945 and is primarily used as a soil fumigant for nematodes. Exposures are reported during production, application, and ingestion.

OCCUPATIONAL EXPOSURE

Chronic subclinical changes in hepatic and renal function have been reported in Dutch flower bulb soil fumigators using dichloropropene.[6] Hematologic cancers including lymphoma and histiocytic lymphoma were reported in firemen after dichloropropene exposure.[32] The threshold limit value (TLV) for dichloropropene is 1 ppm. The Dutch occupational exposure limit is 5 mg/m^3 (equivalent to 1 ppm).

TOXICOKINETICS

Inhalation is the primary method of toxicity for 1,3-dichloropropene. In a human volunteer study, dermal absorption of dichloropropene was only 2% to 5% of inhalational absorption.[28] The metabolism of 1,3-dichloropropene is probably similar to that of other chlorinated hydrocarbon solvents such as carbon tetrachloride and chloroform (see Chap. 106). Glutathione depletion has been documented in the rat model.[21] The dose and route correlate with toxicity and outcome in rodent models of 1,3-dichloropropene toxicity. At 100 mg/kg in mice, hepatotoxicity occurs by the intraperitoneal route, but not after oral gavage. At 700 mg/kg administered by the intraperitoneal route hepatic failure and death resulted.[3] The higher dose correlated with a 130-fold increase in dichloropropene epoxide formation. Interestingly, in a rat hepatocyte model, pretreatment with the antioxidant, α-tocopherol, prevented cell death.[47]

CLINICAL MANIFESTATIONS

There are only a few reports of systemic dichloropropene toxicity. A patient died following the unintentional ingestion of a glass of dichloropropene.[23] Within 2 hours he developed tachycardia, tachypnea, hypotension, sweating, and abdominal pain, followed by hematochezia, acute respiratory distress syndrome (ARDS), rhabdomyolysis, metabolic acidosis, and hyperglycemia prior to death.[23] A hazardous materials incident exposed nine firemen to dichloropropene during cleanup operations. Symptoms included headache, neck pain, nausea, and difficulty breathing.[32] Other exposed individuals developed contact dermatitis and allergies to dichloropropene.[16] Healing of the skin leaves pigmented lesions.

DIAGNOSTIC TESTING

Hepatic and renal function should be monitored following acute poisoning, as autopsy has revealed extensive hepatic and renal necrosis after ingestion.[23] No additional tests are recommended beyond those needed for supportive care. Biomonitoring for exposure to dichloropropene is under development.[6] Hepatic γ-glutamyl transpeptidase (GGTP) concentrations were increased in fumigators, but the increase was not statistically significant. This finding, however, suggests hepatic enzyme induction. In fumigators erythrocyte glutathione S-transferase (GST) and glutathione (GSH) concentrations decreased with increased serum creatinine concentrations and increased urine concentrations of albumin and retinol-binding protein compared with controls.

MANAGEMENT

Because of off-gassing, the patient's clothes should be removed and bagged to avoid continued inhalational and dermal exposure of the patient and the healthcare worker, which demonstrates the benefits of personal protective equipment (PPE). If ingestion occurs, one dose of AC should be administered. There are no data to support specific therapies beyond supportive care, although the use of antioxidant therapy and *N*-acetylcysteine (NAC) warrant further study.

PHOSPHIDES AND PHOSPHINE

HISTORY AND EPIDEMIOLOGY

Phosphides are usually found as powders or pellets, usually in the form of zinc Zn_3P_2 or aluminium phosphide (AlP). Calcium and magnesium phosphides are also available. Phosphine gas (PH_3) is formed from phosphides after contact with water, particularly if acidic. Workers not using respiratory protective equipment may develop toxicity during the manufacturing of phosphides. Phosphide tablets are often placed in grain stores, such as ships, allowing the phosphine to be released once the storage sites are sealed. Phosphine is also available as a compressed gas in metal cylinders. Phosphine exposures and toxicity, both from phosphide salts or from compressed gas, have occurred during grain fumigation in both transport and storage areas, particularly if entry to the storage site occurs prior to proper ventilation. Many reports of serious and fatal phosphide poisonings originate from India, the Middle East, and developing countries. Aluminium phosphide consumption is commonly chosen as a means of suicide in India. In the United Kingdom a review of exposures by the National Poisons Information Service found most cases to be the result of unintentional agricultural exposures.[4] Clandestine methamphetamine laboratories that use the ephedrine/hydriodic acid/red phosphorus manufacturing method may generate phosphine gas at high reaction temperatures. Fatalities at these sites are reported, and first responders have also been exposed to high phosphine concentrations.[8]

TOXICOKINETICS AND PATHOPHYSIOLOGY

Phosphides produce toxicity rapidly, generally within 30 minutes of ingestion, and death may follow in less than 6 hours. The ingestion of fresh, unopened tablets consistently results in death. Toxicity from inhalation of phosphine gas is almost instantaneous. Phosphine disrupts mitochondrial function by blocking cytochrome c oxidase.[45] In addition to producing energy failure in cells, free radical generation increases, resulting in lipid peroxidation.[12,13,45] Phosphine also inhibits cholinesterases in rats, but people do not typically present with a cholinergic syndrome.[34]

CLINICAL MANIFESTATIONS

Phosphide ingestions of over 500 mg are often fatal. Unopened packets are more potent, as once opened, atmospheric moisture may react with tablets to decrease their potency. Phosphides are potent gastric irritants; profuse vomiting and abdominal pain are often the first symptoms to occur following ingestion. Respiratory signs and symptoms include tachypnea, hyperpnea, dyspnea, cough, and chest tightness that may progress to ALI over days. In significant exposures, hypotension and dysrhythmias often develop.[17] Phosphine-induced dysrhythmias include atrial fibrillation and flutter, heart block, and ventricular tachycardia and fibrillation. Echocardiography and electrocardiography have demonstrated reversible myocardial injury (ST elevations and inversions) and left ventricular hypokinesis.[1,26] Central nervous system toxicity includes coma, seizures, and delirium. Pancreatitis and esophageal strictures are occasionally delayed complications of oral exposures. Obstructive airways disease has been reported following occupational inhalational exposure.[5]

DIAGNOSTIC TESTING

The diagnosis is usually established from the history and confirmatory laboratory testing such as elevated lactate concentrations. Further laboratory testing is dictated by the need for supportive care. Headspace gas chromatography with a nitrogen-phosphorus detector was used to detect phosphine gas from postmortem tissue.[35]

MANAGEMENT

Patients who ingest phosphides frequently vomit from the irritant effects. Off-gassing from emesis, theoretically, may expose healthcare workers to phosphine vapor. The emesis should be placed in sealed containers and disposed of properly, as wet phosphides will continue to generate phosphine gas.

The toxicology literature describes many theoretical approaches to prevent the postingestion generation of phosphine gas and its absorption. All of these efforts will be hampered by the vomiting that usually occurs along with the possible aspiration of gastric contents and administered agent. Because the extent to which AC binds phosphides is generally unknown and there is a lack of clinical outcome data for AC, administration of oral AC may be considered appropriate but of uncertain value. Dilution with bicarbonate solution has been recommended, as bicarbonate decreases the gastric hydrochloric acid concentration, which normally assists in the conversion of phosphides to phosphine gas. Also unproven is the use of diluted potassium permanganate to oxidize the phosphides. Case reports from India and Nepal describe the use of vegetable oil for gastric lavage fluid and the use of coconut oil with sodium bicarbonate, based upon the theory that fats and oils are nonmiscible and may prevent the release of phosphine gas.[44] Clinical outcome studies have not been performed for any of these theoretical therapies and therefore cannot be recommended at this time.

Trimetazidine, which is not currently available in the United States, is used elsewhere for the treatment of cardiac toxicity[17] as it may diminish the oxidant stress caused by phosphine.[13] Internationally, trimetazidine is used as an antianginal agent. The drug may improve the energy state within cardiac myocytes by shifting from oxidative metabolism to glucose utilization. Preliminary research using rat models in India suggests possible benefits, including increased survival time with the use of N-acetylcysteine (an antioxidant) and pralidoxime (a cholinesterase reactivator).[2,34] Intravenous magnesium acting as an antiperoxidant has also been proposed as a benefit following aluminium phosphide ingestion. An unblinded trial of 50 subjects reported reduced mortality (42% compared with 20%) in those treated with repeated intravenous doses of magnesium.[14] All of these proposed therapies, however, require further study. At this time the use of NAC and magnesium are of uncertain benefit but appropriate for use.

SULFURYL FLUORIDE

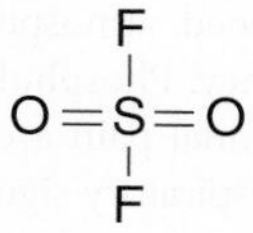

$$F-S(=O)(=O)-F$$

HISTORY AND EPIDEMIOLOGY

Sulfuryl fluoride has been used since 1957 as a structural fumigant insecticide to control wood-boring insects such as termites in homes. Structure or tent fumigation is performed by completely enclosing a house or other structure in plastic or a tarpaulin; the sulfuryl fluoride is pumped in as a compressed gas. Chloropicrin is typically added as a warning agent. Although sulfuryl fluoride is commonly used in Florida, California,[37] and Washington, a 5-year review of fumigant illness did not contain any reports of sulfuryl fluoride toxicity.[8]

TOXICOKINETICS AND PATHOPHYSIOLOGY

Little is known about the toxicokinetics of sulfuryl fluoride in humans. At high concentrations (above 4000 ppm) rats developed seizures followed by respiratory arrest.[36] At lower concentrations and with chronic exposure, rats and rabbits developed respiratory inflammation, renal lesions, and cerebral vacuolation.[18] The mechanism of toxicity is not understood. The measurable fluoride concentrations in patients suggest that the release of fluoride may be a major pathophysiologic mechanism.[37] In models of chronic, low concentration exposures, fluorosis developed. The TLV-TWA for sulfuryl fluoride is 5 ppm; TLV–short-term exposure limit (STEL) is 10 ppm; IDLH (immediately dangerous to life and health) is 200 ppm. Sulfuryl fluoride was not found to be teratogenic in rats or rabbits.[21]

CLINICAL MANIFESTATIONS

Case reports of sulfuryl fluoride exposure describe acute and subacute courses that have many similarities to methyl bromide. As is the case in animal studies, severe exposures in humans affect the cardiopulmonary and nervous systems. Initial symptoms may be gastrointestinal, including nausea, vomiting, diarrhea, and abdominal pain, or respiratory, including cough and dyspnea. Irritation of mucosal surfaces may produce salivation and nasopharyngitis lacrimation with conjunctivitis.

A husband and wife reentered their home after it was cleared by the fumigators, although checks for residual sulfuryl fluoride concentrations were not provided.[37] Within 24 hours both became symptomatic. The husband complained of dyspnea and cough that became severe. Approximately 36 hours after the exposure, he had a seizure followed by cardiopulmonary arrest. His wife initially had nausea and vomiting. Over 3 days she became progressively weaker and unable to walk. She developed severe dyspnea followed by ventricular fibrillation. She had a serum fluoride concentration of 0.5 mg/L (normal is less than 0.2 mg/L) 5 days after the exposure began. Autopsies listed the cause of death as pulmonary edema for both victims. Another report describes suspected suicide by sulfuryl fluoride inhalation.[42] A 19-year-old woman who reentered apparently to retrieve some personal items was found unconscious, but became alert after removal from the home. Her complaints included coughing and chest pain. Approximately 6 hours later she developed carpal/pedal spasm, tetany, and cardiac dysrhythmias followed by death. Her serum fluoride concentration was 20 mg/L. All three autopsies were remarkable for pulmonary edema. Neurotoxicity may also result from low concentrations and acute or chronic exposures. Subclinical effects in memory and dexterity testing were noted in structural fumigation workers exposed to both methyl bromide and sulfuryl fluoride.[10]

DIAGNOSTIC TESTING

Patients with sulfuryl fluoride exposure require frequent monitoring of serum calcium concentrations, as the fluoride complexes with calcium ions as well as potassium and magnesium monitoring (see Chap. 105). Continuous cardiac monitoring should follow the QT interval, as hypocalcemia may precipitate dysrhythmias. Serum fluoride concentrations, although not helpful for the acute management, may help with confirmatory diagnostic testing.

MANAGEMENT

After removal from the scene to fresh air, the patient should be disrobed to avoid further exposure and to avoid the possibility of off-gassing of any sulfuryl fluoride gas. In treating sulfuryl fluoride poisoning, aggressive treatment of hypocalcemia may be needed. Patients should have electrocardiograms (ECGs) performed and be attached to continuous cardiac monitoring to observe for QT interval prolongation. Similar to the management of methyl bromide, supportive care may be needed for the seizures, cardiac dysrhythmias, and management of ALI and bronchospasm (see Chap. 105).

METAM SODIUM

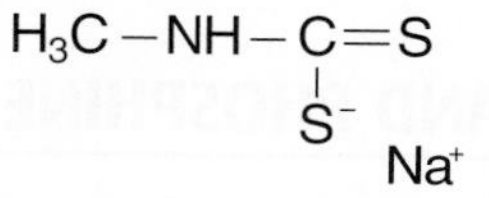

$$H_3C-NH-C(=S)-S^-\ Na^+$$

Metam sodium is used as a soil fumigant to control weeds, nematodes, and fungi, ranking as the third most commonly used agricultural pesticide in the US.[40] It is an agent listed among the more common occupational exposures to fumigants.[9] In Sacramento, California, a train derailment resulted in a metam sodium release with persistent air concentrations for days.[15] Many exposed individuals developed irritant-induced asthma or reactive airways disease syndrome (RADS) following the spill. In the cleanup, prolonged exposure to wet clothing from river water containing 20 to 40 parts per billion (ppb) of metam sodium caused dermatitis.[29] Metam sodium, which breaks down into methyl isothiocyanate, is a potent sensitizer. Off-site drift following soil fumigation to a nearby community produced symptoms in 179 of 200 residents evaluated.[38] Almost all patients complained of ocular tearing or upper respiratory burning. Other less common, nonspecific symptoms included headache, nausea, and vomiting.[33] Subjects complained of lower respiratory tract symptoms including cough, dyspnea, wheezing, and chest pain. Patients with underlying pulmonary disease, especially bronchospastic conditions such as asthma and chronic obstructive pulmonary disease, appeared to be more sensitive.[38] Sheltering in place in homes with central air conditioning compared with window units may have provided some protection by preventing the entry of metam sodium into the homes.

SUMMARY

Exposures to fumigants and their presentations can be highly variable depending on the route and level of exposure. Most unintentional exposures will occur via the inhalational route, while intentional exposures may predominantly be by the oral route with large life-threatening amounts ingested. Low-level inhalational exposures to most of the fumigants may resemble viral syndromes, but manifest delayed neuropsychiatric symptoms. Diagnosis largely relies on the history of exposure, as most confirmatory diagnostic tests are not readily available. Treatment is mainly supportive, often provided in an ICU. The administration of calcium, however, for severe sulfuryl fluoride poisoning may be life-saving. Fumigant use is vital to enhancing crop production in today's global agricultural economy. Extensive research and testing have not yet led to the development of suitable replacements for the toxic compounds described in this chapter.

REFERENCES

1. Akkaoui M, Achour S, Abidi K, et al. Reversible myocardial injury associated with aluminum phosphide poisoning. *Clin Toxicol.* 2007;45:728-731.
2. Azad A, Lall SB, Mittra S. Effect of *N*-acetylcysteine and L-NAME on aluminium phosphide induced cardiovascular toxicity in rats. *Acta Pharmacol Sin.* 2001;22:298-304.
3. Bartels MJ, Brzak KA, Mendrala AL, et al. Mechanistic aspects of the metabolism of 1,3-dichloropropene in rats and mice. *Chem Res Toxicol.* 2000;13:1096-1102.
4. Bogle RG, Theron P, Brooks P, et al. Aluminium phosphide poisoning. *Emerg Med J.* 2006;23:e3.
5. Brautbar N, Howard J. Phosphine toxicity: report of two cases and review of the literature. *Toxicol Ind Health.* 2002;18:71-75.
6. Brouwer EJ, Evelo CTA, Verplanke AJW, et al. Biological effect monitoring of occupational exposure to 1, 3-dichloropropene: effects on liver and renal function and on glutathione conjugation. *Br J Ind Med.* 1991;48:167-172.
7. Buchwald AL, Muller M. Late confirmation of acute methyl bromide poisoning using S-methylcysteine adduct testing. *Vet Hum Toxicol.* 2001;43:208-211.
8. Burgess JL, Morrissey B, Keifer MC, et al. Fumigant-related illness: Washington State's five-year experience. *J Toxicol Clin Toxicol.* 2000;38:7-14.
9. Burgess JL. Phosphine exposure from a methamphetamine laboratory investigation. *J Toxicol Clin Toxicol.* 2001;39:165-168.
10. Calvert GM, Mueller CA, Fajen JM, et al. Health effects associated with sulfuryl fluoride and methyl bromide exposure among structural fumigation workers. *Am J Pub Health.* 1998;88:1774-1780.
11. Chavez CT, Hepler RS, Staatsma BR. Methyl bromide optic atrophy. *Am J Ophthalmol.* 1985;99:715-719.
12. Chefurka W, Kashi KP, Bond EJ. The effect of phosphine on electron transport in mitochondria. *Pesticide Biochem Physiol.* 1976;6:65-84.
13. Chugh SN, Arora V, Sharma A, et al. Free radical scavengers and lipid peroxidation in acute aluminum phosphide poisoning. *Indian J Med Res.* 1996;104:190-193.
14. Chugh SN, Kolley T, Kakkar R et al. A critical evaluation of anti-peroxidant effect of intravenous magnesium in acute aluminium phosphide poisoning. *Magnes Res.* 1997;10:225-230.
15. Cone JE, Wugofski L, Balmes JR, et al. Persistent respiratory health effects after a metam sodium pesticide spill. *Chest.* 1994;106:500-508.
16. Corazza M, Zinna G, Virgili A. Allergic contact dermatitis due to 1,3-dichloropropene soil fumigant. *Contact Dermatitis.* 2003;48:341-342.
17. Duenas A, Perez-Castrillon JL, Cobos MA, et al. Treatment of the cardiovascular manifestations of phosphine with trimetazidine, a new anti-ischemic drug. *Am J Emerg Med.* 1999;17:219-220.
18. Eisenbrandt DL, Nitschke KD. Inhalation toxicity of sulfuryl fluorides in rats and rabbits. *Fundam Appl Toxicol.* 1989;12:540-557.
19. Ferranti P, Sannolo N, Mamone G, et al. Structural characterization by mass spectrometry of hemoglobin adducts formed after in vitro exposure to methyl bromide. *Carcinogenesis.* 1996;17;2662-2671.
20. Goldman LR, Mengle D, Epstein DM, et al. Acute symptoms in persons residing near a field treated with soil fumigants methyl bromide and chloropicrin. *West J Med.* 1987;147:95-98.
21. Hanley TR, Calhoun LL, Kociba RJ, et al. The effects of inhalation exposure to sulfuryl fluoride on fetal development in rats and rabbits. *Fundam Appl Toxicol.* 1989;13:79-86.
22. Hermouet C, Garnier R, Efthymiou M, et al. Methyl iodide poisoning: report of two cases. *Am J Med.* 1996;30:759-764.
23. Hernandez AF, Martin-Rubi JC, Ballesteros JL, et al. Clinical and pathological findings in fatal 1,3-dichloropropene intoxication. *Hum Exp Toxicol.* 1994;13:303-306.
24. Hustinx WNM, van de Laar RTH, van Huffelen AC, et al. Systemic effects of inhalational methyl bromide poisoning: a study of nine cases occupationally exposed due to inadvertent spread during fumigation. *Br J Ind Med.* 1993;50:155-159.
25. Iwasaki K, Ito I, Kagawa J. Biological exposure monitoring of methyl bromide workers by determination of hemoglobin adducts. *Ind Health.* 1989;27:181-183.
26. Kaushik RM, Kaushik R, Mahajan SK. Subendocardial infarction in a young survivor of aluminium phosphide poisoning. *Hum Exp Toxicol.* 2007;26: 457-460.
27. Kawai T, Zhang Z-W, Moon C-S, et al. Comparison of urinary bromide levels among people in East Asia, and the effects of dietary intakes of cereals and marine products. *Toxicol Lett.* 2002;134:285-293.
28. Kezic S, Monster AC, Verplanke AJW, et al. Dermal absorption of cis-1,3 dichloropropene vapour: human experimental exposure. *Hum Exp Toxicol.* 1996;15:396-399.
29. Koo D, Goldman L, Baron R. Irritant dermatitis among workers cleaning up a pesticide spill: California 1991. *Am J Ind Med.* 1995;27:545-553.
30. Letz GA, Pond SM, Osterloh JD, et al. Two fatalities after acute occupational exposure to ethylene dibromide. *JAMA.* 1984;252:2428-2431.
31. Lifshitz M, Gavrilov V. Cental nervous system toxicity and early peripheral neuropathy following dermal exposure to methyl bromide. *J Toxicol Clin Toxicol.* 2000;38:799-801.
32. Markowitz, Crosby WH. Chemical carcinogenesis: a soil fumigant 1,3-dichloropropene, as possible cause of hematologic malignancies. *Arch Intern Med.* 1984;144:1409-1411.
33. Marracinni JV, Thomas GE, Ongley JP, et al. Death and injury caused by methyl bromide, an insecticide fumigant. *J Forensic Sci.* 1983;28:601-637.
34. Mittra S, Peshin SS, Lall SB. Cholinesterase inhibition by aluminium phosphide poisoning in rats and effects of atropine and pralidoxime chloride. *Acta Pharmacol Sin.* 2001;22:37-39.
35. Musshoff F, Preuss J, Lignitz E, et al. A gas chromatographic analysis of phosphine in biological material in a case of suicide. *Forensic Sci Int.* 2008;177:e35-e38.
36. Nitschke KD, Albee RR, Mattsson JL. Incapacitation and treatment of rats exposed to a lethal dose of sulfuryl fluoride. *Fundam Appl Toxicol.* 1986;7:664-670.
37. Nuckolls JG, Smith DC, Walls WE, et al. Fatalities resulting from sulfuryl fluoride exposure after home fumigation—Virginia. *JAMA.* 1987;258: 2041-2042.
38. O'Malley M, Barry T, Ibarra M, et al. Illness related to shank application of metam-sodium, Arvin, California, July 2002. *J Agromedicine.* 2005;10:27-42.
39. Polkowski J, Crowley MS, Moore AM, et al. Unintentional methyl bromide release Florida 1988. *J Toxicol Clin Toxicol.* 1990;28:127-130.
40. Pruett SB, Myers LP, Keil DE. Toxicology of metam sodium. *J Toxicol Environ Health B Crit Rev.* 2001;4:207-222.
41. Robertz-Vaupel GM, Bierl R, von Unruh G. Intravenous methyl iodide poisoning—detoxification using hemoperfusion. *Anasthesiol Intensivmed Notfallmed Schmerzther.* 1991;26:44-47.
42. Scheuerman EH. Case report: suicide by exposure to sulfuryl fluoride. *J Forensic Sci.* 1986;31:1154-1158.
43. Schwartz MD, Obamwonyi AO, Thomas JD, et al. Acute methyl iodide exposure with delayed neuropsychiatric sequelae: report of a case. *Am J Ind Med.* 2005;47:550-556.
44. Shadnia S, Rahimi M, Pajoumand A, et al. Successful treatment of acute aluminium phosphide poisoning: possible benefit of coconut oil. *Hum Exp Toxicol.* 2005;24:215-218.
45. Singh S, Bhalla A, Verma SK, et al. Cytochrome-C oxidase inhibition in 26 aluminum phosphide poisoned patients. *Clin Toxicol.* 2006;44:155-158.
46. Squier MV, Thompson J, Rajgopalan B. Case report: neuropathology of methyl bromide intoxication. *Neuropath Appl Neurobiol.* 1992;18:579-584.
47. Suzuki T, Sasaki H, Komatsu M, et al. Cytotoxicity of 1,3-dichloropropene and cellular phospholipids peroxidation in isolated rat hepatocytes, and its prevention by alpha-tocopherol. *Biol Pharm Bull.* 1994;17:1351-1354.
48. Uncini A, Basciani M, DiMuzio A, et al. Methyl bromide myoclonus: an electrophysiological study. *Acta Neurol Scand.* 1990;81:159-164.
49. Van den Oever R, Roosels D, Lahaye D. Actual hazard of methyl bromide fumigation in soil disinfection. *Br J Ind Med.* 1982;39:140-144.
50. Yamano Y, Nakadate T. Three occupationally exposed cases of severe methyl bromide poisoning: accident caused by a gas leak during fumigation of a folklore museum. *J Occup Health.* 2006;48:129-133.
51. Zatuchni J, Hong K. Methyl bromide poisoning seen initially as psychosis. *Arch Neurol.* 1981;38:529-530.
52. Zwaveling JH, de Kort WL, Meulenbelt J, et al. Exposure of the skin to methyl bromide: a study of six cases occupationally exposed to high concentrations during fumigation. *Hum Toxicol.* 1987;6:491-495.

L.

NATURAL TOXINS AND ENVENOMATIONS

CHAPTER 117

MUSHROOMS

Lewis R. Goldfrank

The diversity of mushroom species is evident in our grocery stores, our restaurant menus, and our environment. The diversity of the American population has led to experimentation by young and old—old citizens and our newest immigrants as well as our young children reaching for what might become an innocuous or a serious ingestion. Rigor in analyzing the possible ingestion is indispensable for poison center staff and emergency physicians treating a patient who has ingested a mushroom of concern. This chapter offers general information of the most consequential toxicologic groups of mushrooms.

EPIDEMIOLOGY

Unintentional exposures to mushrooms represent a small but relatively constant percentage of consultations requested from poison centers (see citations for American Association of Poison Control Centers [AAPCC] data in Chap. 135). A summary of a quarter century of AAPCC data reveals that mushrooms represent far less than 0.5% of the reported human exposures. Combined data accumulated by the AAPCC and the Mushroom Poisoning Registry of the North American Mycological Association indicates that approximately five patient exposures to toxic mushrooms per 100,000 population occur per year. Some variations result from geographic and climatic conditions and mycologic habitats.[109] Although the methods of analysis of patients with mushroom exposures have changed over the past quarter century, cumulative AAPCC data consistently demonstrate the relative benignity of the vast majority of exposures. The inability of most healthcare providers to correctly identify the ingested mushroom and the rarity of lethal ingestions are demonstrated by the accumulated data. In 85% to 95% of cases, the exact species was unidentified.[109] More than 50% of exposed individuals had no symptoms. Most patients were treated at home and rarely had major toxicity. During the quarter century covered by the AAPCC data, fewer than 100 patients died of their ingestions. Of the mushrooms associated with a death, most were *Amanita* spp, and several were hallucinogens, *Boletus* spp, gyromitrin-containing mushroom, while others remained unidentified. All reported deaths occurred in adults. Hallucinogens and gastrointestinal (GI) toxins were the most common exposures yet they accounted for less than 10% of exposures. All other presumed exposures represented less than 2% of the total number of identified. Because 85% to 95% of mushrooms involved in exposures are never identified, a strategy for making significant decisions with incomplete data is essential.

CLASSIFICATION AND MANAGEMENT

This chapter does not address molds, mildews, and yeasts, which in addition to mushrooms are all categorized as fungi. The unifying principle for fungi is the lack of the photosynthetic capacity to produce nutrition. Survival is achieved by the enyzymatic capacity of these organisms to integrate into living materials and digest them. Molds are ubiquitous and often associated with varied adverse health effects such as rhinitis, rashes, headaches, and asthma.[19] An example of a mold-related mycotoxin is discussed in Chap. 132 on biological weapons. All other molds are not associated with toxicologic emergencies and are not addressed in this chapter.

Because mushroom species vary widely with regard to the toxins they contain, and because identifying them with certainty is difficult, a clinical system of classification is more useful than a taxonomic system (Table 117–1). In many cases, management and prognosis can be determined with a high degree of confidence from the history and the geographic origin of the mushroom, the initial signs and symptoms, the organ system or systems involved, and coexistent factors or conditions.[28,53,68,69,95] Groups of toxins are identifiable as cyclopeptides, gyromitrin, muscarine, coprine, ibotenic acid and muscimol, psilocybin, general GI irritants, orellinine, allenic norleucine, acromelic acids, and myotoxins.[28,53,68]

GROUP I: CYCLOPEPTIDE-CONTAINING MUSHROOMS

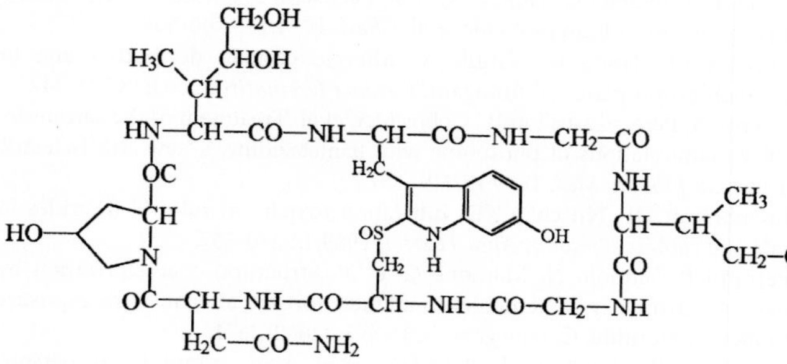

α-Amanitin

Most mushroom fatalities in North America and worldwide are associated with cyclopeptide-containing species.[4,29,121] These mushrooms include a number of *Amanita* species, including *A. verna*, *A. virosa*, and *A. phalloides*; *Galerina* spp, including *G. autumnalis*, *G. marginata*, and *G. venenata*; and *Lepiota* species, including *L. helveola*, *L. josserandi*, and *L. brunneoincarnata* (Figure 117–1).

Early differentiation of cyclopeptide poisonings from other types of mushroom poisoning is difficult. Patients poisoned with cyclopeptides may present to an emergency department (ED) with a seemingly innocuous picture of nausea, vomiting, abdominal pain, and diarrhea, which

TABLE 117–1. Mushroom Toxicity Overview

Representative Genus/Species	Xenobiotic	Time of Onset of Symptoms	Primary Site of Toxicity	Symptoms	Mortality	Specific Therapy[a]
I						
Amanita phalloides, A. tenuifolia, A. virosa *Galerina autumnalis, G. marginata, G. venenata* *Lepiota josserandi, L. helveola*	Cyclopeptides Amatoxins Phallotoxins	5–24 h	Liver	Phase I: GI toxicity—N/V/D Phase II: Quiescent Phase III: N/V/D, jaundice, ↑ AST, ↑ ALT	0%–30%	Activated charcoal Hemoperfusion/hemodialysis Penicillin G *N*-acetylcysteine Silibinin
II						
Gyromitra ambigua, G. esculenta, G. infula	Gyromitrin (metabolite: monomethylhydrazine)	5–10 h	CNS	Seizures, abdominal pain, N/V, weakness, hepatorenal failure	Rare	Benzodiazepines, Pyridoxine 70 mg/kg IV
III						
Clitocybe dealbata, Omphalotus olearius, most *Inocybe* spp	Muscarine	0.5–2 h	Autonomic nervous system	Muscarinic effects—salivation, bradycardia, lacrimation, urination, defecation, diaphoresis	Rare	Atropine— Adults: 1–2 mg Children: 0.02 mg/kg with a minimum of 0.1 mg
IV						
Coprinus atramentarius	Coprine (metabolite: 1-aminocyclopropanol)	0.5–2 h	Aldehyde dehydrogenase	Disulfiramlike effect with ethanol, tachycardia, N/V	Rare	Symptomatic care
V						
Amanita gemmata, A. muscaria, A. pantherina	Ibotenic acid, muscimol	0.5–2 h	CNS	GABAergic effects, rare delirium, hallucinations, dizziness, ataxia	Rare	Benzodiazepines during excitatory phase
VI						
Psilocybe caerulipes, P. cubensis *Gymnopilus spectabilis* *Psathyrella foenisecii*	Psilocybin, psilocin	0.5–1 h	CNS	Ataxia, N/V, hyperkinesis, hallucinations	Rare	Benzodiazepines
VII						
Clitocybe nebularis *Chlorophyllum molybdites, C. esculentum* *Lactarius* spp, *Paxillus involutus*	Various GI irritants	0.5–3 h	GI	Malaise, N/V/D	Rare	Symptomatic care
VIII						
Cortinarius orellanus, C. speciosissimus, C. rainierensis	Orelline, orellanine	>24 h days to weeks	Renal	Phase I: N/V Phase II: Oliguria, renal failure	Rare	Hemodialysis for renal failure
IX						
Amanita smithiana	Allenic norleucine	0.5–12 h	Renal	Phase I: N/V Phase II: Oliguria, renal failure	None	Hemodialysis for renal failure
X						
Tricholoma equestre	Unidentified myotoxin	24–72 h	Muscle (skeletal and cardiac)	Fatigue, nausea, muscle weakness, myalgias, ↑ CPK, facial erythema, diaphoresis, myocarditis	25%	$NaHCO_3$ Hemodialysis for renal failure

(Continued)

TABLE 117–1. Mushroom Toxicity Overview (*Continued*)

Representative Genus/Species	Toxin	Time of Onset of Symptoms	Primary Site of Toxicity	Symptoms	Mortality	Specific Therapy[a]
XI						
Clitocybe acromelalga, C. amoenolens	Acromelic acids	24 h	Peripheral nervous system	Erythromelalgia paresthesias—hands and feet, dysesthesias, erythema, edema	None	Symptomatic care
XII						
Pleurocybella porrigens	Unknown	1–31 days	CNS	Encephalopathy, convulsions, myoclonus in patients with chronic renal failure	High ?30%	Hemodialysis
Hapalopilus rutilans	Polyporic acid	>12 h	GI, CNS	N/V, abdominal pain, vertigo, ataxia, drowsiness, encephalopathy	None	Symptomatic care
XIII						
Paxillus involutus, ? Clitocybe claviceps, ? Boletus luridus	Immune mediated response to involutin	Following repeated exposure 0.5–3 h	Red blood cell kidney	Hemolytic anemia, acute renal failure	Rare	Hemodialysis
XIV						
Lycoperdon perlatum, L. pyriforine, L. gemmatum	Spores	Hours	Pulmonary, GI	Cough, shortness of breath, fever, nausea, vomiting	None	Prednisone

D, diarrhea; N, nausea; V, vomiting.

[a] Supportive care (fluids, electrolyes, and antiemetics) as indicated.

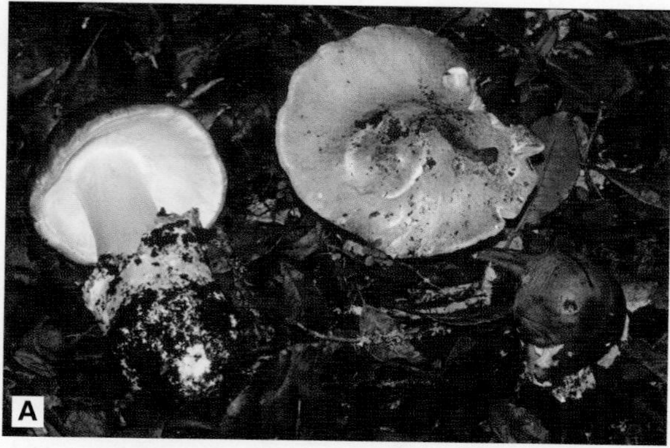

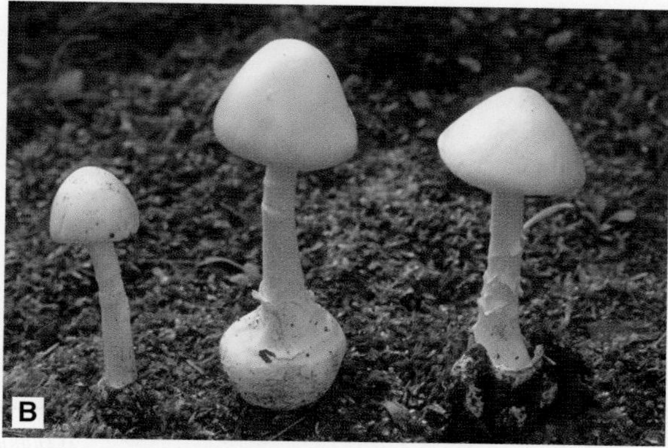

FIGURE 117–1. Group I: Cyclopeptide-containing mushrooms. (**A**) *Amanita phalloides* and (**B**) *Amanita virosa*. *(Images contributed by John Plischke III).*

often is attributed to other causes. Such patients may be sent home, only to return moribund on a subsequent day. The delayed onset of more serious symptoms is typical of cyclopeptide toxicity and is a critical consideration in assessing any potential toxicologic emergency.

A. phalloides contains 15 to 20 cyclopeptides with an approximate weight of 900 Da. The amatoxins (cyclic octapeptides), phallotoxins (cyclic heptapeptides), and virotoxins (cyclic heptapeptides) are the best studied.[32,64,116] There is no evidence for the toxicity of virotoxins in humans. Of these three chemically similar cyclopeptide molecules, phalloidin (the principal phallotoxin) appears to be a rapid-acting toxin, whereas amanitin tends to cause more delayed manifestations.[98] Phalloidin crosses the sinusoidal plasma membranes of hepatocytes by a carrier-mediated process. This process is shared by bile salts and can be prevented in the presence of extracellular bile salts, suggesting a competitive inhibition. A sodium-independent bile salt transporting system may be responsible for phalloidin hepatic uptake, elimination, and detoxification.[76] Phalloidin interrupts actin polymerization and impairs cell membrane function, but because of its limited oral absorption it appears to have minimal toxicity, restricted mostly to GI dysfunction.

The amatoxins are the most toxic of the cyclopeptides, leading to hepatic, renal, and central nervous system (CNS) damage. These polypeptides are heat stable.[32] α-Amanitin is the principal amatoxin responsible for human toxicity following ingestion. Approximately 1.5 to 2.5 mg amanitin can be obtained from 1 g dry *A. phalloides*, and as much as 3.5 mg/g can be obtained from some *Lepiota* spp.[83,87,116] A 20-g mushroom contains well in excess of the 0.1 mg/kg amanitin considered lethal for humans.[31] α-Amanitin and β-amanitin have comparable toxicity in animal models.[31]

α-Amanitin absorption appears to be facilitated by a sodium-dependent bile acid transporter. Several studies demonstrate that the sodium taurocholate cotransporter polypeptide, a member of the organic anion–transporter polypeptide (OATP) family localized in the sinusoidal membranes of human hepatocytes, facilitates hepatocellular α-amanitin uptake.[52,71] Once inside the cells the cytotoxicity of α-amanitin results from its interference with RNA polymerase II, preventing the transcription of DNA.[74,102] The amanitins are poorly but rapidly absorbed from the GI tract,[57] and α-amanitin may be enterohepatically recirculated. Target organs are those with the highest rate of cell turnover, including the GI tract epithelium, hepatocytes, and kidneys. Amatoxins do not appear to cross the placenta, as demonstrated by the absence of fetal toxicity in severely poisoned pregnant women.[6,12,106]

Amatoxins show limited protein binding and are present in the plasma at low concentrations for 24 to 48 hours.[57] In an intravenous radiolabeled amatoxin study in dogs, 85% of the amatoxin was recovered in the urine within the first 6 hours, whereas less than 1% was found in the blood at that time.[33] Amatoxins can be detected by high-performance liquid chromatography,[57] thin-layer chromatography, ion trap mass spectrometry,[37] and radioimmunoassay in gastroduodenal fluid, serum, urine, stool, and liver and kidney biopsies for several days following an ingestion.[31,32,63]

Some of the toxicokinetic analyses following unquantified ingestions demonstrate 12 to 23 μg amatoxin excretion in the urine over 24 to 66 hours, of which 60% to 80% occurred during the first 2 hours of collection. The extreme variabilities of the type and quantity of ingestant, the host, and the management make interpretations exceedingly difficult.[112] In another series, total maximal urinary α- and β-amanitin excreted over 6 to 72 hours were 3.19 and 5.21 mg, respectively. Two-thirds of the patients had total amanitin toxin excretion greater than 1.5 mg.[57] Urinary amanitin excretion concentrations differ by several orders of magnitude. Whether the variation results from exposure dose, time following ingestion, or laboratory technique is unclear. Several techniques for quantitative and qualitative evaluation of urinary amanitin are under investigation. The sensitivity and specificity of these determinations are under investigation.[15,16,87,105]

Clinical Phase I of cyclopeptide poisoning resembles severe gastroenteritis, with profuse watery diarrhea not occurring until 5 to 24 hours after ingestion. Some consider the early onset (less than 8 hours) of diarrhea as a predictive factor for hepatic failure and the need for liver transplantation.[30] Supportive fluid and electrolyte replacement leads to transient improvement during phase II, which occurs between 12 and 36 hours after ingestion.[87,121] However, despite such supportive care, phase III, manifested by hepatic and renal toxicity and death, may ensue 2 to 6 days after ingestion.[4] Pancreatic toxicity may rarely occur.[43] The initial hepatotoxicity begins within the second phase, but clinical hepatotoxicity (Chap. 26) with elevated concentrations of bilirubin, aspartate aminotransferase (AST), and alanine aminotransferase (ALT), hypoglycemia, jaundice, and hepatic coma are not manifest until 2 to 3 days after ingestion. Pathologic manifestations include steatosis, central zonal necrosis, and centrilobular hemorrhage, with viable hepatocytes remaining at the rims of the larger triads. Lobular architecture remains intact (see Fig. 26–2).[4]

Cyclopeptide toxicity alters the hormones that regulate glucose, calcium, and thyroid homeostasis, resulting in widespread endocrine abnormalities.[61] Insulin and C-peptide concentrations are elevated at a stage of poisoning prior to hepatic and renal compromise.[26,61] These findings are suggestive of direct toxicity to pancreatic β cells, resulting in release of preformed hormone or induction of hormone synthesis. This insulin release necessitates vigilance for hypoglycemia prior to hepatocellular damage. Serum calcitonin concentrations may be elevated, and hypocalcemia may be present. Thyroxine concentrations may be depressed and triiodothyronine concentrations undetectable, whereas thyroid-stimulating hormone concentrations may not be elevated. These thyroid-related findings were reported in a single study and merit further investigation.[61]

In a series of 10 patients exposed to diverse *Lepiota* spp, 50% developed a mixed sensory and motor polyneuropathy. Most of the patients spontaneously recovered within 1 year, although a single patient developed progressive clinical and electromyographic deterioration.[89] These neuropathic findings have not been recognized in other case reports.

Treatment The search for treatments has been vigorously pursued in Europe because of the persistently large number of amatoxin victims each year.[42] Survival rates in case series of variable numbers of patients poisoned by *A. phalloides* who received any of the following: supportive care, fluid and electrolyte repletion, high-dose penicillin G, dexamethasone, and thioctic acid, are between 70% and 100%.[42,51,56,79,81,91,121] Many of these case series have excellent survival rates with extremely variable therapeutic interventions, limiting the capacity to determine the need for or efficacy of most of the standard conservative therapeutic regimens.

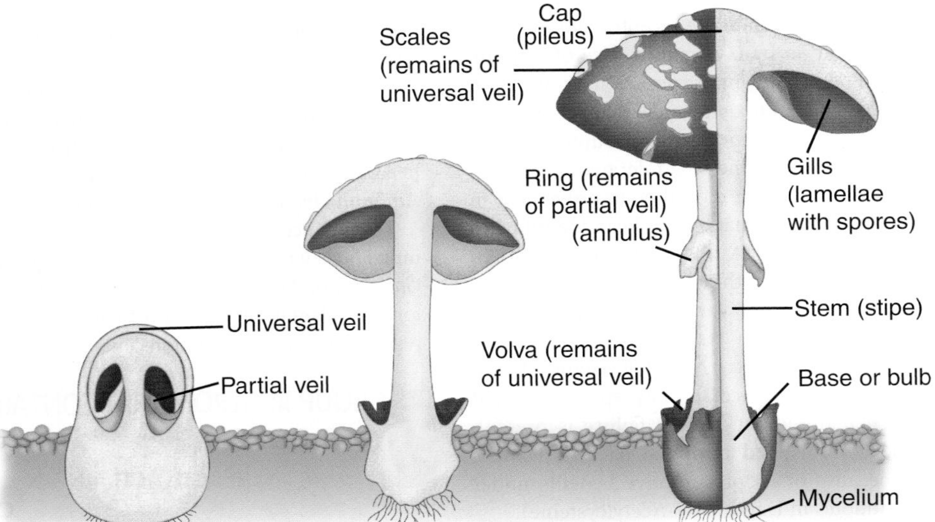

FIGURE 117–2. In the more highly specialized and evolved mushrooms, various protective tissues cover the fruit body and its constituent parts during its development. In the mushroom shown, an *Amanita* species, two veils of tissue are involved–one an outer enclosing bag, the universal veil, which ruptures as the fruit body expands to leave a volva at the base and fragments on the cap; the other an inner partial veil covering the developing gills that is pulled away as the cap opens to leave a ring on the stem. (Redrawn, with permission, from Kibby G: *Mushrooms and Toadstools, A Field Guide.* Oxford, Oxford University Press, 1979, p. 14.)

Fluid and electrolyte repletion and treatment of hepatic compromise are essential. Intravenous 0.9% sodium chloride solution and electrolytes usually are necessary because of substantial fluid loss due to vomiting and diarrhea. Dextrose repletion may be necessary because of nutritional compromise, hepatic failure, or glycogen depletion. Activated charcoal both adsorbs the amanitins and improves survival in laboratory animals.[31] Emesis, lavage, and catharsis are not necessary unless the patient is seen within several hours after the ingestion, because the toxin usually induces emesis and catharsis. Activated charcoal is safe, logical, and a valuable therapeutic strategy. Although the clinical presentation often is delayed, 1 g/kg body weight of activated charcoal should be given orally every 2 to 4 hours (if the patient is not vomiting) or by continuous nasogastric infusion.

Thioctic (α-lipoic) acid initially was reported to be beneficial in treating the amatoxin-induced liver toxicity in several different animal models, and a number of uncontrolled clinical trials in humans followed.[4] Because of its potential effects as a coenzyme in the tricarboxylic acid cycle or as a free radical scavenger, thioctic acid was credited for the survival of 39 of 40 patients reportedly poisoned by *A. phalloides*.[66] Hypoglycemia is a common feature of thioctic acid therapy for *Amanita* poisoning, but whether hypoglycemia results from direct toxicity of the drug or is secondary to hepatic damage is unclear. Despite the initial success, thioctic acid was not effective in various other studies and is no longer recommended.[40,41]

Several laboratory investigations in mice and rats suggest that 1 g/kg penicillin G (1 g = 1,600,000 Units) may have a time- and dose-dependent protective effect.[44,45] These results are limited because the amatoxins were administered intraperitoneally, resulting in the death of untreated animals 12 to 24 hours later. Additional investigations demonstrated that 1 g/kg penicillin G administered 5 hours after sublethal doses of α-amanitin decreased clinical and laboratory toxicity.[44] The mechanisms suggested include displacing α-amanitin from albumin, blocking its uptake from hepatocytes, binding circulating amatoxins, and preventing α-amanitin binding to RNA polymerase. None of these mechanisms is substantiated. Although the hepatoprotective effects of penicillin remain unclear,[29] we recommend a dose of 1,000,000 Units of penicillin G/kg/d intravenously (IV) be used as it is safe and possibly efficacious.[62,63,100]

The active complex of milk thistle (*Silybum marianum*) is silymarin, which is a lipophilic extract composed of three isomeric flavonolignans: silibinin, silychristin, and silydianin. Silibinin represents approximately 50% of the extract, but is 70% to 80% of the marketed product.[55] Silibinin may modify or occupy cell membrane receptor sites, thereby inhibiting hepatocellular penetration by α-amanitin. Use of silibinin 50 mg/kg in dogs 5 and 24 hours following exposure to α-amanitin suppressed chemical evidence of hepatotoxicity and lethality. Although silibinin is routinely available as a nonprescription supplement in most pharmacies and appears to be safe and well tolerated in patients with chronic liver disease, no reduction in mortality, improvement in histology at liver biopsy, or biochemical marker has been identified in a systematic review and meta-analysis.[55] A dose of silibinin 20 to 50 mg/kg/d should be used in humans, even though it is not approved as a therapeutic for hepatic disease by the Food and Drug Administration (FDA) in the United States.[63,115]

Because of its hepatoprotective effects, *N*-acetylcysteine should be given as an antidote, but no evidence for any specific benefit has been demonstrated. When fulminant hepatic failure is present, *N*-acetylcysteine should be administered until the patient recovers from the encephalopathy because of its presumptive benefits under these circumstances (see Antidotes in Depth 4–*N*-Acetylcysteine).

In animals, cimetidine (a potent cytochrome P450 system inhibitor) may have a hepatoprotective effect against α-amanitin by inhibiting metabolism,[96] but it shows no protective effect against phalloidin toxicity.[98] Cimetidine is proposed as a therapeutic intervention,[97] but no available human data support its use.

A recent randomized murine model of α-amanitin intraperitoneal poisoning treated with rescue postexposure *N*-acetylcysteine, benzylpenicillin, cimetidine, thioctic acid, and silybin was unable to show any benefit in hepatotoxicity with regard to aminotransferase concentrations or histologic hepatonecrosis.[107]

Forced diuresis, hemodialysis, plasmapheresis,[58,59] hemofiltration, and hemoperfusion[35] may be effective shortly after ingestion, but most studies offer neither clinical evidence of benefit nor supportive pharmacokinetic data for any of these therapies.[63,86,87,112,114] Most studies suggest that no circulating amatoxins are present by the time the need for transplantation is evident.[27] "Shortly after" is not defined, although these techniques are indicated within 24 hours of a documented ingestion.[36] Plasmapheresis, which is dependent on effective clearance, high plasma protein binding, and a low volume of distribution, does not remove more than 10 μg of amatoxin. Because of the absence of prospective, controlled studies of exposure to amatoxins in addition to the extreme variability of success with many regimens, multiple-dose activated charcoal and supportive care remain the standard therapy. Early recognition of exposure to amanitin is an indication for hemoperfusion, but most patients likely will no longer have the potential for benefit at the time they develop clinical manifestations of toxicity.[59] Future therapeutic interventions may be dependent on improved understanding of the hepatocellular bile acid transporter, which is a member of the OATP family.[52,67,71]

Extracorporal albumin dialysis[34] and molecular absorbent regenerating system[23] are variant detoxification techniques used in patients with fulminant hepatic failure to remove water-soluble and albumin-bound toxins while providing renal support. These two techniques permit time for hepatic regeneration or sufficient bridging time to orthotopic liver transplantation. The criteria and timing for liver transplantation in this setting are far less established than for fulminant viral hepatitis, where grade III or IV hepatic encephalopathy, marked hyperbilirubinemia, and azotemia are the well-established criteria for transplantation (Chap. 26).[85] Successful transplantations were performed in individuals whose resected livers showed 0% to 30% hepatocyte viability. In these cases, the authors did not wait for progression past grade II encephalopathy or for development of azotemia or marked hyperbilirubinemia.[85] Criteria for patient selection are essential to avoid unnecessary risk while offering the potential for survival to appropriate candidates who have no functional liver. The grim prognosis associated with hepatic coma secondary to *Amanita* poisoning has led several transplant groups to consider hepatic transplantation for encephalopathic patients with prolonged international normalized ratios (INRs; greater than 6), persistent hypoglycemia, metabolic acidosis, increased concentrations of serum ammonia and AST, and hypofibrinogenemia.[30,48,49,62,85] There are now case reports of successful liver transplantation for fulminant hepatic failure from presumed *Amanita ocreata*,[62,120] *A. phalloides*,[57,60,85] *Amanita vivosa*,[14] *L. helveola*,[77] and *L. brunneoincarnata* poisoning.[89]

To enhance the likelihood of success, several authors suggest that individuals who manifest symptoms suggestive of hepatotoxic *Amanita*, *Galerina*, or *Lepiota* spp exposure should be told of the potential need for transplantation and, with their consent, be rapidly transferred to a regional liver transplantation center.

GROUP II: GYROMITRIN-CONTAINING MUSHROOMS

$$CH_3-CH=N-N\begin{matrix} CH_3 \\ CHO \end{matrix}$$

Members of the gyromitrin group include *Gyromitra esculenta*, *Gyromitra californica*, *Gyromitra brunnea*, and *Gyromitra infula*. *G. esculenta* enjoys a reputation of being edible in the Western United States but of being toxic in other areas. The most common error occurs in the spring, when an individual seeking the nongilled brainlike

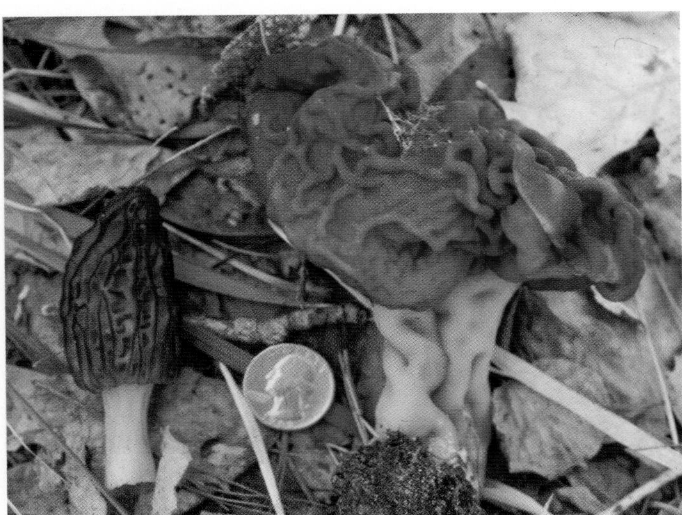

FIGURE 117–3. Group II: Gyromitrin-containing mushrooms. A true morel (*Morchella spp*) on the left is compared to a false morel (*Gyromitra escuelenta*) on the right. (*Image contributed by John Trestrail*).

Morchella esculenta (morel) finds the similar *G. esculenta* (false morel) (Figure 117–3).

These mushrooms are found commonly in the spring under conifers and are easily recognized by their brainlike appearance. Poisonings with these mushrooms are exceptionally uncommon in the United States, representing less than 1% of all recognized events, whereas these poisonings are considered more common in Europe. Certain cooking methods may destroy the toxin, but inhalation of the fumes while cooking may cause toxicity. Because of the potential for toxicity, all members of this mushroom family should be avoided.

Gyromitra mushrooms contain gyromitrin (*N*-methyl-*N*-formyl hydrazone), which on hydrolysis splits into acetaldehyde and *N*-methyl-*N*-formyl hydrazine. Gyromitrin is unstable and therefore unlikely to exist in its free form. Subsequent hydrolysis yields monomethylhydrazine. The hydrazine moiety reacts with pyridoxine, resulting in inhibition of pyridoxal phosphate-related enzymatic reactions. This interference with pyridoxal phosphate disrupts the function of the inhibitory neurotransmitter γ-aminobutyric acid (GABA).[68] The implications of this decrease in GABA, which is thought to contribute to intractable seizures associated with isoniazid or gyromitrin toxicity in a fashion identical to isoniazid toxicity, is discussed in Antidotes in Depth A15–Pyridoxine.

The initial signs of toxicity for these mushrooms occur 5 to 10 hours after ingestion and include nausea, vomiting, diarrhea, and abdominal pain. Patients manifest headaches, weakness, and diffuse muscle cramping. Rarely in the first 12 to 48 hours, patients develop delirium, stupor, convulsions, and coma. Most patients improve dramatically and return to normal function within several days. Infrequently, patients develop a hepatorenal syndrome and require extensive in-hospital care.

Activated charcoal 1 g/kg body weight should be given. Benzodiazepines are appropriate for initial management of seizures. Under most circumstances, supportive care is adequate treatment. Pyridoxine in doses of 70 mg/kg IV up to 5 g in an adult may be useful in limiting seizures (Antidotes in Depth A15–Pyridoxine).

There are no rapid diagnostic strategies in the laboratory, although thin-layer chromatography, gas-liquid chromatography, and mass spectrometry can be used for subsequent identification of the various hydrazine and hydrazone metabolites.

GROUP III: MUSCARINE-CONTAINING MUSHROOMS

H_3C — O — $CH_2{-}N^+(CH_3)_3$
HO
Muscarine

$H_3C - C(=O) - O - CH_2 - CH_2 - N^+(CH_3)_3$
Acetylcholine

Mushrooms that contain muscarine include numerous members of the *Clitocybe* genus, such as *C. dealbata* (the sweater) and *C. illudens* (*Omphalotus olearius*), and the *Inocybe* genus, that in turn include *I. iacera* and *I. geophylla*. *Amanita muscaria* and *Amanita pantherina* contain limited quantities of muscarine (Figure 117–4a, b).

Clinical manifestations, which typically are mild, usually develop within 0.5 to 2 hours and last several additional hours. Muscarine and acetylcholine are similar structurally and have comparable clinical effects at the muscarinic receptors. Peripheral manifestations typically include bradycardia, miosis, salivation, lacrimation, vomiting, diarrhea, bronchospasm, bronchorrhea, and micturition. Central muscarinic manifestations do not occur because muscarine, a quaternary ammonium compound, does not cross the blood–brain barrier. No nicotinic manifestations such as diaphoresis or tremor occur. The effects of muscarine often last longer than those of acetylcholine. Because muscarine lacks an ester bond, it is not susceptible to acetylcholinesterase hydrolysis.

Significant toxicity is uncommon, limiting the need for more than supportive care. Rarely, atropine (1–2 mg given IV slowly for adults or 0.02 mg/kg with a minimum of 0.1 mg IV for children) can be titrated and repeated as frequently as indicated to reverse symptomatology.

No current, clinically available, analytic techniques can identify muscarine, although high-performance liquid chromatography would be appropriate for investigative purposes.

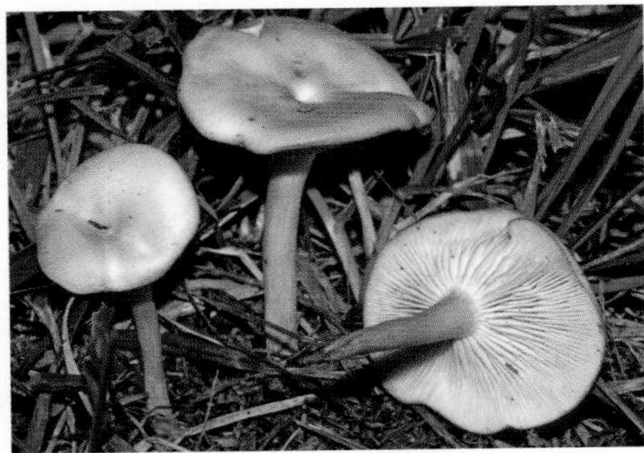

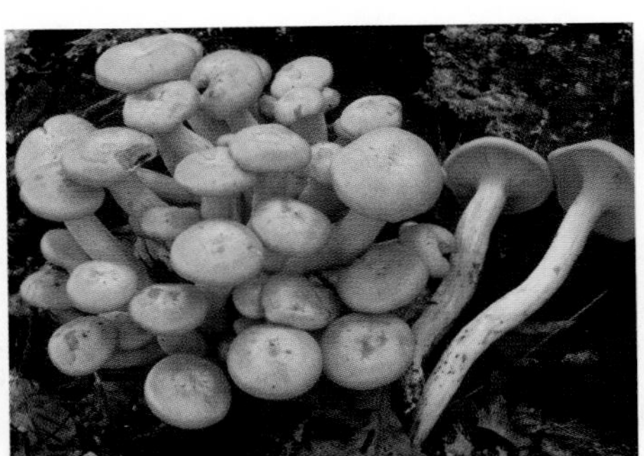

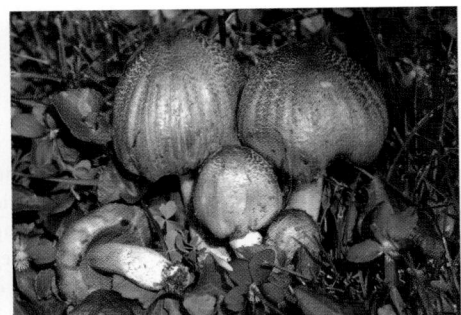

FIGURE 117–4. Group III: Muscarine- and coprine-containing mushrooms. (**A**) Clitocybe dealbata. (**B**) Omphalotus olearius and Group IV: (**C**) Coprinus atramentarius (the inky cap). (*Images contributed by John Plischke III*).

GROUP IV: COPRINE-CONTAINING MUSHROOMS

$$\text{(cyclopropyl)}(OH)-NH-C(=O)-CH_2-CH_2-CH(NH_2)-C(=O)-OH$$

Coprine

$$\text{(cyclopropyl)}(OH)(NH_2)$$

1-Aminocyclopropanol

Coprinus mushrooms, particularly *C. atramentarius*, contain the toxin coprine (Figure 117–4c). These mushrooms grow abundantly in temperate climates in grassy or woodland fields. They are known as "inky caps" because the gills that contain a peptidase autodigest into an inky liquid shortly after picking. The edible member of this group, *Coprinus comatus* (shaggy mane) is nontoxic, and probably its misidentification results in collectors' errors. Coprine, an amino acid, its primary metabolite, 1-aminocyclopropanol,[18,75,108] or, more likely, a secondary in vivo hydrolytic metabolite, cyclopropanone hydrate, has a disulfiramlike effect (see Chap. 79).[119] Although both of these metabolites appear to inhibit aldehyde dehydrogenase, the most stable in vivo inhibitory effect is present in cyclopropane hydrate.[119] Inhibition of acetaldehyde dehydrogenase results in buildup of acetaldehyde and its accompanying adverse effects, which occur if the patient ingests alcohol concomitantly or for as long as 48 to 72 hours after the mushroom ingestion. Within 0.5 to 2 hours of ethanol ingestion, an acute disulfiram effect is noted, with tachycardia, flushing, nausea, and vomiting. Interestingly, alcohol ingested simultaneously does not result in clinical manifestations because inhibition of aldehyde dehydrogenase is slightly delayed during coprine metabolism. Treatment is symptomatic with fluid repletion and antiemetics such as metoclopramide or ondansetron, although clinical manifestations usually are mild and resolve within several hours. Prophylactic use of fomepizole immediately following ingestion of ethanol and coprine-containing mushrooms has a theoretical basis, but no case reports or studies are published. This group of mushrooms rarely causes fatalities.

GROUP V: IBOTENIC ACID– AND MUSCIMOL-CONTAINING MUSHROOMS

Ibotenic acid (isoxazolone ring, N–O, with –CH(COOH)(NH₂) side chain)

Muscimol (isoxazolone ring, N–O, with –C–NH₂ side chain)

GABA (O=C(OH)–CH₂–CH₂–C–NH₂)

Most of the mushrooms in this class are primarily in the *Amanita* genus, which includes *A. muscaria* (fly agaric), *A. pantherina*, and *A. gemmata* (Figure 117–5). They exist singly and are scattered throughout the US woodlands. The brilliant red or tan cap (pileus) is that of the mushroom commonly depicted in children's books and is easily recognized in the fields during summer and fall.

Small quantities of the isoxazole derivatives ibotenic acid and muscimol are found in these mushrooms, which have been used in religious customs throughout history. Ibotenic acid is structurally similar to the stimulatory neurotransmitter glutamic acid. The stereochemistry of muscimol is very similar to that of the neurotransmitter GABA and may act as a GABA agonist.

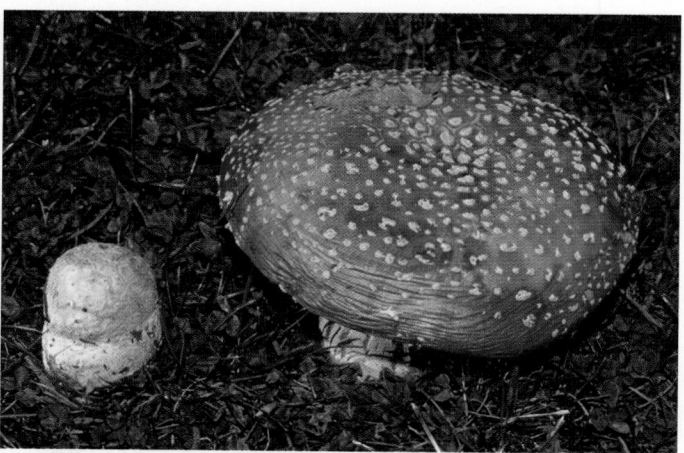

FIGURE 117–5. Group V: Muscimol-containing mushrooms. This image of *Amanita muscaria* highlights different developmental forms and colors. *(Image contributed by John Plischke III).*

Most patients who develop symptoms intentionally ingested large quantities of these mushrooms while seeking a hallucinatory experience. Within 0.5 to 2 hours of ingestion, these mushrooms produce the GABAergic manifestations of somnolence, dizziness, hallucinations, dysphoria, and delirium in adults, the excitatory glutamatergic manifestations of myoclonic movements, seizures, and other neurologic findings predominate in children.[7]

Treatment is invariably supportive. Most symptoms respond solely to supportive care, although a benzodiazepine is appropriate for excitatory CNS manifestations.

GROUP VI: PSILOCYBIN-CONTAINING MUSHROOMS

Psilocybin (indole with 4-O–P(=O)(OH)–OH and $CH_2-CH_2-N(CH_3)_2$)

Psilocin (indole with 4-OH and $CH_2-CH_2-N(CH_3)_2$)

Serotonin (indole with 5-HO and $CH_2-CH_2-NH_2$)

Psilocybin-containing mushrooms include *Psilocybe caerulescens*, *Psilocybe cubensis*, *Conocybe cyanopus*, *Panaeolus foenisecii*, *Gymnopilus spectabilis*, and *Psathyrella foenisecii* (Figure 117–6). These mushrooms have been used for native North and South American religious experiences for thousands of years. They grow abundantly in warm, moist areas of the United States. Drug culture magazines and Internet sources advertise mail-order kits containing *P. cubensis* spores to grow "magic mushrooms" domestically.

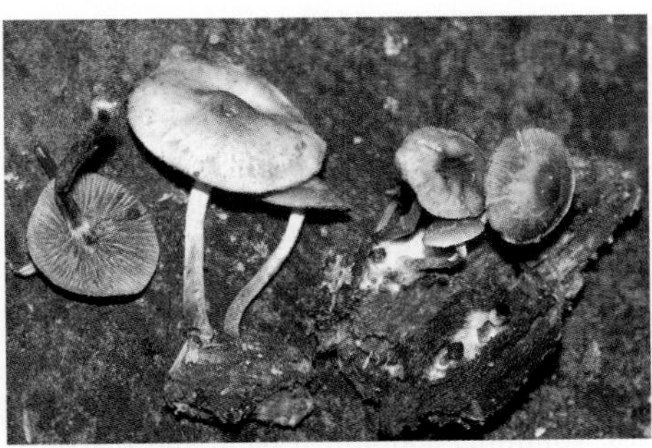
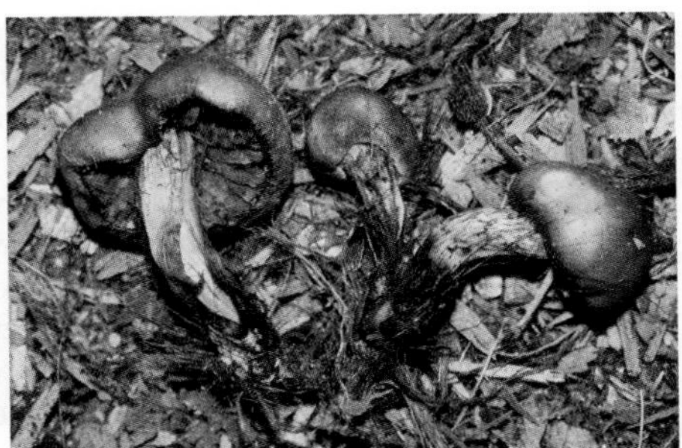
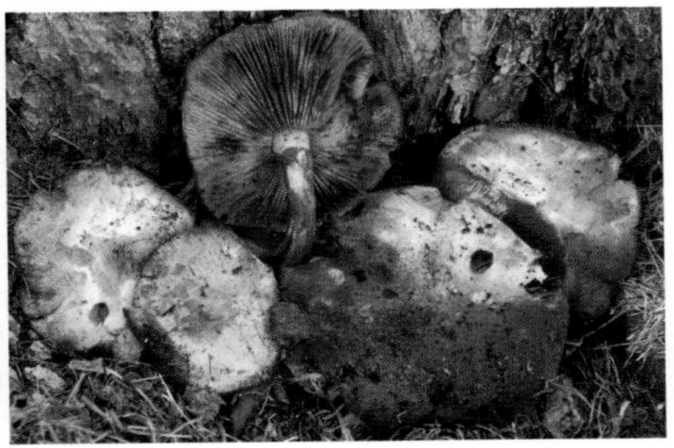

FIGURE 117–6. Group VI: Psilocybin-containing mushrooms. Three examples of hallucinogenic mushrooms: *Psilocybe cyanescens, Psilocybe caerulipes,* and *Gynopilus spectabilis*. *(Images contributed by John Plischke III)*.

Toxicity from this group is common because of the popularity of hallucinogens.[10] The quality, quantity, and variety of mushroom ingested may or may not be related to the hallucinogenic effects. Psilocybin is rapidly and completely hydrolyzed to psilocin in vivo. Serotonin, psilocin, and psilocybin are very similar structurally and presumably act at a similar 5-HT_2 receptor site. The effects of psilocybin as a serotonin agonist and antagonist are discussed in Chaps. 13 and 82.

The psilocybin and psilocin indoles, like those of lysergic acid diethylamide (LSD), rapidly (within 1 hour of ingestion) produce CNS effects, including ataxia, hyperkinesis, visual illusions, and hallucinations.[54] Rare cases of renal failure,[46,88] seizures, and cardiopulmonary arrest[10] are associated with psilocybin-containing species. However, such associations should always be questioned when reported in a substance-using population potentially simultaneously exposed to other xenobiotics.

Some patients manifest tachycardia, anxiety, hallucinations, tremor, agitation, and mydriasis. Anxiety and light-headedness may develop quite rapidly (less than 1 hour), and most manifestations are recognized within 4 hours of ingestion with a return to normalcy within 6 to 12 hours. A single patient who intravenously administered an extract of *Psilocybe* mushrooms experienced chills, weakness, dyspnea, headache, severe myalgias, vomiting associated with hyperthermia, hypoxemia, and mild methemoglobinemia.[24]

Treatment for hallucinations usually is supportive, although a benzodiazepine may be necessary when reassurance proves inadequate.

GROUP VII: GASTROINTESTINAL-TOXIN-CONTAINING MUSHROOMS

By far the largest group of mushrooms is a diverse group that contains a variety of ill-defined GI toxins. Many of the hundreds of mushrooms in this group fall into the "little brown mushroom" category. Some *Boletus, Lactarius* spp, *O. olearius, Rhodophyllus* spp, *Tricholoma* spp, *Chlorophyllum molybdites,* and *Chlorophyllum esculentum* are mistaken for edible or hallucinogenic species. A frequently reported error[3,47,111] is the confusion of the jack-o'-lantern (*Omphalotus illudens*) with the edible species of chanterelle (*Cantharellus cibarius*).

The toxins associated with this group are not identified. The malabsorption of proteins and sugars such as trehalose, and the ingestion of a mushroom infected or partially digested by microorganisms or allergy may be responsible for symptoms. GI toxicity occurs 0.5 to 3 hours after ingestion when epigastric distress, malaise, nausea, vomiting, and diarrhea are evident. Treatment with regard to fluid resuscitation, vomiting, and diarrhea is supportive. The clinical course is brief and the prognosis excellent.

Rarely, clinical presentations are life threatening, with hypovolemic shock necessitating fluids and vasopressors.[103] Resolution of symptoms usually occurs within 6 to 24 hours. The clinical courses associated with specific mushroom ingestions are variable.[7] Death is rare.

GROUP VIII: ORELLANINE- AND ORELLININE-CONTAINING MUSHROOMS

HO, HO, N+, O⁻, ⁻O, +N, OH, OH

Orellanine

Cortinarius mushrooms, such as *Cortinarius speciosissimus* (Figure 117–7) and *Cortinarius orellanus,* are commonly found throughout Europe. *Cortinarius rainierensis* is a common North American species.[17,99] The *C. orellanus* toxin orellanine is reduced by photochemical degradation to orellinine, another bipyridyl agent that is further reduced to the nontoxic orelline.[2,82,92] The toxic compound orellanine is a hydroxylated bipyridine compound activated by its metabolism through the cytochrome P450 system. Toxicologically, these molecules are similar

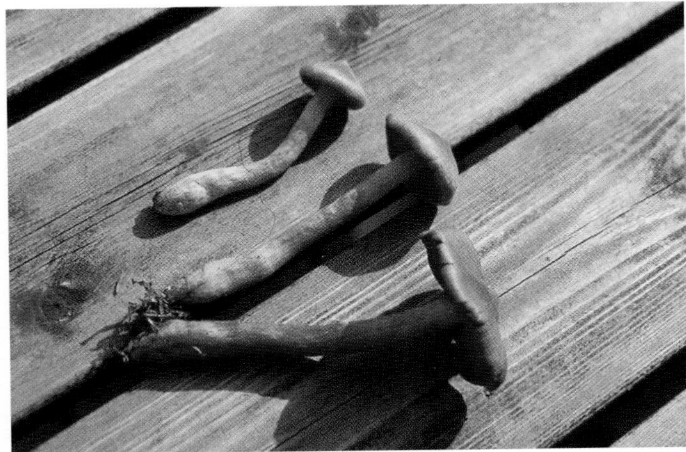

FIGURE 117–7. Group VIII Orellanin- and Orellinine-containing mushrooms: *Cortinarius Speciosissimus*. *(Image contributed by Astrid Holmgren, Swedish Poisons Information Centre)*.

to paraquat and diquat and may have comparable mechanisms of action, although precise knowledge is limited (Chap. 115). Other nephrotoxins, such as cortinarines, are isolated from certain *Cortinarius* species[105] and result in tubular damage, interstitial nephritis, and tubulointerstitial fibrosis.

Orellanine is rapidly removed from the plasma within 48 to 72 hours and concentrated in the urine in a soluble form. It can be detected in the plasma at the time of clinical symptoms by some investigators[90] but not by other investigators.[93] Thin-layer chromatography on renal biopsy material can detect orellanine long after clinical exposure.[90,93]

Initial symptoms occur 24 to 36 hours after ingestion and include headache, chills, polydipsia, anorexia, nausea, vomiting, and flank and abdominal pain. The largest case review demonstrated that numerous patients repetitively ingested the *Cortinarius* spp prior to diagnosis.[25] Oliguric renal failure may develop several days to weeks after initial symptoms.[11] The only initial laboratory abnormalities may be hematuria, leukocyturia, and proteinuria. Nephrotoxicity is characterized by interstitial nephritis with tubular damage and early fibrosis of injured tubules with relative glomerular sparing.[17,99] Hepatotoxicity is rarely reported.[11] Hemoperfusion, hemodialysis, and renal transplantation are used for treatment.[11,25] No evidence suggests that secondary detoxification by plasmapheresis or hemoperfusion is of any benefit in preventing chronic renal failure even when initiated in the first 48 hours.[25,63,90] The data are inadequate to define management or prognosis precisely, as many patients improve rapidly, while some require acute hemodialysis and others require chronic therapy for renal failure.[11] No laboratory or clinical parameters to assist in predicting the individual reactions to the toxins are available. Although case reports in the literature commonly lack definitive proof of ingestion or confirmation of toxin presence, the more rapid the onset of GI and renal manifestations, the greater the risk of both acute and chronic renal failure appear to be.[25]

GROUP IX: ALLENIC NORLEUCINE-CONTAINING MUSHROOMS

$$CH_2{=}C{=}CH{-}CH_2{-}\underset{\underset{NH_2}{|}}{CH}{-}COOH$$

Allenic norleucine

The 13 cases of *Amanita smithiana* poisoning reported have all occurred in the Pacific Northwest (Figure 117–8).[70,110,113] Because the mature specimen often lacks any evidence of a partial or universal veil, these mushrooms are not recognized as *Amanita* species. It appears that all of the poisoned individuals were seeking the edible pine mushroom matsutake (*Tricholoma magnivelare*), a highly desirable look-alike. The *A. smithiana* and *Aminata abrupta* possess two amino acid toxins: allenic norleucine (amino-hexadienoic acid) and possibly 1,2-amino-4-pentynoic acid.[21,84,122] In vitro renal epithelial tissue cultured with allenic norleucine developed necrotic morphologic changes similar to those that occur following *A. smithiana* ingestion.[84] In mice the extract of *A. abrupta* was also demonstrated to be hepatotoxic, which suggests that hepatotoxins and nephrotoxins are present in this species.[122]

Initial symptoms were noted from 30 minutes to 12 hours following ingestion of either raw or cooked specimens. GI manifestations, including anorexia, nausea, vomiting, abdominal pain, and diarrhea, occurred frequently, accompanied by malaise, sweating, and dizziness. In some cases, vomiting and diarrhea persisted. The patients typically presented for care 3 to 6 days after ingestion, at which time they were oliguric or anuric. Acute renal failure manifested 4 to 6 days following ingestion with marked elevation of BUN and creatinine. ALT and lactate dehydrogenase concentrations frequently were elevated, whereas amylase, AST, alkaline phosphatase, and bilirubin were only infrequently abnormal.

Risk of toxicity was greatest in older patients and in patients with underlying renal insufficiency. Patients who required hemodialysis underwent the procedure two to three times per week for approximately 1 month until recovery. None of the patients in the three series died.

There is no known antidote for these nephrotoxins. Activated charcoal, although of no proven benefit, should be used in standard doses when a patient in the Northwest United States presents with early GI manifestations after mushroom ingestions. The clinician will be forced to consider the circumstances of ingestion to assess the probability of *A. smithiana* ingestion as opposed to ingestion of mushrooms containing a GI toxin.

In view of the substantial morbidity associated with *A. smithiana* ingestions, historic, clinical, and/or temporal evidence of this ingestion should lead to activated charcoal hemoperfusion or hemodialysis as a strong consideration when the patient presents in the early phase of exposure. When a patient presents with renal compromise several days, as opposed to weeks, following mushroom ingestion and with a history of early, as opposed to delayed, GI manifestations, the clinician may be able to differentiate *A. smithiana* from *Cortinarius* spp exposure.

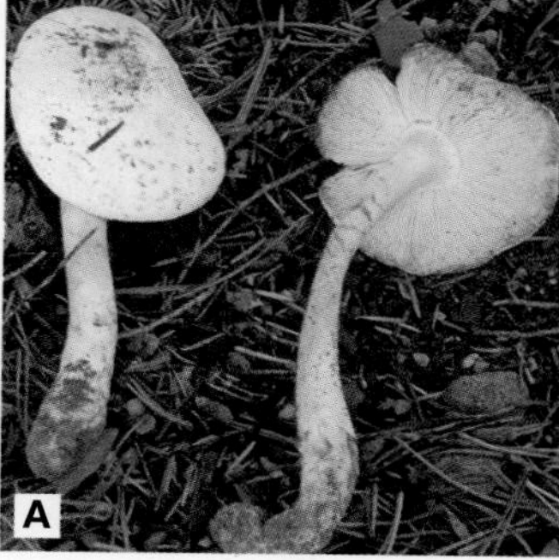

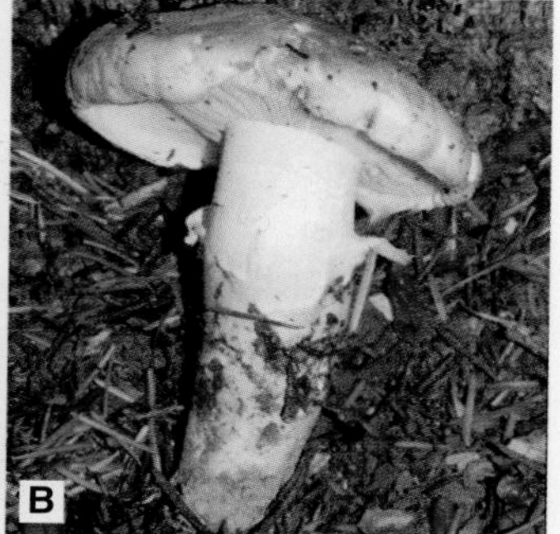

FIGURE 117–8. Group IX Allenic norleucine-containing mushrooms: (**A**) *Amanita smithiana* compared to (**B**) *Tricholoma magnivelare* (*matsutake*, the mushroom with which it has been mistaken). (*Images contributed by John Plischke III*).

GROUP X: RHABDOMYOLYSIS-ASSOCIATED MUSHROOMS

There are several reports of *Tricholoma equestre* (*Tricholoma flavovirens*) ingestions in Europe: in Poland and France, where although this mushroom is considered "edible choice," it has resumed in significant myotoxicity.[22,80] In the first report 12 patients who ingested *T. equestre* mushrooms for 3 consecutive days developed severe rhabdomyolysis that was lethal in three cases.[5] All patients developed fatigue, muscle weakness, and myalgias 24 to 72 hours following the last mushroom meal. The individuals also developed facial erythema, nausea without vomiting, and profuse sweating. The mean maximal creatine phosphokinase (CPK) was 226,067 U/L in women and 34,786 U/L in men, with some values greater than 500,000 U/L. Electromyography revealed muscle injury with myotoxic activity. The biopsies showed myofibrillar injury and edema consistent with an acute myopathy.

Dyspnea, muscle weakness, pulmonary congestion, acute myocarditis, dysrhythmias, cardiac failure, and death ensued in three patients. Autopsy demonstrated myocardial lesions identical to those found in the peripheral muscles. Although muscle toxicity was reproduced using *T. equestre* extracts in a mouse model, the etiology of the toxicity is not defined.[5] All the triterpenoids, sterols, indoles, and acetylenic compounds extracted from these mushrooms previously were assumed to be without toxicity. Currently all the clinical experience originates from Europe where these mushrooms are considered choice and eaten extensively; no cases are reported in the United States.

GROUP XI: ERYTHROMELALGIA–ACROMELIC ACID CONTAINING MUSHROOMS

Acromelic acids D and E
D: R_1 = COOH; R_2 = H
E: R_1 = H; R_2 = COOH

A poorly defined syndrome originally recognized in Japan[78] and more recently in France[8] following the ingestion of various *Clitocybe* species (*C. acromelalga, and C. amaenoleans*). The toxic substances acromelic acids A–E have been isolated. These molecules are similar to kainic acid and are of the pyrrolidine dicarboxylic acid family, which act as ionotropic glutamate receptors. The syndrome typically occurs more than 24 hours following ingestion. Patients typically develop paraesthesias of distal extremities followed by paroxysms of severe burning dysesthesias lasting several hours. The extremities show edema and erythema. These manifestations respond variably to symptomatic and supportive care and resolve completely within several months.

GROUP XII: POLYPORIC ACID AND OTHER MUSHROOM CONSTITUENTS RESULTING IN ENCEPHALOPATHY

Two groupings of toxic mushroom ingestion syndromes result in encephalopathy. In the first group *Pleurocybella porrigens* commonly eaten in Japanese miso soup without any adverse effects when ingested by patients with chronic renal failure resulted in delayed manifestations of encephalopathy.[50] Three quarters (24 of 32) of the affected patients were undergoing hemodialysis at the time of the presumed poisoning. The delay from time of ingestion to the development of an altered consciousness, convulsions, myoclonus, dysarthria, dysesthesias, ataxia, respiratory failure, or death was between 1 and 31 days. No prior toxic link or known toxin in these commonly ingested mushrooms is recognized.

The second group of mushrooms associated with encephalopathy is the *Hapalopilus rutilans* noted in Germany. More than 12 hours after ingestion an adult and two children developed nausea, vomiting, and abdominal pain; aminotransferase and creatine concentration elevations; and CNS abnormalities. Vertigo, ataxia, visual disturbances, and somnolence were reported.[65,95] In each case the urine was a violet color, the color being noted when polyporic acid is placed in an alkaline solution. Polyporic acid, a dehydroquinone derivative (2,5-dihydroxy-3,6-diphenyl-1,4 benzoquinone), a constituent of these mushrooms, is a dehydroorotate dehydrogenase inhibitor that resulted in comparable clinical and biochemical manifestation when administered to rats.[65] Symptomatic treatment is indicated with more specific therapy should hepatic or renal compromise be significant.

GROUP XIII: IMMUNE-MEDIATED HEMOLYTIC ANEMIA

A small number of patients with ingestions of *Paxillus involutus*, and possibly *Clitocybe claviceps* and *Boletus luridus*, develop a mild GI syndrome followed by an immune-mediated hemolytic anemia, hemoglobinuria, oliguria, and renal failure. IgG antibodies to a *Paxillus*-extract-containing involution[63] were detected by a hemagglutination test in these patients.[117,118]

GROUP XIV: LYCOPERDONOSIS

Puffball mushrooms (*Lycoperdon perlatum, Lycoperdon pyriforme*, or *Lycoperdon gemmatum*) are edible in the fall and can (upon decay or drying) release large numbers of spores by compression or agitation (Figure 117–9). Lycoperdonosis is directly related to massive exposure to spores, although many consider the syndrome an allergic bronchoalveolitis. This syndrome occurs in patients following acute inhalation of spores as an alternative or complementary therapy for epistaxis[104] and in adolescents for various experimental reasons.[20] Massive inhalation, insufflation, and chewing of spores can lead to the development of nasopharyngitis, nausea, vomiting, and pneumonitis within hours. Over a period of several days, cough, shortness of breath, myalgias, fatigue, and fever develop. Rarely, patients require intubation because of pulmonary compromise associated with diffuse reticulonodular infiltrates.[20] Lung biopsy demonstrates an inflammatory process with the presence of *Lycoperdon* spores.[104] Patients treated with prednisone and antifungals such as amphotericin B recovered within several weeks without sequelae.

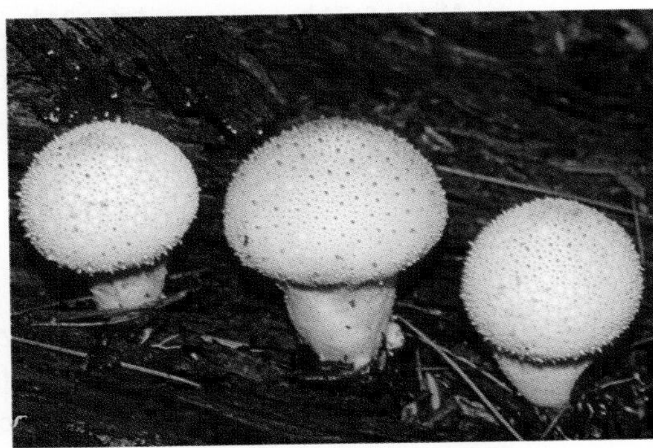

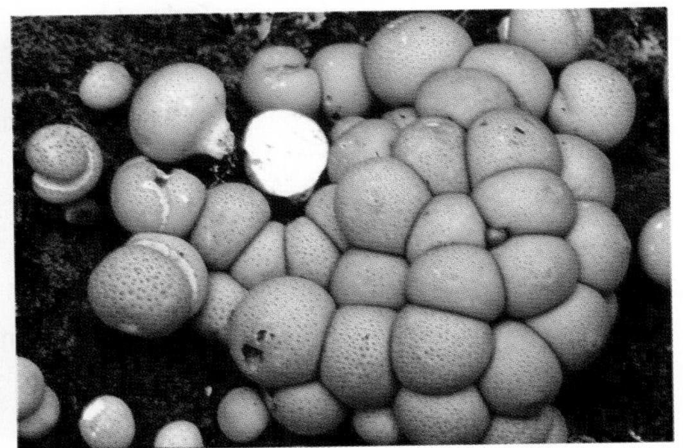

FIGURE 117–9. Puff balls: (**A**) Lycoperdon pyriforme and (**B**) Lycoperdon perlatum. *(Images contributed by John Plischke III).*

MANAGEMENT

Because ingestion of certain mushrooms may lead to toxicity with substantial mortality, patients with suspected mushroom ingestions require rigorous management. A serious effort at precise identification of the genus and species involved will make assessment, management, and follow-up easier and more logical. The basic regimen of adsorption should be initiated if potentially toxic mushrooms are ingested. If nausea and vomiting persist, an antiemetic can be used to ensure that the patient can retain activated charcoal 1 g/kg. Appropriate life support measures should be instituted as necessary. Fluid, electrolyte, and glucose repletion, as needed, are essential.

There is a wide variability in quantity and type of toxin present in mushrooms according to geography, local conditions, and individual susceptibility. The clinical course for *A. smithiana* poisoning has led us to suggest an alteration in the initial approach to patients in the northwest United States who have early onset (0.5–6 hours) of GI distress following mushroom ingestion. Prior to the recognition of this mushroom poisoning, all patients who had early onset of nausea, vomiting, diarrhea, and abdominal cramps were presumed to be poisoned by a member of the groups containing either the GI toxins or muscarine. The routine use of specific antidotes should be avoided because they usually are unnecessary.

DISPOSITION

It is important to remember that many patients with mushroom ingestions present with signs and symptoms suggestive of mixed poisonings. Whereas some ingestions produce "purer" symptom complexes than others, some ingestions, such as those of *A. muscaria,* produce GI and CNS effects, and still other ingestions, such as those of *Cortinarius* spp, have acute GI and delayed renal manifestations. Treatment or partial treatment may further confound the assessment. In addition, it is essential to remember that any acute GI disorder actually may be the manifestation of mushroom toxicity. In the spring and fall, in areas with moderate weather and humidity, it is particularly important to consider intentional or unrecognized exposure to mushroom toxins, although a logical approach to management is impossible in the absence of a precise history.

Because the clinical course of mushroom poisoning can be deceptive, all patients who manifest early symptoms (less than 3 hours) and remain symptomatic despite supportive care (Tables 117–1 and 117–2) should be admitted to the hospital. In this group of patients inhabiting the Pacific Northwest, *A. smithiana* should be of particular concern. Patients whose delayed initial presentation (greater than or equal to 5 hours) is suggestive of amatoxin exposure should be hospitalized, as should any patient postingestion who cannot be followed safely or reliably as an outpatient. Tables 117–1 and 117–2 list the characteristic times of appearance and evolution of symptoms caused by mushroom toxins and groups. Confusion may result from atypical clinical manifestations or, commonly, ingestion of several different mushrooms species, some of which may produce early symptoms and others delayed toxicity. Patients with certain types of ingestions may appear to improve initially with only supportive care. This latency period, which is characteristic of *Amanita* spp, may not be appreciated when several different species are eaten simultaneously. However, because hepatotoxicity leading to death may not appear until 2 to 3 days after ingestion (amatoxins) and nephrotoxicity may not appear for 3 to 21 days (orellanine and allenic norleucine), all patients with symptoms require subsequent follow-up.

IDENTIFICATION

GENERAL

Visualizing and analyzing the gross, microscopic, or chemical characteristics of the ingested mushroom remain vital strategies that are infrequently used. When the whole mushroom or parts are unavailable, the diagnosis must be based on the clinical presentation. No rapidly available studies in EDs or clinical chemistry laboratories are available to assist with management. The development of a rapid clinical test for amatoxins,[15,16,63] gyromitrin, orellanine, and allenic norleucine would be useful and permit early use of hemoperfusion and greater vigilance with regard to use of hemodialysis. We have not yet achieved the ability to use thin-layer chromatography, high-performance liquid chromatography, gas chromatography, or gas chromatography-mass spectrometry for clinically relevant circumstances.

Although mushroom identification is a difficult task, this section may be helpful to the clinician dealing with a suspected case of mushroom toxicity. However, it is generally best to rely on symptomatology,

TABLE 117–2. Mushroom Toxicity: Correlation Between Organ System Affected, Time of Onset of Symptoms, and Mushroom Constituent

Time to Symptoms		Mushroom Constituent		
		Early <3 h	Middle 5–24 h	Late >24 h
Organ systems	Gastrointestinal	Muscarine Gastrointestinal toxins Allenic norleucine	Amatoxin Allenic norleucine Gyromitrin	Orelline and orellanine
	Hepatic			Amatoxin
	Immunologic	Spores Involutin		
	Neurologic	Ibotenic acid and muscimol Psilocybin	Gyromitrin	Gyromitrin Acromelic acid Polyporic acid
	Renal			Orelline and orellanine Allenic norleucine

not mushroom appearances, to confirm a diagnosis. As a general rule, positive identification of the mushroom should be left to the mycologist or toxicologist.[38]

The most important anatomic features of both edible and poisonous mushrooms are their pileus, stipe, lamellae or gills, and volva.

- *Pileus:* Broad, caplike structure from which hang the gills (lamellae), tubes, or teeth.
- *Stipe:* Long stalk or stem that supports the cap; the stipe is not present in some species.
- *Lamellae:* Platelike or gill-like structures on the undersurface of the pileus that radiate out like the spokes of a wheel. The spores are found on the lamellae. Some mushrooms have pores or tooth-like structures on their pili, which contain the spores. The mode of attachment of the lamellae to the stipe is noteworthy in making an identification.
- *Volva:* Partial remnant of the veil found around the base of the stipe in some species.
- *Veil:* Membrane that may completely or partially cover the lamellae, depending on the stage of development. The "universal" veil covers the underside, the spore-bearing surface of the pileus.
- *Annulus:* Ringlike structure that may surround the stipe at some point below the junction, with the cap that is a remnant of the partial veil.
- *Spores:* Microscopic reproductive structures that are resistant to extremes in temperature and dryness, produced in the millions on the spore-bearing surface (see Lamellae). Of all the characteristics of a particular mushroom species, spores are the least variable, although many mushrooms have similar-appearing spores. A spore print is helpful in establishing an identification. A spore print viewed microscopically is comparable to a bacterial Gram stain. Spore colors range from white to black and include shades of pink, salmon, buff, brown, and purple. Spore color in general is constant for a species.

THE UNKNOWN MUSHROOM

1. The most important determinant is whether the ingested mushroom is one of the deadly varieties, especially *Amanita.* Outside of the Pacific Northwest, the onset of GI symptoms within 3 hours of ingestion does not result from amatoxin poisoning. In the Pacific Northwest, symptoms may represent *A. smithiana* (allenic norleucine) poisoning (see Tables 117–1 and 117–2).
2. Attempt to obtain either the collected mushrooms or a detailed description of their features. Arrange for transport of the mushroom in a dry paper bag (not plastic). Ensure that the mushroom is neither moistened nor refrigerated, either of which will alter its structure. Remember that gastric contents may contain spores that can be crucial for analysis.
3. If the mushroom cap is available, make a spore print by placing the pileus spore-bearing surface side down on a piece of paper for at least 4 to 6 hours in a windless area. The spores that collect on the paper can be analyzed for color. White spore prints can be visualized more easily on white paper by tilting the paper and looking at it from an angle.
4. Concomitant with step 3, contact a mycologist and use the best resources available for identification. A botanical garden usually has expert mycologists on staff, or a local mycology club can locate a mycologist. A regional poison center almost always can provide this expertise or locate an expert.
5. If none of the resources in step 4 is accessible, Melzer reagent can be useful in differentiating look-alike species and defining the presence of an amatoxin. A positive reaction is indicated by the development of a dark blue color upon contact with Melzer reagent.[72] Melzer reagent is a solution of 20 mL water, 1.5 g potassium iodide, 0.5 g iodine, and 20 g chloral hydrate. Staining a sample of the spores with one drop of reagent and then viewing the sample under a microscope helps to determine whether the mushroom is a deadly *Amanita,* with bluish-black "amyloid"-reacting round spores.
6. An additional test used by some is the Meixner reaction. Several drops of 10N to 12N hydrochloric acid are applied to an amatoxin-containing mushroom sample squeezed onto newspaper, resulting in a blue reaction.[63] The reliability of this test is doubtful, and most mycologists prefer to use Melzer reagent. Although the Meixner test is sensitive, false-negative and false-positive tests are of concern.[9]

POISONING PRINCIPLES: MYTHS AND SCIENCE

Differentiating myths from science is a difficult task in any field of medicine. This effort is even more complex when discussing mushrooms. The following principles are of great value in developing a logical approach to a potential ingestion.

1. Wild mushrooms should never be eaten unless an experienced mycologist can absolutely identify the mushroom. Even experts have trouble identifying some mushrooms, yet some foragers boldly indicate that distinguishing edible from toxic mushrooms is "as easy as telling brussels sprouts from broccoli." Remember the saying, "There are old mushroom hunters, and bold mushroom hunters; but there are no old, bold mushroom hunters."
2. The toxicology of any species can vary, depending on geographic location.
3. If toxicity is suspected, attempt to obtain samples of the mushrooms eaten and identify them. Every ED should have a readily available resource on mushrooms, such as one of the major mycology field guides.[1,13,72,73,94,101] In any case, identification is best made with the aid of the poison center's consultant mycologist.
4. Mushrooms often are implicated as the cause of an illness when, in fact, infections or other diseases are responsible. Other etiologies include the mode of preparation (the sauce or wine) or the cooking utensil.
5. There are no absolute generic approaches for evaluating the potential toxicity of a mushroom. Myths suggesting the safety or lack of safety by staining of silver, presence of insects or slugs, peeling off the mushroom cap, or the area of mushroom growth are unreliable or false. Neither odor nor taste is a good predictor of toxicity. Pure white mushrooms, little brown mushrooms, large brown mushrooms, and red- or pink-spored boletus (a mushroom without lamellae) should be considered potentially toxic.
6. Cooking may inactivate some toxins but not others. In general, no wild mushroom should be eaten raw or in large quantities. Examples of toxicity associated with lack of cooking include *Armillariella mellea* (honey mushroom), which usually is well tolerated when cooked but not raw, and *Verpa bohemica* (a morel-like mushroom), which is edible but causes illness if eaten in excess.
7. Associated phenomena may be responsible for or contribute to toxicity. Could insecticides have been sprayed on the mushrooms? Is it an alcohol-related response? Besides the well-known disulfiram reaction involving *C. atramentarius,* other good edibles, including the black morel (*Morchella angusticeps*) and the sulfur polypore (*Laetiporus sulfureus*), can cause adverse reactions if consumed with alcohol. The etiology of these adverse reactions is not understood.

8. "Edible" mushrooms that are allowed to deteriorate become toxic. Therefore, only young, recently matured specimens should be eaten when adequate mycologic support is available.
9. The finding that only some people who ate a mushroom species manifested characteristic toxicity should not exclude the diagnosis of mushroom poisoning. The degree of toxicity may be dose related or genetically determined, or a person may have a pathologic predisposition to toxicity.
10. Mushroom allergy can manifest as an anaphylactic reaction.
11. Most poisonous mushrooms resemble edible mushrooms at some phase of their growth. For this reason, even careful examination of the ring, cap, consistency, form, and color may not reliably identify the edible species. Also, characteristic features of specific toxic mushrooms may not be present under certain conditions. Although the deadly *A. phalloides* and *A. virosa* usually have remnant patches of tissue from the universal veil that envelops the mushroom in its "button" stage, rain may wash these remnants away. Similarly, a subterranean basal cup may not be noticed if the mushroom is cut at the ground level by a novice forager (Fig. 117–1).
12. Even the new in-vogue "wild mushrooms" in the specialty markets may not be entirely safe.

REFERENCES

1. Ammirati JF, Traquair JA, Horgen PA. *Poisonous Mushrooms of the Northern United States and Canada.* Minneapolis: University of Minnesota Press; 1985.
2. Antkowiak WZ, Gessner WP. Photodecomposition of orellanine and orellinine, the fungal toxins of *Cortinarius orellanus* fries and *Cortinarius speciosissimus. Experentia.* 1985; 41:769-771.
3. Ayer WA, Browne LM. Terpenoid metabolites of mushrooms and basidiomycetes. *Tetrahedron.* 1981;37:2199-2248.
4. Becker CE, Tong TG, Boerner U. Diagnosis and treatment of *Amanita phalloides*-type mushroom poisoning: use of thioctic acid. *West J Med.* 1976;125:100-109.
5. Bedry R, Baudrimont I, Deffieux G, et al. Wild mushroom intoxication as a cause of rhabdomyolysis. *N Engl J Med.* 2001;345:798-802.
6. Belliardo F, Massano G, Accomo S. Amatoxins do not cross the placental barrier. *Lancet.* 1983;1:1381.
7. Benjamin DR. Mushroom poisoning in infants and children. The *Amanita pantherina/muscaria* group. *J Toxicol Clin Toxicol.* 1992;30:13-22.
8. Bessard J, Saviuc P, Chane-Yene Y, et al. Mass spectrometric determination of acromelic acid A from a new poisonous mushroom: *Clitocybe amoenolens. J Chromatogr A.* 2004;1055:99-107.
9. Beuhler M, Lee DC, Gerkin R. The Meixner test in the detection of α-amanitin and false-positive reactions caused by psilocin and 5-substituted tryptamines. *Ann Emerg Med.* 2004;44:114-120.
10. Borowiak KS, Ciechanowski K, Walosczyk P. Psilocybin mushroom (*Psilocybe semilanceata*) intoxication with myocardial infarction. *J Toxicol Clin Toxicol.* 1998;36:47-49.
11. Bouget J, Bousser J, Pats B, et al. Acute renal failure following collective intoxication by *Cortinarius orellanus. Intensive Care Med.* 1990;16: 506-510.
12. Boyer JC, Hernandez F, Estorc J, et al. Management of maternal *Amanita phalloides* poisoning during the first trimester of pregnancy: a case report and review of the literature. *Clin Chem.* 2001;47:971-974.
13. Bresinsky A, Besl H. *A Colour Atlas of Poisonous Fungi.* Wurzburg, Germany: Wolfe; 1990.
14. Broussard CN, Aggarwal A, Lacey SR, et al. Mushroom poisoning—from diarrhea to liver transplantation. *Am J Gastroenterol.* 2001;96:3195-3198.
15. Butera R, Coccini T, Randine G, et al. Validation of the ELISA test for urinary alpha-amanitin analysis in human Amanita phalloides poisoning (abstract). *J Toxicol Clin Toxicol.* 2004;42:535.
16. Butera R, Locatelli C, Coccini T, Manzo L. Diagnostic accuracy of urinary amanitin in suspected mushroom poisoning: a pilot study. *J Toxicol Clin Toxicol.* 2004;42:901-912.
17. Carder CA, Wojciechlowski NJ, Skoutakis VA. Management of mushroom poisoning. *Clin Toxicol Consult.* 1983;5:103-118.
18. Carlson A, Henning P, Lindberg P, et al. On the disulfiram-like effect of coprine, the pharmacologically active principle of *Coprinus atramentarius. Acta Pharmacol Toxicol.* 1978;42:292-297.
19. Centers for Disease Control and Prevention. Mold prevention strategies and possible health effects in the aftermath of hurricanes and major floods. *MMWR Morb Mortal Wkly Rep.* 2006;55:1-27.
20. Centers for Disease Control and Prevention. Respiratory illness associated with inhalation of mushroom spores. Wisconsin, 1994. *MMWR Morb Mortal Wkly Rep.* 1994;43:525-526.
21. Chilton WS, Tsou G, Kirk L, Benedict RG. A naturally occurring allenic amino acid. *Tetrahedron Lett.* 1968;60:6283-6284.
22. Chodorowski Z, Waldman W, Sein Anand J. Acute poisoning with *Tricholoma equestre. Przegl Lek.* 2002;59:386-387.
23. Covic A, Goldsmith DJA, Gusbeth-Tatomir P, et al. Successful use of molecular absorbent regenerating system (MARS) dialysis for the treatment of fulminant hepatic failure in children accidentally poisoned by toxic mushroom ingestion. *Liver Int.* 2003;23(Suppl 3):21-27.
24. Curry SC, Rose MC. Intravenous mushroom poisoning. *Ann Emerg Med.* 1985;14:900-902.
25. Danel VC, Saviuc PF, Garon D. Main features of *Cortinarius* spp. poisoning: a literature review. *Toxicon.* 2001;39:1053-1060.
26. De Carlo E, Milanesi A, Martini C, et al. Effects of *Amanita phalloides* toxins on insulin release: in vivo and in vitro studies. *Arch Toxicol.* 2003;77:441-445.
27. Detry O, Arkadopoulos N, Ting P, et al. Clinical use of a bioartificial liver in the treatment of acetaminophen-induced fulminant hepatic failure. *Am Surg.* 1999;65:934-938.
28. Diaz JH. Syndromic diagnosis and management of confirmed mushroom poisonings. *Crit Care Med.* 2005;33:427-436.
29. Enjalbert F, Rapior S, Nouguier-Soulé J, et al. Treatment of amatoxin poisoning: 20-year retrospective analysis. *J Toxicol Clin Toxicol.* 2002;40:715-757.
30. Escudié L, Francoz C, Vinel JP, et al. Amanita phalloides poisoning: reassessment of prognostic factors and indications for emergency liver transplantation. *J Hepatol.* 2007;46:466-473.
31. Faulstich H. New aspects of *Amanita* poisoning. *Klin Wochenschr.* 1979;57:1143-1152.
32. Faulstich H. Structure of poisonous components of *Amanita phalloides. Curr Probl Clin Biochem.* 1977;7:2-10.
33. Faulstich H, Talas A, Wellhoener HH. Toxicokinetics of labeled amatoxins in the dog. *Arch Toxicol.* 1985;56:190-194.
34. Faybik P, Hetz H, Baker A, et al. Extracorporeal albumin dialysis in patients with *Amanita phalloides* poisoning. *Liver Int.* 2003;23(Suppl 3):28-33.
35. Feinfeld DA, Mofenson HC, Caraccio T, Kee M. Poisoning by amatoxin-containing mushrooms in suburban New York—report of four cases. *J Toxicol Clin Toxicol.* 1994;32:715-721.
36. Feinfeld DA, Rosenberg JW, Winchester JF. Three controversial issues in extracorporeal toxin removal. *Semin Dial.* 2006;19:358-362.
37. Filigenzi MS, Poppenga RH, Tiwary AK, Puschner B. Determination of α-amanitin in serum and liver by multistage linear ion trap mass spectrometry. *J Agric Food Chem.* 2007;55:2784-2790.
38. Fischbein CV, Mueller GM, Leacock PR, et al. Digital imaging: a promising tool for mushroom identification. *Acad Emerg Med.* 2003;10:808-811.
39. Flammer R. Paxillus syndrome: immunohemolysis following repeated mushroom ingestion. *Schweiz Rundsch Med Prax.* 1985;74:997-999.
40. Floersheim GL. Antagonistic effects against single lethal doses of *Amanita phalloides. Naunyn Schmiedebergs Arch Pharmacol.* 1976;293:171-174.
41. Floersheim GL. Rifampicin and cysteamine protect against the mushroom toxin phalloidin. *Experientia.* 1974;30:1310-1311.
42. Floersheim GL. Treatment of human amatoxin mushroom poisoning: myths and advances in therapy. *Med Toxicol.* 1987;2:1-9.
43. Floersheim GL. Treatment of mushroom poisoning. *JAMA.* 1984;252: 3130-3132.
44. Floersheim GL, Eberhard M, Tschumi P, Buchert F. Effects of penicillin on liver enzymes and blood clotting factors in dogs given a boiled preparation of *Amanita phalloides. Toxicol Appl Pharmacol.* 1978;46:455-462.
45. Floersheim GL, Schneeberger J, Bucher K. Curative potencies of penicillin in experimental *Amanita phalloides* poisoning. *Agents Actions.* 1971;2: 138-141.
46. Franz M, Regele H, Kirchmair M, et al. Magic mushrooms: hope for a "cheap high" resulting in end-stage renal failure. *Nephrol Dial Transplant.* 1996;11:2324-2327.

47. French AL, Garrettson LK. Poisoning with the North American jack-o'-lantern mushroom. *Omphalotus illudens. J Toxicol Clin Toxicol.* 1988;26:81-88.
48. Galler GW, Weisenberg E, Brasitus TA. Mushroom poisoning: the role of orthotopic liver transplantation. *J Clin Gastroenterol.* 1992;15:229-232.
49. Ganzert M, Felgenhauer N, Zilker T. Indication of liver transplantation following amatoxin intoxication. *J Hepatol.* 2005;42:202-209.
50. Gejyo F, Homma N, Higuchi N, et al. A novel type of encephalopathy associated with mushroom Sugihiratake ingestion in patients with chronic kidney diseases. *Kidney Int.* 2005;68:188-192.
51. Giannini L, Vannacci A, Missanelli A, et al. Amatoxin poisoning: a 15-year retrospective analysis and follow-up evaluation of 105 patients. *Clin Toxicol (Phila).* 2007;45:539-542.
52. Gundala S, Wells LD, Milliano MT, et al. The hepatocellular bile acid transporter NTCP facilitates uptake of the lethal mushroom toxin α-amanitin. *Arch Toxicol.* 2004;78:68-73.
53. Hanrahan JP, Gordon MA. Mushroom poisoning: case reports and a review of therapy. *JAMA.* 1984;251:1057-1061.
54. Hatfield GM, Brady LR. Toxins of higher fungi. *Lloydia.* 1975;38:36-55.
55. Jacobs BP, Dennehy C, Ramirez G, et al. Milk thistle for the treatment of liver disease: a systematic review and meta-analysis. *Am J Med.* 2002;113:506-515.
56. Jacobs J, Von Behren J, Kreutzer R. Serious mushroom poisonings in California requiring hospital admission 1990-1994. *West J Med.* 1996;165: 283-288.
57. Jaeger A, Jehl F, Flesch F, et al. Kinetics of amatoxins in human poisoning: therapeutic implications. *J Toxicol Clin Toxicol.* 1993;31:63-80.
58. Jander S, Bischoff J. Treatment of *Amanita phalloides* poisoning: I. Retrospective evaluation of plasmapheresis in 21 patients. *Ther Apher.* 2000;4:303-307.
59. Jander S, Bischoff J, Woodcock BG. Plasmapheresis in the treatment of *Amanita phalloides* poisoning: II. A review and recommendations. *Ther Apher.* 2000;4:308-312.
60. Karakayali H, Ekici Y, Ozcay F, et al. Pediatric liver transplantation for acute liver failure. *Transplant Proc.* 2007;39:1157-1160.
61. Kelner MJ, Alexander NM. Endocrine hormone abnormalities in *Amanita* poisoning. *J Toxicol Clin Toxicol* .1987;25:21-37.
62. Klein AS, Hart J, Brems JJ, et al. *Amanita* poisoning: treatment and the role of liver transplantation. *Am J Med.* 1989;86:187-193.
63. Koppel C. Clinical symptomatology and management of mushroom poisoning. *Toxicon.* 1993;31:1513-1540.
64. Kostansek EC, Lipscomb WN, Yocum RR, et al. The crystal structure of the mushroom toxin β-amanitin. *J Am Chem Soc.* 1977;99:1273-1274.
65. Kraft J, Bauer, S, Keilhoff G, et al. Biological effects of the dihydroorotate dehydrogenase inhibitor polyporic acid, a toxic constituent of the mushroom *Hapalopilus rutilans*, in rats and humans. *Arch Toxicol.* 1998;72:711-721.
66. Kubicka J. Neue Moglichkeiten in der behandlung von vergiftung mit dem grunen Knollenblatterpilz—*Amanita phalloides. Mykol Mitteil.* 1963;7:92-94.
67. Kullak-Ublick GA, Stieger B, Meier PJ. Enterohepatic bile salt transporters in normal physiology and liver disease. *Gastroenterology.* 2004;126:322-341.
68. Lampe KF. Toxic fungi. *Annu Rev Pharmacol Toxicol.* 1979;19:85-104.
69. Lampe KF, McCann MA. Differential diagnosis of poisoning by North American mushrooms with particular emphasis on *Amanita phalloides*-like intoxication. *Ann Emerg Med.* 1987;16:956-962.
70. Leathem AM, Purssell RA, Chan VR, Kroeger PD. Renal failure caused by mushroom poisoning. *J Toxicol Clin Toxicol.* 1997;35:67-75.
71. Letschert K, Faulstich H, Keller D, Keppler D. Molecular characterization and inhibition of amanitin uptake into human hepatocytes. *Toxicol Sci.* 2006;91:140-149.
73. Lincoff GH. *The Audubon Society Field Guide to North American Mushrooms.* New York: Knopf; 1981.
72. Lincoff G, Mitchel DH. *Toxic and Hallucinogenic Mushroom Poisoning: A Handbook for Physicians and Mushroom Hunters.* New York: Van Nostrand Reinhold; 1977.
74. Lindell TJ, Weinberg F, Morris PW, et al. Specific Inhibition of nuclear RNA polymerase II by alpha-amanitin. *Science.* 1970;170:447-449.
75. Marchner H, Tottmar O. A comparative study on the effects of disulfiram, cyanamide, and L-aminocyclopropanol on the acetaldehyde metabolism in rats. *Acta Pharmacol Toxicol.* 1978;43:219-232.
76. Meier-Abt F, Faulstich H, Hagenbuch B. Identification of phalloidin uptake systems of rat and human liver. *Biochim Biophys Acta.* 2004;1664:64-69.
77. Meunier BC, Camus CM, Houssin DP, et al. Liver transplantation after severe poisoning due to amatoxin containing *Lepiota*—report of three cases. *J Toxicol Clin Toxicol.* 1995;33:165-171.
78. Minami T, Matsumura S, Nishizawa M, et al. Acute and late effects on induction of allodynia by acromelic acid, a mushroom poison related structurally to kainic acid. *Br J Pharmacol.* 2004;142:679-688.
79. Moroni F, Fantozzi R, Masini E, Mannaioni PF. A trend in the therapy of *Amanita phalloides* poisoning. *Arch Toxicol.* 1976;36:111-115.
80. Nieminen P, Mustonen AM, Kirsi M. Increased plasma creatine kinase activities triggered by edible wild mushrooms. *Food Chem Toxicol.* 2005;43:133-138.
81. Olson KR, Pond SM, Seward J, et al. *Amanita phalloides*-type mushroom poisoning. *West J Med.* 1982;137:282-289.
82. Oubrahim H, Richard JM, Cantin-Esnault D. Perioxidase mediated oxidation, a possible pathway for activation of the fungal nephrotoxin orellanine and related compounds. *Free Radic Res.* 1998;28:497-505.
83. Paydas S, Kocak R, Erturk F, et al. Poisoning due to amatoxin containing *Lepiota* species. *Br J Clin Pract.* 1990;44:450-453.
84. Pelizzri V, Feifel E, Rohrmoser MM, Gstraunthaler G, Moser M. Partial purification and characterization of a toxic component of *Amanita smithiana. Mycologia.* 1994;86:555-560.
85. Pinson CW, Daya MR, Benner KG, et al. Liver transplantation for severe *Amanita phalloides* mushroom poisoning. *Am J Surg.* 1990;159: 493-499.
86. Piqueras J, Duran-Suarez JR, Massuet L, Hernandez-Sanchez JM. Mushroom poisoning: therapeutic apheresis or forced diuresis. *Transfusion.* 1987;27: 116-117.
87. Pond SM, Olson KR, Woo OF, et al. Amatoxin poisoning in northern California, 1982-1983. *West J Med.* 1986;145:204-209.
88. Raff E, Halloran PF, Kjellstrand CM. Renal failure after eating "magic" mushrooms. *Can Med Assoc J.* 1992;147:1339-1341.
89. Ramirez P, Parrilla P, Sanchez-Bueno F, et al. Fulminant hepatic failure after *Lepiota* mushroom poisoning. *J Hepatol.* 1993;19:51-54.
90. Rapior S, Delpech N, Andary C, Huchard G. Intoxication by *Cortinarius orellanus*: detection and assay of orellanine in biological fluids and renal biopsies. *Mycopathologia.* 1989;108:155-161.
91. Rengstorff DS, Osorio RW, Bonacini M. Recovery from severe hepatitis caused by mushroom poisoning without liver transplantation. *Clin Gastroenterol Hepatol.* 2003;1:392-396.
92. Richard JM, Louis J, Cantin D. Nephrotoxicity of orellanine, a toxin from the mushroom *Cortinarius orellanus. Arch Toxicol.* 1988;62:242-245.
93. Rohrmoser M, Kirchmair M, Feifet E, et al. Orellanine poisonings: rapid detection of the fungal toxin in renal biopsy material. *J Toxicol Clin Toxicol.* 1997;35:63-66.
94. Rumack BH, Salzman E, eds. *Mushroom Poisoning: Diagnosis and Treatment.* Boca Raton, FL: CRC Press; 1978.
95. Saviuc P, Danel V. New syndromes in mushroom poisoning (review). *Toxicol Rev.* 2006;25:199-209.
96. Schneider SM, Borochovitz D, Krenzelok EP. Cimetidine protection against alpha-amanitin hepatotoxicity in mice: a potential model for the treatment of *Amanita phalloides* poisoning. *Ann Emerg Med.* 1987;16: 1136-1140.
97. Schneider SM, Cochran KW, Knenzelok EP. Mushroom poisoning: recognition and emergency management. *Emerg Med Rep.* 1991;12:81-88.
98. Schneider SM, Vanscoy G, Michelson EA. Failure of cimetidine to affect phalloidin toxicity. *Vet Hum Toxicol.* 1991;33:17-18.
99. Schumacher T, Hoiland K. Mushroom poisoning caused by species of the genus *Cortinarius Fries. Arch Toxicol.* 1983;53:87-106.
100. Serné EH, Toorians AW, Geitema JA, et al. *Amanita phalloides*, a potentially lethal mushroom: its clinical presentation and therapeutic options. *Neth J Med.* 1996;49:19-23.
101. Smith AH. *The Mushroom Hunter's Field Guide.* Ann Arbor: University of Michigan Press; 1969.
102. Sperti S, Montanaro L, Fiume L, Mattioli A. Dissociation constants of the complexes between RNA polymerase II and amanitins. *Experientia.* 1973;29:33-34.
103. Stenklyft PH, Augenstein WL. *Chlorophyllum molybdites*: severe mushroom poisoning in a child. *J Toxicol Clin Toxicol.* 1990;28:159-168.
104. Strand RD, Neuhauser EBD, Sornberger CF. Lycoperdonosis. *N Engl J Med.* 1967;277:89-90.
105. Tebbett IR, Caddy B. Mushroom toxins of the genus *Cortinarius. Experientia.* 1984;40:441-446.
106. Tímár L, Czeizel AE. Birth weight and congential anomalies following poisonous mushroom intoxication during pregnancy. *Reprod Toxicol.* 1997;11:861-866.

107. Tong TC, Hernandez M, Richardson WH 3rd, et al. Comparative treatment of alpha-amanitin poisoning with *N*-acetylcysteine, benzylpenicillin, cimetidine, thioctic acid, and silybin in a murine model. *Ann Emerg Med.* 2007;50:282-288.
108. Tottmar O, Lindberg P. Effect on rat liver acetaldehyde dehydrogenases in vitro and in vivo by coprine, the disulfiram-like constituent of *Coprinus atramentarius. Acta Pharmacol Toxicol.* 1977;40:476-481.
109. Trestrail III JH. Mushroom poisoning in the United States: an analysis of 1989 United States Poison Center Data. *J Toxicol Clin Toxicol.* 1991;29:459-465.
110. Tulloss RE, Lindgren JE. *Amanita smithiana*—taxonomy, distribution, and poisonings. *Mycotaxon.* 1992;45:373-387.
111. Vander Hoek TL, Erickson T, Hryhorczuk D, et al. Jack-o'-lantern mushroom poisoning. *Ann Emerg Med.* 1991;20:559-561.
112. Vesconi S, Langer M, Iapichino G, et al. Therapy of cytotoxic mushroom intoxication. *Crit Care Med.* 1985;13:402-406.
113. Warden CR, Benjamin DR. Acute renal failure associated with suspected *Amanita smithiana* mushroom ingestions: a case series. *Acad Emerg Med.* 1998;5:808-812.
114. Wauters JP, Rossel C, Farquet JJ. *Amanita phalloides* poisoning treated by early charcoal hemoperfusion. *Br Med J.* 1978;2:1465.
115. Wellington K, Jarvis B. Silymarin: a review of its clinical properties in the management of hepatic disorders. *Bio Drugs.* 2001;15:465-489.
116. Wieland TH, Faulstich H. Amatoxins, phallotoxins, phallolysin, and antamanide: the biologically active components of poisonous *Amanita* mushrooms. *CRC Crit Rev Biochem.* 1978;5:185-260.
117. Winkelmann M, Borchard F, Stangel W, Grabensee B. Todlich verlaufene immunhamolytische anamie nach genub des kahlen kremplings (*Paxillus involutus*). *Dtsch Med Wschr.* 1982;107:1190-1194.
118. Winkelmann M, Stangel W, Schedel I, Grabensee B. Severe hemolysis caused by antibodies against the mushroom *Paxillus involutus* and its therapy by plasma exchange. *Klin Wochenschr.* 1986;64:935-938.
119. Wiseman JS, Abeles RH. Mechanism of inhibition of aldehyde dehydrogenase by cyclopropanone hydrate and the mushroom toxin coprine. *Biochemistry.* 1979;18:427-435.
120. Woodle ES, Moody RR, Cox KL, et al. Orthotopic liver transplantation in a patient with *Amanita* poisoning. *JAMA.* 1985;253:69-70.
121. Yamada EG, Mohle-Boetani J, Olson KR, Werner SB. Mushroom poisoning due to amatoxin. Northern California, winter 1996-1997. *West J Med.* 1998;169:380-384.
122. Yamaura Y, Fukuhara M, Takabatake E, Ito N, Hashimoto T. Hepatotoxic action of a poisonous mushroom, *Amanita abrupta,* in mice and its toxic component. *Toxicology.* 1986;38:161-173.

CHAPTER 118
PLANTS

Mary Emery Palmer and Joseph M. Betz

Five to ten percent of all human exposures reported to poison centers involve plants. Probably because plants are so accessible and attractive to youngsters, in approximately 80% of these cases the individuals are younger than 6 years of age. As indoor plants have become ever more popular the incidence of plant exposures has increased dramatically. Data compiled by the American Association of Poison Control Centers (AAPCC) give some indication of which plants are more commonly involved (see Chap. 135), but these plants typically have relatively limited toxicity. More than 80% of patients reported to the AAPCC as being exposed were asymptomatic, less than 20% had minor to moderate symptomatology, and less than 7% necessitated a healthcare visit. The benignity of these ingestions is represented by a fatality rate of less than 0.001%. This chapter addresses the toxicologic principles associated with the most potentially dangerous plants.

CLASSIFICATION OF PLANT XENOBIOTICS

Aconitine, from monkshood, exemplifies the rich history of plant toxicology. It was believed by the Greeks to be the first poison—"lycotonum"—created by the goddess Hecate from foam of the river Cerebrus. Alkaloid constituents are responsible for its toxic (and therapeutic) effects. Alkaloids represent one of several classes of organic molecules found in plants as defined by the science of pharmacognosy. The pharmacognosy approach is consistent with the literature of plant efficacy and is applied here to their toxicity (Table 118–1). Unfortunately, the science of pharmacognosy is not always straightforward, and systems of classification may vary depending on the pharmacognosist. Hence our approach borrows primarily from two groups of authors[70,190] to keep the classification as consistent as possible. The major groups are as follows:

1. *Alkaloids:* Molecules that react as bases and contain nitrogen, usually in a heterocyclic structure. Alkaloids typically have strong pharmacologic activity that defines many major toxidromes.
2. *Glycosides:* Organic compounds that yield a sugar or sugar derivative (the glycone) and a nonsugar moiety (the aglycone) upon hydrolysis. The aglycone is the basis of subclassification into saponin or steroidal glycosides (including steroidal cardiac glycosides [defined as cardioactive steroids in Chap. 64], cyanogenic glycosides, anthraquinone glycosides), and others such as atractyloside and salicin.
3. *Terpenes and resins:* Assemblages of five-carbon units (isoprene unit) with many types of functional groups (eg, alcohols, phenols, ketones, and esters) attached. This is the largest group of secondary metabolites; approximately 20,000 are identified. Most essential oils are mixtures of monoterpenes, and the terpene name depends on the number of isoprene assemblages. Monoterpenes have two units ($C_{10}H_{16}$), sesquiterpenes have three isoprene units (C_{15}), diterpenes have four isoprene units (C_{20}), and triterpenes have six (C_{30}). These molecules often play an active role in plant defense mechanisms.
4. *Proteins, peptides, and lectins:* Proteins consist of amino acid units with various side chains, and peptides consist of linkages among amino acids. Lectins are glycoproteins classified according to the number of protein chains linked by disulfide bonds and by binding affinity for specific carbohydrate ligands, particularly galactosamines. The toxalbumins (eg, ricin) are lectins. These components tend to be neurotoxins, hemagglutinins, or cathartics.
5. *Phenols and phenylpropanoids:* Phenols contain phenyl rings and have one or more hydroxyl groups attached to the ring. Phenylpropanoids consist of a phenyl ring attached to a propane side chain. These compounds are devoid of nitrogen, even though some are derived from phenylalanine and tyrosine. They constitute a major group of secondary metabolites and among plant toxins include *coumarins* (lactone side chains), *flavonoids* (built upon a flavan 2,3-dihydro-2-phenylbenzopyran nucleus, such as naringenin and rutin), *lignans* (two linked phenylpropanoids, such as podophyllin), *lignins* (complex polymers of lignans that bind cellulose for woody bark and stem), and *tannins* (polymers that bind to protein and can be further hydrolyzed or condensed).

Plant chemistry is complex. The simplified presentation of one xenobiotic per plant per symptom group used in Table 118–1 overlooks the fact that plants contain multiple xenobiotics that work independently or in concert. Additionally, different plant families may contain similar, if not identical, xenobiotics (either from conservation of biochemical pathways inherited from a common ancestor or through convergent evolution). In some cases, xenobiotics remain unidentified and are grouped in the section Unidentified Toxins.

Dissimilar molecules from diverse pharmacognosy classes that share effects are grouped together for pragmatic purposes in the section Effects Shared Among Different Classes of Xenobiotics. They are further categorized into plant–xenobiotic interactions, sodium channel effects, antimitotic alkaloids and resins, and plant-induced dermatitis.

Our focus is on exposures to flowering plants (angiosperms) related to foraging, dietary, or occupational contact, except for some gymnosperms or algae and, rarely, medicinal contact (medicinal use as herbals is discussed in Chap. 43).[132] Because our understanding of plant toxicity is poor relative to that of pharmaceuticals, animal research is included to provide a more comprehensive foundation for comparison with human experiences that may otherwise go unrecognized without such precedent, or may likewise prove ultimately incorrect. The science of plant toxicology formally began in the United States as a response to significant poisonings of livestock. The overall quality of literature for human exposures is poor and primarily available as case reports. Many of these cases lack clear links between toxin exposure and illness, and qualitative or quantitative analyses are generally unavailable. Uncertainty is compounded by the fact that plants themselves are inherently variable, and potency and type of toxin depend on the season, geography, growing environment, plant part, and methods of processing.

IDENTIFICATION OF PLANTS

Positive identification of the plant species should be attempted whenever possible, especially when the patient becomes symptomatic. Communication with an expert botanist, medical toxicologist, or poison center is highly recommended and can be facilitated by transmission of digital images or a fax.[148] Provisionally, simple comparison of the species in question with pictures or descriptions from a field guide of flora may help exclude the identity of the plant from among the most life-threatening in Table 118–1. A plant identification can also be compared with those searched in the PLANTOX database (http://vm.cfsan.fda.gov/~djw/readme.html) managed by the Food and Drug Administration (FDA). To date, with some exceptions laboratory analysis is generally not timely enough to be useful except as a tool in an investigatory or forensic analysis. As the state of analytical science

TABLE 118–1. Primary Toxicity of Common Important Plant Species

Plant Species (Family)	Typical Common Names	Primary Toxicity	Xenobiotic(s)	Class of Xenobiotic
Abrus precatorius (Euphorbiaceae)[a]	Prayer beans, rosary pea, Indian bean, crab's eye, Buddhist's rosary bead, prayer bead, jequirity pea	Gastrointestinal	Abrin	Protein, lectin, peptide, amino acid
Aconitum napellus and other *Aconitum* spp (Ranunculaceae)[a]	Monkshood and others	Cardiac, neurologic	Aconitine and related compounds	Alkaloid
Acorus calamus (Araliaceae)	Sweet flag, rat root, flag root, calamus	Gastrointestinal	Asarin	Phenol or phenylpropanoid
Aesculus hippocastanum (Hippocastanaceae)	Horse chestnut	Hematologic	Esculoside (6-β-D glucopyranosyloxy-7-hydroxycoumarin)	Phenol or phenylpropanoid
Agave lecheguilla (Amaryllidaceae)	Agave	Dermatitis, photosensitivity in animals	Aglycones, smilagenin, sarsasapogenin	Saponin glycoside
Aloe barbadensis, *Aloe vera*, others (Liliaceae/Amaryllidaceae)	Aloagave	Gastrointestinal	Barbaloin, iso-barbaloin, aloinosides	Anthraquinone glycoside
Anabaena and *Aphanizomenon*[a]	Blue-green algae	Neurologic	Saxitoxin equivalents	Guanidinium compound
Anacardium occidentale, many others (Anacardaceae)	Cashew, many others	Contact dermatitis	Urushiol oleoresins	Terpenoid
Anthoxanthum odoratum (Poaceae)	Sweet vernal grass	Hematologic	Coumarin	Phenol or phenylpropanoid
Areca catechu (Aracaceae)	Betel	Cholinergic	Arecoline	Alkaloid
Argemone mexicana (Papaveraceae)	Mexican pricklepoppy	Gastrointestinal	Sanguinarine	Alkaloid
Argyreia nervosa	Hawaiian baby woodrose seeds	Neurologic	Lysergic acid amide	Alkaloid
Argyreia spp (Convolvulaceae)	Morning glory	Neurologic	Lysergic acid derivatives	Alkaloid
Aristolochia reticulata, *Aristolochia* spp (Aristolochiaceae)[a]	Texan or Red River snake root	Renal, carcinogenic	Aristolochic acid	Alkaloid relative as derivative of isothebaine
Artemisia absinthium (Compositaceae/Asteraceae)[a]	Absinthe	Neurologic	Thujone	Terpenoid
Asclepias spp (Asclepidaceae)[a]	Milk weed	Cardiac	Asclepin and related cardenolides	Cardioactive steroid
Astragalus spp (Fabiaceae)[a]	Locoweed	Metabolic, neurologic	Swainsonine	Alkaloid
Atractylis gummifera (Compositaceae)[a]	Thistle	Hepatic	Atractyloside, gummiferine	Glycoside
Atropa belladonna (Solanaceae)[a]	Belladonna	Anticholinergic	Belladonna alkaloids	Alkaloid
Azalea spp (Ericaceae)[a,b]	Azalea	Cardiac, neurologic	Grayanotoxin	Terpenoid
Berberis spp (Ranunculaceae)	Barberry	Oxytocic, cardiovascular	Berberine	Alkaloid
Blighia sapida (Sapindaceae)[a]	Ackee fruit	Metabolic, gastrointestinal, neurotoxic	Hypoglycin	Protein, lectin, peptide, amino acid
Borago officinalis (Boragniaceae)[a]	Borage	Hepatic (venoocclusive disease)	Pyrrolizidine alkaloids	Alkaloid
Brassaia spp[b]	Umbrella tree	Dermatitis, mechanical and cytotoxic	Oxalate raphides	Carboxylic acid
Brassica nigra (Brassicaceae)	Black mustard	Dermatitis, irritant	Sinigrin	Glucosinolate (isothiocyanate glycoside)
Brassica olearacea var. capitata	Cabbage	Metabolic (precursor to goitrin, antithyroid compound)	Progoitrin	Isothiocyanate glycoside
Cactus spp[b]	Cactus	Dermatitis, mechanical	Nontoxic	None

TABLE 118–1. Primary Toxicity of Common Important Plant Species (*Continued*)

Plant Species (Family)	Typical Common Names	Primary Toxicity	Xenobiotic(s)	Class of Xenobiotic
Caladium spp (Araceae)[b]	Caladium	Dermatitis, mechanical and cytotoxic	Oxalate raphides	Carboxylic acid
Calotropis spp (Asclepidaceae)[a]	Crown flower	Cardiac	Asclepin and related cardenolides	Cardioactive steroid
Camellia sinensis (Theaceae)	Tea, green tea	Cardiac, neurologic	Theophylline, caffeine	Alkaloid
Cannibis sativa	Cannibis, marijuana, Indian hemp, hashish, pot	Neurologic	Tetrahydrocannabinol	Terpenoid, resin, oleoresin
Capsicum frutescens, *Capsicum annuum*, *Capsicum* spp (Solanaceae)[b]	Capsicum, cayenne pepper	Dermatitis, irritant	Capsaicin	Phenol or phenylpropanoid
Cascara sagrada = *Rhamnus purshiana* = *Rhamnus cathartica* (Rhamnaceae)	Cascara, sacred bark, Chittern bark, common buckthorn	Gastrointestinal	Cascarosides, *O*-glycosides, emodin	Anthraquinone glycoside
Cassia senna, *Cassia angustifolia* (Fabaceae)	Senna	Gastrointestinal	Sennosides	Anthraquinone glycoside
Catha edulis (Celastaceae)	Khat	Cardiac, neurologic	Cathinone	Alkaloid
Catharanthus roseus (formerly *Vinca rosea*) (Apocynaceae)	Catharanthus, vinca, madagascar periwinkle	Gastrointestinal	Vincristine	Alkaloid
Caulophyllum thalictroides (Berberidaceae)	Blue cohosh	Nicotinic	*N*-Methylcytisine and related compounds	Alkaloid
Cephaelis ipecacuanha, *Cephaelis acuminata* (Rubiaceae)[a]	Ipecac	Gastrointestinal, cardiac	Emetine/cephaline	Alkaloid
Chlorophytum comosum[b]	Spider plant	Dermatitis, contact and allergic	Urushiol oleoresins	Terpenoid
Chondrodendron spp, *Curarea* spp, *Strychnos* spp[a]	Tubocurare, curare	Neurologic	Tubocurarine	Alkaloid
Chrysanthemum spp, *Taraxacum officinale*, many other Composi-taceae (Asteraceae)[b]	Chrysanthemum, dandelion, other Compositaceae	Contact dermatitis	Sesquiterpene lactones	Terpenoid
Cicuta maculata (Apiaceae/Umbelliferae)[a]	Water hemlock	Neurologic	Cicutoxin	Alcohol
Cinchona spp (Rubiaceae)[a]	Bitter orange	Cardiac, neurologic	Synephrine	Alkaloid
Citrus aurantium (Rutaceae)[a]	Cinchona	Cardiac, cinchonism	Quinidine	Alkaloid
Citrus paradisi (Rutaceae)	Grapefruit	Drug interactions	Bergamottin, naringenin, or naringen	Phenol or phenylpropanoid
Claviceps purpurea, *Claviceps paspali* (Claviceptacea = fungus)[a]	Ergot	Cardiac, neurologic, oxytocic	Ergotamine and related compounds	Alkaloid
Coffea arabica (Rubiaceae)	Coffee	Cardiac, neurologic	Caffeine	Alkaloid
Cola nitida, *Cola* spp (Sterculiaceae)	Kola nut	Cardiac, neurologic	Caffeine	Alkaloid
Colchicum autumnale (Liliaceae)[a]	Autumn crocus	Multisystem	Colchicine	Alkaloid
Conium maculatum (Apiaceae/Umbelliferae)[a]	Poison hemlock	Nicotinic, neurologic, respiratory, renal	Coniine	Alkaloid
Convallaria majalis[a]	Lily of the valley	Cardiac	Convallatoxin, strophanthin (~40 others)	Cardioactive steroid
Coptis spp (Ranunculaceae)	Goldenthread	Oxytocic, cardiovascular	Berberine	Alkaloid

(*Continued*)

TABLE 118–1. Primary Toxicity of Common Important Plant Species (*Continued*)

Plant Species (Family)	Typical Common Names	Primary Toxicity	Xenobiotic(s)	Class of Xenobiotic
Crassula spp[b]	Jade plant	Gastrointestinal	Nontoxic	None
Crotalaria spp (Fabaceae)[a]	Rattlebox	Hepatic (venoocclusive disease)	Pyrrolizidine alkaloids	Alkaloid
Croton tiglium and *Croton* spp (Euphorbiaceae)	Croton	Carcinogen, gastrointestinal	Croton oil	Lipid and fixed oil, also contains tropane alkaloid and diterpene
Cycas circinalis[a]	Queen sago, indu, cycad	Neurologic	Cyacasin	Glycosides
Cytisus scoparius (Fabaceae)[a]	Broom, Scotch broom	Nicotinic, oxytocic	Sparteine	Alkaloid
Datura stramonium (Solanaceae)[a]	Jimson weed, stramonium, locoweed	Anticholinergic	Belladonna alkaloids	Alkaloid
Delphinium spp (Ranunculaceae)[a]	Larkspur, others	Cardiac, neurologic	Methylaconitine	Alkaloid related compounds
Dieffenbachia spp (Araceae)[b]	Dieffenbachia	Dermatitis, mechanical and cytotoxic	Oxalate raphides	Carboxylic acid
Digitalis lanata[a]	Grecian foxglove	Cardiac	Digoxin, lanatosides A–E (contains ~70 cardiac glycosides)	Cardioactive steroid
Digitalis purpurea[a]	Purple foxglove, Grecian foxglove	Cardiac	Digitoxin	Cardioactive steroid
Dipteryx odorata, *Dipteryx oppositifolia* (Fabaceae)	Tonka beans	Hematologic	Coumarin	Phenol or phenylpropanoid
Ephedra spp, especially *sinensis* (Ephedraceae/ Gnetaceae = Gymnosperm)[a]	Ephedra, Ma-huang	Cardiac, neurologic	Ephedrine and related compounds	Alkaloid
Epipremnum aureum (Araceae)[b]	Pothos	Dermatitis, mechanical and cytotoxic	Oxalate raphides	Carboxylic acid
Erythroxylum coca	Coca	Neurologic, cardiac	Cocaine	Alkaloid
Eucalyptus globus or spp[b]	Eucalyptus	Dermatitis, contact and allergic	Eucalyptol	Terpenoid
Euphorbia pulcherrima, *Euphorbia* spp (Eurphorbiaceae)[b]	Poinsettia	Dermatitis, contact and allergic	Phorbol esters	Terpenoid
Galium triflorum (Rubiaceae)	Sweet-scented bedstraw	Hematologic	Coumarin	Phenol or phenylpropanoid
Ginkgo biloba (Ginkgoaceae)	Ginkgo	Dermatitis, contact and allergic	Urushiol oleoresins	Terpenoid
		Hematologic	Ginkgolides A–C, M	Terpenoid
		Neurologic	4-Methoxypyridoxine in seeds only	Alkaloid, pyridine
Gloriosa superba (Liliaceae)[a]	Meadow saffron	Multisystem	Colchicine	Alkaloid
Glycyrrhiza glabra[a]	Licorice	Metabolic, renal	Glycyrrhizin	Saponin glycoside
Gossypium spp	Cotton, cottonseed oil	Metabolic	Gossypol	Terpenoid
Hedeoma pulegioides (Lamiaceae)[a]	Pennyroyal	Hepatic, neurologic, oxytoxic	Pulegone	Terpenoid
Hedera helix (Araliaceae)[b]	Common ivy	Not absorbed	Hederacoside C, α-hederin, hederagenin	Cardioactive steroid
Hedysarium alpinum (Fabiaceae)	Wild potato	Metabolic, neurologic	Swainsonine	Alkaloid
Heliotropium spp (Compositae/Asteraceae)[a]	Ragwort	Hepatic (venoocclusive disease)	Pyrrolizidine alkaloids	Alkaloid
Helleborus niger[a]	Black hellebore, Christmas rose	Cardiac	Hellebrin	Cardioactive steroid

TABLE 118–1. Primary Toxicity of Common Important Plant Species (*Continued*)

Plant Species (Family)	Typical Common Names	Primary Toxicity	Xenobiotic(s)	Class of Xenobiotic
Hydrastis canadensis (Ranunculaceae)[a]	Goldenseal	Neurologic, oxytocic, cardiovascular, respiratory	Hydrastine, berberine	Alkaloid
Hyoscyamus niger (Solanaceae)[a]	Henbane, hyoscyamus	Anticholinergic	Belladonna alkaloids	Alkaloid
Hypericum perforatum (Clusiaceae)	St. John's wort	Dermatitis. photosensitivity, neurologic, hepatic drug interactions	Hyperforin, hypericin	Terpenoid
Ilex paraguariensis (Aquifoliaceae)	Maté, Yerba Maté, Paraguay tea	Cardiac, neurologic	Caffeine	Alkaloid
Ilex spp berries (Aquifoliaceae)[b]	Holly	Gastrointestinal	Mixture. Alkaloids, polyphenols, saponins, steroids, triterpenoids	Unidentified
Illicium anasatum (Illiciaceae)[a]	Japanese Star anise	Neurologic	Anasatin	Terpenoid
Ipomoea tricolor and other *Ipomoea* spp (Convolvulaceae)	Morning glory	Neurologic	Lysergic acid derivatives	Alkaloid
Jatropha curcas (Euphorbiaceae)	Black vomit nut, physic nut, purging nut	Gastrointestinal	Curcin	Protein, lectin, peptide, amino acid
Karwinskia humboldtiana[a]	Buckthorn, wild cherry, tullidora, coyatillo, capulincillo, others	Neurologic, respiratory	Toxin T-514	Phenol or phenylpropanoid
Laburnum anagyroides (syn. *Cytisus laburnum*; Fabaceae)[a]	Golden chain, laburnum	Nicotinic	Cytisine	Alkaloid
Lantana camara (Verbenaceae)	Lantana	Dermatitis, photosensitivity	Lantadene A and B, phylloerythrin	Terpenoid
Lathyrus sativus[a]	Grass pea	Neurologic, skeletal	β-*N*-oxalylamino-L-alanine (BOAA); β-aminopropionitrile (BAPN)	Protein, lectin, peptide, amino acid
Lobelia inflate (Campanulaceae)	Indian tobacco	Nicotinic	Lobeline	Alkaloid
Lophophora williamsii	Peyote or mescal buttons	Neurologic	Mescaline	Alkaloid
Lupinus latifolius and other *Lupinus* spp (Fabaceae)	Lupin	Nicotinic	Anagyrine	Alkaloid
Lycopersicon spp (Solanaceae)[a]	Tomato (green)	Gastrointestinal, neurologic, anticholinergic	Tomatine, tomatidine	Glycoalkaloid
Mahonia spp (Ranunculaceae)	Oregon grape	Oxytocic, cardiovascular	Berberine	Alkaloid
Mandragora officinarum (Solanaceae)[a]	European or true mandrake	Anticholinergic	Belladonna alkaloids	Alkaloid
Manihot esculentus (Euphorbiaceae)[a]	Cassava, manihot, tapioca	Metabolic, neurotoxic, motor spastic paresis and vision disturbance with chronic use	Linamarin	Cyanogenic glycoside
Melilotus spp (Fabaceae/Legumaceae)	Sweet clover (spoiled moldy)	Hematologic	Dicumarol	Phenol or phenylpropanoid
Mentha pulegium (Lamiaceae)[a]	Pennyroyal	Hepatic, neurologic, oxytocic	Pulegone	Terpenoid
Microcystis and *Anabaena* spp	Blue-green algae (cyanobacteria)	Hepatotoxic, dermatitis, photosensitivity	Microcystin	Protein, lectin, peptide, amino acid

(*Continued*)

TABLE 118–1. Primary Toxicity of Common Important Plant Species (*Continued*)

Plant Species (Family)	Typical Common Names	Primary Toxicity	Xenobiotic(s)	Class of Xenobiotic
Myristica fragrans	Nutmeg, pericarp = mace	Neurologic (hallucinations)	Myristicin, elemicin	Terpenoid
Narcissus spp and other (Amaryllidaceae, Liliaceae)	Narcissus	Dermatitis, mechanical and cytotoxic	Lycorine, homolycorin	Alkaloid
Nerium oleander[a]	Oleander	Cardiac	Oleandrin	Cardioactive steroid
Nicotiana tabacum and other *Nicotiana* spp (Solanaceae)[a]	Tobacco	Nicotinic	Nicotine	Alkaloid
Oxytropis spp (Fabiaceae)	Locoweed	Metabolic, neurologic	Swainsonine	Alkaloid
Papaver somniferum	Poppy	Neurologic	Morphine/other opium derivatives	Alkaloid
Paullinia cupana (Sapindaceae)	Guarana	Cardiac, neurologic	Caffeine	Alkaloid
Pausinystalia yohimbe (Rubiaceae)[a]	Yohimbe	Cardiac, cholinergic	Yohimbine	Alkaloid
Philodendron spp (Araceae)[b]	Philodendron	Dermatitis, mechanical and cytotoxic	Oxalate raphides	Carboxylic acid
Phoradendron spp (Loranthaceae or Viscaceae)	American mistletoe	Gastrointestinal	Phoratoxin, ligatoxin	Protein, lectin, peptide, amino acid
Physostigma venenosum (Fabaceae)[a]	Calabar bean, ordeal bean	Cholinergic	Physostigmine	Alkaloid
Phytolacca americana (Phytolaccaceae)[a]	American cancer Pokeweed, poke	Gastrointestinal	Phytolaccotoxin	Protein, lectin, peptide, amino acid
Pilocarpus jaborandi, Pilocarpus pinnatifolius (Rutaceae)[a]	Pilocarpus, jaborandi	Cholinergic effects	Pilocarpine	Alkaloid
Piper methysticum[a]	Kava kava	Hepatic, neurologic	Kawain, methysticine yangonin, other kava lactones	Terpenoid, resin, and oleoresin
Plantago spp	Plantago (seed husks)	Gastrointestinal	Psyllium	Carbohydrate
Podophyllum emodi (Berberidaceae)[a]	Wild mandrake	Multisystem	Podophyllin (lignan)	Phenol or phenylpropanoid
Podophyllum peltatum (Berberidaceae)[a]	Mayapple	Multisystem	Podophyllin (lignan)	Phenol or phenylpropanoid
Populus spp (Salicaceae)	Poplar species	Salicylism	Salicin	Glycoside
Primula obconica (Primulaceae)	Primrose	Dermatitis, contact, allergic	Primin	Phenol or phenylpropanoid
Prunus armeniaca, Prunus spp, *Malus* spp (Rosaceae)[a]	Apricot seed pits, wild cherry, peach plum, pear, almond, apple and other seed kernels	Metabolic, acidosis, respiratory failure, coma, death	Amygdalin, emulsin	Cyanogenic glycoside
Pteridum spp (Polypodiaceae)	Brachen fern	Carcinogen, thiaminase	Ptaquiloside	Terpenoid
Pulsatilla spp (Ranunculaceae)	Pulsatilla	Dermatitis, contact	Ranunculin, protoanemonin	Glycoside
Quercus spp	Oak	Metabolic, livestock toxicity	Tannic acid	Phenol or phenylpropanoid
Ranunculus spp (Ranunculaceae)	Buttercups	Dermatitis, contact	Ranunculin, protoanemonin	Glycoside
Rauwolfia serpentine (Apocynaceae)	Indian snakeroot	Cardiac, neurologic	Reserpine	Alkaloid
Remijia pedunculata (Rubiaceae)[a]	Cuprea bark	Cardiac, cinchonism	Quinidine	Alkaloid
Rhamnus frangula (Rhamnaceae)	Frangula bark, alder buckthorn	Gastrointestinal	Frangulins	Anthraquinone glycoside

TABLE 118–1. Primary Toxicity of Common Important Plant Species (*Continued*)

Plant Species (Family)	Typical Common Names	Primary Toxicity	Xenobiotic(s)	Class of Xenobiotic
Rheum officinale, Rheum spp (Polygonaceae)	Rhubarb	Gastrointestinal	Rhein anthrones	Anthraquinone glycoside
Rheum spp (Polygonaceae)	Rhubarb species	Urologic	Oxalates	Carboxylic acid
Rhododendron spp (Ericaceae)[a]	Rhododendron	Cardiac, neurologic	Grayanotoxins	Terpenoid including resin and oleoresin
Ricinus communus (Euphorbiaceae)[a]	Castor or rosary seeds, purging nuts, physic nut, tick seeds	Gastrointestinal	Ricin, curcin	Protein, lectin, peptide, amino acid
Robinia pseudoacacia (Fabiaceae)[a]	Black locust	Gastrointestinal	Robin (robinia lectin)	Protein, lectin, peptide, amino acid
Rumex spp (Polygonaceae)	Dock species	Urologic	Oxalates	Carboxylic acid
Salix spp (Salicaceae)	Willow species	Salicylism	Salicin	Glycosides, other
Sambucus spp (Caprifoliaceae)	Elderberry	Metabolic	Anthracyanins	Cyanogenic glycoside
Sanguinaria canadensis (Papaveraceae)	Sanguinaria, bloodroot	Gastrointestinal	Sanguinarine	Alkaloid
Schefflera spp (Araceae)[b]	Umbrella tree	Dermatitis, mechanical and cytotoxic	Oxalate raphides	Carboxylic acid
Schlumbergera bridgesii[b]	Christmas cactus	Dermatitis, mechanical	Nontoxic	None
Senecio spp (Compositae/Asteraceae)[a]	Groundsel	Hepatic (venoocclusive disease)	Pyrrolizidine alkaloids	Alkaloid
Sida carpinifolia (Malvaceae)	Locoweed	Metabolic, neurologic	Swainsonine	Alkaloid
Sida cordifolia (Malvaceae)[a]	Bala	Cardiac, neurologic	Ephedrine and related compounds	Alkaloid
Solanum americanum (Solanaceae)[a]	American nightshade	Gastrointestinal, neurologic, anticholinergic	Solasodine, soladulcidine, solanine, chaconine	Glycoalkaloid
Solanum dulcamara (Solanaceae)[a,b]	Bittersweet woody nightshade	Gastrointestinal, neurologic, anticholinergic	Solanine, chaconine, belladonna alkaloids, eg, atropine	Alkaloid
Solanum nigrum (Solanaceae)[a]	Black nightshade, common nightshade	Gastrointestinal, neurologic, anticholinergic	Solanine, chaconine, belladonna alkaloids (atropine)	Alkaloid
Solanum tuberosum (Solanaceae)[a]	Potato (green), leaves	Gastrointestinal, neurologic, anticholinergic	Solanine, chaconine	Alkaloid
Spathiphyllum spp (Araceae)[b]	Peace lily	Dermatitis, mechanical and cytotoxic	Oxalate raphides	Carboxylic acid
Spinacia oleracea (Chenopodiaceae)	Spinach, others	Urologic	Oxalates	Carboxylic acid
Strychnos nux-vomica, Strychnos ignatia (Loganiaceae)[a]	Nux vomica, Ignatia, St. Ignatius bean, vomit button	Neurologic	Strychnine, brucine	Alkaloid
Swainsonia spp (Fabiaceae)	Locoweed	Metabolic, neurologic	Swainsonine	Alkaloid
Symphytum spp (Boragniaceae)[a]	Comfrey	Hepatic (venoocclusive disease)	Pyrrolizidine alkaloids	Alkaloid
Tanacetum vulgare (= *Chrysanthemum vulgare*; Compositaceae/Asteraceae)[a]	Tansy	Neurologic	Thujone	Terpenoid
Taxus baccata, Taxus brevifolia, other *Taxus* spp (Taxaceae)[a]	English yew, Pacific yew, yew	Cardiac	Taxine	Alkaloid
Theobroma cacao (Sterculiaceae)	Cocoa	Cardiac, neurologic	Theobromine	Alkaloid
Thevetia peruviana[a]	Yellow oleander	Cardiac	Thevetin	Cardioactive steroid

(*Continued*)

TABLE 118–1. Primary Toxicity of Common Important Plant Species (*Continued*)

Plant Species (Family)	Typical Common Names	Primary Toxicity	Xenobiotic(s)	Class of Xenobiotic
Toxicodendron radicans, Toxicodendron toxicarium, Toxicodendron diversilobum, Toxicodendron vernix, Toxicodendron spp, many others (Anacardaceae)[b]	Poison ivy, oak, sumac, many others	Dermatitis, contact and allergic	Urushiol oleoresins	Terpenoid
Tribulus terrestris (Fabaceae)	Caltrop, puncture vine	Dermatitis, photosensitivity in animals	Steroidal saponins (aglycones, diosgenin, yamogenin)	Saponin glycoside
Trifolium pratense and other (Fabaceae/ Legumaceae)	Red clover	Phytoestrogen hematologic	Formononetin, Biochanin A coumarin	Phenol (isoflavone)
Tussilago farfara (Compositae/Asteraceae)[a]	Coltsfoot	Hepatic (venoocclusive disease)	Pyrrolizidine alkaloids	Alkaloid
Urginea maritima, Urginea indica[a]	Red, or Mediterranean squill, Indian squill, sea onion	Cardiac	Scillaren A, B	Cardioactive steroid
Veratrum viride, Veratrum album, Veratrum californicum (Liliaceae)[a]	False hellebore, Indian poke California hellbore	Cardiac	Veratridine	Alkaloid
Vicia fava, Vicia sativa (Fabaceae)	Fava bean, vetch	Hematologic	Vicine, convicine	Glycoside
Viscum album (Loranthaceae or Viscaceae)	European mistletoe	Gastrointestinal	Viscumin	Protein, lectin, peptide, amino acid, lignan, polypeptide
Wisteria floribunda (Fabiaceae)	Wisteria	Gastrointestinal	Cystatin	Protein, lectin, peptide, amino acid

[a] Reports of life-threatening effects from plant use.

[b] Plants reported commonly among calls to poison centers.

advances, however, it may soon be possible to confirm a diagnosis once a preliminary hypothesis based on botanical identification or symptomology has been made.

In cases where expert identification cannot be immediately achieved, preliminary recognition of taxonomic families of poisonous plants is the simplest first step to identify or exclude poisonous plants, but is most easily achieved when the plant is in flower or fruit. For instance, if the flower is described or looks like a flower from a tomato or potato, it probably is in the Solanaceae family. Plants of this family typically produce gastroenteritis or anticholinergic findings following ingestion. It then would be appropriate to consider management with a specific antidote such as physostigmine. This approach will be less useful for xenobiotics such as pyrrolizidine alkaloids that occur in numerous different families.

APPROACH TO THE EXPOSED PATIENT AND UNDERSTANDING RISK

Identified plant species most frequently reported to poison centers are indicated in Table 118–1. In most cases, these species provide reassurance because most exposures result in benign outcomes, and only a few among these are regularly life threatening depending on the circumstances of the exposure. Given the relatively poor understanding of toxins and in the absence of complete information about an exposure, expectant management and supportive care are the rule. Even if a plant is not marked as life threatening or commonly reported, the patient should undergo a period of observation and follow-up, given the relatively immature science of plant toxicology relative to that of pharmaceuticals.

The difficult task in human plant toxicology is the lack of adequate data to determine risk (see examples in Chap. 129). Typically, evaluations of risk are based on poison center data and usually cite the numerous calls without clinical consequence as a part of the risk equation (Chap. 135).[117,135,159,244] However, poison center data are dominated by unconfirmed exposures and cases with unsubstantiated clinical manifestations (Chap. 135). These cases often represent small or nonexistent exposures, and their inclusion in the database may mask real risks by diluting "true" hazardous exposures with trivial or nonexistent exposures.[95] Furthermore, misidentification of the plant may occur because of either similar appearance or similar nomenclature.

In summary, basic decontamination and supportive care should be instituted as appropriate for the clinical situation, with consultation to a poison center. The most consequential and dangerous plant xenobiotics for humans are discussed here, and those that can produce life-threatening signs acutely are denoted in Table 118–1.

Potential symptoms listed in Table 118–1 are organized by plant name and the associated *major* organ system effects for quick reference as to the type of symptoms and their potential for morbidity or mortality. For instance, life-threatening symptoms such as dysrhythmias or seizures can be searched by "cardi-" or "neuro-" in the third column and compared with the plant(s) in question. The plants and xenobiotics that present life-threatening symptoms are so noted. Exposures associated with one of these plants or xenobiotics or major organ system symptoms dictate the need for possible prompt gastric emptying, decontamination, individualized therapy, and hospitalization. Note that nonspecific symptoms such as nausea and vomiting are listed only when they are a major cause of morbidity or mortality (toxalbumins such as ricin), but nausea and vomiting are nearly ubiquitous among acute poisonings of clinical consequence.

TOXIC CONSTITUENTS IN PLANTS, TAXONOMIC ASSOCIATIONS, AND SELECTED SYMPTOMS

ALKALOIDS: TOXIC MANIFESTATIONS

The term *alkaloid* refers to nitrogen-containing basic xenobiotics of natural origin and limited distribution. They figure prominently in the history of human–plant interaction, ranging from epidemics of poisoning caused by ergot-infested rye bread in the Middle Ages to dependency on cocaine, heroin, and nicotine in contemporary time. Numerous examples of toxic constituents of these families are given in the following discussion, which begins with a description of the major toxidromes that involves alkaloids. See also Sodium Channel Effects under Effects Shared Among Different Classes of Xenobiotics later in this chapter for descriptions of additional life-threatening alkaloids.

Anticholinergic Effects: Belladonna Alkaloids The belladonna alkaloids are from the family Solanaceae and the plants can be identified as members of this family by their characteristic flowers (most familiar from nightshade, potato, or tomato flowers). The belladonna alkaloids have potent antimuscarinic effects. Ingestion produces classic signs of this toxidrome: tachycardia, hyperthermia, dry skin and mucous membranes, skin flushing, diminished bowel sounds, urinary retention, agitation, disorientation, and hallucinations (Chap. 3). Since the 1970s, the quest for recreational "highs" has surpassed unintentional ingestions as the main source of toxicity. Hallucinatory effects are sought in seeds and teas, especially in late summer, when jimsonweed (*Datura stramonium*) seeds (Figure 118–1) become available.[31,33,91,214] One hundred of these seeds contain up to 6 mg atropine and related alkaloids, and an ingestion of this amount can be fatal.[23]

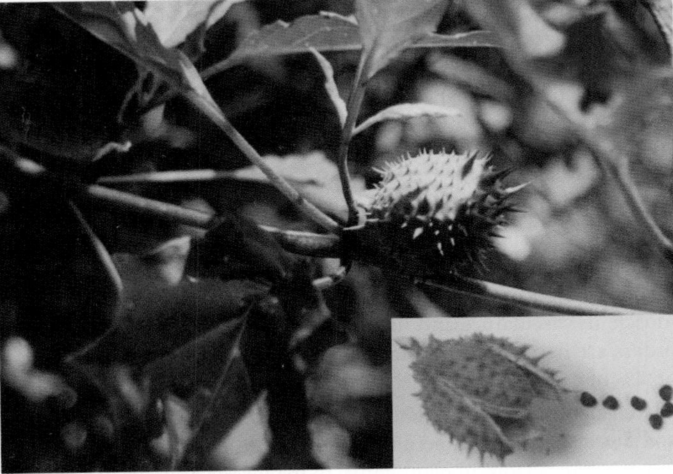

FIGURE 118–1. Jimsonweed, *(Datura stramonium)* initially has a showy white tubular flower which becomes a prickly fruit (pod) following maturation. Inset: The pod (inset) of Jimsonweed holds multiple small seeds containing atropine and scopolamine. *(Image contributed by the New York City Poison Center Toxicology Fellowship Program.)*

Although several anticholinergic alkaloid-containing species and even individual plants within species bear differing concentrations of several different phytochemicals, the clinical manifestations usually are similar. Following ingestions of the plant the onset of symptoms typically occurs 1 to 4 hours postingestion, or more rapidly if the plants are smoked or consumed as a tea infusion. The duration of effect is partly dose dependent and may last from a few hours to days.[31] The course of anticholinergic poisoning is not substantially altered by use of physostigmine, though this may be lifesaving in patients with seizures or an agitated delirium (see Antidotes in Depth A12–Physostigmine Salicylate).[59,200] Although methods for detection of atropine and scopolamine in clinical specimens are improving, anticholinergic toxicity may be observed without detectable atropine, scopolamine, or hyoscyamine concentrations in biological fluids and is better left as a clinical and not a laboratory diagnosis.

Solanine and chaconine are glycoalkaloids contained in many members of the Solanaceae family, but they are structurally and pharmacologically dissimilar to the belladonna alkaloids. The aglycone solanidine is a steroidal alkaloid. Solanine inhibits cholinesterase in vitro, although cholinergic symptoms are not noted clinically. Nonetheless, reports of solanine-induced central nervous system (CNS) toxicity include hallucinations, delirium, and coma.[149,209] However, most symptomatic patients typically develop nausea, vomiting, diarrhea, and abdominal pain that begins 2 to 24 hours after ingestion, which, like CNS toxicity, may persist for several days. Although solanine is present in most of the 1700 species in the genus *Solanum*, solanine toxicity in humans is rarely encountered. The content of glycoalkaloids in tubers is usually 10 to 100 mg/kg and the maximum concentrations do not exceed 200 mg/kg. Green potatoes and the green potato plant itself are most commonly associated with symptoms, which is not surprising because the alkaloids are most concentrated in those items. The ingestion of 1 to 3 mg of glycoalkaloid per kilogram of body weight is likely to produce clinical symptoms.[198] Most reports of death come from the older literature,[3] and consumption of 2 to 5 g of green components of potatoes per kilogram of body weight per day is not predicted to cause acute toxicity.[177]

Nicotine and Alkaloids with Nicotinelike Activity: Nicotine, Anabasine, Lobeline, Sparteine, *N*-Methylcytisine, Cytisine, and Coniine Nicotine toxicity (other than from inhaled sources) occurs via ingestion of leaves of *Nicotiana tabacum*, cigarette remains, organic products, and insecticides, and transdermally among farm workers harvesting tobacco (green tobacco sickness).[182] A topical folk remedy made from the leaf of *Nicotiana glauca* (tree tobacco) caused anabasine toxicity in an infant.[162] The free bases of nicotine and anabasine are pale yellow oils at room temperature and readily penetrate the intact dermis. A dose of nicotine as small as 1 mg/kg of body weight can be lethal to an adult.[145] Overstimulation of the nicotinic receptors by high doses of the alkaloid produces nicotinism, a toxidrome that progresses from gastrointestinal (GI) symptoms to diaphoresis, mydriasis, fasciculations, tachycardia, hypertension, hyperthermia, and seizures, respiratory depression, and death (Chap. 84). Wearing of protective clothing is essential for tobacco farm workers to prevent green tobacco sickness.[8]

These manifestations are also produced by alkaloids other than nicotine.[236] There are no recent reports of nicotinic toxicity from lobeline (found in all parts of *Lobelia inflata*), although its use in the 18th century resulted in morbidity and mortality.

Sparteine from broom (*Cytisus scoparius*) and *N*-methylcytisine from blue cohosh (*Caulophyllum thalictroides*)[184] are examples of alkaloids that produce nicotinelike effects. Laburnum or golden chain (*Cytisus laburnum*) contains cytisine, which reportedly is responsible for mass poisonings and fatalities in children and adults who eat the plants or parts thereof (even as little as 0.5 mg/kg, or a few peas).[158] Unfortunately, such reports have resulted in thousands of unnecessary hospital admissions for patients without morbidity and mortality after ingestion of this plant, demonstrating the difficulty in separating hazard from risk and in obtaining accurate dose–response information in the setting of plant exposures and human variability.[95]

The most famous description of the end stages of nicotinic toxicity dates from approximately 2400 years ago by an observer of Socrates' fatal ingestion of a decoction of poison hemlock (*Conium maculatum*).[187]

> . . . the person who had administered the poison went up to him and examined for some little time his feet and legs, and then squeezing his foot strongly asked whether he felt him. Socrates replied that he did not and said to us when the effect of the poison reached his heart, Socrates would depart.

Birds do not experience coniine toxicity but provide a vector for poisoning. According to the book of Exodus, quail that fed on seeds (presumably from poison hemlock) became toxic and passed the toxicity on to the Israelites who ate the fowl.[20] In the 20th century, people have succumbed to hemlock poisoning following their avian repasts. This is especially well documented in Italy, where the toxic alkaloid coniine subsequently was detected in bird meat, as well as in the blood, urine, and tissue of some individuals.[189,203]

The age of the plant seems to be directly correlated with increasing concentrations of coniine, whereas the toxin γ-coniceine occurs in greater amounts in new growth; hence, the plant remains toxic over the entire growing season.[60] Fatal poisonings are reported on multiple continents, and death may result from respiratory arrest.[18] Of 17 poisoned Italian patients, all had elevated liver aminotransferases and myoglobin concentrations, and five had acute tubular necrosis. Death developed 1 to 16 days following ingestion.[189]

Cholinergic Effects in Alkaloids: Arecoline, Physostigmine, and Pilocarpine Betel chewing has been a habitual practice in the East since ancient times. The "quid" consists of betel nut (*Areca catechu*) and other ingredients. The effects of acute exposure to arecoline, the major alkaloid, include sweating, salivation, hyperthermia, and rarely death.[55] Prolonged use is linked to dental decay and oral cancer. Physostigmine is an alkaloid derived from the Calabar bean (*Physostigma venenosum*), where it is present in concentrations of 0.15% (see Antidotes in Depth A12–Physostigmine Salicylate). Pilocarpine is derived from *Pilocarpus jaborandi* from South America. Its stimulatory effects on muscarinic receptors have proven valuable in the treatment of glaucoma.[70] Reversal of toxicity can be achieved by atropine.

Psychotropic Alkaloids: Lysergic Acid and Mescaline Hallucinations from the direct serotonin effects of lysergic acid diethylamide (LSD) and its derivatives, and from the amphetaminelike serotonin effects of the mescaline alkaloids are reported following ingestion of morning glory seeds (*Ipomoea* spp) and peyote cactus (*Lophophora williamsii*), respectively (Chap. 82). Despite their chemical relatedness to LSD, molecules such as lysergic acid amide and lysergic acid ethylamide, found in Hawaiian baby woodrose seeds (*Argyreia nervosa*) produce anticholinergic symptoms.[22]

Alkaloidal Central Nervous System Stimulants and Depressants: Ephedrine, Synephrine, Cathinone, and Opioids The use of ephedrine-containing *Ephedra* spp. in herbal dietary supplement products was banned by the FDA in 2004 because of the associated cardiovascular toxicity and deaths.[205] Varieties of *Sida cordifolia* also contain ephedrine. Synephrine, a xenobiotic structurally related to ephedrine, occurs in bitter orange (*Citrus aurantium*), which is ingested as a plant, in foods such as marmalades, as a dietary supplement, or as a traditional medicine. Deaths and drug interactions can ensue from their use. Although illegal in the United States, another plant ingested for its CNS stimulant activity is khat (*Catha edulis*). The plant contains cathinone (α-aminopropiophenone) and cathine [(+)-norpseudoephedrine]. In addition, opioids derived from the poppy plant (*Papaver* spp) are prototypic CNS depressants and analgesics (Chap. 38).

Pyrrolizidine Alkaloids Pyrrolizidine alkaloids are widely distributed both botanically and geographically. Approximately half of the 350 different pyrrolizidine alkaloids characterized to date possess the structural characteristics to render them toxic when ingested. Pyrrolizidine alkaloids are found in 6000 plants and in 13 plant families, but are most heavily represented within the Boraginaceae, Compositae, and Fabaceae families. Within these families, the genera *Heliotropium*, *Senecio*, and *Crotalaria*, respectively, are particularly notable for their content of toxic pyrrolizidine alkaloids.[220] These hepatotoxic alkaloids all contain an unsaturated 1-hydroxymethyl pyrrolizidine system.[80] The hepatic cytochrome P450 (CYP) system converts these compounds to highly reactive pyrroles in vivo. Chronic exposures can result in diagnostic hepatic venoocclusive disease (HVOD) by stimulating proliferation of the intima of hepatic vasculature. Poisonings occur as a result of use of pyrrolizidine-rich plants for medicinal purposes[193,194] and by contamination of food grain with seeds of pyrrolizidine-alkaloid-containing plants. Acute poisoning resulting in loss of hepatocellular function can occur following ingestion of 10 to 20 mg of pyrrolizidine alkaloid and is probably caused by an oxidant effect producing hepatic necrosis. An estimated 20% of patients with acute pyrrolizidine alkaloid poisoning die, 50% recover completely, and the rest develop subacute or chronic manifestations of HVOD.[13] Pyrrolizidine alkaloids are teratogenic and are also transmitted through breast milk. Pyrrolizidine alkaloids may be present in bee pollen and have been reported in honey.[21] Other types of plant-associated hepatic disorders are discussed in Effects Shared Among Different Classes of Xenobiotics.

Isoquinoline Alkaloids: Sanguinarine, Berberine, and Hydrastine Adverse effects on human health due to consumption of edible mustard oil adulterated with argemone oil have been reported. The clinical manifestation of the disease are described as dropsy.[48] Sanguinarine was detected in 26 family members who consumed a mustard oil contaminated with seeds of *Argemone mexicana*.[207] All patients suffered GI distress followed by peripheral edema, skin darkening, erythema, skin lesions, perianal itching, anemia, and hepatomegaly. Ascites developed in 12%, and myocarditis and congestive heart failure occurred in approximately a third of affected individuals. Alterations in redox potentials and antioxidants in plasma may be responsible for the histopathological changes including swollen hepatocytes, fluid accumulation in spaces of Disse Kupffer cell hyperplasia.[12] Medicinally, sanguinarine is used for dental hygiene.[99] In North America, sanguinarine is found in blood root (*Sanguinaria canadensis*), which like *Argemone*, is in the Ranuculaceae family.

Berberine is structurally similar to sanguinarine and reportedly also has cardiac depressant effects.[129] A number of medicinal plants contain berberine, including goldenseal (*Hydrastis canadensis*), Oregon grape (*Mahonia* spp), and barberry (*Berberis* spp). It causes myocardial and respiratory depression and contraction of smooth muscle in vasculature and the uterus. Strychninelike movement disorders are described following ingestion of hydrastine, which makes up 4% of goldenseal.

Miscellaneous Other Alkaloids: Emetine/Cephaline, Strychnine/Curare, and Swainsonine Emetine and cephaline are derived from *Cephaelis ipecacuanha*, a tropical plant native to the forests of Bolivia and Brazil. They are the principal active constituents in syrup of ipecac, which produces emesis. Chronic use of syrup of ipecac, typically by patients with eating disorders or Munchausen syndrome by proxy, can lead to cardiomyopathy, smooth muscle dysfunction, myopathies, electrolyte and acid–base disturbances related to excessive vomiting, and death (see Antidotes in Depth A1–Syrup of Ipecac). Poisoning in patients ingesting plant material is not reported.

Curare was used as an arrow poison derived from plants of the genus *Strychnos* as well as *Chondrodendron,* but the plants and their phytochemicals produce very different clinical effects. The convulsant alkaloids strychnine and brucine are found in various members of the genus *Strychnos.* Although used to produce arrow poison, the more widespread use of *Strychnos* spp in Africa was for trial by ordeal.[176] The seeds of *Strychnos nux-vomica* are especially rich in strychnine, which causes muscular spasms and rigidity by antagonizing glycine receptors in the spinal cord and brainstem. The plant is used as an herbal remedy for arthritis pain called "maqianzi," which if improperly processed produces muscle spasm and weakness, including respiratory muscles (Chap. 112).

Curare is the name given to the unstandardized extract of the bark of *Chondrodendron tomentosum* and certain members of the genus *Strychnos.* The physiologically active xenobiotic of curare from *Chondrodendron* is d-tubocurarine chloride, a competitive antagonist of acetylcholine at nicotinic receptors in the neuromuscular junction. The pharmacology and potential applications of curare are great, as it is the molecule from which most nondepolarizing neuromuscular blockers are derived (Chap. 68). Plant poisoning is recorded solely with its traditional use as a hunting poison.[19,181]

Swainsonine has been isolated from *Swainsonia canescens, Astragalus lentiginosis* (spotted locoweed), *Sida carpinifolia,* other species of *Swainsonia* and *Astragalus,* as well as several species in the genera *Oxytropis* and *Ipomoea,* and several fungi.[43] After subsisting on seeds containing swainsonine for nearly 4 months, a naturalist forager manifested profound muscular weakness and died in the wilderness.[116] The compound is teratogenic and causes chronic neurologic disease called "locoism," with weakness and failure to thrive in livestock. Swainsonine inhibits the glycosylation of glycoproteins by α-mannosidase II of the Golgi apparatus, resulting in a lysosomal storage disease. Swainsonine was used with some success in clinical trials for treatment of advanced neoplasms. Adverse effects included hepatic, pancreatic, and respiratory manifestations, as well as lethargy and nausea.

GLYCOSIDES

Glycosides yield a sugar or sugar derivative (the glycone) and a nonsugar moiety (the aglycone) upon hydrolysis. The nonsugar or aglycone group determines the subtype of glycoside. For instance, the cardiac glycosides have saponin (steroid) aglycone groups and are placed among the saponin glycosides.

Saponin Glycosides: Cardiac Glycosides, Glycyrrhizin, Ilex Saponins

Poisoning by virtually all *cardioactive steroidal glycosides* is clinically indistinguishable from poisoning by digoxin (Chap. 64), which itself is a cardioactive steroid derived from *Digitalis lanata.* However, compared with toxicity from pharmaceutical digoxin, toxicity resulting from the cardioactive steroidal glycosides found in plants has markedly different pharmacokinetic characteristics. For example, digitoxin in *Digitalis* species has a plasma half-life as long as 192 hours (average 168 hours).

The pharmacologic properties are true across taxonomic boundaries. Poisonings by *Digitalis* spp,[166,183,188,208] squill (*Urginea* spp),[230] lily of the valley,[119] oleander (*Nerium* spp),[126,130,241] yellow oleander (*Thevetia* spp,[62,64] and *Cerbera manghas*[63] are clinically similar (Figure 118–2). The potency of these effects depends on the specific cardioactive glycoside constituents and their dose. For instance, lily of the valley is rarely

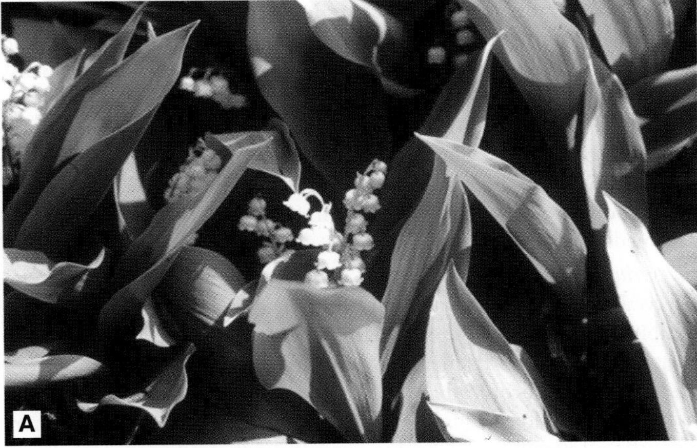

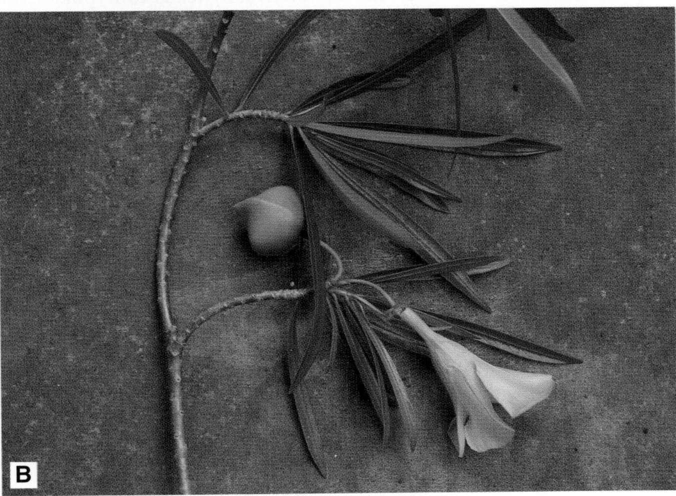

FIGURE 118–2. Saponin-glycoside containing plants: (**A**) Lily of the Valley *(Convallaria majalis)* contains the cardioactive steroid convallatoxin. (**B**) Yellow oleander *(Thevetia peruviana)* contains a cardioactive steroid, thevetin. *(Image contributed by Darren Roberts, M.D.)*

associated with morbidity or mortality, whereas ingestion of only two seeds of yellow oleander by adults can produce severe symptoms, and expected outcome is grave if more than four seeds are consumed.[62] Poisonings by oleander and yellow oleander occur predominantly in the Mediterranean and in the Near and Far East. These two plants are popular attractive ornamentals and commonly result in poisoning in the United States and Europe.

Patients experience vomiting within several hours, followed by hyperkalemia, conduction delays, and increased automaticity (bradycardia and tachydysrhythmias). Interestingly, the cardiac manifestations may be difficult to distinguish from those produced by plants with sodium channel blockers (see section sodium channel effects). Activated charcoal was beneficial in preventing death after suicide attempts with yellow oleander in Sri Lanka and its use should not be delayed in the face of uncertain plant identity.[53] Antibody therapy reduces mortality threefold from yellow oleander poisoning but is too expensive for developing countries where oleander-induced mortality is highest.[64,65] In addition, various cardioactive steroids respond differently to therapeutic use of digoxin-specific antibody fragments (Fab). Use of very large doses of digoxin-specific antibody (up to 37 vials reported in one case[188]) may be necessary to capitalize on the therapeutic cross-reactivity between antibody and the nondigoxin cardioactive steroids. The potential for success should lead to use of antibody therapy without delay when available.[199] Similarly, there is variable cross-reactivity among the individual plant cardioactive steroids with regard to the degree to which each elevates diagnostic polyclonal digoxin assay measurements in clinical laboratories.[49] These measurements can be used only as qualitative proof of exposure but not as quantitative indicators of the exposure, because the elevations can result in marked *underestimation* of the "functional digoxin concentrations." Until more is known, any positive digoxin concentration following exposure to a plant should be assumed to be significant.

Glycyrrhizin. Glycyrrhizin is a saponin glycoside derived from *Glycyrrhiza glabra* (licorice) and other *Glycyrrhiza* spp. Glycyrrhizin inhibits 11-β-hydroxysteroid dehydrogenase, an enzyme that converts cortisol to cortisone.[186] When large amounts of licorice root are consumed chronically, cortisol concentrations rise, resulting in pseudo-hyperaldosteronism because of its affinity for renal mineralocorticoid receptors.[72] Chronic use eventually leads to hypokalemia with muscle weakness, sodium and water retention, hypertension, and dysrhythmias.[106,253] Assessment involves evaluation of the patient's fluid and electrolytes, and electrocardiogram. Potassium replacement is the most common necessary intervention.

***Ilex* Species.** Holly berries from more than 300 *Ilex* spp are a common and attractive ingestant among children, especially during winter holidays. They contain a mixture of alkaloids, polyphenols, saponin glycosides, steroids, and triterpenes.[248] Saponin glycosides appear to be responsible for GI symptoms such as nausea, vomiting, diarrhea, and abdominal cramping that result from ingestion of the berries. Experimental data in animals suggest hemolysis as well as cardiotonic effects, but these are unreported in humans.[243] CNS depression was reported in a case in which a child consumed a "handful" of berries; however, this child was also treated with syrup of ipecac.[192] The toxic quantity is undefined, but one study suggested that no untoward effects are to be expected for ingestions of fewer than six berries.[243] Symptoms may be expected to be restricted to GI effects, and treatment is supportive.

Cyanogenic Glycosides: (S)-Sambunigrin, Amygdalin, Linamarin, and Cyacasin Cyanogenic glycosides yield hydrogen cyanide on complete hydrolysis. These glycosides are represented in a broad range of taxa and in approximately 2500 plant species.[235] The species that are most important to humans are cassava (*Manihot esculenta*), which contains linamarin, and *Prunus* spp, which contain amygdalin. Cycad toxins are neurotoxic or pseudocyanogenic. Rare reports of cyanide poisoning associated with (*S*)-sambunigrin in European elderberry (*Sambucus nigra*; sambunigrin) are more severe when these ingestions include leaves as well as berries.[34]

Many North American species of plants contain cyanogenic compounds, including ornamental *Pyracantha*, *Passiflora*, and *Hydrangea* spp, which either do not release cyanide or are rarely consumed in quantities sufficient to result in toxicity. On the other hand, although the fleshy fruit of *Prunus* spp in the Rosaceae are nontoxic (apricots, peaches, pears, apples, and plums), the leaves, bark, and seed kernels contain amygdalin, which is metabolized to cyanide.[30] Sufficient cyanide can be absorbed to cause acute poisoning.[223] Amygdalin was the active ingredient of Laetrile, an apricot pit extract promoted in the 1970s for its supposed selective toxicity to tumor cells. Its sale was restricted in the United States because it lacked efficacy and safety.[156] However, patients went to other countries for Laetrile therapy, which was marketed as "vitamin B-17," and available through alternative medicine providers.[250] The manifestations of cyanide poisoning and treatment involving use of the cyanide antidote kit are detailed elsewhere (Chap. 126 and Antidotes in Depth: A38 Sodium and amyl nitrite, A39 Sodium Thiosulfate; and A40 Hydroxcobalamin).

Acute and chronic cyanide toxicity (including deaths) associated with consumption of inadequately prepared cassava (*M. esculenta*) are reported worldwide (Chap. 126).[2] Chronic manifestations include visual disturbances (amblyopia), upper motor neuron disease with spastic paraparesis, and hypothyroidism. These findings are associated with protein-deficient states and the use of tobacco and alcohol. The ataxic neuropathy resembles that produced by lathyrism (see section Proteins, Peptides, and Lectins). A unifying hypothesis about the etiology of these two similar diseases from seemingly very different sources is that thiocyanate accumulation may lead to degeneration of the α-amino-3-hydroxy-5-methyl-isoxazole-4-propionic acid (AMPA)-containing neurons that are first stimulated and then destroyed in neurolathyrism.[212]

Similarly, seeds of cycads contain cycasin and neocycasin, which belong to the family of cyanogenic glycosides, as well as neurotoxins associated with consumption of indigenous food. The cyanogenic glycosides of cycads are considered pseudocyanogenic, with little potential to liberate hydrogen cyanide, but most typically produce violent vomiting 30 minutes to 7 hours after ingestion of one to 30 seeds.[40] On the island of Guam, indigenous peoples develop a devastating amyotrophic lateral sclerosis-parkinsonism dementia complex (ALS-PDC) that appears associated with ingestion of *Cycas circinalis* seeds or the flying foxes that feed extensively upon the cycads.[44] The implicated xenobiotic originally was believed to be an excitatory amino acid,[26] but more recently is identified as a sterol glycoside.[217] Research on the mechanism of this cycad-induced disease is ongoing, with the goal of understanding potential mechanisms of this disease and its links to ALS and Parkinson disease.[78]

Anthraquinone Glycosides: Sennoside and Others Anthraquinone laxatives are regulated both as nonprescription pharmaceuticals and as dietary supplements. These glycosides, such as sennoside, are metabolized in the bowel to produce derivatives that stimulate colonic motility, probably by inhibiting Na^+-K^+ adenosine triphosphatase (ATPase) in the intestine, which also promote accumulation of water and electrolytes in the gut lumen, producing fluid and electrolyte shifts that can be life threatening.[216]

Other Glycosides: Salicin, Atractyloside, Carboxyatractyloside, Vicine, Convicine Salicin is an inactive glycoside until it is hydrolyzed to produce salicylic acid (Chap. 35). The glycosidic bond is relatively resistant to stomach acid, and the hydrolysis must be accomplished by gut flora. The ability of individual human flora to produce the necessary enzymes varies significantly, resulting in variable clinical effects for salicin or plant material that contains salicin. However, sufficient hydrolytic capacity for some transformation of the glycoside into salicylic acid occurs in all individuals.

Atractylis gummifera was a favorite agent for homicide during the reign of the Borgias. Atractyloside, the toxic xenobiotic primarily inhibits oxidative phosphorylation in the liver by inhibiting the ADP/ATP antiporter blocking influx of adenosine diphosphate (ADP) into hepatic mitochondria and outflow of ATP to the rest of the cell (Chap. 12). Death or severe illness as a result of liver failure or hepatorenal disease following ingestion is reported.[98] *Callilepis laureola* is a South African medicinal plant that contains atractyloside and carboxyatractyloside and that has been reported to cause human poisonings.[218] Cocklebur (*Xanthium strumarium*) is an herbaceous plant with worldwide distribution. The seeds contain the glycoside carboxyatractyloside. The toxic mechanism is similar to that for atractyloside, and seed ingestion has resulted in human fatalities. Nine patients presented with acute onset abdominal pain, nausea and vomiting, drowsiness, palpitations, sweating, and dyspnea. Three developed convulsions followed by loss of consciousness and death. Laboratory findings showed raised liver enzymes indicating severe hepatocellular damage, raised BUN and creatine levels, and raised creatine phosphokinase-MB (CPK-MB) values indicating myocardial injury.[232]

Favism is a potentially fatal disorder brought about by eating fava beans or vetch seeds (*Vicia faba*, *Vicia sativa*, respectively). These seeds contain the pyrimidine glycosides vicine and convicine (divicine is the aglycone of vicine). Consumption of these compounds by individuals with an inborn error of metabolism (glucose-6-phosphate dehydrogenase deficiency) can cause acute hemolytic crisis (see Chap. 24, "Hematologic Principles").[115,127]

The effects of the glycosides sinigrin (from *Brassica nigra* seed and *Alliaria officinalis* [horseradish] root) and naringen (a polyphenolic glycoside from the grapefruit *Citrus paradisi*) are discussed in the sections on Plant-Induced Dermatitis and Plant–Xenobiotic Interactions, respectively.

TERPENOIDS AND RESINS: GINKGOLIDES, KAVA LACTONES, THUJONE, ANISATIN, PTAQUILOSIDE/THIAMINASE, AND GOSSYPOL

Ginkgolides in *Ginkgo biloba* are associated with antiplatelet aggregation effects. Reports of spontaneous bleeding associated with ingestion of *Ginkgo* leaf products as an herbal medicine are perhaps explained by this property.[196,233] Another xenobiotic found only in the seed, 4-methoxypyridoxine (pyridine alkaloid), is associated with seizures.[112,239] A mechanism similar to isoniazid-induced seizures is plausible, suggesting treatment with pyridoxine phosphate (Chap. 57 and Antidotes in Depth A15–Pyridoxine). The dermal effects of *Ginkgo* are discussed in the section Plant-Induced Dermatitis.

Kava lactones are a family of terpene lactones found in kava (*Piper methysticum*) that cause central and peripheral nervous system effects.[29,42,69] Kava has enjoyed a long, ceremonial history among islanders of the South Pacific, and observers visiting Oceania have recorded its acute and chronic effects (both pleasant and unpleasant) over the centuries. Importation of kava to Australia in 1983 was a measure to assist Aborigines with alcohol abuse problems. However, the kava itself became abused, and its subsequent ban has resulted in the growth of a black market for kava. Proposed mechanisms to explain the effects of kava lactones include effects at γ-aminobutyric acid type A ($GABA_A$) and $GABA_B$ receptors or local anesthetic effects. Acute symptoms following ingestion include peripheral numbness, weakness, and sedation. Chronic use leads to kava dermopathy and weight loss. More than 70 cases of hepatotoxicity, several requiring liver transplantation, are associated with both acute and chronic effects of kava extracts on cytochrome oxygenases or other yet-to-be-defined etiologies and prompted regulatory health measures in Europe and North America.[32,69]

Thujone is one of many terpenes associated with seizures. It is found in the wormwood plant (*Artemisia absinthium*), in absinthe (the liquor flavored with *A. absinthium*), and in some strains of tansy (*Tanacetum vulgare*). The α- and β-isomers of thujone are believed to act much like camphor to produce CNS depression and seizures. Invoking the structural similarity of thujone to tetrahydrocannabinol (THC), one of the terpenoids of marijuana, to explain the psychoactive effects is controversial (Chap. 83).[153]

Absinthism is characterized by seizures and hallucinations, permanent cognitive impairment, and personality changes. Acute and chronic absinthism led to a worldwide ban of the alcoholic beverage absinthe, which contained thujone, in the early 1900s.[172] Over the past several years, there has been a reexamination of the role of absinthe in the seizure disorders previously attributed to this liquor. Modern analytical procedures have been used to analyze the thujone content of vintage absinthe and modern products made using vintage recipes. Results have largely concluded that thujone content in the liquor was likely to be too low to have produced symptoms.[122] However, because the essential oil of wormwood is composed almost exclusively of thujone, it, but not absinthe, is a potent cause of seizures.[172] Wormwood oil for making homemade absinthe is currently available and is responsible for at least two reports of adverse reactions in people seeking its hallucinatory or euphoriant effects.[247]

Anisatin is found in *Illicium* spp. This terpenoid produces seizures as a noncompetitive GABA antagonist. The Chinese star anise (*Illicium verum*) is sometimes used in teas and occasionally is confused or contaminated with other species of *Illicium*, particularly Japanese star anise *Illicium anisatum*.[86] These contaminations have resulted in small epidemics of tonic–clonic seizures, particularly, but not exclusively, in infants after use of the tea to treat their infantile colic. Recently, in the United States, a case series of at least 40 individuals who had consumed teas brewed from "Star anise" experienced seizures, motor disturbances, other neurologic effects, and vomiting.[107] These cases include at least 15 infants treated for infantile colic with this home remedy. This trend prompted the FDA to issue an advisory regarding the health risk from remedies sharing the common name "Star anise."

Ptaquilosides are found in the bracken fern (*Pteridium aquilinum*), a plant that is extending its range and density worldwide. In foraging animals, consumption of ptaquilosides results in acute hemorrhage secondary to profound thrombocytopenia, whereas thiaminases produce cerebral disease.[71] Although no acute human poisonings are reported, these xenobiotics are transmitted through cow's milk and are associated with increased prevalence of gastric and esophageal cancer in areas where fern is endemic and consumed by cows whose milk is not diluted. Chronic toxicity through spore inhalation also produces pulmonary adenomas in animals.[252] More recently, research defined links between alimentary cancer in humans who previously consumed bracken fiddleheads.[4]

Gossypol is a sesquiterpene that is derived from cottonseed oil. It has been used experimentally as a reversible male contraceptive. The mechanism for its spermicidal effect is unclear, but the effects have been attributed to inhibition of plasminogen activation and plasmin activity in acrosomal tissue.[226] These effects are not currently reported to produce systemic bleeding. Gossypol also inhibits 11β-hydroxysteroid dehydrogenase, as does glycyrrhizin, but typically results in only isolated hypokalemia.[186]

PROTEINS, PEPTIDES, AND LECTINS: RICIN AND RICINLIKE, POKEWEED, MISTLETOE, HYPOGLYCIN, LATHYRINS, AND MICROCYSTINS

Lectins are glycoproteins that are classified according to their binding affinity for specific carbohydrate ligands, particularly galactosamines, and by the number of protein chains linked by disulfide bonds. Toxalbumins such as ricin and abrin are lectins that are such potent cytotoxins that they are used as biologic weapons (Chap. 131). Ricin, extracted from the castor bean (*Ricinus communis* (Figure 118–3a), exerts its cytotoxicity by two separate mechanisms. The compound is a large molecule that consists of two polypeptide chains bound by disulfide bonds. It must enter the cell to exert its toxic effect. The B chain binds to the terminal galactose of cell surface glycolipids and glycoproteins. The bound toxin then undergoes endocytosis and is transported via endosomes to the Golgi apparatus and the endoplasmic reticulum.[201] There the A chain is translocated to the cytosol, where it stops protein synthesis by inhibiting the 28S subunit of the 60S ribosome. In addition to the GI manifestations of vomiting, diarrhea, and dehydration, ricin can cause cardiac, hematologic, hepatic, and renal toxicity. All contribute to death in humans and animals.[11] Despite the obvious toxicity of this compound, death probably can be prevented by early and aggressive fluid and electrolyte replacement after oral ingestion (but not injection or inhalation; Chap. 131). Allergic reactions to some of these lectin-bearing plants and their derivates are noted.[50,225]

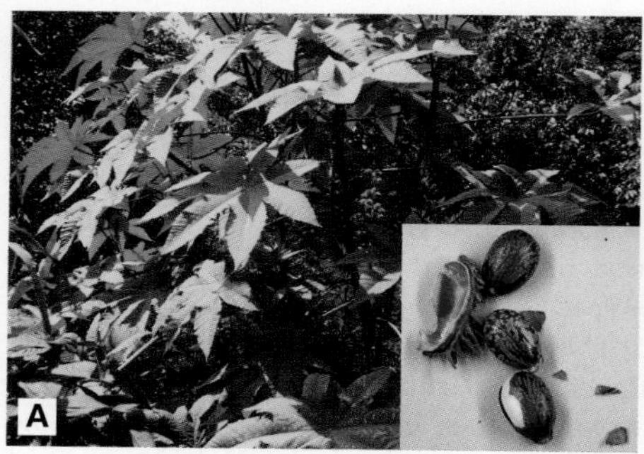

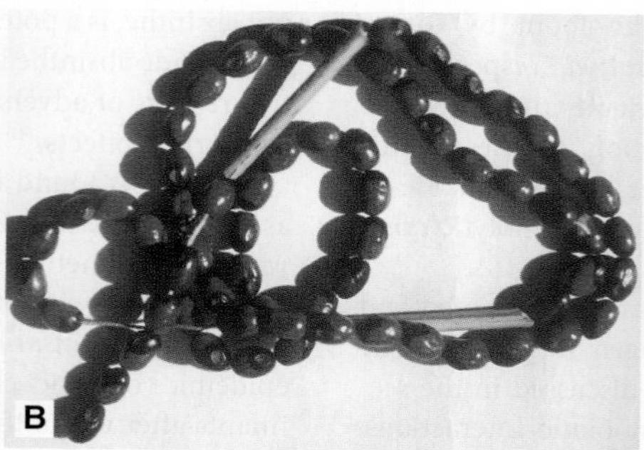

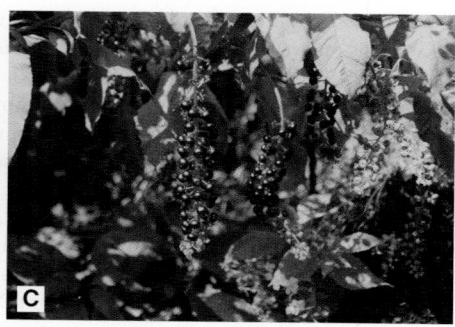

FIGURE 118–3. Protein-, peptide-, and lectin-containing plants: (**A**) The castor bean plant. The seedpods come in bunches, two of which appear near the center of the image. Each seedpod typically contains three seeds. Inset: Castor beans *(Ricinus communus)* which contain the toxalbumin ricin. By interfering with protein synthesis, ricin may cause multiorgan system failure when administered parenterally. However, its oral absorption is poor, and most oral poisonings cause gastroenteritis. (**B**) Rosary pea *(Abrus precatorius)* containing abrin, a toxalbumin that inhibits protein synthesis. The peas are shown strung together as a rosary. (C) Pokeweed *(Phytolacca americana)* has a large rootstock. The unripe berries contain phytolaccatoxin that produces gastroenteritis, but the mature, purple berries are often consumed. *(Images contributed by the New York City Poison Center Toxicology Fellowship Program.)*

Just how lethal are ingestions of the ornamental seeds? The highest concentration of xenobiotic is in the hard, brown-mottled seeds. These seeds are both tempting and available, even to children in the United States, because they are attractive enough to be used to make jewelry, and their parent plants are showy enough to have been exported for horticultural purposes outside of their native India (including to the United States). Although mastication of one seed by a child liberates enough ricin to produce death, this outcome (or even serious toxicity) is uncommon, even if the seeds are chewed, probably because GI absorption of the xenobiotic is poor and supportive care is effective.[7,11] Activated charcoal should be administered promptly.

Other *ricinlike lectins* are found in *Abrus precatorius* (jequirity pea, rosary pea (Figure 118–3b),[56] *Jatropha* spp,[121,131] *Trichosanthes* spp (eg, *T. kirilowii* or Chinese cucumber), *Robinia pseudoacacia* (black locust),[152] *Phoradendron* spp (American mistletoe), *Viscum album* (European mistletoe), and *Wisteria* spp (wisteria).[195] These all produce at least one double-chain lectin that binds to galactose-containing structures in the gut or inhibits protein synthesis in a manner similar to ricin.

The most commonly ingested toxic plant lectins in the United States are from pokeweed (*Phytolacca americana* (Figure 118–3c), which is eaten as a vegetable but rarely causes toxicity or death. The mature, deep purple berries are less toxic. Pokeweed leaves are consumed after boiling without toxic effect if the water is changed between the first and second boiling (parboiling). When this detoxification technique is not followed, as in preparation of poke salad or pokeroot tea, violent GI effects can ensue 0.5 to 6 hours after ingestion. Nausea, vomiting, abdominal cramping, diarrhea, hemorrhagic gastritis, and death may occur. In addition, bradycardia and hypotension, perhaps induced by an increase in vagal tone, may be associated with nausea and vomiting.[96,191] Phytolaccatoxin and pokeweed mitogen are found in all plant parts, but the highest concentrations are found in the plant root. Pokeweed mitogen is a single-chain protein that inhibits ribosomal RNA by removing purine groups.[16,105] It produces a lymphocytosis 2 to 4 days after ingestion that may take up to 10 days to clear, but this is without clinical consequence.[16]

Mistletoe berries, both American and European, can produce severe gastroenteritis, especially when delivered as teas or extracts, or particularly as parenteral antineoplastic medicinal agents in Europe. As festive holiday plants they become seasonally available for children. Poison center data suggest that ingestion of three to five berries or one to five leaves of the American species may not cause toxicity, but these suggestions are based on limited evidence (see Chap. 135). Despite single reports of seizure, ataxia, hepatotoxicity, and death,[118,213] most authors performing such retrospective examinations conclude that mistletoe exposures are not a highly consequential risk.

Hypoglycin A (β-methylene cyclopropyl-L-α-aminopropionic acid) and *hypoglycin B* (dipeptide of hypoglycin A and glutamic acid) are found in the unripe ackee fruit and seeds of *Blighia sapida* (Euphorbiaceae). The tree is native to Africa but was imported to Jamaica in 1778, and subsequently naturalized in Central America, southern California, and Florida. The scientific name of the plant derives from Captain William Bligh, the British explorer.[24] Epidemics of illness (Jamaican vomiting sickness) associated with consumption of the unripe ackee fruit (raw and cooked) occur in Africa but are more common in Jamaica, where ackee is the national dish.[35,111,151] The most toxic part is the yellow oily aril of the fruit,[41] which contains three large, shiny black seeds. Cases may also be associated with canned fruit.[150] Hypoglycin A is metabolized to methylene cyclopropyl acetic acid, which competitively inhibits the carnitine–acyl coenzyme (CoA) transferase system.[1,14,25] This prevents importation of long-chain fatty acids into the mitochondria, preventing their β-oxidation to precursors of gluconeogenesis. β-Oxidation and gluconeogenesis are further arrested by inhibition of various enzymes, such as glutaryl CoA dehydrogenase, which blocks the malate shunt (Chap. 12). In addition, increased concentrations of glutaric acid may inhibit glutamic acid decarboxylase, which produces GABA from glutamic acid. This not only depletes GABA but also increases concentrations of excitatory glutamate to produce seizures. Insulin concentrations remain unaffected by hypoglycin and metabolites.[155] Carboxylic and other organic acid substrates build up in the urine and serum as a result of these metabolic perturbations. Detection of these acids can help corroborate the diagnosis.[14] Jamaican vomiting sickness is characterized by epigastric discomfort and the onset of vomiting starting 2 to 6 hours after ingestion. Convulsions, coma, and death can ensue, with death occurring approximately 12 hours following consumption.[14] Laboratory findings are notable for profound hepatic aminotransferase and bilirubin abnormalities, and aciduria and acidemia without ketonemia. Cholestatic hepatitis can occur and is reported with chronic use.[128] Autopsy reveals fatty degeneration of liver, particularly microvesicular steatosis, and other organs with depletion of glycogen stores. Left untreated, patient mortality reaches 80%, with 85% of the fatal cases suffering seizures. Treatment with glucose and fluid replacement is essential. Benzodiazepines can control seizures, but may fail if the seizures are related to depletion of GABA. L-Carnitine therapy may exert a theoretical therapeutic role similar to that noted with valproic acid toxicity (Chap. 47).[133]

The *lathyrins* β-*N*-oxalylamino-L-alanine (BOAA) and β-aminopropionitrile (BAPN) are peptides from the grass pea (*Lathyrus sativus*) found in the seeds and leaves, respectively. BOAA produces neurolathyrism (seeds) and BAPN produces osteolathyrism (leaves) in individuals with a dietary dependence on this plant. Neurolathyrism is nearly indistinguishable from spastic paresis associated with consumption of improperly prepared cassava (see section Cyanogenic Glycosides: (*S*)-Sambunigrin, Amygdalin, Linamarin, and Cyacasin).[15,45] Thiol oxidation with depletion of nicotinamide adenine dinucleotide (NADH) dehydrogenase at the level of neuronal mitochondria (ie, excitatory AMPA receptors) may be the common etiology.[173,212] Epidemics have occured in Bangladesh, Ethiopia, Israel, and India. Exposure to BOAA results in degeneration of corresponding corticospinal pathways that becomes irreversible if consumption of undetoxified grass peas is not stopped early. BOAA stimulates the AMPA class of glutamate receptors to provide constant neuronal stimulation, eventual degeneration, and hence spasticity.[185] BAPN affects bone matrix and leads to bone pain and skeletal deformities that develop in adulthood.[15] These diseases occur in areas where the plants are endemic, the food is consumed for 2 months or more, and when diets are otherwise poor in protein and possibly in zinc.[85,123]

Microcystins are found in several cyanobacteria (blue-green algae) belonging to various species of the genera *Microcystis*, *Anabaena*, *Nodularia*, *Nostoc*, and *Oscillatoria*. They elaborate a series of peptides called microcystins and nodularins (*Nodularia spumigena*).[58] These compounds produce hepatotoxicity by inhibiting phosphatases and causing deterioration of the microfilament function in hepatocytes, leading to cell shrinkage and bleeding into the hepatic sinusoids.[51,58] Evidence indicates that these peptides are carcinogenic to humans.[57] Although most cases of untoward effects from blue-green algae occur in animals, the potential for harm was demonstrated by use of microcystin-contaminated water in a dialysis unit in Brazil.[110] Unfiltered water was identified as the risk factor for liver disease in 100 patients who attended the dialysis center (Chap. 9). Fifty of these patients died of acute liver failure following early signs of nausea, vomiting, and visual disturbances. Concerningly, certain species of *Cyanobacteria* are harvested and consumed as health foods[87] or may be consumed secondarily in fish.[139]

PHENOLS AND PHENYLPROPANOIDS: COUMARINS, CAPSAICIN, KARWINSKIA TOXINS, NARINGENIN AND BERGAMOTTIN, ASARIN, NORDIHYDROGUAIARETIC ACID, PODOPHYLLIN, PSORALEN, AND ESCULOSIDE

Phenols and phenylpropanoids represent one of the largest groups of plant secondary metabolites. Coumarins and their isomers are phenylpropanoids that are discussed in Chap. 59. Some coumarins are warfarinlike in their activity and are capable of producing a bleeding diathesis when plants are consumed in sufficiently large quantities.[102] Lignans are formed when phenylpropanoid side chains react to form bisphenylpropanoid derivatives. Lignins are high-molecular-weight polymers of phenylpropanoids that bind to cellulose and provide strength to cell walls of stem and bark. Tannins are polymers that bind to proteins and divide into two groups: hydrolyzable and condensed (called proanthocyanidins, eg, karwinol).

Capsaicin is derived from *Capsicum annuum* or other species of chile or cayenne peppers. It is a simple phenylpropanoid that causes release of the neuropeptide substance P from sensory C-type nerve fibers that act upon transient receptor potential (TRP) channels in diverse human tissues.[238] The immediate response to capsaicin is intense local pain and is the rationale for its use as "pepper spray." Eventual depletion of substance P prevents local transmission of pain impulses from these receptors to the spinal cord, blocking perception of pain by the brain, explaining its use in postherpetic neuralgia.

Painful exposures to capsaicin-containing peppers are among the most common plant-related exposures presented to poison centers. They cause burning or stinging pain to the skin.[246] If ingested in large amounts by adults or small amounts by children, they can produce nausea, vomiting, abdominal pain, and burning diarrhea.[229] Eye exposures produce intense tearing, pain, conjunctivitis, and blepharospasm. Fatality is rare, but has occurred after inhalation and infusion.[211]

Skin irrigation, dermal aloe gel, analgesics, and oral antacids are therapeutic agents that may be helpful as appropriate, but patients can be reassured that the effects are transitory and produce no long-term damage. Irritated eyes can be treated with irrigation and local analgesia, but generally resolve without sequelae within 24 hours.

Karwinskia toxins from plants commonly named Buckthorn, coyotillo, tullidora, wild cherry, or capulincillo (*Karwinskia humboldtiana*). These xenobiotics are identified by their molecular weights (T-514, T-496, T-516, T-544). Toxicity has been known for more than 200 years. In 1920, an epidemic of deaths was reported after 20% of 106 Mexican soldiers died following ingestion of foraged *Karwinskia* fruits.[143] Poisonings continue to occur. The fruits are attractive to children; epidemic poisonings have been reported in Central America and are possible wherever the shrub is found (in semidesert areas throughout the southwestern United States and in the Caribbean, Mexico, and Central America).[10] Uncoupling of oxidative phosphorylation or dysfunction of peroxisome assembly and integrity is described as the mechanism of action of T-514 on Schwann cells. Each xenobiotic exhibits similar cytotoxic effects at the cellular level, but with tropism for different organs in animal models.[143]

Within a few days of ingestion, a symmetric motor neuropathy ascends from the lower extremities to produce a bulbar paralysis that may lead to death. Deep-tendon reflexes are abolished in affected areas, but cranial nerve findings are absent. Distinction of this demyelinating motor neuropathy from Guillain-Barré syndrome, poliomyelitis, solvent, and other polyneuropathies is difficult without a history of the fruit ingestion,[168] but can be assisted by detection of T-514 in the blood of affected patients. The other recognized toxins are not detected in blood. Occasionally, axonal damage is observed, but demyelination is the predominant finding on biopsy. Nerve conduction studies always demonstrate loss or abolition of function in fast-conducting axons. Cerebrospinal fluid demonstrates normal protein, glucose, and cytology. Treatment is supportive, with mechanical ventilation as needed, and recovery typically is slow.

Naringin and *naringenin* are flavonoid, while *bergamottin* and *6′,7′-dihydroxybergamottin* are furanocoumarin phenylpropanoids derived from grapefruit that inhibit CYP3A4 in gut and liver.[82] Grapefruit juice consumption can increase circulating concentrations of drugs reliant on 3A4 for metabolic elimination, including carbamazepine, felodipine, and the statins. The most plausible mechanism is inhibition of enteric CYP3A4 and P-glycoprotein.[174] These effects are maximally achieved by a single glass of grapefruit juice.[137]

Comedication with St. John's wort resulted in decreased plasma concentrations of a number of xenobiotics.[138] Hyperforin is a phenylpropanoid found in St. John's wort (*Hypericum perforatum*) and is associated with plant–xenobiotic interactions through strong induction of CYP3A4-mediated drug metabolism as well as induction of P-glycoprotein. These combined mechanisms can cause subtherapeutic concentrations of xenobiotics metabolized via these pathways.[160,161]

Asarin is a term sometimes used for the naturally occurring mixture of α- and β-asarones found in the root of *Asarum europaeum*,

Asarum arifolium, and *Acorus calamus* (sweet flag). Essential oils of the plants have anthelmenthic and nematocidal activity, but putative euphoric and hallucinogenic effects that motivate recreational ingestion are in contrast to confirmed reports of unpleasant GI effects.[234]

Nordihydroguaiaretic acid (NDGA) is associated with hepatotoxicity after ingestion of chaparral (*Larrea tridentata*).[89] Podophyllin and psoralens are phenylpropanoids discussed in the sections Antimitotic Alkaloids and Resins, and Plant-Induced Dermatitis, respectively.

Esculoside (also called *esculin* or *aesculin)* has triterpene saponin side chains and is believed to be the toxic component in horse chestnut (*Aesculus hippocastanum*). Horse chestnut extracts are used medicinally in patients with venous insufficiency. Its therapeutic use at high doses (greater than 340 µg/kg) is associated with renal failure or a lupuslike syndrome.[92] Leaves, twigs, or horse chestnuts ingested by children or infused as teas result in a syndrome that resembles nicotine intoxication. The syndrome consists of vomiting, diarrhea, muscle twitching, weakness, lack of coordination, dilated pupils, paralysis, and stupor.[163] The mechanism of toxicity is not defined, but ingestion of chestnut approximately 1% of a child's weight is suggested to be poisonous to a child.

CARBOXYLIC ACIDS: ARISTOLOCHIC ACIDS, OXALIC ACID, AND OXALATE RAPHIDES

Nitrophenanthrene carboxylic acids, collectively called aristolochic acids, are present in most members of the genus *Aristolochia*, including those used ornamentally and as traditional medicines. Consumption of these compounds can cause aristolochic acid nephropathy (AAN), a progressive renal interstitial fibrosis frequently associated with urothelial malignancies (see Chap. 43).[54] Sources of exposure are via consumption of flour made from wheat contaminated with the seeds of *Aristolochia clematis* or other *Aristolochia* species (so-called Balkan endemic nephropathy),[93] or through use of certain traditional Asian medicines made from *Aristolochia* spp (Chinese herb nephropathy).[52,219]

Oxalic acid is the strongest acid among the carboxylic acids found in living organisms. It forms poorly soluble chelates with calcium and other divalent cations. Higher plants have varying ability to accumulate these include both soluble and insoluble oxalates, and many contain crystals of calcium oxalate called raphides. Certain plant families, such as the Araceae, Chenopodiaceae, Polygonaceae, Amaranthaceae, and several of the grass families, are rich in oxalates. Human dietary sources include rhubarb, spinach, strawberries, chocolate, tea, and nuts.[144] Human consumption of soluble oxalate-rich foods correlates with kidney stone formation.

The insoluble calcium oxalate raphides that are present in certain plants, usually in the Araceae family, are found in conjunction with a protein toxin that increases the painful irritation to skin or mucous membranes. This special manifestation is discussed in greater detail in the section Plant-Induced Dermatitis.

ALCOHOLS: CICUTOXIN

Cicutoxin, a diacetylenic diol, is found in *Cicuta maculata* (water hemlock), *Cicuta douglasii* (western water hemlock), and *Oenanthe crocata* (hemlock water dropwort). *O. crocata* is native to Europe where intoxications have been reported[61] and has been reported to be naturalized to the United States. Ingestion of any part of these plants constitutes the most common form of lethal plant ingestion in the United States. In a series of 83 ingestions from 1900 to 1975, the case fatality rate was 30%, and it dominated plant-related fatalities among the most recent 10-year reviews of the AAPCC data and Centers for Disease Control and Prevention (CDC) plant-poisoning records (Chap. 135).[117] In contrast to most plant exposures in humans, which tend to involve children, these ingestions usually involve adults who incorrectly identify the plant as wild parsnip, turnip, parsley, or ginseng.[36] All plant parts are poisonous at all times, but the tuber is especially toxic, and more so during the winter and early spring. Absorption of cicutoxin is rapid and occurs through the skin as well as through the gut. Although the mechanism is not fully understood, cicutoxin may block potassium channels.[222]

Symptoms of mild or early poisonings consist of GI symptoms (nausea, vomiting, epigastric discomfort) and begin as early as 15 minutes after ingestion. Emesis may diminish the toxic load in the gut. Diaphoresis, flushing, dizziness, excessive salivation, bradycardia, hypotension, bronchial secretions with respiratory distress, and cyanosis occur and rapidly progress to violent seizures. Ingestion of as little as a 2-cm section of the sweet-tasting root of *Cicuta* can produce fatal status epilepticus.[100] Other complications include rhabdomyolysis with renal failure and severe acidemia. Immediate gastric evacuation should be performed if practical, and benzodiazepines should be administered for seizures. No specific antidote exists; supportive and symptomatic care should be provided.

UNIDENTIFIED TOXINS

Consistent with the inherent complexity of plants and the relatively early stage of the science, identification of the active ingredient(s) involved in poisoning is not always possible. An epidemic of the irreversible lung disease bronchiolitis obliterans developed in Taiwan in 1994. It involved more than 200 dieters who had been eating *Sauropus androgynous* as a weight-loss vegetable. The effects were dose related (usually approximately 100 g/d) and manifested by month 7 after approximately 10 weeks of use.[104] The cases were associated with at least four deaths and, in addition to pulmonary disease, included three cases of torsades des pointes.[136] This last complication is consistent with the plant's high concentration of papaverine, a toxin that produces dysrhythmias in animals, but papaverine does not cause the lung disease. Steroid and bronchodilator therapy consistently failed to improve pulmonary symptoms, and lung transplantation remains the only effective treatment for advanced cases.[136] A report of a later outbreak in Japan noted that the plant is eaten in Malaysia and that the case-associated *Sauropus* was consumed in an uncooked state.[171]

Milk sickness is a historic poisoning described by pioneer farmers. It was caused by transmission of the nontoxic ketone tremetone to humans via milk of animals grazing on white snake-root plants (*Eupatorium rugosum*).[206] Tremetone is transformed into an unknown, unstable toxin by hepatic microsomal enzymes.[17] Toxicity is cumulative. Milk sickness can be fatal in 1 to 21 days or is associated with a slow recovery marked by weakness for months or years, relapsing sometimes to death. A delay in the lactating animal's symptoms provided a lag time when xenobiotic-laden milk was taken from presymptomatic animals and thereby transmitted to humans before the problem was detected.

Breynia officinalis,[135] the air potato or bitter yam (*Dioscorea bulbifera*),[227] and commercial black cohosh (*Actaea racemosa*) preparations,[228] are associated with hepatotoxicity. Black cohosh hepatoxicity has come to light primarily through case reports,[140] but causality has been difficult to establish definitively.

Consumption of the food star fruit (*Averrhoa carambola*) and preexisting renal insufficiency are associated with development of intractable hiccups, vomiting, motor disabilities, paresthesias, confusion, seizures, and death unless patients receive supportive care and hemodialysis.[165,231] The unidentified toxin appears to be neuroexcitatory and active in the thalamus and right temporooccipital cortex.[39]

EFFECTS SHARED AMONG DIFFERENT CLASSES OF XENOBIOTICS

PLANT–XENOBIOTIC INTERACTIONS

By increasing the metabolic rate of CYP enzymes and P-glycoprotein, hyperforin in St. John's wort (*H. perforatum*) decreases concentrations of several drugs including amitriptyline, cyclosporine, digoxin, indinavir, irinotecan, warfarin, phenprocoumon, alprazolam, dextrometorphan, simvastatin, theophylline, and oral contraceptives.[108] Bergamottins and naringenin from grapefruit reduce activity of the CYP system enzymes and increase drug concentrations. Other *Citrus* species also appear to increase drug concentrations.[103]

Additive effects may be responsible for serotonin excess or mild serotonin syndrome when St. John's wort is used concurrently with tryptophan or serotonin reuptake inhibitors.[81,108,154] Additive effects also appear to be responsible for increased prothrombin time in patients taking *G. biloba* and various dugs to affect coagulation (eg, warfarin or aspirin) because the ginkgolides have antiplatelet activity.[81,108,154] Hawthorn (*Crataegus* spp), used medicinally for cardiac disorders, may produce an additive effect when taken concomitantly with digoxin, producing bradycardia. Excessive intake of broccoli provides enough vitamin K to competitively inhibit the negative effects of warfarin on vitamin K activation.

SODIUM CHANNEL EFFECTS: ACONITINE, VERATRIDINE, ZYGACINE, TAXINE, AND GRAYANOTOXINS

Several unrelated plants produce xenobiotics that affect the flow of sodium at the sodium channel. For instance, aconitine and veratrum alkaloids tend to open the channels to influx of sodium, whereas others (eg, taxine) tend to block the flow, and grayanotoxins both increase and block sodium flow.[240] The sodium channel opener aconitine from *Aconitum* spp or *Delphinium* spp has the most persistent toxicity and the lowest therapeutic index among the many active alkaloid ingredients of these toxic plants called aconite. Some of the related alkaloids are controlled medicinal substances in the People's Republic of China and Taiwan.[37] Aconite has been abused for its psychoactive "out of body" effects and for suicide and homicide. These alkaloids should be suspected in potentially poisoned patients who manifest cardiac toxicity, paresthesias, and seizures.[134]

The mechanism of action depends on the individual alkaloid.[79] Some compounds block and others activate sodium channels. Aconitine itself opens the voltage-dependent sodium channel at binding site 2 of the α-subunit, initially increasing cellular excitability. By prolonging sodium current influx, neuronal and cardiac repolarization eventually slows. It also has calcium channel–opening effects. Asian prescription medicines use the alkaloids to treat dysrhythmias and pain by reducing the excitability of the cardiac conducting system and sensory neurons, respectively.[5]

Approximately one teaspoon (2–5 mg) of the root may cause death. The aconitine alkaloids are rapidly absorbed from the GI tract, and the calculated half-life of aconitine is 3 hours.[157] CNS symptoms typically progress from paresthesias to CNS depression, respiratory muscle depression, paralysis, and seizures. Nausea, vomiting, diarrhea, and abdominal cramping occur. Cardiotoxicity resembles that caused by cardioactive steroidal glycosides, and typically progress from bradycardia with atrioventricular conduction blockade to increased ventricular automaticity resulting in a variety of rapid ventricular rates. Multifocal premature ventricular contractions, bidirectional ventricular tachycardia,[210] torsades des pointes, and ventricular fibrillation may occur.[134]

A history of paresthesias or muscle weakness may be useful in differentiating aconitine toxicity from that caused by a cardioactive steroids,[38] and hidden aconite poisoning can be diagnosed by detection of the alkaloids in urine by liquid chromatography-mass spectrometry.

Management should not be delayed while awaiting testing. Empiric use of digoxin-specific antibody fragments should be administered if cardioactive steroid poisoning is strongly considered, but these antibodies are ineffectual against aconitine. Antidysrhythmic success with lidocaine is limited, and amiodarone is currently the antidysrhythmic of choice.[134] Orogastric lavage, activated charcoal, and preparation for cardiac pacing, bypass, or balloon pump assist should be used as indicated, given the potential for rapid cardiovascular deterioration.[169]

Ingestion of veratridine and other veratrum alkaloids (from *Veratrum viride* and other *Veratrum* spp) generally results from foraging errors where the root appears similar to leeks (*Allium porrum*) and aboveground parts appear similar to gentian (*Gentiana lutea*) used for teas and wines in Europe.[46,204] Typical symptoms develop within an hour of ingestion and include headache followed by nausea, vomiting, and sometimes diarrhea. Vital signs in one case report were normal except for heart rates of 42 and 45 beats per minute in two patients. Laboratory findings were unremarkable, and electrocardiograms revealed sinus bradycardia.[254] The mechanism of action is similar to that of aconitine (sodium channel opening) but with shorter duration.[240] Although severe toxicity has been reported, management is supportive with fluids, atropine, and pressors. Deaths are rare.[204]

Zygacine from *Zigadenus* spp (death camus) and other members of the lily family produces the same toxic effects as veratridine alkaloids (vomiting, hypotension, and bradycardia).[215] Symptoms begin one to two hours after ingestion and usually result from errors while foraging for onions because of the plant's look-alike bulb.[101] Treatment options are the same as above with Veratrum alkaloids.

Taxine, derived from the yew, is another alkaloid mixture of sodium channel effectors that tend to close the channel (*Taxus baccata*) (Figure 118–4).[251] The toxicity of *Taxus* has been known since antiquity. Toxic alkaloids are contained within the bark, leaves, and hard central seed but not in the surrounding fleshy red aril, which partly explains the low rate of toxicity in reported cases of accidental exposure.[251] Taxine-derived alkaloids (eg, taxine A and B, isotaxine B, paclitaxel), taxane-derived substances (eg, taxol A and B), and glycosides (eg, taxicatine) are responsible for the toxicity of *Taxus* spp. Lethal oral doses (LD_{min}) of yew leaves in humans are estimated to be 0.6 to 1.3 g/kg of

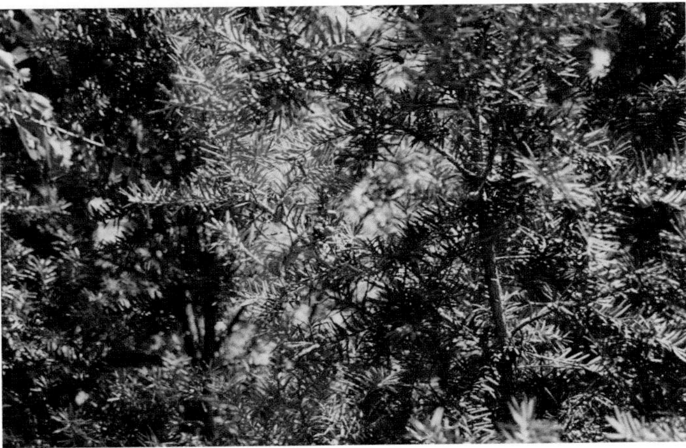

FIGURE 118–4. The Yew (*Taxus sp.*) is a common garden shrub that produces taxine, a cardiotoxin. Though the fleshy red aril is nontoxic, the hard seed it contains is toxic. *(Image contributed by the New York City Poison Center Toxicology Fellowship Program.)*

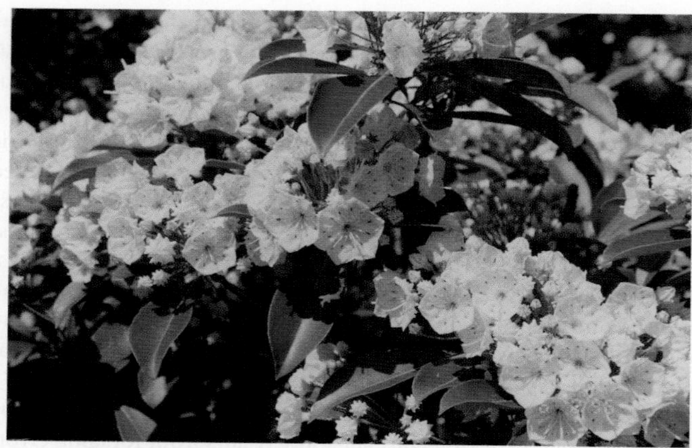

FIGURE 118–5. Mountain laurel (*Kalmia latifolia*), an evergreen shrub, contains the sodium channel opener grayanotoxin, which produces dysrhythmias. *(Image contributed by the New York City Poison Center Toxicology Fellowship Program.)*

body weight, or 3.0 to 6.5 mg taxines/kg of body weight.[249,251] Suicide using leaves is reported despite the large number of leaves required.[245] Clinical manifestations of yew poisoning include dizziness, nausea, vomiting, diffuse abdominal pain, tachycardia (initially), and convulsions followed by bradycardia, respiratory paralysis, and death.[178]

Paclitaxel (Taxol) is an alkaloid component of the relatively rare Pacific yew (*Taxus brevifolia*) that is used as an antitumor chemotherapeutic xenobiotic because of its ability to promote the assembly of microtubules and to inhibit the tubulin disassembly process in mitotic cells. Within 1 hour after ingestion, toxicity progresses from nausea, abdominal pain, bradycardia, and cardiac conduction delays to wide-complex ventricular dysrhythmias, paresthesias, ataxia, and mental status changes.[73] Four prisoners who drank an extract of yew experienced profound hypokalemia, and two died of cardiac arrest.[73] Animal models indicate that bradycardia is responsive to atropine, but wide-complex tachydysrhythmia is unresponsive to sodium bicarbonate.[197]

Grayanotoxins (formerly termed *andromedotoxins*) are a series of 18 toxic diterpenoids present in leaves of various species of *Rhododendron*, *Azalea*, *Kalmia* (Figure 118–5), and *Leucothoe* (Ericaceae). They exert their toxic effects via sodium channels, which they open or close, depending on the toxin.[240] Grayanotoxin I increases membrane permeability to sodium and affected calcium channels in a manner similar to that of veratridine (and batrachotoxin).[94] Grayanotoxins become concentrated in honey made from the plants, mainly in the Mediterranean.[94] Accounts of poisoning by honey date back to at least 401 BC, when Xenophon's troops were incapacitated after they consumed honey made from nectar of *Rhododendron luteum*. These accounts are echoed by modern accounts of toxic honey in the same region.[94] Occasionally, grayanotoxin-containing plants or plant preparations rather than honey cause human poisonings.[180] Bradycardia, hypotension, GI manifestations, mental status changes ("mad honey"), and seizures are described in patients or animals suffering grayanotoxin toxicity.[94,125]

ANTIMITOTIC ALKALOIDS AND RESINS: COLCHICINE, VINCRISTINE, AND PODOPHYLLUM

Consumption of colchicine from plant sources such as autumn crocus (*Colchicum autumnale*) produces a spectrum of symptoms, including nausea, vomiting, watery diarrhea, hypotension, bradycardia, electrocardiographic abnormalities, diaphoresis, alopecia, bone marrow depression, renal failure, hepatic necrosis, hemorrhagic acute lung injury, convulsions, and death.[28,224]

Confusion of the bulbs or leaves of this plant with those of wild onions or garlic occur as a foraging error. Unintentional consumption by children, or ingestion with suicidal intent, accounts for the other cases involving morbidity or mortality. The mechanism of toxicity is disruption of microtubule formation in mitotic cells.

Vincristine and vinblastine are two other indole alkaloids that are used as antineoplastics and are both isolated from the Madagascar periwinkle (*Catharanthus roseus*). No reports of poisoning by these alkaloids following ingestion of the plant could be found (Chap. 37).

Podophyllum resin is the dry, alcoholic extract of the rhizomes and roots of mayapple (*Podophyllum peltatum*) (Figure 118–6). The dry resin consists of up to 20% podophyllotoxin, α- and β-peltatin, desoxy-podophyllotoxin, and dehydropodophyllotoxin. These xenobiotics are originally present in the plant as β-D-glucosides. Podophyllum resin containing podophyllin is available by prescription for topical treatment of venereal warts. Its medicinal derivatives, etoposide, are used for a range of neoplastic diseases. Podophyllum is used as a popular traditional Chinese medicine. Podophyllotoxins make up 20% of the resin from the roots of mayapple (*P. peltatum*). As a group, they disrupt tubulin formation, producing multisystem organ failure. Poisonings are caused by misidentification and adulteration, possibly because the list of common names by which it is known includes mayapple, as well as mandrake, wild mandrake, American mandrake, and European mandrake.[77] Catharsis is prominent after ingestion, but onset of symptoms may be delayed (10 hours in a fatal ingestion). Acute, severe sensorimotor neuropathy and bone marrow suppression following transient leukocytosis can occur even after one-time acute exposures and may be directly related to inhibition of microtubule assembly. Lethargy, confusion, encephalopathy, autonomic instability, sensory ataxia, and death are described following large exposures,[167] but poisoning can also occur after "therapeutic" doses of a popular traditional Chinese medicine.[114]

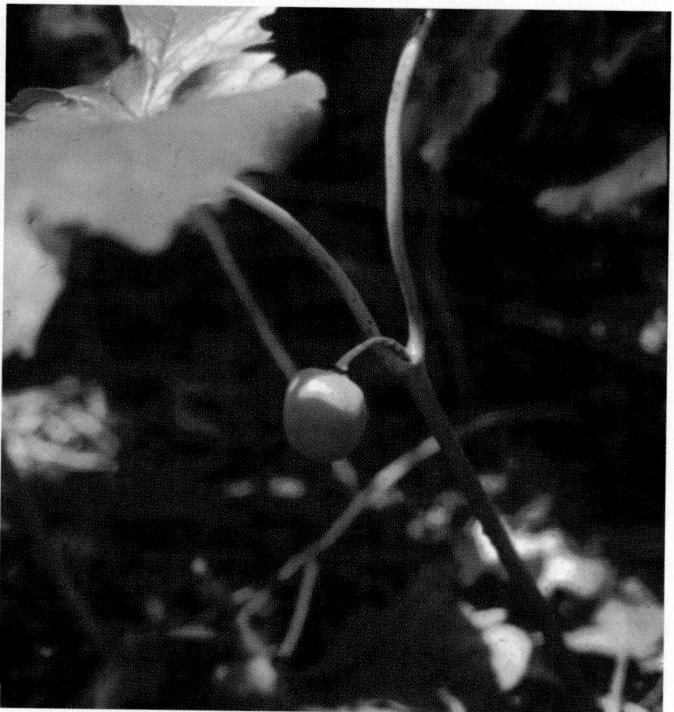

FIGURE 118–6. The Mayapple (*Podophyllum peltatum*) develops from an initial nodding flower that grows from the stem of this low lying ground cover plant. The whole plant contains podophyllotoxin (podophylline), though the apple is generally considered the least toxic part. *(Image contributed by the New York City Poison Center Toxicology Fellowship Program.)*

Glutamic acid has been used to prevent vincristine-induced peripheral neuropathy and would be a reasonable therapy following podophyllin ingestion.[109]

PLANT-INDUCED DERMATITIS

A large number of plants result in undesirable dermal, mucous membrane, and ocular effects (Chap. 29), the most common adverse effects reported to US poison centers and occupational health centers. Plant-induced dermal disorders can be readily categorized into four mechanistic groups, that is, dermatis that results from (1) mechanical injury, (2) irritant molecules that penetrate the skin, (3) allergy, or (4) photosensitivity (direct and hepatogenous) (see Chap. 29).[164,221]

There is much overlap between these categories (some plants can produce all types). Clinicians may have difficulty distinguishing between plant-induced dermatitis and skin disorders[146] or between plant-induced dermatitis and pseudophytodermatitides caused by arthropods, pesticides, or wax (used in fruit and vegetable packaging).[221] Agents that cause adverse skin reactions can also cause eye and local gastric mucosal irritation.

Dermatitis from mechanical injury often is combined with primary or allergic contact dermatitis. Stinging nettles (*Urtica dioica* and other species) have a specialized apparatus in the form of an elongated silicious cell (glandular trichome) that acts like a hypodermic syringe to deliver irritant chemicals into the skin. Contact with these stinging hairs shears off the tip of the hair, producing micromechanical injury and releasing irritant contents: acetylcholine, histamine, and 5-hydroxytryptamine.[170] Acute motor polyneuropathy associated with cutaneous exposure to *Urtica ferox* is reported within 48 hours of walking through a patch of the nettles, with recovery occurring over several weeks.[97] The barbed trichomes (spicules) of *Mucuna pruriens* (velvet bean, cowhage) evoke a histamine-independent itch that is mediated by a cysteine protease, mucunain.[124,221] Workers who handpick pineapples are subject to fissuring and loss of fingerprints after the proteolytic enzyme bromelain is introduced following dermal abrasion by raphides.

Exposures to commonly available household plants such as dumbcane (*Dieffenbachia* spp), *Philodendron* spp, and *Narcissus* bulbs can lead to mechanical injury and painful microtrauma produced by bundles of tiny needlelike calcium oxalate crystals called raphides.[84] Packages of hundreds of raphides called idioblasts contain proteolytic enzymes. *Dieffenbachia* (more than 30 species) (Figure 118–7) exposures are commonly reported household or malicious plant exposures.[179] These exposures are rarely serious.[175] When the leaves are chewed, immediate oropharyngeal pain and swelling occur.[47] Severe oral exposures can be excruciating and progress to profuse salivation, dysphagia, and loss of speech.[84,242] Soothing liquids, ice, parenteral opioids, corticosteroids, and airway protection may be indicated, but antihistamines provide little relief. The edema and pain typically begin to subside after 4 to 8 days. Ocular exposure to the sap may produce chemical conjunctivitis, corneal abrasions, and, rarely, permanent corneal opacifications.

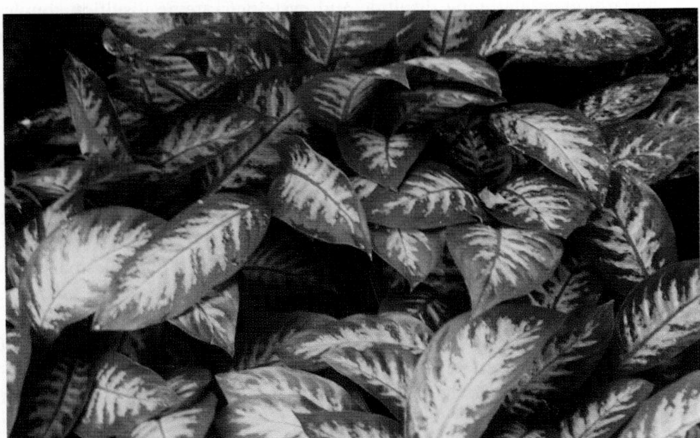

FIGURE 118–7. This Dumbcane (*Dieffenbachia sp.*) plant is representative of the Arum family, which typically have variegated, waxy leaves. Many contain insoluble crystals of calcium oxalate arranged in idioblasts, which may be ejected following trauma to the leaf. *(Image contributed by the New York City Poison Center Toxicology Fellowship Program.)*

Similar exposures to oxalate raphide-containing household plants in the same family (*Philodendron*, *Brassaia*, *Epipremnum aureum*, *Spathiphyllum*, and *Scheflera* spp) are not as painful as those to dumbcane, presumably because the crystals are packaged differently and do not simultaneously deliver proteolytic enzymes.[159] One exception to their lower severity is a report of death in an 11 month old following complications arising from esophageal lesions induced by philodendron.[147]

Irritant dermatitis can result from low-molecular-weight xenobiotics such as phorbol esters (from Euphorbiaceae) that directly penetrate the skin without antecedent mechanical injury. Similar penetrance is achieved by products of glycoside hydrolysis. For instance, hydrolysis of ranunculin gives rise to anemonin in Ranunculaceae, the buttercup family, and hydrolysis of sinigrin in plants in the mustard family Brassicaceae yields allyl isothiocyanate. Exposures to primary irritants in Brassicaceae and Ranuculaceae usually are mild. Alternatively, dermatitis can occur without contact, as in cases of airborne contact dermatitis, in which typically exposed sites are the upper eyelids; neck; uncovered extremities, including antecubital fossae; and other skin folds (Chap. 29).[202]

Phorbol esters found in spurges (Euphorbiaceae) are contained in milky sap that is capable of producing erythema, desquamation, and bullae. The saps of some species are more irritating than others. For instance, the manchineel tree (*Hippomane mancinella*), found in the Caribbean and Florida, once was planted on graves to deter grave robbers, and juice from the tree has been used to brand animals and to blind people. In addition to dermal and ocular injury,[67] ingestion of some spurges can induce severe GI injury. Poinsettia (*Euphorbia pulcherrima*), crown of thorns (*Euphorbia splendens*), candelabra cactus (*Euphorbia lacteal*), and pencil tree (*Euphorbia tirucalli*) are spurges found in the home as holiday or other ornamentation that rarely produce serious injury, despite reputations to the contrary. The poinsettia plant, for instance, gained a reputation of significant toxicity based on a single, inadequately documented case report from Hawaii in 1919, involving the death of a 2-year-old child.[9] In a subsequent case, an 8-month-old child developed oral mucosal burns after chewing poinsettia.[66] Contact dermatitis, irritation of mucous membranes, and GI complaints such as nausea, vomiting, and abdominal pain are rare findings among the many reported exposures to poinsettia.[120]

Allergic contact dermatitis results from type IV hypersensitivity response and, unlike irritant dermatitis, requires repeat exposures to the agent before symptoms manifest. The most infamous of these xenobiotics are the urushiol oleoresins derived from catechols that are found in *G. biloba* (Ginkgoaceae) and members of the Proteaceae (eg, *Macadamia integrifolia*) and the Anacardaceae. The latter family is notable for inclusion of poison ivy (*Toxicodendron radicans*), poison oak (*Toxicodendron toxicarium, Toxicodendron diver-silobum*), and poison sumac (*Toxicodendron vernix*),[88] as well as mango (*Mangifera indica*), pistachio (*Pistacia vera*), cashew (*Anacardium occidentale*), and Indian marking nut "Bhilawanol" (*Semecarpus anacardium*). Upon first exposure, urushiol resins penetrate the skin and react with proteins to form antigens to which the body forms antibodies. Upon reexposure to urushiol resins, inflammatory mediators are released, leading to urticaria, itching, swelling, and pain.[75,76] In extreme cases, these reactions can progress to type I hypersensitivity, as demonstrated by a 6% rate of anaphylaxis to mango among 580 patients who previously had mango-induced contact dermatitis.[6] Cross-reactivity between allergens is possible, and particular vigilance is required in sensitive individuals.[74,164] Prevention by removal of exposed objects that act as fomites for the oils and use of protective linaments are appropriate.[141,237] Therapy includes washing with soap and water and corticosteroid creams and, for those frequently exposed, desensitization (Chap. 29).[75]

Allergic contact dermatitis is the most common plant-induced occupational injury. In the United States, 33% of 462 floral shops surveyed reported that at least one employee had developed contact dermatitis.[202] Reactions are reported following exposure to tulips, *Narcissus*, Peruvian lily (*Alstroemeria* spp), and primroses (*Primula* spp). Exposure to the glycoside tuliposide A results in "tulip fingers," the dry, painfully fissured hyperkeratosis of fingers observed in horticultural workers who chronically handle tulips.[27] Upon hydrolysis, this compound yields α-methylene-butyrolactone, the true allergen. Cross-reactivity is possible among some of these xenobiotics. *Alstroemeria* spp, a common ornamental called *Peruvian lily,* contain tuliposide A and thus can cross-react with antigens in those persons already allergic to tulips, producing an allergic contact dermatitis. Primin (2-methoxy-6-*n*-pentyl-*p*-benzoquinone) from members of the Primulaceae family was responsible for the most frequently reported allergic plant dermatitis in northern Europe until workers refused to stock primroses. The "wood cutters dermatitis" of loggers occurs with development of sensitivity to compounds in liverwort (*Frullania* spp), which is cross-reactive to usnic acid in lichens and mosses found on the wood. Cross-reactivity with common weeds such as ragweed (*Ambrosia* spp) or dandelion (*Taraxacum* spp) initiate the risk of hypersensitivity from members of the Compositae family.[113] A myriad of other types of plants are involved in producing occupational dermatitides.[164,202]

Sensitivity to Compositae (daisy family) involves more than 600 sesquiterpene lactones in at least 200 of the 25,000 species in the family and is as ubiquitous as the distribution of species.[90] *Chrysanthemum* allergy is a common occupational hazard in Europe.

Direct photosensitivity dermatitis is produced when compounds such as psoralen or other linear furocoumarins come into direct contact with the skin or are digested and become bloodborne to dermal capillary beds, where they interact with sunlight.[68] These photosensitizing agents are activated by ultraviolet A radiation (320–400 nm), producing singlet oxygen and DNA adducts. In addition to severe sunburnlike symptoms (erythema, epidermal bullae), hyperpigmentation lasting for several months may result from exposure to these compounds. The mechanism by which this reaction is produced is unknown, but depletion of glutathione is postulated to indirectly stimulate melanogenesis by disinhibiting the normally suppressant tyrosinase.[142] More than 200 of these xenobiotics have been identified in at least 15 plant families, including food sources, such as Apiaceae (anise, caraway, carrot, celery, chervil, dill, fennel, parsley, and parsnip), Rutaceae (grapefruit, lemon, lime, bergamot, and orange), Solanaceae (potato), and Moraceae (figs) family.

Hepatogenous photosensitivity is produced when a xenobiotic that normally is harmlessly ingested, absorbed, and hepatically excreted gains access to the peripheral circulation through failure of a liver excretion or detoxification mechanism. An example is the photosensitivity that occurs when phylloerythrin, a product of chlorophyll digestion normally eliminated in the bile, accumulates in the blood as a result of liver dysfunction. The cyanobacterium *Microcystis aeruginosa*, as well as the plants *Lantana camara*, *Tribulus terrestris*, and *Agave lecheuilla* reportedly cause this type of photosensitization in animals.

SUMMARY

Plant xenobiotics can be organized by the principles of pharmacognosy. Examples are provided in which the xenobiotic has therapeutic use such as colchicine, taxine, physostigmine, and pilocarpine. Some xenobiotics act directly or are metabolized to toxic principals such as tremetone, whereas others are toxic through secondary contact in animal meat or milk such as coniine, tremetone, nitrates, pyrollizidine alkaloids, and ptaquiloside.

This analysis should not lead to the false conclusion that all toxic plants, all xenobiotics in plants, or all toxic mechanisms are known. Some reassurance can be achieved by excluding exposure to most life-threatening plants and plant xenobiotics or ascertaining whether a common exposure is toxic. This determination can be aided by basic taxonomy while awaiting expert input. Management should balance the relative risks of using invasive gastric emptying and use of activated charcoal if the plant induces sedation or vomiting or is nontoxic.

REFERENCES

1. Addae JT, Melvill GN. A re-examination of the mechanism of ackee induced vomiting sickness. *West Ind Med J.* 1988;37:6-8.
2. Akintonwa A, Tunwashe OL. Fatal cyanide poisoning from cassava-based meal. *Hum Exp Toxicol.* 1992;11:47-49.
3. Alexander RF, Forbes GB, Hawkins ES. A fatal case of solanine poisoning. *Br Med J.* 1948;2:518.
4. Alonso-Amelot ME, Avendano M. Human carcinogenesis and bracken fern: a review of the evidence. *Curr Med Chem.* 2002;9:675-686.
5. Ameri A. The effects of Aconitum alkaloids on the central nervous system. *Prog Neurobiol.* 1998;56:211-235.
6. Andre F. Role of new allergens and of allergens consumption in the increased incidence of food sensitizations in France. *Toxicology.* 1994:93:77-83.
7. Aplin PJ, Eliseo T. Ingestion of castor oil plant seeds. *Med J Aust.* 1997;167:260-261.
8. Arcury TA, Vallejos QM, Schulz MR, et al. Green tobacco sickness and skin integrity among migrant Latino farmworkers. *Am J Ind Med.* 2008;51:195-203.
9. Arnold HL. *Poisonous plants of Hawaii.* Honolulu: Tongg Publishing Co;1944.
10. Ascherio A, Bermudez CS, Garcia D. Outbreak of buckthorn paralysis in Nicaragua. *J Trop Pediatr.* 1992;38:87-89.
11. Audi J, Belson M, Patel M, et al. Ricin poisoning: a comprehensive review. *JAMA.* 2005;294:2342-2351.
12. Babu CK, Ansari KM, Mehrotra S, et al. Alterations in redox potential of glutathione/glutathione disulfide and cysteine/cysteine disulfide couples in plasma of dropsy patients with argemone oil poisoning. *Food Chem Toxicol.* 2008;46:2409-2414.
13. Bah M, Bye R, Pereda RM. Hepatotoxic pyrrolizidine alkaloids in the Mexican medicinal plant *Pachera candidissima* (*Asteraceae: Senecioneae*). *J Ethnopharmacol.* 1994;43:19-30.
14. Barceloux DG. Akee fruit and Jamaican vomiting sickness (*Blighia sapida* Köenig). *Dis Mon.* 2009;55:318-326.
15. Barceloux DG. Grass pea and neurolathyrism (*Lathyrus sativus* L.). *Dis Mon.* 2009;55:365-372.
16. Barker BE, Farnes P, LaMarche PH. Peripheral blood plasmacytosis following systemic exposure to *Phytolacca americana* (pokeweed). *Pediatrics.* 1966;38:490-493.
17. Beier RC, Norman JO, Reagor JC, et al. Isolation of the major component in white snakeroot that is toxic after microsomal activation: possible explanation of sporadic toxicity of white snakeroot plants and extracts. *J Nat Toxins.* 1993;1:286-293.
18. Biberci E, Altuntas Y, Cobanoglu A, Alpinar A. Acute respiratory arrest following hemlock (*Conium maculatum*) intoxication. *J Toxicol Clin Toxicol.* 2002;40:517-518.
19. Bisset NG. War and hunting poisons of the New World. Part 1. Notes on the early history of curare. *J Ethnopharmacol.* 1992;36:1-26.
20. Blythe WB. Hemlock poisoning, acute renal failure, and the Bible. *Ren Fail.* 1993;15:653.

21. Boppré M, Colegate SM, Edgar JA, Fischer OW. Hepatotoxic pyrrolizidine alkaloids in pollen and drying-related implications for commercial processing of bee pollen. *J Agric Food Chem.* 2008;56:5662-5672.
22. Borsutzky M, Passie T, Paetzold W, et al. Hawaiian baby woodrose: (psycho-) pharmacological effects of the seeds of *Argyreia nervosa*. A case-orientated demonstration. *Nervenarzt.* 2002;73:892-896.
23. Boumba VA, Mitselou A, Vougiouklakis T. Fatal poisoning from ingestion of *Datura stramonium* seeds. *Vet Hum Toxicol.* 2004;46:81-82.
24. Bressler R. The unripe ackee—forbidden fruit. *N Engl J Med.* 1976;295:500-501.
25. Bressler R, Corredor C, Brendel K. Hypoglycin and hypoglycin-like compounds. *Pharmacol Rev.* 1969;21:105-127.
26. Brownson DM, Mabry TJ, Leslie SW. The cycad neurotoxic amino acid β-N-methylamino-L-alanine (BMAA), elevates intracellular calcium levels in dissociated rats cells. *J Ethnopharmacol.* 2002;82:159-167.
27. Bruynzeel DP. Bulb dermatitis. Dermatological problems in the flower bulb industries. *Contact Dermatitis.* 1997;37:70-77.
28. Brvar M, Kozelj G, Mozina M, Bunc M. Acute poisoning with autumn crocus (*Colchicum autumnale* L.). *Wien Klin Wochenschr.* 2004;116:205-208.
29. Cairney S, Maruff P, Clough AR. The neurobehavioural effects of kava. *Aust N Z J Psychiatry.* 2002;36:657-662.
30. Carter JH, Goldman P. Bacteria-mediated cyanide poisoning by apricot kernels in children from Gaza. *Pediatrics.* 1981;68:5-7.
31. Centers for Disease Control and Prevention (CDC). Anticholinergic poisoning associated with an herbal tea—New York City, 1994. *MMWR Morb Mortal Wkly Rep.* 1995;44:193-195.
32. Centers for Disease Control and Prevention (CDC). Hepatic toxicity possibly associated with Kava-containing products—United States, Germany, and Switzerland, 1999-2002. *MMWR Morb Mortal Wkly Rep.* 2002;51:1065-1067.
33. Centers for Disease Control and Prevention (CDC). Jimson weed poisoning—Texas, New York, California, 1994. *MMWR Morb Mortal Wkly Rep.* 1995;44:41-44.
34. Centers for Disease Control and Prevention (CDC). Poisoning from elderberry juice—California. *MMWR Morb Mortal Wkly Rep.* 1984;33:173-174.
35. Centers for Disease Control and Prevention (CDC). Toxic hypoglycemic syndrome—Jamaica, 1989-1991. *MMWR Morb Mortal Wkly Rep.* 1992;41:53-55.
36. Centers for Disease Control and Prevention (CDC). Water hemlock poisoning—Maine, 1992. *MMWR Morb Mortal Wkly Rep.* 1994;43:229-231.
37. Chan TY. Aconitine poisoning: a global perspective. *Vet Hum Toxicol.* 1994;36:326-328.
38. Chan TY, Tomlinson B, Critchley JA, Cockram CS. Herb-induced aconite poisoning presenting as tetraplegia. *Vet Hum Toxicol.* 1994;36:133-134.
39. Chan YL, Ng HK, Leung CB, Yeung DK. (31)Phosphorous and single voxel proton MR spectroscopy and diffusion-weighted imaging in a case of star fruit poisoning. *AJNR Am J Neuroradiol.* 2002;23:1557-1560.
40. Chang SS, Chan YL, Wu ML, et al. Acute *Cycas* seed poisoning in Taiwan. *J Toxicol Clin Toxicol.* 2004;42:49-54.
41. Chase GW Jr, Landen WO Jr, Soliman AG. Hypoglycin A content in the aril, seeds, husks of ackee fruit at various stages of ripeness. *J Assoc Off Anal Chem.* 1990;73:318-319.
42. Clouatre DL. Kava kava: examining new reports of toxicity. *Toxicol Lett.* 2004;150:85-96.
43. Colodel EM, Gardner DR, Zlotowski P, Driemeier D. Identification of swainsonine as a glycoside inhibitor responsible for *Sida carpinifolia* poisoning. *Vet Hum Toxicol.* 2002;44:177-178.
44. Cox PA, Sacks OW. Cycad neurotoxins, consumption of flying foxes, and ALS-PDC disease in Guam. *Neurology.* 2002;58:956-959.
45. Crone C, Petersen NT, Gimenéz-Roldán S, et al. Reduced reciprocal inhibition is seen only in spastic limbs in patients with neurolathyrism. *Exp Brain Res.* 2007;181:193-197.
46. Crummett D, Bronstein D, Weaver Z 3d. Accidental *Veratrum viride* poisoning in three "ramp" foragers. *N C Med J.* 1985;46:469-471.
47. Cumpston KL, Vogel SN, Leikin JB, Erickson TB. Acute airway compromise after brief exposure to a *Dieffenbachia* plant. *J Emerg Med.* 2003;25:391-397.
48. Das M, Khanna SK. Clinicoepidemiological, toxicological, and safety evaluation studies on argemone oil. *Crit Rev Toxicol.* 1997;27:273-297.
49. Dasgupta A. Therapeutic drug monitoring of digoxin: impact of endogenous and exogenous digoxin-like immunoreactive substances. *Toxicol Rev.* 2006;25:273-281.
50. Davison AG, Britton MG, Forrester JA, et al. Asthma in merchant seamen and laboratory workers caused by allergy to castor beans: analysis of allergens. *Clin Allergy.* 1983;13:553-561.
51. Dawson RM. The toxicology of microcystins. *Toxicon.* 1998;36:953-962.
52. de Jonge H, Vanrenterghem Y. Aristolochic acid: the common culprit of Chinese herbs nephropathy and Balkan endemic nephropathy. *Nephrol Dial Transplant.* 2008;23:39-41.
53. de Silva HA, Fonseka MM, Pathmeswaran A, et al. Multiple-dose activated charcoal for treatment of yellow oleander poisoning: a single-blind, randomised, placebo-controlled trial. *Lancet.* 2003;361:1935-1938.
54. Debelle FD, Vanherweghem JL, Nortier JL. Aristolochic acid nephropathy: a worldwide problem. *Kidney Int.* 2008;74:158-169.
55. Deng JF, Ger J, Tsai WJ, Kao WF, Yang CC. Acute toxicities of betel nut: rare but probably overlooked events. *J Toxicol Clin Toxicol.* 2001;39:355-360.
56. Dickers KJ, Bradberry SM, Rice P, et al. Abrin poisoning. *Toxicol Rev.* 2003;22:137-142.
57. Ding W-X, Shen H-M, Zhur H-G, et al. Genotoxicity of microcystic *Cyanobacteria* extract of a water source in China. *Mutat Res.* 1999;442:69-77.
58. Dittmann E, Wiegand C. Cyanobacterial toxins—occurrence, biosynthesis and impact on human affairs. *Mol Nutr Food Res.* 2006;50:7-17.
59. Doneray H, Orbak Z, Karakelleoglu C. Clinical outcomes in children with hyoscyamus niger intoxication not receiving physostigmine therapy. *Eur J Emerg Med.* 2007;14:348-350.
60. Drummer OH, Roberts AN, Bedford PJ. Three deaths from hemlock poisoning. *Med J Aust.* 1995;162:592-593.
61. Durand MF, Pommier P, Chazalette A, de Haro L. [Child poisoning after ingestion of a wild apiaceae. a case report]. *Arch Pediatr.* 2008;15:139-141.
62. Eddleston M, Ariaratnam CA, Sjostrom L, et al. Acute yellow oleander (*Thevetia peruviana*) poisoning: cardiac arrhythmias, electrolyte disturbances, and serum cardiac glycoside concentrations on presentation to hospital. *Heart.* 2000;83:301-306.
63. Eddleston M, Hagalla S. Fatal injury in eastern Sri Lanka, with special reference to cardenolide self-poisoning with *Cerbera manghas* fruits. *Clin Toxicol (Phila).* 2008;46:745-748.
64. Eddleston M, Rajapakse S, Rajakanthan, et al. Anti-digoxin Fab fragments in cardiotoxicity induced by ingestion of yellow oleander: a randomized controlled trial. *Lancet.* 2000;355:967-972.
65. Eddleston M, Senarathna L, Mohamed F, et al. Deaths due to absence of an affordable antitoxin for plant poisoning. *Lancet.* 2003;362:1041-1044.
66. Edwards N. Local toxicity from a poinsettia plant: a case report. *J Pediatr.* 1983;102:404-405.
67. Eke T, Al-Husainy S, Raynor MK. The spectrum of ocular inflammation caused by *Euphorbia* plant sap. *Arch Ophthalmol.* 2000;118:13-16.
68. Epstein JH. Phototoxicity and photoallergy. *Semin Cutan Med Surg.* 1999;18:274-284.
69. Ernst E. A re-evaluation of kava (*Piper methysticum*). *Br J Clin Pharmacol.* 2007;64:415-417.
70. Evans WC, ed. *Trease and Evans' Pharmacognosy*, 16th ed. London: WB Saunders; 2009.
71. Evans WC, Evans IA, Humphreys DJ, et al. Induction of thiamine deficiency in sheep, with lesions similar to those of cerebrocortical necrosis. *J Comp Pathol.* 1975;85:253-267.
72. Farese RV, Biglieri EG, Shackleton CHL, et al. Licorice-induced hypermineralocorticoidism. *N Engl J Med.* 1991;325:1223-1227.
73. Feldman R, Chrobak J, Liberek Z, Szafewski J. Four cases of poisoning with the extract of yew (*Taxus baccata*) needles. *Pol Arch Med Wewn.* 1988;79:26-29.
74. Fernandez C, Fiandor A, Marinez-Garate A, Martinez Quesada J. Allergy to pistachio: cross-reactivity between pistachio nut and other Anacardiaceae. *Clin Exp Allergy.* 1995;25:1254-1259.
75. Fisher AA. Poison ivy/oak dermatitis. Part I: prevention-soap and water, topical barriers, hyposensitization. *Cutis.* 1996;57:384-385.
76. Fisher AA. Poison ivy/oak dermatitis. Part II: specific features. *Cutis.* 1996;58:22-24.
77. Frasca T, Brett AS, Yoo SD. Mandrake toxicity. A case of mistaken identity. *Arch Intern Med.* 1997;157:2007-2009.
78. Friedland RP, Armon C. Tales of Pacific tangles: cycad exposure and Guamanian neurodegenerative diseases. *Neurology.* 2007;68:1759-1761.
79. Fu M, Wu M, Qiao Y, Wang Z. Toxicological mechanisms of *Aconitum* alkaloids. *Pharmazie.* 2006;61:735-741.

80. Fu PP, Xia Q, Lin G, Chou MW. Pyrrolizidine alkaloids—genotoxicity, metabolism enzymes, metabolic activation, and mechanisms. *Drug Metab Rev.* 2004;36:1-55.
81. Fugh-Berman A. Herb-drug interactions. *Lancet.* 2000;355:134-138.
82. Fugr U. Drug interactions with grapefruit juice. Extent, probable mechanism and clinical relevance. *Drug Saf.* 1998;18:251-272.
83. Fujisawa M, Hori Y, Nakajima M, et al. Gas chromatography-mass spectrometry analysis of 4-O-methylpyridoxine (MPN) in the serum of patients with ginkgo seed poisoning. *J Anal Toxicol.* 2002;26:138-143.
84. Gardner DG. Injury to the oral mucous membranes caused by the common houseplant, dieffenbachia. A review. *Oral Surg Oral Med Oral Pathol.* 1994;78:631-633.
85. Getahun H, Lambein F, Vanhoorne M, Van der Stuyft P. Neurolathyrism risk depends on type of grass pea preparation and on mixing with cereals and antioxidants. *Trop Med Int Health.* 2005;10:169-178.
86. Gil Campos M, Perez Navero JL, Ibarra De La Rosa I. Convulsive status secondary to star anise poisoning in a neonate. *An Esp Pediatr.* 2002;57: 366-368.
87. Gilroy DJ, Kauffman KW, Hall RA, et al. Assessing potential health risks from microcystin toxins in blue-green algae dietary supplements. *Environ Health Perspect.* 2000;108:435-439.
88. Gladman AC. Toxicodendron dermatitis: poison ivy, oak, and sumac. *Wilderness Environ Med.* 2006;17:120-128.
89. Gordon DW, Rosenthal G, Hart J, Sirota R, Baker AL. Chaparral ingestion. The broadening spectrum of liver injury caused by herbal medications. *JAMA.* 1995;273:489-490.
90. Gordon LA. Compositae dermatitis. *Australas J Dermatol.* 1999;40:123-128.
91. Gowdy JM. Stramonium intoxication: a review of symptomatology in 212 cases. *JAMA.* 1972;221:585-587.
92. Grob PJ, Muller-Schoop JW, Hacki MA, Joller-Jemelka HI. Drug-induced pseudolupus. *Lancet.* 1975;2:144-148.
93. Grollman AP, Shibutani S, Moriya M, et al. Aristolochic acid and the etiology of endemic (Balkan) nephropathy. *Proc Natl Acad Sci USA.* 2007;104:12129-12134.
94. Gunduz A, Turedi S, Russell RM, Ayaz FA. Clinical review of grayanotoxin/mad honey poisoning past and present. *Clin Toxicol (Phila).* 2008;46:437-442.
95. Hamilton RJ, Goldfrank LR. Poison center data and the Pollyanna phenomenon. *J Toxicol Clin Toxicol.* 1997;35:21-23.
96. Hamilton RJ, Shih RD, Hoffman RS. Mobitz type I heart block after pokeweed ingestion. *Vet Hum Toxicol.* 1995;37:66-67.
97. Hammond-Tooke GD, Taylor P, Punchihewa S, Beasley M. *Urtica ferox* neuropathy. *Muscle Nerve.* 2007;35:804-807.
98. Hamouda C, Hedhili A, Ben Salah N, et al. A review of acute poisoning from *Atractylis gummifera* L. *Vet Hum Toxicol.* 2004;46:144-146.
99. Harkrader RJ, Reinhart PC, Rogers JA, et al. The history, chemistry and pharmacokinetics of *Sanguinaria* extract. *J Can Dent Assoc.* 1990;56:7-12.
100. Heath KB. A fatal case of apparent water hemlock poisoning. *Vet Hum Toxicol.* 2001;43:35-36.
101. Heilpern KL. Zigadenus poisoning. *Ann Emerg Med.* 1995;25:259-262.
102. Hogan RP III. Hemorrhagic diathesis caused by drinking an herbal tea. *JAMA.* 1983;49:2679-2680.
103. Hou YC, Hsiu SL, Tsao CW, Wang YH, Chao PD. Acute intoxication of cyclosporin caused by coadministration of decoctions of the fruits of *Citrus aurantium* and the Pericarps of *Citrus grandis. Planta Med.* 2000;66:653-655.
104. Hsiue TR, Guo YL, Chen KW, et al. Dose–response relationship and irreversible obstructive ventilatory defect in patients with consumption of *Sauropus androgynus. Chest.* 1998;113:71-76.
105. Hudak KA, Wank P, Tumer NE. A novel mechanism for inhibition of translation by pokeweed antiviral protein: depurination of the capped RNK template. *RNA.* 2000;6:369-380.
106. Isbrucker RA, Burdock GA. Risk and safety assessment on the consumption of licorice root (*Glycyrrhiza* sp.), its extract and powder as a food ingredient, with emphasis on the pharmacology and toxicology of glycyrrhizin. *Regul Toxicol Pharmacol.* 2006;46:167-192.
107. Ize-Ludlow D, Ragone S. Neurotoxicities in infants seen with the consumption of star anise tea. *Pediatrics.* 2004;114:653-656.
108. Izzo AA, Ernst E. Interactions between herbal medicines and prescribed drugs: a systematic review. *Drugs.* 2001;61:2163-2175.
109. Jackson DV, Rosenbaum DL, Carlisle LJ, et al. Glutamic acid modification of vincristine toxicity. *Cancer Biochem Biophys.* 1984;7:245-252.
110. Jochimsen EM, Carmichael WW, An JS, et al. Liver failure and death after exposure to microcystins at a hemodialysis center in Brazil. *N Engl J Med.* 1998;338:873-878.
111. Joskow R, Belson M, Vesper H, Backer L, Rubin C. Ackee fruit poisoning: an outbreak investigation in Haiti 2000-2001, and review of the literature. *Clin Toxicol (Phila).* 2006;44:267-273.
112. Kajiyama Y, Fujii K, Takeuchi H, Manabe Y. *Ginkgo* seed poisoning. *Pediatrics.* 2002;109:325-327.
113. Kanerva L, Alanko K, Pelttari M, Estlander T. Occupational allergic contact dermatitis from Compositae in agricultural work. *Contact Dermatitis.* 2000;42:238-239.
114. Kao WF, Hung DZ, Tsai WJ, et al. Podophyllotoxin intoxication: toxic effect of Bajiaolian in herbal therapeutics. *Hum Exp Toxicol.* 1992;11:480-487.
115. Kaplan M, Vreman HJ, Hammerman C, et al. Favism by proxy in nursing glucose-6-phosphate dehydrogenase-deficient neonates. *J Perinatol.* 1998;18:477-479.
116. Krakauer J. *Into the Wild.* New York: Doubleday; 1996.
117. Krenzelok EP, Jacobsen TD. Plant exposures—a national profile of the most common plant genera. *Vet Hum Toxicol.* 1997;39:248-249.
118. Krenzelok EP, Jacobsen TD, Aronis J. American mistletoe exposures. *Am J Emerg Med.* 1997;15:516-520.
119. Krenzelok EP, Jacobsen TD, Aronis JM. Lily of the valley (*Convallaria majalis*) exposures: are the outcomes consistent with the reputation [abstract]? *J Toxicol Clin Toxicol.* 1996;34:601.
120. Krenzelok EP, Jacobsen TD, Aronis JM. Poinsettia exposures have good outcomes—just as we thought. *Am J Emerg Med.* 1996;14:671-674.
121. Kulkarni ML, Sreekar H, Keshavamurthy KS, Shenoy N. *Jatropha curcas*—poisoning. *Indian J Pediatr.* 2005;72:75-76.
122. Lachenmeier DW, Emmert J, Kuballa T, Sartor G. Thujone—cause of absinthism? *Forensic Sci Int.* 2006;158:1-8.
123. Lambein F, Haque R, Khan JK, et al. From soil to brain: zinc deficiency increases the neurotoxicity of *Lathyrus sativus* and may affect the susceptibility for the motorneuronal disease neurolathyrism. *Toxicon.* 1994;32: 461-466.
124. LaMotte RH, Shimada SG, Green BG, Zelterman D. Pruritic and nociceptive sensations and dysesthesias from a spicule of cowhage. *J Neurophysiol.* 2009;101:1430-1443.
125. Lampe KF. Rhododendrons, mountain laurel, and mad honey. *JAMA.* 1988;259:2009.
126. Langford SD, Boor PJ. Oleander toxicity: an examination of human and animal toxic exposures. *Toxicology.* 1996;109:1-13.
127. Laosombat V, Sattayasevana B, Chotsampancharoen T, Wongchanchailert M. Glucose-6-phosphate dehydrogenase variants associated with favism in Thai children. *Int J Hematol.* 2006;83:139-143.
128. Larson J, Vender R, Camuto P. Cholestatic jaundice due to ackee fruit poisoning. *Am J Gastroenterol.* 1994;89:1577-1578.
129. Lau CW, Yao XQ, Chen ZY, et al. Cardiovascular actions of berberine. *Cardiovasc Drug Rev.* 2001;19:234-244.
130. Le Couteur DG, Fisher AA. Chronic and criminal administration of *Nerium oleander. J Toxicol Clin Toxicol.* 2002;40:523-524.
131. Levin Y, Sherer Y, Bibi H, et al. Rare *Jatropha multifida* intoxication in two children. *J Emerg Med.* 2000;19:173-175.
132. Lewis WH, Elvin-Lewis MPF. *Medical Botany: Plants Affecting Man's Health.* New York: John Wiley & Sons; 1977.
133. Lieu YK, Hsu BY, Price WA, et al. Carnitine effects on coenzyme A profiles in rat liver with hypoglycin inhibition of multiple dehydrogenases. *Am J Physiol.* 1997;272:E359-E366.
134. Lin CC, Chan TY, Deng JF. Clinical features and management of herb-induced aconitine poisoning. *Ann Emerg Med.* 2004;43:574-579.
135. Lin TJ, Su CC, Lan CK, Jiang DD, Tsai JL, Tsai MS. Acute poisonings with *Breynia officinalis*—an outbreak of hepatotoxicity. *J Toxicol Clin Toxicol.* 2003;41:591-594.
136. Luh SP, Lee YC, Chang YL, et al. Lung transplantation for patients with end-stage *Sauropus androgynus*-induced bronchiolitis obliterans (SABO) syndrome. *Clin Transplant.* 1999;13:496-503.
137. Lundahl JU, Regardh CG, Edgar B, Johnsson G. The interaction effect of grapefruit juice is maximal after the first glass. *Eur J Clin Pharmacol.* 1998;54;75-81.
138. Madabushi R, Frank B, Drewelow B, et al. Hyperforin in St. John's wort drug interactions. *Eur J Clin Pharmacol.* 2006;62:225-233.
139. Magalhaes VF, Soares RM, Azevedo SM. Microcystin contamination in fish from the Jacarepagua Lagoon (Rio de Janeiro, Brazil): ecological implication and human health risk. *Toxicon.* 2001;39:1077-1085.
140. Mahady GB, Low Dog T, Barrett ML, et al. United States Pharmacopeia review of the black cohosh case reports of hepatotoxicity. *Menopause.* 2008;15:628-638.

141. Marks JG Jr, Fowler JF Jr, Sheretz EF, Rietschel RL. Prevention of poison ivy and poison oak allergic contact dermatitis by quaternium-18 bentonite. *J Am Acad Dermatol.* 1995;33:212-216.
142. Marrot L, Meunier JR. Skin DNA photodamage and its biological consequences. *J Am Acad Dermatol.* 2008;58(Suppl 2):S139-S148.
143. Martinez HR, Bermudez MV, Rangel-Guerra RA, de Leon Flores L. Clinical diagnosis in *Karwinskia humboldtiana* polyneuropathy. *J Neurol Sci.* 1998;154:49-54.
144. Massey LK, Sutton RAL. Modification of dietary oxalate and calcium reduces urinary oxalate in hyperoxaluric patients with kidney stones. *J Am Diet Assoc.* 1993;93:1305-1307.
145. McGee D, Brabson T, McCarthy J, Picciotti M. Four-year review of cigarette ingestions in children. *Pediatr Emerg Care.* 1995;11:13-16.
146. McGovern TW, LaWarre SR, Brunette C. Is it, or isn't it? Poison ivy look-a-likes. *Am J Contact Dermat.* 2000;11:104-110.
147. McIntire MS, Guest JR, Porterfield JF. Philodendron—an infant death. *J Toxicol Clin Toxicol.* 1990;28:177-183.
148. McKinney PE, Gomez HF, Phillips S, Brent J. The fax machine: a new method of plant identification. *J Toxicol Clin Toxicol.* 1993;31:663-665.
149. McMillan M, Thompson JC. An outbreak of suspected solanine poisoning in schoolboys: examination of solanine poisoning. *QJ Med.* 1979;48:227-243.
150. McTague JA, Forney R Jr. Jamaican vomiting sickness in Toledo, Ohio. *Ann Emerg Med.* 1994;23:1116-1118.
151. Meda HA, Diallo B, Buchet JP, et al. Epidemic of fatal encephalopathy in preschool children in Burkina and consumption of unripe ackee (*Blighia sapida*) fruit. *Lancet.* 1999;353:536-540.
152. Mejia MJ, Morales MM, Llopis A, Martinez I. School children poisoning by ornamental trees. *Aten Primaria.* 1991;8:88, 90-91.
153. Meschler JP, Howlett AC. Thujone exhibits low affinity for cannabinoid receptors but fails to evoke cannabimimetic responses. *Pharmacol Biochem Behav.* 1999;62:473-480.
154. Miller LG. Herbal medicinals: selected clinical considerations focusing on known or potential drug-herb interactions. *Arch Intern Med.* 1998;158: 2200-2211.
155. Mills J, Melville GN, Bennett C, et al. Effect of hypoglycin A on insulin release. *Biochem Pharmacol.* 1987;36:495-497.
156. Moertel CG, Fleming TR, Rubin J, et al. A clinical trial of amygdalin (Laetrile) in the treatment of human cancer. *N Engl J Med.* 1982;306: 201-206.
157. Moritz F, Compagnon P, Kaliszczak IG, et al. Severe acute poisoning with homemade *Aconitum napellus* capsules: toxicokinetics and clinical data. *Clin Toxicol (Phila).* 2005;43:873-876.
158. Morkovsky O, Kucera J. Mass poisoning of children in a nursery school by the seeds of *Laburnum anagyroides*. *Cesk Pediatr.* 1980;35:284-285.
159. Mrvos R, Dean BS, Krenzelok EP. *Philodendron/dieffenbachia* ingestions: are they a problem? *J Toxicol Clin Toxicol.* 1991;29:485-491.
160. Mueller SC, Majcher-Peszynska J, Mundkowski RG, et al. No clinically relevant CYP3A induction after St. John's wort with low hyperforin content in healthy volunteers. *Eur J Clin Pharmacol.* 2009;65:81-87.
161. Mueller SC, Majcher-Peszynska J, Uehleke B, et al. The extent of induction of CYP3A by St. John's wort varies among products and is linked to hyperforin dose. *Eur J Clin Pharmacol.* 2006;62:29-36.
162. Murphy NG, Albin C, Tai W, Benowitz NL. Anabasine toxicity from a topical folk remedy. *Clin Pediatr (Phila).* 2006;45:669-671.
163. Nagy M. Human poisoning from horse chestnuts. *JAMA.* 1973;226:213.
164. Nelson LS, Shih RD, Balick M. *Handbook of Poisonous and Injurious Plants*, 2nd ed. New York: Springer; 2007.
165. Neto MM, da Costa JA, Garcia-Cairasco N, et al. Intoxication by star fruit (*Averrhoa carambola*) in 32 uraemic patients: treatment and outcome. *Nephrol Dial Transplant.* 2003;18:120-125.
166. Newman LS, Feinberg MW, LeWine HE. A bitter tale. *N Engl J Med.* 2004;351:594-599.
167. Ng THK, Chan YW, Yu YL, et al. Encephalopathy and neuropathy following ingestion of a Chinese herbal broth containing podophyllin. *J Neurol Sci.* 1991;101:107-113.
168. Ocampo-Roosens LV, Ontiveros-Nevares PG, Fernández-Lucio O. Intoxication with buckthorn (*Karwinskia humboldtiana*): report of three siblings. *Pediatr Dev Pathol.* 2007;10:66-68.
169. Ohuchi S, Izumoto H, Kamata J, Kawase T, et al. A case of aconitine poisoning saved with cardiopulmonary bypass. *Kyobu Geka.* 2000;53:541-544.
170. Olivera F, Amon EU, Breathnach A, et al. Contact urticaria due to the common stinging nettle (*Urtica dioica*)—histological, ultrastructural and pharmacological studies. *Clin Exp Dermatol.* 1991;16:1-7.
171. Oonakahara K, Matsuyama W, Higashimoto I, et al. Outbreak of Bronchiolitis obliterans associated with consumption of Sauropus androgynus in Japan—alert of food-associated pulmonary disorders from Japan. *Respiration.* 2005;72:221.
172. Padosch SA, Lachenmeier DW, Krööner LU. Absinthism: a fictitious 19th century syndrome with present impact. *Subst Abuse Treat Prev Policy.* 2006;1:14.
173. Pai KS, Ravidranath V. L-BOAA induces selective inhibition of brain mitochondrial enzyme, NADH-dehydrogenase. *Brain Res.* 1993;621: 215-221.
174. Paine MF, Widmer WW, Pusek SN, et al. Further characterization of a furanocoumarin-free grapefruit juice on drug disposition: studies with cyclosporine. *Am J Clin Nutr.* 2008;87:863-871.
175. Pedaci L, Kernzelok EP, Jacobsen TD, Aronis J. Dieffenbachia species exposures: an evidence-based assessment of symptom presentation. *Vet Hum Toxicol.* 1999;41:335-358.
176. Philippe G, Angenot L, Tits M, Frédérich M. About the toxicity of some *Strychnos* species and their alkaloids. *Toxicon.* 2004;44:405-416.
177. Phillips BJ, Hughes JA, Phillips JC, et al. A study of the toxic hazard that might be associated with the consumption of green potato tops. *Food Chem Toxicol.* 1996;34:439-448.
178. Pietsch J, Schulz K, Schmidt U, et al. A comparative study of five fatal cases of *Taxus* poisoning. *Int J Legal Med.* 2007;121:417-422.
179. Pohl RW. Poisoning by *Dieffenbachia*. *JAMA.* 1961;177:812-813.
180. Poon WT, Ho CH, Yip KL, et al. Grayanotoxin poisoning from *Rhododendron simsii* in an infant. *Hong Kong Med J.* 2008;14:450-457.
181. Prance G. The poisons and narcotics of the Amazonian Indians. *JR Coll Physicians Lond.* 1999;33:368-376.
182. Quandt SA, Arcury TA, Preisser JS, et al. Migrant farmworkers and green tobacco sickness: new issues for an understudied disease. *Am J Ind Med.* 2000;37:307-315.
183. Ramlakhan SL, Fletcher AK. It could have happened to Van Gogh: a case of fatal purple foxglove poisoning and review of the literature. *Eur J Emerg Med.* 2007;14:356-359.
184. Rao RB, Hoffman RS. Nicotinic toxicity from tincture of blue cohosh (*Caulophyllum thalictroides*) used as an abortifacient. *Vet Hum Toxicol.* 2002;44:221-222.
185. Rao SD, Banack SA, Cox PA, Weiss JH. BMAA selectively injures motor neurons via AMPA/kainite receptor activation. *Exp Neurol.* 2006;201:244-252.
186. Reidenberg MM. Environmental inhibition of 11beta-hydroxysteroid dehydrogenase. *Toxicology.* 2000;144:107-111.
187. Reynolds T. Hemlock alkaloids from Socrates to poison aloes. *Phytochemistry.* 2005;66:1399-1406.
188. Rich SA, Libera JM, Locke RJ. Treatment of foxglove extract poisoning with digoxin-specific Fab fragments. *Ann Emerg Med.* 1993;22:1904-1907.
189. Rizzi D, Basile L, DiMaggio A, et al. Clinical spectrum of accidental hemlock poisoning: neurotoxic manifestations, rhabdomyolysis and acute tubular necrosis. *Nephrol Dial Transplant.* 1991;6:939-943.
190. Robbers JE, Speedie MK, Tyler VE, eds. *Pharmacognosy and Pharmacobiotechnology.* Baltimore, MD: Williams & Wilkins; 1996.
191. Roberge R, Brader E, Martin ML, et al. The root of evil pokeweed intoxication. *Ann Emerg Med.* 1986;15:470-473.
192. Rodrigues TD, Johnson PN, Jeffrey LP. Holly berry ingestion: case report. *Vet Hum Toxicol.* 1984;26:157-158.
193. Roeder E. Medicinal plants in China containing pyrrolizidine alkaloids. *Pharmazie.* 2000;55:711-726.
194. Roeder E. Medicinal plants in Europe containing pyrrolizidine alkaloids. *Pharmazie.* 1995;50:83-98.
195. Rondeau ES. Wisteria toxicity. *J Toxicol Clin Toxicol.* 1993;31:107-112.
196. Rosenblatt M, Mindel J. Spontaneous hyphema associated with ingestion of *Ginkgo biloba* extract. *N Engl J Med.* 1997;336:1108.
197. Ruha AM, Tanen DA, Graeme KA, et al. Hypertonic sodium bicarbonate for *Taxus media*-induced cardiac toxicity in swine. *Acad Emerg Med.* 2002;9: 179-185.
198. Ruprich J, Rehurkova I, Boon PE, et al. Probabilistic modelling of exposure doses and implications for health risk characterization: glycoalkaloids from potatoes. *Food Chem Toxicol.* 2009;47:2899-2905.
199. Safadi R, Levy I, Amitai Y, et al. Beneficial effect of digoxin-specific Fab antibody fragments in oleander intoxication. *Arch Intern Med.* 1995;155: 2121-2125.
200. Salen P, Shih R, Sierzenski P, Reed J. Effect of physostigmine and gastric lavage in a *Datura stramonium*-induced anticholinergic poisoning epidemic. *Am J Emerg Med.* 2003;21:316-317.

201. Sandvig K, van Deurs B. Endocytosis and intracellular transport of ricin: recent discoveries. *FEBS Lett.* 1999;452:67-70.
202. Santucci B, Picardo M. Occupational contact dermatitis to plants. *Clin Dermatol.* 1992;10:157-165.
203. Scatizzi A, Di Maggio A, Rizzi D, et al. Acute renal failure due to tubular necrosis caused by wildfowl-mediated hemlock poisoning. *Ren Fail.* 1993;15:93-96.
204. Schep LJ, Schmierer DM, Fountain JS. Veratrum poisoning. *Toxicol Rev.* 2006;25:73-78.
205. Schulman S. Addressing the potential risks associated with ephedra use: a review of recent efforts. *Public Health Rep.* 2003;118:487-492.
206. Sharma OP, Dawra RK, Kurade NP, Sharma PD. A review of the toxicosis and biological properties of the genus Eupatorium. *J Nat Toxins.* 1998;6:1-14.
207. Singh R, Faridi MM, Singh K, et al. Epidemic dropsy in the eastern region of Nepal. *J Trop Pediatr.* 1999;45:8-13.
208. Slifman NR, Obermeyer WR, Aloi BK, et al. Contamination of botanical dietary supplements by *Digitalis lanata. N Engl J Med.* 1998;339:806-811.
209. Smith SW, Giesbrecht E, Thompson M, et al. Solanaceous steroidal glycoalkaloids and poisoning by *Solanum torvum*, the normally edible susumber berry. *Toxicon.* 2008;52:667-676.
210. Smith SW, Shah RR, Hunt JL, Herzog CA. Bidirectional ventricular tachycardia resulting from herbal aconite poisoning. *Ann Emerg Med.* 2005;45:100-101.
211. Snyman T, Stewart MJ, Steenkamp V. A fatal case of pepper poisoning. *Forensic Sci Int.* 2001;124:43-46.
212. Spencer PS. Food toxins, AMPA receptors and motor neuron diseases. *Drug Metab Rev.* 1999;31:561-587.
213. Spiller HA, Willias DB, Gorman SE, Sanftleban J. Retrospective study of mistletoe ingestion. *J Toxicol Clin Toxicol.* 1996;34:405-408.
214. Spina SP, Taddei A. Teenagers with Jimson weed (*Datura stramonium*) poisoning. *CJEM.* 2007;9:467-468.
215. Spoerke DG, Spoerke SE. Three cases of *Zigadenus* (death camus) poisoning. *Vet Hum Toxicol.* 1979;21:346-347.
216. Staumont G, Frexinos J, Fioramonti J, Buéno L. Sennosides and human colonic motility. *Pharmacology.* 1988;36(Suppl 1):49-56.
217. Steele JC, McGeer PL. The ALS/PDC syndrome of Guam and the cycad hypothesis. *Neurology.* 2008;70:1984-1990.
218. Steenkamp PA, Harding NM, van Heerden FR, van Wyk BE. Identification of atractyloside by LC-ESI-MS in alleged herbal poisonings. *Forensic Sci Int.* 2006;163:81-92.
219. Stefanovic V, Toncheva D, Atanasova S, Polenakovic M. Etiology of Balkan endemic nephropathy and associated urothelial cancer. *Am J Nephrol.* 2006;26:1-11.
220. Stegelmeier BL, Edgar JA, Colegate SM, et al. Pyrrolizidine alkaloid plants, metabolism and toxicity. *J Nat Toxins.* 1999;8:95-116.
221. Stoner JG, Rasmussen JE. Plant dermatitis. *J Am Acad Dermatol.* 1983;9:1-15.
222. Strauss U, Wittstock U, Schubert R, et al. Cicutoxin from *Cicuta virosa*—a new and potent potassium channel blocker in T lymphocytes. *Biochem Biophys Res Commun.* 1996;219:332-336.
223. Suchard JR, Wallace KL, Gerkin RD. Acute cyanide toxicity caused by apricot kernel ingestion. *Ann Emerg Med.* 1998;32:742-744.
224. Sundov Z, Nincevic Z, Definis-Gojanovic M, et al. Fatal colchicine poisoning by accidental ingestion of meadow saffron-case report. *Forensic Sci Int.* 2005;149:253-256.
225. Szalai K, Schöll I, Förster-Waldl E, et al. Occupational sensitization to ribosome-inactivating proteins in researchers. *Clin Exp Allergy.* 2005;35:1354-1360.
226. Taitzoglou IA, Tsantarliotou M, Kouretas D, Kokolis NA. Gossypol-induced inhibition of plasminogen activator activity in human and ovine acrosomal extract. *Andrologia.* 1999;31:355-359.
227. Tan XQ, Ruan JL, Chen HS, Wang JY. Studies on liver-toxicity in rhigoma of *Dioscorea bulbifera. Zhongguo Zhong Yao Za Zhi.* 2003;28:661-663.
228. Thomsen M, Vitetta L, Sali A, Schmidt M. Acute liver failure associated with the use of herbal preparations containing black cohosh. *Med Aust J.* 2004;180:598-599.
229. Tominack RL, Spyker DA. Capsicum and capsaicin—a review. Case report of the use of hot peppers in child abuse. *J Toxicol Clin Toxicol.* 1987;25:591-601.
230. Tongcok Y, Kozan O, Cavdar C, Guven H, Fowler J. *Urginea maritime* (squill) toxicity. *J Toxicol Clin Toxicol.* 1995;33:83-86.
231. Tse KC, Yip PS, Lam MF, Choy BY, et al. Star fruit intoxication in uraemic patients: case series and review of the literature. *Intern Med J.* 2003;33:314-316.
232. Turgut M, Alhan CC, Gürgöze M, et al. Carboxyatractyloside poisoning in humans. *Ann Trop Paediatr.* 2005;25:125-134.
233. Vale S. Subarachnoid haemorrhage associated with *Ginkgo biloba. Lancet.* 1998;352:36.
234. Vargas CP, Wolf LR, Gamm SR, Koontz K. Getting to the root (*Acorus calamus*) of the problem. *J Toxicol Clin Toxicol.* 1998;36:259-260.
235. Vetter J. Plant cyanogenic glycosides. *Toxicon.* 2000;38:11-36.
236. Vetter J. Poison hemlock (*Conium maculatum* L). *Food Chem Toxicol.* 2004;42:1373-1382.
237. Vidmar DA, Iwane MK. Assessment of the ability of the topical skin protectant (TSP) to protect against contact dermatitis to urushiol (Rhus) antigen. *Am J Contact Dermat.* 1999;10:190-197.
238. Vriens J, Nilius B, Vennekens R. Herbal compounds and toxins modulating TRP channels. *Curr Neuropharmacol.* 2008;6:79-96.
239. Wada K, Ishigaki S, Ueda K, Sakata M, Haga M. An antivitamin B6, 4'-methoxypyridoxine, from seed of *Ginkgo biloba* L. *Chem Pharm Bull.* 1985;33:3555-3557.
240. Wang SY, Wang GK. Voltage-gated sodium channels as primary targets of diverse lipid-soluble neurotoxins. *Cell Signal.* 2003;15:151-159.
241. Wasfi IA, Zorob O, Al katheeri NA, Al Awadhi AM. A fatal case of oleandrin poisoning. *Forensic Sci Int.* 2008;179:e31-e36.
242. Watson JT, Jones RC, Siston AM, et al. Outbreak of food-borne illness associated with plant material containing raphides. *Clin Toxicol (Phila).* 2005;43:17-21.
243. Waud RA. A digitalis-like action of extracts made from holly. *J Pharmacol Exp Ther.* 1932;45:279.
244. Wax PM, Cobaugh DJ, Lawrence RA. Should home ipecac-induced emesis be routinely recommended in the management of toxic berry ingestions? *Vet Hum Toxicol.* 1999;41:394-397.
245. Wehner F, Gawatz O. Suicidal yew poisoning—from Caesar to today—or suicide instructions on the Internet. *Arch Kriminol.* 2003;211:19-26.
246. Weinberg RB. Hunan hand [letter]. *N Engl J Med.* 1981;305:1020.
247. Weisbord SD, Soule JB, Kimmel PL. Poison online—acute renal failure caused by oil of wormwood purchased through the Internet. *N Engl J Med.* 1997;337:825-827.
248. West LG, McLaughlin JL, Eisenbeiss GK. Saponins and triterpenes from *Ilex opaca. Phytochemistry.* 1977;16:1846-1847.
249. Willaert W, Claessens P, Vankelecom B, Vanderheyden M. Intoxication with taxus baccata: cardiac arrhythmias following yew leaves ingestion. *Pacing Clin Electrophysiol.* 2002;25:511-512.
250. Wilson B. The rise and fall of laetrile. *Nutr Forum.* 1988;5:33-40.
251. Wilson CR, Sauer J, Hooser SB. Taxines: a review of the mechanism and toxicity of yew (*Taxus* spp.) alkaloids. *Toxicon.* 2001;39:175-185.
252. Wilson D, Donaldson LJ, Sepai O. Should we be frightened of bracken? A review of the evidence. *J Epidemiol Community Health.* 1998;52:812-817.
253. Yoshida S, Takayama Y. Licorice-induced hypokalemia as a treatable cause of dropped head syndrome. *Clin Neurol Neurosurg.* 2003;105:286-287.
254. Zagler B, Zelger A, Salvatore C, et al. Dietary poisoning with *Veratrum album*—a report of two cases. *Wien Klin Wochenschr.* 2005;117:106-108.

CHAPTER 119
ARTHROPODS

In-Hei Hahn

Arthropoda means "joint-footed" in Latin and describes arthropods' jointed bodies and legs connected to a chitinous exoskelelton.[2] The majority of arthropods are benign to humans and environmentally beneficial. Some clinicians regard bites and stings as inconsequential and more of a nuisance than a threat to life. However, some spiders have toxic venoms that can produce dangerous, painful lesions or significant systemic effects. Important clinical syndromes are produced by bites or stings from animals in the phylum Arthropoda, specifically the classes Arachnida (spiders, scorpions, and ticks) and Insecta (bees, wasps, hornets, and ants) (Table 119–1). Infectious diseases transmitted by arthropods, such as the various encephalitides, Rocky Mountain spotted fever, human anaplasmosis, babesiosis, and Lyme disease, are not discussed in this chapter.

Arthropoda comprises the largest phylum in the animal kingdom. At least 1.5 million species are identified, and half a million or more are yet to be classified. It includes more species than all other phyla combined (Fig. 119–1).[2] Araneism or arachnidism results from the envenomation caused by a spider bite. "Bites" are different from "stings." Bites are defined as creating a wound using the oral pole with the intention for either catching or envenomating prey or blood feeding.[84,185] "Stings" occur from a modified ovipositor at the aboral pole that is also able to function in egg laying as in bees and wasps. Stinging behavior typically is used for defense. Most spiders are venomous, and the venom weakens the prey, enabling the spider to secure, neutralize, and digest their prey. Spiders in general are not aggressive toward humans unless they are provoked. The chelicerae (mouthparts comprised of basal section and hinged fang) of many species are too short to penetrate human skin.

Spiders can be divided into categories based on whether they pursue their prey as hunters or trappers. Trappers snare their prey by spinning webs, feed, and enshrine excess victims in a cocoon silk to be eaten later. The order of spiders (Araneae) differs from other members of the class (Arachnida) because of various anatomic differences best assessed by an entomologist. Simplistically, the arachnids have four pairs of joined legs whereas insects have three pairs. The arachnid's body is divided into two parts (cephalothorax and unsegmented abdomen) connected by a small pedicel, and two, three, or four pairs of spinnerets from which silk is spun. Two pedipalps are attached anteriorly on the cephalothorax on either side of their chelicerae and are used for sensation. Spiders have eight eyes, although there are instances when they have two, four, six, or even no pairs of eyes and are quite myopic. Prey is localized by touch as they land in the spider's web. Most spiders use venom (except for the family Uloboridae) to kill or immobilize their prey. The spiders of medical importance in the United States include the widow spiders (*Latrodectus* spp), the violin spiders (*Loxosceles* spp), and the hobo spider (*Tegenaria agrestis*). In Australia, the funnel web spider (*Atrax robustus*) can cause serious illness and death. In South America, the Brazilian Huntsmen (*Phoneutria fera*) and Arantia Armedeira (*Phoneutria nigriventer*) are threats to humans.

Most information on the clinical presentation of spider bites continues to be unreliable, being based on case reports and case series. Frequently the cases do not have any expert confirmation of the actual spider involved, which can lead to propagation of misinformation about different spiders, particularly with necrotic arachnidism. For example, the white tail spider (*Lampona* spp) was suspected for more than 20 years to cause necrotic lesions. Only recently has a prospective study of confirmed spider bites refuted this myth by reporting more than 700 confirmed spider bites in Australia.[112,113,115] Because most arthropod-focused research involves characterizing the structure of spider toxins rather than verifying clinical presentations, it is important to produce clinical studies that have bites confirmed by the presence of the spider that is identified by an expert. Definite spider bites or stings are defined as the following[113,114]: (1) evidence of a bite or sting soon after the incident or the creature can be seen to bite or sting, (2) collection of the particular creature, either alive or dead, with positive identification of the creature by an expert biologist/taxonomist in the field relating to the creature.

HISTORY AND EPIDEMIOLOGY

Since the time of Aristotle, spiders and their webs were used for medicinal purposes. Special preparations were concocted to cure a fantastic array of ailments, including earache, running of the eyes, "wounds in the joints," warts, gout, asthma, "spasmodic complaints of females," chronic hysteria, cough, rheumatic afflictions for the head, and stopping blood flow.[219]

One *Latrodectus* species has an infamous history of medical concern, hence the name *mactans,* which means "murderer" in Latin.[174] Hysteria regarding spider bites peaked during the 17th century in the Taranto region of Italy. The syndrome tarantism, which is characterized by lethargy, stupor, and a restless compulsion to walk or dance, was blamed on *Lycosa tarantula,* a spider that pounces on its prey like a wolf. Deaths were associated with these outbreaks. Dancing the rapid tarantella to music was the presumed remedy. The real culprit in this epidemic was *Latrodectus tredecimguttatus.*[174] Other epidemics of arachnidism occurred in Spain in 1833 and 1841.[147] In North America, there was a rise of spider exposures during the late 1920s, Rome reported large numbers in 1953, and Yugoslavia reported a large number of cases between 1948 and 1953.[28,147] These epidemics may be related to actual reporting biases as well as climatic variations.[174] Spider bites are more numerous in warmer months, presumably because both spiders and humans are more active during that season.

Approximately 200 species of spiders are associated with envenomations.[182,186] Eighteen genera of North American spiders produce poisonings that require clinical intervention (Table 119–2). In one series of 600 suspected spider bites, 80% were determined to result from arthropods other than spiders, such as ticks, bugs, mites, fleas, moths, butterflies, caterpillars, insects, flies, beetles, water bugs, and *Hymenoptera.* Ten percent of the presumed bites actually were manifestations of other nonarthropod disorders.[184,186]

From 2006 to 2007, an annual average of 14,000 spider exposures and 44,000 insect exposures were reported to US poison centers.[31,32] No more than two fatalities were reported per year. One was from the *Hymenoptera* category and the other was an unknown spider exposure.[31] This could be because of greater public awareness, fewer calls made and recorded by the poison control centers, or some other unknown factor. Arachnophobia is a perceived danger that far exceeds the actual risk. Often the misdiagnosis of spider bites results from the wide presentation of dermatologic conditions. For example, cutaneous anthrax was mistaken for a cutaneous necrotic spider bite.[181] In most cases, mortality is rare if supportive care is available and the patient does not develop an anaphylactoid reaction to the envenomation or antidote.

TABLE 119–1. Insects and Other Arthropods that Bite, Sting, or Nettle Humans

Arthropod	Description
Honeybee (*Apis mellifera*)	Hairy, yellowish brown with black markings
Bumblebee and carpenter bee (*Bombus* spp and *Xylocopa* spp)	Hairy, larger than honeybees and colored black and yellow
Vespids (yellow jackets, hornets, paper wasps)	Short-waisted, robust, black and yellow or white combination
Schecoids (thread-waisted wasps)	Threadlike waist
Nettling caterpillars (browntail, Io, hag, and buck moths, saddleback and puss caterpillars)	Caterpillar shaped
Southern fire ant (*Solenopsis* spp)	Ant shaped
Spiders (*Arachnida*) black widow, brown recluse	Body with 2 regions: cephalothorax, and abdomen; 8 legs
Scorpions (*Centruroides*)	Eight-legged, crablike, stinger at the tip of the abdomen; pedipalps (pincers) highly developed (not a true insect)
Centipedes (*Chilopoda*)	Elongated, wormlike, with many jointed segments and legs; 1 pair of poison fangs behind head

TABLE 119–2. North American Spiders of Medical Importance

Genus	Common Name
Araneus spp	Orb weaver
Argiope aurantia	Orange argiope
Bothriocyrtum spp	Trap door spider
Chiracanthium spp	Running spider
Drassodes spp	Gnaphosid spider
Heteropoda spp	Huntsman spider
Latrodectus spp	Widow spider
Liocranoides spp	Running spider
Loxosceles spp	Brown, violin, or recluse spider
Lycosa spp	Wolf spider
Misumenoides spp	Crab spider
Neoscona spp	Orb weaver
Peucetia viridans	Green lynx spider
Phiddipus spp	Jumping spider
Rheostica (*Aphonopelma*) spp	Tarantula
Steatoda grossa	False black widow spider
Tegenaria agrestis	Hobo spider
Ummidia spp	Trap door spider

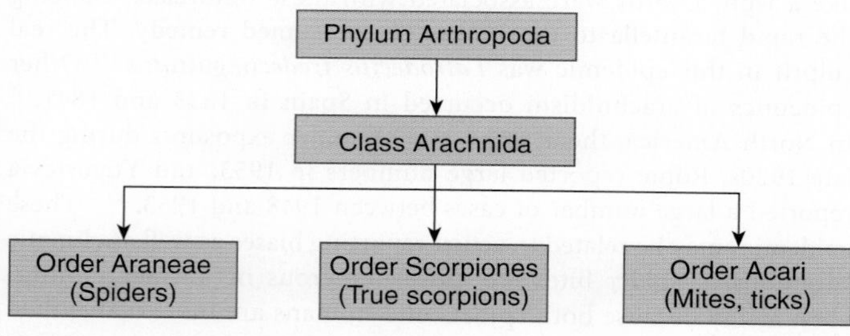

FIGURE 119–1. Taxonomy of the phylum Arthropoda.

BLACK WIDOW SPIDER (*LATRODECTUS MACTANS*; HOURGLASS SPIDER)

Five species of widow spiders are found in the United States: *Latrodectus mactans* (black widow; Figure 119–2a), *Latrodectus hesperus* (Western black widow), *Latrodectus variolus* (found in New England, Canada, south to Florida, and west to eastern Texas, Oklahoma, and Kansas), *Latrodectus bishopi* (red widow of the South), and *Latrodectus geometricus* (brown widow or brown button spider; Figure 119–2b). Dangerous widow spiders in other parts of the world include *L. geometricus* and *Latrodectus tredecimguttatus* (European widow spider found in southern Europe), *Latrodectus hasselti* (red-back widow spider found in Australia, Japan, and India; Figure 119–2c), and *Latrodectus cinctus* (found in

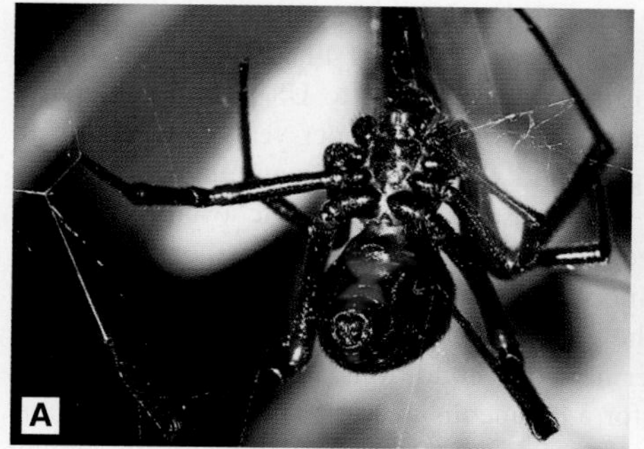

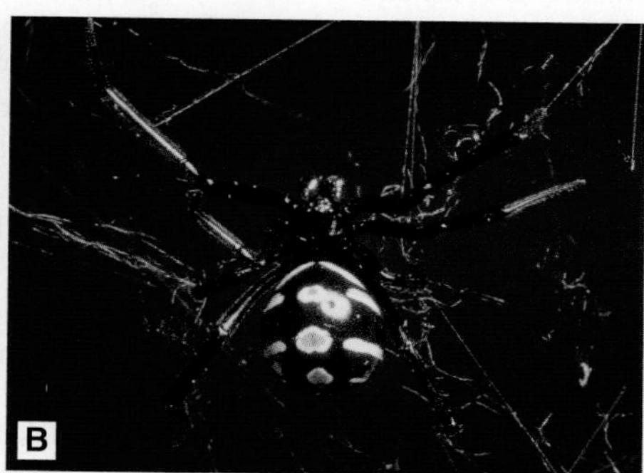

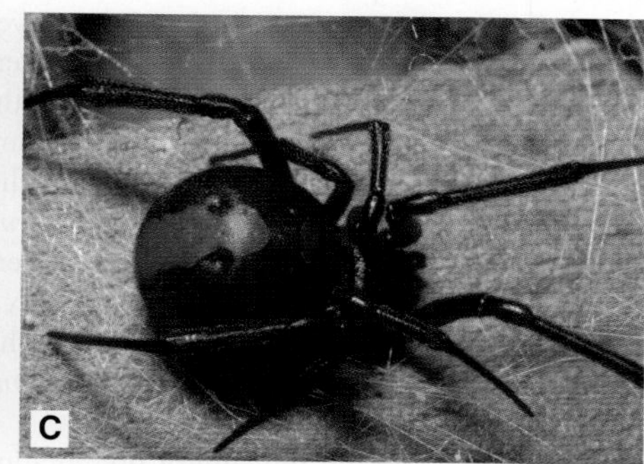

FIGURE 119–2. Widow spiders. (A) The North American Black Widow Spider, *Latrodectus mactans*. Note the hourglass on the abdomen. (B) The Brown Widow Spider, *Latrodectus geometricus*. (C) The Australian redback spider *Latrodectus hasselti*. *(Images contributed by the American Museum of Natural History).*

South Africa). These spiders live in temperate and tropical latitudes in stone walls, crevices, wood piles, outhouses, barns, stables, and rubbish piles. They molt multiple times and as a result can change colors. The ventral markings on the abdomen are species specific, and the classic red hourglass-shaped marking is noted in only *L. mactans.* Other species may have variations on their ventral surface, such as triangles and spots.

Typically, the female *L. mactans* is shiny, jet-black, and large (8–10 mm), with a rounded abdomen and a red hourglass mark on its ventral surface. Her larger size and ability to penetrate human skin with her fangs make her more venomous and toxic than the male spider, which resembles the immature spider in earlier stages of development and is smaller, lighter in color, and has a more elongated abdomen and fangs that usually are too short to envenomate humans (Table 119–3). Black widow females are trappers and inhabit large, untidy, irregularly shaped webs. Webs are placed in or close to the ground and in secluded, dimly lit areas that can trap flying insects, such as outdoor privies, barns, sheds, and garages.[2]

PATHOPHYSIOLOGY

The venom is more potent on a volume-per-volume basis than the venom of a pit viper and contains six active components with molecular weights of 5000 to 130,000 Da.[2] The six components are α-latrotoxin (α-LTX) affecting vertebrates, five latroinsectotoxins (α-, β-, γ-, δ-, ε-LITs) (insect-specific neurotoxin), and α-latrocrustatoxin (α-LCT) (crustacean-specific neurotoxin).[94] α-Latrotoxin binds, with nanomolar affinity, to the specific presynaptic receptors neurexin I-α and Ca^{2+}-independent receptor for α-latrotoxin (CIRL), otherwise known as *latrophilin*.[25,102,111] The binding triggers a cascade of events: conformational change allowing pore formation by tethering the toxin to the plasma membrane, Ca^{2+} ionophore formation, and translocation of the N-terminal domain of α-LTX into the presynaptic intracellular space, and intracellular activation of exocytosis of norepinephrine, dopamine, neuropeptides, and acetylcholine, glutamate, and γ-aminobutyric acid (GABA), respectively.[2,162,165] Neurexin I-α receptors, otherwise known as type I or calcium-dependent receptors, are from a family of neuron-specific cell membrane proteins with one transmembrane domain neuron-specific cell-adhesion molecule.[142,165] Neurexin I-α is not required for the excitotoxic action of α-LTX. Neurexin I-α–deficient mice still are susceptible to α-LTX via stimulation of the CIRL receptor, or the type II receptor.[81] CIRL is a neuronal receptor that belongs to the family of 7-transmembrane domain G-protein–coupled receptors. Type II receptors bind to α-LTX independently of Ca^{2+} in the extracellular media. CIRL is thought to be coupled to phospholipase C, resulting in subsequent phosphoinositide metabolism that couples the function to secretion.[25,130] CIRL-1 and CIRL-3 are high-affinity neuronal receptors. CIRL-2 has 14 times less affinity to α-LTX than CIRL-1 but is expressed ubiquitously, specifically by placenta, kidney, spleen, ovary, heart, lung, and brain.[111] The nervous system is the primary target for α-LTX, but cells from other tissues also are susceptible to the α-LTX because of the presence of CIRL-2.[111]

CLINICAL MANIFESTATIONS

Widow spiders are shy and nocturnal. They usually bite when their web is disturbed or upon inadvertent exposure in shoes and clothing. One patient developed latrodectism following the intentional intravenous injection of a crushed whole black widow spider.[37] A sharp pain typically described as a pinprick occurs as the victim is bitten. A pair of red spots may evolve at the site, although the bite is commonly unnoticed.[43,146] The bite mark itself tends to be limited to a small puncture wound or wheal and flare reaction that often is associated with a halo (see Table 119–3). However, the bite from *L. mactans* may produce *latrodectism,* a constellation of signs and symptoms resulting from systemic toxicity. Some cases do not progress; others may show severe neuromuscular symptoms within 30 to 60 minutes. The effects from the bite spread contiguously. For example, if a person is bitten on the hand, the pain progresses up the arm to the elbow, shoulder, and then toward the trunk during systemic poisoning. Typically, a brief time to symptom onset denotes severe envenomation.

One grading system divides the severity of the envenomation into three categories.[50] Grade 1 envenomations range from no symptoms to local pain at the envenomation site with normal vital signs. Grade 2 envenomations involve muscular pain at the site with migration of the pain to the trunk, diaphoresis at the bite site, and normal vital signs. Grade 3 envenomations include the grade 2 symptoms with abnormal vital signs; diaphoresis distant from the bite site; generalized myalgias to back, chest, and abdomen; and nausea, vomiting, and headache.

Hypertoxic myopathic syndrome of latrodectism involves muscle cramps that usually begin 15 minutes to 1 hour after the bite. The muscle cramps initially occur at the site of the bite but later may involve rigidity of other skeletal muscles, particularly muscles of the chest, abdomen, and face. The pain increases over time and occurs in waves that may cause the patient to writhe. Large muscle groups are affected first. Classically, severe abdominal wall spasm occurs and may be confused with a surgical abdomen, especially in children who cannot relate the history with the initial bite.[35] Muscle pain often subsides within a few hours but may recur for several days. Transient muscle weakness and spasms may persist for weeks to months.

Additional clinical findings include "*facies latrodectismica,*" which consists of sweating, contorted, grimaced face associated with blepharitis, conjunctivitis, rhinitis, cheilitis, and trismus of the masseters.[146] A fear of death, *pavor mortis*, is described.[146] The following symptoms also are reported: nausea, vomiting, sweating, tachycardia, hypertension, muscle cramping, restlessness, and rarely priapism, and compartment syndrome at the site of the bite.[2,51,107,206] The mechanism of compartment syndrome developing after a black widow spider envenomation is unclear, but two postulated theories include rhabdomyolysis and the venom affecting the blood vessels leading to engorgement and obstruction of the venous outflow. The compartment syndrome was treated with antivenom and the patient recovered without the need for a fasciotomy. Recovery usually ensues within 24 to 48 hours, but symptoms may last several days with more severe envenomations. *Life-threatening complications* include severe hypertension, respiratory distress, myocardial infarction, cardiovascular failure, and gangrene.[37,50,51,69,157,170,174] In the past 20 years, more than 40,000 presumed black widow spider bites have been reported to the American Association of Poison Control Centers. Death is rarely reported. There have been two fatalities in Madagascar from envenomation by *L. geometricus,* one from cardiovascular failure and the other from gangrene of the foot.[174] The most recent fatality reported from Greece resulted from myocarditis secondary to envenomation of *L. tredecimguttatus,*[173] confirmed by a local veterinarian. The patient developed severe dyspnea, hypoxemia, cyanosis, cardiomyopathy, and global hypokinesis of the left ventricle confirmed by echocardiography followed by death 36 hours later; antivenom was not available. On autopsy, diffuse interstitial and alveolar edema, with mononuclear infiltrate of the myocardium and degenerative changes, were noted and toxicologic analysis for xenobiotics, as well as all blood, urine, bronchial, and serologic viral cultures, were negative. The paucity of mortalities is presumed to result from the improvement in medical care, the availability of antivenom, or the limited toxicity of the spider.

DIAGNOSTIC TESTING

Laboratory data generally are not helpful in management or predicting outcome. According to one study, the most common findings

TABLE 119–3. Brown Recluse and Black Widow Spiders: Comparative Characteristics

	Brown Recluse *(Loxosceles spp)*	Black Widow *(Latrodectus spp)*
Description	Female brown, 6–20 mm, violin-shaped mark on dorsum of cephalothorax; female greater toxicity than male	Female jet black, 8–10 mm, red hourglass mark on ventral surface, female greater toxicity than male
Major venom component	Sphingomyelinase D	α-Latrotoxin
Pathophysiology of envenomation	Vascular injury, dermatonecrosis, hemolysis	Massive presynaptic discharge of neurotransmitters; lymphatic and hematogenous spread, neurotoxicity
Epidemiology	Bites more common in warmer months	Bites more common in warmer months in subtropical and temperate areas; perennial in tropics
	North America (southern and midwestern states): *L. reclusa*	North America: *L. mactans, L. Hesperus, L. geometricus*
	South America: *L. laeta, L. gaucho*	
	Europe: *L. rufescens*	Europe: *L. tredecimguttatus*
	Africa (southern): *L. parrami, L. spiniceps, L. pilosa, L. bergeri*	Africa (southern): *L. indistinctus*
		Australia: *L. hasselti*
	Asia/Australia: Rare	Asia/South America: Rare
Clinical effects	Cutaneous	Cutaneous
	Initial (0–2 h after bite): painless, erythema, edema	Initial (5 min–1 h after bite): local pain
	2–8 h: Hemorrhagic, ulcerates, painful	1–2 h: Puncture marks
	1 week: Eschar	Hours: Regional lymph nodes swollen, central blanching at bite site with surrounding erythema
	Months: Healing	
		CVS: Initial tachycardia followed by bradycardia, dysrhythmias, initial hypotension followed by hypertension
		GI: Nausea, vomiting, mimic acute abdomen
	Hematologic	Hematologic: Leukocytosis
	Methemoglobinemia, hemolysis, thrombocytopenia, DIC	
		Resolution over several days
		Metabolic
		Hyperglycemia (transient)
		Musculoskeletal: Hypertonia, abdominal rigidity, "facies latrodectismica"
		Neurologic
		CNS: Psychosis, hallucinations, visual disturbance, seizures
		Peripheral nervous system: Pain at the site
		Autonomic nervous system: Increased secretions; sweating, salivation, lacrimation, diarrhea, bronchorrhea, mydriasis, miosis, priapism, ejaculation
	Renal: Renal failure, acute tubular necrosis	Renal: Glomerulonephritis, oliguria, anuria
		Respiratory: Bronchoconstriction, acute lung injury
Treatment	Analgesia	Analgesia
	Wound care	Muscle relaxants
	Dapsone (?)	Antivenom
	Hyperbaric oxygen (local) (?)	
	Antivenom (?) not available universally	
	Corticosteroids	

include leukocytosis and increased creatine phosphokinase and lactate dehydrogenase concentrations.[50] Currently no specific laboratory assay is capable of confirming latrodectism. However, the clinical situation may warrant the need to check laboratory tests and other studies to evaluate the sequelae of the black widow spider envenomation.

MANAGEMENT

Treatment involves establishing an airway and supporting respiration and circulation, if indicated. Wound evaluation and local wound care, including tetanus prophylaxis, are essential.[230] The routine use of antibiotics is not recommended.

Pain management is a substantial component of patient care and depends on the degree of symptomatology. Using the grading system, grade 1 envenomations may require only cold packs and orally administered nonsteroidal anti-inflammatory agents. Grade 2 and 3 envenomations probably require intravenous (IV) opioids and benzodiazepines to control pain and muscle spasm.

Traditionally, 10 mL 10% calcium gluconate solution was given IV to decrease cramping. However, a retrospective chart review of 163 patients envenomated by the black widow concluded that calcium gluconate was ineffective for pain relief compared with a combination of IV opioids (morphine sulfate or meperidine) and benzodiazepines (diazepam or lorazepam).[50,126] Another study found greater neurotransmitter release when extracellular calcium concentrations were increased, suggesting that administration of calcium is irrational in patients suffering from latrodectism.[182] The mechanism of action of calcium remains unknown and its efficacy is anecdotal; therefore, we do not recommend calcium administration for pain management.

Although often recommended, methocarbamol (a centrally acting muscle relaxant) and dantrolene also are ineffective for treatment of latrodectism.[126,187] A benzodiazepine, such as diazepam, is more effective for controlling muscle spasms and achieves sedation, anxiolysis, and amnesia. Management should primarily emphasize supportive care, with opioids and benzodiazepines for controlling pain and muscle spasms, because the use of antivenom risks anaphylaxis and serum sickness.

Latrodectus antivenom is rapidly effective and curative. In the United States, the antivenom formulation is effective for all species but is available as a crude hyperimmune horse serum that may cause anaphylaxis and serum sickness. The morbidity of latrodectism is high, with pain, cramping, and autonomic disturbances, but mortality is low. Hence controversy exists over when to administer the black widow antivenom. The antivenom can be administered for severe reactions (eg, hypertensive crisis or intractable pain), to high-risk patients (eg, pregnant women suffering from a threatened abortion), or for treatment of priapism.[107,174] Use of antivenom probably should not be considered for patients unless systemic symptoms otherwise designated as grade 3 are present.[51] The usual dose is one to two vials diluted in 50 to 100 mL 5% dextrose or 0.9% sodium chloride solution, with the combination infused over 1 hour (Antidotes in Depth A35–Antivenom [Scorpion and Spider]). Skin testing may identify a highly allergic individual but does not eliminate the occurrence of hypersensitivity reactions; therefore, we do not recommend skin testing. Pretreatment with histamine H_1- or H_2-blockers or both, and epinephrine may be beneficial in preventing histamine release and/or anaphylaxis. Patients with allergies to horse serum products and those who have received antivenom or horse serum products are at risk for immunoglobulin IgE-mediated hypersensitivity reactions, and though efficacy is largely unproven may benefit from the pretreatment of antihistamines and steroids.

In Australia, a purified equine-derived IgG-F(ab)$_2$ fragment antivenom for the red-back spider *L. hasselti* (RBS-AV) is available. The RBS-AV (CSL, Melbourne, Australia) is administered intramuscularly and given as first-line therapy to patients presenting with systemic signs or symptoms in Australia. Since its introduction in 1956, there have been no deaths, and the incidence of mild allergic reactions to RBS-AV is reported as 0.54% in 2144 uses.[215]

However, an underpowered prospective cohort study of confirmed red-back spider bites failed to show that intramuscular antivenom was better than no treatment when all patients were followed up over 1 week.[115] This study did note that only 17% of patients were pain-free at 24 hours with antibody treatment. Therefore, intramuscular antivenom appears to be less effective than previously thought, and the route of administration requires review. Recently in Italy, an FM$_1$ Fab fragment specific for the alpha latroxin has been highly effective in neutralizing the toxin in vivo in mice and shows some promise for possible use in humans.[7,36] This single monoclonal antibody shows great promise in the treatment for severe black widow envenomation. Inadvertent use of RBS-AV successfully treated envenomations from the comb-footed spider (*Steatoda* spp).[114] And since the *Steatoda* venom and clinical effects are similar to the *Latrodectus* venom but milder in clinical presentation, the RBS-AV may have a future role in treating black widow spider envenomations in the United States.[92]

BROWN RECLUSE SPIDER (*LOXOSCELES RECLUSA*; VIOLIN OR FIDDLEBACK SPIDER)

Loxosceles reclusa was confirmed to cause necrotic arachnidism in 1957, although reports of systemic symptoms following brown spider bites have appeared since 1872.[6] This spider has a brown violin-shaped mark on the dorsum of the cephalothorax, three dyads of eyes arranged in a semicircle on top of the head, and legs that are five times as long as the body. It is small (6–20 mm long) and gray to orange or reddish brown (see Figure 119–3a). *Loxosceles* spiders weave irregular white, flocculent adhesive webs that line their retreats.[79] Spiders in the genus *Loxosceles* have a worldwide distribution. In the United States, other species of this genus, which include *L. rufescens*, *L. deserta*, *L devia*, and *L. arizonica*, are prominent in the Southeast and Southwest.[4] *L. rufescens* has been introduced and identified in New York City in several old buildings, though it is unclear how they initially arrived there (confirmed by Lou Sorkin BCE, entomologist, American Museum Natural History, New York).[203] They are hunter spiders that live in dark areas (wood piles, rocks, basements), and their foraging is nocturnal. They are not aggressive but will bite if antagonized (see Table 119–3). These spiders live up to 2 years and maybe even longer. They are resilient and can survive up to 6 months without water or food and can tolerate temperatures from 46.4°F to 109.4°F (8°C–43°C).[84] Like the black widow spider, the female is more dangerous than the male. *Loxosceles* venom has variable toxicity, depending on the species, with *Loxosceles intermedia* venom causing more severe clinical effects in humans.[10,11] The peak time for envenomation is from spring to autumn, and most victims are bitten in the morning.

PATHOPHYSIOLOGY

The venom is cytotoxic. The two main constituents of the venom are sphingomyelinase-D and hyaluronidase, though other subcomponents include deoxyribonuclease, ribonuclease, collagenase, esterase, proteases, alkaline phosphatase, and lipase.[59,134,225] Hyaluronidase is a spreading factor that facilitates the penetration of the venom into tissue but does not induce lesion development.[134] Sphingomyelinase-D is the primary constituent of the venom that causes necrosis and red blood cell hemolysis and also causes platelets to release serotonin.[134] Sphingomyelinase also reacts with sphingomyelin in the red blood cell membrane to release choline and *N*-acylsphingosine phosphate, which triggers a chain reaction releasing inflammatory mediators, such as thromboxanes,

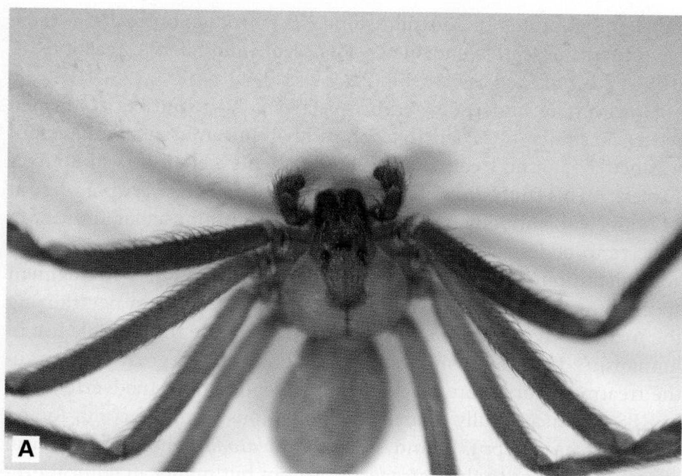

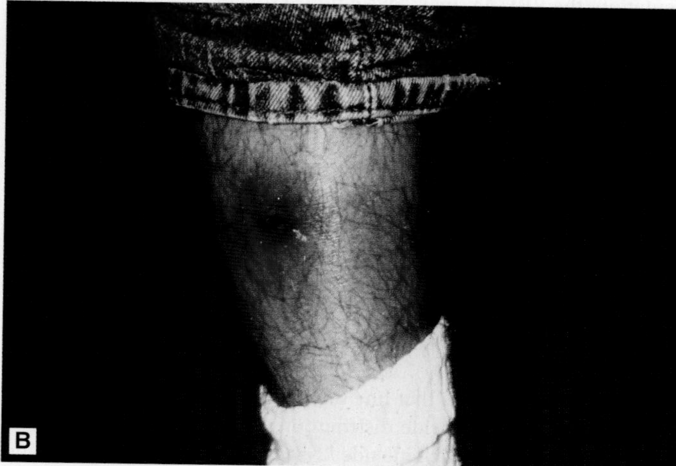

FIGURE 119–3. Brown recluse spider. (**A**) *Loxosceles reclusa*. Note the image of the violin, which gives the spider its common name, "the fiddle back spider". *(Image contributed by Progeny Products, www.brown-recluse.com)* (**B**) A typical envenomation from the Brown Recluse Spider. *(Image contributed by the New York City Poison Center Toxicology Fellowship Program.)*

leukotrienes, prostaglandins, and neutrophils, leading to vessel thrombosis, tissue ischemia, and skin loss.[134] Early perivascular collections of polymorphonuclear leukocytes with hemorrhage and edema progresses to intravascular clotting. Coagulation and vascular occlusion of the microcirculation occur, ultimately leading to necrosis.[198]

CLINICAL MANIFESTATIONS

The clinical spectrum of loxoscelism can be divided into three major categories. The first category includes bites in which very little, if any, venom is injected. A small erythematous papule may be present that becomes firm before healing and is associated with a localized urticarial response. In the second category, the bite undergoes a cytotoxic reaction. The bite initially may be painless or have a stinging sensation but then blisters and bleeds, and ulcerates 2 to 8 hours later (see Table 119–3). The lesion may increase in diameter, with demarcation of central hemorrhagic vesiculation, then ulcerate and develop violaceous necrosis, surrounded by ischemic blanching of skin and outer erythema and induration over 1 to 3 days. This is also known as the "red, white, and blue" reaction (Figure 119–3b).[127,235] Necrosis of the central blister occurs in 3 to 4 days, with eschar formation between 5 and 7 days. After 7 to 14 days, the wound becomes indurated and the eschar falls off, leaving an ulceration that heals by secondary intention. Local necrosis is more extensive over fatty areas (thighs, buttocks, and abdomen).[134] The size of the ulcer determines the time for healing. Large lesions up to 30 cm may require 4 months or more to heal.

Upper airway obstruction was reported in a child who was bitten on his neck and subsequently developed progressive cervical soft tissue edema with airway obstruction and dermatonecrosis 40 hours later.[89] There has been one other report of stridor and respiratory distress following a brown recluse envenomation of the ear. Although the presentation is rare, respiratory compromise should be considered when an envenomation occurs near the airway.[83]

The third category consists of systemic loxoscelism, which is not predicted by the extent of cutaneous reaction, and occurs 24 to 72 hours after the bite. The young are particularly susceptible.[105,188] The clinical manifestations of systemic loxoscelism include fever, chills, weakness, edema, nausea, vomiting, arthralgias, petechial eruptions, rhabdomyolysis, disseminated intravascular coagulation, hemolysis that can lead to hemoglobinemia, hemoglobinuria, renal failure, and death.[22,39,76,144,192,233] However, in North America, the incidence of systemic illness is rare and mortality is low.[3]

DIAGNOSTIC TESTING

Bites from other spiders, such as *Cheiracanthium* (sac spider), *Phidippus* (jumping spider), *Argiope* (orb weaver), and *Tegenaria* (northwestern brown spider), can produce necrotic wounds. These spiders are often the actual culprits when the brown recluse is mistakenly blamed. Definitive diagnosis is achieved only when the biting spider is positively identified. No routine laboratory test for loxoscelism is available for clinical application, but several techniques are presently used for research purposes. The lymphocyte transformation test measures lymphocytes that have undergone blast transformation up to 1 month after exposure to *Loxosceles* venom. The lymphocytes incorporate thymidine into the nucleoprotein, providing a quantitative response.[5] A passive hemagglutination inhibition test (PHAI) has been developed in guinea pigs. The PHAI assay is based on the property of certain brown recluse spider venom components to spontaneously adsorb to formalin-treated erythrocyte membranes and the ability of the brown recluse spider venom to inhibit antiserum-induced agglutination of venom-coated red blood cells.[13] The test is 90% sensitive and 100% specific for 3 days postenvenomation and may prove useful for early diagnosis of brown recluse spider envenomation.[13] An enzyme-linked immunoassay (ELISA) specific for *Loxosceles* venom in biopsied tissue can confirm the presence of venom for 4 days postenvenomation.[13] The drawbacks of using a skin biopsy are the invasive nature of the procedure, which can result in further scarring with an increased potential for infection, and the lack of proof that skin biopsy can diagnose early envenomations prior to the development of dermatonecrosis. Another ELISA utilizing serum for detection of venom antigens has been developed that correctly discriminates the mice inoculated with antigens from *L. intermedia* venom. The ELISA immunoassay and antivenom may become useful diagnostic tools if envenomation can be proved or disproved early.[47] A venom-specific enzyme immunoassay that uses hair, skin biopsies, or aspirated tissue near a suspected lesion to detect the presence of venom up to 7 days after injury is under investigation.[132,152] In Brazil, ELISA is used to detect the venom of *Loxosceles gaucho* in wounds and patient sera, but the technique is not in widespread clinical use.[43]

Clinical laboratory data may be remarkable for hemolysis, hemoglobinuria, and hematuria. Coagulopathy may be present, with laboratory data significant for elevated fibrin split products, decreased fibrinogen levels, and a positive D-dimer assay. Other tests may show increased prothrombin time (PT) and partial thromboplastin time (PTT), leukocytosis (up to 20,000–30,000 cells/mm³), spherocytosis, Coombs-positive hemolytic anemia, thrombocytopenia, or abnormal renal and liver function tests.[2,7,79,184,186,188,231]

TREATMENT

Optimal local treatment of the lesion is controversial. The most prudent management of the dermatonecrotic lesion is wound care, immobilization, tetanus prophylaxis, analgesics, and antipruritics as warranted (Table 119–4).[2,79,228,231] Early excision or intralesional injection of corticosteroids appears unwarranted.[179] Corrective surgery can be performed several weeks after adequate tissue demarcation has occurred. In one case series the use of curettage of the lesion to remove necrotic and indurated tissue from the lesion, thus eliminating any continuing action of the lytic enzymes on the surrounding tissue, showed promising results.[105] These patients had wound healing without further necrosis and minimal scarring. Electric shock delivered via stun guns was not found to be useful in a guinea pig envenomation model.[13] Cyproheptadine, a serotonin antagonist, was not beneficial in a rabbit model.[167] A randomized, controlled study evaluating the efficacy of topical nitroglycerin for envenomated rabbits showed no difference in preventing skin necrosis and suggested the possibility of increased systemic toxicity.[140] Antibiotics should be used to treat cutaneous or systemic infection, but should not be used prophylactically.

Early use of dapsone in patients who develop a central purplish bleb or vesicle within the first 6 to 8 hours may inhibit local infiltration of the wound by polymorphonuclear leukocytes.[127] The dosage recommended is 100 mg twice daily for 2 weeks.[178] However, prospective trials with large numbers of patients are lacking. One study compared the efficacy of erythromycin and dapsone therapy, erythromycin and antivenom therapy, and erythromycin, dapsone, and antivenom therapy (developed in rabbits based on a previous study).[177] Although the treatment groups were very small, all groups showed wound healing at approximately 20 days despite the different therapies used. This study's biggest limitation includes the definition of a spider bite diagnosis (the study used the following criteria: a patient feeling the spider bite, seeing the spider, or having a clinically plausible necrotic lesion). There was no expert confirming the identity of the spider. The study suggests that the use of dapsone may eliminate the need for surgery following bites and that antivenom therapy was most effective clinically if the patient never developed the necrotic lesion. Hence, the use of dapsone in the management of a local lesion should be considered experimental until its use is validated by randomized, controlled clinical trials. Hepatitis,[180] methemoglobinemia, and hemolysis (Chap. 127) are associated with dapsone use. If dapsone therapy is used, a baseline glucose-6-phosphate dehydrogenase and weekly complete blood counts should be performed.

TABLE 119–4. Management of Brown Recluse Spider Bite

General Wound Care	Local Wound Care	Systemic
Clean	Serial observations	Antipruritic/antianxiety and/or analgesics
Tetanus prophylaxis as indicated	Natural healing by granulation	Antibiotics for secondary bacterial infection
Immobilize and elevate bitten extremity	Delayed primary closure	(?) Polymorphonuclear white blood cell inhibitors: dapsone, colchicine
Apply cool compresses; avoid local heat	Delayed secondary closure with skin graft	Antivenom (experimental)
	Gauze packing, if applicable	(?) Hyperbaric oxygen (local)

An underpowered animal study evaluated the effects on the size of skin lesions induced by *Loxosceles* envenomation by treatment with hyperbaric oxygen therapy, dapsone, and combined hyperbaric oxygen therapy and dapsone.[103] The study concluded that there was no clinically significant change in necrosis or induration by these treatment modalities. Further evaluation of these interventions remains appropriate. Another study using hyperbaric oxygen for treatment of *Loxosceles*-induced necrotic lesions in rabbits revealed no clinical improvement in the size of the lesion; however, the histology of the lesions improved. Whether this finding is of value in humans has not been determined.[208] Use of 1.2 mg colchicine, a leukocyte inhibitor, followed at 2-hour intervals with 0.6 mg for 2 days, then 0.6 mg every 4 hours for 2 additional days is sometimes recommended, but we do not advocate this treatment because of potential colchicine toxicity.[184] Rabbit-derived intradermal anti-*Loxosceles* Fab (α-Loxd) fragments attenuated the dermatonecrotic inflammation of rabbits injected with *L. deserta* venom in a time-dependent fashion.[86] At time 0 after envenomation, lesion development was blocked. At time 1 and 4 hours after envenomation, the α-anti-Loxd Fab antivenom continued to suppress the lesion areas, although the longer the delay in treatment, the smaller the difference in treatment and control lesion areas. At time 8 and 12 hours postenvenomation, there was no difference in lesion size. The typical 24-hour delay in lesion development makes the diagnosis difficult, and the antivenom would likely be useless if administered so late in the clinical course. Currently this antivenom is not available for commercial use.

One study shows promise for the treatment of *Loxosceles* envenomations. This preclinical study of a new antiloxoscelic serum was produced using recombinant sphingomyelinase D (SMase D is derived from the sphingomyelinase of the *L. intermedia* and *Loxosceles laeta* spiders). The isolated sphingomyelinase from the respective *Loxosceles* species carried the full biological effects of the entire venom. This antiloxoscelic serum when administered IV into rabbits that were given intradermal injections of the loxoscelic venom from *L. laeta* and *L. intermedia* had greater neutralizing activity then when compared to the existing antiarachnid serum, which is made by hyperimmunizing horses against the venom of *L. gaucho*, *P. nigriventer*, and the scorpion *Tityus serrulatus*. In Brazil and South America, most of the envenomations occur with the *L. laeta* and *L. intermedia*, not *L. gaucho*. Knowing which species envenomated the patient could help determine which antiserum should be used.[63] Patients manifesting systemic loxoscelism or those with expanding necrotic lesions should be admitted to the hospital. All patients should be monitored for evidence of hemolysis, renal failure, or coagulopathy. If hemoglobinuria ensues, increased IV fluids and urinary alkalinization can be used in an attempt to prevent acute renal failure. Hemolysis, if significant, can be treated with transfusions. Patients with a coagulopathy should be monitored with serial complete blood cell count, platelet count, PT, PTT, fibrin split products, and fibrinogen. Disseminated intravascular coagulopathy may require treatment, based on severity.

HOBO SPIDER (*TEGENARIA AGRESTIS*, NORTHWESTERN BROWN SPIDER, WALCKENAER SPIDER)

The hobo spider is native to Europe and was introduced to the northwestern United States (Washington, Oregon, Idaho) in the 1920s or 1930s.[227] These spiders build funnel-shaped webs within wood piles, crawl spaces, basements, and moist areas close to the ground. They are brown with gray markings and 7 to 14 mm long. They are most abundant in the midsummer through the fall. They bite if provoked or threatened, but otherwise retreat quickly with disturbance.[18] The medical literature is sparse in reported hobo spider bites that are verified by a specialist. There is only one confirmed Hobo spider bite resulting in a necrotic lesion.[45] A 42-year-old woman with a history of phlebitis who felt a burning sensation on her ankle rolled her pants and found a crushed brown spider, which was later confirmed (unpublished source cited by MMWR) to be *T. agrestis*. She complained of persistent pain, nausea, and dizziness, and a vesicular lesion developed within several hours. The vesicle ruptured and ulcerated the next day. The lesion initially was 2 mm, but over the next 10 weeks enlarged to 30 mm in diameter and was circumscribed with a black lesion, at which time she sought medical advice. She was given a course of antibiotics, which did not limit the progression of this ulcer. Subsequently, the patient was unable to walk, and she was found to have a deep venous thrombosis. The other cases implicating Hobo spiders as a cause for dermatonecrotic injuries are based on proximity of the Hobo spider or other large brown spiders that are unidentified. *T. agrestis* envenomation induced on rabbit skin can produce hemorrhagic necrotic lesions dermally as well as systemically.[227,228] However, the venom from European Hobo spiders and US Hobo spiders was analyzed using liquid chromatography to address the question of variability between the two spiders. *T. agrestis* originated from Europe and is considered medically harmless. The authors suggest four possibilities for the discrepancy between the European Hobo and American Hobo spiders: (1) an evolutionary change may have accounted for the novel necrotic effects; (2) venom chemistry may be similar but the habitat might account for the difference in behavior; (3) venom chemistry and habitat may be similar but an extrinsic factor such as a bacterium found in the US Hobo spider might be the cause for the necrotic effects; (4) *T. agrestis* do not directly or indirectly cause necrotic arachnidism and have been falsely accused.[23] Liquid chromatography (European Hobo *T. agrestis* from the United Kingdom and American Hobo *T. agrestis* from Washington State, United States) found little variability between the two venoms to account for their differential necrotic effects.[23] The authors suggest that either a bacterium such as *Mycobacterium ulcerans*, known to cause slow-developing ulcers on human skin, might coexist on the chelicerae of the *T. agrestis*, which is highly unlikely because of the presence of antibacterial peptides in the venom,[101,234] or the more likely circumstance that *T. agrestis* has been falsely accused as being a cause for necrotic arachnidism. Misdiagnosis of spider bites is common. Wounds can be misleading and can occur from the reaction of other organisms such as ticks and other arthropods, superinfection with anthrax, and/or underlying medical conditions like diabetes and leukemia. The need to revisit the Hobo spider toxicity syndrome with further studies that show direct evidence of *T. agrestis* causing necrotic arachnidism in humans is warranted before one can conclude that any necrotic arachnidism in the Pacific Northwest is caused by *T. agrestis*.

PATHOPHYSIOLOGY

The toxin has been fractionated, with three peptides identified as having potent insecticidal activity, and no discernible effects in mammalian in vivo assays.[120] The peptide toxins TaITX-1, TaITX-2, and TaITX-3 exhibit potent insecticidal properties by acting directly in the insect central nervous system, and not at the neuromuscular junction.[120] Insects envenomated with *T. agrestis* venom and the insecticidal toxins purified from the venom developed a slowly evolving spastic paralysis. Currently, little is known about the toxin and its mechanism of action in humans.

CLINICAL MANIFESTATIONS

The toxicity of Hobo spider venom is questionable; however, it occasionally causes necrosis secondary to infection. Other causes of dermatonecrotic lesions should be considered. The most common symptom associated with the spider bite is a headache that may persist for 1 week.[45] Other symptoms, including nausea, vomiting, fatigue, memory loss, visual impairment, weakness, and lethargy, are reported.[45,228]

DIAGNOSTIC TESTING

No specific laboratory assay confirms envenomation with *T. agrestis* spider.

TREATMENT

Treatment emphasizes local wound care and tetanus prophylaxis, although systemic corticosteroids for hematologic complications may be of value. Surgical graft repair for severe ulcerative lesions may be warranted when there is no additional progression of necrosis.[45]

TARANTULAS

Tarantulas are primitive mygalomorph spiders that belong to the family Theraphosidae, a subgroup of Mygalomorphae (Greek word *mygale* for field mouse).[49,190] There are more than 1500 species, with 54 species found in the deserts of the western United States.[169] Because of their great size and reputation, tarantulas are often feared. They are the largest and hairiest spiders, popular as pets, and can be found throughout the United States as well as tropical and subtropical areas (Figure 119–4). The lifespan of the female can exceed 15 to 20 years. They have poor eyesight and detect their victims by vibrations. Despite their large size, at least one species is able to ascend vertical surfaces because of silk fibers secreted from their feet.[87] Their defense lies in either their painful bite with erect fangs or by barraging their victim with barbed urticating hairs that are released on provocation.[49] Only the New World tarantulas (tarantulas indigenous to the Americas) use the urticating hairs to defend themselves.[49]

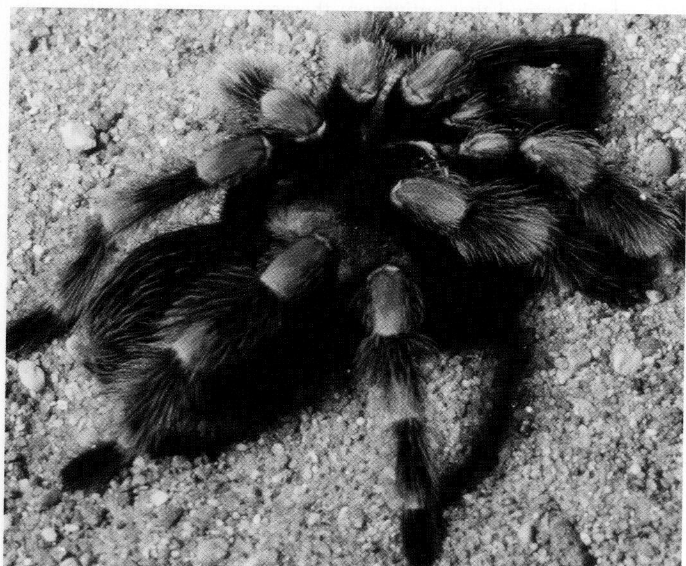

FIGURE 119–4. The Mexican Redknee Tarantula, Brachypelma smithi. *(Image contributed by the American Museum of Natural History.)*

Tarantulas may bite when provoked or roughly handled. Based on the few case reports, their venom has relatively minor effects in humans but can be deadly for canines and other small animals, such as rats, mice, cats, and birds.[35,117] A study from Australia covering a 25-year span reported only nine confirmed bites by theraphosid spiders in humans and seven confirmed bites in canines—in two cases the owner was bitten after the dog.[117] Four genera of tarantulas (*Lasiodora*, *Grammostola*, *Acanthoscurria*, and *Brachypelma*) possess urticating hairs that are released in self-defense when the tarantulas rub their hind legs against their abdomen rapidly to create a small cloud.[84] There are seven different types of urticating hairs. Type 1 hairs are found on tarantulas in the United States and are the only hairs that do not penetrate human skin. Type 2 hairs are incorporated into the silk web retreat but are not thrown off by the spider. Type 3 hairs can penetrate up to 2 mm into human skin. Type 4 hairs belong to the South American *Grammostola* spider and cause severe respiratory inflammation.

PATHOPHYSIOLOGY

Tarantula venom, specifically the venoms of *Aphonopelma hentzi* (synonym *Dugesiella hentzi* [Arkansas tarantula]) and other members of the genus *Aphonopelma* (Arizona or Texas brown tarantula), contains hyaluronidase, nucleotides (adenosine triphosphate [ATP], adenosine diphosphate, and adenosine monophosphate), and polyamines (spermine, spermidine, putrescine, and cadaverine) that are used for digesting their prey.[38,125,190] The role of spermine is unclear, but hyaluronidase is a spreading factor that allows more rapid entrance of venom toxin by destruction of connective tissue and intercellular matrix. ATP potentiates death in mice exposed to the *A. hentzi* venom and lowers the LD_{50} in comparison to venom without ATP.[46,164] Both venoms cause skeletal muscle necrosis when injected intraperitoneally into mice.[78] The primary injury results in rupture of the plasma membrane, followed by the inability of mitochondria and sarcoplasmic reticulum to maintain normal levels of calcium in the cytoplasm leading to cell death. *Aphonopelma* venom is similar to scorpion venom in composition and clinical effects. Novel toxins have been discovered in the venom that can act on potassium channels, calcium channels, and the recently discovered acid-sensing ion channels that may elucidate the molecular mechanism of voltage-dependent channel gating and their respective physiologic roles.[70,71]

CLINICAL MANIFESTATIONS

Although relatively infrequent in occurrence, bites present with puncture or fang marks. They range from being painless to a deep throbbing pain that may last several hours without any inflammatory component.[117] Fever is associated in the absence of infection, suggesting a direct pyrexic action of the venom. Rarely, bites create a local histamine response with resultant itching, and hypersensitive individuals could have a more severe reaction and, less commonly, mild systemic effects such as nausea and vomiting.[84,117] Contact reactions from the urticating hairs are more likely to be the health hazard than the spider bite. The urticating hairs provoke local histamine reactions in humans and are especially irritating to the eyes, skin, and respiratory tract. Tarantula urticating hairs cause intense inflammation that may remain pruritic for weeks. Inflammation can occur at all levels from conjunctiva to retina. An allergic rhinitis can develop if the hairs are inhaled.[125] Tarantula hairs resemble sensory setae of caterpillars: both are type 3 that can migrate relentlessly and cause multiple foci of inflammation at all levels of the eye.[109] Ophthalmia nodosa, a granulomatous nodular reaction to vegetable or insect hairs, is reported with casual handling of tarantulas.[17,21] Other eye findings include setae in the corneal stroma, anterior chamber inflammation, migration into the retina, and secondary glaucoma and cataracts.[26]

TREATMENT

Treatment is largely supportive. Cool compresses and analgesics should be given as needed. All bites should receive local wound care, including tetanus prophylaxis if necessary. If the hairs are barbed, as in some species, they can be removed by using adhesive or cellophane tape followed by compresses or irrigation with 0.9% sodium chloride solution. If the hairs are located in the eye, then surgical removal may be required, followed by medical management of inflammation. Urticarial reactions should be treated with oral antihistamines and topical or systemic corticosteroids.

FUNNEL WEB SPIDERS

Australian funnel web spiders are a group of large Hexathelidae mygalomorphs that can cause a severe neurotoxic envenomation syndrome in humans. The fang positions of funnel web spiders (as well as the tarantulas) are vertical relative to their body, which requires the spider to rear back and lift the body to attack. The length of fangs can reach up to 5 mm. This spider can bite tenaciously and may require extraction from the victim.[154] *Atrax* and *Hadronyche* species have been found along the eastern seaboard of Australia. *A. robustus,* also called the Sydney funnel web spider, is the best known and is located around the center of Sydney, Australia.[154] Funnel web spiders tend to prefer moist, temperate environments.[154] They are primarily ground dwellers and live in burrows, crevices in rocks, and around foundations of houses. They build tubular or funnel-shaped webs.[84] At night, the spiders ascend the tubular web and wait for their prey. The Sydney funnel web spider is considered one of the most poisonous spiders. It was responsible for 14 deaths between 1927 and 1980, at which time the antivenom was introduced.[211,212]

PATHOPHYSIOLOGY

Robustotoxin (atracotoxin or atraxin) is the lethal protein component of *A. robustus* venom and is unique in its toxicity affecting primates and newborn mice in biological doses, although other mammals are susceptible in higher doses.[154,210,211,232] Robustotoxin produces an autonomic storm, releasing acetylcholine, noradrenaline, and adrenaline. A 5 µg/kg intravenous infusion dose of robustotoxin from male *A. robustus* spiders causes dyspnea, blood pressure fluctuations leading to severe hypotension, lacrimation, salivation, skeletal muscle fasciculation, and death within 3 to 4 hours when administered to monkeys.[160] Versutoxin, a toxin from the Blue Mountain funnel web spider, is closely related to robustotoxin and has demonstrated voltage-dependent slowing of sodium channel inactivation.[163]

CLINICAL MANIFESTATIONS

A biphasic envenomation syndrome is described in humans and monkeys.[211,212] Phase 1 consists of localized pain at the bite site, perioral tingling, piloerection, and regional fasciculations (most prominent in the face, tongue, and intercostals). Fasciculations may progress to more overt muscle spasm; masseter and laryngeal involvement may threaten the airway.[210] Other features include tachycardia, hypertension, cardiac dysrhythmias, nausea, vomiting, abdominal pain, diaphoresis, lacrimation, salivation, and acute lung injury, which often is the cause of death in phase 1.[232] Phase 2 consists of resolution of the overt cholinergic and adrenergic crisis; secretions dry up, and fasciculations, spasms, and hypertension resolve. This apparent improvement can be followed by the gradual onset of refractory hypotension, apnea, and cardiac arrest.[211]

TREATMENT

Pressure immobilization using the crepe bandage to limit lymphatic flow and immobilization of the bitten extremity may inactivate the venom and should be applied if symptoms of envenomation are present. Funnel web venom is one of the few animal toxins known to undergo local inactivation. Monkey studies and a human case report suggest the utility of pressure immobilization.[90,214] It has been shown by injecting *A. robustus* venom subcutaneously in monkeys that the pressure-immobilization technique increased survival in these monkeys by retarding the venom movement and also by the local peripheral enzymes inactivating the venom.[212,214] The patient should be transferred to the nearest hospital with the bandage in place and then stabilized and placed in a resuscitation facility with adequate ampules of antivenom readily available before the bandage is removed; otherwise, a precipitous envenomation may occur during the removal of the pressure bandage. A purified IgG antivenom protective against *Atrax* envenomations was developed in rabbits.[212] One ampule of the antivenom contains 100 mg purified rabbit IgG or 125 Units of neutralizing capacity per ampule.[232] It has been effective for more than 40 humans bitten by the *Atrax* species.[214] The starting dose is two ampules if systemic signs of envenomations are present, and four ampules if the patient develops pulmonary edema or decreased mental status. Doses are repeated every 15 minutes until clinical improvement occurs.[232] Up to eight ampules is common in a severe envenomation. Anaphylaxis has not been reported.[214] The manufacturer no longer recommends premedication. Serum sickness is rare after funnel web antivenom administration, with only one reported case in a patient who received five ampules of antivenom.[153]

SCORPIONS

Scorpions are invertebrate arthropods that have existed for more than 400 million years.[52] Of the 650 known living species, most of the lethal species are in the family Buthidae (Table 119–5). The genera of the family Buthidae include *Centruroides, Tityus, Leuirus, Androctonus, Buthus,* and *Parabuthus*.[52] Scorpions envenomate humans by stinging rather than biting. Their five-segmented metasoma (tail) contains a bulbous segment called the *telson* that contains the venom apparatus (Figure 119–5). More than 100,000 medically significant stings likely occur annually worldwide, predominantly in the tropics and North Africa.[1,20,,63,95,118,131] According to American Association of Poison Control Centers data from 1995 to 2003, approximately 11,000 to 14,000 scorpion annual exposures occurred in the United States, mostly in the southwestern region, but no deaths have been reported. These members of the class Arachnida rarely cause mortality in victims older than 6 years.[179] The venomous scorpions in the United States are *Centruroides exilicauda and Centruroides vittatus*. The most important is *C. exilicauda*, previously called *Centruroides sculpturatus* Ewing and *Centruroides gertschii* (bark scorpion; Table 119–6).[74]

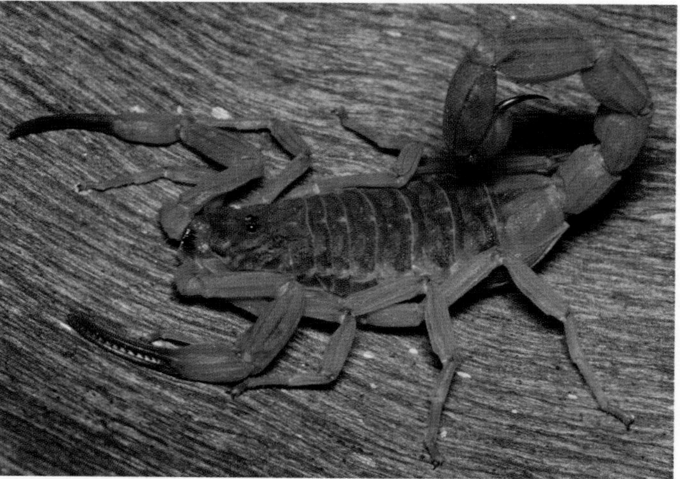

FIGURE 119–5. The Brazilian scorpion, *Tityus serrulatus*, shown here to demonstrate the typical features of scorpions. Note the telson (stinger) located on the tail. *(Image contributed by the American Museum of Natural History.)*

TABLE 119–5. Scorpions of Toxicologic Importance[74,84]

Australia: *Lychas marmoreus, Lychas* spp, *Isometrus* spp, *Cercophonius squama, Urodacus* spp
India: *Buthus tamulus*
Mexico: *Centruroides sufusus*
Middle East: *Androctonus crassicauda, Androctonus Australis, Buthus minax, Androctonus Australis, Buthus occitanus, Leirus quinquestriatus*
Spain: *Buthus occitanus*
South Africa: *Androctonus crassicauda*
South America: *Tityus serrulatus*
United States: *Centruroides exilicauda*

PATHOPHYSIOLOGY

Components of scorpion venom are complex and species specific.[99,172,179,180] Buthidae venom is thermostable and consists of phospholipase, acetylcholinesterase, hyaluronidase, serotonin, and

TABLE 119–6. Envenomation Gradation for *Centruroides exilicauda* (Bark Scorpion)

Grade	Signs and Symptoms
I	Site of envenomation Pain and/or paresthesias Positive tap test (severe pain increase with touch or percussion)
II	Grade I in addition to Pain and paresthesias remote from sting site (eg, paresthesias moving up an extremity, perioral "numbness")
III	One of the following: Somatic skeletal neuromuscular dysfunction: jerking of extremity(ies), restlessness, severe involuntary shaking and jerking, which may be mistaken for seizures Cranial nerve dysfunction: blurred vision, wandering eye movements, hypersalivation, trouble swallowing, tongue fasciculation, upper airway dysfunction, slurred speech
IV	Both cranial nerve dysfunction and somatic skeletal neuromuscular dysfunction

neurotoxins. Components of *C. exilicauda* venoms are primarily neurotoxic. Four neurotoxins, designated toxins I to IV, have been isolated from *C. exilicauda*. Some of the toxins target excitable membranes, especially at the neuromuscular junction, by opening sodium channels. The results are repetitive depolarization of nerves in both sympathetic and parasympathetic nervous systems causing acetylcholine and catecholamine release, increased neurotransmitter release, catecholamine release from the adrenal gland, catecholamine-induced cardiac hypoxia, and action at the juxtaglomerular apparatus, causing increased renin secretion.[68,179] *Tityus* scorpion sting is related to elevated concentrations of interleukin (IL)-1β, IL-6, IL-8, IL-10, and tumor necrosis factor (TNF)-α, which correlate with the severity of envenomation and hyperamylasemia.[56,78] The kinin system participates in the pathogenesis of human *Tityus* envenomation.[77]

CLINICAL MANIFESTATIONS

Scorpion stings produce a local reaction consisting of intense local pain, erythema, tingling or burning, and occasionally discoloration and necrosis without tissue sloughing (see Table 119–6). Depending on the scorpion species involved, systemic effects may occur, including autonomic storm consisting of cholinergic and adrenergic effects. Cardiotoxic effects include myocarditis, dysrhythmias, and myocardial infarction.[60,73,97,150,189] Electrocardiographic (ECG) abnormalities may persist for several days and include sinus tachycardia, sinus bradycardia, bizarre broad notched biphasic T-wave changes with additional ST elevation or depression in the limb and precordial leads, appearance of tiny Q waves in the limb leads consistent with an acute myocardial infarction pattern, occasional electrical alternans, and prolonged QT interval.[97,99] Other reported effects include pancreatitis, coagulation disorders, acute lung injury (ALI), massive hemoptysis, cerebral infarctions in children, seizures, and a shock syndrome that may precede but usually follows the hypertensive phase.[19,66,73,97,98,189,201]

In the United States, *C. exilicauda* stings produce local paresthesias and pain that can be accentuated by tapping over the envenomated area (tap test) without local skin evidence of envenomation.[52,179] Symptoms begin immediately after envenomation, progress to maximum severity in 5 hours, and may persist for up to 30 hours.[52,179] Autonomic symptoms include hypertension, tachycardia, diaphoresis, emesis, and bronchoconstriction. The somatic motor symptoms reported include ataxia, muscular fasciculations, restlessness, thrashing, and opsoclonus; rarely, children require respiratory support (see Table 119–6).[68,172]

TREATMENT

Because most envenomations do not produce severe effects, local wound care, including tetanus prophylaxis and pain management, usually is all that is warranted. In young children or patients who manifest severe toxicity, hospitalization may be required. Treatment emphasizes support of the airway, breathing, and circulation. Corticosteroids, antihistamines, and calcium have been administered without any known benefit.[56]

The severity of envenomation dictates the need to use antivenom. Continuous IV midazolam infusion has been used for *C. exilicauda* scorpion envenomation until resolution of the abnormal motor activity and agitation occurs.[82] Atropine has been used to reverse the excessive oral secretions in *C. exilicauda* scorpion envenomation, with some success in healthy children.[209] Routine use is not recommended and should be limited to species such as such as *Parabuthus transvaalicus* in southern Africa,[209] whose envenomations cause a prominent cholinergic crisis. Potentiation of the adrenergic effects causing cardiopulmonary toxicity is reported.[14] Atropine use to reverse the effects of stings from scorpions from India, South America, the Middle East, and Asia is contraindicated, because these scorpions cause an "autonomic storm" with transient cholinergic stimulation followed by sustained adrenergic hyperactivity.[15,209]

One grading system suggests using antivenom for severe grade III and grade IV envenomations, which include somatic and/or cranial nerve dysfunction (see Table 119–6).[56] A goat serum-derived anti-*Centruroides* antivenom is no longer available and was previously only available in Arizona, but was used successfully in a limited number of severe cases.[29] This approach is not universally accepted because of the safety profile of whole immunoglobins. Proponents believe antivenom may resolve symptoms sooner, whereas opponents cite serum sickness as a substantial concern (Antidotes in Depth 35–Antivenom [Scorpion and Spider]).[29] A retrospective chart review of children younger than 10 years who experienced severe *Centruroides* scorpion envenomation found that anti-*Centruroides* antivenom resulted in rapid resolution of all symptoms in all 12 patients treated.[29] Of the patients treated with antivenom, 3% developed immediate hypersensitivity reactions and 58% had a delayed rash or serum sickness.[139] An equine-derived $F(ab')_2$ product called Alacramyn, developed in Mexico against the *Centruroides limpidus* venom, can be used to treat *C. exilicauda* stings, but US use of this foreign pharmaceutical is controversial.[16,200] A very small randomized double-blind study of a scorpion-specific $F(ab')_2$ antivenom administered to critically ill children with neurotoxicity from scorpion stings demonstrated a rapid resolution of symptoms, decreased need for sedation, and reduced concentrations of circulating unbound venom.[29] These encouraging results will necessitate further generalizability, but are quite comparable to those results of previous uncontrolled Mexican studies with this antivenom.

Scorpion envenomation can be prevented by wearing shoes when walking, particularly at night, because of the nocturnal nature of scorpions. Shoes, sleeping bags, and tents should be shaken out prior to use. Cracks and crevices should be filled, wood piles and rubbish piles eliminated, and insecticides used in infested areas. The bark scorpion (*C. exilicauda*) as do all scorpions, fluoresce in the dark when using a Woods lamp.

TICKS

In 1912, Todd[222] described a progressive ascending flaccid paralysis after bites from ticks. Three families of ticks are recognized: (1) Ixodidae (hard ticks), (2) Argasidae (soft ticks), and (3) Nuttalliellidae (a group that has characteristics of both hard and soft ticks). The terms *hard* and *soft* refer to a dorsal scutum or "plate" that is present in the Ixodidae but absent in the Argasidae. Both types are characteristically soft and leathery, and both have clinical importance. Ixodidae females are capable of enormous expansion up to 50 times their weight in fluid and blood.[80] Ticks have four stages in their life cycle: egg, larva, nymph, and adult. The paralytic syndrome can occur during the larva, nymph, and adult stages and is related to the tick obtaining a blood meal. The following discussion focuses only on tick paralysis or tick toxicosis, and not on any of the infectious diseases associated with tick bites. Most of the major tick-borne diseases in North America are transmitted by Ixodid ticks except for relapsing fever, which is spread by the soft tick of the genus *Ornithodorus* or the *Pediculus* (louse).

In North America, *Dermacentor andersoni* (Rocky Mountain wood tick) and *Dermacentor variabilis* (American dog tick), and *Amblyomma americanum* (Lone Star tick) are the most commonly implicated causes of tick paralysis.[88,222] Typically, tick toxicosis occurs in the Southeastern, Rocky Mountain, and Pacific Northwest regions of the United States, but cases have been reported in the Northeastern area recently.[61] In Australia, the *Ixodes holocyclus* or Australian marsupial tick is the most common offender.[88,222] *I. holocyclus* also seems to be the most potent of the world's paralyzing ticks and has been known to paralyze dogs, cats, sheep, mice, foals, pigs, chickens, and humans.[145]

PATHOPHYSIOLOGY

Venom secreted from the salivary glands during the blood meal is absorbed by the host and systemically distributed. Paralysis results from the neurotoxin "ixobotoxin,"[159] which inhibits the release of acetylcholine at the neuromuscular junction and autonomic ganglia, very similar to botulinum toxin.[91,159] Both botulinum toxin and ixobotoxin demonstrate temperature dependence in rat models and show increased muscular twitching activity as the temperature is reduced.[53,145]

CLINICAL MANIFESTATIONS

Usually the tick must remain on the person for 5 to 6 days in order to cause systemic symptoms. Several days must pass before tick salivary glands begin to secrete significant quantities of toxin. Once secreted, the toxin does not act immediately and may undergo binding and internalization, in a similar sequence to botulinum toxin.[53,122] Ticks typically attach to the scalp but can be found on any part of the body, including the ear canals and anus. Children, particularly girls, and adult men in tick-infested areas are predominantly affected. One large series of 305 cases in Canada reported that 21% were adults older than 16 years.[194] Among the children, 67% were girls; in adults 83% were male. The distribution was attributed to the difficulty of detecting ticks in long hair and the possible greater exposure of adult men to tick-infested environments. Children may appear listless, weak, ataxic, and irritable for several days before they develop an ascending paralysis that begins in the lower limbs. Fever usually is absent. Other manifestations include sensory symptoms such as paresthesias, numbness, and mild diarrhea. These symptoms are followed by absent or decreased deep-tendon reflexes and an ascending generalized weakness that can progress to bulbar structures involving speech, swallowing, and facial expression within 24 to 48 hours, as well as fixed dilated pupils and disturbances of extraocular movements.[91,194] Other atypical presentations are reported and include the following: a child presenting with double vision and being unable to see before the neuromuscular changes occurred, and a healthy elderly male presenting with unilateral weakness and numbness in the left arm for 2 days. Both patients fully recovered after the removal of the tick.[61] If the tick is not removed, respiratory weakness can lead to hypoventilation, lethargy, coma, and death. Unlike the *Dermacentor* spp of North America, removal of the *I. holocyclus* tick does not result in dramatic improvement for several days to weeks. The maximal weakness may not be reached until 48 hours after the tick has been removed or drops off.[91] It is imperative to closely observe patients for possible deterioration.

The differential diagnosis includes Guillain-Barré syndrome (GBS); the Miller-Fisher variant of Guillain-Barré, poliomyelitis; botulism; transverse myelitis; myasthenia gravis; periodic paralysis; acute cerebellar ataxia; and spinal cord lesions. The cerebrospinal fluid remains normal and the rate of progression is rapid, unlike GBS and poliomyelitis.[72,191] The edrophonium test is negative. Nerve conduction studies in patients with tick paralysis may resemble those of patients with early stages of GBS: findings in both conditions include prolonged latency of the distal motor nerves, diminished nerve conduction velocity, and reduction in the amplitudes of muscle and sensory-nerve action potentials.[72] With GBS, there is a prolongation of the F wave, however, which does not occur with tick paralysis, reflecting the more proximal demyelination of the nerve root.[93]

TREATMENT

The most important aspect of treatment is considering tick paralysis in the differential diagnosis of any patient with ascending paralysis. Other than removal of the entire tick, which is curative, treatment is entirely supportive. Since *I. holocyclus* of Australia is considerably more toxic and patients are more likely to deteriorate before they improve, so they must be closely observed for several days until improvement is certain.[72] A hyperimmune serum prepared from dogs is the usual treatment for paralyzed animals, and has been used sparingly in severely ill humans because of the risk of acute reactions and serum sickness.[72]

Prevention of tick bites includes wearing protective clothing and spraying clothes with insect repellant. Diethyltoluamide (DEET) repels ticks, but does not kill them. Permanone is a new tick aerosol spray repellant for use on clothing. It contains permethrin, which kills ticks on contact.[129] According to one study, permethrin in concentrations of 0.036 to 2.276 mg/m^2 induces 90% to 100% tick mortality, with 100% effectiveness for 1 month, and a decrease in effectiveness to 52% after the first washing.[129] Close inspection of all body parts and especially the scalp is important. Proper removal of the tick is very important, otherwise infection or incomplete tick removal may occur. The tick should be grasped as close to the skin surface as possible with blunt curved forceps, tweezers, or gloved hands. Steady pressure without crushing the body should be used; otherwise, expressed fluid may infect the patient and lead to inoculating the patient with a higher dose of toxin or infectious agent. After tick removal, the site should be disinfected. Traditional methods of tick removal using petroleum jelly, topical lidocaine, fingernail polish, isopropyl alcohol, or a hot match head are ineffective and/or may induce the tick to salivate or regurgitate into the wound.[161] It should be remembered that the very same vectors responsible for tick toxicosis can also cause infectious illnesses such as babesiosis, Rocky Mountain spotted fever, anaplasmosis, tularemia, Colorado tick fever, tick-borne relapsing fever, and Lyme disease.

HYMENOPTERA: BEES, WASPS, HORNETS, YELLOW JACKETS, AND ANTS

Within the order Hymenoptera are three families of clinical significance: Apidae (honeybees and bumblebees), Vespidae (yellow jackets, hornets, and wasps), and Formicidae (ants, specifically fire ants). These insects (Fig. 119–6) are of great medical importance because their stings are the most commonly reported and can cause acute toxic and fatal allergic reactions (Table 119–7). An estimated 40 deaths per year are attributed to anaphylaxis secondary to hymenoptera stings.[12,199]

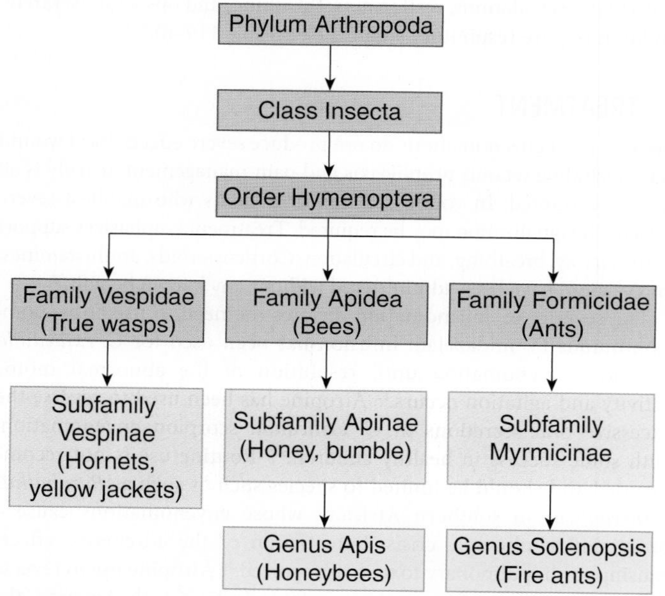

FIGURE 119–6. Taxonomy of the order Hymenoptera.

TABLE 119–7. Classification of Reactions to Hymenoptera Sting

Reaction	Clinical Presentation
Local	
Minimal	Localized pain, pruritus, swelling
	Lesion <5 cm
	Duration several hours
Large	Localized pain and pruritus
	Contiguous swelling and erythema
	Lesion >5 cm
	Duration 1–3 days
Systemic	
Minimal	Localized pain, pruritus, swelling
	Distant and diffuse urticaria, angioedema, pruritus, and/or erythema, conjunctivitis
	Abdominal pain, nausea, diarrhea
Severe	Dermatologic
	Local: Pain, pruritus, and swelling
	Distant: Urticaria, angioedema, pruritus, and/or erythema
	Gastrointestinal
	Nausea, abdominal pain, diarrhea
	Respiratory
	Nasal congestion, rhinorrhea, hoarseness, bronchospasm, stridor, tachypnea, cough, wheezing
	Cardiovascular
	Tachycardia, hypotension, dysrhythmias, myocardial infarction
	Miscellaneous
	Seizures, feeling of impending doom, uterine contractions

Reprinted with permission from Sinkinson CA, French RS, Graft DF, eds. Individualizing therapy for Hymenoptera stings. *Emerg Med Rep.* 1990;11:134.

Apis and *Bombus* species (honeybees and bumblebees) generally build nests away from humans and are passive unless disturbed, but nests of both the honeybees and bumblebees have been found in walls and rodent burrows near homes. Honeybees can only sting once because their stinger is a modified ovipositor that resides in the abdomen. The structure is barbed and has a venom sac attached. Once the stinger embeds into the skin, the stinger disembowels the bee. Bumblebees, however, can sting multiple times. Vespids, on the other hand, are more aggressive and build nests in human living areas, such as in trees and under awnings; yellow jackets inhabit shrubs, trees, and the ground. They, too, are able to sting multiple times.[84] The introduction of the Africanized honeybee in Brazil (because originally they were thought to be a more efficient honey producer) has caused significant economic and health issues. The bees have migrated toward the southern border of the United States, are less productive as a honey producer, and pose a greater threat to humans. African honeybees are characterized by large populations, can make nonstop flights of at least 20 km, and have a tendency toward mass attack with little provocation.[156]

PATHOPHYSIOLOGY

Several allergens (Table 119–8) and pharmacologically active compounds are found in honeybee venom. The three major venom proteins

TABLE 119–8. Composition of Hymenoptera Venom

Vespid (Wasps, Hornets, Yellow Jackets)	Apids (Honeybees)	Formicids (Fire Ants)
Biogenic amines (diverse)	Biogenic amines (diverse)	Biogenic amines (diverse)
Phospholipase A, phospholipase B	Phospholipase A, phospholipase B (?)	Phospholipase A
Hyaluronidase	Hyaluronidase	Hyaluronidase
Acid phosphatase	Acid phosphatase	Piperidines
Mast cell degranulating peptide	Minimine	
Kinin	Mellitin	
	Apamin	
	Mast cell degranulating peptide	

for the honeybee are melittin, phospholipase A_2, and hyaluronidase.[138] Other proteins include apamin, acid phosphatase, and other unidentified proteins. Phospholipase A_2 is the major antigen/allergen in bee venom.[27]

Melittin is the principal component of honeybee venom. It acts as a detergent to disrupt the cell membrane and liberate potassium and biogenic amines.[9] Histamine release by bee venom appears to be largely mediated by mast cell degranulation peptide. Apamin is a neurotoxin that acts on the spinal cord. Apamin binds to the Ca^{+2}-triggered K^{+1} channel and depresses delayed hyperpolarization to cause its toxicity, which is seen in the mouse model as uncoordinated movements leading to spasms, jerks, and convulsions of a spinal origin.[100] Adolapin inhibits prostaglandin synthase and has anti-inflammatory properties that may account for its use in arthritic therapy.[196] Phospholipase A_2 and hyaluronidase are the chief enzymes in bee venom.

Vespid venoms contain three major proteins that serve as allergens and a wide array of vasoactive peptides and amines.[138] The intense pain following by vespid stings is largely caused by serotonin, acetylcholine, and wasp kinins. Antigen 5 is the major allergen in vespid venom.[157] Its biologic function is unknown. Mastoparans have action similar to mast cell degranulation peptide, but weaker.[9] Phospholipase A_2 may be responsible for inducing coagulation abnormalities.[166]

CLINICAL MANIFESTATIONS

Normally, the honeybee sting is manifested as immediate pain, a wheal-and-flare reaction, and localized edema without a systemic reaction. Vomiting, diarrhea, and syncope can occur with a higher dose of venom resulting from multiple stings.[30] Rarely, a sting in the oropharynx produces airway compromise.[199]

Toxic reactions occur with multiple stings (more than 500 stings are described as possibly fatal, and occur with Africanized honeybees)[84] and include gastrointestinal (GI) symptoms, headache, fever, syncope and, rarely, rhabdomyolysis, renal failure, and seizures.[30] Other rare complications include idiopathic intracranial hypertension,[218] cerebral infarction, and ischemic optic neuropathy[193] and Parkinsonism[137] are thought to occur because of the proximity of the sting near the head and neck. Bronchospasm and urticaria are typically absent. This type of toxic reaction is different from the hypersensitivity reactions or anaphylactic reactions because it is not an IgE-mediated response, but rather a direct effect from the venom itself.

Hypersensitivity reactions, including anaphylaxis, occur from hymenoptera stings. These reactions are IgE mediated. The IgE antibodies attach to tissue mast cells and basophils in individuals who have been previously sensitized to the venom. These cells are activated, allowing for progression of the cascade reaction of increased vasoactive substances, such as leukotrienes, eosinophil chemotactic factor-A, and histamine. An anaphylactic reaction is not dependent on the number of stings. Patients who are allergic to hymenoptera venom develop a wheal-and-flare reaction at the site of the inoculum. The shorter the interval between the sting and symptom onset, the more likely the reaction will be severe. Fatalities can occur within several minutes; even initially mild symptoms may be followed by a fulminant course. Generalized urticaria, throat and chest tightness, stridor, fever, chills, and cardiovascular collapse can ensue.

TREATMENT

Application of ice at the site usually is sufficient to halt discomfort. The stinger should be removed by scraping with a credit card or scalpel, as opposed to pulling, which may release additional retained venom. Therapy is aimed at supportive care that includes standard therapy for anaphylaxis with epinephrine, diphenhydramine, and corticosteroids.

Prevention, especially in the allergic person, includes avoiding bright clothing, flowers, scented deodorants and shampoos, perfumes, and barefoot walks outdoors. An emergency kit containing a prefilled spring-loaded epinephrine syringe (EpiPen delivers 0.3 mg, EpiPen Jr. delivers 0.15 mg) with careful instructions from a physician, an antihistamine (diphenhydramine), and an emergency alert card or tag should be carried or worn by the sensitized individual. Individuals with a clear history of anaphylaxis should follow up with an allergist for skin testing and venom immunotherapy for positive results. Immunotherapy significantly reduces the potential risk of anaphylaxis with subsequent stings.[85,110] Commercial preparations of venom from the honeybee, yellow jacket, bald-faced hornet, and wasp can be used for diagnosis and immunotherapy for patients with life-threatening reactions to stings. Several authors have discussed the indications and safety of immunotherapy.[138,236]

FIRE ANTS

There are native fire ants in the United States, but the imported fire ants *Solenopsis invicta* and *Solenopsis richteri* are significant pests that have no natural enemies. They are native to Brazil, Paraguay, Uruguay, and Argentina, but were introduced into Alabama in the 1930s. They have spread rapidly throughout the southern United States, damaging crops, reducing biologic diversity, and inflicting severe stings to humans.[216] *S. invicta,* the most aggressive species, now infests 13 southern states and has been introduced into Australia.[202,205] Allergic reactions to ant stings were limited to the jumper ant (*Myrmecia pilosula*, other *Myrmecia* spp) and the greenhead ant (*Rhytidoponera metallica*; *Odontomachs*, *Cerapachys*, and *Brachyponera* spp) in Australia until February 2001, when the red imported fire ant was identified at two sites in Brisbane.[202] The mode of introduction is unknown but may have originated from the transport of infested sea cargo. Fire ants range from 2 to 6 mm in size. They live in grassy areas, garden sites, and near sources of water. The nests are largely subterranean and have large, conspicuous, dome-shaped above-ground mounds (up to 45 cm above the ground), with many openings for traffic. The mounds can contain 80,000 to 250,000 workers and one or more queens that live for 2 to 6 years and produce 1500 eggs daily.[229] Fire ants are named for the burning pain inflicted after exposure, and necrosis can result at the site. The imported fire ant attacks with little warning. By firmly grasping the skin with its mandibles, both the fire ant and the jumper ant can repeatedly inject venom from a retractile stinger at the end of the abdomen. Pivoting at the head, the fire ant injects an average of seven or eight stings in a circular pattern.[205]

PATHOPHYSIOLOGY

The venom inhibits sodium and potassium adenosine triphosphatases, reduces mitochondrial respiration, uncouples oxidative phosphorylation, adversely affects neutrophil and platelet function, inhibits nitric oxide synthetase, and perhaps activates coagulation.[119,121] Unlike the venoms of wasps, bees, and hornets that contain mostly aqueous-containing proteins, the imported fire ant venom is 95% alkaloid, with a small aqueous fraction that contains soluble proteins.[143] Of the alkaloids, 99% is a 2,6-disubstituted piperidine that has hemolytic, antibacterial, insecticidal, and cytoxic properties.[64] These alkaloids do not cause allergic reactions, but produce a pustule and pain. The aqueous portion of the venom contains the allergenic activity of fire ant venom, *Sol i* I to IV.[104,205] The proteins identified in the venom include a phospholipase, a hyaluronidase, and the enzyme *N*-acetyl-β-glucosaminidase.[65,205]

CLINICAL MANIFESTATIONS

Three categories are suggested based on the reactions to the imported fire ant: local, large local, and systemic.[205] *Local reactions* occur in nonallergic individuals. *Large local reactions* are defined as painful, pruritic swelling at least 5 cm in diameter and contiguous with the sting site. *Systemic reactions* involve signs and symptoms remote from the sting site. The sting initially forms a wheal that is described as a burning itch at the site, followed by the development of sterile pustules. In 24 hours, the pustules umbilicate on an erythematous base. Pustules may last 1 to 2 weeks.[84] Late cutaneous allergic reactions can occur in some persons who experience indurated pruritic lumps at the site of subsequent stings.[64] Large reactions may lead to tissue edema sufficient to compromise blood flow to an extremity. Anaphylaxis occurs in 0.6% to 6% of persons who have been stung.[205] Often, healing occurs with scarring in 10 to 14 days.

DIAGNOSIS

Clinical clues such as pustule development at the sting site after 24 hours, species identification, and history may help to identify fire ant exposure. No laboratory assays to determine exposure are available. Fire ant allergy can be determined by correlating the clinical manifestation of fire ant sting reactions with imported fire ant–specific IgE determined by skin testing or radioallergosorbent test.

TREATMENT

Local reactions require cold compresses and cleansing with soap and water. Some authors recommend topical or injected lidocaine with or without 1:100,000 epinephrine, and topical vinegar and salt mixtures to decrease pain at the site of the bite and sting.[34,108,148,183]

Large local reactions can be treated with oral corticosteroids, antihistamines, and analgesics. Secondary infections should be treated with antibiotics. Systemic reactions should be treated with subcutaneous or intravenous epinephrine.

In the United States, residents of healthcare facilities who are immobile or cognitively impaired are at risk for fire ant attacks, especially when the facility lacks pest control techniques for fire ants.[65] Usually these pests are controlled with traditional insecticides, but there has been a push for environmentally safe insecticides. One study looks at the use of the essential oil from the cinnamon tree, *Cinnamomum osmophloeum* leaf oil, which is similar to the constituents of the cinnamon cassia bark oil that is used for its aroma in the food industry.[48] The indigenous cinnamon leaf essential oil and trans-cinnamaldehyde had an excellent inhibitory effect in controlling the red imported fire ant. The LD_{50} values for both 2% leaf essential oil and 2% trans-cinnamaldehyde after open exposure were 105.0 minutes and 32.2 minutes, respectively; after close exposure they were were 18.5 minutes and 21.2 minutes, respectively, and 100% mortality at 40 minutes in close exposure. This may be a safe alternative for environmental control of the red fire ant.

BUTTERFLIES, MOTHS, AND CATERPILLARS

Butterflies and moths are insects of the order Lepidoptera. Several moth and butterfly families have species whose caterpillars are clinically important, that is, they contain spines or urticating hairs that secrete a poison that is irritating to humans on contact. *Lepidopterism* is a general term that describes the adverse effects to humans when humans are exposed to moths and butterflies.[158] These adverse reactions include urticarial dermatitis, allergic reactions, consumptive coagulopathy, and renal failure. Caterpillar, which means *hairy cat* in Latin, is the larval stage for moths and butterflies. In the United States, several significant stinging caterpillars are of note. The puss caterpillar (*Megalopyge opercularis*) often is considered one of the most important and toxic of the caterpillars in the United States because it has been reported to be such a nuisance, especially in Texas.[207] Other names for the puss caterpillar are woolly/hairy worm, wooly slug, opossum bug, tree asp, Italian asp, and little perrito in Spanish.[207] The caterpillars look furry and are covered in silky tan to brownish hairs that hide short spines containing an urticarial toxin. The spines are yellowish with black tips, and the hairs vary in color ranging from pale yellow and gray to brown.[24] Other significant stinging caterpillars in the United States are the flannel moth caterpillar (*Megalopyge crispata*), the Io moth (*Automeris io*), the saddleback caterpillar (*Sibine stimulata*), and the hickory tussock caterpillar (*Lophocampa caryae*).[136] In South America, especially Brazil, *Lonomia obliqua* caterpillars are notorious for causing severe pain and a hemorrhagic syndrome.[41,58] In Australia several caterpillars are of medical importance: mistletoe brown tail moth (*Euproctis edwardsi*), processionary caterpillars (*Ochrogaster lunifer*), cup moths (*Doratifera* spp), and the white-stemmed gum moth (*Chelepteryx collesi*).[8] Pine processionary caterpillars (*Thaumetopoea pityocampa*) are the most important defoliator of pine forests in the Mediterranean and central European countries, with significant consequential economic and occupational repercussions for workers who frequent these pine forests.[223]

PATHOPHYSIOLOGY

Little is known about the composition of the venom, which probably varies according to the different caterpillar species. Some toxins contain proteins that cause histamine release, such as thaumetopoien isolated from *T. pityocampa* or pine processionary caterpillar.[223,224] Another protein isolated from the *L. obliqua* caterpillar causes coagulopathy; its mechanism of action is not fully known but it somehow activates factors X and II.[67,124] The venom and hair structure of *Lagoa crispata*, which has often been confused with the southern Texas puss caterpillar, has been characterized.[136] The venom is stored at the base of the hollow setae (spines) where the poison sac and nervous tissue are located. Upon contact with these spines, the toxin is released. The toxin may be a protein or a substance that conjugates with proteins.[75] The varying differences of caterpillar venom and their clinical effects emphasize the importance of positive identification of caterpillars.

CLINICAL MANIFESTATIONS

The clinical effects of caterpillar exposure can generally be separated into two types–stinging reaction and pruritic reaction—although overlap may occur. Stinging caterpillars, such as *M. opercularis*, envenomate by contact with their hollow spines containing venom. The reaction is characterized as a painful, burning sensation with local effects and, less commonly, systemic effects. The area may become erythematous and swollen, and papules and vesicles may appear. The classic gridlike pattern develops within 2 to 3 hours of contact. Reported symptoms include nausea, vomiting, fever, headache, restlessness, tachycardia, hypotension, urticaria, seizures, and even radiating lymphadenitis and regional adenopathy.[168] Another stinging caterpillar previously mentioned is the *L. obliqua* caterpillar, which causes the hemorrhagic syndrome that presents as a disseminating intravascular coagulopathy and as secondary fibrinolysis with skin, mucosal, and visceral bleeding, acute renal failure, and intracerebral hemorrhage.[41,124] Pruritic reactions occur upon exposure to the itchy caterpillars that have nonvenomous urticating hairs, which can produce a mechanical irritation, allergic reaction, or a granulomatous reaction from the chronic presence of the hairs. Several species that cause allergic reactions are the white-stemmed moth (*C. collesi*), Douglas fir tussock moth (*Orgyria pseudotsugata*), and gypsy moth caterpillar (*Lymantria dispar*).[158] Caterpillar hairs can cause ocular trauma, otherwise known as *ophthalmia nodosa*.[204] The range of ocular pathology depends on the penetration factor and the effect of the released urticating toxins.[40] The ocular spectrum has been classified into five types by Cadera et al[40]:

Type 1: Brief exposure time of 15 minutes. Symptoms of chemosis, inflammation, epiphora, and foreign body sensation may last for weeks.

Type 2: Chronic mechanical keratoconjunctivitis (hairs in bulbar/palpebral conjunctivitis). Foreign body sensation is relieved by removal of hairs. Cornea abrasions may be present.

Type 3: Gray-yellow nodules or asymptomatic granulomas.

Type 4: Severe iritis with or without iritis nodules. Hairs in the anterior chamber and possible intralenticular foreign body.

Type 5: Vitreoretinal involvement. Hairs may enter through the anterior chamber or iris lens or by transscleral migration. May cause vitreitis, cystoid macular edema, papillitis, or endophthalmitis.

TREATMENT

Treatment of ocular lesions depends upon the exposure classification. Most patients can be classified as type 1 or 2. Irrigation with saline should be followed by meticulous removal of setae, followed by topical steroids and antibiotics. Type 3 requires surgical excision of the nodules. Type 4 requires topical steroids with or without iridectomy for nodules or operative removal of setae. Type 5 requires local treatment with or without systemic steroids. Resistant cases may require vitrectomy with removal of setae. Treatment for dermal contact should be immediate, with removal of the embedded spines using cellophane tape and application of ice. Opioids may be necessary, if minor analgesics do not provide relief. If muscle cramps develop, benzodiazepines should be administered. One study recommended the use of 10 mL 10% calcium gluconate administered IV, which provided pain relief.[151] Topical corticosteroids can be used to decrease local inflammation. Antihistamines such as diphenhydramine (25–50 mg for adults and 1 mg/kg, maximum 50 mg, in children) can be used to relieve pruritus and urticaria.[151,168] Nebulized β-agonists and epinephrine administered subcutaneously may be required for more severe respiratory symptoms and anaphylactoid/anaphylactic-type reactions. For hemorrhagic syndrome resulting from exposure to *L. obliqua* caterpillar, an antidote called the antilonomic serum (SALon) is available and is used for treatment of the hemorrhagic syndrome in Brazil.[58]

BLISTER BEETLES

Blister beetles are plant-eating insects that exude a blistering agent for protection. They can be found in the eastern United States, southern Europe, Africa, and Asia. Most are from the order Coleoptera, family Meloidae. *Epicauta vittata* is the most common of more than 200 blister beetles identified in the United States.[123] When the beetles sense danger, they exude cantharidin by filling their breathing tubes with air, closing their breathing pores, and building up body fluid pressure until fluid is pushed out through one or more leg joints.[84] Cantharidin is a potent blistering agent found throughout all 10 stages of life of the blister beetle.[44] Cantharidin is produced only by the male blister beetle and is stored until mating. The female loses most of her reserves as she matures. In the wild, the female repeatedly acquires cantharidin as copulatory gifts from her mates.[44] Cantharidin, also known popularly as *Spanish fly*, takes its name from the Mediterranean beetle *Cantharis vesicatoria*. It has been ingested as a sexual stimulant for millennia. The aphrodisiac properties are related to the ability of cantharidin to cause vascular engorgement and inflammation of the genitourinary tract upon elimination, hence the reports of priapism and pelvic organ engorgement.[220] Cantharidin has been used for treatment of bladder and kidney infections, stones, stranguria (bladder spasm), and various venereal diseases.[123] In the last century, cantharidin was commonly used for treatment of pleurisy, pneumonia, arthritis, neuralgias, and various dermatitides. A topical 1% commercial preparation can be used for removal of warts and molluscum contagiosum.[54,195] Cantharidin poisoning has been reported by cutaneous exposure,[33] unintentional inoculation,[171] and inadvertent ingestion of the beetle itself.[217] There is one case report of a child being treated for molluscum contagiosum with cantharidin preparation that included podophyllin and salicylic acid, also called Canthacur PS or Canthacur Plus.[195] The child developed varicelliform vesicular dermatitis in the distribution of the application of petrolatum. It is thought that the petrolatum used by the parents to moisturize her skin spread the lipophillic cantharidin preparation to the nearby areas causing the blistering reaction. Canthacur PS should not be used for molluscum contagiosum but is reserved for verrucae vulgaris on acral areas. Canthacur or Cantharone contains plain cantharidin and can be used for the treatment of molluscum contagiosum. Fewer than 30 cases of Spanish fly poisoning have been reported since 1900.[123]

PATHOPHYSIOLOGY

Cantharidin is a natural, defensive, highly toxic terpenoid (lethal dose for humans 0.5 mg/kg) produced by blister beetles and shares a structural similarity with the herbicide Endothall.[149] Endothall causes corrosive effects to the GI tract; cardiomyopathy and vascular permeability lead to shock. A single case report of lethal poisoning with 7 to 8 g of endothall has been reported and the healthy young male died of hemorrhage of the GI tract and lung, which is clinically similar to the cantharidin exposures. Although the mechanism of action has not been elucidated, one mechanism based on an in vitro study suggests that cantharidin inhibits the activity of protein phosphatases type 1 and 2A. This inhibition alters endothelial permeability by enhancing the phosphorylation state of endothelial regulatory proteins and results in elevated albumin flux and dysfunction of the barrier.[128] Enhanced permeability of albumin may be responsible for the systemic effects of cantharidin, which lead to diffuse injury of the vascular endothelium and resultant blistering, hemorrhage, and inflammation.

CLINICAL MANIFESTATIONS

The clinical effects can mostly be attributed to the irritative effects on the exposed organ systems. The secretions of cantharidin from the beetle's leg joints cause an urticarial dermatitis that is manifested several hours later by burns, blisters, or vesiculobullae.[33] Symptoms may be immediate or delayed over several hours. In addition to the local effects, cantharidin can be absorbed through the lipid bilayer of the epidermis and cause systemic toxicity, with diaphoresis, tachycardia, hematuria, and oliguria from extensive dermal exposure.[220] If the periorbital region is contaminated, edema and blistering can evolve. Ocular findings from direct contact with the beetle or hand contamination include decreased vision, pain, lacrimation, corneal ulcerations, filamentary keratitis, and anterior uveitis.[171] Most human exposures involve inadvertent contact with the beetle or its secretions, resulting in dermatitis, keratoconjunctivitis, and periorbital edema secondary to hand–eye involvement, also called the *Nairobi eye*.[171]

When cantharidin is ingested, severe GI disturbances and hematuria can occur. Initial patient complaints may include burning of the oropharynx, dysphagia, abdominal cramping, vomiting, hematemesis followed by lower GI tract hematochezia, and tenesmus. An inadvertent blister beetle ingestion by a child who thought it was the edible *Eulepida mashona* or white grub resulted in hematuria and abdominal cramping.[217] Genitourinary effects include dysuria, urinary frequency, hematuria, proteinuria, and renal impairment. Most symptoms resolved over several weeks. However, death from renal failure with acute tubular necrosis has been reported.[220]

DIAGNOSTIC TESTING

Cantharidin toxicosis has been identified for equine and ruminant exposures by screening urine and gastric contents with high-performance liquid chromatography and gas chromatography-mass spectrometry.[175,176] This method has not been used in clinical practice.

TREATMENT

Treatment is largely supportive. Wound care and tetanus status should be assessed. For keratoconjunctivitis, an ophthalmologist should be consulted early in the clinical course and the patient treated with topical corticosteroids (prednisolone 0.125%), mydriatics (cyclopentolate 1%), and antibiotics (ciprofloxacin 0.3%).

SUMMARY

Healthcare providers should have an extensive knowledge regarding bites and stings by arthropods and arachnids so they can provide optimal care to their patients. And though arachnid envenomation tends to be more of a nuisance than a life threat, good supportive care, rapid identification of the arthropod, and, rarely, antivenom are the keys to the rapid recovery. This includes proper hygiene to prevent secondary infections, avoiding contact with arthropods, decreasing the arthropod population mechanically and/or chemically, and the use of repellents as important measures to decrease morbidity from arthropods. The patient should bring the arthropod to the hospital, if possible, to facilitate identification, and every attempt should be made to describe the evolution of the bite to assist in the differential diagnosis.

ACKNOWLEDGMENT

Neal A. Lewin contributed to this chapter in previous editions of this book.

REFERENCES

1. Abroug F, El Atrous S, Nouira S, Haguiga H, Touzi N, Bouchoucha S. Serotherapy in scorpion envenomation: a randomised controlled trial. *Lancet.* 1999;354:906-9.
2. Allen C. Arachnid envenomations. *Emerg Med Clin North Am.* 1992;10: 269-298.
3. Anderson PC. Missouri brown recluse spider: a review and update. *Mo Med.* 1998;95:318-322.
4. Anderson PC. Spider bites in the United States. *Dermatol Clin.* 1997;15: 307-311.
5. Anderson PC. What's new in loxoscelism? *Mo Med.* 1973;70:711-712 passim.
6. Atkins JA, Wingo CW, Sodeman WA. Probable cause of necrotic spider bite in the Midwest. *Science.* 1957;126:73.
7. Babcock JL, Marmer DJ, Steele RW. Immunotoxicology of brown recluse spider (*Loxosceles reclusa*) venom. *Toxicon.* 1986;24:783-790.
8. Balit CR, Geary MJ, Russell RC, Isbister GK. Prospective study of definite caterpillar exposures. *Toxicon.* 2003;42:657-662.
9. Balit CR, Isbister GK, Buckley NA. Randomized controlled trial of topical aspirin in the treatment of bee and wasp stings. *J Toxicol Clin Toxicol.* 2003;41:801-808.
10. Banks B. Immunotoxicology of the brown recluse spider venom. In: Koiznalik F, Mebs D, ed. *Proceedings of the 7th European Symposium on Animal, Plant, and Microbial Toxins.* Prague; 1986:41.
11. Barbaro KC, Ferreira ML, Cardoso DF, Eickstedt VR, Mota I. Identification and neutralization of biological activities in the venoms of *Loxosceles* spiders. *Braz J Med Biol Res.* 1996;29:1491-1497.
12. Barnard JH. Studies of 400 Hymenoptera sting deaths in the United States. *J Allergy Clin Immunol.* 1973;52:259-264.
13. Barrett SM, Romine-Jenkins M, Blick KE. Passive hemagglutination inhibition test for diagnosis of brown recluse spider bite envenomation. *Clin Chem.* 1993;39:2104-2107.
14. Bawaskar HS, Bawaskar PH. Role of atropine in management of cardiovascular manifestations of scorpion envenoming in humans. *J Trop Med Hyg.* 1992;95:30-35.
15. Bawaskar HS, Bawaskar PH. Management of scorpion sting. *Heart.* 1999;82: 253-254.
16. Belghith M, Boussarsar M, Haguiga H, et al. Efficacy of serotherapy in scorpion sting: a matched-pair study. *J Toxicol Clin Toxicol.* 1999;37:51-57.
17. Belyea DA, Tuman DC, Ward TP, Babonis TR. The red eye revisited: ophthalmia nodosa due to tarantula hairs. *South Med J.* 1998;91:565-567.
18. Bennett RG, Vetter RS. An approach to spider bites. Erroneous attribution of dermonecrotic lesions to brown recluse or hobo spider bites in Canada. *Can Fam Physician.* 2004;50:1098-1101.
19. Berg RA, Tarantino MD. Envenomation by the scorpion *Centruroides exilicauda* (*C sculpturatus*): severe and unusual manifestations. *Pediatrics.* 1991;87:930-933.
20. Bergman NJ. Clinical description of *Parabuthus transvaalicus* scorpionism in Zimbabwe. *Toxicon.* 1997;35:759-771.
21. Bernardino CR, Rapuano C. Ophthalmia nodosa caused by casual handling of a tarantula. *CLAO J.* 2000;26:111-112.
22. Bernstein B, Ehrlich F. Brown recluse spider bites. *J Emerg Med.* 1986;4: 457-462.
23. Binford GJ. An analysis of geographic and intersexual chemical variation in venoms of the spider *Tegenaria agrestis* (Agelenidae). *Toxicon.* 2001;39:955-968.
24. Bishopp F. The puss caterpillar and the effects of its sting on man. In: *Department Circular 288.* Washington, DC: US Department of Agriculture; 1923:1-14.
25. Bittner MA. Alpha-latrotoxin and its receptors CIRL (latrophilin) and neurexin 1 alpha mediate effects on secretion through multiple mechanisms. *Biochimie.* 2000;82:447-452.
26. Blaikie AJ, Ellis J, Sanders R, MacEwen CJ. Eye disease associated with handling pet tarantulas: three case reports. *BMJ.* 1997;314:1524-1525.
27. Blaser K, Carballido J, Faith A, Crameri R, Akdis C. Determinants and mechanisms of human immune responses to bee venom phospholipase A2. *Int Arch Allergy Immunol.* 1998;117:1-10.
28. Bogen E. Arachnidism, a study in spider poisoning. *JAMA.* 1926;86: 1894-1896.
29. Bond GR. Antivenin administration for *Centruroides* scorpion sting: risks and benefits. *Ann Emerg Med.* 1992;21:788-791.
30. Bresolin NL, Carvalho LC, Goes EC, Fernandes R, Barotto AM. Acute renal failure following massive attack by Africanized bee stings. *Pediatr Nephrol.* 2002;17:625-627.
31. Bronstein AC, Spyker DA, Cantilena LR Jr, Green J, Rumack BH, Heard SE. 2006 Annual Report of the American Association of Poison Control Centers' National Poison Data System (NPDS). *Clin Toxicol (Phila).* 2007;45: 815-917.
32. Bronstein AC, Spyker DA, Cantilena LR Jr, Green JL, Rumack BH, Heard SE. 2007 Annual Report of the American Association of Poison Control Centers' National Poison Data System (NPDS): 25th Annual Report. *Clin Toxicol (Phila).* 2008;46:927-1057.
33. Browne S. Cantharidin poisoning due to a blister beetle. *Br Med J.* 1960;2: 1260-1291.
34. Bruce S, Tschen EH, Smith EB. Topical aluminum sulfate for fire ant stings. *Int J Dermatol.* 1984;23:211.
35. Bucherl W. *Spiders.* London: Academic Press; 1971.
36. Bugli F, Graffeo R, Sterbini FP, et al. Monoclonal antibody fragment from combinatorial phage display library neutralizes α-latrotoxin activity and abolishes black widow spider venom lethality, in mice. *Toxicon.* 2008;51:547-554.
37. Bush SP, Naftel J. Injection of a whole black widow spider. *Ann Emerg Med.* 1996;27:532-533.
38. Cabbiness SG, Gehrke CW, Kuo KC, et al. Polyamines in some tarantula venoms. *Toxicon.* 1980;18:681-683.
39. Cacy J, Mold JW. The clinical characteristics of brown recluse spider bites treated by family physicians: an OKPRN Study. Oklahoma Physicians Research Network. *J Fam Pract.* 1999;48:536-542.
40. Cadera W, Pachtman MA, Fountain JA, Ellis FD, Wilson FM 2nd. Ocular lesions caused by caterpillar hairs (ophthalmia nodosa). *Can J Ophthalmol.* 1984;19:40-44.
41. Caovilla JJ, Barros EJ. Efficacy of two different doses of antilonomic serum in the resolution of hemorrhagic syndrome resulting from envenoming by *Lonomia obliqua* caterpillars: a randomized controlled trial. *Toxicon.* 2004;43:811-818.
42. Carbonaro PA, Janniger CK, Schwartz RA. Spider bite reactions. *Cutis.* 1995;56:256-259.
43. Cardoso JL, Wen FH, Franca FO, Warrell DA, Theakston RD. Detection by enzyme immunoassay of *Loxosceles gaucho* venom in necrotic skin lesions caused by spider bites in Brazil. *Trans R Soc Trop Med Hyg.* 1990;84:608-609.
44. Carrel JE, McCairel MH, Slagle AJ, Doom JP, Brill J, McCormick JP. Cantharidin production in a blister beetle. *Experientia.* 1993;49:171-174.
45. Centers for Disease Control and Prevention (CDC). Necrotic arachnidism—Pacific Northwest, 1988-1996. *MMWR Morb Mortal Wkly Rep.* 1996;45: 433-436.
46. Chan TK, Geren CR, Howell DE, Odell GV. Adenosine triphosphate in tarantula spider venoms and its synergistic effect with the venom toxin. *Toxicon.* 1975;13:61-66.
47. Chavez-Olortegui C, Zanetti VC, Ferreira AP, Minozzo JC, Mangili OC, Gubert IC. ELISA for the detection of venom antigens in experimental and clinical envenoming by *Loxosceles intermedia* spiders. *Toxicon.* 1998;36:563-569.
48. Cheng SS, Liu JY, Lin CY, et al. Terminating red imported fire ants using *Cinnamomum osmophloeum* leaf essential oil. *Bioresour Technol.* 2008;99:889-893.
49. Choi JT, Rauf A. Ophthalmia nodosa secondary to tarantula hairs. *Eye.* 2003;17:433-434.
50. Clark RF, Wethern-Kestner S, Vance MV, Gerkin R. Clinical presentation and treatment of black widow spider envenomation: a review of 163 cases. *Ann Emerg Med.* 1992;21:782-787.
51. Cohen J, Bush S. Case report: compartment syndrome after a suspected black widow spider bite. *Ann Emerg Med.* 2005;45:414-416.
52. Connor D, Seldon, BS. Scorpion envenomation. In: Auerbach P, ed. *Wilderness Medicine: Management of Wilderness and Environmental Emergencies.* St. Louis: Mosby; 1995:831-842.

53. Cooper BJ, Spence I. Temperature-dependent inhibition of evoked acetylcholine release in tick paralysis. *Nature.* 1976;263:693-695.
54. Coskey RJ. Treatment of plantar warts in children with a salicylic acid-podophyllin-cantharidin product. *Pediatr Dermatol.* 1984;2:71-73.
55. Curry SC. Black widow spider envenomation. In: Harwood A, Linden, C, Lutten R, et al, eds. *The Clinical Practice of Emergency Medicine.* Philadelphia: JB Lippincott; 1991:617-619.
56. Curry SC, Vance MV, Ryan PJ, Kunkel DB, Northey WT. Envenomation by the scorpion *Centruroides sculpturatus. J Toxicol Clin Toxicol.* 1983;21: 417-449.
57. da Silva GH, Hyslop S, Alice da Cruz-Hofling M. *Lonomia obliqua* caterpillar venom increases permeability of the blood–brain barrier in rats. *Toxicon.* 2004;44:625-634.
58. Da Silva WD, Campos CM, Goncalves LR, et al. Development of an antivenom against toxins of *Lonomia obliqua* caterpillars. *Toxicon.* 1996;34:1045-1049.
59. da Silveira RB, dos Santos Filho JF, Mangili OC, et al. Identification of proteases in the extract of venom glands from brown spiders. *Toxicon.* 2002;40:815-822.
60. Das S, Nalini P, Ananthakrishnan S, Sethuraman KR, Balachander J, Srinivasan S. Cardiac involvement and scorpion envenomation in children. *J Trop Pediatr.* 1995;41:338-340.
61. Daugherty RJ, Posner JC, Henretig FM, McHugh LA, Tan CG. Tick paralysis: atypical presentation, unusual location. *Pediatr Emerg Care.* 2005;21:677-680.
62. de Almeida DM, Fernandes-Pedrosa Mde F, de Andrade RM, et al. A new anti-loxoscelic serum produced against recombinant sphingomyelinase D: results of preclinical trials. *Am J Trop Med Hyg.* 2008;79:463-470.
63. Dehesa-Davila M, Possani LD. Scorpionism and serotherapy in Mexico. *Toxicon.* 1994;32:1015-1018.
64. deShazo RD, Butcher BT, Banks WA. Reactions to the stings of the imported fire ant. *N Engl J Med.* 1990;323:462-466.
65. deShazo RD, Kemp SF, deShazo MD, Goddard J. Fire ant attacks on patients in nursing homes: an increasing problem. *Am J Med.* 2004;116:843-846.
66. Devi CS, Reddy CN, Devi SL, et al. Defibrination syndrome due to scorpion venom poisoning. *Br Med J.* 1970;1:345-347.
67. Donato JL, Moreno RA, Hyslop S, et al. *Lonomia obliqua* caterpillar spicules trigger human blood coagulation via activation of factor X and prothrombin. *Thromb Haemost.* 1998;79:539-542.
68. D'Suze G, Moncada S, Gonzalez C, Sevcik C, Aguilar V, Alagon A. Relationship between plasmatic levels of various cytokines, tumour necrosis factor, enzymes, glucose and venom concentration following *Tityus* scorpion sting. *Toxicon.* 2003;41:367-375.
69. Erdur B, Turkcuer I, Bukiran A, Kuru O, Varol I. Uncommon cardiovascular manifestations after a *Latrodectus* bite. *Am J Emerg Med.* 2007;25:232-235.
70. Escoubas P, Diochot S, Celerier ML, Nakajima T, Lazdunski M. Novel tarantula toxins for subtypes of voltage-dependent potassium channels in the Kv2 and Kv4 subfamilies. *Mol Pharmacol.* 2002;62:48-57.
71. Escoubas P, Diochot S, Corzo G. Structure and pharmacology of spider venom neurotoxins. *Biochimie.* 2000;82:893-907.
72. Felz MW, Smith CD, Swift TR. A six-year-old girl with tick paralysis. *N Engl J Med.* 2000;342:90-94.
73. Fernandez-Bouzas A, Morales-Resendiz ML, Llamas-Ibarra F, Martinez-Lopez M, Ballesteros-Maresma A. Brain infarcts due to scorpion stings in children: MRI. *Neuroradiology.* 2000;42:118-120.
74. Fet V, Sisson, WD, Lowe, G, Braunwalder ME. *Catalog of the Scorpions of the World (1758-1998).* New York: New York Entomological Society; 2000.
75. Foot N. Pathology of the dermatitis caused by the *Megalopyge opercularis*, a Texas caterpillar. *J Exp Med.* 1922;35:737-753.
76. Franca FO, Barbaro KC, Abdulkader RC. Rhabdomyolysis in presumed viscero-cutaneous loxoscelism: report of two cases. *Trans R Soc Trop Med Hyg.* 2002;96:287-290.
77. Fukuhara YD, Dellalibera-Joviliano R, Cunha FQ, Reis ML, Donadi EA. The kinin system in the envenomation caused by the *Tityus serrulatus* scorpion sting. *Toxicol Appl Pharmacol.* 2004;196:390-395.
78. Fukuhara YD, Reis ML, Dellalibera-Joviliano R, Cunha FQ, Donadi EA. Increased plasma levels of IL-1beta, IL-6, IL-8, IL-10 and TNF-alpha in patients moderately or severely envenomed by *Tityus serrulatus* scorpion sting. *Toxicon.* 2003;41:49-55.
79. Gendron BP. *Loxosceles reclusa* envenomation. *Am J Emerg Med.* 1990;8: 51-54.
80. Gentile D. Tick-borne diseases. In: Auerbach P, ed. *Wilderness Medicine: Management of Wilderness and Environmental Emergencies.* St Louis: Mosby; 1995:787-812.
81. Geppert M, Khvotchev M, Krasnoperov V, et al. Neurexin I alpha is a major α-latrotoxin receptor that cooperates in α-latrotoxin action. *J Biol Chem.* 1998;273:1705-1710.
82. Gibly R, Williams M, Walter FG, McNally J, Conroy C, Berg RA. Continuous intravenous midazolam infusion for *Centruroides exilicauda* scorpion envenomation. *Ann Emerg Med.* 1999;34:620-625.
83. Ginsburg CM, Weinberg AG. Hemolytic anemia and multiorgan failure associated with localized cutaneous lesion. *J Pediatr.* 1988;112:496-499.
84. Goddard J. *Physician's Guide to Arthropods of Medical Importance.* 3rd ed. Boca Raton, FL: CRC Press; 2000.
85. Golden DB, Valentine MD, Kagey-Sobotka A, Lichtenstein LM. Regimens of Hymenoptera venom immunotherapy. *Ann Intern Med.* 1980;92: 620-624.
86. Gomez HF, Miller MJ, Trachy JW, Marks RM, Warren JS. Intradermal anti-loxosceles Fab fragments attenuate dermonecrotic arachnidism. *Acad Emerg Med.* 1999;6:1195-1202.
87. Gorb SN, Niederegger S, Hayashi CY, Summers AP, Votsch W, Walther P. Biomaterials: silk-like secretion from tarantula feet. *Nature.* 2006;443:407.
88. Gordon BM, Giza CC. Tick paralysis presenting in an urban environment. *Pediatr Neurol.* 2004;30:122-124.
89. Goto CS, Abramo TJ, Ginsburg CM. Upper airway obstruction caused by brown recluse spider envenomization of the neck. *Am J Emerg Med.* 1996;14:660-662.
90. Grant SJ, Loxton EH. Effectiveness of a compression bandage and antivenene for Sydney funnel-web spider envenomation. *Med J Aust.* 1992;156: 510-511.
91. Grattan-Smith PJ, Morris JG, Johnston HM, et al. Clinical and neurophysiological features of tick paralysis. *Brain.* 1997;120(Pt 11):1975-1987.
92. Graudins A, Gunja N, Broady KW, Nicholson GM. Clinical and in vitro evidence for the efficacy of Australian red-back spider (*Latrodectus hasselti*) antivenom in the treatment of envenomation by a cupboard spider (*Steatoda grossa*). *Toxicon.* 2002;40:767-775.
93. Greenstein P. Tick paralysis. *Med Clin North Am.* 2002;86:441-446.
94. Grishin EV. Black widow spider toxins: the present and the future. *Toxicon.* 1998;36:1693-1701.
95. Groshong TD. Scorpion envenomation in eastern Saudi Arabia. *Ann Emerg Med.* 1993;22:1431-1437.
96. Gueron M, Ilia R, Margulis G. Arthropod poisons and the cardiovascular system. *Am J Emerg Med.* 2000;18:708-714.
97. Gueron M, Ilia R, Sofer S. The cardiovascular system after scorpion envenomation. A review. *J Toxicol Clin Toxicol.* 1992;30:245-258.
98. Gueron M, Sofer S. Vasodilators and calcium blocking agents as treatment of cardiovascular manifestations of human scorpion envenomation. *Toxicon.* 1990;28:127-128.
99. Gueron M, Yaron R. Cardiovascular manifestations of severe scorpion sting. Clinicopathologic correlations. *Chest.* 1970;57:156-162.
100. Habermann E. Apamin. *Pharmacol Ther.* 1984;25:255-270.
101. Haeberli S, Kuhn-Nentwig L, Schaller J, Nentwig W. Characterisation of antibacterial activity of peptides isolated from the venom of the spider *Cupiennius salei* (Araneae:Ctenidae). *Toxicon.* 2000;38:373-380.
102. Henkel AW, Sankaranarayanan S. Mechanisms of α-latrotoxin action. *Cell Tissue Res.* 1999;296:229-233.
103. Hobbs GD, Anderson AR, Greene TJ, Yealy DM. Comparison of hyperbaric oxygen and dapsone therapy for loxosceles envenomation. *Acad Emerg Med.* 1996;3:758-761.
104. Hoffman DR. Allergens in Hymenoptera venom. XVII. Allergenic components of *Solenopsis invicta* (imported fire ant) venom. *J Allergy Clin Immunol.* 1987;80:300-306.
105. Hollabaugh RS, Fernandes ET. Management of the brown recluse spider bite. *J Pediatr Surg.* 1989;24:126-127.
106. Honig PJ. Bites and parasites. *Pediatr Clin North Am.* 1983;30:563-581.
107. Hoover NG, Fortenberry JD. Use of antivenin to treat priapism after a black widow spider bite. *Pediatrics.* 2004;114:e128-e129.
108. Horen WP. Insect and scorpion sting. *JAMA.* 1972;221:894-898.
109. Horng CT, Chou PI, Liang JB. Caterpillar setae in the deep cornea and anterior chamber. *Am J Ophthalmol.* 2000;129:384-385.
110. Hunt KJ, Valentine MD, Sobotka AK, Benton AW, Amodio FJ, Lichtenstein LM. A controlled trial of immunotherapy in insect hypersensitivity. *N Engl J Med.* 1978;299:157-161.

111. Ichtchenko K, Bittner MA, Krasnoperov V, et al. A novel ubiquitously expressed α-latrotoxin receptor is a member of the CIRL family of G-protein-coupled receptors. *J Biol Chem.* 1999;274:5491-5498.
112. Isbister GK. Data collection in clinical toxinology: debunking myths and developing diagnostic algorithms. *J Toxicol Clin Toxicol.* 2002;40: 231-237.
113. Isbister GK, Gray MR. A prospective study of 750 definite spider bites, with expert spider identification. *QJM.* 2002;95:723-731.
114. Isbister GK, Gray MR. Effects of envenoming by comb-footed spiders of the genera Steatoda and Achaearanea (family Theridiidae:Araneae) in Australia. *J Toxicol Clin Toxicol.* 2003;41:809-819.
115. Isbister GK, Gray MR. Latrodectism: a prospective cohort study of bites by formally identified redback spiders. *Med J Aust.* 2003;179:88-91.
116. Isbister GK, Gray MR. White-tail spider bite: a prospective study of 130 definite bites by *Lampona* species. *Med J Aust.* 2003;179:199-202.
117. Isbister GK, Seymour JE, Gray MR, Raven RJ. Bites by spiders of the family Theraphosidae in humans and canines. *Toxicon.* 2003;41:519-524.
118. Ismail M. Treatment of the scorpion envenoming syndrome: 12-years experience with serotherapy. *Int J Antimicrob Agents.* 2003;21:170-174.
119. Javors MA, Zhou W, Maas JW Jr, Han S, Keenan RW. Effects of fire ant venom alkaloids on platelet and neutrophil function. *Life Sci.* 1993;53: 1105-1112.
120. Johnson JH, Bloomquist JR, Krapcho KJ, et al. Novel insecticidal peptides from *Tegenaria agrestis* spider venom may have a direct effect on the insect central nervous system. *Arch Insect Biochem Physiol.* 1998;38:19-31.
121. Jones T, Blum, M, Fales, H. Ant venom alkaloids from *Solenopsis* and *Monomovian* species venom. *Tetrahedron.* 1982;38:1949-1958.
122. Kaire GH. Isolation of tick paralysis toxin from *Ixodes holocyclus. Toxicon.* 1966;4:91-97.
123. Karras DJ, Farrell SE, Harrigan RA, Henretig FM, Gealt L. Poisoning from "Spanish fly" (cantharidin). *Am J Emerg Med.* 1996;14:478-483.
124. Kelen E, Picarelli A, Duarte A. Hemorrhagic sydnrome induced by contact with caterpillars of the genus *Lonomia obliqua. J Toxicol Toxin Review.* 1995;14:283-308.
125. Kelley TD 3rd, Wasserman G. The dangers of pet tarantulas: experience of the Marseilles Poison Centre. *J Toxicol Clin Toxicol.* 1998;36:55-56.
126. Key GF. A comparison of calcium gluconate and methocarbamol (Robaxin) in the treatment of latrodectism (black widow spider envenomation). *Am J Trop Med Hyg.* 1981;30:273-277.
127. King LE Jr, Rees RS. Dapsone treatment of a brown recluse bite. *JAMA.* 1983;250:648.
128. Knapp J, Boknik P, Luss I, et al. The protein phosphatase inhibitor cantharidin alters vascular endothelial cell permeability. *J Pharmacol Exp Ther.* 1999;289:1480-1486.
129. Kocisova A, Para L. Possibilities of long-term protection against blood-sucking insects and ticks. *Cent Eur J Public Health.* 1999;7:27-30.
130. Krasnoperov VG, Bittner MA, Beavis R, et al. α-Latrotoxin stimulates exocytosis by the interaction with a neuronal G-protein-coupled receptor. *Neuron.* 1997;18:925-937.
131. Krifi MN, Kharrat H, Zghal K, et al. Development of an ELISA for the detection of scorpion venoms in sera of humans envenomed by *Androctonus australis garzonii* (Aag) and *Buthus occitanus tunetanus* (Bot): correlation with clinical severity of envenoming in Tunisia. *Toxicon.* 1998;36: 887-900.
132. Krywko DM, Gomez HF. Detection of *Loxosceles* species venom in dermal lesions: a comparison of 4 venom recovery methods. *Ann Emerg Med.* 2002;39:475-480.
133. Kunkel DB, Wasserman GS. Envenomations by miscellaneous animals. *J Toxicol Clin Toxicol.* 1983;21:557-560.
134. Kurpiewski G, Forrester LJ, Barrett JT, Campbell BJ. Platelet aggregation and sphingomyelinase D activity of a purified toxin from the venom of *Loxosceles reclusa. Biochim Biophys Acta.* 1981;678:467-476.
135. Kuspis DA, Rawlins JE, Krenzelok EP. Human exposures to stinging caterpillar: *Lophocampa caryae* exposures. *Am J Emerg Med.* 2001;19: 396-398.
136. Lamdin JM, Howell DE, Kocan KM, et al. The venomous hair structure, venom and life cycle of *Lagoa crispata*, a puss caterpillar of Oklahoma. *Toxicon.* 2000;38:1163-1189.
137. Leopold NA, Bara-Jimenez W, Hallett M. Parkinsonism after a wasp sting. *Mov Disord.* 1999;14:122-127.
138. Lichtenstein LM, Valentine MD, Sobotka AK. Insect allergy: the state of the art. *J Allergy Clin Immunol.* 1979;64:5-12.
139. LoVecchio F, Welch S, Klemens J, Curry SC, Thomas R. Incidence of immediate and delayed hypersensitivity to *Centruroides* antivenom. *Ann Emerg Med.* 1999;34:615-619.
140. Lowry BP, Bradfield JF, Carroll RG, Brewer K, Meggs WJ. A controlled trial of topical nitroglycerin in a New Zealand white rabbit model of brown recluse spider envenomation. *Ann Emerg Med.* 2001;37:161-165.
141. Lundh H. Antagonism of botulinum toxin paralysis by low temperature. *Muscle Nerve.* 1983;6:56-60.
142. Lux SE, John KM, Bennett V. Analysis of cDNA for human erythrocyte ankyrin indicates a repeated structure with homology to tissue-differentiation and cell-cycle control proteins. *Nature.* 1990;344: 36-42.
143. MacConnell JG, Blum MS, Buren WF, Williams RN, Fales HM. Fire ant venoms: chemotaxonomic correlations with alkaloidal compositions. *Toxicon.* 1976;14:69-78.
144. Malaque CM, Castro-Valencia JE, Cardoso JL, Francca FO, Barbaro KC, Fan HW. Clinical and epidemiological features of definitive and presumed loxoscelism in Sao Paulo, Brazil. *Rev Inst Med Trop Sao Paulo.* 2002;44: 139-143.
145. Malik R, Farrow BR. Tick paralysis in North America and Australia. *Vet Clin North Am Small Anim Pract.* 1991;21:157-171.
146. Maretic Z. Latrodectism: variations in clinical manifestations provoked by *Latrodectus* species of spiders. *Toxicon.* 1983;21:457-466.
147. Maretic Z, Stanic M. The health problem of arachnidism. *Bull World Health Organ.* 1954;11:1007-1022.
148. Marshall TK. Wasp and bee stings. *Practitioner.* 1957;178:712-722.
149. McCormick J, Carell JE. Cantharidin biosynthesis and function in meloid beetles. In: Prestwich GD, Blomquist G, eds. *Pheromone Biochemistry.* Orlando, FL: Academic Press; 1987:307-350.
150. Meki AR, Mohamed ZM, Mohey El-deen HM. Significance of assessment of serum cardiac troponin I and interleukin-8 in scorpion envenomed children. *Toxicon.* 2003;41:129-137.
151. Micks DW. Clinical effects of the sting of the "puss caterpillar" (*Megalopyge opercularis* S & A) on man. *Tex Rep Biol Med.* 1952;10:399-405.
152. Miller MJ, Gomez HF, Snider RJ, Stephens EL, Czop RM, Warren JS. Detection of *Loxosceles* venom in lesional hair shafts and skin: application of a specific immunoassay to identify dermonecrotic arachnidism. *Am J Emerg Med.* 2000;18:626-628.
153. Miller MK, Whyte IM, Dawson AH. Serum sickness from funnel web spider antivenom. *Med J Aust.* 1999;171:54.
154. Miller MK, Whyte IM, White J, Keir PM. Clinical features and management of *Hadronyche* envenomation in man. *Toxicon.* 2000;38: 409-427.
155. Minton S, Bechtel HB. Arthropod envenomation and parasitism. In: Auerbach P, ed. *Wilderness Medicine: Management of Wilderness and Environmental Emergencies.* St. Louis: Mosby; 1995:742-768.
156. Monsalve RI, Lu G, King TP. Expression of yellow jacket and wasp venom Ag5 allergens in bacteria and in yeast. *Arb Paul Ehrlich Inst Bundesamt Sera Impfstoffe Frankf A M.* 1999:181-188.
157. Moss HS, Binder LS. A retrospective review of black widow spider envenomation. *Ann Emerg Med.* 1987;16:188-192.
158. Mulvaney JK, Gatenby PA, Brookes JG. Lepidopterism: two cases of systemic reactions to the cocoon of a common moth, *Chelepteryx collesi. Med J Aust.* 1998;168:610-611.
159. Murnaghan MF. Site and mechanism of tick paralysis. *Science.* 1960;131: 418-419.
160. Mylecharane EJ, Spence I, Sheumack DD, Claassens R, Howden ME. Actions of robustoxin, a neurotoxic polypeptide from the venom of the male funnel-web spider (*Atrax robustus*), in anaesthetized monkeys. *Toxicon.* 1989;27:481-492.
161. Needham GR. Evaluation of five popular methods for tick removal. *Pediatrics.* 1985;75:997-1002.
162. Nicholson GM, Graudins A. Spiders of medical importance in the Asia-Pacific: atracotoxin, latrotoxin and related spider neurotoxins. *Clin Exp Pharmacol Physiol.* 2002;29:785-794.
163. Nicholson GM, Willow M, Howden ME, Narahashi T. Modification of sodium channel gating and kinetics by versutoxin from the Australian funnel-web spider *Hadronyche versuta. Pflugers Arch.* 1994;428:400-409.
164. Ownby CL, Odell GV. Pathogenesis of skeletal muscle necrosis induced by tarantula venom. *Exp Mol Pathol.* 1983;38:283-296.
165. Petrenko AG, Kovalenko VA, Shamotienko OG, et al. Isolation and properties of the α-latrotoxin receptor. *EMBO J.* 1990;9:2023-2027.

166. Petroianu G, Liu J, Helfrich U, Maleck W, Rufer R. Phospholipase A2-induced coagulation abnormalities after bee sting. *Am J Emerg Med.* 2000;18:22-27.
167. Phillips S, Kohn M, Baker D, et al. Therapy of brown spider envenomation: a controlled trial of hyperbaric oxygen, dapsone, and cyproheptadine. *Ann Emerg Med.* 1995;25:363-368.
168. Pinson RT, Morgan JA. Envenomation by the puss caterpillar (*Megalopyge opercularis*). *Ann Emerg Med.* 1991;20:562-564.
169. Platnick N. The world spider catalog, version 9.5. In: *American Museum of Natural History*; 2009.
170. Pneumatikos IA, Galiatsou E, Goe D, Kitsakos A, Nakos G, Vougiouklakis TG. Acute fatal toxic myocarditis after black widow spider envenomation. *Ann Emerg Med.* 2003;41:158.
171. Poole TR. Blister beetle periorbital dermatitis and keratoconjunctivitis in Tanzania. *Eye.* 1998;12(Pt 5):883-885.
172. Rachesky IJ, Banner W Jr, Dansky J, Tong T. Treatments for *Centruroides exilicauda* envenomation. *Am J Dis Child.* 1984;138:1136-1139.
173. Ramialiharisoa A, de Haro L, Jouglard J, Goyffon M. Latrodectism in Madagascar. *Med Trop (Mars).* 1994;54:127-130.
174. Rauber A. Black widow spider bites. *J Toxicol Clin Toxicol.* 1983;21: 473-485.
175. Ray AC, Kyle AL, Murphy MJ, Reagor JC. Etiologic agents, incidence, and improved diagnostic methods of cantharidin toxicosis in horses. *Am J Vet Res.* 1989;50:187-191.
176. Ray AC, Post LO, Hurst JM, Edwards WC, Reagor JC. Evaluation of an analytical method for the diagnosis of cantharidin toxicosis due to ingestion of blister beetles (*Epicauta lemniscata*) by horses and sheep. *Am J Vet Res.* 1980;41:932-933.
177. Rees R, Campbell D, Rieger E, King LE. The diagnosis and treatment of brown recluse spider bites. *Ann Emerg Med.* 1987;16:945-949.
178. Rees RS, Altenbern DP, Lynch JB, King LE Jr. Brown recluse spider bites. A comparison of early surgical excision versus dapsone and delayed surgical excision. *Ann Surg.* 1985;202:659-663.
179. Rimsza ME, Zimmerman DR, Bergeson PS. Scorpion envenomation. *Pediatrics.* 1980;66:298-302.
180. Robertson FM OS, Jackson MR. Dapsone hepatitisfollowing treatment of a brown recluse spider. *Comp Surg.* 1992;38:900-923.
181. Roche KJ, Chang MW, Lazarus H. Images in clinical medicine. Cutaneous anthrax infection. *N Engl J Med.* 2001;345:1611.
182. Rosenthal L, Zacchetti D, Madeddu L, Meldolesi J. Mode of action of α-latrotoxin: role of divalent cations in Ca2(+)-dependent and Ca2(+)-independent effects mediated by the toxin. *Mol Pharmacol.* 1990;38:917-923.
183. Ross EV Jr, Badame AJ, Dale SE. Meat tenderizer in the acute treatment of imported fire ant stings. *J Am Acad Dermatol.* 1987;16:1189-1192.
184. Russell FE. Arachnid envenomations. *Emerg Med Serv.* 1991;20:16-47.
185. Russell FE. Venomous animal injuries. *Curr Probl Pediatr.* 1973;3:1-47.
186. Russell FE, Gertsch WJ. For those who treat spider or suspected spider bites. *Toxicon.* 1983;21:337-339.
187. Ryan PJ. Preliminary report: experience with the use of dantrolene sodium in the treatment of bites by the black widow spider *Latrodectus hesperus. J Toxicol Clin Toxicol.* 1983;21:487-489.
188. Sams HH, Dunnick CA, Smith ML, King LE Jr. Necrotic arachnidism. *J Am Acad Dermatol.* 2001;44:561-573; quiz 73-76.
189. Santhanakrishnan BR. Scorpion sting. *Indian Pediatr.* 2000;37:1154-1157.
190. Schanbacher FL, Lee CK, Wilson IB, Howell DE, Odell GV. Purification and characterization of tarantula, *Dugesiella hentzi* (Girard) venom hyaluronidase. *Comp Biochem Physiol B.* 1973;44:389-396.
191. Schaumburg HH, Herskovitz S. The weak child—a cautionary tale. *N Engl J Med.* 2000;342:127-129.
192. Schenone H, Saavedra T, Rojas A, Villarroel F. Loxoscelism in Chile. Epidemiologic, clinical and experimental studies. *Rev Inst Med Trop Sao Paulo.* 1989;31:403-415.
193. Schiffman JS, Tang RA, Ulysses E, Dorotheo N, Singh SS, Bahrani HM. Bilateral ischaemic optic neuropathy and stroke after multiple bee stings. *Br J Ophthalmol.* 2004;88:1596-1598.
194. Schmitt N, Bowmer EJ, Gregson JD. Tick paralysis in British Columbia. *Can Med Assoc J.* 1969;100:417-421.
195. Shah A, Treat J, Yan AC. Spread of cantharidin after petrolatum use resulting in a varicelliform vesicular dermatitis. *J Am Acad Dermatol.* 2008;59:S54-S55.
196. Shkenderov S, Koburova K. Adolapin—a newly isolated analgetic and anti-inflammatory polypeptide from bee venom. *Toxicon.* 1982;20:317-321.
197. Silverman RA, Lucky A. Ken and Katie caterpillar: helpful props for treatment of molluscum contagiosum. *Pediatr Dermatol.* 2003;20:279-280.
198. Smith CW, Micks DW. The role of polymorphonuclear leukocytes in the lesion caused by the venom of the brown spider, *Loxosceles reclusa. Lab Invest.* 1970;22:90-93.
199. Smoley BA. Oropharyngeal hymenoptera stings: a special concern for airway obstruction. *Mil Med.* 2002;167:161-163.
200. Sofer S, Shahak E, Gueron M. Scorpion envenomation and antivenom therapy. *J Pediatr.* 1994;124:973-978.
201. Sofer S, Shalev H, Weizman Z, Shahak E, Gueron M. Acute pancreatitis in children following envenomation by the yellow scorpion *Leiurus quinquestriatus. Toxicon.* 1991;29:125-128.
202. Solley GO, Vanderwoude C, Knight GK. Anaphylaxis due to red imported fire ant sting. *Med J Aust.* 2002;176:521-523.
203. Sorkin L. *Loxosceles rufescens*' presence in New York City. (Personal Communication).
204. Sridhar MS, Ramakrishnan M. Ocular lesions caused by caterpillar hairs. *Eye.* 2004;18:540-543.
205. Stafford CT. Hypersensitivity to fire ant venom. *Ann Allergy Asthma Immunol.* 1996;77:87-95.
206. Stiles AD. Priapism following a black widow spider bite. *Clin Pediatr (Phila).* 1982;21:174-175.
207. Stipetic ME, Rosen PB, Borys DJ. A retrospective analysis of 96 "asp" (*Megalopyge opercularis*) envenomations in central Texas during 1996. *J Toxicol Clin Toxicol.* 1999;37:457-462.
208. Strain GM, Snider TG, Tedford BL, Cohn GH. Hyperbaric oxygen effects on brown recluse spider (*Loxosceles reclusa*) envenomation in rabbits. *Toxicon.* 1991;29:989-996.
209. Suchard JR, Hilder R. Atropine use in *Centruroides* scorpion envenomation. *J Toxicol Clin Toxicol.* 2001;39:595-598; discussion 9.
210. Sutherland S. Genus *Atrax* Cambridge, the funnel web spiders. In: Sutherland S, ed. *Australian Animal Toxins.* Melbourne: Oxford University Press; 1983:255-298.
211. Sutherland SK. Antivenom to the venom of the male Sydney funnel-web spider *Atrax robustus*: preliminary report. *Med J Aust.* 1980;2:437-441.
212. Sutherland SK. The management of bites by the Sydney funnel-web spider, *Atrax robustus. Med J Aust.* 1978;1:148-150.
213. Sutherland SK. Treatment of arachnid poisoning in Australia. *Aust Fam Physician.* 1990;19:47, 50-61, 4.
214. Sutherland SK, Tibballs J, Duncan AW. Funnel-web spider (*Atrax robustus*) antivenom. 1. Preparation and laboratory testing. *Med J Aust.* 1981;2:522-525.
215. Sutherland SK, Trinca JC. Survey of 2144 cases of red-back spider bites: Australia and New Zealand, 1963-1976. *Med J Aust.* 1978;2:620-623.
216. Taber S. *Fire Ants.* College Station, TX: Texas A&M University Press; 2000.
217. Tagwireyi D, Ball DE, Loga PJ, Moyo S. Cantharidin poisoning due to "Blister beetle" ingestion. *Toxicon.* 2000;38:1865-1869.
218. Thapa R, Biswas B, Mallick D. Hymenoptera sting complicated by pseudotumor cerebri in a 9-year-old boy. *Clin Toxicol (Phila).* 2008;46: 1100-1101.
219. Thorp R, Woodson W. *Black Widow, America's Most Poisonous Spider.* Chapel Hill: North Carolina Press; 1945.
220. Till JS, Majmudar BN. Cantharidin poisoning. *South Med J.* 1981;74: 444-447.
221. Todd J. Tick bite in British Columbia. *CMAJ.* 1912;2:1118-1119.
222. Vedanarayanan V, Sorey WH, Subramony SH. Tick paralysis. *Semin Neurol.* 2004;24:181-184.
223. Vega J, Vega JM, Moneo I, Armentia A, Caballero ML, Miranda A. Occupational immunologic contact urticaria from pine processionary caterpillar (*Thaumetopoea pityocampa*): experience in 30 cases. *Contact Dermatitis.* 2004;50:60-64.
224. Vega JM, Moneo I, Armentia A, Vega J, De la Fuente R, Fernandez A. Pine processionary caterpillar as a new cause of immunologic contact urticaria. *Contact Dermatitis.* 2000;43:129-132.
225. Veiga SS, da Silveira RB, Dreyfus JL, et al. Identification of high molecular weight serine-proteases in *Loxosceles intermedia* (brown spider) venom. *Toxicon.* 2000;38:825-839.
226. Verheyden C. Snakebite and spider bite. *Hospital Physician.* 1988;24: 21-32.
227. Vest DK. Envenomation by *Tegenaria agrestis* (Walckenaer) spiders in rabbits. *Toxicon.* 1987;25:221-224.

228. Vest DK. Necrotic arachnidism in the northwest United States and its probable relationship to *Tegenaria agrestis* (Walckenaer) spiders. *Toxicon.* 1987;25:175-184.
229. Vinson S. Invasion of the red imported fire ant (Hymenoptera:Formicidae): spread, biology, and impact. *Ann Entomol.* 1997;43:23-39.
230. Wasserman GS. Wound care of spider and snake envenomations. *Ann Emerg Med.* 1988;17:1331-1335.
231. White J, Hirst, D, Hender, E. Clinical toxicology of spider bites. In: Meier J, White, J, ed. *Handbook of Clinical Toxicology of Animal Venoms and Poisons.* Boca Raton, FL: CRC Press; 1995:259-329.
232. Wiener S. The Sydney funnel-web spider. *Med J Aust.* 1957;2:377-382.
233. Williams ST, Khare VK, Johnston GA, Blackall DP. Severe intravascular hemolysis associated with brown recluse spider envenomation. A report of two cases and review of the literature. *Am J Clin Pathol.* 1995;104: 463-467.
234. Yan L, Adams ME. Lycotoxins, antimicrobial peptides from venom of the wolf spider *Lycosa carolinensis. J Biol Chem.* 1998;273:2059-2066.
235. Yarbrough B. Current treatment of brown recluse spiders. *Curr Concepts Wound Care.* 1987;10:4-6.
236. Youlten LJ, Atkinson BA, Lee TH. The incidence and nature of adverse reactions to injection immunotherapy in bee and wasp venom allergy. *Clin Exp Allergy.* 1995;25:159-165.

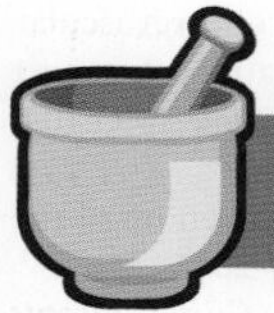

ANTIDOTES IN DEPTH (A35)

ANTIVENOM (SCORPION AND SPIDER)

Richard Franklin Clark

The terms *antivenom* (English) and *antivenin* (French and other countries) often are used interchangeably. In 1981, the World Health Organization determined that the preferred terms for the English language are "venom" and "antivenom." *Venin* is the French word for venom and *antivenin* is traditionally used in certain parts of the world, but Wyeth, the maker of Crotaline and *Micrurus* antivenom, and Merck and Company, the makers of *Latrodectus* antivenom, adopted *antivenin* in the brand names for their products.

Antivenom for spiders and scorpions is prepared in the same manner as other antivenom products by first immunizing animals with nontoxic amounts of venom.[4,35] Monkeys, horses, goats, sheep, chickens, camels, and rabbits have been used as sources of antivenom.[40] The animals are placed on an inoculation schedule to allow gradual production of immunoglobulins, most importantly immunoglobulin IgG. Sufficient antibody production usually takes up to 6 weeks. The choice of animal used to make an immune serum is more often dictated by the availability of a species, financial considerations, and tradition rather than by scientific modeling. Horses are used by the majority of antivenom producers since they are relatively easy to maintain, and large volumes of serum can be obtained at one time without harming the animals. Varying efforts are made during antivenom production to remove animal proteins such as albumin. To date, no studies have compared immune sera of different animals for human compatibility or tolerance.

The antidotal fraction of an antivenom exists as either whole IgG, or only Fab, or $F(ab)_2$. The IgG molecule is composed of two antigen-binding fragments (Fab fragments) that are fused together and attached to two larger complement-binding fragments (Fc fragments). The larger Fc portions are generally considered to be the most antigenic, initiating most of the undesirable histamine release on infusion. Digestion of the disulfide bonds of an IgG molecule with the enzyme pepsin will cleave the Fc fragments, allowing isolation of pure $F(ab)_2$ fragments (two fused Fab fragments). In contrast, digestion with papain cleaves the molecule more distally such that a larger Fc portion is removed from two separate Fab fragments. Both Fab and $F(ab)_2$ molecules can be isolated with affinity chromatography, while the highly antigenic Fc portion is discarded. Although Fab and $F(ab)_2$ are more difficult and more expensive to produce than their whole immunoglobin counterparts, they are generally regarded as less allergenic and therefore safer products.

Whole IgG antivenom has a molecular weight of 150 kDa, the largest of the three antivenom types. Because of its size, IgG is the least filterable at the glomerulus and has the smallest volume of distribution. IgG has a longer elimination half-life than either Fab or $F(ab)_2$.[26]

$F(ab)_2$ has an intermediate size (100 kDa) and elimination half-life. Preliminary pharmacokinetic studies of an $F(ab)_2$ antivenom for scorpions demonstrate a mean time of residence within volunteers of 10 days.[58] While lowering the risk of anaphylaxis compared with whole IgG, the $F(ab)_2$ portion retains much of the allosteric configuration of the original IgG molecule that is lost when Fab are formed. This configuration theoretically allows for tighter binding to venom.

Fab is the smallest (50 kDa) antivenom molecule in size and is eliminated by the kidneys. It has the largest volume of distribution and the greatest ability to reach intracellular compartments. To be effective, antivenoms require similar pharmacokinetic properties to the venom on which they act.[26] Arachnid venoms that affect the central nervous system have low molecular weights and large volumes of distribution. Fab- and $F(ab)_2$-based antivenoms may therefore be best suited for this function.[26]

Immunoglobulin-based antivenoms can be given by the intramuscular (IM), intravenous (IV), or subcutaneous route. Intravenous administration achieves rapid peak serum concentrations, and the infusion can be stopped in the event of an allergic reaction.[27] Intramuscular injection has been used in instances where IV access is unobtainable. In a rabbit model, the elimination half-life of *Buthus occitanus* venom is shorter when antivenom is given by the IV route compared with similar doses given intramuscularly. Pharmacokinetic comparisons of venom and antivenom suggest that the lower-molecular-weight components of scorpion venom are absorbed and distributed faster than antivenom, when administered intramuscularly or given subcutaneously. Therefore, IV antivenom is the preferred route for neutralization of most venoms.[33,36,37]

The unavailability of specific antivenoms often necessitates symptomatic treatment or use of a comparable foreign antivenom. In the United States, *Centruroides* scorpion antivenom has not been available for some time. Similarly, in a study of 72 moderate scorpion stings in Para, Brazil, 33% who met criteria for antivenom administration did not receive treatment because of unavailability of the antivenom.[45] *Latrodectus* antivenom has been in short supply in the past, leading to studies of neutralizing *Latrodectus mactans* and *Latrodectus hesperus* venom with *Latrodectus hasseltii* antivenom.[18]

CENTRUROIDES SPECIES

Centruroides exilicauda (formerly known as *Centruroides sculpturatus*) is the only scorpion of medical importance in the United States. It is indigenous to the deserts of Arizona, but reportedly exists in Texas, New Mexico, California, and Nevada.[17] Occasionally, envenomations occur in nonindigenous areas of the country from "stowaway" scorpions in the luggage of travelers.[57]

Arizona poison centers receive several thousand calls annually for scorpion exposures (Chap. 119). Although the incidence of morbidity from these envenomations is significant, no deaths associated with the toxic effects of scorpion venom have been reported in the United States for almost 50 years. Deaths are associated with anaphylactic reactions to scorpion venom.[10] Antivenom for the *Centruroides* spp was produced in horses in Mexico as early as the 1930s.[17] In 1947, antivenom was produced from rabbits and cats immunized with *C. sculpturatus* and *Centruroides gertschi*.[51] The Antivenom Production Laboratory at Arizona State University (APL-ASU) began producing antivenom to *C. sculpturatus* in goats in 1965. This antivenom was used for treatment of scorpion stings in Arizona until 2004, when production ceased and stockpiles expired. Treatment for *Centruroides* envenomation in this country is now limited predominantly to supportive care with airway maintenance and the administration of analgesics and benzodiazepines as needed. Without antivenom treatment available, hospital admissions following scorpion stings may have increased.[48]

Cross-neutralization of the venom of eight different species of *Centruroides*, including *C. exilicauda*, has been documented in vitro.[22] In Mexico, several antivenoms are used in the treatment of *Centruroides* spp envenomation. The Instituto Bioclon product Alacramyn antivenom may also be effective against North American *Centruroides* stings. Although antibody fragments (Fab) were developed experimentally in the United States from immune goat serum for treatment of *Centruroides* envenomation, they are not commercially available.[8] In June 2000, Silanes Laboratory obtained orphan drug status for a *Centruroides* scorpion antivenom, an equine-derived $F(ab)_2$ from *Centruroides limpidus*, *Centruroides noxius*, *Centruroides suffusus suffusus*, and *Centruroides meisei* (formerly known as *Centruroides elegans*). This product is manufactured by Instituto Bioclon of Mexico, and is at this time referred to as Anascorp. Clinical trials evaluating this scorpion $F(ab)_2$ are being done in Arizona. One vial of this scorpion antivenom contains sufficient $F(ab)_2$ to neutralize 150 mouse LD_{50} of *Centruroides* venom,[41] and its safety and efficacy have been previously documented in both animals and humans.[1,12,24] In a rabbit model, the total serum concentration of scorpion venom increased after administration of $F(ab)_2$, suggesting that $F(ab)_2$ is capable of pulling venom from its site of action into serum.[12] A prospective evaluation of serum venom concentrations in 14 children clinically envenomated by scorpions was performed using enzyme-linked immunosorbent assay. After administration of antivenom, serum venom concentrations fell from 1000 to 4000 pg/mL to less than 200 pg/mL within 30 minutes and were unmeasurable within 2 hours.[24] Anascorp is administered by slow IV infusion, one vial at a time with observation for 30 to 60 minutes, and may be repeated. Dosing is similar in children and adults.

The incidence of allergic reactions to Anascorp is reported to be 2.7%, similar to the 3.4% previously reported for the APL-ASU goat serum product.[9,38] In a study of 15 children stung by *Centruroides* scorpions, 12 who received the APL-ASU antivenom had resolution of neurologic, respiratory, and cardiovascular symptoms within 3 hours of initiating therapy, compared with three patients who did not receive antivenom therapy where symptoms lasted 15 to 24 hours.[9] A current clinical trial of *Centruroides* $F(ab')_2$ in a very small randomized, double blind study in critically ill children with neurotoxicity from scorpion stings demonstrated a rapid resolution of symptoms, decreased need for sedation, and reduced concentration of circulating and bound venom.[11] Should this product prove safe, effective, and appropriate for a general population it may greatly improve treatment for scorpion stings.

LEIURUS SPECIES

The *Leiurus quinquestriatus* scorpion is indigenous to Africa, Asia, and the Middle East, including Egypt, Israel, Jordan, Kuwait, Lebanon, Oman, Qatar, Saudi Arabia, Syria, and Turkey. Antivenom to *L. quinquestriatus* is made in France, Germany, Israel, Saudi Arabia, Egypt, Tunisia, and Turkey. The clinical effects of this scorpion, such as acute lung injury and a variety of neurologic abnormalities, are relatively resistant to treatment with antivenom. The Turkish manufacturer of antiscorpion antivenom recommends a starting dose of 1 mL antivenom for treatment of envenomation. The usual dose for control of symptoms is 5 to 20 mL antivenom administered intravenously.

In observational studies, an IV infusion of 5 to 20 mL was needed to control venom effects, and only patients given antivenom within the first several hours demonstrated significant benefit.[2,32] The rate of allergic reactions for the Turkish antiscorpion antivenom is reported to be 1.6% to 6.6%.[32] The recommended dose of the Israeli *L. quinquestriatus* antivenom is 5 to 15 mL for IV use, although several authors report lack of clinical efficacy of this particular antivenom.[6,25,52]

L. quinquestriatus antivenom was successfully used to treat a 2-year-old boy with envenomation by *Androctonus crassicauda*. Symptoms resolved 2 hours after antivenom administration.[46]

TITYUS SPECIES

Tityus species of scorpions are endemic to South America, particularly Brazil. An $F(ab)_2$ antivenom for *Tityus serrulatus* is available from Fundação Ezequiel Dias (FUNED), in Belo Horizonte, Brazil. The usual dose of the antivenom is 20 mL as an IV infusion.[19]

In a series of 18 patients with *T. serrulatus* envenomation treated with antivenom, vomiting and local pain decreased within 1 hour, and cardiorespiratory manifestations disappeared within 6 to 24 hours in all patients except the two presenting with acute lung injury.[19] Sixteen patients recovered completely by 24 hours. Additionally, the Instituto Buntantan in Brazil produces Soro antiarachnidico and Soro antiscorpionico for treatment of *Tityus* spp.

ANDROCTONUS SPECIES

Scorpion antivenom in South Africa is an equine-derived antivenom available from the South African Vaccine Producers, formerly South African Institute for Medical Research (SAIMR), Johannesburg, South Africa.

Scorpifav, produced by Aventis Pasteur, is produced for treatment of *Androctonus* spp, *B. occitanus*, and *L. quinquestriatus*.

Buthus tamulus monovalent red scorpion antivenom serum produced by Central Research Institute of India is equine-derived lyophilized antivenom for the venom of *Mesobuthus tamulus*. Although the manufacturer recommends a dose of only one vial, five vials decreased mortality significantly in one study.[34,53]

In Pakistan, the treatment of scorpion stings was modified in 1991 to include the administration of five vials of antivenom. A retrospective case series of 950 patients treated with one vial and without antivenom was compared with 968 cases treated after the five-vial protocol was initiated. A statistically significant decrease in mortality resulted from the five-vial regimen. The last recorded death in Pakistan resulting from a scorpion sting occurred in 1991 in a patient who did not receive any antivenom.[53]

Parabuthus spp antivenom from South African Vaccine Producers is equine-derived antivenom to *Parabuthus* spp. In one study antivenom became unavailable, allowing for a unique design of matched pairing of patients. Patients who received antivenom had a significant decrease in hospital stay after receiving one (5-mL) vial. Pain, hypersalivation, fasciculations, tremor, and bladder distension responded best to antivenom, whereas dysphagia, ptosis, and local swelling were more resistent.[7] More recent studies from India show equivocal results for scorpion envenomation treated with antivenom when compared with treatment with prazocin.[5,43]

LATRODECTUS SPECIES (*L. MACTANS, L. HESPERUS, L. BISHOPI, L. GEOMETRICUS, L. INDISTINCTUS*)

The need to use antivenom in the treatment of black widow spider envenomation remains controversial. Although black widow bites are associated with severe muscle pain, cramping, and autonomic disturbances,

TABLE A35–1. Worldwide Availability of Scorpion and Spider Antivenom

Scorpions	*Scorpions*	*Scorpions*	*Spiders*
***Androctonus* species** Algeria: Antiscorpion Serum, Institut Pasteur d'Algerie Egypt: Purified Polyvalent Antiscorpion Serum, Egyptian Organization for Biological Products and Vaccines (VACSERA) France: Pasteur LABS Antiscorpion Venom Serum, Aventis Pasteur France: Scorpifav, Aventis Pasteur Germany: Scorpion Antivenom, Twyford Iran: Polyvalent Scorpion Antivenom, Razi Vaccine and Serum Research Institute Morocco: Antiscorpion Serum Tunisia: Scorpion Antivenom, Institut Pasteur de Tunis Turkey: Antiscorpion ***Buthus* species** Algeria: Antiscorpion Serum (Monovalent), Institut Pasteur d'Algerie Egypt: Purified Polyvalent Antiscorpion Serum, Egyptian Organization for Biological Products and Vaccines (VACSERA) France: Pasteur Labs Antiscorpion Venom Serum, Aventis Pasteur France: Scorpifav, Aventis Pasteur Germany: Scorpion Antivenom, Twyford Morocco: Scorpion Antivenom Saudi Arabia: Polyvalent Scorpion Antivenom–Equine, National Antivenom and Vaccine Production Center (NAVPC) Tunisia: Scorpion Antivenom, Institut Pasteur de Tunis	***Mesobuthus* species** India: Monovalent Scorpion Antivenom Central Research Institute Iran: Polyvalent Scorpion Antivenom, Razi Vaccine and Serum Research Institute Venezuela: Antiscorpion serum, Centro de Biotecnologia ***Odontobuthus doriae*** Iran: Polyvalent Scorpion Antivenom, Razi Vaccine and Serum Research Institute ***Palamnaeus* species** India: Monovalent Red Scorpion Antivenom Serum ***Parabuthus* species** South Africa: SAIMR Scorpion Antivenom, South African Vaccine Producers (Pty) Ltd: (S.A.V.P.) ***Scorpio maurus*** Egypt: Purified Polyvalent Antiscorpion Serum, Egyptian Organization for Biological Products and Vaccines (VACSERA) France: Antiscorpion Serum, Sanofi-Pasteur Iran: Polyvalent Scorpion Antivenom, Razi Vaccine and Serum Research Institute Turkey: Antiscorpion Serum ***Tityus* species** Argentina: Scorpion antivenom, Instituto Nacional de Produccion de Biologicos Brazil: Antiscorpion Serum, Instituto Butantan Brazil: Antiarachnid Serum, Instituto Butantan (contains *Loxosceles* sp, *Tityus* sp, and *Phoneutria* sp: antivenom) Brazil: Antiscorpion serum IVB, Instituto Vital Brazil S.A. Brazil: Antiscorpion Serum, Fundacao Ezequiel Dias (FUNED)	India: Scorpion Venom Antiserum IP, Haffkine Biopharmaceutical Corporation LTD Turkey: Antiscorpion ***Centruroides* species *(elegans, gertschi, limpidus, suffuses, noxius, exilicauda)*** Mexico: Suero Antialacran Alacrmyn, Instituto Bioclon Mexico: Centruroides Scorpion Antivenom, Laboratories MYN ***Euscorpius carpathicus, italicus*** Turkey: Antiscorpion Serum ***Heterometrus* species** India: Monovalent Scorpion Antivenom Central Research Institute ***Leiurus* species** Egypt: Purified Polyvalent Antiscorpion Serum, Egyptian Organization for Biological Products and Vaccines (VACSERA) France: Pasteur Labs Antiscorpion Venom Serum, Aventis Pasteur France: Scorpifav, Aventis Pasteur Germany: Scorpion Antivenom, Twyford Israel: Leiurus quinquestriatus Saudi Arabia: Polyvalent Scorpion Antivenom–Equine, National Antivenom and Vaccine Production Center (NAVPC) Tunisia: Scorpion Antivenom, Institut Pasteur de Tunis Turkey: Antiscorpion	***Atrax* species, *Hadronyche* species (Funnel-web spider)** Australia: Funnel-Web Spider Antivenom, CSL Ltd ***Latrodectus* species (black widow spider, red-backed spider)** Argentina: Antilatrodectus, Antivenom Instituto Nacional de Produccion de Biologicos Australia: Red-backed Spider Antivenom, CSL Ltd Croatia: Antilatrodectus Mactans Tredecimguttatus Serum, Institute of Immunology Mexico: Aracmyn, Instituto Bioclon South Africa: SAIMR Spider antivenom, SAIMR USA: Antivenin *Latrodectus mactans,* Merck ***Loxosceles* species (brown spiders)** Brazil: Antiloxosceles Serum, Centro de Producao e Pesquisas de Imunobiologicos Brazil: Soro Antiarachnidico, Instituto Butantan (contains *Loxosceles* sp, *Tityus* sp, and *Phoneutria* sp: antivenom) Mexico: Aracmyn, Instituto Bioclon Peru: Antiloxosceles Serum, Instituto Nacional de Salud, Centro Nacional de Production de Biologicos

mortality is low.[13,14] Symptomatic treatment with muscle relaxants and opioid analgesics is generally effective, although the duration of symptoms following severe envenomations may necessitate hospitalization for 1 to 2 days or more. The use of *Latrodectus* antivenom may shorten the length of symptoms dramatically, allowing outpatient care in some cases.[14,44,54] However, studies of reported *Latrodectus* envenomated patients in Australia have found little difference in clinical outcome after *Latrodectus* antivenom or placebo.[29] In addition, anaphylaxis is reported following the administration of *Latrodectus* antivenom.[14] These issues have led some authors to question its use.[49] Most toxicologists believe *Latrodectus* antivenom is safe and effective when used appropriately, and that it is generally indicated in cases of severe envenomation when muscle cramping, hypertension, diaphoresis, nausea, vomiting, and respiratory difficulty are present (Chap. 119).[13] *Latrodectus* antivenom has also been reported to successfully treat priapism that complicates severe bites.[28] Although the safety of antivenom has not been clearly established in the developing fetus, pregnancy is suggested as an added consideration for *Latrodectus* antivenom administration as the stress of severe pain and muscle cramps is likely to have adverse effects on fetal well-being.[3,50]

Antivenoms for a number of *Latrodectus* spiders are available worldwide (Table A35–1). *Latrodectus mactans* antivenom is produced by Merck and Company in North America. The Australian red-back spider *L. hasseltii* antivenom is manufactured in horses by CSL Ltd. South Africa (SAFR) produces antivenom for both the black widow (*L. indistinctus*) and the brown widow (*L. geometricus*). Aracmyn, a polyvalent $F(ab)_2$, is an equine-derived antivenom created for *L. mactans* in both Argentina and Mexico that is currently undergoing clinical trials in *Latrodectus* envenomated patients in the United States.

The *Latrodectus* antivenom produced by Merck and Company is equine-derived IgG. Each vial of this product contains 6000 antivenom units standardized by biologic assay in mice. Because the venoms of *Latrodectus* species are virtually identical by immunologic and electrophoretic mechanisms, antivenom created for *L. mactans* is presumed to be effective in other species of *Latrodectus* as well.[39] A recent shortage of Merck antivenom (Merck and Co) prompted the finding that antivenom against *L. hasseltii*, the Australian red-back spider, also neutralizes venom of *L. mactans* in a mouse model.[18] In a review of 163 cases of presumed *L. hesperus* and *mactans* envenomations, antivenom reduced the duration of symptoms from a mean of 22 hours to a mean of 9 hours. Symptoms usually subsided within 1 to 3 hours of administration of the antivenom. The hospital admission rate fell from 52% in those who were managed with opioids and muscle relaxants to 12% in those patients receiving antivenom.[14] Administration of this antivenom is reportedly effective even when given as late as 90 hours after envenomation.[44,54]

The starting dose of Merck antivenom is one vial (2.5 mL) diluted in 50 mL of saline for IV administration. Although black widow spider antivenom can also be given IM, this route carries the disadvantage of slower, more erratic absorption, less control over the rate of administration, and the inability to stop the administration should an allergic reaction occur. In addition, recent studies suggest IM injection of antivenom may not yield significant serum concentrations.[31] For these reasons, the IM route is not routinely recommended.

Despite the apparent efficacy of antivenom, the decision to give horse serum for a disease with limited mortality must be considered. Death from bronchospasm and anaphylaxis is a reported complication of antivenom administration, as is serum sickness.[13] The effect of black widow antivenom use during pregnancy is unknown.

In Australia, antivenom to the red-back spider (*L. hasseltii*, CSL Ltd) is made by immunizing horses for production of $F(ab)_2$. Horse-derived $F(ab)_2$ has a lower reported incidence of allergic reactions than IgG preparations, with early hypersensitivity reactions as low as 0.5% to 0.8%. The incidence of serum sickness is reported to be less than 5%.[55,56]

In a report covering 1995 to 1996, only 20% of patients with *L. hasseltii* (red-back spider) bites required antivenom administration.[59] When treatment was given, one vial was used in 76% of cases, two vials were used in 18% of cases, and three vials were administered in only 6% of cases.[59] In another study, three patients required six to eight vials of antivenom after failing to respond to the usual one to two vials.[30] No antihistamine or epinephrine pretreatment was given, and no allergic or serum sickness complications occurred.

FUNNEL-WEB SPIDER (*ATRAX* AND *HADRONYCHE*) ENVENOMATION

A rabbit IgG-based funnel-web spider (*Atrax robustus* and others) antivenom is available in Australia. Since the introduction of the antivenom, no deaths have been reported.[30] The initial dose is two vials in patients with any signs of envenomation. Patients with evidence of acute lung injury or decreased consciousness should receive four vials.[42] The dosage for children is the same as for adults.

In severe funnel-web spider envenomations, the following protocol should be used.[42] Two vials of (each 5 mL of 2.0% [100-mg] rabbit IgG) antivenom should be administered very slowly intravenously in both adults and children. The dose should be doubled for severe cases and the dose can be repeated in 15 minutes if no improvement occurs. A rapid response should occur. Administration of antivenom should be repeated until symptoms are completely reversed.[21] *Atrax robustus* envenomations may require more than three vials of antivenom.

LOXOSCELES SPECIES (*L. RECLUSA, L. LAETA, L. RUFESCENS, L. ARIZONICA, L. UNICOLOR*)

Envenomation by the brown recluse spider, *Loxosceles reclusa*, is associated with low, but significant, morbidity, particularly in the southeast United States. Anti-*Loxosceles* Fab blocks dermonecrosis in a rabbit model, but only when given within 24 to 48 hours of envenomation.[16,23,47] No commercially available antivenom exists in North America for treatment of *Loxosceles* envenomation; however, antivenom produced against South American *Loxosceles* spiders has cross-reactivity with North American species like *L. reclusa*.[20] The usual late presentation of patients with necrotic lesions from spider bites make antivenom use for *Loxosceles* difficult to study. National laboratories in Brazil and Argentina have produced antivenoms for *L. reclusa*, *L. boneti*, and *L. rufescens*.[4,20]

SUMMARY

The indications for antivenom administration in both spider and scorpion envenomations remain controversial. The decision to use antivenom should be individualized to the patient, weighing the risk of giving an immune serum, the level of available supportive care, the cost of supportive care, and the cost of obtaining or importing antivenom. Scorpion antivenom administration for some species may not improve outcome. When given, the preferred route of administration of these products is intravenous. One to two vials is the recommended dose for most scorpion and spider antivenoms; higher doses may be needed to alleviate symptoms in some cases.

REFERENCES

1. Alagon CA, Gonzalez JC. De la seroterapia a la faboterapia. *Foro Silanes.* 1998;2:8-9.
2. Amitai Y, Mines Y, Aker M, Goitein K. Scorpion sting in children: a review of 51 cases. *Clin Pediatr.* 1985;24:136-140.

3. Bailey B. Are there teratogenic risks associated with antidotes used in the acute management of poisoned pregnant women? *Birth Defects Res A Clin Mol Teratol.* 2003;67:133-140.
4. Barbaro KC, Knysak I, Martins R, Hogan C, Winkel K. Enzymatic characterization, antigenic cross-reactivity and neutralization of dermonecrotic activity of five *Loxosceles* spider venoms of medical importance in the Americas. *Toxicon.* 2005;45:489-499.
5. Bawaskar HS, Bawaskar PH. Utiliy of scorpion antivenin vs prazosin in the management of severe *Mesobuthus tamulus* (Indian red scorpion) envenoming at rural setting. *J Assoc Physicians India.* 2007;55:14-21.
6. Belghith M, Boussarsar M, Haguiga H, et al. Efficacy of serotherapy in scorpion sting: a matched-pair study. *J Toxicol Clin Toxicol.* 1999;37:51-57.
7. Bergman NJ. Clinical description of *Parabuthus transvaalicus* scorpionism in Zimbabwe. *Toxicon.* 1997;35:759-771.
8. Bernstein JN, Dart RC, Garcia R, et al. Efficacy of antiscorpion (*Centruroides exilicauda*) Fab in a mouse model [abstract]. *Vet Hum Toxicol.* 1994;36:346.
9. Bond GR. Antivenin administration for *Centruroides* scorpion sting: risks and benefits. *Ann Emerg Med.* 1992;21:788-791.
10. Boyer L, Heubner K, McNally J. Death from *Centruroides* scorpion sting allergy. *J Toxicol Clin Toxicol.* 2001;39:561.
11. Boyer LV, Theodorou AA, Berg RA, et al. Antivenom for critically ill children with neurotoxicity from scorpion stings. *N Engl J Med.* 2009;360:2090-2098.
12. Calderon-Aranda ES, Riviere G, Choumet V, et al. Pharmacokinetics of the toxic fraction of *Centruroides limpidus limpidus* venom in experimentally envenomed rabbits and effects of immunotherapy with specific Fab_2. *Toxicon.* 1999;37:771-782.
13. Clark RF. The safety and efficacy of antivenin *Latrodectus actans. J Toxicol Clin Toxicol.* 2001;39:125-127.
14. Clark RF, Werthern-Kestner S, Vance MV, Gerkin R. Clinical presentation and treatment of black widow spider envenomation: a review of 163 cases. *Ann Emerg Med.* 1992;21:782-787.
15. Clinical Toxicology Resources. http://www.toxinology.com/ (accessed April 27, 2005).
16. Cole HP 3rd, Wesley RE, King LE Jr. Brown recluse spider envenomation of the eyelid: an animal model. *Ophthal Plast Reconstr Surg.* 1995;11:153-164.
17. Curry SC, Vance MV, Ryan PJ, et al. Envenomation by the scorpion *Centruroides sculpturatus. J Toxicol Clin Toxicol.* 1984;21:417-449.
18. Daly FF, Hill RE, Bogdan GM, Dart RC. Neutralization of *Latrodectus mactans* and *L. hesperus* venom by redback spider (*L. hasseltii*) antivenom. *J Toxicol Clin Toxicol.* 2001;39:119-123.
19. De Rezende NA, Dias MB, Campolina D, et al. Efficacy of antivenom therapy for neutralizing circulating venom antigens in patients stung by *Tityus serrulatus* scorpions. *Am J Trop Med Hyg.* 1995;52:277-280.
20. de Roodt AR, Estevez-Ramirez J, Litwin S, Magana P et al. Toxicity of two North American *Loxoscles* (brown recluse spiders) venoms and their neutralization by antivenoms. *Clin Toixcol.* 2007;45:678-687.
21. Dieckmann J, Prebble J, McDonogh A. Efficacy of funnel-web spider antivenom in human envenomation by *Hadronyche* species. *Med J Aust.* 1989;151:706-707.
22. Estevez JR, Alagon A, Paniagua SJ. Determination of cross-reactivity of Alacramyn against different scorpion venoms of the genus *Centruroides*, using ELISA technique. Presented at the 4th Reunion of Experts in Envenomation by Poisonous Animals, Cuernavaca, 2000.
23. Gomez HF, Miller MJ, Trach JW, et al. Intradermal anti-*Loxosceles* Fab fragments attenuate dermonecrotic arachnidism. *Acad Emerg Med.* 1999;6:1195-1202.
24. Gonzalez C, Cabral J, Reyes S, et al. Development of an immunoenzymatic assay for the quantification of scorpion venom in plasma. Presented at the 4th Reunion of Experts in Envenomation by Poisonous Animals, Cuernavaca, 2000.
25. Gueron M, Yaron R. Cardiovascular manifestations of severe scorpion sting. Clinicopathologic correlation. *Chest.* 1970;57:156-162.
26. Gutierrez JM, Leon G, Lomonte B. Pharmacokinetic-pharmacodynamic relationships of immunoglobulin therapy for envenomation. *Clin Pharmacokinet.* 2003;42:721-741.
27. Heard K, O'Malley GF, Dart RC. Antivenom therapy in the Americas. *Drugs.* 1999;585-515.
28. Hoover NG, Fortenberry JD. Use of antivenin to treat priapism after black widow spider bite. *Pediatrics.* 2004;114:e128-e129.
29. Isbister GK, Brown SG, Miller M, Tankel A, et al. A randomized controlled trial of intramuscular vs. intravenous antivenom for latrodectism—the RAVE study. *QJM.* 2008;188:473-476.
30. Isbister GK, Graudins A, White J, et al. Antivenom treatment in Arachnidism. *J Toxicol Clin Toxicol.* 2003;41:291-300.
31. Isbister GK, O'Leary M, Miller M, Brown SG et al. A comparison of serum antivenom concentrations after intravenous and intramuscular administration of redback (widow) spider antivenom. *Br J Pharmacol.* 2008;65:139-143.
32. Ismail M. The treatment of the scorpion envenoming syndrome: the Saudi experience with serotherapy. *Toxicon.* 19994;32:1019-1026.
33. Ismail M, Abd-Elsalam MA, Al-Ahaidib MS. Pharmacokinetics of 125I-labelled *Walterinnesia aegyptia* venom and its distribution of the venom and its toxin versus slow absorption and distribution of IgG, $F(ab')_2$ and F(ab) of the antivenin. *Toxicon.* 1998;36:93-114.
34. Krifi MN, Amri F, Kharrat H, el Ayeb M. Evaluation of antivenom therapy in children severely envenomed by *Androctonus australis garzonii* (Aag) and *Buthus occitanus tunetanus* (Bot) scorpions. *Toxicon.* 1999;37:1627-1634.
35. Krifi MN, el Ayeb M, Dellagi K. The improvement and standardization of antivenom production in developing countries: comparing antivenom quality therapeutical efficiency and cost. *J Venom Anim Toxins.* 1999;5: 128-141.
36. Krifi MN, Miled K, Abderrazek M, El Ayeb M. Effects of antivenom on *Buthus occitanus tunetanus* (Bot) scorpion venom pharmacokinetics: towards an optimization of antivenom immunotherapy in a rabbit model. *Toxicon.* 2001;39:1317-1326.
37. Krifi MN, Savin S, Debray M, et al. Pharmacokinetic studies of scorpion venom before and after antivenom immunotherapy. *Toxicon.* 2005;45:187-198.
38. LoVecchio F, Welch S, Klemens J, et al. Incidence of immediate and delayed hypersensitivity to *Centruroides* antivenom. *Ann Emerg Med.* 1999;34:615-619.
39. McCrone JD, Netzcoff ML. An immunological and electrophoretical comparison of the venoms of the North American *Latrodectus* spiders. *Toxicon.* 1965;3:107-110.
40. Meddeb-Mouelhi F, Bouhaouala-Zahar B, Benlasfar Z, et al. Immunized camel sera and derived immunoglobulin subclasses neutralizing *Androctonus australis hector* scorpion toxins. *Toxicon.* 2003;42:785-791.
41. *Mexican Pharmacopeia*, 6th ed. 1994;163-164.
42. Miller MK, Whyte IM, White J, Keir PM. Clinical features and management of *Hadronyche* envenomation in man. *Toxicon.* 2000:38:409-427.
43. Natu VS, Murthy RK, Deodhar KP. Efficacy of species-specific anti-scorpion venom serum (AScVS) against severe, serious scorpion stings (*Mesobuthus tamulus concanesis* Pocock)—an experience from rural hospital in western Maharashtra. *J Assoc Physicians India.* 2006;54:283-287.
44. O'Malley GF, Dart RC, Kuffner EF. Successful treatment of latrodectism with antivenin after 90 hours. *N Engl J Med.* 1999;340:657.
45. Pardal PP, Castro LC, Jennings E, et al. Epidemiological and clinical aspects of scorpion envenomation in the region of Santarem, Para, Brazil. *Rev Soc Bras Med Trop.* 2003;36:349-353.
46. Pomeranz A, Amitai P, Braunstein I, et al, Scorpion sting: successful treatment with nonhomologous antivenin. *Isr J Med Sci.* 1984;20:451-452.
47. Rees R, Campbell D, Rieger E, King LE. The diagnosis and treatment of brown recluse spider bites. *Ann Emerg Med.* 1987;16:945-949.
48. Riley BD, LoVecchio F, Pizon AF. Lack of scorpion antivenom leads to increased pediatric ICU admission *Ann Emerg Med.* 2006;47:398-399.
49. Robertson WO. Black widow spider case. *Am J Emerg Med.* 1997;15:211.
50. Russell FE, Marcus P, Streng JA. Black widow spider envenomation during pregnancy. *Toxicon.* 1979;17:188-189.
51. Schnur L, Schnur P. A case of allergy to scorpion antivenin. *Ariz Med.* 1968;25:413-414.
52. Sofer S, Gueron M. Respiratory failure in children following envenomation by the scorpion *Leiurus quinquestriatus*: hemodynamic and neurological aspects. *Toxicon.* 1988:26:931-939.
53. Soomro RM, Andy JJ, Sulaiman K. A clinical evaluation of the effectiveness of antivenom in scorpion envenomation. *J Coll Physicians Surg Pak.* 2001;11:297-299.
54. Suntorntham S, Roberts JR, Nilsen GJ. Dramatic clinical response to the delayed administration of black widow spider antivenom. *Ann Emerg Med.* 1994;24:1198-1199.
55. Sutherland SK. Antivenom use in Australia. Premedication, adverse reactions and the use of venom detection kits. *Med J Aust.* 1992;157:734-739.
56. Sutherland SK, Trinca JC. Survey of 2144 cases of red back spider bites. Australia and New Zealand, 1963-1976. *Med J Aust.* 1978;2:620-623.
57. Trestrail JH. Scorpion envenomation in Michigan: three cases of toxic encounters with poisonous stow-aways. *Vet Hum Toxicol.* 1981;23:8-11.
58. Vazquez H, Chavez-Haro A, Garcia-Ubbelohde W, Mancilla-Nava R, et al. Pharmacokinetics of a $F(ab)_2$ scorpion antivenom in healthy human volunteers. *Toxicon.* 2005;46:797-805.
59. White J. Envenoming and antivenom use in Australia. *Toxicon.* 1998;36: 1483-1492.

CHAPTER 120
MARINE ENVENOMATIONS

D. Eric Brush

Human contact with venomous marine creatures is common and may result in serious injury from biological toxins or mechanical destruction inflicted by the stinging apparatus. Significant morbidity results from envenomation by spiny fish, cone snails, octopi, sea snakes, and several species of jellyfish. Despite significant advances in basic science research regarding the biochemical nature of marine toxins and their mechanisms of action, our knowledge of the pathophysiology related to clinical syndromes in humans and the optimal therapies for human envenomation remain limited. Evidence for effective treatment is primarily derived from in vitro and in vivo animal research without the benefit of controlled human trials. However, current research in toxinology coupled with clinical observations allows the development of cogent treatment guidelines for victims of marine envenomation.

INVERTEBRATES

CNIDARIA

The phylum Cnidaria (formerly Coelenterata) includes more than 9000 species, of which approximately 100 are known to injure humans. They are commonly referred to as *jellyfish*; however, their phylogenetic designations separate "true jellyfish" and other organisms into distinct classes (Table 120–1; Figure 120–1a). All species possess microscopic cnidae (the Greek *knide* means nettle), which are highly specialized organelles consisting of an encapsulated hollow barbed thread bathed in venom. Thousands of these stinging organelles, called *nematocysts* (or *cnidoblasts*), are distributed along tentacles. A trigger mechanism called a *cnidocil* regulates nematocyst discharge. Pressure from contact with a victim's skin, or chemical triggers such as osmotic changes, stimulates discharge of the thread and toxin from its casing. Penetration of flesh leads to intradermal venom delivery. Nematocysts of most Cnidaria are incapable of penetrating human skin, rendering them harmless. Cnidaria causing human envenomation, such as the box jellyfish, discharge threads capable of penetrating into the papillary dermis.[135]

Cubozoa Members of the class Cubozoa are not true jellyfish. Animals in the Cubomedusae order have a cube-shaped bell with four corners, each of which supports between one and 15 tentacles. Species from this order produce the greatest morbidity and mortality of all Cnidaria. The order has two main families of toxicologic importance: Chirodropidae and Carybdeidae.

The Chirodropidae family is well known for the box jellyfish *Chironex fleckeri* (Greek *cheiro* means hand, Latin *nex* means murderer; therefore, "assassin's hand").[131] When full grown, its bell measures 25 to 30 cm in diameter, and 15 tentacles are attached at each "corner" of the bell. These tentacles may extend up to 3 m in length. Another member of this family is *Chiropsalmus quadrigatus*, the sea wasp. Its pale blue color makes detection in water nearly impossible.

The Carybdeidae family is most notable for *Carukia barnesi*, the Irukandji jellyfish.[60] Its small size, with a bell diameter of 2.5 cm, limits detection in open waters.

Hydrozoa The Hydrozoa class, like the Cubozoa, are also not true jellyfish; however, they are capable of inflicting considerable pain and even death in humans. The order Siphonophora (Physaliidae family) includes two unusual creatures of toxicologic concern: *Physalia physalis*, the Portuguese man-of-war, and its smaller counterpart, *Physalia utriculus*, the bluebottle. They are pelagic (floating) colonial Hydrozoa, meaning they exist as a colony of multiple hydroids in a formed mass. The easily recognizable blue sail that floats above the surface of the water is filled with nitrogen and carbon monoxide. Tentacles of *P. physalis* may reach lengths in excess of 30 meters and contain more than 750,000 nematocysts in each of its numerous tentacles (up to 40). *P. utriculus* has only one tentacle, which measures up to 15 m.

The Milleporina order is well known for the sessile *Millepora alcicornis* (fire coral) that exists as a fixed colony of hydroids. It appears much like true coral and has a white to yellow-green lime carbonate exoskeleton. Small tentacles protrude through minute surface gastropores. The overall structure ranges from 10 cm to 2 m.

Scyphozoa True jellyfish belong to the class Scyphozoa and are extremely diverse in size, shape, and color. Common varieties known to envenomate humans are *Cyanea capillata* (lion's mane or hair jelly), *Chrysaora quinquecirrha* (sea nettle), and *Pelagia noctiluca* (mauve stinger). The mauve stinger is easily recognized; it appears pink in daylight and phosphorescent at night. Larvae of certain *Linuche unguiculata* cause sea bather's eruption (SBE). The larvae are pinhead sized and are seen only when they are grouped in large numbers near the surface of the water.

Anthozoa The Anthozoa class has a diverse membership, including true corals, soft corals, and anemones. Only the anemones are of toxicologic importance. They are common inhabitants of reefs and tide pools and attach themselves to rock or coral. Armed with modified nematocysts known as *sporocysts* located on their tentacles, they produce stings similar to those of organisms from other Cnidaria classes.

History and Epidemiology Stings from Cnidaria represent the overwhelming majority of marine envenomations. In Australia, approximately 10,000 stings per year are recorded from *Physalia* spp alone.[55] Most Cnidaria stings occur during the warmer months of the year. Stings occur with greatest frequency on hotter-than-average days with low winds, particularly during times of low precipitation. "Stinger nets" are used in high-risk areas of the Australian coastline; however, one study reported that 63% of stings requiring medical attention occurred within netted waters.[85] Each stinger season, the Royal Darwin Hospital in Australia treats approximately 40 patients with stings.[41] A prospective evaluation of stings presenting to that hospital during a 12-month period from 1999 to 2000 revealed that 70% resulted from the box jellyfish. The remaining 30% involved other Cubozoa such as *C. barnesi*.[106] Although this finding may indicate a predominance of box jellyfish as the cause of stings, it also suggests that stings from box jellyfish are more severe and require medical attention with greater frequency than stings from other species of Cnidaria.

Cases of SBE, a stinging rash evoked by contact with Cnidaria larvae, occur in clusters. Variation in intensity and frequency occurs from year to year as exemplified by a 25-year hiatus during which no cases were reported in Florida.[142] In 1992, more than 10,000 cases of SBE occurred in south Florida, with similar peaks in the 1940s and 1960s. Cases of SBE also are reported in Cuba, Mexico, the Caribbean, and occasionally in Long Island, New York.

Cnidaria common to the United States include the Portuguese man-of-war and sea nettle. Other species are widely distributed throughout the

TABLE 120–1. Characteristics of Common Cnidaria

Latin Name	Common Name	Habitat[a]
Cubozoa class		
Chironex fleckeri[b]	Box jellyfish	Tropical Pacific Ocean, Indian Ocean, Gulf of Oman
Carukia barnesi[b]	Irukandji jellyfish	North Australian coast
Chiropsalmus spp[b]	Sea wasp or fire medusa	North Australian coast, Philippines, Japan, Indian Ocean, Gulf of Mexico, Caribbean
C. quadrigatus		
C. quadrumanus		
Carybdea alata	Hawaiian box jelly fish	Hawaii
Carybdea rastoni	Jimble	Australia
Hydrozoa class		
Physalia physalis[b]	Portuguese man-of-war	Eastern US Coast from Florida to North Carolina, Gulf of Mexico, Australian coastal waters (rare reports)
Physalia utriculus	Bluebottle	Tropical Pacific Ocean, particularly Australia
Millepora alcicornis	Fire coral	Widespread in tropical waters, including Caribbean
Scyphozoa class		
Chrysaora quinquecirrha	Sea nettle	Chesapeake Bay, widely distributed in temperate and tropical waters
Stomolophus meleagris	Cabbage head or cannonball jelly fish	Gulf of Mexico, Caribbean
Stomolophus nomurai[b]		Yellow Sea between China and South Korea
Cyanea capillata	Lion's mane or hair jelly fish	Northwest US coast up to Arctic Sea, Norwegian and British coastlines as well as Australia
Pelagia noctiluca	Mauve stinger or purple-striped jelly fish	Wide distribution in tropical zones
Linuche unguiculata	Thimble jelly fish	Florida, Mexico, and Caribbean
Anthozoa[b] class		
Anemonia sulcata	European stinging anemone	Eastern Atlantic, Mediterranean, Adriatic Sea
Actinodendron plumosum	Hell's fire anemone	South Pacific
Actinia equina	Beadlet anemone	Great Britain, Ireland

[a] Represents most common areas where stings are reported.

[b] Well-documented human fatalities.

tropical and temperate waters of the globe (see Table 120–1). Locations with documented Cnidaria-related deaths include the United States (Florida, North Carolina, Texas), Australia, the Indo-Pacific region (Malaysia, Langkawi Islands, Philippines, Solomon Islands, Papua New Guinea), and the coast of China. Since 1884 the number of deaths in Australia attributed to *C. fleckeri* is approximately 70.[55,84] An estimated two to three deaths per year occur in Malaysia from an unknown species.[55] Approximately 20 to 40 deaths are reported yearly in the Philippines from an unidentified species of the Chirodropidae family.[55] Three deaths are well documented from *P. physalis* in the United States (Florida, North Carolina).[22,55,134] One death from *Chiropsalmus quadrumanus* occurred along the coast of Texas.[12] Eight fatalities in the Bohai waters of China (Yellow Sea) have been reported from *Stomolophus nomurai*.[55,158] Although Chirodropidae are found off the western coast of Africa, no fatalities in that region are documented in the medical literature.

Pathophysiology Cnidaria venoms contain a variety of components that may induce dermatonecrosis, myonecrosis, hemolysis, or cardiotoxicity, depending on the particular species. In rats, *C. fleckeri* venom evokes transient hypertension, followed by hypotension and cardiovascular collapse within minutes.[109] Cardiac effects in animals include negative inotropy, conduction delay, ventricular tachycardia, and decreased coronary artery blood flow.[41] However, experiments using the purest venom extracts without contamination from tentacle material demonstrate cardiovascular collapse without electrocardiographic changes.[109] *C. fleckeri* venom also possesses dermatonecrotic and hemolytic fractions, although hemolysis in humans is not documented.[9] Two myotoxins from *C. fleckeri* cause powerful sustained muscle contractions in isolated muscle fibers.[45] Isolated heart models using *C. fleckeri* venom suggest its mechanism of action is nonspecific enhancement of cation conductance leading to increased Na^+ and Ca^{2+} entry into cells.[101] Other in vitro work confirms increased Na^+ permeability in cardiac tissue.[62]

C. barnesi, the Irukandji jelly, likely induces its dramatic vasopressor effects via catecholamine release. In rats the venom produces a pressor response that is blocked by α_1-adrenergic antagonism.[112] The pressor response is not dose dependent; therefore, catecholamines in the venom would not explain this effect. In vitro experiments suggest a sodium channel modulator effect leading to massive catecholamine release.[153] No electrocardiographic abnormalities occurred in envenomated rats.

Venom from *Physalia* spp blocks neural impulses in isolated frog sciatic nerve[81] and produces ventricular ectopy, cardiovascular collapse, hyperkalemia, and hemolysis in dogs.[71] *Physalia* spp venom inhibits Ca^{2+} entry into the sarcoplasmic reticulum.[81] Similar mechanisms

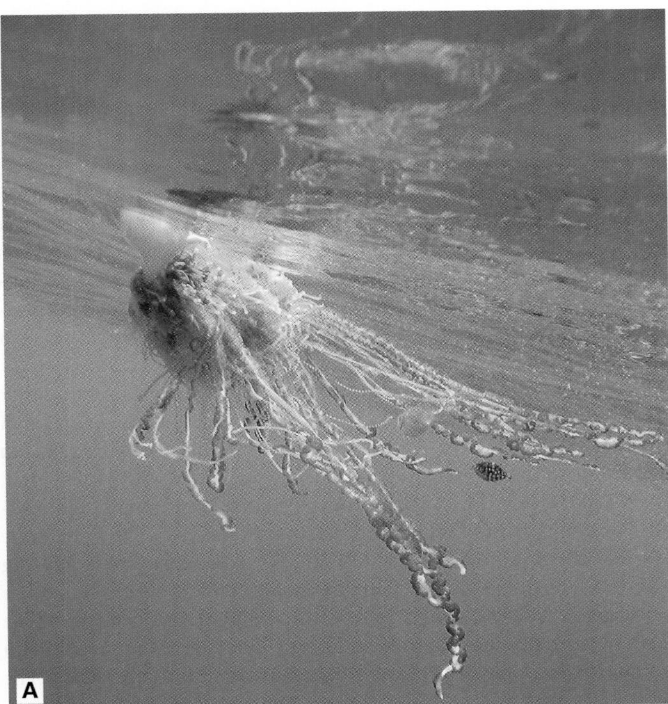

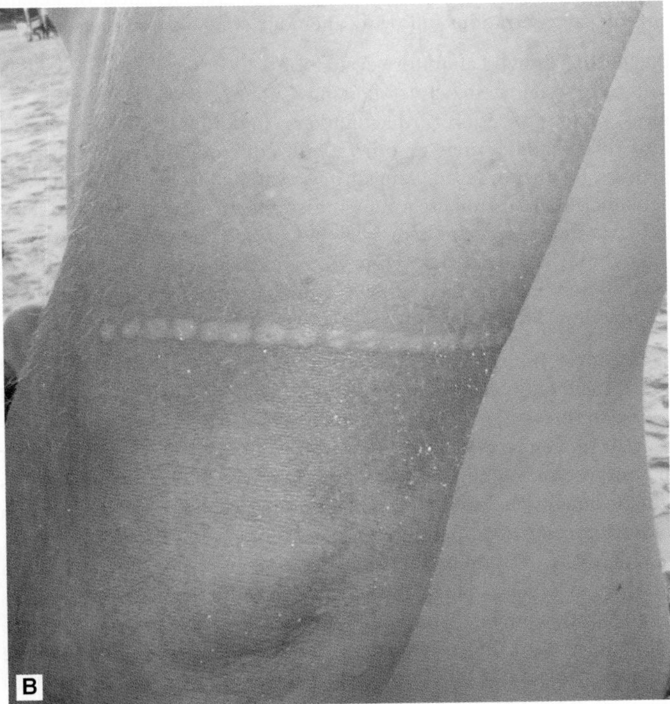

FIGURE 120–1. (A) North Atlantic Portuguese Man-O-War *Physalia physalis* with multiple tentacles dangling in the water. The tentacles filled with venomous nematocysts, and extend several meters in length. *(Image contributed by Adam Laverty Reproduced with permission from Knoop et al., The Atlas of Emergency Medicine, 3e (c) 2010, McGraw-Hill Inc., New York, New York.)* (B) Linear eruption from contact with an unidentified jellyfish in the South Atlantic Ocean. *(Image contributed by David Goldfarb.)*

are proposed for *Chrysaora*, *Chiropsalmus*, and *Stomolophus*. *C. quinquecirrha* venom contains a 150-kDa polypeptide that induces atrioventricular block[19] and produces myocardial ischemia, hypertension, dysrhythmias, and nerve conduction block,[23,24] as well as hepatic and renal necrosis.[100] *C. quinquecirrha*–induced hepatotoxicity is believed to be a direct toxin effect not mediated by pore formation or Ca^{2+} channel effects.[73] Equinatoxin II (EqtII), found in the venom of the anemone *Actinia equina*, creates pores in cell membranes leading to hemolysis.[1] This protein belongs to a group of anemone lysins known as *actinoporins* that bind to cell membranes and form pores via oligimerization.[90]

An immune-mediated response to venom may explain some sting-related symptoms. Elevated serum anti–sea nettle immunoglobulin IgM, IgG, and IgE may persist for years in patients with exaggerated reactions to stings compared with controls.[20] A direct correlation between titers against *Chrysaora* and *Physalia* and severity of a visible skin reaction to envenomation strongly suggests an allergic component.[123] Elevated IgG titers were demonstrated in one death from *P. physalis*.[134] Dermatonecrosis from *C. fleckeri* may involve the release of leukotrienes and other arachidonic acid derivatives as well as direct toxin-mediated cell damage.[42] Postenvenomation syndromes may result from an exaggerated, prolonged, aberrant T-cell response.[25,26] Erythema nodosum following a sting from *P. physalis* lends further support to a immunologic component.[5] SBE displays a characteristic delay in onset of symptoms and can be effectively treated with steroids, suggesting a primary immune-mediated process for this entity. This is further supported by histopathology revealing the presence of perivascular and interstitial infiltrates with lymphocytes, neutrophils, and eosinophils.[154]

Clinical Manifestations Most patients with stings are treated beachside and never require hospitalization. The vast majority of patients with stings who seek medical care have severe pain without evidence of systemic poisoning.[41] However, severe systemic manifestations may develop following stings from *C. fleckeri*, *C. barnesi*, *P. physalis*, and a few other Cnidaria.

Envenomation by *C. fleckeri* inflicts the most severe pain and is frequently associated with systemic toxicity. Common symptoms include immediate severe pain, followed by an erythematous whiplike linear rash with a "frosted ladder" appearance. The pain often is excruciating and may require parenteral analgesia. Systemic symptoms include nausea, vomiting, muscle spasms, headache, malaise, fever, and chills. Pain generally abates over several hours, although the rash may persist for days. In a prospective series of *C. fleckeri* stings, 58% manifested delayed hypersensitivity reactions in the form of an itchy maculopapular rash at 7 to 14 days.[106] Most resolved spontaneously; some were treated with antihistamines and topical corticosteroids.

Fatality is documented to occur with only 4 m of tentacle markings.[135] Death is rapid, preventing many victims from reaching shore. Cardiac arrest and pulmonary edema may develop in young, healthy patients without prior cardiopulmonary disease.[77,89,152] Survival is possible with immediate cardiopulmonary resuscitation (CPR).[151] *C. quadrumanus*, a close relative of the box jellyfish, induces symptoms that parallel *C. fleckeri* stings, including pulmonary edema and death.[12]

Previous reports suggesting a 15% to 20% fatality rate[118] following *C. fleckeri* envenomation likely represent a gross overestimation given the low number of documented fatalities in the context of the extraordinary number of yearly stings. A prospective study of stings from Cubozoa over 1 year in Australia revealed no dysrhythmias, pulmonary edema, or death.[106] No patient received antivenom, and analgesia was the only pharmacotherapy implemented. Hospital admission was not required for any victim. Although most victims suffer only local severe pain, serious systemic toxicity occurs occasionally, and may include vertigo, ataxia, paralysis, delirium, syncope, respiratory distress, pulmonary edema, hypotension, and dysrhythmia. The last 10 reported deaths from *C. fleckeri* occurred in children, suggesting vulnerability due to lower body mass and thinner dermis.[41]

Irukandji syndrome is a severe form of envenomation following Cubozoa stings from *C. barnesi*.[74] However, nematocysts obtained from one fatality could not be identified, suggesting the existence of another causative species. Although the syndrome is considered unique to Australia, an unidentified species produced three cases of Irukandji-like syndrome in the Florida Keys.[68]

Individuals afflicted with Irukandji syndrome often notice a mild sting while they are in the water; however, skin findings typically are absent. Severe systemic symptoms develop within 30 minutes and mimic a catecholamine surge: tachycardia, palpitations, hyperpnea, headache, pallor, restlessness, apprehension, sweating, and a sense of impending doom. A prominent feature is severe whole-body muscle spasms that come in waves and preferentially affect the back. Spasms are described as unbearable and frequently require parenteral analgesia. Symptoms generally abate over several hours. Admission rates in patients presenting to medical care can exceed 50%.[85] Hypertension is universal and may be severe, with systolic blood pressures well over 200 mm Hg. Two fatalities are described involving severe hypertension (systolic 280/150 mm Hg and 230/90 mm Hg) resulting in intracranial hemorrhage.[51,74] Hypotension frequently follows, requiring vasopressor support. Pulmonary edema can develop within hours. Echocardiograms consistently reveal global ventricular dysfunction,[85,87,92] although focal hypokinesis may occur.[74] Restored cardiac function typically returns after several days.[86] A retrospective review of 116 cases of Irukandji presenting to Cairns Base Hospital identified elevated troponin I measurements in 22% of patients,[74] although a higher frequency is documented (78%).[87] Electrocardiographic changes are described as nonspecific.

P. physalis envenomation typically induces severe pain, bullae, and skin necrosis (see Figure 120–1b). Systemic symptoms include weakness, numbness, anxiety, headache, abdominal and back spasms, lacrimation, nasal discharge, diaphoresis, vertigo, hemolysis, cyanosis, renal failure, shock, and rarely death. Some patients experience local numbness and paralysis of the affected extremity that resolves spontaneously.[75] As with serious *C. fleckeri* stings, cardiovascular collapse and death can occur within minutes of envenomation.[22] However, fatalities can be delayed several days following envenomation and relate to complications such as myocardial infarction and aspiration pneumonitis.[134] An unusual presentation is reported of a 4-year-old child who was stung along the North Carolina coast and developed massive hemolysis requiring transfusions, followed by renal failure necessitating temporary dialysis.[69] In contrast to *P. physalis, P. utriculus* stings typically are mild, although systemic toxicity occasionally develops.[57]

M. alcicornis (fire coral) is a common cause of stings in southern United States and Caribbean waters. While a member of the same phylogenetic class as *P. physalis,* it produces far less significant injuries. It is a nuisance to divers who touch the coral and suffer moderate burning pain for hours. Untreated pain generally lessens within 90 minutes, with skin wheals flattening at 24 hours and resolving within 1 week. Hyperpigmentation may persist for up to 8 weeks.[15] The feather hydroid is the most numerous of the Hydrozoa and produces only mild stings.[94]

True jellyfish typically are less harmful to humans than Cubozoa or Hydrozoa. However, systemic toxicity and occasional deaths are reported from certain species such as *S. nomurai, C. capillata, C. quinquecirrha*, and *P. noctiluca*. *Stomolophus meleagris* is a common cause of stings; however, its weak venom produces only minor injury.[4]

Larvae of *Linuche unguiculata* are the primary cause of a pruritic papular eruption on the skin of sea bathers in Florida, occurring mostly in areas covered by a bathing suit as a result of larvae trapped under the garments. Cases were first noted in 1949 and dubbed sea bather's eruption (SBE).[124] The larvae appear as pin-sized brown to green-brown spheres in the upper 2 inches of the water and are typically unnoticed. In a retrospective review, 50% of people reported a stinging sensation while they were in the water, and 25% reported itching upon exiting the water.[154] The remainder of patients developed symptoms within 11 hours. Skin lesions develop within hours of itching and appear as discrete, closely spaced papules, with pustules, vesicles, and urticaria. Most lesions occur in areas covered by the bathing suit where the larvae accumulate; however, folds of skin such as the axilla, breasts, and neck may be affected. Itching often is severe and prevents sleep. New lesions may continue to develop over 72 hours. The average duration of symptoms is just under 2 weeks, and a small percentage of patients experience a recurrence of lesions several days later. Systemic symptoms such as chills, headache, nausea, vomiting, and malaise may occur.

Following stings from sea anemones, victims may develop either immediate or delayed pain. Skin findings range from mild erythema and itching to ulceration. A review of 55 stings from *Anemonia sulcata* presenting to a hospital in Yugoslavia (Adriatic Sea) revealed that, in addition to the local skin findings, many patients suffered nausea, vomiting, muscle aches, and dizziness.[91] Larvae of the anemone *Edwardsiella lineata* also cause SBE among ocean swimmers in Long Island, New York. The hell's fire anemone *Actinodendron plumosum* is native to the South Pacific and produces significant local pain. One death occurred in the Virgin Islands following envenomation from an unknown species described as a "white anemone with blue tips." The onset of hepatic and renal failure was rapid and required transplantation, after which the patient died.[64] Nonfatal elevation of hepatic enzyme concentrations following anemone sting also is reported.[16]

Diagnostic Testing Laboratory evaluation may be warranted in patients suffering systemic toxicity following Cnidaria envenomation. Serial measurement of serum cardiac markers should be obtained from victims of Irukandji stings or others with consequential cardiovascular toxicity. Following severe stings from a variety of Cnidaria, urinalysis, hematocrit, and serum creatinine measurements should be considered to detect the presence of hemolysis and subsequent renal injury. Chest radiography is indicated for complaints of dyspnea or abnormalities in oxygenation. Venom assays are not available, and serum antibody titers are not clinically useful.

Management Initial interventions after Cnidaria envenomation should follow standard management strategies. Secondary measures are directed toward the prevention of further nematocyst discharge, which could intensify pain and enhance toxicity. Many topical therapies have been used for this purpose, including sea water, vinegar, a commercial solution known as Stingose, methylated spirits, ethanol, isopropyl alcohol, dilute ammonium hydroxide, urine, sodium bicarbonate, papain, shaving cream, and sand.

Vinegar is a common first-line treatment for topical application following Cnidaria stings. In vitro trials with *C. fleckeri* tentacles demonstrate complete irreversible inhibition of nematocyst discharge following a 30-second application.[70] Additional study findings include massive nematocyst discharge with application of urine or ethanol, and no effect on discharge with use of sodium bicarbonate. Follow-up in vivo experiments demonstrate that vinegar is effective for other Cubozoa, including Morbakka (large Cubozoan in Australia),[50] *Carybdea rastoni*,[53] and *C. barnesi*.[54] Although massive nematocyst discharge occurs when vinegar is applied to *C. capillata* tentacles in vitro, clinical exacerbation following this treatment is not reported in humans.[49] Massive discharge also occurs with *C. quinquecirrha*.[28] A smaller degree of discharge (30%) occurs with *P. physalis*,[57] whereas nematocysts of *P. utriculus* are unaffected by application of vinegar.[70]

Stingose is a commercially available product designed to counteract venom of insects, bees, stinging plants, and marine stingers. It is an aqueous solution of 20% aluminum sulfate and 1.1% surfactant. Its purported mechanism of action is denaturing of proteins and long-chain polysaccharides via interactions with the Al^{3+} ion, as well as osmotic removal of venom. A human volunteer trial involving stings from live tentacles of *C. fleckeri* demonstrated pain relief within 5 seconds of Stingose application.[72] Similar results were achieved following treatment of stings from *C. quinquecirrha*. Further investigation involved beachside evaluation of 17 *C. fleckeri* and 150 *P. utriculus* sting victims treated with Stingose immediately following injury. All victims reported rapid relief. However, placebo or alternative therapies were not used in this case series. The efficacy of treatment with vinegar, Stingose, methylated spirits, and salt water was measured in human volunteers following forearm application of *P. physalis* tentacles.[145] Vinegar demonstrated superior pain control compared with Stingose, whereas methylated spirits increased pain. The study assessed pain relief only and did not investigate the effects of the treatments on nematocyst discharge or systemic toxicity.

In many cases the identity of the "jellyfish" causing injury is unknown. In those cases, therapy must be guided by geographic location. In the United States, where *P. physalis* and *C. quinquecirrha* are of greatest consequence, sea water should be used to aid in tentacle removal given that vinegar enhances nematocyst discharge in those species. In the Indo-Pacific region, where *C. fleckeri* and *C. barnesi* are of greatest concern, vinegar should be used. Following a 30-second application, adherent tentacles must be carefully removed. This can be accomplished with a gloved or towel-covered hand, or with sand and gentle scraping with a credit card or other blunt, straight-edged tool.

In a nonrandomized trial, ice packs provided rapid, effective relief for patients with mild to moderate pain from Cnidaria stings in Australia.[46] Patients with severe pain were less likely to benefit from ice packs. Some authors suggest that the use of heat is not only ineffective for venom neutralization, but that it increases pain.[17] However, recent controlled trials designed to address this controversy highlight the efficacy of hot water immersion in lieu of cold packs for the treatment of stings from *Carybdea alata* and *Physalia* sp.[57,88,103,140,157] Hot-water immersion therapy for treatment of *C. fleckeri* stings has not been rigorously evaluated.

Pressure immobilization bandaging is a technique that applies sufficient pressure to a wound to impede lymphatic drainage and prevent the entrance of venom into systemic circulation. Its application for snake bites is commonplace, while its role following Cnidaria stings has sparked controversy. Given the rapid onset of symptoms, the utility of a technique that impedes lymphatic drainage is unlikely to provide benefit. Although the technique would be used only after tentacle removal, some microscopic nematocysts remain adherent to the skin after visible tentacles are removed. In vitro data investigating the effect of pressure on discharged nematocysts demonstrate not only that discharged nematocysts still contain venom, but that applying pressure forces more venom down the hollow tube.[108] This finding is correlated clinically as patients can deteriorate following pressure immobilization bandaging.[56] Given the lack of evidence suggesting benefit, coupled with clear in vitro evidence of increased venom delivery with this technique, it should not be implemented for treatment of Cnidaria stings.

Box jellyfish antivenom is sheep-derived whole IgG raised against the "milked" venom of *C. fleckeri*. It has been available in Australia since 1970. Combining *C. fleckeri* venom with box jellyfish antivenom prior to injection into pigs prevents all toxicity.[145] An isolated chick muscle experiment demonstrates that box jellyfish antivenom prevents the neurotoxicity and myotoxicity from *C. fleckeri* following pretreatment; however, there is no "rescue effect."[110] Given that antivenom in humans is always used as a rescue therapy, this research raises concerns regarding efficacy in the clinical setting. Pretreatment of rats with box jellyfish antivenom prevented cardiovascular collapse in 40%, but did not blunt the initial hypertensive effect.[111] In vitro data demonstrate that box jellyfish antivenom neutralizes the dermatonecrotic, hemolytic, and lethal fractions of venom from *Chiropsalmus* spp; however, the venom of *P. physalis* and *C. quinquecirrha* were not neutralized.[10] Other in vitro and in vivo data demonstrate incomplete neutralization of *Chiropsalmus* spp venom.[10,110]

There are no controlled studies in humans evaluating the efficacy of box jellyfish antivenom in the treatment of *C. fleckeri* envenomations, nor is there convincing evidence that its administration has saved human lives. Despite the frequency of hospital visits for stings from *C. fleckeri* in Australia, the use of box jellyfish antivenom is rare.[41] Evidence for its efficacy stems from case reports suggesting that pain abates rapidly after administration.[14,152] Although box jellyfish antivenom may improve pain control, patients still may require parenteral narcotics for analgesia following antivenom administration.[11] Significant morbidity and mortality still occur despite antivenom use.[40,89,135] Case reports of box jellyfish antivenom use for *C. barnesi* stings demonstrate no apparent benefit.[48]

Many serious stings occur in the Northern Territory of Australia, where stinger nets are not commonly used. Distance from medical care limits the ability to obtain antivenom in a timely fashion.[41] Although box jellyfish antivenom can be administered by paramedics via intramuscular (IM) injection,[56] poor IM absorption and incomplete venom neutralization with antivenoms, as well as delayed peak serum concentrations, limit the utility of this approach.[117] The amount of antivenom required to neutralize twice the lethal dose in humans is estimated at 12 vials.[41] The manufacturer recommends treating initially with one ampule intravenously (IV) diluted 1:10 with saline or three undiluted ampules (1.5–4 mL each) IM at three separate sites, if IV access is unavailable. Some authors who have treated multiple patients with antivenom suggest treating coma, dysrhythmia, or respiratory depression with one ampule IV, titrating up to three ampules with continuation of CPR in patients with refractory dysrhythmia until a total of six ampules have been administered.[106] For less serious envenomations, clinicians may consider administering one ampule if ice packs and parenteral analgesia prove ineffective.[106] Serious adverse events or delayed sequelae following the use of IV antivenom are uncommon, although allergic reactions are a consideration.[136]

Verapamil was evaluated as a treatment for *C. fleckeri* stings based on evidence that calcium entry into cells represents an important mechanism of toxicity. One animal model demonstrated synergy with use of verapamil in combination with box jellyfish antivenom,[27] whereas another showed verapamil pretreatment as well as rescue prolonged survival.[18] This is in contrast to other models demonstrating that verapamil negates the benefits of antivenom[111] and increases mortality.[141] Verapamil administration to animals with *C. quinquecirrha* envenomation demonstrated no benefit.[100] Interestingly, addition of magnesium to antivenom for treatment of *C. fleckeri* envenomation in rats prevented cardiovascular collapse in 100%, suggesting that magnesium may have a role in the treatment of stings from this species.[111] Given that animal data are inconsistent with regard to verapamil and that hypotension may develop with severe envenomation, use of calcium channel blockers is not recommended for treatment of *C. fleckeri* stings.

Treatment for Irukandji syndrome should focus on analgesia and blood pressure control. Several modalities for control of severe hypertension have been suggested and include phentolamine, IV magnesium sulfate and nitroglycerin.[39,52] Whereas hypotension may occur in late stages of toxicity, clinicians should also consider short-acting titratable agents such as esmolol, nitroprusside or nicardipine.

MOLLUSCA

The phylum Mollusca (Latin *mollis* meaning soft) includes the classes Cephalopoda (octopus, squid, and cuttlefish) and Gastropoda (cone

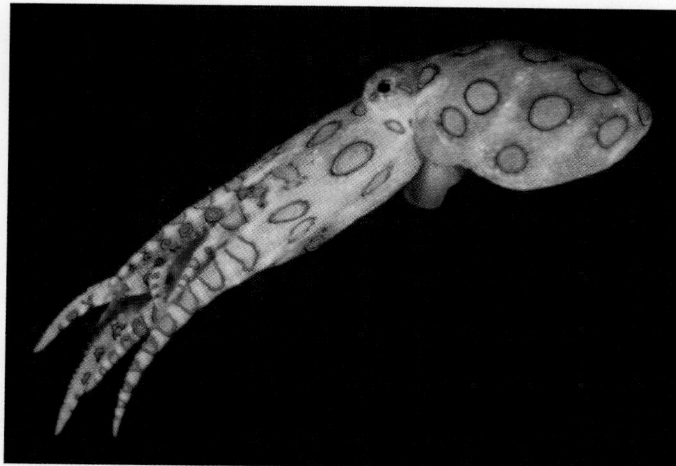

FIGURE 120-2. The Blue Ringed octopus, *Hapalochlaena maculosa*. *(Image contributed by Dr. Roy Caldwell, Professor of Integrative Biology, University of California, Berkeley.)*

snails). Cephalopod species of toxicologic concern are limited to the blue-ringed octopus *Hapalochlaena maculosa* and the greater blue-ringed octopus *Hapalochlaena lunulata*. The blue-ringed and greater blue-ringed octopi are found in the Indo-Pacific region, primarily in Australian waters (Figure 120–2). Of the 400 species of cone snails that belong to the genus Conus, 18 are implicated in human envenomations.

History and Epidemiology The blue-ringed octopus normally displays a yellow-brown color, but develops iridescent blue rings when threatened. The species is not aggressive and only bites humans when handled. A 1983 review of reported octopus envenomations uncovered a total of 14 cases, all of which occurred in Australia.[146] There were two deaths[61,133] and four serious envenomations. Other reviews suggest that up to seven deaths may have occurred prior to 1969, some outside Australia.[44]

Estimates of reported cone snail envenomations suggest only 15 human deaths have occurred worldwide.[47] *Conus geographicus* (fish hunting cone) is the most common species implicated, although *Conus textile* may also cause death in humans. Cone snails predominantly inhabit the Indo-Pacific, including all parts of Australia, New Guinea, Solomon Islands, and the Philippines. Two deaths from *C. geographicus* occurred in Guam.[83]

Pathophysiology The blue ringed octopus salivary gland secretes a toxin originally designated maculotoxin and later identified as tetrodotoxin.[128] The beak of the octopus creates small punctures in human skin through which venom is introduced. Tetrodotoxin blocks Na^+ conductance in neurons, leading to paralysis. Venom also contains serotonin (5-HT), hyaluronidase, tyramine, histamine, tryptamine, octopine, taurine, acetylcholine, and dopamine.[137] Rabbits subjected to bites develop rapid flaccid paralysis without cardiotoxicity and die from asphyxia.[137] Other animal models using venom gland extract demonstrate rapid onset of respiratory muscle paralysis and severe hypotension.[59] Death occurs despite artificial respiration and results from hypotension.

Cone snails have a hollow proboscis that contains a tooth bathed in venom. Envenomations occur when the shells are handled. The proboscis can extend the length of its shell, thereby envenomating the hand of someone touching the opposite end of the shell. Any *Conus* species contains approximately 100 peptides or *conotoxins* in its venom. Targets include voltage- and ligand-gated ion channels as well as G-protein–linked receptors (Table 120–2).[105,139] Many of these

TABLE 120–2. Conus Peptide Targets

Receptor Type	Peptide	Mechanism
Ligand-gated ion channels		
Nicotinic	α-Conotoxin	Competitive antagonism
	M1	Neuromuscular junction
	M2	Neuronal receptors
5-HT_3	σ-Conotoxin	Noncompetitive antagonism
NMDA	Conantokins	Inhibits conductance
Voltage-gated ion channels		
Ca^{2+}	ω-Conotoxin	Channel blockade
Na^+	μ-Conotoxin	Channel blockade
	δ-Conotoxin	Delayed channel activation
K^+	κ-Conotoxin	Channel blockade
G-protein linked		
Vasopressin receptor	Conopressin-G	Receptor agonism
Neurotensin receptor	Contulakin-G	Receptor agonism

peptides are used extensively in laboratory research for their ability to selectively target a variety of specific calcium channel subtypes. Venom from *Conus imperialis* (worm hunter) contains a substantial amount of 5-HT, a component not found in any other *Conus* venom tested thus far.[96] This species also contains a vasopressin-like peptide.[102] The neuropeptide ω- conotoxin, isolated from *Conus magnus*, is valued for its antinociceptive properties that arise from blockade of the N-type voltage-sensitive calcium channel in spinal cord afferents.[95] The Food and Drug Administration approved ziconotide (Prialt, Elan Pharmaceuticals) in 2004 for intrathecal (IT) infusion in patients with severe chronic pain that require IT therapy, and in whom other treatment modalities such as IT morphine are not tolerated or ineffective. Patients reported modest improvements in pain with long-term treatment.[148] Frequent side effects such as dizziness, nausea, confusion, and memory impairment limit the broad application of this novel therapy.

Clinical Manifestations The blue-ringed octopus creates one or two puncture wounds with its chitinous jaws, inflicting only minor discomfort. A wheal may develop with erythema, tenderness, and pruritus. Tetrodotoxin exerts a curarelike effect characterized by paralysis without depressing mental status. Symptoms include perioral and intraoral paresthesias, diplopia, aphonia, dysphagia, ataxia, weakness, nausea, vomiting, flaccid muscle paralysis, respiratory failure, and death. Detailed case reports describe rapid onset of symptoms.[146] Complete paralysis requiring intubation with findings of fixed and dilated pupils is followed within 24 to 48 hours by near-complete recovery of neuromuscular function.[146] In one reported death, a young man placed the octopus on his shoulder. He subsequently noted a small puncture wound, developed dry mouth, dyspnea, inability to swallow, and became apneic. Asystole occurred 30 minutes after arrival at the hospital despite artificial ventilation.[61] Another similar bite resulted in symptom onset at 10 minutes, followed by death at 90 minutes, despite bystander CPR.[137] With less severe envenomations, cerebellar signs may arise without paralysis. Near-total paralysis with intact mentation resolving over 24 hours is described in humans.[137]

Cone snail envenomation results from careless handling of the animal or rummaging through sand. Cone snails are nocturnal feeders, so they may present more of a hazard to night divers. Localized symptoms range from a slight sting to excruciating pain, tissue ischemia, cyanosis, and numbness. Systemic symptoms include weakness, diaphoresis, diplopia, blurred vision, aphonia, dysphagia, generalized muscle paralysis, respiratory failure, cardiovascular collapse, and coma. Death is rapid and occurs within 2 hours. Based on military medical records of more than 30 cases predating 1970, the mortality rate approaches 25%, with *C. geographicus* causing the most deaths.[83] Other estimates suggest that, without medical care, mortality may reach 70%.[156] Given the rarity of severe human envenomation from cone snails, the manner of death, whether purely from respiratory insufficiency or direct cardiovascular toxicity, remains unknown.

Diagnostic Testing Laboratory testing following envenomation from octopi or cone snails should be directed by clinical findings. Coma, respiratory failure, and hypotension merit evaluation of serum metabolic parameters, chest radiography, and electrocardiogram. Although not a widely available assay, tetrodotoxin can be detected in the urine or serum using high-performance liquid chromatography with subsequent fluorescence detection.[104]

Management Primary interventions include maintenance of airway, breathing, and circulation. Some authors recommend hot water (45°–50°C, 113°–122°F) following cone snail stings for pain relief.[83] Unlike Cnidaria envenomations, where nematocysts full of venom can persist on the skin and lead to continued venom delivery, stings from the octopus and cone snail mirror those of snake bites, where venom delivery is an immediate and finite event. Therefore, pressure immobilization bandaging may blunt toxin distribution by decreasing lymphatic spread.[47] Additional measures include local wound care and tetanus prophylaxis. Antivenom is not available for octopus or cone snail venoms.

ECHINODERMATA, ANNELIDA, AND PORIFERA

The Echinodermata phylum includes sea stars,, brittle stars, sea urchins, sand dollars, and sea cucumbers. Annelida are segmented worms that include the Polychaetae family of bristle worms. Sponges are classified in the Porifera phylum. One feature that all three phyla share is the passive envenomation of people who mistakenly handle or step on the animals. Most stings from these creatures are mild.

History and Epidemiology Echinoderms, annelids, and sponges are ubiquitous ocean inhabitants. The crown-of-thorns *Acanthaster planci* is found in the warmest waters of Polynesia to the Red Sea and is a particularly venomous species because of its sharp spines that easily puncture human skin. Sea urchins inhabit all oceans of the world. Bristle worms such as *Hermodice carunculata* typically inhabit tropical waters such as those of Florida and the Caribbean. However, some species thrive in the frigid waters of Antarctica. The fire sponge *Tedania ignis* is a brilliant yellow-orange sponge identified in large numbers off the coast of Hawaii and in the Florida Keys. Other common American sponges are *Neofibularia nolitangere* (poison-bun sponge or touch-me-not sponge) and *Microciona prolifera* (red sponge). *Neofibularia mordens* (Australian stinging sponge) is a common Southern Australian variety. In the Mediterranean, sponges are often colonized with sea anemones that may inflict severe stings.[15]

Pathophysiology Sea urchins are covered in spines and pedicellariae. The pedicellariae are pincerlike appendages used for feeding, cleaning, and defense. They generally contain more venom than the spines and are more difficult to remove from wounds. Urchins laden with pedicellariae can evoke more severe stings than urchins with less pedicellariae. Venom contained within the spines consists of steroid glycosides, serotonin, hemolysin, protease, and acetylcholinelike substances. Some species harbor neurotoxins. The most venomous are species of *Diadema*, *Echinothrix*, and *Asthenosoma*. Sea stars are less noxious because they generally have short, blunt spiny projections. The crown-of-thorns is the exception with its longer, sharp spines containing toxic saponins with hemolytic and anticoagulant effects as well as histaminelike substances.[138] Sea cucumbers excrete holothurin, a sulfated triterpenoid oligoglycoside, from the anus (organs of Cuvier) as a defense. The toxin inhibits neural conduction in fish, leading to paralysis. Some sea cucumbers eat Cnidaria and subsequently secrete their venom.

Bristle worms have many parapodia that have the appearance, but not the function, of legs. Several bristles extend from each parapodium giving the family (Polychaeta) its name (*poly* means many, *chaetae* means bristles). The bristles may penetrate human skin, leading to envenomation with an unknown substance.

Sponges have an elastic skeleton with spicules of silicon dioxide or calcium carbonate. They attach to the sea floor or coral beds. Toxins include halitoxin, odadaic acid, and subcritine, the nature of which is uncertain.[21] Dried sponges are nontoxic; however, on rewetting they may produce toxicity even after several years.[132]

Clinical Manifestations Most injuries from sea urchins are caused by inadvertently stepping on the spines or attempting to handle the animal. An intense burning with local tissue reaction occurs, including edema and erythema. Rarely, with multiple punctures, lightheadedness, numbness, paralysis, bronchospasm, and hypotension may reportedly occur, although this is not documented in the peer-reviewed medical literature.[3] Reports of death are not well substantiated. The Pacific urchin *Tripneustes* has a neurotoxin with a predilection for cranial nerves.[15] Mild elevations of hepatic enzymes are reported in one patient with foot cellulitis from an urchin sting.[155] Small cuts on the skin from handling starfish may allow venom to penetrate, leading to contact dermatitis. The crown-of-thorns may cause severe pain, nausea, vomiting, and muscular paralysis.[94] Cutaneous, scleral, or corneal exposure to sea cucumbers triggers contact dermatitis, intense corneal inflammation, and even blindness. Bristle worms are shrouded with bristles that can produce a reddened urticarial rash. Symptoms typically are mild and resolve over several hours to days.

Contact with the fire sponge, poison-bun sponge, or red-moss sponge causes erythema, papules, vesicles, and bullae that generally subside within 3 to 7 days. Victims may develop fever, chills, and muscle cramps. Skin desquamation occurs at 10 days to 2 months,[4] with chronic skin changes lasting several months.[21] Erythema multiforme and anaphylaxis are uncommon complications associated with *Neofibularia* spp exposure.[15] Contact with sponges that are colonized with Cnidaria can lead to dermatitis with skin necrosis, referred to as *sponge diver's disease*.

Management The primary objective following envenomation from sea urchins and crown-of-thorns starfish is analgesia. Submersion of the affected extremity in hot water (105°F–115°F, 40.6°C–46.1°C) and administration of oral analgesics often is sufficient.[47,94] Puncture wounds require radiographic evaluation to locate potential foreign bodies. Spines frequently crumble with attempted extraction. Intraarticular spines necessitate surgical removal. Decisions regarding spines in other locations should be influenced by ease of removal, presence of infection, and persistent pain. Tetanus immune status must be addressed. Decisions regarding antibiotic prophylaxis should be based on degree of injury and patient factors such as diabetes or other immunocompromise. Although most infections likely are secondary to human skin flora, marine flora such as *Mycobacterium marinum* and *Vibrio parahaemolyticus* are potential wound contaminants. Treatment of sponge exposures usually requires only removal of spicules using adhesive tape or the edge of a credit card. Antihistamines and topical steroids often provide no relief from stinging sponges.[21]

VERTEBRATES

SNAKES

Sea snakes are members of the class Reptilia and are divided into two subfamilies: Hydrophiinae and Laticaudinae. They are close relatives of the cobra and krait. Length typically does not exceed 1 m. Their tails are flattened, and their bodies often are brightly colored. Distinction from eels is made by the presence of scales and the absence of fins and gills. All 52 species of sea snakes are venomous and at least six species are implicated in human fatalities. The most common species cited in human envenomation are *Enhydrina schistosa*, the beaked sea snake and *Pelamis platurus*, the yellow-bellied sea snake.

History and Epidemiology Sea snakes are common to the tropical and temperate Indian and Pacific Oceans, but are also found along the eastern Pacific Coast of Central and South America and the Gulf of California. In the eastern Pacific region, the yellow-bellied sea snake is the only species known. There are no sea snakes in the Atlantic Ocean. The majority of envenomations occur along the coasts of Southeast Asia, the Persian Gulf, and the Malay Archipelago (Malaysia). Snakes tend to inhabit the turbid coastlines and deeper reefs of these regions.

The true incidence of sea snake envenomation is unknown because many bites are not recorded. Worldwide the number of deaths per year may approach 150, with an overall mortality rate estimated at 3%.[47] In a review of 120 documented bites, 51.7% of victims were fisherman handling nets.[116] The remainder of victims were wading or swimming along the coastline. In another review of 101 bites occurring from 1957 to 1964 in Northwest Malaysia, more than 50% of bites were from the beaked sea snake, including seven of the eight fatal bites in that series, bringing the mortality to 8% prior to the availability of antivenom.[114] However, 31 "dry bites" were excluded, suggesting that the overall mortality is somewhat lower. Among the 20% of patients in that series suffering "serious envenomation," half died despite supportive care.[114] A follow-up series of patients after the introduction of antivenom described two deaths out of 11 "serious envenomations," suggesting a decreased mortality resulting from this intervention. These were all retrospective reviews of published or personally communicated cases.

Pathophysiology All sea snakes have small front fangs. Their venom is neurotoxic, myotoxic, nephrotoxic, and hemolytic. Known components of the venom include acetylcholinesterase, hyaluronidase, leucine aminopeptidase, 5′-nucleotidase, phosphodiesterase, and phospholipase A. The neurotoxin is a highly stable 6000- to 8000-Da protein similar to that of the cobra and krait. In mice, beaked sea snake venom is four to five times more potent than cobra venom based on a μg/kg ratio; however, cobra venom yield is greater.[31] Venom homology exists across many species.[76] The neurotoxin targets postsynaptic acetylcholine (ACh) receptors creating a blockade at the neuromuscular junction. Presynaptic effects include initial enhanced ACh release and subsequent inhibition of ACh release.[99,119,147] In vitro research confirms direct nephrotoxicity of crude venom, and may partially explain the nephrotoxicity described clinically.[127] Rhabdomyolysis likely contributes to this clinical finding.

Clinical Manifestations Sea snakes generally are docile, except when provoked, or during the mating season. Bites typically are painless or inflict minimal discomfort. Between one and four fang marks are common; however, up to 20 fang marks are possible as a result of multiple bites. The diagnosis can be obscured, because victims may not associate the slight prick following the bite with later onset of ascending paralysis. Symptoms may progress within minutes, although a delay of up to 6 hours is possible. Neurotoxin-induced paralysis occurs in conjunction with muscle destruction stemming from myotoxic fractions. Painful muscular rigidity and myoglobinuria are hallmarks of sea snake myotoxicity. Myoglobinuria develops between 30 minutes and 8 hours after the bite. Other classic symptoms include ascending flaccid paralysis, dysphagia, trismus, ptosis, aphonia, nausea, vomiting, fasciculations, and ultimately respiratory insufficiency, seizures, and coma.

Diagnostic Testing Laboratory diagnostics are directed toward identifying hemolysis, myonecrosis, hyperkalemia, and renal failure. Serum electrolytes, creatinine, and creatine phosphokinase, as well as hematocrit and urinalysis, should be obtained. Elevated concentrations of hepatic enzymes may indicate severe envenomation. Serial measurement of these parameters is recommended.

Management Prehospital management of sea snake bites mirrors treatment of terrestrial snake bites and includes immobilization of the extremity and consideration of a pressure immobilization bandage to impede lymphatic drainage. Currently no data regarding the efficacy of this technique for sea snake envenomations are available. Tourniquets that impede venous or arterial flow are not recommended and may be detrimental. Airway and respiratory effort require close monitoring because paralysis can develop rapidly.

The most commonly used antivenoms for sea snakes are equine IgG Fab fragments produced using the venom of beaked sea snake (*E. schistosa*) or terrestrial tiger snake (*Notechis scutatus*) (Table 120–3). In vitro experiments demonstrate that sea snake antivenom is effective for neutralizing all species of sea snakes tested (*Praescutata viperina* in Thailand, *P. platurus* in Central America, *Laticauda semifasciata* in the Philippines, *Laticauda laticaudata* in Japan, *Hydrophis cyanocinctus*, *Lapemis hardwickii*).[144] Optimal neutralization occurs within the subfamily Hydrophiinae, which contains *E. schistosa*; however, effective neutralization is demonstrated within the subfamily Laticaudinae. Terrestrial tiger snake antivenom also can neutralize sea snake venom in vitro. Based on the volume of antivenom required, tiger snake antivenom was superior for neutralization of all sea snake venoms tested except that of the beaked sea snake, for which sea snake antivenom was more effective.[7] This finding is expected because sea snake antivenom is raised against beaked sea snake venom. In contrast to volume comparisons, measurements of unit dosing demonstrate sea snake antivenom is more effective for all venoms tested. Another in vitro study comparing tiger snake and sea snake antivenom against venom *E. schistosa* demonstrated tiger snake antivenom was 10 times more effective in terms of milligram of venom neutralized per milliliter of antivenom.[98] In the

TABLE 120–3. Antivenoms

Organism	Derivation	Concentration
Box jellyfish		
C. fleckeri	Ovine, whole IgG	20,000 Units/ampule
Sea snake		
E. schistose (beaked sea snake)	Equine, IgG Fab	1000 Units/ampule
N. scutatus (terrestrial tiger snake)	Equine, IgG Fab	3000 Units/ampule
Stonefish		
S. trachynis	Equine, IgG Fab	2000 Units/ampule

CSL, Commonwealth Serum Laboratories, Melbourne, Australia manufacture these antivenom.

same study, the use of 17 different types of elapid antivenom resulted in poor neutralization of beaked sea snake venom.

In rescue experiments with mice using 11 sea snake venoms and four different antivenoms (*E. schistosa*, *E. schistosa-N. scutatus*, *N. scutatus*, and polyvalent sea snake *L. hardwickii*, *L. semifasciata*, *H. cyanocinctus*), tiger snake antivenom was superior to all others with respect to volume amount required to prevent death.[2,8,63] Another finding of the study was improved efficacy with early administration of antivenom.

No controlled human trials have evaluated the efficacy of sea snake antivenom, although case reports suggest improved outcomes and more rapid recovery with its use.[97,114] Anecdotal experience in Malaysia using sea snake antivenom suggests slow recovery from myalgias and weakness over 48 hours, compared with resolution over 2 weeks without antivenom (two cases, one control).[115]

Based on in vitro and in vivo research, selection of the optimal antivenom for treatment of sea snake bites is unclear. Both sea snake and tiger snake antivenom are effective in neutralizing a wide variety of sea snake venoms. Therefore, the most readily available antivenom should be used when needed. Commonwealth Serum Laboratories manufactures both monovalent sea snake and tiger snake antivenom for use in Australia. However, limited distribution to aquariums and zoos outside Australia occurs. The manufacturer's guidelines for use of monovalent sea snake antivenom recommend administration of one ampule (1000 Units) for systemic symptoms. However, because symptoms may be delayed and early administration is more likely to result in venom neutralization, any evidence of envenomation should prompt the administration of antivenom. The antivenom requires a 1:10 dilution with 0.9% sodium chloride solution followed by administered IV over 30 minutes. A 1:5 dilution can be used for small children. Skin testing is not recommended. Epinephrine and antihistamines should be readily available. No upper limit is suggested for the number of vials to administer, although larger amounts are more likely to result in serum sickness. Patients have received up to 7000 Units without adverse effect directly attributable to the antivenom.[97] One ampule (3000 Units) of tiger snake antivenom can be used as an alternative if sea snake antivenom is unavailable. Other treatments should focus on wound care, tetanus prophylaxis, analgesia, and fluid administration to minimize nephrotoxicity from myoglobinuria.

FISH

Stingrays are members of the class Chondrichthyes (order Rajiformes: skates and rays). Families include Dasyatidae (whip ray or sting ray), Urolophidae (round ray), Myliobatidae (batfish or eagle ray), Gymnuridae (butterfly ray), and Potamotrygonidae (river ray, freshwater).

Spiny fish of the family Scorpaenidae include a variety of venomous creatures (Table 120–4). Fish of the genus *Pterois* are commonly called *lionfish* (*P. volitans* and *P. lunulata*). Stonefish are grouped under the genus *Synanceja* and include *S. trachynis* (Australian estuarine stonefish), *S. horrida* (Indian stonefish), and *S. verrucosa* (reef stonefish). They are unattractively disguised to blend in with the rocky sea bottom (Figure 120–3). Scorpionfish have a similar appearance and belong to the genus *Scorpaena* (eg, *S. guttata*: California sculpin). Other Scorpaenidae include *Notesthes robusta* (bullrout) and *Gymnapistes marmoratus* (cobbler). The European weeverfish produce toxicity similar to members of Scorpaenidae and are classified under the family Trachinidae. This includes *Trachinus vipera* (lesser weever) and *Trachinus draco* (greater weever, aka adderpike, stingfish, seacat). These bottom dwellers are smaller and have fewer spines than Scorpaenidae and are much less ghoulish in appearance. Catfish also may envenomate humans. Although most live in freshwater, marine catfish such as *Plotosus lineatus* can inflict injury. Other venomous spiny fish include rabbitfish, stargazers, toadfish, ratfish, and even some sharks that have spines on their dorsal fins (Port Jackson shark, dogfish shark).

History and Epidemiology There are 11 different species of stingrays in US costal waters (seven in the Atlantic, four in the Pacific). In the southeastern United States, *Dasyatis americana* is a common inhabitant.

TABLE 120–4. Spiny Fish

Latin Name	Common Name	Habitat
Scorpaenidae family		
Pterois		
P. volitans	Lionfish (also zebrafish, turkeyfish, or red firefish)	Indo-Pacific region, coast of Florida to North Carolina (nonnative to US coast)
P. lunulata	Lionfish or butterfly cod	
Synanceja		
S. trachynis	Australian estuarine stonefish	Indo-Pacific region (Pacific and Indian Oceans)
S. horrida	Indian stonefish	
S. verrucosa	Reef stonefish	
Scorpaena		
S. cardinalis	Red rock cod, scorpionfish	Coast of Australia
S. guttata	California sculpin, scorpionfish	Coast of California
Notesthes robusta	Bullrout	Coast of Australia
Gymnapistes marmoratus	Cobbler	Coast of Australia
Trachinidae family		
Trachinus		
T. vipera	Lesser weeverfish	Coasts of Great Britain to Northwest Africa, throughout Mediterranean and Black Seas
T. draco	Greater weeverfish (also adderpike, stingfish, or seacat)	

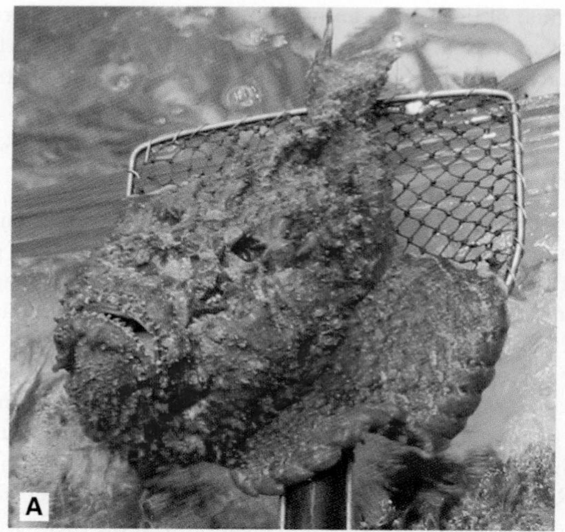

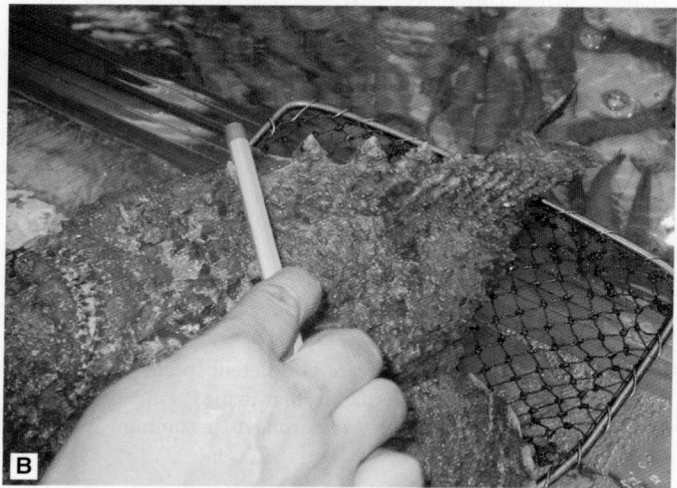

FIGURE 120–3. The Stonefish, *Synanceia spp.* Note the stinging spines on the close-up. *(Images contributed by the New York City Poison Center Toxicology Fellowship Program.)*

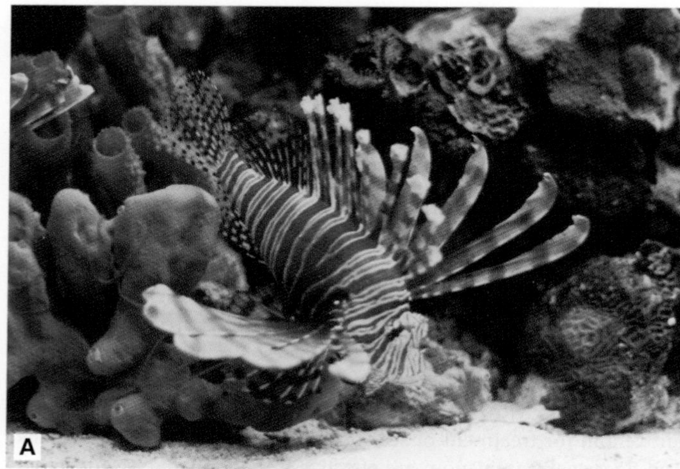

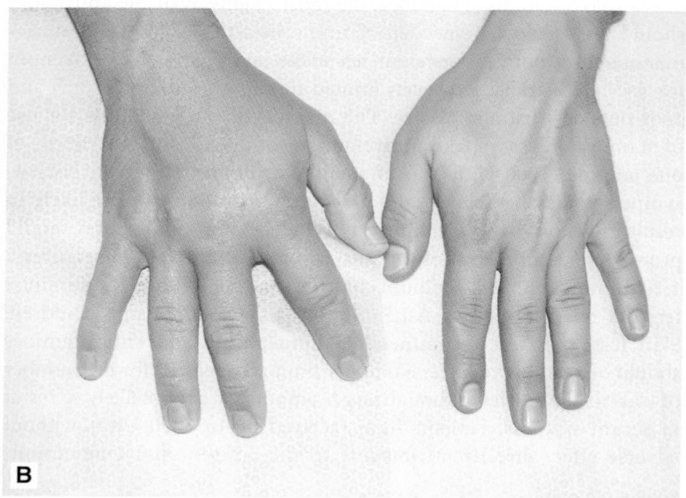

FIGURE 120–4. (**A**) The Lionfish, Pterois volitans. (**B**) This patient's hand was envenomated by his pet lionfish while cleaning his aquarium. *(Images contributed by the New York City Poison Center Toxicology Fellowship Program)*

Urolophus halleri is the most common species on the western coast of the United States. Some estimates suggest 1500 to 2000 stingray injuries occur yearly in the United States. Most envenomations occur when the animal is inadvertently stepped on. In one review a total of 17 fatalities resulting from trunk wounds, hemorrhage, or tetanus were identified worldwide.[47] Another review of 603 cases of stingray injuries identified two deaths resulting from intraabdominal trauma.[121]

Three populations are at highest risk for spiny fish envenomation: fishermen sorting the catch from nets, waders, and aquarium enthusiasts. Only five deaths from Scorpaenidae have been reported; all resulted from stonefish and are poorly documented.[38,47] No deaths from stonefish are reported in Australia, a country where they are commonly found in coastal waters.[41] The incidence of weeverfish stings is unknown, but they are a common occurrence in the summertime among Italian coastal towns.[30,130] Scorpaenidae inhabit waters throughout the tropical and temperate oceans. They exist as far north as the Gulf of Oman and Southern Japan and extend south beyond New Zealand. In the United States, Scorpaenidae stings occur in the Florida Keys, in the Gulf of Mexico, off the coast of California, and in Hawaii. Lionfish (genus *Pterois*) (Figure 120–4) are common to home aquariums and account for most poison center calls involving spiny fish envenomation in the United States. The bullrout inhabits the eastern coast of Australia, along with the cobbler, which is found only in Australia. Weeverfish inhabit shallow temperate waters with sandy or muddy bottoms in the eastern Atlantic and Mediterranean, including the European Coast extending to the southern tip of Norway.[29] The marine catfish lives in the tropical Indo-Pacific waters.

Pathophysiology Tapered, bilaterally retroserrated spines covered by an integumentary sheath emanate from the stingray tail. The ventrolateral groove contains venom glands that saturate the spine with venom and mucus. The venom contains several amino acids, serotonin, 5′-nucleotidase, and phosphodiesterase.[4] In animal models venom induces local vasoconstriction, bradydysrhythmias, atrioventricular nodal block, subendocardial ischemia, seizures, coma, cardiovascular collapse, and death.[3,121] A rabbit model demonstrates initial vasodilation followed by vasoconstriction and cardiac standstill suggesting a direct cardiac effect.[122] Wound specimens reveal necrotic muscle and neutrophilic infiltrates.[6] Other reports show central hemorrhagic necrosis with surrounding lymphoid and eosinophilic infiltrates indicating an immune-mediated cause of delayed wound healing.[66]

Scorpaenidae have 12 to 13 dorsal, two pelvic, and three anal spines that are covered with an integumentary sheath. Glands at the base contain 5 to 10 mg of venom each. Ornate pectoral fins are not venomous. Venom can remain stable for 24 to 48 hours after the fish dies.[93] Three main toxins have been isolated from various species of stonefish: stonustoxin (SNTX), verrucotoxin (VTX), and trachynilysin (TLY). SNTX, from *S. horrida*,[67] has two subunits, α and β (71,000 and 79,000 Da, respectively). It induces formation of hydrophilic pores in cell membranes.[32] Toxicity in animals includes hemolysis, local edema, vascular permeability, platelet aggregation, endothelium-dependent vasodilation, and hypotension. Decreased myocardial contractility occurs in rabbits.[125] Heating stonefish venom to 122°F (50°C) for 5 minutes prevents wound necrosis and hypotension in animal models.[150] VTX, isolated from *S. verrucosa*, shares homology with SNTX. It blocks cardiac Ca^{2+} channels.[65] TLY, isolated from *S. trachynis*, is a 159-kDa protein that forms pores in cell membranes. It allows Ca^{2+} entry and causes Ca^{2+}-dependent release of ACh from nerve endings at motor end plates and increased catecholamine release.[80,107,126] *S. trachynis* venom causes endothelium-dependent vasodilation and cardiovascular collapse in rats, which appears to be mediated by muscarinic and adrenergic receptors.[33] Hemolysis is demonstrated in animals but does not occur in human erythrocytes.[79] Other venoms of Scorpaenidae include hyaluronidase, proteinase, phosphodiesterase, alkaline phosphomonoesterase, arginine esterase, arginine amidinase, 5'-nucleotidase, acetylcholinesterase, and biogenic amines. Crude venom from *G. marmoratus*, *P. volitans*, and *S. trachynis* leads to increased intracellular Ca^{2+} and muscle contracture in vivo.[36] Toxins from other spiny fish include dracotoxin (*T. draco*), trachinine (*T. vipera*), and nocitoxin (*N. robusta*).[35] Effects mirror those of Scorpaenidae toxins.[129]

Clinical Manifestations Stepping on the body of a stingray causes a reflexive whip of the tail leading to wounds in the lower extremity. Intense pain out of proportion to the appearance of the wound is characteristic. Symptoms peak 30 to 90 minutes after injury and may persist for 48 hours. Local edema, cyanosis, erythema, and petechiae may follow rapidly and may lead to necrosis and ulceration. Systemic symptoms include weakness, nausea, vomiting, diarrhea, vertigo, headache, syncope, seizures, muscle cramps, fasciculations, hypotension, and dysrhythmias. Chest and abdominal wounds, as well as tetanus, have caused death.[113]

Stings from stonefish produce immediate, severe pain with rapid wound cyanosis and edema that may progress up the injured extremity. Pain reaches a maximum after 30 to 90 minutes and usually resolves over 6 to 12 hours, although pain may persist for days. Headache, vomiting, abdominal pain, delirium, seizures, limb paralysis, hypertension, respiratory distress, dysrhythmia, congestive heart failure, and hypotension characterize systemic toxicity.[82] Wound healing may require months.

A poison center case series from 1979 to 1988 identified 23 cases of *P. volitans* envenomation.[143] Reported symptoms included pain, swelling, nausea, numbness, joint pain, anxiety, headache, dizziness, and cellulitis. Another Poison Center series identified 51 Scorpaenidae stings (45 *P. pterois*, six *S. guttata*).[78] Intense pain was reported in 98%, extension of pain to the limb in 22%, swelling in 58%, and systemic signs (nausea, diaphoresis, dyspnea, chest pain, abdominal pain, weakness, hypotension, and syncope) in 13%. Thirteen percent of patients in the series developed wound infection; one patient's wound healing was delayed several weeks. Stings from weeverfish are similar to Scorpaenidae envenomation and rarely result in death.[13] Injury from catfish stings is comparable to that of other stinging fish.[43]

Management Wounds inflicted by stingrays and spiny fish should be carefully examined for imbedded foreign material. Radiographs may uncover retained spines. Stingray wounds can be extensive and require surgical attention for vascular or tendonous disruption. Tetanus immune status should be addressed. Prophylactic antibiotics may decrease rates of wound infection.[37] In a series of 51 stings from *P. pterois* and *S. guttata*, 80% of patients had complete relief of local pain with hot water immersion.[78] Hot water produces similar relief for pain from weeverfish stings.[120] A review of 119 stingray envenomations demonstrates comparable efficacy with hot water immersion.[37] Although patients occasionally required a single dose of oral or parenteral analgesia, clinicians rarely prescribed pain medication upon discharge. In a human volunteer study in which subjects received a subcutaneous injection of stingray venom, severe pain developed immediately, and was alleviated with water heated to 122°F (50°C).[121] Pain increased with application of cold water. Local lidocaine infiltration provides an alternate modality for pain control.[58]

Stonefish antivenom, an equine-derived IgG Fab fragment, is raised against the venom of *S. trachynis*. Each ampule contains 2000 Units and neutralizes 20 mg venom. Between 1965 and 1981, antivenom was used in at least 267 cases.[41] Anecdotal reports suggest it provides effective relief from pain.[41,149] In a review of 26 documented cases in Australia where antivenom was administered IM, no acute adverse effects were identified.[136] Two of 15 patients who had follow-up visits suffered serum sickness. Rash may develop several days postinjection.[149] In vitro and in vivo research with the antivenom demonstrates neutralization of venom from *G. marmoratus*[34] and *P. volitans*[35]; however, the application for human therapy remains untested.

The manufacturer recommends IM administration of stonefish antivenom, although IV administration may be considered. Administration is indicated for systemic toxicity or refractory pain. The number of puncture wounds guides therapy: one vial for one to two punctures, two vials for three to four punctures, and three vials for five or more punctures. Epinephrine and diphenhydramine should be readily available for treatment of anaphylactic reactions.

SUMMARY

Fatalities from marine envenomations are rare. However, significant morbidity may result from bites and stings, including severe pain, retained foreign bodies, infection, respiratory compromise, hemodynamic instability, and a variety of other end organ toxicities. Interventions should focus on patient comfort and recognition of potential complications. A thorough understanding of the mechanisms of toxicity and expected clinical course following envenomations from marine creatures will provide clinicians with the ability to manage these injuries effectively.

REFERENCES

1. Anderluh G, Barlic A, Potrich C, et al. Lysine 77 is a key residue in aggregation of equinatoxin II, a pore-forming toxin from sea anemone Actinia equina. *J Membr Biol.* 2000;173:47-55.
2. Audley I. A case of sea-snake envenomation. *Med J Aust.* 1985;143:532.
3. Auerbach PS. Hazardous marine animals. *Emerg Med Clin North Am.* 1984;2:531-544.
4. Auerbach PS. Marine envenomations. *N Engl J Med.* 1991;325:486-493.
5. Auerbach PS, Hays JT. Erythema nodosum following a jellyfish sting. *J Emerg Med.* 1987;5:487-491.
6. Barss P. Wound necrosis caused by the venom of stingrays. Pathological findings and surgical management. *Med J Aust.* 1984;141:854-855.
7. Baxter EH, Gallichio HA. Cross-neutralization by tiger snake (*Notechis scutatus*) antivenene and sea snake (*Enhydrina schistosa*) antivenene against several sea snake venoms. *Toxicon.* 1974;12:273-278.
8. Baxter EH, Gallichio HA. Protection against sea snake envenomation: comparative potency of four antivenenes. *Toxicon.* 1976;14:347-355.
9. Baxter EH, Marr AG. Sea wasp (*Chironex fleckeri*) venom: lethal, haemolytic and dermonecrotic properties. *Toxicon.* 1969;7:195-210.

10. Baxter EH, Marr GM. Sea wasp (*Chironex fleckeri*) antivenene: neutralizing potency against the venom of three other jellyfish species. *Toxicon.* 1974;12:223-229.
11. Beadnell CE, Rider TA, Williamson JA, Fenner PJ. Management of a major box jellyfish (*Chironex fleckeri*) sting. Lessons from the first minutes and hours. *Med J Aust.* 1992;156:655-658.
12. Bengtson K, Nichols MM, Schnadig V, et al. Sudden death in a child following jellyfish envenomation by *Chiropsalmus quadrumanus*. Case report and autopsy findings. *JAMA.* 1991;266:1404-1406.
13. Borondo JC, Sanz P, Nogue S, et al. Fatal weeverfish sting. *Hum Exp Toxicol.* 2001;20:118-119.
14. Boyd W. Sea-wasp antivenom in a toddler. *Med J Aust.* 1984;140:504.
15. Brown CK, Shepherd SM. Marine trauma, envenomations, and intoxications. *Emerg Med Clin North Am.* 1992;10:385-408.
16. Burnett JW. Human injuries following jellyfish stings. *Md Med J.* 1992;41:509-513.
17. Burnett JW, Bloom DA, Imafuku S, et al. Coelenterate venom research 1991-1995: clinical, chemical and immunological aspects. *Toxicon.* 1996; 34:1377-1383.
18. Burnett JW, Calton GJ. Response of the box-jellyfish (*Chironex fleckeri*) cardiotoxin to intravenous administration of verapamil. *Med J Aust.* 1983;2:192-194.
19. Burnett JW, Calton GJ. The chemistry and toxicology of some venomous pelagic coelenterates. *Toxicon.* 1977;15:177-196.
20. Burnett JW, Calton GJ. Use of IgE antibody determinations in cutaneous coelenterate envenomations. *Cutis.* 1981;27:50-52.
21. Burnett JW, Calton GJ, Morgan RJ. Dermatitis due to stinging sponges. *Cutis.* 1987;39:476.
22. Burnett JW, Gable WD. A fatal jellyfish envenomation by the Portuguese man-o'war. *Toxicon.* 1989;27:823-824.
23. Burnett JW, Goldner R. Effect of *Chrysaora quinquecirrha* (sea nettle) toxin on rat nerve and muscle. *Toxicon.* 1970;8:179-181.
24. Burnett JW, Goldner R. Effects of *Chrysaora quinquecirrha* (sea nettle) toxin on the rat cardiovascular system. *Proc Soc Exp Biol Med.* 1969;132:353-356.
25. Burnett JW, Hepper KP, Aurelian L. Lymphokine activity in coelenterate envenomation. *Toxicon.* 1986;24:104-107.
26. Burnett JW, Hepper KP, Aurelian L, et al. Recurrent eruptions following unusual solitary coelenterate envenomations. *J Am Acad Dermatol.* 1987;17:86-92.
27. Burnett JW, Othman IB, Endean R, et al. Verapamil potentiation of *Chironex* (box-jellyfish) antivenom. *Toxicon.* 1990;28:242-244.
28. Burnett JW, Rubinstein H, Calton GJ. First aid for jellyfish envenomation. *South Med J.* 1983;76:870-872.
29. Cain D. Weeverfish sting: an unusual problem. *Br Med J.* 1983;287: 406-407.
30. Carducci M, Mussi A, Leone G, Catricala C. Raynaud's phenomenon secondary to weever fish stings. *Arch Dermatol.* 1996;132:838-839.
31. Carey JE, Wright EA. The toxicity and immunological properties of some sea-snake venoms with particular reference to that of *Enhydrina schistosa*. *Trans R Soc Trop Med Hyg.* 1960;54:50-67.
32. Chen D, Kini RM, Yuen R, Khoo HE. Haemolytic activity of stonustoxin from stonefish (*Synanceja horrida*) venom: pore formation and the role of cationic amino acid residues. *Biochem J.* 1997;325:685-691.
33. Church JE, Hodgson WC. Dose-dependent cardiovascular and neuromuscular effects of stonefish (*Synanceja trachynis*) venom. *Toxicon.* 2000;38:391-407.
34. Church JE, Hodgson WC. Stonefish (*Synanceia* spp.) antivenom neutralises the in vitro and in vivo cardiovascular activity of soldier-fish (*Gymnapistes marmoratus*) venom. *Toxicon.* 2001;39:319-324.
35. Church JE, Hodgson WC. The pharmacological activity of fish venoms. *Toxicon.* 2002;40:1083-1093.
36. Church JE, Moldrich RX, Beart PM, Hodgson WC. Modulation of intracellular Ca^{2+} levels by Scorpaenidae venoms. *Toxicon.* 2003;41:679-689.
37. Clark RF, Girard RH, Rao D, et al. Stingray envenomation: a retrospective review of clinical presentation and treatment in 119 cases. *J Emerg Med.* 2007; 33:33-37.
38. Cooper NK. Historical vignette—the death of an Australian army doctor on Thursday Island in 1915 after envenomation by a stonefish. *J R Army Med Corps.* 1991;137:104-105.
39. Corkeron MA. Magnesium infusion to treat Irukandji syndrome. *Med J Aust.* 2003;178:411.
40. Currie BJ. Clinical toxicology: a tropical Australian perspective. *Ther Drug Monit.* 2000;22:73-78.
41. Currie BJ. Marine antivenoms. *J Toxicol Clin Toxicol.* 2003;41:301-308.
42. Czarnetzki BM, Thiele T, Rosenbach T. Evidence for leukotrienes in animal venoms. *J Allergy Clin Immunol.* 1990;85:505-509.
43. de Haro L, Pommier P. Envenomation: a real risk of keeping exotic house pets. *Vet Hum Toxicol.* 2003;45:214-216.
44. Edmonds C. A non-fatal case of blue-ringed octopus bite. *Med J Aust.* 1969;2:601.
45. Endean R. Separation of two myotoxins from nematocysts of the box jellyfish (*Chironex fleckeri*). *Toxicon.* 1987;25:483-492.
46. Exton DR, Fenner PJ, Williamson JA. Cold packs: effective topical analgesia in the treatment of painful stings by *Physalia* and other jellyfish. *Med J Aust.* 1989;151:625-626.
47. Fenner P. Marine Envenomations: an update—a presentation on the current status of marine envenomations first aid and medical treatments. *Emerg Med.* 2000;12:295-302.
48. Fenner P, Rodgers D, Williamson J. Box jellyfish antivenom and "Irukandji" stings. *Med J Aust.* 1986;144:665-666.
49. Fenner PJ, Fitzpatrick PF. Experiments with the nematocysts of *Cyanea capillata*. *Med J Aust.* 1986;145:174.
50. Fenner PJ, Fitzpatrick PF, Hartwick RJ, Skinner R. "Morbakka," another cubomedusan. *Med J Aust.* 1985;143:550-551, 554-555.
51. Fenner PJ, Hadok JC. Fatal envenomation by jellyfish causing Irukandji syndrome. *Med J Aust.* 2002;177:362-363.
52. Fenner PJ, Lewin M. Sublingual glyceryl trinitrate as prehospital treatment for hypertension in Irukandji syndrome. *Med J Aust.* 2003;179:655.
53. Fenner PJ, Williamson J. Experiments with the nematocysts of *Carybdea rastoni* ("Jimble"). *Med J Aust.* 1987;147:258-259.
54. Fenner PJ, Williamson J, Callanan VI, Audley I. Further understanding of, and a new treatment for, "Irukandji" (*Carukia barnesi*) stings. *Med J Aust.* 1986;145:569, 572-564.
55. Fenner PJ, Williamson JA. Worldwide deaths and severe envenomation from jellyfish stings. *Med J Aust.* 1996;165:658-661.
56. Fenner PJ, Williamson JA, Blenkin JA. Successful use of *Chironex* antivenom by members of the Queensland Ambulance Transport Brigade. *Med J Aust.* 1989;151:708-710.
57. Fenner PJ, Williamson JA, Burnett JW, Rifkin J. First aid treatment of jellyfish stings in Australia. Response to a newly differentiated species. *Med J Aust.* 1993;158:498-501.
58. Fenner PJ, Williamson JA, Skinner RA. Fatal and non-fatal stingray envenomation. *Med J Aust.* 1989;151:621-625.
59. Flachsenberger WA. Respiratory failure and lethal hypotension due to blue-ringed octopus and tetrodotoxin envenomation observed and counteracted in animal models. *J Toxicol Clin Toxicol.* 1986;24:485-502.
60. Flecker H. Irukandji sting to North Queensland bathers without production of wheals but severe general symptoms. *Med J Aust.* 1952;2:89-91.
61. Flecker H, Cotton BC. Fatal bite from octopus. *Med J Aust.* 1955;42:329-331.
62. Freeman SE. Actions of *Chironex fleckeri* toxins on cardiac trans-membrane potentials. *Toxicon.* 1974;12:395-404.
63. Fulde GW, Smith F. Sea snake envenomation at Bondi. *Med J Aust.* 1984;141:44-45.
64. Garcia PJ, Schein RM, Burnett JW. Fulminant hepatic failure from a sea anemone sting. *Ann Intern Med.* 1994;120:665-666.
65. Garnier P, Sauviat MP, Goudey-Perriere F, Perriere C. Cardiotoxicity of verrucotoxin, a protein isolated from the venom of *Synanceia verrucosa*. *Toxicon.* 1997;35:47-55.
66. Germain M, Smith KJ, Skelton H. The cutaneous cellular infiltrate to stingray envenomization contains increased TIA+ cells. *Br J Dermatol.* 2000;143:1074-1077.
67. Ghadessy FJ, Chen D, Kini RM, et al. Stonustoxin is a novel lethal factor from stonefish (*Synanceja horrida*) venom. cDNA cloning and characterization. *J Biol Chem.* 1996;271:25575-25581.
68. Grady JD, Burnett JW. Irukandji-like syndrome in South Florida divers. *Ann Emerg Med.* 2003;42:763-766.
69. Guess HA, Saviteer PL, Morris CR. Hemolysis and acute renal failure following a Portuguese man-of-war sting. *Pediatrics.* 1982;70:979-981.
70. Hartwick R, Callanan V, Williamson J. Disarming the box-jellyfish: nematocyst inhibition in *Chironex fleckeri*. *Med J Aust.* 1980;1:15-20.
71. Hastings SG, Larsen JB, Lane CE. Effects of nematocyst toxin of *Physalia physalis* (Portuguese man-of-war) on the canine cardiovascular system. *Proc Soc Exp Biol Med.* 1967;125:41-45.

72. Henderson D, Easton RG. Stingose. A new and effective treatment for bites and stings. *Med J Aust.* 1980;2:146-150.
73. Houck HE, Lipsky MM, Marzella L, Burnett JV. Toxicity of sea nettle (*Chrysaora quinquecirrha*) fishing tentacle nematocyst venom in cultured rat hepatocytes. *Toxicon.* 1996;34:771-778.
74. Huynh TT, Seymour J, Pereira P, et al. Severity of Irukandji syndrome and nematocyst identification from skin scrapings. *Med J Aust.* 2003;178:38-41.
75. Kaufman MB. Portuguese man-of-war envenomation. *Pediatr Emerg Care.* 1992;8:27-28.
76. Kent CG, Tu AT, Geren CR. Isotachophoretic and immunological analysis of venoms from sea snakes (*Laticauda semifasciata*) and brown recluse spiders (*Loxosceles reclusa*) of different morphology, locality, sex, and developmental stages. *Comp Biochem Physiol B.* 1984;77:303-311.
77. Kingston CW, Southcott RV. Skin histopathology in fatal jellyfish stinging. *Trans R Soc Trop Med Hyg.* 1960;54:373-384.
78. Kizer KW, McKinney HE, Auerbach PS. Scorpaenidae envenomation. A five-year poison center experience. *JAMA.* 1985;253:807-810.
79. Kreger AS. Detection of a cytolytic toxin in the venom of the stone-fish (*Synanceia trachynis*). *Toxicon.* 1991;29:733-743.
80. Kreger AS, Molgo J, Comella JX, et al. Effects of stonefish (*Synanceia trachynis*) venom on murine and frog neuromuscular junctions. *Toxicon.* 1993;31:307-317.
81. Larsen JB, Lane CE. Direct action of *Physalia* toxin on frog nerve and muscle. *Toxicon.* 1970;8:21-23.
82. Lehmann DF, Hardy JC. Stonefish envenomation. *N Engl J Med.* 1993;329:510-511.
83. Linaweaver PG. Toxic marine life. *Mil Med.* 1967;132:437-442.
84. Little M. Is there a role for the use of pressure immobilization bandages in the treatment of jellyfish envenomation in Australia? *Emerg Med (Fremantle).* 2002;14:171-174.
85. Little M, Mulcahy RF. A year's experience of Irukandji envenomation in far north Queensland. *Med J Aust.* 1998;169:638-641.
86. Little M, Mulcahy RF, Wenck DJ. Life-threatening cardiac failure in a healthy young female with Irukandji syndrome. *Anaesth Intensive Care.* 2001;29:178-180.
87. Little M, Pereira P, Mulcahy R, et al. Severe cardiac failure associated with presumed jellyfish sting. Irukandji syndrome? *Anaesth Intensive Care.* 2003;31:642-647.
88. Loten C, Scokes B, Worsley D, et al. A randomized controlled trial of hot water (45°C) immersion versus ice packs for pain relief in blue bottle stings. *Med J Aust.* 2006; 184:329-333.
89. Lumley J, Williamson JA, Fenner PJ, et al. Fatal envenomation by *Chironex fleckeri*, the north Australian box jellyfish: the continuing search for lethal mechanisms. *Med J Aust.* 1988;148:527-534.
90. Malovrh P, Barlic A, Podlesek Z, et al. Structure-function studies of tryptophan mutants of equinatoxin II, a sea anemone pore-forming protein. *Biochem J.* 2000;346:223-232.
91. Maretic Z, Russell FE. Stings by the sea anemone *Anemonia sulcata* in the Adriatic Sea. *Am J Trop Med Hyg.* 1983;32:891-896.
92. Martin JC, Audley I. Cardiac failure following Irukandji envenomation. *Med J Aust.* 1990;153:164-166.
93. McGoldrick J, Marx JA. Marine envenomations. Part 1: vertebrates. *J Emerg Med.* 1991;9:497-502.
94. McGoldrick J, Marx JA. Marine envenomations. Part 2: invertebrates. *J Emerg Med.* 1992;10:71-77.
95. McIntosh JM, Corpuz GO, Layer RT, et al. Isolation and characterization of a novel conus peptide with apparent antinociceptive activity. *J Biol Chem.* 2000;275:32391-32397.
96. McIntosh JM, Foderaro TA, Li W, et al. Presence of serotonin in the venom of *Conus imperialis*. *Toxicon.* 1993;31:1561-1566.
97. Mercer HP, McGill JJ, Ibrahim RA. Envenomation by sea snake in Queensland. *Med J Aust.* 1981;1:130-132.
98. Minton SA Jr. Paraspecific protection by elapid and sea snake antivenins. *Toxicon.* 1967;5:47-55.
99. Mori N, Tu AT. Isolation and primary structure of the major toxin from sea snake, *Acalyptophis peronii*, venom. *Arch Biochem Biophys.* 1988;260:10-17.
100. Muhvich KH, Sengottuvelu S, Manson PN, et al. Pathophysiology of sea nettle (*Chrysaora quinquecirrha*), envenomation in a rat model and the effects of hyperbaric oxygen and verapamil treatment. *Toxicon.* 1991;29:857-866.
101. Mustafa MR, White E, Hongo K, et al. The mechanism underlying the cardiotoxic effect of the toxin from the jellyfish *Chironex fleckeri*. *Toxicol Appl Pharmacol.* 1995;133:196-206.
102. Nielsen DB, Dykert J, Rivier JE, McIntosh JM. Isolation of Lysconopressin-G from the venom of the worm-hunting snail, *Conus imperialis*. *Toxicon.* 1994;32:845-848.
103. Nomura JT, Sato RL, Ahern RM, et al. A randomized paired comparison trial of cutaneous treatments for acute jellyfish (*Carybdea alata*) stings. *Am J Emerg Med.* 2002;20:624-626.
104. O'Leary MA, Schneider JJ, Isbister GK. Use of high performance liquid chromatography to measure tetrodotoxin in serum and urine of poisoned patients. *Toxicon.* 2004;44:549-553.
105. Olivera BM, Cruz LJ, Yoshikami D. Effects of *Conus* peptides on the behavior of mice. *Curr Opin Neurobiol.* 1999;9:772-777.
106. O'Reilly GM, Isbister GK, Lawrie PM, et al. Prospective study of jellyfish stings from tropical Australia, including the major box jelly-fish *Chironex fleckeri*. *Med J Aust.* 2001;175:652-655.
107. Ouanounou G, Malo M, Stinnakre J, et al. Trachynilysin, a neurosecretory protein isolated from stonefish (*Synanceia trachynis*) venom, forms nonselective pores in the membrane of NG108-15 cells. *J Biol Chem.* 2002;277:39119-39127.
108. Pereira PL, Carrette T, Cullen P, et al. Pressure immobilisation bandages in first-aid treatment of jellyfish envenomation: current recommendations reconsidered. *Med J Aust.* 2000;173:650-652.
109. Ramasamy S, Isbister GK, Seymour JE, Hodgson WC. Pharmacologically distinct cardiovascular effects of box jellyfish (*Chironex fleckeri*) venom and a tentacle-only extract in rats. *Toxicol Lett.* 2005;155:219-226.
110. Ramasamy S, Isbister GK, Seymour JE, Hodgson WC. The in vitro effects of two chirodropid (*Chironex fleckeri* and *Chiropsalmus* sp.) venoms: efficacy of box jellyfish antivenom. *Toxicon.* 2003;41:703-711.
111. Ramasamy S, Isbister GK, Seymour JE, Hodgson WC. The in vivo cardiovascular effects of box jellyfish *Chironex fleckeri* venom in rats: efficacy of pre-treatment with antivenom, verapamil and magnesium sulphate. *Toxicon.* 2004;43:685-690.
112. Ramasamy S, Isbister GK, Seymour JE, Hodgson WC. The in vivo cardiovascular effects of the Irukandji jellyfish (*Carukia barnesi*) nematocyst venom and a tentacle extract in rats. *Toxicol Lett.* 2005;155:135-141.
113. Rathjen WF, Halstead BW. Report on two fatalities due to stingrays. *Toxicon.* 1969;6:301-302.
114. Reid HA. Antivenom in sea-snake bite poisoning. *Lancet.* 1975;1:622-623.
115. Reid HA. Sea snake antivenene: successful trial. *Br Med J.* 1962;2:576.
116. Reid HA. Sea-snake bite research. *Trans R Soc Trop Med Hyg.* 1956;50:517-538; discussion, 539-542.
117. Riviere G, Choumet V, Audebert F, et al. Effect of antivenom on venom pharmacokinetics in experimentally envenomed rabbits: toward an optimization of antivenom therapy. *J Pharmacol Exp Ther.* 1997;281:1-8.
118. Rosson CL, Tolle SW. Management of marine stings and scrapes. *West J Med.* 1989;150:97-100.
119. Rowan EG, Harvey AL, Takasaki C, Tamiya N. Neuromuscular effects of a toxic phospholipase A2 and its nontoxic homologue from the venom of the sea snake, *Laticauda colubrina*. *Toxicon.* 1989;27:587-591.
120. Russell FE. Weeverfish sting: the last word. *Br Med J.* 1983;287:981-982.
121. Russell FE, Panos TC, Kang LW, et al. Studies on the mechanism of death from stingray venom: a report of two fatal cases. *Am J Med Sci.* 1958;235:566-584.
122. Russell FE, Van Harreveld A. Cardiovascular effects of the venom of the round stingray, *Urobatis halleri*. *Arch Int Physiol Biochim.* 1954;62:322-333.
123. Russo AJ, Calton GJ, Burnett JW. The relationship of the possible allergic response to jellyfish envenomation and serum antibody titers. *Toxicon.* 1983;21:475-480.
124. Sams W. Seabather's eruption. *Arch Dermatol.* 1949;60:227-237.
125. Saunders PR, Rothman S, Medrano VA, Chin HP. Cardiovascular actions of venom of the stonefish *Synanceja horrida*. *Am J Physiol.* 1962;203:429-432.
126. Sauviat MP, Meunier FA, Kreger A, Molgo J. Effects of trachynilysin, a protein isolated from stonefish (*Synanceia trachynis*) venom, on frog atrial heart muscle. *Toxicon.* 2000;38:945-959.
127. Schmidt ME, Abdelbaki YZ, Tu AT. Nephrotoxic action of rattlesnake and sea snake venoms: an electron-microscopic study. *J Pathol.* 1976;118:75-81.
128. Sheumack DD, Howden ME, Spence I, Quinn RJ. Maculotoxin: a neurotoxin from the venom glands of the octopus *Hapalochlaena maculosa* identified as tetrodotoxin. *Science.* 1978;199:188-189.
129. Skeie E. Toxin of the weeverfish (*Trachinus draco*). Experimental studies on animals. *Acta Pharmacol Toxicol (Copenh).* 1962;19:107-120.
130. Skeie E. Weeverfish stings. Frequency, occurrence, clinical course, treatment and studies on the venom apparatus of the weeverfish, the nature of the toxin and immunological aspects. *Dan Med Bull.* 1966;13:119-121.

131. Southcott R. Studies on Australian cubomedusae including a new genus and species apparently harmful to man. *Aust J Mar Freshw Res.* 1956;7:254-280.
132. Southcott RV, Coulter JR. The effects of the southern Australian marine stinging sponges, *Neofibularia mordens* and *Lissodendoryx* sp. *Med J Aust.* 1971;2:895-901.
133. Starr B. This story must be told—it need never have been. *Austr Skin Diving Spear Fishing Digest* 1960:10.
134. Stein MR, Marraccini JV, Rothschild NE, Burnett JW. Fatal Portuguese man-o'-war (*Physalia physalis*) envenomation. *Ann Emerg Med.* 1989;18:312-315.
135. Strutton G, Lumley J. Cutaneous light microscopic and ultrastructural changes in a fatal case of jellyfish envenomation. *J Cutan Pathol.* 1988;15:249-255.
136. Sutherland SK. Antivenom use in Australia. Premedication, adverse reactions and the use of venom detection kits. *Med J Aust.* 1992;157:734-739.
137. Sutherland SK, Lane WR. Toxins and mode of envenomation of the common ringed or blue-banded octopus. *Med J Aust.* 1969;1:893-898.
138. Taira E, Tananara N, Fanatsu M. Studies on the toxin in the spines of the starfish *Acanthaster planci*. 1. Isolation and properties of the toxin found in spines. *Sci Bull Coll Agr Univ Ryukus.* 1975;22:203-212.
139. Terlau H, Olivera BM. *Conus* venoms: a rich source of novel ion channel-targeted peptides. *Physiol Rev.* 2004;84:41-68.
140. Thomas CS, Scott SA, Galanis DJ, et al. Box jellyfish (*Carybdea alata*) in Waikiki: their influx cycle plus the analgesic effect of hot and cold packs on their stings to swimmers at the beach: a randomized, placebo-controlled clinical trial. *Hawaii Med J.* 2001;60:100-107.
141. Tibballs J, Williams D, Sutherland SK. The effects of antivenom and verapamil on the haemodynamic actions of *Chironex fleckeri* (box jellyfish) venom. *Anaesth Intensive Care.* 1998;26:40-45.
142. Tomchik RS, Russell MT, Szmant AM, Black NA. Clinical perspectives on seabather's eruption, also known as "sea lice." *JAMA.* 1993;269:1669-1672.
143. Trestrail JH 3rd, al-Mahasneh QM. Lionfish string experiences of an inland poison center: a retrospective study of 23 cases. *Vet Hum Toxicol.* 1989;31:173-175.
144. Tu AT, Salafranca ES. Immunological properties and neutralization of sea snake venoms. II. *Am J Trop Med Hyg.* 1974;23:135-138.
145. Turner B, Sullivan P. Disarming the bluebottle: treatment of *Physalia* envenomation. *Med J Aust.* 1980;2:394-395.
146. Walker DG. Survival after severe envenomation by the blue-ringed octopus (*Hapalochlaena maculosa*). *Med J Aust.* 1983;2:663-665.
147. Walker MJ, Peng Nam Y. The in vitro neuromuscular blocking properties of sea snake (*Enhydrina schistosa*) venom. *Eur J Pharmacol.* 1974;28:199-208.
148. Wallace MS, Rauck R, Fisher R, et al. Intrathecal ziconotide for severe chronic pain: safety and tolerability results of an open-label, long-term trial. *Int Anesth Research Soc.* 2008;106:628-637.
149. Wiener S. A case of stone-fish sting treated with antivenene. *Med J Aust.* 1965;191:191.
150. Wiener S. Observations on the venom of the stone fish (*Synanceja trachynis*). *Med J Aust.* 1959;46:620-627.
151. Williamson JA, Callanan VI, Hartwick RF. Serious envenomation by the Northern Australian box-jellyfish (*Chironex fleckeri*). *Med J Aust.* 1980;1:13-16.
152. Williamson JA, Le Ray LE, Wohlfahrt M, Fenner PJ. Acute management of serious envenomation by box-jellyfish (*Chironex fleckeri*). *Med J Aust.* 1984;141:851-853.
153. Winkel KD, Tibballs J, Molenaar P, et al. Cardiovascular actions of the venom from the Irunkandji (*Carukia barnesi*) jellyfish: effects in human, rat and guinea-pig tissues in vitro and in pigs in vitro. *Clin and Exper Pharm and Phys.* 2005;32:777-788.
154. Wong DE, Meinking TL, Rosen LB, et al. Seabather's eruption. Clinical, histologic, and immunologic features. *J Am Acad Dermatol.* 1994;30:399-406.
155. Wu ML, Chou SL, Huang TY, Deng JF. Sea-urchin envenomation. *Vet Hum Toxicol.* 2003;45:307-309.
156. Yoshiba S. An estimation of the most dangerous species of cone shell, *Conus* (Gastridium) *geographus* Linne, 1758, venom's lethal dose in humans. *Nippon Eiseigaku Zasshi.* 1984;39:565-572.
157. Yoshimoto CM, Yanagihara AA. Cnidarian envenomations in Hawaii improve following heat application. *Trans R Soc Trop Med Hyg.* 2002;96:300-303.
158. Zhang M. Investigation of jellyfish *Stomolophus nomurai* sting in Beidaine. *Nat Med J China.* 1988;68:489.

CHAPTER 121

SNAKES AND OTHER REPTILES

Bradley D. Riley, Anthony F. Pizon, and Anne-Michelle Ruha

Snakes in North America are common, but venomous snakes are far more consequential elsewhere in the world. In Africa and Asia, morbidity and mortality remain far higher than in the United States, where most exposures occur among snake handlers and very effective antivenom is readily available. Recognition of the local species, protection of children, and respect for the risk associated with handling a dangerous snake limit injury. If envenomation occurs, appropriate first aid and rapid assessment help avoid substantial iatrogenic morbidity and lead to essential medical care.

HISTORY AND EPIDEMIOLOGY

INCIDENCE OF VENOMOUS SNAKEBITES IN THE UNITED STATES

There are 120 species of snakes native to North America, including approximately 30 venomous species and subspecies from two families, Viperidae and Elapidae (Table 121–1). Viperidae (subfamily Crotalinae) include the rattlesnakes (genera *Crotalus and Sistrurus*) along with the copperheads and water moccasins (genus *Agkistrodon*). The vast majority of venomous snakebites in the United States that occur annually are from Crotalinae, with about 55% of these being rattlesnake bites and the rest from copperheads and water moccasins. The other family of venomous snakes native to the United States is the Elapidae, which includes the coral snakes. Fewer than 5% of poisonous snakebites are from the coral snake.[6]

Venomous snakes are found throughout the United States, except Maine, Alaska, and Hawaii. They are common in the Appalachian states, the South, and the West but are rare in New England and the northern states. There are approximately 6000 to 8000 venomous snakebites per year in the United States. Mortality from snakebite is considered to be quite rare in the United States, with estimates ranging from five to 15 deaths per year.[25] Exact statistics are lacking, but mortality rates can be significantly higher in other countries. There may be as many as 27,000 rattlesnake bites and 100 fatalities per year in Mexico[14] and thousands of deaths per year in some Southeast Asian and African countries.

Because snakes hibernate in the winter, most bites in the United States occur between May and October. Snakebites may occur at night, but the most common time for envenomation is from 2 to 6 P.M.[61] Coral snakes are particularly known for their nocturnal habits. The majority of bites occur in the extremities, but bites to the face and tongue have been reported when snakes are purposefully held near the body. The striking range of a snake is approximately one-half its length.

Children, intoxicated individuals, snake handlers, and collectors are frequent victims. More than half of the bites occur while the individual is purposely handling a known venomous snake. There is a significant market for many illegal and dangerous reptiles, and a number of individuals keep and sell exotic venomous snakes as pets. Some religious groups handle poisonous snakes (usually rattlesnakes) as a routine ceremonial practice.

IDENTIFICATION OF A VENOMOUS SNAKE

Crotalinae The venomous Crotalinae in the United States have a triangular-shaped head, vertically elliptical pupils, and easily identifiable fangs (Fig. 121–1). These fangs are paired, needlelike structures that inject venom and can retract on a hinge-like mechanism into the roof of the mouth. An adult snake usually has two fangs, but the fangs may be single or multiple. Rattlesnakes have the longest fangs, reaching 3 to 4 cm. In addition to fangs, venomous snakes also have rows of small teeth that may cause additional injury during a bite. Snakes of the subfamily Crotalinae are also called pit vipers because of the presence of a pitlike depression of the skin behind the nostril that contains a heat-sensing organ used to locate prey. The undersurface of pit vipers has a single row of plates or scales, as opposed to the double row found on nonvenomous varieties. Rattlesnakes may or may not have rattles, depending on maturity, which are occasionally heard before a strike. Water moccasins are semiaquatic and have a distinct white mouth suggesting their common name (ie, cottonmouths). They are also reported to be quite aggressive and capable of underwater bites. Copperheads are known for their reddish-brown (copper) heads and hourglass markings on their bodies (Fig. 121–2).

Elapidae The coral snakes (genera *Micruroides* and *Micrurus*) are brightly colored Elapids indigenous to North America with easily identifiable red, yellow, and black bands along the length of their bodies. Coral snakes and the similarly colored nonpoisonous scarlet king snake are often confused. In one report, 23% of victims of coral snake bites were envenomated because they erroneously believed they were dealing with the nonpoisonous scarlet king snake.[35] Coral and king snakes can be distinguished by their color patterns. Whereas coral snakes have black snouts, king snakes have red snouts. Both species have red, yellow, and black rings, but in different sequences: the red and yellow rings touch in the coral snake but in are separated by black rings king snakes ("Red on yellow kills a fellow, red on black, venom lack") (Fig. 121–3).

The fangs of coral snakes are much smaller (1–3 mm) than those of rattlesnakes, and discrete fang marks may not be obvious after envenomation. Coral snakes often hang on to a victim or "chew" for a few seconds in an attempt to deliver venom, and a history of this activity may help identify a coral snakebite when the offending reptile cannot be located.

Exact identification of a snake is often not possible unless it is brought to the hospital. This is usually impossible and poses an additional threat to the victim and to prehospital personnel. Because of the excitement generated by the bite, the victim's identification of the snake may not be accurate. Identifying a snake by its color or markings is difficult for the novice. Knowledge of the indigenous venomous snakes is more helpful to medical personnel. Snake handlers and owners of pet snakes usually know the exact species responsible for the bite, but some are reluctant to offer specific information out of fear of prosecution or confiscation of the illegal snake by authorities.

CHARACTERISTICS OF A VENOMOUS SNAKEBITE

The severity and clinical manifestations of envenomation depend on a number of factors, including the number of strikes, depth of envenomation, potency and amount of venom injected, size and underlying health of the victim, and location of the bite. Larger snakes generally inject more venom, but the potency is species variable. Children and small adults, as well as those with underlying medical conditions, such

TABLE 121–1. Medically Important North American Snakes

Genus	Species	Common Name
Crotalinae		
Crotalus	*adamanteus*	Eastern Diamondback rattlesnake
	atrox	Western Diamondback rattlesnake
	cerastes	Sidewinder
	horridus	Timber or canebrake rattlesnake
	lepidus	Rock rattlesnake
	mitchellii	Speckled rattlesnake
	molossus	Northern blacktail rattlesnake
	pricei	Twin-spotted rattlesnake
	ruber	Red diamond rattlesnake
	scutulatus	Mojave rattlesnake
	tigris	Tiger rattlesnake
	oreganus	Western rattlesnake[a]
	viridis	Prairie rattlesnake
	willardi	Ridgenose rattlesnake
Sistrurus	*catenatus*	Massasauga
	miliarius	Pygmy rattlesnake
Agkistrodon	*contortrix*	Copperhead
	piscivorus	Cottonmouth
Elapidae		
Micrurus	*fulvius*	Eastern coral snake
Micrurus	*tener*	Texas coral snake

[a] Subspecies of the Western rattlesnake include the Southern Pacific, Northern Pacific, Great Basin, Coronado Island, Arizona black, midget faded, and Grand Canyon rattlesnakes.

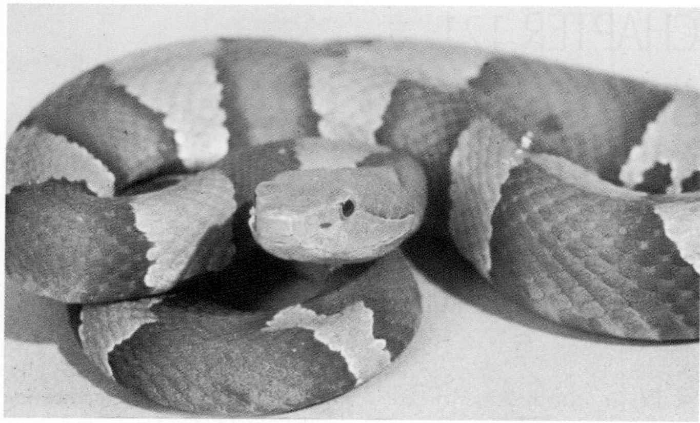

FIGURE 121–2. Copperhead (*Agkistrodon contortrix*). *(Image contributed by Banner Good Samaritan Medical Center Department of Medical Toxicology.)*

as diabetes and cardiovascular disease, may be more seriously affected by envenomation.[45] Envenomation usually occurs in subcutaneous tissues and less commonly in muscle. Systemic absorption occurs as a result of lymphatic and venous drainage of the envenomated sites. One rather bizarre observation is that individuals may be envenomated by rattlesnakes thought to be dead, even up to 60 minutes after decapitation. This is likely because of persistent reflexes in the venom apparatus.[56]

Pit vipers produce a characteristic bite when they strike, and distinct fang marks can usually be identified. The small delicate fangs of coral snakes may not produce easily identifiable fang marks. Fang marks may be single, double, and occasionally multiple. Although most snakes have two fangs, the exact number of fang marks may vary because of glancing blows or multiple strikes. Protection by clothing or shoes can

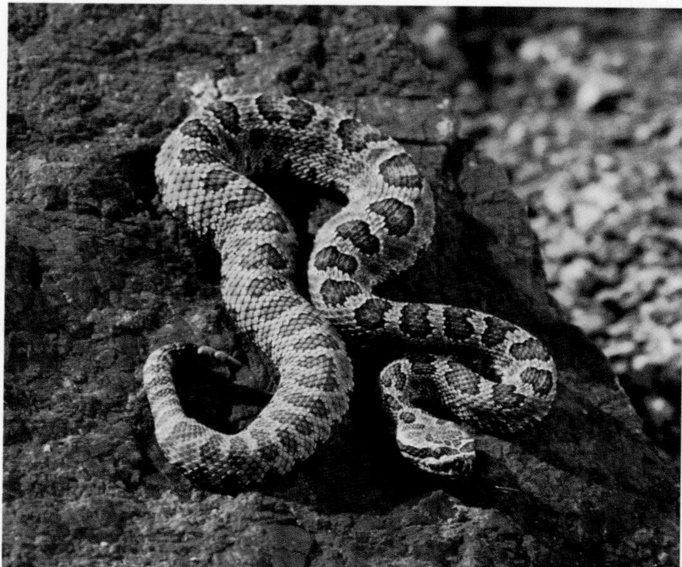

FIGURE 121–1. Pit vipers like the Hopi rattlesnake (*Crotalus viridis nuntius*) have triangular heads, which are distinct from those of nonvenomous species as well as the venomous elapids such as the coral snakes. *(Image contributed by Banner Good Samaritan Medical Center Department of Medical Toxicology.)*

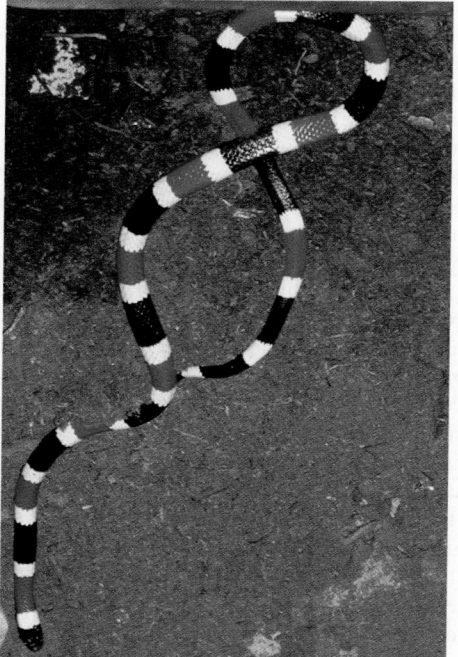

FIGURE 121–3. Sonoran coral snakes (*Micruroides euryxanthus*) demonstrate striking red, yellow, and black banding typical of North American Elapidae. *(Image contributed by Banner Good Samaritan Medical Center Department of Medical Toxicology.)*

alter classical findings. The bites of rodents or lizards and even thorn or cactus injuries may be mistaken for the bite of a poisonous snake.

PHARMACOLOGY AND PATHOPHYSIOLOGY

Snakes use their venom while hunting to incapacitate and kill prey and, when threatened, in a defensive fashion. Crotaline venom also begins the digestive process. With these different functions, it comes as no surprise then that snake venom is a complex heterogeneous solution and suspension of various proteins, peptides, lipids, and carbohydrates, with complex actions that are, in many cases, not fully understood.

The content and potency of venom in any given snake vary with size, age, diet, climate, time of year, and possible crossbreeding between different species. Not every bite from a venomous snake results in the release of venom into the victim, with so called "dry bites" occurring in up to 20% of strikes.[37] Repeat strikes may result in additional envenomation because the snake's entire quantity of venom is not usually exhausted with the first attack. After it has been exhausted, approximately 3 to 4 weeks are necessary for the snake to replenish its supply of venom.[51]

Crotaline venom can simultaneously damage tissue directly, affect blood vessels and cellular elements of blood, and alter the myoneural junction and nerve transmission. It is difficult to attribute specific pathology or pathophysiology to any particular component of snake venom. In fact, clinical effects often occur as the result of action by several venom components (Table 121–2). For instance, local tissue damage results from the action of venom metalloproteinases and hyaluronidase, which both contribute to swelling through disruption of the extracellular matrix and basement membrane surrounding microvascular endothelial cells.[29] As a result of reduced blood flow through damaged capillaries, they may also contribute to myonecrosis, which results primarily from the action of phospholipase A_2 enzymes (PLA_2) on muscle.[29] Additionally, venom metalloproteinases contribute to dermatonecrosis, both directly and through activation of endogenous inflammatory mediators.[29,58]

TABLE 121–2. Major Venom Components of Crotalinae Snakes

General Clinical Effect	Responsible Venom Components
Local tissue damage	Metalloproteinases Phospholipases A_2 Hyaluronidase
Coagulation effects[a]	C-type lectin-like proteins Metalloproteinases[b] Serine proteases[b] Phospholipases A_2
Platelet effects[c]	Disintegrins C-type lectin-like proteins Metalloproteinases Phospholipases A_2
Neurotoxic effects	Phospholipases A_2

[a] Venom contains both pro- and anticoagulants, with anticoagulant effects predominating in North American crotaline envenomation.

[b] Include thrombin-like enzymes as well as fibrino(geno)lytic enzymes.

[c] Venom may contain factors that inhibit, activate, or affect aggregation of platelets.

Venom effects on the hematologic system are especially complex. Numerous components act as anticoagulants, and many others act as procoagulants. Similarly, platelets may be inhibited, activated, agglutinated, aggregated, or inhibited from aggregating by various venom components. Venom components can be grouped according to certain characteristics, such as structure and enzymatic activity, but as noted above with local tissue damage, components within several groups may contribute to similar effects. For instance, anticoagulants in snake venoms are found among the C-type lectin-like proteins (CLPs), PLA_2 enzymes, serine proteases, and metalloproteinases. Conversely, components within a single group may have many different actions. Various CLPs in venom act as anticoagulants, procoagulants, or platelet modulators. PLA_2 enzymes are especially diverse, acting as anticoagulants and platelet modulators in addition to producing myotoxic and neurotoxic effects. Platelet effects result mainly from the action of disintegrins, although CLPs, PLA_2 enzymes and other proteinases also have platelet-modulating effects.[40,64]

Specific hematologic effects are species dependent, with no single venom containing all of the identified hemostatically active components. Of particular importance to North American rattlesnake envenomation are the thrombin-like enzymes and fibrino(geno)lytic enzymes. These are metalloproteinases and serine proteases that preferentially cleave fibrinopeptide A or fibrinopeptide B from fibrinogen. Unlike thrombin, they do not activate factor XIII. The end result is production of a poorly cross-linked fibrin clot that is easily degradable. Multiple other venom components exist, some of which affect the vascular system and contribute to the hypotension sometimes seen clinically after envenomation. Examples include bradykinin-potentiating peptides and vascular endothelial growth factors.

Coral snake venom contains neurotoxins with curare-like effects that produce systemic neurotoxicity as opposed to local tissue injury. Similar to other elapids, an α-neurotoxin binds and blocks acetylcholine receptors at motor endplates, leading to weakness. Phospholipase A_2 can also cause myotoxicity, although this appears to be of less clinical importance.

CLINICAL MANIFESTATIONS

CROTALINE ENVENOMATION

Local Reactions Symptoms may range from mild to severe, but the initial benign presentation of a pit viper bite may be very misleading[33] (Table 121–3). Generally, within minutes after significant envenomation from a pit viper, the area around the bite becomes swollen and painful. Edema may progress to involve an entire extremity within a few hours, and ecchymosis may be evident. Rarely, onset of appreciable swelling is delayed up to 10 hours. This is most often noted in lower extremity envenomations.

Hemorrhagic blisters (blebs) often form at the site of the bite after rattlesnake envenomations. This most commonly occurs after bites to the fingers but may occur at any bite location or even in dependent areas proximal or distal to the bite (Fig. 121–4). Blebs usually do not appear for several hours after the envenomation but can progress for several days. Tissue underlying blebs is often healthy, but extensive bleb development may signify underlying tissue necrosis.

In addition to local myonecrosis, generalized severe rhabdomyolysis may occur in the absence of impressive muscular swelling. This finding is considered characteristic after envenomation by the canebrake rattlesnake (*Crotalus horridus atricaudatus*) found in the Gulf Atlantic states.[11]

Systemic Signs Most bites from pit vipers that occur on the extremities are limited to local or regional pathology, but life-threatening systemic symptoms may develop. In the most severe cases, patients quickly

TABLE 121–3. Evaluation and Treatment of Crotaline Envenomation

Extent of Envenomation	Clinical Observations	Antivenom Recommended[a]	Other Treatment	Disposition
None ("dry bite")	Fang marks may be seen but no local or systemic symptoms after 8–12 hours	No	Local wound care Tetanus prophylaxis	Discharge after 8–12 hours of observation
Minimal	Minor local swelling and discomfort only with no systemic symptoms or hematologic abnormalities	No	Local wound care Tetanus prophylaxis	Admit to monitored unit for 24-hour observation
Moderate	Progression of swelling beyond area of bite with local tissue destruction, hematologic abnormalities, or systemic symptoms	Yes	IV fluids Cardiac monitoring Analgesics Follow laboratory parameters Tetanus prophylaxis	Admit to Intensive Care Unit
Severe	Marked progressive swelling and pain, with blisters, brusing, and necrosis Systemic symptoms such as vomiting, fasciculations, weakness, tachycardia, hypotension, severe coagulopathy	Yes	IV Fluids Cardiac monitoring Analgesics Follow laboratory parameters Oxygen Vasopressors as indicated Tetanus prophylaxis	Admit to Intensive Care Unit

[a] See Antidotes in Depth A36: Antivenom (Crotaline) for dosing recommendations.

develop circulatory shock or airway edema and obstruction. This may be caused by anaphylaxis or anaphylactoid reactions to venom. Rarely, patients may exhibit disseminated intravascular coagulation with spontaneous bleeding along with significant hypotension and multiorgan system failure.[22] This has been reported after intravascular envenomation.[16] Other systemic signs include confusion, vomiting, diarrhea, diaphoresis, tachycardia, metallic taste, and blurred vision. More often, early systemic symptoms are mild and include nausea, nonspecific weakness, or restlessness. Delayed systemic symptoms are also possible because venom travels by lymphatic and superficial venous channels and spreads rather slowly to reach the general circulation. Although crotaline venom may be directly nephrotoxic, renal failure is probably secondary to hemoglobinuria, myoglobinuria, or cardiovascular collapse.

Although local tissue destruction dominates the picture of Crotalinae envenomations, neurotoxic effects occur with certain species of snakes. The Mojave rattlesnake (*Crotalus scutulatus*) produces the neurotoxic Mojave toxin, which may cause weakness, cranial nerve dysfunction, and respiratory paralysis.[34] It acts at presynaptic terminals of the neuromuscular junction by inhibiting acetylcholine release. Mojave toxin is formed by a heterodimer protein made up of an acidic and a basic subunit, both of which need to be present to have a functional neurotoxin.[63] Interestingly, the production of Mojave toxin appears to be geographically distributed.[23] A western population in California produces functional Mojave toxin A, and neurotoxic effects occur but there is little to no tissue destruction. More eastern populations lack the acidic subunit and do not make functional Mojave toxin but do express metalloproteases that lead to necrosis. Mojave toxin has also been found in the venom of the Southern Pacific rattlesnake (*Crotalus halleri*) found in southern California, with envenomations leading to neurologic symptoms.[12,20] The Timber rattlesnake (*Crotalus horridus horridus*) is noted to commonly cause rippling fasciculations of the skin (myokymia), particularly of the facial muscles.[5,38]

Hematologic Significant rattlesnake envenomation may produce rather dramatic hematologic abnormalities secondary to the venom's effects on the blood coagulation pathways, endothelial cells, and platelets.[3,8,50,55] Coagulopathy or thrombocytopenia may be present with a paucity of other local or systemic effects. An initial decrease in fibrinogen levels (to near zero) and platelet count (in the 10,000–50,000/mm^3 range) along with immeasurably high prothrombin time may occur after moderate to severe crotaline envenomation. However, the vast majority of patients, regardless of which snake caused the envenomation, have no clinical bleeding, even with severe laboratory abnormalities. Thrombocytopenia appears to be especially common and often severe after the bite of the Timber rattlesnake (*Crotalus horridus horridus*).[3] The protein crotalocytin that is found in Timber rattlesnake venom causes platelet aggregation and is thought to be at least partially responsible for the thrombocytopenia.

Anaphylaxis Rarely, patients bitten by crotalines may experience classic anaphylaxis from the venom itself that may complicate evaluation or mimic a severe systemic reaction to venom. Previous sensitization to venom results in development of IgE antibodies to venom in these patients. This is thought to more often occur in patients who have previously experienced a snakebite but has also been observed in snake handlers who are thought to be sensitized through inhalation or skin contact with snake proteins. Antivenom is not indicated for the treatment of anaphylaxis, but differentiating anaphylaxis from envenomation is often clinically difficult. The presence of pruritus and urticaria or wheezing, uncommon with envenomation, should suggest anaphylaxis.[11]

Grading of Severity Envenomation is a dynamic and ever-changing process that can rapidly or unpredictably progress to serious local or

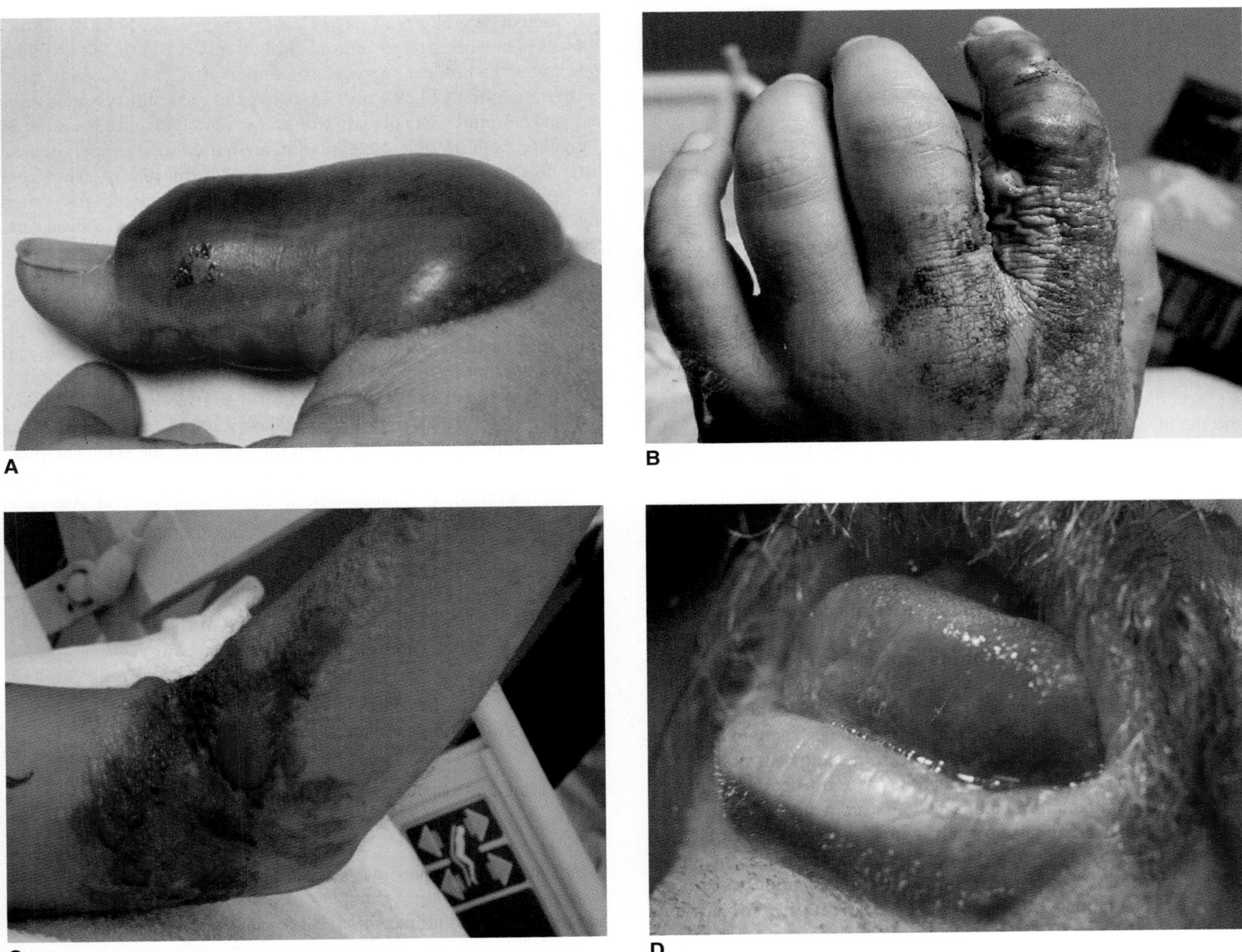

FIGURE 121-4. (**A**) Hemorrhagic bullae 24 hours after a bite by *Crotalus atrox.* (**B**) Hemorrhagic bullae 36 hours after a bite by an unknown rattlesnake. (**C**) Antecubital hemorrhagic bullae and skin necrosis (species unknown). (**D**) Tongue swelling 24 hours after a bite to the tongue by *C. atrox. (Copyright © 2002, Department of Toxicology Good Samaritan Regional Medical Center)*

systemic involvement. It may require a number of hours for the full extent of envenomation to become evident. On rare occasions, symptoms may appear to be resolving, only to return minutes to hours later with greater intensity. As a general rule, however, it may be assumed that if no symptoms develop within 8 to 12 hours from the time of the bite, envenomation from a North American pit viper has not occurred (dry bite).

A major difficulty in objectively grading the severity of crotaline envenomation and following its progress is that no scoring system readily fits the wide range of presentations. Most patients exhibit only a subset of possible consequences, so all, some, or none of the anticipated signs and symptoms may develop in any given individual. In addition, some of the characteristics of envenomation (eg, nausea, tachycardia, restlessness, and tachypnea) may be related to fear rather than to envenomation. A validated severity score for the objective assessment of crotaline envenomation has been developed and can be useful for research and clinical evaluation.[17]

Agkistrodon (water moccasins and copperhead) bites generally tend to produce less severe local and systemic pathology than rattlesnake bites. Copperhead bites in particular rarely cause systemic symptoms, and pathology is usually limited to soft tissue swelling without necrosis.[60] Although serious copperhead bites occasionally occur, no reports of death can be found in the medical literature.

ELAPID ENVENOMATION

Coral snake bites are characterized by a lack of local symptoms but potentially serious systemic symptoms. The effects of elapid envenomation are characteristically delayed for a number of hours. One report described a patient who had an asymptomatic period of 13 hours followed by a sudden and precipitous deterioration severe enough to require ventilatory support.[35] The neurologic abnormalities noted included slurred speech, paresthesias, ptosis, diplopia, dysphagia, stridor, muscle weakness, fasciculations, and respiratory paralysis.[37] The major immediate cause of death from coral snake envenomations is respiratory arrest secondary to neuromuscular weakness, with fewer cardiovascular effects occurring than in crotaline envenomation. Patients may develop total-body paralysis that may take weeks to months to resolve completely. With respiratory support, however, the paralysis is completely reversible. Pulmonary aspiration is a common sequela in the subacute phase.

It is difficult to judge initially which patients bitten by coral snakes will develop symptoms. In general, fewer than 40% of patients bitten by a coral snake are subsequently determined to have been envenomated, with rates for the Eastern coral snake species possibly higher.[35] The venom of the Eastern coral snake (*Micrurus fulvius*) and Texas coral snake (*Micrurus tener*) are more potent than that of the Sonoran coral snake (*Micruroides euryoxanthus*). In fact, there have been no reported cases of serious toxicity after the bite of the Sonoran coral snake, which is found primarily in Arizona and western New Mexico.

DIAGNOSTIC TESTING AND MANAGEMENT

OBJECTIVES FOR TREATMENT OF PATIENTS WITH ENVENOMATION

The specific treatment of a patient with a snakebite is controversial, and the literature contains confusing and contradictory recommendations. Folklore and home remedies abound. The benign natural history of many bites undoubtedly has accounted for many "miraculous cures" from such clearly unhelpful interventions as ethanol, electric shocks, carbolic acid, strychnine, cauterization, and cryotherapy. Many accepted treatment plans are based on anecdotal or biased information with conclusions drawn from animal studies or uncontrolled case reports. There are no universally accepted standards of care for many aspects of treatment.[61] The initial objectives are to determine the presence or absence of envenomation, provide basic supportive therapy, treat the local and systemic effects of envenomation, and limit or repair tissue loss or functional disability (see Table 121-3).

A combination of medical therapy (mainly supportive care and possibly antivenom) and conservative surgical treatment (mainly debridement of devitalized tissue), individualized for each patient, will provide the best results. In general, the more rapidly treatment is instituted, the shorter the period of disability, but no specific standard of care exists for the institution of various interventions.

OBSERVATION OF ASYMPTOMATIC PATIENTS

All patients reporting a history of snakebite from North American crotalines should be observed for 8 to 12 hours after the bite if the skin is broken and the offending snake cannot be positively identified as nonpoisonous. The initial presentation of pit viper bites may be misleading, and significant worsening of a seemingly benign bite may occur as long as 24 hours after presentation,[33] but such cases are unusual. Restlessness, anxiety, abdominal pain, nausea, and tachycardia are nonspecific symptoms but could signal systemic envenomation, and they should not be routinely dismissed as being a result of fear or anxiety. If the patient has been bitten by an exotic or nonnative snake, it would be prudent to extend the period of observation to 12 to 24 hours.

Eastern coral snake bites can initially be misleading with fang marks that are quite subtle and easily mistaken for scratches or teeth marks. Serious delayed neurologic and respiratory symptoms have been specifically noted, so patients bitten by these snakes should be observed for 24 hours regardless of their initial presenting symptoms. Sonoran coral snakes, indigenous to Arizona and California, have never been reported to cause significant toxicity, and bite victims can be discharged if the offending snake has been positively identified.

CROTALINE SNAKE BITES

Field Treatment for Snakebite Victims No first aid measures or specific field treatment has proven to positively affect the outcome from a crotaline envenomation, and undue importance has been placed on the immediate prehospital care of patients with snake bites. When the patient is not in extremis and medical attention is available within a few hours, the prudent approach is a conservative one. The excitement or hysteria generated by a possible poisonous snakebite compels some caregivers to intervene quickly with unproven or harmful procedures. In reality, both death and amputation are quite rare if proper medical attention is available within a few hours. Most morbidity stems from delayed treatment, either because of inaction on the patient's part (often related to alcohol intoxication) or because of inaccessible medical care. Prehospital care should generally be limited to immobilization of the patient's affected limb and rapid transport to a medical facility.[42]

In the past, various methods have been advocated to prevent systemic absorption of venom after snake bites. The traditional tourniquet that occludes venous and arterial flow is contraindicated and may compound the initial insult by increasing edema and aggravating ischemia. A constriction band is not a true tourniquet and is intended to collapse lymphatics and superficial veins; if it is applied properly, a finger may be easily placed between the band and the skin. The pressure immobilization technique with a constriction band has been used in the treatment of nonnecrotizing elapid snakebites in Australia, where systemic toxicity is the major concern and transit times can be prolonged.[62] Utility of this technique for the more necrotizing bite of North American crotalines has not been demonstrated. A randomized, controlled study of pressure immobilization versus observation in a porcine model with intramuscular injection of *Crotalus atrox* venom showed a prolonged time to death in the pressure immobilization group but also markedly increased compartment pressures. With local tissue necrosis, the major morbidity associated with North American crotaline envenomations, not death, the authors concluded that pressure immobilization with a compression bandage cannot be suggested as a routine field procedure.[9]

Incision and suction, whether by mouth or with a commercially available device, cannot be recommended as standard first aid in the field. Incision may lead to damage of underlying structures such as nerves and tendons, and mouth suction is unproven and may introduce bacteria into the wound. Commercially available plunger-type suction devices in human models provide no benefit, and additional injury is possible from the device. Venom extractors are currently unproved therapy and are not recommended.[1,10] Simple suction cups supplied in first aid kits are worthless.

It should be stressed that compression dressings and vacuum extraction should not be considered if the patient can rapidly reach a hospital. Minor pain or swelling is not an indication for zealous field treatment. Furthermore, these treatments are never a substitute for rapid transport, in-hospital evaluation, or antivenom therapy. The bitten area should not be placed in ice because cryotherapy is not effective in neutralizing venom and may compound the initial injury.[41]

Immediate In-Hospital Therapy The initial in-hospital assessment of a patient with a snakebite should focus on airway, breathing, and circulation. Early airway management with endotracheal intubation should be considered in all patients with bites to the face or tongue.[21] Intravenous (IV) lines should be placed and fluid boluses initiated. An epinephrine continuous infusion, starting at 0.1 μg/kg/minute and titrating as needed, is the vasopressor of choice for signs of shock. A complete medical history, including current tetanus immunization status and known allergies, should be obtained. A careful description of the bite and the extent of the local pathology should be documented, including measuring the diameter of the extremity and noting the extent of edema by marking the skin with a pen to help recognize progression of the envenomation. This evaluation should be repeated frequently as required by the clinical condition. A comprehensive physical examination should be done, with emphasis on vital signs, cardiorespiratory and neurologic status, neurovascular status of the extremity, and evaluation for evidence of bleeding. A baseline complete blood count, electrolytes, urinalysis, creatinine, glucose, prothrombin time (PT), fibrinogen level, and platelet count should be obtained initially, with platelets, fibrinogen, and PT repeated in 4 to 6 hours.

Pain and anxiety should be alleviated and tetanus prophylaxis addressed. The extremity should be immobilized in a well-padded splint in near-full extension and elevated to avoid dependent edema. This is especially important with hand bites because significant swelling of the hand and forearm mimicking compartment syndrome may be avoided. The patient should be reassessed frequently with repeat physical examinations, specifically noting any progression of swelling. This may be accomplished by taking measurements of the circumference of the involved extremity at multiple points proximal to the wound.

Antivenom Therapy For Crotalinae envenomations, antivenom should be considered as first line therapy for those patients with moderate to severe envenomations (see Table 121–3). Although each case must be individualized, in the vast majority of patients who have a moderate or severe envenomation, the benefits of antivenom therapy outweigh the risks. Antivenom given in a timely manner can reverse coagulopathy and thrombocytopenia and halt progression of local swelling. There is no evidence, however, that antivenom can prevent the development of tissue necrosis, so patients should be informed of the risk of tissue loss. This is most commonly noted with rattlesnake bites to the fingers, which occasionally lead to amputation of the digit despite appropriate treatment with antivenom.

The only currently available antivenom for North American pit viper envenomations is Crotalidae polyvalent immune Fab (CroFab™, Protherics, Savage Laboratories). CroFab is an ovine-derived Fab fragment antivenom developed from commonly encountered North American pit vipers. It is less allergenic than the previously available equine-derived Antivenin Crotalidae Polyvalent (Wyeth-Ayerst). CroFab is administered IV in an initial dose of four to six vials reconstituted in normal saline. The infusion is initiated at a slow rate, and if no signs of an anaphylactoid reaction develop, increased to complete the infusion over one hour. The patient should be reassessed after completion of the infusion for evidence of continued swelling or coagulopathy, and, if present, an additional four to six vial dose is infused. This process is repeated until control of symptoms is achieved. Control is generally considered cessation of progression of swelling and systemic symptoms in addition to improvement in coagulopathy and thrombocytopenia. After control has been gained, maintenance doses are given as two vials every 6 hours times three, for six total additional vials. Antivenom therapy is discussed in detail in Antidotes in Depth A36: Antivenom (Crotaline and Elapid).

Surgical Therapy Envenomation may mimic a compartment syndrome by producing distal paresthesias, tense soft tissue swelling, pain on passive stretch of muscles within a compartment, and muscular weakness. However, because subfascial envenomation is uncommon, much of the impressive edema produced by envenomation does not occur in compartmentalized areas. Using noninvasive vascular arterial studies and skin temperature determinations in patients with rattlesnake envenomation, one report demonstrated that pulsatile arterial blood flow to an envenomated extremity actually increased after envenomation, even distal to the site of envenomation.[15] Compartment syndrome cannot be reliably diagnosed in envenomated extremities without directly measuring compartment pressures. Although there is little doubt that some crotaline bites may eventually require some surgical debridement or even skin grafting, the initial routine use of tissue excision or "exploration and debridement" is not recommended.[30,57] Fasciotomy is rarely needed and should be done only based on objective data of measured compartment pressures. Successful treatment of documented elevated compartment pressure after rattlesnake evenomation with antivenom and mannitol alone has been reported.[26] Debridement of hemorrhagic blebs and blisters may be performed to evaluate underlying tissue and relieve discomfort. Some patients may require surgical debridement of necrotic tissue or even amputation of a digit 1 to 2 weeks after the bite. Referral to a hand surgeon is most appropriate for patients with evidence of extensive tissue necrosis. Physical therapy should be instituted early to ameliorate joint stiffness and decrease swelling.

Blood Products Immeasurably low fibrinogen levels, prothrombin times greater than 100 seconds, and platelet counts lower than 20,000 are routinely encountered after rattlesnake envenomation, and such abnormal laboratory results alone should not prompt the clinician to treat with blood products in the absence of clinically significant bleeding. The circulating crotaline venom responsible for the initial bleeding diathesis is still present and will likely inactivate any component transfusions. For this reason, the mainstay of treatment for crotaline envenomation–induced coagulopathy is antivenom, not blood products. Correction of laboratory coagulation abnormalities and bleeding can frequently be achieved with antivenom alone. Monitoring trends in the coagulation profile is one objective way of assessing the seriousness of envenomation and the response to antivenom therapy.

Rarely, a patient will have active bleeding, and antivenom alone will not correct the coagulopathy. In such cases, fresh frozen plasma, cryoprecipitate, packed red blood cells, or platelet transfusions may be required. The criteria for the use of blood products appears to be quite arbitrary in clinical practice, but in general, blood products should be administered along with antivenom if the patient is actively bleeding.

Venom-induced thrombocytopenia that occurs after bites by many rattlesnake species is responsive to treatment with antivenom. The Timber rattlesnake, however, is known for producing thrombocytopenia resistant to antivenom. In some cases, thrombocytopenia may be difficult, or impossible, to totally correct with even large amounts of antivenom. The initial correction of platelet counts that occurs after treatment may be transient (lasting only 12–24 hours), with thrombocytopenia sometimes persisting for days to weeks after normalization of other coagulation parameters. In the absence of bleeding, thrombocytopenia is a benign, self-limiting disorder, resolving within 2 to 3 weeks of envenomations. It may be best to closely follow patients with resistant thrombocytopenia who are not bleeding clinically rather than attempt further platelet transfusions or antivenom administration.[13]

COPPERHEAD ENVENOMATIONS

Victims of proven copperhead bites should be observed for 4 to 6 hours and evaluated for signs of systemic involvement, the development of coagulation abnormalities, and progression of the local pathology. In the absence of progression of local symptoms and the lack of any systemic symptoms, this shorter observation period may be sufficient. In many instances, the entire care of a patient with a minimal copperhead envenomation can be accomplished in the emergency department, but a conservative approach is advised. Hospital admission for further observation is warranted for unreliable patients or if there are questions as to the identification of the snake or progression of symptoms.[50]

OTHER CONSIDERATIONS

Prophylactic antibiotics are not needed because studies show extremely low (0%–3%) rates of wound infections.[39] There is no rationale for the use of corticosteroids or antihistamines in the routine treatment of patients with snakebites, except for the rare case of anaphylaxis. Tetanus prophylaxis should be administered as clinically indicated.

Cardiovascular collapse is a life-threatening consequence of severe systemic crotaline envenomation and should be treated aggressively. It may be prudent to use initial doses of eight to 10 vials of antivenom as opposed to the four to six vial doses indicated for mild to moderate envenomations, although this has not been studied. Blood pressure support with epinephrine may be required, and respiratory compromise should be anticipated in severe cases. Because of sudden and unpredictable respiratory paralysis associated with coral snake envenomation, tracheal intubation should be considered at the first sign of bulbar paralysis.

RECURRENCE PHENOMENA OF CROTALINE ENVENOMATION

In a significant proportion of patients treated with Crotalidae polyvalent immune Fab antivenom, a return of swelling, coagulopathy, or thrombocytopenia may be noted after initial successful resolution of the effect after antivenom initial treatment. This has been termed *recurrence of venom effect* and is attributed to the interrelated kinetics and dynamics of venom and antivenom.[4,54] Simply stated, Fab antivenom has a clinical half-life shorter than that of venom. Administration of "maintenance" doses of antivenom are used in an attempt to prevent development of recurrent effects. Anecdotally, this appears to be effective in preventing recurrence of local swelling in most cases, but many patients develop hematologic recurrence within 3 to 4 days of antivenom treatment despite administration of maintenance doses. Additionally, patients who never manifested thrombocytopenia or coagulopathy on their hospital presentation may later develop the effect, presumably because of initial "masking" of the effect by early antivenom. The exact clinical significance of these observations and the need for clinical intervention are uncertain. Currently, the most reasonable way to address possible recurrent hematologic effects of crotaline envenomation is careful outpatient follow-up after hospital discharge. The safest approach is to measure platelets and coagulation studies in all patients with rattlesnake envenomation 3 to 5 days after the last antivenom treatment. If values are abnormal or trending in the wrong direction, the studies should be repeated every few days until normalized. Patients should be advised to avoid surgical procedures and activities that place them at risk for injury. Opinions on when to retreat patients exhibiting recurrence with antivenom vary. Our general approach is to treat any patient with evidence of bleeding and recurrence, as well as patients with severe isolated thrombocytopenia (platelets <30,000/mm^3) or moderate thrombocytopenia (platelets 30,000–50,000 /mm^3) in combination with severe coagulopathy (fibrinogen <80 mg/dL). Many clinicians choose to cautiously observe patients with isolated coagulopathy as outpatients rather than to retreat them with antivenom.

SPECIAL CONSIDERATIONS FOR THE MANAGEMENT OF PREGNANT PATIENTS WITH SNAKEBITES

There is scant information available on the effects of poisonous snakebites during pregnancy. Case series show that although maternal death is rare, fetal demise may be as high as 43%.[18] Proposed mechanisms of injury to the fetus from envenomation include uterine artery hypotension with subsequent hypoxia, hemorrhagic complications such as abruptio placentae, and uterine contractions initiated by venom. As in each case of snakebite, it is prudent to evaluate the need for antivenom carefully during pregnancy. A single case report exists of a woman treated with CroFab in the third trimester of pregnancy without complications.[36] Given the relative safety of this antivenom and the high rate of fetal demise after envenomation, a low threshold for treatment should be considered. Fetal and maternal monitoring should be carried out throughout the patient's care.[19]

Repeated Exposure to Snake Venom. Snake handlers and collectors are at risk for multiple bites over their careers, and questions have been raised about possible immunity. No evidence was established that immunity develops as a result of repeated envenomation in one report of 14 patients with two or more bites.[46] Victims of repeat bites may actually be at greater risk for anaphylaxis because of prior sensitization and the development of IgE antibodies to venom.

TREATMENT OF CORAL SNAKE ENVENOMATION

The benign local effects of coral snake envenomation can be misleading and mistakenly equated with a dry bite.[44] Because it is difficult to judge initially which patients are envenomated, any patient with a confirmed coral snake exposure with fang marks or other evidence of skin penetration is recommended to receive antivenom therapy even in the absence of symptoms. This currently presents a problem because North American Coral Snake Antivenin, produced by Wyeth Pharmaceuticals, has been discontinued. Limited remaining supplies expired in October 2009. Until another antivenom becomes available, patients must be treated supportively with close observation and mechanical ventilation when indicated. Acetylcholinesterase inhibitors, neostigmine 0.5 mg, and edrophonium 10 mg have been successfully used to treat patients with South American coral snake bites, but their use should be considered experimental.[7]

A conservative approach is taken even for patients with less suspicion for envenomation. Any patient in whom coral snake bite cannot be excluded requires 24 hours of observation in a monitored unit where resuscitative measures, including endotracheal intubation, can be performed. Clinical deterioration may be totally unexpected and progress rapidly. In one series, 15% of patients required intubation and ventilation, but none died or suffered tissue loss or permanent neurologic sequelae.[37] Surgery is not a concern because no local tissue destruction is seen. Coral snake venom does not alter coagulation, so no bleeding diathesis is to be expected. Eastern coral snake envenomation can be fatal, but with supportive care and antivenom therapy, if available, patients usually recover completely.

EXOTIC SNAKEBITE

About 3% of poisonous snakebites reported in the United States are from nonnative species.[2,27] Many such snakes are owned by collectors, illegally imported, or stolen from zoos or pet stores. However, private individuals may easily purchase a plethora of vipers, cobras, and adders by mail or at reptile shows. Out of fear of legal retribution, some owners of exotic snakes can be quite vague about the circumstances of their envenomation. If they do not provide accurate identification, the local zoo, regional poison center, or herpetology society may be helpful in identification.

Bites from many nonnative Elapidae snakes, such as mambas, kraits, cobras, and several Australian species, are associated with high morbidity and mortality rates. Approximately one-third of bites from the king cobra are fatal.[27] Bites from these snakes may not display early local or systemic signs; therefore, the grading system developed for North American pit vipers is not helpful. Although local tissue destruction and edema may develop, classically, it is the neurologic signs, such as ptosis, dysphagia, muscular weakness, paresis, ophthalmoplegia, and respiratory failure that are noted. Cobra envenomation usually produces significant local toxicity, and these snakes are the only elapids whose venom possesses hemorrhagic activity.

Compression immobilization of an entire extremity with an elastic bandage (the Sutherland wrap) for the bite of some elapids (eg, sea snakes, kraits, cobras, and brown snakes) experimentally decreases the movement of elapid snake venom from the bite site to the systemic circulation and may be useful when antivenom is not available. This intervention, when it does not delay transport to medical care, has been recommended for bites from exotic elapids.[62] Local incision and suction should be avoided.

After the snake has been identified, attempts should be made to obtain appropriate antivenom. A good place to start is by contacting a regional poison center (800-222-1222) that has access to the Online Antivenom Index, a listing of available antivenoms for exotic snakes. Zoos may also stock exotic antivenoms and may be useful resources. Guidelines for the administration of antivenom for exotic snakes are vague and empiric. In addition, there is little standardization of the antivenoms for the same snake by different manufacturer. Because exotic snakes are generally quite poisonous, if fang marks are present, envenomation is strongly suspected, the snake has been identified, and the specific antivenom has been obtained, many physicians believe that it is logical to proceed with antivenom administration empirically. Antivenom is administered according to the package insert under the same monitoring guidelines as for crotaline antivenom. If the antivenom cannot be obtained then supportive care and close in-hospital observation, with prolonged mechanical ventilation in severe cases, may be all that is possible. Crotalidae polyvalent immune Fab (CroFab) may be effective in South American pit viper envenomations.[49]

One report documents rather dramatic reversal of the neurotoxic effects of a monocellate cobra (*Naja kaouthia*) bite after IV administration of the anticholinesterase neostigmine methyl sulfate (0.5 mg every 20 minutes for four doses).[24] The major neurotoxin from this snake is believed to resemble curare, causing a postsynaptic blockade of nicotinic neuromuscular receptor sites. The neurotoxicity from sea snakes and other elapids has been experimentally reversed with neostigmine.[53] Edrophonium chloride (10 mg administered IV with 0.5 mg of atropine) has also been suggested.

NONVENOMOUS SNAKEBITES

There are approximately 50,000 snakebites annually in the United States, and most (90%–95%) are from nonvenomous snakes.[25] Most snakes in the United States are nonvenomous, and the majority are of the Colubrid family, which are generally considered harmless to humans. However, several authors have reported toxic secretions from Duvernoy glands in many common species, including the hognose snake, garter snake, parrot snake, banded water snake, and ringneck snake.[28,43] Although no deaths have been reported, some victims developed coagulopathies and local edema and hemorrhage that could be confused with early crotaline envenomation.[41] There is no antivenom available to treat bites from these snakes, and serious complications from nonvenomous snakebites are extremely rare.

When there is no sign of envenomation after an appropriate period of observation after a suspected nonpoisonous snakebite, attention should be focused on the basic principles of wound care. Incision and suction, excision, and wide debridement are unnecessary in such bites. The wound should be treated as a contaminated puncture wound because it may contain foreign material, especially broken teeth. Any foreign material should be removed and an appropriate dressing applied. Certain large snakes of the Biodae family (not seen in the United States, except as pets or in zoologic gardens), including boas, pythons, and anacondas, may present a special problem because the force of contraction of their jaws may be great enough to cause severe tissue contusion or fractures and retained teeth. These reptiles also have numerous large, brittle teeth that commonly are broken off and lodged in the wound when the bitten part is forcibly extricated from the snake's mouth. Radiographs of the bitten area are needed to exclude fracture or foreign body.

Antibiotics are not recommended for routine use after nonvenomous snakebites. In one report, no infections occurred after snakebites in 72 patients bitten by a variety of nonpoisonous snakes indigenous to New England and imported boa constrictors and pythons.[59] Although *Clostridium tetani* has not been isolated from the mouths of snakes, the ubiquitous nature of this organism requires prophylaxis after the recommended approach for a contaminated wound. A cogent argument can be made for administering prophylactic antibiotics in nonvenomous snakebites if tooth fragments are retained or if there is significant soft tissue contusion. Outpatient therapy is appropriate; the patient should be instructed with regard to wound care and to seek medical care if signs of infection occur. Minor abrasions from nonvenomous snakes require only local wound care and tetanus prophylaxis. Delayed infection should prompt an investigation for a retained foreign body, especially a tooth fragment.[32]

OTHER POISONOUS REPTILES IN THE UNITED STATES

In North America, there are two indigenous species of venomous lizards that belong to the order Squamata, the same order as venomous snakes: the Gila monster (*Heloderma suspectum*) and the beaded lizard (*Heloderma horridum*). These lizards are found primarily in the desert areas of Arizona, southwestern Utah, southern Nevada, New Mexico, California, and Mexico. They are large, slow-moving, nocturnal, thick-bodied lizards that are prized by collectors and hobbyists. Adults are 30 to 40 cm long and are generally shy creatures, so bites are relatively rare and usually secondary to handling. Gila monsters are known for their forceful bites and propensity to hang on tenaciously during a bite, and they may be difficult to disengage. Some rather innovative anecdotal techniques have been developed to remove a Gila monster from an extremity, including the use of chisels, screwdrivers, and crowbars; pouring gasoline or ammonia into the lizard's mouth; or holding a flame to the animal's jaw. Teeth may break off in the wound.

Gila monster venom is complex, containing components similar to those of snake venoms, including numerous enzymes, hyaluronidase, phospholipase A, kallikrein, and serotonin.[31,52] Helothermine is the suspected toxin. Their venom delivery systems are not as efficient as those of poisonous snakes and consist of venom glands and grooved teeth rather than fangs. Dry bites often occur because of the ineffective mechanism of delivery. After skin puncture and venom release, the victim experiences local tenderness and soft tissue swelling, pain, and edema. There are occasional reports of anaphylactoid reactions; hypotension; angioedema of lip, tongue, and throat; respiratory depression; coagulopathy; and myocardial infarction.[47,48] Significant tissue destruction is unusual, but maceration may occur, and a cyanosis or blue discoloration is noted about the wound. There is no antivenom available against lizard venom. Treatment consists of avoiding overaggressive local treatment and providing supportive care and wound care. Epinephrine, corticosteroids, and antihistamines may be indicated for the treatment of anaphylactoid reactions. Serious morbidity from lizard bites is unusual. The characteristics of the beaded lizard are similar, but their bites are less commonly confronted clinically.

SUMMARY

Clinicians face numerous critical decisions when treating patients with venomous snakebites. These patients should be rapidly assessed for signs and symptoms of envenomation through a careful history and examination along with judicious use of laboratory data. For significant envenomations, supportive care and early use of antivenom, when available, are the mainstays of treatment.

REFERENCES

1. Alberts BM, Shalit M, LoGalbo F. Suction for venomous snakebite: a study of "mock venom" extraction in a human model. *Ann Emerg Med.* 2004;43:181-186.
2. Bey TA, Boyer L, Walter FG, et al. Exotic snakebite: envenomation by an African puff adder. *J Emerg Med.* 1997;15:827-831.

3. Bond GR, Burkhart KK. Thrombocytopenia following timber rattlesnake envenomation. *Ann Emerg Med.* 1997;30:40-44.
4. Boyer LV, Seifert SA, Cain JS. Recurrence phenomena after immunoglobulin therapy for snake envenomations: part 2. Guidelines for clinical management with Crotaline Fab antivenom. *Ann Emerg Med.* 2001;37:196-210.
5. Brick JF, Gutmann L, Brick J, et al. Timber rattlesnake venom-induced myokymia: evidence of peripheral nerve origin. *Neurology.* 1987;37:1545-1546.
6. Bronstein AC, Spyker DA, Cantilena LR. 2006 Annual report of the American Association of Poison Control Centers' National Poison Data Systems (NPDS). *Clin Toxicol.* 2007;45:815-917.
7. Bucaretchi F, Hyslop S, Vieira RJ, et al. Bites by coral snakes (*Micrurus* spp) in Campinas, State of Sao Paulo, Southeastern Brazil. *Rev Inst Trop Sao Paulo.* 2006;48(3):141-145.
8. Burgess JL, Dart RC. Snake venom coagulopathy: use and abuse of blood products in the treatment of pit viper envenomation. *Ann Emerg Med.* 1991;20:795-780.
9. Bush SP, Green, SM, et al. Pressure immobilization delays mortality and increases intracompartmental pressure after artificial intramuscular rattlesnake envenomation in a porcine model. *Ann Emerg Med.* 2004;44:599-604.
10. Bush SP, Hegewald KG, Green SM, et al. Effects of a negative pressure venom extraction device (Extractor) on local tissue injury after artificial rattlesnake envenomation in a porcine model. *Wild Environ Med.* 2000;11:180-188.
11. Bush SP, Jansen PW. Severe rattlesnake envenomation with anaphylaxis and rhabdomyolysis. *Ann Emerg Med.* 1995;25:845-848.
12. Bush SP, Siedenburg E. Neurotoxicity associated with suspected Southern Pacific rattlesnake envenomation. *Wild Environ Med.* 1999;10:247-249.
13. Bush SP, Wu VH, Corbett SW. Rattlesnake venom-induced thrombocytopenia response to Antivenin (*Crotalidae*) Polyvalent: a case series. *Acad Emerg Med.* 2000;7:181-185.
14. Cruz NS, Alvarez RG. Rattlesnake bite complications in 19 children. *Pediatr Emerg Care.* 1994;10:30-33.
15. Curry SC, Kraner JC, Kunkel DB, et al. Noninvasive vascular studies in management of rattlesnake envenomation to extremities. *Ann Emerg Med.* 1985;4:1081-1084.
16. Curry SC, Kunkel DB. Death from a rattlesnake bite. *Am J Emerg Med.* 1985;3:227-235.
17. Dart RC, Hurlbut KM, Garcia R, Bkoren J. Validation of severity score for the assessment of crotaline snakebite. *Ann Emerg Med.* 1996;27:321-326.
18. Dunnihoo DR, Rush BM, Wise RB et al. Snakebite poisoning in pregnancy: a review of the literature. *J Reproductive Med.* 1992;37:653-658.
19. Entman SS, Moise KJ. Anaphylaxis in pregnancy. *South Med J.* 1984;77:402.
20. French WJ, Hayes WK, Bush SP, et al. Mojave toxin in venom of *Crotalus helleri* (Southern Pacific rattlesnake): molecular and geographic characterization. *Toxicon.* 2004;44:781-799.
21. Gerkin R, Sergent K, Curry SC. Life-threatening airway obstruction from rattlesnake bite to the tongue. *Ann Emerg Med.* 1987;16:813-816.
22. Gibly RL, Nowlin SW, Berg RA. Intravascular hemolysis associated with North American crotaline envenomation. *J Toxicol Clin Toxicol.* 1998;36:337-343.
23. Glenn JL, Straight RC, Wolfe MC, Hardy DL. Geographical variation in Crotalus scutulatus scutulatus (Mojave rattlesnake) venom properties. *Toxicon.* 1983;21:119-130.
24. Gold BS. Neostigmine for the treatment of neurotoxicity following envenomation by the Asiatic cobra. *Ann Emerg Med.* 1996;28:87-89.
25. Gold BS, Barish RA: Venomous snakebites: current concepts in diagnosis, treatment and management. *Emerg Med Clin North Am.* 1992; 10:249-267.
26. Gold BS, Barish RA, Dart RC, et al. Resolution of compartment syndrome after rattlesnake envenomation utilizing non-invasive measures. *J Emerg Med.* 2003;24(3):285-288.
27. Gold BS, Pyle P. Successful treatment of neurotoxic king cobra envenomation in Myrtle Beach, South Carolina. *Ann Emerg Med.* 1998; 32:736-738.
28. Gomez HF, Davis M, Phillips S, McKinney P, Brent J. Human envenomation from a wandering garter snake. *Ann Emerg Med.* 1994;23:1117-1118.
29. Gutierrez JM, Lomonte B, Leon G, et al. Trends in snakebite envenomation therapy: scientific, technological and public health considerations. *Curr Pharm Des.* 2007;13:2935-2950.
30. Hall EL. Role of surgical intervention in the management of crotaline snake envenomation. *Ann Emerg Med.* 2001;37:175-180.
31. Hendon RA, Tu AT. Biochemical characterization of the lizard toxin gilatoxin. *Biochemistry.* 1981;20:3517-3522.
32. Herman RS. Nonvenomous snakebite. *Ann Emerg Med.* 1988;17:1262-1263.
33. Hurlbut KM, Dart RC, Spaite D. Reliability of clinical presentation for predicting significant pit viper envenomation. *Ann Emerg Med.* 1988;12:438.
34. Jansen PW, Perkin RM, VanStralen D. Mojave rattlesnake envenomation: prolonged neurotoxicity and rhabdomyolysis. *Ann Emerg Med.* 1992;21:322-325.
35. Kitchens CS, Van Mierop LHS. Envenomation by the eastern coral snake (*Micrurus fulvius fulvius*). *JAMA.* 1987;258:1615-1618.
36. Kravitz J, Gerardo CJ. Copperhead snakebite treated with crotalidae polyvalent immune fab (ovine) antivenom in third trimester pregnancy. *Clin Toxicol (Phila).* 2006;44(3):353-354.
37. Kunkel DB, Curry SC, Vance MV, Ryan PJ. Reptile envenomations. *J Toxicol Clin Toxicol.* 1983-84;21:503-526.
38. Lewis RL, Gutmann L. Snake venoms and the neuromuscular junction. *Semin Neurol.* 2004;24(2)175-179.
39. LoVecchio F, Klemens J, Welch S, Rodriguez R. Antibiotics after rattlesnake envenomation. *J Emerg Med.* 2002;23(4):327-328.
40. Lu Q, Clemetson JM, Clemetson KJ. Snake venoms and hemostasis. *J Thromb Haemost.* 2005;3(8):1791-1799.
41. McCollough N, Gennaro J. Evaluation of venomous snakebite in the southern United States. *J Fla Med Assoc.* 1963;49:959-967.
42. McKinney PE. Out-of-hospital and interhospital management of Crotaline snakebite. *Ann Emerg Med.* 2000;37:168-174.
43. McKinstry DM. Evidence of toxic saliva in some colubrid snakes of the United States. *Toxicon.* 1978;16:523-534.
44. Norris RL, Dart RC. Apparent coral snake envenomation in a patient without visible fang marks. *Am J Emerg Med.* 1989;7(4):402-405.
45. Parrish HM, Goldner JC, Silbert SL. Comparison between snakebites in children and adults. *Pediatrics.* 1965;36:251.
46. Parrish HM, Pollard CB. Effects of repeated poisonous snakebites in man. *Am J Med Sci.* 1959;237, 277-286.
47. Placentine J, Curry SC, Ryan PJ. Life-threatening anaphylaxis following Gila monster bite. *Ann Emerg Med.* 1986;15:147-149.
48. Preston CA. Hypotension, myocardial infarction, and coagulopathy following Gila monster bite. *J Emerg Med.* 1989;7:38-40.
49. Richardson WH 3rd, Tanen DA, Tong TC. Crotalidae polyvalent immune Fab (ovine) antivenom is effective in the neutralization of South American viperidae venoms in a murine model. *Ann Emerg Med.* 2005;45(6):595-602.
50. Roberts JR, Greenberg JI. Ascending hemorrhagic signs after a bite from a copperhead. *N Engl J Med.* 1997;336:1262-1263.
51. Russell FE. *Snake Venom Poisoning.* Philadelphia: JB Lippincott; 1980.
52. Russell FE, Bogert CM. Gila monster: its biology, venom and bite—a review. *Toxicon.* 1981;19:341-359.
53. Sakai A, Junsuke T, Mamoru V. Efficacy of anticholinesterase against paralysis caused by postsynaptic neurotoxic snake venom [abstract]. *Ann Emerg Med.* 1995;26:712-713.
54. Seifert SA, Boyer LV. Recurrence phenomena after immunoglobulin therapy for snake envenomations: part 1. Pharmacokinetics and pharmacodynamics of immunoglobulin antivenoms and related antibodies. *Ann Emerg Med.* 2001;37:189-195.
55. Simon TL, Grace TG. Envenomation coagulopathy in wounds from pit vipers. *N Engl J Med.* 1981;305:443-447.
56. Suchard JR, LoVecchio F. Envenomations by rattlesnakes thought to be dead. *N Engl J Med.* 1999;340:1930.
57. Tanen DA, Danish DC, Grice GA, et al. Fasciotomy worsens the amount of myonecrosis in a porcine model of crotaline envenomation. *Ann Emerg Med.* 2004;44(2):99-104.
58. Teixeira CFP, Fernandes CM, Zuliani JP, and Zamuner SF. Inflammatory effects of snake venom metalloproteinases. *Mem Inst Oswaldo Cruz.* 2005;100(suppl 1):181-184.
59. Weed HG. Nonvenomous snakebite in Massachusetts: prophylactic antibiotics are unnecessary. *Ann Emerg Med.* 1993;22:220-224.
60. Whitley RE. Conservative treatment of copperhead snakebites without antivenom. *J Trauma.* 1996;41:219-221.
61. Wingert WA, Chan L. Rattlesnake bites in southern California and rationale for recommended treatment. *West J Med.* 1988;148:37-43.
62. Winkel KD, Hawdon GM, Levick N. Pressure immobilization for neurotoxic snake bites. *Ann Emerg Med.* 1999;34:294-295.
63. Wooldridge BJ, Pineda G, Banuelas-Ornelas JJ, et al. Mojave rattlesnakes (crotalus scutulatus scutulatus) lacking the acidic subunit DNA sequence lack Mojave toxin in their venom. *Comp Biochem Physiol B Biochem Mol Biol.* 2001;130(2):169-179.
64. Yamazaki Y and Morita T. Sanke venom components affecting blood coagulation and the vascular system: structural similarities and marked diversity. *Curr Pharm Des.* 2007;13:2872-2886.

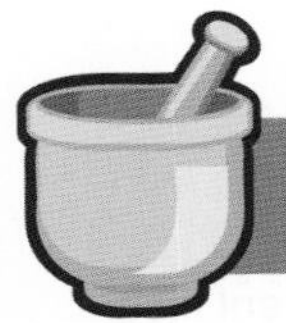

ANTIDOTES IN DEPTH (A36)

ANTIVENOM (CROTALINE)

Anthony F. Pizon, Bradley D. Riley, and Anne-Michelle Ruha

For decades Wyeth-Ayerst (Marietta, PA) manufactured Antivenin Crotalidae Polyvalent (ACP) for treatment of crotaline snakebites in the United States. It was a poorly purified whole IgG product derived from horse serum with significant risk for acute and delayed allergic reactions.[10] ACP was formulated as a freeze-dried powder that required reconstitution before use. Wyeth has since stopped production of ACP, though expired supplies may still be available. Previous editions of this textbook contain details about Wyeth ACP.

In October 2000, the US Food and Drug Administration approved Crotalidae polyvalent immune Fab, manufactured by Protherics Inc (Savage Laboratories, Brentwood, TN). This antivenom is derived from sheep serum and formulated specifically to treat crotaline snakebites found in the United States. It is an effective and less allergenic alternative to the previously manufactured horse serum product and is currently the only crotaline antivenom available in the United States.[10,14]

A limited number of bites from exotic nonnative snakes, kept in zoos and by amateur collectors, occur in North America each year. Numerous antivenoms exist to treat bites from these exotic snakes, but they are of limited availability and difficult to obtain. Poison centers have access to the online Antivenom Index, which is useful when attempting to locate antivenom for a nonnative snake envenomation. Local zoos may also be useful resources when attempting to locate an exotic antivenom. Recommendations for these diverse antivenoms are difficult to make, but any available package instructions should be followed, and preparations should be made to treat life-threatening hypersensitivity reactions when using these unfamiliar products.

CROTALIDAE POLYVALENT IMMUNE Fab (OVINE)

Crotalidae polyvalent immune Fab (ovine), marketed under the brand name CroFab™, is produced by inoculating sheep with the venom of the eastern diamondback rattlesnake (*Crotalus adamanteus*), western diamondback rattlesnake (*Crotalus atrox*), cottonmouth (*Agkistrodon piscivorus*), and Mojave rattlesnake (*Crotalus scutulatus*). The refining process begins with papain digestion of isolated IgG antibodies to eliminate the Fc portion of the immunoglobulin, and then isolation of the antibody fragments [Fab and $F(ab)_2$]. This is followed by affinity purification and lyophilization. The resultant Fab fragments have a smaller molecular weight, are less immunogenic, and have increased tissue penetration compared with whole IgG antivenoms used previously.

CLINICAL USE

After an envenomation, the major indications for administration of antivenom are (1) hemodynamic compromise, (2) significant coagulopathy or thrombocytopenia, (3) neuromuscular toxicity, or (4) progression of swelling. These indications are vague and allow clinical interpretation of the need for antivenom under varying circumstances. Antivenom should not be given prophylactically to patients with minimal symptoms, or in the absence of evidence of envenomation. Patients with only minimal local tissue swelling that is not progressing should not be given antivenom.

When indicated, antivenom should be given as soon as possible to neutralize circulating venom. Animal studies report decreased mortality when antivenom is given immediately after envenomation.[5] Antivenom will not reverse swelling and tissue necrosis that has already occurred, and tissue necrosis may develop despite administration of antivenom. However, since antivenom will halt but will not reverse tissue injury, it makes sense that early administration is expected to reduce the pain and loss of function associated with a significant swelling of an extremity. A delay in treatment lessens the beneficial effects of antivenom in animal models,[7] and it is unknown how long antivenom remains effective following an envenomation. Anecdotally, antivenom may reverse venom-induced coagulopathy even if administered more than 24 hours after the bite.

In addition to halting the progression of local tissue swelling, antivenom can at least temporarily reverse systemic effects, including most coagulation and platelet defects.[2,8,9,11] While there are no studies comparing outcomes of envenomated patients treated with and without antivenom, it is generally agreed that antivenom reduces morbidity in patients with significant crotaline envenomation and in some situations may be a lifesaving therapy.[8]

TECHNIQUE OF ADMINISTRATION

A thorough history regarding asthma, atopy, use of β-adrenergic antagonists, food allergies, and previous use of antivenoms should be obtained. According to the manufacturer, the only absolute contraindication is an allergy to papaya or papain, which can still be present in residual amounts after the manufacturing process. A history of asthma, atopy, or use of β-adrenergic antagonists should be carefully considered when weighing the risks and benefits of antivenom. These conditions should not exclude the use of antivenom if the patient is suffering from a moderate to severe envenomation (see definitions below). Since antivenom is ovine derived, previous reactions to equine-derived antivenoms should not preclude its use. In cases of mild envenomation, the risk of allergic reaction to antivenom or difficulty in effectively treating an allergic reaction in a patient receiving β-adrenergic antagonists might outweigh any benefit of therapy. Antivenom should be administered in a monitored setting where resuscitation can be performed and airway supplies can be quickly accessed. Epinephrine, steroids, and antihistamines should be immediately available in the event a hypersensitivity reaction occurs.

Antivenom is packaged in vials as a lyophilized powder that must be reconstituted. Completely filling each vial with 25 mL of sterile water, rather than the 10 mL advised in the package insert, and then gently hand rolling the vials will result in dissolution times as rapid as 1 minute. Adding the greater volume also reduces foaming of the product.[6,13]

The initial recommended dose is four to six vials, which is mixed in 250 mL 0.9% sodium chloride solution and administered over 1 hour. The exact concentration of antivenom is not critical. For children, the total volume of fluid in which the antivenom is diluted can be decreased when necessary.[12] No dosing adjustment is required for children or small adults because the amount of venom requiring neutralization is not dependent upon the patient's weight. On the other hand, there is no justification for partial doses or infusions of one or two vials in minor cases.

In order to avoid serious adverse reactions, the first dose of antivenom is administered cautiously in an escalating-rate fashion. No skin testing is suggested. The first dose of antivenom (four to six vials diluted in 250 mL 0.9% saline) is infused at an initial rate of 10 mL/h while the patient is observed carefully for evidence of hypersensitivity. If no adverse reactions are witnessed, then the rate is doubled every few minutes, as tolerated by the patient, with the goal of infusing the first dose over 1 hour. If the patient tolerates the initial dose without adverse effects, subsequent doses can be given at a rate of 250 mL/h without need for titration of rate.

The total dose of antivenom required to *control* an envenomation may vary widely, so additional doses may be needed to halt swelling and/or reverse coagulopathy or thrombocytopenia. With the introduction of Crotalidae polyvalent immune Fab (ovine), *control* was defined as arrest of local tissue manifestations and return of coagulation parameters, platelet counts, and systemic signs to normal. However, clinical experience demonstrated that some patients have venom-induced coagulopathy and thrombocytopenia that is resistant to antivenom treatment.[14] Therefore, we advocate *control* to mean clear improvement in hematologic parameters rather than complete normalization.[14] This definition may be more realistic, especially for patients with difficult-to-treat coagulopathy and thrombocytopenia. After each dose of four to six vials, prothrombin time, fibrinogen, and platelet counts are determined, and the patient's local injury is reexamined. Multiple doses are often required to achieve control. If repeat dosing is necessary to control swelling, but fibrinogen, prothrombin time and platelets remain normal, then these laboratory studies do not need to be repeated after each additional control dose. After achieving control, maintenance doses of two vials every 6 hours are given, for a total of three doses. Again, the two vials are added to 250 mL 0.9% sodium chloride solution and administered over 1 hour. Because the duration of action of antivenom is less than that of venom, the maintenance doses are given in an attempt to prevent recurrence of local manifestations, thrombocytopenia, and coagulopathy. An algorithm describing this approach is shown in Fig. A36–1.

Some patients will demonstrate recurrence of swelling during their maintenance infusions. For this reason close monitoring of extremity swelling should occur for 18 to 24 hours after apparent control has been achieved. If recurrent swelling occurs, additional control doses of four to six vials should be given until the swelling again becomes controlled. Likewise, despite successful completion of maintenance antivenom doses, patients may develop a recurrence of coagulopathy and/or thrombocytopenia, in which case additional antivenom should be considered.

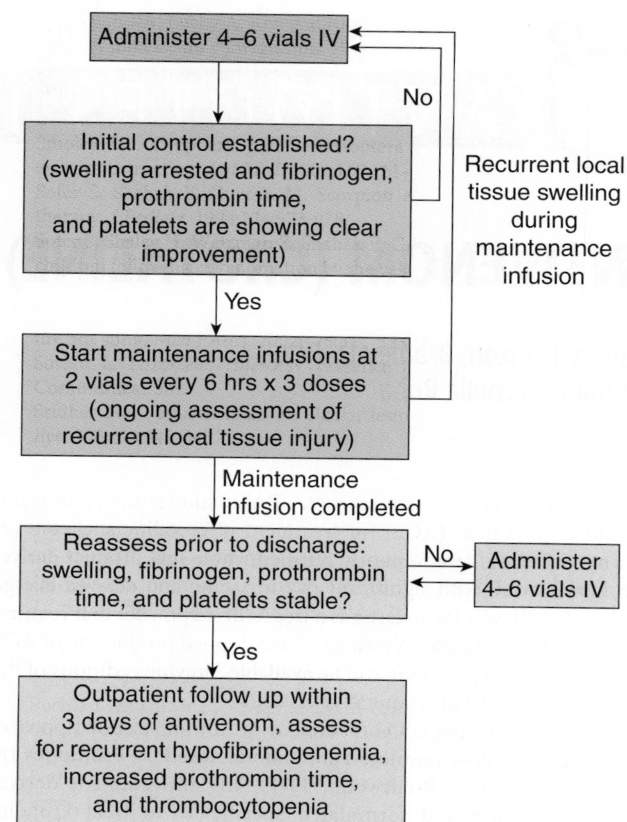

FIGURE A36–1. Algorithm for the administration of Crotalidae polyvalent immune Fab (ovine) antivenom for moderate to severe North American crotaline snake envenomation.

ADVERSE REACTIONS

Despite reduced immunogenicity, acute and delayed hypersensitivity reactions to antivenom are well reported.[3,4] Urticaria, rash, bronchospasm, pruritus, angioedema, anaphylaxis, and delayed serum sickness all are associated with use of this product.[9,14] Acute reactions are reported in 5.4% to 14.3% of patients, while delayed hypersensitivity reactions occur in 16% of patients.[3,8]

When antivenom is administered too rapidly, nonimmunogenically mediated anaphylactoid reactions may occur. In general, patients appear to tolerate four to six vials per hour without developing anaphylactoid reactions. If the patient requires rapid administration of antivenom because of the severity of the envenomation, H_1 and H_2 histamine receptor antagonists may be needed in addition to an epinephrine infusion. Clinically differentiating between anaphylactoid and anaphylactic reactions may be difficult, especially when antivenom is administered rapidly. Regardless, the treatment remains the same.

For acute anaphylactic reactions (which often occur shortly following initiation of even low doses of antivenom), the antivenom should be stopped and intravenous steroids, H_1 and H_2 histamine receptor antagonists, and epinephrine given. Epinephrine 2 to 4 μg/min (0.03–0.06 μg/kg/min for children) can be initiated and then titrated to effect. After the symptoms of hypersensitivity resolve, the antivenom should be restarted only in patients at high risk for significant morbidity or mortality from snake envenomation. In such cases, the antivenom infusion is restarted at 1 to 2 mL/h, while the epinephrine infusion is continued. The antivenom infusion rate can be slowly increased as tolerated. If anaphylaxis recurs, the antivenom should be stopped and the epinephrine infusion increased until symptoms resolve. Antivenom once again can be restarted while epinephrine is continued at the higher rate. With constant monitoring of patients at the bedside and titrating epinephrine and antivenom infusions, most patients with life-threatening envenomation should tolerate the full antivenom dose. Patients have safely received subsequent doses of antivenom after an acute life-threatening reaction.[4]

In addition to acute allergic reactions, delayed hypersensitivity syndromes in the form of serum sickness may occur. Mild cases of serum sickness consist of urticaria, pruritus, and malaise. Occasionally arthritis, lymphadenopathy, and fever develop. Immune-complex glomerulonephritis, neuritis, vasculitis, and myocarditis occur rarely. The syndrome of serum sickness after antivenom use has not been well characterized or studied, but usually it is neither serious nor associated with chronic sequelae.[10] Most patients respond favorably to antihistamines and corticosteroids. Immediately after onset of symptoms, prednisone (2 mg/kg divided into twice daily oral dosing) is given and tapered over 2 to 3 weeks. Oral antihistamines can be used for symptomatic treatment as well. The vast majority of patients can be managed as outpatients.

At the time of discharge, the patient should be informed of the possibility of recurrent venom effects and told to refrain from activities associated with high risk for trauma and to avoid any surgical procedures for 3 weeks. The patient should receive instructions to watch for signs of bleeding, which may be associated with coagulopathy or thrombocytopenia. Recurrence occurs in approximately 25% to 50% of patients with rattlesnake envenomation who receive this antivenom.[1,14] Follow-up prothrombin time, fibrinogen concentration, and platelet count should be obtained within 3 to 5 days of antivenom completion in all patients. In most patients who develop recurrence, the decrease in platelets or increase in prothrombin time is evident within 3 days of the last antivenom therapy. Since early administration of antivenom may have masked the findings in patients who initially did not demonstrate coagulopathy or thrombocytopenia, and these patients still may develop these effects within days of completing antivenom treatment, follow-up coagulation studies are recommended in all cases.

Treatment recommendations vary for delayed recurrence of venom effects. Clinical experience demonstrates that delayed recurrence may be resistant to additional antivenom,[14] so the benefits of retreatment in the absence of active bleeding are unclear. No specific dosing regimen for retreatment is known at this time. In our practice, where we frequently encounter recurrence, our general approach is to only retreat patients who develop (1) severe isolated thrombocytopenia (platelet count less than 20,000–30,000/mm^3), (2) moderate thrombocytopenia (platelet count less than 30,000–50,000/mm^3) with severe coagulopathy (fibrinogen less than 80 mg/dL), or (3) active bleeding. A more conservative approach can be used for patients with additional risk factors for bleeding, such as increased risk for trauma or use of anticoagulants. Other patients with less severe recurrence, or isolated coagulopathy without thrombocytopenia, usually can be managed as outpatients with close follow-up and repeat laboratory tests every few days. Increased local tissue swelling at the time of follow-up usually is not an indication for redosing antivenom and most often is the result of dependent edema from inadequate extremity elevation. In the absence of any recurrence phenomenon, patients should have regular telephone follow-up for 3 weeks to check for signs of serum sickness.

ELAPID ANTIVENOM (EQUINE ORIGIN)

The production of North American Coral Snake Antivenin (Wyeth-Ayerst, Marietta, PA) for treatment of envenomation by the eastern coral snake (*Micrurus fulvius*) and Texas coral snake (*Micrurus tener*) was recently discontinued. Limited supplies are still available with an expiration date of October 2009. This equine-derived coral snake antivenom does not treat envenomation from coral snakes found in Mexico, Central America, or South America. Additionally, toxicity requiring treatment with antivenom has not been reported following bites from the less virulent Arizona (Sonoran, *Micruroides euryoxanthus*) coral snake.

In contrast to the recommendation to withhold crotaline polyvalent antivenom unless signs of significant envenomation are evident, prophylactic use of coral snake antivenom is recommended in any asymptomatic patient where a coral snake bite is assumed or proven.[11] For a number of hours following the bite of a coral snake, little objective evidence suggests envenomation, but systemic symptoms can develop insidiously. Therefore, at least three to five vials of coral snake antivenom are given initially and repeated on the basis of the clinical condition. The caveats for administration of crotaline antivenom discussed above (rate of infusion and treatment of allergic reactions) apply to coral snake antivenom, except less antivenom usually is required for coral snake bites. Up to 10 vials can be administered, but dosing recommendations are vague. Limited supplies of this antivenom may make adherence to this recommendation difficult.

If no antivenom is available, the mainstay of treatment will consist of aggressive supportive care. In particular, respiratory failure requiring intubation may ensue from muscle paralysis. This would require supporting the patient's respirations until recovery. With respiratory support, paralysis is completely reversible. However, it may take weeks to months to resolve completely.

SUMMARY

Antivenom, combined with good supportive care, is effective in the management of North American snake envenomations. All antivenoms are derived from foreign proteins and are capable of producing acute and delayed hypersensitivity reactions in humans. While crotaline polyvalent immune Fab appears to produce fewer hypersensitivity reactions than whole immunoglobulin antivenoms, the healthcare provider must be aware of the possibility of life-threatening reactions resulting from use of this product and be prepared to effectively treat a reaction should one occur.

ACKNOWLEDGMENT

James R. Roberts and Edward J. Otten contributed to this Antidotes in Depth in previous editions.

REFERENCES

1. Boyer LV, Seifert SA, Cain JS. Recurrence phenomena after immunoglobulin therapy for snake envenomations: Part 2. Guidelines for clinical management with Crotaline Fab antivenom. *Ann Emerg Med.* 2001;37:196-210.
2. Buntain WL. Successful venomous snakebite neutralization with massive antivenom infusion in a child. *J Trauma.* 1983;23:1012-1014.
3. Cannon R, Ruha AM, Kashani J. Acute hypersensitivity reactions associated with administration of Crotalidae polyvalent immune Fab antivenom. *Ann Emerg Med.* 2008;51:407-411.
4. Clark RF, McKinney PE, Chase PB, et al. Immediate and delayed allergic reactions to Crotalidae polyvalent immune Fab (ovine) antivenom. *Ann Emerg Med.* 2002;39:671-676.
5. Consroe P, Egen NB, Russell FE, et al. Comparison of a new ovine antigen binding fragment (Fab) antivenin for United States Crotalidae with the commercial antivenin for protection against venom-induced lethality in mice. *Am J Trop Med Hyg.* 1995;53:507-510.

6. CroFab™ [package insert]. Brentwood, TN: Protherics Inc; 2008.
7. Dart RC, Goldner AP, Lindsey D. Efficacy of post envenomation administration of antivenin. *Toxicon.* 1988;26:1218-1221.
8. Dart RC, McNally J. Efficacy, safety, and use of snake antivenom in the United States. *Ann Emerg Med.* 2001;37:181-188.
9. Dart RC, Seifert SA, Boyer LV, et al. A randomized multicenter trial of Crotalinae polyvalent immune Fab (ovine) antivenom for the treatment for crotaline snakebite in the United States. *Arch Intern Med.* 2001;161:2030-2036.
10. Howland MA, Smilkstein MJ. Primer on immunology with applications to toxicology. *Contemp Manage Crit Care.* 1991;1:109-145.
11. Kitchen CS, Mierop LHS. Envenomation by the Eastern coral snake (*Micrurus fulvius fulvius*). *JAMA.* 1987;258:1615-1618.
12. Pizon AF, Riley BD, LoVecchio F, Gill R. Safety and efficacy of Crotalidae polyvalent immune Fab in pediatric crotaline envenomations. *Acad Emerg Med.* 2007;14:373-376.
13. Quan AN, Quan D, Curry SC. Improving CroFab reconstitution times. *J Med Tox.* 2008;4:60-61.
14. Ruha AM, Curry SC, Beuhler M, et al. Initial postmarketing experience with crotalidae polyvalent immune Fab for treatment of rattlesnake envenomation. *Ann Emerg Med.* 2002;39:609-615.

M.

OCCUPATIONAL AND ENVIRONMENTAL TOXINS

CHAPTER 122

INDUSTRIAL POISONING: INFORMATION AND CONTROL

Peter H. Wald

Many important problems are associated with the diagnosis and treatment of occupational and environmentally caused diseases, including (1) the ability to establish correctly the diagnosis, (2) the ability to treat the condition correctly, and (3) the ability to act correctly on any public health issues related to the exposure. The following discussion instructs clinicians on how to assemble adequate information to achieve the appropriate diagnosis and treatment.

TAKING AN OCCUPATIONAL HISTORY

Because time spent at work is a large percentage of many people's day, the occupational health history should be a routine part of any medical history. This is especially true of patients who present to a physician with potential xenobiotic exposures at work or unusual symptoms. The history should include several brief survey questions. Positive responses then lead to a more detailed occupational and environmental history, which is composed of three elements: present work, past work, and nonoccupational exposures.

THE BRIEF OCCUPATIONAL SURVEY

The following three questions should be incorporated into the occupational survey:

Exactly what kind of work do you do?

Are you exposed to any physical (radiation, noise, extremes of temperature or pressure), chemical (liquids, fumes, vapors, dusts, or mists), or biologic hazards at work (Table 122–1)?

Are your symptoms related in any way to starting or being away from work? For example, do the symptoms start when you arrive at work at the beginning of the day or week or when you work at a specific location or during a specific process at work?

PRESENT WORK

Collected data on a person's present job reveal what his or her present exposures may be, which can help formulate the differential diagnosis for the employee's complaints. These data can be systematically collected by focusing on four areas: specifics of the job, hazardous exposures, health effects, and control measures (Table 122–2).

Specifics of the Job It is not sufficient simply to inquire what the patient does for a living. Similar to healthcare professionals, workers in other industries have their own jargon. When asked for a job title, a patient may respond with a title that has meaning only in his or her trade. Even if the job title is recognizable, it may not provide any useful information and, in fact, may be misleading. A secretary working in a small plastics manufacturing plant may have occupational exposures that are quite different from a secretary who works for a law firm.

The important specific information requested should include the name of the employer, type of industry, duration and location of employment, hours and shift changes, process description (including unusual occasional activities), and adjacent processes. The employer may be able to provide information about materials used at the plant. However, clinicians should always obtain the patient's permission before calling the employer. A patient may be fired or otherwise discriminated against (despite legal protections) for suggesting that health problems are work related.

It is important to learn precisely what happens in the patient's immediate work environment because nearby work processes may contribute other exposures. If possible, the patient should be asked for a diagram of the work area. The patient also should be questioned about job process changes. A previously safe job may have been changed to a potentially dangerous job without a change in the patient's job title.

The patient should describe exactly what he or she does on any given day and for how long. Unusual and nonroutine tasks, such as those performed during overtime, maintenance, or in an emergency, should also be described. The primary job may not involve xenobiotics, but the patient may nevertheless perform tasks that entail unprotected exposure to a toxic xenobiotic.

Hazardous Exposures The names or types of all xenobiotic to which the patient may be exposed are important in determining potential adverse effects and any relationship to the patient's complaints. It is important to elicit any recent changes in suppliers of these products because even a slight change in the formulation of a xenobiotic may cause adverse effects in an individual who previously had no problems working with that compound. This information may be obtained from the material safety data sheet (MSDS), an important but not universally reliable source of information about the xenobiotic. In addition to adverse health effects, the MSDS contains information on chemical reactivity, safety precautions, and other data. As an initial step, the MSDS should be requested and reviewed; however, information provided on health effects should be confirmed using other resources. Four major concerns result from relying solely on the MSDS: (1) some MSDS forms are excellent, but others are incomplete and inadequate; (2) components of a product that are regarded as "trade secrets" do not

TABLE 122–1. Hazard Classes, Hazard Types, and Several Common Examples Found in the Workplace

Hazard Class	Hazard Type	Examples
Physical hazards	Human–machine interfaces	Repetitive motion Lifting Vibration Mechanical trauma, electric shock
	Physical environment	Temperature Pressure Long or rotating shifts
	Energy	Ionizing radiation: x-ray, ultraviolet Nonionizing radiation: infrared, microwave, magnetic fields Lasers Noise
Chemical hazards	Solvents	Aliphatics, aromatics, alcohols, ketones, ethers, aldehydes, acetates, peroxides, halogenated compounds
	Metals	Lead, mercury, cadmium
	Gases	Combustion products, irritants, simple and chemical asphyxiants, oxygen-deficient environments
	Dusts	Organic (wood) and inorganic (asbestos or silica)
	Pesticides	Organic chlorine, organic phosphorus, carbamate
	Epoxy resins and polymer systems	Toluene diisocyanate, phthalates
Biologic hazards	Bacteria	*Bacillus anthracis, Legionella pneumophila, Borrelia burgdorferi*
	Viruses	Hepatitis, HIV, Hantavirus
	Mycobacteria	*Mycobacterium tuberculosis*
	Rickettsia and *Chlamydia*	*Chlamydia psittaci, Coxiella burnetii*
	Fungi	*Histoplasma capsulatum, Coccidioides immitis*
	Parasites	*Echinococcus* spp, *Plasmodium* spp
	Envenomations	Arthropod, marine, snake
	Allergens	Enzymes, animals, dusts, insects, latex, plant pollen dusts

TABLE 122–2. Components of an Occupational Health History

- Current work history
  - Specifics of the job
    - Employer's name
    - Type of industry
    - Duration of employment
    - Employment location, hours, and shift changes
    - Description of work process
    - Unusual activities of the job that are occasional (eg, maintenance)
    - Adjacent work processes
  - Hazardous exposures (see Table 122–1)
  - Possible health effects
    - Suspicious health problems
    - Temporality of symptoms
    - Specific distribution of symptoms (rash, paresthesias)
    - Affected coworkers
    - Presence or absence of known risk factors (smoking, alcohol)
  - Workplace sampling and monitoring
    - Individual or area air monitoring
    - Surface sampling
    - Biologic monitoring
    - Medical surveillance records
  - Exposure controls
    - Administrative controls
    - Process engineering controls
      - Enclosure
      - Shielding
      - Ventilation
      - Electrical and mechanically controlled interlocks
    - Personal protective equipment
      - Respirators
      - Protective clothing
      - Earplugs, glasses, gloves, face shields, head and foot protection
- Work history (prior)
  - Review current work history for all past employment
- Nonoccupational exposures
  - Secondary employment
  - Hobbies
  - Outdoor activities
  - Residential exposures
  - Community contamination
  - Habits: tobacco, alcohol, other xenobiotics

have to be revealed; (3) components that have important health effects (eg, solvent or solid carriers of the "active ingredients") often may be grouped together under "inert ingredients" without being specifically named; and (4) process intermediates or unintended byproducts of a manufacturing process may not be identified. However, if a xenobiotic is believed to be related to a health effect, manufacturers are required to release to a physician all information, including trade secrets and inert components.

Exposures to physical and biologic xenobiotics can be elicited during the review of job processes. Most patients know what they are, or have been, exposed to, even if they do not know the exact name of the xenobiotics or its medical effects.

TABLE 122–3. Evidence Supporting Work-Relatedness of Occupational Disease

Known or documented exposure to a causative xenobiotic
Symptoms consistent with suspected workplace exposure
Suggestive or diagnostic physical signs
Similar problems in coworkers or workers in related occupations
Temporal relationship of complaints related to work
Confirmatory environmental or biologic monitoring data
Scientific biologic plausibility
Absence of a nonoccupational etiology
Resistance to maximum medical treatment because employee continues to be exposed at work

Health Effects Significant occupational exposures usually cause medical effects, although some do so only after a substantial latency period. Key areas of inquiry include suspicious health problems, temporality of symptoms, and affected coworkers. These data, combined with workplace monitoring and sampling data, may help in determining whether the patient is experiencing a work-related illness (Table 122–3). Patients may suspect that their illness or complaint is work related, especially when symptoms occur at the workplace and improve or disappear over the weekend or during a vacation. Specific distribution of findings, such as a rash in a bilateral glove pattern, is supportive of an occupational cause. Coworkers with similar complaints (not necessarily of the same severity) should raise suspicion that a workplace exposure is responsible for a particular symptom complex. Diseases such as lung cancer or hepatitis, which occur in the absence of known risk factors such as smoking and alcohol, must be epidemiologically investigated.

Workplace Sampling, Monitoring, and Control Control of workplace hazards begins with an industrial hygiene monitoring program. Employers are required to give results of both area and individual sampling to employees. A medical surveillance program that includes periodic spirometry and respiratory questionnaires usually indicates that the patient works with a potential respiratory toxin. A medical surveillance program that includes biologic monitoring for a specific xenobiotic may also provide an immediate clue to what may be causing the patient's complaints. Finally, if the patient knows exactly what he or she is working with, the physician can usually quickly determine whether any of the xenobiotics are compatible with the patient's complaints. Many companies do not perform routine industrial hygiene monitoring or medical surveillance. Individuals who become sick or ill at work are often sent to local emergency departments. In such situations, emergency physicians may need to perform the type of time-consuming, detailed occupational history outlined here or be able to consult or refer immediately to appropriate physicians or clinics.

Portions of Table 122–2 and the following section on Evaluation and Control of Workplace Hazards detail the types of controls typically used in workplaces. It is important to determine whether the workplace uses any control measures, engineering controls, work practice protocols, administrative controls, or personal protective equipment. The existence of control measures usually indicates that the employer recognizes and has attempted to deal with a hazardous exposure.

PAST WORK

It is important not to limit the occupational history to the patient's current workplace and job. Many occupational diseases have long latency periods between xenobiotic exposure and initial development of clinical symptoms. In addition, patients may have been exposed to xenobiotics at work that make them more sensitive to other environmental xenobiotics. For example, someone who developed asthma secondary to a previous workplace exposure may have asthma attacks upon exposure to simple irritants in the current workplace. When taking an in-depth occupational history, issues that may be relevant to the current work history as well as for each previous job should be explored.

NONOCCUPATIONAL EXPOSURES

Workers may be exposed to toxic xenobiotics in the course of pursuing secondary employment, hobbies, or outdoor activities in contaminated or industrial areas. Residential exposures, such as those from gas and wood stoves, chemically treated furniture and fabrics, and pest control, may be relevant. It is important to ask patients about these potential exposures before focusing entirely on exposures in their primary place of employment. This obviously includes relevant issues from the social history, such as tobacco, alcohol, and licit and illicit drug use.

EVALUATION AND CONTROL OF WORKPLACE HAZARDS

INITIAL WORKPLACE EVALUATION

The Occupational Safety and Health Act (OSHA) places legal responsibility for providing a safe and healthy workplace on the employer. The rationale for this placement of responsibility is that the employer is in the best position to make any modifications necessary to prevent additional work-related illness and injury. The physician may wish to initiate a dialogue with a patient's employer to promote preventive action but should do so only with the patient's informed consent. The initial treating physician may also refer the patient to an occupational medicine specialist, who is specifically trained to manage work-related exposures and diseases and initiate prevention programs.

Because the initial contact may influence subsequent events, it is important to identify an individual with an appropriate administrative role, such as someone in the company's medical department, the patient's supervisor, the plant's safety officer, or the shop manager. If management is willing to examine the hazardous conditions, a plant walk-through inspection can provide unique insight and information usually unavailable in an office setting. A walk-through by an occupational medicine specialist makes it easier to understand the work environment, identify safety and health hazards, assess control measures, and recognize opportunities for prevention. It also facilitates a good working relationship with key personnel in management and labor. The physician who cares for a number of patients who work in the plant or who provides health services to the workers through the company or labor union may wish to be involved in the walk-through. Assistance with plant inspections can be obtained from occupational health specialists, such as occupational physicians or industrial hygienists.

INDUSTRIAL HYGIENE SAMPLING AND MONITORING

Equipment is available to measure airborne concentrations of toxic xenobiotics, noise levels, radiation levels, temperature, and humidity. Employees can be fitted with pumps and other devices to measure individual exposure concentrations at the breathing zone, where, depending on what controls are used, concentrations may vary from those in the general work area. These results then can be compared with OSHA standards and other available standards to help determine the extent of the hazard and to formulate a control plan. OSHA requires that employers monitor the concentrations of only a few specific hazards, including arsenic, asbestos, benzene, cadmium, chromium, cotton dust, ethylene oxide, formaldehyde, lead, noise, and vinyl chloride. A complete listing of all xenobiotics is available in the OSHA standard *29 CFR 1910 Part Z—Toxic and Hazardous Substances* (http://www.osha.gov/pls/oshaweb/owastand.display_standard_group?p_toc_level=1&p_part_number=1910). In addition, monitoring is required for certain operations such as hazardous waste operations or entering a confined space that may have an oxygen-deficient atmosphere. Ongoing sampling of the remaining estimated 60,000 xenobiotics used in the workplace is not required. Where industrial hygiene sampling is performed, OSHA's medical access standard gives any exposed worker or his or her representative the right to review and copy all sampling data.

CONTROL OF WORKPLACE HAZARDS

Workplace hazard control traditionally has relied on a hierarchy of methods to protect workers from exposure. The preferred solution is complete elimination of the hazard by *substitution*. When substitution is not possible, the next preferred method consists of shielding for workers to reduce their exposure. The least favored method is personal protective equipment, which requires a positive action from the worker.

Engineering Controls Health and safety professionals prefer and OSHA regulations require when feasible the use of engineering controls to reduce worker exposure to hazardous xenobiotics. These controls intercept hazards at their source or in the workplace atmosphere before they reach the worker. Engineering controls include redesign or modification of process or equipment to reduce hazardous emissions; isolation of a process through enclosure; automation of an operation; and installation of exhaust systems that remove hazardous dusts, fumes, and vapors. Local exhaust systems, such as hoods, are preferable to general dilution ventilation because the former removes contaminants closer to their source and at relatively high rates.

Engineering controls have several advantages over control measures focused on the worker. Properly installed and maintained engineering controls are reliable and consistent, and their effectiveness does not depend on human supervision or interaction. They can simultaneously limit exposure through several routes, such as inhalation and skin absorption. In addition, engineering controls do not place a burden on the worker or interfere with worker comfort or safety.

Work Practices Work practices are procedures that the worker can follow to limit exposure to hazardous xenobiotics. Examples are the use of high-powered vacuum cleaners instead of compressed air cleaning and pouring techniques that direct hazardous xenobiotics away from the worker. Although not as effective as engineering controls, work practice can be a useful component of an overall hazard control program.

ADMINISTRATIVE CONTROLS

Administrative controls reduce the duration of exposure for any individual worker or reduce the total number of workers exposed to a hazard. Examples are rotating workers into and out of hazardous areas so that no single worker is exposed full time and scheduling procedures likely to generate high levels of exposure, such as cleaning or maintenance activities, during nights or weekends. Administrative controls sometimes have the side effect of exposing more workers to a hazard, albeit at lower doses that are hoped do not cause health effects.

Personal Protective Equipment Personal protective equipment, such as respirators, earplugs, gloves, and hard hats, is the least effective but most commonly used control method. Personal protective equipment may be the only viable protection strategy when other controls are not practical but can also be used as an additional layer of protection in the presence of engineering controls. Some employers may favor personal protective equipment over the institution of more costly engineering and administrative controls.

Respirators and other forms of personal protective equipment often are hot, uncomfortable, and awkward to wear and may make it difficult for workers to breathe, speak, or hear, depending on the equipment involved. Consequently, workers often remove or refuse to wear the protection. Respirators place extra stress on the heart and the lungs. Both respirators and earplugs limit conversation and therefore present a safety hazard in themselves.

Because personal protective equipment does not stop a hazard from entering the environment, the worker is entirely vulnerable to exposure if the equipment fails. In addition, generally only one route of exposure is protected. For example, the commonly used half-mask respirator still leaves the skin and eyes exposed.

Choosing the right piece of personal protective equipment can be difficult and may depend on the nature and extent of the hazard. For example, each type of respirator is rated for the amount of protection it provides; as expected, the cost of a respirator increases with its protection factor. Use of the wrong type of respirator can leave the worker insufficiently protected.

Half-mask respirator cartridges are available in various colors that are coded to the xenobiotic filtered out of the breathing environment. If the wrong cartridge is used, the worker is essentially unprotected from the hazardous contaminant. To be effective, a respirator must be meticulously fit to the individual worker. Failure to achieve a proper seal negates the respirator's usefulness. High cheekbones, dentures, scars, perspiration, talking, head movements, and facial hair can prevent a proper seal. These factors often are ignored or overlooked by an employer who adopts a "one-size-fits-all" policy.

Even if each employee is provided the proper respirator, the respiratory protection program may not be effective. OSHA requires that employers institute a program of proper fit testing, cleaning, maintenance, and storage of respirators, which can be at least as costly as the institution of engineering controls.

In some instances, use of personal protective equipment may be unavoidable. An employer may need to control a hazardous exposure through a combination of measures, such as engineering controls and personal protective equipment. Ideally, the employer is using personal protective equipment as a control of last resort and in strict compliance with OSHA standards.

Worker Education and Training Regardless of the control measures used, workers and supervisors must be educated in the recognition and control of workplace hazards and the prevention of work-related illness and injury. The OSHA Hazard Communication Standard requires that employers train workers in ways to detect the presence or release of hazardous xenobiotics, their physical and health hazards, methods of protection against the hazards, and proper emergency procedures, as well as how to read the labeling system and how to read and use an MSDS.

With the passage of federal, state, and local right-to-know laws, many consulting companies now offer hazard communication training. These programs are of uneven quality. Those that tend to focus on acute hazards, ignore chronic effects, and emphasize personal protective equipment over other control measures may not be effective in training workers to recognize and control hazardous xenobiotics.

Medical Monitoring Together with worker education and industrial hygiene, a medical program can form the foundation of an effective occupational disease prevention regimen. However, medical monitoring is fraught with technical and ethical pitfalls. Medical monitoring encompasses both medical screening and medical surveillance.

Medical screening refers to the cross-sectional testing of a population of workers for evidence of excessive exposure or early stages of disease that may or may not be related to work and that may or may not influence the ability to tolerate or perform work.

Preemployment and preplacement physical examinations are another type of medical screening that are often favored by employers. The Americans with Disabilities Act (ADA) and the new ADA Amendment Act of 2008 (ADAAA) regulate the timing, scope, content, and use of these examinations and the information gathered. Comprehensive resources for information on the ADA are available at http://www.adata.org. The ADA prohibits "preemployment" medical examinations and inquiries. After a job offer has been made, "preplacement" examinations and inquiries can be conducted to determine whether an applicant can perform a job safely and effectively. The physician evaluates the individual's medical history, current symptoms, and physical laboratory findings to determine whether he or she currently has the physical or mental abilities necessary to perform the essential functions of the job and whether the individual can do so without posing a "direct threat" to the health or safety of him- or herself or others. This threat must be more than theoretical and cannot be based on some future time; the threat must be concrete and relatively immediate.

Few tests and few conditions are good predictors of either the ability to perform a task or increased susceptibility to a particular exposure. Many workers and their advocates view preplacement examinations as a way for employers to choose the "fittest" worker and to avoid their legally mandated obligation to provide a safe and healthy workplace for all workers. This is not true for most employers. Physicians asked by an employer to perform preplacement examinations should be sure that each component of the examination relates to the actual job the individual is being hired to perform and the actual risks he or she will encounter on the job. Both the law and sound occupational medical practice dictate that the employer's attention and efforts be directed toward redesign of the job and its hazards so that it is safe and healthy for all workers to perform.

Medical surveillance refers to the ongoing evaluation, by means of periodic examinations, of high-risk individuals or potentially exposed workers to detect early pathophysiologic changes indicative of significant exposure. OSHA requires little in the way of medical surveillance, although several OSHA standards require employers to institute medical surveillance programs, for example, for workers exposed to asbestos, arsenic, cadmium, chromium, vinyl chloride, lead, and ethylene oxide. Depending on the potential exposure, medical surveillance may include a history and physical examination, chest radiography, pulmonary function tests, blood and urine tests, and other laboratory evaluations.

A medical surveillance program may also include biologic monitoring, the purpose of which is not to identify the occurrence of disease but to measure the uptake or presence of a particular xenobiotic or its metabolites in body fluids or organs. Ideally, this occurs before any pathophysiologic damage occurs. Consequently, biologic monitoring is potentially a primary preventive measure. For example, several volatile organic compounds, such as benzene and toluene, if inhaled or absorbed through the skin, produce metabolites that can be measured in urine.

Biologic monitoring can have some advantages over air monitoring because biologic monitoring measures the *actual* absorption of a xenobiotic by the body as opposed to ambient concentrations in the workplace. The amount of a chemical absorbed may not be closely correlated to ambient xenobiotics for several reasons, including differences in individual work habits, use and effectiveness of personal protective equipment, dermal absorption of xenobiotics unrelated to their concentration in the air, and nonoccupational exposures.

Biologic monitoring, however, has several significant limitations. For most xenobiotics, there are no standards of "normal" or "safe" concentrations against which results can be compared. The timing of specimen collection is critical because different xenobiotics have different biologic half-lives. The storage and handling of specimens and interpretation of results are vulnerable to error. Nevertheless, if carefully designed and implemented, biologic monitoring can be a useful complement to a comprehensive industrial hygiene program.

With the exception of biologic monitoring, medical monitoring programs identify disease processes already underway and therefore are, at best, a form of secondary prevention. Employers who use results to remove workers rather than remediating the hazard are abusing medical and biologic monitoring programs. To be an effective preventive measure, these programs must be coordinated with environmental monitoring programs that identify the nature, source, and extent of workplace hazards; implementation of engineering controls and other measures that control hazards as close as possible to the source; and worker education programs that, at a minimum, inform workers of exposures, their effects, and proper control measures.

Both medical monitoring programs and preplacement examinations raise issues of doctor–patient confidentiality. Employee medical records should be available only to the corporate medical or first-aid department and not to the personnel office and general management. Unless required by statute, employers should never be told the results of history, physical, or diagnostic examinations unless the patient gives his or her written consent. The examining physician need only inform the employer that an individual is or is not capable of performing a particular job with or without specified restrictions. The physician should not disclose diagnostic information about medical conditions.

INFORMATION RESOURCES

Healthcare professionals require information on industrial toxins in a number of situations, ranging from caring for an acutely ill patient in an emergency department, when information must be obtained quickly, to caring for a patient with chronic symptoms that may reflect an occupational disease. The American College of Occupational and Environmental Medicine publishes a Recommended Library and Electronic Resources (http://www.acoem.org) that provides reference sources for information on toxicology, acute and chronic health effects, diagnosis, and treatment; assists in screening and surveillance; and provides information on groups at risk, product uses, and sources of further information. However, use of these resources depends on the proper identification of the xenobiotic in question. If the xenobiotic, its generic name, and ingredients are not known, the research process becomes more difficult.

The practitioner should take a logical approach to seeking information about industrial xenobiotics. First, the xenobiotic must be identified by its generic name. This can be done by reviewing the MSDS or by contacting poison centers (PCs), the employer, manufacturer, unions, or government agencies. MSDSs also are available by searching online. A good starting point to find MSDSs on the Internet is http://www.ilpi.com/MSDS/index.html, but typing "MSDS" into any online search engine yields a number of sites offering data sheets.

POISON CENTERS

Regional PCs can provide assistance even when the exact chemical name is unknown because information on xenobiotics and their management may be cross-referenced by trade name and manufacturer. Moreover, PC personnel can usually suggest additional resources. Most PCs have computerized listings of poisons that are updated regularly. The best-known system is POISINDEX (Thompson Healthcare, Greenwood Village, CO). Subscribers to this system receive quarterly updates of an alphabetically organized listing of approximately 500,000 industrial and nonindustrial xenobiotics. The system includes trade names, the components, and the concentrations, when available, of each xenobiotic listed. These elements are then cross-referenced to management protocols. The name of the manufacturer is also listed.

EMPLOYERS AND MANUFACTURERS

Many state and federal laws require manufacturers to generate, retain, and disclose information that may help physicians care for persons with work-related health problems. Scientific information, exposure data, information on health effects, and collected medical data are included in the types of information that must be retained.

The Chemical Transportation Emergency Center (CHEMTREC; 800-262-8200; http://www.chemtrec.com), sponsored by the Chemical Manufacturers Association, has as its primary responsibility providing information to healthcare practitioners responding to hazardous spills. However, it also provides information on commercial products found in patients' workplaces. Employers are required to furnish this information to employees in the form of MSDSs.

WORKER'S COMPENSATION INSURANCE CARRIERS

Smaller companies often lack internal health and safety staffs. Worker's compensation or company risk insurance carriers may have valuable information about exposures and controls in the workplace. As a service to their clients, carriers often do walk-throughs and hazards evaluations for clients that lack these resources and suggest appropriate engineering controls. Healthcare professionals can contact the carrier directly to see what additional information is available.

REGULATORY AGENCIES

OSHA requires chemical manufacturers to create a MSDS for each chemical they produce, and employers who use chemicals must retain the MSDSs in the workplace. Required information includes xenobiotic and common names; physical, safety, and health hazard data; exposure limits; precautions for safe handling and use; generally applicable control measures; and emergency and first-aid procedures. The OSHA Hazardous Communication Standard requires individual employers to provide employees with information on the xenobiotics used in their workplaces. With the patient's permission, a call to the plant manager, foreperson, or safety officer may be all that is necessary to determine the name of the xenobiotic in question. Employers may be able to provide information on exposure concentrations in the patient's work environment. In addition, company medical departments (where they exist) may have results of medical testing done on the patient.

There is an important point to reiterate about MSDSs: healthcare providers should not rely on these sheets as the sole source of information. The MSDSs are created by the chemical manufacturers as they generate scientific and health data during the course of seeking approval from the Environmental Protection Agency (EPA) to manufacture xenobiotics, and they are not a complete product evaluation. In addition, Section 8(c) of the Toxic Substances Control Act (TSCA) requires chemical manufacturers to report records of significant adverse reactions to human health or the environment. When contacting chemical manufacturers, physicians should ask to speak with a toxicologist, chemist, or someone in the products information department.

UNIONS

Labor unions, where they exist, can be excellent sources of information on xenobiotic exposures. At the local level, union officers, health and safety committee members, and shop stewards may be able to provide MSDSs, exposure data, medical and epidemiologic information, and reports of incidents or cases of interest in a particular plant. The health and safety department of the American Federation of Labor and Congress of Industrial Organizations (AFL-CIO), (http://www.aflcio.org) in Washington, DC, can provide information on occupational health and safety activities and advice on which member unions may be of specific help. At the international level, unions often have well-trained health and safety professionals who may provide or suggest sources of helpful information. In addition, some cities have a coalition of occupational safety and health groups that may provide information about other known exposed or affected workers.

GOVERNMENT AGENCIES

A myriad of agencies have some regulatory authority over manufacturing and services industries. These agencies and their important regulatory authority are listed in Table 122–4.

OSHA of the U.S. Department of Labor (http://www.osha.gov) is responsible for setting and enforcing workplace health and safety standards. It is empowered to investigate occupational health and safety complaints and can inspect work sites and levy fines for violations of its standards. In approximately half of the 50 states, the OSHA program is implemented by a state agency. Individual workers, their representatives (unions), or their physicians can file a complaint with the state or federal OSHA program and request an inspection. OSHA regulations protect workers from discrimination and punishment by their employer, who may be angered by their filing a complaint.

Some state OSHA agencies have separate enforcement and consultation arms. Thus, companies can request assistance from the occupational health specialists in the consultation branch without fear of reprisal from the enforcement branch. Healthcare workers should be familiar with the functions of their state agency and workers' rights under the law.

The National Institute for Occupational Safety and Health (NIOSH) of the U.S. Department of Health and Human Services is part of the Centers for Disease Control and Prevention (http://www.cdc.gov/niosh). NIOSH is not a regulatory agency and is responsible for researching the causes of occupational disease and injury and methods for their prevention and control, evaluating workplace conditions, recommending exposure limits to OSHA for standard setting, and training occupational health and safety professionals. It is empowered to conduct onsite evaluations of health hazards in response to requests from employee representatives or employers. After conducting these evaluations, NIOSH investigators immediately contact OSHA, the employees, and the employer if they find that the workers are in imminent danger.

TABLE 122–4. Government Agencies and Their Important Regulatory Authority of the Workplace—A Timeline

Regulation	Agency	Authority
Occupational Safety and Health Act (OSHA, 1970)	Department of Labor	Congress passed OSHA and created the Occupational Safety and Health Administration to ensure worker and workplace safety. The goal was to make sure employers provide their workers a place of employment free from recognized hazards to safety and health, such as exposure to toxic xenobiotics, excessive noise levels, mechanical dangers, heat or cold stress, and unsanitary conditions. To establish standards for workplace health and safety, the Act also created the National Institute for Occupational Safety and Health (NIOSH) as the research institution for the Occupational Safety and Health Administration. Part 1910.1200 of OSHA established the Hazardous Communication Standard (HazCom). The purpose of this section is to ensure that the hazards of all xenobiotics produced or imported are evaluated and that information concerning their hazards is transmitted to employers and employees. This transmittal of information is to be accomplished by means of comprehensive hazard communication programs, which are to include container labeling and other forms of warning, material safety data sheets, and employee training.
Resource Conservation and Recovery Act (RCRA, 1976)	Environmental Protection Agency (EPA)	RCRA (pronounced "rick-rah") gave the EPA the authority to control hazardous waste from "cradle to grave." This includes the generation, transportation, treatment, storage, and disposal of hazardous waste. RCRA also set forth a framework for the management of nonhazardous wastes. The 1986 amendments to RCRA enabled the EPA to address environmental problems that could result from underground tanks storing petroleum and other hazardous xenobiotics. RCRA focuses only on active and future facilities and does not address abandoned or historic sites (see CERCLA). HSWA (pronounced "hiss-wa"), the Federal Hazardous and Solid Waste Amendments, are the 1984 amendments to RCRA that required the phasing out of land disposal of hazardous waste. Some of the other mandates of this strict law include increased enforcement authority for the EPA, more stringent hazardous waste management standards, and a comprehensive underground storage tank program.
Toxic Substances Control Act (TSCA, 1976)	EPA	TSCA was enacted by Congress to give the EPA the ability to track the 75,000 industrial xenobiotics currently produced or imported into the United States. The EPA repeatedly screens these xenobiotics and can require reporting or testing of those that may pose an environmental or human health hazard. The EPA can ban the manufacture and import of xenobiotics that pose an unreasonable risk. Reporting requirements include (1) premanufacturing notification for new xenobiotics, (2) allegation of significant adverse reactions, (3) reporting of health and safety studies, and (4) notification of suspicion of substantial risk to health.
Comprehensive Environmental Response, Compensation, and Liability Act (CERCLA, 1980)	EPA	CERCLA, commonly known as the Superfund, was enacted by Congress on December 11, 1980. This law created a tax on the chemical and petroleum industries and provided broad federal authority to respond directly to releases or threatened releases of hazardous xenobiotics that may endanger public health or the environment. Over 5 years, $1.6 billion was collected, and the tax went to a trust fund for cleaning up abandoned or uncontrolled hazardous waste sites. CERCLA (1) established prohibitions and requirements concerning closed and abandoned hazardous waste sites, (2) provided for liability of persons responsible for releases of hazardous waste at these sites, and (3) established a trust fund to provide for cleanup when no responsible party could be identified. The law authorizes two types of response actions: (1) short-term removals, in which actions may be taken to address releases or threatened releases requiring prompt response, and (2) long-term remedial response actions that permanently and significantly reduce the dangers associated with releases or threats of releases of hazardous xenobiotics that are serious but not immediately life threatening. These actions can be conducted only at sites listed on the EPA's National Priorities List (NPL).
Superfund Amendments and Reauthorization Act (SARA, 1986)	EPA	SARA reflected the EPA's experience in administering the complex Superfund program during its first 6 years and made several important changes and additions to the program. SARA (1) stressed the importance of permanent remedies and innovative treatment technologies in cleaning up hazardous waste sites, (2) required Superfund actions to consider the standards and requirements found in other state and federal environmental

(*Continued*)

TABLE 122–4. Government Agencies and Their Important Regulatory Authority of the Workplace–A Timeline (*Continued*)

Regulation	Agency	Authority
		laws and regulations, (3) provided new enforcement authorities and settlement tools, (4) increased state involvement in every phase of the Superfund, (5) increased the focus on human health problems posed by hazardous waste sites, (6) encouraged greater citizen participation in making decisions on how sites should be cleaned up, and (7) increased the size of the trust fund to $8.5 billion. SARA also required the EPA to revise the Hazard Ranking System (HRS) to ensure that it accurately assessed the relative degree of risk to human health and the environment posed by uncontrolled hazardous waste sites that may be placed on the NPL. Emergency Planning and Community Right-to-Know Act (EPCRA), also known as Title III of SARA, was enacted by Congress as the national legislation on community safety. This law was designated to help local communities protect public health, safety, and the environment from xenobiotic hazards. The law requires manufacturers to report the amount of toxic xenobiotics released each year (Toxic Release Inventory [TRI]).
		To implement EPCRA, Congress required each state to appoint a State Emergency Response Commission (SERC). The SERCs were required to divide their states into Emergency Planning Districts and to name a Local Emergency Planning Committee (LEPC) for each district.
Americans with Disabilities Act (ADA, 1990) and the ADA Amendments Act of 2008 (ADAAA)	Department of Labor	The ADA was enacted by Congress to establish clear and comprehensive prohibition of discrimination on the basis of disability. The act specifically covers discrimination in the areas of (1) employment, (2) public services, (3) public accommodations and services operated by private entities, and (4) telecommunications. The ADAAA reaffirms Congress' initial intent of the 1990 law to (1) broadly define "disability," (2) use the definition of "handicapped individual" under the Rehabilitation Act of 1973 and (3) state that mitigating measures (eg, insulin for diabetes) shall not be a factor when determining whether an impairment substantially limits a major life activity

As part of the process of recommending exposure standards to OSHA, NIOSH develops comprehensive documents that critically evaluate all available scientific data on particular xenobiotics. These "criteria documents" review the chemical's properties, production methods, uses, and workers at risk as well as studies of exposure effects in humans and animals. Methods of screening, surveillance, and control are presented. The agency periodically issues technical reports and special occupational hazard reviews of specific occupations. In conjunction with OSHA, NIOSH develops and disseminates health hazard alerts to inform employers, employees, and healthcare professionals of serious health effects of particular xenobiotics.

The EPA (http://www.epa.gov) is charged with protecting the nation's land, air, and water. The agency administers a number of laws designed to preserve the public health and environment, one of which is the TSCA. This act authorizes the EPA to collect information on xenobiotic risks from manufacturers and processors and to review information on new xenobiotics and new uses of xenobiotics before they are manufactured. Unless designated a trade secret, this information is subject to disclosure and therefore is available. The TSCA assistance office may be most useful when resource materials and government documents contain no information about the xenobiotics or processes in question.

The National Toxicology Program (NTP; http://ntp-server.niehs.nih.gov) is a federal program established in 1978 to develop scientific information on exposure to xenobiotics.

The Agency for Toxic Substances and Disease Registry (ATSDR; http://www.atsdr.cdc.gov) was created by Congress in the Comprehensive Environmental Response, Compensation and Liability Act of 1980 (CERLA; also known as Superfund Act) to implement the health-related sections of laws that protect the public from hazardous wastes and environmental spills of hazardous substances. In 1986, the Superfund Amendments and Reauthorization Act (SARA) made amendments to the initial enabling legislation of 1980 and broadened the ATSDR's responsibilities in the areas of health assessment, toxicologic databases, information dissemination, and medical education. One of its offices, the Division of Health Assessment and Consultation, provides emergency response for toxic and environmental disasters, consults in public health emergencies, assesses hazardous waste sites, provides technical assistance to agencies and organizations, and estimates health risks to humans from exposure to hazardous xenobiotics. The program areas in which ATSDR operates include health assessments, toxicologic profiles, emergency response, and exposure and disease registries.

ONLINE DATABASES

Printed material often is adequate for determining the adverse health effects of xenobiotic exposures, but some resources may be unavailable to physicians, and textbook publications usually lag 2 years or more behind new information. As a result, current findings and reports may be missed if the practitioner relies solely on printed material. The National Library of Medicine (http://www.nlm.nih.gov) now sponsors Internet searching of both Medline (PubMed: http://www.ncbi.nlm.gov/pubmed/) and a number of databases in the Toxicology Data Network (TOXNET: http://www.toxnet.nlm.nih.gov) that are very useful for finding information about industrial xenobiotics. Additional databases are available for searching on the OSHA, NIOSH, EPA, and ATSDR web sites.

OBLIGATIONS OF THE HEALTHCARE PROVIDER TO THE INDIVIDUAL PATIENT, COWORKERS, EMPLOYER, GOVERNMENT, AND COMMUNITY

Occupational diseases and injuries are, in principle, preventable. Physicians who diagnose a work-related disease or injury have an opportunity and an ethical obligation to participate in the identification and control of workplace hazards and the prevention of further occupational illness and injury. Physicians can choose from a range of possible follow-up measures, the goals of which are to prevent recurrence or worsening of the disease or injury in the patient and to prevent the development of disease or injury in other potentially exposed workers. Some of these activities may necessitate contact with occupational medicine physicians, toxicologists, industrial hygienists, lawyers, journalists, government officials, management personnel, and union officials.

OBLIGATIONS TO THE PATIENT

Inform the Patient that the Illness may be Work Related When the workplace is determined to be a factor in the etiology or aggravation of the patient's illness, this fact and its implications should be discussed with the patient. It should never be assumed that the patient is fully aware of the health risks associated with any workplace exposure. He or she should be provided information regarding the nature of workplace hazards, their health risks, preventive measures, and recommendations regarding continued exposure.

Suggest How the Patient Can Reduce the Exposure In some cases, the patient can take steps to reduce exposure. Adjustments in work habits that may be helpful include using a respirator or other personal protective equipment provided by the employer; using workplace shower and dressing rooms to avoid carrying xenobiotics from the workplace to the home; and avoiding ingestion of workplace xenobiotics by careful hand washing before eating or smoking and by taking lunch, coffee, and smoking breaks away from the work station. Obviously, these recommendations assume that the employer provides the appropriate equipment and facilities, which is not always the case. The most effective hazard control measures require significant commitment by, and cooperation from, the employer.

Suggest that the Patient Remove Him- or Herself from the Exposure The employer may be willing to transfer the patient to a location away from the offending hazard. This may result in a reduction in pay, seniority, or other benefits, which may be compensable under workers' compensation. The employment provisions of the ADA require employers to make "reasonable accommodations" for both work- and non–work-related disabilities. Nevertheless, the employer may not be able to accommodate the patient. The patient should be counseled carefully, and other options should be explored.

Advise the Patient to Notify the Employer Patients who are experiencing a work-related illness may be entitled to workers' compensation benefits, Social Security disability, or other government-sponsored benefit programs. In addition, they may have a valid claim against the manufacturer of a xenobiotic, a defective product, or another third party. The degree of disability necessary to bring a successful claim varies.

After a patient is informed that he or she has a work-related illness, strict time limits are set in motion, and failure to meet them can preclude the patient from successfully filing a claim or receiving needed benefits. The patient should be advised to provide written notice immediately to his or her employer of a work-related illness (supported by a physician's letter) and to seek advice about statutes of limitations and other requirements. This information is generally available from the State Workers' Compensation Board and is usually required to be provided to the employee by the employer. If a union is available at the workplace, it may be able to advise and assist the patient.

OBLIGATIONS TO COWORKERS

A patient with a work-related illness should be advised to inform his or her coworkers about the condition. If the patient belongs to a union, he or she should inform the union representative. If there is no union, the patient may contact OSHA or discuss the situation with the employer.

If the patient is a union member and agrees, the physician can contact the union, which may assist in hazard investigation, identify and warn other workers potentially affected by the hazard, and pressure the employer to take corrective action if it is unwilling to do so. The union can help the patient obtain any available benefits. The patient may be able to identify appropriate contacts, such as shop stewards, members of the union's health and safety or workers' compensation committees, an occupational health specialist employed by the union at the local or national level, or an official of the union local.

Committees on Occupational Safety and Health (COSH); coalitions of labor, health, and legal professionals; and community and environmental activists working to prevent job-related illness and injury may be able to help with the diagnosis and follow-up of occupational diseases. These groups provide education and technical assistance nationwide on a range of topics, including the health effects of specific hazards, control measures, how to use government agencies, and the legal rights of disabled workers.

OBLIGATIONS TO NOTIFY THE GOVERNMENT

States may have laws that require direct physician reporting of occupational disease. If management is uncooperative despite notification of a hazardous situation, OSHA should be contacted, with the patient's consent. In addition to the federal agencies specifically empowered to protect worker health and safety, physicians may contact the state or local health department, which may initiate action or refer the problem to one of the federal agencies. Many states also require physicians to report any occupational injury or illness to the workers' compensation carrier.

OBLIGATION TO NOTIFY THE EMPLOYER

When treating a patient with an occupational injury or illness, healthcare providers often are required to report to government agencies, health departments, or insurance carriers. As part of that reporting process, the employer should also be notified. When there is imminent danger to coworkers or the public health, the employer should be contacted to correct the exposure situation.

OBLIGATION TO INFORM COLLEAGUES AND THE PUBLIC

On occasion, an individual primary care physician or specialist is the first person to suspect a link between a workplace exposure and a serious health problem. This is likely to recur in the future, especially if the physician practices in a small town or industrial area or provides healthcare to worker groups through a company or union. Armed with an increased index of suspicion and the occupational history, the physician may be able to alert workers and companies and prevent the occurrence of a major health problem. Even if the physician chooses not to be involved in subsequent investigation or research, it is important that information about suspected problems and hazards be made available to workers and employers in similar industrial settings, government agencies, healthcare professionals, and perhaps the public at large. Case reports discussed in the medical literature, at medical meetings, or through the media can be helpful in this regard.

SUMMARY

Industrial, workplace, and environmental exposures represent a different kind of challenge to primary care and emergency physicians. Patients often present as a diagnostic dilemma or with common symptoms that do not respond to the usual medical treatment. The challenge for nonoccupational health professionals is to correctly establish and treat the condition. This chapter offers a basic approach to all patients that will aid in the diagnosis and treatment of occupational and environmental diseases. This approach uses additional questions applied to the medical history and access to printed and electronic information resources. Exposures to these materials have public health implications. Physicians who make the diagnosis of an occupationally or environmentally related disease have an obligation to prevent further injury. They should work with employee groups, employers, and government agencies to identify the toxic agent and prevent the development of disease in other potentially exposed individuals.

PRIMARY READINGS

1. Hathaway GJ, Proctor NH, Hughes JP, Fischman ML. *Proctor and Hughes' Chemical Hazards in the Workplace*, 5th ed. New York: John Wiley & Sons; 2004.
2. Stellman JM, ed. *Encyclopedia of Occupational Health and Safety*, 4th ed. Geneva, Switzerland: International Labor Organization; 1998.
3. Wald P, Stave G. *Physical and Biological Hazards in the Workplace*, 2nd ed. New York: John Wiley & Sons; 2002.
4. Wallace RB, ed. *Maxcy-Rosenau-Last Public Health and Preventive Medicine*, 15th ed. Stamford, CT: Appleton & Lange; 2007.

ADDITIONAL READINGS

Bingham E, Cohrssen B, Powell CH eds. *Patty's Industrial Hygiene and Toxicology*, 5th ed. New York: Wiley Interscience; 2005.

Burgess WA. *Recognition of Health Hazards in Industry: A Review of Materials and Processes*, 2nd ed. New York: Wiley; 1995.

Gosselin RE, Smith RP, Hodge HC. *Clinical Toxicology of Commercial Products*, 5th ed. Baltimore: Williams & Wilkins; 1984.

Key MM. *Occupational Diseases: A Guide to Their Recognition*. Washington, DC: US Department of Health, Education, and Welfare; 1977.

Lewis RJ. *Hazardous Chemicals Desk Reference*, 6th ed. New York: Wiley Interscience; 2008.

Magos L. Three cases of methylmercury intoxication which eluded correct diagnosis. *Arch Toxicol.* 1998;72:701-705.

Rom WN, Markowitz, S eds. *Environmental and Occupational Medicine*, 4th ed. Philadelphia: Lippincott Williams & Wilkins; 2006.

Sullivan JB, Krieger GR. *Hazardous Materials Toxicology: Clinical Principles in Environmental Health*, 2nd ed. Baltimore: Williams & Wilkins; 2001.

CHAPTER 123
NANOTOXICOLOGY

Silas W. Smith

HISTORY

Humanity has serendipitously used nanotechnology for hundreds of years. In the Greco-Roman period, the mixing of lead oxide and slaked lime with water resulted in the creation of lead sulfite nanocrystals (5 nm), which blackened hair when allowed to accumulate in the hair cuticle and cortex.[293] Gold nanoparticles produce the striking color of ruby glass present in the Roman Lycurgus cup and in later church stained glass windows.[107] Carbon nanotubes (CNTs) and cementite (Fe_3C) nanowires found in 17th century Damascus steel sword blades explain its high-quality mechanical properties.[240] In 1959, the physicist Richard Feynman proposed the theoretical framework for "manipulating and controlling things" all the way down to the atomic level in "There's Plenty of Room at the Bottom."[83] Norio Taniguchi is generally credited with coining the term "nano-technology"—"the processing of separation, consolidation and deformation of materials by one atom or one molecule"—in 1974.[270]

In practical terms, the invention of the scanning tunneling microscope (STM) in 1981 enabled the visualization of individual atoms and allowed the direct physical manipulation of atomic surfaces.[139] In 1985, Kroto and colleagues reported on a novel minute crystalline allotropic form of carbon, apparently conceived of some 15 years previously.[55,154,213] These now-familiar soccer ball–shaped carbon-60 structures were named "buckminsterfullerenes" after Buckminster Fuller. The discovery of CNTs followed in 1991.[123] The 2003 Congress enacted the "21st Century Nanotechnology Research and Development Act" to create a National Nanotechnology Program with a mandate to establish the goals, priorities, and metrics for evaluation of federal nanotechnology research, development, and other activities; to invest in federal research and development programs in nanotechnology and related sciences to achieve those goals; and to provide for federal interagency coordination.[196]

The health and safety impact of nanotoxicology came to fore during the first consumer recall of a purported nano-based invention.[301] In 2006, the bathroom cleaning product "Magic-Nano" was released in Germany. Within days, more than 110 cases of illness were reported, and several patients were hospitalized with severe respiratory complaints, including acute lung injury. No further episodes of illness occurred after product recall only 3 days after introduction.[135] Although it was ultimately determined that "Magic-Nano" contained no nanoparticles, the incident raised many questions about nanotechnology development, regulation, and health risks.[20,21] There are now more than 600 consumer xenobiotics incorporating nanotechnology, with approximately three to four new ones reaching the market weekly.[272] Exposure to nanoparticles is anticipated through a variety of mechanisms that must be considered from a toxicologic perspective.

PHYSIOCHEMICAL PRINCIPLES

Nanotechnology is defined as the "understanding, control, and use of matter at dimensions of roughly 1 to 100 nm, where unique characteristics enable novel applications."[238] The American Society for Testing and Materials (ASTM) International defines an *ultrafine particle* as a particle ranging in size from approximately 0.001 μm (1 nm; 10 Å) to 0.1 μm (100 nm; 1000 Å) and a *nanoparticle* as an ultrafine particle with lengths in two or three dimensions greater than 0.001 μm (1 nm; 1000 Å) and smaller than about 0.1 μm (100 nm; 1000 Å).[12]

For spherical nanoparticles, as particle diameter decreases, the percentage of molecules on the surface of the nanoparticle increases relative to the total number of molecules. This percentage increases quite steeply below 100 nm.[152] This provides a large area (high surface to volume ratio) for chemical reactions to occur and for contact and interaction with biologic systems. Furthermore, as particles reach sizes below 100 nm, quantum mechanical principles become manifest, and thus unique electrical, magnetic, optical, and solubility properties may emerge. Nanoparticles may exist as aggregations (individual particles held together by strong forces) and agglomerations (held together by weak forces such as van der Waals forces, electrostatic and surface tension). The extent of aggregations and agglomerations, particle dispersal, and electrical charge varies, depending on the primary particle constituents and on solvents or media.[304] This imparts additional properties to identical substances even at the nanoparticle level: whereas C_{60} fullerenes are intensely hydrophobic and essentially insoluble in water, colloidal C_{60} clusters remain mono-dispersed in water as long as electrostatic repulsions are not disrupted by salts.[31]

Nanomaterials and nanoparticles include a vast array of structures, such as composite nanodevices, dendrimers, fullerenes, liposomes, nanocrystals, nanogels, nanofibers, nanoshells, nanospheres, nanotubes, nanowires, polymeric micelles, quantum dots (QDs) and quantum rods, supermagnetic particles, and environmentally generated "ultrafine particles" (Fig. 123–1). They are composed of materials as diverse as their applications, including carbon, lipids, metals and metal oxides, nucleic acids, polymers, proteins, and combinations thereof.

CURRENT AND PROJECTED APPLICATIONS

Nanotechnologies are currently or anticipated to be incorporated into an ever-widening range of disciplines and industries, including agriculture; automobile parts; chemical and materials science (alloys, catalysts, ceramics, coatings, and thin films); electronics; energy capture and storage; environmental sensing and remediation; food processing; fuel additives; house-cleaning products; paints, varnishes, and sealants; textiles; and water purification.[238,246,257] Thousands of tons of engineered metal oxide nanoparticles and fullerenes are anticipated to be produced globally.[27] Ongoing areas of exploration and uses for human and biomedical applications include biomaterials, cancer treatments, diagnostics, drug and gene delivery systems, and imaging.[246,251,313]

BIOMATERIALS

Applications include creation of scaffolds for in vivo or ex vivo growth as well as coatings to minimize immunogenicity, inhibit specific tissues or cell types, and allow macromolecular repair. Nanocrystalline hydroxyapatite and β-tricalcium phosphate have been approved for human use, as has a nanoparticle dental restorative. Multiple-walled CNTs (MWCNTs) can be molded into various scaffolds, which can support connective tissue and osteoblast adherence and growth.[54,87] Nanoscale systems have achieved selective human keratinocyte and fibroblast adhesion and stimulation.[247] Implanted self-assembled nanofiber scaffolds have been shown to span transected rat spinal cords and support angiogenesis and migration and differentiation of neural cells.[101] Such self-assembling peptide scaffold structures have allowed actual reconstitution of functional visual pathways after traumatic transection.[76] Neuronal growth and improved neuronal

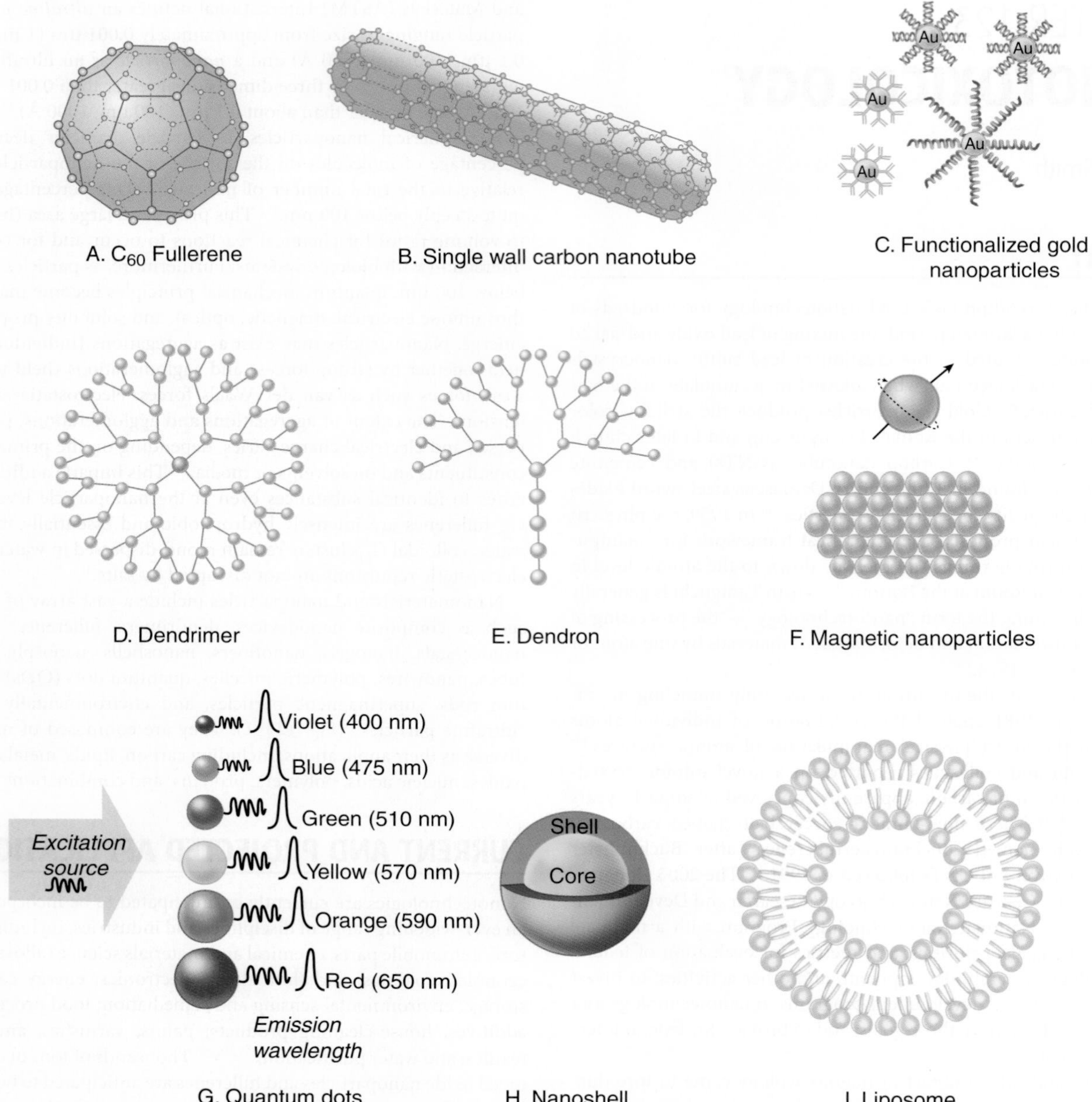

FIGURE 123–1. Nanoparticles (not to scale). **(A)** C_{60} is a prototypical fullerene, or carbon cage, which may enclose additional atoms, ions, or molecular clusters. **(B)** Carbon nanotubes (CNTs) are single-walled (SWCNTs) or multiple-walled (MWCNTs) cylinders, which are capped at each end and can bundle together into longer and wider agglomerates. **(C)** Gold nanoparticles and other nanosized noble metals (eg, silver, copper, platinum) have unusual catalytic, optical, electronic, and (photo)thermal properties and can be conjugated to dyes, antibodies, peptides, and oligonucleotides. **(D)** Dendrimers are branched polymers consisting of a central core, an internal branching region, and surface terminal groups; drugs, genes, and imaging agents can be loaded into the inner protected cavities. **(E)** Dendrons are wedge-shaped sections of dendrimers with an accessible reactive group. **(F)** Magnetic nanoparticles include superparamagnetic iron oxide (SPIO) nanoparticles (Fe_2O_3, Fe_3O_4), pure metals (Fe and Co), and alloys ($CoPt_3$ and FePt). They are usually surrounded by a shell to minimize agglomeration and chemical reactivity. **(G)** Quantum dots (QDs) are semiconductor nanocrystals capable of size-dependent fluorescence with a "tunable" emission spectrum in the 400-nm to 2-μm range. **(H)** Nanoshells contain a dielectric silica core surrounded by thin metal gold shell. **(I)** Liposomes are globular vesicles with hydrophobic and hydrophilic zones composed of phospholipids, sphingolipids, and ceramides or other esters or polymers ranging in size from 25 nm to the micron range. Nanoparticles can be derivatized or bioengineered with a variety of detection, imaging, or targeting molecules.

electrical signaling on purified multiwall nanotubes,[166] and integration of neural tissues with free-standing vertically aligned carbon nanofiber platforms provides a basis for ultimately stable implantable neural devices.[203]

Bioactive coatings in prosthetics provide the opportunity to control fibrous tissue formation and biointegration. With the goal of increased osseointegration of implanted biomaterials, nano-engineered polymethylmethacrylate structures have been created to control cell adhesion, growth, spreading, cytoskeletal development, and production of the osteoblast marker proteins of human bone marrow cells.[57,195] Nanofilm layers (4 nm) containing dexamethasone can suppress immune response to implants.[51]

CANCER THERAPY

Several authors have reviewed nanocarrier-based cancer treatment modalities.[70,148,149,222,279,313] Examples of currently commercial products include albumin-bound paclitaxel nanoparticles, daunorubicin, doxorubicin, and vincristine liposomes; styrene maleic anhydride-neocarzinostatin; and PEG-L-asparaginase. New carriers include hyaluronic acid-PEG-poly(lactide-co-glycolide) nanoparticles copolymers for sustained release (15 days) of doxorubicin.[305]

Because of "leaky" tumor vasculature and poor lymphatic drainage compared with normal tissue, nanoparticles can nonselectively accumulate in tumor tissue. Tumor vascular pores range between 380 and 780 nm compared with normal vasculature (2–4 nm).[149] This can be used either diagnostically or therapeutically for imaging or drug delivery. However, a more selective approach is nanocarriers linked to specific proteins or antibodies targeting malignantly expressed receptors. Functionalized single-walled CNTs (SWCNTs) have targeted cells expressing specific integrins or overexpressing folate receptors.[163,309] Gold particles linked to vascular endothelial growth factor (VEGF) antibodies induced apoptosis in B-cell chronic lymphocytic leukemia.[190] Magnetic resonance imaging (MRI)–detectible magnetic nanoparticles labeled with near-infrared fluorescence dye and linked with short interfering RNA permitted both visualization and silencing of targeted genes in mice implanted with tumors.[178] Nanoparticles can achieve dual tumor imaging and thermal ablation through the ability to separately modify scattering, resonance shifts, and absorption spectrum.[129]

EXTERNAL PRODUCTS

Sunscreens (TiO_2, ZnO) and cosmetic lotions and conditioners are incorporating a range of nanotechnologies.[206] These provide both aesthetic (transparent sunscreen) and clinical (more efficient ultraviolet [UV] filtration) benefit.[238] The Food and Drug Administration (FDA) has permitted titanium dioxide and zinc oxide nanoparticles since 1999.[301] Nanotechnology is also advancing skin and wound care. FDA-approved wound dressings containing nanocrystalline silver delivery systems are currently commercially available. These silver nano-dressings improve wound healing through suppression of infection and inflammation and promotion of epithelialization via upregulation of micronutrients.[195,275,297]

DIAGNOSTICS AND DRUG DELIVERY

Nanotechnology is expected to accelerate medical diagnostic capability. Cancer diagnosis, biochemical monitoring, and pathogen sensing via a range of protein, nucleic acid, ion, and chemical detection techniques are rapidly advancing.[127] Tagged nanoparticles are currently used in commercial genotyping tests for coagulation disorders, folate metabolism, and warfarin metabolism.

Nanoengineering holds the promise of improved pharmacokinetics, delivery, and targeting of pharmaceuticals, proteins, and genes in a cell- or tissue-specific manner. Gram-positive antibacterial activity of rifampin increases when nanoencapsulated into a biodegradable polymer.[80] Encapsulation allows for more efficient drug delivery to intracellular pathogens such as *Mycobacterium tuberculosis*[6,260] and *Toxoplasma gondii*.[58] Gold nanoparticles conjugated with streptomycin and kanamycin showed greater heat stability and improved efficacy against *Escherichia coli, Micrococcus luteus,* and *Staphylococcus aureus*.[245] Antiretroviral drugs can be loaded into nanoparticles allow for improved organ uptake.[130]

In addition to the cancer modalities described above, aprepitant, fenofibrate, megestrol acetate, sirolimus, and topical estrogen preparations have been engineered for nanometer-sized particle delivery. A range of largely unregulated fat-soluble vitamins, carotenoids, phytosterols, minerals, and supplements are currently marketed as nano-based formulations.

IMAGING

Several reviews illuminate the expanding field of nanoparticle incorporation into both targeted and nontargeted approaches to imaging.[38,149,259] Intravenous (IV) superparamagnetic iron oxide (SPIO) and gadolinium chelate are nanotechnologies currently approved for MRI imaging. Specific organ, tumor, and sentinel lymph node imaging is now possible.[77,145,146,258] Iodinated nanoparticle contrast agents permit computed tomography detection of macrophages in atherosclerotic plaques.[122] Imaging at the cellular and molecular level includes differentiation of cellular subcompartments, uptake mechanisms, cell architecture, intracellular trafficking, and single proteins and receptors.[97,268,274]

IMMUNOLOGY

Nanotechnology is being applied to observe or suppress immune system functions to minimize the need for immunosuppressant medications. Thin coatings of cross-linked polyethylene glycol have been reduced to the 20-μm size to allow pancreatic islet cells thus encapsulated to excluded large immunostimulatory molecules while retaining the ability to secrete insulin in response to glucose in vitro.[303] Extending this work, intraperitoneal-delivered islet cells surrounded by a multicomponent capsule of 60 μm or smaller with nanometer-engineered pores maintained insulin independence in pancreatectomized dogs without requiring immunosuppressant drugs.[295] T-cell targeting with nanoparticles is being explored as a mechanisms of treating immune-mediated disease.[82,233]

EXPOSURE AND DISTRIBUTION

Exposure to nanoparticles is anticipated through a variety of mechanisms (Fig. 123–2). Exposure might occur through environmental discharge into air, water, or soil during the primary manufacturing process; disposition of industrial or research waste; engine combustion; or after biologic elimination from a primary target. Sanding, machining, wearing and weathering, or disposing of nanomaterial-containing products could also liberate nanoparticles. Several federal agencies involved in the National Nanotechnology Initiative are attempting to characterize actual exposure data and metrics.[238,267]

DERMAL EXPOSURE

Nanosized liposomes and other formulations for transdermal drug delivery systems have already achieved dermal penetration for therapeutic intent. Various proprietary cosmetics also incorporate nanomaterials. The presumed etiology of podoconiosis (endemic nonfilarial elephantiasis, noninfectious geochemical elephantiasis) is absorption of various colloid-sized elemental particles in irritant clays (aluminum, silicon, magnesium, iron, and possibly beryllium and zirconium), which undergo macrophage phagocytosis to induce collagenization of afferent lymphatics and their ultimate obliteration.[60] A large review summarizing the available studies on dermal penetration of TiO_2 and ZnO nanoparticles found in sunscreens concluded that dermal penetration for those substances was unlikely[206]; however, abraded skin might increase dermal penetration.[243] Lymphatic drainage

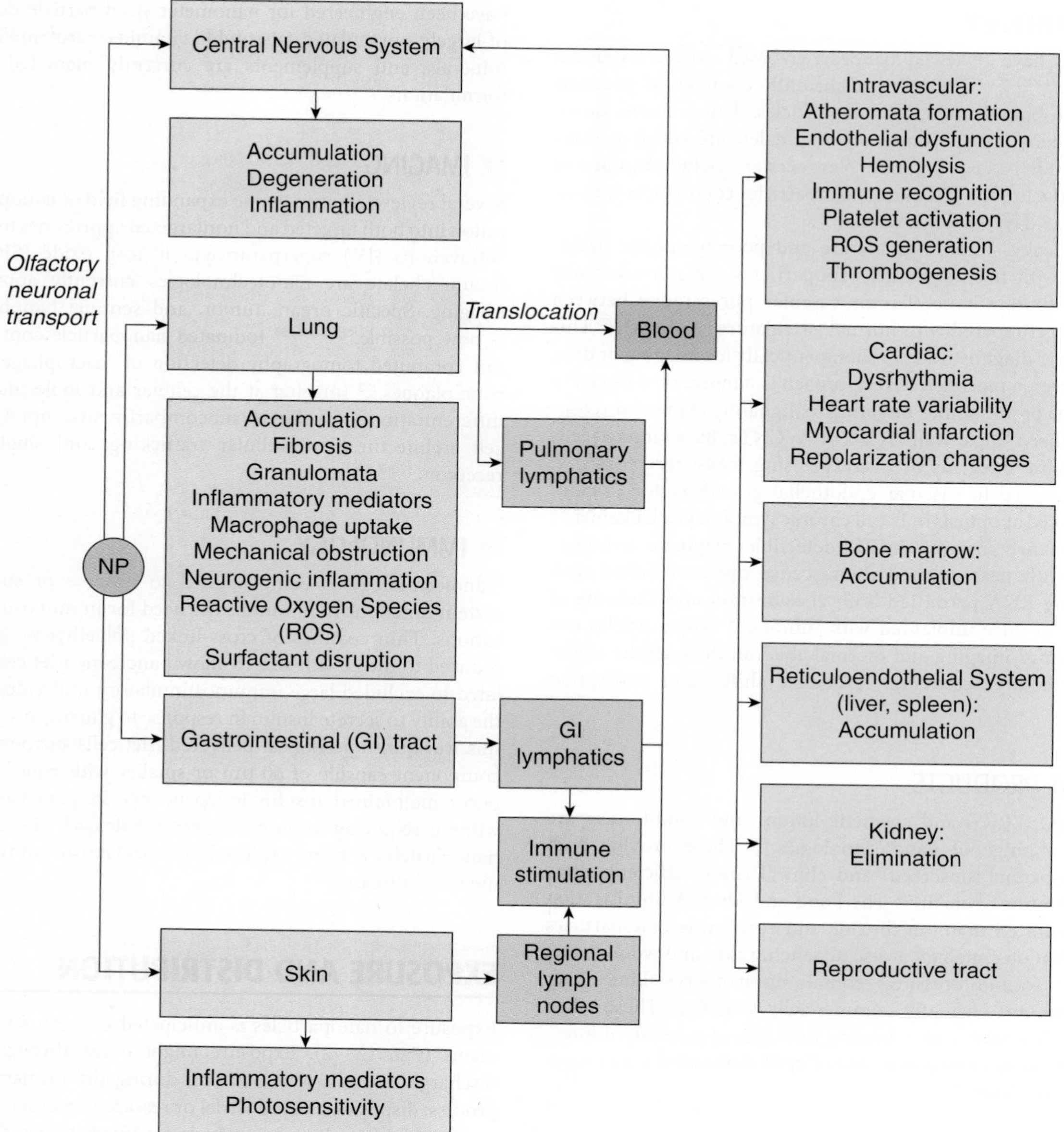

FIGURE 123–2. Potential mechanisms of nanoparticle (NP) toxicity including exposure, distribution, and organ system effects. Accumulation may not be limited to the organ systems depicted.

to sentinel lymph nodes and systemic distribution are possible after the dermis is reached.[99,142]

INHALATION EXPOSURE

Inhalation is expected to be a major route of nanoparticle entry and toxicity. Nanoparticle aerosols may be generated in manufacturing or research environments. Non-engineered ultrafine products are encountered in welding, soldering, cooking fumes, and combustion products (pollution). As the iron-to-carbon (soot) ratio increases in diesel combustion, the number and size of self-nucleated metallic nanoparticles and larger agglomeration of metallic and carbon particles are observed.[159] Carbon fullerenes may be detected in flaming soot after combustion of various hydrocarbon fuels, including benzene, styrene, cyclohexane, cyclopentane, and rarely in charcoal.[262] Secondary nanoparticles may form in the atmosphere via gas-to-particle conversions after nucleation and coagulation or condensation.[27] The tendency of intermediate particles (>80 nm and <200 nm) to remain suspended in air for prolonged periods of time (days to weeks) provides an additional exposure source.[284]

The pulmonary deposition of inhaled particles is affected by various factors, including diffusion and inertial impaction. Gravity contributes to greater particle deposition of fine particles in the central airways instead of the lung periphery.[59] Inhaled particles are transported from the airway duct to the alveoli by convective bulk flow combined with particle motion from sedimentation and diffusion. Alveolar deposition models support peak particle deposition at 30 nm and 4000 nm, with minimal particle deposition at 50 μm.[49] Consistent with diffusion motion theory, the total deposition fraction (TDF) of ultrafine aerosols in healthy young men and women *increased* as median particle diameter *decreased* from

100 nm (TDF, 26%) to 40 nm (TDF, 44%), as tidal volume increased, and as respiratory flow rate decreased (longer respiratory and retention time).[131] Deep breathing increased deposition of inhaled boluses of ^{99m}Tc–radiolabeled ultrafine carbon particles. After deposited, clearance may be affected by mucociliary movement, augmented by macrophages in at the alveolar level. Macrophages may either move particles toward ciliated epithelium, uptake and store particles, or contribute to transepithelial movement, where particles may deposit in the basement membrane or enter the lymphatics or bloodstream.[152,210] Inherently soluble compounds are generally rapidly absorbed. An additional concern is that nanoparticles may actually evade effective clearance. Macrophages inefficiently take up 15 to 80 nm particles (~20%), which are instead retained in epithelial cells or interstitium.[210] Prolonged pulmonary persistence (75% at 24 hours in healthy subjects) was seen in one human ultrafine particle inhalation study, even accounting for (minimal) translocation and urinary elimination.[184] In an animal study, at 60 days, 81% of MWCNTs and 36% of ground CNTs administered intratracheally (0.5 mg/rat) could be recovered.[191]

ORAL

Unintentional oral exposure is expected to be uncommon, although upper aerodigestive tract aerosol exposure could provide particulate matter for subsequent swallowing. Nanoparticles can enter bacteria and living cells, providing a mechanism for food chain bioaccumulation.[23] Therapeutically, multiple nanoparticulate systems are under evaluation for their ability to enhance solubility, permeability, bioadhesion, bioavailability, and efficacy of poorly absorbed drugs, proteins, and vaccines.[9,63,150] Direct uptake of nanoparticles has been observed via single enterocytes at villi and in Peyer's patch regions of the small intestine.[112] Similar to skin, inflamed or infected intestinal mucosa may increase permeability.[158] Macrophages in human gut–associated lymphoid tissue frequently contain multiple microparticles,[237] which correlate with chronic latent granulomatous inflammation in susceptible individuals.

CIRCULATORY ACCESS

Aside from intentional IV administration of nanoparticle pharmaceuticals, pulmonary translocation, intestinal absorption, dermal penetration, or draining lymphatics may provide circulatory access. In human volunteers, inhaled ^{99m}Tc-labeled ultrafine carbon particles (<100 nm) reached the blood within 1 minute, with a peak between 10 and 20 minutes, and persisted for up to 60 minutes.[200] Both hepatic accumulation and urinary excretion occurred. Gold nanomers (30 nm) can be recovered rapidly in blood platelets of the alveolar capillaries after rat intratracheal injection.[18] Aerosolized gold nanoparticles accumulated in more than 20 rat organs and tissues, particularly the lungs, esophagus, kidneys, aorta, spleen, and heart.[311]

ELIMINATION

Tight junctions (<2 nm) between endothelial cells preclude most nanoparticle exit from systemic circulation. However, organ-specific endothelial characteristics (hepatic fenestrations and splenic discontinuity), transcytosis, or leak-inducing disease conditions (inflammation and cancer) may allow exit of large particles.[86] Overall reticuloendothelial system (RES) and renal clearance are particle- and coating-specific.[1,3,161,241] Shielding nanoparticles with neutral compounds is also thought to impair opsonization and subsequent RES clearance.[214]

CELLULAR ENTRY

Applied research provides multiple examples of nanoparticle entry into cells. Although this can be taken advantage of therapeutically to deliver vaccines, genes, and chemotherapy, unwanted cellular introduction of nanoparticles might engender ensuing toxicity. Cellular uptake of nanoparticles involves multiple mechanisms, including phagocytic or endocytic mechanisms (clathrin mediated, scavenger receptor mediated, mannose receptor mediated, Fcγ receptor mediated, complement receptor mediated), potocytosis (caveolin dependent), macropinocytosis—and direct cytoplasmic entry.[41,56,68,86,198,220,263,274,286] CNTs have been observed to pierce and penetrate plasma membranes through largely energy independent mechanisms.[156] Various water-soluble C_{60} fullerene derivatives and native C_{60} are capable of easily penetrating biologic membranes, including those of human erythrocytes and platelets.[5] The mechanism of nanoparticle entry (free diffusion versus endosomal containment) may impact cellular effects.

DETECTION AND DOSE QUANTIFICATION

Development of effective nanomaterial detection methods is a national priority.[267] In the past, sampling of generated aerosols has focused on the average chemical composition and mass of all deposited particles, with the exception of asbestos, for which the number of fibers with a specific shape and composition is important.[176] Measurement approaches have been reviewed and include various devices to assess particle number (concentration), surface area, and mass.[4,88,176,197,204] Importantly, engineered nanoparticles are generally produced as a distribution of sizes as opposed to a uniform product. Dose assessment is further complicated by the multiple differences among nanoparticles and ongoing investigation as to the most appropriate metric: bulk amount (total particulate mass), particle burden (number of particles of a certain size), total surface area, or alternative metrics. In actual industrial settings, mass concentration measurements can vary significantly compared with particle number counts.[81,230]

TOXICITY

The diverse nature of the xenobiotics, compositions, structures, and physical properties involved in nanotechnology prohibits generalization regarding toxic effect. One review reported 428 studies documenting adverse effects of 965 unique nanoparticles.[104] Even reviews of a single "class" of nanoparticles (QDs,[106] fullerenes,[162] CNTs,[126] dendrimers,[71] and gold nanoparticles[162]) have found both adverse and neutral effects. The in vitro nature of many studies does not reliably predict or confirm systemic biologic effects in humans. Differences in experimental methodology, cell line, substance concentration, particle size and geometry, exposure parameters, duration of observation, and end points or surrogate markers have hindered comparison. There is a paucity of data addressing of long-term effects. Cell line–specific, organ-specific, and species-specific toxicities and effects in clinically or genetically susceptible populations are incompletely described. In addition to reported toxic effects, actual exposure assessments are required to appropriately characterize risk.

Several reviews have attempted to address the many real and theoretical issues surrounding nanoparticle toxicity,[27,33,66,67,115,152,162,198,210,212,219,286,299] and various schemes have been proposed to categorize nanoparticles.[104,176] Despite the many unknowns, experiences from previous work with particle toxicology have contributed to a large body of epidemiologic and experimental literature associating airborne particulate matter (PM) from pollution with mortality, cardiovascular, pulmonary, and neurological injury.[35,67,96,105,114,134,140,223,227,229,256] The strength of the association depends on the particle size and type and on the outcome of interest. Similarly, ultrafine particles in home-generated cooking fumes have been implicated in pulmonary disease, inflammation, and genotoxicity.[45,179,180,265,283,291,302]

Genetic or unique susceptibilities to nanoparticles are not well categorized. Preexisting acute or chronic disease (pulmonary disease, cardiac disease, malignancy, infection) or individual genetic variations (resistance to oxidative stress, immune composition, surface or serum proteins) may modify nanoparticle toxicity, specifically by altering deposition rates, clearance, or toxicity thresholds.[36,64,184] Although the following sections generally report "positive" studies in order to highlight nanotoxicity principles, it is important to acknowledge that many other studies have also produced negative results.[16,50,53,142,169,170,188,189,263,290,310]

FACTORS AFFECTING TOXICITY

Composition Ultrafine elemental carbon particles (90 nm) have been shown to be significantly more toxic to macrophages than diesel exhaust particles of comparable size.[183] Acid-functionalized SWCNTs and oxidized MWCNTs produced more murine pulmonary toxicity and human lymphocyte cytotoxicity than their "pristine" counterparts.[29,253] Decay of certain water-soluble fullerenes leads to daughter compounds with increased toxicity in vivo.[19] Gold nanoparticles, asbestos (chrysotile), Al_2O_3, Fe_2O_3, ZrO_2 (zirconia), and TiO_2 have different cytotoxicity in vitro.[266] Uncoated QD core materials (cadmium, lead, selenium) are toxic at relatively low concentrations, damaging the plasma membrane, mitochondrion, and nucleus, and resulting in cell death.[48,106,168]

Coating and Surfactant Materials Coating materials may have inherent toxicity or may shield toxicity of core compounds.[37,43,52] They also mediate the duration of circulation and cell- and organ-specific uptake.[244] Air exposure or photodecomposition can render initially benign coatings cytotoxic.[62] Hydrophilic compounds coating of QDs appear to mediate genotoxicity in human lymphoblast cells.[118] Organic solvents and surfactants used to maintain particle dispersion are frequently cytotoxic.[298] Exposure to protein-rich biologic fluids may change the tendency to agglomerate and therefore produce unique size-dependent effects. Using surfactants (eg, SWCNTs) may decrease protein adherence and therefore alter biological effect or fate.[72,92]

Contaminants Additional toxicity may occur in the presence of contaminants. "Doping" is the intentional process of introducing impurities in order to modify the behavior of materials such as the electrical properties of semiconductors. Similarly, doping may alter the electronic, optical, and magnetic properties of nanocrystals.[207] Doping may also be used to reduce toxicity. MWNTs doped with nitrogen improved biocompatibility and reduced lethality compared with unmodified MWNTs in mice exposed via intranasal, oral, intratracheal, and intraperitoneal routes.[40]

Contamination may unintentionally occur during the manufacturing process and may include atomic or molecular impurities in the nanomaterial structure itself, residual reagents, or byproducts of manufacturing in the final product. "Purified" SWNCTs may retain significant percentages of cobalt, mobolybdenum, iron, nickel, yttrium, and zinc.[157,173] Residual contaminants and impurities of substances used in surface modification of QDs are cytotoxic and genotoxic in vitro.[118] The near-total lethality of a preparation of citrate-, biotin-, cetyltrimethylammonium bromide–modified gold nanoparticles (18 nm) was eliminated by washing off the unbound cetyltrimethylammonium bromide.[53]

Size and Surface Area Size plays an important role in toxicity for certain compounds. Nanoparticles may have different toxicities than the sum of the particles despite a comparable exposure on a mass-for-mass basis. For example, cobalt–ferrite particles reduced in size to 6 nm showed significant increase in cytotoxicity and genotoxicity compared with 10- or 120-μm particles.[53] Ultrafine elemental carbon particles (5–10 nm) induced inflammatory mediators significantly more compared with larger carbon black particles (14 or 51 nm).[17] CoCr nanoparticles generate more superoxide and hydroxyl free radicals and DNA damage than CoCr microparticles.[218] Independent of the concomitant increase in surface area, the small size allows access to protected sites such as the cell nucleus. Gold nanoparticles (1 nm) can penetrate cell and nuclear membranes.[282] QDs (2.1 nm) can rapidly enter the nucleus of human macrophages.[194] Small (2.2 nm) CdTe QDs induced cell death to a far greater extent than equally charged QDs of greater size (5.2 nm).[167]

Shape and Structure Shape and structure may affect toxicity and biologic interactions, even among nanoparticles of similar composition. SWCNTs produce pulmonary granulomata and inflammation, but nanoparticle carbon black does not.[157,173,264] Asbestos-like or mesothelioma-like pathology was seen for "long" MWCNTs (nanometer diameter, >15 μm length) in mice.[234] Compared with 220-nm structures, "long" (825 nm) CNTs increased the degree of inflammatory response in rats; macrophages more easily enveloped 220-nm CNTs.[252] Gold nanorods had significantly less cellular uptake than comparable spherical structures.[47] Toxicity varies with the type of crystalline structure of a given material. The particle shape of asbestos has been considered to constitute an important factor in genotoxicity, and inflammatory and mutagenic properties vary by silica type (crystalline or amorphous).[254] Amorphous TiO_2 crystals were found to generate significantly more reactive oxygen species (ROS) than anatase, mixed anatase and rutile, or rutile crystals, and material surface defects were important for ROS generation.[132]

In vivo, nanoparticles may be associated with layers of surrounding adsorbed biologic proteins or lipids, which may alter their effective size or shape. Curvature of the nanoparticle may affect the extent of this "corona" and influence interactions with bound proteins such as apolipoprotein and albumin, which may effect cells entry or receptor interactions.[171] Binding of albumin; fibrinogen; IgG; Ig light chain; and apolipoproteins A-I, A-IV, C-III and J to polymer nanoparticles was affected by particle hydrophobicity, charge, and functional groups.[89,90,92,249] Bioassociation may also alter nanomaterial properties. SWCNTs adsorbed with serum proteins (primarily albumin) gained an antiinflammatory effect.[72] In contrast, prevention of protein adsorption to amorphous silica particles reduced toxicity.

Charge Surface charge may alter the physical characteristics of the nanoparticle (dispersion, hydrophilicity) or biologic interaction and effect. Neutral SWCNTs aggregate in aqueous solution; introducing a strong negative charge induces dispersal.[253] Negatively charged nanoparticles permeated model pig skin, which excluded positively charged and neutral particles.[147] Increasing surface charge density alters protein absorption.[90] Charged nanoparticles are recognized as important in complement activation.[65] Strongly charged particles can mediate direct membrane damage (hole formation) in the lipid bilayer.[116,117] Positively charged polystyrene nanospheres induced oxidative stress; those with neutral charge did not.[304] Charge-dependent endocytosis was demonstrated in mouse peritoneal macrophages and a human hematopoietic monocytic cell line—the higher the negative or positive surface charge of albumin particles, the greater the uptake cells.[242] Nanoparticle charge and cytotoxicity were positively correlated in human colonic adenocarcinoma cells.[165]

Dose Depending on the xenobiotic, the observed "dose" (particle number or bulk amount) may or may not be relevant. Appropriate dose–response curves (linear, supralinear, biphasic, or threshold) are lacking for most nanoparticles.[210] Cytotoxicity of CdSe/CdS QDs was directly proportional to the number of intracellular particles.[43] Dose-dependent cytotoxicity occurred in human keratinocytes as SWCNT concentration increased from 0.11 to 10 μg/mL.[174] Dose- and time-dependent effects were apparent in human peripheral blood lymphocytes exposed to oxidized or pristine MWCNTs.[29] SWCNT necrotic and apoptotic cytotoxicity to macrophages was dose-dependent starting at 2.5 μg/mL.[235] In zebrafish embryos, silver nanoparticles induced dose-dependent embryotoxicity and multiple developmental abnormalities.[160]

pH Nanoparticles have been engineered to be pH responsive. In the acidic environment of the endosome or lysosome (pH, 4.5), core-shell particles can swell by almost three times, disrupting these structures and allowing cytosolic entry.[120] Alternatively, at altered pH, certain functional groups can be cleaved, resulting in altered charge and improved QDs delivery.[182]

CELLULAR TOXICITY

Ultimately, after cellular–nanoparticle interaction occurs, toxicity may occur via a variety of different mechanisms (Fig. 123–3). Oxidative stress, membrane damage, cytoskeleton alteration, energy failure, cytoplasmic and nuclear protein alteration, photoxicity, and genotoxicity have all been described.

Oxidative Stress Oxidative stress with subsequent lipid peroxidation, DNA damage, and apoptotic or necrotic pathway induction is perceived as a major factor in nanoparticle toxicity. Interpretation of research is complicated by the finding that some particles induce ROS under abiotic conditions but not intracellularly.[304] The biological medium used may also alter ROS generation.[85] C_{60} fullerenes have shown conflicting results. Under visible light irradiation, C_{60} and C_{70} fullerenes induced $O_2^{\cdot -}$ and ·OH, which could induce DNA cleavage.[307] In contrast, C_{60} fullerene and several derivatives have antioxidant activity, preventing radical-related toxicity of carbon tetrachloride in rats[93] and liposome lipid peroxidation induced by superoxide and hydroxyl radicals.[294] Unmodified CdTe QDs induced ROS formation, leading to multiple organelle damage and cell death.[48,168]

Cell Substructure Damage Independent of oxidative stress, nanoparticles may alter or damage multiple cellular substructural components. One of the most important functions that may be disrupted is energy production by mitochondria. Nanoparticles may exert significant toxic effects on mitochondria, including alterations in mitochondrial calcium levels, dissipation of the mitochondrial membrane potential, and lipid membrane destruction.[48,168,304] Gold nanoparticles (3 nm but not 6 nm) cross the mitochondrial membrane by accessing the voltage-dependent anion channel (porin).[248] In a rat liver–derived cell line, molybdenum (30 and 150 nm) and aluminum (30 and 103 nm)

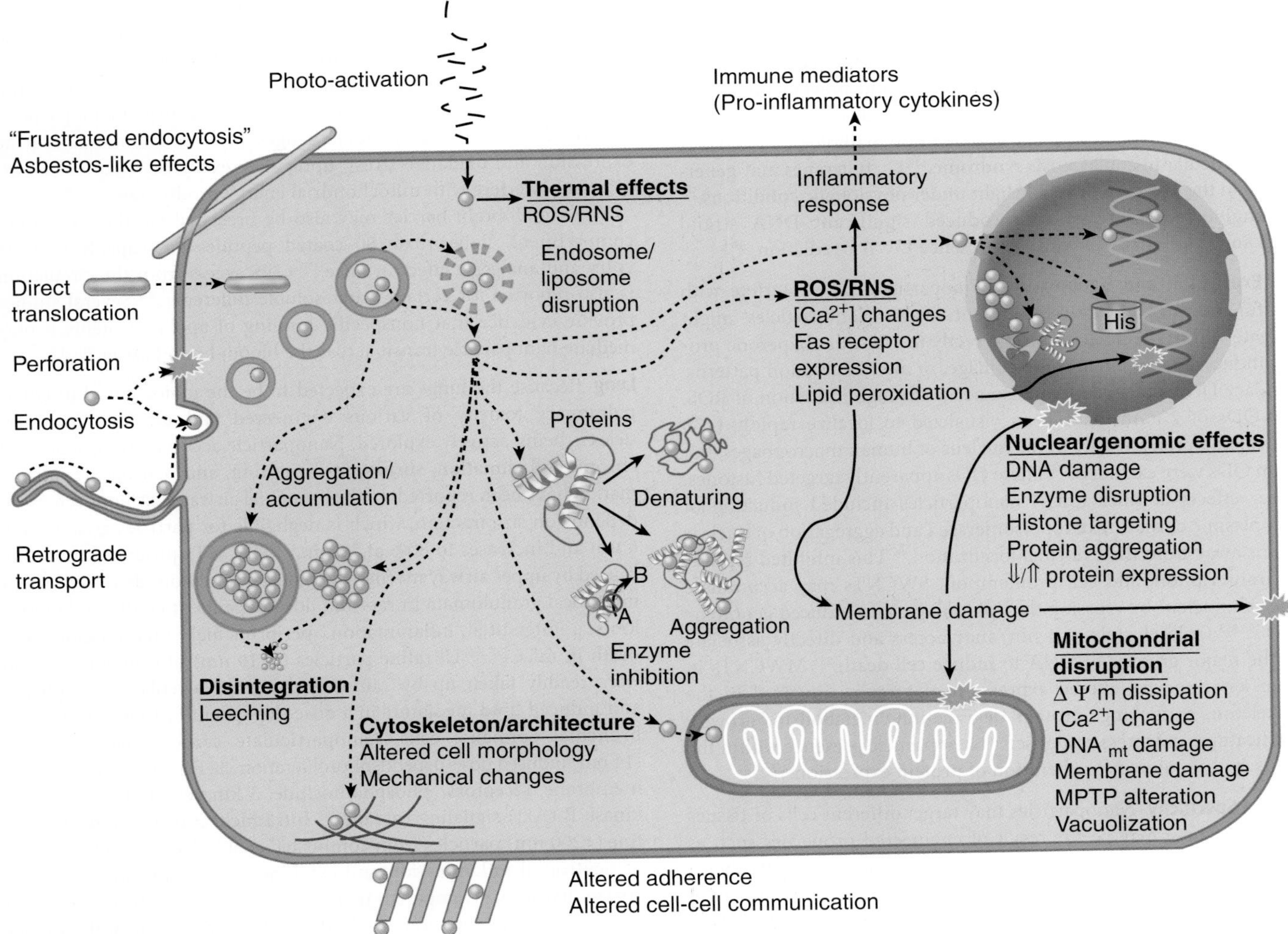

FIGURE 123–3. Potential mechanisms of nanoparticle cellular toxicity. ΔΨm, mitochondrial membrane potential, DNA_{mt}, mitochondrial DNA; His, histone; MPTP, mitochondrial permeability transition pore; RNS, reactive nitrogen species; ROS, reactive oxygen species.

significantly impaired mitochondrial function at high levels of 100 to 250 μg/mL; silver (15 and 100 nm) did so at much lower levels of 5 to 50 μg/mL.[121] Evidence suggests that exposure to MWCNTs may result in mitochondrial DNA damage.[314]

Effects of nanoparticles on extracellular adherence are the subject of bioapplications research. Gold–citrate nanoparticles (13 nm) induced morphologic changes, including loss of adhesion and intracellular actin fiber changes in human dermal fibroblasts.[224] Calcium-mediated cytoskeletal function of murine macrophages was altered by ultrafine carbon particles but not by diesel exhaust or urban dust particles.[183] Superparamagnetic iron oxide nanoparticles rapidly disrupted actin distribution and microtubule structures within cells.[102] In a cell system, iron oxide nanoparticles reduced formation of actin microfilaments and microtubules extension, leading to an impaired ability to extend neurites.[232]

Protein function may also be altered by nanoparticles. Whereas clusters of copper nanoparticles selectively induced unfolding and precipitation of hemoglobin A0 and E, almost none occurred with hemoglobin A2.[22] C_{60} fullerene noncompetitively inhibited glutathione peroxidase in a substrate-specific manner.[125] Although relatively high concentrations were required (250 μM), C_{60} fullerene derivatives selectively inhibited P450 metabolism of progesterone.[84]

Phototoxicity One concern is that nanoparticles could be excited by ambient light to incidentally generate either oxygen radicals or direct thermal injury. One current clinical application uses liposomal verteporfin (benzoporphyrin derivative monoacid ring A) activated by low-intensity nonthermal laser light (689 nm) to efficiently generate singlet oxygen. This is believed to induce cell death and prevent the loss of visual acuity in patients with subfoveal choroidal neovascularization secondary to age-related macular degeneration, pathologic myopia, or presumed ocular histoplasmosis syndrome.[138] C_{60} fullerenes may generate ROS in the presence of visible light under physiologic conditions.[308] TiO_2-engineered nanoparticles produced significant DNA strand breaks and cytotoxicity only in the presence UV A irradiation.[289]

Gene Expression and Genotoxicity Nanoparticles may interfere with gene functioning on several different levels. Nanoparticles might aggregate within the nucleus, bind directly to DNA or chaperone proteins, induce nuclear membrane damage, or alter expression patterns. Secondary DNA damage might also occur through induction of ROS. Small QDs of 2.1 nm have been visualized to localize rapidly (<30 minutes) and preferentially in the nucleus of human macrophages, but 3.4-nm QDs were excluded.[194] These QDs apparently targeted histones. Nuclear effects of silica (SiO_2) nanoparticles included induction of nucleoplasmic clustering of topoisomerase I and aggregation of nuclear proteins away from their normal localization.[46] This inhibited replication, transcription, and cell proliferation. SWCNTs may accumulate in the cell nucleus by crossing the lipid bilayer and induced genotoxic effects.[143,235] Gold clusters (1.4 nm) may access and directly associate with the major grooves of DNA to induce cell death.[282] MWCNTs in human keratinocytes altered expression of proteins involved in the cytoskeleton, trafficking, protein degradation, metabolism, growth, detoxification, and stress response.[300] Nanoparticle presence within the nucleus is not required for alteration of protein expression.[215]

Cell Type Specificity Nanoparticles may target different cells or tissues differently. These may be the result of engineered properties such as antibody linkage, ferritin linkage, properties of nanomaterials themselves (size-dependent RES deposition), or biologic processes of target cells (phagocytosis ability, resistance to oxidative stress, cytoskeletal architecture). Although gold nanoparticles (33 nm) were cytotoxic (via apoptosis induction) to human lung carcinoma type II epithelial cells, human hepatocellular liver carcinoma and baby hamster kidney cells were unaffected.[221] It is precisely because of this differential effect that multiple cell lines are advocated for toxicity testing.[261]

ORGAN SYSTEMS TOXICITY

Brain A significant concern is the ability of nanoparticles to translocate to normally protected spaces. This may be on both the macroscopic scale in organs such as the brain or on the microscopic level such as the ability to penetrate lipid bilayers protecting individual cells or nuclear space. Early studies of the poliomyelitis virus (25–30 nm) provided evidence that small particles could access the brain via the nose.[25,26,119,281] Therapeutically, engineered nanoparticle characteristics for intentional central nervous system (CNS) drug targeting have been reviewed by several authors.[24,128,280] Other compounds successfully transported into the brain using nanoparticles include loperamide, tubocurarine, dalargin (a hexapeptide), kytorphin (a dipeptide), MRZ 2/576 (*N*-methyl-D-aspartic acid receptor antagonist), and doxorubicin.[151] Children and dogs exposed to air pollution showed similar prefrontal white matter hyperintense lesions. These were associated with significant cognitive deficits in children; anatomic correlation in the dogs showed ultrafine particulate matter deposition, vascular pathology, and neuroinflammation.[39] Ultrafine elemental ^{13}C particles translocated into axons of the olfactory nerve in inhalation-exposed rats.[211] Rats exposed to poorly soluble manganese oxide ultrafine particles (30 nm) showed olfactory bulb uptake and CNS delivery to the striatum, frontal cortex, and cerebellum.[73] Cadmium, cobalt, manganese, mercury, nickel, and zinc reach the olfactory bulb when applied intranasally in animal models, and neuronal connections may carry cobalt, manganese, and zinc into deeper brain structures.[7,34,109,225,226,273,278] Entry of nanoparticles may result in CNS inflammatory changes, increase inflammatory gene expression and oxidative stress, upregulate excitatory neurotransmitters, and interfere with mitochondrial energy production.[73,144,164,228,277]

The blood–brain barrier may also be breached via the circulatory compartment. Polysorbate 80–coated peptides are capable of CNS entry and analgesic effect in mice.[150] CNS access from the circulation is also reported for certain water-soluble fullerenes.[306] Several studies provide evidence that nonspecific binding of apolipoproteins E may mediate nanoparticle transit across the blood–brain barrier.[91,151]

Lung Because the lungs are expected to be the major portal of entry, pulmonary toxicity of various engineered and ultrafine nanoparticles is being actively explored. Nanoparticle accumulation, acute and chronic inflammation, surfactant disruption, and neurogenic inflammation have been reported. In the bronchial airways, 24-hour retention depends on size fraction, which is negligible for particles greater than 6 μm and increases to 80% at 30 nm.[153] SWCNTs produced mortality caused by upper airway mechanical blockage and non–dose-dependent multifocal granulomata in rats and dose-dependent epithelioid granulomata, interstitial inflammation, peribronchial inflammation, and death in mice.[157,296] Ultrafine particles (5–10 nm) of elemental carbon were readily taken up by canine and human alveolar macrophages and induced lipid mediators in a dose-dependent fashion.[17] In human bronchial epithelial cells, nanoparticulate carbon black particles (14 nm) induced dose-dependent proliferation via EGF-R and β1-integrin membrane receptors, phosphoinositide 3-kinases, and the protein kinase B (Akt) signaling cascade.[287] Intratracheal instillation of ultrafine (<200 nm) particles from combusted coal induced a higher degree of neutrophil inflammation and cytokine levels than did the fine or coarse particles. Compared with control subjects, mice aspirating native and acid-functionalized SWCNTs had significantly higher bronchoalveolar lavage (BAL) cell counts, PMNs, and cytokines (IL-6, tumor necrosis factor-α, and macrophage-inflammatory protein-2 (MIP2)).[253] The severe toxicity of air-generated polytetrafluorethylene

(PTFE fumes) may be reduced by aging, filtering, and preexposure, suggesting nanoparticle upregulation of pulmonary inflammatory cytokines and antioxidants.[133]

Pulmonary surfactant is a mixture of lipids, phospholipids, and proteins that provides low surface tension and serves to bind and identify targets for phagocytosis. Independent of cellular effects, in vitro lung models suggest that nanoparticle deposition may cause pulmonary surfactant dysfunction during the breathing cycle.[136] Nanosized nickel, cobalt, and TiO_2 create more inflammation than larger metal particles of an equivalent mass concentration. Diesel exhaust particulate matter may be solubilized and dispersed in the major component of pulmonary surfactant (dipalmitoyl phosphatidyl choline) and induce genotoxicity in multiple different assays in bacteria and mammals.[250,292]

Hematological and Cardiovascular Effects Possible hematologic and vascular effects of concern include thrombogenesis, atherogenesis, endothelial dysfunction, hemolysis, and immune stimulation. Epidemiologic studies support an association between exposure to particulate matter of less than 10 μm (PM_{10}) and increased risk of deep venous thrombosis.[13] This is in contrast to larger particles (PM_{10}), which were not statistically associated with mortality from embolism and thrombosis.[113] Diesel exhaust particles (20–50 nm, 200–500 times smaller than PM_{10}) and positively charged polystyrene nanoparticles cause rapid activation of circulating blood platelets and microcirculatory thrombi.[199,201] Healthy volunteers exposed to concentrated ambient air particles had a linear increase in fibrinogen concentrations.[95]

Compared with larger particles, ultrafine particles produced larger atherosclerotic lesions, decreased the antiinflammatory effect of high-density lipoprotein, and induced oxidative stress in a susceptible animal model.[8] Human exposure to wood smoke increased the levels of serum amyloid A, a cardiovascular risk factor, as well as factor VIII in plasma and the factor VIII/von Willebrand factor ratio.[15] At doses that produced no significant pulmonary inflammatory changes, rats exposed to ultrafine TiO_2 aerosols displayed impaired endothelium-dependent arteriolar dilation or outright constriction.[208,209]

Multiple engineered and combustion-derived carbon nanoparticles stimulate human platelet aggregation, activate glycoprotein (GP) IIb/IIIa, and accelerate the rate of vascular thrombosis in rat carotid arteries.[239] Metal nanoparticles (iron, copper, gold, cadmium sulfide) induced dose-dependent platelet aggregation through the P2Y12 ADP receptor.[61] Nickel, cobalt, and titanium dioxide nanoparticles variably induce blood neutrophils to release ROS and reactive nitrogen species.[181] IV administration of ultrafine diesel exhaust particles induced monocyte proliferation, decreased hemoglobin concentrations, and increased pulmonary inflammation.[202]

Dendrimers may alter human erythrocyte shape, induce clustering, and cause significant hemolysis.[2,68,71,172] Polycationic water-soluble fullerene C_{60} derivatives and stabilized poly(lactide-co-glycolide) acid (PLGA) nanoparticles also induce significant hemolysis.[28,141]

The ability of ultrafine particles to alter intracardiac function (decrease heart rate variability and repolarization changes) has been reported by several investigators.[64,98,105,108,276,288,312] Heart rate variability provides a measure of cardiac autonomic control, and a decrease predicts mortality in patients with prior myocardial infarction.[276] Significant pulmonary inflammation is not a prerequisite for this independent effect. At levels that initiated only low-grade pulmonary inflammation but not increased blood coagulability, carbon ultrafine particles (38 nm) increased heart rate and decreased heart rate variability.[105] Autonomic reflexes from pulmonary nerve endings appeared to mediate these effects.[94]

Immune System Nanoparticles may interact with the immune system in complex ways. Depending on their biophysiochemical properties, nanoparticles may stimulate, suppress, or elude the immune responses.[66] Induction of chronic inflammation is of concern because commercially and academically available MWCNTs induced asbestos-like, length-dependent pathology in the abdominal cavity of mice following intraperitoneal exposure in mice,[234] and work in murine macrophage cells lines demonstrates that MWCNTs have a cytotoxic response nearly identical to that of asbestos.[266] Particle specific interactions with macrophages may result in intracellular particle accumulation, antigen-mediated immune stimulation, inflammatory mediator release, or fibrous or granulomata formation. In fact, formation of mouse granulocyte-macrophage colonies is now a standard testing methodology for assessing nanoparticle toxicity.[11] Multiple examples of significant ultrafine and engineered nanoparticle interaction with macrophages and monocytes are detailed throughout this chapter. Other cell lines can be also induced to release inflammatory mediators. Human epidermal cells exposed to SWCNTs release interleukin-8.[185] MWCNTs introduced in human neonatal epidermal keratinocytes increased IL-8 and IL-1β release.[300]

Direct immune stimulation may also occur. Fullerenes may induce a direct IgG response, which is capable of cross-reaction with other fullerenes.[30,44] The degree of induced opsonization by various IgG and complement molecules is thought to explain part of the differences seen in blood clearance and tissue distribution of nanoparticles.[214] CNTs may also act as adjuvants to boost immune response even in the absence of direct immune stimulation.[217]

Antibodies are not the only responses involved. Volunteer exposure to concentrated ambient particles (<200 nm) increased inflammatory blood mediators (intercellular adhesion molecule 1).[98] Given that proteins are known to absorb to nanoparticles, expectedly, CNTs were found to activate human complement via both classical and alternative pathways, and C1q binds directly to CNTs.[249] Complement activation may underlie non–IgE-mediated immediate hypersensitivity reactions seen in PEGylated liposomal doxorubicin administration.[42] $MnFe_2O_4$ magnetic nanoparticles (diameter, 10 nm) induced severe inflammatory reactions in mice.[155] Last, nanoparticles may contribute to "neurogenic inflammation," the process of inflammation by airway nerves, which synthesize various inflammatory mediators (neurokinin A, substance P, calcitonin gene-related peptide, and others) in response to exogenous irritants and contribute to pathology.[75,100,187]

Reproduction and Embryologic Development Research into nanoparticle effects on the reproductive system is sparse. One review of eight articles concluded that nanoparticles are able to cross the blood–testis barrier and locate in the testes.[177] At least one study found dose-dependent mitochondrial impairment cytotoxicity in spermatogonia, particularly silver nanoparticles.[32] In the animal model of organogenesis, fish eggs (*Oryzias latipes*) easily took up 39.4-nm fluorescent particles and concentrated them in the yolk area and gallbladder during embryonic development.[137] More complex interactions, such as endocrine or androgen disruption from leaching or degradation of nanoparticles, are largely unexplored.[110,216,231]

Bioaccumulation and Persistence A final concern is nanoparticle accumulation in cells, tissues, or organs. Repeated exposure would then permit attainment of threshold toxicities. Alternatively, prolonged periods of persistence could allow leaching and toxicity of initially protected materials. Work in small-fiber toxicology (eg, asbestos) has demonstrated that biopersistent particle effects may not manifest for decades.[186] Among different fine particles (fiberglass, rock wool, slag wool, asbestos), biopersistent potential seems to underlie toxic effects.[111] Thus, the independent findings that MWCNTs may induce asbestos-like pathology and mesothelioma is worrisome.[234,269] Bone marrow deposition of nanoparticles[236] could allow for ongoing systemic exposure. Persistence in other compartments could also permit more extensive distribution (eg, translocation from lung tissue).

Dextran-coated ultrasmall superparamagnetic iron oxide particles currently used in clinical trials are retained by human monocyte–macrophages for days.[192,193] QDs persisted at least 4 months in mice, remaining at least 1 month in the liver, lymph nodes, and bone marrow.[14] At the cellular level, nanocrystals can be passed to daughter cells upon mammalian cell division.[103,175] In fact, retained fluorescing QDs have been used experimentally to trace *Xenopus* cells from the embryo to the tadpole stage.[69]

ADMINISTRATIVE, REGULATORY, AND RESEARCH ISSUES

The 21st Century Nanotechnology Research and Development Act guides U.S. nanotechnology policy.[196] Amendments to the National Nanotechnology Initiative (NNI) are currently under Congressional consideration.[271] Elements include establishment of national strategic plans for nanotechnology and triennial review by the National Research Council; establishment of a public database for funded EHS (environmental, health, and safety), educational and societal dimensions, and nanomanufacturing projects; fiscal support for a Nanotechnology Coordination Office; mandates for research in environmental, health, and safety; development of nomenclature and engineered nanoscale standard reference materials standards; development of standards for detection, measurement, monitoring, sampling, and testing of engineered nanoscale materials for environmental, health, and safety impacts; and nanotechnology education. The NNI comprises various federal agencies with funding, research, regulatory, and administrative roles, including the Department of Defense, National Science Foundation, Department of Education, National Institutes of Heath, National Institute for Occupational Safety and Health (NIOSH), FDA, National Institute of Standards and Technology, Environmental Protection Agency (EPA), United States Department of Agriculture, National Aeronautics and Space Administration, and others. In its congressionally mandated role to review federal nanotechnology research and development, the National Nanotechnology Advisory Panel has provided recommendations for continued development of infrastructure, standards, and EHS risk analysis concurrent with applications research.[238]

ENVIRONMENTAL, HEALTH, AND SAFETY

The detailed NNI strategy for EHS research recommends incorporation of many factors in concluding a nanotechnology risk assessment, including nanomaterials synthesis and use; nanomaterial lifecycle stage; transport, transformation, and abiotic effects; environmental concentration; exposure of environmental and biologic systems; internal dose; biologic response; and environmental effects.[267] Identified immediate priority needs included the development of nanomaterial detection methods, certified reference materials, and standardized physiochemical assessments; understanding generalizable toxicologic characteristics of nanomaterials in biologic systems; identification of environmental and occupational exposures; and evaluation of risk management approaches to nanomaterials.

OCCUPATIONAL HEALTH

NIOSH is the coordinating U.S. agency for nanotechnology human and environmental exposures assessment research.[267] At the time of writing, established U.S. government occupational exposure limits, action levels, or disclosure and surveillance guidelines specific for engineered nanoparticles were nonexistent.[255] The general federal statute limiting "particulates not otherwise regulated" (PNOR) (also known as "inert or nuisance dusts") to a respirable fraction of 15 millions of particles per cubic foot of air (5 mg/m^3) would include nanoparticles, although this may provide inadequate protection.[74,157,264] NIOSH has released two reports, "Approaches to Safe Nanotechnology"[204] and "Progress towards Safe Nanotechnology in the Workplace."[205] These identified potential health concerns (nanoparticle dose, deposition, reactivity, toxicity, and translocation) and safety issues (combustion and catalytic potential). Recommendations included epidemiology, surveillance and background nanoaerosol measurements, personnel exposure sampling, engineering controls, implementation of risk management programs, and use of filters and respirators when necessary.[204] NIOSH anticipates that properly fit NIOSH-certified respirators in conjunction with a respiratory control program will protect workers from most inhaled nanoparticles.[205] Other occupational professional guidance can be found in national and international guidelines and reviews.[10,88,124,197,255]

FOOD AND DRUG ADMINISTRATION

The FDA regulates food and color additives, drugs, biologics, devices, blood products, and cosmetics to ensure that they are "safe" and unadulterated. The FDA does not regulate "nanotechnology." Rather, marketing authorization occurs on a product-by-product basis. The FDA can require manufacturers to provide necessary information (eg, chemistry, manufacturing, active ingredients, pharmacologic and toxicologic results, and particle size) to support decisions regarding premarket approval; however, in evaluating the sponsor "claims," the FDA may be unaware that nanotechnology is being used. In general, the FDA has treated nanomaterial ingredients no differently than bulk material ingredients or products. An FDA task force recommended addressing nanotechnology labeling and environmental impact on a case-by-case basis.[285] Cosmetics and dietary supplement nanomaterials claims are largely unevaluated.

ENVIRONMENTAL PROTECTION AGENCY

The EPA is the coordinating agency for human nanomaterials environmental research.[267] Nanomaterial applications for environmental remediation are particularly attractive. Regulation of nanomaterials and the effects of nanotechnology may also come under the EPA's broad authorities under the Clean Air Act (CAA), Pollution Prevention Act (PPA), Clean Water Act (CWA), Safe Drinking Water Act (SDWA), Federal Insecticides and Rodenticides Act (FIFRA), Comprehensive Environmental Response Compensation and Liability Act (CERCLA), Resource Conservation and Recovery Act (RCRA), and Toxic Substances Control Act (TSCA). For example, the EPA determined that (nano) silver ion–generating washing machines marketed with bactericidal claims were subject to registration requirements under FIFRA,[79] and extended the requirement to copper- and zinc-emitting devices and ion generators in swimming pools. The EPA also launched a Nanoscale Materials Stewardship Program (NMSP) for reporting available information on the engineered nanoscale materials to complement its existing programs per TSCA, under which new nanomaterials might be regarded as "chemical substances."[78] The balance of nanotechnology to improve environmental conditions (e.g., improved fuel efficiency and decreased emissions via cerium oxide nanoparticle additives diesel fuel) will need to be carefully weighed against unintended consequences (eg, increased ambient cerium air concentrations and altered diesel emissions composition with increased benzene, 1,3-butadiene, and acetaldehyde concentrations).[284]

The rapid pace of development will mandate constant updating and assessment of available knowledge. A selected list of organizational resources is provided in Table 123–1.

TABLE 123–1. Selected Nanotechnology Organizational Resources[a]

Organization	Website
Center for Biological and Environmental Nanotechnology (CBEN)	http://cben.rice.edu/
Center for Environmental and Human Toxicology (CHET)	http://www.floridatox.org/
Center for Nanoscale System (CNS)	http://www.cns.cornell.edu/
European Commission, Nanotechnology Homepage	http://cordis.europa.eu/nanotechnology/
German Federal Institute for Occupational Safety and Health (BAuA), Nanotechnology	http://www.baua.de/en/Topics-from-A-to-Z/Hazardous-Substances/Nanotechnology/Nanotechnology.html?__nnn=true
International Council on Nanotechnology (ICON)	http://icon.rice.edu/
Nano/Bio Interface Center	http://www.nanotech.upenn.edu/
Nanoscale Science and Engineering Center (NSEC), Nanotechnology Risk Resources	http://www.nsec.wisc.edu/NanoRisks/NS--NanoRisks.php
National Cancer Institute (NCI), Alliance for Nanotechnology in Cancer	http://nano.cancer.gov/
National Center for Learning and Teaching in Nanoscale Science and Engineering (NCLT)	http://www.nclt.us/
Organization for Economic Co-operation and Development (OECD), Work on Nanotechnology	http://www.oecd.org/sti/nano
Project on Emerging Nanotechnologies, Woodrow Wilson International Center for Scholars	http://www.nanotechproject.org/
The Library of Congress, Selected Internet Resources in Science and Technology, Nanotechnology	http://www.loc.gov/rr/scitech/selected-internet/nanotechnology.html
UK Safenano Initiative	http://www.safenano.org/
US Department of Commerce, National Technical Information Service, Nanotechnology	http://www.ntis.gov/nanotech/nano.asp
US Environmental Protection Agency (EPA)	http:/www.epa.gov/; http:/es.epa.gov/ncer/nano/
US Food and Drug Administration (FDA), Nanotechnology	http://www.fda.gov/nanotechnology/
US National Institute for Occupational Safety and Health (NIOSH), Nanotechnology Topic Page	http://www.cdc.gov/niosh/topics/nanotech/
US National Institute of Standards and Technology (NIST), Nanotechnology Portal	http:/www.nist.gov/public_affairs/nanotech.htm
US National Nanotechnology Initiative (NNI)	http:/www.nano.gov/
US National Science Foundation (NSF) National Nanotechnology Initiative	http://www.nsf.gov/crssprgm/nano/
US National Toxicology Program (NTP), Nanotechnology Safety Initiative	http://ntp.niehs.nih.gov/?objectid=7E6B19D0-BDB5-82F8-FAE73011304F542A

[a] Many of these websites are searchable for nano-related developments, policy, research, and toxicology. Websites retrieved August 12, 2008.

SUMMARY

Nanotechnology and nanotoxicology represents new and expanding disciplines. Although the possible applications of nanotechnology are diverse and beneficial at this early stage in nanotoxicology, toxicologic profiles are incomplete. The special physiochemical properties of nanoparticles, which can yield non-intuitive biologic effects, complicate this assessment. Appropriate research methodologies, *in* vitro and in vivo models, risk assessment, and workplace and environmental standards await further exploration and consensus.

REFERENCES

1. Agashe HB, Babbar AK, Jain S, et al. Investigations on biodistribution of technetium-99m-labeled carbohydrate-coated poly(propylene imine) dendrimers. *Nanomedicine.* 2007;3:120-127.
2. Agashe HB, Dutta T, Garg M, Jain NK. Investigations on the toxicological profile of functionalized fifth-generation poly (propylene imine) dendrimer. *J Pharm Pharmacol.* 2006;58:1491-1498.
3. Akerman ME, Chan WCW, Laakkonen P, et al. Nanocrystal targeting in vivo. *PNAS.* 2002;99:12617-12621.
4. American Chemistry Council. *Recommendations from the Toxicology Working Group of the Nanotechnology Panel of the American Chemistry Council for a Reasoned Approach to the Testing of Nanoscale Materials.* Arlington, VA: American Chemistry Council; 2006. Retrieved July 6, 2008, from http://www.americanchemistry.com/s_acc/bin.asp?SID=1&DID=5091&CID=654&VID=109&DOC=File.PDF.
5. Andreev I, Petrukhina A, Garmanova A, et al. Penetration of fullerene c60 derivatives through biological membranes. *Fuller Nanotub Car N.* 2008;16:89.
6. Anisimova YV, Gelperina SI, Peloquin CA, Heifets LB. Nanoparticles as antituberculosis drugs carriers: effect on activity against mycobacterium tuberculosis in human monocyte-derived macrophages. *J Nanopart Res.* 2000;2:165-171.
7. Antonini JM, Santamaria AB, Jenkins NT, et al. Fate of manganese associated with the inhalation of welding fumes: potential neurological effects. *Neurotoxicology.* 2006;27:304-310.
8. Araujo JA, Barajas B, Kleinman M, et al. Ambient particulate pollutants in the ultrafine range promote early atherosclerosis and systemic oxidative stress. *Circ Res.* 2008;102:589-596.
9. Asghar LF, Chandran S. Multiparticulate formulation approach to colon specific drug delivery: current perspectives. *J Pharm Pharm Sci.* 2006;9:327-338.

10. ASTM International. *ASTM E2535-07 Standard Guide for Handling Unbound Engineered Nanoscale Particles in Occupational Settings*. West Conshohocken, PA: ASTM International; 2007. Retrieved June 2, 2008, from http://www.astm.org/Standards/E2535.htm.
11. ASTM International. *ASTM E2525-08 Standard Test Method for Evaluation of the Effect of Nanoparticulate Materials on the Formation of Mouse Granulocyte-Macrophage Colonies*. West Conshohocken, PA: ASTM International; 2008. Retrieved June 2, 2008, from http://www.astm.org/Standards/E2525.htm.
12. ASTM International. *Terminology for Nanotechnology. Designation: E 2456-06*. West Conshohocken, PA: ASTM International; 2006. Retrieved June 3, 2008, from http://www.liu.se/cte/english/Nanotechnology%20terminology.pdf.
13. Baccarelli A, Martinelli I, Zanobetti A, et al. Exposure to particulate air pollution and risk of deep vein thrombosis. *Arch Intern Med*. 2008;168:920-927.
14. Ballou B, Lagerholm BC, Ernst LA, et al. Noninvasive imaging of quantum dots in mice. *Bioconjugate Chem*. 2004;15:79-86.
15. Barregard L, Sallsten G, Gustafson P, et al. Experimental exposure to wood-smoke particles in healthy humans: effects on markers of inflammation, coagulation, and lipid peroxidation. *Inhal Toxicol*. 2006;18:845-853.
16. Beckett WS, Chalupa DF, Pauly-Brown A, et al. Comparing inhaled ultrafine versus fine zinc oxide particles in healthy adults: a human inhalation study. *Am J Respir Crit Care Med*. 2005;171:1129-1135.
17. Beck-Speier I, Dayal N, Karg E, et al. Oxidative stress and lipid mediators induced in alveolar macrophages by ultrafine particles. *Free Radic Biol Med*. 2005;38:1080-1092.
18. Berry JP, Arnoux B, Stanislas G, Galle P, Chretien J. A microanalytic study of particles transport across the alveoli: role of blood platelets. *Biomedicine*. 1977;27:354-357.
19. Beuerle F, Witte P, Hartnagel U, Lebovitz R, Parng C, Hirsch A. Cytoprotective activities of water-soluble fullerenes in zebrafish models. *J Exp Nanosci*. 2007;2:147.
20. BfR (Federal Institute of Risk Assessment). Cause of intoxications with nano spray not yet full elucidated [press release]. Berlin: BfR (Federal Institute of Risk Assessment); April 12, 2006. Retrieved June 10, 2008, from http://www.bfr.bund.de/cms5w/sixcms/detail.php/7750.
21. BfR (Federal Institute of Risk Assessment). Nano particles were not the cause of health problems triggered by sealing sprays [press release]! Berlin: BfR (Federal Institute of Risk Assessment); May 25, 2006. Retrieved June 10, 2008, from http://www.bfr.bund.de/cms5w/sixcms/detail.php/7842.
22. Bhattacharya J, Choudhuri U, Siwach O, Sen P, Dasgupta AK. Interaction of hemoglobin and copper nanoparticles: implications in hemoglobinopathy. *Nanomedicine*. 2006;2:191-199.
23. Biswas P, Wu CY. Nanoparticles and the environment. *J Air Waste Manag Assoc*. 2005;55:708-746.
24. Blasi P, Giovagnoli S, Schoubben A, Ricci M, Rossi C. Solid lipid nanoparticles for targeted brain drug delivery. *Adv Drug Deliv Rev*. 2007;59:454-477.
25. Bodian D, Howe HA. An experimental study of the role of neurones in the dissemination of poliomyelitis virus in the nervous system. *Brain*. 1940;63:135-162.
26. Bodian D, Howe HA. The rate of progression of poliomyelitis virus in nerves. *Bull Johns Hopkins Hosp*. 1941;69:79-85.
27. Borm PJ, Robbins D, Haubold S, et al. The potential risks of nanomaterials: a review carried out for ECETOC. *Part Fibre Toxicol*. 2006;3:11.
28. Bosi S, Feruglio L, Da Ros T, et al. Hemolytic effects of water-soluble fullerene derivatives. *J Med Chem*. 2004;47:6711-6715.
29. Bottini M, Bruckner S, Nika K, et al. Multi-walled carbon nanotubes induce T lymphocyte apoptosis. *Toxico Lett*. 2006;160:121-126.
30. Braden BC, Goldbaum FA, Chen BX, Kirschner AN, Wilson SR, Erlanger BF. X-ray crystal structure of an anti-Buckminsterfullerene antibody fab fragment: biomolecular recognition of C(60). *PNAS*. 2000;97:12193-12197.
31. Brant J, Lecoanet H, Wiesner MR. Aggregation and deposition characteristics of fullerene nanoparticles in aqueous systems. *J Nanopart Res*. 2005;7:545-553.
32. Braydich-Stolle L, Hussain S, Schlager JJ, Hofmann MC. In vitro cytotoxicity of nanoparticles in mammalian germline stem cells. *Toxicol Sci*. 2005;88:412-419.
33. Brayner R. The toxicological impact of nanoparticles. *Nano Today*. 2008;3:48-55.
34. Brenneman KA, Wong BA, Buccellato MA, Costa ER, Gross EA, Dorman DC. Direct olfactory transport of inhaled manganese ((54)MnCl(2)) to the rat brain: toxicokinetic investigations in a unilateral nasal occlusion model. *Toxicol Appl Pharmacol*. 2000;169:238-248.
35. Brook RD, Franklin B, Cascio W, et al. Air pollution and cardiovascular disease: a statement for healthcare professionals from the Expert Panel on Population and Prevention Science of the American Heart Association. *Circulation*. 2004;109:2655-2671.
36. Brown JS, Zeman KL, Bennett WD. Ultrafine particle deposition and clearance in the healthy and obstructed lung. *Am J Respir Crit Care Med*. 2002;166:1240-1247.
37. Byrne SJ, Williams Y, Davies A, et al. "Jelly dots": synthesis and cytotoxicity studies of CdTe quantum dot-gelatin nanocomposites. *Small*. 2007;3:1152-1156.
38. Cai W, Chen X. Nanoplatforms for targeted molecular imaging in living subjects. *Small*. 2007;3:1840-1854.
39. Calderon-Garciduenas L, Mora-Tiscareno A, Ontiveros E, et al. Air pollution, cognitive deficits and brain abnormalities: a pilot study with children and dogs. *Brain Cogn*. 2008;68(2):115-116.
40. Carrero-Sanchez JC, Elias AL, Mancilla R, et al. Biocompatibility and toxicological studies of carbon nanotubes doped with nitrogen. *Nano Lett*. 2006;6:1609-1616.
41. Chan WC, Nie S. Quantum dot bioconjugates for ultrasensitive nonisotopic detection. *Science*. 1998;281:2016-2018.
42. Chanan-Khan A, Szebeni J, Savay S, et al. Complement activation following first exposure to pegylated liposomal doxorubicin (Doxil): possible role in hypersensitivity reactions. *Ann Oncol*. 2003;14:1430-1437.
43. Chang E, Thekkek N, Yu WW, Colvin VL, Drezek R. Evaluation of quantum dot cytotoxicity based on intracellular uptake. *Small*. 2006;2:1412-1417.
44. Chen B, Wilson SR, Das M, Coughlin DJ, Erlanger BF. Antigenicity of fullerenes: antibodies specific for fullerenes and their characteristics. *Proc Natl Acad Sci*. 1998;95:10809-10813.
45. Chen H, Yang M, Ye S. A study on genotoxicity of cooking fumes from rapeseed oil. *Biomed Environ Sci*. 1992;5:229-235.
46. Chen M, von Mikecz A. Formation of nucleoplasmic protein aggregates impairs nuclear function in response to SiO2 nanoparticles. *Exp Cell Res*. 2005;305:51-62.
47. Chithrani BD, Ghazani AA, Chan WC. Determining the size and shape dependence of gold nanoparticle uptake into mammalian cells. *Nano Lett*. 2006;6:662-668.
48. Choi AO, Cho SJ, Desbarats J, Lovric J, Maysinger D. Quantum dot-induced cell death involves Fas upregulation and lipid peroxidation in human neuroblastoma cells. *J Nanobiotechnol*. 2007;5:1.
49. Choi J, Kim CS. Mathematical analysis of particle deposition in human lungs: an improved single path transport model. *Inhal Toxicol*. 2007;19:925.
50. Choi MR, Stanton-Maxey KJ, Stanley JK, et al. A cellular Trojan Horse for delivery of therapeutic nanoparticles into tumors. *Nano Lett*. 2007;7:3759-3765.
51. Chow EK, Pierstorff E, Cheng G, Ho D. Copolymeric nanofilm platform for controlled and localized therapeutic delivery. *ACS Nano*. 2008;2:33-40.
52. Colognato R, Bonelli A, Bonacchi D, Baldi G, Migliore L. Analysis of cobalt ferrite nanoparticles induced genotoxicity on human peripheral lymphocytes: comparison of size and organic grafting-dependent effects. *Nanotoxicology*. 2007;1:301.
53. Connor EE, Mwamuka J, Gole A, Murphy CJ, Wyatt MD. Gold nanoparticles are taken up by human cells but do not cause acute cytotoxicity. *Small*. 2005;1:325-327.
54. Correa-Duarte MA, Wagner N, Rojas-Chapana J, Morsczeck C, Thie M, Giersig M. Fabrication and biocompatibility of carbon nanotube-based 3d networks as scaffolds for cell seeding and growth. *Nano Lett*. 2004;4:2233-2236.
55. Curl RF, Smalley RE, Kroto HW, O'Brien S, Heath JR. How the news that we were not the first to conceive of soccer ball C60 got to us. *J Mol Graph Model*. 2001;19:185-186.
56. Dahan M, Laurence T, Pinaud F, et al. Time-gated biological imaging by use of colloidal quantum dots. *Opt Lett*. 2001;26:825-827.
57. Dalby MJ, McCloy D, Robertson M, Wilkinson CDW, Oreffo ROC. Osteoprogenitor response to defined topographies with nanoscale depths. *Biomaterials*. 2006;27:1306-1315.
58. Dalençon F, Amjaud Y, Lafforgue C, Derouin F, Fessi H. Atovaquone and rifabutine-loaded nanocapsules: formulation studies. *Int J Pharmaceut*. 1997;153:127-130.
59. Darquenne C, Prisk G. Deposition of inhaled particles in the human lung is more peripheral in lunar than in normal gravity. *Eur J Appl Physiol*. 2008;103(6):687-695.
60. Davey G, Tekola F, Newport MJ. Podoconiosis: non-infectious geochemical elephantiasis. *Trans R Soc Trop Med Hyg*. 2007;101:1175-1180.

61. Deb S, Chatterjee M, Bhattacharya J, et al. Role of purinergic receptors in platelet-nanoparticle interactions. *Nanotoxicology*. 2007;1:93.
62. Derfus AM, Chan WCW, Bhatia SN. Probing the cytotoxicity of semiconductor quantum dots. *Nano Lett.* 2004;4:11-18.
63. des Rieux A, Fievez V, Garinot M, Schneider YJ, Preat V. Nanoparticles as potential oral delivery systems of proteins and vaccines: a mechanistic approach. *J Control Release*. 2006;116:1-27.
64. Devlin RB, Ghio AJ, Kehrl H, Sanders G, Cascio W. Elderly humans exposed to concentrated air pollution particles have decreased heart rate variability. *Eur Respir J Suppl.* 2003;40(suppl):76S-80S.
65. Dobrovolskaia MA, Aggarwal P, Hall JB, McNeil SE. Preclinical studies to understand nanoparticle interaction with the immune system and its potential effects on nanoparticle biodistribution. *Mol Pharm.* 2008;5(4):487-495.
66. Dobrovolskaia MA, McNeil SE. Immunological properties of engineered nanomaterials. *Nat Nano*. 2007;2:469-478.
67. Dockery DW, Luttmann-Gibson H, Rich DQ, et al. Association of air pollution with increased incidence of ventricular tachyarrhythmias recorded by implanted cardioverter defibrillators. *Environ Health Perspect.* 2005;113:670-674.
68. Domanski DM, Klajnert B, Bryszewska M. Influence of PAMAM dendrimers on human red blood cells. *Bioelectrochemistry*. 2004;63:189-191.
69. Dubertret B, Skourides P, Norris DJ, Noireaux V, Brivanlou AH, Libchaber A. In vivo imaging of quantum dots encapsulated in phospholipid micelles. *Science*. 2002;298:1759-1762.
70. Duncan R. Polymer conjugates as anticancer nanomedicines. *Nat Rev Cancer*. 2006;6:688-701.
71. Duncan R, Izzo L. Dendrimer biocompatibility and toxicity. *Adv Drug Deliv Rev.* 2005;57:2215-2237.
72. Dutta D, Sundaram SK, Teeguarden JG, et al. Adsorbed proteins influence the biological activity and molecular targeting of nanomaterials. *Toxicol Sci.* 2007;100:303-315.
73. Elder A, Gelein R, Silva V, et al. Translocation of inhaled ultrafine manganese oxide particles to the central nervous system. *Environ Health Perspect.* 2006;114:1172-1178.
74. Electronic Code of Federal Regulations. Title 29 (Labor). Subtitle B (Regulations Relating to Labor). Chapter XVII (Occupational Safety and Health Administration, Department of Labor). Section 1910.1000. Table Z-1—Limits for Air Contaminants. 2008.
75. Elekes K, Helyes Z, Németh J, et al. Role of capsaicin-sensitive afferents and sensory neuropeptides in endotoxin-induced airway inflammation and consequent bronchial hyperreactivity in the mouse. *Regul Pept.* 2007;141:44-54.
76. Ellis-Behnke RG, Liang YX, You SW, et al. Nano neuro knitting: peptide nanofiber scaffold for brain repair and axon regeneration with functional return of vision. *Proc Natl Acad Sci U S A*. 2006;103:5054-5059.
77. Enochs WS, Harsh G, Hochberg F, Weissleder R. Improved delineation of human brain tumors on MR images using a long-circulating, superparamagnetic iron oxide agent. *J Magn Reson Imaging*. 1999;9:228-232.
78. Environmental Protection Agency. Nanoscale Materials Stewardship Program [EPA-HQ-OPPT-2004-0122; FRL-8344-5]. *Fed Reg.* January 28, 2008;73(18). Retrieved October 19, 2009, from http://frwebgate.access.gpo.gov/cgi-bin/getpage.cgi?position=all&page=4861&dbname=2008_register.
79. Environmental Protection Agency. Pesticide registration; clarification for ion-generating equipment [EPA–HQ–OPP–2007–0949; FRL–8149–4]. *Fed Reg.* September 21, 2007;72(183). Retrieved October 19, 2009, from http://frwebgate.access.gpo.gov/cgi-bin/getpage.cgi?dbname=2007_register&position=all&page=54039.
80. Esmaeili F, Hosseini-Nasr M, Rad-Malekshahi M, Samadi N, Atyabi F, Dinarvand R. Preparation and antibacterial activity evaluation of rifampicin-loaded poly lactide-co-glycolide nanoparticles. *Nanomedicine.* 2007;3:161-167.
81. Evans DE, Heitbrink WA, Slavin TJ, Peters TM. Ultrafine and respirable particles in an automotive grey iron foundry. *Ann Occup Hyg.* 2008;52:9-21.
82. Fahmy TM, Schneck JP, Saltzman WM. A nanoscopic multivalent antigen-presenting carrier for sensitive detection and drug delivery to T cells. *Nanomedicine*. 2007;3:75-85.
83. Feynman RP. There's plenty of room at the bottom. An invitation to enter a new field of physics. *Eng Sci (Caltech).* 1960;23:22-36.
84. Foley S, Curtis ADM, Hirsch A, et al. Interaction of a water soluble fullerene derivative with reactive oxygen species and model enzymatic systems. *Fuller Nanotub Car N.* 2002;10:49-67.
85. Foucaud L, Wilson MR, Brown DM, Stone V. Measurement of reactive species production by nanoparticles prepared in biologically relevant media. *Toxicol Lett.* 2007;174:1-9.
86. Garnett MC, Kallinteri P. Nanomedicines and nanotoxicology: some physiological principles. *Occup Med (Lond).* 2006;56:307-311.
87. George JH, Shaffer MS, Stevens MM. Investigating the cellular response to nanofibrous materials by use of a multi-walled carbon nanotube model. *J Exp Nanosci.* 2006;1:1.
88. German Federal Institute for Occupational Safety and Health (Bundesanstalt für Arbeitsschutz und Arbeitsmedizin/BAuA), German Chemical Industry Association (Verband der Chemischen Industrie/VCI). *Guidance for Handling and Use of Nanomaterials at the Workplace.* Berlin: BAuA & VCI, 2007. Retrieve June 4, 2008, from http://www.baua.de/nn_49456/en/Topics-from-A-to-Z/Hazardous-Substances/Nanotechnology/pdf/guidance.pdf.
89. Gessner A, Lieske A, Paulke BR, Muller RH. Functional groups on polystyrene model nanoparticles: influence on protein adsorption. *J Biomed Mater Res A.* 2003;65:319-326.
90. Gessner A, Lieske A, Paulke B, Muller R. Influence of surface charge density on protein adsorption on polymeric nanoparticles: analysis by two-dimensional electrophoresis. *Eur J Pharm Biopharm.* 2002;54:165-170.
91. Gessner A, Olbrich C, Schroder W, Kayser O, Muller RH. The role of plasma proteins in brain targeting: species dependent protein adsorption patterns on brain-specific lipid drug conjugate (LDC) nanoparticles. *Int J Pharm.* 2001;214:87-91.
92. Gessner A, Waicz R, Lieske A, Paulke B, Mader K, Muller RH. Nanoparticles with decreasing surface hydrophobicities: influence on plasma protein adsorption. *Int J Pharm.* 2000;196:245-249.
93. Gharbi N, Pressac M, Hadchouel M, Szwarc H, Wilson SR, Moussa F. [60]Fullerene is a powerful antioxidant in vivo with no acute or subacute toxicity. *Nano Lett.* 2005;5:2578-2585.
94. Ghelfi E, Rhoden CR, Wellenius GA, Lawrence J, Gonzalez-Flecha B. Cardiac oxidative stress and electrophysiological changes in rats exposed to concentrated ambient particles are mediated by TRP-dependent pulmonary reflexes. *Toxicol Sci.* 2008;102:328-336.
95. Ghio AJ, Hall A, Bassett MA, Cascio WE, Devlin RB. Exposure to concentrated ambient air particles alters hematologic indices in humans. *Inhal Toxicol.* 2003;15:1465-1478.
96. Ghio AJ, Kim C, Devlin RB. Concentrated ambient air particles induce mild pulmonary inflammation in healthy human volunteers. *Am J Respir Crit Care Med.* 2000;162:981-988.
97. Giepmans BN, Deerinck TJ, Smarr BL, Jones YZ, Ellisman MH. Correlated light and electron microscopic imaging of multiple endogenous proteins using Quantum dots. *Nat Methods.* 2005;2:743-749.
98. Gong H Jr, Sioutas C, Linn WS. Controlled exposures of healthy and asthmatic volunteers to concentrated ambient particles in metropolitan Los Angeles. *Res Rep Health Eff Inst.* 2003;(118):1-36; discussion 37-47.
99. Gopee NV, Roberts DW, Webb P, et al. Migration of intradermally injected quantum dots to sentinel organs in mice. *Toxicol Sci.* 2007;98:249-257.
100. Groneberg DA, Quarcoo D, Frossard N, Fischer A. Neurogenic mechanisms in bronchial inflammatory diseases. *Allergy*. 2004;59:1139-1152.
101. Guo J, Su H, Zeng Y, et al. Reknitting the injured spinal cord by self-assembling peptide nanofiber scaffold. *Nanomedicine.* 2007;3:311-321.
102. Gupta AK, Gupta M. Cytotoxicity suppression and cellular uptake enhancement of surface modified magnetic nanoparticles. *Biomaterials.* 2005;26:1565-1573.
103. Hanaki K, Momo A, Oku T, et al. Semiconductor quantum dot/albumin complex is a long-life and highly photostable endosome marker. *Biochem Biophys Res Commun.* 2003;302:496-501.
104. Hansen SF, Larsen BH, Olsen SI, Baun A. Categorization framework to aid hazard identification of nanomaterials. *Nanotoxicology*. 2007;1: 243-250.
105. Harder V, Gilmour P, Lentner B, et al. Cardiovascular responses in unrestrained WKY rats to inhaled ultrafine carbon particles. *Inhal Toxicol.* 2005;17:29-42.
106. Hardman R. A toxicologic review of quantum dots: toxicity depends on physicochemical and environmental factors. *Environ Health Perspect.* 2006;114:165-172.
107. Haslbeck S, Martinek K-, Stievano L, Wagner F. Formation of gold nanoparticles in gold ruby glass: The influence of tin. *Hyperfine Interactions.* 2005;165:89-94.

108. Henneberger A, Zareba W, Ibald-Mulli A, et al. Repolarization changes induced by air pollution in ischemic heart disease patients. *Environ Health Perspect.* 2005;113:440-446.
109. Henriksson J, Tjalve H. Manganese taken up into the CNS via the olfactory pathway in rats affects astrocytes. *Toxicol Sci.* 2000;55:392-398.
110. Henson MC, Chedrese PJ. Endocrine disruption by cadmium, a common environmental toxicant with paradoxical effects on reproduction. *Exp Biol Med (Maywood).* 2004;229:383-392.
111. Hesterberg TW, Miiller WC, Musselman RP, Kamstrup O, Hamilton RD, Thevenaz P. Biopersistence of man-made vitreous fibers and crocidolite asbestos in the rat lung following inhalation. *Fundam Appl Toxicol.* 1996;29:269-279.
112. Hillyer JF, Albrecht RM. Gastrointestinal persorption and tissue distribution of differently sized colloidal gold nanoparticles. *J Pharm Sci.* 2001;90:1927-1936.
113. Hoek G, Brunekreef B, Fischer P, van Wijnen J. The association between air pollution and heart failure, arrhythmia, embolism, thrombosis, and other cardiovascular causes of death in a time series study. *Epidemiology.* 2001;12:355-357.
114. Hoek G, Brunekreef B, Goldbohm S, Fischer P, van den Brandt PA. Association between mortality and indicators of traffic-related air pollution in the Netherlands: a cohort study. *Lancet.* 2002;360:1203-1209.
115. Hoet PH, Bruske-Hohlfeld I, Salata OV. Nanoparticles—known and unknown health risks. *J Nanobiotechnol.* 2004 8;2:12.
116. Hong S, Bielinska AU, Mecke A, et al. Interaction of poly(amidoamine) dendrimers with supported lipid bilayers and cells: hole formation and the relation to transport. *Bioconjug Chem.* 2004;15:774-782.
117. Hong S, Leroueil PR, Janus EK, et al. Interaction of polycationic polymers with supported lipid bilayers and cells: nanoscale hole formation and enhanced membrane permeability. *Bioconjug Chem.* 2006;17:728-734.
118. Hoshino A, Fujioka K, Oku T, et al. Physicochemical properties and cellular toxicity of nanocrystal quantum dots depend on their surface modification. *Nano Lett.* 2004;4:2163-2169.
119. Howe HA, Bodian D. Poliomyelitis in the chimpanzee: a clinical-pathological study. *Bull Johns Hopkins Hosp.* 1941;69:149-181.
120. Hu Y, Litwin T, Nagaraja AR, et al. Cytosolic delivery of membrane-impermeable molecules in dendritic cells using pH-responsive core-shell nanoparticles. *Nano Lett.* 2007;7:3056-3064.
121. Hussain SM, Hess KL, Gearhart JM, Geiss KT, Schlager JJ. In vitro toxicity of nanoparticles in BRL 3A rat liver cells. *Toxicol in Vitro.* 2005;19: 975-983.
122. Hyafil F, Cornily JC, Feig JE, et al. Noninvasive detection of macrophages using a nanoparticulate contrast agent for computed tomography. *Nat Med.* 2007;13:636-641.
123. Iijima S. Helical microtubules of graphitic carbon. *Nature.* 1991;354:56-58.
124. International Organization for Standardization (ISO). *Workplace Atmospheres—Ultrafine, Nanoparticle and Nano-structured Aerosols—Inhalation Exposure Characterization and Assessment.* ISO/TR 27628:2007. Geneva, Switzerland: International Organization for Standardization (ISO); 2007. Retrieved July 5, 2008, from http://www.iso.org/iso/iso_catalogue/catalogue_tc/catalogue_detail.htm?csnumber=44243.
125. Iwata N, Mukai T, Yamakoshi YN, et al. Effects of C60, a fullerene, on the activities of glutathione S-transferase and glutathione-related enzymes in rodent and human livers. *Fuller Nanotub Car N.* 1998;6:213.
126. Jain AK, Mehra NK, Lodhi N, et al. Carbon nanotubes and their toxicity. *Nanotoxicology.* 2007;1:167.
127. Jain KK. Applications of nanobiotechnology in clinical diagnostics. *Clin Chem.* 2007;53:2002-2009.
128. Jain KK. Nanobiotechnology-based drug delivery to the central nervous system. *Neurodegener Dis.* 2007;4:287-291.
129. Jain PK, Lee KS, El-Sayed IH, El-Sayed MA. Calculated absorption and scattering properties of gold nanoparticles of different size, shape, and composition: applications in biological imaging and biomedicine. *J Phys Chem B.* 2006;110:7238-7248.
130. Jain SK, Gupta Y, Jain A, Saxena AR, Khare P, Jain A. Mannosylated gelatin nanoparticles bearing an anti-HIV drug didanosine for site-specific delivery. *Nanomedicine.* 2008;4:41-48.
131. Jaques PA, Kim CS. Measurement of total lung deposition of inhaled ultrafine particles in healthy men and women. *Inhal Toxicol.* 2000;12:715-731.
132. Jiang J, Oberdörster G, Elder A, Gelein R, Mercer P, Biswas P. Does nanoparticle activity depend upon size and crystal phase? *Nanotoxicology.* 2008;2:33.
133. Johnston CJ, Finkelstein JN, Mercer P, Corson N, Gelein R, Oberdorster G. Pulmonary effects induced by ultrafine PTFE particles. *Toxicol Appl Pharmacol.* 2000;168:208-215.
134. Kan H, London SJ, Chen G, et al. Differentiating the effects of fine and coarse particles on daily mortality in Shanghai, China. *Environ Int.* 2007;33:376-384.
135. Kanarek MS. Nanomaterial health effects part 3: conclusion—hazardous issues and the precautionary principle. *WMJ.* 2007;106:16-19.
136. Kanno S, Furuyama A, Hirano S. Effects of eicosane, a component of nanoparticles in diesel exhaust, on surface activity of pulmonary surfactant monolayers. *Arch Toxicol.* 2008;82(11):841-850.
137. Kashiwada S. Distribution of nanoparticles in the see-through medaka (Oryzias latipes). *Environ Health Perspect.* 2006;114:1697-1702.
138. Keam SJ, Scott LJ, Curran MP. Verteporfin: a review of its use in the management of subfoveal choroidal neovascularisation. *Drugs.* 2003;63:2521-2554.
139. Kearnes M, Macnaghten P. Introduction: (re)imagining nanotechnology. *Science as Culture.* 2006;15:279-290.
140. Kettunen J, Lanki T, Tiittanen P, et al. Associations of fine and ultrafine particulate air pollution with stroke mortality in an area of low air pollution levels. *Stroke.* 2007;38:918-922.
141. Kim D, El-Shall H, Dennis D, Morey T. Interaction of PLGA nanoparticles with human blood constituents. *Colloids Surf B Biointerfaces.* 2005;40:83-91.
142. Kim S, Lim YT, Soltesz EG, et al. Near-infrared fluorescent type II quantum dots for sentinel lymph node mapping. *Nat Biotechnol.* 2004;22:93-97.
143. Kisin ER, Murray AR, Keane MJ, et al. Single-walled carbon nanotubes: geno- and cytotoxic effects in lung fibroblast V79 cells. *J Toxicol Environ Health A.* 2007;70:2071-2079.
144. Kleinman MT, Araujo JA, Nel A, et al. Inhaled ultrafine particulate matter affects CNS inflammatory processes and may act via MAP kinase signaling pathways. *Toxicol Lett.* 2008;178:127-130.
145. Knapp DW, Adams LG, Degrand AM, et al. Sentinel lymph node mapping of invasive urinary bladder cancer in animal models using invisible light. *Eur Urol.* 2007;52:1700-1708.
146. Kobayashi H, Kawamoto S, Bernardo M, Brechbiel MW, Knopp MV, Choyke PL. Delivery of gadolinium-labeled nanoparticles to the sentinel lymph node: comparison of the sentinel node visualization and estimations of intra-nodal gadolinium concentration by the magnetic resonance imaging. *J Control Release.* 2006;111:343-351.
147. Kohli AK, Alpar HO. Potential use of nanoparticles for transcutaneous vaccine delivery: effect of particle size and charge. *Int J Pharm.* 2004;275:13-17.
148. Kontermann RE. Immunoliposomes for cancer therapy. *Curr Opin Mol Ther.* 2006;8:39-45.
149. Koo OM, Rubinstein I, Onyuksel H. Role of nanotechnology in targeted drug delivery and imaging: a concise review. *Nanomedicine.* 2005;1:193-212.
150. Kreuter J. Nanoparticles and microparticles for drug and vaccine delivery. *J Anat.* 1996;189(Pt 3):503-505.
151. Kreuter J. Nanoparticulate systems for brain delivery of drugs. *Adv Drug Deliv Rev.* 2001;47:65-81.
152. Kreyling W, Semmler-Behnke M, Möller W. Health implications of nanoparticles. *J Nanopart Res.* 2006;8:543-562.
153. Kreyling WG, Semmler-Behnke M, Moller W. Ultrafine particle-lung interactions: does size matter? *J Aerosol Med.* 2006;19:74-83.
154. Kroto HW, Heath JR, O'Brien SC, Curl RF, Smalley RE. C_{60}: Buckminsterfullerene. *Nature.* 1985;318:162-163.
155. Lacava ZGM, Azevedo RB, Martins EV, et al. Biological effects of magnetic fluids: toxicity studies. *J Magn Magn Mater.* 1999;201:431-434.
156. Lacerda L, Raffa S, Prato M, Bianco A, Kostarelos K. Cell-penetrating CNTs for delivery of therapeutics. *Nano Today.* 2007;2:38-43.
157. Lam CW, James JT, McCluskey R, Hunter RL. Pulmonary toxicity of single-wall carbon nanotubes in mice 7 and 90 days after intratracheal instillation. *Toxicol Sci.* 2004;77:126-134.
158. Lamprecht A, Schafer U, Lehr CM. Size-dependent bioadhesion of micro- and nanoparticulate carriers to the inflamed colonic mucosa. *Pharm Res.* 2001;18:788-793.
159. Lee D, Miller A, Kittelson D, Zachariah MR. Characterization of metal-bearing diesel nanoparticles using single-particle mass spectrometry. *Aerosol Sci.* 2006;37:88-110.
160. Lee KJ, Nallathamby PD, Browning LM, Osgood CJ, Xu XN. In vivo imaging of transport and biocompatibility of single silver nanoparticles in early development of zebrafish embryos. *ACS Nano.* 2007;1:133-143.

161. Leu D, Manthey B, Kreuter J, Speiser P, DeLuca PP. Distribution and elimination of coated polymethyl [2-14C]methacrylate nanoparticles after intravenous injection in rats. *J Pharm Sci.* 1984;73:1433-1437.
162. Lewinski N, Colvin V, Drezek R. Cytotoxicity of nanoparticles. *Small.* 2008;4:26-49.
163. Liu Z, Cai W, He L, et al. In vivo biodistribution and highly efficient tumour targeting of carbon nanotubes in mice. *Nat Nano.* 2007;2:47-52.
164. Long TC, Saleh N, Tilton RD, Lowry GV, Veronesi B. Titanium dioxide (P25) produces reactive oxygen species in immortalized brain microglia (BV2): implications for nanoparticle neurotoxicity. *Environ Sci Technol.* 2006;40:4346-4352.
165. Loretz B, Bernkop-Schnürch A. In vitro cytotoxicity testing of non-thiolated and thiolated chitosan nanoparticles for oral gene delivery. *Nanotoxicology.* 2007;1:139.
166. Lovat V, Pantarotto D, Lagostena L, et al. Carbon nanotube substrates boost neuronal electrical signaling. *Nano Lett.* 2005;5:1107-1110.
167. Lovric J, Bazzi HS, Cuie Y, Fortin GR, Winnik FM, Maysinger D. Differences in subcellular distribution and toxicity of green and red emitting CdTe quantum dots. *J Mol Med.* 2005;83:377-385.
168. Lovric J, Cho SJ, Winnik FM, Maysinger D. Unmodified cadmium telluride quantum dots induce reactive oxygen species formation leading to multiple organelle damage and cell death. *Chem Biol.* 2005;12:1227-1234.
169. Lu CW, Hung Y, Hsiao JK, et al. Bifunctional magnetic silica nanoparticles for highly efficient human stem cell labeling. *Nano Lett.* 2007;7:149-154.
170. Lu Q, Moore JM, Huang G, et al. RNA Polymer translocation with single-walled carbon nanotubes. *Nano Lett.* 2004;4:2473-2477.
171. Lynch I, Dawson KA. Protein-nanoparticle interactions. *Nano Today.* 2008;3:40-47.
172. Malik N, Wiwattanapatapee R, Klopsch R, et al. Dendrimers: relationship between structure and biocompatibility in vitro, and preliminary studies on the biodistribution of 125I-labelled polyamidoamine dendrimers in vivo. *J Control Release.* 2000;65:133-148.
173. Mangum JB, Turpin EA, Antao-Menezes A, Cesta MF, Bermudez E, Bonner JC. Single-walled carbon nanotube (SWCNT)-induced interstitial fibrosis in the lungs of rats is associated with increased levels of PDGF mRNA and the formation of unique intercellular carbon structures that bridge alveolar macrophages in situ. *Part Fibre Toxicol.* 2006;3:15.
174. Manna SK, Sarkar S, Barr J, et al. Single-walled carbon nanotube induces oxidative stress and activates nuclear transcription factor-kappaB in human keratinocytes. *Nano Lett.* 2005;5:1676-1684.
175. Mattheakis LC, Dias JM, Choi Y, et al. Optical coding of mammalian cells using semiconductor quantum dots. *Anal Biochem.* 2004;327:200-208.
176. Maynard AD, Aitken RJ. Assessing exposure to airborne nanomaterials: current abilities and future requirements. *Nanotoxicology.* 2007;1:26-41.
177. McAuliffe ME, Perry MJ. Are nanoparticles potential male reproductive toxicants? A literature review. *Nanotoxicology.* 2007;1:204-210.
178. Medarova Z, Pham W, Farrar C, Petkova V, Moore A. In vivo imaging of siRNA delivery and silencing in tumors. *Nat Med.* 2007;13:372-377.
179. Metayer C, Wang Z, Kleinerman RA, et al. Cooking oil fumes and risk of lung cancer in women in rural Gansu, China. *Lung Cancer.* 2002;35:111-117.
180. Mitsakou C, Housiadas C, Eleftheriadis K, Vratolis S, Helmis C, Asimakopoulos D. Lung deposition of fine and ultrafine particles outdoors and indoors during a cooking event and a no activity period. *Indoor Air.* 2007;17:143-152.
181. Mo Y, Zhu X, Hu X, Tollerud DJ, Zhang Q. Cytokine and NO release from peripheral blood neutrophils after exposure to metal nanoparticles: in vitro and ex vivo studies. *Nanotoxicology.* 2008;2:79-87.
182. Mok H, Park JW, Park TG. Enhanced intracellular delivery of quantum dot and adenovirus nanoparticles triggered by acidic pH via surface charge reversal. *Bioconjug Chem.* 2008;19:797-801.
183. Moller W, Brown DM, Kreyling WG, Stone V. Ultrafine particles cause cytoskeletal dysfunctions in macrophages: role of intracellular calcium. *Part Fibre Toxicol.* 2005;2:7.
184. Moller W, Felten K, Sommerer K, et al. Deposition, retention, and translocation of ultrafine particles from the central airways and lung periphery. *Am J Respir Crit Care.* Med 2008;177:426-432.
185. Monteiro-Riviere NA, Inman AO, Wang YY, Nemanich RJ. Surfactant effects on carbon nanotube interactions with human keratinocytes. *Nanomedicine.* 2005;1:293-299.
186. Mossman BT, Churg A. Mechanisms in the pathogenesis of asbestosis and silicosis. *Am J Respir Crit Care Med.* 1998;157:1666-1680.
187. Mostafa GA, Reda SM, Abd El-Aziz MM, Ahmed SA. Sputum neurokinin A in Egyptian asthmatic children and adolescents: relation to exacerbation severity. *Allergy.* 2008;63(9):1244-1247.
188. Mouchet F, Landois P, Flahaut E, Pinelli E, Gauthier L. Assessment of the potential in vivo ecotoxicity of double-walled carbon nanotubes (DWNTs) in water, using the amphibian *Ambystoma mexicanum*. *Nanotoxicology.* 2007;1:149-156.
189. Mouchet F, Landois P, Sarremejean E, et al. Characterisation and in vivo ecotoxicity evaluation of double-wall carbon nanotubes in larvae of the amphibian *Xenopus laevis*. *Aquat Toxicol.* 2008;87:127-137.
190. Mukherjee P, Bhattacharya R, Bone N, et al. Potential therapeutic application of gold nanoparticles in B-chronic lymphocytic leukemia (BCLL): enhancing apoptosis. *J Nanobiotechnology.* 2007;5:4.
191. Muller J, Huaux F, Moreau N, et al. Respiratory toxicity of multi-wall carbon nanotubes. *Toxicol Appl Pharmacol* 2005;207:221-231.
192. Muller K, Skepper JN, Posfai M, et al. Effect of ultrasmall superparamagnetic iron oxide nanoparticles (Ferumoxtran-10) on human monocyte-macrophages in vitro. *Biomaterials.* 2007;28:1629-1642.
193. Muller K, Skepper JN, Tang TY, et al. Atorvastatin and uptake of ultrasmall superparamagnetic iron oxide nanoparticles (Ferumoxtran-10) in human monocyte-macrophages: Implications for magnetic resonance imaging. *Biomaterials.* 2008;29:2656-2662.
194. Nabiev I, Mitchell S, Davies A, et al. Nonfunctionalized nanocrystals can exploit a cell's active transport machinery delivering them to specific nuclear and cytoplasmic compartments. *Nano Lett.* 2007;7:3452-3461.
195. Nair LS, Laurencin CT. Nanofibers and nanoparticles for orthopaedic surgery applications. *J Bone Joint Surg Am.* 2008;90(suppl 1):128-131.
196. National Nanotechnology Program. United States Code. Title 15, Chapter 101, § 7501; December 3, 2003.
197. National Toxicology Program. *NTP Nanotechnology Safety Initiative Fact Sheet.* Research Triangle Park, NC: National Toxicology Program, NIEHS/NIH; 2006. Retrieved June 4, 2008, from http://ntp.niehs.nih.gov/files/NanoColor06SRCH.pdf.
198. Nel A, Xia T, Madler L, Li N. Toxic potential of materials at the nanolevel. *Science.* 2006;311:622-627.
199. Nemmar A, Hoet PH, Dinsdale D, Vermylen J, Hoylaerts MF, Nemery B. Diesel exhaust particles in lung acutely enhance experimental peripheral thrombosis. *Circulation.* 2003;107:1202-1208.
200. Nemmar A, Hoet PH, Vanquickenborne B, et al. Passage of inhaled particles into the blood circulation in humans. *Circulation.* 2002;105:411-414.
201. Nemmar A, Hoylaerts MF, Hoet PH, Vermylen J, Nemery B. Size effect of intratracheally instilled particles on pulmonary inflammation and vascular thrombosis. *Toxicol Appl Pharmacol.* 2003;186:38-45.
202. Nemmar A, Inuwa IM. Diesel exhaust particles in blood trigger systemic and pulmonary morphological alterations. *Toxicol Lett.* 2008;176:20-30.
203. Nguyen-Vu TD, Chen H, Cassell AM, Andrews RJ, Meyyappan M, Li J. Vertically aligned carbon nanofiber architecture as a multifunctional 3-D neural electrical interface. *IEEE Trans Biomed Eng.* 2007;54:1121-1128.
204. NIOSH. *Approaches to Safe Nanotechnology and Information Exchange with NIOSH (version 1.1). Draft for Public Comment.* Cincinnati, OH: U.S. Department of Health and Human Services, Public Health Service, Centers for Disease Control and Prevention, National Institute for Occupational Safety and Health; 2006. Retrieved June 6, 2008, from http://www.cdc.gov/niosh/topics/nanotech/safenano/pdfs/approaches_to_safe_nanotechnology_28november2006_updated.pdf.
205. NIOSH. *Progress Toward Safe Nanotechnology in the Workplace: A Report from the NIOSH Nanotechnology Research Center* (revised). DHHS (NIOSH) Publication No. 2007–123. Cincinnati, OH: U.S. Department of Health and Human Services, Public Health Service, Centers for Disease Control and Prevention, National Institute for Occupational Safety and Health; 2007. Retrieved June 6, 2008, from http://www.cdc.gov/niosh/docs/2007-123/pdfs/2007-123.pdf.
206. Nohynek GJ, Lademann J, Ribaud C, Roberts MS. Grey goo on the skin? Nanotechnology, cosmetic and sunscreen safety. *Crit Rev Toxicol.* 2007;37:251-277.
207. Norris DJ, Efros AL, Erwin SC. Doped nanocrystals. *Science.* 2008;319:1776-1779.
208. Nurkiewicz TR, Porter DW, Barger M, et al. Systemic microvascular dysfunction and inflammation after pulmonary particulate matter exposure. *Environ Health Perspect.* 2006;114:412-419.

209. Nurkiewicz TR, Porter DW, Hubbs AF, et al. Nanoparticle inhalation augments particle-dependent systemic microvascular dysfunction. *Part Fibre Toxicol.* 2008;5:1.
210. Oberdorster G, Oberdorster E, Oberdorster J. Nanotoxicology: an emerging discipline evolving from studies of ultrafine particles. *Environ Health Perspect.* 2005;113:823-839.
211. Oberdorster G, Sharp Z, Atudorei V, et al. Translocation of inhaled ultrafine particles to the brain. *Inhal Toxicol.* 2004;16:437-445.
212. Oberdörster G, Stone V, Donaldson K. Toxicology of nanoparticles: a historical perspective. *Nanotoxicology.* 2007;1:2-25.
213. Osawa E. Superaromaticity. *Kagaku (Kyoto).* 1970;25:854-863.
214. Owens DE 3rd, Peppas NA. Opsonization, biodistribution, and pharmacokinetics of polymeric nanoparticles. *Int J Pharm.* 2006;307:93-102.
215. Palmieri A, Brunelli G, Guerzoni L, et al. Comparison between titanium and anatase miRNAs regulation. *Nanomedicine.* 2007;3:138-143.
216. Panaye A, Doucet JP, Devillers J, Marchand-Geneste N, Porcher JM. Decision trees versus support vector machine for classification of androgen receptor ligands. *SAR QSAR Environ Res.* 2008;19:129-151.
217. Pantarotto D, Partidos CD, Hoebeke J, et al. Immunization with peptide-functionalized carbon nanotubes enhances virus-specific neutralizing antibody responses. *Chem Biol.* 2003;10:961-966.
218. Papageorgiou I, Brown C, Schins R, et al. The effect of nano- and micron-sized particles of cobalt-chromium alloy on human fibroblasts in vitro. *Biomaterials.* 2007;28:2946-2458.
219. Papp T, Schiffmann D, Weiss D, Castranova V, Vallyathan V, Rahman Q. Human health implications of nanomaterial exposure. *Nanotoxicology.* 2008;2:9-27.
220. Parak WJ, Boudreau R, Le Gros M, et al. Cell motility and metastatic potential studies based on quantum dot imaging of phagokinetic tracks. *Adv Mater.* 2002;14:882-885.
221. Patra HK, Banerjee S, Chaudhuri U, Lahiri P, Dasgupta AK. Cell selective response to gold nanoparticles. *Nanomedicine.* 2007;3:111-119.
222. Peer D, Karp JM, Hong S, Farokhzad OC, Margalit R, Langer R. Nanocarriers as an emerging platform for cancer therapy. *Nat Nano.* 2007;2:751-760.
223. Pekkanen J, Peters A, Hoek G, et al. Particulate air pollution and risk of ST-segment depression during repeated submaximal exercise tests among subjects with coronary heart disease: the Exposure and Risk Assessment for Fine and Ultrafine Particles in Ambient Air (ULTRA) study. *Circulation.* 2002;106:933-938.
224. Pernodet N, Fang X, Sun Y, et al. Adverse effects of citrate/gold nanoparticles on human dermal fibroblasts. *Small.* 2006;2:766-773.
225. Persson E, Henriksson J, Tallkvist J, Rouleau C, Tjalve H. Transport and subcellular distribution of intranasally administered zinc in the olfactory system of rats and pikes. *Toxicology.* 2003;191:97-108.
226. Persson E, Henriksson J, Tjalve H. Uptake of cobalt from the nasal mucosa into the brain via olfactory pathways in rats. *Toxicol Lett.* 2003;145:19-27.
227. Peters A, Pope CA 3rd. Cardiopulmonary mortality and air pollution. *Lancet.* 2002;360:1184-1185.
228. Peters A, Veronesi B, Calderon-Garciduenas L, et al. Translocation and potential neurological effects of fine and ultrafine particles a critical update. *Part Fibre Toxicol.* 2006;3:13.
229. Peters A, Wichmann HE, Tuch T, Heinrich J, Heyder J. Respiratory effects are associated with the number of ultrafine particles. *Am J Respir Crit Care Med.* 1997;155:1376-1383.
230. Peters TM, Heitbrink WA, Evans DE, Slavin TJ, Maynard AD. The mapping of fine and ultrafine particle concentrations in an engine machining and assembly facility. *Ann Occup Hyg.* 2006;50:249-257.
231. Piasek M, Laskey JW, Kostial K, Blanusa M. Assessment of steroid disruption using cultures of whole ovary and/or placenta in rat and in human placental tissue. *Int Arch Occup Environ Health.* 2002;75(suppl):S36-S44.
232. Pisanic TR 2nd, Blackwell JD, Shubayev VI, Finones RR, Jin S. Nanotoxicity of iron oxide nanoparticle internalization in growing neurons. *Biomaterials.* 2007;28:2572-2581.
233. Pitsillides CM, Joe EK, Wei X, Anderson RR, Lin CP. Selective cell targeting with light-absorbing microparticles and nanoparticles. *Biophys J.* 2003;84:4023-4032.
234. Poland CA, Duffin R, Kinloch I, et al. Carbon nanotubes introduced into the abdominal cavity of mice show asbestos-like pathogenicity in a pilot study. *Nat Nano.* 2008;3(7):423-428.
235. Porter AE, Gass M, Muller K, Skepper JN, Midgley PA, Welland M. Direct imaging of single-walled carbon nanotubes in cells. *Nat Nano.* 2007;2:713-717.
236. Porter CJH, Moghimi SM, Illum L, Davis SS. The polyoxyethylene/polyoxypropylene block co-polymer Poloxamer-407 selectively redirects intravenously injected microspheres to sinusoidal endothelial cells of rabbit bone marrow. *FEBS Lett.* 1992;305:62-66.
237. Powell JJ, Ainley CC, Harvey RS, et al. Characterisation of inorganic microparticles in pigment cells of human gut associated lymphoid tissue. *Gut.* 1996;38:390-395.
238. President's Council of Advisors on Science and Technology. *The National Nanotechnology Initiative: Second Assessment and Recommendations of the National Nanotechnology Advisory Panel.* Arlington, VA: National Nanotechnology Coordination Office (NNCO); 2008. Retrieved June 22, 2008, from www.nano.gov/PCAST_NNAP_NNI_Assessment_2008.pdf.
239. Radomski A, Jurasz P, Alonso-Escolano D, et al. Nanoparticle-induced platelet aggregation and vascular thrombosis. *Br J Pharmacol.* 2005;146:882-893.
240. Reibold M, Paufler P, Levin AA, Kochmann W, Patzke N, Meyer DC. Materials: carbon nanotubes in an ancient Damascus sabre. *Nature.* 2006;444:286.
241. Roberts JC, Bhalgat MK, Zera RT. Preliminary biological evaluation of polyamidoamine (PAMAM) Starburst dendrimers. *J Biomed Mater Res.* 1996;30:53-65.
242. Roser M, Fischer D, Kissel T. Surface-modified biodegradable albumin nano- and microspheres. II: effect of surface charges on in vitro phagocytosis and biodistribution in rats. *Eur J Pharm Biopharm.* 1998;46:255-263.
243. Rouse JG, Yang J, Ryman-Rasmussen JP, Barron AR, Monteiro-Riviere NA. Effects of mechanical flexion on the penetration of fullerene amino acid-derivatized peptide nanoparticles through skin. *Nano Lett.* 2007;7:155-160.
244. Ryman-Rasmussen JP, Riviere JE, Monteiro-Riviere NA. Variables influencing interactions of untargeted quantum dot nanoparticles with skin cells and identification of biochemical modulators. *Nano Lett.* 2007;7:1344-1348.
245. Saha B, Bhattacharya J, Mukherjee A, et al. In vitro structural and functional evaluation of gold nanoparticles conjugated antibiotics. *Nanoscale Res Lett.* 2007;2:614-622.
246. Sahoo SK, Parveen S, Panda JJ. The present and future of nanotechnology in human health care. *Nanomedicine.* 2007;3:20-31.
247. Salber J, Grater S, Harwardt M, et al. Influence of different ECM mimetic peptide sequences embedded in a nonfouling environment on the specific adhesion of human-skin keratinocytes and fibroblasts on deformable substrates. *Small.* 2007;3:1023-1031.
248. Salnikov V, Lukyanenko YO, Frederick CA, Lederer WJ, Lukyanenko V. Probing the outer mitochondrial membrane in cardiac mitochondria with nanoparticles. *Biophys J.* 2007;92:1058-1071.
249. Salvador-Morales C, Flahaut E, Sim E, Sloan J, Green ML, Sim RB. Complement activation and protein adsorption by carbon nanotubes. *Mol Immunol.* 2006;43:193-201.
250. Salvador-Morales C, Townsend P, Flahaut E, et al. Binding of pulmonary surfactant proteins to carbon nanotubes; potential for damage to lung immune defense mechanisms. *Carbon.* 2007;45:607-617.
251. Sanvicens N, Marco MP. Multifunctional nanoparticles—properties and prospects for their use in human medicine. *Trends Biotechnol.* 2008;26(8):425-433.
252. Sato Y, Yokoyama A, Shibata K, et al. Influence of length on cytotoxicity of multi-walled carbon nanotubes against human acute monocytic leukemia cell line THP-1 in vitro and subcutaneous tissue of rats in vivo. *Mol Biosyst.* 2005;1:176-182.
253. Saxena RK, Williams W, Mcgee JK, Daniels MJ, Boykin E, Gilmour MI. Enhanced in vitro and in vivo toxicity of poly-dispersed acid-functionalized single-wall carbon nanotubes. *Nanotoxicology.* 2007;1:291-300.
254. Schins RP. Mechanisms of genotoxicity of particles and fibers. *Inhal Toxicol.* 2002;14:57-78.
255. Schulte PA, Trout D, Zumwalde RD, et al. Options for occupational health surveillance of workers potentially exposed to engineered nanoparticles: state of the science. *J Occup Environ Med.* 2008;50:517-526.
256. Schwartz J, Marcus A. Mortality and air pollution in London: a time series analysis. *Am J Epidemiol.* 1990;131:185-194.
257. Scientific Committee on Emerging and Newly Identified Health Risks (SCENIHR). *The Appropriateness of Existing Methodologies to Assess the Potential Risks Associated with Engineered and Adventitious Products of Nanotechnologies.* SCENIHR/002/05. European Commission, Health & Consumer Protection Directorate-General, Directorate C—Public Health and Risk Assessment, C7—Risk assessment; 2005. Retrieved June 15, 2008, from ec.europa.eu/health/ph_risk/committees/04_scenihr/docs/scenihr_o_003.pdf.

258. Shamsi K, Balzer T, Saini S, et al. Superparamagnetic iron oxide particles (SH U 555 A): evaluation of efficacy in three doses for hepatic MR imaging. *Radiology*. 1998;206:365-371.
259. Sharma R, Kwon S. New applications of nanoparticles in cardiovascular imaging. *J Exp Nanosci*. 2007;2:115-126.
260. Sharma R, Saxena D, Dwivedi AK, Misra A. Inhalable microparticles containing drug combinations to target alveolar macrophages for treatment of pulmonary tuberculosis. *Pharm Res*. 2001;18:1405-1410.
261. Shaw SY, Westly EC, Pittet MJ, Subramanian A, Schreiber SL, Weissleder R. Perturbational profiling of nanomaterial biologic activity. *PNAS*. 2008;105:7387-7392.
262. Shibuya M, Kato M, Ozawa M, Fang PH, Osawa E. Detection of Buckminsterfullerene in usual soots and commercial charcoals. *Fuller Nanotub Car N*. 1999;7:181-193.
263. Shukla R, Bansal V, Chaudhary M, Basu A, Bhonde RR, Sastry M. Biocompatibility of gold nanoparticles and their endocytotic fate inside the cellular compartment: a microscopic overview. *Langmuir*. 2005;21:10644-10654.
264. Shvedova AA, Kisin ER, Mercer R, et al. Unusual inflammatory and fibrogenic pulmonary responses to single-walled carbon nanotubes in mice. *Am J Physiol Lung Cell Mol Physiol*. 2005;289:L698-L708.
265. Sjaastad AK, Svendsen K, Jorgensen RB. Sub-micrometer particles: their level and how they spread after pan frying of beefsteak: indoor and built environment. *Indoor Built Environ*. 2008;17:230-236.
266. Soto KF, Carrasco A, Powell TG, Garza KM, Murr LE. Comparative in vitro cytotoxicity assessment of some manufactured nanoparticulate materials characterized by transmission electron microscopy. *J Nanopart Res*. 2005;7:145-169.
267. Subcommittee on Nanoscale Science, Engineering and Technology (NSET)—Nanotechnology Environmental and Health Implications (NEHI) Working Group, Committee on Technology (CT), National Science and Technology Council. *The National Nanotechnology Initiative Strategy for Nanotechnology-Related Environmental, Health, and Safety Research*. Arlington, VA: National Nanotechnology Coordination Office; 2008. Retrieved June 13, 2008, from http://www.nano.gov/NNI_EHS_Research_Strategy.pdf.
268. Sundara Rajan S, Vu TQ. Quantum dots monitor TrkA receptor dynamics in the interior of neural PC12 cells. *Nano Lett*. 2006;6:2049-2059.
269. Takagi A, Hirose A, Nishimura T, et al. Induction of mesothelioma in p53+/- mouse by intraperitoneal application of multi-wall carbon nanotube. *J Toxicol Sci*. 2008;33:105-116.
270. Taniguchi N. *On the Basic Concept of "NanoTechnology."* Proceedings of the International Conference of Production Engineering. Part II, Japan Society of Precision Engineering; Tokyo, Japan; 1974:18-23.
271. The Library of Congress. THOMAS [Legislative information from the Library of Congress]. 2008.
272. The Project on Emerging Nanotechnologies, Woodrow Wilson International Center for Scholars. Consumer Products. An inventory of nanotechnology-based consumer products currently on the market. Washington, DC: Woodrow Wilson International Center for Scholars; 2008. Retrieved June 13, 2008, from http://www.nanotechproject.org/inventories/consumer.
273. Thompson K, Molina RM, Donaghey T, Schwob JE, Brain JD, Wessling-Resnick M. Olfactory uptake of manganese requires DMT1 and is enhanced by anemia. *FASEB J*. 2007;21:223-230.
274. Thurn KT, Brown EMB, Wu A, et al. Nanoparticles for applications in cellular imaging. *Nanoscale Res Lett*. 2007;2:430-441.
275. Tian J, Wong KK, Ho CM, et al. Topical delivery of silver nanoparticles promotes wound healing. *Chem Med Chem*. 2007;2:129-136.
276. Timonen KL, Vanninen E, de Hartog J, et al. Effects of ultrafine and fine particulate and gaseous air pollution on cardiac autonomic control in subjects with coronary artery disease: the ULTRA study. *J Expo Sci Environ Epidemiol*. 2006;16:332-341.
277. Tin-Tin-Win-Shwe, Mitsushima D, Yamamoto S, et al. Changes in neurotransmitter levels and proinflammatory cytokine mRNA expressions in the mice olfactory bulb following nanoparticle exposure. *Toxicol Appl Pharmacol*. 2008;226:192-198.
278. Tjalve H, Henriksson J. Uptake of metals in the brain via olfactory pathways. *Neurotoxicology*. 1999;20:181-195.
279. Torchilin VP. Recent advances with liposomes as pharmaceutical carriers. *Nat Rev Drug Discov*. 2005;4:145-160.
280. Tosi G, Costantino L, Ruozi B, Forni F, Vandelli MA. Polymeric nanoparticles for the drug delivery to the central nervous system. *Expert Opin Drug Deliv*. 2008;5:155-174.
281. Trask JD, Paul JR. Experimental poliomyelitis in Cercopithecus aethiops sabaeus (the green African monkey) by oral and other routes. *J Exp Med*. 1941;73:453-459.
282. Tsoli M, Kuhn H, Brandau W, Esche H, Schmid G. Cellular uptake and toxicity of Au55 clusters. *Small*. 2005;1:841-844.
283. Tung YH, Ko JL, Liang YF, Yin L, Pu Y, Lin P. Cooking oil fume-induced cytokine expression and oxidative stress in human lung epithelial cells. *Environ Res*. 2001;87:47-54.
284. U.S. Environmental Protection Agency (EPA) Science Policy Council (Nanotechnology Workgroup). *Nanotechnology White Paper*. EPA 100/B-07/001. Washington, DC: U.S. Environmental Protection Agency; 2007. Retrieved June 13, 2008, from http://www.epa.gov/OSA/pdfs/nanotech/epa-nanotechnology-whitepaper-0207.pdf.
285. U.S. Food and Drug Administration. *Nanotechnology: a report of the U.S. Food and Drug Administration Nanotechnology Task Force*. Rockville, MD: U.S. Food and Drug Administration, Public Health Service, Department of Health and Human Services; 2007. Retrieved June 9, 2008, from http://www.fda.gov/nano-technology/taskforce/report2007.html.
286. Unfried K, Albrecht C, Klotz L, Von Mikecz A, Grether-Beck S, Schins RPF. Cellular responses to nanoparticles: target structures and mechanisms. *Nanotoxicology*. 2007;1:52.
287. Unfried K, Sydlik U, Bierhals K, Weissenberg A, Abel J. Carbon nanoparticle-induced lung epithelial cell proliferation is mediated by receptor-dependent Akt activation. *Am J Physiol Lung Cell Mol Physiol*. 2008;294: L358-L367.
288. Vallejo M, Ruiz S, Hermosillo AG, Borja-Aburto VH, Cardenas M. Ambient fine particles modify heart rate variability in young healthy adults. *J Expos Sci Environ Epidemiol*. 2005;16:125-130.
289. Vevers WF, Jha AN. Genotoxic and cytotoxic potential of titanium dioxide (TiO(2)) nanoparticles on fish cells in vitro. *Ecotoxicology*. 2008;17: 410-420.
290. Voura EB, Jaiswal JK, Mattoussi H, Simon SM. Tracking metastatic tumor cell extravasation with quantum dot nanocrystals and fluorescence emission-scanning microscopy. *Nat Med*. 2004;10:993-998.
291. Wallace LA, Emmerich SJ, Howard-Reed C. Source strengths of ultrafine and fine particles due to cooking with a gas stove. *Environ Sci Technol*. 2004;38:2304-2311.
292. Wallace W, Keane M, Murray D, Chisholm W, Maynard A, Ong T. Phospholipid lung surfactant and nanoparticle surface toxicity: lessons from diesel soots and silicate dusts. *J Nanopart Res*. 2007;9:23-38.
293. Walter P, Welcomme E, Hallegot P, et al. Early use of PbS nanotechnology for an ancient hair dyeing formula. *Nano Lett*. 2006;6:2215-2219.
294. Wang IC, Tai LA, Lee DD, et al. C60 and water-soluble fullerene derivatives as antioxidants against radical-initiated lipid peroxidation. *J Med Chem*. 1999;42:4614-4620.
295. Wang T, Adcock J, Kuhtreiber W, et al. Successful allotransplantation of encapsulated islets in pancreatectomized canines for diabetic management without the use of immunosuppression. *Transplantation*. 2008;85:331-337.
296. Warheit DB, Laurence BR, Reed KL, Roach DH, Reynolds GA, Webb TR. Comparative pulmonary toxicity assessment of single-wall carbon nanotubes in rats. *Toxicol Sci*. 2004;77:117-125.
297. Warriner R, Burrell R. Infection and the chronic wound: a focus on silver. *Adv Skin Wound Care*. 2005;18(suppl 1):2-12.
298. Wick P, Manser P, Limbach LK, et al. The degree and kind of agglomeration affect carbon nanotube cytotoxicity. *Toxicol Lett*. 2007;168:121-31.
299. Wiesner MR, Lowry GV, Alvarez P, Dionysiou D, Biswas P. Assessing the risks of manufactured nanomaterials. *Environ Sci Technol*. 2006;40: 4336-4345.
300. Witzmann FA, Monteiro-Riviere NA. Multi-walled carbon nanotube exposure alters protein expression in human keratinocytes. *Nanomedicine*. 2006;2:158-168.
301. Wolinsky H. Nanoregulation: a recent scare involving nanotech products reveals that the technology is not yet properly regulated. *EMBO Rep*. 2006;7:858-861.
302. Wu M, Che W, Zhang Z. Enhanced sensitivity to DNA damage induced by cooking oil fumes in human OGG1 deficient cells. *Environ Mol Mutagen*. 2008;49:265-275.
303. Wyman JL, Kizilel S, Skarbek R, et al. Immunoisolating pancreatic islets by encapsulation with selective withdrawal. *Small*. 2007;3:683-690.
304. Xia T, Kovochich M, Brant J, et al. Comparison of the abilities of ambient and manufactured nanoparticles to induce cellular toxicity according to an oxidative stress paradigm. *Nano Lett*. 2006;6:1794-1807.

305. Yadav AK, Mishra P, Mishra AK, Mishra P, Jain S, Agrawal GP. Development and characterization of hyaluronic acid-anchored PLGA nanoparticulate carriers of doxorubicin. *Nanomedicine.* 2007;3:246-257.
306. Yamago S, Tokuyama H, Nakamura E, et al. In vivo biological behavior of a water-miscible fullerene: 14C labeling, absorption, distribution, excretion and acute toxicity. *Chem Biol.* 1995;2:385-389.
307. Yamakoshi Y, Sueyoshi S, Fukuhara K, Miyata N, Masumizu T, Kohno M. ·OH and O2·- generation in aqueous C60 and C70 solutions by photoirradiation: an EPR study. *J Am Chem Soc.* 1998;120:12363-12364.
308. Yamakoshi Y, Umezawa N, Ryu A, et al. Active oxygen species generated from photoexcited fullerene (C60) as potential medicines: O2-· versus 1O2. *J Am Chem Soc.* 2003;125:12803-12809.
309. Yang X, Zhang Z, Liu Z, Ma Y, Yang R, Chen Y. Multi-functionalized single-walled carbon nanotubes as tumor cell targeting biological transporters. *J Nanopart Res.* 2008;10:815-822.
310. Yehia HN, Draper RK, Mikoryak C, et al. Single-walled carbon nanotube interactions with HeLa cells. *J Nanobiotechnology.* 2007;5:8.
311. Yu LE, Yung LL, Ong C, et al. Translocation and effects of gold nanoparticles after inhalation exposure in rats. *Nanotoxicology.* 2007;1:235.
312. Yue W, Schneider A, Stolzel M, et al. Ambient source-specific particles are associated with prolonged repolarization and increased levels of inflammation in male coronary artery disease patients. *Mutat Res.* 2007;621: 50-60.
313. Zharov VP, Kim JW, Curiel DT, Everts M. Self-assembling nanoclusters in living systems: application for integrated photothermal nanodiagnostics and nanotherapy. *Nanomedicine.* 2005;1:326-345.
314. Zhu L, Chang DW, Dai L, Hong Y. DNA damage induced by multiwalled carbon nanotubes in mouse embryonic stem cells. *Nano Lett.* 2007;7: 3592-3597.

CHAPTER 124
SIMPLE ASPHYXIANTS AND PULMONARY IRRITANTS

Lewis S. Nelson and Oladapo A. Odujebe

The respiratory system is responsible for gas exchange, elimination of certain xenobiotics, insensible water loss, temperature regulation, and minor metabolic processes. The principle function of the respiratory system is gas exchange, which occurs in the greater than 300 million alveoli that make up approximately 90% of the human lung volume. The average resting adult is exposed to about 8 L/min of air (a tidal volume of about 500 mL) and averages 16 breaths per minute, and this volume can be increased exponentially by increasing the respiratory rate and tidal volume as occurs during exertion. In a 24-hour period, an average adult human at rest will have been exposed to 11,500 L of air. There are a number of protective systems within the respiratory system to prevent exposure to xenobiotics, but these systems can be overwhelmed. The principles of respiratory system function are covered extensively in Chapter 21.

The respiratory tract performs several important physiologic functions. Its most important role involves the transfer of oxygen to hemoglobin across the pulmonary endothelium. This transfer facilitates oxygen distribution throughout the body to permit effective cellular respiration. Diverse xenobiotics may act at unique points in this distribution pathway to limit or impair tissue oxygenation. For example, whereas opioids and neuromuscular blockers may induce hypoventilation, carbon monoxide and methemoglobin inducers prevent binding of oxygen to hemoglobin. Certain xenobiotics prevent adequate oxygenation of hemoglobin at the level of pulmonary gas exchange. Two mechanistically distinct groups of xenobiotics are capable of interfering with gas exchange: simple asphyxiants and pulmonary irritants. Impairment of transpulmonary oxygen diffusion, regardless of the etiology, reduces the oxygen content of the blood and may result in tissue hypoxia.

HISTORY AND EPIDEMIOLOGY

Unlike most xenobiotic exposures, simple asphyxiant and pulmonary irritant poisonings frequently occur on a mass scale because of the nature of the inhalational route. For example, the large-scale emission of carbon dioxide from Lake Nyos, a carbonated volcanic crater lake in Cameroon, West Africa, resulted in nearly 2000 human and many more livestock deaths (see Chap. 2).[15] In this disaster, simple asphyxiation was likely because medical evaluation of both survivors and fatalities demonstrated neither signs of cutaneous or pulmonary irritation nor toxicologic abnormalities.[201] The widespread use of compressed liquefied gases, which expands several hundredfold on depressurization or warming, account for a substantial number of workplace injuries.[123,183]

Irritant gases similarly may result in mass casualties. For this reason, chlorine and phosgene were used in battle during World War I, resulting in thousands of Allied deaths[83] (see Chap. 131). Atmospheric sulfur dioxide and oxides of nitrogen are the primary components of photochemical smog. During the London Fog incident in 1952, 4000 deaths occurred primarily from respiratory causes.[171] Similar smog incidents have occurred across the globe. Relatedly, the diverse irritants found in fire smoke are largely responsible for the development of acute lung injury (ALI) after smoke inhalation.[180]

Unexpected release of other irritant inhalants may lead to large-scale poisoning. In 1984, an inadvertent release of methylisocyanate in Bhopal, India, resulted in immediate and persistent respiratory symptoms in approximately 200,000 local inhabitants, with approximately 2500 deaths.[16,53]

Isolated exposures to individuals occur as well, often in workplaces, and more frequently in contained spaces (eg, indoors). Additionally, the use of simple asphyxiation as a painless and relatively undetectable method for committing suicide and, paradoxically, for euphoric experiences can be found in books, on the Internet, and in the medical literature.[67,75,77,162]

SIMPLE ASPHYXIANTS

Simple asphyxiants work primarily by displacing oxygen from ambient air, unlike chemical asphyxiants, which cause cellular hypoxia and are discussed in Chapters 125 and 126. Virtually every gas, excluding oxygen, is capable of acting as a simple asphyxiant.

PATHOPHYSIOLOGY

Simple asphyxiants displace oxygen from ambient air, thereby reducing the fraction of inspired oxygen (FiO_2) in air to below 21%, and result in a decrease in the partial pressure of oxygen. The partial pressure is a measure of the contribution of oxygen to the total inspired air and is based on both FiO_2 and barometric pressure. For example, because the ambient pressure at sea level (less water vapor, 47 mm Hg) is 713 mm Hg and the percentage of oxygen is 21%, the partial pressure of oxygen in the lungs is 150 mm Hg. Under these typical conditions, the FiO_2 is a suitable surrogate for the partial pressure of oxygen. However, this relationship is not applicable at other barometric pressures. For example, at the summit of a mountain, the reduced barometric pressure results in a decrease in the partial pressure of oxygen despite a near-normal FiO_2. The barometric pressure decreases in a linear fashion with altitude (above sea level) and increases with decent below sea level. This reduced partial pressure may be insufficient to allow adequate oxygen saturation, and supplemental oxygen becomes necessary. As barometric pressure decreases, exposure to simple asphyxiant gases may further reduce the oxygen partial pressure to life-threatening levels. Conversely, underwater divers reduce their FiO_2 to below 21% by adding simple asphyxiant gases, such as helium, to their breathing mixture to avoid oxygen toxicity, yet they still maintain adequate oxygenation. This is because the elevated barometric pressure increases the partial pressure of oxygen to normal levels despite the addition of an asphyxiant gas. However, systemically poisonous gases that enter the breathing mixture would have a magnified effect, given their increased partial pressure at depth.

In general, simple asphyxiants have no pharmacologic activity. For this reason, exceedingly high ambient concentrations of these gases are necessary to produce asphyxia. Asphyxiation typically occurs in confined spaces or with rapid release of concentrated simple asphyxiants.

CLINICAL MANIFESTATIONS

A patient exposed to any simple asphyxiant gas will develop characteristic clinical findings of hypoxia, or lack of oxygen at the cellular level (Table 124–1). These clinical findings are directly related to the

TABLE 124–1. Clinical Findings Associated with Reduction of Inspired Oxygen

FiO_2[a]	Signs and Symptoms
21	None
16–12	Tachypnea, hyperpnea, (resultant hypocapnia), tachycardia, reduced attention and alertness, euphoria, headache, mild incoordination
14–10	Altered judgment, incoordination, muscular fatigue, cyanosis
10–6	Nausea, vomiting, lethargy, air hunger, severe incoordination, coma
<6	Gasping respiration, seizure, coma, death

[a] At sea level, barometric pressure appropriate adjustments must be made for altitude and depth exposures.

FiO_2, fraction of inspired oxygen.

reduction in the partial pressure of oxygen in ambient air, which leads to hypoxemia, or low oxygen content of the blood.[123] Cardiovascular and central nervous system (CNS) complications of simple asphyxiants predominate because these organs have the greatest oxygen requirements. As hypoxemia becomes severe, multisystem organ failure and death from tissue hypoxia may occur.[50] Postmortem findings are generally minimal, hampering the cause of death determination without historical evidence or advanced laboratory testing.[10]

During simple asphyxiation, carbon dioxide exchange is not impaired, and hypercapnia does not occur. Because dyspnea develops more rapidly from hypercapnia than hypoxemia, the breathlessness associated with physical or simple chemical asphyxiation does not develop until severe hypoxemia intervenes.[92,111] In these circumstances, victims may succumb to hypoxemia without ever developing the expected warning symptoms. In the case of carbon dioxide inhalation, hypercapnia may occur very rapidly, which itself may produce acute cognitive impairment.

SPECIFIC AGENTS

Noble Gases: Helium, Neon, Argon, and Xenon Noble gases, which are stored almost exclusively in the compressed form, have numerous industrial and medical roles. Argon is predominantly used as a shielding gas during welding operations. Neon is used in the manufacture of decorative lighting. Xenon, in its radioactive gaseous form, has diagnostic medical applications in ventilation–perfusion scans. Helium has the lowest molecular weight and is the smallest member of the noble gas family of elements. Because of its lower lipid solubility, helium is used by divers to replace nitrogen to prevent nitrogen narcosis at depth (see Nitrogen). Even at diving gas mixtures of 50% helium, divers suffer no adverse effects as long as a normal partial pressure of oxygen is maintained by the mixture at depth. At depth, the quantity (molar quantity, not volume) of air inspired per breath is several-fold greater than that at sea level. The fact that helium has a lower density than nitrogen results in a lower viscosity, or a marked decrease in flow resistance. This property of helium is the basis for its use in patients with increased airway resistance, such as those with asthma.

Helium is also used in magnetic resonance imaging scanners to keep the coils super cooled. During emergency shutdown of a superconducting electromagnet, an operation known as "quenching," the liquid helium is rapidly boiled from the device and vented into the scanner room. This may displace oxygen from the environment and cause asphyxia.[86] Helium is also used in lung imaging studies and pulmonary function tests. Similarly, helium's low viscosity has led to its use as an inflation gas for intraaortic balloons, for which rapid inflation and deflation are critical.

All noble gases, when compressed, form cryogenic liquids, which expand rapidly to their gas phase on decompression. Liberation of these gases in closed spaces may result in asphyxiation or freezing injuries[86] Xenon, unlike the other noble gases, has unique anesthetic properties because of its high lipid solubility and inhibition of *N*-methyl-D-aspartic acid (NMDA)receptors[86] The other noble gases have no known direct toxicity.

Short-Chain Aliphatic Hydrocarbon Gases: Methane, Ethane, Propane, and Butane The short-chain aliphatic hydrocarbon gases are primarily used in the compressed form as fuel. Methane (CH_4) has no known direct toxicity. Animals can breathe a mixture of 80% methane and 20% oxygen without manifesting hypoxic symptoms because their FiO_2, and thus their oxygen content, essentially is normal. Methane, also known as natural gas and "swamp gas," may be present in high ambient concentrations in bogs of decaying organic matter. In addition, compressed natural gas is now used as an alternative fuel for automotive use. Methane exposure is an occupational hazard for miners who historically carried canaries into their workplace as an "early warning" sign for the presence of toxic gases or oxygen deficiency. Theoretically, the higher metabolic and respiratory rates of small animals (and children) make them more rapidly susceptible to gas exposures. Methane is also an explosive risk.

Methane is odorless and undetectable without sophisticated equipment.[34] For this reason, natural gas is intentionally adulterated with a small concentration of ethyl mercaptan, a stenching agent, which is responsible for the well-recognized sulfur odor of natural gas. Cooking with natural gas may lead to increased respiratory symptoms and pulmonary dysfunction.[95] However, methane itself is unlikely to be the cause because its combustion is generally complete and ambient concentrations are negligible. It is likely that exposure to nitrogen dioxide (NO_2), one of the products of combustion of methane in air (70% nitrogen), is the explanation for these symptoms.

Ethane (C_2H_6) is an odorless gas that is a component of natural gas and is used as a refrigerant. It has characteristics similar to methane and has been occasionally implicated as a simple asphyxiant. Propane (C_3H_8) is widely used in compressed, liquefied form both as an industrial and domestic fuel and as an industrial solvent. Butane (C_4H_{10}) is a common fuel and solvent. Deliberate butane inhalation from cigarette lighters or air fresheners for recreational purposes predominantly in adolescents is associated with cardiovascular dysfunction and cerebral damage (see Chap. 81).[59,178]

Carbon Dioxide (CO_2) Although not a simple asphyxiant gas by definition because it produces physiologic effects, carbon dioxide closely resembles simple asphyxiants from a toxicologic viewpoint. Carbon dioxide gas has many practical industrial uses, such as production of carbonation in soft drinks and use as a shielding gas during welding. It is used in laboratories as a painless form of animal euthanasia and as a means of large-scale euthanasia of diseased livestock.[151] Carbon dioxide is widely used to extinguish fires because of its ability to safely displace oxygen from the local environment.[74] Dry ice, the frozen form of carbon dioxide, is an extremely cold substance (−141.3°F [−78.5°C]) that undergoes conversion from solid to gas without liquefaction, a process known as sublimation. Profound poisoning may occur when dry ice is allowed to sublimate in a closed space,[37] such as the cabin of a car or, as in the case above, in a cold storage room at 39.2°F (4°C).[74,57] Furthermore, inadvertent connection of respirable gas hoses to carbon dioxide and other nonrespirable sources has occurred in both industrial[92,184] and medical[96] settings, with resultant worker and patient fatalities. This occurrence is uncommon because of the mandated use of engineering controls to prevent the incorrect connection of hose and source terminals.

Pharmacology and Pathophysiology. Carbon dioxide, an end product of normal human metabolism, dissolves in the plasma and is in equilibrium with carbonic acid (H_2CO_3). The pH at the central chemoreceptors, reflective of the dissolved carbon dioxide (PCO_2), is responsible for our respiratory drive, and PCO_2 is tightly controlled by the CNS through regulation of breathing.[111] For this reason, exogenous carbon dioxide, combined with oxygen, was at one time used medically as a respiratory stimulant in neonates. Under normal conditions, ambient air contains approximately 0.03% CO_2. When ambient concentrations increase above this level, uptake of carbon dioxide occurs, which further stimulates respiration,[148] increasing the uptake of ambient carbon dioxide. Accordingly, closed anesthesia systems use scrubbers containing sodium hydroxide to chemically eliminate exhaled carbon dioxide. Failure of the scrubber system results in increasing depth of anesthesia from hypercapnia-induced hyperventilation.

Clinical Manifestations. Carbon dioxide produces both acute and subacute poisoning syndromes. The latter occurs during hypoventilation when a patient fails to eliminate endogenous carbon dioxide, develops hypercapnia, and typically presents with gradual somnolence. This occurrence may be linked to respiratory failure, as in the case of emphysema or opioid poisoning, or it may be iatrogenic, as occurs during permissive hypercapnia.[133] Alternatively, intense carbon dioxide exposure may produce rapid and lethal poisoning. However, unlike other simple asphyxiants, experimental models of acute carbon dioxide poisoning in which FiO_2 is maintained at normal levels demonstrate that central nervous and respiratory system manifestations occur within seconds.[85,94] This finding suggests that CO_2 is not solely a simple asphyxiant but also possesses a potential for systemic effects.

Nitrogen (N_2) Gas Although nitrogen, like carbon dioxide, may produce clinical effects independently of hypoxemia, most poisonings are characterized by the manifestations of simple asphyxiants. Nitrogen gas is used as a carrier gas for chromatography, as a fertilizer, as a cryogenic gas for surgery, and extensively in manufacturing. Poisoning by nitrogen gas is uncommon but may occur after rapid evaporation of the liquid.[99,100]

Pharmacology and Pathophysiology. Nitrogen is a colorless, odorless, and tasteless gas that makes up 78% by volume of the atmospheric gas. Under standard conditions, it is an inert diatomic gas that has no direct physiologic toxicity.

Clinical Manifestations. Inadvertent connection of air-line respirator hoses to nitrogen and other inert gas sources results in acute asphyxiation, with unconsciousness occurring in approximately 12 seconds[92,123,183] and death shortly thereafter. More indolent inhalational poisoning by nitrogen is characterized by impairment of intellectual function and judgment, giddiness, and euphoria, which is qualitatively similar to ethanol intoxication.[126] More severely poisoned patients may manifest lethargy or coma.[66] Systemic absorption is not rapid, however, and prolonged, high-level exposure is required for poisoning. Nitrogen poisoning, also known as *nitrogen narcosis*, occurs in underwater divers while they are breathing air that contains 70% nitrogen. It has been called *rapture of the deep* (*l'ivresse des grandes profondeurs*) and has led to many deaths in the subaquatic environment. The underlying mechanism of nitrogen narcosis is unknown,[49] but the simple structure and relatively high lipophilicity of nitrogen suggest a mechanism similar to that of the anesthetic gases.[66] To avoid nitrogen narcosis, a less lipid-soluble inert gas such as helium is generally substituted for nitrogen. Substitution with oxygen, although intuitively logical, is inappropriate because of the risk of oxygen toxicity (see Oxygen).

Dermal exposure to liquid nitrogen produces frostbite because of liquid nitrogen's extremely cold temperature.[155] Ingestion of liquid nitrogen similarly produces a freezing injury of the gastrointestinal (GI) tract.[104,203] Rarely, bubbles introduced through the skin embolize through the vascular system and impair organ blood flow.[58]

TREATMENT

Treatment of all individuals poisoned by simple asphyxiants begins with immediate removal of the persons from exposure and provision of ventilatory assistance. Provision of supplemental oxygen is preferable, but room air usually suffices. Hyperbaric oxygen therapy has shown no benefit in the majority of cases. Restoration of oxygenation through spontaneous or mechanical ventilation occurs after only several breaths. Support of vital functions is the mainstay of therapy but is generally unnecessary after a brief exposure.

PULMONARY IRRITANTS

The irritant gases are a heterogeneous group of chemicals that produce toxic effects via a final common pathway: destruction of the integrity of the mucosal barrier of the respiratory tract (Table 124–2).

PATHOPHYSIOLOGY

In the lung, irritant chemicals damage both the more prevalent type I pneumocytes and the surfactant-producing type II pneumocytes.[106] Neutrophil influx, recruited in response to macrophage-derived inflammatory cytokines such as tumor necrosis factor (TNF)-α, releases toxic mediators that disrupt the integrity of the capillary endothelial cells.[116,153] This host defense response results in accumulation of cellular debris and plasma exudate in the alveolar sacs, producing the characteristic clinical findings of ALI. The specific mechanisms by which the irritant gases damage the pulmonary endothelial and epithelial cells vary. Many irritant gases require dissolution in lung water to liberate their ultimate toxicant, which often is an acid, as occurs when hydrogen chloride gas produces hydrochloric acid. The exact mechanism by which acids damage cells and induce an inflammatory response remains uncertain. Oxidation of intracellular proteins may result in rapid cytoskeletal shortening, creating spaces between endothelial cells and allowing fluid movement into the alveolar spaces.[189] Other gases, such as oxygen, induce pulmonary damage solely through free radical–mediated oxidative stress on the cellular membranes. NO_2 and chlorine are characteristic of a group of gases that produce both acid and free radical oxidants. Furthermore, other respirable xenobiotics, such as metals, injure the respiratory tract through oxidant stress and other mechanisms. Because the precise toxicologic and pathophysiologic effects vary widely depending on the physicochemical properties of the xenobiotic, these mechanisms are covered more completely in the following specific discussions.

By virtue of its use as a war agent, phosgene has received more investigation than the other irritant gases. Although the specific mechanisms of toxicity of the other irritants remain poorly defined, they likely cause injury through a similar process. The acids liberated upon dissolution in the mucosal water react with functional groups on epithelial and endothelial cell membranes and, via cellular messengers, result in a complex inflammatory response.[165,140] Phosgene stimulates the synthesis of lipoxygenase-derived leukotrienes and other cytokines such as TNF-α.[165] Leukotrienes are important chemotactic factors for neutrophils, which accumulate, liberate oxidants, and produce ALI.[93] ALI can be prevented in rabbits by tomelukast, a leukotriene receptor antagonist,[81] and by methylprednisolone, which blocks leukotriene

TABLE 124–2. Characteristics of Common Respiratory Irritants

Gas	Source or Exposure	Solubility (g%)[a]	Detection Threshold (ppm)	Regulatory Standard (ppm)[b]	IDLH[c] (ppm)	STEL[d] (ppm)
Ammonia	Fertilizer, refrigeration, synthetic fiber synthesis	90	5	50	300	35
Cadmium oxide fumes	Welding	I	Odorless	0.005 mg/m³	9 mg/m³ (as Cd)	NA
Carbon dioxide	Exhaust, dry ice sublimation	0.2	Odorless	5000	40,000	30,000
Chloramine	Bleach plus ammonia	M	NA	NR	NR	NR
Chlorine	Water disinfection, pulp and paper industry	0.7	0.3	0.5	10	1
Copper oxide fumes	Welding	I	NA	0.1 mg/m³	100 mg/m³ (as Cu)	NA
Ethylene oxide	Sterilant	M	500	1	800	5
Formaldehyde	Chemical disinfection	M	0.8	0.016	20	2
Hydrogen chloride	Chemical	67	1–5	5	50	5
Hydrogen fluoride	Glass etching, semiconductor industry	M	0.042	3 (as F)	30 (as F)	6
Hydrogen sulfide	Petroleum industry, sewer, manure pits	0.4	0.025		100	50
Mercury vapor	Electrical equipment, thermometers, catalyst, dental fillings, metal extraction, heating or vacuuming elemental mercury	I	Odorless	0.1 mg/m³	10 mg/m³	0.05
Methane	Natural heating gas, swamp gas	3.3	Odorless	NR	NR	NR
Methyl bromide	Fumigant	2	20	20	250	NA
Nickel carbonyl	Nickel purification, nickel coating, catalyst	0.05	1-3	0.001	2 (as Ni)	0.1
Nitrogen		0.017	Odorless	NR	NR	NR
Nitrogen dioxide	Chemical synthesis, combustion emission	P	0.12	3	20	5
Nitrous oxide	Anesthetic gas, whipping cream dispensers (abuse), racing fuel additive	0.07	2	25	100	NA
Ozone	Disinfectant, produced by high-voltage electrical equipment	0.001	0.05	0.1	5	0.1
Phosgene	Chemical synthesis, combustion of chlorinated compounds	P	0.5	0.1	2	0.1
Phosphine	Fumigant, semiconductor industry	P	2	0.3	50	1
Propane	Liquified propane gas	0.007	Odorless	1000	2100	NR
Sulfur dioxide	Environmental exhaust	23	1	2	100	5
Zinc chloride fumes	Artificial smoke (no longer in use)	432	NA	1 mg/m³	50 mg/m³	2 mg/m³
Zinc oxide	Welding	0.16	Odorless	5 mg/m³	500 mg/m³	10 mg/m³

[a] g% = grams of gas per 100 mL water; if applicable.

[b] Standards are either; Threshold Limit Value-Time-Weighted Average; (TLV-TWA) set by the American Conference of Governmental Industrial Hygienists (ACGIH); or permissible exposure limits (PELs) set by the Occupational Safety and Heath Administration (OSHA).

[c] Immediately dangerous to life and health: National Institute for Occupational Safety and Health (NIOSH), revised 1995. (Documentation for each IDLH (Immediately Dangerous to Life and Health limit) is available at http://www.cdc.gov/niosh/idlh/idlhintr.html.)

F, fluorine; I, insoluble; M, miscible; NR, no regulatory standard; NA, not available; P, poor; NIOSH and OSHA 15 minute or ceiling. STEL[d], short term exposure limit, synthesis; both xenobiotics also offer postexposure benefit.[81] Ibuprofen, an inhibitor of the arachidonic acid cascade, and xenobiotics capable of reducing neutrophil influx, such as colchicine and cyclophosphamide, reduce lung injury and mortality in mice when they are administered shortly after phosgene exposure.[73,167] Intratracheal dibutyryl cyclic adenosine monophosphate (DBcAMP), a cAMP analog, and other cAMP amplifiers, such as terbutaline or aminophylline, inhibit the release of leukotrienes and reduce toxicity.[98,168] When administered 45 minutes after exposure to phosgene-poisoned rabbits, intratracheal *N*-acetylcysteine (NAC) decreases the formation of leukotrienes by an undefined means and limits the development of ALI.[169] Presumably, administration via nebulization would prove similarly effective. Intravenous administration of NAC to patients with mild to moderate ALI, none of whom had phosgene-induced pulmonary damage, improved systemic oxygenation and reduced their need for ventilatory support.[185] However, progression to pulmonary failure was not altered.

Free radicals are highly reactive molecular derivatives, typically from oxygen or nitrogen that bind to and destroy tissue near their site of generation. Through initiation of a lipid peroxidative cascade, free radicals destroy lipid membranes and inhibit energy production through the electron transport chain (see Chap. 12). Products of lipid peroxidation and cellular damage initiate neutrophilic influx, presumably in an immunologic attempt to combat a pathogen. Ironically, free radicals generated by the invading inflammatory cells contribute to pulmonary damage. Fortunately, the lung has antioxidant systems, both enzymatic (eg, superoxide dismutase, glutathione peroxidase, catalase) and nonenzymatic (eg, glutathione, ascorbate), which detoxify virtually all free radicals present in the lung.[149] However, the oxidant burden imposed by oxidant gases can preempt these detoxifying systems and produce cellular damage. For example, nebulization of manganese superoxide dismutase into the airway 1 hour after smoke inhalation, a form of oxidant lung injury, did not improve lung edema or pulmonary gas exchange.[114] However, the observed benefit of NAC may also be related to improved hemodynamic function (see Antidotes in Depth A4: *N*-Acetylcysteine.[87]

CLINICAL MANIFESTATIONS

Regardless of the mechanism by which the mucosa is damaged, the clinical presentations of patients exposed to irritant gases are similar. Those exposed to gases that result in irritation within seconds generally develop mucosal injury limited to the upper respiratory tract. The rapid onset of symptoms is usually a sufficient signal to the patient to escape the exposure. Patients may present with nasal or oropharyngeal pain in addition to drooling, mucosal edema, cough, or stridor.[188] Conjunctival irritation or chemosis, as well as skin irritation, is often noted because concomitant ocular and cutaneous exposure to the gases usually is unavoidable. Gases that are less rapidly irritating may not provide an adequate signal of their presence and may not prompt expeditious escape by the exposed individual. In this case, prolonged breathing allows entry of the toxic gas farther into the bronchopulmonary system, where delayed toxic effects may subsequently be noted. Tracheobronchitis, bronchiolitis, bronchospasm, and ALI are typical inflammatory responses of the airway and represent the spectrum of acute lower respiratory tract injury.

Experimental models assessing the water solubility of a gas to predict the location of its associated lesions have largely agreed with the clinical data.[101] However, exceptions to this relationship of a gas and its expected toxicity are common. For example, in situations in which escape from ongoing exposure is prevented, patients may develop lower respiratory tract injury after prolonged exposure to acutely irritating gases. Alternatively, rapid onset of upper respiratory irritation may be noted in patients after exposure to concentrated gases that are generally associated with delayed symptomatology. Exposure to exceedingly high concentrations of any gas may produce hypoxemia analogous to that resulting from exposure to a simple asphyxiant gas.

The most characteristic and serious clinical manifestation of irritant gas exposure is ALI.[11,18,157,158] ALI consists of the clinical, radiographic, and physiologic abnormalities caused by pulmonary inflammation and alveolar filling that must be both acute in onset and not attributable solely to pulmonary capillary hypertension as occurs in patients with congestive heart failure.[11,18,157,158] The most severe manifestation of ALI is the acute respiratory distress syndrome (ARDS). The criteria for diagnosis of ARDS is based on the ratio of the partial pressure of dissolved oxygen (PaO_2) to FiO_2, that is, patients with an appropriate history and clinical presentation for ALI with PaO_2/FiO_2 below 200 mm Hg meet the definition of ARDS. Importantly, positive end-expiratory pressure (PEEP) is not part of the oxygenation criteria (see Chap. 21). Both ALI and ARDS are nonspecific syndromes resulting from diverse physiologic insults such as sepsis or trauma. Patients with ALI may present with dyspnea, chest tightness, chest pain, cough, frothy sputum, wheezing or crackles, and arterial hypoxemia. Typical radiographic abnormalities include bilateral pulmonary infiltrates with an alveolar filling pattern and a normal cardiac silhouette that differentiate this syndrome from congestive heart failure.

SPECIFIC XENOBIOTICS

Acid- or Base-Forming Gases Highly Water-Soluble Xenobiotics *Ammonia (NH_3).* Ammonia is a common industrial and household chemical used in the synthesis of plastics and explosives and as a fertilizer, a refrigerant, and a cleaner. The odor is characteristic and may be an effective warning signal of exposure and stimulus to avoid further exposure. Dissolution of NH_3 in water to form the base ammonium hydroxide (NH_4OH) rapidly produces severe upper airway irritation. Patients with exposures to highly concentrated NH_3 or exposures for prolonged periods may develop tracheobronchial or pulmonary inflammation. Experimental inhalation of nebulized high-dose ammonia causes ALI that is manifested by a decrease in oxygen saturation and an increase in airway pressure within 2 minutes of exposure.[174] Ultrastructural study of the lungs from two individuals dying acutely of ammonia inhalation revealed marked swelling and edema of type I pneumocytes consistent with ALI.[33] Chronic inhalation of low concentrations of NH_3 or repetitive exposure to high concentrations of ammonia may cause pulmonary fibrosis.[29]

Chloramines. This series of chlorinated nitrogenous compounds (Fig. 124–1) includes monochloramine (NH_2Cl), dichloramine ($NHCl_2$), and trichloramine (NCl_3). The chloramines are most commonly generated by the admixture of ammonia with sodium hypochlorite (NaOCl) bleach, often in an effort to potentiate their individual cleaning powers.[68] Interestingly, the addition of bleach to septic systems may result in liberation of the chloramines after the reaction of bleach with urinary nitrogenous compounds.[124] On dissolution of the chloramines in the epithelial lining fluid, hypochlorous acid (HOCl), ammonia, and oxygen radicals are generated, all of which act as irritants. Although less water soluble than ammonia, the chloramines typically promptly result in symptoms. Because these initial symptoms are often mild, however, they may not prompt immediate escape, resulting in prolonged or recurrent exposure with pulmonary and ocular symptoms predominating.[38] Exposure to trichloramine occurs at indoor swimming pools[40] and is responsible for inducing permeability changes in the pulmonary epithelium, the consequences of which are not yet understood.[36]

A. $3\,NaOCl + 2\,NH_3 \rightarrow NH_2Cl + NHCl_2 + 3\,NaOH$

B. $NH_2Cl + H_2O \rightarrow HOCl + NH_3$

$HOCl \rightarrow HCl + [O]$

FIGURE 124–1. Chloramine chemistry. (**A**) Sodium hypochlorite (bleach) plus ammonia form monochloramine and dichloramine. (**B**) Chloramine dissolves in water to liberate hypochlorous acid; hydrochloric acid; ammonia; and nascent oxygen [O], an oxidant.

A. $HCl + HOCl \rightarrow Cl_2 + H_2O$

B. $Cl_2 + H_2O \rightarrow 2\,HCl + [O]$

$Cl_2 + H_2O \rightarrow HCl + HOCl$

FIGURE 124–2. Chlorine chemistry. (**A**) Formation of chlorine gas from the acidification of hypochlorous acid. (**B**) Dissolution of chlorine in mucosal water to generate both hydrochloric and hypochlorous acids (HCl and HOCl) and oxidants [O].

Hydrogen Chloride (HCl). The largest and most important use of hydrogen chloride gas is in the production of hydrochloric acid. Dissolution of hydrogen chloride gas in lung water after inhalation similarly produces hydrochloric acid.[32,147] Pyrolysis of polyvinyl chloride (PVC), a plastic commonly used in pipe fabrication, generates HCl and is an occupational hazard for firefighters.[136] By adsorbing to respirable carbonaceous particles generated in the fire, HCl may be deposited at the alveolar level and produce pulmonary toxicity.

Hydrogen Fluoride (HF). Hydrogen fluoride and its aqueous form, hydrofluoric acid, are used in the gasoline, glassware, building renovation, and semiconductor industries. Hydrogen fluoride gas dissolves in epithelial lining fluid to form the weak acid hydrofluoric acid. The intact HF molecule is the predominant form in solution, and few free hydronium ions are liberated. Low-dose inhalational exposures may result in irritant symptoms,[195,207] and large exposures may cause bronchial and pulmonary parenchymal destruction.[28,195] Death after inhalation may result from ALI but usually is related to systemic fluoride poisoning independent of the route of exposure because of the resultant calcium binding and subsequent hypocalcemia and hyperkalemia[24,55] (see Chap. 105).

Sulfur Dioxide and Sulfuric Acid (SO_2 and H_2SO_4). Sulfur dioxide has multiple industrial applications and is a byproduct found in the smelting and oil refinery industries. It may also be generated by the inadvertent mixing of chemicals, such as an acid with sodium bisulfite ($NaHSO_3$). Sulfur dioxide is highly water soluble and has a characteristic pungent odor that provides warning of its presence at concentrations well below those that are irritating. In the presence of catalytic metals (Fe, Mn), environmental sulfur dioxide is readily converted to sulfurous acid (H_2SO_3) within water droplets. Sulfurous acid is a major environmental concern and the cause of "acid rain." Exposure to atmospheric sulfur dioxide results in a roughly dose-related bronchospasm, which is most pronounced and difficult to treat in patients with asthma. Inhalation of sulfurous acid or dissolution of sulfur dioxide in epithelial lining fluid produces typical pathologic and clinical findings associated with ALI.[154] In addition to the effect of acid generation upon dissolution, sulfur dioxide may cause oxidative damage to the lungs.[122] Large acute exposure to either xenobiotic produces the expected acute irritant response of both the upper and lower respiratory tracts,[41] and pulmonary dysfunction (see Asthma and Reactive Airways Dysfunction Syndrome) may persist for several years.[144]

Intermediate Water-Soluble Xenobiotics *Chlorine (Cl_2).* Chlorine gas is a valuable oxidizing agent with various industrial uses, and occupational exposure is common. Chlorine gas was used as a chemical warfare agent by both the French and the Germans in World War I (see Chap. 131). Although chlorine gas is not generally available for use in the home, domestic exposure to chlorine gas is common. The admixture of an acid to bleach liberates chlorine gas (Fig. 124–2).[76,130] Because the anionic component of the acid is not involved in the reaction, combining hypochlorite with virtually any acid, such as phosphoric, hydrochloric, or sulfuric acid, may result in the release of chlorine gas. As such, inappropriate mixing of cleaning agents is the cause of most nonoccupational exposures.[130] Rarely, patients have intentionally generated chlorine gas in this manner for purportedly "pleasurable" purposes.[150] Concentrated chlorine gas may be generated when aging swimming pool chlorination tablets, such as calcium hypochlorite [$Ca(OCl)_2$] or trichloro-*s*-triazinetrione (TST), decompose[113,208] or are inadvertently introduced to a swimming pool while swimmers are present.[13,200] Inadvertent mixture of $Ca(OCl)_2$ and TST results in excessive chlorine gas generation and may also be explosive.[113] Acute chlorine toxicity may occur when there is a failure of the system when compressed chlorine gas is used for direct chlorination of public swimming pools[13,199] or for drinking water systems. Occasional mass poisoning may occur during scientific, industrial, or transportation incidents.[39,193]

The odor threshold for chlorine is low, but distinguishing toxic from permissible air concentrations may be difficult until toxicity is manifest. The intermediate solubility characteristics of chlorine result in only mild initial symptoms after moderate exposure and permit a substantial time delay, typically several hours, before clinical symptoms develop. Chlorine dissolution in lung water generates HCl and hypochlorous (HOCl) acids. Hypochlorous acid rapidly decomposes into HCl and nascent oxygen (O^-). The unpaired nascent oxygen atom produces additional pulmonary damage by initiating a free radical oxidative cascade. Although the majority of life-threatening chlorine poisonings occur after acute, large exposures, patients with chronic, low-concentration exposure or recurrent, moderate concentration poisonings may manifest increased bronchial responsiveness.[5,65,72]

Hydrogen Sulfide (H_2S). Hydrogen sulfide exposures occur most frequently in the waste management, petroleum, and natural gas industries,[88] although poisoning occurs in asphalt, synthetic rubber, and nylon industry workers as well. It is also rarely seen in hospital workers using acid cleaners to unclog drains clogged with plaster of Paris sludge.[143] Hydrogen sulfide is present in natural sources such as volcanic emission, in caves, and in sulfur springs. It is a decay product of organic material found in sewers or manure pits. Hydrogen sulfide, hydrogen fluoride, and phosphine are differentiated from the other irritant gases by their ability to produce significant systemic toxicity. Hydrogen sulfide inhibits mitochondrial respiration in a fashion similar to that of cyanide (see Chap. 126).[60,152]

H_2S has the distinctive odor of "rotten eggs," which, although helpful in diagnosis, is not specific for the agent. Despite a sensitive odor threshold of several parts per billion,[152] rapid olfactory fatigue ensues, providing a misperception that the exposure and its attendant risk have diminished. At low and moderate concentrations (≤500 ppm), upper respiratory tract mucosal irritation occurs and is the principal toxicity.[187] The rapidity of death in patients exposed to high H_2S concentrations makes it likely that either simple asphyxiation or cytochrome oxidase inhibition is causal in most cases.

Phosgene (Carbonyl Chloride [$COCl_2$]). During World War I, phosgene was an important weapon of mass destruction that produced countless deaths (see Chap. 131). Currently, phosgene is used in the synthesis of various organic compounds, such as isocyanates, and it occasionally produces poisoning. It is a byproduct of heating or combustion of various chlorinated organic compounds.[176]

Exposure to phosgene initially may produce limited manifestations but may result in acute mucosal irritation after intense exposure. In fact, the pleasant odor of fresh hay, rather than prompting escape, ironically may promote deep and prolonged breathing of the toxic gas. The most consequential clinical effect related to phosgene exposure is delayed ALI.[25,164] Because of the accumulation of a significant alveolar burden of phosgene, symptoms generally are severe after they occur. The delay in onset may be nearly 1 day, so prolonged observation of patients thought to be phosgene poisoned is warranted. The mechanism of phosgene toxicity is dependent on the dissolution of the gas into the fluid of the epithelial lining with resultant liberation of hydrochloric acid and reactive oxygen species (ROS).[164]

Oxidant Gases Rather than acidic or alkaline metabolites, free radicals mediate the pulmonary toxicity of certain irritant gases. Many of the chemicals discussed participate in both acid–base and oxidant types of injury. However, the clinical distinction between acid- or alkali-forming agents and oxidant gases is difficult but ultimately may prove therapeutically relevant.

Oxygen (O_2). Oxygen toxicity is uncommon in the workplace but, ironically, is common in hospitalized patients. Although O_2 may produce CNS and retinal toxicity, pulmonary damage is more common.[175] Several clinical studies indicate that humans can tolerate 100% O_2 at sea level for up to 48 hours without significant acute pulmonary damage.[35,52] Under hyperbaric conditions (2.0 atmospheres absolute), such as during compressed-air diving or while inside a pressurized hyperbaric chamber, oxygen toxicity may develop within 3 to 6 hours.[44] ALI occurs in approximately 5% of patients administered hyperbaric oxygen for therapeutic purposes.[175] Delayed pulmonary fibrosis, presumably from healing of subclinical injury, may develop in patients breathing lower concentrations of O_2 at sea level for shorter periods.

Although it appears paradoxical that O_2, an essential molecule, may be deleterious at elevated concentrations, it is not. In mitochondria, O_2 plays a critical role as the ultimate acceptor for electrons completing the electron transport chain. It is this same potent oxidizing activity that allows O_2 to remove electrons from other compounds generating the reactive oxygen intermediates.[159]

Generation of ROS, including superoxide (O_2^-), hydroxyl radical (OH·), hydrogen peroxide (HOOH), and singlet oxygen (O·), and nitric oxide (NO) produces cellular necrosis, increases pulmonary capillary permeability, and induces apoptosis.[137,159] NO, produced by inducible NO synthase in the setting of oxidative stress, is directly cytotoxic or may combine with superoxide anions to form the more reactive oxidant peroxynitrite.[89] Experimental prevention of these effects by administration of either parenteral NAC,[160,202] a chemical antioxidant, or superoxide dismutase, an enzymatic antioxidant,[35,194] suggests that the mechanism of toxicity relates to the oxidant, or electrophilic, effects of these ROS (see Chap. 11). Although several other therapies have shown promise in preventing oxygen-mediated toxicity, none has yet proven to be valuable for patients who already manifest pulmonary toxicity. Current techniques for preventing pulmonary oxygen toxicity emphasize reduction of the inspired oxygen concentration by use of PEEP ventilation, although this approach failed to prove beneficial in at least one clinical trial.[12] The potential role of liquid ventilation of the lung with perfluorocarbons to prevent or treat pulmonary oxygen toxicity remains under investigation.[12]

Oxides of Nitrogen (NO_x). Oxides of nitrogen are a series of variably oxidized nitrogenous compounds.[69] The most important substances included in this series are the stable free radicals nitrogen dioxide (NO_2) and nitric oxide (NO), as well as nitrogen tetroxide (dinitrogen tetroxide [N_2O_4]), nitrogen trioxide (N_2O_3), and nitrous oxide (N_2O). The oxides of nitrogen are of limited value in industrial operations, although they may be generated during welding and brazing. NO_2, in addition to hydrogen cyanide, is produced in the pyrolysis of nitrocellulose, which is a substantial component of radiographic film. For example, a fire in the radiology department of the Cleveland Clinic in 1929 resulted in 125 casualties, with virtually all deaths resulting from cyanide or NO_2 gas poisoning.[78] NO_2 toxicity may occur when propane-driven ice-cleaning machines are used in indoor ice skating rinks with poor ventilation, thereby allowing accumulation of the generated NO_2.[109] Military exposure to high NO_2 concentrations may occur during closed-space fires, such as in submarines.[115] NO_2 also causes silo filler's disease, in which the toxic gas generated during decomposition of silage accumulates within the silo shortly after grain storage, eliminating rodents that feast on the grains.[56,210] In the absence of ventilation, high concentrations of NO_2 may accumulate in the silo such that an individual entering the silo is rapidly asphyxiated from the depletion of oxygen.[79] Additionally, substantial quantities of NO_2 remaining after incomplete ventilation may produce the delayed-onset pulmonary toxicity characteristic of silo filler's disease. Chronic indoor exposure to NO_2, generated during cooking[95] or outdoor exposure to photochemical smog, of which the oxides of nitrogen are a component, may predispose individuals to the development or exacerbation of chronic lung diseases.

The various oxides of nitrogen may directly oxidize respiratory tract cellular membranes but more typically generate reactive nitrogen intermediates, or radicals, such as peroxynitrite ($ONOO^-$), which subsequently damage the pulmonary epithelial cells.[141] In addition to generating oxidant cascades, dissolution in respiratory tract water generates nitric acid (HNO_3) and NO, which produce injury consistent with other inhaled acids. In fact, inhalation of HNO_3 produces the same clinical and pathologic syndrome.[82] Antioxidants afford significant protection to human endothelial cells exposed to NO_2, indicating an important role of free radicals in the toxicology of these xenobiotics.[196]

NO, an endogenous compound important as a neurotransmitter and vasorelaxant, is used clinically as exogenous inhalational therapy for pulmonary hypertension and ALI.[190] In patients with ALI not resulting from sepsis (although not specifically from inhalational injury), low concentrations of inhaled NO (5 ppm) did not improve the clinical outcome.[190] However, one patient with NO_2 pulmonary toxicity improved clinically after NO therapy, so further consideration is warranted.[107] Furthermore, its use in premature infants with respiratory distress syndrome is well accepted.[163] NO is less soluble in the fluid lining the epithelial surfaces than are the other oxides of nitrogen and produces irritant effects after large exposures.[84,206] Its pulmonary oxidative toxicity, the manifestations of which are typical of the oxidant gases, is substantially enhanced by conversion to reactive nitrogen intermediates such as $ONOO^-$.[17] This radical selectively interacts with tyrosine to produce nitrotyrosine, which may subsequently serve as a marker for oxidant damage.[84] NO may be absorbed from the lung and is rapidly bound by hemoglobin to form nitrosylhemoglobin and methemoglobin.

Ozone (O_3). Ozone is abundant in the stratospheric region found between 5 and 31 miles above the planet. Ozone is formed by the action of ultraviolet light on oxygen molecules, thus reducing the amount of solar ultraviolet irradiation reaching earth. The ozone concentration in passenger aircrafts may at times be above regulatory limits,[177] although a specific relationship with the development of clinical effects in airline crew members is elusive.[131] Ozone is another important component of photochemical smog and, as such, contributes to chronic lung disease.[30,197] It is produced in significant quantities by welding

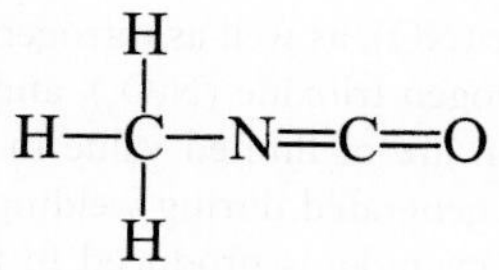

$$H_3C{-}N{=}C{=}O$$

FIGURE 124–3. Methylisocyanate.

and high-voltage electrical equipment and in more moderate doses by photocopying machines and laser printers. Because of its high electronegativity (only fluorine is higher), ozone is one of the most potent oxidizing agents available. For this reason, it is used as a bleaching agent, particularly as an alternative to chlorine in water purification and sewage treatment.

The pulmonary toxicity associated with ozone primarily results from its high reactivity toward unsaturated fatty acids and amino acids with sulfhydryl functional groups.[19,97] Ozonation and free radical damage to the lipid component of the membrane initiate an inflammatory cascade, with resultant influx of inflammatory cells.[20,153] Reactive nitrogen species also are implicated, as NO synthase knockout mice are relatively protected from ozone-induced inflammation and tissue injury.[63] Increased permeability of the pulmonary epithelium results in alveolar filling from the transudation of proteins and fluids characteristic of ALI. Antioxidant agents (eg, vitamin E) that react preferentially with free radicals before membrane damage occurs prevent or limit the pulmonary toxicity of ozone.

Miscellaneous Pulmonary Irritants *Methylisocyanate.* Methylisocyanate (MIC; Figure 124–3) is one of a series of compounds sharing a similar isocyanate (N=C=O) moiety. Toluene diisocyanate (TDI) and diphenylmethane diisocyanate (MDI) are important chemicals in the polymer industry. In those exposed to MIC in Bhopal, ALI was evident both clinically and radiographically.[125] MIC is a significantly more potent respiratory irritant than the other regularly used isocyanate derivatives such as TDI.[6] Cyanide poisoning does not occur, and empiric antidotal therapy is not indicated.

Riot Control Agents: Capsaicin, Chlorobenzylidenemalononitrile, and Chloroacetophenone. Historically, riot control agents (see Fig. 131–5), commonly called Mace, consisted primarily of chloroacetophenone (CN) or chlorobenzylidenemalononitrile (CS).[22] Both are white solids that are dispersed as aerosols. The dispersion is generally accomplished through mixture with a pyrotechnic agent such as a grenade or with a volatile organic solvent in a personal protection canister. Because the delivery systems of these agents are of limited sophistication and are subject to prevailing environmental conditions, dosing is unpredictable, and unintended self-poisoning is common.[22] After low-concentration exposure, ocular discomfort and lacrimation alone are expected, accounting for the common appellation *tear gas.* The effects are transient, and complete recovery within 30 minutes is typical, although long-lasting pulmonary effects may occur (see Asthma and Reactive Airways Dysfunction Syndrome).[156] Closed-space or close-range exposure, as well as physical exertion during exposure, may produce significant ocular toxicity, dermal burns, laryngospasm, ALI,[191] or death[22]. Because of their high potential for severe toxicity, CN and CS were replaced for civilian use by oleoresin capsicum (OC), also known as *pepper spray* or *pepper mace.* Although capsaicin, its active component, is considerably less toxic, it is occasionally responsible for pneumonitis[21] and death.[181]

Capsaicin interacts with the vanilloid receptor-1 (VR1), which was recently renamed the transient receptor potential vanilloid-1 (TRPV1).[186] Stimulation of this receptor invokes the release of substance P, a neuropeptide involved with transmission of pain impulses. Substance P also induces neurogenic inflammation, which, in the lung, results in ALI and bronchoconstriction (see Asthma and Reactive Airways Dysfunction Syndrome).[186] The severe pulmonary toxicity of CS and CN likely is related to their ability to alkylate tissues in a manner similar to mustard agents.[45]

Metal Pneumonitis. Acute inhalational exposures to certain metal compounds produce clinical effects identical to those of the chemical irritants. For example, zinc chloride ($ZnCl_2$) fume is used as artificial smoke because of the dense white character of the fume, and an aqueous solution is still used as a soldering flux. Exposure to zinc chloride fumes for just a few minutes is associated with ALI and death[62,90,91] (see Chap. 101). Cadmium oxide (CdO) is generated during the burning of cadmium metal in an oxygen-containing environment, as occurs during smelting or welding (see Chap. 90). The refining of nickel using carbon monoxide (Mond process) produces nickel carbonyl [$Ni(CO)_4$], a volatile pulmonary oxidant[170] (see Chap. 97). Inhalation of volatilized elemental mercury,[129] which occurs during the vacuuming of mercury spills or home extracting of precious metals, may be toxic. Although at sufficient concentrations, many of these metal exposures produce warning symptoms, severe toxicity may occur even in the absence of warning symptoms. The mechanism of toxicity may relate to overwhelming oxidant stress with a pronounced inflammatory response as measured by serum cytokines (eg, TNF-α) concentrations.[91] Experimental findings suggest a role for inactivation of natural antioxidant systems.[209] Patients with metal-induced pneumonitis present with chest tightness, cough, fever, and signs consistent with ALI. Metal pneumonitis is distinguishable from other causes of ALI only by history or, retrospectively, by elevated serum or urine metal concentrations.[8] In particular, metal pneumonitis should be differentiated from the more common and substantially less consequential metal fume fever, discussed later in this chapter. In addition to standard supportive measures, patients with acute metal-induced pneumonitis should be hospitalized and receive corticosteroids.[91] Chelation therapy has no documented benefit for treatment of patients with ALI but should be used based on conventional indications.

MANAGEMENT

STANDARD AND SUPPORTIVE MEASURES

Management of patients with acute respiratory tract injury begins with meticulous support of airway patency by limiting bronchial and pulmonary secretions and maintaining oxygenation. Although various theoretical and experimental treatment modalities have been proposed, supportive care remains the mainstay of therapy. Supplemental oxygen, bronchodilators, and airway suctioning should be used if clinically indicated. Nitrovasodilators, diuretics, and morphine have little role in the management of patients with ARDS, although low-dose morphine may prove beneficial as an anxiolytic agent.[3,145] Corticosteroid therapy, designed to reduce the inflammatory host defense response, frequently improves surrogate markers of pulmonary damage,[118,119] such as oxygenation status, but generally offers little outcome enhancement in patients with ARDS.[4,142] Importantly, most studies of ARDS involve predominantly septic or traumatized patients, with few patients suffering from inhalational poisoning. Because the inflammatory response initiated by bacterial endotoxin differs from that caused by irritant gases, the applicability of these studies to the treatment of poisoned individuals is limited. There is an interesting report of simultaneous, presumably equivalent chlorine exposure in two sisters, with improved outcome in the sister who received steroid treatment.[42] Most available research evaluates parenterally administered corticosteroids, although animal models demonstrate a beneficial effect of nebulized beclomethasone[80] and nebulized budesonide[204] after acute chlorine poisoning. However, a human pretreatment model of inhaled budesonide fails to document a substantive alteration of the effects of ozone inhalation.[132] Ketoconazole, an antifungal agent with antiinflammatory effects,[1] and nonsteroidal antiinflammatory agents, such as ibuprofen,[166] variably improve experimental lung function or mortality in patients with ALI of various nontoxicologic etiologies and have little current role in the therapeutic armamentarium. Furthermore, most of the aforementioned studies assess acute outcome and not long-term effects in survivors. Because corticosteroids experimentally reduce the late fibroproliferative phase during lung recovery, they ultimately may prove beneficial. Overall, there is little reason to suspect any specific benefit of corticosteroids and other antiinflammatory drugs in most poisoned patients. However, because most studies demonstrate some benefit and little identifiable risk, corticosteroid use appropriately remains routine and based largely on local practices.

The clinical similarities among patients with irritant gas exposure and other etiologies of ALI suggest that similar management principles should be applied. Prone positioning during ventilation,[7,70] PEEP,[64] and inverse-ratio ventilation are successful in enhancing the oxygenation of patients with ALI of various causes but are not necessarily successful in improving outcome. Lower tidal volume mechanical ventilation using 6 mL/kg and plateau pressures 30 cm H_2O attenuated the inflammatory response[138] and resulted in lower mortality and less need for mechanical ventilation than traditional volume ventilation with 12 mL/kg.[2,127] Although not specifically evaluated in any of these studies, there are sound theoretical reasons to believe that all of these modalities should improve oxygenation in poisoned patients as well. Although it is always important to reduce the inspired concentration of oxygen to below 50% as rapidly as possible, patients poisoned by irritant gases may be even more susceptible to oxygen toxicity as a result of depletion of endogenous antioxidant barriers.[173]

NEUTRALIZATION THERAPY

A therapy unique to several of the acid-or base-forming irritant gases is chemical neutralization. Although contraindicated in acid or alkali injury of the GI tract, the large surface area of the lung and the relatively small amount of xenobiotic present allow dissipation of the heat and gas generated during neutralization. Case studies suggest that nebulized 2% sodium bicarbonate may be beneficial in patients poisoned by acid-forming irritant gases.[199] The vast majority of these cases involve chlorine gas exposure, and most patients received other symptomatic therapies as well.[26] Although there appears to be no specific benefit for patients exposed to chloramine, nebulized bicarbonate therapy appears to be safe.[139] A prospective evaluation of patients poisoned with chloramine and chlorine gas did not show any clinically significant difference between the group getting nebulized sodium bicarbonate and the control group, although there was a small but statistical improvement in forced expiratory volume in 1 second (FEV_1) at 120 and 240 minutes in the group that received nebulized sodium bicarbonate.[9] Any sodium bicarbonate solution used should be sufficiently diluted to prevent irritation. Typically, 1 mL of 7.5% or 8.4% sodium bicarbonate solution is added to 3 mL sterile water (resulting in an approximately 2% solution for nebulization).

Whether nebulized sodium bicarbonate therapy alters the natural course of irritant-induced pulmonary damage remains uncertain. The fact that many irritants produce concomitant oxidant injury suggests that it may not. Nebulized 4% sodium bicarbonate administered to chlorine-poisoned sheep improved oxygenation but failed to decrease mortality rates.[43] Therefore, patients receiving nebulized bicarbonate therapy require observation beyond the time of symptom resolution. Because administration of neutralizing acids for alkaline irritants, such as ammonia, has not been attempted, their use cannot be recommended at this time (see Antidote in Depth A5: Sodium Bicarbonate).

ANTIOXIDANTS

Antioxidants include reducing agents such as ascorbic acid, NAC,[102] free radical scavengers such as vitamin E, and enzymes such as superoxide dismutase. Studies in humans have noted both increased[161] and decreased[27] endogenous antioxidant concentrations in bronchoalveolar lavage fluid in patients with ALI. Although the concept of treating pulmonary oxidant stress with antioxidants or free radical scavengers is intriguing, most currently available evidence suggests that these xenobiotics offer negligible benefit.[128,135] The rapid onset of the self-perpetuating destructive effects initiated by redox reactions may hinder any postexposure therapy. This interpretation is supported by pretreatment models in which antioxidants are effective at preventing or at least limiting the pathologic effects. Use of these and other newer therapies targeted against inflammatory mediators or the oxidative cascade are in the earliest investigative stages.

XENOBIOTIC-DIRECTED THERAPY

Patients with inhalational exposure to hydrogen fluoride should undergo frequent electrocardiographic evaluations and correction of serum electrolytes. Administration of nebulized 2.5% calcium gluconate, prepared as 1.5 mL 10% calcium gluconate plus 4.5 mL 0.9% sodium chloride solution or sterile water should be considered to limit systemic fluoride absorption.[103,108,195] By binding fluoride ion locally, nebulized calcium may prevent fluoride-induced cellular and systemic toxicity. Systemic calcium salts should be administered as needed to correct hypocalcemia (see Chap. 105 and Antidotes in Depth A30: Calcium).

Current therapy for inhalation of capsaicin, or of any tear gas, is primarily supportive. Extracorporeal membrane oxygenation has been used in children to maintain oxygenation in the presence of severe pulmonary toxicity resulting from capsaicin exposure.[21] Although no antidotes currently are available, the newly developing insight into the receptor mechanism of capsaicin suggests that a receptor active agent may hold future promise.

ADVANCED PHARMACOLOGIC THERAPY

Perfluorocarbon Partial Liquid Ventilation Partial liquid ventilation involves the intrapulmonary administration of perfluorocarbons, which are inert liquids with low surface tension and excellent oxygen-carrying capacity. Studies in patients with nonchemically induced ARDS suggest that exfoliated tissue, and presumably persistent xenobiotic, may be effectively lavaged from the bronchopulmonary tree with this method.[48] Perfluorocarbons improve oxygenation and may have an antiinflammatory effect, as demonstrated by reduced oxidant lung injury after liquid ventilation in animals.[47] Although this may prove to be a highly useful therapy in the future, their limited availability, high cost, and lack of demonstrated efficacy make them suitable only for academic and research settings.[48]

Exogenous Surfactant Several other recent developments may prove useful in the general management of patients with ARDS. Surfactant replacement therapy initially received attention as a treatment for patients with ARDS because of its beneficial effects in infant respiratory distress syndrome. Although several experimental and clinical studies suggested the safety and efficacy of surfactant therapy in patients with ARDS, large randomized, controlled clinical trials fail to show a benefit on survival.[179] Patients who received surfactant had a greater improvement in gas exchange during the 24-hour treatment period than patients who received standard therapy alone, suggesting the potential benefit of a longer treatment course.[179] But because most studies involved patients with sepsis-related ARDS, the inability to show a beneficial effect may not adequately reflect the potential of surfactant in irritant gas-induced ARDS.[146] Many oxidant gases inactivate endogenous surfactant, although the specific effects on exogenous surfactant are not well understood.[146]

OTHER INHALATIONAL PULMONARY XENOBIOTICS

A particulate, or dust, is a solid dispersed in a gas. Dust is a substantial source of occupational particulate exposure and is an important cause of acute pulmonary toxic syndromes. A respirable particulate must have an appropriately small size (generally <10 μm) and aerodynamic properties to enter the terminal respiratory tree. Nonrespirable particulates, also called *nuisance dusts*, are trapped by the upper airways and are not generally thought to cause pulmonary damage. In distinction from the irritant gases, there is no unifying toxic mechanism among the respirable particulates. Many of the particulate diseases, such as asbestos exposure and its sequelae, are chronic in nature; only the acute or subacute syndromes are discussed here.

INORGANIC DUST EXPOSURE

Silicosis is a range of pulmonary diseases associated with inhalation of crystalline silica (SiO_2), or quartz. It typically occurs in workers involved in occupations in which rock or granite is pulverized, including mining, quarry work, and sandblasting. Although typically a chronic disease, intense subacute exposure may produce acute silicosis in a few weeks and death within 2 years. The mechanism of toxicity probably relates to the relentless inflammatory response generated by the pulmonary macrophages.[134] These cells engulf the indigestible particles and are destroyed, releasing their lytic enzymes and oxidative products locally within the pulmonary parenchyma. Patients present with dyspnea, cor pulmonale, restrictive lung findings, and classic radiographic findings. Treatment is limited and includes steroids and supportive care.

Silica combined with other minerals is referred to as *silicates*, the most important of which include asbestos and talc. Talc, or magnesium silicate [$(Mg_3Si_4)O_{10}(OH)_2$], is widely used in industry, but its use in the home has been curtailed over the past two decades because of cases of severe pulmonary injury.[112] Much of the toxicity of talc is related to free silica or asbestos contamination. Improvement after acute massive exposure may be accompanied by progressive pulmonary fibrosis.

ORGANIC DUSTS

Inhalation of dusts from cotton or similar natural fibers, usually during the refinement of cotton fibers (byssinosis), produces chest tightness, dyspnea, and fever that typically begin within 3 to 4 hours of exposure. Similar reactions may occur after inhalation of hay, silage, grain, hemp, or compost dust. Symptoms often resolve during the work week but return after a weekend hiatus. Byssinosis is probably caused by an endotoxin present on the cotton and is not immunologic in nature.[205] "Grain fever" is caused by a respirable compound associated with grain dust, as occurs during harvesting, milling, and transporting.

HYPERSENSITIVITY PNEUMONITIS

Hypersensitivity pneumonitis, also known as extrinsic allergic alveolitis, is the final common pathway for many different organic dust exposures.[182] The name attached to the individual syndrome typically identifies the associated occupation or substrate. For example, *bagassosis* is the term associated with sugar cane (bagasse), and *farmer's lung* is the term associated with moldy hay, although both conditions are caused by thermophilic *Actinomycetes* spp. When associated with puffball mushroom spores (*Lycoperdon* spp), the syndrome is called *lycoperdonosis* (see Chap. 117); when caused by bird droppings, it is called *bird fancier's lung*. The implicated allergen is capable of depositing in the pulmonary parenchyma and eliciting a cell-mediated (type IV) immunologic response. Clinical findings include fever, chills, and dyspnea beginning 4 to 8 hours after exposure. The chest radiograph usually is normal but may reveal diffuse or discrete infiltrates. Progressive disease is associated with a honeycombing pattern on the radiograph and a restrictive lung disease pattern on formal pulmonary function testing. Treatment includes corticosteroids and avoidance of the antigen.

METAL FUME FEVER AND POLYMER FUME FEVER

Metal fume fever is a recurrent influenza-like syndrome that develops several hours after exposure to metal oxide fumes generated during welding, galvanizing, or smelting. Although most symptoms of metal fume fever are similar to those expected with irritant gas exposures (dyspnea, cough, chest pain), the presence of fever, typically 100.4°F to 102.2°F (38°C–39°C), distinguishes the syndromes.[23] In addition, patients may experience headache, metallic taste, myalgias, and chills. Direct pulmonary toxicity probably does not occur, and patients with metal fume fever generally have normal chest radiographs. Interestingly, acute tolerance develops, so repeat daily exposures produce progressively milder symptoms. However, the tolerance disappears rapidly, and after a short work hiatus such as a weekend, the original intensity resumes, thus accounting for the designation "Monday morning fever." Many metal oxides are capable of eliciting this syndrome, but it is noted most frequently in patients who have welded galvanized steel, which contains zinc. Metal fume fever also occurs commonly after the high-temperature welding of copper-containing compounds, thus accounting for the historical appellation "brass foundry workers ague." There is a strong association between welding-related metal fume fever and welding-related respiratory symptoms suggestive of occupational asthma.[61] Serum and urine metal concentrations typically are not elevated after the acute event, although they may be chronically elevated from daily occupational exposure. The etiology of metal fume fever is debated, but the syndrome has features suggestive of both an immunologic and a toxic etiology.[23] Antigen release with immunologic response appears to be responsible for the induction of symptoms. On subsequent exposure, proinflammatory cytokines, such as TNF-α, and various interleukins can be detected in bronchoalveolar lavage fluid.[105] However, because symptoms may occur with the patient's first exposure to fumes, a direct toxic effect on the respiratory mucosa presumably exists.[117] Exposure to certain metal fumes, such as cadmium oxide or other zinc compounds, may produce direct toxic effects on the pulmonary parenchyma.[117]

The management of patients with metal fume fever is supportive and includes analgesics and antipyretics. There is no specific antidote, and chelation therapy should not be instituted unless otherwise indicated; patients with ALI probably have metal toxicity (eg, cadmium pneumonitis). The natural course of metal fume fever involves spontaneous resolution within 48 hours. Persistent symptoms are rare and should prompt investigation for metal toxicity.

A remarkably similar syndrome occurs subsequent to inhaling pyrolysis products of fluorinated polymers (eg, Teflon), which is aptly termed *polymer fume fever*.[172] Patients develop self-limited viral illness-type symptoms several hours after exposure to the fumes. As with metal fumes, very large exposures to polymer fumes may result in direct pulmonary toxicity. Supportive care is the therapy of choice.

ASTHMA AND REACTIVE AIRWAYS DYSFUNCTION SYNDROME

Asthma, or *reversible airways disease*, is a clinical syndrome that includes intermittent episodes of dyspnea, cough, chest pain or tightness, wheezes on auscultation, and measurable variations in expiratory airflow. Episodes typically are triggered by a xenobiotic or physical stimulus and resolve over several hours with appropriate therapy. The underlying process is immunologic in most cases, with allergen-triggered release of inflammatory mediators causing bronchiolar smooth muscle contraction and subsequent inflammation. Because asthma affects 5% to 10% of the world's population and the triggers often are nonspecific, it is not surprising that work-aggravated asthma is extremely common. The patients are previously sensitized, and the initial irritant exposure causes bronchospasm or similar symptoms. Thus, work-aggravated asthma is discovered early in the worker's employment, and a more appropriate workplace or occupation can be pursued.

Occupational asthma, or asthma occasioned by a workplace exposure to a sensitizing xenobiotic, accounts for perhaps 10% to 17% of all newly diagnosed asthma in adults.[110,192] Casual exposure to one of the 250 or more known sensitizers (Table 124–3) is usually associated with a latency period of weeks or months of exposure before symptom onset. After symptoms begin, however, they recur consistently after reexposure to the inciting trigger agent. Occupational asthma with latency may be IgE dependent, in which case it is identical to allergic asthma, or is IgE independent.[198] The IgE-dependent form is most commonly associated with high-molecular-weight compounds (>5000 daltons) or with certain haptenic low-molecular-weight agents (eg, acetic anhydride). The low-molecular-weight agents (eg, nickel, isocyanates) more typically cause IgE-independent disease, which manifests as the delayed reaction pattern of cell-mediated, or type IV, hypersensitivity. Because contact with a trigger may be difficult to avoid in either case, reassignment or an outright occupational change may be required. Treatment for exacerbations is comparable to standard asthma therapy and includes bronchodilators and corticosteroids.

Acute exposure to irritant gas may result in the development of a persistent asthma-like syndrome also termed *reactive airways dysfunction syndrome* (RADS), *irritant-induced asthma*, or *occupational asthma without latency*. Virtually every irritative xenobiotic is reported to cause this syndrome, and those not yet described probably are simply unrecognized. Although asthma typically is associated with massive inhalational exposure, as occurred after the World Trade Center collapse,[14] occasional patients are susceptible to low-level exposure.[31] RADS is often compared to occupational asthma because both disorders are chemically induced and most frequently occur after chemical exposure in the workplace.[46] However, in comparison with those who develop occupational asthma, patients who develop RADS have a lower incidence of atopy and are exposed to agents not typically considered to be immunologically sensitizing.[31] In addition, the airflow improvement with β_2-adrenergic agonist therapy is significantly better in patients with occupational asthma.[71] Bronchial biopsy performed in patients with RADS generally reveals a chronic inflammatory response.[71] RADS may have a neurogenic etiology[120] as opposed to an immunologic origin, as in patients with occupational asthma, which may differentiate these clinically similar diseases on a mechanistic basis. Neurogenic inflammation results from increased vascular permeability, presumably secondary to release of substance P from unmyelinated sensory neurons (C fibers).[54] Neurogenic inflammation is inhibited by substance P depletors such as capsaicin and enhanced by substances that inhibit neutral endopeptidase, the enzyme responsible for degradation of substance P.[121] The role of corticosteroids is undefined, but animal models suggest an antiinflammatory benefit.[51] Recovery may take months, with the delay related to either ongoing low-level exposures to endopeptidase inhibitors or persistent irritation of impaired tissue by environmental irritants such as pollution.

TABLE 124–3. Common Xenobiotic Sensitizers Producing Occupational Asthma

Molecular Weight	Example	Primary Risk Occupations
High		
Proteins	Crab shell protein	Seafood processors
Low		
Acrylate	–	Adhesives, plastics
Glutaraldehyde	–	Healthcare workers
Isocyanates	Toluene diisocyanate	Polyurethane foam, automobile painters
Metals	Nickel sulfate	Nickel platers
Trimellitic anhydride	–	Chemical workers
Wood dust	Western red cedar (*Thuja plicata*)	Foresters, carpenters

SUMMARY

The overall quality of the air we breathe continues to deteriorate, and fluctuations in environmental pollutants periodically cause epidemic disease. Although the spectrum of xenobiotics capable of causing pulmonary toxicity is large, the pathologic changes are rather limited. Gases that have little or no irritant potential or systemic toxicity cause simple asphyxiation, in which the ambient atmosphere has a diminished oxygen concentration. Parenchymal irritation and ALI occur after exposure to acid-forming or free radical–generating gases and may progress to severe toxicity manifesting as ARDS. RADS is described in patients after exposure to virtually all of the irritant gases. Treatment of all such exposures centers on symptomatic and supportive care.

REFERENCES

1. Acute Respiratory Distress Syndrome Network. Ketoconazole for early treatment of acute lung injury and acute respiratory distress syndrome: a randomized controlled trial. *JAMA*. 2000;283:1995-2002.
2. Acute Respiratory Distress Syndrome Network. Ventilation with lower tidal volumes as compared with traditional tidal volumes for acute lung injury and the acute respiratory distress syndrome. *N Engl J Med*. 2000;342:1301-1308.
3. Adhikari NK, Burns KE, Friedrich JO, Granton JT, Cook DJ, Meade MO. Effect of nitric oxide on oxygenation and mortality in acute lung injury: systematic review and meta-analysis. *Br Med J*. 2007;334:779-786.
4. Adhikari N, Burns KE, Meade MO. Pharmacologic therapies for adults with acute lung injury and acute respiratory distress syndrome. *Cochrane Database Syst Rev*. 2004;CD004477.
5. Agabiti N, Ancona C, Forastiere F, et al. Short term respiratory effects of acute exposure to chlorine due to a swimming pool accident. *Occup Environ Med*. 2001;58:399-404.
6. Alarie Y, Ferguson JS, Stock MF, et al. Sensory and pulmonary irritation of methyl isocyanate in mice and pulmonary irritation and possible cyanide-like effects of methyl isocyanate in guinea pigs. *Environ Health Perspect*. 1987;72:159-167.

7. Alsaghir AH, Martin CM. Effect of prone positioning in patients with acute respiratory distress syndrome: a meta-analysis. *Crit Care Med.* 2008;36:603-609.
8. Ando Y, Shibata E, Tsuchiyama F, Sakai S. Elevated urinary cadmium concentrations in a patient with acute cadmium pneumonitis. *Scand J Work Environ Health.* 1996;22:150-153.
9. Aslan S, Kandiş H, Akgun M, et al. The effect of nebulized NaHCO3 treatment on "RADS" due to chlorine gas inhalation. *Inhal Toxicol.* 2006;18:895-900.
10. Auwaerter V, Perdekamp MG, Kempf J, et al. Toxicological analysis after asphyxial suicide with helium and a plastic bag. *Forensic Sci Int.* 2007;170:139-141.
11. Avecillas JF, Freire AX, Arroliga AC. Clinical epidemiology of acute lung injury and acute respiratory distress syndrome: incidence, diagnosis, and outcomes. *Clin Chest Med.* 2006;27:549-557
12. Babu PB, Chidekel A, Shaffer TH. Hyperoxia-induced changes in human airway epithelial cells: the protective effect of perflubron. *Pediatr Crit Care Med.* 2005;6:188-194.
13. Babu RV, Cardenas V, Sharma G. Acute respiratory distress syndrome from chlorine inhalation during a swimming pool accident: a case report and review of the literature. *J Intensive Care Med.* 2008;23:275-280.
14. Banauch GI, Dhala A, Alleyne D, et al. Bronchial hyperreactivity and other inhalation lung injuries in rescue/recovery workers after the World Trade Center collapse. *Crit Care Med.* 2005;33(suppl):S102-S106.
15. Baxter PJ, Kapila M, Mfonfu D. Lake Nyos disaster, Cameroon, 1986: the medical effects of large scale emission of carbon dioxide? *Br Med J.* 1989;298:1437-1441.
16. Beckett WS. Persistent respiratory effects in survivors of the Bhopal disaster. *Thorax.* 1998;53(suppl 2):S43-S46.
17. Beckman JS, Koppenol WH. Nitric oxide, superoxide, and peroxynitrite: the good, the bad, and ugly. *Am J Physiol.* 1996;271:C1424-C1437.
18. Bernard GR, Artigas A, Brigham KL, et al. The American-European Consensus Conference on ARDS definitions, mechanisms, relevant outcomes, and clinical trial coordination. *Am J Respir Crit Care Med.* 1994;149:818-824.
19. Bhalla DK. Ozone-induced lung inflammation and mucosal barrier disruption: toxicology, mechanisms, and implications. *J Toxicol Environ Health B Crit Rev.* 1999;2:31-86.
20. Bhalla DK, Reinhart PG, Bai C, Gupta SK. Amelioration of ozone-induced lung injury by anti-tumor necrosis factor-alpha. *Toxicol Sci.* 2002;69:400-408.
21. Billmire DF, Vinocur C, Ginda M, et al. Pepper-spray-induced respiratory failure treated with extracorporeal membrane oxygenation. *Pediatrics.* 1996;98:961-963.
22. Blain PG. Tear gases and irritant incapacitants. 1-Chloroacetophenone, 2-chlorobenzylidene malononitrile and dibenz[b,f]-1,4-oxazepine. *Toxicol Rev.* 2003;22:103-110.
23. Blanc P, Wong H, Bernstein MS, Boushey HA. An experimental human model of metal fume fever. *Ann Intern Med.* 1991;114:930-936.
24. Blodgett DW, Suruda AJ, Crouch BI. Fatal unintentional occupational poisonings by hydrofluoric acid in the U.S. *Am J Ind Med.* 2001;40:215-220.
25. Borak J, Diller WF. Phosgene exposure: mechanisms of injury and treatment strategies. *J Occup Environ Med.* 2001;43:110-119.
26. Bosse GM. Nebulized sodium bicarbonate in the treatment of chlorine gas inhalation. *J Toxicol Clin Toxicol.* 1994;32:233-241.
27. Bowler RP, Velsor LW, Duda B, et al. Pulmonary edema fluid antioxidants are depressed in acute lung injury. *Crit Care Med.* 2003;31:2309-2315.
28. Braun J, Stoss H, Zober A. Intoxication following the inhalation of hydrogen fluoride. *Arch Toxicol.* 1984;56:50-54.
29. Brautbar N, Wu MP, Richter ED. Chronic ammonia inhalation and interstitial pulmonary fibrosis: a case report and review of the literature. *Arch Environ Health.* 2003;58:592-596.
30. Bromberg PA, Koren HS. Ozone-induced human respiratory dys-function and disease. *Toxicol Lett.* 1995;82-83:307-316.
31. Brooks SM, Hammad Y, Richards I, et al. The spectrum of irritant-induced asthma: sudden and not-so-sudden onset and the role of allergy. *Chest.* 1998;113:42-49.
32. Burleigh-Flayer H, Wong KL, Alarie Y. Evaluation of the pulmonary effects of HCl using CO2 challenges in guinea pigs. *Fundam Appl Toxicol.* 1985;5:978-985.
33. Burns TR, Mace ML, Greenberg SD, Jachimczyk JA. Ultrastructure of acute ammonia toxicity in the human lung. *Am J Forensic Med Pathol.* 1985;6:204-210.
34. Byard RW, Wilson GW. Death scene gas analysis in suspected methane asphyxia. *Am J Forensic Med Pathol.* 1992;13:69-71.
35. Capellier G, Maupoil V, Boussat S, et al. Oxygen toxicity and tolerance. *Minerva Anestesiol.* 1999;65:388-392.
36. Carbonnelle S, Francaux M, Doyle I, et al. Changes in serum pneumoproteins caused by short-term exposures to nitrogen trichloride in indoor chlorinated swimming pools. *Biomarkers.* 2002;7:464-478.
37. Centers for Disease Control and Prevention. Acute illness from dry ice exposure during hurricane Ivan—Alabama, 2004. *MMWR Morb Mortal Wkly Rep.* 2004;53:1182-1183.
38. Centers for Disease Control and Prevention. Ocular and respiratory illness associated with an indoor swimming pool–Nebraska, 2006. *MMWR Morb Mortal Wkly Rep.* 2007;56:929-932.
39. Centers for Disease Control and Prevention. Public health consequences from hazardous substances acutely released during rail transit—South Carolina, 2005; selected States, 1999–2004. *MMWR Morb Mortal Wkly Rep.* 2005;54:64-67.
40. Centers for Disease Control and Prevention. Respiratory and ocular symptoms among employees of a hotel indoor waterpark resort—Ohio, 2007. *MMWR Morb Mortal Wkly Rep.* 2009;58:81-85.
41. Charan NB, Myers CG, Lakshminarayan S, Spencer TM. Pulmonary injuries associated with acute sulfur dioxide inhalation. *Am Rev Respir Dis.* 1979;119:555-560.
42. Chester EH, Kaimal J, Payne CB Jr, Kohn PM. Pulmonary injury following exposure to chlorine gas. Possible beneficial effects of steroid treatment. *Chest.* 1977;72:247-250.
43. Chisholm C, Singletary E, Okerberg C, Langlinais P. Inhaled sodium bicarbonate for chlorine inhalation injuries [abstract]. *Ann Emerg Med.* 1989;18:466.
44. Clark JM, Lambertsen CJ. Rate of development of pulmonary O2 toxicity in man during O2 breathing at 2.0 ATA. *J Appl Physiol.* 1971;30:739-752.
45. Cucinell SA, Swentzel KC, Biskup R, et al. Biochemical interactions and metabolic fate of riot control agents. *Fed Proc.* 1971;30:86-91.
46. Currie GP, Ayres JG. Assessment of bronchial responsiveness following exposure to inhaled occupational and environmental agents. *Toxicol Rev.* 2004;23:75-81.
47. Dani C, Costantino ML, Martelli E, et al. Perfluorocarbons attenuate oxidative lung damage. *Pediatr Pulmonol.* 2003;36:322-329.
48. Davies MW, Fraser JF. Partial liquid ventilation for preventing death and morbidity in adults with acute lung injury and acute respiratory distress syndrome. *Cochrane Database Syst Rev.* 2004;CD003707.
49. Dean JB, Mulkey DK, Garcia AJ 3rd, et al. Neuronal sensitivity to hyperoxia, hypercapnia, and inert gases at hyperbaric pressures. *J Appl Physiol.* 2003;95:883-909.
50. DeBehnke DJ, Hilander SJ, Dobler DW, et al. The hemodynamic and arterial blood gas response to asphyxiation: a canine model of pulseless electrical activity. *Resuscitation.* 1995;30:169-175.
51. Demnati R, Fraser R, Martin JG, et al. Effects of dexamethasone on functional and pathological changes in rat bronchi caused by high acute exposure to chlorine. *Toxicol Sci.* 1998;45:242-246.
52. Deneke SM, Fanburg BL. Normobaric oxygen toxicity of the lung. *N Engl J Med.* 1980;303:76-86.
53. Dhara VR, Dhara R. The Union Carbide disaster in Bhopal: a review of health effects. *Arch Environ Health.* 2002;57:391-404.
54. Di Maria GU, Bellofiore S, Geppetti P. Regulation of airway neurogenic inflammation by neutral endopeptidase. *Eur Respir J.* 1998;12:1454-1462.
55. Dote T, Kono K, Usuda K, et al. Lethal inhalation exposure during maintenance operation of a hydrogen fluoride liquefying tank. *Toxicol Ind Health.* 2003;19:51-54.
56. Douglas WW, Hepper NG, Colby TV. Silo-filler's disease. *Mayo Clin Proc.* 1989;64:291-304.
57. Dunford JV, Lucas J, Vent N, Clark RF, Cantrell FL. Asphyxiation due to dry ice in a walk-in freezer. *J Emerg Med.* 2009;36(4):353-356.
58. Dwyer DM, Thorne AC, Healey JH, Bedford RF. Liquid nitrogen instillation can cause venous gas embolism. *Anesthesiology.* 1990;73:179-181.
59. Edwards KE, Wenstone R. Successful resuscitation from recurrent ventricular fibrillation secondary to butane inhalation. *Br J Anaesth.* 2000;84:803-805.
60. Eghbal MA, Pennefather PS, O'Brien PJ. H2S cytotoxicity mechanism involves reactive oxygen species formation and mitochondrial depolarisation. *Toxicology.* 2004;203:69-76.
61. El-Zein M, Malo JL, Infante-Rivard C, Gautrin D. Prevalence and association of welding related systemic and respiratory symptoms in welders. *Occup Environ Med.* 2003;60:655-661.

62. Evans EH. Casualties following exposure to zinc chloride smoke. *Lancet.* 1945;246:368-370.
63. Fakhrzadeh L, Laskin JD, Laskin DL. Deficiency in inducible nitric oxide synthase protects mice from ozone-induced lung inflammation and tissue injury. *Am J Respir Cell Mol Biol.* 2002;26:413-419.
64. Ferguson ND, Frutos-Vivar F, Esteban A, et al. Airway pressures, tidal volumes, and mortality in patients with acute respiratory distress syndrome. *Crit Care Med.* 2005;33:21-30.
65. Fleta J, Calvo C, Zuniga J, et al. Intoxication of 76 children by chlorine gas. *Hum Toxicol.* 1986;5:99-100.
66. Fowler B, Ackles KN, Porlier G. Effects of inert gas narcosis on behavior—a critical review. *Undersea Biomed Res.* 1985;12:369-402.
67. Gallagher KE, Smith DM, Mellen PF. Suicidal asphyxiation by using pure helium gas: case report, review, and discussion of the influence of the internet. *Am J Forensic Med Pathol.* 2003;24:361-363.
68. Gapany-Gapanavicius M, Molho M, Tirosh M. Chloramine-induced pneumonitis from mixing household cleaning agents. *Br Med J (Clin Res Ed).* 1982;285:1086.
69. Gaston B, Drazen JM, Loscalzo J, Stamler JS. The biology of nitrogen oxides in the airways. *Am J Respir Crit Care Med.* 1994;149:538-551.
70. Gattinoni L, Tognoni G, Pesenti A, et al. Effect of prone positioning on the survival of patients with acute respiratory failure. *N Engl J Med.* 2001;345:568-573.
71. Gautrin D, Boulet LP, Boutet M, et al. Is reactive airways dysfunction syndrome a variant of occupational asthma? *J Allergy Clin Immunol.* 1994;93:12-22.
72. Gautrin D, Leroyer C, Infante-Rivard C, et al. Longitudinal assessment of airway caliber and responsiveness in workers exposed to chlorine. *Am J Respir Crit Care Med.* 1999;160:1232-1237.
73. Ghio AJ, Kennedy TP, Hatch GE, Tepper JS. Reduction of neutrophil influx diminishes lung injury and mortality following phosgene inhalation. *J Appl Physiol.* 1991;71:657-665.
74. Gill JR, Ely SF, Hua Z. Environmental gas displacement: three accidental deaths in the workplace. *Am J Forensic Med Pathol.* 2002;23:26-30.
75. Gilson T, Parks BO, Porterfield CM. Suicide with inert gases: addendum to Final Exit. *Am J Forensic Med Pathol.* 2003;24:306-308.
76. Gorguner M, Aslan S, Inandi T, Cakir Z. Reactive airways dysfunction syndrome in housewives due to a bleach-hydrochloric acid mixture. *Inhal Toxicol.* 2004;16:87-91.
77. Grassberger M, Krauskopf A. Suicidal asphyxiation with helium: report of three cases. *Wien Klin Wochenschr.* 2007;119(9-10):323-325.
78. Gregory KL, Malinoski VF, Sharp CR. Cleveland Clinic Fire Survivorship Study, 1929–1965. *Arch Environ Health.* 1969;18:508-515.
79. Groves JA, Ellwood PA. Gases in forage tower silos. *Ann Occup Hyg.* 1989;33:519-535.
80. Gunnarsson M, Walther SM, Seidal T, Lennquist S. Effects of inhalation of corticosteroids immediately after experimental chlorine gas lung injury. *J Trauma.* 2000;48:101-107.
81. Guo YL, Kennedy TP, Michael JR, et al. Mechanism of phosgene-induced lung toxicity: role of arachidonate mediators. *J Appl Physiol.* 1990;69:1615-1622.
82. Hajela R, Janigan DT, Landrigan PL, et al. Fatal pulmonary edema due to nitric acid fume inhalation in three pulp-mill workers. *Chest.* 1990;97:487-489.
83. Haller JS Jr. Gas warfare: military-medical responsiveness of the Allies in the Great War, 1914–1918. *N Y State J Med.* 1990;90:499-510.
84. Hallman M, Bry K, Turbow R, et al. Pulmonary toxicity associated with nitric oxide in term infants with severe respiratory failure. *J Pediatr.* 1998;132:827-829.
85. Halpern P, Raskin Y, Sorkine P, Oganezov A. Exposure to extremely high concentrations of carbon dioxide: a clinical description of a mass casualty incident. *Ann Emerg Med.* 2004;43:196-199.
86. Harris PD, Barnes R. The uses of helium and xenon in current clinical practice. *Anaesthesia.* 2008;63:284-293.
87. Harrison PM, Wendon JA, Gimson AE, et al. Improvement by acetylcysteine of hemodynamics and oxygen transport in fulminant hepatic failure. *N Engl J Med.* 1991;324:1852-1857.
88. Hendrickson RG, Chang A, Hamilton RJ. Co-worker fatalities from hydrogen sulfide. *Am J Ind Med.* 2004;45:346-350.
89. Hesse AK, Dorger M, Kupatt C, Krombach F. Proinflammatory role of inducible nitric oxide synthase in acute hyperoxic lung injury. *Respir Res.* 2004;5:11.
90. Hsu HH, Tzao C, Chang WC, et al. Zinc chloride (smoke bomb) inhalation lung injury: clinical presentations, high-resolution CT findings, and pulmonary function test results. *Chest.* 2005;127:2064-2071.
91. Huang KL, Chen CW, Chu SJ, Perng WC, Wu CP. Systemic inflammation caused by white smoke inhalation in a combat exercise. *Chest.* 2008;133:722-728.
92. Hudnall JB, Suruda A, Campbell DL. Deaths involving air-line respirators connected to inert gas sources. *Am Ind Hyg Assoc J.* 1993;54:32-35.
93. Hyde DM, Miller LA, McDonald RJ, et al. Neutrophils enhance clearance of necrotic epithelial cells in ozone-induced lung injury in rhesus monkeys. *Am J Physiol.* 1999;277:L1190-L1198.
94. Ikeda N, Takahashi H, Umetsu K, Suzuki T. The course of respiration and circulation in death by carbon dioxide poisoning. *Forensic Sci Int.* 1989;41:93-99.
95. Jarvis D, Chinn S, Luczynska C, Burney P. Association of respiratory symptoms and lung function in young adults with use of domestic gas appliances. *Lancet.* 1996;347:426-431.
96. Jawan B, Lee JH. Cardiac arrest caused by an incorrectly filled oxygen cylinder: a case report. *Br J Anaesth.* 1990;64:749-751.
97. Kelly FJ, Mudway IS. Protein oxidation at the air-lung interface. *Amino Acids.* 2003;25:375-396.
98. Kennedy TP, Michael JR, Hoidal JR, et al. Dibutyryl cAMP, aminophylline, and beta-adrenergic agonists protect against pulmonary edema caused by phosgene. *J Appl Physiol.* 1989;67:2542-2552.
99. Kernbach-Wighton G, Kijewski H, Schwanke P, et al. Clinical and morphological aspects of death due to liquid nitrogen. *Int J Legal Med.* 1998;111:191-195.
100. Kim DH, Lee HJ. Evaporated liquid nitrogen-induced asphyxia: a case report. *J Korean Med Sci.* 2008;23:163-165.
101. Kimbell JS, Gross EA, Joyner DR, et al. Application of computational fluid dynamics to regional dosimetry of inhaled chemicals in the upper respiratory tract of the rat. *Toxicol Appl Pharmacol.* 1993;121:253-263.
102. Koksel O, Cinel I, Tamer L, et al. N-acetylcysteine inhibits peroxynitrite-mediated damage in oleic acid-induced lung injury. *Pulm Pharmacol Ther.* 2004;17:263-270.
103. Kono K, Watanabe T, Dote T, et al. Successful treatments of lung injury and skin burn due to hydrofluoric acid exposure. *Int Arch Occup Environ Health.* 2000;73(suppl):S93-S97.
104. Koplewitz BZ, Daneman A, Fracr S, et al. Gastric perforation attributable to liquid nitrogen ingestion. *Pediatrics.* 2000;105:121-123.
105. Kuschner WG, D'Alessandro A, Wong H, Blanc PD. Early pulmonary cytokine responses to zinc oxide fume inhalation. *Environ Res.* 1997;75:7-11.
106. Laskin DL, Heck DE, Laskin JD. Role of inflammatory cytokines and nitric oxide in hepatic and pulmonary toxicity. *Toxicol Lett.* 1998;102-103:289-293.
107. Leavey JF, Dubin RL, Singh N, Kaminsky DA. Silo-filler's disease, the acute respiratory distress syndrome, and oxides of nitrogen. *Ann Intern Med.* 2004;141:410-411.
108. Lee DC, Wiley JF 2nd, Synder JW 2nd. Treatment of inhalational exposure to hydrofluoric acid with nebulized calcium gluconate. *J Occup Med.* 1993;35:470.
109. Levy JI, Lee K, Yanagisawa Y, et al. Determinants of nitrogen dioxide concentrations in indoor ice skating rinks. *Am J Public Health.* 1998;88:1781-1786.
110. Malo JL, Chan-Yeung M. Occupational asthma. *J Allergy Clin Immunol.* 2001;108:317-328.
111. Manning HL, Schwartzstein RM. Pathophysiology of dyspnea. *N Engl J Med.* 1995;333:1547-1553.
112. Marchiori E, Souza Junior AS, Muller NL. Inhalational pulmonary talcosis: high-resolution CT findings in 3 patients. *J Thorac Imaging.* 2004;19:41-44.
113. Martinez TT, Long C. Explosion risk from swimming pool chlorinators and review of chlorine toxicity. *J Toxicol Clin Toxicol.* 1995;33:349-354.
114. Maybauer MO, Kikuchi Y, Westphal M, et al. Effects of manganese superoxide dismutase nebulization on pulmonary function in an ovine model of acute lung injury. *Shock.* 2005;23:138-143.
115. Mayorga MA. Overview of nitrogen dioxide effects on the lung with emphasis on military relevance. *Toxicology.* 1994;89:175-192.
116. McDonald DM, Thurston G, Baluk P. Endothelial gaps as sites for plasma leakage in inflammation. *Microcirculation.* 1999;6:7-22.
117. McNeilly JD, Heal MR, Beverland IJ, et al. Soluble transition metals cause the pro-inflammatory effects of welding fumes in vitro. *Toxicol Appl Pharmacol.* 2004;196:95-107.

118. Meduri GU. Levels of evidence for the pharmacologic effectiveness of prolonged methylprednisolone treatment in unresolving ARDS. *Chest.* 1999;116(suppl):116S-118S.
119. Meduri GU, Headley AS, Golden E, et al. Effect of prolonged methylprednisolone therapy in unresolving acute respiratory distress syndrome: a randomized controlled trial. *JAMA.* 1998;280:159-165.
120. Meggs WJ. Hypothesis for induction and propagation of chemical sensitivity based on biopsy studies. *Environ Health Perspect.* 1997;105(suppl 2): 473-478.
121. Meggs WJ. RADS and RUDS—the toxic induction of asthma and rhinitis. *J Toxicol Clin Toxicol.* 1994;32:487-501.
122. Meng Z, Qin G, Zhang B, et al. Oxidative damage of sulfur dioxide inhalation on lungs and hearts of mice. *Environ Res.* 2003;93:285-292.
123. Miller TM, Mazur PO. Oxygen deficiency hazards associated with liquefied gas systems: derivation of a program of controls. *Am Ind Hyg Assoc J.* 1984;45:293-298.
124. Minami M, Katsumata M, Miyake K, et al. Dangerous mixture of household detergents in an old-style toilet: a case report with simulation experiments of the working environment and warning of potential hazard relevant to the general environment. *Hum Exp Toxicol.* 1992;11:27-34.
125. Misra NP, Pathak R, Gaur KJ, et al. Clinical profile of gas leak victims in acute phase after Bhopal episode. *Ind J Med Res.* 1987;86(suppl):11-19.
126. Monteiro MG, Hernandez W, Figlie NB, et al. Comparison between subjective feelings to alcohol and nitrogen narcosis: a pilot study. *Alcohol.* 1996;13:75-78.
127. Moran JL, Bersten AD, Solomon PJ. Meta-analysis of controlled trials of ventilator therapy in acute lung injury and acute respiratory distress syndrome: an alternative perspective. *Intensive Care Med.* 2005;31:227-235.
128. Morcillo EJ, Estrela J, Cortijo J. Oxidative stress and pulmonary inflammation: pharmacological intervention with antioxidants. *Pharmacol Res.* 1999;40:393-404.
129. Moromisato DY, Anas NG, Goodman G. Mercury inhalation poisoning and acute lung injury in a child. Use of high-frequency oscillatory ventilation. *Chest.* 1994;105:613-615.
130. Mrvos R, Dean BS, Krenzelok EP. Home exposures to chlorine/chloramine gas: review of 216 cases. *South Med J.* 1993;86:654-657.
131. Nagda NL, Koontz MD. Review of studies on flight attendant health and comfort in airliner cabins. *Aviat Space Environ Med.* 2003;74:101-109.
132. Nightingale JA, Rogers DF, Chung KF, Barnes PJ. No effect of inhaled budesonide on the response to inhaled ozone in normal subjects. *Am J Respir Crit Care Med.* 2000;161:479-486.
133. O'Croinin D, Ni Chonghaile M, Higgins B, Laffey JG. Bench-to-bedside review: permissive hypercapnia. *Crit Care.* 2005;9:51-59.
134. O'Reilly KM, Phipps RP, Thatcher TH, et al. Crystalline and amorphous silica differentially regulate the cyclooxygenaseprostaglandin pathway in pulmonary fibroblasts: implications for pulmonary fibrosis. *Am J Physiol Lung Cell Mol Physiol.* 2005;288:L1010-L1016.
135. Ortolani O, Conti A, De Gaudio AR, et al. Protective effects of N-acetylcysteine and rutin on the lipid peroxidation of the lung epithelium during the adult respiratory distress syndrome. *Shock.* 2000;13:14-18.
136. Orzel RA. Toxicological aspects of firesmoke: polymer pyrolysis and combustion. *Occup Med.* 1993;8:414-429.
137. Pagano A, Barazzone-Argiroffo C. Alveolar cell death in hyperoxia-induced lung injury. *Ann NY Acad Sci.* 2003;1010:405-416.
138. Parsons PE, Eisner MD, Thompson BT, et al. Lower tidal volume ventilation and plasma cytokine markers of inflammation in patients with acute lung injury. *Crit Care Med.* 2005;33:1-6.
139. Pascuzzi TA, Storrow AB. Mass casualties from acute inhalation of chloramine gas. *Mil Med.* 1998;163:102-104.
140. Pauluhn J, Carson A, Costa DL, et al. Workshop summary: phosgene-induced pulmonary toxicity revisited: appraisal of early and late markers of pulmonary injury from animal models with emphasis on human significance. *Inhal Toxicol.* 2007;19:789-810.
141. Persinger RL, Poynter ME, Ckless K, Janssen-Heininger YM. Molecular mechanisms of nitrogen dioxide induced epithelial injury in the lung. *Mol Cell Biochem.* 2002;234-235:71-80.
142. Peter JV, John P, Graham PL, et al. Corticosteroids in the prevention and treatment of acute respiratory distress syndrome (ARDS) in adults: meta-analysis. *Br Med J.* 2008;336:1006-1009.
143. Peters JW. Hydrogen sulfide poisoning in a hospital setting. *JAMA.* 1981;246: 1588-1589.
144. Piirila PL, Nordman H, Korhonen OS, Winblad I. A thirteen-year follow-up of respiratory effects of acute exposure to sulfur dioxide. *Scand J Work Environ Health.* 1996;22:191-196.
145. Pino F, Puerta H, D'Apollo R, et al. Effectiveness of morphine in non-cardiogenic pulmonary edema due to chlorine gas inhalation. *Vet Hum Toxicol.* 1993;35:36.
146. Podgorski A, Sosnowski TR, Gradon L. Deactivation of the pulmonary surfactant dynamics by toxic aerosols and gases. *J Aerosol Med.* 2001;14:455-466.
147. Promisloff RA, Lenchner GS, Phan A, Cichelli AV. Reactive airway dysfunction syndrome in three police officers following a roadside chemical spill. *Chest.* 1990;98:928-929.
148. Putnam RW, Filosa JA, Ritucci NA. Cellular mechanisms involved in CO(2) and acid signaling in chemosensitive neurons. *Am J Physiol Cell Physiol.* 2004;287:C1493-C1526.
149. Quinlan T, Spivack S, Mossman BT. Regulation of antioxidant enzymes in lung after oxidant injury. *Environ Health Perspect.* 1994;102(suppl 2):79-87.
150. Rafferty P. Voluntary chlorine inhalation: a new form of self-abuse? *Br Med J.* 1980;281:1178-1179.
151. Raj M. Humane killing of nonhuman animals for disease control purposes. *J Appl Anim Welf Sci.* 2008;11:112-124.
152. Reiffenstein RJ, Hulbert WC, Roth SH. Toxicology of hydrogen sulfide. *Annu Rev Pharmacol Toxicol.* 1992;32:109-134.
153. Reinhart PG, Bassett DJ, Bhalla DK. The influence of polymorphonuclear leukocytes on altered pulmonary epithelial permeability during ozone exposure. *Toxicology.* 1998;127:17-28.
154. Riechelmann H, Maurer J, Kienast K, et al. Respiratory epithelium exposed to sulfur dioxide—functional and ultrastructural alterations. *Laryngoscope.* 1995;105:295-299.
155. Roblin P, Richards A, Cole R. Liquid nitrogen injury: a case report. *Burns.* 1997;23:638-640.
156. Roth VS, Franzblau A. RADS after exposure to a riot-control agent: a case report. *J Occup Environ Med.* 1996;38:863-865.
157. Rubenfeld GD, Caldwell E, Peabody E, et al. Incidence and outcomes of acute lung injury. *N Engl J Med.* 2005;353:1685-1693.
158. Rubenfeld GD, Herridge MS. Epidemiology and outcomes of acute lung injury. *Chest.* 2007;131:554-62.
159. Sanders KA, Huecksteadt T, Xu P, et al. Regulation of oxidant production in acute lung injury. *Chest.* 1999;116(suppl):56S-61S.
160. Sarnstrand B, Tunek A, Sjodin K, Hallberg A. Effects of N-acetylcysteine stereoisomers on oxygen-induced lung injury in rats. *Chem Biol Interact.* 1995;94:157-164.
161. Schmidt R, Luboeinski T, Markart P, et al. Alveolar antioxidant status in patients with acute respiratory distress syndrome. *Eur Respir J.* 2004;24:994-999.
162. Schön CA, Ketterer T. Asphyxial suicide by inhalation of helium inside a plastic bag. *Am J Forensic Med Pathol.* 2007;28(4):364-367.
163. Schreiber MD, Gin-Mestan K, Marks JD, et al. Inhaled nitric oxide in premature infants with the respiratory distress syndrome. *N Engl J Med.* 2003;349:2099-2107.
164. Sciuto AM. Assessment of early acute lung injury in rodents exposed to phosgene. *Arch Toxicol.* 1998;72:283-288.
165. Sciuto AM, Clapp DL, Hess ZA, Moran TS. The temporal profile of cytokines in the bronchoalveolar lavage fluid in mice exposed to the industrial gas phosgene. *Inhal Toxicol.* 2003;15:687-700.
166. Sciuto AM, Hurt HH. Therapeutic treatments of phosgene-induced lung injury. *Inhal Toxicol.* 2004;16:565-580.
167. Sciuto AM, Stotts RR, Hurt HH. Efficacy of ibuprofen and pentoxifylline in the treatment of phosgene-induced acute lung injury. *J Appl Toxicol.* 1996;16:381-384.
168. Sciuto AM, Strickland PT, Kennedy TP, et al. Intratracheal administration of DBcAMP attenuates edema formation in phosgene-induced acute lung injury. *J Appl Physiol.* 1996;80:149-157.
169. Sciuto AM, Strickland PT, Kennedy TP, Gurtner GH. Protective effects of N-acetylcysteine treatment after phosgene exposure in rabbits. *Am J Respir Crit Care Med.* 1995;151:768-772.
170. Scott JA. Fog and deaths in London, December 1952. *Public Health Rep.* 1953;68:474-479.
171. Scott LK, Grier LR, Arnold TC, Conrad SA. Respiratory failure from inhalational nickel carbonyl exposure treated with continuous high-volume hemofiltration and disulfiram. *Inhal Toxicol.* 2002;14:1103-1109.
172. Shusterman DJ. Polymer fume fever and other fluorocarbon pyrolysis-related syndromes. *Occup Med.* 1993;8:519-531.

173. Sinclair SE, Altemeier WA, Matute-Bello G, Chi EY. Augmented lung injury due to interaction between hyperoxia and mechanical ventilation. *Crit Care Med.* 2004;32:2496-2501.
174. Sjoblom E, Hojer J, Kulling PE, et al. A placebo-controlled experimental study of steroid inhalation therapy in ammonia-induced lung injury. *J Toxicol Clin Toxicol.* 1999;37:59-67.
175. Smerz RW. Incidence of oxygen toxicity during the treatment of dysbarism. *Undersea Hyperb Med.* 2004;31:199-202.
176. Snyder RW, Mishel HS, Christensen GC 3rd. Pulmonary toxicity following exposure to methylene chloride and its combustion product, phosgene. *Chest.* 1992;101:860-861.
177. Spengler JD, Ludwig S, Weker RA. Ozone exposures during transcontinental and trans-Pacific flights. *Indoor Air.* 2004;14(suppl 7):67-73.
178. Spiller HA. Epidemiology of volatile substance abuse (VSA) cases reported to US poison centers. *Am J Drug Alcohol Abuse.* 2004;30:155-165.
179. Spragg RG, Lewis JF, Walmrath HD, et al. Effect of recombinant surfactant protein C-based surfactant on the acute respiratory distress syndrome. *N Engl J Med.* 2004;351:884-892.
180. Stefanidou M, Athanaselis S, Spiliopoulou C. Health impacts of fire smoke inhalation. *Inhal Toxicol.* 2008;20:761-6.
181. Steffee CH, Lantz PE, Flannagan LM, et al. Oleoresin capsicum (pepper) spray and "in-custody deaths." *Am J Forensic Med Pathol.* 1995;16:185-192.
182. Story RE, Grammer LC. Hypersensitivity pneumonitis. *Allergy Asthma Proc.* 2004;25(suppl):S40-S41.
183. Suruda A, Agnew J. Deaths from asphyxiation and poisoning at work in the United States 1984–6. *Br J Ind Med.* 1989;46:541-546.
184. Suruda A, Milliken W, Stephenson D, Sesek R. Fatal injuries in the United States involving respirators, 1984–1995. *Appl Occup Environ Hyg.* 2003;18:289-292.
185. Suter PM, Domenighetti G, Schaller MD, et al. N-acetylcysteine enhances recovery from acute lung injury in man. A randomized, double-blind, placebo-controlled clinical study. *Chest.* 1994;105:190-194.
186. Szolcsanyi J. Forty years in capsaicin research for sensory pharmacology and physiology. *Neuropeptides.* 2004;38:377-384.
187. Tanaka S, Fujimoto S, Tamagaki Y, et al. Bronchial injury and pulmonary edema caused by hydrogen sulfide poisoning. *Am J Emerg Med.* 1999;17:427-429.
188. Tanen DA, Graeme KA, Raschke R. Severe lung injury after exposure to chloramine gas from household cleaners. *N Engl J Med.* 1999;341:848-849.
189. Tatsumi T, Fliss H. Hypochlorous acid and chloramines increase endothelial permeability: possible involvement of cellular zinc. *Am J Physiol.* 1994;267:H1597-H1607.
190. Taylor RW, Zimmerman JL, Dellinger RP, et al. Low-dose inhaled nitric oxide in patients with acute lung injury: a randomized controlled trial. *JAMA.* 2004;291:1603-1609.
191. Thomas RJ, Smith PA, Rascona DA, et al. Acute pulmonary effects from o-chlorobenzylidenemalonitrile "tear gas": a unique exposure outcome unmasked by strenuous exercise after a military training event. *Mil Med.* 2002;167:136-139.
192. Torén K, Blanc PD. Asthma caused by occupational exposures is common—a systematic analysis of estimates of the population-attributable fraction. *BMC Pulm Med.* 2009;9:7-17.
193. Traub SJ, Hoffman RS, Nelson LS. Case report and literature review of chlorine gas toxicity. *Vet Hum Toxicol.* 2002;44:235-239.
194. Tsan MF. Superoxide dismutase and pulmonary oxygen toxicity: lessons from transgenic and knockout mice [review]. *Int J Mol Med.* 2001;7:13-19.
195. Tsonis L, Hantsch-Bardsley C, Gamelli RL. Hydrofluoric acid inhalation injury. *J Burn Care Res.* 2008;29:852-855.
196. Tu B, Wallin A, Moldeus P, Cotgreave I. The cytoprotective roles of ascorbate and glutathione against nitrogen dioxide toxicity in human endothelial cells. *Toxicology.* 1995;98:125-136.
197. Uysal N, Schapira RM. Effects of ozone on lung function and lung diseases. *Curr Opin Pulm Med.* 2003;9:144-150.
198. Vandenplas O, Malo JL. Definitions and types of work-related asthma: a nosological approach. *Eur Respir J.* 2003;21:706-712.
199. Vinsel PJ. Treatment of acute chlorine gas inhalation with nebulized sodium bicarbonate. *J Emerg Med.* 1990;8:327-329.
200. Vohra R, Clark RF. Chlorine-related inhalation injury from a swimming pool disinfectant in a 9-year-old girl. *Pediatr Emerg Care.* 2006;22:254-257.
201. Wagner GN, Clark MA, Koenigsberg EJ, Decata SJ. Medical evaluation of the victims of the 1986 Lake Nyos disaster. *J Forensic Sci.* 1988;33:899-909.
202. Wagner PD, Mathieu-Costello O, Bebout DE, et al. Protection against pulmonary O2 toxicity by N-acetylcysteine. *Eur Respir J.* 1989;2:116-126.
203. Walsh MJ, Tharratt SR, Offerman SR. Liquid nitrogen ingestion leading to massive pneumoperitoneum without identifiable gastrointestinal perforation. *J Emerg Med.* 2008. Epub 2008
204. Wang J, Zhang L, Walther SM. Administration of aerosolized terbutaline and budesonide reduces chlorine gas-induced acute lung injury. *J Trauma.* 2004;56:850-862.
205. Wang XR, Eisen EA, Zhang HX, et al. Respiratory symptoms and cotton dust exposure; results of a 15 year follow up observation. *Occup Environ Med.* 2003;60:935-941.
206. Weinberger B, Heck DE, Laskin DL, Laskin JD. Nitric oxide in the lung: therapeutic and cellular mechanisms of action. *Pharmacol Ther.* 1999;84:401-411.
207. Wing JS, Brender JD, Sanderson LM, et al. Acute health effects in a community after a release of hydrofluoric acid. *Arch Environ Health.* 1991;46:155-160.
208. Wood BR, Colombo JL, Benson BE. Chlorine inhalation toxicity from vapors generated by swimming pool chlorinator tablets. *Pediatrics.* 1987;79:427-430.
209. Yoshida M, Satoh M, Shimada A, et al. Pulmonary toxicity caused by acute exposure to mercury vapor is enhanced in metallothionein-null mice. *Life Sci.* 1999;64:1861-1867.
210. Zwemer FL Jr, Pratt DS, May JJ. Silo filler's disease in New York State. *Am Rev Respir Dis.* 1992;146:650-653.

CHAPTER 125
CARBON MONOXIDE

Christian Tomaszewski

Carbon Monoxide (CO)

MW	=	28.01 daltons
Gas density	=	0.968 (air = 1.0)
Blood carboxyhemoglobin level		
Nonsmokers	=	1–2%
Smokers	=	5–10%
Action level	>	10%
TLV–TWA	=	50 ppm

Carbon monoxide (CO) is a leading cause of poisoning morbidity and mortality in the United States. It is formed during the incomplete combustion of virtually any carbon-containing compound. Because it is an odorless, colorless, and tasteless gas, it is remarkably difficult to detect in the environment even when present at high ambient concentrations. The clinical findings are protean, making diagnosis difficult, and even objective data, such as elevated carboxyhemoglobin (COHb) concentrations, are not highly prognostic unless at one of the extremes. Hyperbaric oxygen (HBO) therapy, if practical to perform, remains the treatment of choice. However, the necessity for HBO therapy remains controversial, in large part related to the controversy over the incidence and significance of the long-term clinical effects of CO exposure.

HISTORY AND EPIDEMIOLOGY

Based on U.S. national death certificate data, there were 439 annual deaths from unintentional non-fire exposure to CO from 1999 to 2004.[20,107] The groups with the highest risk were male gender and elderly age, possibly because of occupational exposure and inability to discern CO symptoms, respectively. CO-related mortality remained essentially unchanged in 2002 despite increased CO detector use.[21,22,23] In that time period, 2001 to 2003, there were 15,200 patients treated annually in emergency departments (EDs) for nonfatal, unintentional, non–fire-related CO exposure. More than half of these cases (64%) occurred in homes with faulty furnaces, usually in the fall or winter months. Despite increased awareness for CO poisoning, in 2004 to 2006, there were still an average of 20,636 nonfatal, unintentional, non–fire-related CO exposures treated annually in the United States.[22] More than 40% of cases occurred in the winter, with almost 75% occurring in residences. However, exclusion of intentional and fire-related cases severely underestimates the extent of the problem. Based on firsthand hospital data, a minimum of 50,000 CO cases present to U.S. EDs each year.[67]

The more significant problem with CO poisoning may be the morbidity rather than mortality. The most serious complication is persistent or delayed neurologic or neurocognitive sequelae, which occurs in up to 50% of patients with symptomatic acute poisonings.[58,128,171] To date, there is still no completely reliable method of predicting who will have a poor outcome, suggesting that the threshold for HBO therapy for CO poisoning should be appropriately low.

Potential sources of CO abound in our society, often resulting in unintentional poisoning[22] (Table 125–1). Although CO is found naturally in the body as a byproduct of hemoglobin degradation by heme oxygenase found in the liver and spleen,[32] it is readily available for inhalation from the incomplete combustion of virtually any carbonaceous fuel. Alternatively, absorption—dermal, ingestion, or inhalation—of methylene chloride may result in CO toxicity after hepatic metabolism[112] (see Chap. 106). Despite catalytic converters and other emission controls, more than 50% of unintentional CO deaths are still caused by motor vehicle exhaust.[31,107] Occupants of motor vehicles are not the only victims of exhaust gases; CO poisoning is also reported in occupants of the beds of pickup trucks and on boats.[19,66] Workers can become symptomatic from use of propane-powered equipment indoors such as ice skating rink resurfacers[16] and forklifts.[45] For optimal performance, propane-powered forklifts are typically adjusted to produce no less than 10,000 ppm of CO in exhaust and in fact average more than 30,000 ppm.[46] In an enclosed warehouse with poor ventilation, even with proper emission control, CO levels could exceed safe concentration within 1 hour.

In the past 10 years, non-vehicular sources of CO have increasingly accounted for most unintentional poisonings.[107] Predominantly, these have involved the burning of charcoal, wood, or natural gas for heating and cooking.[63] Propane burning furnaces for heating are often implicated, especially when the flue is blocked.[70,71] Gas kitchen stoves are also an important source of CO in indigent populations with marginal heating systems.[71] In fact, the use of gas stoves for supplemental heat is predictive of CO poisoning in patients who present to the ED with headache and dizziness.[71] During ice storms and other natural disasters, the indoor use of gasoline-powered generators and charcoal burning grills, the latter particularly in immigrant populations, has resulted in epidemic CO poisoning outbreaks.[18,21,179]

Fires are another important source of CO exposure, contributing substantially to the approximate 5613 smoke inhalation deaths each year.[31] CO is considered to be the most common hazard to smoke inhalation victims.[51,138]

TOXICOKINETICS

CO is readily absorbed after inhalation. The Coburn-Forster-Kane (CFK) model allows the prediction of COHb concentrations based on exposure history.[33] This model has been simplified to allow estimation of the equilibrium based on the ambient concentration of CO in ppm: $\text{COHb}(\%) = 100/[1 + (643/\text{ppm CO})]$.[163] This assumes that the individual weighs 70 kg and is not anemic. With exponential uptake, it may take more than 4 hours for equilibrium to be attained. Therefore, within minutes of high CO exposures, the arterial COHb concentration may actually overshoot predicted estimates before equilibration.[7,12] Endogenous production of CO is not factored in because its contribution to COHb is only 2%.

After it has been absorbed, CO is carried in the blood, primarily bound to hemoglobin. The Haldane ratio states that hemoglobin has approximately a 200 to 250 times greater affinity for CO than for oxygen. Therefore, CO is primarily confined to the blood compartment, but eventually up to 15% of total CO body content is taken up by tissue, primarily bound to myoglobin.[33] Therefore, the dissolved CO concentration in the serum may better reflect the ultimate potential for poisoning because it is available for diffusion into all tissue compartments, including the muscle and brain.[92]

Elimination of CO, like absorption, from the blood can be modeled mathematically using the CFK model. The equation predicts a half-life of 252 minutes. In actual volunteer studies, means of 249 and 320 minutes breathing room air are reported.[124] With 100% oxygen, these half-lives can be reduced significantly to means of 47, 78, and 80 minutes in studies of volunteers who attain COHb concentrations of 10% to 12%.[124,146] Patients poisoned with CO showed actual mean half-lives of 74 and 131 minutes when treated with 100% oxygen.

TABLE 125–1. Sources of Carbon Monoxide Implicated in Poisonings[168]

Anesthetic absorbents[82]
Banked blood
Boats[19]
Camp stoves and lanterns
Charcoal grills[50]
Coffee roasting[114]
Gasoline-powered equipment (eg, generators, power washers)[17,18]
Ice resurfacing machines[16]
Methylene bromide
Methylene chloride
Natural gas combustion furnaces (water heaters, ranges and ovens)
Propane-powered forklifts[46]
Underground mine explosions[98]
Wood pellet storage

Methylene chloride, a paint stripper, is another source of CO. It is readily absorbed through the skin or by ingestion or inhalation and is metabolized in the liver to CO.[141] Reaching peak COHb concentrations may take 8 hours or longer and may range from 10% to 50%.[91,131] Because of ongoing production of CO, the apparent COHb half-life is prolonged to 13 hours in these patients.[129] COHb concentrations after methylene chloride exposure appear to be proportional to the concentration and duration of exposure.[129]

PATHOPHYSIOLOGY

The most obvious deleterious effect of CO is binding to hemoglobin, rendering it incapable of delivering oxygen to the cells. Therefore, despite adequate partial pressures of oxygen in blood (PO_2), there is decreased arterial oxygen content. Further insult occurs because CO causes a leftward shift of the oxyhemoglobin dissociation curve, thus decreasing the offloading of oxygen from hemoglobin to tissue[133] (see Fig. 21–2). This may result in part from a decrease in erythrocyte 2,3-bisphosphoglycerate (2,3-BPG) concentration. The net effect of all these processes is the decreased ability of oxygen to be delivered to tissue.

CO toxicity cannot be attributed solely to COHb-mediated hypoxia. Neither clinical effects nor the phenomena of delayed neurologic deficits can be completely predicted by the extent of binding between hemoglobin and CO.[159] Furthermore, such a model fails to explain why even minimal levels of COHb (4%–5%) may result in cognitive impairment. An early study showed that dogs breathing 13% CO died within 1 hour and had COHb levels of 54% to 90%. However, exchange transfusion of this same blood into healthy dogs to reach similar COHb levels caused no untoward effects.[52] Hemorrhaging the dogs to comparable degrees of anemia also produced no adverse effects. The appropriate conclusion was that inherent to CO toxicity is its delivery to target organs such as the brain and heart and that although COHb is easily measured, it rarely has a significant contribution to clinical toxicity. For CO to reach tissue, it had to be dissolved in the plasma rather than bound to hemoglobin.[56,57]

CO interferes with cellular respiration by binding to mitochondrial cytochrome oxidase. Initial studies show that this binding is especially exaggerated under conditions of hypoxia and hypotension. In vitro rat models demonstrate that this oxidative stress causes mitochondrial damage with protein oxidation and lipid peroxidation, particularly in the hippocampus and corpus striatum.[147] In vivo models reveal that CO poisoning causes cell loss in the frontal cortex, which is associated with decrements in learning and memory.[125] Although no comparable brain studies exist in humans, the peripheral lymphocytes of CO-poisoned patients show cytochrome oxidase inhibition accompanied by increased lipid peroxidation.[103] In a small clinical series of CO-poisoned patients, normalization of this cytochrome activity lagged behind and seemed to agree better with symptom severity than COHb concentrations.[104]

Inactivation of cytochrome oxidase may be only an initial part of the cascade of inflammatory events that results in ischemic reperfusion injury to the brain after CO poisoning (see Fig. A37–1). During recovery from the initial poisoning, white blood cells are attracted to and adhere to the damaged brain microvasculature.[152,153,154] This attraction may be partly attributable to endothelial changes from initial cytochrome oxidase dysfunction, mediated primarily through the free radical nitric oxide (NO).[152,157] CO displaces NO from platelets that in turn form peroxynitrites, which are even stronger inactivators of cytochrome oxidase.[157] Multiple animal studies demonstrate that NO is ultimately responsible for much of the endothelial damage from CO and that NO synthase inhibitors can prevent toxicity.[156,157] The NO formation promotes platelet–neutrophil aggregates that in turn leads to neutrophil adhesion to the brain microvasculature.[153] Myelin peroxidase activation in the area may further promote neutrophil adhesion with degranulation and release of proteases that convert xanthine dehydrogenase to xanthine oxidase, an enzyme that promotes formation of oxygen free radicals.[151] The end result of this process is delayed lipid peroxidation of the neurons, and the extent of destruction may be correlated with decrements in learning in rodents.[151] Rats depleted of xanthine oxidase through a tungsten modified diet show no changes in myelin basic protein and cognitive function after CO poisoning.[69]

Simultaneously, with all this perivascular oxidative stress in the brain, there is activation of excitatory amino acids, which ultimately may be responsible for the subsequent neuronal cell loss.[157] In fact, in rat brains, glutamate concentrations increase after CO poisoning. Glutamate is an excitatory amino acid that can bind at *N*-methyl-D-aspartate (NMDA) receptors and cause intracellular calcium release, resulting in delayed neuronal cell death (see Chap. 18). Blockade of NMDA receptors may prevent the neuronal death and learning deficits that accompany serious CO poisoning in mice.[77] Increases in the glutamate concentrations in rat brain in the first hour after severe CO poisoning are followed by a later increase in hydroxyl radicals.[125] Ultimately, at 1 to 3 weeks, the animals show histologic evidence of both neuronal necrosis and apoptosis in the frontal cortex, globus pallidus, and cerebellum that are accompanied by deficits in learning and memory.

Ultimately, CO neuronal cell death may be caused by apoptosis, and this has been confirmed in various models. In bovine pulmonary artery cells, CO exposure is accompanied by activation of caspase-1, a protease implicated in delayed cell death.[155] Confirmatory evidence was provided in the same study because both caspase-1 and NO synthase inhibitors blocked apoptosis. The end result of all these cellular processes is brain injury, particularly in the basal ganglia and hippocampus, resulting in learning impairment. Thus, animal models correlate well with what ultimately occurs in victims of serious CO poisoning, namely, persistent or delayed deficits in learning and memory associated with structural changes in the brain.

Myoglobin, another heme protein, binds CO with an affinity about 60 times greater than it binds oxygen.[34] About 10% to 15% of the total body store of CO is extravascular, primarily binding to myoglobin.[12,33] A dog model demonstrates that this binding is enhanced under hypoxic conditions.[34] This binding may partially explain the myocardial impairment that occurs in both animal studies and low-level exposures in patients with ischemic heart disease. The combination of COHb formation, which decreases oxygen-carrying capacity, and the production of reduced myoglobin in the heart, which decreases oxygen extraction, may explain the preterminal dysrhythmias that occur in animals.

Several studies suggest that CO effects on the cardiovascular system are necessary for ischemic reperfusion injury of the brain. Hypotension is an essential component and results from a combination of myocardial depression and vasodilation. CO, perhaps because of its similarity to NO, activates guanylate cyclase, which in turn relaxes vascular smooth muscle. Also, CO may further displace NO from platelets, resulting in additional vasodilation.[156] These factors contribute to the hypotension that occurs in animal experiments with exposure to high concentrations of CO.[52] Such an episode of hypotension may present clinically as syncope, and this finding portends a worse clinical outcome.[28] In rhesus monkeys, cerebral white matter lesions correlate better with decreases in blood pressure than with COHb level.[55] Lipid peroxidation of the brain in rats develops 1 hour after a CO exposure that has produced syncope and hypotension.[150] This delay is comparable to the time that is necessary to produce mitochondrial destruction from oxidative stress in rats exposed to CO. In a feline model, central nervous system (CNS) damage from CO can be reproduced only when hypoxia is accompanied by one interval of ischemia, confirming the ischemic-reperfusion model.[116]

Endogenous CO behaves like NO, binding to guanylate cyclase and thereby increasing cGMP concentrations.[78] Although low endogenous concentrations are physiologic, excessive concentrations of CO from exogenous sources may be problematic because CO persists much longer than NO. CO appears to be a neuronal messenger by virtue of the fact that as a gas, it can diffuse and signal adjacent cells.[97]

CLINICAL MANIFESTATIONS

EFFECTS OF ACUTE EXPOSURE

The earliest symptoms associated with CO poisoning are often nonspecific and readily confused with other illnesses, typically a viral syndrome[175] (Table 125–2). The initial symptom reported by volunteers within 4 hours of exposure to 200 ppm COHb levels (15%–20%) is headache; shorter exposures at 500 ppm also produces nausea.[143] The incidence of CO poisoning in symptomatic patients presenting to EDs in the winter with an influenzalike illness ranges from 3% to 24% in some series.[41,71] The typical presenting complaints include headache, dizziness, and nausea, and the most frequent exposures occur during the winter, explaining why influenza is the most common misdiagnosis.[41] The most common symptom, headache, is usually described as dull, frontal, and continuous. CO poisoning is also frequently misdiagnosed as food poisoning, gastroenteritis, and even colic in infants. Similar to adults, children tend to develop nonspecific symptoms, complicating identification of the diagnosis.

Continued exposure to CO may lead to symptoms attributable to oxygen deficiency in the heart. Low-level exposures, leading to COHb levels of 2% to 4%, in volunteers with stable angina results in decreased exercise tolerance as well as signs and symptoms of myocardial ischemia.[2] At higher levels (COHb 6%), there is a greater frequency of premature ventricular contractions during exercise. Myocardial infarction and dysrhythmias are described in victims of CO poisoning, and acute mortality from CO is usually a result of ventricular dysrhythmias.[1,2] Prolonged exposure to CO or high levels of COHb is associated with temporary myocardial stunning, lasting usually less than 24 hours and reflected by a decrease in left ventricular ejection fraction (LVEF).[80] This stunning is reflected by a decrease in LVEF and is correlated with increased B-type natriuretic peptide. Troponin may be elevated as well in the absence of any coronary artery disease. These patients have an increased propensity for cardiac mortality, with almost one-third dying within 8 years after serious CO poisoning.[72]

The CNS is the organ system that is most sensitive to CO poisoning. Acutely, otherwise healthy patients may manifest headache, dizziness, and ataxia at COHb levels as low as 15% to 20%; with higher levels or longer exposures, syncope, seizures, or coma may result.[175] Patients may present with focal neurologic symptoms suggestive of a cerebrovascular accident. The electroencephalogram (EEG) may show diffuse frontal slow-wave activity. Within 1 day of exposures that result in coma, computed tomography (CT) and magnetic resonance imaging (MRI) may show decreased density in the central white matter and globus pallidus (Fig. 125–1).[93] Autopsies show involvement of other areas, including the cerebral cortex, hippocampus, cerebellum, and substantia nigra.[89]

Metabolic changes may reflect CO's toxic effects better than any particular COHb concentration. Patients with mild CO poisoning

TABLE 125–2. Clinical Manifestations of CO Poisoning

Ataxia	Myocardial ischemia
Cardiac dysrhythmias	Nausea
Chest pain	Syncope
Confusion	Tachypnea
Dizziness	Visual blurring
Dyspnea	Vomiting
Headache	Weakness

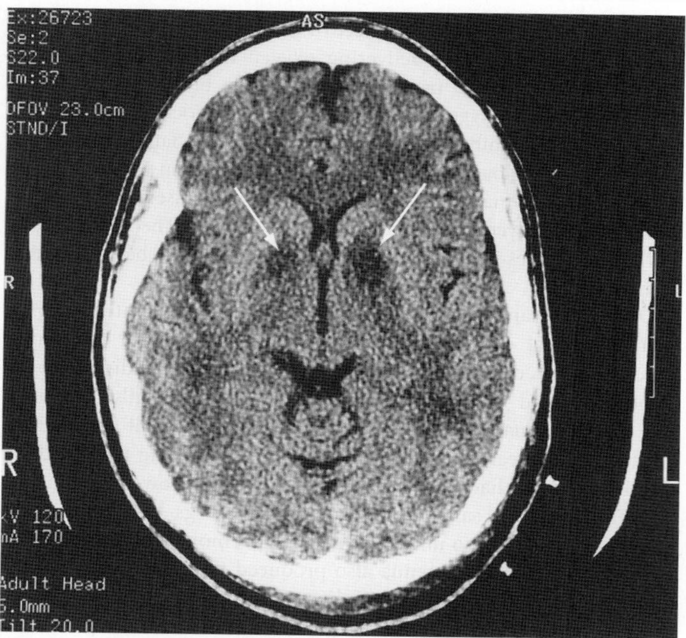

FIGURE 125–1. Computed tomography of the brain showing bilateral lesions of the globus pallidus (arrows) in a patient with poor recovery from severe carbon monoxide poisoning. *(Image contributed by New York City Poison Center Fellowship in Medical Toxicology.)*

may develop respiratory alkalosis in an attempt to compensate for the reduction in oxygen-carrying capacity and delivery. More substantial exposures result in metabolic acidosis with lactate production that accompanies tissue hypoxia.[140] The importance of metabolic acidosis is highlighted by the findings of a retrospective series of 48 CO-poisoned patients, in which hydrogen ion concentration was a better predictor of poor recovery during initial hospitalization than was COHb concentration.[167]

Although the brain and heart are the most sensitive, other organs may also manifest the effects of CO poisoning. One-fifth to one-third of patients with severe CO poisoning—those who required endotracheal intubation—develop pulmonary edema.[59] This does not appear to be a direct effect of CO on lung tissue because sheep with prolonged exposure to CO, resulting in COHb levels greater than 50%, showed no anatomic or physiologic changes in lung function.[137] Although myonecrosis and even compartment syndromes occur, patients rarely develop renal failure. Retinal hemorrhages may develop with exposures greater than 12 hours.[81] Cherry-red skin coloration occurs only after excessive exposure (2%–3% of cases referred to one hyperbaric center) and may represent a combination of CO-induced vasodilation, concomitant tissue ischemia, and failure to extract oxygen from arterial blood.[132] Another classic but uncommon phenomenon is the development of cutaneous bullae after severe exposures. These bullae are thought to be caused by a combination of pressure necrosis and possibly direct CO effects in the epidermis.

DELAYED NEUROCOGNITIVE SEQUELAE

The persistent or delayed effects of CO poisoning are varied and include dementia, amnestic syndromes, psychosis, parkinsonism, paralysis, chorea, cortical blindness, apraxia and agnosia, peripheral neuropathy, and incontinence.[90] Neurologic deterioration is typically preceded by a lucid period of 2 to 40 days after the initial poisoning.[28] In patients admitted to an intensive care unit for severe CO poisoning and treated with 100% oxygen, 14% of survivors had permanent neurologic impairment.[85] In a Korean series of 2360 CO-poisoned patients, 3% continued to show memory failure or parkinsonian features 1 year after exposure.[28] Another series of 63 seriously poisoned patients showed memory impairment in 43% and deterioration of personality in 33% at 3 year follow-up.[140] Children also develop behavioral and educational difficulties after severe poisoning.[88] However, patients older than 30 years of age appear to be more susceptible to the development of delayed sequelae.[28,173] Most cases of delayed neurocognitive sequelae are associated with loss of consciousness in the acute phase of toxicity.[28]

Delayed or persistent neurocognitive sequelae probably involve lesions of the cerebral white matter.[53] Weeks after exposure, autopsies show necrosis of the white matter, globus pallidus, cerebellum, and hippocampus. MRI studies confirm the damage to the white matter and hippocampus.[48,93,175] Animal studies show that having a markedly elevated COHb concentration alone cannot cause similar white matter lesions but that there must also be an episode of hypotension.[55,116] The fact that the areas permanently damaged in serious CO poisoning cases are the areas with the poorest vascular supply in the brain is consistent with these findings.

EFFECTS OF CHRONIC EXPOSURE

Often, patients complain of persistent headaches and cognitive problems after long-term exposure to low concentrations of CO. Unfortunately, to date, there have been no controlled studies demonstrating that in the absence of a severe acute poisoning episode, this type of exposure results in any long-term sequelae. Warehouse workers who are chronically exposed to CO from propane combustion have intermittent problems with headache, nausea, and lightheadedness.[45] Fortunately, unless there has been an episode of severe poisoning with acute deterioration, most workers go on to have resolution of their symptoms.[46] One series of chronic CO poisoning demonstrates a high incidence of headache and memory complaints along with motor slowing and memory problems on neuropsychologic testing.[109] Although many of the objective deficits improved with elimination of the exposure and HBO treatment, many continued to have posttraumatic stress and conversion disorders. Although it is unclear that chronic exposure to low concentrations of CO can cause permanent damage, healthcare providers still should be vigilant for symptomatic individuals to prevent continued or catastrophic outcomes.

DIAGNOSTIC TESTING

The most useful diagnostic test obtainable in a suspected CO poisoning is a COHb level. Normal levels of COHb range from 0% to 5%. Levels at the high end of this range occur in neonates and patients with hemolytic anemia because CO is a natural byproduct of the breakdown of protoporphyrin to bilirubin.[33] COHb levels average 6% in one-pack-per-day smokers but may range as high as 10%.[142] Although high COHb levels confirm exposure to CO, particular levels are not necessarily predictive of symptoms or outcome.

The usual method for measuring COHb is with a co-oximeter, a device that spectrophotometrically reads the percentage of total hemoglobin saturated with CO. Traditionally, arterial blood is used for this determination; however, venous blood levels are accurate.[166] Refrigerated heparinized samples yield accurate COHb levels for months and at room temperature for 28 days, making retrospective clinical and postmortem evaluations possible.[62,87]

Bedside tests using ammonia or sodium hydroxide are unable to differentiate reliably various levels of COHb versus control subjects.[118] Because of the similarities in extinction coefficients, COHb is misinterpreted as oxyhemoglobin on most types of pulse oximetry (see Chap. 21).[6] Thus, the pulse oximetry reading is usually normal in the setting of even severe CO poisoning.[61] Some newer pulse oximeters, called pulse co-oximeters, have the ability to measure COHb noninvasively.[4] A study in 10 healthy volunteers who inhaled CO at 500 ppm until they reached a peak COHb level of 15% found good agreement between pulse co-oximetry and cooximetry.[5] Because the test is noninvasive, it may be useful in screening ED patients who present with nonspecific symptoms for occult CO poisoning.[26] In addition, it may be used in the field for screening fire victims, patients with potential CO exposure, and rescuers.

Breath-sampling methods may be used for screening patients.[35,37,43] A cutoff of 53 ppm in patients breathing air and 43 ppm in those breathing oxygen has an approximate reliability of approximately 80% in predicting COHb concentrations above 10%.[47] Breath sampling for CO has been advocated as quick screening device for detecting recent exposure to CO in ED patients.

Some clinical laboratories measure CO directly in blood samples rather than COHb. This technique involves assaying CO directly with infrared spectrophotometry after it is extracted from the blood sample with a manometer. Based on calculations rather than true experimental data, the assumption has been made that for a patient with a normal hemoglobin, a CO concentration of 1 mmol/L corresponds to an 11% COHb concentration. A simpler method to measure serum CO content is to add a known solution of hemoglobin followed by sodium dithionite to form COHb. The resulting COHb is measured spectrophotometrically with the assumption that 1 mole of hemoglobin binds 4 moles of CO. Interestingly, in one study, serum CO ranged 0.14 to 0.6 mg/L but was the same in smokers (average,

4.6% COHb) and nonsmokers (average, 1% COHb).[177] At this time, further research is required to determine the clinical importance of serum CO content.

Additional laboratory tests may be useful in severe poisoning cases. An arterial or venous blood gas analysis will confirm the presence of metabolic acidosis, and a measurement of serum lactate concentration should be performed simultaneously. Metabolic acidosis with elevated lactate concentration may serve as a more reliable index of severity than a measurement of the COHb concentration.[140] Unfortunately, arterial pH does not correlate well with either initial neurologic examination or the COHb level, making it a poor criterion for deciding the need for HBO treatment.[108]

Cardiac monitoring and a 12-lead electrocardiography (ECG) are essential to identify ischemia or dysrhythmias in symptomatic patients with preexisting coronary artery disease or severe exposure. Mild elevations of creatine phosphokinase are common (ranging 20–1315 IU/L in one series of 65 cases), usually because of rhabdomyolysis rather than cardiac sources.[136] However, because CO may cause myocardial infarction in the presence of normal coronaries,[80] it is not surprising to see nonspecific increases in troponin concentrations, which may reflect diffuse cardiac myonecrosis rather than focal coronary artery disease.[24] Congestive heart failure or hypotension can be evaluated with a B-type natriuretic peptide or echocardiography (or both), looking for evidence of myocardial stunning.[80] Because of the potential for increased cardiovascular mortality,[72] patients with ECG changes or elevated cardiac enzymes may benefit from further cardiac testing, a stress test, or angiography.

The problem with using COHb levels to base treatment is that there is a wide variation in clinical manifestations with identical COHb levels. Furthermore, particular COHb levels are not predictive of symptoms or final outcome.[99,115,140] In a large prospective study of CO poisoning, COHb levels did not correlate with loss of consciousness and were not predictive of delayed neurologic sequelae.[128] The admission COHb levels are inaccurate predictors of peak levels, and the use of nomograms to extrapolate to earlier levels has not been validated. Their credibility is also suspect because of the great variability in COHb half-lives and differences in treatment with oxygen.

Because of the inherent unreliability of COHb levels in predicting outcome, researchers have been searching for other surrogate markers. Rats have early increases in glutathione released from erythrocytes, a potential marker for CO oxidative stress that could ultimately lead to brain injury.[158] Another promising marker is serum S100B, a structural protein in astroglia that is released from the brain after hypoxic stress. A series of 38 consecutive patients poisoned with CO showed that those who presented with normal neurologic findings and no loss of consciousness had normal S100B concentrations.[14] Patients who presented with loss of consciousness and neurologic deficits all had elevated concentrations. CO-poisoned rats treated with HBO did not develop elevated S100B concentrations unlike those treated with ambient oxygen therapy.[13] However, other studies have failed to find a difference between CO-poisoned patients and control subjects with respect to such markers as the S-100B protein and neuron-specific enolase.[130]

NEUROPSYCHOLOGIC TESTING

The extent of neurologic insult from CO can be assessed with a variety of tests. The most basic is documentation of the normal neurologic examination with a quick mini mental status examination. A more sensitive indicator of the acute effects of CO on cortical function is a detailed neuropsychologic test battery developed specifically for CO patients.[102] The advantages of such testing, which usually takes about 30 minutes, are that it can reliably distinguish 79% of the time between CO-poisoned patients and control subjects, and it shows improvement with appropriate HBO treatment.[102] Unfortunately, such testing shows a sensitivity of only 77% and specificity of 80% for CO poisoning. There may be practice effects as well if repeated testing is performed. Another study suggested that the degree of impairment CO patients had on a test of short-term rote and context-aided verbal memory correlated well with the number of HBO treatments needed.[100] The biggest problem with such neuropsychiatric testing is that it is unclear if deficits in the test during the acute CO poisoning phase are at all predictive of the development of neurologic sequelae and therefore the necessity of HBO treatment.

NEUROIMAGING

Acute changes on CT scans of the brain occur within 12 hours of CO exposure that resulted in loss of consciousness.[93,105] Symmetric low-density areas in the region of the globus pallidus, putamen, and caudate nuclei are frequently noted.[75] Changes in the globus pallidus and subcortical white matter early within the first day after poisoning are associated with poor outcomes[120] (see Fig. 125–1). Alternatively, in one series of 18 patients, a negative CT within a week of admission was associated with favorable outcome.[164] The use of contrast may enhance early isodense changes not visible on initial CT scan[182] but is not routinely performed.

MRI appears to be superior in detecting basal ganglia lesions after CO poisoning.[93] One study found a much higher incidence of periventricular white matter changes on MRIs done within the first day after exposure. However, such changes had no correlation with COHb level or cognitive sequelae.[120] These periventricular changes are more common and probably more sensitive than globus pallidus lesions. However, globus pallidus lesions were present on MRI in only one patient (1.4%) in a prospective study of CO-poisoned patients, half of whom had loss of consciousness.[75] Diffusion-weighted MRI may have more promise in detecting changes in subcortical white matter within hours of serious CO poisoning.[148] Regardless, neuroimaging usually does not influence patient management and can be reserved for patients who show poor response or have an equivocal diagnosis.

The most promising area of neuroimaging after CO poisoning is in assessing regional cerebral perfusion.[30,119] Single-photon emission CT (SPECT) gauges regional blood flow noninvasively using an iodine or technetium tracer. In one series of 13 patients with delayed neurologic sequelae, all cases showed patchy hypoperfusion throughout the cerebral cortex within 11 days of poisoning.[29] These changes in perfusion may occur as early as 1 day after poisoning and primarily involve watershed regions such as the temporoparietooccipital area.[40] Perfusion defects on SPECT scanning appear to be associated with neuropsychological impairment months after serious CO poisoning.[48] Unfortunately, because of the scant availability of the procedure and the lack of comprehensive studies, SPECT scanning is not the definitive tool at this time for determining prognosis or need for HBO.

Positron emission tomography (PET) can also be used to evaluate regional blood flow as well as oxygen metabolism in the brain after CO exposure. In one series of severely CO-poisoned patients, PET examination after HBO treatment showed increased oxygen extraction and decreased blood flow in the frontal and temporal cortices.[38] Of note, patients with permanent deficits persisted in showing these abnormalities on PET scanning. One delayed PET study demonstrated that increases in dopamine D2 receptor binding in the caudate and putamen after CO poisoning were improved with bromocriptine, at which time neuropsychiatric symptoms resolved.[181] Although PET scanning cannot be used to predict outcome, abnormalities that persist on the scan may be indicative of patients with permanent neurologic sequelae.

To complement perfusion studies, EEG mapping has also been performed on CO-poisoned patients. Although initial studies demonstrate that many patients have regional EEG abnormalities after poisoning, it is unknown if these are predictive of persistent or delayed neurologic problems. EEG mapping may be discrepant relative to SPECT scanning because EEG preferentially demonstrates subcortical lesions.

MANAGEMENT

The mainstay of treatment is initial attention to the airway. One hundred percent oxygen should be provided as soon as possible by either non-rebreather face mask or endotracheal tube. It is important to remember that a non-rebreathing mask only delivers 70% to 90% oxygen; a positive pressure mask or an endotracheal tube is necessary to achieve higher oxygen concentrations. The immediate effect of oxygen is to enhance the dissociation of COHb.[133] In volunteers, the half-life of COHb is reduced from a mean of 5 hours (range, 2–7 hours) when breathing room air (21% oxygen) to approximately 1 hour (range, 36–137 minutes) when breathing 100% oxygen at normal atmospheric pressure.[124] Actual poisonings show a range in half-lives of 36 to 137 minutes (mean, 85 minutes) when breathing 100% oxygen; the longer elimination half-lives appear to be most often associated with long, low-level exposures.[110,172] With oxygenation and intensive care treatment, hospital mortality rates for serious exposures range from 1.0 to 30%. The duration of treatment is unclear, with a valid end point being the resolution of symptoms, usually accompanied by a COHb below 5%.

Cardiac monitoring and intravenous (IV) access are necessary in any patient with systemic toxicity from CO poisoning. Hypotension can initially be treated with IV fluids; inotropes may also be necessary to treat myocardial depression. An evaluation for cardiac ischemia, including ECG and cardiac enzymes, should be considered in symptomatic patients at risk. Standard advanced cardiac life support protocols can be followed for the treatment of patients with life-threatening dysrhythmias. Patients with a depressed mental status should have a rapid blood glucose checked. Animal studies of CO poisoning suggest that hypoglycemia can be deleterious.[122] Correction of any acidemia with bicarbonate is controversial and may result in further cellular injury secondary to a left shift of the oxyhemoglobin dissociation curve.

HYPERBARIC OXYGEN

HBO therapy appears to be the treatment of choice for patients with significant CO exposures.[160] One hundred percent oxygen at ambient pressure reduces the half-life of COHb to 40 minutes; at 2.5 atmospheres absolute (ATA), it is reduced to 20 minutes.[124] Actual CO-poisoned victims treated with HBO have half-lives ranging from 4 to 86 minutes.[110] HBO also increases the amount of dissolved oxygen by about 10 times, which is sufficient alone to supply metabolic needs in the absence of hemoglobin.[9] This is rarely an important clinical issue because most patients have already been stabilized and have appreciably decreased COHb with ambient oxygen alone and the time required for transport to an HBO facility.

HBO is more than just a modality to clear COHb more quickly than ambient oxygen (see Antidotes in Depth A37: Hyperbaric Oxygen for more details). More importantly, in rats after loss of consciousness from CO exposure, hyperbaric, but not normobaric, oxygen therapy prevents brain lipid peroxidation.[149] HBO appears to prevent ischemic reperfusion injury by a variety of mechanisms. First, in animal models, HBO accelerates regeneration of inactivated cytochrome oxidase, which may be the initiating site for CO neuronal damage.[11] Second, HBO also prevents β integrin mediated neutrophil adhesion to brain microvascular endothelium, a process essential for amplification of CNS damage from CO.[160] This may explain why HBO, but not 100% oxygen at atmospheric pressure, prevented delayed deficits in a learning and memory maze model.[153]

Clinical studies of the effectiveness of HBO in preventing neurologic damage from CO are not as convincing as basic science studies would suggest. In uncontrolled human clinical series, the incidence of persistent neuropsychiatric symptoms, including memory impairment,

TABLE 125–3. Favorable Cognitive Outcome at 4 to 6 Weeks After Exposure to Carbon Monoxide in Randomized Clinical Trials of Hyperbaric Oxygen

Study	Design	Max HBO Pressure	Time to Treatment	Syncope (%)	Suicide (%)	Treatment	Control	Odds Ratio (95% CI)
Mathieu[101]	HBO 90 min vs 12-hr NBO	2.5 ATA	<12 h	N/A	N/A	69/299	73/276	0.83(0.57–1.22)
Raphael[128]	HBO 2 hr vs 6-hr NBO	2.0 ATA	Mean, 7.1 h	0	N/A	51/159	50/148	0.93(0.57–1.49)
Thom[162]	HBO 2 hr vs 100% NBO until asymptomatic	2.8 ATA	Mean, 2.0 h	0	N/A	0/30	7/30	0.05(0.00–0.95)
Scheinkestel[135]	HBO 1 hr vs NBO 100 min	2.8 ATA	Mean, 7.1 h	53%	69%	30/48	25/40	1.00(0.42–2.38)
Weaver[171]	HBO 2 hr (x3) vs NBO 2 hr (x1)	3.0 ATA	Mean, 5.6 h	53%	31%	19/76	35/76	0.39(0.20–0.78)
Raphael[127]	HBO at 2.0 ATA 60 min vs 6-hr NBO	2.0 ATA	<12 h	N/A	N/A	33/79	29/74	1.11(0.58–2.12)

Adapted from Juurlink D, Buckley N, Stanbrook M, et al. Hyperbaric oxygen for carbon monoxide poisoning. *Cochrane Database Syst Rev*. 2005:CD002041 and Tomaszewski C. The case for the use of hyperbaric oxygen in carbon monoxide poisoning. In: Penney DG, ed. *Carbon Monoxide Poisoning*. New York: CRC Press; 2008:375-390.

ATA, atmospheres absolute; CI, confidence interval; HBO, hyperbaric oxygen; N/A, not applicable; NBO, normobaric oxygen.

ranged from 12% to 43% in patients treated with 100% oxygen and was as low as 0% to 4% in patients treated with HBO.[59,99,111,115]

More recently, several controlled clinical trials have evaluated the efficacy of HBO in CO poisoning (Table 125–3). The first randomized study of CO poisoning included more than 300 patients and failed to show a benefit from HBO in patients who had no initial loss of consciousness.[128] Unfortunately, seriously ill patients were not randomized to surface pressure oxygen; they received either one or three treatments of HBO. Flaws in the study included significant delays to treatment and the use of suboptimal pressure of 2.0 ATA. A smaller ($n = 60$) controlled study avoided some of these flaws and showed that HBO was able to decrease delayed neurologic sequelae from 23% to 0% in CO-poisoned patients without loss of consciousness.[162] However, all patients with syncope, a marker of serious poisoning, were excluded. A very small study ($n = 26$) of patients presenting with Glasgow Coma Scores (GCS) above 12 after CO poisoning included almost half with loss of consciousness.[42] Randomization to HBO versus 100% normobaric oxygen resulted in decreased EEG abnormalities and less reduction in blood flow reactivity to acetazolamide at 3 weeks. Unfortunately, all of these studies failed to definitively study all CO-poisoned patients, including those with syncope or coma.

The first randomized trial to directly address the issue of HBO efficacy in seriously CO-poisoned patients evaluated 191 CO-poisoned patients referred for HBO treatment.[135] Patients were randomized to a minimum of three daily treatments of HBO (2.8 ATA for 60 minutes) or 100% oxygen at 1.0 ATA for 3 days. Although the HBO group had a higher incidence of persistent neurologic sequelae at 1 month, there was no significant difference between the two groups; more than two-thirds of each group had persistent problems. This study, although the largest controlled, randomized study to date, suffered from several flaws. Fewer than half of the patients had follow-up at 1 month. Disproportionate numbers of suicide cases (about two-thirds) and drug toxicity (44%), with accompanying neuropsychologic defects, could have confounded any beneficial effect from HBO. Finally, HBO treatment was delayed for 6 hours, making it much less likely to be effective.[59,128]

A more recent randomized, double-blind, placebo-controlled study identified a beneficial effect of HBO in CO-poisoned patients.[171] Most of these patients were ill, with a mean initial COHb level of 25% and a 50% incidence of loss of consciousness. Patients were all treated within a 24-hour window after exposure, but the success of the study might be partially attributable to the rapid mean time to treatment of less than 2 hours. Patients received HBO three times at intervals of 6 to 12 hours, each at 2.0 ATA, except for the first hour of the first treatment, which was at 3.0 ATA. Control patients received sham treatments in the HBO chamber with 100% oxygen at 1.0 ATA. At 6 weeks, the HBO group had a 24% incidence of cognitive sequelae versus 46% in the control group. Based on these data, the number of patients needed to treat to prevent one case of cognitive impairment is only five. Critics of this study point out that the neuropsychiatric tests were not significantly different between the groups except for digit spam and trail making, and there was no difference in activities of daily living. However, untreated patients had increased self-reported memory problems at 6 weeks (28% versus 51%), and the beneficial effect on cognitive sequelae lasted well into 12 months.

Based on the above studies, it is not surprising that the Underwater and Hyperbaric Medical Society (UHMS) recommends HBO treatment for all CO patients with signs of serious toxicity.[49] With the low risk of this procedure,[134,139] almost 1500 patients are treated with HBO for CO poisoning in the United States each year.[61] Therefore, HBO has become the standard of care for serious CO poisoning, even though that there is substantial disagreement in the interpretation of the existing evidence.[70,94,178]

TABLE 125–4. Suggested Indications for Hyperbaric Oxygen[a]

Syncope (loss of consciousness)
Coma
Seizure
Altered mental status (GCS<15) or confusion
Carboxyhemoglobin >25%
Abnormal cerebellar function
Age ≥36 years
Prolonged CO exposure (≥24 hours)
Fetal distress in pregnancy

[a] These are criteria that are potential risk factors for cognitive sequelae, suggesting that such patients have the most to benefit from HBO treatment)[174] GCS, Glasgow Coma Score.

Indications for Hyperbaric Oxygen Therapy Although specific indications for HBO after acute CO poisoning are listed (Table 125–4), they have not been prospectively evaluated. The patients most likely to benefit are those most at risk for persistent or delayed neurologic sequelae, such as those presenting in coma or with a history of syncope.[173] These may be clinical markers for the episode of hypotension that are necessary for causing neuronal damage from CO-induced ischemic–reperfusion injury in animal models.[55,117] However, syncope is neither particularly sensitive nor specific marker for cognitive sequelae. Patients with long exposures, or "soaking" periods, are also at greater risk for neurologic sequelae.[10] The presence of a significant metabolic acidosis may be a surrogate marker.[140,167] Some authors advocate ongoing myocardial ischemia as an indication for HBO; however, in our experience, these patients usually already meet neurologic criteria for treatment, such as loss of consciousness or ongoing mental status changes. Isolated cardiac ischemia, more importantly, deserves immediate proven myocardial salvaging therapy rather than delayed treatment with an unproven therapy such as HBO.

Some authors advocate treating all patients with COHb levels of 40% or greater with HBO. Many HBO centers arbitrarily use a more conservative level of 25% as an indication for HBO.[65] More important than the actual level are patient history and examination. Further analysis of data from the most recent controlled trial demonstrates that in patients not treated with HBO, there were no reliable factors—COHb level, loss of consciousness, or base excess—for predicting who progressed to cognitive sequelae.[173] This recent multivariate analysis showed that of all factors—loss of consciousness, age, exposure time, and COHb levels—only age of 36 years or older and CO exposure duration of 24 hours or longer predicted risk factor for cognitive dysfunction at 6 week follow-up. More problematic is the incidence of cognitive sequelae in patients without those risk factors: 32% in those younger than age 36 years and 36% in those with less than 24 hours of exposure. In conclusion, it appears that there are no reliable predictors for screening out patients who will do well and not develop cognitive sequelae, thereby avoiding HBO treatment in patients with mild CO poisoning.

Therefore, at this time, it is prudent to refer for HBO patients with the most serious neurologic symptoms, regardless of their COHb concentration. Such symptoms include coma, seizures, focal neurologic deficits, altered mental status (GCS <15), and although controversial, loss of consciousness. Patients who have had cardiac arrest from CO poisoning and had the return of spontaneous circulation may be poor candidates for HBO therapy because all of these cases have been fatal.[68]

Excluding patients with milder symptoms after CO poisoning may be problematic because they are susceptible to neurocognitive sequelae. One series of 55 patients with mild poisoning as defined by no LOC and highest reported COHb level below 15% found that even one-third of these individuals had neurocognitive sequelae up to 12 months after exposure.[25] This was no different than that occurring in the severely poisoned group, although the milder group had a much longer duration of exposure as well as a greater delay to COHb level drawn. Brain imaging studies have confirmed that mild exposures, marked by no LOC and COHb levels lower than 15%, may result in visible changes.[48,126] Taken to its logical but impractical conclusion, because even apparently mild cases of CO poisoning may have poor neurocognitive outcomes, HBO treatment of every CO-exposed patient, regardless of severity, could be justified.

It is still unclear if mild neurologic symptoms, such as confusion, headache, dizziness, visual blurring, or abnormal mental status testing on initial presentation after CO poisoning, are prognostic for cognitive sequelae. These symptoms simply represent CO poisoning, which, at COHb levels approaching 10% in volunteers, may cause temporary impairment of learning and memory.[3] In a recent prospective clinical trial of CO poisoning, the incidence of cerebellar dysfunction portended a higher incidence of cognitive sequelae (odds ratio, 5.7 [95% confidence interval, 1.7–19.3]).[171] Therefore, difficulty with finger-to-nose, heel-to-shin, rapid alternating hand movements, or even ataxia, should be considered indications for HBO. Patients with other mild neurologic findings, such as headache, warrant at least several hours of oxygen by non-rebreather face mask until symptoms resolve. If symptoms do not resolve, HBO may be considered; however, any delay in HBO may decrease its efficacy.

A more promising track to try to discern patients who may respond to HBO may be the genotype, apolipoprotein E, specifically the isoform ε4.[76] This particular polymorphism allele is present in up to one quarter of the population and its presence is associated with worse neurologic outcome from trauma and stroke. In the presence of CO poisoning, it is associated with lack of response to HBO for the prevention of neurocognitive sequelae. Further studies may support not treating patients with this particular allele, focusing on those with the potential for response to HBO therapy.

Because of the confusion in determining which CO poisoned patients really need HBO treatment, several professional societies have developed evidence-based guidelines. As alluded to previously, the American College of Emergency Physicians has noted that no clinical variable can be used to predict patients at risk of cognitive sequelae and therefore most likely to benefit from HBO.[178] Similarly, the Cochrane Collaboration review on the use of HBO in CO poisoning concluded that because of so much conflicting data, there is really no ability to recommend HBO for CO poisoning at this time.[79] The most recent guidelines from the UHMS states that CO-poisoned patients should be referred for HBO if they have serious poisoning, such as unconsciousness, whether it is transient or persistent; age 36 years or older; or CO exposure duration of 24 hours or longer, even if intermittent.[174] This is all consistent with the prior studies discussed earlier. The UHMS guidelines also state that many physicians treat when neuropsychologic testing is abnormal or COHb levels are greater than 25% to 30%.

Some authors recommend selective use of HBO because of cost and difficulties in transport if the primary facility lacks a chamber. However, complications that may make such transfers and treatment unsafe are rare.[139] Although HBO cannot be recommended for every patient with CO poisoning, it is a relatively safe treatment that should be considered in all patients with significant findings by history or clinical examination. Fortunately, even without HBO, anywhere from one-third to three-quarters of cases with persistent cognitive sequelae resolve over the subsequent year.[28,171]

Delayed Administration of Hyperbaric Oxygen The optimal timing and number of HBO treatments for CO poisoning is unclear. Patients treated later than 6 hours after exposure tend to have worse outcomes in terms of delayed sequelae (30% versus 19%) and mortality (30% versus 14%).[59] This may explain the failure of one of the first randomized trials on HBO in CO, which had a mean time to treatment of over 6 hours after poisoning.[135] Meanwhile, HBO treatments delivered within 6 hours after poisoning in patients with loss of consciousness after CO seem to be almost completely preventive of neurologic sequelae.[183] However, patients may benefit if they are treated even later. In the most recent randomized clinical trial showing beneficial effects of HBO, although all patients were treated within 24 hours of exposure, 38% of patients were treated later than 6 hours after exposure. Therefore, it is not unreasonable to consider HBO, contingent on transport limitations, within 24 hours of presentation for symptomatic acute poisoning.

One case series suggests beneficial effects for HBO used up to 21 days after exposure, even after patients have developed neuropsychologic sequelae.[111] The problem with studies showing HBO benefits days after an acute poisoning or after chronic poisoning is that these cases are all anecdotal and lack control subjects. In fact, delayed neurocognitive sequelae frequently resolve within 2 months in patients with mild CO poisoning[162] and in those with serious CO poisoning who survive to HBO treatment, one-third resolve within 1 year.[171] It is possible that these delayed or chronic cases may simply represent the beneficial effects of HBO.

Repeat Treatment with Hyperbaric Oxygen A randomized clinical trial demonstrated that three HBO treatments within the first 24 hours improves cognitive outcome.[171] Unfortunately, there was no group treated with only one or two HBO sessions. Regardless, multiple treatments are advocated for patients who have persistent symptoms, particularly coma, and do not clear after their first HBO session. In a nonrandomized retrospective study, CO-poisoned patients who received a second HBO treatment had a reduction in delayed neurologic sequelae from 55% to 18% compared with control subjects who had only one treatment.[58] Prospective studies comparing single versus multiple courses of HBO therapy have failed to confirm any benefit from repeated HBO treatment, so multiple treatments cannot be recommended routine at this time. The most recent clinical guidelines from the UHMS state that the optimal number of HBO treatments for CO poisoning is unknown at this time and that one should consider reserving multiple treatments for patients who fail to fully recover after one treatment.[49]

TREATMENT OF PREGNANT PATIENTS

The management of CO exposure in the pregnant patient is difficult because of the potential adverse effects of both CO and HBO. A literature review of all CO exposures during pregnancy revealed a high incidence of fetal CNS damage and stillbirth after severe maternal poisonings.[169] A series of three severely symptomatic patients who did not receive HBO had adverse fetal outcomes: two stillbirths and one case of cerebral palsy.[84] There have even been cases of limb malformations, cranial deformities, and a variety of mental disabilities in children poisoned in utero.[15,95,96]

Traditionally, it was thought that fetal hemoglobin had a high affinity for CO. Pregnant ewe studies show a delayed but substantive increase in COHb levels in fetuses, exceeding the level and duration of those in the mothers.[96] Thus, it appeared that fetuses are a sink for CO and could be poisoned at levels lower than mothers. However, such data may not apply to humans because in vitro work shows that as opposed to sheep, human fetal hemoglobin actually has less affinity for CO than maternal hemoglobin, at a ratio of 0.8. Under conditions of low oxygenation and high 2,3-BPG, as in serious CO poisoning, the affinity of human fetal hemoglobin starts to approach that of maternal.[176] The more important issue with maternal CO exposure is the precipitous decrease in fetal arterial oxygen content that occurs within minutes at CO concentrations of 3000 ppm.[54] Therefore, the ensuing hypoxia of the fetus, rather than increase in fetal COHb, is of more concern.

Maternal COHb levels do not accurately reflect fetal hemoglobin or tissue levels.[36] In primate studies, a single CO exposure insufficient to cause clinical disease in the mother led to intrauterine hypoxia, fetal brain injury, and increased rate of fetal death.[54,55] In humans, there are a few cases of fetal demise with maternal levels of COHb less than 10%.[15] However, in that series, some mothers were treated with oxygen before obtaining their COHb levels. Another issue with some of these data is that often the mother has been chronically "soaked" with CO, making levels difficult to interpret. Rodent studies show that chronic low level CO exposure in pregnant mothers may result in permanent cognitive deficits in the subsequent progeny.[39]

Because maternal COHb does not necessarily predict fetal demise, clinicians must direct their attention to maternal symptoms of CO toxicity. Multiple case series demonstrate that pregnant women who present with normal mental status and no loss of consciousness have excellent outcomes in terms of normal deliveries.[15,84] These infants have no subsequent delay in attaining their developmental milestones. Therefore, it appears that mothers who appear well after acute CO poisoning will have good outcomes with respect to their pregnancies.

The bigger dilemma for clinicians is the approach to treatment of seriously symptomatic CO-poisoned pregnant patients. All patients should receive 100% oxygen by face mask, at least until the mother is asymptomatic. However, CO absorption and elimination are slower in the fetal circulation than in the maternal circulation.[96] A mathematical model predicts that elimination of CO from fetuses takes 3.5 times longer than maternal CO elimination.[73] However, based on the fact that some of these data are based on sheep fetal hemoglobin kinetics, the optimum time for treatment of the mother cannot be recommended at this time.

For exposed pregnant women with a loss of consciousness or high COHb levels, HBO might be considered. Unfortunately, pregnant patients were excluded from all prospective trials documenting efficacy of HBO. However, treatment of pregnant patients with HBO is not without theoretical risk. Animal studies show conflicting results on the effects of HBO on fetal development. Some studies have shown that HBO causes developmental abnormalities in the central nervous, cardiovascular, and pulmonary systems of rodent fetuses. This is in marked contrast to the extensive Russian experience, in which hundreds of pregnant women were treated with HBO, apparently without significant perinatal complications and with improvement in fetal and maternal status for their underlying conditions of toxemia, anemia, and diabetes.[106] Cases in the United States have been published in which HBO used for mild CO poisoning resulted in infants who were normal at birth. However, less than optimal outcomes have occurred in cases of sicker patients in which the mother has had loss of consciousness or presented comatose.[44] Thus, it appears that HBO should be safe and have the same efficacy for pregnant patients as in nonpregnant patients. However, its effect in preventing adverse fetal outcomes is unclear.

There currently is no scientific validation for an absolute level at which to provide HBO therapy for a pregnant patient with CO exposure. Arbitrarily, COHb levels greater than 20% are recommended as an indication in a pregnant patient regardless of symptoms. Pregnant patients should not be treated any differently if they meet criteria for HBO that have already been mentioned (see Table 125–4). Additional criteria include any signs of fetal distress, such as abnormal fetal heart rate.

TREATMENT OF CHILDREN

It has been suggested that children are more sensitive to the effects of CO because of their increased metabolic rate.[27] Epidemiologic studies suggest that children can become symptomatic at COHb levels less that 10%, which is lower than commonly expected in adults.[83] The other problem is that these patients may have unusual presentations. Most children manifest nausea, headache, or lethargy. But an isolated seizure or vomiting may be the only manifestation of CO toxicity in an infant or child.

In drawing COHb levels in infants, clinicians must be aware of two confounding factors. First, many co-oximeters give falsely elevated COHb levels in proportion to the amount of fetal hemoglobin present.[170] Second, CO is produced during breakdown of protoporphyrin to bilirubin. Therefore, infants normally have higher levels of COHb, which are even higher in the presence of kernicterus. Thus, before it is assumed that an elevated COHb level implies CO poisoning in an infant, the contribution of jaundice and fetal hemoglobin must be considered in the final analysis.

Although children may be more susceptible to acute toxicity with CO, their long-term outcomes appear to be more favorable than adults. In a series of 2360 serious CO cases, all incidences of delayed neurologic sequelae were in adults older than age 30 years.[28] Pediatric series of CO poisoning demonstrated an incidence of delayed neurologic sequelae of 10% to 20% of children after severe CO poisoning.[27] This low incidence, in patients treated only with 100% oxygen at 1.0 ATA, has been used as an argument to avoid HBO. However, there still is a real risk of such sequelae, and HBO has been used successfully to prevent it.[180] If the use of surface-pressure oxygen is selected to treat a child, it is comforting to know that the COHb half-life is approximately 44 minutes, which is comparable to that in adults.[83]

NOVEL NEUROPROTECTIVE TREATMENTS

A variety of neuroprotective agents have been tested in animal models. They are targeted primarily at preventing the delayed neurologic sequelae associated with serious CO poisoning. One of the simplest treatments tested is insulin. Hyperglycemia has been shown to exacerbate neuronal injury from stroke as well as in arrest situations. In CO poisoning of rodents, it is associated with worse neurologic outcome.[122] However, insulin, independent of its glucose-lowering effect, may be the protective agent after ischemia. In rodent studies, improved neurologic outcome, as measured by locomotor activity, occurs after those with CO poisoning treated with insulin. In light of these findings, it is reasonable to aggressively treat documented hyperglycemia with insulin in serious CO poisoning.

Many neuroprotective agents involve blockage of excitatory amino acids that are implicated in neuronal cell death after CO poisoning. Pretreatment of mice with dizocilpine (MK-801), which blocks the action of glutamate at *N*-methyl-D-aspartate receptors, ameliorates learning, memory, and hippocampal deficits with CO poisoning.[77] Ketamine, another glutamate antagonist, decreases the mortality rate of rats poisoned with CO after carotid ligation.[123] Treatment of mice with various glutamate antagonists prevents learning and memory deficits in a model of CO poisoning.[52] Blockage earlier in the immunologic cascade, with a neuronal NO synthase inhibitor also prevented NMDA receptor activation, thus protecting mice from learning deficits after CO poisoning.[157] One exciting approach is the use of antioxidants, such as dimethyl sulfoxide and disulfiram, that prevent learning and memory deficits when given after CO poisoning in mice.[52] Use of these or related therapeutics, although promising, awaits further animal testing because of potential adverse effects.

Other modalities have been tested in preventing neuronal damage from CO without much success. Hypothermia, rather than being beneficial, actually increases mortality in animals.[145] Allopurinol has been shown to prevent formation of free radicals through xanthine oxidase. This xenobiotic, when given prior to exposure, inhibits lipid peroxidation in CO poisoning.[151] This strategy has not been promising because of the necessity for pretreatment.

PREVENTION

Early diagnosis prevents much of the morbidity and mortality associated with CO poisoning, especially in unintentional exposures. The increased quality of home CO-detecting devices allows personal intervention in the prevention of exposure.[86] If a patient presents complaining that his or her CO alarm sounded, it is important to realize that the threshold limit for the alarm is set roughly to approximate a COHb level of 10% at worst. Therefore, manufacturers must have their alarms activate within 189 minutes at 70 ppm CO, 50 minutes at 150 ppm, and 15 minutes at 400 ppm (Underwriters Laboratories, UL2034). Alarms are not to activate for prolonged exposures below 30 ppm to prevent epidemic alarms during winter inversions in large cities.[8] Government ordinances for obligatory CO alarms could potentially prevent many poisonings, particularly during winter storms.[21,60]

Routine laboratory screening of ED patients during the winter is not very efficacious in diagnosing unsuspected CO poisoning; the yield is less than 1% when patients are tested in whom the diagnosis of CO exposure was already excluded by history. Instead, selecting patients with CO-related complaints, such as headache, dizziness, or nausea, increases the yield to 5% to 11%.[43,144] During the winter, risk factors such as gas heating or symptomatic cohabitants in patients with influenzalike symptoms such as headache, dizziness, or nausea, particularly in the absence of fever, is the most useful method for deciding when to obtain COHb levels for potential patient.

The issue of symptomatic cohabitants is especially important from a preventive standpoint. Alerting other cohabitants to this danger and effecting evacuation may prevent needless morbidity and mortality. Most communities have multiple resources for onsite evaluation. Usually the local fire department or utility company can either check home appliances or measure ambient CO concentrations with portable monitoring equipment. Current workplace standard for ambient CO exposures is 35 ppm averaged over 8 hours with a ceiling limit of 200 ppm (measured over a 15-minute period).[113] Just a 4-hour exposure to 100 ppm of CO may result in COHb level greater than 10% with symptoms.

SUMMARY

Unintentional exposures to CO may easily be missed or misdiagnosed. Patients with a suspected influenzalike illness should be screened for potential home sources of CO, and symptomatic cohabitants should be alerted. CO should also be considered in patients with unexplained coma, acidosis, or signs of cardiac ischemia, especially if attempted suicide is suspected. Fire victims, in addition to airway problems and potential cyanide toxicity, may succumb to CO toxicity. The mainstay of treatment in all these cases is good supportive care with early oxygenation to increase the elimination of CO. Because of the overwhelming clinical successes with HBO and its limited risks, early use of this treatment modality in severe exposures is encouraged. Discussion with a regional poison center or hyperbaric facility will help in identifying patients who are most likely to benefit from such treatment.

REFERENCES

1. Allred EN, Bleecker ER, Chaitman BR, et al. Effects of carbon monoxide on myocardial ischemia. *Environ Health Perspect.* 1991;91:89-132.
2. Allred EN, Bleecker ER, Chaitman BR, et al. Short-term effects of carbon monoxide exposure on the exercise performance of subjects with coronary artery disease. *N Engl J Med.* 1989;321:1426-1432.
3. Amitai Y, Zlotogorski Z, Golan-Katzav V, et al. Neuropsychological impairment from acute low-level exposure to carbon monoxide. *Arch Neurol.* 1998;55:845-848.
4. Barker SJ, Badal JJ. The measurement of dyshemoglobins and total hemoglobin by pulse oximetry. *Curr Opin Anaesthesiol.* 2008;21:805-810.
5. Barker SJ, Curry J, Redford D, et al. Measurement of carboxyhemoglobin and methemoglobin by pulse oximetry: a human volunteer study. *Anesthesiology.* 2006;105:892-897.
6. Barker SJ, Tremper KK. The effect of carbon monoxide inhalation on pulse oximetry and transcutaneous PO2. *Anesthesiology.* 1987;66:677-679.
7. Benignus VA, Hazucha MJ, Smith MV, et al. Prediction of carboxyhemoglobin formation due to transient exposure to carbon monoxide. *J Appl Physiol.* 1994;76:1739-1745.
8. Bizovi KE, Leikin JB, Hryhorczuk DO, et al. Night of the sirens: analysis of carbon monoxide-detector experience in suburban Chicago. *Ann Emerg Med.* 1998;31:737-740.
9. Boerema I, Meyne I, Brummelkamp WH, et al. Life without blood. *Arch Chir Neer.* 1959;11:70-83.
10. Bogusz M, Cholewa L, Pach J, et al. A comparison of two types of acute carbon monoxide poisoning. *Arch Toxicol.* 1975;33:141-149.
11. Brown SD, Piantodosi CA. Recovery of energy metabolism in rat brain after carbon monoxide hypoxia. *J Clin Invest.* 1991;89 666-672.
12. Bruce EN, Bruce MC. A multicompartment model of carboxyhemoglobin and carboxymyoglobin responses to inhalation of carbon monoxide. *J Appl Physiol.* 2003;95:1235-1247.
13. Brvar M, Finderle Z, Suput D, et al. S100B protein in conscious carbon monoxide-poisoned rats treated with normobaric or hyperbaric oxygen. *Crit Care Med.* 2006;34:2228-2230.
14. Brvar M, Mozina H, Osredkar J, et al. S100B protein in carbon monoxide poisoning: a pilot study. *Resuscitation.* 2004;61:357-360.
15. Caravati EM, Adams CJ, Joyce SM, et al. Fetal toxicity associated with maternal carbon monoxide poisoning. *Ann Emerg Med.* 1988;17 714-717.
16. Centers for Disease Control and Prevention. Carbon monoxide poisoning at an indoor ice arena and bingo hall—Seattle, 1996. *MMWR Morbid Mortal Wkly Rep.* 1996;45:265-267.
17. Centers for Disease Control: Carbon monoxide poisoning from use of gasoline-fueled power washers in an underground parking garage—District of Columbia, 1994. *MMWR Morb Mortal Wkly Rep* 1995; 44: 356-357.
18. Centers for Disease Control and Prevention. Carbon monoxide poisoning from hurricane-associated use of portable generators—Florida, 2004. *MMWR Morb Mortal Wkly Rep.* 2005;54:697-700.
19. Centers for Disease Control and Prevention. Carbon-monoxide poisoning resulting from exposure to ski-boat exhaust—Georgia, June 2002. *MMWR Morbid Mortal Wkly Rep.* 2002;51:829-830.
20. Centers for Disease Control and Prevention. Carbon monoxide-related deaths—United States, 1999–2004. *MMWR Morbid Mortal Wkly Rep.* 2007;56:1309-1312.
21. Centers for Disease Control and Prevention. Epidemic carbon monoxide poisoning despite a CO alarm law. Mecklenburg County, NC, December, 2002. *MMWR Morbid Mortal Wkly Rep.* 2004.
22. Centers for Disease Control and Prevention. Nonfatal, unintentional, non-fire related carbon monoxide exposures—United States, 2004–2006. *MMWR Morbid Mortal Wkly Rep.* 2008;57:896-899.
23. Centers for Disease Control and Prevention. Unintentional non-fire-related carbon monoxide exposures—United States, 2001–2003. *MMWR Morb Mortal Wkly Rep.* 2005;54:36-39.
24. Chamberland DL, Wilson BD, Weaver LK. Transient cardiac dysfunction in acute carbon monoxide poisoning. *Am J Med.* 2004;117:623-625.
25. Chambers CA, Hopkins RO, Weaver LK, et al. Cognitive and affective outcomes of more severe compared to less severe carbon monoxide poisoning. *Brain Injury.* 2008;22:387-395.
26. Chee KJ, Nilson D, Partridge R, et al. Finding needles in a haystack: a case series of carbon monoxide poisoning detected using new technology in the emergency department. *Clin Toxicol.* 2008;46:461-469.

27. Cho CH, Chiu NC, Ho CS, et al. Carbon monoxide poisoning in children. *Pediatr Neonatol.* 2008;49:121-125.
28. Choi IS. Delayed Neurological Sequelae in Carbon Monoxide Intoxication. *Arch Neurol.* 1983;40 433-435.
29. Choi IS, Kim SK, Lee SS. Evaluation of outcome of delayed neurologic sequelae after carbon monoxide poisoning by technetium-99m hexamethylpropylene amine oxime brain single photon emission computed tomography. *Eur Neurol.* 1995;35:137-142.
30. Chu K, Jung KH, Kim HJ, et al. Diffusion-weighted MRI and 99mTc-HMPAO SPECT in delayed relapsing type of carbon monoxide poisoning: evidence of delayed cytotoxic edema. *Eur Neurol.* 2004;51:98-103.
31. Cobb N, Etzel RA. Unintentional carbon monoxide related deaths in the United States, 1979 through 1988. *JAMA.* 1991;266:659-663.
32. Coburn RF. Endogenous carbon monoxide production. *N Engl J Med.* 1970;282:207-209.
33. Coburn RF. The carbon monoxide body stores. *Ann N Y Acad Sci.* 1970;174: 11-22.
34. Coburn RF, Mayers LB. Myoglobin O2 tension determined from measurement of carboxymyoglobin in skeletal muscle. *Am J Physiol.* 1971;220: 66-74.
35. Cone DC, MacMillan DS, Van Gelder C, et al. Noninvasive fireground assessment of carboxyhemoglobin levels in firefighters. *Prehosp Emerg Care.* 2005;9:8-13.
36. Copel JA, Bowen F, Bolognese RJ. Carbon monoxide intoxication in early pregnancy. *Obstet Gynecol.* 1982;59(suppl):26S-28S.
37. Cunnington AJ, Hormbrey P. Breath analysis to detect recent exposure to carbon monoxide. *Postgrad Med J.* 2002;78:233-237.
38. De Reuck J, Decoo D, Lemahieu I, et al. A positron emission tomography study of patients with acute carbon monoxide poisoning treated by hyperbaric oxygen. *J Neurol.* 1993;240:430-434.
39. De Salvia MA, Cagiano R, Carratù MR, Di Giovanni, Trabace L, Cuomo V: Irreversible impairment of active avoidance behavior in rats prenatally exposed to mild concentration of carbon monoxide. *Psychopharmacology.* 1995; 122:66–71.
40. Denays R, Makhoul E, Dachy B, et al. Electronencephalographic mapping and Tc HMPAO single-photon emission computed tomography in carbon monoxide poisoning. *Ann Emerg Med.* 1994;24:947-952.
41. Dolan MC, Haltom TL, Barrows GH, et al. Carboxyhemoglobin levels in patients with flu-like symptoms. *Annn Emerg Med.* 1987;16 782-786.
42. Ducasse JL, Celsis P, Marc-Vergnes JP. Non-comatose patients with acute carbon monoxide poisoning: hyperbaric or normobaric oxygenation? *Undersea Hyperb Med.*1995;22:9-15.
43. Eberhardt M, Powell A, Bonfante G, et al. Noninvasive measurement of carbon monoxide levels in ED patients with headache. *J Med Toxicol.* 2006;2:89-92.
44. Elkharrat D, Raphael JC, Korach JM, et al. Acute carbon monoxide intoxication and hyperbaric oxygen in pregnancy. *Intensive Care Med.* 1991;17: 289-292.
45. Ely EW, Moorehead B, Haponik EF. Warehouse workers' headache: emergency evaluation and management of 30 patients with carbon monoxide poisoning. *Am J Med.* 1995;98:145-155.
46. Fawcett TA, Moon RE, Fracica PJ, et al. Warehouse workers' headache. Carbon monoxide poisoning from propane-fueled forklifts [see comments]. *J Occup Med.* 1992;34:12-15.
47. Fife CE, Otto GH, Koch S, et al. A noninvasive method for rapid diagnosis of carbon monoxide poisoning. *Intern J Emerg Intensive Care Med.* 2001;5:1-8.
48. Gale SD, Hopkins RO, Weaver LK, et al. MRI, quantitative MRI, SPECT, and neuropsychological findings following carbon monoxide poisoning. *Brain Injury.* 1999;13:229-243.
49. Gesell LB, ed. *Hyperbaric Oxygen 2009. Indications and Results. The Hyperbaric Oxygen Therapy Committee Report.* Durham, NC. Undersea and Hyperbaric Medical Society; 2008.
50. Ghim M, Severance HW: Ice storm–related poisonings in North Carolina: A reminder. *South Med J.* 2005;97:1060-1065.
51. Gill JR, Goldfeder LB, Stajic M. The happy land homicides: 87 deaths due to smoke inhalation. *J Forensic Sci.* 2003;48:161-163.
52. Gilmer B, Thompson C, Tomaszewski C, et al. The protective effects of experimental neurodepressors on learning and memory following carbon monoxide poisoning. *J Toxicol Clin Toxicol.* 1999;37 606.
53. Ginsberg MD. Carbon monoxide intoxication. Clinical features, neuropathology, and mechanisms of injury. *J Toxicol Clin Toxicol.* 1985;23: 281-288.
54. Ginsberg MD, Myers RE. Fetal brain injury after maternal carbon monoxide intoxication. Clinical and neuropathologic aspects. *Neurology.* 1976;26:15-23.
55. Ginsberg MD, Myers RE, McDonagh BF. Experimental carbon monoxide encephalopathy in the primate. II. Clinical aspects, neuropathology, and physiologic correlation. *Arch Neurol.* 1974;30:209-216.
56. Goldbaum LR, Orellano T, Dergal E. Mechanism of the toxic action of carbon monoxide. *Ann Clin Lab Sci.* 1976;6:372-376.
57. Goldbaum LR, Ramirez RG, Absalon KB. What is the mechanism of carbon monoxide toxicity? *Aviat Space Environ Med.* 1975;46:1289-1291.
58. Gorman DF, Clayton D, Gilligan JE, et al. A longitudinal study of 100 consecutive admissions for carbon monoxide poisoning to The Royal Adelaide Hospital. *Undersea Hyperb Med.* 1992;20 311-316.
59. Goulon M, Barios A, Rapin M. Carbon monoxide poisoning and acute anoxia due to breathing coal gas and hydrocarbons. *J Hyperbar Med.* 1986;1 23-41.
60. Graber JM, Macdonald SC, Kass DE, et al. Carbon monoxide: the case for environmental public health surveillance. *Public Health Rep.* 2007;122:138-144.
61. Hampson NB. Pulse oximetry in severe carbon monoxide poisoning. *Chest.* 1998;114:1036-1041.
62. Hampson NB. Stability of carboxyhemoglobin in stored and mailed blood samples. Am *J Emerg Med.* 2008;26:191-195.
63. Hampson NB, Kramer CC, Dunford RG, et al. Carbon monoxide poisoning from indoor burning of charcoal briquets. *JAMA.* 1994;271:52-53.
64. Hampson NB, Little CE. Hyperbaric treatment of patients with carbon monoxide poisoning in the United States. *Undersea Hyperb Med.* 2005;32:21-26.
65. Hampson NB, Mathieu D, Piantadosi CA, et al. Carbon monoxide poisoning: interpretation of randomized clinical trials and unresolved treatment issues. *Undersea Hyperb Med.* 2001;28:157-164.
66. Hampson NB, Norkool DM. Carbon monoxide poisoning in children riding in the back of pickup trucks. *JAMA.* 1992;267:538-540.
67. Hampson NB, Weaver LK. Carbon monoxide poisoning: a new incidence for an old disease. *Undersea Hyperb Med.* 2007;34:163-168.
68. Hampson NB, Zmaeff JL. Outcome of patients experiencing cardiac arrest with carbon monoxide poisoning treated with hyperbaric oxygen. *Ann Emerg Med.* 2001;38:36-41.
69. Han S, Bhopale VM, Thom SR. Xanthine oxidoreductase and neurological sequelae of carbon monoxide poisoning. *Toxicol Lett.* 2007;170:111-115.
70. Heckerling PS, Leikin JB, Maturen A. Occult carbon monoxide poisoning: validation of a prediction model. *Am J Med.* 1988;84 251-256.
71. Heckerling PS, Leikin JB, Maturen A, et al. Predictors of occult carbon monoxide poisoning in patients with headache and dizziness. *Ann Intern Med.* 1987;107 174-176.
72. Henry CR, Satran D, Lindgren B, et al. Myocardial injury and long-term mortality following moderate to severe carbon monoxide poisoning. *JAMA.* 2006;295:398-402.
73. Hill EP, Hill JR, Power GG, et al. Carbon monoxide exchanges between the human fetus and mother: a mathematical model. *Am J Physiol.* 1977;232:H311-323.
74. Hon KL, Yeung WL, Ho CH, et al. Neurologic and radiologic manifestations of three girls surviving acute carbon monoxide poisoning. *J Child Neurol.* 2006;21:737-741.
75. Hopkins RO, Fearing MA, Weaver LK, et al. Basal ganglia lesions following carbon monoxide poisoning. *Brain Injury.* 2006;20:273-281.
76. Hopkins RO, Weaver LK, Valentine KJ, et al. Apolipoprotein E genotype and response of carbon monoxide poisoning to hyperbaric oxygen treatment. *Am J Resp Crit Care Med.* 2007;176:1001-1006.
77. Ishimaru H, Katoh A, Suzuki H, et al. Effects of *N*-methyl-D-aspartate receptor antagonists on carbon monoxide-induced brain damage in mice. *J Pharmacol Exp Ther.* 1992;261:349-352.
78. Jackson EB Jr, Mukhopadhyay S, Tulis DA. Pharmacologic modulators of soluble guanylate cyclase/cyclic guanosine monophosphate in the vascular system—from bench top to bedside. *Curr Vasc Pharmacol.* 2007;5:1-14.
79. Juurlink D, Buckley N, Stanbrook M, et al. Hyperbaric oxygen for carbon monoxide poisoning. *Cochrane Database Syst Rev.* 2005:CD002041.
80. Kalay N, Ozdogru I, Cetinkaya Y, et al. Cardiovascular effects of carbon monoxide poisoning. *Am J Cardiol.* 2007;99:322-324.
81. Kelley JS, Sophocleus GJ. Retinal hemorrhages in subacute carbon monoxide poisoning. Exposures in homes with blocked furnace flues. *JAMA.* 1978;239:1515-1517.
82. Kharasch ED, Powers KM, Artu AA: Comparison of Amsorb, Sodalime, and Baralyme degradation of volatile anesthetics and formation of carbon monoxide and compound A in swine in vivo. *Anesthesiology.* 2002;96:173-182.

83. Klasner AE, Smith SR, Thompson MW, et al. Carbon monoxide mass exposure in a pediatric population. *Acad Emerg Med.* 1998;5:992-996.
84. Koren G, Sharav T, Pastuszak A, et al. A multicenter, prospective study of fetal outcome following accidental carbon monoxide poisoning in pregnancy. *Reprod Toxicol.* 1991;5 397-403.
85. Krantz T, Thisted B, Strom J, et al. Acute carbon monoxide poisoning. *Acta Anaesthesiol Scand.* 1988;32:278-282.
86. Krenzelok EP, Roth R, Full R. Carbon monoxide. . . the silent killer with an audible solution. *Am J Emerg Med.* 1996;14:484-486.
87. Kunsman GW, Presses CL, Rodriguez P. Carbon monoxide stability in stored postmortem blood samples. *J Analyt Toxicol.* 2000;24:572-578.
88. Lacey DJ. Neurologic sequelae of acute carbon monoxide intoxication. *Am J Dis Child.* 1981;135:145-147.
89. Lapresle J, Fardeau M. The central nervous system and carbon monoxide poisoning. II. Anatomical study of brain lesions following intoxication with carbon monoxide (22 cases). *Prog Brain Res.* 1967;24:31-74.
90. Lee MS, Marsden CD. Neurological sequelae following carbon monoxide poisoning: clinical course and outcome according to the clinical types and brain computed tomography scan findings. *Mov Disord.* 1996;9: 550-558.
91. Leikin JB, Kaufman D, Lipscomb JW, et al: Methylene chloride report of 5 exposures and 2 deaths. *Am J Emerg Med.* 1990;8:534-537.
92. Levasseur L, Galliot-Guilley M, Richter F, et al. Effects of mode of inhalation of carbon monoxide and of normobaric oxygen administration on carbon monoxide elimination from the blood. *Hum Exp Toxicol.* 1996;15: 898-903.
93. Lo CP, Chen SY, Lee KW, et al. Brain injury after acute carbon monoxide poisoning: early and late complications. *AJR Am J Roentgenol.* 2007;189:W205-211.
94. Logue CJ. An inconvenient truth? *Ann Emerg Med.* 2008;51:339-340; author reply 340-332.
95. Longo LD. Carbon monoxide poisoning in the pregnant mother and fetus and its exchange across the placenta. *Ann NY Acad Sci.* 1970;174 313-341.
96. Longo LD, Hill EP. Carbon monoxide uptake in fetal and maternal sheep. *Am J Physiol.* 1977;232:H324-330.
97. Mannaioni PF, Vannacci A, Masini E. Carbon monoxide: the bad and the good side of the coin, from neuronal death to anti-inflammatory activity. *Inflamm Res.* 2006;55:261-273.
98. Markey MA, Zumwalt RE: Fatal carbon monoxide poisoning after the detonation of explosives in an underground mine: A case report. *Am J Forensic Med Pathol.* 2001;22:387-390.
99. Mathieu D, Nolf M, Durocher A. Acute carbon monoxide poisoning: risk of late sequelae and treatment by hyperbaric oxygen. *J Toxicol Clin Toxicol.* 1985;23 315-324.
100. McNulty JA, Maher BA, Chu M, et al. Relationship of short-term verbal memory to the need for hyperbaric oxygen treatment after carbon monoxide poisoning. *Neuropsychiatry Neuropsychol Behav Neurol.* 1997;10: 174-179.
101. Mathieu D, Wattel F, Mathieu-Nolf M et al. Randomized prospective study comparing the effect of hyperbaric oxygen versus twelve hours normobaric oxygen in non-comatose carbon monoxide poisoned patients. *Undersea Hyperbaric Med.* 1996;23(suppl):7-8.
102. Messier LD, Myers RAM. A neuropsychological screening battery for emergency assessment of carbon-monoxide-poisoned patients. *J Clin Psychol.* 1991;47:675-684.
103. Miro O, Alonso JR, Casademont J, et al. Oxidative damage on lymphocyte membranes in increased in patients suffering from acute carbon monoxide poisoning. *Toxicol Lett.* 1999;110:219-223.
104. Miro O, Casademont J, Barrientos A, et al. Mitochondrial cytochrome c oxidase inhibition during acute carbon monoxide poisoning. *Pharmacol Toxicol.* 1998;82:199-202.
105. Miura T, Mitomo M, Kawai R, et al. CT of the brain in acute carbon monoxide intoxication: characteristic features and prognosis. *AJNR Am J Neuroradiol.* 1985;6:739-742.
106. Molzhaninov EV, Chaika VK, Domanova AI, et al. Experience and prospects of using hyperbaric oxygenation in obstetrics. *Proceedings of the 7th International Congress on Hyperbaric Medicine.* Moscow: Nauka; 1981:139-141.
107. Mott JA, Wolfe MI, Alverson CJ, et al. National vehicle emissions policies and practices and declining US carbon monoxide-related mortality. *JAMA.* 2002;288:988-995.
108. Myers RA, Britten JS. Are arterial blood gases of value in treatment decisions for carbon monoxide poisoning? *Crit Care Med.* 1989;17:139-142.
109. Myers RA, DeFazio A, Kelly MP. Chronic carbon monoxide exposure: a clinical syndrome detected by neuropsychological tests. *J Clin Psychol.* 1998;54:555-567.
110. Myers RA, Jones DW, Britten JS, et al. Carbon monoxide half-life study. *Proceedings of the 9th International Congress on Hyperbaric Medicine.* Flagstaff, AZ: Best Publishing; 1987:263-266.
111. Myers RAM, Snyder SK, Emhoff TA. Subacute sequelae of carbon monoxide poisoning. *Ann Emerg Med.* 1985;14:1167.
112. Nager EC, O'Connor RE. Carbon monoxide poisoning from spray paint inhalation. *Acad Emerg Med.* 1998;5:84-86.
113. National Institute for Occupational Safety and Health: NIOSH Pocket Guide to Chemical Hazards, Department of Health and Human Services, Centers for Disease Control. Publication Number 2005-149, U.S. Government Printing Offices, Washington D.C., 2005.
114. Nishimura F, Abe S, Fukunaga T. Carbon monoxide poisoning from industrial coffee extraction. *JAMA.* 2003;290:334.
115. Norkool DM, Kirkpatrick JN. Treatment of acute carbon monoxide poisoning with hyperbaric oxygen: a review of 115 cases. *Ann Emerg Med.* 1985;14:1168-1171.
116. Okeda R, Funata N, Song SJ, et al. Comparative study on pathogenesis of selective cerebral lesions in carbon monoxide poisoning and nitrogen hypoxia in cats. *Acta Neuropathol.* 1982;56:265-272.
117. Okeda R, Runata N, Takano T, et al. The pathogenesis of carbon monoxide encephalopathy in the acute phase—physiological and morphological conditions. *Acta Neuropathol.* 1981;54:1-10.
118. Otten EJ, Rrosenberg JM, Tasset JT. An evaluation of carboyxhemoglobin spot tests. *Ann Emerg Med.* 1985;14 850-852.
119. Ozyurt G, Kaya FN, Kahveci F, et al. Comparison of SPECT findings and neuropsychological sequelae in carbon monoxide and organophosphate poisoning. *Clin Toxicol (Phila).* 2008;46:218-221.
120. Parkinson RB, Hopkins RO, Cleavinger HB, et al. White matter hyperintensities and neuropsychological outcome following carbon monoxide poisoning. *Neurology.* 2002;58:1525-1532.
121. Pelham TW, Holt LE, Moss MA: Exposure to carbon monoxide and nitrogen dioxide in enclosed ice arenas. *Occup Environ Med.* 2002; 59: 224-233.
122. Penney DG. Acute carbon monoxide poisoning in an animal model: the effects of altered glucose on morbidity and mortality. *Toxicology.* 1993;80:85-101.
123. Penney DG, Chen K. NMDA receptor-blocker ketamine protects during acute carbon monoxide poisoning, while calcium channel-blocker verapamil does not. *J Appl Toxicol.* 1996;16:297-304.
124. Peterson JE, Stewart RD. Absorption and elimination of carbon monoxide by inactive young men. *Arch Environ Health.* 1970;21:165-171.
125. Piantadosi CA, Zhang J, Levin ED, et al. Apoptosis and delayed neuronal damage after carbon monoxide poisoning in the rat. *Exp Neurol.* 1997;147:103-114.
126. Porter SS, Hopkins RO, Weaver LK, et al. Corpus callosum atrophy and neuropsychological outcome following carbon monoxide poisoning. *Arch Clin Neuropsychol.* 2002;17:334-337.
127. Raphael JC, Chevret S, Driheme A, Annane D: Managing carbon monoxide poisoning with hyperbaric oxygen. *J Toxicol Clin Toxicol.* 2004;42:455-456.
128. Raphael JC, Elkharrat D, Jars-Guincestre MC, et al. Trial of normobaric and hyperbaric oxygen for acute carbon monoxide intoxication. *Lancet.* 1989;334:414-419.
129. Ratney RS, Wegman DH, Elkins HB: In vivo conversion of methylene chloride to carbon monoxide. *Arch Environ Health.* 1974;28:223-236.
130. Rasmussen LS, Poulsen MG, Christiansen M, et al. Biochemical markers for brain damage after carbon monoxide poisoning. *Acta Anaesthesiol* Scand. 2004;48:469-473.
131. Rioux JP, Myers RAM: Hyperbaric oxygen for methylene chloride poisoning: Report on two cases. *Ann Emerg Med.* 1989;18:691-695.
132. Risser D, Bonsch A, Schneider B. Should coroners be able to recognize unintentional carbon monoxide-related deaths immediately at the death scene? *J Forensic Sci.* 1995;40:596-598.
133. Roughton FJW, Darling RC. The effect of carbon monoxide on the hemoglobin dissociation curve. *Am J Physiol.* 1944;141:17-31.
134. Sanders RW, Katz KD, Suyama J, et al. Seizure during hyperbaric oxygen therapy for carbon monoxide toxicity: a case series and five-year experience. *J Emerg Med.* 2009;Apr 14. [Epub ahead of print].

135. Scheinkestel CD, Bailey M, Myles PS, et al. Hyperbaric or normobaric oxygen for acute carbon monoxide poisoning: a randomised controlled clinical trial. *Med J Aust.* 1999;170:203-210.
136. Shapiro AB, Maturen A, Herman G, et al. Carbon monoxide and myonecrosis: a prospective study. *Vet Hum Toxicol.* 1989;31:136-137.
137. Shimazu T, Ikeuchi H, Hubbard GB, et al. Smoke inhalation injury and the effect of carbon monoxide in the sheep model. *J Trauma.* 1990;30: 170-175.
138. Shusterman D, Alexeeff G, Hargis C, et al. Predictors of carbon monoxide and hydrogen cyanide exposure in smoke inhalation patients. *J Toxicol Clin Toxicol.* 1996;34:61-71.
139. Sloan EP, Murphy DG, Hart R, et al. Complications and protocol considerations in carbon monoxide-poisoned patients who require hyperbaric oxygen therapy: report from a ten-year experience. *Ann Emerg Med.* 1989;18:629-634.
140. Sokal JA, Kralkowska E. The relationship between exposure duration, carboxyhemoglobin, blood glucose, pyruvate and lactate and the severity of intoxication in 39 cases of acute carbon monoxide poisoning in man. *Arch Toxicol.* 1985:196-199.
141. Stewart RD: Paint remover hazard. *JAMA.* 1976;235:398-401.
142. Stewart RD, Baretta ED, Platte LR, et al. Carboxyhemoglobin levels in American blood donors. *JAMA.* 1974;229:1187-1195.
143. Stewart RD, Peterson JE, Fisher TN, et al. Experimental human exposure to high concentrations of carbon monoxide. *Arch Environ Health.* 1973;26:1-7.
144. Suner S, Partridge R, Sucov A, et al. Non-invasive pulse co-oximetry screening in the emergency department identifies occult carbon monoxide toxicity. *J Emerg Med.* 2008;34:441-450.
145. Sutariya BB, Penney DG, Nallamothu BG: Hypothermia following acute carbon-monoxide poisoning increases mortality. *Toxicol Lett.* 1990;52:201-208.
146. Takeuchi A, Vesely A, Rucker J, et al. A simple "new" method to accelerate clearance of carbon monoxide. *Am J Respir Crit Care Med.* 2000;161: 1816-1819.
147. Taskiran D, Nesil T, Alkan K. Mitochondrial oxidative stress in female and male rat brain after ex vivo carbon monoxide treatment. *Hum Exp Toxicol.* 2007;26:645-651.
148. Teksam M, Casey SO, Michel E, et al. Diffusion-weighted MR imaging findings in carbon monoxide poisoning. *Neuroradiology.* 2002;44: 109-113.
149. Thom SR. Antagonism of carbon monoxide-mediated brain lipid peroxidation by hyperbaric oxygen. *Toxicol Appl Pharmacol.* 1990;105:340-344.
150. Thom SR. Carbon monoxide-mediated brain lipid peroxidation in the rat. *J Appl Physiol.* 1990;68:997-1003.
151. Thom SR. Dehydrogenase conversion to oxidase and lipid peroxidation in brain after carbon monoxide poisoning. *J Appl Physiol.* 1992;73:1584-1589.
152. Thom SR. Leukocytes in carbon monoxide-mediated brain oxidative injury. *Toxicol Appl Pharmacol.* 1993;123:234-247.
153. Thom SR, Bhopale VM, Fisher D, et al. Delayed neuropathology after carbon monoxide poisoning is immune-mediated. *Proc Natl Acad Sci U S A.* 2004;101:13660-13665.
154. Thom SR, Bhopale VM, Han S, et al. Intravascular neutrophil activation due to carbon monoxide poisoning. *Am J Respir Crit Care Med.* 2006;174:1236-1248.
155. Thom SR, Fisher D, Xu YA, et al. Adaptive responses and apoptosis in endothelial cells exposed to carbon monoxide. *Proc Natl Acad Sci U S A.* 2000;97:1305-1310.
156. Thom SR, Fisher D, Xu YA, et al. Role of nitric oxide-derived oxidants in vascular injury from carbon monoxide in the rat. *Am J Physiol Heart Circ Physiol.* 1999;276:H984-H992.
157 Thom SR, Fisher D, Zhang J, et al. Neuronal nitric oxide synthase and *N*-methyl-D-aspartate neurons in experimental carbon monoxide poisoning. *Tox Appl Pharmacol.* 2004;194:280-295.
158. Thom SR, Kang M, Fisher D, et al. Release of glutathione from erythrocytes and other markers of oxidative stress in carbon monoxide poisoning. *J Appl Physiol.* 1997;82:1424-1432.
159. Thom SR, Keim LW. Carbon monoxide poisoning: a review of epidemiology, pathophysiology, clinical findings, and treatment options including hyperbaric oxygen. *J Toxicol Clin Toxicol.* 1989;27:141-156.
160. Thom SR, Mendiguren I, Hardy KR, et al. Inhibition of human neutrophil B2 integrin-dependent adherence by hyperbaric oxygen. *Am J Physiol (Cell Physiol).* 1997;272:C770-C777.
161. Thom SR, Ohnishi ST, Ischiropoulos H. Nitric oxide release by platelets inhibits neutrophil B2 integrin function following acute carbon monoxide poisoning. *Toxicol Appl Pharmacol.* 1994;128:105-110.
162. Thom SR, Taber RL, Mendiguren II, et al. Delayed neuropsychologic sequelae after carbon monoxide poisoning: prevention by treatment with hyperbaric oxygen. *Ann Emerg Med.* 1995;25:474-480.
163. Tikuisis P, Penney DG. *Modeling the Uptake and Elimination of Carbon Monoxide. Carbon Monoxide.* Boca Raton: CRC Press; 1996:45-67.
164. Tom T, Abedon S, Clark RI, et al. Neuroimaging characteristics in carbon monoxide toxicity. *J Neuroimaging.* 1996;6:161-166.
165. Tomaszewski C. The case for the use of hyperbaric oxygen in carbon monoxide poisoning. In: Penney DG, ed. *Carbon Monoxide Poisoning.* New York: CRC Press; 2008:375-390.
166. Touger M, Gallagher EJ, Tyrell J. Relationship between venous and arterial carboxyhemoglobin levels in patients with suspected carbon monoxide poisoning. *Ann Emerg Med.* 1995;25:481-483.
167. Turner M, Esaw M, Clark RJ. Carbon monoxide poisoning treated with hyperbaric oxygen: metabolic acidosis as a predictor of treatment requirements. *J Acad Emerg Med.* 1999;16:96-98.
168. Vagts SA: Non-Fire Carbon Monoxide Deaths Associated with the Use of Consumer Products: 1999 and 2000 Annual Estimates. Bethesda, MD, US Consumer Products Safety Commission, 7-31-2003.
169. Van Hoesen KB, Camporesi EM, Moon RE, et al. Should hyperbaric oxygen be used to treat the pregnant patient for acute carbon monoxide poisoning? A case report and literature review. *JAMA.* 1989;261: 1039-1043.
170. Vreman HJ, Mahoney JJ, Stevenson DK. Carbon monoxide and carboxyhemoglobin. *Adv Pediatr.* 1995;42:303-334.
171. Weaver LK, Hopkins RO, Chan KJ, et al. Hyperbaric oxygen for acute carbon monoxide poisoning. *N Engl J Med.* 2002;347:1057-1067.
172. Weaver LK, Howe S, Hopkins R, et al. Carboxyhemoglobin half-life in carbon monoxide-poisoned patients treated with 100% oxygen at atmospheric pressure. *Chest.* 2000;117:801-808.
173. Weaver LK, Valentine KJ, Hopkins RO. Carbon monoxide poisoning: risk factors for cognitive sequelae and the role of hyperbaric oxygen. *Am J Respir Crit Care Med.* 2007;176:491-497.
174. Weaver LK, Gesell LB. Carbon Monoxide Poisoning. In: Gesell LB, ed. *Hyperbaric Oxygen 2009: Indications and Results The Hyperbaric Oxygen Therapy Committee Report.* Durham: Underwater and Hyperbaric Medical Society; 2008:19-28.
175. Weaver LK. Clinical practice. Carbon monoxide poisoning. *N Engl J Med.* 2009;360:1217-1225.
176. Westphal M, Weber TP, Meyer J, et al. Affinity of carbon monoxide to hemoglobin increases at low oxygen fractions. *Biochem Biophys Res Commun.* 2002;295:975-977.
177. Widdop B. Analysis of carbon monoxide. *Ann Clin Biochem.* 2002;39: 378-391.
178. Wolf SJ, Lavonas EJ, Sloan EP, et al. Clinical policy: critical issues in the management of adult patients presenting to the emergency department with acute carbon monoxide poisoning. *Ann Emerg Med.* 2008;51: 138-152.
179. Wrenn K, Conners GP. Carbon monoxide poisoning during ice storms: a tale of two cities. *J Emerg Med.* 1997;15:465-467.
180. Yarar C, Yakut A, Akin A, et al. Analysis of the features of acute carbon monoxide poisoning and hyperbaric oxygen therapy in children. *Turk J Pediatr.* 2008;50:235-241.
181. Yoshii F, Kozuma R, Takahashi W, et al. Magnetic resonance imaging and 11C-N-methylspiperone/positron emission tomography studies in a patient with the interval form of carbon monoxide poisoning. *J Neurol Sci.* 1998;160:87-91.
182. Zeiss J, Brinker R. Role of contrast enhancement in cerebral CT of carbon monoxide poisoning. *J Comput Assist Tomogr.* 1988;12:341-343.
183. Ziser A, Shupak A, Halpern P, et al. Delayed hyperbaric oxygen treatment for acute carbon monoxide poisoning. *Br Med J (Clin Res Ed).* 1984;289:960.

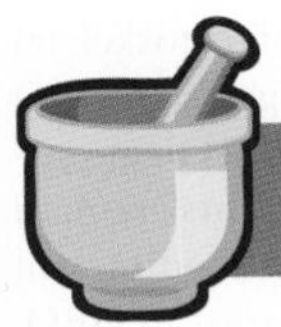

ANTIDOTES IN DEPTH (A37)

HYPERBARIC OXYGEN

Stephen R. Thom

Hyperbaric oxygen (HBO) therapy is a treatment modality whereby a person breathes 100% O_2 while exposed to increased atmospheric pressure. Treatments are performed in either a monoplace (single patient) or a multiplace (typically two to 14 patients) chamber. Pressures applied while patients are in the chamber usually are two to three atmospheres absolute (ATA). Treatments vary from 1.5 to 8 hours, depending on the indication, and may be performed one to three times daily. Monoplace chambers usually are compressed with pure oxygen. Multiplace chambers are pressurized with air, and patients breathe pure oxygen through a tight-fitting face mask, a head tent, or endotracheal tube.

Therapeutic mechanisms of action for HBO are based on elevation of both hydrostatic pressure and the partial pressure of oxygen. Elevation of the hydrostatic pressure causes a reduction in the volume of gas according to Boyle's law. This action has direct relevance to pathologic conditions in which gas bubbles are present in the body, such as arterial gas embolism and decompression sickness. During treatment, the arterial oxygen tension typically exceeds 1500 mm Hg, and tissue oxygen tensions of 200 to 400 mm Hg.[153] Under normal environmental conditions, hemoglobin is virtually saturated with oxygen on passage through the pulmonary microvasculature, so the primary effect of HBO is to increase the dissolved oxygen content of plasma. Application of each additional atmosphere of pressure while breathing 100% oxygen increases the dissolved oxygen concentration in the plasma by 2.2 mL O_2/dL (vol%) (Chap. 21).

Mechanisms of HBO relevant to its use as an antidote are its ability to diminish hypoxic stress by increasing tissue oxygen tension and decreasing the production of reactive oxygen species (ROS) and reactive nitrogen species (RNS).[74,130,142,150,151] Reactive species are recognized to serve as signaling molecules in transduction cascades.[2,25,166] Reactive species have positive and negative effects depending on their concentration and intracellular localization. Hence, with regard to HBO as with any xenobiotic, one must contend with a dosing issue in order to achieve benefit versus injury. Because exposure to hyperoxia in typical clinical HBO protocols is rather brief, studies show that antioxidant defenses are adequate so that tissue injuries can be avoided.[44,45,123,164]

Although elevating tissue O_2 tension is a primary effect of HBO, lasting benefits are related to abatement of the underlying pathophysiological processes. In the context of an antidote, HBO is most commonly used for treatment of carbon monoxide (CO) poisoning. Experience using HBO for life-threatening poisonings from cyanide (CN), hydrogen sulfide (H_2S), or carbon tetrachloride (CCl_4) and in patients with high methemoglobin levels is limited. HBO has been suggested for management of diverse poisonings, but discussion of these applications is beyond the scope of this Antidotes in Depth because supporting clinical and experimental evidence is sparse.[161]

CARBON MONOXIDE

Administration of supplemental oxygen is the cornerstone for treatment of CO poisoning. Historically, its use was based on the affinity of CO for heme proteins and formation of carboxyhemoglobin (COHb). Elevated COHb can result in tissue hypoxia, and exogenous oxygen both hastens dissociation of CO from hemoglobin and provides enhanced tissue oxygenation directly through the increased Po_2. HBO causes COHb dissociation to occur at a rate greater than that achievable by breathing 100% O_2 at sea-level pressure.[113] Additionally, HBO accelerates restoration of mitochondrial oxidative processes.[20] CO poisoning causes perivascular inflammatory injuries, especially in the brain, and animal studies have shown that HBO ameliorates this process by impeding neutrophil adherence to the vasculature.[28,76,82,152,157]

Survivors of CO poisoning are faced with potential impairments to cardiac and neurological function. CO poisoning can cause acute cardiac compromise and survivors exhibit an increased risk for cardiovascular-related death in the subsequent 10 years.[65,126] With regard to neurological impairments, there is a historical precedence for dividing disorders into "acute/persistent" and "delayed" forms. Some patients exhibit acute abnormalities wherein they have an abnormal level of consciousness and/or focal neurological findings from the time of initial presentation and never recover.[4,34,37,54] Other patients seemingly recover from acute poisoning but then manifest neurological or neuropsychiatric abnormalities from 2 days to about 5 weeks after poisoning.[29,46,56,68,92,98,101,108,119,133,136,158,175] Events occurring after a clear or "lucid" interval have been termed "delayed" neurological sequelae.

Results from animal studies do not provide a clear distinction between mechanisms responsible for "acute/persistent" and "delayed" sequelae. Several animal studies indicate that "acute/persistent" sequelae arise because of neuronal necrotic or apoptotic death, but this does not mean that injuries are mediated solely by hypoxia/ischemia versus processes such as excitotoxicity and perivascular oxidative stress that have been linked to more slowly evolving "delayed" brain disorders.[53,71,99,109,149,155,156] Because the different pathological processes occur in close proximity and in some cases concurrently, one can expect that pathological insults for "acute/persistent" and "delayed" sequelae overlap. Thus, there may be more of a continuum of clinical disorders as opposed to distinctly different syndromes.

Vascular abnormalities occur in animal models of CO poisoning. Among the earliest events that occur in both animal models and humans is platelet-neutrophil adherence that mediates intravascular neutrophil activation. These changes precipitate neutrophil adherence that initiates a cascade of events that ultimately causes neurological dysfunction (Fig. A37–1).[70,155,156] Animals poisoned with CO then treated with HBO have more rapid improvement in cardiovascular status,[47] lower mortality,[115] and lower incidence of neurological sequelae.[154] Benefits are likely based on both improved oxygenation and secondary effects pertaining to inhibition of neutrophil adhesion. The ability of HBO to inhibit function of neutrophil β_2-integrin adhesion molecules in animal models forms the basis for amelioration of encephalopathy resulting from CO poisoning and decompression sickness, smoke-induced lung injury, as well as reperfusion injuries of brain, heart, lung, liver, and skeletal muscle.[7,79,95,146,147,152,160,165,169,178–180]

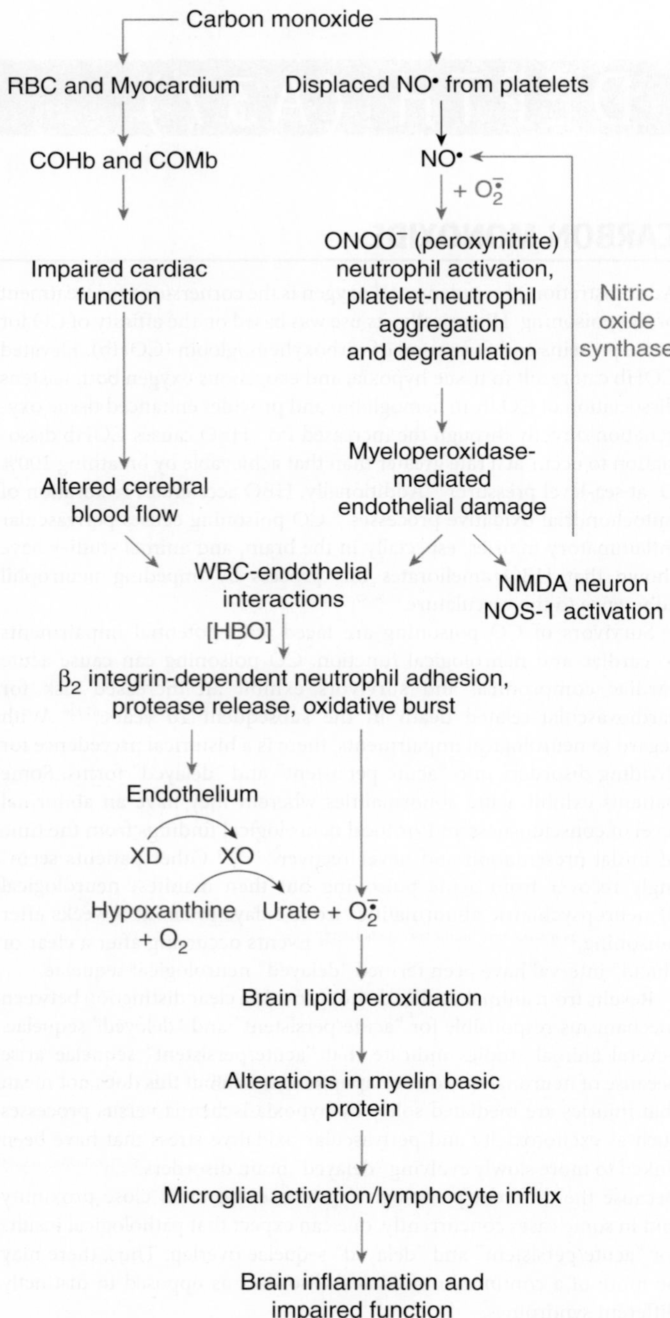

FIGURE A37–1. This figure demonstrates concurrent events leading to vascular injury with CO poisoning and the sequence of events leading to neurological injuries. RBC, erythrocyte; ONOO-, peroxynitrite; ·NO, nitric oxide; $O_2^{\bullet -}$, superoxide radical; COHb, carboxyhemoglobin; COMb, carboxymyoglobin; NMDA, *N*-methyl-D-aspartate; NOS-1, neuronal nitric oxide synthase; NO_2, nitrite (major oxidation product of ·NO); WBC, leukocytes; XD, xanthine dehydrogenase; XO, xanthine oxidase.

Exposure to 2.8 to 3.0 ATA O_2 for 45 minutes temporarily inhibits neutrophil adherence mediated by the activation-dependent β_2-integrins on the neutrophil membrane in both rodents and humans.[28,76,82,152,157] Exposure to HBO *inhibits* β_2-integrins of neutrophils, but not other circulating leukocytes, because hyperoxia increases synthesis of RNS derived from type-2 nitric oxide synthase and myeloperoxidase (see A37–1). This leads to excessive S-nitrosylation of cytoskeletal β actin, which in turn impedes the function of β_2 integrins.[150] HBO does not reduce neutrophil viability, and functions such as degranulation and oxidative burst, in response to chemoattractants, remain intact.[152,157] Inhibiting β_2-integrins with monoclonal antibodies will also ameliorate ischemia-reperfusion injuries, but in contrast to HBO, antibody therapy causes profound immunocompromise.[102,103]

Since 1960, HBO has been used with increasing frequency for severe CO poisoning because clinical recovery appeared to improve beyond that expected with ambient-pressure oxygen therapy. Support for HBO use comes from this experience.[56,57,69,83,97,108,111,122] The clinical efficacy of HBO for acute CO poisoning has been assessed in five prospective, randomized trials published in peer-reviewed journals. Only one clinical trial satisfies all items deemed to be necessary for the highest quality of randomized, controlled trials.[175] This double-blind, placebo-controlled clinical trial involved 152 patients. All patients received treatment with either three sessions of HBO therapy or normobaric O_2 (NBO) with sham pressurization to maintain blinding. Critically ill patients were included, with half of enrolled patients having lost consciousness and 8% requiring intubation. The follow-up rate was 95%. The definition of neurological sequelae, defined a priori, was fulfilled in symptomatic patients by an aggregate performance on six neuropsychological tests. The pretreatment characteristics of the 152 patients enrolled in the trial were similar except that cerebellar dysfunction was more frequent in the NBO treatment group. The group treated with HBO had a lower incidence of cognitive sequelae than the group treated with NBO after adjustment for pretreatment cerebellar dysfunction and stratification (odds ratio 0.45, 95% confidence interval 0.22–0.92, $p = 0.03$). Post hoc subgroup analysis incorporating risk factors showed that HBO reduced cognitive sequelae in patients with any of the following: unconsciousness, COHb greater than or equal to 25%, age greater than or equal to 50 years, or base excess less than or equal to 2 mEq/L. HBO did not improve outcome in patients with none of these criteria.

The only other blinded, prospective, randomized trial was published in 1999 and it involved 191 patients of different severity treated with either daily HBO (3.0 ATA for 60 minutes) with intervening high-flow oxygen for 3 or 6 days versus high-flow NBO for 3 or 6 days.[128] Additional HBO treatments (up to six daily) were performed in patients without neurological recovery. The primary outcome measure for this trial was testing performed at completion of treatment (3–6 days) and not from long-term follow-up. This study had a high rate of adverse neurological outcomes in all patients, regardless of treatment assignment. Neurological sequelae were reported in 74% in HBO-treated patients and 68% in controls. No other clinical trial has described this magnitude of neurological dysfunction. The high incidence is likely to be related to the assessment tool, which could not discern true neurological impairments from poor test-taking related to depression.[129] Suicide attempts with CO represented 69% of cases in this trial. Moreover, 54% of subjects were lost to follow-up. Outcomes at 1 month were not reported, but were stated to show no difference. Multiple statistical comparisons were reported without apparent planning or the requisite statistical correction. Both treatment arms received continuous supplemental mask O_2 for 3 days between their hyperbaric treatments (both true HBO and "sham"), resulting in greater overall O_2 doses than conventional therapy. Multiple flaws in the design and execution of this study are discussed in the literature, so it is impossible to draw meaningful conclusions from the data.[60,106] Despite these issues, conclusions from the trial have been accepted by some as a negative outcome for HBO therapy.[75]

The first prospective clinical trial involving HBO therapy did not demonstrate therapeutic benefits.[119] This study has been criticized because the authors used a low oxygen partial pressure (2 ATA) versus the more usual protocols with 2.5 to 3 ATA and because nearly half of the patients received hyperbaric treatments more than 6 hours after they were discovered.[19] In 1969, a retrospective study indicated that HBO reduced mortality and morbidity only if HBO was administered within 6 hours of CO poisoning.[57] HBO was effective in several other prospective investigations. In a trial involving mildly to moderately poisoned patients, 23% of patients (seven of 30) treated with ambient-pressure oxygen developed neurologic sequelae, whereas no patients (zero of 30; $p < 0.05$) treated with HBO (2.8 ATA) developed sequelae.[158] In another prospective, randomized trial, 26 patients were hospitalized within 2 hours of discovery and were equally divided between two treatment groups: ambient-pressure oxygen or 2.5 ATA O_2.[46] Three weeks later, patients treated with HBO had significantly fewer abnormalities on electroencephalogram, and single-photon emission computed tomography (SPECT) scans showed that cerebral vessels had nearly normal reactivity to carbon dioxide, in contrast to diminished reactivity in patients treated with ambient-pressure oxygen.

In conclusion, published clinical trials span a broad range in quality. Efficacy of HBO for acute CO poisoning is well supported in animal trials and studies provide a mechanistic basis for treatment. In this era of evidence-based medicine a great deal of emphasis has been placed on systematic reviews, although flaws in this approach are increasingly recognized. Treatment of CO poisoning has undergone a number of systematic reviews, but the analytical fidelity has been poor. For example, profound flaws in two successive Cochrane Library Reviews have been identified but, to date, are not corrected.[88]

Several recent reports have provided additional insight into risks for neurological sequelae post-CO poisoning and the benefit of HBO. One such study reported on a cohort of 238 patients and found that independent risk factors for developing neurological sequelae include age greater than or equal to 36 years, exposure for 24 hours or longer (with or without intermittent CO exposures), and acute complaints of memory abnormalities.[174] The only risk factor where HBO demonstrated a reduction in incidence of sequelae was for the group greater than or equal to 36 years. The trial was underpowered to reliably assess the benefit of HBO in those with long-duration CO exposure, but none of five patients exposed for 24 hours or longer manifested neurological sequelae.

Another study has shown that HBO is only beneficial in reducing neurological sequelae among patients who do not possess the apolipoprotein ε4 allele.[66] Because genotype is typically unknown this report does not provide treatment guidelines, but it will become important for future research. Although the basic mechanisms are unknown, it is well established that the apolipoprotein genotype can have profound effects on risk for a variety of neuropathological events.[1,50,100,127] Whether apolipoprotein ε4 modifies the primary pathophysiological insults of CO or mechanisms of HBO is currently unknown. As yet no objective method is available for staging the severity of CO poisoning, although preliminary reports suggest plasma markers may be used in the future.[149] Psychometric screening tests have not proved reliable because abnormalities during the initial screening do not correlate with development of delayed sequelae.[158] The optimal dose of HBO, the number of treatments, treatment pressure, and the time after which it is no longer effective therapy are not clearly defined. Randomized trials have treated patients as soon as possible after CO poisoning based on work suggesting the existence of a 6-hour window of greatest opportunity.[57] However, it is possible that the time of potential benefit goes beyond what has been investigated for some patients. The requisite number of treatments also remains unclear. Clinical indications for HBO in CO poisoning are reviewed in greater detail in Chap. 125 and specifically in Table 125-4.

METHYLENE CHLORIDE

Methylene chloride (CH_2Cl_2) is an organic solvent used commercially in aerosol sprays as a solvent in plastics manufacturing, photographic film production, and food processing; as a degreaser; and as a paint stripper. It is readily absorbed through the skin or by inhalation. It is metabolized by the cytochrome P450 oxidase system to yield CO.[144] This process is slow, and peak COHb levels of 10% to 50% may not be reached for 8 hours or more.[27,48,77,84,93,135,144] Methylene chloride toxicity can have many of the same acute manifestations as CO poisoning.[144] Acute signs and symptoms are attributable to the direct effects of this solvent on the central nervous system (CNS) and to concomitant hypoxia. Effects that are present after 1 hour or more, particularly if the COHb level is elevated, may be partially caused by CO toxicity. There are anecdotal reports of treatment with HBO.[67,121,124,125]

COMBINED CARBON MONOXIDE AND CYANIDE

CO and CN poisonings can occur concomitantly in victims of smoke inhalation.[5,6,10–12,15,30,36,81,89,91,104,134,137,171,176] Experimental evidence suggests that they can produce synergistic toxicity.[9,107,112,113,116] Animal studies demonstrate that ambient-pressure 100% O_2 can enhance protection from CN toxicity[132] and can also enhance CN metabolism to thiocyanate when thiosulfate is used concomitantly.[17] HBO may have either direct effects on reducing CN toxicity[35,72,73,138,148] or augment other antidote treatments.[24,132,173] However, not all animal studies have found that HBO improved outcome,[172] and clinical experience regarding CN treatment with HBO is sparse.[4,55,131] In a series of smoke-inhalation victims with both toxic CO and CN concentrations who received both HBO and treatment for CN involving sodium nitrite and sodium thiosulfate, four of five patients survived without apparent neurologic damage.[63] Clinical case reports where HBO was used along with standard antidote treatment (sodium nitrite plus sodium thiosulfate) for isolated CN poisonings are equivocal.[55,87,131,162] One case showed dramatic improvement,[162] but another showed no response.[87] Methemoglobin formation with the standard antidote treatment involving nitrite is not thought to generate seriously high methemoglobin concentrations, but in the face of concomitant COHb the additional reduction of oxygen carrying capacity may pose a risk. In this regard, there is a report of a patient with 75% methemoglobin due to isobutyl nitrite poisoning who was successfully treated with toluidine-blue and HBO.[86] Further research in this area is necessary. Because CN is among the most lethal poisons and toxicity is rapid, standard antidotal therapy for isolated CN poisoning is of primary importance. Hyperbaric oxygen may be an adjunct for consideration in refractory cases. Consideration for possible use of HBO therapy may also change as the role of hydroxocobalamin alters the use of nitrites (see Chaps 126 and 127).

HYDROGEN SULFIDE

Hydrogen sulfide (H_2S) binds to cytochrome a-a_3 and hence it is similar to CN, although it is more readily dissociated by O_2.[145] Clinical manifestations of toxicity are also similar to those with CO and CN.[145] Management of patients with serious H_2S poisoning principally involves oxygenation and cardiovascular support, as well as consideration of sodium nitrite.[51,59,110] HBO may be more effective than sodium nitrite in preventing mortality in animals.[16] In several instances, HBO appeared to be beneficial.[13,23,58,140,177] Relatively late treatment with HBO (eg, over 10 hours after poisoning) is reported to be beneficial in some[168] but not all cases.[3,141] No definitive data regarding use of HBO for H_2S poisoning are available, but HBO should be considered in refractory cases.

CARBON TETRACHLORIDE

Carbon tetrachloride (CCl_4) hepatotoxicity may be diminished by HBO. Mortality was decreased in a number of animal studies,[14,22,105,120] and there are several case reports of patients surviving potentially lethal ingestions with HBO therapy.[85,143,163,181] HBO appears to inhibit the cytochrome P450 oxidase system responsible for conversion of CCl_4 to hepatotoxic free radicals.[21,96] Because there are no proven antidotes for CCl_4 poisoning, HBO should be considered for potentially severe CCl_4 exposures. However, there may be a delicate balance between oxidative processes that are therapeutic and those that mediate hepatotoxicity.[18] Therefore, when HBO is being considered, it should be instituted before the onset of liver function abnormalities.

PATIENT MANAGEMENT

A fundamental aspect to emergency patient management and treatment is the knowledge and training of the healthcare team. HBO treatment centers typically have the ability to manage patients who require critical care support. Plans for treatment begin while the patient is still in the emergency department, before transport to the hyperbaric chamber is initiated. Issues to be addressed include informed consent, determination that all intravenous/arterial lines and nasogastric tubes/Foley catheters are secured, capping all unnecessary intravenous catheters, placing chest tubes to suction venting apparatus or one-way Heimlich valves, replacing air in endotracheal tube cuffs with water to prevent excessive air leakage at pressure, and adequately sedating or paralyzing the patient as clinically indicated. Substantial clinical experience demonstrates that patients can be transported without adverse events.[94,139]

HBO therapy should never be considered unless proper supportive medical care can be delivered. Most chamber facilities today have equipment and treatment protocols analogous to an intensive care unit. Intensive care support for pediatric cases also can be achieved.[78,170] The inherent toxicity of O_2 and potential for injury resulting from elevations of ambient pressure must be addressed whenever HBO is used therapeutically. Preexisting conditions that require evaluation for possible management before initiation of HBO include claustrophobia, sinus congestion, and patients with scarred or noncompliant structures in the middle ear, such as otosclerosis.[80]

Middle ear barotrauma is the most common adverse effect of HBO treatment.[26] As the ambient pressure within the hyperbaric chamber increases, the patient must be able to equalize the pressure within the middle ear by autoinsufflation. When autoinsufflation fails, tympanostomies can be performed. The incidence of aural barotrauma has been reported to be between 1.2% and 7%.[33,117,164] Pulmonary barotrauma during HBO treatment is rare but should be suspected if any chest or hemodynamic alterations occur during or shortly after decompression. If pneumothorax is suspected, placement of a chest tube is appropriate. Preexisting pneumothorax should be treated with chest tube insertion prior to initiating therapy.

Toxicity resulting from O_2 can be manifested by injuries to the CNS, lungs, and eyes. CNS O_2 toxicity is manifested as a grand mal seizure and occurs at an incidence of approximately one to four per 10,000 patient treatments.[39,62,117] The complex pathophysiology of CNS oxygen toxicity involves production of ROS, RNS, and an imbalance of excitatory and inhibitory neurotransmitters.[8,41,43] The risk of CNS oxygen toxicity is higher in hypercapnic patients and possibly in those who are acidotic or have compromise resulting from sepsis, as an incidence of 7% (23 of 322 patients) was reported in case series of HBO treatment of gas gangrene.[38,61] Pulmonary oxygen toxicity involves local free radical production as well as a neurogenic mechanism involving adrenergic/cholinergic pathways.[40,42] Pulmonary insults can impair mechanics (elasticity), vital capacity, and gas exchange (reviewed in reference[31]). These conditions typically do not arise when standard treatment protocols are followed.[32,49,64,118] There is one report of reversible small airways changes in four of 21 patients treated daily for 90 minutes at 2.4 ATA for 21 days.[159] Progressive myopia may occur in patients undergoing prolonged daily therapy but typically reverses within 6 weeks after treatments are terminated.[90] Nuclear cataracts can form with excessive treatments, exceeding a total of 150 to 200 hours, and they may rarely develop with standard treatment protocols.[52,114] Although there is a theoretical risk for retrolental fibroplasia in neonates, experimental and clinical evidence does not indicate that typical HBO therapy protocols have detrimental effects on neonates or the unborn fetus.[167]

SUMMARY

In conclusion, the mechanisms of action and efficacy of HBO in toxicology continue to be investigated. Some research findings are provocative because they highlight the fact that traditional assessments of mechanisms for toxicity of some agents are incomplete. Questions persist on many issues. Further investigation is required to discern those cases where clear benefit arises with HBO treatment and to define the constraints that may limit its efficacious use.

REFERENCES

1. Aamar S, Saada A, Rotshenker, S. Lesion-induced changes in the production of newly synthesized and secreted apo-E and other molecules are independent of the concomitant recruitment of blood-borne macrophages into injured peripheral nerves. *J Neurochem.* 1992;59:1287-1292.
2. Allen R, Balin A. Oxidative influence on development and differentiation: an overview of a free radical theory of development. *Fr Radic Biol Med.* 1989;6:631-661.
3. Al-Mahasneh QM, Cohle SD, Haas E. Lack of response to hyperbaric oxygen in a fatal case of hydrogen sulfide poisoning (abstract). *Vet Hum Toxicol.* 1989;31:353.
4. Anderson E, Andelman R, Strauch J, Fortuin N, Knelson J. Effects of low-level carbon monoxide exposure on onset and duration of angina pectoris. *Ann Intern Med.* 1973;79:46-50.
5. Anderson RA, Harland WA. Fire deaths in the Glasgow area. III. The role of hydrogen cyanide. *Med Sci Law.* 1982;22:35-40.
6. Anderson RA, Thomson I, Harland WA. The importance of cyanide and organic nitriles in fire fatalities. *Fire Materials.* 1979;3:91-99.
7. Atochin D, Fisher D, Demchenko I, Thom S. Neutrophil sequestration and the effect of hyperbaric oxygen in a rat model of temporary middle cerebral artery occlusion. *Undersea Hyperbaric Med.* 2000;27:185-190.
8. Atochin DN, Demchenko IT, Astern J, Boso AE, Piantadosi CA, Huang PL. Contributions of endothelial and neuronal nitric oxide synthases to cerebrovascular responses to hyperoxia. *J Cereb Blood Flow Metab.* 2003;23(10):1219-1226.
9. Ballantyne B. Hydrogen cyanide as a product of combustion and a factor in morbidity and mortality from fires. In: Ballantyne B, Marrs T, eds: *Clinical and Experimental Toxicology of Cyanides.* Bristol, UK: John Wright; 1987:248-291.
10. Barillo DJ, Goode R, Esch V. Cyanide poisoning in victims of fire: analysis of 364 cases and review of the literature. *J Burn Care Rehabil.* 1994;15:46-57.
11. Barillo DJ, Goode R, Rush BF, Lin R, Freda A, Anderson J. Lack of correlation between carboxyhemoglobin and cyanide in smoke inhalation injury. *Current Surg.* 1986:421-423.
12. Baud FJ, Barriot P, Toffis V, et al. Elevated blood cyanide concentrations in victims of smoke inhalation. *N Engl J Med.* 1991;325:1761-1766.

13. Belley R, Bernard N, Cote M, Paquet F, Poitras J. Hyperbaric oxygen therapy in the management of two cases of hydrogen sulfide toxicity from liquid manure. *Can J Emerg Med.* 2005;7:257-261.
14. Bernacchi A, Myers R, Trump BF, Margello L. Protection of hepatocytes with hyperoxia against carbon tetrachloride induced injury. *Toxicol Pathol.* 1984;12:315-323.
15. Birky MM, Paabo M, Brown JE. Correlation of autopsy data and materials in the Tennessee jail fire. *Fire Safety J.* 1979;2:17-22.
16. Bitterman N, Talmi Y, Lerman A. The effect of hyperbaric oxygen on acute experimental sulfide poisoning in the rat. *Toxicol Appl Pharmacol.* 1986 84:325-328.
17. Breen PH, Isserles SA, Westley J, Roizen MF, Taitelman UZ. Effect of oxygen and sodium thiosulfate during combined carbon monoxide and cyanide poisoning. *Toxicol Appl Pharmacol.* 1995;134:229-234.
18. Brent JA, Rumack BH. Role of free radicals in toxic hepatic injury: I. Free radical biochemistry. *J Toxicol Clin Toxicol.* 1993;31:173-196.
19. Brown SD, Piantadosi CA. Hyperbaric oxygen for carbon monoxide poisoning. *Lancet.* 1989:1032-1033.
20. Brown SD, Piantadosi CA. Recovery of energy metabolism in rat brain after carbon monoxide hypoxia. *J Clin Invest.* 1991;89:666-672.
21. Burk RF, Lane JM, Patel K. Relationship of oxygen and glutathione in protection against carbon tetrachloride-induced hepatic microsomal lipid peroxidation and covalent binding in the rat. *J Clin Invest.* 1984;74:1996-2001.
22. Burk RF, Reiter R, Land JM. Hyperbaric oxygen protection against carbon tetrachloride hepatotoxicity in the rat: association with altered metabolism. *Gastroenterology.* 1986;90:812-818.
23. Burnett WW, King EG, Grace M. Hydrogen sulfide poisoning: review of 5 years' experience. *Can Med Assoc J.* 1977;117:1277-1280.
24. Burrows GE, Way JL. Cyanide intoxication in sheep: therapeutic value of oxygen or colbalt. *Am J Vet Res.* 1977;38:223-227.
25. Calabrese V, Mancuso C, Calvani M, Rizzarelli E, Butterfield D, Stella A. Nitric oxide in the central nervous system: neuroprotection versus neurotoxicity. *Nat Rev Neurosci.* 2007;8:766-775.
26. Carlson S, Jones J, Brown M. Prevention of hyperbaric-associated middle ear barotrauma. *Ann Emerg Med.* 1992;21:1468-1471.
27. Chang YL, Yang CC, Deng JF. Diverse manifestations of oral methylene chloride poisoning: report of 6 cases. *J Toxicol Clin Toxicol.* 1999;37:497-504.
28. Chen Q, Banick PD, Thom SR. Functional inhibition of rat polymorphonuclear leukocyte B2 integrins by hyperbaric oxygen is associated with impaired cGMP synthesis. *J Pharmacol Exp Therap.* 1996;276:929-933.
29. Choi S. Delayed neurologic sequelae in carbon monoxide intoxication. *Arch Neurol.* 1983;40:433-435.
30. Clark CJ, Campbell D, Reid WH. Blood carboxyhaemoglobin and cyanide levels in fire survivors. *Lancet.* 1981;1:1332-1335.
31. Clark J, Thom S. Oxygen under pressure. In: Brubakk AO, Neuman TS, eds. *Physiology and Medicine of Diving.* Philadelphia: Saunders; 2003:358-418.
32. Clark JM, Lambersten CJ. Rate of development of pulmonary O_2 toxicity in man during O_2 breathing at 2.0 atm absolute. *J Appl Physiol.* 1971;30: 739-768.
33. Clements KS, Vrabec JT, Mader JT. Complications of tympanostomy tubes inserted for facilitation of hyperbaric oxygen therapy. *Arch Otolaryngol Head Neck Surg.* 1998;124:278-280.
34. Coburn RF, Forman HJ. Carbon monoxide toxicity. In: Fishman AP, Farki LE, Geiger SR, eds. *Handbook of Physiology.* Baltimore: Williams & Wilkins; 1987:439-456.
35. Cope C. The importance of oxygen in the treatment of cyanide poisoning. *JAMA.* 1961;175:1061-1064.
36. Copeland AR. Accidental fire deaths: the 5-year metropolitan Dade County experience from 1979 to 1983. *Z Rechtsmed.* 1985;94:71-79.
37. Cramlet SH, Erickson HH, Gorman HA. Ventricular function following acute carbon monoxide exposure. *J Appl Physiol.* 1975;39:482-486.
38. Darke SG, King AM, Slack WK. Gas gangrene and related infection: classification, clinical features and aetiology, management and mortality. A report of 88 cases. *Br J Surg.* 1977;64:104-112.
39. Davis JC, Dunn JM, Heimbach RD. Hyperbaric medicine: patient selection, treatment procedures, and side-effects. In: Davis JC, Hunt TK, eds. *Problem Wounds.* New York: Elsevier; 1988:225-235.
40. Demchenko I, Atochin D, Gutsaeva D, et al. Contributions of nitric oxide synthase isoforms to pulmonary oxygen toxicity, local vs. mediated effects. *Am J Physiol Lung Cell Mol Physiol.* 2008;294:L984-L990.
41. Demchenko I, Piantadosi C. Nitric oxide amplifies the excitatory to inhibitory neurotransmitter imbalance accelerating oxygen seizures. *Undersea Hyperbaric Med.* 2006;33:169-174.
42. Demchenko I, Welty-Wolf K, Allen B, Piantadosi C. Similar but not the same: normobaric and hyperbaric pulmonary oxygen toxicity, the role of nitric oxide. *Am J Physiol Lung Cell Mol Physiol.* 2007;293:L229-L238.
43. Demchenko IT, Oury TD, Crapo JD, Piantadosi CA. Regulation of the brain's vascular responses to oxygen. *Circ Res.* 2002;91:1031-1037.
44. Dennog C, Gedik C, Wood S, Speit G. Analysis of oxidative DNA damage and HPRT mutations in humans after hyperbaric oxygen treatment. *Mutation Res.* 1999;431:351-359.
45. Dennog C, Hartmann A, Frey G, Speit G. Detection of DNA damage after hyperbaric oxygen (HBO) therapy. *Mutagenesis.* 1996;11:605-609.
46. Ducasse JL, Celsis P, Marc-Vergnes JP. Non-comatose patients with acute carbon monoxide poisoning: hyperbaric or normobaric oxygenation? *Undersea Hyperbaric Med.* 1995;22:9-15.
47. End E, Long CW. Oxygen under pressure in carbon monoxide poisoning. *J Ind Hyg Toxicol.* 1942;24:302-306.
48. Fagin J, Bradley J, Williams D. Carbon monoxide poisoning secondary to inhaling methylene chloride. *Br Med J.* 1980;281:1461.
49. Fisher AB, Forman HJ, Glass M. Mechanisms of pulmonary oxygen toxicity. *Lung.* 1984;162:255-259.
50. Friedman G, Froom P, Sazbon L. Apolipotrotein E-epsilon 4 genotype predicts a poor outcome in survivors of traumatic brain injury. *Neurology.* 1999;52:244-248.
51. Gerasimon G, Bennett S, Musser J, Rinard J. Acute hydrogen sulfide poisoning in a dairy farmer. *Clin Toxicol (Phila).* 2007;45:420-423.
52. Gesell L, Trott A. De novo cataract development following a standard course of hyperbaric oxygen therapy. *Undersea Hyperbaric Med.* 2007;34:389-392.
53. Gilmer B, Kilkenny J, Tomaszewski C, Watts JA. Hyperbaric oxygen does not prevent neurologic sequelae after carbon monoxide poisoning. *Acad Emerg Med.* 2002;9:1-8.
54. Ginsberg MD, Myers RE. Experimental carbon monoxide encephalopathy in the primate. I. Physiologic and metabolic aspects. *Arch Neurol.* 1974;30:202-208.
55. Goodhart GL. Patient treated with antidote kit and hyperbaric oxygen survives cyanide poisoning. *South Med J.* 1994;87:814-816.
56. Gorman DF, Clayton D, Gilligan JE, Webb RK. A longitudinal study of 100 consecutive admissions for carbon monoxide poisoning to the Royal Adelaide Hospital. *Anaesth Intens Care.* 1992;20:311-316.
57. Goulon M, Barois A, Rapin M, Nouailhat F, Grosbuis S, Labrousse J. Carbon monoxide poisoning and acute anoxia due to breathing coal gas and hydrocarbons. *Ann Med Interne (Paris).* (*J Hyperbaric Med.* 1986;1:23-41) 1969;120:335-349.
58. Gunn B, Wong R. Noxious gas exposure in the outback: two cases of hydrogen sulfide toxicity. *Emerg Med (Fremantle).* 2001;13:240-246.
59. Hall AH, Rumack BH. Hydrogen sulfide poisoning: an antidotal role for sodium nitrate? *Vet Hum Toxicol.* 1997;39:152-154.
60. Hampson N. Hyperbaric oxygen for carbon monoxide poisoning. *MJA.* 2000;172:141-142.
61. Hart GB, Lamb RC, Strauss MB. Gas gangrene: I. A collective review. *J Trauma.* 1983;23:991-1000.
62. Hart GB, Strauss MB. Central nervous system oxygen toxicity in a clinical setting. In: Bove AA, Bachrack AJ, Greenbaum LJ, eds. *Undersea and Hyperbaric Physiology IX.* Bethesda: Undersea and Hyperbaric Med Soc; 1987:695-699.
63. Hart GB, Strauss MB, Lennon PA, Whitcraft DD. Treatment of smoke inhalation by hyperbaric oxygen. *J Emerg Med.* 1985;3:211-215.
64. Hart GB, Strauss MB, Riker J. Vital capacity of quadriplegic patients treated with hyperbaric oxygen. *J Am Paraplegia Soc.* 1984;7:113-114.
65. Henry CR, Satran D, Lindgren B, Adkinson C, Nicholson CI, Henry TD. Myocardial injury and long-term mortality following moderate to severe carbon monoxide poisoning. *JAMA.* 2006;295:398-402.
66. Hopkins R, Weaver L, Valentine K, Mower C, Churchill S, Carlquist J. Apolipoprotein E genotype and response of carbon monoxide poisoning to hyperbaric oxygen treatment. *Am J Respir Crit Care Med.* 2008;176:1001-1006.
67. Horowitz BZ. Carboxyhemoglobinemia caused by inhalation of methylene chloride. *Am J Emerg Med.* 1986;4:48-51.
68. Hsiao. Delayed encephalopathy after carbon monoxide intoxication-long term prognosis and correlation of clinical manifestations and neuroimages. *Acta Neurol Taiwan.* 2004;13:64-70.
69. Hsu LH, Wang JH. Treatment of carbon monoxide poisoning with hyperbaric oxygen. *Chinese Med J.* 1996;58:407-413.
70. Ischiropoulos H, Beers MF, Ohnishi ST, Fisher D, Garner SE, Thom SR. Nitric oxide production and perivascular tyrosine nitration in brain after carbon monoxide poisoning in the rat. *J Clin Invest.* 1996;97:2260-2267.

71. Ishimaru H, Katoh A, Suzuki H, Fukuta T, Kameyama T, Nabeshima T. Effects of *N*-methyl-d-aspartate receptor antagonists on carbon monoxide-induced brain damage in mice. *J Pharmacol Exp Ther*. 1992;261:349-352.
72. Isom GE, Way JL. Effect of oxygen on cyanide intoxication. VI. Reactivation of cyanide inhibited glucose metabolism. *J Pharmacol Exp Ther*. 1974;189: 235-243.
73. Ivanov KP. The effect of elevated oxygen pressure on animals poisoned with potassium cyanide. *Pharmacol Toxicol*. 1959;22:476-479.
74. Jamieson D, Chance B, Cadenas E, Boveris A. The relation of free radical production to hyperoxia. *Annu Rev Physiol*. 1986;48:703-719.
75. Juurlink DN, Buckley NA, Stanbrook MB, Isbister GK, Bennett M, McGuigan MA. Hyperbaric oxygen for carbon monoxide poisoning. 2005;CD002041.
76. Kalns J, Lane J, Delgado A, et al. Hyperbaric oxygen exposure temporarily reduces Mac-1 mediated functions of human neutrophils. *Immunol Lett*. 2002;83:125-131.
77. Leikin JB, Kaufman D, Lipscomb JW. Methylene chloride: report of 5 exposures and 2 deaths. *Am J Emerg Med*. 1990;8:534-537.
78. Keenan H, Bratton S, Norkool D, Brogan T, Hampson N. Delivery of hyperbaric oxygen therapy to critically ill, mechanically ventilated children. *J Crit Care*. 1998;13:7-12.
79. Kihara K, Ueno S, Sakoda M, Aikou T. Effects of hyperbaric oxygen exposure on experimental hepatic ischemia reperfusion injury: relationship between its timing and neutrophil sequestration. *Liver Transpl*. 2005;11:1574-1580.
80. Kindwall EP. *Hyperbaric Medicine Practice*. Flagstaff, AZ: Best Publishing; 1994.
81. Kirk MA, Gerace R, Kulig KW. Cyanide and methemoglobin kinetics in smoke inhalation victims treated with the cyanide antidote kit. *Ann Emerg Med*. 1993;22:1413-1418.
82. Labrouche S, Javorschi S, Leroy D, Gbikpi-Benissan G, Freyburger G. Influence of hyperbaric oxygen on leukocyte functions and haemostasis in normal volunteer divers. *Thromb Res*. 1999;96:309-315.
83. Lamy M, Hauguet M. Fifty patients with carbon monoxide intoxication treated with hyperbaric oxygen therapy. *Acta Ahes Belgica*. 1969;1:49-53.
84. Langehennig PL, Seeler RA, Berman E. Paint removers and carboxyhemoglobin. *N Eng J Med*. 1981;295:1137.
85. Larcan A, Lambert H. Current epidemiological, clinical, biological, and therapeutic aspects of acute carbon monoxide intoxication. *Bull Acad Natl Med (Paris)*. 1981;165:471.
86. Lindenmann J, Matzi V, Kaufmann P, et al. Hyperbaric oxygenation in the treatment of life-threatening isobutyl nitrite-induced methemoglobinemia-a case report. *Inhalation Toxicol*. 2006;18:1047-1049.
87. Litovitz TL, Larkin RF, Myers RAM. Cyanide poisoning treated with hyperbaric oxygen. *Am J Emerg Med*. 1983;1:94-101.
88. Logue C. Hyperbaric Oxygen for Carbon Monoxide Poisoning, in Letter to the Editor, *C. Review*, Editor. 2006.
89. Lundquist P, Lennart R, Sorbo B. The role of hydrogen cyanide and carbon monoxide in fire casualties: a prospective study. *Forensic Sci Int*. 1989;43:9-14.
90. Lyne AJ. Ocular effects of hyperbaric oxygen. *Trans Ophthalmol Soc UK*. 1978;98:66-68.
91. Madden MR, Finkelstein JL, Goodwin CW. Respiratory care of the burn patient. *Clin Plast Surg*. 1986;13:29-38.
92. Maeda Y, Kawasaki Y, Jibiki I, Yamaguchi N, Matsuda H, Hisada K. Effect of therapy with oxygen under high pressure on regional cerebral blood flow in the interval form of carbon monoxide poisoning: observation from subtraction of technetium-99m HMPAOSPECT brain imaging. *Eur Neurol*. 1991;31:380-383.
93. Mahmud M, Kales S. Methylene chloride poisoning in a cabinet worker. *Environ Health Perspectives*. 1999;107:769-772.
94. Maloney G, Pakiela J. Characteristics of patients transported by an aeromedical service for acute toxicologic emergencies: a 5-year experience. *Air Med J*. 2008;27:48-50.
95. Martin JD, Thom SR. Vascular leukocyte sequestration in decompression sickness and prophylactic hyperbaric oxygen therapy in rats. *Aviat Space Environ Med*. 2002;73:565-569.
96. Marzella L, Muhvich K, Myers RAM. Effect of hyperoxia on liver necrosis induced by hepatotoxins. *Virchows Arch*. 1986;51:497-507.
97. Mathieu D, Nolf M, Durocher A, et al. Acute carbon monoxide poisoning risk of late sequelae and treatment by hyperbaric oxygen. *Clin Toxicol*. 1985;23:315-324.
98. Mathieu D, Wattel F, Mathieu-Nolf M, et al. Randomized prospective study comparing the effect of HBO versus 12 hours NBO in non-comatose CO poisoned patients. *Undersea Hyperbaric Med*. 1996;23(suppl):7.
99. Maurice T, Hiramatsu M, Kameyama T, Hasegawa T, Nabeshima T. Cholecystokinin-related peptides, after systemic or central administration, prevent carbon monoxide-induced amnesia in mice. *J Pharmacol Exp Ther*. 1994;269:665-673.
100. McCarron M, Muir K, Nicoll J. Prospective study of apolipoprotein E genotype and functional outcome following ischemic stroke. *Arch Neurol*. 2000;57:1480-1484.
101. Meyer BC. Experimentelle erfahrungen uber die kohlenoxydverguftung des zentralnervens systems. *Z Ges Neurol Psychiatr*. 1928;112:187-212.
102. Mileski WJ, Sikes P, Atiles L, Lightfoot E, Lipsky P, Baxter C. Inhibition of leukocyte adherence and susceptibility to infection. *J Surg Res*. 1993;54:349-354.
103. Mileski WJ, Winn RK, Vedder NB, Pohlman TH, Harlan JM, Rice CL. Inhibition of CD18-dependent neutrophil adherence reduces organ injury after hemorrhagic shock in primates. *Surgery*. 1990;108:206-212.
104. Mohler SR. Air crash survival: injuries and evacuation toxic hazards. *Aviat Space Environ Med*. 1975;46:86-88.
105. Montani S, Perret C. Oxygenation hyperbare dans l'intoxication experimentale au tetrachlorure de carbon. *Rev Fr Etudes Clin Biol*. 1967;12:274-278.
106. Moon R, DeLong E. Hyperbaric oxygen for carbon monoxide poisoning. *MJA*. 1999;170:197-198.
107. Moore SJ, Norris JC, Walsh DA, Hume AS. Antidotal use of methemoglobin forming cyanide antagonists in concurrent carbon monoxide/cyanide intoxication. *J Pharmacol Exp Ther*. 1987;242:70-73.
108. Myers R, Snyder S, Emhoff T. Subacute sequelae of carbon monoxide poisoning. *Ann Emerg Med*. 1985;14:1163-1167.
109. Nabeshima T, Katoh A, Ishimaru H, et al. Carbon monoxide-induced delayed amnesia, delayed neuronal death and change in acetylcholine concentration in mice. *J Pharm Exp Ther*. 1991;256:378-384.
110. Nikkanen H, Burns M. Severe hydrogen sulfide exposure in a working adolescent. *Pediatrics*. 2004;113:927-929.
111. Norkool DM, Kirkpatrick JN. Treatment of acute carbon monoxide poisoning with hyperbaric oxygen: a review of 115 cases. *Ann Emerg Med*. 1985;14:1168-1171.
112. Norris JC, Moore SJ, Hume AS. Synergistic lethality induced by the combination of carbon monoxide and cyanide. *Toxicology*. 1986;40:121-129.
113. Pace N, Strajman E, Walker EL. Acceleration of carbon monoxide elimination in man by high pressure oxygen. *Science*. 1950;111:652-654.
114. Palmquist BM, Philipson BO, Barr PO. Nuclear cataract and myopia during hyperbaric oxygen therapy. *Br J Ophthalmol*. 1984;68:113-117.
115. Peirce EC 2nd, Zacharias A, Alday JM Jr, Hoffman BA, Jacobson JH 2nd. Carbon monoxide poisoning: experimental hypothermic and hyperbaric studies. *Surgery*. 1972;72:229-237.
116. Pitt BR, Radford EP, Gurtner GH, Traystman RJ. Interaction of carbon monoxide and cyanide on cerebral circulation and metabolism. *Arch Environ Health*. 1979;34:354-359.
117. Plafki C, Peters P, Almeling M, Welslau W, Busch R. Complications and side effects of hyperbaric oxygen therapy. *Aviat Space Environ Med*. 2000;71:119-124.
118. Pott F, Westergaard P, Mortensen J, Jansen EC. Hyperbaric oxygen treatment and pulmonary function. *Undersea Hyperbaric Med*. 1999;26:225-228.
119. Raphael JC, Elkharrat D, Guincestre MCJ, et al. Trial of normobaric and hyperbaric oxygen for acute carbon monoxide intoxication. *Lancet*. 1989:414-419.
120. Rapin M, Got C, Le Gall JR. Effect de l'oxygene hyperbare sur la toxicite tetrachlorure de carbone chez le rat. *Rev Fr Etudes Clin Biol*. 1967;12:594-599.
121. Rioux J, Myers R. Hyperbaric oxygen for methylene chloride poisoning: report on two cases. *Ann Emerg Med*. 1989;18:691-695.
122. Roche L, Bertoye A, Vincent P. Comparison de deux groupes de vingt intoxications oxycarbonees traitees par oxygene normobare et hyperbare. *Lyon Med*. 1968;49:1483-1499.
123. Rothfuss A, Radermacher P, Speit G. Involvement of heme oxygenase-1 (HO-1) in the adaptive protection of human lymphocytes after hyperbaric oxygen (HBO) treatment. *Carcinogenesis*. 2001;22:1979-1985.
124. Rudge F. Treatment of methylene chloride induced carbon monoxide poisoning with hyperbaric oxygenation. *Mil Med*. 1990;155:570-572.
125. Rudge FW. Treatment of methylene chloride induced carbon monoxide poisoning with hyperbaric oxygen. *Mil Med*. 1990;155:570-572.
126. Satran D, Henry CR, Adkinson C, Nicholson CI, Bracha Y, Henry TD. Cardiovascular manifestations of moderate to severe carbon monoxide poisoning. *J Am Coll Cardiol*. 2005;45:1513-1516.
127. Saunders A, Strittmatter W, Schmechel D. Association of apolipoprotein E allele epsilon 4 with late-onset familial and sporadic Alzheimer's disease. *Neurology*. 1993;43:1467-1472.

128. Scheinkestel C, Bailey M, Myles P, et al. Hyperbaric or normobaric oxygen for acute carbon monoxide poisoning: a randomised controlled clinical trial. *MJA*. 1999;170:203-209.
129. Schiltz KL. Failure to assess motivation, need to consider psychiatric variables, and absence of comprehensive examination: a skeptical review of neuropsychologic assessment in carbon monoxide research. *Undersea Hyperbaric Med*. 2000;27:48-50.
130. Schmetterer L, Findl O, Strenn K, et al. Role of NO in the O_2 and CO_2 responsiveness of cerebral and ocular circulation in humans. *Am J Physiol (Regulatory Integrative Comp Physiol)*. 1997;273:R2005-R2012.
131. Scolnick B, Hamel D, Woolf AD. Successful treatment of life-threatening propionitrile exposure with sodium nitrite/sodium thiosulfate followed by hyperbaric oxygen. *J Occup Med*. 1993;35:577-580.
132. Sheehy M, Way JL. Effect of oxygen on cyanide intoxication: III Mithridate. *J Pharmacol Exp Ther*. 1968;161:163-168.
133. Shimosegawa E, Hatazawa J, Nagata K, et al. Cerebral blood flow and glucose metabolism measurements in a patient surviving one year after carbon monoxide intoxication. *J Nucl Med*. 1992;33:1696-1698.
134. Shusterman D, Alexeeff G, Hargis C, et al. Predictors of carbon monoxide and hydrogen cyanide exposure in smoke inhalation patients. *J Toxicol Clin Toxicol*. 1996;34:61-71.
135. Shusterman D, Quinlan P, Lowengart R, Cone J. Methylene chloride intoxication in a furniture refinisher. *J Occup Med*. 1990:451-454.
136. Silverman CS, Brenner J, Murtagh FR. Hemorrhagic necrosis and vascular injury in carbon monoxide poisoning: MR demonstration. *AJNR*. 1993;14:168-170.
137. Silverman SH, Purdue GF, Hunt JL, et al. Cyanide toxicity in burned patients. *J Trauma*. 1988;28:171-176.
138. Skene WG, Norman JN, Smith G. Effect of hyperbaric oxygen in cyanide poisoning. In: Brown IW, Cox B, eds. *Proceedings of the Third International Congress on Hyperbaric Medicine*. Washington, DC: National Academy of Sciences, National Research Council; 1966:705-710.
139. Sloan EP, Murphy DG, Hart R, et al. Complications and protocol considerations in carbon monoxide-poisoned patients who require hyperbaric oxygen therapy: report from a ten-year experience. *Ann Emerg Med*. 1989;18:629-634.
140. Smilkstein MJ, Bronstein AC, Pickett HM. Hyperbaric oxygen therapy for severe hydrogen sulfide poisoning. *J Emerg Med*. 1985:27-30.
141. Snyder J, Safir E, Summerville G, Middleberg R. Occupational fatality and persistent neurological sequelae after mass exposure to hydrogen sulfide. *Am J Emerg Med*. 1995;13:199-203.
142. Stamler JS, Jia L, Eu JP, et al. Blood flow regulation by S-nitrosohemoglobin in the physiological oxygen gradient. *Science*. 1997;276:2034-2037.
143. Stewart RD, Boettner EA, Southworth RR. Acute carbon tetrachloride intoxication. *JAMA*. 1963;183:994-997.
144. Stewart RD, Hake CL. Paint remover hazard. *JAMA*. 1976;235:398-401.
145. Stine RJ, Slosberg B, Beacham BE. Hydrogen sulfide intoxication. *Ann Intern Med*. 1976;85:756-758.
146. Tahepold P, Vaage J, Starkopf J, Valen G. Hyperoxia elicits myocardial protection through a nuclear factor kB-dependent mechanism in the rat heart. *J Thorac Cardiovasc Surg*. 2003;125:650-660.
147. Tahepold P, Valen G, Starkopf J, Kairane C, Zilmer M, Vaage J. Pretreating rats with hyperoxia attenuates inschemia-reperfusion injury of the heart. *Life Sci*. 2001;68:1629-1640.
148. Takano T, Miyazaki Y, Nashimoto I, Kobayashi K. Effect of hyperbaric oxygen on cyanide intoxication: in situ changes in intracellular oxidation reduction. *Undersea Biomed Res*. 1980;7:191-197.
149. Thom S, Bhopale V, Han S-T, Clark J, Hardy K. Intravascular neutrophil activation due to carbon monoxide poisoning. *Am J Respir Crit Care Med*. 2006;174:1239-1248.
150. Thom S, Bhopale V, Mancini J, Milovanova T. Actin S-nitrosylation inhibits neutrophil beta-2 integrin function. *J Biol Chem*. 2008;283:10822-10834.
151. Thom S, Bhopale V, Velazquez O, Goldstein L, Thom L, Buerk D. Stem cell mobilization by hyperbaric oxygen. *Am J Physiol Heart Circ Physiol*. 2006;290:H1378-H1386.
152. Thom SR. Functional inhibition of leukocyte B2 integrins by hyperbaric oxygen in carbon monoxide-mediated brain injury in rats. *Toxicol Appl Pharmacol*. 1993;123:248-256.
153. Thom SR. Hyperbaric oxygen therapy. *J Intensive Care Med*. 1989;4:58-74.
154. Thom SR. Learning dysfunction and metabolic defects in globus pallidus and hippocampus after CO poisoning in a rat model. *Undersea Hyperbaric Med*. 1997;23(Suppl):20.
155. Thom SR, Bhopale VM, Fisher D, Zhang J, Gimotty P. Delayed neuropathology after carbon monoxide poisoning is immune-mediated. *Proc Natl Acad Sci U S A*. 2004;101:13660-13665.
156. Thom SR, Fisher D, Zhang J, Bhopale VM, Cameron B, Buerk DG. Neuronal nitric oxide synthase and *N*-methyl-d-aspartate neurons in experimental carbon monoxide poisoning. *Toxicol Appl Pharmacol*. 2004;194:280-295.
157. Thom SR, Mendiguren I, Hardy K, et al. Inhibition of human neutrophil β_2-integrin-dependent adherence by hyperbaric O_2. *Am J Physiol*. 1997;272:C770-C777.
158. Thom SR, Taber RL, Mendiguren II, Clark JM, Hardy KR, Fisher AB. Delayed neuropsychologic sequelae after carbon monoxide poisoning: prevention by treatment with hyperbaric oxygen. *Ann Emerg Med*. 1995;25:474-480.
159. Thorsen E, Aanderud L, Aasen TB. Effects of a standard hyperbaric oxygen treatment protocol on pulmonary function. *Eur Respir J*. 1998;12:1442-1445.
160. Tjarnstrom J, Wikstrom T, Bagge U, Risberg B, Braide M. Effects of hyperbaric oxygen treatment on neutrophil activation and pulmonary sequestration in intestinal ischemia-reperfusion in rats. *Eur Surg Res*. 1999;31:147-154.
161. Tomaszewski CA, Thom SR. Use of hyperbaric oxygen in toxicology. *Emerg Med Clin N Am*. 1994:437-459.
162. Trapp WG, Lepawsky M. 100% survival in five life-threatening acute cyanide poisoning victims treated by a therapeutic spectrum including hyperbaric oxygen. Paper presented at the First European Conference on Hyperbaric Medicine, Amsterdam, 1983.
163. Truss CD, Killenberg PG. Treatment of carbon tetrachloride poisoning with hyperbaric oxygen. *Gastroenterology*. 1982;82:767-769.
164. Trytko B, Bennett M. Hyperbaric oxygen therapy: complication rates are much lower than authors suggest. *Br Med J*. 1999;318:1077-1078.
165. Ueno S, Tanabe G, Kihara K, et al. Early post-operative hyperbaric oxygen therapy modifies neutrophile activation. *Hepato Gastroenterology*. 1999;46:1798-1799.
166. Ushio-Fukai M, Alexander R. Reactive oxygen species as mediators of angiogenesis signaling. *Mol Cell Biochem*. 2004;264:85-97.
167. Van Hoesen K, Camporesi EM, Moon RE, et al. Should hyperbaric oxygen be used to treat the pregnant patient for acute carbon monoxide poisoning? A case report and literature review. *JAMA*. 1989;261:1039-1043.
168. Vicas I, Fortin S, Uptigrove OF. Hydrogen sulfide exposure treated with hyperbaric oxygen. *Vet Hum Toxicol*. 1989;31:353.
169. Wada K, Ito M, Miyazawa T, et al. Repeated hyperbaric oxygen induces ischemic tolerance in gerbil hippocampus. *Brain Res*. 1996;740:15-20.
170. Waisman D, Shupak A, Weisz G, Melamed Y. Hyperbaric oxygen therapy in the pediatric patient: the experience of the Israel Naval Medical Institute. *Pediatrics*. 1998;102:1-9.
171. Way JL. Cyanide intoxication and its mechanism of antagonism. *Annu Rev Pharmacol Toxicol*. 1984;24:451-481.
172. Way JL, End E, Sheehy MH, et al. Effect of oxygen on cyanide intoxication. *Toxicol Appl Pharmacol*. 1972;22:415-421.
173. Way JL, Gibbon SL, Sheehy M. Effect of oxygen on cyanide intoxication. I. Prophylactic protection. *J Pharmacol Exp Ther*. 1966;13:381-382.
174. Weaver L, Valentine K, Hopkins R. Carbon monoxide poisoning: risk factors for cognitive sequelae and the role of hyperbaric oxygen. *Am J Respir Crit Care Med*. 2007;176:491-497.
175. Weaver LK, Hopkins RO, Chan KJ, et al. Hyperbaric oxygen for acute carbon monoxide poisoning. *N Engl J Med*. 2002;347:1057-1067.
176. Wetherill HR. The occurrence of cyanide in the blood of fire victims. *J Forensic Sci*. 1966;11:167-173.
177. Whitcraft DD, Bailey TD, Hart GB. Hydrogen sulfide poisoning treated with hyperbaric oxygen. *J Emerg Med*. 1985;3:23-25.
178. Wong HP, Zamboni WA, Stephenson LL. Effect of hyperbaric oxygen on skeletal muscle necrosis following primary and secondary ischemia in a rat model. *Surgical Forum*. 1996:705-707.
179. Yang ZJ, Bosco G, Montante A, Ou XI, Camporesi EM. Hyperbaric O_2 reduces intestinal ischemia-reperfusion-induced TNF-alpha production and lung neutrophil sequestration. *Eur J Appl Physiol*. 2001;85:96-103.
180. Zamboni WA, Roth AC, Russell RC, Graham B, Suchy H, Kucan JO. Morphologic analysis of the microcirculation during reperfusion of ischemic skeletal muscle and the effect of hyperbaric oxygen. *Plast Reconstr Surg*. 1993;91.
181. Zearbaugh C, Gorman DF, Gilligan JE. Carbon tetrachloride/chloroform poisoning: case studies of hyperbaric oxygen in the treatment of lethal dose ingestion. *Undersea Biomed Res*. 1988;15:44.

CHAPTER 126

CYANIDE AND HYDROGEN SULFIDE

Christopher P. Holstege, Gary E. Isom, and Mark A. Kirk

Cyanide (CN)		
MW	=	26.02 daltons
Whole blood	<	1 μg/mL (38.5 μmol/L)
Concentrations: Airborne		
Immediately fatal	=	270 ppm
Life threatening	=	110 ppm (>30 min)
Hydrogen Sulfide (H_2S)		
MW	=	34.08 daltons
Concentrations: Airborne		
Odor threshold	=	0.02–0.13 ppm
Olfactory fatigue	=	100–150 ppm
Immediately fatal	=	700 ppm

CYANIDE POISONING

An emergency involving the diagnosis and management of patients exposed to cyanide is a potential scenario for any healthcare facility. Cyanide exposure is associated with smoke inhalation, laboratory mishaps, industrial incidents, suicide attempts, and criminal activity. Cyanide is a chemical group that consists of one atom of carbon bound to one atom of nitrogen by three molecular bonds (C≡N). Inorganic cyanides (also know as cyanide salts) contain cyanide in the anion form (CN^-) and are used in numerous industries, such as metallurgy, photographic developing, plastic manufacturing, fumigation, and mining. Common cyanide salts include sodium cyanide (NaCN) and potassium cyanide (KCN). Sodium salts react readily with water to form hydrogen cyanide. Organic compounds that have a cyano group bonded to an alkyl residue are called nitriles. For example, methyl cyanide is also known as acetonitrile (CH_3CN). Hydrogen cyanide (HCN) is a colorless gas at standard temperature and pressure with a reported bitter odor. Cyanogen gas, a dimer of cyanide, reacts with water and breaks down into the cyanide anion.

Many plants, such as *Manihot* spp, *Linum* spp, *Lotus* spp, *Prunus* spp, *Sorghum* spp, and *Phaseolus* spp, contain cyanogenic glycosides.[112] The *Prunus* species consisting of apricots, bitter almond, cherry, and peaches have pitted fruits containing the glucoside amygdalin. When ingested, amygdalin is biotransformed by intestinal β-*d*-glucosidase to glucose, aldehyde, and cyanide (Fig. 126–1). Laetrile, which contains amygdalin, has been inappropriately suggested to have antineoplastic properties. When laetrile is administered by intravenous (IV) infusion, amygdalin bypasses the necessary enzymes in the gastrointestinal (GI) tract to liberate cyanide and does not cause toxicity. However, when ingested, laetrile may cause cyanide poisoning.[48] Despite data demonstrating its lack of utility in the treatment of cancer, laetrile is still available via the Internet.

Cassava (*Manihot esculenta*) root is a major source of food for millions of people in the tropics. It is a hardy plant that can remain in the ground for up to 2 years and needs relatively little water to survive. Because the shelf life of a cassava root is very short after it is removed from the stem, cassava root must be processed and sent to market as soon as it is harvested. However, proper processing must occur to ensure the food's safety. Processed cassava is called *Gari.* Linamarin (2-hydroxyixo-butynitrite-β-D-glycoside) is the major cyanogenic glycoside in cassava roots. It is hydrolyzed to hydrogen cyanide and acetone in two steps during the processing of cassava roots.[126] Whereas soaking peeled cassava in water for a single day releases approximately 45% of the cyanogens, soaking for 5 days causes 90% loss. If processing is inefficient, linamarin and cyanohydrin, the immediate product of hydrolysis of linamarin, remain in the food.[87,88] Consumed linamarin is hydrolyzed to cyanohydrins by β-glucosidases of the microorganisms in the intestines. Cyanohydrins present in the food and formed from linamarin then dissociate spontaneously to cyanide in the alkaline pH of the small intestines.

Iatrogenic cyanide poisoning may occur during use of nitroprusside as a vasodilator given to reduce blood pressure and afterload. Each nitroprusside molecule contains five cyanide molecules, which are slowly released in vivo. If endogenous sulfate stores are depleted, as in a malnourished or postoperative patient, cyanide may accumulate even with therapeutic nitroprusside infusion rates (2–10 μg/kg/min).

HISTORY AND EPIDEMIOLOGY

In 1782, the Swedish chemist Carl Wilhelm Scheele first isolated hydrogen cyanide. He reportedly died from the adverse health effects of cyanide poisoning in 1786. Napoleon III was the first to use hydrogen cyanide in chemical warfare, and it was subsequently used on World War I battlefields. During World War II, cyanide (Zyklon B) caused more than 1 million deaths in Nazi gas chambers at Auschwitz, Buchenwald, and Majdanek. In 1978, KCN was used in a mass suicide led by Jim Jones of the People's Temple in Guyana, resulting in 913 deaths. Other notorious suicide cases include Wallace Carothers, Herman Goring, Heinrich Himmler, and Ramon Sampedro. In 1982, seven deaths resulted from consumption of cyanide-tainted acetaminophen in Chicago that subsequently led to the requirement of tamper-resistant pharmaceutical packaging.[30,38] Cyanide has also been used for illicit euthanasia.[18]

Cyanide poisoning accounted for 242 of the more than 2 million exposures reported to the American Association of Poison Control Centers (AAPCC) in 2007.[23] The majority of reported cyanide exposures are unintentional. These events frequently involve chemists or technicians working in laboratories where cyanide salts are common reagents.[17] The potential for cyanide poisoning also exists after smoke inhalation.[6,31,107] The combustion of materials such as wool, silk, synthetic rubber, and polyurethane releases cyanide. Ingestion of cyanogenic chemicals (ie, acetonitrile, acrylonitrile, and propionitrile) is another source of cyanide poisoning.[116] Acetonitrile (C_2H_3N) and acrylonitrile (C_3H_3N) are themselves nontoxic, but biotransformation via cytochrome P450 liberates cyanide (see Fig. 126–1).[128]

PHARMACOLOGY

The dose of cyanide required to produce toxicity is dependent on the form of cyanide (ie, gas or salt), the duration, and the route of exposure. However, cyanide is an extremely potent toxin with even small exposures lead to symptoms. For example, an adult oral lethal dose of KCN is approximately 200 mg. An airborne concentration of 270 ppm (μg/mL) of hydrogen cyanide (HCN) may be immediately fatal, and exposures above 110 ppm for more than 30 minutes are generally considered life threatening. The current Occupational Safety and Health Administration (OSHA) permissible exposure limit (PEL) for both hydrogen cyanide and cyanogen is 10 ppm as an 8-hour time-weighted average (TWA) concentration. The American Conference of

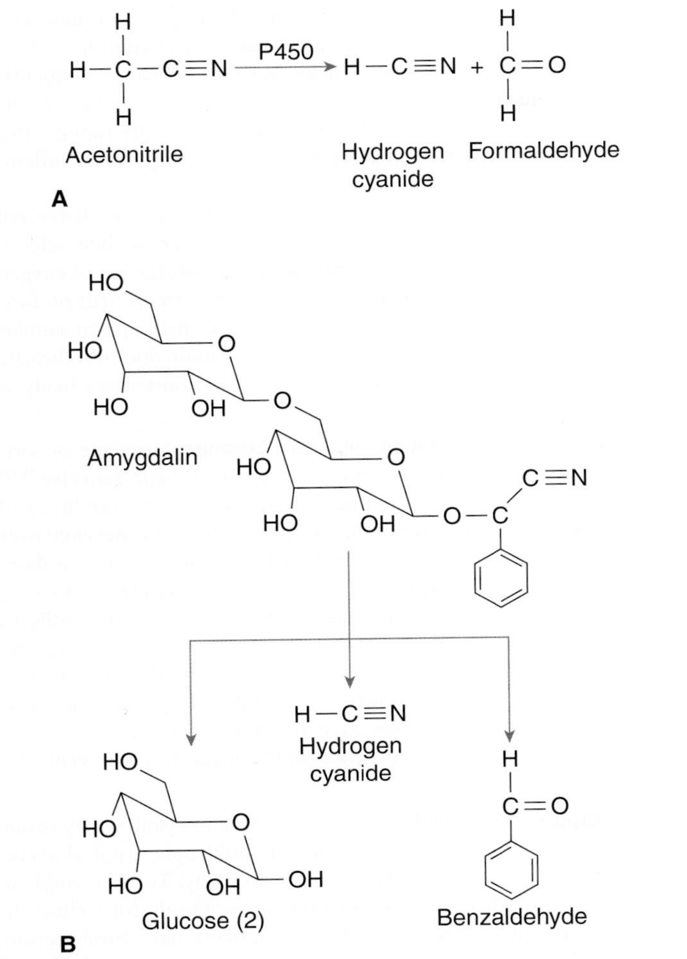

Acetonitrile —P450→ Hydrogen cyanide + Formaldehyde

A

Amygdalin → Glucose (2) + Hydrogen cyanide + Benzaldehyde

B

FIGURE 126–1. Biotransformation of cyanogens (**A**) acetonitrile and (**B**) amygdalin to cyanide.

Governmental Industrial Hygienists has assigned a ceiling limit value of 4.7 ppm, which should not be exceeded during any part of the working exposure.

Acute toxicity occurs through a variety of routes, including inhalation, ingestion, dermal, and parenteral. Hydrogen cyanide readily crosses membranes because it has a low molecular weight (27 daltons) and is nonionized. After absorption and dissolution in blood, cyanide exists in equilibrium as the cyanide anion (CN^-) and undissociated HCN. Hydrogen cyanide is a weak acid with a pK_a of 9.21. Therefore, at physiologic pH 7.4, it exists primarily as HCN. Rapid diffusion across alveolar membranes followed by direct distribution to target organs accounts for the rapid lethality associated with HCN inhalation.

PHARMACOKINETICS AND TOXICOKINETICS

Cyanide is eliminated from the body by multiple pathways. The major route for detoxification of cyanide is the enzymatic conversion to thiocyanate. Two sulfur transferase enzymes, rhodanese (thiosulfate-cyanide sulfurtransferase) and β-mercaptopyruvate-cyanide sulfurtransferase, catalyze this reaction. The primary pathway for metabolism is rhodanese, which is widely distributed throughout the body and has the highest concentration in the liver. This enzyme catalyzes the transfer of a sulfane sulfur from a sulfur donor, such as thiosulfate, to cyanide to form thiocyanate. In acute poisoning, the limiting factor in cyanide detoxification by rhodanese is the availability of adequate quantities of sulfur donors. The endogenous stores of sulfur are rapidly depleted, and cyanide metabolism slows. Hence, the efficacy of sodium thiosulfate as an antidote stems from its normalization of the metabolic inactivation of cyanide. The sulfation of cyanide is essentially irreversible, and the sulfation product thiocyanate has relatively little inherent toxicity. Thiocyanate is eliminated in urine. A number of minor pathways of metabolism (<15% of total) account for cyanide elimination, including conversion to 2-aminothiazoline-4-carboxylic acid, incorporation into the one-carbon metabolic pool, or in combination with hydroxocobalamin to form cyanocobalamin.

Limited human data regarding the cyanide elimination half-life are available. Elimination appears to follow first-order kinetics,[69] although it varies widely in reports (range, 1.2–66 hours).[6,47,69] Disparity in values may result from the number of samples used to perform calculations and the effects of antidotal treatment. The volume of distribution of the cyanide anion varies according to species and investigator, with 0.075 L/kg reported in rats.[35]

PATHOPHYSIOLOGY

Cyanide is an inhibitor of multiple enzymes, including succinic acid dehydrogenase, superoxide dismutase, carbonic anhydrase, and cytochrome oxidase.[130] Cytochrome oxidase is an iron-containing metalloenzyme essential for oxidative phosphorylation and hence aerobic energy production. It functions in the electron transport chain within mitochondria, converting catabolic products of glucose into adenosine triphosphate (ATP). Cyanide induces cellular hypoxia by inhibiting cytochrome oxidase at the cytochrome a_3 portion of the electron transport chain (Fig. 126–2).[93,130] Hydrogen ions that normally would have combined with oxygen at the terminal end of the chain are no longer incorporated. Thus, despite sufficient oxygen supply, oxygen cannot be used, and ATP molecules are no longer formed.[72] Unincorporated hydrogen ions accumulate, contributing to acidemia.

Hyperlactemia occurs after cyanide poisoning because of failure of aerobic energy metabolism. During aerobic conditions, when the electron transport chain is functional, lactate is converted to pyruvate by mitochondrial lactate dehydrogenase. In this process, lactate donates hydrogen moieties that reduce nicotinamide adenine dinucleotide (NAD^+) to nicotinamide adenine dinucleotide (NADH). Pyruvate then enters the tricarboxylic acid cycle, with resulting ATP formation. When cytochrome a_3 within the electron transport chain is inhibited by cyanide, there is a relative paucity of NAD^+ and predominance of NADH, favoring the reverse reaction, in which pyruvate is converted to lactate.[108]

Cyanide is a potent neurotoxin. It exhibits a particular affinity for regions of the brain with high metabolic activity.[96,135] Central nervous system (CNS) injury occurs via several mechanisms, including impaired oxygen utilization, oxidant stress, and enhanced release of excitatory

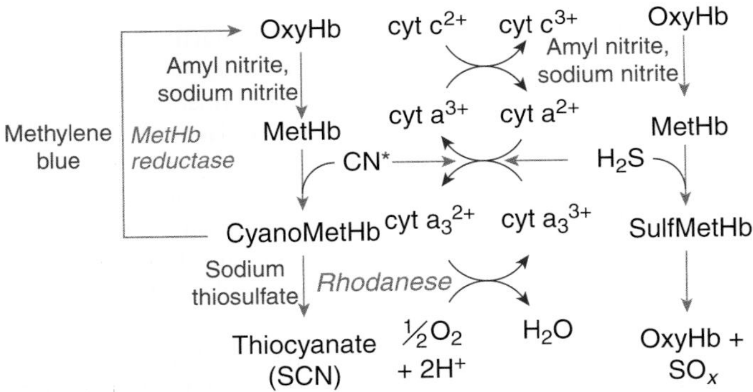

FIGURE 126–2. Pathway of cyanide and hydrogen sulfide toxicity and detoxification. * = hydroxocobalamin.

neurotransmitters. Cranial imaging of survivors of cyanide poisoning reveals that injury occurs in the most oxygen-sensitive areas of the brain, such as the basal ganglia, cerebellum, and sensorimotor cortex.[104]

Cyanide enhances *N*-methyl-D-aspartate (NMDA) receptor activity and directly activates the NMDA receptor,[3,91] which increases release of glutamate[90] and inhibits voltage-dependent magnesium blockade of the NMDA receptor.[136] This NMDA receptor stimulation results in Ca^{2+} entry into the cytosol of neurons. Cyanide also activates voltage-sensitive calcium channels[59] and mobilizes Ca^{2+} from intracellular stores.[73,97] As a result, cytosolic Ca^{2+} increases and activates a series of biochemical reactions that lead to the generation of reactive oxygen species (ROS) and nitrous oxide.[66,77,105] These ROS initiate peroxidation of cellular lipids, which together with cyanide-induced inhibition of the respiratory chain adversely affect mitochondrial function, initiating cytochrome c release and execution of apoptosis, necrosis, and subsequent neurodegeneration.[5,59,95,106] Experimental studies demonstrate that NMDA inhibitors such as dextrorphan and dizocilpine, antioxidants, and cyclooxygenase inhibitors protect neurons against cyanide-induced damage.[56,71,127]

Sulfurtransferase metabolism via rhodanese is crucial for detoxification. However, the aforementioned cyanide-induced metabolic derangement may decrease enzyme detoxification. Decreased ATP and ROS and increased cytosolic calcium stimulate protein kinase C activity, which in turn inactivates rhodanese.[2]

CLINICAL MANIFESTATIONS

Acute Exposure to Cyanide The amount, duration of exposure, route of exposure, and premorbid condition of the individual influence the time to onset and severity of illness. A critical combination of these factors overwhelms endogenous detoxification pathways, allowing cyanide to diffusely affect cellular function within the body. No reliable pathognomonic symptom or toxic syndrome is associated with acute cyanide poisoning.[45] Clinical manifestations reflect rapid dysfunction of oxygen-sensitive organs, with CNS and cardiovascular findings predominating. The time to onset of symptoms typically is seconds with inhalation of gaseous HCN or IV injection of a water-soluble cyanide salt and several minutes after ingestion of an inorganic cyanide salt. The clinical effects of cyanogenic chemicals often are delayed, and the time course varies among individuals (range, 3–24 hours), depending on their rate of biotransformation.[116] Clinically apparent cyanide toxicity may occur within hours to days of initiating nitroprusside infusion, although concurrent administration of thiosulfate or hydroxocobalamin may prevent toxicity (see Chap. 62).[102]

CNS signs and symptoms are typical of progressive hypoxia and include headache, anxiety, agitation, confusion, lethargy, seizures, and coma. A centrally mediated tachypnea occurs initially followed by bradypnea.

Cardiovascular responses to cyanide are complex. Studies of isolated heart preparations and intact animal models show that the principal cardiac insult is slowing of rate and loss of contractile force. Several reflex mechanisms, including catecholamine release and central vasomotor activity, may modulate myocardial performance and vascular response in patients with cyanide poisoning. In laboratory investigations, a brief period of increased inotropy caused by reflex compensatory mechanisms occurs before myocardial depression. Clinically, an initial period of bradycardia and hypertension may occur followed by hypotension with reflex tachycardia, but the terminal event is consistently bradycardia and hypotension. Ventricular dysrhythmias do not appear to be an important factor.

Pulmonary edema is found at necropsy.[45] In cyanide poisoning, acute lung injury (ALI) may be neurogenic in origin or result from membrane leak from direct pneumocyte toxicity. Inhalation of HCN may be associated with mild corrosive injury to the respiratory tract mucosa.

GI toxicity may occur after ingestion of inorganic cyanide and cyanogens and includes abdominal pain, nausea, and vomiting. These symptoms are caused by hemorrhagic gastritis, which is frequently identified on necropsy, and are thought to be secondary to the corrosive nature of cyanide salts. However, if death occurs rapidly, this gastritis may not be present at autopsy because development of inflammation occurs over time.[45]

Cutaneous manifestations may vary. Traditionally, a cherry-red skin color is described as a result of increased venous hemoglobin oxygen saturation, which results from decreased utilization of oxygen at the tissue level.[108] This phenomenon may be more evident on funduscopic examination, where veins and arteries may appear similar in color. Despite the inference in the name, cyanide does not directly cause cyanosis. The occurrence of cyanosis in some cases likely is secondary to shock.[123]

Delayed Clinical Manifestations of Acute Exposure Survivors of serious, acute poisoning may develop delayed neurologic sequelae.[75,104] Parkinsonian symptoms, including dystonia, dysarthria, rigidity, and bradykinesia, are most common. Symptoms typically develop over weeks to months, but subtle findings may be present within a few days. Head computed tomography (CT) and magnetic resonance imaging (MRI) consistently reveal basal ganglia damage to the globus pallidus, putamen, and hippocampus, with radiologic changes appearing several weeks after onset of symptoms. Whether delayed manifestations result from direct cellular injury or secondary hypoxia is unclear. Extrapyramidal manifestations may progress or resolve. Response to pharmacotherapy with antiparkinsonian medications is generally disappointing.

Chronic Exposure to Cyanide Chronic exposure to cyanide may result in insidious syndromes, including tobacco amblyopia, tropical ataxic neuropathy, and Leber hereditary optic neuropathy. Tobacco amblyopia is a progressive loss of visual function that occurs almost exclusively in men who smoke cigarettes. Affected smokers have lower serum cyanocobalamin and thiocyanate concentrations than unaffected smoking counterparts, suggesting a reduced ability to detoxify cyanide. Cessation of smoking and administration of hydroxocobalamin often reverse symptoms.

Tropical ataxic neuropathy is a demyelinating disease associated with improperly processed cassava consumption.[86,113] Neurologic manifestations include Parkinson's disease, spastic paraparesis, sensory ataxia, optic atrophy, and sensorineural hearing loss.[124] Concomitant dermatitis and glossitis suggest an association of high dietary cassava with low vitamin B_{12} intake. Elevated thiocyanate concentrations in affected individuals further implicate cyanide as the cause. Removal of dietary cassava and institution of vitamin B_{12} therapy alleviates symptoms. Leber hereditary optic atrophy, a condition of subacute visual failure affecting men, is thought to be caused by rhodanese deficiency.[41]

Chronic exposure to cyanide is associated with thyroid disorders.[1] Thiocyanate is a competitive inhibitor of iodide entry into the thyroid, thereby causing the formation of goiters and the development of hypothyroidism.[65] Chronic exposure to cyanide in animals is associated with hydropic degeneration in hepatocytes and epithelial cells of the renal proximal tubules; however, these morphologic lesions are not linked to functional alternations.[112]

DIAGNOSTIC TESTING

Because of nonspecific symptoms and delay in laboratory cyanide confirmation, clinicians must rely on historical circumstances and some initial findings to raise suspicion of cyanide poisoning and institute therapy (Table 126–1).

TABLE 126–1. Cyanide Poisoning: Emergency Management Guidelines

When to suspect cyanide poisoning
- Sudden collapse of a laboratory or industrial worker
- Fire victim with coma or metabolic acidosis
- Suicide attempt with unexplained coma or metabolic acidosis
- Ingestion of artificial nail remover
- Ingestion of seeds or pits from *Prunus* spp.
- Patient with altered mental status, metabolic acidosis, and tachyphylaxis to nitroprusside

Supportive care
- Control airway, ventilate, and give 100% oxygen
- Crystalloids and vasopressors for hypotension
- Administer $NaHCO_3$; titrate according to blood gas analysis and serum HCO_3^-

Antidotes
1. *Hydroxycobalamin*
   - Initial adult dose: 5 g IV over 15 minutes
2. *Cyanide antidote kit*
   - Amyl nitrite pearls are included in the kit for prehospital use; for hospital management, sodium nitrite is the preferred methemoglobin inducer and is given in lieu of the pearls
   - Give sodium nitrite ($NaNO_2$) as a 3% solution over 2–4 minutes IV:
     - Adult dose: 10 mL (300 mg)
     - Pediatric dose: See Table 126-2; if hemoglobin is unknown, presume 12-g dosing

Caution: Monitor blood pressure frequently and treat hypotension by slowing the infusion rate and giving crystalloids and vasopressors. Obtain methemoglobin level 30 minutes after dose and consider possible excessive methemoglobin formation if the patient deteriorates during therapy.

Give sodium thiosulfate (NaS_2O_3) as a 25% solution IV: Adult dose: 50 mL (12.5 g) Pediatric dose: 1.65 mL/kg

Decontamination
- Protect healthcare providers from contamination
- Cutaneous: Carefully remove all clothing and flush the skin
- Ingestion: Lavage with an orogastric tube and instill 1 g/kg of activated charcoal

Laboratory
- Arterial blood gas
- Electrolytes and glucose concentrations
- Blood lactate concentrations
- Whole-blood cyanide concentration (for later confirmation only)
- Consider a central venous blood gas for AV O_2 difference

ABG, arterial blood gas; AV, arteriovenous; IV, intravenous.

Laboratory findings suggestive of cyanide poisoning reflect the known metabolic abnormalities, which include metabolic acidosis, elevated lactate concentration, and increased anion gap. Elevated venous oxygen saturation results from reduced tissue extraction.[60] A venous oxygen saturation above 90% from superior vena cava or pulmonary artery blood indicates decreased oxygen utilization. This finding is not specific for cyanide and may represent cellular poisoning from other xenobiotics such as carbon monoxide, clenbuterol, hydrogen sulfide, and sodium azide or medical conditions such as sepsis, high-output cardiac syndromes, and left-to-right intracardiac shunts.

Lactic acidosis is found in numerous critical illnesses and typically is a nonspecific finding. However, a significant association exists between blood cyanide and serum lactate concentrations.[11] In a small group of patients in whom the diagnosis of cyanide poisoning was strongly suspected clinically, a serum lactate concentration above 72 mg/dL (8 mmol/L) was associated with sensitivity of 94%, specificity of 70%, positive predictive value of 64%, and negative predictive value of 98% for a blood cyanide concentration above 1.0 μg/mL. Arterial blood gas (ABG) analysis of whole blood may provide additional information. Arterial pH correlates inversely with cyanide concentration.[7] The finding of a narrow arterial–venous oxygen difference also may suggest cyanide toxicity.

Cyanide results in nonspecific electrocardiographic findings. Bradycardia, tachycardia, myocardial injury pattern, or atrioventricular conduction block may occur.

Blood cyanide determination can confirm toxicity, but this determination is not available in a sufficiently rapid manner to affect initial treatment. Whole blood or serum usually is analyzed. In mammals, including primates, whole-blood concentrations are twice serum concentrations[9] as a result of cyanide sequestration in red blood cells. Background whole-blood concentrations in nonsmokers range between 0.02 and 0.5 μg/mL.[49,54] Higher blood concentrations suggest toxicity. Coma and respiratory depression are associated with concentrations above 2.5 μg/mL, and death is associated with concentrations above 3 μg/mL. Detecting urinary cyanide is difficult, and urinary thiocyanate is a more readily detectable and useful marker of cyanide exposure. Serum thiocyanate concentrations are of little value in assessing patients with acute poisoning because of little correlation with symptoms but are useful in confirming exposure.

A semiquantitative assay that uses calorimetric paper test strips may immediately detect cyanide. Cyantesmo test strips currently are used by water treatment facilities to detect cyanide. An investigation of the utility of these strips in clinical practice found that the test strips incrementally increased to a deep blue color over a progressively longer portion of the test strip with increasing concentrations of cyanide.[100] These strips accurately and rapidly detected CN concentrations above 1 μg/mL in a semiquantifiable manner.

MANAGEMENT

Because cyanide poisoning is rare, it is easy to overlook the diagnosis unless there is an obvious history of exposure. Thus, the most critical step in treatment is considering the diagnosis in high-risk situations (see Table 126-1) and initiating empiric therapy with 100% oxygen and either hydroxocobalamin or the cyanide antidote kit. The initial care (see Table 126-1) of a cyanide-poisoned patient begins by directing attention to airway patency, ventilatory support, and oxygenation. Acidemia should be treated with adequate ventilation and sodium bicarbonate administration.[26]

IV access should be rapidly obtained and blood samples sent for renal function, glucose, and electrolyte determinations. A whole-blood cyanide concentration can be obtained for later confirmation of exposure. ABG analysis and serum lactate concentration will help assess the patient's acid–base status. Initiation of crystalloid and infusion of vasopressor for hypotension are warranted.

First responders should exercise extreme caution when entering potentially hazardous areas such as chemical plants and laboratories where a previously healthy person is "found down." Exposure to cyanide may occur by multiple routes, including ingestion, inhalation, dermal, and parenteral. For patients with inhalation exposure, removal from the area of exposure is critical. Further decontamination is generally unnecessary. Decontamination of the cyanide-poisoned patient occurs concurrently with initial resuscitation. The healthcare provider should always be protected from potential dermal contamination by using personal protective devices such as water-impervious gowns, gloves, and eyewear. For patients with cutaneous exposure, the healthcare provider should remove the patient's clothing, brush off any powder from the skin, and flush the skin with water. Particular attention should be given to open wounds because CN^- or HCN is readily absorbed through abraded skin.

Instillation of activated charcoal often is considered ineffective because of low binding of cyanide (1 g of activated charcoal only adsorbs 35 mg of cyanide). However, a potentially lethal oral dose of cyanide (ie, a few hundred milligrams) is within the adsorptive capacity of a 1-g/kg dose of activated charcoal. Prophylactic activated charcoal administration improved survival in animals given an LD_{100} dose of KCN.[70] Based on the potential benefits and minimal risks, activated charcoal may be considered in the patient with an intact protected airway.

Either hydroxocobalamin or the cyanide antidote kit should be administered as soon as cyanide poisoning is suspected. Hydroxocobalamin, a vitamin B_{12} precursor, is now available in multiple countries for cyanide poisoning.[16] In 2006, it was approved by the U.S. Food and Drug Administration (FDA). Hydroxocobalamin is a metalloprotein with a central cobalt atom that complexes cyanide, forming cyanocobalamin (vitamin B_{12}). Cyanocobalamin is eliminated in the urine or releases the cyanide moiety at a rate sufficient to allow detoxification by rhodanese. One molecule of hydroxocobalamin binds one molecule of cyanide, yielding a molecular weight binding ratio of 50:1. The adult starting dose is 5 g administered by IV infusion over 15 minutes. Depending on the severity of the poisoning and the clinical response, a second dose of 5 g may be administered by IV infusion for a total dose of 10 g. Hydroxocobalamin has few adverse effects, which include allergic reaction and a transient reddish discoloration of the skin, mucous membranes, and urine.[19,24,50] No hemodynamic adverse effects other than a potential transient increase in blood pressure are observed[10,103] (see Antidotes in Depth A40: Hydroxocobalamin).

The cyanide antidote kit contains amyl nitrite, sodium nitrite, and sodium thiosulfate. Both thiosulfate and nitrite individually have antidotal efficacy when given alone in animal models of cyanide poisoning, but they have even greater benefit when they are given in combination.[31a] Thiosulfate donates the sulfur atoms necessary for rhodanese-mediated cyanide biotransformation to thiocyanate. The mechanism of nitrite is less clear. The traditional rationale relies on the ability of nitrite to generate methemoglobin. Because cyanide has a higher affinity for methemoglobin than for cytochrome a_3, cytochrome oxidase function is restored. However, improved hepatic blood flow and nitric oxide formation are alternate explanations (Antidotes in Depth A38: Sodium and Amyl Nitrites, A39: Sodium Thiosulfate, and A40: Hydroxocobalamin). Amyl nitrite is contained within glass pearls that are crushed and intermittently inhaled or intermittently introduced into the ventilator system to initiate methemoglobin formation. The amyl nitrite pearls are reserved for cases in which IV access is delayed or not possible. IV sodium nitrite is preferred and is supplied as a 10-mL volume of 3% solution (300 mg). The outdated goal of IV nitrite therapy is to achieve a methemoglobin concentration of 20% to 30%. This concentration is not based on cyanide treatment data but represents the maximum tolerated concentration without adverse symptoms from methemoglobinemia in a healthy individual. Clinical response is reported at lower methemoglobin concentrations of 3.6% to 9.2%. These reports are not conclusive because levels typically are not drawn serially, and peak concentrations may be misrepresented. Also, methemoglobin concentrations do not include cyanmethemoglobin. Therefore, lower-than-expected methemoglobin concentrations may represent indirect evidence of cyanide poisoning. Adverse effects of nitrites include excessive methemoglobin formation and, because of potent vasodilation, hypotension and tachycardia. Avoiding rapid infusion, monitoring blood pressure, and adhering to dosing guidelines limit adverse effects. Because of the potential for excessive methemoglobinemia during nitrite treatment, pediatric dosing guidelines are available.[11] Based on the premise that nitrite oxidizes hemoglobin on a mole-for-mole basis, doses were calculated for various hemoglobin concentrations (Table 126–2). These values are useful if the patient is known to be anemic. However, when giving nitrite empirically, treatment is based on a presumed 12-g hemoglobin concentration. The practitioner should not delay treatment while awaiting a hemoglobin measurement. Sodium thiosulfate is the second component of the cyanide antidote kit. It is supplied as 50 mL of 25% solution (12.5 g). It is a substrate for the reaction catalyzed by rhodanese that is essentially irreversible, converting a highly toxic entity to a relatively harmless compound. However, thiocyanate does have its own toxicity in the presence of renal failure, including abdominal pain, vomiting, rash, and CNS dysfunction.[34] Thiosulfate itself is not associated with significant adverse reactions. The pediatric dose of thiosulfate is adjusted for weight.

TABLE 126–2. Cyanide Management: Pediatric Sodium Nitrite Guidelines[a]

Hemoglobin (g)	$NaNO_2$ (mg/kg)	3% $NaNO_2$ solution (mL/kg)
7.0	5.8	0.19
8.0	6.6	0.22
9.0	7.5	0.25
10.0	8.3	0.27
11.0	9.1	0.30
12.0	10.0	0.33
13.0	10.8	0.36
14.0	11.6	0.39

[a] Pediatric thiosulfate dose: 1.65 mL/kg of 25% solution.

In Europe, 4-dimethylaminophenol (4-DMAP), rather than sodium nitrite, is the methemoglobin-inducer of choice. It generates methemoglobin more rapidly than sodium nitrite, with peak methemoglobin concentrations at 5 minutes after 4-DMAP rather than 30 minutes after sodium nitrite. The dose of 4-DMAP is 3 mg/kg and is coadministered with thiosulfate. As with sodium nitrite, its major adverse effect is excessive methemoglobin formation and the potential for hypotension. Cobalt in the form of dicobalt edetate has been used as a cyanide chelator, but its usefulness is limited by serious adverse effects such as hypotension, cardiac dysrhythmias, decreased cerebral blood flow, and angioedema.[21,79] Stroma-free methemoglobin, oxidized hemoglobin from which the cell membrane has been removed, is an investigational therapy. It attenuates lethality and prevents hemodynamic changes in animal models.[20,115] The advantage of this treatment lies in providing exogenous methemoglobin to bind cyanide without compromising the oxygen-carrying capacity of native hemoglobin, and removal of the cell membrane eliminates antigenicity. Dihydroxyacetone (DHA) is an investigational antidote that restores mitochondrial respiration inhibited by cyanide in isolated rat hepatocytes.[81] It also diminishes cyanide lethality in animal models and has synergistic effects with thiosulfate.[80,82] DHA binds readily to cyanide to form a cyanohydrin, but this binding is reversible, and cyanide's clinical effects reappear between 1 and 24 hours without readministration.[80] α-Ketoglutarate is another investigational antidote.[14,52] It rapidly complexes cyanide to form a cyanohydrin.[103] Pretreatment with α-ketoglutarate reduced lethality and increased sodium thiosulfate efficacy in animal studies.[15,37,58,83]

The advantage of α-ketoglutarate is direct binding of cyanide without generation of methemoglobin. Preliminary evidence demonstrates that α-ketoglutarate at a dose offering maximum antidotal efficacy is nontoxic and potentially safe for treatment of patients with cyanide poisoning.[13] Cobalamin has been used both prophylactically and therapeutically to treat experimental cyanide toxicity, and when given at high enough doses, it has rescued animals from cyanide-induced apnea and coma.[22] Cobalamin has been used in France to treat human cyanide exposure, either alone or combined with sodium thiosulfate. Cobinamide has a much greater affinity for cyanide ion than cobalamin.[80]

In animal models, the antioxidant vitamins A, C, and E diminish the extent of tissue damage caused by subacute cyanide intoxication.[85] This is especially important in the tropics, where the majority of dietary staples are cyanophoric crops such as cassava.

Patients who do not survive cyanide poisoning are suitable organ donors. The heart, liver, kidneys, pancreas, cornea, skin, and bone have been successfully transplanted after cyanide poisoning.[40]

HYDROGEN SULFIDE POISONING

HISTORY AND EPIDEMIOLOGY

Hydrogen sulfide (H_2S) exposures are often dramatic and can be fatal. The AAPCC's National Poison Data System reported only 1229 exposures in 2007 (see Chap. 135). Only 317 of these exposures required evaluation at a healthcare facility, 77 reported moderate or major effects, and 13 deaths occurred.[23] Over a 10-year period from 1983 to 1992, 5563 exposures and 29 deaths attributed to hydrogen sulfide were reported in the national poison center database.[111] Most often, serious consequences of hydrogen sulfide exposures occur through workplace exposures but are also implicated in environmental disasters and most recently in suicides.

Hydrogen sulfide is produced naturally by bacterial decomposition of proteins and is used or produced in many industrial activities. Industrial sources of hydrogen sulfide include pulp paper mills, heavy-water production, the leather industry, roofing asphalt tanks, vulcanizing of rubber, viscose rayon production, and coke manufacturing from coal.[32] Hydrogen sulfide is a major industrial hazard in oil and gas production, particularly in sour gas fields (natural gas containing sulfur). Decay of sulfur-containing products such as fish, sewage, and manure also produces hydrogen sulfide. Several farm workers and rescuers have died from exposure to hydrogen sulfide generated in liquid manure pits. OSHA records show 80 occupationally related fatalities between 1984 and 1994.[42] Between 1990 and 1999, hydrogen sulfide poisoning was associated with the deaths of 18% of U.S. construction workers killed by toxic inhalation.[36] Many died while working in confined spaces. Poisoned workers are "knocked down," which prompts coworkers to attempt a rescue. Numerous case reports describe multiple victims because the would-be rescuers often themselves become victims when they attempt a rescue in an environment having high concentrations of hydrogen sulfide.[36,84,111] Studies report that up to 25% of fatalities involve rescuers.[36,42,53] OSHA and a variety of occupational organizations, such as the American Industrial Hygiene Association, National Institute of Occupational Safety and Health, American Shipbuilding Association, and U.S. Chemical Safety Board, recognize the serious dangers of hydrogen sulfide exposures in the workplace and continue to promote safety alerts and educational programs.[89]

Natural sources of hydrogen sulfide are volcanoes, caves, sulfur springs, and underground deposits of natural gas,[32,99] and it has been implicated in several environmental disasters. In 1950, 22 people died and 320 were hospitalized in Poza Rica, Mexico, when a local natural gas facility inadvertently released hydrogen sulfide into the air.[74] Hydrogen sulfide claimed nine lives when a sour gas well failed, releasing a cloud of the poisonous gas into the Denver City, Texas, community in 1975.[78] In 2003, a gas drilling incident in southwest China released natural gas and a cloud of hydrogen sulfide into a populated area. More than 200 people died, 9000 were treated for injuries, and more than 40,000 were evacuated.[131]

Recently, a large number of suicides have been attributed to mixing common household chemicals such as fungicides and toilet bowl cleaners to create hydrogen sulfide gas.[117,120] In Japan, it is reported that more than 500 people killed themselves in the first half of 2008 by this means.[133] Information resources on the Internet are implicated for the widespread practice and prompted police to request purging the suicide recipes from Internet sites.[51] One suicidal incident in Japan caused 90 people to become ill from the toxic gas as it permeated an apartment building.[120] Also in 2008, the Pasadena hazmat team evacuated an area surrounding the scene of a man found dead in his car and a note on the vehicle warning first responders of the hazardous chemicals he used.[117]

PHARMACOLOGY AND TOXICOKINETICS

Hydrogen sulfide is a colorless gas, more dense than air, with an irritating odor of "rotten eggs." It is highly lipid soluble, a property that allows easy penetration of biologic membranes. Systemic absorption usually occurs through inhalation, and it is rapidly distributed to tissues.[99]

The tissues most sensitive to hydrogen sulfide are those with high oxygen demand. The systemic toxicity of hydrogen sulfide results from its potent inhibition of cytochrome oxidase, thereby interrupting oxidative phosphorylation.[32,67] Hydrogen sulfide binds to the ferric (Fe^{3+}) moiety of cytochrome a_3 oxidase complex with a higher affinity than does cyanide (see Fig. 126-2). The resulting inhibition of oxidative phosphorylation produces cellular hypoxia and anaerobic metabolism.[32,134]

Cytochrome oxidase inhibition is not the sole mechanism of toxicity. Other enzymes, such as carbonic anhydrase and monoamine oxidase, are inhibited by hydrogen sulfide and may contribute to its toxic effects.[99] Besides producing cellular hypoxia, hydrogen sulfide alters brain neurotransmitter release and transmission through potassium channel–mediated hyperpolarization of neurons and other neuronal inhibitory mechanisms.[99] A proposed mechanism of death is poisoning of the brainstem respiratory center through selective uptake by lipophilic white matter in this region.[129] The olfactory nerve is a specific target of great interest. Not only does the toxic gas cause olfactory nerve paralysis but it is also thought to be a portal of entry into the CNS because of its direct contact with the brain.[134] It is also cytotoxic through formation of reactive sulfur and oxygen species. It may also react with iron to fuel the Fenton reaction, causing free radical injury[118] (see Chaps. 11 and 12).

In addition to systemic effects, hydrogen sulfide reacts with the moisture on the surface of mucous membranes to produce intense irritation and corrosive injury. The eyes and nasal and respiratory mucous membranes are the tissues most susceptible to direct injury.[70,134] Despite skin irritation, it has little dermal absorption.

Inhaled hydrogen sulfide enters the systemic circulation, where it dissociates into hydrosulfide ions (HS^-), sulfide (S^{-2}), and sulfate (SO_2^{-4}). After it has been absorbed, hydrogen sulfide and dissociation products are metabolized by oxidation, methylation, and binding to metalloproteins. The major pathway of detoxification is enzymatic and nonenzymatic oxidation of sulfides and sulfur to thiosulfate and polysulfides.[134] Other pathways, such as methylation to dimethyl sulfide and conversion to sulfite or sulfate by oxidized glutathione, may also play a role in detoxification and elimination.[32,134] Hydrosulfide ions interact with metalloproteins, disulfide-containing enzymes, and thio dimethyl S transferase.[33] Sulfhemoglobin is not found in significant concentrations in the blood of animals or fatally poisoned humans.[94]

CLINICAL MANIFESTATIONS

Acute Manifestations Hydrogen sulfide poisoning should be suspected whenever a person is found unconscious in an enclosed space, especially if the odor of rotten eggs is noted. The primary target organs of hydrogen sulfide poisoning are those of the CNS and respiratory system. The clinical findings reported in two large series are listed in Table 126–3.[4,25]

The intensity of exposure likely accounts for the diverse clinical findings in the reports. A distinct dose response to hydrogen sulfide is identified. The odor threshold is between 0.02 and 0.13 ppm, and a strong, intense odor is noted at 20 to 30 ppm. Mild mucous membrane irritation occurs at 50 to 100 ppm, and olfactory fatigue occurs at 100 to 150 ppm. The ability to perceive the odor is rapidly extinguished at higher concentrations because of olfactory nerve paralysis. Prolonged exposure may occur when the extinction of odor recognition is misinterpreted as dissipation of the gas. Strong irritation of the upper respiratory tract and eyes and ALI occur at 200 to 300 ppm. At above 500 ppm, H_2S produces systemic effects. Rapid unconsciousness and cardiopulmonary arrest occur at concentrations above 700 ppm.[8,99]

Hydrogen sulfide reacts with the moisture on the surface of mucous membranes to produce intense irritation and corrosive injury. Mucous membrane irritation of the eye produces keratoconjunctivitis. If exposure persists, damage to the epithelial cells produces reversible corneal ulcerations ("gas eye") and, rarely, irreversible corneal scarring.[70,125] The irritant effects on the respiratory tract include rhinitis, bronchitis, and ALI.[4,25,134]

Neurologic manifestations are common and may be severe. Hydrogen sulfide's rapid and deadly onset of clinical effects have been termed the *slaughterhouse sledgehammer effect*. In a series, 75% of 221 patients with acute hydrogen sulfide exposure lost consciousness at the time of exposure.[25] In acute, massive exposures, rapid loss of consciousness ("knockdown") results from loss of central respiratory drive.[76] If the patient is rapidly removed from the exposure, recovery may be prompt and complete. Hypoxia from respiratory compromise may cause secondary neurologic effects.[8,32,134] Neurologic outcomes are quite variable, ranging from no neurologic impairment to permanent sequelae. Delayed neuropsychiatric sequelae may occur after acute exposures.[27] Most evidence suggests that whereas the early rapid CNS effects are direct neurotoxic effects of hydrogen sulfide, the permanent neurologic sequelae result from hypoxia secondary to respiratory insufficiency.[8,134] Reported neuropsychiatric changes include memory failure (amnestic syndrome), lack of insight, disorientation, delirium, and dementia.[32,134] Neurosensory abnormalities include transient hearing impairment, vision loss, and anosmia. Motor symptoms are likely caused by injury to the basal ganglia and result in ataxia, position or intention tremor, and muscle rigidity.[121] Common neuropathologic findings observed on neuroimaging and at autopsy are subcortical white matter demyelination and globus pallidus degeneration.[27,122]

Acute exposures affect other organ systems. Myocardial hypoxia or direct toxic effects of hydrogen sulfide on cardiac tissue may cause cardiac dysrhythmias, myocardial ischemia, or myocardial infarction.[46] Because unresponsiveness is rapid, trauma from falls should not be overlooked.[4,43] In a report, 7% of patients experiencing a "knockdown" had associated traumatic injuries.[4]

TABLE 126–3. Hydrogen Sulfide Poisoning

When to suspect hydrogen sulfide poisoning

- Person rapidly loses consciousness ("knocked down")
- Rotten eggs odor
- Rescue from enclosed space, such as sewer or manure pit
- Multiple victims with sudden death syndrome
- Collapse of a previously healthy worker at work site

Clinical Manifestations

System	Signs and Symptoms
Cardiovascular	Chest pain, bradycardia
Central nervous	Headache, weakness, dysequilibrium, convulsions, coma
Gastrointestinal	Pharyngitis, nausea, vomiting
Ophthalmic	Conjunctivitis
Pulmonary	Dyspnea, cyanosis, hemoptysis, crackles

Chronic Manifestations Most data about chronic, low-level exposures to hydrogen sulfide come from oil and gas industry workers. Mucous membrane irritation seems to be the most prominent problem in patients with low-concentration exposures. Workers report nasal, pharyngeal, and eye irritation; fatigue; headache; dizziness; and poor memory with low-concentration, chronic exposures. The chronic irritating effects of hydrogen sulfide were thought to be the cause of reduced lung volumes observed in sewer workers.[101] Volunteer studies have not demonstrated significant cardiovascular effects after long-term exposure to concentrations less than 10 ppm.[12] The liver, kidneys, and endocrine system are unaffected. No studies demonstrate increased incidences of cancer with low-level exposures.[32]

Rapid loss of consciousness from hydrogen sulfide exposure was a well-known and, amazingly, accepted part of the workplace in the gas and oil industry for many years.[55] Some workers experienced repeated "knockdowns," and these workers reported an increased incidence of respiratory diseases and cognitive deficits. Single or repeated high-concentration exposures resulting in unconsciousness may cause serious cognitive dysfunction. The acute effects of rapid loss of consciousness are most likely caused by hydrogen sulfide neurotoxicity. Although a clear association exists between knockdown and chronic neurologic sequelae, many of the case reports are complicated by associated apnea or hypoxemia from respiratory failure, asphyxia or exposure to other xenobiotics in a confined space, head injury from a fall, or near drowning in liquid manure or sludge.[134] The association of neurotoxic sequelae is less clear with protracted low-concentration exposures. Case series suggest that low-concentration exposures may cause subtle changes that can be measured by only the most sensitive neuropsychiatric tests.[68]

Epidemiologic data regarding the effects of low-concentration environmental exposures to hydrogen sulfide are clouded in populations exposed to complex mixtures of pollutants. Other malodorous sulfur compounds (eg, methyl mercaptan and methyl sulfide) are generated as byproducts of pulp mills. Study populations exposed to this complex mixture of pollutants demonstrate a dose-related increase in nasal symptoms, cough, nausea, and vomiting.[32]

These changes are nonspecific, and many of the patients have a poorly documented exposure assessment. Currently, the association of protracted and low-concentration hydrogen sulfide exposure with chronic neurologic sequelae remains controversial and needs further study.[134]

The strong odor of low concentrations of hydrogen sulfide can magnify irritant effects by triggering a strong psychological response.[134] Hydrogen sulfide has been the alleged source of mass psychogenic illness cases.[44] Clinical, epidemiologic, and toxicologic analyses suggested that 943 cases of illness in Jerusalem were caused by the odor of low concentrations of hydrogen sulfide gas. The most frequent associated symptoms are headaches; faintness; dizziness; nausea; chest tightness; dyspnea and tachypnea; eye, nose, and throat irritation; weakness; and extremity numbness.[29] Low-concentration exposure to hydrogen sulfide may produce nonspecific signs and symptoms that could closely mimic psychogenic illness. Attempting to identify true toxicity from a powerful emotional reaction can be extremely difficult.[44] Therefore, symptomatic patients must be assessed for toxicity even when mass psychogenic illness is suspected.

DIAGNOSTIC TESTING

In hydrogen sulfide poisoning, diagnostic testing is of limited value for clinical decision making after acute exposures, confirmation of acute exposures, occupational monitoring, and forensic analysis after fatal accidents.

Because no available rapid method of detection is of clinical diagnostic use, management decisions must be made based on the patient's history, clinical presentation, and diagnostic tests that infer the presence of hydrogen sulfide. Circumstances surrounding the patient's illness often provide the best evidence for hydrogen sulfide poisoning (see Table 126-3). At the bedside, the smell of rotten eggs on clothing or emanating from the blood, exhaled air, or gastric secretions suggests hydrogen sulfide exposure. In addition, darkening of silver jewelry is a clue to exposure. Paper impregnated with lead acetate changes color when exposed to hydrogen sulfide and is used to detect its presence in the patient's exhaled air but is not rapidly available.[32]

Specific tests for confirming hydrogen sulfide exposure are not readily available in clinical laboratories. Therefore, the presence of hydrogen sulfide is best confirmed by directly measuring the gas in the environment. It can be detected in atmospheric air samples by monitoring devices such as colorimetric tubes or xenobiotic-specific air sampling devices. Many emergency response teams investigate the toxic environment of a hazardous materials incident with detection devices that measure hydrogen sulfide with electrochemical sensors.

In acute poisoning, readily available diagnostic tests that are biomarkers of hydrogen sulfide poisoning may be useful but are nonspecific. ABG analysis demonstrating metabolic acidosis with an associated elevated serum lactate concentration is expected, and oxygen saturation should be normal unless ALI is present. Hydrogen sulfide, similar to cyanide, decreases oxygen consumption and is reflected as an elevated mixed venous oxygen measurement. Because sulfhemoglobin typically is not generated in patients with hydrogen sulfide poisoning, an oxygen saturation gap is not expected.[94]

After serious injury from hydrogen sulfide, diagnostic testing for neurologic structure and function may show abnormalities for weeks or months. Brain MRI and head CT studies demonstrate structural changes such as globus pallidus degeneration and subcortical white matter demyelination. Neuropsychologic testing after serious hydrogen sulfide poisoning demonstrates specific abnormalities in cortical functions, such as concentration, attention, verbal abstraction, and short-term retention. Single-photon emission CT (SPECT) or positron emission tomography brain scans define neurotoxin-induced lesions that correlate well with clinical neuropsychologic testing.[28]

Whole-blood sulfide concentrations above 0.05 mg/L are considered abnormal. Reliable measurements are ensured only if the concentration is obtained within 2 hours after the exposure and analyzed immediately.[99]

In acute exposures, blood and urine thiosulfate concentrations may be reflective of exposure.[64] Urinary thiosulfate excretion is used to monitor chronic low-concentration exposure in the workplace.

One study attempted to establish background concentrations of urinary thiosulfate in an occupational environment with low-level and short-term hydrogen sulfide exposure with a reported mean increase from preexposure concentrations of 4.6 μm/L to postexposure concentrations of 11.5 μm/L.[39] These concentrations provide a comparison for concentrations obtained from fatal and nonfatal victims after exposure. However, the study could not demonstrate a correlation between the degree of exposure and change in urine thiosulfate. Another study analyzed the value of blood and urine thiosulfate from data collected in case series of fatal and nonfatal hydrogen sulfide victims.[61,63] Because thiosulfate was detected in the urine but sulfide and thiosulfate were not detected in the blood of nonfatal exposures, this report concluded that thiosulfate in the urine is the only indicator to prove hydrogen sulfide poisoning in nonfatal cases. In addition, measuring sulfide and thiosulfate in the blood are helpful in forensic investigations.

Sulfide concentrations obtained in postmortem investigations may be useful, but their use requires rapid sample collection because sulfide concentrations increase with tissue decomposition.[99] In addition to blood sulfide concentrations, sulfide and thiosulfate concentrations are at their highest in the lung and brain.[62] If death is rapid, urinary thiosulfate concentrations may be nondetectable despite blood sulfide and thiosulfate concentrations 10-fold or greater than normal concentrations.[61] During the autopsy, a greenish discoloration of the gray matter, viscera, and bronchial secretions may be noted.[62,84]

MANAGEMENT

The initial treatment (Table 126–4) is immediate removal of the victim from the contaminated area into a fresh air environment. High-flow oxygen should be administered as soon as possible. Optimal supportive care has the greatest influence on the patient's outcome. Because death from inhalation of hydrogen sulfide is rapid, limited patients reaching the hospital for treatment are reported in the literature. Most patients experience significant delays before receiving treatment. Therefore, specific treatments and antidotal therapies do not show definitive improvement in patient outcome.

TABLE 126–4. Hydrogen Sulfide Poisoning: Emergency Management

Supportive care
Prehospital
Attempt rescue only if using SCBA
Move victim to fresh air
Administer 100% oxygen
During extrication, consider traumatic injuries from falls
Apply ACLS protocols as indicated
Emergency department
Maximize ventilation and oxygenation
Consider PEEP for ALI
Treat metabolic acidosis based on arterial pH and serum bicarbonate analysis
Administer crystalloid and vasopressors for hypotension
Antidote
Give sodium nitrite (3% $NaNO_2$) IV over 2–4 minutes
Adult dose: 10 mL (300 mg)
Pediatric dose: See Table 126-2; if hemoglobin is unknown, presume 12 g dosing
Caution:
Monitor blood pressure frequently
Obtain methemoglobin level 30 minutes after dose
Consider HBO if immediately available

ACLS, advanced cardiac life support; ALI, acute lung injury; HBO, hyperbaric oxygen; IV, intravenous; PEEP, positive end-expiratory pressure; SCBA, self-contained breathing apparatus.

The proposed toxic mechanisms, animal studies, and human case reports suggest that oxygen therapy is beneficial for hydrogen sulfide poisoning.[32,98,134] Proposed mechanisms for the beneficial effects of oxygen are competitive reactivation of oxidative phosphorylation by inhibiting hydrogen sulfide–cytochrome binding, enhanced detoxification by catalyzing oxidation of sulfides and sulfur, and improved oxygenation in the presence of ALI. All patients suspected of hydrogen sulfide poisoning should receive supplemental oxygen. In case reports, poisoned patients receiving hyperbaric oxygen (HBO) had favorable clinical outcomes.[57,109] However, no clinical data are available to suggest HBO is superior to normobaric oxygen for acute poisoning or preventing delayed neurologic sequelae.

The similarities in the toxic mechanism between hydrogen sulfide and cyanide created an interest in the use of nitrite-induced methemoglobin as an antidote. Methemoglobin protects animals from toxicity of hydrogen sulfide poisoning in both pretreatment and postexposure models.[110] Nitrite-generated methemoglobin acts as a scavenger of sulfide. The affinity of hydrogen sulfide for methemoglobin is greater than that for cytochrome oxidase. When hydrogen sulfide binds to methemoglobin, it forms sulfmethemoglobin.[9] Because hydrogen sulfide poisoning is rare, no studies have evaluated the clinical outcomes of patients treated with sodium nitrite. Animal studies suggest that nitrite must be given within minutes of exposure to ensure effectiveness.[9] However, several human case reports showed a rapid return of normal sensorium when nitrites were administered soon after exposure.[57,92,114] Patients with suspected hydrogen sulfide poisoning who have altered mental status, coma, hypotension, or dysrhythmias should receive sodium nitrite by slow infusion at the same dose given for cyanide poisoning. Sodium thiosulfate is of no benefit in the treatment of patients with hydrogen sulfide poisoning. In addition, only a single in vivo mouse model is published to suggest a beneficial effect of hydroxocobalamin as an antidote for hydrogen sulfide poisoning.[119] Additional research is warranted to determine its usefulness for hydrogen sulfide poisoning.

Treatment of patients with hydrogen sulfide poisoning requires optimal supportive care. Treatments and antidotes beyond supportive care are not of proven clinical benefit. Because hydrogen sulfide toxicity is severe and research studies suggest potential benefits of nitrite therapy, it should be considered for seriously ill patients exposed to hydrogen sulfide. This therapy should be initiated after optimum supportive care has been ensured.

Only a few inhalation risks are similar to that of hydrogen sulfide in their ability to rapidly "knock down" victims. Some examples include low oxygen environments in an enclosed space, hydrogen cyanide, volatile nerve agents, and carbon monoxide. The cause may be unclear early in the patient's emergency care, requiring clinicians to make treatment decisions without confirmatory evidence of poisoning. Clinicians faced with victims of knockdown syndrome should search for clues such as a victim's activities such as working at a manure pit, reports of chemicals detected at the scene by first responders, or suggestive clinical signs. The critical decision is whether to empirically administer specific antidotes. Vapor exposure to volatile nerve agents would likely result in miosis and require antidotes such as atropine, pralidoxime, and benzodiazepines. Which, if any, cyanide antidotes to administer in a "knockdown" situation is most difficult. The basic aims are to gather as many facts and suggestive clues as possible, weigh the risk benefits for treatment or not, and treat early in the course. Again, meticulous attention to optimal supportive care is required.

SUMMARY

Both cyanide and hydrogen sulfide are highly toxic xenobiotics. Cyanide is of great concern with regard to homicide and suicide. There are particular metabolic risks and concerns with regard to exposure to both xenobiotics because they bind specifically to the ferric moiety of the cytochrome a_3 oxidase complex. Odor recognition is unreliable and is not a definitive approach to diagnosis. The laboratory evaluation usually is not timely for diagnostic purposes. Decontamination, removal from the site of exposure, and oxygen are essential. The controversies over the ideal therapeutic modalities for these agents are substantial, and extensive research continues.

REFERENCES

1. Adewusi SR, Akindahunsi AA. Cassava processing, consumption, and cyanide toxicity. *J Toxicol Environ Health*. 1994;43:13-23.
2. Ardelt BK, Borowitz JL, Maduh EU, et al. Cyanide-induced lipid peroxidation in different organs: subcellular distribution and hydroperoxide generation in neuronal cells. *Toxicology*. 1994;89:127-137.
3. Arden SR, Sinor JD, Potthoff WK, et al. Subunit-specific interactions of cyanide with the *N*-methyl-D-aspartate receptor. *J Biol Chem*. 1998;273: 21505-21511.
4. Arnold IM, Dufresne RM, Alleyne BC, et al. Health implication of occupational exposures to hydrogen sulfide. *J Occup Med*. 1985;27:373-376.
5. Atlante A, de Bari L, Bobba A, et al. Cytochrome c, released from cerebellar granule cells undergoing apoptosis or excytotoxic death, can generate proton motive force and drive ATP synthesis in isolated mitochondria. *J Neurochem*. 2003;86:591-604.
6. Baud FJ, Barriot P, Toffis V, et al. Elevated blood cyanide concentrations in victims of smoke inhalation. *N Engl J Med*. 1991;325:1761-1766.
7. Baud FJ, Borron SW, Megarbane B, et al. Value of lactic acidosis in the assessment of the severity of acute cyanide poisoning. *Crit Care Med*. 2002;30:2044-2050.
8. Beauchamp RO Jr, Bus JS, Popp JA, et al. A critical review of the literature on hydrogen sulfide toxicity. *Crit Rev Toxicol*. 1984;13:25-97.
9. Beck JF, Bradbury CM, Connors AJ, et al. Nitrite as antidote for acute hydrogen sulfide intoxication? *Am Ind Hyg Assoc J*. 1981;42:805-809.
10. Beregi JP, Riou B, Lecarpentier Y. Effects of hydroxocobalamin on rat cardiac papillary muscle. *Intensive Care Med*. 1991;17:175-177.
11. Berlin CM Jr. The treatment of cyanide poisoning in children. *Pediatrics*. 1970;46:793-796.
12. Bhambhani Y, Burnham R, Snydmiller G, et al. Effects of 10-ppm hydrogen sulfide inhalation on pulmonary function in healthy men and women. *J Occup Environ Med*. 1996;38:1012-1017.
13. Bhattacharya R, Kumar D, Sugendran K, et al. Acute toxicity studies of alpha-ketoglutarate: a promising antidote for cyanide poisoning. *J Appl Toxicol*. 2001;21:495-499.
14. Bhattacharya R, Tulsawani R. In vitro and in vivo evaluation of various carbonyl compounds against cyanide toxicity with particular reference to alpha-ketoglutaric acid. *Drug Chem Toxicol*. 2008;31:149-161.
15. Bhattacharya R, Vijayaraghavan R. Cyanide intoxication in mice through different routes and its prophylaxis by alpha-ketoglutarate. *Biomed Environ Sci*. 1991;4:452-460.
16. Bismuth C, Baud FJ, Pontal PG. Hydroxocobalamin in chronic cyanide poisoning. *J Toxicol Clin Exp*. 1988;8:35-38.
17. Blanc P, Hogan M, Mallin K, et al. Cyanide intoxication among silver-reclaiming workers. *JAMA*. 1985;253:367-371.
18. Blanco PJ, Rivero AG. First case of illegal euthanasia in Spain: fatal oral potassium cyanide poisoning. *Soud Lek*. 2004;49:30-33.
19. Borron SW, Baud FJ, Megarbane B, et al. Hydroxocobalamin for severe acute cyanide poisoning by ingestion or inhalation. *Am J Emerg Med*. 2007;25:551-558.
20. Breen PH, Isserles SA, Tabac E, et al. Protective effect of stroma-free methemoglobin during cyanide poisoning in dogs. *Anesthesiology*. 1996;85:558-564.
21. Brian MJ. Cyanide poisoning in children in Goroka. *P N G Med J*. 1990;33:151-153.
22. Broderick KE, Potluri P, Zhuang S, et al. Cyanide detoxification by the cobalamin precursor cobinamide. *Exp Biol Med (Maywood)*. 2006;231:641-649.
23. Bronstein AC, Spyker DA, Cantilena LR, et al. 2007 Annual Report of the American Association of Poison Control Centers' National Poison Data System (NPDS): 25th Annual Report. *Clin Toxicol*. 2008;46:927-1057.
24. Brouard A, Blaisot B, Bismuth C. Hydroxocobalamine in cyanide poisoning. *J Toxicol Clin Exp*. 1987;7:155-168.
25. Burnett WW, King EG, Grace M, et al. Hydrogen sulfide poisoning: review of 5 years' experience. *Can Med Assoc J*. 1977;117:1277-1280.

26. Burrows GE, Way JL. Cyanide intoxication in sheep: therapeutic value of oxygen or cobalt. *Am J Vet Res.* 1977;38:223-227.
27. Byungkuk N, Hyokyung K, Younghee C, et al. Neurologic Sequela of Hydrogen Sulfide Poisoning. *Ind Health.* 2004 42:83-87.
28. Callender TJ, Morrow L, Subramanian K, et al. Three-dimensional brain metabolic imaging in patients with toxic encephalopathy. *Environ Res.* 1993;60:295-319.
29. Centers for Disease Control and Prevention. Acute illness epidemic. West Bank—Jerusalem. *MMWR Morb Mortal Wkly Rep.* 1983;32:205-208.
30. Centers for Disease Control and Prevention. Cyanide poisonings associated with over-the-counter medication—Washington State, 1991. *MMWR Morb Mortal Wkly Rep.* 1991;40:167-168.
31. Chaturvedi AK, Smith DR, Canfield DV. Blood carbon monoxide and hydrogen cyanide concentrations in the fatalities of fire and non-fire associated civil aviation accidents, 1991–1998. *Forensic Sci Int.* 2001;121:183-188.
31a. Chen KK, Rose CL: Nitrite and thiosulfate therapy in cyanide poisoning. *JAMA.* 1952;149:113-119.
32. Chou S, Fay M, Keith S, et al. *Toxicological Profile for Hydrogen Sulfide.* US Department of Health and Human Services: ATSDR; 2006
33. Chou SJ. *Hydrogen Sulfide. Human Health Aspects.* Geneva: World Health Organization; 2003. Retrieved October 19, 2009, from www.who.int/ipcs/publications/cicad/en/cicad53.pdf.
34. Curry SC, Arnold-Capell P. Toxic effects of drugs used in the ICU. Nitroprusside, nitroglycerin, and angiotensin-converting enzyme inhibitors. *Crit Care Clin.* 1991;7:555-581.
35. Djerad A, Monier C, Houze P, et al. Effects of respiratory acidosis and alkalosis on the distribution of cyanide into the rat brain. *Toxicol Sci.* 2001;61:273-282.
36. Dorevitch S, Forst L, Conroy L, et al. Toxic inhalation fatalities of US construction workers, 1990 to 1999. *J Occup Environ Med.* 2002;44:657-662.
37. Dulaney MD Jr, Brumley M, Willis JT, et al. Protection against cyanide toxicity by oral alpha-ketoglutaric acid. *Vet Hum Toxicol.* 1991;33:571-575.
38. Dunea G. Death over the counter. *Br Med J (Clin Res Ed).* 1983;286:211-212.
39. Durand M, Weinstein P. Thiosulfate in human urine following minor exposure to hydrogen sulfide: implications for forensic analysis of poisoning. *Forensic Toxicol.* 2007;25:92-95.
40. Fortin JL, Ruttimann M, Capellier G, et al. Successful organ transplantation after treatment of fatal cyanide poisoning with hydroxocobalamin. *Clin Toxicol (Phila).* 2007;45:468-471.
41. Freeman AG. Optic neuropathy and chronic cyanide toxicity. *Lancet.* 1986;1:441-442.
42. Fuller DC, Suruda AJ. Occupationally related hydrogen sulfide deaths in the United States from 1984 to 1994. *J Occup Environ Med.* 2000;42:939-942.
43. Gabbay DS, De Roos F, Perrone J. Twenty-foot fall averts fatality from massive hydrogen sulfide exposure. *J Emerg Med.* 2001;20:141-144.
44. Gallay A, Van Loock F, Demarest S, et al. Belgian coca-cola-related outbreak: intoxication, mass sociogenic illness, or both? *Am J Epidemiol.* 2002;155:140-147.
45. Gill JR, Marker E, Stajic M. Suicide by cyanide: 17 deaths. *J Forensic Sci.* 2004;49:826-828.
46. Gregorakos L, Dimopoulos G, Liberi S, et al. Hydrogen sulfide poisoning: management and complications. *Angiology.* 1995;46:1123-1131.
47. Hall AH, Doutre WH, Ludden T, et al. Nitrite/thiosulfate treated acute cyanide poisoning: estimated kinetics after antidote. *J Toxicol Clin Toxicol.* 1987;25:121-133.
48. Hall AH, Linden CH, Kulig KW, et al. Cyanide poisoning from laetrile ingestion: role of nitrite therapy. *Pediatrics.* 1986;78:269-272.
49. Hall AH, Rumack BH. Clinical toxicology of cyanide. *Ann Emerg Med.* 1986;15:1067-1074.
50. Hall AH, Rumack BH. Hydroxycobalamin/sodium thiosulfate as a cyanide antidote. *J Emerg Med.* 1987;5:115-121.
51. Harden B. Japan's latest suicide recipe purged from internet at police request. *The Irish Times*; May 30, 2007. Retrieved October 19, 2009, from http://www.irishtimes.com/newspaper/world/2008/0530/1212095650051.html.
52. Hariharakrishnan J, Satpute RM, Prasad GB, et al. Oxidative stress mediated cytotoxicity of cyanide in LLC-MK2 cells and its attenuation by alpha-ketoglutarate and N-acetyl cysteine. *Toxicol Lett.* 2009;185:132-141.
53. Hendrickson RG, Chang A, Hamilton RJ. Co-worker fatalities from hydrogen sulfide. *Am J Ind Med.* 2004;45:346-350.
54. Hernandez T, Lundquist P, Oliveira L, et al. Fate in humans of dietary intake of cyanogenic glycosides from roots of sweet cassava consumed in Cuba. *Nat Toxins.* 1995;3:114-117.
55. Hessel PA, Herbert FA, Melenka LS, et al. Lung health in relation to hydrogen sulfide exposure in oil and gas workers in Alberta, Canada. *Am J Ind Med.* 1997;31:554-557.
56. Himori N, Tanaka Y, Kurasawa M, et al. Dextrorphan attenuates the behavioral consequences of ischemia and the biochemical consequences of anoxia: possible role of *N*-methyl-D-aspartate receptor antagonism and ATP replenishing action in its cerebroprotecting profile. *Psychopharmacology (Berl).* 1993;111:153-162.
57. Hoidal CR, Hall AH, Robinson MD, et al. Hydrogen sulfide poisoning from toxic inhalations of roofing asphalt fumes. *Ann Emerg Med.* 1986;15:826-830.
58. Hume AS, Mozingo JR, McIntyre B, et al. Antidotal efficacy of alpha-ketoglutaric acid and sodium thiosulfate in cyanide poisoning. *J Toxicol Clin Toxicol.* 1995;33:721-724.
59. Jensen MS, Ahlemeyer B, Ravati A, et al. Preconditioning-induced protection against cyanide-induced neurotoxicity is mediated by preserving mitochondrial function. *Neurochem Int.* 2002;40:285-293.
60. Johnson RP, Mellors JW. Arteriolization of venous blood gases: a clue to the diagnosis of cyanide poisoning. *J Emerg Med.* 1988;6:401-404.
61. Kage S, Ikeda H, Ikeda N, et al. Fatal hydrogen sulfide poisoning at a dye works. *Leg Med (Tokyo).* 2004;6:182-186.
62. Kage S, Ito S, Kishida T, et al. A fatal case of hydrogen sulfide poisoning in a geothermal power plant. *J Forensic Sci.* 1998;43:908-910.
63. Kage S, Kashimura S, Ikeda H, et al. Fatal and nonfatal poisoning by hydrogen sulfide at an industrial waste site. *J Forensic Sci.* 2002;47:652-655.
64. Kage S, Takekawa K, Kurosaki K, et al. The usefulness of thiosulfate as an indicator of hydrogen sulfide poisoning: three cases. *Int J Legal Med.* 1997;110:220-222.
65. Kamalu BP, Agharanya JC. The effect of a nutritionally-balanced cassava (Manihot esculenta Crantz) diet on endocrine function using the dog as a model. 2. Thyroid. *Br J Nutr.* 1991;65:373-379.
66. Kanthasamy AG, Ardelt B, Malave A, et al. Reactive oxygen species generated by cyanide mediate toxicity in rat pheochromocytoma cells. *Toxicol Lett.* 1997;93:47-54.
67. Khan AA, Schuler MM, Prior MG, et al. Effects of hydrogen sulfide exposure on lung mitochondrial respiratory chain enzymes in rats. *Toxicol Appl Pharmacol.* 1990;103:482-490.
68. Kilburn KH, Warshaw RH. Hydrogen sulfide and reduced-sulfur gases adversely affect neurophysiological functions. *Toxicol Ind Health.* 1995;11:185-197.
69. Kirk MA, Gerace R, Kulig KW. Cyanide and methemoglobin kinetics in smoke inhalation victims treated with the cyanide antidote kit. *Ann Emerg Med.* 1993;22:1413-1418.
70. Lambert RJ, Kindler BL, Schaeffer DJ: The efficacy of superactivated charcoal in treating rats exposed to a lethal oral dose of potassium cyanide. *Ann Emerg Med.*1988;17:595–598.
71. Li L, Prabhakaran K, Shou Y, et al. Oxidative stress and cyclooxygenase-2 induction mediate cyanide-induced apoptosis of cortical cells. *Toxicol Appl Pharmacol.* 2002;185:55-63.
72. Maduh EU, Borowitz JL, Isom GE. Cyanide-induced alteration of the adenylate energy pool in a rat neurosecretory cell line. *J Appl Toxicol.* 1991;11:97-101.
73. Mathangi DC, Namasivayam A. Calcium ions: its role in cyanide neurotoxicity. *Food Chem Toxicol.* 2004;42:359-361.
74. McCabe L, Clayton GD. Air pollution by hydrogen sulfide in Poza Rica, Mexico; an evaluation of the incident of Nov. 24, 1950. *Arch Ind Hyg Occup Med.* 1952;6:199-213.
75. Messing B, Storch B. Computer tomography and magnetic resonance imaging in cyanide poisoning. *Eur Arch Psychiatry Neurol Sci.* 1988;237:139-143.
76. Milby TH, Baselt RC. Hydrogen sulfide poisoning: clarification of some controversial issues. *Am J Ind Med.* 1999;35:192-195.
77. Mills EM, Gunasekar PG, Pavlakovic G, et al. Cyanide-induced apoptosis and oxidative stress in differentiated PC12 cells. *J Neurochem.* 1996;67:1039-1046.
78. Morris J. The Brimstone Battles: death came from a cloud: a silent killer took 9 lives in 1975. Could it happen again? *Houston Chronicle (Special Report)*; Nov. 9, 1997.
79. Nagler J, Provoost RA, Parizel G. Hydrogen cyanide poisoning: treatment with cobalt EDTA. *J Occup Med.* 1978;20:414-416.
80. Niknahad H, Ghelichkhani E. Antagonism of cyanide poisoning by dihydroxyacetone. *Toxicol Lett.* 2002;132:95-100.
81. Niknahad H, Khan S, Sood C, et al. Prevention of cyanide-induced cytotoxicity by nutrients in isolated rat hepatocytes. *Toxicol Appl Pharmacol.* 1994;128:271-279.

82. Niknahad H, O'Brien PJ. Antidotal effect of dihydroxyacetone against cyanide toxicity in vivo. *Toxicol Appl Pharmacol.* 1996;138:186-191.
83. Norris JC, Utley WA, Hume AS. Mechanism of antagonizing cyanide-induced lethality by alpha-ketoglutaric acid. *Toxicology.* 1990;62:275-283.
84. Oesterhelweg L, Puschel K. "Death may come on like a stroke of lightening": phenomenological and morphological aspects of fatalities caused by manure gas. *Int J Legal Med.* 2008;122:101-107.
85. Okolie NP, Iroanya CU. Some histologic and biochemical evidence for mitigation of cyanide-induced tissue lesions by antioxidant vitamin administration in rabbits. *Food Chem Toxicol.* 2003;41:463-469.
86. Oluwole OS, Onabolu AO, Sowunmi A. Exposure to cyanide following a meal of cassava food. *Toxicol Lett.* 2002;135:19-23.
87. Onabolu A, Bokanga M, Tylleskar T, et al. High cassava production and low dietary cyanide exposure in mid-west Nigeria. *Public Health Nutr.* 2001;4:3-9.
88. Onabolu AO, Oluwole OS, Bokanga M, et al. Ecological variation of intake of cassava food and dietary cyanide load in Nigerian communities. *Public Health Nutr.* 2001;4:871-876.
89. OSHA Alliance Program. *Safety Alert. Deadly Hydrogen Sulfide and Shipyard Sewage;* 2006. Retrieved October 26, 2009, http://www.osha.gov/dcsp/alliances/aiha/aiha.html.
90. Patel MN, Yim GK, Isom GE. *N*-methyl-D-aspartate receptors mediate cyanide-induced cytotoxicity in hippocampal cultures. *Neurotoxicology.* 1993;14:35-40.
91. Patel MN, Peoples RW, Yim GK, et al. Enhancement of NMDA-mediated responses by cyanide. *Neurochem Res.* 1994;19:1319-1323.
92. Peters JW. Hydrogen sulfide poisoning in a hospital setting. *JAMA.* 1981;246:1588-1589.
93. Pettersen JC, Cohen SD. Antagonism of cyanide poisoning by chlorpromazine and sodium thiosulfate. *Toxicol Appl Pharmacol.* 1985;81:265-273.
94. Policastro MA, Otten EJ. Case files of the University of Cincinnati fellowship in medical toxicology: two patients with acute lethal occupational exposure to hydrogen sulfide. *J Med Toxicol.* 2007;3:73-81.
95. Prabhakaran K, Li L, Borowitz JL, et al. Caspase inhibition switches the mode of cell death induced by cyanide by enhancing reactive oxygen species generation and PARP-1 activation. *Toxicol Appl Pharmacol.* 2004;195:194-202.
96. Rachinger J, Fellner FA, Stieglbauer K, et al. MR changes after acute cyanide intoxication. *AJNR Am J Neuroradiol.* 2002;23:1398-1401.
97. Rajdev S, Reynolds IJ. Glutamate-induced intracellular calcium changes and neurotoxicity in cortical neurons in vitro: effect of chemical ischemia. *Neuroscience.* 1994;62:667-679.
98. Ravizza AG, Carugo D, Cerchiari EL, et al. The treatment of hydrogen sulfide intoxication: oxygen versus nitrites. *Vet Hum Toxicol.* 1982;24:241-242.
99. Reiffenstein RJ, Hulbert WC, Roth SH. Toxicology of hydrogen sulfide. *Annu Rev Pharmacol Toxicol.* 1992;32:109-134.
100. Rella J, Marcus S, Wagner BJ. Rapid cyanide detection using the Cyantesmo kit. *J Toxicol Clin Toxicol.* 2004;42:897-900.
101. Richardson DB. Respiratory effects of chronic hydrogen sulfide exposure. *Am J Ind Med.* 1995;28:99-108.
102. Rindone JP, Sloane EP. Cyanide toxicity from sodium nitroprusside: risks and management. *Ann Pharmacother.* 1992;26:515-519.
103. Riou B, Gerard JL, La Rochelle CD, et al. Hemodynamic effects of hydroxocobalamin in conscious dogs. *Anesthesiology.* 1991;74:552-558.
104. Rosenow F, Herholz K, Lanfermann H, et al. Neurological sequelae of cyanide intoxication—the patterns of clinical, magnetic resonance imaging, and positron emission tomography findings. *Ann Neurol.* 1995;38:825-828.
105. Shou Y, Gunasekar PG, Borowitz JL, et al. Cyanide-induced apoptosis involves oxidative-stress-activated NF-kappaB in cortical neurons. *Toxicol Appl Pharmacol.* 2000;164:196-205.
106. Shou Y, Li L, Prabhakaran K, et al. p38 Mitogen-activated protein kinase regulates Bax translocation in cyanide-induced apoptosis. *Toxicol Sci.* 2003;75:99-107.
107. Silverman SH, Purdue GF, Hunt JL, et al. Cyanide toxicity in burned patients. *J Trauma.* 1988;28:171-176.
108. Singh BM, Coles N, Lewis P, et al. The metabolic effects of fatal cyanide poisoning. *Postgrad Med J.* 1989;65:923-925.
109. Smilkstein MJ, Bronstein AC, Pickett HM, et al. Hyperbaric oxygen therapy for severe hydrogen sulfide poisoning. *J Emerg Med.* 1985;3:27-30.
110. Smith L, Kruszyna H, Smith RP. The effect of methemoglobin on the inhibition of cytochrome c oxidase by cyanide, sulfide or azide. *Biochem Pharmacol.* 1977;26:2247-2250.
111. Snyder JW, Safir EF, Summerville GP, et al. Occupational fatality and persistent neurological sequelae after mass exposure to hydrogen sulfide. *Am J Emerg Med.* 1995;13:199-203.
112. Sousa AB, Soto-Blanco B, Guerra JL, et al. Does prolonged oral exposure to cyanide promote hepatotoxicity and nephrotoxicity? *Toxicology.* 2002;174:87-95.
113. Spencer PS. Food toxins, ampa receptors, and motor neuron diseases. *Drug Metab Rev.* 1999;31:561-587.
114. Stine RJ, Slosberg B, Beacham BE. Hydrogen sulfide intoxication. A case report and discussion of treatment. *Ann Intern Med.* 1976;85:756-758.
115. Ten Eyck RP, Schaerdel AD, Ottinger WE. Stroma-free methemoglobin solution: an effective antidote for acute cyanide poisoning. *Am J Emerg Med.* 1985;3:519-523.
116. Thier R, Lewalter J, Selinski S, et al. Possible impact of human CYP2E1 polymorphisms on the metabolism of acrylonitrile. *Toxicol Lett.* 2002;128: 249-255.
117. Tricarico T. New hazmat threat comes to the US. Hydrogen sulfide is a new method of suicide. *Trics of the Trade.* 2009. Retrieved October 26, 2009, from http://cms.firehouse.com/web/online/Hazardous-Materials/Trics-of-the-Trade--New-Hazmat-Threat-Comes-to-the-US/18$61765.
118. Truong DH, Eghbal MA, Hindmarsh W, et al. Molecular mechanisms of hydrogen sulfide toxicity. *Drug Metab Rev.* 2006;38:733-744.
119. Truong DH, Mihajlovic A, Gunness P, et al. Prevention of hydrogen sulfide (H2S)-induced mouse lethality and cytotoxicity by hydroxocobalamin (vitamin B(12a)). *Toxicology.* 2007;242:16-22.
120. Truscott A. Suicide fad threatens neighbours, rescuers. *CMAJ.* 2008;179: 312-313.
121. Tvedt B, Edland A, Skyberg K, et al. Delayed neuropsychiatric sequelae after acute hydrogen sulfide poisoning: affection of motor function, memory, vision and hearing. *Acta Neurol Scand.* 1991;84:348-351.
122. Tvedt B, Skyberg K, Aaserud O, et al. Brain damage caused by hydrogen sulfide: a follow-up study of six patients. *Am J Ind Med.* 1991;20:91-101.
123. van Heijst AN, Douze JM, van Kesteren RG, et al. Therapeutic problems in cyanide poisoning. *J Toxicol Clin Toxicol.* 1987;25:383-398.
124. Van Heijst AN, Maes RA, Mtanda AT, et al. Chronic cyanide poisoning in relation to blindness and tropical neuropathy. *J Toxicol Clin Toxicol.* 1994;32:549-556.
125. Vanhoorne M, de Rouck A, de Bacquer D. Epidemiological study of eye irritation by hydrogen sulphide and/or carbon disulphide exposure in viscose rayon workers. *Ann Occup Hyg.* 1995;39:307-315.
126. Vetter J. Plant cyanogenic glycosides. *Toxicon.* 2000;38:11-36.
127. Vornov JJ, Tasker RC, Coyle JT. Delayed protection by MK-801 and tetrodotoxin in a rat organotypic hippocampal culture model of ischemia. *Stroke.* 1994;25:457-464; discussion 464-455.
128. Wang H, Chanas B, Ghanayem BI. Cytochrome P450 2E1 (CYP2E1) is essential for acrylonitrile metabolism to cyanide: comparative studies using CYP2E1-null and wild-type mice. *Drug Metab Dispos.* 2002;30:911-917.
129. Warenycia MW, Goodwin LR, Benishin CG, et al. Acute hydrogen sulfide poisoning. Demonstration of selective uptake of sulfide by the brainstem by measurement of brain sulfide levels. *Biochem Pharmacol.* 1989;38: 973-981.
130. Way JL, Leung P, Cannon E, et al. The mechanism of cyanide intoxication and its antagonism. *CIBA Found Symp.* 1988;140:232-243.
131. Weaver L, Jiang S. China seals gas well after leak. *CNN International*; 2003. Retrieved October 26, 2009, from http://edition.cnn.com/2003/WORLD/asiapcf/east/12/26/china.gas/index.html.
132. Willets JM, Lambert DG, Lunec J, et al. Studies on the neurotoxicity of 6,7-dihydroxy-1-methyl-1,2,3,4-tetrahydroisoquinoline (salsolinol) in SH-SY5Y cells. *Eur J Pharmacol.* 1995;293:319-326.
133. Wiseman P. Suicide epidemic grips Japan. *USA Today.* 2008. Retrieved October 26, 2009, from http://www.usatoday.com/news/world/2008-07-20-japan-suicides_N.htm.
134. Woodall GM, Smith RL, Granville GC. Proceedings of the Hydrogen Sulfide Health Research and Risk Assessment Symposium, October 31–November 2, 2000. *Inhal Toxicol.* 2005;17:593-639.
135. Zaknun JJ, Stieglbauer K, Trenkler J, et al. Cyanide-induced akinetic rigid syndrome: clinical, MRI, FDG-PET, beta-CIT and HMPAO SPECT findings. *Parkinsonism Relat Disord.* 2005;11:125-129.
136. Zeevalk GD, Nicklas WJ. NMDA receptors, cellular edema, and metabolic stress. *Ann N Y Acad Sci.* 1992;648:368-370.

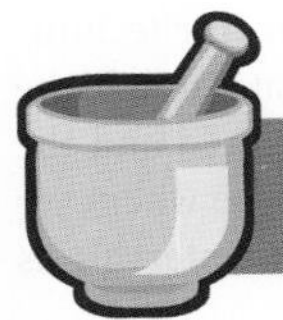

ANTIDOTES IN DEPTH (A38)

SODIUM AND AMYL NITRITE

Mary Ann Howland

Amyl and sodium nitrite are effective cyanide antidotes when they are administered in a timely fashion. Amyl nitrite is volatile and available in ampules that can be broken and administered by inhalation while sodium nitrite is being prepared to administer intravenously. Although the exact mechanism of action of the nitrites is unclear, the production of methemoglobin is both therapeutic in cyanide poisoning and potentially life threatening if nitrites are administered to a patient with impaired oxygen-carrying capacity, from smoke inhalation or elevated concentrations of carboxyhemoglobin or methemoglobin from any cause. In the latter cases, sodium thiosulfate and/or hydroxocobalamin can still be administered intravenously without causing harm.

HISTORY

Expanding on earlier work that demonstrated the limited role of methylene blue and the efficacy of sodium nitrite in cyanide-poisoned animals, inhaled amyl nitrite prevented and protected against cyanide-induced seizures and muscular rigidity in dogs.[3] Amyl nitrite administered by inhalation protected dogs from up to four minimum lethal doses of sodium cyanide (a total of 24 mg/kg subcutaneously). In the regimen used, therapy started within 5 to 7 minutes of exposure and continued for several hours. The frequency of inhalations was based on clinical response. These experimental results led to the use of inhaled amyl nitrite for patients poisoned by cyanide. The same authors discovered that intravenous (IV) use of sodium thiosulfate alone protected against three minimum lethal doses of cyanide in dogs and that the combination of sodium thiosulfate with either inhaled amyl nitrite or IV sodium nitrite protected against 10 and 13 to 18 minimum lethal doses, respectively.[2,4]

CHEMISTRY

The chemical formula for sodium nitrite is $NaNO_2$ and for amyl nitrite is $C_5H_{11}NO_2$. Sodium nitrite has a molecular weight of 69 daltons and amyl nitrite 117 Da. Amyl nitrite is volatile even at low temperatures, and is highly flammable.

Cyanide quickly and reversibly binds to the ferric iron in cytochrome oxidase, inhibiting effective energy production throughout the body. The ferric iron in methemoglobin preferentially combines with cyanide, producing cyanomethemoglobin. This drives the reaction toward cyanomethemoglobin and liberates cyanide from cytochrome oxidase. Stroma-free methemoglobin is effective against four minimum lethal doses of cyanide in rats.[17] Nitrites oxidize the iron in hemoglobin to produce methemoglobin. Because nitrites are accepted antidotes for cyanide poisoning, for many years methemoglobin formation was assumed to be their sole antidotal mechanism of action.[13,21] Other, faster methemoglobin inducers, such as 4-dimethyaminophenol and hydroxylamine, also are effective as cyanide antidotes.[13,19] The production of methemoglobin by nitrite is slow, but when methylene blue is administered to prevent methemoglobin formation, nitrite still is an effective antidote.[13,21] Reasoning that nitrite-induced vasodilation might be part of the mechanism of action, investigators considered the antidotal actions of other vasodilators. Only the α-adrenergic antagonists and ganglionic blockers demonstrate antidotal activity, and only when they are administered with sodium thiosulfate.[21] It is possible that the benefits of nitrites given shortly after cyanide result from reversal of cyanide-induced circulatory effects rather than reversal of the effects of cyanide on cytochrome oxidase.[18] Experimental evidence in organ damage induced by hypoxia or hypotension suggest that the benefits of nitrite may be related to its ability to be converted to nitric oxide, a potent vasodilator. The conversion to nitric oxide appears to occur only in tissues or blood with the lowest oxygen concentrations.[5,14]

PHARMACOKINETICS AND PHARMACODYNAMICS

The pharmacokinetics of sodium nitrite are not established. Most studies have been directed at measuring methemoglobin levels rather than nitrite concentrations.[19]

Sodium nitrite administered intramuscularly to dogs is not effective as a cyanide antidote unless atropine is given as pretreatment.[20] Most likely the rapid reversal of cyanide-induced bradycardia by atropine allows sufficiently rapid absorption of sodium nitrite, which then can be effective.[20] In healthy adults, 300 mg IV sodium nitrite can produce peak methemoglobin concentrations of 10% to 18%.[2] Inhalation of crushed amyl nitrite ampules in human volunteers produces insignificant amounts of methemoglobin but does cause headache, fatigue, dizziness, and hypotension.[12]

CLINICAL USE

Maximal benefits of sodium nitrite are realized experimentally when sodium nitrite is given prophylactically, but benefits are still evident even when sodium nitrite is administered following cyanide poisoning. Regardless of the exact mechanism of action, amyl and sodium nitrite clearly are effective soon after administration, even when methemoglobin concentrations are low. Thus a target methemoglobin concentration should not be used to determine the correct dose of sodium nitrite, although care must be taken to avoid excessive methemoglobinemia.[11] Administration of sodium nitrite should always be followed by sodium thiosulfate. Sodium thiosulfate donates a sulfur, which, with the help of rhodanese (cyanide sulfur transferase) and mercaptopyruvate sulfurtransferase, carries sulfane sulfur to bind to cyanide, producing thiocyanate. Thiocyanate is a much less toxic substance than cyanide and is renally eliminated.[3]

As early as 1952, the literature reported 16 cyanide-poisoned patients who survived with administration of nitrites and sodium thiosulfate.[2]

Even patients who were unconscious or apneic have survived when given timely cardiopulmonary resuscitation and antidotal therapy.[2] Case reports attest to the ability of amyl nitrite, sodium nitrite, and sodium thiosulfate to reverse the effects of cyanide if they are administered in a timely fashion.[8,22] A 34-year-old man who ingested 1 g potassium cyanide became comatose within 45 minutes. One hour after ingestion, he arrived in the emergency department, became apneic, and was intubated. His blood pressure was 134/84 mm Hg and pulse 84 beats/min; his pupils were dilated. Seizure activity that began just prior to sodium nitrite infusion resolved rapidly, and by the time the sodium thiosulfate had finished infusing, his pupils were reactive and spontaneous respirations had returned.[8] At 1 hour 15 minutes, he was given 300 mg sodium nitrite intravenously over 20 minutes, followed by 12.5 g sodium thiosulfate.

In another case, a 4-year-old boy ingested twelve 50-mg tablets of laetrile (amygdalin), became unresponsive, and developed seizures within 90 minutes.[10] Upon arrival at a second hospital, the patient required intubation, had no blood pressure, and had dilated pupils that were minimally responsive. Arterial blood gas analysis revealed pH, 6.85; Pco_2, 15 mm Hg; Po_2, 169 mm Hg on 100% oxygen. The anion gap was 26 mEq/L. The patient's vital signs improved with intermittent inhalation of amyl nitrite pearls. Six hours after ingestion (and 1 hour 45 minutes after amyl nitrite administration), sodium nitrite and sodium thiosulfate obtained from another hospital were administered. Within 30 minutes of completion of 5 mL (0.33 mL/kg) 3% sodium nitrite solution by IV infusion, spontaneous respirations returned, and his blood pressure and pulse normalized. Over the next 3 hours, the patient's mental status and acid–base balance improved. By 15 hours after ingestion, he was alert, oriented, and extubated. Elevated whole blood cyanide concentrations verified the ingestion.

ADVERSE EFFECTS

Amyl nitrite and sodium nitrite work by inducing methemoglobinemia, but excessive methemoglobinemia is potentially lethal. Therefore, nitrite dosages must be carefully calculated and nitrites administered to avoid excessive methemoglobinemia, especially in cases where other coexisting conditions, such as carboxyhemoglobin, sulfhemoglobin, and anemia, might compromise hemoglobin oxygen saturation.[9,15] Children are particularly at risk for medication errors because of dosage miscalculations. A reported death from methemoglobinemia was caused by the administration of an adult dose of sodium nitrite to a 17-month-old child suspected of ingesting a toxic amount of cyanide.[1]

Nitrites are potent vasodilators, so transient hypotension may occur. Other adverse effects include headache, nausea and vomiting.[2]

ADMINISTRATION AND DOSING

CYANIDE

Adults Amyl nitrite can be used prior to IV administration of sodium nitrite, but only as a temporizing measure until IV sodium nitrite can be administered. Break one amyl nitrite ampule and hold it in front of the patient's mouth for 15 seconds on and 15 seconds off.[7,16] Inhalation of amyl nitrite should be discontinued prior to sodium nitrite administration. The healthcare provider should be extremely careful not to inhale the amyl nitrite to prevent light-headedness and syncope. Sodium nitrite 300 mg (10 mL of 3% solution) should be injected intravenously at a rate of 2.5 to 5 mL/min. The dose can be repeated at half the initial dose if manifestations of cyanide toxicity reappear or at 2 hours as prophylaxis.[6,16]

Immediately following the completion of the sodium nitrite infusion, 12.5 g (50 mL of 25% solution) sodium thiosulfate should be infused intravenously. The same needle and vein can be used and the dose of the thiosulfate can be repeated at half the initial dose whenever manifestations of cyanide toxicity reappear or at 2-hour intervals as prophylaxis.[6,16]

In situations where additional methemoglobin formation would be harmful, as in patients with smoke inhalation from a fire, it may be safer to withhold the nitrite and only administer the sodium thiosulfate and/or IV hydroxocobalamin. Sodium thiosulfate can be administered through a separate IV line following the hydroxocobalamin. The initial dose of hydroxocobalamin in adults is 5 g (2 × 2.5 g vials) IV over 15 minutes (7.5 min/vial) with a second dose administered if warranted.[7]

Children As for adults, amyl nitrite can be used prior to IV administration of sodium nitrite, but only as a temporizing measure until IV sodium nitrite can be administered. Break one amyl nitrite ampule and hold it in front of the patient's mouth for 15 seconds on and 15 seconds off.[6,16] Inhalation of amyl nitrite should be discontinued prior to sodium nitrite administration.

Intravenously inject 6 to 8 mL/m^2 (approximately 0.2 mL/kg) of 3% sodium nitrite solution, not to exceed 10 mL or 300 mg.[6,16] A 0.2-mL/kg dose of 3% sodium nitrite solution is 6 mg/kg sodium nitrite. Based on an in vitro calculation, this dose would be safe for a child with a hemoglobin of 7 g/dL in the absence of other factors that could compromise hemoglobin oxygen saturation, such as carboxyhemoglobin or sulfhemoglobin.[1] The dose can be repeated at half the initial dose if manifestations of cyanide toxicity reappear or at 2 hours after the first dose as prophylaxis (see Table 126–2).[16]

Immediately following sodium nitrite infusion, 7 g/m^2 or 0.5 g/kg (2 mL/kg) of 25% solution of sodium thiosulfate, not to exceed the adult dose of 12.5 g (50 mL of 25% solution) sodium thiosulfate, should be infused intravenously. The same needle and vein can be used. The dose can be repeated at half the initial dose if manifestations of cyanide toxicity reappear or at 2 hours as prophylaxis.[6,16]

In situations where additional formation of methemoglobin would be harmful, as in patients with smoke inhalation from a fire in which other toxic gases may coexist, the nitrite can be withheld and only the sodium thiosulfate administered. Since hydroxocobalamin is now available in the United States, combined therapy with hydroxocobalamin and sodium thiosulfate would be synergistic and ideal. Although there is no approved US pediatric dose of hydroxocobalamin, 70 mg/kg has been used outside of the United States.[7] Care must be taken not to administer the hydroxocobalamin and sodium thiosulfate through the same IV line since a physical incompatibility occurs, inactivating the hydroxocobalamin.

AVAILABILITY

Sodium nitrite is available in ampules containing 300 mg in 10 mL (3% concentration) water for injection (USP). It contains no additives or preservatives. It is also available in a kit containing two ampules of sodium nitrite (300 mg in 10 mL) with 12 ampules of amyl nitrite inhalants (0.3 mL) and two vials of sodium thiosulfate 12.5 g in 50 mL water for injection (USP), with boric acid or sodium hydroxide added to adjust the pH.[6]

REFERENCES

1. Berlin CM Jr. The treatment of cyanide poisoning in children. *Pediatrics.* 1970;46:793-796.
2. Chen KK, Rose C. Nitrite and thiosulfate therapy in cyanide poisoning. *JAMA.* 1952:149:113-119.

3. Chen KK, Rose C, Clowes G. Amyl nitrite and cyanide poisoning. *JAMA.* 1933;100:1921-1922.
4. Chen KK, Rose C, Clowes G. Methylene blue, nitrites, and sodium thiosulphate against cyanide poisoning. *Proc Soc Exp Biol Med.* 1933;31:250-252.
5. Cosby K, Partovi KS, Crawford JH. Nitrite reduction to nitric oxide by deoxyhemoglobin vasodilates the human circulation. *Nat Med.* 2003;9:1498-1505.
6. Cyanide Antidote [package insert]. Decatur, IL: Taylor Pharmaceuticals; Feb 2006.
7. Cyanokit [package insert]. Napa, CA: Dey, LP; Dec 2006.
8. Hall AH, Doutre WH, Ludden T, et al. Nitrite/thiosulfate treated acute cyanide poisoning: estimated kinetics after antidote. *J Toxicol Clin Toxicol.* 1987;25:121-133.
9. Hall AH, Kulig KW, Rumack BH. Suspected cyanide poisoning in smoke inhalation: complications of sodium nitrite therapy. *J Toxicol Clin Exp.* 1989;9:3-9.
10. Hall AH, Linden CH, Kulig KW, et al. Cyanide poisoning from laetrile ingestion: role of nitrite therapy. *Pediatrics.* 1986;78:269-272.
11. Johnson WS, Hall AH, Rumack BH. Cyanide poisoning successfully treated without therapeutic methemoglobin levels. *Am J Emerg Med.* 1989;7:437-440.
12. Klimmek R, Krettek C, Werner HW. Ferrihaemoglobin formation by amyl nitrite and sodium nitrite in different species in vivo and in vitro. *Arch Toxicol.* 1988;62:152-160.
13. Marrs TC. The choice of cyanide antidotes. In: Ballantyne B, Marrs TC, eds. *Clinical and Experimental Toxicology of Cyanides.* Bristol: Wright; 1987:383-401.
14. Modin A, Bjorne H, Herulf M. Nitrite-derived nitric oxide: a possible mediator of "acidic-metabolic" vasodilation. *Acta Physiol Scand.* 2001;171:9-16.
15. Moore SJ, Norris JC, Walsh DA, et al. Antidotal use of methemoglobin forming cyanide antagonists in concurrent carbon monoxide/cyanide intoxication. *J Pharmacol Exp Ther.* 1987;242:70-73.
16. Sodium Nitrite [package insert]. Scottsdale, AZ: Hope Pharmaceuticals; July 2003.
17. Ten Eyck RP, Schaerdel AD, Ottinger WE. Stroma-free methemoglobin solution: an effective antidote for acute cyanide poisoning. *Am J Emerg Med.* 1985;3:519-523.
18. Vick JA, Froehlich HL. Studies of cyanide poisoning. *Arch Int Pharmacodyn Ther.* 1985;273:314-322.
19. Vick JA, Froehlich HL. Treatment of cyanide poisoning. *Mil Med.* 1991;156:330-339.
20. Vick JA, Von Bredow JD. Effectiveness of intramuscularly administered cyanide antidotes on methemoglobin formation and survival. *J Appl Toxicol.* 1996;16:509-516.
21. Way JL. Cyanide intoxication and its mechanism of antagonism. *Annu Rev Pharmacol Toxicol.* 1984;24:451-481.
22. Wurzburg H. Treatment of cyanide poisoning in an industrial setting. *Vet Hum Toxicol.* 1996;38:44-47.

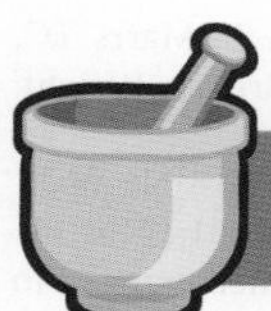

ANTIDOTES IN DEPTH (A39)

SODIUM THIOSULFATE

Mary Ann Howland

Sodium thiosulfate is a safe and effective antidote that detoxifies cyanide by donating a sulfur moiety to form thiocyanate. Thiocyanate is much less toxic than cyanide and is renally eliminated. Sodium thiosulfate works synergistically with nitrites and hydroxocobalamin in the detoxification of cyanide. Because sodium thiosulfate does not compromise hemoglobin oxygen saturation, it can be used without nitrites in circumstances where the formation of methemoglobin would be detrimental, as in patients who have elevated concentrations of carboxyhemoglobin or preexistent methemoglobinemia from smoke inhalation from fires. Sodium thiosulfate is used prophylactically with nitroprusside to prevent cyanide toxicity. Sodium thiosulfate is also used to treat calciphylaxis (calcific uremic arteriolopathy) by forming the very water-soluble calcium thiosulfate.[4,21]

HISTORY

In 1933 Chen et al.[6] noted that preexposure treatment with intravenous (IV) sodium thiosulfate protected dogs against three minimum lethal doses of sodium cyanide, and even more remarkable was the synergistic effects obtained by combining sodium thiosulfate with either inhaled amyl nitrite or IV sodium nitrite, which protected the dogs against 10 to 18 minimum lethal doses of cyanide.[5,6]

CHEMISTRY

The chemical formula of sodium thiosulfate is $Na_2S_2O_3$. The molecular weight of sodium thiosulfate is 248 Da including the pentahydrate. It is a pentahydrate that is highly water soluble. Sodium hyposulfite is a synonym.

MECHANISM OF ACTION

The sulfur provided by sodium thiosulfate binds to cyanide with the help of rhodanese (cyanide sulfur transferase) and mercaptopyruvate sulfur transferase.[6,27,29] This sulfur, a sulfane sulfur (a divalent sulfur bound to one other sulfur), is the only type of sulfur that reacts with cyanide to produce thiocyanate, which is minimally toxic and renally eliminated. In many different animal models, sodium thiosulfate protects against several minimum lethal doses of cyanide.[14,17] The addition of rhodanese increases the efficacy of sodium thiosulfate, but the use of rhodanese is impractical in the clinical setting.[17,28] The cationic site on rhodanese is crucial to cleaving the sulfur–sulfur bond of thiosulfate and forming a sulfur–rhodanese complex that readily reacts with cyanide.[29]

Rhodanese is probably not solely responsible for sulfur–sulfur bond cleavage, as rhodanese is largely a mitochondrial enzyme found in the liver and skeletal muscle, and sodium thiosulfate is a divalent ion that poorly crosses membranes.[11,17,22,27,29] An additional theory proposes that both mercaptopyruvate sulfurtransferase and rhodanese are involved in the formation of sulfane sulfur in the liver from sodium thiosulfate, and that serum albumin then carries the sulfane sulfur from the liver to other organs. When cyanide is present, albumin delivers this sulfur to cyanide, forming thiocyanate.[15,27–29]

PHARMACOKINETICS AND PHARMACODYNAMICS

ANIMAL STUDIES

Sodium thiosulfate is a large divalent anion. Canine studies suggest that sodium thiosulfate rapidly distributes into the extracellular space and then slowly into the cell, perhaps with a carrier facilitating entry into the mitochondria.[13,22] When administered prior to cyanide, thiosulfate converted more than 50% of the cyanide to thiocyanate within 3 minutes and increased the endogenous conversion rate more than 30 times.[26] One study in canines, using a continuous IV infusion model of cyanide toxicity to induce a respiratory arrest, demonstrated that the IV administration of 500 mg/kg of sodium thiosulfate brought the serum cyanide concentration down and with it restored respiration within 3 minutes.[8] Thiosulfate is filtered and secreted in the kidney. At low serum concentrations, thiosulfate is largely reabsorbed. At high serum concentrations, filtration and secretion predominate.[12,22]

HUMAN VOLUNTEERS

A volunteer study examined the pharmacokinetics of sodium thiosulfate and the fate of thiosulfate.[14,22] After injection of 150 mg/kg, volume of distribution (Vd) was 0.15 L/kg, distribution half-life was 23 minutes, and elimination half-life was 3 hours. The peak serum thiosulfate concentration rose 100-fold. Approximately 50% of the drug was eliminated in 18 hours, most of it within 3 hours. Baseline thiosulfate concentrations were higher in starved patients and children, presumably because of their higher protein utilization and metabolism to thiosulfate.[14] Normally, the kidney actively reabsorbs thiosulfate, but this study found that with exogenous administration, thiosulfate clearance equaled creatinine clearance.[14]

Another report researching the effects of thiosulfate as a cisplatin neutralizer found that thiosulfate had a half-life of 80 minutes, and that renal clearance accounted for only 30% of the total clearance.[25] Oral sodium thiosulfate is poorly absorbed and acts as a laxative.[22]

CLINICAL USE

CYANIDE TOXICITY

In 1952, 16 cyanide-poisoned patients survived with administration of nitrites and sodium thiosulfate.[5] Even patients who were unconscious or apneic survived when given timely cardiopulmonary resuscitation and antidotal therapy.[5]

Case reports attest to the ability of sodium nitrite and sodium thiosulfate to reverse the effects of cyanide with timely administration.[7,20,22]

In the few reported cases of cyanide ingestion treated with sodium thiosulfate alone all patients had favorable outcomes.[22] Prior to sodium thiosulfate administration, we advocate the use of amyl or sodium nitrite, or hydroxocobalamin if available. As noted, nitrites would be relatively contraindicated for patients who have elevated carboxyhemoglobin or methemoglobin concentrations from smoke inhalation from a fire.

CALCIFIC UREMIC ARTERIOLOPATHY (CALCIPHYLAXIS)

Case reports attest to sodium thiosulfate ameliorating calcification of the medial layer of arteries leading to subcutaneous nodules that progress to necrotic skin ulcers, a rare manifestation of vascular disease in chronic renal failure patients.[1,2,4,21] The dose of sodium thiosulfate is usually 5 to 25 g IV in adults after or during hemodialysis.[21] Thiosulfate is always used in concert with other therapies for this condition since the mechanism of action is unclear, although the increased water solubility of calcium thiosulfate is proposed.[23] In a uremic rat model, sodium thiosulfate was able to prevent vascular calcifications but also induced a metabolic acidosis and reduced bone strength.[24]

ADVERSE EFFECTS

The toxicity of sodium thiosulfate is low. The LD_{50} (median lethal dose in 50% of test subjects) for animals is approximately 3 to 4 g/kg, with death attributed to metabolic acidosis, elevated sodium concentration, and decreased blood pressure and Po_2.[17] Sodium thiosulfate delivers a significant sodium load and is hyperosmolar. Administering the infusion over 10 to 30 minutes attenuates some of these adverse effects.[22]

Adverse effects associated with therapeutic dosing include hypotension, nausea, and vomiting. The osmotic and diuretic effects presumably result from both the formation of thiocyanate and the intrinsic osmotic properties of the drug.[22]

ADMINISTRATION AND DOSING

CYANIDE TOXICITY

Adults In a patient with presumed cyanide poisoning, the adult dose of sodium thiosulfate is 12.5 g (50 mL of 25% solution) administered intravenously either as a bolus injection or infused over 10 to 30 minutes, depending on the severity of the situation.[9] The dose of sodium thiosulfate can be repeated at half the initial dose if manifestations of cyanide toxicity reappear or at 2 hours as prophylaxis.[9]

In situations where the formation of methemoglobin by a nitrite would not be harmful, intravenously inject 300 mg sodium nitrite (10 mL of 3% solution) at a rate of 2.5 to 5 mL/min prior to administration of sodium thiosulfate. The same needle and vein can be used. The dose of sodium nitrite can be repeated at half the initial dose if manifestations of cyanide toxicity reappear or at 2 hours as prophylaxis.[9]

Amyl nitrite can be used prior to IV administration of sodium nitrite, but only as a temporizing measure until IV sodium nitrite can be administered. Break one amyl nitrite ampule and hold it in front of the patient's mouth for 15 seconds on and 15 seconds off.[9] Inhalation of amyl nitrite should be discontinued prior to administration of sodium nitrite.

In situations where the additional formation of methemoglobin would be harmful, as in patients in whom carboxyhemoglobin or methemoglobin may be present from smoke inhalation from a fire, the nitrite can be withheld and only the sodium thiosulfate administered. Since hydroxocobalamin is now available in the United States, combined therapy of hydroxocobalamin with sodium thiosulfate, which is synergistic, would be ideal. The initial dose of hydroxocobalamin in adults is 5 g (2 × 2.5 g vials) IV over 15 minutes with a second dose administered if warranted.[10] Care must be taken not to administer the hydroxocobalamin and sodium thiosulfate through the same IV line since a physical incompatibility occurs, inactivating the hydroxocobalamin.

Children The dose of sodium thiosulfate in children is 7 g/m^2 up to the adult dose[9] or 0.5 g/kg (2 mL/kg of 25% solution) up to the adult dose of 12.5 g (50 mL of 25% solution).[22] The dose can be repeated at half the initial dose if manifestations of cyanide toxicity reappear or at 2 hours as prophylaxis.[9]

In situations where the formation of methemoglobin by a nitrite would not be harmful, intravenously inject 3% sodium nitrite solution at 6 to 8 mL/m^2 (approximately 0.2 mL/kg), not to exceed 10 mL or 300 mg, prior to administration of sodium thiosulfate.[9] The same needle and vein can be used. A 0.2-mL/kg dose of 3% sodium nitrite solution is approximately 6 mg/kg sodium nitrite. Based on an in vitro calculation, this dose would be safe for a child with a hemoglobin of 7 g/dL in the absence of other factors that could compromise hemoglobin oxygen saturation, such as carboxyhemoglobin, methemoglobin, or sulfhemoglobinemia.[3] The dose of sodium nitrite can be repeated at half the initial dose if manifestations of cyanide toxicity reappear or at 2 hours after the first dose as prophylaxis.[9]

Amyl nitrite can be used prior to IV administration of sodium nitrite, but only as a temporizing measure until IV sodium nitrite can be administered. Break one amyl nitrite ampule and hold it in front of the patient's mouth for 15 seconds on and 15 seconds off. Amyl nitrite inhalation should be discontinued prior to administration of sodium nitrite. The healthcare provider must not inhale the amyl nitrite.

In situations where additional formation of methemoglobin would be harmful, as in patients with smoke inhalation from a fire, the nitrite can be withheld and only the sodium thiosulfate administered. Since hydroxocobalamin is now available in the United States, combined therapy of hydroxocobalamin with sodium thiosulfate, which is synergistic, would be ideal. Although there is no approved US pediatric dose, 70 mg/kg of hydroxocobalamin has been used outside of the United States.[10] Care must be taken not to administer the hydroxocobalamin and sodium thiosulfate through the same IV line since a physical incompatibility occurs, inactivating the hydroxocobalamin.

NITROPRUSSIDE-INDUCED CYANIDE TOXICITY

Nitroprusside Canine experiments reveal that when the nitroprusside infusion rate is greater than 0.5 mg/kg/h, cyanide concentrations in the blood begin to rise. Coadministration of sodium thiosulfate with sodium nitroprusside in a 5:1 molar ratio (because nitroprusside contains five cyanide ions) prevents the rise in cyanide concentration.[22] The usual dosage of sodium nitroprusside is 3 μg/kg/min (range 0.25–10 μg/kg/min).[18] Each mole of nitroprusside has a molecular weight of 298 Da including the sodium dehydrate and contains five cyanide ions. A 70-kg person administered 3 μg/kg/min would receive 12.6 mg/h of nitroprusside. This would require 52.4 mg of sodium thiosulfate per hour to detoxify the five cyanide ions liberated from nitroprusside. Prolonged infusion or doses in excess of the body's detoxifying capability may lead to thiocyanate or cyanide toxicity. Some authors recommend adding 0.5 g sodium thiosulfate to each 50 mg of nitroprusside.[19] This dose of sodium thiosulfate usually is sufficient to prevent cyanide toxicity from nitroprusside; however, thiocyanate may accumulate, especially in patients with renal insufficiency. Although thiocyanate is relatively nontoxic compared to cyanide it may produce dose-dependent tinnitus, miosis, hyperreflexia, and hypothyroidism, especially at serum concentrations greater than 60 μg/mL,[18] and thiocyanate is hemodialyzable. Nitroprusside-induced cyanide toxicity should be treated like cyanide toxicity from any other cause: stop the nitroprusside dosage and administer sodium thiosulfate, sodium nitrite, or hydroxocobalamin (if available) according to the doses and precautions listed.

AVAILABILITY

Sodium thiosulfate is available in 50-mL vials containing 12.5 g in water for injection (USP), with boric acid or sodium hydroxide added to adjust the pH. It is also available in a kit containing two ampules of sodium nitrite (300 mg in 10 mL water for injection) with 12 ampules of amyl nitrite inhalants (0.3 mL) and two vials of sodium thiosulfate 12.5 g in 50 mL water for injection, with boric acid or sodium hydroxide added to adjust the pH.[9]

REFERENCES

1. Ackermann F, Levy A, Daugas E, et al. Sodium thiosulfate as first line therapy for calciphylaxis. *Arch Derm.* 143:1336-1337.
2. Baker B, Fitzgibbons C, Buescher L. Calciphylaxis responding to sodium thiosulfate therapy. *Arch Derm.* 2007;143:269-270.
3. Berlin CH Jr. The treatment of cyanide poisoning in children. *Pediatrics.* 1970;46:793-796.
4. Brucculeri M, Cheigh J, Bauer G, et al. Long term intravenous sodium thiosulfate in the treatment of a patient with calciphylaxis. *Semin Dialysis.* 2005;18:431-434.
5. Chen KK, Rose C. Nitrite and thiosulfate therapy in cyanide poisoning. *JAMA.* 1952:149:113-119.
6. Chen KK, Rose C, Clowes G. Methylene blue, nitrites, and sodium thiosulphate against cyanide poisoning. *Proc Soc Exp Biol Med.* 1933;31:250-252.
7. Chin RG, Calderon Y. Acute cyanide poisoning: a case report. *J Emerg Med.* 2000;18:441-445.
8. Christel D, Eyer P, Hegemann M, et al. Pharmacokinetics of cyanide in poisoning of dogs and the effect of 4-dimethylaminophenol or thiosulfate. *Arch Toxicol.* 1977;38:177-189.
9. Cyanide [package insert]. Decatur, IL: Taylor Pharmaceuticals; July 1998.
10. Cyanokit [package insert]. Napa, CA: Dey, LP; Dec 2006.
11. Devlin DJ, Mills JW, Smith RP. Histochemical localization of rhodanese activity in rat liver and skeletal muscle. *Toxicol Appl Pharmacol.* 1989;97:247-255.
12. Foulks J, Brazeau P, Koelle ES, et al. Renal secretion of thiosulfate in the dog. *Am J Physiol.* 1952;168:77-85.
13. Ivankovich AD, Braverman B, Kanuru RP, et al. Cyanide antidotes and methods of their administration in dogs: a comparative study. *Anesthesiology.* 1980;52:210-216.
14. Ivankovich AD, Braverman B, Stephens TS, et al. Sodium thiosulfate disposition in humans: relation to sodium nitroprusside toxicity. *Anesthesiology.* 1983;58:11-17.
15. Jarabak R, Westley J, Dungan JM, et al. A chaperone-mimetic effect of serum albumin on rhodanese. *J Biochem Toxicol.* 1993;8:41-48.
16. Mannaioni G, Vannacci A, Marzocca C, et al. Acute cyanide intoxication treated with a combination of hydroxycobalamin, sodium nitrite, and sodium thiosulfate. *J Toxicol Clin Toxicol.* 2002;40:181-183.
17. Marrs TC. The choice of cyanide antidotes. In: Ballantyne B, Marrs TC, eds. *Clinical and Experimental Toxicology of Cyanides.* Bristol: Wright; 1987:383-401.
18. McEvoy GE, ed. *AHFS Drug Information 2005. Nitroprusside.* Bethesda, MD: American Society of Health-System Pharmacists; 2005.
19. Megarbane B, Delahaye A, Goldgran-Toledano D, et al. Antidotal treatment of cyanide poisoning. *J Chin Med Assoc.* 2003;66:193-203.
20. Mehta C. Antidotal effect of sodium thiosulfate in mice exposed to acrylonitrile. *Res Commun Mol Pathol Pharmacol.* 1995;87:155-165.
21. Meissner M, Kaufmann R, Gille J. Sodium thiosulfate: a new way of treatment for caliphylaxis? *Dermatology.* 2007;214:278-282.
22. Meredith TJ, Jacobsen D, Haines JA, et al, eds. *Antidotes for Poisoning by Cyanide.* New York: Cambridge Press; 1993.
23. O'Neill C. Treatment of vascular calcification. *Kid Internat.* 2008;74:1376-1388.
24. Pasch A, Schaffner T, Huynh-Do U, et al. Sodium thiosulfate prevents vascular calcifications in uremic rats. *Kid Internat.* 2008;74:1444-1453.
25. Shea M, Koziol JA, Howell SB. Kinetics of sodium thiosulfate, a cisplatin neutralizer. *Clin Pharmacol Ther.* 1984;35:419-425.
26. Sylvester DM, Hayton WL, Morgan RL, et al. Effects of thiosulfate on cyanide pharmacokinetics in dogs. *Toxicol Appl Pharmacol.* 1983;69:265-271.
27. Way JL. Cyanide intoxication and its mechanism of antagonism. *Annu Rev Pharmacol Toxicol.* 1984;24:451-481.
28. Westley J. Mammalian cyanide detoxification with sulphane sulphur. *Ciba Found Symp.* 1988;140:201-218.
29. Westley J, Adler H, Westley L, et al. The sulfurtransferases. *Fundam Appl Toxicol.* 1983;3:377-382.

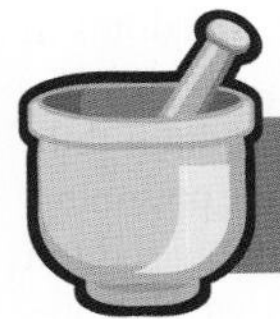

ANTIDOTES IN DEPTH (A40)

HYDROXOCOBALAMIN

Mary Ann Howland

Hydroxocobalamin is a relatively new antidote for cyanide toxicity in the United States. Cyanocobalamin, vitamin B_{12}, is formed when hydroxocobalamin combines with cyanide. Nitrites and sodium thiosulfate have traditionally been used to treat patients with cyanide toxicity. Nitrites have the disadvantage of producing methemoglobin, which is dangerous in a patient with coexistent elevated carboxyhemoglobin concentrations, such as would be found in fire victims suspected of having cyanide toxicity. Unfortunately, there are no controlled studies comparing sodium thiosulfate with hydroxocobalamin in these circumstances.

HISTORY

The antidotal actions of cobalt as a chelator of cyanide were recognized as early as 1894.[12,35] Hydroxocobalamin has been used as a cyanide antidote in France for many years, first as a sole agent and then in combination with sodium thiosulfate.[19] In the United States, hydroxocobalamin was finally approved by the Food and Drug Administration (FDA) in December 2006 and is available under the trade name Cyanokit.[11,13]

Hydroxocobalamin subsequently was shown to be successful in protecting against several minimum lethal doses of cyanide as long as an equimolar ratio of hydroxocobalamin to cyanide was used.[1,7,28,33]

CHEMISTRY

The molecule is porphyrinlike in structure and has a cobalt ion at its core. The only difference between cyanocobalamin (vitamin B_{12}) and hydroxocobalamin (referred to as vitamin B_{12a}) is the replacement of the CN group with an OH group at the active site in the latter.[24,30]

MECHANISM OF ACTION

The cobalt ion in hydroxocobalamin combines with cyanide to form the nontoxic cyanocobalamin.[27,28] One mole of hydroxocobalamin binds 1 mole of CN. Given the molecular weights of each, 52 g of hydroxocobalamin are needed to bind 1 g of cyanide.[19] An ex vivo study using human skin fibroblasts demonstrates that hydroxocobalamin penetrates intracellularly to form cyanocobalamin.[2] In the setting of cyanide poisoning, hydroxocobalamin removes cyanide from the mitochondrial electron transport chain, allowing oxidative metabolism to proceed. Hydroxocobalamin also binds nitric oxide, a vasodilator, causing vasoconstriction, particularly in the absence of cyanide. This same property potentially contributes to its beneficial effects by increasing systolic and diastolic blood pressure and improving the hemodynamic status of cyanide-poisoned patients.[7,16] Other cobalt chelators, such as dicobalt ethylenediaminetetraacetic acid (EDTA), have been used both experimentally and clinically in other countries, but their therapeutic index is narrow, especially in the absence of cyanide. Additionally, idiosyncratic adverse effects make these compounds less advantageous.[27,35] Use of hydroxocobalamin with sodium thiosulfate is synergistic and comparable to the sequential use of sodium nitrite with sodium thiosulfate.[19,33]

PHARMACOKINETICS AND PHARMACODYNAMICS

Under an FDA Investigational New Drug permit, the first pharmacokinetic study of intravenous (IV) hydroxocobalamin was performed in the United States and published in 1993.[13,14] Adult volunteers who were heavy smokers were given 5 g hydroxocobalamin (5%) intravenously, obtained from a French manufacturer. The first four patients received the dose undiluted over 20 minutes.[14] They then received 12.5 g (50 mL of 25% solution) of sodium thiosulfate intravenously infused over 20 minutes. The next 11 patients received the same dose of hydroxocobalamin but diluted with 100 mL water for injection (USP) and infused over 30 minutes. The serum and urine sampling of hydroxocobalamin differed in the two patient groups, yielding somewhat different half-lives (4 hours versus 1.27 hours). The α distribution half-life was 0.52 hours in the group 1 patients. Peak hydroxocobalamin concentration averaged 813 μg/mL (604 μmol/L), and volume of distribution (Vd) averaged 0.38 L/kg. A mean dose of 62% was recovered in the urine in 24 hours. Whole-blood cyanide concentrations significantly decreased in all subjects following hydroxocobalamin. A problem with this study was the short collection time for serum hydroxocobalamin concentrations of only 6 hours, making the pharmacokinetic analysis imprecise.[20,21]

A pharmacokinetic study performed in adult victims of smoke inhalation in France[19] was conducted with very different patients given hydroxocobalamin 5 g (5%) by IV infusion over 30 minutes, starting within 30 minutes of their removal from the fire.[20,21] The α distribution half-life of hydroxocobalamin was 1.86 hours, elimination half-life was 26.2 hours based on sampling up to 6 days, and Vd was 0.45 L/kg. The peak serum cyanocobalamin concentration was 287 μg/mL (212 μmol/L). In the one patient who was subsequently determined not exposed to cyanide, the hydroxocobalamin elimination half-life was 13.6 hours and Vd was 0.23 L/kg. Renal clearance of hydroxocobalamin was 37% in the cyanide-exposed patients compared with 62% in the unexposed patient.

In a study of 12 fire victims in France who were suspected of having cyanide poisoning, the patients received IV hydroxocobalamin 5 g in 100 mL sterile water (USP) over 30 minutes.[23] Pretreatment and posttreatment cyanide concentrations and cyanocobalamin concentrations were analyzed. In patients with cyanide concentrations less than 1.04 μg/mL (less than 40 μmol/L), a linear relationship existed between the blood cyanide concentration and the formation of cyanocobalamin. In the three patients with blood cyanide concentration greater than 1.04 μg/mL (greater than 40 μmol/L), the formation of cyanocobalamin reached a plateau, implying that all of the hydroxocobalamin was consumed. In the one patient with a blood cyanide concentration greater than 1.04 μg/mL (greater than 40 μmol/L) who received a second 5-g dose of hydroxocobalamin, the cyanocobalamin concentration subsequently rose.[3,23]

The protein binding and tissue distribution of cyanide, hydroxocobalamin, and cyanocobalamin likely are different.[22] In addition, hydroxocobalamin probably causes redistribution of cyanide from the intracellular to the intravascular space.[22]

CLINICAL USE

Many case reports and studies in France document the efficacy of hydroxocobalamin combined with sodium thiosulfate for treatment of cyanide toxicity.[6,8,18] An observational case series reviewed 69 adult smoke inhalation victims suspected of cyanide poisoning who were treated either at the scene of the fire or in the intensive care unit (ICU). They received a median dose of 5 g of hydroxocobalamin, up to a maximum of 15 g, infused as a 5% solution in sterile water for injection over 15 to 30 minutes. Cardiopulmonary arrest occurred in 15 patients, with a mean blood cyanide concentration of 123 μmol/L (greater than 100 μmol/L = greater than 2.7 μg/mL and potentially fatal), and a mean carboxyhemoglobin of 30%. Two of these patients survived with normal neurologic function. Of 42 patients with confirmed cyanide concentrations greater than 39 μmol/L (1 μg/mL), 28 (67%) survived. The contribution to toxicity of carboxyhemoglobin is difficult to sort out in this study. Of the 69 patients in this study, 57 also received hyperbaric oxygen, complicating the interpretation of the outcome results.[7]

An 8-year retrospective analysis of the use of hydroxocobalamin in the prehospital setting concluded that the risk-benefit ratio favors its use in smoke inhalation victims suspected of cyanide poisoning.[15] Of 72 patients in whom survival status could be determined, 30 (42%) survived. Cyanide blood concentrations were not measured in these patients. Of 38 patients found in cardiac arrest, 21 had hemodynamic improvement; however, survival was dismal with only two patients ultimately surviving. The neurologic function of those two patients was not revealed.

Hydroxocobalamin also prevented the rise in cyanide concentration following nitroprusside infusion compared with patients who just received nitroprusside.[9] When nitroprusside is administered, use of concomitant hydroxocobalamin prevents cyanide accumulation and toxicity in both animal models and in humans.[8,9,36] Sodium thiosulfate also prevents nitroprusside-induced cyanide toxicity (see Antidotes in Depth A39: Sodium Thiosulfate).

There are currently no studies comparing the nitrite plus sodium thiosulfate regimen with hydroxocobalamin in patients with cyanide poisoning. There are no studies comparing hydroxocobalamin with or without sodium thiosulfate to sodium thiosulfate alone in smoke inhalation victims presumed cyanide toxic. Most animal studies demonstrate a synergistic effect of hydroxocobalamin and thiosulfate on the elimination of cyanide.[18]

ADVERSE EFFECTS

Hydroxocobalamin has a wide therapeutic index.[7,15,34] Large doses have been administered to animals with no adverse effects.[27,31,32] The LD_{50} (median lethal dose in 50% of test subjects) in mice is 2 g/kg.

Red discoloration of mucous membranes, serum, and urine may occur and last from 12 hours to days after therapy.[7,15] Allergic reactions including anaphylaxis and angioedema are reported, but serious allergic reactions are rare.[5,6,8,30] Prior chronic exposure to hydroxocobalamin or cyanocobalamin for treatment of vitamin B_{12} deficiency is associated rarely with development of anaphylaxis.[19] A study in 102 healthy volunteers demonstrated that chromaturia is universal, and as the dose increases from 2.5 g to 10 g, the incidence of skin erythema, pustular rash, headache, injection site reaction, nausea, pruritus, chest discomfort, dysphagia, and papular rash increases.[34] Two patients developed allergic reactions that required therapy. Skin rash lasted up to 9 days, while the pustular rash appeared most often on the face and neck after a delay of 1 to 3 weeks and lasted 1 to 4 weeks. Of 102 volunteers randomized to receive hydroxocobalamin, 24 experienced a clinically significant rise in diastolic blood pressures, up to 124 mm Hg. However, only three of them also had a clinically significant rise in systolic blood pressure up to 188 mm Hg. These elevations in blood pressure resolved within 4 hours of the end of the infusion.

The hydroxocobalamin solution should not be administered through the same infusion site or at the same time as the thiosulfate solution because sodium thiosulfate binds to hydroxocobalamin and renders it inactive.[29]

An in vitro study found statistically significant alterations in serum concentrations of aspartate aminotransferase (AST), total bilirubin, creatinine, magnesium, and iron after hydroxocobalamin administration.[10] Colorimetric assays are most likely to be adversely affected because both hydroxocobalamin and cyanocobalamin have an intensely red color. Although an in vitro study demonstrated a considerable false increase in carboxyhemoglobin concentrations by hydroxocobalamin when measured by cooximetry, other authors suggest that the interference is minimal and results in slight overestimates depending on the instrument and the concentration of hydroxocobalamin.[4,17,25] Inconsequential increases of 1% to 5.7% in the carboxyhemoglobin concentration occurred in another study.[17]

ADMINISTRATION AND DOSING

CYANIDE TOXICITY

The starting dose of hydroxocobalamin in adults is 5 g (two 2.5-g vials). Each vial is reconstituted with 100 mL of 0.9% sodium chloride and administered intravenously over 15 minutes (7.5 min/vial). Each vial should be inverted or rocked (not shaken) for 30 seconds prior to administration. The reconstituted solution should be dark red and free of particulate matter, and should be used within 6 hours of reconstitution.[11] A second dose of 5 g can be repeated as clinically necessary and infused over 15 minutes to 2 hours depending on patient status.[11]

In children, a dose of 70 mg/kg of hydroxocobalamin up to the adult dose has been used in places outside of the United States.[11]

Sodium thiosulfate can be administered in addition to hydroxocobalamin. It is expected to be synergistic and has been used extensively in conjunction with hydroxocobalamin.[26] Care must be taken not to administer the hydroxocobalamin and sodium thiosulfate simultaneously through the same IV line since this may inactivate the hydroxocobalamin. The adult dose of sodium thiosulfate is 12.5 g (50 mL of 25% solution) and should be administered intravenously as either a bolus injection or infused over 10 to 30 minutes, depending on the severity of the situation. The dose of sodium thiosulfate in children is 7 g/m^2 up to the adult dose, or 0.5 g/kg (2 mL/kg of 25% solution) up to the adult dose of 12.5 g. The dose of sodium thiosulfate can be repeated at half the initial dose if manifestations of cyanide toxicity persist or reappear, or empirically at 2 hours as prophylaxis.

NITROPRUSSIDE INDUCED CYANIDE TOXICITY

The dose of hydroxocobalamin to prevent cyanide toxicity from the IV infusion of nitroprusside is not precisely known, but a dose of hydroxocobalamin of 25 mg/h in one study was sufficient to decrease the red cell and serum cyanide concentrations and to prevent the development of a metabolic acidosis while the nitroprusside continued to be administered.[36] These authors recommend possibly continuing the hydroxocobalamin for 10 hours after the discontinuation of the nitroprusside. Hydroxocobalamin could also be used as rescue therapy in the typical dosage, as could sodium thiosulfate (see Antidotes in Depth A39: Sodium Thiosulfate).

AVAILABILITY

Each Cyanokit contains two 250 mL glass vials, each containing 2.5 g of lyophilized dark red, hydroxocobalamin crystalline powder for injection.[11] The kit also contains two sterile transfer spikes, one sterile IV infusion set, one quick reference guide and one package insert, but no diluent.

REFERENCES

1. Anonymous. Editorial comment: hydroxocobalamin analysis. *J Toxicol Clin Toxicol.* 1997;35:417.
2. Astier A, Baud FJ. Complexation of intracellular cyanide by hydroxocobalamin using a human cellular model. *Hum Exp Toxicol.* 1996;15:19-25.
3. Astier A, Baud FJ. Simultaneous determination of hydroxocobalamin and its cyanide complex cyanocobalamin in human plasma by high-performance liquid chromatography. Application to pharmacokinetic studies after high-dose hydroxocobalaminas an antidote for severe cyanide poisoning. *J Chromatogr B Biomed Appl.* 1995;667:129-135.
4. Baud F. Clarifications regarding interference of hydroxocobalamin with carboxyhemoglobin measurements in victims of smoke inhalation. *Ann Emerg Med.* 2007;50:625-626.
5. Baud FJ, Barriot P, Toffis V, et al. Elevated blood cyanide concentrations in victims of smoke inhalation. *N Engl J Med.* 1991;325:1761-1766.
6. Beasley DM, Glass WI. Cyanide poisoning: pathophysiology and treatment recommendations. *Occup Med (Lond).* 1998;48:427-431.
7. Borron SW, Baud F, Barriot P, et al. Prospective study of hydroxocobalamin for acute cyanide poisoning in smoke inhalation. *Ann Emerg Med.* 2007;49:794-801.
8. Braitberg G, Vanderpyl M. Treatment of cyanide poisoning in Australasia. *Emerg Med.* 2000;12:232-240.
9. Cottrell JE, Casthely P, Brodie JD. Prevention of nitroprusside-induced cyanide toxicity with hydroxocobalamin. *N Engl J Med.* 1978;298:809-811.
10. Curry SC, Connor DA, Raschke RA. Effect of the cyanide antidote hydroxocobalamin on commonly ordered serum chemistry studies. *Ann Emerg Med.* 1994;24:65-67.
11. Cyanokit [package insert]. Columbia, Md: manufactured for King Pharmaceuticals, Inc. by Merck Sante and distributed by Meridian Medical Technolgies, Inc; August, 2009.
12. Evans CL. Cobalt compounds as antidotes for hydrocyanic acid. *Br J Pharmacol.* 1964;23:455-475.
13. Food and Drug Administration. Listing of Orphan Drugs. http://www.fda.gov/orphan/designat/alldes.rtf (accessed November 18, 2005).
14. Forsyth JC, Mueller PD, Becker CE, et al. Hydroxocobalamin as a cyanide antidote: safety, efficacy and pharmacokinetics in heavily smoking normal volunteers. *J Toxicol Clin Toxicol.* 1993;31:277-294.
15. Fortin JL, Giocanti JP, Ruttimann M, Kowalski JJ. Prehospital administration of hydroxocobalamin for smoke inhalation-associated cyanide poisoning: 8 years of experience in the Paris Fire Brigade. *Clin Toxicol.* 2006;44:37-44.
16. Gerth K, Ehring T, Braendle M, Schelling P. Nitric oxide scavenging by hydroxocobalamin may account for its hemodynamic profile. *Clin Toxicol.* 2006;44:29-36.
17. Gourlain H, Buneaux F, Levillain P. Mesure du CO et de la COHb dans le sang: interferences de l'hydroxocobalamine et du bleu de methylene en CO-oxymetre. *Revue Francaise des Laboratoires.* 1996;282:144-148.
18. Hall AH, Rumack BH. Hydroxycobalamin/sodium thiosulfate as a cyanide antidote. *J Emerg Med.* 1987;5:115-121.
19. Hall AH, Rumack BH, Schaffer MI, et al. Clinical toxicology of cyanide: North American experiences. In: Ballantyne B, Marrs TC, eds. *Clinical and Experimental Toxicology of Cyanides.* Bristol: Wright; 1987:313-333.
20. Houeto P, Borron SW, Sandouk P, et al. Hydroxocobalamin analysis and pharmacokinetics. Authors' response. *J Toxicol Clin Toxicol.* 1997;35:413-415.
21. Houeto P, Borron SW, Sandouk P, et al. Pharmacokinetics of hydroxocobalamin in smoke inhalation victims. *J Toxicol Clin Toxicol.* 1996;34:397-404.
22. Houeto P, Hoffman JR, Imbert M, et al. Authors' reply to: Monitoring of cyanocobalamin and hydroxocobalamin during treatment of cyanide intoxication. *Lancet.* 1995;346:1706-1707.
23. Houeto P, Hoffman JR, Imbert M, et al. Relation of blood cyanide to plasma cyanocobalamin concentration after a fixed dose of hydroxocobalamin in cyanide poisoning. *Lancet.* 1995;346:605-608.
24. Kaczka EA, Wolf DE, Kuehl FA Jr, Folkers K. Vitamin B_{12}: reactions of cyano-cobalamin and related compounds. *Science.* 1950;112:354-355.
25. Lee J, Mukai D, Kreuter K, et al. Potential interference by hydroxocobalamin in cooximetry hemoglobin measurements during cyanide and smoke inhalation treatments. *Ann Emerg Med.* 2007;49:802-805.
26. Leybell I, Hoffman R, Boron S. Toxicity, Cyanide. http://emedicine.medscape.com/article/814287-overview (accessed February 1, 2009).
27. Marrs TC. Antidotal treatment of acute cyanide poisoning. *Adverse Drug React Acute Poisoning Rev.* 1988;7:179-206.
28. Marrs TC. The choice of cyanide antidotes. In: Ballantyne B, Marrs TC, eds. *Clinical and Experimental Toxicology of Cyanides.* Bristol: Wright; 1987:383-401.
29. Mengel K, Kramer W, Isert B. Thiosulphate and hydroxocobalamin prophylaxis in progressive cyanide poisoning in guinea-pigs. *Toxicology.* 1989;54:335-342.
30. Meredith TJ, Jacobsen D, Haines JA, et al, eds. *Antidotes for Poisoning by Cyanide.* New York: Cambridge Press; 1993.
31. Posner MA, Tobey RE, McElroy H. Hydroxocobalamin therapy of cyanide intoxication in guinea pigs. *Anesthesiology.* 1976;44:157-160.
32. Riou B, Berdeaux A, Pussard E, et al. Comparison of the hemodynamic effects of hydroxocobalamin and cobalt edetate at equipotent cyanide antidotal doses in conscious dogs. *Intensive Care Med.* 1993;19:26-32.
33. Rose CL, Worth RM, Chen KK. Hydroxo-cobalamine and acute cyanide poisoning in dogs. *Life Sci.* 1965;4:1785-1789.
34. Uhl W, Nolting A, Golor G, et al. Safety of hydroxocobalamin in healthy volunteers in a randomized, placebo controlled study. *Clin Toxicol.* 2006;44:17-28.
35. Way JL. Cyanide intoxication and its mechanism of antagonism. *Annu Rev Pharmacol Toxicol.* 1984;24:451-481.
36. Zerbe NF, Wagner BK. Use of vitamin B_{12} in the treatment and prevention of nitroprusside-induced cyanide toxicity. *Crit Care Med.* 1993;21:465-467.

CHAPTER 127
METHEMOGLOBIN INDUCERS

Dennis P. Price

Methemoglobin occurs when the iron atom in hemoglobin loses one electron to an oxidant, and the ferrous (Fe^{2+}) or oxidized state of iron is transformed into the ferric (Fe^{3+}) state. Although methemoglobin is always present at low concentrations in the body, methemoglobinemia is defined herein as an abnormal elevation of the methemoglobin level above 1%.

The widespread utilization of pulse oximetry in clinical medicine has made it easier to recognize low oxygen saturation, consequently increasing our recognition of methemoglobinemia. The ubiquity of oxidants both in the environment and in the hospital has increased the number of case reports associated with methemoglobin. It is also evident that host factors play a crucial role in the development of methemoglobinemia in many individuals.

Biologic systems have protective cell membrane and intracellular mechanisms that are protective with regard to oxidant stresses. Some are enzyme systems that involved electron transport mechanisms, and others are simple reducers such as ascorbic acid and reduced glutathione. When fully functional, these systems maintain methemoglobin levels under 1%, but with acute and/or chronic stress, they may be overwhelmed, allowing methemoglobin level to increase.

The cellular systems that protect the individual from oxidant stress involve cytochrome b reductase, flavin, nicotinamide adenine dinucleotide (NADH)methemoglobin reductase, nicotinamide adenine dinucleotide phosphate (NADPH) methemoglobin reductase, reduced glutathione and ascorbic acid are interrelated and incompletely understood. Depletion of the reducing power of these systems leads to methemoglobinemia and other disorders of oxidant stress such as hemolysis.

Underlying illnesses,[47,57,72,74] the treatment with xenobiotics for these illnesses,[3,17,58,73] and the therapeutic and diagnostic modalities involved[47,72] in patient care all predispose patients to methemoglobinemia. For many individuals, methemoglobinemia is not caused by one oxidant stressor but rather a series of stressors that makes methemoglobinemia clinically apparent and potentially predictable.

Reduced hemoglobin functions reliably as an oxygen transporter because in its protected heme pocket, it shares an outer valence electron with the oxygen it transports. Normally reduced hemoglobin releases this oxygen without giving up an electron, but occasionally, this electron is lost to the departing oxygen in the process of autooxidation. Oxidation is increased in the presence of some hereditary conditions such as hemoglobin M disease. However, oxidizing xenobiotics may produce methemoglobin by direct interaction with the Fe^{2+} moiety. These exogenous products are a major source of oxidant stress to the individual and the most frequent cause of methemoglobinemia. Although typically not life threatening, methemoglobinemia may produce symptoms of cellular hypoxia and should be considered in the differential diagnosis of cyanotic patients who do not have an apparent cardiovascular cause. In the cases of methemoglobinemia, cyanosis is not caused by deoxyhemoglobin but rather by the color imparted to the skin as a result of oxidized hemoglobin.

HISTORY AND EPIDEMIOLOGY

Methemoglobin was first described by Felix Hoppe-Seyler in 1864.[29] Subsequently, in 1891, a case of transient drug-induced methemoglobinemia was described.[65] In the late 1930s, methemoglobinemia was recognized as a predictable adverse effect of sulfanilamide use, and methylene blue was recommended for treatment of the ensuing cyanosis.[39] Some authors even recommended concurrent use of methylene blue when sulfanilamides were used.[93] Methylene blue has been used prophylactically during general surgery to treat an individual with congenital methemoglobinemia.[6] In 1948, an enzyme defect was reported in twin brothers. The defect caused cyanosis in the absence of cardiopulmonary disease and responded to ascorbic acid. [31]

Methemoglobinemia may be hereditary or acquired. The hereditary types are rare, with only several hundred cases reported.[40,89] Although the frequency with which xenobiotic-induced methemoglobinemia occurs is unknown, the American Association of Poison Control Centers' annual data show approximately 100 uses of methylene blue as an antidote. These data substantially underestimate the incidence of this poisoning because poison centers are not notified in most cases (see Chap. 135).

Methemoglobinemia is relatively common and generally produces no clinical findings. Co-oximetry data collected at two teaching hospitals noted a significant number of elevated methemoglobin levels.[4] Of a total of 5248 co-oximetry tests over 28 months on 1267 patients, 660 tests revealed methemoglobin levels above 1.5% in 414 patients (some patients had more than one test). Thus, 12.5% of all tests and 19.1% of all patients who had co-oximetry performed had an abnormal methemoglobin level. A total of 138 patients with peak methemoglobin levels greater than 2% were identified. The mean peak methemoglobin level was 8.4% (range, 2.1%–60.1%), and the ages of the patients ranged from 4 days to 86 years old.

Benzocaine spray accounted for the most seriously poisoned patients ($n = 5$), with a mean peak methemoglobin level of 43.8% (range, 19.1–60.1%). Dapsone accounted for the largest number of cases ($n = 58$), with a mean peak of 7.6% (range, 2.1–34.1%). Of the 33 of 35 patients who had elevated methemoglobin levels, 8% had symptomatic methemoglobinemia, and 12 received methylene blue. One fatality and three near fatalities were directly attributed to methemoglobinemia. These data likely represent an underestimation of the true number of cases of methemoglobinemia at these institutions because co-oximetry was performed only upon physician orders for suspected dyshemoglobinemia, and 25% of cases with levels above 2% were found incidentally when co-oximetry was performed in the catheterization laboratory to provide data on oxyhemoglobin and deoxyhemoglobin. Also, not all patients taking dapsone were tested.[4] Extrapolating these data throughout the country would suggest underreporting and substantial under recognition of this entity with its potential danger.

The incidence of induced methemoglobinemia in the workplace is poorly documented. A number of reports document several hundred such cases of methemoglobinemia and several more workplace exposures.[15,61,86] Underreporting and underrecognition occur because of the limited symptoms associated with low concentrations of methemoglobin in most cases.

HEMOGLOBIN PHYSIOLOGY

Hemoglobin consists of four polypeptide chains noncovalently attracted to each other. Each of these subunits carries one heme molecule deep within the structure. The polypeptide chain protects the iron moiety of the heme molecule from inappropriate oxidation (Fig. 127–1).

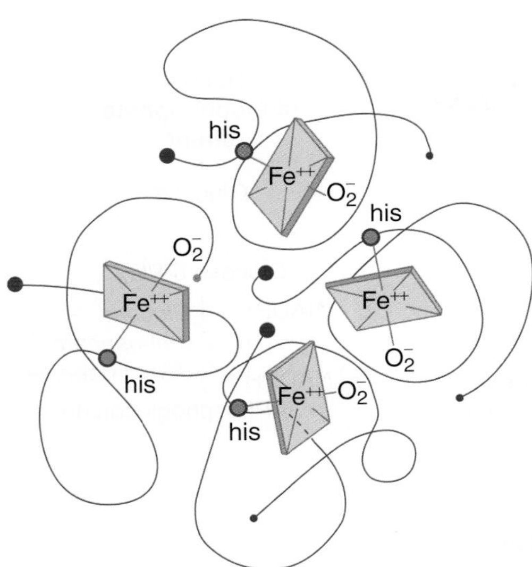

FIGURE 127–1. Hemoglobin molecule symbolically represented with its heme center surrounded by the globin portion of the molecule. his = histidine.

The iron is held in position by six coordination bonds. Four of these bonds are between iron and the nitrogen atoms of the protoporphyrin ring with the fifth and sixth bond sites lying above and below the protoporphyrin plane. The fifth site is occupied by histidine of the polypeptide chain. A variety of hemoglobin mutations are attributable to changes in the amino acid sequence of the polypeptide chain, as occur in the hemoglobin M diseases. This influences this protective "pocket," allowing easier iron oxidation (Fig. 127–2), or hemoglobin auto-oxidation. The sixth coordination site is where most of the activity within hemoglobin occurs. Oxygen transport occurs here, and this site is involved with the formation of methemoglobin or carboxyhemoglobin (Fig. 127–3). It is at this site that an electron is lost to oxidant xenobiotics, transforming iron from its ferrous (Fe^{2+}) to its ferric (Fe^{3+}) state.

Hemoglobin transports an oxygen molecule only when its iron atom is in the reduced ferrous state (Fe^{2+}). During oxygen transport, the iron atom actually transfers an electron to oxygen, thus transporting oxygen as a superoxide charged particle $Fe^{3+}O^{2-}$. When oxygen is released, the ferrous state is restored, and hemoglobin is ready to accept another oxygen molecule. Interestingly, a small percentage of oxygen is released from hemoglobin with its shared electron (forming superoxide $O^{2\cdot}$), leaving iron oxidized (Fe^{3+}). This sixth coordination site becomes occupied by a water molecule. This abnormal unloading of oxygen contributes to the steady-state level of approximately 1% methemoglobin found in normal individuals.

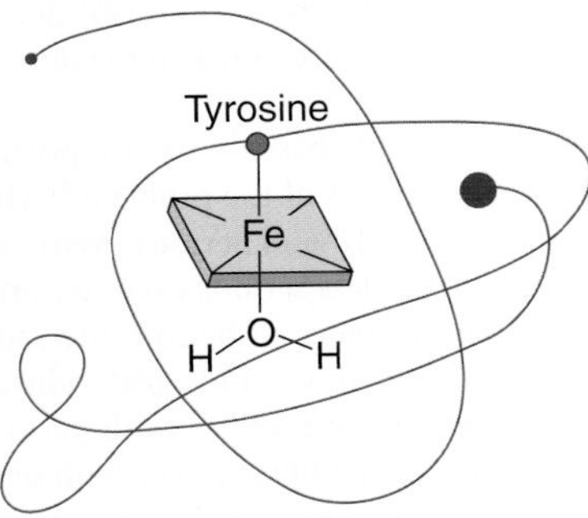

FIGURE 127–2. Hemoglobin M occurs when histidine is replaced by tyrosine in the amino acid sequence of the polypeptide chain. Hemoglobin M is more easily auto-oxidized (as shown) to methemoglobin.

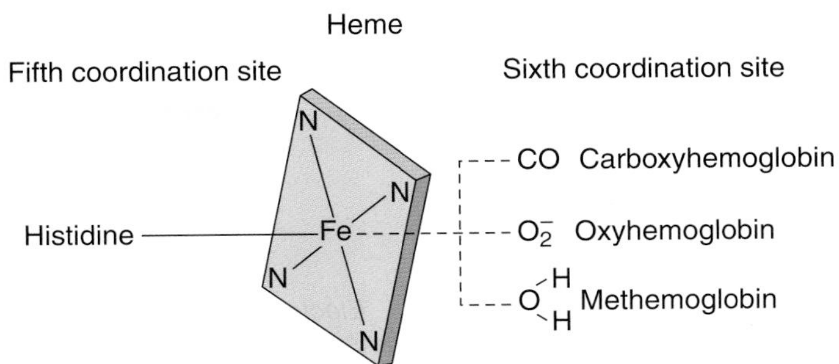

FIGURE 127–3. Heme molecule depicted with its bonding sites. Oxyhemoglobin, carboxyhemoglobin, and methemoglobin all involve the sixth coordination bonding site of iron.

METHEMOGLOBIN PHYSIOLOGY AND KINETICS

Because of the spontaneous and xenobiotic-induced oxidation of iron, the erythrocyte has developed multiple mechanisms to maintain a normal concentration of methemoglobin.[12] All of these systems donate an electron to the oxidized iron atom. Because of these effective reducing mechanisms, the half-life of methemoglobin acutely formed as a result of exposure to oxidants is between 1 and 3 hours.[44,64] With continuous exposure to the oxidant, the apparent half-life of methemoglobin is prolonged.

Quantitatively the most important reductive system requires NADH, which is generated in the Embden-Meyerhof glycolytic pathway (Fig. 127–4). NADH serves as an electron donor, and along with the enzyme NADH methemoglobin reductase, reduces Fe^{3+} to Fe^{2+}. There are numerous cases of hereditary deficiencies of the enzyme NADH methemoglobin reductase.[40] Individuals who are homozygotes for this enzyme deficiency usually have methemoglobin levels of 10% to 50% under normal conditions without any clinical or xenobiotic stressors. Individuals who are heterozygotes do not ordinarily demonstrate methemoglobinemia except when they are subject to oxidant stress. Additionally, because this enzyme system lacks full activity until approximately 4 months of age, even genetically normal infants are more susceptible than adults to oxidant stress.[69,95]

Oxidized iron can be reduced nonenzymatically using either ascorbic acid or reduced glutathione as electron donors, but this method is slow and quantitatively less important under normal circumstances.

Within the red cell is another enzyme system for reducing oxidized iron that is dependent on the NADPH generated in the hexose monophosphate shunt pathway (see Fig. 127–4). Although it is generally accepted that this NADPH-dependent system reduces only a small percentage of methemoglobin under normal circumstances, it may play a more prominent role in maintaining oxidant balance in the cell.[53] Patients with an isolated deficiency of NADPH methemoglobin reductase do not exhibit methemoglobinemia under normal circumstances,[85] perhaps because of the prominence of other cellular protective mechanisms.

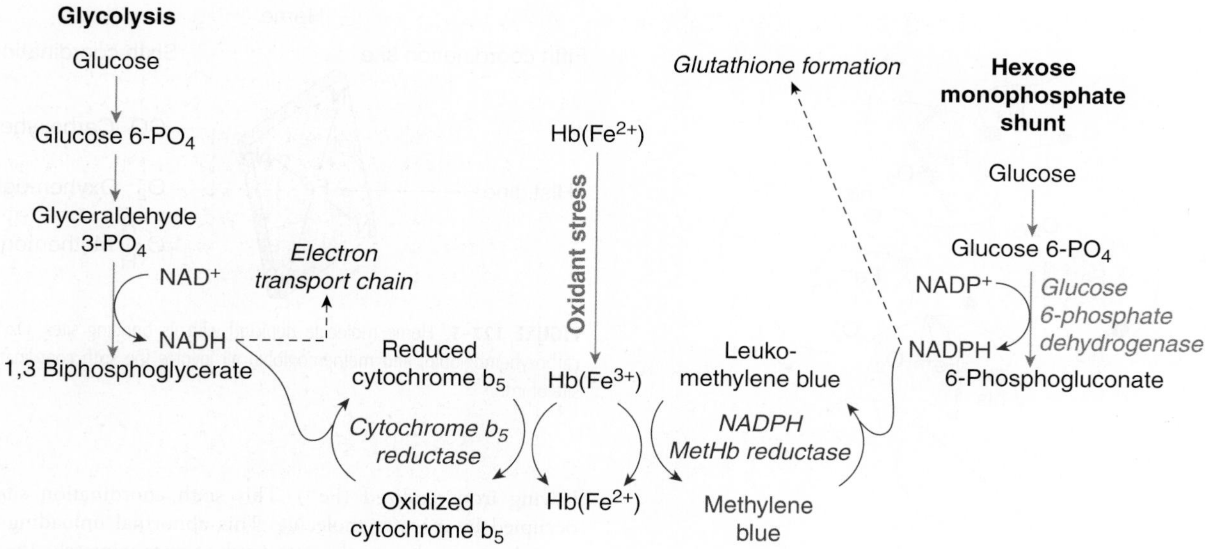

FIGURE 127–4. Role of glycolysis in the Embden-Meyerhof pathway and the role of methylene blue in the reduction of methemoglobin using NADPH generated by the hexose monophospate shunt. Hb(Fe^{3+}) is methemoglobin.

However, when the NADPH methemoglobin reductase system is provided with an exogenous electron carrier, such as methylene blue, this system is accelerated and may assist in the reduction of oxidized hemoglobin (see Antidotes in Depth A41: Methylene Blue).

XENOBIOTIC INDUCED METHEMOGLOBINEMIA

Nitrates and nitrites are powerful oxidizing agents that are two of the most common methemoglobin-forming compounds. Sources of nitrates and nitrites include well water, food, industrial compounds, and pharmaceuticals. Nitrogen-based fertilizers and nitrogenous waste from animal and human sources may contaminate shallow rural wells. The contamination of drinking water occurs mainly with nitrates because nitrites are easily oxidized to the highly soluble nitrates in the environment. Furthermore, foods such as cauliflower, carrots, spinach, and broccoli have high nitrate content, as do preservatives in meat products such as hot dogs and sausage.[5] Dietary nitrates are generally converted by intestinal bacteria to nitrates before absorption.

The reactions of nitrates that occur both in vivo and in vitro are complex and poorly understood. Ingested nitrates are reduced to nitrites by bacteria in the gastrointestinal (GI) tract (especially in infants) and then can be absorbed, ultimately leading to methemoglobin production. This conversion is not essential, however, because nitrates themselves can oxidize hemoglobin.[27,38,88] Some question whether well water consumption alone can cause serious methemoglobinemia in the absence of comorbid disease.[24]

In the past, nitrate-contaminated well water was associated with infant fatalities because of methemoglobinemia.[55,63] A number of reports from the Midwest United States demonstrated the problems of poorly constructed shallow wells that permit contamination by surface waters containing chemicals, pesticides, fertilizers, and microorganisms.[66] In several South Dakota studies, 20% to 50% of wells contained both coliform bacteria and water that exceeded the Environmental Protection Agency standards for permissible quantities of nitrogen as nitrates (10 ppm or 10 mg/L).[46] In New York State, 419 wells from rural farms demonstrated elevated concentrations of nitrogen compounds, and 15.7% were found to have well water nitrate concentrations >10 mg/L.[30]

Nitroglycerin (glyceryl trinitrate) and organic nitrates are more effectively absorbed through mucous membranes and intact skin than from the GI tract. Their onset of action is more rapid, and the total effect is much greater, when mucous membrane or cutaneous absorption occurs.[20,43,,75] Aromatic amino and nitro compounds indirectly produce methemoglobin.[49] These xenobiotics do not form methemoglobin in vitro; therefore, they are assumed to do so by in vivo metabolic chemical conversion to some active intermediates.[14,51]

Elevated methemoglobin and carboxyhemoglobin level are found in victims of fires and automobile exhaust fume poisoning.[11,43,48,59] Heat-induced hemoglobin denaturation in burn patients and the inhalation of oxides of nitrogen from combustion are suggested to be causative factors for methemoglobin formation.

Topical anesthetics are widely used to facilitate multiple procedures and are implicated in the most serious of toxic methemoglobin cases.[1,36] Cetacaine spray (14% benzocaine, 2% tetracaine, 2% butylaminobenzoate) and 20% benzocaine sprays commonly produce of methemoglobinemia. The dosing recommendations are difficult to comprehend (eg, 0.5-second spray repeat once) and are often ignored. One study showed that the dose is dependent on the residual volume in the canister and the physical orientation of the canister as the spray is being applied.[52]

A review of 52 months of data from the Food and Drug Administration (FDA) Adverse Event Reporting System demonstrated 132 cases of benzocaine-induced methemoglobinemia. Benzocaine spray was implicated in 107 severe adverse events and two deaths. In 123 cases, the product was a spray. In 69 cases in which the dose was specified, 37 patients received a single spray.[67]

This FDA effort is exclusively based on self-reporting and probably greatly underestimates the extent of the problem.[34] The FDA itself has estimated that approximately 10% of serious events are reported and that some studies show 1% or less serious event reporting.[67]

In one institution, the incidence of benzocaine-induced methemoglobinemia occurring during transesophageal echocardiograms was determined in 28,478 patients over a 90-month period. The incidence was low at 0.067% (one case per 1499 patient), with sepsis, anemia, and hospitalization suggested as predisposing factors.[47] During a 32-months period at another institution, an incidence of 0.115% (five of 4336) of benzocaine-induced methemoglobinemia was observed.[72] There were no cases of methemoglobinemia in a study of 154 patients receiving

TABLE 127–1. Factors That May Predispose an Individual to Methemoglobinemia

Acidosis[84,96]
Advanced age[72]
Age younger than 36 months[21,69,95]
Anemia[47]
Concomitant oxidant use[3,58,73]
Diarrhea[37,77]
Hospitalization[47,72]
Malnutrition
Renal insufficiency[33]
Sepsis[47,57,72,74]

lidocaine for bronchoscopy at doses as high as 15 mg/kg. Lidocaine is a much weaker oxidant than benzocaine and is a reasonable substitute in susceptible individuals.

Nitric oxide (NO) delivered by inhalation is used to treat persistent pulmonary hypertension of newborns and other cardiopulmonary diseases associated with pulmonary hypertension because it is a potent vasodilator.[82] Despite being a potent oxidant, if NO is used in doses of less than 40 ppm, most patients will maintain methemoglobin levels under 4%.[41,92] Some cases of serious toxicity have occurred because of intentional and unintentional overdoses.

Dapsone has been implicated as a cause of methemoglobinemia and is used in patients with AIDS. Cases of prolonged methemoglobinemia from dapsone ingestion are related to the long half-life of dapsone and the slow conversion to its methemoglobin-forming hydroxylamine metabolites.[23] Patients receiving dapsone should be carefully monitored for methemoglobinemia.[94] The bladder anesthetic phenazopyridine is a commonly reported causes of methemoglobinemia.[19,26,30,68] For this reason, its use should be limited to short periods of time and at the lowest dose to improve symptoms. This approach is particularly pertinent in the presence of renal failure. Predispositions for methemoglobinemia are listed in Table 127–1.

Infants who are bottled fed with well water may be exposed to nitrates and nitrites. Additionally, infants have a relatively large body surface area, making dermal and mucosal absorption of oxidants more of a threat to them than adults.

Methemoglobinemia of unknown origin is often reported in infants.[77,84,96] These patients are usually ill for other reasons such as dehydration, acidosis, or diarrhea.[37] These infants may have methemoglobin levels in the 20% to 67% range with severe consequences.[42] As noted above, young children are relatively deficient in the enzyme glucose-6-phosphate dehydrogenase (G-6-PD), accounting for their high incidence of methemoglobinemia.

METHEMOGLOBINEMIA AND HEMOLYSIS

The enzyme defect responsible for most instances of oxidant-induced hemolysis is G-6-PD deficiency. Reviews of hemolysis addressed the confusion regarding the relationship between hemolysis and methemoglobinemia.[9,10,28]

Both hemolysis and methemoglobinemia are caused by oxidant stress, and hemolysis may occur after episodes of methemoglobinemia.[10] Certain protective mechanisms involving NADPH and reduced glutathione nonspecifically reduce the oxidant burden and prevent the development of both disorders. Another source of confusion concerning hemolysis and methemoglobinemia is that reduced glutathione is required to protect against both toxic manifestations. Erythrocytes are able to withstand hemolytic oxidant damage as long as they can maintain adequate concentrations of reduced glutathione, the principal cellular antioxidant. Glutathione is maintained in its reduced form by using NADPH as its reducing agent. Cells with reduced capacity to produce NADPH (ie, erythrocytes of patients with G-6-PD deficiency or cells with depleted reduced glutathione or NADPH) are thus susceptible to hemolysis. In the presence of methemoglobinemia, reduced glutathione plays a minor role as a reducing agent, but NADPH is necessary for successful antidotal therapy with methylene blue. This codependence on the reducing power of NADPH links the two disorders. Competition for NADPH by oxidized glutathione and exogenously administered methylene blue is postulated to be the cause of methylene blue-induced hemolysis (ie, competitive inhibition of glutathione reduction). Methylene blue itself is an oxidant, but in an assessment of the hemolytic potency of varied drugs, methylene blue in doses of 390 to 780 mg proved to be only a moderate hemolytic agent.[50] The clinical importance of this phenomenon is uncertain. It may be easier to consider hemolysis and methemoglobin formation as subclasses of disorders of oxidant stress. They should be considered separate clinical entities sharing limited characteristics.

However, oxidative damage to erythrocytes occurs at different locations in the two disorders. Hemolysis occurs when oxidants damage the hemoglobin chain acting directly as electron acceptors or through the formation of hydrogen peroxide or other oxidizing free radicals. This results in oxidants forming irreversible bonds with sulfhydryl group of hemoglobin cause denaturation and precipitation of the globin protein to form Heinz bodies within the erythrocyte (Figure 127–5). Cells with large numbers of Heinz bodies are removed by the reticuloendothelial system, producing hemolysis. Alternatively, a limited number of oxidants can destroy the erythrocyte membrane directly, causing non–Heinz body hemolysis. Methemoglobinemia does not necessarily progress to hemolysis, even if untreated (Table 127–2).

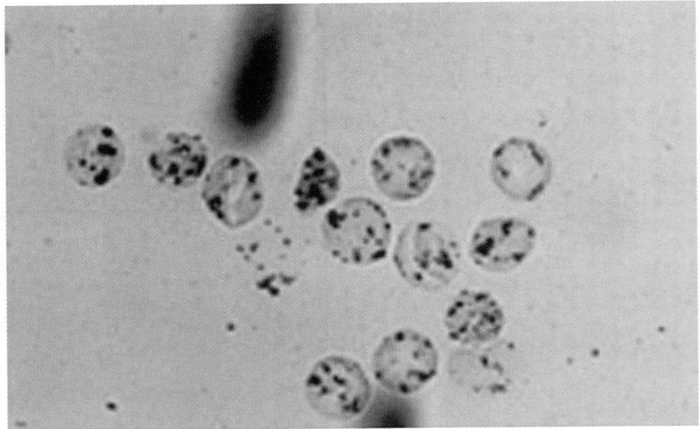

FIGURE 127–5. Heinz bodies are particles of denatured hemoglobin, usually attached to the inner surface of the red cell membrane. Xenobiotics that result in the oxidative denaturation of hemoglobin in normal (eg, phenylhydrazine) or glucose-6-phosphate dehydrogenase–deficient (primaquine) individuals and unstable hemoglobin mutants are prone to develop these bodies. The Heinz bodies can be identified when blood is mixed with a supravital stain, notably crystal violet. The Heinz bodies appear as purple inclusions. (Reproduced with permission from Lichtman MA, Shafer MS, Felgar RE, Wang N. *Lichtman's Atlas of Hematology*, 1st ed. New York: McGraw-Hill, Inc; 2007.)

Numerous cases describe the occurrence of hemolysis after methemoglobinemia. The combined occurrence is reported with dapsone,[23] phenazopyridine,[19,26,32,68] amyl nitrite,[16] and aniline.[46,49] These instances of combined syndromes may represent the incidental toxicity of an oxidizing agent at both locations or may represent the depletion of all cellular defenses against oxidants. Currently, it is not possible to predict when hemolysis will occur after methemoglobinemia with any degree of certainty.

CLINICAL MANIFESTATIONS

The clinical manifestations of methemoglobinemia are related to impaired oxygen-carrying capacity and delivery to the tissue. The clinical manifestations of acquired methemoglobinemia are usually more severe than those produced by a corresponding degree of anemia. This discordance occurs because methemoglobin not only decreases the available oxygen-carrying capacity but also increases the affinity of the unaltered hemoglobin for oxygen. This shifts the oxygen hemoglobin dissociation curve to the left, which further impairs oxygen delivery[22] (see Chap. 21). This effect is attributed to the formation of heme compounds intermediate between normal reduced hemoglobin (all four iron atoms are ferrous) and methemoglobin, in which one or more of the iron moieties are in the ferric state.[22] The degree to which this high oxygen affinity hemoglobin reduces oxygen delivery to the tissue from arterial blood is unclear but is clinically significant.[18]

Because the symptoms associated with methemoglobinemia are related to impaired oxygen delivery to the tissues, concurrent diseases such as anemia, congestive heart failure, chronic obstructive pulmonary disease, and pneumonia may greatly increase the clinical effects of methemoglobinemia (Fig. 127–6). Predictions of symptoms and recommendations for therapy are based on methemoglobin percentage in previously healthy individuals with normal total hemoglobin concentrations.

Cyanosis is a consistent physical finding in patients with substantial methemoglobinemia and is caused by the deeply pigmented color of methemoglobin. Cyanosis typically occurs when just 1.5 g/dL of methemoglobin is present. This represents only 10% conversion of hemoglobin to methemoglobin if the baseline hemoglobin is 15 g/dL. In contrast, 5 g/dL of deoxyhemoglobin (which represents 33% of hemoglobin) is needed to produce the same degree of cyanosis from hypoxia.

In previously healthy individuals, methemoglobin levels of 10% to 20% usually result in cyanosis without apparent adverse clinical manifestations. At 20% to 50% methemoglobin levels, dizziness, fatigue, headache, and exertional dyspnea may develop. At about 50% methemoglobin, lethargy and stupor usually appear. The lethal percent probably is greater than 70% (Table 127–3).

The cyanosis associated with methemoglobinemia is both peripheral and central. Patients often appear in less distress or less ill than patients with cyanosis secondary to cardiopulmonary causes.

The symptoms of methemoglobinemia are determined not only by the absolute percent of methemoglobin but also by its rates of formation and elimination. A percentage of methemoglobin that may be clinically benign when caused by hereditary defects or maintained chronically likely will produce more severe signs when acutely acquired. Healthy subjects lack the compensatory mechanisms that develop over a lifetime in individuals with hereditary compromise, such as erythrocytosis and increased 2,3-bisphosphoglyceric acid (2,3 BPG).

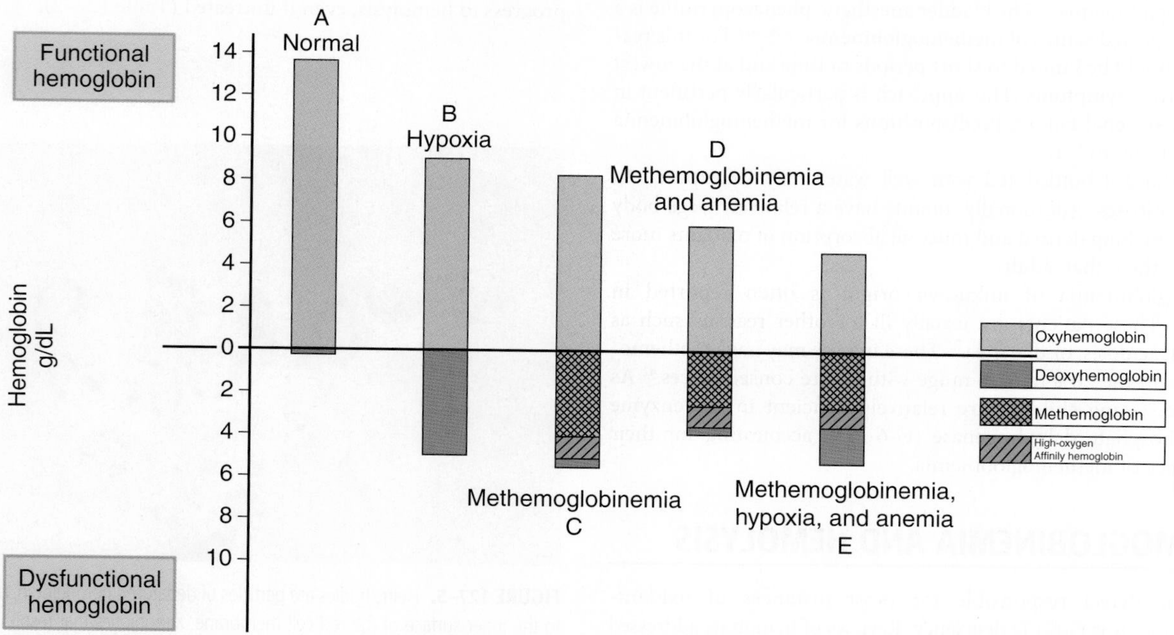

FIGURE 127–6. Clinical manifestations of methemoglobinemia depend on the level of methemoglobin and on host factors such as preexisting disease, anemia, and hypoxemia. Five examples of arterial blood gas and co-oximeter analyses are presented. **(A)** Blood gas from a normal individual with 14 g/dL of hemoglobin. Almost all hemoglobin is saturated with oxygen. **(B)** Blood gas from a patient with cardiopulmonary disease producing cyanosis in which only 9 g/dL of hemoglobin is capable of oxygen transport. **(C)** Methemoglobin level of 28% in an otherwise normal individual will reduce hemoglobin available for oxygen transport to less than 9 g/dL (~4 g/dL of methemoglobin and 1.3 g/dL of high oxygen affinity hemoglobin because of the left shift of the oxyhemoglobin dissociation curve). **(D)** Same degree of methemoglobin as in *C* but in a patient with a hemoglobin of 10 g/dL. Only 6 g/dL of hemoglobin would be capable of oxygen transport. **(E)** Methemoglobinemia and anemia to the same degree as *D* but in a hypoxic patient.

TABLE 127–2. Common Causes of Methemoglobinemia

Hereditary
- Hemoglobin M
- Cytochrome b_5 reductase deficiency (homozygote and heterozygote)

Acquired
- A. Medications
  - Amyl nitrite
  - Benzocaine
  - Dapsone
  - Lidocaine
  - Nitric oxide
  - Nitroglycerin
  - Nitroprusside
  - Phenazopyridine
  - Prilocaine
  - Quinones (chloroquine, primaquine)
  - Sulfonamides (sulfanilamide, sulfathiazide, sulfapyridine, sulfamethoxazole)
- B. Other xenobiotics
  - Aniline dye derivatives (shoe dyes, marking inks)
  - Chlorobenzene
  - Fires (heat-induced denaturation)
  - Organic nitrites (eg, Isobutyl nitrite, butyl nitrite)
  - Naphthalene
  - Nitrates (eg, well water)
  - Nitrites (eg, foods)
  - Nitrophenol
  - Nitrous gases (seen in arc welders)
  - Silver nitrate
  - Trinitrotoluene

Pediatric
- Reduced NADH methemoglobin reductase activity in infants (<4 months)
- Associated with low birth weight, prematurity, dehydration, acidosis, diarrhea, and hyperchloremia

DIAGNOSTIC TESTING

For an individual in whom methemoglobinemia is suspected, a source for the oxidant stress should be sought. Arterial blood gas sampling may reveal blood with a characteristic chocolate brown color. However, in patients who are clinically stable and not in need of an arterial puncture, a venous blood gas will be accurate in demonstrating the methemoglobin level. The arterial PO_2 should be normal, reflecting the adequacy of pulmonary function to deliver dissolved oxygen to the blood. However, arterial PO_2 does not directly measure the hemoglobin oxygen saturation (SaO_2) or oxygen content of the blood. When the partial pressure of oxygen is known and oxyhemoglobin and deoxyhemoglobin are the only species of hemoglobin, oxygen saturation can be calculated accurately from the arterial blood gas. If, however, other hemoglobins are present, such as methemoglobin, sulfhemoglobin, or carboxyhemoglobin, then the fractional saturation of the different hemoglobin species must be determined by co-oximetry.

The co-oximeter is a spectrophotometer that identifies the absorptive characteristics of several hemoglobin species at different wavelengths. Because oxyhemoglobin, deoxyhemoglobin, methemoglobin, and carboxyhemoglobin all have different absorptions at the different measuring points of the co-oximeter, their proportions and concentrations can be determined. Some newer co-oximeters have an expanded spectrum at which they read and are also able to read fetal hemoglobin and sulfhemoglobin.[97]

The pulse oximeter applied to a patient's finger at the bedside was developed to estimate oxygen saturation trends in critically ill patients. The device takes advantage of the unique absorptive characteristics of oxyhemoglobin and deoxyhemoglobin and the different concentrations of these two hemoglobin species during different phases of the pulse. Each manufacturer has calibrated its oximeter using volunteers breathing progressively increasing hypoxic gas mixtures in the absence of a dyshemoglobinemia.[78,87,91] In other words, the oxygen saturation values displayed on the pulse oximeter are derived independently by each manufacturer, which develops a formula using their own hardware and sensor. The manufacturer then compares this value with a set of validation data derived from an experimental population.

Most pulse oximeters in use today use two different wavelengths to determine O_2, saturation and the manufactures do not provide validation data for situation where any dyshemoglobin is present. These manufactures disclaim accuracy under such circumstances. Similar to co-oximetry, the dual-wavelength pulse oximeter reads absorbance of light at wavelengths of 660 and 940 nm, which are selected to efficiently separate oxyhemoglobin and deoxyhemoglobin. However, methemoglobin absorption at these wavelengths is greater than that of either oxyhemoglobin or deoxyhemoglobin.[8,70] Therefore, when methemoglobin is present, the readings become inaccurate. The degree of inaccuracy is unique for each brand of instrument and may be influenced by signal quality, skin temperature, refractive error induced by blood cells, and other factors (eg, finger thickness and perfusion).[80]

In the dog model, the pulse oximeter oxygen saturation (SpO_2) values decrease with increasing methemoglobin levels. This decrease in SpO_2 is not exactly proportional to the percentage of methemoglobin. However, the pulse oximeter overestimates the level of actual oxygen saturation. For example, in a case in which the methemoglobin level measured in the blood using a co-oximeter was 20%, the pulse oximeter indicated an SpO_2 of 90%.[8,90] However, as the methemoglobin concentration approached 30%, the pulse oximeter saturation values decreased to about 85% and then leveled off, regardless of how much higher the methemoglobin level became.[8,90]

From our experience and that of others,[35,79] in humans, much lower levels of oxygen saturation (SpO_2) than 85% can occur by pulse oximetry when methemoglobin levels increase above 30%.[45] These differences result from variations in the way different model pulse oximeters deal with methemoglobin interference.[78,79] The clinician, therefore, must understand how the particular pulse oximeter measures oxygen saturation when methemoglobin levels are elevated and recognize that co-oximetry determination is needed when methemoglobinemia is suspected.

Although the pulse oximeter reading in patients with methemoglobinemia may not be as accurate as desired, it may be helpful when it is compared with that of the arterial blood gas: if there is a difference between the *measured* oxyhemoglobin saturation of the pulse oximeter (SaO_2) and the *calculated* oxyhemoglobin saturation of the arterial blood gas (SpO_2), then a "saturation gap" exists. The calculated SaO_2 of the blood gas will be greater than the measured SpO_2 if methemoglobin is present (Table 127–4).

Recently, a pulse oximeter has been developed that reads at eight different wavelengths. This pulse oximeter displays methemoglobin and carboxyhemoglogin. Validation experiments were performed using volunteers with varying degrees of methemoglobinemia.[7]

TABLE 127–3. Signs and Symptoms Typically Associated with Methemoglobin Levels in Healthy Patients with Normal Hemoglobin Concentrations

Methemoglobin Level (%)	Signs and Symptoms
1–3 (normal)	None
3–15	Possibly none
	Slate gray cutaneous coloration
	Pulse oximeter reads low SaO_2
15–20	Cyanosis
	Chocolate brown blood
20–50	Dyspnea
	Exercise intolerance
	Headache
	Fatigue
	Dizziness, syncope
	Weakness
50–70	Tachypnea
	Metabolic acidosis
	Dysrhythmias
	Seizures
	CNS depression
	Coma
>70	Grave hypoxic symptoms
	Death

MANAGEMENT

For most patients with mild methemoglobinemia of approximately 10%, no therapy is necessary other than withdrawal of the offending xenobiotic because reduction of the methemoglobin will occur by normal reconversion mechanisms (NADH methemoglobin reductase). However, in some patients, even small elevations of methemoglobin should be considered problematic because they suggest the individual is at a point where further oxidant stress may cause methemoglobin levels to increase. An individual receiving dapsone with a small elevation of methemoglobin level may be more susceptible to clinically significant methemoglobinemia if challenged with a benzocaine-containing anesthetic or an increase in dapsone dose. In the clinical setting, continued absorption, prolonged half-life, and toxic intermediate metabolites may prolong methemoglobinemia. Patients should be examined carefully for signs of physiologic stress related to decreased oxygen delivery to the tissue (Fig. 127–7). Obviously, changes in mental status or ischemic chest pain necessitate immediate treatment, but subtle changes in behavior or inattentiveness may be signs of global hypoxia and should be treated. Patients with abnormal vital signs tachycardia and tachypnea or an elevated lactate concentration thought to be caused by tissue hypoxia or the functional anemia of methemoglobinemia should be treated aggressively. An elevated methemoglobin level alone generally is not an adequate indication of need for therapy.

The most widely accepted treatment of methemoglobinemia is administration of one to two mg/kg body weight of methylene blue infused intravenously (IV) over 5 minutes. This is 0.1 to 0.2 mL/kg of 1% solution. The use of a slow 5-minute infusion helps prevent painful local responses from rapid infusion. When a painful reaction occurs, it can be minimized by flushing the IV rapidly with a bolus of at least 15 to 30 mL of fluid after the infusion. Clinical improvement should be noted within minutes of methylene blue administration. If cyanosis has not disappeared within 1 hour of the infusion, a second dose should be given and other factors considered (see Fig. 127–7). Methylene blue causes a transient decrease in the pulse oximetry reading because its blue color has excellent absorbance at 660 mm.[54,60]

The use of methylene blue in patients with G-6-PD deficiency is controversial. Deficiency of this enzyme is an estimated 200 million people worldwide. Its incidence in the United States is highest among African Americans (11%),[9] among whom the disease has different degrees of severity. For this reason, G-6-PD–deficient patients have been excluded from most treatment protocols because methylene blue is a mild oxidant and case reports have suggested methylene blue's toxicity. However, because of the lack of immediate availability of G-6-PD testing, most patients who need treatment receive methylene blue therapy before their G-6-PD status is known. Although many patients with G-6-PD deficiency undoubtedly have been treated unknowingly, few case reports of toxicity have been described.

Even the authors of the review most frequently cited as a rationale for withholding methylene blue treatment were unsure whether the methylene blue given to their G-6-PD–deficient patient produced hemolysis[83]; the dose of methylene blue given to the patient was small, and the patient had taken other xenobiotics capable of producing hemolysis. Patients with G-6-PD deficiency have variable activity of the enzyme and manifest different degrees of disease in response to oxidant stress. For all of these reasons, the judicious use of methylene blue is warranted in most patients with G-6-PD deficiency and symptomatic methemoglobinemia.

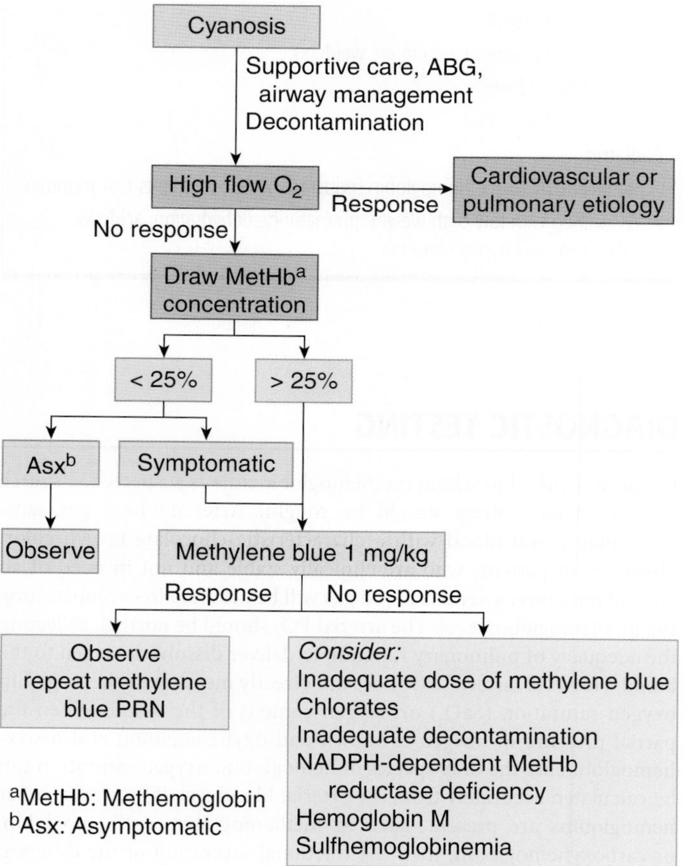

FIGURE 127–7. Toxicologic assessment of a cyanotic patient.

If methylene blue treatment fails to significantly relieve the methemoglobinemia, a number of possibilities should be considered. The cause of the oxidant stress may not have been identified and adequately removed, allowing for continuing oxidation. In such situations, decontamination of the gut and skin cleansing must be assured. Additional doses of methylene blue are also indicated. Patients who have sulfhemoglobinemia, or are deficient in NADPH methemoglobin reductase, may not improve after methylene blue therapy (see Antidotes in Depth A41: Methylene Blue).

Theoretically, exchange transfusion or hyperbaric oxygen (HBO) may be beneficial when methylene blue is ineffective. Both interventions are time consuming and costly, but HBO allows the dissolved oxygen time to protect the patient while endogenous methemoglobin reduction occurs. Ascorbic acid is not indicated in the management of acquired methemoglobinemia if methylene blue is unavailable because the rate at which ascorbic acid reduces methemoglobin is considerably slower than the rate of normal intrinsic mechanisms.[13] Methylene blue has no therapeutic benefit in the presence of sulfhemoglobinemia.[76]

Treatment with dapsone deserves special consideration because of its tendency to produce prolonged methemoglobinemia. *N*-hydroxylation of dapsone to its hydroxylamine metabolite by a cytochrome P450–mediated reaction is partly responsible for methemoglobin formation in both therapeutic and overdose situations. Both the parent compound and its metabolites are oxidants with long half-lives. Cimetidine is a competitive inhibitor in the cytochrome p450 metabolic pathway and reduces methemoglobin concentrations during therapeutic dosing because less dapsone will be metabolized by the route.[81] In overdose situations, cimetidine may exert some protective effects and should be used with methylene blue. When dapsone is therapeutically indicated but low levels of methemoglobin are found, cimetidine should be considered as a method for reducing oxidant stress.

SULFHEMOGLOBIN

Sulfhemoglobin is a hemoglobin variant in which a sulfur atom is incorporated into the heme molecule but is not attached to iron. The exact location of the sulfur atom in the porphyrin ring is unclear. Sulfhemoglobin is a darker pigment than methemoglobin, producing cyanosis when only 0.5 g/dL of blood is affected. The cyanosis produced is similar to that produced by methemoglobinemia. Sulfhemoglobin also reduces the oxygen saturation determined by the pulse oximeter[2,71] and is characterized in the laboratory by its spectrophotometric appearance and its lack of reaction when cyanide is added to the mixture. Cyanide does not react with sulfhemoglobin but does react with methemoglobin, forming cyanomethemoglobin, which has no adsorption at the spectrums tested. In contrast, the methemoglobin absorption peak will no longer be present after the addition of cyanide. Using conventional co-oximetery, sulfhemoglobin is misidentified as methemoglobin. However, the addition of cyanide to the blood sample eliminates the methemoglobin peak (through conversion to cyanomethemoglobin) but not the methemoglobin peak caused by sulfhemoglobin. This technique is not routinely done in the clinical laboratory, and the diagnosis often is made based on the patient's failure to improve with methylene blue.[2,56,62,71] In the laboratory, isoelectric focusing techniques further define sulfhemoglobin.

Sulfhemoglobin is an extremely stable compound that is eliminated only when red blood cells are removed naturally from circulation. Although the oxygen-carrying capacity of hemoglobin is reduced by sulfhemoglobinemia, unlike methemoglobinemia there is a decreased affinity for oxygen in the remaining "unaltered" hemoglobin. The oxyhemoglobin dissociation curve is shifted to the right (see Fig. 21-2). This makes oxygen more available to the tissues. This phenomenon reduces the clinical effect of sulfhemoglobin in the tissues.

Sulfhemoglobin can be produced experimentally in vitro by the action of hydrogen sulfide on hemoglobin and was produced in dogs fed elemental sulfur.[76] A number of xenobiotics induce sulfhemoglobin in humans, including acetanilid, phenacetin, nitrates, trinitrotoluene, and sulfur compounds. Most of the xenobiotics that produce methemoglobinemia have been reported in various degrees to produce sulfhemoglobinemia. Sulfhemoglobinemia is also recognized in individuals with chronic constipation and in those who abuse laxatives.[76]

Sulfhemoglobinemia usually requires no therapy other than withdrawal of the offending xenobiotic. It appears that patients come to the

TABLE 127–4. Hemoglobin Oxygenation Analysis

Measuring Device	Source	What is Measured?	How Are Data Expressed?	Benefits	Pitfalls	Insight
Blood gas analyzer	Blood	Partial pressure of dissolved oxygen in whole blood	PO_2	Also gives information about pH and PCO_2	Calculates SaO_2 from the partial pressure of oxygen in blood; inaccurate if forms of Hb other than OxyHb and DeoxyHb are present	An abnormal Hb form may exist if gap exists between ABG and pulse oximeter
Co-oximeter	Blood	Directly measures absorptive characteristics of oxyhemoglobin, deoxyhemoglobin, methemoglobin, and carboxyhemoglobin at different wavelength bands in whole blood	SaO_2, %MethHb, %CoHb, %OxyHb, %DeoxyHb	Directly measures hemoglobin species	Provides data on hemoglobin only; most instruments will not measure sulfhemoglobin, HbM, and some other forms of Hb	Most accurate method of determining the oxygen content of blood
Pulse oximeter	Monitor sensor on patient	Absorptive characteristics of oxyhemoglobin in pulsatile blood assuming the presence of only OxyHb and DeoxyHb in vivo	SpO_2	Moment-to-moment bedside data	Inaccurate data if interfering substances are present (methemoglobin, sulfhemoglobin, carboxyhemoglobin, methylene blue)	Maximum depression, 75%–85% regardless of how much methemoglobin is present

ABG, arterial blood gas; Hb, hemoglobin; HbM, hemoglobin M; SaO_2, hemoglobin oxygen saturation; SpO_2, pulse oximeter oxygen saturation.

attention of clinicians earlier because sulfhemoglobinemia produces more cyanosis than does methemoglobinemia. There is no antidote for sulfhemoglobinemia because it results from an irreversible chemical bond that occurs within the hemoglobin molecule. Exchange transfusion would lower the sulfhemoglobin concentration, but this approach usually is unnecessary.

SUMMARY

Oxidation of hemoglobin is a less common but rapidly treatable cause of cyanosis. In the absence of findings of cardiopulmonary disease, methemoglobinemia is likely the cause of cyanosis. The diagnosis is confirmed by evaluation of blood by co-oximetry. When treatment is clinically indicated, methylene blue is the treatment of choice. The source of oxidant stress should be sought and eliminated. Patients with low methemoglobin levels should be considered to be under oxidant stress and at risk for more serious methemoglobinemia if oxidant stressors persist or increase in their environment. Methemoglobinemia should be considered to be a disease state sometimes caused by an acute, overwhelming oxidant protective mechanism of the host by an oxidant or more commonly and importantly, as a final clinical manifestation of multiple oxidant stressors.

REFERENCES

1. Aepfelbacher FC, Breen P, Manning WJ. Methemoglobinemia and topical pharyngeal anesthesia. *N Engl J Med.* 2003;348:85-86.
2. Aravindhan N, Chisholm DG. Sulfhemoglobinemia presenting as pulse oximetry desaturation. *Anesthesiology.* 2000;93:883-884.
3. Arrivabene Caruy CA, Cardoso AR, Cespedes Paes F, Ramalho Casta L. Perioperative methemoglobinemia. *Minerva Anestesiol.* 2007;73:377-379.
4. Ash-Bernal R, Wise R, Scott M. Acquired methemoglobinemia: a retrospective series of 138 cases at two teaching hospitals. *Medicine.* 2004;83:265-273.
5. Bacon R. Nitrate preserved sausage meat causes an unusual food poisoning incident. *Commun Dis Rep CDR Rev.* 1997;7:R45-R47.
6. Baraka A, Ayoub C, Yazabeck-Karam V, et al. Prophylactic methylene blue in a patient with congenital methemoglobinemia. *Can J Anesth.* 2005;52:258-261.
7. Barker SJ, Curry J, Redford D, Morgan S. Measurement of carboxyhemoglobin and methemoglobin by pulse oximetry: a human volunteer study. *Anesthesiology.* 2006;105:892-897.
8. Barker SJ, Tremper KK, Hyatt J. Effects of methemoglobinemia on pulse oximetry and mixed venous oximetry. *Anesthesiology.* 1989;70:112-117.
9. Beutler E. Glucose-6-phosphate dehydrogenase deficiency. *N Engl J Med.* 1991;324:169-174.
10. Beutler E. The hemolytic effect of primaquine and related compounds: a review. *J Hematol.* 1959;14:103-139.
11. Birky M, Malek D, Paabo M. Study of biological samples obtained from victims of MGM Grand Hotel fire. *J Anal Toxicol.* 1983;7:265-271.
12. Bodansky O. Methemoglobinemia and methemoglobin producing compounds. *Pharmacol Rev.* 1951;3:144-196.
13. Bolyai JZ, Smith RP, Gray CT. Ascorbic acid and chemically induced methemoglobinemias. *Toxicol Appl Pharmacol.* 1972;21:176-185.
14. Bower PJ, Peterson JN. Methemoglobinemia after sodium nitroprusside therapy. *N Engl J Med.* 1975;293:865.
15. Bradberry SM, Aw TC, Williams NR, et al. Occupational methemoglobinemia. *Occup Environ Med.* 2001;58:611-616.
16. Brandes JC, Bufill JA, Pisciotta AV. Amyl nitrite-induced hemolytic anemia. *Am J Med.* 1989;86:252-254.
17. Brar R, Eshaghian S, Eshaghian S, Miles P. Acute Dapsone-induced methemoglobinemia in a 24-year-old woman with ulcerative colitis. *Hosp Phys.* 2007;43:54-58.
18. Caprari P, Bozzi A, Ferroni L, et al. Membrane alterations in G6PD and PK-deficient erythrocytes exposed to oxidizing agents. *Biol Med Metab Biol.* 1991;45:16-27.
19. Cohen BL, Bovasso GJ. Acquired methemoglobinemia and hemolytic anemia following excessive Pyridium (phenazopyridine hydrochloride) ingestion. *Clin Pediatr.* 1971;10:537-540.
20. Craun GF, Greathouse DG, Gunderson DH. Methemoglobin levels in young children consuming high nitrate well water in the United States. *Int J Epidemiol.* 1981;10:309-317.
21. Dahshan A, Donovan K. Severe methemoglobinemia complicating topical benzocaine use during endoscopy in a toddler: a case report and review of the literature. *Pediatrics.* 2006;117:e806-e809
22. Darling RC, Roughton FJW. The effect of methemoglobin on the equilibrium between oxygen and hemoglobin. *Am J Physiol.* 1942;137:56-66.
23. Dawson AH, Whyte IM. Management of dapsone poisoning complicated by methemoglobinemia. *Med Toxicol Adverse Drug Exp.* 1989;4:387-392.
24. Fewtrell L. Drinking water nitrate, methemoglobinemia, and burden of disease: a discussion. *Environ Health Perspect.* 2004;112:1371-1374.
25. Fibuch EE, Cecil WT, Reed WA. Methemoglobinemia associated with organic nitrate therapy. *Anesth Analg.* 1979;58:521-523.
26. Fincher ME, Campbell HT. Methemoglobinemia and hemolytic anemia after phenazopyridine hydrochloride (Pyridium) administration in end-stage renal disease. *South Med J.* 1989;82:372-374.
27. Fung H. Pharmacokinetic determinants of nitrate action. *Am J Med.* 1984;76:22-27.
28. Gaetani GD, Parker JC, Kirkman HN. Intracellular restraint: a new basis for the limitation in response to oxidative stress in human erythrocytes containing low-activity variants of glucose-6-phosphate dehydrogenase. *Proc Natl Acad Sci U S A.* 1974;9:3584-3587.
29. Garrison FH. *An Introduction to the History of Medicine*, 4th ed. Philadelphia: WB Saunders; 1929:566-567.
30. Gelberg KH, Church L, Casey G, et al. Nitrate levels in drinking water in rural New York State. *Environ Res.* 1999;80:34-40.
31. Gibson QH. The reduction of methaemoglobin in red blood cells and studies on the causes of idiopathic methemoglobin. *Biochem J.* 1948;42:13.
32. Greenberg MS, Wong H. Methemoglobinemia and Heinz body hemolytic anemia due to phenazopyridine hydrochloride. *N Engl J Med.* 1964;271:431-435.
33. Guay J. Methemoglobinemia related to local anesthetics: a summary of 232 episodes. *Anesthesiology.* 2007;107:A640
34. Gunter JB. Benefits and risks of local anesthetics in infants and children. *Paediatr Drugs.* 2002;4:649-672.
35. Gupta PM, Lala DS, Arsura E. Benzocaine-induced methemoglobinemia. *South Med J.* 2000;93:83-86.
36. Hahn IH, Hoffman RS, Nelson LS. EMLA-induced methemoglobinemia and systemic topical anesthetic toxicity. *J Emerg Med.* 2004;26:85-88.
37. Hanukoglo A, Danon PN. Endogenous methemoglobinemia associated with diarrheal disease in infancy. *J Pediatr Gastroenterol Nutr.* 1996;23:1-7.
38. Harris JC, Rumack BH, Peterson RG, McGuire BM. Methemoglobinemia resulting from absorption of nitrates. *JAMA.* 1979;242:2869-2871.
39. Hartman AF, Perley AM, Barnett HL. A study of some of the physiological effects of sulfanilamide. II. Methemoglobin formation and its control. *J Clin Invest.* 1938;17:699-710.
40. Hegesh E, Hegesh J, Kaftory A. Congenital methemoglobinemia with a deficiency of cytochrome b5. *N Engl J Med.* 1985;314:757-761.
41. Hermon MM, Burda G, Golej J, et al. Methemoglobin formation in children with congenital heart disease treated with inhaled nitric oxide after cardiac surgery. *Intensive Care Med.* 2003;29:447-452.
42. Hjelt K, Lund JT, Scherling B, et al. Methemoglobinemia among neonates in a neonatal intensive care unit. *Acta Paediatr.* 1995;84:365-370.
43. Hoffman RS, Sauter D. Methemoglobinemia resulting from smoke inhalation. *Vet Hum Toxicol.* 1989;31:40-42.
44. Horne MK, Waterman MR, Simon LM, Garriott JC, Foerster EH. Methemoglobinemia from sniffing butyl nitrite. *Ann Intern Med.* 1979;91:417-418.
45. Huang A, Terry W, Guido F, et al. Methemoglobinemia following unintentional ingestion of sodium nitrite—New York, 2002. *MMWR Morbid Mortal Wkly Rep.* 2002;51;639-642.
46. Johnson CJ, Bonrud PA, Dosch TL, et al. Fatal outcome of methemoglobinemia in an infant. *JAMA.* 1987;257:2796-2797.
47. Kane G, Hoehn S, Behrenbeck T, et al. Benzocaine-Induced methemoglobinemia based on the mayo clinic experience from 28 478 transesophageal echocardiograms. *Arch Intern Med.* 2007;167:1977-1982.
48. Katsumata Y, Aoki M, Oya M, et al. Simultaneous determination of carboxyhemoglobin and methemoglobin in victims of carbon monoxide poisoning. *J Forensic Sci.* 1980;25:546-549.
49. Kearney TE, Manoguerra AS, Dunford JV. Chemically induced methemoglobinemia from aniline poisoning. *West J Med.* 1984;140:282-286.

50. Kellermeyer RW, Tarlov AR, Brewer GJ, et al. Hemolytic effect of therapeutic drugs: clinical considerations of the primaquine-type hemolysis. *JAMA.* 1962;180:128-134.
51. Kelly KJ, Neu J, Camitta BM, Honig GR. Methemoglobinemia in an infant treated with the folk remedy glycerited asafoetida. *Pediatrics.* 1984;73:717-719.
52. Khorasani A, Candido KD, Ghaleb AH, et al. Canister tip orientation and residual volume have significant impact on the dose of benzocaine delivered by Hurricane(r) Spray. *Anesth Analg.* 2001;92:379-383.
53. Kinoshita A, Nakayama Y, Kitayama T, et al. Simulation study of methemoglobin reduction in erythrocytes. *FEBS J.* 2007;274:1449-1458.
54. Kirlangitis JJ, Middaugh RE, Zablocki A, Rodriquez F. False indication of arterial oxygen desaturation and methemoglobinemia following injection of methylene blue in urological surgery. *Mil Med.* 1990;155:260-262.
55. Knobeloch L, Salna B, Hogan A, et al. Blue babies and nitrate-contaminated well water. *Environ Health Perspect.* 2001;109:12-14.
56. Kouides PA, Abboud CN, Fairbanks VF. Flutamide-induced cyanosis refractory to methylene blue therapy. *Br J Haematol.* 1996;94:73-75.
57. Kraft-Jacobss B, Brilli, R, Szabo C, et al. Circulating methemoglobin and nitrite/nitrite concentrations as indicators of nitric oxide overproduction in critically ill children with septic shock. *Crit Care Med.* 1997;25;1588-1593.
58. Kreeftenberg H, Braams R, Nauta Piet. Methemoglobinemia after low-dose prilocaine in an adult patient receiving barbiturate comedication. *Anesth Analg.* 2007;104:459-460.
59. Laney RF, Hoffman RS. Methemoglobinemia secondary to automobile exhaust fumes. *Am J Emerg Med.* 1992;10:426-428.
60. Larsen VH, Freudendal-Pedersen A, Fogh-Andersen NF. The influence of patent blue V on pulse oximetry and haemoximetry. *Acta Anesthesiol Scand.* 1995;39:53-55.
61. Linz A, Greenham R, Fallon, L. Methemoglobinemia: an industrial outbreak among rubber molding workers. *J Occ Environ Med.* 2006;48:523-528.
62. Lu HC, Shih RD, Marcus S, et al. Pseudomethemoglobinemia: a case report and review of sulfhemoglobinemia. *Arch Pediatr Adolesc Med.* 1998;152:803-805.
63. Lukens JN. The legacy of well water methemoglobinemia. *JAMA.* 1987;257:2793-2795.
64. Machabert R, Testud F, Descotes J. Methaemoglobinemia due to amyl nitrite inhalation: a case report. *Hum Exp Toxicol.* 1994;13:313-314.
65. Mansouri A, Lurie AA. Concise review: methemoglobinemia. *Am J Hematol.* 1993;42:7-12.
66. Methemoglobinemia in an infant—Wisconsin. *MMWR Morbid Mortal Wkly Rep.* 1993;42:217-219.
67. Moore TJ, Walsh CS, Cohen MR. Reported adverse event cases of methemoglobinemia associated with benzocaine products. *Arch Intern Med.* 2004;164:1192-1196.
68. Nathan DM, Siegel AJ, Bunn F. Acute methemoglobinemia and hemolytic anemia with phenazopyridine. *Arch Intern Med.* 1977;137:1636-1638.
69. Nathan GD, Oski FA. *Hematology of Infancy and Childhood*, 4th ed. Philadelphia: WB Saunders; 1993:698-731.
70. Nijland R, Jongsma HW, Nijhuis JG, et al. Notes on the apparent discordance of pulse oximetry and multiwavelength hemoglobin photometry. *Acta Anaesthesiol Scand.* 1995;107:49-52.
71. Noor M, Beutler E. Acquired sulfhemoglobinemia an underreported diagnosis? *West J Med.* 1998;169:386-389.
72. Novaro G, Aronow H, Militello M, et al. Benzocaine-induced methemoglobinemia. Experience from a high-volume transesophageal echocardiography laboratory. *J Am Soc Echocardiogr.* 2003;16:170-175.
73. Noyes C, Olufolabi A, Habib A. Subtle desaturation and preoperative methemoglobinemia. The need for continued vigilance. *Can J Anesth.* 2005;52:771-772.
74. Ohashi k, Yukioka H, Hayashi M, et al. Elevated methemoglobin in patient with sepsis. *Acta Anaesthesiol Scand.* 1998;48:713-716
75. Paris PM, Kaplan RM, Steward RD, Weiss LD. Methemoglobin levels following sublingual nitroglycerin in human volunteers. *Ann Emerg Med.* 1986;15:171-173.
76. Park CM, Nagel RL. Sulfhemoglobinemia: clinical and molecular aspects. *N Engl J Med.* 1984;310:1579-1584.
77. Pollack ES, Pollack CV. Incidence of subclinical methemoglobinemia in infants with diarrhea. *Ann Emerg Med.* 1994;24:652-656.
78. Ralston AC, Webb RK, Runchiman WB. Potential errors in pulse oximetry. *Anaesthesia.* 1991;46:291-295.
79. Rausch-Madison S, Mohsenifar Z. Methodologic problems encountered with cooximetry in methemoglobinemia. *Am J Med Sci.* 1997;314:203-206.
80. Reynolds KJ, Palayiwa E, Moyle JTB, et al. The effects of dyshemoglobins on pulse oximetry: part 1, theoretical approach and part II, experimental results using an in vitro test system. *J Clin Monit.* 1993;9:81-90.
81. Rhodes LE, Tingle MD, Park BK, et al. Cimetidine improves the therapeutic/toxic ratio of dapsone in patients on chronic dapsone therapy. *Br J Dermatol.* 1995;132:257-262.
82. Roberts JD, Fineman JR, Morin FC, et al. Inhaled nitric oxide and persistent pulmonary hypertension of the newborn. *N Engl J Med.* 1997;336:605-610.
83. Rosen PJ, Johnson C, Mcgehee WG, Beutler E. Failure of methylene blue treatment in toxic methemoglobinemia. *Ann Intern Med.* 1971;76:83-86.
84. Sager S, Garyson GH, Feig SA. Methemoglobinemia associated with acidosis of probable renal origin. *J Pediatr.* 1995;126:59-61.
85. Sass MD, Caruso CJ, Farhangi M. TPNH-methemoglobin reductase deficiency: a new red-cell enzyme defect. *J Lab Clin Med.* 1967;5:760-767.
86. Sekimpi DK, Jones RD. Notifications of industrial chemical cyanosis poisoning in the United Kingdom 1961–80. *Br J Ind Med.* 1986;43:272-279.
87. Sinex JE. Pulse oximetry: principles and limitations. *Am J Emerg Med.* 1999;17:59-66.
88. Smith ER, Smiseth IK, Maryari D, et al. Mechanism of action of nitrates. *Am J Med.* 1984;76:14-22.
89. Sugahara K, Sadohara T, Kawaguchi T, et al. NADH-diaphorase deficiency identified in a patient with congenital methaemoglobinaemia detected by pulse oximetry. *Intensive Care Med.* 1998;24:706-708.
90. Tremper KK, Barker SJ. Using pulse oximetry when dyshemoglobin levels are high. *J Crit Illness.* 1988;11:103-107.
91. Watcha MF, Connor MT, Hing AV. Pulse oximetry in methemoglobinemia. *Am J Dis Child.* 1989;143:845-847.
92. Weinberger B, Laskin DL, Heck DE, et al. The toxicology of inhaled nitric oxide. *Toxicol Sci.* 2001;59:5-16.
93. Wendel WB. The control of methemoglobinemia with methylene blue. *J Clin Invest.* 1939;18:179-185.
94. Williams S, MacDonald P, Hoyer JD, et al. Methemoglobinemia in children with acute lymphoblastic leukemia (ALL) receiving dapsone for *Pneumocystis carinii* pneumonia (PCP) prophylaxis: a correlation with cytochrome b5 reductase (Cb5R) enzyme levels. *Pediatr Blood Cancer.* 2005;44:55-62.
95. Wintrobe MM, Lee GR. Unstable hemoglobin disease. In: Lee GR, ed. *Wintrobe's Clinical Hematology*, 10th ed. Baltimore: Williams & Wilkins; 1999:1046-1055.
96. Yano SS, Danish EH, Hsia YE. Transient methemoglobinemia with acidosis in infants. *J Pediatr.* 1982;100:415-418.
97. Zijlstra WG, Buursma A, Zwart A. Performance of an automated six-wavelength photometer (Radiometer OSM3) for routine measurement of hemoglobin derivatives. *Clin Chem.* 1988;34:149-152.

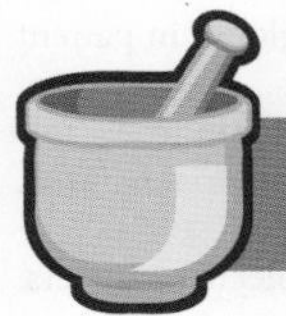

ANTIDOTES IN DEPTH (A41)

METHYLENE BLUE

Mary Ann Howland

Methylene blue is an extremely effective antidote for acquired methemoglobinemia. Methylene blue also has other actions, including inhibition of nitric oxide synthase and guanylyl cyclase, and inhibition of the generation of oxygen free radicals. These effects are offered as explanations of the beneficial effects of methylene blue in the hepatopulmonary syndrome, treatment of priapism, modulation of streptozocin-induced insulin deficiency, prevention and treatment of ifosfamide-induced encephalopathy, use in sepsis, treatment of refractory hypotension, and reduction of development of postsurgical peritoneal adhesions.[14,15,19,22,28,34,42,50]

HISTORY

Methylene blue was initially recommended as an intestinal and urinary antiseptic and subsequently recognized as a weak antimalarial.[18] In 1933, Williams and Challis successfully used methylene blue for treatment of aniline-induced methemoglobinemia.[54]

PHARMACOLOGY

Methylene blue is tetramethylthionine chloride,[18] a basic thiazin dye. Methylene blue is an oxidizing agent, which, in the presence of nicotinamide adenine dinucleotide phosphate (NADPH) and NADPH methemoglobin reductase, is reduced to leukomethylene blue (see Fig. 127–4). Leukomethylene blue then becomes available to reduce methemoglobin to hemoglobin.[10,18,51] Reduction of methemoglobin via this NADPH pathway is limited under normal circumstances. However, in the presence of methylene blue, the role of the NADPH pathway is dramatically increased (four to five times in dogs) and becomes the most efficient means of methemoglobin reduction. This property makes methylene blue the treatment of choice for methemoglobinemia.

PHARMACOKINETICS

The pharmacokinetics of methylene blue were studied in animals and human volunteers following intravenous (IV) and oral administration of 100 mg.[10–12,35] Methylene blue exhibits complex pharmacokinetics consistent with extensive distribution into deep compartments, followed by a slower terminal elimination with a half-life of 5.25 hours. Peak concentrations after oral administration were reached in 1 to 2 hours, but were approximately 80 to 90 nmol/L, as opposed to 8000 to 9000 nmol/L following IV administration. The substantial differences in whole-blood concentrations achieved by these routes of administration can be attributed to extensive first-pass organ distribution into the intestinal wall and liver, following oral administration.[35] Total urinary excretion at 24 hours accounts for 28.6% of the drug following IV administration versus 18.5% after oral administration. In both cases, one-third was in the leukomethylene blue form.

ADVERSE EFFECTS

Reports of the paradoxical induction of methemoglobinemia by methylene blue suggest an equilibrium between the direct oxidization of hemoglobin to methemoglobin by methylene blue and its ability (through the NADPH and NADPH-methemoglobin-reductase pathway, and leukomethylene blue production) to reduce methemoglobin to hemoglobin.[5,6] Methylene blue does not produce methemoglobin at doses of 1 to 2 mg/kg. The equilibrium seems to favor the reducing properties of methylene blue, unless excessively large doses of methylene blue are administered[4,17,53] or the NADPH methemoglobin reductase system is abnormal. This equilibrium constant may vary substantially, as 20 mg/kg IV in dogs and 65 mg/kg intraperitoneally in rats failed to produce methemoglobinemia.[45] In the earliest studies, 50 to 100 mL of a 1% concentration (500–1000 mg) of methylene blue was used intravenously in volunteers[30] and to treat patients with aniline dye-induced methemoglobinemia.[54] In these studies, methemoglobin levels, measured when symptoms were most pronounced, were approximately 1.0 g/dL (0.4%–8.3% of total hemoglobin), and unlikely to be solely responsible for the adverse effects demonstrated. Other consequential adverse effects included shortness of breath, tachypnea, chest discomfort, burning sensation of the mouth and stomach, initial bluish-tinged skin and mucous membranes, paresthesias, restlessness, apprehension, tremors, nausea and vomiting, dysuria, and excitation. Urine and vomitus make take on a blue color. These studies with limited evidence led to the recommendation to avoid doses greater than 7 mg/kg.

In high doses, methylene blue can induce an acute hemolytic anemia independent of the presence of methemoglobinemia.[17,27] In dose–response studies in glucose-6-phosphate dehydrogenase (G6PD)-deficient homozygous African American men, daily doses of 390 to 780 mg (5.5–11 mg/kg) of methylene blue produced hemolysis,[26] which was comparable with the results following exposure to 15 mg of primaquine base.[26] Because of the sensitivity of neonates (hemoglobin F [HbF] and diminished NADH reductase) to these risks, the smallest effective dose of methylene blue should be used.[21,25] Because oxidizing agents can independently induce Heinz body hemolytic anemia, the specific contribution of methylene blue often is difficult to elucidate.[25]

Since methylene blue is a dye it will alter pulse oximeter readings.[7] Large doses may interfere with the ability to detect a clinical decrease in cyanosis; therefore, repeat cooximeter measurements and arterial blood gas analysis should be used in conjunction with clinical findings to evaluate improvement.

Intraamniotic injection of methylene blue may result in a number of adverse effects, including infants born with skin dyed blue (with resultant inaccurate pulse oximetry readings),[43] methemoglobinemia, hemolysis, phototoxic skin reactions,[36] or intestinal obstruction.[7,9,24,27,29,32,38,48] One infant exposed in utero at 5.5 weeks was normal at birth.[24] An excessive dose of enterally administered methylene blue that subsequently leaked into the peritoneum of a premature neonate most likely was responsible for a hemolytic anemia appearing 3 days later.[1]

Methylene blue leads to a bluish-green discoloration of the urine and may cause dysuria.[37] Intravenous methylene blue is irritating and exceedingly painful. It may cause local tissue damage even in the absence of extravasation.[38] Subcutaneous and intrathecal administrations are contraindicated.[38]

Two recent reviews reveal an association between an encephalopathy and the use of methylene blue for localization of parathyroid tumors in women on serotonin reuptake inhibitors.[31,47] Five out of 132 patients in the first review developed one or more of the following: confusion, expressive aphasia, lethargy, and vertigo which lasted from 2 to 3 days. The second review detailed seven patients with signs and symptoms consistent with serotonin toxicity. It should be noted that these patients usually received 3 to 5 mg/kg of methylene blue as a continuous infusion over 1 hour. A subsequent in vitro study documented the ability of methylene blue to competitively bind to monoamine oxidase A (MAO_A), raising the possibility that methylene blue might interact with serotonergic xenobiotics by acting as a monamine oxidase inhibitor (MAOI).[39]

XENOBIOTIC-INDUCED METHEMOGLOBINEMIA

Sulfanilamide-induced methemoglobinemia was reversed by methylene blue doses of 1 to 2 mg/kg intravenously or 65 to 130 mg orally every 4 hours.[20,52] With these regimens, a very rapid fall in methemoglobin was accompanied by disappearance of cyanosis. Subsequent investigations confirmed the effectiveness and safety of IV doses of 1 to 2 mg/kg methylene blue in reversing the methemoglobinemia produced by sulfanilamide,[52] aniline dye,[13] silver nitrate, benzocaine, nitrites, phenazopyridine and among other xenobiotics.[46,49]

USE IN PATIENTS WITH GLUCOSE-6-PHOSPHATE DEHYDROGENASE DEFICIENCY

Methylene blue is frequently hypothesized to be ineffective in reversing methemoglobinemia in patients with G6PD deficiency[41] because G6PD is essential for generation of NADPH (Chap. 24) and without NADPH, methylene blue cannot reduce methemoglobin. However, G6PD deficiency is an X-linked hereditary deficiency with more than 400 variants. The red cells containing the more common G6PD A^- variant found in 11% of African Americans retain 10% residual activity, mostly in younger erythrocytes and reticulocytes. In contrast, the enzyme is barely detectable in those of Mediterranean descent who have inherited the defect. Therefore, it is impossible to predict before the use of methylene blue who will or will not respond, and to what extent. Currently, it appears that most individuals have adequate G6PD and express deficiency states in relative terms. This variable expression of their deficiency allows an effective response to most oxidant stresses. In addition, in theory, normal cells might convert methylene blue to leukomethylene blue, which might diffuse into G6PD-deficient cells and effectively reduce methemoglobin to hemoglobin.[3]

Before it is assumed that G6PD deficiency is responsible for a continued elevation of methemoglobin levels despite administration of methylene blue, ongoing xenobiotic absorption and/or continued methemoglobin production must be excluded. On the other hand, when therapeutic doses of methylene blue fail to have an impact on the methemoglobin concentration, the possibility of G6PD deficiency should be considered, and further doses of methylene blue should not be administered because of the risk of methylene blue–induced hemolysis. In these cases, exchange transfusion and hyperbaric oxygen are potential alternatives for treating methemoglobinemia (Chap. 127).

DOSING

Methylene blue is indicated in patients with symptomatic methemoglobinemia. This usually occurs at methemoglobin levels greater than 20%, but may occur at lower levels in anemic patients or those with cardiovascular, pulmonary, or central nervous system compromise.

In most cases, doses of 1 to 2 mg/kg given intravenously over 5 minutes, followed immediately by a fluid flush of 15 to 30 mL to minimize local pain, is both effective and relatively safe. In neonates, 0.3 to 1 mg/kg doses often are effective.[16,23] The onset of action is rapid, and maximal effects usually occur within 30 minutes.

Repetitive dosing of methylene blue may be required in conjunction with efforts to decontaminate the gastrointestinal (GI) tract when there is continued absorption or slow elimination of the xenobiotic producing the methemoglobinemia, such as with dapsone.[44] Additionally, cimetidine is indicated to prevent further formation of the methemoglobin-inducing metabolite of dapsone.[8,40]

A continuous IV infusion of methylene blue at 0.1 mg/kg/h or 3 to 7 mg/h (in a concentration of 0.05% in 0.9% sodium chloride solution) also has been used.[2,44] However, this method of administration is not adequately studied.

Intraosseous administration of 0.3 mL of 1% solution (1 mg/kg) of methylene blue over 3 to 5 minutes into the anterior tibia of a 6-week-old infant was well tolerated.[21,33] Methylene blue is ineffective in treating sulfhemoglobinemia (Chap. 127).

AVAILABILITY

Methylene blue is available in 10-mL 1% ampules containing 10 mg/mL.

SUMMARY

Methylene blue is an effective reducing agent for patients with acquired induced methemoglobinemia. When used in the proper dose, its onset of action is rapid and adverse reactions are limited. Repeat doses often are required when methemoglobin-producing drugs with a long duration of effect such as dapsone are ingested.

REFERENCES

1. Albert M, Lessin MS, Gilchrist BF. Methylene blue: dangerous dye for neonates. *J Pediatr Surg.* 2003;38:1244-1245.
2. Berlin G, Brodin B, Hilden J, Martensson J. Acute dapsone intoxication. A case treated with continuous infusion of methylene blue, forced diuresis and plasma exchange. *J Toxicol Clin Toxicol.* 1984-1985;22:537-548.
3. Beutler E, Baluda M. Methemoglobin reduction: studies of the interaction between cell populations and of the role of methylene blue. *Blood.* 1963;22:323-333.
4. Blass N, Fung D. Dyed but not dead—methylene blue overdose. *Anesthesiology.* 1976;45:458-459.
5. Bodansky O. Mechanism of action of methylene blue in treatment of methemoglobinemia. *JAMA.* 1950;142:923.
6. Bodansky O. Methemoglobinemia and methemoglobin-producing compounds. *Pharmacol Rev.* 1951;3:144-196.
7. Coleman MD, Coleman NA. Drug-induced methaemoglobinemia. *Drug Saf.* 1996;14:394-405.
8. Coleman MD, Rhodes LA, Scott AK, et al. The use of cimetidine to reduce dapsone-dependent methemoglobinemia in dermatitis herpetiformis patients. *Br J Clin Pharmacol.* 1992;34:244-249.
9. Crooks J. Haemolytic jaundice in a neonate after intra-amniotic injection of methylene blue. *Arch Dis Child.* 1982;57:872-886.
10. DiSanto AR, Wagner JG. Pharmacokinetics of highly ionized drugs. I: methylene blue—whole blood, urine and tissue assays. *J Pharm Sci.* 1972;61:598-602.

11. DiSanto AR, Wagner JG. Pharmacokinetics of highly ionized drugs. II: methylene blue—absorption, metabolism and excretion in man and dog after oral absorption. *J Pharm Sci.* 1972;61:1086-1090.
12. DiSanto AR, Wagner JG. Pharmacokinetics of highly ionized drugs. III: methylene blue—blood levels in the dog and tissue levels in the rat following intravenous administration. *J Pharm Sci.* 1972;61:1090-1094.
13. Etteldorf JN. Methylene blue in the treatment of methemoglobinemia in premature infants caused by marking ink. *J Pediatr.* 1951;38:24-27.
14. Fallon MB. Methylene blue and cirrhosis: pathophysiologic insights, therapeutic dilemmas. *Ann Intern Med.* 2000;133:738-740.
15. Galili Y, Ben-Abraham R, Rabau M, et al. Reduction of surgery-induced peritoneal adhesions by methylene blue. *Am J Surg.* 1998;175:30-32.
16. Geiger JC. Cyanide poisoning in San Francisco. *JAMA.* 1932;99:1944-1945.
17. Goluboff N, Wheaton R. Methylene blue-induced cyanosis and acute hemolytic anemia complicating the treatment of methemoglobinemia. *J Pediatr.* 1961;58:86-89.
18. Goodman LS, Gilman A. *The Pharmacological Basis of Therapeutics.* New York: Macmillan; 1941:869.
19. Haluzik M, Neduidkova J, Skrha J. Treatment with the NO-synthase inhibitor, methylene blue, moderates the decrease in serum leptin concentration in streptozotocin-induced diabetes. *Endocr Res.* 1999;25:163-171.
20. Harman A, Perley A, Barnett H. A study of some of the physiological effects of sulfanilamide. II: methemoglobin formation and its control. *J Clin Invest.* 1938;17:699-710.
21. Herman M, Chyka P, Butler A, Rieger S. Methylene blue by intraosseous infusion for methemoglobinemia. *Ann Emerg Med.* 1999;33:111-113.
22. Hubler J, Szanto A, Konyves K. Methylene blue as a means of treatment for priapism caused by intracavernous injection to combat erectile dysfunction. *Int Urol Nephrol.* 2003;35:519-521.
23. Hjelt K, Lund JT, Scherling B, et al. Methemoglobinemia among neonates in a neonatal intensive care unit. *Acta Pediatr.* 1995;84:365-370.
24. Katz Z, Lancet M. Inadvertent intrauterine injection of methylene blue in early pregnancy. *N Engl J Med.* 1981;304:1427.
25. Kearney T, Manoguerra A, Dunford JV. Chemically induced methemoglobinemia from aniline poisoning. *West J Med.* 1984;140:282-286.
26. Kellermeyer RW, Tarlov A, Brewer G, et al. Hemolytic effect of therapeutic drugs. *JAMA.* 1962;180:128-134.
27. Kirsch I, Cohen M. Heinz body hemolytic anemia from the use of methylene blue in neonates. *J Pediatr.* 1980;96:276-278.
28. Kwok E, Howes D. Use of methylene blue in sepsis: a systematic review. *J Intensive Care Med.* 2006;21:359-363.
29. McEnerney JK, McEnerney LN. Unfavorable neonatal outcome after intra-amniotic injection of methylene blue. *Obstet Gynecol.* 1983;61:35S-37S.
30. Nadler JE, Green M, Rosenbaum A. Intravenous injection of methylene blue in man with reference to its toxic symptoms and effect on the electrocardiogram. *Am J Med Sci.* 1934;188:15-21.
31. Ng B, Cameron A, Fanza R, Rahman H. Serotonin syndrome following methylene blue during parathyroidectomy: a case report and literature review. *Can J Anesth.* 2008;55:36-41.
32. Nicolini U, Monni G. Intestinal obstruction in babies exposed in utero to methylene blue. *Lancet.* 1990;336:1258-1259.
33. Orlowski JP, Porembka DT, Gallagher JM, et al. Comparison study of intraosseous, central intravenous, and peripheral intravenous infusions of emergency drugs. *Am J Dis Child.* 1990;144:112-117.
34. Pelgrims J, De Vos F, Van den Brande J, et al. Methylene blue in the treatment and prevention of ifosfamide-induced encephalopathy: report of 12 cases and a review of the literature. *Br J Cancer.* 2000;82:291-294.
35. Peter C, Hongwan D, Kupfer A, Lauterburg BH. Pharmacokinetics and organ distribution of intravenous and oral methylene blue. *Eur J Clin Pharmacol.* 2000;56:247-250.
36. Porat R, Gilbert S, Magilner D. Methylene blue-induced phototoxicity: an unrecognized complication. *Pediatrics.* 1996;97:717-721.
37. Prischl F, Hofinger I, Kramar R. Fever, shivering … and blue urine. *Nephrol Dial Transplant.* 1999;14:2245-2246.
38. Raimer S, Quevedo E, Johnston R. Dye rashes. *Cutis.* 1999;63:103-106.
39. Ramsay B, Dunford C, Gillman PK. Methyelene blue and serotonin toxicity: inhibition of monoamine oxidase A (MAO A) confirms a theoretical prediction. *Br J Pharmacol.* 2007;152:946-951.
40. Rhodes LE, Tingle MD, Park BK, et al. Cimetidine improves the therapeutic/toxic ratio of dapsone in patients on chronic dapsone therapy. *Br J Dermatol.* 1995;132:257-262.
41. Rosen PJ, Johnson C, McGehee WG, Beutler E. Failure of methylene blue treatment in toxic methemoglobinemia. *Ann Intern Med.* 1971;76:83-86.
42. Schenk P, Madl C, Rezaie-Majd S, et al. Methylene blue improves hepatopulmonary syndrome. *Ann Intern Med.* 2000;133:701-706.
43. Serota FT, Bernbaum JC, Schwartz E. The methylene blue baby. *Lancet.* 1979;2:1142-1143.
44. Southgate HJ, Masterson R. Lessons to be learned: a case study approach. Prolonged methemoglobinemia due to inadvertent dapsone poisoning; treatment with methylene blue and exchange transfusion. *J R Soc Health.* 1999;119:52-55.
45. Stossel TP, Jennings RB. Failure of methylene blue to produce methemoglobinemia in vivo. *Am J Clin Pathol.* 1966;45:600-604.
46. Strauch B, Buch W, Grey W, et al. Successful treatment of methemoglobinemia secondary to silver nitrate therapy. *N Engl J Med.* 1969;281: 257-258.
47. Sweet G, Standiford S. Methylene blue associated encephalopathy. *J Am Coll Surg.* 2007;204:454-458.
48. Troche BI. The methylene blue baby. *N Engl J Med.* 1989;320:1756-1757.
49. Umbreit J. Methemoglobin—it's not just blue: a concise review. *Am J Hematology.* 2007;134-144.
50. Weinbroum AA. Methylene blue attenuates lung injury after mesenteric artery clamping/unclamping. *Eur J Clin Invest.* 2004;34:436-442.
51. Wendel WB. The control of methemoglobinemia with methylene blue. *J Clin Invest.* 1939;18:179-185.
52. Wendel WB. Use of methylene blue in methemoglobinemia from sulfanilamide poisoning. *JAMA.* 1937;109:1216.
53. Whitwam JG, Taylor AR, White JM. Potential hazard of methylene blue. *Anesthesiology.* 1979;34:181-182.
54. Williams JR, Challis FE. Methylene blue as an antidote for aniline dye poisoning. *J Lab Clin Med.* 1933;19:166-171.

CHAPTER 128 SMOKE INHALATION

Nathan Phillip Charlton and Mark A. Kirk

Smoke is generated as a result of thermal degradation of a material; it is a complex mixture of heated air, suspended solid and liquid particles (aerosols), gases, fumes, and vapors. Particulates and aerosols typically make these thermal degradation products visible to the naked eye, resulting in the black, acrid substance so often thought of as "smoke;" however, thermal decomposition also results in generation of gaseous substances that are invisible to the naked eye. The ever-growing variety of materials used in our environment contributes to the broad spectrum of products present in typical smoke.[30] The chemical composition of the parent materials, oxygen availability, and temperature at the time of decomposition determine the combustion products found in smoke (Table 128–1).[11,29,30,44,54,66,112,122,132,133,156] As a result of these variabilities, specific thermal degradation products resulting from a fire are difficult to predict; in fact, even the composition of smoke is quite variable within the same fire environment.[11,38,122]

Smoke inhalation is a complex medical syndrome involving diverse toxicologic injuries, making care of smoke-injured patients very challenging. Victims of smoke inhalation exhibit a spectrum of illness induced by tissue hypoxia. Importantly, smoke inhalation, not burns, is the leading cause of death from fires. However, cutaneous burns found concurrently with smoke inhalation complicate airway management and fluid resuscitation and increase infection risk. Consequently, burn victims with smoke inhalation injury have higher morbidity and mortality than those with burns alone.[41,148,154,158,171] Treatment of smoke inhalation should be aimed at correcting tissue hypoxia by maximizing oxygen delivery while avoiding unnecessary therapies that delay or hinder oxygenation.

HISTORY AND EPIDEMIOLOGY

Disastrous fires are frequent reminders of the role of inhalation injuries in fire deaths.[38,86] Throughout the United States, a fire department responds to a fire every 20 seconds.[79] In 2007, the National Fire Protection Agency reported 1,557,500 fire incidents in the United States, with 3430 fire deaths and 17,675 fire injuries.[79] A civilian fire death occurred every 153 minutes on average in 2007.[79] Compared with other countries, the United States has one of the highest fire death rates in the world.[99] An estimated 50% to 80% of these fire deaths result from smoke inhalation injuries rather than dermal burns or trauma.[17,67,112,173] More than 30% of patients hospitalized in burn units develop concomitant pulmonary complications, and 75% of these patients die.[70,155] World Health Organization data show that in developing countries, indoor smoke from heating and cooking fuel is one of the four most common causes of death and disease.[16]

Fire injuries may result from an array of inhaled toxic xenobiotics or thermal burns. Before 1942, toxic inhalation from dwelling fires was not considered in the pathophysiology of morbidity and mortality in fire victims. However, in that year, a fire at the Cocoanut Grove Night Club in Boston resulted in a number of fatalities in which victims had no cutaneous burns. This led to the observation that toxic gases are generated in typical structure fires and may result in significant pathology.[121] From 1955 to 1972, death from smoke inhalation injury increased threefold and was attributed to abundant use of newer synthetic materials for building and furnishings.[17] Despite improved firefighting resources, mass casualties from smoke inhalation continue. On November 11, 2000, 170 deaths occurred when a cable train carrying skiers caught fire in a tunnel in Austria. Most of the victims apparently managed to escape the burning train but were killed by "acrid smoke" as they tried to flee.[3] A fire in a crowded Rhode Island nightclub on February 20, 2003, killed 100 people and injured more than 200 people, with the majority suffering from smoke inhalation.[37] On December 31, 2004, a fire at an Argentina night club killed 175 people and injured more than 700. Most of the victims died of smoke inhalation.[4] Forty-five women died in a fire on December 9, 2006, at a state-sponsored drug treatment facility in Moscow, Russia. The majority of these women were patients and were unable to escape the building because the windows had been barred. Most died from smoke inhalation.[5]

PATHOPHYSIOLOGY

Toxic combustion products are classified into three categories: simple asphyxiants, irritant toxins, and chemical asphyxiants (Table 124–2). Simple asphyxiants such as carbon dioxide exert a space-occupying effect; they simply displace oxygen.[38,44,151,171] In addition, combustion uses oxygen, potentially resulting in an oxygen-deprived environment (see Chap. 124).[38]

Irritant gases are chemically reactive compounds that exert a local effect on the respiratory tract, primarily through the production of any combination of acids, alkalis, or reactive oxygen species (ROS) (see Chap. 124). For example, high concentrations of acrolein are measured in air samples from fire environments and in the blood of fire victims.[2,95,163] Acrolein penetrates cell membranes easily because it is lipid soluble, injuring cells by denaturing intracellular proteins and nucleic acids.[55,173] Ammonia is generated when wool, silk, nylon, or synthetic resins are burned. It reacts with the mucosal moisture to produce the alkaline agent ammonium hydroxide.[31,90] Sulfur dioxide, an oxidation product of sulfur-containing material, is found in more than 50% of air samples from fires.[24] Sulfurous acid forms when sulfur dioxide reacts with the water of the respiratory mucosa. Hydrogen chloride, chlorine, and phosgene are formed from the thermal degradation of polyvinyl chloride (PVC), a plastic widely used in home and office furnishings, floor coverings, and electrical insulation.[18,20,38,44,97] In the presence of mucosal water, these combustion products generate damaging hydrogen chloride and ROS.[39] Phosgene produces delayed alveolar injury.[21] Isocyanates, combustion products generated from burning foam furniture padding, cause intense irritation of the upper and lower respiratory tracts.[128]

Thermal degradation of organic material produces finely divided carbonaceous particulate matter (soot) suspended in hot air and gases. These particles are not just composed of carbon; organic acids, aldehydes, heavy metals, and reactive chemicals such as sulfur dioxide, hydrogen chloride, chlorine, and phosgene are adsorbed to their surfaces.[24,44,71,97,151,171] Soot adheres to the mucosa of the airways, allowing adsorbed irritant xenobiotics to react with the mucosal surface moisture and often enhancing and prolonging exposure to irritants in a fire environment. The deposition of these particles in the respiratory tract depends on their size, with particles of 1 to 3 μm reaching the alveoli.[105] Experimental animals have markedly decreased lung injury when they are exposed to toxic gas from smoke that was filtered to remove particulates.[83] Irritant gases can also "piggyback" on aerosol droplets and alter the site of gas deposition.[68]

Water solubility is the most important chemical characteristic in determining the timing and anatomic level of respiratory tract injury. Highly water-soluble xenobiotics primarily injure the upper airway

TABLE 128–1. Common Materials and Their Thermal Degradation Xenobiotics

Material	Thermal Degradation Xenobiotics
Wool	Carbon monoxide, hydrogen chloride, phosgene, chlorine, cyanide, ammonia
Silk	Sulfur dioxide, hydrogen sulfide, ammonia, cyanide
Nylon	Ammonia, cyanide
Wood, cotton, paper	Carbon monoxide, acrolein, acetaldehyde, formaldehyde, acetic acid, formic acid, methane
Petroleum products	Carbon monoxide, acrolein, acetic acid, formic acid
Polystyrene	Styrene
Acrylic	Acrolein, hydrogen chloride, carbon monoxide
Plastics	Cyanide, hydrogen chloride, aldehydes, ammonia, nitrogen oxides, phosgene, chlorine
Polyvinyl chloride	Carbon monoxide, hydrogen chloride, phosgene, chlorine
Polyurethane	Cyanide, isocyanates
Melamine resins	Ammonia, cyanide
Rubber	Hydrogen sulfide, sulfur dioxide
Sulfur-containing material	Sulfur dioxide
Nitrogen-containing material	Cyanide, isocyanates, oxides of nitrogen
Fluorinated resins	Hydrogen fluoride
Fire-retardant materials	Hydrogen chloride, hydrogen bromide

by damaging mucosal cells, which subsequently release mediators of inflammation or ROS.[22,91,107,132] These xenobiotics deposit rapidly in the upper airway by combining with mucosal water and leaving little of the parent compound to travel farther down the airway. The rapidity with which these xenobiotics exert their effects provides a warning that the environment is unsafe and prompts escape. After more than

TABLE 128–2. Toxic Thermal Degradation Xenobiotics

Asphyxiants	Irritants
Simple	**High water solubility** (upper airway injury)
Carbon dioxide	Ammonia
Chemical	Hydrogen chloride
Carbon monoxide	Sulfur dioxide
Hydrogen cyanide	**Intermediate water solubility**
Hydrogen sulfide	(upper and lower respiratory tract injury)
Oxides of nitrogen (methemoglobinemia)	Chlorine
	Isocyanates
	Low water solubility
	(pulmonary parenchymal injury)
	Oxides of nitrogen
	Phosgene

a trivial exposure, the intense inflammatory response increases microvascular permeability and allows movement of fluid from the intravascular space into the tissues of the upper airway. The loosely attached underlying tissue of the supraglottic larynx may become markedly edematous, causing upper airway obstruction within minutes to hours.[74] The obstruction may progress such that the upper airway is completely occluded.[140] Xenobiotics with low water solubility react with the upper respiratory mucosa very slowly and do not elicit an escape response. These xenobiotics reach the distal lung parenchyma, where they react slowly to create a delayed toxic effect. Xenobiotics, such as chlorine, with intermediate water solubility are more likely to result in damage to both the upper and lower respiratory tracts. Other factors, such as concentration of the substance inhaled, duration of exposure, particle size, respiratory rate, absence of protective reflexes, and preexisting disease, influence the region of respiratory tract injury. For example, as the concentration of a highly water-soluble irritant gas increases, more chemical is presented to the lower airway, possibly leading to damage of the lower respiratory tract. In addition, patients with loss of consciousness may increase their exposure secondary to their loss of protective reflexes.

Damage to the tracheobronchial tree is mediated by many of the same mechanisms as those of the pharynx and hypopharynx. Inhaled particulates and toxic gases result in deposition of acids, alkalis, and oxidative agents. Direct thermal injury is less likely to occur secondary to the efficient cooling ability of the upper airways.[107] Injury to the tracheobronchial tree leads to an increase in airway resistance from mucosal edema, bronchoconstriction, and accumulation of intraluminal debris and airway secretions.[28,96,159] Increased tracheobronchial vascular permeability contributes to interstitial edema of the airways and increased airway resistance. Bronchoconstriction and subsequent wheezing are caused by a reflex response to toxic mucosal injury and a response to mediators of inflammation.[63,161] Damaged cells release chemotactic factors that stimulate production of an exudate rich in protein, including fibrin and inflammatory cells.[46,165] This injury eventually results in sloughing of the mucosa; sloughed epithelial cells and inflammatory cells combined with the exudate to create casts of the airways.[46] In victims of smoke inhalation, casts block both the small and large airways, increasing airway resistance and mechanically preventing passage of oxygen to the alveoli.[28,34,110,159,165]

Irritant xenobiotics that reach the alveoli injure the lung parenchyma.[116] Caustics, proteolytic enzymes, reactive free radicals, and mediators of inflammation all contribute to acute lung injury (ALI).[82,85,127,161,171] Pathophysiologic changes of ALI decrease lung compliance and bacterial defenses and lead to ventilation–perfusion mismatch with intrapulmonary shunting, increased extravascular lung water, and microvascular permeability.[28,56,161,165,169] Lung compliance is further decreased from atelectasis when toxic chemicals deactivate pulmonary surfactant.[28,116,124,165] In animals, patchy atelectasis occurs rapidly after smoke is inspired.[28,116,165] In addition, ventilation–perfusion mismatch occurs when pulmonary blood flow is diverted by hypoxia and vasoactive mediators of inflammation.[92,93,115,161] Xenobiotics cause additional injury by impairing mucociliary clearance, altering alveolar macrophage function, and impairing phagocytosis of bacteria, which all contribute to development of pulmonary infections and sepsis.[13,14,51,69,139] The combination of delayed toxic effects of some inhaled xenobiotics and slowly developing inflammatory response may explain the limited initial manifestations of parenchymal injury during the first 24 hours after smoke exposure.

Nitric oxide plays a significant role in the pathogenesis of smoke inhalation induced lung injury.[49,102,166] Combined smoke inhalation and burn injury results in an upregulation of inducible nitric oxide synthase (iNOS) mRNA synthesis in animal models and subsequently results in increased activity of iNOS.[47,48,50,102,149] Elevation of nitric oxide may result in myocardial contractile dysfunction with subsequent hypotension.[149] It also appears to play a role in increased vascular permeability and resultant edema.[102] A possible mechanism is the formation of the highly reactive peroxynitrite ($ONOO^-$) radical from the combination of nitric oxide and ROS, which may lead to alveolar capillary membrane damage and subsequent ALI.[47,102] Inhibition of iNOS reduced lung injury in combined smoke inhalation and burn injury in an ovine model.[49]

Chemical asphyxiants exert their toxic effects at extrapulmonary sites. Incomplete combustion of organic materials generates carbon monoxide, which is considered the most common serious acute hazard to victims of smoke inhalation injury (see Chap. 124).[1,15,38,163,173] Carbon monoxide prevents oxygen from binding to hemoglobin, creating a functional anemia. It also hinders the release of oxygen at the tissues by shifting the oxyhemoglobin dissociation curve to the left. In addition, CO binds myoglobin in cardiac and skeletal muscle[25] and cytochrome oxidase in all tissues.[75] The combination of these features impairs oxygen utilization by the myocardium and contributes to myocardial dysfunction. Other mechanisms of toxicity include induction of oxidative stress and lipid peroxidation (see Chap. 124).[157] Cyanide is produced from combustion of organic nitrogen-containing products such as plastics, melamine resins, polyurethanes, wool, silk, nylon, nitrocellulose, polyacrylonitriles, synthetic rubber, and paper.[122] High concentrations of cyanide are measured in air samples from fires, and elevated blood cyanide concentrations occur in both fire survivors as well as those who die in fires.[6,10,11,28,38,65,78,146,147,153,167] Cyanide has at least an additive, if not synergistic, effect with carbon monoxide in smoke inhalation toxicity (see Chaps. 125 and 126).[10,104,119,130,133] Combustion of nitrogen-containing materials generate oxides of nitrogen, which are irritants and methemoglobin inducers (see Chap. 127).

Depending on the fuel, other combustion products are aerosolized and act by local irritation or systemic toxicity. Metal oxides, hydrocarbons, hydrogen fluoride, and hydrogen bromide may contribute to toxicity. Antimony, bromine, cadmium, chromium, cobalt, gold, iron, lead, and zinc often are recovered from air samples taken during fires and from soot removed from the surface of the trachea and bronchi of fire victims.[15,38] Fires at industrial sites, clandestine drug laboratories, transportation incidents, and natural disasters such as erupting volcanoes produce additional unique toxic inhalants.

CLINICAL MANIFESTATIONS

The primary clinical problem in smoke inhalation victims is respiratory compromise; therefore, clinical evaluation should specifically address this issue. Initially, patients may complain of mucous membrane, ocular, and pharyngeal irritation. They may have voice changes, and their speech may progressively worsen as the airway becomes increasingly edematous. Cough, chest tightness, and dyspnea are common. Stridor and acute respiratory arrest may develop. Patients may have difficulty managing their airway secretions, with expectoration of copious quantities of soot containing sputum. The oropharynx and nares may be erythematous, coated with soot, or have progressing edema. Visualization of the vocal cords by direct laryngoscopy is sometimes difficult secondary to soot accumulation, secretions, or edema. Conjunctival injection, corneal ulcerations, marked lacrimation, and blepharospasm may be noted on ophthalmologic examination.

Auscultation of the chest may reveal rhonchi, rales, and wheezing suggestive of ALI.[61] Bronchospasm may occur, particularly in patients with underlying reactive airway disease. Breath sounds, including wheezing, may become virtually inaudible in patients with severe bronchospasm. ALI is a common complication and is defined as diffuse alveolar filling of acute onset with hypoxemia but without left atrial hypertension.[12] The most severe manifestation of ALI is the acute respiratory distress syndrome (ARDS), which is defined based on the patient's ability to oxygenate at a given FiO_2 (see Chaps. 21 and 124).

Tachycardia and tachypnea may be pronounced, and hypotension may occur, with faint or no peripheral pulses noted.[149] Smoke inhalation victims may develop an altered mental status, including agitation, confusion, or coma. This is most likely attributable to hypoxia from either pulmonary compromise or cellular hypoxia.

DIAGNOSTIC TESTING

Because smoke inhalation injury causes pulmonary and airway damage, diagnostic studies should focus on assessing oxygenation and ventilation. Therefore, arterial blood gas (ABG) analysis, carboxyhemoglobin and methemoglobin concentrations, and chest radiography are the most important tests to obtain.

ABG analysis assesses both pulmonary function and blood pH. The presence of metabolic acidosis may be an early clue to tissue hypoxia or cyanide poisoning. Serial measurements of arterial oxygenation and alveolar ventilation are helpful in identifying hypoxemia or ventilatory failure. The accuracy of oxygen saturation measurement depends on the method used. Oxygen saturation calculated from ABG analysis may be unreliable in the setting of an elevated blood carbon monoxide concentration, but measured oxygen saturation determined by co-oximeter accurately reflects the percent saturation of hemoglobin. Transcutaneous measurement of oxygen saturation by pulse oximetry is unreliable in patients with smoke inhalation because the test overestimates oxygen saturation in the presence of carboxyhemoglobin.[8,45,118,164]

A carboxyhemoglobin concentration should be obtained for all smoke inhalation victims.[27,172] When using blood sampling, either arterial or venous samples can be used to accurately measure carboxyhemoglobin concentrations.[94,160] Noninvasive bedside pulse co-oximetry may be a rapid screening tool for the detection of carbon monoxide, and its use is becoming more prevalent in clinical practice.[131,152] The carboxyhemoglobin concentration alone is a poor predictor of the severity of smoke inhalation because a low or nondetectable concentration does not exclude the possibility of developing inhalation injury.[101,150] Rarely, elevated methemoglobin levels are reported in fire victims. Because methemoglobin can further reduce oxygen-carrying capacity and is part of standard co-oximetry measurement, methemoglobin concentrations, along with carboxyhemoglobin concentrations, should also be obtained in the initial laboratory evaluation.[72,144] Blood cyanide analysis is of little clinical use because results of analysis are not available for hours, and therapy should never await laboratory confirmation of the presence of cyanide. Accurate measurement depends on acquiring the sample soon after exposure because cyanide is rapidly eliminated from the blood.[10,80] A plasma lactate level greater than 10 mmol/L in the setting of smoke inhalation suggests cyanide poisoning and should be enough evidence to support empiric antidotal treatment of critically ill patients.[10,108]

A chest radiograph obtained early in the course of smoke inhalation is an insensitive indicator of pulmonary injury.[27,61,129,170] The most frequent abnormal findings on initial chest radiography are diffuse alveolar and interstitial changes, found in up to 34% of patients admitted to the intensive care unit (ICU) with smoke inhalation after dwelling fires followed by focal abnormalities

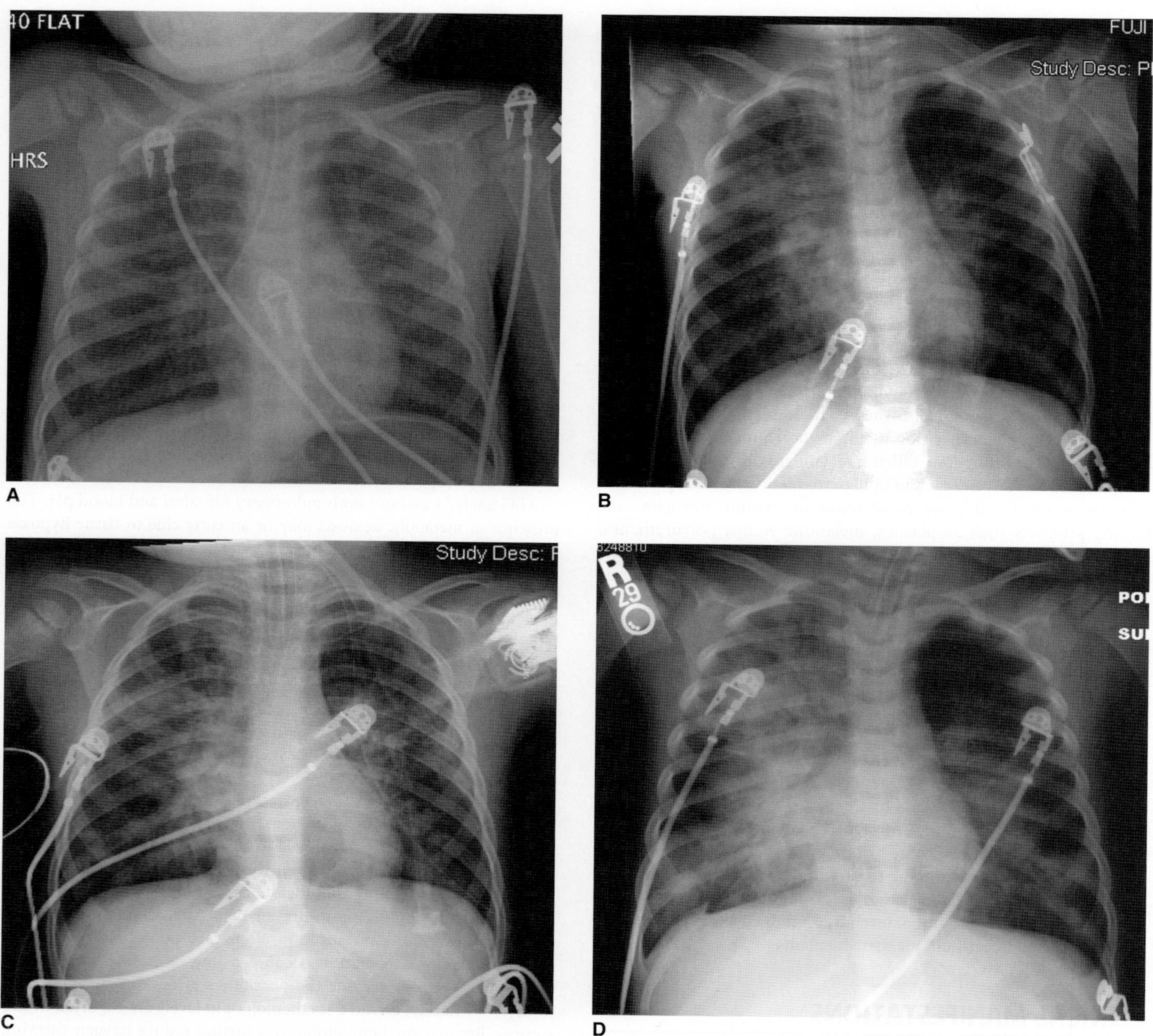

FIGURE 128–1. (A) to (D) Progression over 72 hours of diffuse alveolar and interstitial infiltrates representative of inhalation induced acute lung injury. *(Images contributed by the University of Virginia Medical Toxicology Fellowship Program.)*

in 12% of patients.[61] In one series, no significant differences in the duration of either ventilation or duration in the ICU stay were observed between smoke inhalation victims who exhibited abnormal findings on the first chest radiographic examination and those without any abnormalities.[61] Subtle findings within 24 hours of exposure include perivascular haziness, peribronchial cuffing, bronchial wall thickening, and subglottic edema.[87,155] Serial chest radiographs (Fig. 128–1) done after a baseline study are helpful in detecting pulmonary injury after smoke inhalation.[63] Widespread airway disease usually occurs more than 24 hours after inhalation injury and may represent ALI, aspiration, volume overload, infection, or cardiogenic pulmonary edema.[155] Computed tomography (CT) of the lungs appears to be a more sensitive modality than plain radiography for detecting early pulmonary injury after smoke inhalation.[81,126,137] However, no data are available to support improved patient outcomes when using this radiographic modality.

MANAGEMENT

From oxygen acquisition to cellular utilization, the final common pathophysiologic effect resulting from smoke's injury is hypoxia. Basic critical care strategies that optimize oxygen delivery and oxygen utilization take priority over other treatments. High-flow oxygen, preferably humidified, should accompany initial resuscitation and will begin to correct hypoxia induced by smoke inhalation. To aid in oxygen delivery, hypotensive patients should have two large-bore intravenous (IV) lines placed and receive aggressive fluid resuscitation. Because smoke is a complex mixture of xenobiotics, it is recommended that treatments beyond basic critical care are focused on symptom-based therapy based on recognized toxidromes. Specific antidotes available for common xenobiotics found in smoke should be considered if they are relatively safe and their antidotal effects comply with this strategy. Because many of these treatments are empiric, the risks of treatment must be weighed against the potential benefits.

Critical airway compromise may be present upon the patient's arrival at the hospital, or it may develop subsequently.[35,62,140] A major pitfall in managing a patient with smoke inhalation is failing to appreciate the possibility of rapid deterioration. The history and physical findings help to determine significant smoke exposure and the potential for clinical deterioration. The clinical effects of smoke exposure and their appropriate treatment are described in Figure 128–2 .Upper airway patency must be rapidly established. When obvious oropharyngeal burns are observed, upper airway injury almost certainly is present, even if overt injuries are not visualized, and distal injury may be present and underestimated.[62] Direct evaluation of the upper airway, preferably with fiberoptic endoscopy, is essential for assessing patients at high risk for inhalation airway injury.[35,62,63,74] When evidence of upper airway injury exists, early endotracheal intubation should be performed under controlled circumstances. Other indications for early intubation include coma, stridor, and full-thickness circumferential neck burns.[9,62,63,140] Edema of injured tissue, including that of the airway, is worsened with massive fluid resuscitation in burned patients.[62,63,111,140] Therefore, early intubation may be necessary for patients with dermal burns undergoing aggressive fluid management.[62]

Pathophysiologic changes in the lung may cause progressive hypoxia over hours to days. Treatment of progressive respiratory failure includes mechanical ventilation, continuous positive airway pressure, positive end-expiratory pressure (PEEP), and vigorous clearing of pulmonary secretions.[113] Decreased lung compliance is common secondary to cast formation, tissue damage, and atelectasis.[46,103,113] Recommendations for limiting barotrauma in mechanically ventilated patients include using a low tidal volume (6–8 mL/kg), PEEP, and allowing permissive hypercapnia as necessary.[103] FiO_2 should be weaned to below 0.4 as rapidly as tolerated to limit oxygen toxicity.[103] Frequent airway suctioning, chest physiotherapy, and therapeutic bronchoscopy can clear inspissated secretions, plugs, and casts.[34,103,110] High-frequency percussive ventilation (HFPV) may be considered as an alternative to conventional forms of ventilation in patients with inhalational injury. Several studies have investigated the use of HFPV in ventilated patients with inhalational injury. Although limited, some evidence suggests that HFPV may decrease peak pulmonary pressures, limit barotrauma, decrease the incidence of pneumonia, and improve mortality.[32,58,103,136,143] Experimental treatment has examined percutaneous arteriovenous carbon dioxide removal, perfluorocarbons, inhaled nitric oxide, extracorporeal membrane oxygenation, instillation of natural surfactant into the lung, and deferoxamine–hetastarch complex for improving inhalation injury.[26,33,40,64,76,84,109,117,120,123,134,135] However, none of these modalities has been definitively proven to improve outcome.

The initial treatment of carbon monoxide poisoning consists of supplemental oxygen therapy. Oxygen can be administered by a high-flow tight-fitting mask, endotracheal tube, or hyperbaric oxygen therapy. Hyperbaric oxygen has been recommended as a modality for treatment in certain situations involving carbon monoxide exposure; however, smoke inhalation injury is much more complex than poisoning with carbon monoxide alone (eg, a furnace leak).[60] In victims of smoke inhalation, other clinical requirements, such as maintaining a secure airway and the need for additional resuscitative measures, should be taken to account when determining the appropriate therapy (see Chap. 125 and Antidotes in Depth A37: Hyperbaric Oxygen).

Cyanide poisoning should be suspected in seriously ill patients with smoke inhalation and metabolic acidosis with an elevated lactic acid level, particularly if the carboxyhemoglobin concentration is low.[53,138] Serum lactate concentrations at the time of hospital admission correlate closely with blood cyanide concentrations, with serum lactate concentrations of 10 mmol/L reported to be a sensitive indicator of cyanide toxicity.[10] Treatment of cyanide toxicity should be considered while other life support measures, including 100% oxygen therapy, are instituted.[10,104,119,130,132,147] Treatment options include supportive care alone, administration of all or part of the traditional cyanide antidote kit, or administration of hydroxocobalamin. The risks of antidote administration should be weighed against the benefits because patients have survived potentially lethal cyanide concentrations with simply oxygen therapy and supportive care[19,142] (see Chap. 126 and Antidotes in Depth A38: Sodium and Amyl Nitrite and A40: Hydroxocobalamin).

The amyl nitrite and sodium nitrite components of the classic cyanide antidote kit should be used with caution in victims of smoke inhalation. Amyl nitrite and sodium nitrite produce methemoglobinemia, which binds cyanide to form cyanmethemoglobin (see Chap. 126 and Antidotes in Depth A38: Sodium and Amyl Nitrite). Unfortunately, methemoglobin is a dysfunctional hemoglobin that is unable to carry oxygen. In addition, its presence increases the affinity of the remaining hemoglobin for oxygen, which prevents its release to the tissues.[36] Impairing oxygen-carrying capacity and oxygen delivery to tissues with nitrite-induced methemoglobinemia is a valid concern in the presence of tissue hypoxia from carboxyhemoglobinemia, lung injury, or other factors. Furthermore, rapid infusion of sodium nitrite may cause hypotension secondary to vasodilation.[57]

Inhaled β_2-adrenergic agonists are effective and considered first-line therapy for acute reversible bronchoconstriction resulting from asthma or chronic obstructive pulmonary disease. Pathophysiologic changes induced by irritant toxins in smoke are partially reversible, suggesting that β_2-adrenergic agonists improve airflow obstruction.[77,100] β_2-adrenergic agonists also possess antiinflammatory properties, partially through interaction with β receptors on immune cells.[98,168] β_2-adrenergic agonists may also enhance resolution of alveolar edema by modulating the flow of sodium and potassium across cell membranes.[98,168] Limited data in an ovine model suggest that nebulized albuterol may improve pulmonary function after smoke inhalation and burn injury.[125] Although human data on the efficacy of β_2-adrenergic agonists specifically in smoke inhalation injury are lacking, their role is well established in conditions with reversible brochoconstriction; animal studies[125,168] lend support for their use and the potential benefits greatly outweigh any risks.

Corticosteroids have been used after smoke inhalation in an attempt to limit inflammation and improve outcome. One argument for the use of corticosteroids is for the treatment of lung injury induced by oxides of nitrogen. Pulmonary sequelae, including bronchiolitis obliterans, are known to occur after significant exposure to oxides of nitrogen, which may be a prominent composition of smoke.[52,73,88] Although data regarding efficacy are limited, corticosteroids are often used in treatment of nitrogen oxide exposure in relation to industrial exposure and silo filler's disease to prevent bronchiolitis obliterans.[73,145] The mixed xenobiotic exposure from smoke inhalation appears to further complicate the outcome. One early rat study showed a trend toward reduced mortality in animals given supraphysiologic doses (25–100 mg/kg) of methylprednisolone; however, other tested steroids (hydrocortisone, dexamethasone, cortisone) failed to demonstrate similar improvement. Consequently, this study failed to effectively prove that steroids reduce mortality after rat exposure to white pine smoke.[43] Subsequent human studies have been quite limited in size and design. The results of these human studies have also failed to show an improvement in

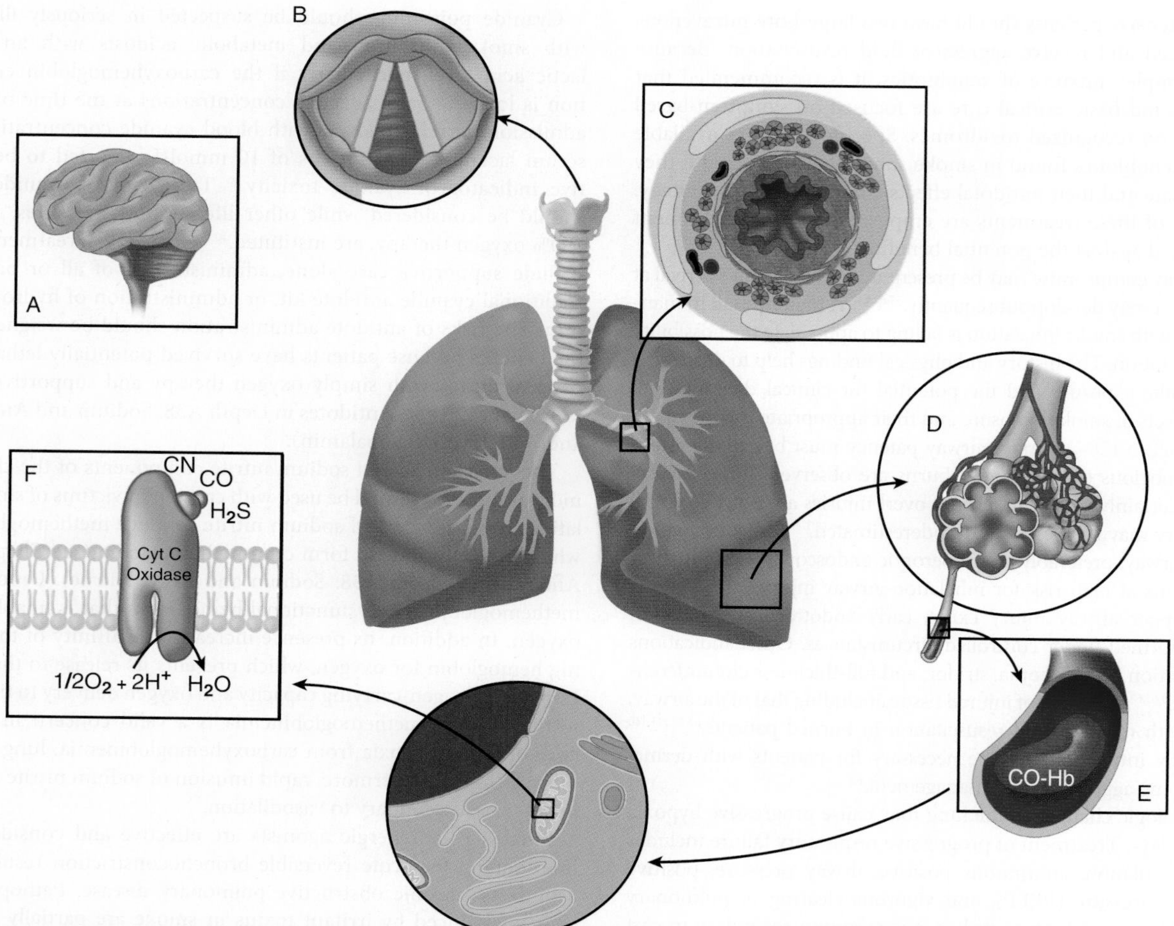

Pathophysiology	Signs and symptoms	Management
A) Direct CNS toxic effects	Coma Hypoventilation	Oxygen; secure unprotected airway
B) Upper airway edema	Hypoxemia; respiratory distress Stridor Hoarse voice	Oxygen Direct visualization of vocal cords Endotracheal intubation
C) Bronchiolar airway obstruction Mucosal edema Intraluminal debris and casts Inspissated secretions Bronchospasm	Respiratory distress Hypoxemia Wheezes Cough Increased peak airway pressures	Oxygen Removal of debris and secretions Chest physiotherapy Frequent airway suctioning Therapeutic bronchoscopy Inhaled β-adrenergic agonists
D) Atelectasis Surfactant destruction Acute lung injury (ALI)	Respiratory distress Hypoxemia Crackles Chest radiographic changes	Oxygen Continuous positive airway pressure Mechanical ventilation Positive end–expiratory pressure
E) Impaired oxygen–carrying capacity (carbon monoxide or methemoglobinemia)	CNS depression or seizures Myocardial ischemia Dysrhythmias Metabolic acidosis	Oxygen Consider hyperbaric oxygen Consider methylene blue
F) Impaired oxygen use at tissues (cyanide, hydrogen sulfide, or carbon monoxide)	CNS depression or seizures Myocardial ischemia Dysrhythmias Metabolic acidosis	Oxygen Assure adequate tissue perfusion Consider treating suspected cyanide toxicity with cyanide antidote Consider hyperbaric oxygen

FIGURE 128–2. The final common pathway from all pathophysiologic changes that occur in smoke inhalation is hypoxia. All treatments should be focused on improving oxygen delivery and oxygen utilization.

clinical outcome and may trend toward worsening outcome.[23,89,114,141] Consequently, limited available literature does not support the use of corticosteroids for treatment of patients with smoke inhalation.

A significant amount of pulmonary injury after smoke inhalation is attributable to free radical damage. Smoke inhalation decreases systemic levels of the antioxidant vitamin E in sheep models.[162] Two animal models demonstrate a decrease in smoke inhalation induced pulmonary injury after treatment with nebulized vitamin E (α- and γ-tocopherol).[59,106] Nebulized heparin and *N*-acetylcysteine (NAC) are used by some centers to limit pulmonary toxicity. Heparin is a glycosaminoglycan with anticoagulant and antiinflammatory properties also occasionally used both topically and IV in burn treatment. Nebulized heparin combined with NAC appeared to attenuate lung injury in pediatric patients.[42] In an ovine model of combined cutaneous burn and smoke inhalation, nebulized heparin combined with recombinant human antithrombin reduced airway obstruction and improved gas exchange.[46] The mechanism is likely attributable to deceased airway inflammation and decreased fibrin deposition and, consequently, decreased cast formation in the airway.[46] Although limiting free radical damage appears to be a promising area of future research, human data are currently limited regarding each of these modalities, and all are considered experimental at this time. Victims from fires may have respiratory compromise and other pathology not directly related to smoke inhalation but rather from trauma or underlying medical problems. Trauma from falls or explosions must be suspected and treatment started simultaneously with treatment of burns and inhalation injury. Comatose patients should be considered to have other causes for their injuries and should receive naloxone, thiamine, and hypertonic dextrose as indicated. Inhaled xenobiotics, such as carbon monoxide, may directly cause altered mental status, but drug and ethanol intoxication contribute significantly to fire fatalities and injuries. Blood ethanol concentrations correlate with elevated concentrations of carbon monoxide and cyanide, implying that intoxication impairs escape and prolongs toxic smoke exposure.[7,15,112] Intracranial pathology should be considered and CT scans obtained as indicated.

Xenobiotics may injure the skin or mucous membranes in addition to the respiratory mucosa.[31] The duration of contact of a xenobiotic with tissue is an important factor in determining the extent of chemical injury to the skin and eyes. Rapid removal of soot from the skin or eyes may prevent continued injury. The eyes should be evaluated for corneal burns caused by thermal or irritant chemical injury. Patients with signs of ocular irritation should have their eyes irrigated. Dermal decontamination should be considered to prevent burns from toxin-laden soot adherent to the skin.

SUMMARY

Smoke inhalation continues to contribute significantly to the morbidity and mortality of fire victims. Clinicians caring for these patients must have a basic knowledge of the pathophysiology of smoke inhalation injury. Smoke inhalation is a complex syndrome involving diverse toxicologic injury. A spectrum of damage may occur, ranging from rapid upper airway occlusion to delayed ALI and ARDS. The end result of toxicity is tissue hypoxia. Goals of treatment should focus on maximizing oxygen delivery while avoiding unnecessary therapies that may hinder oxygenation. Early airway management should be implemented for patients with airway compromise. High-flow oxygen will help reverse tissue hypoxia, and fluid resuscitation should be instituted to improve cardiovascular status. Definitive therapies are available and should be considered in appropriate cases to help stabilize the patient. There are still many controversies regarding the care of these patients. Treatments are still evolving, and further research is warranted.

ACKNOWLEDGMENT

Christopher P. Holstege, MD contributed to this chapter in a previous edition.

REFERENCES

1. Alarie Y. Toxicity of fire smoke. *Crit Rev Toxicol.* 2002;32:259-289.
2. Anderson RA, Cheng KN, Harland WA. The toxicology of fire deaths. *Acta Med Leg Soc.* 1984;34:110-121.
3. Anonymous. Cable car fire kills about 170. *Richmond Times-Dispatch.* November 12, 2000:A1.
4. Anonymous. Locked doors prevented escape from fire. *Richmond Times-Dispatch.* January 1, 2005:A4.
5. Anonymous. Tight security blamed for deaths in Moscow fire. Associated Press; December 6, 2006. Retrieved October 27, 2009, from http://www.msnbc.msn.com/id/16116136/.
6. Ansell M, Lewis FA. A review of cyanide concentrations found in human organs. *J Forensic Med.* 1970;17:148-155.
7. Barillo DJ, Goode R, Rush BF, et al. Lack of correlation between carboxyhemoglobin and cyanide in smoke inhalation. *Curr Surg.* 1986:421-423.
8. Barker SJ, Tremper KK. The effect of carbon monoxide inhalation on pulse oximetry and transcutaneous PO2. *Anesthesiology.* 1987;66:677-679.
9. Bartlett RH, Niccole M, Tavis MJ, et al. Acute management of the upper airway in facial burns and smoke inhalation. *Arch Surg.* 1976;111:744-749.
10. Baud FJ, Barriot P, Toffis V, et al. Elevated blood cyanide concentrations in victims of smoke inhalation. *N Engl J Med.* 1991;325:1761-1766.
11. Becker CE. The role of cyanide in fires. *Vet Hum Toxicol.* 1985;27:487-490.
12. Bernard G, Artigas A, Brigham K, et al. The American-European Consensus Conference on ARDS. Definitions, mechanisms, relevant outcomes, and clinical trial coordination. *Am J Respir Crit Care Med.* 1994;149:818-824.
13. Bidani A, Wang C, Heming T. Cotton smoke inhalation primes alveolar macrophages for tumor necrosis factor-alpha production and suppresses macrophage antimicrobial activities. *Lung.* 1998;176:325-336.
14. Bidani A, Wang CZ, Heming TA. Early effects of smoke inhalation on alveolar macrophage functions. *Burns.* 1996;22:101-106.
15. Birky MM, Clarke FB. Inhalation of toxic products from fires. *Bull NY Acad Med.* 1981;57:997-1013.
16. Bosch X. Report highlights hazard of smoke from indoor fires. *Lancet.* 2003;362:1902.
17. Bowes PC. Casualties attributed to toxic gas and smoke at fires: a survey of statistics. *Med Sci Law.* 1976;16:104-110.
18. Brandt-Rauf PW, Fallon LF, Tarantini T. Health hazards of fire fighters: exposure assessment. *Br J Ind Med.* 1988;45:606-609.
19. Brivet F, Delfraissy JF, Duche M, et al. Acute cyanide poisoning: recovery with non-specific supportive therapy. *Intensive Care Med.* 1983;9:33-35.
20. Brown JE, Birky MM. Phosgene in the thermal decomposition products of poly(vinyl chloride): generation, detection and measurement. *J Anal Toxicol.* 1980;4:166-174.
21. Brown RF, Jugg BJ, Harban FM, et al. Pathophysiological responses following phosgene exposure in the anaesthetized pig. *J Appl Toxicol.* 2002;22:263-269.
22. Cahalane M, Demling RH. Early respiratory abnormalities from smoke inhalation. *JAMA.* 1984;251:771-773.
23. Cha SI, Kim CH, Lee JH, et al. Isolated smoke inhalation injuries: acute respiratory dysfunction, clinical outcomes, and short-term evolution of pulmonary functions with the effects of steroids. *Burns.* 2007;33:200-208.
24. Charan NB, Meyers CG, Lakshminarayan S, et al. Pulmonary injuries associated with acute sulfur dioxide inhalation. *Am Rev Resp Dis.* 1979;119:555-560.
25. Chung Y, Huang S-J, Glabe A, et al. Implication of CO inactivation on myoglobin function. *Am J Physiol Cell Physiol.* 2006;290:C1616-1624.
26. Cioffi WG, deLemos RA, Coalson JJ, et al. Decreased pulmonary damage in primates with inhalation injury treated with high-frequency ventilation. *Ann Surg.* 1993;218:328-337.
27. Clark WR, Bonaventura M, Meyers W. Smoke inhalation and airway management at a regional burn unit: 1974–1983. *J Burn Care Rehabil.* 1989;10:52-62.
28. Clark CJ, Campbell D, Reid WH. Blood carboxyhaemoglobin and cyanide levels in fire survivors. *Lancet.* 1981;1:1332-1335.

29. Clark WR, Nieman GF. Smoke inhalation. *Burns.* 1988;14:473-494.
30. Clarke FB. Toxicity of combustion products: current knowledge. *Fire J.* 1983;77:84-101.
31. Close LG, Catlin FI, Cohn AM. Acute and chronic effects of ammonia burns of the respiratory tract. *Arch Otolaryngol.* 1980;106:151-158.
32. Cortiella J, Mlcak R, Herndon D. High frequency percussive ventilation in pediatric patients with inhalation injury. *J Burn Care Rehabil.* 1999;20:232-235.
33. Cox CS, Zwischenberger JB, Traber DL, et al. Heparin improves oxygenation and minimizes barotrauma after severe smoke inhalation in an ovine model. *Surg Gynecol Obstet.* 1993;176:339-349.
34. Cox RA, Burke AS, Soejima K, et al. Airway obstruction in sheep with burn and smoke inhalation injuries. *Am J Respir Cell Mol Biol.* 2003;29:295-302.
35. Crapo RO. Smoke-inhalation injuries. *JAMA.* 1981;246:1694-1696.
36. Curry S. Methemoglobinemia. *Ann Emerg Med.* 1982;11:214-221.
37. Dacey MJ. Tragedy and response—the Rhode Island nightclub fire. *N Engl J Med.* 2003;349:1990-1992.
38. Davies JW. Toxic chemicals versus lung tissue—an aspect of inhalation injury revisited. *J Burn Care Rehab.* 1986;7:213-222.
39. Decker WJ, Koch HF. Chlorine poisoning at the swimming pool: an overlooked hazard. *Clin Toxicol.* 1978;13:377-381.
40. Demling R, LaLonde C, Ikegami K. Fluid resuscitation with deferoxamine hetastarch complex attenuates the lung and systemic response to smoke inhalation. *Surgery.* 1996;119:340-348.
41. Demling RH, Knox J, Youn Y, et al. Oxygen consumption early postburn becomes oxygen delivery dependent with the addition of smoke inhalation injury. *J Trauma.* 1992;32:593-599.
42. Desai MH, Mlcak R, Richardson J, et al. Reduction in mortality in pediatric patients with inhalation injury with aerosolized heparin/*N*-acetylcysteine therapy. *J Burn Care Rehabil.* 1998;19:210-212.
43. Dressler DP, Skornik WA, Kupersmith S. Corticosteroid treatment of experimental smoke inhalation. *Ann Surg.* 1976;183:46-52.
44. Dyer RF, Esch VH. Polyvinyl chloride toxicity in fires: hydrogen chloride toxicity in fire fighters. *JAMA.* 1976;235:393-397.
45. Eisenkraft JB. Pulse oximeter desaturation due to methemoglobinemia. *Anesthesiology.* 1988;68:279-282.
46. Enkhbaatar P, Cox RA, Traber LD, et al. Aerosolized anticoagulants ameliorate acute lung injury in sheep after exposure to burn and smoke inhalation. *Crit Care Med.* 2007;35:2805-2810.
47. Enkhbaatar P, Murakami K, Shimoda K, et al. Inducible nitric oxide synthase dimerization inhibitor prevents cardiovascular and renal morbidity in sheep with combined burn and smoke inhalation injury. *Am J Physiol Heart Circ Physiol.* 2003;285:H2430-2436.
48. Enkhbaatar P, Murakami K, Shimoda K, et al. Ketorolac attenuates cardiopulmonary derangements in sheep with combined burn and smoke inhalation injury. *Clin Sci (Lond).* 2003;105:621-628.
49. Enkhbaatar P, Murakami K, Shimoda K, et al. The inducible nitric oxide synthase inhibitor bbs-2 prevents acute lung injury in sheep after burn and smoke inhalation injury. *Am J Respir Crit Care Med.* 2003;167:1021-1026.
50. Enkhbaatar P, Traber DL. Pathophysiology of acute lung injury in combined burn and smoke inhalation injury. *Clin Sci (Lond).* 2004;107:137-143.
51. Fein A, Leff A, Hopewell PC. Pathophysiology and management of the complications resulting from fire and the inhaled products of combustion: review of the literature. *Crit Care Med.* 1980;8:94-98.
52. Fleetham JA, Munt PW, Tunnicliffe BW. Silo-filler's disease. *Can Med Assoc J.* 1978;119:482-484.
53. Fortin JL, Ruttiman M, Domanski L, et al. Hydroxocobalamin: treatment for smoke inhalation-associated cyanide poisoning. Meeting the needs of fire victims. *JEMS.* 2004;29(suppl):18-21.
54. Guzzardi L. Toxic products of combustion. *Topics Emerg Med.* 1985;7:45-51.
55. Hales CA, Barkin PW, Jung BW, et al. Synthetic smoke with acrolein but not HCL produces pulmonary edema. *J Appl Physiol.* 1988;64:1121-1133.
56. Hales CA, Musto SW, Janssens S, et al. Smoke aldehyde component influences pulmonary edema. *J Appl Physiol.* 1992;72:555-561.
57. Hall AH, Kulig KW, Rumack BH. Suspected cyanide poisoning in smoke inhalation: complications of sodium nitrite therapy. *J Toxicol Clin Exp.* 1989;9:3-9.
58. Hall JJ, Hunt JL, Arnoldo BD, et al. Use of high-frequency percussive ventilation in inhalation injuries. *J Burn Care Res.* 2007;28:396-400.
59. Hamahata A, Enkhbaatar P, Kraft ER, et al. [gamma]-Tocopherol nebulization by a lipid aerosolization device improves pulmonary function in sheep with burn and smoke inhalation injury. *Free Radic Biol Med.* 2008;45:425-433.
60. Hampson N, Hauff N. Risk factors for short-term mortality from carbon monoxide poisoning treated with hyperbaric oxygen. *Crit Care Med.* 2008;36:2523-2527.
61. Hantson P, Butera R, Clemessy JL, et al. Early complications and value of initial clinical and paraclinical observations in victims of smoke inhalation without burns. *Chest.* 1997;111:671-675.
62. Haponik EF, Meyers DA, Munster AM, et al. Acute upper airway injury in burn patients. *Am Rev Resp Dis.* 1987;135:360-366.
63. Haponik EF, Summer WR. Respiratory complications in burned patients: diagnosis and management of inhalation injury. *J Crit Care.* 1987;2:121-143.
64. Harrington DT, Jordan BS, Dubick MA, et al. Delayed partial liquid ventilation shows no efficacy in the treatment of smoke inhalation injury in swine. *J Appl Physiol.* 2001;90:2351-2360.
65. Hart GB, Strauss MB, Lennon PA, et al. Treatment of smoke inhalation by hyperbaric oxygen. *J Emerg Med.* 1985;3:211-215.
66. Hartzell GE. Overview of combustion toxicology. *Toxicology.* 1996;115:7-23.
67. Harwood B, Hall JR. What kills in fires: smoke inhalation or burns? *Fire J.* 1989;84:29-34.
68. Henderson RF, Schlesinger RB. Symposium on the importance of combined exposures in inhalation toxicology. *Fund Appl Toxicol.* 1989;12:1-11.
69. Herlihy JP, Vermeulen MW, Joseph PM, et al. Impaired alveolar macrophage function in smoke inhalation injury. *J Cell Physiol.* 1995;163:1-8.
70. Herndon DN, Barrow RE, Linares HA, et al. Inhalation injury in burned patients: effects and treatment. *Burns Incl Therm Inj.* 1988;14:349-356.
71. Hill IR. Particulate matter of smoke inhalation. *Ann Acad Med Singapore.* 1993;22:119-123.
72. Hoffman RS, Sauter D. Methemoglobinemia resulting from smoke inhalation. *Vet Hum Toxicol.* 1989;31:168-170.
73. Horvath EP, doPico GA, Barbee RA, et al. Nitrogen dioxide-induced pulmonary disease: five new cases and a review of the literature. *J Occup Med.* 1978;20:103-110.
74. Hunt JL, Agee RN, Pruitt BA. Fiberoptic bronchoscopy in acute inhalation injury. *J Trauma.* 1975;15:641-649.
75. Iheagwara KN, Thom SR, Deutschman CS, et al. Myocardial cytochrome oxidase activity is decreased following carbon monoxide exposure. *Biochim Biophys Acta.* 2007;1772:1112-1116.
76. Jackson MP, Philp B, Murdoch LJ, et al. High frequency oscillatory ventilation successfully used to treat a severe paediatric inhalation injury. *Burns.* 2002;28:509-511.
77. Jagoda A, Shepherd SM, Spevitz A, et al. Refractory asthma, part 1: epidemiology, pathophysiology, pharmacologic interventions. *Ann Emerg Med.* 1997;29:262-274.
78. Jones J, Mcmullen MJ, Dougherty J. Toxic smoke inhalation: cyanide poisoning in fire victims. *Am J Emerg Med.* 1987;5:318-321.
79. Karter M. (National Fire Protection Association). *Fire Loss in the United States in 2007.* Retrieved May 15, 2009, from http://www.nfpa.org/assets/files/PDF/OS.fireloss.pdf.
80. Kirk MA, Gerace R, Kulig KW. Cyanide and methemoglobin kinetics in smoke inhalation victims treated with the cyanide antidote kit. *Ann Emerg Med.* 1993;22:1413-1418.
81. Koljonen V, Maisniemi K, Virtanen K, et al. Multi-detector computed tomography demonstrates smoke inhalation injury at early stage. *Emerg Radiol.* 2007;14:113-116.
82. Laffon M, Pittet J-F, Modelska K, et al. Interleukin-8 mediates injury from smoke inhalation to both the lung endothelial and the alveolar epithelial barriers in rabbits. *Am J Respir Crit Care Med.* 1999;160:1443-1449.
83. LaLonde C, Demling R, Brain J, et al. Smoke inhalation injury in sheep is caused by the particle phase, not the gas phase. *J Appl Physiol.* 1994;77:15-22.
84. LaLonde C, Ikegami K, Demling R. Aerosolized deferoxamine prevents lung and systemic injury caused by smoke inhalation. *J Appl Physiol.* 1994;77:2057-2064.
85. LaLonde C, Nayak U, Hennigan J, et al. Plasma catalase and glutathione levels are decreased in response to inhalation injury. *J Burn Care Rehabil.* 1997;18:515-519.
86. Layton TR, Elhauge ER. U.S. fire catastrophes of the 20th century. *J Burn Care Rehab.* 1982;3:21-28.

87. Lee MJ, O'Connell DJ. The plain chest radiograph after acute smoke inhalation. *Clin Radiol.* 1988;39:33-37.
88. Lehnert BE, Archuleta DC, Ellis T, et al. Lung injury following exposure of rats to relatively high mass concentrations of nitrogen dioxide. *Toxicology.* 1994;89:239-277.
89. Levine BA, Petroff PA, Slade CL, et al. Prospective trials of dexamethasone and aerosolized gentamicin in the treatment of inhalation injury in the burned patient. *J Trauma.* 1978;18:188-193.
90. Levy DM, Divertie MB, Litzow TJ, et al. Ammonia burns of the face and respiratory tract. *JAMA.* 1964;190:873-876.
91. Lin YS, Kou YR. Acute neurogenic airway plasma exudation and edema induced by inhaled wood smoke in guinea pigs: role of tachykinins and hydroxyl radical. *Eur J Pharmacol.* 2000;394:139-148.
92. Loick HM, Traber LD, Stothert JC, et al. Smoke inhalation causes a delayed increase in airway blood flow to primarily uninjured lung areas. *Intensive Care Med.* 1995;21:326-333.
93. Loick HM, Traber LD, Tokyay R, et al. The effects of dopamine on pulmonary hemodynamics and tissue damage after inhalation injury in an ovine model. *J Burn Care Rehabil.* 1992;13:305-315.
94. Lopez DM, Weingarten-Arams JS, Singer LP, et al. Relationship between arterial, mixed venous, and internal jugular carboxyhemoglobin concentrations at low, medium, and high concentrations in a piglet model of carbon monoxide toxicity. *Crit Care Med.* 2000;28:1998-2001.
95. Mahut B, Delacourt C, de Blic J, et al. Bronchiectasis in a child after acrolein inhalation. *Chest.* 1993;104:1286-1287.
96. Mallory TB, Brickley WJ. Management of the Cocoanut Grove burns at Massachusetts General Hospital. Pathology: with special reference to the pulmonary lesions. *Ann Surg.* 1943;117:865-884.
97. Markowitz JS, Gutterman EM, Schwartz S, et al. Acute health effects among firefighters exposed to a polyvinyl chloride (PVC) fire. *Am J Epidemiol.* 1989;129:1023-1031.
98. Matthay MA, Abraham E. Beta-adrenergic agonist therapy as a potential treatment for acute lung injury. *Am J Respir Crit Care Med.* 2006;173:254-255.
99. McNeil DG. Why so many more Americans die in fires? *The New York Times.* December 22, 1991:3.
100. Mellins RB, Park S. Respiratory complications of smoke inhalation in victims of fires. *J Pediatr.* 1975;87:1-7.
101. Meyer GW, Hart GB, Strauss MB. Hyperbaric oxygen therapy for acute smoke inhalation injuries. *Postgrad Med.* 1991;89:221-223.
102. Mizutani A, Enkhbaatar P, Esechie A, et al. Pulmonary changes in a mouse model of combined burn and smoke inhalation-induced injury. *J Appl Physiol.* 2008;105:678-684.
103. Mlcak RP, Suman OE, Herndon DN. Respiratory management of inhalation injury. *Burns.* 2007;33:2-13.
104. Moore SJ, Ho IK, Hume AS. Severe hypoxia produced by concomitant intoxication with sublethal doses of carbon monoxide and cyanide. *Toxicol Appl Pharm.* 1991;109:412-420.
105. Morgan WK. The respiratory effects of particles, vapours, and fumes. *Am Ind Hyg Assoc J.* 1986;47:670-673.
106. Morita N, Traber MG, Enkhbaatar P, et al. Aerosolized alpha-tocopherol ameliorates acute lung injury following combined burn and smoke inhalation injury in sheep. *Shock.* 2006;25:277-282.
107. Moritz A, Henriques F. The effects of inhaled heat on the air passages and lungs: an experimental investigation. *Am J Pathol.* 1945;21:311-331.
108. Morocco AP. Cyanides. *Crit Care Clin.* 2005;21:691-705.
109. Murakami K, Enkhbaatar P, Shimoda K, et al. High-dose heparin fails to improve acute lung injury following smoke inhalation in sheep. *Clin Sci (Lond).* 2003;104:349-356.
110. Nakae H, Tanaka H, Inaba H. Failure to clear casts and secretions following inhalation injury can be dangerous: report of a case. *Burns.* 2001;27:189-191.
111. Navar PD, Saffle JR, Warden GD. Effect of inhalation injury on fluid requirements after thermal injury. *Am J Surg.* 1985;150:716-720.
112. Nelson GL. Regulatory aspects of fire toxicology. *Toxicology.* 1987;47:181-199.
113. Nieman GF, Clark WR, Goyette DA. Positive end expiratory pressure (PEEP) efficacy following wood smoke inhalation (abstract). *Am Rev Resp Dis.* 1986;133:A347.
114. Nieman GF, Clark WR, Hakim T. Methylprednisolone does not protect the lung from inhalation injury. *Burns.* 1991;17:384-390.
115. Nieman GF, Clark WR, Paskanik AM, et al. Unilateral smoke inhalation increases pulmonary blood flow to the injured lung. *J Trauma.* 1994;36:617-623.
116. Nieman GF, Clark WR Jr, Wax SD, et al. The effect of smoke inhalation on pulmonary surfactant. *Ann Surg.* 1980;191:171-181.
117. Nieman GF, Paskanik AM, Fluck RR, et al. Comparison of exogenous surfactants in the treatment of wood smoke inhalation. *Am J Respir Crit Care Med.* 1995;152:597-602.
118. Nijland R, Jongsma HW, Nijhuis JG, et al. Notes on the apparent discordance of pulse oximetry and multi-wavelength haemoglobin photometry. *Acta Anaesthesiologica Scand Suppl.* 1995;107:49-52.
119. Norris JC, Moore SJ, Hume AS. Synergistic lethality induced by the combination of carbon monoxide and cyanide. *Toxicology.* 1986;40:121-129.
120. Ogura H, Saitoh D, Johnson AA, et al. The effects of inhaled nitric oxide on pulmonary ventilation-perfusion matching following smoke inhalation injury. *J Trauma.* 1994;37:893-898.
121. Oliver O. Management of the Cocoanut Grove burns at the Massachusetts General Hospital. *Ann Surg.* 1943;117:801-802.
122. Orzel RA. Toxicologic aspects of firesmoke: polymer pyrolysis and combustion. *Occup Med.* 1993;8:414-429.
123. O'Toole G, Peek G, Jaffe W, et al. Extracorporeal membrane oxygenation in the treatment of inhalational injuries. *Burns.* 1998;24:562-565.
124. Oulton MR, Janigan DT, MacDonald JM, et al. Effects of smoke inhalation on alveolar surfactant subtypes in mice. *Am J Pathol.* 1994;145:941-950.
125. Palmieri TL, Enkhbaatar P, Bayliss R, et al. Continuous nebulized albuterol attenuates acute lung injury in an ovine model of combined burn and smoke inhalation. *Crit Care Med.* 2006;34:1719-1724.
126. Park MS, Cancio LC, Batchinsky AI, et al. Assessment of severity of ovine smoke inhalation injury by analysis of computed tomographic scans. *J Trauma.* 2003;55:417-427; discussion 427-419.
127. Park MS, Cancio LC, Jordan BS, et al. Assessment of oxidative stress in lungs from sheep after inhalation of wood smoke. *Toxicology.* 2004;195:97-112.
128. Pauluhn J. Pulmonary irritant potency of polyisocyanate aerosols in rats: comparative assessment of irritant threshold concentrations by bronchoalveolar lavage. *J Appl Toxicol.* 2004;24:231-247.
129. Peitzman AB, Shires GT, Teixidor HS, et al. Smoke inhalation injury: evaluation of radiographic manifestations and pulmonary dysfunction. *J Trauma.* 1989;29:1232-1239.
130. Pitt BR, Radford EP, Gurtner GH, et al. Interaction of carbon monoxide and cyanide on cerebral circulation and metabolism. *Arch Environ Health.* 1979;34:354-355.
131. Plante T, Harris D, Savitt J, et al. Carboxyhemoglobin monitored by bedside continuous CO-oximetry. *J Trauma.* 2007;63:1187-1190.
132. Prien T. Toxic smoke compounds and inhalation injury—a review. *Burns.* 1988;14:451-460.
133. Purser DA, Woolley WD. Biological studies of combustion atmospheres. *J Fire Sci.* 1983;1:118-144.
134. Qi S, Sun W. The effects of inhaled nitric oxide on cardiac pathology and energy metabolism in a canine model of smoke inhalation injury. *Burns.* 2004;30:65-71.
135. Reper P, Van Bos R, Van Loey K, et al. High frequency percussive ventilation in burn patients: hemodynamics and gas exchange. *Burns.* 2003;29:603-608.
136. Reper P, Wibaux O, Van Laeke P, et al. High frequency percussive ventilation and conventional ventilation after smoke inhalation: a randomised study. *Burns.* 2002;28:503-508.
137. Reske A, Bak Z, Samuelsson A, et al. Computed tomography—a possible aid in the diagnosis of smoke inhalation injury? *Acta Anaesthesiol Scand.* 2005;49:257-260.
138. Riddle K. Hydrogen cyanide: fire smoke's silent killer. *JEMS.* 2004;29 (suppl):5.
139. Riyami BM, Kinsella J, Pollok AJ, et al. Alveolar macrophage chemotaxis in fire victims with smoke inhalation and burns injury. *Eur J Clin Invest.* 1991;21:485-489.
140. Robinson L, Miller RH. Smoke inhalation injuries. *Am J Otolaryngol.* 1986;7:375-380.
141. Robinson NB, Hudson LD, Riem M, et al. Steroid therapy following isolated smoke inhalation injury. *J Trauma.* 1982;22:876-879.
142. Saincher A, Swirsky N, Tenenbein M. Cyanide overdose: survival with fatal blood concentration without antidotal therapy. *J Emerg Med.* 1994;12:555-557.
143. Salim A, Martin M. High-frequency percussive ventilation. *Crit Care Med.* 2005;33:S241-245.
144. Schwerd W, Schulz E. Carboxyhaemoglobin and methaemoglobin findings in burnt bodies. *Forensic Sci Int.* 1978;12:233-235.
145. Seifert SA, Von Essen S, Jacobitz K, et al. Organic dust toxic syndrome: a review. *J Toxicol Clin Toxicol.* 2003;41:185-193.

146. Shusterman D, Alexeeff G, Hargis C, et al. Predictors of carbon monoxide and hydrogen cyanide exposure in smoke inhalation patients. *J Toxicol Clin Toxicol.* 1996;34:61-71.
147. Silverman SH, Purdue GF, Hunt JL, et al. Cyanide toxicity in burned patients. *J Trauma.* 1988;28:171-176.
148. Soejima K, Schmalstieg FC, Sakurai H, et al. Pathophysiological analysis of combined burn and smoke inhalation injuries in sheep. *Am J Physiol Lung Cell Mol Physiol.* 2001;280:L1233-1241.
149. Soejima K, Schmalstieg FC, Traber LD, et al. Role of nitric oxide in myocardial dysfunction after combined burn and smoke inhalation injury. *Burns.* 2001;27:809-815.
150. Sokal JA, Kralkowska E. The relationship between exposure duration, carboxyhemoglobin, blood glucose, pyruvate and lactate and the severity of intoxication in 39 cases of acute carbon monoxide poisoning in man. *Arch Toxicol.* 1985:196-199.
151. Stone JP, Hazlett RN, Johnson JE, et al. The transport of hydrogen chloride by soot from burning polyvinyl chloride. *J Fire Flammability.* 1973;4:42-51.
152. Suner S, Partridge R, Sucov A, et al. Non-invasive pulse co-oximetry screening in the emergency department identifies occult carbon monoxide toxicity. *J Emerg Med.* 2008;34:441-450.
153. Symington IS, Anderson RA, Oliver JS, et al. Cyanide exposures in fires. *Lancet.* 1978;2:90-92.
154. Tasaki O, Goodwin C, Saitoh D, et al. Effects of burns on inhalational injury. *J Trauma Inj Inf Crit Care.* 1997;43:603-607.
155. Teixidor HS, Rubin E, Novick GS, et al. Smoke inhalation: radiologic manifestations. *Radiology.* 1983;149:383-387.
156. Terrill JB, Montgomery RR, Reinhardt CF. Toxic gases from fires. *Science.* 1978;200:1343-1347.
157. Thom SR. Carbon monoxide mediated brain lipid peroxidation in the rat. *J Appl Physiol.* 1990;63:997-1003.
158. Thom SR, Mendiguren I, Van Winkle T, et al. Smoke inhalation with a concurrent systemic stress results in lung alveolar injury. *Am J Respir Crit Care Med.* 1994;149:220-226.
159. Thorning DR, Howard ML, Hudson LD, et al. Pulmonary responses to smoke inhalation: morphologic changes in rabbits exposed to pine wood smoke. *Hum Pathol.* 1982;13:355-364.
160. Touger M, Gallagher EJ, Tyrell J. Relationship between venous and arterial carboxyhemoglobin levels in patients with suspected carbon monoxide poisoning. *Ann Emerg Med.* 1995;25:481-483.
161. Traber DL, Linares HA, Herndon DN. The pathophysiology of inhalation injury—a review. *Burns.* 1988;14:357-364.
162. Traber MG, Shimoda K, Murakami K, et al. Burn and smoke inhalation injury in sheep depletes vitamin E: kinetic studies using deuterated tocopherols. *Free Radic Biol Med.* 2007;42:1421-1429.
163. Treitman RD, Burgess WA, Gold A. Air contaminants encountered by firefighters. *Am Ind Hyg Assoc J.* 1980;41:796-802.
164. Tremper KK, Barker SJ. Using pulse oximetry when dyshemoglobin levels are high. *J Crit Illness.* 1988;3:103-107.
165. Wang CZ, Li A, Yang ZC. The pathophysiology of carbon monoxide poisoning and acute respiratory failure in a sheep model with smoke inhalation injury. *Chest.* 1990;97:736-742.
166. Westphal M, Enkhbaatar P, Schmalstieg FC, et al. Neuronal nitric oxide synthase inhibition attenuates cardiopulmonary dysfunctions after combined burn and smoke inhalation injury in sheep. *Crit Care Med.* 2008;36:1196-1204.
167. Wetherell HR. The occurrence of cyanide in the blood of fire victims. *J Forensic Sci.* 1966;11:167-173.
168. Wiener-Kronish JP, Matthay MA. Beta-2-agonist treatment as a potential therapy for acute inhalational lung injury. *Crit Care Med.* 2006;34:1841-1842.
169. Willey-Courand DB, Harris RS, Galletti GG, et al. Alterations in regional ventilation, perfusion, and shunt after smoke inhalation measured by PET. *J Appl Physiol.* 2002;93:1115-1122.
170. Wittram C, Kenny JB. The admission chest radiograph after acute inhalation injury and burns. *Br J Radiol.* 1994;67:751-754.
171. Youn Y, Lalonde C, Demling R. Oxidants and the pathophysiology of burn and smoke inhalation injury. *Free Radic Biol Med.* 1992;12:409-415.
172. Zawacki BE, Jung RC, Joyce J, et al. Smoke, burns, and the natural history of inhalation injury in fire victims: a correlation of experimental and clinical data. *Ann Surg.* 1977;185:100-110.
173. Zikria BA, Ferrer JM, Floch HF. The chemical factors contributing to pulmonary damage in "smoke poisoning." *Surgery.* 1972;71:704-709.

N.

DISASTER PREPAREDNESS

CHAPTER 129
RISK ASSESSMENT AND RISK COMMUNICATION

Charles A. McKay

Certified Specialists in Poison Information (CSPIs) and clinical and medical toxicologists are confronted by a range of patient presentations daily. The spectrum ranges from an anxious parent with questions about a child's potentially toxic exposure, an urgent consultation for a critically ill patient in the emergency department or intensive care unit and media requests for information about environmental public health issues, and biopreparedness education. Toxicologists and CSPIs must establish rapport and provide information; instructions; and when appropriate, reassurance, typically by telephone or in short face-to-face interactions. For CSPIs, attribution of the patient's complaints to one or more potential exposures and ascertaining the true reason or concern behind a call are also difficult given the limited information and time and lack of visual clues that are usually available during a clinical evaluation. All of these situations require a knowledgeable, compassionate, and well-reasoned response. This chapter focuses on two particular components of this response: risk assessment and risk communication. These principles apply to both individual calls to poison control centers as well as interactions with the public and medical professionals in educational outreaches, occupational and environmental exposure evaluations, and supportive roles with other public health agencies, as in bioterrorism preparedness, environmental public health tracking programs, and research.

RISK ASSESSMENT

Risk assessment is the process of determining the likelihood of toxicity for an individual or group after a perceived exposure to some substance, generally referred to as a xenobiotic. It involves determining the nature and extent of the exposure (ie, xenobiotic, dose, duration, route) and its specific clinical effects, defining an exposure pathway, and assessing the likelihood of effects from a given situation. A published body of knowledge can be applied to some components of risk characterization or assessment. An overview and a number of tools can be accessed through the websites of the Environmental Protection Agency (EPA) and the Agency for Toxic Substance and Disease Registry (ATSDR) of the Centers for Disease Control and Prevention (CDC).[1,9] However, any given risk assessment is often based on incomplete information. This may include such features as uncertainty regarding the exposure xenobiotic or mixture, whether there has been an actual exposure or just proximity to the xenobiotic (completion of an exposure pathway), lack of the exact dose, or unpredictable features such as host factors (underlying medical conditions or genetic polymorphisms) that could modify the response to a potential exposure. Unfortunately, those conducting a risk assessment are affected by their own biases and assumptions in the interpretation of their results, as are the people to whom a risk assessment is communicated. The emotional response to being "poisoned" makes this process even more difficult.

A good example of the practical difficulties involved in a risk assessment is evident from a published description of mass psychogenic illness.[17] In this incident, many individuals at a school complained of odor-triggered symptoms that spread in a so-called "line of sight" transmission with no evident dose–response pattern. Extensive testing demonstrated the possibility of potential sources of exposure, such as dry floor drain traps, but identified no actual release. The extent of investigation of these events can be profound, highlighting the difficulty in appropriately applying potentially unlimited laboratory technology to a situation. Also, our ability to assess a "no-risk" situation is limited, as can be noted in the letters to the editor to this publication criticizing the methods or conclusions in this event and "subsequent and comparable" outbreaks.[4,15,22]

The response of individuals to uncertainty correlates with their affinity for one component of the negative data paradigm—"the absence of evidence of harm" versus "evidence of absence of harm." Both of these positions have at their core the continued evaluation of evidence as it becomes available, with subsequent refinement of a resulting risk assessment. Unfortunately, these potentially converging points on a spectrum of knowledge and research have been polarized in debate and policy as two opposing principles: the *Kehoe principle* and the *precautionary principle*. The Kehoe principle is best summarized as "prove something is harmful before excluding a product with known benefits because of concern about potential, unproven future adverse effects." A common example of the use of this principle is the continued marketing of a xenobiotic after another member of the class has been removed because of safety issues. More intense scrutiny may be indicated, but a class-wide medication recall without evidence of some level of harm by an individual therapeutic drug is very rare. This principle has been misused in the past to minimize known risks attributable to environmental lead pollution to delay removal of lead additives from gasoline.[24] Critics of the Kehoe principle have suggested that waiting for evidence of harm from a substance results in costly or irreparable damage.

The alternative position of the precautionary principle is often summarized as "where there are threats of serious or irreversible damage, lack of full scientific certainty shall not be used as a reason to postpone cost-effective measures to prevent environmental degradation."[20,28] Critics of the precautionary principle often cite the lack of attention paid to the "cost" component of the principle, complaining that devotees stifle economic growth and prosperity with unfounded fears rather than reasoned consideration of known data. This principle is commonly extended to potentially harmful situations other than the

TABLE 129–1. Components of Risk Assessment

Hazard Identification
Name and amount of suspected xenobiotic (or general use category if the xenobiotic is unknown)
Exposure Pathway
Proposed route of exposure
Consistency with the nature of the xenobiotic (eg, water-soluble liquid)
Modifying Factors
Environmental factors that would influence systemic availability of the xenobiotic
Patient characteristics (susceptibility or resistance factors), such as:
Chronic medical conditions
Possible xenobiotic–drug or other interactions
Genetic polymorphisms in hepatic or other metabolic pathways
Toxicity Assessment
Compare and contrast organ effects expected from the particular xenobiotic with existing symptoms

environment. A common criticism of the precautionary principle is the degree to which alternative actions have been evaluated for safety. As an example, concern about thimerosal safety (as a vaccine preservative and source of ethylmercury exposure) in young children led many parents to forego childhood vaccinations. Vaccine manufacturers have removed the thimerosal preservative from most routine childhood vaccines. Although this process was accelerated by the theoretical—and ultimately unfounded—concerns regarding this source of mercury exposure in young children, the cost of delayed or omitted vaccination was a number of real and preventable infectious diseases, including hepatitis B.[5,6]

Although the Kehoe and precautionary principles originated as policy approaches to public health issues, they underlie the automatic or subconscious biases that each individual brings to his or her own personal risk assessment or tolerance. The response to uncertain situations is derived from one's framing of belief systems and assumptions about life, justice, and eternity.[3,10,13] These underlying world views should be explicitly recognized and addressed in a formal risk assessment. Table 129–1 lists components of a risk assessment.

DIFFERENTIATING PUBLIC HEALTH FROM INDIVIDUAL RISK ASSESSMENT

It is difficult to translate public health risk assessment done for populations by entities such as the EPA to the individual level. Simplistically, the iterative process of adjusting known noncancer adverse exposure outcome limits in an animal model (eg, lowest observed adverse effect level [LOAEL] or no observed effect level [NOEL]) to a safe level of exposure for all humans (including so-called "sensitive subpopulations") has been arbitrarily set at repetitive multiplicative factors of 10 for each of these extrapolations. These are called "uncertainty factors" and are used in the absence of specific information about human exposure to identify a conservative human "safe dose." This would be set at 0.001 times the animal model LOAEL, reflecting a 10-fold reduction in dose for extrapolation from LOAEL to NOEL, another 10-fold reduction for extrapolation from animal to human, and another 10-fold reduction for potentially "sensitive" human populations. These "uncertainty factors" are actually safety factors for the adverse effect of interest. When individuals exceed these limits, they remain protected by very robust safety factors, and are not—as it is often portrayed—exposing themselves to a defined harm. An example of this is the dietary guidelines (also known as "fish health advisories") for fish consumption based on concern about exposure to methylmercury and polychlorinated biphenyls (PCBs). These dietary recommendations are based on epidemiologic studies that suggest subtle neuropsychiatric abnormalities in maternal–fetal pairs (in at least some populations) from levels of consumption 10 to 100 times that of the "usual" American diet. Clinical mercury toxicity requires still higher levels of consumption. Although it seems reasonable for pregnant women to limit their intake of certain high mercury-containing fish species, it is inappropriate to avoid fish and the nutrients contained therein because of a misplaced fear of mercury exposure. Furthermore, these risk assessments do not apply to nonpregnant women, children, or men, although they are often generalized to all humans.[2]

The public health modeling concept for cancer health effects risk assessment is even more complex and often misunderstood. In this setting, modeling assumes a linear, no-threshold carcinogenic effect from exposure to a given xenobiotic. Cancer risk from small exposures is extrapolated from data in cancer-prone animal models with exposures so large that they are only likely in the experimental setting. This experimental construct ignores incremental dosing of small amounts over a protracted period of time, and potential metabolic and self-repair mechanisms in the human. The "acceptable risk" in this setting is then taken as "one excess cancer in a population of 1,000,000 exposed individuals." Although a limitation of this model is explicit in the statement that this represents "a plausible upper bound estimate of risk at low dose where true risk may be lower, including zero,"[11] this important caveat is rarely communicated, resulting in the common response by individuals that "an extra cancer may be acceptable for you, but not when it is my child."

As this brief review of the principles of regulatory approaches to noncancer and cancer effects demonstrates, risk assessment is often imprecise. Risk characterization for the individual should avoid unfamiliar statistical concepts, aiming instead to communicate the likelihood of significant risk for the exposure actually experienced. The CDC has codified this approach for a community using such escalating terms as "no public health concern," "public health concern," "public health threat," and "immediate risk." Although there is debate about the general use of these terms in isolation (without explicit explanations), a similar approach with an individual could summarize the risk assessment using the terms "safe"; "don't expect any adverse effects"; "may be of concern—we will need to do some follow-up testing"; and "this might be (or is) a problem—let's do the following studies or treatments."

RISK COMMUNICATION

Risk communication is an exchange of facts and opinions to allow an individual or a group of individuals to make an informed decision regarding a course of action or treatment. Practically, risk communication is a way of translating incomplete knowledge in a manner such that individuals can achieve informed decision making. During a one-on-one interaction with a poisoned individual and his or her family or a caller to the poison center, there is a need to gain the fullest attention or cooperation of the individual. After this has occurred, the discussion is usually focused on the risks and benefits of various treatment options (eg, gastrointestinal decontamination) or possible diagnostic modalities (eg, observation versus neuroimaging versus antidote administration). The group dynamics of environmental exposure risk communication at a public meeting are very different.

TABLE 129–2. Principles of Risk Communication[7] and Applicability to the Poison Center

Principle	Applications
Accept and involve the individual as a partner.	The caller must be involved to obtain the best information possible.
Plan carefully and evaluate your efforts.	There is a very short time to establish rapport with the caller; do not increase the caller's anxiety by asking irrelevant questions or arguing. Monitor your tone; ask for repetition of key information or recommendations.
Listen to the individual's specific concerns.	Why did the person call? Was it for information, treatment recommendations, or reassurance? Make sure the underlying reason has been addressed.
Be honest, frank, and open.	If there is uncertainty or there are unknowns, indicate that uncertainty while providing a workable plan.
Work with other credible sources.	Involve medical toxicology backup and other consultants, particularly for questions regarding chronic exposure or effects.
Meet the needs of the media.	If calls involve media notification or contact, make sure the critical information is stated frequently, provide a human context, and avoid sensationalism.
Speak clearly and compassionately.	Remember that the caller was concerned enough to initiate the contact; make sure the call is completed with a clear plan; provide follow-up appropriate to the situation.

Federal agencies that interact with communities in "Superfund" sites (eg, the EPA and the ATSDR) have promulgated principles and practical recommendations for risk communication in this setting. Table 129–2 summarizes general principles of risk communication.

Although some of these recommendations are more applicable to longer-term deliberations and interactions, much of the individual communication done by the poison center and medical toxicologists succeeds or fails based on these same principles (see Table 129–2). Lacking the opportunity for repeated interactions over time to identify and discuss assumptions and biases, toxicologists need to establish credibility, listen to concerns and respond empathetically, admit areas of insufficient knowledge, and commit to follow-up interactions to effectively convey a risk characterization for an individual based on the available knowledge and experience. The scientific terms, rationale, and any extrapolation from modeling (eg, animal data or case series) should be conveyed in an understandable manner to show that appropriate safety factors are incorporated into areas of uncertainty as a risk-diminishing step. The patient or audience should leave the interaction with a clear understanding of the difference between a short-term risk of symptoms that will resolve or result in serious illness and the degree of certainty about the potential for a long-term consequence.

An example of poor risk communication can be found in the immediate aftermath of the World Trade Center disaster in September 2001. The mass rescue and recovery response was largely voluntary and heroic; however, inadequate attention was paid to the importance of respiratory protection against the heavy particulate and alkaline dust in the early hours after the towers collapsed. The high incidence and persistence of cough and other respiratory symptoms in responders has been attributed to this exposure. Communication of the real risk of respiratory symptoms to early responders would have emphasized the critical importance of appropriate use of personal protective equipment. This would have been balanced against the time-limited possibility of saving lives of those potentially trapped in largely inaccessible locations. Since 2001, a proliferation of other associations to World Trade Center dust exposure (including low birthweight) are reported, which are of doubtful validity.[29] Appropriate risk communication to people concerned about these reports should emphasize the important role of confounders, the investigational nature of the study hypothesis, and the lack of relevant risk to any given individual.

Effective risk communication must therefore address several questions. After the best information has been obtained about the identification of the xenobiotic and the nature of the exposure, the following must be conveyed:

- The likely **magnitude** of the risk. This includes information on the process by which the person would be exposed (ie, the exposure pathway), such as airborne inhalation or drinking water delivery via a contaminated plume in the ground water and dose–response, such as: "Does the reported exposure to a particular xenobiotic (amount and duration) approach the exposure amounts reported to cause symptoms?"
- The **urgency** of the risk must also be conveyed along with practical recommendations for simple actions consistent with the level of urgency.
- The **applicability** of a risk characterization might also need to be addressed. Are the animal data applicable to humans? Is the exposure something of concern for an individual?
- The **uncertainties** of the risk assessment. This could include a "worst-case scenario" approach to unknown exposures or uncertainties in the quantity of an absorbed dose. The need for continued observation or follow-up for clinical changes would be expressed here. Individual risk tolerance may vary greatly. The same information may be interpreted differently by risk-averse versus risk-tolerant people. A variety of comparisons or communication techniques may be used to provide an adequate characterization of risk.
- **Management options.** In addition to follow-up and repeated evaluations by a medical toxicologist, the range of choices, associated with their relative benefits or risks, would be presented to the individual or group of individuals. A summary recommendation or opinion from the presenter should emphasize specific steps people can take to decrease exposure or potential toxicity if indicated by the level of risk. This last step is important because uncertainty significantly impacts the ability of an individual to take appropriate action. People should not leave the meeting with the impression that "no one knows what is going on or what we should do."

APPLICATION OF RISK ASSESSMENT AND COMMUNICATION PRINCIPLES TO TOXICOLOGY

Although it has long been recognized that many home-initiated poison center calls concern nontoxic or minimally toxic xenobiotics ingested by children,[23] the frequent lack of documented ingestion raises the possibility of under-triage based on misplaced confidence based on prior experience. It is generally assumed that the sheer volume of calls provides some reassurance regarding the accuracy of our risk assessment of these xenobiotics, but we should remain cautious in our interpretation of poison center data[5,16,25] (see Chap. 135). Moreover, even calls about nontoxic xenobiotics require communication between the caller and CSPI beyond simple substance identification. The importance of risk assessment and communication principles can be seen in the joint Position Statement on the Prehospital Management of "Minimally Toxic Substances" crafted by the American Association of Poison Control Centers (AAPCC), American Academy of Clinical Toxicology (AACT), and American College of Medical Toxicology (ACMT).[21] According to the position statement, for a CSPI to make a risk assessment that an exposure is benign or minimally toxic, the following characteristics must be true:

- "The information specialist has confidence in the accuracy of the history obtained and the ability to communicate effectively with the caller.
- "The information specialist has confidence in the identity of the product(s) or substance(s) and a reasonable estimation of the maximum amount involved in the exposure.
- "The risks of adverse reactions or expected effects are acceptable to both the information specialist and the caller based on available medical literature and clinical experience.
- "The exposure does not require a healthcare referral because the worst potential effects are benign and self-limited."[21]

The position statement further notes that patient disposition decisions can be altered by many additional factors, including intent, environment, presence of symptoms (possibly unrelated to the xenobiotic in question), and ongoing review of current recommendations in the face of more data. These points emphasize both the dependence of the CSPI on information derived from the caller and his or her confidence in the level of comprehension of the caller. The caller should understand that his or her exposed child is safe; the conversation with the toxicology experts should alleviate concern as the nature of the assessment process is explained to whatever degree is necessitated by the caller's risk tolerance.

In the case of a symptomatic patient or a hospital- or physician-initiated contact to a poison center or medical toxicologist, the caller should expect more than just xenobiotic-related information; he or she also expects knowledge and expertise that will provide reassurance or direction for improving the patient's health status. However, merely relaying information regarding the diagnosis, course, and predicted outcome is insufficient. There is often another underlying reason for the call. This could be anxiety, uncertainty, or misinformation established by an individual's previous experiences or knowledge base. A sense of guilt may underlie a parent's call for an inadvertent exposure occurring when a child was unsupervised. A physician may have had significant difficulties previously in the management of a poisoned patient. If these issues are not addressed, the caller may continue seeking reassurance by repeated calls to the poison control center or by seeking additional input from other sources, such as family, friends, primary physicians, other healthcare providers. Any variance in the information obtained from these sources may be construed as inconsistencies between supposed experts rather than differences in emphasis with regard to the same information, leading to further uncertainty for the caller. Of further concern, the Internet has become a common source of second opinion for healthcare. Although many sites are useful, there is no quality control or filter to sort good information from bad or even harmful advice.[12] Table 129–3 lists some barriers to effective risk assessment and communication.

TABLE 129–3. Factors That Affect Appropriate Risk Assessment and Effective Risk Communication

Nature of previous encounters with poison center or healthcare field
Lack of prior patient–healthcare provider relationship
Incomplete or inadequate response to a prior question
The provision of information contrary to "popular understanding" or media representation
Loss of credibility
Lack of appreciation of individual or cultural differences in the perception of risk or the applicability of data
Incomplete or limited comprehension of scientific or statistical principles

INTERPRETING PUBLIC HEALTH CONCERNS FOR THE INDIVIDUAL

CSPIs and medical toxicologists frequently encounter callers or individuals at community events or interact with the media regarding public health–related issues, such as heavy metal exposures involving mercury, lead, or arsenic or concerns about "toxic mold" and other environmental xenobiotics. Often these people are concerned that their symptoms or future health or family health may be adversely impacted by such exposures. Such supposed exposures are usually poorly documented, sometimes also driven by popular media descriptions or litigation, and the risk is virtually impossible to ascertain during a short telephone or personal interaction. In these situations, the individual is best served by referral to a primary care physician with toxicology consultation or directly to a medical toxicology clinic. In such a setting, the data and perceptions can be reviewed completely and a more appropriate risk assessment communicated. These interactions are very difficult because they are often emotionally and politically charged.

In general, the communication of and response to information depend on a preexisting world view and prevailing circumstances. The same possible outcome will be perceived as more or less severe depending on several factors other than the nature of the outcome itself. Several authors have characterized the perceived tolerance to different risks, stratified by features such as familiarity and personal control[10,27] (Table 129–4). The emotional response of individuals confronted with these risks is sometimes characterized as "outrage." One communications specialist has posited that "Risk = Hazard + Outrage."[26]

TABLE 129–4. Factors That Alter the Acceptability of Perceived Risk[10]

More Acceptable	Less Acceptable
Natural	Human-made
Associated with a trusted source	Not associated with a trusted source
Familiar	Unfamiliar
Voluntary	Involuntary
Potentially beneficial	Limited or absent potential benefit
Statistical (low harm likelihood)	Catastrophic (high harm likelihood)
Fairly distributed or shared by all	Unfairly distributed ("injustice")
Affects adults	Affects children

He characterizes situations in which there is a significant hazard but little outrage as requiring "precaution advocacy," essentially informing the relevant parties of the need for more action or involvement to reduce risk. On the other end of the spectrum is a situation with little hazard but significant outrage, which requires "outrage management" to address fear or anger that is dissociated from the actual hazard posed by the situation. Although not necessarily applicable to the initial "fight-or-flight" response to an emergency, these concepts are certainly applicable to the aftermath of these events. The greater the degree of familiarity with the particular exposure situation and the greater the voluntary nature of the exposure, the less fear or outrage will be expressed for a given adverse outcome, whether this is an appropriate response or not. Of note, although risk communicators use analogies to place exposures into a context familiar to their audience, one must be careful to avoid equating voluntary and involuntary risk assumption or equating those exposures or risks assumed by one segment of the population unequally. An example of this is the use of a smoking risk analogy for a nonsmoker versus for a smoker.

Risk communication has become very important in the setting of preparedness for terrorism. Although a great deal of attention and money have been directed to improvement of public health infrastructure, reporting and surveillance mechanisms, and response to perceived and actual terrorist acts, less attention has been directed to the process of communicating risk to the individual.[8,19] Although some countries practice public health emergency drills regularly, the United States has concentrated on development of organizational structures and lines of authority, with attention to the importance of outcome-based exercises only recently emphasized.

Maintaining a readiness for catastrophic terrorist events (or natural occurrences such as pandemic influenza) should use the same risk assessment and communication techniques that are appropriate for other urgent public health matters. Unfortunately, many factors affect the characterization of risk other than the facts. The importance of presentation or the role of the communicator's own biases are exemplified by these two composite articles describing the same events:

1. Unknown assailants have infiltrated the mail delivery system, resulting in severe illness and death of children, healthy adults, and elderly people throughout the country. The initial symptoms can be nonspecific but rapidly progress to death if treatment is not begun early. The medical community routinely fails to diagnose the conditions early, and the government has no system in place to detect this threat after it occurs. The long-ignored public health system is not prepared to deal with the huge burden of preventing illness in those who may have been or will be exposed. Anyone who receives regular mail may be at risk. Tens of thousands of our citizens are taking prophylactic antibiotics "just in case." If you receive any unusual packages or see collections of powder that do not have an obvious explanation, call the police. If you develop a fever, cough, chest pain, or unusual rash, which may not be painful, seek medical attention at once. Tune in to your local news station for more information on this burgeoning threat to our nation's security.
2. A small number of individuals in isolated exposure settings have developed illnesses after bioterrorism events. Most people have survived these exposures, particularly with early and proper medical care. The government has developed a case definition, and medical experts have disseminated information to assist the medical community and public in the early recognition of symptoms and signs that are consistent with this exposure. Prophylactic treatment within days of exposure of those in high-risk professions, such as mail handlers at major postal sorting facilities, prevents illness. Unfortunately, there have been a large number of hoaxes and false alarms about possible terrorist events and a lot of understandable fear in the community about nonspecific symptoms. For more information, contact your local health department or use the CDC website: http://www.bt.cdc.gov/agent/anthrax/needtoknow.asp.

Both of these paragraphs describe the 2001 anthrax bioterrorism events within the United States during which a total of 22 people become ill of whom five died from anthrax exposure. The first communication suggests that everyone is at risk and the situation is dire; the communication in the second paragraph is that the risk is isolated (a single individual died who was not in what was recognized as an at-risk setting from the seven identified mailings) and there is a plan and process being developed to respond to the threat. Whereas the first is sensationalistic, imparting a helpless victim role to the reader, the second provides a framework in which to assess one's personal risk and access to sources of reliable information. Both types of reports were prevalent after the 2001 anthrax attacks. Which report seems more complete, accurate, or useful is determined by the assumptions and perspectives of the reader in addition to the message the author wishes to deliver or response desired. Some would say that communicating a high degree of risk is important to gain the attention of the reader and to ensure that no one ignores a warning. However, the lack of a risk perspective prevents the reader from placing this information in context with the myriad other risk communication messages conveyed on a daily basis. In general, risk communication messages that do not provide a context or comparison to generally familiar activities or risks are more prone to misinterpretation or misapplication. As biopreparedness moves from public health infrastructure development and surveillance improvement to planning and response drills, appropriate message development and risk communication to the public become increasingly important.

SUMMARY

High-quality risk assessment and effective risk communication are the hallmarks of a successful interaction between the public and poison centers and between a toxicologist and an individual patient, the media, or the public health community. Adherence to general principles include obtaining the best information possible regarding potential exposures and conveying in an understandable fashion as complete as possible a risk characterization of the hazard, likelihood of a completed exposure pathway (thus, the likelihood of an actual exposure), possible health effects, and treatment options. It is important to clarify the difference between public health standards and individual exposure risks, with an understanding of the many psychosocial issues that influence perception. Information should be provided in a context that allows the individual to prioritize his or her response based on a factual and balanced presentation with respect to his or her health literacy and health numeracy (ie, the ability of the listener to understand quantitative concepts and interpret data that relies on numbers).[14]

REFERENCES

1. Agency for Toxic Substance and Disease Registry, Environmental Protection Agency. *A Citizen's Guide to Risk Assessments and Public Health Assessments at Contaminated Sites.* Retrieved August 18, 2008, from http://www.atsdr.cdc.gov/publications/01-0930CitizensGuidetoRiskAssessments.pdf.
2. Agency for Toxic Substance and Disease Registry. *Toxicological Profile for Mercury*; March 1999. Retrieved October 29, 2009, from http://www.atsdr.cdc.gov/toxprofiles/tp46.html.
3. Ames BN, Profet M, Gold LS. Nature's chemicals and synthetic chemicals: comparative toxicology. *Proc Natl Acad Sci.* 1990;87:7782-7786.
4. Black D, Murray V. Mass psychogenic illness attributed to toxic exposure at a high school. *N Engl J Med.* 2000;342:1674.

5. Centers for Disease Control and Prevention. A comprehensive immunization strategy to eliminate transmission of hepatitis B virus transmission in the United States. *MMWR Morbid Mortal Wkly Rep.* 2005;54(RR16):1-23. Retrieved December 12, 2008, from http://www.cdc.gov/mmwr/preview/mmwrhtml/rr5416a1.htm.
6. Centers for Disease Control and Prevention. Impact of the 1999 AAP/USPHS joint statement on thimerosal in vaccines on infant hepatitis B vaccination practices. *MMWR Morbid Mortal Wkly Rep* 2001;50(6):94-97. Retrieved December 12, 2008, from http://www.cdc.gov/mmwr/preview/mmwrhtml/mm5006a3.htm.
7. Covello V, Allen F. *Seven Cardinal Rules of Risk Communication*. Washington, DC: US Environmental Protection Agency, Office of Policy Analysis; 1988.
8. Durodié B. Facing the possibility of bioterrorism. *Curr Op Biotech.* 2004;15:264-268.
9. Environmental Protection Agency. *Risk Assessment Website Portal.* Retrieved August 18, 2008, from http://www.epa.gov/risk/.
10. Fischhoff B, Lichtenstein S, Slovic P, Keeney D. *Acceptable Risk*. Cambridge, MA: Cambridge University Press; 1981.
11. Fowle JR III, Dearfield KL. *Risk Characterization Implementation Core Team. Risk Characterization Handbook*. Washington, DC: Environmental Protection Agency, Science Policy Council; December 2000. Retrieved August 24, 2008, from http://www.epa.gov/OSA/spc/pdfs/rchandbk.pdf.
12. Fox S. *The Engaged E-Patient Population*. Washington, DC: Pew Internet & American Life Project; 2008. Retrieved December 14, 2008, from http://www.pewinternet.org/pdfs/PIP_Health_Aug08.pdf.
13. Glassner B. *The Culture of Fear: Why Americans Are Afraid of the Wrong Things*, 2nd ed. New York City: Basic Books; 2004.
14. Golbeck AL, Ahlers-Schmidt CR, Paschal AM, Dismuke SE. A definition and operational framework for health numeracy. *Am J Prev Med.* 2005;29(4):375-376.
15. Goode MD. Mass psychogenic illness attributed to toxic exposure at a high school. *N Engl J Med.* 2000;342:1673-1674.
16. Hamilton RJ, Goldfrank LR. Poison center data and the Pollyanna phenomenon. *J Toxicol Clin Toxicol.* 1997;35:21-23.
17. Jones TF, Craig AS, Hoy D, et al. Mass psychogenic illness attributed to toxic exposure at a high school. *N Engl J Med.* 2000;342:96-100.
18. Longo LD. Environmental pollution and pregnancy: risks and uncertainties for the fetus and infant. *Am J Ob Gynecol.* 1980;137:162-173.
19. Manning FJ, Goldfrank L, eds. *Preparing for Terrorism: Tools for Evaluating the Metropolitan Medical Response System Program*. Washington, DC: Committee on Evaluation of the Metropolitan Medical Response System Program, Board on Health Sciences Policy, Institute of Medicine; 2002.
20. Martuzzi M, Tickner JA, eds. *The Precautionary Principle: Protecting Public Health, the Environment and the Future of Our Children*. Budapest: Fourth Ministerial Conference on Environment and Health, World Health Organization; 2004. Retrieved August 24, 2008, from http://www.euro.who.int/document/eehc/ebakdoc09.pdf.
21. McGuigan MA. Guideline Consensus Panel. Guideline for the out-of-hospital management of human exposures to minimally toxic substances. *J Toxicol Clin Toxicol.* 2003;41:907-917.
22. Miller CS, Ashford NA. Mass psychogenic illness attributed to toxic exposure at a high school. *N Engl J Med.* 2000;342:1673.
23. Mofenson HC, Greensher J. The nontoxic ingestion. *Pediatr Clin North Am.* 1970;17:583-590.
24. Nriagu JO. Clair Patterson and Robert Kehoe's paradigm of "show me the data" on environmental lead poisoning. *Environ Res.* 1998;78:71-78.
25. Robertson WO. Poison center data and the Pollyanna phenomenon disputed. *J Toxicol Clin Toxicol.* 1998;36:139-141.
26. Sandman P. *The Peter Sandman Risk Communication Website*. Retrieved December 14, 2008, from http://www.psandman.com/index.htm.
27. Slovic P. Perception of risk. *Science.* 1987;236:280-285.
28. Tickner JA, Kriebel D, Wright S. A compass for health: rethinking precaution and its role in science and public health. *Int J Epidemiol.* 2003;32:489-492.
29. World Trade Center Medical Working Group of New York City. *2008 Annual Report on 9/11 Health*; September 2008. Retrieved September 12, 2008, from http://www.nyc.gov/html/om/pdf/2008/2008_mwg_annual_report.pdf.

CHAPTER 130
HAZMAT INCIDENT RESPONSE

Bradley J. Kaufman

A hazardous material (hazmat) can be any xenobiotic (solid, liquid, or gas) with the potential to harm. Typically, we are most concerned about xenobiotics that can harm people, although a hazmat may only harm other living organisms, the environment, or property. Outside of the United States, hazardous materials are often referred to as *dangerous goods*.

A "hazmat incident" implies that there was an unplanned or uncontrolled release of or exposure to a hazardous material. Although there are no specific requirements for an event to be considered a hazmat incident, typically there will be the potential for many people or a large area to be affected; otherwise, all toxicologic exposures would fall into this category. Therefore, a hazmat incident falls within the larger disaster management framework within a community.

Hazardous materials include chemical, biologic, and radiologic xenobiotics. In fact, a single event could provide exposure to multiple xenobiotics. Complicating matters, the incident response required for chemical, biologic, or radiologic xenobiotics may differ substantially depending on many factors. For instance, an envelope containing a white powder suspicious for containing anthrax spores that is opened in an office might require decontamination of the exposed people and environment. However, the release of the same anthrax spores surreptitiously at multiple sites may not be recognized until days later because of the delayed onset of symptoms. Certainly, a very different emergency response would be required. Emergency managers and healthcare providers must consider all possibilities and adjust the incident response based on the specific xenobiotics involved. This chapter discusses the basic principles used for a confined and quickly identifiable hazmat incident.

In general, a hazmat incident response focuses on the care of patients exposed to xenobiotics in the prehospital setting, prepares for multiple casualties, and emphasizes patient decontamination while at the same time trying to prevent exposure and contamination of healthcare providers.

DISASTER MANAGEMENT AND RESPONSE

Disaster management has four phases: mitigation, planning, response, and recovery. *Mitigation* measures are plans and efforts that attempt to prevent or reduce the effects of a potential hazard from becoming a disaster or minimizing the effects of a disaster if it has already occurred. One example of a mitigation measure is to use a secure container to prevent leakage of a chemical that is to be stored. *Preparedness* requires the planning of actions to be taken when a disaster occurs, as well as the practicing with mock exercises of these actions. Pre-planning is critical to limit damage from an event, and numerous such hazmat incident response plans exist. The *recovery* phase occurs after the immediate needs and threats to human life are addressed in the response phase and entail the restoration of property, infrastructure, and the environment.

The *response* phase includes the mobilization of appropriate resources and the coordinated management of the incident. Hazmat incident response must include the containment of the xenobiotic followed by neutralization, removal, or both. Typically, such a response includes multiple trained professionals from various agencies, often including the emergency medical services (EMS), fire departments, police departments, environmental protection agencies, and other first responder emergency services personnel. In fact, major hazmat events, especially those considered purposeful or terrorist related, may have responders from multiple federal, state, and local agencies, each with equipment and vehicles, and hundreds of personnel at the scene. These events can be chaotic until control and coordination are achieved.

Initial disaster management is provided by local resources and agencies with progressive escalation to county, state, and federal agencies as necessary. The Federal Emergency Management Agency (FEMA) within the Department of Homeland Security is the lead federal agency for emergency management in the United States.

Medical providers are a necessary part of all hazmat incident responses because patient assessment and treatment are typically the highest priority. However, as with all mass casualty events, physicians and other healthcare providers, even those highly trained in emergency medicine, toxicology, or hazmat response, must not respond to the location of the event unless they are part of a planned response team that has been requested to respond to the incident. Unsolicited medical personnel at the scene of a hazmat incident, although well intentioned, may actually harm the coordinated response and lifesaving efforts.

Limiting the loss of life is dependent on all responding agencies and personnel working efficiently and effectively together. The coordination of federal, state, and local governments is mandated by a National Incident Management System (NIMS).[9] Interoperability and compatibility among on-scene assets is dictated by the Incident Command System (ICS), which consists of an organizational hierarchy and defines the necessary management components of the overall incident, including mechanisms necessary for controlling personnel, operations, communications, and so on.

The request for mobilization, management, and utilization of volunteer medical personnel at the scene of a disaster should be planned for in advance for those events that might benefit from these resources.[29] Unsolicited medical providers lack the communications equipment necessary to work within a multi-agency coordinated operation. They often function outside the organized ICS. They may lack or be unaware of the necessary personal protective equipment (PPE). The medical treatments they provide may lack the oversight and protections required for the provision of medical care. These environments are, by definition, hazardous, and freelance medical personnel may in turn become patients themselves, thereby adding to the burden of on-scene rescuers. Furthermore, although a patient affected by a specific hazardous material may have the same physical findings and treatment indications whether at the hazmat scene or at the hospital and although the same toxicologic principles apply, these differences in location often require variation to the medical decisions made and care provided. Typically, disaster plans incorporate the utilization of local medical assets such as hospitals and clinics. Therefore, communities are best served if medical providers respond to their respective institutions during an incident.

RESPONSE COMPONENTS

After the release of a hazardous material, there must be a notification to emergency response personnel. Typically, someone witnesses the incident itself, such as a motor vehicle collision in which a road trailer is breached, or some resultant effects of the release, such as a fire, and the individual then activates the emergency response system by calling 911. Alternatively, an established detector may activate an emergency response to a hazmat incident even before there are easily observable results of the release.

The first responders may not be aware that an incident is hazmat related when responding. For instance, they may be assigned to respond to an unconscious patient, unaware that the cause of the medical emergency was a chemical exposure. Although every emergency response cannot be assumed to have a hazmat etiology, emergency responders must always remain vigilant for such situations.

Extensive knowledge, training, and judgment are required for all emergency personnel who respond to hazmat incidents. There are some basic paradigms followed for a hazmat response. Personnel should approach the scene from uphill and upwind if possible. They should not rush in to try to help patients because the rescuer may become an additional victim if exposed. It is important to establish a perimeter to secure the scene while evacuating those not contaminated, thereby preventing additional people from being exposed or contaminated. The identification of material, establishment of zones, wearing of PPE, decontamination, and medical management of patients are discussed later. Other considerations include hazmat resources available, the need for escalation to other emergency response agencies, weather conditions, terrain, whether the release is confined to a specific area or has potential for further dissemination, whether the release was intentional or unintentional, and the need for rapid rescue and evacuation of casualties.

IDENTIFICATION OF THE HAZMAT

If the identity of the xenobiotic(s) is known before arrival at the scene, research can begin while the responders are still en route with reviews of the physical, chemical, and toxicologic properties of the xenobiotic. If the xenobiotic is not known before arrival at the scene, efforts to obtain this information should begin as soon as safely possible.

The identification of the specific xenobiotic(s) involved is of highest priority because many of the response components depend on the properties and potential health effects of the xenobiotic itself. Whether the incident involves a transportation element such as a rail car or road trailer or is at a fixed location such as a factory or medical facility, all available information must be used toward material identification, including placards, container labels, shipping documents, material safety data sheets (MSDS), detector devices, knowledgeable persons at the scene, patient symptomatology, and even odors at the scene such as the rotten egg smell of hydrogen sulfide.

Because many hazardous materials are transported via rail car or road trailer, emergency response personnel must always maintain a high index of suspicion when responding to a transportation incident. In the United States, first responders are required to be familiar with the use of the *Emergency Response Guidebook*, which is an aid for quickly identifying the hazards of the material(s) involved in a transportation incident.[43]

Hazardous materials may be categorized in various ways, often grouped by their harm-causing property. For instance, hazmats may be radioactive, flammable, explosive, asphyxiating, pathogenic and biohazardous.

The substances most commonly encountered at hazmat incidents vary from one locale to another and are predominately determined by the major industries in a particular area.[46,47] For example, pesticides are the most commonly encountered class of hazardous materials in Fresno County, California, whose major industry is agribusiness.[47] Although most hazmat incidents involve only one hazardous material, more than one hazardous material may be encountered at a given incident. One study described 107 hazmat incidents involving a total of 156 materials.[47]

The vast majority of consequential hazmat incidents are caused by gases, vapors, or aerosols. In one study, four of the five most commonly encountered individual chemicals were ammonia, phosphine, sulfur oxides, and hydrogen sulfide.[8] The important implication for decontamination is that gases do not usually contaminate people secondarily because they do not adhere to patients. Therefore, patients exposed only to gases generally do not require skin decontamination to prevent secondary contamination, and much greater efficiency is possible in patient care at gas, vapor, and aerosol hazmat incidents. Inhalation is the most common route of exposure at hazmat incidents and was the route of exposure at 73% of the hazmat incidents, accounting for 76% of the exposed patients described in one study.[7,8]

Because the number of hazardous materials is so large, it is efficient to group hazardous materials according to their toxicological characteristics. Various classification systems have been devised. The International Hazard Classification System (IHCS) is the most commonly used system (Table 130–1).[43,46] Individual hazmat studies commonly use their own classification systems, emphasizing the toxicodynamic effects of hazardous materials such as systemic asphyxiants or highlighting individual chemicals such as ammonia or chlorine or general classes of chemicals such as acids, bases, or volatile organic compounds.[7,8]

TABLE 130–1. International Hazard Classification System

Class 1: Explosives
Division 1.1: Mass explosion hazard
Division 1.2: Projection hazard
Division 1.3: Predominantly a fire hazard
Division 1.4: No significant blast hazard
Division 1.5: Very insensitive explosives
Division 1.6: Extremely insensitive detonating articles
Class 2: Gases
Division 2.1: Flammable gases
Division 2.2: Nonflammable compressed gases
Division 2.3: Poisonous gases
Division 2.4: Corrosive gases (Canada)
Class 3: Flammable/combustible liquids
Class 4: Flammable solids
Division 4.1: Flammable solid
Division 4.2: Spontaneously combustible materials
Division 4.3: Dangerous when wet materials
Class 5: Oxidizers and organic peroxides
Division 5.1: Oxidizers
Division 5.2: Organic peroxides
Class 6: Poisonous materials and infectious substances
Division 6.1: Poison materials
Division 6.2: Infectious substances
Class 7: Radioactive substances
Class 8: Corrosive materials
Class 9: Miscellaneous hazardous materials

Chemical Names and Numbers Chemical compounds may be known by several names, including the chemical, common, generic, or brand (proprietary) name.[4,5] A chemical may be the sole substance in a given hazardous material or one of several compounds in a mixture.

The Chemical Abstracts Service (CAS) of the American Chemical Society (ACS) numbers chemicals to overcome the confusion regarding multiple names for a single chemical. The CAS assigns a unique CAS registry number (CAS#) to atoms, molecules, and mixtures. For example, the CAS# of methanol is 67–56–1.[34,35] These numbers provide a unique identification for chemicals and a means for crosschecking chemical names. Identifying a chemical by name and CAS# is critical because one must be as specific as possible about the hazardous material in question. Trade or brand names can be misleading. The MSDS describing a product usually lists the chemical name, the CAS#, and the brand name.[28]

Vehicular Placarding: UN Numbers, NA Numbers, and PIN Substances in each hazard class of the IHCS (see Table 130-1) are assigned four-digit identification numbers, which are known as United Nations (UN), North American (NA), or Product Identification Numbers (PINs) and are displayed on characteristic vehicular placards. This system is used by the U.S. Department of Transportation in the *Emergency Response Guidebook*.[43] The IHCS assigns a chemical to a hazard class based on its most dangerous physical characteristic, such as explosiveness or flammability. Other potential hazards of an agent, such as its ability to cause cancer or birth defects, are not considered. This system provides very little guidance in treating poisonings caused by hazardous materials.

National Fire Protection Association 704 System for Fixed Facility Placarding Fixed facilities, such as hospitals and laboratories, use a placarding system that is different from the vehicular placarding system. The National Fire Protection Association (NFPA) 704 system is used at most fixed facilities.[30] The NFPA system uses a diamond-shaped sign that is divided into four color-coded quadrants; red, yellow, white, and blue. This system gives hazmat responders information about the flammability, reactivity, and health effects, as well as other information, such as the water reactivity, oxidizing activity, or radioactivity.

The red quadrant on top indicates flammability; the blue quadrant on the left indicates health hazard; the yellow quadrant on the right indicates reactivity; and the white quadrant on the bottom is for other information, such as OXY for an oxidizing product, W for a product that has unusual reactivity with water, and the standard radioactive symbol for radioactive substances.

Numbers in the red, blue, and yellow quadrants indicate the degree of hazard: numbers range from 0, which is minimal, to 4, which is severe, and indicate specific levels of hazard.

Similar to all placarding systems, this one also has limitations. It does not name the specific hazardous substances in the facility and gives no information about the quantities or locations of the materials.

United Nations Recognizing that the transport of chemicals often occurs internationally and that the labels and MSDS often have different information in different countries, the United Nations developed a chemical classification system in an attempt to harmonize an approach to classification and labeling. The Globally Harmonized System of Classification and Labelling of Chemicals (GHS) classifies substances and mixtures by their health, environmental, and physical hazards.

CHEMTREC is a service of the Chemical Manufacturers Association with regard to shippers, products, and manufacturers and CHEMTREC is available at 800–424–9300 or at http://www.chemtrec.org at no charge, 24 hours a day. Details of an incident are relayed to the shipper's or manufacturer's 24-hour emergency contact, and they, in turn, are linked to hazmat incident responders. Technical data are available on handling the substance(s) involved, including the physical characteristics, transportation, and disposal.

A regional poison center is another valuable source of information. Other information sources include local and state health departments, the American Conference of Governmental and Industrial Hygienists (ACGIH), Occupational Safety and Health Administration (OSHA), National Institutes of Occupational Safety and Health (NIOSH), Agency for Toxic Substances and Disease Registry (ASTDR), and Centers for Disease Control and Prevention (CDC).[1,2,3,34,35,37]

Exact identification is desirable but not always possible. Hazmat responders may be able to classify the hazardous material into one of several major toxicologic classes by identifying a hazmat toxidrome that allows them to reasonably treat the patients and protect themselves and others. For example, do patients have irritation of the mucous membranes and upper airway caused by a highly water-soluble irritant gas? Do the patients exhibit signs of asphyxia with major central nervous system (CNS) or cardiopulmonary signs and symptoms? Do patients exhibit signs of cholinergic excess caused by organic phosphorus compounds or carbamate poisoning? Do patients exhibit chemical burns compatible with corrosives? Do patients have the odor of solvents with signs of CNS depression and cardiac irritability compatible with exposure to hydrocarbons or halogenated hydrocarbons?

Also, even when the exact identity of the hazardous material is not known, what is usually known is the physical state of the material, that is, solid, liquid, or gas. Airborne xenobiotics potentially mean many more victims. Airborne xenobiotics include not only gases and vapors but also the liquid suspensions (fog and mists) and the solid suspensions (smoke, fumes, and dusts).

EXPOSURE AND CONTAMINATION

A person may have received an external *exposure* to a hazmat and may be at risk for the resultant health consequences even though he or she may not to be contaminated by the hazmat. For instance, a person may be temporarily irradiated by an exposure to a radioactive source. After exposure, a hazardous material may remain on a victim (external) or within a victim (internal). For instance, if radioactive materials (usually in the form of dust particles) are on the body surface or clothing (ie, contamination has occurred), then the person will continue to have exposure until decontamination occurs.

Primary contamination is contamination of people or equipment caused by direct contact with the initial release of a hazardous material by direct contact at its source of release. Primary contamination may occur whether the hazardous material is a solid, a liquid, or a gas. *Secondary contamination* is contamination of healthcare personnel or equipment caused by direct contact with a patient or equipment covered with adherent solids or liquids that have been removed from the source of the hazardous material spill.

The state of matter will help healthcare providers determine whether the hazardous material presents a significant risk of secondary contamination and whether decontamination of the skin and mucous membranes is necessary. Secondary contamination generally occurs only with solids or liquids. In general, patients or equipment covered with adherent solid or liquid hazardous materials, including chemical, biologic, or radiologic agents, should be decontaminated before transportation to prevent downstream contamination of healthcare providers and equipment. An exception to the principles of limited need for cutaneous decontamination for those exposed to gas is a patient whose sweaty skin was exposed to a highly water-soluble irritant gas such as ammonia that dissolves in sweat to produce corrosive ammonium hydroxide. In this case, the primary purpose of decontamination is to prevent or treat the patient's chemical burns caused by the caustic action of aqueous ammonium hydroxide on perspiring skin rather than to prevent secondary contamination of rescuers. Aerosols are airborne xenobiotics that are not gases. Aerosols are suspensions of solids or liquids in air, such as solid dusts or liquid mists, that can cover victims with these adherent solids or liquids, which can effect secondary contamination. These patients do require decontamination to prevent secondary contamination.

Emergency personnel and equipment can become contaminated at hazmat incidents.[11,19,20,21,46,47,50] For example, in one study, contamination occurred to one ambulance that drove through a puddle of liquid organic phosphorus pesticides that had spilled from a crashed exterminator truck. This ambulance was responding to a call for a "motor vehicle crash."[47]

HAZMAT SITE OPERATIONS

Limiting dispersion of the hazardous material is critical to prevent further ill consequences. The physical state of a material determines how it will spread through the environment and gives clues to the potential route(s) of exposure for the material. Unless moved by physical means such as wind, ventilation systems, or people, solids will usually stay in one area. Solids can cause exposures by inhalation of dusts, by ingestion, or rarely by absorption through skin and mucous membranes. Solids that undergo sublimation, changing directly from a solid into a gas without passing through the liquid state, can give off vapors that may cause airborne exposure. Only two commonly encountered solids sublime, dry ice (CO_2) and naphthalene. A vapor is defined as a gaseous dispersion of the molecules of a substance that is normally a liquid or a solid at standard temperature and pressure (STP), that is, 32°F (0°C = 273°K) and 1 atm (760 torr = 760 mm Hg = 14.7 psi). Uncontained liquids will spread over surfaces and flow downhill. Liquids may evaporate, creating a vapor hazard.

The vapor pressure (VP) is useful to estimate whether enough of a solid or liquid will be released in the gaseous state to pose an inhalation risk. VP is defined essentially as the quantity of the gaseous state overlying an evaporating liquid or a subliming solid. The lower the VP, the less likely the xenobiotics will volatilize and generate a respirable gas. Conversely, the higher the VP of a chemical, the more likely it will volatilize or generate a respirable gas. Water has a VP of approximately 20 mm Hg at 70°F (21°C), and acetone has a VP of 250 mm Hg at the same temperature. Therefore, acetone evaporates more rapidly than water and poses more of an inhalation risk. Standard reference texts (eg, *NIOSH Pocket Guide to Chemical Hazards Merck Index*) list VPs for commonly encountered chemicals.[34,35,43]

Hazmat Scene Control Zones Scene management is a fundamental feature at a hazmat incident. It is almost always necessary to isolate the scene, deny access to the public and the media, and limit access to emergency response personnel to prevent needless contamination. Three control zones are established around a scene and are described by "temperature," "color," or "explanatory terminology" (Table 130–2 and Fig. 130–1). NIOSH, the U.S. Environmental Protection Agency (EPA), and most U.S. prehospital and hospital healthcare professionals use the temperature terminology system.[35]

The hot zone is the area immediately surrounding a hazardous materials incident. It extends far enough to prevent the primary contamination of people and materials outside this zone. Primary contamination may occur to those who enter this zone. In general, evacuation—but no decontamination or patient care—is carried out in this zone, except for opening the airway and placing the patient on a backboard with spine precautions. This is because rescuers are generally hazmat technicians who wear level A or B suits that severely limit their visibility and dexterity. In specific situations, antidotes may be administered via autoinjectors (eg, nerve agent antidotes).

TABLE 130–2. The Nomenclatures of the Hazmat Control Zones

Temperature Terminology System[a]	Color Terminology System	Explanatory Terminology System
Hot zone	Red zone	Exclusion or restricted zone
Warm zone	Yellow zone	Decontamination or contamination reduction zone
Cold zone	Green zone	Support zone

[a]From the National Institutes of Occupational Safety and Health and the Environmental Protection Agency.

The warm zone is the area surrounding the hot zone and contains the decontamination or access corridor, where victims and the hazmat entry team members and their equipment are decontaminated. It includes two control points for the access corridor. Many consider initiating therapy at this stage, particularly for chemical weapons, events where multiple casualties are involved.

The cold zone is the area beyond the warm zone. Contaminated victims and hazmat responders should be decontaminated before entering this area from the warm zone. Equipment and personnel are not expected to become contaminated in this zone. This is the area in which resources are assembled to support the hazmat emergency response. The incident command center is usually located in the cold zone, and there is greater ability to provide patient care there. Care provided in this zone includes the primary survey and resuscitation with management of airway (with cervical spine control), breathing, circulation, disability, and exposure with evaluation for toxicity and trauma (ABCDE). Definitive care also includes antidotal treatment for specific poisonings.

PERSONAL PROTECTIVE EQUIPMENT

A critical goal of hazmat emergency responders is protecting themselves and the public. Safeguarding hazmat responders includes wearing appropriate PPE to prevent exposure to the hazard and prevent injury to the wearer from incorrect use of or malfunction of the PPE equipment.[25,36]

PPE can create significant health hazards, including loss of cooling by evaporation, heat stress, physical stress, psychological stress, impaired vision, impaired mobility, and impaired communication. Because of these risks, individuals involved in hazmat emergency response must be trained regarding the appropriate use, decontamination, maintenance, and storage of PPE. This training includes instruction regarding the risk of permeation, penetration, and degradation of PPE. PPE with a self-contained breathing apparatus (SCBA) has a fixed supply of air that significantly limits the amount of time the wearer can operate in the hot zone, usually about 20 minutes.

Levels of Protection The EPA defines four levels of protection for PPE: levels A (highest) through D (lowest). The different levels of PPE are designed to provide a choice of PPE, depending on the hazards at a specific hazmat incident (Table 130–3).

Level A provides the highest level of both respiratory and skin (clothing) protection and provides vapor protection to the respiratory tract, mucous membranes, and skin. This level of PPE is airtight, fully encapsulating and the breathing apparatus must be worn under the suit.

Level B provides the highest level of respiratory protection and skin splash protection by using chemical-resistant clothing. It does not

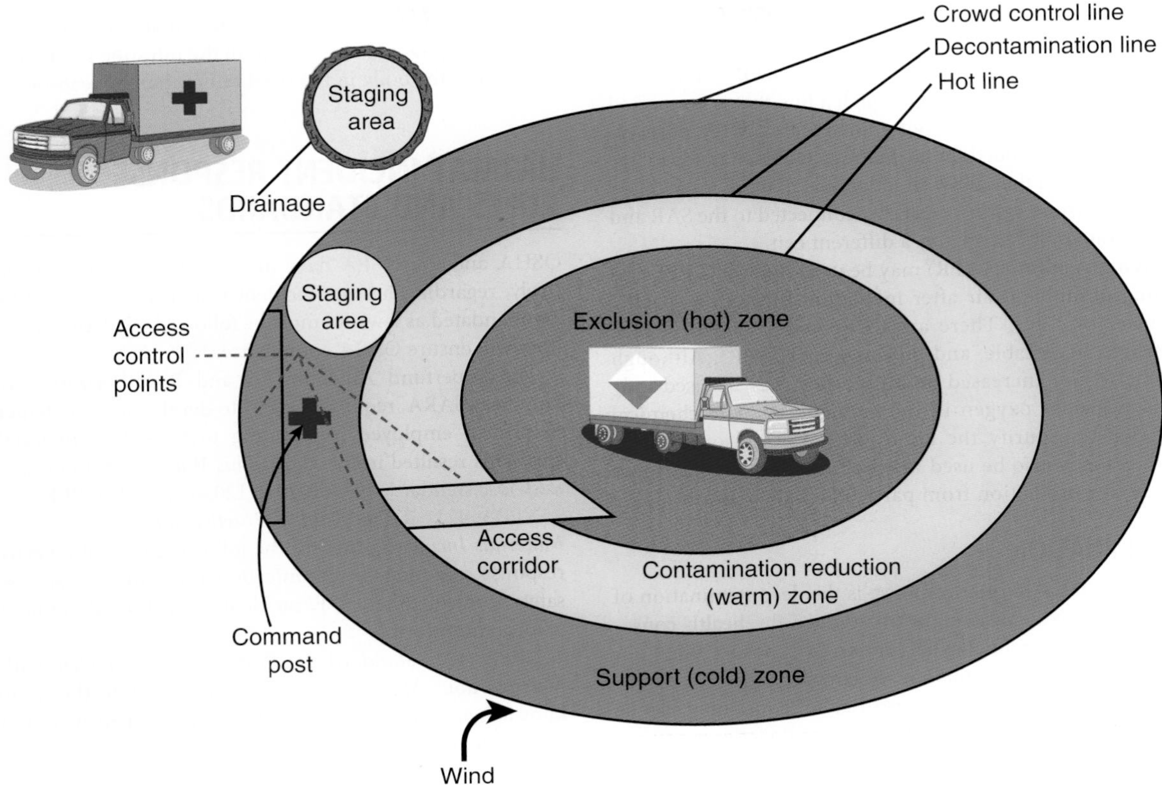

FIGURE 130–1. NIOSH/OSHA recommended control zones.

provide skin vapor protection but does provide respiratory tract vapor protection. Some hospitals have specially trained healthcare professionals who wear level B PPE when decontaminating patients presenting to the hospital. However, the majority of hospitals are training their frontline emergency department (ED) healthcare professionals to wear level C PPE when decontaminating contaminated patients who present to the hospital.

TABLE 130–3. Personal Protective Equipment

	Protects Skin and Eyes from:			Protects Respiratory System from:	
Level[a]	Select Vapors and Aerosols	Gases, Vapors, and Aerosols	Oxygen-Deficient Atmospheres	Liquids and Solids	Gases and Vapors
D					
C	+			+	
B	+		+	+	+
A	+	+	+	+	+

[a]Level A is a self-contained breathing apparatus (SCBA) worn under a vapor-protective, fully encapsulated, airtight, chemical-resistant suit. Level B is a positive-pressure supplied-air respirator with an escape SCBA worn under a hooded, splash-protective, chemical-resistant suit. Level C is an air-purifying respirator worn with a hooded, splash-protective, chemical-resistant suit. Level D is regular work clothing (offers no protection).

Level C protection should be used when the type of airborne substance is known, its concentration can be measured, the criteria for using air-purifying respirators are met, and skin and eye exposures are unlikely. Level C provides skin splash protection, the same as level B; however, level C has a lower level of respiratory protection than levels A and B.

Level D is basically a regular work uniform. It should not be worn when significant chemical respiratory or skin hazards exist. It provides no respiratory protection and minimal skin protection. Level D was specifically developed to show *what not to wear* for chemical protection.

Personal Protective Equipment Respiratory Protection Personnel must be fit tested before using any respirator. A tiny space between the edge of the respirator and the face of the hazmat responder could permit exposure to an airborne hazard. Contact lenses cannot be worn with any respiratory protective equipment. Corrective eyeglass lenses must be mounted inside the face mask of the PPE. The only exception to these general rules are the use of hooded level C powered air purifying respirators (PAPRs) that do not require fit testing and allow individuals to wear their own eyeglasses within the hooded PAPR. This is the reason that the majority of U.S. hospitals prefer hooded PAPRs for their ED personnel who must decontaminate patients.

Level A PPE mandates the use of a SCBA. An SCBA is composed of a face piece connected by a hose to a compressed air source. An open-circuit, positive-pressure SCBA is used most often in emergency response and provides clean air from a cylinder to the face piece of the wearer, who exhales into the atmosphere. Thus, a higher air pressure is maintained inside the face piece than outside. This affords the SCBA wearer the highest level of protection against airborne hazards because any leakage will force air out of the face piece and not allow airborne hazards to enter against the higher pressure within the face piece. Disadvantages of the SCBA include its bulkiness and heaviness and a limited time period of respiratory protection because of the limited amount of air in the tank.

A supplied-air respirator (SAR) may be used in level B PPE and differs from SCBA in that air is supplied through a line that is connected to a source located away from the contaminated area. Only positive-pressure SARs are recommended for hazmat use. One major advantage of SARs over SCBA is that they allow an individual to work for a longer period. However, a hazmat worker must stay connected to the SAR and cannot leave the contaminated area by a different exit.

An air-purifying respirator (APR) may be used in level C PPE and allows breathing of ambient air after inhalation through a specific purifying canister or filter. There are three basic types of APRs: chemical cartridge, disposable, and powered air (PAPR). Although APRs afford the wearer increased mobility, they may be used only where there is sufficient oxygen in the ambient air. The chemical cartridges or canisters purify the air by filtration, adsorption, or absorption. Filters may also be used in combination with cartridges to provide increased protection from particulates such as asbestos.

DECONTAMINATION

A major goal of the initial hazmat response is the decontamination of contaminated victims. Not only might this reduce the health consequences for the victim (by reducing absorption or exposure time) but also prevents secondary contamination. Decontamination of equipment, the environment, and the entire area (ie, hot zone) may also be necessary but is secondary to the decontamination of victims.

An estimated 75% to 90% of contaminants may be removed simply by removing the victim's clothing and garments. Subsequent decontamination is most commonly accomplished by using water to copiously irrigate the skin of a victim, thereby physically washing off, diluting, or hydrolyzing the agent. However, the water solubility of a hazardous material must be considered to determine whether water alone is sufficient for skin decontamination or whether a detergent must also be used. The general rule regarding solubility is that "like dissolves like." In other words, a polar solvent, such as water, will dissolve polar substances such as salts. For example, the herbicide paraquat is actually a salt, paraquat dichloride, that is miscible in water. Therefore, if a patient's skin is contaminated with paraquat, copious water irrigation is sufficient for skin decontamination. A mild liquid detergent is acceptable but is not necessary. On the other hand, a nonpolar solvent, such as toluene, is not water soluble and is immiscible.[34,35] Therefore, if a patient's skin is contaminated with toluene, water irrigation alone may be insufficient for decontamination, and a mild liquid detergent is also necessary.[34,35] Furthermore, copious water may not be available at the site, thereby requiring rescuers to ration the supply and minimize irrigation using the least amount of water necessary. Some solid chemical contaminants may react with water and thereby cause an increased hazard if water used for decontamination. Such xenobiotics may be better removed mechanically by physically wiping it from the skin while avoiding smearing the agent or abrading the skin. Some contaminants may be chemically 'inactivated' by applying another chemical, such as a 0.5% hypochlorite solution.

When performing decontamination, close attention should be paid to all exposed skin, particularly, the skin folds, axillae, genital area, and feet. Lukewarm water should be used with gentle water pressure to reduce the risk of hypothermia. Water should be applied systematically from head to toe while the patient's airway is protected.

Exposed, symptomatic eyes should be continuously irrigated with water throughout the patient contact, including transport, if possible. Remember to check for and remove contact lenses.

Removal of internal contamination is often much more problematic. In some cases, specific medications may be administered to enhance elimination or inactivate the hazardous material. For instance, Prussian blue can trap radioactive cesium in the intestine so that it can be eliminated from the body in the stool rather than be reabsorbed.

HAZMAT INCIDENT RESPONSE RULES AND STANDARDS

OSHA and the NFPA have developed rules and guidelines, respectively, regarding hazmat incident response.[23,30,31,32,33,39,44] OSHA's rules are mandated as law and must be followed.[23,39,44] Meeting NFPA guidelines will ensure OSHA compliance.[23,30,31,33,36,39]

The Superfund Amendments and Reauthorization Act of 1986, known as SARA, required OSHA to develop and implement standards to protect employees responding to hazardous materials emergencies. This resulted in the *Hazardous Waste Operations and Emergency Response* standard, 29 CFR 1910.120, or HAZWOPER.[44]

NFPA 471, *Recommended Practice for Responding to Hazardous Materials Incidents*, outlines the following tactical objectives: incident response planning, communication procedures, response levels, site safety, control zones, PPE, incident mitigation, decontamination, and medical monitoring.[31]

NFPA 472, *Standard on Professional Competence of Responders to Hazardous Materials Incidents*, helps define the minimum skills, knowledge, and standards for training outlined in HAZWOPER for three types of responders.[32]

PREHOSPITAL HAZMAT EMERGENCY RESPONSE TEAM COMPOSITION, ORGANIZATION, AND RESPONSIBILITIES

First Responder at the Awareness Level First responders at the awareness level could be first on the scene at an emergency incident involving hazardous material. They are expected to recognize the presence of hazardous materials, protect themselves, secure the area, and call for better trained personnel. They must take a safe position and keep other people from entering the area. They must recognize that the level of mitigation exceeds their training and call for a hazmat response team. Most basic curricula of emergency medical technicians (EMTs) include this level of first responder training.

First Responder at the Operational Level These individuals are trained in all competencies of the awareness level and are additionally trained to protect nearby persons, the environment, and exposed property from the effects of hazmat releases. Operational-level certified individuals are expected to assume a defensive posture, control the release from a safe distance, and keep the hazardous material from spreading. Operational-level individuals are trained to perform absorption of liquids, containment of the spill, vapor suppression, and vapor dispersion. They do not operate within the hot zone.

Hazardous Materials Technician Hazardous materials technicians respond to hazmat releases, or potential releases, for the purpose of controlling the release. They are trained in the use of chemical-resistant suits, air-monitoring equipment, mitigation techniques, and the interpretation of physical properties of hazardous materials. Technicians are capable of containing an incident, making safe entry into a hazardous environment, determining the appropriate course of action, victim rescue, and cleaning up or neutralizing the incident to return the property to a safe and usable status, if possible. These individuals are trained to operate within the hot zone to mitigate the incident. This certification level includes knowledge of hazardous material chemistry, air-monitoring equipment, tools used within the hot zone, and more.

ADVANCED HAZMAT COMPONENTS

Advanced Hazmat Providers Paramedics should be trained in the recognition of signs and symptoms caused by exposure to hazardous materials and the delivery of antidotal therapy to victims of hazmat poisonings.[23]

The inclusion of such training into a department's hazmat response team is beneficial, not only for the needs of the public but also to protect hazmat technicians who make entry into hazardous atmospheres.[23] Ideally, hazmat technicians' entry into hazardous atmospheres should not be performed until appropriately trained paramedics are on the scene with resuscitative equipment in place, including a drug box containing essential antidotes for specific hazardous materials.[23]

Patient Care Responsibilities of the Prehospital Decontamination Team and the Hazmat Entry Team Hazmat responders should identify the entry and exit areas by controlling points for the access corridor (decontamination corridor) from the hot zone, through the warm zone, to the cold zone (see Fig. 130–1). This corridor should be upwind, uphill, and upstream from the hot zone, if possible. Hazmat technician entry team members should remove victims from the contaminated hot zone and deliver patients to the inner control point of the access (decontamination) corridor. Hazmat decontamination team members decontaminate patients in the decontamination (access) corridor of the contamination reduction (warm) zone.[10,13,17,18,23,26,27,41]

The primary responsibility of the prehospital hazmat medical sector is the protection of the hazmat entry team personnel. This is accomplished by researching and recording clinically pertinent information about the hazardous material, remaining available on scene for medical treatment, and assessing individuals before entry into and on exit from a hazardous environment.[23] Documentation of each assessment should be recorded on a prepared form and compared with the exclusion criteria defined by NFPA 471.[23,31]

In some systems, the hazmat entry team may include specialized providers who have the ability to provide lifesaving patient care within the hot zone. The ability to perform triage or cardiopulmonary resuscitation or to provide any medical care is greatly limited by the PPE being worn. Therefore, only immediately lifesaving procedures should be considered, such as intubation/ventilation or antidote administration using an autoinjector.

Patient Care Responsibilities of Emergency Medical Services Providers at Hazmat Incidents EMS providers who are not part of the hazmat team should report to the incident staging area and await direction from the incident commander. They should approach the site from upwind, uphill, and upstream, if possible.

EMS providers should remain in the cold zone until properly protected hazmat incident responders arrive, decontaminate, and deliver patients to them for further triage and treatment. Then EMS providers should evaluate each patient, triage as appropriate, and move the patient to the appropriate casualty collection point or rapidly transport to the hospital as resources allow. Exposed victims who are initially asymptomatic should continue to be observed and reassessed for the delayed development of symptoms, and the EMS provider should be prepared to upgrade the triage category for the patient. All EMS systems should have protocols in place that direct operations at hazmat scenes. Ideally, the EMS response matrix for such events includes the response of an EMS physician or contact with online medical control, who will coordinate appropriate care with the regional poison center, toxicologists, and hospitals.

Transportation of patients from the hazmat incident is ultimately under the control of the incident commander but is usually delegated to the prehospital hazmat medical sector and EMS providers. In general, no victim with skin contamination should be transported from the hazmat site without being properly decontaminated. Before transportation, EMS should notify the receiving hospital of the number of victims being transported and their toxicologic history, patient assessments, and treatment rendered.

HOSPITAL RESPONSIBILITIES FOR HAZMAT VICTIMS

Ideally, the local or regional ED physicians and personnel will receive advanced notification about a hazmat incident before any victims arrive at the hospital. This notification to the hospital should occur as early in the event as possible to allow for maximum "ramp-up" time. The notification should include, if known, information regarding the event, hazmat involved, number and condition of casualties to be transported to the hospital, as well as information regarding the decontamination completed.

Victims may leave an incident scene on their own and subsequently present to a hospital. The hospital must have a preestablished protocol by which hospital response teams will decontaminate patients who arrive at the hospital if they have not been previously decontaminated or if field decontamination is believed to be insufficient.[6,14,15,16,22,24,38,40,42,45,48,49] Hazmat patients who require skin decontamination should be denied entry to the ED until they are decontaminated by an appropriately trained and equipped hazmat response team. The emergency physician will determine when the patient is safe to enter the ED after carefully assessing the risks and benefits to the decontaminated patient, the other patients in the ED, and the ED healthcare personnel.

SUMMARY

Hazmat incident response is an integrated, interdisciplinary approach involving prehospital, hospital, poison center, and public health professionals. Most patients at hazmat incidents are exposed through inhalation of a gas, a solid, or a liquid aerosol. Prehospital and hospital healthcare professionals must use appropriate PPE when caring for patients who have not been decontaminated. Decontamination is critical to alter absorption for patients and to prevent secondary contamination of downstream healthcare providers and equipment.

The general principles of toxicology apply regardless of whether a patient is at a hazmat incident in a prehospital or hospital setting. Although patient care resources vary among these treatment settings, the fundamental principles of patient care remain the same. All patients should receive a primary survey and resuscitation, emphasizing airway, breathing, and circulation.

ACKNOWLEDGMENT

Frank G. Walter, MD contributed to this chapter in previous editions.

REFERENCES

1. Agency for Toxic Substances and Disease Registry. Retrieved May 20, 2009, from http://www.atsdr.cdc.gov.
2. American Conference of Governmental Industrial Hygienists. Retrieved May 20, 2009, from http://www.acgih.org/home.htm.
3. American Conference of Governmental Industrial Hygienists (ACGIH). *2005, TLVs and BEIs*. Cincinnati, OH: ACGIH; 2005.
4. Borak J, Callan M, Abbott W. *Hazardous Materials Exposure*. Englewood Cliffs, NJ: Brady Publications; 1991.
5. Bronstein AC, Currance PL. *Emergency Care for Hazardous Materials Exposure*, 2nd ed. St. Louis: Mosby-Year Book; 1994.
6. Burgess JL, Blackmon GM, Brodkin CA, Robertson WO. Hospital preparedness for hazardous materials incidents and treatment of contaminated patients. *West J Med*. 1997;167:387-391.

7. Burgess JL, Keifer MC, Barnhart S, et al. Hazardous materials exposure information service: development, analysis, and medical implications. *Ann Emerg Med.* 1997;29:248-254.
8. Burgess JL, Pappas GP, Robertson WO. Hazardous materials incidents: the Washington Poison Center experience and approach to exposure assessment. *J Occup Environ Med.* 1997;39:760-766.
9. Bush GW. *Homeland Security Presidential Directive/HSPD-5.* Washington, DC: The White House; February 28, 2003.
10. Cancio LC. Chemical casualty decontamination by medical platoons in the 82d Airborne Division. *Mil Med.* 1993;158:1-5.
11. Centers for Disease Control and Prevention. Public health consequences among first responders to emergency events associated with illicit methamphetamine laboratories, selected states 1996–1999. *MMWR Mortal Morbid Wkly Rep.* 2000;49:1021-1024.
12. CHEMTREC. Retrieved May 20, 2009, from http://www.chemtrec.org.
13. Domestic Preparedness Program, Defense Against Weapons of Mass Destruction. *Technician-Hospital Provider Course Manual.* Aberdeen, MD: US Army CBDCOM, Domestic Preparedness Office; 1997.
14. Gough AR, Markus K. Hazardous materials protections in practice ED, laws and logistics. *J Emerg Nurs.* 1989;15:477-480.
15. Hall SK. Management of chemical disaster victims. *J Toxicol Clin Toxicol.* 1995;33:609-616.
16. Huff JS. Lessons learned from hazardous materials incidents. *Emerg Care Q.* 1991;7:17-22.
17. Hurst C. Decontamination. In: Zatchuk R, ed. *Textbook of Military Medicine.* Washington, DC: Borden Institute, US Dept of Army, Surgeon General; 1997:351-359.
18. Kales SN, Christiani DC. Acute chemical emergencies. *N Engl J Med.* 2004;350:800-808.
19. Kales SN, Mendoza PJ, Hill JM, et al. Spirometric surveillance in hazardous materials firefighters: does hazardous materials duty affect lung function? *J Occup Environ Med.* 2001;43:1114-1120.
20. Kales SN, Polyhronopoulos GN, Christiani DC. Medical surveillance of hazardous materials response fire fighters: a two-year prospective study. *J Occup Environ Med.* 1997;39:238-247.
21. Kelly KJ, Connelly E, Reinhold GA, et al. Assessment of health effect in New York City firefighters after exposure to polychlorinated biphenyls (PCBs) and polychlorinated dibenzofurans (PCDFs). The Staten Island transformer fire health surveillance project. *Arch Environ Health.* 2002;57:282-293.
22. Kirk MA, Cisek J, Rose SR. Emergency department response to hazardous materials incidents. *Emerg Med Clin North Am.* 1994;12:461-481.
23. Klein R, Criss EA. Establishing and organizing a hazmat response team. In: Walter FG, Klein R, Thomas RG, eds. *Advanced Hazmat Life Support Provider Manual*, 3rd ed. Tucson, AZ: Arizona Board of Regents; 2003:125-177.
24. Lavoie FW, Coomes T, Cisek JE, Fulkerson L. Emergency department external decontamination for hazardous chemical exposure. *Vet Hum Toxicol.* 1992;34:61-64.
25. Lehmann J. Considerations for selecting personal protective equipment for hazardous materials response. *Disaster Manag Response.* 2002;1:21-25.
26. Leonard RB. Hazardous materials accidents: initial scene assessment and patient care. *Aviat Space Environ Med.* 1993;64:546-551.
27. Levitin HW, Siegelson HJ. Hazardous materials. Disaster medical planning and response. *Emerg Med Clin North Am.* 1996;14:327-348.
28. MSDS SEARCH. Retrieved May 20, 2009, from http://www.msdssearch.com.
29. National Association of EMS Physicians (NAEMSP) and the American College of Emergency Physicians (ACEP) Joint Position Statement. *Unsolicited Medical Personnel Volunteering at Disaster Scenes*; 2002.
30. National Fire Protection Association (NFPA). Retrieved October 29, 2009, from http://www.nfpa.org.
31. Technical Committee on Hazardous Materials Response Personnel. *NFPA 471 Recommended Practice for Responding to Hazardous Materials Incidents.* Quincy, MA: National Fire Protection Association; 1997.
32. National Fire Protection Association Technical Committee on Hazardous Materials Response Personnel. *NFPA 472 Standard on Professional Competence of Responders to Hazardous Materials Incidents.* Quincy, MA: National Fire Protection Association; 2002.
33. National Fire Protection Association Technical Committee on Hazardous Materials Response Personnel. *NFPA 473 Standard for Competencies for EMS Personnel Responding to Hazardous Materials Incidents.* Quincy, MA: National Fire Protection Association; 1997.
34. National Institute for Occupational Safety and Health (NIOSH). *NIOSH Pocket Guide to Chemical Hazards.* Washington, DC: US Government Printing Office for the US Department of Health and Human Services (DHHS) and the National Institute of Occupational Safety and Health (NIOSH); 2004.
35. National Institute of Occupational Safety and Health. Retrieved May 20, 2009, from http://www.cdc.gov/niosh.
36. Noll G, Hildebrand M, Yvorra J. Personal protective clothing and equipment. In: Daly P, ed. *Hazardous Materials.* Oklahoma State University: Stillwater, Oklahoma, Fire Protection Publications; 1995:285-322.
37. Occupational Safety and Health Administration. Retrieved May 20, 2009, from http://www.osha.gov.
38. Pons P, Dart RC. Chemical incidents in the emergency department: if and when. *Ann Emerg Med.* 1999;34:223-225.
39. Rubin JN. Roles and responsibilities of medical personnel at hazardous materials incidents. *Semicond Saf Assoc J.* 1998;12:25-30.
40. Shapira Y, Bar Y, Berkenstadt H, et al. Outline of hospital organization for a chemical warfare attack. *Isr J Med Sci.* 1991;27:616-622.
41. Sullivan F, Wang R, Jenouri I. Principles and protocols for prevention, evaluation, and management of exposure to hazardous materials. *Emerg Med Rep.* 1998;19:21-32.
42. Tur-Kaspa I, Lev EI, Hendler I, et al. Preparing hospitals for toxico-logical mass casualties events. *Crit Care Med.* 1999;27:1004-1008.
43. U.S. Department of Transportation (DOT), Transport Canada (TC), Secretariat of Communications and Transportation of Mexico (SCT). *2008 Emergency Response Guidebook.* Washington, DC: DOT, TC, SCT; 2008. Retrieved May 18, 2009, from http://www.phmsa.dot.gov/staticfiles/PHMSA/DownloadableFiles/Files/erg2008_eng.pdf
44. U.S. Government. *Title 29, Code of Federal Regulations 1986, Parts 1910.120.*
45. Waldron RL 2d, Danielson RA, Shultz HE, et al. Radiation decontamination unit for the community hospital. *Am J Roentgenol.* 1981;136:977-981.
46. Walter FG, Bates G, Criss EA, et al. Hazardous materials incidents in a mid-sized metropolitan area. *Prehosp Emerg Care.* 2003;7:214-218.
47. Walter FG, Dedolph R, Kallsen G, et al. Hazardous materials incidents: a one-year retrospective review in central California. *Prehospital Disaster Med.* 1992;7:151-156.
48. Young CF, Persell DJ. Biological, chemical, and nuclear terrorism readiness: major concerns and preparedness for future nurses. *Disaster Manag Response.* 2004;2:109-114.
49. Zavotsky KE, Valendo M, Torres P. Developing an emergency department based special operations team: Robert Wood Johnson University Hospital's experience. *Disaster Manag Response.* 2004;2:35-39.
50. Zeitz P, Berkowitz Z, Orr MF. Frequency and type of injuries in responders of hazardous substances events 1996, to 1998. *J Occup Environ Med.* 2000;42:1115-1120.

CHAPTER 131
CHEMICAL WEAPONS

Jeffrey R. Suchard

Recent years have witnessed an enormous resurgence of interest in chemical and biological weapons (CBW). Although "unconventional" warfare with chemical and biological agents has been practiced since antiquity, it was not until the 20th century that such weapons were manufactured and used on a mass scale. In addition to battlefield use, chemical weapons may appeal to terrorist groups, in that the technology and financial outlay required to produce them is much less than for nuclear weapons, although the potential morbidity, mortality, and societal impact remain high (Table 131–1).

Chemical weapons clearly fall within the purview of medical toxicology. Indeed, unlike the many drugs and chemicals widely studied by toxicologists that may incidentally cause poisonings, these compounds were specifically designed to kill, injure, or incapacitate. Some compounds generally considered nonlethal, such as tear gas and pepper spray, are therefore also considered chemical weapons. Biological warfare agents share some characteristics with chemical agents (Table 131–2) and are covered in Chap. 132, although the issues common to both chemical and biological weapons are discussed in this chapter.

This chapter focuses on the acute and long-term clinical effects of exposure to chemical weapons, their mechanisms of toxicity, and the medical treatment of individual casualties, based on published human case experience. There are many other potential subtopics related to chemical (and biological) weapons that are not specifically reviewed here, including disaster incident command (see Hazmat Incident Response, Chap. 130), CBW agent detection, provision of medical care in a chemically contaminated environment, and the ever-growing body of evidence accumulated from in vitro and ex vivo models of chemical warfare agent poisoning.

HISTORY

The first well-documented intentional use of chemicals as weapons occurred in 423 B.C. when Spartans besieging Athenian cities burned pitch-soaked wood and brimstone to produce sulfurous clouds.[88] Chemical weapons were sporadically used, or their use considered, up through the 19th century.[49]

Large-scale chemical warfare began in World War I when the Germans released chlorine near Ypres, Belgium killing hundreds and forcing 15,000 troops to retreat.[20,49] Both sides rapidly escalated the use of toxic gases, released from cylinders or by artillery shells that included various pulmonary irritants, lacrimators, arsenicals, and cyanides.

The Germans first used sulfur mustard in 1917, again near Ypres, and caused over 20,000 deaths or injuries.[49] Unlike prior war gases, mustard was persistent in the environment and vesicated the skin in addition to injuring the lungs and mucous membranes. The Allies soon responded in kind. Sulfur mustard was unequaled in its ability to incapacitate opponents.[9] Injuries far outweighed fatalities, tying up manpower and resources to care for the wounded. By the end of the war, chemical weapons had caused over 1.3 million casualties and approximately 90,000 deaths.[20]

Only one major chemical weapon event occurred during World War II when German planes bombed American ships carrying chemical munitions in Bari, Italy releasing the contents of 2000 mustard bombs and causing over 600 Allied military and an unknown number of civilian casualties.[9,49]

Germany began producing nerve agents just before World War II. Tabun was developed in 1936 by Gerhard Schrader when conducting insecticide research for IG Farbenindustrie,[30,77] but was abandoned as an insecticide because of its overwhelming human toxicity. Sarin was synthesized in 1938, and named after its developers: ***S***chrader, ***A***mbrose, ***R***udringer, and Van der L***in***de.[30] Between 10,000 and 30,000 tons of tabun and 5–10 tons of sarin were produced during World War II. Soman was synthesized in 1944, but no large-scale production facilities were developed. When the Allies discovered these nerve agents at the end of the war, code names were designated based on the order of their development. Tabun was called GA (the letter G standing for German), sarin was GB, and soman was GD.[30]

In 1952, the British synthesized an even more potent nerve agent while searching for a dichlorodiphenyltrichloroethane (DDT) replacement. This substance was given to the United States for military development, and was named VX. A VX leak killed 6000 sheep near a military base in Skull Valley, Utah in 1968.[30,44,77] The Russians developed a similar nerve agent, variably referred to as VR or "Russian VX."[40] The United States used defoliants and riot-control agents in Vietnam and Laos. Iraq used sulfur mustard, tabun, and soman during its war with Iran in the 1980s, and may have also used cyanide against the Kurds.[49]

More recently, terrorist groups have begun to employ chemical weapons. Sarin was released twice by the Aum Shinrikyo cult in Japan. The first release occurred in Matsumoto in 1994, killing 7 and injuring over 600.[51] A more highly publicized sarin attack occurred in the Tokyo subway system in 1995, killing 12 and resulting in over 5000 persons seeking medical attention.[74] Cult members have also used VX in assassinations.[50]

GENERAL CONSIDERATIONS

PHYSICAL PROPERTIES

The term *war gas* is generally a misnomer. Sulfur mustard and nerve agents are liquids at normal temperatures and pressures, and many riot-control agents are solids. These weapons are most efficiently dispersed as aerosols, which probably leads to the confusion with gases. Some chemical weapons (eg, chlorine, phosgene, hydrogen cyanide) are truly gases, and although they are generally considered obsolete for battlefield use, they might still be used as improvisational agents, especially in terrorist attacks.

Liquid chemical weapons have a certain degree of volatility and may evaporate into poisonous vapors. Volatility is inversely related to persistence, the tendency to remain in the environment. Persistent agents, such as mustard or VX, can contaminate an area for prolonged periods, denying the enemy free movement and use of contaminated material. The toxic hazard from semipersistent agents like sarin or nonpersistent agents like hydrogen cyanide dissipates more rapidly.

Aerosols, gases, and vapors are highly subject to local atmospheric conditions. Less dispersion occurs with atmospheric inversion layers and in the absence of wind, as typically occurs at night or in the early morning. Enclosed spaces also prevent wind dispersion and even simple dilution. Except for hydrogen cyanide, CW gases and vapors are all denser than air and will pool in low-lying areas.

An example was the use of sarin in the Tokyo subway where the number of fatalities could have been much higher had the nerve agent

TABLE 131–1. Unconventional Weapons: Definitions and Acronyms

Chemical warfare	Intentional use of weapons designed to kill, injure, or incapacitate on the basis of toxic or noxious chemical properties
Biological warfare	Intentional use of microorganisms or xenobiotics derived from living organisms to cause death, disability, or damage in humans, animals, or plants
Terrorism	The unlawful use of force against persons or property to intimidate or coerce a government, the civilian population, or any segment thereof, in furtherance of political or social objectives
CW	Chemical warfare, or chemical weapon
BW	Biological warfare, or biological weapon
CBW	Chemical and/or biological warfare, or weapons
NBC	Nuclear, biological and/or chemical; usually in reference to weapons
CBRNE	Chemical, biological, radiological, nuclear, and explosive; usually in reference to weapons
WMD	Weapon of mass destruction; nuclear, radiologic, chemical, or biological weapon intended to produce mass casualties

been effectively aerosolized instead of simply allowed to evaporate. Photos from the attack show severely affected or deceased victims in very close proximity to mildly affected, ambulatory individuals. Presumably, sarin concentrations decreased so rapidly with distance from the source, that few victims, if any, were actually contaminated. After removal from high-concentration areas, the victims' bodies posed less threat to bystanders because of dilution and improved ventilation. Even so, some healthcare providers were secondarily exposed, as the victims were not disrobed prior to entering the hospitals. Up to 46% of hospital staff in areas with poor ventilation reported symptoms consistent with mild acute poisoning, although cholinesterase levels were not reported.[55,56,59] About one-third of rescue workers in the 1994 Matsumoto sarin incident also developed mild toxicity. Rescuers arriving at the scene later were less likely to develop symptoms,[52] suggesting that the vapor had dissipated over time.

PREPARATION FOR CBW INCIDENTS

A rational medical response to CBW events differs from the common response to isolated toxicologic incidents. Healthcare providers must learn about these unconventional weapons and the expected "toxidromes" that may occur.[1] In addition, healthcare providers must protect themselves and their facilities first, or ultimately no one will receive care. New medicolegal and ethical considerations will arise in CBW mass-casualty events that are otherwise infrequently seen. The greatest good for the greatest number of victims may preclude heroic

TABLE 131–2. Chemical versus Biological Weapons: Comparison and Contrast[27]

Similarities

Xenobiotics most effectively dispersed in aerosol or vapor forms
Delivery systems frequently similar
Movement of xenobiotics highly subject to wind and weather conditions
Appropriate personal protective equipment prevents illness

Differences	Chemical Weapons (CW)	Biological Weapons (BW)
Rate at which attack results in illness	Rapid, usually minutes to hours	Delayed, usually days to weeks
Identifying release	*Easier*: Rapid clinical effects Possible chemical odor Commercially available chemical detectors	*Harder*: Delayed effects Lack of color, odor, or taste Limited development of real-time detectors
Xenobiotic persistence	Variable Liquids semipersistent to persistent Gases nonpersistent	Generally nonpersistent most BW agents degraded by sunlight, heat, desiccation (exception: anthrax spores)
Victim distribution	Near and downwind from release point	Victims may be widely dispersed by time disease is apparent
First responders	EMTs, Hazmat teams, firefighters, law enforcement officers	Emergency physicians and nurses, primary care practitioners, infectious disease physicians, epidemiologists, public health officials (but may be same as CW if release is identified immediately)
Decontamination	Critically important in most cases	Not needed in delayed presentations; less important for acute exposures
Medical treatment	Chemical antidotes, supportive care	Vaccines, antibiotics, supportive care
Patient isolation	Unnecessary after adequate decontamination	Crucial for easily communicable diseases (eg, smallpox, pneumonic plague); however, many BW agents are not easily transmissible

interventions in a few critical patients. Charges of negligence may later arise regarding delays in treatment or failure to diagnose subtle signs of disease, even if such actions were unavoidable at the time. Even if physicians become well versed in the appropriate response to CBW incidents, the question remains of how many will be willing to continue working in case of an actual public health disaster.[31]

The responses to chemical and biological agents will also differ.[27] Chemical weapons, like conventional explosives, generally produce clinical effects within seconds to hours, making a "scene" or "hot zone" evident. The first responders for a chemical event will be fire and police authorities, hazmat teams, and emergency medical services. Patients will be brought to local healthcare facilities and the disease process, although perhaps not the specific diagnosis, will be recognized rapidly. With biological agents, the victims will not all present for care at the same time in the same place. First responders will be local and distant emergency departments and primary care offices, highlighting the need for training in these specialties.

Recommendations for sustained healthcare facility domestic preparedness include improved training to promptly recognize CBW mass casualty events, efforts to protect healthcare providers, and establishing decontamination and triage protocols.[43] Table 131–3 lists some specific recommendations. Several facets of the response to a CBW event are still being refined, such as the optimal choice of personal protective equipment, determining who needs decontamination and by what means, and what is to be done with wastewater produced by mass decontamination.[39,43] On a tactical level, communication can be severely impaired by personal protective gear, which points out the need for loudspeakers or some other form of public address.[43,87]

Individual clinicians and hospitals caring for victims of known or suspected CBW incidents should contact their local department of health, who may in turn report the incident to outside agencies such as the Federal Bureau of Investigation (FBI) and the Centers for Disease Control and Prevention (CDC) (Table 131–4).

TABLE 131–3. Recommendations for Healthcare Facility Response to CBW Incidents

- Immediate access to personal protective equipment (PPE) for healthcare providers
- Decontamination facilities that can be made operational within minimal delay 2 to 3 minutes (Rational? Realistic?)
- Triage of victims into those able to decontaminate themselves (decreasing the workload for healthcare providers) and those requiring assistance
- Decontamination facilities permitting simultaneous use by multiple persons and providing some measure of visual privacy
- A brief sign-in process where patients are assigned numbers and given identically numbered plastic bags to contain and identify their clothing and valuables
- Provision of food, water, and psychological support for staff, who may be required to perform for extended periods
- Secondary triage to separate persons requiring immediate medical treatment from those with minor or no apparent injuries who are sent to a holding area for observation
- Providing victims with written information regarding the agent involved, potential short- and long-term effects, recommended treatment, stress reactions, and possible avenues for further assistance
- Careful handling of information released to the media to prevent conflicting or erroneous reports
- Instituting postexposure surveillance

TABLE 131–4. CBW Phone Numbers/Contacts

CDC Emergency Preparedness & Response
www.bt.cdc.gov
Contact number for health professionals or government officials (770) 488–7100
CDC Bioterrorism Preparedness and Response Program
(404) 639–0385
Federal Bureau of Investigation (FBI)
Find your local FBI field office at: www.fbi.gov/contact/fo/fo.htm
National Response Center
For reporting releases of hazardous substances: www.nrc.uscg.mil/
(800) 424–8802, or (202) 267-2675

DECONTAMINATION

Decontamination serves two functions: (1) to prevent further absorption and spread of a noxious substance on a given casualty, and (2) to prevent spread to other persons. Decontamination is critical for some chemical weapons exposures, but is less crucial for biologic agents. Victims of an occult biological weapon agent release will not present for medical care until they become symptomatic, usually several days later when decontamination will be futile. Also, chemical weapon agents can be dispersed as liquids, which are more amenable to decontamination than gases or aerosols, and are more likely to spread on a person or between persons. Decontamination issues specific to biological weapon agents are discussed in the following chapter.

Chemical weapons that are exclusively gases at normal temperatures and pressures such as chlorine, phosgene, or hydrogen cyanide require as decontamination only removing the victim from the area of exposure. Isolated vapor exposures, as from volatilized nerve agents or sulfur mustard, are also terminated by leaving the area and may require no skin decontamination of the victims.[49,75] Japanese experience with sarin suggests that clothing should be removed from victims of nerve agent vapor exposure and placed in airtight receptacles, such as sealed plastic bags. Some of the secondary exposures to sarin were thought to have occurred as nerve agent that had condensed on the victims' clothing revaporized into the ambient air, and this caution probably holds true also for sulfur mustard vapor exposures.

Chemical weapons dispersed as liquids present the greatest need for decontamination. Because nerve agents are highly potent and have rapid onset of effects, some victims with significant dermal contamination may not survive to reach medical care.[75] Liquid-contaminated clothing must be removed, and if able, victims should remove their own clothing to prevent cross-contamination.

Decontamination should be done as soon as practicable, to prevent progression of disease, and should occur outside of healthcare facilities to prevent contamination of the working environment and secondary casualties. Decontamination near the incident scene would be ideal in terms of timeliness, although logistically this will not be possible in many situations. Evidence supports the likelihood that contaminated victims will present at healthcare facilities on their own, or be transported for care without decontamination.[39] In mass-casualty incidents, decontamination efforts may benefit from separating victims into those who can remove their own clothing and shower themselves with minimal direction and assistance, and the more seriously affected who will require full assistance. The degree of protective gear required by the decontamination personnel cannot be predicted in advance, and may not be easy to objectively determine at the time of the incident. Level C personal protective equipment may be sufficient for most hospital settings when the source is defined (eg, receiving and decontamination areas); however, if healthcare workers begin to develop symptoms, level B gear with supplied air would become necessary[57] (see Chap. 130). When the source of the contamination is not yet known, level B gear should be used. Chemically contaminated victims presenting to a healthcare facility should, if possible, be denied entrance until decontaminated. Patients who have already entered a healthcare facility and are only later determined to be a contamination hazard present a more difficult problem. If the situation allows, such patients should be taken outside for decontamination before returning, and the previous care area cordoned off until any remaining safety hazard has been assessed and eliminated. In a mass-casualty disaster, however, such efforts at remediation may not be practical.

Nerve agents are hydrolyzed and inactivated by solutions that release chlorine, such as household bleach or solutions that are sufficiently alkaline. To avoid potential dermal and mucous membrane injury, a 1:10 dilution of household bleach in water (producing a 0.5% sodium hypochlorite solution) has been recommended, not only for nerve agents, but also for sulfur mustard and many biological agents.[43,47,77] Alternatives include regular soap and water or copious water alone. Rapid washing is more important than the choice of cleaning solution because 15–20 minutes is necessary for hypochlorite solutions to inactivate chemical agents.[43] Care should be taken to clean the hair, intertriginous areas, axillae, and groin.[77]

Decontamination after sulfur mustard exposure is more problematic than for nerve agents. First, it is more likely that significantly contaminated victims will survive to reach medical care, and they may remain asymptomatic for several hours. Also, the biochemical damage becomes irreversible long before symptoms develop. Decontamination within 1–2 minutes is the only effective means of limiting tissue damage from mustard.[79] The actual means of mustard decontamination, however, are identical to those for nerve agents. Victims must be disrobed and thoroughly showered. Dilute hypochlorite solutions (eg, 0.5% sodium hypochlorite, a 1:10 dilution of household bleach) have been advocated to inactivate mustard, but copious water irrigation will also suffice.[49] Symptomatic victims of mustard exposure should still be decontaminated, even though it is unlikely to benefit that particular casualty, to prevent the spread of agent to others.[79] Lewisite and phosgene oxime must also be decontaminated quickly, although they produce immediate symptoms, making it more likely that victims will present promptly when decontamination is most effective.

Water irrigation is generally recommended for riot control agent exposures because hypochlorite solutions may exacerbate skin lesions.[49] Inadequately decontaminated patients exposed to lacrimator agents can produce secondary cases among healthcare providers, so any contaminated clothing should be removed and bagged.

Significant issues remain regarding decontamination measures. The number of people potentially requiring decontamination may easily outstrip capacity. Incidents with hundreds or thousands of victims may necessitate communal showers and/or selective decontamination. Decontamination wastewater should ideally be contained and treated, but few facilities have the capability or funds to do this. Wastewater may, however, be a minor issue. In biological weapon incidents there is only a temporary risk because of rapid environmental degradation, and in large-scale chemical weapon events the wastewater poses only a small percentage of the total environmental impact.[43]

RISK OF EXPOSURE

The actual release of CBW agents can be characterized as a low-probability, high-consequence event. Potential sources for civilian exposure include terrorist attacks, inadvertent releases from domestic stockpiles, direct military attacks, and industrial events. Terrorists may sabotage military or industrial stockpiles or directly attack the populace. Experience has shown that physicians are much more likely to encounter hoaxes,[12] isolated cases,[66] or limited incidents with a modest number of casualties.[86] Riot control agents are exceptions, in that treating riot control agent and pepper spray victims is a routine occurrence in many urban emergency departments (EDs).

Technical and organizational obstacles decrease the chance of major CBW terrorist events. Obtaining or producing chemical or biological weapons, although simpler than for nuclear weapons, is only part of the process. Effective dissemination is difficult if the goal is to maximize casualties. Proper milling of biologic agents to produce stable, respirable aerosols requires technical sophistication probably only attainable with governmental research support.[81] Illustrating this point is the ineffectiveness of the Aum Shinrikyo's biological weapon releases and the limited number of sarin fatalities, despite large amounts of funds available to support these attacks.[61] Low-technology attacks such as food contamination, poisoning of livestock, and enclosed-space weapons dispersal appear more likely to occur than attacks resulting in hundreds, thousands, or millions of casualties.[81] Smaller attacks, or merely threatening use of CBW agents, may be equally consequential from a terrorist's perspective if they exert the same political influence.

Nevertheless, even inefficiently dispersed agents of sufficient toxicity can produce multiple casualties and terrorize the populace, as occurred in the Matsumoto and Tokyo sarin attacks. Impact estimates of efficiently dispersed biological weapons are alarming. Fifty kilograms of anthrax spores disseminated along a 2-km line upwind of 500,000 people would be expected to kill 95,000 and incapacitate another 125,000 people—nearly a 50% casualty rate.[18] The societal economic impact of bioterrorist attacks ranges from $477.7 million per 100,000 persons exposed for brucellosis to $26.2 billion per 100,000 exposed for anthrax.[35]

The chemicals most likely to be used militarily appear to be sulfur mustard and the nerve agents. A "low-tech" terrorist attack could involve the release of industrial chemicals, such as chlorine, phosgene, or ammonia gas. Although the list of potential biological weapon agents is long, only a handful of pathogens have credible risk of producing public health disasters by overwhelming healthcare resources and causing high mortality, widespread panic, and massive disruption of commerce.[13] Topping this list are anthrax, smallpox, and plague, followed by botulinum toxin, hemorrhagic fever viruses, and tularemia.

PSYCHOLOGICAL EFFECTS

Either the threat or the actual use of CBW agents presents unique psychologic stressors. Even among trained persons, a CBW-contaminated environment will produce high stress through the necessity of wearing protective gear, potential exposure to agents, high workload intensity, and interactions with the dead and dying. Disorders of mood, cognition, and behavior will be common among exposed or potentially exposed victims as a result of the uncertainty, fear, and panic that may accompany a CBW incident, even a hoax. The psychological casualties will probably outnumber victims requiring medical treatment. Civilians without training, including some healthcare providers, are likely to confuse somatic symptoms with true exposure. Medical resources may easily be overwhelmed unless triage can identify those who will benefit most from appropriate counseling, education, and psychologic support. Psychiatrists should be enlisted in plans to manage CBW incidents for their expertise in treating anxiety, fear, panic, somatization, and grief.[15]

In Israel during the Gulf War, anxiety-related somatic reactions to missile attacks were reported in 18%–38% of persons surveyed,[10] and over 500 people sought medical attention in emergency departments for anxiety.[63] Among 5510 people seeking medical attention after the Tokyo subway sarin release, only about 25% were hospitalized.[74] Some of the "victims" presented days or even weeks after the incident, apparently feeling unwell and thinking they had been exposed.[56,60] Civilian survivors of chemical attacks in the 1980–1988 Iran–Iraq war report increased symptoms of depression, anxiety, and posttraumatic stress disorder compared to those exposed to low-intensity conventional warfare.[24] In one longitudinal study of American Persian Gulf War veterans, 4.6% reported their belief that they were exposed to CBW agents, despite the lack of any convincing evidence of deliberate exposures, nor of unintended exposure to any significant levels of chemical agents. Greater combat stress was associated with a higher incidence in belief in such exposures.[82] Another study reported a 64% incidence in belief of CBW agent exposure among Gulf War veterans.[8] Reported indicators supporting these beliefs included receiving an alert, having physical symptoms, and being told to use protective gear. Belief in exposure to biological agents correlated with having received an alert about chemical agents, suggesting that CW alerts can spread misinformation and confusion among recipients.

Uncontrolled release of information may compound terror and increase psychologic casualties. Imagine the influx of patients resulting from a news report suggesting that anyone with dizziness or nausea be checked for nerve agent toxicity, or that fever and cough indicate infection with anthrax.

THE ISRAELI EXPERIENCE DURING THE GULF WAR

Israel as a country is probably best prepared for CBW disasters. In late 1990, the civilian population was supplied with rubber gas masks, atropine syringes, and Fuller's earth decontamination powder.[63] Major Israeli hospitals conduct chemical practice drills every 3–5 years.[87] These drills identify several key lessons, including designating specific hospitals for chemical casualties, blocking hospital access to a single guarded entrance to prevent internal contamination, and extending nurses' authority to initiate treatment by established protocols. The Israeli plan provides two tiers of triage. The first triage occurs outside of the hospital by protected medical personnel who perform only life-saving interventions, such as intubation, hemorrhage control, and antidotal therapy. Patients are then decontaminated and enter the hospital. Afterward, patients are triaged again according to severity of illness into separate areas in which dedicated healthcare teams provide the appropriate interventions.[68,87]

Thirty-nine ballistic missiles with conventional warheads were launched against Israel from Iraq in early 1991, with only six missiles causing direct casualties. Many more "injuries" resulted from CBW defensive measures and psychologic stress than from physical trauma. Out of 1060 injuries reported from EDs during this time period, 234 persons were directly wounded in explosions (most injuries were minor), and there were only 2 fatalities from trauma.[34,63] Over 200 people presented for medical evaluation after self-injection of atropine, a few requiring admission to the hospital.[3,34,63] About 540 people sought care for acute anxiety reactions. Some suffocated from improperly used gas masks, fell and injured themselves when rushing to rooms sealed against CBW agents, or were poisoned by carbon monoxide in these airtight rooms.[34,63] Increased rates of myocardial infarction and cerebrovascular accidents were also observed.[63] A survey of hospital staff members found that only 42% would report for duty following a chemical weapon attack.[69]

SPECIAL POPULATIONS

Pregnancy does not appear to be a significant factor in the treatment of women victims of chemical weapons. In the Tokyo subway sarin attack, five victims were identified at one hospital as being pregnant. These women were only mildly affected and were admitted for observation. All had healthy babies, the first one born 3 weeks after the incident.[56,58,60] In Israel, no obstetric complications occurred among women wearing gas masks during labor and delivery.[19,63]

Children have important differences from adults regarding chemical weapon effects and decontamination efforts. Children breathe at a lower elevation above the ground and at a higher rate than adults. Because nearly all chemical weapon gases and vapors are heavier than air, children will be exposed to higher concentrations than adults in the same exposure setting, and will likely exhibit symptoms earlier.[4,65,92] Children may also be more susceptible to vesicants and nerve agents than adults with equivalent exposures.[64,92] Children have thinner and more delicate skin, allowing for more systemic absorption and more rapid onset of injury with sulfur mustard. The pediatric blood–brain barrier may also be less resistant than in adults and the activity of endogenous detoxifying enzymes, such as paraoxonase, is less, allowing for greater toxicity with nerve agents. Additionally, children with organic phosphorus compound poisoning less frequently exhibit a muscarinic toxic syndrome than adults, and often present with isolated CNS depression.[64]

The decontamination of children is another feature that requires an age-adjusted approach. Children have a larger surface area-to-mass ratio and may be more likely to carry a toxic or fatal dose of a chemical weapon on their skin. Most children will need assistance and supervision during decontamination procedures; keeping a mother or other adult guardian with a child should help with both decontamination and thermoregulation.[65]

NERVE AGENTS

Physical Characteristics and Toxicity Nerve agents (Fig. 131–1) are extremely potent organic phosphorus compound cholinesterase inhibitors, and are the most toxic of the known chemical weapons.[49] For example, sarin is 1000-fold more potent in vitro than the pesticide parathion.[75] Aerosol doses of nerve agents causing 50% human mortality (LD_{50}) range from 400 mg-min/m^3 for tabun down to 10 mg-min/m^3 for VX, compared to 2500–5000 mg-min/m^3 for hydrogen cyanide. Dermal exposure LD_{50}s for nerve agents range from 1700 mg for sarin down to only 6–10 mg for VX.[49,75] Pure nerve agents are clear and colorless. Tabun has a faint fruity odor, and soman has been variably described as smelling sweet, musty, fruity, spicy, nutty, or like camphor. Most subjects exposed to sarin and VX have been unable to describe the odor.[44,75] The G-agents tabun (GA), sarin (GB), and soman (GD) are volatile and present a significant vapor hazard. Sarin is the most volatile, only slightly less so than water. VX is an oily liquid with low volatility and higher environmental persistence.[44,49,75] Other G- and V-agents have been developed, including cyclosarin (GF) and Russian VX (VR).

Pathophysiology The pathophysiology of nerve agents is essentially identical to that from organic phosphorus compound insecticides (see Chap. 113), differing only in terms of potency and physical characteristics of the toxins. The resultant toxic syndrome includes muscarinic (salivation, lacrimation, urination, defecation, GI cramping, emesis, or SLUDGE syndrome) and nicotinic (muscle fasciculation, weakness, paralysis) signs, and central effects (loss of consciousness, seizures, respiratory depression).[30,73,77]

Clinical Effects Nerve agent vapor exposures produce rapid effects, within seconds to minutes, whereas the effects from liquid exposure may be delayed as the agent is absorbed through the skin.[47,75] Vapor

Military Designation	Common Name	Proper Name	Chemical Formula
GA	Tabun	Ethyl-*N,N*-dimethylphosphoramidocyanidate	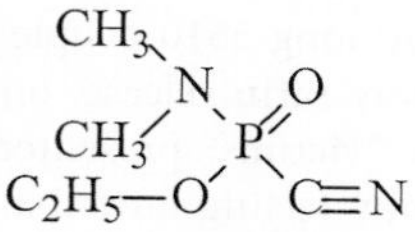 $(CH_3)_2N-P(=O)(OC_2H_5)(C\equiv N)$
GB	Sarin	Isopropyl-methylphosphonofluoridate	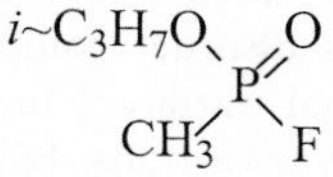 $i\text{-}C_3H_7O-P(=O)(CH_3)F$
GD	Soman	Pinacolyl-methylphoshonofluoridate	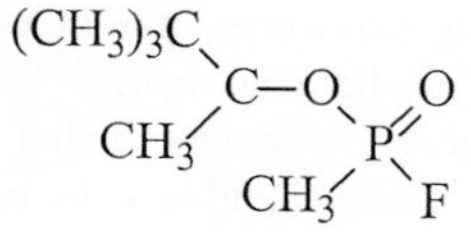 $(CH_3)_3C-CH(CH_3)-O-P(=O)(CH_3)F$
VX	-	*O*-Ethyl-*S*-[2-(diisopropylamino)ethyl]-methylphosphonothiolate	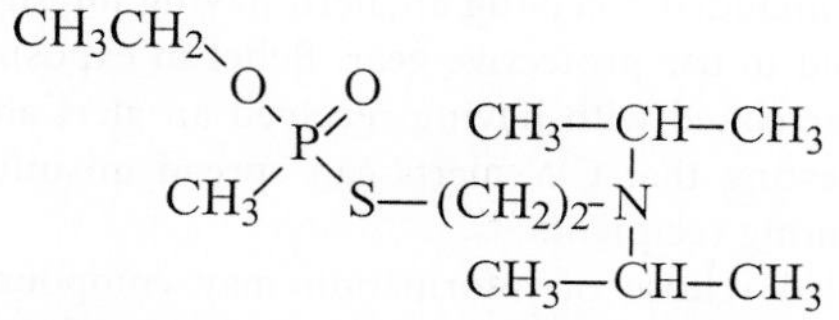 $CH_3CH_2O-P(=O)(CH_3)-S-(CH_2)_2-N[CH(CH_3)_2]_2$

FIGURE 131–1. Nerve agents.

or aerosol exposures have historically been more common, whether through experiments or from unintentional releases in the laboratory[73] or in terrorist attacks.[51,60] Aerosol or vapor exposure initially affects the eyes, nose, and respiratory tract. Miosis is common, resulting from direct contact of nerve agent with the eye, and may persist for several weeks.[73,77] Other ocular effects include conjunctival injection and blurring and dimming of the vision. Dim vision is often ascribed to pupillary constriction, but central neural mechanisms also play a role.[75] Ciliary spasm produces ocular pain, headache, nausea, and vomiting, often exacerbated by near-vision accommodation.[30] Rhinorrhea, airway secretions, bronchoconstriction, and dyspnea occur with increasing exposures. With a large vapor exposure, one or two breaths may produce loss of consciousness within seconds, followed by seizures, paralysis, and apnea within minutes.[47]

In the 1995 Tokyo subway sarin incident, ocular effects were most common after sarin vapor exposure, with miosis (89%–99% of symptomatic victims), eye pain, dim vision, and decreased visual acuity.[30,60] Other common complaints were cough, throat tightness, nausea, headache, dizziness, chest discomfort, and abdominal cramping.[46,84] Among 111 patients admitted to one hospital, the most common presenting signs and symptoms were miosis (99%), headache (74.8%), dyspnea (63.1%), nausea (60.4%), eye pain (45%), blurred vision (39.6%), dim vision (37.8%), and weakness (36.9%).[56,60] Excessive secretions were less common, with rhinorrhea seen in about one-quarter of patients admitted at one hospital,[60] and in none of 58 patients at another.[84] Secondary exposures occurred among emergency medical technicians (EMTs) and hospital personnel in both the Tokyo[46,55,56] and Matsumoto[51,52] terrorist sarin releases, apparently from evaporation of nerve agent that had condensed on the primary victims' clothing.

Liquid nerve agents can permeate ordinary clothing, allowing for percutaneous absorption and rendering patients as potential hazards to healthcare personnel prior to proper decontamination. Mild dermal exposure produces localized sweating and muscle fasciculations after an asymptomatic period lasting up to 18 hours. Moderate skin exposure produces systemic effects with nausea, vomiting, diarrhea, and generalized weakness. Substantial dermal contamination will produce earlier and more severe symptoms, often with abrupt onset. Severe toxicity from any route of exposure causes loss of consciousness, seizures, generalized fasciculations, flaccid paralysis, apnea, and/or incontinence.[49,75,77] Cardiovascular effects are less predictable, as either bradycardia (muscarinic) or tachycardia (nicotinic) may occur.[47] In the Tokyo sarin event, tachycardia and hypertension were more common than bradycardia.[54,84] Subtle CNS effects may continue for weeks, but typically resolve if no anoxic brain injury occurred.

Long-term effects from nerve agent exposure have mostly been limited to psychologic sequelae.[71] Neither delayed peripheral neuropathy nor the intermediate syndrome has been reliably described in humans exposed to nerve agents.[77,78] Followup studies from the Japanese sarin incidents show that neuropathy and ataxia, when initially present, resolved within 3 days to 3 months.[91] The main persistent sequela is posttraumatic stress disorder, found in up to 8% of victims.[29,91]

TREATMENT OF NERVE AGENT EXPOSURE

Decontamination In critically ill patients, antidotal treatment may be necessary before or during the decontamination process; but generally, decontamination should occur before other treatment is instituted.

Atropine Atropine is the standard anticholinergic antidote for the muscarinic effects of nerve agents.[17] Atropine does not reverse nicotinic effects but does have some central effects and may thus assist in halting seizure activity.[30,44,75]

Atropine is administered parenterally, either by the intravenous (IV) or intramuscular (IM) route, and the dose is determined by titration to effect. The standard adult dose determined by the American military is 2 mg, an amount expected to produce substantial benefit in reversing nerve agent toxicity but one that should be tolerated by a healthy unexposed adult unintentionally receiving the drug.[75] Current recommendations place the minimum initial dose of atropine in adults at 2 mg; dosing in children begins at 0.05 mg/kg for mild to moderate symptoms and 0.1 mg/kg for severe symptoms.[4] Severely poisoned adult patients receive an initial dose of 5–6 mg.[30,75] Repeat doses are given every 2–5 minutes until resolution of muscarinic signs of toxicity. Therapeutic endpoints are, drying of respiratory secretions and resolution of bronchoconstriction, bradycardia, and/or seizures (if initially present). Neither reversal of miosis nor development of tachycardia is a reliable marker to guide atropine therapy.[30] The total amount of atropine necessary to treat nerve agent poisoning is often much less than required for organic phosphorus insecticide toxicity of a similar degree. Typically, less than 20 mg is required in the first 24 hours, even in severe cases.[30,75,77] Fewer than 20% of moderately ill patients admitted to one hospital for sarin poisoning in Tokyo required more than 2 mg atropine.[60]

American troops in the Gulf War were issued 3 MARK I kits for immediate field treatment of nerve agent poisoning. Each kit contains two autoinjectors: an AtroPen containing 2 mg of atropine in 0.7 mL diluent, and a ComboPen containing 600 mg of pralidoxime chloride (pyridine-2-aldoxime, 2-PAM) in 2 mL diluent (Survival Technology, Rockville, MD).[75] These autoinjectors permit rapid IM injections of antidote through protective clothing and are given in the lateral thigh.[17] Treatment algorithms guided the number of MARK I kits to administer. In general, conscious casualties not in severe distress self-administer one kit (2 mg atropine), moderate to severe cases receive three kits (6 mg atropine) initially, and all receive additional doses as necessary, every 5–10 minutes[17,49,75](Antidotes in Depth A34: Atropine).

In a nerve agent mass casualty incident, a hospital's intravenous atropine supplies may be rapidly depleted. Alternative sources include atropine from ambulances, ophthalmic and veterinary preparations, or substituting an antimuscarinic such as glycopyrrolate.[30] Atropine might also be stored as a bulk powder formulation and rapidly reconstituted for injection when needed.[21]

Oximes Oximes are nucleophilic compounds that reactivate organic phosphorus compound-inhibited cholinesterase enzymes by removing the dialkylphosphoryl moiety. The only oxime approved in the United States by the FDA is 2-PAM, a monopyridinium compound. Other pralidoxime salts are used elsewhere, such as the methanesulfonate salt of pralidoxime (P2S) in the United Kingdom and 2-PAM methiodide in Japan. Other oximes include the bispyridinium compounds trimedoxime (TMB4) and obidoxime (toxogonin) used in other European countries.[44,60,75] Oximes should be given in conjunction with atropine, as they are not particularly effective in reversing muscarinic effects when given alone. Oximes are the only available nerve agent antidotes that can reverse the neuromuscular nicotinic effects of fasciculations, weakness, and flaccid paralysis (see Antidotes in Depth A33: Pralidoxime).

Oximes are effective only if administered before irreversible dealkylation, or "aging," of the organic phosphorus compound-cholinesterase complex occurs. Soman has an aging half-life of 2–6 minutes in humans.[16] It is unlikely that soman-poisoned victims will reach medical care early enough for oxime therapy to be of great benefit. For comparison, tabun has an aging half-life of about 14 hours, sarin 3–5 hours, and VX 48 hours.[16,80] Pralidoxime is effective against sarin and VX in animal studies but not against tabun because of ineffective nucleophilic attack against that particular agent, and not because of aging issues. Obidoxime also is effective against sarin but not against tabun.[44]

The bispyridinium Hagedorn (H-series) oximes, particularly HI-6 and HLö-7, have also been studied in the context of nerve agent toxicity.[44] HI-6 appears beneficial against soman poisoning (possibly through direct pharmacological action and/or reactivation of aged soman-inhibited ChE) but is not very effective against tabun. HLö-7 has reactivating activity for both soman- and tabun-inhibited ChE and may thus represent a universal oxime antidote for nerve agents. Administration of HI-6 and HLö-7 by autoinjector is difficult because they are not stable in aqueous solution.

For more details about pralidoxime administration, dosing, and side effects, see Antidotes in Depth A33: Pralidoxime. The ComboPen autoinjector in MARK I kits contains 600 mg pralidoxime, which produces a therapeutic maximal serum concentration of 6.5 μg/mL in average human subjects.[75] When possible, however, pralidoxime is optimally administered IV. Repeat pralidoxime dosing or continuous infusions are less likely to be needed for nerve agents than for organic phosphorus compound insecticides because severe effects are shorter-lived in properly decontaminated patients.[30]

Anticonvulsants Severe human nerve agent toxicity rapidly induces convulsions, which persist for a few minutes until the onset of flaccid paralysis. Diazepam is more beneficial than other anticonvulsants and simple γ-aminobutyric acid (GABA) channel agonists due to its effects on choline transport across the blood–brain barrier and acetylcholine turnover.[44] Current American military doctrine is to administer 10 mg diazepam IM by autoinjector at the onset of severe toxicity whether seizures are present or not. Thus, whenever 3 MARK I kits are used, a victim is given diazepam as well. Additional autoinjectors are given by medical personnel as necessary for seizures.[49] The reason for the IM route of diazepam suggested above is related to timely administration under field conditions. If intravenous access is feasible, IV diazepam in 5-mg doses IV every 15 minutes (up to 15 mg) is recommended[44] (see Antidote in Depth A24: Benzodiazepines)

Although diazepam is the most well-studied benzodiazepine in the treatment of nerve agent toxicity, other medications in the same class such as lorazepam and midazolam should have similar beneficial effects. Armed service personnel of the United Kingdom are supplied with ComboPens containing atropine sulfate (2 mg), pralidoxime mesylate (P2S; 30 mg), and avizafone (10 mg), a water-soluble prodrug of diazepam.[90]

Pyridostigmine Pretreatment The first large-scale use of pyridostigmine as a pretreatment for nerve agent toxicity occurred during Operation Desert Storm.[36] Pyridostigmine is a carbamate acetylcholinesterase inhibitor that is freely and spontaneously reversible, whereas nerve agent inhibition is permanent once "aging" occurs. Toxicity from rapidly aging nerve agents such as soman (GD) can probably not be reversed by standard oxime therapy in realistic clinical situations. Almost paradoxically, then, a carbamate can occupy cholinesterase, blocking access of nerve agent to the active site, and thereby protect the enzyme from permanent inhibition. Following nerve agent exposure, pyridostigmine is rapidly hydrolyzed from acetylcholinesterase and can also be easily displaced by oximes, regenerating functional enzyme. Between 20% and 40% cholinesterase inhibition is desired to protect against nerve agents.[17] Sixty-milligram doses of pyridostigmine bromide reduces cholinesterase activity by 28.4% in healthy individuals. Asthmatics taking 30 mg doses had a mean 24.3% reduction in cholinesterase activity without significant reductions in respiratory function or in response to inhaled atropine.[62] In animal studies, pyridostigmine confers a benefit against soman and tabun, but not against sarin or VX.[17] Also, it must be recognized that pyridostigmine is not an antidote, but is instead a pretreatment adjunct that greatly enhances the efficacy of atropine and oxime therapy.[77]

American troops in the Gulf War took 30 mg pyridostigmine bromide orally every 8 hours when under threat of nerve agent attack. Cholinergic side effects, mostly gastrointestinal, were common but rarely required treatment or discontinuing therapy.[36] Israeli soldiers taking the same dose also reported a range of mostly cholinergic symptoms but also a high incidence (71.4%) of dry mouth, which may be more related to environmental and psychological stressors.[70] Nine Israeli patients were hospitalized during the Gulf War for acute intentional pyridostigmine overdoses.[2] All patients recovered fully, including one patient who self-treated with atropine autoinjectors and presented with anticholinergic toxicity and another who suffered cardiac arrest, apparently from co-ingesting 4000 mg propranolol.

VESICANTS

Vesicants are agents that cause blistering of skin and mucous membranes (Fig. 131–2).

Sulfur Mustard Sulfur mustard is bis(2-chloroethyl) sulfide, a vesicant alkylating compound similar to nitrogen mustards used in chemotherapy. Nineteenth-century scientists described the compound as smelling like mustard, tasting like garlic, and causing blistering of the skin on contact. The Allies of World War I called it Hun Stoffe (German Stuff), abbreviated as HS and later as just H. Distilled, nearly pure mustard is designated HD. The French called it Yperite, after the site where it was first used, and the Germans called it LOST after the two chemists who suggested its use as a chemical weapon, **Lo**mmel and **St**einkopf. It was also called "yellow cross" after the markings on German artillery shells filled with mustard.[9,14,79] Sulfur mustard caused over one million casualties in World War I,[22] and has since been use by the Italians and Japanese in the 1930s, by Egypt in the 1960s, and by Iraq in the 1980s.[49] About 100,000 Iranians from both military and civilian backgrounds were exposed to chemical warfare agents during the latter years of the Iran–Iraq war (1984–1988), many of whom are still suffering long-term effects.[23] Nonbattlefield exposures have also occurred among Baltic Sea fishermen while recovering corroding shells dumped after WWII, and to persons unearthing or handling old chemical warfare ordinance.[22,53,66,79]

Physical Characteristics Sulfur mustard is a yellow to brown oily liquid with an odor resembling mustard, garlic, or horseradish. Mustard has relatively low volatility and high environmental persistence. Nonetheless, most historical mustard injuries occurred from vapor exposure, a danger that increases in warmer climates. Mustard vapor is 5.4 times denser than air. Mustard freezes at 57°F (13.9°C), so it is sometimes mixed with other substances, including chemical weapon agents like chloropicrin or Lewisite, to lower the freezing point and permit dispersion as a liquid.[14,49,79]

Pathophysiology Sulfur mustard toxicity occurs through several mechanisms. First, mustard is an alkylating agent. Mustard spontaneously undergoes intramolecular cyclization to form a highly reactive sulfonium ion that alkylates sulfhydryl (–SH) and amino ($-NH_2$) groups.[9,14,49,79] The most important acute manifestation is indirect inhibition of glycolysis. Sulfur mustard rapidly alkylates and crosslinks purine bases in nucleic acids (see Fig. 131–3). DNA repair mechanisms are activated, including the activation of the enzyme poly(ADP-ribose) polymerase,[45] depleting NAD^+, which in turn inhibits glycolysis, and ultimately leads to cellular necrosis from adenosine triphosphate (ATP) depletion.[9] Other mechanisms are probably involved, since the inhibition of glycolysis only partially correlates with the depletion of NAD^+; sulfur mustard may also inhibit glycolysis directly through undetermined mechanisms.[45] Mustard also depletes glutathione, leading to loss of protection against oxidant stress, dysregulation of calcium homeostasis, and further inactivation of sulfhydryl-containing enzymes.[79] Sulfur mustard is also a weak cholinergic agonist.[49,79]

Clinical Effects The organs most commonly affected by mustard are the eyes, skin, and respiratory tract. During WWI, 80%–90% of American mustard casualties had cutaneous lesions, 86% had ocular involvement, and 75% had airway injury. Iranian soldiers had more airway (95%) and ocular injuries (92%), and 83% had cutaneous lesions, probably because of the more extensive vaporization occurring in the warmer environment.[9,79] Incapacitation may be severe in terms of number of lost man-days, time for lesions to heal, and increased risk of infection. In contrast, mortality is rather low. In WWI, only 2%–3% of British mustard casualties and fewer than 2% of American casualties died. Fatality rates of 3%–4% were reported from the Iran–Iraq War.[9] Most deaths occur several days after exposure, either from respiratory failure, secondary bacterial pneumonia, or bone marrow suppression.

Dermal exposure produces dose-related injury. After a latent period of 4–12 hours, victims develop erythema that may progress to vesicles and/or bullae formation and skin necrosis. Warm, moist, and thin skin is at increased risk of mustard injury, in particular the perineum, scrotum, axillae, antecubital fossae, and neck. The vesicle fluid does not contain mustard because all chemical reactions are complete within a few minutes. If decontamination is not performed immediately after exposure, injury cannot be prevented. Later decontamination may, however, limit the severity of lesions and further spread of the agent.

Military Designation	Common Name	Proper Name	Chemical Formula
H, HD	Sulfur mustard	Bis-(2-Chloroethyl) sulfide 2,2'-Dichloroethyl sulfide	$S(CH_2CH_2Cl)_2$
L	Lewisite	2-Chlorovinyldichloroarsine β-Chlorovinyldichloroarsine	$Cl_2AsCH{=}CHCl$
CX	Phosgene oxime	Dichloroformoxime	$Cl_2C{=}N{-}OH$

FIGURE 131–2. Vesicants.

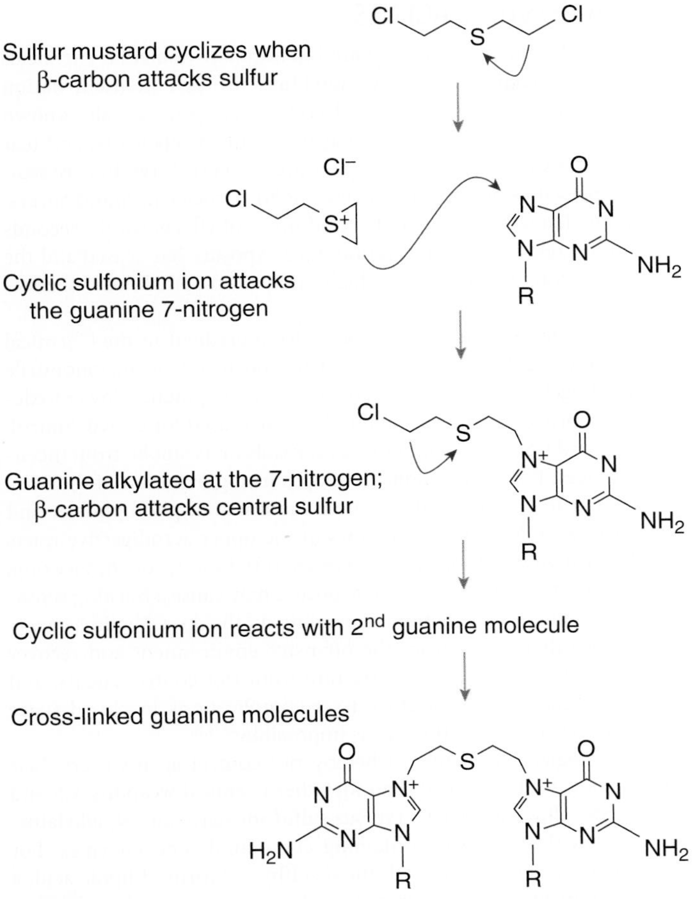

Sulfur mustard cyclizes when β-carbon attacks sulfur

Cyclic sulfonium ion attacks the guanine 7-nitrogen

Guanine alkylated at the 7-nitrogen; β-carbon attacks central sulfur

Cyclic sulfonium ion reacts with 2nd guanine molecule

Cross-linked guanine molecules

FIGURE 131–3. Mechanism of sulfur mustard toxicity: alkylation and DNA cross-linking.

Skin exposure to vapor typically results in first- or second-degree burns, although liquid exposure may result in full-thickness burns.[79] Mustard easily penetrates normal clothing and uniforms, and many soldiers received gluteal, perineal, and scrotal burns from sitting on contaminated objects.

Latency of several hours also occurs following ocular and respiratory tract exposures. Ocular effects include pain, miosis, photophobia, lacrimation, blurred vision, blepharospasm, and corneal damage. Permanent blindness is rare, with recovery generally occurring within a few weeks. Inhalation of mustard results in a chemical tracheobronchitis. Hoarseness, cough, sore throat, and chest pressure are common initial complaints. Bronchospasm and obstruction from sloughed membranes occur in more serious cases, but lung parenchymal damage occurs only in the most severe inhalational exposures. Productive cough associated with fever and leukocytosis is common 12–24 hours after exposure, and represents a sterile bronchitis or pneumonitis. Nausea and vomiting are common within the first few hours. High-dose exposures may also cause bone marrow suppression.[9,10,49,79]

Various long-term sequelae have been associated with sulfur mustard. Factory workers chronically exposed to mustard have increased risk of respiratory tract carcinomas, although the carcinogenic risk from battlefield exposures is more controversial.[22,23,78] Respiratory sequelae include chronic bronchitis, emphysema, tracheobronchomalacia, and bronchiolitis obliterans.[23] Mustard victims may also develop a delayed and often recurrent keratitis.[22,72] Chronic dermatologic complications include scarring, pigmentation changes, and chronic, neuropathic pain and pruritus.[22,72] Among approximately 34,000 Iranians with confirmed exposure to sulfur mustard during the war with Iraq, chronic pulmonary sequelae were noted in 42.5%, ocular lesions in 39.3%, and dermatologic lesions in 24.5%.[38]

Treatment Decontamination is essential in treating the sulfur mustard exposures, even among asymptomatic victims. Further treatment is largely supportive and symptomatic.[9,49,79] Victims may become blinded because of a combination of blepharospasm and corneal edema, which completely resolves in most cases; patients should be informed that this condition is very likely temporary.[32]

Several xenobiotics have been investigated as treatments for sulfur mustard injury. Antiinflammatory and sulfhydryl-scavenging agents have shown benefit in animals as prophylactic therapy or if given immediately after exposure.[79] *N*-acetyl cysteine appears to be a promising therapeutic agent in cell culture and animal studies, although most of the evidence for its use relates to inhalational aerosol exposures to mustard.[7] Neutropenia can be treated with granulocyte colony–stimulating factor.[48]

Lewisite Lewisite (2-chlorovinyldichloroarsine) was developed as a less persistent alternative to avoid some shortcomings in the use of sulfur mustard in World War I. Lewisite was never used in combat because the first shipment was en route to Europe when the war ended, and it was intentionally destroyed at sea. British anti-Lewisite (BAL, dimercaprol) was developed as a specific antidotal agent and remains in use for chelation of arsenic and other heavy metals.[44,79]

Pure Lewisite is an oily, colorless liquid. Impure preparations are colored from amber to blue-black to black and have the odor of geraniums. Lewisite is more volatile than mustard and is easily hydrolyzed by water and by alkaline aqueous solutions such as sodium hypochlorite. These properties increase safety for offensive battlefield use, but make maintaining a potent vapor concentration difficult.

Lewisite toxicity is similar to that of sulfur mustard, resulting in dermal and mucous membrane damage, with conjunctivitis, airway injury, and vesiculation. An important clinical distinction is that Lewisite is immediately painful, whereas initial contact with mustard is not. Other differences are faster onset of inflammatory response and healing of lesions from Lewisite, less secondary infection of Lewisite lesions, and less subsequent pigmentation changes.[79] The mechanisms of Lewisite toxicity are not completely known, but appear to involve glutathione depletion and arsenical interaction with enzyme sulfhydryl groups. Nevertheless, Lewisite toxicity is qualitatively and quantitatively different from the arsenic it contains. Treatment consists of decontamination with copious water and/or dilute hypochlorite solution, supportive care, and BAL. BAL is given parenterally for systemic toxicity and is also used topically for dermal or ophthalmic injuries. Alternative heavy metal chelators that may be used as Lewisite antidotes include dimercaptopropane sulfonate (DMPS) and succimer (2,3-dimercaptosuccinic acid).[44]

Phosgene Oxime Although classified as a vesicant, phosgene oxime (dichloroformoxime, or CX) does not cause vesiculation of the skin. CX is more properly an urticant or "nettle" agent, in that it produces erythema, wheals, and urticaria likened to stinging nettles. Phosgene oxime produces immediate irritation of the skin and mucous membranes. CX has never been used in battle, and little is known about its mechanism or effects on humans.[49,79]

CYANIDES (BLOOD AGENTS)

Several cyanides have been used as chemical weapons. During World War I, the French used hydrogen cyanide (HCN) and cyanogen chloride (CNCl), designated as agents AC and CK, respectively, without great success; the Austrians introduced cyanogen bromide (CNBr).

Cyanide weapons are relatively ineffective because of rapid dispersion and their "all or nothing" biological activity. An exposed individual either rapidly succumbs to cyanide toxicity, or will rapidly recover with minimal sequelae. Mass casualty events from cyanide CW agents have been reported during the Iran–Iraq War and from Iraq's suppression of the Kurds.[5,49]

The clinical effects and treatment of cyanide toxicity are covered elsewhere (Chap. 126) and do not differ significantly if used as a weapon. Hydrocyanic acid gas persists for only a few minutes in the atmosphere, because it is lighter than air and rapidly disperses. Cyanogen chloride additionally causes ophthalmic and respiratory tract irritation and can produce delayed acute lung injury in victims who are not rapidly killed.[5,49]

PULMONARY AGENTS

Both chlorine and phosgene were used as war gases in World War I. Chlorine, phosgene, various organohalides, and nitrogen oxides belong to a group of toxic chemicals designated "pulmonary agents" because they can all induce delayed pulmonary edema from increased alveolar-capillary membrane permeability.[44,49,88] Although pulmonary agents have not been used militarily since 1918, the risk of chlorine and phosgene exposure remains because of their extensive use in industry, or possibly as a terrorist weapon. (See Chap. 124 for clinical details, as the remainder of this section highlights mass-casualty issues regarding these agents.)

When released on the battlefield, chlorine forms a yellow-green cloud with a distinct pungent odor detectable at levels that are not immediately dangerous. Phosgene is either colorless or seen as a white cloud as a result of atmospheric hydrolysis. Phosgene, which is reported to smell like grass, sweet newly mown hay, corn, or like moldy hay, accounted for about 85% of all WWI deaths attributed to chemical weapons.[9,44] Phosgene produces injury by hydrolysis in the lungs to hydrochloric acid and by forming diamides that cross-link cell components (Fig. 131–4). Similar cross-linking reactions may occur with hydroxyl and thiol groups. Battlefield exposure triggers cough, chest discomfort, dyspnea, lacrimation, and the peculiar complaint that smoking tobacco produces an objectionable taste. WWI phosgene fatalities were noted to develop a mushroom-shaped efflux of pink foam at their mouths from pulmonary edema fluid. Prolonged observation after phosgene exposure is the rule, as some casualties have initially appeared well and have been discharged, only to return in severe respiratory distress a few hours later.[44,49,88] Exercise appeared to precipitate pulmonary edema in phosgene casualties.[67] For American soldiers in WWI, the average time spent recovering away from the front was 60 days for chlorine and 45.5 days for phosgene.[20]

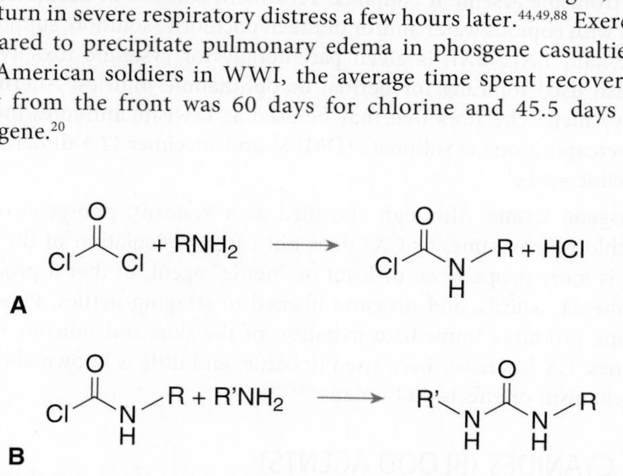

FIGURE 131–4. Proposed mechanism of phosgene toxicity. **A.** Phosgene reacts with amine group to form an amide, releasing hydrochloric acid. **B.** A second reaction cross-links two amine equivalents, forming a diamide.

RIOT CONTROL AGENTS

Riot control agents (Fig. 131–5) are intentionally nonlethal chemicals that temporarily disable exposed individuals through intense irritation of exposed mucous membranes and skin. These agents are also known as lacrimators, irritants, harassing agents, human repellents, and tear gas. They are solids at normal temperatures and pressures, but are typically dispersed as aerosols or as small solid particles in liquid sprays. Common characteristics include rapid onset of effects within seconds to minutes, relatively brief duration once exposure has ceased and the victim is decontaminated, and a high safety ratio (lethal dose vs. effective dose).[44,49,76]

Chloroacetophenone (CN) is the active ingredient in the Chemical Mace brand nonlethal weapon.[83] *o*-Chlorobenzilidene malononitrile (CS) has largely replaced CN because of its higher potency, lower toxicity, and improved chemical stability.[41,76] When used for crowd control, both CN and CS are disseminated as aerosols or as smoke from incendiary devices. Exposed persons develop burning irritation of the eyes, progressing to conjunctival injection, lacrimation, photophobia, and blepharospasm. Mucous membranes of the upper aerodigestive tracts can also be involved. Inhalation causes chest tightness, cough, sneezing, and increased secretions. Dermal exposure may cause a burning sensation, erythema, or vesiculation, depending on the dose. Victims generally remove themselves from the offensive environment and recover within 15–30 minutes. Deaths are rare from riot control agents, and typically occur from respiratory tract complications in closed-space exposures where exiting the area is impossible.[44,49,76]

The biological mechanism whereby riot-control agents exert their effects is less well described than for other chemical weapons. CS and CN are SN_2 alkylating agents (versus sulfur mustard, an SN_1 alkylator) and react with sulfhydryl-containing compounds and enzymes. For instance, CS reacts rapidly with the disulfhydryl form of lipoic acid, a coenzyme for pyruvate decarboxylase. Tissue *injury* may be related to inactivation of certain enzyme systems. Pain in the absence of tissue injury may be bradykinin mediated.[49]

Personal protective devices dispensing lacrimator substances also cause chemical injuries in the absence of war or civil unrest. Law enforcement agencies and private citizens may have access to products containing CS, CN, and/or OC (oleoresin capsicum, or pepper spray). OC is the essential oil derived from pepper plants (*Capsicum anuum* species) which contains capsaicin (trans-8-methyl-*N*-vanillyl-6-noneamide), a naturally occurring lacrimator. Capsaicin activates heat-dependent nociceptors, explaining why exposures are experienced as "hot."[11] Severe respiratory tract injuries and fatalities are occasionally reported from exposures to these devices, typically only with prolonged or highly concentrated exposures. A new capsaicin-containing riot control device called Pepperball Tactical Powder has caused severe localized skin injuries.[26] This device is a pellet of powdered capsaicin (and carrier substances) pressurized within a thin plastic shell fired as a munition.

Chloropicrin (trichloronitromethane, or nitrochloroform) is another lacrimator that occasionally causes human toxicity through its use as a fumigant and soil insecticide.[85] DM (10-chloro-5,10-dihydrodiphenarsazine, or diphenylaminearsine) is a vomiting agent. Clinical effects are delayed for several minutes after exposure, by which time the victim may have absorbed a significant amount. In addition to upper respiratory and ocular irritation, diphenylaminearsine causes more prolonged systemic effects with headache, malaise, nausea, and vomiting.[49,76]

The primary treatment for all riot-control agents is removal from exposure. Contaminated clothing should be removed and placed in airtight bags to prevent secondary exposures.[41] Skin irrigation with copious cold water is used for significant dermal exposures.[6,41,42]

Military Designation	Common Name	Proper Name	Chemical Formula
CN	Chemical mace	1-Chloroacetophenone 2-Chloroacetophenone 2-Chloro-1-phenylethanone	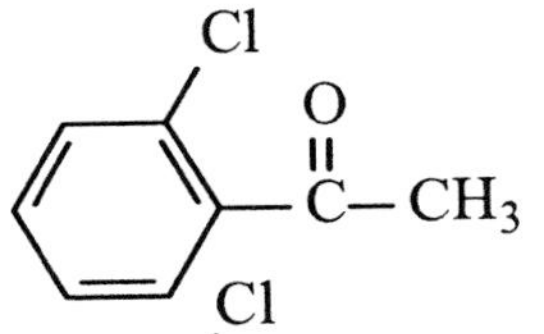
CS	Tear gas	O-Chlorobenzylidene malonitrile 2-Chlorobenzalmalonitrile	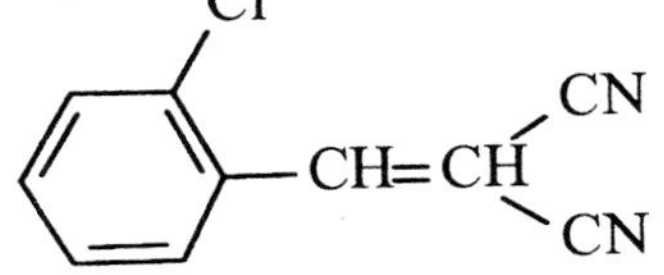
DM	Adamsite	10-Chloro-5,10-dihydrophenarsazine Diphenylaminechlorarsine	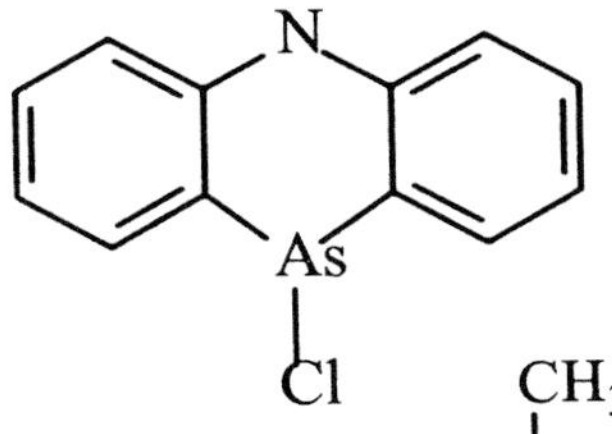
OC	Pepper spray, capsaicin	*trans*-8-Methyl-*N*-vanillyl-6-noneamide Oleoresin capsicum	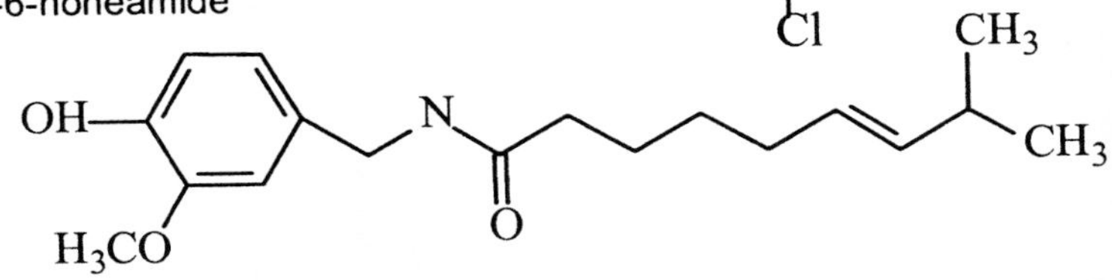

FIGURE 131–5. Riot control agents.

Symptomatic treatments, such as with topical ophthalmic anesthetics, nebulized bronchodilators, or oral antihistamines and corticosteroids, are indicated as appropriate in more severely affected victims.[6] Capsaicin-induced dermatitis has been treated variably with immersion in water or oil, vinegar, bleach, lidocaine gel, and topical antacid suspensions.[28,33,83] Cold water produces earlier symptomatic relief, but oil immersion has longer-lasting benefit.[33]

INCAPACITATING AGENTS

3-Quinuclidinyl benzilate (BZ or QNB; Fig. 131–6) is an antimuscarinic compound that has been developed as an incapacitating CW agent. BZ is 25-fold more potent centrally than atropine, with an ID_{50} (dose that incapacitates 50% of those exposed) of about 0.5 mg. Clinical effects are characteristic for anticholinergics, with drowsiness, poor coordination, and slowing of thought processes progressing to delirium. BZ takes at least an hour to produce initial manifestations, peaks at 8 hours, continues to incapacitate for 24 hours, and takes 2–3 days to fully resolve.[37] During the recent Balkan wars, allegations were made that Bosnian Serbs used BZ against civilians, who reported hallucinations associated with attacks by artillery shells emitting smoke.[25]

Ultrapotent opioids may also be used as incapacitating CW agents. In 2002, Russian security forces used a fentanyl derivative (possibly carfentanil or remifentanil) to end a 3-day standoff with terrorists in a Moscow theater in which Chechen rebels held more than 800 hostages.[89] A "gas" was introduced into the theater ventilation system, which quickly subdued the occupants. Over 650 of the hostages were hospitalized, and 128 died. Initial news reports suggested the use of BZ, although the clinical findings were more consistent with a CNS depressant. Within a few days, Russian officials stated that the agent used was a fentanyl derivative and was not expected to cause fatalities. The relatively high case fatality rate could be because of multiple factors, including variability in dose, displacement of oxygen by rapid introduction of gas into the building, failure to adequately notify healthcare teams and supply them with antidotes, and poor physical condition of the hostages.

Lysergic acid diethylamide (LSD) has also been investigated as an incapacitating agent.[37] Although effective at very low doses, battlefield use of LSD is impractical since intoxication will not reliably prevent a soldier from participation in combat.

Table 131–5 describes the various toxic syndromes that may be seen from use of CW agents.

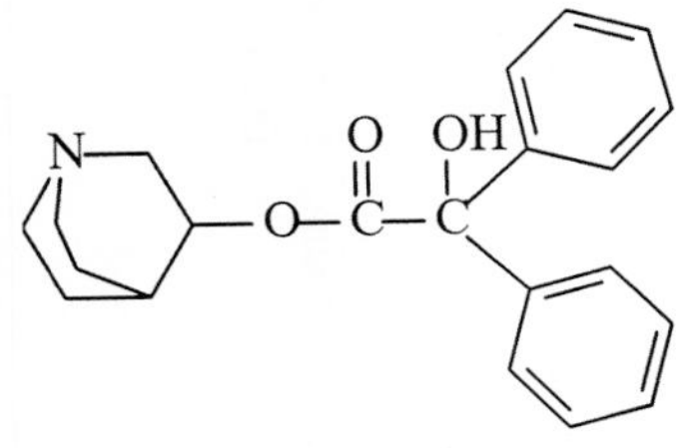

FIGURE 131–6. Incapacitating agent BZ (3-quinuclidinyl benzilate, QNB).

TABLE 131–5. Chemical Weapons Toxic Syndromes

		Organ System						
Chemical Weapon	Onset	Eyes	Upper Airways and Mucous Membranes	Lungs	Skin	CNS	GI Tract	Other
Nerve Agents								
Tabun (GA), Sarin (GB) Soman(GD), VX								
Aerosol/vapor (Mild/moderate exposure)	Rapid (sec-mins)	Miosis, eye pain, dim or blurred vision	Rhinorrhea, ↑ secretions	Dyspnea, cough, wheezing, bronchorrhea	–	Headache	Nausea, vomiting, abdominal cramps	–
Dermal exposure (Mild/moderate exposure)	Delayed (min-hrs)	–	–	–	Localized sweating	–	Nausea, vomiting, diarrhea, cramping	Subjective weakness local muscle fasciculations generalized fasciculations, weakness, flaccid paralysis
Severe exposure (Any route)	As above (by route)	Miosis	↑ Secretions	Apnea	–	Sudden collapse, seizures	Incontinence	
Vesicants								
Sulfur Mustard (H, HD)	Delayed (hrs)	Conjunctivitis, eye pain, blurred vision, blindness (temporary)	Irritation, hoarseness barky cough, sinus tenderness tracheobronchitis	(More severe exposures) Productive cough, pseudomembrane formation, airway obstruction	Erythema, vesicles, bullae, necrosis	–	Nausea, vomiting	Bone marrow suppression (in severe exposures)
Lewisite (L)	Immediate irritation Delayed vesication	Pain, blepharo-spasm conjunctivitis, lid edema	(Same as Sulfur Mustard)	(Same as Sulfur Mustard)	Erythema, vesicles	–	–	Shock (in severe exposures)
Phosgene Oxime (CX)	Immediate irritation Delayed urtication	Pain, corneal damage	Irritation	Acute lung injury	Pain blanching, erythema, urticaria Necrosis	–	–	–

Pulmonary Agents								
Phosgene (CG), Chlorine (CL)	Immediate Irritation Delayed ALI	Irritation	Irritation stridor (Chlorine)	Dyspnea, cough Acute lung injury	–	–	–	Chlorine effects more rapid than phosgene
Cyanides								
Hydrogen Cyanide (AC)	Rapid (sec-mins)	–	–	Hyperpnea then apnea	–	Anxiety, agitation, sudden collapse, seizures	–	–
Cyanogen Chloride (CK)	Rapid (sec-mins)	Irritation	Irritation	Hyperpnea then apnea	–	Anxiety, agitation, sudden collapse, seizures	–	–
Riot Control Agents								
Lacrimators (CN, CS) Capsaicin (OC)	Immediate	Pain, lacrimation, blepharospasm conjunctivitis	Irritation	Cough, chest pain	Burning pain, erythema Vesiculation severe exposures	–	Nausea, retching (may occur with CN/CS)	–
Adamsite (DM)	Rapid (min)	Irritation	Irritation, sneezing	Cough, chest pain	–	Headache	Nausea, vomiting, abdominal cramps	–
Incapacitating Agent								
3-quinuclidinyl benzilate (BZ)	Delayed (hrs)	Mydriasis	Dry mouth	–	–	Anticholinergic delirium	–	–
Ultra-potent opioids	Rapid (sec-min)	Miosis	–	Hypoventilation	–	CNS depression	–	–

SUMMARY

Unconventional weapons of mass destruction continue to pose a threat to public safety. Chemical and biologic weapons releases are considered more likely to occur than thermonuclear weapons incidents, as CBW agents use resources subject to less governmental control and require less sophisticated technology and financial outlay than nuclear weapons. CBW agents are appealing to terrorist groups because the impact in terms of death, disability, economic losses, and panic remains high. The psychological impact of CBW terrorism may well exceed that for conventional or nuclear weapons. Although the probability of incidents resulting in widespread public health disasters appears low, the consequences are high, and substantial preparations must be made in advance. Smaller CBW incidents, unintentional releases, and hoaxes have occurred and will probably continue to occur. Toxicologists and associated healthcare professionals occupy a unique position to impact preparedness and response through familiarity with chemical hazards and biologic toxins.

REFERENCES

1. Alexander GC, Larkin GL, Wynia MK. Physicians' preparedness for bioterrorism and other public health priorities. *Acad Emerg Med.* 2006;13:1238-1241.
2. Almog S, Winkler E, Amitai Y, et al. Acute pyridostigmine overdose: a report of nine cases. *Isr J Med Sci.* 1991;27:659-663.
3. Amitai Y, Almog S, Singer R, et al. Atropine poisoning in children during the Persian Gulf crisis: a national survey in Israel. *JAMA.* 1992;268:630-632.
4. Baker MD. Antidotes for nerve agent poisoning: should we differentiate children from adults? *Curr Opin Pediatr.* 2007;19:211-215.
5. Baskin SI, Brewer TG. Cyanide poisoning. In Sidell FR, Takafuji ET, Franz DR, eds. *Medical Aspects of Chemical and Biological Warfare.* Washington, DC: Office of the Surgeon General; 1997:271-286.
6. Blaho K, Winbery S. "Safety" of chemical batons. *Lancet.* 1998;352:1633.
7. Bobb AH, Arfsten DP, Jederberg WW. *N*-acetyl-L-cysteine as prophylaxis against sulfur mustard. *Mil Med.* 2005;170:52-56.
8. Brewer NT, Lillie SE, Hallman WK. Why people believe they were exposed to biological or chemical warfare: a survey of Gulf War veterans. *Risk Analysis.* 2006;2:337-345.
9. Borak J, Sidell FR. Agents of chemical warfare: sulfur mustard. *Ann Emerg Med.* 1992;21:303-308.
10. Carmell A, Liberman N, Mevorach L. Anxiety-related somatic reactions during missile attacks. *Isr J Med Sci.* 1991;27:677-680.
11. Caterina MJ, Schumacher MA, Tominaga M, et al. The capsaicin receptor: Aa heat-activated ion channel in the pain pathway. *Nature.* 1997;389:816-824.
12. Centers for Disease Control and Prevention. Bioterrorism alleging use of anthrax and interim guidelines for management—United States 1998. *MMWR Morbid Mortal Wkly Rep.* 1999;48:69-74.
13. Centers for Disease Control and Prevention. Biological and chemical terrorism: strategic plan for preparedness and response. *MMWR Morbid Mortal Wkly Rep.* 2000;49(RR04):1-14.
14. Dacre JC, Goldman M. Toxicology and pharmacology of the chemical warfare agent sulfur mustard. *Pharmacol Rev.* 1996;48:289-326.
15. DiGiovanni C. Domestic terrorism with chemical or biological agents: psychiatric aspects. *Am J Psychiatr.* 1999;156:1500-1505.
16. Dunn MA, Hackley BE, Sidell FR. Pretreatment for nerve agent exposure. In Sidell FR, Takafuji ET, Franz DR, eds. *Medical Aspects of Chemical and Biological Warfare.* Washington, DC: Office of the Surgeon General; 1997:181-196.
17. Dunn MA, Sidell FR. Progress in medical defense against nerve agents. *JAMA.* 1989;262:649-652.
18. Eitzen EM. Use of biological weapons. In Sidell FR, Takafuji ET, Franz DR. eds. *Medical Aspects of Chemical and Biological Warfare.* Washington, DC: Office of the Surgeon General; 1997:437-450.
19. Elchalal U, Lurie S, Goldshmit C, et al. Delivery with gas mask during missile attack. *Lancet.* 1991;337:242.
20. Fitzgerald GJ. Chemical warfare and medical response during World War I. *Am J Public Health.* 2008;98:611-625.
21. Geller RJ, Lopez GP, Cutler S, et al. Atropine availability as an antidote for nerve agent casualties: validated rapid reformulation of high concentration atropine from bulk powder. *Ann Emerg Med.* 2003;41:453-456.
22. Geraci M. Mustard gas: imminent danger or eminent threat? *Ann Pharmacother.* 2008;42:237-246.
23. Ghanei M, Harandi AA. Long term consequences from exposure to sulfur mustard: a review. *Inhal Toxicol.* 2007;19:451-456.
24. Hashemian F, Khoshnood K, Desai MM, et al.. Anxiety, depression, and posttraumatic stress in Iranian survivors of chemical warfare. *JAMA.* 2006;296;560-566.
25. Hay A. Surviving the impossible: the long march from Srebrenica. An investigation of the possible use of chemical warfare agents. *Med Confl Surviv.* 1998;14:120-155.
26. Hay A, Giacaman R, Sansur R, Rose S. Skin injuries caused by new riot control agent used against civilians on the West Bank. *Med Confl Surviv.* 2006;22:283-291.
27. Henderson DA. The looming threat of bioterrorism. *Science.* 1999;283:1279-1282.
28. Herman LM, Kindschuh MW, Shallash AJ. Treatment of mace dermatitis with topical antacid suspension. *Am J Emerg Med.* 1998;16:613-614.
29. Hoffman A, Eisenkraft A, Finkelstein A, et al.. A decade after the Tokyo sarin attack: a review of neurological follow-up of the victims. *Mil Med.* 2007;172:607-610.
30. Holstege CP, Kirk M, Sidell FR. Chemical warfare nerve agent poisoning. *Crit Care Clin.* 1997;13:923-942.
31. Iserson KV, Heine CE, Larkin GL, et al.. Fight or flight: the ethics of emergency physician disaster response. *Ann Emerg Med.* 2008;51:345-353.
32. Anonymous. Chemical casualties: vesicants (blister agents). *J R Army Med Corps.* 2002:148:358-370.
33. Jones LA, Tandberg D, Troutman WG. Household treatment for "chile burns" of the hands. *J Toxicol Clin Toxicol.* 1987;25:483-491.
34. Karsenty E, Shemer J, Alsech I, et al. Medical aspects of the Iraqi missile attacks on Israel. *Isr J Med Sci.* 1991;27:603-607.
35. Kaufmann AF, Meltzer MI, Schmid GP. The economic impact of a bioterrorist attack: are prevention and postattack intervention programs justifiable? *Emerg Infect Dis.* 1997;3:83-94.
36. Keeler JR, Hurst CG, Dunn MA. Pyridostigmine used as a nerve agent pretreatment under wartime conditions. *JAMA.* 1991;266:693-695.
37. Ketchum JS, Sidell FR. Incapacitating agents. In Sidell FR, Takafuji ET, Franz DR, eds. *Medical Aspects of Chemical and Biological Warfare.* Washington, DC: Office of the Surgeon General; 1997:287-305.
38. Khateri S, Ghanei M, Keshavarz S, et al. Incidence of lung, eye, and skin lesions as late complications in 34,000 Iranians with wartime exposure to mustard agent. *J Occup Environ Med.* 2003;45:1136-1143.
39. Koenig KL, Boatright CJ, Hancock JA, et al.. Health care facility-based decontamination of victims exposed to chemical, biological, and radiological materials. *Am J Emerg Med.* 2008;26:71-80.
40. Kuca K, Jun D, Cabal J, et al.. Russian VX: inhibition and reactivation of acetylcholinesterase compared with VX agent. *Basic Clin Pharm Tox.* 2006;98:389-394.
41. "Safety" of chemical batons. [editorial]. *Lancet.* 1998;352:159.
42. Lee BH, Knopp R, Richardson ML. Treatment of exposure to chemical personal protection agents. *Ann Emerg Med.* 1984;13:487-488.
43. Macintyre AG, Christopher GW, Eitzen E, et al. Weapons of mass destruction events with contaminated casualties: effective planning for health care facilities. *JAMA.* 2000;283:242-249.
44. Marrs TC, Maynard RL, Sidell FR. Chemical warfare agents. *Toxicology and Treatment.* Chichester, UK: John Wiley & Sons, 1996.
45. Martens ME, Smith WJ. The role of NAD$^+$ depletion in the mechanism of sulfur mustard-induced metabolic injury. *Cutan Ocul Toxicol.* 2008;27:41-53.
46. Masuda N, Takatsu M, Morinari H, Ozawa T. Sarin poisoning in Tokyo subway. *Lancet.* 1995;345:1446.
47. Treatment of nerve gas poisoning. *Med Lett Drugs Ther.* 1995;37:43-44.
48. Prevention and treatment of injury from chemical warfare agents. *Med Lett Drugs Ther.* 2002;44:1-4.
49. *Medical Management of Chemical Casualties Handbook, 3rd ed.* US Army Medical Research Institute of Chemical Defense, Chemical Casualty Care Division, Aberdeen Proving Ground, MD, 1999. Available at http://www.brooksidepress.org/Products/OperationalMedicine/DATA/

operationalmed/Manuals/RedHandbook/001TitlePage.htm. Accessed May 8, 2008.
50. Morimoto F, Shimazu T, Yoshioka T. Intoxication of VX in humans. *Am J Emerg Med.* 1999:17:493-494.
51. Morita H, Yanagisawa N, Nakajima T, et al. Sarin poisoning in Matsumoto, Japan. *Lancet.* 1995;346:290-293.
52. Nakajima T, Sato S, Morita H, Yanagisawa. Sarin poisoning of a rescue team in the Matsumoto sarin incident in Japan. *Occup Environ Med.* 1997;54:697-701.
53. Newmark J, Langer JM, Capacio B, et al. Liquid sulfur mustard exposure. *Mil Med.* 2007;172:196-198.
54. Nozaki H, Aikawa N. Sarin poisoning in Tokyo subway. *Lancet.* 1995;345:1446-1447.
55. Nozaki H, Hori S, Shinozawa Y, et al. Secondary exposure of medical staff to sarin vapor in the emergency room. *Intensive Care Med.* 1995;21: 1032-1035.
56. Ohbu S, Yamashina A, Takasu N, et al. Sarin poisoning on Tokyo subway. *South Med J.* 1997;90:587-593.
57. Okumura S, Okumura T, Ishimatsu S, et al.. Clinical review: Tokyo—protecting the health care worker during a chemical mass casualty event: an important issue of continuing relevance. *Crit Care.* 2005;9:397-400.
58. Okumura T. Organophosphate poisoning in pregnancy. *Ann Emerg Med.* 1997;29:299.
59. Okumura T, Suzuki K, Fukuda A, et al. The Tokyo subway sarin attack: disaster management, part 2: Hospital response. *Acad Emerg Med.* 1998;5:618-624.
60. Okumura T, Takasu N, Ishimatsu S, et al. Report of 640 victims of the Tokyo subway sarin attack. *Ann Emerg Med.* 1996;28:129-135.
61. Olson KB. Aum Shinrikyo: once and future threat? *Emerg Infect Dis.* 1999;5:513-516.
62. Ram Z, Molcho M, Danon YL, et al. The effect of pyridostigmine on respiratory function in healthy and asthmatic volunteers. *Isr J Med Sci.* 1991;27:664-668.
63. Rivkind A, Barach P, Israeli A, et al. Emergency preparedness and response in Israel during the Gulf War. *Ann Emerg Med.* 1998;32:224-233.
64. Rotenberg JS. Diagnosis and management of nerve agent exposure. *Pediatr Ann.* 2003;32:242-250.
65. Rotenberg JS, Burklow TR, Selanikio JS. Weapons of mass destruction: the decontamination of children. *Pediatr Ann.* 2003;32:260-267.
66. Ruhl CM, Park SJ, Danisa O, et al. A serious skin sulfur mustard burn from an artillery shell. *J Emerg Med.* 1994;12:159-166.
67. Russell D, Blaine PG, Rice P. Clinical management of casualties exposed to lung damaging agents: a critical review. *Emerg Med J.* 2006;23:421-424.
68. Shapira Y, Bar Y, Berkenstadt H, et al. Outline of hospital organization for a chemical warfare attack. *Isr J Med Sci.* 1991;27:616-622.
69. Shapira Y, Marganitt B, Roziner I, et al. Willingness of staff to report to their hospital duties following an unconventional missile attack: a state-wide survey. *Isr J Med Sci.* 1991;27:704-711.
70. Sharabi Y, Danon YL, Berkenstadt H, et al. Survey of symptoms following intake of pyridostigmine during the Persian Gulf war. *Isr J Med Sci.* 1991;27:656-658.
71. Sharp D. Long-term effects of sarin. *Lancet.* 2006;367:95-97.
72. Shorati M, Davoudi M, Ghanei M, et al. Cutaneous and ocular late complications of sulfur mustard in Iranian veterans. *Cutan Ocul Toxicol.* 2007;26:73-81.
73. Sidell FR. Clinical effects of organophosphorus cholinesterase in hibitors. *J Appl Toxicol.* 1994;14:111-113.
74. Sidell FR. Chemical agent terrorism. *Ann Emerg Med.* 1996;28:223-224.
75. Sidell FR. Nerve agents. In Sidell FR, Takafuji ET, Franz DR, eds. *Medical Aspects of Chemical and Biological Warfare.* Washington, DC: Office of the Surgeon General; 1997:129-179.
76. Sidell FR. Riot control agents. In Sidell FR, Takafuji ET, Franz DR, eds. *Medical Aspects of Chemical and Biological Warfare.* Washington, DC: Office of the Surgeon General; 1997:307-324.
77. Sidell FR, Borak J. Chemical warfare agents: II. Nerve agents. *Ann Emerg Med.* 1992;21:865-871.
78. Sidell FR, Hurst CG. Long-term health effects of nerve agents and mustard. In: *Medical Aspects of Chemical and Biological Warfare.* In Sidell FR, Takafuji ET, Franz DR, eds. Washington, DC: Office of the Surgeon General; 1997:229-246.
79. Sidell FR, Urbanetti JS, Smith WJ, Hurst CG. Vesicants. In Sidell FR, Takafuji ET, Franz DR, eds. *Medical Aspects of Chemical and Biological Warfare.* Washington, DC: Office of the Surgeon General; 1997:197-228.
80. Solano MI, Thomas JD, Taylor JT, et al. Quantification of nerve agent VX-butyrylcholinesterase adduct biomarker from an accidental exposure. *J Anal Tox.* 2008;32:68-72.
81. Stern J. The prospect of domestic bioterrorism. *Emerg Infect Dis.* 1999;5: 517-522.
82. Stuart JA, Ursano RJ, Fullerton CS, Wessely S. Belief in exposure to chemical and biological agents in Persian Gulf War soldiers. *J Nerv Ment Dis.* 2008;196:122-127.
83. Suchard JR. Treatment of capsaicin (Mace?) dermatitis. *Am J Emerg Med.* 1999;17:210-211.
84. Suzuki T, Morita H, Ono K, et al. Sarin poisoning in Tokyo subway. *Lancet.* 1995;345:980.
85. TeSlaa G, Kaiser M, Biederman L, Stowe CM. Chloropicrin toxicity involving animal and human exposure. *Vet Hum Toxicol.* 1986;28:323-324.
86. Török TJ, Tauxe RV, Wise RP, et al. A large community outbreak of salmonellosis caused by intentional contamination of restaurant salad bars. *JAMA.* 1997;278:389-395.
87. Tur-Kaspa I, Lev EI, Hendler I, et al. Preparing hospitals for toxicological mass casualties events. *Crit Care Med.* 1999;27:1004-1008.
88. Urbanetti JS. Toxic inhalational injury. In Sidell FR, Takafuji ET, Franz DR, eds. *Medical Aspects of Chemical and Biological Warfare.* Washington, DC: Office of the Surgeon General; 1997:247-270.
89. Wax PM, Becker CE, Curry SC. Unexpected "gas" casualties in Moscow: a medical toxicology perspective. *Ann Emerg Med.* 2003;41:700-705.
90. Wetherell J, Price M, Mumford H, et al.. Development of next generation medical countermeasures to nerve agent poisoning. *Toxicology.* 2007;233:120-127.
91. Yanagisawa N, Morita H, Nakajima T. Sarin experiences in Japan: acute toxicity and long-term effects. *J Neurol Sci.* 2006;249:76-85.
92. Yu CE, Burklow TR, Madsen JM. Vesicant agents and children. *Pediatr Ann.* 2003;32:254-257.

CHAPTER 132
BIOLOGICAL WEAPONS

Jeffrey R. Suchard

Expertise in dealing with biological weapons requires specific knowledge from the fields of infectious disease, epidemiology, toxicology, and public health. Biological and chemical warfare agents share many characteristics in common, including intent of use, some dispersion methods, and initial defense based on adequate personal protective equipment and decontamination (see Tables 131–2 and 131–3). Key differences between biological and chemical weapons, however, involve a greater delay in onset of clinical symptoms after exposure to biological weapons; that is, the incubation period for most biological warfare (BW) agents is greater than the latent period for most chemical warfare (CW) agents. Decontamination is less crucial for victims exposed to BW agents than to CW agents. Additionally, a few BW agents can reproduce in the human host and cause secondary casualties, and disease following exposure to several of these agents can be prevented by the timely administration of prophylactic medications.

Biological weapons may be bacteria, fungi, viruses, or toxins derived from microorganisms. Some fungi are listed as potential BW agents, although to date, none are known to have been developed into weapons.[84] Because toxin weapons do not contain living organisms, some authorities classify them as chemical, rather than biological, weapons. For the purposes of discussion in this chapter, toxin weapons derived from microorganisms will be considered biological weapons. Most of the bacterial BW agents exert their effects by elaborating protein toxins.

A majority of the diseases caused by biological weapons are either infrequently encountered in modern clinical medicine, such as anthrax and plague, or no longer occur naturally, such as smallpox. Healthcare personnel therefore require specific training in the recognition and management of biological warfare victims. Potential BW agents have been categorized by the risk of mass-casualty outbreaks resulting from deployment and exposure.[17] The high-risk agents are easily disseminated or transmitted and may cause high mortality and potentially a public health disaster; these agents include smallpox, anthrax, plague, botulism, tularemia, and several hemorrhagic fever viruses. The moderate-risk agents include Q fever, brucellosis, the equine encephalitis viruses, ricin, and staphylococcal enterotoxin B, all of which are briefly discussed in this chapter.

HISTORY

Biological warfare has ancient roots. Missile-type weapons poisoned with natural toxins were used as early as 18,000 years ago (Chap. 1). Excavation of an Egyptian tomb, from about 2100 B.C., yielded arrows coated with cardioactive steroids and paralytic toxins.[62] The first recorded intentional spread of infectious disease in warfare occurred in the Anatolian war of 1320–1318 B.C. and appears to have involved tularemia.[81] Around 600 B.C., the Athenians used hellebore, and the Assyrians used ergot alkaloids, to poison enemy water supplies. In 200 B.C., the Carthaginian general Maharbal tainted wine consumed by African rebel forces with the anticholinergic herb mandragora and then ambushed the intoxicated troops. In 184 B.C., Hannibal ordered earthen pots filled with "serpents of every kind" hurled onto enemy ships, thereby winning the naval battle of Eurymedon against King Eumenes of Pergamon.[32] In 67 B.C., King Mithridates VI of Pontus was retreating from the Roman General Pompey near Trebizond, modern northeast Turkey. At the advice of a physician-counselor, Mithridates maneuvered Pompey's troops into a region where the honey was contaminated with grayanotoxins from rhododendron nectar. The Romans ate the poisoned honey and were effectively ambushed.[52]

From 1344 to 1346 A.D., the Tartars besieged the Genoan trade city of Kaffa on the Black Sea coast. When the Tartars began to die of bubonic plague, the dead bodies were hurled over the battlements. Within the city, plague forced the Genoans to flee, and they then disseminated the disease to other trade ports and eventually to the rest of Europe, causing the Black Death.[86] In 1763, Sir Jeffrey Amherst, the commander of British forces during the French and Indian War, instituted a policy of spreading smallpox to Native Americans by giving them contaminated blankets and handkerchiefs.[26]

During World War I, Germany was the only combatant nation with an active BW program. German agents infected Allied livestock with anthrax and glanders.[85] Eighty years after the capture of a German device used to disseminate anthrax, viable spores were recovered.[70]

Shiro Ishii, a Japanese army doctor, headed an active BW program throughout Japan's war with China and World War II.[41] Several centers were founded, the most famous being Unit 731 in Manchuria, where human experiments on prisoners of war and imprisoned civilians occurred. Several field trials with bubonic plague were performed on Chinese civilians and Russian troops. The Soviet Union, Germany, France, Britain, and Canada all started BW research facilities in the period between the World Wars.

BW research program in the United States was founded at Camp Detrick, Maryland in 1942. Fort Detrick, as it is now known, remains the home of the United States Army Medical Research Institute of Infectious Diseases (USAMRIID). Anthrax and botulinum toxin were the foci of weapons development during WWII; it is estimated that the United States could have manufactured 1,000,000 anthrax bombs and 275,000 botulinum bombs by 1945 had full-scale production been implemented.[7]

In 1940 the British BW program was established at Porton Down, but most of the field testing of anthrax occurred on Gruinard Island off the northern coast of Scotland. In 1979, the soil was still found to be contaminated with viable anthrax spores.[53] The island was decontaminated with 5% formaldehyde in sea water, and was deemed safe by the British government in 1988.[1]

During the Cold War, the US military maintained active research into biological weapons, including field trials with bacterial simulants. In 1950, ships in San Francisco harbor released aerosols of *Serratia marcesans* and other simulants, which resulted in a minor outbreak of Serratia sepsis. In 1966, light bulbs filled with *Bacillus subtilis* var *globigii* were shattered in the New York City subway system, confirming the hypothesis that the piston-like action of the subway trains could rapidly disperse the bacterial aerosol throughout the city.[26,73]

In London, in 1978, the Bulgarian exile Georgi Markov was assassinated by a tiny metal pellet fired from a gun designed to appear like an umbrella. He was thought to have died from sepsis until the pellet was found at autopsy.[27] After the fall of the Soviet Union, government officials confirmed that the KGB used umbrella guns firing ricin pellets to assassinate Markov and others.

In 1979, an outbreak of human anthrax caused at least 66 fatalities in the Russian city of Sverdlovsk. Autopsies revealed that the deaths were from inhalational anthrax, and epidemiologic investigation demonstrated that almost all of the cases occurred downwind from a military facility. These data are consistent only with a release of aerosolized anthrax, which has since been confirmed by Russian authorities.[59]

In the late 1970s and early 1980s, many reports came from Southeast Asia and Afghanistan that Soviet-supported troops were using a biological weapon known as Yellow Rain.[83] Some samples of Yellow Rain were found to contain trichothecene mycotoxins, although controversy remains regarding whether this finding represents intentional biological warfare or a naturally occurring phenomenon.[74]

During the 1990s there was a great deal of concern about the use and possible stockpiling of weapons of mass destruction (WMD) by Saddam Hussein in Iraq.[51] As part of the WMD program, Iraq had a very active BW research program, investigating at least five bacteria, one fungus, five viruses, four toxins, simulants, and a variety of dispersion methods.[75,88] Thousands of liters of anthrax spores, botulinum toxin, and aflatoxin were produced and weaponized into bombs and as payloads for SCUD missiles.

Biological terrorism and the threat of bioterrorism are now recognized as worldwide, growing public health concerns.[42] In the United States in 1984, a large outbreak of salmonellosis was traced to intentional contamination of restaurant salad bars by the Rajneeshee cult in Oregon.[80] The Aum Shinrikyo cult based in Japan investigated the use of cholera and Q fever, unsuccessfully released anthrax spores and botulinum toxin, and even sent members to Africa to obtain the Ebola virus.[64,78] The mere threat of biologic agent release can terrorize a city. At the end of the 1990s, there was a huge increase in false anthrax threats, which paralyzed Los Angeles and cities in Indiana, Kentucky, and Tennessee among many others.[15] Because of heightened concern for bioterrorism, even naturally occurring disease outbreaks have raised suspicion of biological terrorism. In 1999, an outbreak of West Nile-like virus encephalitis in New York and a case of brucellosis in New Hampshire acquired under suspicious circumstances were investigated as potential BW agent releases.[16,71] Similarly, a 1999–2000 epidemic of tularemia in war-torn Kosovo was scrutinized as the potential result of an intentional BW agent release.[40]

GENERAL CONSIDERATIONS

DIFFERENCES BETWEEN BW INCIDENTS AND NATURALLY OCCURRING OUTBREAKS

Because the clinical effects of bioweapons are often delayed for several days after exposure to the agents, it may be difficult to differentiate occult BW releases from naturally occurring disease outbreaks. Several epidemiologic criteria are proposed to aid in such determinations,[63] many of which should be identifiable in a BW incident (Table 132–1).

To avoid early detection, terrorists might choose to release an agent causing endemic infection, or a disease that mimics an endemic infection, during its season of peak incidence. In some areas of the United States, for example, a few cases of bubonic plague would not attract notice; that is, until dozens or hundreds of cases were identified. An outbreak of inhalational anthrax during the influenza season may similarly be hidden among patients with similar early symptoms until an unusually high mortality was evident.[22] By the time the BW outbreak was recognized, the perpetrators could dispose of any physical evidence and flee the area. On the other hand, even a single case of smallpox (anywhere in the world), Ebola virus infection, or Congo-Crimean hemorrhagic fever (in nonendemic areas) should immediately raise suspicion of a BW attack.

TABLE 132–1. Epidemiologic Clues Suggesting Biological Weapon Release

- Large epidemic with unusually high morbidity and/or mortality
- Epidemic curve (number of cases versus time) showing an "explosion" of cases, reflecting a point source in time rather than insidious onset
- Tight geographic localization of cases, especially downwind of potential release site
- Predominance of respiratory tract symptoms because most BW agents are transmitted by aerosol inhalation
- Simultaneous outbreaks of multiple unusual diseases
- Immunosuppressed and elderly persons more susceptible
- Nonendemic infection ("impossible epidemiology")
- Nonseasonal time for endemic infection
- Organisms with unusual antimicrobial resistance patterns, reflecting BW genetic engineering
- Animal casualties from same disease outbreak
- Absence of normal zoonotic disease host
- Low attack rates among persons incidentally working in areas with filtered air supplies or closed ventilation systems, using HEPA masks, or remaining indoors during outdoor exposures
- Delivery vehicle or munitions discovered
- Law enforcement or military intelligence information
- Claim of BW release by belligerent force

PREPAREDNESS

Many BW agents initially produce nonspecific symptoms, and diseases that are rarely, if ever, seen in clinical practice. Inhalational anthrax and pneumonic plague, for example, could easily be misdiagnosed as influenza or acute bronchitis. Providers in emergency departments (EDs) and primary care medicine must be educated to recognize the signs, symptoms, and clinical progression of diseases caused by BW agents.[72] Clear identification, isolation, and aggressive treatment early after exposure within the first 24–48 hours are the best and only means of reducing mortality and, in the case of smallpox or plague, preventing secondary or tertiary cases.[31] However, even with increasing awareness and educational efforts, many physicians remain inadequately prepared.

DECONTAMINATION

Biological warfare agents are most effective when dispersed by aerosol. Shortly after a known or suspected release of bioaerosols, decontamination is a relatively minor concern, because aerosols sized to reach the lower respiratory tract (<5-μm particles) produce little surface contamination. However, simple removal of clothing will eliminate a high proportion of deposited particles, and subsequent showering with soap and water will probably remove 99.99% of any remaining organisms on the skin.[50] Thus, decontamination after BW aerosol exposure, when needed, is achieved through disrobing and showering with soap and water. This can be done onsite or in the victims' homes and away from healthcare facilities, thereby reducing strain on disaster response manpower and material in multiple-victim exposures.[31,42,50,72] When there is gross, visible evidence of skin exposure to biological agents, the patient should be decontaminated by thorough irrigation, and, if available, sterilizing the skin with a sporicidal/bactericidal solution (eg, 0.5% sodium hypochlorite), and a final water rinse.[50,72] After occult bioweapons releases, victims are identified late after exposure; decontamination will obviously not be helpful and may only serve to delay care.

BIOLOGICAL WARFARE AGENTS

BACTERIA

Anthrax Anthrax is caused by *Bacillus anthracis*, a Gram-positive spore-forming bacillus found in soil worldwide. *B. anthracis* causes disease primarily in herbivorous animals. Human anthrax cases generally occur in farmers, ranchers, and among workers handling contaminated animal carcasses, hides, wool, hair, and bones.[37]

Clinical Manifestations. A few clinically distinct forms of anthrax may occur, depending on the route of exposure. Cutaneous anthrax results from direct inoculation of spores into the skin via abrasions or other wounds and accounts for about 95% of endemic (naturally occurring) human cases. Patients develop a painless red macule that vesiculates, ulcerates, and forms a 1- to 5-cm brown-black eschar surrounded by edema.[56] The eschar color gave rise to the name anthrax, from the Greek *anthrakos* meaning "coal." Most skin lesions heal spontaneously, although 10%–20% of untreated patients progress to septicemia and death. Cutaneous anthrax when treated with antibiotic therapy rarely results in fatalities. Anthrax is not transmissible among humans.

Gastrointestinal anthrax results from ingesting insufficiently cooked meat from infected animals. Patients develop nausea, vomiting, fever, abdominal pain, and mucosal ulcers, which can cause GI hemorrhage, perforation, and sepsis. Mortality from gastrointestinal anthrax is at least 50%, even with antibiotic treatment.[37]

Inhalational anthrax results from exposure to aerosolized *B. anthracis* spores. Although this form of anthrax is very rare, it is so closely associated with occupational exposures that it has been called "woolsorter's disease." Inhalational anthrax is also likely to be the form that occurs in a BW attack, because the anthrax spores would be most effectively disseminated by aerosol. After an incubation period of 1–6 days, the patient develops fever, malaise, fatigue, nonproductive cough, and mild chest discomfort, which may be easily mistaken for community acquired pneumonia.[22] The initial symptoms may briefly improve for 2–3 days or the patient may abruptly progress to severe respiratory distress with dyspnea, diaphoresis, stridor, and cyanosis. Bacteremia, shock, metastatic infection such as meningitis, which occurs in about 50% of cases, and death may follow within 24–36 hours. Prior to the 2001 bioterrorist outbreak, mortality from inhalational anthrax was expected to be nearly 100%, even with antibiotics, once symptoms develop.[35,37] With appropriate antibiotic therapy and supportive care, 5 of 11 patients with inhalational anthrax in 2001 died, and although this is still a high mortality rate, it is less than that previously predicted.[46]

Pathophysiology. Inhalational anthrax causes a mediastinitis. Diagnostic imaging typically shows mediastinal widening from enlarged hilar lymph nodes and pleural effusions, although pulmonary parenchymal infiltrates may also be seen.[46] Inhaled spores are taken up into the lymphatic system where they germinate and the bacteria reproduce. *B. anthracis* produces three toxins: protective antigen, edema factor, and lethal factor. Protective antigen (PA) is so named because antibodies against it protect the subject from the effects of the other two toxins. PA forms a heptamer that inserts into plasma membranes, facilitating endocytosis of the other two toxins into target cells (see Figure 132–1). Edema factor is a calmodulin-dependent adenylate cyclase. Increased intracellular cyclic adenosine monophosphate (AMP) upsets water homeostasis, leading to massive edema and impaired neutrophil function. Lethal factor is a zinc metalloprotease

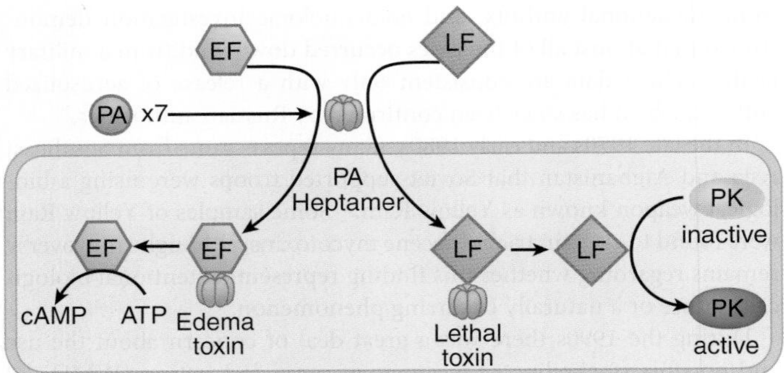

FIGURE 132–1. Model of action of anthrax toxins. PA = protective antigen; EF = edema factor; LF = lethal factor; PK = Protein Kinase. EF and LF are unable to enter cells until they complex with a PA heptamer, forming edema toxin and lethal toxin respectively. Once intracellular, release from PA allows EF and LF to exert their intracellular effects. Antibodies against PA confer resistance to the toxic effects of anthrax.

that stimulates macrophages to release tumor necrosis factor α and interleukin-1β, contributing to death in systemic anthrax infections.[29] The combination of PA plus edema factor is called *edema toxin*, while PA plus lethal factor is *lethal toxin*.[39]

Treatment. The primary antibiotics recommended to treat anthrax are ciprofloxacin and doxycycline. Although other fluoroquinolones would be expected to have similar activity against anthrax, only the manufacturer of ciprofloxacin applied for and received a Food and Drug Administration (FDA)-approved indication for use in this infection. In a mass-casualty setting or for postexposure prophylaxis, adults should be treated with ciprofloxacin 500 mg PO every 12 hours. Alternate therapies are doxycycline 100 mg PO every 12 hours, or amoxicillin 500 mg PO every 8 hours, if the anthrax strain is proven susceptible.[46] The recommended duration of therapy is 60 days, stemming from case experience in Sverdlovsk where some patients developed disease several (6–7) weeks after the spore release.[59] Children can also be treated with ciprofloxacin (15 mg/kg; maximum 500 mg/dose) or amoxicillin (80 mg/kg/d divided every 8 hours; maximum 500 mg/dose). The relative pediatric contraindication to fluoroquinolones is outweighed by the risk of potentially fatal disease. Cutaneous anthrax is treated with the same drugs and doses as for postexposure prophylaxis.

Inhalational anthrax should be treated initially with intravenous antibiotics. Adults should receive ciprofloxacin 400 mg IV or doxycycline 100 mg IV every 12 hours, along with one or two additional antibiotics with in vitro activity against anthrax (eg, rifampin, vancomycin, penicillin, ampicillin, chloramphenicol, imipenem, clindamycin, clarithromycin). Children should be given ciprofloxacin 10 mg/kg IV (max. 400 mg/dose), or doxycycline 2.2 mg/kg IV (max. 100 mg/dose), and additional antibiotics as above.[46] In a true mass-casualty event, however, when resources are strained and inpatient care is not available for every victim, oral therapy, as described above, may be instituted. When clinically appropriate, oral antibiotic therapy can be substituted for IV, with a total treatment duration of 60 days. Some patients in the 2001 outbreak were specifically treated with additional antibiotics that inhibit protein synthesis in attempts to reduce bacterial production of toxins.

Anthrax Vaccine. An effective vaccine against anthrax is available.[38,58,89] In the United States, the Bioport Corporation (formerly Michigan Biologic Products Institute) is licensed by the FDA to produce anthrax vaccine adsorbed (AVA). The vaccine consists of a membrane-sterilized culture filtrate of *B. anthracis* V770-NP1-R, an avirulent, nonencapsulated strain that produces protective antigen, adsorbed to aluminum hydroxide, formulated with benzethonium chloride (preservative) and formaldehyde (stabilizer).[89] In human and animal experiments, the vaccine is highly effective in preventing all forms of anthrax (including inhalational), and the vaccine is recommended for workers in high-risk occupations. As in the case of any vaccine, local reactions to AVA occur in some recipients (up to 20% with mild, local reactions), and self-limited systemic reactions occur more rarely (<1.5%). Women have been noted to have more frequent injection-site reactions and other adverse events, although this sex difference is also noted with other common vaccines.[39] Serious adverse events are very rare, with only 22 potentially related cases of serious adverse events from over 1 million doses administered to US armed forces.[38] The dosage schedule for AVA is 0.5 mL subcutaneously at 0, 2, and 4 weeks and 6, 12, and 18 months, followed by yearly boosters.

The 2001 Bioterrorist Anthrax Outbreak. Starting on September 27, 2001 a 63-year-old Florida man developed malaise, fatigue, fever, chills, anorexia, and diaphoresis. He was admitted to a local hospital on October 2, after presenting with additional complaints of nausea, vomiting, and confusion. Chest radiography showed cardiomegaly, a left perihilar infiltrate, small left pleural effusion, and a prominent superior mediastinum. Lumbar puncture revealed hemorrhagic meningitis with many Gram-positive bacilli. *Bacillus anthracis* was isolated from the cerebrospinal fluid after only a 7-hour incubation and from blood cultures within 24 hours. The patient had progressive clinical deterioration and died on hospital day four.[12,48]

On October 4, the Centers for Disease Control and Prevention (CDC) released a public health message regarding this case, which initially appeared to be an isolated, perhaps naturally occurring sporadic event; another case of anthrax was reported in Texas earlier the same year.[18] Nevertheless, the rarity of inhalational anthrax especially outside of a high-risk occupation, combined with increased suspicion in the wake of events on September 11, 2001, led to intense investigation of a potential bioterrorist event. Within days, epidemiologic investigation suggested workplace exposure to anthrax spores, and personnel working in the same building were started on prophylactic ciprofloxacin.[19] On October 12, a case of cutaneous anthrax was reported in New York City associated with a suspicious letter opened on September 25.[20] Anthrax cases and environmental contamination were also soon detected in Washington DC and in a New Jersey postal facility. The public response to the reports of these serious and fatal cases included misuse and hoarding of antibiotics, purchasing gas masks (often with inappropriate filtering mechanisms for biological weapons), reporting numerous miscellaneous powdery substances, and perpetrating or reporting copycat hoaxes.

By November 7, 2001, a total of 22 cases of anthrax were reported: 10 inhalational and 12 cutaneous.[21] One additional death from inhalational anthrax occurred on November 21, 2001,[5] and a case of cutaneous anthrax also occurred in a laboratory worker analyzing samples obtained during the investigation.[23] In two of the fatal cases, no contact with contaminated letters could be established.[5,61] One infant hospitalized in New York City with cutaneous anthrax was initially misdiagnosed as suffering from a brown recluse spider envenomation.[36] The total number of medical victims of anthrax by the Spring of 2002 was 23: 11 cases of inhalational anthrax (with 5 fatalities), and 12 cases of cutaneous anthrax (8 confirmed and 4 suspected).[23]

Although the overall morbidity and mortality from this bioterrorist event were relatively low, the psychosocial-economic impact was high. Several hundred postal and other facilities were tested for *B. anthracis* spore contamination, and public health authorities recommended antibiotic prophylaxis be initiated for approximately 32,000 persons.[21] Additional indirect costs and effects are more difficult to quantify, including the number of persons self-initiating antibiotic treatment without an evident indication, lost production and wages, environmental and biologic sample testing, decontamination efforts, and an international sense of unease.

Published estimates of tens of thousands of deaths from a military-style anthrax attack[49] depend on efficient BW agent dispersion. The technically easier anthrax letter has clearly proven itself to be a "weapon of mass disruption." As predicted, the psychological impact far exceeded the actual medical emergency, and events with a modest number of medical patients are probably more likely than true mass-casualty BW incidents. On the other hand, prior assumptions regarding the clinical aspects of anthrax were not as reliable. The mortality rate among the 11 cases of inhalational anthrax was 45%, considerably lower than expected and probably because of earlier diagnosis, improved supportive care measures, and a wider choice of antibiotics, compared to historical controls. Presentation with fulminant illness, such as sepsis, still appears to be predictive of a fatal outcome, yet the initial phase of illness does not necessarily lead to death, if treated with appropriate antibiotics.[8,48,54] Pleural effusions were the most common radiographic abnormality, rather than a widened mediastinum, and pulmonary parenchymal infiltrates were seen in seven patients, whereas earlier teaching had been that pneumonia does not commonly occur with inhalation anthrax.[37,48]

Plague *Yersinia pestis* is a Gram-negative bacillus responsible for over 200 million human deaths and 3 major pandemics in recorded history.[56,57] Naturally occurring plague is transmitted by flea vectors from rodent hosts, or by respiratory droplets from infected animals or humans. Bubonic plague could result from an intentional release of plague-infested fleas. Plague is a particularly frightening BW agent because it can be released as an aerosol to cause a fulminant communicable form of the disease for which no effective vaccine exists. Antibiotics must be initiated early after exposure because once symptoms develop, mortality is extremely high.

Clinical Presentation. Plague occurs in three clinical forms: bubonic, septicemic, and pneumonic. Bubonic plague has an incubation period of 2–10 days followed by fever, malaise, and painful, enlarged regional lymph nodes called buboes. The inguinal nodes are most commonly affected, presumably because the legs are more prone to flea bites, although cervical or axillary buboes are more common in children.[69] In the United States, 85%–90% of human plague patients have the bubonic form, 10%–15% have a primary septicemic form without lymphadenopathy, and about 1% present with pneumonic plague. Secondary septicemia occurs in 23% of patients presenting with bubonic plague.[57] Various skin lesions at the site of inoculation (pustules, vesicles, eschars, or papules) occur in some patients, although the petechiae and ecchymoses that occur in advanced cases may resemble meningococcemia.[56] Distal gangrene may occur from small artery thrombosis, explaining why plague pandemics are sometimes called "The Black Death." If left untreated, bubonic plague carries a 60% mortality rate.[56]

Pneumonic plague is an infection of the lungs with *Y. pestis*. Between 5% and 15% of bubonic plague patients develop secondary pneumonic plague through septicemic spread of the organism.[57] Primary pneumonic plague occurs from inhalation of infected respiratory droplets or an intentionally disseminated BW aerosol. The incubation period of pneumonic plague after inhalation is 2–3 days. The onset of disease is acute and often fulminant. Patients develop fever, malaise, and cough productive of bloody sputum, rapidly progressing to dyspnea, stridor, cyanosis, and cardiorespiratory collapse. Plague pneumonia is almost always fatal unless treatment is begun with 24 hours of symptom onset.[35]

Diagnosis and Treatment. Plague can be diagnosed by various staining techniques, immunologic studies, or by culturing the organism from blood, sputum, or lymph node aspirates. When gram stained, *Y. pestis* appears as a Gram-positive safety pin–shaped bipolar coccobacillus.[35,69] Chest radiographs in pneumonic plague reveal patchy or consolidated bronchopneumonia. Leukocytosis with a left shift is common, as are markers of low-grade disseminated intravascular coagulation (DIC) and elevations of unconjugated bilirubin and hepatic aminotransferases.[35]

Antibiotic treatment options are similar to those for anthrax. In a mass-casualty setting or for postexposure prophylaxis, adults are treated with doxycycline 100 mg PO twice daily or ciprofloxacin 500 mg orally twice daily. Children receive doxycycline 2.2 mg/kg or ciprofloxacin 20 mg/kg, up to a maximum of the adult doses. Chloramphenicol 25 mg/kg orally four times daily is an alternative. The duration of treatment is 7 days for postexposure prophylaxis, and 10 days for mass-casualty incidents.[45] Patients with pneumonic plague need to be isolated to prevent secondary cases. Respiratory droplet precautions are necessary in pneumonic plague until the patient has received antibiotics for 3 days.[35] In a contained-casualty setting, pneumonic plague is treated with parenteral streptomycin or gentamicin; alternative antibiotics include doxycycline, ciprofloxacin, and chloramphenicol.[45] A killed whole-cell vaccine effective against bubonic plague is available, but does not reliably protect against pneumonic plague in animal studies.[56,58]

Tularemia *Francisella tularensis* is a small, aerobic, Gram-negative coccobacillus weaponized by the United States and probably other countries as well. Tularemia occurs naturally as a zoonotic disease spread by bloodsucking arthropods or by direct contact with infected animal material. Tularemia in humans may occur in ulceroglandular or typhoidal forms, depending on the route of exposure. Ulceroglandular tularemia is more common, occurring after skin or mucous membrane exposure to infected animal blood or tissues. Patients develop a local ulcer with associated lymphadenopathy, fever, chills, headache, and malaise. Typhoidal tularemia presents with fever, prostration, and weight loss without adenopathy. Exposure to aerosolized bacteria, as employed in BW, will most likely result in typhoidal tularemia with prominent respiratory symptoms such as a nonproductive cough and substernal chest discomfort. Diagnosing tularemia is often difficult, as the organism is hard to isolate by culture and the symptoms are nonspecific. Chest radiography may demonstrate infiltrates, mediastinal lymphadenopathy, or pleural effusions.[28,33,35,58]

Antibiotic treatment options are again similar to those for anthrax and plague. In mass-casualty settings, or for postexposure prophylaxis, adults are treated with doxycycline 100 mg twice daily or ciprofloxacin 500 mg orally twice daily for 14 days; pediatric dosing for doxycycline is 2.2 mg/kg or ciprofloxacin 15 mg/kg (maximum = adult dose) twice daily. When dealing with a limited number of casualties, the preferred antibiotics are streptomycin 1 g IM twice daily, or gentamicin 5 mg/kg IM/IV once daily. Alternatives include parenteral doxycycline, chloramphenicol, and ciprofloxacin.[28]

Brucellosis Brucellosis could potentially be used as an incapacitating BW agent, because it causes disease with low mortality but significant morbidity. Indeed, the initial attraction of brucellosis as a weapon was its ability to induce chronic disease.[65] Brucellae (*Brucella melitensis, abortus, suis,* and *canis*) are small, aerobic, Gram-negative coccobacilli that generally cause disease in ruminant livestock. Humans develop brucellosis by ingesting contaminated meat and dairy products or by aerosol transmission from infected animals. The United States weaponized *B. suis* and other countries are also believed to have developed *Brucella* bioweapons. Brucellosis commonly presents with nonspecific symptoms such as fever, chills, and malaise, with either an acute or insidious onset. Because brucellae are facultative intracellular parasites that localize in the lung, spleen, liver, CNS, bone marrow, and synovium, organ-specific signs and symptoms may occur. Diagnosis is made by serologic methods or culture. Because single-drug treatment often results in relapse, combined therapy is indicated. Treatments of choice (adult doses) are doxycycline 200 mg/d orally, plus rifampin 600–900 mg/d orally for 6 weeks, or doxycycline 200 mg/d orally for 6 weeks with either streptomycin 15 mg/kg twice daily IM or gentamicin 1.5 mg/kg IM q8h for the first 10 days.[35,44,58]

Rickettsiae Features of rickettsiae favoring their use as BW agents include environmental stability, aerosol transmission, persistence in infected hosts, low infectious dose, and high associated morbidity and mortality. Rickettsiae that have been weaponized include *Coxiella burnetti*, the causative organism of Q Fever, and *Rickettsia prowazekii*, the causative organism of louseborne typhus. Release of *R. prowazekii* into a crowded louse-infested population might induce a typhus outbreak with rapid transmission and high mortality.[4]

Q Fever Q fever was first described in 1937, and was given its name—Q for "query"—because the causative organism was not then known. Q fever occurs naturally as a self-limited febrile, zoonotic disease contracted from domestic livestock. Q fever is now known to be caused by *Coxiella burnetti*, a unique rickettsia-like organism that can persist on inanimate objects for weeks to months and can cause clinical disease with the inhalation of only a single organism. These features are of obvious benefit for use as a potential BW agent. After a 10- to 40-day incubation period, Q fever manifests as an undifferentiated febrile illness, with headache, fatigue, and myalgias. Patchy pulmonary infiltrates on chest radiography that resemble viral or atypical bacterial pneumonia occur in 50% of cases, although only half of patients have cough and even fewer have pleuritic chest pain. Uncommon complications include hepatitis, endocarditis, meningitis, encephalitis, and osteomyelitis. Patients are generally not critically ill, and the disease can last as long as 2 weeks. Treatment with antibiotics will shorten the course of acute Q fever and can prevent clinically evident disease when given during the incubation period. Tetracyclines are the mainstay of therapy, and either tetracycline 500 mg PO q6h or doxycycline 100 mg PO q12h should be given for 5–7 days.[13,35]

VIRUSES

Smallpox Smallpox is caused by the variola virus, a large DNA orthopoxvirus with a host range limited to humans. Prior to global World Health Organization (WHO) efforts to eradicate naturally occurring smallpox by immunization, recurrent epidemics were common and the disease carried roughly a 30% fatality rate in unvaccinated populations.[43,55] Smallpox is highly contagious. Outbreaks during the 1960s and 1970s in Europe often resulted in 10–20 secondary cases per index case. One German smallpox patient with a cough, isolated in a single room, infected persons on three floors of a hospital.[43] The overwhelming majority of secondary infections, however, occur among close family contacts, especially those sleeping in the same room or even in the same bed.[30]

In 1980, the United Nations' WHO certified that smallpox had been eradicated from the world, and recommended ceasing vaccinations and either destroying or transferring remaining stocks of variola virus to one of two designated biosafety level 4 facilities: the CDC in Atlanta, or the Russian State Research Center of Virology and Biotechnology.[11] All remaining known variola stocks were scheduled for destruction in 1999; however, before this was done, a WHO resolution called for a delay based on an Institute of Medicine report concluding that live virus should be retained to develop new antiviral agents or vaccines to protect against any potential future release of smallpox.[76] The Soviet Union is known to have weaponized smallpox, and other countries are believed to maintain stocks of variola virus. In addition to the known stockpiles of smallpox vaccine, several types of new vaccines are being produced.[66,87] Smallpox vaccination for military personnel was reinstated in 2002 and was made available for some civilians in 2003.[24,25]

Pathophysiology. Transmission of smallpox typically occurs through inhalation of droplets or aerosols, but may also occur through contaminated fomites. The infectious dose is not known, but is probably only a few virions. After a 12- to 14-day incubation period, the patient develops fever, malaise, and prostration with headache and backache. Oropharyngeal lesions appear, shedding virus into the saliva. Two to three days after the onset of fever, a papular rash develops on the face and spreads to the extremities. The fever continues while the rash becomes vesicular and then pustular. Scabs form from the pustules and eventually separate, leaving pitted and hypopigmented scars. Deaths usually occur during the second week of the illness. Vaccination before exposure, or within 2–3 days after exposure, provides almost complete protection against smallpox. The disease most likely to be confused with smallpox is chickenpox (varicella). Although the individual lesions of smallpox and varicella are physically indistinguishable, the person infected with smallpox may still be differentiated clinically. The lesions of smallpox should all appear at the same stage of development (synchronous), whereas chickenpox lesions occur at varying stages (asynchronous). Smallpox lesions tend to be found in a centrifugal distribution (face and distal extremities), whereas chickenpox lesions are more centripetal and tend to appear first on the trunk.

Two antiviral drugs commercially available in the United States, cidofovir and ribavirin, are effective in vitro against variola.[58] Current evidence suggests, however, that although cidofovir may prevent smallpox when given within 1 or 2 days of exposure, it is unlikely to be effective once symptoms develop.[43] Even a single case of smallpox should be considered a potential international health emergency and immediately reported to the appropriate public health authorities.

Smallpox Vaccination. Rapid postexposure vaccination confers excellent protection against smallpox. The smallpox vaccine employs a live vaccinia virus (derived from cowpox vaccine) rather than the actual variola virus that causes smallpox. Although contracting smallpox from the vaccine is therefore impossible, other adverse reactions may occur. The two most serious reactions are postvaccinal encephalitis and progressive vaccinia. Postvaccinal encephalitis occurs in about three cases per million primary vaccinees. Forty percent of cases are fatal, and some survivors are left with permanent neurologic sequelae. Progressive vaccinia can occur in immunosuppressed individuals and is treated with vaccinia immune globulin (VIG).[87] Another historically common complication of smallpox vaccination was ocular vaccinia, which typically occurred among healthcare personnel administering vaccine when it was inadvertently placed in the eye. Ocular vaccinia is also treated with VIG. Because smallpox was eradicated before the emergence of HIV, there is limited clinical experience with smallpox vaccination in AIDS patients, who theoretically are at increased risk of progressive vaccinia.[43,55] However, among 10 individuals with undiagnosed HIV at the time of recent smallpox vaccination, none developed complications.[79] Routine vaccination is contraindicated in the immunosuppressed, persons with a history or evidence of eczema and other chronic dermatitis, close household or sexual contacts of patients with these contraindications, and during pregnancy. Because the vaccine is a live virus, it can be transmitted from the vaccinee to close contacts. Thirty secondary and tertiary cases of vaccinia were reported resulting from recent US military vaccinations.[24] The number of serious adverse events from modern smallpox vaccination is very low;[25] however, rare cardiac complications not reported in previous decades were noted with the recent re-institution of smallpox vaccination in the early 2000s. More than one million military vaccinations by 2006 resulted in 120 cases of myopericarditis, while 21 cases of myopericarditis occurred among nearly 40,000 civilian vaccine recipients between 2002 and 2003.[66] The number of cardiac ischemic events among vaccinees was not significantly higher than age-matched controls. After a true exposure to variola, most authorities would agree that the only absolute contraindication to smallpox vaccination is significant impairment of systemic immunity. Concomitant administration of VIG would be recommended for pregnant women and persons with eczema.[55]

Viral Hemorrhagic Fevers Several taxonomically diverse RNA viruses produce acute febrile illnesses characterized by malaise, prostration, and increased vascular permeability that can result in bleeding manifestations in the more severely affected patients. Viral hemorrhagic fevers (VHF) are all highly infectious by the aerosol route, making them candidates for use as BW agents. These agents include the viruses causing Lassa fever, dengue, yellow fever, Crimean-Congo hemorrhagic fever, and the Marburg, Ebola, and Hanta viruses. Clinical features, such as the extent of renal, hepatic, and hematologic involvement, vary according to the infectious agent, but they all carry the risk of secondary infection through droplet aerosols. Ribavirin has been used for some VHFs, but supportive care is the mainstay of therapy.[9,35,47]

Viral Encephalitides Three antigenically related alpha viruses of the *Togaviridae* family pose risks as BW agents: western equine encephalitis (WEE), eastern equine encephalitis (EEE), and Venezuelan equine encephalitis (VEE). Birds are the natural reservoir of these viruses, and natural outbreaks occur among equines and humans by mosquito transmission. Eastern equine encephalitis infections are the most severe in humans, with a 50%–70% fatality rate and high incidence of neurologic sequelae among survivors. WEE is less neurologically invasive, and severe encephalitis from VEE is rare, except in children. Adults infected with VEE usually develop an acute, febrile, incapacitating disease with prolonged recovery. The equine encephalitides have many properties helpful for weaponization, in that they can be produced in large quantities, they are relatively stable and highly infectious to humans as aerosols, and a choice is available between lethal or incapacitating infections.[77]

Venezuelan equine encephalitis is considered the most likely BW threat among the viral encephalitides. After a 1- to 5-day incubation period, victims experience the sudden onset of malaise, myalgias, prostration, spiking fevers, rigors, severe headache, and photophobia. Nausea, vomiting, cough, sore throat, and diarrhea may follow. This acute phase lasts 24–72 hours. Between 0.5% and 4% of cases develop overt encephalitis, with meningismus, seizures, coma, and paralysis, which carries up to a 20% fatality rate. The diagnosis is usually established clinically, although the virus can sometimes be isolated from serum or from throat swabs, and serologic tests are available. The white blood cell count often shows a striking leukopenia and lymphopenia. Treatment is supportive. Person-to-person transmission can theoretically occur from droplet nuclei. Recovery takes 1–2 weeks.[35,77]

TOXINS

Several toxins derived from bacteria, plants, fungi, and algae could theoretically be used as BW agents, if produced in sufficient quantities. Because of their high potency, only small amounts of these agents would be needed to kill or incapacitate exposed victims. Fortunately, obstacles in manufacturing weaponizable amounts limit the number of toxins that are practical for use as biological weapons. Discussion here is limited to those toxins known or highly suspected to have been weaponized. Toxins themselves are not living organisms and therefore can not reproduce; for this reason, they are arguably equivalent to chemical weapons. But because toxin weapons are derived from living organisms, they are categorized here as biological weapons.

Botulinum Toxin Botulinum toxin has been developed as a biological weapon in the United States and other countries.[2,64,75,88] The two most likely means of employing botulism as a BW agent are by food contamination or by aerosol. Either method would result in the clinical syndrome of botulism (Chap. 46), characterized by multiple bulbar nerve palsies and a symmetric descending paralysis, ending in death from respiratory failure. Inhalation botulism from laboratory incidents has occurred rarely in humans and has also been investigated in animal experiments.[60]

Ricin Ricin is derived from the castor bean plant (*Ricinus communis*) and is the only biological toxin to exist naturally in macroscopic quantities, comprising 1%–5% of the beans by weight.[10] Its easy accessability, relative ease of preparation, and low cost may make ricin an attractive biological weapon for terrorists or poor countries.[68] Although ricin has never been used in battle, it has attracted the attention of domestic extremists and terrorists and has been used in politically motivated assassinations.[3,27,34] Ricin is a glycoprotein lectin (or toxalbumin) composed of two protein chains linked by a disulfide bond. The B chain facilitates cell binding and entry of the A chain into cells. The A chain inhibits protein synthesis, inactivating eukaryotic ribosomes by removing an adenine residue from ribosomal RNA.[3]

Clinical toxicity from ricin will vary depending on the dose and route of exposure. Inhalation of aerosolized ricin results in increased alveolar-capillary permeability and airway necrosis following a latent phase of 4–8 hours. Ingestion causes gastrointestinal hemorrhage with necrosis of the liver, spleen, and kidney. Intramuscular administration produces severe local necrosis with extension into the lymphatics. In the absence of specific immunologic testing, differentiating ricin poisoning from sepsis may be difficult, because of the presence of leukocytosis and fever. Vaccination of laboratory animals with an investigational toxoid is protective.[34]

Staphylococcal Enterotoxin B Staphylococcal enterotoxin B (SEB) is one of seven enterotoxins produced by *Staphylococcus aureus*. SEB is recognized as a "superantigen," because of its profound activation of the immune system on exposure to even minute quantities. As a BW agent, SEB could be ingested through contaminated food or water, resulting in acute gastroenteritis identical to classic staphylococcal food poisoning. If inhaled as an aerosol, SEB produces fever, myalgias, and a pneumonitis after a 3- to 12-hour latent period. SEB inhalation can be fatal, but more often would simply be incapacitating for several days to weeks. Treatment is supportive.[82]

Trichothecene Mycotoxins The trichothecene mycotoxins are low-molecular-weight (250–500 Da) nonvolatile compounds produced by filamentous fungi (molds) of various genera, including *Fusarium, Myrothecium, Phomopsis, Trichoderma, Tricothecium*, and *Stachybotrys*.[6,83] Tricothecene mycotoxins are unusual among potential BW agents in that toxicity can occur with exposure to intact skin. Naturally occurring trichothecene toxicity results from ingesting contaminated grains or by inhaling toxin aerosolized from contaminated hay or cotton. Outbreaks of ingested trichothecene toxins result in a clinical syndrome called alimentary toxic aleukia, characterized by gastroenteritis, fevers, chills, bone marrow suppression with granulocytopenia, and secondary sepsis—a syndrome similar to acute radiation poisoning. Survival beyond this stage is characterized by the development of GI and upper airway ulceration, and intradermal and mucosal hemorrhage. Trichothecene toxins are potent inhibitors of protein synthesis in eukaryotic cells, producing widespread cytotoxicity, particularly in rapidly proliferating tissues; different tricothecene toxins interfere with initiation, elongation, and termination stages of protein synthesis.[6] Exposure to any mucosal surface results in severe irritation. Dermal exposure can produce inflammatory lesions lasting for 1–2 weeks, vesiculation, and, in higher doses, death.[83]

Several reports from the 1970s and 1980s suggested that Soviet-supported forces were using trichothecene mycotoxins, particularly the toxin T-2 (Fig. 132–2), as BW agents. Aerosol and droplet clouds called Yellow Rain were associated with mass casualty incidents in southeast Asia.[83] Such incidents would involve multiple routes of exposure, with skin deposition likely being the major site. Early symptoms included nausea, vomiting, weakness, dizziness, and ataxia. Diarrhea would then ensue, at first watery and then becoming bloody. Within 3–12 hours victims would develop dyspnea, cough, chest pain, sore mouths, bleeding gums, epistaxis, and hematemesis. Exposed skin areas would become intensely inflamed, with the appearance of vesicles, bullae, petechiae, ecchymoses, and frank necrosis.[83]

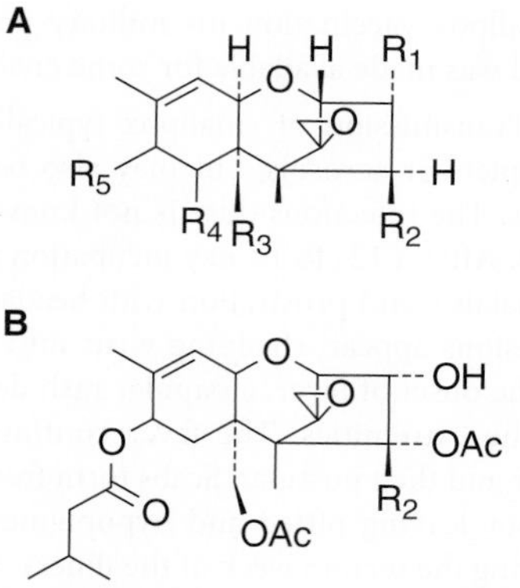

FIGURE 132–2. Trichothecene mycotoxins. (A) Tetracyclic trichothecene nucleus (B) T-2 toxin.

Nonetheless, evidence that trichothecene mycotoxins were used as BW agents was mostly circumstantial. Although T-2 toxin was found in victims' blood and urine, it was also found in samples from unexposed individuals, probably from baseline ingestion of contaminated foods. Environmental samples containing Yellow Rain droplets were inconsistently found to contain mycotoxins. Eyewitness accounts of Yellow Rain attacks varied widely (including various descriptions of the alleged agent's color), and, despite the large number of such attacks, no contaminated ordinance or dispersal device was ever recovered.[74] It was also discovered that Yellow Rain droplets were composed mostly of pollen grains. Supporters of the Yellow Rain as BW theory retorted that pollen grains would be an ideal carrier for biotoxins, given that their size is ideal for aerosolization. However, the pollen in Yellow Rain samples did not contain protein, similar to pollen that has been digested by bees. Further, the distribution of pollen species found in Yellow Rain was indistinguishable from the contents of feces of the Asian honeybee, and mass bee defecation resulting in showers of yellow droplets has been observed.[74] The Yellow Rain as bee feces theory assumes that any mass-casualty incidents were from endemic disease outbreaks, other CBW agents not yet identified, or a combination of both.

FUNGI AND OTHER FUNGAL TOXINS

Fungi may at first appear to be ideal BW agents, given their relative ease of handling, dissemination, and resistance of spores to physical stressors.[14] The only fungi to be included on lists of microbes with potential use as biological weapons are *Coccidioides* species, probably based on the high incidence of symptomatic infection in endemic areas. Nevertheless, the risk of serious disease is low, limiting the utility of *Coccidioides* as an effective weapon.[14,67]

Fungal toxins considered to have potential use as biological weapons include tricothecene mycotoxins (above), aflatoxins, and amanita toxins. Although α-amanitin is extremely potent, water soluble, and heat stabile, its use as a weapon would be limited by difficulties in mass production.[67] Aflatoxin would be ineffective on the battlefield, since its acute toxicity is uncertain and the carcinogenetic potential is too delayed.[6] Both of these agents may, however, still be effective as terror agents.

SUMMARY

Although biological weapons have been used intermittently for centuries, only recently has their danger in potentially causing mass casualties been commonly recognized. Even with multinational bans against their development and use, the threat of biological weapons remains because the financial outlay in developing biological weapons is low compared to other weapons of mass destruction, and because even the threat of their use may aid some parties in furthering their political goals. Currently, the risk of a medical catastrophe from BW agents producing thousands or millions of victims appears low, with inhalational anthrax or smallpox being the most likely agents in such a scenario. Nevertheless, incidents with limited numbers of casualties, or just threats of employing BW agents, can have significant social impact.

REFERENCES

1. Aldhous P. Gruinard Island handed back. *Nature*. 1990;344:801.
2. Arnon SS, Schechter R, Inglesby TV, et al. Botulinum toxin as a biological weapon: medical and public health management. *JAMA*. 2001;285:1059-1070.
3. Audi J, Belson M, Patel M, et al. Ricin poisoning: a comprehensive review. *JAMA*. 2005;294:2342-2351.
4. Azad AF. Pathogenic rickettsiae as bioterrorism agents. *Clin Infect Dis*. 2007;45:S52-55.
5. Barakat LA, Quentzel HL, Jernigan JA, et al. Fatal inhalational anthrax in a 94-year-old Connecticut woman. *JAMA*. 2002;287:863-868.
6. Bennett JW, Klich M. Mycotoxins. *Clin Microbiol Rev*. 2003;16:497-516.
7. Bernstein BJ. The birth of the US biological-warfare program. *Sci Am*. 1987;256:116-121.
8. Borio L, Frank D, Mani V, et al. Death due to bioterrorism-related inhalational anthrax: report of 2 patients. *JAMA*. 2001;286:2554-2559.
9. Borio L, Inglesby T, Peters CJ, et al. Hemorrhagic fever viruses as biological weapons: medical and public health management. *JAMA*. 2002;287:2391-2405.
10. Bradberry SM, Dickers KJ, Rice P, et al. Ricin poisoning. *Toxicol Rev*. 2003;22:65-70.
11. Bremen JG, Henderson DA. Poxvirus dilemmas—monkeypox, smallpox, and biologic terrorism. *N Engl J Med*. 1998;339:556-559.
12. Bush LM, Abrams BH, Beall A, et al. Index case of fatal inhalational anthrax due to bioterrorism in the United States. *N Engl J Med*. 2001;345:1607-1610.
13. Byrne WR. Fever Q. In: Sidell FR, Takafuji ET, Franz DR (eds). *Medical Aspects of Chemical and Biological Warfare*. Washington, DC: Office of the Surgeon General; 1997:523-537.
14. Casadevall A, Pirofski LA. The weapon potential of human pathogenic fungi. *Med Mycol*. 2006;44:689-696.
15. Centers for Disease Control and Prevention. Bioterrorism alleging use of anthrax and interim guidelines for management—United States 1998. *MMWR Mort Morbid Wkly Rep*. 1999;48:69-74.
16. Centers for Disease Control and Prevention. Suspected brucellosis case prompts investigation of possible bioterrorism-related activity—New Hampshire and Massachusetts 1999. *MMWR Morbid Mortal Wkly Rep*. 2000;49:509-512.
17. Centers for Disease Control and Prevention. Biological and chemical terrorism: strategic plan for preparedness and response. *MMWR Morbid Mortal Wkly Rep*. 2000;49(RR04):1-14.
18. Centers for Disease Control and Prevention. Public health message regarding anthrax case. October 4, 2001. Available from http://www.cdc.gov/od/oc/media/pressrel/r011004.htm. Accessed May 6, 2008.
19. Centers for Disease Control and Prevention. Update: public health message regarding Florida anthrax case. October 7, 2001. Available from http://www.cdc.gov/od/oc/media/pressrel/r011007.htm. Accessed May 6, 2008.
20. Centers for Disease Control and Prevention. Update: public health message regarding anthrax. October 12, 2001. Available from http://www.cdc.gov/od/oc/media/pressrel/r011012.htm. Accessed May 6, 2008.
21. Centers for Disease Control and Prevention. Update: investigation of bioterrorism-related anthrax and adverse events from antimicrobial prophylaxis. *MMWR Morbid Mortal Wkly Rep*. 2001;50:973-976.
22. Centers for Disease Control and Prevention. Notice to readers: considerations for distinguishing influenza-like illness from inhalational anthrax. *MMWR Morbid Mortal Wkly Rep*. 2001;50:984-986.
23. Centers for Disease Control and Prevention. Update: cutaneous anthrax in a laboratory worker—Texas 2002. *MMWR Morbid Mortal Wkly Rep*. 2002;51:482.
24. Centers for Disease Control and Prevention. Secondary and tertiary transfer of vaccinia virus among US military personnel—United States and worldwide 2002-2004. *MMWR Morbid Mortal Wkly Rep*. 2004;53:103-105.
25. Centers for Disease Control and Prevention. Update: adverse events following civilian smallpox vaccination—United States 2004. *MMWR Morbid Mortal Wkly Rep*. 2004;53:106-107.
26. Christopher GW, Cieslak TJ, Pavlin JA, Eitzen EM. Biological warfare. A historical perspective. *JAMA*. 1997;278:412-417.
27. Crompton R, Gall D. Georgi Markov—death in a pellet. *Med Leg J*. 1980;48:51-62.
28. Dennis DT, Inglesby TV, Henderson DA, et al. Tularemia as a biological weapon: medical and public health management. *JAMA*. 2001;285:2763-2773.
29. Dixon TC, Meselson M, Guillemin J, Hanna PC. Anthrax. *N Engl J Med*. 1999;314:815-826.
30. Eichner M: Case isolation and contact tracing can prevent the spread of smallpox. *Am J Epidemiol*. 2003;158:118-128.
31. Eitzen EM. Education is the key to defense against bioterrorism. *Ann Emerg Med*. 1999;34:221-223.
32. Eitzen EM, Takafuji ET. Historical overview of biological warfare. In: Sidell FR, Takafuji ET, Franz DR, eds. *Medical Aspects of Chemical and Biological Warfare*. Washington, DC: Office of the Surgeon General; 1997:415-423.
33. Evans ME, Friedlander AM. Tularemia. In: Sidell FR, Takafuji ET, Franz DR, eds. *Medical Aspects of Chemical and Biological Warfare*. Washington, DC: Office of the Surgeon General; 1997:503-512.
34. Franz DR, Jaax NK. Ricin toxin. In: Sidell FR, Takafuji ET, Franz DR, eds. *Medical Aspects of Chemical and Biological Warfare*. Washington, DC: Office of the Surgeon General; 1997:631-642.
35. Franz DR, Jahrling PB, Friedlander AM, et al. Clinical recognition and management of patients exposed to biological warfare agents. *JAMA*. 1997;278:399-411.
36. Freedman A, Afonja O, Chang MW, et al. Cutaneous anthrax associated with microangiopathic hemolytic anemia and coagulopathy in a 7-month-old infant. *JAMA*. 2002;287:869-874.
37. Friedlander AM. Anthrax. In: Sidell FR, Takafuji ET, Franz DR, eds. *Medical Aspects of Chemical and Biological Warfare*. Washington, DC: Office of the Surgeon General; 1997:467-478.
38. Friedlander AM, Pittman PR, Parker GW. Anthrax vaccine: evidence for safety and efficacy against inhalational anthrax. *JAMA*. 1999;282:2104-2106.
39. Grabenstein JD. Countering anthrax: vaccines and immunoglobulins. *Clin Infect Dis*. 2008;46:129-136.
40. Grunow R, Finke EJ. A procedure for differentiating between the intentional release of biological warfare agents and natural outbreaks of disease: its use in analyzing the tularemia outbreak in Kosovo in 1999 and 2000. *Clin Microbiol Infect*. 2002;8:510-521.
41. Harris S. Japanese biological warfare research on humans: a case study of microbiology and ethics. *Ann NY Acad Sci*. 1992;666:21-52.
42. Henderson DA. The looming threat of bioterrorism. *Science*. 1999;283:1279-1282.
43. Henderson DA, Inglesby TV, Bartlett JG, et al. Smallpox as a biological weapon: medical and public health management. *JAMA*. 1999;281:2127-2137.
44. Hoover DL, Friedlander AM. Brucellosis. In: Sidell FR, Takafuji ET, Franz DR, eds. *Medical Aspects of Chemical and Biological Warfare*. Washington, DC: Office of the Surgeon General; 1997:513-521.
45. Inglesby TV, Dennis DT, Henderson DA, et al. Plague as a biological weapon: medical and public health management. *JAMA*. 2000;283:2281-2290.
46. Inglesby TV, O'Toole T, Henderson DA, et al. Anthrax as a biological weapon 2002: updated recommendations for management. *JAMA*. 2002;287:2236-2252.

47. Jahrling PB. Viral hemorrhagic fevers. In: Sidell FR, Takafuji ET, Franz DR, eds. *Medical Aspects of Chemical and Biological Warfare.* Washington, DC: Office of the Surgeon General; 1997:591-602.
48. Jernigan JA, Stephens DS, Ashford DA, et al. Bioterrorism-related inhalational anthrax: the first 10 cases reported in the United States. *Emerg Infect Dis.* 2001;7:933-944.
49. Kaufmann AF, Meltzer MI, Schmid GP. The economic impact of a bioterrorist attack: are prevention and postattack intervention programs justifiable? *Emerg Infect Dis.* 1997;3:83-94.
50. Keim M, Kaufmann AF. Principles for emergency response to bioterrorism. *Ann Emerg Med.* 1999;34:177-182.
51. Knudson GB. Operation Desert Shield: medical aspects of weapons of mass destruction. *Mil Med.* 1991;156:267-271.
52. Lampe KF. Rhododendrons, mountain laurel, and mad honey. *JAMA.* 1988;259:2009.
53. Manchee RJ, Broster MG, Melling BJ, et al. Bacillus anthracis on Gruinard Island. *Nature.* 1981;294:254-255.
54. Mayer TA, Bersoff-Matcha S, Murphy C, et al. Clinical presentation of inhalational anthrax following bioterrorism exposure: report of 2 surviving patients. *JAMA.* 2001;286:2549-2553.
55. McClain DJ. Smallpox. In: Sidell FR, Takafuji ET, Franz DR (eds). *Medical Aspects of Chemical and Biological Warfare.* Washington, DC: Office of the Surgeon General; 1997:539-559.
56. McGovern TW, Christopher GW, Eitzen EM. Cutaneous manifestations of biological warfare and related threat agents. *Arch Dermatol.* 1999;135:311-322.
57. McGovern TW, Friedlander AM. Plague. In: Sidell FR, Takafuji ET, Franz DR, eds. *Medical Aspects of Chemical and Biological Warfare.* Washington, DC: Office of the Surgeon General; 1997:479-502.
58. Med Lett Drugs Ther. Ed. Abramowicz M. Drugs and vaccines against biological weapons. 1999;41:15-16.
59. Meselson M, Guillemin J, Hugh-Jones M, et al. The Sverdlovsk anthrax outbreak of 1979. *Science.* 1994;266:1202-1208.
60. Middlebrook JL, Franz DR. Botulinum toxins. In: Sidell FR, Takafuji ET, Franz DR, eds. *Medical Aspects of Chemical and Biological Warfare.* Washington, DC: Office of the Surgeon General; 1997:643-654.
61. Mina B, Dym JP, Kuepper F, et al. Fatal inhalational anthrax with unknown source of exposure in a 61-year-old woman in New York City. *JAMA.* 2001;287:858-862.
62. Neuwinger HD. *African Ethnobotany-Poisons and Drugs: Chemistry, Pharmacology, Toxicology.* New York: Chapman and Hall; 1996.
63. Noah DL, Sobel AL, Ostroff SM, Kildew JA. Biological warfare training: infectious disease outbreak differentiation criteria. *Mil Med.* 1998;163:198-201.
64. Olson KB. Aum Shinrikyo: once and future threat? *Emerg Infect Dis.* 1999;5:513-516.
65. Pappas G, Panagopoulou P, Christou L, Akritidis N. Brucella as a biological weapon. *Cell Mol Life Sci.* 2006;63:2229-2236.
66. Parrino J, Graham BS. Smallpox vaccines: past, present, and future. *J Allergy Clin Immunol.* 200;118:1320-1326.
67. Paterson RR. Fungi and fungal toxins as weapons. *Mycol Res.* 2006;110: 1003-1010.
68. Patočka J, Středa L. Protein biotoxins of military significance. *Acta Medica (Hradec Králové).* 2006;49:3-11.
69. Prentice MB, Rahalison L. Plague. *Lancet.* 2007;369:1196-1207.
70. Redmond C, Pearce MJ, Manchee RJ, Berdal BP. Deadly relic of the Great War. *Nature.* 1998;393:747-748.
71. Reuters. NY outbreak not work of terrorists, experts say. *LA Times.* October 12, 1999, p. A21.
72. Richards CF, Burstein JL, Waeckerle JF, Hutson HR. Emergency physicians and biological terrorism. *Ann Emerg Med.* 1999;34:183-190.
73. Robertson AG, Robertson LJ. From asps to allegations: biological warfare in history. *Mil Med.* 1995;160:369-373.
74. Seeley TD, Nowicke JW, Meselson M, et al. Yellow rain. *Sci Am.* 1985;253: 128-137.
75. Seelos C. Lessons from Iraq on bioweapons. *Nature.* 1999;398:187-188.
76. Shalala DE. Smallpox: setting the research agenda. *Science.* 1999;285:1011.
77. Smith JF, Davis K, Hart MK, et al. Viral encephalitides. In: Sidell FR, Takafuji ET, Franz DR, eds. *Medical Aspects of Chemical and Biological Warfare.* Washington, DC: Office of the Surgeon General; 1997: 561-589.
78. Takahashi H, Keim P, Kaufmann AF, et al. Bacillus anthracis incident, Kameido, Tokyo 1993. *Emerg Infect Dis.* 2004;10:117-120.
79. Tasker SA, Schnepf GA, Lim M, et al. Unintended smallpox vaccination of HIV-1-infected individuals in the United States military. *Clin Infect Dis.* 2004;38:1320-1322.
80. Török TJ, Tauxe RV, Wise RP, et al. A large community outbreak of salmonellosis caused by intentional contamination of restaurant salad bars. *JAMA.* 1997;278:389-395.
81. Trevisanato SI. The 'Hittite plague', an epidemic of tularemia and the first record of biological warfare. *Med Hypoth.* 2007:69:1371-1374.
82. Ulrich RG, Sidell S, Taylor TJ, et al. Staphylococcal enterotoxin B and related pyrogenic toxins. In: Sidell FR, Takafuji ET, Franz DR, eds. *Medical Aspects of Chemical and Biological Warfare.* Washington, DC: Office of the Surgeon General; 1997:621-630.
83. Wannemacher RW, Wiener SL. Trichothecene mycotoxins. In: Sidell FR, Takafuji ET, Franz DR, eds. *Medical Aspects of Chemical and Biological Warfare.* Washington, DC: Office of the Surgeon General; 1997:655-676.
84. Weinstein RS, Alibek K. *Biological and Chemical Terrorism.* New York: Thieme Medical Publishers; 2003.
85. Wheelis M. First shots fired in biological warfare. *Nature.* 1998;395:213.
86. Wheelis M. Biological warfare at the 1346 siege of Caffa. *Emerg Infect Dis.* 2002;8:971-975.
87. Wittek R. Vaccinia immune globulin: current policies, preparedness, and product safety and efficacy. *Int J Infect Dis.* 2006;10:193-201.
88. Zilinskas RA. Iraq's biological weapons: the past as future? *JAMA.* 1997;278:418-424.
89. Zoon KC. Vaccines, pharmaceutical products, and bioterrorism: challenges for the US Food and Drug Administration. *Emerg Infect Dis.* 1999;5:534-536.

CHAPTER 133
RADIATION

Joseph G. Rella

Over the last century, radiation injuries and the nature of radiation itself have been vigorously studied as a result of its expanding role in our society. Today, radionuclides are used for a wide variety of medical and nonmedical purposes ranging from detecting smoke to diagnostic testing to powering spacecraft. Although useful, radionuclides can present a danger to humans both through their metallic nature and through the process of radioactive decay. This ionizing radiation may cause injury to multiple cellular structures and critical molecules, such as DNA, resulting in mutations, neoplasms, or cell death. The particles of radiation, their sources, and the mechanisms by which they pose a health risk are the subjects of the following discussion.

HISTORICAL EXPOSURES

Radiation became a concern for scientists as a toxin only a year following the discovery of x-rays by Wilhelm Roentgen in 1895.[91] Soon after, Thomas Edison reported corneal injuries in several of his workers conducting experiments using his newly invented x-ray generator. Eight years later, Clarence Dally, one of Edison's most dependable assistants, became the first radiation-related death in the United States.[32] Fortunately, the medical community recognized the utility of Edison's fluoroscope and began to use x-ray machines to help diagnose various illnesses. For example, the British army developed and used mobile x-ray machines to find bullets and shrapnel in wounded soldiers in Sudan in the early 1900s.

Over the next 10–15 years, radioactive substances also found their way into society as objects of fascination and as a means of alternative medical therapies. Aggressively marketed as "cure-alls," advertisements for products such as the Revigator and Radithor enticed people to drink water "charged" with radon or radium. These products ushered in 20 years of "health" products containing radioactive materials.[60,61]

In 1915, the British Roentgen Society, recognizing the potential hazards of radiation, proposed standards for radiation protection of workers, which included shielding, restricted work hours, and medical examinations. Unfortunately, no dose limits were implemented because dose quantitation was unavailable.

The opening of the Radium Luminous Materials Corporation in Orange, New Jersey, in 1917 represented the first of several companies to profit from the novelty and popularity of the bluish glow of radium. In an industry that employed over 4000 workers at its peak, nearly all of whom were women, the radium was hand-painted onto watch and instrument dials. These young women were instructed to obtain a fine tip on their paintbrushes using a technique called "lip pointing," which meant using their lips and tongues to shape their paintbrushes. Unaware of the danger, some of these women also painted their nails, lips, and eyelids with the radioactive paint. By 1927, about 100 of them died from osteosarcoma of the jaw, brain tumors, and developed other noncancerous lesions of the mouth, all related to radium exposure.[63,74]

The only occasions nuclear bombs were used against humans occurred in August 1945 when the United States dropped bombs on Hiroshima and Nagasaki, Japan.[30] One contained a uranium core and liberated energy equivalent to 12,500 tons of TNT. The other contained a plutonium core and liberated an energy equivalent to 20,000 tons of TNT. Estimates of dead and injured for both cities are well over 200,000.[38] Most of the deaths were from the bomb blast, but many thousands died from acute radiation syndrome (ARS) and subsequently from radiation-induced cancers. In addition to the people of those cities who were victims of the bombs, at least 20,000 men and women from Britain, Australia, New Zealand, and India who formed the British Commonwealth Occupation Forces (BCOF) were also exposed to residual radiation as they were involved in security and clean-up tasks. Published memoirs even include photographs of Australian soldiers playing football on the flattened hypocenter of Hiroshima. Data concerning the health effects of the BCOF in postwar Japan are less well known than those reported by the British Nuclear Tests Veterans Association (BNTVA). The BNTVA is a group of 20,000 men who were required to attend United Kingdom nuclear weapons tests in Australia and at Christmas Island between 1952 and 1963. Over two thirds of this cohort died of neoplasms at ages of 50–65 years, irrespective of the individual's age at the time of the witnessed explosion.[83,84] Since that time there have been thousands of nuclear bomb tests around the world in the atmosphere, underground, and underwater.

With the beginning of the nuclear age also came unintentional criticality events of varying kinds in which individuals were exposed to large amounts of radiation. Criticality refers to the chain reaction of fissionable atoms that results in the release of energy. It is the basic operating principle behind fission bombs and nuclear reactors and is an efficient means of generating energy. Two criticality events occurred in Los Alamos in the 1940s during experiments in which scientists performed what was called "tickling the dragon." In that era, determining the amount of fissionable material necessary to precipitate a chain reaction was not precisely defined mathematically. Harry Daghlian and Louis Slotin, two scientists involved in the development of the first atomic bomb, were to bring subcritical amounts of fissionable material together to see if a reaction would occur. Both men died of acute radiation sickness (ARS) following exposure to high levels of radiation released during these experiments. Since 1945 numerous criticality events have occurred, the most recent in Tokaimura, Japan in 1999. In that instance, workers making fuel for nuclear reactors allowed excess uranium to enter the reaction container. The criticality event that resulted killed one worker and caused the evacuation of all the people living within 350 meters of the manufacturing plant.

During the late 1920s, radiologists used a thorium-containing contrast agent called Thorotrast. During that time when imaging modalities were limited, this opacifying xenobiotic, given intravascularly in a colloidal suspension, provided essential medical information during the early development of angiography. Unfortunately, physicians did not appreciate the dangers and only later discovered its very slow elimination rate and propensity to accumulate in hepatic tissue. Because of emission of α particles, cases of thorium-induced hepatic carcinomas and angiosarcomas led to its eventual discontinuance in 1952.

Although many nuclear reactor incidents have occurred around the world, the most serious occurred at Chernobyl in the Ukraine in 1986. In this instance, a series of errors led to a fire at the reactor core, several explosions, and a meltdown of the reactor. Over the first 10 days following the incident, a cloud carrying radioactive material (predominantly ^{131}I and ^{137}Cs) spread to the Baltic States, Scandinavia, and Europe. In addition to the 31 people who died of ARS in the first few weeks following the event, nearly 250 others in the surrounding area were hospitalized, and an unknown number suffered other long-term sequelae.[31,37,48]

Not all radiation events occur at nuclear facilities. In September 1987 in Goiânia, Brazil, two men scavenged the contents of an abandoned medical clinic and unwittingly handled a source of ^{137}Cs. As in the early part of the century with radium, the fascinating bluish glow contributed to many radiation exposures, some of them quite extensive. In the end, the government monitored approximately 113,000 individuals and found nearly 250 contaminated individuals. Forty-six patients were treated with a chelating agent, 19 were found to have localized radiation burns, and 4 died in the month following the initial exposure with another dying several years afterward from radiation-induced injuries.[69]

Perhaps one of the most notorious deaths from radiation was that of Alexander Litvinenko, a former Soviet KGB operative who was living in London. On November 1, 2006, shortly after meeting with several men in a public restaurant, Litvinenko experienced nausea and vomiting prompting a visit to the emergency department. He was treated and released only to return 3 days later for continued vomiting and worsening abdominal pain. Physicians were puzzled by his rapid deterioration, including weight loss, alopecia, hypotension, kidney failure, and leukopenia. He was initially thought to have been poisoned by thallium, and later by radioactive thallium. Litvinenko died on November 23; it was only after his death that ^{210}Po was discovered to be the cause, heralding what some consider to be a new era of nuclear terrorism.

THE PRINCIPLES OF RADIOACTIVITY

Dating from the 15th century, *radiation* is defined as energy sent out in the form of waves or particles. Although considered by physicists as incomplete, the particle-wave theory remains a useful model by which to understand the toxic aspects of radiation. Despite the strong nuclear force that holds the basic building blocks of atoms together, many isotopes are unstable. Several other forces, most notably the weak nuclear force, may tip the balance toward instability and an isotope will transform. This process may be intentional, as with the criticality events in a nuclear reactor or nuclear bomb, but mainly occurs spontaneously in nature as the process called radioactive decay.

RADIOACTIVE DECAY

In 1900, Marie Curie discovered that unstable nuclei decay or transform into more stable nuclei (daughters) via the emission of various particles or energy. Radioactive decay occurs through five mechanisms: emission of γ-rays, α-particles, β-particles, positrons, or by capture of an electron. The emission of these various particles makes radioactive decay dangerous because these particles form ionizing radiation. These emitted particles are released with specific decay energies depending on the isotope undergoing the process.

The half-life ($t_{1/2}$), a term first used by Ernest Rutherford in 1904, is the period of time it takes for a radioisotope to lose half of its radioactivity. Every radioisotope has a characteristic half-life. Some isotopes exist for only millionths of a second, whereas others last billions of years. In every case, the activities of radioactive isotopes diminish exponentially with time. The equation $R = R_0e^{-\lambda}t$ describes radioactive decay, in which R is the activity, R_0 is initial activity, t is time, and λ is the decay constant. Each radioisotope has its own decay constant (Table 133–1).

Photons are massless particles that travel at the speed of light and mediate electromagnetic radiation. Depending on the energy of the particles, and therefore their wavelength, they are given (or have) different names. Radiation having the lowest energy and the longest wavelength are called radio waves. As photons become more energetic and have shorter wavelengths, they are called, sequentially, microwaves, heat or infrared, visible light, and ultraviolet rays. X-rays and γ-rays have greater energy than ultraviolet rays and can penetrate deeply into the body, which makes them both deadly and beneficial as radiation therapy.

TABLE 133–1. Physical Properties of Common Radioisotopes

Isotope	Half-Life	Mode of Decay	Decay Energy (MeV)[a]
^{14}C	5730 y	β^-	0.156
^{47}Ca	4.53 d	β^-	1.979
^{57}Co	270 d	electron capture	0.837
^{51}Cr	27.8 d	electron capture	0.752
^{137}Cs	30.23 y	β^-	1.176
^{67}Cu	61.8 h	β^-	0.576
^{3}H	12.26 y	β^-	0.02
^{123}I	13.3 h	electron capture	1.4
^{131}I	8 d	β^-	0.970
^{40}K	1.28×10^9 y	β^-/β^+ electron Capture	1.35/1.505
^{32}P	14.3 d	β^-	1.710
^{210}Po	138 d	α	5.297
^{222}Rn	3.8 d	α	5.587
^{85}Sr	64 d	electron capture	1.11
^{201}Tl	73 h	electron capture	0.41
^{238}U	4.51×10^9 y	α	4.268
^{133}Xe	5.27 d	β^-	0.427

[a]MeV = mega-electron volts.

X-rays and γ-rays are essentially the same and are only distinguishable by their source. γ-radiation is emitted by unstable atomic nuclei in the process of radioactive decay. A given γ-ray will have a fixed wavelength depending on the energy that formed it; the greater the energy of the decay, the smaller the wavelength of the γ-radiation. X-rays come from atomic processes outside the nucleus. For example, an x-ray machine generates x-rays by accelerating electrons through a large voltage and colliding them into a heavy metal target. The rapid deceleration of electrons in the target generates x-rays. This process is also known as *bremsstrahlung* or braking radiation. In general, the higher the voltage, the greater the energy of the x-rays generated along a spectrum of wavelengths. X-rays and γ-rays may have the same energy. Once an x-ray and γ-ray of the same energy leave their respective sources they cannot be distinguished from one another. They behave in exactly the same way, including the types of biological effects they may cause. Because of their nature, high-energy γ- and x-rays can penetrate several feet of insulating concrete.

β-particles are also called electrons. They are emitted during β-decay from an unstable radionuclide, which is an atom that disintegrates by emitting a particle, electromagnetic radiation, or both. Positrons, positively charged electrons, may also be emitted during decay processes. Because of their mass, electrons have less penetration than γ-radiation but may still pass several centimeters into human skin.[90] For this reason, β-particles cause health problems chiefly through incorporation into living organisms, which occurs when a radionuclide is inhaled, ingested, or deposited on a wound.[6]

α-particles are helium nuclei (two protons and two neutrons) stripped of their electrons. These relatively massive particles are emitted during α-decay. They are the most easily shielded of the emitted particles and are stopped by a piece of paper, skin, or clothing. Like β-particles, α-particles principally cause health effects only when they are incorporated.

Neutrons are primarily released from nuclear fission, although high-energy photon beams used in radiotherapy may also produce them. The natural decay of radionuclides does not include emission of neutrons. This is mainly a health hazard for workers in a nuclear power facility or victims of a nuclear explosion. Unique among the particles of radioactivity, when neutrons are stopped or captured they can cause a previously stable atom to become radioactive.

Cosmic rays complete the group of various kinds of radiation to which an individual may be exposed. Cosmic rays are streams of electrons, protons, and α-particles thought to emanate from stars and supernovas. They rain down on the earth from all directions only to give up their energy as they strike the nuclei of oxygen and nitrogen in the upper reaches of the earth's atmosphere. By the time it reaches the earth, the energy of cosmic radiation is reduced by several orders of magnitude. Traveling or living at altitude where the atmosphere shields relatively less cosmic radiation naturally means greater exposure to cosmic rays but in general is not considered a toxic threat to humans.

Isotope, nuclide, radioisotope, and radionuclide atoms that have the same number of protons but different numbers of neutrons, contributing to a different atomic mass, are isotopes (eg, 123^{I}, 125^{I}, 127^{I}, 131^{I}). A nuclide is a species of atom that is characterized by the number of protons, neutrons, and the energy state of the nucleus. (eg, 99_{mTc} vs. 99_{Tc}) The term nuclide is not synonymous with isotope, which is any member of a set of nuclides having the same atomic number but a different atomic mass. Radioisotopes are isotopes that are radioactive, that is, they spontaneously decay and emit energy. Of the iodine isotopes listed previously, 123^{I} , 125^{I}, and 131^{I} are radioisotopes. The isotope 127^{I} is stable. Finally, radionuclides are simply nuclides that are radioactive.

IONIZING RADIATION VERSUS NONIONIZING RADIATION

Ionizing radiation refers to any radiation with sufficient energy to disrupt an atom or molecule with which it impacts. In this interaction, an electron is removed or some other decay process occurs, leaving behind a changed atom. Depending on the specifics of the interaction, these atoms may now be ionized or highly reactive free radicals. Hydroxyl free radicals, formed by ionizing water, are responsible for biochemical lesions that are the foundation of radiation toxicity.

The space between collisions of ionizing radiation and their target molecules varies with the particle type and its energy. A heavy charged particle, such as an α-particle, loses kinetic energy through a series of small energy transfers to other atomic electrons in the target medium, such as tissues. Most of the energy deposition occurs in the "infratrack," a narrow region around the particle track extending about 10 atomic distances. The energy loss per unit length of particle track is called the linear energy transfer (LET), which is expressed in kiloelectron volts per micrometer (keV/μm; see Table 133–1). Heavy charged particles, such as α-particles, are referred to as high-LET radiation, whereas x-rays, γ-rays, and fast electrons are low-LET radiation.

Because of its large size, collisions along the path of an α-particle are clustered together, limiting its ability to penetrate tissue. By comparison, collisions along the path of γ-rays are spread out, increasing their ability to penetrate tissue. It is this ability to penetrate tissue and transfer energy that accounts for the relative dangers of the forms of radiation and tissue susceptibility.

For a source of radiation to pose a threat to tissue, the ionizing particle must be placed in close proximity to vital components of tissue that can sustain damage. High-energy photons penetrate deeply and so pose a similar risk whether they come from an external source or from an incorporated source. As noted previously, α- and β-particles have much more limited tissue penetration and thus radionuclides that radiate these particles must first be incorporated to pose a threat to tissue.

Nonionizing radiation spans a wide spectrum of electromagnetic radiation frequencies. Generally, nonionizing radiation consists of relatively low-energy photons and is used safely in cell phone and television signal transmission, radar, microwaves, and magnetic fields that emanate from high-voltage electricity and metal detectors. Although these are all considered radiation in that they are all energies released from a source, these photons lack the necessary energy required to cause ionization and cellular damage.

RADIATION UNITS OF MEASURE

The amount of radiation to which an object is exposed, that is, the amount emitted from a source that falls on an object, is given in units called roentgens (R). A roentgen is a unit for measuring the quantity of γ- or x-radiation by measuring the amount of ionization produced in air. It may be loosely defined as the amount of x-radiation that produces 1 electrostatic unit of charge in 1 cubic centimeter of air at standard temperature and pressure. As an example, an individual standing at a given distance from the x-ray–generating tube of a particular x-ray machine is exposed, on the skin, to a particular number of roentgens of x-rays (Fig. 133–1).

Not all roentgens to which an individual is exposed pose a risk for cellular damage. Much of the radiation passes through the body and does not cause harm. Only the fraction that is absorbed by the tissue has a probability of causing cellular damage. The unit that describes absorbed radiation is the rad (radiation-absorbed dose), which corresponds to an absorption of energy in any medium of 100 ergs/g. The units of the International System (SI), first introduced in the 1970s, have largely replaced the older units. The gray (Gy) is the corresponding SI unit to the rad and is equivalent to 100 rads.

To measure the risk of biological damage regardless of the type of radiation, the effective dose is given in rem (roentgen equivalent man) and Sv (sievert, in SI). This calculation is an overall indicator that enables all types of exposures (external or internal, partial or total) to be measured on the same scale. These units are also useful for comparing the effects of different radiations or evaluating the danger of a mixture of radiations, such as in radioactive decay, in which some isotopes emit more than one kind of radiation at a time (eg, β and γ). In defining rem, x-rays are the standard radiation for comparison. One rem may be defined as the dose of radiation that produces damage equivalent to one rad of x-rays (or 0.01 Sv). Thus, for x-rays, one Sv is equivalent to100 rem. The effective dose is calculated according to the following equation:

$$E = D \times W_R \times W_T$$

E is the dose in sieverts, D is the absorbed dose in grays, W_R is the radiation weighting factor, also called Q, and W_T is the tissue weighting factor indicating the radiosensitivity of each organ.

To perform the normalization, the dose in grays is multiplied by a relative biologic effectiveness-dependent quality factor (Q). This factor Q multiplies the amount of radiation by 1 for x-rays, γ-rays, and β-particles, 2 for α-particles, and by 5 or more for neutron radiation. Thus, 1 Sv is equivalent to 1 Gy of x-rays. As a very coarse reference point, a regular chest radiograph imparts about 20 to 40 mrem or 0.2 to 0.4 mSv to an individual, but it must be remembered that this radiation dose is delivered very quickly to a limited portion of the body and is quite different from a similar amount delivered over a longer period of time to a worker through an occupational exposure.

In 1910, the curie (Ci) became the unit defining the activity of radioactive decay, although it does not give information regarding what is released or the risk of exposure. One curie equals 3.7×10^{10} disintegrations per second, based on the decay of 1 g of radium. The SI unit is the becquerel (Bq), named for Antoine Henri Becquerel, who in 1896 first reported invisible emanations from naturally occurring minerals that

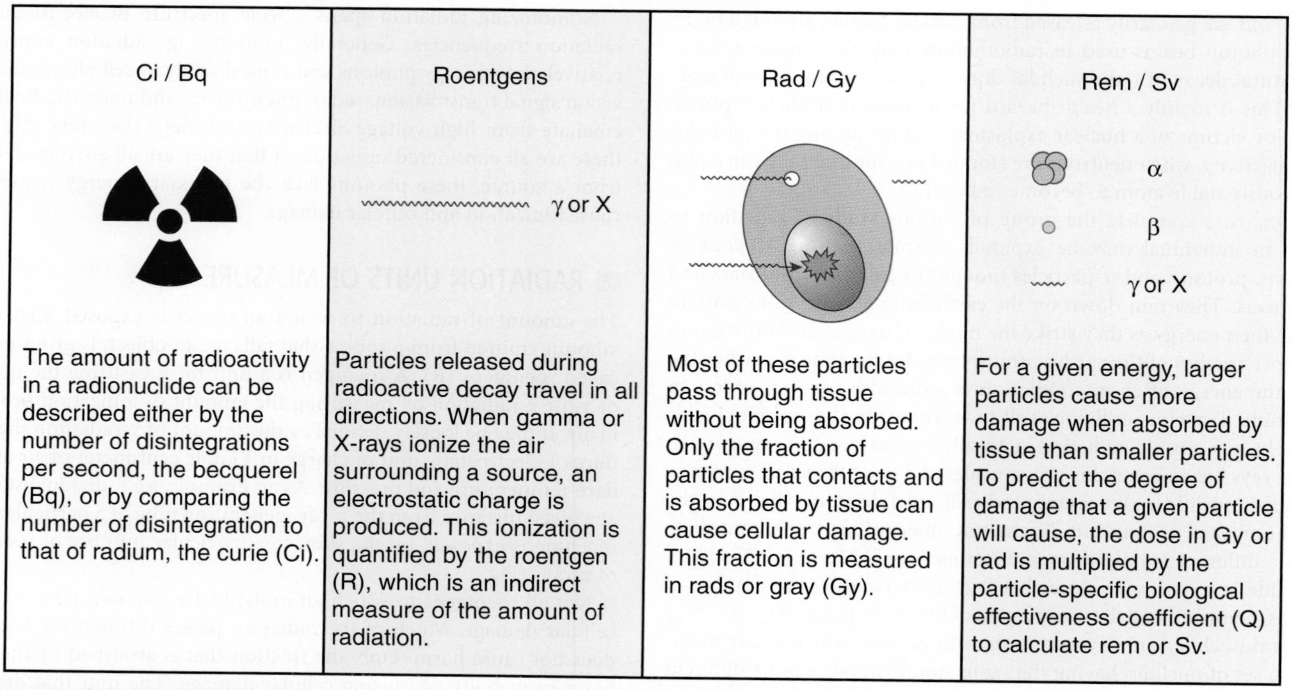

Ci / Bq	Roentgens	Rad / Gy	Rem / Sv
	γ or X		α β γ or X
The amount of radioactivity in a radionuclide can be described either by the number of disintegrations per second, the becquerel (Bq), or by comparing the number of disintegration to that of radium, the curie (Ci).	Particles released during radioactive decay travel in all directions. When gamma or X-rays ionize the air surrounding a source, an electrostatic charge is produced. This ionization is quantified by the roentgen (R), which is an indirect measure of the amount of radiation.	Most of these particles pass through tissue without being absorbed. Only the fraction of particles that contacts and is absorbed by tissue can cause cellular damage. This fraction is measured in rads or gray (Gy).	For a given energy, larger particles cause more damage when absorbed by tissue than smaller particles. To predict the degree of damage that a given particle will cause, the dose in Gy or rad is multiplied by the particle-specific biological effectiveness coefficient (Q) to calculate rem or Sv.

FIGURE 133–1. The definitions associated with radiation. Both curie and bequerel describe a quantity of radionuclide in terms of the number of disintegrations rather than mass. Roentgens describes the amount of air ionized by either gamma (γ) or x-rays, which indirectly quantifies the amount of radiation in the air around a source. Rad and gray (Gy) describe the fraction of radiation that actually interacts with cellular material and potentially causes injury. Roentgen equivalent man (Rem) and sievert (Sv) calculate the effective dose taking into account the different particles. For example, a 100 keV alpha (α) particle causes more damage to cellular material than a 100 keV beta (β) particle.

fogged photographic plates. One becquerel is equivalent to 1 disintegration per second. Thus, 1 Ci is equivalent to 3.7×10^{10} Bq. This number corresponds to an amount of radioactivity in a source. For example, following the Chernobyl incident, 1.2×10^7 TBq (terabecquerel) or 1.2×10^{19} disintegrations per second of radioactive material was released into the atmosphere. By comparison, the men who removed the source of ^{137}Cs in Goiânia found 50.9 TBq (50.9×10^{12} Bq or 13.7×10^5 mCi) of cesium. A thallium stress test uses 111×10^6 Bq (3 mCi) of ^{201}Tl, and the average indoor concentration of ^{222}Rn in the United States is 55 Bq/m^3 (14.8×10^{-6} mCi). To illustrate further, a stress test's dose of ^{201}Tl provides a dose of 0.018 Gy (1.8 rad) and 0.018 Sv (1.8 rem).

PROTECTION FROM RADIATION

Shielding refers to the process by which one may limit the amount of unwanted ionizing radiation in a given setting. Placing a specific material between a radiation source and a target will limit the amount of ionizing radiation that will interact with the target and possibly cause harm. When a particle of ionizing radiation is incident on a material, there exists some probability that it will interact with the material and be attenuated. What happens as a result of this interaction is dependent upon several factors, including the type of particle, its energy, and the atomic number of the target material. The photoelectric effect for photons, Bremsstrahlung for β-particles, and elastic scattering for neutrons are several examples of specific interactions. The shielding equation below allows calculation of the efficacy of shielding.

$$I = I_0 e^{-\mu x}$$

I is the radiation intensity after shielding; I_0 is the radiation intensity before shielding; μ is the linear attenuation coefficient; x is the thickness material in centimeters. The linear attenuation coefficient is defined as the fraction of photons removed from the radiation field per centimeter of absorber through which it passes. Examples of shielding materials are Lucite, lead, and concrete.

Distance is an important safety factor in limiting radiation exposure. Because of their greater interaction with the atmosphere particle radiation, such as α- and β-particles, do not travel more than a few centimeters through air. Generally, moving a few feet from the source of this kind of radiation is enough protection by distance. X-rays and γ-rays, however, have an unlimited range in space and their intensity is only reduced by interactions with matter. Photon radiation that is emitted from a point source diverges from that source to cover an increasingly wider area. The intensity of this radiation follows the inverse square law:

$$\frac{I_1}{I_2} = \frac{(r_2)^2}{(r_1)^2}$$

where I_1 is the initial intensity; I_2 is the final intensity; r_1 is the initial distance from the source; r_2 is the final distance from the source. For example, if the intensity of radiation one meter from a source is 1 Gy, its intensity would be 0.11 Gy at 3 meters from the source.

Time of exposure is another important safety factor in limiting radiation exposure. Obviously the longer a person is exposed to radiation the greater the exposure. Federal and state regulations based on National Council on Radiation Protection and Measurement and FDA recommendations specify the limits of occupational exposure as well as exposure to patients designed to limit the potentially damaging effects of radiation.

IRRADIATION, CONTAMINATION, AND INCORPORATION

An object that is irradiated is exposed to ionizing radiation. This type of exposure includes handling radioactive isotopes, medical diagnostic imaging modalities such as x-ray machines and CT scanners, and rare exposures to criticality events. These sources of ionizing radiation can generate high-energy photons, which penetrate tissue well and cause tissue damage. A whole-body irradiation is one in which the entire body is exposed at once, whereas more commonly shielding devices, such as lead aprons, and collimation techniques used in radiotherapy limit the amount of exposed tissue to the intended target. The risk of tissue damage depends on the total amount of radiation and the tissue type because different tissue types have their own intrinsic resistance to radiation damage. An irradiated object does not become radioactive itself, unless exposed to neutrons.

The Food and Drug Administration (FDA) approved irradiation of wheat and flour in 1963. They have concluded from 40 years of study that irradiation is a safe and effective process for many foods to control bacteria such as *Escherichia coli*, *Salmonella spp*, and *Campylobacter spp*. Irradiation does not make food radioactive, compromise nutritional quality, or noticeably change the taste, texture, or appearance of food, as long as it is applied properly to a suitable product. Organizations that support irradiation of food include the American Medical Association (AMA), the Centers for Disease Control and Prevention (CDC), and the World Health Organization (WHO).

Contamination occurs when a radioactive substance covers an object completely or in part. Several examples include a laboratory or industrial worker who unintentionally spills a radionuclide on clothing or skin or a victim of a radiologic dispersing device, a "dirty bomb," in which a radionuclide is packaged with a conventional explosive and the resultant explosion disperses the radionuclide. In these similar cases, the source of radiation is the nuclide undergoing its normal decay process, and the individual is exposed to particles such as those mentioned in Table 133–1. The risk for tissue damage from the radiation particles is usually quite low, assuming that the contamination is detected and appropriate measures for decontamination are instituted.

Incorporation occurs when a radionuclide assimilates into a patient's body tissue. It generally follows exposure via the inhalational, enteral, or parenteral route, but may occur via any route that permits a radionuclide to enter the body. This principle is used in many diagnostic and therapeutic procedures such as a thallium stress test, bone scan, gallium scan, liver and spleen scan, and strontium therapy.[93] Depending on the dose and type of radionuclide, incorporation may lead to tissue damage, as was the situation for many people following the event at Chernobyl. In this instance, inhalation and subsequent absorption of ^{131}I allowed this radionuclide access to the thyroid, resulting in an increase in thyroid cancer among children and adolescents in the most contaminated regions of Ukraine and Belarus.[11,46,96]

REGULATION AND REPORTING

The use of ionizing radiation, radiation sources, and the byproducts of nuclear energy are among the most heavily regulated processes worldwide. Regulations for medical use of radiation derive from six international organizations and three national organizations. Among the international groups are: United Nations Scientific Committee on the Effects of Atomic Radiation (UNSCEAR), International Commission on Radiological Protection (ICRP), Biological Effects of Ionizing Radiation Committee (BEIR), International Commission on Radiological Units and Measurements (ICRU), Radiation Effects Research Foundation (RERF), and International Radiation Protection Association (IRPA). Since international organizations do not have the authority to enforce their recommendations worldwide, most countries have their own regulatory groups that cooperate internationally. The agencies in the United States are the National Council on Radiation Protection and Measurement (NCRP), Nuclear Regulatory Commission (NRC), and the Food and Drug Administration (FDA). The NCRP issues reports called the Biological Effects of Ionizing Radiation (BEIR reports), which have direct standards for ionizing radiation use. For medical imaging standards, recommendations from the NCRP are considered to be guidelines with which all radiology departments must comply. The goal is to foster a radiation protection program that prevents deterministic effects (see below)

The Nuclear Regulatory Commission (NRC), the Environmental Protection Agency (EPA), and many state governments share the responsibility of licensing and regulating radionuclides in the United States. The Oak Ridge Institute for Science and Education's (ORISE) supports the NRC by maintaining the NRC's website for Radiation Exposure Information and Reporting System (REIRS) and the database of radiation exposure from NRC licensees. http://www.reirs.com/ Individual states regulate radioactive substances that occur naturally or are produced by machines, such as linear accelerators or cyclotrons. The FDA regulates the manufacture and use of linear accelerators, but the individual states regulate their operation. The NRC regulates medical, academic, and industrial uses of nuclear materials generated by or from a nuclear reactor.

ORISE's Radiation Emergency Assistance Center/Training Site (REAC/TS) and the International Atomic Energy Agency (IAEA) both maintain radiation incident registries that track US and foreign radiation incidents. However, recognizing that both these registries are limited in their data collection regarding individual patient's clinical conditions and their therapy, the Moscow Ulm Radiation Accident Clinical History Database (MURAD) was formed in 1990. The International Computer Database for Radiation Exposure Case Histories (ICDREC) succeeded MURAD and seeks to gather as many cases of ARS as possible to develop research and management strategies for the scientific community.[18]

Exposures to man-made sources of radiation are not required to be reported to poison centers and in general do not result in significant morbidity. However, the American Association of Poison Control Centers Toxic Exposure Surveillance System (AAPCC-TESS) reported a total of 2950 exposures to radioactive isotopes over the last 14 years, increasing from 166 in 1993 to 314 in 2007. This increase in reported exposures was commensurate with the overall increase in reports to poison centers. Of the 2007 reported cases, 219 (69%) were unintentional, and 24 (7%) involved children younger than 6 years of age. There were no deaths reported to poison centers from exposure to radioisotopes over the last 14 years[12] (see Chap. 135).

EPIDEMIOLOGY

Everyone is exposed to radiation in one form or another each day (Table 133–2). There are naturally occurring sources of radiation in the earth's crust that make the largest annual contribution to radiation exposure, and man-made sources of radiation that make a relatively smaller contribution to our average annual exposure.

NATURAL SOURCES OF RADIATION

A wide variety of natural sources expose humans on a daily basis to ionizing radiation. In the United States, the estimated annual dose equivalent of radiation is 3.6 mSv, and natural sources contribute about 80% of that annual dose.[15,32] Terrestrial sources of radiation originate from radionuclides in the earth's crust that move into the air and water. These primordial radionuclides, so named because their physical half-lives are comparable to the age of the earth, include uranium, actinium, and thorium. Geographic areas vary regarding the content of these radionuclides.

Radon, a radioactive noble gas, accounts for most of the human exposure to radiation from natural sources. This gas, a natural decay product of uranium and thorium, enters homes and other buildings from the building materials themselves or through microscopic cracks

TABLE 133–2. Average Effective Annual Ionizing Radiation Dose Equivalent in the United States

Source	Dose[a]	
	mSv[b]	% of Total
Natural		
Cosmic	0.27	8
Internal	0.39	11
Radon[c]	2.0	55
Terrestrial	0.28	8
Subtotal	**2.94**	**82**
Man-made		
Consumer products	0.10	3
Nuclear medicine	0.14	4
Occupational	<0.01	<0.3
X-ray diagnostic imaging	0.39	11
Subtotal	**0.63**	**18**
Total	**3.6**	**100**

[a] All doses are averages and contain some variability within the measurement.
[b] mSv = millisieverts.
[c] Average effective dose to bronchial epithelium.

in the building's structures. With a relatively short half-life of 3.82 days, ^{222}Rn poses a health risk if decay occurs while in the respiratory space and deposits on respiratory tissue as one of its daughter isotopes, which are solids. These radon daughters emit α-particles as they decay and are the principle causes in the associated increased incidence of lung cancer in those exposed to radon[76] (Table 133–2).

Additionally, radon daughters are charged and can attach to larger aerosols to be inhaled primarily. Radon daughters can also remain unattached to aerosols and form smaller-sized aggregates, enabling them to penetrate to smaller airspaces. There is a complex relationship between exposure to radon progeny and dose to target cells. Influencing physiologic factors include tidal volume, minute ventilation, mucus thickness, and mucociliary clearance. The risk of lung cancer is increased in heavy smokers who additionally expose their lungs to 200 mSv from ^{210}Po (a radon daughter) that is naturally found in tobacco smoke.

Areas of New York, New Jersey, and Pennsylvania, called the Reading Prong, have particularly high concentrations of radon as a result of a richer concentration in the earth's crust of primordial radionuclides that liberate radon. The EPA has recommended household level intervention when ambient radon concentrations exceed 147 Bq/m^3 (4 pCi/L). Individuals can test their own homes for radon with either short-term (less than 90 days) or long-term (greater than 90 days) commercially available measurement devices.

The second largest natural source of radiation originates from ingested radionuclides, of which ^{40}K, a naturally occurring isotope, is the most abundant. Potassium is the seventh most abundant element in the earth's crust and ^{40}K represents about 0.012% of this naturally occurring element. With a half-life of 1.3 billion years, ^{40}K decays via beta emission and electron capture. Since it is part of the environment, the average amount of ^{40}K in the body is about 3700 Bq, delivering about 1.8×10^{-4}Sv and 1.4×10^{-4} Sv to soft tissue and bone, respectively. The lifetime cancer mortality risk has been calculated for ^{40}K to be 5.9×10^{-6} per Bq ingested or 4 in 100,000 from external exposure (compared to 1 in 5 from the group predicted to die of cancer from all other causes per US average.) Together with other primordial radionuclides in our diet, this source of internal radiation accounts for about 12% of the annual dose of absorbed radiation.

MAN-MADE SOURCES

As mentioned earlier, man-made sources of radiation can be found in many consumer products and in many different types of industry (Table 133–3). The National Council on Radiation Protection and

TABLE 133–3. Uses of Radioisotopes

Radioisotope	Use
^{241}Americium	Smoke detectors, to measure lead concentrations in paint, steel, and paper production
^{109}Cadmium	Analyze metal alloys
^{47}Calcium	Biomedical research of cell function and bone formation
^{252}Californium	Inspect luggage for explosives, gauge moisture content of soil and silo materials
^{14}Carbon	Pharmaceutical research, radiometric dating
^{137}Cesium	Measure dosages of radioactive pharmaceuticals, oil industry to measure flow in pipelines
^{51}Chromium	Red blood cell survival studies
^{57}Cobalt	Nuclear medicine
^{67}Copper	Chemotherapy
^{244}Curium	Mining industry
^{123}Iodine	Diagnosis of thyroid disorders
^{129}Iodine	Check some radioactivity counters in vitro diagnostic testing
^{131}Iodine	Treatment of thyroid disorders
^{192}Iridium	Test the integrity of pipeline welds, boilers, and aircraft parts
^{55}Iron	Analyze electroplating solutions
^{85}Krypton	Indicator lights, textile industry
^{63}Nickel	Detect explosives, voltage regulators, surge protectors
^{32}Phosphorus	Molecular biology and genetics research
^{238}Plutonium	Power source for NASA spacecraft
^{210}Polonium	Photographic film production
^{147}Promethium	Thermostats, textile industry
^{226}Radium	Lightning rods
^{75}Selenium	Protein studies
^{24}Sodium	Industrial pipelines integrity
^{85}Strontium	Study bone formation and metabolism
^{99}Technetium	Nuclear medicine
^{201}Thallium	Cardiac imaging
^{229}Thorium	Fluorescent lights
^{230}Thorium	Coloring and fluorescence in colored glazes and glassware
^{232}Thoriated Tungsten	Electric arc welding
^{3H}Tritium	Basic science and pharmaceutical studies, for self- luminous signs, luminous dials, gauges and wrist watches, luminous paint
^{234}Uranium	Dental fixtures, military projectiles
^{235}Uranium	Fuel for nuclear power plants and naval nuclear propulsion systems, fluorescent glassware, colored glazes, and wall tiles
^{133}Xenon	Nuclear medicine

Measurements estimates the annual number of workers occupationally exposed to radiation to be nearly a million, although worldwide this number is several million.[32,82] On average, those occupations with the highest exposures (about 4 mSv/yr) are uranium miners and millers, nuclear power operators, and sailors in close proximity to nuclear reactors. Those with lesser additional exposures (about 0.5–1 mSv/yr) include physicians, x-ray technologists, nuclear fuel processing workers, and workers in other industries that use radionuclides.

Medical occupational exposure principally includes physicians, nurses, and x-ray technologists, who receive an additional annual effective dose of about 1 mSv. This dose can range up to 17 mSv with certain techniques such as fluoroscopy but are only partial body exposures because of the appropriate use of lead aprons and other protective barriers. Medical procedures also account for substantial annual exposure to man-made radiation for patients. In 1989, the NCRP estimated the annual number of various diagnostic procedures involving radiation in the United States to exceed 250 million, although the number has increased quite rapidly over the last decade. Medical sources of exposure to patients account for about 0.5 mSv or 15% of the average annual exposure.

Exposures have been studied in emergency physicians, orthopedists, and interventional cardiologists.[33,45,99,105] Each of these fields uses different modalities of radiation, which pose different risks to the individual performing the procedure. Two studies examining exposure to physicians assisting in cervical spine radiographs found the calculated whole-body exposure ranged up to 0.027 mSv per procedure, or 0.75% of the estimated annual dose equivalent of radiation in the United States.[45,105] This exposure annualized over a year neared the NCRP upper limits of safety, but this exposure should decrease as these studies have decreased with the increased use of CT of the cervical spine for diagnostic purposes. Two other studies examined physician exposure to radiation by fluoroscopy used in interventional cardiology and orthopedic procedures. These doses ranged from 0.05 to 0.3 mSv per procedure. In each of these four studies, appropriate shielding was used, and dosimeters measured individual areas of exposed body parts such as extremities and the head. Radiation was undetectable beneath a lead apron. Estimated whole-body exposures to these procedures were considered not to exceed the limits established by OSHA of 50 mSv per year. Although the likelihood of exceeding established radiation limits is low regardless of the procedure, and even assuming a reasonable increase in the number of procedures performed, appropriate shielding and safety training are emphasized to minimize the risk of exposure.

Various medical scans use radionuclides to study various disease processes (Table 133–4). Other radionuclides used in medical diagnostics include ^{111}In, ^{67}Ga, and ^{51}Cr. Other scientific research uses tritium (3H) and ^{32}P. These radionuclides decay through β-particle capture or emission. In general, unintentional topical exposure to these radionuclides in this setting is not considered hazardous because skin and clothing provide adequate barriers against the poorly penetrating particles emitted. In the case of unintentional incorporation, it is highly unlikely that the amount infused will be sufficient to cause a serious health risk.

Depleted uranium (DU) is used by the US military and by several other governments as an armor-piercing alloy ammunition. Munitions made of this material are favored because it is pyrophoric, sharpens on impact, has a high density (about 1.7 times that of lead), and is less expensive than tungsten, which was used for this purpose until 1973. DU can be obtained from the enrichment process of natural uranium in the development of nuclear fuel, the reprocessing of spent nuclear fuel, or developed directly for military purposes. DU is mainly ^{238}U, but contains approximately 0.2% of other isotopes of uranium and several other transuranic elements as well depending on its origin. Consequently, DU's α- and β-activity is about 40% less radioactive than naturally occurring uranium. When DU munitions strike a hard target, it is dispersed as an aerosol and contaminates a limited area. Radiation exposure is derived from incorporation of the aerosolized material as well as from retained shrapnel.[34] Thus, as a radiation hazard, external exposure to solid ^{238}U is considered to be negligible although currently many studies are investigating the potential link between DU and the incidence of leukemias, other cancers, and birth defects.[5,14,21,27,44,66,67,71,72,75] One study examined a cohort of over 50,000 service personnel from the United Kingdom who served in Gulf War I but found no increase in the incidence of any cancers over 6 years following the end of the war.[59] Another study examining a cohort of Gulf War I veterans over 16 years found only subtle bone differences and few clinically significant uranium-related health effects despite ongoing exposure from embedded DU fragments.[65]

TABLE 133–4. Diagnostic Imaging Procedures: Type and Amount of Radionuclide or Radiation

Test	Radionuclide	Amount
Whole body bone scan	^{99}Tc	25mCi(9.25 × 10^8 Bq)
Radionuclide cerebral angiogram	^{99}Tc-DTPA	15mCi(5.55 × 10^8 Bq)
Cardiac ejection scan (MUGA)	^{99}TcO$_4$	20mCi(7.4 × 10^8 Bq)
DISIDA/Hepatobiliary scan	^{99}Tc-DISIDA	5mCi(18.5 × 10^7 Bq)
Ventilation/Perfusion scan	^{133}Xe	10mCi(37 × 10^7 Bq)
	^{99}Tc	4mCi(14.8 × 10^7 Bq)
Thyroid scan	^{123}I	0.2mCi(0.74 × 10^7 Bq)
Myocardial perfusion	^{201}Tl	3mCi(11.1 × 10^7 Bq)
scan (exercise)	^{99}Tc	20mCi(7.4 × 10^8 Bq)
Strontium therapy	^{89}Sr	4mCi(14.8 × 10^7 Bq)
Venogram	^{99}Tc	20mCi(7.4 × 10^8 Bq)
Chest radiograph	60 mrad or 0.06 mGy in a collimated field[a]	
Abdominal radiograph	100–1500 mrad or 1–5 mGy in a collimated field	
CT-head	1–2 rads or 0.01–0.02 Gy per slice[b]	
CT-body	1 rad or 0.01 Gy per slice[2b]	

[a] Collimation is the act of restricting the size of the useful x-ray field to the region of clinical interest. These skin-entry doses are approximations dependent on equipment and technique.

[b] The dose per each examination is about the same as the dose per slice and not the sum of the slices.

EXPOSURE LIMITS

The various agencies involved in regulating radiation exposures to both workers and the public include OSHA, the NRC, and the Department of Transportation (DOT). The NRC has established "Standards for

Protection against Radiation," which regulates radiation exposures using a 2-fold system of dose limitation: doses to individuals shall not exceed limits established by the NRC, and all exposures shall be kept *as low as reasonably achievable* (ALARA). The total effective dose equivalent may not exceed 50 mSv/yr to reduce the risk of stochastic effects (see Stochastic Versus Deterministic Effects of Radiation later in the chapter). The dose to the fetus of a pregnant radiation worker may not exceed 5 mSv over 9 months and should not substantially exceed 0.5 mSv in any 1 month, although this amount is not carefully defined.[43,86]

PATHOPHYSIOLOGY

Ionizing radiation causes damage to tissue by several mechanisms depending on its energy. Radiation with high LET predominantly causes direct damage, which is when incoming radiation impacts a target molecule directly. This occurs because high LET radiation, such as an α particle, has a high statistical probability of impacting an important molecule, such as DNA.[32] If this occurs, a mutation may arise, which may then result in alteration of a germ line, development of a neoplasm, or cell death. The risk of these consequences overall, however, is low because of the relative paucity of DNA within a cell and the even smaller percentage of active DNA within a given cell.

Low LET radiation, x-rays, γ-rays, and fast electrons, predominantly cause indirect damage. The likelihood that radiation will cause cell damage is a function of its LET and reaches a peak at about 100 keV/μm. At this energy, the average separation between ionization events coincides with the diameter of the DNA helix and allows for the greatest probability of double-strand breaks, which is the basis for most biologic effects. Greater or lesser energies correlate to a lower probability of DNA impacts, and so the rest of the cell media becomes the energy absorber.[40]

Indirectly, radiation impacts a molecule and creates a reactive species, which then chemically reacts with organic molecules in cells, altering their structure or function. These radiation-induced ions are quite unstable, however, and usually convert to free radicals. Most importantly, radiation may impact a water molecule, which is in great abundance, to generate a hydroxyl radical (OH·).[32] The hydroxyl radical diffuses only a short distance through the cell because of its highly reactive nature and itself causes molecular damage.

The bystander effect refers to cellular damage in unirradiated cells that neighbor irradiated cells. As early as the 1940s, there were reports of inactivation of cells by ionization of the surrounding medium. Recently, the use of a single-particle microbeam (a device that can fire a predefined exact number of α-particles through a particular cell nucleus) demonstrated that cultured cells that were not hit by radiation showed increased chromosome damage, rearrangement, and rate of death. The bystander effect is demonstrated using proton beams and x-rays, and in cells cultured with DU.[68,77] Communication from cell to cell via gap junctions is an important factor in cell death and mutations, which are observed in these experiments. In one experiment, when 10% of cells on a dish were exposed to two or more α-particles, the resulting frequency of induced oncogenic transformation was indistinguishable from that when all the cells on the dish were exposed to the same number of α-particles.[88]

Genomic instability is when a gene responsible for the stability of the genome and the consistency of replication is altered, resulting in a cascade of other mutations and the subsequent development of a neoplasm. Several studies demonstrate that, in addition to direct radiation damage to genetic material, radiation causes perturbations in intracellular oxidation-reduction reactions and far outlast radiation-generated hydroxyl radicals, which exist only for fractions of a second. These changes in oxidation–reduction reactions, in turn, cause other changes in signaling pathways leading to apoptosis, transformation, and other bystander effects that manifest as delayed or lethal mutations and chromosomal instability. Studies are ongoing that investigate specific causes of cellular injury and the precise mechanisms that may be responsible.[40,58]

Although any molecule may be damaged in a variety of ways that may lead to cell injury of varying severity, double-stranded breaks in DNA are the type of damage most likely to cause chromosomal aberrations or cell death. The radiosensitivity of the cell is directly related to its rate of proliferation and inversely related to its degree of differentiation.[47,80] Thousands of these types of lesions occur daily in the human body from natural environmental radiation.

For this reason, there are several mechanisms that protect and repair damage that may result from either direct or indirect means of radiation damage. Estimates are that up to 90% of all chromosomal breaks heal by adhesion in a process known as "restitution." All that is required for DNA to heal is oxygen and time, which forms the basis for fractionated radiation therapy. This therapy takes advantage of the inefficient repair mechanisms of cancerous cells compared to normal cells. Thus, by giving the radiation dose over several sessions, radiation damage will accumulate in cancer cells during radiation therapy, and more cancer cells are killed. Sulfhydryl-containing molecules, such as glutathione, and other scavengers provide protection against free radicals. These molecules react with free radicals and inactivate them quickly, thus limiting the potential damage. Following a large radiation exposure, however, both restitution and the protection provided by free-radical scavengers may be overwhelmed, and damage may occur.

STOCHASTIC VERSUS DETERMINISTIC EFFECTS OF RADIATION

The radiation damage just described has two consequential results: it kills cells or it alters cells and causes cancer. Injuries that do not require a threshold limit to be exceeded include mutagenic and carcinogenic changes to individual cells where DNA is the critical and ultimate target. This is the stochastic effect of radiation. Theoretically, there is no dose of radiation too small to have the potential of causing cancer in an exposed individual.[16] Theories suggesting that a single dose of radiation can cause a change in the genome that potentially alters the structure of a protooncogene, control of an oncogene, or activates oncogenic viruses in hosts are supported by a growing body of work investigating bystander effects and genomic instability.[40] These effects may take several months to years to manifest, as happened with Japanese survivors of the nuclear bombs who suffered a spectrum of malignancies many years after the event.

Whereas the stochastic effects of radiation may follow less severe exposures, such as prolonged exposure to low-concentrations of radon gas, the deterministic effects of radiation usually follow a large whole-body exposure, such as a Chernobyl- or Tokaimura-type event. In terms of cell death, a relatively large number of cells of an organ system must be killed before an effect becomes clinically evident. This number of killed cells constitutes a threshold limit that must be exceeded, and this is what is known as the deterministic or nonstochastic effects of radiation.

To illustrate the differences between stochastic and nonstochastic effects, consider a single alpha particle from ^{210}Po incorporated in a radon-contaminated household may impact an active segment of DNA in a patient's respiratory tract, ultimately giving rise to a cancer—the stochastic effect. In Tokaimura, the most severely injured worker received 17 Sv of neutron- and γ-radiation and experienced so much cell death across so many systems in his body that he died well before any injured yet surviving cells could develop into a cancer—the deterministic effect.

ACUTE RADIATION SYNDROME

The Army Medical Corps first described ARS in 1946 when victims of the explosions at Hiroshima and Nagasaki were admitted for treatment at Osaka University Hospital.[50] Understanding the features of ARS is essential for managing a patient who is exposed to massive whole-body irradiation, generally considered to be 1 Gy (250 times the average annual exposure) or more. In many cases, a reliable estimate of the radiation dose is difficult, thus making it more practical to focus on the clinical features of radiation injury and their prognostic utility.

The acute radiation syndrome involves a sequence of events that varies with the severity of the exposure.[29,97,104] Generally, more severe exposures lead to more rapid onset of symptoms and more severe clinical features. Four classic clinical stages are described, which begin with the early prodromal stage of nausea and vomiting. These symptoms begin anywhere from hours to days postexposure. Although the time to onset postexposure is inversely proportional to the dose received, the duration of the prodromal phase is directly proportional to the dose. That is, the greater the dose received, the more rapid the onset of symptoms, and the longer their duration, except in cases in which death follows rapidly.[80] The latent period follows next as an apparent improvement of symptoms, during which time the patient appears to have recovered and has no clinically apparent difficulties. The duration of this stage is inversely related to dose and may last from several days to several weeks. The third stage usually begins in the third to fifth week after exposure and consists of manifest illness described in subsequent paragraphs. If the person survives this stage, recovery, the fourth stage, is likely, but may take weeks to months before it is completed. Those exposed to supralethal amounts of radiation may experience all the phases in a few hours prior to a rapid death.

These four stages describe the clinical manifestations that may be observed as a result of massive exposure, but the various systems of the body manifest their own injuries, which constitute several subsyndromes.[29,104] These subsyndromes are not mutually exclusive of one another and may overlap as cell death or damage progresses.

The cerebrovascular syndrome describes the manifestations of injury to the central nervous system following massive irradiation. This syndrome, following exposure to doses of about 15 to 20 Gy or greater, is characterized by rapid or immediate onset of hyperthermia, ataxia, loss of motor control, apathy, lethargy, cardiovascular shock, and seizures. The mechanism of this injury may be a combination of radiation-induced vascular lesions and free radical–induced neuronal death and cerebral edema.

Despite autopsy evidence of some radiation-induced inflammatory changes to the heart, animal experiments demonstrate that the heart is relatively resistant to high doses of radiation. Cardiovascular shock is more likely because of systemic vascular damage, which may later compound shock resulting from other subsyndromes should the patient survive to that point. A "vascular radiation subsyndrome" might be considered to help explain the hemodynamic changes a patient experiences following a massive dose of radiation. Once these subsyndromes are manifest, they may be irreversible.[23,29,80,87]

The gastrointestinal syndrome begins following an exposure to about 6 Gy or more when gastrointestinal mucosal cell injury and death occur. Symptoms include anorexia, nausea, vomiting, and diarrhea. As the mucosal lining is sloughed, there is persistent bloody diarrhea, hypersecretion of cellular fluids into the lumen, and a loss of peristalsis, which may progress to abdominal distension and dehydration. Destruction of the mucosal lining allows for colonization by enteric organisms with ensuing sepsis.

The hematologic changes that occur following an exposure to about 1 Gy or greater are called the hematopoietic syndrome. Hematopoietic stem cells are highly radiosensitive, in contrast to the more mature erythrocytes and platelets. Lymphocytes are also radiosensitive and can die quickly from cell lysis following an exposure. This contrasts with granulocytes, which endure radiation better. In addition to stem cell death and white cell depletion with immunodeficiency, platelets are consumed in gingival and gastrointestinal microhemorrhages. The main effect of radiation-induced hematopoietic syndrome is pancytopenia leading to death from sepsis complicated by hemorrhage. A lymphocyte nadir typically occurs 8–30 days postexposure, with higher doses achieving earlier nadir.[17,28]

The pulmonary system is not spared injury from irradiation. Pneumonitis may occur within 1–3 months following a dose of 6–10 Gy. This may lead to respiratory failure, pulmonary fibrosis, or cor pulmonale months to years later.

DOSE ESTIMATION

Determining the dose received by an individual who was irradiated is important in providing appropriate therapy and establishing a prognosis. However, estimating the dose received is difficult for a number of reasons, such as the absence of a radiation-monitoring device, exposure to radiation of mixed form (such as γ and neutron radiation), and partial shielding of various body parts.[87]

In cases of whole-body irradiation, it is the ARS itself that allows for an estimate of the radiation dose received. The Biological Assessment Tool available at the Armed Forces Radiobiology Research Institute's web site, and guidelines from the International Atomic Energy Agency (IAEA), use clinical signs and symptoms, including the time to onset of vomiting after an exposure to radiation, to calculate the exposure dose and may be the clinician's best dosimeter.[80] Use of this kind of timing may be limited, however, because most exposures cannot be perceived by human senses.

As previously mentioned, lymphopenia is common following an exposure to 1 Gy or more. The observed predictability of lymphopenia has led to the development of several models for biodosimetry. It is important to note that dosimetry models have been validated and already take into account other potential modifiers of lymphocyte count, such as trauma or burns. However, discrepancies between the models suggest that more than one element of dosimetry be used whenever possible.[104]

The broad ranges of radiation doses that correlate with lymphocyte count are described in the classic Andrews nomogram of 1965 (Fig. 133–2). Using historical data from exposed patients, a lymphocyte depletion constant was calculated using the equation:

$$L(t) = L_0 e^{-K(D)\,t}$$

in which $L(t)$ is the lymphocyte count at time t, L_0 is the lymphocyte count prior to the exposure—the population mean taken as 2.45×10^9 cells/L, K is the rate constant for a given dose of radiation, and D is the dose of radiation. Solving for $K(D)$ will allow for an accurate estimate of a rapidly delivered, whole body exposure[35] (Table 133–5).

The currently accepted standard criteria for biodosimetry are chromosome aberration bioassays. Introduced in 1966, this technique analyzes the number of dicentric chromosomes that occur following an exposure to radiation. An exposure to radiation can cause breakage of the DNA molecule in two nonhomologous chromosomes and produce "sticky ends" that recombine end-to-end. In metaphase, these appear as a single chromosome with two centromeres and are called dicentric. The number of dicentrics in lymphocytes correlates reliably with a given dose of radiation. Additionally, if the number of dicentric chromosomes follows a Poisson distribution, a uniform exposure can be assumed (see Table 133–5).[2,53,78]

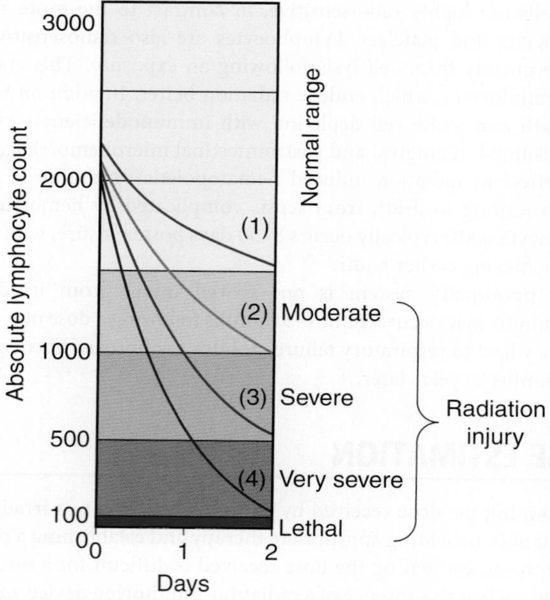

FIGURE 133–2. Classic Andrews lymphocyte depletion curves with accompanying clinical severity curves. Curves 1–4 correspond to whole body exposures of 3.1, 4.4, 5.6, and 7.1 Gy, respectively. (Adapted from Goans RE, Holloway EC, Berger ME, Ricks RC. Early dose assessment following severe radiation accidents. *Health Phys.* 1997:72:513–518.)

Even though there is no currently accepted standard for performance, analysis of dicentric chromosomes in peripheral blood lymphocytes is the only method routinely used in biodosimetry. Unfortunately, because proliferative death of cells containing aberrant chromosomes reduces the number of such cells available for analysis over time, and the migration of lymphocytes into tissue and the lymphatic system, a limited period is available to use this test to perform dose calculations retrospectively.[49,52] A recent development in molecular biology, the fluorescence *in situ* hybridization (FISH) chromosome-painting technique, has opened the possibility for accurate recognition of translocations and thus retrospective determination of dose. Unlike dicentrics, complete translocations persist in cell division and enable dose estimation over years following exposure.[51] In fact, this technique was employed to evaluate the radiation dose experienced by clean-up workers at Chernobyl. These authors concluded that it is likely that recorded doses for these cleanup workers overestimate their average bone marrow doses, perhaps substantially.[55] Unfortunately, these techniques are not widely available, require incubation times of 48–72 hours, and cannot assess for doses greater than 5 Gy, although new methods for high-exposure assessments are being developed.

TABLE 133–5. Biodosimetry Tools[104]

Dose Estimate (Gy)	Time to Onset of Vomiting (Hours)	Rate Constant for Lymphocyte Depletion	Dicentric Chromosomes in Human Peripheral Blood Lymphocytes (per 1000 Cells)
0	n/a	–	1–2
1	>24	0.126	88
2	4.5	0.252	234
3	2.5	0.378	439
4	1.75	0.5	703
5	1.25	0.63	1024

PROGNOSIS

The prognosis of those exposed to radiation varies with the amount of the exposure, the type of medical care received, and the number of casualties in a given exposure scenario. Survival is inversely proportional to the radiation dose absorbed, and even the relatively radioresistant cell types can be killed by high amounts of radiation. For these reasons, an acute dose of 20 Gy or more is considered supralethal.[90] Historically, those who were exposed to greater than 10 Gy died despite care. This includes one worker at Tokaimura who was exposed to 17 Gy who died 3 months postexposure, and 20 of 21 workers who were exposed to radiation in the 6- to16-Gy range at Chernobyl. Some authors suggest that those exposed to 10 Gy or greater be given supportive and comfort care only because their survival is considered to be unlikely.[104]

Within the group exposed to 5–10 Gy, depending on the dose received, there may be milder forms of CNS and cardiovascular syndromes that last for prolonged periods of time. A severe GI syndrome in which high fever and persistent hematochezia are present suggests a poor prognosis. This syndrome may overlap with a severe form of the hematopoietic syndrome in which damage to bone marrow stem cells is so severe that bone marrow function may not recover for weeks or months. These patients will likely require bone marrow transplantation and multiple transfusions of platelets and red blood cells, optimal supportive care, and infection control to survive.

Patients exposed to radiation in the range of 2–5 Gy will likely survive with medical care. Although the median lethal dose of radiation for humans is estimated to be 4.5 Gy, the manifestations of ARS will be similar to those noted previously but will likely be delayed and less severe. Many patients will survive without bone marrow transplantation if supportive care optimizes fluid and electrolyte replacement and controls bleeding and infection.

Survival is expected for those patients acutely exposed to less than 2 Gy with little medical intervention necessary. Mild forms of GI and hematopoietic syndromes may occur in delayed fashion compared to more severe exposures.

CARCINOGENESIS

Radiation increases the incidence of specific cancers in humans. One of the most important evidentiary sources is life-span studies of atomic bomb survivors in Japan.[22] This group of people is extensively studied over the last half-century, and although the relative risks assigned to specific cancers are modified over the years and subject to interpretation, there is a general agreement that the incidences of leukemia (except chronic lymphocytic leukemia, CLL), female breast carcinoma, and thyroid cancer increase following a sufficient exposure. This risk is largely extrapolated from models of high-dose exposures, but is also supported by data for persons exposed to radon.[22] These cancers usually do not appear until many years after the exposure. Because of technical and logistical difficulties in performing appropriate epidemiological studies, quantifying the cancer risk from exposure to low-dose (less than 10 mSv) radiation is difficult, leading some to question the validity of the linear–no threshold theory.[9,16] For those exposed while they are young, the excess incidence of cancer occurs only when they are at the age when those cancers otherwise appear in the unirradiated population, as was discussed earlier with the BNTVA group.[32,83]

Pulmonary exposure to radon has been studied extensively in the last few years. Both uranium miners and household residents in areas with high ambient radon concentrations, such as New Jersey and Sweden are at increased risk for developing lung cancer from exposure to radon gas. A cohort of nonsmoking uranium miners showed a 12-fold increased risk of lung cancer over controls, which is similar to the estimates of the increased risk of lung cancer caused by radiation exposure in atomic bomb survivors.[15,85] The increased risk of lung cancer from exposure to radon gas is modified by concurrent cigarette smoking, which may have a multiplicative effect rather than an additive effect.[73]

COMMONLY ENCOUNTERED RADIONUCLIDES

Most exposures that come to medical attention are not large, whole-body irradiations but are rather small spills in the laboratory or inadvertent exposures from one of many products that are commercially available. With the notable exception of a well-known case of massive americium contamination in Oak Ridge, Tennessee, and the cesium exposure in Goiânia, Brazil, the vast majority of these types of cases are not reported in the medical literature.[28,95]

Americium (symbol Am, atomic number 95, and atomic weight 243) was discovered in 1944 in Chicago during the Manhattan Project. Its most stable isotope, ^{243}Am, has a half-life of over 7500 years, although ^{241}Am, with a half-life of 470 years, was the first americium isotope to be isolated. It decays by α-activity and γ-emissions and will accumulate in bone if incorporated.[53] It is used to test machinery integrity, glass thickness, and in smoke detectors (about 0.26 μg per detector), where it ionizes the air between 2 electrodes and generates an electric current that soot may impede. α-Particles from these detectors are easily absorbed within a few centimeters of the surrounding air and pose little risk. One g of americium dioxide provides enough americium for more than 5000 smoke detectors. In 1976, a worker at the Hanford Plutonium Finishing Plant, suffered a large ^{241}Am contamination in an explosion at the site. One hundred grams (500,000 smoke detectors' worth) of ^{241}Am was involved, contaminating the victim's face with 70 MBq, but there was likely some inhalational exposure as well. He was treated with long-term diethylenetriaminepentaacetic acid (DTPA), and despite some leukopenia from the radiation, he survived for 11 years before dying from unrelated cardiac disease.[95]

Cesium (symbol Cs, atomic number 55, and atomic weight 132): Bunsen discovered Cs spectroscopically in 1860. It decays by β activity and γ emissions and tends to follow the potassium cycle in nature, providing a whole-body dose if incorporated. It is used as a radiation source in radiation therapy and as a radionuclide source for atomic clocks. Cesium, the radionuclide of the Goiânia incident, comes in the form of a powder, which would make dispersal relatively easy if used in a dirty bomb. Insoluble Prussian blue is the FDA-approved chelator for patients contaminated with cesium (see Antidotes in Depth A29: Prussian Blue).[20,54]

Cobalt (symbol Co, atomic number 27, and atomic weight 58.9) was discovered in 1735 by Brandt. ^{60}Co is an artificially made isotope and is an important source of γ-rays for radiotherapy, and detecting weld seam integrity. ^{60}Co was the source of a significant radiation incident that took place in North America in 1983.[62] A radiotherapy source containing 16.65×10^{12}Bq (450 Ci) of ^{60}Co in the form of thousands of millimeter-sized pellets was opened and spilled onto a truck in a junk yard in Juarez, Mexico. At least 200 people were exposed to the contaminated truck and the materials subsequently made from the contaminated scrap metal in the junk yard.

Iodine (symbol I, atomic number 53, and atomic weight 126.9): Courtois discovered iodine in 1811. There are 23 isotopes of iodine; ^{127}I is the only one that is stable. ^{125}I is used in thyroid studies and decays by γ emissions. ^{131}I is used in metastatic thyroid surveys and decays by β activity and γ emissions. ^{129}I and ^{131}I are also products of fission in nuclear reactors that may be released into the environment during an event. These isotopes will accumulate in thyroid tissue if incorporated and can cause local damage to thyroid tissue. It is this potential for incorporation that prophylaxis with potassium iodide (KI) is indicated in the event of a large exposure.

Phosphorus (symbol P, atomic number 15, and atomic weight 30) was discovered in 1669 by Brand. ^{32}P has a half-life of 14 days and decays by β-activity. The maximum range of decay particles in air is 20 feet, and in tissue, one-third of an inch. For soluble ^{32}P compounds, bone receives approximately 20% of the dose following ingestion or inhalation. Shielding for ^{32}P and other β-emitters should be made of material with atomic numbers of less than 13 (aluminum) to reduce the generation of x-rays, electromagnetic radiation produced by the rapid change of velocity of a fast-moving particle as it approaches an atomic nucleus and is deflected. This is best accomplished by Lucite or other plastics and not by lead or even glass. Pharmacodynamics of sodium [^{32}P] phosphate, given to patients with polycythemia vera include whole body distribution within the phosphate pool. Five percent to 10% is excreted in the urine within the first 24 hours and about 20% during the first week. After 3 days, ^{32}P is deposited primarily in bone marrow, liver, and spleen. Whole body retention curves show a mean biological half-life of 39.2 days.

Polonium (symbol Po, atomic number 84, and atomic weights range from 192 to 218) was discovered by Marie Curie while searching for the cause of radioactivity of pitchblende (uranium ore). It was named after her native country, Poland. Po has 27 isotopes; the most isotopes of all the elements and all are radioactive. Po is a very rarely occurring natural element where only 100 mcg is found in a ton of uranium ore. Po is chiefly manufactured by bombarding ^{210}Bi with neutrons in nuclear reactors, but can also be extracted from commercially produced devices that are used to remove dust and control static charge by a chemical process.[1] ^{210}Po exhibits several properties that make it extremely dangerous. The short half-life of ^{210}Po and high specific activity of 4490 Ci/g means it emits a great deal of high energy alpha particles (5.3 MeV) that produce 140 W/g. A capsule containing 500 mg of ^{210}Po reaches a temperature of 500°C. It also demonstrates a high volatility where 50% vaporizes in 45 hours at 55°C and can contaminate a relatively large area even when left alone. Although only a small fraction of absorbed ^{210}Po accumulates in tissue, cumulative doses of radiation can lead to organ systems failure and death. Animal data estimate an LD_{50} of 1.3MBq/kg, and that various mammalian species die within 20 days following in ingestion of 1–3 GBq. Because of the extreme specific activity of ^{210}Po this corresponds to a dose of about 0.01 μg/kg. Currently there are no specific chelating agents for ^{210}Po although development of new agents continues.[7,81,102] While there are limited data regarding the effects of ^{210}Po on humans, Alexander Litvinenko's death within 22 days of his poisoning is similar to animal survival data.

Radon (symbol Rn, atomic number 86, and atomic weights range from 204 to 224) was discovered in 1900 by Dorn, and was first called *radium emanation*, then *niton*, and finally radon in 1923. Radon is the heaviest noble gas. Radon is also a decay product of radium and a decay product of thorium and actinium, where it is also called thoron and actinon, respectively. ^{222}Rn decays by α-activity and γ-emissions. Exposure of radon gas to the pulmonary epithelium is associated with an increased incidence of lung cancer in both uranium miners and in those who dwell in residences with increased concentrations of radon. Damage to bronchial epithelium results from the α emissions of radon and radiation from radon daughters that precipitate as solids and remain in the lungs. Good enclosed space ventilation, abstinence from cigarette smoking, and monitoring of radon concentrations will help to minimize this risk.

Technetium (symbol Tc, atomic number 43, and atomic weight 98.9) was discovered in 1937, and was the first element to be produced artificially. Unusual among the lighter elements, Tc has no stable isotopes and is therefore rarely found on earth as a product of spontaneous uranium fission. The majority of technetium is extracted from nuclear fuel rods and is a byproduct of fission of ^{235}U. ^{99m}Tc is used in nuclear medicine for imaging and immunoscintigraphy because of several favorable attributes. ^{99m}Tc (the *m* is for metastable referring to an intermediate energy state), emits γ-rays of similar energy to diagnostic x-rays for easy detection, and has a brief half-life of 6 hours. The daughter isotope, ^{99}Tc, has a half-life of 2.1×10^5 years and allows the isotope to be eliminated before it decays. Most human contact with Tc is in medical scans where Tc has a biological half-life of about a day. There are no reports of adverse effects resulting from overdose with Tc, and no specific therapy is recommended in that event. Chelation with DTPA may be effective.

Thallium (symbol Tl, atomic number 81, and atomic weight 204): Crookes discovered thallium spectroscopically in 1861. ^{201}Tl is used for cardiac imaging, has a half-life of 73 hours, and decays by electron capture and γ emission. Pharmaceutical ^{201}Tl comes as thallous chloride and is created in a cyclotron by bombarding thallium with protons creating ^{201}Pb. It is shipped in this form, which decays into ^{201}Tl. Since the radioactive decay process is continual, it is recommended to administer the ^{201}Tl close to its calibration time to minimize the presence and effects of other radionuclidic contaminants. Chelation can be accomplished with Prussian blue (see Antidotes in Depth A29: Prussian Blue).

Tritium is an isotope of hydrogen whose nucleus contains 1 proton and 2 neutrons, and its symbol is ^{3}H.[103] Tritium decays by β activity and is used in basic science research as a radioactive label, for luminous dials, and self-powered exit signs, which may contain as much as 9.3×10^{11} Bq (25Ci). Tritium has a half-life of 12.3 years. Tritium emits very weak radiation in the form of 18.6 KeV beta particles, which are very easily stopped by thin layers of material and is safe for glow-in-the-dark watches. Tritium is not absorbed as a hydrogen gas, although in contact with oxygen forms tritiated water, which can be absorbed via inhalation or transdermally. The estimated LD_{50} is 3.7×10^{11} Bq (10 Ci) given its extreme specific activity of 9649 Ci/g. When absorbed as tritiated water, tritium tends to follow the water cycle in humans, providing a whole-body dose if incorporated. However, its biological half-life is 10–12 days, which can be decreased by increasing urine output, greatly limiting its potential toxicity.

MANAGEMENT

INITIAL ASSESSMENT

The initial management of patients exposed to radiation will obviously depend on a number of different factors, including the amount of radiation in the exposure and the number of casualties in the event. These important factors will describe to a great extent the amount of resources, such as hospital beds or relatively rarely used medications, which will be required in managing those who were exposed. In a mass-casualty event, established prehospital plans should be followed to provide the best management for the large numbers of variously injured given that the radiation exposure may also be accompanied by an explosion of potentially catastrophic size.

Each patient should have stabilization of the airway, breathing, and circulation. Field triage protocols, according to the kind of event, will designate patients as minor, delayed, immediate, or deceased depending on their burns or physical trauma and will not be altered because of their radiation exposure. Decontamination should proceed in the field taking care not to contaminate prehospital providers or equipment. Prehospital personnel should use personal protective equipment appropriate to the situation, although most events will only require C- or D-level protection, and Geiger counters.

INITIAL EMERGENCY DEPARTMENT MANAGEMENT

When one or more patients who have been exposed to massive irradiation present to the emergency department (ED), attention must first be paid to the more conventional injuries that may also be present.[80,97,104] Many times radiation exposures occur with fires or explosions, and patients may have burns, smoke inhalation injuries, or traumatic injuries. This scenario would be the same for the explosion of the "dirty bomb," a conventional explosive designed to disperse a radionuclide. Most survivable radiation injuries require prompt treatment but are not life-threatening in the first few hours post-event. Thus, there is time to determine if the nature of the exposure was an irradiation or contamination by a radionuclide. Routine considerations of airway, breathing, and circulation take priority for these patients as with all others. If a patient should require surgery, the Armed Forces Radiobiology Research Institute (AFRRI) recommends that surgery proceed immediately because of the delayed and impaired wound healing associated with irradiated tissue.

For large-scale radiation incidents, it is likely that a number of individuals will be involved in developing the best management plan for the casualties. Locally, the radiation safety officer, the medical toxicologist, and the medical oncologist will lend their expertise to the emergency physician to determine the risk of the contaminant, begin appropriate testing to determine the biological effect, and to initiate medical therapy if warranted. Additionally, the local or regional Department of Health should be notified. Larger or complex exposures may require the expertise of the Radiation Emergency Assistance Center based in Oak Ridge, Tennessee (865-576-3131 Monday–Friday 8 am–4:30 pm EST, after hours call 865-576-1005), which can provide valuable support.

Smaller-scale exposures to radiation still require at least a brief evaluation for burns and trauma, depending on the circumstances surrounding the nature of the exposure. Calls to the poison center from a residence require referral to emergency services for an expert evaluation of the extent of the contamination of the site and appropriate decontamination measures. Exposures in the laboratory or nuclear medicine suites require referral to the radiation safety officer in the building for a similar evaluation.

DECONTAMINATION

Patients exposed to radionuclides may be contaminated either externally or internally or both. Historically no medical personnel have ever developed ARS through exposure to a contaminated patient, although caution must be exercised when performing decontamination to minimize exposure to care providers. Unless there is active ongoing radiation, many authors recommend decontamination at the site of exposure to minimize the spread of radioactive materials.[80] All clothing should be removed, and patients should be thoroughly washed with soap and water. In the past, green soap, phosphate-based detergents, and chelating agents such as ethylenediaminetetraacetic acid (EDTA) and DTPA were used.[87] This approach can remove up to 95% of radioactive material from the patient. Open wounds should be carefully scrubbed to minimize the risk of internal contamination. A portable dosimeter may assist in external decontamination. If the patient was exposed to neutron radiation such as from a nuclear reactor, blood samples testing for induced ^{24}Na by γ-spectrophotometric analysis may help as an additional indicator of total dose received. Collected emesis and feces may also be analyzed to help estimate total body dose. All clothing and liquid used to decontaminate must be collected and be clearly marked as radioactive waste. Obviously, there should be no eating, drinking, or smoking at the scene of decontamination.

For patients with smaller exposures to radionuclides, such as laboratory workers, decontamination is often the only management technique required to limit injury. Portable dosimeters will identify contaminated areas, which may be sealed off to limit spread of exposure, especially if the radionuclide is in gaseous form. As with larger exposures, contaminated clothing must be removed and collected. Contaminated skin must be washed with lukewarm soap and water, repeatedly if needed, with care taken not to abrade intact skin and risk inadvertent incorporation. Washing may also be guided by a portable dosimeter. The cesium-exposed patients in Goiânia received repeated baths in warm water and neutral soap over the first 2 days of their hospitalization, as did the patient exposed to americium at Hanford.[95] If the patient is still contaminated after repeated washing, it is recommended to use a cream hand cleaner that contains no abrasives. Some of the Goiânia patients habitually walked barefoot and had developed hyperkeratosis. The palms and soles that were heavily contaminated were treated with titanium dioxide mixed with hydrated lanolin. The paste was rubbed into the contaminated area and then gently abraded to try to remove more cesium.[69]

In evaluating an area in which a spill of radioactive material has occurred, a judgment must be made regarding the severity of the incident so that appropriate steps are taken. If a major incident has occurred involving large amounts of radioactive material, a large contaminated area, airborne radioactivity, or spread of radiation outside an authorized area, evacuation, notification of the radiation safety officer in an institutional setting, and calling local or regional emergency response personnel are recommended. Minor incidents involve small amounts of radioactive material where the individual knows how to clean the site, has appropriate decontamination material on hand, and can clean the area in a reasonably short time. Several different decontaminating agents are commercially available from general stores and many scientific suppliers. These agents come in the form of concentrated detergents or foaming sprays where a small spill is quickly wiped clean and disposed of in an appropriate container.

TRIAGE

It is critical for patients exposed to a large dose of radiation to be triaged according to the dose so that a management plan can be created for them. There are many proposed stages of the various subsyndromes of ARS to help with this dosimetry, but in general we may consider three groups: exposure to less than 2 Gy, exposure to 2–4 Gy, and exposure greater than 4 Gy. Those exposed to less than 2 Gy may experience some of the hematopoietic syndrome, but may be followed as outpatients with or without cytokine therapy. Between 2 and 4 Gy, the hematopoietic syndrome is likely and may be severe, but at this dose the GI syndrome is not likely to be a major complication. Hospitalization is recommended at least initially for more accurate dosimetry and supportive care, including the early initiation of cytokine therapy. Exposure to greater than 4 Gy will mean a severe hematopoietic syndrome and likely a severe GI syndrome as well. These patients will likely require an intensive care setting and substantial supportive care for their survival.

MEDICAL MANAGEMENT

In the ED, after airway and breathing have been managed appropriately, intravenous access should be established. As in the case of patients with thermal burns, peripheral IVs are more prone to infection, and central venous access is recommended. Fluid replacement may begin with crystalloid solution where the rate will be modified by recorded inputs and outputs and assessment of surface area burns if any.

Emergency management of emesis and pain may be difficult in those patients who received a high dose of radiation. Many types of antiemetics are used to control an irradiated patient's vomiting. The 5-HT_3 antagonists are particularly effective in this setting. Mild pain may be managed with acetaminophen, but nonsteroidal antiinflammatory medications are not recommended as they may exacerbate gastric bleeding in a patient for whom bleeding may soon become difficult to control. Morphine is recommended for the management of more severe pain, which may develop within a few hours after the injury from burns, mucositis, and other complications. Prophylactic use of antibiotics is not recommended as is the case with burned patients.

In the ED, it is important to obtain a complete blood count as soon as possible after exposure to begin biodosimetry estimation, and for blood typing. The timing of prodromal signs, such as vomiting, and calculation of the rate constant for lymphocyte depletion help to estimate the dose of radiation to which the patient was exposed. Ideally, a CBC is obtained every 4–6 hours on the first day and then daily following exposure.[36] Some authors recommend initiation of cytokine therapy as soon as possible if the estimated exposure dose is 3 Gy or greater. A threshold of 2 Gy may be used for children younger than 12 years and adults older than 60 years because these patients may be relatively more sensitive to the toxic effects of radiation. Blood typing early is important because the patient may require transfusions of red blood cells and platelets. Use of irradiated cells is recommended to avoid graft-versus-host disease.

For patients who survive the acute period, sepsis is the leading cause of death. To maximize survival, patients with a severe radiation exposure should be treated as other severely burned or immunocompromised patients regarding their risk of infection. Rigorous attention must be paid to the proper use of H_2 antagonists, antibiotics, antifungals, antivirals, and cultures of body fluids.

SPECIAL MANAGEMENT TECHNIQUES

Some patients may require supportive measures to boost their immune system and decrease the risk of infection.[80,104] The colony-stimulating factors, granulocyte colony-stimulating factor, and granulocyte macrophage colony-stimulating factor prime neutrophil microbicidal activity and accelerate neutrophil recovery. Spared hematopoietic stem cells in patients with significant whole body or partial radiation exposures can be stimulated to proliferate in this manner. Although these cytokines only have approval by the FDA for treatment of myelosuppression resulting from cancer treatments, the rationale for their use in the setting of radiation-induced myelosuppression is based on positive results obtained in treating cancer patients and a small number of radiation incident victims and experiments with nonhuman primates.[24,25,104] Colony-stimulating factors were used successfully at Goiânia and decreased the period of leukocyte depression while raising the nadir. Although there is no conclusive evidence that early administration is critical for best outcome for these patients, colony-stimulating-factor therapy should be initiated as early as possible following the diagnosis of a 3-Gy exposure or greater. These factors should be continued until the absolute neutrophil count exceeds 1000 cells/mm^3. However, in the setting of a mass casualty event, it may be prudent to withhold these resources from those with large dose exposures or those with significant concurrent traumatic injuries.

Following Chernobyl, 13 patients received bone marrow transplantation for hematopoietic support until their irradiated bone marrow could recover.[2,80] Unlike patients who undergo bone marrow suppression for clinical reasons, patients involved in a radiation exposure may have incomplete exposure and are usually partially shielded, which may allow for survival of some stem cells. Eleven of these bone marrow transplantation patients at Chernobyl died, complicating the interpretation of the efficacy of transplantation. Bone marrow transplantation does not change the mortality risk from the other subsyndromes of ARS. The ability of bone marrow transplantation to improve the clinical course of an irradiated patient depends on how likely the patient was to die from hematopoietic syndrome alone. Some authors consider that there is limited indication for stem cell transplantation when there is also severe radiation injury to organ systems other than the hematopoietic system.[18] This remains a controversial mode of treatment for irradiated patients.

Probiotics is the introduction of selective nonpathogenic strains of *Lactobacillus* and *Bifidobacteria* into the gastrointestinal tract to suppress the number of pathogens.[80,98] Experimentally, this technique increases survival in canine and rodent models. Probiotics was also used in Chernobyl on three men whose survival time was prolonged, although it was not statistically significant when compared, respectively, to case controls.

Incorporation of radionuclides presents a challenge to the treating physicians in which the goal is removing an internal store of the radioactive material. Beginning in 1966, experiments with beagle dogs treated with DTPA showed decreased incidences of bone cancer when exposed to ^{241}Am.[56,57] Both Ca-DTPA and Zn-DTPA were approved in August 2004 by the FDA for human use for decontamination of plutonium, americium, and curium (see Antidotes in Depth A43: DTPA) Currently, Oak Ridge Associated Universities (ORAU) distributes DTPA under contract with the US Department of Energy (DOE). Additionally, rat experiments with LIHOPO demonstrate decreased retention of plutonium and uranium even after incorporation into bone.[21,101]

Prussian blue, ferric hexacyanoferrate, has been used for many years to treat thallium poisoning. Because it absorbs cesium ions, it is used in fission product recovery and is therefore useful in chelation therapy for patients contaminated with cesium. The two forms of Prussian blue, soluble and insoluble, have been used somewhat interchangeably as antidotes for thallium. However, it is the insoluble form that has the advantage when increasing elimination of cesium from the body (see Antidotes in Depth A29: Prussian Blue).[20,94,100]

As was mentioned earlier, ^{131}I is one of the key fission products that may be released from a nuclear power facility in an accident such as happened at Chernobyl. Additionally, much discussion is currently devoted to the potential for a terrorist attack either on a nuclear power facility or using a radiological dispersal device (ie, "dirty bomb") in which there could be environmental dispersal of radioactive iodine, although the 8-day half-life of ^{131}I theoretically limits its effectiveness as an environmental contaminant. The increase of thyroid cancer observed in atomic bomb survivors and in those contaminated from the Chernobyl event prompted the International Atomic Energy Agency (IAEA) to establish intervention criteria for a radiation emergency of an effective dose equivalent of 100 mSv. The detrimental effects of radioactive iodine can be limited through the use of supplemental potassium iodide (see Antidotes in Depth A42: Potassium Iodide).

PREGNANCY AND RADIATION

In the normal course of events, uncertainty exists regarding the normal viability of the fertilized ovum, and there is a naturally high rate of embryo loss during the early weeks of pregnancy. When exposure to radiation via medical examination is possible, pregnant women and physicians have exhibited extreme concern over its potential teratogenic effects, even though maternal exposures to less than 0.05 Gy (5 rad) is not considered to be teratogenic.[4,39,79] Additionally, risk of direct harm to the fetus from cosmic radiation during casual airline travel is thought to be negligible.[3] Unfortunately, there is little direct information concerning the effects of radiation in early human pregnancy. Experimental data using rats and mice show increased mortality rates both in vitro and in vivo following irradiation and a dose-response curve that depicts incremental increases in radiation dose corresponding to increasingly greater effects in causing malformations.[92] Experimental human data from the 1930s show increased lethality and induction of abortion when pregnant women were exposed to 3.6 Gy and 5 Gy for a therapeutic abortion by x-ray.[42,64]

The most important sources of information concerning the teratogenic effects of fetal irradiation are the survivors of the nuclear bomb blasts of World War II. The three principal risks to a fetus following radiation exposure are congenital abnormalities, severe mental retardation, and the late development of a neoplasm. The embryo is at particular risk because of its rapid development, and there are several periods of particular sensitivity so that irradiation at specific times is associated with increased risk of specific problems. Roughly speaking, uterine absorption of 0.1–0.15 Sv during the first 2 weeks postconception risks fetal lethality. During the third to seventh weeks postconception, uterine doses of 0.05–0.5 Sv risks congenital abnormalities, growth retardation, and small head size that may be accompanied by mental retardation. During the time between weeks 8 and 25 postconception, the risk is severe mental retardation, though that risk decreases at the 16th week.[26,89,92]

Accurate specification of the risks from fetal doses is difficult especially at doses less than 0.2 Sv. Different models consider dose-response relationships for developmental complications and cancer development as linear or linear-quadratic, and with or without a threshold limit. A risk of congenital abnormalities of 5% following exposure to 0.2 Sv compares to a widely accepted average incidence for congenital abnormality of 6% for newborns throughout the world.[92] Patients receiving various diagnostic procedures in the hospital may be exposed to these doses.[41] Clearly, pregnant women who are exposed to radiation are at some risk for a fetal complication, although that risk may be difficult to quantify at the low doses expected with routine radiologic procedures.[13] That low-level intrauterine exposure to radiation increases subsequent cancer risk is not the question, but rather the etiologic significance of the radiation. For many years, studies have been plagued with incomplete data, biological implausibility, and other problems that confound an explanation.[8] Consideration should always be given to the potential maternal benefit of the radiologic procedure and the potential risk to the fetus.[86] However, the vast majority of routine diagnostic imaging procedures imparts less than 0.05 Sv to the fetus and so is considered to be of negligible risk.

PEDIATRICS AND RADIATION

The use of CT scanning in children has markedly increased over the last 20 years. One hospital survey showed a 92% increase in abdominal and pelvic CT examinations from 1996 to 1999 for children younger than 15 years old. Although it is difficult to estimate the increased incidence of cancer rates because of LET radiation, there are reports that attribute a greater lifetime risk for cancer mortality resulting from CT examination in children. This risk is compounded by the tendency not to adjust the radiation dose given to a child during a CT examination from the amount given to adults. Together, these trends may mean increased radiation-induced mortality over the lifetime of the patient resulting from medical evaluation.[10,19,70]

SUMMARY

The danger of ionizing radiation to humans is through the disruption of cellular structure and function. Cell death and mutagenesis are the destructive consequences of an exposure to radiation. Fortunately, large exposures of radiation to the general population are rare outside of the setting of an armed conflict, and most contaminations that occur are small and easily controlled.

In general, recognition of the exposure and thorough decontamination are the critical steps to minimizing the potential toxicity of an exposure. Careful attention to storage of radioactive waste and contaminated materials and good supportive care are usually all that are required to care for most patients.

REFERENCES

1. Azure M, Howell R. Simple isolation of polonium-210 from silver. *Appl Radiat Isot.* 1994;45:637-638.
2. Baranov A, Gale RP, Guskova A, et al. Bone marrow transplantation after the Chernobyl nuclear accident. *N Engl J Med.* 1989;321:205-212.
3. Barish RJ. In-flight radiation exposure during pregnancy. *Obstet Gynecol.* 2004;103:1326-1330.
4. Bentur Y, Horlatsch N, Koren G. Exposure to ionizing radiation during pregnancy: perception of teratogenic risk and outcome. *Teratology.* 1991;43:109-112.
5. Birchard K. Does Iraq's depleted uranium pose a health risk? *Lancet.* 1998;351:657.
6. Blattmann H. Radiation physics. *Experientia.* 1989;45:2-5.
7. Bogdan G, Aphoshian H. N-(2,3-dimercaptopropyl)phthalamidic acid (DMPA) increases polonium-210 excretion. *Biol Metals.* 1990;3:232-236.
8. Boice JD, Miller RW. Childhood and adult cancer after intrauterine exposure toionizing radiation. *Teratology.* 1999;59:227-233.
9. Brenner DJ, Doll R, Goodhead DT, et al. Cancer risks attributable to low doses of ionizing radiation: Assessing what we really know. *Proc Nat Acad Sci.* 2003;100:13761-13766.
10. Brenner DJ, Elliston CD, Hall EJ, et al. Estimated risks of radiation-induced fatal cancer from pediatric CT. *AJR.* 2001;176:289-296.
11. Broga DW, Gilbert MA. A review of three incidents involving the release of 125I from seeds interstitially implanted within the prostate gland. *Health Phys.* 1983;45:593-597.
12. Bronstein A, Spyker D, Cantilena L, et al. 2007 Annual report of the American Association of Poison Control Centers' National Poison Data System (NPDS). *Clin Toxicol.* 2008;46:927-1057.
13. Castronovo FP. Teratogen update: Radiation and Chernobyl. *Teratology.* 1999;60:100-106.
14. Clancy T. Armored Cav. *A Guided Tour of an Armored Cavalry Regiment.* New York: Berkley Publishing Group; 1994.
15. Clarke RH, Southwood TR. Risks from ionizing radiation. *Nature.* 1989;338:197-198.
16. Cohen BL. A test of the linear-no threshold theory of radiation carcinogenesis. *Environmental Res.* 1990;53:193-220.
17. Dainiak N. Hematologic consequences of exposure to ionizing radiation. *Exp Hematol.* 2002;30:513-528.
18. Densow D, Kindler H, Baranov A, et al. Criteria for the selection of radiation accident victims for stem cell transplantation. *Stem Cells.* 1997;15(Suppl 2):287-297.
19. Donnelly LF, Emery KH, Brody AS, et al. Minimizing radiation dose for pediatric body applications of single-detector helical CT: strategies at a large children's hospital. *AJR.* 2001;176:303-306.
20. Dresow B, Nielsen P, Fischer R, et al. In vivo binding of radiocesium by two forms of Prussian blue by ammonium iron hexacyanoferrate (II). *J Toxicol Clin Toxicol.* 1993;31:563-569.
21. Durakovic A. Medical effects of internal contamination with uranium. *Croat Med J.* 1999;40:49-66.
22. Fabrikant JI. The carcinogenic risks of low-LET and high-LET ionizing radiations. *J Radiat Res.* 1991;32:143-164.
23. Fanger H, Lushbaugh CC. Radiation death from cardiovascular shock following a criticality accident. *Arch Path.* 1967;83:446-460.
24. Farese AM, MacVittie TJ, Roskos L, et al. Hematopoietic recovery following autologous bone marrow transplantation in a nonhuman primate: effect of variation in treatment schedule with PEG-rHuMGDF. *Stem Cells.* 2003;21:79-89.
25. Farese AM, Yang BB, Roskos L, et al. Pegfilgrastim, a sustained-duration form of filgrastim, significantly improves neutrophil recovery after autologous marrow transplantation in rhesus macaques. *Bone Marrow Transplant.* 2003;32:399-404.
26. Fattibene P, Mazzei F, Nuccetelli C, et al. Prenatal exposure to ionizing radiation: sources, effects and regulatory aspects. *Acta Pediatrica.* 1999;88:693-702.
27. Fetter S, von Hippl FN. The hazard posed by depleted uranium munitions. *Scientific Global Security.* 1999;8:125-161.
28. Filipy RE, Toohey RE, Kathren RL, et al. Deterministic effects of ^{241}Am exposure in the Hanford americium case. *Health Phys.* 1995;69:338-345.
29. Finch SC. Acute radiation syndrome. *JAMA.* 1987;258:664-667.
30. Forrow L, Sidel VW. Medicine and nuclear war. *JAMA.* 1998;280:456-461.
31. Franic Z, Lokobauer N, Marovic G. Radioactive contamination of cistern waters along the Croatian coast of the Adriatic sea by 90_{Sr}. *Health Phys.* 1999;77:62-66.
32. Fry RJ, Fry SA. Health effects of ionizing radiation. *Med Clin North Am.* 1990;74:475-488.
33. Fuchs M, Schmid A, Eiteljörge T, et al. Exposure of the surgeon to radiation during surgery. *Int Orthoped.* 1998;22:153-156.
34. Giannardi C, Dominci D. Military use of depleted uranium: assessment of prolonged population exposure. *J Environ Radioact.* 2003;64:227-236.
35. Goans RE, Holloway EC, Berger ME, et al. Early dose assessment following severe radiation accidents. *Health Phys.* 1997;72:513-518.
36. Goans RE, Waselenko JK. Medical management of radiological casualties. *Health Phys.* 2005;89:505-512.
37. Golosov VN, Walling DE, Panin ED, et al. The spatial variability of Chernobyl-derived 137Cs inventories in a small agricultural drainage basin in central Russia. *Appl Radiat Isot.* 1999;51:341-352.
38. Groves LM. *Now It Can Be Told.* New York: Da Capo;1983.
39. Haigh F, Given-Wilson R. Current working practices during pregnancy in British radiologists. *Clin Radiol.* 1991;44:108-112.
40. Hall EJ, Hei TK. Genomic instability and bystander effect induced by high-LET radiation. *Oncogene.* 2003;22:7032-7042.
41. Harding LK. Pregnancy and ionizing radiation. *Br Med J.* 1993;306:146-147.
42. Harris W. Therapeutic abortion produced by the roentgen ray. *AJR.* 1932;27:415-419.
43. Hart GC. Diagnostic medical exposures to ionizing radiation during pregnancy. *Nucl Med Commun.* 1994;15:403-404.
44. Hooper FJ, Squibb KS, Siegel EL, et al. Elevated urine uranium excretion by soldiers with retained uranium shrapnel. *Health Phys.* 1999;77:512-519.
45. Ingegno M, Nahabedian M, Tominaga GT, et al. Radiation exposure from cervical spine radiographs. *Am J Emerg Med.* 1994;12:15-16.
46. Jacob P, Kenigsberg Y, Zvonova I. Childhood exposure due to the Chernobyl accident and thyroid cancer risk in contaminated areas of Belarus and Russia. *Br J Cancer.* 1999;80:1461-1469.
47. Jaspers NG, Zdzienicka MZ. Inhibition of DNA synthesis by ionization radiation. *Methods Mol Biol.* 1999;113:535-542.
48. Jonsson B, Forseth T, Ugedal O. Chernobyl radioactivity persists in fish. *Nature.* 1999;400:417.
49. Kanda R. Improvement of accuracy of chromosome aberration analysis for biological radiation dosimetry. *J Radiat Res.* 2000;41:1-8.
50. Keller PD. A clinical syndrome following exposure to atomic bomb explosions. *JAMA.* 1946;131:504-506.
51. Lindholm C, Edwards A. Long-term persistence of translocations in stable lymphocytes from victims of a radiological accident. *Int J Radiat Biol.* 2004;80:559-566.
52. Lindholm C, Luomahaara S, Koivistoinen A, et al. Comparison of dose-response curves for chromosomal aberrations established by chromosome painting and conventional analysis. *Int J Radiat Biol.* 1998;74:27-34.
53. Lindholm C, Salomaa S, Tekkel M, et al. Biodosimetry after accidental radiation exposure by conventional chromosome analysis and FISH. *Int J Radiat Biol.* 1996;70:647-656.
54. Lipsztein JL, Bertelli L, Oliveira CA, et al. Studies of Cs retention in the human body related to body parameters and Prussian blue administration. *Health Phys.* 1991;60:57-61.

55. Littlefield LG, McFee AF, Salomaa SI, et al. Do recorded doses overestimate true doses received by Chernobyl cleanup workers? Results of cytogenetic analyses of Estonian workers by fluorescence in situ hybridization. *Radiat Res.* 1998;150:237-249.
56. Lloyd RD, Taylor GN, Angus W, et al. Soft tissue tumors in beagles injected with ^{241}Am citrate. *Health Phys.* 1995;68:225-233.
57. Lloyd RD, Taylor GN, Mays CW. ^{241}Am removal by DTPA vs. occurrence of skeletal malignancy. *Health Phys.* 1998;75:640-645.
58. Lorimore SA, Coates PJ, Wright EG. Radiation-induced instability and bystander effects: inter-related nontargeted effects of exposure to ionizing radiation. *Oncogene.* 2003;22:7058-7069.
59. Macfarlane GJ, Biggs AM, Maconochie N, et al. Incidence of cancer among UK Gulf war veterans: cohort study. *Br Med J.* 2003;327:1373-1375.
60. Macklis RM. The great radium scandal. *Sci Am.* 1993;269:94-99.
61. Macklis RM, Bellerive MR, Humm JL. The radiotoxicology of radithor. Analysis of an early case of iatrogenic poisoning by a radioactive patent medicine. *JAMA.* 1990;264:619-621.
62. Marshall E. Juarez: an unprecedented radiation accident. *Science.* 1984;223:1152-1154.
63. Martland HS. Occupational poisoning in manufacture of luminous watch dials. *JAMA.* 1929;92:466-473.
64. Mayer M, Harris W, Wimpfheimer S. Therapeutic abortion by means of x-ray. *Am J Obstet Gynecol.* 1936;32:945-957.
65. McDiarmid MA, Engelhardt S, Dorsey C, et al. Surveillance results of depleted uranium-exposed Gulf War I veterans: sixteen years of follow-up. *J Toxicol Environ Health.* 2009;72:14-29.
66. McDiarmid MA, Hooper FJ, Squibb K, et al. The utility of spot collection for urinary uranium determinations in depleted uranium exposed Gulf War veterans. *Health Phys.* 1999;77:261-264.
67. McDiarmid MA, Keogh JP, Hooper FJ, et al. Health effects of depleted uranium on exposed Gulf War veterans. *Environ Res.* 2000;82:168-180.
68. Miller AC, Brooks K, Stewart M, et al. Genomic instability in human osteoblast cells after exposure to depleted uranium: delayed lethality and micronucei formation. *J Environ Radioact.* 2003;64:247-259.
69. Oliveira AR, Hunt JG, Valverde NJL, et al. Medical and related aspects of the Goiânia accident: an overview. *Health Phys.* 1991;60:17-24.
70. Patterson A, Frush DP, Donnelly LF. Helical CT of the body: are settings adjusted for pediatric patients? *AJR.* 2001;176:297-301.
71. Pellmar TC, Fuciarelli AF, Ejnik JW, et al. Distribution of uranium in rats implanted with depleted uranium pellets. *Toxicol Sci.* 1999;49:29-39.
72. Pellmar TC, Keyser DO, Emery C, et al. Electrophysiological changes in hippocampal slices isolated from rats embedded with depleted uranium fragments. *Neurotoxicology.* 1999;20:785-792.
73. Pershagen G, Åkerblom G, Axelson O. Residential radon exposure and lung cancer in Sweden. *N Engl J Med.* 1994;330:159-164.
74. Polednak AP, Stehney AF, Rowland RE. Mortality among women first employed before 1930 in the US radium dial-painting industry. *Am J Epidemiol.* 1978;107:179-195.
75. Priest ND. Toxicity of depleted uranium. *Lancet.* 2001;357:244-245.
76. Prime D. Exposure to radon decay product in dwellings. *J R Soc Health.* 1987;107:228-230.
77. Prise KM, Belyakov OV, Folkard M, et al. Studies of bystander effects in human fibroblasts using a charged particle microbeam. *Int J Radiat Biol.* 1998;74:793-798.
78. Ramalho AT, Nascimento AC, Littlefield LG, et al. Frequency of chromosomal aberrations in a subject accidentally exposed to 137Cs in the Goiânia (Brazil) radiation accident: intercomparison among four laboratories. *Mutat Res.* 1991;252:157-160.
79. Ratnapalan S, Bona N, Chandra K, et al. Physicians' perceptions of teratogenic risk associated with radiography and CT during early pregnancy. *AJR.* 2004;182:1107-1109.
80. Reeves GI. Radiation injuries. *Crit Care Clin.* 1999;2:457-473.
81. Rencova J, Svoboda V, Holusa R, et al. Reduction of subacute lethal radiotoxicity of polonium-210 in rats by chelating agents. *Int J Radiat Biol.* 1997;72:341-348.
82. United Nations Scientific Committee on the Effects of Atomic Radiation (UNSCEAR). Report of the United Nations Scientific Committee on the Effects of Atomic Radiation to the General Assembly. http://www.unscear.org/unscear/en/publications/2000_1.html Published 2000. Accessed January 6, 2009
83. Roff SR. Mortality and morbidity of members of the British Nuclear Tests Veterans Association and the New Zealand Tests Veterans Association and their families. *Med Confl Surviv.* 1999;15:1-51.
84. Roff SR. Residual radiation in Hiroshima and Nagasaki. *Lancet.* 1996;348:620.
85. Roscoe RJ, Steenland K, Halperin WE, et al. Lung cancer mortality among nonsmoking uranium miners exposed to radon daughters. *JAMA.* 1989;262:629-633.
86. Russell JG. Pregnancy and ionizing radiation. *Br Med J.* 1992;305:1172-1173.
87. Saenger EL. Radiation accidents. *Ann Emerg Med.* 1986;15:1061-1066.
88. Sawant SG, Randers-Pehrson G, Geard CR, et al. The bystander effect in radiation oncogenesis: I. Transformation in C3H 10T1/2 cells in vitro can be initiated in the unirradiated neighbors of irradiated cells. *Radiat Res.* 2001;155:397-401.
89. Schull WJ, Otake M. Cognitive function and prenatal exposure to ionizing radiation. *Teratology.* 1999;59:222-226.
90. Shipman TL. Acute radiation death resulting from an accidental nuclear critical excursion. *J Occup Med.* 1961;3:146-192.
91. Spiers FW. A note on Roentgen's x-ray absorption measurements in 1895. *Br J Radiol.* 1986;59:1109-1110.
92. Stovall M, Blackwell CR, Cundiff J. Fetal dose from radiotherapy with photon beams: report of AAPM radiation therapy committee task group no. 36. *Med Phys.* 1995;22:63-83.
93. Takamura N, Nakamura Y, Ishigaki K, et al. Thyroid blockade during a radiation emergency in iodine-rich areas: effect of a stable-iodine dosage. *J Radiat Res.* 2004;45:201-204.
94. Thompson DF, Callen ED. Soluble or insoluble Prussian blue for radiocesium and thallium poisoning. *Ann Pharmacother.* 2004;38:1509-1514.
95. Toohey RE, Kathren RL. Overview and dosimetry of the Hanford americium accident case. *Health Phys.* 1995;69:310-317.
96. Tronko MD, Bogdanova TI, Komissarenko IV, et al. Thyroid carcinoma in children and adolescents in Ukraine after the Chernobyl nuclear accident. *Cancer Res.* 1999;86:149-156.
97. Turai I, Veress K, Günalp B, et al. Medical response to radiation incidents and radionuclear threats. *Br Med J.* 2004;328:568-572.
98. Urbancsek H, Kazar T, Mezes I, et al. Results of a double-blind, randomized study to evaluate the efficacy and safety of *Antibiophilus* in patients with radiation-induced diarrhoea. *Eur J Gastroenterol Hepatol.* 2001;13:391-396.
99. Vañó E, González L, Guibelalde E, et al. Radiation exposure to medical staff in interventional and cardiac radiology. *Br J Radiol.* 1998;71:954-960.
100. Verzijl JM, Joore JC, van Dijk A, et al. In vitro binding characteristics for cesium of two qualities of Prussian blue, activated charcoal, and resonium-a. *J Toxicol Clin Toxicol.* 1992;30:215-222.
101. Volf V, Burgada R, Raymond KN, et al. Chelation therapy by DFO-HOPO and 3,4,3-LIHOPO for injected Pu-238 and Am-241 in the rat: effect of dosage, time, and mode of chelate administration. *Int J Radiat Biol.* 1996;70:765-772.
102. Volf V, Rencova J, Jones MM, et al. Combined chelation treatment for polonium after simulated wound contamination in rat. *Int J Radiat Biol.* 1995;68:395-404.
103. Wang B, Takeda H, Gao WM, et al. Induction of apoptosis by beta radiation from tritium compounds in mouse embryonic brain cells. *Health Phys.* 1999;77:16-23.
104. Waselenko JK, MacVittie TJ, Blakely WF, et al. Medical management of the acute radiation syndrome: recommendations of the Strategic National Stockpile Radiation Working Group. *Ann Int Med.* 2004;140:1037-1051.
105. Weiss EL, Singer CM, Benedict SH, et al. Physician exposure to ionizing radiation during trauma resuscitation: a prospective clinical study. *Ann Emerg Med.* 1990;19:134-138.

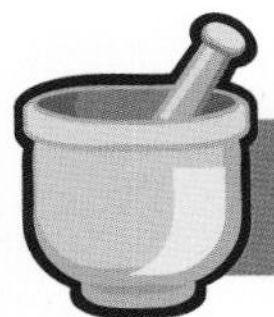

ANTIDOTES IN DEPTH (A42)

POTASSIUM IODIDE

Joseph G. Rella

When a nuclear reactor experiences a catastrophic failure, an uncontrolled release of nuclear fission products such as radioactive iodine (eg, ^{131}I) may occur (Fig. A42–1). Monitoring of the exposed population of Belarus, Russia, following the Chernobyl meltdown of the reactor in 1986 revealed almost a 100-fold increase in the incidence of thyroid cancer among children, echoing similar long-term effects of the nuclear destruction of Hiroshima and Nagasaki in 1945.[4] Iodine is a solid, bimolecular halogen that sublimates under standard conditions. Potassium iodide (KI), the most commonly available iodide salt, has been "generally recognized as safe" by the Food and Drug Administration (FDA) for nearly 40 years. Potassium iodide is recommended to prevent the uptake of radioactive iodine into the thyroid in order to reduce the future risk of thyroid cancer.

IODINE PHYSIOLOGY

Iodine, or its ionic form iodide (I^-), is an essential nutrient present in humans in minute amounts of 15 to 25 mg. Iodine is required for the synthesis of the thyroid hormones l-triiodothyronine (T_3) and L-thyroxine (T_4), which in turn regulate metabolic processes and determine early growth of most organs, especially the brain. Radioactive tracer iodine is distributed in the neck only 3 minutes after ingestion in a fasting subject. Iodide is actively transported with sodium into thyroid follicular cells where it is concentrated 20- to 40-fold compared with its serum concentration. It is then transported into the follicular lumen where it iodinates thyroglobulin to form T_3 and T_4 (see Chap. 49). Thyroid hormones are metabolized in hepatic and other peripheral, extrathyroid tissues by sequential deiodination. Iodide is then excreted in sweat, feces, and urine, and the presence of iodine in the urine is considered a reliable indicator of adequate iodine intake.

PATHOPHYSIOLOGY OF INADEQUATE OR EXCESS IODINE CONCENTRATIONS

Iodine deficiency is a worldwide health problem with large geographic areas deficient in iodine in the foods; this occurs predominantly in mountainous areas and regions far from the world's oceans. In 2003 the World Health Organization (WHO) estimated there were 1.9 billion people with insufficient iodine intake despite universal salt iodization.[22] Iodine deficiency disorders include spontaneous abortions, congenital anomalies, endemic cretinism, goiter, subclinical or overt hypothyroidism, mental retardation, retarded physical development, decreased fertility, and increased susceptibility of the thyroid gland to radiation.

During the critical, immediate postnatal period and the prepubertal and pubertal growth periods, there is a progressive growth of the thyroid gland as well as an increase in thyroglobulin and iodothyronine stores. Insufficient iodine supply in the diet results in increased iodine trapping by the thyroid gland. That is, the thyroid gland accumulates a larger percentage of exogenous ingested iodide and more efficiently reuses iodine that is released by the thyroid or generated by degraded thyroid hormones. These periods of increased iodine uptake explain why children are at greater risk than adults for developing thyroid cancer following exposure to radioactive iodine, especially in endemic areas or areas of relative iodine deficiency.

IODINE EXCESS

Because the effect of iodine on the thyroid is complex, problems may arise as a result of iodine excess as well. The Wolff-Chaikoff effect is a well-known phenomenon where high concentrations of iodine or iodide inhibit the synthesis of thyroid hormones. While this phenomenon is transient and adults generally tolerate it well, its effect may be devastating to a fetus or neonate as it progresses through critical stages of its development. Both the prevalence of goiter and subclinical hypothyroidism can increase when iodine intake is chronically high.[17] Historically, the introduction of iodized salt to iodide-deficient areas increased the incidence of thyrotoxicosis from three to seven per 100,000 in one study,[19] and from 25 to 125 per 100,000 in another study.[5] The majority of these patients were over 40 years old and had autonomous thyroid nodules. The incidences of thyroid autoantibodies and thyroiditis are increased in populations that are iodine replete rather than iodine deficient.[2] One study where subjects began a daily intake of 50 mg of iodide, which was continued for 32 weeks, reported sharply increased thyroid antibody levels in 14% of the studied population.[12]

PATHOPHYSIOLOGY OF RADIOACTIVE IODINE

Exposure via inhalation of gaseous molecular iodine, gaseous organic iodine, and particulate iodine (iodine adherent to suspended particles) may occur when a plume of radioactive material passes overhead. Deposition of radioactive iodine either in the upper respiratory tissue or the digestive tract leads to rapid absorption. The major pathway to toxicity following the Chernobyl incident was ingestion of food contaminated by radioactive iodine, specifically via milk from cows grazing on contaminated grass.[11] For reasons mentioned above, patients with relative iodine deficiency and all children are at increased risk of radioactive iodine uptake. Once incorporated into the thyroid gland, ^{131}I exposes tissue to relatively low energy β and γ emissions, potentially leading to genetic alterations and cancer. This is the stochastic effect of radiation. Although there is some controversy regarding whether the increased number of post-Chernobyl patients with thyroid cancer were due to increased screening[7,8] several reports bear out the increased risk of thyroid cancer,[1,9,11] and it is notable that genetic analysis can distinguish radiation-induced cancers from sporadic papillary cancers.[13,14]

$$^{235}U + ^{1}n \longrightarrow ^{131}In \xrightarrow{0.28\ s} ^{131}Sn \xrightarrow{56\ s} ^{131}Sb \xrightarrow{23\ m} ^{131}Te \xrightarrow{25\ m} \boxed{^{131}I} \xrightarrow{8.02\ d} \boxed{^{131}Xe}$$

FIGURE A42–1. The decay pathway that describes how ^{131}I derives from nuclear fuel, whether in a bomb or a reactor, ultimately decaying to stable xenon.

BENEFITS AND RISKS OF POTASSIUM IODIDE FOR RADIOACTIVE IODINE EXPOSURE

BENEFITS

The principle behind prophylaxis with KI is isotopic dilution where KI competes with radioactive iodine for the active iodine transport system. Similar to the Wolff-Chaikoff effect where excess iodine decreases the synthesis of thyroid hormone, KI prophylaxis blocks thyroid uptake of radioactive iodine by direct competition, although potentially putting some vulnerable populations at risk for hypothyroidism. In nuclear radiology, administration of iodine-containing contrast media can contain up to 45 times the recommended daily intake of free iodine and delay the uptake of therapeutic ^{131}I for several weeks.[10,15,20] Limitation of radioactive iodine incorporation in this situation reduces the risk of developing thyroid cancer. Although radioactive iodine may still be incorporated into thyroid tissue by diffusion from blood (to a much smaller degree), administration of KI limits the recycling of radioactive iodine, diminishes its chemical half-life, and increases its rate of excretion.

RISKS

Adverse reactions can be described in terms of thyroidal and extrathyroidal effects. The thyroidal effects, both hyper- and hypothyroidism, including the Wolff-Chaikoff effect, are described above. Pregnant women with hyperthyroidism must not take KI because of the same effect. Many extrathyroidal effects of KI have been described. Sialadenitis, or iodide mumps, is an inflammation of the salivary glands and appears to be unpredictable. Ioderma is a rare and reversible acneiform eruption related to iodine ingestion that may result from nonspecific immune stimulation.[16] Other reactions reported in association with KI use include gastrointestinal disturbances, fever, and shortness of breath.

Although some reports use imprecise definitions when attributing adverse reactions to iodine or iodide-containing medications, *allergy* refers to a specific immune response to target proteins via an IgE-triggered release of cell mediators, such as histamine. There are no studies that demonstrate IgE antibodies to small molecules such as iodine or iodide.

"Allergy" to radiocontrast media is actually an anaphylactoid response to the high osmolarity of the xenobiotics. Anaphylactoid responses manifest by release of similar mediators to anaphylactic response but via non–IgE-mediated pathways. An anaphylactoid response to iodine-containing medications or iodinated contrast materials may be predicted in patients with asthma, allergic rhinitis, and food allergies to chocolate, eggs, and milk. While seafood may contain iodine, allergy to fish or shellfish is due to specific marine proteins and not sensitivity to iodine. Patients manifesting allergic contact dermatitis resulting from iodine-containing cleaning preparations, such as povidone-iodine, do not react to patch testing with KI. Therefore, when physicians consider the safety of KI dosing in the event of radioactive iodine exposure, reactions to radiocontrast media, seafood, and povidone-iodine should not be interpreted as an allergy to KI. Physicians must also consider that there are inactive ingredients or diluents of the KI formulation.[17]

RECOMMENDATIONS FOR DOSING POTASSIUM IODIDE

CONSIDERATION FOR DIFFERENT EXPOSED GROUPS[6,23]

Adults over 40 years face a near-zero risk of developing thyroid cancer from exposure to radioactive iodine. For this group, the complications from iodide supplementation, including nodular goiter, Grave disease, and autoimmune thyroiditis, outweigh any benefit. Therefore, iodide prophylaxis is not indicated for this age group unless the risk from inhalation rises to 5 Gy or greater, which is unlikely at a substantial distance from the site of nuclear origin. The exact safe distance regarding the likelihood of an exposure greater than 5 Gy is uncertain but is probably about 10 miles from the release site. Beyond this distance, dispersal of the radioactive material in the environment should decrease any exposure to less than 5 Gy.

Adults 18 to 40 years of age have risk of developing thyroid cancer that is approximately equal to the risks of side effects of a single dose of iodide supplementation, although it should be understood that both risks are very small. The decision to treat should be based upon the threshold criteria used as well as the risks of iodine supplementation, such as iodine allergy or a history of past thyroid disease. Repeat administration of KI is not indicated in this group because of increased risk of side effects. Control of food intake should be used to limit any further exposure to radioactive iodine.

Lactating mothers pass as much as 25% of absorbed iodine to their milk within 24 hours. Iodide supplementation will limit this to some extent, but there are several potential complications. Repeat dosing of lactating mothers carries the same risk of repeat doses for other adults 18 to 40 years. Additionally, while stable iodine will be delivered to the nursing newborn, it is possible to cause functional blocking of iodine uptake by an overload of iodine via the Wolff-Chaikoff effect. Therefore, the FDA recommends that lactating mothers not receive repeated doses except during continuing, severe contamination, which would generally be defined by health officials.

Pregnant women have increased thyroid uptake of iodine, especially in the first trimester, compared with other adults. The developing fetus also has increased iodine uptake during the second and third trimesters. Since iodine passes across the placenta, the fetus potentially may be exposed to radioactive iodine. Thus supplementation with KI is recommended at appropriate thresholds. At this critical point in the fetus' development there is a risk of blocking fetal thyroid function by repeat dosing, and the principle of using the minimum effective dose should be followed. While there is no need to vary dosing between pregnant women in different trimesters, if KI is given late in pregnancy, thyroid function should be monitored in the newborn. Repeat dosing of pregnant women is generally not recommended.

Children 1 month to 18 years are at high risk of thyroid cancer from exposure to radioactive iodine and are at low risk of side effects from supplementation with KI. Supplementation for children in this age group should therefore begin promptly following official notification of a potential radioactive iodine release and may continue daily if continued risk warrants it.

Neonates are at significantly increased risk from exposure to radioactive iodine because of a marked increase in uptake of iodine resulting from neonatal body cooling in the immediate postdelivery period. At the same time, neonates are susceptible to functional blocking by overloading with stable iodine. Therefore, when supplementation is indicated, KI should promptly be given to neonates paying critical attention to dosing. The WHO recommends the KI solution be available for maternity wards in the precise dosing for newborns. Since the most critical time period for thyroid blockage is within the first postpartum week, dosing neonates who are older than 1 week may be performed at home via dividing, crushing, or suspending tablets in milk, formula, or water. Repeat dosing of neonates is not recommended. Neonates who are treated with KI in the first weeks of life should be monitored for thyroid-stimulating hormone and free T_4.

DIFFERENCES BETWEEN WHO AND FDA RECOMMENDATIONS

There are several differences between the FDA and the WHO recommendations for dosing adolescents, and also regarding radiation intervention levels. For adolescents 12 to 18 years old, the WHO recommends 130-mg doses based on their perception of this age group's high risk of cancer from exposure instead of the FDA recommended dose of 65 mg. The FDA does allow for a 130-mg dose in adolescents in this age range who approach adult size. Treatment recommendations made by the FDA and the WHO are shown in Table A42–1.

For those exposed in childhood and for lactating women, the WHO additionally recommends a lower intervention threshold of 0.01 Gy rather than the 0.05 Gy threshold used by the FDA. This recommendation is derived from a basic safety standard generic intervention level of 0.1 Gy regardless of age and an estimated incidence of thyroid cancer following a severe event resulting in 20 to 50 new patients with thyroid cancer per million children per year. To decrease this estimate of additional thyroid cancer patients from 20 to 50 to two to five new patients per million per year, compared with an estimated one case per million per year background risk, the WHO recommends decreasing the intervention threshold to 0.01 Gy.

TABLE A42–1. Food and Drug Administration and World Health Organization Guidance for Threshold Thyroid Radioactive Exposures and Recommended Doses of KI for Different Risk Groups

	Predicted Thyroid Exposure (Gy)		KI dose (mg)		No of 130-mg Tablets
	FDA	WHO	FDA	WHO	
Adults > 40 years	≥5	≥5	130	130	1
Adults 18–40 years	≥0.1	≥0.1	130	130	1
Pregnant or lactating women	0.05	0.01	130	130	1
Adolescents 12–18 years			65	130	1/2-1
Children 3–12 years			65	65	1/2
Children 1 month to 3 years			32	32	1/4
Birth to 1 month			16	16	1/8

FORMULATION

Potassium iodide is preferred over potassium iodate (KIO_3) since KI produces less gastrointestinal irritation. When stored in a cool, dry place, tablets packed in their foil should remain fresh for 5 years. These tablets are nonprescription and may be purchased online from multiple vendors. They are sold under such trade names as KI4U, Iosat, Nuke pills, Rad-block, and others, and are available in 65-mg and 130-mg tablets. A liquid formulation also exists with a concentration of 65 mg KI per mL.

TIMING OF ADMINISTRATION

For full blocking effect, KI should be administered shortly before exposure or as soon as possible afterwards. Some models describe the blockade of only 50% of iodine uptake when there is a delay of several hours following an exposure.[23] Depending on the duration and type of risk, administration of KI months after an exposure may also partially reduce thyroid cancer risk.[7] One study from Poland shows that following the Chernobyl disaster the incidence of thyroid cancers increased with the degree of radioactive contamination as well as the degree of iodine deficiency. Young people aged 19 years old or younger accounted for only 1.6% of the new cancers compared with women over 40 years old who comprised nearly 80% of the new cancers in this group. No mention was made regarding KI prophylaxis for patients in this group.[18]

AVAILABILITY, DISTRIBUTION, AND OTHER PROTECTIVE MEASURES

The degree of regulation of KI by the government has changed several times over the last few years. Although the US government began stockpiling iodine for defense purposes following the end of World War II, it reduced its KI stockpile from 3700 to 1629 metric tons by 2001. Following the incident at Three Mile Island in 1979, the federal government established the Federal Radiological Preparedness Coordinating Committee (FRPCC) to ensure a consolidated federal position on preparedness, which recommended KI only be stockpiled for emergency workers and institutionalized persons within a 10-mile *plume exposure pathway emergency planning zone* (EPZ) for emergencies near nuclear power plants. In 2001, the FRPCC supported a Nuclear Regulatory Commission (NRC) rule change extending KI to the general public within a 10-mile EPZ as a prudent adjunct to sheltering and evacuation. Section 127 of the Public Health Security and Bioterrorism Preparedness and Response Act of 2002 stated the federal government would make KI available to state and local governments for populations within 20 miles of a nuclear power plant. As of October 2006, 21 of 34 states with commercial nuclear power facilities requested and/or received KI tablets, and 11 also requested or received liquid preparations. These supplies are made available through the Strategic National Stockpile to local governments that may distribute KI from various distribution centers. A waiver of Section 127 of the Public Health Security and Bioterrorism Preparedness and Response Act of 2002 was invoked in July 2007 reducing the radius of federally supported KI to 10 miles, favoring evacuation and food interdiction for those living outside that area.[3]

The perception of the nature of the threat is varied. The FRPCC considers a significant exposure to radioactive iodine a very low risk and has determined that state and local governments should decide on stockpiling and distribution plans for themselves. One survey of public health officials in New York State reported that 65% of those surveyed were not in favor of taking any steps to plan or act to protect the public's health against the potential dangers from local nuclear plant even though 62% of the same group considered a Chernobyl-type event could occur in the United States.[21]

Despite an experience in Poland following the Chernobyl event where a single age-appropriate dose was given to more than 18 million people over a period of 3 days, drills to distribute KI to homes within five miles of a nuclear power plant in the United States were considered too slow to provide adequate protection, supporting the argument of having KI distributed prior to any potential event. In 2002, the New Jersey Department of Health and Senior Services (NJDHSS) distributed KI to interested persons living within 10 miles of two nuclear reactors and surveyed the recipients regarding indications and usage of KI. Whereas the study demonstrated the need for a significant education and outreach program, 40% of respondents indicated they might use KI regardless of an announcement from a government agency, which may herald an epidemic of inappropriate use of KI. Additionally, the study found that emergency departments and primary care physicians would likely receive large volumes of patients seeking KI pills during a nuclear event.[3]

EVACUATION AND FOOD INTERDICTION

KI is not a panacea for radiation exposure. Even if appropriately used during a release of ^{131}I, KI will not protect against direct radiation exposure or against other radioactive elements that may be included in fallout. Depending on radiation levels, communities may be evacuated from areas immediately surrounding a nuclear power plant experiencing a release of radioactive material. Evacuation is most effective if implemented before the passage of a radioactive plume, but this should be guided by realistic dose estimates.

The FDA and WHO both recommend food interdiction and food control as the principle means to limit public exposure to contamination. Exposed canned food from affected areas may ultimately pose no risk to the population if they are stored for weeks to months, which would allow the radioactive iodine to decay completely. The WHO considers food control to be preferable to iodine prophylaxis and removal of milk from the diet of some populations to be merely inconvenient.[6,23]

SUMMARY

KI is a safe and effective means of blocking the uptake of ^{131}I following a nuclear catastrophe. Firm reliance on health officials' evaluation of the risk of exposure is vital since the overall likelihood of exposure to the critical radiation threshold is very low except for those living within 10 miles of a nuclear reactor. Exposed persons should strictly adhere to dosing guidelines to minimize the potential risks of KI dosing, especially in pregnant women and newborn children. It should be recognized that food interdiction and evacuation or avoidance of the radioactive plume are preferable to KI prophylaxis in the event of a potential exposure and may obviate the need for KI completely.

REFERENCES

1. Astakhova LN, Anspaugh LR, Beebe GW, et al. Chernobyl-related thyroid cancer in children of Belarus: a case-control study. *Radiat Res.* 1998;150:349-356.
2. Baltisberger B, Minder C, Bürgi H. Decrease in incidence of toxic nodular goitre in a region of Switzerland after full correction of mild iodine deficiency. *Eur J Endocrinol.* 1995;132:546-549.
3. Blando J, Robertson C, Pearl K, et al. Assessment of potassium iodide (KI) distribution program among communities within the emergency planning zones (EPZ) of two nuclear power plants. *Health Phys.* 2007;(suppl 1):S18-S26.
4. Cardis E, Kesminiene A, Ivanov V, et al. Risk of thyroid cancer after exposure to ^{131}I in childhood. *J Natl Cancer Inst.* 2005;97:724-732.
5. Connolly R, Vidor G, Stewart J. Increase in thyrotoxicosis in endemic goitre area after iodation of bread. *Lancet.* 1970;i:500-502.
6. Food and Drug Administration. Guidance. Potassium iodide as a thyroid blocking agent in radiation emergencies. http://wwwfdagov/cder/guidance/4825fnl.pdf. Published 2001. Accessed February 2009.
7. Holm L. Thyroid cancer after exposure to radioactive ^{131}I. *Acta Oncol.* 2006;45:1037-1040.
8. Jaworowski Z. Lessons of Chernobyl—with particular reference to thyroid cancer. *Australasian Radiat Protect Soc Newsletter.* 2004;30.
9. Kazakov VS, Demidchik EP, Astakhova LN. Thyroid cancer after Chernobyl. *Nature.* 1992;359:21.
10. Laurie A, Lyon S, Lasser E. Contrast material iodides: potential effects on radioactive iodine thyroid uptake. *J Nucl Med.* 1992;33:237-238.
11. Mahoney MC, Lawvere S, Falkner KL, et al. Thyroid cancer incidence trends in Belarus: examining the impact of Chernobyl. *Int J Epidemiol.* 2004;33:1-9.
12. Pearce E, BGerber A, Gootnick D, et al. Effects of chronic iodine excess in a cohort of long-term American workers in West Africa. *J Clin Endocrinol Metab.* 2002;87:5499-5502.
13. Port M, Boltze C, Wang Y, et al. A radiation-induced gene signature distinguishes post-Chernobyl from sporadic papillary thyroid cancers. *Radiat Res.* 2007;168:639-649.
14. Robbins J, Schneider A. Radioiodine-induced thyroid cancer. studies in the aftermath of the accident at Cherobyl. *Trends Endocrinol Metab.* 1998;3:87-94.
15. Rogers W, Robbins L. Iodiamide (cholografin) administration. Its effect on the thyroid uptake of I-131 and the serum precipitable iodine in euthyroid persons. *N Engl J Med.* 1955;253:424-425.
16. Sicherer SH. Risk of severe allergic reactions from the use of potassium iodide for radiation emergencies. *J Allergy Clin Immunol.* 2004;114:1395-1397.
17. Suzuki H, Higuchi T, Sawa K, et al. Endemic coast goiter in Hokkaido, Japan. *Acta Endocrinol (Copenh).* 1965;50:161-176.
18. Szybinski Z, Huszno B, Zemla B, et al. Incidence of thyroid cancer in the selected areas of iodine deficiency in Poland. *J Endocrinol Invest.* 2003;26(suppl 2):63-70.
19. Todd C, Allain T, Gomo Z, et al. Increase in thyrotoxicosis associated with iodine supplements in Zimbabwe. *Lancet.* 1995;346:1563-1564.
20. van der Molen A, Thomsen H, Morcos S. Effect of iodinated contrast media on thyroid function in adults. *Eur Radiol.* 2004;14:902-907.
21. Winder AE, Hossain Z, Reddy S. The health effects of ionizing radiation: a survey of local health officials in New England and New York. *Public Health Rep.* 1994;109:219-225.
22. World Health Organization, Department of Nutrition for Health and Development. Iodine status worldwide. WHO database on global iodine deficiency. http://whqlibdoc.who.int/publications/2004/9241592001.pdf. Published 2004. Accessed January 13, 2009.
23. World Health Organization. Guidelines for iodine prophylaxis following nuclear accidents—update 1999. http://www.who.int/ionizing_radiation/pub_meet/Iodine_Prophylaxis_guide.pdf. Published 1989. Updated 1999. Accessed February 2009.

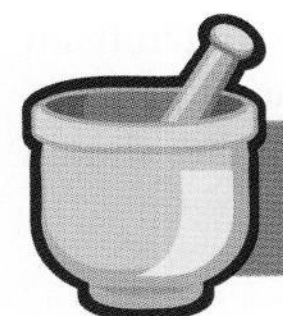

ANTIDOTES IN DEPTH (A43)

DTPA [PENTETIC ACID OR PENTETATE (ZINC OR CALCIUM) TRISODIUM]

Joseph G. Rella

Pentetate zinc trisodium and pentetate calcium trisodium (zinc or calcium diethylenetriaminepentaacetate), Zn-DTPA and Ca-DTPA, are chelators approved for the treatment of internal contamination with plutonium (Pu), americium (Am), and curium (Cm). Both xenobiotics were first used investigationally in 1955 to enhance elimination of these transuranic elements.[3] DTPA has also been used for the extraction of metals from soil,[20] as a treatment for iron overload and lead toxicity,[2,9] and as a chelator for Food and Drug Administration (FDA)-approved nuclear medical studies to prevent incorporation of injected radioisotopes.

CHEMISTRY

DTPA is a synthetic polyamino polycarboxylic acid with a molecular weight of 522 daltons. It is water soluble and bonds stoichiometrically with a central metal ion through the formal donation of one or more of its electrons. In addition to the use of DTPA to chelate the transuranic elements Am, Pu, and Cm, there are also reports of its use in chelating patients contaminated with californium (Cf),[17] and berkelium (Bk). The transuranic elements displace the calcium or zinc ion forming a stable DTPA-chelate complex (Fig. A43–1), which is then excreted in urine. DTPA has specific stability coefficients for the various elements that it chelates, which presumably explains the different binding efficacies of the calcium and zinc salts.

DTPA is not recommended or approved for treating patients contaminated with uranium (U) or neptunium (Np) for several reasons. DTPA mobilizes uranium from tissue stores but does not increase urinary elimination.[6,15] Chelating incorporated Np is somewhat dependent on its valence Np^{+4} versus Np^{+5} but because it forms very stable complexes with transferrin it is very difficult to decorporate, and Np currently remains the subject of in vitro experiments combining DTPA with other chelators.[7,14] While a systematic evaluation of all available data on DTPA efficacy for decorporation of transuranics has not been reported, it is nevertheless clear from many case reports that DTPA is very effective.

PHARMACOKINETICS

DTPA is rapidly absorbed via intramuscular, intraperitoneal, and intravenous routes. Animal studies show that DTPA is poorly (less than 5%) absorbed by the gastrointestinal tract. Absorption from the lungs is about 20% to 30%. Its volume of distribution is small (0.14 L/kg in humans) and is distributed throughout the extracellular space. It does not appear to penetrate well into erythrocytes or other cells. There is no binding of the chelate in the renal parenchyma, which is important to note since animal data showed severe lesions in the kidneys when exposed to 100-fold overdoses.[5] The serum half-life is 20 to 60 minutes, although a small fraction is bound to plasma proteins with a half-life of more than 20 hours. DTPA undergoes minimal, if any, metabolism. Only a minimal release of acetate has been demonstrated, and splitting of ethylene groups was not detected.

Elimination is via glomerular filtration with more than 95% excreted within 12 hours and 99% by 24 hours. There are no data regarding dosing or clearance changes in patients with renal impairment. For patients with renal impairment, hemodialysis increases the rate of elimination of Tc-99m DTPA and Gd-DTPA.[13,21] Less than 3% is excreted via stool.

ADVERSE EFFECTS AND SAFETY

No serious toxicity has been reported among humans after over 4500 Ca-DTPA administrations at recommended doses.[3] Adverse reactions have included nausea, vomiting, diarrhea, chills, fever, pruritus, and muscle cramps. Transient anosmia was observed in one individual after repeated treatments with Ca-DTPA. The specific mechanisms for these adverse reactions remain undefined.

Mice given 60 times the recommended dose of Ca-DTPA developed severe injuries to kidneys, liver, and intestines, and deaths occurred.[5] Toxicity was correlated to the total dose and dosing schedule, where fractionated doses were more fatal than similar doses given as a single injection. The injuries were believed to result from significant depletion of Zn and Mn, since Zn-DTPA did not show the same toxicity at the same dose and schedule. These mouse data were interpreted to suggest that Zn-DTPA is approximately 30-fold less toxic than Ca-DTPA. Acutely lethal doses of Zn-DTPA were estimated to be 10 g/kg in the adult male mouse.

INDICATIONS, DOSING, AND ADMINISTRATION

DTPA is indicated for suspected contamination with Pu, Am, and Cm, and should be strongly considered for contaminations involving californium and berkelium. A registry of persons treated with DTPA was established in 1977 at the Oak Ridge Associated Universities (ORAU), and to date all recipients were contaminated while working with transuranics except for one deliberate overdose of uranium acetate.[15] This is important in that the treated patients were aware of their exposure, whereas a member of the general public exposed to a radiation dispersal device would not necessarily have this knowledge. Additionally, the assessment of the severity of contamination is measured not by mass but in disintegrations (becquerel), which may not be readily available at the time of the patient's initial presentation. Thus, these surreptitiously contaminated patients present the additional challenge of determining if their exposure is severe enough to warrant administration of the chelator, which will require consultation with a radiation safety officer.

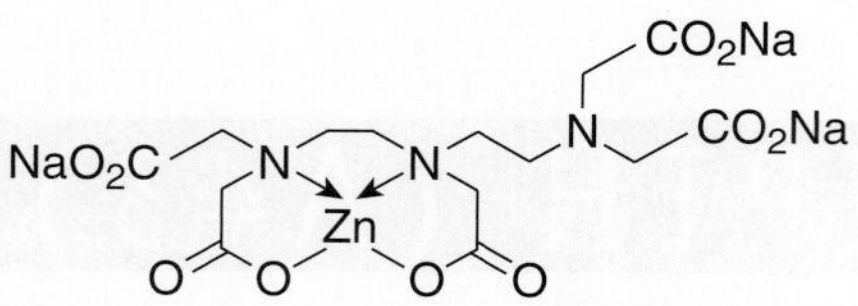

FIGURE A43–1. Trisodium zinc diethylenetriaminepentaacetate, where a transuranic element (Am, Pu, Cm) is substituted for Zn forming a stable chelate.

Treatment of contaminated patients includes attention to vital signs and simultaneous superficial decontamination of the radioactive material. Baseline blood and urine samples (for urine radioassay) should be obtained. Administration of DTPA is recommended to begin within the first 24 hours following the exposure, preferably within the first hour. By 24 hours postexposure soluble Pu and Am are deposited in bone, theoretically rendering DTPA ineffective (in the absence of bone remodeling).[8] Historical data concerning contaminated workers at nuclear materials production facilities include those who received both prolonged and delayed treatments and demonstrated greatly increased urinary excretion of radioactive material.[1,10-12,18,19]

If the route of contamination is oral, mixed, or unknown, then Ca-DTPA should be administered intravenously. The intravenous dose of Ca-DTPA is 1 g in adults and 14 mg/kg up to the adult dose in children under 12 years, administered either undiluted over 3 to 4 minutes, or diluted in 100 to 250 mL D_5W, Ringer's lactate, or 0.9% sodium chloride, over 30 minutes. On the basis of animal studies it should not be given more slowly.[5] Maintaining normal volume status and frequent voiding should be encouraged to dilute the radioactive chelate and minimize exposure to the bladder. If contamination occurred only via inhalation, Ca-DTPA may be diluted 1:1 with sterile water and administered via nebulization.[16]

Although Ca-DTPA is recommended as the initial chelator, Zn-DTPA should be used after the first 24 hours. Studies in rodents show a 10-fold increased rate of elimination of Pu with Ca-DTPA compared with Zn-DTPA, and Ca-DTPA has its greatest effect when given within 24 hours of contamination. Additionally, there is concern that trace metals, such as zinc, are excessively removed with continued treatment with Ca-DTPA. After this period, Zn-DTPA given daily at the same dose is recommended for any continuing therapy because of its relatively diminished depletion of trace metals and the absence of liver, kidney, and intestinal injury.

The decision to continue therapy should be based on radioassay data. Historically, about 55% of all patients treated with DTPA required only one dose. This assessment should include collection of 24-hour urine samples, whole body or chest counting, and close consultation with the hospital radiation safety officer. Assistance is also available from the Oak Ridge Institute for Science and Education (ORISE) and its training center, the Radiation Assistance Center/Training Site (REAC/TS) at (865) 576–3131, or (865) 576–1005 after hours. These calculations involve radioassay by alpha spectroscopy for actinides and, using intake retention factors and dose conversion coefficients, one can calculate the residual body activity and resultant committed effective dose to a relevant organ system. Current recommendations are to continue chelation until the deposition of contaminant is less than 5% of the maximum permissible body burden for a given contaminant.[3]

If continued therapy is indicated, a regimen of Zn-DTPA may continue the following day. The FDA recommends daily dosing of 1 g. ORISE recommends 1 g daily for up to 5 days per week, for the first week. If continuing chelation therapy is indicated a two-dose per week regimen should be initiated until the excretion rate of the contaminant does not increase with Zn-DTPA administration.[4,16,22] For all patients, data regarding vital signs, adverse effects, and bioassay studies should be reported to the drug manufacturer and also to ORAU.

AVAILABILITY

DTPA is available as Ca-DTPA or Zn-DTPA as a sterile solution in 5-mL ampules containing 200 mg/mL (1 g per ampule). It should be stored in a cool, dry place with an ambient temperature of between 15°C and 30°C (59°F–86°F) away from sunlight. The available solution is a clear hyperosmolar solution (1260 mOsm/kg).[16]

USE IN PREGNANCY AND CHILDREN

These chelators do not cross the placental barrier. There are no human pregnancy outcome data from which to draw conclusions regarding the risk of DTPA. Likewise, there are no data regarding safety in lactating women, and data regarding the use in children are extrapolated. Mouse studies involving doses up to 10 times recommended dosage for Ca-DTPA did not produce harmful effects; however, higher doses of greater than 20 times recommended dosage produced teratogenicity and fetal death. Studies have not been conducted on pregnant women or on children. Conversely, these same studies showed only a slight weight reduction in mouse fetuses when given similar overdoses of Zn-DTPA.

SUMMARY

Ca-DTPA, started within the first 24 hours, and Zn-DTPA, which may continue after 24 hours, enhance urinary excretion of Am, Cu, and Pu, and should be considered as chelators for Cf and Bk. Fifty years of experience accompanies the use of these xenobiotics, which have been shown experimentally and historically to be very safe to use in humans. Recommended doses should not be exceeded and adequate hydration is recommended. Dialysis may be considered for contaminated patients with renal insufficiency.

REFERENCES

1. Bailey B, Eckerman K, Townsend L. An analysis of a puncture wound case with medical intervention. *Radiat Prot Dosimetry.* 2003;105:509-512.
2. Barry M, Cartei G, Sherlock S. Quantitative measurement of iron stores with diethylenetriamene penta-acetic acid. *Gut.* 1970;11:891-898.
3. Breitenstein B, Fry S, Lushbaugh CC. DTPA therapy: the US experience 1958-1987. In: Ricks RC, Fry S, eds. *The Medical Basis for Radiation Accident Preparedness II: Clinical Experience and Follow-Up Since 1979.* New York: Elsevier; 1990:397-414.
4. Calcium DTPA [package insert]. Oak Ridge: Radiation Emergency Assistance Center/Training Site; 2002. http://orise.orau.gov/reacts/ca-dtpa.htm. Accessed January 15, 2009.
5. Calder S, Mays CW, Taylor GN, et al. Zn-DTPA safety in the mouse fetus. *Health Phys.* 1979;36:524-526.
6. Domingo J, de la torre A, Belles M, et al. Comparative effects of the chelators sodium 4,5-dihydroxybenzene-1,3-disulfonate (Tiron) and diethylenetriaminepentaacetic acid (DTPA) on acute uranium nephrotoxicity in rats. *Toxicol Appl Pharmacol.* 1997;118:49-59.
7. Fritsch P, Ramounet B, Burgada R, et al. Experimental approaches to improve the available chelator treatments for Np decorporation. *J Alloys Compd.* 1998;271:89-92.
8. Guilmette R, Lindhorst P, Hanlon L. Interaction of Pu and Am with bone mineral in vitro. *Radiat Prot Dosimetry.* 1998;79:453-458.

9. Jackson M, Brenton D. DTPA therapy in the management of iron overload in thalassaemia. *J Inher Metab Dis.* 1983;6(suppl 2):97-98.
10. Khokhryakov V, Belyaev A, Kudryavtseva T, et al. Successful DTPA therapy in the case of ^{239}Pu penetration via injured skin exposed to nitric acid. *Radiat Prot Dosimetry.* 2003;105:499-502.
11. Lagerquist C, Hammond S, Putzier E, et al. Effectiveness of early DTPA treatments in two types of plutonium exposures in humans. *Health Phys.* 1965;11:1177-1180.
12. Ohlenschlager L, Schieferdecker H, Schmidt-Martin W. Efficacy of Zn-DTPA and Ca-DTPA in removing plutonium from the human body. *Health Phys.* 1978;35:694-698.
13. Okada S, Katagiri K, Kumazaki T, et al. Safety of gadolinium contrast agent in hemodialysis patients. *Acta Radiol.* 2001;42:339-341.
14. Paquet F, Metivier H, Poncy J, et al. Evaluation of the efficiency of DTPA and other new chelating agents for removing neptunium from target organs. *Int J Radiat Biol.* 1997;71:613-621.
15. Pavlakis N, Polock C, McLean G, et al. Deliberate overdose of uranium: toxicity and treatment. *Nephron.* 1996;72:313-317.
16. Pentetate zinc trisodium injection [package insert—instructions for use]. Food and Drug Administration; 2004. http://www.fda.gov/cder/foi/label/2004/021751lbl.pdf. Accessed January 9, 2009.
17. Poda G, Hall R. Two californium-252 inhalation cases. *Health Phys.* 1975;29:407-409.
18. Rosen J, Gur D, Pan S, et al. Long-term removal of Am-241 using DTPA. *Health Phys.* 1980;39:601-609.
19. Schofield G, Howells H, Ward F, et al. Assessment and management of a plutonium contaminated wound case. *Health Phys.* 1974;26:541-554.
20. Soltanpour P, Schwab A. A new soil test for simultaneous extraction of macro- and micro-nutrients in alkaline soils. *Commun Soil Sci Plant Anal.* 1977;8:195-207.
21. Wainer E, Boner G, Lubin E, et al. Clearance of Tc-99m DTPA in hemodialysis and peritoneal dialysis: concise communication. *J Nucl Med.* 1981;22:768-771.
22. Zinc-DTPA [package insert]. Oak Ridge: Radiation Emergency Assistance Center/Training Site; 2002. http://orise.orau.gov/reacts/zinc-dtpa.htm. Accessed January 15, 2009.

SECTION 2 POISON CENTERS AND EPIDEMIOLOGY

CHAPTER 134 POISON PREVENTION AND EDUCATION

Lauren Schwartz

Unintentional poisonings are a global health concern. According to the World Health Organization (WHO), in 2002 approximately 350,000 people died worldwide from unintentional poisoning. WHO has undertaken initiatives in many countries including China, Trinidad and Tobago, Ghana, the Bahamas, Myanmar, Senegal, and Lebanon to establish Poison Centers (PC) and raise awareness about poison prevention.[28] This chapter focuses on programs in North America that aim to prevent unintentional poisonings and improve access to PC services.

Healthy People 2010 is a US federal program that outlines the health goals for the nation. The goals reflect the input of public health individuals and organizations and consist of 28 areas to reach 2 main goals: increasing quality and years of healthy life, and eliminating health disparities. Two objectives in the Injury and Violence Prevention section relate to poison prevention. Objective 15–7 is to reduce nonfatal poisonings and Objective 15–8 is to reduce deaths caused by poisoning. Objective 1–12 under Access to Quality Health Services recommends establishing a single toll-free telephone number for access to PCs on a 24-hour basis throughout the United States.[26] This objective was achieved in 2002. Community-based public education programs at PCs are designed to help meet these other public health objectives.

LEGISLATION AND POISON PREVENTION

Since the first PC was established in 1953, a number of legislative events have improved poison prevention and awareness efforts and reduced the number of unintentional poisonings in children. Public education programs at PCs have been influenced by these federal measures.[71]

NATIONAL POISON PREVENTION WEEK

In 1961, President John F. Kennedy signed Public Law 87–319, designating the third week of March as National Poison Prevention Week (PPW)[6] to raise awareness of the dangers of unintentional poisonings. Each year, during PPW, PCs and other organizations around the country organize events and activities to promote poison prevention.

CHILD-RESISTANT PACKAGING ACT

In 1970, the Poison Prevention Packaging Act was passed. This law requires that the Consumer Product Safety Commission (CPSC) mandate the use of child-resistant containers for toxic household substances. In 1974, oral prescription medications were included in this requirement. A review of mortality data in children younger than age 5 shows a significant decrease in deaths after enforcement of the child-resistant packaging legislation.[59,71,74]

TASTE-AVERSIVE XENOBIOTICS AND POISON PREVENTION

Nontoxic taste-aversive xenobiotics are frequently added to products such as shampoo, cosmetics, cleaning products, automotive products, and rubbing alcohol to discourage ingestion.[25] Except in the case of rubbing alcohol, this is done primarily to prevent poisoning in children. The most common taste-aversive xenobiotics are the denatonium salts, particularly denatonium benzoate (Bitrex, benzyldiethyl[(2,6-xylylcarbamoyl)methyl] ammonium benzoate), one of the most bitter-tasting xenobiotics known. The bitter taste of denatonium benzoate can be detected at 50 parts per billion (ppb). This aversive xenobiotic is used in concentrations of 6–50 parts per million (ppm), typically 6 ppm in cosmetic products and ethanol and 30–50 ppm in methanol and ethylene glycol.[12,52] Only limited data are available on the usefulness of taste-aversive xenobiotics for prevention of poisoning. Studies using denatonium benzoate added to liquid detergent and orange juice demonstrate that it can decrease the amount ingested by children.[10,67] However, the degree of taste aversion is not universal; in one study, some children were noted to take more than one sip of denatonium benzoate-laced orange juice.[67] Taste aversion is partially a learned response; frequently young children do not find a bitter taste as offensive as do adults.[11] It seems unlikely that taste-aversive xenobiotics will eliminate unintentional ingestions in children, because oral ingestion is required for aversive effects to occur. Taste-aversive xenobiotics may be most beneficial in the prevention of poisoning by toxic and nonaversive xenobiotics, such as ethylene glycol, methanol, paraquat, certain pesticides, acetonitrile, and bromate-containing cosmetics, where more than one or two sips of the product must be ingested to cause toxicity. In 1995, Oregon became the first state to mandate the addition of an aversive xenobiotic to ethylene glycol- or methanol-containing car products in their 1995 Toxic Household Products statute. Analysis on the incidence and severity of ethylene glycol and methanol exposures before and after the mandate could not demonstrate any difference.[48] Taste-aversive xenobiotics are not and cannot be substitutes for other poison prevention modalities.

TOLL-FREE ACCESS TO POISON CENTERS

In 2000, the Poison Control Center Enhancement and Awareness Act was enacted with a goal of nationwide access to PCs. A toll-free number (1–800-222–1222) was established in January 2002 for all US

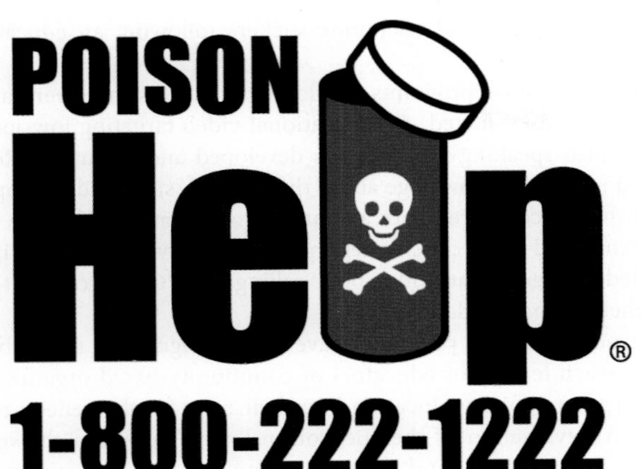

FIGURE 134–1. National toll-free number logo.

PCs. Callers are connected to a regional PC based on the area code and telephone number exchange. Figure 134–1 displays the national logo incorporated into educational efforts.

THE ROLE OF PUBLIC EDUCATORS IN POISON CENTERS

Poison Center educators encompass a range of educational backgrounds including nurses, pharmacists, health educators, and teachers. The role of the public educator is based on social marketing concepts and encompasses two objectives: health promotion to change behavior and marketing the PC.[69] Public education programs at PCs teach poison prevention techniques (primary prevention) and raise awareness about available services should a poisoning occur (secondary prevention). Education programs may utilize primary or secondary teaching or a combination of both.[9,29,36,42] Public educators at PCs provide a range of community-based programs ranging from workshops and health fairs to producing print materials, videos, and awareness campaigns through public service advertising using radio, television, print, and mass transit venues. Additionally, the use of the Internet has provided a new medium for educators to provide information and materials that can be rapidly updated and downloaded without cost.[6] Educators also participate in community health coalitions, working in conjunction with other injury prevention groups such as National Safe Kids, and collaborate with a wide range of community health agencies. Caregivers of children younger than age 6 are often deemed the most important group to reach with education programs. Educators often work with national programs for families including Women, Infant and Children (WIC), Head Start, and the Red Cross. Additionally, programs for grandparents offer an educational opportunity to reach this large high-risk population. Collaborative programs with the American Association of Retired Persons (AARP), senior centers, and Department for the Aging offer an opportunity to provide programs focused on poison prevention for older adults.

The membership of the American Association of Poison Control Center's Public Education Committee (PEC) includes the educators from PCs across the United States and Canada. The mission of the PEC is to provide poison prevention awareness programs in an effort to reduce morbidity and mortality associated with poisoning.[5] Each year, the PEC provides educational sessions at the North American Congress of Clinical Toxicology. PEC workshops focus on program development, evaluation, grant writing, strategic planning, and other topics of interest to PC educators.[6,29]

NEEDS ASSESSMENTS

To develop successful poison education programs, educators must first analyze demographic data, call volume rates, cultural and language issues, and barriers to calling a PC. Geographic information systems (GIS) software offers a way for PCs to visually map demographic data. The use of this type of software is increasing in public health and can be applied to PC efforts. The coordination of data retrieval from various data entry programs and the use of GIS software by PC staff provide access to call rates by zip codes, counties, census tracts, or congressional districts to be used for planning programs. Health and social services for the targeted community may also be presented using GIS maps. Using GIS for population-based programs is recommended for developing social marketing campaigns, health education programs, outreach efforts, and coalition building.[58] The study of geographic areas with low call rates enhances the potential for targeted educational programs.

Focus groups provide a useful qualitative method for PC educators to identify caregivers' and seniors' perceptions about calling the PC. Barriers regarding PC utilization include not knowing the PC number, preference for calling 911 rather than the PC; fear of being reported to child welfare agencies; concerns with regard to confidentiality; language difficulties; lack of direct contact with health providers; low self-efficacy; and concerns regarding the cost of the call.[1,8,13,31,32,64,73] Each of these barriers must be considered and creatively addressed when planning new programs for reaching caregivers of young children. In one study, 51% of caregivers interviewed in a low-income urban pediatric clinic said that they would immediately take their children to the emergency department (ED) after a possible poisoning exposure.[61] In a separate study, focus group participants stated they would not call the PC in the case of a poison emergency. Their responses ranking was (1) call the pediatrician; (2) go to the ED, (3) read the label; and (4) call a friend after a poisoning exposure.[31] Historically, seniors have not been a priority population for PC education resources. However, this group represents the majority of fatalities reported nationally to PCs.[14,29] Focus groups conducted with seniors show that most do not perceive the PC as an appropriate service for their concerns, but rather as a service for children and parents. Additionally, the participants expressed a very narrow view of what was considered a poison such as bleach and household products. Similar to caregivers of children, seniors repeatedly state that they would call 911 in an emergency.[15]

A focus group with parents provided information to refine a telephone survey focusing on hazardous household materials and health risks. Feedback from caregivers resulted in a more concise instrument with more targeted questions. In addition, perceptions of the PC and suggestions for future educational interventions were also gathered from participants.[31]

Followup surveys are an additional way to analyze factors related to PC access. English- and Spanish-speaking caregivers in Texas were contacted after an ED visit related to a child's poisoning exposure. Findings showed that more than half had spoken to PC staff prior to the hospital visit. Of those who did not call the PC, 68% claimed prior knowledge of the PC, yet failed to use it. Significant demographic variables associated with a failure to call the PC were Hispanic (schooled in Mexico) and African American ethnicities.[34] Findings from an ethnographic study of 50 Mexican mothers with children younger than 5 years demonstrated that none had the PC number in their home.[46]

POISON EDUCATION PROGRAMS

Of the two million annual calls to PCs nationally, more than one million involve children younger than age 6.[14] As a result, programs to teach caregivers about primary and secondary prevention techniques have

TABLE 134–1. Poison Prevention Tips

- Identify all potential poisons inside and outside the home
- Keep all potential poisons out of reach in a locked cabinet
- Keep all products in their original containers
- Never keep food and nonfood items together
- Install carbon monoxide detectors in all sleeping areas
- Keep plants out of reach of children and pets
- Use child-resistant containers
- Post the poison center number on all telephones and store in cell phones

been the focus of education efforts. Typically, these programs focus on teaching poison prevention (Table 134–1) and raising awareness of PC services. Poison education programs designed to reach individuals (caregivers, pediatricians, children, and seniors) through community-wide interventions are reported in the literature. Interventions have reported an increase in knowledge about PC messages and poison prevention.[33,41]

INTERVENTIONS TARGETING HEALTH BEHAVIOR

Unintentional poisonings frequently happen when children are left unattended for a brief period of time (<5 minutes) and a toxic product in use or recently purchased is left within reach of the unattended child.[50] A qualitative study conducted with 65 parents, some whose children had experienced an unintentional poisoning, showed that poison prevention strategies were not consistently implemented in the home. Recommendations included ongoing parent education to reemphasize that "child resistant" is not "childproof," and reinforce safe storage of potentially toxic products, particularly those that are often used.[23] When knowledge and behavior were measured through telephone surveys conducted after a poison prevention intervention, caregivers were more likely to have the PC number posted in the home.[33,75]

In the past, syrup of ipecac was distributed as a component of poison prevention programs for parents. However, this has drastically changed since the American Academy of Pediatrics' (AAP) policy statement in 2003. The AAP recommends that healthcare providers disseminate poison prevention information but no longer supports the public's use of syrup of ipecac for poisoning exposures that happen in the home.[3]

The ED presents an opportunity for poison education programs to work with families to prevent further poisoning exposure situations.[19] An injury prevention program provided to caregivers of young children after a home injury was shown to be effective, particularly regarding retention of poison prevention information and the use of safety devices.[54] The use of a computer kiosk in an ED to provide personalized child safety information including poison storage for parents showed increased knowledge scores on followup telephone surveys.[24]

The effectiveness of poison prevention education for families that called the PC following a potential exposure in a young child was also studied. Poison prevention instructions, telephone stickers, and a cabinet lock were sent to the family one week after the initial call. Followup telephone interviews showed that intervention group recipients reported a higher use of the cabinet lock (59%) and were significantly more likely to post the telephone number for the PC (78%) than those in the control group who did not receive any poison prevention materials within 2 weeks of the incident.[75] Similar results were found during followup telephone calls made to WIC participants receiving a free cabinet lock and telephone stickers following an educational workshop.[63]

Poison education programs developed to address caregiver barriers have also been evaluated. An educational video targeting low-income and Spanish-speaking mothers was developed and evaluated. Results showed increased knowledge about the services, staff, and appropriate use of the PC compared with a control group that attended the regularly scheduled WIC class. After the video intervention, participants reported changes in attitude about calling the PC and comfort level with their recommendations.[33]

Instructor training programs have been designed by a number of PCs to reach leaders or educators of community-based organizations to incorporate poison education into their roles for the general population. An evaluation of the "Be Poison Smart" program showed an increase in knowledge and behavior change among service providers after a standardized training session. These reported changes included having the PC number visibly posted and keeping hazardous products out of reach.[53] Working with community-based services such as WIC presents an opportunity to reach the target population. Pretests and posttests administered to WIC staff and public health nurses showed increased understanding about poison prevention and increased awareness of PC services.[55]

Focus group participants have identified pediatricians as a trusted source of health information for parents.[31,64] The AAP includes a poison prevention counseling recommendation as part of The Injury Prevention Program (TIPP). TIPP is a safety education program for parents of children newborn through age 12. The TIPP Age-Related Safety Sheets include poison prevention advice for parents of children 6–12 month olds, 1–2 years, and 2–4 years.[4] In each, parents are encouraged to call the toll-free number for PCs if the child ingests a potentially poisonous product. It is important that the AAP continues its support for efforts by PCs to prevent childhood poisonings.[42] In another study, family practitioners and pediatricians were surveyed with respect to poison prevention counseling for parents. Although more than 80% of both groups reported that this was an important topic, family practitioners were less likely than pediatricians to provide poison information during a visit.[22]

Education programs are designed for school-age curricula. The effectiveness of MORE HEALTH, a program to teach kindergarten and third-grade students about poison prevention, was studied.[41] Posttests administered 1–2 weeks after the intervention showed increased knowledge in the intervention group of children. Parents of children in the intervention group also reported that their homes were more likely to be "poison-proofed."

The population at highest risk for poisoning fatalities is older adults. As mentioned previously, there is a paucity of poison education research targeting this group. Recommendations have been made to educate older adults, particularly about potential problems with medication use and storage.[29,40,68] Efforts to teach nursing home staff about potential poisoning exposures is also recommended.[40] There has been a shift in the priority of poison education programs to address this target population. An ED study of patients greater than 65 years of age showed that seniors had poor knowledge of their current medications. Also, patients taking more medications were less likely to know the proper dose, name, and purpose of the medications.[17]

COMMUNITY-WIDE INTERVENTIONS

In a recent review of pediatric literature focusing on community-based poisoning prevention programs, only four studies could be found using poisoning rates as the outcome measure. Additional creative studies to measure community-based poison prevention efforts will be essential to determine the importance of these efforts.[49]

In general, mass mailing has not been proven to be an effective effort to increase call volume for poison exposure or information requests.[21,38] Likewise, a distribution of textbook covers with the national logo and PC information to elementary and secondary schools in low PC utilization counties was not an effective method for increasing PC calls.[77] However, a few studies have shown an increase in call volume after mass mailing programs. A mailing that combined primary (poison prevention tips) and secondary (telephone stickers) messages and was included in a family health initiative showed increased call volume in areas where at least 5% of the residents received the information.[36] In addition, another study showed that overall call volume increased by 11.2% after more than one million pieces of literature containing the toll-free number were distributed in another mass mailing effort.[37]

An increased number of information calls to the PC was attributed to a campaign developed to raise community awareness.[70] Media provide a venue for conducting educational activities. Direct mail, radio, television, newspapers, and magazines were incorporated into a media campaign developed to raise awareness in a particular Latino community. A telephone survey conducted pre- and postmedia campaign showed an increase in awareness about the PC.[1] Developing this type of program is often costly compared with other education efforts; however, the potential audience is extensive. Mass media campaigns are powerful tools used in health promotion and disease prevention efforts. Research shows that media campaigns combined with community-based interventions and health education materials influence health behaviors and raise awareness. Additional factors that contribute to successful mass media include influencing the information environment to maximize exposure, using social marketing strategies, creating a supportive environment for the target audience to make health changes, and theory-based and process analyses to make changes mid-campaign and assess outcomes.[56] News stations often provide a way to broadcast poison prevention messages through the media during PPW and during periods associated with perceived increased risks to a community. Free and confidential services at poison centers provide caregivers with access to general information or in response to emergencies.

MULTILINGUAL POPULATIONS

Language and culture must be addressed when planning community-based programs. Quantitative and qualitative research examining Latino communities and calls to the PC have been conducted. The findings from interviews with 206 Latino parents at a WIC site showed that 62% had not heard of the local PC and 77% did not know the PC services were free and offered in Spanish.[73] Two other studies examined the call rates in communities with significant Latino populations. These areas had lower call rates than comparable areas with high Caucasian populations.[18,72] Furthermore, a number of studies demonstrate that Spanish-speaking caregivers are less likely to call the PC because of concerns including confidentiality and language barriers.[1,8,18,32,46] In a study conducted with 100 Mexican mothers of children younger than age 5, 32% reported that a doctor or nurse would be the initial contact for health advice. Other sources include friends and family (29%), mother, grandmother, mother-in-law (21%), and spouses (17%). The majority of mothers (81%) acknowledged the use of home remedies to treat their children's illnesses.[44] New immigrant families from Mexico and Latin America are at high risk for poisoning exposures. PC education programs should target populations in communities where the impact has the potential to be consequential.[66] Caution should be used when planning programs based on census data for demographic information as this data may not reflect the specific population or characteristic under study in community-based programs. When ethnicity information is not collected from callers who contact the PC, there are severe limitations to the value of the data.[18,65]

Qualitative research can help to identify cultural issues when planning targeted education efforts. Monolingual Spanish mothers were more likely to report poor storage of household products and lack of protective placement of plants.[1] Mexican-born mothers of children younger than 5 were interviewed in their homes about poison prevention techniques. Safe storage was clearly a problem in these homes with 64% of homes having bleach stored within reach of children. Housing made up of multiple families living in the same home further impedes safe storage practices. In this study, families stored all personal products including medications and household cleansing agents with them in their bedrooms rather than in common areas such as the bathroom.[46]

It is important to consider employment of bilingual staff as public educators when attempting to expand public awareness. The benefits of a bilingual educator include the ability to provide programs directly to an audience and eliminate the need for a translator. A lack of bilingual providers was the most significant barrier identified for Latina women interviewed about injury prevention techniques.[27] Recommendations for more effective outreach to Latino populations include television advertisements and distribution of written information at schools, churches, and doctor's offices.[73] Health education programs including mass media campaigns, designed to accurately reflect the cultural identity—language, beliefs, roles—of the targeted population are more likely to be accepted. Field testing concepts and materials are important for the development and distribution of appropriate information for multicultural populations. Further work is needed to examine cultural beliefs related to poison prevention and an individual's use of and access to the PC. It is important to address cultural beliefs related to use of herbal and other complementary medicines.[33] New education programs are needed to reach targeted populations including Latino and Asian communities across the country. Programs may be more successful if individuals trust and view a source as credible, particularly when cultural attitudes and beliefs closely resemble their own.[39]

LITERACY/HEALTH LITERACY

Literacy is another area of consideration when designing poison education programs. Health literacy is defined as "the degree to which individuals have the capacity to obtain, process, and understand basic health information and services needed to make appropriate health decisions."[57] This encompasses the ability to read, understand, and discuss medical information.[51] It is estimated that approximately 90 million Americans—half the adult population—have limited literacy skills and are often unable to understand health information and complete the tasks essential for navigating the healthcare system. Older adults, minority groups, immigrants, and low-income individuals are at highest risk for low health literacy.[35] People with low functional health literacy abilities are less likely to understand written and verbal health information, medicine labels, and appointment information.[76] This type of health information is often written at reading levels of at least 10th grade or higher.[20] The recommended reading level for written information is sixth grade. The majority of Americans are able to understand medical information at this level. In addition to reading level, use of graphics, font style, color, type size, and layout are important components when developing print material.[20] Recommendations for nonprint methods for communicating health information include audiotapes, visuals (posters, fotonovelas, pictographs), action-oriented activities (role-play, theater, storytelling), and audiovisuals (videos, CDs).[2,20,51,76]

The inability to read warning labels in English presents a literacy issue for those who are not native English speakers regardless of age.[46] Household product labels are also a concern. Identification of products often includes brand recognition.[45] Instructions for proper use and warnings may not be understood from the label itself.

The effects of health numeracy as a distinct component of health literacy have been presented in the literature.[47,62] Health numeracy involves one's ability to use numeric information to make effective decisions in daily life. This also includes concepts of risk, probability, and the communication of scientific evidence.[47,60,62] Health-related tasks including measuring medications, scheduling appointments, and refilling prescriptions rely on applied numeracy skills.[60,62] Because of their extensive use of medications, older adults are at high risk for medication errors.[68] Working with this population requires educators to understand the importance of interventions that accurately assess numeracy literacy levels and appropriately address health outcomes.

APPLYING HEALTH EDUCATION PRINCIPLES TO POISON EDUCATION PROGRAMS

Health education involves planning, implementing, and evaluating programs based on theories and models. These models offer direction for educators with health promotion planning.[43] There is a need to increase the number of poison educational programs incorporating health education principles. This includes educational efforts designed to reach individuals through community-based programs and media campaigns.

Both the Health Belief Model (HBM) and Social Cognitive Theory (SCT) incorporate the concept of "self-efficacy" and are applicable when designing poison prevention interventions and mass media campaigns. Self-efficacy is the individual's belief that he or she will be able to accomplish the task requested.[7,20,30,56] Many health educators believe that self-efficacy is necessary for changing behavior. The SCT suggests that individuals, the environment, and behavior are intimately and inextricably interrelated.[7] The HBM suggests that individuals are more likely to make health behavior changes based on perceived risk susceptibility, severity, potential barriers, and self-efficacy. These decisions are made when actions are seen as potentially more beneficial to the individual than the perceived risks associated with surmounting the current barriers.[30]

In one study, the HBM approach was used as a framework for poison prevention and for the assessment of barriers to PC use. Questions for focus group participants were developed based on the principles of HBM—that is, perceived susceptibility, severity, benefits, barriers, and self-efficacy related to the health action requested. The majority of mothers viewed poisoning as an emergency and felt it was a health concern for their children. Cues to action are also a component of the model and involve discussions about poison prevention or related information. Participants recommended using community-based venues and culturally appropriate information to expand awareness about poison prevention and the poison center.[13]

The HBM and SCT approaches were used to develop the questions for focus groups in both English and Spanish. These questions addressed issues related to poison prevention (severity and susceptibility), the services of the PC (including barriers), and suggestions for education. Focus group participants suggested the use of modeling to reinforce real-life scenarios in which a mother handles the poisoning emergency with the staff at the PC with a positive outcome.[32] As a result, a video was developed addressing these ideas. Two poisoning situations in which a mother calls the center are depicted. One involves home management (ingestion of bleach) and the second involves taking the child to the emergency department (swallowing grandmother's antihypertensive pill). The video and correlated teaching guides are available in English and Spanish.[33]

It is important to develop questionnaires that will be accepted and understood by the target population.[27] A Spanish-language instrument that addresses home safety beliefs using the HBM framework was developed and tested. Low-income monolingual Spanish-speaking mothers of children younger than 4 years of age were interviewed about perceived susceptibility, severity, barriers, and self-efficacy factors affecting unintentional home injuries including poison prevention measures. Barriers identified include literacy skills and access to bilingual health information.[27]

The HBM supports the idea that a "teachable moment" may be the ideal opportunity to present poison prevention interventions.[24,54] People may be more open to health information after experiencing a traumatic experience.[16] Events such as an unintentional poisoning exposure may motivate individuals to behavioral change. Applying HBM principles suggests that individuals will make changes in terms of poison prevention when or if they view the severity and susceptibility of a poisoning to be high in the home.

SUMMARY

Poison center public education efforts encompass needs assessments, program development, implementation, and evaluation. Two populations, children younger than 6 years and older adults, are at highest risk for unintentional poisoning exposures. Focus groups with caregivers of young children conducted across the country have consistently identified barriers to calling poison centers. These include calling 911, fear of being reported to child welfare agencies, and lack of confidence in handling poisoning emergencies. Using health education theories and models, programs should be developed that address these barriers and encourage caregivers to use the services of the PC appropriately. Education programs focusing on the needs of seniors addressing multigenerational living conditions should be designed. Cultural, health literacy, health numeracy and language needs of target populations are important considerations when planning poison education programs.

REFERENCES

1. Albertson TE, Tharratt RS, Alsop J, et al. Regional variations in the use and awareness of the California poison control system. *J Toxicol Clin Toxicol.* 2004;42:625-633.
2. AMC Cancer Research Center. Beyond the brochure: alternative approaches to effective health communication 1994. AMC Cancer Center and Centers for Disease Control and Prevention. Denver, Colorado.
3. American Academy of Pediatrics, Committee on Injury, Violence and Poison Prevention. Poison treatment in the home. *Pediatrics.* 2003;112:1182-1185.
4. American Academy of Pediatrics. The injury prevention program (TIPP). Available from http://www.aap.org. Accessed May 14, 2009.
5. American Association of Poison Control Centers. Public Education Committee. Mission, Structure and Resources. April 1999. Available at http://www.aapcc.org.
6. American Association of Poison Control Centers. Available at http://www.aapcc.org. Accessed May 14, 2009.
7. Baranowski T, Perry CL, Parcel GS. How individuals, environments, and health behavior interact: Social Cognitive Theory model. In: Glanz K, Rimer BK, Lewis FM, eds. *Health Behavior and Health Education Theory, Research, Practice*, 3rd ed. San Francisco, CA: Josey-Bass; 2002:165-184.
8. Belson M, Kieszak S, Watson W, et al. Childhood pesticide exposures on the Texas-Mexico border: clinical manifestations and poison center use. *Am J Public Health.* 2003;93:1310-1315.
9. Berlin R. Poison prevention—where can we make a difference? *Acad Emerg Med.* 1997;4:163-164.
10. Berning CK, Griffith JF, Wild JE. Research on the effectiveness of denatonium benzoate as a deterrent to liquid detergent ingestion by children. *Fundam Appl Toxicol.* 1982;2:44-48.
11. Bernstein IL, Webster MM. Learned taste aversions in humans. *Physiol Behav.* 1980;25:363-366.
12. Bitrex Product Information. Edinburgh: Macfarlan Smith; 1989.
13. Brannan JE. Accidental poisoning of children: barriers to resource use in a black, low-income community. *Public Health Nurs.* 1992;9:81-86.

14. Bronstein AC, Spyker DA, Cantilena JR, Louis R, et al. Annual report of the American Association of Poison Control Centers' National Poison Data System (NPDS). *Clin Toxicol.* 2007;46:927-1057.
15. C & R Research. Seniors' perceptions of the Illinois poison center. Report. May 2002. Illinois Poison Center: Chicago.
16. Caliva M, Stork C, Cantor R. Frequency of post-poisoning exposure information provided to patients requiring emergency care. *Vet Human Toxicol.* 1998;40:305-306.
17. Chung MK, Bartfield JM. Knowledge of prescription medications among elderly emergency department patients. *Ann Emerg Med.* 2002;39:605-608.
18. Clark RF, Phillips M, Manoguerra AS, Chan TC. Evaluating the utilization of a regional poison center by Latino communities. *J Toxicol Clin Toxicol.* 2002;40:855-860.
19. Demorest RA, Posner JC, Osterhoudt KC, Henretig FM. Poisoning prevention education during emergency department visits for childhood poisoning. *Pediatr Emerg Care.* 2004;20:281-284.
20. Doak CC, Doak LG, Root JH. Teaching patients with low literacy skills. Philadelphia: JB Lippincott Company; 1996.
21. Everson G, Rondeau ES, Kendrick M, Garza I. Ineffectiveness of a mass mailing campaign to improve poison center awareness in a rural population. *Vet Human Toxicol.* 1993;35:165-167.
22. Gerard JM, Klasner AE, Madhok M, et al. Poison prevention counseling: a comparison between family practitioners and pediatricians. *Arch Pediatr Adolesc Med.* 2000;154:65-70.
23. Gibbs L, Waters E, Sherrard J, Ozanne-Smith J, et al. Understanding parental motivators and barriers to uptake of child poison safety strategies: a qualitative study. *Inj Prev.* 2005;11:373-377.
24. Gielen AC, McKenzie LB, McDonald EM, et al. Using a computer kiosk to promote child safety: results of a randomized, controlled trial in an urban pediatric emergency department. *Pediatrics.* 2007;120:330-339.
25. Hansen SR, Janssen C, Beasley VR. Denatonium benzoate as a deterrent to ingestion of toxic substances: toxicity and efficacy. *Vet Hum Toxicol.* 1993;35:234-236.
26. Healthy People 2010. Available at http://www.healthypeople.gov. Accessed May 14, 2009.
27. Hendrickson SG. Beyond translation...cultural fit. *West J Nurs Res.* 2003;25:593-608.
28. The International Programme on Chemical Safety (IPCS). World Health Organization. Poisoning Prevention and Management. Available at http://www.who.int/ipcs/poisons/en. Accessed May 14, 2009.
29. Institute of Medicine. *Forging a Poison Prevention and Control System.* Washington, DC: The National Academies Press; 2004.
30. Janz NK, Champion VL, Strecher VJ. The health belief model In: Glanz K, Rimer BK, Lewis FM, eds. *Health Behavior and Health Education Theory, Research, Practice.* 3rd ed. San Francisco, CA: Josey-Bass; 2002:45-65.
31. Kaufman MM, Smolinske S, Keswick D. Assessing poisoning risks to storage of household hazardous materials: using a focus group to improve a survey questionnaire. *Environ Health.* 2005;4:16.
32. Kelly NR, Groff JY. Exploring barriers to utilization of poison centers: a qualitative study of mothers attending an urban women, infants, and children (WIC) clinic. *Pediatrics.* 2000;106:199-204.
33. Kelly NR, Huffman LC, Mendoza FS, Robinson TN. Effects of a videotape to increase use of poison control centers by low-income and Spanish-speaking families. *Pediatrics.* 2003;111:21-26.
34. Kelly NR, Kirkland RT, Holmes SE, et al. Assessing parental utilization of the poison center: an emergency center-based survey. *Clin Pediatr.* 1997;36:467-473.
35. Kirsch IS, Jungelut A, Jenkins L, Kolstad A. Adult literacy in America: a first look at the results of the national adult literacy survey. Washington, DC: National Center for Education Statistics, US Department of Education; 2002.
36. Krenzelok E, Mrvos R, Mazo E. Combining primary and secondary poison prevention in one initiative. *Clin Toxicol.* 2008;46:101-104.
37. Krenzelok EP, Mrvos R. Initial impact of toll-free access on poison center call volume. *Vet Human Toxicol.* 2003;45:325-327.
38. Krenzelok EP, Mrvos R. Is mass-mailing an effective form of passive poison center awareness enhancement? *Vet Human Toxicol.* 2004;46:155-156.
39. Kreuter MW, McClure SM. The role of culture in health communication. *Annu Rev Public Health.* 2004;25:439-455.
40. Kroner BA, Scott RB, Waring ER, Zanga JR. Poisoning in the elderly: characterization of exposures reported to a poison control center. *J Am Geriatr Soc.* 1993;41:842-846.
41. Liller KD, Craig J, Crane N, McDermott RJ. Evaluation of a poison prevention lesson for kindergarten and third grade students. *Inj Prev.* 1998;4: 218-221.
42. Lovejoy FH, Robertson WO, Woolf AD. Poison centers, poison prevention, and the pediatrician. *Pediatrics.* 1994;220-224.
43. McKenzie JF, Smeltzer JL. Planning, implementing, and evaluating health promotion programs: a primer. Needham Heights, MA: Allyn and Bacon; 2001.
44. Mikhail BI. Hispanic mothers' beliefs and practices regarding selected children's health problems. *West J Nurs Res.* 1994;16:623-638.
45. Mrvos R, Krenzelok EP. Illiteracy: a contributing factor to poisoning. *Vet Human Toxicol.* 1993;35:325-327.
46. Mull DS, Agran PF, Winn DG, et al. Household poisoning exposure among children of Mexican-born mothers: an ethnographic study. *West J Med.* 1999;171:16-19.
47. Nelson W, Reyna VF, Fagerlin A, et al. Clinical implications of numeracy: theory and practice. *Am Behav Med.* 2008;35:261-274.
48. Neumann CM, Giffin S, Hall S, et al. Oregon's toxic household products law. *J Public Health Policy.* 2000;21:342-359.
49. Nixon J, Spinks A, Turner C, McClure R. Community-based programs to prevent poisoning in children 0-15 years. *Inj Prev.* 2004;10:43-46.
50. Ozanne-Smith J, Day L, Parsons B, et al. Childhood poisoning: access and prevention. *J Paediatr Child Health.* 2001;37:262-265.
51. Parker RM, Ratzan SC, Lurie N. Health literacy: a policy challenge for advancing high-quality health care. *Health Aff.* 2003;22:147-153.
52. Payne HAS, Smalley HM, Tracy MJ. Denatonium benzoate as a bitter aversive additive in ethylene glycol and methanol-based automotive products. SAE Technical Paper Series. Presented at the 23rd International Conference on Environmental Systems, Colorado Springs, CO, July 1993, pp. 125-131.
53. Polivka BJ, Casavant MJ, Malis E, Baker D. Evaluation of the Be Poison Smart ¯ poison prevention intervention. *Clin Toxicol.* 2006;44:109-114.
54. Posner JC, Hawkins LA, Garcia-Espana F, Durbin DR. A randomized clinical trial of a home safety intervention based in an emergency department setting. *Pediatrics.* 2004;113:1603-1608.
55. Purello PL, Oransky SH, Fisher L. An outreach program to low-income, high risk populations through WIC. *Vet Human Toxicol.* 1990;32:130-132.
56. Randolph W, Viswanath K. Lessons learned from public health mass media campaigns: marketing health in a crowded media world. *Annu Rev Public Health.* 2004;25:419-437.
57. Ratzan SC, Parker RM. Introduction. In: Selden CR, Zorn M, Ratzan SC, Parker RM, eds. National Library of Medicine Current Bibliographies in Medicine: Health Literacy. Washington, DC: National Institutes of Health, US Department of Health and Human Services; 2000. Available at http://www.nlm.nih.gov/archive//20061214/pubs/cbm/hliteracy.html. Accessed May 14, 2009.
58. Riner ME, Cunningham C, Johnson A. Public health education and practice using geographic information system technology. *Public Health Nurs.* 2004;21:57-65.
59. Rodgers GB. The safety effects of child-resistant packaging for oral prescription drugs. *JAMA.* 1996;275:1661-1665.
60. Rothman RL, Montori VM, Cherrington A, Pignone MP. Perspective: the role of numeracy in health care. *J Health Commun.* 2008;13:583-595.
61. Santer LJ, Stocking CB. Safety practices and living conditions of low-income urban families. *Pediatrics.* 1991;88:1112-1118.
62. Schapira MM, Fletcher KE, Gilligan MA, et al. A framework for health numeracy: how patients use quantitative skills in health care. *J Health Commun.* 2008;13:501-517.
63. Schwartz L, Howland MA, Mercurio-Zappala M, Hoffman RS. Follow up survey with parents given cabinet safety locks. *J Toxicol Clinic Toxicol.* 2000;38:559.
64. Schwartz L, Howland MA, Mercurio-Zappala M, Hoffman RS. The use of focus groups to plan poison prevention educations for low-income populations. *Health Promot Pract.* 2003;4:340-346.
65. Schwartz L, Mercurio-Zappala M, Howland MA, et al. Is regional ethnicity related to poison center utilization? *J Toxicol Clin Toxicol.* 2004;42:778.
66. Shepherd G, Larkin GL, Velez LI, Huddleston L. Language preferences among callers to a regional poison center. *Vet Human Toxicol.* 2004;46:100-101.
67. Sibert JR, Frude N. Bittering agents in the prevention of accidental poisoning: children's reactions to denatonium benzoate (Bitrex). *Arch Emerg Med.* 1991;8:1-7.

68. Skarupski KA, Mrvos R, Krenzelok EP. A profile of calls to a poison information center regarding older adults. *J Aging Health*. 2004;16:228-247.
69. Spiller HA, Mowry JB. Evaluation of the effect of a public educator on calls and poisonings related to a regional poison center. *Vet Human Toxicol*. 2004;46:206-208.
70. Sumner D, Hudak C, Rouse A, Langley R. A project to reduce accidental pediatric poisonings in North Carolina. *Vet Human Toxicol*. 2003;45:266-269.
71. Swartz MK. Poison prevention. *J Pediatr Health Care*. 1993;7:143-144.
72. Vassilev ZP, Marcus S, Jennis T, et al. Rapid communication: sociodemographic differences between counties with high and low utilization of a regional poison control center. *J Toxicol Environ Health A*. 2003;66:1905-1908.
73. Vassilev ZP, Shiel M, Lewis MJ, Marcus SM, Robson MG. Assessment of barriers to utilization of poison centers by Hispanic/Latino populations. *J Toxicol Environ Health*. 2006;69:1711-1718.
74. Walton WW. An evaluation of the poison prevention packaging act. *Pediatrics*. 1982:69:363-370.
75. Woolf AD, Saperstein A, Forjuoh S. Poisoning prevention knowledge and practices of parents after a childhood poisoning incident. *Pediatrics*. 1992;90:867-870.
76. Youmans SL, Schillinger D. Functional health literacy and medication use: the pharmacist's role. *Ann Pharmacother*. 2003;37:1726-1729.
77. Yudizky M, Grisemer P, Shepherd G, et al. Can textbook covers be used to increase poison center utilization? *Vet Human Toxicol*. 2004;46:285-286.

CHAPTER 135
POISON CENTERS AND POISON EPIDEMIOLOGY

Robert S. Hoffman

Regional poison centers are staffed by highly trained and certified health professionals who are assisted by extensive information systems. Support is provided by 24-hour access to board-certified medical toxicologists and consultants from diverse medical disciplines, the natural sciences, and industry. The American poison center (PC) is charged with maintaining a database, providing information to the public and to health professionals, collecting epidemiologic data on the incidence and severity of poisoning, preventing unnecessary hospitalizations following exposure, and educating healthcare professionals on the diagnosis and treatment of poisoning. This chapter explores some of the critical roles of poison centers and attempts to offer a vision of the future. Unique issues facing poison centers in other countries are discussed in Chap. 136.

HISTORY

In 1950, the American Academy of Pediatrics (AAP) created a Committee on Accident Prevention to explore methods to reduce injuries in young children. A subsequent survey by that committee demonstrated that injuries resulting from unintentional poisoning were a significant cause of childhood morbidity. Simultaneously came the realizations that a source of reliable information on the active ingredients of common household xenobiotics was lacking and that there were few accepted methods for treating poisoned patients. In response to this void, the first PC was created in Chicago in 1953.[72] Although initially designed to provide information to healthcare providers, both the popularity and the success of this center stimulated a PC movement, which rapidly spread across the country. The myriad of new PCs not only offered product content information to healthcare providers, but also began to offer first aid and prevention information to members of the community.

In the 60 years that have since passed, countless achievements have been realized by a relatively small group of remarkably altruistic individuals. Throughout this time, poison services have remained free to the public, highlighting their essential role in the American public health system. Many of the legislative and educational accomplishments, which are chronicled in Chap. 1, have directly reduced the incidence and severity of poisoning in children.[69,77,82] Concurrently, the number, configuration, and specific role of PCs has shifted in response to public and professional needs.[32,90] However, a crucial test of the utility of modern PCs will be their ability help reverse the US current trend of increased adult mortality from poisoning.[16] Additional metrics, such as ICU admissions, length of stay in hospitals, and total healthcare expenditures might serve as other indicators of PC success. The basic functions of PCs are discussed in the following sections.

MAINTAINING A DATABASE ON PRODUCT CONTENTS AND POISON MANAGEMENT

The first toxicology database created in the United States was a set of cumbersome 5″ × 8″ index cards produced in the 1950s by the US National Clearinghouse of Poison Control Centers.[72] When it grew to include more than 16,000 cards, the sheer volume of space required to store this information, and the extensive time necessary to manually search these cards created the necessity of a central repository, such as a PC. As available information grew, a rapid expansion of information technology occurred, and the unwieldy index card database was privatized and transformed into microfiche. Although this resource was physically smaller, specialized equipment was required, and a search was still time-consuming. Numerous encyclopedic and clinical textbooks were written to supplement the database and provide resources for the office or the bedside. With the growth of the computer age and the Internet, the computer product known as POISINDEX was established to replace the microfiche format as the major source of data on the contents of innumerable household and industrial products, drugs, and plant and animal xenobiotics. POISINDEX also provides uniform management strategies for many potentially toxic exposures.

With this evolution of information technology, PCs are no longer perceived as the sole guardians of toxicology information. Although these services are still essential for the public at large, and those professionals away from their computers or mobile phones, a predictable decline in PC utilization has paralleled this growth in availability of information. A 1991 study in Utah demonstrated that 82.6% of emergency physicians who had POISINDEX available in their institutions no longer routinely consulted the PC.[15] A similar 1994 New York State study suggested that 76% of physicians who had POISINDEX in their emergency departments (EDs) perceived that this decreased their own use of their PC.[87]

An initial analysis might suggest that this is an acceptable trend for healthcare professionals in that it both allows physicians to respond more rapidly to patient needs and for PCs to be more available to those individuals, especially nonhealthcare professionals, who do not have access to this information system. However, this practice of "not calling" not only undermines the efforts of PCs to gather epidemiologic data (see later) but also creates an understanding gap. In other words, the interpretation of the data is as essential (or more essential) than the data itself. For example, some commonly used sources of toxicology information such as the Physicians' Desk Reference (PDR) and material safety data sheets (MSDS) occasionally provide information that may be inaccurate, potentially misleading, or severely limited.[35,64] Likewise, two reviews of drug interaction programs designed for mobile devices demonstrated significant variability between individual programs.[2,68] Although POISINDEX routinely provides more accurate information regarding overdose, it cannot be expected to adapt to ongoing epidemiological trends such as regional variations in substance use and is currently updated only periodically.

The best source for essential new information is skilled professionals who specialize in poisoning. Also, because most databases are designed to provide information about known entities, they perform poorly when dealing with unknown and unclear scenarios—especially long and complicated differential diagnoses. For example, consider the case of a clinician caring for a lethargic child whose only medication is Zantac syrup. After the other causes of altered mental status have been excluded, the clinician considers drug toxicity. Consultation with standard references suggests that altered consciousness would not be expected with use of this medication. However, a certified poison specialist at a regional PC recognizes the potential for drug error, has the physician review the syrup bottle in question, and then calls the pharmacy where the drug was provided. The poison specialist learns that although the prescription was written for Zantac (ranitidine), the bottle actually contains Zyrtec syrup (cetirizine) which could account for the child's symptoms.

Thus, although originally designed as providers of information, PCs must now be considered more as valued consultants, with staff who not only provide content information but also interpret clinical material and link both to appropriate management strategies. This goal can only be achieved through rigorous training and certification and recertification criteria designed to provide valued up-to-date interactions with healthcare professionals. Access to computer programs can never be considered a substitute for a thoughtful human analysis. Computers do not recognize anxiety, inappropriate questions, and other subtle issues that can only be appreciated with human interactions.

Another illustrative example of the value of PCs can be drawn from the use of flumazenil for benzodiazepine overdose (Chap. 74). Although it may easily be determined by anyone capable of using an index that flumazenil is an antidote for benzodiazepine overdoses, many subtle characteristics of the patient or the overdose often contraindicate its use. A prospective study determined that when flumazenil was used before consultation with the PC, contraindications were present in 10 of 14 (71%) cases, resulting in one serious adverse event.[12] In the study mentioned earlier, although physicians with access to POISINDEX were less likely to call the PC, 86.7% still felt that using the PC to gain access to a physician toxicologist was a valued resource.[15] Many PCs are linked with centers for poison treatment (CPT), which are healthcare facilities that can provide both bedside consultation and unique diagnostic and therapeutic interventions for a subset of patients with severe or complex poisoning.[1] The benefits of consultation are discussed later under Health Care Savings.

COLLECTING POISON EPIDEMIOLOGY DATA

Recent data demonstrate that poisoning is the second leading cause of injury-related fatalities, ranking only behind motor vehicle crashes and recently surpassing firearm use.[16] Understanding the evolving trends in poisoning is essential to the development of enhanced surveillance, prevention, and education programs designed to reduce unintentional poisoning. Although data can be analyzed from numerous sources such as death certificates, hospital discharge coding records, and PCs, it is essential to recognize the biases that are inherent in each of these reports. Because not all significant poisonings result in either hospitalization or fatality, data from PCs appear to offer a unique perspective.

Unfortunately, the term "poisoning" is often defined differently and therefore may be confusing. In this text, "poisoning" is used to denote any exposure to any xenobiotic (drug, toxin, chemical, or naturally occurring substance) that results in injury. Yet the data collected and disseminated by PCs are defined by the term "exposures."[10,49,53–57,83–85] Many exposures are of no toxicologic consequence either because of the properties of the xenobiotic involved, the magnitude or duration of the exposure, or the uncertainties regarding whether an actual exposure has occurred; therefore, data collected by PCs represent a limited and ill-defined measure of poisoning.

The situation is further confounded by multiple biases that are introduced by the actual reporting process, which first and foremost is voluntary and passive. Because the majority of calls concern self-reported data that come from the home and are never subsequently confirmed, a significant percentage of the data generated to date may actually represent only potential or possible exposures, potentially resulting in large statistical errors introduced into the database. For example, although a recent study evaluated all children with a history of methanol or ethylene glycol ingestion over more than 2 years, only 21 of 102 children analyzed actually demonstrated the presence of a toxic alcohol concentration.[51] Nevertheless, all 102 of these cases were entered into the database as exposures. If these figures are representative of the rest of the data set, they suggest that ingestion does not actually occur in the vast majority of reported unintentional exposures in children. Also, current events, hoaxes, and media awareness campaigns all may influence self-reporting rates.[58] Furthermore, in order to report a possible exposure a caller must have a telephone and probably speak English. Although telecommunications devices for the hearing impaired and translation services exist, they are rarely used. Enhancement of technology to facilitate the accurate exchange of information between poison specialists and either hearing impaired callers or those who do not speak English is essential to the success of PCs. Another would be to entertain more active reporting systems automatically triggered directly by hospital laboratory values.

Under the present passive system, when hospitals report exposures to the PC, a comparison of the hospital chart with the PC record shows good agreement, demonstrating an accurate exchange of information.[40] Unfortunately, a reporting bias similar to that described above is well recognized regarding professional utilization of poison centers and has been called the *Pollyanna phenomenon*.[36] For example, in the spring of 1995, PCs in the northeast United States began to receive numerous reports of severe psychomotor agitation and other manifestations of anticholinergic syndrome in heroin users. In the initial phase of the epidemic, most of the callers requested assistance in establishing a diagnosis, determining possible etiologies, and raised questions regarding treatment with physostigmine.[37] Although the epidemic continued for many months, once the media announced that the heroin supply was tainted with scopolamine, and clinicians became familiar with the indications and administration of physostigmine, call volume decreased. Stated simply, healthcare professionals are less likely to call the PC regarding issues with which they are familiar, are of little clinical consequence, or are not recognized as being related to a poison. Thus, a bias is introduced that results in a relative overreporting of new and serious events and a relative underreporting of the familiar or very common, unrecognized poisoning, and those exposures or poisonings that are apparently inconsequential. Numerous comparisons support this contention. Investigators who rely on published data from PCs as a sole source of epidemiological information demonstrate a failure to understand the complexity of poisoning data and the aforementioned consequential limitations of PC-derived data.

FATAL POISONING

A 4-year study compared deaths from poisoning reported to the Rhode Island medical examiner with those reported to the area PC.[52] Not surprisingly, the medical examiner reported many more deaths: 369 compared to 45 reported by the PC. Although the majority of the cases not reported to the PC were victims who died at home, were pronounced dead on arrival to the hospital, or those in whom poisoning was not suspected until the postmortem analysis, 79 patients who subsequently became unreported fatalities were actually admitted to the hospital with a suspected poisoning. In 10 of these cases, the authors concluded that a toxicology consultation might have altered the outcome. Examples of interventions that, if recommended and performed, might have resulted in a more favorable outcome included the proper use of antidotes such as naloxone, *N*-acetylcysteine for acetaminophen poisoning, the cyanide antidote kit, sodium bicarbonate for a cyclic antidepressant overdose, hyperbaric oxygen for carbon monoxide poisoning, hemoperfusion for a theophylline overdose, and hemodialysis for a lithium overdose.

Likewise, when medical examiner data were analyzed in Massachusetts, over 47% of poison fatalities had not been reported to the PC.[75] A California study evaluating 358 poisoning fatalities reported to the medical examiner showed that only 10 PC fatalities had been reported over a similar time period, demonstrating an even more consequential reporting gap.[4] Once again in this study, whereas the majority of underreporting was with respect to prehospital deaths (68%), only 5 of 113 hospitalized patients who ultimately died were reported to the PC. Additionally, a cross-sectional comparison of national mortality data with PC data for agricultural chemical poisoning demonstrated a similar trend of underreporting to PCs of seriously poisoned admitted patients who became fatalities.[46] Furthermore, when data for an entire year from the National Center for Health Statistics (NCHS) were compared to the same year of data from the American Association of Poison Control Centers (AAPCC), it was apparent that the AAPCC data captured only about 5% of annual poison fatalities.[39]

More recent analyses have highlighted a remarkable trend. When 11 states evaluated trends in poison-related mortality from 1990 to 2001, an average increase of 145% was noted.[17] A more comprehensive investigation of the National Vital Statistics System (NVSS) accessed via the Centers for Disease Control and Prevention's (CDC) Web-based Injury Statistics Query and Reporting System (WISQARS) database demonstrated a 5.5% increase in injury related mortality from 1999 to 2004. Mortality from poisoning accounted for 61.95 of the increase in unintentional injury, 28% of the increase in suicide, 81.2% of the increase in death from undetermined intent, and more than half of the total increase injury-related mortality.[16] As of 2004 death from poisoning surpassed firearms and became the second most common cause of injury-related fatality. Focusing on PC data alone would produce the erroneous assumption that poisoning-related fatalities were not a significant public health concern. In actuality, poisoning is a significant concern in that other programs designed to reduce deaths from motor vehicle crashes and firearms have been largely successful.

It is logical to assume that similar disparities exist regarding the reporting of nonfatal poisonings. The resultant gap in public health data needs to be addressed through improved definitions, epidemiology, reporting, and analysis of poison-related data systems. This inequity has developed through a long-standing tradition of PCs to focus attention and concentrate on the largely benign exposures in children. The emphasis needs to be redirected toward seriously ill poisoning, ICU utilization, and other markers of actual poisoning rather than healthcare utilization for benign events.

NONFATAL POISONING

An outreach study in Massachusetts determined that hospitals geographically close to a PC reported their cases almost twice as often as hospitals remotely located (46% vs. 27% of total cases).[18] Additionally, the authors noted that private physicians were less likely to report cases than residents in training. A 1-year retrospective review demonstrated that only 26% (123/470) of poisoned patients who were treated in a particular ED were reported to the PC.[38] Interestingly, only 3% of inhalational exposures were reported, compared with 95% of cyclic antidepressant ingestions. The authors also noted, as suggested above, that reporting decreased when comparable exposures occurred over a short period of time. Finally, in the physician survey study cited earlier, physicians reported that they would "almost never" contact the PC for asymptomatic exposures (62.9%), chronic toxicity (50.4%), or simply to assist in establishing a reliable database (90.2%).[15] This statement is most likely accurate even in jurisdictions where reporting of all or select exposures is incorporated into public health laws.

OCCUPATIONAL EXPOSURES

Xenobiotic exposure occurs commonly in the workplace. As a result of the long-recognized association between occupational exposure and illness, a number of federal and state government-funded agencies, such as the National Institute for Occupational Safety and Health (NIOSH), Occupational Safety and Health Act (OSHA), and the Agency for Toxic Substances and Disease Registry (ATSDR), exist to prevent occupational illness, to educate the public, and to collect data on exposures to occupational xenobiotics. Legislation provides for mandatory reporting in some instances and offers workers job protection for voluntary reporting. PCs also provide information on occupational exposures and collect data. Once again, there are discrepancies between the poison information data and the data collected by governmental agencies. A 6-month survey in California noted that only 15.9% of the occupational cases reported to the PC were captured by a state occupational reporting system.[6] The most common occupational toxicologic illness—dermatitis—was underrepresented in these cases. A follow-up study by the same authors demonstrated that over a third of calls came directly from the individual worker, 70% of whom were unaware of the link between their occupation and their symptoms.[5] Although these data suggest that PCs can provide substantial assistance following occupational exposures, one author expressed concern, noting in a followup study that the PC failed to provide an adequate epidemiological assessment in that it did not identify an average of 12 other people per workplace who were also potentially exposed in addition to the index case.[9] A 1999 survey of PCs concluded that PCs' "responses to work-related calls are inadequate," and suggested that written protocols might be helpful.[8] Additional efforts need to address the abilities of poison centers to respond to other events that generate multiple patients such as hazardous materials releases, malicious acts, and natural disasters.

ADVERSE DRUG EVENTS AND XENOBIOTIC ERRORS

Although the actual numbers are a source of controversy, data suggest that a striking number of adverse drug events (ADEs) occur each year in the United States, with many resulting in death.[23,50] The ease of 24-hour telephone access, combined with the ability to consult with a health professional, make PCs ideal resources for reporting of ADEs.[24] Yet, over 76% of physicians surveyed stated that they would "almost never" contact the PC regarding adverse drug events.[15] Moreover, 30 of 56 (53.6%) PCs surveyed stated that they had not submitted any of their ADE data to the FDA's Med-Watch program.[22] Many of the other centers reported only partial compliance with the MedWatch system.[22]

Prescription drug errors are another source of potential poisoning. Retrospective review of PC data suggests that many of these errors are reported. In one report, the PC provided valuable feedback to pharmacists and physicians about these errors. Ideally, reporting to the state board of pharmacy would ensure that proper surveillance and counseling continue. The PC would seem to be ideally suited to perform this function.[74]

DRUGS OF ABUSE

PCs also collect data on exposures to drugs of abuse and misuse. These data consist largely of calls for information from the concerned public and reports of overdose requiring healthcare intervention. Although ethanol, tobacco, and caffeine are the most common xenobiotics used in society, these cases are rarely reflected in poison center data, with the exception of unintentional exposures in children. In fact, because most substance abuse does not result in immediate interactions with the healthcare system, other databases such as the National Institute of Drug Abuse (NIDA) Household Survey (now referred to as the Monitoring the Future Study) might better reflect substance abuse trends.[22] Yet even this database has significant limitations.[3,34] Because PCs are more focused on immediate healthcare effects of exposures, it could be argued that only those cases in which healthcare interaction is required are of value in the database. Whereas PC data are collected passively, the Drug Abuse Warning Network (DAWN) provides an active surveillance system of a sample of hospital visits and deaths that relate to substance misuse. Unfortunately, because DAWN data use hospital chart "mentions," which are infrequently validated, the data have been significantly criticized.[78] Clearly none of these three systems accurately encompasses the entire scope of the substance abuse problem.

GROSSLY UNDERREPORTED XENOBIOTICS

As discussed above, there is little doubt that ethanol and tobacco are the most common xenobiotics intentionally used and misused in our society. Although their toxicologic manifestations can be acute and severe, chronic subclinical poisoning often goes unnoticed for many years. Similarly, more than one million American children have lead concentrations above 10 μg/dL and polychlorinated biphenyls (PCBs) can be found in countless adults and children. We must remain cognizant of these large-scale exposures when we read that plants, cleaning products, and cosmetics comprise the most common exposures to xenobiotics;[10] rather, these are the most common "reported" exposures.

USING THE EXISTING DATA

With the current limitations of the PC data, it should be clear that neither the numerator nor the denominator of the actual number of poisonings can be easily appreciated. However, analysis of these data for trends may be more useful because the inherent biases involved in PC reporting are probably consistent over many years. Efforts should be directed to encourage reporting by such enhanced access methods as Web-based forms for passive reporting, a direct interface between laboratory and hospital databases that actively transmits data to PCs and linkages to other agencies that collect reports of poisoning such as state and local health departments. Additional resources should be directed at improved case definitions (distinguishing asymptomatic exposure from poisoning) and integration with other essential databases such as MedWatch, National Vital Statistics System (NVSS), and the National Center for Health Statistics (NCHS).

Despite its limitations, PC data have significant utility. It is often an exposure rather than an actual poisoning that provides the impetus for contact with healthcare. For those exposures that are unlikely to be consequential, the PC can intervene to prevent potentially harmful attempts at home decontamination and costly unnecessary visits to healthcare providers. Interaction with parents at a time of perceived crisis also provides a "teachable moment" (Chap. 134) that may help prevent a more consequential exposure in the future. For those exposures that may result in poisoning, the period of time immediately following exposure is an ideal moment to initiate first aid measures designed to prevent or lessen the severity of poisoning. For both of these reasons the cost, benefits, and efficacy of PCs especially regarding home calls must be measured in terms of exposures and not poisonings.

HEALTHCARE SAVINGS

When visits to pediatric EDs for acute poisoning were analyzed, one study demonstrated that 95% of parents had not contacted the PC before coming to the hospital and 64% of those children required no hospital services.[19] In contrast, when parents called the PC first, fewer than 1% sought emergency services afterward. When 589 callers to one PC were surveyed, 464 (79%) stated that they would have used the emergency care system if the PC were unavailable.[43] In a similar, more recent study 36% of callers would have selected a more costly alternative if the PC were unavailable.[7] Poison center data confirm that approximately 75% of reported exposures that originate outside of healthcare facilities can be safely managed onsite with limited telephone followup. Suggesting simple techniques or reassurance can successfully reduce hospital visits for patients who typically call PCs which, as defined, may only represent a potential exposure. Unfortunately, this approach is less applicable to adults and the population as a whole. Limited data suggest that direct bedside consultation and care help reduce length of hospital stay and healthcare costs.[26] In a recent assessment, consult with a PC for patients already in hospital is associated with a significant decrease in length of stay and total health care costs.[11,80]

The national average cost to the PC for a single human exposure call is on the order of $35.[90] A federally funded study concluded that in 1 year PCs reduced the number of patients who were treated but not hospitalized by 350,000 and reduced hospitalizations by an additional 40,000 patients.[63] Each call to a PC prevented at least $175 in subsequent medical costs, providing strong theoretical evidence to support the cost efficacy of PCs. In fact, two natural experiments support these calculations: In 1988, Louisiana closed its state-sponsored PC. During the year that followed, the cost of emergency medical services for poisoning in Louisiana increased by more than $1.4 million. This additional expenditure represented a greater than 3-fold increase above the operating cost of that center.[45] Similarly, because of financial disputes in California, direct access to the San Francisco PC was electronically restricted for one major county, with a recording referring callers instead to the 911 system for assistance.[67] The result of each blocked call was to increase healthcare costs by approximately $33. Moreover, these calculations cannot account for the unmeasured benefits to society from PC interventions that reduce waiting times for ambulance availability and hospital treatments because of lower volumes, money saved by the prevention or reduction of injury from early intervention, or lives saved by enhancing access to or utilization of the healthcare system for seriously poisoned patients.

However, many barriers prevent a person from calling a PC, including lack of familiarity with its available services, intellectual and cultural factors, language difficulties, and confidentiality concerns.[25,44,81] Epidemiological studies demonstrate that areas of increased population density with high percentages of minority inhabitants have lower utilization of PC services.[79] Additional barriers include the absence of caregiver comfort with the extensive personal contact provided by the healthcare system and a concern regarding implications of child abuse or neglect when reporting to agencies such as PC, many of which have governmental ties.[73] Data demonstrate that public educators can help overcome some of these barriers.[76] One good example of an effort to overcome reporting barriers was the institution of a single national toll-free number for poisoning (1-800-222-1222). Although it is clear that this intervention improved access and increased total calls to the PC,[48] it has yet to be determined if this has altered the patterns of use.

PROVIDING EDUCATION FOR THE PUBLIC AND HEALTH PROFESSIONALS

Poison center staff work closely with physicians, community health educators, community support groups, and parent–teacher associations to develop poison prevention activities.[59] Table 135–1 lists common strategies advocated to prevent poisoning. PCs are also actively involved in enhancing training programs for paramedics,[31] medical students,[42] pharmacy students,[28] and resident physicians[28,66,88] and are an integral part of postgraduate training programs in medical toxicology fellowships.

As stated previously, there is an inherent risk in both enhanced public and professional education programs. Currently, the decreased telephone utilization of a PC could be both the result of a decrease in the incidence of exposure or poisoning or an enhanced understanding of the prevention, diagnosis, and treatment of poisoning. Although

TABLE 135–1. Common Strategies Advocated to Help Prevent Poisoning

All xenobiotics should be kept in their original containers. Food and drink containers should never be used for the excess of a xenobiotic.
Never store xenobiotics in unlocked cabinets under the sink. Apply locks to medicine cabinets that are within the reach of a child.
In the absence of a lock, the more toxic xenobiotics should be stored on the highest shelves.
Xenobiotics should never be left in the glove compartment of the family car.
Parents should buy or accept medication only if it is in a child-resistant container.
Medication should be considered as medicine, not a plaything and certainly not candy.
Adults should not take their medications in front of children:
This will limit exposure to drug-taking role models that may become objects of imitative behavior.
Unused portions of prescription medications should be discarded.
Activated charcoal should be readily available in the home for use if directed by a poison specialist or clinician.
Children who have ingested a poison will do so again within a year, these children should receive an enhanced level of supervision.

education should never be viewed as detrimental, programs must include an emphasis on the continued use of PCs to ensure access to current information in a rapidly changing discipline. In actuality, as a result of the ongoing analysis of incoming calls, the knowledge base has the potential to change as rapidly as the calls are reported. This is far more rapid than can occur in any published literature or electronic database. Thus, additional emphasis should be applied to routine utilization of the PC as a public health tool to improve the accuracy of epidemiological data. Reporting of rare or suspected events can serve as sentinel efforts that help identify consequential adverse drug opportunities long before normal postmarketing surveillance tools identify areas of concern.

On the other hand, outreach programs that advise the public to access free services for inconsequential events can easily overwhelm an already stressed system of responding to incoming calls by demanding an immediate response to the less serious calls in an appropriate time frame. Public education and public health must both be considered to assure that PCs are staffed with the appropriate number of skilled individuals to respond not only to daily events, but also to address surges in calls that may be the result of true epidemics or responses to media announcements. Increasing calls to demonstrate increased utilization offers no public health advantage if the utilization is inappropriate or if seriously ill or potentially ill callers lose access to timely responses.

DEVELOPMENT OF PUBLIC HEALTH INITIATIVES

The initial public health efforts of poison centers focused on attempts to alter product concentration and to enhance product labeling and packaging. These clearly beneficial endeavors should continue and must evolve. However, current events have also increased PC activities in preparedness for disasters resulting from radiological, biological, and chemical terrorism.[33,47] Additional links with governmental agencies such as the CDC and ATSDR will expand the role of medical toxicology in community health.[86] The need for 24-hour rapid access to centralized information, existing data entry and retrieval systems, and links to experts in medical toxicology and emergency medicine helps to place PCs in critical roles in both local and national initiatives. Important contributions have included development of triage and treatment protocols and assessments of antidote supplies.[13,14,20,21,27,29,30,60–62,65,70,71,89]

SUMMARY

Poison centers provide unique benefits to society. Public education efforts help reduce the likelihood of exposure. Provision of basic management advice helps to diminish the consequences of a poisoning once an exposure has occurred. Reassurance and proper basic management help to curtail unnecessary utilization of expensive healthcare. Interactions with healthcare professionals streamline the care of poisoned patients and improve access to toxicologically specific antidotes and the services of medical toxicologists. Data on exposures are used effectively to create legislation to further limit poisoning by altering contents or improving packaging or labeling.

TABLE 135–2. Goals for Improving Poisoning Epidemiology Data

Identify and remove barriers to reporting
Create multiple methods of reporting:
Telephone, Facsimile, Internet based or e-mail
Simplify communications devices for the hearing impaired
Allow rapid access to translation services
Enhance awareness of the public health role of PCs
Enhance education of caregivers and healthcare professionals
Establish public health legislation requiring professional reporting of exposures
Distinguish possible exposures from actual exposures to improve the integrity of the database
Create a category for unconfirmed exposures in the database and encourage its use
Divide confirmed exposures by certainty:
Confirmed by history
Confirmed by physical examination
Confirmed by quantitative and qualitative laboratory analysis
Integrate AAPCC database with other databases (such as the ICD and "E" code systems) and utilize a standardized data collection instrument
Automatically interact with hospital and commercial laboratories
Uplink pharmacy ADE reports, hospital discharges, public health department reports (similarly available with lead screening programs), fire departments and hazardous materials responders, industry workplace exposures, death certificates, and drug abuse monitoring systems
Provide real-time analysis of incoming data
Enhance the speed of data collection and reporting
Analyze data as it is reported to identify emerging trends
Mandate the use of accepted epidemiological and statistical analyses of data
Provide rapid and regular feedback to primary reporters
Issue timely analyses and reports

Successes include the establishment of a single nationwide toll-free number to assure easy access to poison services, the development of new databases with enhanced near real-time surveillance system,[10] and the creation of a more stable stream of federal funding. Goals for the continued success of PCs must involve maintaining a uniformly high quality of service, and working to improve the accuracy of the PC database, a shift in emphasis toward active reporting, active involvement in the care of those in need of ICU care and more appropriate utilization of critical services such as ICU admissions and critical resources such as complex and costly antidotes prevention of fatal poisoning, and prevention of medical error. Many experts believe that part of this success will be through development of uniform practice guidelines, which has already begun. Poison centers must publicize the need for reporting all poisonings including ADEs and strive to improve systems of active surveillance. Although mandated reporting may somewhat improve surveillance, barriers to utilization and reporting must be identified and overcome. Poison center reporting must be integrated with other databases so that the true numerators and denominators of poisoning can be understood and so that a concerted response to poisoning and poison prevention can be made. Finally, the causes of the recently identified dramatic rise in poison-related deaths must be identified and addressed. Table 135–2 summarizes these and other initiatives, which are also discussed extensively in a recent report from the Institute of Medicine.[41]

ACKNOWLEDGMENT

Richard S. Weisman, PharmD, contributed to Table 135-1 in a previous edition of this book.

REFERENCES

1. American Academy of Clinical Toxicology. Facility assessment guidelines for regional toxicology treatment centers. American Academy of Clinical Toxicology. *J Toxicol Clin Toxicol.* 1993;31:211-217.
2. Barrons R. Evaluation of personal digital assistant software for drug interactions. *Am J Health-Syst Pharm.* 2004;61:380-385.
3. Biemer PP, Witt M. Repeated measures estimation of measurement bias for self-reported drug use with applications to the national household survey on drug abuse. *NIDA Res Monogr.* 1997;167:439-476.
4. Blanc PD, Kearney TE, Olson KR. Underreporting of fatal cases to a regional poison control center. *West J Med.* 1995;162:505-509.
5. Blanc PD, Maizlish N, Hiatt P, et al. Occupational illness and poison control centers. Referral patterns and service needs. *West J Med.* 1990;152:181-184.
6. Blanc PD, Olson KR. Occupationally related illness reported to a regional poison control center. *Am J Public Health.* 1986;76:1303-1307.
7. Blizzard JC, Michels JE, Richardson WH, et al. Cost-benefit analysis of a regional poison center. *Clin Toxicol (Phila).* 2008;46:450-456.
8. Bresnitz EA, Gittleman JL, Shic F, et al. A national survey of regional poison control centers' management of occupational exposure calls. *J Occup Environ Med.* 1999;41:93-99.
9. Bresnitz EA. Poison control center follow-up of occupational disease. *Am J Public Health.* 1990;80:711-712.
10. Bronstein AC, Spyker DA, Cantilena LR, Jr, et al. 2006 annual report of the American Association of Poison Control Centers' National Poison Data System (NPDS). *Clin Toxicol (Phila).* 2007;45:815-917.
11. Bunn TL, Slavova S, Spiller HA, et al. The effect of poison control center consultation on accidental poisoning inpatient hospitalizations with preexisting medical conditions. *J Toxicol Environ Health A.* 2008;71:283-288.
12. Burda T, Leikin JB, Fischbein C, et al. Emergency department use of flumazenil prior to poison center consultation. *Vet Hum Toxicol.* 1997;39:245-247.
13. Caravati EM, Erdman AR, Christianson G, et al. Elemental mercury exposure: an evidence-based consensus guideline for out-of-hospital management. *Clin Toxicol (Phila).* 2008;46:1-21.
14. Caravati EM, Erdman AR, Scharman EJ, et al. Long-acting anticoagulant rodenticide poisoning: an evidence-based consensus guideline for out-of-hospital management. *Clin Toxicol (Phila).* 2007;45:1-22.
15. Caravati EM, McElwee NE. Use of clinical toxicology resources by emergency physicians and its impact on poison control centers. *Ann Emerg Med.* 1991;20:147-150.
16. Centers for Disease Control and Prevention (CDC). Increases in age-group-specific injury mortality—United States, 1999-2004. *MMWR Morb Mortal Wkly Rep.* 2007;56:1281-1284.
17. Centers for Disease Control and Prevention (CDC). Unintentional and undetermined poisoning deaths—11 states, 1990-2001. *MMWR Morb Mortal Wkly Rep.* 2004;53:233-238.
18. Chafee-Bahamon C, Caplan DL, Lovejoy FH, Jr. Patterns in hospitals' use of a regional poison information center. *Am J Public Health.* 1983;73:396-400.
19. Chafee-Bahamon C, Lovejoy FH, Jr. Effectiveness of a regional poison center in reducing excess emergency room visits for children's poisonings. *Pediatrics.* 1983;72:164-169.
20. Chyka PA, Erdman AR, Christianson G, et al. Salicylate poisoning: an evidence-based consensus guideline for out-of-hospital management. *Clin Toxicol (Phila).* 2007;45:95-131.
21. Chyka PA, Erdman AR, Manoguerra AS, et al. Dextromethorphan poisoning: an evidence-based consensus guideline for out-of-hospital management. *Clin Toxicol (Phila).* 2007;45:662-677.
22. Chyka PA, McCommon SW. Reporting of adverse drug reactions by poison control centres in the US. *Drug Saf.* 2000;23:87-93.
23. Chyka PA. How many deaths occur annually from adverse drug reactions in the United States? *Am J Med.* 2000;109:122-130.
24. Chyka PA. Role of US poison centers in adverse drug reactions monitoring. *Vet Hum Toxicol.* 1999;41:400-402.
25. Clark RF, Phillips M, Manoguerra AS, Chan TC. Evaluating the utilization of a regional poison center by Latino communities. *J Toxicol Clin Toxicol.* 2002;40:855-860.
26. Clark RF, Williams SR, Nordt SP, et al. Resource-use analysis of a medical toxicology consultation service. *Ann Emerg Med.* 1998;31:705-709.
27. Cobaugh DJ, Erdman AR, Booze LL, et al. Atypical antipsychotic medication poisoning: an evidence-based consensus guideline for out-of-hospital management. *Clin Toxicol (Phila).* 2007;45:918-942.
28. Cobaugh DJ, Goetz CM, Lopez GP, et al. Assessment of learning by emergency medicine residents and pharmacy students participating in a poison center clerkship. *Vet Hum Toxicol.* 1997;39:173-175.
29. Dart RC, Goldfrank LR, Chyka PA, et al. Combined evidence-based literature analysis and consensus guidelines for stocking of emergency antidotes in the United States. *Ann Emerg Med.* 2000;36:126-132.
30. Dart RC, Stark Y, Fulton B, et al. Insufficient stocking of poisoning antidotes in hospital pharmacies. *JAMA.* 1996;276:1508-1510.
31. Davis CO, Cobaugh DJ, Leahey NF, Wax PM. Toxicology training of paramedic students in the United States. *Am J Emerg Med.* 1999;17:138-140.
32. Felberg L, Litovitz TL, Soloway RA, Morgan J. State of the nation's poison centers: 1994 American Association of Poison Control Centers Survey of US Poison Centers. *Vet Hum Toxicol.* 1996;38:214-219.
33. Geller RJ, Lopez GP. Poison center planning for mass gatherings: the Georgia poison center experience with the 1996 centennial olympic games. *J Toxicol Clin Toxicol.* 1999;37:315-319.
34. Gfroerer J, Lessler J, Parsley T. Studies of nonresponse and measurement error in the national household survey on drug abuse. *NIDA Res Monogr.* 1997;167:273-295.
35. Greenberg MI, Cone DC, Roberts JR. Material safety data sheet: a useful resource for the emergency physician. *Ann Emerg Med.* 1996;27:347-352.
36. Hamilton RJ, Goldfrank LR. Poison center data and the Pollyanna phenomenon. *J Toxicol Clin Toxicol.* 1997;35:21-23.
37. Hamilton RJ, Perrone J, Hoffman R, et al. A descriptive study of an epidemic of poisoning caused by heroin adulterated with scopolamine. *J Toxicol Clin Toxicol.* 2000;38:597-608.
38. Harchelroad F, Clark RF, Dean B, Krenzelok EP. Treated vs reported toxic exposures: discrepancies between a poison control center and a member hospital. *Vet Hum Toxicol.* 1990;32:156-159.
39. Hoppe-Roberts JM, Lloyd LM, Chyka PA. Poisoning mortality in the United States: comparison of national mortality statistics and poison control center reports. *Ann Emerg Med.* 2000;35:440-448.
40. Hoyt BT, Rasmussen R, Giffin S, Smilkstein MJ. Poison center data accuracy: a comparison of rural hospital chart data with the TESS database. Toxic Exposure Surveillance System. *Acad Emerg Med.* 1999;6:851-855.

41. Institute of Medicine. *Forging a Poison Prevention and Control System.* Washington, DC: National Academies Press; 2004.
42. Jordan JK, Dean BS, Krenzelok EP. Poison center rotation for health science students. *Vet Hum Toxicol.* 1987;29:174-175.
43. Kearney TE, Olson KR, Bero LA, et al. Health care cost effects of public use of a regional poison control center. *West J Med.* 1995;162:499-504.
44. Kelly NR, Huffman LC, Mendoza FS, Robinson TN. Effects of a videotape to increase use of poison control centers by low-income and spanish-speaking families: a randomized, controlled trial. *Pediatrics.* 2003;111:21-26.
45. King WD, Palmisano PA. Poison control centers: can their value be measured? *South Med J.* 1991;84:722-726.
46. Klein-Schwartz W, Smith GS. Agricultural and horticultural chemical poisonings: mortality and morbidity in the United States. *Ann Emerg Med.* 1997;29:232-238.
47. Krenzelok EP, Allswede MP, Mrvos R. The poison center role in biological and chemical terrorism. *Vet Hum Toxicol.* 2000;42:297-300.
48. Krenzelok EP, Mrvos R. Initial impact of toll-free access on poison center call volume. *Vet Hum Toxicol.* 2003;45:325-327.
49. Lai MW, Klein-Schwartz W, Rodgers GC, et al. 2005 annual report of the American Association of Poison Control Centers' National Poisoning and Exposure Database. *Clin Toxicol (Phila).* 2006;44:803-932.
50. Lazarou J, Pomeranz BH, Corey PN. Incidence of adverse drug reactions in hospitalized patients: a meta-analysis of prospective studies. *JAMA.* 1998;279:1200-1205.
51. Levy A, Bailey B, Letarte A, et al. Unproven ingestion: an unrecognized bias in toxicological case series. *Clin Toxicol (Phila).* 2007;45:946-949.
52. Linakis JG, Frederick KA. Poisoning deaths not reported to the regional poison control center. *Ann Emerg Med.* 1993;22:1822-1828.
53. Litovitz TL, Klein-Schwartz W, Caravati EM, et al. 1998 annual report of the American Association of Poison Control Centers Toxic Exposure Surveillance System. *Am J Emerg Med.* 1999;17:435-487.
54. Litovitz TL, Klein-Schwartz W, Dyer KS, et al. 1997 annual report of the American Association of Poison Control Centers Toxic Exposure Surveillance System. *Am J Emerg Med.* 1998;16:443-497.
55. Litovitz TL, Klein-Schwartz W, Rodgers GC,Jr, et al. 2001 annual report of the American Association of Poison Control Centers Toxic Exposure Surveillance System. *Am J Emerg Med.* 2002;20:391-452.
56. Litovitz TL, Klein-Schwartz W, White S, et al. 1999 annual report of the American Association of Poison Control Centers Toxic Exposure Surveillance System. *Am J Emerg Med.* 2000;18:517-574.
57. Litovitz TL, Klein-Schwartz W, White S, et al: 2000 annual report of the American Association of Poison Control Centers Toxic Exposure Surveillance System. *Am J Emerg Med.* 2001;19:337-395.
58. LoVecchio F, Katz K, Watts D, Pitera A. Media influence on poison center call volume after 11 September 2001. *Prehospital Disaster Med.* 2004; 19:185.
59. Lovejoy FH,Jr, Robertson WO, Woolf AD. Poison centers, poison prevention, and the pediatrician. *Pediatrics.* 1994;94:220-224.
60. Manoguerra AS, Cobaugh DJ, Guidelines for the Management of Poisoning Consensus Panel: guideline on the use of ipecac syrup in the out-of-hospital management of ingested poisons. *Clin Toxicol.* 2005;43:1-10.
61. Manoguerra AS, Erdman AR, Wax PM, et al. Camphor poisoning: an evidence-based practice guideline for out-of-hospital management. *Clin Toxicol (Phila).* 2006;44:357-370.
62. McGuigan MA, Guideline Consensus Panel. Guideline for the out-of-hospital management of human exposures to minimally toxic substances. *J Toxicol Clin Toxicol.* 2003;41:907-917.
63. Miller TR, Lestina DC. Costs of poisoning in the United States and savings from poison control centers: a benefit-cost analysis. *Ann Emerg Med.* 1997;29:239-245.
64. Mullen WH, Anderson IB, Kim SY, et al. Incorrect overdose management advice in the physicians' desk reference. *Ann Emerg Med.* 1997;29:255-261.
65. Nelson LS, Erdman AR, Booze LL, et al. Selective serotonin reuptake inhibitor poisoning: an evidence-based consensus guideline for out-of-hospital management. *Clin Toxicol (Phila).* 2007;45:315-332.
66. Nelson LS, Gordon PE, Simmons MD, et al. The benefit of houseofficer education on proper medication dose calculation and ordering. *Acad Emerg Med.* 2000;7:1311-1316.
67. Phillips KA, Homan RK, Hiatt PH, et al. The costs and outcomes of restricting public access to poison control centers. Results from a natural experiment. *Med Care.* 1998;36:271-280.
68. Robinson RL, Burk MS. Identification of drug-drug interactions with personal digital assistant-based software. *Am J Med.* 2004;116:357-358.
69. Rodgers GB. The safety effects of child-resistant packaging for oral prescription drugs. Two decades of experience. *JAMA.* 1996;275:1661-1665.
70. Scharman EJ, Erdman AR, Cobaugh DJ, et al. Methylphenidate poisoning: an evidence-based consensus guideline for out-of-hospital management. *Clin Toxicol (Phila).* 2007;45:737-752.
71. Scharman EJ, Erdman AR, Wax PM, et al. Diphenhydramine and dimenhydrinate poisoning: an evidence-based consensus guideline for out-of-hospital management. *Clin Toxicol (Phila).* 2006;44:205-223.
72. Scherz RG, Robertson WO. The history of poison control centers in the United States. *Clin Toxicol.* 1978;12:291-296.
73. Schwartz L, Howland MA, Mercurio-Zappala M, Hoffman RS. The use of focus groups to plan poison prevention education programs for low-income populations. *Health Promot Pract.* 2003;4:340-346.
74. Seifert SA, Jacobitz K. Pharmacy prescription dispensing errors reported to a regional poison control center. *J Toxicol Clin Toxicol.* 2002;40:919-923.
75. Soslow AR, Woolf AD. Reliability of data sources for poisoning deaths in Massachusetts. *Am J Emerg Med.* 1992;10:124-127.
76. Spiller HA, Mowry JB. Evaluation of the effect of a public educator on calls and poisonings reported to a regional poison center. *Vet Hum Toxicol.* 2004;46:206-208.
77. Temple AR. Testing of child-resistant containers. *Clin Toxicol.* 1978;12: 357-365.
78. Ungerleider JT, Lundberg GD, Sunshine I, Walberg CB. DAWN: drug abuse warning network or data about worthless numbers? *J Anal Toxicol.* 1980;4:269-271.
79. Vassilev ZP, Marcus S, Jennis T, et al. Rapid communication: sociodemographic differences between counties with high and low utilization of a regional poison control center. *J Toxicol Environ Health A.* 2003;66:1905-1908.
80. Vassilev ZP, Marcus SM. The impact of a poison control center on the length of hospital stay for patients with poisoning. *J Toxicol Environ Health A.* 2007;70:107-110.
81. Vassilev ZP, Shiel M, Lewis MJ, et al. Assessment of barriers to utilization of poison centers by Hispanic/Latino populations. *J Toxicol Environ Health A.* 2006;69:1711-1718.
82. Walton WW. An evaluation of the poison prevention packaging act. *Pediatrics.* 1982;69:363-370.
83. Watson WA, Litovitz TL, Klein-Schwartz W, et al. 2003 annual report of the American Association of Poison Control Centers Toxic Exposure Surveillance System. *Am J Emerg Med.* 2004;22:335-404.
84. Watson WA, Litovitz TL, Rodgers GC, Jr, et al. 2002 annual report of the American Association of Poison Control Centers Toxic Exposure Surveillance System. *Am J Emerg Med.* 2003;21:353-421.
85. Watson WA, Litovitz TL, Rodgers GC, et al. 2004 annual report of the American Association of Poison Control Centers Toxic Exposure Surveillance System. *Am J Emerg Med.* 2005;23:589-666.
86. Wax PM, Nelson LS, Kosnett M. A nation-wide consultative network between medical toxicology fellowship programs and ATSDR regional offices. *J Toxicol Clin Toxicol.* 203;41:707.
87. Wax PM, Rodewald L, Lawrence R. The arrival of the ED-based POISINDEX: perceived impact on poison control center use. *Am J Emerg Med.* 1994;12:537-540.
88. Wolf LR, Hamilton GC. Objectives to direct the training of emergency medicine residents of off-service rotations: toxicology. *J Emerg Med.* 1994;12:391-405.
89. Woolf AD, Erdman AR, Nelson LS, et al. Tricyclic antidepressant poisoning: an evidence-based consensus guideline for out-of-hospital management. *Clin Toxicol (Phila).* 2007;45:203-233.
90. Youniss J, Litovitz T, Villanueva P. Characterization of US poison centers: a 1998 survey conducted by the American Association of Poison Control Centers. *Vet Hum Toxicol.* 2000;42:43-53.

CHAPTER 136

INTERNATIONAL PERSPECTIVES ON MEDICAL TOXICOLOGY

Michael Eddleston

Poisoning and envenomations are worldwide problems but the major effects are felt in the developing world. At least 250,000–350,000 people die every year from acute pesticide poisoning[59] and many more suffer from acute or chronic occupational exposure,[38,74] hundreds of thousands of people are affected by groundwater arsenic contamination in Bangladesh and India,[116] and an estimated 20,000–94,000 humans die each year from snake bites.[80] Outbreaks of plant food–derived poisoning affect whole communities,[32] and leaks from poorly regulated chemical plants affect urban areas as the Bhopal disaster did in 1984.[112]

The resources for dealing with these problems are limited. Public health education about poisons and laws limiting access to the most highly toxic chemicals are practically absent in much of the developing world. Rudimentary public health infrastructures make the western model of a toxicology consult service impractical. Clinical toxicology is frequently not a recognized specialty and patients are evaluated by general physicians with little training, although often with great experience. Diagnostic facilities are few, effective treatment options even rarer. Where antidotes exist, there is rarely enough knowledge or experience to know how to use them.[23] Intensive care beds for long-term ventilation are scarce.

Variations in poisoning patterns within any given country may be significant, especially when comparing wealthier urban centers with agrarian, often poorer, rural areas. While the majority of healthcare and academic resources are concentrated in urban centers, it is in the countryside where much of the mortality from acute poisoning occurs. The accessibility of pesticides to rural people, and their lethality, has a profound influence on global poisoning patterns.

EPIDEMIOLOGY OF ACUTE POISONING GLOBALLY

PESTICIDES

A systematic review suggested that at least 250,000, and probably 350,000, deaths occur each year from acute pesticide self-poisoning around the world.[59] The annual number of deaths from occupational or unintentional poisoning is unknown but was estimated 20 years ago at 20,000.[73] The majority of self-harm deaths occur in Asia, particularly in China and India.[59] Around 3000–6000 ventilators are required each day for ventilation of pesticide-poisoned patients,[59] with many patients requiring ventilation for weeks.[46] The World Health Organization now considers pesticide poisoning to be the single most important global means of suicide, accounting for more than one-third of all suicides.[17]

While many classes of pesticides are implicated in fatal self-poisonings, organic phosphorous (OP) insecticides appear to be responsible for the majority of pesticide-related deaths.[42] Deliberate self-poisoning with OP insecticides puts a high cost on the healthcare system. In one study examining the experience in Sri Lanka, OP insecticide poisoning was responsible for 943 of 2559 (36%) admissions to a secondary hospital for poisoning.[48] The case fatality for OP poisoning was 21%, and pesticide poisoned patients occupied 41% of all medical intensive care beds. Similar situations have been reported from across the world.[42] In all likelihood, such studies underestimate the mortality associated with intentional pesticide ingestion as most are hospital based and do not include patients who die prior to hospital presentation.[3]

Factors that contribute to the high mortality in self-poisoning with pesticides in the developing world include the intrinsic lethality of many pesticides and healthcare systems that are poorly prepared to handle such critically ill patients (Table 136–1). Pesticides are easily available in highly concentrated preparations in rural communities throughout the developing world. The ease of drinking liquid pesticides is also a factor facilitating massive intentional ingestions.

Inadequate pesticide storage systems are also implicated,[83] particularly in unintentional ingestions in children. Outbreaks of unintentional poisoning from contaminated flour or old pesticide containers used to store food still occur in rural areas.[40] The extraordinarily high human, economic, and social costs of pesticide-related mortality in the developing world reinforce the importance of developing strategies specifically designed to care for acutely poisoned patients in resource-poor environments. Treatment protocols should be simple, economical, and evidence based.[23]

Patients die from other pesticides. Poisoning with organic chlorine insecticides was a common problem in many countries[42] and remains one in Turkey[41,79] (see Chap. 114). However, recent international bans, in particular the *Stockholm Convention on Persistent Organic Pollutants*, have generally reduced their use in agriculture and self-harm. Carbamate insecticides are also a frequent means of fatal self-harm[2,18,78] and may become more common as agricultural use of organic phosphorus insecticides decreases. Avermectin poisoning is reported from Taiwan.[36] The fumigant aluminum phosphide is the most important cause of fatal self-poisoning in Northern India,[115] with a case fatality over 60%.[62] Fatal aluminum phosphide poisoning is also common in children.[117]

Dipyridyl herbicides, particularly paraquat, are common methods of self-harm in some countries, particularly Korea and Sri Lanka.[57,137] Glyphosate-containing herbicides are widely used for agriculture and self-harm;[131] human toxicity appears to relate to the salt and surfactant present in the formulation rather than the actual herbicide itself.[22] Other herbicides reported to be important local self-harm problems include propanil, causing methemoglobinemia and hemolysis anemia,[47] chlorphenoxy compounds, possibly causing oxidative uncoupling in severe cases,[109] and alachlor and butachlor, causing CNS depression[90] (see Chap. 115).

As pesticides are developed[25] and integrated into agricultural practices, their emergence as a means of self-harm is likely to occur. The avermectins and phenylpyrazoles affect the CNS in opposing ways, the former causing coma,[36] the latter seizures.[93] Both have a low case fatality. Other new pesticides, including chitin synthesis inhibitors and neonicotinoids,[25,132] appear to have very low toxicity in overdose compared to the older OP insecticides. Many patients will survive poisoning with only careful supportive care.

CAUSTICS

Caustics are common in the developing world in both industry and the home. Poisoning with these chemicals is distinct from other common poisonings in two respects. First, gastric decontamination is generally contraindicated due to direct damage to the oropharynx, esophagus, and stomach. Second, if the acute phase of caustic poisoning is survived, there is a high rate of delayed complications, primarily esophageal strictures. These delayed complications may require surgical

TABLE 136–1. Factors Contributing to High Mortality from Self-Poisoning with Pesticides in the Developing World

1. Ease of access to pesticides in rural, agrarian households
2. Poor storage practices
3. Inadequate labeling of lethal pesticide products
4. High potency of pesticides
5. Lack of evidence-based practice guidelines appropriate for resource poor areas
6. Lack of clear guidelines
7. Distance from and time to health care facilities and resources available at healthcare facilities

intervention, balloon dilatation of the esophagus (bouginage), or feeding tube placement. These treatments are expensive, require significant hospital resources, and have inherent morbidity and mortality. While some patients may die acutely from the original exposure, others die from complications of later reparative surgery (see Chap. 104).

The common form of caustic ingested varies between countries. In Taiwan and Morocco, self-poisoning with hydrochloric or sulfuric acids is a major problem.[4,87,122,139]

Formic and acetic acids are used in the manufacture of rubber, and case series are reported from areas surrounding rubber factories in India and Sri Lanka.[107] In Surinam and Curacao, concentrated acetic acid was an important means of self-harm in the 1970s.[39,100] *Rubigine* is a domestic cleaning product containing hydrofluoric acid and ammonium difluoride that is used for self-harm in the Caribbean.[69] Car battery acid ingestion occurs in Africa, Papua New Guinea, and the Caribbean[138] while ingestion of sodium hydroxide is common in Malaysia.[13] All the caustics have high case fatality, usually well over 10%.

INDUSTRIAL PRODUCTS

While many xenobiotics used in industrial processes have been used for self-harm, a complete review of intentional or occupational poisoning is beyond the scope of this chapter. However, two xenobiotics commonly used in self-poisoning require mention. Copper sulfate causes direct damage to the GI tract, hepatorenal failure, and hemolysis[111] (see Chap. 93). Once widely used for self-poisoning in South Asia, there has been a resurgence in cases in Bangladesh in recent years.[8] Cyanide has become a commonly used method in Korea over the last 20 years[88] (see Chap. 126).

Occupational and environmental poisoning from industrial xenobiotics is a significant problem in the developing world. As the world becomes increasingly more industrialized, laws to regulate access to industrial xenobiotics and ensure their safe labeling in developing countries have lagged behind the expansion of exposure. Furthermore, industrial factories are often placed in urban areas, or the areas around factories are rapidly urbanized, placing large numbers of people at risk of poisoning from industrial errors[12] and facilitating easy access to poisons in cases of intentional ingestion.

DOMESTIC XENOBIOTICS

Patterns of self-harm using domestic xenobiotics appear to have significant intracountry variability. In one Zimbabwean case series of 1192 cases, the majority of exposures were unintentional ingestions of kerosene in children under the age of 6.[99] However, self-harm was cited in 19% of cases and was responsible for many deaths. Poor storage of kerosene and paraffin, typically in soda or water containers and in easily accessible locations, is a major factor in the high incidence of poisoning in children[50] (see Chap. 106).

In Hong Kong, significant morbidity is associated with self-poisoning using detergent products such as dettol (4.8% chloroxylenol, pine oil and isopropyl alcohol) and savlon (cetrimide).[26,29,31,37] Common use of potassium permanganate for self-harm has been reported from Hong Kong.[1021,140] While cosmetics are not cited as a major source of poisoning, fatal poisoning with hair dye (paraphenylenediamine) is known in the Middle East and north Africa.[21,49,66,119] Barium sulfide, arsenic sulfide, and calcium oxide are contained in hair removal preparations;[114] ingestion of such preparations has been reported from India and Iran.[6]

ANIMAL ENVENOMATION

Snake bites and envenomation by other animals represent a significant cause of morbidity and mortality in the developing world. Venomous snakes are found on all continents, with the exception of Antarctica, although the majority of species are found in equatorial, tropical or subtropical environments.[134,136] The epidemiology of snake bites and therefore the health impact is determined by the species of snake in a given area, lethality of venom from these species, snake behavior, human activities, and access to healthcare. Snakebites from members of the Elapidae and Viperidae families are responsible for the majority of deaths worldwide, although several other families are medically important (Colubridae and Atractaspididae species, in particular)[134,136] (see Chap. 121).

Snakebite is most commonly an occupational hazard in the rural tropics. Victims are just as likely to be women as men, reflecting rural farming practices. Working in large plantations and subsistence farms places rural people in frequent contact with venomous snakes. With simultaneous changes in global climate and expansion of human settlements, it is likely that the range of venomous snakes will enlarge to include urban areas and regions previously considered too temperate to support them.[67,98]

Few countries mandate the reporting of animal bites, making it difficult to estimate snakebite incidence, severity and outcome. Because the majority of rural people in the developing world first consult traditional healers, hospital-based studies of mortality and morbidity associated with snakebites may underestimate the scope of the problem.[33,118] A study of rural Philippine rice farmers found that only 8% of cobra (*Naja philippinensis*) bite victims reached a hospital in the 1980s.[135] However, changes in treatment seeking can occur. Studies over the last decade in Sri Lanka have shown that patients have started going to the hospital rapidly after common krait (*Bungarus caeruleus*) snake bite, bypassing traditional healers.[85]

Taking into account these caveats, a recent study has estimated that 20,000–94,000 deaths occur globally each year from snake bite.[80] The vast majority of deaths and serious envenomations occur in the developing world. In contrast, less than 100 snakebite deaths per year are estimated to occur in Europe, the United States, Canada, and Australia combined.[33,80]

The burden of snake envenomation on local resources can be substantial. During the rainy season in Benin, snakebites account for up to 20% of all hospital admissions.[34] The case fatality is estimated to be 3%–6%. In this region, the annual incidence of snake envenomation ranges from 200–100,000 in rural villagers to 1300–100,000 in sugar cane plantation workers.[34] One study conducted in Nigeria in the late 1970s noted an incidence of 497 per 100,000 and a 12% case fatality (primarily due to envenomation by the carpet viper, *Echis occelatus*).[104] Difficulty with accessing healthcare facilities was responsible in part for the high mortality noted in one Nepalese community study.[113]

The mainstay of effective therapy is antivenom, which must be safe, effective, economical, available, and widely distributed.[130] Currently available antivenoms are prohibitively expensive, ineffective, or have a high rate of adverse reactions. Equally important, some antivenoms must be refrigerated, making them impractical therapies in the developing world. The most important challenge to treating patients with snakebites is this lack of antivenom availability in the developing world.[129] Critical evaluation of existing antivenoms and development of new products are desperately needed.[15,64,87,129,130,1376]

After snakebites, the second most common cause of mortality and morbidity from venomous animals is scorpion stings[70,134] (see Chap. 119). Medically important scorpion species are widely distributed throughout the tropics, being particularly common causes of morbidity in North Africa, Mexico, India, and Brazil.[35] The total number of medically significant scorpion stings that occur annually is unknown; a recent review estimated 1.2 million stings, leading to more than 3250 deaths (case fatality 0.27%).[35] The majority of these deaths occur in children and elderly people in rural areas where access to healthcare and antivenom is limited. The role of antivenom therapy is widely accepted in many countries, although evidence for its efficacy is scant and there is still some debate.[5,58,70,71]

Other venomous insects, such as Arachnida (spiders) and Hymenoptera (bees, ants, and wasps) are rarely sources of significant mortality on a global scale[70] (see Chap. 119). Most deaths are associated with anaphylactic reactions to Hymenoptera venom.[53] Effective antivenom is available to widow spiders (*Lactrodectus* ssp), the Brazilian banana or armed spider (*Phoneutria* ssp), and the Australian funnel spider (*Atrax robustus*).[70]

XENOBIOTICS

In the developing world, the use of pharmaceuticals for self-harm is more common in urban areas where access is easier and more people have the financial means to buy them. The pharmacopeia available in the developing world is smaller than in the industrialized world, with the exception of drugs to treat tropical diseases that may be common in particular areas.

One important medicine for self-harm in the developing world is the antimalarial chloroquine.[42] Chloroquine self-harm was widely reported from west Africa during the 1960s and 1970s;[19,96] recently a rising number of cases have been reported from Zimbabwe[14,105] (see Chap. 58). Cases of intentional and unintentional poisoning with the leprosy drug dapsone, as well as the tuberculosis drug isoniazid, have been reported[102,1265,126,133] (see Chap. 57).

Criminal poisoning of commuters to aid robbery is a common problem across south Asia.[72,97,1043] However, it appears to be particularly common around Dhaka in Bangladesh. In the 1970s and 1980s, drinks containing extracts of *Datura stramonium* were given to unsuspecting commuters, resulting in anticholinergic poisoning.[82] Practice has changed recently so that benzodiazepines are now given to sedate commuters.[90] As many as 300 people are admitted unconscious with this problem to a single university medical unit in Dhaka each year.[90]

HERBAL AND TRADITIONAL MEDICINES

Much is known about the use or the potential toxicity of traditional medicines in the developing world. Large schools of traditional medical theory and practice exist throughout China and India (Ayurvedic medicine). In other countries, traditional medical theory is learned through an apprenticeship process. In Mexico, for example, the National Ethnobotanical herbarium catalogues more than 14,000 different plants used in traditional medical practices.

While traditional medicinal preparations have been tested by generations of practitioners and the concentrations of active ingredients are generally low, both intentional and unintentional poisonings are common.[30,77,121,124] Adulterants are also common in traditional Ayurvedic medicines (particularly steroids[63]) and Asian medicines (particularly synthetic pharmaceuticals and heavy metals[28]) (see Chap. 43). A Taiwanese study of 2609 samples found that 23% were adulterated with pharmaceutical products such as caffeine, NSAIDS, acetaminophen, and diuretics.[68]

PLANTS

Poisonous plants have been used therapeutically and for harm throughout human history. Typically, they are used to induce abortion, for recreational intoxication, in homicidal acts, or for self-harm. Plants have also been the source of unintentional poisoning, either through direct toxicity or due to a toxic contaminant. This section briefly mentions toxic plants that are commonly used in self-poisoning or have caused epidemic poisoning in the developing world.[136]

Self-poisoning with seeds of two plants containing cardioactive steroids are important clinical problems in Asia. Yellow oleander (*Thevetia peruviana*) kills hundreds of people each year in Sri Lanka and India[20,43] (see Chap. 64). Sea mango (*Cerbera manghas*) has killed hundreds of people in Kerala, India,[56], and is a focal problem in eastern Sri Lanka.[44] Oduvan (*Cleistanthus collinus*) leaf contains the glycosides cleistanthin A and B, which produce severe hypokalemia and cardiac dysrhythmias.[11] Self-poisoning has killed hundreds of people in Tamil Nadu, India.[10,123]

Ackee tree fruit (*Blighia sapida*), which contains hypoglycin when unripe, is widely consumed as a food source. Epidemics of fatal poisoning with unripe Ackee fruit have occurred throughout the Caribbean and in Africa.[51,75,91,94] The superb lily (*Gloriosa superba*) contains colchicine alkaloids and has been used for self-harm in south Asia[7,9,92] (see Chap. 37).

Numerous plant species contain atropine like alkaloids, causing an anticholinergic syndrome when ingested. Reports of intentional ingestion of *Datura* species have been reported from Africa, Asia, and Latin America.[65,110,120] Most commonly, the seeds are ingested as a recreational drug for their hallucinatory effects,[55,106] or as part of traditional medical preparations.[27] Poisoning by castor beans (*Ricinus communis*) or other lectin-containing plants such as *Jatropha* spp (African purging nut) has been reported from Africa and South Asia[1,52,65,76] (see Chap. 118).

Unintentional ingestion of *Karwinskia humboldtiana* (buckthorn, coyotillo in Mexico, wild cherry or tullidora) causes a demyelinating polyneuropathy, clinically similar to Guillain-Barré syndrome.[16,24] Contamination of wheat with pyrrolizidine alkaloid-containing *Heliotropium* spp and *Crotalaria* spp in India, Tadjikistan, and Afghanistan has resulted in chronic veno-occlusive liver disease.[32,127,128]

REDUCING POISONING MORTALITY GLOBALLY

Recognition that self-poisoning with pesticides is responsible for the majority of poisoning deaths worldwide compels us to act to reduce the associated mortality. Ironically, some programs to remove the most environmentally persistent and toxic pesticides have inadvertently replaced them with pesticides that are highly toxic to humans, for example, the replacement of persistent organic chlorine compounds with carbamates in malaria control programs. The opposite has also occurred when pyrethroids replaced OP insecticides in an effort to reduce human toxicity.[84] Strategies to reduce the health effects of pesticides should take into account concerns regarding both environmental and human toxicity, and anticipate which xenobiotics will replace the most highly toxic chemicals as they are phased out of use.[108] A strategy

TABLE 136–2. Hierarchical Strategies to Reduce Pesticide Poisoning Mortality in the Developing World[108]

Most	Eliminate the most highly toxic pesticides Substitute with less toxic, equally effective alternatives
Efficacy	Reduce use through improved equipment Isolate people from the hazard Label products and train applicators in safe handling practices Promote use of personal protection equipment
Least	Institute administrative controls

based on industrial hygiene models of hierarchy of controls has been proposed by several authors (see Table 136–2).[95,108]

Voluntary interventions include international policy statements and industrial pesticide initiatives. In 1985, the Food and Agriculture Organization (FAO) of the United Nations issued a strongly worded document, the *Code of Conduct on the Distribution and Use of Pesticides*.[54] The pesticide industry has also worked in cooperation with the FAO to remove or destroy large stockpiles of obsolete or banned pesticides in the developing world. CropLife International is an industry-sponsored initiative that aims to reduce the health burden of pesticide poisoning through Safe Use and Integrated Pest Management (IPM) programs (www.croplife.org). The cost effectiveness of industry sponsored Safe Use of Pesticides programs, however, has been questioned.[95] Voluntary initiatives also suffer from a lack of resources, a shortage of political will, and nonexistent enforcement mechanisms.[84]

Restricting access to pesticides is the critical step in reducing the number of cases and the mortality of intentional ingestions. National programs that remove specific WHO-defined high-risk pesticides demonstrate this effect on mortality. The most dramatic illustration of the effectiveness of this approach is provided by Sri Lanka where banning of all WHO high-risk OP insecticides and the organic chlorine endosulfan resulted in an arrest in the previously exponential increase in incidence of pesticide poisoning and a halving of the national suicide rate between 1995 and 2005.[60] The program was estimated to have saved at least 20,000 lives over 10 years.[60]

A minimum pesticide list, based on the WHO essential xenobiotic list initiative, has been proposed.[45] Such a list would provide policy makers and farmers with a source of unbiased information, and remove the most dangerous and obsolete pesticides from everyday use. Programs to restrict the availability of pesticides reduce mortality, although careful consideration of alternative self-harm xenobiotics is necessary to prevent the public from simply switching to another, equally deadly, xenobiotic.[108]

SUMMARY

Poisoning is a common cause of death throughout the developing world. While many different xenobiotics exist in the developing world, pesticides are the most important source of mortality. In particular, organic phosphorous compounds, aluminum phosphide, and paraquat are responsible for a disproportionate number of deaths. Conservative estimates suggest that at least 3 million cases of pesticide poisoning occur annually, resulting in 250,000–350,000 deaths.[59] The majority of deaths occur in the context of acts of deliberate self-poisoning. Envenomation is another significant problem; an estimated 5 million snakebites occur each year, resulting in 20,000–94,000 additional deaths.[80]

Epidemiologic information about regional and local poisoning patterns is needed to guide public health interventions. At present, poisoning epidemiology represents estimates derived from a minority of developing world countries. Assumptions regarding the generalization of these data may not be true. Efforts to develop epidemiologic surveillance systems and establish harmonized definitions of poisonings will yield a more complete picture of global poisonings.

Lack of evidence to support many treatment interventions hinders public health policy in the developing world. Randomized controlled trials need to be conducted to critically evaluate accepted toxicology dogma.[61] Economic analysis must also be conducted prior to recommending expensive, yet unproven, therapies. Pending the implementation of such studies, proven therapies, such as atropine and pralidoxime for organic phosphorous pesticide poisoning and snake antivenins, should be made available and affordable. In the case of pesticide poisoning, a coordinated international effort to restrict access to the most lethal xenobiotics is of paramount importance.[45]

ACKNOWLEDGMENT

Aaron Hexdall contributed to this chapter in a previous edition.

REFERENCES

1. Abdu-Aguye I, Sannusi A, Alafiya-Tayo RA, Bhusnurmath SR. Acute toxicity studies with Jatropha curcas L. *Hum Toxicol.* 1986;5:269-274.
2. Abdullat EM, Hadidi MS, Alhadidi N, et al. Agricultural and horticultural pesticides fatal poisoning; the Jordanian experience 1999-2002. *J Clin Forensic Med.* 2006;13:304-307.
3. Abeyasinghe R, Gunnell D. Psychological autopsy study of suicide in three rural and semi-rural districts of Sri Lanka. *Soc Psychiatry Psychiatr Epidemiol.* 2008;43:280-285.
4. Abi F, El Fares F, El Moussaoui A, et al. Les lesions caustiques du tractus digestif superieur. A propos de 191 observations. *J Chir (Paris).* 1986;123:390-394.
5. Abroug F, Elatrous S, Nouira S, et al. Serotherapy in scorpion envenomation: a randomised controlled trial. *Lancet.* 1999;354:906-909.
6. Agarwal SK, Bansal A, Mani NK. Barium sulfide poisoning. *J Assoc Physicians India.* 1986;34:151.
7. Agunawela RM, Fernando HA. Acute ascending polyneuropathy and dermatitis following poisoning by tubers of *Gloriosa superba*. *Ceylon Med J.* 1971;233-234.
8. Ahasan HAMN, Chowdhury MAJ, Azhar MA, Rafiqueuddin AKM. Copper sulphate poisoning. *Trop Doct.* 1994;24:52-53.
9. Aleem HM. Gloriosa superba poisoning. *J Assoc Physicians India.* 1992;40:541-542.
10. Annapoorani KS, Damodaran C, Chandra Sekharan P. A promising antidote to Cleistanthus collinus poisoning. *J Forensic Sci Soc India.* 1986;2:3-6.
11. Annapoorani KS, Periakali P, Ilangovan S, et al. Spectrofluorometric determination of the toxic constituents of Cleistanthus collinus. *J Anal Toxicol.* 1984;8:182-186.
12. Anon. Calamity at Bhopal. *Lancet.* 1984;2:1378-1379.
13. Balasegaram M. Early management of corrosive burns of the oesophagus. *Br J Surg.* 1975;62:444-447.
14. Ball DE, Tagwireyi D, Nhachi CF. Chloroquine poisoning in Zimbabwe: a toxicoepidemiological study. *J Appl Toxicol.* 2002;22:311-315.
15. Bawaskar HS. Snake venoms and antivenoms: critical supply issues. *J Assoc Physicians India.* 2004;52:11-13.
16. Bermudez-de Rocha MV, Lozano-Melendez FE, Tamez-Rodriguez VA, Diaz-Cuello G, Pineyro-Lopez A. Frecuencia de intoxicacion con Karwinskia humboldtiana en Mexico. *Salud Publica Mex.* 1995;37:57-62.

17. Bertolote JM, Fleischmann A, Eddleston M, Gunnell D. Deaths from pesticide poisoning: a global response. *Brit J Psychiat.* 2006;189:201-203.
18. Bond GR, Pieche S, Sonicki Z, et al. A clinical decision aid for triage of children younger than 5 years and with organophosphate or carbamate insecticide exposure in developing countries. *Ann Emerg Med.* 2008;52:617-622.
19. Bondurand A, N'Dri KD, Coffi S, Saracino E. L'intoxication a la chloroquine au C.H.S.Abidjan. *Afr Med.* 1980;19:239-242.
20. Bose TK, Basu RK, Biswas B, et al. Cardiovascular effects of yellow oleander ingestion. *J Indian Med Assoc.* 1999;97:407-410.
21. Bourquia A, Jabrane AJ, Ramdani B, Zaid D. Toxicite systemique de la paraphenylene diamine. Quatre observations. *Presse Med.* 1988;17:1798-1800.
22. Bradberry SM, Proudfoot AT, Vale JA. Glyphosate poisoning. *Toxicol Rev.* 2004; 23:159-167.
23. Buckley NA, Karalliedde L, Dawson A, et al. Where is the evidence for the management of pesticide poisoning—is clinical toxicology fiddling while the developing world burns? *J Toxicol Clin Toxicol.* 2004;42: 113-116.
24. Carrada T, Lopez H, Vazquez Y, Ley A. Brote epidemico de poliradiculoneuritis por tullidora (Karwinskia humboldtiana). *Bol Med Hosp Infant Mex.* 1983;40:139-142.
25. Casida JE, Quistad GB. Golden age of insecticide reserch: past, present, or future? *Annu Rev Entomol.* 2005;43:1-16.
26. Chan TY. Poisoning due to Savlan (cetrimide) liquid. *Hum Exp Toxicol.* 1994;13:681-682.
27. Chan TY. Anticholinergic poisoning due to Chinese herbal medicines. *Vet Hum Toxicol.* 1995;37:156-157.
28. Chan TY, Critchley JA. Usage and adverse effects of Chinese herbal medicines. *Hum Exp Toxicol.* 1996;15:5-12.
29. Chan TY, Critchley JA, Lau JT. The risk of aspiration in Dettol poisoning: a retrospective cohort study. *Hum Exp Toxicol.* 1995;14:190-191.
30. Chan TY, Lee KK, Chan AY, Critchley JA. Poisoning due to Chinese proprietary medicines. *Hum Exp Toxicol.* 1995;14:434-436.
31. Chan TYK, Leung KP, Critchley JAJH. Poisoning due to common household products. *Singapore Med J.* 1995;36:285-287.
32. Chauvin P, Dillon JC, Moren A: An outbreak of Heliotrope food poisoning, Tadjikistan, November 1992-March 1993. *Sante.* 1994;4:263-268.
33. Chippaux JP. Snake-bites: appraisal of the global situation. *Bull World Health Organ.* 1998;76:515-524.
34. Chippaux JP. Snake bite epidemiology in Benin. *Bull Soc Pathol Exot.* 2002;95:172-174.
35. Chippaux JP, Goyffon M. Epidemiology of scorpionism: a global appraisal. *Acta Trop.* 2008;107:71-79.
36. Chung K, Yang CC, Wu ML, et al. Agricultural avermectins: an uncommon but potentially fatal cause of pesticide poisoning. *Ann Emerg Med.* 1999;34:51-57.
37. Chung SY, Luk SL, Mak FL. Attempted suicide in children and adolescents in Hong Kong. *Soc Psychiatry.* 1987;22:102-106.
38. de Silva HJ, Samarawickrema NA, Wickremasinghe AR. Toxicity due to organophosphorus compounds: what about chronic exposure? *Trans R Soc Trop Med Hyg.* 2006;100:803-806.
39. de Vries RR, Sitalsing AD, Schipperheyn JJ, Sedney MI. Klinische aspecten van azijnzuurintoxicatie. *Ned Tijdschr Geneeskd.* 1977;121:862-866.
40. Dewan A, Patel AB, Pal RR, et al. Mass ethion poisoning with high mortality. *Clin Toxicol.* 2008;46:85-88.
41. Durukan P, Ozdemir C, Coskun R, et al. Experiences with endosulfan mass poisoning in rural areas. *Eur J Emerg Med.* 2009;16:53-56.
42. Eddleston M. Patterns and problems of deliberate self-poisoning in the developing world. *Q J Med.* 2000;93:715-731.
43. Eddleston M, Ariaratnam CA, Meyer PW, et al. Epidemic of self-poisoning with seeds of the yellow oleander tree (*Thevetia peruviana*) in northern Sri Lanka. *Trop Med Int Health.* 1999;4:266-273.
44. Eddleston M, Haggalla S. Fatal injury in eastern Sri Lanka, with special reference to cardenolide self-poisoning with *Cerbera manghas* fruits. *Clin Toxicol.* 2008;46:745-748.
45. Eddleston M, Karalliedde L, Buckley N, et al. Pesticide poisoning in the developing world—a minimum pesticides list. *Lancet.* 2002;360: 1163-1167.
46. Eddleston M, Mohamed F, Davies JOJ, et al. Respiratory failure in acute organophosphorus pesticide self-poisoning. *Q J Med.* 2006;99: 513-522.
47. Eddleston M, Rajapakshe M, Roberts DM, et al. Severe propanil [N-(2,3-dichlorophenyl) propanamide] pesticide self-poisoning. *J Toxicol Clin Toxicol.* 2002;40:847-854.
48. Eddleston M, Sheriff MHR, Hawton K. Deliberate self-harm in Sri Lanka: an overlooked tragedy in the developing world. *BMJ.* 1998;317: 133-135.
49. El Ansary EH, Ahmed MEK, Clague HW. Systemic toxicity of paraphenylenediamine. *Lancet.* 1983;i:1341.
50. Ellis JB, Krug A, Robertson J, et al. Paraffin ingestion — the problem. *S Afr Med J.* 1994;84:727-730.
51. Escoffery CT, Shirley SE. Fatal poisoning in Jamaica: a coroner's autopsy study from the University Hospital of the West Indies. *Med Sci Law.* 2004;44:116-120.
52. Fernando R, Fernando D. Poisoning with plants and mushrooms in Sri Lanka: a retrospective hospital based study. *Vet Hum Toxicol.* 1990;32: 579-581.
53. Fitzgerald KT, Flood AA. Hymenoptera stings. *Clin Tech Small Anim Pract.* 2006;21:194-204.
54. Food and Agriculture Organization of the United Nations. International Code of Conduct on the Distribution and Use of Pesticides (Revised Version, adopted by the Hundred and Twenty-third Session of the FAO Council in November 2002), 0 edn. Rome: FAO; 2002.
55. Francis PD, Clarke CF. Angel trumpet lily poisoning in five adolescents: clinical findings and management. *J Paediatr Child Health.* 1999;35:93-95.
56. Gaillard Y, Krishnamoorthy A, Bevalot F. Cerbera odollam: a 'suicide tree' and cause of death in the state of Kerala, India. *J Ethnopharmacol.* 2004;95:123-126.
57. Gil HW, Kang MS, Yang JO, et al. Association between plasma paraquat level and outcome of paraquat poisoning in 375 paraquat poisoning patients. *Clin Toxicol (Phila).* 2008;46:515-518.
58. Gueron M, Ilia R. Is antivenom the most successful therapy in scorpion victims? *Toxicon.* 1999;37:1655-1657.
59. Gunnell D, Eddleston M, Phillips MR, Konradsen F. The global distribution of fatal pesticide self-poisoning: systematic review. *BMC Public Health.* 2007;7:357.
60. Gunnell D, Fernando R, Hewagama M. The impact of pesticide regulations on suicide in Sri Lanka. *Int J Epidemiol.* 2007;36:1235-1242.
61. Gunnell D, Ho DD, Murray V. Medical management of deliberate drug overdose—a neglected area for suicide prevention? *Emerg Med J.* 2004;21:35-38.
62. Gupta S, Ahlawat SK. Aluminium phosphide poisoning—a review. *J Toxicol Clin Toxicol.* 1995;33:19-24.
63. Gupta SK, Kaleekal T, Joshi S. Misuse of corticosteroids in some of the drugs dispensed as preparations from alternative systems of medicine in India. *Pharmacoepidemiol Drug Saf.* 2000;9:599-602.
64. Gutierrez JM, Theakston RDG, Warrell DA. Confronting the neglected problem of snake bit envenoming: the need for a global partnership. *PLoS Med.* 2006;3:727-731.
65. Hamouda C, Amamou M, Thabet H, et al. Plant poisonings from herbal medicines admitted to a Tunisian toxicological intensive care unit, 1983-1998. *Vet Hum Toxicol.* 2000;42:137-141.
66. Hashim M, Hamza YO, Yahia B, et al. Poisoning from henna dye and paraphenylenediamine mixtures in children in Khartoum. *Ann Trop Paediatr.* 1992;12:3-6.
67. Hon KL, Kwok LW, Leung TF. Snakebites in children in the densely populated city of Hong Kong: a 10-year survey. *Acta Paediatr.* 2004;93: 270-272.
68. Huang WF, Wen KC, Hsiao ML. Adulteration by synthetic therapeutic substances of traditional Chinese medicines in Taiwan. *J Clin Pharmacol.* 1997;37:344-350.
69. Hulin A, Presles P, Desbordes JM. Les intoxications volontaires dans l'ile de Cayenne en 1979, 1980 et 1981. *Med d'Afrique Noire.* 1983;30: 267-271.
70. Isbister GK, Graudins A, White J, Warrell D. Antivenom treatment in arachnidism. *J Toxicol Clin Toxicol.* 2003;41:291-300.
71. Ismail M. Treatment of the scorpion envenoming syndrome: 12-years experience with serotherapy. *Int J Antimicrob Agents.* 2003;21:170-174.
72. Jain A, Bhatnagar MK. Changing trends of poisoning at railway stations. *J Assoc Physicians India.* 2000;48:1036.
73. Jeyaratnam J. Acute pesticide poisoning: a major global health problem. *World Health Stat Q.* 1990;43:139-144.

74. Jeyaratnam J, Lun KC, Phoon WO. Survey of acute pesticide poisoning among agricultural workers in four Asian countries. *Bull World Health Organ*. 1987;65:521-527.
75. Joskow R, Belson M, Vesper H, et al. Ackee fruit poisoning: an outbreak investigation in Haiti 2000-2001, and review of the literature. *Clin Toxicol (Phila)*. 2006;44:267-273.
76. Joubert PH, Brown JM, Hay IT, Sebata PD. Acute poisoning with Jatropha curcas (purging nut tree) in children. *S Afr Med J*. 1984;65:729-730.
77. Joubert PH, Mathibe L. Acute poisoning in developing countries. *Adverse Drug React Acute Poisoning Rev*. 1989;8:165-178.
78. Kanchan T, Menezes RG. Suicidal poisoning in Southern India: gender differences. *J Forensic Leg Med*. 2008;15:7-14.
79. Karatas AD, Aygun D, Baydin A. Characteristics of endosulfan poisoning: a study of 23 cases. *Singapore Med J*. 2006;47:1030-1032.
80. Kasturiratne A, Wickremasinghe AR, De Silva N, et al. The global burden of snakebite: a literature analysis and modelling based on regional estimates of envenoming and deaths. *PLoS Med*. 2008;5:e218.
81. Kenmore PE. Integrated pest management. Introduction. *Int J Occup Environ Health*. 2002;8:173-174.
82. Khan NI, Sen N, al Haque N. Poisoning in a medical unit of Dhaka Medical College Hospital in 1983. *Bangladesh Med J*. 1985;14:9-12.
83. Konradsen F, Dawson AH, Eddleston M, Gunnell D. Pesticide self-poisoning: thinking outside the box. *Lancet*. 2007;369:169-170.
84. Konradsen F, van der Hoek W, Cole DC, Hutchinson G, et al. Reducing acute poisoning in developing countries — options for restricting the availability of pesticides. *Toxicology*. 2003;192:249-261.
85. Kularatne SAM. Common krait (Bungarus caeruleus) bite in Anuradhapura, Sri Lanka: a prospective clinical study, 1996-98. *Postgrad Med J*. 2002;78:276-280.
86. Lai KH, Huang BS, Huang MH, et al. Emergency surgical intervention for severe corrosive injuries of the upper digestive tract. *Chinese Med J*. 1995;56:40-46.
87. Lalloo DG, Theakston RD, Warrell DA. The African challenge. *Lancet*. 2002;359:1527.
88. Lee JB, Hwang JJ. Analysis of suicide in legal autopsy during the period of 1981-1984. *Seoul J Med*. 1985;26:325-330.
89. Lo YC, Yang CC, Deng JF. Acute alachlor and butachlor herbicide poisoning. *Clin Toxicol (Phila)*. 2008;46:1-6.
90. Majumder MM, Basher A, Faiz MA, et al. Criminal poisoning of commuters in Bangladesh: prospective and retrospective study. *Forensic Sci Int*. 2008;180:10-16.
91. Meda HA, Diallo B, Buchet JP, et al. Epidemic of fatal encephalopathy in preschool children in Burkino Faso and consumption of unripe ackee (Blighia sapida) fruit. *Lancet*. 1999;353:536-540.
92. Mendis S. Colchicine cardiotoxicity following ingestion of *Gloriosa superba* tubers. *Postgrad Med J*. 1989;65:752-755.
93. Mohamed F, Senarathna L, Azhar S, et al. Acute human self-poisoning with the N-phenylpyrazole insecticide fipronil—a GABA-gated chloride channel blocking pesticide. *J Toxicol Clin Toxicol*. 2004;42:955-963.
94. Moya J. Ackee (Blighia sapida) poisoning in the Northern Province, Haiti, 2001. *Epidemiol Bull*. 2001;22:8-9.
95. Murray DL, Taylor PL. Claim no easy victories: evaluating the pesticide industry's Global Safe Use campaign. *World Dev*. 2000,;28:1735-1749.
96. N'Dri KD, Palis R, Saracino E, et al. A propos de 286 intoxications a la chloroquine. *Afr Med*. 1976;15:103-105.
97. Nagaraj A. Watch out for a friendly stranger at railway station. *Indian Express*. 06 April 1999.
98. Nhachi CFB, Kasilo OMJ. The pattern of poisoning in urban Zimbabwe. *J Appl Toxicol*. 1992;12:435-438.
99. Nhachi CFB, Kasilo OMJ. Household chemical poisoning admissions in Zimbabwe's main urban centres. *Hum Exp Toxicol*. 1994;13:69-72.
100. Nossent JD, Vismans FJFE. Azijnzuurintoxicatie op Curacao. *Ned Tijdschr Geneeskd*. 1982;126:1180-1183.
101. Ong KL, Tan TH, Cheung WL. Potassium permanganate poisoning—a rare cause of fatal self poisoning. *J Accident Emerg Med*. 1997;14:43-45.
102. Prasad R, Singh R, Mishra OP, Pandey M. Dapsone induced methemoglobinemia: intermittent vs continuous intravenous methylene blue therapy. *Indian J Pediatr*. 2008;75:245-247.
103. Press Trust of India. Inter-state gang involved in train robbery busted. *Indian Express*. 01 August 1999.
104. Pugh RN, Theakston RD. Incidence and mortality on snake bite in savanna Nigeria. *Lancet*. 1980;2:1181-1183.
105. Queen HF, Tapfumaneyi C, Lewis RJ. The rising incidence of serious chloroquine overdose in Harare, Zimbabwe: emergency department surveillance in the developing world. *Trop Doct*. 1999;29:139-141.
106. Quek KC, Cheah JS. Poisoning due to ingestion of the seeds of kechubong (Datura fastuosa) for its ganja-like effect in Singapore. *J Trop Med Hyg*. 1974;77:111-112.
107. Rajan N, Rahim R, Kumar SK. Formic acid poisoning with suicidal intent: a report of 53 cases. *Postgrad Med J*. 1985;61:35-36.
108. Roberts DM, Karunarathna A, Buckley NA, et al. Influence of pesticide regulation on acute poisoning deaths in Sri Lanka. *Bull World Health Organ*. 2003;81:789-798.
109. Roberts DM, Seneviratne R, Mohamed F, et al. Deliberate self-poisoning with the chlorphenoxy herbicide 4-chloro-2-methylphenoxyacetic acid (MCPA). *Ann Emerg Med*. 2005;46:275-284.
110. Rwiza HT. Jimson weed food poisoning. An epidemic at Usangi rural government hospital. *Trop Geogr Med*. 1991;43:85-90.
111. Saravu K, Jose J, Bhat MH, et al. Acute ingestion of copper sulphate: a review of its clinical manifestations and management. *Ind J Crit Care Med*. 2007;11:74-80.
112. Sharma DC. Bhopal: 20 years on. *Lancet*. 2005;365:111-112.
113. Sharma SK, Chappuis F, Jha N, et al. Impact of snake bites and determinants of fatal outcomes in southeastern Nepal. *Am J Trop Med Hyg*. 2004;71:234-238.
114. Sigue G, Gamble L, Pelitere M, et al. From profound hypokalemia to life-threatening hyperkalemia: a case of barium sulfide poisoning. *Arch Intern Med*. 2000;160:548-551.
115. Singh D, Tyagi S. Changing trends in acute poisoning in Chandrigah zone. A 25-year autopsy experience from a tertiary care hospital in northern India. *Am J Forensic Med Pathol*. 1999;20:203-210.
116. Singh N, Kumar D, Sahu AP. Arsenic in the environment: effects on human health and possible prevention. *J Environ Biol*. 2007;28:359-365.
117. Singh S, Singhai S, Sood NK, et al. Changing pattern of childhood poisoning (1970-1989): experience of a large north Indian hospital. *Indian Pediatr*. 1995;32:331-336.
118. Snow RW, Bronzan R, Roques T, et al. The prevalence and morbidity of snake bite and treatment-seeking behaviour among a rural Kenyan population. *Ann Trop Med Parasitol*. 1994;88:665-671.
119. Sood AK, Yadav SP, Sood S, Malhotra RC. Hair dye poisoning. *J Assoc Physicians India*. 1996;44:69.
120. Srivastava A, Peshin SS, Kaleekal T, Gupta SK. An epidemiological study of poisoning cases reported to the National Poisons Information Centre, All India Institute of Medical Sciences, New Delhi. *Hum Exp Toxicol*. 2005;24:279-285.
121. Stewart MJ, Steenkamp V, Zuckerman M. The toxicology of African herbal remedies. *Ther Drug Monitor*. 1998;20:510-516.
122. Su JM, Hsu HK, Chang HC, Hsu WH. Management for acute corrosive injury of upper gastrointestinal tract. *Chinese Med J*. 1994;54:20-25.
123. Subrahmanyam DKS, Mooney T, Raveendran R, Zachariah B. A clinical and laboratory profile of Cleistanthus collinus poisoning. *J Assoc Physicians India*. 2003;51:1052-1054.
124. Tagwireyi D, Ball DE, Nhachi CF. Traditional medicine poisoning in Zimbabwe: clinical presentation and management in adults. *Hum Exp Toxicol*. 2002;21:579-586.
125. Tai DY, Yeo JK, Eng PC, Wang YT. Intentional overdosage with isoniazid: case report and review of the literature. *Singapore Med J*. 1996;37:222-225.
126. Taldukar MQK, Azad K, Kawser CA. Acute isoniazid poisoning: a case report and review of the literature. *Bangladesh Med J*. 1983;12:112-115.
127. Tandon BN, Tandon HD, Tandon RK, et al. An epidemic of veno-occlusive disease of liver in central India. *Lancet*. 1976;2:271-272.
128. Tandon HD, Tandon BN, Mattocks AR. An epidemic of veno-occlusive disease of the liver in Afghanistan. Pathologic features. *Am J Gastroenterol*. 1978;70:607-613.
129. Theakston RDG, Warrell DA. Crisis in snake antivenom supply for Africa. *Lancet*. 2000;356:2104.
130. Theakston RDG, Warrell DA, Griffiths E. Report of a WHO workshop on the standardization and control of antivenoms. *Toxicon*. 2003;41:541-557.
131. Tominack RL, Yang GY, Tsai WJ, et al. Taiwan National Poison Center Survey of glyphosate-surfactant herbicide ingestions. *Clin Toxicol*. 1991;29:91-109.

132. Tomizawa M, Casida JE. Selective toxicity of neonicotinoids attributable to specificity of insect and mammalian nicotinic receptors. *Annu Rev Entomol*. 2003;48:339-364.
133. Tracqui A, Gutbub AM, Kintz P, Mangin P. A case of dapsone poisoning: toxicological data and review of the literature. *J Anal Toxicol*. 1995;19:229-235.
134. Warrell DA. Venomous bites and stings in the tropical world. *Med J Aust*. 1993;159:773-779.
135. Watt G, Padre L, Tuazon ML, Hayes CG. Bites by the Philippine cobra (Naja naja philippinensis): an important cause of death among rice farmers. *Am J Trop Med Hyg*. 1987;37:636-639.
136. White J, Warrell D, Eddleston M, et al. Clinical toxinology—where are we now? *J Toxicol Clin Toxicol*. 2003;41:263-276.
137. Wilks MF, Fernando R, Ariyananda PL, et al. Improvement in survival after paraquat ingestion following introduction of a new formulation in Sri Lanka. *PLoS Med*. 2008;5:e49.
138. Wilson DAB, Wormald PJ. Battery acid—an agent of attempted suicide in black South Africans. *S Afr Med J*. 1994;84:529-531.
139. Wu MH, Lai WW. Surgical management of extensive corrosive injuries of the alimentary tract. *Surg Gynecol Obstet*. 1993;177:12-16.
140. Young RJ, Critchley JA, Young KK, et al. Fatal acute hepatorenal failure following potassium permanganate ingestion. *Hum Exp Toxicol*. 1996;15:259-261.

CHAPTER 137
PRINCIPLES OF EPIDEMIOLOGY AND RESEARCH DESIGN

Kevin C. Osterhoudt

Advances in medical toxicology are achieved through the scientific method using observations, derived from cases of poisoning and nonpoisoning due to xenobiotic exposures, to generate hypotheses. Subsequent research questions are analyzed with epidemiological investigation, and preliminary studies are examined with methodological scrutiny. Initial analytical techniques are improved, and confirmatory studies are performed. Ultimately, models relating cause to effect are formulated.

To optimize patient care, it is useful to grade the quality of available scientific evidence used to justify treatment recommendations. Decisions about how strongly to recommend a medical action will be based upon the careful consideration of the risks of leaving a patient untreated, the potential benefits and harms of treatment, the quality of the guiding evidence, a balanced view of resource utilization, and the values of the person to be treated. The Grading of Recommendations Assessment, Development, and Evaluation (GRADE) Working Group has provided a framework for assessing and communicating levels of scientific evidence (Table 137–1).[15] An understanding of basic principles of research design and epidemiology is required to interpret published studies and to lay the groundwork for future investigation in toxicology.

EPIDEMIOLOGIC TECHNIQUES AVAILABLE TO INVESTIGATE CLINICAL PROBLEMS

Table 137–2 lists different study formats.

OBSERVATIONAL DESIGN: DESCRIPTIVE

A staggering array of xenobiotics are able to injure people, necessitating reliance of toxicologists on good descriptive data regarding toxic outcomes. Through 2007, the National Poison Data System (NPDS) of the American Association of Poison Control Centers (AAPCC) has amassed a database of more than 45 million human exposures.[5] Descriptive case reporting serves a valuable purpose in describing the characteristics of a medical condition or procedure and remains a fundamental tool of epidemiological investigation. A *case report* is a clinical description of a single patient or procedure with respect to a situation. Case reports are most useful for hypothesis generation. However, single case reports are not always generalizable, as the reported situation may be atypical. A number of case reports can be grouped, on the basis of similarities, into a *case series*. Case series can be used to characterize an illness or syndrome, but without a control group they are severely limited in proving cause and effect. In 1966, a case series of two patients with "acute liver necrosis following overdose of paracetamol"[12] was accompanied by a case report of "liver damage and impaired glucose tolerance after paracetamol overdosage"[36] which led to further study and the eventual creation of the Rumack-Matthew nomogram (Chap. 34). Similarly, a 1979 case report of "hypertension and cerebral hemorrhage after trimolets ingestion"[22] led to subsequent animal studies, experimental human studies, and epidemiological studies culminating in the decision by the US Food and Drug administration to remove phenylpropanolamine from nonprescription cold remedies and appetite suppressants. The important role for descriptive data in guiding clinical research, focusing educational efforts, and formulating public policy are often underappreciated.

Cross-sectional studies assess a population for the presence or absence of an exposure and condition simultaneously. Such data often provide estimates of prevalence—the fraction of individuals in a population sharing a characteristic or condition at a point in time. These studies are particularly helpful in public health planning and have been extremely useful in monitoring common environmental exposures, such as childhood lead poisoning, or population-wide drug use, such as occurs with tobacco, marijuana, and alcohol. The US National Health and Nutrition Examination Survey investigations demonstrated that the percentage of children with blood lead concentration greater than 10 μg/dL decreased from 88.2% to 4.4% between 1976 and 1991, with the highest rates of plumbism among African American, low-income, or urban children.[4]

An *analysis of secular trends* is a study type that compares changes in illness over time or geography to changes in risk factors. These analyses often lend circumstantial support to a hypothesis; however, because of the ecological nature of their design, individual data on risk factors are not available to allow exclusion of alternative hypotheses also consistent with the data. A prime example of an analysis of secular trends is the finding that reports of Reye Syndrome declined between 1980 and 1985, coincident with a fall in sales of, or physician recommendations of, children's aspirin products.[3] This investigation suggested an etiologic role of aspirin in the development of Reye Syndrome but could not exclude alternative hypotheses such as a change in viral epidemic patterns.

OBSERVATIONAL DESIGN: ANALYTICAL

Hypotheses generated by theoretical reasoning or anecdotal association require analytical testing. Case-control studies and cohort studies are analytical techniques that use observational data, and each technique has its own advantages and disadvantages (Table 137–3). *Case-control studies* compare affected, treated, or diseased patients (cases) to nonaffected patients (controls) and look for a difference in prior risk factors or exposures (Fig. 137–1A). Because subjects are recruited into the study based on prior presence or absence of a particular outcome, case-control studies are always retrospective in nature. They are especially useful when the outcome being studied is rare, and they enable the investigation of any number of potential etiologies for a single disease.

The hypothesis, derived from multiple case reports and case series, that phenylpropanolamine might increase risk for hemorrhagic stroke was well suited to case-control study. Exposure to ingested phenylpropanolamine, as an ingredient in cold remedies and appetite suppressants, was common; but hemorrhagic stroke is rare among children and young adults. Other putative risk factors such as tobacco use, hypertension history, family history, cocaine use, and contraceptive use were identifiable and could be studied simultaneously. In a case-control analysis of 702 subjects with hemorrhagic stroke and 1376 controls, the use of appetite-suppressant doses of phenylpropanolamine were found to be independently associated with the occurrence of hemorrhagic stroke.[21]

Cohort studies compare patients with certain risk factors or exposures to those patients without the exposure, then follow these cohorts to see which subjects develop the outcome of interest (see Fig. 137–1B).

TABLE 137–1. GRADE System for Evaluating Clinical Recommendations[15]

Strength of Recommendation	Quality of Evidence
Strong	High
Weak	Moderate
	Low or very low

TABLE 137–3. Advantages of Case-Control versus Cohort Study Designs

Case-control Study	Cohort Study
Smaller sample required when outcome is rare	Provides more robust evidence of association
Reduced bias in outcome data	Reduced bias in exposure data
Can study many exposures simultaneously	Can study many outcomes simultaneously
Allows estimation of relative risk	Allows direct calculation of incidence
May obviate need for long followup period	Allows direct calculation of relative risk

In this respect, they allow the comparison of *incidence* (the number of new outcomes occurring within a population initially free of disease over a period of time) between populations who share an exposure and populations who do not. They may be retrospective or prospective and enable the study of any number of outcomes from a single exposure. They are particularly well suited to investigations in which the outcome of interest is relatively common. In circumstances when an outcome of interest is very uncommon, such as the case with stroke after phenylpropanolamine use, the large number of study subjects required might make a cohort study impractical. A cohort of 981 acetaminophen overdose subjects was used retrospectively to investigate whether administration of activated charcoal might be beneficial therapy for acetaminophen poisoning.[8] Subjects were separated on the basis of whether or not they were treated with activated charcoal and were subsequently followed to see if they developed concentrations deemed toxic by the Rumack-Matthew nomogram. Perhaps the most famous and ambitious cohort study is the Framingham Heart Study in which 5209 residents of Framingham, MA, ages 30–62 years, were followed for over 50 years. This study provided a useful tool for studying the incidence of lung cancer, stroke, and cardiovascular disease in those exposed to cigarette smoke[13] and other hazardous xenobiotics.

EXPERIMENTAL DESIGN

Experimental studies are those in which the treatment, risk factor, or exposure of interest can be controlled by the investigator to study differences in outcome between the groups (Fig. 137–2). The prototype is the randomized, blinded, controlled clinical trial. Among epidemiologic study types, these provide the most convincing demonstration of causality. Clinical trials are used to measure the *efficacy* (the treatment effect within a controlled experimental setting) of treatment regimens and to draw inferences about the *effectiveness* of a treatment applied to the general population. Unfortunately, interventional studies are the most complex to perform, and several questions must be addressed by investigators before performing a clinical trial (Table 137–4). Human clinical trials have been especially difficult to apply to the practice of toxicology. Table 137–5 lists characteristics of poisoned patients, which hamper attempts at clinical trials. Volunteer studies, using nontoxic xenobiotics or nontoxic doses, are often used to circumvent many of the problems in controlling human poisoning studies; but it is typically difficult to apply results from these studies to the actual physiology of toxic overdose. In an experimental study, activated charcoal was found to result in a 57% reduction in absorption of ampicillin in a nontoxic

TABLE 137–2. Types of Epidemiologic Study Designs[a]

Experimental
Clinical trial
Observational: Analytical
Cohort
Case-control
Observational: Descriptive
Analysis of secular trends
Cross-sectional
Case series
Case report

[a] Study designs are listed in descending order from the design that offers the best epidemiologic evidence for association to that which offers the least.

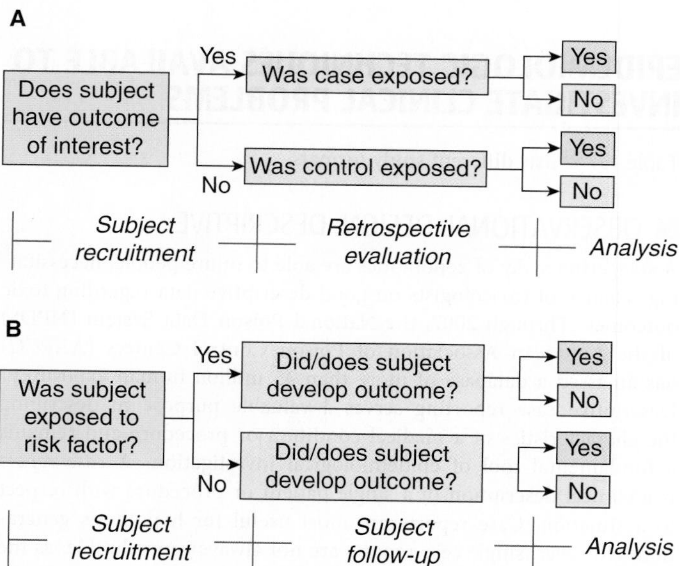

FIGURE 137–1. **A.** Schematic representation of the case-control study design. Subjects with an outcome or condition of interest are selected, along with control subjects, and then are evaluated for previous exposure to a risk factor of interest. **B.** Schematic representation of the cohort study design. Subjects are recruited based on the presence or absence of a risk factor or exposure, then followed to see if they develop an outcome.

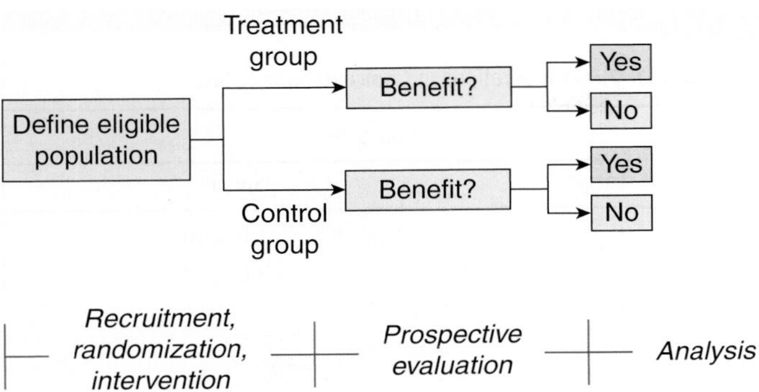

FIGURE 137–2. Schematic representation of the design of a randomized clinical trial.

TABLE 137–5. Difficulties in Utilizing Clinical Trials to Study Human Poisoning

It is unethical to intentionally "poison" subjects.
Poisoned patients represent a broad spectrum of demographic patterns.
A wide variety of xenobiotics exist.
Exposures to any single xenobiotic are usually limited.
A limited number of poisoned patients are available at any one study site.
Uncertainty often exists as to type, quantity, and timing of most xenobiotic exposures.
Poisoning typically results in a relatively short course of illness.

model using human volunteers.[35] Taken out of this artificial setting, a trial of single-dose oral activated charcoal was unable to prove benefit to outcome among 1479 heterogenous subjects presenting to an emergency department (ED) for possible poisoning.[26] Neither study was able to answer whether activated charcoal reduces morbidity from ingestion of dangerous xenobiotics if given while the xenobiotic is still in the stomach and amenable to adsorption.

As toxicologists strive to find evidence for, or against, the traditions of clinical practice, several important clinical trials have been published. Among them are many important examples and lessons in epidemiologic study design. One trial attempted to evaluate whether or not corticosteroids might be beneficial in preventing esophageal strictures secondary to circumferential caustic injury of the esophagus.[2] Because of the inherent difficulty in recruiting eligible patients from a single institution, only a small sample of 60 patients with esophageal injury were recruited over an 18-year period. Another study randomized hyperbaric oxygen therapy versus sham (placebo) therapy, among 152 victims of carbon monoxide poisoning, to investigate its effect on the development of neurocognitive injury.[38] Certain concerns with the methodology and analyses of clinical studies are examined later in this chapter to illustrate epidemiologic concepts, and must be carefully considered when trying to apply the results of any clinical trial into the patient care setting.

TABLE 137–4. Considerations in Designing a Clinical Trial

What is the question of interest?
What is the target patient population?
How will the safety of subjects be assured?
What is a suitable control group?
How will outcomes be measured?
What difference in outcomes between groups is considered important?
What is the analysis plan?
How many subjects will be required?
How will randomization and blinding be achieved and maintained?
How long a followup period will be required?
How will loss of study subjects be addressed?
How will treatment compliance be evaluated?

MEASURES USED TO QUANTIFY THE STRENGTH OF AN EPIDEMIOLOGIC ASSOCIATION

The objective of analytical studies is to define and quantify the degree of statistical dependence between an exposure and an outcome. Such associations are ideally represented by the relative risk of developing an outcome if exposed in comparison to being unexposed. Thus, the *relative risk* can be defined as the incidence of outcome in exposed individuals compared to the incidence of outcome in unexposed individuals. The relative risk can be calculated directly from cohort or interventional studies. However, in a case-control study, an investigator chooses the numbers of cases and controls to be studied, so true incidence data are not obtained. In case-control studies an *odds ratio* can be calculated, and the odds ratio will provide an estimate for relative risk in situations in which the outcome is rare, such as when the outcome occurs in fewer than 10% of exposed individuals. Figure 137–3 demonstrates the calculation of relative risk or odds ratio from analytic studies.

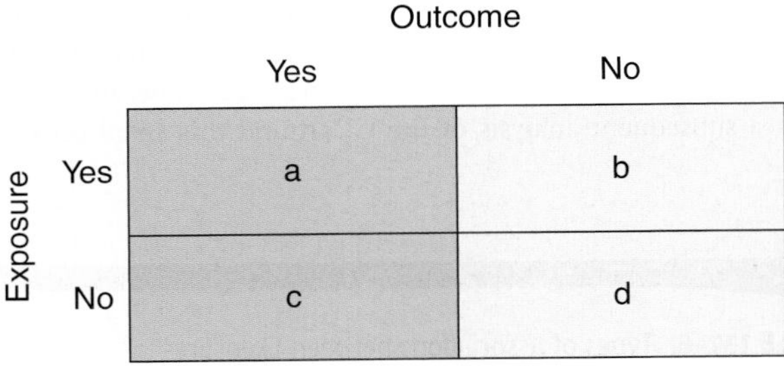

Cohort study

$$\text{Relative risk} = \frac{a}{a+b} \Big/ \frac{c}{c+d}$$

Case control study

$$\text{Odds ratio} = ad/bc$$

FIGURE 137–3. Use of a 2 × 2 table to calculate or estimate relative risk from analytic studies. In cohort studies, study subjects are selected on the basis of exposure. In case-control studies, subjects are selected on the basis of outcome. The letters a, b, c, and d represent the number of subjects either exposed or unexposed to a "risk factor" or treatment, with or without the outcome of interest. The odds ratio estimates the relative risk if the outcome of interest is rare.

A relative risk of 1.0 signifies that an outcome is equally likely to occur whether an individual either is exposed or is not exposed and implies that no association exists between the exposure and the outcome. A relative risk approaching 0 suggests that an exposure is a marker of protection regarding the outcome, and a relative risk approaching infinity suggests the exposure predicts a tendency toward the outcome. Among men and women using phenylpropanolamine appetite suppressants the odds ratio for development of hemorrhagic stroke was 15.9 which suggests a strong association.[21]

MEASURES USED TO QUANTIFY THE SIGNIFICANCE OF AN EPIDEMIOLOGIC ASSOCIATION

Analytical studies are performed to test hypotheses, typically that an exposure is associated with an outcome. The presence of such association in any given study has a number of possible explanations, as detailed in Table 137–6. The goal of statistical analysis is to determine the degree to which chance can be excluded as the true reason the results of the study were obtained. By convention, statistical analysis typically tests the *null hypothesis*—the hypothesis that there is no association between exposure and outcome.

Because analytic studies involve only a sample of the total population, they contain two types of inherent error. *Type I error*, also referred to as alpha (α) error, is the likelihood that an investigator may conclude that an association exists when none truly does. *Type II error*, or beta (β) error, is the possibility that an investigator will be unable to find an association when one is really present. The most commonly reported measures of type I error in published toxicology studies are the *p-value* and the *confidence interval* (CI). Statistical significance has customarily, but not necessarily, been defined as having less than a 1 in 20 chance of conducting a false-positive study. Therefore, a type I error of less than 5%, which corresponds to a *p*-value of less than 0.05, is usually deemed "statistically significant."

Perhaps a more informative description of the significance of an association is provided through the CI. The CI not only provides a test of statistical significance, it also offers information pertaining to the degree (and possible range) of differences observed. In an unbiased study, the 95% CI provides a range between which, if the study could be repeated an infinite number of times, the observed magnitude of effect would lie 95% of the time. One study reported that no toddlers ingesting one or two calcium channel blocker tablets became seriously ill, but a subsequent analysis of the CI around this small set of data demonstrated that the true incidence could be as high as 18%.[29] A CI around a relative risk or odds ratio is not statistically significant if it includes 1.0, and the narrower the CI the more precise the estimate of the magnitude of effect.

The likelihood that a study will find a difference if one truly exists is termed statistical *power* and relates to the likelihood of a false-negative study (type II error). Power is usually artificially set by an investigator before a study is performed and is typically set at 80% or 90% to practically limit the number of study subjects needed. Table 137–7 lists considerations applicable to choice of sample size. The sample size of a study is determined by the frequency of the exposure and outcome within the study population, the strength of association deemed clinically relevant, and the amount of error deemed acceptable in the study. Because power is often set relatively low, it is difficult to state that an association does not exist. It is more appropriate to state that a study was unable to reject the null hypothesis to find an association.

The finding of a low *p*-value indicates a statistically high level of confidence that a difference between study groups exists but offers no indication that the difference is clinically important. The interpretation of statistical versus clinical significance is often facilitated through calculation of confidence intervals. Small actual differences between two groups can become statistically significant if large numbers of subjects are studied. Likewise, impressive associations of cause and effect can seem trivial if few subjects are in a study. The clinical significance of an association is left to the judgment of the individual interpreting a study. Ideally, a working definition of clinical significance is developed before a study is performed.

TABLE 137–6. Types of Associations between Exposures and Outcomes That May Be Found with a Clinical Study

No Association	The outcome is independent of exposure.
Artifactual Association	
Chance	The association demonstrated by the study resulted from random error.
Bias	Systematic error in the study led to the noted association.
Indirect Association	The association is real, but not truly cause and effect (confounding).
Causal Association	The outcome is dependent on the exposure.

TABLE 137–7. Considerations in Choice of Sample Size

	Sample Size	
	Large	Small
Pros	• Able to detect associations of small magnitude • Less susceptible to some biases • More robust analysis	• Less work • Less cost
Cons	• More work and more cost	• Might not detect associations of small magnitude • More susceptible to biases associated with patient differences

METHODOLOGICAL PROBLEMS FOUND WITHIN CLINICAL STUDIES

Calculation of a *p*-value or confidence interval does nothing to assess the adequacy of study design. These measures are used to quantify the influence of random error, or chance, on research findings. Clinical research involving patients is particularly susceptible to *bias*, which can be defined as systematic error in the collection or interpretation of data. Because such error can lead to an inappropriate estimate of the association between an exposure and an outcome, careful evaluation of potential biases affecting a clinical study is of paramount importance.

Selection bias refers to error introduced into a study by the manner in which subjects are selected for inclusion in the study. This type of bias is most problematic for retrospective studies in which exposures and outcomes have both occurred at the time of subject recruitment. Selection bias may be introduced into a prospective clinical study if the study fails to enroll potential subjects, or if potential subjects refuse to participate, on a systematic basis. Selection bias may even influence the results of clinical trials. In a 1995 trial that found no difference in outcome between acutely poisoned patients treated with gastric emptying and patients from whom gastric emptying was withheld, all patients presenting to the ED after acute overdose were enrolled.[32] Because most patients with poisoning exposure are likely to do well with minimal support,[5] selection of patients on this basis might be expected to bias this study to find no effect. Reasoning suggests that the patients most likely to benefit from gastric emptying are those with life-threatening toxic ingestion presenting within the first hour after overdose. Indeed, subgroup review of the results of this paper suggests clinical benefit within this group of patients, but without conclusive power.

Information bias refers to error introduced into a study as a result of systematic differences in the quality of data obtained between exposed and unexposed groups, or between those with and without the outcome of interest. Several distinct types of information bias may exist. Affected and nonaffected individuals may have differential memories regarding exposures, so recall bias is a concern in retrospective studies. The potential for *recall bias* may be cited as criticism of retrospective case-control studies of the association between phenylpropanolamine and hemorrhagic stroke, in which families were asked to recollect phenylpropanolamine use history. Stroke victims and their families might be more vigorous in their recall of exposures than control subjects. Similarly, *interviewer bias* may occur if study personnel differ in how they solicit, record, or interpret information as a result of knowledge of the subjects' status regarding exposures or outcomes.

Prospective studies may be troubled by loss to followup, especially if subjects are lost from the study for reasons relating to either exposure or outcome such as when subjects withdraw from a study because they are feeling better, or are "lost" because they die. *Misclassification bias* occurs when investigators incorrectly categorize subjects with respect to exposure or outcome. In a retrospective study of 378 children regarding the predictability of caustic esophageal injury from clinical signs and symptoms, it was found that 11 of 80 asymptomatic children had significant burns.[14] There is a possibility that these "asymptomatic" children were misclassified because of lack of rigorous written documentation of symptoms or signs within the medical charts.

Bias is best minimized through careful study design. It is important to precisely define the study question and the population at risk and to carefully define rigorous inclusion and exclusion criteria. The outcome should also be defined precisely. During data acquisition the best way to reduce bias may be to keep study personnel gathering exposure data blinded to outcome, and vice versa. Often, it may also be advisable to keep study subjects unaware of their status within a study to the extent that it is ethical (thus, "double-blinded"—neither investigators nor subjects are aware of the subjects' status within a study). Use of *placebos* or "sham treatments" is a way to facilitate blinding. One of the strongest criticisms of a 1995 trial of HBO for the prevention of delayed neurologic syndromes after CO poisoning[33] has been the failure to blind patients and investigators to the treatment in question,[28] a flaw that was corrected in a followup study published in 2002.[38] It is inevitable that some degree of potential bias will be present in any clinical study. Such bias should be reviewed in analysis, and estimations of its magnitude and direction (bias toward or away from rejection of the null hypothesis) should be considered.

Unlike selection and information biases, which are errors introduced into studies primarily by the investigators or subjects, *confounding* is a special type of problem that may occur within a study as a result of interrelationships between the exposure of interest and another exposure. Confounding is a bias wherein an observed association is not a product of cause and effect but instead results from linking of the exposure of interest to another associated exposure. Studies pertaining to adverse effects of drugs of abuse are especially prone to confounding by variables such as concomitant caffeine use, alcohol use, tobacco use, nutritional deficiency, and/or psychiatric illness. Analytic studies may restrict characteristics of enrolled subjects or match subject characteristics between comparison groups in an effort to reduce confounding. Accordingly, it has been suggested that future studies on delayed neuropsychiatric manifestations following CO poisoning control for potential confounding from depression and cyanide exposure.[24] Randomization is an important method to assure that unsuspected confounding factors are equally distributed between treatment groups within interventional studies. During data analysis, confounding can often be controlled through stratification of data into subgroups or through multivariate analysis techniques.

In order to improve the reporting of clinical trials, and to improve the recognition and interpretation of biases within them, guidelines referred to as the Consensus Standards of Reporting Trials (CONSORT) have been adopted by many medical journals.[27] The CONSORT guidelines provide a checklist to allow authors to systematically and uniformly report data and limitations. When interpreting published studies, it is also important to consider the potential for *publication bias*. Publication bias refers to the tendency for researchers, editors, and pharmaceutical companies to handle the reporting of studies with positive results differently from those with negative or inconclusive results.[34] Many journals now require that researchers register all planned clinical trials into a registry as a prerequisite for subsequent publication.

BIASES INHERENT IN STUDIES USING THE AMERICAN ASSOCIATION OF POISON CONTROL CENTERS DATABASE

The NPDS database of the AAPCC is an ambitious effort to catalog and describe the epidemiology of poisoning in the United States and Canada. These data serve to help identify new poisoning epidemics, focus prevention and education efforts, guide demographic and economic poisoning analyses, and guide implementation of public health policies. It is a desirable goal to use this database in defining the scope of toxicity for particular xenobiotics and as a clinical research tool. In this regard, it is important to understand the biases inherent in the current database.

It has been suggested that *selection bias* might exist within poison center (PC) data if poisoning is unrecognized as a cause of illness or if a caregiver has no questions pertaining to the management of a recognized poisoning.[16] Indeed, a survey of 170 emergency physicians in Utah found that 53% admitted to using a PC for symptomatic acute overdoses, and only 10% contacted PC for the purposes of reporting cases to the national database.[10] Such selection might result in a bias of PC data toward more severe cases. On the other end of the spectrum, investigation has found selection bias in PC data suggesting that fatal poisonings may be severely underrepresented.[18] It is interesting to note that in a 2004 report of the Institute of Medicine,[20] the estimated range of annual fatal poisonings in the United States was from approximately 1000, derived from AAPCC data, to over 30,000, derived from other databases. A study of potential spectrum bias in PC utilization found that one ED reported 95% of cyclic antidepressant overdoses, 33% of venomous snakebites, and only 3% of inhalation exposures.[17] Further complicating the interpretation of PC data are the findings that such data may also be biased regarding geographic distribution of callers,[1] age,[31] ethnicity,[1,11,31,37] and socioeconomic status.[37]

Knowledge of *information bias* within NPDS data is less well characterized. Phone interviews of callers, many under duress, are certain to be subject to *recall* and *interviewer bias*. A comparison of rural hospital chart data to the NPDS database demonstrated deficiencies in PC reporting and in clinical information transfer to the NPDS database.[19] Loss to followup remains a problem for many PCs, and misclassification of poisonings by healthcare providers inadequately trained in medical toxicology remains too common. The clinical conundrum of the unwitnessed ingestion frequently becomes an issue in poison center–derived studies designed to create triage policies. Some children having never ingested a xenobiotic of concern may be misclassified as an exposure and may be improperly analyzed.[23]

Despite the large volume of descriptive poisoning data available, it has proven difficult to derive valid, clinically useful conclusions from either the NPDS database or from published case reports.[6] One suggested means through which to minimize information bias in descriptive toxicology is through the use of improved data collection charts.[7] Other researchers have found it useful in clinical studies to transform PC data collection from a passive to an active process through use of specific research instruments.[25] Further efforts are required to reduce and to quantify the impact of selection, interviewer, recall, misclassification, and information biases within PC data to optimize the value of this important resource.

EVIDENTIARY CRITERIA USED TO LINK CAUSE AND EFFECT

As was illustrated in Table 137-6, association of an exposure to an illness does not necessarily equate to cause and effect. In assessing causation it must be determined if bias is present in the selection or measurement of exposure or outcome. If a study is unbiased, the role of chance in the occurrence of the observed association must be explored. If an association is unbiased, unlikely to result from random error, and is not subject to confounding, then assumptions regarding to causation can be derived. Table 137–8 provides a list of evidentiary criteria that are often used to support causation.

TABLE 137–8. Questions to Consider When Determining Causation

Study design	Was the association demonstrated in a well-designed study?
Temporality	Does the cause precede the effect?
Strength	What degree of relative risk was demonstrated in the analysis?
Dose response	Does an increased presence of risk factor correlate to greater or more frequent effect?
Consistency	Does the cause and effect hold true in different studies, locations, and populations?
Plausibility	Is the association in accordance with current scientific knowledge?
Specificity	Does the effect occur without the cause in question, or vice versa?

Many toxicologists deem clinical trials indicating a lack of benefit from gastric emptying, or indicating a therapeutic benefit of HBO therapy for CO intoxication, unconvincing because of the degree of bias present in all relevant published clinical trials. In medical toxicology it is virtually impossible to prove causal relationships beyond any doubt. The goal is to build empiric evidence so that associations can be confirmed or refuted with conviction.

EVALUATION OF DIAGNOSTIC TESTS AND CRITERIA

In clinical practice it is often useful to have a test, which may be a laboratory result or clinical paradigm, to help arrive at a diagnosis or predict an outcome. For instance, historical questionnaires, capillary blood lead concentrations, and venous blood lead concentrations might all be used to identify children at risk of neurocognitive injury from plumbism.[9] However, each of these approaches is likely to have certain disadvantages in terms of effort, cost, discomfort, and/or accuracy. Targeting lead evaluation and therapy at children on the basis of exposure history is expected to be easy and inexpensive, but may not identify some children with significant poisoning; thus, the test may be susceptible to being falsely negative. Capillary blood testing is more costly and uncomfortable and may be susceptible to false-positive test results because of environmental lead dust present on fingertips. The possibility of false-positive or false-negative results must be considered with any diagnostic test (Fig. 137–4).

The utility of diagnostic testing is often described in terms of sensitivity, specificity, predictive value of a positive test (PPV), and predictive value of a negative test (NPV). A cross-sectional design is often

Test result	Presence of disease +	Presence of disease −
+	True positive (a)	False positive (b)
−	False negative (c)	True negative (d)

$$\text{Sensitivity} = \frac{a}{a+c} = \frac{\text{True positives}}{\text{True positives + False negatives}}$$

$$\text{Specificity} = \frac{d}{b+d} = \frac{\text{True negatives}}{\text{False positives + True negatives}}$$

$$\text{PPV} = \frac{a}{a+b} = \frac{\text{True positives}}{\text{True positives + False positives}}$$

$$\text{NPV} = \frac{d}{c+d} = \frac{\text{True negatives}}{\text{False negatives + True negatives}}$$

PPV = Positive predictive value
NPV = Negative predictive value

FIGURE 137–4. Possible results of diagnostic testing and the statistical characteristics used to describe the utility of diagnostic tests. The letters a, b, c, and d represent the numbers of tested individuals with or without the disease of interest.

TABLE 137–9. Questions to Consider When Evaluating a Study

Research objectives
What is the study question?
What is the studied population?
Study design
What type of study was performed?
How were subjects recruited and enrolled? Why were subjects excluded?
What was the nature of the comparison group?
Data accrual
How were the data collected?
Are the exposures and outcomes clearly defined?
Are the observations reliable and reproducible?
Was randomization and/or blinding used?
Were subjects lost to followup?
Analysis
Are the results statistically significant?
Are the results clinically significant?
Are potential confounding variables controlled?
Was the study powered to detect important differences?
Conclusions
Are the conclusions justified by data?

used to study diagnostic tests, as we seek to determine the prevalence of positive tests among the diseased (*sensitivity*), and the prevalence of negative tests among the healthy (*specificity*). A perfect test would be highly sensitive and specific, but this is seldom possible in medical toxicology. A highly sensitive test is often used in screening programs because they rarely lead to false-negative diagnoses. Specific tests are typically used to "rule-in" a diagnosis, as they rarely yield false-positive results. Whereas sensitivity and specificity are inherent properties of a diagnostic test applied to a given population; the probability of disease, based on the results of a test, is highly dependent on the prevalence of disease within the population being tested. *The PPV is the probability of having disease in a patient with a positive test; the NPV is the probability of not having disease when the test result is negative.* A number of studies have tried to examine the utility of vomiting, leukocytosis, hyperglycemia, total iron-binding capacity, and radiographic findings in predicting toxicity after acute iron overdose. In a retrospective assessment of 40 adults with oral iron overdose, vomiting was found to predict a serum iron concentration above 300 μg/dL with a sensitivity of 84%, specificity of 50%, NPV of 44%, and PPV of 87%.[30] This suggested that the presence of vomiting should raise concern for iron toxicity but that the lack of vomiting was not particularly reassuring. Figure 137–4 illustrates the calculation of the sensitivity, specificity, PPV, and NPV. It is important to remember that these calculations, too, are subject to bias and are best presented with confidence intervals.

SUMMARY

Medical toxicology has embraced the vision of incorporating "evidence-based, or literature-based, medicine" into practice. Randomized clinical trials, although a noble goal, are rare and have proven difficult to perform within the discipline. As toxicologists move beyond descriptive data reporting, there remains great potential for scientific advancement in the field of toxicology via observational, hypothesis-testing, clinical research. Clinical investigators are charged with the imperative to perform studies based on sound epidemiologic principles. All studies, by nature of population sampling, are at the mercy of chance, but such random error can be quantified using statistical techniques. Systematic error (bias) can be limited, but not entirely excluded, through careful study design. Clinicians interpreting published toxicologic research need to thoroughly evaluate a study's research objectives, design, data acquisition, analysis, and conclusions before applying the results to patient care (Table 137–9). Future epidemiological investigation should allow more valid conclusions to be drawn regarding the associations between exposures and outcomes, or regarding the value of treatments for poisonings, discussed in the preceding chapters of this text.

Galen, an influential physician from the second century, remarked of his clinical trial, "All who drink of this remedy recover in a short time, except those whom it does not help, who all die. Therefore, it is obvious that it fails only in incurable cases." Unfortunately, error in contemporary clinical investigation of poisoning tends to be more insidious than the error in logic in Galen's conclusion, and skillful scrutiny of published research remains an important endeavor.

REFERENCES

1. Albertson TE, Tharratt RS, Alsop J, et al. Regional variations in the use and awareness of the California Poison Control System. *J Toxicol Clin Toxicol.* 2004;42:625-633.
2. Anderson KD, Rouse TM, Randolph JG. A controlled trial of corticosteroids in children with corrosive injury of the esophagus. *N Engl J Med.* 1992;323:637-640.
3. Arrowsmith JB, Kennedy DL, Kuritsky JN, et al. National pattern of aspirin use and Reye's syndrome reporting, United States 1980 to 1985. *Pediatrics.* 1987;79:858-863.
4. Brody DJ, Pirkle JL, Kramer RA, et al. Blood lead levels in the population US, Phase 1 of the third Health and Nutrition Examination Survey (NHANES III 1988–1991). *JAMA.* 1994;272:277-283.
5. Bronstein AC, Spyker DA, Cantilena LR, et al. 2007 annual report of the American Association of Poison Control Centers Toxic Exposure Surveillance System. *Clin Toxicol.* 2008;46:927-1057.
6. Buckley NA, Smith AJ. Evidence based medicine in toxicology: where is the evidence? *Lancet.* 1996;347:1167-1169.
7. Buckley NA, Whyte IM, Dawson AH, et al. Preformatted admission charts for poisoning admissions facilitate clinical assessment and research. *Ann Emerg Med.* 1999;34:476-482.
8. Buckley NA, Whyte IM, O'Connell DL, Dawson AH. Activated charcoal reduces the need for n-acetylcysteine treatment after acetaminophen overdose. *Clin Toxicol.* 1999;37:753-757.
9. Campbell C, Osterhoudt KC. Prevention of childhood lead poisoning. *Curr Opin Pediatr.* 2000;12:428-437.
10. Caravati EM, McElwee NE. Use of clinical toxicology resources by emergency physicians and its impact on poison control centers. *Ann Emerg Med.* 1991;20:147-150.
11. Clark RF, Phillips M, Manoguerra AS, et al. Evaluating the utilization of a regional poison center by Latino communities. *J Toxicol Clin Toxicol.* 2002;40:855-860.
12. Davidson DGD, Eastham WN. Acute liver necrosis following overdose of paracetamol. *BMJ.* 1966;2:497-499.
13. Freund KM, Belanger AJ, D'Agostino RB, et al. The health risks of smoking. The Framingham Study: 34 years of follow-up. *Ann Epidemiol.* 1993;3:417-424.
14. Gaudreault P, Parent M, McGuigan MA, et al. Predictability of esophageal injury from signs and symptoms: a study of caustic ingestion in 378 children. *Pediatrics.* 1983;71:767-770.
15. Guyatt GH, Oxman AD, Vist GE, et al. GRADE: an emerging consensus on rating quality of evidence and strength of recommendations. *BMJ.* 2008;336:924-926.

16. Hamilton RJ, Goldfrank LR. Poison center data and the Pollyanna phenomenon. *J Toxicol Clin Toxicol.* 1998;35:21-23.
17. Harchelroad F, Clark RF, Dean B, et al. Treated vs. reported toxic exposures: discrepancies between a poison control center and a member hospital. *Vet Hum Toxicol.* 1990;32:156-159.
18. Hoppe-Roberts JM, Lloyd LM, Chyka P. Poisoning mortality in the United States: comparison of national mortality statistics and poison control center reports. *Ann Emerg Med.* 2000;35:440-448.
19. Hoyt BT, Rasmussen R, Giffin S, et al. Poison center data accuracy: a comparison of rural hospital chart data with Tdatabase ESS, *Acad Emerg Med.* 1999;6:851-855.
20. Institute of Medicine of the National Academies. *Forging a Poison Prevention and Control System.* Washington, DC: The National Academies Press; 2004.
21. Kernan WN, Viscoli CM, Brass LM, et al. Phenylpropanolamine and the risk of hemorrhagic stroke. *N Engl J Med.* 2000; 343: 1826-1832.
22. King J. Hypertension and cerebral hemorrhage after trimolets ingestion. *Med J Aust.* 1979;2:258.
23. *Lévy A, Bailey B, Letarte A*, et al. Unproven ingestion: an unrecognized bias in toxicological case series. *Clin Toxicol (Phila).* 2007;45:946-949.
24. Martin JD, Osterhoudt KC, Thom SR. Recognition and management of carbon monoxide poisoning in children. *Clin Pediatr Emerg Med.* 2000; 1:244-250.
25. McFee RB, Caraccio TR, Mofensen HC. The granny syndrome and medication access as significant causes of unintentional pediatric poisoning [abstract]. *J Toxicol Clin Toxicol.* 1999;37:593.
26. Merigian KS, Blaho KE. Single-dose activated charcoal in the treatment of the self-poisned patient: a prospective, randomized, controlled trial. *Am J Ther.* 2002;9:301-308.
27. Moher D, Schulz KF, Altman D. The CONSORT statement: revised recommendations for improving the quality of reports of parallel-group randomized trials. *JAMA.* 2001;285:1987-1991.
28. Olson KR, Seger D. Hyperbaric oxygen for carbon monoxide poisoning: does it really work? *Ann Emerg Med.* 1995;25:535-537.
29. Osterhoudt KC, Henretig FM. How much confidence that calcium channel blockers are safe? [letter]. *Vet Hum Toxicol.* 1998;40:239.
30. Palatnick W, Tenenbein M. Leukocytosis, hyperglycemia, vomiting, and positive x-rays are not indicatiors of severe iron overdose in adults. *Am J Emerg Med.* 1996;14:454-455.
31. Polivka BJ, Elliott MB, Wolowich WR. Comparison of poison exposure data: NHIS and Tdata ESS. *J Toxicol Clin Toxicol.* 2002;40:839-845.
32. Pond SM, Lewis-Driver DJ, Williams GM, et al. Gastric emptying in acute overdose: a prospective randomised controlled trial. *Med J Aust.* 1995;163:345-349.
33. Scheinkestel CD, Bailey M, Myles PS, et al. Hyperbaric or normobaric oxygen for acute carbon monoxide poisoning: a randomised controlled clinical trial. *Med J Aust.* 1999;170:203-210.
34. Sutton AJ, Duval SJ, Tweedie RL, et al. Empirical assessment of effect of publication bias on meta-analyses. *BMJ.* 2000;320:1574-1577.
35. Tenenbein M, Cohen S, Sitar DS. Efficacy of ipecac-induced emesis, orogastric lavage, and activated charcoal for acute drug overdose. *Ann Emerg Med.* 1987;16:838-841.
36. Thomson JS, Prescott LP. Liver damage and impaired glucose tolerance after paracetamol overdosage. *BMJ.* 1966;2:506-507.
37. Vassilev ZP, Marcus S, Jennis T, et al. Rapid communication: socioeconomic differences between counties with high and low utilization of a regional poison control center. *J Toxicol Env Health.* 2003;66:1905-1908.
38. Weaver LK, Hopkins RO, Chan KJ, et al. Hyperbaric oxygen for acute carbon monoxide poisoning. *N Engl J Med.* 2002;347:1057–1067.

CHAPTER 138
ADVERSE DRUG EVENTS AND POSTMARKETING SURVEILLANCE

Louis R. Cantilena

This chapter focuses on drug-induced disease resulting from adverse drug events (ADEs) caused by either inherent drug toxic effects, drug–disease adverse interactions or as a consequence of unintentional drug–drug interactions. Additional topics covered in this chapter include a discussion about the diagnosis of drug-induced disease, an overview of the Food and Drug Administration (FDA) process for drug approval, postmarketing surveillance of ADEs, and the role of the medical toxicologist in the discovery, reporting, and prevention of ADEs.

ADEs are defined as untoward effects or outcomes associated with use of a drug. In this chapter, the word "drug" will be used for a pharmaceutical product and includes prescription and nonprescription medications, and dietary supplements.

In the United States, all new prescription and nonprescription medications must be shown to be both safe and effective in order to achieve approval by the FDA, a prerequisite for marketing and sale. Dietary supplements fall outside of this legal requirement.

HISTORY OF THE UNITED STATES DRUG APPROVAL PROCESS

Prior to 1900, there was no requirement for a drug or medical device manufacturer to demonstrate that the product actually worked (efficacy), was safe when used as directed, or was made to be within precise specifications. In addition, no laws existed that required labeled claims be proven valid. Anyone could sell any product desired and it was left to the consumer or healthcare worker to determine if the products actually worked and were safe. Initiation of medicinal product regulation and the overall evolution of the US drug law and regulations are closely linked to specific medical product disasters that occurred during the 20th century in the United States. Relatively recent changes in US drug approval law further changed drug review timelines and prioritization of drug application reviews.

Examples of the pre-1900 regulation of medicinal products include the lack of a legal requirement for a company to test a product for safety or efficacy or even to make valid claims in the drug label. Products such as aspirin-containing heroin were sold as cough syrup. Wine with cocaine was marketed to enhance sales of the alcoholic beverage. Further, there was no legal requirement for systematic testing of products to determine content or the presence of possible adulterants in product formulations. The Food and Drug Act of 1906 required pharmaceutical manufacturers to meet a standard for the concentration and purity of the drugs they marketed. However, the burden of proof was on the FDA to show that the drug was incorrectly labeled or that the advertising or label was false or misleading.

The Food, Drug and Cosmetic Act of 1938 resulted from a tragedy in which more than 100 patients (mostly children) died from poisoning by an excipient of an oral solution of sulfanilamide. A pharmaceutical company, in an attempt to improve the palatability of a sulfanilamide product for pediatric formulations, introduced the solvent diethylene glycol into the formulation. Diethylene glycol is a sweet-tasting but nephrotoxic hydrocarbon. Only after almost a full year of marketing were cases of renal failure and death reported in sufficient numbers to alert authorities to the extremely toxic nature of the product. The Food Drug and Cosmetic Act of 1938 accomplished the following:

1. Required companies to list the ingredients of the product on the product label.
2. Required companies to provide the known risks concerning use of the product to physicians or pharmacists.
3. Made illegal the misbranding of food or medical products.
4. For the first time required companies to test their products for safety before being sold.

Drugs already marketed before 1938 were exempt from the requirement (see Chap. 1).

An application in the early 1960s for the approval of α-*N*-phthalylglutaramide (thalidomide), a sedative that had already been marketed in Europe, was submitted to the FDA. The sedative drug had a rapid onset and short duration of action, did not affect ventilation, did not cause a morning-after effect, and was inexpensive. Dr. Frances Kelsey, a medical officer at the FDA, delayed approval by asking the sponsor to clarify several issues in the reportedly poorly organized new drug application (NDA). In the interim, an unusual teratogenic effect, phocomelia, or limb misdevelopment, was linked in Europe to the use of thalidomide. Congressional hearings resulted in the Kefauver-Harris Act of 1968, which required a drug manufacturer or sponsor to do the following:

1. File an investigational new drug application (IND) before beginning a clinical study with a drug in humans.
2. Demonstrate that the drug was effective for the condition that it was being marketed to treat.
3. Provide adequate directions for safe usage of the drug.

Once again, the act was not retroactive and drugs that were already on the market were exempt from these new requirements.

Subsequent US laws that affect FDA review and approval of products include the following:

1. The Orphan Drug Act of 1983, which provides financial incentives to drug manufacturers to develop drugs for the treatment of rare diseases and conditions (see http://www.fda.gov/ orphan/designat/list.htm for a list of drugs that have been approved under the Orphan Drug Act). A rare disease is defined as one in which there are less than 200,000 affected persons in the United States, or one affecting more people, but in which the cost of drug development is likely to exceed any potential sales of the drug (http://www.fda.gov/orphan/oda.htm).
2. The Prescription Drug User Fee Act (PDUFA) of 1992, which required manufacturers to pay user fees to the FDA for NDAs and supplements, to enable the FDA to hire additional reviewers and accelerate the review process. This Act, which has undergone several revisions (the latest in 2007), has proven to be controversial due to the new working relationship it creates between industry and regulators, and the concern that it may force compromises that are not in the best interest of public health.

The overall question as to whether or not the introduction of user fees and their associated mandate for shorter FDA review times for new drug applications (NDAs) have negatively impacted safety remains controversial.[15,31,39] While some believe that the shorter review times for FDA approval appear to be associated with an increased likelihood of drug withdrawal and black box label modification of the drug label postapproval,[2] others have not yet reached that conclusion.[40] The debate on this issue intensified during the controversy involving the cyclooxygenase-2 (COX-2) inhibitor anti-inflammatory drugs. This widely publicized withdrawal and press coverage of the related litigation resulted in congressional hearings on the review practices and monitoring of drug safety by the FDA.

3. The Dietary Supplement Health and Education Act (DSHEA amendment) of 1994, which removed from FDA the authority to require proof of safety or efficacy prior to marketing of products considered dietary supplements (including herbal remedies). Only when a specific health claim is made by the manufacturer of a product does the FDA have premarketing approval authority. Furthermore, rather than placing on the manufacturers the burden of proof for safety and efficacy of a product, the FDA is required to determine that a product is unsafe to prevent sale and distribution in the United States.
4. Section 112 of the FDA Modernization Act of 1997, which allowed for an accelerated drug approval process for the treatment of life-threatening illnesses such as AIDS and cancer if the drug has the potential to address medical needs unmet by currently available drugs. Many of the accelerated drug approvals rely on efficacy results derived from surrogate markers linked to the ultimate indication for the drug. For example, the protease inhibitors were approved on the accelerated track for the treatment of AIDS because of their ability to reduce HIV viral load.
5. The Pediatric Research Equity Act of 2003, which requires manufacturers to study drugs being submitted for approval for a claimed indication in children. The FDA provides incentives such as patent extension and marketing exclusivity for performing these evaluations. As a result more data from children are being provided to guide therapeutic use of medication in this patient group.
6. Recent FDA funding renewal legislation has added specified deadlines for drug application reviews as well as established a priority for FDA review based on indication and potential benefit of the candidate drug for a disease population. In 2007 the United States signed into law legislation referred to as Food and Drug Administration Amendments Act (FDAAA) which increased FDA responsibilities and authorizations primarily aimed at improving product safety.

Four of the provisions of FDAAA reauthorize past legislation: the Prescription Drug User Fee Act (PDUFA) of 2007, the Medical Device User Fee Amendments of 2007 (MDUFA), the Pediatric Research Equity Act of 2007 (PREA), and the Best Pharmaceuticals for Children Act of 2007 (BPCA).

Other important actions coming from FDAAA include a requirement for FDA to ensure that clinical trial information is provided to the National Institute of Health's ClinicalTrials.gov web site. FDAAA gives authorization to FDA to require postmarketing studies, primarily of drug safety, including surveillance and clinical trials as well as to require that sponsors incorporate Risk Evaluation and Mitigation Strategies (REMS) in their proposed marketing activities as a prerequisite for product approval. The goal of these latter components was to enhance the regulatory authority of the FDA to require active risk surveillance for newly approved products and make it easier for the FDA to take regulatory action if safety signals are detected. The elements of REMS vary considerably among products, and may be applied to both safety concerns and the potential for misuse, as in the case of prescription opioids.[38] The impact of these new regulations will be measured and in time, it should be clear as to whether or not newly approved drugs are better monitored and by extension, the public health is at less risk for unintended drug-induced disease from FDA approved medications.

A complete listing of the laws and statutes enforced by the FDA is found on the FDA Web site.[14]

Recent legislative action suggests that Congress has, for the time being, chosen to provide FDA with increased postmarketing authority rather than reconsider PDUFA for new drug applications. The short- and long-term implications of this decision are not yet fully known.

THE DRUG DEVELOPMENT PROCESS

Figure 138–1 shows a schematic overview of the process for drug development of a new molecular entity (NME). The process begins with the preclinical evaluation of the candidate drug. During this evaluation, toxicologic testing is performed in more than one animal species and other testing includes stability of the product, manufacturing methods, purity, and initiation of testing for possible carcinogenicity. Dose–response relationships in animal models and in vitro receptor binding or surrogate marker effects are often determined at this phase of the evaluation. Also, this is the time when many manufacturers determine the metabolism of the drug in animal and in vitro human systems. Following this preclinical testing, the sponsor submits an IND application to the FDA for approval to initiate human testing. This application contains all relevant data concerning animal and in vitro toxicology testing, product manufacturing and purity, and a protocol for using the drug in initial human investigation. Within 30 days, the FDA must review the IND application and either allow the proposed human study to proceed or inform the sponsor that additional data or preclinical work is required before clinical testing of the candidate drug can begin.

The clinical study of new candidate medications is divided into four basic phases. Phase 1 clinical testing involves a relatively small number of subjects with the primary aim of determining the safety and toxicity of the drug. Many phase 1 studies will also determine the human pharmacokinetics and metabolism of the drug. Phase 1 studies are normally conducted in 20–100 healthy volunteer subjects with the

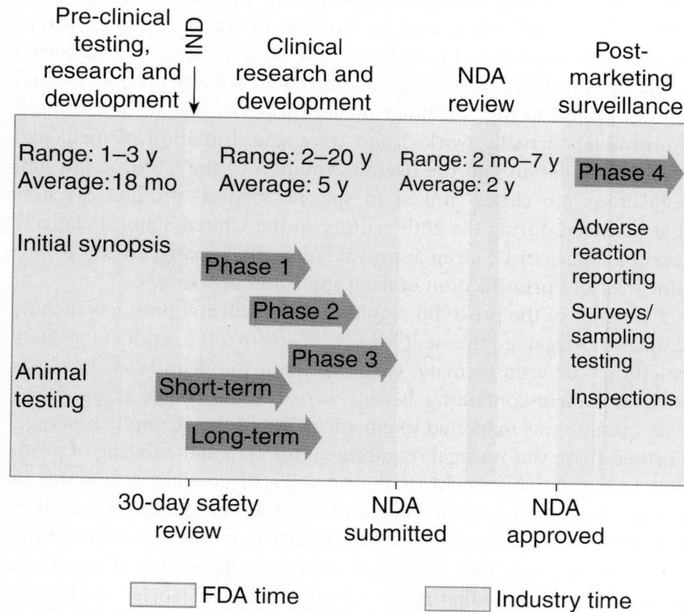

FIGURE 138–1. Schematic representation of new drug development. (From www.fda.gov.) NDA = New Drug Application; IND = Investigational New Drug; FDA = Food and Drug Administration.

notable exception of phase 1 studies for cancer chemotherapeutics, which enroll only patients with cancer.

Phase 2 clinical testing is designed to determine the potential efficacy of the drug product in humans and sometimes explores the range of effective drug dosages. In this phase, approximately 100–300 subjects are usually studied. In phase 2 clinical trials, subjects generally have the diseases for which the drug is intended or are capable of demonstrating the appropriate, validated, biologic surrogate marker to indicate response to the drug. An example of this would be a drug intended for early treatment of the acute coronary syndrome is tested to show that it can inhibit in vivo platelet function after oral dosing in human study subjects.

Phase 3 clinical drug studies usually involve large-scale clinical trials in the actual population for which the drug use is intended. Typically, this phase of drug development will involve testing a treatment cohort of several hundred to several thousand patients who have the target disease, depending on both the prevalence of the disease and effectiveness of the drug. The primary goal of phase 3 studies is to determine the safety and efficacy of the candidate drug in the actual intended patient population in question, under conditions similar to the anticipated medical use. At the completion of phase 3, an NDA (request for approval to market) is submitted to the FDA. A candidate drug completing phases 1, 2, and 3 can thus be approved for marketing after study in only 2000–4000 patients. In the setting of a fast-track approval or under the Orphan Drug regulations, substantially fewer patients will receive the drug before its approval for marketing. The relatively small number of human exposures to a new chemical or biologic entity prior to approval for marketing is an important factor that limits the sensitivity of the drug approval process to detect uncommon ADEs. There are additional considerations that set a drug review priority based on the PDUFA classification of the candidate drug. This classification also determines the review deadline for FDA. For example, a drug application given a "priority" review status is targeted to complete FDA review in 6 months as compared to the now standard review cycle of 10 months.

The FDA sometimes seeks the external advice of its constituted advisory committees prior to approval, especially in the setting of an uncertain risk–benefit profile of a candidate drug. FDA advisory committees generally are organized by therapeutic areas and are composed of medical professionals, usually from academia, as well as a patient representative and a nonvoting industry representative. These same advisory committees also convene to consider postapproval safety or efficacy data when FDA is considering an important change to a drug label or other postapproval regulatory action. Generally the FDA prepares questions for the committee members and provides an FDA briefing document containing a detailed data analysis and background of the issue from the FDA perspective as well as a briefing document prepared by the manufacturer containing analogous information. Committee members comment and vote on the FDA questions during the proceedings. For a new drug approval one question generally includes a yes or no answer as to whether or not the advisor believes that the drug can be marketed with an adequate risk–benefit profile. The advisory committee vote is technically nonbinding for the FDA, but the FDA generally follows the committee advice. A recent issue of concern is the fact that some members of FDA advisory committees with perceived conflicts of interest are granted waivers by FDA to participate. The appearance of conflict of interest on an advisory committee can have a significant impact on the drug approval process and the FDA has begun to decrease the number of committee member waivers.

At the conclusion of the NDA review and at times an Advisory Committee meeting on the application, the FDA may issue an approval for marketing the new product. On occasion, the FDA issues an "approvable" letter, indicating that the product is potentially approvable but additional data will be needed before final approval can be granted. Examples of additional data required in this setting include further clinical study of a specific drug interaction, use of the drug in a specific patient population, or extension of the submitted drug stability testing. Once approval of the drug is given by FDA, the next phase of drug development begins as discussed separately below.

PHASE 4 DRUG DEVELOPMENT: POSTMARKETING SURVEILLANCE

Every drug, therapeutic biologic product, or medical device carries with it some potential risk.[40] If society required that only "completely" safe drug products were allowed to be marketed, the drug approval process would likely take decades and few if any new drugs would be made available. The FDA and the pharmaceutical industry therefore significantly rely on postmarketing surveillance for further safety information regarding the toxicity of a medical product after approval. A postmarketing surveillance system is in place to monitor postapproval drug safety that is intended to detect instances in which the safety profile appears different following marketing. Individual pharmaceutical manufacturers are responsible for monitoring the safety of their products and regularly reporting any detected ADEs to the FDA. The FDA postmarketing surveillance (MedWatch Program) for all medical products is a parallel system in place to monitor drug and medical device safety.[21] This system relies on spontaneous reports by healthcare professionals or patients regarding the occurrence of deleterious effects associated with the use of a medical product. Because manufacturers are also required by law to report ADEs associated with use of their products to MedWatch, the FDA database contains one complete data set called the Adverse Event Reporting System (AERS database). Because the MedWatch system is passive in nature, the estimated overall rate for adverse event reporting is estimated at only 1%–10%.[17,27,30]

The primary goals of the MedWatch system are the following:

1. To increase awareness of drug- and device-induced disease.
2. To clarify what should (and should not) be reported to the agency.
3. To facilitate reporting of adverse effects by creating a single system for health professionals to use in reporting ADEs and product problems to the agency.
4. To provide regular feedback to the healthcare community about safety issues involving medical products.[24]

Establishing causality for a specific medical product is not required before submission of a MedWatch report. The FDA is primarily interested in the report of a serious adverse event, or an ADE previously not associated with the drug being administered, whether or not a causal relationship is established. Although any potential ADE should be reported, an event is considered serious and should be reported when the patient outcome is one of the following:

1. Death, if the death is suspected to be a direct result of the adverse event.
2. Life threatening, if the patient was considered to be at substantial risk of dying at the time of the adverse event or the use or continued use of the product would result in the patient's death. (Examples include gastrointestinal hemorrhage, bone marrow suppression, pacemaker failure, and infusion pump failure that permits uncontrolled free flow and results in excessive drug dosing.)
3. Hospitalization (initial or prolonged), if admission to the hospital or prolongation of a hospital stay resulted from the adverse event. (Examples include anaphylaxis, pseudomembranous colitis, or bleeding causing or prolonging hospitalization.)

4. Disability, if the adverse event resulted in a significant, persistent, or permanent change, impairment, damage, or disruption in the patient's body function/structure, physical activities, or quality of life. (Examples include cerebrovascular accident caused by drug-induced coagulopathy, toxicity, and peripheral neuropathy.)
5. Congenital anomaly, if there are suspicions that exposure to a medical product before conception or during pregnancy resulted in an adverse effect on the child. (Examples include vaginal cancer in female offspring from exposure to diethylstilbestrol during pregnancy or limb malformations in the offspring from thalidomide use during pregnancy.)
6. Requires intervention to prevent permanent impairment or damage if use of a medical product is suspected to result in a condition requiring medical or surgical intervention to preclude permanent impairment or damage to a patient. (Examples include acetaminophen overdose–induced hepatotoxicity requiring treatment with *N*-acetylcysteine to prevent permanent damage, or burns from radiation equipment requiring drug therapy.[24])

MedWatch reports are easily done through the MedWatch Web site, or by facsimile, telephone, or mail. Physician reports are given priority for review by the FDA in the MedWatch system. A well-documented case of a serious adverse event is a significant and useful contribution to the MedWatch system.

Reports of serious ADEs to the FDA or to the manufacturer can become an epidemiologically detectable signal that can result in more detailed investigations, several examples of which are provided later in this chapter. On occasion serious ADEs detected in the AERS database have led to the withdrawal of products from the US market without conducting additional studies.

Reporting serious ADEs has periodically been encouraged by various healthcare groups in conjunction with the FDA. Currently, the MedWatch program is supported by over 140 organizations, representing health professionals and industry that have agreed to be MedWatch Partners to help achieve these goals. These organizations include medical societies and organizations such as the American Medical Association (AMA), the American College of Medical Toxicology (ACMT), and the American Academy of Pediatrics (AAP) that have encouraged their members to report to the MedWatch system. As a requirement for hospital accreditation, the Joint Commission mandates hospitals to collect, analyze, and report significant and unexpected ADEs to the FDA.

The primary limitation of the MedWatch system is the exclusive reliance on spontaneous reporting of ADEs. The system is passive in nature and therefore has several important limitations. Significant underreporting is known to occur in such systems. The uncertainty about the significance of a signal in the AERS database is aided by the low estimated rate for adverse event reporting and the fact that the true incidence of the reported ADE is almost never precisely known because the denominator, which is the number of actual exposures to the drug, is rarely accurately known.[17,27,30] Despite these limitations, the MedWatch system has detected significant ADEs during the postmarketing period.

Drug regulators must rely on passive surveillance systems like the AERS database to detect potential uncommon or rare but serious ADEs postapproval. This is primarily because a relatively small number of patients or subjects are exposed to the drug during phases 1–3 prior to before approval for marketing. For example, to detect an uncommon ADE occurring in approximately 1 of 5000 individuals exposed to a drug with 95% probability that the ADE resulted from exposure to that drug, approximately 15,000 patients would have to be exposed to the drug.[13] In a balanced (equal numbers of drug and placebo recipients) placebo-controlled clinical trial, 30,000 subjects would need to be enrolled. Premarketing clinical studies (phase 1, 2, and 3) are usually inadequate to detect rare ADEs, ADEs that are incorrectly diagnosed, or ADEs that result from a drug interaction that may not have been tested in the development program.

An example of a rare ADE not detected until postmarketing involves the drug felbamate, which was approved by the FDA in September 1993 and subsequently found to be associated with aplastic anemia during postmarketing surveillance. Felbamate-induced aplastic anemia had not been detected during the drug development program for the agent. By July 1994, 9 cases had been reported from an estimated 100,000 patients exposed to felbamate in the United States. Most of the aplastic anemia cases occurred in patients who had taken the drug for less than 1 year. The 9 cases represented an approximate 50-fold increase in aplastic anemia over the expected rate in the population with the very low background rate of 2–5 cases per million per previous year[1,34] allowing the FDA to attribute this rare condition to exposure to felbamate.

The primary role of the MedWatch system is to generate a hypothesis for potential association of an ADE with a specific drug. These hypotheses are sometimes further tested in subsequent phase 4 investigations. An example of this "hypothesis generation" function of MedWatch was the question of whether phenylpropanolamine (PPA) caused hemorrhagic stroke in patients using nonprescription diet suppressants or cough and cold preparations containing PPA. In the early 1990s, the Spontaneous Reporting System (SRS, now AERS) detected a potential association of hemorrhagic stroke and nonprescription use of PPA. An industry-sponsored prospective, case-controlled study was designed, to determine if such an association existed. The multicenter study demonstrated that an association did exist, especially for women ages 18–49. The Nonprescription Drug Advisory Committee (NDAC) of FDA reviewed this study and the associated MedWatch data in the fall of 2000 and decided that the evidence supported such an association. The committee advised the FDA to remove PPA from the market, which occurred a short time later. Although the entire process of signal identification from MedWatch to presentation of results from the prospective epidemiologic study required nearly a decade for PPA, the process demonstrates the value of the hypothesis-generating ability of the MedWatch system.

Potential outcomes of a safety signal detection for a marketed drug include dose reduction in all or certain high risk patient populations, restriction of the sale of the specific drug to a more medically supervised environment or with a patient registry to more closely monitor use, and removal of the drug from the market. These are further discussed later in this chapter.

Other types of phase 4 investigations include clinical studies, marketing-type studies, comparative studies with the new drug versus a competitor, or a special population study or drug interaction study when suspicion is raised for a potentially different risk–benefit relationship in certain clinical settings. The enhancement of safety information is the primary goal of most phase 4 studies. Other than the specific prospective study in patient subpopulations, the methods by which phase 4 safety studies are usually conducted are primarily observational and epidemiologic studies. Main sources of data for the postapproval monitoring of the safety of a drug are the spontaneous reports gathered by both the pharmaceutical manufacturer and FDA. The fields of pharmacovigilance and pharmacoepidemiology are typically employed in the conduct of phase 4 studies.[25] Attributing a serious ADE to a drug solely from MedWatch reports does occur but is it much more common for the AERS database to produce a signal suggesting a possible drug-related safety problem.

ESTABLISHING THE DIAGNOSIS OF DRUG-INDUCED DISEASE

The recognition and diagnosis of a drug-induced disease, or an ADE, is an essential skill for all practitioners, and especially for medical toxicologists and clinical pharmacologists. The diagnosis of an ADE is

TABLE 138–1. Questions to Consider When Establishing the Diagnosis of an Adverse Drug Event

1. Was the timing of the adverse event appropriate relative to the exposure to the drug?
2. Has the effect noted, which is the suspected ADE, been previously reported?
3. Is there evidence of excessive exposure to the drug?
4. Are there other more likely etiologies responsible for the condition suspected as being an ADE?
5. What is the patient's response to cessation of a suspect drug (dechallenge)?
6. What is the patient's response to rechallenge?

typically established as a result of a systematic medical evaluation. One approach to establishing the diagnosis of drug-induced disease involves consideration of six related questions concerning the patient's clinical presentation and available medical data, as shown in Table 138–1.

The first question concerns the timing of the onset of the adverse event in relationship to the reported exposure to the drug. Perhaps because of publicity or word of mouth, ADEs are sometimes reported to the FDA MedWatch system even when the onset of the adverse event occurs before the first exposure to the suspect drug. A careful reconstruction of the time course of drug exposure and onset of adverse effects is extremely important in assessing causality. The time course differs considerably for different adverse clinical events. An anaphylactic reaction to a drug usually occurs within minutes of exposure, whereas renal insufficiency caused by a drug is not likely to be clinically detectable for up to several days after the exposure. A drug that causes cancer (a carcinogen) may not produce a clinically detectable effect for decades. Establishing a time course is an essential first step in the process of making the diagnosis of drug-induced disease.

The second question is whether or not this adverse effect has been reported previously for the suspect drug. An adverse drug effect that occurs commonly is likely to be known before the approval of the drug and therefore is typically found on the initial drug label. For example, respiratory depression and mental status changes were well known before the approval of fentanyl, an opioid agonist. Less common ADEs for drugs that have been on the market for a period of time are sometimes found in case reports in the literature, included in various medical databases, and in some cases will appear in a revised drug label for the medical product. Previous reports linking the observed adverse effect to drug exposure are very helpful to the physician trying to establish a significant level of probability for causality in the setting of an ADE.

However, in the setting of a newly approved drug or a previously unreported possible ADE, neither previous reports/medical literature nor the drug label will help establish causality. In this setting, the clinician must rely more on what is known of the pharmacology, the pharmacokinetics, and the anticipated pharmacodynamics of the suspect drug and the timing of the appearance and observed time course of the adverse event. It is important to put "drug-induced disease" in the differential diagnosis for most patients presenting for medical care. Someone has to be the first to report what is ultimately recognized as an adverse effect. Appropriate vigilance for the possibility of a new ADE significantly increases the probability that a finding can be made early after introduction of a new drug to prevent more widespread drug-induced morbidity or mortality.

The next question to consider is, "Is there evidence of excessive exposure to the drug?" The majority of ADEs that occur are predictable on the basis of the known pharmacology of the specific drug. Such ADEs are referred to as *type A* ADEs.[5] For example, antihistamines such as diphenhydramine are known to cause significant anticholinergic effects. When a patient presents with mental status changes and clinical findings consistent with the anticholinergic toxidrome after significant exposure to an antihistamine-containing product, the observed effects are consistent with an ADE attributable to the antihistamine. Occasionally, proof of drug excess can come from measurement of the drug in serum. In the case of the patient with a history of atrial fibrillation who exhibits nausea, vomiting, vision changes, and ventricular dysrhythmias, the measurement of an elevated serum digoxin concentration supports the diagnosis of digoxin toxicity or an ADE attributable to digoxin perhaps as an inadvertent or intentional overdose, drug interaction, or change in patient renal function resulting in excessive circulating digoxin concentration. In any case, knowing the pharmacology of the drug is important for establishing the diagnosis of an ADE.

When an ADE is caused by an allergic mechanism or another mechanism unrelated to extent of the exposure to the drug, ie, a type B ADE, evidence of drug excess usually does not contribute to the diagnosis. In this setting, other factors such as allergy history or pharmacogenetic background are weighed more heavily to support the diagnosis of an ADE. Patients are usually not aware of their genetically determined ability to metabolize or react to medications but most patients will recall a previously experienced allergic reaction.

The next issue to address in considering possible causality is whether there are other more likely etiologies that could be responsible for the observed effects. Although it is important to be appropriately vigilant for possible ADEs, it is equally important not to miss an alternative cause for the patient's condition. There are certain clinical settings in which establishing an ADE becomes a diagnosis of exclusion. For example, in the case of persistent fever, the assignment of the diagnosis "drug fever" should not be made until a complete search for infectious causes has excluded this etiology.

A very important factor to consider in contemplating a diagnosis of ADE is "What is the patient's response to cessation of a suspect drug (*dechallenge*)?" In this case, the pharmacokinetics of the drug and the timing of resolution of the specific condition must be carefully considered. In some instances, the resolution of a type A ADE closely follows the pharmacokinetics of the suspect drug. For example, in the case of acute β adrenergic antagonist intoxication, cardiac effects resolve in association with decreasing serum concentrations of the drug in question. However, in other instances, onset and resolution of the ADE may not correlate with drug concentrations in the body, for example, in the case of a penicillin rash, which may develop within 1 or 2 days or longer after starting the medication, but may take several days to weeks to completely resolve. In this example of a type B ADE, the resolution of the condition (rash) occurs over a much longer time period than would be predicted by the pharmacokinetics of the drug. When a suspected ADE resolves after discontinuation of exposure to the offending drug, along a predictable time course, the result of this dechallenge would support the diagnosis of ADE.

Lastly, the clinician may have the opportunity or need to *rechallenge* the patient with the suspect agent. If the rechallenge results in the identical response or effect, this would be considered strong evidence to support a causal relationship for the suspect drug and the adverse event. In the setting of a serious or life-threatening adverse event, it is too dangerous to perform a rechallenge with the suspect drug, in which case the response to rechallenge will not be known. In this setting, the weight of evidence previously discussed will then be the only factors available to assign the probability of causality.

FDA REGULATORY ACTIONS REGARDING SAFETY

When new information about a safety issue for an already marketed drug raises concern at FDA, several regulatory options are available to either attempt to improve the safety of the drug or remove the drug from the US market. The most common regulatory action taken by the FDA is modification of the drug label. These modifications can include restrictions as to whom should receive the drug, what doses should be given for which indications or to which patient populations, what type of monitoring should be performed during therapy, and how long treatment should be administered. When potentially life-threatening safety information is discovered, and the FDA believes that the risk–benefit relationship remains in favor of continued availability of the drug, the FDA can require that a "black box" warning be carried in the label. A black box warning is the most serious warning placed in the label of a prescription medication. If a black box warning is established, healthcare professional advertisements regarding product availability are no longer permitted. Additionally, the manufacturer is required in most cases to send a "Dear Doctor" letter to potential prescribers informing them of the new black box warning. Dear Doctor letters may also be required when the FDA requires that prescribers be notified about a significant change in the drug label warning. An example of current medications with recently added black box warnings is antidepressant medication that now must warn about the increased risk of suicidality if children and adolescents are prescribed antidepressants.

Another option sometimes employed by the FDA is the implementation of restricted availability measures to permit continued availability of the drug but only with specified restrictions. For example, use of the drug isotretinoin (Accutane) requires compliance with a multiple component risk evaluation and mitigation program (REMS) program called iPLEDGE that includes informed consent, prescriber and dispensing pharmacy registration, serial pregnancy testing if applicable, documentation of patient education, and completion of risk management programs by patients who will receive the medication.[10] The FDA authority to require companies to submit, prior to drug approval, and execute, postapproval, an effective risk management plan is intended to improve both the monitoring and prevention of postapproval adverse drug events and their consequences.

When the FDA believes that a drug can no longer be safely used despite modification of the drug label or any of the aforementioned restrictions, the regulatory threshold is reached to initiate removal of the drug from the market. This occurs when an acceptable risk–benefit relationship for continued availability of a drug product is no longer possible. Table 117-2 in the seventh edition of *Goldfrank's Toxicologic Emergencies* contains a compilation of products that were withdrawn or removed from the market in the United States for reasons of safety or efficacy. Some recent additions to that list of drugs include valdecoxib (marketed as Bextra) and rofecoxib (marketed as Vioxx), withdrawn because of recognition of elevated cardiovascular risk associated with their use.[15] Table 138–2 contains a listing of drugs that were withdrawn from the US market during the years 2006, 2007, and 2008. In the case of the COX-2 inhibitor withdrawals, the precipitating factor for withdrawal was the findings of a strong safety signal for excess cardiovascular mortality and morbidity during the conduct of efficacy studies for other potential therapeutic indications for these drugs. The postmarketing surveillance system did not serve as the initial, precipitating data set for regulatory action in this instance.[6,11,22,28,29] The manufacturers voluntarily withdrew these COX-2 inhibitors and the majority of the drugs from the United States market. In many cases, the manufacturer ceases marketing the specific drug after notification by the FDA that regulatory action is being initiated to remove their drug from the market. Only very rarely has the FDA itself actually removed a drug from the market. One example where the FDA did implement removal is the drug phenformin, which was removed by the FDA after due process was completed. In the case of ephedra-containing dietary supplements, the FDA removed these products from the market based on their analysis of safety data obtained from the medical literature and from analysis of cases reported to the MedWatch system. In some cases, the pharmaceutical manufacturers file suit against the FDA to fight or delay the planned regulatory action against the product. The manufacturer's legal action generally prolongs the time the product remains on the market because the drug usually continues to be sold while the legal proceedings and appeals proceed through the courts.

TABLE 138–2. US Drug Withdrawals for Safety Concerns: 2006, 2007, and 2008

Year	Drug
2006	Gatifloxacin–manufacturer discontinued marketing. Hyper/hypoglycemia
2007	Pergolide–manufacturer discontinued marketing. Heart valve damage
	Aprotinin–manufacturer discontinued marketing. Possible increased risk of death
	Tegaserod–manufacturer discontinued marketing. Increased risk of cardiac adverse events
2008	Colchicine (injection)–manufacturer discontinued marketing. Safety concerns and unapproved status
	Papain (topical)–manufacturer discontinued marketing. Safety concerns and unapproved status
	Edetate sodium–manufacturer discontinued marketing. Inappropriate off-label use and name confusion with edetate calcium disodiuim

Some feel that approval of a drug by FDA should preempt legal action for safety issues identified in the drug labeling. However, the FDA decision-making process regarding drug approval is largely reliant on efficacy and safety data provided by the manufacturer or in the publicly available medical literature. Plaintiff actions, taken against drug and device manufacturers, are sometimes a source of significant publicity and confidential disclosures regarding questionable behaviors practiced by companies that market medicinal products. The patient's right to tort action against a product's manufacturer provides an important mechanism to assure drug safety following approval and marketing.[4,16,20] Recent Supreme Court appeals have challenged this position seeking to reinforce the legal position of federal preemption. In the case of *Wyeth v. Levine*, the manufacturer appealed to the US Supreme Court to uphold the federal preemption status for FDA approved drugs. On March 4, 2009, the US Supreme Court ruled that federal law does not preempt this particular plaintiff from seeking and obtaining a judgment from the product manufacturer because the product was approved by the FDA. The case provided the opportunity to debate the extent of protection afforded by the FDA approval status and the issue of product liability litigation as a part of postmarketing surveillance of drug products in the United States. At the current time, medical devices are governed under a distinct statute in which FDA approval does preempt many forms of litigation.

In addition to the highly publicized COX-2 withdrawals, where an elevated risk of cardiovascular ADEs was cited, the past several years have seen drug withdrawals from the US market because of postmarketing recognition of ADEs in three general areas:

1. Prolongation of the QTc interval
2. Significant drug–drug interactions
3. Hepatotoxicity

PROLONGATION OF THE QT INTERVAL

Three significant drug withdrawals in the mid- to late 1990s exemplified a serious drug safety issue with regard to drug-related prolongation of the QT interval when administered alone or as the result of increasing plasma concentrations due to inhibition of its metabolism by other medications. The three examples in this category are terfenadine (Seldane), astemizole (Hismanal),[7] and cisapride (Propulsid).[8,33] Numerous deaths were reported to the MedWatch system for patients taking these medications. The FDA funded small prospective clinical studies to confirm a previously unrecognized ability of terfenadine to dramatically alter cardiac repolarization, which can lead to torsades de pointes. The drug was marketed in 1985, cardiac toxicity detected in clinical use in 1990,[26] the FDA-funded clinical cardiac safety research performed in 1991,[19] and ultimately the drug was withdrawn from the market in 1998. The medicolegal course of the other two is quite similar and these experiences have led to greater rigor by manufacturers and the FDA.

In addition to the drug–drug interactions that led to accumulation of toxic cardiac parent drugs as in the case of terfenadine, astemizole, and cisapride, drugs shown to inhibit multiple metabolic pathways, especially of drugs with narrow therapeutic indices, have been removed from the market. These three drug withdrawals demonstrated that the pre-approval assessment of cardiac repolarization effects at that time was incapable of detecting even the most potent dysrhythmogenic drugs during their respective development and FDA review. Based on this dramatic systematic failure, FDA (as well as the European and Japanese drug regulatory agencies) now requires a thorough QT study (tQT) for all new molecular entities. These studies are designed to detect as little as a 5-millisecond increase in the corrected QT interval in healthy volunteer subjects and must include a positive control to demonstrate the sensitivity of the study to detect this low-level change reliably. Thus far, since this new requirement has been put in place, no newly approved drugs have subsequently been removed from the US market for QT safety reasons.[32]

SIGNIFICANT DRUG–DRUG INTERACTIONS

Removal of mibefradil (Posicor) from the US market is an example of drug withdrawn from the US market because of postmarketing discovery of a plethora of drug–drug interactions. Mibefradil, a pharmacologically unique calcium channel blocker, was approved by the FDA for the treatment of patients with hypertension and chronic stable angina. The FDA approved mibefradil for marketing in 1997 with the knowledge that the compound possessed the ability to inhibit certain hepatic CYP isozymes; these facts were included on the drug label. The initial labeling for mibefradil specifically listed three drug–drug interactions: astemizole, cisapride, and terfenadine (CYP3A pathway interactions). During the 1 year that mibefradil was marketed, information accumulated regarding drug–drug interactions with many other drugs and CYP pathways. As the in vitro and in vivo drug interaction data continued to accumulate for mibefradil, the FDA made labeling changes and issued a public warning for these potential drug interactions within 5 months of its initial approval. Additionally, the sponsor distributed a letter to healthcare professionals warning of drug–drug interactions. In the face of a growing and significant list of drug–drug interactions, and a 3-year international study demonstrating no clinical benefit of mibefradil over placebo for congestive heart failure, the FDA initiated regulatory action. In an unprecedented step for a drug with numerous drug interactions, the FDA requested that it be withdrawn from the market approximately 1 year after it was approved.[12] The FDA felt that the diversity of drug–drug interactions could not be addressed by standard drug label instructions and additional public warnings.[9]

DRUG-INDUCED HEPATOTOXICITY

Another category of ADE of recent concern is those drugs that cause hepatotoxicity. In June 1998, the manufacturer of the NSAID bromfenac sodium (Duract) withdrew this agent from the US market. The NDA was submitted for review to the FDA in 1994 and after 28 months of review was approved. The drug was withdrawn approximately 11 months later after postmarketing discovery of significant hepatotoxicity. Although no cases of serious liver injury were reported during premarketing clinical trials, after introduction to the market a higher incidence of liver enzyme elevation was found in patients who were being treated with the drug. Postapproval exposure of patients to bromfenac generally resulted in longer periods of treatment than that of the subjects in the clinical trials. Because of a preapproval concern by the FDA that long-term exposure to bromfenac could cause hepatotoxicity, bromfenac labeling specified that the product was to be used for 10 days or less. This dosing limitation appeared to be inconsistent with the initial approved drug indication for treatment of a chronic condition (eg, osteoarthritis). Information concerning elevated hepatic enzymes was actually included in the original product labeling. The postmarketing surveillance of this product identified rare cases of hepatitis and liver failure, including some patients who required liver transplantation, among those using the drug for more than the 10 days specified on the label. In February 1998, approximately 6 months after approval for marketing, the FDA added a black box warning indicating that the drug should not be taken for more than 10 days. Nonetheless, severe injury and death from long-term use of bromfenac sodium continued to be reported, and ultimately, the sponsor agreed to voluntarily withdraw bromfenac sodium from the market. The withdrawal of bromfenac sodium raised several important questions concerning interpretation of "safety laboratories," such as liver enzymes during the drug development program, and also raised questions concerning the effectiveness of drug labeling.

Another example of a drug withdrawn for safety concerns related to hepatotoxicity is the oral antidiabetic agent troglitazone (Rezulin). It was approved in the mid-1990s and severe liver toxicity was detected by postmarketing surveillance in 1997. Increasingly serious labeling changes and warnings to prescribers recommending close monitoring of liver function tests in patients taking troglitazone were issued over the next 2 years. In March 1999, an FDA advisory committee reviewed the status of troglitazone and its risk of liver toxicity and recommended continued marketing of this drug in patients with type II diabetes who were not well controlled by other drugs. When two newer agents for type II diabetes, rosiglitazone and pioglitazone, became available, the FDA concluded that the risk profile for troglitazone was significantly worse than these newer agents and asked the manufacturer to remove troglitazone from the market.[18] Analogous to the example with mibefradil, this FDA-initiated drug withdrawal was based on a change in the risk–benefit profile for the specific agent in light of new safety information discovered during the postapproval phase for the drug.

OTHER EXAMPLES OF POSTMARKETING SAFETY PROBLEMS LEADING TO DRUG WITHDRAWAL

One voluntary withdrawal of two separate drugs used in combination serves as an important example of the discovery and publicizing of an unusual adverse event occurring years after individual drug approval but after a significant increase in the prescription use of the combination product. The drug fenfluramine was approved in 1973 after an FDA review period of 75 months. A significant increase in prescription use of a combination product of fenfluramine with phentermine, another weight loss agent (referred to as "fen-phen"), began to occur in the 1990s when clinical data suggested that this drug combination was effective in a weight loss program.[35–37] Use of the fen-phen drug combination, however, was never fully approved by the FDA and was therefore considered an "off-label usage" of the product. The number of prescriptions for the drug combination soared in the mid-1990s. In July 1997, research from the Mayo Clinic reported 24 cases[3] of an unusual form of cardiac valvular disease causing aortic and mitral regurgitation in patients using the fen-phen combination. The publicity surrounding the potential linkage of this drug combination to an unusual adverse event led to a significant increase in reports of possible adverse events associated with this drug combination. The FDA issued a public health advisory and initiated further epidemiologic studies to ascertain its prevalence. The FDA also encouraged echocardiographic studies of valvular diseases in patients taking fenfluramine or dexfenfluramine either alone or in combination with phentermine. Although at the onset the FDA, the product manufacturers, and the medical community did not expect valvular lesions to be associated with either fenfluramine or dexfenfluramine, the epidemiologic evidence suggested a possible association, leading the FDA to conclude that these agents should be removed from the US market. The potential association of valvular heart disease with these agents is an example of the use of a case-control study to explore a possible causal relationship between drug exposure and an ADE. In this case, it is unclear what the strength of the MedWatch signal was for the possible association of cardiac valvular disease with exposure to the fen-phen combination. The association between cardiac valvular lesions and exposure to the drug combination serves as an example of elucidation of a rare, unexpected ADE as the result of a dramatic increase in the number of exposed patients using a product.

THE ROLE OF THE TOXICOLOGIST IN THE DETECTION AND PREVENTION OF ADVERSE DRUG EVENTS

Toxicologists can play an extremely important role in ADE diagnosis and prevention, through efforts in patient care, education, and administrative functions. In patient care, it is common for the medical toxicologist to be the first medical specialist to be consulted for a patient with a potential ADE. Perhaps more than any other medical specialty, medical toxicologists are likely to include a thorough medication history that also includes prescription and nonprescription products, as well as dietary supplements. The medical toxicologist's active involvement in the clinical arena, especially in settings in which the initial diagnosis of ADEs can be made, also serves to provide an important role model: the medical toxicologist as an educator to promote the detection and prevention of ADEs often in the academic setting of a medical school and affiliated teaching hospitals. Here, the academic toxicologist can champion the inclusion of education in therapeutics in the curriculum for medical students and house officers and take an active role in the implementation of the instruction. Assuring that the curriculum in therapeutics includes recognition and prevention of ADEs and medical errors that lead to ADEs could have a significant beneficial impact on the ultimate outcome of the education process toward reduction of preventable ADEs. In addition to making sure that quality information is presented in the curriculum for trainees, the medical toxicologist can often create a special teaching opportunity for this type of education by establishing an elective or, in some cases, required experience in the curriculum for training in therapeutics. Participation in a quality learning experience can significantly impact on the graduates' knowledge of and attitudes toward therapeutics and risk reduction in the practice of medicine. Although the 2000 Institute of Medicine report on medical errors[23] did not focus on education initiatives in its main recommendations for reduction of medical errors in United States, it seems logical that education be considered an important (yet incomplete) tool to improve medication use and prevent ADEs and medical errors with therapeutic agents.

In the private practice setting, medical toxicologists educate fellows in training in the medical specialty and medical staff peers. In this setting, a consistent approach to the patient that includes the listing of drug-induced disease, drug excess, or potential drug–drug interactions in the differential diagnosis as well as incorporating available pharmacologic knowledge about the drugs in question to explain an unexpected drug response can provide an example for medical colleagues.

The administrative functions that the medical toxicologist can perform could have a beneficial impact on detection and prevention of ADEs. Service on hospital or healthcare organization committees, such as the local pharmacy and therapeutics, ADE-monitoring or Medication Safety Committees are important opportunities to impact on the drug-induced disease problem. These committees systematically analyze ADE trends and recommend interventions for medical, nursing, and pharmacy staff to reduce the risk of ADEs. These interventions include targeted education programs, system modifications to reduce error rates, or a limitation of a specific drug usage to certain units of the organization or by certain specialties.

ADEs are known to be significantly underreported in the United States.[17,27,30] Despite efforts to encourage filing of ADE reports, the overall reporting rates do not appear to have changed significantly. A well-documented, complete report to MedWatch made by a healthcare professional is given priority review by the FDA. The toxicologist is likely to encounter a significant number of drug-induced disease cases from a diagnostic and management standpoint, therefore practitioners of the specialty can make a significant impact on ADE reporting. All staff including medical toxicologists and their trainees should always submit an adverse event report locally for appropriate cases they encounter. Hospitals generally do not mandate or request that the reported event be "serious" as a requirement. The FDA MedWatch system requests that reported events be serious in nature or not previously associated with the medication involved. In addition to reporting of the ADE, the medical toxicologist should promote publication of case reports of all new adverse events or adverse events occurring with newly approved products. Such publication often stimulates appropriate reporting of ADEs from other practitioners and generally raises awareness concerning a new ADE.

An additional and very important role for medical toxicologists who work with Poison Centers is to facilitate the accurate reporting of poison center data to the National Poison Data System (NPDS). Poison center data are invariably considered in the overall safety evaluation of approved and marketed drug. This is especially true for drugs with the potential for abuse and misuse. Accurate information and causality assignment for fatalities by the poison centers' medical directors can greatly aid regulatory decisions and guide efforts to improve drug safety at the national and international level. The recent review regarding the safety concerns associated with the use of nonprescription cough and cold preparations in the pediatric age group is an example of an important regulatory use of poison center data in FDA decision making (http://www.fda.gov/cder/drug/advisory/cough_cold_2008).

SUMMARY

Drug-induced disease is common in both inpatient and outpatient settings in the practice of medicine. Despite significant advances in medical science applied to drug development and regulation, ADEs continue to occur and will continue to do so for the foreseeable future. ADEs have a significant impact on patient mortality and morbidity in addition to producing a significant burden on the healthcare system. ADEs caused by newly approved drugs and ADEs resulting from a previously unrecognized association with drugs with a long marketing history continue to be a significant cause of mortality and morbidity. The rapidly expanding number of approved drugs requires that the medical toxicologist and other practitioners have a continuing commitment to reduce the risk for ADEs in medical practice. Active participation in clinical, teaching, and administrative roles that can improve ADE detection, analysis and accurate reporting at the local and national levels by medical toxicologists has led to important advances in patient safety. Maintaining a high level of commitment to these tasks as individuals and as a specialty will ultimately improve patient safety and benefit society.

REFERENCES

1. Alter BP. Bone marrow failure disorders. *Mt Sinai J Med.* 1991;58:521-534.
2. Carpenter D, Zucker EJ, Avorn J. Drug-review deadlines and safety problems. *N Engl J Med.* 2008;358:1354-1361.
3. Connolly HM, Crary JL, McGoon MD, et al. Valvular heart disease associated with fenfluramine-phentermine. *N Engl J Med.* 1997;337:581-588.
4. DeAngelis CD, Fontanarosa PB. Prescription drugs, products liability, and preemption of tort litigation. *JAMA.* 2008;300:1939-1941.
5. Edwards IR, Aronson JK. Adverse drug reactions: definitions, diagnosis and management. *Lancet.* 2000;356:1255-1259.
6. Eisenberg RS. Learning the value of drugs—is rofecoxib a regulatory success story? *N Engl J Med.* 2005;352:1285-1287.
7. FDA Talk Paper. Janssen pharmaceutical announces the withdrawal of Hismanal from the market. June 21, 1999. http://www.fda.gov/bbs/topics/answers/ans00961.html. Last accessed April 17, 2009.
8. FDA Talk Paper. Janssen pharmaceutical stops marketing cisapride in the US. March 23, 2000. http://www.fda.gov/bbs/topics/answers/ans01007.html. Last accessed April 17, 2009.
9. FDA Talk Paper. Roche Labotatories announces withdrawal of Posicor from the market. Available at http://www.fda.gov/bbs/topics/answers/ans00876.html. Last accessed April 17, 2009.
10. FDA Talk Paper. FDA announces enhancement to isotretinoin risk management program. Available at http://www.fda.gov/bbs/topics/answers/2004/ans01328.html. Last accessed April 17, 2009.
11. FDA Talk Paper. Analysis and recommendations for Agency action regarding non-steroidal anti-inflammatory drugs and cardiovascular risk. Available at http://www.fda.gov/cder/drug/infopage/COX2/ NSAIDdecisionMemo.pdf. Last accessed April 17, 2009.
12. FDA Talk Paper. Center for Drug Evaluation & Research. Available at http://www.fda.gov/cder/foi/nda/2001/20689_Posicor_biopharmr.pdf. Last accessed April 17, 2009.
13. FDA Talk Paper. Betaseron (Interferon Beta-1b). Available at http://www.fda.gov/medwatch/SAFETY/2005/safety05.htm#Betaseron. Last accessed April 17, 2009.
14. FDA Talk Paper. Laws enforced by the FDA and related statutes. Available at http://www.fda.gov/opacom/laws. Last accessed April 17, 2009.
15. Friedman MA, Woodcock J, Lumpkin MM, et al. The safety of newly approved medicines. Do recent market removals mean there is a problem? *JAMA.* 1999;281:1728-1734.
16. Gostin LO. The deregulatory effects of preempting tort litigation: FDA regulation of medical devices. *JAMA.* 2008;299(19):2313-2316.
17. Griffin JP, Weber JC. Voluntary systems of adverse reaction reporting. Part II. *Adverse Drug React Acute Poisoning Rev.* 1986;5:23-55.
18. Health and Human Services News, P00–8. Rezulin to be withdrawn from the Market. March 21, 2000. http://www.fda.gov/bbs/topics/news/new00721.html. Last accessed April 17, 2009.
19. Honig PK, Wortham DC, Zamani K, et al. Terfenadine-ketoconazole interaction study, pharmacokinetic and electrocardiographic consequences. *JAMA.* 1993;269:1513-1518.
20. Kesselheim AS, Avorn J. The role of litigation in defining drug risks. *JAMA.* 2007; 297:308-311.
21. Kessler DA. Introducing MEDWatch: a new approach to reporting medications and device adverse effects and product problems. *JAMA.* 1993;269:2765-2768.
22. Kim PS, Reicin A S, Villalba L, et al. Rofecoxib, Merck, and the FDA. *N Engl J Med.* 2004:351:2875-2878.
23. Kohn LT, Corrigan JM, Donaldson MS. To Err Is Human: Building a Safer Health System. Washington, DC; Committee on Quality of Health Care in America, Institute of Medicine: 2000.
24. MedWatch Web site. Available at http://www.fda.gov/medwatch/partner.htm. Last accessed April 17, 2009.
25. Meyboom RHB, Egberts ACG, Gribnau FWJ, Hekster YA. Pharmacovigilance in perspective. *Drug Saf.* 1999;21:429-447.
26. Monahan BP, Ferguson CL, Killeavy ES, et al. Torsade de pointes occurring in association with terfenadine use. *JAMA.* 1990;264:2788-2790.
27. Moride Y, Harambaru F, Requejo AA, Bejaud B. Underreporting of adverse drug reactions in general practice. *Br J Clin Pharmacol.* 1997;43:177-181.
28. Okie S. Raising the safety bar—the FDA's coxib meeting. *N Engl J Med.* 2005:352:1283-1285.
29. Okie S. What ails the FDA? *N Engl J Med.* 2005;352:1707-1709.
30. Rogers AS, Israel E, Smith CR, et al. Physician knowledge, attitudes and behavior related to reporting adverse drug events. *Arch Intern Med.* 1988;148:1596-1600.
31. Schwartz J. Is FDA too quick to clear drugs? Growing recalls, side-effect risks raise questions. *Washington Post*, March 23, 1999, p. A01.
32. United States Food and Drug Administration document. http://www.fda.gov/oc/pdufa/FDADrugAppSafetyData_files/NMESafetySumm.html. Last accessed April 17, 2009.
33. van Haarst AD, van't Klooster GA, van Gerven JM, et al. The influence of cisapride and clarithromycin on QT intervals in healthy volunteers. *Clin Pharmacol Ther.* 1998;64:542-546.
34. Wallace Laboratories. Express telegram to physicians. Cranbury, NJ: Wallace Laboratories, August 1, 1994.
35. Weintraub M. Long-term weight control: The National Heart, Lung, Blood Institute–funded multimodal intervention study. *Clin Pharmacol Ther.* 1992;51:581-585.
36. Weintraub M, Sundaresan PR, Madan M, et al. Long-term weight control study (weeks 0–34): the enhancement of behavior modification, caloric restriction, and exercise by fenfluramine plus phentermine versus placebo. *Clin Pharmacol Ther.* 1992;51:586-594.
37. Weintraub M, Sundaresan PR, Schuster B, et al. Long-term weight control study (weeks 34–104): an open-label study of continuous fenfluramine plus phentermine versus targeted intermittent medication as adjuncts to behavior modification, caloric restriction, and exercise. *Clin Pharmacol Ther.* 1992;51:595-601.
38. Wright C, Schnoll S Bernstein D. Risk evaluation and mitigation strategies for drugs with abuse liability: public interest, special interest, conflicts of interest, and the industry perspective. *Ann NY Acad Sci.* 2008;1141:284-303.
39. Wood AJJ. The safety of new medicines: the importance of asking the right questions. *JAMA.* 1999;281:1753.
40. Woodcock J. Drug safety and the drug approval process: hearings before the Senate Committee on Health, Education, Labor and Pensions, March 3, 2005. Washington, DC: Department of Health and Human Services. Available at http://www.hhs.gov/asl/testify/t050303b.html. Last accessed April 17, 2009.

CHAPTER 139

MEDICATION SAFETY AND ADVERSE DRUG EVENTS

Brenna M. Farmer

A medication error is "any preventable event that may cause or lead to inappropriate medication use or patient harm while the medication is in the control of the health care professional, patient, or consumer."[74] An adverse drug event (ADE) is an untoward event or outcome associated with the use of a drug. The definition of ADEs includes medication errors as well as adverse reaction to a drug, drug interactions, and reactions. A medication error is a preventable ADE and vice versa. An adverse drug reaction is defined as "any noxious, unintended, and undesired effect of a medication, which occurs at doses used for prophylaxis, diagnosis, or therapy, excluding therapeutic failures, intentional and unintentional poisoning, and medication abuse, and also excluding ADEs because of medication administration errors, or noncompliance."[98] Therefore, a medication error is not an adverse drug reaction but both are ADEs. This chapter will address medication errors and ADEs with a focused analysis of the relevant history and epidemiology, special at-risk populations, possible solutions, and the role of the medical toxicologist.

Patient safety is an area of great interest to many regulatory groups, such as the Joint Commission, hospital administrations, healthcare providers, and the general public. The interest has continued to grow since the publication of the Institute of Medicine report in 1999 which focused on the measures necessary to insure a safer healthcare system including medication errors and adverse effects.[52] Medications errors represent up to 25% of all medical errors.[42] The importance of medication errors is highlighted in another Institute of Medicine report that focused solely on medication errors.[4] Many hospitals focus on medication safety through their pharmaceutical and therapeutics committees, patient safety committees, and medication safety committees.

HISTORY AND EPIDEMIOLOGY

Although medication safety developments have occurred throughout history, in the 1990s they became a major cause of concern. Table 139–1 shows a timeline of some important developments for medication safety.

Studies of medical errors and medication are of a highly variable quality as they deal with different populations, the definitions utilized vary, and the methods employed a variety of data collection techniques including observational studies and voluntary reporting.

One recent study estimates that 180,000 people die each year of iatrogenic injury[58] and 60% of these injuries are probably preventable.[16] Another study estimates that an additional 44,000–98,000 people die each year from medical errors.[52] The difference between these studies may be due to variance of populations, inclusion and exclusion criteria, or case definitions. However, despite the statistical differences both studies establish that medical errors cause thousands of deaths each year. Over 1.5 million preventable ADEs (ie, medication errors) may occur each year,[4] with 3% of adverse events occurring in the emergency department (ED).[60] Those ADEs and medication errors with serious effects lead to 3.1%–6.2% of all hospital admissions.[57]

In 1997, the cost of a single ADE was estimated to be $2000–$5000.[9,21] In the same era, other studies estimated that the annual cost of ADE morbidity and mortality was greater than $77–177 billion in the ambulatory care setting,[29,44] $2 billion in hospitals,[9,21] and $4 billion in nursing homes.[15] Another study estimated that the annual cost of drug-related morbidity and mortality in the United States in 1997 was $76 billion with a significant part being due to hospitalizations.[45] These costs exclude legal or other costs that accrue to the patient or their families.

DEATHS FROM MEDICATION ERRORS AND ADES

Although medication errors are the most common cause of iatrogenic patient injury, less than 2% results in injuries. Nevertheless, the incidence of ADEs in hospitalized patients is estimated to range from 2% to 20%[20] resulting in 7000 deaths annually in the United States.[52] A retrospective review of hospital death certificates by ICD 9 and ICD 10 codes from 1983 to 2004 revealed an increase of 361% in fatal medication errors and a 33% increase in deaths from ADEs occurring in a patient's home.[78] It also revealed a 3196% increase in fatal medication errors when prescription medications were combined with alcohol and or illicit drugs.[78] According to voluntary MedWatch reports to the FDA, 17% of ADEs were associated with death, 7% were associated with permanent disability, and many others had serious complications. Women and elderly patients were at the highest risk.[72] Reports suggest that 2.5%–21% of all ED visits are for ADEs.[18,37,79] The patients identified in these studies were typically older, triaged to higher severity/acuity levels, and had increased numbers of drug exposures.[79]

NATIONAL COORDINATING COUNCIL FOR MEDICATION ERROR REPORTING AND PREVENTION TAXONOMY

A useful medication error taxonomy, developed by the National Coordinating Council for Medication Error Reporting and Prevention (NCC MERP), classifies medication errors according to severity (Fig. 139–1).[74] Importantly, the categories of least severity (A and B) describe circumstances or events in which the potential to cause error exists, or the error occurs, but does not affect the patient. These "near misses," or "near hits" more correctly, are so frequent that they serve as a critical source of information and education about medication error, but are typically underreported and underappreciated. In one study of 154,816 errors reported by hospitals and health systems to MEDMARX from 1999 to 2001, the majority of the errors were in Category C (47%) and resulted in no patient injury, whereas there were 19 errors in category I, contributing to or resulting in patient death, comprising 0.01%.[84] See Figure 139–1 for definitions of categories. The top four types of the errors were omission (30%), improper dose/quantity (21%), unauthorized medication (13%), and incorrect prescribing (12%). Performance deficit was the most frequently reported cause of error in each of the 3 years of study. It accounted for 43% of all errors, and was more than double nonadherence to established procedures and protocols (20%), the next most frequent cause.[84] See Figure 139–2 for a comparison of errors in the inpatient versus the ED setting. A performance deficit means that the individual making the error had the prerequisite knowledge to avoid the error but failed to do so. There are numerous variables that contribute to performance deficit, including many ergonomic issues such as workload, distractions, resource limitations and staff shortages.[84] Documentation was the third cause of error at 12% and knowledge deficit was fourth at 10%.[84]

TABLE 139–1. Historical Timeline of Medication Safety

1820	United States Pharmacopeia (USP) is established in Washington, DC
1906	The Pure Food and Drugs Act is passed by Congress.
1927	The Bureau of Chemistry is reformed into Food, Drug, and Insecticide Administration and the Bureau of Chemistry and Soils.
1930	The Food, Drug, and Insecticide Administration was renamed the Food and Drug Administration (FDA).
1962	Kefauver-Harris Drug Amendments passed to ensure drug efficacy and greater drug safety.
	President Kennedy proclaims the Consumer Bill of Rights which includes the right to safety, right to be informed, and right to choose.
1963	Representatives from FDA, USP, AMA and American Pharmacists Association form the United States Adopted Names Council to establish drug nomenclature.
1968	The FDA is placed in the Public Health Service after reorganization of the federal government health programs.
1970	The FDA requires the first patient package insert.
1975	The Institute of Safe Medication Practices's (ISMP) work officially begins with a continuing column in *Hospital Pharmacy*.
1987	The first ISMP list of dangerous drug abbreviations is printed in *Nursing '87*.
1989	Agency for Health Care Policy and Research (AHCPR) is established as an agency in the Public Health Service in the Dept. of Health and Human Services.
1991	Institute for Healthcare Improvement is founded as a not-for-profit organization to aid in improvement of healthcare quality.
	USP and ISMP create Medication Error Reporting Program (MERP).
1993	A consolidation of several adverse reaction reporting systems is launched as MedWatch, the FDA voluntary reporting system for problems associated with medical products.
1996	The National Coordinating Council for Medication Error Reporting and Prevention (NCC MERP) is formed.
1997	National Patient Safety Foundation is established with patient safety as its sole purpose.
	ISMP founds a subsidiary, Medical Error Recognition and Revision Strategies (Med. E.R.R.S.), to work with drug companies to predict problems with names, labels, and packaging.
1998	USP launches MEDMARX, an internet-accessible medication errors reporting system for hospitals.
	Founding members of The Leapfrog Group meet to discuss ways to purchase healthcare to influence its quality and affordability.
	ISMP publishes a list of high alert medications.
1999	IOM Report *To Err is Human: Building a Safer Health System*[52] is published.
	The Leapfrog Group founding members establish the reduction of preventable medical errors as their initial focus.
	The National Quality Forum is created as the President's Advisory Commission on Consumer Protection and Quality in the Health Care Industry.
	Agency for Health Care Policy and Research is renamed Agency for Healthcare Research and Quality (AHRQ).
2006	IOM Report *Preventing Medication Errors*[4] is published.
2007	USP and Quantros, a company that collects data on healthcare quality, patient safety and accreditation, partner to run MEDMARX.

MEDICATIONS INVOLVED

FDA reports suggest that opioid analgesics and immune modulators are the commonest medications in which errors resulted in death.[72] The medications most frequently involved in errors and ADEs reported to MEDMARX were insulin, anticoagulants, morphine, and potassium chloride.[84] These medications are considered high alert drugs according to the sentinel event alert system of the Joint Commission. Identifying characteristics of high-risk drugs include low therapeutic index, those with pharmacokinetic interactions, inherent undesirable effects, interactions, classifications as an opioid, newly approved or "off-label" use, and direct-to-consumer promotion.[12] Table 139–2 lists medications commonly reported and their classes of errors.

THE MEDICATION PROCESS

The Medication Process comprises the five stages in the sequence of ordering a medication to its delivery to the patient. The steps are prescribing, transcribing, dispensing, administering, and monitoring.[5] For patients discharged from the ED or hospital, discharging and followup were added.[27] Although the medicating process has only six stages, there are multiple steps within each stage and so the potential for error is high, increasing proportionately as the number of steps and their complexity increases. Figure 139–3 describes typical errors that occur at each stage in the process, along with prevention strategies.

The greatest number of errors resulting in preventable ADEs (medication errors) occurs at the first or prescribing stage.[6] In a study of serious medication errors, 39% were found to occur at the prescribing stage, 12% at transcription, 11% at dispensing, and 38% at administration.[59] In one study of 17,808 inpatient and ED medication orders, 6.2% of orders written involved a prescribing error and 30% of these were likely to harm the patient if they were not discovered.[14] Transcribing errors usually involve poor communication due to illegible handwriting, the use of trailing zeroes, or inappropriate abbreviations. Poor handwriting can lead to confusion, particularly with regard to look-alike and sound-alike medications. The dispensing step is one of the last phases of the medication process where correction and prevention

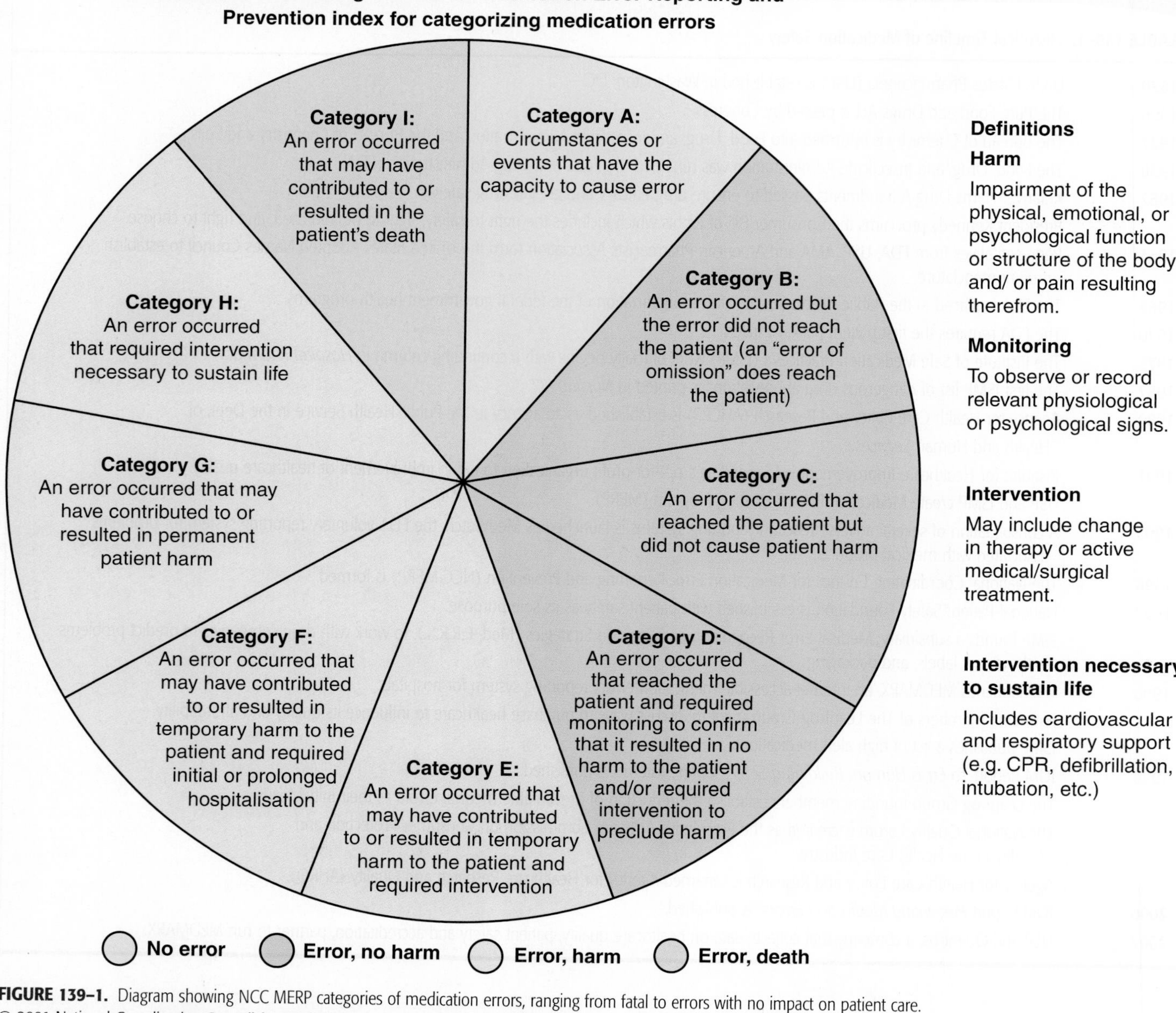
National Coordinating Council for Medication Error Reporting and Prevention index for categorizing medication errors
Category A: Circumstances or events that have the capacity to cause error
Category B: An error occurred but the error did not reach the patient (an "error of omission" does reach the patient)
Category C: An error occurred that reached the patient but did not cause patient harm
Category D: An error occurred that reached the patient and required monitoring to confirm that it resulted in no harm to the patient and/or required intervention to preclude harm
Category E: An error occurred that may have contributed to or resulted in temporary harm to the patient and required intervention
Category F: An error occurred that may have contributed to or resulted in temporary harm to the patient and required initial or prolonged hospitalisation
Category G: An error occurred that may have contributed to or resulted in permanent patient harm
Category H: An error occurred that required intervention necessary to sustain life
Category I: An error occurred that may have contributed to or resulted in the patient's death
Definitions
Harm
Impairment of the physical, emotional, or psychological function or structure of the body and/ or pain resulting therefrom.
Monitoring
To observe or record relevant physiological or psychological signs.
Intervention
May include change in therapy or active medical/surgical treatment.
Intervention necessary to sustain life
Includes cardiovascular and respiratory support (e.g. CPR, defibrillation, intubation, etc.)
No error
Error, no harm
Error, harm
Error, death

FIGURE 139–1. Diagram showing NCC MERP categories of medication errors, ranging from fatal to errors with no impact on patient care.

of an error can occur.[77] A retrospective review suggests that substitution and labeling errors are the most common pharmacy dispensing errors.[86] Errors at the stage of administering medications include incorrect drug, incorrect dose, incorrect route, and a drug given to the wrong patient.

Monitoring and discharging with followup are associated with fewer errors. This phase involves attention to hepatic and renal function, checking xenobiotic concentrations, and attention to and evaluation of drug interactions and pharmacokinetic interactions.[27] Monitoring must be an ongoing process that begins when the patient receives the medication, wherever the patient is in the healthcare system, and continues as long as the individual continues to have the medication prescribed. In the acute stages of treatment, such as in the hospital or ED, the process is especially important and requires optimal three-way linkage between the pharmacy, laboratory, and physician.[85] This process must continue throughout the individual's continued relationship with the healthcare system. In the primary care setting, 17 separate tasks were identified from the initial decision to order a laboratory test through to getting the result to the patient.[39]

Communication issues are very important at all stages in this process. All information, whether printed, spoken, or otherwise communicated, must be transmitted in a clear, unambiguous, and timely fashion with avoidance of abbreviations. Physician's handwriting is still an important issue. Furthermore, in its 2004 National Patient Safety Goals, the Joint Commission developed a minimum list of five sets of dangerous abbreviations, acronyms, and symbols that should not be used, and proposed preferred terms.[47] The Institute for Safe Medication Practices (ISMP) also published a comprehensive list.[43] Communication is also especially important between physicians and patients. In a study of 661

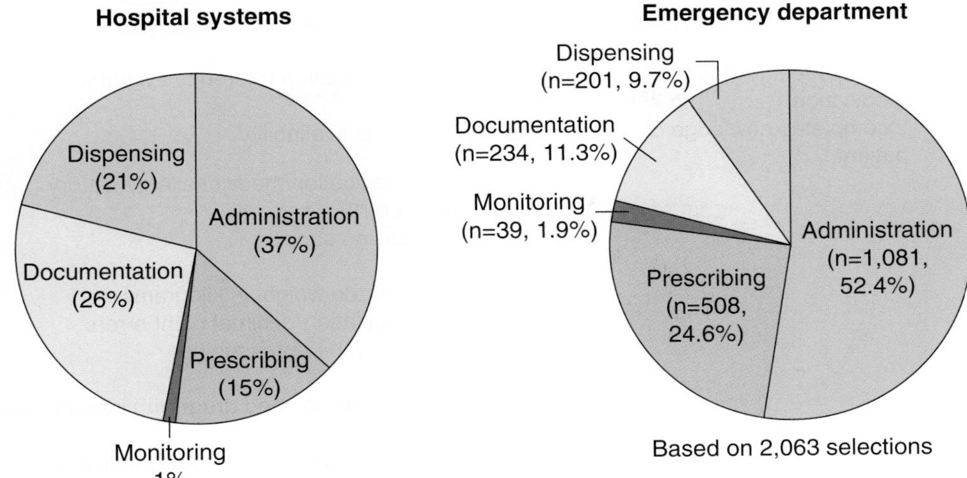

FIGURE 139–2. Diagram showing MEDMARX data for (A) hospital systems and (B) specifically for the Emergency Department. Adapted from United States Pharmacopeial Convention, www.usp.org.

patients in four primary care practices, patient reports of medication side effects to their physicians led to changed therapies in 76% of cases. A failure to identify medication-related symptoms and change therapy resulted in 21% ameliorable and 2% preventable ADEs. Ameliorable ADEs were defined as those in which "the severity or duration could have been reduced substantially had different actions been taken."[95] The study illustrates the "Swiss Cheese Model of Error."[80] The first error of a preventable ADE is compounded by the second error of failing to identify it.

TABLE 139–2. Medications or Classes Commonly Responsible for Medication Errors

Acetaminophen	Electrolyte replacement:
Albuterol	Potassium chloride
Antibiotics:	Fluid replacement therapies
Amoxicillin	Furosemide
Cefazolin	Insulin, other antidiabetics
Cephalexin	Opioids:
Levofloxacin	Fentanyl
Penicillin	Meperidine
Vancomycin	Methadone
Anticoagulants:	Morphine
Heparin	Opioid-acetaminophen combinations
Warfarin	Oxycodone
Antineoplastics	Sedatives
Aspirin	Benzodiazepines
Cardiovascular:	
Clopidogrel	
Digoxin	
Inotropes	
Vasopressors	

SPECIAL AT-RISK POPULATIONS

Important medication safety issues exist for children and older adults, a problem that is exacerbated by their underrepresentation or exclusion from clinical trials. It is estimated, for example, that only a third of the medications used to treat children have been adequately tested in this population.[24] Similar concerns apply to medications used in older adults.[41]

PEDIATRIC CONSIDERATIONS

Adverse exposure to medications may occur during pregnancy and lactation and subsequent errors may occur in all settings: the home, in ambulatory care, the ED, hospital floor, pediatric intensive care unit (PICU), and neonatal intensive care unit (NICU). Approximately 1 in 6.4 pediatric orders results in an error that reaches the patients.[68] In particular, one study showed that 31% of errors in a pediatric population resulted in harm or death compared to 13% in adults.[28] More errors can occur at each stage of the medication process in children and are likely related to calculation requirements and weight-based dosing.[48] Errors occur in the home environment with nonprescription medications, but the true incidence is unknown. In one survey, the errors associated with home antipyretic use were estimated at almost 50%.[69] These errors are typically associated with underdosing, which can be harmless although the converse may be life threatening.[83] In the ambulatory setting, the incidence is unknown but one study identified "numerous" errors in prescription writing in a pediatric clinic.[93] In the ED setting, the error rate was estimated at 10% of all charts.[54] One study showed an increased risk of errors in nonacademic or rural EDs.[51] A retrospective chart review of 177 pediatric charts in 4 rural EDs revealed that 69 of the 135 patients who received medications had 84 different medication errors identified. The outcomes of these errors were in NCCMERP Categories A-D (see Fig. 139–1).[67] Hospitalized children experience up to three times the rate of medication errors and potential ADEs as do adults.[50] The incidence for medication errors of hospitalized children is estimated at about 6% for all orders written; the majority (74%) of these occurred at the prescribing stage and approximately 20% were classified as potentially harmful.[33] Generally, children in the intensive care unit appear to be at higher risk for errors,

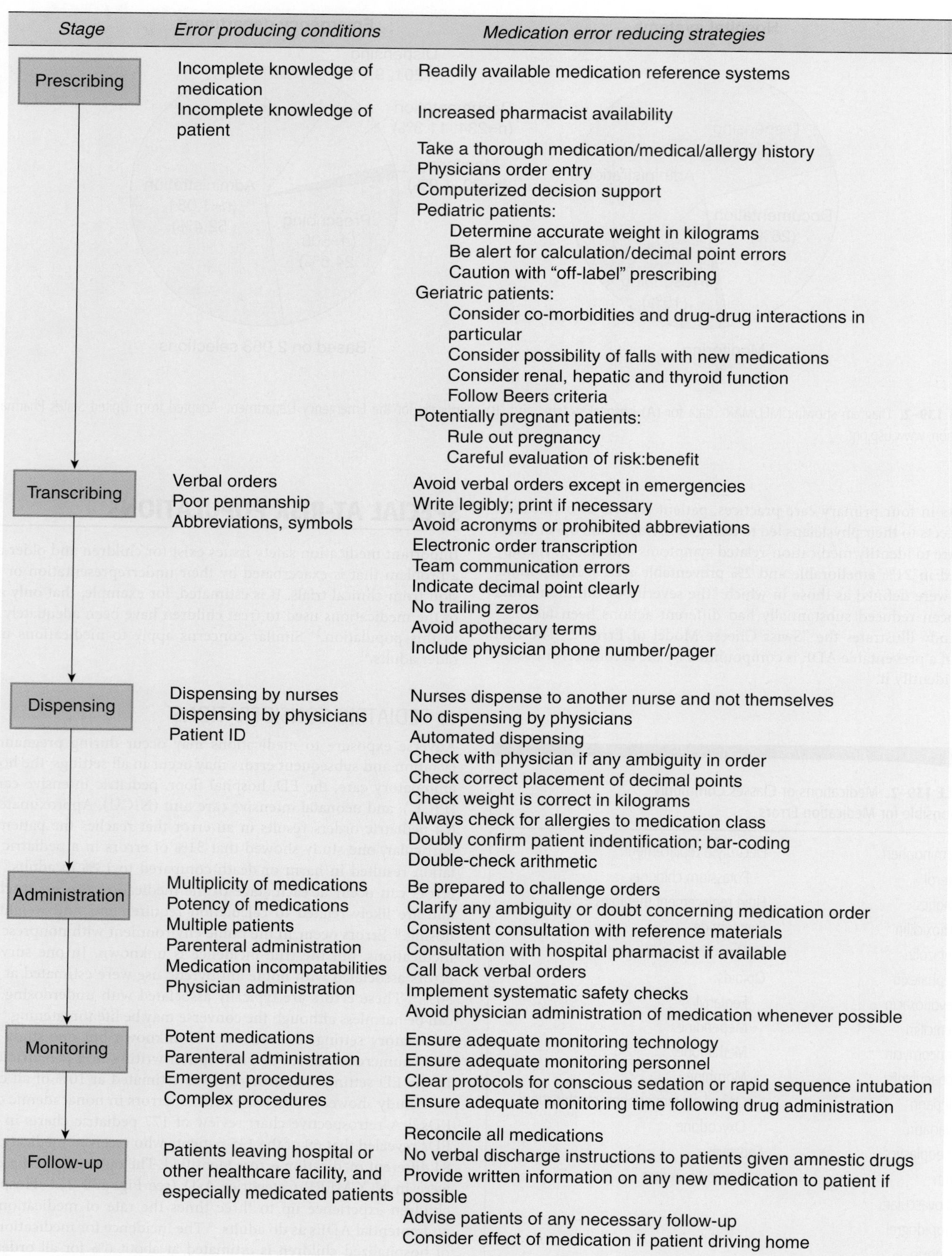

Stage	Error producing conditions	Medication error reducing strategies
Prescribing	Incomplete knowledge of medication Incomplete knowledge of patient	Readily available medication reference systems Increased pharmacist availability Take a thorough medication/medical/allergy history Physicians order entry Computerized decision support Pediatric patients: Determine accurate weight in kilograms Be alert for calculation/decimal point errors Caution with "off-label" prescribing Geriatric patients: Consider co-morbidities and drug-drug interactions in particular Consider possibility of falls with new medications Consider renal, hepatic and thyroid function Follow Beers criteria Potentially pregnant patients: Rule out pregnancy Careful evaluation of risk:benefit
Transcribing	Verbal orders Poor penmanship Abbreviations, symbols	Avoid verbal orders except in emergencies Write legibly; print if necessary Avoid acronyms or prohibited abbreviations Electronic order transcription Team communication errors Indicate decimal point clearly No trailing zeros Avoid apothecary terms Include physician phone number/pager
Dispensing	Dispensing by nurses Dispensing by physicians Patient ID	Nurses dispense to another nurse and not themselves No dispensing by physicians Automated dispensing Check with physician if any ambiguity in order Check correct placement of decimal points Check weight is correct in kilograms Always check for allergies to medication class Doubly confirm patient indentification; bar-coding Double-check arithmetic
Administration	Multiplicity of medications Potency of medications Multiple patients Parenteral administration Medication incompatabilities Physician administration	Be prepared to challenge orders Clarify any ambiguity or doubt concerning medication order Consistent consultation with reference materials Consultation with hospital pharmacist if available Call back verbal orders Implement systematic safety checks Avoid physician administration of medication whenever possible
Monitoring	Potent medications Parenteral administration Emergent procedures Complex procedures	Ensure adequate monitoring technology Ensure adequate monitoring personnel Clear protocols for conscious sedation or rapid sequence intubation Ensure adequate monitoring time following drug administration
Follow-up	Patients leaving hospital or other healthcare facility, and especially medicated patients	Reconcile all medications No verbal discharge instructions to patients given amnestic drugs Provide written information on any new medication to patient if possible Advise patients of any necessary follow-up Consider effect of medication if patient driving home

FIGURE 139–3. Stages in the ordering and delivery of a medication, and typical errors associated with each stage. (Croskerry P, Shapiro M, Campbell S, et al. Profiles in patient safety: medication errors in the emergency department. *Acad Emerg Med*. 2004;11:298).

presumably reflecting the increased complexity of disease and the medications used.[51] Dosing errors and the intravenous route are the most commonly reported errors with dosing of antimicrobials and intravenous fluids being the most common medications involved.[28,32,50] Errors and discrepancies found in hospital discharge instructions could lead to patient harm[46] (see Chap. 31).

GERIATRIC CONSIDERATIONS

Medication errors in older adults occur throughout the healthcare continuum: the home, ambulatory care, in nursing homes, in the assisted-living setting, and in the hospital (Chap. 32). Adults over 65 years of age have a relative risk of 2.37 for drug complications and 4.12 for medication errors compared to patients younger than age 65.[16] The incidence of medication error at home with nonprescription medications is unknown but, for reasons outlined below, would be expected to exceed that of the younger adult population. Using a variety of methodologies, ADEs were evaluated for a 12-month period in a multispeciality ambulatory care practice in a cohort of 27,617 Medicare enrollees, equivalent to over 30,000 person-years of observation. Extrapolating their findings, to the estimated 38 million Medicare enrollees (those 65 or older), would predict nearly 2 million ADEs annually, of which >25% would be considered preventable and about 180,000 fatal or life threatening.[36]

Of the more than 1.5 million nursing home residents in the United States, the average resident uses six different medications, and 20% use ten or more.[13] Extrapolating from the findings of a study of 18 community-based nursing homes in Massachusetts over a 1-year period would predict 350,000 ADEs annually, more than half of which would be preventable.[35] Fatal or life-threatening ADEs would represent 20,000 of these predicted events of which 80% would be preventable. Approximately one million other seniors live in assisted-living facilities, and are vulnerable to medication errors for a variety of reasons including inadequate physician support, inadequately trained staff, and staffing shortages. ADEs cause 10.5% of hospital admissions for geriatric patients and are the most common type of adverse event occurring in hospitalized elderly patients.[60,97] Medications prescribed leading to ADEs and ED visits include oral anticoagulants and antiplatelet medications, antidiabetics, and those medications with narrow therapeutic indexes.[19] These xenobiotics result in nearly 50% of ADE-related visits to the ED but are only prescribed during 9.4% of outpatient visits.[19]

Addressing these issues is becoming increasingly important as the US Census Bureau predicts an increase of 62 million in the number of Americans 65 years or older by the year 2025 and a 68% increase in the 85 or older population that may be at an even higher risk.[3]

Advancing age brings with it several important considerations from the point of view of medication safety:

1. There is an increasing morbidity with age, and therefore an increasing likelihood of receiving medication. Comorbidities and chronic disease increase the number of concurrent medications, and therefore the number of potential interactions.
2. Frailty and cognitive decline in older adults may result in errors following self-administration and may require the assistance of family members or others to achieve proper use.
3. Alterations in medication absorption, metabolism, distribution, and elimination may all affect the efficacy of the medication (see Chaps. 8 and 32).

Criteria were developed in both the United States[10,11,31] and Canada[70] to determine appropriateness of medication prescribing for nursing home residents. Forty-eight medications or classes of medications to avoid, and medications to avoid in the presence of 20 diseases/conditions were identified.[31] The prevalence of inappropriate medication use in older adults has been and continues to be estimated in the 12%–40% range.[87] Older adult patients medicated with benzodiazepines, for example, have a 4-fold increase in falls. Significant differences within the class of benzodiazepines were found: the risk of injury associated with benzodiazepine use generally appeared to be independent of half-life; there was no increase associated with long-acting diazepam use, nor was there a dose-effect, whereas there was an increased risk associated with the use of the short-acting oxazepam. Flurazepam and chlordiazepoxide (both long-acting) were associated with a 50%–60% increase in risk of injury.[88] There is an alternate approach to develop specific clinical indicators of preventable medication-related morbidity (PMRM) in older adults. The four unique elements of a PMRM include that it be recognizable, foreseeable, identifiable, and controllable as developed by an expert consensus on 52 clinical indicators.[66] In a followup study, the top five indicators were found to account for almost half of all PMRMs.[65] These indicators included four or more diagnoses, four or more prescribers, six or more prescription medications used, antihypertensive drug use, and male gender[65] (see Chap. 32).

RESPONSE TO MEDICATION ERROR

One of the leading causes of medication errors is human performance deficit. Invariably a human action will precede the ADE, and this temporal contiguity of action and consequence inevitably generates a tendency to blame someone; this will usually be the last person to have had contact with the patient. In recent years, however, a consensus has emerged that blaming people for errors is counterproductive. The number of ADEs that result from truly egregious behavior is very small, and more often than not the explanation will be found within the system. Root cause analysis (RCA), a term originally used to investigate major industrial events, is a technique that provides a structured, process-oriented analysis of sentinel events. Its use was mandated by the Joint Commission in accredited hospitals in 1997. It is a time-consuming process requiring multidisciplinary teams with specialized training, and is subject to bias and methodologic limitations.[91] Nevertheless, a judiciously conducted RCA may provide insights into systemic failures underlying the ADE, and identify areas that require change. An alternative approach, a clinical incident analysis protocol, was developed that more appropriately shifts the emphasis from the individual to the system.[90] The clinical incident analysis protocol utilizes seven factors as the basis for an investigation. Some organizations have developed a hybrid combining these two approaches. Both RCA and clinical incident analysis are conducted retrospectively, and therefore subject to retrospective bias.

An alternative approach is failure mode and effect analysis (FMEA), which proactively attempts to identify potential errors, to initiate preventive measures. A multidisciplinary group is utilized in the FMEA approach to identify a process or subprocess that needs analysis to identify the steps of the process and determine the risk/likelihood/severity of failure of each step. Once this phase is accomplished, the team prioritizes a high risk step and conducts a root-cause analysis to make recommendations on redesigning the step. The establishment modifications are analyzed in their performance to determine change and decrease in risk. This process is designed as a quality control and assurance in order to protect the proceedings from legal investigation.[2]

REDUCING ERRORS

In order to reduce medication errors, each hospital should simplify, standardize, and stratify processes and communication. The medication process should be carefully automated with computer order entry and bar coding as extensively as the system will allow. Limitations of attention and vigilance should be understood and the reporting of errors in a nonpunitive environment should be encouraged.[59] Improving information access, error proofing, reducing reliance on memory, training, and the use of buffers or redundancy to prevent inevitable errors should also be encouraged.[58] Each time a medication is given the focus should be "right drug, right dose, right route, right patient, at the right time." Regulatory agencies such as the US FDA and the European Medicines Agency (EMEA) have developed initiatives to evaluate drug names for their error potentials.

In 2003, the American Academy of Pediatrics Committees on Drugs and on Hospital Care developed a position statement regarding the reduction of medication errors in the pediatric population. The recommendations can be adapted to all hospital settings to patients of all ages. Appropriate staffing was encouraged in addition to dependency on the resources of the pharmacy, standardization of hospital equipment and protocols, and the development of a nonpunitive barrier-free system to report and easily track errors. The committee encouraged improved communication skills and an enhanced team environment such that any member of the team should be able to calculate the dose of a medication and confirm that the dose prescribed is the correct dose for the particular child.[22]

For older adults, prescribers should review medication indications and avoid age bias. Polypharmacy should be limited, but medications should be prescribed as necessary. Dosing should be adjusted as needed based on renal and hepatic function. Computer physician order entry with decision support and bar coded medication administration should be implemented.[81]

HUMAN FACTORS/HUMAN PERFORMANCE DEFICIT

Human factors lead to many medication errors. In fact, it is not surprising that human performance deficits are the primary causes of medication errors in such an extremely complex medical environment. This environment is both burdened and enriched by many inherited properties. Human factors and ergonomics theory draws on a variety of disciplines including industrial engineering, industrial psychology, cognitive psychology, and information technology. Much can be done to optimize the interface between humans and the work environment and to ensure that systems operate more efficiently. As a general principle, it would be preferable if the dominant purpose in designing medical devices and processes was that they fit human users, and not the converse.

Human performance deficits such as diminished memory, sleep deprivation, depression, and distractions contribute to errors. Table 139–3 lists some of the more common human performance deficits. Such errors often manifest as simple slips of action, or execution failures, arising from distraction or attentional capture by something other than the task at hand.[80] Vigilance is better maintained in individuals who are well rested and working without interruption or distraction in a well-designed environment. Fewer medication errors occur in optimally designed environments.[59]

Another factor that contributes to errors is the assignment of a new role to a provider such as asking physicians to dispense or administer medications. Pharmacists are the only professional group formally trained in dispensing medication, and not surprisingly, their presence is associated with a lower medication-dispensing error rate.[61] Nurses administer medications because they receive such training and the administration should be restricted to them except during certain

TABLE 139–3. Common Factors That may Adversely Affect Human Performance[26,84]

Fatigue
Sleep deprivation/debt
Fragmentation, transitions of care
Interruptions
Distractions
Attentional capture
Diminished motivation/morale
Increased work acuity/cognitive load
Poor workplace ergonomics
Inadequate resource availability (RACQITO)[a]
Inexperience

[a] RACQITO refers to Resource Availability Continuous Quality Improvement Trade-Off.[26]

circumstances such as procedural sedation.[27] Depressed residents made 6.2 times as many medication errors as nondepressed residents.[30] Sleep deprivation and improper supervision, both human performance deficit problems, were highlighted intially after the Libby Zion case, in which a patient on phenelzine developed a fatal serotonin syndrome following the administration of meperidine by a sleep-deprived and inadequately supervised intern. Previous interns working a traditional schedule of call every third night with extended work shifts (36 hours) made 35.9% more serious medical errors than those with the current reduced work schedule.[56] In particular, there were 20.8% more serious medication errors during the older work schedules compared with the current reduced hour schedule.[56] In 2008, an Institute of Medicine study addressed resident work hours and patient safety. This report recommended residents be provided with designated sleep time during each day and rest periods each week in order to decrease the risk of fatigue-related medical errors.[89]

A particularly important goal for human performance deficit is the reduction of cognitive load. Many medication errors originate from cognitive failings because of interruptions, distractions, inexperience, or simple overloading—referred to as performance deficit. Further efforts must be directed at strategies to reduce cognitive failure. The adoption of some very simple strategies based on human factors engineering principles will reduce error, such as simplification of the number of steps involved, reducing reliance on memory, applying cognitive forcing strategies,[26] and using cognitive aids. One particularly useful aid is the color-coded Broselow-Luten system, for pediatric medication dosing.[63] This approach has the potential for further development to improve the safety of nonprescription medications and other potentially dangerous products used in the home. A universal standard color-coding drug labeling system has been proposed in anesthesia to reduce between-class medication errors.[1,76]

KNOWLEDGE DEFICITS

The two most common factors contributing to prescribing errors are related to knowledge deficits. These deficits include lack of knowledge about the drug and lack of knowledge about the patient.[59,62] Knowledge deficits are also likely due to the number of medications that have been introduced to providers. With the large number of medications prescribed and the continuing release of new medications, it is difficult to know all medication interactions, side effects, and contraindications. References should be contemporaneously available to healthcare providers to assist in decreasing prescribing errors.[77]

Knowledge deficits may also effect dosing calculations and drug ordering. This may be related in part to the lack of formal education regarding the medication process during undergraduate medical training. Only 10% of medical students answered dose calculation questions correctly.[96] However, students in their final year of training performed much better than students in the lower years.[96] It is unclear where the knowledge was obtained by the students in the higher years. Specific training is needed in both of these areas of calculation and order-writing. Improvements have been demonstrated following a short educational intervention,[75] but it is unclear how long this knowledge is retained. Generally, there appears to be a tacit assumption that these skills will be acquired during clinical training, but this study suggested that this knowledge might not be acquired independently and that specific training is indicated.

The prevailing emphasis in physician training is on knowledge acquisition. Less time is spent inculcating critical thinking skills and/or teaching reasoning, the assumption being made that these are passively acquired during the process of training. Although this is partially true it does not exclude opportunities to improve these cognitive faculties by direct intervention.[25]

COMMUNICATION

Improved team communication should result in fewer medication errors. Orders should be written clearly, or computerized physician order entry (CPOE, discussed in detail in Information Technology section) should be used. Orders should optimally include the indications for the medication. Both generic and trade names should be included in orders so that confusion with look-alike/sound-alike drugs may be avoided. Abbreviations should have limited use and trailing zeros should be eliminated. Verbal orders should be used sparingly due to the high risk of sound-alike medications and confusion with dosing.[77] If a verbal order is necessary, it should be restated to the physician prior to administration to ensure that it is correct.

Communication theory should receive more emphasis in healthcare training. Good communication skills both within and among disciplines and especially between practitioners and their patients will limit errors. As patients are admitted, transferred within, and discharged from healthcare facilities it is essential that precise communication as to what medications, strengths, and doses the patient is receiving occurs. Any changes that have occurred must be accurately recorded in the process of medication reconciliation. This effort was adopted by the Joint Commission in 2005 and continues to be an important National Patient Safety Goal. As with other aspects of patient safety, these issues should be formally introduced into the education curriculum.

INFORMATION TECHNOLOGY: COMPUTER PRESCRIBER ORDER ENTRY AND BARCODING

Information technology (IT) in healthcare has been ponderously slow to develop compared with its use in other organizations, but it is now gathering momentum and has obvious potential to improve patient safety.[7] On the other hand, as considerable gains may be made, new technology can also be expected to introduce new types of errors. The US Pharmacopeia announced in 2004 that nearly 20% of 235,159 medication errors reported to MEDMARX involved computerization or automation.[84] One study evaluating CPOE in a tertiary care hospital found that the system actually facilitated a wide variety of medication error risks.[38] Another study identified 24 different types of failures associated with CPOE but suggested that many could be easily corrected, in particular by concentrating on organizational factors.[53] However, more detailed insights have been offered into why process-supporting IT systems fail.[94] Much of the data involved in the medication process are relatively straightforward, amenable to rapid and efficient processing, including cross-checking with patient medication history and evaluating for drug interactions (an example of decision support).

Computerized order entry with decision support has been shown to reduce the incidence of serious medication errors by 50%–55% once the transitional instability has passed.[8,64] This approach mainly reduces errors at the prescribing stage of the medication process and, while likely to prevent 80% of prescribing errors that led to no patient harm, the errors most likely to cause patient harm may not be as amenable to reduction as these errors may be related to dispensation, administration, or monitoring.[14]

In high risk populations, CPOE reduces medication errors. In children, CPOE with substantive decision support reduced ADEs (including medication errors) and potential ADEs in an inpatient pediatrics ward.[40] It also decreased the rate of nonintercepted medication errors by 7% although there was no change in the rate of patient harm.[50,92] In the neonatal ICU, CPOE eliminated all calculation errors as decision support included an automatic dosage calculator.[23] In geriatric medication errors, CPOE resulted in less potentially inappropriate medication prescribing through decision alerts which led to a pharmacist call to the prescriber that offered alternative choices of medications if possible.[71]

Use of barcoding for dispensing and administration of medication ensures that the correct drug is given to the intended patient at the dose intended. Barcoding significantly decreased the relative risk of targeted, preventable ADEs by 47%–50% in a neonatal Intensive Care Unit.[73]

Unit dose dispensing systems, usually in association with CPOE and barcoding of medications, reduced monthly errors from five to none in the inpatient setting.[34] The package sent from pharmacy is prepared to administer to a specific patient at the appropriate dose, eliminating the need for the nurse to draw up medications resulting in fewer errors.

SERVICE-BASED CLINICAL PHARMACISTS

Clinical pharmacists are being stationed in high-risk areas such as the ICUs, the pediatrics services, and EDs to indentify and prevent medication errors. In one ICU study, the input of a clinical pharmacist during rounds saved an estimated $270,000 annually in costs of rehospitalization due to ADEs.[61] The involvement of a clinical pharmacist in work rounds of an adult ICU reduced preventable ADEs by 66%.[61] The introduction of clinical pharmacists in pediatric services has been credited with a 94% reduction of potential ADEs and medication errors.[50] In particular, the addition of pharmacists in the Pediatric Intensive Care Units (PICU) reduced the serious medication error rate by 80%.[49] One study showed that pharmacists in three EDs identified 2200 interventions with an estimated savings of $488,000. This savings came from lower-cost medications, reduced length of stay, and fewer readmissions.[82] Another study showed that there were 16 errors per 100 medication orders in the control group (without a pharmacist) while the intervention group (pharmacist present in the ED) only had 5 errors per 100 medication orders, resulting in a 67% reduction.[17]

However, fiscal restrictions will inevitably mitigate against the expansion of service pharmacists as cost-benefit arguments will be applied. An unintended consequence of having a clinical pharmacist present may be that nurses, residents, and attending physicians will always defer to them and consequently spend less time developing and maintaining their own skills for off-hour periods when such help may not be available.

MEDICAL TOXICOLOGIST IN MEDICATION SAFETY

Medical toxicologists are in a unique position to investigate causes and help decrease the incidence of both medication errors and ADEs in the institutions where they work. With their specialized knowledge and training in pharmacology, poisoning, and clinical medicine, medical toxicologists can also aid in the prediction, identification, and management of ADEs. Medical toxicologists should optimally be involved in Pharmacy and Therapeutics and Medication Safety committees at their institutions. They should educate the providers at their hospitals on ways to reduce errors and encourage diligent reporting of medication errors to the hospital and the national databases such as MedWatch at FDA. They should also encourage drug manufacturers to be diligent in alerting physicians with regard to identified problems.[55]

SUMMARY

Medications are the principal commerce of modern medicine, and medication safety is of paramount importance to healthcare systems. The delivery of medications safely to patients is a more complex process than was originally imagined. It affects patients of all ages but is particularly important in pediatrics and geriatrics. With a new industrywide focus on patient safety, renewed attention and energy has been directed to the problem. Healthcare providers should be aware of why errors occur and how they can be prevented in order to improve patient and medication safety. Many innovations, especially in the field of information technology, hold promise for significant improvement. Focus should be on computerized order entry (CPOE), barcoding, unit dose dispensing, avoidance of look-alike/sound-alike medications, and education. Resource utilization such as use of a clinical pharmacist and reference textbooks or handbooks should be encouraged. Most of all, in order to learn from errors when they occur and to prevent them in the future, communication and nonpunitive local and national reporting must be encouraged.

The process can no longer be perceived as a simple tripartite relationship between the patient, healthcare providers, and pharmacist. Patient safety requires a collaborative effort particularly with the medication manufacturer, but also federal regulation authorities, independent research organizations, error theorists, hospital administrators and managers, information technologists, nurses, cognitive psychologists, human factors ergonomists, and chronobiologists and all of the physicians involved with a patient's care. Input from the medical toxicologist can also improve medication safety. A new multidisciplinary approach may considerably reduce current error rates in the future. In this way tangible and measurable gains can be made in this area of patient safety.

ACKNOWLEDGMENTS

Patrick Crosskerry, MD, PhD contributed to this chapter in a previous edition.

REFERENCES

1. Abeysekera A, Bergman IJ, Kluger MT, Short TG. Drug error in anaesthetic practice: a review of 896, reports from the Australian Incident Monitoring Study database. *Anaesthesia.* 2005;60:220-227.
2. American Society for Healthcare Risk Management. *Strategies and Tips of Maximizing Failure Mode Effects Analysis in Your Organization.* Chicago, IL: American Society for Healthcare Risk Management; 2002.
3. Arnett RH III, Blank LA, Brown AP, et al. National Health Expenditures 1988: Office of National Cost Estimates. Health Care Finance Rev. 1990;11:1-41.
4. Aspen P, Wolcott J, Bootman JL, et al. Committee on Identifying and Preventing Medication Errors Eds. Preventing Medication Errors. Washington DC: National Academy Press; 2006.
5. Bates DW. Using information technology to reduce rates of medication errors in hospitals. *BMJ.* 2000;320:788-791.
6. Bates DW, Boyle DL, Vander Vliet MB, et al. Relationship between medication errors and adverse drug events. *J Gen Intern Med.* 1995;10:199-205
7. Bates DW, Gawande AA. Improving safety with information technology. *N Engl J Med.* 2003;348:2526-2534.
8. Bates DW, Leape LL, Cullen DJ, et al. Effect of computerized physician order entry and a team intervention on prevention of serious medication errors. *JAMA.* 1998;280(15):1311-131.
9. Bates DW, Spell N, Cullen DJ, et al. The costs of adverse drug events in hospitalized patients. Adverse Drug Events Prevention Study Group. *JAMA.* 1997;277:307-311.
10. Beers MH. Explicit criteria for determining potentially inappropriate medication use by the elderly. *Arch Intern Med.* 1997;157:1531-1536.
11. Beers MH, Ouslander JG, Rollingher J, et al. Explicit criteria for determining inappropriate medication use in nursing home residents. *Arch Intern Med.* 1991;151:1825-1832.
12. Benjamin DM. Reducing Medication errors and increasing patient safety: case studies in clinical pharmacology. *J Clin Pharmacol..* 2003;43:768-783.
13. Bernabei R, Gambassi G, Lapane K, et al. Characteristics of the SAGE database: a new resource for research on outcomes in long-term care. *J Gerontol A, Biol Sci Med Sci.* 1999;54:M25-M33.
14. Bobb A, Gleason K, Husch M, et al. The epidemiology of prescribing errors. The potential impact of computerized prescriber order entry. *Arch Intern Med.* 2004;164:785-792.
15. Bootman JL, Harrison DL, Cox E. The health care cost of drug-related morbidity and mortality in nursing facilities. *Arch Intern Med.* 1997;157:2089-2096.
16. Brennan TA, Leape LL, Laird NM. Incidence of adverse events and negligence in hospitalized patients. Results of the Harvard Medical Practice Study I. *N Engl J Med.* 1991;324:370-376.
17. Brown JN, Barnes CL, Beasley B, et al.. Effect of pharmacists on medication errors in an emergency department. *Am J Health-Syst Pharm.* 2008; 65: 330-333.
18. Budnitz DS, Pollock DA, Weidenbach KN, Mendelsohn AB, Schroeder TJ, Annest JL. National surveillance of emergency department visits for outpatient adverse drug events. *JAMA.* 2006;296(15):1858-1866.
19. Budnitz DS, Shehab N, Kegler SR, et al. Medication use leading to emergency department visits for adverse drug events in older adults. *Ann Intern Med.* 2007;147:755-765.
20. Classen D. Medication safety: moving from illusion to reality. *JAMA.* 2003;289:1154-1156.
21. Classen DC, Pestotnick SL, Evans RS, et al. Adverse drug events in hospitalized patients: excess length of stay, extra costs, and attributable mortality. *JAMA.* 1997;277:301-306.
22. Committee on Drugs and Committee on Hospital Care. American Academy of Pediatrics Policy Statement. Prevention of medication errors in the pediatric inpatient setting. *Pediatrics.* 2003;112:431-436.
23. Cordero L, Kuehn L, Kumar RR, Mekhjian HS Impact of computerized physician order entry on clinical practice in a newborn intensive care unit. *J Perinatol.* 2004;24(2):88-93.
24. Cote C, Kaufmann R, Troendle G, Lambert H. Is the "therapeutic orphan" about to be adopted? *Pediatrics.* 1996;98:118-123.
25. Croskerry PG, The Cognitive Imperative: thinking about how we think. *Acad Emerg Med.* 2000;7:1223-1231.
26. Croskerry P. The importance of cognitive errors in diagnosis and strategies to prevent them. *Acad Med.* 2003;78:1-6.
27. Croskerry P, Shapiro M, Campbell S, et al. Profiles in patient safety: medication errors in the emergency department. *Acad Emerg Med.* 2004;11:289-299.
28. Crowley E, Williams R, Cousins D. Medication errors in children: a descriptive summary of medication error reports submitted to the United States Pharmacopeia. *Curr Ther Res.* 2001;26:627-640.
29. Ernst FR, Grizzle AJ. Drug-related morbidity and mortality: updating the cost-of-illness model. *J Am Pharm Assoc.* 2001;41:192-199.
30. Fahrenkopf AM, Sectish TC, Barger LK, et al. Rates of medication errors among depressed and burnt out residents: prospective cohort study. *BMJ.* 2008;336:488-491.
31. Fick DM, Cooper JW, Wade WE, et al. Updating the Beers criteria for potentially inappropriate medication use in older adults. *Arch Intern Med.* 2003;163:2716-2724.

32. Folli HL, Poole RL, Benitz WE, Russo JC. Medication error prevention by clinical pharmacists in two children's hospitals. *Pediatrics.* 1987;79(5):718-722.
33. Fortescue EB, Kaushal R, Landrigan CP, et al. Prioritizing strategies for preventing medication errors and adverse drug events in pediatric inpatients. *Pediatrics.* 2003;111:722-729.
34. Gard JW, Starnes HM, Morrow EL Sanchez PJ, Perlman JM Reducing antimicrobial dosing errors in a neonatal intensive care unit. *Am J Health Syst Pharm.* 1995;15;52(14):1508, 1512-1513.
35. Gurwitz JH, Field TS, Avorn J, et al. Incidence and preventability of adverse drug events in nursing homes. *Am J Med.* 2000;109:87-94.
36. Gurwitz JH, Field TS, Harrold LR, et al. Incidence and preventability of adverse drug events among older persons in the ambulatory setting. *JAMA.* 2003;289:1107-1116.
37. Hafner JW, Belknap SM, Squillante MD, et al. Adverse drug events in the emergency department. *Ann Emerg Med.* 2002;39:258-267.
38. Hersh W. Health care information technology: progress and barriers. *JAMA.* 2004;292:2273-2274.
39. Hickner JM, Fernald DH, Harris DM, et al. Issues and initiatives in the testing process in primary care physician offices. *Jt Comm J Qual Patient Saf.* 2005;31:81-89.
40. Holdsworth MT, Fichtl RE, Raisch DW, Hewryk A, Behta M, Mendez-Rico E, Wong CL, Cohen J, Bostwick S, Greenwald BM. Impact of computerized prescriber order entry on the incidence of adverse drug events in pediatric inpatients. *Pediatrics.* 2007;120(5):1058-1066.
41. Hutchins LF, Unger JM, Crowley JJ, et al. Underrepresentation of patients 65, years of age or older in cancer-treatment trials. *N Engl J Med.* 1999;341: 2061-2067.
42. ISMP Medication Safety Alert! 19, April 2000;5:8.
43. ISMP Medication Safety Alert! Error-prone abbreviations, symbols, and dose designations 27, November 2003;8:24.
44. Johnson JA, Bootman JL. Drug-related morbidity and mortality: a cost-of-illness model. *Arch Intern Med.* 1995;155:1949-1956.
45. Johnson JA, Bootman JL. Drug-related morbidity and mortality and the economic impact of pharmaceutical care. *Am J Health Syst Pharm.* 1997;54(5):554-558.
46. Johnson KB, Butta JK, Donohue PK, et al. Discharging patients with prescriptions instead of medications: sequelae in a teaching hospital. *Pediatrics.* 1996;97:481-485.
47. Joint Commission on Accreditation of Healthcare Organizations, National Patient Safety Goal #2: Communication—Prohibited abbreviations, 2004.
48. Kaushal R, Barker KN, Bates DW. How can information technology improve patient safety and reduce medication errors in children's health care? *Arch Pediatr Adolesc Med.* 2001;155(9):1002-1007.
49. Kaushal R, Bates D, Mckenna KJ, et al. Ward-based clinical pharmacists and serious medication errors in pediatric inpatients. Paper presented at the Proceedings of the Annual Meeting of the National Academy of Health, June 28, 2003, Nashville, TN.
50. Kaushal R, Bates DW, Landrigan C, et al. Medication errors and adverse drug events in pediatric inpatients. *JAMA.* 2001;285:2114-2120.
51. Kaushal R, Jaggi T, Walsh K, et al. Pediatric medication errors: what do we know? What gaps remain? *Ambul Pediatr.* 2004;4:73-81.
52. Kohn LT, Corrigan JM, Donaldson MS. Committee on Safety of Medicines, eds. *To Err is Human: Building a Safer Health System.* Washington, DC: National Academy Press;, 1999.
53. Koppel R, Metlay JP, Cohen A, et al. Role of computerized physician order entry systems in facilitating medication errors. *JAMA.* 2005;293:1197-1203.
54. Kozer E, Scolnick D, Macpherson A, et al. Variables associated with medication errors in pediatric emergency medicine. *Pediatrics.* 2002;110:737-742.
55. Kulig K. American College of Medical Toxicology Position Statement: medication errors and adverse drug reactions or events. *Int J Med Toxicol.* 2001;4:11.
56. Landrigan CP, Rothschild JM, Cronin JW, et al. Effect of reducing interns' work hours on serious medical errors in intensive care units. *N Engl J Med.* 2004;351:1838-1848.
57. Lazarou J, Pomeranz BH, Corey PN. Incidence of adverse drug reactions in hospitalized patients: a meta-analysis of prospective studies. *JAMA.* 1998;279:1200-1205.
58. Leape LL. Error in medicine. *JAMA.* 1994;272:1851-1857.
59. Leape LL, Bates DW, Cullen DJ, et al. For the ADE Prevention Study Group. Systems analysis of adverse drug events. *JAMA.* 1995;274:35-43.
60. Leape LL, Brennan TA, Laird N, et al. The nature of adverse events in hospitalized patients. Results of the Harvard Medical Practice Study II. *N Engl J Med.* 1991;7;324(6):377-84.
61. Leape LL, Cullen DJ, Clapp MD, et al. Pharmacist participation on physician rounds and adverse drug events in the intensive care unit. *JAMA* 1999;282:267-270.
62. Lesar TS, Briceland L, Stein DS. Factors related to errors in medication prescribing. *JAMA.* 1997;277(4):312-317.
63. Luten R, Wears R, Broselow J, et al. Managing the unique size related issues of pediatric resuscitation: reducing cognitive load with resuscitation aids. *Acad Emerg Med.* 2002;9:840-847.
64. Lykowski G, Mahoney D. Computerized provider order entry improves workflow and outcomes. *Nurs Manage.* 2004;35(2):40G-H.
65. MacKinnon NJ, Hepler CD. Indicators of preventable drug-related morbidity in older adults 2. Use within a managed care organization. *J Managed Care Pharmacy.* 2003;9:134-141.
66. MacKinnon NJ, Hepler CD. Preventable drug-related morbidity in older adults 1. Indicator development. *J Managed Care Pharmacy.* 2002;8: 365-371.
67. Marcin JP, Dharmar M, Cho M, et al. Medication errors among acutely ill and injured children treated in rural emergency departments. *Ann Emerg Med.* 2007;50:361-367.
68. Marino BL, Reinhardt K, Eichelberger WJ, Steingard R. Prevalence of errors in a pediatric hospital medication system: implications for error proofing. *Outcomes Manag Nurs Pract.* 2000;4(3):129-135.
69. McErlean MA, Bartfield JM, Kennedy DA, et al. Home antipyretic use in children brought to the emergency department. *Ped Emerg Care.* 2001;17:249-251.
70. McLeod JP, Huang AR, Tamblyn RM. Defining inappropriate practices in prescribing for elderly people: a national consensus panel. *CMAJ.* 1997;156:385-391.
71. Monane M, Matthias DM, Nagle BA, Kelly MA. Improving prescribing patterns for the elderly through an online drug utilization review intervention: a system linking the physician, pharmacist, and computer. *JAMA.* 1998;280(14):1249-1252.
72. Moore TJ, Cohen MR, Furberg CD. Serious adverse drug events reported to the Food and Drug Administration, 1998-2005. *Arch Intern Med.* 2007;167:1752-1759.
73. Morriss FH Jr, Abramowitz PW, Nelson SP, Milavetz G, Michael SL, Gordon SN, Pendergast JF, Cook EF. Effectiveness of a barcode medication administration system in reducing preventable adverse drug events in a neonatal intensive care unit: a prospective cohort study. *J Pediatr.* 2008 Sep 27. [Epub ahead of print]
74. National Coordinating Council for Medication Error Reporting and Prevention (NCC MERP). About medication errors: medication error category index. Available at http://www.nccmerp.org/medError CatIndex. html.
75. Nelson LS, Gordon PE, Simmons MD, et al. The benefit of houseofficer education on proper medication dose calculation and ordering. *Acad Emerg Med.* 2000;7:1311-1316.
76. Orser BA, Chen RJ, Yee DA. Medication errors in anesthetic practice: a survey of 687, practitioners. *Can J Anaesthes.* 2001;48:139-146.
77. Peth HA. Medication errors in the emergency department. A systematic approach to minimizing risk. *Emerg Med Clin N Am.* 2003;21:141-158.
78. Phillips DP, Barker GEC, Eguchi MM. A steep increase in domestic fatal medication errors with use of alcohol and/or street drugs. *Arch Intern Med.* 2008;168:1561-1566.
79. Queneau P, Bannwarth B, Carpentier F, et al. Emergency department visits caused by adverse drug events. Results of a French survey. *Drug Saf.* 2007;30:81-88.
80. Reason J. *Human Error.* New York: Cambridge University Press; 1990.
81. Rothschild JM, Bates DW, Leape LL. Preventable medical injuries in older patients. *Arch Intern Med.* 2000;160(18):2717-2728.
82. Runy LA. Pharmacists in the ED help reduce errors. *H&HN.* 2008;82: 12-14.
83. Russell FM, Shann F, Curtis N, Mulholland K. Evidence on the use of paracetamol in febrile children. *Bull World Health Organ.* 2003;81:367-372.
84. Santell JP, Hicks RW, McMeekin J, et al. Medication errors: experience of the United States Pharmacopeia (USP) MEDMARX reporting system. *J Clin Pharmacol.* 2003;43:760-767.
85. Schiff GD, Klass D, Peterson J, et al. Linking laboratory and pharmacy: opportunities for reducing errors and improving care. *Arch Intern Med.* 2003;163:893-900.
86. Seifert SA, Jacobitz K. Pharmacy prescription dispensing errors reported to a regional poison control center. *Clin Toxicol.* 2002;40:919-923.

87. Simon SR, Chan KA, Soumerai SB, et al. Potentially inappropriate medication use by elderly persons in US health maintenance organizations 2000-2001. *J Am Geriatr Soc.* 2005;53:227-232.
88. Tamblyn R, Abrahamowicz M, du Berger R, et al. A 5-year prospective assessment of the risk associated with individual benzodiazepines and doses in new elderly users. *J Am Geriatr Soc.* 2005;53:233-241.
89. Ulmer C, Wolman DM, Johns MME, eds. Committee on Optimizing Graduate Medical Trainee (Resident) Hours and Work Schedule to Improve Patient Safety. National Research Council. Washington DC: National Academy Press; 2008.
90. Vincent C, Taylor-Adams S, Chapman EJ, et al. How to investigate and analyse clinical incidents: clinical risk unit and association of litigation and risk management protocol. *BMJ.* 2000;320:777-781.
91. Wald H, Shojania KG. Root cause analysis. In: Shojania KG, Duncan BW, McDonald KM, Watcher RM, eds. *Making Health Care Safer: A Critical Analysis of Patient Safety Practices.* Evidence Report/ Technology Assessment No. 43 (prepared by the University of California at San Francisco-Stanford Evidence-based Practice Center under Contract No 209-97-0013), AHRQ Publication No 01-E058. Rockville, MD: Agency for Healthcare Research and Quality, 2001: 51-56.
92. Walsh KE, Landrigan CP, Adams WG, et al. Effect of computer order entry on prevention of serious mediation errors in hospitalized children. *Pediatrics.* 2008;121:e421-e427.
93. Walson PD, Martin R, Endow E, Sakata A. Prescription writing in a pediatric clinic. *Pediatr Pharmacol.* 1981;1:239-244.
94. Wears RL, Berg M. Computer technology and clinical work: still waiting for Godot. *JAMA.* 2005;293:1261-1263.
95. Weingart SN, Gandhi TK, Seger AC, et al. Patient-reported medication symptoms in primary care. *Arch Inter Med.* 2005;165:234-240.
96. Wheeler DW, Remoundos DD, Whittlestone KD, et al. Calculations of doses of drugs in solution. Are medical students confused by different means of expressing drug concentrations? *Drug Saf.* 2004;27: 729-734.
97. Williamson J, Chopin JM. Adverse reactions to prescribed drugs in the elderly: a multicentre investigation. *Age Ageing.* 1980;9(2):73-80.
98. World Health Organization. International Drug Monitoring. The Role of the Hospital. Geneva, Switzerland: WHO Technical Report Series, No. 425; 1966.

CHAPTER 140

RISK MANAGEMENT AND LEGAL PRINCIPLES

Barbara M. Kirrane and Dainius A. Drukteinis

The number and diversity of toxicologic emergencies faced by emergency department (ED) staff has increased steadily since the early 1970s, and continues to rise today. This chapter discusses the medical-legal management of patients who are intoxicated or exposed to xenobiotics that may affect their thinking. It also addresses the legal and ethical dilemmas routinely encountered by emergency medicine practitioners.

Patients with toxicologic emergencies require immediate care, and yet are often unable to give consent because their impaired consciousness prevents them from making informed decisions. Treating patients who present with an acute organic impairment manifested by confusion, irrational thought, or even dangerous behavior is very challenging. Emergency physicians must recognize the medical-legal problems created when the impaired patient refuses treatment and insists on leaving against medical advice. The issue is further complicated by the variations in relevant laws from state to state. Emergency physicians must become familiar with the legal requirements of informed consent and the essential management necessary to avoid liability for negligence and abandonment within the state that they practice. Of particular concern are the risk management and liability issues that relate to impaired patients attempting to leave the ED before medical care is complete. The legal requirements of informed consent in emergency settings, the duty to treat, medical malpractice, battery, and negligence, are examined here. Guidelines based on generally accepted common law principles are suggested for developing appropriate patient care plans and departmental policies. These issues and principles are best illustrated by case examples.

INFORMED CONSENT

Patient 1 An 18-year-old college student was brought by ambulance to the emergency department (ED) after a friend reported seeing her in the bathroom with slit wrists and an empty bottle of acetaminophen. In the ED, the patient was alert and oriented to person, place, and time. Vital signs were: blood pressure 120/65 mm Hg; pulse 95 beats/min; respiratory rate 16 breaths/min; and temperature 99.1°F (37.3°C). A rapid bedside glucose concentration was 120 mg/dL. The patient stated that she ingested the acetaminophen approximately 5 hours earlier. The healthcare team wished to measure an acetaminophen concentration to determine whether *N*-acetylcysteine should be administered. The patient refused venipuncture and stated that she would refuse any medications. The physicians informed the patient that she might suffer irreparable damage to her liver and possibly die if not treated immediately.

Medically treating patients against their will poses a difficult problem. Forcible treatment violates a patient's autonomy and right to privacy. However, harm may be caused to the patient if the appropriate evaluation and treatment is not performed. As an example, in the case above, the patient gives a history of ingesting a large amount of acetaminophen, which may cause hepatotoxicity and even death if not treated (Chap. 34). Her refusal for this evaluation highlights the important issue of whether a physician is ever justified in performing an assessment of someone who is alert and oriented, yet poisoned, and who refuses treatment. Do most patients suffering from a mental illness such as depression need to be treated against their will? If the harm that faces the patient is not immediate, but certain in the near future, does the physician have the authority to treat? General principles of patient autonomy and informed consent will be elucidated here.

A patient's right to choose the course of medical treatment was first recognized in the early 20th century in a landmark case decided by the NYS Court of Appeals in *Schloendorff v Society of New York Hospital.*[16] Mary Schloendorff was admitted for abdominal pain and was found to have a mass on physical examination. Her physicians offered her a more thorough examination under anesthesia and the option for surgery. She consented only to the exploratory surgery; however, during the procedure the mass was removed. Postoperatively, Schloendorff developed an infection, gangrene and the amputation of several fingers. She sued the hospital. In its decision, the Court upheld Schloendorff's right to self-determination, and the right to refuse treatment. It stated:

> "Every human being of adult years and sound mind has a right to determine what shall be done with his own body and a surgeon who performs an operation without his patient's consent commits an assault, for which he is liable in damages, except in cases of emergency in which the patient is unconscious and it is necessary to operate before consent can be obtained."[16]

This decision became the foundation for the "Doctrine of Informed Consent." Informed consent serves to protect a patient's autonomy, the concept that each individual has the right to choose a personal course of medical treatment.[27] This includes the right to refuse care, and the right to terminate care already in process. In a nonemergent situation, it is the physician's responsibility to obtain approval from the patient or surrogate before rendering treatment.

Generally accepted components to the informed consent process consist of (1) an explanation of the treatment/procedure, (2) alternative choices to the proposed intervention, and (3) relevant risks, benefits, and uncertainties associated with each alternative. This discussion must take place whether the patient is consenting to a procedure, or refusing a recommended procedure. A patient does not automatically assume the risks of rejecting a physician's recommendations if the patient has not been fully apprised of the consequences of his or her decision.[29] Furthermore, it is the duty of the physician to assess how well the patient understands the above information. Before a physician may accept a patient's approval or refusal of care the patient must demonstrate adequate understanding of the information discussed.

State courts may apply one of two standards to determine if the information communicated by the physician was sufficient. The reasonable person standard requires a physician to disclose information that a reasonable person in the same position as the patient would need to make an informed decision.[5] The alternative is the reasonable physician standard, which requires a physician to reveal information that a reasonable physician in a similar circumstance would disclose.[5] States vary on which standard they apply.

Courts recognize that the requirement for informed consent is not absolute, and that there are exceptions in which a physician does not need to obtain permission before rendering treatment. In *Schloendorff v. Society of New York Hospital*, the Court recognized that consent is not required in emergency situations. Situations are generally considered emergent if a patient's care would be compromised if there were a delay in treatment. In New York, an emergency is defined as a situation that includes both the immediate endangerment of life or health, or the need for the immediate alleviation of pain.[19] Physicians need to determine the specific requirements of informed consent in their respective states.

Often a physician's well-intended efforts to communicate treatment information to an impaired patient prove ineffectual and present the practitioner with a medical-legal dilemma. The physician may be unable to discuss in a meaningful way the implications of the proposed treatment with the patient; nevertheless, there is a duty to treat the patient who presents with a life-threatening condition or the potential for permanent disability. In these situations, consent is considered to be implied, and emergent treatment should be provided. The principle of implied consent is a general tenet of tort law.[14]

RISK MANAGEMENT CONSIDERATION AND DOCUMENTATION

Patient 2 A 28-year-old woman was brought to the ED by police who believed she might be a "bodystuffer" (an individual who swallows drugs to avoid arrest and prosecution). The triage nurse helped the patient onto a stretcher and brought her to the treatment area and recorded normal vital signs. The patient became combative and uncooperative as the phyisician initiated the examination and he verbally ordered that the patient be restrained. The patient was given 40% oxygen via face mask, cardiac monitoring was begun, and an intravenous line was started with 0.9% sodium chloride at 125 mL/h; a bolus of 100 mL of $D_{50}W$ and 100 mg of thiamine were administered IV. Orogastric lavage was then performed, and 50 g of activated charcoal (AC) was administered.

An hour after arrival the patient's vital signs were: blood pressure 120/70 mmHg; pulse 82 beats/min; and respiratory rate 24 breaths/min. The patient was noted to be stable and transferred to an observation unit. Oxygen and cardiac monitoring were discontinued. No further orders were written, and the patient remained restrained. Three hours later the vital signs were: blood pressure, 110/60 mm Hg; pulse 92 beats/min; and respiratory rate 18 breaths/min. A nurse's note stated the patient was resting comfortably.

Forty-five minutes later, the initial physician completed his shift at midnight and informed his replacement that the patient was stable and resting in the holding area.

At 4:20 am the patient was found unresponsive and hypotensive, with agonal respirations and a weakly palpable pulse. She felt very hot to the touch and had a rectal temperature of 108°F (42.4°C). Resuscitative efforts were initiated but unsuccessful; 30 minutes later the patient was pronounced dead.

Several important risk management questions frequently arise in medical malpractice litigation involving the ED. To prove that a case constitutes medical malpractice, a plaintiff's attorney must show clear and convincing evidence of a departure from good practice by the physician. The attorney must further demonstrate that the negligent act or omission by the physician proximately caused the patient's injury. Courts have held that where "there is substantial probability that the [defendant physician's] negligent conduct caused the resulting injury, that sufficient evidence has been developed against [the] physician."[26]

The problems associated with an improperly documented ED record are numerous, but they can be minimized if the practitioner is cognizant of risk management principles. When the attorney for the patient (plaintiff's attorney) introduces evidence to prove the case, the central document in the medical malpractice trial is likely to be the ED record. Thus, every entry in that record is scrutinized with great care by both parties (plaintiff and defendants), and the importance of completing it with knowledge of risk management implications should be a concern for all healthcare providers.

The physician is required to write a medical record that will amply support the basis for the medical judgments exercised. When a physician chooses to write only a summary statement on the record without noting supporting clinical data or patient history, claims alleging failure to diagnose will be extremely difficult, if not impossible, to defend. One of the basic elements of the defense in a medical malpractice case is that the physician's judgment was appropriate, given the clinical facts and the patient's history available at that time. Therefore, physicians who do not record supporting clinical data and history deprive themselves of a strong "medical judgment" defense.

Inappropriate entries or markings on the medical record can weaken the defense in a liability case. For example, in attempting to correct an error in entering a PO_2 value, if the physician or nurse totally obliterates the number, an attorney representing a patient may suggest to the jury that the obliteration was done intentionally to conceal clinical data harmful to the position of the defense. If a physician must correct a prior entry made on the record, the preferable method is to draw a single line through the value or word to be changed, insert the correct information directly above and initial the correction. Timing and dating the correction also precludes potentially difficult questions of chronology and responsibility in a courtroom setting. By following these suggestions, the physician can avoid any accusations of intentionally concealing an error in judgment (Fig. 140–1).

A frequent claim is that the patient was abandoned or improperly monitored. For the above patient, although the chart appears to document repeated vital signs at appropriate intervals, no temperature is included after the first set until the patient is moribund; nor is any mention made again of the continued use of restraints, the patient's continued need for these restraints, or any adverse effects developing from the use of restraints. Additionally, documentation of physician assessment of the patient's medical condition is incomplete. For example, there is no mention in the physician's notes of the possible cause of the patient's change in mental status. Likewise, there is no documentation regarding the police officers' concerns that the patient was a "body stuffer." Body stuffers quickly ingest a drug to avoid detection, which can result in life-threatening toxicity (see Special Considerations SC-4: Body Packers and Body Stuffers). Documentation of the physician's review of this concern is necessary.

Quality assurance reviews of ED records often demonstrate inadequate charting by physicians and nurses monitoring patients who remain in the department for prolonged periods of time. Under any circumstances, a lapse of documentation of the patient's clinical condition for 4 hours or more after the initial physician and nursing assessment creates a potential risk management problem. In a lawsuit, the plaintiff's attorney would undoubtedly use such a record to develop the theory that no care whatsoever was given to the patient during this time interval, and that the patient was abandoned.

Monitoring notations in the patient's record are considered inadequate when they do not offer insight into the patient's clinical status. Thus, any monitoring note for a patient who must be restrained in the ED for a lengthy period of evaluation, observation, or until an inpatient bed becomes available must include specific clinical data and

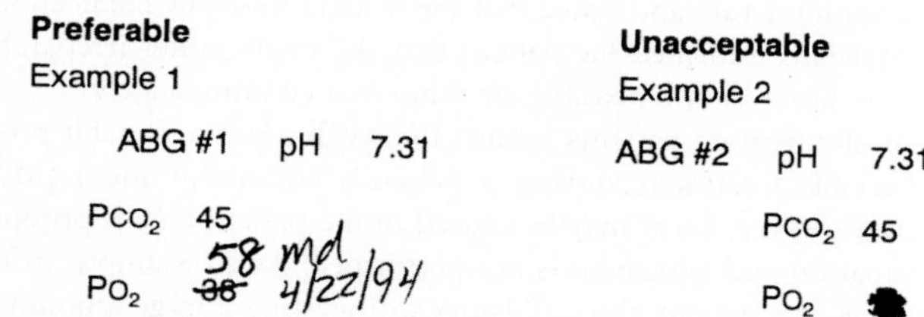

FIGURE 140–1. Examples of the preferred and an unacceptable procedure for correcting an error in the medical record.

observations (laboratory results, radiographic findings, hemodynamic changes, and infusion of medications and solutions). All of these deficiencies would undoubtedly be noticed and highlighted at trial by a plaintiff's expert, who frequently is a board-certified physician in the same specialty.

Documentation supporting the restraint of an impaired patient against his will must include a clinical description to support such a forcible impediment to the patient's right to liberty and freedom of movement. Such a clinical description should specifically describe any manifestation of agitation and uncooperative behavior. The record should refer to the specific uncooperative acts of the patient and, most importantly, should comment on the difficulties in providing care to the patient because of the patient's actions.

Physicians who order restraints for patients must exercise extreme caution in the language used to describe such patients. A judgmental physician's note stating that a patient is "a chronic drunk and obnoxious" could undermine the support for the use of restraints. Poorly written physician's notes can become an issue in a medical malpractice action, with the plaintiff's attorney focusing on the derogatory nature of such a statement and suggesting a less-than-caring attitude by the doctor toward the patient. A plaintiff's appeal criticizing the ethical and social consciousness of the physician could very likely be seized upon by a jury and result in a punitive verdict against the physician. As a general rule, all healthcare professionals should depict a compassionate and professional manner when describing patient behavior and life styles in objective and concrete terms. An alternative and more appropriate description of a patient comparable to the one above would note that the patient had a "history of alcohol dependence and was agitated and/or combative."

To summarize, a well-documented ED record consistent with the accepted risk management principles set forth is the best course for the physician managing a difficult overdose situation in which legal principles may appear to present problems in providing proper medical management.

FORCIBLE RESTRAINT OF THE IMPAIRED PATIENT

Patient 3 A 31-year-old woman was found unresponsive on the street and brought to the ED by ambulance. Friends on the scene reported that the patient used methadone. In the ED she was unresponsive and apneic. Oxygen was immediately administered by bag-valve mask and intravenous access was obtained. Naloxone was administered, and shortly thereafter the patient regained consciousness. After 20 minutes of care in the ED, the patient became fully alert and oriented, with no evidence of hypoxia or other clinical signs to suggest impaired judgment. The patient stated that she had taken methadone and demanded to be discharged immediately.

The right of a hospital to retain and physically restrain a person who has an altered level of consciousness for evaluation and emergency intervention is generally well supported by states and case law.[6] Reasonably clear guidelines for the management of such impaired patients have evolved from legal precedents governing appropriate medical assessment, from risk management considerations, and from the predictability of patient injury in the event of premature discharge.

A staff decision to allow a treated or partially treated patient with a drug overdose who subsequently becomes alert to return to the community must be based on an assessment of several factors. The initial concern is the patient's capacity to comprehend. Before the patient can be permitted to leave the hospital, a determination would have to be made that the patient is capable of understanding the information presented and has neither a medical nor a psychiatric problem preventing such a voluntary decision. The next consideration is that of medical stability. Has the initial process that caused the clinical scenario completed its course? The history of drug use in this patient is cause for concern that the underlying toxic metabolic process is not yet resolved, and alteration in mental status, significant respiratory compromise, or other medical symptoms may recur when the naloxone is metabolized, again placing the patient at risk.

Common ED practice and sound legal principles suggest that both the hospital and its staff have a duty to prevent such a person from leaving if the duration of the effect of the involved xenobiotic is longer than that expected for the antidote. Because the duration of effect for naloxone is considerably shorter than that of methadone, the physician can predict with reasonable certainty that coma or apnea will reoccur in the near future. The physician has the duty to inform the individual of the life-threatening nature of the condition, and then to retain, with restraints if necessary to retain, the patient in the hospital until medically stable.

Liability in this situation is further reduced when the chart substantiates the medical judgment that was the basis for the decision to retain the patient and, if applicable, the use of restraints. Such documentation should specifically note the likely relapse of the patient into a symptomatic state and that this occurrence could place the patient in a life-threatening situation. When documented in a clear manner, legal challenges to the decision to restrain the patient have a limited chance of success. Sound risk management principles support treatment and detainment. Conversely, prematurely releasing a patient with a significant overdose exposes both the physician and the hospital to a claim of negligence on the grounds of failure to foresee a likely and harmful event.

BLOOD ALCOHOL CONCENTRATION AND EVIDENCE COLLECTION

Patient 4 A 41-year-old man who was a driver involved in a motor vehicle collision was taken to the ED by ambulance. Two motorists in another vehicle were killed. The patient had no physical complaints, but was brought to the hospital for medical clearance. On arrival, he was alert and oriented, responded appropriately to all commands, and demonstrated normal motor function and had a normal gait. Police officers suspected that he was driving while intoxicated, but he refused a breath alcohol test at the scene.

The police officers informed the ED staff that he was arrested and might be charged with vehicular homicide. The officers then requested that the emergency physician draw a blood specimen to determine the blood alcohol concentration. The patient stated that he would not allow the ED staff to draw blood for a determination of an alcohol concentration.

In 2005, 16,885 people died in alcohol-related motor vehicle crashes, which was 39% of all traffic-related deaths in the United States.[9] An alcohol-related motor vehicle crash kills someone every 31 minutes and nonfatally injures someone every 2 minutes.[9] Drugs other than alcohol (eg, marijuana and cocaine) are involved in about 18% of motor vehicle driver deaths.[9,10] The judicial system has historically been one of the most effective tools to combat drunk driving, and its effectiveness depends on the ability to identify and punish individuals who violate the law. It is essential, however, that the collection of evidence does not violate the rights afforded by the US Constitution. Does forced phlebotomy for patients suspected of driving while intoxicated violate these protected rights? This has long been debated in the courts, and issues specifically brought into question include the Fourth Amendment,[22] the right against unreasonable search and seizure; the

Fifth Amendment,[23] the right against self-incrimination; and the Due Process clause of the Fourteenth Amendment.[24] Past decisions on these issues help guide current laws and practices.

Every state, and the District of Columbia, has driver "implied consent" laws. When a person obtains a driver's license, he or she consents at the time of acquisition to a chemical alcohol test if suspected of driving while intoxicated. Under implied consent laws, when a person suspected of driving while intoxicated refuses to take an alcohol test, a penalty is imposed. Specific penalties for refusals vary from state to state. At a minimum, the refusal results in suspension or revocation of a driver's license. Some states assign additional fines and penalties for this action. A few states allow the refusal itself to be submitted at trial in support of the prosecution, making it possible to be convicted of an intoxication charge without chemical evidence.[1] Certain states, for example Texas and Illinois, allow blood tests to be performed on patients as ordered by an officer of the law, when there is probable cause of driving while intoxicated resulting in severe injury.[13,21] Other states, such as New York and California, allow forced blood samples with a warrant issued by a judge.[3,11] State laws regarding the approach to this situation vary and it is important that the ED staff be familiar with the specific requirements of the law of that state.

How much force may be used to collect chemical evidence? Does a physician violate human dignity and privacy in obtaining evidence for the State? These issues have been addressed by the United States Supreme Court. In *Rochin v California*,[15] the Court overturned a conviction of drug possession based on violation of the Fourteenth Amendment. In this case, police were informed that Rochin was selling drugs. While entering the defendant's home, the police witnessed the defendant swallow two pills that were lying on the nightstand. When the officers failed to recover the pills on the scene, the officers took Rochin to the ED, where they directed the physician to administer an emetic through a nasogastric tube. The capsules were recovered from the vomit, and *Rochin* was convicted by the trial court for possessing morphine.[1,15] The Supreme Court reversed this decision, based on the Fourteenth Amendment, "nor shall any State deprive any person of life, liberty or property, without due process of law...."[25] The term *due process* is vague, and is defined on a case-by-case basis, but it essentially means that states must use fair legal procedures when depriving an individual of life, liberty, or property. In *Rochin*, the court concluded that forced emesis by a physician was believed to violate Due Process, stating:

> This is conduct that shocks the conscience. Illegally breaking into the privacy of the petitioner, the struggle to open his mouth and remove what was there, the forcible extraction of stomach contents—this course of proceeding by agents of government to obtain evidence is bound to offend even hardened sensibilities. They are methods too close to the rack and the screw to permit constitutional differentiation.[15]

The Supreme Court revisited the issues presented in *Rochin* 4 years later in *Breithaupt v Abram*.[2] Breithaupt was the driver of a truck that killed three occupants of another vehicle. In the ED, a police officer requested that a blood alcohol concentration be drawn. The blood, drawn while the patient was unconscious, was above the legal limit for alcohol and the patient was convicted of involuntary manslaughter. Breithaupt argued that the blood draw, as in forced emesis in *Rochin*, violated due process as he did not consent to its collection. Justice Clark disagreed, stating "the distinction rests on the fact that there is nothing 'brutal' or 'offensive' when done, as in this case, under the protective eye of a physician" and that the "blood test procedure has become routine in our everyday life."[1,2] Phlebotomy while the patient is unconscious and unable to give consent was determined not to violate the due process clause of the Fourteenth Amendment.

The Supreme Court continued to expand the scope of permissible phlebotomy in *Schmerber v California*.[17] Schmerber was involved in a motor vehicle crash in which the police officer suspected he was intoxicated. Unlike in *Breithaupt*, Schmerber was not unconscious, and a physician drew a blood sample at the officer's request despite the patient's verbal refusal. The attorney for Schmerber asserted that forced phlebotomy violated several constitutional rights. Specifically, it violated the Fourth, Fifth, and Fourteenth Amendments of the United States Constitution. He alleged that forced phlebotomy denied him due process of the law, it violated his privilege against self-incrimination, and it violated his right against unreasonable search and seizure.[1,17] The Supreme Court rejected all of these arguments. The phlebotomy did not violate the due process clause because "the extraction was made by a physician in a simple, medically acceptable manner in a hospital environment.... we cannot see that it should make any difference whether one states unequivocally that he objects or resorts to physical violence in protest or is in such condition that he is unable to protest."[17] Furthermore, the forced blood draw did not violate the Fifth Amendment's Privilege Against Self-incrimination because the Fifth Amendment only protects evidence of a "testimonial or communicative nature," such as writings or speech. Finally, there was no violation of the Fourth and Fourteenth Amendments' protections against unreasonable search and seizure:

> The delay necessary to obtain a warrant, under the circumstances, threatened the destruction of evidence.... Similarly, we are satisfied that the test chosen to measure petitioner's blood-alcohol level was a reasonable one. Extraction of blood samples for testing is a highly effective means of determining the degree to which a person is under the influence of alcohol. Such tests are a commonplace in these days of periodic physical examinations and experience with them teaches that the quantity of blood extracted is minimal, and that for most people the procedure involves virtually no risk, trauma, or pain.

To ensure compliance with standards set forth in *Schmerber*, the states have tailored laws and regulations governing the seizure of blood for the purpose of blood alcohol testing. Laws generally require the procedure be (1) done in a reasonable, medically approved manner, (2) incident to a lawful arrest, and (3) based on the belief that the arrestee is intoxicated. It should be remembered that the issues raised by any one case are complex, and the application in real situations is difficult. Laws and regulations governing blood draws for alcohol testing vary from state to state and are the subject of frequent restructuring and amendment. Medical staff should review with hospital counsel the local laws and regulations that pertain to these issues. However, physician and patient safety must always be the priority. The benefits of determining a patient's alcohol concentration must be weighed against the risks of the procedure. For example, drawing blood in an agitated patient may place the staff at risk for a needle stick and the patient at risk of vascular injury.

CONFIDENTIALITY

Patient 5 A 32-year-old woman was fired from her job as a high school mathematics teacher. The school board called for her termination after learning that she had a history of alcohol dependence and had a previous hospitalization for detoxification at the local community hospital. A parent on the school board was also employed as a nurse at the hospital, where the teacher had received therapy. The school board member (and nurse) had inadvertently accessed the teacher's medical record while caring for a patient with the same last name.

The Health Insurance Portability and Accountability Act (HIPAA) was created in 1996. Initially, the purpose of HIPAA was to increase the portability of health insurance, and allow employees to maintain insurance when they changed jobs. The Act called for the establishment of several provisions, among them an electronic database designed to facilitate the exchange of information between healthcare providers, insurance companies, and those involved in financial and administrative transactions.[8] However, the idea of developing an electronic database brought to light already growing concerns regarding the maintenance of patient privacy. For the first time, patients' medical records would be accessible to an unlimited number of people working in healthcare, from bill processors to pharmacists to clinicians. Could a patient's right to privacy be jeopardized by a system designed to increase efficiency?

Prior to HIPAA, individual hospitals or physician offices designed their own methods for maintaining confidential patient information. Records were maintained on computers in some circumstances and on paper in others. Accessibility to that information was largely regulated by state laws, and supported by some federal regulations and ethical codes of conduct. During the 1990s, however, the weaknesses of the existing systems gained attention as multiple high profile breeches of confidentiality surfaced. For example, the medical records of a congresswoman were released to the media during her campaign, making her history of depression and a past suicide attempt public knowledge.[18] There were also several cases of the medical records of hospital employees being read by staff members not involved in the employees' care, health insurance companies releasing heath care information to employers without permission, and physicians releasing information to pharmaceutical companies that subsequently solicited the patient.[28] These breaches of ethics were each a testament to the fact that a patient's right to privacy needed more stringent regulation. If these examples could occur in the previous systems for recording information, then it could be assumed that further violations would occur with increased access through an electronic database.

The Privacy Rule of HIPAA has become the most well-publicized aspect of this Act among healthcare personnel. The Privacy Rule governs the use and disclosure of protected health information in the hands of healthcare providers, health plans, and healthcare clearinghouses.[8] The terminology used in the Privacy Rule is extensively defined. The following is a brief summary of the terms used:

Protected Health Information: This includes any individually identifiable information concerning the past, present, or future health of an individual; medical information pertaining to assessment and treatment of an individual; in addition to payment and billing information. All forms of information, written, oral, or electronic, are protected by this rule.

Covered Entities: This includes any person or business that provides health-related services or products. All those providing health-related services, for example, clinicians, pharmacists, medical equipment providers, and other healthcare providers, are considered covered entities. Companies that provide disability insurance, car insurance, or casualty insurance are not included in the rule.[8,25]

Healthcare Clearinghouses: These are entities that compile healthcare information, such as billing companies or data processing centers.

Institutions are required to provide all individuals with written notice of their privacy policy when they first seek medical care. Patients must be informed of how the institution may use and disclose information. The notice must also describe patients' rights, including the right to access their medical information and their right to file a complaint if they believe their rights are violated. The notice must be written in plain language, and the patient must be written acknowledgement of receipt of the information in the notice.

The Privacy Rule of HIPAA was not intended to impede healthcare. There are several exceptions to the rule. A covered entity is permitted to use and disclose protected health information for the purposes of evaluation and treatment. Physicians have the freedom to consult with each other, both within and outside their own institution in order to provide clinical care. Additionally, there are several specific exceptions to the Privacy Rule listed within the document—situations in which protected health information may and often must be disclosed, and may be done without an individual's permission. For example, activities related to public health, such as reporting communicable diseases, information necessary to report actual or suspected abuse, neglect or domestic violence, or information pertaining to cadaver organ or tissue donation are specifically exempt from the Privacy Rule.[7]

The HIPAA Privacy Rule specifically addresses consultations with poison centers (PCs). It states: "We consider the counseling and follow-up consultations provided by poison control centers with individual providers regarding patient outcomes to be treatment. Therefore, poison control centers and other healthcare providers can share protected health information about the treatment of an individual without a business associate contract."[7]

Violations of the Privacy Rule are subject to penalties, the severity of which is dependent on the type of infraction. Simple noncompliance may result in financial penalties; however, more significant or intentional disclosures of information may incur steeper fines in addition to criminal charges and potential imprisonment.[28]

OTHER LEGAL CONSIDERATIONS FOR POISON CENTERS AND POISON SPECIALISTS

Patient 6 The Poison Center (PC) received a call from a concerned mother that her daughter might have ingested one of the grandmother's diabetes medications. The mother stated that the child was acting normally all day at the grandmothers' house, but when the family returned home the child had become drowsy. When contacted, the grandmother had confirmed that one pill was missing from her purse although she did not know the name of her medication. The PC advised that the parents give the child juice and closely observe her for the next 6 hours. Approximately 2 hours later, while sleeping, the child had a seizure. The child continued to seize in the hospital, where medical evaluation revealed hypoglycemia. The patient subsequently suffered permanent neurological damage. The medication was later identified as glyburide. Action was brought against the PC, alleging inappropriate advice and failure to recommend transport to a hospital.

As a general rule, any physician who decides to treat a patient enters into a physician–patient relationship that creates well-established legal duties. Courts have ruled that the physician–patient encounter need not be a face-to-face interaction to have legal consequences. For example, the absence of physical contact between a physician and patient as in the practice of radiology and pathology does not preclude a patient from asserting that a duty of care exists.[4] More particularly and quite relevant to the practice of a PC, a New York State court ruled that an initial telephone call from a patient to a physician can be sufficient basis to hold that physician responsible for inappropriate advice or a significant error in judgment.[12] Given the legal precedents previously stated, it is eminently clear that contact with a poison information specialist is a sufficient foundation for a subsequent legal action if inappropriate advice was given.

STANDARDS OF CARE APPLICABLE IN POISON CENTERS

Standards of care applicable to toxicologists are examined under the same legal framework as other medical specialists. The basic medical malpractice concepts are universal with some variations from state to state. Generally, for patients to prevail in medical malpractice cases they must demonstrate "by a preponderance of the evidence: (1) that the doctor's treatment fell below the ordinary standard of care expected of a physician in his [or her] medical specialty, and (2) the existence of a causal relationship between the alleged negligent treatment and the injury sustained.[30]" While standard of care is recognized not to be one of perfection, what constitutes the "ordinary standard of care" has much room for interpretation.

In the 19th century, courts determined what the "ordinary standard of care" was by introducing testimony from physicians practicing in the community where the event occurred. This was known as the strict locality rule.[31] The strict locality rule was intended to prevent the inequities of comparing rural physicians working with limited resources and under exigent conditions from physicians working in large urban hospital settings.[32] In many jurisdictions, however, the strict locality rule was rejected because: (1) it was difficult to find an expert witness in a small community to testify against another physician in the community, and (2) the strict locality rule permitted some small medical communities to set unacceptably low standards of care.[33] In response, some states adopted the modified locality rule, which compares the physician in question with physicians practicing "in similar localities."[31] Over time, the basis for the modified locality rule was also questioned. Advances in transportation, communication, and education continued to minimize the disparity between rural and urban medical practice. Many states abandoned the locality rule altogether, permitting evidence of nationwide medical practices, as described by one court:

> [A] physician must exercise that degree of care, skill, and proficiency exercised by reasonably careful, skillful, and prudent practitioners in the same class to which he [or she] belongs, acting under the same or similar circumstances. Rather than focusing on different standards for different communities, this standard uses locality as but one of the factors to be considered in determining whether the doctor acted reasonably.[34]

While there is movement toward reviewing nationwide medical practices, depending on the jurisdiction where the event occurs, any one of the above rules may apply. In New York, courts allow evidence from the specific locality where the event occurred, from statewide practice, or from nationwide practice.[35]

A discussion of standard of care for poison control specialists should also mention several operational aspects of poison centers. Poison information specialists are required to have rapid and accurate access to a standard information resource system that contains both basic information and recommendations to deal with most toxic exposures. If a patient were to bring an action, the negligence theory against the poison center might rely on deviations from the standard recommendations in these resources.

It would be inaccurate to suggest, however, that the duty of care owed by a poison information specialist can be measured only by how closely the advice given compares with these standard resources. Frequently, a poison specialist may encounter situations that cannot be managed in accordance with an information system alone, and may seek counsel from a clinical pharmacist or a medical toxicologist working with the poison control center. If this were to occur, any subsequent legal proceeding would also review carefully the content of the information given to the consultant regarding accuracy and appropriateness of treatment for the underlying toxicologic problem.

PRACTICES OF REGIONAL POISON CENTERS THAT CAN REDUCE POTENTIAL LIABILITIES

Clearly there are some inherent risks of potential liability for a PC. To minimize such risk and the risk of civil actions against a PC, quality assurance and risk management programs should be a regular function. Daily audits or monitoring of the advice given by poison information specialists should be done. Such interactions enhance care and ensure patient safety for the individual and establish a higher general standard.

The medical toxicologists and clinical pharmacists responsible for supervising the poison information specialists must be able to adequately assess the competence and capabilities of the staff and to make recommendations, take corrective actions, and provide suggestions for improvement to involved members. This process is facilitated by such actions as audiotaping calls made to the PC and the subsequent advice given, and reviewing written records maintained by the information specialist on each particular case. Documentation is extremely important, because in the event of a lawsuit, the most likely area of dispute will be what was actually said to the patient.

SUMMARY

The risk management and legal issues of an active ED have implications for many patients. The ability of providers to function responsibly is dependent on an understanding of these constantly evolving principles. Those patients whose consciousness is abnormal because of a xenobiotic represent an acute complex medicolegal emergency. A well-organized hospital is dependent on a close working relationship among the legal, risk management, and medical personnel. Only in this manner can they learn, cooperate, and meet the needs of the ever-evolving clinical dilemmas they confront.

ACKNOWLEDGMENTS

Walter LeStrange, RN, MPH, MS, and Kevin Porter, Esq, contributed to this chapter in previous editions.

REFERENCES

1. Beauchamp, RB. "Shed thou no blood": the forcible removal of blood samples from drunk driving suspects. *South Calif Law Rev.* 1987:V(60): 1115–1141.
2. *Breithaupt v. Abram* 352, US 432(1957).
3. California Vehicle Code 23612 (West 1996).
4. *Capunao v. Jacobs* 33, AD 2d 743, 305, NY State 2d 837 (1960).
5. Gatter, R. Informed Consent law and the forgotten duty of physician inquiry. *Loyola Univ Chicago Law J.* 1999;31:557–597.
6. *Gonzalez v. State* 110, AD 2d 810, 488, NY 2d 231, 67, NY 2d 647 (1985).
7. Health Insurance Portability and Accessibility Act of 1996, Pub. No L 104–191, 110, Stat 1936(1996). See also 45 CFR 160, 164 (2002).
8. Kutzko D, Boyer GL, Thoman DJ, et al. HIPAA in real time: practical implications of the federal privacy rule. Drake Law Rev. 2003;51:403–450.
9. Dept of Transportation (US), National Highway Safety Administration (NHTSA). Traffic safety facts 2005: alcohol. Washington (DC): NHTSA; 2006.
10. Jones RK, Shinar D, Walsh JM. State of knowledge of drug-impaired driving. Department of Transportation (US), National Highway Traffic Safety Administration, (NHTSA): 2003, Report DOT HS 809 642.
11. NY Vehicle and Traffic Law 1194 (McKinney's Consolidated Laws of NY 1996).
12. *O'Neil v. Montefiore Hospital* 11AD 2d 132, 202, NY State 2d 436 (1960).
13. *People v. Ruppel* 303, I11. App.3d 885, 708, NE2d 824 (4 Dist 1999).
14. Prosser WL. *The Law of Torts. Implied Consent.* St. Paul, MN: West; 1984.
15. *Rochin v. California* 342, US 165 (1952).
16. *Schloendorff v. Society of New York Hospital* 211, NY 125, 105, NE (1914).
17. *Schmerber v. California* 384, US 757 (1966).
18. Statement of Janlori Goldman, Deputy Director before Senate Committee on Labor and Human Resources S1360. The Medical Records Confidentiality Act of 1995. http://www.cdt.org/testimony/951114goldman. shtml.
19. *Sullivan v. Montegomery* 279, NYS:575 (1935).

20. *Surgical Consultants v. Ball* 447, NW2d 676 (1989).
21. Texas Transportation Code Ann 724 (Vernon 1991).
22. US Constitution 4th Amendment. http://www.archives.gov/national-archives-experience/charters/bill_of_rights_transcript.html.
23. US Constitution 5th Amendment. http://www.archives.gov/national-archives-experience/charters/bill_of_rights_transcript.html.
24. US Constitution 14th Amendment. http://www.archives.gov/national-archives-experience/charters/constitution_amendments_11-27.html.
25. United States Department of Health and Human Services: Office of Civil Rights. "Summary of the HIPAA Privacy Rule." Available at http://www.hhs.gov/ocr/privacysummary.pdf. Last accessed April 25, 2005.
26. *Vialva v. City of New York* 118, AD 2d.701, 499, NY 2d 977 (2nd dept 1986).
27. Walter P. The doctrine of informed consent: to inform or not to inform? *St. John's Law Rev.* 1997;71:543–589.
28. White RJ, Hoffman CA. The privacy standard under the health insurance portability and accountability act: a practical guide to promote order and avoid potential chaos. *West VA Law Rev.* 2004;106:709–779.
29. *Truman v. Thomas*, 611 P.2d 902 (1980).
30. *Wainwright v. Leary*, 623 So.2d 233 (La. 1993).
31. *Vergara v. Doan*, 593 N.E.2d 185 (Ind. 1992).
32. *See* John Kimbrough Johnson, Jr., *An Evaluation in the Medical Standard of Care*, 23 *Vand Law Rev.* 729, 731-732 (1970).
33. *Vergara v. Doan*, 593 N.E.2d 185 (Ind. 1992), *Pederson v. Dumouchel*, 72 Wash. 2d 73, 431 P.2d 973, 977 (Wash. 1967).
34. *See Bates v. Meyer*, 565 So.2d 134 (Ala. 1990); *Mann v. Cracchiolo*, 38 Cal. 3d 18, 694 P.2d 1134, 210 Cal. Rptr. 762 (Cal. 1985); *Hyles v. Cockrill*, 169 Ga. App. 132, 312 S.E.2d 124 (Ga.App. 1983); *Speed v. State*, 240 N.W.2d 901 (Iowa 1976); *Blair v. Eblen*, 461 S.W.2d 370 (Ky. 1970); *Shilkret v. Annapolis Emergency Hosp.*, 276 Md. 187, 349 A.2d 245 (Md. 1975); *Brune v. Belinkoff*, 354 Mass. 102, 235 N.E.2d 793 (Mass. 1968); *Hall v. Hilbun*, 466 So.2d 856 (Miss. 1985); *Schueler v. Strelinger*, 43 N.J. 330, 204 A.2d 577 (N.J. 1964); *Wiggins v. Piver*, 276 N.C. 134, 171 S.E.2d 393 (N.C. 1970); *Pharmaseal Lab., Inc., v. Goffe*, 90 N.M. 753, 568 P.2d 589 (N.M. 1977); *King v. Williams*, 276 S.C. 478, 279 S.E.2d 618 (S.C. 1981); *Peterson v. Shields*, 652 S.W.2d 929 (Tx. 1983); *Farrow v. Health Services Corp.*, 604 P.2d 474 (Utah 1979); *Brown v. Koulizakis*, 229 Va. 524, 331 S.E.2d 440 (Va. 1985); *Paintiff v. Parkersburg*, 345 S.E.2d 564 (W.Va. 1986); *Pederson v. Dumouchel*, 72 Wash. 2d 73, 431 P.2d 973 (Wash. 1967); *Shier v. Freedman*, 58 Wis. 2d 269, 206 N.W.2d 166 (Wis. 1973), modified on other grounds and rehearing denied, 58 Wis. 2d 269, 208 N.W.2d 328.
35. *Hock v. United Presbyterian Home*, 236 N.Y.L.J 106 (2006).

INDEX

Common Toxicology Laboratory Concentrations (serum unless otherwise noted)

	Conventional	SI
Acetaminophen#	10–30 μg/mL	66–199 μmol/L
Arsenic (blood)	<5 μg/L	<0.665 μmol/L
Arsenic (urine)	<50 μg/day	<6.65 μmol/day
Caffeine	1–10 μg/mL	5.2–51 μmol/L
Carbamazepine	4–12 mg/L	17–51 μmol/L
Carboxyhemoglobin (blood)	<2%	<2%
Cyanide (blood)	<1 μg/mL	<38.5 μmol/L
Digoxin	0.8–2 ng/mL	1.1–2.6 nmol/L
Ethanol	100 mg/dL	22 mmol/L
Ethlyene glycol*	<25 mg/dL	<4 mmol/L
Iron	80–180 μg/dL	14–32 μmol/L
Lead (blood)	<10 μg/dL	<0.48 μmol/L
Lidocaine	1.5–5 μg/mL	6.4–21.4 μmol/L
Lithium	0.6–1.2 mEq/L	0.6–1.2 mmol/L
Mercury (blood)	<10 μg/L	<50 nmol/L
Mercury (urine)	<20 μg/L	<100 nmol/L
Methanol*	<25 mg/dL	<7.8 mmol/L
Methemoglobin	<3%	<3%
Phenobarbital	15–40 mg/L	65–172 μmol/L
Phenytoin	10–20 mg/L	40–79 μmol/L
Salicylates*	15–30 mg/dL	1.1–2.2 mmol/L
Thallium (blood)	<2.0 μg/L	<9.78 nmol/L
Thallium (urine)	<5.0 μg/L	<24.5 nmol/L
Theophylline	5–15 μg/mL	27.8–83 μmol/L
Thiocyanate	<30 μg/mL	<100 μmol/L
Valproic acid	50–120 mg/L	347–833 μmol/L

Therapeutic or generally accepted normal concentrations are listed. Please see the appropriate chapter for details regarding specific situations. Normal ranges may vary by laboratory.
* = Concentration must be interpreted with respect to the patient's serum pH and clinical status
# = See acetaminophen nomogram (page 486).

Common Standard Blood/Serum Laboratory Concentrations

	Conventional	SI
Ammonia	10–80 μg/dL	6–47 μmol/L
Bicarbonate	18–24 mEq/L	18–24 mmol/L
BUN	7–18 mg/dL	2.5–6.4 mmol/L
Calcium	8.4–10.2 mg/dL	2.10–2.55 mmol/L
Chloride	98–106 mEq/L	98–106 mmol/L
Creatinine	0.6–1.2 mg/dL	0.053–0.106 mmol/L
Glucose	60–110 mg/dL	3.3–6.1 mmol/L
Lactate	18 mg/dL	<2 mmol/L
Magnesium	1.3–2.1 mEq/L	0.65–1.05 mmol/L
PCO_2 (art)	35–45 mm Hg	4.7–6 kPa
PCO_2 (ven)	45–55 mm Hg	6.0–7.33 kPa
pH (art)	7.35–7.45	7.35–7.45
pH (ven)	7.33–7.40	7.33–7.40
PO_2 (art)	90–100 mm Hg	12–13.3 kPa
PO_2 (ven)	30–50 mm Hg	4.0–6.67 kPa
Phosphorus	3–4.5 mg/L	1–1.4 mmol/L
Potassium	3.5–5.0 mEq/L	3.5–5 mmol/L
Sodium	135–145 mEq/L	135–145 mmol/L

art = arterial; ven = venous